Textbook of Therapeutics

Drug and Disease Management

EIGHTH EDITION

Textbook of Therapeutics
Drug and Disease Management
EIGHTH EDITION

EDITORS

Richard A. Helms, PharmD, BCNSP
Professor and Chair
Department of Pharmacy
College of Pharmacy
Professor of Pediatrics
University of Tennessee Health Sciences Center
Memphis, Tennessee

Eric T. Herfindal, PharmD, MPH
Professor Emeritus
School of Pharmacy
University of California
San Francisco, California

David J. Quan, PharmD, BCPS
Assistant Clinical Professor
School of Pharmacy
University of California San Francisco
Pharmacist Specialist
UCSF Medical Center
San Francisco, California

Dick R. Gourley, PharmD
Professor and Dean
College of Pharmacy
University of Tennessee Health Sciences Center
Memphis, Tennessee

SECTION EDITORS

Kimberly A. Bergstrom / Paul M. Beringer /Ali J. Olyaei /
W. Nathan Rawls / P. David Rogers / Timothy H. Self

CASE EDITORS

Joanna K. Hudson / Greta K. Gourley / Caroline S. Zeind

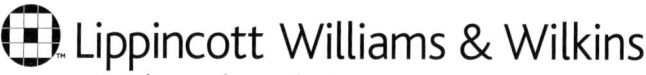

Lippincott Williams & Wilkins
a Wolters Kluwer business
Philadelphia · Baltimore · New York · London
Buenos Aires · Hong Kong · Sydney · Tokyo

Acquisitions Editor: David P. Troy
Managing Editor: Matthew J. Hauber
Developmental Editor: Andrea M. Klinger
Associate Production Manager: Kevin P. Johnson
Creative Director: Doug Smock
Marketing Manager: Marisa O'Brien
Production Services: Maryland Composition Inc
Printer: QuebecorWorld Versailles

Library of Congress Cataloging-in-Publication Data

Textbook of therapeutics : drug and disease management. — 8th ed.
   / editors, Richard A. Helms, David J. Quan.
      p. ; cm.
   Includes bibliographical references and index.
   ISBN 0-7817-5734-7
   1. Chemotherapy.   2. Therapeutics.   I. Helms, Richard A.
II. Quan, David J.
   [DNLM: 1. Drug Therapy.   2. Therapeutics.   WB 330 T3555
2006]
RM262.C5 2006
615.5'8—dc22
                                                      2005034101

To purchase additional copies of this book, call our customer service department at (800) 638-3030 or fax orders to (301) 223-2320. International customers should call (301) 223-2300.

Visit Lippincott Williams & Wilkins on the Internet at LWW.com. Lippincott Williams & Wilkins customer service representatives are available from 8:30am to 6pm, EST.

10 9 8 7 6 5 4 3 2 1

Preface

As the new editors for the *Textbook of Therapeutics: Drug and Disease Management,* we are convinced the release of the eighth edition could not be more timely. The publication of the *Textbook* has spanned more than three decades, during which time health care has continued to evolve, often in dramatic ways. Since the seventh edition was published, the Human Genome Project (HGP) was completed. The project goals were to discover an estimated 25,000 human genes and to sequence the 3 billion DNA subunits. (The importance of the project deserves more extensive review. We encourage you to review the April 11, 2003 issue of *Science.*) The HGP has resulted in a new era of molecular medicine that investigates the fundamental causes of disease. More specific diagnostic tests will allow for the early detection and treatment of many common disorders. The HGP has enabled biotechnology to develop novel pharmacotherapeutic agents based on rational drug design.

One might assume that world health and the health care system would be improving as a result of innovative science and technology. However, in the United States, health care practitioners are confronted with growing numbers of individuals with obesity, diabetes, dyslipidemias, cardiovascular disease, neurological and psychiatric illnesses, and select cancers. Health care spending continues to skyrocket in the United States, reaching $1.7 trillion in 2003. In 2004, employer health insurance premiums increased by 11.2% with annualized cost to employers of nearly $10,000 per year for a family of four. Workers' contributions have risen to nearly $2,700 per year, a 10% increase in 2004. In 2006, health insurance premiums will increase to nearly $14,500 per year according to the National Coalition on Health Care. These alarming trends are making U.S. employers less competitive in the global marketplace, and have resulted, in part, in the financial failure of companies in the airline and automobile industries. Skyrocketing health care costs have also resulted in an increasing number of Americans not being covered by any health care plan as employers restructure their relationships with current and previous employees.

Within U.S. health care, other concerning trends have been identified. Spending for prescription drugs grew from $40.3 billion in 1990 to $179.2 billion in 2003. While drug cost is a relatively finite percentage of total health care spending (~11%), it is among the fastest growing components. The Kaiser Foundation reports private health insurance has seen a substantial increase in prescription drug cost (nearly doubled as a percent of total national prescription drug expenditures), whereas more modest gains were seen in government programs over the period 1990 through 2003. However, this changed with the passage of the Medicare Modernization Act in November 2003. The Congressional Budget Office estimates suggest the cost of Medicare Part D to U.S. tax payers will be $558 billion for the period 2004 through 2013.

These societal trends and governmental directives suggest, more than ever, the need for well-trained clinicians in therapeutics. By using the scientific, economic, and humanistic strategies of disease management as outlined in this book, we will go a long way toward achieving the goal of optimal, rational, and affordable medical care by a society that places a strong emphasis on health and wellness. Disease management is the process of caring for patients using standardized treatment strategies that ensure appropriate utilization and high quality care across the continuum (The Disease Management Strategies Research Study & Resource Guide, published by NMHCC, 1998). Disease management is a highly effective strategy in controlling health care costs and improving outcomes. It focuses on chronic, costly disease states with high co-morbidity as well as acute, catastrophic episodes of care. By basing therapeutic decisions on scientific and clinical evidence clearly delineated in treatment algorithms and protocols, bias is reduced and the arbitrary and heavy-handed managed care strategies that have failed in the past can be eliminated. Finally, a major impetus for change in drug use policy since the last edition of the *Textbook* was the Institute of Medicine's report ''To err is human: building a safer health system.'' Released on November 1, 1999, this report was a wake-up call to all health care providers regarding the prevalence of medical and medication errors. The report resulted in JCAHO medication management standards for 2004. These expanded the definition of medication and resulted in changes in standards related to patient-specific information, medication selection and procurement, medication storage, medication preparation and dispensing, medication administration and monitoring, high-risk medications, and a new standard for medication ordering and transcription. Medical centers are now directing much more attention to medication errors.

As disease and medication management have matured as a concept, so have the requirements of a textbook that attempts to provide the student and practitioner with sufficient information organized in a useful and logical way. For the eighth edition, we have made extensive changes in our list of contributors to bring you the most knowledgeable leaders in therapeutics and disease and drug management. We have continued the format changes of the seventh edition and have included treatment goals, pharmacoeconomic considerations, psychosocial issues, and key points in each chapter. We have provided the user with extensive chapter bibliographies so the reader can access original papers related to the subject matter.

We've also included an insert of full-color illustrations and photographs found throughout the text chapters to help the students recognize and understand disease states.

We have incorporated cases into the *Textbook* to make the eighth edition a very useful teaching tool in the classroom and clinics. Cases are found at the end of each section in the *Textbook*. The cases refer the student and practitioner to specific chapters in the *Textbook* for further information to assist them in understanding and resolving questions related to the cases. All cases have a consistent format and are categorized as Level 1, 2, or 3 based on their degree of therapeutic difficulty. Case questions are based on identifiable educational objectives from the Universal Set of Educational Objectives. All cases have disease or drug management questions, and most cases have questions relating to psychosocial issues, pharmacoeconomics, and key points from the *Textbook*. (See the Case Instructions for further information.)

We have wonderful ancillaries included with this new edition, including online case studies, a full color image bank, and a student CD-ROM that houses an electronic version of the book and pathophysiological animations. In addition to these items, we have added a bank of questions for the students to use in their review and study. We think these changes make the *Textbook of Therapeutics* among the best therapeutics teaching and practice texts available.

Editorial Team for the *Textbook*

The eighth edition marks a change in the editorial management of the *Textbook*. Drs. Eric Toby Herfindal and Dick R. Gourley have stepped aside after 25 years and seven editions of the *Textbook*. As new editors, we have come to understand the enormous energy and commitment of these two men. Their names will always be associated with the *Textbook* as founding editors, and now emeritus editors. We thank them for their trust in us to continue the fine tradition of the *Textbook*, and we hope that we can build upon the excellence initiated and propagated over the last three decades.

We are pleased to have the assistance of six section and three case editors. These colleagues bring a breadth of experience in practice, education, and research to the editorial team of the *Textbook* and its cases. The editors, section and case editors, and staff have worked together to redesign the structure of the book, as well as providing editorial review throughout the editorial process. The Section Editors for the *Textbook* are Drs. Kim Bergstrom, Paul Beringer, Ali Olyaei, Nathan Rawls, David Rogers, and Timothy Self. Our Case Editors are Drs. Greta Gourley, Joanna Hudson, and Caroline Zeind. Dr. Greta Gourley will step away from the *Textbook* with this edition, but all of us want to express our appreciation for her hard work and guiding influence. We want to especially thank our contributing authors, for they are the individuals who bring content to the *Textbook*. As new editors, we want to thank the editorial staff at Lippincott Williams & Wilkins. Without their support, this *Textbook* would never have reached publication. A special thank you to David Troy, Matthew Hauber, Andrea Klingler at Lippincott Williams & Wilkins, and Heidi Pongratz at Maryland Composition.

R.A.H. and D.J.Q.

Textbook of Therapeutics Case Instructions

In this eighth edition, case studies have been incorporated within the textbook with the intent of facilitating the learning process. The case editors have selected cases that address a variety of disease states and have asked authors to incorporate specific disease states in addition to the primary disease state within the case. The intent is to expose the students to disease states other than that of the primary focus of the case. The format of the case and guidelines are based on the same format that was used in the seventh-edition casebook.

Cases are categorized based on their degree of therapeutic difficulty as simple (Level 1), moderately complex (Level 2), or highly complex (Level 3). The three-level classification system allows the user to identify the level of knowledge and problem-solving required to design a pharmaceutical care plan and answer pertinent questions for each case. The ascending level of complexity of the cases provides the student with an opportunity to increase problem-solving ability and helps students develop self-efficacy in many therapeutic areas while building their disease management knowledge base. The case levels are described below.

LEVEL 1 CASES

1. Involve *simple* therapeutic and disease management problems.
2. Require application of baseline (fundamental) knowledge of therapeutics, pathophysiology, and disease management expected of the *beginner* student.
3. Include development of a pharmaceutical plan of care for such therapeutic related problems as:

   - Epidemiologic considerations and other factors contributing to the condition.
   - Pharmacokinetic differences.
   - Physical assessment parameters (including signs and symptoms), laboratory, diagnostic tests, serum drug concentrations, and pharmacokinetic abnormalities.
   - Actual/potential drug interactions.
   - Adverse drug effects.
   - Nonoptimal pharmacologic and nonpharmacologic treatment regimens.
   - Nonadherance to therapy.
   - Psychosocial problems.
   - Potential or actual pharmacoeconomic problems.

4. Provide for analysis of 2 or 3 case problems.
5. Require summarization of therapeutic, pathophysiologic, and disease management concepts for a given condition utilizing a key points format.
6. Provide opportunity for *beginning* level application of knowledge for problem-solving.

LEVEL 2 CASES

1. Include *moderately complex* therapeutic and disease management problems.
2. Require application of intermediate (median) knowledge of therapeutics, pathophysiology, and disease management expected of the *intermediate* student.
3. Include development of a pharmaceutical plan of care for such therapeutic-related problems listed under the Level 1 cases with an emphasis on application of a broader knowledge base.
4. Provide for analysis of 4 to 5 case problems.
5. Require summarization of therapeutic, pathophysiologic, and disease management concepts for a given condition utilizing a key points format.
6. Provide opportunity for *intermediate level* application of knowledge for problem-solving.

LEVEL 3 CASES

1. Include *highly complex* therapeutic and disease management problems.
2. Require application of a superior (outstanding) knowledge of therapeutics, pathophysiology, and disease management expected of the *advanced* student.
3. Include development of a pharmaceutical plan of care for such therapeutic related problems as depicted for level 1 and 2 cases with a greater emphasis on critical thinking.
4. Provide for analysis of more than 5 case problems.
5. Require summarization of therapeutic, pathophysiologic, and disease management concepts for a given condition utilizing a key points format.
6. Provide opportunity for *advanced level* application of knowledge for problem-solving and critical thinking.

After the case scenarios, multiple choice questions (with a single correct answer) and open-ended questions are presented. The case questions are developed using the universal set of Educational Objectives (EOs; see below), which correspond to the following areas of learning: knowledge acquisition, application, problem-solving, and critical thinking. The EOs from the Universal Set of Objectives that correspond to the case questions are shown in parentheses after each question. This assists the educator planning to use the cases for a seminar/class by providing both specific evaluation questions and the corresponding objectives. It also helps the student doing a self-directed study to determine which educational objectives they have accomplished. Though the case study is generally viewed as a problem-solving teaching and learning strategy, the case questions may be written to assess knowledge attained, application of knowledge, problem-solving, and critical thinking ability.

Every aspect of each disease and every potential therapeutic problem cannot be discussed in the case studies. Therefore, the cases cannot be used to ensure understanding of all the material in the textbook. However, it is likely that a student who is able to analyze the case, prioritize the problems, document pharmaceutical care using the SOAP note format, and answer the case questions has a good grasp of the material presented in the cases and the corresponding textbook chapter(s).

UNIVERSAL SET OF EOS

For the conditions presented, the student should be able to:

1. Describe the etiology and pathophysiology, including sequelae.
2. Identify signs and symptoms.
3. Discuss epidemiologic considerations such as incidence, prevalence, demographics (e.g., age, sex, racial and ethnic groups), and other contributing factors.
4. Analyze pharmacokinetic differences as they relate to age, gender, genetic factors (racial and ethnic groups), environment and cultural factors, disease states, alcohol consumption, and smoking.
5. Evaluate pertinent physical assessment parameters, laboratory studies, diagnostic tests, serum drug concentrations, and pharmacokinetics for abnormal findings.
6. Apply general principles of clinical pharmacokinetics, including calculations, as required.
7. Describe the mechanism of action of pharmacologic and nonpharmacologic interventions employed in the treatment.
8. Analyze factors that should be considered when selecting pharmacologic and nonpharmacologic therapy.
9. Identify potential or actual drug interactions (e.g., drug–drug, drug–food, drug–disease, etc.).
10. Recognize common adverse effects of pharmacologic treatments.
11. Evaluate present pharmacologic and nonpharmacologic treatment for problems.
12. Suggest recommendations for optimizing pharmacologic and nonpharmacologic treatment to achieve optimal control of the disease state(s) (e.g., through use of treatment algorithms found in the eighth edition textbook chapters).
13. Use the Problem List and SOAP note format to analyze, synthesize, and prioritize pertinent data to develop a pharmaceutical care plan. (This objective will not be used to develop case questions; however, it is met in each case through use of the Problem List and SOAP note.)
14. Develop a detailed education plan for the patient, including necessary lifestyle changes, medication counseling information, specific counseling (communication) techniques, and adherence strategies. (This objective may be met in each case through use of the Plan portion of the SOAP Note or by use of specific case questions.)
15. Analyze psychosocial factors that may affect patient adherence to both pharmacologic and nonpharmacologic therapy (e.g., influence of family, significant others, and/or peer group(s); financial resources; perceived susceptibility or severity of long-term consequences; interference with lifestyle).
16. Describe the health care provider's role relative to psychosocial factors.
17. Evaluate the pharmacoeconomic considerations relative to the patient's pharmaceutical plan of care.
18. Summarize therapeutic, pathophysiologic, and disease management concepts for a given condition using a Key Points format.

PROBLEM-ORIENTED APPROACH

To use the cases, it is necessary to become familiar with the Problem-Oriented Medical Record (POMR). In 1964, Lawrence E. Weed published the problem-oriented approach to medical records, patient care, and medical education. The method differed from the previously used method in which health care providers approached the patient from the point of view of their medical specialties. Before 1964, a physician would write a note in the chart about one of the patient's diseases, usually stating the condition of the patient at that time; if a procedure was performed, the note would describe the procedure and its results. The note usually did not summarize previous data and rarely outlined a thorough process about how a diagnosis was made or how a particular treatment was chosen. Many notes were contradictory. This so-called "Source Method" was cited as a cause of fragmented patient care, and Dr. Weed suggested that this form of record keeping was inappropriate for more sophisticated health care where the medical record was used as a means of communication between health care providers. The problem-oriented method, in addition to being comprehensive because of better communication among everyone contributing to health care, allows auditing of care to assure quality. Today, nearly all health care providers use some from of the problem-oriented method for documentation patient care in the medical record.

Clinicians should learn the problem-oriented method of health care so that a systemic, disciplined approach to each patient is used and so no important therapeutic considerations are missed. The approach should always be the same regardless of the simplicity or complexity of the problem.

TWO MAIN COMPONENTS OF THE PROBLEM-ORIENTED APPROACH

Problem List. A problem is defined as a patient concern, a health professional concern, or a concern of both. Many problems are diseases that have been fully worked-up and diagnosed, but all problems are not diagnoses. A problem may be a patient complaint (i.e., a symptom); a social or financial situation; a psychological concern; or a physical limitation. A problem is identified as generally or as specifically as possible, based on available information. A symptom may result in a sign after a physical examination is completed, which may lead to a diagnosis after the completion of the appropriate diagnostic test. The diagnosed disease may then be cured by treatment. For example, a patient may complain of cough and fever, and a sputum culture and chest x-ray lead to the diagnosis of pneumococcal pneumonia. Penicillin is administered and the pneumonia is cured. Thus, problems are dynamic: problems are resolved and new problems develop. Patients frequently have some stable and some inactive problems, but they usually have one problem that is the most severe or that demands attention before the others.

The problem list is developed from the data in a medical record, which would typically include the chief complaint, history of the present illness, medical history, surgical history, family history, social history, medication and allergy history, physical examination, review of systems, results of laboratory tests, serum drug concentration, and diagnostic procedures such as electrocardiogram and radiographs. Health care providers gather information to contribute to the data and organize the data to develop the problem list (see the figure below). However, health care providers may not interpret the data in exactly the same manner, nor will they consider each problem in the same rank of importance; ranking will depend on the health care provider's perspective. The problem list is the table of contents of the medical record and the framework for patient care.

SOAP Note. The second component of the problem-oriented medical record is the organization of the data into the SOAP (subjective, objective, assessment, and plan) note. Each record entry is recorded in this format. A generally accepted clinical practice is the use of a single SOAP note per patient encounter. *Therefore, a single SOAP Note versus a note per problem is to be used to analyze the cases in this textbook.* The subjective and objective data are recorded for the problem(s). Assessments, along with their etiologies,

should be numbered as in the problem list (in priority order), and the plan(s) should also allow such numbering. A blank SOAP sheet is included at the end of this section. Students should use copies of this sheet for writing each of their SOAP notes. The SOAP note components include:

Subjective (S)—Subjective data record how the patient feels or what can be observed about the patient. Subjective data are descriptive in nature and usually cannot be confirmed by procedures or tests. The primary way to obtain subjective data is to listen to the patient's descriptions of complaints or symptoms and responses to questions that are asked in a systematic fashion as a review of systems. Subjective data are also obtained by observing how the patient looks, talks, acts, responds, etc.

Objective (O)—Objective data include the history, as documented in the medical record, and the results of various tests, procedures, and assessments. Objective data may include vital signs, physical examination findings, laboratory test results, and findings for diagnostic procedures such as radiographs, CT scans, and electrocardiograms. Current medications are included as objective data (this is to remind the clinician what the patient is receiving for each problem). Every medication that the patient is receiving should correspond to a problem. If a patient is receiving mediations for an unidentified problem, the problem list is incomplete. Note that some drugs may treat more than one problem.

Assessment (A)—The clinician uses the subjective and objective data to assess therapy or develop a therapeutic plan. A systematic method for assessing each problem should be developed so that the assessment is complete. There are three components to the assessment of each problem.

1. *Etiology:* The clinician should first assess whether this is a drug-induced problem. Many problems are not diseases, but adverse reactions to drugs. Under etiology, the

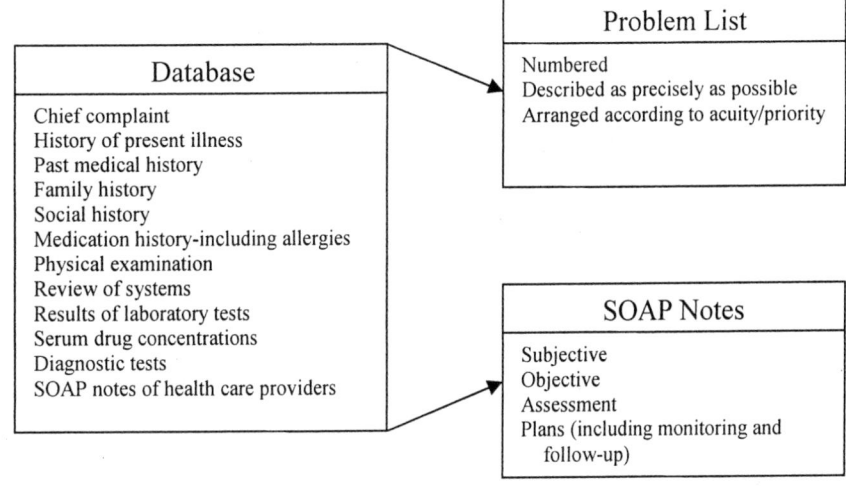

clinician should also identify any risk factors or predisposing factors for a problem in the patient. Modification or reduction of these factors may be a part of the treatment plan and may be as important as drug therapy.

2. *Assessment if therapy is indicated:* Problems may be mild, moderate, or severe; they may be acute or chronic; and they may be stable or progressing. Obviously, the need and urgency of treatment varies with each of these. For acute, severe problems emergency aggressive therapy may be required, while for mild stable problems, a wait-and-watch approach may be more appropriate. Some problems may not be severe enough for drug treatment, and non-drug therapy may be more appropriate for some problems. At times, the diagnosis may not yet be established; more data may be required for diagnosis for an isolated abnormal value may not be a rational basis for drug therapy.

3. *Assessment of current therapy and/or new therapy:* Patients frequently have multiple chronic problems and are therefore already receiving drug therapy. However, this therapy may not be the best possible choice for this patient. New therapy may be initiated for new or old problems. The clinician must systematically evaluate the patient's current therapy as well as the new therapy. The same process applies to both situations. The SOAP note should list all of the reasons for the current assessment. The reasons are important for all health care providers to understand why therapy was changed, for auditing the quality of care, and for helping the healthcare professional remember the reasons for the changes.

■ *Optimal therapy (i.e., drug of choice):* The clinician should determine that this is the optimal therapy for this patient. This does not necessarily mean that it is the usual "drug of choice" for this disease. There may be patient-specific reasons why the usual "drug of choice" would be contraindicated or inappropriate for this patient. The drug should be chosen considering the patient's other problems (drug-disease interactions), other drugs (drug-drug interactions), age, renal and hepatic function, allergies (considering cross-sensitivities), risk factors for adverse reactions or side effects, convenience, compliance, and cost.

■ *Correct dose:* The clinician should determine the correct dose of the drug for this patient considering the patient's age, sex, weight, renal and hepatic functions, other drugs that the patient is taking, and any other pertinent factors. The pharmacist on the team should always perform pharmacokinetic calculations based on population parameters or previous drug levels.

■ *Correct dosage form:* The correct dosage form, route, and schedule of administration should be determined. Patient-specific factors, convenience, compliance, costs, and lifestyle should be considered.

■ *Correct duration:* The correct duration of therapy should be determined. Patient-specific factors may require that therapy be longer or shorter than what is usually recommended for this problem. Some problems require that therapy be continued for lifetime or until circumstances change, while other problems are cured by a single course of therapy. Unfortunately, patients are frequently started on therapy that is never discontinued, although the problem has resolved. Some patients need to be treated longer because the disease is severe and they have certain predisposing factors. Other patients may need to be treated only during an acute exacerbation of their disease. Thus, the duration of therapy is patient specific.

■ *Drug(s) required:* A determination should be made as to whether or not all the drugs that the patient is taking are required. All drugs taken by the patient should be for problems identified on the problem list. The patient should not be taking additional drugs; if there are additional drugs, the problem list is incomplete. Duplication of drugs from the same therapeutic category frequently occurs, and some of these drugs may be discontinued. A higher dose of a single agent may be preferred to two drugs for the same problem. At times, a single drug may be used to treat more than one problem. Some problems do not require drug therapy. Health care professionals should always try to minimize the number of drugs that a patient is taking.

■ *Additional monitoring parameters:* For current therapy, in addition to the above, the following should be determined.

○ **Response to therapy:** If the patient is responding appropriately to therapy. Patient-specific factors should be considered and include the items discussed under goals and monitoring parameters below.

○ **Untoward reactions:** If the patient is having adverse reactions, side effects, or drug interactions. Obviously, the plan will be influenced by the occurrence of any of these.

○ **Medication adherence issues:** If the medications have been taken as prescribed. Drugs that are not taken as prescribed are usually not effective. The plan for treatment of a patient who is non-adherent to his/her medications is different from the plan for a patient who is adherence to therapy but is not responding. Serious consequences can occur in a patient who is non-adherent to therapy when therapy is altered based on the assumption that the patient has been taking his/her medications as prescribed. Questions must be phrased carefully to obtain accurate information about medication adherence.

Plan (P)—After the assessment of the subjective and objective data and therapy, a plan is developed.

1. Therapeutic: Current therapy must be either continued or discontinued. The reasons for continuing or discontinuing current therapy should have been stated in the assessment portion of the SOAP note. If new therapy is initiated, the clinician should state the drug, dose, dosage form, route, schedule, duration, and exactly how therapy will be initiated. Therapy may be initiated at full doses or the dose may be titrated depending on the drug and the patient or

problem. If the drug is to be titrated, the size and the frequency of the dosage changed should be stated. Precise instructions for drug administration should be included. The reasons for selecting the drug, dose, dosage form, route schedule, and duration should have been stated in the assessment portion of the soap note.

2. Drugs to be avoided: The clinician should list all drugs that could potentially be used to treat this problem but that should be avoided in this patient for patient-specific reasons. If the patient is likely to receive a drug for another problem which would interact with the therapy for this problem, it should be stated that it, too, should be avoided. If these drugs are not documented in the POMR as ones to avoid, other health care providers may inadvertently prescribe them. The clinician should list the reasons why these drugs are being avoided, such as allergies, age, drug-disease interactions, drug-drug interactions, renal or hepatic dysfunction, risk factors for adverse reactions or side effects, convenience, adherence issues, or cost, if these reasons were not already stated in the assessment portion of the SOAP note.

3. Goals: Each treatment plan should have a long-term goal that should be both problem- and patient-specific. Some problems are cured, while others are controlled or relieved. In some patients, the subjective and objective evidence of the problem will return to normal; in other patients with severe problems the subjective and objective evidence will only return toward normal. Other appropriate goals include preventing acute complications, preventing long-term morbidity and mortality, avoiding adverse drug reactions or drug interactions, improving compliance, improving quality of life, and decreasing health care costs.

4. Therapeutic and toxicity monitoring parameters: Each therapeutic plan should be monitored by specific parameters to assess response and to document that no adverse drug reactions or side effects are occurring. When selecting *therapeutic monitoring parameters*, the clinician must select the appropriate subjective and objective data that will be followed to assess response to therapy. These parameters should be chosen carefully, considering cost, invasiveness, risks of the procedure, sensitivity, and reliability. Usually the same subjective and objective data that were used to diagnose the disease are used to monitor therapy, except expensive or invasive tests are not always repeated as monitoring parameters. The frequency for monitoring these parameters should be stated. Some critically ill patients should be monitored every 5 minutes, while other tests may be performed only yearly in stable patients. End points should be established for each therapeutic plan. The end points should be patient-, drug-, and problem-specific. Like the goals, the monitoring parameters may return to normal or toward normal, depending upon the patient, drug, or problem. The end point may indicate that therapy is complete or has been inadequate. If the end point shows that therapy is complete,

then it should be stated that the drugs will be discontinued. If the end point shows that therapy is inadequate, additional or alternative therapy may be prescribed.

When considering *toxicity monitoring parameters*, each therapeutic plan should be monitored for adverse drug reactions, side effects, and drug interactions. The clinician must select the appropriate subjective and objective data that will be observed for assessment of toxicity. The intervals for monitoring these data should be stated. Any abnormalities that would be revealed by routine screening tests and that would indicate a drug-induced problem should also be identified in the plan. Along with the frequency of these observations the plan should include how serious or frequently encountered adverse effects should be handled.

5. Patient education: The plan will be useless unless it is implemented correctly. All patients should know the name(s), dose, indication, schedule, storage, precautions, duration, and side effect/adverse reactions of the drugs that they are using. Some plans involve no-drug therapy or lifestyle changes as well as drug therapy. Some dosage forms require more detailed instruction for administration than others. Specific information or techniques to enhance patient adherence to therapy should be discussed and documented in the POMR. Any patient concerns about the medication should be addressed. Any information required for the safe and proper use of the drug should be discussed.

6. Future plans: It is likely that the patient will be seen again, so some plans should be made for follow-up. Another clinic visit may be scheduled, additional tests may be required to establish a baseline before treatment is initiated, or contingency plans may be made in case the patient does not respond to therapy or develop a drug-induced problem. The clinician should document what future plans are needed for this patient.

Using the SOAP format is a systematic way to critique or plan pharmacologic and nonpharmacologic therapy for a patient. Because it is a systematic approach if it is employed in a disciplined way for each patient only patient-specific treatment decisions will be made.

For the sake of saving space, all information from the record has been abbreviated and condensed. The laboratory data have been reported in SI units followed by standard units in parenthesis. Abbreviations have been used less frequently than they are used in medical charts, but common abbreviations are used to save space and familiarize the student with these abbreviations.

CONCLUSION

The SOAP format allows a systematic approach to therapy and is widely used in medical education and practice. However, individual practitioners may analyze a case slightly differently. In many cases, the correct therapy for an individual patient will be agreed upon by all who analyze the case, because in these situations there is only one possible therapy based upon the contraindications or other patient variables. In other cases, the correct therapy is not so straightforward and two or three alternatives may be equally acceptable. In these cases, the choice of therapy frequently rests with the individual practitioner's preference. In other cases, there may be one therapy that would be the best for the patient, but other alternatives may be acceptable because of extenuating circumstances such as a history of non-adherence to therapy. Therefore the student should use the case primarily to learn a method of analyzing cases. The answers given in these cases may not be the only acceptable answers, and other available alternatives would be equally efficacious and safe. In addition, the therapy and information given in these cases may become incorrect as new knowledge is accumulated. In some cases, the available literature is conflicting or controversial, and two practitioners may have different opinions based on the available information. In all cases, the case analysis and answers to the questions pertain only to the patient involved. The information may or may not be applicable to other patients with the same problem. Therefore, the student is warned against memorizing these cases. This case allows the students to practice analyzing cases and making decisions concerning therapeutics in a situation that cannot harm a patient. By this process the student should develop skill in therapeutics. If these cases are used as intended, the student will make a commitment to a method of analyzing the patient's case. This will be useful in developing the skills that are necessary for performance in a clinical setting. Thus, the student is highly encouraged to write the SOAP notes. A single book cannot be responsible for the development of critical evaluation skills, but the cases incorporated within the 8th edition of *Textbook of Therapeutics: Drug and Disease Management,* along with the guidance of faculty in appropriate courses, will aid in preparing students in therapeutics.

PROBLEM LIST and SOAP NOTE FOR CASE_____
Problem List:
SUBJECTIVE:
OBJECTIVE:
ASSESSMENT:
PLAN:

Section Editors

Kimberly A. Bergstrom, PharmD
Chief Clinical Officer
Oncology Therapeutics Network
South San Francisco, California
Adjunct Assistant Professor
University of California San Francisco
San Francisco, California

Paul M. Beringer, PharmD, BCPS, FASHP
Associate Professor of Clinical Pharmacy
School of Pharmacy
University of Southern California
Los Angeles, California

Ali J. Olyaei, PharmD, BCPS
Associate Professor of Medicine
Director of Clinical Research
Nephrology and Hypertension
Clinical Pharmacotherapist
Oregon Health & Sciences University
Portland, Oregon

W. Nathan Rawls, PharmD
Professor
Department of Pharmacy
College of Pharmacy
University of Tennessee Health Sciences Center
Clinical Pharmacy Specialist
Veterans Affairs Medical Center
Memphis, Tennessee

P. David Rogers, PharmD, PhD, FCCP
Associate Professor of Pharmacy
Assistant Professor of Pharmaceutical Sciences and
Pediatrics
Colleges of Pharmacy and Medicine
University of Tennessee Health Sciences Center
Children's Foundation Research Center of Memphis
Le Bonheur Children's Medical Center
Memphis, Tennessee

Timothy H. Self, PharmD
Professor of Pharmacy
Department of Pharmacy
University of Tennessee Health Sciences Center
Memphis, Tennessee

Contributors

Brian K. Alldredge, PharmD
Professor of Clinical Pharmacy and Clinical Professor of
Neurology
School of Pharmacy
University of California, San Francisco
San Francisco, California

Kristan A. Augustin, PharmD, BCOP
Clinical Pharmacist
Bone Marrow Transplantation and Leukemia
Barnes-Jewish Hospital at Washington University in St.
Louis Medical Center
St. Louis, Missouri

Lisa M. Avery, PharmD
Clinical Pharmacist
St. Joseph's Hospital
Princeton, New Jersey

Lamar E. Bailey, MD
Assistant Professor of Medicine and Psychiatry
University of Tennessee
Certified Addictionologist
American Society of Addiction Medicine
Memphis, Tennessee

Jeffrey N. Baldwin, PharmD, FAPha, FASHP
Associate Professor of Pharmacy Practice
University of Nebraska Medical Center
Omaha, Nebraska

Carol Balmer, PharmD, BCOP
Assistant Dean for Postgraduate Professional Education
Associate Professor of Pharmacy
University of Colorado at Denver Health Sciences Center
Denver, Colorado

Jennifer W. Beall, PharmD
McWhorter School of Pharmacy
Samford University
St. Vincent's Hospital
Birmingham, Alabama

Rosemary R. Berardi, PharmD, FCCP, FASHP, FAPHA
Professor of Pharmacy
University of Michigan College of Pharmacy
Clinical Pharmacist
Gastrointestinal and Liver Diseases
Department of Pharmacy
University of Michigan Health System
Ann Arbor, Michigan

Kimberly A. Bergstrom, PharmD
Chief Clinical Officer
Oncology Therapeutics Network/Onmark
South San Francisco, California
Adjunct Assistant Professor
University of California San Francisco
San Francisco, California

Paul M. Beringer, PharmD, BCPS, FASHP
Associate Professor of Clinical Pharmacy
School of Pharmacy
University of Southern California
Los Angeles, California

Kathryn Blake, PharmD
Senior Research Scientist
Center for Clinical Pediatric Pharmacology Research
Nemours Children's Clinic
Jacksonville, Florida

Rebecca Florez Boettger, PharmD
Assistant Clinical Professor
University of California San Francisco
San Francisco, California

Michael Bottorff, PharmD, FCCP
Professor of Clinical Pharmacy
University of Cincinnati College of Pharmacy
Cincinnati, Ohio

Bradley A Boucher, PharmD, FCCP, FCCM
Professor of Pharmacy
University of Tennessee Health Sciences Center
Clinical Pharmacist
Regional Medical Center at Memphis
Memphis, Tennessee

Eric G. Boyce, PharmD
Professor of Clinical Pharmacy
Philadelphia College of Pharmacy
University of the Sciences in Philadelphia
Philadelphia, Pennsylvania

Ronald L. Braden, PharmD
Associate Professor of Pharmacy
University of Tennessee Health Sciences Center
Clinical Pharmacy Specialist, Critical Care
Veterans Affairs Medical Center
Memphis, Tennessee

Geneva C. Briggs, PharmD, BCPS
President, Briggs Associates
Richmond, Virginia

Bernadette K. Brown, PharmD
Associate Professor of Pharmacy Practice
Butler University College of Pharmacy and Health
Sciences
Indianapolis, Indiana

J. Richard Brown, PharmD, BCPS, FASHP
Professor of Pharmacy and Medicine
University of Tennessee Health Sciences Center
Clinical Pharmacy Specialist
Veterans Affairs Medical Center
Memphis, Tennessee

Rex O. Brown, PharmD, BCNSP, FCCP
Professor and Executive Vice-Chair Department of
Pharmacy
College of Pharmacy
University of Tennessee Health Sciences Center
Memphis, Tennessee

Howard A. Burris, III
The Sarah Cannon Research Institute
Nashville, Tennessee

Kristina L. Butler, PharmD, BCPS, CDE
Affiliate Faculty Member
Oregon State University College of Pharmacy
Clinical Pharmacy Specialist, Primary Care
Providence Medical Group
Portland, Oregon

R. Keith Campbell, BPharm, MBA, CDE
Professor of Pharmacotherapy
Washington State University
St. Louis, Missouri

Diane M. Cappelletty, PharmD
University of Toledo
College of Pharmacy
Toledo, Ohio

Judy L. Chase, PharmD, FASHP
Clinical Pharmacy Specialist
University of Texas MD Anderson Cancer Center
Houston, Texas

Jack J. Chen, PharmD, BCPS, CGP, FASCP
Associate Professor of Neurology
School of Pharmacy
Clinical Associate Professor of Neurology
Movement Disorders Clinic
Loma Linda University
Loma Linda, California

Cinda L. Christensen, PharmD
Assistant Clinical Professor of Pharmacy
University of California, San Francisco
San Francisco, California
Clinical Specialist in Infectious Diseases
Department of Pharmaceutical Services
University of California, Davis Medical Center
Sacramento, California

Bruce D. Clayton, PharmD, RPh
Professor of Pharmacy Practice
Butler University College of Pharmacy and Health
Sciences
Indianapolis, Indiana

G. Dennis Clifton, PharmD, FCCP
Vice President, INGfertility
Valleyford, Washington

Jennifer Cocohoba, PharmD
Health Sciences Assistant Clinical Professor
Department of Clinical Pharmacy
School of Pharmacy
University of California, San Francisco
San Francisco, California

L. Brian Cross, PharmD, CDE
Assistant Professor of Pharmacy and Family Medicine
University of Tennessee Health Science Center
Memphis, Tennessee
Director, Center of Excellence in Primary Care and Rural
Health
Kingsport, Tennessee

Kristin L. Hennenfent, PharmD, MBA
Ortho Biotech Clinical Affairs
Manager of Clinical Affairs
St. Louis, Missouri

Michael B. Doherty, PharmD
Director of Experiential Training
Assistant Professor of Pharmacy Practice
University of Cincinnati College of Pharmacy
Cincinnati, Ohio

Betty J. Dong, PharmD
Professor of Clinical Pharmacy
University of California, San Francisco
San Francisco, California

Vicky Dudas, PharmD
Assistant Clinical Professor of Pharmacy
Clinical Pharmacist
Infectious Diseases
University of California San Francisco Medical Center
San Francisco, California

Shareen El-Ibiary, PharmD, BCPS
Assistant Professor of Clinical Pharmacy
Women's Health Pharmacy Specialist
Drug Information Analysis Service
University of California, San Francisco
San Francisco, California

Erika J. Ernst, PharmD, BCPS
Department of Clinical and Administrative Pharmacy
University of Iowa
Iowa City, Iowa

William E. Evans, PharmD
Professor of Pharmacy, Pediatrics, and Pharmaceutical Services
University of Tennessee Health Sciences Center
Director and CEO
St. Jude Children's Research Hospital
Memphis, Tennessee

Rebecca S. Finley, PharmD, MS, FASHP
President, Meniscus Educational Institute
West Conshohocken, Pennsylvania

Douglas N. Fish, PharmD, FCCM, BCPS
Associate Professor and Vice Chair of Clinical Pharmacy
University of Colorado Health Sciences Center
Clinical Specialist in Infectious Diseases/Critical Care
University of Colorado Hospital
Denver, Colorado

Stephan L. Foster, PharmD, BSPharm
Associate Professor of Pharmacy and Family Medicine
Director, Office of Community Health
University of Tennessee Health Sciences Center
Memphis, Tennessee

Andrea S. Franks, PharmD, BCPS
Assistant Professor of Pharmacy
University of Tennessee Health Sciences Center
Director, Pharmacotherapy Education
University of Tennessee Family Practice Center
St. Francis Hospital
Memphis, Tennessee

Laurie H. Fukushima, PharmD
Ambulatory Care Clinical Pharmacist
Internal Medicine
Kaiser Permanente
Wailuku, Hawaii

Michael P. Gabay, BS, PharmD, BCPS
Clinical Assistant Professor of Pharmacy
University of Illinois at Chicago
Assistant Director, Drug Information Center
Chicago, Illinois

Marie E. Gardner, PharmD
Associate Professor of Pharmacy Practice
University of Arizona College of Pharmacy
Tucson, Arizona

Kevin W. Garey, PharmD
Assistant Professor of Pharmacy
University of Houston College of Pharmacy
Houston, Texas

Jody Sheehan Garey, PharmD
Clinical Pharmacy Specialist
Thoracic/Head and Neck Medical Oncology
University of Texas MD Anderson Cancer Center
Houston, Texas

Christa M. George, PharmD, BCPS, CDE
Assistant Professor of Pharmacy
University of Tennessee Health Sciences Center
Ambulatory Care Clinical Pharmacist
Regional Medical Center at Memphis
Memphis, Tennessee

Laura N. Gerard, PharmD
University of Houston College of Pharmacy
St. Luke's Episcopal Hospital
Houston, Texas

Jane M. Gervasio, PharmD, BCNSP
Assistant Professor of Pharmacy Practice
Butler University
Nutrition Support Pharmacist
Methodist Hospital at Clarian Health Partners
Indianapolis, Indiana

Jacob P. Gettig, PharmD, BCPS
Assistant Professor of Pharmacy Practice
Midwestern University
Chicago College of Pharmacy
Downers Grove, Illinois
Drug Information Specialist
Edward Hospital
Naperville, Illinois

Mark A. Gill, PharmD, FASHP, FCCP
Professor of Clinical Pharmacy
University of Southern California
Los Angeles, California

Edgar R. Gonzalez, PharmD, FASHP
President and CEO
Capital Pharmacy Consultant
Mechanicsville, Virginia

Dick R. Gourley, PharmD
Professor and Dean
College of Pharmacy
University of Tennessee
Memphis, Tennessee

Greta K. Gourley, MSN, PhD, PharmD
Associate Professor of Pharmacy Practice and
Pharmacoeconomics
College of Pharmacy
University of Tennessee Health Sciences Center
Memphis, Tennessee

Mary A. Gutierrez, PharmD
Associate Professor of Clinical Pharmacy
University of Southern California School of Pharmacy
Los Angeles, California

Emily B. Hak, PharmD, BCNSP, BCPS
University of Tennessee Health Sciences Center
Departments of Pharmacy, Pediatrics, and Pharmacology
Le Bonheur Children's Medical Center
Memphis, Tennessee

Emily E. Han, PharmD
Assistant Professor of Clinical Pharmacy
University of Southern California
Los Angeles, California

Scott D. Hanes, PharmD
College of Pharmacy
University of Illinois at Chicago
University of Illinois Medical Center
Chicago, Illinois

Helene Hardy, PharmD
Assistant Professor of Pharmacy Practice
Boston School of Pharmacy
Massachusetts College of Pharmacy and Health Sciences
HIV Pharmacotherapy Services, Director
Center for HIV/AIDS Care and Research
Boston Medical Center
Boston, Massachusetts

Mary F. Hebert, PharmD, FCCP
Professor of Pharmacy
University of Washington, School of Pharmacy
Seattle, Washington

Richard A. Helms, PharmD
Professor and Chair of Pharmacy
Professor of Pediatrics
Director, Center for Pediatric Pharmacokinetics and
Therapeutics
University of Tennessee Health Sciences Center
Director of Clinical Pharmacy
Le Bonheur Children's Medical Center
Memphis, Tennessee

Richard N. Herrier, PharmD
Assistant Professor of Pharmacy Practice
University of Arizona College of Pharmacy
Tucson, Arizona

Timothy J. Heuring, PharmD
Infectious Disease Clinical Specialist
Saint Louis University Hospital
St. Louis, Missouri

Michael D. Hogue, PharmD
McWhorter School of Pharmacy
Samford University
Jefferson County Department of Health
Birmingham, Alabama

Valerie W. Hogue, PharmD, CDE
Associate Professor of Clinical and Administrative
Pharmacy Sciences
College of Pharmacy, Nursing, and Allied Health
Sciences
Howard University
Ambulatory Care Pharmacist
Veterans Affairs Medical Center
Washington, District of Columbia

Joanna Q. Hudson, PharmD, BCPS
Associate Professor of Pharmacy
Assistant Professor of Medicine
University of Tennessee Health Sciences Center
Memphis, Tennessee

Heather J. Johnson, PharmD
Assistant Professor of Pharmacy Practice
University of Pittsburgh Medical Center
Pittsburgh, Pennsylvania

Jannifer L. Johnson, PharmD
Medical Science Liaison
Science Oriented Solutions
Decatur, Georgia

Richard P. Johnson, MD
Associate Professor of Psychiatry
University of Tennesse
Director, Mental Health Sciences
Veterans Affairs Medical Center
Memphis, Tennessee

Suzanne Fields Jones, PharmD
The Sarah Cannon Cancer Center
Nashville, Tennessee

Paul W. Jungnickel, PhD, RPh
Professor of Pharmacy Practice
Associate Dean for Academic and Student Affairs
Harrison School of Pharmacy
Auburn University
Auburn, Alabama

Charles M. Karnack, PharmD, BCNSP
Assistant Professor of Clinical Pharmacy
Duquesne University
Clinical Pharmacy Specialist
Mercy Hospital of Pittsburgh
Pittsburgh, Pennsylvania

H. William Kelly, PharmD
Professor Emeritus of Pediatrics
University of New Mexico
Albuquerque, New Mexico

Wendy Klein-Schwartz, PharmD, MPh
Department of Pharmacy Practice and Science
Maryland Poison Center
University of Maryland School of Pharmacy
Baltimore, Maryland

Maria D. Kostka-Rokosz, PharmD
Assistant Professor of Pharmacy Practice
Director, Drug Information Center
School of Pharmacy, Boston
Massachusetts College of Pharmacy and Health Sciences
Boston, Massachusetts

Susan Krikorian, MS
Associate Professor of Pharmacy Practice
Massachusetts College of Pharmacy and Health Sciences
Clinical Pharmacy Specialist in Nephrology
Beth Israel Deaconess Medical Center
Boston, Massachusetts

S. Casey Laizure, PharmD
Associate Professor of Pharmacy
College of Pharmacy
University of Tennessee Health Sciences Center
Memphis, Tennessee

Andreas Katsoya Lauer, MD
Residency Program Director
Assistant Professor of Ophthalmology
Casey Eye Institute
Oregon Health & Science University
Devers Eye Institute
Legacy Good Samaritan Hospital
Portland, Oregon

Russell E. Lewis, PharmD, BCPS, FCCP
Associate Professor of Pharmacy
University of Houston
The University of Texas M.D. Anderson Cancer Center
Houston Texas

Richard D. Lozano, RPh
Clinical Practitioner
Department of Pharmacy
University of Texas MD Anderson Cancer Center
Houston, Texas

Sherry A. Luedtke, PharmD
Associate Dean of Professional Affairs
Associate Professor of Pharmacy Practice
Texas Tech University Health Sciences Center
School of Pharmacy
Amarillo, Texas

Harold J. Manley, PharmD, BCPS
Associate Professor of Pharmacy Practice
Albany College of Pharmacy
Albany, New York

Leisa L. Marshall, PharmD, FASCP, CGP
Clinical Associate Professor of Clinical and
Administrative Sciences
Mercer University Southern School of Pharmacy
Atlanta, Georgia

Hewitt W. Matthews, PhD
Dean and Hood-Meyer Professor
Department of Pharmaceutical Sciences
Mercer University School of Pharmacy
Atlanta, Georgia

Monique Mayo, PharmD
Oncology Pharmacist Consultant
Solano Beach, California

Dayna L. McCauley, PharmD, BCOP
Long Island Gynecological Oncologists, PC
Smithtown, New York

William W. McCloskey, PharmD
Associate Professor of Pharmacy Practice
Massachusetts College of Pharmacy and Health Sciences
Boston, Massachusetts

John N. McCormick, PharmD, BCNSP
University of Tennessee School of Pharmacy
Department of Pharmaceutical Services
St. Jude Children's Research Hospital
Memphis, Tennessee

Yolanda B. McKoy-Beach, PharmD
Minority Faculty Fellow in Pharmacy
College of Pharmacy, Nursing, and Allied Health
Sciences
Howard University
Clinical Pharmacist
Family Medical and Counseling Services
La Clinic Del Pueblo
Washington, District of Columbia

Bernd Meibohm, PhD, FCP
Department of Pharmaceutical Sciences
College of Pharmacy
University of Tennessee Health Sciences Center
Memphis, Tennessee

Helen Meldrum, EdD
Associate Professor of Social and Administrative Sciences
Massachusetts College of Pharmacy and Health Sciences
Boston, Massachusetts

Robert Keith Middleton, PharmD
Saint Clare's Hospital
Weston, Wisconsin

Susan W. Miller, PharmD, FASCP, CGP
Department of Clinical and Administrative Sciences
Mercer University Southern School of Pharmacy
Atlanta, Georgia

Tammi T. Miyahara, PharmD
Oncology Medical Writing Consultant
San Jose, California

Susannah E. Motl, PharmD
Assistant Professor
University of Tennessee Health Sciences Center
Memphis, Tennessee

Myrna Y. Munar, PharmD, BCPS
Associate Professor of Phamacotherapy
Department of Pharmacy Practice
Oregon Health & Science University
Portland, Oregon

Brien L. Neudeck, PharmD
Assistant Professor of Pharmacy
University of Tennessee College of Pharmacy
Memphis, Tennessee

Tien M.H. Ng, BSPharm, PharmD
Assistant Professor of Clinical Pharmacy
University of Southern California
Los Angeles, California

David E. Nix, PharmD
Associate Professor of Pharmacy Practice
University of Arizona College of Pharmacy
Tucson, Arizona

Paul E. Nolan, Jr., PharmD
Associate Professor of Pharmacy
University of Arizona College of Pharmacy
Tucson, Arizona

Diane Nykamp-McCarter, PharmD
Professor of Pharmacy Practice
Mercer University Southern School of Pharmacy
Atlanta, Georgia

Ali J. Olyaei, PharmD, BCPS
Associate Professor of Medicine
Director of Clinical Research
Nephrology and Hypertension
Clinical Pharmacotherapist
Oregon Health & Sciences University
Portland, Oregon

Michael A. Oszko, PharmD, BCPS, FASHP
Department of Pharmacy Practice
University of Kansas Pharmacy Practice
Kansas City, Kansas

Brian R. Overholser, PharmD
Associate Professor of Pharmacy Practice
School of Pharmacy and Pharmaceutical Sciences
Purdue University
Adjunct Assistant Professor of Medicine
Indiana University
Indianapolis, Indiana

Amy L. Pakyz, PharmD, MS
Assistant Professor of Pharmacy
Virginia Commonwealth University
Richmond, Virginia

Shirley Palmer-Murrow, BS, PharmD
Senior Scientific Liaison
Ortho-McNeil Janssen Scientific Affairs, LLC
Denver, Colorado

Beth Logsdon Pangle, PharmD, BCNSP
Senior Clinical Pharmacy Specialist
Cook Children's Medical Center
Fort Worth, Texas

Louise Parent-Stevens, PharmD, BCPS
Clinical Assistant Professor of Pharmacy Practice
Clinical Pharmacist
Family Medical Center
University of Illinois at Chicago
Chicago, Illinois

Dina K. Patel, BS, PharmD
University of Texas MD Anderson Cancer Center
Houston, Texas

Jennifer L. Pauley, PharmD
University of Tennessee College of Pharmacy
Department of Pharmaceutical Services
St. Jude Children's Research Hospital
Memphis, Tennessee

Constance M. Pfeiffer, PharmD, BCPS, BCOP
Clinical Assistant Professor of Pharmacy Practice and Administration
Rutgers University College of Pharmacy
Piscataway, New Jersey

Stephanie J. Phelps, PharmD
Professor of Pharmacy and Pediatrics
Vice-Chair of Professional Experience Program
University of Tennessee Health Sciences Center
Director of Pharmacokinetic Service
Le Bonheur Children's Medical Center
Memphis, Tennessee

Kalen B. Porter, PharmD, BCPS
Clinical Assistant Professor of Pediatrics
Department of Clinical and Administrative Services
Mercer University Southern School of Pharmacy
Atlanta, Georgia

Talia Puzantian, PharmD, BCPP
Associate Clinical Professor of Pharmacy
University of California, San Francisco
San Francisco, California

David J. Quan, PharmD, BCPS
Assistant Clinical Professor
School of Pharmacy
University of California San Francisco
Pharmacist Specialist
UCSF Medical Center
San Francisco, California

R. Chris Rathbun, PharmD, BCPS-ID
Associate Professor of Pharmacy
University of Southern California School of Pharmacy
Infectious Diseases Pharmacist
Huntington Hospital
Los Angeles, California

W. Nathan Rawls, PharmD
Professor of Pharmacy
University of Tennessee Health Sciences Center
Clinical Pharmacist Specialist
Veterans Affairs Medical Center
Memphis, Tennessee

Lori A. Reisner, PharmD
Associate Clinical Professor of Clinical Pharmacy
University of California, San Francisco
San Francisco, California

Beth H. Resman-Targoff, PharmD
Clinical Associate Professor of Pharmacy Practice
University of Oklahoma College of Pharmacy
Oklahoma City, Oklahoma

Ted L. Rice, MS, FASHP, BCPS
Associate Professor of Pharmacy and Therapeutics
University of Pittsburgh
School of Pharmacy
Clinical Pharmacy Specialist
Critical Care, University of Pittsburgh Medical Center
Pittsburgh, Pennsylvania

P. David Rogers, PharmD, PhD, FCCP
Associate Professor of Pharmacy
Assistant Professor of Pharmaceutical Sciences and Pediatrics
Colleges of Pharmacy and Medicine
University of Tennessee Health Sciences Center
Children's Foundation Research Center of Memphis
Le Bonheur Children's Medical Center
Memphis, Tennessee

Charles F. Seifert, PharmD, FCCP, BCPS
Professor of Pharmacy Practice
Regional Dean for Lubbock Programs
Texas Tech University Health Sciences Center
Specified Professional Personnel
University Medical Center
Lubbock, Texas

Cindy C. Selzer, PharmD, BCPS
Assistant Professor of Pharmacy Practice
Butler University
Clinical Pharmacist
Indiana University Hospital of Clarian Health Partners
Indianapolis, Indiana

Stephen M. Setter, PharmD, CDE, CGP, DVM
Associate Professor of Pharmacotherapy
Elder Services/Visiting Nurses Association
Washington State University
Spokane, Washington

Amy Heck Sheehan, PharmD
Associate Professor of Pharmacy Practice
Purdue University School of Pharmacy and Pharmaceutical Sciences
Drug Information Specialist
Clarian Health Partners
Indianapolis, Indiana

Sam K. Shimomura, PharmD
Professor of Clinical Pharmacy
Western University of Health Sciences College of Pharmacy
Pomona, California

Stephen D. Silberstein, MD
Professor of Neurology
Jefferson Medical College
Thomas Jefferson University
Director, Jefferson Headache Center
Thomas Jefferson University Hospital
Philadelphia, Pennsylvania

J. Jason Sims, PharmD
Principal Scientist
Medtronic Cardiac Rhythm Management
Minneapolis, Minnesota

Harleen Singh, PharmD
Assistant Professor of Pharmacy Practice
College of Pharmacy
Oregon Health & Science University
Portland, Oregon

Renu F. Singh, PharmD
Assistant Clinical Professor
University of California, San Diego School of Pharmacy
and Pharmaceutical Sciences
La Jolla, California

Douglas Slain, PharmD, BCPS
Associate Professor
West Virginia University School of Pharmacy
West Virginia University Hospitals
Morgantown, West Virginia

Ralph E. Small, PharmD
Professor Emeritus of Pharmacy and Medicine
Virginia Commonwealth University
Richmond, Virginia

Kelly M. Smith, PharmD
Associate Professor of Pharmacy Practice Science
University of Kentucky College of Pharmacy
Lexington, Kentucky

Kevin M. Sowinski, PharmD, BCPS
Assistant Professor of Pharmacy Practice
Purdue University School of Pharmacy and
Pharmaceutical Sciences
Indianapolis, Indiana

Joan M. Stachnik, PharmD, BCPS
Department of Pharmacy Practice
College of Pharmacy
University of Illinois Medical Center at Chicago
Chicago, Illinois

Robert J. Stagg, PharmD
Vice President, Regulatory and Drug Safety
PDL BioPharma, Inc.
Fremont, California

Gregory V. Stajich, PharmD
Associate Professor of Pharmacy Practice
Mercer University Southern School of Pharmacy
Atlanta, Georgia

Robert C. Stevens, PharmD, FCCP, BCPS
Associate Professor of Pharmacy
Clinical College of Pharmacy
University of Tennessee Health Sciences Center
Memphis, Tennessee

Glen L. Stimmel, PharmD, BCPP
Professor of Clinical Pharmacy and Psychiatry
University of Southern California Schools of Pharmacy
and Medicine
Los Angeles, California

Wendy Gattis Stough, PharmD
Assistant Clinical Professor in Medicine
Duke University Medical Center
Durham, North Carolina

Janice L. Stumpf, PharmD
Clinical Associate Professor of Pharmacy
University of Michigan
Clinical Pharmacist, Drug Information Service
University of Michigan Health System
Ann Arbor, Michigan

Paula A. Thompson, MS, PharmD, BCPS
Assistant Professor of Pharmacy
McWhorter School of Pharmacy
Samford University
Birmingham, Alabama

Karen J. Tietze, BS, PharmD
Professor of Clinical Pharmacy
Philadelphia College of Pharmacy
University of Sciences in Philadelphia
Philadelphia, Pennsylvania

Sarah R. Tomasello, PharmD, BCPS
Clinical Assistant Professor of Pharmacy Practice
Piscataway, New Jersey
Clinical Specialist in Nephrology
Robert Wood University Hospital
New Brunswick, New Jersey

Kevin A. Townsend, MS, PharmD, BCPS
Adjunct Clinical Associate Professor of Pharmacy
University of Michigan
Clinical Education Consultant
Pfizer, Inc.
Ann Arbor, Michigan

VanAnh Trinh, PharmD
Clinical Pharmacy Specialist
Melanoma and Sarcoma
Medical Oncology
Department of Pharmacy
University of Texas MD Anderson Cancer Center
Houston, Texas

Candy Tsouronis, PharmD
Associate Professor of Clinical Pharmacy
University of California, San Francisco
San Francisco, California

Jeanne Hawkins Van Tyle, MS, PharmD
Professor of Pharmacy Practice
Butler University College of Pharmacy and Health
Sciences
Indianapolis, Indiana

Linh Khanh Vuong, PharmD
Clinical Adjunct Professor
Clinical Hospital Pharmacist
Jackson Memorial Hospital
Miami, Florida

Mary L. Wagner, MS, PharmD
Associate Professor
Ernest Mario School of Pharmacy
Rutgers University
Piscataway, New Jersey

Deborah A. Ward, PharmD, BCOP
Assistant Professor of Pharmacy
University of Tennessee
Clinical Pharmacist
St. Jude Children's Research Hospital
Memphis, Tennessee

John F. Weaver, PhD
Psychologist
Clinical Supervisor
Chemical Dependency Center
Veterans Affairs Medical Center
Memphis, Tennessee

James W. Wheless, MD
Professor and Chief of Pediatric Neurology
University of Tennessee Helath Sciences Center
Director, Le Bonheur Comprehensive Epilepsy Program
and Neuroscience
Le Bonheur Children's Medical Center
Clinical Chief and Director of Pediatric Neurology
St. Jude Children's Research Hospital
Memphis, Tennessee

John R. White, Jr., PA-C, PharmD
Department of Pharmacotherapy
College of Pharmacy
Washington State University
Spokane, Washington
Indian Health Service Clinic
Wellpinit, Washington

Kimberly Bardel Whitlock, PharmD
Manager, Clinical Services
National Oncology Alliance, Inc.
San Rafael, California

Dennis M. Williams, PharmD, FCCP
Associate Professor of Pharmacotherapy and Experimental
Therapeutics
UNC School of Pharmacy
Chapel Hill, North Carolina

Michael Z. Wincor, PharmD, BCPP
Associate Professor of Clinical Pharmacy
Psychiatry and the Behavioral Sciences
Associate Dean of External Programs
University of Southern California Schools of Pharmacy
and Medicine
Los Angeles, California

Annie Wong-Beringer, PharmD
Associate Professor of Pharmacy
University of Southern California School of Pharmacy
Infectious Diseases Pharmacist
Department of Pharmacy
Huntington Hospital
Los Angeles, California

J. Douglas Wurtzbacher, PharmD, PhD
Adjunct Instructor of Pharmacy
The Ohio State College of Pharmacy
The Medicine Shoppe Pharmacy
Kettering, Ohio

Courtney W. Yuen, PharmD, BCOP
Assistant Clinical Professor of Pharmacy
University of California, San Francisco Medical Center
San Francisco, California

Dawn G. Zarembski, PharmD
Assistant Professor of Pharmacy Practice
Midwestern University Chicago College of Pharmacy
Downers Grove, Illinois

Caroline S. Zeind, PharmD
Chair of Pharmacy Practice
Associate Professor of Pharmacy Practice
Boston School of Pharmacy
Massachusetts College of Pharmacy and Health Sciences
Boston, Massachusetts

Case Editors

Joanna Q. Hudson, PharmD, BCPS
Associate Professor of Pharmacy
Assistant Professor of Medicine
University of Tennessee
Memphis, Tennessee

Greta K. Gourley, MSN, PhD, PharmD
Associate Professor of Pharmacy Practice and
Pharmacoeconomics
University of Tennessee Health Sciences Center
College of Pharmacy
Memphis, Tennessee

Caroline S. Zeind, PharmD
Chair of Pharmacy Practice
Associate Professor of Pharmacy Practice
Boston School of Pharmacy
Massachusetts College of Pharmacy and Health Sciences
Boston, Massachusetts

Case Contributors

Michael Angelini, PharmD, BCPP
Assistant Professor of Pharmacy Practice
Boston School of Pharmacy
Massachusetts College of Pharmacy and Health Sciences
Boston, Massachusetts

Snehal Bhatt, PharmD, BCPS
Assistant Professor of Pharmacy Practice
Boston School of Pharmacy
Massachusetts College of Pharmacy and Health Sciences
Boston, Massachusetts

Kathryn Blake, PharmD
Senior Research Scientist
Department of Biomedical Research
Nemours Children's Clinic
Jacksonville, Florida

Bradley A Boucher, PharmD, FCCP, FCCM
Professor of Pharmacy
University of Tennessee
Clinical Pharmacist
Regional Medical Center at Memphis
Memphis, Tennessee

Eric G. Boyce, PharmD
Professor of Clinical Pharmacy

Philadelphia College of Pharmacy
University of the Sciences in Philadelphia
Philadelphia, Pennsylvania

Kristina L. Butler, PharmD, BCPS, CDE
Affiliate Faculty Member
Oregon State University College of Pharmacy
Clinical Pharmacy Specialist, Primary Care
Providence Medical Group
Portland, Oregon

Joseph M. Calomo, PharmD, MBA
Assistant Dean for Experiential Education
Assistant Professor of Pharmacy Practice
Boston School of Pharmacy
Massachusetts College of Pharmacy and Health Sciences
Boston, Massachusetts

Jack J. Chen, PharmD, BCPS, CGP, FASCP
Associate Professor of Neurology
School of Pharmacy
Clinical Associate Professor of Neurology
Movement Disorders Clinic
Loma Linda University
Loma Linda, California

Susan Crecco, PharmD
Assistant Professor of Pharmacy Practice
Boston School of Pharmacy
Massachusetts College of Pharmacy and Health Sciences
Boston, Massachusetts

Trisha L. Ford, PharmD, BCPS
Assistant Professor of Pharmacy Practice
Boston School of Pharmacy
Massachusetts College of Pharmacy and Health Sciences
Boston, Massachusetts

Rebecca S. Finley, PharmD, MS, FASHP
President, Meniscus Educational Institute
West Conshohocken, Pennsylvania

Rowena S. Gascon, PharmD Candidate
College of Pharmacy
Western University of Health Sciences
Pomona, California

Kathleen Gura, PharmD, BCNSP
Clinical Pharmacist GI/Nutrition
Team Leader, Surgical Pharmacy Programs
Children's Hospital Boston
Boston, Massachusetts

Helene Hardy, PharmD
Assistant Professor of Pharmacy Practice
Boston School of Pharmacy
Massachusetts College of Pharmacy and Health Sciences
HIV Pharmacotherapy Services, Director
Center for HIV/AIDS Care and Research
Boston Medical Center
Boston, Massachusetts

Maryann Cooper, PharmD, BCPS
Assistant Professor of Pharmacy Practice
Boston School of Pharmacy
Massachusetts College of Pharmacy and Health Sciences
Boston, Massachusetts

Julie Hixson-Wallace, PharmD, BCPS
Clinical Associate Professor
Assistant Dean for Administration
Mercer University Southern School of Pharmacy
Atlanta, Georgia

Brian M. Hodges, PharmD, BCPS, BCNSP
Assistant Professor of Pharmacy
West Virginia University School of Pharmacy
Morgantown, West Virginia

Collin A. Hovinga, PharmD
Neuropharmacologist
Miami Children's Hospital Research/Brain Institute
Miami, Florida

Jason L. Iltz, PharmD
Clinical Assistant Professor of Pharmacotherapy
College of Pharmacy
Washington State University
Clinical Pharmacy Specialist
Group Health Cooperative
Spokane, Washington

Sarah Karish, PharmD
Assistant Professor of Pharmacy Practice
Boston School of Pharmacy
Massachusetts College of Pharmacy and Health Sciences
Boston, Massachusetts

Mark Klee, PharmD
Clinical Pharmacy Specialist (SICU)
Tufts-New England Medical Center
Boston, Massachusetts

Susan A. Krikorian, MS, RPh
Associate Professor of Pharmacy Practice
Boston School of Pharmacy
Massachusetts College of Pharmacy and Health Sciences
Boston, Massachusetts

Paul J. Kritsy, MS, RPh
Assistant Professor of Pharmacy Practice
Boston School of Pharmacy
Massachusetts College of Pharmacy and Health Sciences
Boston, Massachusetts

Karen W. Lee, PharmD
Assistant Professor of Pharmacy Practice
Boston School of Pharmacy
Massachusetts College of Pharmacy and Health Sciences
Boston, Massachusetts

Matthew Machado, PharmD
Assistant Professor of Pharmacy Practice
Boston School of Pharmacy
Massachusetts College of Pharmacy and Health Sciences
Boston, Massachusetts

Hewitt W. Matthews, PhD
Dean and Hood-Meyer Professor
Department of Pharmaceutical Sciences
Mercer University School of Pharmacy
Atlanta, Georgia

Harold J. Manley, PharmD, BCPS
Associate Professor of Pharmacy Practice
Albany College of Pharmacy
Albany, New York

Lisa McDevitt, PharmD, BCPS
Assistant Professor of Pharmacy Practice
Boston School of Pharmacy
Massachusetts College of Pharmacy and Health Sciences
Boston, Massachusetts

Susan W. Miller, PharmD, FASCP, CGP
Department of Clinical and Administrative Sciences
Mercer University Southern School of Pharmacy
Atlanta, Georgia

Erica Murrell, PharmD, CGP
Assistant Professor of Pharmacy Practice
Boston School of Pharmacy-Boston
Massachusetts College of Pharmacy and Health Sciences
Boston, Massachusetts

Brian R. Overholser, PharmD
Assistant Professor of Pharmacy Practice
School of Pharmacy and Pharmaceutical Sciences
Purdue University
Adjunct Assistant Professor of Medicine
Indiana University
Indianapolis, Indiana

Beth Logsdon Pangle, PharmD, BCNSP
Senior Clinical Pharmacy Specialist
Cook Children's Medical Center
Fort Worth, Texas

Kalen B. Porter, PharmD, BCPS
Clinical Assistant Professor of Pediatrics
Department of Clinical and Administrative Services
Mercer University Southern School of Pharmacy
Atlanta, Georgia

Dorothea C. Rudorf, PharmD, MS
Associate Professor of Pharmacy Practice
Boston School of Pharmacy
Massachusetts College of Pharmacy and Health Sciences
Boston, Massachusetts

Laurie J. Schmitt, PharmD, BCPS
Assistant Professor of Pharmacy Practice
Boston School of Pharmacy
Massachusetts College of Pharmacy and Health Sciences
Boston, Massachusetts

Cindy C. Selzer, PharmD, BCPS
Assistant Professor of Pharmacy Practice
Butler University
Clinical Pharmacist
Indiana University Hospital of Clarian Health Partners
Indianapolis, Indiana

Stephen M. Setter, PharmD, CDE, CGP, DVM
Associate Professor of Pharmacotherapy
Elder Services/Visiting Nurses Association
Washington State University
Spokane, Washington

Sam K. Shimomura, PharmD
Professor of Clinical Pharmacy
Western University of Health Sciences College of Pharmacy
Pomona, California

Richard J. Silvia, PharmD, BCPP
Assistant Professor of Pharmacy Practice
Boston School of Pharmacy
Massachusetts College of Pharmacy and Health Sciences
Boston, Massachusetts

Douglas Slain, PharmD, BCPS
Associate Professor
West Virginia University School of Pharmacy
West Virginia University Hospitals
Morgantown, West Virginia

Ralph E. Small, PharmD
Professor Emeritus of Pharmacy and Medicine
Virginia Commonwealth University
Richmond, Virginia

Helen E. Smith, PhD, RPh
Department of Pharmaceutics
University of Washington
Seattle, Washington

Kelly M. Smith, PharmD
Associate Professor of Pharmacy Practice Science
University of Kentucky College of Pharmacy
Lexington, Kentucky

Kevin M. Sowinski, PharmD, BCPS
Assistant Professor of Pharmacy Practice
Purdue University School of Pharmacy and Pharmaceutical Sciences
Indianapolis, Indiana

Gregory V. Stajich, PharmD
Associate Professor of Pharmacy Practice
Mercer University Southern School of Pharmacy
Atlanta, Georgia

Joseph M. Swanson, PharmD, BCPS
Critical Care Fellow
The University of Tennessee
Health Science Center
Department of Pharmacy
Memphis, Tennessee

Lynne Sylvia, PharmD
Associate Professor of Pharmacy Practice
Boston School of Pharmacy
Massachusetts College of Pharmacy and Health Sciences
Boston, Massachusetts

Jeanne Hawkins Van Tyle, MS, PharmD
Professor of Pharmacy Practice
Butler University College of Pharmacy and Health Sciences
Indianapolis, Indiana

Beth Ellen Welch, PharmD
Director, Non-Traditional PharmD Program
Assistant Professor of Pharmacy Practice
Boston School of Pharmacy
Massachusetts College of Pharmacy and Health Sciences
Boston, Massachusetts

Phillip I. Wizwer, MS, RPh
Associate Professor of Pharmacy Practice
Boston School of Pharmacy
Massachusetts College of Pharmacy and Health Sciences
Boston, Massachusetts

J. Douglas Wurtzbacher, PharmD, PhD
Adjunct Instructor of Pharmacy
The Ohio State College of Pharmacy
The Medicine Shoppe Pharmacy
Kettering, Ohio

Acknowledgments

We would like to express our appreciation to our colleagues at Lippincott Williams & Wilkins for being tolerant, responsive, and helpful to these two rookie editors. We want to thank Drs. Toby Herfindal and Dick Gourley, again and again, for their support and trust in us.

We want to thank our families for their perpetual support, for none of this would be possible without them. Without their patience and understanding during countless late nights of writing and editing, this endeavor would not have been possible. Our love and thanks to Susan Helms and Lori Quan.

Contents

Clinical Pharmacodynamics and Pharmacokinetics

1

Bernd Meibohm and William E. Evans

In applied pharmacotherapy, usage of medications is adjusted to the individual need of the patient to maximize efficacy and safety, i.e., to achieve the maximum therapeutic response with a minimum likelihood of adverse events. The rational use of drugs and the design of effective dosage regimens are facilitated by the appreciation of the relationships among the administered dose of a drug, the resulting drug concentrations in various body fluids and tissues, and the intensity of pharmacologic effects caused by these concentrations. These relationships and thus the dose of a drug required to achieve a certain effect are determined by the drug's pharmacokinetic and pharmacodynamic properties. Thus, pharmacokinetic (PK) and pharmacodynamic (PD) information form the scientific basis of modern pharmacotherapy.[1,2]

Pharmacokinetics describes the time course of the concentration of a drug in a body fluid, preferably plasma or blood that results from the administration of a certain dosage regimen. In simple terms, pharmacokinetics is *"what the body does to the drug."* Pharmacodynamics describes the intensity of a drug effect in relation to its concentration in a body fluid, usually at the site of drug action. It can be simplified to *"what the drug does to the body."*[3]

The plasma concentration-time profile resulting from drug administration is determined by pharmacokinetic parameters and the administered dosage regimen. While the pharmacokinetic parameters are characteristic for the disposition or handling of a drug in a specific patient and thus usually cannot be altered during pharmacotherapy, the dosage regimen is the clinician's tool to affect drug concentrations for maximum therapeutic benefit. For most drugs, therapeutic response and/or toxicity are related to free concentration of the drug at the site of action. However, drug concentrations at the site of action (e.g., heart tissue for β_1-blockers) often cannot be practically measured. Thus, drug concentrations in accessible body fluids such as plasma are often related to the observed effect under the assumption that the drug concentrations in the measured body fluid and at the site of action are in a constant relationship. Even though this assumption frequently is not accurate, it has proven to be a useful simplification that allows most drugs to achieve the desired effect levels via modulation of their plasma concentration, especially during prolonged pharmacotherapy with multiple dose regimens.

THERAPEUTIC RANGE

The relationship between dosage regimen and effects of a drug, also known as the dose–concentration–response relationship, or exposure–response relationship, is not identical for all patients. Biologic variability in pharmacokinetics and pharmacodynamics as well as their modification by physiologic, pathophysiologic, and environmental factors result in different effect intensities when the same dosage regimen of a drug is given to different patients. Thus, different patients may require different dosage regimens to achieve the same effect intensity. Factors that contribute to variability in the relationship between dose and effect intensity include age, weight, ethnicity and genetics, gender, disease type and severity, concomitant drug therapy, and environmental factors.

The variability in the relationship between dosage regimen and effect intensity is caused by pharmacokinetic variability, pharmacodynamic variability, or a combination of both. Knowledge about the variability in the plasma drug-concentration-effect relationship allows establishing a drug-specific *therapeutic range*. A therapeutic range is a range of drug concentrations within which the *probability* of desired clinical response in the considered patient population is relatively high and the probability of unacceptable toxicity is relatively low. The therapeutic range approach combines between-patient pharmacodynamic variability with the therapeutic as well as toxic effects of a drug. It is important to note that the therapeutic range should not be considered in absolute terms as the limits for this probability range are oftentimes chosen arbitrarily. In addition, the therapeutic range is not well defined for a large fraction of the drugs that are used clinically.

The left panel in Figure 1.1 *(see color insert)* shows a drug concentration-effect relationship. The probability of achieving the desired response is very low when drug concentrations are less than 5 mg per L, as is the chance of observing toxicity. As drug concentrations increase from 5 to 20 mg per L, the probability of desired response increases significantly, while the probability of toxicity increases more slowly. One could select a therapeutic range of 10 to 20 mg per L, where the minimum probability of a therapeutic response is at least 50% and the probability of toxicity is less than 10%. An optimal dosage regimen can be defined as one that maintains the plasma concentration of the drug within the therapeutic range. The right panel in Figure 1.1 demonstrates this concept by comparing two dosage regimens. The dosing interval (time between doses; in this case 8 hours) is the same, but the discrete doses given in regimen B are twice as large as those given in regimen A. As shown, drug accumulates in the body during multiple dosing. Regimen A keeps the concentration-time profile within the therapeutic range, which will result in the majority of patients with adequate therapeutic efficacy with only rare occurrence of undesired toxicity. Regimen B will likely result in most patients with only a marginal increase in efficacy compared to regimen A, but with a much larger likelihood of undesired toxicity. It should, however, be stressed, that despite having plasma concentrations within the therapeutic range at all times, some of the patients treated with regimen A may not experience an adequate drug response or may experience drug-related toxicity.

CLINICAL PHARMACOKINETICS

The utility of pharmacokinetics does not lie in diagnosing the disease or selecting the ''drug of choice,'' but in deciding the best way to administer a given drug to achieve its therapeutic objective. The manner in which a drug is taken is referred to as the *dosage regimen*. The dosage regimen tells us ''how much'' and ''how often'' a drug must be taken to achieve the desired result. It is these two questions (how much?, how often?) that form the basis for the discipline of pharmacokinetics.[4,5]

Clinical pharmacokinetics is the application of pharmacokinetic principles in a patient care setting for the design of optimum dosage regimens for the individual patient. Probably the most difficult aspect of clinical pharmacokinetics is understanding the full potential and practical limitations and pitfalls of using specific pharmacokinetic models of drug disposition to attain target concentrations based on only a limited number (usually 1–2) of drug concentration measurements. Although a good understanding of common pharmacokinetic concepts is crucial, the competent clinician will have knowledge of not only the mathematics of these concepts, but also the principles, assumptions, and potential errors underlying their application in a clinical setting. Furthermore, a broad therapeutic knowledge is also necessary because measured drug concentrations must be interpreted with respect to the patient's clinical condition and the pharmacodynamic profile of the therapeutic agent.

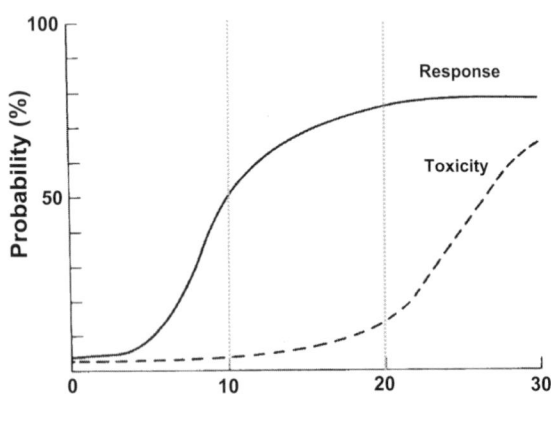

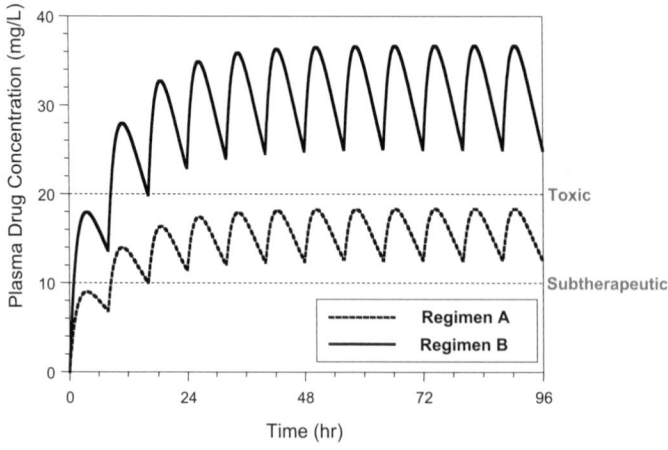

FIGURE 1.1 The concept of a therapeutic range. The **left panel** shows a relationship between the probability of achieving the desired response as well as the chance of observing toxicity in relation to drug concentration in plasma. A therapeutic range of 10 to 20 mg/L could be defined as a range of concentration with relatively high probability of a therapeutic response but low probability of drug-related toxicity. The **right panel** demonstrates the application of the therapeutic range concept in designing multiple dose regimens. In the concentration-time plot, regimen A keeps drug concentrations within the therapeutic range, whereas regimen B results in concentrations exceeding the therapeutic range. Regimen B will likely result in most patients with only a marginal increase in efficacy compared to regimen A, but with a much larger likelihood of drug-related toxicity.

PRIMARY PHARMACOKINETIC PARAMETERS

Pharmacokinetic parameters are characteristic for the disposition and uptake of drug into the body of one specific drug in a specific patient. Pharmacokinetic parameters are usually not accessible for therapeutic manipulation by the clinician, but may be modulated by physiologic or pathophysiologic processes in the patient as well as concomitant drug therapy (drug-drug interactions) and environmental factors.

The most important pharmacokinetic parameters are clearance (CL), volume of distribution (V), and bioavailability (F) (Fig. 1.2; *see color insert*). CL is reflective for the drug-eliminating capacity of the body, especially liver and kidneys, V refers to the distribution of drug within the body including uptake into specific organs and tissues as well as binding to proteins and other macromolecules. Based on these underlying physiologic processes, CL and V are independent of each other and are called *primary pharmacokinetic parameters*. Bioavailability (F) refers to the extent of drug uptake into the systemic circulation. Although being at least partially dependent on hepatic CL via the so-called first-pass effect, bioavailability may also be considered as a primary parameter.

Clearance. CL quantifies the elimination of a drug. It is the volume of body fluid, blood, or plasma that is cleared of the drug per time unit. Thus, it measures the removal of drug from the plasma or blood. For simplicity, only plasma CLs will be considered in the following. CL does not indicate how much drug is being removed, but it represents the volume of plasma from which the drug is completely removed, or cleared, in a given time period. The unit of CL is volume per time, e.g., liters per hour or milliliters per minute. It may also be normalized to body size, e.g., L/hr/kg. CL is an independent pharmacokinetic parameter, and is the most important pharmacokinetic parameter because it determines the dosing rate.

The overall total body CL is the sum of individual organ CLs that contribute to the elimination of a drug:

$$CL = CL_R + CL_H + CL_{Other} \qquad (1\text{-}1)$$

CL_R is the renal clearance representing elimination via the kidneys, CL_H hepatic clearance representing elimination via the liver, and CL_{other} the clearance of other elimination organs (e.g., gastrointestinal tract, lungs) that contribute to the elimination of a specific drug.

Organ CLs can be defined by a flow rate Q that represents the volume of plasma that flows through the organ per time unit and the extraction ratio E, a measure of the extraction efficiency of the organ. E provides the fraction of the volume of plasma that is completely cleared of drug per passage through the organ. The extraction ratio can be assessed as ratio of the difference between the drug concentration in the plasma entering (C_{in}) and leaving (C_{out}) the elimination organ compared to C_{in}. In other words, it gives the percent of Q that is completely cleared from the drug during passage through the organ.

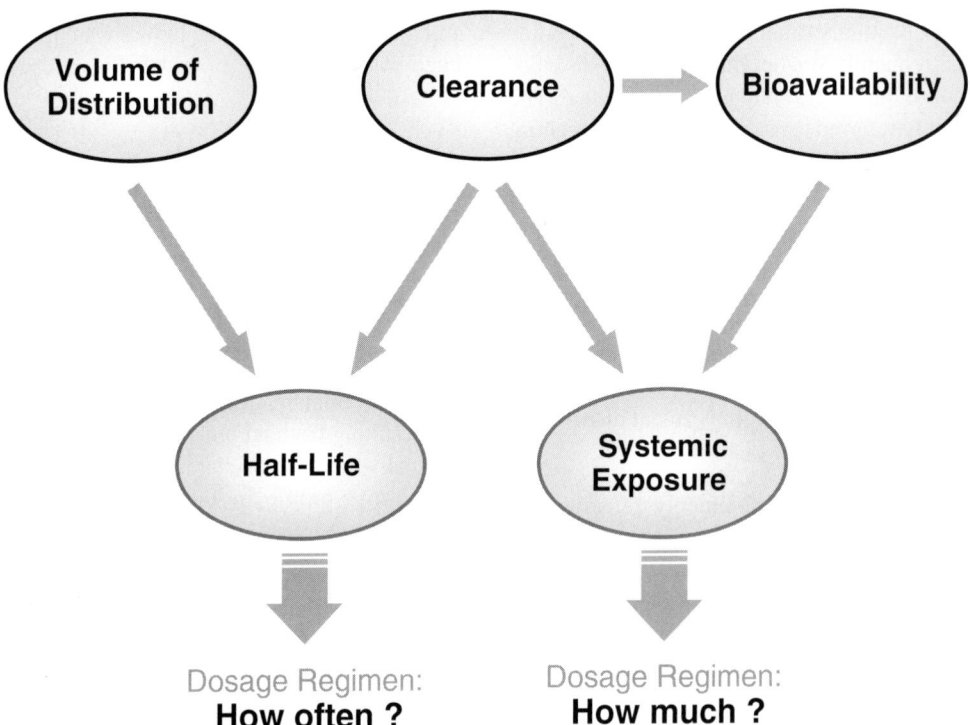

FIGURE 1.2 Interrelationship of primary pharmacokinetic parameters (clearance, volume of distribution, and bioavailability) and their relevance for determining dosage regimens. (Modified from van de Waterbeemd H, Gifford E. ADMET in silico modelling: towards prediction paradise? Nat Rev Drug Discov 2:192–204, 2003.)

Volume of Distribution. V quantifies the extent of distribution of a drug throughout the body. Drug distribution means the reversible transfer of drug from one location to another within the body. The concentration achieved in plasma after distribution depends on the dose and the extent of distribution. The V relates the amount of drug in the body to the plasma concentration. It is an apparent volume, which is calculated upon the simplifying assumption that the plasma concentration is present in all body compartments. The unit of V is volume, e.g., liter or milliliter. It may also be normalized to body size, e.g., liter per kilogram. The larger the V, the smaller the fraction of the dose that resides in the plasma.

Once drug has entered the vascular system, it becomes distributed throughout the various tissues and body fluids. However, most drugs do not distribute uniformly throughout the various organs and tissues of the body. This heterogeneous distribution is based on tissue-specific differences in rate and extent of drug uptake, including blood flow, i.e., the delivery of drug to the tissues, the ability for the drug to cross biomembranes, partitioning into the tissue, and drug binding to tissue elements including binding to proteins and other macromolecules. As a consequence, V is an apparent volume that acts as a proportionality factor between drug amount in the body and measured concentration in plasma and can range between 3 L for a typical 70-kg subject representing the plasma volume and up to values like 5,000 L for amiodarone, i.e., far in excess of the total body size.

For most drugs, distribution throughout the body is not instantaneous, but a time-consuming process. Thus, the initial drug distribution volume after intravenous (IV) bolus administration is frequently smaller than that after distribution equilibrium throughout the body has been reached. The initial V is frequently referred to as the volume of the central compartment V_C, representing well-perfused organs and tissues for which drug distribution for a specific drug is nearly instantaneous. Differentiation between the postequilibrium V and the volume of the central compartment V_C becomes especially important for loading dose calculations. Drugs with instantaneous and homogenous distribution are referred to in the following as having one-compartment distribution characteristics, those with differences between V_C and the postequilibrium V as having multicompartment distribution characteristics.

Bioavailability. Bioavailability commonly refers to the rate and extent of drug absorption into the systemic circulation. In the following, however, the term bioavailability (F) will be limited to the extent of absorption, i.e., the fraction of the administered dose that reaches the systemic circulation. By definition, F is 100% for intravascular administrations, e.g., IV dosing.

Absolute bioavailability is the fraction (or percent) of a dose administered extravascularly which is systemically available as compared to an IV dose. If given orally, absolute bioavailability (F) is:

$$F = \frac{AUC_{oral}}{AUC_{IV}} \times \frac{D_{IV}}{D_{oral}} \qquad (1\text{-}2)$$

where AUC is the area-under-the-plasma-concentration-time curve after oral or IV administration, respectively, and D is the administered dose (e.g., in milligrams) of the two respective administration routes.

Relative bioavailability does not compare an extravascular with an IV administration, but two formulations given via extravascular routes. It is the fraction of a dose administered as a test formulation that is systemically available as compared to a reference formulation:

$$F = \frac{AUC_{test\ formulation}}{AUC_{reference}} \times \frac{D_{reference}}{D_{test\ formulation}} \qquad (1\text{-}3)$$

Bioavailability can be viewed as the result of a combination of processes that reduce the amount of extravascularly administered drug that reaches the systemic circulation. Components that describe these processes for an oral dose administration include the fraction of drug that is absorbed from the gastrointestinal tract (F_a), the fraction of drug that escaped presystemic gut wall metabolism (F_G), and the fraction of the drug that escaped hepatic first-pass metabolism (F_H).

$$F = F_a \times F_G \times F_H \qquad (1\text{-}4)$$

First-pass metabolism refers to the phenomenon that drug absorbed in the gastrointestinal tract first undergoes transport through the portal vein, then passage through the capillary bed of the liver before it reaches the systemic circulation. Metabolism during this first liver passage may, depending on the drug, dramatically reduce the fraction of the administered dose that reaches the systemic circulation. F_H is interrelated with CL_H via the hepatic extraction ration E_H:

$$F_H = 1 - E_H = 1 - \frac{CL_H}{Q_H} \qquad (1\text{-}5)$$

where Q_H is the hepatic flow rate of plasma.

INTERRELATIONSHIP BETWEEN PRIMARY PHARMACOKINETIC PARAMETERS AND THEIR EFFECT ON PLASMA CONCENTRATION-TIME PROFILES

The primary pharmacokinetic parameters CL, V, and F are major determinants for the plasma concentration-time profile resulting from administration of a dosage regimen. The clinically most useful characteristics of the resulting concentration-time profile are the elimination half-life $t_{1/2}$, as well as the average steady-state concentration $C_{ss,av}$ and the area under the plasma concentration-time curve AUC as measures of systemic exposure (Fig. 1.2).

Half-Life. Half-life ($t_{1/2}$) characterizes the monoexponential decline in drug concentration after drug input processes have been completed. Half-life is the time required for the plasma concentration to decrease by one-half. It is a transformation of the first-order elimination rate constant K that characterizes drug removal from the body if the elimination process follows first-order kinetics. Drug concentration C at any time t during a monoexponential decrease can be described by

$$C = C_0 \times e^{-K \times t} \tag{1-6}$$

where C_0 is the initial drug concentration at time t = 0 hours. Half-life is then given as

$$t_{1/2} = \frac{ln\ 2}{K} \tag{1-7a}$$

or

$$t_{1/2} = \frac{0.693}{K} \tag{1-7b}$$

The elimination rate constant K is the negative slope of the plasma concentration-time profile in a plot of the natural logarithm (*ln*) of the concentration versus time. Half-life can thus be calculated from two concentrations C_1 and C_2 during the monoexponential decline of drug concentration via the relationship

$$K = \frac{ln\left(\dfrac{C_1}{C_2}\right)}{t_2 - t_1} \tag{1-8}$$

Half-life is a secondary pharmacokinetic parameter that is defined by the primary parameters CL and V. The elimination rate constant K as a transform of half-life can be seen as a proportionality factor between CL and V:

$$CL = K \times V \tag{1-9A}$$

or

$$K = \frac{CL}{V} \tag{1-9B}$$

Thus, half-life is given by

$$t_{1/2} = \frac{0.693 \times V}{CL} \tag{1-10}$$

Because CL and V are determined by unrelated underlying physiologic processes as described earlier, they are independent of each other. If V, for example is increased due to a pathophysiologic process, then CL remains unaffected. According to Equation 1-9A, change in V would result in a compensatory change in the elimination rate constant K without affecting CL. Vice versa, an increase or decrease in CL will only result in a corresponding change in the elimination rate constant K, but V would remain unaffected.

Half-life provides important information about specific aspects of a drug's disposition, such as how long it will take to reach steady-state once maintenance dosing is started and how long it will take for "all" the drug to be eliminated from the body once dosing is stopped (usually considered five half-lives). Also, the relationship between half-life and dosing interval of a multiple dose regimen determines the fluctuation between peak and trough plasma concentration levels for this dosage regimen.

Systemic Exposure. Exposure to drug in the systemic circulation is a time-integrated or time-averaged measure of drug concentration that is secondary to the administered dosage regimen and the primary parameters CL and bioavailability (F).

The area-under-the-concentration-time curve (AUC) is the integrated concentration over time as a measure of overall exposure to a drug resulting from a specific dosage regimen. It is given by

$$AUC = \frac{F \times D}{CL} \tag{1-11}$$

where D is the administered dose.

The average steady-state concentration $C_{ss,av}$ is the average concentration over one dosing interval in a multiple dose regimen. It is related to CL and bioavailability (F) via

$$C_{ss,av} = \frac{F \times D}{\tau \times CL} = \frac{AUC}{\tau} \tag{1-12}$$

where τ is the dosing interval between two consecutive doses of the multiple dose regimen. The ratio D/τ is also referred to as *dosing rate*.

As indicated in Eqs. 1-11 and 1-12, systemic exposure assessed as AUC or $C_{ss,av}$ is only dependent on the bioavailable dose or dosing rate and CL, but not the extent of drug distribution as quantified by V. Table 1.1 summarizes the interrelationship between the primary pharmacokinetic parameters CL, V, and F and the secondary parameters half-life, AUC, and $C_{ss,av}$.

TABLE 1.1	Effect of Changes in Primary Pharmacokinetic Parameters on Secondary Parameters					
Independent (primary) Parameters			**Dependent (secondary) Parameters**			
CL	**V**	**F**	**$t_{1/2}$**	**C_{ssav}***	**AUC**	
↑	↔	↔	↓	↓	↓	
↓	↔	↔	↑	↑	↑	
↔	↑	↔	↑	↔	↔	
↔	↓	↔	↓	↔	↔	
↔	↔	↑	↔	↑	↑	
↔	↔	↓	↔	↓	↓	
↑	↑	↔	*	↓	↓	
↑	↓	↔	↓	↓	↓	
↓	↑	↔	↑	↑	↑	
↓	↓	↔	*	↑	↑	

The '*' in the table indicates that the effect on the secondary parameter cannot be determined without knowing the extent of changes in CL, V, and F.

↑, increase; ↔, little or no change; ↓, decrease.

THERAPEUTIC DOSAGE REGIMENS

For a lot of drugs to be therapeutically effective, drug concentrations of a certain level have to be maintained within the therapeutic range for a prolonged period of time (e.g., β-lactam antibiotics, antiarrhythmics). To continuously maintain drug concentrations in a certain therapeutic range over a prolonged period of time, two basic approaches to administer the drug can be applied:

1. Drug administration at a constant input rate (i.e., a continuous, constant supply of drug; zero-order input)
2. Sequential administration of discrete single doses (multiple dose regimens)

Constant Input Rate Regimens. Administration of constant input rate regimens can be via intravascular or via extravascular administration. Intravascular administration is most frequently accomplished by IV infusion of drug via a drip or an infusion pump. Although IV drug administration provides a high level of control and precision, its major limitation is that it is restricted primarily to clinical settings. Extravascular administration with a constant input rate has become available only recently and is now widely used in constant release rate devices that deliver drug for an extended period of time at a constant rate. Best known examples for constant rate release devices are transdermal therapeutic systems in patch format and oral therapeutic systems in capsule form. Here, absorption is an additional prerequisite to attain effective plasma concentrations. An example for the resulting concentration-time profile of such a dosage form [oxybutynin chloride (OROS)] is given in Figure 1.3. For understanding the principles involved in constant rate regimens, administration by constant release rate devices in the following are assumed to be equivalent to constant rate IV infusions.

At any time during an infusion, the rate of change in the amount of drug in the body and subsequently the drug

concentration is the difference between the input rate (infusion rate R_0) and the output rate (CL $\times$ concentration C). At time t = 0 hours, when the infusion is started, the concentration and the output rate are both zero. Thus, the rate of change in plasma concentration has its maximum value. With increasing time, the output rate increases as the plasma concentration C is rising while the input rate remains constant. Thus, the rate of change in drug concentration gets smaller with increasing time, but drug concentrations continue to increase as the rate of change is still positive. Finally, the plasma concentration has risen enough that the output rate is equal to the input rate. At this time, the so-called steady-state C_{ss} has been reached, where the rate of change in drug plasma concentration is zero and a constant steady-state concentration C_{ss} has been achieved. At steady-state, input rate is equal to output rate.

$$R_0 = CL \times C_{ss} \qquad (1\text{-}13)$$

Hence, the steady-state concentration C_{ss} is only determined by the infusion rate R_0 and the CL.

$$C_{ss} = \frac{R_0}{CL} \qquad (1\text{-}14)$$

An increase in the infusion rate will result in a proportional increase in the steady-state concentration C_{ss}, as shown in Figure 1.4. For therapeutic purposes, it is often of critical importance to know how long it will take after initiation of an infusion to finally reach a targeted steady-state concentration C_{ss}. The rise in drug concentration during a constant rate infusion before steady-state is exponential in nature and is determined by the elimination process (elimination rate constant K), *not* the infusion rate R_0:

$$C = \frac{R_0}{CL} \times \left(1 - e^{-K \times t}\right) \qquad (1\text{-}15)$$

After initiation of a constant rate infusion, it takes one elimination half-life to reach 50% of C_{ss}, two elimination half-lives to reach 75% of C_{ss}, and three elimination half-

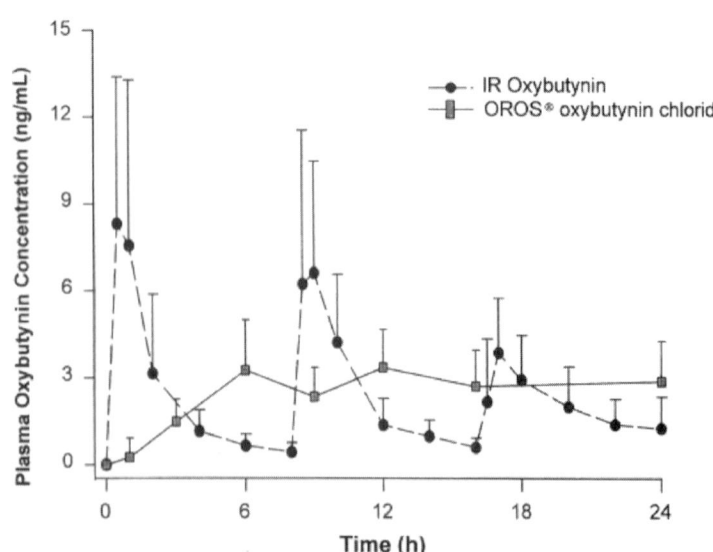

FIGURE 1.3 Oral dosage form with constant input rate. Mean (SD) oxybutynin plasma concentrations in 13 subjects after oral administration of either 15 mg OROS oxybutynin chloride once a day or 5 mg immediate release oxybutynin every 8 hours. OROS is an orally administered constant release rate dosage form. (From Gupta SK, Sathyan G. Pharmacokinetics of an oral once-a-day controlled-release oxybutynin formulation compared with immediate-release oxybutynin. J Clin Pharmacol 39: 289–296, 1999.)

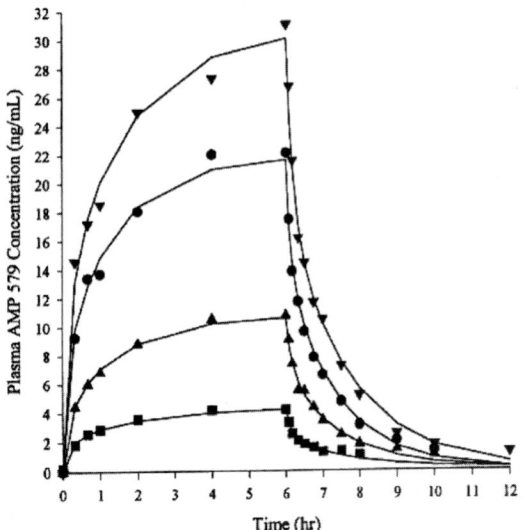

FIGURE 1.4 Linear relationship between steady-state concentration and infusion rate. Mean AMP 579 concentrations in six subjects after single intravenous infusions of 20, 50, 100, or 150 μg/kg AMP 579 administered as 6-hour constant rate infusions. AMP 579 is an investigational adenosine agonist for the treatment of paroxysmal supraventricular tachycardia. (From Zannikos PN, Baybutt RI, Boutouyrie BX, et al. Pharmacokinetics, safety, and tolerability of single intravenous infusions of an adenosine agonist, AMP 579, in healthy male volunteers. J Clin Pharmacol 39:1044–1052, 1999.)

lives to reach 87.5% of C_{ss}. Assuming for clinical purposes that a concentration of more than 95% of C_{ss} is therapeutically equivalent to the final steady-state concentration, it takes approximately five elimination half-lives ($t_{1/2}$) to reach steady-state after initiation of an infusion.

The decline in drug concentration after cessation of an infusion can be described by Equation 1-6 where C_0 is the concentration at the end of the infusion as determined by Equation 1-15 and t is the postinfusion time, the time increment between end of infusion and the time of the observed plasma concentration C.

During therapy it sometimes becomes necessary to change the input rate of a constant rate regimen, e.g., because of drug-related toxicity or inadequate therapeutic effect. After each change in the infusion rate it again takes five half-lives $t_{1/2}$ before more than 95% of the change in the steady-state concentration C_{ss} has occurred. An increase in the infusion rate R_0 is best imagined by the sum of two independent infusions. The first one has the same infusion rate as before the change in R_0. The second one has an infusion rate equal to the incremental increase in R_0. The resulting plasma concentration profile is the sum of the concentrations independently produced by the two infusions (Fig. 1.5). Similarly, a decrease in the infusion rate R_0 can be imagined as the result of two concomitant infusions of which one has been stopped.[4]

Loading Dose and Maintenance Dose. Because the time to reach steady-state concentrations after initiation of a constant rate infusion is determined by the elimination half-life of the drug, depending on the drug's half-life, it may

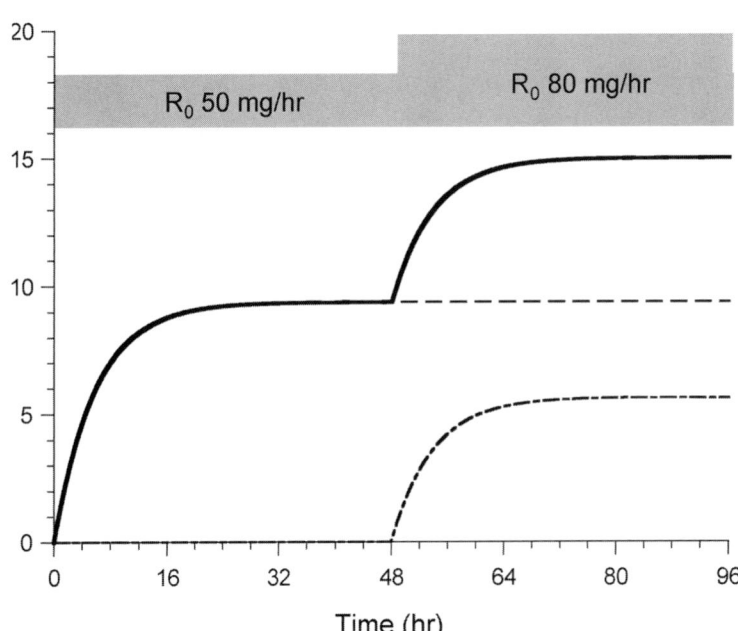

FIGURE 1.5 Increase in infusion rate. An increase in the infusion rate R_0 is best imagined by the sum of two independent infusions, where a second infusion with the incremental infusion rate (in this case 30 mg/hour) is initiated at the time of change in R_0. The resulting plasma concentrations (*bold line*) are the sum of the concentrations independently produced by the two infusions (*dashed lines*).

take a long time until the targeted steady-state concentration C_{target} is reached. For a drug with an elimination half-life of 8 hours, approximately 40 hours (5 × 8 hours) will be needed to reach more than 95% of C_{ss}. Clinical situations sometimes demand that the C_{target} is reached more rapidly.

A solution for this problem is to give a bolus dose and start an infusion at the same time. The resulting plasma concentration is additive from the two modes of administration. The loading dose (LD) is supposed to immediately reach the desired target concentration C_{target}. It is administered as an IV bolus injection or, more frequently, as a short-term infusion. The maintenance dose (MD) is intended to sustain C_{target}. It is administered as a constant rate infusion. When the LD and the MD are exactly matched, the concentrations of drug associated with LD and MD exactly complement each other (Fig. 1.6; *see color insert*). The gain in concentration of MD offsets the loss of the concentration that was initially achieved with LD. In clinical practice, IV dosage regimens are often performed as a sequential combination of LD and MD. But also oral constant rate release systems often contain a LD to facilitate a more rapid achievement of therapeutic concentrations.

The LD for a certain target concentration, C_{target} for a drug with one-compartment distribution characteristics is solely determined by V. It has the unit of an amount, e.g., milligrams.

$$LD = C_{target} \times V \qquad (1\text{-}16)$$

The MD necessary to sustain the target concentration C_{target} is solely determined by the CL. It has the unit of an amount per time, e.g., milligrams per hour:

$$MD = R_0 = C_{target} \times CL \qquad (1\text{-}17)$$

Multicompartment Characteristics and Loading Dose. When applying clinical pharmacokinetics to design and optimize dosage regimens for patients, it is generally assumed for practical purposes that the drug considered follows one-compartment characteristics. In reality, however, most drugs show at least after IV administration multicompartment characteristics. For those drugs, plasma concentrations resulting from an LD based on the postequilibrium V are initially always higher than predicted by a one-compartment model, which may lead to toxicity. The reason is that the volume of the central compartment V_C in which the drug is initially distributed is always smaller than postequilibrium V. Approaches to overcome this problem are to base the LD on V_C instead of V or to give a LD based on V as a short-term infusion rather than as bolus injection.

A patient shall be started on a combination dosing regimen consisting of a LD and a MD. A drug's postequilibrium V in a patient is V = 50 L. A LD of 500 mg was calculated to achieve a target plasma concentration of 10 mg per L. If the drug follows multicompartment characteristics and has a volume of the central compartment of V_C = 10 L, the concentration immediately after drug administration via bolus injection would be 50 mg per L—far beyond the target concentration and potentially toxic. If the LD of 500 mg, however, is slowly administered into the V_C of 10 L, the drug has time to distribute into peripheral tissues and high peak levels are avoided. Basing the LD calculation on V_C would give a LD of 50 mg. Although this LD would initially provide the target concentration, plasma concentrations would consequently drop temporarily below the target concentration because of concurrent distribution and elimination processes, for which only the elimination is offset by the MD.

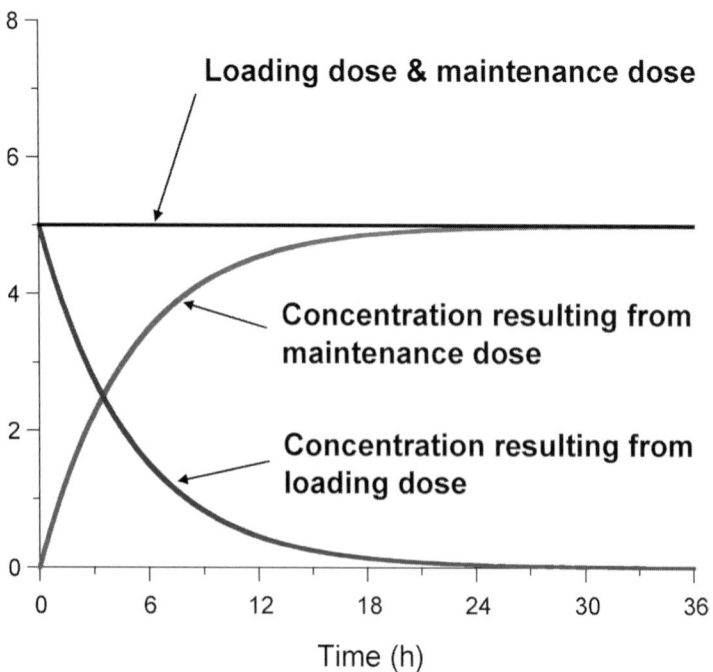

FIGURE 1.6 Loading dose and maintenance dose. When the loading dose and maintenance dose are exactly matched, the drug concentrations associated with the two modes of administration complement each other, maintaining a constant target concentration.

Dosage Regimen Adjustment for Constant Rate Regimen. A 53-year-old male, 85-kg patient, was admitted to the coronary care unit with acute myocardial infarction. Besides other standard treatment, lidocaine therapy was started for the treatment of his symptomatic ventricular arrhythmia. He was given an IV LD of 85 mg and simultaneously started on a constant rate infusion of 2 mg per min (= 120 mg/hour). As recurrent arrhythmia episodes occurred after several hours, a plasma level was drawn 10 hours after initiation of the therapy to determine whether lidocaine was underdosed or the ventricular arrhythmia was refractory to lidocaine treatment. The plasma drug concentration was 1.15 mg/L. The therapeutic concentration range for lidocaine is 1.5–5 mg per L. The population mean pharmacokinetic parameters for lidocaine are V = 1 L per kg and CL = 0.55 L/hr/kg. A LD and a MD shall be recommended to increase the patient's levels from 1.15 mg per L to a target concentration of 3 mg per L.

Based on the population pharmacokinetic parameters of lidocaine, the population estimate for half-life was calculated as 1.3 hours:

$$t_{1/2} = \frac{ln\ 2}{K} = \frac{ln\ 2 \times V}{CL}$$

$$= \frac{0.693 \times 1\ L\ /\ kg}{0.55\ L\ /\ hr\ /\ kg} = 1.3\ hr \qquad (1\text{-}18)$$

Because the time to reach steady-state after initiation of the infusion based on population estimates is approximately 5 × 1.3 hours = 6.5 hours, it can be expected that the plasma concentration measured 10 hours after initiation of the infusion was the steady-state concentration. Thus, the patient's individual CL can be calculated as

$$CL = \frac{R_0}{C_{ss}} = \frac{120\ mg\ /\ hr}{1.15\ mg\ /\ L} = 104\ L\ /\ hr \qquad (1\text{-}19)$$

The new MD to reach the target concentration of 3 mg per L is then

$$\begin{aligned} MD &= CL \times C_{target} \\ &= 104\ L\ /\ hr \times 3\ mg\ /\ L \\ &= 312\ mg\ /\ hr \approx 300\ mg\ /\ hr \end{aligned} \qquad (1\text{-}20)$$

The LD for the incremental increase in drug concentration from 1.15 to 3 mg/L is based on the population estimate of V as follows:

$$\begin{aligned} LD &= \left(C_{target} - C_{measured}\right) \times V \\ &= \left(3 - 1.15\right) mg\ /\ L \times 1\ L\ /\ kg \times 85\ kg \\ &= 157\ mg \approx 150\ mg \end{aligned} \qquad (1\text{-}21)$$

Multiple Dose Regimens. As discussed in the previous section, steady drug concentrations for a prolonged therapy can be maintained by drug administration at a constant input rate or by sequential administration of discrete single doses via multiple dose regimens. The latter one is the more frequently used approach and can be applied for extravascular as well as intravascular routes of administration.

Multiple dose regimens are defined by two components, the *dose D* that is administered at each dosing occasion, and the *dosing interval τ*, the time period between the administrations of two consecutive doses. The ratio of dose and dosing interval can be summarized in the *dosing rate DR*. The dosing rate DR for multiple dose regimens can be seen as an analogue to the infusion rate R_0 for constant rate regimens. Multiple dose regimens are most commonly designed in such a way that a fixed dose is given in fixed time intervals, known as the dosing interval τ. In the following, the pharmacokinetic principles associated with such multiple dose regimens will be discussed.

When a drug is administered during multiple dosing before the previous dose has completely been eliminated, the doses are no longer independent from each other and accumulation takes place, i.e., the plasma concentration resulting after administration of the new dose is the sum of the drug concentrations produced by the new dose and the remainder of the previous doses that is still in the body at the time of administration of the new dose. Thus, the plasma concentration after administration of a dose during multiple dosing is not only dependent on that dose, but also on the dosing history. The drug accumulation observed during multiple dosing follows the *principle of superposition*, i.e., the observed drug concentration is the additive result of the concentration resulting from each individual dose administered (Fig. 1.7). This principle holds true for all drugs that follow linear PK, i.e., when primary PK parameters are constant and independent of dose and time. In this chapter, only cases of linear PK are considered.

On repeated drug administration, the plasma concentration will accumulate to finally reach a steady-state condition. Analogous to constant-rate regimens, at steady-state, the rate of drug input per dosing interval is equal to the rate of drug output. However, the drug concentration within each dosing interval is no longer constant, but is fluctuating between a

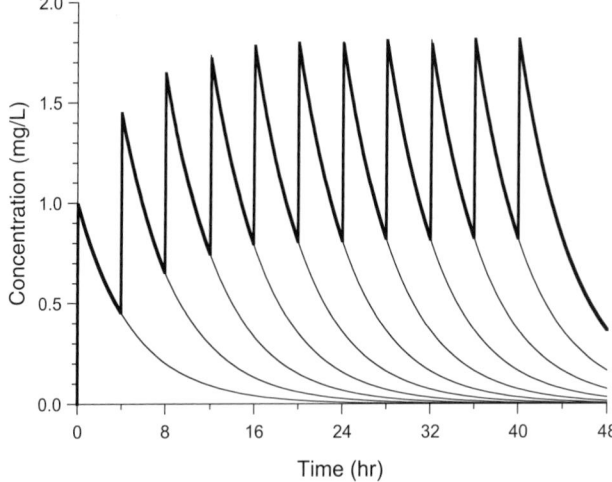

FIGURE 1.7 Principle of superposition. During multiple dose regimens, the resulting plasma concentration-time profile is the sum of the concentrations resulting from each individual dose administered during the dosing history of the regimen.

maximum or peak value $C_{ss,max}$ and a *minimum or through value* $C_{ss,min}$.

The plasma concentrations at any time point during a multiple dose regimen can be calculated as the sum of the plasma concentrations resulting from each individual dose at that time point. However, the calculation of this concentration might be very tedious work if numerous individual doses are involved. An easier way to calculate the drug concentrations during a fixed dose/fixed dosing interval multiple dose regimen (e.g., 300 mg every 8 hours) is to use the so-called accumulation factor (AF).

The AF can be used for calculating drug concentrations once steady-state has been reached:

$$AF = \frac{1}{1 - e^{-K \times \tau}} \qquad (1\text{-}22)$$

where K is the respective elimination rate constant of the drug and τ the dosing interval.

The concentration-time profile during each dosing interval of a multiple dose regimen at steady-state can now be calculated by using the equation that describes the concentration profile after a single dose and multiplying each exponential expression in the equation with the respective AF. Thus, the extent of accumulation during multiple dosing at steady-state is determined by the dosing interval τ and the half-life of the drug $t_{1/2}$ (or the elimination rate constant, K). Thus, the extent of accumulation is not only dependent on the pharmacokinetic properties of a drug, but also on the multiple dose regimen chosen.

Multiple Dose Regimens with Intravenous Input (IV Bolus). For the first dosing interval of an IV bolus multiple dose regimen, the peak $C_{1,max}$, trough $C_{1,min}$, and any concentration C are based on Equation 1-6 described by the following relationships:

$$C_{1,max} = \frac{D}{V} \qquad (1\text{-}23a)$$

$$C_{1,min} = \frac{D}{V} \times e^{-K \times \tau} \qquad (1\text{-}23b)$$

$$C = \frac{D}{V} \times e^{-K \times t} \qquad (1\text{-}23c)$$

Thus, peak and trough at steady-state can be expressed as the peak and trough after the first dose multiplied by the AF:

$$C_{ss,max} = \frac{C_{1,max}}{1 - e^{-K \times \tau}} = \frac{D}{V \times (1 - e^{-K \times \tau})} \qquad (1\text{-}24a)$$

$$C_{ss,min} = \frac{C_{1,min}}{1 - e^{-K \times \tau}} = \frac{D \times e^{-K \times \tau}}{V \times (1 - e^{-K \times \tau})} \qquad (1\text{-}24b)$$

Any other concentration during one dosing interval at steady-state is given by

$$C = \frac{D}{V} \times \frac{e^{-K \times t}}{1 - e^{-K \times \tau}} \qquad (1\text{-}25)$$

where t is the time elapsed within the dosing interval.

A less detailed, but also less computationally intensive view of accumulation is the calculation of the average concentration for a dosing interval τ. By definition, the average drug input rate is equal to the average drug output rate at steady-state. While the average input rate is the drug amount entering the systemic circulation per dosing interval, the average output rate is equal to the product of CL and the average plasma concentration within one dosing interval $C_{ss,av}$.

$$\frac{D}{\tau} = CL \times C_{ss,av} \qquad (1\text{-}26)$$

Thus, the average steady-state concentration $C_{ss,av}$ during multiple dosing is only determined by the dose, the dosing interval τ (or both together as dosing rate DR = D/τ), and the CL:

$$C_{ss,av} = \frac{D}{\tau \times CL} \qquad (1\text{-}27)$$

$C_{ss,av}$ is not the mean of $C_{ss,max}$ and $C_{ss,min}$. Due to the exponential decrease in plasma concentrations from peak to trough within each dosing interval, $C_{ss,av}$ is arithmetically closer to $C_{ss,min}$ than $C_{ss,max}$.

The average steady-state concentration $C_{ss,av}$ rises during multiple dosing just as it does following a constant-rate IV infusion. In contrast to a constant-rate infusion, however, concentrations are fluctuating within each dosing interval. Analogous to constant-rate infusions, the rate of drug accumulation is only determined by the elimination half-life of the drug. Thus, it takes one elimination half-life to reach 50% of $C_{ss,av}$, and two to reach 75% of $C_{ss,av}$.

Consequently, accumulation is complete after *five elimination half-lives* and more than 95% of the final average concentration at steady-state $C_{ss,av}$ is reached. In addition, the change in average concentration $C_{ss,av}$ after every change in dose rate, i.e., in dose D or dosing interval τ, also takes approximately five elimination half-lives. This is true for increases as well as decreases in τ or D, respectively.

The degree of fluctuation between peak and trough concentrations during one dosing interval, i.e., $C_{ss,max}$ and $C_{ss,min}$, can be expressed as

$$Fluctuation = \frac{C_{ss,max} - C_{ss,min}}{C_{ss,min}} \qquad (1\text{-}28)$$

Fluctuation is determined by the relationship between elimination half-life $t_{1/2}$ and dosing interval τ. If the dosing interval τ is equal to the half-life $t_{1/2}$, then the trough concentration is exactly one half of the peak concentration and the degree of fluctuation is 100%. If $\tau > t_{1/2}$, the degree of fluctuation is more than 100%; if $\tau < t_{1/2}$, the degree of fluctuation is less than 100%. The same DR, i.e., the same amount of drug administered in a certain time period, always results in the same average steady-state concentration $C_{ss,av}$, independent of the number of doses into which it was divided. Dose frequency, however, determines the degree of fluctuation (Fig. 1.8).

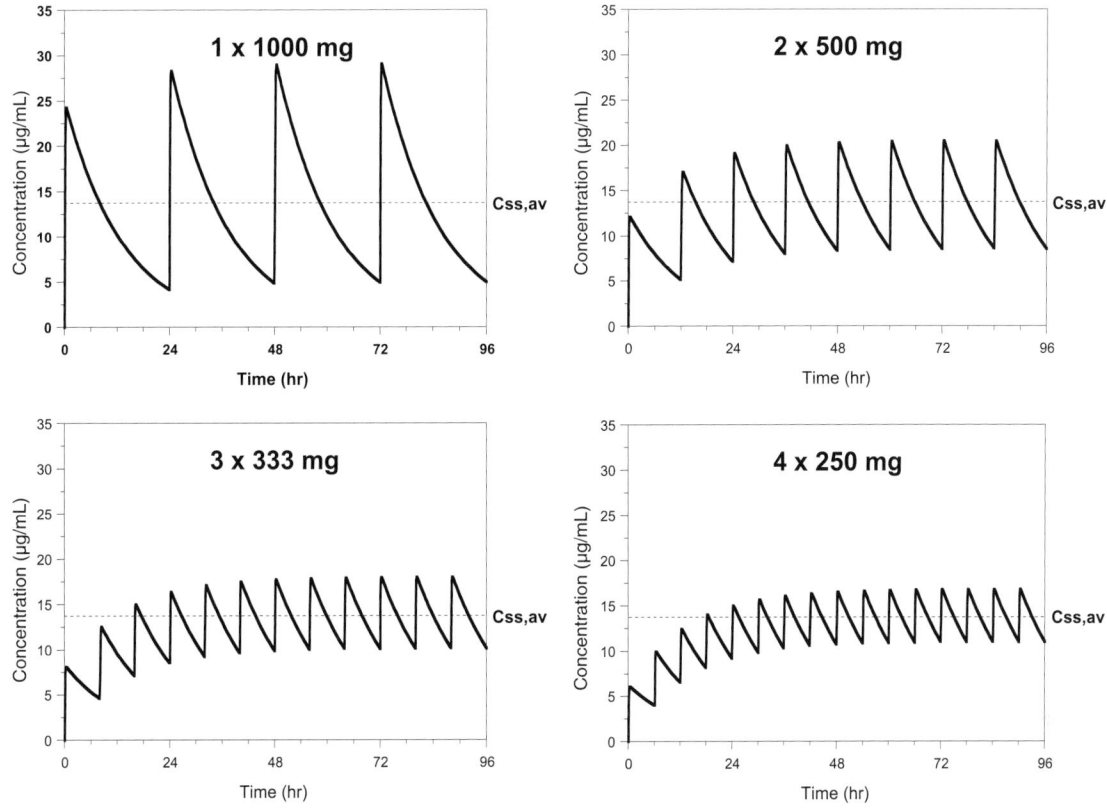

FIGURE 1.8 Fluctuation and dosing interval. In all four panels, a dosing rate of 1,000 mg daily or 41.7 mg/hour was given (CL = 3 L/hour, V = 40 L). This dosing rate is given once daily (1,000 mg QD), twice daily (500 mg BID), three times daily (333 mg TID), or four times daily (250 mg QID). The shorter the dosing interval, the less fluctuation is observed and the more $C_{ss,min}$ and $C_{ss,max}$ approximate $C_{ss,av}$.

Multiple Dose Regimens with First-Order Input (Oral Dosing). In clinical practice, most multiple dose regimens use dosage forms from which the drug enters the systemic circulation through a first-order or similar absorption process. Oral administration is the most predominant example for such multiple dose regimens, but other administration pathways also follow these principles, for example intramuscular (IM) administration.

The concepts of multiple dose regimens introduced for IV bolus multiple dosing are also applicable for multiple dose regimens of dosage forms with first-order drug input, e.g., oral dosage forms. It should be noted that the average steady-state concentration $C_{ss,av}$ is now determined by the bioavailable fraction F of the dose D administered per dosing interval τ and the CL:

$$C_{ss,av} = \frac{F \times D}{\tau \times CL} \quad (1\text{-}29)$$

Given that absorption is virtually instantaneous, oral administration can be approximated more easily using IV bolus doses. The calculated peak and trough values at steady-state can then be used as reasonable approximations during oral multiple dosing at steady-state upper and lower limits for the expected peaks and troughs, respectively. This concept

is shown in Figure 1.9 where the same dosage regimen is given as a multiple IV bolus dose regimen (equivalent to oral multiple dose regimens with very rapid absorption process; dotted line) or as dosage regimens with much slower absorption rate constants. Only the following differences have to be taken into account when dealing with multiple oral dosing compared to IV bolus dosing:

1. The dose has to be corrected for the extent of bioavailability F.
2. The rate of absorption affects the fluctuation of drug concentration, but not the value of the average steady-state concentration $C_{ss,av}$.
3. With increasing accumulation of drug, the concentration within one dosing interval at steady-state becomes relatively insensitive to variations in the rate of absorption.

Prediction of Concentration During a Multiple Dose Regimen. A patient is started on a therapy with 0.25 mg oral digoxin given once daily for the treatment of atrial fibrillation. Digoxin has a narrow therapeutic range (0.8–2 µg/L) and a long half-life (24–48 hours). Therefore, it is of particular interest to know early during therapy, whether the applied multiple dose regimen will ensure therapeutic plasma concentrations throughout the dosing interval at steady-state.

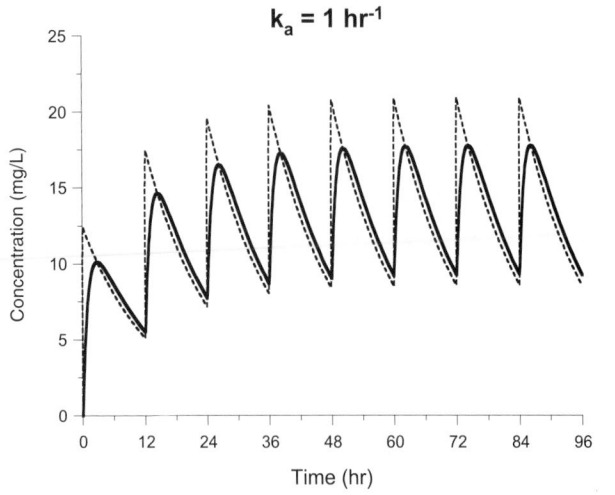

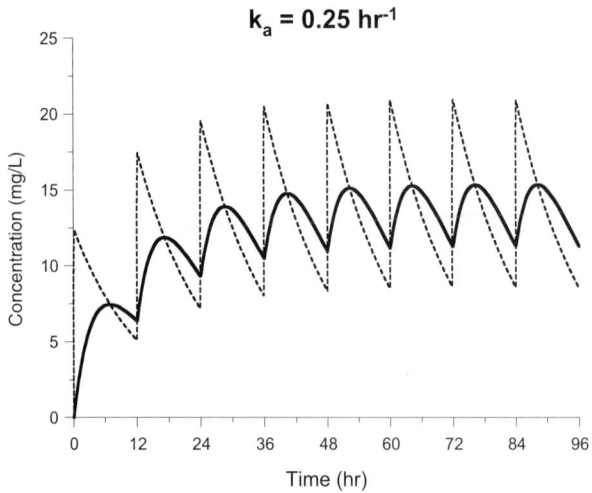

FIGURE 1.9 Comparison of IV and extravascular multiple dose regimens. The same multiple dose regimen is given by IV bolus dosing (*dashed line*) or by extravascular administration (*bold line*) with a fast ($k_a = 1$ hour^{-1}) and a slow ($k_a = 0.25$ hour^{-1}) first-order absorption rate constant (assuming F=1). The slower the absorption process, the less pronounced is the peak-to-trough fluctuation. Peak and trough concentrations after IV bolus dosing define the upper limit of peaks and the lower limit of troughs possible after multiple oral dosing.

The concentrations of digoxin 12 and 24 hours after administration of the first dose were measured and were 0.39 and 0.31 μg per L.

As the trough concentration is the lowest concentration during one dosing interval, the trough during multiple dosing at steady-state $C_{ss,min}$ should be higher than the lower limit of the therapeutic range.

Assuming that digoxin is rapidly absorbed and oral drug absorption has been completed by the time the first concentration was measured (12 hours), the elimination rate constant K can be estimated as

$$K = \frac{ln\left(\dfrac{0.39\ \mu g\,/\,L}{0.31\ \mu g\,/\,L}\right)}{24\ hr\ -\ 12\ hr} = 0.019\ hr^{-1} \quad (1\text{-}30)$$

Thus, the accumulation factor for the multiple dose regimen is

$$AF = \frac{1}{1\ -\ e^{-K \times \tau}}$$

$$= \frac{1}{1\ -\ e^{-0.019\ hr^{-1} \times 24\ hr}} = 2.7 \quad (1\text{-}31)$$

$C_{ss,min}$ can then be predicted from the measured trough after the first dose (0.31 μg/L) and the accumulation factor:

$$C_{ss,min} = C_{1,min} \times AF$$
$$= 0.31\ \mu g\,/\,L \times 2.7 \quad (1\text{-}32)$$
$$= 0.84\ \mu g\,/\,L$$

Dosage Regimen Adjustment for Multiple Dose Regimen. A patient with chronic obstructive pulmonary disease (COPD) will be started on a therapy with oral theophylline as part of the pharmacotherapeutic management of the disease. The recommended therapeutic range for theophylline in

COPD is 8–12 mg per L. The population values for CL and V are CL = 2 L per hour and V = 35 L. The oral bioavailability of the immediate release tablet used was reported as 90%. A step-wise approach can be used to design a dosage regimen for achieving a target concentration of 10 mg per L.

Step 1: Necessary DR. In Step 1, the dose rate necessary to achieve the target concentration as $C_{ss,av}$ is determined based on the known values for bioavailability of the theophylline oral dosage form and the population average for theophylline CL:

$$DR_{necessary} = \frac{C_{target} \times CL}{F}$$
$$= \frac{10\ mg\,/\,L \times 2\ L\,/\,hr}{0.90} \quad (1\text{-}33)$$
$$= 22.2\ mg\,/\,hr$$
$$= 533\ mg\,/\,day$$

Step 2: Maximum dosing interval. In Step 2, a maximum dosing interval τ_{max} is calculated to keep the plasma drug concentrations within the therapeutic range of 8 to 12 mg per L, again using population averages for theophylline CL and V:

$$\tau_{max} = \frac{ln\left(\dfrac{C_{ss,max}}{C_{ss,min}}\right)}{K} = \frac{ln\left(\dfrac{C_{ss,max}}{C_{ss,min}}\right) \times V}{CL}$$
$$\quad (1\text{-}34)$$
$$= \frac{ln\left(\dfrac{12}{8}\right) \times 35\ L}{2\ L\,/\,hr} = 7.1\ hr$$

Step 3: Practical dosage regimen. In Step 3, a clinically practical dosing interval smaller than τ_{max} is chosen and the dose per dosing interval is calculated based on the necessary dose rate:

Practical dosing interval $<\tau_{max}$: 6 hours

$$\begin{aligned} D &= DR_{necessary} \times \tau \\ &= 22.2 \; mg \,/\, hr \times 6hr \\ &= 133.2 \; mg \end{aligned} \qquad (1\text{-}35)$$

Available dosage form: 125 mg

Recommended dosing regimen: 125 mg Q6hr

Step 4: Calculation of expected $C_{ss,max}$, $C_{ss,min}$, and $C_{ss,av}$. The optional Step 4 checks whether the dosage regimen chosen in Step 3 results in the desired peak, trough, and average concentrations at steady-state:

$$\begin{aligned} C_{ss,max} &= \frac{D \times F}{V} \times \frac{1}{1 - e^{-CL\,/\,V \,\times\, \tau}} \\ &= \frac{125 \; mg \times 0.9}{35 \; L} \times \frac{1}{1 - e^{-2\,L\,/\,hr\,/\,35\,L \times 6hr}} \quad (1\text{-}36) \\ &= 11.1 \; mg\,/\,L \end{aligned}$$

$$\begin{aligned} C_{ss,min} &= C_{ss,max} \times e^{-CL\,/\,V \times \tau} \\ &= 11.1 \; mg\,/\,L \times e^{-2\,L\,/\,hr\,/\,35\,L \,\times\, 6hr} \quad (1\text{-}37) \\ &= 7.9 \; mg\,/\,L \end{aligned}$$

$$C_{ss,av} = \frac{D \times F}{\tau \times CL} = \frac{125 \; mg \times 0.9}{6 \; hr \times 2 \; L\,/\,hr} \qquad (1\text{-}38)$$

$$= 9.4 \; mg\,/\,L$$

In clinical practice, oral sustained release dosage forms instead of immediate release dosage forms are frequently used in theophylline therapy to allow a longer dosing interval, i.e., less frequent dosing per day.

It should also be stressed that the calculated values for $C_{ss,max}$ and $C_{ss,min}$ are upper and lower limits, respectively, based on the assumption that absorption is instantaneous. Because absorption after oral administration of theophylline is likely to be a time-consuming process, actual peaks and troughs during multiple dosing at steady-state will be within the limits calculated. The slower the absorption process, the less fluctuation between $C_{ss,max}$ and $C_{ss,min}$ will be present.

Effect of Compliance on Multiple Dose Regimens. Because some medication regimens can be complex and many are self-administered by the patient, dosing errors can easily occur. The effect of dosing errors is different for drugs with similarly narrow therapeutic range dependent on their degree of accumulation. Generally, the more accumulation occurs, the less important compliance is. In other words, the smaller the ratio between dosing interval to half-life, the larger the degree of accumulation and the less impact a dosing error will have (Fig. 1.10).

PHYSIOLOGIC VARIABLES AFFECTING DRUG CLEARANCE

Clearance is one of the most important pharmacokinetic parameters for clinical pharmacokinetics as it determines the systemic exposure of a drug resulting from a therapeutic dosage regimen. Thus, any factors changing drug CL will also result in changes in the systemic exposure to the drug,

which may ultimately be relevant for the efficacy and/or toxicity of the respective pharmacotherapeutic intervention.

As pointed out in Equation 1-1, total CL is the sum of individual organ CLs. The most important organs involved with drug elimination are the liver and the kidneys. The fractional contribution of excretion via the kidneys to overall drug CL can be expressed as f_e, the fraction of drug excreted unchanged into the urine. Thus, f_e is the fraction that renal CL contributes to overall CL:

$$CL_R = f_e \times CL \qquad (1\text{-}39)$$

The parameter f_e can be used to describe the primary route of elimination for a drug and whether a change in the drug eliminating capacity of an elimination organ may likely affect the specific drug. Vancomycin is nearly exclusively eliminated by renal excretion ($f_e \sim 1$). Thus, any change in renal function is likely to affect vancomycin CL and thus systemic exposure. In contrast, nifedipine's route of elimination is nearly exclusively via hepatic metabolism ($f_e \sim 0$). Thus, nifedipine systemic exposure is likely to be affected by changes in hepatic function.

Protein Binding. Before further discussing the determinants and processes involved in the CL of drugs, the importance of free, unbound drug concentrations should be stressed. In therapeutic drug monitoring, drug concentrations in plasma are generally determined as total concentrations, i.e., bound and unbound drug. Drug molecules are to a variable extent bound to circulating proteins in plasma. Major binding proteins include albumin, α_1-acid glycoprotein (AAG), and lipoproteins. Drug bound in plasma, however, is not pharmacologically active, for some drugs is not accessible for metabolism and excretion, and is not able to pass biomembranes. In contrast, free drug is relevant for the pharmacologic effects, can be metabolized and excreted, and is able to pass biomembranes. Thus, only free drug concentrations are ultimately relevant in pharmacotherapy. Free drug concentrations are generally not measured by clinical laboratories, because their measurement involves advanced analytic techniques and is usually more expensive. Therapeutic ranges are therefore expressed as total concentration ranges. However, they can be related to therapeutic ranges for free, unbound concentrations.

Protein Binding and Therapeutic Range. The therapeutic range for total quinidine concentrations is 1 to 4 mg per L. As quinidine is approximately 90% bound to plasma proteins in normal patients, the corresponding therapeutic range for free quinidine concentrations is 0.1 to 0.4 mg per L.

Using total instead of the pharmacologically active free drug concentrations is valid as long as the degree of binding and thus the ratio between free and total drug concentrations remains constant. If the degree of binding changes, for example by drug-drug interactions or certain disease states, then the total drug concentration no longer provides a valid substitute for the free drug concentration. In these cases, measured total drug concentrations have to be carefully inter-

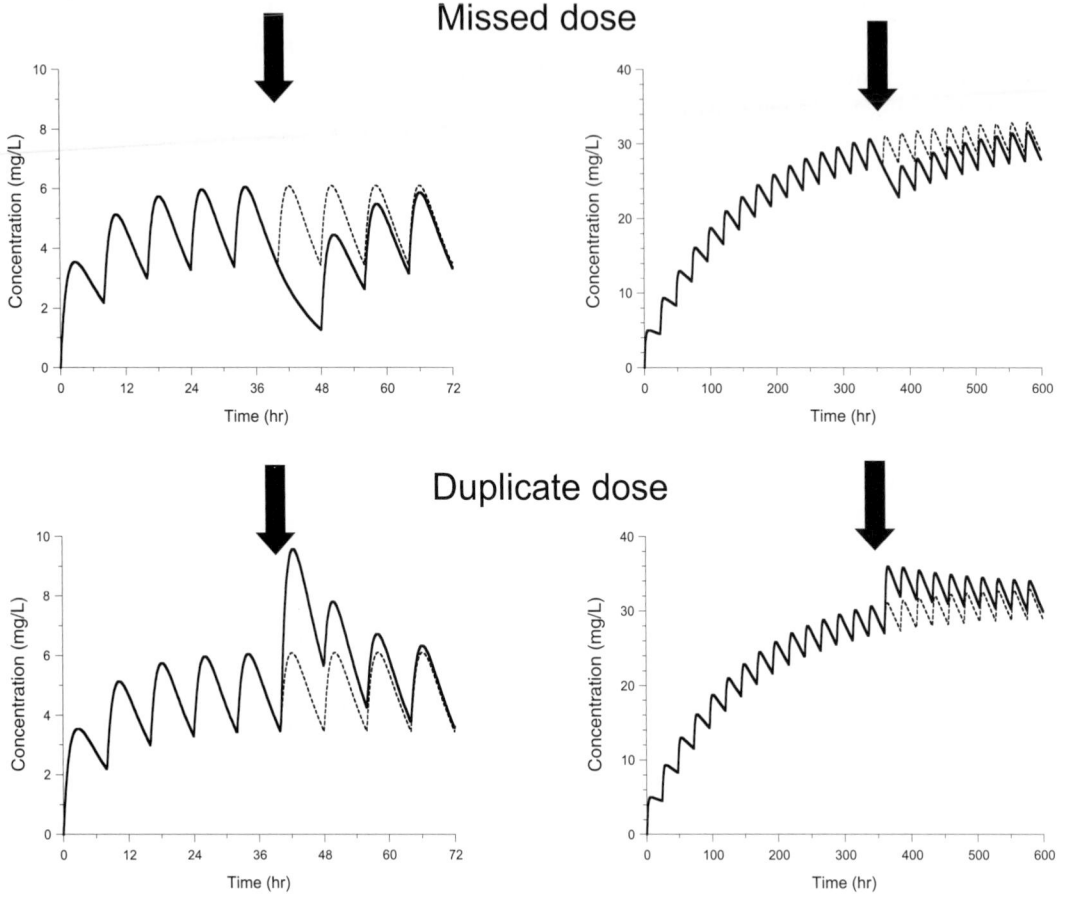

Disopyramide
200 mg /8 hr, $t_{1/2}$ = 5.5 hr, AF = 1.6

Phenobarbital
200 mg /24 hr, $t_{1/2}$ = 100 hr, AF = 6.5

Missed dose

Duplicate dose

FIGURE 1.10 Effect of compliance on multiple dose regimens. Disopyramide and phenobarbital dosage regimens are used to compare the effect of compliance on multiple dose regimens with a small compared to a large ratio of half-life and dosing interval (disopyramide: 0.69; phenobarbital 4.2). The phenobarbital regimen results in substantial drug accumulation (AF 6.5), with only a small effect of each discrete dose on the plasma concentration-time profile. Thus, the effect of a duplicate of a missed dose on the average concentration is very limited and probably not clinically significant. The disopyramide regimen results only in relatively little accumulation (AF 1.6). Duplicate or missed doses have a substantial effect on the concentration-time profile and are likely to play a more important role than for phenobarbital.

preted and a different range of total drug concentrations may be therapeutically necessary.

In plasma, the total drug concentration C is the sum of the concentration of drug bound to plasma proteins C_b and the concentration of unbound, free drug C_u.

$$C = C_b + C_u \tag{1-40}$$

The degree of binding to plasma proteins is expressed as fraction unbound f_u. The fraction unbound f_u is a dimensionless number between 0 and 1, or 0% and 100%. It is defined as:

$$f_u = \frac{C_u}{C} \tag{1-41}$$

Thus, with the fraction unbound f_u, free drug concentrations can easily be assessed from total concentrations as

$$C_u = f_u \times C \tag{1-42}$$

Renal Clearance. Drug elimination of unchanged drug via the kidneys is the net result of three processes, glomerular filtration, tubular secretion, and tubular reabsorption. Renal CL is equal to the plasma volume that is cleared per minute by renal excretion. It is composed of the CLs related to glomerular filtration, tubular reabsorption, and tubular secretion:

$$CL_R = CL_{filtration} + CL_{secretion} - CL_{reabsorption} \tag{1-43}$$

Renal CL values can range from 0 mL/min for substances like glucose that are completely reabsorbed up to values approaching renal plasma flow for compounds like p-amino-hippuric acid that are highly secreted.

Glomerular filtration is a passive process that removes all molecules of low molecular weight (MW $< \sim$20,000) out of plasma. However glomerular filtration is limited to the fraction of drug not bound to plasma proteins. Thus, changes in plasma protein binding can modulate the glomerular filtration CL ($CL_{filtration}$) and thus CL_{ren} of a drug:

$$CL_{filtration} = f_u \times GFR \qquad (1\text{-}44)$$

where GFR is the glomerular filtration rate, approximately 125 mL per min (7.5 L/hour) in a young, healthy individual, and f_u is the fraction of drug not bound to plasma proteins. Tubular secretion is an active secretion process that can occur against a concentration gradient and involves various drug transporters, specific membrane proteins that facilitate transport or actively transport drug molecules from one side of a biomembrane to the other. Tubular secretion is not limited by plasma protein binding. Tubular reabsorption may either occur by passive diffusion or by active transport.

For a drug that is only filtered and not reabsorbed or secreted, renal CL is only determined by plasma protein binding (f_u) and the glomerular filtration rate (GFR). GFR can clinically be estimated by measuring the CL of compounds that are not plasma protein bound ($f_u = 1$) and are exclusively eliminated via renal excretion ($f_e \sim 1$) with no contribution of tubular secretion and tubular reabsorption (e.g., creatinine, inulin, ^{51}Cr-EDTA).

Creatinine Clearance. Creatinine CL (CL_{cr}) is frequently used to estimate GFR in a clinical setting. Creatinine is an endogenous compound that is produced by muscle metabolism in the body with a production rate dependent on age, weight, and sex of the patient. It is predominantly excreted by glomerular filtration and shows only minor plasma protein binding, tubular secretion, or reabsorption. In stable patients, creatinine plasma concentration is determined by the equilibrium between creatinine formation controlled by muscle metabolism and creatinine excretion dependent on GFR. Under the assumption of constant muscle metabolism, creatinine concentrations (serum creatinine concentration S_{cr}) increase with decreasing renal function and vice versa.

$$CL_{cr} = \frac{Creatinine\ formation\ rate}{S_{cr}} \qquad (1\text{-}45)$$

Creatinine CL can be estimated from various empirical relationships. The most frequently used is the equation of Cockcroft and Gault:

$$CL_{cr} = \frac{(140 - age) \times IBW}{72 \times S_{cr}} \qquad (1\text{-}46)$$
$$(\times\ 0.85\ for\ female\ patients)$$

The Cockcroft and Gault equation provides the CL_{cr} in mL per min. It requires using the ideal body weight (IBW) in kilograms, age in years, and creatinine plasma concentration in milligrams per deciliter. It is only valid for adult patients. IBW can be calculated by the following relationships:

IBW (male) = 50 kg (1-47)
+ 2.3 kg for every inch over 5 ft

IBW (female) = 45.5 kg (1-48)
+ 2.3 kg for every inch over 5 ft

Renal Impairment. Although creatinine CL is mechanistically only related to GFR, it is also often used clinically as a measure of global renal function. This approach assumes that only a fraction of the kidney's nephron population is affected by the impairment, and that the unaffected fraction is fully functional. The fraction of normal renal function RF is then determined as ratio of creatinine CL in a patient with impaired renal function compared to the normal creatinine CL. Because creatinine CL is body size dependent, is it usually corrected for body surface area to allow comparisons among different individuals. The creatinine CL of a normal adult is 125 mL/min/1.73 m^2. Renal function as a fraction of normal can then be determined as

$$RF = \frac{CL_{cr}^{impaired}}{125\ mL\,/\,min\,/\,1.73\ m^2 \times BSA} \qquad (1\text{-}49)$$

where $CL_{Cr}^{impaired}$ is the creatinine CL in the individual with impaired renal function and BSA is the individual's body surface area. Body surface area can be estimated based on the individual's height and body weight via nomograms or empirical relationships such as the one by Dubois [*BSA = (Total body weight in kg)$^{0.425}$ × (Height in cm)$^{0.725}$ × 0.007184*].

The effect of renal impairment on the CL of a drug undergoing renal excretion can then be estimated as

$$CL_{renal\ impairment} = CL \times \left[1 - f_e \times (1 - RF) \right] \quad (1\text{-}50)$$

where f_e is the fraction of drug excreted unchanged via the kidneys and CL is the drug's CL in the absence of renal impairment.

Dosage Adjustment in Renal Impairment. A female patient (61 years old; total body weight: 63.5 kg; height: 5′3″; BSA 1.66 m^2; serum creatinine 1.1 mg/dL) will be started on digoxin therapy. The therapeutic range of digoxin is 0.8–2.0 μg per L. The population value for CL is 2.7 mL/min/kg total body weight, f_e is 0.65, and the oral bioavailability of the dosage form is 72%. What dose rate is necessary to achieve an average steady-state concentration of 1.2 μg per L?

IBW (female) = 45.5 kg + 2.3 kg × 3 = 52.4 kg

$$CL_{cr} = \frac{(140 - 61) \times 52.4}{72 \times 1.1} \times 0.85$$
$$= 44.4\ mL\,/\,min \qquad (1\text{-}51)$$

$$RF = \frac{44.4\ mL\,/\,min}{125\ mL\,/\,min\,/\,1.73\ m^2 \times 1.66\ m^2}$$
$$= 0.37 \qquad (1\text{-}52)$$

$$CL_{renal\ impairment} = 63.5\ kg \times 2.7\ mL\ /\ min\ /\ kg$$
$$\times \left[1 - 0.65 \times (1 - 0.37)\right] \quad (1\text{-}53)$$
$$= 101\ mL\ /\ min = 6\ L\ /\ hr$$

$$DR = \frac{C_{target} \times CL_{renal\ impairment}}{F}$$
$$= \frac{1.2\ \mu g\ /\ L \times 6\ L\ /\ hr}{0.72} \quad (1\text{-}54)$$
$$= 10\ \mu g\ /\ hr$$

In clinical practice, a dose of 250 μg daily (10 μg/hour × 24 hours/day = 240 μg/day rounded off to 250 μg) can be given.

Hepatic Clearance

Hepatic Drug Elimination Processes. Hepatic drug elimination is mediated by two primary routes: biliary drug excretion, and hepatic drug metabolism. Drugs may be excreted into the bile either in unchanged form or after metabolism, especially by conjugation reactions such as glucuronidation. Biliary excretion is an active excretion process that is known to involve multiple drug transporters, including P-glycoprotein (MDR1, ABCB1), MRP2 (ABCC2), and BCRP (ABCG2).

Hepatic drug metabolism can be divided into two broad groups: phase I reactions, which involve chemical alteration of the drug structure (e.g., hydrolysis, reduction, or oxidation); and phase II reactions, in which the drug molecule is conjugated (e.g., by glucuronidation, sulfation, acetylation,

etc.). Metabolism patterns generally consist of one or several phase I reactions and may be followed by phase II reactions. However, both reaction groups may also occur in isolation. An overview of the major phase I and phase II drug-metabolizing enzymes and their relative importance for drug disposition is described in Figure 1.11 *(see color insert)*.

The best-researched enzyme family, and perhaps the most important based on the proportion of drugs which are metabolized by it, is the cytochrome (CYP) P450-system, which is involved in the oxidative metabolism of many endogenous compounds, environmental chemicals, herbal components, and drugs. The family of CYP enzymes is divided into various subfamilies of enzymes that have different substrate specificity and may be involved in different chemical reactions. Major CYP enzymes that are relevant for drug metabolism include CYP1A2, CYP2B6, CYP2C8, CYP2C9, CYP2C19, CYP2D6, and the CYP3A subfamily with CYP3A4, CYP3A5, and CYP3A7. The activity of CYP enzymes as well as other drug-metabolizing enzyme systems is dependent on genetic and environmental factors including nutrition, age, concomitant drug therapy (drug-drug interactions), and other host or environmental variables.

CYP enzymes demonstrate a high degree of substrate specificity, i.e., a drug is often a good substrate for one CYP enzyme but not others. Although many drugs rely heavily on a specific CYP enzyme for their metabolism, some drugs are metabolized by more than one CYP enzyme. The overall

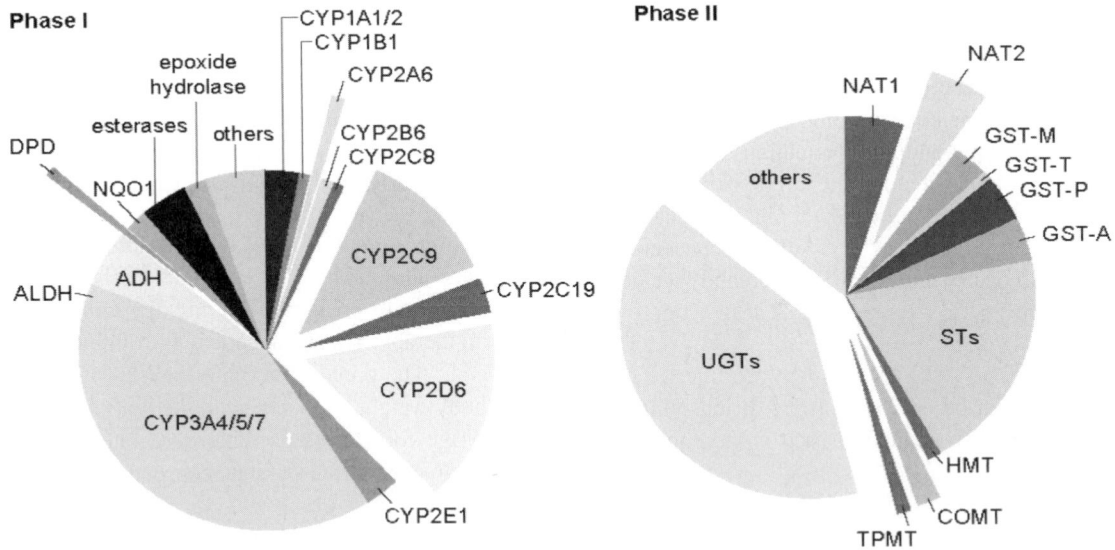

FIGURE 1.11 Major drug-metabolizing enzymes *(see color insert)*. The percentage of phase I and phase II metabolism of drugs that each enzyme contributes is estimated by the relative size of each section of the corresponding chart. Essentially all of the major human enzymes responsible for modification of functional groups [classified as phase I reactions **(left)**] or conjugation with endogenous substituents [classified as phase II reactions **(right)**] exhibit genetic polymorphisms; those enzyme polymorphisms that have already been associated with changes in drug effects are separated from the corresponding pie charts. ADH, alcohol dehydrogenase; ALDH, aldehyde dehydrogenase; CYP, cytochrome P450; DPD, dihydropyrimidine dehydrogenase; NQO1, NADPH:quinone oxidoreductase or DT diaphorase; COMT, catechol O-methyltransferase; GST, glutathione S-transferase; HMT, histamine methyltransferase; NAT, N-acetyltransferase; STs, sulfotransferases; TPMT, thiopurine methyltransferase; UGTs, uridine 5′-triphosphate glucuronosyltransferases. (From Evans WE, Relling MV. Pharmacogenomics: translating functional genomics into rational therapeutics. Science 286:487–491, 1999.)

metabolism, and therefore metabolic CL, of a drug is the sum of all its metabolic pathways.

A frequently updated table that indicates which commonly used drugs are major substrates, inducers, and inhibitors for various CYP enzymes is available at: http://medicine.iupui.edu/flockhart/table.htm

Knowledge of the substrates, inhibitors, and inducers of individual CYP enzymes assists in predicting clinically significant drug interactions and allows part of the frequently observed interindividual variability in pharmacokinetics and thus drug response to be explained and predicted. Refer to Chapter 3 for a further discussion of drug-drug interactions.

Venous Equilibrium Model of Hepatic Clearance. Based on the previously discussed organ CL model, CL_H can be expressed by

$$CL_H = Q_H \times E_H \qquad (1\text{-}55)$$

where Q_H is the liver flow rate (for blood: 1.5 L/min or 90 L/hour in a normal, 70 kg individual; for plasma: 0.825 L/min or 50 L/hour) and E_H is the hepatic extraction ratio. E_H is an indicator of the efficiency of the processes responsible (e.g., metabolism) for eliminating drug from the blood or plasma as it passes through the liver. E_H can range from 0 to 1. An E_H of 1 means 100% of the drug entering the liver is eliminated, and an E_H of 0 means none of the drug entering the liver is eliminated.

Based on the venous equilibrium model for hepatic CL,[6] the hepatic extraction ratio E_H is defined as

$$E_H = \frac{CL_{int} \times f_u}{Q_H + CL_{int} \times f_u} \qquad (1\text{-}56)$$

where f_u is the unbound fraction as a measure of protein binding and CL_{int} is the intrinsic CL. CL_{int} is the theoretic value for a drug's CL by the liver if it were not protein bound, and it is an indication of the liver's enzymatic capacity to eliminate a drug if access is not impeded by protein binding or liver flow rate. Hepatic CL is then given as

$$CL_H = E_H \times Q_H = \frac{Q_H \times CL_{int} \times f_u}{Q_H + CL_{int} \times f_u} \quad (1\text{-}57)$$

and the fraction escaping hepatic first-pass metabolism F_H as

$$F_H = 1 - E_H = 1 - \frac{CL_{int} \times f_u}{Q_H + CL_{int} \times f_u} \quad (1\text{-}58)$$
$$= \frac{Q_H}{Q_H + CL_{int} \times f_u}$$

Conceptually, two basic classes of drugs can be distinguished based on the venous equilibrium model, drugs with high hepatic extraction ratio and drugs with low hepatic extraction ratio. This approach has been useful to predict changes in hepatic CL or steady-state drug concentrations secondary to changes in protein binding (f_u), hemodynamics (Q_H), and drug-metabolizing activity (CL_{int}), for example

by drug-drug interactions resulting in induction or inhibition of drug-metabolizing enzymes. Table 1.2 summarizes the effect of changes in f_u, Q_H, and CL_{int} on total and unbound steady-state concentration C_{ss} and $C_{ss,u}$.

High-Extraction Drugs. A high-extraction drug is one that has an extraction ratio greater than or equal to 0.7. In this case, the product of CL_{int} and f_u is much larger than Q_H as transport of drug to the liver is the limiting factor for hepatic CL. Thus, high-extraction drugs have a flow-limited hepatic CL. As $f_u \times CL_{int} >> Q_H$, the expressions for CL_H and F_H simplify to

$$CL_H \cong Q_H \qquad (1\text{-}59)$$

$$F_H \cong \frac{Q_H}{CL_{int} \times f_u} \qquad (1\text{-}60)$$

For the purpose of qualitative prediction of the effect of changes in f_u, CL_{int}, and Q_H on total and unbound steady-state concentrations (C_{ss} and $C_{ss,u}$), F_a and F_G are assumed to be 1 for extravascular administrations.

For IV administration with dose rate DR:

$$C_{ss} \cong \frac{DR}{Q_H} \qquad (1\text{-}61a)$$

$$C_{ss,u} \cong \frac{f_u \times DR}{Q_H} \qquad (1\text{-}61b)$$

For extravascular (oral) administration with dose rate DR:

$$C_{ss} \cong \frac{F_H \times DR}{Q_H} = \frac{Q_H \times DR}{CL_{int} \times f_u \times Q_H} \quad (1\text{-}62a)$$
$$= \frac{DR}{CL_{int} \times f_u}$$

$$C_{ss,u} \cong \frac{f_u \times F_H \times DR}{Q_H} = \frac{DR}{CL_{int}} \qquad (1\text{-}62b)$$

High-extraction drugs are characterized by route-dependent differences in the effect of f_u, Q_H, and CL_{int}. For a high-extraction drug given by the IV route, alterations in liver flow rate result in inverse changes in C_{ss} and $C_{ss,u}$. When given orally, changes in liver flow rate are offset by changes in bioavailability, resulting in no net change in C_{ss} or $C_{ss,u}$.

Changes in intrinsic clearance (CL_{int}) have no effect on C_{ss} and $C_{ss,u}$ after IV administration. When given orally, changes in CL_{int} result in inverse changes in C_{ss} and $C_{ss,u}$ due to changes in F_H.

Changes in protein binding do not affect C_{ss} after IV administration, but affect $C_{ss,u}$ proportionally. After oral administration, changes in f_u would be expected to result in changes in C_{ss} but not $C_{ss,u}$ based on changes in F_H. However, since high-extraction drugs are generally nonrestrictively cleared, i.e., protein binding is not a CL limiting factor, it might also be expected that hepatic first-pass metabolism is not affected by the degree of protein binding for high-extraction drugs.

TABLE 1.2	Predicted Effect of Perturbations on Free and Total Steady-State Concentrations Using the Venous Equilibrium Model for Hepatic Clearance			
Perturbation	CL_H	F_H	C_{ss}	$C_{ss,u}$
High-Extraction Drugs – IV Administration				
$Q_H \uparrow$	$\uparrow$	–	$\downarrow$	$\downarrow$
$Q_H \downarrow$	$\downarrow$	–	$\uparrow$	$\uparrow$
$f_u \uparrow$	$\leftrightarrow$	–	$\leftrightarrow$	$\uparrow$
$f_u \downarrow$	$\leftrightarrow$	–	$\leftrightarrow$	$\downarrow$
$CL_{int} \uparrow$	$\leftrightarrow$	–	$\leftrightarrow$	$\leftrightarrow$
$CL_{int} \downarrow$	$\leftrightarrow$	–	$\leftrightarrow$	$\leftrightarrow$
High-Extraction Drugs – Oral Administration				
$Q_H \uparrow$	$\uparrow$	$\downarrow$	$\leftrightarrow$	$\leftrightarrow$
$Q_H \downarrow$	$\downarrow$	$\uparrow$	$\leftrightarrow$	$\leftrightarrow$
$f_u \uparrow$	$\leftrightarrow$	$\leftrightarrow$ (?)		
$f_u \downarrow$	$\leftrightarrow$	$\leftrightarrow$ (?)		
$CL_{int} \uparrow$	$\leftrightarrow$	$\downarrow$	$\downarrow$	$\downarrow$
$CL_{int} \downarrow$	$\leftrightarrow$	$\uparrow$	$\uparrow$	$\uparrow$
Low-Extraction Drugs – IV and Oral Administration				
$Q_H \uparrow$	$\leftrightarrow$	$\leftrightarrow$	$\leftrightarrow$	$\leftrightarrow$
$Q_H \downarrow$	$\leftrightarrow$	$\leftrightarrow$	$\leftrightarrow$	$\leftrightarrow$
$f_u \uparrow$	$\uparrow$	$\leftrightarrow$	$\downarrow$	$\leftrightarrow$
$f_u \downarrow$	$\downarrow$	$\leftrightarrow$	$\uparrow$	$\leftrightarrow$
$CL_{int} \uparrow$	$\uparrow$	$\leftrightarrow$	$\downarrow$	$\downarrow$
$CL_{int} \downarrow$	$\downarrow$	$\leftrightarrow$	$\uparrow$	$\uparrow$

$\uparrow$, increase; $\leftrightarrow$, little or no change; $\downarrow$, decrease.

High-Extraction Drug and Congestive Heart Failure. A 53-year-old patient recently developed congestive heart failure (CHF) due to a myocardial infarction. The patient has been on oral propranolol therapy for several years for the management of hypertension. Propranolol is almost exclusively eliminated by hepatic metabolism and can be classified as a high-extraction drug based on its high hepatic CL of 1,100 mL per min combined with its low oral bioavailability (25%). Mild-to-moderate CHF is known to reduce the hepatic flow rate, Q_H. Severe CHF may additionally result in liver damage, i.e., a reduction in CL_{int}. What are the expected effects on total and unbound propranolol concentrations C_{ss} and $C_{ss,u}$?

$$C_{ss} \cong \frac{DR}{CL_{int} \times f_u} \quad \text{(1-63a)}$$

$$C_{ss,u} \cong \frac{DR}{CL_{int}} \quad \text{(1-63b)}$$

The effect of Q_H on CL is predicted to be offset by its effect on bioavailability. Thus, C_{ss} and $C_{ss,u}$ would not be affected in mild-to-moderate CHF, but would increase if CL_{int} is reduced in more severe cases of CHF.

Low-Extraction Drugs. A low-extraction drug is one that has an extraction ratio less than or equal to 0.3. In this case, the product of CL_{int} and f_u is much smaller than Q_H as the capacity of drug-metabolizing enzymes is the limiting factor for hepatic CL. Thus, low-extraction drugs have a capacity-limited hepatic CL:

As $f_u \times CL_{int} << Q_H$, the expressions for CL_H and F_H simplify to

$$CL_H \cong f_u \times CL_{int} \quad \text{(1-64)}$$

$$F_H \cong 1 \quad \text{(1-65)}$$

For IV administration with dose rate DR:

$$C_{ss} \cong \frac{DR}{f_u \times CL_{int}} \quad \text{(1-66a)}$$

$$C_{ss,u} \cong \frac{f_u \times DR}{f_u \times CL_{int}} = \frac{DR}{CL_{int}} \quad \text{(1-66b)}$$

For extravascular (oral) administration with dose rate DR:

$$C_{ss} \cong \frac{F_H \times DR}{f_u \times CL_{int}} \cong \frac{DR}{f_u \times CL_{int}} \quad (1\text{-}67a)$$

$$C_{ss,u} \cong \frac{f_u \times F_H \times DR}{f_u \times CL_{int}} \cong \frac{DR}{CL_{int}} \quad (1\text{-}67b)$$

For low-extraction drugs, there are no route-dependent differences in the effect of alterations in CL_{int}, Q_H, or f_u. Changes in liver blood flow rate have no relevant effect on C_{ss} and $C_{ss,u}$. Changes in CL_{int} result in inversely proportional changes in both C_{ss}, and $C_{ss,u}$.

Changes in f_u have no effect on the pharmacologically active $C_{ss,u}$, but result in inversely proportional changes in C_{ss}. Acknowledging this change in the relationship between $C_{ss,u}$ and C_{ss} becomes especially important if concentration measurements for therapeutic drug monitoring are based on total rather than unbound drug. Although C_{ss} changes, no dosage adjustment is necessary as the pharmacologically active $C_{ss,u}$ remains unchanged. Misinterpretation of changes in total drug concentration under these conditions, especially if no unbound drug concentration is available, could result in unnecessary changes in the dosing regimen and subsequent toxicity or lack of efficacy. This is illustrated in Figure 1.12.

Low-Extraction Drug and Change in Plasma Protein Binding. The antiepileptic phenytoin is primarily eliminated via hepatic metabolism and is a low-extraction drug. It is 90% bound to plasma proteins ($f_u = 0.1$) with albumin as the major binding protein. The therapeutic range for phenytoin is 10–20 mg per L.

A patient with chronic renal failure has a steady-state phenytoin level of 8.4 mg per L and a serum albumin of 2.2

g per dL. One might be tempted to increase the daily dose of phenytoin to achieve a target concentration of 15 mg per L. However, this would likely result in toxicity.

When the patient developed chronic renal failure, renal loss of albumin resulted in a decrease in albumin concentrations from the normal value of approximately 4.3 g per dL to 2.2 g per dL. This led to an increase in f_u from 0.1 to 0.18. Because phenytoin is an orally administered low-extraction drug, the increase in f_u resulted in a decrease in C_{ss}, but $C_{ss,u}$ remained unchanged.

$$\downarrow C_{ss} \cong \frac{DR}{\uparrow f_u \times CL_{int}} \quad (1\text{-}68a)$$

$$\leftrightarrow C_{ss,u} \cong \frac{DR}{CL_{int}} \quad (1\text{-}68b)$$

This is the reason for the low total phenytoin concentration of 8.4 mg per L that was measured. It corresponds to an unbound concentration of

$$C_u = f_u \times C = 0.18 \times 8.4\ mg/L = 1.5\ mg/L \quad (1\text{-}69)$$

As the therapeutic range for total phenytoin concentrations is 10 to 20 mg per L and f_u is 0.1 in normal individuals, the therapeutic range for unbound concentrations is 1 to 2 mg per L. Thus, the patient's unbound phenytoin concentrations are within the therapeutic range and the dose rate of phenytoin in this patient should not be increased despite total phenytoin levels below the therapeutic range.

Alterations in Plasma Protein Binding. The extent of plasma protein binding of a drug may be affected by several different mechanisms. Under numerous physiologic and

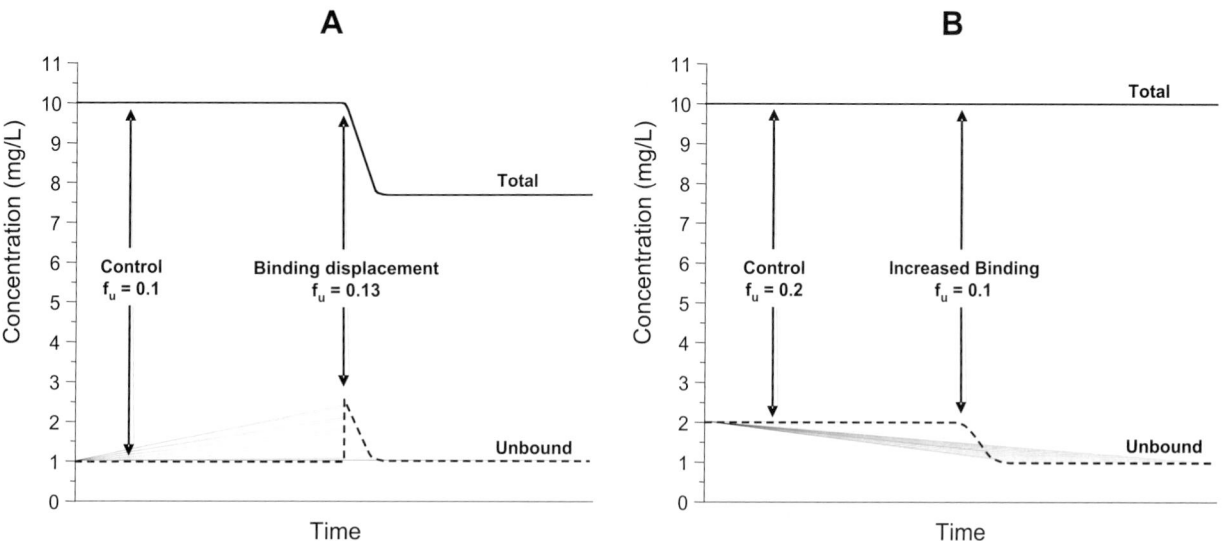

FIGURE 1.12 Effect of plasma protein binding displacement on steady-state plasma concentrations during a constant IV infusion. For a low extraction drug **(A)**, binding displacement has no effect on the unbound concentration $C_{ss,u}$ except for a transient increase, but total concentrations will be reduced. For a high extraction drug **(B)**, increase in binding results in a decrease in unbound concentration $C_{ss,u}$, but total concentrations C_{ss} remain unaffected. Solid lines, total drug concentrations; dashed lines,: unbound concentration. (From MacKichan JJ, Comstock TJ. General pharmacokinetic principles. In: Taylor WJ, Diers Cavinness M, eds. A textbook for the clinical application of therapeutic drug monitoring. Irving, TX: Abbott Laboratories, 1986.)

pathologic conditions, synthesis or degradation of binding proteins is modified, thereby increasing or decreasing the binding capacity for the drug in plasma and thus changing the fraction unbound, f_u. In addition, binding displacements may occur either through endogenous substances competing for the same binding sites or exogenous compounds such as concomitantly administered drugs. The latter mechanism is the typical case of a drug-drug interaction via binding displacement.

One prerequisite for protein displacements to be clinically relevant is that the displaced drug must be extensively protein bound (i.e., >90% bound to plasma proteins), because only then will displacement result in a substantial increase in the fraction unbound.

Decreasing the binding of a drug that is 99% protein bound by 1% will result in doubling the fraction unbound (from 1% to 2%) and thus the unbound, pharmacologically active concentration of the drug. Decreasing the binding of a drug that is 60% protein bound by 1% will result in an increase of the fraction unbound from 40% to 41%, i.e., an increase in the unbound concentration of 2.5%.

The clinical importance of protein binding displacement interactions is frequently overstated.[7,8] Very specific conditions have to be fulfilled before protein displacement becomes therapeutically relevant. These are summarized in Figure 1.13. One can distinguish between long-term effects at steady-state and transient effects shortly after binding displacement.

Long-Term Effects of Displacement. The influence of displacement on the unbound concentration at steady-state $C_{ss,u}$ depends on the extraction ratio and the route of administration of the affected drug. As discussed in the previous section, $C_{ss,u}$ is unaffected by changes in f_u for low-extraction drugs. For high-extraction drugs given by IV administration, however, changes in f_u affect $C_{ss,u}$, but not total concentrations. These relationships are summarized in Figure 1.12.

Transient Effects of Displacement. Protein displacements for low-extraction drugs result in a transient increase in free concentration C_u while the body re-equilibrates. During this period, drug distribution and drug elimination will change to compensate for the increased C_u, but a relevant increase in C_u is only likely to occur for drugs with a small V (<10 L), for which most of the drug resides in the plasma. This transient increase in C_u becomes acutely relevant only if C_u increases above the corresponding therapeutic range, a situation that is relatively uncommon.

CLINICAL PHARMACODYNAMICS

This chapter has focused on the time course of drug concentrations in blood or plasma as a function of the administered dosage regimen, assuming that these concentrations are representative of or functionally related to the concentration at the sites of action for therapeutic as well as toxic effects. What is really of interest in clinical pharmacotherapy, however, is not the time course of concentrations, but the time course of therapeutic and toxic effects. Therefore, not only the PK of a drug have to be considered, but also its PD.

PHARMACOKINETIC VERSUS PHARMACODYNAMIC VARIABILITY

PK can be seen as the translator of dose to concentration over time, whereas PD links concentration to drug effects.

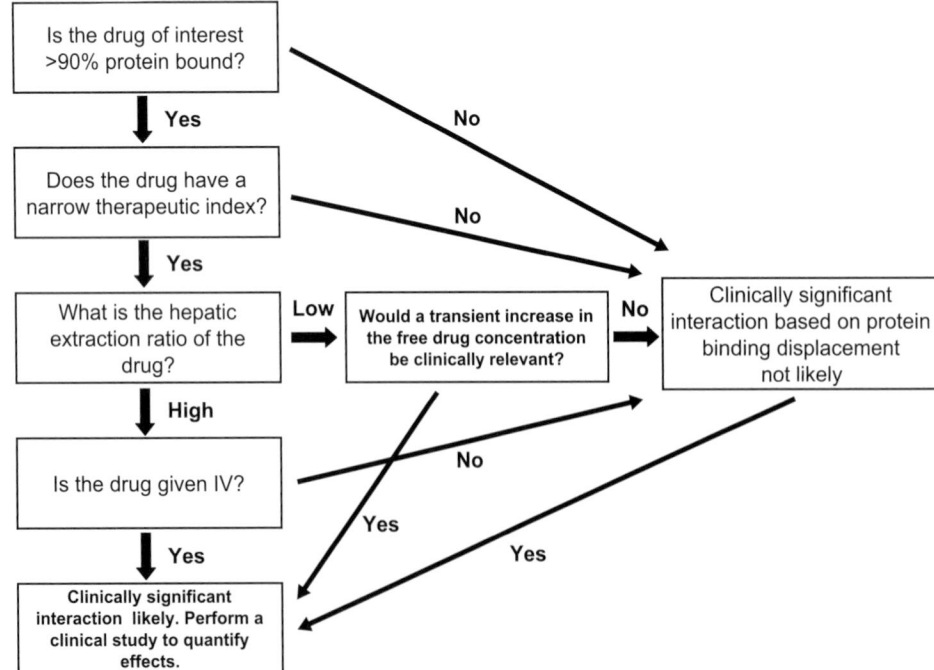

FIGURE 1.13 Algorithm for determining clinical significance of potential protein binding displacement interactions. (From Rolan PE. Plasma protein binding displacement interactions—why are they still regarded as clinically important? Br J Clin Pharmacol 37: 125–128, 1994.)

Together, they determine the time course of drug effects. Note that while PK and PD are essentially predetermined by the physiochemical properties of the drug and physiologic and/or pathophysiologic conditions of the body, manipulating the dose, route of administration, and frequency of dosing can result in optimized targeted effects by controlling concentrations.

Variability in response to the same dosage regimen of a drug given to different patients is the result of variability in PK and PD characteristics among patients. Empirical dosing without any knowledge about the PK and PD of individual patients leaves PK and PD variability uncontrolled. Thus, if PK and /or PD variability are high, the observed effect resulting from an administered dosage regimen is only poorly predictable in an individual patient.

Concentration-based dosing controls PK variability between different patients by determining individual PK based on plasma concentration measurements. Subsequent individualization of the dosage regimen allows a certain target concentration in all individuals to be maintained. However, the PD variability still is uncontrolled, which may lead to different magnitudes of effect in different patients despite the same target concentration. Concentration-based dosing is clinically used via therapeutic drug monitoring and is applicable for drugs for which PK variability is higher than PD variability. Thus, effectively controlling for PK variability may significantly reduce the variability in response to a drug therapy among patients.

For numerous drugs, however, PD variability is much higher than PK variability. In these cases, plasma concentration monitoring is of limited benefit, as the plasma concentration is a poor predictor for the patient's therapeutic response to the dosage regimen. Also, when drug concentrations required to achieve a desired therapeutic effect are much lower than concentrations that produce serious toxicity, then it may be feasible to treat all patients with a high enough dose so that essentially all patients achieve therapeutic drug concentrations, despite PK variability, without toxicity. These are among the major reasons why therapeutic drug monitoring is only performed for a limited number of drugs.

Theophylline and warfarin are drugs with a narrow therapeutic range and high interindividual variability in response. For theophylline, therapeutic drug monitoring by plasma level measurements is performed as theophylline plasma concentrations are a good predictor for its effects and PK variability is higher than PD variability. For warfarin, PD variability is higher than PK variability. Thus, warfarin plasma concentrations would only be a poor predictor for its effect and thus, patients are monitored for warfarin efficacy (prothrombin time or INR) instead of its plasma concentration.

PK/PD-based dosing would overcome the drawbacks of controlling only one component of pharmacologic variability by controlling for PK as well as PD variability. This would require determining the individual patient's PK parameters (i.e., CL and V) and the patient's PD parameters (i.e., E_{max} and EC_{50}). Individual assessment of pharmacodynamic parameters, however, currently is rarely performed in clinical settings. One example for clinically applied PK/PD-based dosing is antibiotic pharmacotherapy, for example with vancomycin, where the in vitro sensitivity of the pathogen is routinely assessed as minimum inhibitory concentration (MIC), a typical PD parameter characterizing the concentration-effect relationship. The MIC together with the site of infection is used to guide the selection of an appropriate target therapeutic range that can then be achieved by concentration-controlled dosing using plasma concentration measurements and therapeutic drug monitoring.

PHARMACODYNAMIC MODELS

PK relationships are linear for most drugs, i.e., follow the principle of superposition. In contrast, the relationship between plasma concentration and effect for most drugs is not linear, but follows a nonlinear relationship that levels off at a maximum effect being reached with a specific drug therapy.[9]

The most widely used pharmacodynamic model for concentration-dependent, reversible drug effects that are directly mediated is the E_{max}-model. The E_{max}-model is an empirically derived relationship that relates the effect (E) to the concentration (C) by the following relationship:

$$E = \frac{E_{max} \times C}{EC_{50} + C} \qquad (1\text{-}70)$$

where E_{max} is the maximum effect possible with the specific drug and EC_{50} is the concentration that causes 50% of E_{max}, the half-maximum effect. E_{max} refers to the intrinsic activity of a drug, EC_{50} to its potency.

Although the E_{max}-model is an empiric relationship, its value lies in the fact that it can be related to the receptor theory of drug action. Under the assumption that the observed effect E is directly proportional to the number of occupied receptors, E_{max} is equivalent to the number of receptors available, and EC_{50} is equivalent to the affinity constant of the drug to the receptor, i.e., the concentration at which half of the receptor sites are occupied.

The E_{max}-model describes the concentration-effect relationship over a wide range of concentrations from zero effect in the absence of drug to the maximum effect at concentrations much higher than EC_{50} ($C \gg EC_{50}$). The clear nonproportional concentration-effect relationship of the E_{max}-model is presented in Figure 1.14 *(see color insert)* in linear and semilogarithmic plots. Whereas small increases in concentration may result in significant increases of the effect for low concentrations, this is much less pronounced for higher concentrations where only small changes in effect will result from changes in concentration. From the semilogarithmic presentation, it is apparent that in the range from 20% to 80% of the maximum effect, the relationship between effect and the logarithm of the concentration is linear. This is consistent with a log-linear concentration-effect relationship

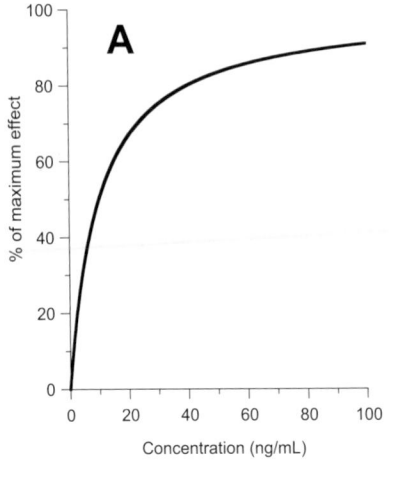

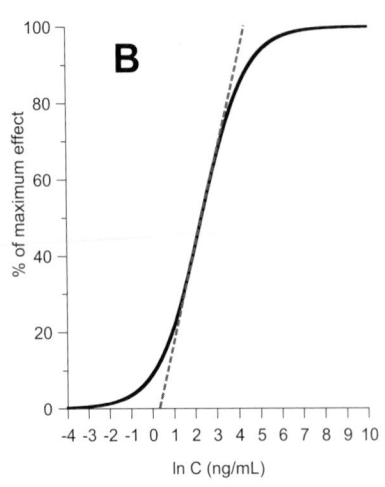

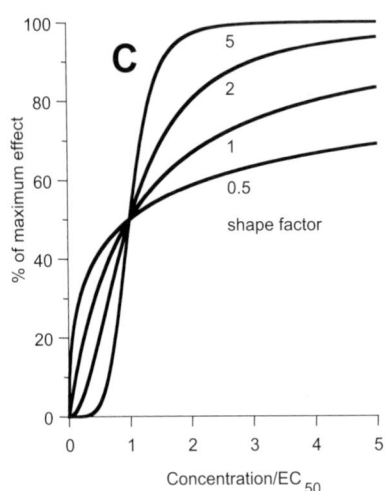

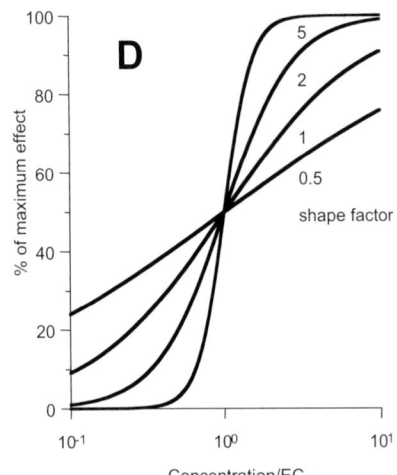

FIGURE 1.14 E_{max} and sigmoid E_{max}-model. Effect versus concentration (linear: **A,C**; and logarithmic: **B,D**) relationship defined by an E_{max}-model **(A,B)** and a sigmoid E_{max}-model **(C,D)**. The *dotted line* in **B** indicates the log-linear range of the concentration-effect relationship between 20% to 80% of the maximum effect. Numerals next to the curves in **C** and **D** indicate different values for the shape factor in the sigmoid E_{max}-model.

clinically observed for many drugs. Thus, in this range, the E_{max}-equation can be rewritten for a log-linear model as

$$E = \frac{E_{max}}{4} \times \ln C + \frac{E_{max}}{4} \times (\ln EC_{50} + 2) \quad (1\text{-}71)$$

where $E_{max}/4$ is the slope in the log-linear relationship. For concentrations much smaller than EC_{50} ($C \ll EC_{50}$), the E_{max}-model reduces to a linear relationship between concentration and effect with a slope of E_{max}/EC_{50}. Hence, both, a log-linear as well as the linear model for the concentration-effect relationship may be interpreted as special cases of the E_{max}-model.

Often, the effect of a drug therapy is the change in a physiologic parameter, e.g., mean arterial blood pressure. In these cases, a baseline value E_0, i.e., a measure for the physiologic response variable in the absence of drug dosing, has to be considered in the E_{max}-relationship:

$$\text{For stimulating effects: } E = E_0 + \frac{E_{max} \times C}{EC_{50} + C} \quad (1\text{-}72)$$

$$\text{For inhibitory effects: } E = E_0 - \frac{E_{max} \times C}{EC_{50} + C} \quad (1\text{-}73)$$

The sigmoid E_{max}-model is an expansion of the E_{max}-model, including a so-called shape factor or Hill-coefficient n.

$$E = \frac{E_{max} \times C^n}{EC_{50}^n + C^n} \quad (1\text{-}74)$$

Addition of the shape factor n increases the versatility of the model to describe concentration-effect relationships. The simple E_{max}-model can be seen as a special case of the sigmoid E_{max}-model with $n = 1$. The effect of different values of n on the concentration-effect curves for a sigmoid E_{max}-model are shown in Figure 1.14. The larger n, the steeper the curve in the log-linear phase from 20% to 80% of the maximum effect, with the respective slope given by $n \times E_{max}/4$.

Figure 1.15 shows the use of an inhibitory sigmoid E_{max}-model in relating the antiarrhythmic activity of tocainide measured as reduction of premature ventricular heart contractions (PVCs) per hour in relation to its plasma concentration. The range of slope factor in individual subjects was $n = 2.3\text{-}20.6$. As the maximum effect is total suppression of PVCs, $E_{max} = E_0$, the resulting model can be simplified as

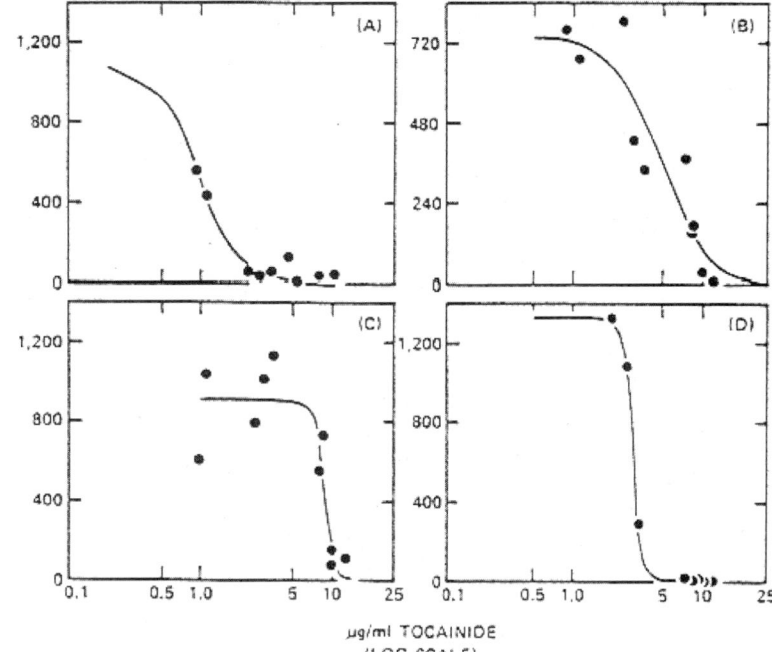

FIGURE 1.15 Inhibitory sigmoid E_{max}-model. Antiarrhythmic activity of tocainide measured as reduction of premature ventricular heart contractions (PVCs) per hour in relation to its plasma concentration. Shown are the concentration-effect relationships of four representative patients (measured data as dots), modeled with an inhibitory sigmoid E_{max}-model (solid lines). (From Meffin PJ, Winkle RA, Blaschke TF, et al. Response optimization of drug dosage: antiarrhythmic studies with tocainide. Clin Pharmacol Ther 22:42–57, 1977.)

$$E = E_0 - \frac{E_{max} \times C^n}{EC_{50}^n + C^n} \qquad (1\text{-}75)$$

$$= E_0 \times \left(1 - \frac{C^n}{EC_{50}^n + C^n}\right)$$

DOSING BASED ON PHARMACOKINETIC AND PHARMACODYNAMIC PARAMETERS

PK/PD modeling combines both approaches, PK and PD, and establishes models to describe the time course of the effect directly resulting from the administration of a certain dosage regimen. Thus, a so-called integrated PK/PD model consists of a PK model component that describes the time course of drug in plasma and a PD model component that relates the plasma concentration to the drug effect (Fig. 1.16).

Two simple, characteristic parameters can be used to translate PK and PD data into dosage recommendations. Both parameters, D_{50} and DR_{50} assume equilibrium between plasma and effect-site concentrations and can be based on $EC_{50,u}$ for free drug concentrations or EC_{50} for total drug concentrations.[10]

D_{50} is the amount of drug that has to be in the body to produce 50% of the maximum effect. It is the LD to be given to achieve 50% of E_{max}:

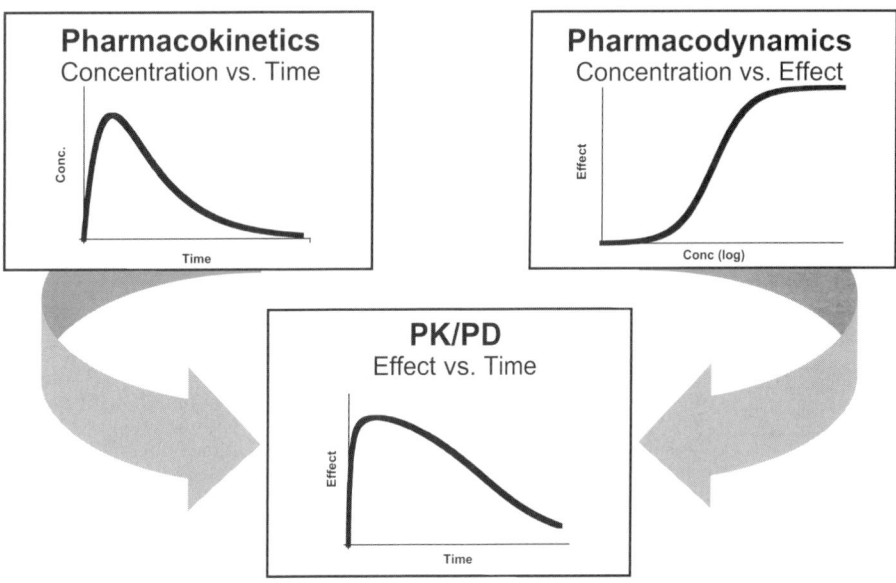

FIGURE 1.16 General concept of PK/PD-modeling. Pharmacokinetic/pharmacodynamic (PK/PD) modeling combines a PK model component that describes the time course of drug in plasma and a PD model component that relates the plasma concentration to the drug effect in order to describe the time course of the effect intensity resulting from the administration of a certain dosage regimen. (From Derendorf H, Meibohm B. Modeling of pharmacokinetic/pharmacodynamic (PK/PD) relationships: concepts and perspectives. Pharm Res 16:176–185, 1999.)

$$D_{50} = EC_{50} \times V \quad (1\text{-}76a)$$

or

$$D_{50} = \frac{EC_{50,u} \times V}{f_u} \quad (1\text{-}76b)$$

The second, more important parameter is DR_{50}, the dose rate that produces 50% of the maximum effect. It is the MD to be given to maintain 50% of E_{max}:

$$DR_{50} = EC_{50} \times CL \quad (1\text{-}77a)$$

or

$$DR_{50} = \frac{EC_{50,u} \times CL}{f_u} \quad (1\text{-}77b)$$

The dosing rate DR_{50} (as well as D_{50}) can easily be converted to a dosing rate for any other fraction (x%) of E_{max} as:

$$DR_x = \frac{x}{100 - x} \times DR_{50} \quad (1\text{-}78)$$

A patient (53 years old, female, 5'4", 66 kg) will be started on an oral theophylline dosage regimen with an immediate release dosage form to control her asthma. The effect of theophylline on respiratory function was reported as an improvement in peak expiratory flow rate from baseline (PEFR) using an E_{max}-model. The reported population average parameters are $E_{max} = 344$ L per min and $EC_{50} = 11$ mg per L. For the pharmacokinetic parameters of theophylline, a CL of 0.04 L/hr/kg, a V_{ss} of 0.5 L/kg, and an oral bioavailability of F = 1 are assumed. If PEFR improvement of at least 200 L/min from baseline is targeted, the corresponding LD and MD to achieve this target can be calculated:

Step 1: Determine the D_{50} and DR_{50} for the PEFR improvement by theophylline:

$$D_{50} = EC_{50} \times V_{ss} = 11 \ mg/L \times 0.5 \ L/kg$$
$$\times \ 66 \ kg = 363 \ mg \quad (1\text{-}79)$$

$$DR_{50} = EC_{50} \times CL = 11 \ mg/L \times 0.04 \ L/hr/kg$$
$$\times \ 66 \ kg = 29 \ mg/hr \quad (1\text{-}80)$$

Step 2: Determine the $\%E_{max}$ for the targeted effect level:

$$\%E_{max} = \frac{E}{E_{max}} = \frac{200 \ L/min}{344 \ L/min} = 58\% \quad (1\text{-}81)$$

Step 3: Convert D_{50} and DR_{50} to the targeted effect level:

$$D_{58} = \frac{58}{100 - 58} \times D_{50} = \frac{58}{42} \quad (1\text{-}82)$$
$$\times \ 363 \ mg = 501 \ mg$$

$$DR_{58} = \frac{58}{100 - 58} \times DR_{50} = \frac{58}{42} \quad (1\text{-}83)$$
$$\times \ 29 \ mg/hr = 40 \ mg/hr$$

HYSTERESIS

For the previously discussed PK/PD models, the drug concentrations were directly linked to the observed effect. That means that the same drug concentration will always cause the same effect intensity. For some drugs, however, the relationship between concentration and effect is also dependent on the time point after drug administration. For these drugs, the relationship between concentration and effect is not defined by a curve like in the sigmoid E_{max}-model, but by a hysteresis loop (Fig. 1.17). Hysteresis in the concentration-effect relationship means that the same drug concentration

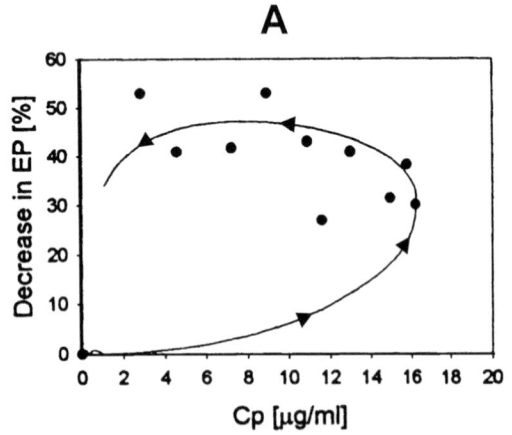
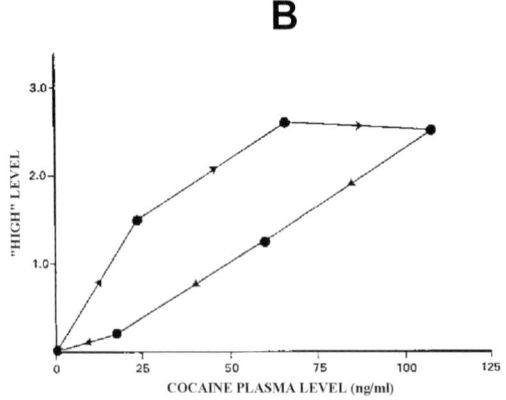

FIGURE 1.17 Hysteresis in the concentration-effect relationships. **(A)** Counterclockwise hysteresis loop for the relationship between plasma concentration of S-ibuprofen and its analgesic effect quantified as a decrease in evoked potential amplitudes (EP) attributed to a distributional delay between plasma and effect site concentration. **(B)** Clockwise hysteresis loop for the subjective psychologic effect ("high" levels) versus plasma concentrations after 1.5 mg/kg cocaine intranasally attributed to development of functional tolerance. (From Suri A, Grundy BL, Derendorf H. Pharmacokinetics and pharmacodynamics of enantiomers of ibuprofen and flurbiprofen after oral administration. Int J Clin Pharmacol Ther 35:1–8, 1997; Van Dyke C, Ungerer J, Jatlow P, et al. Intranasal cocaine: dose relationships of psychological effects and plasma levels. Int J Psychiatry Med 12:1–13, 1982.)

in plasma will result in different effect levels at different time points after drug administration. A hysteresis loop may be clockwise or counterclockwise, depending on the mechanisms involved in the temporal dissociation between plasma concentration and effect profile.

The major reasons for counterclockwise hysteresis loops include a distributional delay to the effect site, a time-consuming indirect response mechanism, agonistically acting active metabolites of a drug that are not quantified, or sensitization, i.e., an increase in effect over time despite constant drug concentration. Major reasons for clockwise hysteresis loops include functional tolerance and antagonistically acting active metabolites of a drug that are not quantified. Some of these causes of hysteresis will be discussed in detail.

Distributional Delay to the Effect Site. While the measurement of drug concentrations is usually performed in plasma, the input in the response system mediating the effect is provided by the concentration at the effect site, the site of action. For the previously described PK/PD models, the measured concentration in plasma is directly related to the effect site concentration. Equilibrium between concentrations is assumed to be rapidly achieved, and thus their ratio is constant, under PK steady-state as well as non-steady–state conditions. Hence, the measured concentrations can be directly linked to the observed effect. In that case, concentration and effect maxima would occur at the same time and effect versus concentration plots would lack any hysteresis. An example for this kind of concentration-effect relationship is the effect of tocainide measured on premature ventricular heart contractions (Fig. 1.15).

The equilibration between the plasma and the effect site concentrations, however, may be slow for some drugs due to time-consuming distribution processes involved. As a consequence of such a distributional delay, the ratio between plasma and effect site concentration would change with time resulting in a temporal dissociation between the time courses of measured plasma concentration and observed effect. For example, concentration maxima would occur before effect maxima, effect intensity might increase despite decreasing plasma concentrations and may persist beyond the time drug concentrations in plasma are no longer detectable. A counterclockwise hysteresis loop would be the consequence in an effect versus concentration plot. The muscle relaxant effect of d-tubocurarine is an example of a temporal dissociation between the concentration and effect-time courses (Fig. 1.18).

Tolerance. Development of tolerance to a drug therapy is characterized by diminishing effects in response to repeated administration of the same drug dose. Two major categories of tolerance can be distinguished based on the underlying causal mechanisms:

Metabolic tolerance, also called PK tolerance, is characterized by decreasing drug concentrations after repeated administration of the same dose, which consequently results in diminishing drug effects in response to these doses. The mechanistic basis for metabolic tolerance is a time-dependent change in PK parameters of the drug, most frequently caused by induction of the capacity of drug-metabolizing enzymes (i.e., an increase in CL_{int}).

Functional tolerance, also called PD tolerance, is characterized by a reduction in effect intensity at concentrations that earlier produced a greater effect or a decrease in drug effect over time despite constant drug concentrations at the effect site. The mechanistic basis for functional tolerance is a time-dependent change in

FIGURE 1.18 Temporal dissociation between the concentration and effect-time courses. Muscle relaxant effect of d-tubocurarine (DTC) after infusion of 16.8 μg/kg/min for 10 min followed by 1.2 μg/kg/min for 150 min. Shown are plasma concentration and effect versus time courses for one patient (lines are modeled). The temporal dissociation between concentration and effect is the result of a distributional delay between the concentrations in plasma and at the effect site. (From Sheiner LB, Stanski DR, Vozeh S, et al. Simultaneous modeling of pharmacokinetics and pharmacodynamics: application to d-tubocurarine. Clin Pharmacol Ther 25:358–371, 1979.)

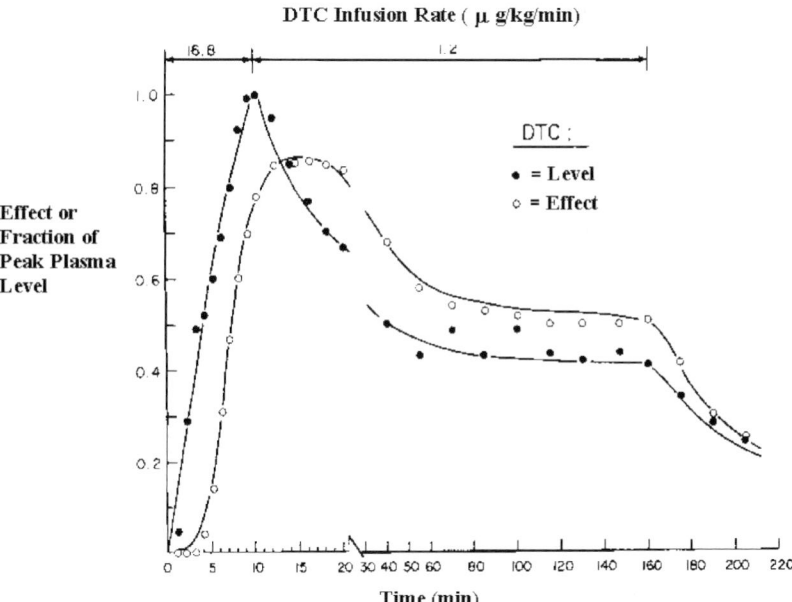

one or several pharmacodynamic parameters, e.g., E_{max} and EC_{50}. The diminishing response with rechallenging stimulus (i.e., concentrations) may be caused, for example, by downregulation of the number of receptors or a decrease in the receptor binding affinity for the drug. Functional tolerance results in a clockwise hysteresis loop in a plot of effect versus concentration (Fig. 1.17).

PHARMACOGENOMICS

Differences in efficacy as well as toxicity between patients in response to a medication are frequently much greater than the variations in efficacy and toxicity within the same person at different times. This discrepancy between large differences among members of a population and small intraindividual variability is consistent with inheritance as a major determinant of drug response. It is estimated that, depending on the drug, genetics can account for 20% to 95% of variability in drug disposition and effect. The phenotype, or clinically observable characteristics of a drug response, however, is a function of genetics (i.e., genotype), as well as nongenetic factors. Nongenetic factors include age, organ function, concomitant therapy, drug interactions, and nature and severity of the patient's disease. Unlike other factors influencing drug response, however, inherited determinants generally remain stable throughout a person's lifetime.[11]

Pharmacogenomics aims to identify the inherited basis for interindividual differences in drug response, and to translate this knowledge into molecular diagnostics that can be used to individualize drug therapy. While classic pharmacogenetics addresses the effect of polymorphic expression of a single gene on a drug's response profile, pharmacogenomics is a polygenic approach that assesses the effect of the concurrent interplay of multiple polymorphically expressed genes on an individual's response to a specific drug. Most drug effects are determined by multiple genes encoding drug-metabolizing enzymes, drug transporters, and drug targets (e.g., receptors).

PHARMACOGENETICS AFFECTING PHARMACOKINETIC PROCESSES

Genetic variations affecting functional activity have been identified for several drug-metabolizing enzymes and drug transporters. Functionally relevant polymorphisms have been described for genes encoding for multiple phase I and phase II enzymes including *CYP2B6, CYP2C9, CYP2C19, CYP2D6,* and *CYP3A5* as well as *NAT2, COMT,* and *TPMT* (see Fig. 1.11). For drug transporters, the effect of genetic variants has been described most extensively for *MDR1* (*ABCB1*), the gene encoding for the exsorption transporter P-glycoprotein.

CYP2D6. Metabolism via CYP2D6 is the major elimination pathway for numerous widely used medications, including beta-blockers such as carvedilol, metoprolol, and proprano-

lol; antidepressants such as amitriptyline, desipramine, imipramine, and fluoxetine; and antipsychotics such as haloperidol and risperidone. *CYP2D6* is a highly polymorphic gene for which more than 70 variant alleles have been described. A series of genetic variants is responsible for low levels of CYP2D6 activity or no activity. Carriers of these variant alleles are characterized by impaired metabolism for CYP2D6 substrates, which is referred to as a "poor metabolizer" status. In comparison, "extensive metabolizer" status refers to normal CYP2D6 activity. Approximately 5% to 10% of the white population has a relative deficiency in their CYP2D6-mediated metabolism, i.e., are poor metabolizers with regard to CYP2D6. These patients are likely to experience high levels of systemic exposure after standard doses of CYP2D6 substrates, which depending on the drug may lead to an increased likelihood of drug-induced toxicity. In addition, some subjects have multiple copies of the *CYP2D6* gene, resulting in ultrarapid metabolism. These patients are likely to have inadequate therapeutic response to standard doses of drugs that are metabolized by CYP2D6. The frequency of genetic variants in *CYP2D6* is ethnically diverse. Ultrarapid metabolizers are relatively rare in Northern European populations (1% to 3%), but more frequent in Mediterranean (7% to 10%) and African populations (20% to 30%).[12]

The effect of the variable number of *CYP2D6* functional alleles is shown in Figure 1.19 for the systemic exposure of nortriptyline. The higher the number of functional *CYP2D6* alleles, the lower the systemic exposure that was observed after administration of the same 25-mg nortriptyline dose to groups of subjects with different genotypes. Correspondingly, systemic exposure to 10-hydroxynortriptyline, the metabolite formed from nortriptyline via CYP2D6, was highest in the group with the highest number of functional *CYP2D6* alleles.[13]

TPMT. The genetic polymorphism of thiopurine-S-methyltransferase (TPMT) is a prime example for genetic variations used to adjust pharmacotherapy in individual patients. TPMT is the predominant inactivation mechanism for thiopurine drugs like mercaptopurine and azathioprine in hematopoietic tissues, two drugs that are clinically used as antineoplastic and immunosuppressant agents, respectively. TPMT activity is highly variable and polymorphic: approximately 90% of individuals have high activity, 10% have intermediate activity, and 0.3% (1 in 300) have low or undetectable enzyme activity. Patients with inherited TPMT deficiency accumulate excessive amounts of the active thioguanine nucleotides in blood cells when treated with thiopurines, resulting in potentially fatal hematopoietic toxicity. TPMT-deficient patients can be treated successfully with much lower doses of thiopurines (5% to 10% of the conventional dose), thereby avoiding the hematopoietic toxicity. Molecular diagnostic tests have recently become clinically available to detect the inactivating genetic variations in the *TPMT* gene before treatment initiation to adjust dosing a priori to the TPMT activity status of the patient. This approach of dosage individualization based on a genetic test is cost-effective in avoiding serious drug-associated toxicity.[14]

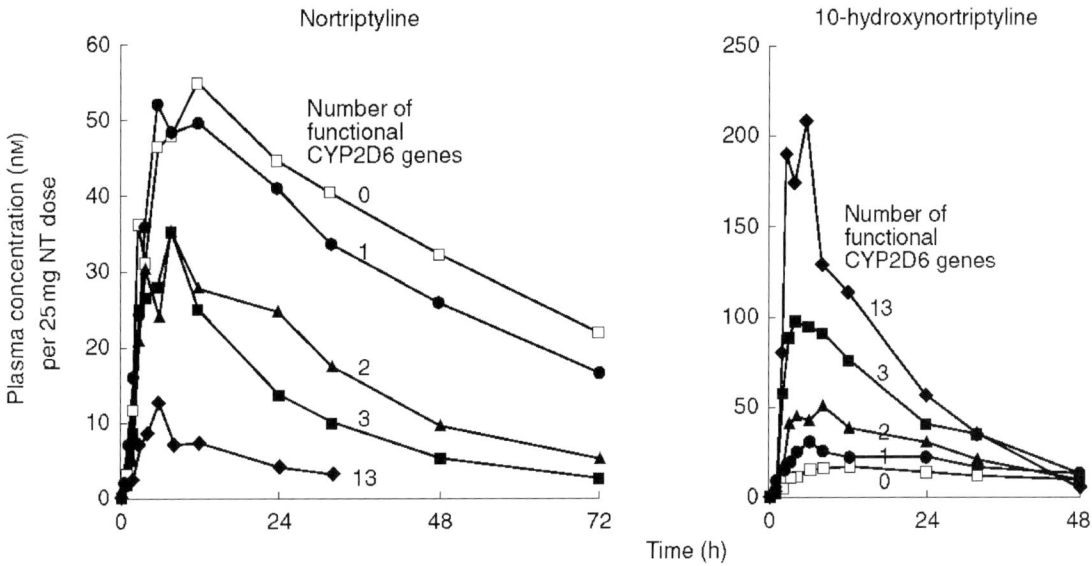

FIGURE 1.19 Effect of the variable number of *CYP2D6* functional alleles on the systemic exposure of nortriptyline. Mean plasma concentration of nortriptyline **(left)** and 10-hydroxynortriptyline **(right)** in different *CYP2D6* genotype groups after a single oral dose of nortriptyline. The numerals close to the curves represent the number of functional *CYP2D6* genes in each genotype group. In groups with 0–3 functional genes, there were five subjects in each group while there was only one subject with 13 functional genes. (From Dalen P, Dahl ML, Ruiz ML, et al. 10-Hydroxylation of nortriptyline in white persons with 0, 1, 2, 3, and 13 functional CYP2D6 genes. Clin Pharmacol Ther 63:444–452, 1998.)

PHARMACOGENETICS AFFECTING PHARMACODYNAMIC PROCESSES

Genetic variations leading to polymorphisms may not be limited to drug-metabolizing enzymes and drug transporters affecting the PK of a drug. They might also affect drug targets such as receptors, enzymes, ion channels, or other endogenous proteins, thereby altering the concentration-effect relationship for a drug, i.e., its PD. Therapeutically relevant polymorphisms have been described for numerous

drug targets, including angiotensin-converting enzymes (ACE inhibitors), arachidonate 5-lipoxygenase (leukotriene inhibitors), dopamine receptors (antipsychotics), estrogen receptor-α (estrogen hormone replacement therapy), and the serotonin transporter (antidepressants).

Polymorphisms for the β_2-adrenergic receptor (*ADRB2*) are a well-investigated example of the effect of genetic variations on a drug's PD. Single nucleotide polymorphisms (SNPs) leading to sequence changes in the ADRB2 protein

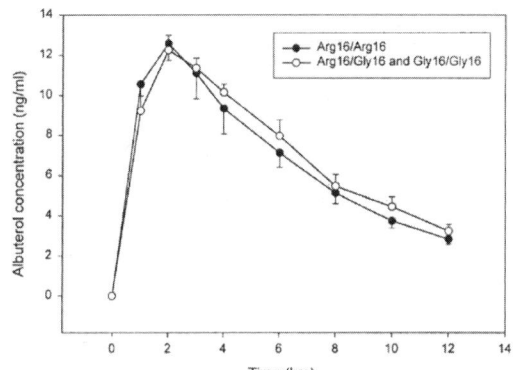

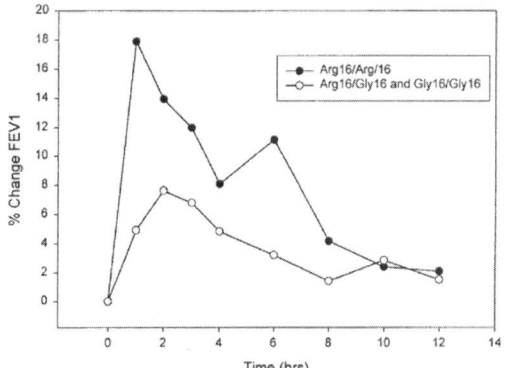

FIGURE 1.20 Effect of genetic polymorphism in the β_2-adrenergic receptor (*ADRB2*) on bronchodilator response to albuterol in asthmatics. Comparison of median FEV_1 **(right)** and mean ± SE albuterol plasma concentrations **(left)** versus time after administration of a single 8-mg oral dose of albuterol in Arg16 homozygotes (solid circles) and in heterozygotes and Gly16 homozygotes (open circles). (From Lima JJ, Thomason DB, Mohamed MH, et al. Impact of genetic polymorphisms of the beta2-adrenergic receptor on albuterol bronchodilator pharmacodynamics. Clin Pharmacol Ther 65:519–525, 1999.)

at amino acid positions 16, 27, and 164 have been found to significantly alter receptor function. In in vitro experiments, the Thr-to-Ile amino acid change at position 164 displays altered coupling to adenyl cyclase, the Arg-to-Gly change at position 16 results in enhanced agonist-promoted downregulation of *ADRB2* expression, and the form with the Gln-to-Glu change at position 27 is resistant to downregulation.

Therapeutic relevance of the genetic variations in *ADRB2* has been shown for the response to β₂-agonists in asthma. The frequencies of these various *ADRB2* genetic variants are not different in asthmatics compared to normal individuals, but albuterol-evoked FEV₁ (forced expiratory volume

in one second) was higher and the bronchodilatory response was more rapid in Arg16 homozygotes than in a group of carriers of the Gly16 variant. In addition, an association has been demonstrated between the Arg16Gly variant and susceptibility to bronchodilator desensitization in moderately severe, stable asthmatics. Figure 1.20 shows the time courses of albuterol plasma concentrations and change in FEV₁ in subjects that are homozygous wild-type or a carrier of at least one variant allele with respect to codon 16 of the *ADRB2* gene. Although there is no pharmacokinetic difference between the two groups as indicated by the superimposable concentration-time profiles for albuterol, the Arg16Gly

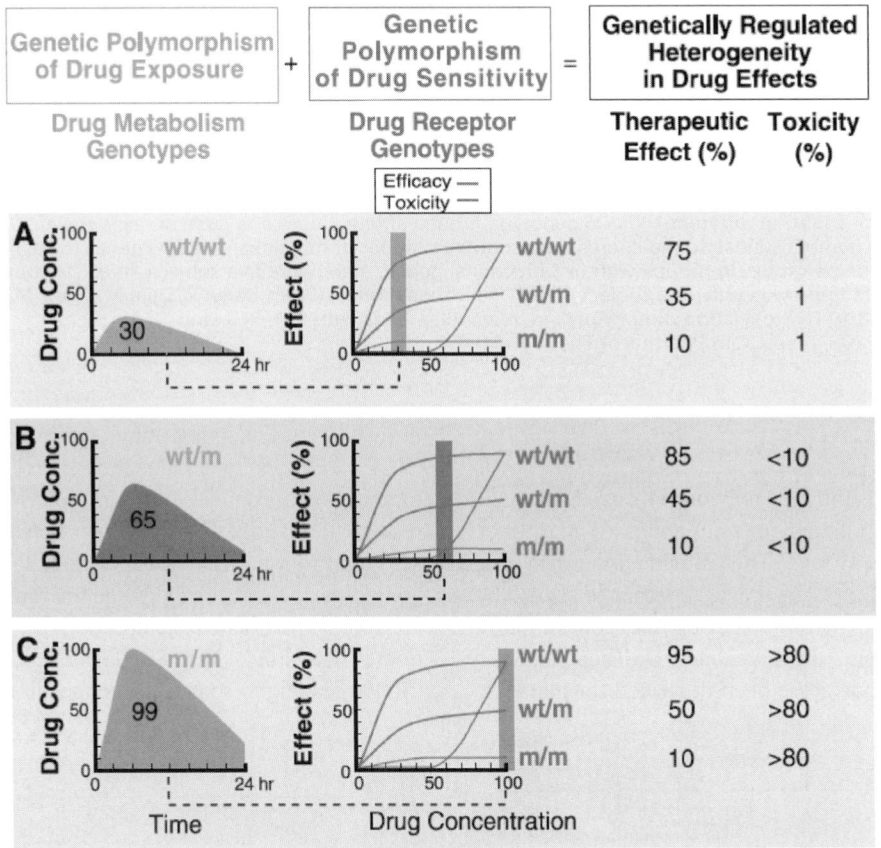

FIGURE 1.21 Polygenic determinants of drug effects *(see color insert)*. The potential consequences of administering the same dose of a medication to individuals with different drug metabolism genotypes and different drug-receptor genotypes is illustrated. Active drug concentrations in systemic circulation are determined by the individual's drug-metabolism genotype (green lettering), with **(A)** homozygous wild type (wt/wt) patients converting 70% of a dose to the inactive metabolite, leaving 30% to exert an effect on the target receptor. **(B)** For the patient with heterozygous (wt/m) drug-metabolism genotype, 35% is inactivated, whereas **(C)** the patient with homozygous mutant (m/m) drug metabolism inactivates only 1% of the dose by the polymorphic pathway, yielding the three drug concentration-time curves. Pharmacologic effects are further influenced by different genotypes of the drug receptor (blue lettering), which have different sensitivity to the medication, as depicted by the curves of drug concentration versus effects (middle). Patients with a wt/wt receptor genotype exhibit a greater effect at any given drug concentration in comparison to those with a wt/m receptor genotype, whereas those with m/m receptor genotypes are relatively refractory to drug effects at any plasma drug concentration. These two genetic polymorphisms (in drug metabolism and drug receptors) yield nine different theoretical patterns of drug effects **(right)**. The therapeutic ratio (efficacy: toxicity) ranges from a favorable 75 in the patient with wt/wt genotypes for drug metabolism and drug receptors to <0.13 in the patient with m/m genotypes for drug metabolism and drug receptors. (From Evans WE, Relling MV. Pharmacogenomics: translating functional genomics into rational therapeutics. Science 286:487–491, 1999.)

variant was associated with a difference in the concentration-effect relationship, i.e., a pharmacodynamic difference, between the groups: Asthmatics who were homozygous for the Arg 16 allele (Arg16/Arg16) showed more rapid increases in response and a higher bronchodilator response ($\%\Delta FEV_1$) 1 hour after drug administration than asthmatics that carried at least one variant allele (Arg16/Gly16 or Gly16/Gly). These results suggest that the genetic variation at codon 16 of the *ADRB2* gene is a major determinant of bronchodilator response to albuterol in asthmatics.

POLYGENIC EFFECTS ON PHARMACOKINETICS AND PHARMACODYNAMICS

Pharmacogenetics influences the pharmacologic response to drug therapy by determining both the dose-concentration relationship (i.e., PK) as well as the concentration-effect relationship (i.e., PD). Most genetic effects on pharmacotherapy and drug response that have been described are monogenic and highly penetrant, with clearly recognizable drug-induced phenotypes. A more likely frequent situation, however, is a scenario in which several polymorphisms influence simultaneously the pharmacologic response observed after administration of a therapeutic dosage regimen. The simplest case of such a polygenic effect on pharmacotherapy with only two polymorphic genes involved is exemplified in a hypothetical example in Figure 1.21 *(see color insert)*. Here, PK and PD of a drug are influenced by one polymorphism each, including high, intermediate, and low activity for each polymorphism for homozygous wild-type, heterozygous, and homozygous variant (nonfunctional or low-activity/sensitivity) individuals, respectively. The resulting nine different genotype combinations from only two polymorphisms illustrate the multitude of effect levels that may be expected from a polygenic modulation of pharmacotherapy. A future challenge will be to define these genetic determinants of drug response when 6 or 12 or even more genes are involved.

CONCLUSION

This chapter highlights some basic concepts in PK and PD as well as some pharmacogenetic aspects that are relevant to applied pharmacotherapy and determine the selection of an optimum dosage regimen for the individual patient. These concepts also provide the basis for the clinically applied interpretation of drug concentration measurements in patients and for therapeutic drug monitoring. It should be viewed as the starting point toward acquiring the skills and knowledge needed to become a competent clinical pharmacist with regard to clinical PK and PD.

KEY POINTS

■ The systemic exposure to a drug is only determined by dose, bioavailability, and CL.

■ Dosing regimens, i.e., how much and how often a dose needs to be administered, are determined by half-life and the targeted systemic exposure.

■ If half-life changes, it is because CL or V changed.

■ The therapeutic range is a range of concentrations with high probability of the desired therapeutic success and low probability of unacceptable toxicity.

■ Loading dose is determined by the target concentration and the V, MD by the target concentration and the CL of the drug.

■ The extent of drug accumulation is a function of drug properties and dosing regimen, namely the half-life of the drug and the dosing interval of the dosage regimen.

■ Free, unbound drug concentrations need to be considered in dosing adjustments if the degree of plasma protein binding is changed.

■ Renal and hepatic CL models can be used to guide dosage adjustments in case of changes in physiologic variables affecting the systemic exposure to a drug.

■ Pharmacodynamic responses usually follow a nonlinear relationship with concentration, which levels off at high concentrations.

■ Pharmacodynamic parameters like EC_{50} can be used together with pharmacokinetic parameters to guide dosage selection.

■ Pharmacogenomics may explain between-subject variability in drug effects on the level of drug disposition (PK) and/or drug response (PD).

SUGGESTED READINGS

Atkinson AJ, Daniels CE, Dedrick RL, et al., eds. Principles in clinical pharmacology. San Diego, CA: Academic Press, 2001.

Rowland M, Tozer TN. Clinical pharmacokinetics: Concepts and applications. Media, PA: Williams & Wilkins, 1995.

Pharmacogenomics: applications to patient care. Kansas City, MO: American College of Clinical Pharmacy, 2004.

REFERENCES

1. Evans WE, Schentag JJ, Jusko WJ, eds. Applied pharmacokinetics: principles of therapeutic drug monitoring. Media, PA: Lippincott Williams & Wilkins, 1992.

2. Atkinson AJ, Daniels CE, Dedrick RL, et al., eds. Principles in clinical pharmacology. San Diego: Academic Press, 2001.

3. Holford NH, Sheiner LB. Kinetics of pharmacologic response. Pharmacol Ther 16:143–166, 1982.

4. Rowland M, Tozer TN. Clinical Pharmacokinetics: Concepts and Applications. Media, PA: Williams & Wilkins, 1995.

5. Gibaldi M, Perrier D. Pharmacokinetics. New York: Marcel Dekker, 1982.

6. Wilkinson GR, Shand DG. Commentary: a physiological approach to hepatic drug clearance. Clin Pharmacol Ther 18:377–390, 1975.

7. Benet LZ, Hoener BA. Changes in plasma protein binding have little clinical relevance. Clin Pharmacol Ther 71:115–121, 2002.

8. Rolan PE. Plasma protein binding displacement interactions—why are they still regarded as clinically important? Br J Clin Pharmacol 37:125–128, 1994.

9. Meibohm B, Derendorf H. Basic concepts of pharmacokinetic/pharmacodynamic (PK/PD) modelling. Int J Clin Pharmacol Ther 35: 401–413, 1997.

10. Derendorf H, Hochhaus G, eds. Handbook of pharmacokinetic/pharmacodynamic correlation. Boca Raton, FL: CRC Press, 1995.

11. Evans WE, McLeod HL. Pharmacogenomics—drug disposition, drug targets, and side effects. N Engl J Med; 348:538–549, 2003.

12. Bertilsson L, Dahl ML, Dalen P, et al. Molecular genetics of CYP2D6: clinical relevance with focus on psychotropic drugs. Br J Clin Pharmacol 53:111–122, 2002.

13. Dalen P, Dahl ML, Ruiz ML, et al. 10-Hydroxylation of nortriptyline in white persons with 0, 1, 2, 3, and 13 functional CYP2D6 genes. Clin Pharmacol Ther 63:444–452, 1998.

14. Evans WE, Relling MV. Moving towards individualized medicine with pharmacogenomics. Nature 429:464–468, 2004.

Adverse Drug Reactions and Drug-Induced Diseases

2

Candy Tsouronis

TREATMENT GOALS: ADVERSE DRUG REACTIONS AND DRUG-INDUCED DISEASES

- Identify potential risk factors for the development of adverse drug reactions and drug-induced diseases.
- Recognize the elements of a preventable adverse drug reaction.
- Participate in national and, when appropriate, institutional reporting systems.
- Implement early recognition and prevention programs.

BACKGROUND

Adverse drug reactions (ADRs) contribute to overall health care costs by increasing morbidity and even mortality in severe cases.[1] A meta-analysis of prospective ADR studies estimates the ADR fatality rate to be 0.32%, resulting in 106,000 deaths in 1994, placing it as the fourth leading cause of death in the United States after heart disease, cancer, and stroke.[2] The Joint Commission on Accreditation of Healthcare Organizations (JCAHO) and the US Food and Drug Administration (FDA) place a high priority on the recognition and reporting of ADRs by health care professionals to improve the quality of life of patients who are receiving drug therapy.

The impact of ADRs on the cost of health care can be demonstrated by the number of hospital admissions that are drug related. Approximately 5% of reported hospitalizations are a result of an ADR, and the incidence has not changed over the past 30 years.[2,3] Many ADRs are acute and necessitate expensive emergency department care. Drug classes often involved in ADR-related admissions include antibiotics, anticoagulants, anticonvulsants, cardiovascular agents, respiratory drugs, and pain medications.[3,4] ADRs may also occur in hospitalized patients and may increase length of stay and necessitate medical and pharmacologic interventions. It is estimated that 11% of hospitalized patients experience an ADR, with 2.1% of these considered serious.[2]

DEFINITION

Discussion regarding definitions of the terms *ADR, side effect,* and *drug allergy* is ongoing. The World Health Organization (WHO) endorses an ADR definition that many health care practitioners have also adopted: ''any response to a drug that is noxious and unintended, and that occurs at doses used in man for prophylaxis, diagnosis, or treatment.''[5] An ADR may therefore include an exaggerated drug response, an unwanted effect on an organ system different from that being treated, an allergic or hypersensitivity reaction, an idiosyncratic reaction, or a drug interaction that causes an increased or diminished response.[6] A side effect and a drug allergy are both types of ADRs. A side effect, also called a type A reaction, is an example of a dose-related, predictable reaction to a drug.[1,7] It is typically accepted that a side effect of a drug is known to occur in a given percentage of the population and has been observed with regular frequency. A side effect is also expected on the basis of the pharmacologic activity of the agent. A drug allergy is an example of a non–dose-related, unpredictable adverse effect to a drug and is called a type B reaction. Other type B reactions include idiosyncratic, immunologic, carcinogenic, and teratogenic effects.[1] Side effects that are not drug allergies may be inappropriately classified as such. For example, nausea secondary to narcotic use is not immunologically mediated and should not be considered an allergy; however, an anaphylactic reaction to penicillin is an adverse reaction that should be categorized as a true allergic reaction.[8] Unfortunately, reactions reported to health care professionals by patients or caregivers during the course of history taking often are mislabeled as allergies. This mislabeled diagnosis is often perpetuated throughout the patient's medical record. Left uncorrected, inaccurate allergy information may result in inappropriate medical care in future circumstances.

ADRs must be further classified in terms of severity, causality, and preventability. Most institutions and community providers follow published algorithms that assist in this task.[9–11] Preventable ADRs should be a focus of any ADR reporting system in both ambulatory care and hospital settings. Most preventable ADRs involve administration of drugs or related compounds to which documented allergies exist, drugs that affect coagulation, drugs that require therapeutic drug monitoring, and drug dosages that have not been adjusted for renal impairment.[11] By identifying trends, risk factors, and circumstances that contribute to a preventable ADR, practitioners can implement programs to decrease its occurrence.[12,13] Refer to Table 2.1 for severity definitions and Table 2.2 for preventable reactions.

TABLE 2.1	Severity Definitions
Severity	**Definition**
Minor	No antidote, therapy, or prolongation of hospitalization
Moderate	Change in drug therapy or specific treatment, or increased hospitalization by at least 1 day
Severe	Potentially life threatening, causing permanent damage or requiring intensive medical care
Lethal	Directly or indirectly contributing to the death of the patient

(From Anonymous. ASHP Guidelines on adverse drug reaction monitoring and reporting. Am J Hosp Pharm 49:336–337, 1989.)

TABLE 2.2	Elements of a Preventable Adverse Drug Reaction

Inappropriate drug use according to the patient's clinical condition

Inappropriate dosage, route, or frequency of administration on the basis of patient-specific variables (e.g., age, weight, underlying disease)

Omission of appropriate laboratory monitoring, including therapeutic drug monitoring

Previous allergy or drug reaction history

Known drug–drug interaction

Known administration technique error (e.g., rapid intravenous vancomycin administration leading to red man syndrome)

(From Schumock GT, Thornton JP. Focusing on preventability of adverse drug reactions. Clin Pharmacol Ther 30:239–245, 1992.)

REPORTING

NATIONAL ADVERSE DRUG REACTION REPORTING SYSTEM

The FDA requirements on ADR reporting vary depending on the source of the report. Pharmaceutical manufacturers are legally required to report to the FDA all ADRs, including severe reactions. However, the manufacturers do not fulfill this reporting requirement through information submission alone. Manufacturers must also use the reported data to verify the reaction and analyze additional reports for trends.[14–16] Although clinicians are viewed as critical in monitoring drugs for safety issues after approval, participation in the monitoring structure is voluntary. It is important to note that hospitals are under a federal mandate to report problems with medical devices.[17]

The question of what constitutes a reportable ADR can be answered through examination of the FDA's definition of an ADR and the types of reactions the FDA is most interested in reviewing. With the increasing speed of some drug approvals, the FDA has become increasingly dependent on postmarketing surveillance to monitor reactions involving new chemical entities. Thus, any reaction to a new drug (e.g., a drug on the market 3 years or less), whether or not it is included in the product labeling and regardless of its severity, should be reported. The FDA places particular emphasis on unexpected and serious reactions. Reactions of these types should be reported for any medication, not only those that are newly approved.[18,19] Because of the complex nature of adverse event reporting for drugs, biologicals, and devices, the FDA launched the MedWatch program in 1993 (Figs. 2.1 and 2.2). The goals of the MedWatch Program are to simplify the reporting process, clarify what should be reported to the FDA, enhance awareness of serious adverse drug or device reactions, and provide feedback to health

MEDWATCH

THE FDA MEDICAL PRODUCTS REPORTING PROGRAM

For **VOLUNTARY** reporting
by health professionals of adverse
events and product problems

Page _____ of _____

Form Approved: OMB No. 0910-0291 Expires:12/31/94
See OMB statement on reverse

FDA Use Only

Triage unit
sequence #

A. Patient information

1. Patient identifier
In confidence

2. Age at time
of event:
or
Date
of birth:

3. Sex
☐ female
☐ male

4. Weight
_____ lbs
or
_____ kgs

B. Adverse event or product problem

1. ☐ Adverse event and/or ☐ Product problem (e.g., defects/malfunctions)

2. Outcomes attributed to adverse event
(check all that apply)
☐ death (mo/day/yr)
☐ life-threatening
☐ hospitalization – initial or prolonged
☐ disability
☐ congenital anomaly
☐ required intervention to prevent permanent impairment/damage
☐ other: _____

3. Date of
event
(mo/day/yr)

4. Date of
this report
(mo/day/yr)

5. Describe event or problem

6. Relevant tests/laboratory data, including dates

7. Other relevant history, including preexisting medical conditions (e.g., allergies, race, pregnancy, smoking and alcohol use, hepatic/renal dysfunction, etc.)

C. Suspect medication(s)

1. Name (give labeled strength & mfr/labeler, if known)
#1
#2

2. Dose, frequency & route used
#1
#2

3. Therapy dates (if unknown, give duration)
from/to (or best estimate)
#1
#2

4. Diagnosis for use (indication)
#1
#2

5. Event abated after use stopped or dose reduced
#1 ☐ yes ☐ no ☐ doesn't apply
#2 ☐ yes ☐ no ☐ doesn't apply

6. Lot # (if known)
#1
#2

7. Exp. date (if known)
#1
#2

8. Event reappeared after reintroduction
#1 ☐ yes ☐ no ☐ doesn't apply
#2 ☐ yes ☐ no ☐ doesn't apply

9. NDC # (for product problems only)
– –

10. Concomitant medical products and therapy dates (exclude treatment of event)

D. Suspect medical device

1. Brand name

2. Type of device

3. Manufacturer name & address

4. Operator of device
☐ health professional
☐ lay user/patient
☐ other:

5. Expiration date
(mo/day/yr)

6.
model #
catalog #
serial #
lot #
other #

7. If implanted, give date
(mo/day/yr)

8. If explanted, give date
(mo/day/yr)

9. Device available for evaluation? (Do not send to FDA)
☐ yes ☐ no ☐ returned to manufacturer on _____ (mo/day/yr)

10. Concomitant medical products and therapy dates (exclude treatment of event)

E. Reporter (see confidentiality section on back)

1. Name, address & phone #

2. Health professional?
☐ yes ☐ no

3. Occupation

4. Also reported to
☐ manufacturer
☐ user facility
☐ distributor

5. If you do NOT want your identity disclosed to the manufacturer, place an " X " in this box. ☐

FDA

Mail to: MEDWATCH
5600 Fishers Lane
Rockville, MD 20852-9787

or FAX to:
1-800-FDA-0178

FDA Form 3500 (6/93) Submission of a report does not constitute an admission that medical personnel or the product caused or contributed to the event.

FIGURE 2.1 MedWatch form for reporting adverse drug reactions.

ADVICE ABOUT VOLUNTARY REPORTING

Report experiences with:
- medications (drugs or biologics)
- medical devices (including in-vitro diagnostics)
- special nutritional products (dietary supplements, medical foods, infant formulas)
- other products regulated by FDA

Report SERIOUS adverse events. An event is serious when the patient outcome is:
- death
- life-threatening (real risk of dying)
- hospitalization (initial or prolonged)
- disability (significant, persistent or permanent)
- congenital anomaly
- required intervention to prevent permanent impairment or damage

Report even if:
- you're not certain the product caused the event
- you don't have all the details

Report product problems – quality, performance or safety concerns such as:
- suspected contamination
- questionable stability
- defective components
- poor packaging or labeling

How to report:
- just fill in the sections that apply to your report
- use section C for all products except medical devices
- attach additional blank pages if needed
- use a separate form for each patient
- report either to FDA or the manufacturer (or both)

Important numbers:
- 1-800-FDA-0178 to FAX report
- 1-800-FDA-7737 to report by modem
- 1-800-FDA-1088 for more information or to report quality problems
- 1-800-822-7967 for a VAERS form for vaccines

If your report involves a serious adverse event with a device and it occurred in a facility outside a doctor's office, that facility may be legally required to report to FDA and/or the manufacturer. Please notify the person in that facility who would handle such reporting.

Confidentiality: The patient's identity is held in strict confidence by FDA and protected to the fullest extent of the law. The reporter's identity may be shared with the manufacturer unless requested otherwise. However, FDA will not disclose the reporter's identity in response to a request from the public, pursuant to the Freedom of Information Act.

The public reporting burden for this collection of information has been estimated to average 30 minutes per response, including the time for reviewing instructions, searching existing data sources, gathering and maintaining the data needed, and completing and reviewing the collection of information. Send your comments regarding this burden estimate or any other aspect of this collection of information, including suggestions for reducing this burden to:

Reports Clearance Officer, PHS
Hubert H. Humphrey Building,
Room 721-B
200 Independence Avenue, S.W.
Washington, DC 20201
ATTN: PRA

and to:
Office of Management and
Budget
Paperwork Reduction Project
(0910-0230)
Washington, DC 20503

Please do NOT
return this form
to either of these
addresses.

FDA Form 3500-back   **Please Use Address Provided Below – Just Fold In Thirds, Tape and Mail**

**Department of
Health and Human Services**
Public Health Service
Food and Drug Administration
Rockville, MD 20857

Official Business
Penalty for Private Use $300

NO POSTAGE
NECESSARY
IF MAILED
IN THE
UNITED STATES
OR APO/FPO

BUSINESS REPLY MAIL
FIRST CLASS MAIL   PERMIT NO. 946   ROCKVILLE, MD

POSTAGE WILL BE PAID BY FOOD AND DRUG ADMINISTRATION

MEDWATCH
**The FDA Medical Products Reporting Program
Food and Drug Administration
5600 Fishers Lane
Rockville, MD 20852-9787**

FIGURE 2.2 MedWatch form for reporting adverse drug reactions.

care providers about issues related to product safety. The MedWatch system should be used to report cases involving death; life-threatening hazards; hospitalization (admission or prolongation); disability; birth defects, miscarriages, stillbirths, or birth with disease; the need for medical or surgical treatment to prevent impairment; or any combination of these. It is not necessary that a direct causal relationship be demonstrated.[20] The FDA also oversees ADR reporting for biologic agents (e.g., vaccines) and devices, and any reaction to these agents or products should be reported as well.

To simplify the reporting process, MedWatch uses one telephone number, so that health care practitioners can report events efficiently and do not have to identify a particular department to call (e.g., devices, drugs, biologicals). Methods for submitting information to the FDA via MedWatch are as follows: by using a prepaid US mail reporting form (FDA 3500), by calling 1-800-FDA-1088, by facsimile transmission to 1-800-FDA-0178, and via Internet on the FDA Web site (http://www.fda.gov/medwatch/).

The Vaccine Adverse Event Reporting System (VAERS) is a national program that monitors the safety of vaccines after they are licensed. VAERS is managed by the US Centers for Disease Control and Prevention (CDC) and the FDA.[21,22] The system is the MedWatch equivalent for vaccines. VAERS receives about 12,000 reports per year, of which 14% are serious.[21]

HEALTH CARE ORGANIZATION–BASED REPORTING SYSTEMS

The JCAHO, an independent health care accrediting body, places a great deal of emphasis on ADR reporting and analysis. In addition, the FDA recognizes that hospitals play an important role in postmarketing surveillance.[20,23,24]

Although adverse reaction monitoring is a joint responsibility of medical, pharmacy, and nursing personnel, it often becomes the obligation of the pharmacy department to develop, initiate, and manage the ADR reporting system. This function is often carried out under the auspices of the Pharmacy and Therapeutics Committee.[17]

Most effective ADR programs contain four fundamental components: a definition of an ADR that clearly describes reportable ADRs; a concurrent method of monitoring and reporting adverse drug events; a system for reviewing and evaluating ADRs for severity, causality, probability, and preventability; and a system for using the results of the ADR program to educate health care providers and patients alike, to ultimately improve patient care. The Pharmacy and Therapeutics Committee should review each of these components. In general, three types of surveillance systems have been described: prospective, concurrent, and retrospective. Prospective surveillance may include providing ADR information at the time a drug is prescribed to a patient, before he or she experiences an ADR. Prospective systems are effective in that they are preventative; however, they are labor intensive, and, if they are to function successfully, the active participation of health care providers is required, to identify patients who would most benefit from preventative counseling.[25] Concurrent systems involve the active participation of all health care professionals when an ADR occurs. For example, a pharmacist may notice the use of an antidote or tracer drug (epinephrine, naloxone, diphenhydramine), the sudden discontinuation of a long-term drug, or an urgent order for a drug level.[26] All of these suggest that the patient may have experienced an ADR, thus allowing the pharmacist to intervene, recommend an alternative drug, and document the ADR in the medical record. Many computerized systems

are now readily able to identify similar signals in the patient's profile, thereby simplifying the process. Retrospective surveillance is the most popular method used to characterize ADRs in hospitals and health care systems. Retrospective surveillance involves a review of medical records based on defined coding of adverse events.[27] Although this method may be useful, it may not include all ADRs in that many ADRs go uncoded, may be miscoded, or are not documented in the medical record.

Approval by the Pharmacy and Therapeutics Committee of any ADR program should be obtained before implementation because the JCAHO requires that hospitals and health care organizations follow written procedures in reporting ADRs.[24]

OUTPATIENT-BASED REPORTING SYSTEMS

Because more patients are being cared for in the ambulatory setting, the detection of ADRs in this arena is important. Patients are now taking more prescription drugs than in previous years, largely due to a trend in preventative health, but also as a result of increased use of drugs for chronic conditions. In addition, some prescription-only drugs have been changed to over-the-counter (OTC) status, and the use of dietary supplements has increased the need for health care professionals to acquire complete medication histories. Postmarketing surveillance continues to detect clusters of ADRs and to develop ADR profiles for newly released drugs. Given that OTC drugs, dietary supplements, and prescription drugs are all widely used, ambulatory care professionals must closely monitor and inquire about ADRs associated with all types of medications.

PHARMACOVIGILANCE

Safety profiles are an important aspect of a drug submission that must be reviewed before FDA approval of a new molecular entity is granted. However, generating sufficient numbers to detect rare and serious ADRs is difficult. Even phase 3 trials may not enroll enough patients or be carried out over a long enough period to detect a rare ADR that may occur in fewer than 1 in 1,000 patients.[1,28–30] In addition to the fact that small numbers of subjects are enrolled in clinical trials as compared with the general population that will use the drug, clinical trials often do not include patient populations that may be at higher risk of developing an ADR. Such populations include children, older adults, adults with compromised organ function, and those taking multiple medications.

When a drug is approved, it is quickly used in thousands of patients with concomitant diseases and medications. As a result, there is a high level of probability that within the first year of marketing of a new drug, previously unidentified ADRs and drug interactions will become apparent.[1] If a problem is identified from these spontaneous reports, the FDA has several options by which to protect the public, including letters or safety alerts to health professionals, labeling changes, initiation of epidemiologic studies, postmarketing surveillance, inspection of manufacturers' practices, or, ultimately, product withdrawal.[20] Examples of these occurrences are plentiful. Felbamate was approved for treating tonic-clonic seizures in 1993, and within 6 months, it was implicated in numerous cases of aplastic anemia. Troglitazone, an oral antidiabetic agent marketed in 1997, required labeling changes regarding hepatic dysfunction and relevant patient monitoring within the first year; it was subsequently withdrawn from the market.[31] Mibefradil, a calcium channel blocker, was approved in August of 1997, and within 6 months, serious drug interactions were identified. Following that, numerous other drugs were found to interact with mibefradil, leading to its voluntary withdrawal in June of 1998.[32] Bromfenac, a nonsteroidal anti-inflammatory drug (NSAID), was approved in July of 1997; after reports of severe liver dysfunction, a black box warning was placed in the labeling in February of 1998. Because of continued reports of toxicity and death, the drug was voluntarily withdrawn in June of 1998.[33] Tolcapone, an antiparkinson agent approved in August of 1997, underwent labeling changes regarding severe hepatotoxicity and death, as well as a black box warning in November of 1998.[34] In September of 2004, rofecoxib, a cyclooxygenase-2 inhibitor was voluntarily withdrawn from the market by the manufacturer.[35] This removal was a result of increased cardiovascular risks, such as heart attack, stroke, and heart failure. These risks occurred when rofecoxib was used for longer than 18 months for the prevention of colorectal cancer. Dose-related cardiovascular risks were also identified with celecoxib. Two other cyclooxygenase-2 inhibitors, valdecoxib and its intravenous prodrug parecoxib, were found to increase cardiovascular risks in patients following heart bypass surgery. The impact of these warnings and the removal of rofecoxib led to widespread concern among consumers and among the medical community regarding the FDA drug approval process and the effectiveness of the current postmarketing surveillance process. In response to these concerns, the FDA established a new independent Drug Safety Oversight Board to oversee the management of safety issues related to drugs. The FDA also plans to improve communication of safety information to health care providers and the public, in part by developing a new Drug Watch Internet site for emerging risk information.[36]

VARIABLES THAT AFFECT THE INCIDENCE AND SEVERITY OF ADVERSE DRUG REACTIONS

Certain variables predispose individuals to the development of ADRs. These variables may be patient or drug focused. In terms of patient variables, age, underlying conditions (including metabolic dysfunction), and genetic factors may influence the likelihood that a patient will experience an ADR.

Efforts are being made to promote the inclusion of particular subgroups of the population in clinical trials. Drug variables that also may affect the incidence of adverse reactions are route of administration, product formulation, and duration of therapy.

PATIENT VARIABLES

Older Adults. ADRs in older adults may lead to very serious clinical consequences. In a study by Mannesse and colleagues, 42% of hospitalized older adults (70 years or older) evaluated in the study had one or more ADRs, and 24% had severe reactions.[37] A significant correlation was noted between severe ADRs and a fall before admission, gastrointestinal (GI) bleeding or hematuria, and the use of three or more drugs. Serious ADRs can be life threatening, especially because older adults are better able to identify and correlate mild ADRs with drug therapy than more serious ADRs.[37]

Because hepatic and renal function decline with age, older adults are subject to changes in metabolism that affect the clearance of drugs and active metabolites.[38] Decreased hepatic blood flow may lead to increased bioavailability and ultimately increased serum concentrations of certain drugs with high first-pass clearance. Drugs that do not undergo high hepatic clearance may be affected by decreased microsomal enzyme activity, especially of the phase I metabolism type. The result is a generally decreased metabolism, which may lead to increased serum concentrations.[39,40]

A decline in renal function is common in older adults. A decline in glomerular filtration rate (GFR) of approximately 35% is not uncommon.[41] The GFR may be low despite a normal serum creatinine level, which can be misleading. For drugs that are excreted unchanged in the urine, doses should be adjusted and carefully monitored to avoid excessive serum drug concentrations.

Age-related changes in metabolism and clearance should be correlated with the therapeutic index of the drug that is being used. Clinicians should be especially concerned about agents that have a narrow therapeutic index and should monitor drug concentrations, if appropriate (e.g., warfarin, digoxin, quinidine, theophylline, phenytoin). Even with agents that have a high therapeutic index, clinicians should exercise appropriate caution in monitoring patients.[39]

Neonates. Neonates experience ADRs through primary and secondary exposures. Several reasons for these ADRs include placental transfer of drugs, which results in exposure in utero; lack of information on drug use in neonates; altered drug disposition, metabolism, and excretion profiles; multiple drug administration; and exposure through breast milk.[42–44] Furthermore, many neonates are born in critical condition with multiple-organ compromise. Neonates are also susceptible to adverse reactions that result from percutaneous absorption of environmental agents that are not meant for therapeutic use (e.g., antiseptics containing phenol, alcohol, other disinfectants).

The pediatric population—neonates specifically—are at increased risk for ADRs that may affect short- and long-term growth and development. Neurodevelopmental ADRs are of particular concern because of the susceptibility of the central nervous system (CNS). Psychoactive drugs can cause significant defects (e.g., sleep disturbances, hyperactivity and irritability, behavioral disturbances). Drugs may also affect somatic development. Some examples in the literature include the effects of tetracycline on tooth enamel and phenytoin-induced gingival hyperplasia. Adverse neurodevelopmental and somatic outcomes are difficult to predict because of insufficient studies and interindividual variability.[44]

Drug metabolism and excretion are crucial components of successful drug therapy in neonates. The neonate is born without a full capacity to process exogenous substrates. For example, it may take the hepatic glucuronyl transferase system up to 4 weeks postpartum to become fully functional. Gray baby syndrome may develop if agents dependent on the glucuronyl transferase pathway (e.g., chloramphenicol) are administered to neonates. Specific dosage adjustments are required.[45] The demethylation and hydroxylation pathways necessary for theophylline metabolism may take a year to develop fully.[46] A full-term newborn has approximately 33% of the GFR of an adult. Kidney function continues to improve rapidly, and by the time a child is approximately 9 to 12 months of age, his or her kidney function is equivalent to that of an adult. Until the organ systems have a chance to develop, neonates and infants are at higher risk of developing ADRs because of the immaturity of their organs.[2] (See Chapter 15.)

Patients with Human Immunodeficiency Virus.
The incidence of ADRs in patients infected with the human immunodeficiency virus (HIV) appears to be higher than in the general population.[47–49] Several factors appear to increase the risk of ADRs, including an advanced stage of HIV disease, an increased number of medications, and prolonged hospitalization.[50] In particular, patients with HIV appear to be at greater risk for skin rashes.[50] Severe immunosuppression, development of drug-specific antibodies, and impaired capacity to clear drugs and unchanged metabolites result in an increased sensitivity to drug toxicity. In most cases, drug reactions are not life threatening, but they often lead to suboptimal changes in therapy, which may limit the number of effective treatment plans. A classic example of increased hypersensitivity in patients infected with HIV is illustrated by the use of trimethoprim/sulfamethoxazole (TMP/SMX). In a study conducted at San Francisco General Hospital, 83% (29/35) of patients experienced some level of toxicity to TMP/SMX as they were being treated for *Pneumocystis carinii* pneumonia (PCP).[51] This figure is much higher than was reported in a group of hospitalized patients with no known HIV history (2% to 8%; Table 2.3).[52]

Because of the current practice of treating patients with HIV with combination drug therapy, the clinician must remember that the patient may be at risk for additive drug toxicity and drug–drug interactions, all of which are superimposed on the underlying disease.[53]

TABLE 2.3	Combined Rates of Hypersensitivity Reactions in Patients with the Human Immunodeficiency Virus
Drug	**Rate of Occurrence, %**
Amoxicillin	17–40
Amphotericin B	4–15
Antituberculosis medication	3–20
Ciprofloxacin	5–7
Clindamycin and pyrimethamine	21–33
Trimethoprim-sulfamethoxazole	37–69
Fluconazole	6–13
Pentamidine	5–15
Sulfadiazine-pyrimethamine	13–34

(From Harb GE, Jacobson MA. Human immunodeficiency virus (HIV) infection: does it increase susceptibility to adverse drug reactions? Drug Saf 9:1–8, 1993.)

Genetics. Rates of metabolism and elimination of various substances may be influenced by genetic factors (e.g., glucose-6-phosphate dehydrogenase [G6PD] deficiency resulting in drug-induced hemolytic anemia; acetylator status and drug-induced systemic lupus erythematosus [SLE]).[54] It has been reported that some degree of polymorphism is present in up to 50% of the enzyme systems involved in drug metabolism. Enzyme systems that have been evaluated include acetylation, oxidation, and hydroxylation. Some phenotypes may be predicted from a single blood sample through available genotyping methods.[55] In many cases, however, screening tests for genetically susceptible patients are not easily performed, and clinical decisions must be based on available epidemiologic data. (See Chapter 1.)

DRUG VARIABLES
Route of Administration. Route of administration and drug formulation are variables that are associated with the likelihood that a patient will experience an ADR.[56] Intravenous administration may be associated with adverse effects local to the site of injection, such as phlebitis and extravasation, as well as with systemic adverse effects secondary to rapid increases in drug–blood concentrations and accelerated clinical response. Oral administration, which is generally associated with decreased bioavailability, may be associated with somewhat milder adverse effects.[55] Variability in absorption of oral agents subsequent to drug–drug or drug–food interactions also may change adverse effect profiles. Local adverse effects, such as irritation to the GI mucosa, may also result from oral administration. Topically applied medications may cause systemic toxicity (e.g., ophthalmic β-blockers).

Product Formulation. Product formulations that alter the extent and rate of absorption may also affect the incidence of ADRs. Sustained-release products may avoid the potential for adverse effects from excessive peaks and inadequate trough levels associated with immediate-release products. For example, sustained-release antihypertensive agents produce more consistent serum drug concentrations and, therefore, fewer potentially suboptimal trough periods and lower peak concentrations that may be associated with lightheadedness and other side effects.[55] Flushing secondary to niacin has been a major contributor to noncompliance and therapeutic failures with this agent. The sustained-release product, which avoids the peak serum concentrations of the immediate-release preparations, is associated with a decreased incidence of flushing. However, sustained-release niacin products have been implicated as a cause of hepatic dysfunction.[57] Although sustained-release products may help to limit certain ADRs, in some cases, disturbing the sustained-release preparation may also cause an ADR. A common concern regarding these formulations is that the product may be split, crushed, or chewed, which would disturb the sustained-release properties. Consumers and health care professionals must be informed regarding the release characteristics of a particular sustained-release product so that unwanted ADRs can be prevented.

Duration of Therapy. The duration of therapy may also be a causative factor in ADRs. For example, in patients older than 60 years of age, an increased duration of therapy with NSAIDs was associated with an increased risk of upper GI toxicity.[58] Similarly, the prolonged use of oral corticosteroids like prednisone increases the risks for osteoporosis and

many other conditions. The active metabolite of meperidine, normeperidine, accumulates in patients with renal dysfunction, which may result in seizures. This is more likely to occur with long-term administration than with single-dose or intermittent therapy.[59]

DRUG-INDUCED DISEASES

Disease state management, which refers to the collective management of all aspects of a patient's disease, is rapidly becoming the standard practice in health care. ADR monitoring and management should be part of this process. It is impossible to consider the desired outcomes of drug therapy without taking into account potential adverse consequences of treatment. The remaining sections of this chapter focus on the major organ systems that are most commonly associated with adverse pharmacologic reactions. The reader will be referred to other chapters in this book that describe in detail the mechanisms of specific drug-induced diseases.

HYPERSENSITIVITY REACTIONS

Many drug reactions are erroneously called *hypersensitivity* or *allergic reactions*.[60,61] A common error occurs when a patient is identified as having an allergic response to a specific medication, when, in reality, he or she is intolerant to the medication because of nausea or vomiting. True hypersensitivity reactions are immunologically mediated through a series of reproducible steps. The four classic hypersensitivity reactions are outlined in Table 2.4.[62]

TABLE 2.4	Classic Hypersensitivity Reactions		
Type	Antibody	Mechanism	Examples and Causative Agents
I	IgE	Anaphylactic	True systemic anaphylactic reaction
		Antigen-antibody reaction on mast cells leading to histamine, leukotriene, platelet-activating factor release	Penicillin and cephalosporins. Classic example of the hapten hypothesis
II	IgG, IgM	Cytotoxic	Hemolytic anemia
		Antigen-specific antibodies directed against antigens on cell surface	Penicillin and quinine are examples of causative agents
III	IgG, IgM	Immune complex mediated	Serum sickness
		Immune complexes interact with antibodies	Penicillin, cephalosporins, isoniazid, phenytoin, etc.
IV	T-cells	Delayed hypersensitivity	Typically seen with topical therapies rather than systemic
		Generally takes longer than 12 hours to develop. Antigen interacts directly with sensitized T-cells	Characterized clinically by rash that worsens on subsequent or repetitive administration

Ig, immunoglobulin.
(From Lachmann PJ, Peters DK, eds. Clinical aspects of immunology. 4th ed. Boston: Blackwell Scientific, 1982.)

Type I hypersensitivity reactions are most often associated with β-lactam antibiotics, which include penicillins and cephalosporins.[63,64] Although allergic reactions to penicillin have been reported to occur in 0.7% to 8% of the general population, anaphylaxis occurs in only 0.01% of identified treatment courses. The true immunochemistry of the penicillin reaction has been characterized, and cross sensitivity to cephalosporins has been postulated on the basis of chemical structure and similarities—typically, a four-member β-lactam ring. Most of the cross reactions between penicillins and cephalosporins involve first- and second-generation cephalosporins, as a result of structural similarities between these agents. It is important to consider that even though the β-lactam ring is closely related to cross-sensitivity reactions, a similarity in side chains is another critical consideration, as in the cases of aztreonam and ceftazidime. Therefore, when the potential for cross-sensitivity between two antibiotics is considered, one must note not only the presence of a β-lactam ring, but also a similarity in side chains. Hypersensitivity reactions that are mediated by immunoglobulin E show clinical cross reactivity between penicillins and cephalosporins in approximately 5% of patients.[65] Imipenem (a carbapenem antibiotic) has a bicyclic nucleus and is associated with cross reactivity in approximately 50% of penicillin-allergic patients.[66] Meropenem (a new carbapenem antibiotic) also cross-reacts in penicillin allergy.[67] Aztreonam, a monocyclic β-lactam antibiotic, is poorly immunogenic. β-Lactam-allergic patients have been given aztreonam and have not demonstrated any clinical signs of cross sensitivity. Structural differences may therefore be a significant determinant in the incidence of hypersensitivity reactions.

Hypersensitivity reactions may manifest as acute urticaria, rhinitis, bronchial asthma, or angioedema. Depending on the severity of the reaction, peripheral circulatory collapse may occur; therefore, immediate medical care should be sought. The offending agent should be removed. Epinephrine should be administered and repeated every 15 to 20 minutes as needed, up to three doses. Oxygen should be administered if available. Because the patient may be experiencing vascular collapse, fluid resuscitation should be initiated as needed to maintain blood pressure. If the patient is unresponsive to fluid replacement, a vasopressor infusion may be needed. β-Agonists, diphenhydramine, and a corticosteroid should also be administered after the emergent situation is brought under control.

HEPATOTOXICITY

Drug-induced hepatotoxicity has been associated with more than 800 drugs. Hepatotoxicity can be difficult to diagnose because correlation to a specific drug may be difficult, and injury may occur acutely or after prolonged drug administration.[68] The severity of drug-induced hepatotoxicity can range from mild alteration in liver function test results to fulminant hepatic failure. Table 2.5 lists some of the risk factors associated with hepatotoxic reactions. When acetaminophen is used as an example, it can be seen that chronic

TABLE 2.5	Risk Factors Associated with Hepatotoxic Reactions
Factor	**Example**
Age	
Adults > children	Isoniazid, halothane
Older adults > others	Nonsteroidal anti-inflammatory drugs
Children > adults	Valproic acid, aspirin
Sex	
Female > male	Methyldopa, drug-induced chronic active hepatitis
Drugs	
Alcohol, phenobarbital	May induce cytochrome P-450 system and enhance the toxicity of agents converted to active metabolites
Disease	
AIDS	Increased susceptibility to hepatotoxic effects of sulfamethoxazole/trimethoprim
Diabetes	Enhances toxicity of carbon tetrachloride
Hyperthyroidism	Enhances toxicity of carbon tetrachloride
Arthritis	Active rheumatoid arthritis, rheumatic fever, and systemic lupus erythematosus enhance the hepatic effects of aspirin

(From Zimmerman HJ. Hepatotoxicity. Dis Mon 39:675–787, 1993.)

ethanol ingestion may induce the cytochrome P-450 enzyme systems, and deplete glutathione stores. Thus, patients with chronic ethanol ingestion may be at increased risk for liver toxicity following therapeutic dosages of acetaminophen.[69,70]

Acute liver injury may be cytotoxic or cholestatic. Cytotoxic injury involves direct injury to the hepatocytes, with necrosis that can be localized or diffuse throughout the liver. Following the acute insult, aminotransferase concentrations may be elevated to up to 500 times normal values. What is important to consider is that after immediate injury to the hepatocytes occurs, aminotransferase concentrations begin to decline, either because of clearance of aminotransferases from the serum, or because of the massive injury, results in few hepatocytes available to produce aminotransferases. If the offending agent is not removed, this decline in aminotransferase may be misinterpreted as an improvement in liver function when indeed, it may be a sign of worsening organ damage. A rising prothrombin time (PT) due to decreased synthesis of clotting factors is useful in assessing hepatic function. Prominent signs and symptoms of cytotoxic liver injury include fatigue, anorexia, nausea, and jaundice. Drug-induced cytotoxic injury may progress to fulminant hepatic failure. Acetaminophen, isoniazid, methyldopa, and phenytoin have been associated with direct cytotoxic reactions that have led to mortality rates of 10% or higher.[71,72]

Cholestatic injury results in a characteristic decrease in bile flow. Hepatic injury of this type leads to jaundice and pruritus, with aminotransferase concentrations only moderately elevated. Cholestatic hepatic injury has a much better prognosis than does cytotoxic injury, with a mortality rate of less than 1%.[71]

Chronic liver damage consists of a group of disorders that includes chronic hepatitis, steatosis, pseudoalcoholic liver disease, granulomatous disease, and cirrhosis. Chronic lesions may result from continued or repeated exposure to hepatotoxic agents. Table 2.6 lists a number of drugs that have been implicated as a cause of chronic hepatitis.[71]

Most cases of drug-induced hepatotoxicity involve transformation of the parent drug to an active intermediate that may be inherently toxic or may evoke an immune response. Some drugs implicated in hepatic injury include anesthetic agents (e.g., halothane), chlorpromazine, anticonvulsants (e.g., phenytoin, valproic acid), NSAIDs, and allopurinol. Herbal products and teas have also been implicated in several cases of severe hepatotoxicity.[73] The specific hepatotoxicity profiles associated with each of these agents are beyond the scope of this chapter. Health care practitioners should be aware that a plethora of agents may cause hepatotoxicity and that careful history taking is crucial in a patient who presents with nonspecific symptoms.[71] (See Chapter 49 for further discussion.)

PANCREATITIS

Pancreatitis may be characterized as acute or chronic. An acute attack of pancreatitis may result in severe abdominal pain and tenderness, accompanied by a rise in the levels of amylase and lipase (pancreatic digestive enzymes) in the blood to greater than three times the upper limit of normal.[74] Serum lipase is specific to pancreatic origin, and levels remain elevated for a longer time than those of amylase, which may be normal in up to one third of patients with acute pancreatitis.[74] Both amylase and lipase are measured, however, in patients with suspected disease. Chronic pancreatitis

TABLE 2.6	Drugs Implicated in Causing Chronic Active Hepatitis
Dantrolene	
Diclofenac	
Isoniazid	
Nitrofurantoin	
Methyldopa	
Papaverine	

(From Zimmerman HJ. Hepatotoxicity. Dis Mon 39:675–787, 1993.)

TABLE 2.7	Drug-Induced Pancreatitis

Criteria for Drug-Induced Pancreatitis

Pancreatitis developed during treatment with the drug.

Pancreatitis disappeared upon withdrawal of the drug.

Pancreatitis recurred upon rechallenge with the drug.

Elements of Classification

Definite	Literature report met all three criteria.
Probable	Literature reports did not meet all three criteria, but an association was thought to exist.
Doubtful	Published evidence was inadequate or contradictory.

(From Mallory A, Kern F. Drug-induced pancreatitis: a critical review. Gastroenterology 78:813–820, 1980.)

is associated with abdominal pain, steatorrhea, and weight loss, which may become debilitating over time. A literature review by Underwood and Frye[75] described that a large number of medications may cause acute pancreatitis, whereas few cause chronic pancreatitis, with the most common cause being alcohol. Morphologic changes in the pancreas itself are minor or absent. On the basis of a system originally developed by Mallory and Kern,[76] implicated drugs may be classified into three categories (Table 2.7). Table 2.8 summarizes the agents that have been shown to have a definite association with pancreatitis.[75-77] (See Chapter 51 for further discussion about drug-induced pancreatitis.)

NEPHROTOXICITY

Drug-induced nephrotoxicity varies according to the concentration of drug presented to the kidney and the biochemical or physiologic effects of the drug on tissue.[78] Factors that influence the concentration of given drugs in the kidney include mechanisms for the transport of drugs across the tubular epithelium, rate of water versus drug reabsorption, plasma protein binding, and rate of urine flow. Some of the drugs most commonly associated with nephrotoxicity include the aminoglycosides, amphotericin B, cisplatin, cyclosporine, and NSAIDs.[79-83]

Four types of lesions are used to describe drug-induced kidney damage: acute tubular necrosis (ATN), acute tubulointerstitial disease (ATID), chronic tubulointerstitial disease (CTID), and glomerulonephritis (GN). A list of drugs associated with each of these lesions is provided in Table 2.9. A discussion of drug-induced nephrotoxicity can be found in Chapter 42, ''Acute Renal Disease.''

From an ADR reporting system standpoint, drug-induced nephrotoxicity should be monitored closely because most of these ADRs are preventable. For example, underlying renal dysfunction necessitates a dosage adjustment of many drugs. Carefully monitoring drug concentrations and altering drug dosages accordingly can minimize damage to the nephron.

TABLE 2.8	Examples of Drugs Suspected in Drug-Induced Pancreatitis
Drug	**Comments**
Asparaginase	Frequently reported to cause pancreatitis. Possible direct cytotoxic effect
Azathioprine	Mechanism of injury unknown but thought to be related to the immunosuppressive effects of azathioprine
Didanosine	Pancreatitis detected in 3% to 23% of patients in clinical reports. Dosages higher than 10 mg/kg/day are more likely to cause pancreatitis
Estrogens	Estrogen use is known to cause hyperlipidemia, a risk factor for development of pancreatitis
Furosemide	Suggested direct toxic effect. A similar outcome was observed with bumetanide administration
Mercaptopurine	Mechanism may be type II or type IV hypersensitivity reaction
Pentamidine	Mechanism may be direct toxic effect. Toxicity may be related to cumulative dose. Also often administered after exposure to sulfonamides
Sulfonamides	Pancreatitis accompanied by fever, chills, pruritus, and rash. Possible allergic reaction
Sulindac	Most reports received through the voluntary reporting system. Strong correlation with rechallenge
Tetracyclines	Occurred primarily in patients with preexisting liver disease
Thiazides	Among the first class of drugs to be associated with pancreatitis. Possible direct toxic effect or electrolyte abnormalities (e.g., hypercalcemia)
Valproic acid	May occur within normal dosages of the drug. Has occurred in children. Possible direct toxic effect or idiosyncratic reaction

(From Underwood TW, Frye CB. Drug-induced pancreatitis. Clin Pharm 12:440–448, 1993; Mallory A, Kern F. Drug-induced pancreatitis: a critical review. Gastroenterology 78:813–820, 1980; Wilmink T, Fric TW. Drug induced pancreatitis. Drug Saf 14:406–423, 1996.)

HEMATOLOGIC DISORDERS

One of the most common hematologic ADRs involves platelet inhibition and the risk for bruising or bleeding. Aspirin and the other cyclooxygenase-1 (COX-1) NSAIDs have antiplatelet effects, which may prevent clotting and the formation of a thrombus. Aspirin irreversibly inhibits COX-1, and a single daily dose of aspirin is sufficient to inhibit platelet function for the life of the platelet (10 days).[84] The dose of

| TABLE 2.9 | Drugs Associated with Nephrotoxicity |

Acute Tubular Necrosis
Antibiotics:
  Aminoglycosides
  Amphotericin B
  Cephalosporins
  Quinolones
  Nitrofurantoin
  Sulfonamides
  Tetracycline (outdated)
  Pentamidine
Radiocontrast media
Miscellaneous agents:
  Acetaminophen
  Carbamazepine
  Cisplatin
  Cyclosporine
  Mephenytoin
  Quinine
  Quinidine
  Tacrolimus
  Diazepam
  Barbiturates
  Codeine
  Ethanol
  Lovastatin
  Ifosfamide
  Mithramycin
  Foscarnet
  IVIG
  Hydralazine
  Methotrexate
  Methoxyflurane
  Streptozocin

Acute Tubulointerstitial Disease
Penicillins
Other antibiotics:
  Cephalosporins
  Rifampin
  Sulfonamides
  Ciprofloxacin
NSAIDs
Miscellaneous:
  Allopurinol
  Cytosine arabinoside
  Interferon
  Azathioprine
  Captopril
  Cimetidine
  Clofibrate
  Furosemide
  Phenytoin
  Thiazides

Glomerulonephritis
Allopurinol
Ampicillin
Captopril
Cyclophosphamide
Daunorubicin
Gold
Heroin
Mercury
Methicillin
NSAIDs
Penicillamine
Penicillin
Rifampin
Sulfonamides
Thiazides
Trimethadione

Chronic Tubulointerstitial Disease
Acetaminophen
Aspirin
Lithium
Methyl-CCNU
Phenacetin
NSAIDs
Cyclosporine
Tacrolimus

Miscellaneous Mechanisms
Prerenal azotemia
NSAIDs

Renal Tubular Acidosis and Concentration Defects
Lithium
Amphotericin B

Postrenal Obstruction
Methysergide
Acyclovir
Methotrexate
Ergotamine
Sulfonamides
Hydralazine
Methyldopa
Pindolol
Atenolol

IVIG, intravenous immunoglobulin; NSAIDs, nonsteroidal anti-inflammatory drugs. (From Underwood TW, Frye CB. Drug-induced pancreatitis. Clin Pharm 12:440–448, 1993; Mallory A, Kern F. Drug-induced pancreatitis: a critical review. Gastroenterology 78:813–820, 1980; Wilmink T, Fric TW. Drug-induced pancreatitis. Drug Saf 14:406–423, 1996; Walker RJ, Duggin GG. Drug nephrotoxicity. Annu Rev Pharmacol Toxicol 28:331–345, 1988; Schlondorff D. Renal complications of nonsteroidal anti-inflammatory drugs. Kidney Int 44:643–653, 1993.)

aspirin required to inhibit platelet function is relatively low compared with that required to achieve an anti-inflammatory effect.[84] The antithrombotic effect of aspirin is maximal at a dose of 100 mg. NSAIDs, however, are reversible inhibitors of COX-1 that produce a weaker antiplatelet effect, thus allowing for a return of platelet function following discontinuation within 2 to 3 days.[84] In addition, evidence suggests that NSAIDs may antagonize the antiplatelet effects of low-dose aspirin. Given the widespread use of aspirin, particularly for the prevention of stroke and heart attack, the risk for developing a serious ADR is relatively low. It is estimated that a major gastrointestinal bleed will occur in 1 to 2 patients of 1,000 treated for 1 year.[84] This risk is considered to be acceptable given the greater risk of dying from heart attack or stroke. Also, it is important for clinicians to identify those patients who are at high risk for bleeding to ensure they are appropriately educated and monitored. Drug-induced hematologic disorders encompass a wide variety of disorders, only some of which are mechanistically understood. The reader is referred to the chapters in this book that describe anemias for discussions of aplastic anemia, agranulocytosis, hemolytic anemia, megaloblastic anemia, and thrombocytopenia. All these hematologic disorders have been associated with ADRs.

CARDIOVASCULAR EFFECTS

The scope of this topic is too large for it to be covered in a chapter that focuses on ADRs. The reader is referred to the chapters in this book that discuss cardiovascular disorders and critical care issues. Cardiovascular adverse reactions require specific management.

ADRs that involve the cardiovascular system are not specifically limited to agents used to treat patients with cardiovascular disease. For example, bronchodilator therapy and sympathomimetic effects of various cough and cold remedies may negatively affect cardiac rate and rhythm regulation. Many antiarrhythmic agents may also be proarrhythmic.[85,86] A tricyclic antidepressant overdose may cause electrocardiographic changes and can be life threatening.[87] Bradycardia may be induced by certain cardiac medications, as well as by agents such as carbamazepine, methyldopa, and H_2 antagonists.[88–90] Certain chemotherapeutic agents such as the anthracyclines (e.g., doxorubicin) may cause a dose-limiting cardiomyopathy.[91] Additionally, some diuretics and β-blockers may adversely affect lipid risk profiles, the clinical outcome of which remains to be elucidated.[92] In addition to the known risks of primary pulmonary hypertension,[93] recent concerns about valvular abnormalities associated with appetite-suppressant drugs[94] have led to withdrawal from the market of dexfenfluramine and fenfluramine. Careful monitoring of patients for cardiovascular ADRs is crucial because the potential for negative sequelae is enormous.

PULMONARY EFFECTS

Pulmonary injury secondary to pharmacologic treatment has been associated with more than 150 medications.[95–97] Table 2.10 lists agents that are known to cause pulmonary disease. Four mechanisms of drug-induced pulmonary disease have been described: direct cytotoxic effect on alveolar endothelial cells, deposition of phospholipid within the alveolar macrophages, oxidized injury by drugs, and immune-mediated injury (e.g., drug-induced SLE).[98]

Bronchospasm occurs commonly as a drug-induced effect. This ADR has been identified with use of any of the β-blockers and is reversible within 1 to 7 days of discontin-

TABLE 2.10	Agents Known to Cause Pulmonary Disease	
Cardiovascular	**Anti-Inflammatory**	**Chemotherapy**
Amiodarone	Aspirin	Azathioprine
Angiotensin-converting enzyme inhibitors	Gold	Bleomycin
Anticoagulants	Methotrexate	Busulfan
β-Blockers	Nonsteroidal anti-inflammatory drugs	Chlorambucil
Dipyridamole	Penicillamine	Cyclophosphamide
Tocainide		Etoposide
	Miscellaneous	Melphalan
Antibiotics	Bromocriptine	Mitomycin
Amphotericin B	Dantrolene	Nitrosourea
Nitrofurantoin	Oral contraceptives	Procarbazine
Sulfasalazine	Hydrochlorothiazide	Vinblastine
Sulfonamides	Tricyclic antidepressants	Ifosfamide
Pentamidine		

(From Rosenow EC. Drug-induced pulmonary disease. Dis Mon 5:258–310, 1994.)

uation. Symptoms include a dry, unproductive cough.[98] β-Blockade can precipitate asthmatic attacks. Even a cardioselective agent, such as atenolol or metoprolol, may precipitate bronchospasms and should be avoided in asthmatic patients if possible.[99] Aggravation of chronic obstructive pulmonary disease with subsequent death has been reported secondary to topical timolol because the drug can be systemically absorbed.[100] Angiotensin-converting enzyme (ACE) inhibitors cause cough in approximately 15% of the population, with a 2:1 ratio of affected women to affected men. Aspirin administration leads to bronchospasm in approximately 4% to 20% of all patients with asthma.[101] The pathogenesis is believed to be related to cyclooxygenase inhibition and subsequent destabilization of mast cells and bronchial smooth muscle constriction.[102] All NSAIDs, which inhibit cyclooxygenase, can also produce this reaction, and the degree of cross reactivity is related to the degree of cyclooxygenase inhibition. Patients may also have increased levels of cysteinyl leukotrienes and increased airway reactivity to these agents. Supporting information indicates that 5-lipoxygenase inhibitors may improve pulmonary function in these patients.[103]

Noncardiogenic pulmonary edema may develop secondary to narcotic use, as cases have been reported with heroin, methadone, and propoxyphene administration. The mechanism of this reaction is unclear, but could be related to a direct toxic effect on the alveolar-capillary membrane. Other possible mechanisms include hypoxemia, CNS effects that result in neurogenic pulmonary edema, and immunologic activation. Pulmonary edema generally improves within 24 to 48 hours, and radiologic clearing results after approximately 2 to 4 days.[104]

SEXUAL DYSFUNCTION

Normal sexual function is mediated by various physiologic mechanisms, including neurogenic, psychogenic, vascular, and hormonal factors. These functions are coordinated by the hypothalamus, limbic system, and cerebral cortex. It is expected, then, that medications that interfere with any of these systems may also impair sexual function.[105]

Sexual dysfunction is often associated with antihypertensive and antipsychotic medications. Antihypertensive agents, more than any other type of drug, are reported to be associated with sexual dysfunction. However, most associations between antihypertensive therapy and sexual dysfunction are observed from case reports.[106] Furthermore, many incidents go unreported because sexual dysfunction may be an uncomfortable topic for patients to discuss with a health care provider. Thiazide diuretics, peripheral and central sympatholytics, and β-blockers have all been associated with a decline in sexual function. Adverse events include impotence, loss of libido, ejaculatory failure, and anorgasmia. Calcium channel blockers and ACE inhibitors appear to have lower potential for causing sexual dysfunction.[107] Combination therapy appears to be associated with a higher incidence of sexual dysfunction than is monotherapy.

Antipsychotic and antidepressant medications are also associated with a variety of effects on sexual function (e.g., impotence, priapism, anorgasmia, diminished libido); however, ejaculatory failure is the most frequently reported.[107,108] All classes of antidepressants have been associated with some degree of sexual dysfunction.[109] These agents may impair sexual function through anticholinergic and sympatholytic activity, through effects on neurotransmitters or hormonal secretion (e.g., increased serum prolactin concentrations secondary to amoxapine), or by causing sedation.[107]

It is important to note that the disease states for which these medications are prescribed may independently be associated with an alteration in normal sexual function. For example, sexual dysfunction has been shown to occur frequently (up to 17%) in untreated hypertensive men.[110] Hypertensive diabetic patients have an even higher incidence of impotence (25% to 60%).[111] With regard to the psychiatric population, the rate of impotence in untreated patients may be as high as 70% and varies with the particular diagnosis. The high incidence of sexual dysfunction associated with these conditions is an important consideration when one is evaluating the relationship of drug administration to altered sexual function, and baseline data on sexual function before the institution of therapy may be helpful in differentiating disease from drug effects.

Additional medications that have been associated with sexual dysfunction, although less often than the aforementioned agents, are the H_2 antagonists (e.g., cimetidine, ranitidine, famotidine, nizatidine), anticonvulsants (e.g., carbamazepine, phenytoin, phenobarbital, primidone), antiarrhythmic agents (e.g., amiloride, disopyramide, digoxin), NSAIDs (e.g., indomethacin, naproxen), benzodiazepines (e.g., alprazolam, diazepam, lorazepam), baclofen, bromocriptine, clofibrate, ketoconazole, metoclopramide, and opioids, when used on a long-term basis.[107]

PHARMACOECONOMICS

Drug-related morbidity and mortality cost $30 billion to $136 billion annually in the United States,[1,112] making it one of the more costly diseases.[112] Given the number of new drugs that are entering the market, the popularity of dietary supplements, and the number of drugs being switched from prescription to OTC status, it is not surprising that these cost estimates will likely increase over the next few years. It has been estimated that in hospitalized patients, ADRs increase length of stay by approximately 2 days and increase hospital costs by $2,000.[1] Furthermore, aging of the population and the use of multiple drugs will likely contribute to the overall costs of adverse drug reactions over the next 20 to 30 years. The cost of drug-related morbidity and mortality in nursing facilities alone has been estimated to be $7.6 billion.[113] It has also been estimated that consultant pharmacy services may decrease this cost by 47%.[113]

CONCLUSION

ADRs are an important cause of morbidity and mortality. Drug-induced disease is common in certain patient populations, such as older adults, newborns, HIV-infected patients, and patients with impaired hepatic or renal function. Many ADRs are both reversible and preventable. Because they are reversible, early identification and treatment are of great importance. The preventable nature of adverse reactions is the motivation for current reporting programs. It is through reporting that high-risk patient populations are identified, so that certain medications can be avoided. The monitoring programs currently in place rely on voluntary reporting from health care professionals and mandatory reporting from pharmaceutical manufacturers. The increased complexity of drug therapy requires increased vigilance on the part of health care practitioners. In many cases, the pharmacist is in a unique position to safeguard the patient from preventable ADRs.

KEY POINTS

- An ADR is any response to a drug that is noxious and unintended and occurs at normal doses
- ADRs significantly increase patient morbidity and mortality
- Virtually every organ system in the body may be affected by an ADR
- Recognition and reporting of ADRs are high priorities of the JCAHO and the FDA
- MedWatch is the FDA reporting system for ADRs
- ADRs must be classified in terms of severity, causality, and preventability
- Patient variables that influence the likelihood of an ADR include age, underlying disorder, and genetic factors
- Drug classes frequently involved in ADRs include antibiotics, anticoagulants, anticonvulsants, cardiovascular agents, respiratory treatments, and pain medications
- Many drug reactions are erroneously called *hypersensitivity* or *allergic reactions*

SUGGESTED READINGS

Ajayi FO, Sun H, Perry J. Adverse drug reactions: a review of relevant factors. J Clin Pharmacol 40:1093–1101, 2000.

Bennett CL, Nebeker JR, Lyons EA, et al. The Research on Adverse Drug Events and Reports (RADAR) project. JAMA 293:2131–2140, 2005.

Brewer T, Colditz GA. Postmarketing surveillance and adverse drug reactions: current perspectives and future needs. JAMA 281:824–829, 1999.

Brown SD, Landry FJ. Recognizing, reporting, and reducing adverse drug reactions. South Med J 94:370–373, 2001.

Thurmann PA. Methods and systems to detect adverse drug reactions in hospitals. Drug Saf 24:961–968, 2001.

REFERENCES

1. Holland EG, De Gruy FA. Drug-induced disorders. Am Fam Physician 56:1781–1788, 1997.
2. Lazarou J, Pomeranz BH, Corey PN. Incidence of adverse drug reactions in hospitalized patients. A meta-analysis of prospective studies. JAMA 279:1200–1205, 1998.
3. Einarson TR. Drug-related hospital admissions. Ann Pharmacother 27:832–840, 1993.
4. Prince BS, Goetz CM, Rihn TL, et al. Drug-related emergency department visits and hospital admissions. Am J Hosp Pharm 49:1696–1700, 1992.
5. Karch FE, Lasagna L. Adverse drug reactions: a critical review. JAMA 234:1236–1241, 1975.
6. Fincham JE. An overview of adverse drug reactions. Am Pharm NS 31:47–52, 1991.
7. Berkow R, ed. The Merck manual of diagnosis and therapy. 16th ed. Rahway, NJ: Merck Research Laboratories, 1992:2642–2644.
8. Anderson JA. Allergic reactions to drugs and biological agents. JAMA 268:2845–2857, 1992.
9. Anonymous. ASHP guidelines on adverse drug reaction monitoring and reporting. Am J Hosp Pharm 46:336–337, 1989.
10. Naranjo CA, Busto U, Sellers EM, et al. A method for estimating the probability of adverse drug reactions. Clin Pharmacol Ther 30:239–245, 1981.
11. Pearson TF, Pittman DG, Longley JM, et al. Factors associated with preventable adverse drug reactions. Am J Hosp Pharm 51:2268–2272, 1994.
12. Burnum JF. Preventability of adverse drug reactions [letter]. Ann Intern Med 85:80, 1976.
13. Melmon KL. Preventable drug reactions—causes and cures. N Engl J Med 284:1361–1368, 1971.
14. Faich GA. National adverse drug reaction reporting: 1984–1989. Arch Intern Med 151:1645–1647, 1991.
15. Rossi AC, Knapp DE. Discovery of new adverse drug reactions. A review of the Food and Drug Administration's spontaneous reporting system. JAMA 252:1030–1033, 1984.
16. McQueen K. ADR monitoring: rationale, impact and cost issues. Calif J Hosp Pharm 2:5–7, 1990.
17. Goldman SA, Kennedy DL. MedWatch: FDA's medical products reporting program. A joint effort toward improved public health. Postgrad Med 103:13–16, 1998.
18. Edlavitch SA. Adverse drug event reporting. Improving the low US reporting rates [editorial]. Arch Intern Med 148:1499–1503, 1998.
19. Baum C, Anello C. The spontaneous reporting system in the United States. In: Strom BL, ed. Pharmacoepidemiology. New York: Churchill Livingstone, 1989:107–118.
20. White GG, Love L. The MedWatch program. Clin Toxicol 36:145–149, 1998.
21. Surveillance for Safety After Immunization: Vaccine Adverse Event Reporting System (VAERS), United States. Morb Mortal Wkly Rep 52:1–24, 2003.
22. Ellenberg SS, Chen RT. The complicated task of monitoring vaccine safety. Public Health Rep 112:10–20, 1997.
23. Johnson JM. Contributing to drug safety [editorial]. Am J Hosp Pharm 47:1280, 1990.
24. Hoffman RP. Adverse drug reaction revisited—JCAHO. Hosp Pharm 23:685–686, 1988.
25. Seeger JD, Kong SX, Shumock GT. Characteristics associated with ability to prevent adverse drug reactions in hospitalized patients. Pharmacotherapy 18:1284–1289, 1998.
26. Raschkle RA, Gollihare B, Wunderlich TA, et al. A computer alert system to prevent injury from adverse drug events. Development and evaluation in a community teaching hospital. JAMA 280:1317–1320, 1998.
27. Corr K, Stoller R. Adverse drug event reporting at Veterans Affairs facilities. Am J Health Syst Pharm 53:314–315, 1996.
28. Stang PE, Fox JL. Adverse drug events and the Freedom of Information Act: an apple in Eden. Ann Pharmacother 26:238–243, 1992.
29. Edwards IR, Biriell C. Harmonisation in pharmacovigilance. Drug Saf 10:93–102, 1994.
30. Auriche M, Loupi E. Does proof of causality ever exist in pharmacovigilance? Drug Saf 9:230–235, 1993.

31. Sigmund W. Dear Healthcare Professional Letter: Rezulin, December 1, 1997. Available at: http://www.FDA.gov/medwatch/safety/1997/rezul3.html. Accessed December 1, 1998.

32. Roche Laboratories announces withdrawal of Posicor from the market. FDA Talk Paper, June 8, 1998. Available at: http://www.fda.gov/bbs/topics/ANSWERS/ANS00876.html. Accessed December 1, 1998.

33. Wyeth-Ayerst Laboratories announces the withdrawal of Duract from the market. FDA Talk Paper 1998, June 22, 1998. Available at: http://www.fda.gov/bbs/topics/ANSWERS/ANS00876.html. Accessed December 1, 1998.

34. Ellison RH. Written communication, November 17, 1998. Nutley, NJ: Roche Laboratories.

35. FDA issues public health advisory on Vioxx as its manufacturer voluntarily withdraws the product. FDA News, September 30, 2004. Available at: http://www.fda.gov/bbs/topics/news/2004/NEW01122.html.

36. Questions and answers on FDA's New Drug Safety Initiative, May 5, 2005. Available at: http://www.fda.gov/cder/drug/DrugSafety/drugSafetyQA.htm#b-1.

37. Mannesse CK, Derkx FHM, de Ridder MAJ, et al. Adverse drug reactions in elderly patients as contributing factor for hospital admission: cross sectional study. BMJ 315:1057–1058, 1997.

38. French EH. ADRs and metabolic changes in the elderly. US Pharmacist 5:H1–H28, 1994.

39. Greenblatt DJ, Sellers EM, Shader RI. Drug disposition in old age. N Engl J Med 306:1081–1088, 1982.

40. Brawn LA, Castleden CM. Adverse drug reactions: an overview of special considerations in the management of the elderly patient. Drug Saf 5:421–435, 1990.

41. Rowe JW, Andres R, Tobin JP, et al. The effects of age on creatinine clearance in man: a cross sectional and longitudinal study. J Gerontol 31:155–163, 1976.

42. Knight M. Adverse drug reaction in neonates. J Clin Pharmacol 34:128–135, 1994.

43. Toddywalla VS, Patel SB, Betrabet SS, et al. Can chronic maternal drug therapy alter the nursing infant's hepatic drug metabolizing enzyme pattern? J Clin Pharmacol 35:1025–1029, 1995.

44. Gupta A, Waldhauser LK. Adverse drug reactions from birth to early childhood. Pediatr Clin North Am 44:79–92, 1997.

45. Kapusnik-Uner JE, Sande MA, Chambers HF. Tetracyclines, chloramphenicol, erythromycin, and miscellaneous antibacterial agents. In: Hardman JG, Gilman AG, Limbird LE, eds. Goodman and Gilman's the pharmacological basis of therapeutics. New York: McGraw-Hill, 1996:1123–1154.

46. Hendeles L, Jenkins J, Temple R. Revised FDA labeling guideline for theophylline oral dosage forms. Pharmacotherapy 15:409–427, 1995.

47. Bayard PJ, Berger TG, Jacobson MA. Drug hypersensitivity reactions and human immunodeficiency virus disease. J Acquir Immune Defic Syndr 5:1237–1257, 1992.

48. Peters BS, Carlin E, Weston RJ, et al. Adverse effects of drugs used in the management of opportunistic infections associated with HIV infection. Drug Saf 10:439–454, 1994.

49. Harb GE, Jacobson M. Human immunodeficiency virus (HIV) infection. Does it increase susceptibility to adverse drug reactions? Drug Saf 9:1–8, 1993.

50. Harb GE, Alldredge BK, Coleman R, et al. Pharmacoepidemiology of adverse drug reactions in hospitalized patients with human immunodeficiency virus disease. J Acquir Immune Defic Syndr 6:919–926, 1993.

51. Gordin FM, Simon GL, Wofsy CB, et al. Adverse reactions to trimethoprim-sulfamethoxazole in patients with the acquired immunodeficiency syndrome. Ann Intern Med 100:495–499, 1984.

52. Jick H. Adverse reactions to trimethoprim-sulfamethoxazole in hospitalized patients. Rev Infect Dis 4:426–428, 1982.

53. Anonymous. Drugs for HIV infection. Med Lett Drugs Ther 39:111–116, 1997.

54. Goedde HW. Ethnic differences in reactions to drugs and other xenobiotics: outlooks of a geneticist. In: Kalow W, Goedde HS, Agerwal DP, eds. Ethnic differences in reactions to drugs and xenobiotics. New York: Alan R. Liss, 1986.

55. Benetz LZ, Kroetz DL, Sheiner LB. Pharmacokinetics. The dynamics of drug absorption, distribution, and elimination. In: Hardman JG, Gilman AG, Limbird LE, eds. Goodman and Gilman's the pharmacological basis of therapeutics. New York: McGraw-Hill, 1996: 3–28.

56. Florence AT, Jani PU. Novel oral drug formulation. Their potential in modulating adverse effects. Drug Saf 10:233–266, 1994.

57. Witztum JL. Drugs used in the treatment of hyperlipoproteinemias. In: Hardman JG, Gilman AG, Limbird LE, eds. Goodman and Gilman's the pharmacological basis of therapeutics. New York: McGraw-Hill, 1996:875–897.

58. Carson JL, Willett LR. Toxicity of nonsteroidal anti-inflammatory drugs: an overview of the epidemiological evidence. Drugs 46(Suppl 1):243–248, 1993.

59. Meperidine. In: McEvoy GK, ed. AHFS drug information. Bethesda, Md: American Society of Health-System Pharmacists, 1998.

60. Preston SL, Briceland LL, Lesar TS. Accuracy of penicillin allergy reporting. Am J Hosp Pharm 51:79–84, 1994.

61. Lin RY. A perspective on penicillin allergy. Arch Intern Med 152:930–937, 1992.

62. Lachmann PJ, Peters DK, eds. Clinical aspects of immunology. 4th ed. Boston: Blackwell Scientific, 1982.

63. Kishiyama JL, Adelman DC. The cross-reactivity and immunology of beta-lactam antibiotics. Drug Saf 10:318–327, 1994.

64. Madaan A, Li JTC. Cephalosporin allergy. Immunol Allergy Clin North Am 24:463–476, 2004.

65. Thompson JW, Jacobs RF. Adverse effects of newer cephalosporins. An update. Drug Saf 9:132–142, 1993.

66. Saxon A, Adelman DC, Patel A, et al. Imipenem cross-reactivity with penicillin in humans. J Allergy Clin Immunol 82:213–217, 1988.

67. Merrem (meropenem) package insert. Wilmington, Del: Zeneca, 1998.

68. Døssing M, Sonne J. Drug-induced hepatic disorders. Incidence, management and avoidance. Drug Saf 9:441–449, 1993.

69. Maddrey WC. Hepatic effects of acetaminophen: enhanced toxicity in alcoholics. J Clin Gastroenterol 9:180–185, 1987.

70. Anker AL, Smilkstein MJ. Acetaminophen. Concepts and controversies. Emerg Med Clin North Am 12:335–349, 1994.

71. Zimmerman HJ. Hepatotoxicity. Dis Mon 39:675–787, 1993.

72. Lee WM. Drug-induced hepatotoxicity. N Engl J Med 333:1118–1127, 1995.

73. Larrey D, Vial T, Pauwels A, et al. Hepatitis after germander (Teucrium chamaedrys) administration: another instance of herbal medicine hepatotoxicity. Ann Intern Med 117:129–132, 1992.

74. Apte MV, Wilson JS. Alcohol-induced pancreatic injury. Best Pract Res Clin Gastroenterol. 17:593–612, 2003.

75. Underwood TW, Frye CB. Drug-induced pancreatitis. Clin Pharm 12:440–448, 1993.

76. Mallory A, Kern F. Drug-induced pancreatitis: a critical review. Gastroenterology 78:813–820, 1980.

77. Wilmink T, Fric TW. Drug-induced pancreatitis. Drug Saf 14:406–423, 1996.

78. Walker RJ, Duggin GG. Drug nephrotoxicity. Annu Rev Pharmacol Toxicol 28:331–345, 1988.

79. Schlondorff D. Renal complications of nonsteroidal anti-inflammatory drugs. Kidney Int 44:643–653, 1993.

80. Clive DM, Stoff JS. Renal syndromes associated with nonsteroidal antiinflammatory drugs. N Engl J Med 310:563–572, 1984.

81. Whelton A, Hamilton CW. Nonsteroidal anti-inflammatory drugs: effects on kidney function. J Clin Pharmacol 31:588–598, 1991.

82. Humes HD. Aminoglycoside nephrotoxicity. Kidney Int 33:900–911, 1988.

83. Choudhury D, Ahmed Z. Drug induced nephrotoxicity. Med Clin North Am 81:705–717, 1997.

84. Messmore HL, Jeske WP, Wehrmacher W et al. Antiplatelet agents: current drugs and future trends. Hematol Oncol Clin 19:87–117, 2005.

85. CAST (Cardiac Arrhythmia Suppression Trial) Investigators. Preliminary report: effect of encainide or flecainide on mortality in a randomized trial of arrhythmia suppression after myocardial infarction. N Engl J Med 321:406–412, 1989.

86. Roden DM. Risks and benefits of antiarrhythmic therapy. N Engl J Med 331:785–791, 1994.

87. Pellinen TJ, Farkkilae M, Keikrila J, et al. Electrocardiographic and clinical factors of tricyclic antidepressant intoxication. Ann Clin Res 19:12, 1987.

88. Benassi E, Bo G, Cocito L, et al. Carbamazepine and cardiac conduction disturbances. Ann Neurol 22:280–281, 1987.

89. Rosen B, Ovsyshcher IA, Zimlichman R. Complete atrioventricular block induced by methyldopa. PACE Pacing Clin Electrophysiol 11:1555–1558, 1988.

90. Hart A. Cardiac arrest associated with ranitidine. BMJ 299:519, 1989.

91. Rhoden W, Hasleton P, Brooks N. Anthracyclines and the heart. Br Heart J 70:499–502, 1993.

92. Henkin Y, Como JA, Oberman A. Secondary dyslipidemia. Inadvertent effects of drugs in clinical practice. JAMA 267:961–968, 1992.

93. Abenhaim A, Moride Y, Brenot F, et al. Appetite-suppressant drugs and the risk of primary pulmonary hypertension. N Engl J Med 335:609–619, 1996.

94. Khan MA, Herzog CA, St Peter JV, et al. The prevalence of cardiac valvular insufficiency assessed by transthoracic echocardiography in obese patients treated with appetite-suppressant drugs. N Engl J Med 339:713–718, 1998.

95. Rosenow EC, Myers JL, Swensen SJ, et al. Drug-induced pulmonary disease: an update. Chest 102:239–250, 1992.

96. Gregory AS, Grippi MA. The clinical diagnosis of drug-induced pulmonary disorders. J Thorac Imaging 6:8–18, 1991.

97. Goodwin SD, Glenny RW. Nonsteroidal anti-inflammatory drug-associated pulmonary infiltrates with eosinophilia. Review of literature and Food and Drug Administration adverse drug reaction reporting. Arch Intern Med 152:1521–1524, 1992.

98. Rosenow EC. Drug-induced pulmonary disease. Dis Mon 5:258–310, 1994.

99. Hoffman BB, Lefkowitz RJ. Catecholamines, sympathomimetic drugs, and adrenergic receptor antagonists. In: Hardman JG, Gilman AG, Limbird LE, eds. Goodman and Gilman's the pharmacological basis of therapeutics. New York: McGraw-Hill, 1996: 199–248.

100. Dunn TL, Gerber MJ, Shen AS, et al. The effect of topical ophthalmic instillation of timolol and betaxolol on lung function in asthmatic subjects. Am Rev Respir Dis 133:264–268, 1986.

101. Setipane GA. Aspirin and allergic disease: a review. Am J Med 74(Suppl 6a):102–109, 1983.

102. Szczeklik A, Grylewski RJ. Asthma and anti-inflammatory drugs. Mechanisms and clinical patterns. Drugs 25:533–543, 1983.

103. Holgate ST, Bradding P, Sampson AP. Leukotriene antagonists and synthesis inhibitors: new directions in asthma therapy. J Allergy Clin Immunol 98:1–13, 1996

104. Cooper JAD, White DA, Matthay RA. Drug-induced pulmonary disease. Part 2: noncytotoxic drugs. Am Rev Respir Dis 133: 488–505, 1986.

105. Smith PJ, Talbert RL. Sexual dysfunction with antihypertensive and antipsychotic agents. Clin Pharm 5:373–384, 1986.

106. Prisant LM, Carr AA, Bottini PB, et al. Sexual dysfunction with antihypertensive drugs. Arch Intern Med 154:730–736, 1994.

107. Anonymous. Drugs that cause sexual dysfunction: an update. Med Lett Drugs Ther 34:73–78, 1992.

108. Deamer RL, Thompson JF. The role of medications in geriatric sexual function. Clin Geriatr Med 7:95–110, 1991.

109. Woodrum ST, Brown CS. Management of SSRI-induced sexual dysfunction. Ann Pharmacother 32:1209–1215, 1998.

110. Bulpitt CJ, Dollery CT, Carne S. Change in symptoms of hypertensive patients after referral to hospital clinic. Br Heart J 38: 121–128, 1976.

111. Buvat J, Lamaire A, Buvat-Herbaut M, et al. Comparative investigations in 26 impotent and 26 nonimpotent diabetic patients. J Urol 133:34–38, 1985.

112. Johnson JA, Bootman JL. Drug-related morbidity and mortality. A cost-of-illness model. Arch Intern Med 155:1949–1956, 1995.

113. Bootman JL, Harrison DL, Cox E. The health care cost of drug-related morbidity and mortality in nursing facilities. Arch Intern Med 157:2089–2096, 1997.

Drug Interactions

3

Robert Keith Middleton

DEFINITION

A drug interaction is defined as the "pharmacologic or clinical response to the administration of a drug combination different from that anticipated from the known effects of the two agents."[1] The interaction may result in a change in the nature or type of response to a drug (i.e., *pharmacodynamic* interaction), or a change in the magnitude or duration of response to a drug (i.e., *pharmacokinetic* interaction).[2]

Most commonly, a drug interaction is taken to mean an interaction between two or more medicines, which is a drug–drug interaction. However, a "drug interaction" can have many causes. For example, several food–drug interactions have been well documented,[3] and within this category, enteral feeding–drug interactions,[4] nutrient–drug interactions,[5] alcohol–drug interactions,[6] and tobacco–drug interactions[7] are all well established. With the rising use of alternative medicines, herbal– or botanical–drug interactions are increasingly being reported.[8] Furthermore, drug–disease interactions, drug–laboratory interactions, and parenteral–drug interactions may result in physical and chemical incompatibility. Drug–disease interactions are discussed throughout this text under the specific disease states. Readers interested in drug–laboratory interactions and parenteral–drug compatibilities are referred to specialized references on these subjects.[9,10]

EPIDEMIOLOGY

In 2004 in the United States, more than 3,500 drugs could be prescribed, and any five of these drugs could be used in 5.2×10^{17} different combinations.[11] When the large number of alternative medicines (e.g., herbs, botanicals), vitamins, and foods with pharmacologically active ingredients (e.g., caffeinated beverages, calcium-fortified drinks, herbal teas, "naturally" fortified beverages) that are available are factored into this, the number of possible combinations is even more staggering. A review of drug usage in the United States found that more than 81% of persons in a given week take at least one medication [prescription drug, over-the-counter (OTC) product, vitamin, mineral, or herbal supplement], and 25% take at least five such medications.[12] Clearly, the *potential* for an interaction between two or more agents is large.

The reported frequency of drug interactions varies greatly depending upon the population studied (outpatients vs. hospitalized patients vs. nursing home residents), the type of interaction reported (any interaction vs. only interactions that cause an adverse event), the study design (prospective vs. retrospective), and the demographics of the population studied (e.g., elderly vs. young patients). The Boston Collaborative Drug Surveillance program reported 83,200 drug exposures in almost 10,000 patients and found 3,600 adverse drug reactions, of which 6.5% resulted from drug interactions.[13] A review of the adverse event literature in 1993 found that up to 2.8% of hospitalizations resulted from drug–drug interactions[14]: another study found almost double that rate in Australian hospitals.[15] A US study found that drug–drug interactions accounted for 4.6% of adverse events *during* hospitalization,[16] and a recent literature review reported that 2.8% of preventable adverse drug events in the hospitalized population were due to drug–drug interactions.[17] A recent study of medication use by residents of three nursing homes found drug interactions with 5.8% of all drugs being taken.[18] The occurrence of drug–drug interactions in the ambulatory setting is reported to be as high as 70.3%.[19] However, a recent study that applied successive filters to screen out inconsequential drug combinations found that clinically relevant interactions occurred in only 0.04% of ambulatory patients.[20] Finally, in a retrospective review of adverse event reports, it was noted that drug interactions accounted for 10.5% of all drug-related events that would likely result in patient death if no intervention was made.[21]

CONSEQUENCES OF DRUG INTERACTIONS

Drug interactions touch all facets of health care.[11] Their effect on patients can vary greatly, from no untoward effects to the most extreme result of severe morbidity or death. Physicians face medical-legal liability if a poor patient outcome is the result of a known drug interaction. Health care facilities face increased consumption of resources and increased costs for diagnosing and treating patients with significant drug interactions. One study found that hospitalized patients who received interacting drugs had a longer and more costly hospitalization than patients who did not experience such interactions.[22] The pharmaceutical industry faces loss of investment, time, and financial resources if a drug is removed from the market, as well as potential litigation. Notably, five of the ten drugs removed from the US market between 1998 and 2001 were removed because of significant drug–drug interactions.[23]

RISK FACTORS

A high degree of variability has been observed in patient response to two or more interacting compounds. Plainly put, not every patient reacts the same way or to the same degree when exposed to the same interacting drugs. Several factors, both patient specific and drug specific, influence the risk of drug interactions (Table 3.1). Intuitively, it has been noted that the risk of drug interaction increases as the number of pharmacologically active compounds used increases. A retrospective study of patients who presented to two emergency departments found that significant drug interactions increased from 34% among patients taking two medications to 82% in patients taking seven or more medicines.[24] Use of multiple prescribers and/or multiple pharmacies increases the odds that health professionals will have incomplete medical and drug information available to them, and raises the chance that a potential drug interaction may go undetected. The genetic makeup of an individual determines his or her complement of metabolizing enzymes and other proteins. Patients classified as slow metabolizers appear to be at less risk for drug interactions than extensive metabolizers or ultrarapid metabolizers (see Pharmacogenetics, below).[25] Specific populations are at increased risk of experiencing drug interactions. For example, the elderly, because of a greater

---

TABLE 3.1 | Risk Factors for Drug Interactions[24–30]

Polypharmacy

Multiple prescribers

Multiple pharmacies

Genetic makeup

Specific populations
- Females
- Elderly
- Obese
- Malnourished
- Critically ill patients
- Transplant recipients

Specific illnesses
- Cardiovascular disease (CHF, arrhythmias)
- Diabetes
- Epilepsy
- Gastric illness (ulcer disease, dyspepsia)
- Hepatic disease
- Hyperlipidemia
- Hypothyroidism
- Infection (HIV, fungal infection)
- Psychiatric illness
- Renal dysfunction
- Respiratory illness (asthma, COPD)

Drug dose

Narrow therapeutic index drugs
- Aminoglycosides
- Antiarrhythmics (quinidine, lidocaine, procainamide)
- Carbamazepine
- Cyclosporine
- Digoxin
- Insulin
- Lithium
- Oral sulfonylureas
- Phenytoin
- Theophylline
- Tricyclic antidepressants
- Unfractionated heparin
- Valproic acid
- Warfarin

CHF, congestive heart failure; HIV, human immunodeficiency virus; COPD, chronic obstructive pulmonary disease.

number of chronic illnesses, increased drug usage to manage those illnesses, and age-related physiologic changes (e.g., decreased renal function, decreased protein binding), are at higher risk for drug interactions and adverse events.[26] A number of studies have found females to be at greater risk for drug interactions.[26,27] Obese patients have altered levels of metabolizing enzymes, making them more susceptible to drug interactions, as do malnourished patients.[28,29] Other populations at risk include critically ill patients, patients with autoimmune disorders, and transplant recipients.[30] Drugs with a narrow therapeutic index, a steep dose-response curve, or potent pharmacologic effects have been associated with greatest risk for significant drug interactions. Aminoglycosides, cyclosporine, some medicines for human immunodeficiency virus (HIV), many anticonvulsants, many antiarrhythmics, and anticoagulants fall into this category.[30] Several diseases seem to predispose patients to drug interactions. This is due to a combination of factors. For example, some disease states such as congestive heart failure, acquired immunodeficiency syndrome (AIDS), epilepsy, or psychiatric illness may require multiple medications for effective management. Many of the drugs used to treat some illnesses, such as tuberculosis, epilepsy, and AIDS, are potent enzyme inducers or inhibitors and therefore predispose patients to drug interactions. Some illnesses are treated with a narrow therapeutic index drug. Lithium, used for bipolar disorder, has a very narrow therapeutic range, for instance. Consequently, even minor changes in its blood level caused by a drug interaction could lead to toxicity. Finally, many drug interactions are concentration dependent. Thus, the occurrence of the interaction and its outcome are often dictated by the dose of the drug and its pharmacokinetics.

CLINICAL RELEVANCE

For an interaction to be clinically meaningful, it must result in a change in patient response or outcome and ultimately in prescribing behavior. Thus, an in vitro or an in vivo drug interaction may be *statistically* significant but still not therapeutically significant. Two key factors to consider when one is evaluating the clinical relevance of a drug interaction are the magnitude of the effect and the therapeutic index of the drug, which is graphically shown in Figure 3.1. Even small changes in drug level may have significant clinical impact if the drug has a narrow therapeutic margin, as is the case with digoxin. On the other hand, a doubling or even tripling of drug concentration for drugs with a wide therapeutic window, such as ceftriaxone, may have no clinical effect. Ultimately, the patient's clinical outcome determines the significance of a drug interaction.

NOMENCLATURE

When one is discussing drug interactions, it is necessary to distinguish between the compound that is causing the interaction (referred to as the precipitant drug, or perpetrator drug) and the agent that is being affected (referred to as the object, or victim drug). Additionally, a drug can be a *substrate* for a particular enzyme, meaning that that enzyme or family of enzymes metabolizes the drug. *Inhibitors* are agents that block the action of an enzyme or transport protein; *inducers* are compounds that stimulate the action of an enzyme or transport protein.

Before proceeding, it is important to review the key processes involved in drug metabolism, as well as the significant

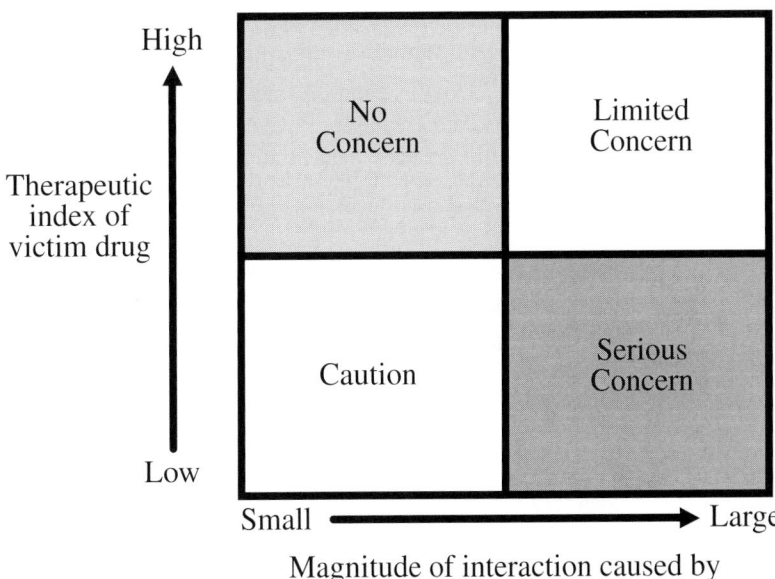

FIGURE 3.1 Evaluating the clinical relevance of drug interactions. Drugs with a high therapeutic index are less of a concern in drug interactions. The most relevant interactions are those in which the victim drug has a low therapeutic index and is subject to a moderate-to-large interaction. The same reasoning can be applied to induction drug interactions if the absence of the drug effect results in therapeutic failure and serious progression of disease. (Modified from Obach RS. Drug-drug interactions: an important negative attribute in drugs. Drugs Today 39: 301–338, 2003, with permission.)

advances that have been made in pharmacogenetics and in active drug transport.

BIOTRANSFORMATION

Drug biotransformation is divided into two general processes: phase I and phase II reactions. Phase I reactions involve intramolecular changes such as oxidation, reduction, and hydrolysis that increase the polar nature of the compound. Phase II reactions generally involve combining a parent compound or, more commonly, a phase I product with an endogenous substance (e.g., glucuronic acid, acetic acid, sulfate) to increase its water solubility and enhance its elimination. Compounds such as drugs, chemicals, and toxins (collectively called *xenobiotics*) can undergo repetitive phase I and phase II reactions until a water-soluble metabolite is reached that favors excretion. Table 3.2 lists the major enzymes involved in drug biotransformation[31–33]

The major drug-metabolizing systems in phase I reactions are the cytochrome P-450 enzymes. Cytochrome P-450 was named for its spectrophotometric absorption peak at 450 nm when bound to a molecule of carbon monoxide. This superfamily of heme-containing isoenzymes is subdivided into families and subfamilies on the basis of amino acid sequence homology. For example, in the isoenzyme named CYP3A4, "CYP" designates the cytochrome P-450 enzyme system, the numeral "3" names the family, "A" designates the subfamily, and the numeral "4" identifies the individual enzyme.[34] Thus, the isoenzymes CYP2C9 and CYP2C19 are closely related (same family and subfamily), 2C9 and 2D6 are somewhat related (same family), and 2C9 and 3A4 are not closely related (different families).[35] Each enzyme shows distinct but overlapping substrate specificity with occasionally overlapping selectivity—a characteristic of many drug-metabolizing enzymes. Of the more than 100 human cytochrome enzymes that belong to 17 gene families and 42 subfamilies, three—CYP1, CYP2, and CYP3— are responsible for most known phase I reactions.[36] Within these families, CYP1A2, 2C9, 2C19, 2D6, 2E1, and 3A4 account for more than 90% of CYP-mediated reactions.[28] Cytochrome P-450 enzymes are located in greatest concentration in the endoplasmic reticulum of hepatocytes and in the enterocytes

and crypt cells of the small intestine, but also in lesser concentrations in the kidneys, lung, brain, and placenta.[28,35]

Drugs may be substrates for more than one enzyme. Imipramine, for instance, is a substrate of CYP1A2, CYP2C19, and CYP2D6. A drug may sometimes inhibit or induce the activity of a specific enzyme that is not involved in its own metabolism. For example, mexiletine is an inhibitor of the CYP1A2 isoenzyme but is a substrate for CYP2D6. Furthermore, some drugs may act as both inhibitor and inducer. Omeprazole is a CYP1A2 inducer but an inhibitor of CYP2C19.

In addition to the cytochrome P-450 enzymes, several other enzymes participate in phase I reactions (Table 3.2). As the biochemistry and genetics of these enzymes become better understood, their involvement in drug interactions will become clearer.

Generally speaking, the enzymes involved in phase II reactions (Table 3.2) are less involved in drug interactions than are phase I enzymes. As with the CYP enzymes, there are superfamilies of phase II enzymes, for example, the uridine diphosphate (UDP) glucuronyltransferases (UGT) and the sulfonotransferases.[37] Although most phase II reactions involve the end product of phase I biotransformation, for some compounds, direct conjugation may be the primary route of metabolism, as is the case with morphine. Similar to the cytochrome P-450 enzymes, phase II enzymes are primarily located in the liver but may also be found at several extrahepatic sites, including the gastrointestinal (GI) tract.[37]

PHARMACOGENETICS

As has already been stated, a high degree of variability has been seen in responses to drug interactions. Some of this variability can be attributed to differences in the genes that encode for drug-metabolizing enzymes or drug transporters. The study of these differences is called *pharmacogenetics*.[38] Several of the major CYP families display genetic polymorphism, that is, the presence of a variant gene with a frequency greater than 1% in the general population. For example, 11 2C9 variants, 15 2C19 variants, and more than 70 2D6 variants have been identified.[39] Consequently, metabolic capabilities vary considerably in the general population. Most

TABLE 3.2	Major Enzymes Involved in Drug Biotransformation[31–33]	
Clearance Mechanism	Phase of Metabolism	Enzymes/Proteins Involved
Oxidative metabolism	Phase I	CYP, MAO, FMO, Mo-CO, aldehyde oxidase, xanthine oxidase, peroxidases
Hydrolytic metabolism	Phase I	Esterases, amidases, epoxide hydrolases
Conjugative metabolism	Phase II	UGT, ST, MT, NAT, GST

CYP, cytochrome P450 enzymes; MAO, monoamine oxidases; FMO, flavin-containing monooxygenases; Mo-CO, molybdenum-containing oxidases; UGT, uridine diphosphate–glucuronyltransferases; ST, sulfotransferases; MT, methyltransferase; NAT, N-acetyltransferase; GST, glutathione-S-transferase.

individuals are extensive metabolizers (EMs), meaning that they encompass the "normal" complement of functional enzymes and metabolize substrates "normally." A small group of individuals are classified as poor metabolizers (PMs) because they lack functional genes that code for one or more CYP enzymes. These individuals have a low or completely absent level of enzyme and do not metabolize certain substrates well. Last, some individuals have duplicate or multiple copies of CYP-encoding genes and are classified as ultrarapid metabolizers (UMs) because they have a higher than average amount of enzyme and rapidly metabolize substrates.[35].

Ethnicity influences metabolizer status. For example, 4% of whites and 8% of African-Americans are poor metabolizers for CYP2D6, and approximately 5% of whites and 20% of Asians and African-Americans are poor metabolizers for 2C19.[28,35] Phase II enzymes are also subject to genetic polymorphism.[23,40] In fact, one of the earliest studied polymorphisms was the phase II enzyme, N-acetyltransferase.[38] The impact of pharmacogenetics on drug interactions is now being realized and is being incorporated into drug information. For example, the prescribing information for the newly approved attention-deficit disorder drug atomoxetine (Strattera) states: "Atomoxetine is primarily metabolized by the CYP2D6 pathway to 4-hydroxyatomoxetine. In EMs, selective inhibitors of CYP2D6 increase atomoxetine steady-state plasma concentrations to exposures similar to those observed in PMs. Dosage adjustment of Strattera may be necessary when coadministered with CYP2D6 inhibitors, e.g., paroxetine, fluoxetine, and quinidine. In EM individuals treated with paroxetine or fluoxetine, the AUC of atomoxetine is approximately 6- to 8-fold and $C_{ss,max}$ is about 3- to 4-fold greater than atomoxetine alone."[41]

DRUG TRANSPORTERS

Over the past few years, knowledge of the role that drug transporters play in drug absorption, distribution, and excretion has dramatically increased. Several families of drug transporters have been identified (Table 3.3).[42–53] Similar to phase I and II enzymes, drug transporters are genetically determined and polymorphisms for many transporters have been discovered.[42] Given the number of different transporters, their ubiquity, and the broad range of substrates carried, transport proteins may rival metabolic enzymes in terms of importance in drug handling. The best studied family of transport proteins is the adenosine triphosphate (ATP)-binding cassette (ABC) transporter superfamily, which includes P-glycoprotein (Pgp), several multidrug resistance–associated proteins (MRP1–MRP6), breast cancer resistance protein (BCRP), and sister-Pgp (SPGP).[43] All ABC transporters are secretory proteins that are principally located in the plasma membrane of cells, where they extrude a variety of compounds from the cellular interior to the exterior. ABC proteins transport a wide variety of substrates, including

drugs, drug conjugates from phase II reactions, metabolites, steroids, and other compounds. Hydrolysis of ATP provides the energy for this process, which can take place against a significant concentration gradient. Pgp is the best characterized of the ABC transporters and was originally identified by its ability to confer chemotherapeutic resistance to cancer cells. Pgp is located in the apical surface of mucosal cells in the large and small intestine, the renal proximal tubules, the biliary membrane of hepatocytes, and the capillary endothelial cells of the brain and testes, where it is a key component of the blood–brain and blood–testes barrier, the adrenal gland, and the endometrium of the pregnant uterus.[54] Pgp is able to transport a wide range of diverse substances that do not share any structural similarity, making it a significant transport protein.

ETIOLOGY

PHARMACOKINETICS

Most drug interactions are pharmacokinetic in nature, that is, the perpetrator drug affects the absorption, distribution, metabolism, or excretion of the object drug.

Absorption. After oral administration, most drug absorption takes place in the proximal small intestine, where the large surface area facilitates this process. However, drug interactions that alter absorption may occur throughout the GI tract through a variety of mechanisms, including complexation (adsorption or chelation), changes in pH, changes in GI motility, altered drug transport, and enzymatic metabolism. The net effect of one or more of these processes is a change in the *rate* of drug absorption, or a change in the *extent* of drug absorption. In the former situation, the total amount of drug absorbed remains the same, only the speed with which it is absorbed is changed. Generally speaking, for medicines given over the long term as multiple doses, this is not a clinically significant effect. However, for drugs given as a single dose, whose effect may depend upon achieving a desired serum level (e.g., analgesics, hypnotics), a change in the rate of absorption may lead to therapeutic failure or possibly an adverse event.

Complexation. Agents that form chemical complexes with drugs may cause lower rates of drug absorption. Cholestyramine or colestipol lowers cholesterol by binding bile acids in the intestine, inhibiting their reabsorption and enterohepatic recirculation, and increasing their fecal excretion. This same action affects numerous drugs when they are coadministered with one of these bile acid–binding resins, including digoxin, warfarin, levothyroxine, furosemide, and mycophenolate. The result is lowered serum concentration and reduced effectiveness. Divalent and trivalent metallic ions such as magnesium, aluminum, calcium, zinc, bismuth, and iron can form insoluble complexes with drugs, also resulting in reduced serum levels and possibly therapeutic failure. The quinolone antibiotics are highly susceptible to chelation by

TABLE 3.3	Major Drug-Transporting Proteins[43–54]

ATP-Binding Cassette (ABC) Family

Name (alternative name)	Location	Drug Substrates
P-glycoprotein (Pgp, MDR1)	Brain, intestine, kidney, placenta, testes	Multiple: see Table 3.4
MRP1 (MRP, GS-X, ABCC1)	Brain, intestine, kidney	Chemotherapeutic drugs, glutathione, sulfate, or glucuronide conjugates of several drugs
cMOAT (cMRP, MRP2, ABCC2)	Intestine	Pravastatin, methotrexate, grepafloxacin, irinotecan, glutathione, sulfate, or glucuronide conjugates of several drugs
MRP3 (MOAT-D, cMOAT–2)	Adrenal gland, intestine, liver	Chemotherapeutic drugs
MRP4 (MOAT-B)	Kidney, liver	Monophosphate analogs of zidovudine, didanosine, zalcitabine, lamivudine, methotrexate, intracellular active metabolite of 6-mercaptopurine
MRP5 (MOAT-C, pABC11)	Intestine, kidney	Intracellular active metabolite of 6-mercaptopurine
MRP6	Intestine, liver	Anionic conjugates
BCRP (MXR, ABCP)	Intestine, liver	Anticancer drugs
Sister-Pgp (SPGP, BSEP, ABCB11)	Liver	Not determined

Organic Anion–Transporting Polypeptide (OATP) Family

Name	Location	Drug Substrates
OATP-A	Brain	Fexofenadine, rocuronium, D-penicillamine
OATP-B	Intestine, kidney, liver, lung, placenta	Estrone, fexofenadine
OATP-C	Liver	Conjugated steroids, thyroid hormones, pravastatin, rifampin, benzylpenicillin
OATP-E	Ubiquitous	Not determined
OATP–8	Liver	Digoxin, D-penicillamine, methotrexate, thyroid hormone
PGT	Ubiquitous	Not determined

Organic Anion Transport (OAT) Family

Name	Location	Drug Substrates
OAT1	Brain, kidney	Nonsteroidal anti-inflammatory drugs (NSAIDs), methotrexate, β-lactam antibiotics, cidofovir, adefovir
OAT2	Kidney, liver	Salicylate
OAT3	Brain, kidney	Cimetidine, estrone
OAT4	Kidney, placenta	

Organic Cationic Transport (OCT) Family

Name	Location	Drug Substrates
OCT1	Brain, intestine, kidney, liver	Dopamine
OCT2	Brain, kidney, placenta	Dopamine
OCT3	Brain, kidney, liver, placenta	Dopamine, norepinephrine, clonidine, imipramine, procainamide
OCTN1	Kidney	L-carnitine, quinidine, verapamil
OCTN2	Brain, kidney, liver, placenta	L-carnitine

(continued)

TABLE 3.3	continued

Proton-Dependent Oligopeptide Transporter (POT) Family

Name	Location	Drug Substrates
PEPT1	Intestine, kidney	β-Lactam antibiotics, valacyclovir, angiotensin-converting enzyme (ACE) inhibitors, valganciclovir, levodopa
PEPT2	Brain, lung, kidney	β-Lactam antibiotics, ACE inhibitors
Concentrative Nucleoside Transporter (CNT) Family		
CNT1	Kidney	Pyrimidine nucleosides
CNT2	Kidney	Purine nucleosides
CNT3	Kidney	Pyrimidine and purine nucleosides
Equilibrative Nucleoside Transporter (ENT) Family		
ENT1	Kidney	Pyrimidine and purine nucleosides
ENT2	Kidney	Pyrimidine and purine nucleosides

sucralfate, most antacids, calcium acetate, and ferrous sulfate (including iron in multivitamins), as are many of the tetracycline antibiotics and penicillamine. The bisphosphonates alendronate and risedronate are rendered ineffective if taken with any calcium-containing compound.

Gastric Acidity. Some drugs, for example, ketoconazole, itraconazole, atazanavir, and iron supplements, require an acidic environment for optimal dissolution and absorption. Compounds that raise gastric pH such as H_2 receptor blockers (e.g., cimetidine, ranitidine), proton pump inhibitors (e.g., omeprazole, lansoprazole), or antacids can reduce the absorption of these drugs, thereby decreasing their effectiveness.

Gastric Motility. Many drugs alter gastrointestinal motility. For example, narcotics or drugs with anticholinergic effects (e.g., tricyclic antidepressants, phenothiazines, oxybutynin, tolterodine) can slow GI motility. On the other hand, metoclopramide, erythromycin, and some laxatives can increase GI motility. How altered GI motility affects drug absorption is difficult to predict, however. Slowing motility may lead to enhanced drug absorption by allowing more time for drug dissolution and prolonged contact with the absorptive surface of the small intestine. Alternatively, slowed motility may prolong exposure to intestinal enzymes, reducing the amount of drug available for absorption. Enhanced motility may speed the transit of drugs through the GI tract, decreasing medication absorption. This is particularly important for drugs that require prolonged contact with the absorptive surface, or those drugs that have an ''absorption window.'' Sustained-release products and enteric-coated drugs may also undergo decreased absorption if GI motility is increased.

Altered Drug Transport. Two types of transport proteins are present in the intestinal mucosa—those that are involved in the transport of compounds from the lumen of the intestine into the portal bloodstream, and those that are involved in the efflux of compounds from the intestinal mucosa back into the gut lumen. Of these, efflux transporters, particularly Pgp, are the most studied and are a source of drug interactions. Pgp is located on the apical surface of mucosal cells in the intestine, generally in increasing concentration from the stomach to the colon, and is oriented to pump compounds from the inside of the cell back into the gut lumen.[37] Several drugs are substrates of Pgp (Table 3.4), meaning that these drugs are normally transported from intestinal cells back into the intestinal lumen after oral administration.[28,42–44,49,55] Also, several drugs are now known to block the action of Pgp (i.e., they are Pgp inhibitors; Table 3.4). Coadministration of a Pgp substrate and an inhibitor increases the amount of substrate available for absorption and may elevate the serum drug concentration. Similarly, some compounds such as rifampin are known to increase expression of Pgp (Table 3.4). Administration of a substrate with a Pgp inducer leads to enhanced efflux of the substrate into the gut lumen, and lower serum levels of the substrate.

Intestinal Metabolism. The intestinal mucosa is now appreciated to be much more than an organ for passive drug diffusion. As has been stated, many phase I and phase II enzymes are present in the small and large intestines, conferring the gastrointestinal mucosal a significant role in drug metabolism and the first-pass effect. The highest concentration of mucosal enzymes is found in the duodenum, followed by the jejunum, ileum, and colon.[37] CYPs 1A1, 2C, 2D6, and 3A4 have been identified in the human small intestine; of these, CYP3A4 is the most prevalent oxidative enzyme and the most important. In most individuals, the amount of CYP3A4 in the intestine is 10% to 50% lower than that found in the liver, although exceptions have been documented.[37] Thus, drugs that are substrates of CYP3A4 can undergo significant metabolism in the small intestine during

TABLE 3.4	P-glycoprotein Substrates, Inhibitors, and Inducers[28,42–44,49,55,150]

Substrates		Inhibitors	Inducers
Analgesics	Corticosteroids	Antimicrobials	Clotrimazole
Fentanyl	Dexamethasone	Clarithromycin	Dexamethasone
Methadone	Hydrocortisone	Erythromycin	Reserpine
Morphine	Triamcinolone	Itraconazole	Rifampin
Antiemetics	HIV Protease Inhibitors	Ivermectin	Ritonavir
Ondansetron	Amprenavir	Ketoconazole	St. John's wort
Antihistamines	Indinavir	Mefloquine	
Cimetidine	Lopinavir	Ofloxacin	
Fexofenadine	Nelfinavir	Cardiac Drugs	
Ranitidine	Ritonavir	Amiodarone	
Antimicrobials	Saquinavir	Carvedilol	
Erythromycin	Lipid Lowering Drugs	Diltiazem	
Fluoroquinolones	Atorvastatin	Dipyridamole	
Ivermectin	Lovastatin	Felodipine	
Rifampin	Pravastatin	Nifedipine	
Cardiac Drugs	Simvastatin	Propranolol	
Amiodarone	Immunosuppressants	Propafenone	
Digoxin	Cyclosporine	Verapamil	
Diltiazem	Tacrolimus	Immunosuppressants	
Lidocaine	Proton Pump Inhibitors	Cyclosporine	
Losartan	Omeprazole	Tacrolimus	
Nadolol	Pantoprazole	Pharmaceutical Excipients	
Propranolol	Rheumatologic Drugs	Cremophor EL	
Quinidine	Methotrexate	PEG 400	
Timolol	Quinine	Tween 80	
Verapamil	Miscellaneous	Psychotropic Drugs	
Anticancer Agents	Colchicine	Amitriptyline	
Dactinomycin	Cimetidine	Chlorpromazine	
Daunorubicin	Loperamide	Desipramine	
Docetaxel	Octreotide	Disulfiram	
Doxorubicin		Doxepin	
Epirubicin		Fluphenazine	
Etoposide		Haloperidol	
Fluorouracil		Imipramine	
Mitomycin C		Steroids	
Mitoxantrone		Progesterone	
Paclitaxel		Testosterone	
Tamoxifen		Miscellaneous	
Topotecan		Grapefruit juice (intestinal 3A4)	
Vinblastine		Seville orange juice (intestinal 3A4)	
Vincristine			

HIV, human immunodeficiency virus.

cellular transport before ever reaching the hepatic circulation. It is important to note that CYP3A4 and Pgp have similar areas of distribution along the GI tract, and most substrates of Pgp are CYP3A4 substrates as well, suggesting a cooperative role in drug metabolism.[37] This model is supported at the molecular level by the recognition that the nuclear receptor, SXR, synchronizes transcription of both CYP3A4 and Pgp.[56] For example, a compound (also called a *ligand*) such as phenobarbital binds to the SXR receptor and stimulates transcription of both CYP3A4 and Pgp coordinately (see Hepatic Metabolism for more discussion on nuclear receptors). A system of ''intestinal recycling'' is proposed, wherein drug diffuses into the intestinal cell and is then secreted by Pgp back into the gut lumen; this process is followed by oxidation by CYP3A4. The process of diffusion, extrusion, and metabolism is repeated as the drug travels along the GI tract. The net effect is an increase in the intracellular residence time of the drug, a decrease in its rate of absorption, and increased drug metabolism relative to crossing of the intestine by the unmetabolized drug.[57] Inhibitors of CYP3A4 will interfere with the metabolism of drugs that are CYP3A4 substrates, resulting in greater absorption and elevated serum levels. On the other hand, a CYP3A4 inducer will increase enzyme activity, causing increased metabolism of CYP3A4 substrates and lower serum levels. Just as CYP3A4 and Pgp have common substrates, they also have common inhibitors (e.g., erythromycin, ketoconazole) and inducers (e.g., rifampin). Administration of a drug that is a substrate of both CYP3A4 and Pgp with another drug that is an inhibitor of both can lead to a significant increase in plasma levels, in that the efflux action of Pgp is blocked (i.e., more drug is absorbed by the intestinal mucosa) and the metabolic ability of CYP3A4 is reduced (allowing more unmetabolized drug to be absorbed). The exact opposite occurs when a Pgp/3A4 substrate is administered with an inducer of both, that is, significantly reduced plasma levels of drug are observed. For a more detailed discussion of metabolic drug interactions, see Hepatic Metabolism.

Distribution

Protein Displacement. Following administration and absorption, drugs are quickly distributed throughout the body. Some drugs have near-complete dissolution in the plasma, but many are bound to circulating proteins—acidic drugs generally to albumin and basic drugs to α_1-glycoprotein.[58] The degree of protein binding is variable, ranging from less than 10% to 99% or greater. Regardless of the extent of protein binding, equilibrium is established between bound and unbound drug, and it is only the unbound or free fraction of the drug that is capable of exerting a pharmacologic effect. Competition between drugs for the same protein-binding site can lead to displacement of bound drug and an increase in its unbound or free fraction. Displacement occurs only if both drugs are highly protein bound (>90%). Such drug interactions, however, most often are not clinically meaningful for several reasons. First, following displacement, the free fraction of the drug rises, transiently increasing its serum level and possibly its pharmacologic action.[58] However, the newly unbound drug is also available for distribution, metabolism, and excretion, and equilibrium is reestablished between bound and unbound drug, thus maintaining a constant serum level. Second, many drugs have a large therapeutic index; thus, even a doubling of the serum level will not result in clinically observable effect.[59] Third, the time between the pharmacokinetic interaction of displacement and the pharmacodynamic response can be too great for the interaction to be relevant. For example, warfarin is highly protein bound and can be displaced by many drugs such as phenytoin, phenylbutazone, and disulfiram. This displacement occurs quickly with rapid changes in serum warfarin levels. However, the anticoagulant action of warfarin takes several days to change because of the long half-lives of some of the vitamin K–dependent clotting factors that it inhibits. Before a new steady state can be reached for these clotting factors, warfarin equilibrium is reestablished and no effect from protein displacement is observed.[59] Note, however, that these drugs do have clinically significant interactions with warfarin because of changes in warfarin metabolism. In a review of the relevance of protein binding to drug interactions, Benet and Hoener show that only a small percentage of drugs may be influenced by changes in protein binding.[59]

Altered Drug Transport. The degree to which transporters control the distribution of drugs has become better appreciated with advances in this field, which can now explain the pharmacology of many compounds. For example, Pgp in the endothelial cells of brain capillaries is oriented to pump drug out of the cell and into the blood, thus limiting distribution of many drugs, chemicals, and toxins. Fexofenadine is a nonsedating antihistamine by virtue of the fact that it is a Pgp substrate and does not reach the central nervous system (CNS). First-generation antihistamines are not Pgp substrates, resulting in CNS exposure and sedation.[42] Although clinically significant drug interactions such as these are few, they can occur. Loperamide is an opiate antidiarrheal that has minimal CNS effects because Pgp prevents its distribution into the CNS. When it is combined with the Pgp inhibitor quinidine, however, CNS loperamide concentrations can reach levels that produce respiratory depression.[60]

Hepatic Metabolism

Cytochrome P-450. Pharmacokinetic interactions that involve changes in metabolism account for most therapeutically important drug interactions. As has already been reviewed, some metabolism occurs in the intestine. Other metabolic sites include the kidneys, the lungs, and the blood itself, but by and large, most metabolic activity occurs in the endoplasmic reticulum of hepatocytes in the liver.[35] The main enzymes responsible for drug metabolism are the CYP450 enzymes; of these, CYP1A2, 2C9, 2C19, 2D6, 2E1,

TABLE 3.5	Factors Influencing Cytochrome P-450 Enzymes[28,38]				
	1A2	**2C**	**2D6**	**2E1**	**3A4**
Nutrition	+			+	+
Smoking	+				
Alcohol		+		+	
Drugs	+	+	+	+	+
Environmental factors	+			+	+
Genetics	+	+			+

(Modified from Shapiro LE, Shear NH. Drug interactions: proteins, pumps, and P-450s. J Am Acad Dermatol 47:467–484, 2002, with permission.)

and 3A4 are most often involved in drug metabolism. Table 3.5 lists the factors that influence each of these enzyme systems.[28,38] Table 3.6 lists the substrates, inhibitors, and inducers for these enzyme systems.[28,33–36] Metabolic drug interactions occur when enzymes responsible for metabolism are inhibited or induced by another drug. The most common and important mechanism for drug interactions is inhibition, because of its potential to elevate drug levels, increase drug response, and cause toxicity.[36] Drug-induced inhibition occurs quickly, usually within hours after introduction of the inhibitor.[30] However, the full effect is concentration dependent and is determined by the half-life of the inhibitor. For example, fluoxetine, an inhibitor of CYP2D6, has a half-life of 4 to 6 days after long-term administration. Although inhibition of 2D6 will begin shortly after fluoxetine therapy starts, its full impact on 2D6, and on any drugs metabolized by this enzyme, will not be realized for approximately 1 month. On the other hand, quinidine, also a 2D6 inhibitor, has a half-life of 6 to 8 hours. Subsequently, the full effect of its interaction with a 2D6 substrate will be evident within 2 days. In the same way, the offset of an inhibition interaction will depend on the half-life of the inhibitor. Continuing with the fluoxetine example, it has been observed that inhibition interactions are possible for up to 4 to 6 weeks after the last dose is taken, which is the length of time it will take before fluoxetine levels are negligible.

Inhibition of drug metabolism occurs when a drug (the inhibitor) slows down the metabolic activity of the enzyme responsible for metabolism of a substrate drug. Inhibition can be reversible or irreversible, with the former being the more common process. Reversible inhibition occurs by one of three mechanisms: competitive inhibition (competition between the inhibitor and the substrate for the active site on the enzyme; this prevents substrate binding), noncompetitive inhibition (binding of the inhibitor with no effect on the binding of the substrate to the active site), or uncompetitive inhibition (binding of the inhibitor to the enzyme–substrate complex; this renders it ineffective).[33,36] Irreversible inhibition occurs when the perpetrator drug forms a reactive inter-

mediate with the enzyme that permanently inactivates the enzyme. Drug interactions that result from irreversible inhibition tend to be more profound than those caused by reversible inhibition.[33] Drugs known to cause irreversible inhibition interactions include erythromycin, diltiazem, paroxetine, and spironolactone.[28,33,36] Following irreversible inhibition, the return of normal enzyme activity is dependent on both the half-life of the perpetrator drug and the synthesis of new enzyme molecules.

The opposite of inhibition is induction, whereby the inducing drug boosts the synthesis of the enzyme(s) responsible for metabolism of the substrate drug. Mechanistically, the inducer usually does not interact directly with the enzyme itself. Instead, inducers bind to specific sites on the genes that regulate enzyme synthesis, called *nuclear receptors*; these stimulate gene transcription and enzyme production.[36] Similar to inhibition, enzyme induction is dose dependent. Thus, the onset of an induction interaction is gradual because it depends on accumulation of the inducer, as well as on new enzyme synthesis. Consequently, the full effect of the inducing drug may not be seen for several weeks after the inducer is introduced, in contrast to the impact of inhibition interactions, which may be fully evident within days.[28,35,36] The offset of induction interactions is also gradual because it depends upon the elimination of both the inducer and the metabolizing enzyme(s) until a return to the baseline rate of enzyme production is achieved. Less common mechanisms of enzyme induction include stabilization of the enzyme–substrate complex, processing of messenger RNA (mRNA), stabilization of mRNA, and increased translation.[33,36]

Induction interactions tend to be less prominent than inhibition interactions because elevated drug levels, and therefore drug toxicity, rarely occur. However, therapeutic failure from lowered plasma levels following enzyme induction is well documented and can be significant. For example, rifampin, a potent inducer of CYP3A4, can lower levels of the CYP3A4 and Pgp substrate cyclosporine, leading to acute organ graft rejection. Rifampin affects hepatic and intestinal 3A4, as well as intestinal Pgp. Consequently, rifampin interacts with cyclosporine by all three mechanisms—increased intestinal and hepatic metabolism and increased efflux via Pgp.

Amplified drug metabolism can also lead to increased production of active metabolites or toxic intermediates. For example, isoniazid is an inducer of CYP2E1 that causes increased production of a hepatotoxic metabolite of acetaminophen.[36]

First-Pass Effect. The first-pass effect describes the metabolism of a drug before it reaches the systemic circulation and is a key determinant of bioavailability. From the preceding discussions, it can be seen that the intestine and liver work coordinately to affect drug metabolism. Subsequently, the extent and rate of intestinal metabolism affect the extent and rate of hepatic metabolism. Notably, although these two

TABLE 3.6	Substrates, Inhibitors, and Inducers of the Major Cytochrome P-450 Enzymes[28,33–36,149,150]

Substrates	Inhibitors	Inducers	Substrates	Inhibitors	Inducers
1A2			**2C19**		
Amitriptyline	Amiodarone	Broccoli	Amitriptyline	Cimetidine	Carbamazepine
Caffeine	Cimetidine	Brussels sprouts	Carisoprodol	Felbamate	Norethindrone
Clomipramine	Ciprofloxacin	Charbroiled foods	Citalopram	Fluconazole	Prednisone
Clozapine	Clarithromycin	Modafinil	Clomipramine	Fluoxetine	Rifampin
Cyclobenzaprine	Erythromycin	Nafcillin	Cyclophosphamide	Fluvoxamine	
Desipramine	Fluvoxamine	Omeprazole	Diazepam	Indomethacin	
Estradiol	Ketoconazole	Phenobarbital	Imipramine	Ketoconazole	
Fluvoxamine	Methoxsalen	Phenytoin	Indomethacin	Lansoprazole	
Haloperidol	Norfloxacin	Ritonavir	Lansoprazole	Modafinil	
Imipramine	Paroxetine	Tobacco	R-Mephobarbital	Omeprazole	
Mexiletine	Ticlopidine		S-Mephenytoin	Paroxetine	
Naproxen			Moclobemide (investigational)	Probenecid	
Ondansetron			Nelfinavir	Ticlopidine	
Propranolol			Nilutamide	Topiramate	
Riluzole			Omeprazole	Voriconazole	
Ropivacaine			Pantoprazole		
Tacrine			Phenobarbital		
Theophylline			Phenytoin		
Verapamil			Primidone		
R-warfarin			Progesterone		
Zileuton			Proguanil		
Zolmitriptan			Propranolol		
			Teniposide		
2C9			Voriconazole		
Amitriptyline	Amiodarone	Carbamazepine	R-warfarin		
Celecoxib	Cimetidine	Ethanol	**2D6**		
Diclofenac	Fluconazole	Phenobarbital			
Fluoxetine	Fluvastatin	Rifampin	Amiodarone	Amiodarone	Dexamethasone
Fluvastatin	Fluvoxamine	Secobarbital	Amitriptyline	Amitriptyline	Rifampin
Glipizide	Isoniazid		Amphetamine	Bupropion	
Glyburide	Ketoconazole		Atomoxetine	Celecoxib	
Ibuprofen	Lovastatin		Captopril	Chlorpheniramine	
Irbesartan	Omeprazole		Carvedilol	Chlorpromazine	
Losartan	Paroxetine		Chlorpheniramine	Cimetidine	
Meloxicam	Phenylbutazone		Chlorpromazine	Clomipramine	
Phenytoin	Probenecid		Clomipramine	Cocaine	
Piroxicam	Ritonavir		Clozapine	Desipramine	
Rosiglitazone	Sertraline		Codeine	Doxepin	
Sulfonamides	Sulfamethoxazole		Desipramine	Doxorubicin	
Tamoxifen	Teniposide		Dexfenfluramine	Fluoxetine	
Tolbutamide	Trimethoprim		Dextromethorphan	Halofantrine	
Torsemide	Voriconazole		Diphenhydramine	Haloperidol	
Valproic acid	Zafirlukast		Encainide	Imatinib	
Vardenafil			Flecainide	Indinavir	
Voriconazole			Fluoxetine	Methadone	
S-warfarin					

(continued)

TABLE 3.6	continued

Substrates	Inhibitors	Inducers	Substrates	Inhibitors	Inducers
2D6 (continued)			**3A Family (3A4, 3A5, 3A7) (continued)**		
Fluvoxamine			Atorvastatin	Delavirdine	Modafinil
Haloperidol	Metoclopramide		Busulfan	Diltiazem	Nevirapine
Imipramine	Moclobemide (investigational)		Buspirone	Erythromycin	Phenobarbital
			Cafergot	Fluconazole	Phenytoin
Lidocaine	Nortriptyline		Caffeine	Fluoxetine	Pioglitazone
Maprotiline	Paroxetine		Carbamazepine	Fluvoxamine	Primidone
MDMA ("Ecstasy")	Propafenone		Cerivastatin	Gestodene	Rifabutin
	Quinidine		Chlorpheniramine	Grapefruit juice (intestinal)	Rifampin
Metoclopramide			Cisapride		Rifampin
S-Metoprolol	Ranitidine		Clarithromycin	Imatinib	St. John's wort
Mexiletine	Ritonavir		Cocaine	Indinavir	
Mianserin (investigational)	Sertraline		Codeine	Itraconazole	
	Terbinafine		Cyclophosphamide	Ketoconazole	
Norfluoxetine			Cyclosporine	Metronidazole	
Nortriptyline	Thioridazine		Dapsone	Mifepristone	
Ondansetron	Ticlopidine		Dextromethorphan	Nefazodone	
Oxycodone	Venlafaxine		Diazepam	Nelfinavir	
Paroxetine			Diltiazem	Nifedipine	
Perphenazine			Docetaxel	Norfloxacin	
Propafenone			Doxorubicin	Norfluoxetine	
Propranolol			Enalapril	Paroxetine	
Risperidone			Eplerenone	Quinine	
Tamoxifen			Erythromycin	Quinopristin/ dalfopristin	
Thioridazine			Estradiol		
Timolol			Ethosuximide	Ritonavir	
Trimipramine			Etoposide	Saquinavir	
Tramadol			Felodipine	Sertraline	
Venlafaxine			Fentanyl	Seville oranges (intestinal)	
			Fexofenadine		
2E1			Finasteride	Tacrolimus	
			Flutamide	Telithromycin	
Benzene	Disulfiram	Ethanol	Haloperidol	Verapamil	
Chlorzoxazone	Ethanol	Isoniazid	Hydrocortisone	Voriconazole	
Enflurane			Imatinib		
Ethanol			Indinavir		
Halothane			Irinotecan		
Isoflurane			Ifosfamide		
Methoxyflurane			Isradipine		
Sevoflurane			Lidocaine		
Theophylline			Losartan		
			Lovastatin		
3A Family (3A4, 3A5, 3A7)			Methadone		
			Midazolam		
Acetaminophen	Amiodarone	Carbamazepine	Nelfinavir		
Alfentanil	Atazanavir	Efavirenz	Nifedipine		
Alprazolam	Cannabinoids	Ethosuximide	Nisoldipine		
Amlodipine	Cimetidine	Glucocorticoids	Nitrendipine		
Amiodarone	Ciprofloxacin	Griseofulvin			
Atazanavir	Clarithromycin	Isoniazid			

(continued)

TABLE 3.6	continued		
Substrates		**Inhibitors**	**Inducers**
3A Family (3A4, 3A5, 3A7) (continued)			
Omeprazole	Sirolimus		
Ondansetron	Tacrolimus		
Oral contraceptives	Tadalafil		
Paclitaxel	Tamoxifen		
Pimozide	Telithromycin		
Progesterone	Testosterone		
Propafenone	Theophylline		
Propranolol	Trazodone		
Quinidine	Triazolam		
Quinine	Vardenafil		
Retinoic acid	Verapamil		
Rifampin	Vinblastine		
Ritonavir	Vincristine		
Salmeterol	Voriconazole		
Saquinavir	Warfarin		
Sildenafil	Zaleplon		
Simvastatin	Zolpidem		
	Zileuton		

MDMA, 3,4-methylenedioxymethamphetamine

organs work together, their metabolic capabilities are independently controlled and regulated.[37] Drug interactions that affect the cytochrome P-450 system and/or intestinal transporters like Pgp can alter the oral bioavailability of the target drug, either by increasing its first-pass metabolism (enzyme induction causing low bioavailability) or by lowering its first-pass metabolism (enzyme inhibition causing increased bioavailability).

Non–Cytochrome P-450 Metabolism—Phase I Reactions. Many other phase I enzymes are responsible for drug metabolism (Table 3.2). With the few exceptions outlined in Table 3.7, these are not major sources of drug interactions.[32,36,61–68] This is largely because many drugs do not use these enzymes as the sole vehicle for metabolism, there are far fewer known inhibitors and inducers for these enzymes, and many of the drugs metabolized by these proteins have a wide therapeutic index.

Non–Cytochrome P-450 Metabolism—Phase II Reactions. Phase II reactions are conjugations whereby a transferase attaches a polar molecule such as glucuronic acid, sulfate, or a methyl group to a drug to enhance its elimination. Generally speaking, the enzymes involved in phase II reactions, similar to those catalyzing non–cytochrome P-450 metabolism, are not a major source of drug interactions for many of the same reasons. As has previously been stated, most phase II reactions involve a product of phase I metabolism. Compared with phase I reactions, fewer drugs undergo a phase II reaction as the initial or primary metabolic route. There are some notable exceptions, however. For example, morphine, zidovudine, epinephrine, norepinephrine, hydralazine, isoniazid, and azathioprine are metabolized principally by phase II reactions (Tables 3.7 and 3.8).Of the phase II processes, glucuronidation via UDP-glucuronyltransferase (UDPGT) is the most common and most studied.[69,70] Analogous to the cytochrome P-450 enzymes, the UGTs are a superfamily of enzymes. More than 33 families of UDPGTs have been identified, and these are subdivided into families and subfamilies on the basis of amino acid sequence homology, similar to the cytochrome P-450 system. Nomenclature similar to that of the P-450 system has been adopted for the UGTs. Thus, just as CYP3A4 and CYP2D6 represent different enzymes in the same cytochrome family, UGT1A1 and UGT2B7 are different enzymes in the UGT family. Among the UGTs, the UGT1 and UGT2 families are the most important in human drug metabolism (Table 3.8). Similar to the CYP enzymes, some of the UGT enzymes, most notably, UGT1A1, 1A6, 2B4, 2B7, and 2B15, display polymorphism.[31] Table 3.8 lists the most important UGTs in terms of drug metabolism and their substrates and inducers. Many of the drugs that induce the CYP enzymes coinduce the UGT enzymes such as phenobarbital, phenytoin, and rifampin. Specific inhibitors of the UGT system have not been identified; however, any substrate for UDPGT has the potential for competitive inhibition of another substrate metabolized by the same enzyme. Many UGT drug interactions

TABLE 3.7	Substrates, Inhibitors, and Inducers of Non-Cytochrome P-450 Enzymes[31,32,62–68]			
Enzyme	**Substrates**	**Inhibitors**	**Inducers**	**Comment**
Phase I Transformation				
Aldehyde oxidase	Famciclovir Zaleplon Ziprasidone Zonisamide	Amitriptyline Chlorpromazine Cimetidine Clomipramine Estradiol Ethinyl estradiol Felodipine Menadione Nortriptyline Perphenazine Promethazine Raloxifene Thioridazine Trifluoperazine	Not determined	The only reported interaction is elevated zaleplon levels by cimetidine
Xanthine oxidase	Azathioprine 6-mercaptopurine	Allopurinol	Not determined	Allopurinol inhibits xanthine oxidase metabolism of 6-mercaptopurine (azathioprine is converted to 6-mercaptopurine in vivo), leading to severe hematologic toxicities
MAO-A	Almotriptan Rizatriptan Sumatriptan Zolmitriptan	Moclobemide (investigational) Propranolol	Not determined	Therapeutically relevant interactions have not been reported, although pharmacokinetic studies show that propranolol and moclobemide (a MAO-A inhibitor) can decrease the clearance and increase levels of many triptan drugs
Phase II Transformation				
GST	Azathioprine 6-mercaptopurine Nitroglycerin Organophosphates	Not determined	St. John's wort	
MT	Apomorphine Bitolterol Dobutamine Dopamine Epinephrine Isoproterenol Levodopa 6-mercaptopurine Norepinephrine Serotonin	Entacapone Olsalazine Sulfasalazine Tolcapone	Not determined	Few clinically important drug–drug interactions involving MT documented. Tolcapone and entacapone are used therapeutically with levodopa
NAT	Dapsone Hydralazine Isoniazid Phenelzine Procainamide	Not determined	Not determined	Clinically important drug–drug interactions involving NAT not reported. Genetic polymorphisms (slow acetylators vs. fast acetylators) important
ST	Acetaminophen Albuterol Terbutaline Methyldopa	Not determined	Glucocorticoids Phenobarbital Rifampin	

UGT: See Table 3.8.

MAO, monoamine oxidase; UGT, uridine diphosphate–glucuronyltransferases; ST, sulfotransferases; GST, glutathione S-transferase; NAT, N-acetyltransferase; MT, methyltransferase.

TABLE 3.8 | Substrates, Inhibitors, and Inducers of the Major UGT Enzymes[31,32,69,70,150]

Substrates	Inhibitors	Inducers	Substrates	Inhibitors	Inducers
1A1	Not determined	Clofibrate	**1A6**	Not determined	Dexamethasone
Atorvastatin		Dexamethasone	Acetaminophen		
Buprenorphine		Phenobarbital	Aspirin		
Carvedilol		Phenytoin	Ketoprofen		
Cerivastatin		Rifampin	Methylsalicylate		
Ethinyl estradiol		Ritonavir	Naproxen		
Etoposide					
Ezetimibe			**1A9**	Not determined	Phenobarbital
Gemfibrozil			Acetaminophen		Rifampin
Irinotecan			Clofibric acid		
Naltrexone			Dapsone		
Raloxifene			Diclofenac		
Simvastatin			Diflunisal		
Telmisartan			Entacapone		
			Ethinyl estradiol		
1A3	Not determined	Rifampin	Furosemide		
Amitriptyline			Ibuprofen		
Atorvastatin			Ketoprofen		
Buprenorphine			Labetalol		
Cerivastatin			Mefenamic acid		
Chlorpromazine			Mycophenolate		
Clofibrate			Naproxen		
Clozapine			R-oxazepam		
Cyproheptadine			Propranolol		
Diclofenac			Propofol		
Diflunisal			Retinoic acid		
Diphenhydramine			Tolcapone		
Doxepin					
Ezetimibe			**2B7**	Not determined	Phenobarbital
Fenoprofen			Buprenorphine		Phenytoin
Gemfibrozil			Carvedilol		Rifampin
Hydromorphone			Chloramphenicol		
Ibuprofen			Codeine		
Imipramine			Clofibric acid		
Ketoprofen			Cyclosporine		
Ketotifen			Epirubicin		
Losartan			Ezetimibe		
Loxapine			Fenoprofen		
Morphine			Hydromorphone		
Naloxone			Ibuprofen		
Naproxen			Ketoprofen		
Promethazine			Lorsartan		
Simvastatin			Morphine		
Valproic acid			Nalmefene		
			Naloxone		
1A4	Not determined	Carbamazepine	Naltrexone		
Amitriptyline		Methsuximide	S-naproxen		
Chlorpromazine		Oral contraceptives	Oxazepam		
Clozapine		Oxcarbazepine	Oxycodone		
Cyproheptadine		Phenobarbital	Oxymorphone		
Diphenhydramine		Phenytoin	Propranolol		
Doxepin		Primidone	Tacrolimus		
Imipramine		Rifampin	Temazepam		
Ketoprofen			Valproic acid		
Lamotrigine			Zidovudine		
Loxapine					
Olanzapine			**2B15**	Not determined	Phenobarbital
Promethazine			Dienestrol		
Trifluoperazine			Diethylstilbesterol		
Tripelennamine			Ezetimibe		

UGT, uridine diphosphate–glucuronyltransferases.

have been identified from in vitro and in vivo studies but have not been clinically validated. There are some exceptions, however. For example, the combination of lamotrigine and valproic acid has led to CNS toxicity in four cases.[71,72] Glucuronidation of lamotrigine was felt to be competitively inhibited by valproic acid, leading to elevated lamotrigine levels and neurotoxicity. A similar explanation has been offered for a case of coma following the combination of valproic acid and lorazepam,[73] and for a case of anemia following valproic acid and zidovudine.[74] Induction reactions with UGTs have also been reported, although again such reactions with clinical relevance are few.[75–77] As genetic and molecular research techniques improve, drug interactions involving all phase II enzymes will likely grow in clinical importance as well.

Elimination. With the exception of inhaled anesthetics, most drugs or drug metabolites are eliminated from the body via the urine or the bile. Other means of elimination are possible, for example, via sweat, saliva, or in the breast milk of nursing mothers. By and large, however, these are insignificant compared with the biliary and renal routes.

Renal Elimination. To review, blood enters the kidney via the renal artery, traveling first to the glomeruli. Pores in the glomerular membrane allow water, salts, and some drugs into the lumen of the tubules, while larger molecules and proteins such as albumin are retained. Blood flow then passes to the remaining portions of the kidney, where transport proteins can actively secrete endogenous substances, as well as drugs, into the tubular lumen. Tubular cells in the lumen also have the capacity for active and passive reabsorption of these substances. From this brief description, it can be seen that a drug interaction may occur at several points, namely, interference with the passive diffusion, active secretion, or active reabsorption of drugs.

Passive Diffusion. Drugs in the kidney tubule may be reabsorbed back into the plasma by passive diffusion. This process is optimal when the drug is in its nonionized form, that is, in its most lipid-soluble state. Thus, the pKa of the drug and the pH of the urine influence the extent of passive reabsorption that a drug undergoes. Weakly acidic drugs exposed to alkaline urine are in their most ionized state, have minimal reabsorption, and are excreted in the urine. The same holds true for weakly basic drugs in acidic urine. On the other hand, reabsorption is enhanced for acidic drugs in acidic urine and alkaline drugs in alkaline urine. Drugs that alter urinary pH may therefore influence renal elimination. For example, magnesium-containing antacids may elevate urine pH sufficiently to increase reabsorption of the basic antiarrhythmic drug quinidine, causing potentially toxic serum levels.[78] Similarly, aspirin effectiveness may be decreased by concurrent antacid use owing to enhanced elimination.[79] Despite these examples, drug interactions that result from changes in urinary pH are generally not clinically important. This is because most drugs undergo some metabolism before being eliminated in the urine. Also, many drugs that are excreted unchanged and may be affected by drug-induced

changes in urine pH have a wide therapeutic index, such that an elevated plasma level has a negligible clinical impact.

Active Transport. The renal proximal tubule is the primary site of active transport for a wide variety of substrates, including organic anions/cations, peptides, nucleosides, and drugs. Many drug transporters are responsible for both the active secretion and the reabsorption of drugs in the kidney; several of these proteins have been identified and characterized (Table 3.3). However, information on the substrates, inducers, and inhibitors of each transporter is still emerging. Drug interactions can arise from many of the mechanisms already described, including competitive inhibition between two or more drugs for the same transport protein, and induction or inhibition of transporter production or function. Inhibition of renal P-glycoprotein has been well researched, particularly with the Pgp substrate digoxin. Located at the brush border membrane of the nephron, Pgp drives hydrophobic substances, such as digoxin, into the renal proximal tubule, aiding in their elimination.[45] Blocking of the action of renal Pgp by known Pgp inhibitors such as clarithromycin, quinidine, itraconazole, and ritonavir decreases digoxin excretion into the proximal tubule and elevates plasma digoxin levels.[54,80–84] Some drug interactions can now be explained by the impact of the perpetrator drug on Pgp at multiple locations. Quinidine, for example, blocks intestinal Pgp, thus increasing oral digoxin bioavailability; it also inhibits renal Pgp, thus blocking renal elimination of digoxin and causing elevated plasma levels. One might anticipate that induction of renal Pgp may lead to enhanced renal elimination of Pgp substrates, although this has not yet been well documented.

Organic anion and cation transporters in the kidney are involved in several notable drug interactions. The organic anion transport (OAT) inhibitor probenecid, for example, blocks the tubular secretion of the OAT substrates ciprofloxacin, many penicillins and cephalosporins, zalcitabine, acyclovir, ganciclovir, methotrexate, and angiotensin-converting enzyme (ACE) inhibitors, causing increased plasma levels and drug exposure.[42,45,85,86] This interaction may be used to therapeutic benefit, as with coadministration of probenecid and a penicillin to increase plasma penicillin levels, or probenecid given with cidofovir to minimize cidofovir nephrotoxicity. However, significant toxicity may also occur from such interactions. Competitive inhibition between methotrexate and a nonsteroidal anti-inflammatory drug (NSAID) or a penicillin antibiotic for an OAT can produce elevated methotrexate levels and bone marrow suppression in patients receiving high-dose methotrexate therapy.[86]

Fewer drug interactions have been reported that involve organic cation transporter (OCT) proteins. However, cimetidine and triamterene are potent inhibitors of OCT that block the secretion of procainamide and its active metabolite N-acetylprocainamide (NAPA), potentially causing cardiac toxicity due to elevated procainamide and NAPA levels.[45]

Despite these noteworthy examples, clinically important interactions involving renal transport proteins remain relatively few. However, information on the specific substrates, inducers, and inhibitors of the numerous renal transport proteins thus far discovered is still emerging, and their role in drug interactions is yet to be fully appreciated.

Biliary Elimination. Hepatobiliary elimination is the primary means of elimination for many drugs and drug metabolites. Drugs in the blood enter hepatocytes by crossing the sinusoidal membrane. Within the hepatocyte, a drug may be transported to a metabolic site (e.g., the cytochrome P-450 system in the endoplasmic reticulum) or carried to the biliary canalicular membrane of the hepatocyte. Finally, a drug, its metabolite(s), or both cross the canalicular membrane into the bile for excretion in the feces or possibly for enterohepatic recirculation.[42] Each stage of this three-step process can occur by passive diffusion or active transport. Several of the transport proteins involved in each stage and their drug substrates have been identified (Table 3.3). The organic anion–transporting polypeptide (OATP) family plays a significant role in transport of substances across the sinusoidal membrane of the hepatocyte. Although the name suggests that substrates are limited to organic anions, in fact, this family of proteins has broad substrate specificity that includes both neutral and basic compounds. Drug substrates include digoxin, pravastatin, fexofenadine, and rocuronium, as well as many drug metabolites such as N-methylquinidine and estradiol glucuronide.[42,85] Among the several proteins that make up this family, OATP-C and OATP-8 are the most important and are linked to significant drug interactions. For example, cyclosporine, a known inhibitor of OATP-C, has been shown to increase rosuvastatin exposure by more than sevenfold in transplant recipients compared with historical controls not receiving cyclosporine.[87] Using an in vitro model, the same investigators established that rosuvastatin is an OATP-C substrate and proposed that cyclosporine inhibited the OATP-C–mediated transport of rosuvastatin across hepatocytes, leading to elevated drug levels. This is important clinically in that myopathy and rhabdomyolysis from statin drugs are in part concentration dependent. The interaction between cyclosporine and statin drugs is well documented and has previously been explained by cyclosporine-mediated inhibition of statin metabolism via CYP3A4 because many of these compounds are 3A4 substrates. Rosuvastatin, though, undergoes very little metabolism through the CYP2C9 pathway and is not significantly affected by CYP inhibitors such as cyclosporine, thus supporting that it is inhibition of OATP-C that is the cause of the interaction. Because other statins such as atorvastatin and cerivastatin are also OATP-C substrates, the interaction between these drugs and cyclosporine may involve inhibition of CYP3A4 metabolism, as well as OATP-C uptake.[88,89] The combination of gemfibrozil and a statin is also known to increase the risks of myopathy and rhabdomyolysis. A recent study found that gemfibrozil inhibited OATP-C–mediated uptake of rosuvastatin in vitro and caused a twofold elevation in plasma rosuvastatin exposure in healthy volunteers, suggest-

ing a possible role in gemfibrozil–statin interactions.[90] Although the antitubercular drugs rifampin and rifamycin SV are best known as enzyme inducers, they are also both inhibitors of human OATP-C and OATP-8 in vitro, and their role in drug interactions via this mechanism is being studied.[91]

Members of the ABC family of transporters, including P-glycoprotein, canalicular multispecific organic anion transporter (cMOAT), MRP1, and sister-Pgp, are the primary proteins involved in movement of substances across the canalicular membrane of the hepatocyte and into the bile. Canalicular Pgp substrates include cyclosporine, paclitaxel, vincristine, vinblastine, digoxin, loperamide, and doxorubicin.[42] In vitro studies have shown that Pgp inhibitors can decrease biliary excretion of drugs.[92] although therapeutically meaningful drug interactions via this mechanism have not been documented. Similar to the field of renal transport proteins, the study of hepatobiliary transport of drugs is still developing, as is an understanding of their role in drug interactions.

PHARMACODYNAMICS

Although most significant drug interactions involve a pharmacokinetic mechanism, numerous pharmacodynamic interactions are clinically important as well. Pharmacodynamic interactions can be divided into one of two mechanisms: synergistic and antagonistic.

Synergistic Interactions. Two drugs with similar pharmacologic profiles when taken together can produce a response greater than that of either drug alone. This can occur independent of changes to any pharmacokinetic parameter. This is an example of a synergistic (also called *additive*) pharmacodynamic interaction. For example, a patient taking amitriptyline for depression who is prescribed benztropine for Parkinson's disease may experience additive anticholinergic effects. These can manifest as severe constipation, dry mouth, worsening vision, or psychosis. The synergistic mechanism may not always be clear, however. For instance, the combination of an erectile dysfunction drug such as sildenafil, vardenafil, or tadalafil and a nitrate such as isosorbide mononitrate causes profound hypotension. The former drugs reverse erectile dysfunction by inhibiting phosphodiesterase type 5 (PDE5), which is responsible for the metabolism of cyclic guanosine monophosphate (cGMP). Although PDE5 is primarily located in the corpus cavernosum of the penis, it is also present in the systemic vasculature, where elevated cGMP causes vasodilation. Nitric oxide donors such as isosorbide mononitrate, nitroglycerin, or isosorbide dinitrate exert their vasodilatory effects by ultimately increasing cGMP levels. Because these two drug classes have additive effects on cGMP and blood pressure, the combination of a PDE5 inhibitor and any nitrate is contraindicated.[93–97]

Antagonistic Interactions. As the name implies, the end result of an antagonistic pharmacodynamic interaction is a degradation or blunting of the response to one or both interacting drugs. For example, corticosteroids can cause hyperglycemia, worsening blood glucose control for diabetic patients, which may require changes in insulin dosing. Similarly, the antidepressant mirtazapine has been reported to block α-receptors, causing loss of hypertensive control in patients taking clonidine.[98,99]

Frequently, a pharmacodynamic interaction may be difficult to detect and may be interpreted as loss of drug effect or worsening of disease. Take the case of a patient with Alzheimer dementia who is receiving treatment with the cholinesterase inhibitor donepezil and is prescribed the anticholinergic drug tolterodine for urinary incontinence.[100] Without a complete understanding of the pharmacodynamic principles, the patient's deteriorating mental state could simply be attributed to worsening Alzheimer's disease, instead of to the loss of cholinergic effect of donepezil caused by tolterodine, especially because this is a progressive illness. It is therefore essential that clinicians be vigilant for pharmacodynamic interactions and fully evaluate any change in patient symptoms or disease state after drug therapy is added or deleted.

THE NATURE OF DRUG INTERACTIONS

Up to this point, drug interactions have been discussed from a generally negative standpoint, highlighting the potential for toxicity or loss of efficacy that can occur. It is important to realize, however, that many drug interactions are beneficial and are used for therapeutic purposes. Numerous pharmacodynamic examples exist, such as combinations of antihypertensives to lower blood pressure; two or more antimicrobials to treat an infection; use of epinephrine with lidocaine to prolong local anesthesia; the combination of a statin drug such as atorvastatin with a fibrate, bile acid–binding resin, or ezetimibe to enhance cholesterol lowering; and the variety of hypoglycemic agents used in combination to manage type 2 diabetes. Antidotes such as naloxone and flumazenil are also examples of beneficial pharmacodynamic interactions. Generally speaking, examples of therapeutically used pharmacokinetic drug interactions are fewer than pharmacodynamic ones. The already mentioned interaction of probenecid with penicillin to elevate serum penicillin levels is one well-known case. Ketoconazole and diltiazem have been used in combination with both cyclosporine and tacrolimus to elevate serum levels of these immunosuppressants, subsequently requiring lower doses to maintain therapeutic levels and reduce treatment costs.[101–103] Notably, these interactions involve inhibition of both CYP3A4 and intestinal Pgp. Significant research is being devoted to identifying and developing inhibitors of many of the transport proteins to enhance drug therapy, especially Pgp. Pgp inhibitors may improve the response of tumor cells to chemotherapy[104]; enhance CNS penetration of protease inhibitors in HIV treatment[105]; and improve response to anticonvulsants in refractory epilepsy.[106,107] Additionally, development of Pgp modulators to improve oral bioavailability is being actively pursued.[44]

FOOD–DRUG INTERACTIONS

Food–drug interactions are extensive and in some ways more complex than drug–drug interactions. The presence or absence of food, the composition of the meal and its size, the formulation of the drug, and even the age of the patient all factor into food–drug interactions. Moreover, not only must the impact of food and diet on a drug be considered, but the effect of a drug on diet and nutrition must be evaluated as well. For example, any drug that induces nausea or vomiting can influence oral intake and the nutritional state of the patient. Antineoplastic drugs are among the most notorious emetogenic agents, and many also severely affect the gastric mucosa, which alters the absorptive processes of foods and nutrients. Drugs that affect taste, such as metronidazole, captopril, or penicillamine, may cause decreased appetite, decreased oral intake, and poor nutrition. Vitamins and minerals that are dependent upon an acidic environment for absorption can be affected by proton pump inhibitors, H_2-receptor blockers, and antacids, leading to deficiencies. Hypertriglyceridemia from propofol, parenteral nutrition, cyclosporine, or tacrolimus is well known. Last, numerous drugs cause electrolyte losses, including diuretics, many antineoplastics, laxatives, and antimicrobials. Clearly, the impact of drugs on nutrition should not be overlooked.[5,108]

The impact of food on drugs may be pharmacokinetic or pharmacodynamic in nature, with the former being the most common. Table 3.9 lists significant examples of both and the mechanisms involved.[3,109,110] As with drug–drug interactions, the clinical importance of a food–drug interaction is determined by the magnitude of the interaction and the therapeutic index of the drug.

The most important pharmacokinetic food–drug interactions are those that alter the absorption of a drug. This may occur through one of the mechanisms previously described for drug–drug interactions, namely, chelation, adsorption, changes in gastric pH, altered GI motility, altered gut metabolism, or altered transport across the gastric mucosa.

How food influences drug absorption is not easily predicted. The presence of food in the GI tract can increase, decrease, or have no effect on the absorption of a drug. Food stimulates gastric acid secretion, thus reducing gastric pH, increases gastric emptying, and slows small intestine transit time, any of which may affect drug solubility and/or absorption.[111] The protease inhibitor saquinavir, for instance, has negligible absorption when taken on an empty stomach, which can lead to therapeutic failure. Taken with food, however, its bioavailability increases by 600% to 1,800%. Furthermore, a heavy meal increases bioavailability to a greater extent than does a light meal. Meal composition can change drug bioavailability. A high-fat meal significantly reduces the absorption of the protease inhibitor indinavir compared with the fasting state, but a low-fat meal has no major effect

TABLE 3.9	Examples of Significant Food–Drug Interactions[3-5,109-111]		
Food	Drug(s)	Mechanism	Effect
Pharmacokinetic Interactions			
Dairy products Nutritional supplements (e.g., Boost) Calcium-fortified drinks Fortified cereals	Quinolone antibiotics Tetracycline antibiotics	Chelation	Decreased absorption and lower blood and tissue levels
High-fiber foods	Digoxin Antidepressants	Adsorption	Decreased absorption and lower blood and tissue levels
Any food	Alendronate Risedronate Penicillamine	Chelation	Decreased absorption and loss of therapeutic effect
Enteral feeds	Phenytoin Ciprofloxacin Warfarin	Chelation	Decreased absorption and loss of therapeutic effect
Any food	Azithromycin capsules Didanosine Erythromycin enteric coated	Increased degradation from lowered pH	Decreased absorption with therapeutic failure
Grapefruit juice	Multiple drugs (see Table 3.10)	Inhibition of intestinal CYP3A4 metabolism Inhibition of OATP	Improved oral bioavailability from 3A4 inhibition Decreased oral bioavailability from OATP inhibition
Pharmacodynamic Interactions			
Vitamin K–rich foods (spinach, kale, Brussels sprouts, broccoli) Green tea Canola, soy oils	Warfarin	Loss of anticoagulant effect	Vitamin K antagonizes the anticoagulant effect of warfarin
Tyramine-containing foods (aged cheeses, avocado, banana, liver, Chianti wine)	MAO inhibitors (phenelzine, tranylcypromine, isoniazid, linezolid)	Pressor effect causing potentially serious hypertension	Inhibition of gut and liver monoamine oxidase prevents metabolism of tyramine, a pressor-like substance
Caffeinated beverages (tea, coffee, soft drinks)	Sedatives, hypnotics	Loss of sedative effect	Antagonism of pharmacologic effect
Potassium salt substitutes	ACE inhibitors Angiotensin receptor blockers	Hyperkalemia	Additive effect with potassium-retaining properties of these drugs
Potassium-rich foods	Potassium-sparing diuretics		
Salt	Lithium	Fluctuating lithium levels	Lithium is reabsorbed from the kidney after a low-salt diet, and excretion is enhanced following high salt intake

OATP, organic anilon-transporting polypeptide; ACE, angiotensin converting enzyme; MAO, monoamine oxidase.

on its absorption.[112] Drug dosage form can also be important in determining the effect of food. Azithromycin capsules should be taken 1 hour before or 2 hours after a meal because food significantly lowers its bioavailability; azithromycin tablets and suspension may be taken without regard to a meal.[113] Given the unpredictability of the effects of food on

medicines, it is essential that clinicians avoid generalizations and instead review prescribing information and pertinent pharmacokinetic literature, especially for new drugs and dosage forms.

Foods that affect distribution, metabolism, and elimination of drugs are uncommon and usually are not clinically significant, with some notable exceptions. Cruciferous vegetables such as cabbage, broccoli, and Brussels sprouts induce CYP1A2, as do charbroiled or smoked foods.[109] Consequently, significant increases or decreases in the consumption of these foods may affect CYP1A2 substrates.

The most important metabolic food–drug interaction is the so-called ''grape juice'' effect. First reported in 1991, a single glass of grapefruit juice was found to cause a twofold to threefold increase in the plasma concentration of the oral calcium channel blocker felodipine.[114] Since that time, numerous drugs have been found to have significantly improved bioavailability when given with grapefruit juice.[115] Among several ingredients, grapefruit juice contains bergamottin and 6'7'-dihydroxybergamottin, furanocoumarins that selectively inhibit intestinal CYP3A4 but have little effect on hepatic 3A4.[116] Subsequently, drugs with poor oral availability due to significant first-pass metabolism in the gut tend to be substrates for grapefruit juice (Table 3.10). Furanocoumarins inhibit intestinal 3A4 by three mechanisms: competitive inhibition, irreversible inhibition, and actual loss of 3A4 through degradation of the enzyme.[117] These effects can occur after a single glass of grapefruit juice and can last for up to 3 days.[118] With the exception of Seville (sour) oranges, other citrus fruits do not appear to affect intestinal CYP3A4.[119]

Besides inhibiting intestinal 3A4, grapefruit juice appears to affect transport proteins. The effect of grapefruit juice on Pgp has been studied extensively with conflicting conclusions.[119–121] Although it seems clear that bergamottin and 6'7'-dihydroxybergamottin do not inhibit Pgp, it has not yet been determined whether other as yet unidentified components may have this effect. Recent evidence suggests that grapefruit juice and 6'7'-dihydroxybergamottin inhibit OATPs, which on the luminal side of cells in the GI mucosa actively transport substances from the lumen into the cell, that is, in the opposite direction to Pgp.[122] One study reported that grapefruit juice and 6'7'-dihydroxybergamottin significantly reduced intestinal absorption of the OATP substrate fexofenadine. Orange juice and apple juice were found to have similar effects.[123] Further research on the role of these juices in OATP and the potential for food–drug interactions is under way.

The clinical relevance of grapefruit juice–drug interactions has been disputed. Although adverse events have been reported [one review examining cases up to 2002 found 36 such reports to the US Food and Drug Administration (FDA)[23]], such occurrences are by and large uncommon for two reasons. First, with few exceptions, most of the drugs affected by grapefruit juice have a large therapeutic index. Second, the extent of the response to grapefruit juice depends upon an individual's intestinal CYP3A4 activity. Those with low 3A4 activity have relatively high exposure to a substrate drug before they ingest grapefruit juice. Following ingestion, there is little 3A4 activity to inhibit, and drug exposure is not likely to change significantly. Those with the highest 3A4 activity will experience the greatest degree of inhibition and the largest increase in drug exposure of the victim drug

TABLE 3.10	Drugs Affected by Grapefruit Juice[37,115,120]
Drug	**Effect on Absorption**
Albendazole	Increase
Alprazolam	Increase
Amiodarone	Increase
Atorvastatin	Increase
Buspirone	Increase
Carbamazepine	Increase
Carvedilol	Increase
Cisapride (no longer marketed)	Increase
Cyclosporine	Increase
Dextromethorphan	Increase
Diazepam	Increase (theoretical)
Diltiazem	Increase
Erythromycin	Increase
Ethinyl estradiol	Increase
Etoposide	Decrease
Felodipine	Increase
Fexofenadine	Decreased
Fluoxetine	Increase
Fluvoxamine	Increase
Halofantrine	Increase
Indinavir	Decrease
Itraconazole	Decrease
Lovastatin	Increase
Methylprednisolone	Increase
Midazolam	Increase
Nicardipine	Increase
Nifedipine	Increase
Nimodipine	Increase
Nisoldipine	Increase
Praziquantel	Increase
Quinidine	Increase
Saquinavir	Increase
Scopolamine	Increase
Sertraline	Increase
Sildenafil	Increase
Simvastatin	Increase
Sirolimus	Increase
Tacrolimus	Increase
Tadalafil	Increase (theoretical)
Terfenadine (no longer marketed)	Increase
Theophylline	Decrease
Triazolam	Increase
Vardenafil	Increase (theoretical)
Verapamil	Increase

and are more likely to experience an important clinical effect.[117] Other factors to be considered are the timing of the ingestion relative to drug administration, the amount of grapefruit juice ingested, and the variable furanocoumarin content of differing grapefruit juice preparations.[28] Nevertheless, given the potential for interactions, it may be prudent to err on the side of caution and suggest to patients that grapefruit juice be avoided, especially in those patients who may have risk factors that predispose them to drug interactions.

RECREATIONAL DRUGS AND DRUG INTERACTIONS

Recreational drugs, including ethanol, tobacco, MDMA ("Ecstasy"), cocaine, and marijuana, can have both pharmacokinetic and pharmacodynamic interactions with medicines. Ethanol and tobacco interactions are the best documented and the most studied of these. A complete review of this topic is beyond the scope of this chapter. Interested readers are referred to more detailed references for additional information.[6,7,124–126]

ALTERNATIVE MEDICINE–DRUG INTERACTIONS

The use of herbs, dietary supplements, nutraceuticals, phytochemicals, natural substances, megadose vitamins, and so forth (collectively referred to hereafter as *alternative medicines*, or *AM*), has been steadily increasing. A survey in 1993 found that one in three Americans used some form of alternative medicine and 14% used herbs.[127] A follow-up survey conducted 6 years later found that the percentage of AM users was over 40%, and that 18% of adults used herbs regularly.[128] Sales of alternative medicines increased from $8.8 billion in 1994 to $15.7 billion in 2000.[8] Given their widespread use, as well as the more recent introduction of beverages and foods fortified with "natural" substances (e.g., energy drinks with ginkgo, ginseng, guarana, caffeine), interactions with mainstream or traditional medicines have been widely reported and seem to be increasing.[129] These interactions occur through the same pharmacokinetic and pharmacodynamic principles already reviewed. Although most interactions are modest at best, some may be significant with potentially serious consequences. These tend to be pharmacokinetic in nature and involve inhibition or induction of metabolic or transport systems. As an example, the herb St. John's wort (*Hypericum perforatum*), which is commonly used for depression, has been found to be a potent inducer of CYP3A4 (intestinal to a greater extent than hepatic), CYP1A2, and intestinal P-glycoprotein.[130–133] Preliminary studies also suggest that it is an inducer of UGT1A and glutathione S-transferase.[131] Documented important interactions with St. John's wort include reduced serum levels of digoxin, oral contraceptives, warfarin, cyclosporine, tacrolimus, theophylline, phenytoin, carbamazepine, phenobarbital, and HIV protease inhibitors.[8,133,134] Cases of breakthrough bleeding and unintended pregnancy from presumed contraceptive failure in women using birth control pills and St. John's wort have been reported.[133] The interaction between protease inhibitors and St. John's wort is so significant, and the potential for therapeutic failure so great, that the FDA issued a Public Health Advisory warning against their combined use, and also advised against using St. John's wort with nonnucleoside reverse transcriptase inhibitors.[135] Additionally, there are reports of serotonin syndrome from the combination of St. John's wort and serotonin reuptake inhibitors and the triptan antimigraine drugs—examples of pharmacodynamic interactions.[133] Additional alternative medicines that may have significant interaction potential include ginkgo (inhibition of CYP2C9), ginseng (induction of CYP2C9), ipriflavone (inhibition of CYP1A2), ephedra (additive adrenergic effect, now unavailable in the United States), Cat's claw, chamomile, goldenseed (all inhibition of CYP3A4), Echinacea (inhibition of CYP3A4 and CYP1A2), and garlic (inhibition of platelet aggregation). Readers are referred to detailed reviews for more in-depth information on such alternative medicine–drug interactions.[8,136–140]

Despite the apparent potential that exists, the true occurrence of clinically meaningful AM–drug interactions is unknown and has not been extensively investigated. One study, however, suggests that the risks of a severe interaction are small. A review of two outpatient veteran populations found that 197 (43%) of patients surveyed were taking at least one dietary supplement. Among these, an interaction of any significance between the dietary supplement and a traditional medicine was found in 89 (45%) subjects; of this subset, only 5 (6%) were potentially severe.[141]

At first glance, AM–drug interactions may seem straightforward. In fact, this area of study and research is far more complex than that of drug–drug interactions for several reasons. First, drug–drug interactions generally deal with single-ingredient products that are standardized with respect to the concentration of the active ingredient. Mainstream medicines are also generally "pure," that is they are produced under controlled conditions at facilities that meet government manufacturing standards and do not contain unlabeled chemically active substances. By contrast, alternative medicines commonly contain several active ingredients, any of which either singly or in combination may contribute to the product's pharmacologic effects and drug interactions. St. John's wort has at least 9 groups of compounds that add to its pharmacologic activity, many of which have not been fully characterized. One of the active constituents, hypericin, is responsible for induction of CYP1A2, and another, hyperforin, induces 3A4.[133] Second, there can be tremendous variability in the quality and potency of alternative medicines between manufacturers of the same product, and remarkable lot-to-lot variations within the same manufacturer have been reported.[117] Third, there have been several reports of "natural'' products that have been adulterated or contaminated with known pharmacologic substances such as indomethacin, caffeine, corticosteroids, and diuretics—an occurrence that has been noted with some fortified beverages as well.[136,142] Taken together, these problems make the interpretation of drug interaction studies and case reports difficult. This points to another deficiency involving alternative medicines: the lack of carefully conducted and designed trials to support therapeutic claims and investigate drug interaction potential. The Dietary Supplement Health and Education Act (DSHEA), passed in 1994, removed natural products from stringent FDA oversight. Consequently, in contrast to traditional medicines, natural product manufacturers are not required to demonstrate human safety or efficacy before they reach market, or to conduct any studies to establish drug interactions. A survey of leading pharmaceutical/herbal companies conducted in 2003 sought to assess the importance these firms place on conducting drug interaction research. Only 35% of the companies surveyed responded to the questionnaire. Although 67% of respondents considered herb–drug interactions to be an important concern, only 20% of this subset conducted studies to examine this issue, and only 13% regularly devoted funds for such research.[143] Furthermore, the DSHEA does not require manufacturers to follow strict manufacturing guidelines or to provide product labeling that fully discloses ingredients (active and inactive) or known or potential drug interactions. Should a natural product be suspected of significant public harm, for example from a drug interaction, the burden of proof is on the FDA to demonstrate this risk before the product can be removed from the market. Such action was taken when the FDA prohibited the sale of ephedra-containing products in the United States in 2004 after several deaths were reported.[144] Notably, this is the opposite of mainstream medicine, wherein manufacturers are required to demonstrate that their products are effective and safe before use and during marketing.[141] As already stated, many of the drugs taken off the US market were removed because of significant drug interactions. The above factors, taken as a whole, clearly indicate that assessing a drug regimen that includes one or more alternative medicines for drug interactions can be perilous. A statement published by the American Society of Health-System Pharmacists provides guidance on the use of alternative medicines in the hospital setting and can be used as a basis for establishing institutional guidelines on complementary and alternative medicines in general.[129]

IMPROVING OUTCOMES FROM DRUG INTERACTIONS

It should be clear by now that the *potential* for drug interactions is large. It must be borne in mind, however, that most interactions that do occur do not result in a severe outcome. Nevertheless, the clinician has a responsibility to optimize patient drug therapy and minimize all risks associated with that therapy. It should also be clear that no person can possibly keep abreast of all drug interactions; as has been stated, the number of drug combinations for a patient taking only five of the more than 3,500 currently marketed US drugs is unimaginably large (5.2×10^{17}).[11] The number of possible drug interactions is equally staggering.

Certainly, computerization for screening of drug interactions can help clinicians deal with this information overload. However, the inadequacies of such programs have been well documented.[145] These systems often include so many interactions of all levels of importance that users are desensitized to the alerts and simply ignore or override the warnings (''alert fatigue'').[145,146] Computer programs often attribute interactions to a class of drugs, rather than to individual members of the drug class, which is clearly inappropriate for many medicines. For example, among the H_2-receptor blockers, cimetidine interacts to a far greater degree than does ranitidine, famotidine, or nizatidine. Among the macrolide antibiotics, erythromycin has a greater interaction potential than does clarithromycin, and both have more interaction potential than either azithromycin or dirithromycin. Other shortcomings of drug interaction software include use of inadequate systems to classify drug interactions, use of literature that has not been evaluated or reviewed as the basis of warnings, and failure to include alternative medicines as part of the screening process.[145,147] These issues are slowly being addressed, but it will take time for an acceptable program to be developed. Even if drug interaction software is created that addresses all of these issues, clinical judgment cannot be abrogated. A computer cannot take into account the myriad factors that must be considered when an *individual's* risk of interaction is assessed, such as drug dose, dosage form, route of administration, duration of administration, concurrent disease states, pharmacogenetics, and so forth.

So, how can drug interactions best be minimized?[2,145,147,148]

KEY POINTS

■ Evaluate drug interaction risk on a patient-specific basis

■ Use computerized drug interaction programs as a screening tool only

■ Use additional sources of drug interaction information to supplement the program

■ Develop and regularly update a list of ''red flag'' drugs made up of highly potent inducers and inhibitors, as well as narrow therapeutic index drugs

■ Ask patients about all medicines—traditional, over-the-counter, and alternative—before you start any new medicines. Questioning specifically about alternative medicines is especially important because many patients are reluctant to freely offer such information. Many patients are also under the misconception that alternative medicines are ''weak'' and will not interact with traditional drugs; that alternative medicines are free of adverse effects because they are ''natural,'' or ''they must be safe or they would be regulated''; or that alternative medicines are not medicines at all. Education is critical to these patients

■ Offer noninteracting alternatives to victim or perpetrator drugs whenever possible

■ If noninteracting alternatives are unavailable, use low-risk perpetrator drugs and/or find a victim drug with parallel metabolic pathways

■ If interacting drugs must be used concomitantly, take steps to mitigate the interaction, such as staggering administration times or changing dosage forms

■ Monitor the patient if it appears that the chance of interaction is high and the outcome is likely to be clinically meaningful

■ Look at any sudden change in patient status as a potential result of a drug interaction, and investigate. Remember that starting *or* stopping a perpetrator drug can affect a victim drug and patient status

■ Educate other clinicians and patients about the risks of drug interactions and what signs and symptoms to watch out for

SUGGESTED READINGS

Bjornsson TD, Callaghan JT, Einolf HJ, et al. The conduct of in vitro and in vivo drug-drug interaction studies: a PhRMA perspective. Clin Pharmacol Ther 43:443–469, 2003.

Huang SM, Lesko LJ. Drug-drug, drug-dietary supplement, and drug-citrus fruit and other food interactions: what have we learned? J Clin Pharmacol 44:559–569, 2004.

Lee W, Kim RB. Transporters and renal drug elimination. Ann Rev Pharmacol Toxicol 44:137–166, 2004.

Obach RS. Drug-drug interactions: an important negative attribute in drugs. Drugs Today 39:301–338, 2003.

Schmidt LE, Dalhoff K. Food-drug interactions. Drugs 62:1481–1502, 2002.

Shapiro LE, Shear NH. Drug interactions: proteins, pumps, and P-450s. J Am Acad Dermatol 47:467–484, 2002.

REFERENCES

1. Tatro DS, ed. Drug interaction facts. St. Louis, Mo: Facts and Comparisons, 2004.
2. Preskorn SH, Flockart DF. 2004 guide to psychiatric drug interactions. Prim Psychiatry 11:39–60, 2004.
3. Schmidt LE, Dalhoff K. Food-drug interactions. Drugs 62: 1481–1502, 2002.
4. Au Yeung SCS, Ensom MHH. Phenytoin and enteral feedings: does evidence support an interaction? Ann Pharmacother 34: 896–905, 2000.
5. Lourenco R. Enteral feeding: drug/nutrient interaction. Clin Nutr 20:187–193, 2001.
6. Matilla MJ. Alcohol and drug interactions. Ann Med 2:363–369, 1990.
7. Shoaf SE, Linnolia M. Interaction of ethanol and smoking on the pharmacokinetics and pharmacodynamics of psychotropic medications. Psychopharmacol Bull 27:577–594, 1991.
8. Scott GN, Elmer GW. Update on natural product-drug interactions. Am J Health Syst Pharm 59:339–347, 2002.
9. Trissel LA. Handbook on injectable drugs. 13th ed. Bethesda, Md: American Society of Health-System Pharmacists, 2004.
10. Tietz NW, ed. Clinical guide to laboratory tests. 3rd ed. Philadelphia, Pa: WB Saunders, 1995.
11. Preskorn SH. How drug-drug interactions can impact managed care. Am J Manag Care 10 (Suppl):S186–S198, 2004.
12. Kaufman DW, Kelly JP, Rosenberg L, et al. Recent patterns of medication use in the ambulatory adult population of the United States. JAMA 287:337–344, 2002.
13. Boston Collaborative Drug Surveillance Program. Adverse drug interactions. JAMA 220:1238–1239, 1972.
14. Jankel CA, Fitterman LK. Epidemiology of drug-drug interactions as a cause of hospital admissions. Drug Saf 9:51–59, 1993.
15. Stanton LA, Peterson GM, Rumble RH, et al. Drug-related admissions to an Australian hospital. J Clin Pharm Ther 19:341–347, 1994.
16. Classen DC, Pestotnik SL, Evans RS, et al. Adverse drug events in hospitalized patients. JAMA 277:301–306, 1997.
17. Kanjanarat P, Winterstein AG, Johns TE, et al. Nature of preventable adverse drug events in hospitals: a literature review. Am J Health Syst Pharm 60:1750–1759, 2003.
18. Mamun K, Lien CT, Goh-Tan CY, et al. Polypharmacy and inappropriate medication use in Singapore nursing homes. Ann Acad Med Singapore 33:49–52, 2004.
19. Jankel CA, Speedie SM. Detecting drug interactions: a review of the literature. DICP 24:982–989, 1990.
20. Peng CC, Glassman PA, Marks IR. Retrospective drug utilization review: incidence of clinically relevant drug-drug interactions in a large ambulatory population. J Manag Care Pharm 9:513–522, 2003.
21. Marcellino K, Kelly WN. Potential risks and prevention, part 3: drug-induced threats to life. Am J Health Syst Pharm 58: 1399–1405, 2001.
22. Jankel CA, McMillan JA, Martin BC. Effect of drug interactions on outcomes of patients receiving warfarin or theophylline. Am J Hosp Pharm 5:661–666, 1994.
23. Huang SM, Lesko LJ. Drug-drug, drug-dietary supplement, and drug-citrus fruit and other food interactions: what have we learned? J Clin Pharmacol 44:559–569, 2004.
24. Goldberg RM, Mabee J, Chan L, et al. Drug-drug and drug-disease interactions in the ED: analysis of a high-risk population. Am J Emerg Med 14:447–450, 1996.
25. Trujillo TC, Nolan PE. Antiarrhythmic agents. Drug interactions of clinical significance. Drug Saf 23:509–532, 2000.
26. Costa AJ. Potential drug interactions in an ambulatory geriatric population. Fam Pract 8:234–236, 1991.
27. Gorski JC, Jones DR, Hachner-Daniels BD. The contribution of intestinal and hepatic CYP3A4 to the interaction between midazolam and clarithromycin. Clin Pharmacol Ther 64:133–143, 1998.
28. Shapiro LE, Shear NH. Drug interactions: proteins, pumps, and P-450s. J Am Acad Dermatol 47:467–484, 2002.
29. McCabe BJ. Prevention of food-drug interactions with a special emphasis on older adults. Curr Opin Clin Nutr Metabol Care 7:21–26, 2004.
30. Brown CH. Overview of drug interactions—Part 1. US Pharmacist 25:HS3–HS30, 2000.
31. Bjornsson TD, Callaghan JT, Einolf HJ, et al. The conduct of in vitro and in vivo drug-drug interaction studies: a PhRMA perspective. Clin Pharmacol Ther 43:443–469, 2003.
32. Obach RS, Huynh P, Allen MC, et al. Human liver aldehyde oxidase: inhibition by 239 drugs. J Clin Pharmacol 44:7–19, 2004.
33. Obach RS. Drug-drug interactions: an important negative attribute in drugs. Drugs Today 39:301–338, 2003.
34. Graham AS. Cytochrome P450 drug interactions. RX Consultant 8: 1–7, 1999.
35. Brown CH. Overview of drug interactions modulated by cytochrome P450—Part 3. US Pharmacist 26:HS3–HS13, 2001.
36. Weaver RJ. Assessment of drug-drug interactions: concepts and approaches. Xenobiotica 31:499–538, 2001.
37. Doherty MM, Charman WN. The mucosa of the small intestine. How clinically relevant as an organ of drug metabolism? Clin Pharmacokinet 41:235–253, 2002.
38. Ma MK, Woo MH, McLeod HL. Genetic basis of drug metabolism. Am J Health Syst Pharm 59:2061–2069, 2002.

39. Ma JD, Nafziger AN, Bertino LS. Genetic polymorphisms of cytochrome P450 enzymes and the effect on interindividual pharmacokinetic variability in extensive metabolizers. J Clin Pharmacol 44: 447–456, 2004.

40. Ando Y, Saka H, Ando M, et al. Polymorphisms of UDP-glucuronyltransferase gene and irinotecan toxicity: a pharmacogenetic analysis. Cancer Res 60:6921–6926, 2000.

41. Strattera® (atomoxetine HCl) prescribing information. Indianapolis, Ind: Eli Lilly, September 2003.

42. Ayrton A, Morgan P. Role of transport proteins in drug absorption, distribution and excretion. Xenobiotica 31:469–497, 2001.

43. Schinkel AH, Jonker JW. Mammalian drug efflux transporters of the ATP binding cassette (ABC) family: an overview. Adv Drug Deliv Rev 55:3–29, 2003.

44. Wagner D, Spahn-Langguth H, Hanafy A, et al. Intestinal drug efflux: formulation and food effects. Adv Drug Deliv Rev 50: S13–S31, 2001.

45. Inui K, Masuda S, Saito H. Cellular and molecular aspects of drug transport in the kidney. Kidney Int 58:944–958, 2000.

46. Kim RB. Organic anion-transporting polypeptide (OATP) transporter family and drug disposition. Eur J Clin Invest 33 (Suppl 2): 1–5, 2003.

47. You G. The role of organic ion transporters in drug disposition: an update. Curr Drug Metab 5:55–62, 2004.

48. Kunta JR, Sinko PJ. Intestinal drug transporters: in vivo function and clinical importance. Curr Drug Metab 5:109–124, 2004.

49. Wu X, Huang W, Ganapathy, et al. Structure, function, and regional distribution of the organic cation transporter OCT3 in the kidney. Am J Physiol Renal Physiol 279:F449–F458, 2000.

50. Kool M, Van der Linden M, de Haas, et al. MRP3, an organic anion transporter able to transport anti-cancer drugs. Proc Natl Acad Sci USA 96:6914–6919, 1999.

51. Sampath J, Adachi M, Haste S, et al. Role of MRP4 and MRP5 in biology and chemotherapy. AAPS pharmSci 2002; 4 (article 14). Available at: http://www.aapspharmsci.org. Accessed July 30, 2004.

52. Lee W, Kim RB. Transporters and renal drug elimination. Ann Rev Pharmacol Toxicol 44:137–166, 2004.

53. Mangravite LM, Badagnani I, Giacomini KM. Nucleoside transporters in the disposition and targeting of nucleoside analogs in the kidney. Eur J Pharmacol 31:269–281, 2003.

54. Tanigawara Y. Role of P-glycoprotein in drug disposition. Ther Drug Monit 22:137–141, 2000.

55. Sun J, He ZG, Cheng G. Multidrug resistance P-glycoprotein: crucial significance in drug disposition and interaction. Med Sci Monitor 10:RA5–RA14, 2004. Available online at: www.Medscimonit.com. Accessed June 2, 2004.

56. Synold TW, Dussault I, Forman BM. The orphan nuclear receptor SXR coordinately regulates drug metabolism and efflux. Nat Med 7:584–590, 2001.

57. Cummins CL, Jacobsen W, Benet LZ. Unmasking the dynamic interplay between intestinal P-glycoprotein and CYP3A4. J Pharmacol Exp Ther 300:1036–1045, 2002.

58. Gilman AG, Rall TW, Nies AS, et al, eds. Goodman and Gilman's the pharmacological basis of therapeutics. 8th ed. New York, NY: McGraw-Hill, 1993:71.

59. Benet LZ, Hoener BA. Changes in plasma protein binding have little clinical relevance. Clin Pharmacol Ther 71:115–121, 2002.

60. Sadeque AJ, Wandel C, He H, et al. Increased drug delivery to the brain by P-glycoprotein inhibition. Clin Pharmacol Ther 68: 231–237, 2000.

61. Sonata® (zaleplon) Capsules prescribing information. Bristol, Tenn: King Pharmaceuticals Inc, October 2002.

62. Kennedy DT, Hayney MS, Lake KD. Azathioprine and allopurinol: the price of an avoidable drug interaction. Ann Pharmacother 30: 951–954, 1996.

63. Zimm S, Collins JM, O'Neill D, et al. Inhibition of first-pass metabolism in cancer chemotherapy: interaction of 6-mercaptopurine and allopurinol. Clin Pharmacol Ther 34:810–817, 1983.

64. Obach RS. Potent inhibition of human liver aldehyde oxidase by raloxifene. Drug Metab Dispos 32:89–97, 2004.

65. Goldberg MR, Sciberrs D, De Smet M, et al. Influence of β-adrenoceptor antagonists on the pharmacokinetics of rizatriptan, a

66. Rolan P. Potential drug interactions with the novel antimigraine compound zolmitriptan (Zomig, 311C90). Cephalagia 17 (Suppl 18):21–27, 1997.

67. Fleishaker JC, Ryan KK, Jansat JM, et al. Effect of MAO-A inhibition on the pharmacokinetics of almotriptan, an antimigraine agent in humans. Br J Clin Pharmacol 52:437–441, 2001.

68. Van Haarst AD, Van Gerven JM, Cohen AF, et al. The effects of moclobemide on the pharmacokinetics of the 5-HT$_{1B}$/$_{1D}$ agonist rizatriptan in healthy volunteers. Br J Clin Pharmacol 48:190–196, 1999.

69. Liston HL, Markowitz JS, DeVan CL. Drug glucuronidation in clinical psychopharmacology. J Clin Psychopharmacol 21:500–515, 2001.

70. Williams JA, Hyland R, Jones, BC, et al. Drug-drug interactions for UGT substrates: a pharmacokinetic explanation for typically observed low exposure (AUCi/AUC) ratios. Drug Metab Dispos, August 10, 2004 [Epub ahead of print]. Available at: http:// dmd.aspetjournals.org/cgi/reprint/dmd.104.000794v1. Accessed September 6, 2004.

71. Burneo JG, Limdi N, Kuzniecky RI, et al. Neurotoxicity following addition of intravenous valproate to lamotrigine therapy. Neurology 60:1991–1992, 2003.

72. Mueller TH, Beeber AR. Delirium from valproic acid with lamotrigine. Am J Psychiatry 161:1128–1129, 2004.

73. Lee SA, Lee JK, Heo K. Coma probably induced by lorazepamvalproate interaction. Seizure 11:124–125, 2002.

74. Antoniou T, Gough K, Young D, et al. Severe anemia secondary to a possible drug interaction between zidovudine and valproic acid. Clin Infect Dis 38:e38–e40, 2004.

75. Sabers A, Ohman I, Christensen J, et al. Oral contraceptives reduce lamotrigine plasma levels. Neurology 61:570–571, 2003.

76. Gallicano KD, Sahal J, Shukla VK, et al. Induction of zidovudine glucuronidation and amination pathways by rifampicin in HIV-infected patients. Br J Clin Pharmacol 48:168–179, 1999.

77. Fromm MF, Eckhardt K, Li S, et al. Loss of analgesic effect of morphine due to coadministration with rifampin. Pain 72:261–267, 1997.

78. Sadowski DC. Drug interactions with antacids. Mechanisms and clinical significance. Drug Saf 11:395–407, 1994.

79. Hansten PD, Hayton WL. Effect of antacid and ascorbic acid on serum salicylate concentration. J Clin Pharmacol 20:326–331, 1980.

80. Fromm MF, Kim RB, Stein CM, et al. Inhibition of P-glycoprotein-mediated drug transport: a unifying mechanism to explain the interaction between digoxin and quinidine. Circulation 99:552–557, 1999.

81. Jalava KM, Partanen J, Neuvonen PJ. Itraconazole decreases renal clearance of digoxin. Ther Drug Monit 19:609–613, 1997.

82. Wakasugi H, Yano I, Ito T, et al. Effect of clarithromycin on renal excretion of digoxin: interaction with P-glycoprotein. Clin Pharmacol Ther 64:123–128, 1998.

83. Phillips EJ, Rachils AR, Ito S. Digoxin toxicity and ritonavir: a drug interaction mediated through P-glycoprotein. AIDS 17: 1577–1578, 2003.

84. Ding R, Tayrouz Y, Riedel KD, et al. Substantial pharmacokinetic interaction between digoxin and ritonavir in healthy volunteers. Clin Pharmacol Ther 76:73–84, 2004.

85. Mizuno N, Niwa T, Yotsumoto Y, et al. Impact of drug transporter studies on drug discovery and development. Pharmacol Rev 55: 425–461, 2003.

86. Eraly SA, Blantz RC, Bhatngar V, et al. Novel aspects of renal organic anion transporters. Curr Opin Nephrol Hypertens 12: 551–558, 2003.

87. Simonson SG, Raza A, Martin PD, et al. Rosuvastatin pharmacokinetics in heart transplant recipients administered an antirejection regimen including cyclosporine. Clin Pharmacol Ther 76:167–177, 2004.

88. Lennernas H. Clinical pharmacokinetics of atorvastatin. Clin Pharmacokinet 42:1141–1160, 2003.

89. Shitara Y, Itoh T, Sato H, et al. Inhibition of transporter-mediated hepatic uptake as a mechanism for drug-drug interaction between

cerivastatin and cyclosporin A. J Pharmacol Exp Ther 304:610–616, 2003.

90. Schneck DW, Birmingham BK, Zalikowski JA, et al. The effect of gemfibrozil on the pharmacokinetics of rosuvastatin. Clin Pharmacol Ther 75:455–463, 2004.

91. Vavricka SR, Van Montfoort J, Ha HR, et al. Interactions of rifamycin SV and rifampicin with organic anion uptake systems of human liver. Hepatology 36:164–172, 2002.

92. Milne RW, Larsen LA, Jorgensen KL, et al. Hepatic disposition of fexofenadine: influence of the transport inhibitors erythromycin and dibromosulphthalein. Pharmaceut Res 17:1511–1515, 2000.

93. Viagra® (sildenafil) prescribing information. New York, NY: Pfizer Inc, September 2002.

94. Cialis® (tadalafil) prescribing information. Indianapolis, Ind: Eli Lilly, November 2003.

95. Levitra® (vardenafil) prescribing information. West Haven, Conn: Bayer Healthcare, August 2003.

96. Webb DJ, Muirhead GJ, Wulff M, et al. Sildenafil citrate potentiates the hypotensive effects of nitric oxide donor drugs in male patients with stable angina. J Am Coll Cardiol 36:25–31, 2000.

97. Tran D, Howes LG. Cardiovascular safety of sildenafil. Drug Saf 26:453–460, 2000.

98. Abo-Zena RA, Bobek MB, Dweik RA. Hypertensive urgency induced by an interaction of mirtazapine and clonidine. Pharmacotherapy 20:476–478, 2000.

99. Troncoso AL, Gill T. Hypertensive urgency with clonidine and mirtazapine. Psychosomatics 45:449–450, 2004.

100. Siegler EL, Reidenberg M. Treatment of urinary incontinence with anticholinergics in patients taking cholinesterase inhibitors for dementia. Clin Pharmacol Ther 75:484–488, 2004.

101. el-Agroudy AE, Sobh MA, Hamdy AF, et al. A prospective, randomized study of coadministration of ketoconazole and cyclosporine A in kidney transplant recipients: ten-year follow-up. Transplantation 77:1371–1376, 2004.

102. el-Dahshan KF, Bakr MA, Donia AF, et al. Co-administration of ketoconazole to tacrolimus-treated kidney transplant recipients: a prospective randomized study. Nephrol Dial Transplant 19:1613–1617, 2004.

103. Martin JE, Daoud AJ, Schroeder TJ, et al. The clinical and economic potential of cyclosporin drug interactions. Pharmacoeconomics 15:317–337, 1999.

104. Thomas H, Coley HM. Overcoming multidrug resistance in cancer: an update on the clinical strategy of inhibiting p-glycoprotein. Cancer Control 10:159–165, 2003.

105. Kim RB. Drug transporters in HIV therapy. Top HIV Med 11:136–139, 2003.

106. Loscher W, Potschka H. Role of multidrug transporters in pharmacoresistance to antiepileptic drugs. J Pharmacol Exp Ther 301:7–14, 2002.

107. Summers MA, Moore JL, McAuley JW. Use of verapamil as a potential P-glycoprotein inhibitor in a patient with refractory epilepsy. Ann Pharmacother 38:1631–1634, 2004.

108. Strausburg KM. Drug interactions in nutrition support. In: McCabe BJ, Frankel EH, Wolfe JJ, eds. Handbook of food-drug interactions. Boca Raton, FL: CRC Press, 2003:145–165.

109. Sørensen JM. Herb-drug, food-drug, nutrient-drug, and drug-drug interactions: mechanisms involved and their medical implications. J Altern Complement Med 8:293–308, 2002.

110. McCabe BJ. Prevention of food-drug interactions with special emphasis on older adults. Curr Opin Clin Nutr Metabol Care 7:21–26, 2004.

111. Burton PS, Goodwin JT, Vidmar TJ, et al. Predicting drug absorption: how nature made it a difficult problem. J Pharmacol Exp Ther 303:889–895, 2002.

112. Yeh KC, Deutsch PJ, Haddix H, et al. Single-dose pharmacokinetics of indinavir and the effect of food. Antimicrob Agents Chemother 42:332–338, 1998.

113. Zithromax® (azithromycin tablets, azithromycin capsules, and azithromycin suspension) prescribing information. New York, NY: Pfizer Inc, 2003.

114. Bailey DG, Spence JD, Munoz C, et al. Interaction of citrus juices with felodipine and nifedipine. Lancet 337:268–269, 1991.

115. Drug interactions with grapefruit juice. Med Lett Drugs Ther 46:2–4, 2004.

116. Kakar SM, Paine MF, Stewart PW, et al. 6′7′-Dihydroxybergamottin contributes to the grapefruit juice effect. Clin Pharmacol Ther 75:569–579, 2004.

117. Huang SM, Hall SD, Watkins P, et al. Drug interactions with herbal products and grapefruit juice: a conference report. Clin Pharmacol Ther 75:1–12, 2004.

118. Greenblatt DJ, von Moltke LL, Harmatz JS, et al. Time course of recovery of cytochrome p450 3A function after single doses of grapefruit juice. Clin Pharmacol Ther 74:121–129, 2003.

119. Malhotra S, Bailey DG, Paine MF, et al. Seville orange juice-felodipine interaction: comparison with dilute grapefruit juice and involvement of furanocoumarins. Clin Pharmacol Ther 69:14–23, 2001.

120. Parker RB, Yates CR, Soberman JE, et al. Effects of grapefruit juice on intestinal P-glycoprotein: evaluation using digoxin in humans. Pharmacotherapy 23:979–987, 2003.

121. Becquemont L, Verstuyft C, Kerb R, et al. Effect of grapefruit juice on digoxin pharmacokinetics in humans. Clin Pharmacol Ther 70:311–316, 2001.

122. Dresser GK, Bailey DG. The effects of fruit juices on drug disposition: a new model for drug interactions. Eur J Clin Invest 33 (Suppl 2):10–16, 2003.

123. Dresser GK, Bailey DG, Leake BF, et al. Fruit juices inhibit organic anion transporting polypeptide-mediated drug uptake to decrease the oral availability of fexofenadine. Clin Pharmacol Ther 71:11–20, 2002.

124. Kuykendall JR, Houle MD, Rhodes RS. Possible warfarin failure due to interaction with smokeless tobacco. Ann Pharmacother 38:595–597, 2004.

125. Zevin S, Benowitz NL. Drug interactions with tobacco smoking. An update. Clin Pharmacokinet 36:425–438, 1999.

126. Oesterheld JR, Armstrong SC, Cozza KL. Ecstasy: pharmacodynamic and pharmacokinetic interactions. Psychosomatics 45:84–87, 2004.

127. Eisenberg DM, Kessler RC, Foster C, et al. Unconventional medicine in the United States. Prevalence, costs, and patterns of use. N Engl J Med 328:246–252, 1993.

128. Eisenberg DM, Davis RB, Ettner SL, et al. Trends in alternative medicine use in the United States, 1990–1997: results of a follow-up national survey. JAMA 280:1569–1575, 1998.

129. American Society of Health-System Pharmacists. ASHP statement on the use of dietary supplements. Am J Health Syst Pharm 61:1707–1711, 2004.

130. Hennessy M, Kelleher D, Spiers JP, et al. St John's Wort increases expression of P-glycoprotein: implications for drug interactions. Br J Clin Pharmacol 53:75–82, 2002.

131. Tannergren C, Engman H, Knutson L, et al. St John's wort decreases the bioavailability of R- and S-verapamil through induction of first-pass metabolism. Clin Pharmacol Ther 75:298–309, 2004.

132. Mueller SC, Uehleke B, Woehling H, et al. Effect of St John's wort dose and preparations on the pharmacokinetics of digoxin. Clin Pharmacol Ther 75:546–557, 2004.

133. Henderson L, Yie QY, Berquist C, et al. St John's wort (*Hypericum perforatum*): drug interactions and clinical outcomes. Br J Clin Pharmacol 54:349–356, 2002.

134. Hebert MF, Park JM, Chen YL, et al. Effects of St. John's wort (*Hypericum perforatum*) on tacrolimus pharmacokinetics in healthy volunteers. J Clin Pharmacol 44:89–94, 2004.

135. Lumpkin MM, Alpert S. Risk of drug interactions with St John's wort and indinavir and other drugs. FDA Public Health Advisory, February 10, 2000. Available at: http://www.fda.gov/cder/drug/advisory/stjwort.htm. Accessed September 4, 2004.

136. Fugh-Bergman A. Herb-drug interactions. Lancet 355:134–138, 2000.

137. Ang-Lee MK, Moss J, Yuan CS. Herbal medicines and perioperative care. JAMA 286:208–216, 2001.

138. Heck AM, DeWitt BA, Lukes AL. Potential interactions between alterative therapies and warfarin. Am J Health Syst Pharm 57:1221–1230, 2000.

139. Zhou S, Gao Y, Jiang W, et al. Interactions of herbs with cytochrome P450. Drug Metab Rev 35:35–98, 2003.

140. Sparreboom A, Cox MC, Acharya MR, et al. Herbal remedies in the United States: potential adverse interactions with anticancer agents. J Clin Oncol 22:2489–2503, 2004.

141. Peng CC, Glassman PA, Trilli LE, et al. Incidence and severity of potential drug-dietary supplement interactions in primary care patients. An exploratory study of 2 outpatient practices. Arch Intern Med 164:630–636, 2004.

142. Consumer Report.org. SoBe recalls beverages tainted with cough medicine, December, 2002. Available at: http://www.consumerreports.org/main/detailv2.jsp?CONTENT%3C%3Ecnt_id = 298963&FOLDER%3C%3Efolder_id = 162689&bmUID = 1041386961044. Accessed September 5, 2004.

143. Coon JT, Pittler M, Ernst E. Herb-drug interactions: survey of leading pharmaceutical/herbal companies. Arch Intern Med 163:1371, 2003.

144. Dietary Supplements Containing Ephedrine Alkaloids, Final Rule Summary, February 11, 2004. Available at: http://www.fda.gov/oc/initiatives/ephedra/february2004/finalsummary.html. Accessed September 10, 2004.

145. Horn JR, Hansten PD. Computerized drug-interaction alerts: is anybody paying attention? Pharmacy Times, February 2004:56–58.

146. Glassman PA, Simon B, Belperio P, et al. Improving recognition of drug interactions. Benefits and barriers to using automated drug alerts. Med Care 40:1161–1171, 2002.

147. Horn JR, Hansten PD. Drug interaction classification systems. Pharmacy Times, August 2004:60.

148. Horn JR, Hansten PD. Sources of error in drug interactions: the Swiss cheese model. Pharmacy Times, March 2004:53–54.

149. Cytochrome P450 Interactions. Available at: http://medicine.iupui.edu/flockhart/

150. P450, UGT and P-gp Drug Interactions. Available at: http://mhc.com/Cytochromes/.

Clinical Toxicology

Wendy Klein-Schwartz

TREATMENT GOALS

- To minimize poisoning morbidity and mortality through prompt initiation of supportive care, decontamination, enhancement of elimination, and administration of antidotes
- To provide up-to-date therapy by consulting a poison center
- To prevent poisonings by identifying patients at high risk for poisoning and instituting prevention strategies

DEFINITION

Toxicology is the study of adverse effects of exogenous agents on biologic systems. The term *poison* refers to agents that cause harmful effects. Clinical toxicology deals with the assessment and treatment of patients exposed acutely or chronically to potentially harmful agents. Because of the diverse nature of the substances involved in poisonings and the wide range of clinical manifestations and their treatment, optimal management is achieved by an interdisciplinary approach using the expertise of physicians, nurses, pharmacists, and prehospital professionals.

The term *toxicokinetics* is used to describe the rates of absorption (or entry into the body), distribution, metabolism, and excretion of toxic agents or toxic doses of therapeutic agents. In the setting of an overdose, the manner in which the body handles a drug may be altered compared with therapeutic doses. Examples of altered toxicokinetic parameters in an overdose include prolonged absorption of aspirin with delayed peak serum concentrations and formation of the toxic metabolite of acetaminophen due to increased cytochrome P-450 metabolism.

Toxicology is an important consideration during drug development. Predicting drug safety during drug development requires addressing potential toxicity due to the pharmacologic properties of the drug (e.g., drug-organ toxicity), performing acute and chronic toxicity studies in animals as well as mutagenicity, carcinogenicity and reproductive studies, evaluating drug metabolism and pharmacokinetics, and determining risk factors that may increase a patient's susceptibility to toxicity. Attention to drug safety during the drug development process could lessen the likelihood of unacceptable adverse effects observed postmarketing.

ETIOLOGY

Children are at risk for unintentional poisonings, while adolescents and adults are more likely to experience intentional exposures from suicide attempts or substance abuse or misuse. Pediatric poisonings can happen as a result of an interplay between the children's exploration of their environment, developing physical abilities (walking, climbing), and accessibility of harmful substances. Other factors include improper storage of products, child's thirst or hunger, child's imitation of adult behaviors, and inadequate caregiver supervision. Unintentional adult poisoning, caused by therapeutic errors, inadvertent product misuse, or occupational or environmental exposure also can occur. Older adults experience physiologic changes (e.g., decreased vision, memory loss, dementia, altered renal and hepatic function) that place them at increased risk for unintentional poisonings or adverse drug reactions and interactions. Older patients also frequently experience depression which increases the risk of suicide attempts by overdoses, especially in women.[1,2] Less frequent reasons for exposure to harmful substances at any age include malicious acts and contamination or tampering. A growing public health concern is terrorist attacks with weapons of mass destruction including chemical warfare agents such as nerve agents (e.g., sarin).

Toxic exposures from drugs are responsible for approximately 50% of cases reported to poison centers in the United States, with the most common drugs being analgesics, sedative, hypnotics, neuroleptics, topical preparations, cough and cold products, antidepressants, antihistamines, cardiovascular drugs, antimicrobials, and vitamins.[3] The most frequent nonpharmaceuticals include cleaning substances, cosmetics and personal care products, pesticides, plants, alcohols, hydrocarbons, and chemicals. Other common causes are food poisoning and bites/envenomations. The most common route of exposure is ingestion, but other routes include dermal, inhalation, ocular, and parenteral.

Individuals can be exposed to toxins for varying lengths of time before toxicity is evident (i.e., acute, chronic, acute-on-chronic). Sometimes chronic intoxications cause more serious symptomatology than acute overdoses at lower serum concentrations (e.g., salicylates, lithium, theophylline), warranting more aggressive use of therapies such as hemodialysis or hemoperfusion.

EPIDEMIOLOGY

Poisoning is a major cause of injury-related morbidity in the United States, especially in children. Unintentional poisonings are one of the primary causes of injury-related hospitalizations in school-age children. Poisoning-related fatalities in children have declined markedly since the 1940s and 1950s. While children less than 6 years of age are the victims of 52% of poison exposures reported to poison centers nationally, only 3.1% of the fatalities occur in this age group.[3] In contrast, adults 20 to 49 years of age are the victims of 20.8% of poison exposures reported to poison centers, but account for 58% of fatalities. The National Center for Health Statistics (NCHS) mortality data for 2001 report 72,107 poisoning deaths, of which 14,078 were accidental. In children 4 years of age and younger; there were 27 accidental poisoning deaths by drugs, medicaments, and biologic substances (data from http://wonder.cdc.gov/mortICD10J.html; accessed 5/20/04).

In 2003, 64 poison centers serving the entire population of the United States and Puerto Rico (294.7 million) reported 2,395,582 cases to the American Association of Poison Control Centers' (AAPCC) Toxic Exposure Surveillance System (TESS).[3] The actual number of poison exposures in the United States is unknown because reporting to poison centers is voluntary.

For children under 13 years of age, the majority of poison exposures reported to poison centers are unintentional resulting in minimal or no toxicity and can be managed at the site of exposure, usually a residence. Health care facility management occurs in only 10.1% and 13.1% of children under 6 years of age and between 6 and 12 years of age, respectively.[3] For adolescents 13 to19 years of age, the proportion of unintentional and intentional exposures is similar (49.0% unintentional versus 45.9% intentional). Adolescents

experience a higher frequency of more serious toxic effects and 48.1% are managed in a health care facility. Adults fall in between children and adolescents with 68.4% unintentional, 24.0% intentional, and 36.4% managed in a health care facility.

PATHOPHYSIOLOGY

Depending on the toxin, the target organs for toxicity can be the nervous system, cardiovascular, respiratory, liver, kidneys, blood, eye, skin, endocrine, reproductive, and/or immune systems. For some toxins, one organ system is the main target [e.g., central nervous system (CNS) depression from benzodiazepines], but for others multiorgan system involvement is evident [e.g., gastrointestinal (GI), CNS, metabolic, cardiovascular, pulmonary, and hematologic from salicylates). Patients may develop clinical manifestations immediately (e.g., inhalation of chlorine fumes), shortly after exposure (e.g., cyclic antidepressants), or following a latent period. Delayed absorption due to formulation of the product (e.g., sustained or controlled release), decreased GI motility (e.g., anticholinergics), or formation of bezoars or concretions (e.g., meprobamate) can delay symptom onset. Other reasons for delayed toxicity include metabolism of parent compound to active metabolites (e.g., levothyroxine, sulfasalazine, methanol) or time required for the substance to interfere with cellular function or deplete organ reserve capacity (e.g., acetaminophen).[4]

When evaluating the potential for toxicity after an exposure, the site of toxicity should be considered. Some toxins produce local effects at the site of exposure. A splash on the skin of corrosives, such as sulfuric acid and sodium hydroxide, will cause injury to that area of skin. Systemic toxicity is unlikely. In contrast, dermal exposure to a carbamate or organophosphate pesticide may cause some local irritation, usually related to the solvent, but most of the toxicity is due to absorption through the skin and the development of systemic cholinergic effects.

Mechanisms of toxicity vary. Toxicity may be due to agonist or antagonist activity at a receptor including the adrenergic, cholinergic, opioid, serotonin, glutamate, glycine, and GABA (gamma-aminobutyric acid) receptors.[5] Other agents act at channels (e.g., cyclic antidepressants at fast sodium channels in heart) or pumps (e.g., digoxin at Na_+, K_+-ATPase). Toxins can also impair cellular function by interfering with mitochondrial ATP synthesis.[5] Cyanide interferes with cytochrome oxidase, which inhibits electron transport. Nitrites, benzocaine, and other methemoglobin-forming chemicals inhibit delivery of oxygen to the electron transport chain by oxidation of hemoglobin to methemoglobin. Salicylates impair ATP formation by uncoupling oxidative phosphorylation. Acetaminophen's toxic metabolite covalently binds with hepatocytes, inhibiting calcium export from the cytoplasm, and leading to cell death.

CLINICAL PRESENTATION AND DIAGNOSIS

Often the patient presents with a history of exposure to a drug, household product, chemical, biologic, or other possibly harmful substance. To assess the potential for toxicity, the following information should be elicited (Fig. 4.1):

■ *Substance.* Pertinent information includes the quantity of each ingredient in the product. The history may be unreliable or unavailable in suicidal patients or substance abusers; patients with altered mental status or those exposed to a substance in an unmarked container or who ingest an unidentified plant may be unable to provide a history.

■ *Amount.* If an accurate determination of the amount ingested is not possible and the substance is toxic, a potentially toxic dose should be assumed. For intentional exposures, the patient's report of the dose is suspect.

■ *Time since exposure.* This information coupled with information on the onset and duration of action of the substance, allows assessment of whether clinical manifestations are consistent with the history of dose and time since exposure. Whether to institute some therapeutic options, including GI decontamination, is determined by time since ingestion.

■ *Clinical manifestations.* Evaluate if clinical effects are consistent with the substance(s); if not, evaluate for other substances and/or medical conditions. Severe effects (re-

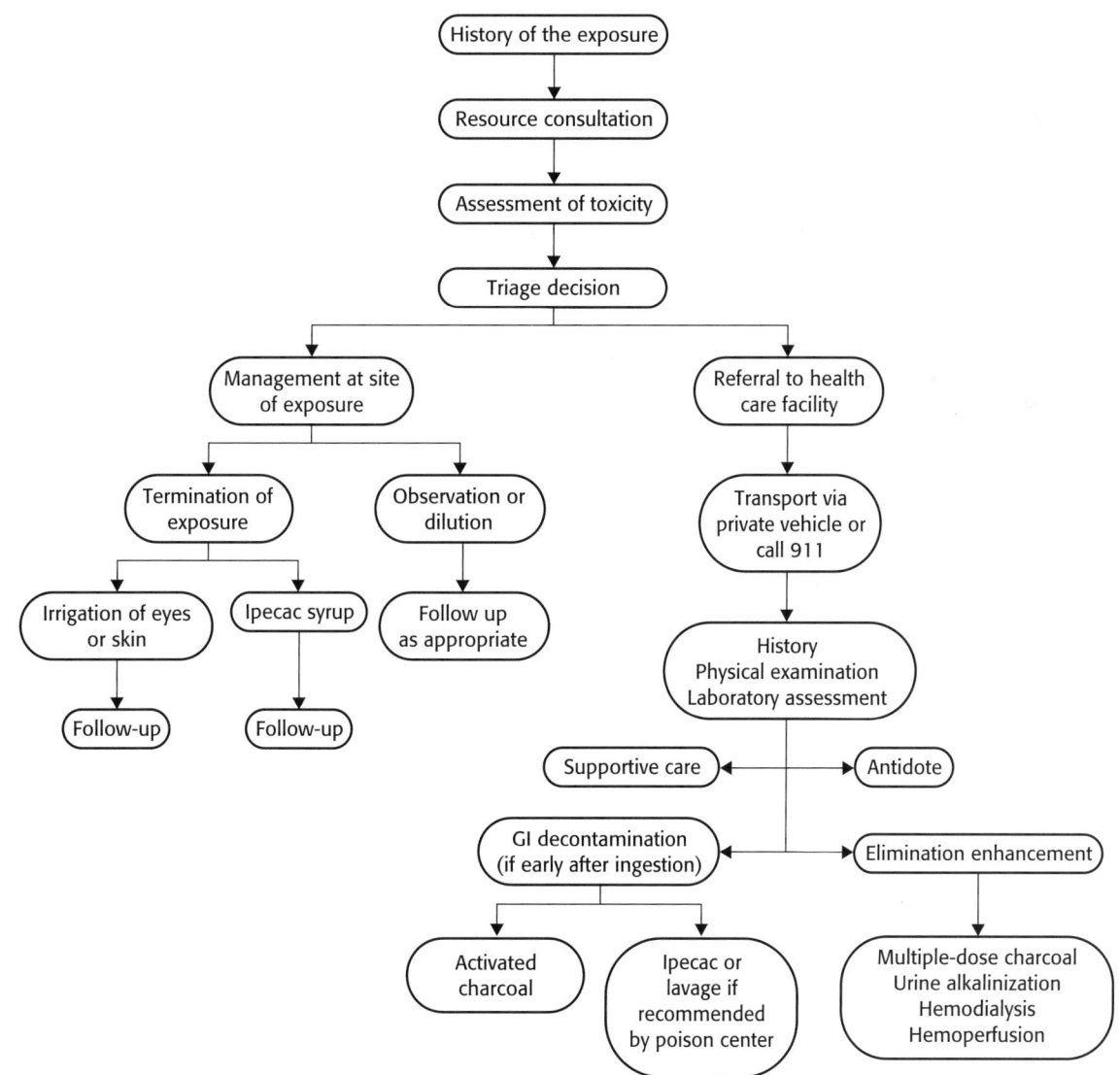

FIGURE 4.1 Algorithm for assessment and treatment of a poison exposure.

spiratory and cardiovascular depression) necessitate immediate treatment.

■ *Patient's age and weight.* Determine the toxicity of the substance, dosing of antidotes, and likely reason for the exposure based on this information.

■ *Past medical history and prior therapy.* The patient's medical history can influence the treatment or severity of the intoxication. Prior treatment may impact subsequent recommendations or may complicate or alter the clinical picture. Examples include development of potentially life-threatening toxicity when salt water emetic is given or altered findings on mental status exam if naloxone was administered by prehospital providers.[6]

In some patients, exposure to a toxic substance is not elucidated on initial history. Poisoning should be considered in the differential diagnosis whenever there is an abrupt onset of illness involving multiple organ systems, especially in children. Delayed recognition of intoxication is a problem in older patients who present with chronic therapeutic overdose. For example, salicylate intoxication in older patients can be missed since clinical effects mimic other illnesses, including encephalopathy, cardiopulmonary disease, diabetic ketoacidosis, and alcohol withdrawal.[7] Patients presenting with unexplained hepatic injury should be evaluated for chronic acetaminophen intoxication. Patients attempting suicide or abusing illicit substances may purposely or unwittingly provide misleading histories, especially if the illicit substance was purchased from a 'street' source. Further complicating the clinical picture is the possibility that the patient's symptoms are related in part or wholly to drug withdrawal.

The toxicology laboratory tests can confirm the history or the suspicion that the history is inaccurate. Qualitative urine screens for amphetamines, benzodiazepines, barbiturates, cocaine, opioids, and cyclic antidepressants, and quantitative serum assays for acetaminophen, salicylates, iron, lithium, theophylline, and digoxin are emergently available at many toxicology labs. An acetaminophen concentration should be obtained in all patients with intentional exposure to rule out acetaminophen as an unnamed intoxicant because early acetaminophen poisoning causes minimal toxic effects.[8]

Finally, recognition of a toxidrome can help clinicians identify the most likely substances for those patients lacking clear-cut histories or with histories inconsistent with clinical findings.[4] A toxidrome is defined by a grouping of vital signs, mental status, clinical findings, and, in some instances, laboratory or ECG evidence. Table 4.1 provides examples of some toxidromes.

THERAPEUTIC PLAN

Components of the therapeutic plan are triage and treatment. The first consideration is where the victim should be treated based on assessment of the intent and potential severity of the intoxication. Minimally toxic unintentional exposures

TABLE 4.1	Examples of Toxidromes	
Toxin	**Vital Signs***	**Clinical Findings/Lab/ECG**
Amphetamines/cocaine	↑ RR, HR, BP, T	Hyperactivity, agitation, mydriasis, diaphoresis
Anticholinergics	↑ HR, T	Agitation, hallucinations, lethargy, dry mucous membranes, flushed, mydriasis, ↓ GI motility; urinary retention
Cholinergics (carbamates, organophosphates, nerve agents)	↓ HR (but tachycardia possible)	DUMBELS (<u>d</u>iarrhea, <u>u</u>rination, <u>m</u>iosis, <u>b</u>ronchorrhea, <u>e</u>mesis, <u>l</u>acrimation, <u>s</u>alivation)
Cyclic antidepressants	↑ HR, ↓ BP, ↓ RR	Lethargy, coma, seizures; prolonged PR, QRS, QT intervals
Opioids**	↓ HR, BP, RR, T	Lethargy, coma, miosis, ↓ GI motility
Salicylates	↑ RR, HR, T	Vomiting, tinnitus, agitation, lethargy; respiratory alkalosis and metabolic acidosis
Toxic alcohols (ethylene glycol; methanol)	↓BP, ↑ RR	Lethargy, coma, abdominal pain; metabolic acidosis; (renal failure, ethylene glycol),(hyperemic discs, visual disturbance, methanol)

* RR, respiratory rate; HR, heart rate; BP, blood pressure; T, temperature.

** Similar for clonidine, except possible hypertension; similar for olanzapine, except resting tachycardia.

can be managed outside of a health care facility. In these cases, therapies usually consist of dilution, dermal or ocular irrigation, or possibly GI decontamination. All patients with intentional exposures and/or serious intoxications should be referred to a health care facility and transported by private vehicle or emergency medical services (EMS) transport, depending on the situation. In a health care facility, the treatment plan includes provision of supportive care; decontamination of skin, eyes, or GI tract; enhancement of elimination; and administration of antidotes.

The poison center should be consulted for assessment and treatment advice when formulating the therapeutic plan. Poison centers provide telephone information 24 hours a day to the public and health professionals, use comprehensive information sources and management guidelines, and have access to regional treatment facilities for patient referral and transport. All US poison centers can be accessed from anywhere in the country by calling 1-800-222-1222.

TREATMENT

SUPPORTIVE CARE

Supportive care is the most important part of treating the seriously intoxicated patient. Attention to airway, breathing, level of consciousness, and blood pressure is critical. In serious intoxications, supportive care sustains the patient while the toxin is being detoxified by liver metabolism or renal elimination, or prior to and during antidotal therapy or while preparations are being made for instituting procedures such as hemodialysis, hemoperfusion, or organ transplantation.

All patients with CNS depression should be given naloxone in case altered mental status is the result of opioid intoxication. Naloxone rapidly reverses CNS depression from opioids and helps identify opioids as responsible to some degree for the intoxication, but has no serious consequences if given to patients without opioid intoxication. Blood glucose should be assessed rapidly by fingerstick glucometer and intravenous (IV) dextrose [50 mL D50W (50% dextrose in water)] administered for hypoglycemia. Flumazenil, the benzodiazepine antagonist, is not routinely recommended in overdose cases because of potential adverse consequences, including seizures and dysrhythmias, especially in patients who are physically dependent or ingest multiple substances.

Airway and breathing should be assessed immediately. If respirations are compromised, the patient should be intubated and placed on a ventilator. IV diazepam or lorazepam is first-line therapy for seizures. Hypotension is treated initially with IV fluids. If blood pressure remains low, vasopressors such as dopamine or norepinephrine should be administered. A patient with an overdose of potentially cardiotoxic agents or unknown agents should be on a cardiac monitor. Fluid and electrolyte status should be monitored and intravenous fluids adjusted accordingly. Decisions about extubation and discontinuing vasopressors are based on continued assessment of the patient's level of consciousness and blood pressure.

DECONTAMINATION

Ocular and Skin Irrigation. For ocular and dermal exposures, the initial goal is to decrease contact time by removing the harmful substance. Eye exposures are managed by irrigating immediately with water or saline for 10 to 15 minutes. For strong acids or bases, irrigation for 20 to 30 minutes is recommended. For skin exposures, contaminated clothing should be removed and the skin washed with soap and water. Depending on the substance and the extent of injury, other therapies include topical steroids, antibiotics, dressings, or patches.

Inhalation. Following inhalation of a potentially toxic gas or fume, the exposure is terminated by moving the patient from the contaminated environment to fresh air. If respiratory irritation is significant, the patient may require oxygen, PEEP, bronchodilators, or intubation to maintain a patent airway and/or ventilation to support respirations.

Gastrointestinal Decontamination. The goal of GI decontamination is to minimize absorption of the ingested toxin. Ideally, GI decontamination should be performed within an hour of ingestion. Examples of drugs for which delayed GI decontamination may be beneficial include salicylates (up to 12 hours after ingestion), which delay gastric emptying; anticholinergics, which decrease GI motility; and phenytoin, which is slowly and erratically absorbed from the GI tract.

Although most clinical toxicologists consider GI decontamination standard care for recent oral overdoses, controversy continues regarding the benefits relative to risks.[9–16] Position papers on GI decontamination procedures uniformly note the lack of conclusive evidence of improved outcome.[9–14] A retrospective study found no worsening in patient outcomes with decreasing use of GI decontamination.[15] A prospective, randomized trial found that activated charcoal provided no additional benefit compared with supportive care only and that patients given charcoal had a higher incidence of vomiting and longer length of emergency department (ED) stay.[16]

Activated charcoal is the primary treatment modality for decreasing absorption of ingested toxins in the ED, despite conflicting evidence and problems with existing outcome studies. Syrup of ipecac is no longer recommended in the ED, and use in the home setting is infrequent.[10] The use of ipecac syrup has decreased from 13.4% of all exposures reported to AAPCC TESS in 1983 to 0.4% of all exposures in 2003, whereas use of activated charcoal increased from 4.0% to 5.9% over the same time period.[3] In 2003, the American Academy of Pediatrics Committee on Injury, Violence and Poison Prevention published a position statement that ipecac should no longer be used routinely as a home treatment strategy.[17] Given these events, home use of ipecac will likely disappear over the next few years. Gastric lavage may cause significant morbidity but may have limited indications in life-threatening overdoses if given early.[11] Whole bowel irrigation (WBI) may be considered for overdoses with delayed release formulations.[14]

Comparison of Gastrointestinal Decontamination Modalities: Activated Charcoal Versus Other Modalities. Why is activated charcoal the primary method of GI decontamination? Many volunteer studies comparing ipecac or lavage with activated charcoal have found activated charcoal superior.[12] Several ED-based studies have compared the effect of procedures on patient outcome. A prospective, randomized, unblinded trial in 70 children found a statistically significantly longer time in the ED before receiving charcoal, higher proportion of patients who vomited charcoal, and longer duration of time discharged patients spend in the ED in the ipecac plus charcoal group compared with the charcoal-only group.[18] There was no difference between groups in the proportion of children admitted or the proportion who improved in the ED. A prospective randomized study of ipecac or lavage plus activated charcoal and a cathartic compared with activated charcoal and a cathartic in 592 acute oral drug overdose cases found no difference in the number of hospital days, number of days in the intensive care unit (ICU), clinical deterioration, morbidity, and mortality between the two groups.[19] Lavage improved outcome if performed in obtunded patients within 1 hour of ingestion. A study in 876 patients, which was designed to replicate the preceding study, found no difference between any of the groups in any of the outcome measures and recommended against using gastric emptying procedures (ipecac or lavage) in adults after acute overdose even if they present with toxicity within 1 hour.[20]

In another prospective study, patients with a symptomatic overdose were randomly assigned to receive gastric emptying and activated charcoal or only activated charcoal, whereas asymptomatic patients were just observed or were given activated charcoal.[21] Activated charcoal provided no benefit in asymptomatic patients, and gastric emptying in symptomatic patients did not improve outcome (length of stay in ED, length of time intubated, or length of stay in ICU) and increased the likelihood of aspiration pneumonitis and ICU admission. Albertson et al, in a study of 200 overdosed patients, also found a higher risk of aspiration in patients receiving ipecac syrup and activated charcoal than in patients receiving activated charcoal alone.[22] There was no difference in the percentage hospitalized, the percentage admitted to an ICU, or the number of hospital or ICU days, but mean time the patients spent in the ED was higher for those receiving ipecac. A comparison of three methods of GI decontamination (activated charcoal alone, saline lavage with activated charcoal, and activated charcoal with saline lavage and activated charcoal) in 51 patients presenting to an ED with tricyclic antidepressant overdose demonstrated no statistically significant differences in clinical effects or outcome measures.[23]

Activated Charcoal. Activated charcoal is an odorless, tasteless, fine black powder that is an effective nonspecific adsorbent of a wide variety of drugs and chemicals. Table 4.2 lists substances not adsorbed by charcoal. Two characteristics of activated charcoal are small particle size with large surface area and low mineral content (vegetable origin). The toxin becomes bound in the internal surface of the pores of the charcoal molecule so it cannot be absorbed. The surface area usually ranges from 950 to 2,000 m^2 per g and higher surface areas products more effectively reduce absorption.[12,24]

Adult and pediatric doses are presented in Table 4.3. Activated charcoal is mixed with water to the consistency of a slurry and administered orally or by nasogastric tube. Charcoal does not mix well with water and must be shaken vigorously. This usually is not a problem with commercially packaged products, which contain sorbitol and/or a suspending agent.

Given the widespread use of activated charcoal, serious adverse effects are uncommon. The most frequent adverse effects are vomiting and black stools. Vomiting occurs in 12% to 20% of patients.[12,25,26] Administration of a sorbitol-containing charcoal product increases the frequency of vomiting.[18,27] A less frequent, but more serious complication is pulmonary aspiration. A retrospective cohort study of poisoning admissions designed to characterize the frequency of aspiration pneumonitis found that administration of activated charcoal was not associated with aspiration pneumonitis.[28] However, there are case reports in which aspiration of charcoal may have contributed to the patients' death or to the development of acute lung injury.[9] There is a case report of GI perforation with charcoal peritoneum and two case reports of corneal abrasions occurring in combative overdose patients in which charcoal got in the patient's eyes.[29,30]

Activated charcoal is most effective when administered soon after ingestion. In human volunteer studies using 50 g of activated charcoal or more, drug absorption was decreased 88.6% when charcoal was given within 30 minutes and 37.3% when charcoal was administered within 1 hour.[12]

TABLE 4.2	Substances Not Adsorbed by Activated Charcoal
Substance	
Alcohols (ethanol, isopropanol, methanol)	
Cyanide	
Boric acid	
Corrosives (acids, alkali)	
Ethylene glycol	
Hydrocarbons	
Iron	
Lithium	

TABLE 4.3	Therapies for GI Decontamination and Augmenting Elimination		
Procedure	**Adult Dose**	**Pediatric Dose**	**Adverse Effects**
Activated charcoal (single dose)	1 g/kg; 50–100 g	1 g/kg; 15–30 g	Vomiting; aspiration pneumonia
Ipecac syrup	30 mL	≥ 1 year: 15 mL < 1 year: 10 mL	Drowsy; diarrhea
Lavage	200–300 mL/wash (several liters total)	10 mL/kg (50–100 mL) per wash	Aspiration, epistaxis, cyanosis, perforation, fluid/electrolyte disturbance
Whole bowel irrigation	2 L/hr	0.5 L/hr	Nausea, vomiting, abdominal cramps
Activated charcoal (multidose)	12.5 g/hr (usually 30–50 g every 4 hr)	10–25 g every 4 hr	Aspiration, bowel obstruction
Sodium bicarbonate (Urine alkalinization)	1–2 mEq/kg IV; repeat boluses or administer as infusion	1–2 mEq/kg IV; repeat boluses or administer as infusion	Systemic alkalosis, hypernatremia

Human volunteer studies designed to evaluate late administration of activated charcoal have conflicting findings. Comparing activated charcoal with control (no activated charcoal), one study found activated charcoal had a significant effect at 1 hour but not at 2 and 3 hours after acetaminophen ingestion, while another study showed that activated charcoal had a significant effect when given 3 hours after acetaminophen ingestion.[31,32]

For drugs and other toxins that form bezoars, have delayed release properties, or alter GI motility, a second dose of activated charcoal can be administered several hours after the initial dose. Examples of drugs for which a second dose of activated charcoal should be considered are salicylates, meprobamate, phenytoin, and valproic acid. If whole bowel irrigation is not being instituted, a second dose of charcoal should be administered for large overdoses of extended, controlled, sustained release or enteric-coated drugs.

Prehospital administration of charcoal is encouraged. A review of prehospital charts of patients who were transported to an ED showed that GI decontamination was done in 6 of 361 patients (2%), all of whom received ipecac.[33] Follow-up data at a single hospital showed that 30 of 43 (70%) patients who might have been suitable candidates for activated charcoal received it in the ED. Median time to administration of activated charcoal in the ED was 82 minutes, a significant delay compared to starting it in the field. In a similar study, the average time for prehospital activated charcoal administration was 5 minutes after first encounter with the paramedics, as compared with 51.4 minutes for those receiving it in the ED.[34] Studies investigating time intervals between ingestion, EMS arrival, and time of EMS arrival at

the ED conclude that prehospital administration of activated charcoal could result in more efficacious use of activated charcoal in a selected subset of patients.[35,36]

The role of activated charcoal in home management of poisoning is controversial because of its poor palatability. In one study in which activated charcoal was used at home in 115 young children with potentially toxic ingestions, a mean of 12.1 g of activated charcoal was administered, and the investigators concluded that home use significantly decreased time to charcoal administration compared to its administration in the ED.[37] In contrast, a study in 15 young children designed to evaluate whether they would consume a therapeutic dose in a simulated home environment found that most children did not drink the full dose.[38] Given the likely demise of ipecac use in the home, studies exploring efficacy of activated charcoal in this setting are warranted.

Cathartics. The rationale for giving cathartics is that by shortening the transit time of the activated toxin complex in the GI tract, the likelihood of absorption of toxin is further diminished. There is no place for cathartics alone and data regarding use with charcoal are conflicting.[13] In a prospective clinical trial in children 1 to 5 years of age with acute ingestions treated with activated charcoal, shorter time to first stool and greater number of stools were noted with sorbitol compared with magnesium citrate, magnesium sulfate, or water.[27] Many charcoal products are formulated with sorbitol, which enhances the palatability of the charcoal. The appearance of charcoal stools indicates that the charcoal (and perhaps the toxic agent) has passed through the GI tract. Although unlikely to cause problems with single doses, hydration and electrolyte status should be monitored. Hypermagnesemia has been reported after a single 17.5-g dose of magnesium citrate in a 77-year-old woman with theophylline toxicity and poor renal function.[39]

Syrup of Ipecac. Syrup of ipecac induces vomiting by local and central mechanisms. It is contraindicated in patients with CNS depression (severe lethargy, loss of the gag reflex, or unconsciousness), patients who are seizing or in whom toxin-induced seizures are believed to be imminent, and in patients who have ingested a hydrocarbon because these patients are all at increased risk of aspiration. Corrosive ingestion is another contraindication because vomiting would re-expose the oropharynx and esophagus. Syrup of ipecac currently is available without a prescription but is no longer routinely recommended. There is no evidence that ipecac syrup-induced emesis improves patient outcomes. An analysis of poison center data comparing centers with low and high rates of home ipecac use in children <6 years of age found no difference in referral rates to emergency departments or adverse outcome rates and concluded that any benefit of ipecac remains to be proven.[40]

If recommended by a poison center, ipecac syrup should be given as soon after the ingestion as possible at the doses in Table 4.3. If vomiting does not occur in 20 to 30 minutes, the initial dosage may be repeated once. The most common side effects of therapeutic dosages of ipecac are diarrhea and mild drowsiness.[45] Although adverse effects are mild with therapeutic doses,[41] with large ipecac doses GI injury and cardiac toxicity including reversible depression of T waves, bradycardia, atrial fibrillation, and hypotension can occur. Fatalities have been reported in adolescents and adults with bulimia or anorexia nervosa who ingest large amounts of ipecac chronically to purge after eating.[42]

Gastric Lavage. Gastric lavage may have limited clinical use within 1 hour of a life-threatening ingestion or for overdoses where the substance is not adsorbed by activated charcoal.[11] A tube is inserted into the stomach through the nose or the mouth, lavage fluid (water, saline) is instilled, and then removed via the same tube multiple times (Table 4.3). In comatose patients, the airway should be protected by prior insertion of a cuffed endotracheal tube to prevent aspiration. Lavage is contraindicated in the setting of caustic ingestions because the lavage tube can result in additional esophageal and gastric damage when it is inserted. The size of the lavage tube is one of the most important factors determining effectiveness. Optimally, a 36 Fr (12 mm, or about 0.5 inch in diameter) or larger Ewald or Lavacuator tube should be used by the oral route in adults. Smaller tubes (16 to 18 Fr) used in children are ineffective. In children, the preferred lavage fluid is normal saline rather than water because of limited tolerance for electrolyte-free solutions. Water intoxication, tonic-clonic seizures, and coma can result from a 5% increase in body water from absorption of electrolyte-free solutions.

Whole Bowel Irrigation. Whole bowel irrigation (WBI) involves administration of large amounts of an osmotically balanced polyethylene glycol electrolyte solution with the goal of decreasing drug absorption by flushing the drug from the GI tract (Table 4.3). WBI is a therapeutic option for toxic ingestions of sustained-release or enteric-coated drugs; data on its use for overdoses of agents not adsorbed by charcoal, such as iron, lead, or zinc, or for packets of illicit drugs are insufficient to support or exclude their use.[14] WBI should be continued until the rectal effluent is clear unless radiographs show persistent presence of the toxin in the GI tract. WBI is contraindicated in patients with bowel perforation, bowel obstruction, ileus, GI hemorrhage, and intractable vomiting.

ENHANCING ELIMINATION

For removal from the body once a toxin has been absorbed, multiple-dose activated charcoal, alteration of urine pH, or extracorporeal procedures, such as hemodialysis and hemoperfusion, can be considered. These procedures are not warranted in the majority of patients exposed to toxic substances. Of 525,710 cases reported to poison centers in 2003 that were managed in a health care facility, multidose activated charcoal was administered in 5,793, hemodialysis in 1,509, hemoperfusion in 27, and other extracorporeal procedures in 22 cases.[3]

Multiple-Dose Activated Charcoal. Elimination via the GI tract can be augmented for drugs that are secreted into the stomach or undergo biliary secretion. Another term used to describe multiple doses of activated charcoal is GI dialysis. Multiple-dose activated charcoal enhances elimination of drugs with a prolonged distributive phase, nonrestrictive protein binding, a small volume of distribution, a long half-life, and a low intrinsic clearance.[43] A review of studies on multiple-dose charcoal found that increased clearance from multiple-dose charcoal has been demonstrated for only a few drugs, and improved outcome has not been demonstrated for any drugs.[44]

Multiple doses of activated charcoal are considered for management of patients ingesting a life-threatening amount of carbamazepine, dapsone, phenobarbital, quinine, or theophylline.[45] A randomized trial in patients with phenobarbital overdose demonstrated a shorter phenobarbital half-life in the multiple-dose than in the single-dose charcoal group, but found no differences in the time course or patient outcome.[46] For salicylates, conflicting evidence is available, but multidose activated charcoal currently is not recommended.[45]

In multiple-dose regimens, activated charcoal usually is given every 4 hours (Table 4.3); a sorbital containing charcoal product can be administered for the first dose but not with subsequent doses. When multiple doses of cathartics have been administered, fluid and electrolyte problems, including hypernatremia and hypermagnesemia, have been reported.[47–50] A 55-year-old salicylate-poisoned patient died after inadvertently receiving 30 g of magnesium sulfate every 6 hours for four doses, 120 cc 70% sorbitol for two doses, and an activated charcoal preparation containing 70% sorbitol for four doses.[51] Postmortem revealed a profoundly dilated bowel containing fluid and activated charcoal, with a perforation at the hepatic flexure. Charcoal aspiration and charcoal-induced bowel obstruction are potential complications of multidose charcoal regimens. A retrospective chart review of 878 patients who received multidose activated charcoal reported pulmonary aspiration in 5 patients, no cases of GI obstruction, but hypernatremia in 53 and hypermagnesemia in 27 patients.[52] A 39-year-old woman on methadone maintenance therapy administered multiple doses of activated charcoal for an amitriptyline overdose developed a 4-cm perforation in the sigmoid colon and a 120-g obstructing charcoal mass.[53]

Alteration of Urine pH. Alteration of urine pH increases the amount of drug in the ionized form, thereby decreasing tubular reabsorption and increasing elimination. IV sodium bicarbonate is administered to produce urine with a pH of 7.5 or greater (Table 4.3). Despite the theoretical advantages of removing the drug from the body more quickly, urine alkalinization has a limited role. No controlled trials have documented changes in patient outcome.

Urine alkalinization increases the renal elimination of chlorpropamide, 2,4-dichlorophenoxyacetic acid, diflunisal, fluoride, mecoprop, methotrexate, phenobarbital, and salicylate. Insufficient evidence is available to recommend urine alkalinization for most of these substances. A review of the evidence and position statement on urine alkalinization concluded that urine alkalinization and high urine flow (600 mL/hour) should be considered in poisonings with the herbicides 2,4-dichlorophenoxyacetic acid and mecoprop.[54] In patients with moderately severe salicylate poisoning who do not meet the criteria for hemodialysis, urine alkalinization is considered first-line treatment. Severely salicylate intoxicated patients should receive hemodialysis. Although urine alkalinization enhances renal elimination of phenobarbital, it is not recommended since multidose activated charcoal is more effective.

Urine alkalinization is contraindicated in patients with renal failure. Significant pre-existing heart disease is a relative contraindication. After an IV line is established, fluid deficits and hypokalemia should be corrected, and urine pH measured. A bolus dose of 1 to 2 mEq per kg of sodium bicarbonate is administered IV. Subsequent dosing can be with additional 1 to 2 mEq per kg boluses or by infusion starting with 3 amps (44 mEq/50 mL ampoule) in 850 mL of D5W infused over 4 hours. Monitoring parameters include urine pH (every 15–30 minutes until pH is 7.5–8.5, then hourly), hourly plasma potassium, arterial blood gases, central venous pressure, and urine output. Plasma salicylate concentrations should be monitored every hour until below

25 to 35 mg per dL (1.8–2.5 mmol/L), at which time urine alkalinization can be discontinued.[54]

Urine acidification increases the renal elimination of amphetamines, phencyclidine, and strychnine; however, it is no longer recommended. Overdoses with these drugs, especially phencyclidine, can produce muscle injury, resulting in rhabdomyolysis and myoglobinuria. In the presence of acidic urine, myoglobin can precipitate in the tubules, leading to acute renal failure.

Hemodialysis and Hemoperfusion. In the severely intoxicated patient, hemodialysis or hemoperfusion may be considered to rapidly remove toxins from the blood. Hemodialysis removes drugs from the blood by diffusion across a synthetic semipermeable membrane. Substances removed by hemodialysis include ethanol, isopropanol, methanol, ethylene glycol, lithium, phenobarbital, theophylline, and salicylates. Early hemodialysis for methanol and ethylene glycol poisoned patients can prevent toxicity by removing the parent compound before it is metabolized to more toxic metabolites. Methanol is metabolized to formaldehyde and formic acid; ethylene glycol is metabolized to glycoaldehyde, glycolate, glyoxylate, and oxalic acid. While some of the toxic metabolites are also dialyzable, if methanol and ethylene glycol can be removed by dialysis before metabolism, toxicity is minimized.

Hemoperfusion involves pumping blood from the patient through a cartridge containing coated activated charcoal or uncoated activated charcoal in a fixed-bed system. Hemoperfusion is effective for removing theophylline, producing a marked drop in blood levels and a rapid improvement in the clinical picture.[55] Potential complications include bleeding, destruction of blood cells (including a significant drop in the platelet count immediately after the procedure), removal of plasma proteins, and hypothermia.[56]

ANTIDOTES

Antidotes, when available, can be lifesaving in severe intoxications and may be required to stabilize the critically ill patient or to prevent or reverse toxicity. Antidotes act by a variety of mechanisms to antagonize the effects of a systemically absorbed toxin. Some examples of different mechanisms include reversal of the toxin's action at the receptor (e.g., naloxone for opioids, flumazenil for benzodiazepines, atropine and pralidoxime for organophosphate pesticides), chelation to enhance removal from the body (e.g., deferoxamine for iron), detoxification of the toxic substances or toxic metabolite (e.g., acetylcysteine for acetaminophen), or prevention of metabolism to toxic metabolites (e.g., ethanol or fomepizole for ethylene glycol).

Antidotes play an important role in treating the poisoned patient but for most poisonings do not replace supportive care. If an antidote is available for a particular intoxicant, specific indications should be considered before its use to ensure maximum benefit with minimal adverse effects. Table 4.4 is a list of major systemic antidotes. Several antidotes are discussed in more detail because of frequency of use (i.e., naloxone, acetylcysteine), controversy surrounding use (i.e., flumazenil), emergently life-threatening nature of the intoxication (i.e., digoxin immune Fab), or relatively recent introduction of the antidote (i.e., fomepizole, octreotide, IV acetylcysteine).

Naloxone. Naloxone is one of the most frequently used antidotes. Naloxone can be used for diagnostic and therapeutic purposes in patients presenting with altered mental status. Naloxone is a pure opioid antagonist without agonist properties, so it is safe if administered to patients in whom coma is not opioid-induced. Naloxone competes at the μ, κ, δ, and σ receptors, antagonizing naturally occurring and synthetic opioids, including heroin, morphine, codeine, meperidine, propoxyphene, pentazocine, diphenoxylate, and dextromethorphan.

The goal of naloxone therapy is reversal of respiratory depression. Naloxone has a short elimination half-life of 1 hour, and its duration of action of between 30 minutes to up to 4 hours is often shorter than the duration of action of the opioid, especially with methadone. After administration of naloxone, patients must be monitored closely for re-emergence of CNS and respiratory depression so that naloxone can be readministered or a naloxone infusion started.

The usual adult dose is 0.4 to 2 mg IV; the adult dose or 0.1 mg per kg can be given to children. If no response is seen, the dose should be repeated until at least 10 mg of naloxone has been administered before opioids are ruled out as the cause of toxicity. Following reversal with bolus doses, a continuous infusion of naloxone can be considered for overdoses for which repeated doses of naloxone are needed for recurring toxicity; those involving long-acting agents such as methadone; poorly antagonized agents such as propoxyphene or pentazocine; sustained- release products (e.g., Oxycontin, MS Contin) or packets of illicit heroin (i.e., body stuffers or packers). After reversal of respiratory depression with the bolus, the infusion is initiated at two-thirds of the bolus dose per hour.[57] At 15 minutes after initiation of the infusion, half of the bolus dose is readministered. If the patient becomes symptomatic at a given infusion rate, toxicity should again be reversed with a naloxone bolus and the infusion rate should be increased. In adults, the naloxone concentration in D5W usually is adjusted to deliver the dose in 100 mL of solution per hour.

An alternative to using a naloxone infusion is the longer-acting opioid antagonist nalmefene.[58] With an elimination half-life of 8 hours, nalmefene's prolonged duration of action, ease of administration, and safety may prove beneficial. Patients are less likely to experience resedation than with naloxone. The initial IV dose of nalmefene is 0.1 mg in opioid-dependent patients; if withdrawal does not occur, 0.5 to 1 mg can be given.

Few adverse effects are caused by naloxone. Isolated case reports of adverse reactions generally have occurred in perioperative patients. The most common adverse effect is acute opioid withdrawal, characterized by vomiting, abdominal pain, diaphoresis, piloerection, and agitation. To avoid withdrawal in suspected opioid dependent patients, begin with smaller naloxone doses (0.2 to 0.4 mg) and then titrate up as needed.

Flumazenil. Flumazenil is a competitive antagonist at the GABA-benzodiazepine receptor, available as a 0.1 mg per mL solution in 5 mL and 10 mL vials. Its main use is to reverse sedation after benzodiazepines are used for conscious sedation during a diagnostic or therapeutic procedure. For this indication, 0.2 mg doses of flumazenil are given intravenously every minute until the patient is alert; usually 1 mg is required.

Flumazenil's use in patients with benzodiazepine overdoses is controversial. The benefit-risk analysis is influenced by the relative safety of benzodiazepine overdoses on the one hand, and the potential risks of flumazenil in patients who are physically dependent on benzodiazepines or with mixed overdoses. Most benzodiazepine overdoses are characterized by mild CNS depression, including lethargy or stupor but still responsive to painful stimuli. Severely poisoned patients can experience respiratory depression, hypothermia, hypotension, and bradycardia, but these effects are uncommon in patients overdosing on benzodiazepines only. Benzodiazepine-induced respiratory insufficiency in comatose patients can result from an increase in upper airway resistance and work of breathing.[59] Although severe toxicity is usually related to co-ingestants, there are differences in the inherent toxicities of different benzodiazepines, with greater risk of severe toxicity with short- or intermediate-acting benzodiazepines (i.e., alprazolam, temazepam) than with long-acting drugs.[60,61] Fatalities are rare, but can occur.[62]

Flumazenil administration can result in seizures, most likely as a result of reversing the anticonvulsant effect of the benzodiazepine or by precipitating a severe benzodiazepine withdrawal in benzodiazepine-dependent patients. Benzodiazepine overdoses in adults are often the result of suicide attempts and, in many instances, the benzodiazepine is their own medication.[63] Benzodiazepine withdrawal is characterized by irritability, anxiety, headache, hallucinations, tremors, and seizures. If the patient has a mixed overdose with a drug that causes seizures and/or arrhythmias, flumazenil administration can result in seizures and/or dysrhythmias. Seizures have been reported when flumazenil has been administered for mixed overdoses with tricyclic antidepressants; co-ingestion of cocaine, lithium, theophylline, isoniazid, bupropion, and other proconvulsive agents is considered a contraindication.[64] Dysrhythmias, including ventricular tachycardia, bradycardia, and asystole, have been reported when flumazenil was administered to patients with co-ingestion of a tricyclic antidepressant or chloral hydrate.[65–67]

TABLE 4.4	**Major Systemic Antidotes**		
Antidote	**Poison**	**Usual Dosage and Route**	**Comments**
Acetylcysteine	Acetaminophen	140 mg/kg orally as a loading dose, then 70 mg/kg every 4 hr for a total of 17 maintenance doses. (See text for IV dosing.)	Dilute 20% solution 1:3 and administer orally as 5% solution. Most effective when initiated within 10 hr.
Atropine	Carbamate insecticides	Test dose of 2 mg IV in an adult and 0.05 mg/kg in a child up to 2 mg.	In severe organophosphate ingestions it is usually given in combination with pralidoxime.
	Organophosphate insecticides Nerve agents (e.g., sarin)	If anticholinergic symptoms are seen, the patient is probably not seriously poisoned. Doses are repeated as needed (up to 2,000 mg/day in severe cases), with the end point being cessation of secretions.	
British anti-Lewisite (dimercaprol; BAL)	Arsenic, gold, mercury, lead	Given by deep IM injection. Dosage variable depending on the agent being chelated and severity of intoxication. Usually 3–5 mg/kg/ dose.	Contraindicated in iron, cadmium, or selenium because complex is toxic. For lead, used in combination with other agents.
Calcium	Calcium channel blockers	Adult: calcium chloride (10%) 1 g IV over 5 min; may be repeated.	Monitor serum calcium if more than one dose is administered; produces positive inotropic effect; less effective for atrioventricular block or hypotension; less useful in massive intoxications.
Deferoxamine	Iron	15 mg/kg/hr IV	Indications: serum iron ≥63 μmol/L (≥350 μg/dL) and symptomatic or ≥90 μmol/L (≥500 μg/dL) regardless of symptoms. Orange-red urine indicates the presence of the deferoxamine-iron chelate; urine color change is not always present.
Digoxin immune Fab	Digoxin Digitoxin	Administered IV. Dosage = body load (mg)/0.5 (mg bound/vial). See package insert for dosing based on amount ingested or serum digoxin levels.	Indicated in severe cases unresponsive to standard antiarrhythmics (see text). Total serum digoxin increases after administration, but digoxin is bound to the Fab fragment and is not toxic.
Diphenhydramine	Phenothiazine-induced extrapyramidal symptoms	Adults: 50 mg IV. Children: 1–2 mg/kg up to a total of 50 mg IV.	
Ethanol	Ethylene glycol, methanol	Ethanol is given to maintain a 22 mmol/L (100 mg/dL) blood level. Loading dose (oral) is 0.8 mL/kg of 95% ethanol given over 30 min followed by an average maintenance dosage of 0.15 mL/kg/hr PO. Loading dose (IV) of 10% ethanol is 7.6 mL/kg IV over 30–60 min followed by an average maintenance dosage of 1.4 mL/kg/hr IV. Monitor blood levels of ethanol and adjust accordingly.	Chronic drinkers may need higher dosages and nondrinkers may require lower dosages. Dosage must be increased if dialysis is used. Glucose usually is administered simultaneously.

(continued)

TABLE 4.4 continued

Antidote	Poison	Usual Dosage and Route	Comments
Flumazenil	Benzodiazepines	Initial dosage 0.2 mg IV. If adequate consciousness not obtained in 30 sec, inject another 0.3 mg IV over 30 sec. Further doses of 0.5 mg may be administered IV at 1-min intervals to a maximum total dosage of 3 mg. Most patients respond to 1–3 mg.	Contraindicated in patients who have taken tricyclic antidepressants or have been given benzodiazepines to treat a life-threatening condition. Seizures may occur if patients have benzodiazepine dependence.
Fomepizole	Ethylene glycol, Methanol	Administer as slow IV infusion over 30 min. Loading dose of 15 mg/kg followed by 10 mg/kg every 12 hr for 4 doses; then 15 mg/kg every 12 hr. Increase dosing to every 4 hr during dialysis.	Administer until ethylene glycol or methanol <20 mg/dL (3.2 mmol/L for ethylene glycol; 6.3 mmol/L for methanol).
Glucagon	β-Blockers; calcium channel blockers	50–150 µg/kg IV bolus initially (5–10 mg in adults); 2–5 mg/hr as needed.	Increases myocardial contractility.
Methylene blue	Nitrates and nitrites	0.2 mL/kg IV of a 1% solution over 5 min.	Reverses methemoglobinemia.
Naloxone	Opioids	0.1 mg/kg/dose IV in children; 0.4–2 mg in adults (see text).	If no IV access, can give IM, ET, nebulized; give several times if no effect before opioids are ruled out. Short duration of action.
Octreotide	Sulfonylurea	50–100 µg SQ	Decreases dextrose requirement.
Oxygen	Carbon monoxide	Inhalation	Consider hyperbaric oxygen.
d-Penicillamine	Copper, gold, mercury, lead, arsenic	Children 20–100 mg/kg/day (depends on the metal being chelated). Adults: 1–1.5 g/day.	Avoid in patients with penicillin allergy. Inhibits enzymes that are pyridoxal-dependent, so pyridoxine usually is given concurrently (10–25 mg/day).
Physostigmine	Anticholinergics	Children: 0.5 mg slow IV. If no response and no cholinergic symptoms, give 0.5 mg every 5 min until a response is seen or 2 mg is reached. Repeat lowest effective trial dosage if severe symptoms recur. Adults: 1–2 mg slow IV. May repeat up to 4 mg total if no response and no cholinergic symptoms. 1–4 mg may be needed for severe symptoms.	Short duration of action. Atropine should be available to reverse any cholinergic effects. Must be given slowly. Of limited usefulness. Avoid when cyclic antidepressants may be involved or in patients with cardiac conduction defects.
Pralidoxime	Organophosphates, severe carbamate ingestions, but not carbaryl	Adults: 1 g IV over 2 min. Children: 25–50 mg/kg slow IV. Either dose may be repeated every 8–12 hr as needed.	Given in combination with atropine. Little benefit if administered more than 36 hr after poisoning.
Pyridoxine	Isoniazid, monomethyl-hydrazine mushrooms	1 g pyridoxine IV per g of isonicotinic acid hydrazide ingested at a rate of 1 g every 2–3 min. If amount is unknown, administer 5 g. May be repeated.	Indicated for management of seizures and correction of acidosis.
Sodium bicarbonate	Cyclic antidepressants	1–2 mEq/kg IV bolus, then IV drip to maintain serum pH of 7.5.	For cardiac arrhythmias, conduction disturbances, and hypotension.

(continued)

Antidote	Poison	Usual Dosage and Route	Comments
Succimer (DSMA)	Lead	Children: 10 mg/kg every 8 hr for 5 days; then every 12 hr for 14 days.	Monitor liver function at least weekly.
Vitamin K₁	Oral anticoagulants (e.g., warfarin, brodifacoum)	Oral: 5–10 mg/day for warfarin and 10–25 mg/day for long-acting agents; doses of 100–125 mg daily and higher have been needed. Intravenous infusion preferable in severe cases at a rate of not more than 1 mg/min.	May need weeks to months of therapy depending on dosage and type of anticoagulant ingested.

TABLE 4.4 continued

Given the potential for adverse events, flumazenil is not indicated as a diagnostic tool for the unknown overdose with altered mental status. Flumazenil may safely reverse CNS depression (but not respiratory depression) in some patients with benzodiazepine overdose who are not chronically using benzodiazepines, do not have a seizure history, and who are without ECG evidence (prolonged QRS or QT intervals) of a tricyclic antidepressant overdose. However, supportive care usually is sufficient in these patients.

Digoxin Immune Fab. Digoxin-specific antibodies or digoxin immune Fab (Digibind) can be lifesaving in digitalis glycoside poisoning.[68] Digoxin immune Fab was used in the management of 446 (31%) of the 1,454 cardiac glycoside exposures treated in a health care facility reported to the AAPCC TESS in 2003.[3] Digoxin immune Fab's high binding affinity for digoxin is greater than digoxin's affinity for the sodium-potassium ATPase. Digoxin immune Fab's affinity for digitoxin is approximately one tenth its affinity for digoxin.

Digoxin immune Fab is indicated in patients with acute or chronic cardiac glycoside intoxication who have life-threatening arrhythmias (e.g., ventricular arrhythmias), conduction defects or progressive bradyarrhythmias (e.g., severe sinus bradycardia), third-degree heart block, or severe hyperkalemia (usually more than 5.0 mEq/L) resistant to treatment. Life-threatening digitalis toxicity was reversed in 21 of 26 patients in one series and 52 of 56 patients in another series with digoxin immune Fab administration.[68,69] Other studies in adults and children have reported complete or partial response in 74% to 93% of patients.[70,71]

Digoxin immune Fab is administered as an IV infusion over 30 minutes in normal saline but may be given as a bolus injection if cardiac arrest is imminent. Each vial contains 38 mg, which binds 0.5 mg of digoxin or digitoxin. The dose is based on body load, which is determined from amount of digoxin or digitoxin ingested in acute poisonings and serum digoxin concentration in chronic intoxications. Tables to determine the dosage in children and adults are included in the product package insert. The total serum digoxin concentration increases markedly after administration of digoxin immune Fab, but digoxin is bound to the Fab fragment and is not active or toxic. In patients with renal failure, elimination of the digoxin immune Fab complex is delayed, so some patients develop a rebound in free digoxin concentration due to the release of Fab fragment-digoxin complex.

Allergic reactions are rare, but skin testing is recommended for patients with known allergy to sheep proteins or previous treatment with digoxin immune Fab. Serum potassium levels, which are elevated in acute digoxin intoxication, drop when digoxin immune Fab reverses toxicity. Patients with digoxin poisoning have a potassium deficit as a result of the loss of intracellular potassium to the extracellular space and subsequent renal elimination. A potential complication of digoxin immune Fab is heart failure in patients with intrinsically poor cardiac function who depend on digoxin's inotropic effect.

Acetylcysteine. In 2003, 127,171 acetaminophen exposures were reported to the AAPCC TESS, of which 65,030 (51%) were treated in a health care facility.[3] Therapy included oral and IV acetylcysteine in 14,710 and 1,886 instances, respectively. The major toxic effect of acetaminophen overdose is hepatic necrosis, which results from saturation of the enzymes in the nontoxic sulfate and glucuronide conjugation pathways and increased formation of the toxic metabolite by the cytochrome P-450 mixed function oxidase system. Glutathione, which detoxifies the toxic metabolite under normal conditions, is depleted in overdose situations. The protective effect of N-acetylcysteine relates to its activity as a glutathione substitute or precursor as well as providing substrate for the sulfate conjugation pathway.

In adults, the generally accepted hepatotoxic acetaminophen dose is 10 to 15 g. However, toxicity has been reported with lower doses, so patients with acute ingestions of more than 7.5 g are considered at risk and should be evaluated in a health care facility. Chronic therapy with more than 4 g of acetaminophen per day, especially in patients who chronically use alcohol, are treated with cytochrome P-450 enzyme inducers or are malnourished, places the adult patient at risk for toxicity. In children, acute overdoses of more than 200 mg per kg and chronic therapy with 150 mg/kg/day for 2 or more days are usually considered potentially hepatotoxic, although toxicity is possible with lower daily doses in some children.[72,73]

N-acetylcysteine is indicated if the plasma acetaminophen concentration at 4 hours or longer after the overdose is at or above the treatment line on the Rumack-Matthew nomogram. (Fig. 4.2) Since N-acetylcysteine is most effective if started early, therapy is sometimes initiated based on history of toxic acetaminophen dose, if the patient presents late, or turnaround time for the acetaminophen concentration is delayed. A study of 2,540 patients with acetaminophen overdoses treated with oral N-acetylcysteine reported that N-acetylcysteine therapy is most efficacious if initiated within 8 hours of the ingestion.[74] A better survival rate and fewer complications have been demonstrated after late administration of N-acetylcysteine in patients with acetaminophen-induced hepatic failure.[75] A 4-hour plasma acetaminophen concentration of 992 μmol per L (150 μg/mL) or higher is possibly hepatotoxic. If the plasma acetaminophen concentration is below the lower line, N-acetylcysteine is not necessary. For chronic therapeutic overdoses, N-acetylcysteine should be administered based on daily dose history, presence of elevated transaminases, and/or above therapeutic plasma acetaminophen concentration on presentation.

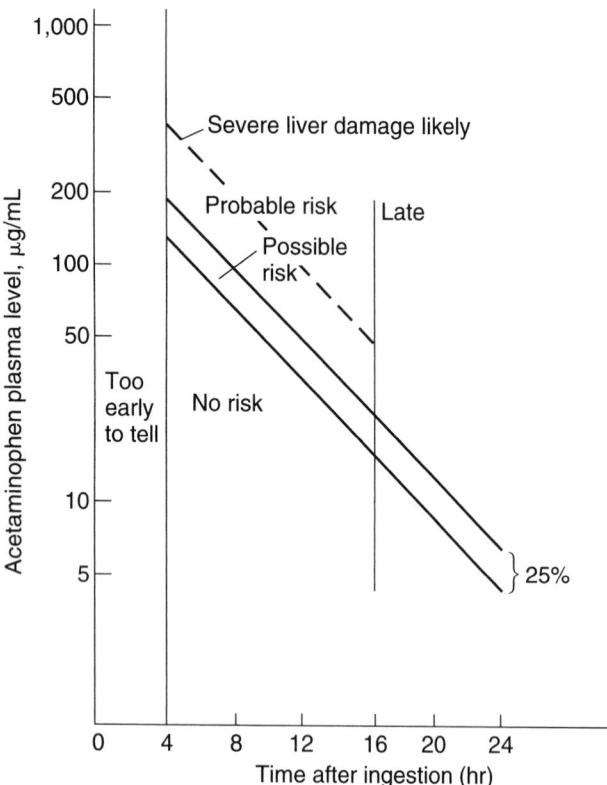

FIGURE 4.2 Rumack-Matthew nomogram for acetaminophen poisoning. Plasma levels drawn before 4 hours may not represent peak levels. The nomogram should be used for single acute ingestions only. (Adapted with permission from Rumack BH, Peterson RC, Koch GG, et al. Acetaminophen overdose. 662 cases with evaluation of oral acetylcysteine treatment. Arch Intern Med 141:380–385, 1981.)

Until 2004, oral dosing was the only approved route for N-acetylcysteine in the United States with a dosing regimen that provides a total dosage of 1,330 mg per kg over 68 hours (Table 4.4). Available in a 10% or 20% concentration, the solution is diluted to a 5% solution before the patient drinks it or it is administered by nasogastric tube. The main side effects of N-acetylcysteine are nausea and vomiting. Patients may have difficulty retaining N-acetylcysteine, which should be readministered if the patient vomits within 1 hour of the dose. Antiemetics such as metoclopramide or ondansetron can be administered prior to subsequent dosing.

In February 2004, the Federal Drug Administration (FDA) approved an IV formulation of N-acetylcysteine (Acetadote). Available in single dose 30-mL vials (200 mg/mL), the loading dose is 150 mg per kg in 200 mL D5W infused over 15 minutes, followed by 50 mg per kg in 500 mL of D5W over 4 hours and then 100 mg per kg in 1,000 mL D5W over 16 hours (total dose, 300 mg/kg). Therapy should be initiated within 8 to 10 hours after acetaminophen overdose. The IV route has been reported to cause hypotension and allergic reactions including rash, urticaria, bronchospasm, angioedema, and anaphylactoid reaction.

There are theoretical advantages for oral acetylcysteine when intrahepatic levels are higher and for IV acetylcysteine when blood concentrations are higher. Duration of therapy and total dose are different for the oral and IV regimens. Patients who present early with plasma acetaminophen concentrations just above the lines on the nomogram are at low risk for toxicity and could probably be adequately treated with a shorter course, regardless of route. A retrospective case series of 75 patients in which oral N-acetylcysteine was discontinued when the acetaminophen concentration was no longer detectable concluded that a shorter course of oral NAC was effective in patients without evidence of hepatotoxicity within 36 hours.[76] High-risk patients are those with markedly elevated plasma acetaminophen concentrations and delayed presentations. These patients should be continued on oral or intravenous N-acetylcysteine if transaminases and/or INR are continuing to increase or have not yet returned to close to normal. Patients with chronic therapeutic overdose should remain on N-acetylcysteine until acetaminophen concentrations are no longer detectable and transaminases and/or INR are close to normal.

Octreotide. Octreotide, a synthetic analog of somatostatin that inhibits release of growth hormone, insulin, and glucagons, is used for the treatment of acromegaly, pituitary adenomas, pancreatic islet cell tumors, and secretory diarrhea. It can also be used for the treatment of recurring hypoglycemia due to sulfonylurea toxicity.

Sulfonylureas are used for the management of hyperglycemia in type 2 diabetes mellitus, lowering blood glucose by depolarizing pancreatic beta cells, which facilitates preformed insulin release. Overdoses of sulfonylureas produce profound hypoglycemia, which can present early or delayed and can recur. Longer duration of hypoglycemia is associated with ingestion of larger doses, with specific sulfonylureas (e.g., chlorpropamide, glyburide) and with extended-release products (e.g., Glucotrol XL). Hypoglycemia has been reported after ingestion of a single tablet of chlorpropamide, glipizide, or glyburide in children and adults.[77–79]

Patients with a history of sulfonylurea ingestion who are asymptomatic and normoglycemic can be observed and encouraged to eat. Patients with sulfonylurea-induced hypoglycemia are initially treated with IV hypertonic glucose (10%) infusion. In some patients hypoglycemia is refractory to IV glucose alone, hypoglycemia recurs after initial response to IV glucose or rebound hypoglycemia develops from pancreatic insulin release in response to hyperglycemia from glucose therapy. Octreotide is indicated in these situations in conjunction with supplemental glucose. Evaluation of octreotide in sulfonylurea-induced hypoglycemia in human volunteers and patients with overdoses have shown that the number of hypoglycemic events and supplemental dextrose requirements are significantly less after octreotide is administered.[80–82] Octreotide usually is administered as a subcutaneous injection at a dose of 50 to 100 µg in adults every 6 to12 hours. Pediatric dose is 4 to 5 µg/kg/day divided every 6 hours; a 25-µg dose has also been suggested for children. Octreotide can also be administered as a continuous IV infusion. Duration of therapy varies, but several days may be required. Adverse effects include nausea, abdominal cramps, flatulence, diarrhea, and pain at the site of injection.

Fomepizole. Fomepizole (Antizol) is approved for the management of methanol and ethylene glycol poisonings, but also prevents metabolism of diethylene glycol, isopropanol, ethanol, and 1,4-butanediol (a precursor of gamma hydroxybutyrate). Fomepizole is a potent inhibitor of the enzyme alcohol dehydrogenase, preventing formation of the more toxic metabolites of methanol and ethylene glycol. The dose can be diluted in 100 mL of normal saline or D5W and then infused over 30 minutes (Table 4.4). Approved indications for its use in methanol and ethylene glycol poisonings are: serum methanol or ethylene glycol concentrations of 20 mg per dL (3.2 mmol/L for ethylene glycol; 6.3 mmol/L for methanol) or more; history of toxic exposures, pending serum concentrations; presence of clinical toxicities associated with these agents (e.g., metabolic acidosis, osmolal gap more than 10 mOsm/L; CNS depression, end-organ injury); prevention of toxicity if serum concentrations are unavailable. Most common adverse effects of fomepizole are headache, nausea, and dizziness.

In 19 patients with ethylene glycol overdoses and 11 patients with methanol overdoses, toxic metabolite concentrations decreased and metabolic acidosis resolved soon after initiation of fomepizole therapy.[83,84] Toxicokinetic analysis of ethylene glycol in these patients found that the elimination of ethylene glycol was significantly slower during fomepizole therapy (half-life of 19.7 ± 1.3 hours) compared to when fomepizole was not administered (half-life of 8.6 ± 1.1 hours).[85] Because patients with normal serum creatinines

eliminated ethylene glycol more rapidly, a conclusion of this study was that an ethylene glycol concentration of more than 50 mg per dL (8.1 mmol/L) should no longer be an absolute indication for hemodialysis if the patient is being treated with fomepizole. The median half-life of methanol during fomepizole in patients who did not undergo hemodialysis was 54 hours; in another study in which patients were treated with ethanol, the median half-life was 43.1 hours. Both of these studies recommended that patients with very high methanol concentrations receive hemodialysis in addition to fomepizole or ethanol to prevent long hospitalizations.[84,86]

Before fomepizole was approved in 1997, continuous IV infusions of ethanol were used to block the metabolism of methanol and ethylene glycol. Treatment with ethanol is more difficult, requiring monitoring of blood ethanol concentrations with frequent readjustment of doses. Blood ethanol concentrations are often well below or well above the desired concentration of 100 mg per dL (21.7 mmol/L). Ethanol-managed patients require ICU admission and frequent monitoring for ethanol-induced CNS depression and hypoglycemia. The only advantage of ethanol is that it is less expensive than fomepizole. Fomepizole is preferred over ethanol because it is a better inhibitor of alcohol dehydrogenase, easier to dose and administer, does not require ICU admission, may eliminate the need for hemodialysis in ethylene glycol poisoned patients, and has a low toxicity profile.

IMPROVING OUTCOMES

POISON PREVENTION

Strategies for injury prevention include education, engineering and technology, and legislation/regulation. The main focus of poison prevention activities is decreasing the number of unintentional poisonings and minimizing severity when an exposure occurs. The target group is usually children, but unintentional exposures in adults, especially older adults, are potentially amenable to poison prevention efforts. Intentional exposures in adolescents and adults are harder to impact with poison prevention efforts.

Education. A major component of poison center activity is poison prevention education. Poison prevention education often is targeted to parents and caretakers of young children, with emphasis on poison prevention and treatment strategies. For children, poison prevention education stresses the importance of limiting access to drugs, household products, personal care products, and other harmful substances by storing these products out of reach and being careful while products are being used. Other messages include: don't call drugs candy, don't take drugs in front of children, leave products in their original containers (don't transfer contents to food containers), be cautious about look-a-like products (e.g., lemon-scented cleaner looking and smelling like lemonade) and dispose of *empty* containers properly.

Health professionals outside of poison centers can promote poison prevention by distributing educational materials and encouraging contact with the poison center if an exposure occurs. Whether products such as activated charcoal should be kept in the home in case of a poisoning would depend on the recommendations of the regional poison center. If activated charcoal is available in the home, parents and other caregivers should be reminded to contact the poison center prior to administering it to be sure it is indicated.

Child-Resistant Packaging. Technologic advances that have had a major impact on childhood poisonings include child-resistant closures (CRCs) and child-resistant blister packs. Legislation and regulations on warning labels and CRCs have played key roles in the decline of serious poisonings in children. Child-resistant packaging of many household products and prescription drugs was mandated by the Poison Prevention Packaging Act in 1970. An annual reduction of 1.40 deaths per million children 4 years of age and younger was attributed to the use of child-resistant packaging, yielding approximately 460 fewer deaths from 1974 through 1992.[87] While aspirin was the leading cause of unintentional poisonings and poisoning deaths in children under 5 years of age, the rate for aspirin deaths decreased by 34% due to CRCs.[88] In 2003, ingestion of aspirin alone by children under 6 years of age accounted for only 0.4% of exposures in this age group reported to poison centers.[3] A unit dose packaging requirement enacted in 1997 for iron products containing 30 mg or more of elemental iron has contributed to a decline in iron poisonings reported to the National Electronic Injury Surveillance System.[89] Whether lifting of these regulations in 2004 impacts on the frequency and severity of childhood iron poisonings remains to be seen.

Pharmacists play a critical role in enforcing drug packaging legislation and regulations. All prescription drugs should be dispensed in CRCs unless specifically excluded by law. If a patient requests a non-CRC, the pharmacist should warn the patient to store the container properly to avoid an unintentional poisoning. Older adults who request non-CRCs should be cautioned regarding proper storage when grandchildren visit.

PHARMACOECONOMICS

Poisoning-related morbidity resulting in ED treatment and inpatient treatment leads to significant expenditures of health care dollars. Almost $1 million in charges at one urban hospital were due to pediatric admissions for poisoning in 1 year.[90] Unnecessary health care cost may be incurred when patients are emergently taken to the hospital for treatment without consulting the poison center to determine if management outside of a health care facility is an option. Poison centers manage 74.5% of reported cases at a non-health care facility, usually the site of exposure.[3]

A benefit-cost analysis found that poison centers reduced the number of patients who were medically treated but not hospitalized by 24% and the number of hospitalizations by 12%.[91] For every dollar spent on poison center services, almost $8 in savings is realized. A study found that the average cost per successful outcome with poison center services was approximately half of that without the services of a regional poison center.[92]

CONCLUSION

Poisoning is a common injury which can be life threatening. Given the diverse nature of toxic substances, intoxications can present with diverse clinical manifestations and levels of severity. Based on history, physical findings, and laboratory evaluation, potential for toxicity is assessed. The management plan includes determining the need for supportive care, decontamination, enhancement of elimination, and antidote administration. A poison center should be consulted for assistance with assessment and treatment. The poison center can also provide assistance with poison prevention activities.

KEY POINTS

- Clinical toxicology provides a challenging opportunity for health care providers in patient care, but requires keeping current with new developments in this growing field.
- Although poison exposures occur more commonly in children under 6 years of age, more serious poisonings often occur in adolescents and adults.
- Thorough patient evaluation and application of these general treatment principles to the specific poisoning situation are essential for definitive treatment.
- Poisoning should be considered in the differential diagnosis whenever there is an abrupt onset of illness with multiple organ system involvement, especially in young children.
- Supportive care is the most important component of treating the seriously intoxicated patient.
- Minimizing absorption of the toxin from the GI tract is most effective if performed early, ideally within the first hour after ingestion.
- Ipecac syrup is no longer used in the ED, and home use is rare as it is no longer a universally accepted therapy.
- Numerous studies have demonstrated that activated charcoal is as effective as or more effective than other GI decontamination modalities. Therefore, activated charcoal is considered the primary method of preventing absorption in ED-treated patients.
- Enhancing elimination from the body by multiple dose activated charcoal, urine alkalinization, hemodialysis, or hemoperfusion may be considered for some toxins.

- Antidotes can be lifesaving in some intoxications, and it is important to be familiar with specific indications, dosing and administration, and potential adverse effects.
- Pharmacists play a critical role in enforcing legislation and regulations related to drug packaging with CRCs.
- Consult the poison center for triage and treatment advice; poison centers improve poisoning outcomes and reduce health care costs.

SUGGESTED READINGS

American College of Emergency Physicians. Clinical policy for the initial approach to patients presenting with acute toxic ingestion or dermal or inhalation exposure. Ann Emerg Med 33:735–761, 1999.

Bond GR. The role of activated charcoal and gastric emptying in gastrointestinal decontamination: a state-of-the-art review. Ann Emerg Med 39:273–286, 2002.

Shannon M. Ingestion of toxic substances by children. N Engl J Med 342:186–191, 2000.

REFERENCES

1. Klein-Schwartz W, Oderda GM, Booze L. Poisoning in the elderly. J Am Geriatr Soc 31:195–199, 1983.
2. Spicer RS, Miller TR. Suicide acts in 8 states: incidence and case fatality rates by demographics and method. Am J Public Health 90:1885–1891, 2000.
3. Watson WA, Litovitz TL, Klein-Schwartz W. 2003 Annual report of the American Association of Poison Control Centers Toxic Exposure Surveillance System. Am J Emerg Med 22:335–404, 2004.
4. Bosse GM, Matyunas NC. Delayed toxidromes. J Emerg Med 7:679–690, 1999.
5. Gregus Z, Klaassen CD. Mechanisms of toxicity. In: Klaassen CD, Watkins JB, eds. Casarett and Doull's essentials of toxicology. New York: McGraw-Hill, 2003: 21–45.
6. Casavant MJ, Fitch JA. Fatal hypernatremia from saltwater used as an emetic. J Toxicol Clin Toxicol 41:861–863, 2003.
7. Durnas C, Cusack BJ. Salicylate intoxication in the elderly. Recognition and recommendations on how to prevent it. Drugs Aging 2:20–34, 1992.
8. Lucanie R, Chiang WK, Reilly R. Utility of acetaminophen screening in unsuspected suicidal ingestions. Vet Human Toxicol 44:171–173, 2002.
9. Seger D. Single-dose activated charcoal-backup and reassess. J Toxicol Clin Toxicol 42:101–110, 2004.
10. American Academy of Clinical Toxicology; European Association of Poisons Centres and Clinical Toxicologists. Position statement: ipecac syrup. J Toxicol Clin Toxicol 42:133–143, 2004.
11. American Academy of Clinical Toxicology; European Association of Poisons Centres and Clinical Toxicologists. Position statement: gastric lavage. J Toxicol Clin Toxicol 35:711–719, 1997.
12. American Academy of Clinical Toxicology; European Association of Poisons Centres and Clinical Toxicologists. Position statement: single-dose activated charcoal. J Toxicol Clin Toxicol 35:721–741, 1997.
13. American Academy of Clinical Toxicology; European Association of Poisons Centres and Clinical Toxicologists. Position statement: cathartics. J Toxicol Clin Toxicol 1997 35:743–752, 1997.
14. American Academy of Clinical Toxicology; European Association of Poisons Centres and Clinical Toxicologists. Position Statement: Whole Bowel Irrigation. J Toxicol Clin Toxicol 35:753–762, 1997.
15. Ardagh M, Flood D, Tai C. Limiting the use of gastrointestinal decontamination does not worsen the outcome from deliberate self-poisoning. N Z Med J 114:423–425, 2001.
16. Merigian KS, Blaho KE. Single-dose oral activated charcoal in the treatment of the self-poisoned patient: a prospective, randomized, controlled trial. Am J Ther 9:301–308, 2002.
17. American Academy of Pediatrics Committee on Injury, Violence, and Poison Prevention. Poison treatment in the home. Pediatrics 112:1182–1185, 2003.
18. Kornberg AE, Dolgin J. Pediatric ingestions: charcoal alone versus ipecac and charcoal. Ann Emerg Med 20:648–651, 1991.
19. Kulig K, Bar-Or D, Cantrill SV, et al. Management of acutely poisoned patients without gastric emptying. Ann Emerg Med 14:562–567, 1985.
20. Pond SM, Lewis-Driver DJ, Williams GM, et al. Gastric emptying in acute overdosage: a prospective randomized controlled trial. Med J Aust 163:345–349, 1995.
21. Merigian KS, Woodward M, Hedges JR, et al. Prospective evaluation of gastric emptying in the self-poisoned patient. Am J Emerg Med 8:479–483, 1990.
22. Albertson TE, Derlet RW, Foulke GE, et al. Superiority of activated charcoal alone compared with ipecac and activated charcoal in the treatment of acute toxic ingestions. Ann Emerg Med 18:56–59, 1989.
23. Bosse GM, Barefoot JA, Pfeifer MP, et al. Comparison of three methods of gut decontamination in tricyclic antidepressant overdose. J Emerg Med 13:203–209, 1995.
24. Roberts JR, Greely EJ, Schoffstall JM. Advantage of high-surface area charcoal in a human acetaminophen ingestion model. Acad Emerg Med 4:167–174, 1997.
25. McFarland AK, Chyka PA. Selection of activated charcoal products for the treatment of poisonings. Ann Pharmacother 27:358–361, 1993.
26. Osterhoudt KC, Durbin D, Alpern ER, et al. Risk factors for emesis after therapeutic use of activated charcoal in acutely poisoned children. Pediatrics 113:806–810, 2004.
27. James LP, Nichols MH, King WD. A comparison of cathartics in pediatric ingestions. Pediatrics 96:235–238, 1995.
28. Isbister GK, Downes F, Sibbritt D, et al. Aspiration pneumonitis in an overdose population: frequency, predictors, and outcomes. Crit Care Med 32:88–93, 2004.
29. Mariani PJ, Pook N. Gastrointestinal tract perforation with charcoal peritoneum complicating orogastric intubation and lavage. Ann Emerg Med 22:606–609, 1993.
30. McKinney P, Phillips S, Gomez HF, et al. Corneal abrasions secondary to activated charcoal. Vet Hum Toxicol 34:336, 1992.
31. Green R, Grierson R, Sitar DS, et al. How long after drug ingestion is activated charcoal still effective? J Toxicol Clin Toxicol 39:601–605, 2001.
32. Sato RL, Wong JJ, Sumida SM, et al. Efficacy of superactivated charcoal administered late (3 hours) after acetaminophen overdose. Am J Emerg Med 21:189–191, 2003.
33. Wax PM, Cobaugh DJ. Prehospital gastrointestinal decontamination of toxic ingestions: a missed opportunity. Am J Emerg Med 16:114–116, 1998.
34. Crockett RC, Krishel SJ, Manoguerra A, et al. Prehospital use of activated charcoal: a pilot study. J Emerg Med 14:335–338, 1995.
35. Thakore S, Murphy N. The potential role of prehospital administration of activated charcoal. Emerg Med J 19:63–65, 2002.
36. Allison TB, Gough JE, Brown LH, et al. Potential time savings by prehospital administration of activated charcoal. Prehosp Emerg Care 1:73–75, 1997.
37. Spiller HA, Rodgers GC. Evaluation of administration of activated charcoal in the home. Pediatrics108:E100, 2001.
38. Scharman EJ, Cloonan HA, Durback-Morris LF. Home administration of charcoal: can mothers administer a therapeutic dose? J Emerg Med 21:357–361, 2001.
39. Weber CA, Santiago R. Hypermagnesemia: a potential complication during treatment of theophylline intoxication with oral activated charcoal and magnesium-containing cathartics. Chest 1989 95:56–59, 1989.
40. Bond GR. Home syrup of ipecac use does not reduce emergency department use or improve outcome. Pediatrics 112:1061–1064, 2003.
41. Litovitz TL, Klein-Schwartz W, Oderda GM, et al. Safety and efficacy of ipecac administration in children younger than one year of age. Pediatrics 76:761–764, 1985.
42. Adler AG, Walinsky P, Krall RA, et al. Death resulting from ipecac syrup. JAMA 243:1927–1928, 1980.

43. Chyka PA, Holley JE, Mandrell TD, et al. Correlation of drug pharmacokinetics and effectiveness of multiple dose activated charcoal therapy. Ann Emerg Med 25:356–362, 1995.

44. Tennenbein M. Multiple doses of activated charcoal: time for reappraisal? Ann Emerg Med 20:529–531, 1991.

45. American Academy of Clinical Toxicology; European Association of Poisons Centres and Clinical Toxicologists. Position statement and practice guidelines on the use of multi-dose activated charcoal in the treatment of acute poisoning. J Toxicol Clin Toxicol 37: 731–751, 1999.

46. Pond SM, Olson KR, Osterloh JD, et al. Randomized study of the treatment of phenobarbital overdose with repeated doses of activated charcoal. JAMA 251:3104–3108, 1984.

47. Caldwell JW, Nowa AJ, Dehaass DD. Hypernatremia associated with cathartics in overdose management. West J Med 147:593–596, 1987.

48. Garrelts JC, Watson WA, Sweet DE, et al. Magnesium toxicity secondary to catharsis during management of theophylline poisoning. Am J Emerg Med 7:34–37, 1989.

49. Grean J, Woolf A. Hypermagnesemia associated with catharsis in a salicylate-intoxicated patient with anorexia nervosa. Ann Emerg Med 8:200–203, 1989.

50. McCord MM. Toxicity of sorbitol-charcoal suspension. J Pediatr 111:307–308, 1987.

51. Brent J, Kulig K, Rumack BH. Iatrogenic death from sorbitol and magnesium sulfate during treatment for salicylism [abstract]. Vet Hum Toxicol 31:334, 1989.

52. Dorrington CL, Johnson DW, Brant R and the Multiple dose activated charcoal complication study group. The frequency of complication associated with the use of multiple-dose activated charcoal. Ann Emerg Med 41:370–377, 2003.

53. Gomez HF, Brent JA, Munoz DC, et al. Charcoal stercolith with intestinal perforation in a patient treated for amitriptyline ingestion. J Emerg Med 12:57–60, 1994.

54. Proudfoot AT, Krenzelok EP, Vale JA. Position paper on urine alkalinization. J Toxicol Clin Toxicol 41:1–26, 2004.

55. Russo M. Management of theophylline intoxication with charcoal-column hemoperfusion. N Engl J Med 300:24–26, 1979.

56. Pond S, Rosenberg J, Benowitz NL, et al. Pharmacokinetics of hemoperfusion for drug overdose. Clin Pharmacokinet 4:329–354, 1979.

57. Goldfrank L, Weisman RS, Errick JK, et al. A dosing nomogram for continuous infusion of intravenous naloxone. Ann Emerg Med 15: 566–570, 1986.

58. Kaplan JL, Marx JA. Effectiveness and safety of intravenous nalmefene for emergency department patients with suspected narcotic overdose: a pilot study. Ann Emerg Med 22:187–190 1993.

59. Gueye PN, Lofaso F, Borron SW, et al. Mechanism of respiratory insufficiency in pure or mixed drug-induced coma involving benzodiazepines. J Toxicol Clin Toxicol 40:35–47, 2002.

60. Buckley NA, Dawson AH, Whyte IM, et al. Relative toxicity of benzodiazepines in overdose. BMJ 310:219–221, 1995.

61. Isbister GK, O'Regan L, Sibbritt D, et al. Alprazolam is relatively more toxic than other benzodiazepines in overdose. J Toxicol Clin Toxicol 41:715, 2003.

62. Drummer OH, Syrjanen ML, Cordner SM. Deaths involving the benzodiazepine flunitrazepam. Am J Forensic Med Pathol 14:238–243, 1993.

63. Buckley NA, Whyte IM, Dawson AH, et al. Self-poisoning in Newcastle, 1987–1992. Med J Aust 162:190–193, 1995.

64. Spivey WH. Flumazenil and seizures: analysis of 43 cases. Clin Ther 15:292–305,1992.

65. Short TG, Maling T, Galletly DC. Ventricular arrhythmias precipitated by flumazenil. BMJ 296:1070–1071, 1988.

66. Burr W, Sandham P, Judd A. Death after flumazenil. BMJ 298: 1713, 1989.

67. Marchant B, Wray R, Leach A, et al. Flumazenil causing convulsions and ventricular tachycardia. Br Med J 299:860, 1989.

68. Smith TW, Butler VP, Habert E, et al. Treatment of life-threatening digitalis intoxication with digoxin-specific Fab antibody fragments. Experience in 26 cases. N Engl J Med 307:1357–1362, 1982.

69. Wenger TL, Butler VP, Haber E, et al. Treatment of 63 severely digitalis-toxic patients with digoxin-specific antibody fragments. J Am Coll Cardiol 5:118A–123A, 1985.

70. Smith TW. Review of clinical experience with digoxin immune Fab. Am J Emerg Med 9:1–5, 1991.

71. Woolf AD, Wenger T, Smith TW, et al. The use of digoxin-specific Fab fragments for severe digitalis intoxication in children. N Engl J Med 326:1739–1744, 1992.

72. Henretig FM, Selbst SM, Forrest C, et al. Repeated acetaminophen overdosing causing hepatotoxicity in children. Clinical reports and literature review. Clin Pediatr 28:525–528, 1989.

73. Heubi JE, Barbacci MB, Zimmerman HJ. Therapeutic misadventures with acetaminophen: hepatotoxicity after multiple doses in children. J Pediatr 132:22–27, 1998.

74. Smilkstein MJ, Knapp GL, Kulig KW, et al. Efficacy of oral N-acetylcysteine in the treatment of acetaminophen overdose. Analysis of the national multicenter study (1976 to 1985). N Engl J Med 319: 1557–1562, 1988.

75. Keays R, Harrison PM, Wendon JA, et al. Intravenous acetylcysteine is paracetamol induced fulminant hepatic necrosis: a prospective controlled trial. Br Med J 303:1026–1029, 1991.

76. Woo OF, Mueller PD, Olson KR, et al. Shorter duration of oral N-acetylcysteine therapy for acute acetaminophen overdose. Ann Emerg Med 35:363–368, 2000.

77. Quadriani DA, Spiller HA, Widder P. Five year retrospective evaluation of sulfonylurea ingestion in children. J Toxicol Clin Toxicol 34: 267–270, 1996.

78. Sketris I, Wheeler D, York S. Hypoglycemic coma induced by inadvertent administration of glyburide. Drug Intell Clin Pharm 18: 142–143, 1984.

79. Szlateny CS, Capes KF, Wang RY. Delayed hypoglycemia in a child after ingestion of a single glipizide tablet. Ann Emerg Med 31: 773–776, 1998.

80. Boyle PJ, Justice K, Drentz AJ, et al. Octreotide reverses hyperinsulinemia and prevents hypoglycemia induced by sulfonylurea overdoses. J Clin Endocrinol Metab 76:752–756, 1993.

81. McLaughlin SA, Crandall CS, McKinney PE. Octreotide: an antidote for sulfonylurea-induced hypoglycemia. Ann Emerg Med 36: 133–138, 2000.

82. Carr R, Zed PJ. Octreotide for sulfonylurea-induced hypoglycemia following overdose. Ann Pharmacother 36:1727–1732, 2002.

83. Brent J, Mc Martin K, Phillips S, et al. Fomepizole for the treatment of ethylene glycol poisoning. N Engl J Med 340:832–838, 1999.

84. Brent J, McMartin K, Phillips S, et al. Fomepizole for the treatment of methanol poisoning. N Engl J Med 344:424–429, 2001.

85. Sivilotti MLA, Burns MJ, McMartin DI, et al. Toxicokinetics of ethylene glycol during fomepizole therapy: implications for management. Ann Emerg Med 36:114–125, 2000.

86. Palatnick W, Redman LW, Sitar DS, et al. Methanol half-life during ethanol administration: Implications for management of methanol poisoning. Ann Emerg Med 26:202–207, 1995.

87. Rodgers GB. The safety of child-resistant packaging for oral prescription drugs. Two decades of experience. JAMA 275:1661–1665, 1996.

88. Rodgers GB. The effectiveness of child-resistant packaging for aspirin. Arch Pediatr Adolesc Med 156:929–933, 2002.

89. Morris CC. Recent trends in pediatric iron poisonings. South Med J 93:1229, 2000.

90. Woolf A, Wieler J, Greenes D. Costs of poison-related hospitalizations at an urban teaching hospital for children. Arch Pediatr Adolesc Med 151:719–723, 1997.

91. Miller T, Lestina DC. Costs of poisoning in the United States and savings from poison control centers: a benefit-cost analysis. Ann Emerg Med 29:239–245, 1997.

92. Harrison DL, Draugalis JR, Slack MK, et al. Cost-effectiveness of regional poison control centers. Arch Intern Med 156:2601–2608, 1996.

Clinical Laboratory Tests and Interpretation

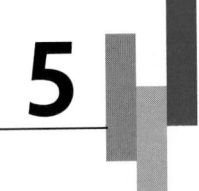

5

Charles F. Seifert and Beth H. Resman-Targoff

Patient assessment should be based on information obtained through laboratory data and a good history and physical examination. If the laboratory data is not consistent with the history and physical examination, the results should be suspect and the tests repeated. There are several steps involved in the collection, evaluation, and reporting of laboratory data. These multiple steps may result in an increased chance of error. Therapeutic and management decisions may be made based on a misleading laboratory value. Examples of errors of this type include estimations of creatinine clearances based on non-steady–state serum creatinine values, or a normal hematocrit in a dehydrated patient, or the evaluation of total phenytoin concentrations in hypoalbuminemic patients. This chapter reviews routinely encountered laboratory tests not thoroughly covered in other parts of this textbook, including their regulation, critical ranges, clinical application, and drug interference. Sodium, potassium, chloride, carbon dioxide content, calcium, magnesium, phosphate, and urinalysis are thoroughly covered in Chapter 28 and Section VIII.

DEFINITIONS

Laboratory test abnormalities are values outside of the normal range for a population. True abnormalities are reproducible, and they are usually associated with signs and symptoms consistent with a disease state. Laboratory test abnormalities are not in themselves diseases, but increases or decreases in values are associated with various diseases. Abnormal values may be caused by drugs, including test interference, side effects, or therapeutic effects. Diseases associated with laboratory tests discussed include, but are not limited to, renal and liver dysfunction, diabetes mellitus, hyperuricemia/gout, myocardial infarction (MI), pancreatitis, malnutrition, ma-

TREATMENT GOALS

- Laboratory test values are generally not treated.
- Treatment goals depend on the specific disease causing the laboratory test abnormality, and they are usually focused on modifying the underlying disease process rather than on changing the laboratory test value. These diseases and their treatment are discussed elsewhere in the textbook.
- An example of a laboratory test goal includes treatment of hyperuricemia in a patient with gout where the goal may be to decrease the uric acid value to between 5 and 6 mg per dL. Another is when warfarin is used in the treatment of a patient with deep venous thrombosis and the dosing goal is an international normalized ratio of 2.0 to 3.0.

lignancies, inflammatory diseases, anemia, blood dyscrasias, infections, and bleeding/clotting disorders.

GENERAL PRINCIPLES

SPECIMEN COLLECTION

Blood and urine are the most common body fluids used for analytic purposes. Phlebotomists should be familiar with the test being performed, know the appropriate container for collection, and how the collection procedure may affect the results. Verification that computer-printed labels match requisitions at the nurses' station and the patient's wristband is essential. Specimens should never be drawn without first identifying the patient. Proper techniques help avoid hemolysis and bacterial contamination. Particular attention should be given to tests where timing is important (e.g., in relation to ingestion of food or drugs). Special precautions are necessary for blood cultures and specimens obtained from indwelling catheters, especially central venous access catheters. Urine collection must also follow a very strict procedure to insure valid results. A freshly obtained urine specimen is crucial when testing for bilirubin, red blood cells, and white blood cells, as these undergo decomposition if left standing at room temperature. Nonpreserved urine specimens are also predisposed to microbial overgrowth at room temperature. A good rule for all specimens is to deliver them to the laboratory within 1 hour of collection or refrigerate them. Proper techniques for performing each method of collection can be found in Henry's *Clinical Diagnosis and Management by Laboratory Methods*[1] or other textbooks on laboratory methods.

METHODS OF ANALYSIS

Several methods are available in the clinical laboratory to assay desired substances in body fluids. Two commonly used techniques are chromatography and immunoassays. The type of compound to be measured determines which assay is used. Certain methods are used for qualitative measurements and others for quantitative measurements. Qualitative measurements only detect that the substance is present and not the quantity of the substance. A urine toxicology screen is an example of a qualitative test in which knowing if a substance is present is usually more important than knowing its amount. Sensitivity and specificity are important aspects of a clinical laboratory test. Sensitivity is commonly defined as the lowest detectable value of a substance, and specificity as the ability to differentiate the substance of interest in the presence of other interfering substances. Sensitivity and specificity are calculated by the formulas below.

$$\text{Sensitivity} = \frac{\text{True positives}}{\text{True positives} + \text{False negatives}} \times 100$$

$$\text{Specificity} = \frac{\text{True negatives}}{\text{True negatives} + \text{False positives}} \times 100$$

Ideally, sensitivity and specificity should each be at least 95%. Most clinical laboratories have strict performance criteria set for their assay techniques. These criteria vary widely among institutions and can greatly affect the interpretation of individual patient results. Most clinical laboratories use the most accurate method with the best automation at a reasonable cost. For each individual clinical laboratory, particular attention to accuracy, precision, and quality control are essential for reliable reproducible results.[2]

REFERENCE VALUES

Normal ranges are provided as a guideline, but individual laboratory results may vary considerably. Values outside of the quoted normal range may be considered abnormal but not clinically important, whereas certain values in the normal range with a particular disease state are actually abnormal (e.g., normal hemoglobin in a patient with chronic obstructive airway disease). Laboratories may evaluate substances with different assays that are more or less precise. Certain tests are time dependent and the time the sample is drawn is crucial in determining if the patient sample is truly within the reference range. This is especially true for most serum drug concentrations. Most of the normal reference ranges quoted in this chapter are reproduced with permission from D.S. Young.[3]

DRUG INTERFERENCE

Medications affect laboratory test results in two major ways. Due to a drug's intrinsic pharmacokinetic, pharmacologic, or toxicologic properties, it may alter the formation, regulation, release, or elimination of the substance being tested (e.g., hydrochlorothiazide blocks the tubular secretion of uric acid, exogenous insulin affects serum glucose, or toxic acetaminophen concentration affects serum transaminases). Medications may also directly interfere with the assay used to detect the substance (e.g., ascorbic acid causes false-negative results with urine glucose by the glucose oxidase method). Each laboratory test discussed in this chapter will include a brief section on common medications that affect the test results.

SYSTÈME INTERNATIONALE D'UNITÉS

The basis for converting all measurements of body fluid substances to a molar concentration unit is that substances in the body interact on a molar basis. It also standardizes units internationally. Certain societies including the American College of Physicians and their official journal (*Annals of Internal Medicine*) have adopted the Système Internationale d'Unités (SI units) as their preferred reference standard. Other journals still accept both sets of units. Reference laboratories in most hospitals and most clinicians in the United States have not accepted this change willingly and still use the old conventional reference standards. For each laboratory test in this chapter, conventional and SI units with conversion factors will be given. To convert from conventional units to SI units, multiply the results in conventional units by the conversion factor.

SPECIFIC LABORATORY TESTS

SERUM CREATININE

[men = 0.6 to 1.2 mg/dL, 0.1 mg/dL lower for women (SI units: males = 50 to 110 μmol/L, women = 10 μmol/L lower), conversion factor (CF) = 88.40]

Serum creatinine (SCr) is a peptide formed as a waste product of creatine, an important energy storage substance in muscle metabolism. Creatinine is an anhydride of creatine and is not used in the body.[4] Formation of creatinine is relatively constant with about 1.6% to 1.7% of creatine transformed to creatinine each 24 hours (Fig. 5.1). This in turn depends on the total muscle content of creatine and creatine

phosphate. Factors that affect creatine levels, such as diet, fever, and muscle damage, do not readily influence SCr level. The serum concentration of creatinine is also relatively constant, and urinary excretion is the result of glomerular filtration and proximal tubular secretion. The SCr level is a more reliable indicator of renal function than the blood urea nitrogen (BUN).

SCr concentration increases in the presence of impaired renal function. Since up to 50% of renal function is lost before the SCr level becomes abnormally elevated, it is not a good indicator of early renal dysfunction. Even with its pitfalls, creatinine clearance based on 24-hour urinary excretion of creatinine is the most reliable readily available clinical test to evaluate glomerular filtration. Several methods exist for the rapid estimation of creatinine clearance based on the patient's age, ideal body weight, and SCr level. The methods are discussed in more detail in Chapter 1 and Section XII. A steady-state SCr level is necessary for an accurate

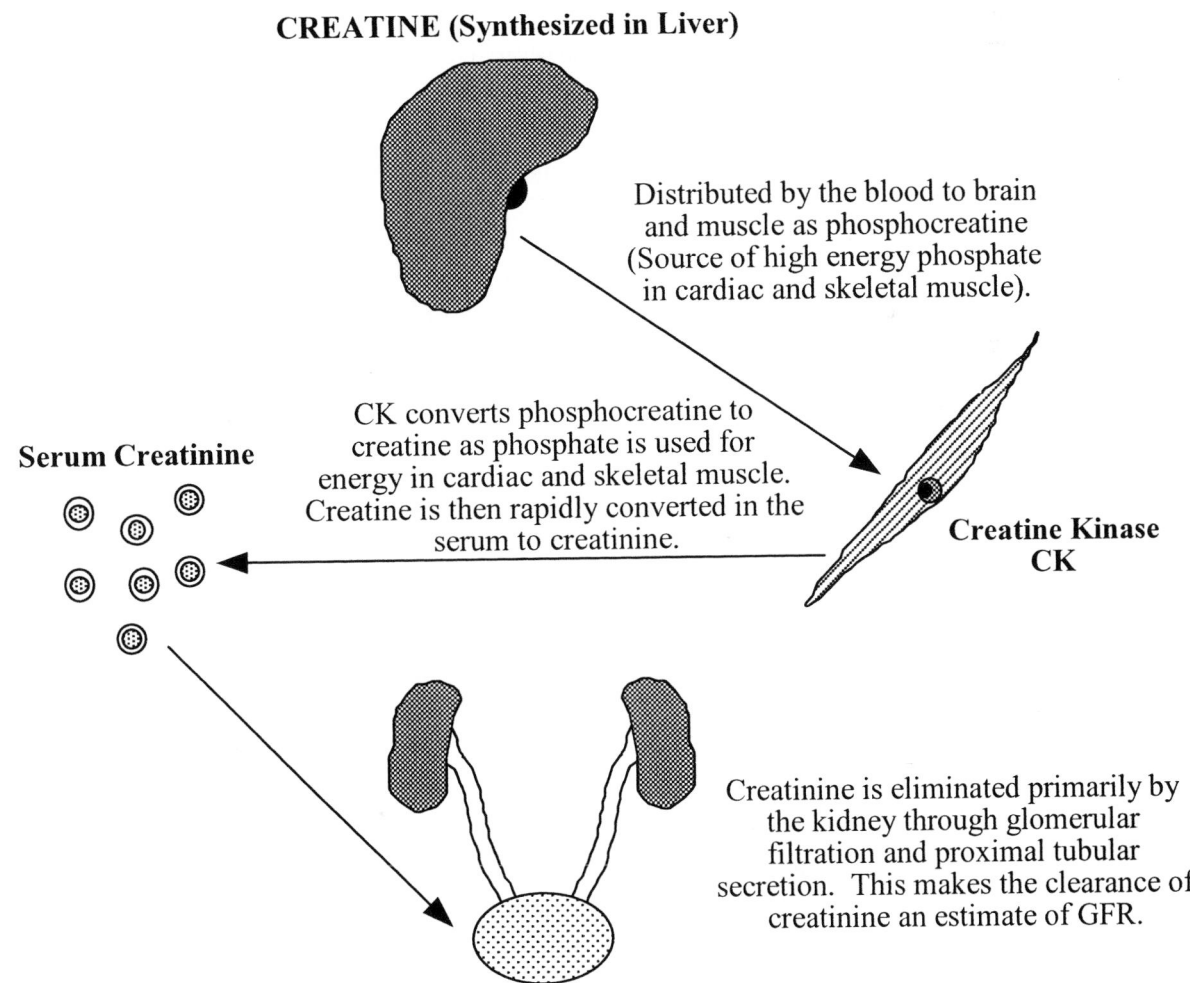

FIGURE 5.1 Creatinine production.

estimation. Certain methods are more inaccurate in the elderly and in patients with decreased muscle mass.[5]

Drugs that may cause an increased SCr level due to interference with tubular secretion of creatinine are cephalosporins, cimetidine, salicylates, and trimethoprim. Drugs such as acetohexamide, ascorbic acid, flucytosine, levodopa, lidocaine, methyldopa, p-aminohippurate, and phenolsulfonphthalein may cause increases by interference with the analytical methodology of the SCr determination.[6]

BLOOD UREA NITROGEN

[8 to 18 mg/dL (SI units = 3.0 to 6.5 mmol/L), CF = 0.357]

Urea is the predominant product of protein and amino acid catabolism and is made in the liver through the urea cycle. It is the main nonprotein nitrogen (NPN) constituent in the blood. Other NPN substances include amino acids, uric acid, creatinine, and ammonia. Total NPN determinations are no longer used clinically. Urea is distributed to all intra- and extracellular fluids and is freely diffusible across most cell membranes.[4] Urea is excreted mostly by the kidneys, with only small amounts excreted in sweat and in the intestines.

When there is a large increase of nonprotein compounds, such as urea in the blood, the condition of azotemia is present. Azotemia can be categorized as prerenal, renal, and postrenal. Prerenal azotemia is the result of inadequate perfusion of the kidneys with otherwise normal renal function. Causes of prerenal azotemia include dehydration, decreased blood volume, shock, and heart failure. Renal azotemia refers to decreased glomerular filtration because of acute or chronic renal disease including glomerulonephritis, interstitial nephritis, and tubular necrosis. Postrenal azotemia is most commonly the result of urinary tract obstruction. The extreme form of azotemia, known as uremia, is a constellation of symptoms resulting from severe elevations in BUN (100 to 200 mg/dL) and other substances not adequately cleared by the kidney. Uremic symptoms include acidosis, water and electrolyte imbalance, nausea, vomiting, and neuropsychiatric changes including stupor or deep coma.[4] Agents that are noted for causing acute interstitial nephritis usually accompanied with an allergic reaction include allopurinol, cephalosporins, penicillins, nonsteroidal antiinflammatory agents, and phenytoin.[7] Common agents that may cause acute tubular necrosis include aminoglycosides, amphotericin B, angiotensin converting enzyme (ACE) inhibitors, carboplatin, cisplatin, cyclosporine, diuretics, gold salts, ifosfamide, intravenous contrast media, lithium, pentamidine, tacrolimus, tetracyclines, and vancomycin.[7] Agents that may increase the risk of urolithiasis include allopurinol, calcium salts, carbonic anhydrase inhibitors, indinavir, sulfonamides, triamterene, and zonisamide.[7] Nephrolithiasis occurs in 1% to 3% with lamivudine-zidovudine combination, but may increase to as high as 4 to 12% with the addition of indinavir.[8,9]

BUN can be used as an estimate of renal function. As with creatinine levels, a clinically important elevation will not be observed until glomerular filtration is decreased by at least 50%. A decreased BUN is usually not clinically significant; however, a few conditions may cause a significant decrease. These include poor nutrition, high fluid intake, and severe liver disease where urea synthesis is decreased. Drugs that may increase BUN by methodologic interference are chloral hydrate, ammonium salts, acetohexamide, and sulfonylureas, while those that decrease it include chloramphenicol and streptomycin.[6]

BUN and SCr concentrations may be evaluated simultaneously. To yield more information than either alone, the BUN is divided by the SCr. This is termed the BUN to creatinine ratio; the normal ratio ranges from 10 to 20:1. Table 5.1 indicates clinical causes of elevated BUN and SCr with increased or normal BUN:creatinine ratios.[10] Specific causes of prerenal, renal, and postrenal azotemia can be further delineated using the BUN to SCr ratio, fractional excretion of sodium (FENa), free water clearance, and urinalysis.[10]

PLASMA GLUCOSE

[70 to 110 mg/dL (fasting SI units = 3.9 to 6.1 mmol/L), however normal ranges depend on the method, CF = 0.05551]

Laboratory determinations of glucose level are usually performed on venous plasma specimens. Whole blood determinations are used only for capillary blood used in finger stick devices. Serum and plasma glucose concentrations are identical and are 10% to 15% higher than whole blood measurements. Glucose is one of the clinically important carbohydrates along with fructose and galactose. Disorders of carbohydrate metabolism such as diabetes are evaluated in part by measurement of plasma glucose in the fasting state or after suppression or stimulation. The concentration of glucose in the blood is regulated within narrow limits by hormones produced by the pancreas and through other mecha-

TABLE 5.1	**BUN to Creatinine Ratio in Clinical Conditions with Elevated BUN and Serum Creatinine**
≥20:1	Prerenal azotemia (e.g., heart failure, dehydration)
	Postrenal azotemia (e.g., obstructive uropathy)
	Impaired renal function plus excess protein intake or tissue breakdown
	Drugs such as tetracycline and glucocorticosteroids
<20:1	Prerenal azotemia in hepatic cirrhosis
	Renal dialysis
	Renal failure in muscular patients
	Decreased urea production (e.g., low protein intake, severe diarrhea or vomiting)

nisms mediated by the adrenergic and cholinergic nervous systems.[11] Glucose is a major source of energy for brain, muscle, and fat. The brain is the only tissue that does not require insulin for glucose utilization. If glucose is not available exogenously (fasting state), the body, using hormonal mechanisms (counter-regulatory hormones: glucagon, epinephrine, cortisol, and somatostatin), will form its own glucose by tissue and hepatic gluconeogenesis and hepatic glycogenolysis. Glucose is therefore carefully regulated by glucagon and insulin secretion, which compensate for food ingestion and fasting states. (Please refer to Chapter 40 for a detailed discussion of carbohydrate metabolism in normal and diabetic patients.)

Methods for clinical determination of glucose are chemical or enzymatic. Chemical analysis is based on the reducing properties of glucose, and uses a color change reaction that is measured spectrophotometrically. The enzymatic method is based on the reaction of glucose and glucose oxidase. This is a very specific method and is generally inexpensive. Ascorbic acid can interfere with this method and result in decreased values.

Elevated plasma glucose concentrations, or hyperglycemia, can be caused by a number of syndromes and diseases. The classification of hyperglycemia is shown in Table 5.2.[7,11] A fasting plasma glucose of 126 mg per dL (7.0 mmol/L) or greater is considered abnormal.

Hypoglycemia is a syndrome of low plasma glucose with related symptoms. In the adult, an overnight fasting plasma glucose <45 mg per dL (2.5 mmol/L) is considered abnormal and more than 55 mg per dL (3.0 mmol/L) is considered the lower limit of normal. In neonates, less than 35 mg per dL (1.9 mmol/L) is abnormal and in infants and children, less than 45 mg per dL (2.5 mmol/L) is abnormal. Table 5.3

TABLE 5.2	Classification of Hyperglycemia

Primary
 Insulin-dependent diabetes mellitus
 Noninsulin-dependent diabetes mellitus
Secondary
 Hyperglycemia resulting from disease of the pancreas
  Inflammation
   Acute pancreatitis (rare)
   Chronic pancreatitis
   Pancreatitis due to mumps
   ? Cell damage due to coxsackievirus B_4 infection
   ? Autoimmune disease
  Pancreatectomy
  Pancreatic infiltration
   Hemochromatosis
   Tumors
  Trauma to pancreas (rare)
 Hyperglycemia related to other major endocrine diseases
  Acromegaly
  Cushing's syndrome
  Thyrotoxicosis
  Pheochromocytoma
  Hyperaldosteronism
  Glucagonoma
  Somatostatinoma
 Hyperglycemia caused by drugs
  Corticosteroids, acetazolamide, thiazide diuretics, and beta agonists
  Pentamidine (late), tacrolimus, and protease inhibitors
 Hyperglycemia related to other major disease states
  Chronic renal failure
  Chronic liver disease
  Infection
 Miscellaneous hyperglycemia
  Pregnancy
  Related to insulin receptor antibodies (acanthosis nigricans)

TABLE 5.3	Classification of Common Causes of Hypoglycemia

No anatomic lesion present
Fasting plasma glucose normal
 Reactive hypoglycemia
  Functional hypoglycemia
  Alimentary hypoglycemia
  Diabetic and impaired glucose tolerance
Fasting plasma glucose low
 Drug-induced hypoglycemia
  Oral hypoglycemic agents
  ACE inhibitors
  Insulin
  Ethanol
  Salicylates (late in overdose)
  Pentamidine (early in therapy)
  Combinations of the above
 Factitious-fasting glucose normal or low
Anatomic lesion present
 Insulinoma
 Extrapancreatic neoplasms
 Adrenocortical insufficiency
 Hypopituitarism
 Acute liver failure

ACE, angiotensin-converting enzyme.

shows the classification of common causes of hypoglycemia.[7,11]

URIC ACID

[2.0 to 7.0 mg/dL (SI units = 120 to 420 μmol/L), CF = 59.48] (Refer to Chapter 67.)

Uric acid is the end product of purine metabolism. The major rate-limiting step in the synthesis of uric acid is the intracellular concentration of 5-phosphoribosyl-1-pyrophosphate (PRPP). Uric acid serves no biologic function. Approximately two thirds of uric acid is excreted by the kidneys and one-third through the gastrointestinal tract. Assuming that the uric acid filtered through the glomerulus equates to 100%, 98% to 100% of this glomerular filtrate is reabsorbed in the proximal portion of the proximal convoluted tubule (Fig. 5.2).[12] Fifty percent of the original amount is secreted into the distal portion of the proximal convoluted tubule, but 40% to 44% is subsequently reabsorbed, and 6% to 12% of the original glomerular filtrate eventually excreted.

Hyperuricemia is due to an overproduction of uric acid (increased destruction of nucleoproteins, high protein diet, or inborn enzymatic defects) or an underexcretion (renal defect). Since the serum is saturated with urate at a concentration of 7 mg per dL (420 μmol/L), as serum urate concentrations exceed this saturation point, monosodium urate crystals deposit in and around the joints and cartilage and in the kidneys, sometimes eliciting the disease known as gout. As urinary pH is increased, the solubility of uric acid is increased; decreasing urinary pH may precipitate urate nephrolithiasis in patients with high urine uric acid concentrations. Asymptomatic hyperuricemia is classified as an elevated serum uric acid without symptoms of acute gouty arthritis.[12] With increasing uric acid levels, there is an increased risk of developing acute gout. There is a 2.0% to 4.1% 5-year cumulative incidence of gouty arthritis in men with serum urate levels ranging from 7.0 to 8.9 mg per dL (416 to 529 μmol/L) as compared to a 5-year cumulative incidence of 0.5% to 0.6% with serum urate levels of less than 6.9 mg per dL (≤410 μmol/L). The incidence of gouty arthritis increases tremendously as urate levels rise above 9.0 mg per dL (535 μmol/L). The 5-year cumulative incidence for men with serum urate levels of 9.0 to 9.9 mg per dL (535 to 589 μmol/L) and more than 10.0 mg per dL (≥595 μmol/L) were 19.8% and 30.5%, respectively.[13] After one attack of gout, a patient may never have another or may have a recurrence from 3 to 42 years later (mean 11.4 years).[13]

Agents that have a cytotoxic effect causing an increased turnover of nucleic acids may increase uric acid concentrations (e.g., antimetabolite and chemotherapeutic agents used to treat neoplastic diseases, such as methotrexate, busulfan, vincristine, prednisone, and azathioprine).[6] Agents that decrease the renal clearance or block tubular secretion may cause a substantial elevation in serum urate concentrations (e.g., thiazide and loop diuretics, pyrazinamide, and ethambutol).[6,14] Diuretic-induced hyperuricemia accounts for 95% of acute attacks of gout in women older than 60 years of age and 56% of men.[15] Some agents, such as salicylates, probenecid, and sulfinpyrazone, inhibit the tubular secretion of urate at low doses, but at high doses also inhibit tubular reabsorption, inducing a marked uricosuric effect.[4] Tacrolimus and cyclosporine may cause hyperuricemia in more than 3% of patients through an unknown mechanism.[16] Allopurinol therapeutically lowers serum uric acid by inhibiting xanthine oxidase (enzyme that converts xanthine to uric acid in purine metabolism), while uricosuric agents, such as probenecid, are also used therapeutically to lower serum uric acid by blocking proximal tubular reabsorption. Ascorbic acid, caffeine, glucose, levodopa, methyldopa, and theophylline may interfere with the analytical technique and cause false high results.[4,6]

ENZYMES

Enzymes are located in all body tissues and are responsible for the organic catalytic conversion of chemicals throughout the body. When enzymatically active cells are lysed or destroyed, certain enzymes are released into the serum. These enzymes are measured to assess which tissue is damaged. Only active cells release high quantities of enzymes in the serum. The more acute and extensive tissue injury is, the greater the rise in enzymes released from that tissue. Chronic smoldering damage causes moderate release of similar enzymes, with patterns usually different from those in acute injury.

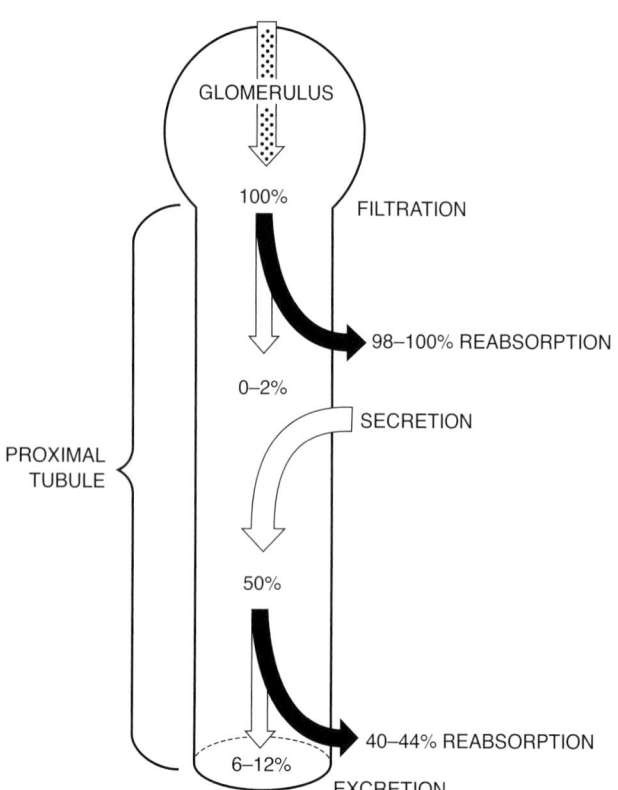

FIGURE 5.2 Uric acid excretion.

Isoenzymes are proteins with different amino acid sequences, arising primarily from different tissues, which have the same enzymatic action. Clinically, these isoenzyme fractions are used to determine which tissue is damaged, and by using their particular patterns, clinical diagnoses are made. Isoenzymes are usually separated by gel electrophoresis. Even though two isoenzymes have the same enzymatic activity, they are of different sizes and electronegativity, and predominate in different tissues.[17]

Enzymatic units are determined on a micromolar catalytic basis. One international unit (IU) is the amount of enzyme that catalyzes the conversion of 1 μmol of substrate per minute. The SI unit for enzymatic activity is known as the katal (kat). One katal is equal to 1 mol catalyzed per second.[17] One μkat is equal to 1 μmol of substrate catalyzed per second, therefore, 1 μkat = 60 IU.

CREATINE KINASE

[0 to 130 IU/L (SI units = 0 to 2.16 μkat/L), however, normal ranges vary considerably with method, CF = 0.01667]

Creatine kinase (CK), formerly known as creatine phosphokinase, catalyzes the conversion of phosphocreatine to creatine releasing high-energy phosphate to skeletal and cardiac muscle (Fig. 5.1). Creatine is an unstable molecule and is converted very rapidly to creatinine. CK is a dimer consisting of two subunits, M and B. Brain tissue yields approximately 90% BB (CK$_1$) and 10% MM (CK$_3$), cardiac tissue yields approximately 40% MB (CK$_2$) and 60% MM, whereas, normal serum contains virtually 100% MM as does skeletal muscle. Clinical conditions causing elevated serum CK primarily involve skeletal muscle or cardiac tissue. The brain fraction is almost never observed in serum, even after a cerebrovascular accident, since the enzyme does not readily cross the blood–brain barrier.[17]

Almost any damage to skeletal muscle will cause an elevation in serum CK. Severe acute rhabdomyolysis secondary to trauma, prolonged coma, or overdoses of various drugs may cause dramatic rises of CK, ranging from 10,000 to 100,000 IU per L (167 to 1,670 μkat/L).[18] Other conditions damaging skeletal muscle such as progressive muscular dystrophy, polymyositis/dermatomyositis, delirium tremens, seizures, or hypothyroidism may cause significant elevations in CK.

CK serum concentrations begin to rise approximately 4 to 8 hours after acute myocardial injury, peak at 12 to 24 hours, and may persist throughout the initial 72-hour period.[19] An MB fraction more than 6% of the total is indicative of myocardial injury.[20] Several studies have shown that patients with a history of angina compatible with acute MI in whom total peak CK serum concentrations were normal, but MB isoenzyme fractions were more than 6% of the total had true acute infarctions.[21–23]

Intramuscular injections of medications may cause a variable increase in CK of 2 to 6 times the normal concentration. These elevations return to normal within 48 hours after cessation of the injections. CK rises in over 50% of patients receiving countershock or defibrillation but usually returns to normal in 48 to 72 hours.[6] Several medications have been reported to cause rhabdomyolysis in therapeutic and overdose situations, including opiates, cocaine, phencyclidine, amphetamines, theophylline, antihistamines, fibric acid derivatives, barbiturates, aminocaproic acid, certain antibiotics, chloroquine, colchicine, corticosteroids, HMG-CoA reductase inhibitors, and vincristine.[17,18] Patients receiving therapeutic doses of neuroleptics may rarely experience the neuroleptic malignant syndrome, which may cause severe elevations in CK.[24]

LACTATE DEHYDROGENASE

[100 to 190 IU/L (SI units = 1.67 to 3.17 μkat/L), CF = 0.01667]

Lactate dehydrogenase (LDH) catalyzes the conversion of pyruvate to lactate anaerobically to generate adenosine triphosphate (ATP).[25] LDH is in high concentrations in cardiac and skeletal muscle, liver, kidney, lung parenchyma, and erythrocytes. It is essential to have prompt analysis of the sample, which has to be hemolysis free for an accurate LDH measurement. LDH can be separated into five distinct components. The five LDH isoenzymes all have approximately the same molecular weight but have different charges. LDH$_5$ has the greatest mobility and LDH$_1$ the least. Table 5.4 lists the LDH isoenzymes and their relative activity in each tissue.[17]

Serum LDH is almost always increased after an acute MI. The serum LDH begins to rise 10 to 12 hours after the acute event, reaching a peak in 48 to 72 hours with prolonged elevation for up to 10 to 14 days.[6] Increased serum LDH level, with LDH$_1$ greater than LDH$_2$ (flipped enzymes), occurs in acute MI in approximately 80% of patients, but also occurs in acute renal infarction, pernicious anemia, and hemolysis.[6] In a large MI with biventricular failure, LDH$_5$ levels may also be elevated due to liver congestion.

LDH$_5$ may be markedly increased in hepatitis and may also be increased in other hepatic disorders. LDH elevations may occur 50% of the time with malignant tumors, usually with a nonspecific isoenzyme pattern. LDH is elevated in approximately 60% of patients with lymphomas and 90% of patients with leukemias. Marked increases in LDH$_5$ levels are seen in patients with skeletal muscle damage, extensive burns, and trauma. Pulmonary embolus and infarction may cause elevations in LDH$_2$ and LDH$_3$; if cor pulmonale is present, LDH$_5$ will also rise. In nephrotic syndrome, LDH$_4$ and LDH$_5$ will rise, but in nephritis and renal infarction, LDH$_1$ and LDH$_2$ rise. All forms of hemolysis, including sickle cell crisis and drug-induced hemolysis, will cause elevations in LDH$_1$ and LDH$_2$.[26,27]

Serum LDH is usually elevated in patients with *Pneumocystis carinii* pneumonia particularly in human immunodeficiency virus (HIV) patients.[28] However, LDH can also be

| TABLE 5.4 | Lactate Dehydrogenase Isoenzymes Nomenclature |

Nomenclature of Isoenzyme Starting with Most Anodic	Composition: Proportion of Monomers in Each Isoenzyme	Relative Percentage of LD Isoenzymes in Various Tissues					
		Myocardium	Liver	Skeletal Muscle	Lung	Renal Cortex	RBC
1	HHHH	45	0	0	10	35	40
2	HHHM	40	5	0	15	30	35
3	HHMM	10	10	10	40	25	15
4	HMMM	5	15	30	30	20	10
5	MMMM	0	70	60	5	0	0

Adapted from Table 15.7 from Dufour D, Lott JA, Henry JB. Clinical Enzymology. In: Henry JB, ed. Clinical diagnosis and management by laboratory methods. 20th ed. Philadelphia: WB Saunders, 2001:295. Adapted with permission of the publisher.

LD, lactate dehydrogenase; Monomer H, myocardial; Monomer M, skeletal muscle; RBC, red blood cell.

elevated in multiple other pulmonary conditions including tuberculosis and bacterial pneumonia.[28]

All drugs causing damage to the above-mentioned tissues will cause elevations in LDH. Hepatotoxic agents and agents inducing hemolysis will increase serum LDH concentrations.[27,29]

TROPONINS

[Troponin I (cTnI) 0.7 to 1.5 ng/mL
(SI units = 0.7 to 1.5 µg/L), CF = 1.0]

Troponin is a complex of three proteins, troponin T, troponin C, and troponin I.[17] Each troponin has its own specific function in the regulation of myosin and actin in the contractile process. cTnI is very sensitive and specific for myocardial tissue. After acute myocardial injury, cTnI starts to rise approximately 2 hours after myocardial damage (2 to 6 hours faster than myocardial bound CK [CKMB]) with peak elevations occurring at about 24 to 36 hours. There is a 13-fold greater concentration of cTnI than CKMB in the heart and is at least as sensitive for the clinical detection of cardiac injury as CKMB.[30] Cardiac troponin I is much more specific than CKMB for cardiac tissue and is not elevated in skeletal muscle injury, chronic muscle disease, hypothyroidism, after endurance exercise, chronic renal failure, and postoperative patients without myocardial injury.[30,31] An elevation of cTnI greater than 2.0 ng per mL is indicative of acute myocardial injury.[30–32] Unlike CKMB, cTnI can also detect acute myocardial injury for up to 10 to 12 days without the lack of specificity and necessary isoenzyme separation of LDH.[32] Hamm et al, studied two troponin I levels at least more than 4 hours apart and at least 6 hours after the onset of pain in 773 consecutive patients who had acute chest pain for less than 12 hours without ST-segment elevation on their electrocardiograms presenting to the emergency room.[33] Among 47 patients with evolving MI, troponin I was positive in all

47. The cardiac event rates in patients with negative troponin I during 30 days of follow-up was only 0.3%. Several authors are recommending cTnI as the gold standard serologic test to quickly diagnose acute myocardial injury and have developed protocols for its use in this diagnosis.[30,31]

BRAIN NATRIURETIC PEPTIDE

[<100 pg/mL (SI units = <100 ng/L), CF = 1.0]

The natriuretic peptide system is composed of three major proteins: (a) atrial natriuretic peptide, (b) brain natriuretic peptide (BNP), and (c) C-type natriuretic peptide.[34] All three peptides are associated with vasodilating, natriuretic, diuretic, lusitropic, and antiproliferative/antifibrotic properties to counterregulate the pathophysiologic influences of the renin-angiotensin-aldosterone system. BNP is the most commonly measured peptide clinically. Recombinant human BNP is approved clinically as nesiritide for use in decompensated heart failure. BNP measurements are used clinically to assess patients with congestive heart failure (CHF).[35] Young healthy individuals have low levels of BNP (<20 pg/mL), however, the elderly, patients with hypertensive renal disease, and patients with CHF can have elevated BNP levels. Over 20% of patients with established chronic symptomatic CHF can have BNP levels lower than 100 pg/mL.[36] BNP levels of 100 pg/mL or higher imply left ventricular dysfunction, however, this needs to be verified using the patient's history, physical, and other tests, such as an echocardiography.[35]

ASPARTATE AMINOTRANSFERASE

[0 to 35 IU/L (SI units = 0 to 0.58 µkat/L), CF = 0.01667]

Aspartate aminotransferase (AST), formerly known as serum glutamic oxaloacetic transaminase (SGOT) is one of several transaminases responsible for transfer of amino groups in gluconeogenesis. AST is responsible for transferring an amino group from aspartate to α, β-glutaric acid forming glutamate and oxaloacetate.[25] The highest concentrations of AST are located in cardiac and hepatic tissues.

AST usually appears within 6 to 8 hours after myocardial injury, peaking in 24 hours, and returning to baseline in 4 to 6 days.[6] AST rises in virtually all types of hepatic diseases. Its peak concentration and ratio to other enzymes reflect the type of hepatic damage. These differences will be discussed later under bilirubin.

Several medications may cause elevations in AST levels by direct hepatocellular damage or cholestasis.[7,29,37,38] Cholinergic drugs and opioids cause elevation of transaminases due to spasm of the sphincter of Oddi.[39] Several agents (commonly isoniazid and rifampin) may cause transient elevations in transaminase levels.[29,40,41] Initially, dye-binding techniques were used to assay for transaminases, which accounted for several drug interferences including isoniazid, but with newer ultraviolet techniques, there is very little interaction with the assay.[39]

ALANINE AMINOTRANSFERASE

[0 to 35 IU/L (SI units = 0 to 0.58 μkat/L), CF = 0.01667]

Alanine aminotransferase (ALT), formerly known as serum glutamate pyruvate transaminase (SGPT), transfers an amino group from alanine to α-ketoglutarate forming glutamate and pyruvate.[25] ALT is very specific for hepatic tissue and is almost always absent in acute MI. It is much more sensitive to hepatic damage, and levels rise faster and higher than those of AST in most types of hepatocellular damage.

γ-GLUTAMYL TRANSFERASE

[SI units = 0 to 0.50 μkat/L (0 to 30 IU/L), CF = 0.01667]

γ-Glutamyl transferase (GGT) catalyzes the transfer of a γ-glutamyl group from one peptide to another.[25] The kidneys, liver, and pancreas contain large quantities of GGT. Several isoenzymes of GGT have been isolated, but to date, no clinical use for them has been found.[17]

The elevation of GGT parallels that of alkaline phosphatase and rises higher in cholestatic and obstructive diseases than in acute hepatocellular diseases. It is always elevated in acute pancreatitis, and its rise is faster and greater than that of alkaline phosphatase in obstructive jaundice. GGT is the most sensitive biochemical indicator of alcohol exposure, since elevation exceeds that of other commonly monitored liver enzymes. In alcoholic hepatitis, GGT is usually the enzyme that rises fastest and has the highest peaks. Agents such as phenytoin and phenobarbital that induce the cytochrome P450 enzyme system may cause elevations in GGT.[6]

PHOSPHATASES

Phosphatases are primarily responsible for catalyzing cleavage of monophosphate esters and may be acid or alkaline.[25]

Acid phosphatases have optimal enzymatic activity at a pH of 5, and alkaline phosphatases have an optimal enzymatic activity at a pH of 9.[17] Acid phosphatase [0 to 5.5 IU/L (SI units = 0 to 90 nkat/L), CF = 16.67] is primarily found in prostate, erythrocytes, and platelets. Approximately 60% to 75% of men with prostate cancer have elevated acid phosphatase concentrations.[6]

Alkaline phosphatase (ALP), [30 to 120 IU/L (SI units = 0.5–2.0 μkat/L), CF = 0.01667] is found in most tissues but is derived predominantly from hepatic, osseous, and intestinal cells.[6] The placenta produces high concentrations of ALP in the third trimester because of high fetal osteoblastic activity. Children in the active growth phase produce ALP at two to five times adult rates. The osseous and hepatic isoenzymes of ALP can be readily identified in electrophoretic patterns of serum.[42]

ALP is elevated in most disorders of bone involving osteoblastic activity. Metastatic disease to bone may cause substantial elevations in ALP levels. ALP is also elevated in acute fractures, hyperparathyroidism, renal bone disease, osteogenic sarcoma, and Paget disease.[17]

ALP is secreted into bile, and an elevation may be the first clue to intra- or extrahepatic cholestasis.[43] The diagnosis of intra- or extrahepatic disease cannot be determined by the peak height of the serum ALP concentration.[43] When biliary obstruction is complete, ALP serum concentrations are almost always three to eight times normal; whereas, with incomplete obstruction, concentrations are only two to three times normal.[44]

AMYLASE

[0 to 70 Somogyi units/dL; 0 to 130 IU/L (SI units = 0 to 2.17 μkat/L), CF: Somogyi to IU = 1.85, Somogyi to SI units = 0.031, IU to SI units = 0.01667]

Amylase enzymatically cleaves large polysaccharides into oligo- and monosaccharides in the gastrointestinal tract through salivary and pancreatic secretions. Amylase is present as α-, β-, and γ-amylase, but only α-amylase is of clinical interest. Amylase is present in a variety of human tissues including the pancreas, salivary glands, muscle, adipose tissue, kidney, brain, lung, fallopian tubes, intestine, spleen, and heart.[45] Normal serum amylase is composed of approximately 40% pancreatic isoenzyme (P-type isoamylase) and 60% salivary isoenzyme (S-type isoamylase).[46] This percentage changes with age so that after the age of 70, P-type isoamylase comprises only 20% of total serum amylase.[45]

Serum amylase concentrations rise within 6 to 48 hours after the onset of acute pancreatitis in >80% of patients.[46] Values over four times the upper limit of normal are highly suggestive of the diagnosis.[45] This is a sensitive measure of acute pancreatitis, but it is not highly specific, since several other conditions may present with acute abdominal pain and elevated serum amylase levels, including biliary colic, perforated peptic ulcer, and mesenteric infarction.[46] In acute pancreatitis, the urinary clearance of amylase is increased, possibly because of altered renal tubular function. A urinary amylase to creatinine ratio >0.04 suggests acute pancreatitis; however, this method is unreliable since elevated ratios may also be seen with other conditions, such as burns, renal insufficiency, and ketoacidosis.[45,46] The usefulness of isoenzyme separation is limited since other intestinal sources also account for P-type isoamylase. Patients with acute alcoholic pancreatitis have normal serum amylase levels approximately 30% of the time.[46]

Parotitis and mumps cause elevations of S-type isoamylase. Chronic alcohol consumption may also increase S-type isoamylase. This is an important consideration because alcohol is the most common cause of acute pancreatitis. Macroamylase is a circulating complex of normal amylase bound to either IgG or IgA.[45] Analysis of macroamylase reveals variable amounts of P-type and S-type isoamylase. Macroamylasemia is an acquired benign condition that must be separated from other causes of hyperamylasemia.

Medications that cause spasm of the sphincter of Oddi, such as narcotics and cholinergic agents, may cause elevations in serum amylase.[6] Agents definitely associated with causing pancreatitis include 5-aminosalicylic acid, asparaginase, azathioprine, didanosine, estrogens, furosemide, 6-mercaptopurine, methyldopa, metronidazole, pentamidine, sulfonamides, sulindac, tetracycline, thiazide diuretics, and valproic acid.[47] Certain pancreatic enzyme preparations contain amylase and lipase that may elevate serum amylase and lipase values.[6]

LIPASE

[0 to 0.6 Cherry-Crandall units/mL; 0 to 160 IU/L (SI units = 0 to 2.66 μkat/L), CF: Cherry-Crandall to IU = 278, Cherry-Crandall to SI units = 4.63]

Lipase hydrolyzes glycerol esters of long chain fatty acids at the one and three positions, producing β-monoglyceride and 2 mol of free fatty acid. Serum lipase should not be confused with lipoprotein lipase, since these are entirely different enzymes. Lipase is located in stomach, intestine, leukocytes, fat cells, and milk, but predominates in the pancreas.[45] Serum lipase concentrations are usually elevated in patients with acute pancreatitis and are more predictive than amylase.[45,46] Serum lipase increases at approximately the same time as amylase in acute pancreatitis, but elevations may persist for much longer than serum amylase (7 to 10 days).[45] Serum lipase concentrations may also be elevated in other acute abdominal illnesses.[46] Medications that may elevate serum lipase concentrations are very similar to those that elevate serum amylase.

BILIRUBIN

[Total 0.1 to 1.0 mg/dL, Direct 0 to 0.2 mg/dL (SI units = Total 2 to 18 μmol/L, Direct 0 to 4 μmol/L), CF = 17.10]

Bilirubin is a metabolic byproduct of the lysis of heme by the reticuloendothelial system (RES). This production is predominantly from senescent erythrocytes (>85%) (Fig. 5.3).[44] The RES catabolizes heme into free iron, globin, and biliverdin, which is rapidly converted to bilirubin. Unconjugated bilirubin is poorly soluble in serum; therefore, it is transported to the liver bound to albumin. This unconjugated form is also known as indirect or prehepatic bilirubin. In the liver, glucuronyl transferase conjugates bilirubin with two molecules of glucuronic acid forming bilirubin diglucuronide.[44] This form of bilirubin is highly soluble in serum and is known as direct or hepatic bilirubin. Direct bilirubin is transported through the biliary tree with bile acids and stored in the gall bladder as bile. When bile is released during the digestive process, intestinal bacteria convert bilirubin into several compounds, collectively referred to as urobilinogen. An estimated 10% of urobilinogen is reabsorbed from the intestine into the bloodstream and resecreted by the liver. Small amounts of urobilinogen are then excreted in the urine, accounting for the urine's straw color. However, most urobilinogen is converted to stercobilin and eliminated in the feces, accounting for their characteristic dark brown color. The presence of bilirubin in the urine implies direct bilirubin, since indirect bilirubin is bound to serum albumin, which should normally not be filtered by the glomerulus.[43] δ-bilirubin is a protein-bound pigment that may falsely raise total bilirubin measurements during hepatobiliary disease. Agents that may interfere with the bilirubin assay include ascorbic acid, dextran, intravenous contrast agents, propranolol, and rifampin.[7]

Causes of hyperbilirubinemia can be classified into three broad categories: (a) prehepatic (hemolysis), (b) hepatic (defective removal of bilirubin from the blood or defective conjugation), and (c) posthepatic (obstruction of the extrahepatic biliary tree), also referred to as cholestatic or obstructive.[44] As serum bilirubin concentrations rise above approximately 2 mg per dL (34 μmol/L), classic scleral icterus and jaundice develop. Table 5.5 summarizes the enzymatic patterns of the common etiologies of hyperbilirubinemia.

Hemolytic jaundice results from the rapid destruction of erythrocytes overwhelming the ability of the liver to process excess bilirubin. Tissue hematomas or collection of blood in body cavities may increase the serum bilirubin. Severe sepsis or malignancy-induced disseminated intravascular coagulation, sickle cell crisis, or certain medications may induce hemolytic anemia. Drug-induced hemolytic anemia may also occur and is discussed later in this chapter under the section, ''Erythrocytes.''

Hepatocellular injury from viral hepatitis, alcoholic hepatitis, toxin-mediated hepatitis, or cirrhosis may elevate serum bilirubin concentrations. Viral hepatitis usually causes elevations in direct bilirubin levels. Viral hepatitis may cause extreme elevations in transaminases (10,000 to 20,000 IU/L, 167 to 334 μkat/L), with ALT levels usually greater than those of AST. Medications commonly reported to cause direct hepatocellular damage include acetaminophen, amio-

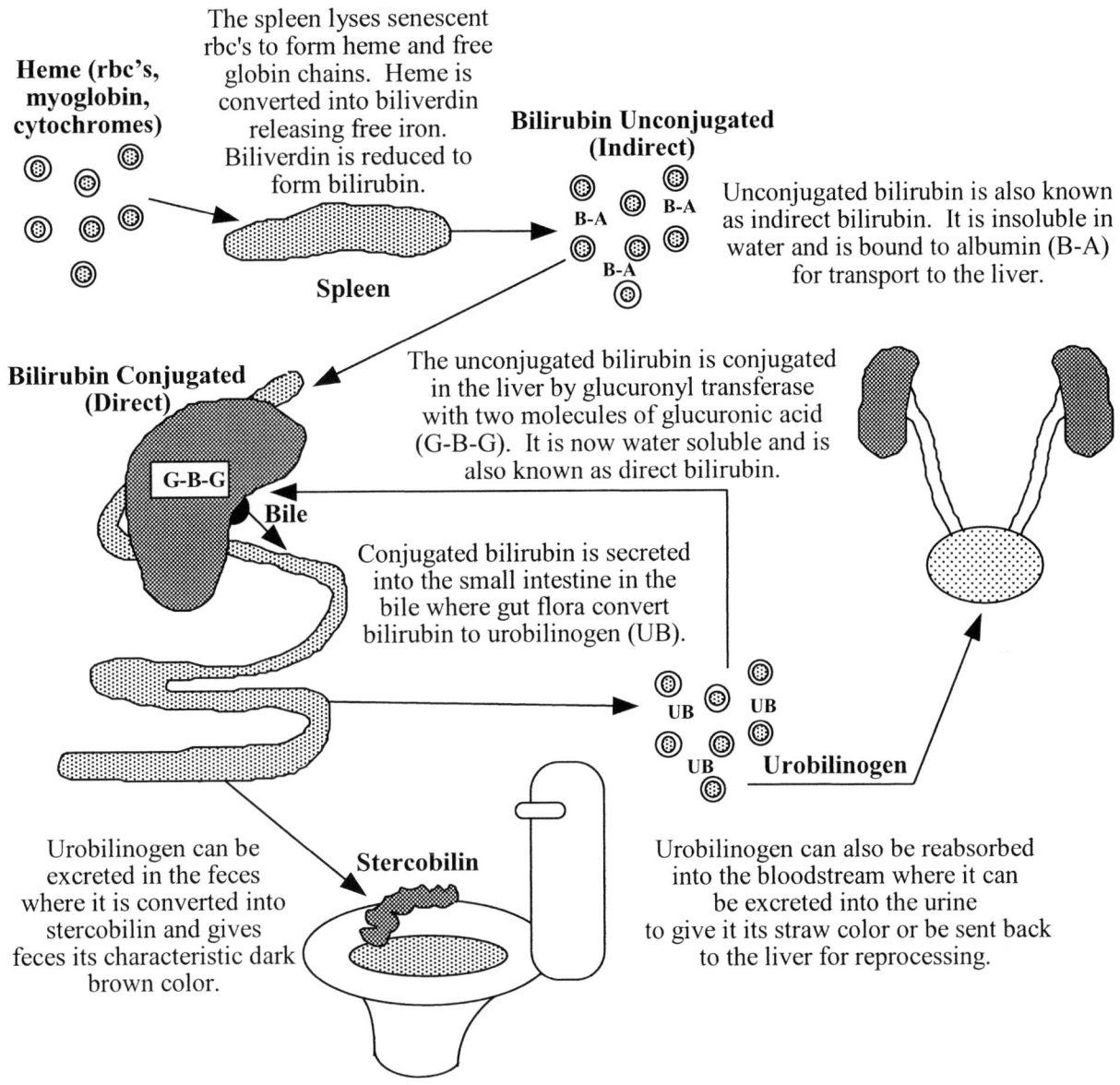

FIGURE 5.3 Bilirubin formation, metabolism, and excretion.

darone, amsacrine, halothane, indinavir, irinotecan, tetracycline, valproic acid, isoniazid, rifampin, methyldopa, labetalol, and tacrine.[7,29,37,38] Drug-induced hepatocellular damage may be indistinguishable from acute viral hepatitis. Alcoholic hepatitis presents in patients with acute or chronic alcohol ingestion. Transaminase elevations are only a fraction of those seen in viral or toxin-induced hepatitis. AST concentration is usually greater than ALT, but GGT levels may be markedly elevated due to the effects of alcohol on GGT release.

Patients with obstructive jaundice usually present with light clay-colored stools and dark cola-colored urine due to reabsorption of conjugated bilirubin from the biliary ducts with redistribution to the urine and lack of stercobilin in the stool. The lack of bile acids in the gastrointestinal tract because of obstruction may cause steatorrhea. Transaminase levels are usually only mildly elevated unless severe obstruction occurs causing hepatocellular damage. ALP and GGT concentrations are usually quite high. The most common cause of biliary obstruction is choledocholithiasis (gallstones) obstructing the common bile duct. Obese, middle-aged women are highly predisposed to choledocholithiasis; however, it may occur in both sexes at any age. Other causes of obstructive jaundice include pancreatitis, carcinoma of the head of the pancreas, or other neoplastic invasion of the papilla of Vater. Cholestatic changes may be due to an intrahepatic defect of the transport of bilirubin into hepatic canaliculi.[44] Cholestatic jaundice closely resembles posthe-

TABLE 5.5	Usual Enzymatic Patterns in Hyperbilirubinemia							
	Fecal Bilinogen	Urine Bilirubin	Direct Bili (% total)	AST	ALT	ALP	GGT	LDH
Hemolysis	↑	–	<20%	nl	nl	nl	nl	↑↑↑
Hepatocellular damage (Viral or Toxin)	↓	+	>40%	↑↑↑↑	↑↑↑↑↑	↑↑	↑↑	LDH₁ > LDH₂ ↑↑ LDH₅
Alcoholic hepatitis	↓	+	<30%	↑↑	↑	↑	↑↑↑	nl
Obstructive or cholestatic jaundice	↓	+	>50%	↑	↑	↑↑↑	↑↑↑	↑ LDH₅
Alcoholic cirrhosis	nl	±	<30%	↑↑ nl (25%)	↑ nl (50%)	↑	↑	nl

AST, aspartate aminotransferase; ALT, alanine aminotransferase; ALP, alkaline phosphatase; GGT, γ-glutamyl transferase; LDH, lactate dehydrogenase; nl, normal; ↑, increased; ↓, decreased.

patic biliary obstruction, except the stools are only somewhat lighter than normal due to less exclusion of bilirubin from the duodenum. Common medications that induce obstructive or cholestatic jaundice include C-17 alkyl steroids, estrogens, chlorpromazine, and erythromycin estolate. Other medications may cause a mixed picture of hepatic injury by an atypical (phenytoin) or granulomatous pattern (quinidine, allopurinol).[29]

Common pitfalls in the application of liver function tests in the etiology of hyperbilirubinemia include: (a) dependence on single tests rather than patterns of abnormality; (b) normal results, implying no disease (AST is normal in 25% and ALT is normal in 50% of cirrhotic patients); (c) abnormal liver function tests, suggesting only liver disease; (d) failure to recognize hepatocellular disease with low transaminase and high ALP levels, or failure to recognize cholestasis or obstruction with high transaminase and low ALP levels; or (e) failure to repeat tests that did not correlate with clinical results.[44]

SERUM PROTEINS
Total Protein.
[6.0 to 8.0 g/dL (SI units = 60 to 80 g/L), CF = 10]

Serum proteins are separated by serum protein electrophoresis into prealbumin, albumin, and globulin fractions.

Prealbumin.
[0.15 to 0.36 g/dL (SI units = 1.5 to 3.6 g/L), CF = 10]

Prealbumin makes up a small percentage of total protein (<1%) and is not widely used for clinical management. Prealbumin contains retinol-binding protein, which plays a role in the transport and metabolism of vitamin A.[48] Prealbumin is exquisitely sensitive to nutritional intake and has a short half-life in the circulation. Measurements of prealbumin, therefore, have clinical utility as a marker for nutritional status.

Albumin.
[4.0 to 6.0 g/dL (SI units = 40 to 60 g/L), CF = 10]

Albumin is by far the most abundant serum protein. Albumin is synthesized in the liver and accounts for up to 65% of total protein. Albumin has three major functions: (a) controlling oncotic pressure in the plasma, (b) transporting amino acids synthesized in the liver to other tissues, and (c) transporting poorly soluble organic and inorganic ligands.[48]

Albumin accounts for 80% of the oncotic pressure of the plasma. Capillary hemodynamics are controlled by four major forces, including intravascular oncotic pressure, interstitial oncotic pressure, capillary hydrostatic pressure, and interstitial hydrostatic pressure (Fig. 5.4). Intravascular oncotic pressure and interstitial hydrostatic pressure are the forces holding fluid in the intravascular space, while capillary hydrostatic pressure and interstitial oncotic pressure force fluid into tissue spaces. Normally intravascular oncotic pressure overrides capillary hydrostatic pressure having a net hemodynamic flow into the vasculature. These forces may be disrupted causing local edema, ascites, or anasarca. Malnutrition, malignancy, severe trauma, or burns cause a net catabolic state, decreasing serum albumin and oncotic pressure. In hepatic cirrhosis, there is decreased synthesis of albumin and increased portal capillary pressure resulting in ascites. In severe sepsis, toxin-mediated increases in capil-

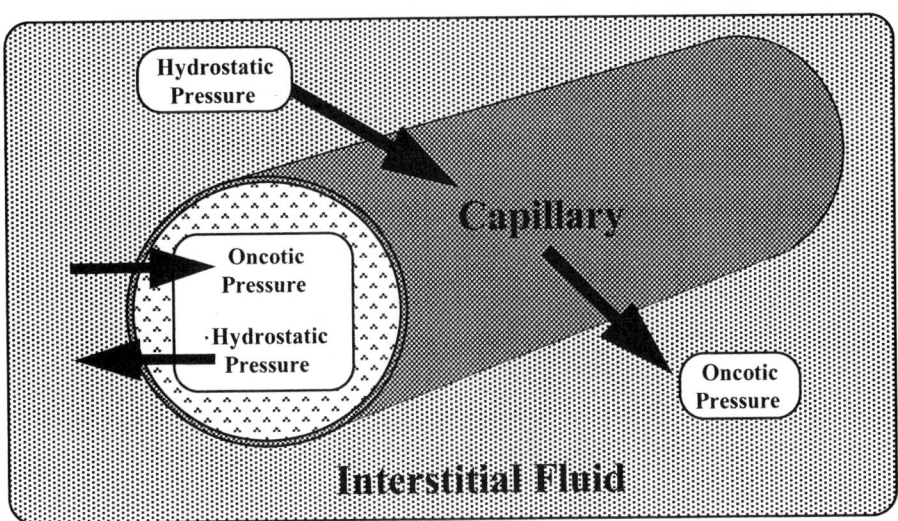

FIGURE 5.4 Capillary hemodynamic forces.

lary permeability allow intravascular albumin to escape into the interstitial tissues, accounting for increases in interstitial oncotic pressure. Nephrotic syndrome and protein-losing enteropathies cause increased losses of serum albumin resulting in anasarca. CHF alters pulmonary capillary hydrostatic pressure, resulting in pulmonary edema. Table 5.6 summarizes changes in capillary hemodynamics, resulting from various disease states. Dehydration and hemodilution may increase or decrease serum albumin concentrations respectively.

Albumin acts as a carrier protein for organic and inorganic molecules, which may bind ionically or covalently.[48,49] Several common medications, which are highly insoluble in serum, bind over 90% to albumin, including phenytoin, salicylates, first generation sulfonylureas, valproic acid, warfarin, and certain sulfonamides.[49] Since free drug is thought to be the active portion, changes in serum albumin concentrations may have a large influence on drug distribution and pharmacologic effect.[50]

Globulin.
[2.0 to 4.0 g/dL (SI units = 20 to 40 g/L), CF = 10]

The globulin fraction comprises one third of total protein and is composed of four major components including α-1, α-2, β, and γ.[48] Important proteins located in the α-1 fraction are α-1 antitrypsin, which is a scavenger enzyme for lysosomal proteases, and α-1 acid glycoprotein (AAG). Young patients with homozygous α-1 antitrypsin deficiency develop severe pulmonary emphysema due to protein lysis by elastase. AAG is an acute-phase reactant that acts as a carrier protein for poorly soluble medications. AAG is increased transiently in a variety of clinical conditions, including burns, chronic pain, enzyme induction, rheumatoid arthritis, morbid obesity, MI, malignancy, surgery, or trauma. Several common medications bind to AAG, including amitriptyline, chlorpromazine, dipyridamole, disopyramide,

erythromycin, imipramine, lidocaine, meperidine, methadone, nortriptyline, propranolol, and quinidine.[49] The transient elevations in AAG levels during the previously mentioned conditions may cause important changes in the binding and pharmacologic effect of these medications.

The α-2 portion consists primarily of α-2-macroglobulin, haptoglobin, and ceruloplasmin. α-2 Macroglobulin is another major protease inhibitor; haptoglobin is a carrier protein for hemoglobin; and ceruloplasmin is a copper-binding protein. The β portion is composed of low-density lipoprotein (LDL), transferrin, C_3, and fibrinogen.[48] LDL is the major transport protein for cholesterol to tissues; transferrin transports ferric iron stores to bone marrow for erythropoiesis; C_3 is a major component of the complement system; and fibrinogen is a coagulation precursor for fibrin. The gamma globulin portion is composed of antibody immunoglobulins IgA, IgE, IgG, and IgM. IgA is responsible for surface immunity; IgE binds to mast cells and is responsible for hypersensitivity reactions; IgM is responsible for initial humoral immunity; and IgG for sustained humoral immunity.[48] The primary disorder associated with hypergammaglobulinemia is multiple myeloma.

COMPLETE BLOOD COUNT WITH DIFFERENTIAL
The complete blood count provides information about the erythrocytes, leukocytes, and platelets. The number of parameters provided with a CBC depends on the type of machine used for the analysis. Any other desired tests may be ordered separately.

In the normal adult, blood cells are predominantly made in the bone marrow of the sternum, skull, ribs, vertebrae, pelvis, and the proximal ends of the long bones (humerus and femur). The pathways of hematopoiesis from the pluripotential stem cell and the relationship between the different cell lines are shown in Figure 5.5.[51]

TABLE 5.6	Common Disease States Resulting in Altered Capillary Hemodynamics			

Disease	Mechanism	Serum Albumin	Capillary Hydrostatic Pressure	Interstitial Oncotic Pressure
Malnutrition	Decreased protein synthesis; increased protein catabolism	↓↓↓[a]	nl	nl
Malignancy	Increased protein catabolism	↓↓	nl, ↑ Tumor compression	nl
Burns	Increased protein catabolism; altered skin capillary permeability	↓↓↓	nl	↑↑, Skin
Hepatic cirrhosis	Decreased albumin synthesis; increased portal capillary hydrostatic pressure	↓↓↓	↑↑↑, Portal	nl,↑
Sepsis	Toxin altered capillary permeability	↓↓↓	nl	↑↑↑
Congestive heart failure	Increased pulmonary and systemic capillary hydrostatic pressure due to biventricular failure	nl, ↓ Malnutrition due to cardiac cachexia	↑↑↑, Pulmonary and/or systemic	nl
Nephrotic syndrome	Loss of albumin into the urine due to glomerular damage and leakage	↓↓↓	nl	nl

nl, normal; ↓, decreased; ↑, increased.

Erythrocytes.
[Men = 4.3 to 5.9 × 10⁶/mm³ (4.3 to 5.9 × 10¹²/L); women = 3.5 to 5.0 × 10⁶/mm³ (3.5 to 5.0 × 10¹²/L); CF = 1]

The main functions of erythrocytes, or red blood cells (RBC), are to carry oxygen from the lungs to the tissues and transport carbon dioxide back to the lungs.[51] Anemia occurs when the hemoglobin, hematocrit, and/or erythrocyte count are below the normal range. This can be a result of impaired erythrocyte production, increased erythrocyte destruction, blood loss, or increased plasma volume.[52] The extent of anemia is generally described by the hemoglobin or hematocrit values. The RBC indices may be used to further characterize the anemia by cell morphology or color. Normal-sized RBC are called normocytes, small ones are microcytes, and large RBC are macrocytes. If there is abnormal variation in size, the patient is said to have anisocytosis, which is a feature of most anemias. Those with normal amounts of hemoglobin are said to be normochromic; those with decreased, hypo-

chromic; and those with increased hemoglobin, hyperchromic. Abnormally shaped cells are poikilocytes.[53] Polycythemia means ''many blood cells'' but usually refers to an increased RBC mass and/or an elevated hematocrit value.[52]

Red cell production is regulated by tissue oxygenation. Tissues receive inadequate oxygen if there is an insufficient supply in inspired air, impaired oxygen transport from the alveoli into the blood stream, hypoventilation, inadequate hemoglobin to carry oxygen, decreased arterial oxygen saturation, abnormal blood flow, or a failure of hemoglobin to release bound oxygen at tissue sites.[54] This can occur in diseases such as anemia, in cardiac or pulmonary disease, or with decreased oxygen tension in the air, such as at high altitudes.[51] Smokers tend to have a stimulation of erythrocyte production.[53] Hypoxia or decreased oxygenation stimulates the production of erythropoietin, with most being produced by the kidneys. A small amount of erythropoietin is produced by the liver. Erythropoietin stimulates erythroid

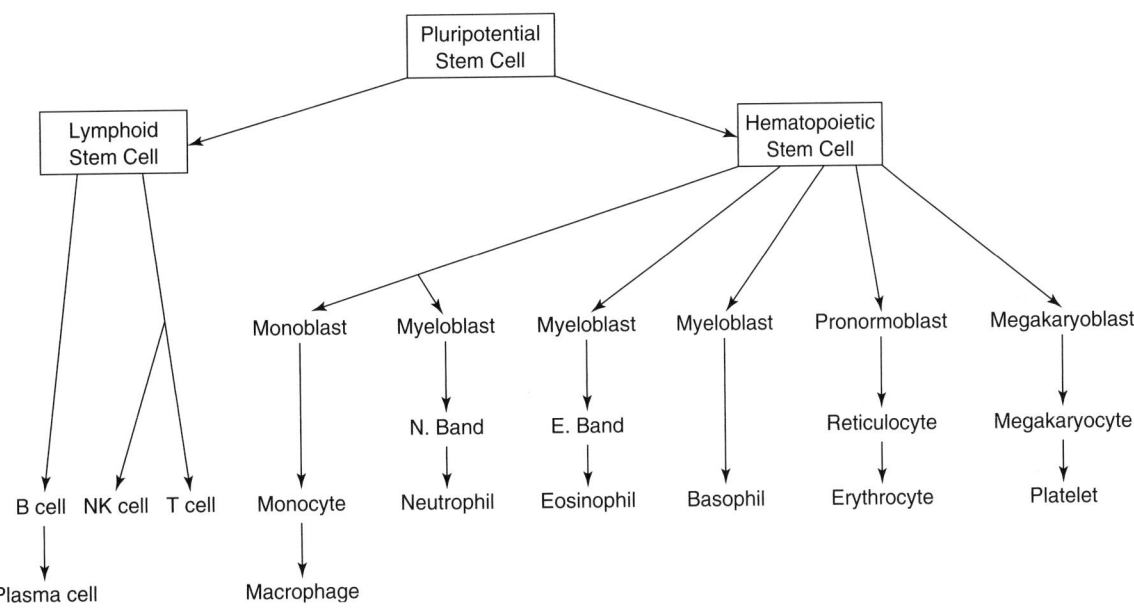

FIGURE 5.5 Hematopoiesis.

differentiation and survival.[55] Erythropoietin increases in most anemias, but its production and effects may be impaired in those associated with chronic diseases.[52] If tissue oxygen concentrations are perceived as inadequate, erythrocyte production continues, regardless of the erythrocyte count or hemoglobin concentration, resulting in a secondary or reactive polycythemia.[54]

The life span of erythrocytes in circulation is 120 days. They are removed by the RES.[51] Normally, most RBC destruction occurs in the spleen, liver, and bone marrow by phagocytosis by macrophages.[56] With an abnormally large spleen, there is increased destruction of normal cells. The spleen may be enlarged in conditions such as liver disease, CHF, leukemias, lymphomas, or protozoal infections.[57] There can be accelerated destruction of erythrocytes by a normal spleen when they contain abnormal hemoglobin or have abnormal membranes or enzymes. Increased destruction can also occur with abnormal physical, chemical, microbiologic, or immunologic conditions.[52]

Hemolysis refers to the disruption of the mature erythrocyte membrane and release of hemoglobin before the end of the usual life span. It can take place in the spleen (or other RES organs) or vasculature. This accelerated destruction of cells can occur in response to physical trauma or massive exertion, severe burns, infections such as malaria, mycoplasmal pneumonia, or mononucleosis, or toxic insults such as *Clostridium* infections or brown recluse spider bites. Hemolysis can also occur with drugs and chemicals, such as arsine gas, lead, or copper salts. With oxidizing drugs, such as nitrates, methemoglobin can be formed and lead to severe cases of erythrocyte destruction.[52,58]

Destruction of erythrocytes may be mediated by antibodies. Various types of antibody-mediated hemolysis are associated with drugs. Penicillins and cephalosporins can tightly bind to erythrocyte membranes and stimulate production of IgG antibodies and hemolysis. Cephalosporins can also change erythrocyte membranes leading to nonspecific adsorption of proteins. Methyldopa can directly induce a positive antiglobulin reaction and hemolysis. In the immune complex type of drug-induced hemolytic anemia, the drug loosely combines with the RBC membrane to form a neoantigen that then binds an antibody. Complement is attracted and cell lysis occurs. Only a small amount of drug is needed for this to occur. The reaction can be abrupt and severe and may be accompanied by renal failure. In the past, the RBC was considered to be an "innocent bystander" on which the drug-antibody complex settled, but now it is thought to be an essential component in promulgating this reaction. This has been reported with quinidine, quinine, p-aminosalicylic acid, phenacetin, rifampin, antihistamines, chlorpromazine, sulfonylureas, sulfonamides, and insecticides.[52,59]

Patients with chronic diseases, such as infections, renal or liver disease, various endocrine disorders, rheumatoid arthritis, or neoplasms, often have anemia. Aplastic anemia involves a pancytopenia or a depression of erythrocytes, neutrophils, and platelets. About 11% to 20% of cases can be attributed to drug or chemical exposure, and about 2% to 9% to infectious hepatitis.[52] It can occur secondary to infections; thymoma; ionizing radiation; pregnancy; drugs such as chloramphenicol, cimetidine, gold salts, indomethacin, ibuprofen, sulfonamides, thioamides, anticonvulsants, or antineoplastic drugs; or chemicals such as benzene, mercury, or DDT.[52,60] About 70% of aplastic anemia cases are primary or idiopathic, where there is no known predisposing cause. Patients with aplastic anemia may later develop acute leukemia, paroxysmal nocturnal hemoglobinuria, or myelodysplastic syndrome.[52] Polycythemia vera is a myeloproliferative syndrome in which there is a spontaneous increase in erythrocytes. The predominant picture is one of erythrocyte proliferation, but other elements of the blood are also hyperactive. It most commonly presents in middle age. Thrombosis and hemorrhage are common complications.[61]

Hemoglobin.

[Men = 13.6 to 17.2 g/dL (8.45 to 10.65 mmol/L or 136 to 172 g/L); women = 12.0 to 15.0 g/dL (7.45 to 9.30 mmol/L or 120 to 150 g/L); CF = 0.6206 for mmol/L and 10 for g/L)

Hemoglobin (Hb), the primary component of erythrocytes, transports oxygen and carbon dioxide.[53] Hemoglobinopathies occur when genes code for abnormal amino acid sequences. The most common abnormal hemoglobin is sickle hemoglobin. Thalassemias are characterized by decreased synthesis of globin chains.[62]

The preferred assay for hemoglobin is the cyanmethemoglobin method. Errors in venipuncture technique can lead to hemoconcentration, which results in falsely elevated values for hemoglobin and cell counts. The difference in the normal range between men and women is thought to result mainly from androgen stimulation of erythropoiesis in the marrow. Estrogen may slightly suppress erythrocyte production.[53] Menstrual blood loss is also a contributing factor.[63] In older men, the hemoglobin tends to fall. This occurs to a lesser extent in women, who may even have a slight increase in the value. As a result, there is a <1 g per dL (0.62 mmol/L) sex difference in hemoglobin in older individuals. There is a diurnal variation of approximately 8% to 9% in hemoglobin concentrations, with the highest value in the morning and the lowest in the evening.[53] Hemoglobin values are approximately 0.5 to 0.6 g per dL (0.31 to 0.37 mmol/L) lower in blacks than in whites. Some attribute this to a higher incidence of iron deficiency anemia in blacks.[63,64]

Hematocrit.

[Men = 39% to 49% (0.39 to 0.49); women = 33% to 43% (0.33 to 0.43); CF = 0.01]

The hematocrit (Hct) is the ratio of the volume of erythrocytes to that of whole blood or the packed erythrocyte volume.[53] It increases when more fluid is lost than erythrocytes and volume depletion occurs, as is seen in patients with vomiting, diarrhea, burns, prolonged fever, or those taking diuretics. An inappropriate polycythemia occurs with renal cancer, hepatomas, pheochromocytomas, or adrenal cortical neoplasms where there is increased erythropoietin and increased hematocrit.[52,54] The hematocrit is unreliable for patient assessment immediately after blood loss or transfusion.[53]

Reticulocytes.

[10,000 to 75,000 mm^{-3} (10–75 × 10^9/L); CF = 0.001; or 0.1 to 2.4% erythrocytes (0.001–0.024); CF = 0.01]

Reticulocytes are immature erythrocytes. Generally, the absolute reticulocyte count is more useful than the percentage

of erythrocytes. Reticulocytes provide an estimate of erythrocyte production; however, as the hematocrit drops, increasingly immature reticulocytes are released into the blood. These cells take longer to mature in circulation as indicated below:

Hct (%)	Reticulocyte Maturation Time (days)
45	1.0
35	1.5
25	2.0
15	2.5

To accurately estimate erythrocyte production in response to anemia, a correction factor must be used to account for this longer maturation time and avoid overestimating the erythropoietic response. The reticulocyte production index (RPI) can be calculated by:

$$RPI = \frac{Patient's\ reticulocyte\ count}{Normal\ reticulocyte\ count} \times \frac{Patient's\ Hct}{Normal\ Hct} \div Maturation\ time$$

In general, an RPI >2 represents an adequate response to anemia and an RPI <2 indicates an inadequate increase in RBC production.[51,52] The reticulocytes are most markedly increased in patients with hemolysis or acute blood loss and also increase when iron or vitamin B_{12} is administered to a deficient patient. If the reticulocyte count is normal, but the hemoglobin low, there is an inadequate response to anemia, such as what may be seen in iron deficiency. If the reticulocyte count is increased, but the hemoglobin is normal, there is probably some destruction or loss of erythrocytes occurring, and the body is appropriately compensating for the loss.[57]

Erythrocyte Indices. The size and hemoglobin content of erythrocytes can be quantified by the erythrocyte indices.

The mean corpuscular volume (MCV) is the average volume of erythrocytes. It can be measured by machines or calculated by the formula MCV = Hct per RBC.[6] The normal range is 76 to 100 μm^3 or 76 to 100 femtoliters (fL) in SI units (a femtoliter is 10^{-15} L).[3] The MCV is decreased in microcytic anemia and increased in macrocytic anemia. Young erythrocytes and reticulocytes are larger than mature cells, so when there is rapid erythrocyte production, the MCV will be increased. This type of macrocytosis can be observed in compensated hemolytic conditions or when a patient is recovering from acute blood loss. Megaloblastic changes can occur when DNA production is impaired but RNA production is normal. This causes nuclear maturation to lag behind cytoplasmic maturation. This change occurs in all cells, but is most dramatic and can be most easily diagnosed in erythrocyte precursors. It is distinguished by the presence of oval macrocytes and hypersegmented neutrophils. The most common causes of megaloblastosis are deficiencies of vitamin B_{12} or folic acid, which are required for DNA synthesis.[52,63] Drugs that interfere with DNA synthesis by blocking folate metabolism (e.g., methotrexate or trimethoprim), interfering with vitamin B_{12} absorption (e.g., colchicine, metformin, neomycin, or cholestyramine), inhibiting purine synthesis (e.g., 6-mercaptopurine) or pyrimidine synthesis (e.g., cytarabine), or alkylating agents (e.g., cyclophosphamide) may also cause megaloblastosis.[52,63,65] It may also result from drugs that decrease folate absorption such as oral contraceptives, sulfasalazine, phenytoin, phenobarbital, and primidone.[52,65] Megaloblastic anemias can be seen with inherited disorders of DNA synthesis such as Lesch-Nyhan syndrome. Excessive alcohol intake is associated with macrocytosis due to poor nutrition, impaired folic acid absorption and metabolism, and direct effects on the bone marrow. Macrocytic anemia can also be associated with hypothyroidism, liver disease, multiple myeloma, myelodysplastic syndromes, and aplastic anemia.[52,63] A microcytic anemia is associated with iron deficiency, thalassemias, sideroblastic anemia, and sometimes chronic diseases.[52]

The mean corpuscular hemoglobin (MCH) is the weight of the hemoglobin in the average RBC. It is calculated by MCH = Hb per RBC.[53] The normal range is 27 to 33 pg.[3] In microcytic anemia it is decreased, and increased in macrocytic anemia.[53] Hypochromic cells are associated with iron deficiency anemia, thalassemias, sideroblastic anemia, and sometimes anemia of chronic disease.[52]

The mean corpuscular hemoglobin concentration (MCHC) is the average concentration of hemoglobin in a given volume of packed erythrocytes and is described by MCHC = Hb per Hct.[53] The normal range is 33 to 37 g per dL or 330 to 370 g per L in SI units (CF = 10).[3] In microcytic anemia it is decreased. In macrocytic anemia it may be normal or decreased. In hypochromic anemias, both the MCH and MCHC are decreased.[53]

The red cell distribution width (RDW) quantifies the extent of variation in the size of erythrocytes. The reference value is 11.5 to 14.5. It may be calculated by RDW = (standard deviation of RBC size) per MCV.[6]

Erythrocyte Sedimentation Rate.

[Men = 0 to 20 mm/h; females = 0 to 30 mm/h, Westergren technique]

The erythrocyte sedimentation rate (ESR) is the rate of fall from the top of a column of erythrocytes in anticoagulated blood over a given period. It is directly proportional to the weight of the cell aggregates, and is inversely proportional to the surface area. Microcytes settle slower than macrocytes. The ESR generally increases in anemia and decreases if there are abnormal or irregularly shaped erythrocytes. The ESR gradually increases with age and moderately increases during pregnancy. The ESR is used mainly as an indicator of active inflammatory diseases (e.g., rheumatoid arthritis), chronic infection (e.g., tuberculosis, osteomyelitis, hepatitis, bacterial endocarditis), collagen disease, or neoplastic disease (e.g., multiple myeloma) and may be used to monitor the disease course. It may have some prognostic value in sickle cell disease, stroke, prostate cancer, and coronary artery disease. It is particularly useful in the diagnosis and monitoring of temporal arteritis and polymyalgia rheumatica. The Westergren technique is widely used as the standard for determining ESR. Alternatives are the Wintrobe method and the Zeta Sedimentation Ratio.[6,53]

Leukocytes.
[3,200 to 9,800 mm^3 (3.2 to 9.8 × 10^9/L); CF = 0.001]

Laboratories commonly report six types of leukocytes or white blood cells (WBC) found in the peripheral blood: neutrophils, bands, lymphocytes, monocytes, eosinophils, and basophils. Less mature or abnormal forms may be observed in certain disease states. The differential white count indicates the percentage of the total leukocyte count that is accounted for by each type (addition of the differential should total 100%). The leukocyte and differential counts can change within minutes to hours of stimulation.[57] Cigarette smokers have a higher average leukocyte count. It is about 30% higher in heavy smokers who inhale, with an increase in neutrophils, lymphocytes, and monocytes. In leukocytosis, the total WBC count is increased above the normal range. Exercise can lead to a leukocytosis with an increase in neutrophils due to shifting of cells and lymphocyte drainage into blood.[53]

The leukocyte count and/or the differential count may be abnormal in patients with sepsis. However, this is not always the case and normal or low values would not rule out an infection.[61] If nucleated RBC are present, they may be read as leukocytes.[53]

Leukemias are malignant diseases characterized by abnormal leukocytes, which may be greatly increased in number (although they may also be decreased). A massive increase in leukocytes as a systemic response to various conditions (e.g., tuberculosis, severe burns, eclampsia, hemolysis, hemorrhage) is called a leukemoid reaction because the hematologic picture strongly resembles that seen in chronic leukemia. Different WBC lines may predominate depending on the etiology.[61]

Granulocytes. Granulocytes are leukocytes with granules in their cytoplasm. They develop from the same precursor cell as monocytes in the bone marrow (Fig. 5.5). Their synthesis is stimulated by the hormone colony-stimulating factor for granulocytes (G-CSF) and granulocytes-monocytes (GM-CSF). Unlike erythrocytes, granulocytes retain their nuclei. There are three main types of granulocytes: neutrophils (including bands), eosinophils, and basophils.[51]

Neutrophils.

[1,800 to 7,000 mm^3 (1.8 to 7.0 × 10^9/L); CF = 0.001]

In normal adults, about 56% of leukocytes are neutrophils, also called polymorphonuclear (meaning many forms of nuclei) leukocytes (PMN), polys, segmented neutrophilic granulocytes, or segs. The lower limit of the normal range is 1,800 mm^3 (1.8 × 10^9/L) for white adults and 1,100 mm^3 (1.1 × 10^9/L) for blacks. There is some diurnal variation in neutrophils, with the highest values in the afternoon and lowest in the morning. The nuclei of neutrophils have two to five lobes connected by thin filaments.[53] Their cytoplasm is packed with enzyme-containing granules that react with acidic and basic stains.[57] Bands or stabs are the immature form of neutrophils.[51] They have thicker strands connecting their nuclear lobes or U-shaped nuclei that look such as curved bands. Band neutrophils normally average 3% of leukocytes. A "shift to the left" means there is an increase in the number of bands and immature neutrophils in the blood.[53] The term is derived from a time when the differential was reported on a grid that listed the immature forms on the left and the mature neutrophils on the right.[57] Neutrophils remain in the "maturation and storage pool" in the marrow for about 6 to 7 days. Neutrophils usually spend less than a day in circulating blood. Their primary site of activity is in tissues.[51] When tissue is damaged or foreign material enters the body, substances are released that stimulate neutrophils to move to that area. This is called chemotaxis. Chemotaxis can be abnormal in some diseases such as Hodgkin's disease, cirrhosis, rheumatoid arthritis, and diabetes mellitus. The neutrophils then phagocytize and destroy microorganisms and other materials at the site enzymatically.[57]

The neutrophils must attach to the particles before they can engulf them. This attachment is enhanced by the presence of antibodies or complement coating the surface of the particles. It is decreased by exposure to alcohol, aspirin, prednisone, or nonsteroidal antiinflammatory drugs.[57] This action of neutrophils is important in host defense against infection, but when enzymes are released outside the cell, it may also play a part in causing tissue damage to the host in other diseases. Neutrophils are stored in the bone marrow and in the marginal granulocyte pool along the vessel walls or in capillary beds.[51] In response to stress, they can be released from these sites into the circulating pool, resulting in a neutrophilia. In an acute infection, the neutrophils leave the circulation and migrate into the tissues. Production of neutrophils will also increase, in which case, more immature forms will be seen. If supply cannot keep up with demand, a neutropenia may occur. A toxic suppression of the bone marrow may also be involved in this process.[61]

An increase in neutrophils is associated with some infections (especially bacterial), various inflammatory diseases (e.g., rheumatoid arthritis, vasculitis), tissue destruction or necrosis (e.g., as in trauma, surgery, MI, or burns), metabolic disorders (e.g., uremia, diabetic ketoacidosis, gout, hemorrhage, hemolysis), and solid tumors. Endogenous or exogenous adrenal corticosteroids cause lymphocytes and eosinophils to disappear from circulation within 4 to 8 hours, with circulating granulocytes increasing due to release from the marrow storage pool.[57,61] Prolonged use of corticosteroids can lead to chronic neutrophilia by decreasing the rate at which neutrophils leave circulation.[61] Epinephrine can cause granulocytosis within minutes and probably is the mediator of neutrophilic leukocytosis associated with physiologic stimuli such as exercise, emotional stress, or exposure to extreme temperatures. Other drugs that can stimulate neutro-

philia include lithium, histamine, heparin, digitalis, and many toxins, venoms, and heavy metals (e.g., lead, mercury).[57,61]

Neutropenia is a result of impaired production, increased removal from blood, or altered distribution of neutrophils. It occurs when the absolute neutrophil count is below the normal range and is associated with certain bacterial (e.g., typhoid, tularemia, brucellosis), viral (e.g., measles, rubella), and protozoal (e.g., malaria) infections, or an overwhelming infection of any kind. This can occur when demand exceeds supply and neutrophils leave circulation and migrate to tissues faster than they can be replaced by the bone marrow. It can be caused by drugs interfering with DNA synthesis (e.g., lamivudine, zidovudine, phenothiazines, anticonvulsants, antibiotics, sulfonamides), idiosyncratic drug reactions (e.g., chloramphenicol, gold salts, antithyroid drugs, indomethacin, quinidine), or treatment with cytotoxic drugs or ionizing radiation.[6,7,61] There can be increased destruction of neutrophils through immunologic mechanisms in patients receiving drugs such as aminopyrine, phenylbutazone, or sulfapyridine.[61] Neutropenia is also seen with hypersplenism due to liver or storage diseases, some collagen-vascular diseases (e.g., lupus erythematosus), and folic acid or vitamin B_{12} deficiency.[6,57]

A more severe form of neutropenia is agranulocytosis, in which the granulocytes suddenly disappear. Often other blood elements are also affected.[61] Agranulocytosis can occur as a complication of drug therapy (e.g., clozapine and ticlopidine).[7,66] The absolute neutrophil count (ANC) is calculated by multiplying the total leukocyte count by the sum of the percentage of mature neutrophils (segs) plus the percentage of immature neutrophils (bands): ANC = Total WBC × (% segs + % bands).[6] When the ANC is <1,000 mm³ (1.0×10^9/L), there is an increased risk of infection, and when it is <500 mm³ (0.5×10^9/L), this risk is even higher.[61]

Eosinophils.

[0 to 500 mm⁻³ (0 to 0.5×10^9/L); CF = 0.001]

Eosinophils are structurally similar to neutrophils but their cytoplasm contains larger round or oval granules that contain enzymes and have a strong affinity for acid (red) stains. Their nuclei usually contain two connected segments. Eosinophils normally average 3% of leukocytes. The count is higher in individuals with allergic conditions.[51,53] Eosinophils are capable of phagocytosis but are not bactericidal.[57] They modulate activities associated with immunologically mediated inflammation and can destroy some helminth parasites.[51] Eosinophils are increased in allergic diseases (e.g., asthma, hay fever), parasitic infections (e.g., trichinosis), infectious diseases (e.g., scarlet fever, human immunodeficiency virus infection), certain skin disorders (e.g., atopic dermatitis, eczema, pemphigus), neoplastic diseases, collagen vascular diseases, adrenal cortical hypofunction, ulcerative colitis, and "hypereosinophilic" syndrome.[57,61,67] Eosinophilia may also be associated with drug use (e.g., pilocarpine, digitalis, sulfonamides). Eosinophils are decreased during acute stress or other conditions with increased epinephrine secretion or elevated levels of adrenal corticosteroids, and in acute inflammatory states.[61]

Basophils.

[0 to 200 mm^3 (0 to 0.2 × 10^9/L); CF = 0.001]

Basophils look similar to neutrophils except that their nuclei are less segmented and their cytoplasmic granules are larger and have a strong affinity for basic (blue) stains. They average about 0.5% of total leukocytes.[53] They show diurnal variation, with levels highest during the night and lowest in the morning.[61] Tissue mast cells have some characteristics and functions similar to basophils. Both basophils and mast cells bind immunoglobulin E on their cell membranes. They react with antigens and cause release of histamine, slow-reacting substance of anaphylaxis, and other substances from the basophil granules, producing immediate hypersensitivity reactions.[51] Basophils may be increased in allergic reactions, myeloproliferative disorders, chronic hemolytic anemia, hypothyroidism, and following splenectomy. They may be decreased with chronic corticosteroid therapy, acute infection or stress, or in patients with hyperthyroidism.[61]

Lymphocytes.

[1,000 to 4,800 mm^3 (1.0 to 4.8 × 10^9/L); CF = 0.001]

Lymphocytes are mononuclear cells without cytoplasmic granules. They average 34% of leukocytes in adults.[53] They may form plasma cells which are not normally present in blood. Plasma cells may be found in patients with neoplasms (e.g., multiple myeloma), viral or chronic infections, allergic states, and other conditions with increased gamma-globulin concentrations.[51,61] Lymphocytes and plasma cells are important for the immune defenses of the body. Normally, the majority of circulating lymphocytes are T cells, which are responsible for cell-mediated immunity including delayed hypersensitivity, graft rejection, graft-versus-host reactions, defense against intracellular organisms, and defense against neoplasms. They have a life span of months to years. They are named for the thymus gland, where they differentiate. Natural killer (NK) cells share a precursor with T cells and develop in the bone marrow. They target virus-infected cells and participate in antibody-dependent cell lysis.[51]

B-lymphocytes (B cells) account for 10% to 20% of circulating lymphocytes and are responsible for humoral immunity. They are named for the bursa of Fabricius, where they develop in birds. In humans, the bursal equivalent is thought to be in fetal liver and bone marrow, with further differentiation occurring in secondary lymphoid organs. These organs, important for postnatal lymphocyte production, include the spleen, lymph nodes, and intestine. B-cells have a life span of days and can differentiate into antibody-producing plasma cells.[51]

There are also "null" or unmarked (non-T, non-B) lymphocytes that cannot be classified. Although lymphocytes can be found in circulation, they mainly concentrate in the lymph nodes, spleen, mucosa of alimentary and respiratory tracts, bone marrow, liver, skin, and chronically inflamed tissue.[57,61]

Changes in the proportion of lymphocytes in the total leukocyte count usually reflect changes in numbers of granulocytes.[57] An absolute or relative increase in lymphocytes occurs with some viral or other infections (e.g., tuberculosis, infectious mononucleosis, cytomegalovirus, pertussis, toxoplasmosis, hepatitis, mumps, chickenpox), thyrotoxicosis, Addison disease, inflammatory bowel disease, vasculitis, and hypersensitivity reactions to drugs (e.g., phenytoin, para-aminosalicylic acid).[6,61] When the number of lymphocytes is decreased abnormally (lymphocytopenia) or function is impaired, the patient suffers from immunodeficiency. This can be an inherited disorder or may be associated with immunodeficiency syndromes (e.g., acquired immune deficiency syndrome [AIDS]).[61] Lymphocytopenia may occur with diseases such as CHF, renal failure, miliary tuberculosis, myasthenia gravis, systemic lupus erythematosus, or with defects of lymphatic drainage.[6] Lymphocytopenia can also occur after irradiation or administration of antineoplastic drugs, or with high concentrations of adrenocortical hormones. Lymphocyte dysfunction may be observed with chronic lymphocytic leukemia, multiple myeloma, Hodgkin disease, sarcoidosis, leprosy, malnutrition, or terminal malignancy.[61]

Monocytes.

[0 to 800 mm^3 (0 to 0.8 × 10^9/L); CF = 0.001]

Monocytes are the largest cells in normal blood with a diameter two to three times that of erythrocytes. They have a single nucleus that is partly lobulated and may appear round, oval, or horseshoe shaped. Their cytoplasm contains fine granules. Monocytes average 4% of leukocytes.[53] After circulating briefly, they enter the tissues and transform into the larger macrophages, and remain there for several months. Macrophages are capable of motility, phagocytosis, killing microorganisms and malignant cells, and interactions with the immune system. They synthesize and secrete many biologically active molecules. They have important functions in host defense and control of hematopoiesis. They remove old or defective blood cells in the marrow and inhaled particles in the lungs.[51] Monocytes are increased in some infectious diseases (e.g., mycotic, rickettsial, protozoal, viral infections; tuberculosis, subacute bacterial endocarditis), leukemias, lymphomas, sarcoidosis, inflammatory bowel disease, and connective tissue disorders.[6,61] The circulating monocytes and tissue macrophages together compose the mononuclear phagocyte or RES.[51]

Platelets.

[130 to 400 × 10^3/mm^3 (130 to 400 × 10^9/L); CF = 1]

Platelets maintain the integrity of blood vessels and play

a key role in hemostasis. The precursors of platelets are megakaryocytes (Fig. 5.5). Their proliferation, differentiation, and maturation are controlled by megakaryocyte colony-stimulating factor (Meg-CSF) and thrombopoietin. Normally, about two thirds of platelets are in circulation and one third in the spleen. However, when the spleen is enlarged up to 80% to 90% may be sequestered there. In patients without a spleen, all are in circulation. Platelets circulate for about 8 to 11 days.[51]

Platelets are removed from circulation by the mononuclear phagocytic system.[51] Antibodies may also destroy platelets. They may be directed against the platelets, or the platelets may be "innocent bystanders" that are destroyed when an immune complex attaches to them. Immune destruction of platelets may occur with exposure to drugs such as platelet glycoprotein IIb/IIIa antagonists (abciximab, eptifibatide, tirofiban), carbamazepine, quinine, quinidine, gold salts, sulfonamides, or heparin.[7,68]

Thrombocytopenia, a reduced number of circulating platelets, can occur as a congenital or acquired disorder. It may result from decreased production, abnormal distribution or dilution, or increased destruction of platelets. These may be associated with factors such as malignancies, immune processes, infections, exposure to drugs or chemicals, or an enlarged spleen, and may be combined with abnormalities of other blood elements such as in aplastic anemia. Thrombocytosis, an increased number of circulating platelets, can be part of a reactive process (e.g., infections, chronic inflammation, severe trauma) or a myeloproliferative disorder.[6,68] Half of patients with an otherwise unexplained increase in platelets are found to have a malignancy.[6]

Platelets are activated at times of vascular injury by exposure to substances such as collagen and thrombin. They adhere to exposed surfaces and aggregate in the presence of calcium. They release adenosine diphosphate (ADP) that promotes further aggregation. When platelets are activated, glycoprotein IIb/IIIa receptors on their membranes undergo conformational changes that allow binding of fibrinogen and von Willebrand factor. This leads to cross-linkage of platelets and formation of a platelet plug.[68,69] Aggregation is also stimulated by thromboxane A_2 from platelets and inhibited by prostacyclin (prostaglandin I_2) from vascular endothelium. Both are products of arachidonic acid metabolism mediated by cyclooxygenase (Fig. 5.6).[70] Platelets also release various substances that activate or allow progression of the clotting cascade. These actions lead to the formation of thrombi. Overall platelet function may be assessed by the bleeding time. Various in vitro techniques using activator substances may also be used to assess platelet aggregation. Platelet contraction within thrombi is responsible for clot retraction.[68]

If the platelet count is 20 to 50 × 10^3/ mm³ (20 to 50 × 10^9/L), the patient is at a high risk for minor spontaneous bleeding and bleeding after surgery, and if it is less than 20 × 10^3/mm³ (20 × 10^9/L), the patient is at risk for more serious bleeding.[6] Platelet function is impaired in various

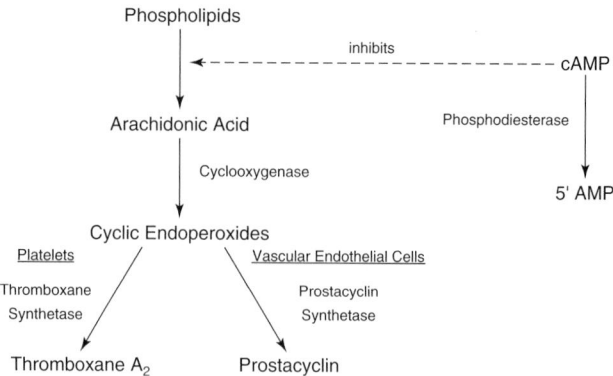

FIGURE 5.6 Arachidonic acid pathway.

diseases such as uremia, myeloproliferative or lymphoproliferative disorders, myeloma, systemic lupus erythematosus, chronic immunologic thrombocytopenic purpura, or disseminated intravascular coagulation. Numerous drugs can also interfere with platelet function. Most affect the arachidonic pathway shown in Figure 5.6. Aspirin irreversibly acetylates platelet cyclooxygenase, thus inhibiting aggregation for the life of the platelet by decreasing formation of thromboxane A_2. This effect is observed for up to 10 days following ingestion of aspirin. Most other nonsteroidal antiinflammatory drugs will also affect platelet cyclooxygenase, but it is a reversible effect observed only while the drug is present. Other drugs inhibit platelet effects by activating adenylate cyclase (e.g., prostaglandins) or inhibiting phosphodiesterase (e.g., dipyridamole), both of which result in increased cyclic adenosine monophosphate (CAMP). Ticlopidine and clopidogrel are drugs that inhibit ADP-induced platelet aggregation. Abciximab, a monoclonal antibody, is a platelet glycoprotein IIb/IIIa receptor antagonist. Examples of additional drugs that may inhibit aggregation include dextran, antimicrobial agents (e.g., penicillins, cephalosporins), psychotropics (e.g., imipramine, chlorpromazine), clofibrate, and beta-adrenergic blocking agents (e.g., propranolol).[68] Synthesis of platelets is inhibited by flucytosine, interferons, thiazide diuretics, chloramphenicol, and numerous antineoplastic agents Ethanol can inhibit the synthesis and function of platelets.[7,71]

COAGULATION TESTS

Clotting Cascade. The clotting cascade involves the progressive activation of clotting factors, with the end result of a stable fibrin clot. Platelets and other substances help or accelerate this process. A simplified diagram of the traditional clotting cascade is shown in Figure 5.7. The process is actually much more complex, with additional clotting factor interactions not shown. The clotting factors are identified by Roman numerals, although they also have other names. Each factor must be activated before it can in turn activate other factors in the cascade. The active forms of most factors are serine proteases, except V and VIII that act as cofactors. Factors II, VII, IX, and X require vitamin K for their synthe-

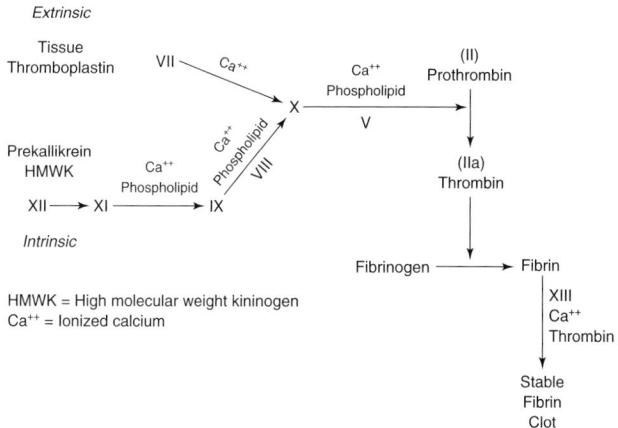

Extrinsic

Intrinsic

HMWK = High molecular weight kininogen
Ca^{++} = Ionized calcium

FIGURE 5.7 Clotting cascade.

sis. The main source of phospholipid is platelets. Ionized calcium is required for some of the steps to proceed. The intrinsic pathway is initiated by contact activation, for example, by exposure to damaged vascular endothelium. The extrinsic pathway is stimulated by factors released from damaged tissue. The two pathways come together at factor X to form the common pathway.[72,73]

Different tests are used to assess the body's ability to form a clot, by evaluating the function of different parts of the clotting cascade. They can also be used to monitor anticoagulant drug therapy. For most coagulation tests, the blood is centrifuged to remove platelets. Citrate is added to bind calcium and thus prevent the cascade from progressing.[74] Patients with defective or deficient clotting factors can experience bleeding. This may be a congenital disorder such as hemophilia, where there is a deficiency of factor VIII or IX, an acquired disorder such as the impaired factor synthesis seen in liver disease, vitamin K deficiency, or an effect of drugs.[72]

Activated Partial Thromboplastin Time.

[25 to 38 seconds.]

The activated partial thromboplastin time (aPTT) is used to assess the integrity of the intrinsic and common coagulation pathways. It is performed by adding a contact activating agent (e.g., kaolin, ellagic acid, silica, or celite), phospholipid, and calcium to citrated plasma, then measuring the time required for a clot to form. It will be prolonged if there is a deficiency of factor XII, XI, IX, VIII, X, V, II, fibrinogen, prekallikrein, high molecular weight kininogen, or if an inhibitor of one of those is present. A mixing study can be used to distinguish between a factor deficiency and presence of a factor inhibitor (e.g., lupus anticoagulant) in patients with a prolonged aPTT. Patient and normal plasma are mixed together. If the aPTT corrects, there is a factor deficiency. If the aPTT remains abnormal, a factor inhibitor is present.[72,75] The aPTT is not affected by abnormal factor VII or XIII.[6] The aPTT usually is prolonged when the plasma concentration of the clotting factors is less than 15% to 30% of normal.[75] It is sometimes abnormal in those with liver failure, since many clotting factors are synthesized in the liver. It may be shortened in an active coagulopathy. It is the most common test used to monitor unfractionated heparin therapy, and can be prolonged in the presence of thrombolytic drugs or coumarin derivatives.[72,75]

Prothrombin Time.

[11 to 16 seconds]

The prothrombin time (PT) is used to evaluate the extrinsic and common pathways. Tissue thromboplastin (e.g., brain, lung, or placenta extract or recombinant human tissue factor with phospholipid) and calcium are added to citrated plasma, and the time to clot formation is measured.[72,76] The PT is prolonged if there is a deficiency of factor VII, X, V, or II, or fibrinogen, (concentrations <10% of normal), or the presence of an inhibitor to one of those factors. It is not affected by abnormal factor VIII, IX, XI, or XII.[72,75] For standardization of test results, the PT is expressed as the International Normalized Ratio (INR). This is calculated by the formula INR = PT ratio$^{(ISI)}$, where the PT ratio is the ratio of the patient's PT to mean normal PT, and ISI is the International Sensitivity Index, which relates an individual batch of thromboplastin to the World Health Organization international reference preparation.[76] The PT is prolonged in liver disease, in patients with a vitamin K deficiency, and in disseminated intravascular coagulation. It is used to monitor coumarin (e.g., warfarin) treatment, but may be prolonged by the presence of heparin or a thrombolytic drug.[72] An extensive discussion of drugs that affect the clotting tests is found in Chapter 25.

Antifactor Xa Activity Assay.

[0.6 to 1.0 IU/mL]

Antifactor Xa activity can be used to gauge the concentration of heparin or danaparoid present in plasma. The chromogenic antifactor Xa assay method is preferred for monitoring low molecular weight heparin. The patient's citrated plasma is mixed with excess antithrombin, then a known amount of factor Xa. After a substrate is added, residual factor Xa is measured. For most patients, it is not necessary to monitor low molecular weight heparin with laboratory tests. It is, however, useful in pediatric and pregnant patients, very obese or underweight patients, or those with renal dysfunction or malignancy. It may also be monitored in those at high risk for thromboembolism or bleeding. Antifactor Xa activity should be checked at peak concentrations of the low-molecular-weight heparin, 4 hours after a subcutaneous injection. The desired range is 0.6 to 1.0 IU per mL if dosed every 12 hours and 1.0 to 2.0 IU per mL for once a day administration.[77,78]

Thrombin Time.

[12 to 18 seconds]

The thrombin time (TT) is used to assess the body's ability to convert fibrinogen to fibrin. Thrombin is added to citrated plasma, and the time for clotting is measured. The thrombin time is prolonged if there is a deficiency or abnormality of fibrinogen, or if heparin, hirudin, or fibrin degradation products are present.[6,72] It can also be increased in patients with uremia, high concentrations of monoclonal immunoglobulins (e.g., myeloma or macroglobulinemia), or antithrombin antibodies.[6] It may also be used in monitoring thrombolytic therapy (e.g., streptokinase or urokinase).[79]

Bleeding Time.

[120 to 480 seconds]

The bleeding time may be used as a screening test to assess platelet function, although it is imprecise. It may be useful in evaluating a patient with a history of increased bleeding but does not appear to predict risk for perioperative bleeding. It is performed by making a uniform incision on the arm while a blood pressure cuff on the upper arm is inflated to maintain a constant pressure of 40 mm Hg. Blood that beads up is removed every 30 seconds by filter paper with care taken not to touch the wound and disturb platelet plugs. The blood is removed to prevent fibrin from forming and stopping the bleeding. The endpoint of the test is when there is no longer a spot on the filter paper after blotting. The test is prolonged when there is platelet dysfunction, when the number of platelets is less than $100 \times 10^3/mm^3$ ($100 \times 10^9/L$), or when a platelet-inhibiting drug, such as aspirin, is present. It also is prolonged in patients with uremia or von Willebrand disease.[68] If the bleeding time is shorter than expected, many young, active platelets may be present.[57]

D-Dimer.

[<0.5 µg/mL (<0.5 mg/L); CF = 1]

D-dimer fragments are produced when crossed-linked fibrin is lysed by plasmin. Their presence provides evidence of a physiologic response to venous thrombosis.[80] The various D-dimer assays all use monoclonal antibodies but they vary in their sensitivity and specificity.[81] For example, the enzyme-linked immunosorbent assay (ELISA) and automated latex immunoassay have high sensitivity (96% to 99%) and low specificity (~40%) for detecting venous thrombosis. This means that most patients with pulmonary embolism or deep vein thrombosis will have elevated D-dimer concentrations, but so will many patients with other disorders (e.g., malignancy, infections, MI, heart failure, or recent surgery). D-dimer values also increase with age and pregnancy. A normal D-dimer concentration can be used to rule out a thromboembolic disorder in patients with low clinical probability of pulmonary embolism or deep vein thrombosis. The test is more useful in outpatients than those who are hospitalized since the latter are more likely to have one or more of the other conditions that can increase D-dimer values.[80,82] An elevated D-dimer test is also an important component in establishing a diagnosis of disseminated intravascular coagulation (DIC), also called consumption coagulopathy. Other typical laboratory findings in DIC include decreased platelets and fibrinogen, prolonged PT and aPPT, and increased fibrin degradation products.[72]

IMPROVING OUTCOMES

Several studies have been done to evaluate the effects of various strategies to alter clinician practice involving diagnostic test ordering. Oxman et al[83] reviewed 102 trials of interventions to improve professional practice. Of these 102 trials, 12 involved attempts to alter physician behavior with regard to test ordering. The following types of interventions were included in the evaluation: educational materials, conferences, outreach visits, local opinion leaders, patient-mediated interventions, audit and feedback, reminders, marketing, multifaceted interventions, and local consensus processes. Oxman et al[83] concluded that there was no ideal strategy (''magic bullet'') for altering physician behavior regarding test ordering. A wide range of interventions exists, that if used appropriately based on the best evidence available, could lead to dramatic improvements in the care of patients. Chapters in this textbook will discuss various strategies to improve the diagnosis and management of individual disease states. Outcome evaluations will be reviewed based on these strategies. Appropriate clinical laboratory test ordering, monitoring, and interpretation will be an important component of these strategies to improve patient outcomes.

CONCLUSION

This chapter has reviewed commonly encountered clinical laboratory tests including SCr, BUN, plasma glucose, uric acid, enzymes, bilirubin, serum proteins, clotting tests, and CBC with differential. Reliable measurements are an integral component in the management of any patient. Laboratory test values that do not correlate with a patient's clinical picture should be questioned and repeated. Reference values used should be those provided by the clinical laboratory in which the test was performed. Critical or treatment values for a given test in a clinical situation should be considered rather than just normal or abnormal values. Drugs may alter a particular laboratory test, and medication histories and administration profiles should be thoroughly reviewed for potential drug causes of these alterations. Clinical laboratory tests are a major component of the diagnosis and treatment of patients. Understanding their regulation, critical ranges, clinical applications, and limitations is vital.

KEY POINTS

- Laboratory test values that do not correlate with a patient's clinical picture should be questioned and repeated.
- Reference values used should be those provided by the clinical laboratory in which the test was performed.
- Critical or treatment values for a given test in a clinical situation should be considered rather than just normal or abnormal values.

- Drugs may alter a particular laboratory test, and medication histories and administration profiles should be thoroughly reviewed for potential drug causes of these alterations.
- The more acute and extensive tissue injury is, the greater the rise in enzymes released from that tissue. Chronic smoldering damage causes moderate release of similar enzymes, with patterns usually different from those in acute injury.
- Azotemia is a rise in BUN and can be categorized as prerenal (inadequate renal perfusion), renal (decreased glomerular filtration), and postrenal (urinary tract obstruction). To yield more information about the category of renal dysfunction, the BUN is divided by the SCr (BUN to creatinine ratio); the normal ratio ranges from 10 to 20:1.
- Troponin-I (cTnI), CK, AST, and LDH are the enzymes that rise after an acute MI. cTnI and CK are the first to rise but CK falls to normal values within 72 hours. LDH is slower to rise but can stay elevated such as cTnI for up to 10 to 14 days.
- Causes of hyperbilirubinemia can be classified into three broad categories: (a) prehepatic (hemolysis), (b) hepatic (defective removal of bilirubin from the blood or defective conjugation), and (c) posthepatic (obstruction of the extrahepatic biliary tree), also referred to as cholestatic or obstructive.
- Common pitfalls in the use of liver function tests to assess the etiology of hyperbilirubinemia include: (a) dependence on single tests rather than patterns of abnormality; (b) normal results, implying no disease (AST is normal in 25% of patients with cirrhosis and ALT in 50%); (c) abnormal liver function tests, suggesting only liver disease; or (d) failure to recognize hepatocellular disease with low transaminase and high ALP levels, or failure to recognize cholestasis or obstruction with high transaminase and low ALP levels.
- Albumin has three major functions: (a) controlling oncotic pressure in the plasma, (b) transporting amino acids synthesized in the liver to other tissues, and (c) transporting poorly soluble organic and inorganic ligands.
- The main function of erythrocytes, or RBC, is to carry oxygen from the lungs to the tissues and transport carbon dioxide back to the lungs. Anemia occurs when the hemoglobin, and/or hematocrit are below the normal range. This can be a result of impaired erythrocyte production, increased erythrocyte destruction, or blood loss.
- Laboratories commonly report six types of leukocytes or WBC found in the peripheral blood: neutrophils, bands, lymphocytes, monocytes, eosinophils, and basophils. The differential white count indicates the percentage of the total leukocyte count that is accounted for by each type (addition of the differential should total 100%). A ''shift to the left'' means there is an increase in the number of bands and immature neutrophils in the blood.
- Neutropenia is a result of impaired production, increased destruction, or altered distribution of neutrophils. It occurs when the ANC is below the normal range. When the neutrophil count is $<1,000$ mm^3, there is an increased risk of infection, and when it is <500 mm^3, this risk is even higher.
- Thrombocytopenia, a reduced number of circulating platelets, can occur as a result of decreased production, abnormal distribution or dilution, or increased destruction of platelets. If the platelet count is 20 to 50 $\times$ 10^3/mm^3, the patient is at a high risk for minor spontaneous bleeding and bleeding after surgery, and if it is less than 20 $\times$ 10^3 per mm^3, the patient is at risk for more serious bleeding.
- The aPTT is the most common test used to monitor unfractionated heparin therapy, and the PT, expressed as the INR, is used to monitor coumarin (e.g., warfarin) treatment.

REFERENCES

1. Henry JB, Kurec AS. The clinical laboratory; organization, purposes, and practice. In: Henry JB, ed. Clinical diagnosis and management by laboratory methods. 20th ed. Philadelphia: WB Saunders, 2001:3–39.
2. Pincus MR, Abraham NZ. Interpreting laboratory results. In: Henry JB, ed. Clinical diagnosis and management by laboratory methods. 20th ed. Philadelphia: WB Saunders, 2001:92–107.
3. Young DS. Implementation of SI units for clinical laboratory data. Style specifications and conversion tables. Ann Intern Med 106:114–129, 1987.
4. Hristova EN, Henry JB. Metabolic intermediates, inorganic ions and biochemical markers of bone metabolism. In: Henry JB, ed. Clinical diagnosis and management by laboratory methods. 20th ed. Philadelphia: WB Saunders, 2001:180–210.
5. Smith CL, Hampton EM. Using estimated creatinine clearance for individualizing drug therapy: a reassessment. DICP Ann Pharmacother 24:1185–1190, 1990.
6. Wallach J. Interpretation of diagnostic tests. 7th ed. Philadelphia: Lippincott Williams & Wilkins, 2000.
7. Klasco RK, ed. DRUGDEX® System. Greenwood Village, CO: Thomson MICROMEDEX, (Vol. 121 expires 9/2004).
8. Hammer SM, Squires KE, Hughes MD, et al. A controlled trial of two nucleoside analogues plus indinavir in persons with human immunodeficiency virus infection and CD4 cell counts of 200 per cubic millimeter or less. N Engl J Med 337:725–733, 1997.
9. Gulick RM, Mellors JW, Havlir D, et al. Treatment with indinavir, zidovudine, and lamivudine in adults with human immunodeficiency virus infection and prior antiretroviral therapy. N Engl J Med 337:734–739, 1997.
10. Dufour DR. Evaluation of renal function, water, electrolytes, acid-base balance, and blood gases. In: Henry JB, ed. Clinical diagnosis and management by laboratory methods. 20th ed. Philadelphia: WB Saunders, 2001:159–179.
11. Knudson PE, Weinstock RS, Henry JB. Carbohydrates. In: Henry JB, ed. Clinical diagnosis and management by laboratory methods. 20th ed. Philadelphia: WB Saunders, 2001:211–223.
12. Stanaszek WF, Seifert CF. Arthritis in the elderly: presentation, treatment and monitoring aspects. J Geriatric Drug Ther 3:5–89, 1989.
13. Campion EW, Clynn RJ, DeLabry LO. Asymptomatic hyperuricemia. Risks and consequences in the normative aging study. Am J Med 82:421–426, 1987.
14. Steele MA, Des Prez RM. The role of pyrazinamide in tuberculosis chemotherapy. Chest 94:845–850, 1988.

15. Borg EJT, Rasker JJ. Gout in the elderly. A separate entity? Ann Rheum Dis 46:72–76, 1987.
16. Van Thiel DH, Iqbal M, Jain A, et al. Gastrointestinal and metabolic problems associated with immunosuppression with either CyA or FK 506 in liver transplantation. Transplant Proc 22 (Suppl 1): 37–40, 1990.
17. Dufour DR, Lott JA, Henry JB. Clinical enzymology. In: Henry JB, ed. Clinical diagnosis and management by laboratory methods. 20th ed. Philadelphia: WB Saunders, 2001:281–303.
18. Koppel C. Clinical features, pathogenesis and management of drug-induced rhabdomyolysis. Med Toxicol Adverse Drug Experience 4: 108–126, 1989.
19. Zeller FP, Bauman JL. Current concepts in clinical therapeutics: acute myocardial infarction. Clin Pharm 5:553–572, 1986.
20. Holland EG, Young LH. Interpretation of clinical laboratory tests. In: Koda-Kimble MA, Young LY, eds. Applied therapeutics: the clinical use of drugs. 7th ed. Philadelphia: Lippincott Williams & Wilkins, 2001:2-1–2-21.
21. Hong RA, Licht JD, Wei JY, et al. Elevated CK-MB with normal total creatine kinase in suspected myocardial infarction: associated clinical findings and early prognosis. Am Heart J 111:1041–1047, 1986.
22. Lee TH, Weisberg MC, Cook F, et al. Evaluation of creatine kinase and creatine kinase-MB for diagnosing myocardial infarction. Clinical impact in the emergency room. Arch Intern Med 147:115–121, 1987.
23. Yusuf S, Collins R, Lin L, et al. Significance of elevated MB isoenzyme with normal creatine kinase in acute myocardial infarction. Am J Cardiol 59:245–250, 1987.
24. Pearlman CA. Neuroleptic malignant syndrome: a review of the literature. J Clin Psychopharmacol 6:257–273, 1986.
25. Montgomery R, Dryer RL, Conway TW, et al. Biochemistry. A Case-Oriented Approach. 2nd ed. Saint Louis, MO: CV Mosby, 1977.
26. Diggs LW. Sickle cell crises. Am J Clin Pathol 44:1–19, 1965.
27. Petz LD. Drug-induced immune haemolytic anaemia. Clin Haematol 9:455–483, 1980.
28. Quist J, Hill AR. Serum lactate dehydrogenase (LDH) in pneumocystis carinii pneumonia, tuberculosis, and bacterial pneumonia. Chest 108:415–418, 1995.
29. Kaplowitz N, Aw TY, Simon FR, et al. Drug-induced hepatotoxicity. Ann Intern Med 104:826–839, 1986.
30. Keffer JH. The cardiac profile and proposed practice guideline for acute ischemic heart disease. Am J Clin Pathol 107:398–409, 1997.
31. Jaffe AS. In search of specificity: the troponins. ACC Curr J Rev 3: 29–33, 1995.
32. Alexander RW, Pratt CM, Roberts R. Diagnosis and management of patients with acute myocardial infarction. In: Alexander RW, Schlant RC, Fuster V, eds. Hurst's The heart arteries and veins. 9th ed. New York, NY: McGraw-Hill, 1998:1345–1433.
33. Hamm CW, Goldmann BU, Heeschen C, et al. Emergency room triage of patients with acute chest pain by means of rapid testing for cardiac troponin T or troponin I. N Engl J Med 337:1648–1653, 1997.
34. McFarlane SI, Winer N, Sowers JR. Role of the natriuretic peptide system in cardiorenal protection. Arch Intern Med 163:2696–2704, 2003.
35. Packer M. Should B-type natriuretic peptid be measured routinely to guide the diagnosis and management of chronic heart failure? Circulation 108:2950–2953, 2003.
36. Wilson Tang WH, Girod JP, Lee MJ, et al. Plasma B-type natriuretic peptide levels in ambulatory patients with established chronic symptomatic systolic heart failure. Circulation 108:2964–2966, 2003.
37. Clark JA, Zimmerman HJ, Tanner LA. Labetalol hepatotoxicity. Ann Intern Med 113:210–213, 1990.
38. Davis KL, Thal LJ, Gamzu ER, et al. A double-blind, placebo-controlled multicenter study of tacrine for Alzheimer's disease. N Engl J Med 327:1253–1259, 1992.
39. Sher PP. Drug interferences with clinical laboratory tests. Drugs 24: 24–63, 1982.
40. Girling DJ. The hepatic toxicity of antituberculosis regimens containing isoniazid, rifampicin, and pyrazinamide. Tubercle 59:13–32, 1978.
41. Mitchell JR, Zimmerman HJ, Ishak KG, et al. Isoniazid liver injury: clinical spectrum, pathology, and probable pathogenesis. Ann Intern Med 84:181–192, 1976.
42. Moss DW. Diagnostic aspects of alkaline phosphatase and its isoenzymes. Clin Biochem 20:225–230, 1987.
43. Chopra S, Griffin PH. Laboratory tests and diagnostic procedures in evaluation of liver disease. Am J Med 79:221–230, 1985.
44. Dufour DR. Evaluation of liver function and injury. In: Henry JB, ed. Clinical diagnosis and management by laboratory methods. 20th ed. Philadelphia: WB Saunders, 2001:264–280.
45. Heisig DG, Threatte GA, Henry JB. Laboratory diagnosis of gastrointestinal and pancreatic disorders. In: Henry JB, ed. Clinical diagnosis and management by laboratory methods. 20th ed. Philadelphia: WB Saunders, 2001:462–476.
46. Geokas MC, Baltaxe HA, Banks PA, et al. Acute pancreatitis. Ann Intern Med 1985;103:86 100, 1985.
47. Berardi RR, Montgomery PA. Pancreatitis. In: Dipiro JT, Talbert RL, Yee GC, et al., eds. Pharmacotherapy a pathophysiologic approach. 5th ed. New York, NY: McGraw-Hill, 2002:701–715.
48. McPherson RA. Specific proteins. In: Henry JB, ed. Clinical diagnosis and management by laboratory methods. 20th ed. Philadelphia: WB Saunders, 2001:249–263.
49. MacKichan JJ. Influence of protein binding and use of unbound (free) drug concentrations. In: Evans WE, Schentag JJ, Jusko WJ, eds. Applied pharmacokinetics principles of therapeutic drug monitoring. 3rd ed. Vancouver, WA: Applied Therapeutics, Inc., 1992: 5-1–5-48.
50. Zini R, Riant P, Barre J, et al. Disease-induced variations in plasma protein levels. Implications for drug dosage regimens (Part I). Clin Pharmacokinet 19:147–159, 1990.
51. Davey FR, Hutchison RE. Hematopoiesis. In: Henry JB, ed. Clinical diagnosis and management by laboratory methods. 20th ed. Philadelphia: WB Saunders, 2001:520–541.
52. Elghetany MT, Davey FR. Erythrocytic disorders. In: Henry JB, ed. Clinical diagnosis and management by laboratory methods. 20th ed. Philadelphia: WB Saunders, 2001:542–585.
53. Morris MW, Davey FR. Basic examination of blood. In: Henry JB, ed. Clinical diagnosis and management by laboratory methods. 20th ed. Philadelphia: WB Saunders, 2001:479–519.
54. Means Jr RT. Erythrocytosis. In: Greer JP, Foerster J, Lukens JN, et al., eds. Wintrobe's clinical hematology. 11th ed. Philadelphia: Lippincott Williams & Wilkins, 2004:1495–1508.
55. Dessypris EN, Sawyer ST. Erythropoiesis. In: Greer JP, Foerster J, Lukens JN, et al., eds. Wintrobe's clinical hematology. 11th ed. Philadelphia: Lippincott Williams & Wilkins, 2004:195–216.
56. Glader B. Destruction of erythrocytes. In: Greer JP, Foerster J, Lukens JN, et al., eds. Wintrobe's clinical hematology. 11th ed. Philadelphia: Lippincott Williams & Wilkins, 2004:249–265.
57. Sacher RA, McPherson RA. Widmann's clinical interpretation of laboratory tests. 10th ed. Philadelphia: FA Davis, 1991.
58. Jeng MR, Glader B. Acquired nonimmune hemolytic disorders. In: Greer JP, Foerster J, Lukens JN, et al., eds. Wintrobe's clinical hematology. 11th ed. Philadelphia: Lippincott Williams & Wilkins, 2004:1223–1246.
59. Neff AT. Autoimmune hemolytic anemias. In: Greer JP, Foerster J, Lukens JN, et al., eds. Wintrobe's clinical hematology. 11th ed. Philadelphia: Lippincott Williams & Wilkins, 2004:1157–1182.
60. Guinan EC, Shimamura A. Acquired and inherited aplastic anemia syndromes. In: Greer JP, Foerster J, Lukens JN, et al., eds. Wintrobe's clinical hematology. 11th ed. Philadelphia: Lippincott Williams & Wilkins, 2004:1397–1419.
61. Hutchison RE, Davey FR. Leukocytic disorders. In: Henry JB, ed. Clinical diagnosis and management by laboratory methods. 20th ed. Philadelphia: WB Saunders, 2001:586–622.
62. Lukens JN. Abnormal hemoglobins: general principles. In: Greer JP, Foerster J, Lukens JN, et al., eds. Wintrobe's Clinical Hematology. 11th ed. Philadelphia: Lippincott Williams & Wilkins, 2004: 1247–1262.
63. Glader B. Anemia: general considerations. In: Greer JP, Foerster J, Lukens JN, et al., eds. Wintrobe's clinical hematology. 11th ed. Philadelphia: Lippincott Wiliams & Wilkins, 2004:947–978.
64. Shapiro MF, Greenfield S. The complete blood count and leukocyte differential count. An approach to their rational application. Ann Intern Med 106:65–74, 1987.

65. Carmel R. Megaloblastic anemias: disorders of impaired DNA synthesis. In: Greer JP, Foerster J, Lukens JN, et al., eds. Wintrobe's clinical hematology. 11th ed. Philadelphia: Lippincott Williams & Wilkins, 2004:1367–1395.

66. Alvir JMJ, Lieberman JA, Safferman AZ, et al. Clozapine–induced agranulocytosis: incidence and risk factors in the United States. N Engl J Med 329:162–167, 1993.

67. Lacy P, Becker AB, Moqbel R. The human eosinophil. In: Greer JP, Foerster J, Lukens JN, et al., eds. Wintrobe's clinical hematology. 11th ed. Philadelphia: Lippincott Williams & Wilkins, 2004: 311–333.

68. Miller JL. Blood platelets. In: Henry JB, ed. Clinical Diagnosis and Management by Laboratory Methods. 20th ed. Philadelphia: WB Saunders, 2001:623–641.

69. Abrams CS, Brass LF. Platelet signal transduction. In: Colman RW, Hirsh J, Marder VJ, et al., eds. Hemostasis and thrombosis: basic principles and clinical practice. 4th ed. Philadelphia, PA: Lippincott Williams & Wilkins, 2001:541–559.

70. Patrono C, Coller B, Dalen JE, et al. Platelet-active drugs: the relationships among dose, effectiveness, and side effects. Chest 119(Suppl 1):39S–63S, 2001.

71. Levine SP. Miscellaneous causes of thrombocytopenia. In: Greer JP, Foerster J, Lukens JN, et al., eds. Wintrobe's clinical hematology. 11th ed. Philadelphia: Lippincott Williams & Wilkins, 2004: 1565–1572.

72. Van Cott EM, Laposata M. Coagulation, fibrinolysis and hypercoagulation. In: Henry JB, ed. Clinical diagnosis and management by laboratory methods. 20th ed. Philadelphia: WB Saunders, 2001: 642–659.

73. Colman RW, Clowes AW, George JN, et al. Overview of hemostasis. In: Colman RW, Hirsh J, Marder VJ, et al., eds. Hemostasis and thrombosis: basic principles and clinical practice. 4th ed. Philadelphia: Lippincott Williams & Wilkins, 2001:3–16.

74. Brown BA. Hematology: principles and procedures. 6, ed. Philadelphia: Lea and Febiger, 1993.

75. Rodgers GM. Diagnostic approach to the bleeding disorders. In: Greer JP, Foerster J, Lukens JN, et al., eds. Wintrobe's clinical hematology. 11th ed. Philadelphia: Lippincott Williams & Wilkins, 2004:1511–1528.

76. Hirsh J, Dalen JE, Anderson DR, et al. Oral anticoagulants: mechanism of action, clinical effectiveness, and optimal therapeutic range. Chest 119 (Suppl 1):8S–21S, 2001.

77. Laposata M, Green D, VanCott EM, et al. College of American Pathologists Conference XXXI on laboratory monitoring of anticoagulant therapy: the clinical use and laboratory monitoring of low-molecular-weight heparin, danaparoid, hirudin and related compounds, and argatroban. Arch Pathol Lab Med 122:799–807, 1998.

78. O'Shea SI, Ortel TL. Issues in the utilization of low molecular weight heparins. Semin Hematol 39:172–178, 2002.

79. Hyers TM, Agnelli G, Hull RD, et al. Antithrombotic therapy for venous thromboembolic disease. Chest 119 (Suppl 1):176S–193S, 2001.

80. Frost SD, Brotman DJ, Michota FA. Rational use of D-dimer measurement to exclude acute venous thromboembolic disease. Mayo Clic Proc 78:1385–1391, 2003.

81. Keeling DM, Mackie IJ, Moody A, et al. The Haemostasis and Thrombosis Task Force of The British Committee for Standards in Haematology. The diagnosis of deep vein thrombosis in symptomatic outpatients and the potential for clinical assessment and D-dimer assays to reduce the need for diagnostic imaging. Br J Haematol 124:15–25, 2004.

82. Perrier A. D-dimer for suspected pulmonary embolism: whom should we test? Chest 125:807–809, 2004.

83. Oxman AD, Thomson MA, Davis DA, et al. No magic bullets: a systematic review of 102 trials of interventions to improve professional practice. Can Med Assoc J 153:1423–1431, 1995.

Racial, Ethnic, and Sex Differences in Response to Drugs

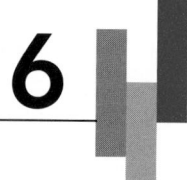

Hewitt W. Matthews and Jannifer L. Johnson

TREATMENT GOALS

- Consider factors affecting drug response in different racial, ethnic, and sex groups.
- Identify drug-metabolizing enzymes that show genetic polymorphism in drug metabolism.
- List the incidence of poor or slow metabolizers in different racial groups.
- Identify the incidence of slow acetylators in some racial and ethnic groups.
- Predict racial and ethnic differences in response to antihypertensive agents, psychotropic agents, and certain miscellaneous agents.
- Consider sex-related differences in pharmacokinetic properties; however, the clinical significance of these differences has not been clearly established.
- Be aware of possible sex differences in response to cardiovascular and psychotropic agents.

For a growing number of drugs, the percentage of patients who react differently or adversely is determined by their racial and ethnic background and sex differences. The adage that ''one size does not fit all'' illustrates the increasingly recognized fact that racial, ethnic, and sex differences must be taken into account when prescribing drug therapy. Factors that affect drug response based on racial, ethnic, and sex differences fall into three major categories: environmental, cultural (psychosocial), and genetic. The major drugs and classes that show varying effects among racial, ethnic, and sex groups are the antipsychotics, benzodiazepines, antidepressants, cardiovascular agents and antihypertensives, atropine, analgesics, antidiabetic agents, alcohol, immunology-related agents, anesthetics, antibiotics, and coronary agents. Even though therapeutic response, metabolism, and side effects may differ with various medicines due to racial, ethnic, and sex differences, clinical significance is oftentimes not established. This chapter will focus primarily on the effects that racial, ethnic, and sex differences have on drug responses.

FACTORS AFFECTING DRUG RESPONSE

ENVIRONMENTAL

Environmental factors may have significant influences on drug response, metabolism, disposition, and excretion. Some of these factors are shown in Table 6.1. It is well known that ethnic variations in diet may play a major role in the absorption and, therefore, plasma levels of a drug. Studies comparing the metabolism of antipyrine between Asian Indians and Indian immigrants in England revealed that as immigrants adopted the lifestyle and dietary habits of the British, their drug metabolism became more rapid.[1] Similar findings were observed among Sudanese and Western Africans.[2,3] Cigarette smoking and heavy drinking are known to induce liver enzymes, thus increasing drug metabolism.[4] Pregnancy, stress, diurnal rhythms, and fever may operate independently or simultaneously in the same person, thus affecting in different ways and to different degrees the processes

TABLE 6.1	Factors Affecting Drug Responses in Different Racial, Ethnic, and Gender Groups
Environmental	**Cultural (psychosocial)**
Chronic alcohol ingestion	Attitudes
Multiple disease states	Beliefs
Diet	Family influence
Fever	Therapy expectations
Cigarette smoking	
Pregnancy	**Genetic**
Stress	Pharmacogenetics
Diurnal rhythms	Genetic polymorphism

of drug absorption, distribution, biotransformation, and excretion.

CULTURAL (PSYCHOSOCIAL)

Drug efficacy and compliance are affected by cultural or psychosocial factors like beliefs, attitudes, therapy expectations, communication skills, and family influences. Noncompliance with medication regimens is a major problem in the treatment of chronic medical conditions. Contrasting cultural beliefs across ethnic groups can affect medication compliance and, hence, drug effectiveness. For example, Kinzie et al[5] reported that 61% of depressed medicated refugee patients from Southeast Asia showed no evidence of tricyclic antidepressants (TCA) in the blood, although they were all adequately treated with TCA. The majority of these patients reported not taking the prescribed TCA and pretended to comply with medication regimens for a number of reasons. In a South African study involving a long-term regimen of oral phenothiazines among black, white, and other patients of color, rates of compliance varied between 33% for black, 50% for colored, and 75% for white patients.[6]

Expectations of medications also play an important role in patient compliance. Clinicians working with refugees and other Asian populations report that these patients typically expect medicines from the Western culture to work quickly, to have a high potential for severe side effects, and to be effective only for the control of the ''superficial'' manifestations, not underlying conditions of the diseases.[7] The investigators concluded that Asian refugees, unless carefully counseled, often have difficulty appreciating the need for maintenance therapy for most psychiatric conditions.[7]

PHARMACOGENETICS

Pharmacogenetics is the study of genetically determined variations in drug response.[8] In healthy individuals, genetically controlled differences in the way individuals metabolize (e.g., oxidize and acetylate) drugs are major determinants of racial and ethnic differences in response to medicines. Genetic polymorphisms (variations in DNA sequences) account for interindividual differences in their ability to meta-

bolize drugs that are controlled by a single gene. The focus of this discussion will be on genetic polymorphisms of drug-metabolizing enzymes. The major polymorphic phase I (e.g., oxidation, reduction, and hydrolysis) enzymes that catalyze drug metabolism are the cytochrome P-450 (CYP) isozymes (existing in multiple forms). The major genetically polymorphic phase II (e.g., acetylation, glucuronidation, and methylation) conjugating enzymes are catechol O-methyltransferase, thiopurine S-methyltransferase, UDP-glucuronosyltransferase, and N-acetyltransferase (NAT); however, this section will be limited to a discussion on NAT.

Pharmacogenetics of Phase I Metabolizing Enzymes. The cytochrome P-450 enzymes represent a superfamily of over 50 heme-containing microsomal drug metabolizing isozymes. It is one of the widely studied and important enzyme systems that catalyze phase I drug metabolism.[9] Its name is derived from the characteristic maximum spectral absorbance at 450 nm, when it is in the reduced state. The recommended nomenclature for these enzymes is now CYP to designate human cytochrome P-450, followed by an Arabic number to designate the family, followed by a capital letter to designate the subfamily, followed by an Arabic number to indicate the individual gene (allele), and sometimes followed by an Arabic number(s) with an asterisk to indicate allelic variant(s). For example, CYP2D6*3 belongs to the family 2 and subfamily D; the gene encoding for the isozyme is 6; and the allelic variant is the last Arabic number 3 with an asterisk preceding it. Some clinically significant genetic polymorphisms in the CYP isozymes will be discussed.

CYP2D6 Polymorphism. CYP2D6 isoenzyme metabolizes 25% to 30% of all clinically used medications, including antidepressants, β-blockers, antipsychotics, morphine derivatives, and many other drugs (Table 6.2). Genetic polymorphisms in CYP2D6 is responsible for the variability in interindividual responses to these agents. This is also termed the debrisoquine/sparteine genetic polymorphism in reference to the drugs metabolized that led to the discovery of the CYP2D6 polymorphic enzyme.[13]

Debrisoquine is an antihypertensive agent that was found to exhibit a genetic polymorphism in its oxidative metabolism.[13] Two distinct phenotypes were observed in the population with a urinary ratio of debrisoquine to its main 4-hydroxy metabolite. Those individuals who were deficient in their ability to oxidize the substrate are called poor metabolizers (PMs), whereas extensive metabolizers (EMs) biotransform a substantial amount of the drug to its metabolite. Therefore, debrisoquine represents a ''probe drug,'' which is a compound used to classify individuals as having either poor or extensive metabolism.[14]

PMs and EMs may experience problems when being treated with the previously mentioned agents. PMs do not metabolize the drugs in question well and will often develop elevated plasma concentrations leading to adverse effects. EMs, however, do not respond to recommended doses be-

Enzyme	CYP2D6	CYP2C19	CYP2C9	CYP3A4
Substrate	Amitriptyline	Omeprazole	Celecoxib	Diltiazem
	Imipramine	Diazepam	Ibuprofen	Nimodipine
	Nortriptyline	Imipramine	Piroxicam	Nifedipine
	Fluoxetine	Lansoprazole	Diclofenac	Verapamil
	Risperidone	Nelfinavir	Losartan	Cyclosporine A
	Thioridazine	Voriconazole	Warfarin	Cortisol
	Paroxetine		Phenytoin	Progesterone
	Haloperidol		Tolbutamide	Testosterone
	Metoprolol		Tamoxifen	Clarithromycin
	Timolol			Erythromycin
	Propranolol			Cyclophosphamide
	Codeine			Tamoxifen
	Dextromethorphan			Vincristine
				Vinblastine
				Alprazolam
				Triazolam
				Fentanyl
				Sufentanil
				Lovastatin
				Simvastitin
				Atorvastatin
				Indinavir
				Saquinavir
				Quindine
				Sildenafil
				Ziprasidone

TABLE 6.2   Some Drugs Metabolized by Cytochrome Isozymes

(From Ma MK, Wood MH, McLeod HL. Genetic basis of drug metabolism. Am J Health-Syst Pharm 59:2061–2069, 2002; Bertilsson L, Dahl ML, Dalén P, et al. Molecular genetics of CYP2D6: Clinical relevance with focus on psychotropic drugs. Br J Clin Pharmacol 53:111–122, 2002; Drug interactions. Medical Lett 45:46–47, 2003, with permission.)

cause drug concentrations are too low.[8] The prevalence of the PM phenotype in all ethnic groups studied ranges on an average between 2% and 10%, with <1% of Asians, 2% to 5% of African Americans, and 5% to 10% of whites being identified as poor metabolizers (Table 6.3).[10,15]

CYP2C19 Polymorphism. CYP2C19 isozyme metabolizes several clinically important therapeutic agents, including antidepressants and antianxiety agents (Table 6.2). Genetic polymorphisms in CYP2C19 is also termed the mephenytoin polymorphism in reference to the use of mephenytoin as a probe drug in the phenotyping (i.e., determination of drug metabolism and response) of CYP2C19.

The polymorphism of mephenytoin varies according to racial and ethnic differences. The incidence of poor metabolizers (PM) is 3% to 5% among whites and 12% to 23% of most Asian populations (Table 6.3).[10,16] A study in an el-

derly unmedicated population showed a higher incidence of slow metabolizers among African Americans (18.5%) as compared to whites (4.1%).[17] It was not determined if these differences were due to genetic or environmental factors.

CYP2C9 Polymorphism. CYP2C9 isozyme metabolizes nonsteroidal antiinflammatory drugs (NSAIDS), losartan, and some narrow therapeutic index drugs, like warfarin, phenytoin, and tolbutamide (Table 6.2). Genetic polymorphisms in CYP2C9 are responsible for interindividual differences in response to these agents. CYP2C9*2 and CYP2C9*3 are the two most common CYP2C9 allelic variants that are found in poor metabolizers. CYP2C9*3 occurs in approximately 6% to 9% of whites and Asians whereas CYP2C9*2 occurs in approximately 8% to 20% of whites, less frequently in African Americans and is virtually absent in Asians (Table 6.3).[10,18]

TABLE 6.3	Generic Polymorphisms Known to Influence Drug Response			
Enzyme	Variant Allele(s)	Frequency of PM	Representative Drugs Metabolized	Effects of Polymorphism
NAT	NAT*5B	40%–70% of whites and African Americans	Isoniazid, sulfonamides, procainamide, hydralazine	Increased relative risk of cancers and drug toxicity
CYP2D6	CYP2D*2A, CYP2D6*3, *4, *5, *6, *10, *17	6%–10% of whites, 2%–5% of African Americans, 1% of Asians	β-receptor antagonists, antiarrhythmics, antidepressants, antipsychotics, morphine derivatives	Lack of analgesic effects from codeine, standard antidepressant dosage ineffective
CYP2C9	CYP2C9*2, CYP2C9*3	6%–8% of whites	Warfarin, phenytoin, glipizide, tolbutamide, losartan, NSAIDS	Increased bleeding episodes from standard warfarin dose, low blood sugar levels in PM
CYP2C19	CYP2C19*2, CYP2C19*3	3%–5% of whites, 12%–23% of Asians	S-mephenytoin, omeprazole, diazepam, propranolol, imipramine, amitriptyline	Increased omeprazole AUC and higher H. pylori eradication rate in PM, prolonged half-life of diazepam and increased risk of diazepam toxicity in Asians
CYP3A4	CYP3A4*1B	Under Investigation	Under Investigation	......
CYP3A5	CYP2A5*1, CYP2A5*3, CYP2A5*6	Under Investigation	Under Investigation	Increased CYP3A5*1 activity, loss of CYP3A5*3, lower CYP3A5*6 activity

NAT, N-acetyltransferase; CYP, cytochrome P-450 isoenzyme system; PM, poor metabolizers; NSAIDS, nonsteroidal antiinflammatory drugs; AUC, area-under-the-concentration-time curve.

(Adapted from Ma MK, Wood MH, McLeod HL. Genetic basis of drug metabolism. Am J Health-Syst Pharm 59:2061–2069, 2002, with permission.)

CYP3A Subfamily Polymorphism. CYP3A isozymes are the predominant subfamily of CYP enzymes. CYP3A activities are the sum of activities of at least three CYP3A isoenzymes: CYP3A4, CYP3A5, and CYP3A7.[19,20] Hepatic CYP3A4 isozyme metabolizes about 50% of currently used drugs (Table 6.2). The frequency of PM and drugs with affected metabolisms by CYP3A isozymes are under investigation (Table 6.3).

Pharmacogenetics of Phase II Acetylation Metabolizing Enzymes.

Acetylation Polymorphism. Polymorphic N-acetylation was first studied when serum concentrations of isoniazid showed substantial interindividual variability.[21] Patients were classified as slow acetylators (SA) or rapid acetylators (RA) according to their ability to metabolize isoniazid. American and European whites and American blacks have approximately equal numbers of SA and RA, whereas in Japanese and Canadian Eskimo subjects, the percentage of RA is high and SA is low (Table 6.4).[22,23] SA will often develop elevated concentrations leading to enhanced drug effects. RAs may not respond to drug therapy because drug

TABLE 6.4	Incidence of Slow Acetylators in Some Racial and Ethnic Groups
Group	Acetylators (%)
Whites	50
American Blacks	50
Japanese	10
Canadian Eskimo	5
Egyptians	80–90
Moroccans	80–90
Chinese (Mainland)	15

(From references Weber WW, Hein DW. N-acetylation pharmacogenetics. Pharmacol Rev 37:25–79, 1985; Wood AJ, Zhou HH. Ethnic differences in drug disposition and responsiveness. Clin Pharmacokinet 20:350–373, 1991, with permission.)

concentration may be too low. Commonly prescribed medications that are metabolized by this pathway include isoniazid, procainamide, hydralazine, sulfonamides, phenelzine, and clonazepam (Table 6.2).

DRUG RESPONSE TO RACIAL AND ETHNIC DIFFERENCES

The drug categories that have been studied the most and shown to be most clinically significant in their actions with regard to racial and ethnic differences are cardiovascular (antihypertensives) and central nervous system agents (psychotropics).

VARIATIONS IN EFFECTS OF CARDIOVASCULAR DRUGS

Antihypertensive Agents. Essential hypertension is considered to be a multifactorial disorder. Recent studies have identified characteristics that may help predict the efficacy of monotherapy in controlling this disease. These characteristics include physiologic factors, like sodium sensitivity, plasma renin activity, sympathetic nervous system activity, and demographic environmental factors.[24] These characteristics of individual patients are important considerations in antihypertensive drug selection because of the increasing numbers and classes of antihypertensive agents and the difference in response among varied ethnic and racial groups.

Although all antihypertensive agents can be effective in the general population, in specific racial and ethnic racial groups, some are more predictable than others and some require different doses for an equivalent effect (Table 6.5).

Diuretics. The pathophysiology of hypertension in a large segment of the black population is characterized by enhanced sodium retention and expanded plasma volume. Diuretics are useful as monotherapy and in combination with other agents in the treatment of hypertension in black patients. Diuretics are effective in this racial group, because they reduce plasma volume and intracellular sodium concentrations. The reduction in blood pressure with diuretics results from decrease in total peripheral resistance that is related to a decreased sensitivity of the vascular wall to pressor substances and possibly to stimulation of the prostacyclin and kallikrein-kinin vasodilator systems.[25]

TABLE 6.5	Racial and Ethnic Differences in Response to Antihypertensive Agents		
Comparison Groups	**Drug Class or Agent**	**Clinical Response**	**References**
African American and white	Calcium channel blockers	African Americans respond to monotherapy as well as whites.	25
Asian American and whites	Calcium channel blockers	Asian Americans experience more side effects.	41
Korean and whites	Nifedipine	Koreans showed significantly lower oral clearance.	42
African American and whites	β-Blockers	African American respond less than whites; no difference if diuretic is added.	26, 36
African American and whites	Propranolol	African Americans have a higher renal clearance.	33
Chinese and whites	Propranolol	Chinese are twice as sensitive to the effects on blood pressure.	37
African American and whites	Diuretics	African Americans respond better.	25, 26
African American and whites	Labetolol (combined α- and β-blocker)	African Americans respond the same as whites.	34
African American and whites	ACE inhibitors	Monotherapy more effective in whites; no difference if diuretic is added.	38
Asian American and Caucasian	ACE inhibitors	Asian Americans experience more side effects.	41

ACE, angiotensin-converting enzyme.

Monotherapy with diuretics tends to cause a greater reduction in blood pressure in black than in white hypertensive patients. Studies by the Veterans Administration documented an average decrease in blood pressure in black males of approximately 20/13 mm Hg as opposed to an average decrease of 15/11 mm Hg in white men, despite a lower dose of diuretic in the black male hypertensive patients.[26]

β-Blockers. The Veterans Administration Cooperative Study Group on Antihypertensive Agents showed that fewer black than white subjects reached their blood pressure goal while taking β-blockers.[27] It has also been shown that differences in plasma renin activity are believed to underlie many of the cross-racial and ethnic differences in response to β-blockers. A greater proportion of white than black people have elevated plasma renin activity, thus requiring lower therapeutic doses of a β-blocker. The reasons for these differences may be differences in renal physiology that may be genetically determined. For example, the renin-angiotensin system is more often suppressed relative to sodium intake and excretion in blacks than in whites.[28] It has been shown that 36% to 62% of black hypertensive patients have relatively suppressed plasma renin activities as compared to 19% to 55% of white hypertensive patients.[29] Even in normotensive patients, plasma renin activity is lower in blacks than in whites.[30,31] Therefore, β-blockers, which are believed to work in part by lowering plasma renin, would be less effective in blacks, who already have lowered renin levels. Even though blacks tend to fall into the low-renin category, with a volume-dependent, salt-sensitive type of hypertension, there are subgroups within the black population that do respond to β-blockers.

Pharmacokinetic and pharmacodynamic factors may also explain the difference in response to β-blockers. Racial differences in affinity for the lymphocyte β-receptor may explain documented differences in response. For example, a study by Johnson[32] showed that the affinity of the β-receptor for propranolol was greater in white than in black patients. Another study concluded that black patients may be less responsive to the effects of β-blockers than whites because of observed higher renal clearance of propranolol.[33]

Evidence exists that black patients may even respond differently to different β-blockers. For example, labetolol (a combined α-β-blocker), unlike propranolol, is equally effective in controlling blood pressure in black and white patients.[34] It was also shown that bisoprolol produced significant decreases in systolic and diastolic blood pressure in black patients, and there also was a trend for atenolol to decrease blood pressure.[35] Also, blacks respond to β-blockers in combination with diuretics equally as well as whites.[26,36] Therefore, pharmacotherapy with β-blockers must be specifically directed toward the individual patient.

Chinese patients seem also to exhibit altered sensitivity to β-blockers but conversely to that of black Americans. A study involving the pharmacokinetics and pharmacodynamics of propranolol compared men of Chinese descent and white American men.[37] The Chinese patients exhibited a 200% higher sensitivity to the effect of propranolol on blood pressure and heart rate as compared to white patients. The investigators concluded that the increased sensitivity to β-blockers may result from the β–receptor-mediated suppression of plasma renin activity, and this increased sensitivity to plasma renin activity suppression in Chinese men may partially explain their greater sensitivity to the hypotensive effects of propranolol.

Angiotensin-Converting Enzyme Inhibitors. Angiotensin-converting enzyme (ACE) inhibitors act using a renin-dependent mechanism. Therefore, the major determinant in response to ACE inhibitors in hypertensive patients is their renin activity. Patients with high plasma renin show much greater response to the antihypertensive effects of ACE inhibitors than do low renin patients. Therefore, one would generally expect the ACE inhibitors to be less effective in black than white patients. This difference was observed with captopril and enalapril; however, when the diuretic hydrochlorothiazide was added, the racial difference in response was eliminated.[38]

A review of the literature was conducted to assess the differences in response to ACE inhibitors and β-blockers in black patients compared with the response in nonblack patients in the management of heart failure.[39] Retrospective reanalyses of major heart failure trials have suggested that black patients may not realize a significant benefit in morbidity or mortality when heart failure is managed with ACE inhibitors or β-blockers. It has also been suggested that black patients may respond more favorably than nonblack patients to the combination of hydralazine and isosorbide dinitrate. The authors conclude that published reanalyses of ACE inhibitor and β-blocker trials in heart failure provide weak data to support a lack of benefit in black patients, and that published literature on this topic is limited by its retrospective nature. Firm conclusions regarding the influence of race on the effectiveness of ACE inhibitors and β-blockers cannot be made until prospective trials, with planned analysis of the effect of race, have been performed.[39]

Calcium Channel Blockers. The hypotensive effect of calcium channel blockers as monotherapy in black patients is comparable to that observed in white patients and significantly greater than that observed in black patients treated with β-blockers or ACE inhibitors.[25] Blacks, elderly, and low-renin hypertensive patients tend to have an enhanced calcium influx-dependent vasoconstriction.[40] This may explain, in part, the excellent antihypertensive effectiveness of monotherapy with calcium channel blockers in black patients.

Comparison of hypertension management in Asian Americans with white patients, using calcium channel blockers or ACE inhibitors, showed that dose reduction and side effects were more common in Asian patients than in white patients.[41] Furthermore, Koreans showed significantly lower oral clearance of nifedipine than white patients.[42] These findings point out the need for additional studies on the outcome of hypertension management in Asian and Asian American patients.

In summary, the low-renin profile, salt retention, expanded plasma volume, and increased intracellular concentrations of sodium and calcium found in many black hypertensive patients may provide the pathophysiologic basis for the significant differences observed in response to antihypertensive agents. When used as monotherapy to treat black hypertensive patients, diuretics and calcium channel blockers tend to produce a greater reduction in blood pressure than do β-blockers and ACE inhibitors.

Coronary Agents. It was found that intracoronary infusion of L-arginine provides significantly greater augmentation of endothelium-dependent vascular relaxation in African American patients when compared with matched white patients drawn from a cohort referred for elective coronary angiography.[43] Therefore, supplemental L-arginine may be of therapeutic value in improving microvascular endothelial dysfunction in African Americans.[43]

VARIATION IN EFFECTS OF CENTRAL NERVOUS SYSTEM DRUGS

Psychotropic Agents. Racial and/or ethnic differences need to be considered in decisions regarding the use of psychotropic drugs (Table 6.6). Growing evidence seems to indicate that the pharmacodynamic and pharmacokinetic influences of these agents differ between races, and these differences can affect clinical outcome.

Antipsychotic Agents. Comparisons of antipsychotic activity among different racial groups reveal similarities and potentially important differences (Table 6.6). Blacks, whites, and Hispanics do not differ in their pharmacokinetics or dose requirements of antipsychotic drugs; however, Asians seem to have a lower threshold than whites for the therapeutic and adverse effects of these agents.[44] Increased absorption, reduced hepatic hydroxylation, and pharmacodynamic factors all play a role in dosage differences.[45] Midha et al[46] and Jann et al[47] reported that Chinese patients showed higher haloperidol plasma concentrations than in white, Hispanic, and black patients. Lam et al[48] showed intra- and interethnic variability among black, white, Chinese, and Mexican-American patients in reduced haloperidol: haloperidol ratios; compared with the other three ethnic groups, the Chinese patients had the lowest ratio. In addition, the haloperidol dose required for the black and white groups was significantly greater than that required for the Chinese group to achieve comparable plasma levels. This observation that Asian patients require lower dosages than do other groups is strengthened by pharmacokinetic studies that report higher plasma or serum drug concentrations in Asian patients, even when controlled for weight and body surface area.[47] In addition, other investigators have reported that lower antipsychotic doses are required in Asian populations when compared to white patients.[49–51] Cultural, environmental, and genetic factors may all be involved in this difference in dose requirement.[1] Therefore, it seems prudent to use lower than usual initial doses of antipsychotic drugs in the treatment of Asian patients.

Ethnic variations in clozapine pharmacokinetics have been studied in Korean Americans and Chinese (Taiwanese) subjects.[52,53] Initial results showed that Korean American patients achieved significantly lower mean clozapine concentrations than white patients, even after controlling differences in daily doses.[52] In contrast to the Korean American patient population, Chinese patients had 30% to 50% higher plasma concentrations than those reported for white patients, suggesting a slower rate of clozapine metabolism in Chinese patients.[53] It should be noted that in these clozapine studies, other confounding variables, like diet and enzyme inducers or inhibitors, may have been present.[54] It has also been found that the use of antipsychotics in blacks is more common than in other racial groups.[55] This may be explained, in part, by the fact that black patients generally receive more severe diagnoses, like schizophrenia, rather than an anxiety or mood disorder.[56] Perhaps for similar reasons, black patients tend to receive substantially higher doses of antipsychotics. This may also result from the stereotype that blacks are more difficult to manage and less compliant.[55]

Raskin and Cook[57] studied the effects of chlorpromazine and imipramine in black and white inpatients. In general, black patients showed greater clinical improvement than whites on measured psychiatric illnesses, irrespective of treatment. However, these differences were more apparent early in treatment. Significant differences were found in drug effects when comparing black men and women. Chlorpromazine was more efficacious for treating black women; and black men were therapeutically more responsive to imipramine. Methodologic concerns include an overrepresentation of patients with the diagnosis of schizophrenia among African Americans (especially black men), and the fact that black patients were much younger and significantly more educationally and economically disadvantaged than their white counterparts.

Lieberman et al[58] observed a genetically determined increased risk of agranulocytosis during clozapine therapy in about 20% of Ashkenazi Jewish patients. This adverse reaction developed only in about 1% of chronic schizophrenic patients. The investigators used human leukocyte antigen typing to identify the haplotype (a cluster of genes that are involved in immune recognition and autoimmunity) that is associated with the development of clozapine-induced agranulocytosis.

Antidepressant Agents. There is not much published information about differences in antidepressant pharmacology among African American, white, Hispanic, and Asian patients. In addition, controlled pharmacokinetic and pharmacodynamic studies with these classes of drugs need to be carried out before clinical applications of TCA in different racial groups can be made.

TABLE 6.6	Racial and Ethnic Differences in Response to Psychotropic Agents		
Comparison Groups	**Drug Class or Agent**	**Clinical Response**	**References**
Chinese, African American, Hispanic, and whites	Haloperidol	Chinese showed higher plasma concentrations.	61
Asian and whites	Antipsychotics	Lower doses are required in Asian population.	63–65
African American and whites	Chlorpromazine	African Americans showed more rapid improvement.	68
African American and whites	Nortriptyline	African Americans had steady-state plasma concentrations ≥50% higher.	71
African American and whites	Imipramine	African Americans showed more rapid improvement.	68
Hispanic and whites	Antidepressants	Hispanics appeared to experience more overall side effects.	73
Asian and whites	Antidepressants	Asians achieved significantly higher plasma concentrations and had lower clearance rates.	77
Chinese, whites, and Hispanics	Antidepressants	Chinese and Hispanic require lower doses; side effects greater in Hispanics than whites.	28
Asian and whites	Alprazolam	Asians exhibit higher serum concentrations, lower clearance, and longer half-lives.	66
Chinese and whites	Diazepam	Chinese showed smaller volume of distribution and higher mean serum concentrations.	78
Asian and whites	Diazepam	Whites showed higher clearance rates.	1
Japanese and Swedish	Clomipramine	Japanese had lower clearance.	65
Korean American and whites	Clozapine	Korean American showed lower mean concentrations.	52
Chinese and whites	Clozapine	Chinese had 30%–50% higher plasma concentrations.	53

General findings seem to indicate that, for a given dosage of TCA, African American patients show higher blood levels and faster therapeutic response than white patients. Also, black patients tend to manifest a greater degree of toxic effects compared to white patients.[55] An often cited study by Ziegler and Biggs[59] reports that steady-state plasma levels of nortriptyline in patients treated with equal oral dosages were 50% higher in black patients than in white patients. It should be noted, however, that the study has been criticized for improper correction of plasma concentrations on the basis of weight.[60] Also, the investigator did not use a fixed-dose protocol, or clearly outline diagnostic criteria or description of sex distribution.[55]

Although many studies indicate that Hispanic and Asian patients required lower dosages of TCA, the results are inconsistent. Hispanic patients also appear to experience more overall side effects with antidepressants than white patients. However, a single-dose study comparing plasma nortriptyline levels and clearance rates in healthy Hispanic and white volunteers failed to demonstrate any major differences between the two groups.[61,62]

Survey data collected from multiple Asian countries indicate that imipramine and amitriptyline are used in much lower dosage ranges than is typical in the United States.[63] In addition, single-dose pharmacokinetic studies indicated that Asians achieve significantly higher plasma concentrations of TCA and have lower clearance rates than do whites.[64] Shimoda et al[65] compared the disposition of the TCA clomipramine in Japanese and Swedish patients receiving continuous treatment. Findings revealed a lower oral clearance of clomipramine in Japanese patients compared with that in Swedish patients. This difference was not accounted for by the lower body weight in Japanese patients or by concomitant treatment with benzodiazepines and is likely to be a true ethnic difference. However, it should be noted that some of the research did not adjust for patient weight.[64] Therefore, the role of racial and ethnic differences in response to antidepressants remains unclear because of limited, and sometimes conflicting, data.

Antianxiety Agents. A single-dose pharmacokinetic study using alprazolam showed that Asians manifested significantly higher plasma concentrations, lower clearance, and longer half-lives than did white patients.[66] Lin et al[67] showed that the clearance rate of diazepam was higher in whites, suggesting that diazepam is metabolized at a significantly higher rate in whites than Asians. Another study showed that healthy male Chinese subjects showed smaller volumes of distribution and higher mean serum concentrations than their white counterparts.[66] Pharmacokinetic differences in the metabolism of these benzodiazepines may result from the fact that there is a higher incidence of PMs among Asians (e.g., Japanese) than among whites.[1]

Based on the data observed, it is suggested that Asian psychiatric patients require smaller initial and maintenance doses of benzodiazepines (i.e., alprazolam and diazepam) for similar clinical effects than do white patients.[67]

Bipolar Agents. There is some evidence for claims of racial and ethnic differences in response to lithium. However, one study reports that African Americans have a significantly longer plasma half-life of lithium than do whites and Chinese.[68] It has also been reported that Japanese patients require lower dosages of lithium and respond to lower plasma lithium levels than their U.S. counterparts for the treatment of bipolar illness.[69] Honda and Suzuki[70] report that whites in the United States have higher lithium clearances and larger volumes of distribution than do Japanese patients.

In summary, Asians in general need lower doses and exhibit adverse effects at lower dosages than do whites when given psychotropic drugs. Hispanics tend to require less antidepressant medication and report more adverse effects at lower doses than whites. Blacks, in general, respond better

than whites to antidepressants, have higher plasma levels, and show a greater degree of adverse effects.

Miscellaneous Agents.

Analgesics. Racial and ethnic differences have been demonstrated for the metabolism of codeine. Wood and Zhou[23] showed that Chinese patients were less able to metabolize codeine than white patients. Another study comparing Swedish white and Chinese subjects revealed that the excretion of unchanged codeine was significantly higher in Chinese subjects than in Swedish white patients.[71] The clinical consequences of these differences in the pharmacokinetics of codeine must be considered in establishing dosing levels for the treatment of pain.

Mucklow et al[72] observed racial and ethnic differences in the metabolism of paracetamol (acetaminophen). Asian immigrants had lower acetaminophen clearance and longer half-life than did whites. It has also been observed that the mean combined recovery of paracetamol metabolites in whites was twice that observed in Ghanians and Kenyan blacks.[36] These findings were attributed to a reduced level of microsomal oxidation in Africans and Asians.

Interethnic differences were found to exist in the disposition of and response to morphine between Chinese and white subjects.[73] Chinese subjects had a significantly higher clearance of morphine than did white subjects. The higher clearance was caused by a higher glucuronidation to morphine-3-glucuronide and morphine-6-glucuronide. In contrast, Chinese subjects were less sensitive than white subjects to the respiratory and vasodepressant effect but not to the nausea-producing effects of morphine.

Furthermore, it was concluded that ethnicity influences the response to morphine when Native Indians were found to be more susceptible to morphine depression of the ventilatory response than white patients, despite higher serum morphine-6-glucuronide levels in whites.[74]

In an open trial of low-dose buprenorphine in treating methadone withdrawal, four white responders required 1 to 2 hours to respond, whereas the two African American responders required only 10 to 20 minutes.[75] This finding suggests that there are racial differences in the metabolism of buprenorphine.

Alcohol. North American Indian, Chinese, and Japanese subjects show a faster rate of alcohol metabolism (i.e., conversion to the aldehyde) and less tolerance than whites.[76] Asians of Mongoloid heritage, American Indians, Japanese, and Chinese subjects show more symptoms of intoxication after alcohol use than do whites and are much more sensitive to its adverse effects, including facial flushing, palpitations, and tachycardia. Facial flushing occurs in 45% to 85% of Asians versus 3% to 29% of whites.[77] The flushing is caused by the accumulation of acetaldehyde due to an unusual less active liver aldehyde dehydrogenase.[36,77] An atypical alcohol dehydrogenase that has higher alcohol metabolism is present in 85% to 90% of Asians and may also contribute to increased blood levels of acetaldehyde.[77]

Jewish men and women have one of the lowest percentages of severe alcohol-related problems of any group. One reason proposed is that Jewish men may have an increased sensitivity to relatively low doses of alcohol. This internal checkpoint might lead Jewish men to avoid high intake of alcoholic beverages.[78]

Atropine. In 1921, Paskind[79] reported that initial bradycardia, attributed to central vagal stimulation before peripheral cholinergic blockade, after parenteral administration of atropine does not occur in African Americans at dose that cause bradycardia in white patients. Similar results were reported in a study from South Africa.[80] However, the black patients were more susceptible to the late bradycardia effect, which occurs about 1 hour after administration. They also observed that the tachycardia effect was significantly more pronounced in African blacks than in whites.[80]

Zhou and Wood[81] reported that healthy Chinese subjects showed a greater increase in heart rate than whites after receiving intravenous atropine. There was no difference in the bradycardia effect that occurred in both groups.

Insulin. Relative to whites, African American children and adults have lower insulin sensitivity and a higher acute insulin response to glucose. The results of this study suggest that greater acute insulin response to glucose among African Americans is due to greater insulin secretion and lesser hepatic insulin extraction.[82]

Antivirals. Black patients with chronic hepatitis C have a lower rate of response to treatment with peginterferon alfa-2b and ribavirin than non-Hispanic white patients. The reason for the differences in response remains unclear; however, they are not explained by differences in viral genome.[83]

Immunosuppressives. Black American heart transplant recipients receiving cyclosporine-based primary immunoprophylaxis suffer higher rates of allograft rejection with hemodynamic compromise, infections, and posttransplant coronary artery disease than do white patients.[84,85] Compared with cyclosporine, an immunosuppressive strategy using tacrolimus in black Americans achieves superior efficacy with regard to allograft rejection, higher allograft survival, and similar safety. Furthermore, tacrolimus-based immunosuppression is similar in immunologic efficacy and safety in black Americans and white heart transplant recipients.[86] The pharmacokinetics and metabolic disposition of tacrolimus were compared among African American, Latin American, and whites. Significant differences in tacrolimus pharmacokinetics were found among the three ethnic groups.[87]

Agents Used in Anesthesia. A study was designed to comparatively investigate the anesthetic requirements of two different ethnic groups: whites and Senegalese African blacks.[88] This study demonstrated statistically significant differences between whites and African blacks in the arousal time from intravenous anesthesia with propofol and remifen-

tanil. Recovery from general anesthesia with propofol was slower in African blacks compared to white patients.[88]

Antibiotics. Yu et al[42] observed racial differences in the oral pharmacokinetics of erythromycin. Koreans showed greater bioavailabilty and significantly lower oral clearance of erythromycin than whites.

DRUG RESPONSE TO SEX DIFFERENCES

Sex is an individual factor that can often lead to interindividual differences in the metabolism of drugs.[89] Studies done to assess sex differences in drug metabolism are inconclusive. Confounding factors like menstrual cycle, pregnancy, lactation, menopause, and the use of oral contraceptives, frequently were not taken into consideration.[90,91] In studies where sex differences in metabolism and pharmacokinetics exist, women generally tend to have lower absorption rates than men (Table 6.7).

In general, drugs that are metabolized by hepatic oxidation have lower metabolic clearance and longer elimination half-lives in women who are on oral contraceptives than those who are not.[90] The clinical significance of sex-related differences in the pharmacokinetic properties of some drugs has not been clearly established. Giudicelli and Tillement[89] concluded that it is unnecessary to change dosage or frequency of administration of a drug based on sex-related differences in metabolism.

Physiologic differences between the sexes in hormone and enzyme levels and basal metabolism influence the metabolism of various drugs.[92] For example, sex differences in muscle mass, disposition of muscle tissue, and vascular resistance could cause variation in response to intramuscular injections. Sex differences in gastric motility, secretion, and metabolic rate may influence plasma levels of orally admin-

TABLE 6.7	Sex Differences in Pharmacokinetic Properties
Parameter	**Observation**
Absorption	Generally, absorption is lower in women.
Volume of distribution	Volume of distribution of lipophilic drugs is higher and volume of distribution of hydrophilic drugs is lower in women.
Protein binding	No clinically significant difference.
Elimination half-life	Longer in women than in men.
Renal elimination	Renal clearance via tubular secretion but not by glomerular filtration may be lower in women.

(From Xie CX, Piecoro LT, Wermeling DP. Gender-related considerations in clinical pharmacology and drug therapeutics. Crit Care Nurs Clin North Am 9: 459–468, 1997, with permission.)

TABLE 6.8	Sex Differences in Response to Cardiovascular Agents	
Drug Class or Agents	**Clinical Response**	**References**
Bisoprolol	In congestive heart failure, there is a decrease in all causes of death in women.	97
Verapamil	Mean plasma concentration higher in women.	94
	Intravenous administration has increased clearance in women.	98, 99
	Causes greater heart rate increase in women.	98, 99
Angiotensin-converting enzyme (ACE) inhibitors	Cough is 2 to 3 times greater in women.	100
Quinidine	Torsade de Pointes more common in women.	101
Procainamide	Drug-induced antinuclear antibody and systemic lupus erythematosus more common in women.	102
Heparin	Women develop higher levels and higher activated partial thromboplastin time.	103
Thiazides	More likely to cause hyponatremia and hypokalemia in women.	104
Guanethidine	Orthostatic hypotension more common in women.	105
Hydralazine	Systemic Lupus Erythematosus more common in women.	106

istered drugs. However, it must be pointed out that the clinical significance of these influencing factors has not been established.

VARIATIONS IN EFFECTS OF CARDIOVASCULAR DRUGS

Treatment of mild to moderate hypertension in young and middle-aged women produces more adverse effects from antihypertensive agents than in men.[93] In a study using a controlled-release form of verapamil, the mean plasma concentration was higher in women than in men.[94] Men and women may respond differently to anticoagulant therapy. A study showed that the use of anticoagulant agents in women

resulted in no significant improvement in reinfarction mortality.[95] This same study reported that women given thrombolytic agents had a relatively lower reduction in mortality than did men. However, another study suggested that women had higher mortality than men due to decreased effectiveness of thrombolytic agents.[96] Additional sex differences in response to cardiovascular drugs are shown in Table 6.8.

VARIATION IN EFFECTS OF CENTRAL NERVOUS SYSTEM DRUGS

Psychotropic Agents. Sex differences in drug therapy probably have been studied the most with the psychotropic agents (Table 6.9). This could result in part from the observa-

TABLE 6.9	Sex Differences in Response to Psychotropic Agents	
Drug Class or Agents	**Clinical Response**	**References**
Chlorpromazine	Women show greater improvement in response.	110,111
Monoamine oxidase inhibitors	Depressed women with panic attacks respond better.	117
Tricyclic antidepressants	Depressed men with panic attacks respond better.	117
Imipramine	Men respond better than women.	115,116
	Depressed women are less responsive than unipolar and bipolar men.	117
Oxazepam, Temazepam	Women eliminate more slowly than men.	119,120
Alprazolam, Diazepam	Renal clearance is higher in women.	121,122
Triazolam, Lorazepam	Renal clearance is same in men and women.	123,126

tion that women have higher admission rates than men for mental disorders, and a greater severity of symptoms.[107,108]

Antipsychotic Agents. There are conflicting reports of sex differences in response to antipsychotic agents. Pinals et al[109] concluded that there were no significant sex differences in response to antipsychotic drugs; however, another study demonstrated that women had greater improvement than men in response to agents like pimozide and chlorpromazine.[110,111] In one study, male schizophrenic patients required less medication than female patients.[112] Another study showed that male schizophrenic patients generally require less medication, at lower dosages, and have a more favorable outcome of psychotropic therapy than female patients.[113] However, findings from Yonkers et al[111] indicate that women seem to experience greater efficacy with antipsychotic agents and a greater likelihood of adverse reactions. Xie et al[91] suggest that women may require a lower dose of antipsychotic agents than men.

Antidepressant Agents. Despite the prevalence of depression in women, data on sex and response to antidepressants are sparse. Also, conflicting data on sex differences in TCA are conflicting.[114]

Studies of imipramine seem to indicate a preferential response in men.[115,116] Risch et al[117] reported that depressed women are less responsive to imipramine than are bipolar women, unipolar men, or bipolar men.

Davidson and Pelton reported that depressed women who suffered from panic attacks responded better to monoamine oxidase inhibitors than men. However, the report also indicated that depressed men with panic attacks responded better to TCA than women.[118]

Antianxiety Agents. Most of the literature on sex differences related to benzodiazepines focuses primarily on pharmacokinetics. In a review by Yonkers et al,[111] it seems as though benzodiazepines that undergo conjugation are eliminated more slowly in women. The clearance of oxazepam, temazepam, and chlordiazepoxide has been reported to be lower in women than men.[119,120] The clearance of alprazolam, diazepam, and demethyldiazepam, which undergo oxidative metabolism, has been shown to be higher in women than men.[121,122] The clearance of nitrazepam, bromazepam, triazolam, and lorazepam, which undergo reduction, has not been found to be influenced by sex.[123–126]

Miscellaneous Agents.
Analgesics. To determine if sex differences are associated with κ-opioid agonism, the analgesic efficacy of two other predominantly κ-opioid analgesics, nalbuphine and butorphanol, was compared in men and women who underwent surgery for removal of third molar teeth. Both nalbuphine and butorphanol produced significantly greater analgesia in women than in men. This observation may result from a difference in κ-opioid-activated endogenous pain modulating circuits.[127]

A lysine salt of aspirin was absorbed more quickly in women than in men (mean absorption times of 16.4 and 21.3 minutes, respectively, although the bioavailability, 54%, was the same in both groups). In contrast, after intramuscular administration, aspirin was absorbed more slowly in women than in men (mean absorption time of 97 and 53 minutes, respectively) but again the bioavailability, 89%, was the same in both groups.[128]

After acute cocaine administration, women reported greater ''nervousness'' but not ''high'' and did not differ from men on cardiovascular indices. On a ''nervousness'' scale, the peak effects were twice as great in the women and, during the 45 minutes after cocaine use, these levels decreased only 18% compared to a 60% decrease in men.[129]

CONCLUSION

The premise that a drug will act identically in people of different races, ethnic groups, sexes, or cultures has been challenged and found to be flawed. Therefore, racial, ethnic, and sex representation in clinical trials must be broadened. For a growing number of drugs, the percentage of patients who react differently or adversely is determined by their racial and ethnic background and sex. The study of racial, ethnic, and sex differences in response to medicines has been limited primarily to a few classes of drugs; however, future studies will likely reveal significant data about these differences in the action of many additional drugs.

Formulary development and management represent a strategic attempt to control drug therapy costs. However, the formulary must not be so restrictive that it ignores the fact that patients in specific groups metabolize drugs differently, have different clinical responses, and experience different side effects. Therefore, racial, ethnic, and sex differences require us to balance control of drug cost with the need for individualized therapy.

More rigorous and carefully designed studies are needed to confirm observed differences across racial, ethnic, and sex groups. Furthermore, systematic investigation of the effects of ethnicity on biologic correlates may aid in the understanding of patient treatments and further application to the clinical setting.

KEY POINTS

- Therapeutic response, metabolism, and side effects may differ with various medicines because of racial, ethnic, and sex differences.
- The pathways of drug metabolism are classified as phase I and phase II reactions.
- Genetically controlled differences in the way individuals metabolize drugs are major determinants of racial and ethnic differences in response to medicines.

- Drug categories that have been shown to be most clinically significant in their actions with regard to racial and ethnic differences are cardiovascular and central nervous system agents.
- When used as monotherapy to treat black hypertensive patients, diuretics and calcium channel blockers tend to produce a greater reduction in blood pressure than β-blockers and ACE inhibitors.
- Asians in general need lower doses of psychotropic drugs and exhibit adverse effects at lower dosages than do white patients.
- Hispanics tend to require less antidepressant medication and report more adverse effects at lower doses than do white patients.
- Blacks, in general, respond better than white patients to antidepressants, have higher plasma levels, and show a greater degree of adverse effects.
- North American Indians, Chinese, and Japanese patients show a faster rate of alcohol metabolism (i.e., conversion to the aldehyde) and less tolerance than do whites.
- The clinical significance of sex-related differences in the pharmacokinetic properties of some drugs has not been clearly established.
- In studies where sex differences in metabolism and pharmacokinetics exist, women generally tend to have lower absorption, greater volume of distribution of lipophilic drugs, no differences in protein binding, longer half-lives, and possibly lower renal clearance than men.
- Physiologic differences between men and women in hormone and enzyme levels and basal metabolism influence the metabolism of various drugs.
- Sex differences in drug therapy have been studied the most with the psychotropic agents.
- In general, women tend to have a greater likelihood of adverse effects from cardiovascular agents than men.
- In general, women show greater improvement in response to psychotropic agents and a greater likelihood of adverse reactions than men. However, women seem less responsive to imipramine than men.

SUGGESTED READINGS

Ma MK, Wood MH, McLeod HL. Genetic basis of drug metabolism. Am J Health-Syst Pharm 59:2061–2069, 2002.
Schaefer BM, Caracciolo V, Frishman WH, et al. Gender, ethnicity, and genes in cardiovascular disease. Part 2: implications for pharmacotherapy. Heart Dis 5:202–204, 2003.
Wood AJ, Zhou HH. Ethnic differences in drug disposition and responsiveness. Clin Pharmacokinet 20:350–373, 1991.

REFERENCES

1. Lin KM, Poland RE, Lesser IM. Ethnicity and psychopharmacology. Cult Med Psychiatry 10:151–165, 1986.
2. Branch RA, Salih SY, Homeida M. Racial differences in drug metabolizing ability: a study with antipyrine in the Sudan. Clin Pharmacol Ther 24:283–286, 1978.
3. Fraser HS, Mucklow JC, Bulpitt CJ, et al. Environmental effects on antipyrine half-life in man. Clin Pharmacol Ther 22:799–808, 1977.
4. Robinson R. Individualization of drug therapy: considering ethnic differences. The Consult Pharm 5:328–334, 1990.
5. Kinzie JD, Leung P, Boehnlein JK, et al. Antidepressant blood levels in Southeast Asians. Clinical and cultural implications. J Nerv Ment Dis 175:480–485, 1987.
6. Gillis LS, Trollip D, Lakoet A, et al. Noncompliance with psychotropic medication. S Afr Med 172:602–606, 1987.
7. Lin KM, Shen WW. Pharmacotherapy for Southeast Asian psychiatric patients. J Nerv Ment Dis 179:346–350, 1991.
8. Meyer UA. Drugs in special patient groups: clinical importance of genetics in drug effects. In: Melman KL, Morrelli HP, Hoffman BB, et al., eds. Melman and Morrelli clinical pharmacology: basic principles in therapeutics. 3rd ed. New York: McGraw-Hill, 1992: 875–894.
9. Wilkinson GR. Pharmacokinetics: the dynamics of drug absorption, distribution, and elimination. In: Hardeman JG, Limbird LE, Goodman AG, eds. Goodman and Gilman's the pharmacological basis of therapeutics.10th ed. New York: McGraw-Hill, 2001:34–43.
10. Ma MK, Wood MH, McLeod HL. Genetic basis of drug metabolism. Am J Health-Syst Pharm 59:2061–2069, 2002.
11. Bertilsson L, Dahl ML, Dalén P, et al. Molecular genetics of CYP2D6: Clinical relevance with focus on psychotropic drugs. Br J Clin Pharmacol 53:111–122, 2002.
12. Drug interactions. Med Lett Drug Ther 45:46–47, 2003.
13. Mahgoub A, Idle JR, Dring LG, et al. Polymorphic hydroxylation of debrisoquine in man. Lancet 2:584–586, 1977.
14. Weinshilboum R. Inheritance and drug response. N Engl J Med 348:529–549, 2003.
15. Kalow W, Otton SV, Kadar D, et al. Ethnic difference in drug metabolism: debrisoquine 4-hydroxylation in Caucasians and Orientals. Can J Physiol Pharmacol 58:1142–1144, 1980.
16. Nakamura K, Goto F, Ray WA, et al. Interethnic differences in genetic polymorphism of debrisoquine and mephenytoin hydroxylation between Japanese and Caucasian populations. Clin Pharmacol Ther 38:402–408, 1985.
17. Pollock BG, Perel JM, Kirshner M, et al. S-mephenytoin 4-hydroxylation in older Americans. Eur J Clin Pharmacol 40:609–611, 1991.
18. Sullivan-Klose TH, Ghanayem BI, Bell DA, et al. The role of the CYP2C9-Leu359 allele variant in the tolbutamide polymorphism. Pharmacogenetics 6:341–349, 1996.
19. Schuetz JD, Beach DL, Guselian PD, et al. Selective expression of cytochrome P450 CYP3A mRNAs in embryonic and adult human liver. Pharmacogenetics 4:11–20, 1994.
20. Kolars JC, Lown KS, Schmiedlin-Ren P, et al. CYP3A gene expression in human gut epithelium. Pharmacogenetics 4:247–259, 1994.
21. Mitchell RS, Bell JC. Clinical implications of isoniazid blood levels in pulmonary tuberculosis. N Engl J Med 257:1066–1071, 1957.
22. Weber WW, Hein DW. N-acetylation pharmacogenetics. Pharmacol Rev 37:25–79, 1985.
23. Wood AJ, Zhou HH. Ethnic differences in drug disposition and responsiveness. Clin Pharmacokinet 20:350–373, 1991.
24. Weinberger MH. Racial differences in antihypertensive therapy: evidence and implications. Cardiovasc Drugs Ther 4:379–382, 1990.
25. Hall WD. Pathophysiology of hypertension in blacks. Am J Hypertens 3:366S–371S, 1991.
26. Veterans Administration Cooperative Study Group on Antihypertensive Agents. Comparison of propranolol and hydrochlorothiazide for the initial treatment of hypertension: I. Results of short-term titration with emphasis on racial differences in response. JAMA 248:1996–2003, 1982.
27. Veterans Administration Cooperative Study Group on Antihypertensive Agents. Racial differences in response to low-dose captopril are abolished by the addition of hydrochlorothiazide. Br J Clin Pharmacol 14:97S–101S, 1982.
28. Gillum RF. Pathophysiology of hypertension in blacks and whites. Hypertension 1:468–475, 1979.
29. Wisenbaugh PE, Garst JB, Hull C, et al. Renin, aldosterone, sodium and hypertension. Am J Med 52:175–186, 1972.

30. Levy SB, Lilley JJ, Frigon RP, et al. Urinary kallikrein and plasma renin activity as determinants of renal blood flow. The influence of race and dietary sodium intake. J Clin Invest 60:129–138, 1977.

31. Luft PC, Grim CE, Higgins JT Jr, et al. Differences in response to sodium administration in normotensive white and black subjects. J Lab Clin Med 90:555–562, 1977.

32. Johnson JA. Racial differences in lymphocyte beta-receptor sensitivity to propranolol. Life Sci 53:297–304, 1993.

33. Johnson JA, Burlew BS. Racial differences in propranolol pharmacokinetics. Clin Pharmacol Ther 51:495–500, 1992.

34. Oster G, Huse DM, Delea TE, et al. Cost effectiveness of labetalol and propranolol in the treatment of hypertension among blacks. J Natl Med Assoc 79:1049–1055, 1987.

35. Neutel JM, Smith DH, Ram CV, et al. Comparison of bisoprolol with atenolol for systemic hypertension in four population groups (young, old, black and nonblack) using ambulatory blood pressure monitoring. Am J Cardiol 72:41–46, 1993.

36. Kitler ME. Clinical trials and trans ethnic pharmacology. Drug Saf 11:378–391, 1994.

37. Zhou H, Koshakji RP, Silberstein DJ, et al. Altered sensitivity to and clearance of propranolol in men of Chinese descent as compared with American whites. N Engl J Med 320:565–570, 1989.

38. 1988 report of the Joint National Committee on Detection, Evaluation, and Treatment of High Blood Pressure. Arch Intern Med 148:1023–1038, 1988.

39. Kalus JS, Nappi JM. Role of race in the pharmacotherapy of heart failure. Ann Pharmacother 36:471–478, 2002.

40. Buhler FR. Antihypertensive treatment according to age, plasma renin and race. Drugs 35:495–503, 1988.

41. Hui KK, Pasic J. Outcome of hypertension management in Asian Americans. Arch Intern Med 157:1345–1348, 1997.

42. Yu K, Cho J, Shon J, et al. Ethnic differences and relationships in the oral pharmacokinetics of nifedipine and erythromycin. Clin Pharmacol Ther 70:228–236, 2001.

43. Houghton JL, Philbin EF, Strogatz DS, et al. The presence of African American race predicts improvement in coronary endothelial function after supplementary L-arginine. J Am Coll Cardiol 39:1314–1322, 2002.

44. Bond WS. Ethnicity and psychotropic drugs. Clin Pharm 10:467–470, 1991.

45. Jann MW, Grimsley SR. Pharmacogenetics of agents on the central nervous system. J Pharm Pract 6:2–16, 1993.

46. Midha KK, Chakraborty BS, Ganes DA, et al. Intersubject variation in the pharmacokinetics of haloperidol and reduced haloperidol. J Clin Psychopharmacol 9:98–104, 1989.

47. Jann MW, Chang WH, Lam YW, et al. Comparison of haloperidol and reduced haloperidol plasma levels in four different ethnic populations. Prog Neuro- Psychopharmacol Biol Psychiatry 16:193–202, 1992.

48. Lam YW, Jann MW, Chang WH, et al. Intra- and interethnic variability in reduced haloperidol to haloperidol ratios. J Clin Pharmacol 35:128–136, 1995.

49. Lin KM, Finder E. Neuroleptic dosage for Asians. Am J Psychiatry 140:490–491, 1983.

50. Potkin SG, Shen Y, Pardes H, et al. Haloperidol concentrations elevated in Chinese patients. Psychiatry Res 12:167–172, 1984.

51. Lin KM, Lau JK, Smith R, et al. Comparison of alprazolam plasma levels in normal Asian and Caucasian male volunteers. Psychopharmacology 96:365–369, 1988.

52. Matuda KT, Cho MC, Lin K-M, et al. Clozapine dosage, serum levels, efficacy, and side-effects profiles: a comparison of Korean-American and Caucasian patients. Psychopharmacol Bull 32:253–257, 1996.

53. Chang WH, Lin SK, Lane H Y, et al. Clozapine dosages and plasma drug concentrations. J Formos Med Assoc 96:599–605, 1997.

54. Poolsup N, Po AL, Knight TL. Pharmacogenetics and pyschopharmacotherapy. J Clin Pharm Ther 25:197–220, 2000.

55. Strickland TL, Ranganath V, Lin KM, et al. Psychopharmacologic considerations in the treatment of black American populations. Psychopharmacol Bull 27:441–448, 1991.

56. Bell CC, Mehta H. Misdiagnosis of black patients with manic depressive illness: second in a series. J Natl Med Assoc 73:101–107, 1981.

57. Raskin A, Cook TH. Antidepressants in black and white inpatients. Arch Gen Psychiatry 32:643–649, 1975.

58. Lieberman JA, Yunis J, Egea E, et al. HLA-B38, DR4, DQw3 and clozapine-induced agranulocytosis in Jewish patients with schizophrenia. Arch Gen Psychiatr 47:945–948, 1990.

59. Ziegler VE, Biggs JT. Tricyclic plasma levels: effects of age, race, sex, and smoking. JAMA 238:2167–2169, 1977.

60. Rifkin A, Klein DF, Quitkin F. Possible effect of race on tricyclic plasma levels [Letter]. JAMA 239:1845–1846, 1978.

61. Mendoza R, Smith MW, Poland RE, et al. Ethnic psychopharmacology: the Hispanic and Native American perspective. Psychopharmacol Bull 27:449–461, 1991.

62. Gaviria M, Gil AA, Javaid I. Nortriptyline kinetics in Hispanic and Anglo subjects. J Clin Psychopharmacol 6:227–231, 1986.

63. Yamashita I, Asano Y. Tricyclic antidepressants: therapeutic plasma level. Psychopharmacol Bull 15:40–41, 1979.

64. Rudorfer MY, Lane EA, Chang WH, et al. Desipramine pharmacokinetics in Chinese and Caucasian volunteers. Br J Clin Pharmacol 17:433–440, 1984.

65. Shimoda K, Jerling M, Böttiger Y, et al. Pronounced differences in the disposition of clomipramine between Japanese and Swedish patients. J Clin Psychopharm 19:393–400, 1999.

66. Kumana CR, Lauder IJ, Chan M, et al. Differences in diazepam pharmacokinetics in Chinese and white Caucasians -relation to body lipid stores. Eur J Clin Pharmacol 32:211–215, 1987.

67. Lin KM, Poland RE, Smith MW, et al. Pharmacokinetic and other related factors affecting psychotropic responses in Asians. Psychopharmacol Bull 27:427–439, 1991.

68. Chang SS, Pandey GN, Zhang MY, et al. Racial differences in plasma and RBC lithium levels. Paper presented at: American Psychiatric Association; Los Angeles, CA. Continuing Medical Education Syllabus and Scientific Proceedings; 1984:239–240.

69. Takahashi R. Lithium treatment in affective disorders: therapeutic plasma level. Psychopharmacol Bull 15:32–35, 1979.

70. Honda Y, Suzuki T. Transcultural pharmacokinetic study on Li concentration in plasma and saliva. Psychopharmacol Bull 15:37–39, 1979.

71. Yue QY, Svensson JO, Alm C, et al. Interindividual and interethnic differences in the demethylation and glucuronidation of codeine. Br J Clin Pharmacol 28:629–637, 1989.

72. Mucklow JC, Fraser HS, Bulpitt CJ, et al. Environmental factors affecting paracetamol metabolism in London factory and office workers. Br J Clin Pharmacol 10:67–74, 1980.

73. Zhou HH, Sheller JR, Nu H, et al. Ethnic differences in response to morphine. Clin Pharmacol Ther 54:507–513, 1993.

74. Cepeda MS, Farrar JT, Roa JH, et al. Ethnicity influences morphine pharmacokinetics and pharmacodynamics. Clin Pharma Ther 351–361, 2001.

75. Banys P, Clark HW, Tusel DJ, et al. An open trial of low dose buprenorphine in treating methadone withdrawal. J Subst Abuse Treat 11:9–15, 1994.

76. Kalow W. Ethnic differences in drug metabolism. Clin Pharmacokinet 7:373–49, 1982.

77. Chan AW. Racial differences in alcohol sensitivity. Alcohol 21:93–104, 1986.

78. Monteiro MG, Klein JL, Schuckit MA. High levels of sensitivity to alcohol in young adult Jewish men: a pilot study. J Stud Alcohol 52:464–469, 1991.

79. Paskind HA. Some differences in response to atropine in white and colored races. J Lab Clin Med 7:104–108, 1921.

80. Meyer EC, Sommers DK, Schoeman HS. The effect of atropine on heart rate: a comparison between two ethnic groups. Br J Clin Pharmacol 25:776–777, 1988.

81. Zhou HH, Wood AJ. Atropine produces a greater increase in heart rate in Chinese than Caucasians [abstract]. Clin Res 38:7A, 1990.

82. Gower BA, Grander WM, Frankin F, et al. Contribution of insulin secretion and clearance to glucose-induced insulin concentration in African-American and Caucasian children. J Clin Endocrinol Metab 87:2218–2224, 2002.

83. Muir AJ, Bornstein JD, Killenbert PG. Peginterferon Alfa-2b and ribavirin for the treatment of chronic hepatitis C in Blacks and Non-Hispanic Whites. N Engl J Med 350:2265–2271, 2004.

84. Mills RM, Naftel DC, Kirlin JK, et al. Heart transplant rejection with hemodynamic compromise: a multi-institutional study of the

role of endomyocardial cellular infiltrate. Cardiac Transplant Research Database. J Heart Lung Transplant 16:813–821, 1997.

85. Costanzo MR, Naftel DC, Pritzker MR, et al. Heart transplant coronary artery diseases detected by coronary angiography: a multi-institutional study of preoperative donor and recipient risk factors. Cardiac Transplant Research Database. J Heart Lung Transplant 17: 744–753, 1998.

86. Mehra MR, Uber PA, Scott RL, et al. Ethnic disparity in clinical outcome after heart transplantation in abrogated using tacrolimus and mycophenolate mofetil-based immunosuppression. Transplantation 74:1568–1573, 2002.

87. Mancinelli LM, Frassetto LY, Floren LC, et al. The pharmacokinetics and metabolic disposition of tacrolimus: a comparison across ethnic groups. Clin Pharm Ther 69:24–31, 2001.

88. Ortolani O, Cont A, Sall/Ka B, et al. The recovery of Senegalese African Blacks from intravenous anesthesia with propofol and remifentanil is slower than that of Caucasians. Anesth Analog 93: 1222–1226, 2001.

89. Giudicelli JF, Tillement JP. Influences of sex on drug kinetics in man. Clin Pharmacokinet 2:157–166, 1977.

90. Bonate PL. Gender-related differences in xenobiotic metabolism. J Clin Pharmacol 31:684–690, 1991.

91. Xie CX, Piecoro LT, Wermeling DP. Gender-related considerations in clinical pharmacology and drug therapeutics. Crit Care Nurs Clin North Am 9:459–468, 1997.

92. Proksch RA, Lamy PP. Sex variation and drug therapy. Drug Intell Clinical Pharm 11:398–406, 1977.

93. Shapiro AP, Rytan GH. Hypertension in women: differences and implications. In: Eaka E, Packard B, Wenger N, et al, eds. Coronary heart disease in women: reviewing the evidence, identifying the needs. New York: Haymarket Doyma, 1987:172–176.

94. Gupta S, Atkinson L, Tu T, et al. Age and gender-related changes in stereoselective pharmacokinetics and pharmacodynamics of verapamil and norverapamil. Br J Clin Pharmacol 40:325–331, 1995.

95. Rice-Wray E. An assessment of long-term anticoagulant administration after cardiac infarction. Second report of the working party on anticoagulant therapy in coronary thrombosis to the medical research council. Br Med J 2:837–843, 1964.

96. Woodfield SL, Lundergan CL, Reiner JS, et al. Gender and acute myocardial infarction: is there a different response to thrombolysis. J Am Coll Cardiol 29:35–41, 1997.

97. Simon T, Mary-Krause M, Fenck-Brentanoc C, et al. Sexual differences in the prognosis of congestive heart failure: result from the Cardiac Insufficiency Bisoprolol Study (CIBIS II). Circulation 103: 378–380, 2001.

98. Krecic-Shepard ME, Barnas CR, Slimko J, et al. Faster clearance of sustained release verapamil in men versus women: continuing observations on sex-specific differences after oral administration of verapamil. Clin Pharmacol Ther 68:286–292, 2000.

99. Krecic-Shepard ME, Barnas CR, Slimko J, et al. Gender specific effects on verapamil pharmacokinetics and pharmacodynamics in humans. J Clin Pharmacol 40:219–230, 2000.

100. Os I, Bratland B, Dahlof B, et al. Female sex as an important determinant of lisinopril-induced cough. Lancet 339:372, 1992.

101. Schaefer BM, Caracciolo V, Frishman WH, et al. Gender, ethnicity, and genes in cardiovascular disease. Part 2: implications for pharmacotherapy. Heart Dis 5:202–204, 2003.

102. Wilson JD. Antinuclear antibodies and cardiovascular drugs. Drugs 19: 292–305, 1980.

103. Campbell NR, Hull RD, Bant R, et al. Different effects of heparin in males and females. Clin Invest Med 21:71–78, 1998.

104. August P, Oparil S. Hypertension in women. J Clin Endocronol Metab 84:1862–1866, 1999.

105. Talbot S, Smith AJ. Factors predisposing to postural hypotensive symptoms in the treatment of high blood pressure. Br Heart J 37: 1059–1063, 1975.

106. Batchelor JR, Welsh KI, Tioco RM, et al. Hydralazine-induced systemic lupus erythematosus: influence of HLA-DR and sex on susceptibility. Lancet 1:1107–1009, 1980.

107. Kramer M. Cross-national study of diagnosis of the mental disorders: origins of the problem. Am J Psychiat 125(Suppl 10):1–11, 1969.

108. Weich MJ. Behavioral differences between groups of acutely psychotic (schizophrenic) males and females. Psychiatr Q 42:107–122, 1968.

109. Pinals DA, Malhotra AK, Missar CD, et al. Lack of gender differences in neuroleptic response in patients with schizophrenia. Schizophr Res 22:215–222, 1996.

110. Chouinard G, Annable L. Pimozide in the treatment of newly admitted schizophrenic patients. Psychopharmacology 76:13–19, 1982.

111. Yonkers KA, Kando JC, Cole JO, et al. Gender differences in pharmacokinetics and pharmacodynamics of psychotropic medication. Am J Psychiatry 149:587–595, 1992.

112. Taylor MA, Levine R. Influence of sex of hospitalized schizophrenics on therapeutic dosage levels of neuroleptics. Dis Nerv Syst 32: 131–134, 1971.

113. Demer HC, Bird EG. Chlorpromazine in the treatment of mental illness. IV Final results with analysis of data on 1,523 patients. Am J Psychiatry 113:972–978, 1957.

114. Dawkins K. Gender differences in psychiatry: Epidemiology and drug response. CNS Drugs 3:393–407, 1995.

115. Perel JM, Irani F, Hurwic M, et al. Tricyclic antidepressants: Relationships among pharmacokinetics, metabolism, and clinical outcomes. In: Garattini S, ed. Depressive disorders. Stuttgart: FK Schattauer, 1978:325–336.

116. Prange A. Discussion. (Published discussion following a paper by Feighner, et al.) Am J Psychiatry 128:1230–1238, 1972.

117. Risch SC, Huey LY, Janowsky DS. Plasma levels of tricyclic antidepressants and clinical efficacy: review of the literature. Part II J Clin Psychiatry 40:58–69, 1979.

118. Davidson J, Pelton S. Forms of atypical depression and their response to antidepressant drugs. Psychiatry Res 17:87–95, 1986.

119. Divoll M, Greenblatt DJ, Harmatz JS, et al. Effect of age and gender on disposition of temazepam. J Pharm Sci 10:1104–1107, 1981.

120. Greenblatt DJ, Divoll MK, Abernethy DR, et al. Age and gender effects on chlordiazepoxide kinetics: relation to antipyrine disposition. Pharmacology 38: 327–334, 1989.

121. Allen MD, Greenblatt DJ, Harmatz JS, et al. Desmethyldiazepam kinetics in the elderly after oral prazepam. Clin Pharmacol Ther 28:196–202, 1980.

122. Kristjansson F, Thorsteinsson SB. Disposition of alprazolam in human volunteers: differences between genders. Acta Pharm Nord 3:249–250, 1991.

123. Divoll M, Greenblatt DJ. Effect of age and sex on lorazepam protein binding. J Pharm Pharmacol 34:122–123, 1982.

124. Jochemsen R, van der Graaff M, Boeijinga JK, et al. Influence of sex, menstrual cycle and oral contraceptives on the disposition of nitrazepam. Br J Clin Pharmacol 13:319–324, 1982.

125. Ochs HR, Greenblatt DJ, Friedman H, et al. Bromazepam pharmacokinetics: influence of age, gender, oral contraceptives, cimetidine and propranolol. Clin Pharmacol Ther 41:562–570, 1987.

126. Smith RB, Divoll M, Gillespie WR, et al. Effect of subject age and gender on the pharmacokinetics of oral triazolam and temazepam. J Clin Psychopharmacol 3:172–176, 1983.

127. Gear RW, Miaskowski C, Gordon NC, et al. Kappa-opioids produce significantly greater analgesia in women than in men. Nat Med 2:1248–1250, 1996.

128. Aarons L, Hopkins K, Rowland M, et al. Route of administration and sex differences in the pharmacokinetics of aspirin, administered as its lysine salt. Pharm Res 6:660–666, 1989.

129. Kosten TR, Kosten T A, McDougle C, et al. Gender differences in response to intranasal cocaine administration to humans. Biol Psychiatry 39:147–148, 1996.

Biotechnology

Kimberly Bergstrom and Monique Mayo

Since October 1982, when the first recombinant human insulin was approved by the U.S. Food and Drug Administration (FDA), over 65 medicines and vaccines have been developed and approved by companies involved in biotechnology. The race to complete the mapping of our genetic makeup has yielded exciting breakthroughs in our understanding of important disease processes, which we are beginning to address at the genetic and chromosomal levels. This chapter focuses on biotechnology and the use of biologic processes to manufacture products. These include the use of recombinant DNA (rDNA) technology and hybridoma technology (for monoclonal antibody production).

To understand what makes biotechnology possible, it is important to first understand the microenvironment in which biotechnological processes are applied. This requires an understanding of the structure and function of human cells and the DNA within them that provides the genetic instructions for cell replication and protein synthesis.

CHROMOSOMES AND GENES

Within the nucleus of all eukaryotic cells are chromosomes that contain regions of DNA called genes. Each gene encodes a single protein. Human cells contain 24 pairs of chromosomes containing a total of 20,000 to 25,000 genes, a much smaller number of genes than originally thought. Each cell in the human body has an identical set of chromosomes and genes. What makes these cells act differently in different cell types in the body is their selective repression of different genetic functions. While most cells produce 8,000 to 9,000 unique proteins, they each have the potential to produce over 100,000 proteins if all the genes were functional.

DNA plays two important roles in the life of an organism. One function is cell replication and the other is protein synthesis. To make a protein the cell must first read the message coded in the gene responsible for that protein. To synthesize a protein, the double-stranded DNA unwinds with the help of many proteins and separates at the site of the gene responsible for producing the desired protein. Once the double helix has separated, messenger RNA (mRNA) is synthesized by other proteins (e.g., RNA polymerase) along that portion of the single-stranded DNA gene in a process known as transcription. Once mRNA has been formed along the DNA blueprint, it travels out of the nucleus of the cell to the ribosomes where protein synthesis occurs. Transfer RNA (tRNA) collects amino acids from the cytoplasm and brings them to the ribosomes where the amino acids are linked together in a sequence that is dictated by the mRNA to form the intended protein. Once this chain of polypeptides (protein) is formed, weak chemical interactions between specific amino acids in the chain cause it to fold up into a unique three-dimensional pattern. The shape that the protein assumes after folding is quite unique to that protein and can significantly affect its function. If inappropriate amino acids are present, the peptide chain may not fold up to form the properly shaped cavity, and the enzyme may not be able to function.

RECOMBINANT DNA TECHNOLOGY

Recombinant DNA technology utilizes the natural genetic processes that occur in mammalian, bacterial, and yeast cells to produce human proteins. With this technology, the cells can be manipulated to produce human proteins, such as erythropoietin (EPO), in large enough quantities to be useful for the treatment of human disease. Recombinant DNA technology entails isolating the specific gene that contains the genetic code for a desired protein and inserting it into a cell that can reproduce that protein rapidly. The result is the production of large quantities of the desired protein.

Yeast cells, *Escherichia coli* bacteria, and mammalian cells (Chinese hamster ovary [CHO] cells, human myeloma cells) are used most commonly to reproduce human proteins. These cell types are used because they can be genetically manipulated easily and quickly, they multiply and divide rapidly, and they provide large quantities of protein.[1]

E. coli cells are genetically simple and well-understood cell types, which makes them ideal host cells for rDNA molecules. However, they cannot perform some of the more complicated processes of fine-tuning proteins, such as glycosylation, that the more advanced mammalian cells can perform. If glycosylation is not necessary, as with interferons, *E. coli* is a less expensive and simpler choice for a host cell.[2]

To produce a specific protein, the gene responsible for the production of that protein must be isolated. A gene can be isolated easily if the nucleic acid sequence of the desired gene is known. If not, a DNA probe may be used to isolate the specific gene. A DNA probe is usually a homologous gene to the gene that you want to produce, but it is from a different species. Once the DNA is identified it can be isolated directly from a cell or by creating a ''copy'' DNA segment. In the latter case, a DNA synthesizer and polymerase chain reaction (PCR) can be used to make a copy of the gene if the complete gene is known. The desired gene is then cut precisely from the DNA molecule by restriction enzymes.

The isolated gene is then inserted into the host cell with a plasmid or viral vector to produce the desired protein (Fig. 7.1). A vector is a DNA molecule that is capable of replicating independently of the host chromosome in at least one organism, and additional DNA can be inserted into it. There are two major types of vectors used in rDNA technology: the plasmid vector and the viral vector. A plasmid vector is a circular strand of DNA that can replicate freely inside a host cell. Plasmids are found in bacteria (e.g., *E. coli*) or yeast, where they are isolated and cut open.[1] The human gene is then spliced to the plasmid by DNA ligase to form the rDNA molecule. The DNA molecule is moved into the host cell by a process called ''transformation'' (the uptake of foreign DNA into a cell) or electroporation.[1] The final step in rDNA production involves fermentation and harvesting of the desired protein. Ideal conditions must exist for the host cell to replicate. As host cell division and replication take

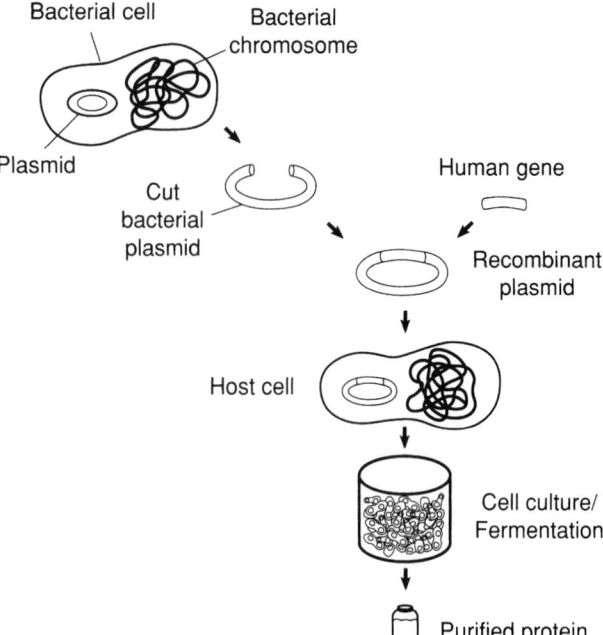

FIGURE 7.1 Summary of the steps typically involved in the formation of a recombinant DNA molecule. (From An introduction to pharmaceutical biotechnology. Regents of the University of Wisconsin System, 1990, with permission.)

place, the vector-containing human gene is also replicated. The host cell replicates into millions of genetically identical cells capable of producing the desired protein. On an industrial scale, this often takes place in a vessel holding thousands of gallons of culture medium. The protein is then harvested from the culture medium, purified, and formulated into the final product.

HOST SYSTEMS FOR PROTEIN PRODUCTION

Traditionally, there have been three host systems commonly used to produce industrial scale proteins. These include (a) yeasts and filamentous fungi (e.g., *Saccharomyces cerevisiae*, *Pichia pastoris*, and *Aspergillus niger*), (b) bacteria (*E. coli*), and (c) mammalian cells (CHO cells). The benefits of bacteria, yeast, and fungi are that they are easy to grow and can secrete large amounts of recombinant protein at relatively modest expense. However, the choice of which system to use is often dictated by where the product will be used and the requirements of glycosylation. Bacteria and some yeasts cannot glycosylate proteins that are needed for their functioning, so often mammalian cells, in particular CHO cells, are used when complex human glycoproteins need to be developed. Currently about 60% of therapeutic proteins are glycoproteins and that number is growing rapidly.[3,4] Many proteins, especially humanized proteins, require glycosylation as a final step in protein synthesis. While yeasts are able to glycosylate proteins, the nonhuman nature of yeast glycans can negatively impact on the half-life of the proteins, producing less desirable proteins for human use. Therefore, it has been primarily mammalian cells, in particular CHO cells, that have been most widely used to produce complex human glycoproteins. And while glycoproteins produced by mammalian cell culture most closely mimic human proteins, they are still an inherently heterogeneous mixture of glycoforms that have inherently different activity levels. This makes production a challenge.

A purified protein preparation derived from a mammalian cell culture process is essentially a mixture of individual drugs, each with its own pharmacokinetic, pharmacodynamic properties, and efficacy profile. An example of the importance of controlled glycosylation is with the drug EPO, a drug used in the treatment of anemia. The production of recombinant EPO is highly sensitive to the glycosylation process and can yield a fivefold difference in function from batch to batch when the environment is not well controlled.

Scientists are now focusing on using the positive attributes of yeast and fungal systems that include producing high-protein titers in fermentation processes that last a few days and are scalable to the 100 m^3 scale, which allows for rapid turnaround from gene to protein. Some are investigating the possibility of humanizing the glycosylation pathways in these hosts to produce humanlike glycoproteins. Yeast cells can create highly uniform glycoproteins less expensively than with mammalian cells, therefore significant research is being conducted to develop these humanized yeast systems.[3]

Transgenic Systems for Protein Production. Manufacturing of biotechnology products has evolved from bacterial, yeast, fungal, and mammalian systems to transgenic systems which use animals or plants to secrete desired proteins. While transgenic systems are still being tested, protein production in transgenic animals is just around the corner. GTC Biotherapeutics has applied for European marketing approval of a recombinant human antithrombin III product, ATryn, which acts as an anticoagulant and anti-inflammatory agent for patients with hereditary antithrombin deficiency (HD). The indication for ATryn in HD patients is for prophylaxis of deep vein thrombosis (DVT) and thromboembolism in clinical risk situations such as surgical procedures or during labor and delivery.

This product is expressed in the milk of transgenic goats and, if approved, would be the first commercially approved therapeutic in the world produced using a transgenic platform. The well-cared for herd of goats have the appropriate human therapeutic gene linked to a milk protein promoting gene. This approach provides a unique opportunity to produce highly purified and well-characterized recombinant forms of these biologic medicines. Current trials have been approved to test this drug in the United States. Transgenic animals, in this case goats, are genetically engineered to produce a specified protein, antithrombin III, in their milk. The process works when a human gene encoding for production of antithrombin III and a promoter gene, which ensures the protein is produced in the goat's milk, are inserted into a fertilized egg and implanted in a surrogate mother goat.

Five months later a kid, carrying the human gene, is born. These goats can then be bred to produce more genetically engineered goats. The female goats will then go on to secrete the protein in their milk. The protein is purified and separated out from the milk.[2]

It is unclear if transgenic systems will become more cost effective than traditional yeast, bacterial, or mammalian cell systems because there are many hidden costs including the need to keep animals or crops secure from contamination. In addition, transgenic crops or animal milk must still be purified before a final product is achieved and some require additional processing or purification steps downstream from production. However, one advantage to transgenic systems is that some proteins are recalcitrant to expression in mammalian cell lines, yet they can be produced with efficiency in transgenic animals. Transgenic plants may find a niche in the production of proteins such as gamma-interferon, which requires glycosylation and protein folding that bacterial cells cannot handle and which cannot be produced in mammalian cell lines because they have receptors to the very cell regulatory protein that they are trying to produce which shuts down production.

RECOMBINANT DNA PRODUCTS

With the advent of biotechnology, new therapeutic classes of products and diagnostic agents have emerged that would not have been made possible using traditional chemical synthesis. Over 50 products based on rDNA technology and another 20 products based on monoclonal antibody technology have been created over the last 20 plus years (Fig. 7.2 and Table 7.1)[5,6] and will be described in further detail below.

BLOOD FACTORS
Antihemophilic factor and Coagulation factor IX were traditionally produced through donor pooled blood, but in the 1970s and 1980s, thousands of hemophiliacs were infected with the human immunodeficiency virus (HIV) and/or hepatitis, due to contaminated clotting factor blood products. The risk of infection with HIV, hepatitis B (HB), or hepatitis C (HCV) and other blood borne viruses and diseases has been completely eliminated with these recombinant products. Recombinant activated factor VII (rVIIa) is used for the treatment of bleeding episodes in hemophilia A and B patients with inhibitors against factors VII and IX.

ANTICOAGULANTS
Alteplase, reteplase, and tenecteplase are all recombinant forms of human tissue plasminogen activator that in the presence of fibrin, converts plasminogen to plasmin. In patients suffering from an acute myocardial infarction, these agents bind to the fibrin in a clot, and convert entrapped plasminogen to plasmin, thus initiating fibrinolysis.[7–9] These products are used to reduce the incidence of heart failure and mortality

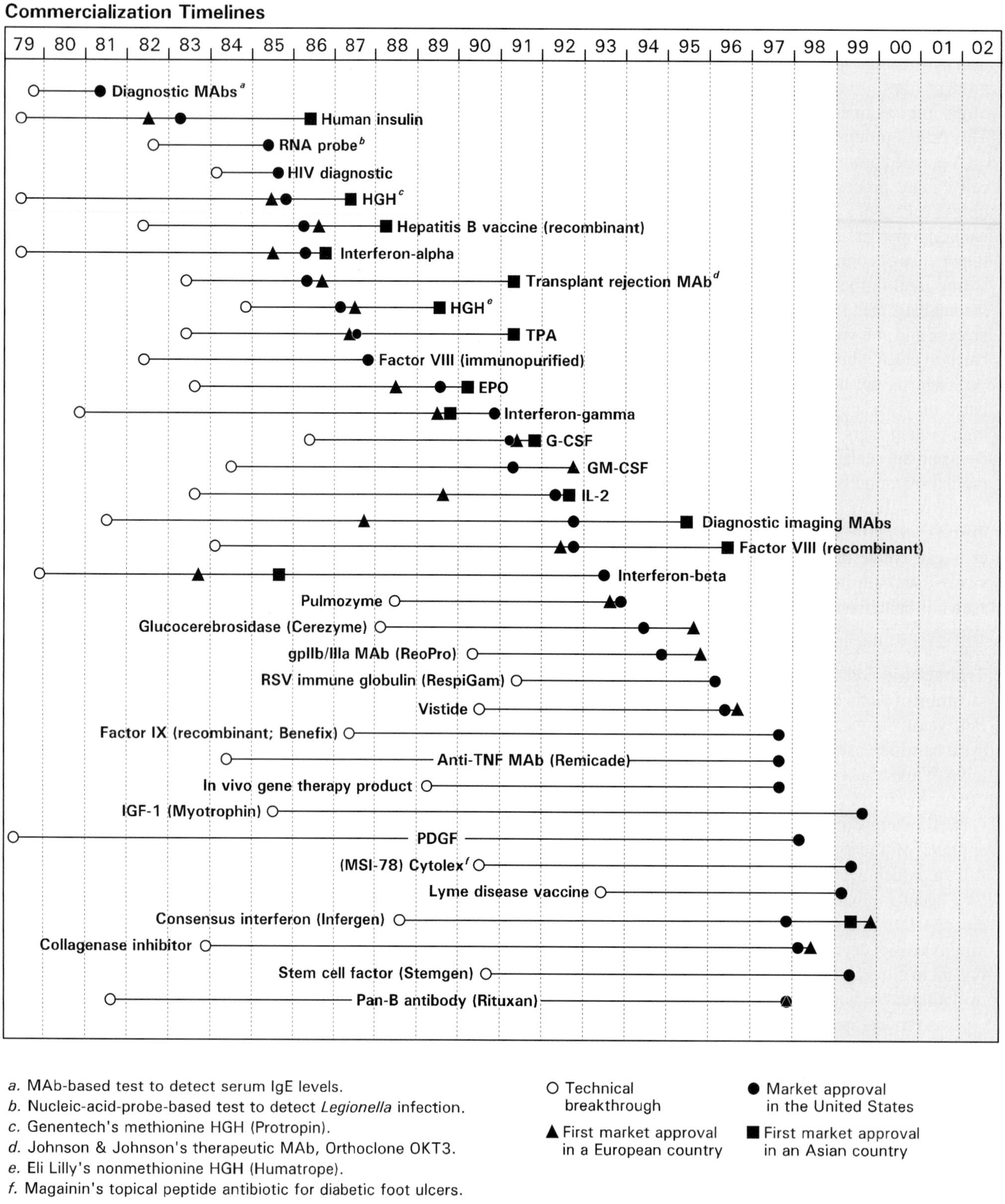
Commercialization Timelines
79 80 81 82 83 84 85 86 87 88 89 90 91 92 93 94 95 96 97 98 99 00 01 02
Diagnostic MAbs[a]
Human insulin
RNA probe[b]
HIV diagnostic
HGH[c]
Hepatitis B vaccine (recombinant)
Interferon-alpha
Transplant rejection MAb[d]
HGH[e]
TPA
Factor VIII (immunopurified)
EPO
Interferon-gamma
G-CSF
GM-CSF
IL-2
Diagnostic imaging MAbs
Factor VIII (recombinant)
Interferon-beta
Pulmozyme
Glucocerebrosidase (Cerezyme)
gpIIb/IIIa MAb (ReoPro)
RSV immune globulin (RespiGam)
Vistide
Factor IX (recombinant; Benefix)
Anti-TNF MAb (Remicade)
In vivo gene therapy product
IGF-1 (Myotrophin)
PDGF
(MSI-78) Cytolex[f]
Lyme disease vaccine
Consensus interferon (Infergen)
Collagenase inhibitor
Stem cell factor (Stemgen)
Pan-B antibody (Rituxan)
a. MAb-based test to detect serum IgE levels.
b. Nucleic-acid-probe-based test to detect Legionella infection.
c. Genentech's methionine HGH (Protropin).
d. Johnson & Johnson's therapeutic MAb, Orthoclone OKT3.
e. Eli Lilly's nonmethionine HGH (Humatrope).
f. Magainin's topical peptide antibiotic for diabetic foot ulcers.
○ Technical breakthrough
● Market approval in the United States
▲ First market approval in a European country
■ First market approval in an Asian country

FIGURE 7.2 Commercialization timelines for biomedical products. (From Vivian Lee and Associates and Decision Resources, Inc. 1998 Update: commercialization timelines for biomedical products. SPECTRUM pharmaceutical industry dynamics portfolio, December 1998, with permission.) (*continues*)

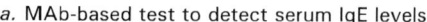

Commercialization Timelines (continued)

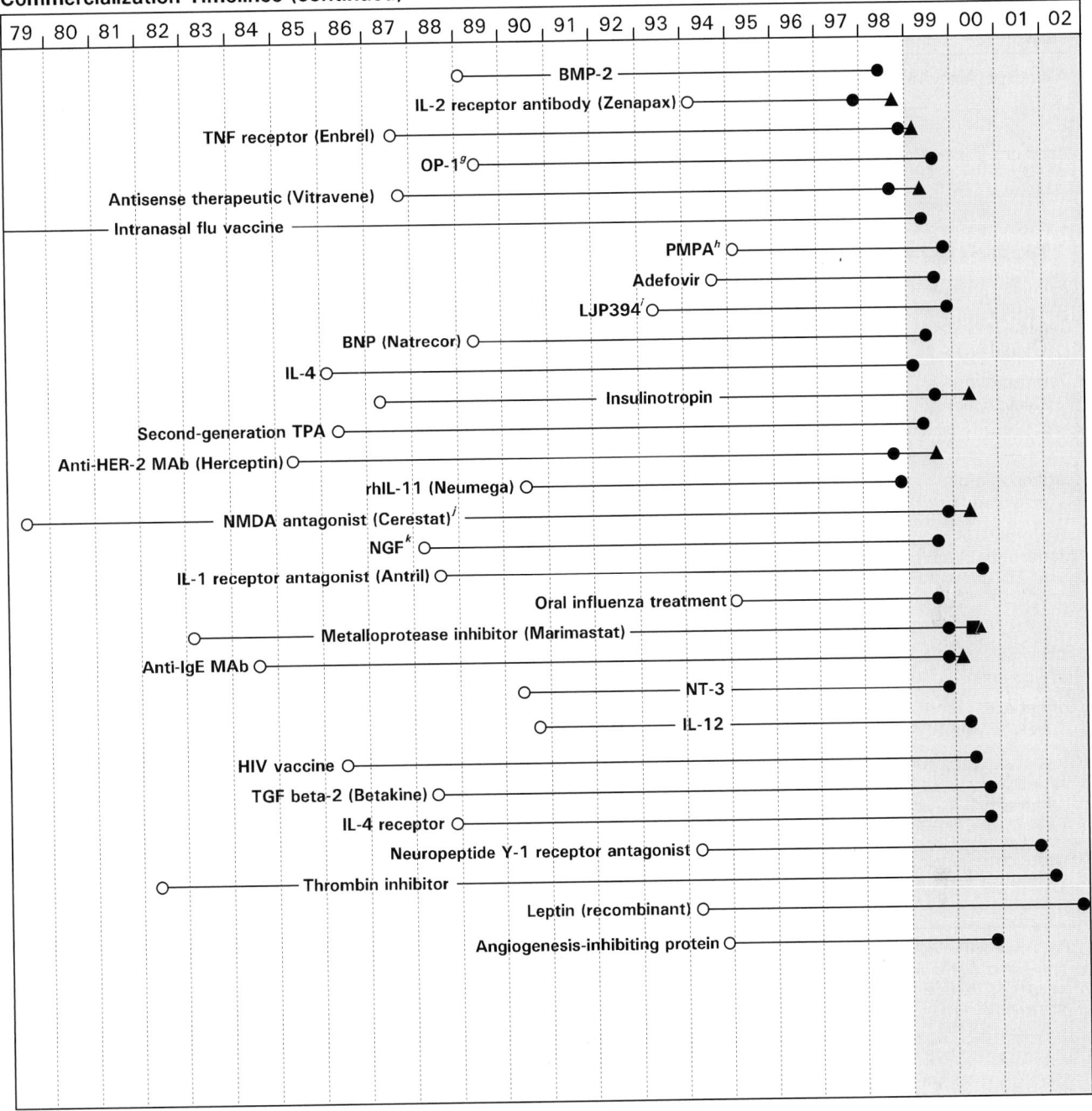

g. Creative Biomolecules' osteogenic protein for treatment of osteoporosis.

h. Gilead Sciences' reverse transcriptase inhibitor.

i. La Jolla Pharmaceutical's anti-dSDNA antibody drug for lupus.

j. Cambridge NeuroScience's NMDA receptor antagonist for stroke.

k. Genentech's nerve growth factor.

Sources: Vivian Lee & Associates and Decision Resources, Inc.

Decision Resources, Inc.

FIGURE 7.2 (continued)

TABLE 7.1	Selected Recombinant DNA Products and Indications for Use
Product	**Indication**
Alefacept (Amevive)	Alefacept is a human fusion protein designed to modulate the activity of T-cells that play a critical role in the pathogenesis of autoimmune diseases and psoriasis. Alefacept currently has FDA approval for use in the management of psoriasis.
Anakinra (Kineret)	Recombinant protein used to reduce the signs and symptoms of moderately to severely active rheumatoid arthritis patients who are 18 years of age or older and who have failed one or more disease modifying antirheumatic drugs (DMARDS).
Becaplermin (Regranex)	Used in the management of diabetic ulcers, becaplermin is a recombinant platelet-derived growth factor (rhPDGF-BB) that is formulated into a gel for topical administration. It acts by promoting recruitment and proliferation of cells involved in wound repair and enhancing the formation of granulation tissue.
Denileukin diftitox (Ontak)	Denileukin diftitox binds to the CD25 component of the interleukin-2 (IL-2) receptor on T-cells in patients with T-cell lymphoma and prevents their proliferation.
Dornase alfa (Pulmozyme)	Dornase alfa is a recombinant human deoxyribonuclease I (rhDNase), an enzyme which selectively cleaves DNA. It is administered by inhalation via a nebulizer system to patients with cystic fibrosis (CF). Dornase alfa hydrolyzes the DNA in sputum of CF patients and reduces sputum viscoelasticity, thereby reducing the incidence of pulmonary infections.
Drotrecogin alfa (activated (Xigris)	Drotrecogin alfa, a recombinant form of human Activated Protein C, is used to help reduce mortality in adult patients with severe sepsis (associated with acute organ dysfunction), by exerting anti-inflammatory and antithrombotic activity.
Etanercept (Enbrel)	Etanercept is used in adult and juvenile rheumatoid arthritis patients to reduce signs and symptoms, and delay structural damage. Etanercept is a dimeric fusion protein consisting of tumor necrosis factor (TNF) receptor linked to the Fc portion of human IgG1 antibody. By blocking TNF binding to cell surfaces, it prevents the inflammatory response processes of rheumatoid arthritis.
Fomivirsen sodium (Vitravene)	Fomivirsen sodium is an antisense molecule that is used to prevent progression of CMV retinitis in patients with HIV infection.
Laronidase (Aldurazyme)	Laronidase is used to improve pulmonary function and walking capacity in patients with Hurler and Hurler-Scheie forms of mucopolysaccharidosis I and for patients with the Scheie form who have moderate to severe symptoms.
Nesiritide (Natrecor)	Nesiritide is a recombinant form of B-type natriuretic peptide that produces hemodynamic and symptomatic improvement in patients with decompensated congestive heart failure (CHF) by balancing vasodilatory effects, neurohormonal suppression, and enhancing natriuresis and diuresis.
Rasburicase (Elitek)	Rasburicase is used in pediatric patients with leukemia, lymphoma, and solid tumors who are receiving anticancer drug therapy which is expected to result in significant tumor lysis and subsequent elevation of plasma uric acid levels.

FDA, Food and Drug Administration; IgG, immunoglobulin G; CMV, cytomegalovirus; HIV, human immunodeficiency virus.
(From Avidor Y, Mabjeesh NJ, Matzkin H. Biotechnology and drug discovery: from bench to bedside, South Med J 96:1174–1186, 2003; Kleinberg M, Mosdell KW. Current and future considerations for the new classes of biologicals. Am J Health-Syst Pharm 61:695–708, 2004, with permission.)

associated with myocardial infarction, and are also used to restore catheter function in occluded indwelling central venous catheters (Cathflo Alteplase), presumably due to thrombus formation. Lepirudin (Refludan) is a recombinant anticoagulant used to manage heparin-induced thrombocytopenia associated with thromboembolic events.[10]

VACCINES

Currently, three genetically engineered vaccines are licensed for human use: (a) the HB vaccine, (b) Haemophilus b Influenza plus HB surface antigen vaccine (Comvax), and (c) the Lyme disease vaccine (LYMErix).[11] The HB vaccine was developed by incorporating the gene that encodes the HB surface antigen polypeptide into a plasmid and cloning it

in yeast, E coli, and mammalian cells. The ability of the recombinant HB vaccine to confer immunity is similar to that of the plasma-derived vaccine. The combination Haemophilus b influenza and HB surface antigen vaccine was developed to protect primarily infants in certain high risk categories (low socioeconomic groups, blacks, Native Americans, day care attendees, etc.) from developing Haemophilus b meningitis and HB.

The Lyme disease vaccine (LYMErix) was approved by the FDA in December 1998 and was the second recombinant vaccine to become licensed for human use. However, as of February 2002, the manufacturer of this vaccine announced that LYMErix will no longer be commercially available because of low demand for the product. However, concern over the drug's side effect profile and efficacy may have also prompted its discontinuation.[12] Lyme disease is caused by an infection with the bacteria *Borrelia burgdorferi*, which is carried by ticks that transmit the infection from animals to humans. The Lyme disease bacteria can affect the joints, tendons, heart, or nervous system, resulting in arthritis, heart abnormalities, and paralysis of one or both sides of the face. This genetically engineered vaccine contains an outer surface protein of *B burgdorferi* called OspA. The vaccine works by stimulating antibodies that specifically target this outer surface protein. When the tick begins sucking a vaccinated person's blood, it ingests these antibodies, which then neutralize the bacteria inside the tick, thereby preventing transmission of the bacteria to the host.

INSULINS

As previously mentioned, human insulin was the first product to be developed utilizing rDNA technology. Since then, insulin aspart, insulin lispro, and insulin glargine have been added to the list of insulins produced via recombinant technology. Insulin glargine was developed with modifications to the human insulin molecule at position A21 and at the C-terminus of the B-chain, resulting in a stable compound that forms amorphous microprecipitates that slowly leak from subcutaneous tissue allowing for once daily injections. Comparisons of insulin glargine to Neutral Protamine Hagedorn (NPH) insulin in patients with type I and II diabetes show comparable or better glycemic control and significantly greater improvement in glycosylated hemoglobin levels.[13] Insulin aspart and insulin lispro have a faster absorption, a faster onset of action, and a shorter duration of action than regular human insulin. This quick onset of blood sugar lowering after injection allows people with diabetes to inject themselves immediately before eating, offering flexibility to the patients. Insulin aspart and insulin lispro still require use of a long-acting insulin, such as insulin glargine, for basal control.[14]

HORMONES

Growth Hormones. Recombinant human growth hormone, Somatrem (Protropin) (no longer commercially available) or Somatropin (Humatrope, Nutropin, Genotropin, Norditropin, Nutropin AQ, Serostim) has been commercially available since 1985 for the treatment of growth hormone deficiency in pediatric and adult patients. Since these recombinant growth hormones came onto the market, they have found additional use in treating short stature in patients with Turner syndrome and idiopathic short stature syndrome in children with open epiphyses, Prader-Willi Syndrome (a rare genetic disorder with short stature as a component), and HIV wasting syndrome or cachexia. Unfortunately, human growth hormone has also been used outside of approved labeling and structured clinical trial settings for a myriad of uses including building muscle mass in competitive athletes and to improve cognitive functioning in the elderly. Placebo-control trials have looked at growth hormone in elderly pa-

tients to prevent or reverse aging. Unfortunately, while growth hormone has been shown to improve lean body mass over placebo, none of these studies showed a reversal of the aging process. In addition, growth hormone replacement in appropriate adult indications is expensive, costing between $7,500 and $10,000 yearly, and estimates suggest that one third of prescriptions for growth hormone in the United States are for indications for which it is not approved by the FDA. This leads to increasing societal health care costs for no benefit. Growth hormone has many useful benefits to appropriate patient candidates, however, it is not a magic bullet to prevent or reverse aging.[15,16]

Other Hormones. Several other recombinant hormones have recently been produced, including the follicle-stimulating hormones follitropin alfa (Gonal-F) and follitropin beta (Follistim), glucagon (GlucaGen), thyrotropin alfa (Thyrogen), teriparatide (Forteo), and choriogonadotropin alfa (Ovidrel). Follitropin alpha and beta are gonadotropins. They are recombinant versions of naturally occurring follicle stimulating hormones (FSHs), secreted by the pituitary gland to stimulate ovulation and follicle development and are, thus, used by women with functional infertility. Follitropin alpha and beta are also used to stimulate spermatogenesis in men with primary or secondary hypogonadotropic hypogonadism. Choriogonadotropin alfa (Ovidrel) is a recombinant human chorionic gonadotropin that works in tandem with FSH to induce final follicular maturation and early luteinization in women undergoing in vitro fertilization or similar programs. It can also be used to induce ovulation and pregnancy in anovulatory infertile patients caused by functional infertility.[17]

Teriparatide (Forteo) is a recombinant human parathyroid hormone (PTH). PTH is the primary regulator of calcium and phosphate metabolism in bone and kidney. PTH regulates bone metabolism, renal tubular resorption of calcium and phosphate, and intestinal calcium absorption. Teriparatide is used to treat postmenopausal women with osteoporosis who are at high risk for fracture and to increase bone mass in men with primary or hypogonadal osteoporosis who are at risk for fracture.[18]

Thyrotropin alfa (Thyrogen) is a recombinant human thyroid stimulating hormone (TSH). In patients with thyroid cancer who undergo total or near total thyroidectomy, they are placed on synthetic thyroid hormone supplements to replace the endogenous hormone and to suppress serum levels of TSH to avoid TSH-stimulated tumor growth. Afterwards, patients are tested for remnants of cancer cells by thyroglobulin (TG) testing while they remain on thyroid hormone suppressive therapy and are euthyroid. Thyrotropin is an exogenous source of TSH that is used as a diagnostic tool in follow-up of thyroid cancer patients.[19]

BIOLOGIC RESPONSE MODIFIERS

Cytokines are responsible for the growth and differentiation of the cells of the immune system (Fig. 7.3). Cytokines that

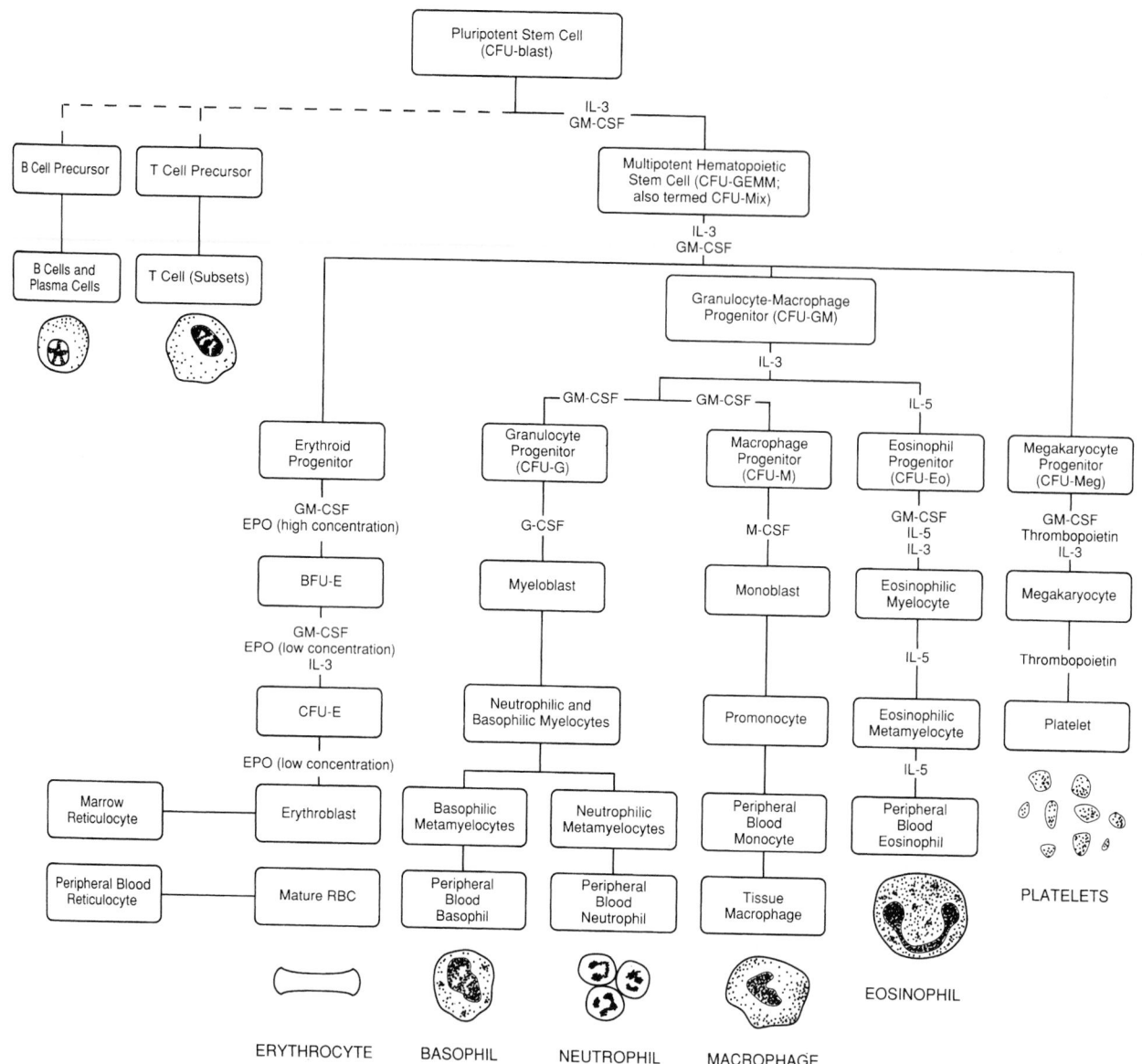

FIGURE 7.3 Differentiation of the hematopoietic stem cell from the pluripotent form to the highly differentiated macrophages, lymphocytes, erythrocytes, and granulocytes and growth factors responsible for their differentiation. (From Shriner DA. Colony-stimulating factors: clinical trials in humans. Highlights on Antineoplastic Drugs 8:6–14, 1990, with permission.)

are products of monocytes and macrophages are called monokines; those derived from lymphocytes are called lymphokines. Cytokines have a broad range of overlapping immunologic, inflammatory, and physiologic properties. The cytokines that have been produced through rDNA technology are broadly called biologic-response modifiers. They include interleukins, colony stimulating factors (CSFs) or growth factors (GFs), and interferons. These immunomodulators may be specific (e.g., target identifiable tumor antigens) or nonspecific (alter the response and function of the immune system against a stimulus without reference to a specific antigen).

Interleukins. The interleukins have been called the hormones of the immune system. They are the molecular media-

tors of immune system cells and induce replication and differentiation of those cells and activate the expression of certain functions. At least 14 different interleukins have been identified, each with its own cell targets and functions. Several of these interleukins have been cloned through rDNA technology and two interleukins, interleukin-2 (IL-2) and interleukin-11 (IL-11), have been approved by the FDA for clinical use. IL-2 is approved for use in the treatment of metastatic renal cell carcinoma and metastatic malignant melanoma. IL-11 is approved for the prevention of chemotherapy-induced thrombocytopenia in patients with nonmyeloid malignancies.

Interleukin-2. IL-2, or Aldesleukin (Proleukin), was the first of the interleukins to receive FDA approval with an initial indication as a treatment for metastatic renal cell carcinoma. More recently, IL-2 has been approved for the treatment of metastatic malignant melanoma. Also known as T-cell growth factor, IL-2 has been shown to increase the proliferation of a subset of T lymphocytes called lymphocyte-activated killer (LAK) cells, which lyse a broad range of tumor targets. In patients with metastatic renal cell carcinoma, IL-2 has an objective response rate of 20%, with 5% of patients achieving a complete response. Response duration varies but can be prolonged (>12 months), with some patients remaining in complete remission for more than 60 months.[20] IL-2 given in combination with LAK cells has shown similar clinical results. The combination of IL-2 and LAK cells is called ''adoptive immunotherapy,'' which means the transfer of active immunologic reagents (LAK cells stimulated by IL-2) to a tumor-bearing host. The goal of adoptive immunotherapy is to have the tumor-targeted immunologic agents destroy the tumor specifically.[20]

In metastatic malignant melanoma, IL-2 monotherapy has shown an objective response of 16%, with 6% of patients achieving a complete response. The median duration of response was 9 months.[21] The FDA-recommended dosing schedule for renal cell carcinoma and metastatic melanoma is 6×10^5 IU per kilogram given intravenously as a 15-minute bolus every 8 hours for up to 14 doses.[20] After 9 days of rest, the schedule is repeated for another 14 doses to a maximum of 28 doses per course, as tolerated. The major drawback to IL-2 therapy is its toxicity. Patients treated with the original IL-2 regimens required intensive care, and in clinical trials the treatment was associated with mortality rates of 1% to 6%. IL-2 can produce a severe capillary leak syndrome that leads to fluid retention, prerenal azotemia, respiratory distress, and interstitial edema. A great deal of effort has been expended in managing and limiting the side effects of IL-2 treatment. More recently developed regimens with moderate and low dosages and subcutaneous rather than intravenous administration have resulted in better tolerability.[20]

Interleukin-11. IL-11, or Oprelvekin (Neumega), was the second interleukin to receive FDA approval. IL-11 is indicated for the secondary prevention (i.e., in patients who have experienced thrombocytopenia in a prior course of chemotherapy) of chemotherapy-induced thrombocytopenia and for the reduction of the need for platelet transfusions in patients with nonmyeloid malignancies. Patients who are receiving chemotherapy frequently develop thrombocytopenia in addition to neutropenia and anemia. Platelet transfusions may be required to decrease the risk of bleeding. Platelet transfusions, though safe, carry the risk of infectious disease transmission, just as other blood products do. In addition, transfusions often must be repeated frequently and can cause delays in administering chemotherapy. IL-11 is a unique thrombopoietic growth factor produced by the bone marrow stromal cells. It causes the proliferation of hematopoietic stem cells and megakaryocytic progenitors and induces megakaryocytic maturation.[22] Two randomized, double-blind, placebo-control clinical trials have evaluated the efficacy of IL-11 in the prevention of thrombocytopenia after single or repeated sequential cycles of various chemotherapy regimens. The first clinical trial was performed in patients with solid tumors or lymphoma who had received a prophylactic platelet transfusion for severe thrombocytopenia during their previous chemotherapy cycles. This study found that at 50 μg per kilogram daily (given subcutaneously), IL-11 allowed a significant number of these patients to avoid platelet transfusions during a subsequent chemotherapy cycle.[23] The second clinical trial was done in patients with advanced breast cancer who were undergoing dose-intensive chemotherapy with cyclophosphamide plus doxorubicin. This group of patients had not previously experienced severe chemotherapy-induced thrombocytopenia. This study concluded that administering IL-11 significantly reduced the platelet transfusion requirement for these patients and allowed maintenance of the planned dosage over repeated cycles.[22] Adverse reactions reported with IL-11 include edema (59%), tachycardia (20%), palpitations (14%), atrial fibrillation or flutter (12%), dyspnea (48%), and pleural effusions (10%).[21] The recommended dose of IL-11 is 50 μg per kilogram given once daily as a subcutaneous injection. IL-11 should be initiated 6 to 24 hours after the completion of chemotherapy and continued until postnadir platelet counts are greater than $50,000 \times 10^9$ per liter. Treatment should be continued for no more than 21 days and should be discontinued at least 2 days before the next planned cycle of chemotherapy.[21]

Colony-Stimulating Factors. The CSFs are the most promising of the cytokines because of their broad range of clinical applications.[24] These glycoproteins have been cloned through DNA technology, and five (granulocyte-macrophage [GM]-CSF, granulocyte [G]-CSF, pegylated G-CSF, darbepoetin alfa, and epoetin alfa) are currently available for clinical use. CSFs help to regulate the growth and differentiation of hematopoietic cells. There are two main CSF classes. Class 1 CSFs, such as GM-CSF, act at the partially committed stem cell level to cause differentiation and proliferation of multiple cell lines (monocytes, granulocytes, eosinophils, etc.). Class 2 CSFs, such as G-CSF, pegylated G-CSF, darbepoetin alfa, and epoetin alfa, act on already differentiated cell lines to stimulate proliferation of more specific cell types.[25]

Granulocyte-Macrophage Colony-Stimulating Factor. GM-CSF supports the expansion of monocytic and granulocytic cell lines and also cell lines containing myeloid, erythroid, and megakaryocytic cells when combined with epoetin alfa. GM-CSF received FDA approval for use in bone marrow transplantation (BMT) on the basis of a pivotal randomized, placebo-control, multicenter trial of 128 patients. Patients receiving high-dose chemotherapy and autologous

BMTs for lymphoid malignancies were randomized to receive placebo or 250 μg/m²/day of GM-CSF administered as a 2-hour infusion for 21 days after transplant. The patients receiving GM-CSF experienced a neutrophil recovery 7 days earlier than the placebo-treated group (19 vs. 26 days). It was also noted that days of hospitalization, days of antibiotic use, and the incidence of documented infection were lower in the GM-CSF treated group. In addition to its indication for accelerating myeloid recovery in patients with lymphoid cancers undergoing autologous BMT, it has received FDA approval for use in patients who have BMT failure or engraftment delay in the allogeneic and the autologous setting. In the setting of peripheral stem cell transplantation, GM-CSF has also received approval to help mobilize peripheral blood progenitor cells for transplant and for use after peripheral blood progenitor cell transplantation.

GM-CSF has been used to accelerate myeloid recovery in patients undergoing chemotherapy for acute myeloid leukemia (AML).[26–28] In one uncontrolled trial, GM-CSF reduced the median recovery time of neutrophils by 4 days in patients receiving 6-thioguanine, standard-dose cytarabine, and daunorubicin and by 9 days in patients receiving high-dose cytarabine and mitoxantrone.[27] In a larger, randomized, placebo-control trial, 124 patients undergoing induction and consolidation therapy for AML were randomized to receive GM-CSF or placebo on day 11 if a day 10 bone marrow sample was aplastic. The median time to recover an absolute neutrophil count of 0.5×10^9 per liter or more was 11 days in the GM-CSF group and 14 days in the placebo group ($P = 0.01$). The median survival time was 325 days in the GM-CSF group and 135 days in the placebo group ($P = 0.035$). GM-CSF is being studied in a variety of clinical areas to reduce the incidence and severity of mucositis, stomatitis, and diarrhea in patients undergoing chemotherapy treatment, to reduce fungal infections in patients with cancer, to promote wound healing, and as an HB adjuvant. The most commonly reported adverse effects of GM-CSF include injection site reactions, slight temperature elevations after injection, bone pain, and myalgias.

Granulocyte Colony-Stimulating Factor and Pegylated Granulocyte Colony-Stimulating Factor (Pegfilgrastim). G-CSF is a cell lineage-specific CSF that stimulates granulocyte progenitor cells to differentiate into granulocytes. G-CSF received FDA approval following a phase III trial in which 211 patients were randomized to receive 200 μg/m² of G-CSF or placebo after chemotherapy with cyclophosphamide, doxorubicin, and etoposide. G-CSF reduced the duration of neutropenia from 6 days to 3 days in the first cycle, the incidence of febrile neutropenia (57% vs. 28% in cycle 1), the length of first cycle hospital stay, and the days of intravenous antibiotic use.[28] Additional studies consistently show a significantly shorter duration of leukopenia than in placebo controls.[29–31] Small studies of G-CSF show reductions in infection, mucositis, and fever and greater adherence

to scheduled chemotherapy regimens.[30,32] G-CSF has also received approval to reduce the duration of neutropenia and neutropenia-related clinical sequelae in patients with non-myeloid malignancies who are undergoing myeloablative chemotherapy followed by marrow transplantation. It has also received approval to reduce the incidence and duration of sequelae of neutropenia (e.g., fever, infection, and oropharyngeal ulcers) in symptomatic patients with congenital neutropenia, cyclic neutropenia, or idiopathic neutropenia. G-CSF has also been approved for use in patients who fail to engraft after receiving an autologous BMT and for mobilization of autologous peripheral blood progenitor cells after chemotherapy.

Pegylated G-CSF, or pegfilgrastim (Neulasta), is the most recent white blood cell growth factor to be approved by the FDA. The filgrastim molecule is modified by adding a covalent 20 kDa polyethylene glycol (peg) moiety to the n-terminus. The addition of the peg moiety decreases systemic clearance, resulting in sustained drug levels. Pegfilgrastim and filgrastim have an identical mechanism of action, however, because pegfilgrastim is pegylated, it has a much longer elimination half-life and can be dosed once per chemotherapy cycle to prevent neutropenia from occurring.

The American Society of Clinical Oncology (ASCO), National Comprehensive Cancer Network, and the National Oncology Alliance, Inc. all have published CSF use guidelines. Recent updates to two of the guidelines state that in consideration of efficacy and cost-modeling analyses, the primary administration of CSFs should be used as a prophylactic measure only when the chemotherapy being administered is expected to have an incidence of febrile neutropenia more than 20% of the time. However, some high-risk patients, including those with bone marrow compromise, preexisting neutropenia, substantial irradiation of the pelvic area, history of recurrent febrile neutropenia during previous chemotherapy exposure, and open wounds, would benefit from treatment with CSFs even when a less myelosuppressive chemotherapy regimen is used.[33,34]

Erythropoietin Alfa and Darbepoetin Alfa. EPO is the primary regulator of red blood cell production, and thus, it is an important cytokine for the erythroid cell line. Recombinant human epoetin alfa (rHuEPO) (Epogen, Procrit), and darbepoetin alfa (Aranesp) are approved for use in the treatment of anemia associated with chronic renal failure in patients on dialysis and predialysis, severe anemia associated with zidovudine (AZT) therapy in acquired immune deficiency syndrome (AIDS), anemic patients scheduled to undergo elective noncardiac, nonvascular surgery, and anemia in patients with cancer receiving chemotherapy.

Epoetin alfa (rHuEPO) was the first recombinant stimulating factor to be approved for use in humans, and many trials have confirmed its benefit in transfusion-dependent patients. The use of rHuEPO in anemia in patients with renal failure and AIDS is discussed in Chapters 14 and 84; it is important to be aware of the studies of its use in treating the anemia of patients undergoing cancer chemotherapy. In double-blind trials involving 124 patients with cancer-induced anemia, 132 patients receiving a cisplatin-containing regimen, and 157 patients receiving other chemotherapy not containing cisplatin, the mean weekly hematocrit level in epoetin alfa-treated patients in all three treatment groups increased from 28.6% to 32.1%. The mean weekly hematocrit level for the placebo-treated group remained essentially unchanged over the same time period (28.4%–28.8%). The transfusion requirements during the second and third months of therapy for erythro-poietic-treated patients were less than for placebo patients, although the difference did not reach statistical significance.[24]

Recently, a new erythro-poietic growth factor, darbepoetin alfa (Aranesp), received FDA approval for the treatment of anemia in patients with chronic renal failure (on or off dialysis) or who are receiving chemotherapy for nonmyeloid malignancies. Darbepoetin alfa binds to the same receptor as rHuEPO, and stimulates erythropoiesis by the same mechanism as endogenous EPO. Compared with rHuEPO, darbepoetin has two additional N-linked carbohydrate chains. These additional carbohydrates were added by changing five amino acids within the protein sequence of rHuEPO distal from the receptor binding site. These extra carbohydrate chains allow for the addition of up to eight sialic acid molecules, and increases the maximum number of sialic acid molecules from 14 to 22. Because of these additional carbohydrates and sialic acid molecules, darbepoetin has an increased molecular weight (~37,100 daltons) compared with rHuEPO (~30,400 daltons) and due to its size difference, decreases its renal clearance and thus increases its half-life. While rHuEPO is usually given weekly in patients undergoing cancer chemotherapy, darbepoetin alfa can be administered every other week, to improve patient convenience.

The common adverse effects associated with the erythropoietic agents are generally mild, and include hypertension, rash, headache, arthralgias, and nausea and vomiting. A rapid rise in red blood cell count caused by EPO administration can also result in severe hypertension, thrombosis, and seizures.

Interferons. The interferons are a group of naturally occurring glycoproteins produced by a variety of cell types in response to viral, antigenic, or mitogenic stimuli. They were originally discovered in 1957 when Isaacs and Lindenmann observed that virus-infected cells produced a protein that rendered them resistant to other viruses.[35] In addition to their antiviral action, interferons affect a number of vital cellular and body functions, including hormone stimulation, immunity, metabolism, and tumor development.

Interferons have been categorized into two classes: type 1 (IFN-α, IFN-β, and IFN-ω) and type 2 (IFN-γ). Many cell types in response to many different factors, including infectious agents, produce the type 1 interferons. The type 2 interferons are produced only by T lymphocytes and natural killer (NK) cells stimulated by antigens or mitogens and IL-2.[36] Whereas naturally occurring interferons are glycosylated, recombinant interferons produced in *E coli* are not. However, activity does not seem to be diminished by their unglycosylated state. While IFN-α and IFN-β are similar in structure, cell receptor site interactions, and biologic effects, IFN-γ interacts at a different receptor site, has a different structure, and appears to have greater antitumor, immunomodulatory, and cytolytic effects.[37]

To date, IFN-α has been approved for use in the treatment of chronic viral HB and HCV, condyloma acuminata, hairy cell leukemia, AIDS-related Kaposi's sarcoma, follicular non-Hodgkin's lymphoma, chronic malignant melanoma, and Philadelphia chromosome positive chronic myelogenous leukemia (CML). IFN-β has been approved for use in ambulatory patients with relapsing-remitting multiple sclerosis to reduce the frequency of clinical exacerbations of the disease. IFN-γ is approved by the FDA to reduce the frequency and severity of serious infections associated with chronic granulomatous disease.

Interferon Alpha. IFN-α was the first of the interferons to be approved for clinical use. It has been widely used as first-line or adjuvant treatment for several other solid tumors and hematologic malignancies. Hairy cell leukemia was the first malignancy for which IFN-α was found to have significant activity. Although up to 90% of patients respond to IFN-α treatment, up to 50% relapse within a short period. Studies show that continuous treatment with IFN-α leads to a long-term survival up to 6 years in 82% of patients when doses of 2×10^6 U/m^2 are used.[38]

In the early 1980s, IFN-α was recognized as an effective agent in the treatment of CML. The mechanism of action of interferon in CML is not completely understood. CML is caused by a specific chromosomal abnormality, the Philadelphia chromosome. It is thought that IFN-α not only is antiproliferative to normal and leukemic stem cells, but may suppress the oncogene responsible for the Philadelphia chromosomal translocation, thus restoring normal adherence to marrow stromal cells, preventing their premature release into the peripheral blood. By selectively repressing the Philadelphia-positive stem cells, IFN-α encourages the repopulation of the bone marrow with normal Philadelphia-negative stem cells.

Two studies, one by the Cancer and Leukemia Group B (CALGB) and another by the Italian Cooperative Study Group on Chronic Myeloid Leukemia, confirm the efficacy of IFN-α in the management of chronic phase CML. In the CALGB trial, 107 patients received IFN-α at a dose of 5 MU/m^2 daily (given subcutaneously) until progression of disease; 59% of patients achieved at least a partial remission for a median of 52 months, and a complete cytogenetic response (complete disappearance of all Philadelphia-positive cytology) was achieved in 14 patients (13%).[39] In the Italian study, the doses of interferon used were lower than the CALGB trial, 3 MU daily for the first 2 weeks, 6 MU daily for the second 2 weeks, and 9 MU daily thereafter. In this study, 322 patients were randomized to IFN-α (218 patients) or conventional-dose hydroxyurea (104 patients). Complete cytogenetic responses occurred in 8% of IFN-α patients and none occurred in the hydroxyurea group. The time to progression to an accelerated or blast crisis phase was longer in the IFN-α group than the hydroxyurea group (median >72 vs. 45 months, respectively; $P < 0.001$), and overall survival was longer with IFN-α than with hydroxyurea (72 vs. 45 months, respectively; $P = 0.002$).[40] Interferon has clearly shown a survival benefit over conventional treatment for patients with CML.

In solid tumors, efficacy of IFN-α has been clinically documented in malignant melanoma, metastatic renal cell carcinoma, bladder cancer, and AIDS-related Kaposi's sarcoma. Since 1978, more than 12 phase II trials have documented the antitumor activity of IFN-α against malignant melanoma. Response rates of up to 16% have been reported. In a phase III, randomized, controlled trial of 287 patients with deep primary tumors or regional lymph node involvement, adjuvant IFN-α was compared with observation alone in patients who had previously undergone surgical removal of their primary tumor. Doses of 20 MU/m² daily (given intravenously) for 1 month followed by 10 MU/m² three times weekly (subcutaneously) for 48 weeks resulted in a median relapse-free survival significantly greater in the IFN-α group (1.7 vs. 0.98 years) and an overall median survival of 3.82 versus 2.78 years for the control group.[41] This was the first trial in almost 20 years to show that an adjuvant agent could alter the natural progression of malignant melanoma.

IFN-α has been studied in the treatment of renal cell cancer, with response rates of 10% to 15% (2% complete response rates). When IFN-α is combined with IL-2, response rates of 38% have been observed.[36] The role of sequential IFN-α followed by IFN-γ is also being studied. IFN-α has also been studied in breast cancer, ovarian cancer, colorectal cancer, and superficial bladder cancer. Although response rates of only 5% to 10% have been seen in breast cancer and ovarian cancer, three trials in colorectal cancer combining 5 fluorouracil (5FU) and IFN-α have produced response rates of 26% to 63%, and trials in superficial bladder cancer have produced response rates of 43%.[42] These encouraging results have led to other trials of gastrointestinal malignancies with this combination of products. In a review of IFN-α, Spiegel[43] reports the incidence of adverse effects in 1403 patients (Table 7.2).

Pegylated formulations of interferon alfa-2a (Pegasys) and alfa-2b (PEG-Intron) have been developed. Both pegylated interferons are indicated for the treatment of chronic HCV infection in adults with compensated liver disease either alone or in combination with ribavirin. Several studies have shown that pegylated interferon is superior to conven-

TABLE 7.2	Incidence of Adverse Experiences with Interferon-α	
	All Patients (n ≤ 1,403)	
Adverse Effects	Any Severity (%)	Grades III, IV (%)
Flulike symptoms	96	37
Nausea/vomiting	42	5
Other gastrointestinal symptoms	24	2
Central nervous system	33	7
Cardiovascular	12	2
Skin	13	1
Respiratory	6	1
Alopecia	6	<1
Weight loss	5	1
Hepatic	<1	0

(From Spiegel RJ. The alpha interferons: clinical overview. Semin Oncol 14:1–12, 1987, with permission.)

tional interferon (nonpegylated), and the combination of pegylated interferon and ribavirin superior to conventional interferon and ribavirin in improving virologic response rates (loss of detectable serum HCV RNA) after treatment and follow-up in patients with chronic HCV.[44,45] Pegylation of the interferon molecule increases its size, causing slower absorption, decreased systemic clearance, and a longer elimination half-life. The longer elimination half-life results in sustained drug levels and increases the duration of its biologic activity. Newer studies have evaluated triple combination therapy with pegylated interferon, ribavirin, and amantadine for HCV infection. This triple combination has been shown to produce sustained virological responses in up to 74.4% of patients at the end of therapy compared to 44.6% in patients treated with the same triple therapy using conventional interferon alpha.[46] Peginterferon alfa-2a monotherapy is also approved for the treatment of patients with chronic HB. Refer to Chapter 49 for further discussion on the clinical use of peginterferons.

Interferon Beta. IFN-β was approved in 1994 for the treatment of exacerbating-remitting ambulatory multiple sclerosis based on the results of a multicenter, randomized, double-blind, placebo-control trial. In that trial, IFN-β resulted in fewer exacerbations, fewer severe exacerbations, and less progression of T2 signal abnormalities seen on yearly magnetic resonance imaging scans.[47]

In solid and hematologic malignancies, IFN-β has shown modest results overall. Its activity against renal cell, melanoma, and colorectal cancers, and its activity in hairy cell leukemia, CML, or non-Hodgkin's lymphoma does not seem to offer any advantage over IFN-α.[37] The best clinical responses to IFN-β have been seen in Kaposi's sarcoma[48] (40%–50% response rate) and glioma brain tumors (10%–20% response rate).[37]

Interferon-Gamma. IFN-γ has been approved by the FDA to reduce infectious complications in patients with chronic granulomatous disease, an inherited immunodeficiency syndrome. A study of 128 patients who received IFN-γ or placebo (subcutaneously 3 times a week for 1 year) had two study end points. The first was the time to serious infection (defined as a clinical event leading to hospitalization and parenteral antibiotic administration), and the second was the number of serious infections, length of hospitalization, and effect on existing infection. After 1 year, 77% of patients treated with IFN-γ were infection-free, compared to 30% in the placebo-treated group. There were 50% fewer serious infections in the IFN-γ group (compared with placebo).

The toxicities of IFN-γ are similar to those of IFN-α and IFN-β, although headaches appear to be more severe and may be dose-limiting. IFN-γ has also been shown to increase serum triglyceride levels by inhibiting lipoprotein lipase.

Other Recombinant Products. Several other important biological proteins manufactured using rDNA technology have been approved by the FDA over the last two decades. Their use spans many therapeutic areas including cardiovascular, endocrine, and pulmonary. Table 7.1 provides a list of additional rDNA products and their uses.[5,6]

MONOCLONAL ANTIBODIES

The most diverse and best studied of the biologicals, the monoclonal antibodies, have been commercially successful with far-reaching therapeutic applicability for the treatment of cancers, transplantation rejection, drug toxicities, Crohn's disease, rheumatoid arthritis, and other diseases. The clinical applications of monoclonal antibodies for diagnostic imaging are also extensive, particularly for cancer, infectious diseases, and heart disease. This has led to the FDA approval of monoclonal imaging agents to detect the presence, location, and extent of myocardial necrosis in acute ischemic heart disease and the detection of colorectal, ovarian, and prostate cancers. Although the theoretical applications seem endless, the practical applications have been somewhat slow in developing, partly because of the difficulties inherent in monoclonal antibody production.

Monoclonal antibody production begins with the identification of the B lymphocyte responsible for the production of a specific antibody to a specific antigen.[49] An antigen to which the desired antibody will respond is first injected into a mouse (Fig. 7.4). The antigen stimulates B lymphocytes (the precursor of the antibody-secreting plasma cell) to produce a specific antibody against that antigen. B lymphocytes

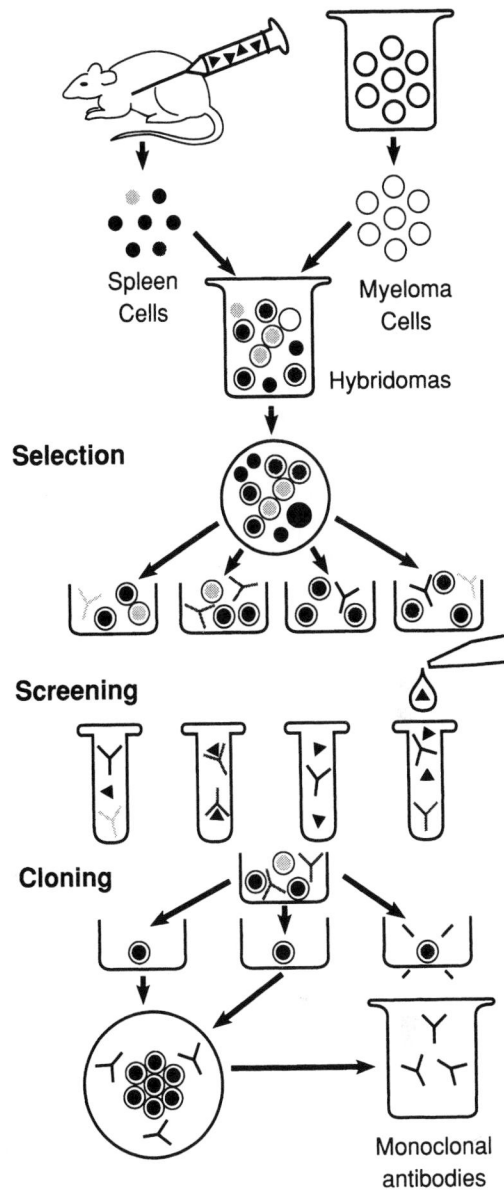

FIGURE 7.4 Summary of the steps involved in the production of monoclonal antibodies. (From Chisolm R. On the trail of the magic bullet. High Technology Business 3:57–63, 1983, with permission.)

are then recovered from the spleen of the mouse. Only a few of the B lymphocytes recovered from the mouse spleen actually secrete the desired antibody. The B lymphocytes are then mixed with myeloma cells (a cell line that can live forever in culture) in polyethylene glycol, resulting in the membranes of the two cell types being fused together.

The technique of fusing myeloma cells and B lymphocytes, developed by Kohler and Milstein in the mid-1970s, results in a hybridoma. The hybridomas are grown for several weeks. Enzyme-linked immunoabsorbent assay (ELISA) or radioimmunoassay (RIA) methods then are used to select the appropriate antibody-secreting hybridoma. The target antigen is chemically bound to the bottom of the testing tray in wells, and the hybridoma cells are added to each of the wells. Antibodies produced inside the wells that are specific for the target antigen bind to the antigen at the bottom of the wells. Radioactive or enzyme-labeled secondary antibodies that are specific for the primary antibodies are then added to the wells, and the mixture is incubated and rewashed. The wells that show radioactivity or a color reaction due to the enzyme are those that contain the desired antibody. Once identified, the hybridomas containing the desired antibody can be cloned.

Monoclonal antibodies exert their killing effect on cells in three primary ways. The first is through antibody-dependent cell-mediated cytotoxicity. As with the rest of the immune system, when an antibody attaches to an antigen, effector cells, such as monocytes, macrophages, granulocytes, and some lymphocytes, bind to the constant region (Fc) of the antibody and cause enzymatic puncture of the antigenic cell membrane, ultimately resulting in cell death.

A second mechanism of monoclonal antibody action is to target molecules on the cell surface that are critical to that cell's growth or differentiation. For example, monoclonal antibodies have been prepared against a growth factor receptor HER-2-neu, found over abundantly on the cell surface of up to one third of patients with breast cancer. The HER-2-neu antibody, when combined with chemotherapy, improves the duration of treatment response and overall survival in women with metastatic breast cancer and more recently has been found to improve disease-free survival and overall survival in the setting of adjuvant therapy.

A third method of killing is through complement-mediated cytotoxicity. Monoclonal antibodies, primarily immunoglobulin M (IgM), invoke the release of complement, which sets off the complement cascade to mediate cell destruction.

Researchers have also been able to augment the effectiveness of monoclonal antibodies by conjugating them with radioisotopes, toxins, chemotherapeutic agents, and drug-filled liposomes (Fig. 7.5). Radioconjugates used in the treatment of malignancies have been successful because they do not have to enter the cells to induce a killing effect. Instead, they can exert their energy over several cells (the field effect). Nearby healthy tissue, especially in areas in which the conjugate may be detained, such as the liver and spleen, may be injured.[50] A radioconjugate monoclonal ^{131}I anti-B1 antibody that targets the CD20 antigen on the cell surface of B cells is FDA-approved for the treatment of low-grade non-Hodgkin's lymphoma. Monoclonal antibodies fused with all or part of plant or bacterial toxins are called immuno-conjugates. Monoclonal antibodies conjugated with ricin-A, a plant toxin, have been used to treat melanoma, lymphoma, rheumatoid arthritis, and leukemia.

Antineoplastic monoclonal antibody conjugates are also being used to deliver antineoplastics to specific areas of the

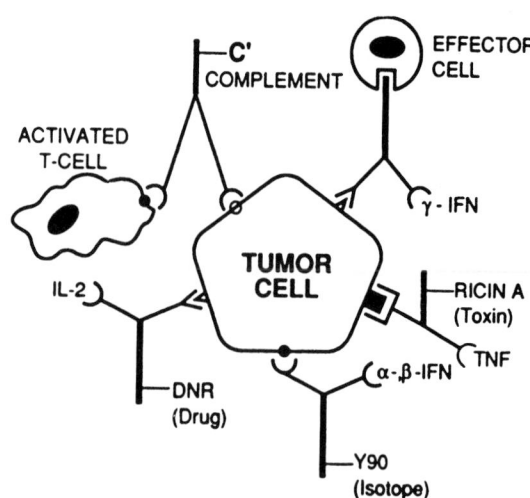

FIGURE 7.5 Various uses of monoclonal antibodies. C', complement; DNR, daunorubicin; IFN, interferon; IL-2, interleukin-2; TNF, tumor necrosis factor. (From Dillman R. Monoclonal antibodies for treating cancer. Ann Intern Med 111:592–603, 1989, with permission.)

body. This helps to improve the therapeutic to toxic ratio of systemic chemotherapy. Antineoplastic conjugates have been tried in colorectal, breast, and ovarian cancers and in malignant melanoma and glioma. Researchers have developed a doxorubicin-conjugated monoclonal antibody yielding a drug that is 10 times more cytotoxic than doxorubicin alone. Liposome-carrying drugs conjugated to monoclonal antibodies also show promise. The liposomes concentrate the drug in cells of the reticuloendothelial system, liver, and spleen and thus reduce drug uptake to other critical organs, such as the heart, kidneys, and gastrointestinal tract. Liposome-containing doxorubicin and daunorubicin have been developed to reduce the cardiotoxic potential of these drugs. They are both used for treatment of HIV-related Kaposi's sarcoma.

Another advance in the mechanistic development of monoclonal antibodies is the engineering of bispecific monoclonal antibodies, which can be bidirected to a tumor cell and an effector cell such as a monocyte or lymphocyte. Bispecific monoclonal antibodies can bind two different antigenic determinants simultaneously to bring effector cells into close contact with tumor cells for improved cellular cytotoxicity. These monoclonal antibodies have been developed by cross-linking hybridomas. Antibodies directed against the CD3 T-cell receptor subunit of cytotoxic T cells help to trigger the effector function once it is brought into contact with the tumor cell. These bispecific antibodies have been tested in clinical trials against Hodgkin's lymphoma and are very promising.

Genetically engineered monoclonal antibody fragments directed to site-specific antigens have also been developed. The rationale for developing these fragments is based on their greater ability to gain access to tumors because of their smaller size and more rapid clearance from the circulation.[51] Digoxin-specific Fab antibody fragments are commercially available for the treatment of digitalis toxicity. The digoxin antibody fragments bind specifically to unbound (free) digoxin in the intravascular space, preventing and reversing the glycoside's toxic effect. The Fab has advantages over the intact antibody in that it causes less immunogenicity because it lacks the antigenic Fc portion and is cleared from the circulation more rapidly.

Eternacept (Enbrel), a dimeric fusion protein consisting of tumor necrosis factor (TNF) receptor linked to the Fc portion of human IgG1 antibody, has been FDA approved for the management of rheumatoid arthritis in patients in whom disease-modifying antirheumatic drugs had failed. Eternacept is a soluble, free-floating molecule that binds to TNF to block its binding to cell surface TNF receptors. By blocking TNF binding to cell surfaces, it prevents the inflammatory response processes of rheumatoid arthritis.[52]

Refer to Chapter 65 for further discussion on the management of rheumatoid arthritis.

MONOCLONAL ANTIBODIES IN TRANSPLANTATION

Muromonab-CD3 (Orthoclone OKT3, Ortho) is the only commercially available monoclonal antibody for the treatment of acute renal, cardiac, and hepatic allograft rejections. It has also been used prophylactically to prevent acute rejection. Muromonab-CD3 is a murine (mouse) IgG monoclonal antibody that directs its action against the CD3 molecule present on the surface of thymocytes and mature T-lymphocytes. CD3 forms a complex with the T-cell antigen receptor (TCR) to induce T-cell function (activation and proliferation) and activation of cytotoxic cells that contribute to allograft rejection. It has been shown in vivo that administering this antibody results in the coating of circulating T-cells and their subsequent disappearance from the circulation. By interfering with the CD3, muromonab-CD3 does not allow the complex to form, rendering the T cells inactive.

In the first controlled trial in 123 patients with acute rejection of deceased donor transplants, the rejection reversal rate was 94% with muromonab-CD3, compared to 75% with high-dose steroids. The 1-year graft survival rate was also higher with muromonab CD3 (62%) than with high-dose steroids (45%).

Side effects of muromonab-CD3 include fever, dyspnea, headache, nausea, vomiting, and diarrhea. These effects (also referred to as cytokine release syndrome) generally begin within 1 hour of administering the first dose of the drug and diminish over the next several hours. On days 2 through 5 of treatment, pruritus, rash, aseptic meningitis, and altered mental status have been reported to occur. The side effects are probably caused by muromonab–CD3-induced increases in TNF and IL-2.

The most serious side effect of muromonab-CD3 therapy is dyspnea caused by complement activation resulting in neutrophil sequestration in the lungs. Different attempts at mitigating this side effect have met with some success. Dose reduction and the use of methylprednisolone all help to attenuate the first-dose dyspnea seen with conventional doses and administration of the drug.[53–55]

Patients can also develop human antimouse antibodies (HAMA) to the monoclonal antibody, which can lead to an abrogated therapeutic response.

Two additional humanized (part human and part murine) monoclonal antibodies have FDA approval for the prevention of acute organ rejection in patients receiving renal transplants. Daclizumab (Zenapax) is a humanized (90% human, 10% murine) antibody that was approved in 1997, while basiliximab (Simulect) is a chimeric (70% human, 30% murine) antibody that was approved in 1998. However because these agents are part human monoclonal antibodies, they do not produce the HAMA response seen with muromonab-CD3, which is completely murine derived. Severe side effects associated with basiliximab and daclizumab include hypersensitivity reactions including anaphylaxis. In addition, the use of daclizumab has been associated with a higher incidence of death from infection. Refer to Chapter 27 for further discussion on the clinical use of these antibodies.

MONOCLONAL ANTIBODIES IN CANCER TREATMENT

The initial studies involving monoclonal antibodies in the treatment of cancers involved primarily hematologic malignancies. More than 25 small phase I trials in 135 patients resulted in complete remission in approximately 5% of patients, partial response in 16%, and minor response in an additional 17% of patients.[51]

Most patients treated in these studies had refractory disease and were immunocompromised, making it difficult for them to respond to immunotherapy. In addition, these earlier studies were conducted using mouse monoclonal antibodies, leading to a significant HAMA response that limited the duration of treatment. Other problems identified in these earlier trials included heterogeneous antigens expressed on the surface of tumor cells; immune complex formation between free, circulating antigens and monoclonal antibodies; disappearance or modulation of antigens on the tumor cell surface; and the short half-life of the mouse monoclonal in the human circulation.

With these problems identified, researchers set out to minimize these problems, achieve site-specific delivery of monoclonals to the tumor cells with minimal disruption to normal tissue, and produce a more stable monoclonal conjugate, resulting in a longer half-life of the monoclonal antibody.[51]

The first monoclonal antibody approved for cancer treatment was rituximab (Rituxan). Rituximab was approved in early 1998 for the treatment of refractory or recurrent low-grade (follicular) non-Hodgkin's lymphoma. Rituximab is a chimeric anti-CD20 monoclonal antibody that targets CD20 antigens, which are expressed on more than 90% of normal and malignant B cells, and are required for cell cycle initiation and differentiation. When rituximab binds to the CD20 antigen on the cell's surface, it induces complement-mediated and antibody-dependent cytotoxicity, which results in cell death.

The phase III pivotal trial evaluated 166 patients with low-grade follicular lymphoma that was recurrent or resistant to chemotherapy.[56] Rituximab at a dose of 375 mg/m^2 weekly for 4 weeks yielded overall response rates of 50% (6% complete responses and 44% partial responses) in 151 evaluable patients. The mean time to progression was not reached at more than 9 months. Side effects were mostly mild and included fever, chills, nausea, and headache. More recently, in Europe, eight fatal cases of a severe cytokine release syndrome have accompanied initial doses of rituximab.[57] Severe cytokine release syndrome usually manifests within 1 or 2 hours of the first infusion of the drug and is characterized by severe dyspnea, bronchospasm, or hypoxia with or without fever, chills, rigors, urticaria, and angioedema. Refer to Chapter 95 for further discussion on the use of rituximab in the treatment of lymphomas.

Trastuzumab (Herceptin), the first monoclonal antibody used in the treatment of advanced breast cancer, was approved in September 1998 for the treatment of women with metastatic breast cancer whose tumors over-express the epidermal growth factor receptor 2 protein (HER2). As a result of a genetic alteration in the HER2 gene, approximately one third of all breast cancer tumors over-express HER2 on the cell surface. Trastuzumab, a mouse monoclonal engineered to closely resemble a human antibody, binds to the HER2 receptors on the cell surface of the tumor cells and through this binding mechanism inhibits tumor cell growth.

Trastuzumab has been studied in clinical trials in combination with chemotherapy. In a randomized, controlled clinical trial, 469 patients with HER2 overexpressing metastatic breast cancer were randomized to trastuzumab plus chemotherapy or chemotherapy alone. In this trial, patients who received trastuzumab combination therapy had a median time to disease progression of 7.2 months, compared to 4.5 months for those receiving chemotherapy alone. In addition, the 1-year survival rate for the trastuzumab combination arm was 79%, compared to 68% for chemotherapy alone.[58] Trastuzumab was also studied alone in women who had relapsed after chemotherapy for metastatic disease. The overall response rate was 14% (3% complete responses) and the median response time was 9 months. The biggest risk of using trastuzumab is its potential for causing a weakening of the heart muscle, leading to congestive heart failure. This side effect was most pronounced when trastuzumab was used in combination with doxorubicin and cyclophosphamide. Therefore, trastuzumab is not approved for use with that combination of chemotherapy drugs. Other side effects include neutropenia, anemia, abdominal pain, and diarrhea.

Also, fever, nausea, vomiting, pain, weakness, and headache can occur with about one half of all first infusions of the drug.[59]

Refer to Chapter 96 for further discussion on the therapeutic options in the management of breast cancer.

Other studies of monoclonal antibodies used to treat malignancies have focused on the use of immunoconjugates, radioconjugates, and chemotherapy conjugates. Iodine ^{131}I tositumomab (Bexxar) is a monoclonal antibody conjugated with the radioisotope ^{131}I. This anti-CD20 monoclonal antibody targets CD20 antigens on the cell surface of B lymphocytes. Therefore, it has the same immunotoxic effect as rituximab with the added benefit of a radioisotope that can be delivered directly to the tumor.[60]

More recently, two new monoclonal antibodies, bevacizumab (Avastin) and cetuximab (Erbitux), have FDA approval for use in the first-line treatment of metastatic colon cancer. Cetuximab is a monoclonal antibody that targets a protein called the epidermal growth factor receptor found on some colon cancer cells. Bevacizumab, a second humanized monoclonal antibody, prevents the binding of vascular endothelial growth factor (VEGF) to receptors on tumor cells, which prevents microvascular growth of blood vessels and causes existing vessels to regress in the tumor and inhibits tumor growth.

MONOCLONAL ANTIBODIES IN CARDIOVASCULAR THERAPEUTICS

In 1994 the FDA approved abciximab (ReoPro, Centocor B.V. and Eli Lilly) for the prevention of acute ischemic complications in patients with percutaneous transluminal coronary angioplasty (PTCA) who were at high risk for abrupt closure of the treated vessel. Abciximab is the Fab of the chimeric human-murine monoclonal antibody 7E3, with antiplatelet activity designed to reduce arterial thrombus formation after PTCA. Abciximab is one agent in a class of agents called platelet glycoprotein IIb/IIIa receptor inhibitors, which bind to an adhesion receptor involved in platelet aggregation and preventing the binding of fibrinogen, von Willebrand factor, and other adhesive molecules to receptor sites on activated platelets.[61]

Abciximab was studied in a multicenter, double-blind, placebo-control trial in 2,099 patients who were at high risk for abrupt closure of the treated coronary vessel. The primary end point was the occurrence of any of the following events within 30 days of PTCA: death, myocardial infarction, or the need for urgent intervention for recurrent ischemia. There was a 4.5% lower incidence of the primary end point in the monoclonal antibody-treated group than in the placebo group. This difference was statistically significant.[61] Its indications for use have since been widened to include the reduction of acute blood clot complications for all patients undergoing any coronary intervention and the treatment of unstable angina not responding to conventional medical therapy when percutaneous coronary intervention is planned within 24 hours. In addition, it has recently shown long-term mortality benefit when used in combination with coronary stents compared with stenting alone.

Abciximab is associated with a greater frequency of major bleeding complications, which limits its use in patients who are at high risk for bleeding. It has also been shown to cause allergic reactions (anaphylaxis), thrombocytopenia, hypotension (mostly caused by bleeding complications), anemia, pleural effusions, pain at the injection site, and peripheral edema.[61]

MONOCLONAL ANTIBODIES IN GASTROINTESTINAL THERAPEUTICS

In 1999, the FDA approved the first monoclonal antibody for the treatment of Crohn's disease. Infliximab (Remicade) is a part-human, part-mouse antibody that acts by binding to TNF-α, thereby reducing its production and the associated intestinal inflammation seen with Crohn's disease. Infliximab is also the only drug approved for fistulizing Crohn's disease. In a randomized, double-blind, placebo-control dose-ranging study, 108 patients with moderate to severe active Crohn's disease were randomized to receive a single intravenous dose of placebo or 5, 10, or 20 mg per kilogram infliximab.[62] The primary end point of the study was a reduction in the Crohn's disease activity index (CDAI) at week 4. Secondary end points included the proportion of patients who were in clinical remission at week 4 (CDAI <150) and clinical response over time. Sixteen percent of the placebo patients achieved a clinical response compared to 82% of the patients receiving 5 mg per kilogram infliximab (p <0.001), and 48% of patients receiving 5 mg per kilogram infliximab were in clinical remission at week 4, compared to only 4% of placebo-treated patients.

Patients with fistulizing Crohn's disease of at least a 3-month duration were also studied. Ninety-four patients received three doses of placebo or 5 or 10 mg per kilogram infliximab at weeks 0, 2, and 6 and were followed for up to 26 weeks. Again the primary end point was the proportion of patients experiencing a clinical response, defined as a reduction of 50% or more in the number of draining fistulas on gentle compression without an increase in other medications or surgery for Crohn's disease. Of placebo-treated patients, 26% achieved a clinical response, compared to 68% of patients in the 5 mg per kilogram infliximab-treated group (p = 0.002).[63] Long-term treatment studies are under way to determine the safety and efficacy of infliximab beyond the established number of doses for Crohn's disease and fistulizing Crohn's disease. Refer to Chapter 46 for a discussion on the management of Crohn's disease.

MONOCLONAL ANTIBODIES IN RHEUMATOID ARTHRITIS

Although infliximab was first approved for use in Crohn's disease, it is probably most used in the treatment of moderate to severe rheumatoid arthritis. While rheumatoid arthritis has traditionally been treated with disease-modifying antirheumatic drugs (DMARDs), newer evidence suggests that a DMARD, such as methotrexate, in combination with a biologic agent with TNF–α-blocking activity is more effective than DMARDs alone. Infliximab binds to soluble TNF monomers and trimers, and membrane-bound TNF-alpha to form a stable complex which prevents TNF-α from binding to its receptor and triggering a biological response.

In a study of 1,049 patients with rheumatoid arthritis of up to 3 years, methotrexate alone was compared to a combination of methotrexate plus infliximab at two dose schedules (3 mg/kg or 6 mg/kg). Results at 54 weeks of therapy showed that the median percentage of American College of Rheumatology improvement (ACR-N) was higher for the MTX-3 mg per kilogram infliximab and MTX-6 mg per kilogram infliximab groups than for the MTX alone group (38.9% and 46.7% vs., 26.4%, respectively; p <0.001 for both comparisons).[64] Physical functioning also improved significantly more in the combination groups than in the methotrexate alone group. Conversely, there was a significantly higher incidence of serious infections associated with the combination therapy. Tuberculosis reinfection is a rare but serious side effect of infliximab therapy and a thorough medical history regarding TB, tuberculin skin testing, and radiographic examination (if indicated) should be an essential component of infliximab therapy.

GENE THERAPY

The underlying cause of many human diseases can be traced to genetic abnormalities. Whether the abnormality is the lack of a receptor, a defective feedback loop, or the overproduction or underproduction of some pharmacologically active substance, many times the cause is a defect in the genetic code. Traditional therapeutic approaches focus on providing the missing substance or blocking the action of a substance that is overproduced or to which the body is overly sensitive. The aim of gene therapy is to correct the underlying defect in the genetic code.

Gene therapy involves the introduction of foreign genetic material into selected cells in the body to treat disease. It has been made possible by developing effective ways to transfer DNA into mammalian cells and by advances in rDNA technologies.[65] Current approaches in gene therapy do not involve reproductive germ cells (i.e., ovum and spermatozoan). Gene therapy is performed only on nonreproductive cells, therefore its therapeutic effects are not passed on to future generations.

Genetic material can be introduced into mammalian cells by viral and nonviral vectors. Nonviral vectors used in gene transfer consist primarily of liposomes and molecular conjugates.[66] Viral vectors most commonly used in gene transfer include adenoviruses and retroviruses. The major difference between retroviruses and adenoviruses is that retroviruses permanently introduce genes into the chromosomes of infected cells and adenoviruses do not.[67] Retroviruses and adenoviruses are the most commonly used vehicles for transferring genes into human cells.[68] In addition, some other types of viruses, including adeno-associated virus (AAV) and herpes viruses, are being modified in the laboratory for use in gene therapy.[69] Because each of these vector systems have unique advantages and disadvantages, each has applications for which it is best suited.

NONVIRAL VECTORS

Nonviral vectors are primarily synthetic vectors such as liposomes and molecular conjugates. Liposomes, when combined with DNA of any size, can form a lipid-DNA complex capable of delivering genes to many cell types.[66] However, liposomes cannot target specific cell types, so gene transfer occurs primarily in cells that are near the site of administration.[66] Molecular conjugates consisting of protein or synthetic ligands can be coupled with DNA to form a protein-DNA complex. This type of gene delivery system can target different cell types because ligands are target-cell specific.[66]

VIRAL VECTORS

Adenoviral Vectors. Adenoviral vectors are DNA viruses that can infect dividing and nondividing cells. To construct adenoviral vectors, a portion of the viral genome called the E1 region is deleted.[70] This creates space for the therapeutic gene to be inserted, and it renders the virus incapable of self-replication, which prevents viral spread.[71] Adenoviral vectors are efficient in transferring genes into most tissues; unfortunately, gene expression lasts for only a short time (5–10 days post-infection).[71] Enthusiasm for adenoviral vectors has been tempered by the discovery that a significant immune response can be produced by the host against the transduced cells.[71] Today, adenoviral vectors are used in suicide gene therapy, in gene-based immunotherapy, in gene replacement strategies, and in approaches that combine gene therapy with chemotherapy.[72]

Retroviral Vectors. Retroviruses are the most commonly used vectors for ex vivo gene transfer (Fig. 7.6).[73] This ex vivo approach has been favored for early trials because it is technically less complicated, and the modified cells can be monitored and controlled before they are given to a patient. One of the primary advantages of retroviral vectors is their ability to integrate in a stable manner into the host genome, which provides the possibility of long-term gene expression. In addition, retroviruses do not elicit an immune response in the host, as adenoviral vectors do. The main disadvantages of retroviral vectors are that their titers are too low for efficient in vivo gene transfer. In addition, theoretical safety concerns surround the use of retroviral gene delivery. There

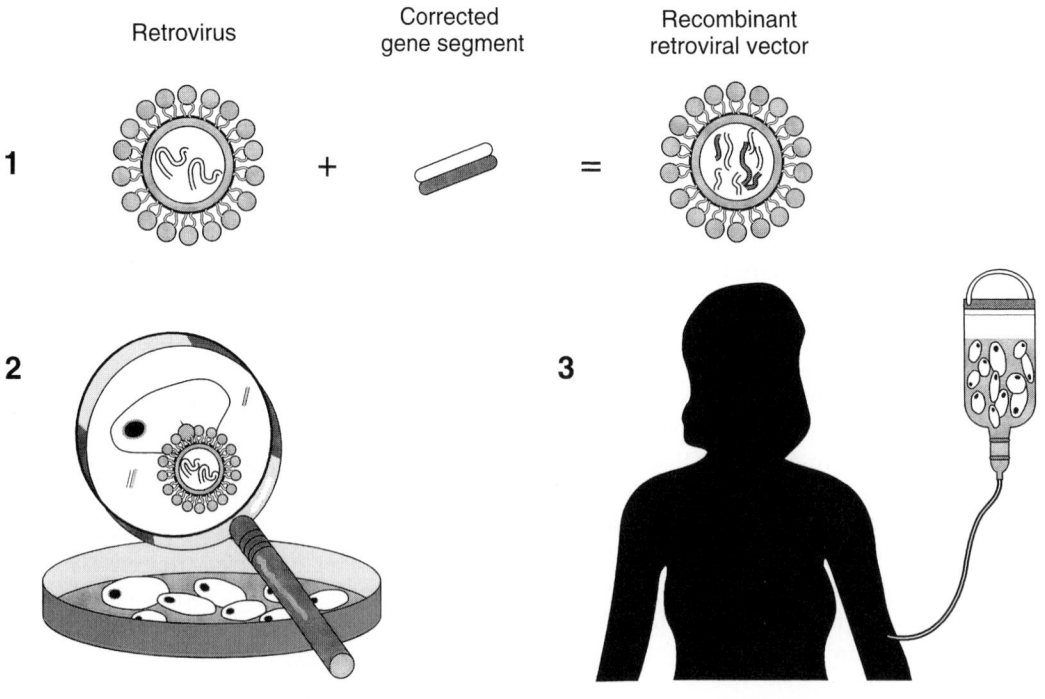

Retrovirus Corrected gene segment Recombinant retroviral vector

1

2 Incubation of target cells with retroviral vector.

3 Introduction of "infected" cells into patient's body, including new gene sequence.

FIGURE 7.6 Ex vivo gene transfer process. **1.** The retrovirus is altered through recombinant DNA technology to add the gene sequence that is to be delivered to the patient. **2.** The retroviral vector is incubated with the target cells, and the desired gene is inserted into the target cells. **3.** The target cells with the desired gene are infused into the patient.

is a risk of generating replication competent retroviruses (RCRs) (i.e., retroviruses that can replicate in the host to cause viral infections) and the risk of inducing insertional mutations through the random integration of the provirus into the host genome.[71]

Adeno-Associated Virus Vectors. AAV vectors contain small, single-stranded DNA genomes and have been shown to transduce brain, skeletal, muscle, and liver when they are injected into the tissue or vasculature.[74] AAVs do not appear to cause an inflammatory response by the host as adenoviruses do.[71] Unfortunately, these vectors have a disadvantage in that there is a limit in the amount of DNA that can be packaged into them. As a result, larger genes cannot be used with this vector.[74]

Herpes Virus Vectors. Herpes virus vectors are DNA viruses that have a large capacity to hold at least 30 kilobase (kb) pairs of exogenous DNA.[72] This large packaging capacity could be very useful for gene therapy purposes to deliver complex genes and regulatory sequences, or to deliver multiple copies of the transgene.[68] Herpes viruses are successful in multiple animal models for cancer and neural tissue gene therapy, and hold promise for intradermal application to sensory neurons.[72] The major problem with herpes virus vectors is their cytopathic effect and the induction of an immune response by viral gene expression.[75]

MANUFACTURE OF VIRAL VECTORS

Pharmaceutical companies face significant issues when determining how to manufacture mass quantities for gene therapy. Good manufacturing practice and quality control procedures, as required by the FDA, are difficult to ensure when working with biologic systems such as viral vectors. With retroviral vectors, the primary safety concern is that an RCR could arise during the manufacturing process. This issue has been analyzed extensively by the National Institutes of Health (NIH) Recombinant DNA Advisory Committee (RAC) and the FDA. The two groups concluded in the late 1990s that with the current FDA-required quality control procedures, it is highly unlikely that a patient would ever receive sufficient RCR to produce a retroviremia or malignancy. However, the manufacturing and testing process that ensures this degree of safety is complex and costly[76] and since that time two infants treated with gene therapy for severe combined immunodeficiency syndrome (SCIDS) have developed malignancies from a retrovirus. Although viral gene delivery systems are considered an efficient form of gene delivery, two factors suggest that nonviral gene delivery systems will be preferred: safety and ease of manufacturing. A synthetic gene delivery system would eliminate the danger of producing a recombinant RCR or other toxicity that could occur with the use of biologically active viral particles.[76]

ETHICAL CONSIDERATIONS IN GENE THERAPY

Although genetic cloning is not considered gene therapy, one particular study attracted considerable attention. In February

1997, scientists in Scotland published an article in *Nature* that described the successful breeding of cloned sheep. An udder cell from a 6-year-old adult sheep was cultured in vitro and the nucleus of this cell was transferred to an enucleated egg, which was then implanted into a surrogate mother. This process led to the birth of a healthy lamb, Dolly, which was genetically identical to the sheep from which the udder cell was taken. This work demonstrated that the process responsible for the normal differentiation of cells could be overcome by nuclear transfer of a differentiated cell into an enucleated egg.[77] Dolly was the first mammal to develop from a cell that was derived from adult tissue and since that time, a dog has been successfully cloned as well as several other species. This experiment attracted worldwide attention and has led to speculation about the possibility of cloning humans.[77]

In March, 1997, then President of the United States, Bill Clinton issued a memorandum that stated: ''Recent accounts of advances in cloning technology, including the first successful cloning of an adult sheep, raise important questions. They potentially represent enormous scientific breakthroughs that could offer benefits in such areas as medicine and agriculture. But the new technology also raises profound ethical issues, particularly with respect to its possible use to clone humans.''[78] The memorandum explicitly prohibited federal funding for cloning of a human being, and also directed the National Bioethics Advisory Commission (NBAC) to thoroughly review the legal and ethical issues associated with the use of cloning technology to create a human being.[79] The report put together by the NBAC was published in September 1999 and is called the ''Ethical Issues in Human Stem Cell Research.''

In March 2001, the FDA clarified its position on cloning with a letter to the research community reminding them that the FDA has jurisdiction over clinical research using cloning technology. The FDA letter states that ''Clinical research using cloning technology to clone a human being is subject to FDA regulation under the Public Health Service Act and the Federal Food, Drug, and Cosmetic Act. Under these statutes and FDA's implementing regulations, before such research may begin, the sponsor of the research is required to: submit to FDA an IND describing the proposed research plan; obtain authorization from a properly constituted institutional review board (IRB); and obtain a commitment from the investigators to obtain informed consent from all human subjects of the research.'' Such research may proceed only when an Investigational New Drug Application (IND) is in effect. Because the FDA believes that there are major unresolved safety questions pertaining to the use of cloning technology to clone a human being, until those questions are appropriately addressed in an IND, FDA would not permit any such investigation to proceed.[80]

CLINICAL APPLICATIONS OF GENE THERAPY

Inhibition of Oncogene Expression. Oncogenes, or tumor-promoting genes, have been implicated in a number of cancers. Oncogenes cause uncontrolled cell growth when mutated or overexpressed, so neutralization of these genes could reverse the malignant phenotype.[71] Methods to replace or deactivate overexpressed tumor-promoting genes have been pursued by a number of researchers. The most common method is to introduce antisense RNA into the cell to stop expression of the oncogene. More recent efforts have included antisense RNA to stop the activity of the tumor-promoting oncogene and a mutant antisense resistant oncogene with the desired activity. This method is theorized to inhibit the expression of the endogenous oncogene, and the "corrected" oncogene restores regulated DNA synthesis.[81]

Introduction of Tumor Suppressor Genes. Tumor suppressor genes, such as p53, are responsible for maintaining normal cell replication. A malfunctioning or missing tumor suppressor gene results in the uncontrolled proliferation of certain malignancies. By introducing a suppressor gene, it may be possible to reverse the malignant potential of the tumor cells.[81] A number of phase I and phase II clinical trials have been performed in patients with a variety of cancers, including ovarian cancer,[82] bladder cancer,[83] brain tumors,[84] hepatobiliary cancers,[85] and lung cancers.[86] Although the results of these studies suggest that gene therapy using tumor suppressor genes can be given safely and may have some antitumor effect, the number of patients in each of these trials is too small to draw any significant conclusions. Additional studies must be done to determine if tumor suppressor gene therapy is safe and effective in larger numbers of patients and if gene therapy is superior to currently available treatments.

Suicide Gene Therapy. Because retroviral DNA is incorporated into rapidly dividing cancer cells more rapidly than normal cells, it is possible to preferentially introduce genetic material into cancer cells. By introducing genes that make the tumor susceptible to substances that will not normally harm cells or cause them to metabolize harmless substances into toxic substances, tumor cells can be killed preferentially. An example of a common suicide gene is the herpes simplex thymidine kinase gene. Nucleoside analogs, such as acyclovir and ganciclovir, bind to this gene product but not to endogenous thymidine kinase. This type of gene therapy was used in a large phase III trial in patients with glioblastoma multiforme (see Clinical Trials: Cancer, below).[87]

Another example of a suicide gene is the *E coli* cytosine deaminase *(cd)* gene. This gene, which is not present in normal mammalian cells, causes the cell to metabolize 5-fluorocytosine, a nontoxic substance, into 5FU, which is toxic to cells. If this gene is inserted into cancer cells, they become susceptible to a substance that will not harm normal cells.[81,88] The first clinical trial using the *cd* gene was done in 12 breast cancer patients. Overexpression of erbB-2 is observed in approximately 20% of breast cancers, and is associated with a reduced relapse-free and overall patient survival. Overexpression of erbB-2 in breast cancer is a re-

sult of increased gene transcription and gene amplification. The activity of the erbB-2 promoter is enhanced in overexpressing cells. Patients in this study received gene therapy using direct intratumoral injection of a plasmid containing an erbB-2 promoter combined with the *cd* gene and then received systemic infusion of the prodrug 5-fluorocytosine. The idea behind this protocol is that fluorocytosine will be activated into fluorouracil within the tumor cells that expressed the oncogene. This study resulted in evidence of gene transfer and expression in 11 of 12 patients, and, importantly, expression seemed to be highly selective for tumor cells.[89] A number of other clinical trials are currently underway evaluating the role of suicide gene therapy in the treatment of brain tumors,[90] ovarian cancer,[91] prostate cancer,[92,93] melanoma,[94] and malignant mesothelioma.[95]

Immunomodulatory Gene Therapy. Introducing tumor-killing cytokines into tumor cells can enhance the host immune response. This can be accomplished in vivo, where the genes for cytokine production are introduced into the tumor, or in vitro, where the cytokine gene is introduced into the tumor cells in culture, then the tumor cells are reinfused into the patient. In a number of preclinical cancer models, injection with tumor cells expressing cytokines such as IL-2, GM-CSF, or IFN-γ can generate cellular immunologic activity against tumors, and in many cases can cure or significantly control the growth of established local or metastatic tumors.[96] A combined cytokine and costimulatory molecule vaccination shows promise as a way to increase the efficiency of tumor vaccines.[96] The most widely studied costimulatory molecule, B7, binds to the CD28 receptor on T-cells and enhances T-cell activation. Transfection of B7 alone into tumor cells inhibits tumor growth through immunologic activity.[96] Covaccination of B7 with IL-2 markedly enhances this activity and may define future approaches to the improvement of vaccination strategies.[96] Another gene therapy approach is to enhance the tumor-killing ability of tumor-infiltrating lymphocytes (TIL) by inserting the gene for TNF into harvested TIL cells and then reinfusing them. This localizes the therapeutic effect of TNF and limits systemic exposure.[97]

RNA Interference. A recent advancement that may help researchers discover new targets to gene therapy is called RNA interference. RNA interference occurs when small pieces of double-stranded RNA (small interfering RNA [siRNA]) suppress the expression of target genes. The discovery of this cellular gene silencing mechanism has already proven itself as a powerful tool for the study of gene function in mammals. The therapeutic potential for RNA interference is enormous, with applications for a wide spectrum of diseases, including some that have thus far proven intractable.[98,99]

CLINICAL TRIALS

Therapeutic trials of gene therapy have been undertaken in cancer, genetic diseases, and infectious diseases. Genetic diseases that have been targeted include SCIDS, Gaucher's disease, Franconia's anemia, cystic fibrosis, and hypercholesterolemia.[67] The primary infectious disease targeted by gene therapy is AIDS, however there are some clinical trials evaluating the effectiveness of gene therapy in the treatment of Epstein-Barr virus infection and cytomegalovirus infection. The FDA has not yet approved for sale any human gene therapy product. However, gene-related research and development continues to grow. Between 1989 and 2003, over 900 gene therapy clinical trials were approved worldwide.[100] In the United States, as of March 2005, 680 gene therapy protocols were submitted to the NIH and FDA for approval: 446 for cancer, 60 for monogenic diseases (cystic fibrosis, familial hypercholesteremia, Gaucher's disease, hemophilia, SCID), 42 for infectious diseases, and 79 for other diseases, including peripheral artery disease, coronary artery disease, arthritis, heart failure, and eye disorders. There are 50 protocols that are for marker or nontherapeutic trials.[101]

Although gene therapy showed early promise in the treatment or prevention of disease, it has not delivered the promised results.[102] While the concept of gene therapy is relatively simple, the reality of translating this new technology into the clinic has proven to be more difficult than first imagined.[100] The main reasons for the relatively disappointing results in gene therapy include inadequacies of the gene delivery systems (or vectors), poor expression of the recombinant genes, and induction of immune response to the gene-modified cells or the gene delivery vectors.[100] In fact, a massive immune response to an adenoviral vector resulted in the tragic death of an 18-year-old patient by the name of Jesse Gelsinger. This case stunned the scientific community and caused many to question the safety of gene therapy.[100]

The patient suffered from ornithine transcarbamylase (OTC) deficiency, a rare genetic defect in the liver that leaves the body unable to clear ammonia from the blood. In September 1999, the patient entered a phase I gene therapy trial at the University of Pennsylvania's Institute of Human Gene Therapy in Philadelphia. In this particular study, an adenoviral vector which contained human OTC cDNA was infused into the patient's right hepatic artery. Within 4 days of receiving the treatment, the patient died.[103] The authors concluded ultimately that Gelsinger had a systemic inflammatory response to the gene therapy treatment, followed by disseminated intravascular coagulation and multiple organ system failure. The FDA, along with the NIH launched several investigations into gene therapy studies all over the country. Later, the University of Pennsylvania investigators were cited for multiple protocol violations in the trial. In addition, the NIH revealed that only 6% of all serious events observed in patients during past and current clinical gene therapy trials were reported to the NIH. These findings triggered a series of corrective actions by the FDA and the NIH.[104]

In March 2001, the Department of Health and Human Services announced two initiatives by the FDA and the NIH.

The first was the Gene Therapy Clinical Trial Monitoring Plan that was designed to increase the level of scrutiny with additional reporting required for study sponsors. Monitors are selected by and report to the sponsor or the sponsor's designee. These monitors verify that the rights and well-being of the subjects are being protected, that the conduct of the trial is in accordance with the protocol and regulatory requirements, and that data reporting (including safety reporting to IRB, FDA, and NIH) is accurate and complete. The second initiative was a series of Gene Transfer Safety Symposia, designed to bring together leading experts in gene transfer research and give them an opportunity to discuss the medical and scientific data. These symposia are supposed to address such gene transfer topics as monitoring of data safety, cardiovascular complications of vector administration, good clinical practice in research, cell and gene therapy, guidance development for product quality control and assurance, entry criteria and informed consent for participants in gene transfer research, and use of drugs to control promoters in gene therapy vectors.

The ''Gelsinger'' case was quickly followed by the first reported ''success'' of gene therapy in 2000.[105] Researchers in Paris successfully corrected the immune defect in infants with life-threatening X-linked severe combined immune deficiency (SCID-X) with gene therapy (see Clinical Trials: Genetic Diseases, below). Following this, Italian investigators reported equally impressive results in children with SCIDS due to adenosine deaminase (ADA) deficiency.[106] Although these results suggest that gene therapy has the potential to fulfill its early promise, researchers have a long way to go before gene therapy becomes a ''standard'' therapy in the treatment of any disease.

Cancer Gene Therapy. The first human trial of gene therapy conducted in the United States began in May 1989 and was designed not as a direct therapeutic trial, but as a method of marking cells critical to the treatment of cancer. The trial used a retroviral vector to genetically mark TILs in patients with cancer.[65] In TIL therapy, which is used for metastatic melanoma and renal cell carcinoma, part of the tumor is removed, and the lymphoid cells that had successfully infiltrated the tumor are harvested. These TIL cells are then cultured with IL-2 to stimulate growth. The large numbers of TIL cells are then reinfused into the patient. The TIL cells were marked by inserting the genetic code for the bacterial antibiotic resistance gene neomycin phosphotransferase, which makes it possible to track them.[81]

One multicenter phase III trial was completed in patients with glioblastoma multiforme, a malignant brain tumor. The goal of this trial was to insert a gene capable of directing cell killing to the tumor cells while protecting the normal brain cells. In the case of glioblastoma multiforme, the only dividing cells in the area of a brain tumor are tumor cells and the vascular endothelial cells which supply blood to the tumor. However, because retroviral vectors transduce only into dividing cells, only tumor cells and tumor blood vessel cells would be targeted. Retroviral vectors were then modified to carry the herpes simplex thymidine kinase gene. This gene adds a phosphate group to nonphosphorylated nucleosides, whereas the endogenous human thymidine kinase cannot. Thus, when an abnormal nucleoside, such as the drug ganciclovir, is given to a patient, only the cells that express the herpes simplex thymidine kinase gene will phosphorylate the drug, incorporate it into their DNA, and be killed. This clinical trial included 248 patients with newly diagnosed glioblastoma multiforme. Patients received standard therapy (surgical resection and radiation therapy) or standard therapy plus adjuvant gene therapy during surgery. The gene therapy was given during surgery into the wall of the resection cavity and into any accessible residual tumor. This study found that adjuvant gene therapy provided no significant differences in terms of progression free survival, median survival, or 12-month survival rates. Despite the results, this study did show that this gene therapy was feasible and had a good safety profile in this group of patients.[107,108]

There are a number of other clinical trials underway evaluating gene therapy in various types of cancers, including brain tumors, pancreatic cancer, prostate cancer, ovarian cancer, head and neck (oropharyngeal) cancer, nonsmall cell lung cancer, melanoma, and renal cell carcinoma.[109] A few of these trials are phase III studies, while most are phase I and phase II. It is important to note that a number of these clinical trials are evaluating gene therapy in combination with chemotherapy, rather than evaluating gene therapy alone. Over the past decade, there has been a growing appreciation of the broader scope of gene therapy, and the potential for gene-based approaches to complement conventional therapies in diseases such as cancer.

Genetic Diseases. In September 1990, a therapeutic trial designed to treat ADA deficiency in children with SCIDS was initiated.[65] This was the first therapeutic human gene therapy trial. The protocol called for the isolation of peripheral lymphocytes from an ADA-deficient patient. The human ADA gene was then introduced into the lymphocytes with a retroviral vector in vitro. The modified lymphocytes were multiplied and then reintroduced into two young girls. The patients were retreated at 6- to 8-week intervals.[65] Both girls have gene-engineered T lymphocytes in their circulation after more than 10 years, expressing transgenic adenosine deaminase, however, the therapeutic effect of gene therapy remained difficult to assess in these cases because of the concomitant treatment with polyethylene glycol-ADA (PEG-ADA).[110]

In April 2000, Cavazzana–Calvo[105] in Paris reported successful correction of the immune defect in infants with life-threatening X-linked SCID-X with gene therapy.[105] The immune reconstitution in gene therapy-treated infants was impressive and far exceeded the results of matched unrelated or haplo-identical transplantation, which are the only treat-

ment options for these types of patients.[100] Unfortunately, 2 of the 14 infants treated developed acute leukemia as a complication of the gene therapy. Although both patients responded to conventional therapy, this illustrates the dangers of genetic manipulation, and has raised serious doubts regarding the potential of this treatment modality.[100] The breakthrough reported by Cavazzana–Calvo was followed by equally impressive results in two children with SCIDS because of ADA deficiency.[106] However, as a result of the development of leukemia in two of the patients in the Paris study, the FDA initially put on hold all gene therapy trials using retroviral vectors to insert new genes in blood stem cells.[111] However, in March, 2003, the NIH RAC sent a memorandum to principal investigators that concluded that although the development of leukemia in those two patients was directly caused by the gene therapy, the committee members felt that there was not sufficient data or reports of adverse events directly attributable to the use of retrovirals at this time to warrant the cessation of other retroviral human gene transfer studies.[112]

Gene therapy is under evaluation as a potential treatment option for cystic fibrosis. Cystic fibrosis is a recessive genetic disease caused by mutations in the cystic fibrosis transmembrane conductance regulator (CFTR) gene. The normal CFTR gene codes for a protein (CFTR) that plays a key part in epithelial transport of salt and water. Mutations in the CFTR gene result in abnormal secretions that obstruct and damage the epithelium in many areas of the body.[106] Patients who are homozygous for mutations in the CFTR gene have defective cyclic AMP (cAMP) regulated secretion of chloride and increased absorption of sodium in the airway epithelium. This leads to thickening of airway secretions, impaired mucociliary clearance, leading to chronic bacterial infections in the airway.[113] Individuals who are carriers of a mutation in the CFTR gene, versus those who are homozygous for mutations, do not have lung disease. This suggests that a single copy of the normal CFTR gene is sufficient for normal defense of the lung. Gene therapy has potential in the treatment of cystic fibrosis because the transfer of a single copy of the normal CFTR gene into the epithelial cells affected by cystic fibrosis may correct airway function.[113] Numerous investigators have studied the possibility of introducing a normal copy of the CFTR gene into the airway of the epithelium of cystic fibrosis patients. One study done in 12 cystic fibrosis patients involved the administration of an adenoviral vector containing the normal CFTR gene given via the nasal epithelium. The results showed that adenoviral vector mediated transfer of the CFTR gene did not correct the defects in the nasal epithelium and that the local inflammatory response limited the dose of adenovirus that could be given.[113] A more recent phase I trial was done in 25 cystic fibrosis patients in which a recombinant adeno-associated virus serotype 2 (rAAV2) expressing the CFTR gene was given intranasally and into the lower lobe of the right lung. The results of this study showed that gene transfer, as measured by DNA PCR, did occur to some extent, suggesting that the rAAV2 vector should continue to be evaluated in additional clinical trials of cystic fibrosis patients.[114]

Familial hypercholesterolemia, a disease characterized by extraordinarily high levels of cholesterol, has also been treated with gene therapy. The disease is caused by defective or absent receptors for low-density lipoprotein (LDL). One gene therapy study, published in 1996, evaluated five patients with homozygous familial hypercholesterolemia. Patients underwent removal of a portion of their liver and placement of a portal venous catheter. Hepatocytes obtained from the liver were then transduced with a recombinant retrovirus encoding the gene for the human LDL receptor. The genetically modified cells were then transplanted into the liver through a portal venous catheter.[115] The authors concluded that this type of gene therapy is safe in humans and may be effective in some patients. However, the number of patients in this particular study was relatively small, and no studies in this patient group have been done since that time.

GENOMICS AND PROTEOMICS

In the past, drug discovery and development has been costly, complicated, and viewed as a series of trial and error processes with most conventionally developed drugs never making it to human phase III clinical studies. However, the advent of genomic and proteomic technologies, has allowed for the development of new therapeutic approaches to proceed at a more rapid pace. The genome is the full complement of an organism's genetic information and includes coding and noncoding DNA sequences. The proteome is the set of encoding DNA regions that result in protein production.[116] The role then of functional genomics is to "prioritize targets" found through the sequencing of the human genome and translate that knowledge into new drug discovery. Now that the human genome has been fully sequenced, we know that there are approximately 25,000 genes and thousands of splice variants of mRNA transcripts within it. To effectively and completely explore the entire genome, we must use technologies capable of identifying, validating, and prioritizing thousands of genes to determine the best "targets" to try to isolate.

GENOMICS

One approach to exploring the human genome is to mine the genetic sequence for similarly known gene families with a range of sequence-search methods. The focus of this approach is to mine for additional members of gene families that are already known to contain drug targets. All sequence search methods start with identifying homologues that share 30% or greater base pair sequences. Another is the utilization of comparative genomics whereby sequences of known genomes of different organisms are compared with similar human genome sequences. There is speculation that approximately 40% of human genes have biological functions that

are unknown and that there could be many disease targets in this pool of unknown genes.

One of the most effective methods used to mine the human genome to date is RNA profiling using high-density arrays of DNA on glass. With this methodology, over 500,000 short DNA sequences (probes) are attached to a glass surface smaller than 2 cm. Different RNA sequences extracted from cells or tissues are converted into cDNA and fluorescently labeled. The fluorescently labeled cDNA is hybridized to the probes and is thus identified. These technologies can be used to compare RNA and DNA levels in diseased tissues with those from normal tissues. RNA profiling has been used in the classification of cancers by reflecting the identity of the source tissue. It may also be useful in predicting drug responsiveness.[116]

Pharmacogenomics. One way in which an understanding of variations in the human genome is advancing science, is through pharmacogenomics: the study of how genetic inheritance influences response to drugs. A better understanding of how individual genetics determines drug response has a great potential to revitalize the use of many drugs. One example of this is with the cancer drug, thioguanine, used to treat acute myelogenous leukemia. Thioguanine acts as a prodrug which is incorporated into DNA to turn off DNA synthesis and prevent cell growth. Thioguanine must be metabolized to thioguanine nucleotide (TGN) to exert its effect. If thioguanine is not metabolized but instead methylated by thiopurine methyltransferase (TPMT), the thioguanine does not produce TGNs. It has been found that TPMT activity is highly variable and polymorphic in human populations with 90% having high activity, 10% having intermediate activity, and 0.3% having low or no activity. Many studies have now shown that patients who are TPMT deficient are at high risk of developing severe hematopoietic toxicity if treated with conventional doses of thioguanine. By using a relatively inexpensive and rapid assay, more than 90% of all mutant alleles can be detected and toxicities with thioguanine can be avoided. With advances being made in genomics, it is hopeful that some day individualized cancer therapy may be utilized based on a patient's specific genetic profile.[117]

PROTEOMICS

While the genome in each cell determines the potential for gene and protein expression, it does not specify which proteins will be expressed, to what level they are expressed, or the extent of their posttranslational modifications. In addition, it is difficult to determine cellular protein levels because they are constantly being upregulated, down regulated, cleaved, and phosphorylated. Proteomics is the study of protein function, which includes protein to protein interactions and the study of protein expression. Many laboratories around the world are busy utilizing different methodologies to identify proteins for drug targets. The most often used tools for protein identification include mass spectrometry, the use of two-dimensional gel electrophoresis, and x-ray crystallography. To identify specific protein expression within cells, specimens of extracted proteins from a given cell (normal or tumor cells) are put onto a two-dimensional gel, which is then fed via robotic systems through an electrophoresis machine and spots of interest are excised. These protein spots are then fed into a mass spectrometer. Mass spectrometry works on the principle that substances carrying a net electric charge can be made to move in a predictable way in an electromagnetic field. Ions are sorted by their charge to mass ratio and from there a "fingerprint" of the sample can be derived. That fingerprint is then matched to a protein database for identification. The resulting differentially expressed or modified protein(s) represent the potential target(s) in a tumor or diseased cell.[118]

GENERIC BIOTECHNOLOGICALS

There is debate between generic drug manufacturers and biotechnology companies over whether the FDA should allow "biogenerics" or "biosimilars." At the core of the debate is the issue of whether a biotechnologically produced drug can ever be "generically created" because biotechnology products are produced by cells in culture and in microorganisms that are very sensitive to the external environment and conditions to which they are exposed. The biotechnology companies state that even under their most stringently controlled culture conditions, proteins will show a high degree of heterogeneity with respect to glycosylation and folding. Any altered step in the process can cause changes to clinical properties or biological activity. And because of this, production is highly controlled with an emphasis on the genetic stability of the cellular expression system and the reproducibility of the production process which includes hundreds of control steps. The biotech companies believe that the process of biotechnologically produced products is the actual product and that the process cannot be reproduced by generic manufacturers.

However, the generic companies argue that while the process is much more complex, it is not impossible to reproduce. They believe that they should be able to use surrogate markers to demonstrate therapeutic equivalency and safety. In addition, there is currently an example of a biogeneric product on the market, interferon α-2b, that is manufactured via a different fermentation and purification process at a different manufacturing site from the original biotechnologically produced product and that over 9 million doses of the product have been made that is equivalent to the original.

Under the current regulatory environment, when a small-molecule drug goes off patent, then a generic company can file for the ability to market a generic version of the product by filing a more limited submission with the FDA. The generic manufacturer only has to show that the product is physicochemically identical to the innovator drug and a bioequivalence study must be performed in a limited crossover schema in human volunteers. These kinds of studies are not possible with biotechnologically produced proteins. For the FDA, some key questions that will need to be answered before this debate is resolved include: how similar do the physicochemical properties of the biogeneric and the innovator product need to be for the biogeneric to be granted a marketing authorization from the FDA; does the biogeneric product have to have the same gene sequence, vector, host cell line, culture conditions, and purification methods as the innovator product, or can a totally different manufacturing process be used if it creates a protein that is comparable to the innovator protein. In the mean time, several biopharmaceuticals are already off patent (imiglucerase, alglucerase, interferon α-2b, human insulin, and epoetin alfa) and several more will be going off patent in the next few years. With health care costs rising at such a rapid rate, the FDA will need to resolve this debate and find a way to bring generic biopharmaceuticals to market.[119]

CONCLUSION

Biotechnology used to be synonymous with the emergence of rDNA technology, which was capable of producing human proteins to replace what had been turned off by disease processes (insulin, Factor VIII, growth hormone). That technology evolved to an understanding of antigen-antibody interactions, and monoclonal antibodies were born to target specific cell receptors (trastuzumab, rituximab). Today, the mapping of the human genome and gene therapy is taking us back inside the human cell to transfer rDNA to create desired proteins to turn on or off disease processes. Biotechnology has come a long way since the discovery of the double helix with many products in the pipeline. We continue to be on the cusp of biotechnological discovery, which will impact many diseases that have up to now eluded effective intervention.

KEY POINTS

- Our understanding of rDNA technology and gene therapy is fundamentally changing the way we will treat diseases in the future
- Biotechnology products are being produced at a remarkably rapid pace and are providing new therapies for some diseases that previously had no treatment (Table 7.3)
- Gene therapy can offer a cure for many previously incurable diseases if the techniques for its production are refined and safety concerns are addressed
- Pharmacists must have a working knowledge of new methods of drug delivery, and of the different biotechnologically produced therapeutic products that will be the drugs of the future

(*text continues on page 158*)

TABLE 7.3	Selected Biotechnology Products in the Marketplace		
Therapeutic Category	**Product (Trade Name), Company**	**Application**	**Approval Year**
Autoimmune disorders	Recombinant interferon-β1B (Betaseron), Berlex Labs/Chiron	Relapsing, remitting multiple sclerosis	1993
	Recombinant interferon-β1B (Avonex), Biogen	Relapsing forms of multiple sclerosis	1996
Blood disorders	Human antihemophilic factor (Alphanate), Alpha Therapeutic Corp.	Treatment of hemophilia A or acquired factor VII deficiency	1997
	Recombinant factor VIIa (NovoSeven), Novo Nordisk	Treatment of hemophilia A or B with inhibitors to factors VIII or IX	1999
	Human coagulation factor IX (virus-filtered) (AlphaNine SD), Alpha Therapeutic Corp.	To prevent and control bleeding in patients with factor IX defiency caused by hemophilia B	1996
	Coagulation factor IX (recombinant) (BeneFix), Genetics Institute	Treatment of hemophilia B	1997
	Recombinant antihemophilic factor (Bioclate Helixate), Centeon, (Kogenate), Bayer (Recombinate), Baxter Healthcare (Genetics Institute)	Blood-clotting factor VIII for the treatment of hemophilia A	1993, 1994 1989, 1986
	Epoetin-α (Epogen), Amgen	Treatment of anemia associated with chronic renal failure and anemia in AZT-treated HIV-infected patients	1989, 1990 (AZT indication only)
	Epoetin-α (Procrit), Ortho Biotech	Anemia in patients on cancer chemotherapy	1993, 1996
		Use in anemic patients scheduled to undergo elective noncardiac, nonvascular surgery	
	Immune globulin (Venoglobulin-S), Alpha Therapeutic Corp.	Primary immunodeficiency	1995 1991
		Idiopathic thrombocytopenic purpura	
		Kawasaki disease	
	Granulocyte-macrophage colony-stimulating factor (Leukine), Berlex	Neutrophil recovery after autologous and allogeneic BMT	1991, 1995
		Treatment of neutropenia after induction chemotherapy in older patients with acute myeloid leukemia	
		Mobilization of peripheral progenitor cells for peripheral stem cell transplant	
	Granulocyte colony-stimulating factor (Neupogen), Amgen	Chemotherapy-induced neutropenia	1994, 1994 1995, 1995
		BMT accompanied by neutropenia	1991
		Severe chronic neutropenia	
		Autologous BMT engraftment or failure	
		Mobilization of autologous peripheral blood progenitor cells after chemotherapy	

(continued)

TABLE 7.3	continued		

Therapeutic Category	Product (Trade Name), Company	Application	Approval Date
Cancer	Interleukin-11 (Neumega), Genetics Institute	Prevention of severe chemotherapy-induced thrombocytopenia	1/97
	Liposomal daunorubicin (DaunoXome), NeXstar Pharmaceuticals Inc.	Treatment for HIV-related Kaposi's sarcoma	1996
	Pegylated liposomal doxorubicin hydrochloride (Doxil STEALTH), SEQUUS Pharmaceuticals Inc.	Second-line therapy for Kaposi's sarcoma in patients with AIDS (liposomal drug delivery)	1995
	Interferon-α (Intron A), Schering-Plough	Hairy cell leukemia	1986, 1988 1992, 1997
		AIDS-related Kaposi's sarcoma	
	(Roferon-A), Hoffmann-La Roche Inc.	Malignant melanoma Follicular lymphoma with chemotherapy	
	2-CDA (Leustatin), Ortho Biotech	Hairy cell leukemia	1993
	Pegasparginase (Oncaspar), Enzon	Pegylated asparaginase for the treatment of acute lymphoblastic leukemia	1994
	Porfimer sodium (Photofrin), Ligand Pharmaceuticals	Palliative treatment of totally and partially obstructing cancers of esophagus	1995
	Interleukin-2 (Proleukin), Chiron	Treatment of renal carcinoma	1992, 1998
		Treatment of metastatic melanoma	
	Rituximab (Rituxin), Biogen-IDEC Pharmaceuticals/Genentech	Relapsed or refractory low-grade or follicular CD20-positive B-cell non-Hodgkin's lymphoma	1997
Cardiovascular disorders	Tissue plasminogen activator (Activase),	Treatment of acute myocardial infarction	1987, 1996 1990, 1996
	Genentach (Retavase), Centocor, Inc.	Treatment of acute massive pulmonary embolism	
		Treatment of acute ischemic stroke within 3 hours of onset	
	Human albumin (Albutein), Alpha Therapeutic Corp.	Treatment of hypovolemic shock	1986
		Use in cardiopulmonary bypass procedures	
	Abciximab (ReoPro), Centocor, Inc./Eli Lily	Reduce acute blood clot-related complications in high-risk PTCA patients	1994, 1997
		Reduce acute blood clot-related complications for all patients undergoing any coronary intervention	
		Treatment of unstable angina not responding to conventional treatment when PTCA is planned within 24 hours	

(continued)

TABLE 7.3	continued		
Therapeutic Category	**Product (Trade Name), Company**	**Application**	**Approval Date**
Endocrine disorders	Recombinant insulin (Humalog), Eli Lily	Treatment of diabetes	1996 1982
	(Humulin-human), Eli-Lily		1982
	(Novolin-human), Novo Nordisk		
	Repaglinide (Prandin), Novo Nordisk	Antidiabetic agent for the treatment of type 2 diabetes	1997
Genetic disorders	Growth hormone (BioTroin), Biotech General	Growth hormone deficiency in children	1995 1985 1997
	(Protropin), Genentech	Growth hormone deficiency in children and adults	1995 1997
	(Norditropin), Novo Nordisk		1996
	(Geref), Serono labs	Somatotropin deficiency syndrome in adults	
	(GenoTropin), Pharmacia and Upjohn		
	(Humatrope), Eli Lily		
	Somatropin rDNA (Nutropin/Nutropin AQ), Genentech	Growth hormone deficiency in children and adults	1993, 1994 1996
		Growth failure associated with chronic renal insufficiency before kidney transplantation	
		Short stature associated with Turner syndrome	
	Dornase, α recombinant (Pulmozyme), Genentech	Mild to moderate cystic fibrosis	1993 ,1996
		Advanced cystic fibrosis	
	Ceredase, Genzyme	Treatment of type I Gaucher's disease	1991
Infectious diseases	Liposomal amphotericin B (Abelcet), The Liposome Company	Treatment of invasive fungal infections in patients who are refractory to or intolerant of conventional amphotericin B	1995 1997 1996
	(AmBisome), NeXstar Pharmaceuticals Inc.	Second-line treatment of invasive aspergillosis infections	
	(AMPHOTEC), SEQUUS Pharmaceuticals		
	Interferonalphacon-1 (Infergen)	Hepatitis C	1997
	Immune globulin-enriched in antibodies against respiratory syncytial virus (RespiGam), MedImmune, Inc.	Prevention of respiratory syncytial virus in infants under 2 with bronchopulmonary dysplasia or history of prematurity	1996
Immune function disorders	Interferon-γ1b (Actimmune), Genentech	Treatment of chronic granulomatous disease	1990
	Adenosine deaminase (Adagen), Enzon	Treatment of severe combined immunodeficiency disease	1990

(continued)

TABLE 7.3	continued		
Therapeutic Category	**Product (Trade Name), Company**	**Application**	**Approval Date**
Reproductive disorders	Follicle-stimulating hormone (Follistim), Organon Inc. (Fertinex), Serono Labs	Recombinant hormone for treatment of infertility	1997 1996
	Follitropin-α (Gonal-F)	Functional infertility not caused by primary ovarian failure	1997
Transplant	CMV immune globulin (CytoGam), MedImmune Inc.	Prevention of cytomegalovirus in patients undergoing kidney transplant	1990
	Muromonab-CD-3 (Orthoclone OKT3), Ortho Biotech	Reversal of acute kidney, heart, and liver transplant rejection	1986
	Daclizumab (Zenapax), Hoffmann-La Roche	Humanized monoclonal antibody for the prevention of kidney transplant rejection	1997
	Basiliximab (Simulect), Novartis Pharmaceutical Corp.		1998
Vaccines	Recombinant hepatitis B vaccine (Recombivax-HB), Merck	Hepatitis B vaccine for adolescents and high-risk infants/adults/ dialysis/pediatrics	1987 1989 1993 1989
	(Engerix-B), SmithKline Beecham		
Other	Platelet-derived growth factor becaplermin (Regranex-Gel), Ortho-McNeil/Chiron	Treatment of diabetic foot ulcers	1997

AZT, azidothymidine; HIV, human immunodeficiency virus; BMT, bone marrow transplantation; AIDS, acquired immune deficiency syndrome; CDA, congenital dyserythropoietic anemia; IDEC, inflammatory dendritic epidermal cells; PTCA, percutaneous transluminal coronary angioplasty; CMV, cytomegalovirus.

SUGGESTED READINGS

Ratledge C, Kristiansen B. Basic biotechnology. New York: Cambridge University Press, 2001.
Smith JE. Biotechnology. 4th ed. New York: Cambridge University Press, 2004.

REFERENCES

1. Regents of the University of Wisconsin System. An introduction to pharmaceutical biotechnology, 1990.
2. Eckelbecker L. From Goat to Champion. Sunday Telegram, Worcester, MA, May 8, 2005.
3. Gerngross TU. Advances in the production of human therapeutic proteins in yeasts and filamentous fungi. Nat Biotechnol 22: 1409–1414, 2004.
4. Wurm FM. Production of recombinant protein therapeutics in cultivated mammalian cells. Nat Biotechnol 22:1393–1398, 2004.
5. Avidor Y, Mabjeesh NJ, Matzkin H. Biotechnology and drug discovery: from bench to bedside, South Med J 96:1174–1186, 2003.
6. Kleinberg M, Mosdell KW. Current and future considerations for the new classes of biologicals. Am J Health-Syst Pharm 61: 695–708, 2004.
7. Alteplase [package insert]. San Francisco, CA: Genentech; August, 2001
8. Wooster MB, Luzier AB. Reteplase: a new thrombolytic for the treatment of acute myocardial infarction. Ann Pharmacother 33: 318–324, 1999.
9. TNKase [package insert]. San Francisco, CA: Genentech; June, 2004.
10. Lepirudin [package insert]. Montville, NJ: Berlex; October, 2004.
11. Dertzbaugh MT. Genetically engineered vaccines: a review. Plasmid 39:100–113, 1998.
12. Center for Disease Control. Lyme disease vaccine information. Available at: http://www.cdc.gov/nip/menus/vaccines.htm#lyme. Accessed December 7, 2005.
13. Dunn CJ, Plosker GL, Keating GM, et al. Insulin glargine: an updated review of its use in the management of diabetes mellitus. Drugs 63:1743–1778, 2003.
14. Noble SL, Johnston E, Walton B. Insulin Lispro: a fast-acting insulin analog. Am Fam Physician 57:279–286, 289–292, 1998.
15. Vance ML. Can growth hormone prevent aging? N Eng J Med 348:779–780, 2003.
16. Mulligan K, Grunfeld C, Hellerstein MK, et al. Anabolic effects of recombinant human growth hormone in patients with wasting associated with human immunodeficiency virus infection. J Clin Endocrinol Metab 77:956–962, 1993.
17. Ovidrel [package insert]. Rockland, MA: Serono Labs; 2000.
18. Forteo [package insert]. Indianapolis, IN: Eli Lilly; 2002.
19. Thyrogen [package insert]. Cambridge, MA: Genzyme; 2003.

20. Whittington R, Faulds D. Interleukin-2, a review of its pharmacological properties and therapeutic use in patients with cancer. Drugs 46:446–514, 1993.
21. Oprelvekin (IL-11; Neumega) [package insert]. Cambridge, MA: Genetics Institute; 1998.
22. Isaacs C, Roberg NJ, Bailey FA, et al. Randomized placebo-controlled study of recombinant human interleukin-11 to prevent chemotherapy-induced thrombocytopenia in patients with breast cancer receiving dose-intensive cyclophosphamide and doxorubicin. J Clin Oncol 15:3368–3377, 1997.
23. Tepler I, Elias L, Smith JW, et al. A randomized placebo-controlled trial of recombinant human interleukin-11 in cancer patients with severe thrombocytopenia due to chemotherapy. Blood 87:3607–3614, 1996.
24. Gabrilove J. Introduction and overview of hematopoietic growth factors. Semin Hematol 26:1–4, 1989.
25. Yee GC. Focus on GM-CSF and G-CSF: promising biotherapeutics for use in hematology and oncology. Hosp Formul 25:943–948, 1990.
26. Bettelheim P, Muhm M, Valent P, et al. GM-CSF in combination with cytotoxic chemotherapy in AML patients. Bone Marrow Transplant 1:127–130, 1990.
27. Buechner T, Hiddemann W, Koenigsmann M, et al. Recombinant human GM-CSF following chemotherapy in high-risk AML. Bone Marrow Transplant 1:131–133, 1990.
28. Vose JM, Armitage JO. Clinical applications of hematopoietic growth factors. J Clin Oncol 13:1023–1035, 1995.
29. Moore M. Hematopoietic growth factors in cancer. Cancer 65: 836–844, 1990.
30. Appelbaum FR. The clinical use of hematopoietic growth factors. Semin Hematol 26:7–14, 1989.
31. Morstyn G, Lieschke G, Sheridan W, et al. Clinical experience with recombinant human granulocyte colony-stimulating factor and granulocyte macrophage colony-stimulating factor. Semin Hematol 26:9–13, 1989.
32. Glaspy J, Golde D. Clinical applications of the myeloid growth factors. Semin Hematol 26:14–17, 1989.
33. NCCN Web site for growth factor guidelines. Available at: http://www.nccn.org/professionals/physician_gls/PDF/myeloid_growth.pdf. Accessed December 7, 2005.
34. NOA Website for growth factor guidelines. Available at: http://guidelines.noainc.com/main.cfm?LoadId=161052. Accessed December 7, 2005.
35. Tyring SK. Interferons: biochemistry and mechanisms of action. Am J Obstet Gynecol 172:1350–1353, 1995.
36. Agarwala S, Kirkwood J. Interferons in the therapy of solid tumors. Oncology 51:129–136, 1994.
37. McManus BC. Clinical use of biologic response modifiers in cancer treatment. Ann Pharmacother 24:761–767, 1990.
38. Takaku F. Clinical application of cytokines for cancer treatment. Oncology 51:123–128, 1994.
39. Ozer H, George SL, Schiffer CA, et al. Prolonged subcutaneous administration of recombinant alpha 2b interferon in patients with previously untreated Philadelphia chromosome-positive chronic-phase chronic myelogenous leukemia: effect on remission duration and survival: Cancer and Leukemia Group B Study 8583. Blood 82: 2975–2984, 1993.
40. Tura S, Baccarani M, Zuffa E, et al. Interferon alpha 2a as compared with conventional chemotherapy for the treatment of chronic myeloid leukemia. N Engl J Med 330:820–825, 1994.
41. Kirkwood JM, Strawderman MH, Ernstoff MS, et al. Interferon alfa-2b adjuvant therapy of high-risk resected cutaneous melanoma: the Eastern Cooperative Oncology Group Trial EST 1684. J Clin Oncol 14:7–17, 1996.
42. Urabe A. Interferons for the treatment of hematological malignancies. Oncology 51:137–141, 1994.
43. Spiegel RJ. The alpha interferons: clinical overview. Semin Oncol 14:1–12, 1987.
44. Moreno L, Quereda C, Moreno A, et al. Pegylated interferon alpha2b plus ribavirin for the treatment of chronic hepatitis C in HIV-infected patients. AIDS 18:67–73, 2004.
45. Lindsay KL, Trepo C, Heintges T, et al. A randomized, double-blind trial comparing pegylated interferon alfa-2b to interferon alfa-2b as initial treatment for chronic hepatitis C). Hepatology 34: 395–403, 2001.
46. Mangia A, Ricci GL, Persico M. A randomized controlled trial of pegylated interferon alpha-2a (40KD) or interferon alpha-2a plus ribavirin and amantadine vs. interferon alpha-2a and ribavirin in treatment-naïve patients with chronic hepatitis C. J Viral Hepat 12: 292–299, 2005.
47. Weinstock-Guttman B, Ransohoff RM, Kinkel RP, et al. The interferons: biological effects, mechanisms of action and use in multiple sclerosis. Ann Neurol 37:7–13, 1995.
48. Triozzi P, Rinehart J. The role of IFN-beta in cancer therapy. Cancer Surv 8:799–807, 1989.
49. Vaickus L. Antitumor antibodies as therapeutic reagents. Pharmacol Ther 15:143–161, 1990.
50. Dillman RO. Monoclonal antibodies for treating cancer. Ann Intern Med 111:592–603, 1989.
51. Reisfeld RA. Monoclonal antibodies in cancer immunotherapy. Clin Lab Med 12:201–216, 1992.
52. ENBREL [package insert]. Seattle, WA: Immunex Corporation and Wyeth-Ayerst Laboratories; 1998.
53. Bysmann S, Hack CE, van Diepen FN, et al. Administration of OKT3 as a two-hour infusion attenuates first-dose side effects. Transplantation 64:1620–1623, 1997.
54. Peces R, Urra JM, Escalada P, et al. High-dose methylprednisolone inhibits the OKT3-induced cytokine-related syndrome. Nephron 63: 118, 1993.
55. Bemelman FJ, Parlevliet KJ, Schellekens PT, et al. Sequestration of labelled granulocytes in the lungs following administration of OKT3 is dose-dependent. Transpl Immunol 2:47–51, 1994.
56. McLaughlin P, Cabanillas AJ, Grillo-Lopez A. IDEC-C2B8 anti CD20 antibody: final report on a phase III pivotal trial in patients with relapsed low-grade or follicular lymphoma. Blood 88:90a, 1996.
57. Roche Rituximab warnings strengthened in European labeling. Health News Daily via NewsEdge Corporation. December 1, 1998.
58. Slamon D, Leyland-Jones B, Shak S, et al. Addition of Herceptin (humanized anti-HER2 antibody) to first line chemotherapy for HER2 overexpressing metastatic breast cancer (HER2+/MBC) markedly increases anti-cancer activity: a randomized, multi-national controlled phase III trial. Proc ASCO 377:98a, 1998.
59. Herceptin [package insert]. San Francisco, CA: Genentech; 1998.
60. Tang K, Harp DR. Bexxar phase II/III enrollment complete: BLA submission on schedule for 4Q 1998. BT Alex Brown Research, 1998.
61. ReoPro [package insert]. Malvern, PA: Centocor, Eli Lilly & Company; 1995.
62. Targan SR, Hanauer SR, van Deventer SJH, et al. A short-term study of chimeric monoclonal antibody cA2 to tumor necrosis factor alpha for Crohn's disease. N Engl J Med 337:1029–1035, 1997.
63. Remicade [package insert]. Malvern, PA: Centocor; 1998.
64. St. Clair EW, van der Heijde DM, Smolen JS, et al. Combination of infliximab and methotrexate therapy for early rheumatoid arthritis: a randomized, controlled trial. Arthritis Rheum 50:3432–3443, 2004.
65. Tolstoshev P. Gene therapy, concepts, current trials and future direction. Annu Rev Pharmacol 32:573–596, 1993.
66. Roth JA, Cristiano RJ. Gene therapy for cancer: what have we done and where are we going? J Natl Cancer Inst 89:21–39, 1997.
67. Kerr WG, Mule JJ. Gene therapy: current status and future prospects. J Leukemia Biol 56:210–214, 1994.
68. Edelstein ML, Abedi MR, Wixon J, et al. Gene therapy clinical trials worldwide 1989–2004-an overview. J Gene Med 6:597–602, 2004.
69. Robbins PD, Ghivizzani SC. Viral vectors for gene therapy. Pharmacol Ther 80:35–47, 1998.
70. Weichselbaum RR, Kufe D. Gene therapy of cancer. Lancet 349: 10–12, 1997.
71. Kay MA, Liu D, Hoogerbrugge PM. Gene therapy. Proc Natl Acad Sci USA 94:12744–12746, 1997.
72. Vorburger SA, Hunt KK. Adenoviral gene therapy. The Oncologist 7:46–59, 2002.
73. Blattner WA. Retroviruses that cause human disease. In: Wyngaarden JB, Smith LH, Bennett JC. Cecil textbook of medicine. 19th ed. Philadelphia: WB Saunders, 1992:1845.

74. Kay MA, Liu D, Hoogerbrugge PM. Gene therapy. Proc Natl Acad Sci USA 94:12744–12746, 1997.

75. Kootstra NA, Verma IM. Gene therapy with viral vectors. Annu Rev Pharmacol Toxicol 43:413–439, 2003.

76. Anderson WF. Human gene therapy. Nature 392:25–30, 1998.

77. Wilmut I, Schnieke AE, McWhir J, et al. Viable offspring derived from fetal and adult mammalian cells. Nature 385:810–813, 1997.

78. Memorandum for the Heads of Executive Departments and Agencies. Available at: http://grants.nih.gov/grants/policy/cloning_directive.htm. Accessed December 7, 2005.

79. Use of Cloning Technology to Clone a Human Being. Available at: http://www.fda.gov/cber/genetherapy/clone.htm. Accessed December 7, 2005.

80. ''10-26-98 Dear Colleague Letter about Human Cloning.'' Available at: http://www.fda.gov/oc/ohrt/irbs/irbletr.html. Accessed December 7, 2005.

81. Tolaza EM, Economou JS. Gene therapy of cancer. In: Haskell CM. Cancer treatment. 4th ed. Philadelphia: WB Saunders, 1995:305.

82. Wolf JK, Bodurkin DC, Gano JD, et al. A phase I study of ADP53 (INGN 201; ADVEXIN) for patients with platinum- and paclitaxel-resistant epithelial ovarian cancer. Gynecol Oncol 94:442–448, 2004.

83. Pagliaro LC, Keyhani A, Williams D, Repeated intravesical instillations of an adenoviral vector in patients with locally advanced bladder cancer: a phase I study of *p53* gene therapy. J Clin Oncol 21:2247–2253, 2004.

84. Lang FF, Bruner JM, Fuller GN, et al. Phase I trial of adenovirus-mediated p53 gene therapy for recurrent glioma: biological and clinical results. J Clin Oncol 21:2508–2518, 2003.

85. Makower D, Rozenblit A, Kaufman H, et al. Phase II clinical trial of intralesional administration of the oncolytic adenovirus ONYX-015 in patients with hepatobiliary tumors with correlative *p53* studies. Clin Cancer Res 9:693–702, 2003.

86. Schuler M, Herrmann R, DeGreve JLP. Adenovirus-mediated wild-type p53 gene transfer in patients receiving chemotherapy for advanced non-small-cell lung cancer: results of a multicenter phase II study. J Clin Oncol 19:1750–1758, 2001.

87. Rainov NG. A phase III clinical evaluation of herpes simplex virus type 1 thymidine kinase and ganciclovir gene therapy as an adjuvant to surgical resection and radiation in adults with previously untreated glioblastoma multiforme. Hum Gene Ther 11:2389–2401, 2000.

88. Rosenberg SA. Immunotherapy and gene therapy of cancer. Cancer Res 51:5074s–5079s, 1991.

89. Pandha HS, Martin LA, Rigg A, et al. Genetic prodrug activation therapy for breast cancer: a phase I clinical trial of erbB-2-directed suicide gene expression. J Clin Oncol 17:2180–2189, 1999.

90. Klatzmann D, Valery CA, Bensimon G. A phase I/II study of herpes simplex virus type 1 thymidine kinase ''suicide'' gene therapy for recurrent glioblastoma. Study Group on Gene Therapy for Glioblastoma. Hum Gene Ther 9:2595–604, 1998.

91. Alvarez RD, Gomez-Navarro J, Wang M, Adenoviral-mediated suicide gene therapy for ovarian cancer. Mol Ther 2:524–530, 2000.

92. Freytag SO, Stricker H, Pegg J, et al. Phase I study of replication-competent adenovirus-mediated double-suicide gene therapy in combination with conventional-dose three-dimensional conformal radiation therapy for the treatment of newly diagnosed, intermediate- to high-risk prostate cancer. Cancer Res 63:7497–7506, 2003.

93. Freytag SO, Khil M, Stricker H. Phase I study of replication-competent adenovirus-mediated double suicide gene therapy for the treatment of locally recurrent prostate cancer. Cancer Res 62:4968–4976, 2002.

94. Klatzmann D, Cherin P, Bensimon G. A phase I/II dose-escalation study of herpes simplex virus type 1 thymidine kinase ''suicide'' gene therapy for metastatic melanoma. Study Group on Gene therapy of Metastatic Melanoma. Hum Gene Ther 9:2585–2594, 1998.

95. Molnar-Kimber KL, Sterman DH, Chang M. Impact of preexisting and induced humoral and cellular immune responses in an adenovirus-based gene therapy phase I clinical trial for localized mesothelioma. Hum Gene Ther 9:2121–2133, 1998.

96. Hall SJ, Chen S, Woo SL. Gene therapy '97: the promise and reality of cancer gene therapy. Am J Hum Genet 1:785–790, 1997.

97. Culver KW. Clinical applications of gene therapy for cancer. Clin Chem 40:510–512, 1994.

98. Ge Q, Filip L, Bai A. Inhibition of influenza virus production in virus-infected mice by RNA interference; JAMA 293:1367–1373, 2005.

99. Hannon GJ, Rossi JJ. Unlocking the potential of the human genome with RNA interference. Nature 431:371–378, 2004.

100. Nathwani AC, Davidoff AM, Linch DC. A review of gene therapy for haematological disorders. Br J Haematol 128:3–17, 2004.

101. Recombinant DNA and Gene Transfer – Office of Biotechnology Activities – National Institutes of Health – ''Human Gene Transfer Protocols'' – Available at: http://www4.od.nih.gov/oba/rac/PROTO-COL.pdf. Accessed December 7, 2005.

102. Rubanyi GM. The future of human gene therapy. Mol Aspects Med 22:113–142, 2001.

103. Raper SE, Chirmule N, Lee FS. Fatal systemic inflammatory response syndrome in a ornithine transcarbamylase deficient patient following adenoviral gene transfer. Genet Metab 80:148–158, 2003.

104. The Last Word – Researchers React to Gene Therapy's Pitfalls and Promises. FDA Consumer Magazine – September-October 2000 – Available at: http://www.fda.gov/fdac/departs/2000/500_word.html. Accessed December 7, 2005

105. Cavazzano-Calvo M. Gene therapy of human severe combined immunodeficiency (SCID)-X1 disease. Science 288:669–672, 2000.

106. Aiuti A, Slavin S, Aker M, et al. Correction of ADA-SCID by stem cell gene therapy combined with nonmyeloablative conditioning. Science 296:2410–2413, 2002.

107. Rainov NG. A phase III clinical evaluation of herpes simplex virus type 1 thymidine kinase and ganciclovir gene therapy as an adjuvant to surgical resection and radiation in adults with previously untreated glioblastoma multiforme. Hum Gene Ther 11:2389–2401, 2000.

108. Anderson WF. Human gene therapy. Nature 392 (Suppl):25–30, 1998.

109. Genetic Modification Clinical Research Information System – NIH. Available at: http://www.gemcris.od.nih.gov/. Accessed December 7, 2005.

110. Aiuti A, Ficara F, Cattaneo F. Gene therapy for adenosine deaminase deficiency. Curr Opin Allergy Clin Immunol 3:461–466, 2003.

111. FDA Talk Paper 2003; FDA places temporary halt on gene therapy trials using retroviral vectors in blood stem cells. Available at: http://www.fda.gov/bbs/topics/ANSWERS/2003/ANS01190.html. Accessed December 7, 2005.

112. Memorandum to Principal Investigators for Human Gene Transfer Trials Employing Retroviral Vectors. Available at: http://www4.od.nih.gov/oba/rac/XSCID_letter2.pdf. Accessed

113. Knowles MR, Hohneker KW, Zhou Z. A controlled study of adenoviral-vector-mediated gene transfer in the nasal epithelium of patients with cystic fibrosis. N Engl J Med 333:823–831, 1995.

114. Flotte TR, Zeitlin PL, Reynolds TC. Phase I trial of intranasal and endobronchial administration of a recombinant adeno-associated virus serotype 2 (rAAV2)-CFTR vector in adult cystic fibrosis patients: a two-part clinical study. Hum Gene Ther 14:1079–1088, 2003.

115. Raper SE, Grossman M, Rader DJ. Safety and feasibility of liver-directed ex vivo gene therapy for homozygous familial hypercholesterolemia. Ann Surg 223:116–126, 1996.

116. Kramer R, Cohen D. Functional genomics to new drug targets. Nat Rev 3:965–969, 2004.

117. McLeod HL. Integrating the genome into cancer care. Proc Am Soc Clin Onc 826–833, 2005.

118. Wichware P. Proteomics technology: character references. Nature 413:869–878, 2001.

119. Herrera S. Biogenerics Standoff. Nat Biotechnol 22:1343–1346, 2004.

Patient Communication in Clinical Pharmacy Practice

8

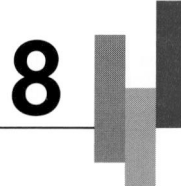

Richard N. Herrier, Marie E. Gardner, and Helen Meldrum

DEFINITION

Patient communication in clinical practice is defined as the dialog between a pharmacist and patient for the purpose of obtaining information needed to assess patient status, provide patient education, and support the patient's attempts to comply with the therapeutic regimen.

TREATMENT GOALS

- Obtain an accurate medication history.
- Evaluate the patient's symptoms.
- Verify the patient understanding of key information about disease and treatment.
- Assess the status of chronic diseases.
- Identify and address the factors that may reduce compliance.
- Verify existing patient compliance practices.

The health care professions are founded on strong technical and people skills. Although all health professionals are well versed in the technical aspects of their profession, most are not as skilled in interpersonal communication. In contemporary clinical practice, good communication skills are critical to achieving optimal patient outcomes. The goal of this chapter is to briefly summarize some of the communication skills necessary to provide high-quality pharmaceutical care. These techniques are very important in improving outcomes for the patient and for increasing practitioners' satisfaction with their professional roles. Although this is a broad topic, the focus of this chapter is limited to a review of essential communication skills, clinical interviewing and medication history guidelines, symptom assessment, basic medication consultation skills, and strategies for interviewing to improve compliance and monitor clinical progress.

In this era of technological advances, clear, direct, and sensitive communication between people seems to be in short supply. Extensive research on customer service and patient education shows that when providers communicate well, patients are more likely to comply with treatment plans and are less likely to complain or entertain thoughts of legal retribution because of perceived mistreatment. In addition, Bolton[1] states that 80% of professionals who fail at their jobs do so because of poor human relations skills. Humanistic psychologist Carl Rogers[2] concludes that people seek counseling because of poor communication with others in their lives. Effective interpersonal communication may be the most important skill we can develop. To function as professionals, pharmacists must not only maintain an open attitude of ongoing learning about human relations, but also master the specific skills of questioning, empathic response, responsible language use, assertiveness, and conflict management.

SKILLS IN ASKING QUESTIONS

Most people are not very conscious about the types of questions they ask. Questions can be organized on a continuum from highly open to restricted to leading. Closed questions narrow the patient's options and evoke minimal recall levels of information instead of thoughtful elaborated responses (Table 8.1 shows examples).

When seeking information from most patients it is best to begin with open-ended questions. These start with *who, what, where, when,* and *how.* Such questions allow the patient to answer in any number of ways. For example, a question such as ''How have you been feeling since starting this new medication?'' can elicit a response that the patient is feeling better (and is happy with the medication) or that side effects are present (and presumably the patient is unhappy with the medication). This type of question is preferred over ''Are you feeling better?'' and ''The medicine hasn't made you sick, has it?'' In medication history interviews, handling over-the-counter (OTC)/self-care requests and consultation regarding prescription medications, the use of open-ended questions is of paramount importance.

It is important to remember that not all open questions are equally effective. ''Why didn't you finish your antibiotic?'' implies strong criticism and will provoke a defensive reaction from the patient. In most cases, when trying to elicit the patient's reasoning, it is better to start with a universal statement and move to an open question (e.g., ''Most people don't realize how important it is to finish an antibiotic because an infection can appear to be gone but actually be lingering. What has been your experience in trying to take antibiotics?''). Although many pharmacists fear that this approach will consume too much time, when quick questions are asked in ways that produce defensiveness, patients learn to hide the real and truthful answers because they do not trust their health care providers.

TABLE 8.1	Open-ended and Closed-ended Questions
Very open	How have you been feeling since starting this new medication?
Open	What exactly has changed since you have started taking this medication?
Moderately open	Of the drugs we have tried, which do you think works best for you?
Highly closed	You're not having any side effects, are you?

WHAT IS EMPATHIC RESPONDING AND WHY IS IT ESSENTIAL?

Many pharmacists have had no coursework in basic counseling and communication skills. Providers often are fearful that they will not know what to do if the patient has a deeply emotional reaction. ''I'm sorry'' sounds empty and inadequate in the face of such feeling. However, empathic communication is a key skill that helps patients open up and share their concerns. Specifically, empathic communication means using reflective responding, a type of active listening that reflects the thought or feeling of the speaker's communication. Practitioners fear opening up Pandora's box by encouraging patients to elaborate on issues that they might not otherwise discuss in a direct fashion. However, if pharmacists do not use this essential skill, patients may conclude that the provider is not interested or that the discussion is bothersome or too time-consuming. Extensive research links empathic communication to patient satisfaction, improved diagnostic assessment, less litigation, and better outcomes.[3–5]

Sometimes, the professional demeanor of pharmacists appears to be cultivated to protect the provider from his or her own discomfort. Unfortunately, such a demeanor prevents genuine communication with the patient. Every provider has heard mentors and colleagues say, ''Don't let it get to you.'' On some level, this advice could be translated as ''Don't have feelings about the patient.'' Without use of empathy skills, which include reflective responding, effective paraphrasing, summarizing, and using words that mirror the patient's thoughts and feelings, providers often report feeling overwhelmed by their patients' or coworkers' emotional reactions with no idea about how to handle the situation.

Effective empathy skills help patients feel safe in discussing their concerns with providers. When trust is established, the patient is more likely to reveal clinically relevant data. Much of the theory on empathic facilitation is based on the work of Carl Rogers.[2,6] Rogers and colleagues came to believe that three conditions were necessary for the maintenance of mental health: (a) congruence (patients would not need to develop a protective facade), (b) unconditional positive regard (patients would feel warmth, interest, respect, and fondness from their providers), (c) and nonjudgmental understanding (patients benefit most when they feel that they can share their perceptions, which will be accepted as valid without feedback that communicates approval or disapproval).

Because these conditions often are lacking, most people express their feelings indirectly. Indirect messages are hard to decode, and the listener's interpretation of the speaker's message generally goes unspoken. Indirect communication is one reason why needs and expectations often are not met.

This indirect expression of concerns is replicated in patients' patterns of questions about medications. For instance, they may present secondary concerns (''What if I forget to take this with food?'') that mask a deeper concern (''What if this makes me sicker?''). The presentation of peripheral concerns may test the provider. If the provider heedlessly launches into a lecture about how to remember to take the medicine at mealtime, then he or she is missing the deeper meaning. Given this response, the patient may be afraid to ask if the medicine will cause illness because such a question could be interpreted as an insult to the pharmacist who is providing the medicine. Reflective responding reduces the emotional charge present during medication counseling. With the emotional tone decreased, the patient is able to process the information in a more conscious manner.[7] Patients who are upset may need repeated demonstrations of empathy to relax to the point that information can be exchanged. Often, it is easier to learn about this type of reflective listening by examining what is *not* an empathic response. For instance, if the patient says to the pharmacist, ''Do you think I'm getting the right medicine?'' a variety of responses are possible. Table 8.2 shows examples of responses.

Judgmental responses imply judgment against what the patient is saying, diverting responses change the subject, advice giving moves to problem solving before the real concern is even known, and questioning seeks to probe the issue but neglects the emotional tone. All four of these responses avoid an open, nonjudgmental discussion of what is really bothering the patient. A fifth type of response, the reflecting or empathic response, attempts to open the discussion of the problem as perceived by the patient.

Making a reflective response initially is difficult for some pharmacists because most of us have not been taught these skills. Reflective responding attempts to reflect in words what the patient is saying or feeling. The reflection may be based on the content or thought expressed by the patient or the feelings associated with it, which are often not expressed overtly. Reflecting responses are especially useful when the patient is demonstrating emotions. Angry looks, pounding fists, averted eye contact, and head drooping all convey certain emotional states. Hesitating gestures or remarks such as ''Well, I *guess* I could try it'' all suggest concerns that must be brought to light gently. The first step in reflective re-

sponding is to identify and label the emotional state. The four basic emotional states are *mad, sad, glad,* and *afraid*. When communicating with patients, observe nonverbal signs or verbal cues (e.g., hesitating words) that suggest one of the four feeling states. The second step is to put the word describing the feeling state into a sentence. Some basic structures for sentences include ''Sounds like you're frustrated by that,'' ''That would be frustrating,'' and ''I can see that you're frustrated by it.'' Remarks such as these let patients know that you are listening and truly attempting to understand their concerns. Patients and their concerns remain the focus of the encounter. It is important to remember that skills in empathy do not come naturally. Rubin et al[8] showed that untrained allied health students could not recognize what constitutes an empathic response. If health care providers do not master the skill of expressing empathy, communication will remain controlled by and centered on the practitioner. Patients are more likely to feel empowered and retain a sense of personal control if they can express their feelings in an atmosphere of acceptance.[9]

RESPONSIBLE LANGUAGE USE

In everyday discussion it is all too easy to blame other people for negative feelings or to pretend that emotions and thoughts are not important. The goal of communicators is to take responsibility for their messages and analyze them for suggestions of blame or denial. Pharmacists have high visibility as part of the interdisciplinary medical team, and each member of the team is responsible for analyzing breakdowns in communication and assessing their own roles in causing and solving the problem. Particularly when one is offering advice or making a complaint, or when there is a conflict of views, careless language choices can create a destructive communication climate. For example, when working with a patient who is noncompliant with an asthma control regimen, the pharmacist could say, ''You are trying to overuse your medication now to make up for not using it correctly when you should have known better'' (blaming) or ''Oh, well, I guess as long as your attacks aren't too serious'' (denial). Responsible language is the appropriate alternative. For example, the pharmacist could say, ''I'm concerned about your having three more asthma attacks this month than last. Let's look at how you have been using the medication.'' Responsible language incorporates a statement of concern citing specifics of the case and a statement or question about what to do next. Notice that the pharmacist's comment neither places blame nor denies that a potentially serious situation exists. It focuses on the problem (more frequent attacks) as perceived by the pharmacist and proposes a joint effort to solve the problem. The skills of responsible ownership of language and specificity come together when we attempt to send assertive messages.

TABLE 8.2	Possible Responses to Emotional Content in Patient Consultation
Judgmental response	"Of course this is the right medication. I wouldn't question the doctor on this."
Diverting response	"Oh, yes. When is your next appointment with the doctor?"
Advice giving	"I'd give this a good try if I were you."
Questioning/probing	"What did you see the doctor about?"
Reflective responding	"You sound concerned about taking this."

ASSERTIVENESS

With patients and coworkers alike, pharmacists must sometimes set limits on behavior that is too demanding, inappropriate, or uncompromising. For example, a consultant pharmacist to a nursing home recently had a case in which a 26-year-old drug-dependent man was admitted for total parenteral nutrition after a bout of alcoholic pancreatitis. The pharmacist was present at the nursing station and had to deal with his constant demands for intravenous narcotics, which were not clinically indicated. The pharmacist decided to use the CLEAR system, an acronym for the steps in formulating an assertive message.[10]

Clear description: "This is the fifth time this hour you have asked for morphine."
Listen: "I'm ready to listen if something new has come up."
Emotional reaction: "I'm finding it difficult to get my work done with the disruptions."
Assert: "I need you to not keep asking."
Results expected: "If you can do this for us, we will be able to work with you more during the time that you are here" or " . . . we will be able to respond more quickly when you really need us."

This assertive message incorporates the elements of a specific description of the problem behavior, a sharing of feelings that the behavior provokes, and a description of the consequences if the behavior does not stop. Sending clear, responsible messages are usually enough to help patients understand what kind of problems such behavior creates.

CONFLICT MANAGEMENT

When faced with an emotionally charged situation most professionals try to avoid the other person, become too passive and accommodating, give in to the urge to fight in a competitive fashion, or compromise their needs prematurely. It is difficult to lower the emotional temperature of an interpersonal conflict so that the two parties can collaborate effectively. The assertiveness and empathy skills discussed previously are helpful in situations when used with appropriate timing and with sensitivity to the setting. In addition, pharmacists have the option of deflection, which is a strategy of partial agreement. For example, it is more effective to say to a nurse, "You've got a good point. It would be great if we had more technicians; then we could get special orders up to you much faster" than to aggressively be defensive in the face of accusations about slow response.

Also, some of the criticism directed at the pharmacy is very vague. "You guys have got to get your act together" is a typical annoying criticism to which it is too easy to respond in kind. Instead, a strategy of inquiry is needed. A question such as "What is it exactly that makes it hard for you to do your job?" can go a long way toward eliciting useful information. When colleagues provide the information, empathic responding can address their concerns. As a

last resort, if tempers are running too high, defer further discussion until after a cooldown period.

With improved skills of empathic and reflective responding, assertiveness, deflection, and inquiry, a strategy of deferral rarely is needed. Using an appropriate combination of these conflict management skills will keep difficult situations from escalating. Additional case studies on conflict resolution in pharmacy practice can be found in other sources.[10]

CLINICAL INTERVIEWING SKILLS

Many of the skills discussed in the previous section apply to clinical interviewing and medication consultation processes. This section discusses clinical interviewing skills as they relate to pharmacy practice. The term "interviewing" here means "bringing into view" the patient's problems and associated issues. The skills associated with interviewing can be applied to a highly structured, complete assessment of medication use, assessing symptom severity before recommending OTC medications, or to a brief conversation with the patient about an adverse drug reaction. Each of these is discussed in more detail in this section.

MEDICATION HISTORY

A thorough, detailed, up-to-date medication history provides the necessary background for consultation with the patient. Pharmacists have the most knowledge about patients' medication use patterns and outcomes. This allows them to communicate effectively with patients and medical providers on matters of drug therapy. Obtaining a detailed history of medication use entails more than giving the patient a form to complete. Knowledge of what history content to obtain and which process skills to use is fundamental to providing good pharmaceutical care in this area. Research shows that skills in medication history interviewing are improved with training on specific techniques.[11,12] The following is a step-by-step guide to conducting a comprehensive medication history.

Opening the Interview. The first of the core skills is opening the interview. Depending on the setting, the interview may have been requested, or perhaps this is a service offered to all patients. Greet the patient warmly. Identify yourself to the patient. Verify the patient's identity and that of others (e.g., caregivers) who are present. Caregivers may be needed to assist in clarifying information. However, if the patient is alert and oriented and can give valid information, address your remarks to the patient. State the purpose of the interview and relate it to expected outcomes for the patient. For example, you might start by saying, "Mrs. Smith, Dr. Welch asked me to speak with you about your medications so we can get a complete picture of what medications you are taking and how they are working."

Setting the Stage for Good Communication. Let the patient know about how long the interview will take to determine if the interview can be completed at that time. Arrange furniture to allow face-to-face communication at eye level. Sit 2 to 4 feet from the patient, if possible. One study showed patients perceived pharmacists who used these nonverbal skills as more available to them, thus facilitating good rapport and better information exchange.[13] Maintain good nonverbal communication throughout the interview: lean slightly forward and maintain an open body posture and good eye contact. These skills are associated with patient satisfaction with care.[4]

Controlling the Flow of Information. The pharmacist must maintain the direction of the interview without appearing brusque or asking questions in an authoritarian style. Using appropriate questioning skills and having a structured framework are imperative to obtaining complete information in a manner that facilitates dialog while allowing the pharmacist to maintain control. Use open-ended, broad questions to start data gathering, and proceed to closed-ended and forced-choice questions for discriminating details. Recall that open-ended questions start with *who, what, where, when, why,* and *how*. These questions cannot be answered with a *yes* or *no*. If the patient answers inappropriately, the pharmacist should suspect some barrier to communication, such as language differences, hearing difficulties, or diminished mental capacity. Use as many open-ended questions as possible, minimizing the use of closed-ended questions. For example, ask "What medications for diabetes have you taken in the past?" rather than "Have you ever taken tolazamide? Or glipizide?" It may be necessary to ask such specific questions, but they should not be used to start discussion of past medications because they limit the patient's responses and do not elicit other important information. However, such questions are helpful if the patient admits to taking medication but cannot recall the name. Using a closed-ended statement such as "Have you ever taken tolazamide?" at that time is appropriate. It can also be very helpful to ask such questions at the very end of an interview in which you may be asked to help select therapy. If you are planning to suggest a specific medication for the patient, ask the patient if he or she has ever taken it. Patients with chronic conditions often have taken numerous medications with good and disastrous results. It is not uncommon for the patients to forget their past medications, only to recall having had a particular one when asked directly. The patient may then respond that he or she has taken the medication in question and that it did not help or caused a problem. This will change your recommendation.

After obtaining a block of related information, such as present medications, give a brief summary or paraphrase of pertinent points (e.g., "Mrs. Smith, you've told me you currently take hydrochlorothiazide and digoxin for your heart, and you used to take potassium, but you're not on it now and you're concerned that you need it. Is that correct?"). Between subsections of the history, use transitional statements to let the patient know that you are asking about a different type of information. After making the preceding statement, the pharmacist might say, "Now I'd like to ask about any allergies or reactions to medications you've had." Again, open the discussion with an open-ended statement such as "Tell me about your allergies." Keep using open-ended statements such as "What other reactions have you had?" to obtain further information. When clarification is needed, it is often necessary to use closed-ended questions. For example, the pharmacist might say, "You mentioned being allergic to 'mycin' but can't recall the name of the medication. Could it be erythromycin?"

The pharmacist needs to keep control of the interview to maximize effort while being efficient. When a long interview is expected, invariably the dialog strays from the topic at hand. The patient may ramble or ask a lot of questions or want to discuss matters not related to drug therapy. The pharmacist must keep the framework of questioning in mind, know what must be asked, and politely defer topics that are not germane to the drug history. Look for openings to bring the subject into focus (e.g., "Mr. Jones, you've been telling me how unpleasant it is to be in the hospital and I'd like to focus on how this medicine can help you stay out of the hospital."). When it is necessary to interrupt, address the patient by name and simply state your need to ask a certain question. Remember that the goal is not to have a social conversation with the patient but to obtain the medication history.

OBTAINING COMPLETE INFORMATION

Table 8.3 shows a suggested order of content for a complete medication history. Begin by asking "What diseases or conditions do you have that you take medication for?" This disease-based approach helps the patient focus on all the medications they use for a particular disease. For each disease, use a broad opening question that allows the patient to list all the medications currently prescribed for that disorder (e.g. "What medications do you take for your asthma?") For each medication, ask specifically for the dose, duration of use, some assessment of how the drug is working, and any drug-related problems the patient perceives. For medications taken as needed, question the patient to determine the amount used per day and per dose. Also, it is important to know what symptoms or in what context the patient uses the as-needed medications. Be attentive to vague responses. For example, a patient may state that he uses the β-agonist inhaler "only when I really need it." Question specifically how much the patient uses and how many times per day. Similarly, when the patient's responses include words such as "sometimes," "not often," or "occasionally," probe for more specifics and document amounts of medications used.

After summarizing information regarding present medications for a specific disease directly, ask about past medications for that disease. "So you are taking albuterol and beclomethasone and they are working well. What medications have you taken in the past for your asthma?" This is impor-

TABLE 8.3	Content Items for a Comprehensive Medication History
Major Category of Information	**Specific Areas to Probe**
Current prescribed medications	Drug name
	Purpose
	Dosage
	Duration
	Beneficial effects
	Adverse effects
Past medication usage	Drug name
	Purpose
	Time period of use
	Reason for discontinuation
Current nonprescription medications	Drug name
	Purpose or symptoms treated
	Dosage and frequency of use
	Duration
	Assessment of effects
Drug allergies and adverse reactions	Drug name
	Date of reaction
	Type and severity of reaction
Lifestyle factors	Herbal remedies used
	Nicotine usage
	Alcohol usage
	Illicit drug usage
	Dietary habits
	Occupation
	Stressors

tant because the pharmacist would not want to recommend medications that were ineffective or caused adverse reactions. It is useful to ask, ''Why was that medication stopped?'' or ''Who stopped that medication?'' It is helpful to know whether the physician advised stopping the medication or the patient made the decision alone.

Once you have finished the present and past medications for one disease, move on to the next, repeating the process until all the disease states and medications are covered. This approach may also elicit history of use of nonprescription medications and nutritional and herbal medications and if they are used to help with a particular disease or symptom.

After asking about prescribed routine and as-needed medications, ask about nonprescription medications used regularly. Because patients may not perceive vitamins or cold products as medications, it may be necessary to specifically ask, ''What medications do you take for a cold? For stomach problems? For a headache?'' Another approach is to query the patient using an approach similar to the review of sys-

tems used by physicians. Begin by asking about medications used for disorders of the head, eyes, ears, nose, and throat. Next, ask about products for respiratory, gastrointestinal, genitourinary, and skin conditions. When the patient mentions using any medication, ask specifically about the amounts used, duration of use, and outcome of treatment. Ask about herbal remedies and alternative treatments and obtain sufficient detail.

Next, obtain complete information on negative drug reactions the patient has had. Because patients may not perceive side effects as allergies it is necessary to ask about negative reactions in multiple ways to assure accuracy. The use of three open-ended questions in a specific order helps maximize the accuracy of any adverse events related to medications. First ask ''What kind of bad reactions have you had to medications?'' Next ask ''What medications has a doctor told you never to take again?'' Finally, ask ''What medications are you allergic to?'' For positive responses ask for details of the reaction (when it occurred, what exactly happened) using the symptom-based interview format to provide a clear picture of the event.

Last, ask about lifestyle issues that may affect drug therapy. These include dietary habits, tobacco and alcohol consumption, and illicit drug use. Because nicotine and alcohol are factors in response to many drug therapies, it is important to quantify their intake, even though it may be uncomfortable for the pharmacist to do so. A useful suggestion is to open the discussion with a statement describing the importance of that information to you (e.g., ''Mr. Smith, I'd like to ask about your intake of alcohol and tobacco because these can affect the way your medicines work. How much alcohol do you drink?''). Specify the amount and type of alcohol used. Note whether the patient smokes and how much.

CLOSING THE INTERVIEW

When you believe you have obtained all the vital information, it is time to close the interview. Begin with a brief summary of only the most important points, not every specific detail. Note any concerns that you or the patient has about the medications and review recommendations for resolution of problems. Ask the patient to verify agreement on the issues and tell the patient what to expect next. Ask the patient if there is anything he or she wants to add and if he or she has any other questions. If not, the interview is ended. Here is an example of a good closure: ''Mr. Smith, we've talked about your heart and diabetes medications, and you mentioned some 'weak spells,' which I think may be caused by one of your medications. You're concerned about them, too. I am going to discuss them with your doctor. Is there anything else you would like to add or discuss?''

SYMPTOM-BASED INTERVIEW

During a disease management visit, at the bedside, over the telephone, during a self-care consultation, or at the prescription counter, the patient may mention symptoms that they are concerned about. Knowing how to explore the patient's symptoms and evaluate their relationship to a disease or its treatment is a key component of the pharmacist's assessment skills. The first step is to get the patient to reveal more information about the symptom. An introductory statement such as "Tell me more about that" will get the patient to provide more detail. The key symptom questions are used to explore the symptom. The following specific, open-ended questions seek specifics that help define if the symptom is related to drug therapy or to an illness.[14,15] Depending on the patient's response to your statement, it may not be necessary to ask all seven questions used in traditional chief complaint history taking.

Location: Where does it hurt?
Timing: When did it start? How long have you had this problem? How frequently does it occur?
Severity: How bad is it?
Context: Under what circumstances does this symptom appear?
Quality: What does it feel like?
Modifying factors: What makes it better? What makes it worse? What have you been doing about it?
Associated symptoms: What other symptoms are you having?

Insufficient recognition and symptom probing is common, especially among inexperienced pharmacists. Without proper symptom probing, pharmacists can jump to erroneous conclusions that the symptom is caused by a disease state or recommend a treatment without knowing the real cause. For example, a patient taking a nonsteroidal antiinflammatory drug (NSAID) complains of fatigue. The pharmacist may simply recommend a vitamin to help fatigue. However, the patient's responses to the key symptom questions could reveal that the fatigue started soon after the medication, and that the patient has gastric distress and has tried vitamins without success. These answers suggest a different cause for the fatigue.

The key symptom questions are important also when there is a tendency to attribute every symptom to a medication, as patients may be inclined to do. For instance, a pharmacy student reviewed the chart of a patient with bipolar illness, seizures, and Parkinsonism. The patient was on several medications, including carbamazepine and carbidopa/levodopa. The patient complained of blurred vision and insomnia, which the student believed were caused by the medications. When the patient was interviewed using the questioning technique just described, she indicated that she had blurred vision only out of the left eye, and that she had insomnia "since the day I was born." Answers to further questions suggested that her symptoms probably were not related to her drug therapy.

Knowledge of each drug's side effect profile and the disease state symptoms is essential in determining if the symptom is a drug-related adverse effect. Onset of the symptom is very important to ascertain. If the symptom began or worsened after starting a new medication, then it is more likely that the problem is drug related.

BASIC MEDICATION CONSULTATION

Consultation on medication use is one of the pharmacist's most important activities, whether in a community pharmacy, clinic, or institutional site. Consultation on new medications is mandated by the Omnibus Budget Reconciliation Act of 1990, and most states require counseling for all patients on new or both new and refill prescriptions.[16,17] The traditional method of consultation involved providing information: The pharmacist "told" and the patient "listened." There was little true dialog because the pharmacist often asked closed-ended questions such as "Do you understand?" or "Do you have any questions?" Such closed-ended questions tend to restrict the flow of information. When the pharmacist merely provides information, there is no opportunity to ascertain what the patient knows or thinks about the medication.

The pharmacist-patient consultation techniques developed by the Indian Health Service three decades ago, and further refined in collaboration with colleagues around the country, teach an interactive method of consultation that seeks to verify what the patient knows about using the medication and fill in the gaps with only the most basic information when needed.[18] Research shows that people forget 90% of what they hear within 60 minutes of hearing it.[1] Any counseling technique that is based on the pharmacist speaking most of the time will be ineffective in promoting patient understanding because patients almost immediately forget what they hear. If the patient is an active participant in the process, he or she will learn more. Engaging patient participation in the exchange entails the use of specific, open-ended questions that seek to determine what the patient already knows about the medication; then the practitioner provides new information to the patient and summarizes at the end of the consultation.

BASIC MEDICATION CONSULTATION SKILLS: THE PRIME QUESTION TECHNIQUE

The interactive technique for consulting on medications consists of two sets of open-ended questions. One set is for a new prescription (prime questions), and the other is for refill prescription consultation (show-and-tell questions), as shown in Table 8.4. Using these questions makes counseling an interactive process that engages the patient, thereby making him or her an active participant. The questions provide an organized approach to ascertain what the patient already knows about the medication. Such a systematic approach is associated with improved recall of prescription instructions.[19] The pharmacist can praise the patient for information correctly recalled, clarify points misunderstood, and add new information when needed. It spares the pharmacist from re-

TABLE 8.4	**Medication Consultation Skills**	
Prime Questions for New Prescriptions	**Related Probes**
What did your doctor tell you the medication is for?	What were you told the medication is for?
(Name and purpose of medication)	What symptom is it supposed to help?
	What is it supposed to do?
How did your doctor tell you to take the medication?	How were you told to take the medication?
(Dose, dose frequency, duration, storage techniques for use)	How much? How often?
	What does three times a day mean to you?
	What did your doctor say to do when you miss a dose?
What did your doctor tell you to expect?	What were you told to expect?
(Expected outcomes and what to do if they don't occur)	What good effects are you supposed to notice?
(Possible untoward effects and what to do if they occur)	What bad effects did the doctor say to watch for?
	What should you do if a bad reaction occurs?
Show-and-Tell Questions for Refill Prescriptions	**Related Probes**
What are you taking this medication for?	How is your medication working?
How do you take it?	How many of these did you take yesterday?
What kind of problems are you having with this medication?	What bad effects have you noticed from taking this medication?

peating information already known by the patient, which is an inefficient use of time. The steps in the consultation process are described in detail here.

Open the Consultation. When the prescription is ready and the patient is called for counseling, establish rapport by introducing yourself by name and stating the purpose of the consultation. Verify the patient's identity by asking for identification or at least asking, "And you are?" after you identify yourself. If the patient does not speak English, has difficulty hearing, or otherwise cannot answer, you must overcome this barrier before discussing the medication.

If time and help permit and a private space is available, suggest that the consultation be conducted there and move to that area. This will be important for patients who have hearing problems or those wanting extra privacy. Sit facing the patient and maintain the appropriate interpersonal distance (1.5–2 feet) during the consultation.

Conduct the Counseling Session. Begin by asking the prime questions if the prescription is new or the show-and-tell questions for a refill prescription. If the patient is able to tell you what the medication is for, you may choose to probe further or move to the next question. Probing further may be helpful when the patient answers in broad or vague

terms. An example would be the patient receiving a β-blocker who tells you the medication is for "my heart." You may want to ask in an open-ended fashion, "What is it supposed to do for your heart?" Avoid asking "Is it for chest pains?" or similar closed-ended questions because you may alarm the patient by your suggestions and you might waste time if multiple questions are needed. If the patient does not know what the medication is for or asks, "Don't you know?" you should then ask why he or she visited the physician. The patient may describe symptoms of a condition known to be treatable with the medication in question. If so, indicate which symptoms the medication will help. If the patient is totally unaware, a referral back to the physician is indicated, lest the pharmacist judge in error the indication for the medication.

After verifying that the patient knows what the medication is for, ask the second prime question. Often, patients are unaware of the dosage instructions or say, "It's on the label, isn't it?" Be aware of the optimal dosing instructions; the patient may respond correctly "twice a day," but you may need to advise on exact timing or indicate whether to take the drug with meals. Other questions to include under the second prime question are how long to take the medication, exactly how much or how often to take as-needed medications, what to do when a dose is missed, and how to store the medication. When possible, rather than providing facts, ask the patient, "What did the doctor say about how long to take this medication?" or "What will you do if you miss a dose?" Remember, asking a question of the patient prompts his or her attention, whereas talking at the patient is passive and the patient may not listen. Think of the counseling session as an opportunity to find out what the patient knows rather than a place to showcase your knowledge. Keep the information you provide brief and to the point, limited to filling in the gaps and providing extra knowledge needed to ensure proper medication use.

After reviewing information about how to take the medication, proceed to the third prime question. Often patients have been told little about expected beneficial effects or potential unwanted effects. Other questions subsumed under the third prime question relate to how the patient will know if the medication is working, what precautions to take while taking the medication, and what to do if the medication does not work. If the patient's answer notes expected beneficial effects, follow up by asking, "What side effects were you warned about?" to determine his or her knowledge of potential side effects.

If the patient is unaware of adverse drug effects, mention the most common and the rare, but potentially serious adverse effects and what to do if they occur. Research shows that patients want information about their medications, especially adverse effects, and that providing such information does not lead to the development of those reactions in most cases.[20–23] Recent work on communicating about risk, in this case risk of drug reactions, suggests a four-quadrant model in which each quadrant requires specific communication skills.[24] The quadrants are shown having a combination of high or low probability of occurrence with high or low magnitude. An example of high probability and high magnitude would be the common and severe toxicities of cancer chemotherapy. Use empathic communication in discussing the risks of therapy in this case. High probability and low magnitude is exemplified by gastric complaints from erythromycin. Many commonly prescribed medications have common, bothersome, but not serious side effects. Useful communication skills include providing information about how the medication will work, why it is a good therapy, and how to manage expected side effects. In the third quadrant, where there is low probability but high magnitude (e.g., stroke with an oral contraceptive), careful assessment of the patient's perceptions about the possible side effects is needed. Be aware of how the patient's perceptions may differ from your own. When discussing serious potential adverse effects, some patients may hear "This is unlikely to happen" and tune out the specifics about the toxicity. Therefore, ask the patient for feedback on the discussion of toxicity. In the fourth case, the low probability and low magnitude of risk may be associated with a perception that the medication may have little value to the patient. Again, heavy-handed tactics to convince, scare, or otherwise threaten the patient are not

effective. Questioning patients to determine their view of the possible benefits of taking the medication is needed. Follow with comments to match the patient's assessment. For example, when a patient says, "Well, I could get an allergic reaction from this," the issue of the adverse effect is first and foremost in their mind, whereas the pharmacist may think, "I've never seen anyone allergic to this." Respond to, but don't minimize, the patient's concern. Rather than trying to convince the patient that no one becomes allergic to it, the pharmacist could say "Yes, that's possible. Which do you think is worse: putting up with the pain or taking a chance on the medication?" This brings into the open the discussion of the risks and benefits of treatment. If the pharmacist can effectively explain the potential benefits, the patient may decide to try the medication. At times, the authors have found it useful to contract with the patient (e.g., "Mr. Jones, we've discussed the good and bad about taking this medicine, and I know you still have concerns about side effects. I really think this medicine is best for you. Would you be willing to try it for a week and I will check in with you after a few days to see how things are going?") More often than not, the anticipated adverse effects do not appear.

Using effective consultation skills to address adverse reactions sets the stage for better patient compliance. However, the mere act of taking a medication when one is not used to doing so poses a problem for compliance. After asking the prime questions, use a universal statement to address compliance. A universal statement describes the situation for a group, then narrows down to focus on the individual (e.g., "Mrs. Green, a lot of patients have trouble fitting a time for taking medications into their daily schedule. What problems do you foresee in taking this?") It may be necessary to probe daily habits and suggest a way to tie taking medication into a particular activity. For instance, if the patient always makes coffee in the morning, having the medication nearby may be a sufficient reminder to promote compliance. A partnership approach is an effective way to address compliance issues.

Close the Consultation. Most consultations are a combination of the patient knowing some information and the pharmacist providing additional information as the prime questions are reviewed. For this reason, it is important to close the consultation with the final verification. Think of the final verification as asking the patient to play back everything he or she has learned to check that the information is complete and accurate. Say to the patient, "Just to make sure I didn't leave anything out, please go over with me how you are going to use the medication." Although the language seems bulky, if the question were phrased "Just to make sure you've got this . . ." the patient may feel embarrassed if he or she does not recall important facts. At this point, the patient should describe correct use of the medication. Any errors can be corrected and any omissions clarified. Then, ask the patient if there is anything else he or she needs, and offer help as needed.

A similar process is used for refill prescriptions. The show-and-tell questions verify patient understanding of proper use of chronic medications or medications that the patient has used in the past. The pharmacist begins the process by showing the medication to the patient (i.e., opening the bottle and displaying the contents). Then the patient tells the pharmacist how he or she uses the medication by answering the questions shown in Table 8.4. Note that the doctor is omitted as a reference because the patient should have been counseled properly before this and should have all the information needed for proper medication usage. The show-and-tell technique allows the pharmacist to detect problems with compliance or unwanted drug effects. If the patient answers the second question (how the medication is taken) incorrectly, the patient may be noncompliant or the physician may have changed the dose. The pharmacist must further define the reason for the discrepancy. The second show-and-tell question also allows the pharmacist to ask the patient to demonstrate use of an inhaler or injectable or how to measure liquid doses to ensure proper usage.

Some pharmacists have difficulty asking the third question (on side effects), fearing that they may arouse suspicion in the patient. However, research discounts this notion. If potential adverse effects were discussed when the patient was counseled initially, it seems natural, and certainly relevant, to ask the patient about adverse effects at the refill visit. If new symptoms are present, explore this further using the key symptom questions. Clinical judgment will dictate if the problem is medication related and how it should be managed.

BARRIERS TO THE CONSULTATION

The clinical skills just described are easily applied when there are few or no barriers in communication between patient and pharmacist. In reality, there are often obstacles to overcome in the environment or within the pharmacist or patient. Examples of problems in the pharmacy environment include lack of privacy, interruptions, high workload, and insufficient staff. Barriers within the pharmacist include lack of desire or skills to adequately counsel patients, stereotyping patients and problems, and personal stress. A detailed analysis of these barriers is beyond the scope of this discussion but can be found elsewhere.[18] Barriers that the patient brings to the encounter are discussed here.

The structured approach for obtaining a medication history, symptom interviewing, and medication counseling can be likened to knowing the road on which one is traveling. Unforeseen events happen on every path. During the clinical encounter, unforeseen issues may arise at any time. Just as one must remove or negotiate around obstacles on the highway, the pharmacist must recognize and manage barriers during the encounter if the consultation is to reach the desired end. Patient-related barriers can be categorized into two types: functional and emotional. Functional barriers include

problems with hearing and vision, which make it difficult for the patient to absorb information during the consultation. Language barriers and illiteracy are formidable obstacles to proper consultation. Recognizing these usually is not difficult because the signs of poor vision are easy to observe. Likewise, language problems become apparent early in the consultation. Strategies specific to each barrier are needed. For instance, moving to a quiet area, repeating information, and asking feedback of the patient are important when hearing is a problem. Giving clear verbal instructions and using large-type print materials are helpful when the patient has vision difficulties. Using translators and picture diagrams and involving English-speaking caregivers are important when language problems exist. Many functional barriers are permanent.

Emotional barriers may be long-standing if mental illness is involved; however, many emotional barriers are transitory, but have a profound impact on the consultation.

Emotional barriers are common in everyday interactions, including pharmacist-patient communication. When improperly handled, they contribute to further aggravation, breakdown of communication, and thus inhibit effective consultation. Patients may directly or indirectly express anger, hostility, sadness, depression, fear, anxiety, and embarrassment during consultation with the pharmacist. They may also give the attitude of a ''know-it-all,'' be suspicious of medications, or seem unmotivated or uninterested. Some of these barriers are momentary, such as the frustration experienced when the prescription cannot be filled because the medication is unavailable. The patient with a chronic pain syndrome may have a varying interest level because he or she is uncomfortable or in pain. The attitude of the patient who ''knows'' all about his or her medications probably will not change in time. This patient needs understanding and a nonjudgmental attitude to maintain an open dialog for consultation.

Emotional barriers can be difficult to discern. Most patients will not say, ''I'm angry and frustrated about feeling so ill'' or ''I'm upset that my doctor didn't spend that much time with me.'' Instead, their feelings surface in statements such as ''I don't know why it takes all day to put a few pills in the bottle!'' and ''I don't know why I have to take this stupid medicine.'' Unfortunately, we usually respond to the content of the message (e.g., ''I'll have this ready for you as soon as I can'') and in doing so overlook the opportunity to respond to the issues behind the statement, which affect the encounter and, more importantly, the patient's decision to comply with therapy. At the beginning of this chapter, several nonverbal and verbal clues were mentioned that suggest different emotional tones (e.g., pounding fists associated with anger). It takes patience and practice to listen *beyond* the words. The first step is to notice these nonverbal and verbal clues, identify the feeling state they represent, and respond with a reflecting or empathic statement. To the patient in the second example, the pharmacist might use the reflective response such as, ''Sounds like you've been frustrated with other things you've tried," rather than "This is a good medicine, Joe, and I really think it will help." Recall that a statement such as this can occur at any time in the consultation and that this barrier of frustration should be dealt with before the consultation is closed. Embarrassment is a factor when vaginal preparations, condom use, and similar topics are the subject of the consultation. Again, observe for signs of embarrassment, such as averted gaze or fidgeting, and respond with "This can be hard to talk about, but we need to discuss it." Be matter-of-fact, move to a private space, and speak in a normal tone of voice to alleviate the embarrassment. Additional strategies can be found in other references.[25]

Once these barriers are removed, consultation can proceed, with both parties devoting attention to the primary issues of drug therapy and usage rather than to any interpersonal difficulties. These skills are also applicable during the medication history interview and discussion of medication compliance, which is covered in the next section.

PSYCHOSOCIAL ASPECTS

Psychosocial factors play an important role in all pharmacist-patient interactions. Success or failure of patient care depends on the recognition of these factors, several of which are discussed in some depth here. Patient health beliefs, both cultural and noncultural, influence their interpretation of pharmacist communication and the appropriateness and accuracy of patient responses. Using open-ended questions helps the pharmacist elicit culture-specific beliefs and advise patients whose English skills are insufficient to enable effective communication. Second, patient readiness to comply with a therapeutic regimen and receptivity to education efforts varies according to psychological, emotional, and cultural factors that accompany the diagnosis of an acute or chronic disease. These important issues must be addressed to achieve effective patient education and compliance. Finally, compliance with therapeutic regimens in chronic disease requires significant long-term behavioral changes. Pharmacists must recognize that these changes are difficult to initiate and to maintain over time. To improve compliance, pharmacists must demonstrate their understanding of the inherent difficulty of change and use an empathic, caring approach.

COMPLIANCE AND DISEASE MONITORING

The pharmacist's role in monitoring and managing medication use is most vital in the case of patients requiring chronic drug therapy, especially with diseases that are asymptomatic. Many factors contribute to the pharmacist's success in ensuring beneficial outcomes. Among them are practice site, pharmacist competence, support of administration, and breadth of responsibilities, including prescriptive authority. Hatoum

and Akhras[26] have documented extensively the value of pharmacists' contributions to ambulatory care sites such as community group practices and the patient's home. The Indian Health Service has provided a full range of pharmaceutical care services to its patients for more than three decades. Besides the traditional dispensing role, Indian Health Service pharmacists offer private consultations to all patients and have prescriptive authority for refilling chronic medications based on their assessment of the patient's needs.[27,28] Some pharmacists have been educated to provide primary care as pharmacist practitioners, and this movement has spread to other practice sites. Currently, over 40 states have passed regulations that allow pharmacists to prescribe.[15] Whether the practice is a sophisticated one or more typical of contemporary community pharmacy, providing pharmaceutical care to patients requiring chronic drug therapy can have significant positive outcomes. To effectively provide long-term pharmaceutical care, several important factors must be considered.

WHOSE DISEASE IS IT, ANYWAY?

One of the most common misperceptions held by health professionals regarding chronic disease is that the professional manages the disease. Nothing could be further from the truth, and this medical myth is probably one of the major contributors to compliance problems among patients with chronic diseases. In the traditional model, health professionals perceive their roles to be in diagnosing, treating, and managing disease. As drug therapy managers, clinical pharmacists focus on blood levels, pharmacokinetic dosage calculations, and drug interactions. Guided by this focus on technical aspects of patient care, health professionals often get frustrated and angry when patients do not follow instructions or, despite the provider's best efforts, achieve only partially satisfactory results. In reality, the only time the health professional manages the treatment is during an office visit or institutionalization in a hospital or long-term care facility. Most of the time, the patient controls the treatment of his or her disease, especially those that require continuous medication. Failure to recognize this basic truth creates considerable tension in patient-provider relationships, provider frustration and anger, poor communication, negative provider attitudes toward individual patients, poor patient outcomes, patient distrust of providers, and legal consequences that contribute to rising health care costs.[29-32]

One author strongly suggests that noncompliance in diabetes mellitus is caused largely by the failure of providers to recognize that their goal is not treating the disease, but helping the patient treat the disease.[33] That contention is supported by current medical literature that links good communication and a partnership style of provider-patient relationship to increased satisfaction, increased compliance, and better patient outcomes.[4,31,32]

To be successful in helping patients achieve good outcomes, the pharmacist must eschew the traditional medical myth about who manages the disease and adopt a partnership approach, acting as a facilitator. Remember that it is the *patient's* disease; the provider's job is to help the patient manage it.

GO SLOW AND USE INTERACTIVE TECHNIQUES

Patients can absorb only a limited amount of new information at each encounter. Too many times, in an attempt to do a thorough job, health professionals inadvertently overwhelm the patient with information at or near the time of diagnosis or treatment initiation. A patient's active listening abilities last less than a minute during a monolog; therefore, he or she retains only a few pieces of information from a prolonged discussion and may miss key facts. In addition, a large volume of technical information may confuse or frighten patients, leading to the poor outcomes that educational efforts are intended to prevent.[34]

Successful patient educators do two things: give patients information in small, manageable increments and actively involve the patient in the educational process by creating an interactive dialog and using other hands-on approaches that are consistent with adult learning principles.[34] For the pharmacist, at the time of the initial prescription, this means verifying that the patient understands how to take the medicine and is aware of its most common side effects. For example, with hydrochlorothiazide 25 mg daily for hypertension, the pharmacist should verify that the patient knows what it is for, knows to take it once daily in the morning, understands that it takes a while before any changes in blood pressure occur, and knows that he or she will notice increased urination during the first week that should lessen after that. Discussions about diet, exercise, and related issues can wait until later visits. Giving the patient a handout on hypertension and diuretics would be appropriate and can lead to questions and subsequent educational efforts.

SET THE STAGE FOR FUTURE ENCOUNTERS

Many providers initially explain to patients how they are going to monitor them for disease control and progression so that patients view subsequent questions, lab tests, and examinations as a normal part of their care. However, few providers follow a similar process regarding compliance. Therefore, without previous explanations, provider questions about compliance are likely to be associated with parent-type sanctions from the provider. To avoid this ''punishment,'' patients may avoid disclosing compliance problems when asked. Providers can prevent this common problem by remembering who ultimately manages the disease and using specific strategies during the initial patient contact. Explain that compliance is very important for successful outcomes, but that you know how hard it is to remember to take medication every day. Tell the patient that you expect that he or she will be like most patients and experience some difficulties remembering to take the medication. Ask patients to keep track of those instances, if possible, and explain that you will be asking them at each visit about what kinds of problems they have had with the medicine (the third show-and-tell question). Remind them that the purpose of your questions is to help them adopt behaviors that help them get the optimal benefit from the medication. This can easily be done in association with explanations about how the progress of the disease will be monitored.

MONITORING AND EDUCATION AT RETURN VISITS

Organizing an effective approach to evaluating and educating patients with chronic disease at return visits may be problematic in a busy practice setting. One simple way to look at all patients returning for follow-up of a chronic disease is to assess the three *C*s: control, complications, and compliance. The first *C* refers to control of the chronic disease. To evaluate the control, objective findings such as blood pressure and range of motion can be coupled with subjective findings from the consultation, such as reports of dizziness, nocturnal voiding, and morning stiffness. The second *C* refers to complications caused by both disease progression and drug effects. A combination of subjective findings from the patient interview and objective findings from the health record or patient profile, physical findings during examination, and pertinent lab and other test results can be used to evaluate the presence of potential complications quickly. For example, a patient with hypertension, diabetes mellitus, and osteoarthritis who takes captopril, chlorpropamide, and ibuprofen can be asked about the presence of cough, difficulty sleeping, and poor exercise tolerance. These questions are intended primarily to detect congestive heart failure or renal failure caused by hypertension or diabetes, but they also will help detect drug-related problems such as cough caused by the angiotensin-converting enzyme (ACE) inhibitor and renal effects from the ibuprofen. Checking recent lab values for creatinine, electrolytes, and blood glucose will help detect diabetes, hypertension-induced or NSAID-induced renal impairment, excessive chlorpropamide dosage, and ACE inhibitor hyperkalemia.

The third *C* relates to compliance problems. The pharmacist's actions can be broken up into three steps: (a) Recognize potential compliance problems, (b) identify probable causes, and (c) manage the problem with specific steps. This recognize, identify, and manage (RIM) model is an easy way to enhance patient compliance.[35] In this model (Table 8.5), subjective and objective findings are used to detect potential compliance problems. The provider reviews the health record or drug profile for objective evidence of potential compliance problems before talking with the patient. During profile review, three items should alert the pharmacist to potential compliance problems. The first, and most common, is a discrepancy between the number of doses that should have been taken and the number of doses dispensed. Second, incomplete refill requests (e.g., only one or two out of more chronic medications due at the same time) raise suspicion

TABLE 8.5	Steps in the Recognize, Identify, and Manage Model for Compliance Counseling	
Step	**Example**
Recognize potential noncompliance	
For objective signs, use a supportive compliance probe.	"I noticed that this refill was due 3 weeks ago."
For subjective signs, use a reflecting response.	"It sounds like you're unsure about taking this medication."
Identify cause of noncompliance and manage problem	
Knowledge deficits	Provide verbal and written information and verify patient's understanding.
Practical impediments (complicated dosing schedule, adverse reaction, forgetfulness)	Simplify dosing regimen, use medication boxes, obtain history about adverse reactions, and manage appropriately.
Attitudinal barriers	Maintain nonjudgmental attitude, use empathy, use open-ended and universal statements.

for noncompliance. Third is the prescribing of a new medication that may be taken to offset adverse effects from another medication, if the effect is unrecognized as such. Patients often present to the medical provider with a new complaint. If the provider does not make the connection between the new symptom and the side effect, it may eventually result in compliance or therapeutic problems. If a patient on ACE inhibitors has a new or repeat prescription for cough suppressants or antibiotics for bronchitis, the pharmacist should suspect ACE inhibitor-induced cough. In extreme cases, patients may stop the needed drug and continue with the drug used to treat the side effects, which is unnecessary and could pose risks.

Care must be given in interpreting these signs. Positive findings during profile or chart review call for further exploration before a definite compliance problem can be ascertained. In some cases there are rational explanations for the objective findings. The patient may be getting refills at another location, or the doctor may have told the patient to change the dosage schedule or to stop the drug altogether.

When the profile suggests noncompliance, the best approach is to begin consultation using the show-and-tell technique for refill prescriptions. The patient may provide clues to confirm the pharmacist's suspicions. If not, the pharmacist must initiate a more direct approach using a supportive compliance probe. This is a specific type of statement in which the pharmacist uses "I" language, describes specifically what he or she sees, and asks a question to probe the discrepancy (e.g., "I noticed when I reviewed your profile that you hadn't had your prednisone refilled in about 2 weeks. I was concerned that there might have been some changes that I'm not aware of."). This combination of "I noticed" and "I'm concerned" can be very effective in getting a dialog started in a nonthreatening manner. Another useful approach is the universal statement (e.g., "Most of my patients have prob-

lems remembering to take every dose of their medication. What kinds of problems are you having?"). Open the discussion of compliance problems with nonthreatening language and there is a greater likelihood that the patient will disclose the problems.

During the consultation, the patient may provide the pharmacist with clues to compliance problems not revealed by patient record review. Indeed, patients may refill their medications on time but actually take only some of the doses. Patients who tell the pharmacist that they are taking their medication differently than prescribed provide a strong indication of a potential compliance problem. Some may be quite obvious, such as when the patient asks, "Why do I have to keep taking this medicine?" This is a red flag because it seems fairly obvious that the patient does not want to take the prescription. However, many statements are more subtle. Examples of these vague clues, called "pink flags," include "My doctor says I should take it," "My doctor wants me to take it," or "I'm supposed to be taking it." These statements usually are made in response to the first two show-and-tell questions. Other pink flags are more closely associated with the third question, such as when a long pause occurs during the patient's reply, which may indicate potential problems. For example, "What kinds of problems are you having with the medication?" may prompt the following pink flag responses: "Well, none, really" or a hesitation before saying, "No, none." Reflecting responses are appropriate (e.g., "Seems like you're not too sure about taking that" or "Sounds like you think there may be a problem."). These open the dialog in a nonthreatening manner and focus on the patient's perceptions or suggestion that a problem exists.

Patients may ask, "Does this medicine have any side effects? What kind of side effects does this have? Is this anything like (specific drug)?" More often than not, pharmacists simply answer the question without really listening to the underlying concern. An appropriate response would be "Why do you ask?" especially if the patient looks hesitant or the intonation of the question suggests doubt about taking the medication. Often, when the authors use this question, patients disclose that a relative had it or something like it, or the media reports problems with it. These indirect experiences create enough doubt that the patient wavers about taking the medication. Obviously, if the pharmacist does not recognize these pink flags, the consultation will be in vain because the patient will leave without having the underlying doubt resolved. Therefore, it is crucial to develop keen active listening skills to identify the presence of the pink flags and use reflecting responses to probe the problem. During the show-and-tell questioning, patients may disclose symptoms that may indicate an adverse drug effect. This is sometimes a reason for premature discontinuation of treatment or for skipping doses. When this appears to be the case, use of the key symptom questions will help identify the exact nature of the problem. Resolution of the problem will be dictated by clinical urgency.

Once the presence of the compliance problem has been confirmed, further use of reflecting and other responses can identify the nature of the problem. Compliance problems can be categorized in three groups. The first is a knowledge deficit. In these cases, patients have insufficient information, lack skills, or have misinformation that prevents compliance. Examples are a patient who put contraceptive jelly on toast and the patient who was never shown or has forgotten how to use an inhaler. The second group involves practical impediments or barriers, such as complex drug regimens involving multiple drugs or different dosage schedules, difficulty in developing routines that facilitate medication compliance, difficulty in opening containers, or insufficient mental aptitude to comply. The final category is attitudinal barriers. Among the most difficult to identify and manage, these include patient beliefs about health, disease, or treatment that are inconsistent with the prescribed regimen. These may reflect differences in cultural beliefs.[36–38] Perceived severity of risk in relation to the perceived benefit of treatment plays a large role in determining patient compliance.[38] Other factors, such as the patient's desire to be in control and the belief that he or she can successfully implement the recommended treatment, also strongly influence compliance.[34] Finally, the most prevalent and potentially the most difficult belief differences to overcome are patients' lay theories.[38] Common lay theories held by patients include "You need to give your body a rest from medicine or it will become immune to it," "You only need to take medicine when you feel sick, not when you feel okay," or "If one pill is good, then two must be better."

Once the specific cause is identified, a specific strategy to manage that problem can be attempted. Most knowledge and skill deficiencies can be corrected with education or training. Practical impediments respond well to specific measures such as simplifying regimens, use of easy-open containers, and the aid of a spouse or caregiver. Attitudinal

issues tend to be the most complex and difficult to solve. Even lay theories, which seem to be easily debunked, are extremely difficult to overcome because the nature of lay theories makes them highly resistant to change. Again, it takes practice, careful listening, repeated conversations, and a supportive climate to help patients acknowledge these barriers. They will only do so when they feel that the pharmacist will not denigrate them or argue against their beliefs. Partnership language and gentle confrontation on the facts are indicated. Over time, repeated efforts to enlighten may change the patient's view.

CONCLUSION

Contemporary pharmacy practice is changing rapidly. Pharmaceutical care, which focuses on the patient's outcomes of drug therapy, is the founding principle for practitioners. New systems for pharmaceutical care delivery are appearing almost daily. From the pioneering work done by the Indian Health Service, which uses pharmacists across the spectrum of care, model clinical pharmacy practices that incorporate their principles into community pharmacies are evolving.[39–41] Whether one practices in a community, hospital, or other setting, the delivery of high-quality pharmaceutical care involves the skills and techniques discussed in this chapter, and others that support the pharmacist-patient interaction. As direct patient contact and responsibility for drug therapy outcomes become the main tasks for the pharmacist, the skills of interpersonal communication, medication history interview and consultation, and compliance monitoring and enhancement become the tools of the trade. The consistent application of a high degree of interpersonal and clinical skill by the pharmacist will lead to optimal outcomes for the patient.

KEY POINTS

- Patient communication skills are essential tools for successful clinical practice
- Successful pharmacist-patient communication requires the creation of a dialog, active involvement of the patient in the interview or education process, good pharmacist listening skills, and pharmacist feedback to verify correct interpretation of patient information and emotions
- Effective interviewing begins with broad open-ended questions and consists largely of focused open-ended questions. Closed-ended questions should be limited to clarifying patient responses and verifying the absence of important clinical information not elicited by open-ended questions
- The primary goal of patient education activities, such as patient consultation, is to verify patient understanding of key points

- During patient consultation and education, the pharmacist must identify and deal with informational deficiencies, patient emotions, and functional limitations to ensure that patients understand and can carry out therapeutic recommendations
- It is important for the pharmacist to remember that her or his job is to help the patient achieve optimal results from treatment, not ensure them
- Patients can absorb only limited amounts of information at one time. Therefore, give information gradually so patients do not become overwhelmed
- When evaluating the status of patients with chronic diseases, focus attention on three important aspects: control of the disease, compliance with therapeutic regimens, and the presence of complications caused by the disease state or drug therapy
- During all types of pharmacist-patient communication, listen carefully to the patient's responses. Many times they contain subtle clues that can lead the pharmacist to the correct assessment or reveal unspoken concerns or emotions that may interfere with education and compliance

SUGGESTED READINGS

Boyce RW, Herrier RN. Obtaining and using patient data. Am Pharm NS35:12–16, 1991.

Foster SL, Smith EB, Seybold MR. Advanced counseling techniques: integrating assessment and intervention. Am Pharm NS35:40–48, 1995.

Herrier RN. Medication compliance in the elderly. J Pharm Pract 8: 232–244, 1995.

Miller WR, Rollnick S. Motivational interviewing. 2nd ed. New York: The Guilford Press, 2002.

Pharmacist-patient Consultation Program, An interactive approach to patient consultation. New York: Pfizer U.S. Pharmaceuticals, 2003.

Smith M. Medication, quality of life and compliance: the role of the pharmacist. Pharmacoeconomics 1:225–230, 1992.

REFERENCES

1. Bolton R. People skills. New York: Simon & Schuster, 1979.
2. Rogers C. On becoming a person. Boston: Houghton Mifflin, 1961.
3. McWhinney I. The need for a transformed clinical method. In: Steward M, Roter D, eds. Communicating with medical patients. Thousand Oaks, CA: Sage, 1989:25–40.
4. Roter D, Hall J. Doctors talking with patients, patients talking with doctors. New York: Auburn House, 1992.
5. Henbest RJ, Stewart M. Patient-centeredness in the consultation, 2: does it really make a difference? Fam Prac 7:28–33, 1980.
6. Lickhart W. Rogers' necessary and sufficient conditions revisited. Br J Guid Counsel 12:113–123, 1984.
7. Barrett-Lennard GT. The empathy cycle: refinement of a nuclear concept. J Counsel Psychol 28:91–100, 1981.
8. Rubin FL, Judd MM, Conine TA. Empathy: can it be learned and retained? Phys Ther 57:644–647, 1977.
9. Kalisch B. What is empathy? Am J Nurs 73:1541–1552, 1973.
10. Meldrum H. Interpersonal communication in pharmaceutical care. New York: Pharmaceutical Products Press, 1994.
11. Gardner ME, Burpeau-DiGregorio MY. Objective assessment of pharmacy students' interviewing skills. Am J Pharm Educ 49: 137–144, 1985.
12. Gardner ME, McGhan WF. Objective assessment of interviewing skills: a comparison of two history types. Am J Pharm Educ 50: 165–169, 1986.
13. Ranelli PL. The utility of nonverbal communication in the profession of pharmacy. Soc Sci Med 13A:733–736, 1979.
14. Billings JA, Stoeckle JD. The clinical encounter. Chicago: Year Book Medical Publishers, 1989.
15. Boyce RW, Herrier RN. Obtaining and using patient data. Am Pharm NS31:65–71, 1991.
16. Meade V. OBRA '90: how has pharmacy reacted? Am Pharm NS35:12–16, 1995.
17. Pugh CB. PreOBRA '90 Medicaid survey: how community pharmacy practice is changing. Am Pharm NS35:17–23, 1995.
18. Boyce RW, Herrier RN, Gardner ME. Pharmacist-patient consultation program, unit 1: an inteactive approach to verify patient understanding. New York: Pfizer, Inc., 1991.
19. Gardner ME, Hurd PD, Slack MK. Effect of information organization on recall of medication instructions. J Clin Pharm Ther 14:1–7, 1989.
20. Morris LA, Grossman R, Barkdoll GL, et al. A survey of patient sources of prescription drug information. Am J Public Health 74: 1161–1162, 1984.
21. Lamb GC. Can physicians warn patients of potential side effects without fear of causing those side effects? Arch Intern Med 154: 2753–2756, 1994.
22. Howland JS, Baker MG, Poe T. Does patient education cause side effects? J Fam Pract 31:62–64, 1980.
23. Gardner ME, Rulien N, McGhan WF, et al. A study of perceived importance of medication information provided in a health maintenance organization setting. Drug Intell Clin Pharm 22:596–598, 1988.
24. Meldrum H, Hardy M. Challenges in communication about risk. Proc U S Pharmacopeial Conv 1995:36–49, 1995.
25. Pharmacist-patient consultation program, unit 2: counseling patients in challenging situations. New York: Pfizer, Inc., 1993.
26. Hatoum HT, Akhras K. 1993 Bibliography: a 32-year literature review on the value and acceptance of ambulatory care provided by pharmacists. Ann Pharmacother 27:1106–1119, 1993.
27. Church RM. Pharmacy practice in the Indian Health Service. Am J Hosp Pharm 44:771–775, 1987.
28. Herrier RN, Boyce RW, Apgar DA. Pharmacist-managed patient care services and prescriptive authority in the U.S. Public Health Service. Hosp Form 25:67–80, 1990.
29. Beckman HB, Markakis KM, Suchman AL, et al. The doctor patient relationship and malpractice: lessons from plaintiff depositions. Arch Intern Med 154: 1365–1370, 1994.
30. Anderson LA, Zimmerman MA. Patient and physician perceptions of their relationship and patient satisfaction: a study in chronic disease management. Patient Educ Counsel 20:27–36, 1993.
31. DiMatteo MR. The physician-patient relationship: effects on quality of health care. Clin Obstet Gynecol 37:149–161, 1994.
32. Viinamake H. The patient-doctor relationship and metabolic control in patients with type I (insulin dependent) diabetes mellitus. Int J Psychiatry Med 23:265–274, 1993.
33. Anderson RM. Is the problem of noncompliance all in our heads? Diabetes Educ 11:31–34, 1985.
34. Herrier RN, Boyce RW. Compliance with prescribed drug regimens. In: Bressler R, Katz M, eds. Geriatric pharmacology. New York: McGraw-Hill, 1993:63–77.
35. Pharmacist-patient consultation program, unit 3: counseling to enhance compliance. New York: Pfizer, Inc., 1985.
36. Eraker SA, Kirscht JP, Becker MH. Understanding and improving patient compliance. Ann Intern Med 100:258–268, 1984.
37. Becker MH. Patient adherence to prescribed therapies. Med Care 23: 539–555, 1985.
38. Leventhal H. The role of theory in the study of adherence to treatment and doctor patient interactions. Med Care 23:556–563, 1985.
39. Meade V. Adapting to providing pharmaceutical care. Am Pharm NS34:37–42, 1994.
40. Meade V. Pharmacist in Richmond launches pharmaceutical care program. Am Pharm NS34:43–45, 1994.
41. Meade V. Helping pharmacists provide disease-based pharmaceutical care. Am Pharm NS35:45–48, 1995.

CASE STUDIES

CASE 1

TOPIC: Adverse Drug Reactions and Drug-Induced Diseases

THERAPEUTIC DIFFICULTY: Level 2
Lynne M. Sylvia

CHAPTER 2: Adverse Drug Reactions and Drug-Induced Diseases

■ Scenario

Patient and Setting: MM, a 68-year-old male; primary care clinic

Chief Complaint: Fever, arthralgias, and a total body rash consisting of itchy, red, slightly raised papules; pain rated as 5 out of 10

■ History of Present Illness

Started on allopurinol approximately 7 weeks ago for the prevention of gouty attacks; most recent gouty attack occurred 8 weeks ago and was treated with indomethacin; pain score reported 2 weeks ago at PMD visit was 1 out of 10; admits to discontinuing one of his blood pressure medications (lisinopril) on his own last week due to a bothersome cough

Medical History: Diagnosed with gout 6 months ago; experienced 3 gouty attacks within the past 6 months that were each treated with indomethacin; hypertension for 5 years

Surgical History: None

Family/Social History: Family History: Mother died at age 75 with stroke; father alive at 92 with type 2 diabetes, hypertension, coronary artery disease (CAD) and gout
Social History: Single, retired postal worker who lives with his sister, nonsmoker, admits to alcohol use (4–5 beers per night) and frequent intake of junk food

Medications
Allopurinol, 300 mg PO QD
Indomethacin, 50 mg PO TID at onset of gout attack for 2 days; 25 mg PO TID until resolution of attack
Lisinopril, 10 mg PO QD
Hydrochlorothiazide (HCTZ), 25 mg PO QD

Allergies: Nausea and sour stomach with Percocet; penicillin VK: shortness of breath and hives

Review of Systems: Denies any difficulty breathing, headache, nausea, vomiting, or pain associated with gout. Admits to achy muscles and joints, oral pain, and a sensation that his skin "feels like ants are crawling"

■ Physical Examination

GEN: Elderly male appearing older than his stated age; complaining of itchy rash and generalized pain
VS: BP 150/95, HR 80, RR 22, T 39°C, Wt 75 kg, Ht 163 cm
HEENT: Ulcerations noted in the buccal mucosa and conjunctiva bilaterally
COR: nl S1, nl S2, − MRG
CHEST: Clear to A and P
ABD: WNL
GU: No mucosal lesions noted
RECT: Deferred
EXT: Left great toe is slightly enlarged with minimal erythema
NEURO: Alert and oriented × 3
SKIN: Diffuse, symmetrical maculopapular rash on the abdomen, arms, and legs; urticarial plaques noted on the upper chest and neck

■ Results of Pertinent Laboratory Tests, Serum Drug Concentrations, and Diagnostic Tests

Na 134 (134)	Hgb 13 (13)	Alk phos 1.6 (95)	Glu 6.1 (110)
K 3.5 (3.5)	Hct 0.35 (35)	T bili 17.1 (1.0)	
Cl 98 (98)	Lkcs 12×10⁹ (12×10³)	Alb 40 (4.0)	
HCO₃ 26 (26)	Plts 150×10⁹ (150×10³)		
BUN 15 (42)	AST 2.5 (150)		
Scr 186 (2.1)	ALT 3.3 (200)		

Lkc differential: 60% neutrophils, 20% lymphocytes, and 20% eosinophils
Complement 4 (C4): 10 mg/dL (20–50 mg/dL; 0.2 to 0.5 g/L)
ESR 85 (85 mm/hr)
Uric acid 357 (6 mg/dL)
Antinuclear antibodies −
Blood, urine, and throat cultures −

■ Problem List

Identify principal problems from the scenario in priority order (see Answers in back of book for correct list of problems).

■ SOAP Note

To be completed by the student (see Answers in back of book for correct SOAP Note).

■ QUESTIONS

(See Answers in back of book for correct responses.)

1. What signs and symptoms in MM are clinical markers of an allergic or hypersensitivity reaction? (EO-2)

2. MM presents with an elevated erythrocyte sedimentation rate (ESR). Based on the presence of an elevated ESR, which of the following can be concluded with confidence? (EO-5)
   a. MM is experiencing an allergic drug reaction.
   b. MM has an active bacterial infection.
   c. MM has increased concentrations of circulating inflammatory proteins.
   d. MM has an active viral infection.

3. MM is experiencing substantial pain relating to the progression of his skin rash and hypersensitivity syndrome. His physician would like to initiate morphine; however, MM's allergy profile reveals nausea and sour stomach related to Percocet. Which of the following statements best describes MM's documented reaction to Percocet? (EO-8, 10)
   a. The reaction is the result of a true hypersensitivity reaction to an opioid.
   b. The reaction is most likely a predictable effect of an opioid on the GI mucosa.
   c. The reaction is an uncommon idiosyncratic effect of specific opioids, not including morphine.
   d. The reaction is most likely related to the acetaminophen component in Percocet rather than the opioid.

4. Inappropriate dosing of allopurinol has been recognized as a risk factor for the development of allopurinol hypersensitivity syndrome. The guidelines for allopurinol dosing are listed below:

Creatinine clearance (mL/min as determined using the Cockcroft and Gault equation)	Dose of allopurinol
Crcl >60 mL/min	300 mg PO QD
Crcl 40–60 mL/min	200 mg PO QD
Crcl 20–39 mL/min	150 mg PO QD
Crcl <20 mL/min	100 mg PO QD or QOD

   At the time that allopurinol was initiated in MM, his serum creatinine concentration was 1.5 mg/dL, and his weight and height were 75 kg and 5'5", respectively. Based on the dosing guidelines, what dose of allopurinol would have been most appropriate for MM? (EO-6)
   a. 300 mg PO QD
   b. 200 mg PO QD
   c. 150 mg PO QD
   d. 100 mg PO QD

5. Further investigation of MM's medical history indicates that his liver tests (AST. ALT, Alk Phos and bilirubin) were within normal limits 8 weeks ago when allopurinol was initiated. Which type of liver injury do MM's current liver test results demonstrate? (EO-5)
   a. Acute cytotoxic liver injury
   b. Acute cholestatic injury
   c. Acute mixed injury (both cytotoxic and cholestatic)
   d. Chronic liver injury

6. On the second day of MM's hospitalization, a stool guaiac test is positive. Which of MM's chronic medications is most likely to cause a positive stool guaiac test? (EO-10)
   a. Allopurinol
   b. Lisinopril
   c. HCTZ
   d. Indomethacin

7. MM's pruritus is relieved by oral diphenhydramine; however, MM tells you that this medication makes him feel drowsy and confused. MM's physician asks you for a recommendation on an alternative agent to treat the pruritus. Which of the following agents is the most appropriate to recommend for this patient? (EO-8, 12)
   a. Hydroxyzine
   b. Chlorpheniramine
   c. Doxepin
   d. Cetirizine

8. MM complained of an unrelenting cough, which he associated with lisinopril therapy. Which of the following terms best describes this type of adverse drug reaction? (EO-7, 10)
   a. Hypersensitivity reaction
   b. Predictable reaction
   c. Idiosyncratic reaction
   d. Unpredictable reaction

9. For control of MM's high blood pressure, a decision is made to start losartan 50 mg PO QD. Develop a monitoring plan for MM to prevent the occurrence of adverse outcomes to this medication and provide counseling points for the patient. (EO-10, 14)

10. MM experienced a severe hypersensitivity syndrome to allopurinol. The syndrome initially presented as a maculopapular rash, which is a rather common skin reaction to medications. Analyze MM's initial presentation and identify those signs and/or symptoms that were indicative of the development of a severe hypersensitivity reaction. (EO-2, 5)

11. A decision was made to discontinue HCTZ as part of his antihypertensive drug regimen. This decision was based on the fact that thiazides may interfere with the management of gout. Describe the mechanism by which thiazides may aggravate gout. (EO-7, 9)

12. During MM's hospitalization, he develops pneumonia that requires antibiotic therapy. The physician caring for MM would like to initiate ceftriaxone, a third-generation cephalosporin; however, MM has a documented allergy to penicillin. Which of the following statements is correct regarding the risk of a cross reaction to ceftriaxone in this patient? (EO-8, 10)
    a. The risk of a cross reaction to ceftriaxone is 50%.
    b. The risk of a cross reaction to ceftriaxone is 10%–15%.
    c. The risk of a cross reaction to ceftriaxone is <5%.
    d. There is no risk of a cross reaction between these agents.

13. Summarize therapeutic, pathophysiologic, and disease management concepts for adverse drug reactions and drug-induced diseases utilizing a key points format. (EO-18)

CASE 2

TOPIC: Racial, Ethnic, and Gender Differences in Response to Drugs

THERAPEUTIC DIFFICULTY: Level 2
Julie A. Hixson-Wallace and Hewitt W. Matthews

Chapter 6: Racial, Ethnic, and Gender Differences in Response to Drugs

■ Scenario

Patient and Setting: DP, a 57-year-old African American male; hepatitis C clinic

Chief Complaint: Irritability, "edginess," headaches, insomnia, fatigue, and generalized body aches over the past month

■ History of Present Illness

Diagnosed with chronic hepatitis C 6 months ago and began therapy with peg-interferon and ribavarin 1 month ago; presents for routine follow-up in hepatitis C clinic; has been self-medicating with acetaminophen 1 g up to 4 times a day for body aches

Medical History: Hypertension × 12 years, hyperlipidemia × 5 years, chronic hepatitis C diagnosed 6 months ago

Surgical History: Appendectomy at age 11

Family/Social History: Family History: Noncontributory
Social History: Married; smokes 1/2 PPD, social ETOH consumption; IVDA × 32 years, clean × last 5 years

Medications:
Enalapril, 40 mg every day
Simvastatin, 40 mg every evening
Pegylated interferon alfa-2b, 150 μg SC every Friday evening
Ribaviran, 400 mg BID

Allergies: No known medication allergies

■ Physical Examination

GEN: Well-developed, well-nourished male in no apparent distress
VS: BP 156/92, HR 78, RR 18, T 37°C, Wt 95 kg, Ht 178 cm
HEENT: PERRLA, mild AV nicking
COR: NL S_1 and S_2
CHEST: WNL
ABD: Splenomegaly; otherwise soft without masses
GU: Deferred
RECT: Heme (−)
EXT: WNL
NEURO: Intact, alert, and oriented × 3

■ Results of Pertinent Laboratory Tests, Serum Drug Concentrations, and Diagnostic Tests

Na 142 (142)	Hct 0.45 (45)	Alk Phos 0.70 (42)
K 3.7 (3.7)	Hgb 150 (15)	Alb 34 (3.4)
Cl 101 (101)	Plts 333 × 10^9	T. Bili 22.23 (1.3)
BUN 7.14 (20)	(333 × 10^3)	AST 0.63 (38)
SCr 97.2 (1.1)	TG 1.60 (142)	Glu 5.99 (108)
HDL 0.98 (38)	ALT 0.60 (36)	LDH 1.86 (112)
LDL 3.41 (132)	TC 5.12 (198)	
INR 1.0		
HCV RNA 2100		

■ Problem List

Identify principal problems from the scenario in priority order (see Answers in back of book for correct list of problems).

■ SOAP Note

To be completed by the student (see Answers in back of book for correct SOAP Note).

■ QUESTIONS

(See Answers in back of book for correct responses.)

1. Which of the following racial or ethnic groups show more symptoms of intoxication after alcohol ingestion due to their less active liver aldehyde dehydrogenase? (EO-3)
   a. Caucasians
   b. African Americans
   c. Hispanics
   d. Asians

2. Which of the following polymorphic isozymes is responsible for the metabolism of antipsychotics? (EO-4)
   a. CYP2C9
   b. CYP2C19
   c. CYP2D6
   d. CYP3A4

3. Polymorphisms in CYP2C19 leading to individuals being poor metabolizers are most prevalent in which racial or ethnic group? (EO-4)
   a. Caucasians
   b. African Americans
   c. Hispanics
   d. Asians

4. As monotherapy in the treatment of hypertension, which of the following classes of agents is most effective in African Americans? (EO-8)
   a. Diuretics
   b. Angiotensin receptor blockers
   c. Beta-blockers
   d. ACE inhibitors

5. Lower doses of antipsychotic medications are generally required in which racial or ethnic group? (EO-8)
   a. Caucasians
   b. African Americans
   c. American Indians
   d. Asians

6. Pharmacokinetic and metabolic parameters in women compared to men generally demonstrate: (EO-4)
   a. Higher absorption
   b. Lower volume of distribution for lipophilic drugs
   c. No differences in protein binding
   d. Shorter half-lives

7. The likelihood of adverse effects from cardiovascular agents is generally: (EO-8)
   a. Greater in women than in men
   b. Less in women than in men
   c. Equally likely in women and men
   d. Greater in elderly men than in women

8. Which drug categories have been shown to be most clinically significant in their actions with regard to racial and ethnic differences? (EO-8)
   a. Antidepressants and antihyperlipidemics
   b. Cardiovascular and central nervous system agents
   c. Antidiabetics and antihypertensives
   d. Pulmonary and gastrointestinal agents

9. List some commonly prescribed medications that are metabolized via N-acetylation. (EO-4)

10. Outline the differences in the incidence of slow acetylators based on racial and ethnic groups. (EO-3)

11. In general, compare and contrast the response of African Americans, Asians, and Hispanics to antidepressant medications. (EO-8)

12. Outline gender differences in response to various psychotropic agents. (EO-8)

13. Summarize therapeutic, pathophysiologic, and disease management concepts for this case utilizing a key points format. (EO-18)

Allergic and Drug-Induced Skin Diseases

9

Kelly M. Smith

Allergic and drug-induced skin diseases encompass a wide variety of conditions, acute and chronic, with varying morphology. The most commonly encountered allergic skin diseases are atopic dermatitis, contact dermatitis, and urticaria. In addition, ingestion of a number of drugs can produce varied dermatological reactions, some of which result in significant morbidity.

TREATMENT GOALS

Therapy for allergic and drug-induced skin diseases primarily consists of removing any causative factor, determining if the disease stage is acute or chronic, and then implementing treatment, which is generally symptomatic in nature. General therapeutic goals include:

■ Identify and remove the cause of the reaction when possible, or eliminate exacerbating factors (e.g., atopic dermatitis).

- Use nonfluorinated or low-potency fluorinated topical steroids in conditions that require long-term therapy.
- Use high-potency fluorinated topical steroids or topical calcineurin inhibitors for short-term treatment during acute phases.
- Reserve systemic steroids for acute, severe cases with extensive involvement, with use limited to 5 to 14 days.
- Treat dry skin with baths and lubricating lotions (particularly atopic dermatitis).
- Promptly diagnose drug-induced skin disease, identify and remove underlying causes, and implement supportive therapeutic measures.
- Educate patients about the proper use of topical measures in treating their condition.
- Educate patients about issues related to their condition to prevent recurrence.

SKIN STRUCTURE AND FUNCTION

The skin, the largest organ of the body, is divided into three (main) distinct layers, the epidermis, the dermis, and the hypodermis (subcutaneous tissue) as indicated in Figure 9.1 (*see color insert*).[1] The epidermis is nonvascular and consists of stratified squamous epithelial cells that are of two distinct types, keratinocytes and dendritic cells. The epidermis consists of five distinct layers, beginning with the innermost:

1. Stratum germinativum (basal)
2. Stratum spinosum (prickle)
3. Stratum granulosum (granular)
4. Stratum lucidum (lucid)
5. Stratum corneum (horny)

The keratinocytes are located in the basal layer and serve as stem cells that differentiate into other cells in the upper layers of the epidermis. As the keratinocytes migrate toward the surface they undergo gradual transformation from living cells to dead, thick-walled flat cells that contain keratin. The

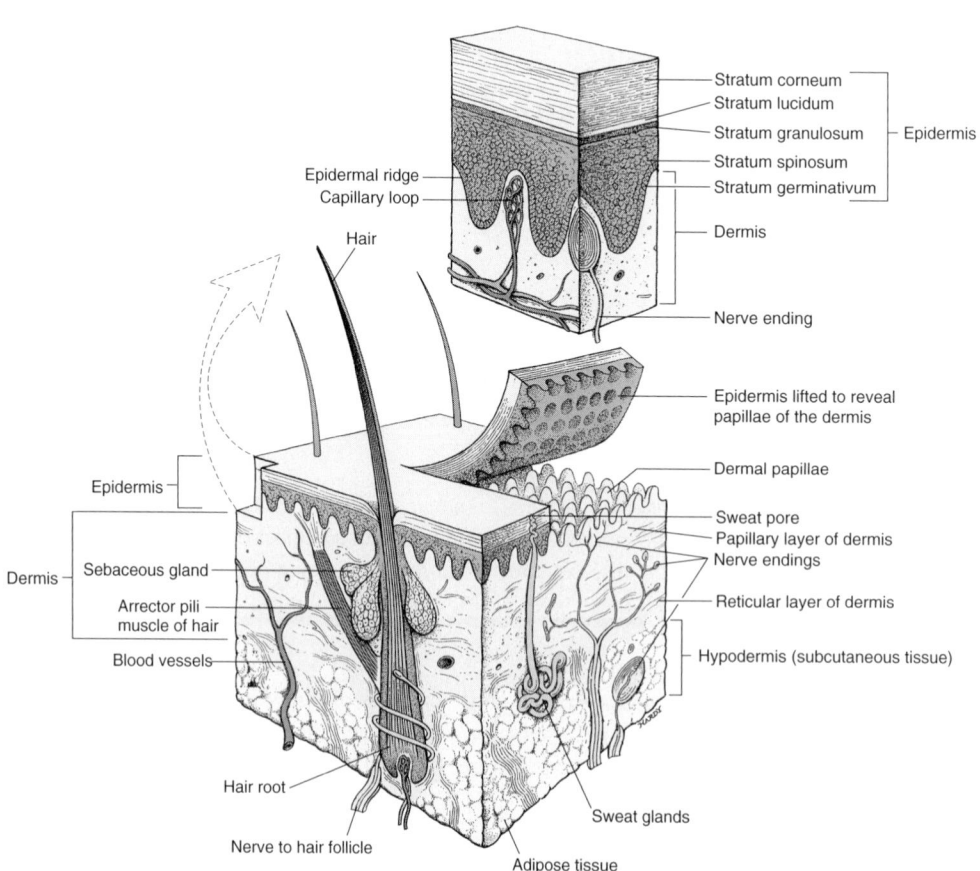

FIGURE 9.1 Skin structure and components (*see color insert*). (With permission from Stedman's Medical Dictionary. 27th ed. Baltimore: Lippincott Williams & Wilkins, 2000.)

basal layer also contains melanocytes, which are the pigment forming cells. The prickle layer also contains keratinocytes and melanocytes. The granular layer consists of several thicknesses of flattened cells with protein granules containing keratohyaline. These granules are changed to keratin, a fibrous substance in the outermost layers.

The lucid layer, which appears as a translucent line, is present only in thicker skin, like on the palms and soles. The outermost horny layer or the stratum corneum consists of flat, scaly dead tissue layers that are constantly shedding. The horny layer is the dead end product while the other four layers are considered the living epidermis. A continual process occurs throughout the sublayers of the epidermis in that new cells from the lower layers push older cells toward the top where they eventually become filled with keratin and die. The epidermis under normal conditions can replicate itself in 3 to 4 weeks.

The dermis consists of connective tissue, cellular elements, and ground substance with a rich blood and nerve supply. The sebaceous glands and shorter hair follicles originate in the dermis that can be divided into two distinct sublayers, the papillary and reticular units. The papillary layer is adjacent to the epidermis and has a rich supply of blood vessels. The reticular sublayer contains coarser tissue that connects the dermis and subcutaneous tissue (hypodermis).

The connective tissue of the dermis is comprised of collagen fibers, elastic fibers, and reticular fibers that provide support and elasticity of the skin. The cellular elements include fibroblasts, histiocytes, and mast cells, the latter of which are increased in itching dermatoses, like contact or atopic dermatitis. Histiocytes normally are present in small numbers around blood vessels. In pathologic conditions, these cells migrate in the dermis as monocytes with an evolution to macrophages. Polymorphonuclear leukocytes and eosinophils, members of the myeloid group, are quite common in dermatoses, particularly where an allergic component is involved. Lymphocytes from the lymphoid group are common in inflammatory lesions of the skin.

The hypodermis is composed of relatively loose connective tissue. In most areas, it contains a unit for formation and storage of fat. The fat layer functions in thermal control, food reserve, and cushioning. The hypodermis also supports the blood vessels and nerves that pass from tissues beneath to the dermis. Deeper hair follicles and sweat glands originate in the hypodermis.

The skin confines underlying tissue and provides a barrier between the body and environment. It prevents harm from external agents like ultraviolet radiation, pathogenic organisms, and chemicals. Various factors can alter the effectiveness of the barrier including age, underlying disease states, use of medications (topical or systemic), and the integrity of the stratum corneum. Other skin functions involve sensation, temperature control, development of pigment, synthesis of some vitamins, and moisture regulation.

MECHANISMS OF ALLERGIC SKIN DISEASE

While many of the conditions discussed in this chapter are believed to result from allergy, nonimmunologic mechanisms are also believed to play a role.[2,3] For example, contact dermatitis may be caused by immunologic mechanisms or result from direct irritant properties. However, the clinical presentation is essentially identical.[3]

Allergic reactions are classified in four categories that are based on immunologic mechanisms.[4] Type I (immediate or anaphylactic reaction) and Type IV (cell-mediated reaction) allergic reactions are most commonly involved in allergic skin manifestations. Immediate or anaphylactic reactions (Type I) result from the production of IgE antibodies that attach to the surface of basophils or mast cells. With reexposure, the offending substance binds to the antibodies on the cell surface causing release of chemical mediators, including histamine, serotonin, peptides, leukotrienes, and prostaglandins.[4,5] The subsequent clinical effects seen are determined by the interaction of mediators with various target organs and may include pruritus, urticaria, bronchospasm, laryngeal edema, and hypotension. Type IV reactions are termed cell-mediated, delayed, or tuberculin type reactions. The offending substance interacts with skin proteins evoking a cell-mediated immune response. Sensitized T lymphocytes release cytokines and lymphokines that cause local edema and inflammation.[4]

ATOPIC DERMATITIS

DEFINITION

Commonly known as eczema, atopic dermatitis is a chronic pruritic skin disorder most commonly associated with a personal or family history of allergic diseases, including rhinitis, asthma, or conjunctivitis.[6–9] Most patients experience mild to moderate symptoms, while up to 10% have severe manifestations.[10] The inflammatory disorder generally presents in early infancy with onset before age 5. However, atopic dermatitis may develop at any age.

ETIOLOGY

The exact cause of atopic dermatitis is unknown. Immunologic and physiologic abnormalities can occur.[6,7] Several factors support the involvement of immunologic functions: (a) the association of atopic dermatitis with other allergic disorders; (b) substantial elevations of serum IgE; (c) positive wheal and flare reactions to a wide variety of scratch tests; (d) increased susceptibility to bacterial, viral, and fungal infections; and (e) association with immunodeficiency disorders. Physiologic abnormalities include evidence of altered adrenergic and cholinergic responses.[6–8] Heredity plays a role with a possible inherited defect in some bone marrow-derived cells.

EPIDEMIOLOGY

Atopic dermatitis occurs in 10% to 20% of children and 1% to 3% of adults.[11] The prevalence of the disease has increased severalfold in industrialized countries over the last 30 to 40 years, and is more commonly noted in urban regions and members of higher social classes.[10,12] Such variations in occurrence suggest the role of environment in disease expression or manifestation.

PATHOPHYSIOLOGY

Genetic susceptibility, environmental factors, pharmacologic features, and immunologic mechanisms may all contribute to the development of atopic dermatitis.[12] Immunologic mechanisms have received the most investigation but the primary event that initiates the reaction is yet to be identified. Abnormalities of humoral- and cell-mediated immunity are present. Two of the most important immunologic alterations identified are an impairment of the delayed hypersensitivity response and an increased production of IgE. Identification of cytokines (interferons and interleukins) has allowed further delineation of possible mechanisms and development of possible new treatment strategies. For example, mononuclear leukocytes in patients with atopic dermatitis produce lower levels of interferon gamma (IFN-γ) and higher levels of interleukin-4 (IL-4). IFN-γ mediates delayed hypersensitivity reactions and IL-4 stimulates IgE synthesis.[7] Other interleukins, like IL-5 and IL-13, may also be involved.[9] IgE apparently is stimulated by specific antigens, attaches to mast cells, and triggers release of mast cell inflammatory mediators (including histamine) that are released on reexposure to the antigens.[6,7] However, other factors must play a role since atopic dermatitis occurs in patients with a deficiency of immunoglobulins, including agammaglobulinemia or Weskott-Aldrich syndrome. Primary T-cell deficiencies, which frequently result in increased concentrations of serum IgE, and eczematoid lesions often resolve following bone marrow transplantation. The demonstration of decreased numbers of T-lymphocytes may indicate lack of sufficient T-cells to control B-cell production of immuno-

globulin, thus producing high levels of IgE. In addition, phagocytic capacity is decreased and chemotaxis of neutrophils and monocytes is impaired.[8]

The immunologic basis of the disease is also demonstrated by the significant numbers of *Staphylococcus aureus* bacteria on the diseased and normal skin of atopic patients.[7,8] Exacerbations of eczema have developed secondary to *S. aureus* skin infections. Increased binding of the microbe to skin is thought to be related to the inflammation associated with atopic dermatitis.[12] Patients with atopic dermatitis also often have increased susceptibility to and recurrence of viral infections, which include herpes simplex, molluscum contagiosum, and warts.[6–8] The influence of genetics in atopic dermatitis cannot be discounted, as the skin disorder is transmitted familially, predominantly through the maternal influence.[9] A potential genotypic association has been identified in the IL-4 gene promoter region, along with a host of other potential genetic influences.

Pharmacologic abnormalities in atopic patients are evident in a number of cutaneous responses. Exaggerated constrictor response of cutaneous vessels, white dermographism, delayed blanch to cholinergic stimuli, and paradoxical response to application of nicotinic acid are examples.[8] A defect in the β-adrenergic receptor was once theorized when cyclic adenosine monophosphate (AMP) responses in atopic patients were noted to be subnormal to isoproterenol, prostaglandin E_1, and histamine agents, which would normally activate cyclic AMP. Decreased cyclic AMP levels accentuate the release of inflammatory mediators from mast cells and basophils.[6] Evidence suggests cyclic AMP phosphodiesterase activity (responsible for degradation of cyclic AMP) is increased, accounting for diminished cyclic AMP responsiveness upon challenge. This enzymatic abnormality might be a primary defect in patients with atopic dermatitis and is not dependent on the β-receptor.

CLINICAL PRESENTATION AND DIAGNOSIS

SIGNS AND SYMPTOMS

Pruritus and eczematous lesions of a chronic or relapsing nature are the hallmark symptoms of atopic dermatitis.[12] Pruritus generally worsens throughout the day and leads to scratching, papule development, and lichenification. Environmental factors, including allergens, reduced humidity, and diaphoresis (sweating) may compound the pruritus. Regardless of the disease stage, nearly all patients will have dry skin.

The skin lesions of atopic dermatitis, like those depicted in Figure 9.2 (*see color insert*), are often intensely pruritic.[6,12] The erythematous papules often bear evidence of excoriation and subsequent serous exudate. Lesion location is typically dictated by patient age. The face, scalp, and extensor surfaces of the extremities are most often affected

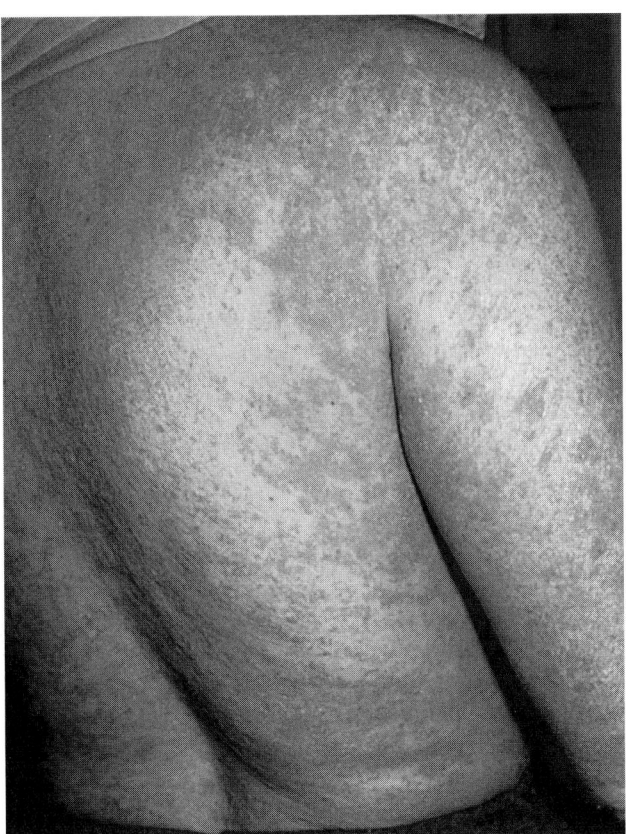

FIGURE 9.2 Atopic Dermatitis (*see color insert*). (With permission from Goodheart HP. Goodheart's photoguide of common skin disorders. 2nd ed. Philadelphia: Lippincott Williams & Wilkins, 2003.)

TABLE 9.1	Flare Factors in Atopic Dermatitis
Dry skin (xerosis)	
Sweating	
Exercise	
Infection	
Anxiety	
Scratching	
Light touch	
Prickly clothes (wool and acrylic)	
Heat	
Cold	
Temperature change	
Allergic contact dermatitis	
Allergies to foods or inhalants	
Coexisting diseases (e.g., scabies)	
Greasy ointments	

during infancy. The eruption generally begins as erythematous patches on the cheeks and spreads to the extensor surfaces of the extremities, while the diaper area is usually spared.[6] Intense itching is evident as the infant scratches constantly and rubs against garments and bedding. Many infantile cases clear over a period of months to years. With increasing age and disease duration, the lesions undergo lichenification and affect the flexural extremity folds. The lichenoid plaques are poorly marginated and vary in color from bright pink-red to brown or gray-brown. Areas commonly involved are the neck, eyelids, forehead/scalp, anterior chest, and wrists. Dorsal areas of the fingers, toes, and feet are often affected as well.

DIAGNOSIS AND CLINICAL FINDINGS

In addition to patient-reported symptoms, a number of diagnostic features may be present.[6,12] A family history of atopy is common, as are elevated serum IgE concentrations, dermatographism, delayed blanch response, orbital darkening, facial erythema or pallor, and numerous cutaneous infections. Environmental factors, also termed "flare factors," may induce or exacerbate atopic dermatitis (Table 9.1). A strong relationship exists between food allergy and atopic

disease, primarily in children.[6,9] Conversely, inhalant allergens, like dust mites, seem to be more of a factor for adults. Foods can exacerbate the dermatitis with evidence that elimination of food allergens results in improvement. The types of foods most commonly involved include eggs, peanuts, milk, soy, wheat, and fish. The disease should be differentiated from a number of other conditions, including cutaneous T-cell lymphoma, seborrheic dermatitis, contact dermatitis, nummular (coin-like) dermatitis, scabies, and psoriasis.

TREATMENT

Management strategies include a variety of nondrug and drug treatment measures depending on the duration of the condition. The most common approaches include environmental change, skin maintenance care techniques, topical antiinflammatory agents, systemic antihistamines, topical or systemic antibiotics and, selectively, systemic corticosteroids. The therapeutic goals are to decrease skin inflammation, eliminate exacerbating factor(s), and relieve itch and dry skin. Topical and systemic therapies are directed at relieving the symptoms of pruritus and dry skin, and reducing inflammation.

TOPICAL THERAPY

Several forms of topical therapy, the majority of which are antiinflammatory in nature, are available. Patients with mild or localized atopic dermatitis may require treatment only with a topical corticosteroid ointment or cream. For patients with extensive disease, a combination of topical measures may be necessary. Topical antihistamines and local anesthetics are not recommended, as they may be associated with patient sensitization.[13]

Topical Corticosteroids. These antiinflammatory agents are commonly used to control acute flares or exacerbations. Acutely, high potency topical steroids can be used for 7 to 10 days. Once control is achieved, the regimen may be changed to twice-weekly application to eczema-prone areas.[14] Nonfluorinated (hydrocortisone 1% or desonide 0.05%) or low potency fluorinated preparations (triamcinolone 0.025%) are preferred for long-term use.[9,15] In general, topical corticosteroid use should be minimized by application only during acute flares, by applying only to the most problematic areas, or by once daily or alternate day application. Long-term use of fluorinated corticosteroids, particularly high-potency agents, causes thinning of the skin and can lead to atrophy and telangiectasia, particularly on the face and skinfold areas.

Corticosteroid creams or ointments can be used and are best applied within a few minutes after bathing. Patient preference or environmental conditions may influence choice. Creams are most often a suitable emollient for the typical eczema lesion, which may be slightly moist. Ointments are better suited for extremely dry skin areas, or for use during the dry months of winter.[10]

Topical Immunosuppressants. Due to the extensive experience clinicians have with topical corticosteroids, their use is still considered a mainstay of treatment. However, the role of topical immunosuppressants is growing. Topical calcineurin inhibitors, including pimecrolimus and tacrolimus, inhibit several mechanisms of atopic dermatitis manifestations, including T-cell, mast cell, and dendritic cell activation.[16] Both agents are generally effective and safe for short-term use in adults and children and are commercially available in topical formulations. Patient response is generally evident within 3 days of drug initiation, with continued use leading to a reduction in number of flares and corticosteroid requirements and diminished potential for skin atrophy associated with topical corticosteroid administration.[12] Local burning is the most frequently reported adverse effect of this class. Though the potential is minimal, tacrolimus and pimecrolimus may be absorbed systemically, particularly if applied over large surface areas with altered skin integrity. Lesions that are unresponsive to topical corticosteroids, that affect the face and neck or extensive surface areas, and those occurring in patients hesitant to use corticosteroids are situations in which topical calcineurin inhibitors may be particularly advantageous.

Reports of dose-related cancer in animals and humans have prompted an FDA public health advisory to warn healthcare professionals and patients about the potential cancer risk. Topical pimecrolimus and tacrolimus should only be used short-term or intermittently, as labelled, in patients unresponsive to or intolerant of other treatments. The true nature of this safety concern is unclear, and the propensity of related compounds to cause similar effects is not known.

However, potential carcinogenicity may temper the enthusiasm clinicians have about topical pimecrolimus and tacrolimus. Reports of dose-related cancer in animals and humans prompted the incorporation of a black box warning in the product labeling for both medications. The revised labels note approved use only for short-term and intermittent periods in patients unresponsive to or intolerant of other treatment approaches. Patients with immune system compromise are not appropriate candidates for topical calcineurin inhibitors, and long-term or first-line treatment is not recommended. The true nature of this safety concern is unclear, and the propensity of related compounds to cause similar effects is not known.

Tar Preparations. Coal tar products may have antiinflammatory properties, although not as pronounced as those of topical corticosteroids and immunosuppressants.[12,13] Use of coal tar products can be problematic, as they often stain clothing and may result in photosensitivity and folliculitis. However, they do reduce the need for topical corticosteroids when administered chronically. Preparations are readily available in shampoos and bath products and may also be compounded in water-soluble bases for application on other skin areas. The administration of the latter products may be more practical at night to limit staining of clothes, and application to acutely inflamed skin areas should be avoided.

Topical Antibacterial Agents. Secondary skin infections, which are frequently due to *Staphylococcus aureus*, can be treated with topical antibiotics if the skin involvement is somewhat limited.[9,15] One- to 2-week treatment with preparations containing erythromycin or bacitracin are preferred because of less sensitization than with agents like neomycin. Mupirocin is another effective agent.

Phototherapy. Treatment with ultraviolet A and B phototherapy can be a useful adjunct in the management of severe disease.[17] Combination use with psoralen may also be considered in patients with severe, widespread disease.[10,12] Patients may initially experience local irritation with phototherapy prior to the realization of any symptomatic benefits. Other short-term effects of phototherapy include erythema, pruritus, skin pain, and pigmentary changes. Premature skin aging and malignancies are potential adverse effects of long-term exposure.

SYSTEMIC THERAPY

Oral Antihistamines. Antihistamines may be useful under limited circumstances. Two possible benefits from oral administration of antihistamines include relief of pruritus and sedation, the latter of which appears to be the predominant benefit, as demonstrated in clinical trials.[10,13] If sedation and anxiolysis are the desired goals, then patients should benefit more from the traditional H_1-blockers, rather than second-generation agents.[18]

Oral Corticosteroids. Oral corticosteroids may be used for acute flares to break the itch-scratch cycle.[9,15] Duration of use should be short-term, generally no more than 5 to 7 days. Oral corticosteroid therapy generally is discouraged except in the case of refractory episodes, particularly since rebound flaring may occur following corticosteroid discontinuation.[12,13] To minimize the potential rebound effects, corticosteroid dosage reduction (i.e., tapering) should be implemented, along with an intensified skin care regimen, including topical corticosteroids, appropriate bathing habits, and the use of emollients.

Oral Antimicrobials. Systemic antibiotic therapy may be indicated to treat secondary bacterial infections (e.g., folliculitis) that can develop.[9,15] Therapy is directed toward Gram-positive cocci, particularly *S. aureus*. A 7-day course of an antistaphylococcal agent (e.g., dicloxacillin) often is used.[9] Antiviral treatment of cutaneous herpes simplex infection is also important in patients with disseminated atopic dermatitis. Left untreated, the viral condition may disseminate and become life-threatening. Fungal infections, particularly with *Malassezia furfur,* may also develop and warrant appropriate treatment.

Other Systemic Options. Cyclosporine inhibits T–lymphocyte-dependent immune responses and down regulates cytokine production. Oral administration of cyclosporine has resulted in improved symptoms and quality of life in adults and children with refractory disease.[19] Treatment response does not correlate with blood concentration, thus, routine blood concentration monitoring is not necessary. After initiating drug therapy at a dose of 5 mg/kg, the dose can be tapered to 1 to 2 mg/kg, minimizing the potential for dose-related adverse effects.[19,20] Reduction to maintenance doses ranging from 0.5 to 2 mg/kg/day or 5 mg/kg given every 5 days has been successful in maintaining response. Hypertension, nephrotoxicity, and serious drug interactions limit the drug to no longer than 2 years of use.[6,9] Discontinuation results in relapse in a high percentage of patients (50% to 75%). Other immunosuppressants, including mycophenolate mofetil, methotrexate, and azathioprine, may be of value to patients with refractory disease.[10,12,21]

NONPHARMACOLOGIC THERAPY

Where environmental factors are identified as contributory, avoidance is advised. This may include avoiding extremes of temperature and humidity, strenuous exercise, rough scratchy clothing, bathing with harsh soaps and hot water, irritating chemicals, and allergens.[6,15] These factors and others can precipitate or perpetuate the itch-scratch cycle (Table 9.1). Stress, anger, or anxiety may contribute to exacerbations of atopic dermatitis and should be managed appropriately. Swimming may be a suitable alternative to other physical activities since the diaphoresis disease trigger is avoided. However, the chlorine in pool water should be rinsed off immediately after swimming, followed by skin lubrication.[12]

Baths. Itching can be relieved at least temporarily by tepid baths; showers are less effective. Oatmeal (Aveeno, plain or oilated), bath oils, or tar preparations may be added. Bathing also assists with rehydration of the skin. However, using hot water and scrubbing with a washcloth or brush will cause irritation, and strong soaps should be avoided in favor of mild soaps with a neutral pH and minimal defatting activity. A lubricating lotion (Cetaphil, Lubriderm, or Nutraderm) can be used for cleansing instead of soap. To aid dry skin, applying a water-in-oil emulsion (e.g., Eucerin) to skin that is still wet from a lukewarm water soak assists in rehydrating the keratin layers.[15] In general, the use of emollients is a core principle of recommended skin care.

Wet Dressings. In the acute setting when lesions are oozing, acute, and possibly infected, wet dressings like Burow solution (aluminum acetate) 1:20 or tap water can be used. Compresses are applied generally for 20 to 60 minutes 3 to 6 times a day. The dressings will cool and dry by evaporation thus stimulating vasoconstriction. In very acute situations, compresses can be applied continuously. Dressings may also effectively prevent persistent scratching, which can facilitate the healing of excoriated lesions.[12]

ALTERNATIVE THERAPIES

In patients who fail to respond despite aggressive treatment, the next step is to break the cycle of scratching. To help achieve this goal, one approach is a major intervention of a "simulated hospitalization."[22] That is, the patient is required to stop the usual routine of school or work, have complete bed rest in a semidarkened room for a few days (e.g., Friday PM to Monday AM), given light sedation, and a short course (≤1 week) of an oral corticosteroid to reduce inflammation. In addition, if the patient has folliculitis, a course of antibiotics is given. After this intense few days of therapy to break the cycle of scratching, the major challenge is to keep the skin clear by eliminating the urge to scratch. If the worst scratching is during sleep, a higher dose of a sedating antihistamine may be used. If sedating antihistamines are not sufficient, other sedating therapies may be considered for a few days or weeks in the most severe cases where quality of life is being affected to a great degree.

Concurrent with a major intervention like medications, another critically important step should be initiated. That intervention involves dealing with the psychology of atopic dermatitis. Clearly, emotional stress is a major trigger for scratching in some patients. In children, hostility or family discord can trigger the itch-scratch cycle. Dealing with these factors can be very helpful. Other techniques that may also be considered include behavioral and cognitive intervention, biofeedback, relaxation training, and learning to properly express anger and be assertive.[12,15,23] Traditional Chinese herbs have also been administered to patients with recalcitrant disease. However, the potential for hepatic and cardiac toxicity, and idiosyncratic reactions, limits the utility of these remedies.[23]

A reduced rate of conversion from linoleic acid to gamma-linolenic acid (GLA), dihomo-gamma-linolenic acid, and arachidonic acid has been identified in some patients with atopic dermatitis.[25] GLA supplementation, via the administration of topical evening primrose oil or borage oil, has been investigated. Study results have been equivocal, and a metaanalysis demonstrating the benefits of GLA supplementation has been criticized for its methodology. However, further investigation in this area is warranted.

FUTURE THERAPIES

Case reports and small studies provide preliminary support for the use of the leukotriene antagonist montelukast as a steroid-sparing and symptom-relieving agent.[25] Daily subcutaneous injections of interferon-γ have demonstrated benefits in a small number of patients.[6,7,20] However, relapse

following discontinuation was very common, and potential side effects include flu-like symptoms, leukopenia, and thrombocytopenia. IL-2 has received limited study but did show benefit in one group of six patients with severe disease.[20] Intravenous immunoglobulin may also have antiinflammatory utility.[26] Phosphodiesterase (PDE) activity may be increased in the leukocytes of patients with atopic dermatitis. The resultant clinical effects of an investigational topical PDE4 inhibitor was demonstrated in 20 patients.[27] Another unique approach is the administration of systemic azole antifungals, including itraconazole and fluconazole. The rationale for such use is to decrease fungal colonization of the skin and gastrointestinal tract.[28] Future investigation will include these and other agents that target the various pathophysiologic mechanisms of atopic dermatitis.

CONTACT DERMATITIS

ETIOLOGY

Contact dermatitis is an inflammatory response of the skin categorized based on origin (i.e., allergic and irritant). Allergic contact dermatitis is a delayed hypersensitivity reaction with an immunologic basis, while irritant contact dermatitis results when a substance has a direct toxic effect on tissue with no immunologic basis.[3,29] The disease spectrum is wide, as all adverse cutaneous reactions rising from direct skin contact with a foreign agent can be classified as contact dermatitis.[30]

Causes of allergic contact dermatitis are varied and commonly include metallic salts, plants, rubber compounds (latex), and cosmetics containing preservatives and fragrances.[29,30] Soaps, detergents, petroleum solvents, acids, and alkalis are frequent offenders in irritant contact dermatitis. Often the dermatitis is related to occupational exposure. The origin, whether allergic or irritant, usually cannot be differentiated by the clinical presentation.[9,30,31] In addition, irritants may also serve as allergens, compounding the diagnostic difficulty.

EPIDEMIOLOGY

Irritant contact dermatitis accounts for about 80% of the reactions, with allergic contact dermatitis responsible for the remainder.[9,30] The occurrence of contact dermatitis is widespread partly due to the large variety of substances implicated as causes (Table 9.2). The prevalence within the general population is also not well documented. According to patch testing, the prevalence of allergy to specific substances in the normal population is nickel (5.8%), neomycin (1.1%), ethylenediamine (0.43%), and benzocaine (0.17%).[32] Sex

differences are observed regarding specific allergies. For example, nickel allergy is more frequent in women than in men, a figure likely explained by a higher rate of contact from the wearing of jewelry and clothing. Contact dermatitis has been identified as a leading cause of occupational allergy, and it is of great concern to individual patients and employers alike.[33]

PATHOPHYSIOLOGY

Allergic contact dermatitis represents a typical delayed hypersensitivity reaction that requires penetration of the stratum corneum by the allergen, interaction with epidermal or dermal cells, interaction with the immune system, and activation of the inflammatory response.[3,9] Sensitizing stimuli (haptens) usually have a low molecular weight, are lipid soluble, and are highly reactive. The Langerhans cells process haptens that then migrate to regional lymph nodes. The processed hapten interacts with T-cells with resulting activation of the Langerhans cells and T-cells. Langerhans cells secrete IL-1, thus stimulating the T-cells to secrete IL-2. Specific T-cells capable of interacting with the antigen proliferate, completing the sensitization phase. A period of 8 to 10 days is generally required for allergy presentation once sensitization has begun.[32]

In the elicitation phase, the T-cells then circulate and penetrate into skin.[9] When the skin is exposed to the hapten again, interaction occurs initially with Langerhans cells. The processed hapten interacts with the antigen-specific T-cells located in the skin. IL-1 and IL-2 are secreted with further production of antigen-specific T-cells. The activated T-cells also secrete cytokines, interferon-γ, and tumor necrosis factor. The former activates keratinocytes, starting a complex

TABLE 9.2	Common Causes of Contact Dermatitis

Pharmaceutical Agents	**Rubber Materials**
Corticosteroids	Gloves
Neomycin	Finger protectors
"Caine" anesthetics	**Hobby Materials**
Merbromin	Epoxy glues
Thimerosal	Paints
Transdermal patches	Solvents
	Occupational Exposure
Lubricants	Chrome
Lotions	Epoxy glues
Hand creams	Other glues
Face creams	Formaldehyde
Bath oils	Nickel
	Cobalt
	Solvents
Cosmetics and Fragrances	Resins
Deodorants	Dyes
Hair dyes	Oils and greases
Makeup	Solvents and waterless
Perfumes	cleaners
	Metals
Surfactants	Jewelry
Hand, bath, and shower soaps	**Plants**
Soaps used at work	Poison oak/ivy
Kitchen and laundry soaps	Algerian ivy
Waterless cleaners	Chrysanthemums
	House plants

(From Wollenberg A, Sharma S, von Bubnoff D, et al. Topical tacrolimus (FK506) leads to profound phenotypic and functional alterations of epidermal antigen-presenting dendritic cells in atopic dermatitis. J Allergy Clin Immunol 107:519–525, 2001; Reynolds NJ, Franklin V, Gray JC et al. Narrow-band ultraviolet B and broad-band ultraviolet A phototherapy in adult atopic eczema: a randomised controlled trial. Lancet 357:2012–2016, 2001; Advenier C, Queille-Roussel C. Rational use of antihistamines in allergic dermatological conditions. Drugs 38:634–644, 1984, with permission.)

cascade of interaction with leukocytes and secretion of other cytokines (IL-1, IL-6, granulocyte macrophage stimulating factor). Mast cells and macrophages are activated by release of eicosanoids from keratinocytes. The result is the classic inflammatory response.

CLINICAL PRESENTATION AND DIAGNOSIS

SIGNS AND SYMPTOMS

Allergic contact reactions are most commonly manifested in an eczematous form, but may occasionally include an urticarial component. Irritant reactions may be dermatitic, acneiform, pigmentary, purpuric, or atrophic in nature.[34]

DIAGNOSIS AND CLINICAL FINDINGS

Contact dermatitis is classified as acute, subacute, or chronic.[9,32] Acute contact dermatitis involves erythema, edema, and formation of highly pruritic papules, vesicles, and bullae (Fig. 9.3, *see color insert*). The subacute form presents with erythema (smaller, superficial vesicles) and minimal pruritus. In chronic forms, the skin may be cracked and scaly with excoriations and plaque formations.[9,31] Severe itching in the acute phase is prominent and may persist into the other phases.

The history and physical examination can provide critical information to establish the diagnosis. An acute dermatitis of the extremities that is of a patchy and streaky nature, coupled with a recent history of outdoor plant exposure, might lead to a diagnosis of poison ivy/oak dermatitis. A dermatitis occurring on the eyelids or face of a woman might be associated with the use of cosmetics, perfumes, or hair sprays. A careful and thorough history regarding general activities, occupation, hobbies, known allergies or previous skin disorders, family history, and careful examination of the distribution and extent of the lesions, may suggest possible causes.[9] Common causes of contact dermatitis are listed in Table 9.2, and the substances most likely involved with reactions in certain body areas are indicated in Table 9.3. In many patients, the diagnosis remains unclear and patch testing may be indicated, particularly in conditions that become chronic, are relatively resistant to treatment or are suspected to be occupationally related.

Patients may not report a problem associated with the previous handling of a material sometimes for prolonged periods (years). Generally, a latent period can be identified, when the latest exposure results in an eruption which is termed the "elicitation dose."[31] An earlier exposure resulted in the initial sensitization. In the case of irritant contact dermatitis, direct cellular damage occurs with no latent period.

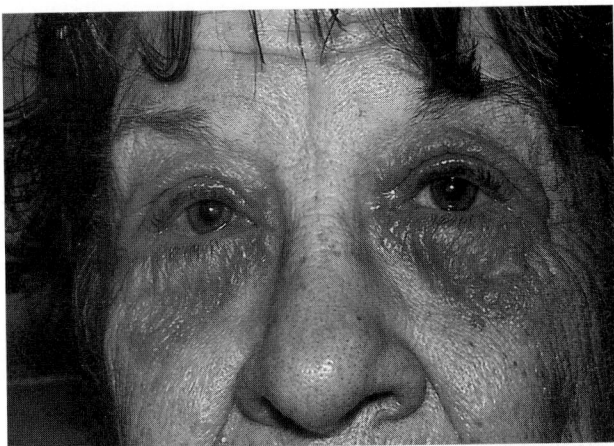

FIGURE 9.3 Allergic dermatitis following use of neomycin ophthalmic ointment (*see color insert*). (With permission from Tasman W, Jaeger E. The Wills Eye Hospital atlas of clinical ophthalmology. 2nd ed. Lippincott Williams & Wilkins, 2001.)

TABLE 9.3	Causes of Contact Dermatitis by Body Region
Scalp:	Hair dyes (paraphenylenediamine, a permanent dye), hair lotions, permanents (glyceryl thioglycolate), nickel in hair pins, wig attachments/adhesives
Face:	Cosmetics, topical medicaments, plants, preshave and aftershave lotions, airborne allergens
	Forehead: hatbands, any hair products
	Eyes: eyelids affected by cosmetics, face creams, lubricants, hair spray, nail polish
	Conjunctivitis: thimerosal
	Lips and perioral areas: lipstick, lip protectants, toothpastes, mouthwashes, mangos
Ears:	Nickel (earrings), perfume, earplugs, earphones, telephone receiver
Neck:	Perfume, nickel (necklace), hair cosmetics, clothing; clothing labels, buttons, zippers
Armpits:	Deodorants, depilatories, clothing, perfumes
Hands:	Materials encountered at work and/or home (e.g., foods, chemicals, topical medicaments, hand lotions and lubricants, rubber gloves, rubber bands, jewelry, plants)
Body (trunk, chest, waist):	
	Dyes, formaldehyde (fabric finisher), resins, rubber in elastic of clothing, perfumes, scarves
Genitalia:	Bubble bath, antiseptic cleansers, condoms, contraceptive creams or jellies, deodorant douches, scented menstrual pads or tampons
Feet:	Shoes, shower sandals, fabrics, metal eye holes, sole inserts, adhesives, colorants, athlete's foot remedies.

(From Reynolds NJ, Franklin V, Gray JC et al. Narrow-band ultraviolet B and broad-band ultraviolet A phototherapy in adult atopic eczema: a randomised controlled trial. Lancet 357:2012–2016, 2001, with permission.)

Damage is proportional to the toxic properties of the irritant, but may depend on repeated exposure for some substances that are mild irritants. With irritant contact dermatitis, those exposed to the same dose under the same conditions for the same length of time would be expected to react. Reduction of the irritant dose (i.e., exposure) often results in a good prognosis.[30]

Patch testing may assist in diagnosis of delayed hypersensitivity contact dermatitis. Standardized methods and concentrations for testing for a variety of substances have been recommended.[30,32] Even with standardized approaches, false-positive and false-negative reactions may occur.[30,31] An irritant reaction may be difficult to differentiate from a weak allergic reaction.

The histopathologic features of contact dermatitis include perivascular infiltrates of lymphocytes and monocytes in the upper dermis. Edema is usually present and may involve intracellular and intercellular edema in the epidermis with a condition called ''spongiosis.'' Basophils and mast cells are present in the cellular infiltrate and may participate in the inflammatory reaction. Hyperkeratosis, acanthosis, and a cellular infiltrate in the superficial dermis containing basophils are often present in the chronic setting.[29]

THERAPEUTIC PLAN

Contact dermatitis may become a chronic, serious condition that interferes with activities of daily living. This is particularly true if the offending agent cannot be identified and further contact then eliminated. Treatment focuses on allergen (irritant) avoidance and treatment of the underlying dermatologic reaction. This may be accomplished more easily in the case of poison ivy dermatitis than in the case of dermatitis due to industrial exposure.

TREATMENT

PHARMACOTHERAPY

Specific drug therapy depends more on the stage and the extent of the dermatitis than on the cause.[32] Severe, acute reactions characterized by blistering, swelling, and oozing may require systemic corticosteroids, for which various regimens are recommended.[9,31,32] An initial dose of 60 mg (range 40–100 mg) of prednisone or equivalent is common, or 1 mg/kg in a single daily dose with treatment recommended for periods of 7 to 14 days. Most clinicians recommend tapering the dose during the treatment period to avoid rebound.[9] Specific doses and duration of treatment are probably best determined by the presentation of the patient. Topical corticosteroids are of little benefit in acute edematous blistering dermatitis because of inadequate tissue penetration. Soothing compresses or baths with water, aluminum acetate, or saline may be beneficial in providing relief at this stage.[9,32] As the acute symptoms are controlled, topical corticosteroids applied once or twice a day can be instituted with treatment continued after the conclusion of oral therapy. Ointments are usually preferred because cream preparations have a greater variety of ingredients, including fragrances and preservatives, that may cause an allergic reaction.[31] Oral antihistamines provide little if any benefit other than sedation since they do not suppress contact allergy.[9,32] Calamine and other shake lotions, topical antihistamines, and topical anesthetics are best avoided because of lack of benefit and potential sensitization.[9,30,32]

For subacute (moderate) or chronic dermatitis, topical corticosteroid therapy is used rather than systemic therapy. A high-potency agent may be applied twice daily in subacute conditions. Ointment or cream preparations of corticosteroids are often preferred due to the likelihood that patients will have dry skin. In chronic situations low-, medium-, or high-potency corticosteroid preparations are selected based on the degree of skin thickening (lichenification). Overnight occlusion with plastic enhances penetration of the steroid.

However, caution should be exercised when applying corticosteroids to the face and in skinfold areas. Skin lubrication is also often needed with frequent application in a thin layer. White petrolatum is a good choice. If secondary infection is present, systemic antibiotic therapy is usually preferred as topical antimicrobial agents can be sensitizing.[9,32]

About 3% of patients treated with corticosteroids will experience contact allergy to the steroid. The occurrence is sometimes difficult to recognize due to several factors: the antiinflammatory property of the steroid may mask the allergic reaction; the steroid may have been used topically for some time; and the dermatitis may be only slightly worse or fail to improve. Budesonide and hydrocortisone are the most frequent offenders, with the fewest reactions caused by betamethasone, dexamethasone, and mometasone furoate. Classification of the steroids based on chemical/molecular structure helps identify potential alternative agents, but there is some cross-reactivity across classes.[31]

Photochemotherapy may be used effectively but is indicated only in carefully selected patients who can comply or do not respond to standard therapy. Such treatment does not incur the systemic adverse effects of corticosteroids, however, it requires office-based treatment several times each week.[30] Topical immunosuppressants (e.g., tacrolimus, pimecrolimus) have been used as well, but not thoroughly studied.[35]

NONPHARMACOLOGIC THERAPY

Beyond preventing exposure to the antigenic stimulus, treatment focuses primarily on pharmacologic management. However, cold compresses applied to the site of the reaction may provide symptomatic relief. They should be used sparingly, as they may cause skin drying. Barrier creams and gloves may also be of value in preventing future antigen exposure. A variety of products (Tecnu Outdoor Skin Cleanser®, Ivy Stat®, Ivy Block®, and Ivy Cleanse®) can prevent or minimize the absorption of urushiol oil, the antigenic component of poison ivy, oak, and sumac.[36]

URTICARIA

Urticaria (hives) and angioedema are edematous vascular reactions of the skin.[9] Extension of the vascular reactions, particularly edema, into the dermis and hypodermis is termed "angioedema." The two conditions occur concurrently in almost half of patients (Fig. 9.4, *see color insert*); another 40% experience only urticaria, and approximately 10% experience angioedema only.[37] Many cases of urticaria are acute, but if the episodes continue for longer than 6 to 8 weeks, the condition is termed "chronic."[9,38]

EPIDEMIOLOGY

Urticaria is estimated to occur in 15% to 25% of the population at some time in life.[38,39] All age groups can be affected, with acute reactions occurring more often in children and young adults. Chronic urticaria occurs more often in adults, particularly middle-aged women.[38]

ETIOLOGY

The etiology of urticaria is varied and often obscure. Urticaria may be associated with or caused by drugs, serums, foods, inhalants, insect bites/stings, contact substances, connective tissue diseases, neoplasms, infections, endocrine disorders, and physical agents.[9] The latter often include cold, heat, sunlight, pressure, and dermographism. The urticaria may be linked to cholinergic or adrenergic factors. Hereditary angioedema, characterized by recurrent, self-limited attacks, is transmitted by autosomal-dominant inheritance with incomplete penetrance. In addition to childhood onset and family history, a specific test for C1-esterase inhibitor, a complement component, can be used to confirm the condition. A cause cannot be specifically identified in 70% to 80% of chronic cases and is thus termed idiopathic.

PATHOPHYSIOLOGY

At least five pathophysiologic mechanisms have been proposed for urticaria and angioedema: (a) IgE-mediated, (b) complement-mediated, (c) direct mast cell-releasing agents, (d) alteration of arachidonic acid metabolism, and (e) idiopathic.[9,37] Skin biopsies of urticarial lesions show edema in the upper dermis, vascular dilation, and cellular infiltrates in the dermis around the small vessels due to leakage.

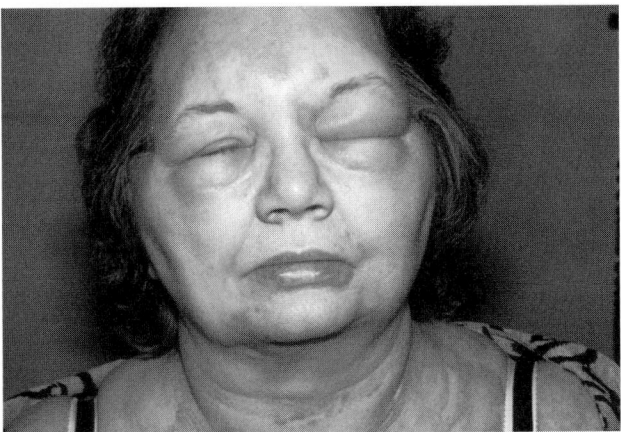

FIGURE 9.4 Urticaria with angioedema of the face and eyelids (*see color insert*). (With permission from Goodheart HP. Goodheart's photoguide of common skin disorders. 2nd ed. Philadelphia: Lippincott Williams & Wilkins, 2003.)

The histologic nature of the infiltrate may vary and have some relation to clinical course. Some infiltrates are predominantly lymphocytic, while others involve polymorphonuclear (PMN) cells (neutrophils, eosinophils, and mononuclear cells). Vasculitis is usually absent with the latter infiltrate. Patients with lymphocytic infiltrates generally respond to antihistamines and constitute most of the patients with chronic urticaria. Those with PMN predominant infiltrates tend to be resistant to antihistamines and exhibit a more severe clinical course.[38] Histamine, an identified mediator in the urticarial response, is produced and stored in dermal mast cells. When activated, the mast cells release histamine and other vasoactive substances including kinins, leukotrienes, and prostaglandins. Kinins are vasoactive peptides that may be an important factor in the development of urticaria. They diminish smooth muscle contraction, cause vasodilation, and increase vascular permeability. Leukotriene C_4 and prostaglandin D_2 cause urticarial reactions when injected into the skin, but their effects are not blocked by antihistamines. Antibodies of the IgE class can interact with antigen on the mast cell surface, as do complement-fixing antibodies, resulting in histamine release. Direct histamine release may also be caused by certain drugs (e.g., radiocontrast media, opiates), and chemicals.[9]

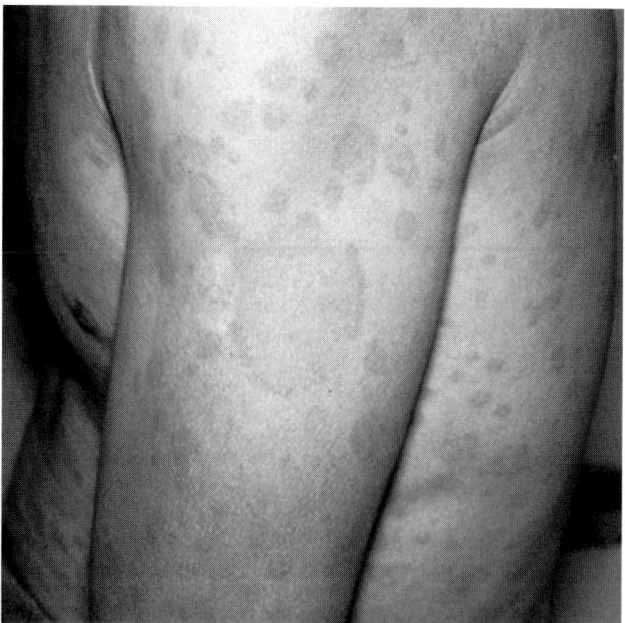

FIGURE 9.5 Urticarial drug eruption (*see color insert*). (With permission from Goodheart HP. Goodheart's photoguide of common skin disorders. 2nd ed. Philadelphia: Lippincott Williams & Wilkins 2003.)

CLINICAL PRESENTATION AND DIAGNOSIS

SIGNS AND SYMPTOMS

Patients generally present with pruritic, erythematous, circumscribed, or coalescent wheals (Fig. 9.5, *see color insert*).[39] Lesions may appear throughout the body, but more commonly involve the extremities and trunk. Angioedema generally results in deeper subcutaneous swelling of loose connective tissues, including the face, eyelids, and mucous membranes of the lips and tongue. Figure 9.6 (*see color insert*) depicts a typical angioedema presentation, with involvement of the lips and tongue. The lesions may be painful if there is tissue distention involving sensory nerves. Urticarial lesions may not be manifested in patients with angioedema. With urticaria and angioedema, symptoms may be sudden in onset or evolve slowly.

DIAGNOSIS AND CLINICAL FINDINGS

Urticarial skin lesions are pruritic, circumscribed, elevated, erythematous areas (wheals) of edema.[9,37] The size of the wheal can vary from 1 mm to many centimeters, and groups of lesions may be localized or generalized. Individual lesions tend to resolve in 24 hours but new lesions will eventually appear. Angioedema may lead to respiratory, gastrointestinal, or cardiovascular symptoms. Laboratory and skin testing is of limited value in establishing a diagnosis or cause. Autoimmune antibodies have been detected in 40% to 50% of

patients with chronic urticaria.[40] Basophil activation and histamine release from mast cells are of particular concern for these patients.

A careful history that describes the pattern of attacks, precipitating causes, duration of wheals, associated symptoms, and atopic background should be taken. As a result, the presence or absence of the following can be established: relationship to any ingested, inhaled, or injected substance;

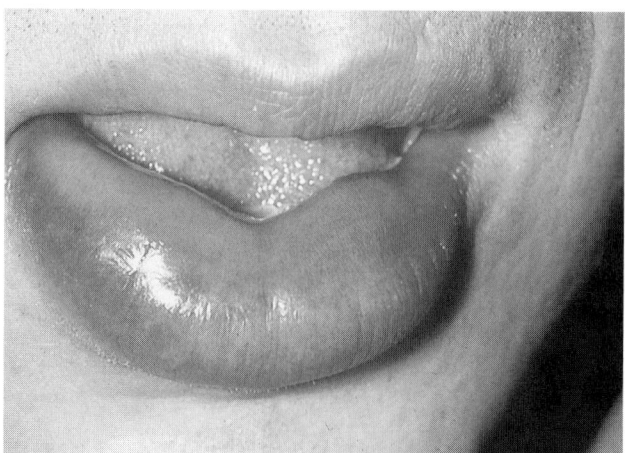

FIGURE 9.6 Angioedema. Note swelling of the lower lip and protruding tongue (*see color insert*). (With permission from Neville B, et al. Color atlas of clinical oral pathology. Philadelphia: Lea & Febiger, 1991.)

a contact reaction; a systemic disease; a hormonal influence; an emotional cause; or infection. While the basic mechanism may still be unknown, the above factors can serve as triggers. Idiopathic urticaria is often worsened by aspirin or nonsteroidal antiinflammatory drugs.[38] Thyroid disease, lymphoma, and systemic lupus erythematosus (SLE) have been linked to urticaria.[9]

TREATMENT

The best treatment of urticaria is identification and removal of the cause. Yet, in the large majority of cases this approach is unsuccessful because the cause cannot be identified or multiple factors are involved.[9,37] Treatment then is directed toward the effector cells and inflammatory mediators to block release or effect. Therapy may also focus on receptor sites on target tissues involving the cutaneous microvasculature and cells. Prompt assessment of angioedema is important, as it may be also indicative of anaphylaxis.

PHARMACOTHERAPY

Due to the large influence of histamine in the pathophysiology of urticaria, antihistamines are the cornerstone of treatment. Antihistamines provide relief in about 65% to 70% of patients with urticaria or angioedema.[18,41] They should be administered on a scheduled basis rather than as needed since antihistamines are more effective in preventing the actions of histamine rather than reversing the effects.[41] Second-generation H_1 receptor antihistamines are currently the drugs of choice, yet occasional doses of first-generation agents may be necessary to provide symptomatic relief. The second-generation agents are chosen due to their lower propensity for daytime sedation. If one agent is ineffective or not tolerated, a second agent from a different chemical group might be effective. Once treatment with H_1-receptor antagonists is successful, the agent should be tapered to prevent flares.[37]

Administered alone, the H_2-receptor blockers have little if any demonstrated benefit in urticaria. Yet, approximately 15% of histamine receptors in the skin are H_2 in nature. Therefore, H_2-receptor antagonists, like cimetidine, may be combined with H_1-receptor antagonists in treating urticaria.[37,41] This practice has been assessed in several studies with equivocal results.[38] The H_2-receptor antagonists may be useful only in certain types of urticaria (e.g., cold, angioedema). If a case does not respond to H_1 receptor antihistamines, a trial of combination therapy may be appropriate.[18] Doses of cimetidine have ranged from 400 to 1,600 mg/day. Ranitidine has been used in standard oral doses.[41]

The tricyclic antidepressant doxepin exhibits H_1 and H_2 histamine receptor blocking activity and is particularly potent against H_1 receptors.[38,41] While it has shown benefit in chronic urticaria, sedative effects may limit it to nighttime use. Doxepin (10 mg tid) compared to diphenhydramine (25 mg tid) resulted in greater efficacy, less sedation, and more dry mouth.

Leukotriene modifiers, including montelukast and zafirlukast, have demonstrated positive effects in chronic urticaria.[39,42] However, any additive effects of these agents once maximal histamine blockade has been induced by antihistamines have yet to be fully demonstrated. One controlled study demonstrated the benefit of montelukast added to a regimen of antihistamines in patients with refractory chronic urticaria. In the study, 20% to 50% of patients unresponsive to antihistamines may experience disease control with leukotriene antagonists. Some experts hypothesize that such response may be linked to the coexistence of aspirin or other additive intolerance.

Corticosteroids are not routinely used for chronic urticaria because of the potential length of therapy and associated adverse effects. Short-term use to control acute disease may benefit selected patients.[37,38] Oral prednisone at doses of 20 to 30 mg/day for 5 days provides symptomatic control. Exacerbation of urticaria occurs on withdrawal in some patients treated for >5 days. Patients with chronic disease may require corticosteroids administered every other day, a regimen that may minimize dose-related adverse effects.

Patients with recurrent angioedema should always have immediate access to an emergency epinephrine injector.[39] In addition to epinephrine administration, the acute appearance of angioedema should be managed with systemic antihistamines, parenteral corticosteroids, and oxygen supplementation as needed.

NONPHARMACOLOGIC THERAPY

As with contact dermatitis, the best method for managing urticaria and angioedema is avoidance of triggering antigens. Agents that aggravate symptoms, including cyclooxygenase inhibitors (e.g., aspirin, ibuprofen, celecoxib) and alcohol, should also be removed from potential exposure.

FUTURE THERAPIES

Other potential treatments include β-adrenergic agonists (e.g., terbutaline) and calcium channel blockers (e.g., nifedipine).[37,41] Sulfasalazine, dapsone, and cyclosporine have received anecdotal support.[39] Plasmapheresis and intravenous immunoglobulin supplementation have yielded positive effects in patients with circulating IgG autoantibodies to IgE. Patients with chronic idiopathic urticaria have benefitted from these treatments but studies with these agents are limited. Use of these or related alternate therapies (e.g., tacrolimus, mycophenolate) should be limited to refractory cases until further data is available.

DRUG-INDUCED SKIN DISEASES

Cutaneous drug reactions are frequent events in all patient types, and they are generally not influenced by age or sex. Proper management relies on prompt diagnosis and identification of underlying causes, drug discontinuation, and therapeutic intervention.

ETIOLOGY AND PATHOPHYSIOLOGY

Cutaneous reactions to drugs result from immunologic or non-immunologic mechanisms. The role of immunologic mechanisms, which require activation of host pathways, is supported by a number of features, including: occurrence in a small percentage of patients; lack of a dose-dependency; rash onset within 1 to 2 weeks after initiation of therapy; presence of other signs and symptoms (e.g., fever, pruritus, eosinophilia); and resolution on withdrawal of the agent and recurrence following rechallenge.[2] Host ability to mount an immune reaction is, therefore, a critical feature of many cutaneous drug reactions. Sensitization can occur by any route, yet the greatest risk occurs with topical drug application and the least risk with oral administration.[43] High molecular weight drugs (e.g., insulin, antisera) are more likely to cause allergy. Low molecular weight drugs act as haptens and must combine with protein carriers before an allergic response can occur.

Cutaneous reactions caused by nonimmunologic mechanisms are more common than allergic reactions.[5] Nonimmunologic mechanisms associated with cutaneous drug reactions in-clude activation of effector pathways, overdosage, cumulative toxicity, side effects, drug interactions, metabolic changes, and exacerbation of existing dermatologic conditions. The most relevant of these, the activation of effector pathways, is not antibody-dependent, is usually indistinguishable from IgE mediated reactions, and actually involves at least three different mechanisms. The first involves direct release of mediators, like histamine from mast cells, which can present as urticaria or angioedema. Drugs implicated in this mechanism include opiates, thiamine, and radiographic contrast media. Second, radiographic contrast media can activate complement in the absence of antibody, again resulting in urticaria. The third mechanism involves alteration of arachidonic acid metabolism, the most notable example being anaphylactic-like responses to aspirin and nonsteroidal antiinflammatory drugs (NSAIDs). Urticaria, as discussed previously, may be induced by drug exposure and accounts for nearly 25% of drug-induced skin reactions. However, drug-induced skin diseases present through a variety of other clinical manifestations (Table 9.4).

DRUG EXANTHEM

CLINICAL PRESENTATION AND DIAGNOSIS

Often referred to as morbilliform or maculopapular reactions, drug exanthems comprise nearly 50% of skin reactions to drugs.[4] Eruptions generally begin on the trunk or in areas where pressure or trauma occur. The rash is frequently pruritic, symmetric, and consists of erythematous macules and

TABLE 9.4	Features of Selected Drug-Induced Skin Diseases			
Condition	Non-Drug Causes	Skin Lesions	Other Common Signs and Symptoms	Mucosal Involvement
Angioedema	Foods, insect stings	Urticaria or swelling of lips, tongue, eyes	Respiratory distress, urticaria, cardiovascular collapse	Common
Drug hypersensitivity syndrome (DRESS)	Lymphomatous conditions	Severe exanthematous rash, exfoliative dermatitis	Fever, lympadenopathy, internal organ inflammation, eosinophilia	Uncommon
Stevens-Johnson Syndrome	Infection, particularly herpes simplex and mycoplasma	Blisters, purpuric macules, confluence is infrequent; detachment <10% of BSA	Fever	Lesions at several sites
Toxic epidermal necrolysis	Not reported	Purpuric macules, confluence is common; large sheet necrotic epidermis; detachment >30% of BSA	Fever, leukopenia	Lesions at several sites

DRESS, Drug rash with eosinophilia and systemic symptoms; BSA, body surface area. (From Stern RS, Chosidow OM, Wintraub BU. Cutaneous drug reactions. In: Braunwald E, Fauci AS, Kasper DL, et al, ed. Harrison's principles of internal medicine. 15th ed. New York: McGraw-Hill, 2001:336–342, with permission.)

papules that may become confluent.[2,5] Fever and eosinophilia may be present, as well as involvement of mucous membranes, palms, and plantar surface. Some agents (e.g., ciprofloxacin, vancomycin, succinylcholine) can cause IgE-mediated or non–IgE-mediated systemic reactions. In general, reactions typically manifest within 1 week of drug initiation with an estimated duration of 1 to 2 weeks. Penicillin and other drugs with long half-lives may result in a delayed reaction onset and duration.[44] Rashes associated with allopurinol can occur for ≥3 weeks.

Some factors contribute to a higher risk of drug exanthem. Women have a 35% higher risk than men.[43] While estimates have varied from as much as 50% to 80%, a high percentage of patients with Epstein-Barr virus (including infectious mononucleosis) taking ampicillin (amoxicillin is also implicated) experience a rash.[2,43] Patients with cytomegalovirus infections, chronic lymphocytic leukemia, hyperuricemia, or those taking the combination of ampicillin and allopurinol experience a higher frequency of rashes. Patients that are human immunodeficiency virus (HIV)-seropositive more commonly experience drug exanthems. A drug-induced exanthem must be differentiated from reactions of viral origin, although this is difficult since definitive diagnostic tests are lacking.

TREATMENT

The mainstay of treatment is drug discontinuation. Most reactions can be expected to disappear within 1 to 2 weeks after discontinuing the offending agent. Symptomatic control may be achieved with tepid water baths or cool compresses. Oral antihistamines and emollients provide pruritic relief. Some severe reactions may warrant systemic corticosteroids.[44]

FIXED DRUG ERUPTION

CLINICAL PRESENTATION AND DIAGNOSIS

Fixed drug eruptions account for approximately 10% of drug-induced skin disorders. These reactions involve the development of a lesion, often solitary, that appears as an erythematous macule and subsequently becomes an edematous plaque (Fig. 9.7, *see color insert*).[2,5,45] After resolution of the acute phase, hyperpigmentation remains with colors varying from brown to violet-brown or even black.[45] Lesions most often occur on the face, lip, sacral region, and genitalia. Pruritus and burning may accompany the reaction with the severity reflecting the intensity of the inflammatory response.

The term "fixed drug eruption" reflects the hallmark lesion recurrence in the same location upon reexposure. Symptoms recur usually between 30 minutes and 8 hours on reexposure. With repeated exposure, the number of lesions may gradually increase. Although rare, systemic symptoms may range from malaise to severe prostration.[45] Drugs most often implicated are tetracyclines, sulfonamides, NSAIDs, and barbiturates. Patch testing may be used to establish a definitive etiology.

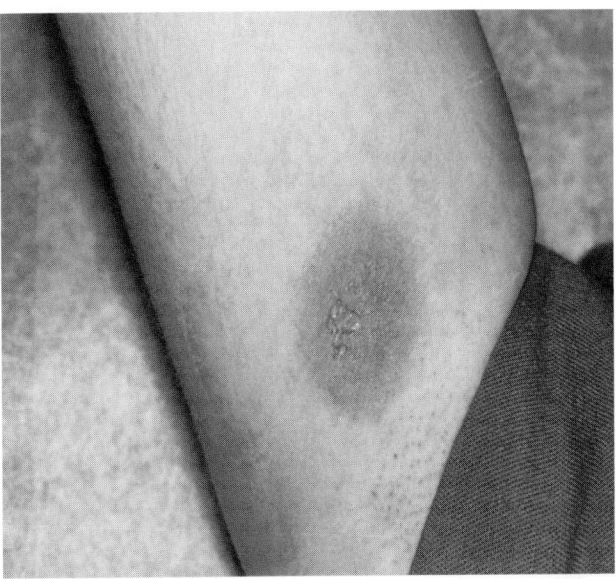

FIGURE 9.7 Fixed drug eruption. Lesion reappeared at original site after subsequent exposure to sulfonamide antibiotic (*see color insert*). (With permission from Goodheart HP. Goodheart's photoguide of common skin disorders, 2nd ed. Philadelphia: Lippincott Williams & Wilkins, 2003.)

TREATMENT

Foremost in management is elimination of subsequent exposure to the offending substance. Failure to do so may result in extension of the eruption to mucous membranes and bullae formation.[2,45] Cool water compresses may provide some acute relief, while systemic corticosteroids and antihistamines appear to be of minimal value. Bleaching creams may reduce the pigmentary changes that follow the acute phase.

PHOTOSENSITIVITY

CLINICAL PRESENTATION AND DIAGNOSIS

A collective term describing reactions to light sources, "photosensitivity," consists of two types, photoallergy and phototoxicity.[5] Phototoxic reactions are the most frequent and can occur with the first exposure to a drug, even within a few hours, and are dose-related. Symptoms of phototoxicity result from exposure to a drug that absorbs ultraviolet (UV) light, which causes tissue damage. The reaction resembles sunburn and can in some cases progress to blister. Such reactions occur in most patients given adequate amounts of drug and exposure to UV light. Chlorpromazine, amiodarone, and doxycycline are examples of drugs implicated in this type of reaction.

Photoallergy involves the combination of the drug, immune system, and light. Such reactions occur in only a small percentage of exposed patients.[2] The delayed hypersensitivity reaction suspected in photoallergy entails the reaction of UV light with a drug or its metabolites in the skin, resulting in hapten formation. An allergic reaction then results on subsequent drug exposure. The delayed rash, recovery from which is generally slow, is usually eczematous but may involve lichenoid, urticarial, bullous, or purpuric lesions. The reaction typically

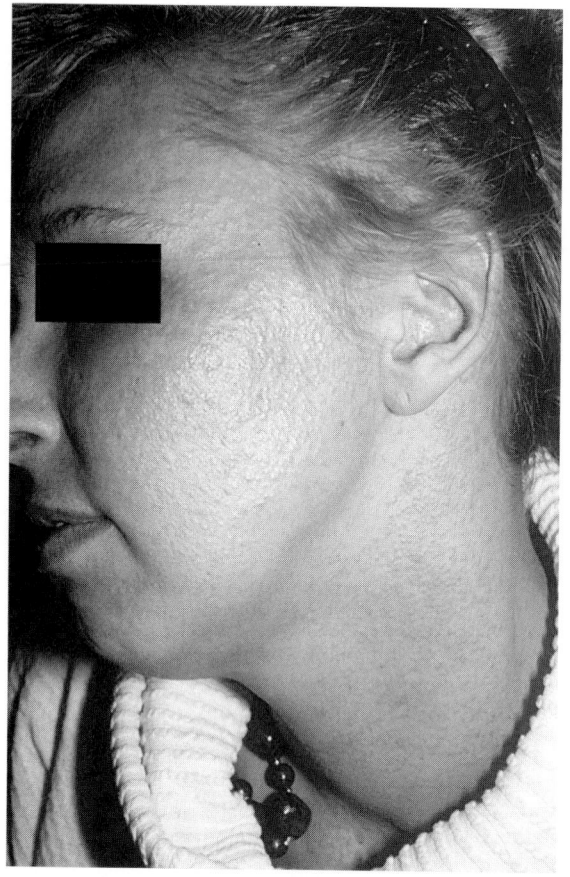

FIGURE 9.8 Photoallergic reaction to nonsteroidal antiinflammatory drug. Two days after initiating piroxicam, patient developed eruption after sun exposure at beach. Note the lack of involvement of unprotected area under the jaw (*see color insert*). (With permission from Goodheart HP. Goodheart's photoguide of common skin disorders. 2nd ed. Philadelphia: Lippincott Williams & Wilkins, 2003.)

occurs in sun-exposed areas but in severe cases may involve areas that are normally protected (Fig. 9.8, *see color insert*). Causative drugs include tetracyclines, thiazide diuretics, sulfonamides, phenothiazines, NSAIDs, and antihistamines.[2,5]

TREATMENT

Removal of the offending agent usually brings resolution to phototoxic reactions, while photoallergic reactions may persist for some time after the drug is withdrawn. Systemic and topical corticosteroids and antihistamines have no role in phototoxic reaction management. Rather, principles similar to the care of sunburn should be used. Topical corticosteroids and antihistamines may provide relief in photoallergy. Further sun exposure should be avoided in both types of reactions.

ERYTHEMA MULTIFORME

CLINICAL PRESENTATION AND DIAGNOSIS

Usually considered an acute, self-limited inflammatory disorder involving skin and mucous membranes, erythema mul-

tiforme (EM) may have a wide spectrum of sequelae.[2,5] A prodrome, consisting of malaise, sore throat, and possibly fever with skin lesions developing over 2 to 7 days, may occur. Lesions have a distinctive iris or target appearance and are erythematous plaques with dusky centers, a surrounding ring of edema, and a darker erythematous outer border. The plaques are most profuse peripherally and develop in groups over a period of a few days, fading after 1 to 2 weeks. Postinflammatory hyperpigmentation may also develop. Sites most commonly affected by EM are the backs of the hands, palms, wrists, forearms, feet, elbows, and knees.

In the most severe form, bullous or vesicular lesions accompanied by mucosal involvement and systemic symptoms is termed "Stevens-Johnson syndrome" (SJS). Usually, mucosal and conjunctival lesions occur (Fig. 9.9, *see color insert*).[2,45] High fevers, arthralgias, myalgias, vomiting, and diarrhea are often present. Healing of SJS lesions, which affect <10% of the body surface area, usually occurs within 6 weeks. SJS complications include keratitis, conjunctival scarring and blindness, esophagitis, and pneumonia.

The exact causes of EM are unknown, with current theories focusing on immunologic and drug metabolism disturbances. Drugs are associated in approximately 50% of EM cases with antibacterial sulfonamides, anticonvulsants, NSAIDs (particularly oxicams), and allopurinol accounting for two thirds of the reactions.[43,46] Diagnosis centers on history, clinical presentation, and histologic confirmation of eosinophil involvement.

TREATMENT

Withdrawal of the suspected triggering drug must first occur. Mild EM treatment is limited to symptomatic therapy. Compresses, diluted hydrogen peroxide gargles for oral lesions, and antihistamines for pruritic symptoms are common ap-

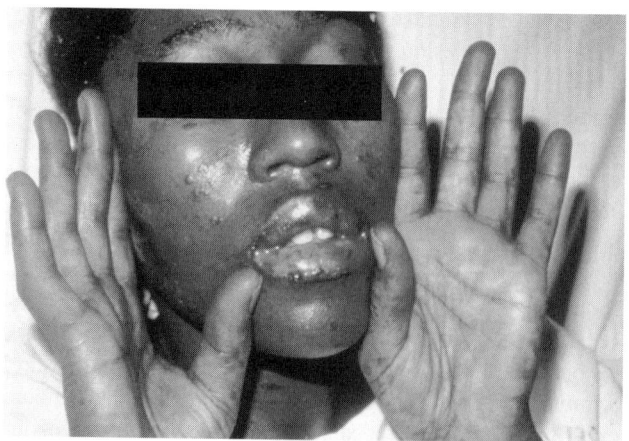

FIGURE 9.9 Erythema multiforme major. Extensive hemorrhagic crusting of mucous membranes and erythematous lesions were accompanied by fever (*see color insert*). (With permission from Goodheart HP. Goodheart's photoguide of common skin disorders. 2nd ed. Philadelphia: Lippincott Williams & Wilkins, 2003.)

proaches. Early corticosteroid use is recommended to prevent visceral involvement and shorten the intensity and duration.[43] However, an increased risk of occurrence has been associated with exposure to corticosteroids.[46]

TOXIC EPIDERMAL NECROLYSIS

CLINICAL PRESENTATION AND DIAGNOSIS

Although uncommon, toxic epidermal necrolysis (TEN) is associated with significant morbidity and mortality and is characterized by many as the most serious cutaneous drug reaction. Symptoms may occur within hours to weeks of exposure to the triggering agent. A brief prodrome of sore throat, malaise, fever, and chills occurs with skin involvement within 24 hours. Small, dusky, necrotic macules with early and extensive involvement of perioral areas and mucous membranes develop within 1 to 3 days. The lesions progressively enlarge to produce large confluent areas of necrosis with extensive subepidermal sloughing of more than 30% of the body surface area within 2 to 5 days. Such sheet-like skin separation is fairly characteristic of the disorder. TEN may also be distinguished from SJS by its extent of body surface area involvement. Lesions may appear anywhere throughout the body, with the exception of the scalp.[44] Gastrointestinal involvement, pneumonia, nephritis, and myocardial damage may ensue, in addition to hematologic disturbances. Patients can become quite ill with mortality ranging from 30% to 40%.[43]

In addition to SJS, staphylococcal scalded skin syndrome (SSSS), a condition that occurs in children or immunocompromised patients, must be considered in the differential diagnosis. Some differentiating factors for SSSS are that epidermal separation is superficial (e.g., intraepidermal, usually the granular layer), perioral and mucous membrane involvement is absent or mild, and skin pain is absent.

Risk factors for TEN include advanced age, systemic lupus erythematosus, HIV or acquired immune deficiency syndrome (AIDS), and bone marrow transplantation. The same agents that cause SJS are involved in the majority of cases of TEN and include NSAIDs, sulfonamides, anticonvulsants, barbiturates, and allopurinol.[5,43,46] With allopurinol, TEN with concomitant renal/hepatic failure often affects patients with renal insufficiency receiving normal doses. Allopurinol doses should be reduced in patients with renal insufficiency to avoid the potential for this reaction.[47]

TREATMENT

Exposure to the precipitating factor must be discontinued immediately. However, removal of the offending substance may not result in prompt clearing of lesions, particularly for drugs with a long elimination half-life. Skin sloughing increases the risk of life-threatening infection, fluid and electrolyte loss, and subsequent hypothermia and shock. Such similarities to extensive skin burns often result in a similar management approach (e.g., fluid and electrolyte replacement, infection prevention and treatment, nutritional support, and prevention of ophthalmic complications).[48] Intravenous immune globulin, oral corticosteroids, and immunosuppressants have also been used, but their effects have not been formally assessed. Thalidomide increased mortality in one clinical trial and should not be used.

DRUG HYPERSENSITIVITY SYNDROME

CLINICAL PRESENTATION AND DIAGNOSIS

Drug rash with eosinophilia and systemic symptoms (DRESS) describes a constellation of symptoms resulting from drug exposure.[44] A severe skin eruption on the face and upper trunk typically progresses to affect the lower extremities with progression from morbilliform eruption to erythroderma. Sterile pustules, of a follicular or nonfollicular nature, may develop. The skin eruption may also include exfoliative dermatitis and angioedema. Other systemic symptoms include lymphadenopathy, fever, hepatitis, and hematologic disturbances (e.g., eosinophilia). Internal organs may also be affected. Symptoms of phenytoin-associated DRESS generally present within 1 to 6 weeks of drug exposure, recur on rechallenge, and may also be associated with related drugs (i.e., cross-reactivity).

DRESS is suspected to arise from alterations in a variety of drug metabolic pathways (e.g., cytochrome P-450 isozyme alterations, slow acetylation). A subsequent immune response leads to the reaction, which is fatal in approximately 10% and results in a median survival rate of 24 to 30 months.[49] Rapid diagnosis and treatment is, therefore, essential. The syndrome has been linked to a variety of drugs, including anticonvulsants, sulfonamides, other antiinfectives, and allopurinol.

TREATMENT

Drug discontinuation is the first step in patient management.[44] However, symptoms may persist for weeks following drug withdrawal. High-potency topical corticosteroids may be used to manage dermatologic manifestations, but may also require systemic administration (e.g., prednisone 0.5 to 1 mg/kg). The resultant immune disturbance is of greatest concern, as fatality is most commonly attributed to subsequent infection. Lymphoma may also be a complication of DRESS. Patient management should, therefore, include prevention, detection, and aggressive treatment of such complications.

ANTIHISTAMINES

The antihistamines (H_1-receptor antagonists) may be categorized according to chemical structure: ethanolamines, ethylenediamines, alkylamines, phthalazinones, piperazines, piperidines, and phenothiazines.[50] However, this classification generally provides little information regarding expected pharmacodynamic and pharmacokinetic properties. A more useful classification involves the terminology of first-generation (classic) and second-generation (nonsedating) H_1-receptor antagonists. Comparison in this fashion more clearly distinguishes differences in pharmacodynamic properties and subsequent pharmacologic effects (Table 9.5).

H_1-receptor antagonists are reversible competitive inhibitors of the actions of histamine on H_1-receptors. The antihistamines block the bronchopulmonary and vasoactive effects of histamine resulting in decreased vascular permeability, decreased pruritus, and relaxation of smooth muscle.[50] While differences in potency exist, the antihistaminic activity of the various agents is considered similar when equipotent doses are given. This effect is demonstrated by suppression of the wheal/flare reactions induced by histamine or allergens. The duration of effect varies among agents, which

is reflected in the corresponding dosing interval for each drug (Table 9.5). In addition, some agents also prevent release of inflammatory mediators from IgE-sensitized mast cells and basophils. An effect on calcium by inhibiting influx across the cell membrane or inhibiting intracellular release is probably responsible. These agents may inhibit late phase allergic reactions by effects on leukotrienes or prostaglandins.

Classic H_1-receptor antagonists possess anticholinergic activity and produce a central nervous system (CNS) depressant effect. While sedation is generally undesirable, in many patients with some type of skin disorder (e.g., atopic dermatitis), sedation can be helpful in reducing nocturnal scratching. These effects are clinically apparent at doses used therapeutically. In general, second-generation agents are devoid of clinically apparent anticholinergic activity or CNS effects at therapeutic doses. These agents penetrate poorly into the

TABLE 9.5	Dosage and Clinical Effects of Antihistamines				
Drug	Dose (mg)	Dosing Interval (h)	Antihistaminic Activity	Anticholinergic Activity	Sedative Effects
First Generation					
Alkylamine					
Brompheniramine	4	4–6	+++	++	+
Chlorpheniramine	4	4–6	++	++	+
Dexchlorpheniramine	2	4–6	+++	++	+
Ethanolamine					
Clemastine	1	12	+ / ++	+++	++
Diphenhydramine	25–50	6–8	+ / ++	+++	+++
Phenothiazine					
Promethazine	12.5–25	6–24	+++	+++	+++
Piperazines					
Hydroxyzine	25–100	4–8	++ / +++	++	+++
Piperidine					
Azatadine	1–2	12	++	++	++
Cyproheptadine	4	8	++	++	+
Phenindamine	25	4–6	++	++	±
Second Generation					
Phthalazinone					
Azelastine	0.5	12	++ / +++	±	±
Piperazine					
Cetirizine	5–10	24	++ / +++	±	±
Piperidine					
Desloratadine	5	24	++ / +++	±	±
Fexofenadine	60	12	–	±	±
Loratadine	10	24	++/+++	±	±

±, low to none; +, low; ++, moderate; +++, high; ++++, very high; − no data.
(From Wickersham RM, ed. Drug Facts and Comparisons. St. Louis: JB Lippincott Co 2004:699, with permission.)

CNS and levels are insufficient to block central H_1 or cholinergic receptors. Binding is preferential for peripheral H_1-receptors.[19,50]

PHARMACOKINETICS

All of the agents are generally well absorbed after oral administration with peak serum levels reached at around 2 hours.[37,50] Most agents undergo metabolism through the cytochrome P-450 system in the liver with clearance and elimination half-lives varying substantially. The duration of response is related to dose and the serum elimination half-life. Children usually exhibit shorter half-lives than adults, while half-lives are expected to be prolonged in elderly patients and those with liver disease.[50]

ADVERSE EFFECTS/DRUG INTERACTIONS

The adverse effect profile of first-generation agents includes CNS and anticholinergic effects. The CNS effects can be divided into depressant, stimulatory, and neuropsychiatric reactions.[50,51] The primary CNS depressant effects are sedation, impaired cognitive function, diminished alertness, difficulty in concentrating, dizziness, and tinnitus. Sedation or drowsiness occurs in 10% to 25% of antihistamine users. Some first-generation agents like diphenhydramine also cause dystonic reactions. Some patients, particularly children, may experience stimulatory effects that involve appetite or muscles or produce nervousness, insomnia, and irritability. Neuropsychiatric effects reported are anxiety, confusion, depression and, rarely, hallucinations. The common anticholinergic effects include dry mouth, blurred vision, and urinary retention. The second-generation agents generally are devoid of sedative and anticholinergic effects, with the exception of cetirizine. In some of the skin diseases discussed, sedation may be a desired property of antihistamines and the only benefit in some allergic diseases, at least in the opinions of some experts.

Adverse effects can be additive when the first-generation antihistamines are given with other drugs that have CNS depressant effects (e.g., alcohol, hypnotics, anxiolytics, antipsychotics, analgesics) or anticholinergic activity (e.g., antispasmodics, tricyclic antidepressants, antipsychotics, anti-Parkinson drugs).[18] Loratadine can interact with some drugs metabolized by the cytochrome P450 system. The clinical significance of these interactions is not known.

Antihistamines should be selected for use in allergic and drug-induced skin diseases based on a variety of factors: drug safety, patient convenience, and cost. Patients that fail to respond to one agent may respond to another of a different chemical class. Patients with conditions that may also benefit from the sedative effects of antihistamines should receive first-generation antihistamines. However, they should be aware of the effects of the drugs on their daytime functions, and adjust their activities (e.g., driving or operating heavy machinery) accordingly. Tolerance to the sedative effects eventually develops, although it may not be seen in the short courses commonly administered to this corresponding group of patients.

IMPROVING OUTCOMES

PATIENT EDUCATION

Effective patient education is critical to the successful management of allergic and drug-induced skin conditions. The need to withdraw exposure to the offending agent and avoid future exposure illustrates this importance. Patients should determine the exact substances to avoid, synonyms for those substances, and related products that may cause similar reactions. In addition, patients should understand the nature of the treatments they will receive, as many require a component of patient judgment regarding drug administration in response to symptomatic worsening or improvement.

METHODS TO IMPROVE ADHERENCE TO DRUG THERAPY

The majority of pharmacotherapeutic interventions previously discussed have minimal adverse reaction potential (e.g., judicious use of topical corticosteroids) or occur in patients with such disease acuity that treatment is administered in an acute care setting (e.g., erythema multiforme). However, many patients may receive antihistamines on an acute or chronic basis. Agents should be selected based on their desired effect, adverse reaction profile, and convenience of administration. First-generation antihistamines administered at bedtime may be desired for use in patients with atopic dermatitis, as the sedation and anxiolysis contribute to management of the dermatologic condition. However, the sedation associated with first-generation agents is not easily tolerated by most patients receiving a short course of therapy. It is in these patients that second-generation antihistamines may be more desirable. Such agents are typically administered less frequently, as well, thus improving the potential for patient adherence.

P H A R M A C O E C O N O M I C S

Few formal pharmacoeconomic analyses of management principles for allergic and drug-induced skin diseases have been conducted. However, a number of factors are certainly pertinent for consideration. Allergic diseases tend to have a chronic component that may require long-term management. As such, medications that are highly effective, well tolerated, and have minimal economic burden are highly desired. Contact dermatitis may also be a result of occupational exposure and may, thus, alter patient employability. Many of the medications used in management of these skin disorders have few differences in their costs or availability within classes. However, the majority of agents in the traditional antihistamine receptor class are available without a prescription, including the second-generation agent, loratadine. Improved access to these drugs may perhaps benefit patients that lack health insurance. One analysis of pimecrolimus and tacrolimus identified the latter to be the more cost-effective agent for the treatment of atopic dermatitis.[52] However, this study

TABLE 9.6	Glossary
Acanthosis	increased thickness of the prickle layer of the skin.
Angioedema	an allergic skin disease characterized by patches of circumscribed swelling involving the skin and its subcutaneous layers, the mucous membranes, and sometimes the viscera. Also called angioneurotic edema, giant urticaria.
Bullae	large vesicles or blisters.
Confluence	a joining together or merging of skin lesions; lesions that are not distinct or discrete from one another.
Dermographism	pressure or friction on the skin gives rise to a transient, raised usually reddish mark, sometimes white, so that a word traced on the skin becomes visible.
Desquamation	peeling of skin in the form of scales.
Eczema	Inflammation of the skin characterized by redness, itching, and oozing vesicular lesions which become scaly, crusted, or hardened.
Erythema	abnormal redness of the skin due to capillary congestion.
Exanthem	an eruptive skin disease (as measles) or its (exanthematous) symptomatic eruption.
Excoriation	a raw irritated lesion; the act of abrading or wearing off the skin.
Exfoliation	the peeling of the horny layer of the (exfoliative) skin.
Hyperkeratosis	an overgrowth of the horny layer of the epidermis.
Lichenoid	resembling lichen which is characterized by the eruption of flat papules.
Macule	a patch of skin that is altered in color but usually not elevated.
Maculopapular	combining the characteristics of macules and papules.
Morbilliform	resembling the eruption of measles.
Papule	a small solid usually conical elevation of the skin caused by inflammation, accumulated secretion, or hypertrophy of tissue elements.
Plaque	a localized abnormal patch on a body part or surface and especially on the skin.
Pruritus	localized or generalized itching due to irritation of sensory nerve endings from organic or psychogenic causes.
Spongiosis	intercellular edema of the epidermis.
Urticaria	an allergic disorder marked by raised edematous patches (wheals) of skin or mucous membrane and usually intense itching. Also called hives.
Vesicle	a small abnormal elevation of the outer layer of skin enclosing a watery liquid; blister.
Wheal	temporary, small, raised area of the skin usually accompanied by itching or burning.

was based only on relative treatment efficacy as demonstrated by previously published trials.

KEY POINTS

- Allergic and drug-induced skin diseases encompass a varied spectrum of diseases.
- Although allergy is suspected in many cases, the specific allergen may be difficult to identify. Other mechanisms operate in some diseases, but the clinical presentation does not distinguish the etiology. Drug-induced conditions tend to be acute and resolve, particularly when the offending agent is removed. However, some cutaneous reactions to drugs result in serious medical conditions that require prompt treatment. Atopic dermatitis, contact dermatitis, and idiopathic urticaria tend to be more chronic with exacerbations and remissions. Topical corticosteroids, occasional short-term systemic corticosteroids in severe conditions, and antihistamines are the mainstay of drug therapy in addition to other nonspecific topical treatments. See Table 9.6 for a glossary.

SUGGESTED READINGS

deShazo RD, Kemp SF. Allergic reactions to drugs and biologic agents. JAMA 278:1895–1906, 1997.

Leung DY, Diaz LA, Deleo V, et al. Allergic and immunologic skin disorders. JAMA 278:1914–1923, 1997.

Roujeau JC, Stern RS. Severe adverse cutaneous reactions to drugs. N Engl J Med 331:1272–1285, 1994.

REFERENCES

1. Sauer GC. Manual of Skin Diseases. 6th ed. Philadelphia: JB Lippincott Co., 1991:1–8.
2. Bigby M, Stern RS, Arndt KA. Allergic cutaneous reactions to drugs. Primary Care 16:713–727, 1989.
3. Thestrup-Pedersen K, Larsen CG, Ronnevig J. The immunology of contact dermatitis. Contact Dermatitis 20:81–92, 1989.
4. Pratt WB. Drug allergy. In: Pratt WB, Taylor P, ed. Principles of drug action: the basis of pharmacology. New York: Churchhill Livingstone, 1990:533–548.
5. Wintroub BU, Stern R. Cutaneous drug reactions: pathogenesis and clinical classification. J Am Acad Dermatol 13:167–179, 1985.
6. Rothe MJ, Grant-Kels JM. Atopic dermatitis: an update. J Am Acad Dermatol 35:1–13, 1996.
7. Chan SC, Hanifin JM. Immunologic aspects of atopic dermatitis. Clin Rev Allergy 11:523–541, 1993.
8. Sampson HA. Pathogenesis of eczema. Clin Exp Allergy 20:459–467, 1990.
9. Leung DY, Diaz LA, Deleo V, et al. Allergic and immunologic skin disorders. JAMA 278:1914–1923, 1997.
10. Thestrup-Pedersen K. Treatment principles of atopic dermatitis. J Eur Acad Dermatol Venereol 16:1–9, 2002.
11. Schultz-Larsen F, Hanifin JM. Epidemiology of atopic dermatitis. Immunol Allergy Clin North Am 22:1–24, 2002.
12. Leung DYM, Bieber T. Atopic dermatitis. Lancet 361:151–160, 2003.
13. Boguniewicz M, Nicol N. Conventional therapy for atopic dermatitis. Immunol Allergy Clin North Am 22:107–124, 2002.
14. Van der Meer JB, Glazenburg EJ, Mulder PG, et al for the Netherlands Adult Atopic Dermatitis Study Group. The management of moderate to severe atopic dermatitis in adults with topical fluticasone propionate. Br J Dermatol 140:1114–1121, 1999.
15. Hanifin JM. Atopic dermatitis. In: Middleton E, et al. Allergy. principles and practice. 4th ed. St. Louis: Mosby, 1993:1595–1600.
16. Wollenberg A, Sharma S, von Bubnoff D, et al. Topical tacrolimus (FK506) leads to profound phenotypic and functional alterations of epidermal antigen-presenting dendritic cells in atopic dermatitis. J Allergy Clin Immunol 107:519–525, 2001.
17. Reynolds NJ, Franklin V, Gray JC et al. Narrow-band ultraviolet B and broad-band ultraviolet A phototherapy in adult atopic eczema: a randomised controlled trial. Lancet 357:2012–2016, 2001.
18. Advenier C, Queille-Roussel C. Rational use of antihistamines in allergic dermatological conditions. Drugs 38:634–644, 1984.
19. Berth-Jones J, Graham-Brown RA, Marks R, et al. Long-term efficacy and safety of cyclosporin in severe adult atopic dermatitis. Br J Dermatol 140:685–688, 1997.
20. Brehler R, Hildebrand A, Luger TA. Recent developments in the treatment of atopic eczema. J Am Acad Dermatol 36:983–994, 1997.
21. Grundmann-Kollmann M, Podda M, Ochsendorf F, et al. Mycophenolate mofetil is effective in the treatment of atopic dermatitis. Arch Dermatol 137:870–873, 2001.
22. Noren P, Melin L. The effect of combined topical steroids and habit-reversal treatment in patients with atopic dermatitis. Br J Dermatol 121:359–366, 1989.
23. Koo J, Arain S. Traditional Chinese medicine for the treatment of dermatologic disorders. Arch Dermatol 134:1388–1393, 1998.
24. Levin C, Maibach H. Exploration of ''alternative'' and ''natural'' drugs in dermatology. Arch Dermatol 138:207–211, 2002.
25. Rackal JM, Vender RB. The treatment of atopic dermatitis and other dermatoses with leukotriene antagonists. Skin Therapy Lett 9:1–5, 2004.
26. Jolles S. A review of high-dose intravenous immunoglobulin treatment for atopic dermatitis. Clin Exp Dermatol 27:3–7, 2002.
27. Hanifin JM, Chan SC, Cheng JB, et al. Type 4 phosphodiesterase inhibitors have clinical and in vitro anti-inflammatory effects in atopic dermatitis. J Invest Dermatol 107:51–56, 1996.
28. Nikkels AF, Pierard GE. Framing the future of antifungals in atopic dermatitis. Dermatology 206:398–400, 2003.
29. Mozzanica N. Pathogenic aspects of allergic and irritant contact dermatitis. Clin Dermatol 10:115–121, 1992.
30. Beltrani VS, Beltrani VP. Contact dermatitis. Ann Allergy Asthma Immunol 78:160–175, 1997.
31. Morren M, Dooms-Goossens A. Contact allergy to corticosteroids. Clin Rev Allergy Immunol 14:199–208, 1996.
32. Maibach H, Epstein E. Allergic contact dermatitis. In: Demis DJ. Clinical dermatology. Philadelphia: JB Lippincott Company, 1988:1–46.
33. Marrakachi S, Maibach HI. What is occupational contact dermatitis? Dermatol Clin 12:477–479, 1994.
34. Fisher AA. Noneczematous contact dermatitis. In: Fisher AA, ed. Contact dermatitis. 3rd ed. Philadelphia: Lea & Febiger, 1986:100–118.
35. Bruckner AL, Weston WL. Allergic contact dermatitis in children: a practical approach to management. Skin Therapy Lett 7:3–5, 2002.
36. Wickersham RM, ed. Drug Facts and Comparisons. St. Louis: JB Lippincott Co, 2004:699.
37. Soter NA. Urticaria: Current therapy. J Allergy Clin Immunol 86:1009–1014, 1990.
38. Tharp MD. Chronic urticaria: Pathophysiology and treatment approaches. J Allergy Clin Immunol 98:S325–S330, 1996.
39. Joint Task Force on Practice Parameters. The diagnosis and management of urticaria: a practice parameter. Ann Allergy Asthma Immunol 85:521–524, 2000.
40. Kaplan AP. Chronic urticaria and angioedema. N Engl J Med 346:175–179, 2002.
41. Kennard CD, Ellis CN. Pharmacologic therapy for urticaria. J Am Acad Dermatol 25:176–187, 1991.
42. Tedeschi A, Airaghi L, Lorini M et al. Chronic urticaria: a role for

newer immunomodulatory drugs? Am J Clin Dermatol 4:297–305, 2003.

43. deShazo RD, Kemp SF. Allergic reactions to drugs and biologic agents. JAMA 278:1895–1906, 1997.
44. Stern RS, Chosidow OM, Wintraub BU. Cutaneous drug reactions. In: Braunwald E, Fauci AS, Kasper DL, et al, ed. Harrison's principles of internal medicine. 15th ed. New York: McGraw-Hill, 2001: 336–342.
45. Korkij W, Soltani K. Fixed drug eruption. A brief review. Arch Dermatol 120:520–524, 1984.
46. Hande KR, Noone RM, Stone WJ. Severe allopurinol toxicity. Am J Med 76:47–56, 1984.
47. Roujeau JC, Kelly JP, Naldi L et.al. Medication use and the risk of Stevens-Johnson syndrome or toxic epidermal necrolysis. N Engl J Med 333:1600–1607, 1995.

48. Majumdar S, Mockenhaupt M, Roujeau JC, et al. Interventions for toxic epidermal necrolysis (Cochrane Review). In: The Cochrane Library, Issue 1, 2004. Chichester, UK: John Wiley & Sons, Ltd.
49. Bocquet H, Bagot M, Roujeau JC. Drug-induced pseudolymphoma and drug hypersensitivity syndrome (drug rash with eosinophilia and systemic symptoms: DRESS). Semin Cutan Med Surg 132: 1315–1321, 1996.
50. DuBuske LM. Clinical comparison of histamine H_1-receptor antagonist drugs. J Allergy Clin Immunol 98:S307–S318, 1996.
51. Meltzer EO. Performance effects of antihistamines. J Allergy Clin Immunol 86:613–619, 1990.
52. Abramovits W, Boguniewicz M, Prendergast MM, et al. Comparisons of efficacy and cost-effectiveness of topical immunomodulators in the management of atopic dermatitis. J Med Econ 5:1–14, 2003.

Common Skin Disorders

10

Rebecca Florez Boettger and Laurie H. Fukushima

The skin is the largest organ of the body. Its primary functions are to protect the body from the external environment and maintain the homeostatic milieu of the internal environment. Proper function and integrity of the skin are essential for life.

Many disease processes can affect this organ system. In addition, skin manifestations can give important clues to underlying systemic disorders, many of which are discussed elsewhere. This chapter describes some common skin dermatoses that pose therapeutic challenges.

TREATMENT GOALS

- Prevent the development of new acne lesions using topical and systemic medications.
- Differentiate between inflammatory and noninflammatory acne to direct specific treatment toward each.
- Prevent acute and chronic damage to the skin by ultraviolet radiation (UVR).
- Treat warts (verrucae) to prevent them from spreading.
- Treat seborrheic dermatitis effectively and help prevent recurrences.
- Treat psoriasis, a chronic, inflammatory disorder, aggressively because of its significant morbidity and potential life-threatening complications.

ACNE

DEFINITION

Acne is a chronic disorder of the hair follicle and sebaceous gland. It is a skin condition characterized by the excess production of oil from sebaceous glands in which the hair follicles become plugged, leading to blackheads, pimple outbreaks, cysts, infected abscesses, and (sometimes) scarring.

EPIDEMIOLOGY

Acne vulgaris is a chronic but usually self-limited disorder that, left untreated, can leave physical and emotional scars. It is the most common skin disorder in adolescents and young adults aged 10 to 30 and is estimated to occur to some degree in 80% of this population.[1,2] The peak age of occurrence is between 16 and 19, and it tends to resolve in the vast majority of patients by age 25. The incidence of acne is similar among the sexes. Girls tend to develop acne at an earlier age because of an earlier onset of puberty.[3] However, boys tend to develop a more severe form of the disorder.

PATHOPHYSIOLOGY

The pathogenesis of acne is multifactorial and complex. The pathophysiology involves four primary events: increased sebum production, follicular hyperkeratinization, proliferation of *Propionibacterium acnes*, and inflammation.[1] Genetic factors may also play a role, particularly in more severe forms of acne.[4] However, the high prevalence and the multi-

factorial origin of the disorder make genetic factors difficult to assess.

Active sebaceous glands and increased sebum production are prerequisites for the development of acne. This is primarily because escalated sebum production leads to the formation of a microcomedo by occluding the follicle and providing an optimal environment for the proliferation of *P. acnes*. Acne patients tend to secrete more sebum than patients without acne, and increased sebum secretion correlates with acne severity.[1]

The maturation of these glands is regulated by hormonal control and commences at puberty.[5] At this time, androgens are produced in the testes in boys, and in the ovaries and adrenal glands in girls. Circulating testosterone is converted at the tissue level by 5-α-reductase to dihydrotestosterone, a potent stimulator of sebum production. These androgens play an important role in the pathogenesis of acne through (a) the stimulation of sebum secretion, (b) increased sebaceous gland size, and (c) increased follicular hyperkeratinization.[6] Acne-prone skin has been shown to have abnormally high 5-α-reductase activity in vitro. In women, estrogens decrease sebum production by suppressing gonadotropin release and subsequent androgen production. Therefore, women with biochemical androgen excess often have more severe acne.

Follicular keratinization is another pathologic change associated with acne formation and occurs when keratinocyte hyperproliferation results in the abnormal shedding of cells in the follicle lumen.[2] The accumulation and adherence of keratinocytes and sebum to the follicular canal plugs the follicle. This occlusion prevents further elimination of follicular material and causes dilation of the follicle below the surface of the skin. This precursor lesion is called a microcomedo and will ultimately progress to form a noninflammatory lesion (open or closed comedo).[7,8] If the follicular opening dilates enough to extrude this material, a blackhead (also known as an open comedo) results. If the follicular opening does not dilate sufficiently, the resultant lesion is a whitehead (as known as a closed comedo) and is often the site of an inflammatory lesion. Conversely, an open comedo is a mature lesion that does not typically become inflamed. The black color is attributed to the impacted keratinous material and is neither dirt nor oxidized sebum or melanin.[9]

The occluded follicle in primarily closed comedos provides an optimal environment for *P. acnes* to proliferate, which ultimately leads to the inflammation of the follicle. The bacterium secretes chemotactic factors that attract polymorphonuclear leukocytes (PMNs) that invade the follicle. The cytotoxic effect of these PMNs leads to the disruption and eventual collapse of the follicle wall.[10] Rupture of the follicular wall allows the contents to spill into the surrounding dermis, further increasing the inflammatory response. In addition, *P. acnes* produces lipases that hydrolyze the triglycerides of sebum into glycerol and free fatty acids (FFAs). These FFAs have been shown to contribute to the inflammatory response. Figure 10.1 shows the four pathogenic factors important in the development of an acne lesion.[1] The magnitude of an individual's inflammatory response determines the severity of the clinical presentation.

A number of exogenous factors can make existing acne worse. Oil-based makeup, pomades, oily soaps, and hair products may occlude the follicle, initiating a comedo. Physical pressure from a headband or hat can induce localized acne. Although exposure to excessive heat and humidity can exacerbate acne, the mechanism is not clear. The ingestion of certain drugs may also aggravate acne. Danazol and birth control pills with a high progesterone component produce increased androgenic activity and may exacerbate acne. Table 10.1 lists other medications that have these untoward effects. However, the underlying mechanism for most of these medications is not understood. Diet and stress often are implicated, but controlled studies are lacking. No food, including chocolate, needs to be eliminated from the diet unless a patient implicitly believes a particular food is aggravating the condition.[1]

CLINICAL PRESENTATION AND DIAGNOSIS

Acne lesions occur within the specialized sebaceous hair follicular units found principally on the face and to a lesser degree on the chest, shoulders, and back. The two basic lesions are noninflammatory and inflammatory. Noninflammatory lesions consist of open comedones (blackheads) and closed comedones (whiteheads) (Fig. 10.2). Comedones develop because of an impaction of keratin and sebum within a dilated follicle and are considered the primary lesions in

acne. Mild acne consists of mostly noninflammatory lesions, but most patients will progress beyond this point.

The depth and magnitude of the inflammatory response corresponds with the clinical development of papules, pustules, nodules, and cysts. Papules are inflammatory lesions with a pink-red dome-shaped appearance. Pustules are papules with an accumulation of white blood cells (pus) on top of the superficial inflammatory lesion. A preponderance of these lesions constitutes at least moderate acne. Deep-seated, exaggerated inflammatory lesions include nodules and cysts (Fig. 10.3). These types of lesions typically affect more than one pilosebaceous unit (pore) and are present in the more severe cases of acne. Patients with nodulocystic acne often have extensive involvement of the chest and back.

Scarring may occur, particularly in the deeper inflammatory forms of acne. It is the most devastating clinical feature prompting early aggressive therapy. The most common scar is the atrophic (ice-pick) form, which is permanent. Hypertrophic or thickened mounded-appearing scars also occur and are more commonly seen on the trunk (Fig. 10.4). These tend to flatten in time.

Often overlooked is the residual pigmentary alteration seen after inflammatory lesions resolve. This is particularly noticeable in patients with dark complexions, in whom hyperpigmentation predominates and is often what prompts a visit to the physician (Fig. 10.5). There is no effective treatment for the pigmentary alteration beyond preventing further inflammatory lesions. The majority of the pigmented lesions fade, but it can take from 6 months to a year for this to occur.

PSYCHOSOCIAL ASPECTS

Although acne is not a serious health threat, it can have a major impact on quality of life. People with acne tend to be more socially withdrawn and have a higher unemployment rate than people without acne. Significant psychological harm can occur in individuals with disfiguring, permanent scarring. Clinicians need to understand the psychosocial aspects to the disease to treat their patients appropriately. For example, a patient who may only have mild to moderate disease but has significant psychological damage may be an appropriate candidate for more aggressive therapy, which would normally be reserved for more severe forms of the disease.[1]

THERAPEUTIC PLAN

Combination therapy should be used as early as possible because no single topical agent is effective against all four of the pathophysiologic features of acne. However, monotherapy with topical retinoids is considered the treatment of choice for mild acne, which includes primarily noninflammatory acne and acne with only a few inflammatory lesions.

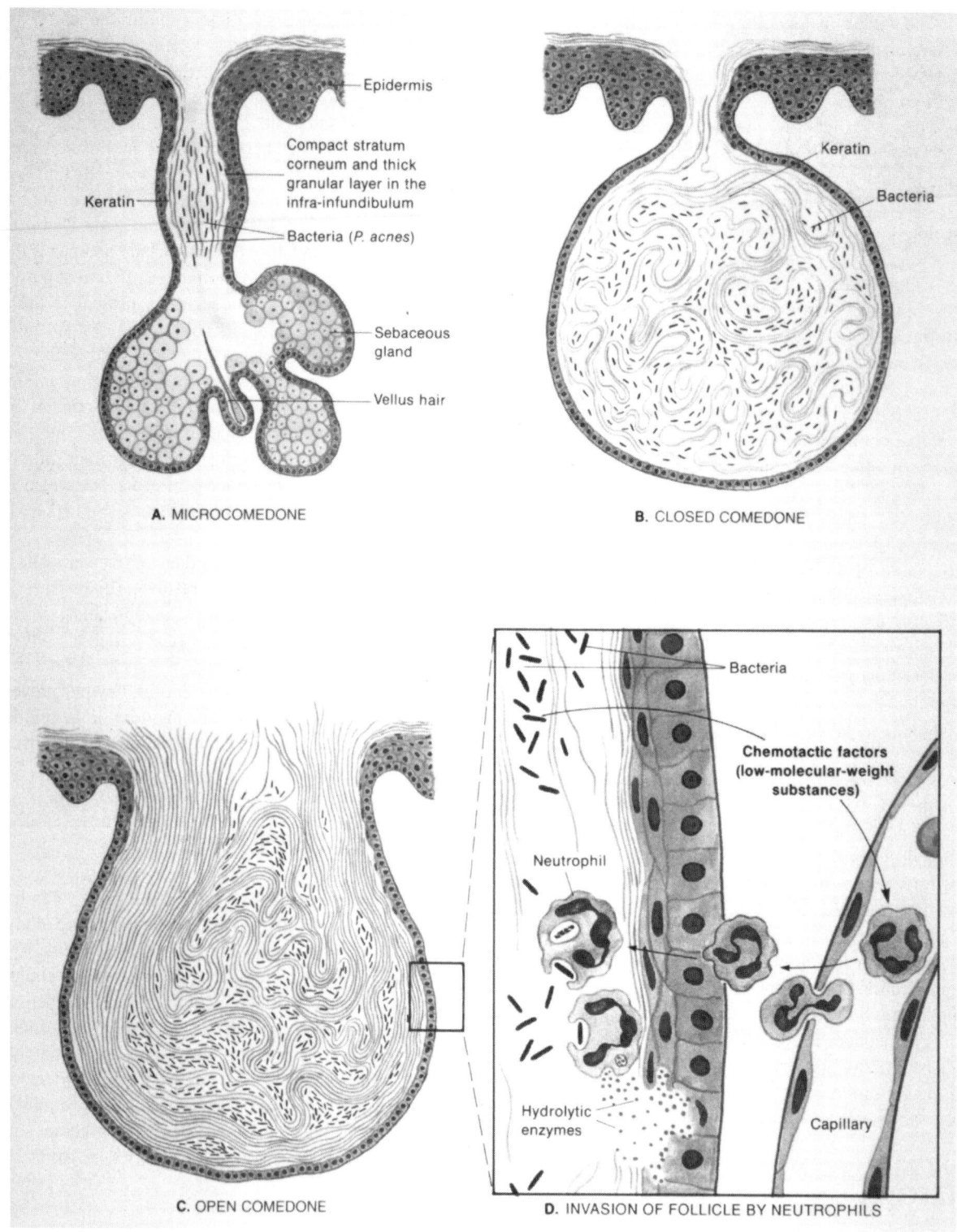

A. MICROCOMEDONE

Epidermis

Compact stratum corneum and thick granular layer in the infra-infundibulum

Keratin

Bacteria (*P. acnes*)

Sebaceous gland

Vellus hair

B. CLOSED COMEDONE

Keratin

Bacteria

C. OPEN COMEDONE

D. INVASION OF FOLLICLE BY NEUTROPHILS

Bacteria

Chemotactic factors (low-molecular-weight substances)

Neutrophil

Hydrolytic enzymes

Capillary

FIGURE 10.1 Pathogenesis of follicular distention, rupture, and inflammation in acne vulgaris. Acne is a disease of the follicular canal of a sebaceous follicle. A compact stratum corneum and a thickened granular layer in the infrainfundibulum are the beginning of the formation of a comedone. Microcomedones **(A)** and closed **(B)** and open **(C)** comedones form. Excessive sebum secretion occurs, and the bacterium *P. acnes* proliferates. The organism produces chemotactic factors, leading to neutrophil migration into the intact comedone. Neutrophilic enzymes are released and the comedone ruptures, inducing a cycle of chemotaxis and intense neutrophilic inflammation **(D,E)** (*see color insert*). (From Rubin E, Farber JL. Pathology. 3rd ed. Philadelphia: Lippincott Williams & Wilkins, 1999.)

TABLE 10.1	**Medications That Aggravate Acne**
Hormonal	**Nonhormonal**
Anabolic steroids	Azathioprine
Danazol	Bromides
Gonadotropins	Cyanocobalamin
High-progesterone oral contraceptive pills	Disulfiram
	Ethambutol
Prednisone	Gold
	Hydantoin drugs
	Iodides
	Isoniazid
	Maprotiline
	Quinidine
	Quinine
	Rifampin
	Thiouracil

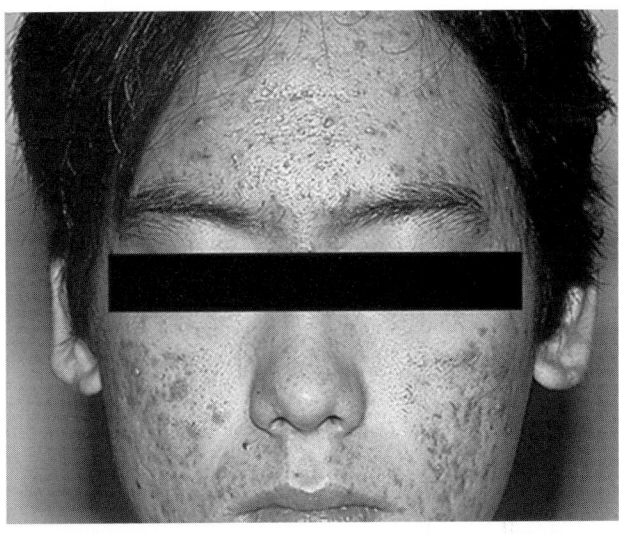

FIGURE 10.3 Severe cystic acne. This patient was subsequently treated with isotretinoin (Accutane) (*see color insert*). (From Goodheart HP. Goodheart's Photoguide of Common Skin Disorders, 2nd ed. Philadelphia: Lippincott Williams & Wilkins, 2003.)

Although benzoyl peroxide was once considered first-line treatment, topical retinoids have proven to be more effective in mild acne. Topical retinoids decrease comedones and, thus, inflammatory lesions by inhibiting follicular keratinization and microcomedo formation. For patients intolerant to topical retinoids, azelaic acid and salicylic acid are viable alternatives, although they are not as effective.

For mild to moderate inflammatory (papular/pustular) acne, the combination of topical retinoids, benzoyl peroxide, and/or topical antibiotics has proven to clear inflammatory lesions effectively. For moderate to severe inflammatory acne, oral antibiotics combined with topical retinoids and/ or benzoyl peroxide are often used as first-line therapy. Anti-

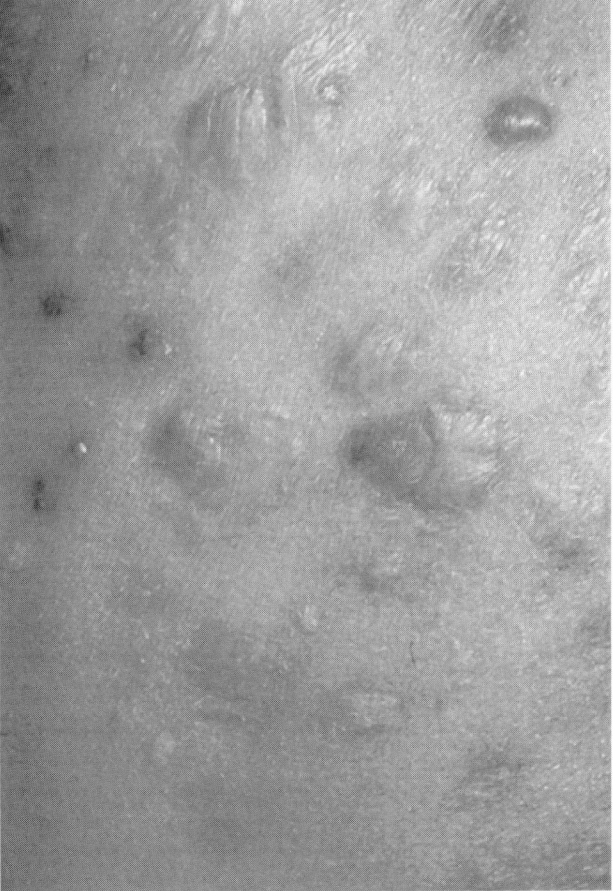

FIGURE 10.4 Acne scars. Hypertrophic scars. These lesions are characteristic of acne scars that occur on the trunk (*see color insert*). (From Goodheart HP. Goodheart's photoguide of common skin disorders. 2nd ed. Philadelphia: Lippincott Williams & Wilkins, 2003.)

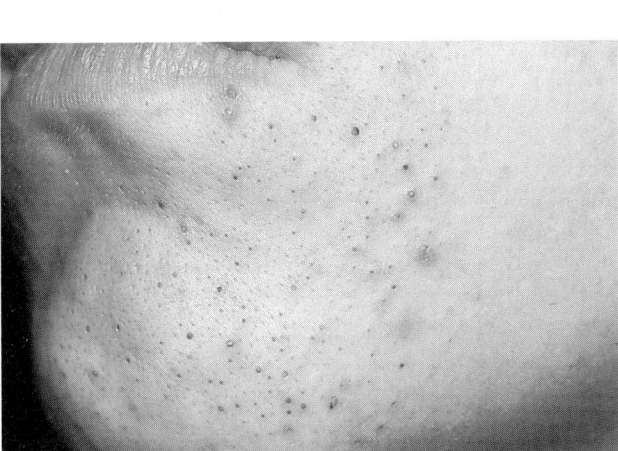

FIGURE 10.2 Noninflammatory lesions. The combination of open and closed comedones, as seen here, is most common in younger patients (*see color insert*). (From Goodheart HP. Goodheart's photoguide of common skin disorders. 2nd ed. Philadelphia: Lippincott Williams & Wilkins, 2003.)

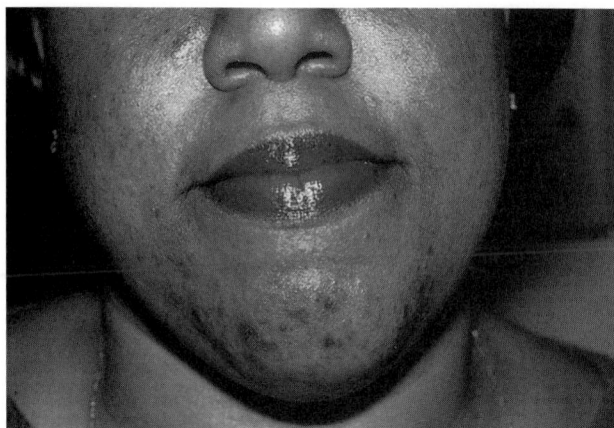

FIGURE 10.5 Postinflammatory hyperpigmentation is seen in this African-American patient (*see color insert*). (From Goodheart HP. Goodheart's photoguide of common skin disorders. 2nd ed. Philadelphia: Lippincott Williams & Wilkins, 2003.)

TABLE 10.2	Summary of Therapeutic Agents in Acne and Principal Mode of Activity
Topical Therapy	**Oral Therapy**

Antimicrobial (*P. acnes*)

Benzoyl peroxide	
Antibiotics	**Antibiotics**
Clindamycin	Clindamycin
Erythromycin	Erythromycin
Tetracycline	Tetracycline
Meclocycline	Minocycline
Azelaic acid	Trimethoprim–sulfamethoxazole
Sulfur	Isotretinoin
Salicylic acid	

Comedolytics — **Comedolytics**

Tretinoin	Isotretinoin
Adapalene	**Decreased Sebaceous Gland Activity**
Tazarotene	
Azelaic acid	Isotretinoin
Benzoyl peroxide (minor)	Hormonal therapy
	Estrogen
Salicylic acid (minor)	Cyproterone acetate
Resorcin (minor)	Spironolactone

androgenic hormonal therapy is also a possibility for female patients with moderate to severe acne as adjunctive therapy.

Monotherapy with oral isotretinoin is the treatment of choice in severe and refractory inflammatory acne, provided there are no contraindications. In women with refractory disease, hormonal therapy can be used adjunctively.[2] Maintenance therapy with either topical or oral agents should follow isotretinoin treatment to maintain remission.[11] Topical retinoids are considered first line for maintenance therapy. The use of benzoyl peroxide in the morning and tretinoin before bedtime is an option when monotherapy with retinoids has failed. Antibiotics are not recommended for maintenance therapy primarily because of the development of antibiotic resistance.[12]

TREATMENT

The treatment of acne can be difficult and disappointing. Acne is a chronic condition, and at times many months or even years of individualized treatment are needed to achieve control. Nevertheless, if the patient is committed and compliant, it is certainly a treatable disease, and acne control should be expected. Compliance is enhanced if the patient understands both the nature of the disease and the rationale behind the therapy. Virtually all therapy is preventive, with little or no effect on the inflammatory lesions present at the outset. For that reason, maximum efficacy is not reached for several months, even with the most effective treatment. Once acne control is achieved, the patient should understand that maintenance therapy will be needed as long as the tendency for acne persists.

Important factors in the pathogenesis of acne are pilosebaceous obstruction by sebum and keratin, androgen-stimulated sebum production, inflammation, and proliferation of *P. acnes*. Acne therapy is directed at correcting each of these factors. As in other diseases without a single best treatment,

many therapies exist, each with specific merits. Many topical therapies are readily available over the counter, and although they are effective in some patients when used properly, they are subject to misuse by uninformed patients. Compliance with a single regimen, whether it is self-initiated or physician-prescribed, should be emphasized for optimal results. A summary of therapeutic agents in acne with their principal mode of activity is shown in Table 10.2.

GENERAL SKIN CARE

There is no evidence that excessive cleansing offers therapeutic benefit. In fact, overcleansing can be an irritant. In addition, surface sebum and bacteria do not play a role in the development of lesions. When choosing a type of soap, the patient should avoid those with high oil content. These are usually reserved for dry, sensitive skin and can be counterproductive in acne. Expensive medicated soaps usually are not indicated as a supplement to other treatment plans. Astringents are alcohol-based cleansers that are easy to use and leave the face feeling cool and refreshed; unfortunately, they are of limited value in treating acne.[7]

In noninflammatory acne, a mildly abrasive cleanser may be of some benefit by inducing a superficial exfoliation of the skin. In inflammatory acne or in the patient with dry skin from previous acne therapy, a gentle soap is indicated. Avoidance of all cosmetics is best, but complete avoidance may be an unrealistic expectation. If cosmetics are to be used, they should be water-based and should not clog pores. Noncomedogenic products, which are less likely to clog pores and aggravate skin, should be recommended. Antibacterial soaps other than those containing benzoyl peroxide have no activity against *P. acnes* and should not be used.[1]

PHARMACOTHERAPY

Topical Therapy. Topically applied medications remain the cornerstone of acne therapy. They are often effective alone in mild to moderate acne and are important adjuncts to oral antibiotics in more severe acne. The most widely used topical preparations are benzoyl peroxide and antibiotics, which inhibit the growth of *P. acnes*, and topical retinoids, which reverse the abnormal follicular keratinization.

Benzoyl Peroxide. Benzoyl peroxide was first formulated for dermatologic use in 1905 and was recognized as useful for acne in 1934. However, the original ointment vehicle was unsuitable for acne therapy. It was not until the mid-1960s that a stable preparation of benzoyl peroxide in a hydrous medium was formulated. Since that time, it has become the most widely used topical medication for acne because of its effectiveness, and is readily available both over the counter and by prescription. When used properly, it can be effective as monotherapy for mild acne and may be used as an adjunct to other therapies in more severe forms of the condition.

The principal mode of action of benzoyl peroxide is thought to be its rapid bacteriostatic and possibly even bactericidal activity against *P. acnes* and *Staphylococcus aureus* on the skin surface. Subsequently, a decrease of about 90% of the organisms and 40% of the FFAs on the skin surface can be observed after a few days.[7] Benzoyl peroxide is metabolized to benzoic acid in the skin, and its lipophilic properties allow it to penetrate better than other topical antimicrobials.[13] Once it penetrates the follicle, the release of nascent oxygen from the peroxide exerts its effect on the bacteria. When the *P. acnes* bacterial load is reduced, FFAs, which contribute to the comedonal plug and inflammation, are also reduced. Benzoyl peroxide has also been thought to have comedolytic and exfoliative properties.[7] However, reports of these effects are contradictory, and these actions are considered minor. Benzoyl peroxide has no effect on sebum production or concentration.

In 11 double-blind clinical trials comparing topical antibiotics with 5% benzoyl peroxide, none of the topical antibiotics were shown to be more effective than benzoyl peroxide against inflamed lesions.[14–16] Even though benzoyl peroxide may be superior to other topical antibiotics when used as monotherapy, benzoyl peroxide used with erythromycin or clindamycin has been shown to be more effective in combination.[17–19] In addition, benzoyl peroxide does not develop the antimicrobial resistance to *P. acnes* compared to other topical antibiotics, and may even decrease the rate of resistance to topical antibiotics when used in combination.[20,21]

Benzoyl peroxide is available over the counter in various strengths, between 2.5% and 10.0%, and in various vehicles, with creams, lotions, washes, and soaps being the most common. It is available in the same concentrations by prescription, usually in various gel vehicles. Selecting the appropriate vehicle for each patient is important. Gels are considered more effective vehicles for consistent release of active ingredient, but they may be more irritating. Although less effective, a wash or lotion may be all that can be tolerated in a patient with more sensitive skin. During the winter, when dry skin can be a problem, switching from the gels to a cream or lotion may be necessary.

There is no difference among the various concentrations of benzoyl peroxide in reducing *P. acnes* numbers in the skin.[2] Therefore, when initiating therapy with benzoyl peroxide, it is reasonable to begin with a low concentration (2.5% to 5.0%) to minimize irritation. Therapy should be initiated with once-daily application. The patient should be reminded to apply the product to the entire affected area, not only to the visible lesions, being careful to avoid the periorbital, perinasal, and perioral skin. Patients may experience mild erythema, burning, or stinging on initial application, and they should be instructed to expect these conditions. If the patient applies the medication at night, the erythema should be minimal by morning. If irritation persists, switching to every-other-night therapy is appropriate.

Tolerance to these side effects usually develops as therapy continues. Once tolerance is achieved, the patient should increase the frequency of application to twice a day. Switching to a more potent vehicle or a higher concentration should be initiated only after tolerance is achieved and there is a lack of significant improvement in the acne after 4 to 8 weeks. As a general rule, the incidence of side effects increases more than the efficacy with increasing concentrations of benzoyl peroxide.

The most common side effect of benzoyl peroxide is skin irritation, which may in part be responsible for its efficacy. It is known that 1% to 2% of people are allergic to this compound.[22] At this point, allergic contact dermatitis should be ruled out. In these cases, stopping the medication is all that is needed, and an alternative therapy is necessary. Patients should be warned that benzoyl peroxide can bleach hair, linens, and clothes, and this could become a major deterrent to its use. Allowing the preparation to dry completely before coming in contact with fabrics can minimize this problem. The question of whether benzoyl peroxide is carcinogenic has been raised. Earlier studies on rodents have supported this finding, but case-controlled studies in humans have not. To date, it is considered completely safe for use in humans, with no reports of adverse effects that could be related to skin carcinogenesis.[23,24]

Topical Retinoids. Since being introduced for acne in 1969, the derivatives of vitamin A have become the most effective agent for treating acne. It was originally thought that their mode of action was related to their ability to promote erythema and skin peeling. It is now known that their activity is directed at reducing the cohesiveness of keratinocytes within the sebaceous follicle, independent of clinical peeling.[25] For this reason, topical retinoids are superior to all other topical or oral therapies for comedonal acne because they prevent the development of the microcomedo, the precursor to all lesions. Because inflammatory lesions are ultimately derived from the microcomedo, topical retinoids can also prevent inflammatory lesions from developing. Current guidelines recommend that retinoids be used in combination with benzoyl peroxide or topical antibiotics to treat mild to moderate inflammatory acne as well as noninflammatory acne.[1]

There are currently three topical retinoids on the market: tretinoin, adapalene, and tazarotene. All three are effective at reducing the number of comedones and inflammatory lesions, but clinical trials have shown that adapalene may have better tolerability, while tazarotene appears to be most effective in reducing papules and open comedones.[26–28] Tretinoin (Retin-A) is available in a 0.025%, 0.05%, and 0.1% cream; a 0.01% and 0.025% gel; a 0.04% and 0.1% microgel; and a 0.05% lotion. Adapalene (Differin) is available as 0.1% cream, gel, and topical solution. Tazarotene (Tazorac) comes in 0.05% and 0.1% cream and gel formulations. Therapy is usually initiated with the lowest-strength cream in all the formulations because the irritation is typically much less and the efficacy is only slightly lower.[26]

The patient should be aware that topical retinoids might cause mild to severe irritation of the skin, which is more common at initiation of therapy. This is manifested by erythema, dryness, and peeling and is influenced by the formulation used. Retinoids in general should not be applied more than once daily initially. They should be applied to completely dry skin because moisture increases the permeability of the retinoids and therefore its irritant potential. The patient should avoid the periorbital, perinasal, and perioral skin. The erythema and dryness is not necessary for effectiveness, so if side effects continue to be a problem, using retinoids every other night or every third night is recommended. As tolerance develops, the frequency can be increased.

Many patients treat the side effects of topical retinoids with heavy emollients, but this is counterproductive in acne treatment and should be discouraged. The use of other harsh skin care products such as astringents can increase the irritant potential of topical retinoids and should be eliminated if possible. A gentle soap should be used, and a mild noncomedogenic lotion if necessary.

Patients may experience a modest exacerbation of their acne upon initiation of therapy. This is secondary to the ability of topical retinoid to release the retained products of comedones to the skin surface. Patients should understand that this is expected, so that they do not discontinue the therapy unnecessarily. This flare should resolve in 3 to 6 weeks.

Topical retinoids decrease the thickness of the stratum corneum, the most superficial layer of the skin.[2] This layer helps protect the skin from solar damage. Patients should be counseled to apply the medication around bedtime and to avoid long exposure to UVR. If exposure is unavoidable, patients should use a sunscreen with a sun protection factor (SPF) of at least 15. The thinned stratum corneum also allows better permeability of other topical agents, which is an advantage when used in conjunction with topical antibiotics. Systemic toxicity, as potentially seen with oral retinoids, is not a problem with topical retinoids even when applied in high concentrations.

Even though topical preparations of retinoids are thought to have minimal percutaneous absorption and have not been directly associated with birth defects, experts agree that they should not be used in pregnant patients. Although there have been case reports of infants born with birth defects to mothers who were using the topical preparation, controlled studies with topical tretinoin used during pregnancy conclude that there is no increased risk of congenital malformations to the fetus.[29–35]

Topical Antibiotics. Topical antibiotics are used in mild to moderate inflammatory acne and as an adjunct in more severe nodulocystic acne. They have weak comedolytic activity and therefore are not useful alone in comedonal acne. When used in more severe types of acne, topical antibiotics are especially useful when tapering oral therapy. The most common topical antibiotics used are clindamycin and erythromycin, formulated in a variety of vehicles and strengths. Topical tetracycline and meclocycline are still available but are not often used. In general, topical antibiotics have a slower onset of action and are less effective than oral antibiotics.[1]

The principal action of topical antibiotics is their bacteriostatic effect against *P. acnes*. In addition to clindamycin, erythromycin, and tetracycline's antibacterial effects against *P. acnes*, they also have antiinflammatory activities through inhibition of lipase production by *P. acnes* as well as inhibition of leukocyte chemotaxis.[2,16] Clindamycin is more lipophilic than erythromycin and appears to be more effective at reducing *P. acnes* counts. However, similar results are obtained when examining the clinical efficacy of the two agents, implying that other factors may play a primary role.

Topical antibiotics usually are applied twice a day to moist skin after washing with soap and water. As with other topical products, the vehicle is important. Vehicles with high alcohol content allow better absorption but may be more drying. A cream or ointment may be better tolerated initially in patients with more sensitive skin or during the winter.

Improvement is often noted after 4 to 6 weeks of therapy, although maximum efficacy may not be seen for at least 12 weeks. Once a clinical response has been achieved and outbreaks have stabilized, topical antibiotic use should be tapered down to decrease the development of resistant organisms. If no improvement is observed within 6 to 8 weeks, the antibiotic should be discontinued and a therapeutic switch considered.[1]

Owing to the development of resistant organisms to these antibiotics, topical antibiotics should not be used alone. Recolonization by susceptible strains of *P. acnes* is seen quickly upon discontinuation of therapy. Current guidelines recommend concurrent use of benzoyl peroxide to reduce the rate of resistance of topical antibiotics and to alleviate recolonization.[11] Benzoyl peroxide also shows benefit when topical antibiotics need to be discontinued. It is recommended that the patient continue using benzoyl peroxide after stopping the topical antibiotics to sustain the decreased colonization of *P. acnes* and prevent future outbreaks.[1,36]

The most common side effect of topical antibiotics is mild erythema and stinging caused by the vehicle. Commercially available topical clindamycin preparations are of the phosphate form and are less readily absorbed through the skin. However, 10% of a daily application does reach the bloodstream, and cases of pseudomembranous colitis have been described with topical use.[37] This is a rare but possible side effect, particularly when clindamycin is applied to a large surface area of skin. Topical meclocycline can impart a faint yellow tint to the skin, which can be washed off.

Combined Topical Therapies. Combination therapy enhances efficacy, counteracts the emergence of bacterial resistance, and helps decrease unwanted side effects.[1,36] Because the pathogenesis of acne is multifactorial, combining two topical therapies directed at different factors in the pathogenesis of acne increases efficacy. Combination topical therapies should be the standard of practice, especially if the patient with mild or noninflammatory acne has not responded to either benzoyl peroxide or tretinoin monotherapy or if the patient's acne is classified as moderate or severe. The most commonly used combination is tretinoin, with its comedolytic activity, and topical antibiotics or benzoyl peroxide. As discussed earlier, by thinning the stratum corneum, tretinoin permits better absorption of the antimicrobials.

The combination of tretinoin and benzoyl peroxide appears to be more effective than each used individually. Therapy is generally initiated with low concentrations of each on an alternate-day basis. When tolerance to the irritant effect is acquired, each may be used daily. The patient usually is instructed to apply benzoyl peroxide in the morning and tretinoin at night. This should be followed strictly because the irritant potential is additive when used concurrently. If the patient cannot tolerate benzoyl peroxide, a topical antibiotic may be used.

Combining a topical antibiotic such as erythromycin or clindamycin with benzoyl peroxide not only increases the bacteriostatic effects of the antibiotic but also reduces the potential for resistance.[36] Erythromycin is more active than benzoyl peroxide against *P. acnes* but is not lipid soluble, making penetration into the skin difficult. The combination is proven to be more effective, because benzoyl peroxide may facilitate the transport of the more active erythromycin to the target tissue.[13] In addition, the antiinflammatory effect of erythromycin is believed to reduce the irritancy of the

benzoyl peroxide.[38] When treating noninflammatory acne, the combination of two antibacterials with little comedolytic properties is not ideal and should not be used.[12]

Other Topical Therapies. Azelaic acid, a naturally occurring dicarboxylic acid molecule, is effective for both noninflammatory and inflammatory acne and is commercially available by prescription as a 20% cream (Azelex) and a 15% gel (Finacea). The dicarboxylic acids initially were found to have a beneficial effect on hyperpigmentary disorders. When patients reported a coincidental improvement in their acne, studies were initiated to investigate azelaic acid's potential as an acne treatment. The result of one such study showed that a 20% azelaic acid cream was as effective as 0.05% tretinoin cream in reducing comedones, with less irritation.[39,40] The best results with azelaic acid cream were seen in papulopustular acne from one study of moderate to severe acne patients. Twenty-percent azelaic acid resulted in an 83% reduction in inflammatory lesions compared to an 86% reduction with oral tetracycline.[41] A more recent study compared the combination of azelaic acid cream plus oral minocycline with oral isotretinoin. The results showed that even though the combination was not as effective as isotretinoin monotherapy, the combination therapy may be an alternative for patients unable to take oral retinoids.[42] Azelaic acid's efficacy is explained by both a strong comedolytic property and a bacteriostatic effect on *P. acnes*.[43] Adverse reactions reported in clinical trials were generally mild and transient and included pruritus, burning, tingling, local irritation, erythema, rash, small depigmented spots, and redness.

Traditional topical therapies using salicylic acid (0.5% to 6%), sulfur (2% to 10%), zinc, or resorcin (2% to 6%) are used less frequently now that other therapies tend to be more efficacious. Their effectiveness is correlated with their ability to reduce erythema and induce desquamation. Salicylic acid is a keratolytic and has weak comedolytic activity. Tretinoin has been shown to be more effective than salicylic acid but could be a safe alternative in patients intolerant to retinoids.[1] However, salicylic acid is an irritant and could cause exacerbation of inflammatory lesions.[44] Sulfur, with its antibiotic properties, appears to hasten the resolution of inflammatory lesions. The combination of sulfur and salicylic acid is synergistic, so they are often formulated together. Zinc is also used in acne medications, but again more conventional agents are more effective. In one controlled study, the combination of benzoyl peroxide 5% and erythromycin 3% gel was significantly more effective than erythromycin 4% and zinc 1.2% solution.[38]

There have been a number of attempts to use topical antiandrogens to treat acne. Topical cyproterone acetate was found to be ineffective, and the results of studies with spironolactone cream have been equivocal. A nonsteroidal antiandrogen, inocoterone acetate (RU882), in a 10% solution, exerted a modest (26%) reduction in the number of inflammatory papules and pustules in treated men after 16 weeks of therapy.[45] However, this compares unfavorably with the results expected using established preparations such as benzoyl peroxide or topical antibiotics (50% to 75% reduction in lesions at 2 months).[46] Another topically active antiandrogen, RU58841, has been shown to have a high affinity for androgen receptors and minimal systemic effects in hamsters.[47]

Systemic Therapy.

Antibiotics. Oral antibiotics should be used at the outset of therapy for patients with moderate to severe inflammatory acne.[1] They should be used in conjunction with either topical benzoyl peroxide or tretinoin and occasionally with topical antibiotics. To optimize results, antibiotics should be used with topical retinoids to increase efficacy, shorten treatment duration, and help prevent antibiotic resistance.[1] It has also been found that benzoyl peroxide or azelaic acid treatment used in combination with antimicrobials may reduce the potential of developing *P. acnes* resistance.[1,11] Tetracycline and its derivative, minocycline, usually are the drugs of first choice. Erythromycin and doxycycline are common alternatives, and trimethoprim-sulfamethoxazole is sometimes prescribed as a third-line agent. These agents inhibit *P. acnes*, resulting in decreased chemotactic factor and lipase production. They also exert a direct antiinflammatory response independent of their effects on bacteria. This is seen more with tetracycline and erythromycin than with other antibiotics.[10,12]

In general, clinical improvement is usually noted within 6 to 8 weeks of oral antibiotic therapy. Once an adequate response is noted, tapering the dose over several weeks is recommended. The goal is to discontinue oral therapy while maintaining control with topical therapy alone. Oral antibiotics should not be used for more than 3 to 6 months unless alternative therapies are not an option; only then can oral antibiotics be continued indefinitely.[1]

Tetracycline, in a dose of 1 g per day in two to four divided doses, is usually tried first. Occasionally, doses of up to 2 g are necessary in nodulocystic acne. Tetracycline is best absorbed if not taken with food, dairy products, iron, or antacids. The patient should be instructed to take the medication 1 hour before or 2 hours after a meal. Tetracycline on an empty stomach may cause nausea in some patients, and in these instances it can be taken with a small amount of food.[7]

A common side effect of tetracycline is vaginal yeast infection, which can be controlled with topical antifungal preparations. Tetracycline can also cause photosensitivity eruptions, so patients should wear a sunscreen with an SPF of at least 15 if planning to spend time in the sun. Tetracycline and its derivatives should never be administered during pregnancy because they can cause liver toxicity in the mother and bone and teeth abnormalities in the fetus.

If cost were not a factor, minocycline would be the antibiotic of first choice in acne treatment. It is more lipophilic than tetracycline and doxycycline, allowing it to accumulate more readily in the sebaceous follicle, and its clinical efficacy is also better than either antibiotic.[14,48] It is better absorbed with food and is less likely to cause nausea than tetracycline. It is also less likely to cause photosensitivity reactions. The usual initial dose is 50 mg twice a day.[49]

Minocycline can cause esophagitis secondary to reflux, so it should not be taken just before bedtime. A dose-dependent vestibular dysfunction can occur, leading to vertigo, ataxia, nausea, and vomiting. Lowering the dose can circumvent these effects, but often the medication must be discontinued. A blue-gray pigmentation of skin and mucous membranes has also been reported with minocycline use. This is more common in sun-exposed areas and may take up to 7 months to resolve.[49] Doxycycline, another derivative of tetracycline, has demonstrated therapeutic equivalence to minocycline but is used less often to treat acne because of a much higher incidence of photosensitivity reactions.[7]

If a patient cannot take tetracycline, erythromycin is an effective alternative. It is as effective as tetracycline, but the higher incidence of gastrointestinal problems and the more frequent development of resistant strains of *P. acnes* make it the second choice.[11] Advantages of erythromycin include the lower rate of monilial overgrowth, the lack of photosensitivity, and maintenance of efficacy when taken with food. It is considered safe for use during pregnancy. However, consulting with the obstetrician is wise before initiating long-term therapy with any medication during pregnancy. Dosing is the same as for tetracycline.

The safety of long-term antibiotics in treating acne is well established.[50] Concern about possible serious superinfections has not been borne out clinically. There is also concern that broad-spectrum antibiotics can decrease the effectiveness of oral contraceptives.[51] Although this remains controversial, this possibility should be discussed with patients and additional forms of birth control considered.

Antibiotic resistance is a real concern.[52] Isolates of resistant strains of *P. acnes* have significantly increased in numbers since the 1970s and are now found in 50% of cases in Europe and the United Kingdom.[53] An international congress of experts stressed the significance of these resistant stains and formulated guidelines to help decrease the rate of resistance. Their consensus statements were (a) long-term use of oral antibiotics should be discouraged and cessation of oral antibiotic should occur as soon as acne control is gained; (b) the combination of topical and oral antibiotics breeds resistance and should be discouraged; (c) concurrent treatment with benzoyl peroxide in addition to in-between oral antibiotic therapies can reduce colonization of resistant strains; and (d) maintenance therapy should be continued with the same oral antibiotic, and switching of antibiotics should occur only after treatment failure has been documented.[1]

Isotretinoin. Oral isotretinoin (13-cis-retinoic acid) is the most effective agent in treating acne. This synthetic derivative of vitamin A was introduced in 1982. It was formerly indicated primarily for treating resistant nodulocystic acne, but the majority of treated patients today have therapy-resistant moderate acne. It should also be considered early in the therapy of patients who experience scarring. Dramatic improvement can be seen with isotretinoin, and in contrast to other acne therapies, prolonged remission can be expected. The teratogenicity and multiple potential side effects associated with isotretinoin preclude its use in less severe acne.

The mechanism of action of isotretinoin is multifactorial. It is the only known therapeutic agent that affects all the major factors associated with the pathogenesis of acne.[54] Its most profound effect is on reduction of sebaceous gland size and sebum production. A 50% to 90% reduction in sebaceous gland size can be expected. As a result, *P. acnes* levels decrease substantially.[55] It has no direct antibacterial properties, but isotretinoin reduces *P. acnes* counts indirectly by reducing sebum. This inhibition continues in most patients for more than a year after therapy is discontinued. Isotretinoin also normalizes the keratinization process in the follicle. Isotretinoin also has direct antiinflammatory properties as a result of its ability to inhibit the chemotaxis of neutrophils and monocytes.

The usual starting dose of isotretinoin is 0.5 to 1 mg per kg orally per day. Treatment is usually started at the lower dose and then the dosage is gradually increased, based on clinical response and tolerability, after 4 to 8 weeks. Therapy is continued for 16 to 20 weeks. In some cases, a longer treatment period (24 to 32 weeks) might be necessary. Oral antibiotics and topical medications that can further dry the skin are not routinely used concurrently and should be discontinued before starting isotretinoin therapy. Improvement usually is noted within 2 months, and continued improvement can be seen for up to 6 months after therapy.

Relapse is not uncommon. In one study, only 38% of patients were shown to have no acne 3 years after a course of isotretinoin. The majority of those who do relapse, however, will have a much milder form than the initial disease.[56] Relapse is seen more often in those treated with lower doses, women older than 25 at initiation of therapy, those with severe acne, and patients with a long history of uncontrolled acne. Relapse is common after the first year of therapy and is relatively uncommon after 3 years.[57] If relapse occurs, a second course can be given, but this is not recommended until 6 months have elapsed because of the delayed improvement that can be seen.

Nearly all patients who receive isotretinoin experience mucocutaneous side effects. These consist primarily of dryness of the skin, eyes, nose, and mouth. Moisturizers can be used to treat the dry skin and cheilitis. An antibiotic ointment is recommended for the nasal passages to prevent cracking, bleeding, and potential colonization by *S. aureus*. Conjunctivitis is common, and corneal opacities can occur but usually resolve within 6 weeks after cessation of therapy. During this period, patients may not tolerate contact lenses. Artificial tears can be used to offset this problem.

The most common laboratory abnormality associated with isotretinoin is a dose-related elevation of serum triglyceride levels. Hyperlipidemia occurs in about 25% of patients and is likely to occur in patients with predisposing factors such as obesity, alcoholism, nicotine use, diabetes, or familial hyperlipidemia, and those receiving concomitant β-blocker, contraceptive, and thiazide therapy. Increased serum triglyceride levels (19%) are seen more often than increased cholesterol levels (12%).[25,39,58] Less common is a decrease in high-density lipoprotein levels (15%). Alterations in the lipid panel are usually not a problem in the young patient treated for acne, but precautions should be taken. Previous recommendations included a baseline lipid profile, with repeat samples obtained after 1 week of therapy and every 2 weeks until levels stabilized. New guidelines suggest monitoring triglycerides and cholesterol values every 4 weeks for the first 2 to 3 months of therapy, then every 8 weeks thereafter.[25] Close monitoring should be done in an obese or diabetic patient. Hyperlipidemia is reversible, with lipid levels returning to baseline within 8 weeks after discontinuing therapy. Practically speaking, pretreatment laboratory tests usually are performed to exclude high-risk patients with hyperlipidemia or with diseases such as mononucleosis. These usually are repeated once during the course of therapy. If an elevation in lipid levels is noted after therapy is initiated, the patient is advised to eat a low-fat diet and therapy is continued.

Approximately 15% of patients will experience an elevation in their hepatic enzymes; this usually normalizes by reducing the dose by 50%.[25] Hepatic enzymes rarely become elevated to the extent that therapy discontinuation is necessary, but periodic monitoring of serum transaminases is recommended.[54,59] In rare instances, a decreased white blood cell count or hypercalcemia is seen. The need for laboratory monitoring of these parameters should be discussed with patients before therapy with isotretinoin. Synthetic retinoid therapy has been associated with skeletal abnormalities, including osteoporosis and osteophyte formation, in a small percentage of patients.[60] In patients with acne treated for 20 weeks, significant clinical changes are rare. Patients treated with either repeated short courses or greater than 20 weeks of therapy may require monitoring for skeletal toxicity. Most common symptoms are muscle and bone discomfort, which respond to mild analgesic therapy.[1]

Less than 10% of patients notice some hair loss during therapy, usually late in the course. Regrowth is expected. Photosensitivity can occur, and patients should wear at least an SPF 15 sunscreen before prolonged exposure to the sun. Benign intracranial hypertension is a rare side effect of isotretinoin administration. This usually manifests by headache, nausea, vomiting, and visual disturbances. If this occurs, the patient should see a physician immediately. Isotretinoin may cause depression, psychosis, mood swings, violent behavior, and, rarely, suicidal ideation and attempted suicide. For these reasons, extensive counseling of patient and family members is critical before therapy is initiated.[59,61]

Isotretinoin should be taken with food to increase the bioavailability of the drug from 20% to 40%. A new micronized formulation has improved bioavailability and less dependence on food; therefore, this formulation can be taken on an empty stomach. In addition, two randomized controlled trials showed that the new formulation may have a lower incidence of side effects and severity of adverse events, particularly hypertriglyceridemia and dryness of mucous membranes.[62,63]

The most serious potential side effect of isotretinoin is its teratogenicity. Miscarriage and stillbirth are common, and a 25-fold increase in major congenital abnormalities is seen.[64] These involve the cranium, face, heart, brain, and thymus during organogenesis. Women must understand the teratogenic potential and the consequences of becoming pregnant while taking this medication. Two pregnancy tests should be performed before the start of therapy and monthly throughout treatment before the patient receives the next month's supply of medication. The first pregnancy test should be taken at the time the decision is made to initiate therapy and the second should be taken no more than 5 days into the menstrual cycle preceding the beginning of therapy. Using two methods of contraception is a must beginning 1 month before therapy and continuing without interruption until 1 month after discontinuation.[39] The yellow Accutane qualification sticker documents that a female patient understands the risks and is qualified to receive the medication; the sticker must be placed on the prescription before it can be dispensed. In addition, only prescriptions written within the last 7 days can be filled, and the prescription is limited to a 30-day supply. Although teratogenic, isotretinoin is not mutagenic, and future pregnancies should not be affected.[64] The drug has no known effect on spermatogenesis.

Hormonal Therapy. The goal of hormonal therapy is to block androgenic activity on the sebaceous glands located in the follicles. By blocking androgens, specifically dihydrotestosterone, sebum production is decreased, leading to better acne control. There are different types of hormonal therapy. Estrogen therapy, found in oral contraceptives (OCs), blocks ovarian and adrenal androgen production, while antiandrogens, such as spironolactone and cyproterone, are androgen receptor blockers.[1]

Estrogen therapy has long been noted to improve acne in women and is an excellent option for women who require treatment of acne and desire an OC for birth control.[1] This hormone counteracts the androgenic stimulation of the sebaceous gland, decreasing sebum production. Various combinations of estrogens and progestins in OCs are effective in treating acne. Higher doses of estrogens are more effective in reducing sebum production and improving acne but are associated with a higher frequency of estrogen-related side effects. Preparations containing progestins with low androgenic activity and low doses of estrogens are generally effective and should be chosen.

There are currently four OCs (Ortho Tri-Cyclen, Alesse, Yasmin, and Estrostep) proven by randomized controlled trials (RCTs) to treat acne vulgaris effectively. The first OC approved for treating acne in women was a triphasic contraceptive containing norgestimate plus ethinyl estradiol (Ortho Tri-Cyclen). In two RCTs, Ortho Tri-Cyclen reduced inflammatory lesions by approximately 50% compared to 30% with placebo.[39,65,66] The results from studies of the other three OCs are considered comparable, and patients can expect anywhere from a 40% to more than 70% improvement in acne lesions with OCs alone.[28] Patients should be made aware that it might take several months before noticeable improvement is obtained. Androgen-dominant OCs containing norgestrel can worsen acne and should be avoided.[6]

Side effects of OC therapy are common and include nausea, weight gain, spotting, breast tenderness, and amenorrhea. Less common are brown pigmentation of the skin (melasma), depression, allergic reactions, headaches, hypertension, hyperlipidemia, deep-vein thrombosis, and alopecia. The risk of cardiovascular events increases in women over 40 years of age. In women over 35 years of age who smoke more than 15 cigarettes a day, the risks are even greater; therefore, smoking cessation should be strongly advocated.[67] Gynecomastia and decreased libido prevent its use in male patients.

Antiandrogens or androgen receptor blockers used in acne include cyproterone acetate and spironolactone. Both drugs prevent androgen activity at the target sites by competing with dihydrotestosterone for the receptor.[68] This therapy is used most commonly in women with hyperandrogenism secondary to polycystic ovarian disease and adrenal hyperactivity manifested by hirsutism and acne.

Excellent results are obtained in women using a combination of low-dose cyproterone acetate (2 mg/day) and ethinyl estradiol (35 μg/day). This combination was twice as effective in reducing acne lesions compared to OCs alone. Seborrhea improves first, but by the end of 3 months, acne lesions also regress.[69] Beneficial effects are maintained for many months after therapy is withdrawn. A higher dosage of cyproterone acetate (25 to 50 mg/day) may be needed in the resistant patient who also has hirsutism.[70] Side effects of cyproterone are uncommon but include headache, dizziness, nausea, and menstrual irregularity. These tend to improve with continued therapy. Cyproterone acetate is not available in the United States.

Spironolactone is a weak potassium-sparing aldosterone antagonist diuretic with antiandrogenic properties usually reserved for cases resistant to conventional therapy. It has been used as monotherapy in female patients in doses of 100 to 200 mg per day, with excellent results achieved in acne regression at 4 to 6 months,[71,72] although 40% of patients relapse 6 to 12 months after therapy. Spironolactone has been used in male patients without development of gynecomastia and decreased libido at these doses. However, these adverse effects have been seen with spironolactone therapy for other disorders, and therefore spironolactone should be used mainly in female patients. Potassium levels were not altered at this dosage in subjects of one study. However, spironolactone should be reserved for patients with normal renal function. Periodic evaluation of electrolytes should be performed in any patient taking long-term spironolactone therapy. Because spironolactone is an antiandrogen, there is a considerable risk of feminization of the male fetus; therefore, spironolactone is not recommended for women who wish to become pregnant. Concomitant use of OCs with spironolactone is not only beneficial to the treatment of acne but also recommended to prevent unplanned pregnancies.[1]

PHOTODERMATOLOGY AND PHOTODERMATOSES

DEFINITION

"Photodermatology" is the study of photobiology as it relates to the skin. "Photodermatoses" is a general term that encompasses all types of abnormal skin responses to ultraviolet radiation (UVR).

GENERAL OVERVIEW

Exposure to sunlight plays an essential role in the development of many dermatologic diseases. These effects range from acute damage (including sunburn and photosensitive skin disorders) to chronic skin damage (including photoaging and carcinogenesis). These conditions usually occur on sun-exposed skin, which should be a clue to their recognition by the clinician, who can then proceed with an evaluation to determine the exact cause and appropriate treatment.

SOLAR RADIATION

The sun emits a broad spectrum of electromagnetic radiation, but at the earth's surface, the solar spectrum consists of wavelengths between 290 and 3000 nm. These are divided into UVR (290 to 400 nm), visible radiation (400 to 760 nm), and near-infrared radiation (wavelengths greater than 760 nm), as shown in Table 10.3. UVR is the spectrum that most often affects the skin and is divided into three main categories: UVC (200 to 290 nm), UVB (290 to 320 nm), and UVA (320 to 400 nm).[73]

ULTRAVIOLET C

Wavelengths between 200 and 290 nm are called UVC or germicidal radiation, and they are lethal to microorganisms. Mercury vapor lights and xenon lamps are artificial light sources that produce UVC for bacterial sterilization.[73] UVC is attenuated during its passage through the atmosphere, where it is largely absorbed by the ozone layer.

ULTRAVIOLET B

UVB radiation is often called the "sunburn spectrum" and includes wavelengths between 290 and 320 nm. This spectrum reaches the earth's surface, and on the skin it is largely absorbed within the epidermis. UVB is a strong inducer of erythema or sunburn and can also produce delayed pigmentation or tanning. UVB contributes to chronic sun-damaged skin and skin carcinogenesis. A physiologic role of UVB is its importance as a mediator of vitamin D_3 synthesis in the skin. UVB is produced by many artificial light sources for therapeutic purposes and can be blocked by window glass.[74]

ULTRAVIOLET A

Although the amount of UVA (320 to 400 nm) reaching the earth is about 10 times greater than UVB, it is 1000-fold less potent than UVB in producing erythema.[75] In artificially high doses, UVA radiation can produce erythema and immediate pigment darkening of the skin. UVA is emitted by numerous therapeutic appliances used to treat dermatologic diseases and is not blocked by untinted window glass.[76] UVA is now thought to be as major of a contributor as UVB to both the acute and chronic effects of UVR. UVA is not only the solar spectrum that most often evokes photoallergy, phototoxicity, and other photosensitive disorders, but it is

TABLE 10.3	Parts of the Electromagnetic Spectrum	
Radiation		**Wavelength (nm)**
X-rays		10
Ultraviolet	UVC	200–290
	UVB	290–320
	UVA	320–400
Visible	Violet	400–760
	Blue	430–500
	Green	520–565
	Yellow	565–590
	Red	625–740
Infrared	Near	760–1,000,000
	Middle	
	Far	
Microwave, radiowave		>1,000,000

also now thought that UVA may play an equal or even larger role than UVB in the development of chronic skin damage and skin cancer.[77,78]

ACUTE EFFECTS OF ULTRAVIOLET RADIATION

The acute effects of UVR on the skin include sunburn, pigmentation, phototoxicity, and photoallergy.

SUNBURN

EPIDEMIOLOGY

UVB is the major cause of sunburn and is much more erythemogenic than UVA. Factors that may modify the effects of UVR on the skin include time of day, season, latitude, clouds, surface reflection, and altitude. Skin type is also important in determining the effects of UVR on the skin.[79,80]

PATHOPHYSIOLOGY

Damage to DNA and cell membranes, with resulting amplification of inflammatory mediators, is thought to be involved in the skin's response to sun damage. Elevated histamine levels have been detected in blisters, and prostaglandin levels have been elevated in the skin after UVB irradiation.[75] Figure 10.6 illustrates the skin's response to ultraviolet radiation.

CLINICAL PRESENTATION AND DIAGNOSIS

Erythema is the first visible sign of sunburn and may be associated with skin tenderness, pain, swelling, and, in severe cases, blistering, chills, fevers, nausea, and vomiting. Erythema produced by UVB occurs 12 to 24 hours after exposure, whereas UVA-induced erythema is more immediate, within the first 6 hours after exposure.[75]

TREATMENT

Generally, a patient with sunburn must suffer through the course of the sunburn. Clinical evidence has shown that corticosteroids, antihistamines, and nonsteroidal anti-inflammatory drugs (NSAIDs) have little effect on erythema caused by sunburns.[81] Palliative therapy may be helpful and includes wet dressings, soothing zinc lotions, topical anesthetics, and systemic analgesics such as acetaminophen or NSAIDs.

TANNING

There are two components of tanning: a pigment darkening produced by UVA, which occurs immediately after exposure, and delayed pigmentation stimulated by UVB, which occurs 24 to 72 hours after exposure.[82] Immediate pigment darkening results from the darkening of melanin, the pigment produced by melanocytes, already present in skin. Generally, this hyperpigmentation fades within minutes after sun exposure. Delayed pigmentation is a type of neomelanogenesis in which the actual number and size of melanocytes are increased.[82] The increased proliferation of melanocytes is stimulated by UVR-induced DNA damage in the cell nucleus.[83] Increased melanin content is thought to be photoprotective against future sun damage; however, tanned skin is actually a sign that skin injury has already occurred.

PHOTOSENSITIVE DERMATOSES

DEFINITION

Photosensitivity is an abnormal reaction in sun-exposed skin, as seen in Figures 10.7 and 10.8. It may be provoked by a number of substances that come in contact with the skin or substances taken internally (Table 10.4). These are divided into phototoxic, photoallergic, and miscellaneous disorders. Phototoxic and photoallergic reactions involve the presence of a photosensitizer and UVR to the skin. Phototoxic reactions are nonimmunologic and occur 2 to 6 hours after sun exposure, causing a severe sunburn type of reaction including bumps, hives, blisters, and red blotches. Photoallergic reactions occur only in people previously sensitized by a photoallergen and typically occur 24 to 48 hours after sun exposure. Photoallergic reactions produce an eczematoid reaction confined to sun-exposed areas, usually the face, neck, and dorsum of hands (refer to Chapter 9). Cutaneous porphyria falls in the genetic/inherited photodermatoses classification and is thought to result from a reaction between light and the byproduct of abnormal porphyrin metabolism. Another miscellaneous skin disorder, systemic lupus erythematosus (SLE), is a chronic autoimmune disease that can present with skin manifestations exacerbated by exposure to light.

CHRONIC EFFECTS OF ULTRAVIOLET RADIATION

The chronic effects of UVR on the skin include photoaging and cancer.

PATHOPHYSIOLOGY

The gradual deterioration of cutaneous structure and function seen in photoaging results in the loss of skin elasticity

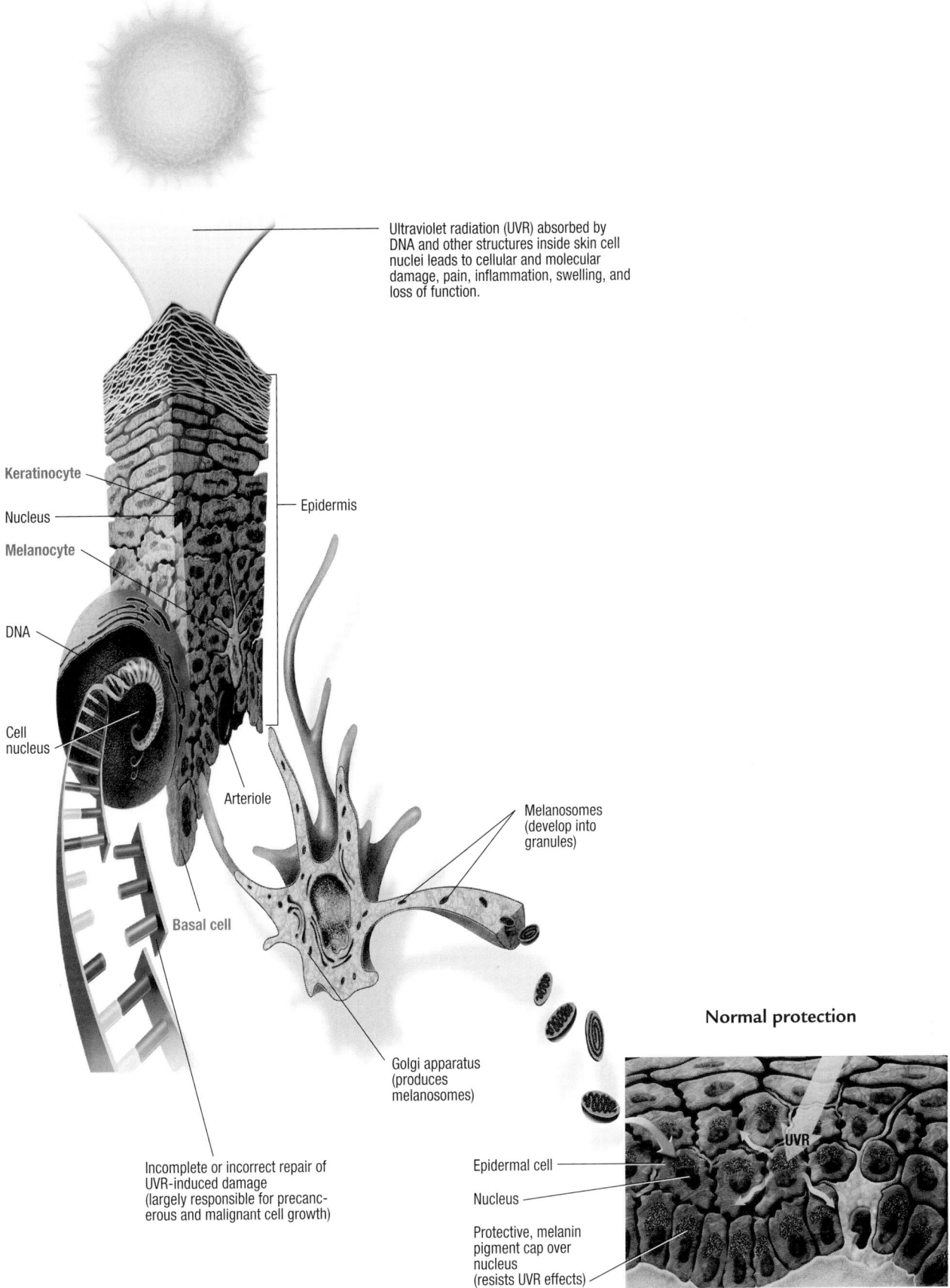

Ultraviolet radiation (UVR) absorbed by DNA and other structures inside skin cell nuclei leads to cellular and molecular damage, pain, inflammation, swelling, and loss of function.

Keratinocyte

Nucleus

Melanocyte

DNA

Cell nucleus

Epidermis

Arteriole

Basal cell

Melanosomes (develop into granules)

Golgi apparatus (produces melanosomes)

Incomplete or incorrect repair of UVR-induced damage (largely responsible for precancerous and malignant cell growth)

Normal protection

Epidermal cell

Nucleus

Protective, melanin pigment cap over nucleus (resists UVR effects)

UVR

FIGURE 10.6 Skin response to ultraviolet radiation (*see color insert*). (Provided by Anatomical Chart Co.)

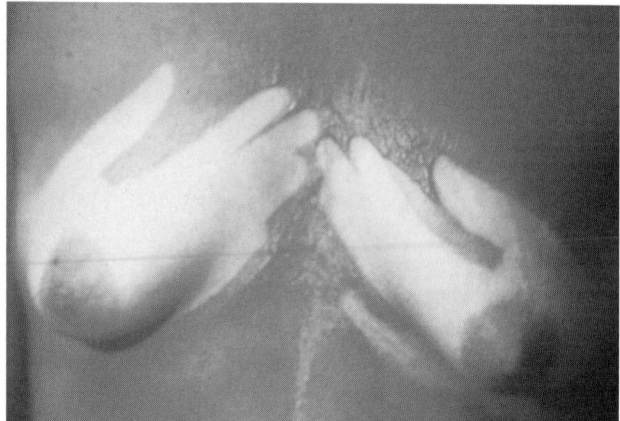

FIGURE 10.7 Drug photosensitivity eruption (*see color insert*). Erythematous (exaggerated sunburn) reaction in a person who was taking demeclocycline (Declomycin) and fell asleep on the beach. (Courtesy of the Albert Einstein College of Medicine, Division of Dermatology, Bronx, NY)

and the formation of coarse wrinkles. Long-term and recurrent UVA and UVB exposure also causes DNA damage, which can lead to the development of DNA mutations and ultimately skin cancer if the mutations are not repaired.[77]

PHOTOAGING

Chronic sun exposure induces prominent changes in the skin. Clinical symptoms include skin that appears deeply wrinkled, rough, inelastic, coarse, and leathery, with associated pigment changes, freckling, telangiectasias (dilation of preexisting blood vessels, creating small, focal, red lesions), easy bruising, and, ultimately, premalignant and malignant skin lesions. Premalignant lesions such as actinic keratoses (solar keratoses) are the most common premalignant, sun-induced lesions usually seen in patients with fair complexions who have had excessive sun exposure.[84] They are small, rough, ill-defined erythematous lesions covered by adherent scales (Fig. 10.9). They are most prominent in sun-exposed areas of the skin, especially the face, neck, and hands. However, the location of actinic keratoses varies according to the location of the sun exposure, and people who sunbathe can develop lesions anywhere. When present on the lips, these lesions are called actinic cheilitis (Fig. 10.10). Individuals with actinic keratoses or actinic cheilitis may have an increased risk of squamous cell carcinoma.[85] Therefore, individuals with significant photoaging should be checked regularly for both actinic keratoses and skin cancers. Risk factors for both photoaging and skin cancer include fair skin, skin that burns easily and tans poorly, severe burns occurring at an early age, and advancing age.[86]

PHOTOCARCINOGENESIS

Skin cancer is the most common of all cancers, accounting for almost half of all cancer cases in the United States. Skin

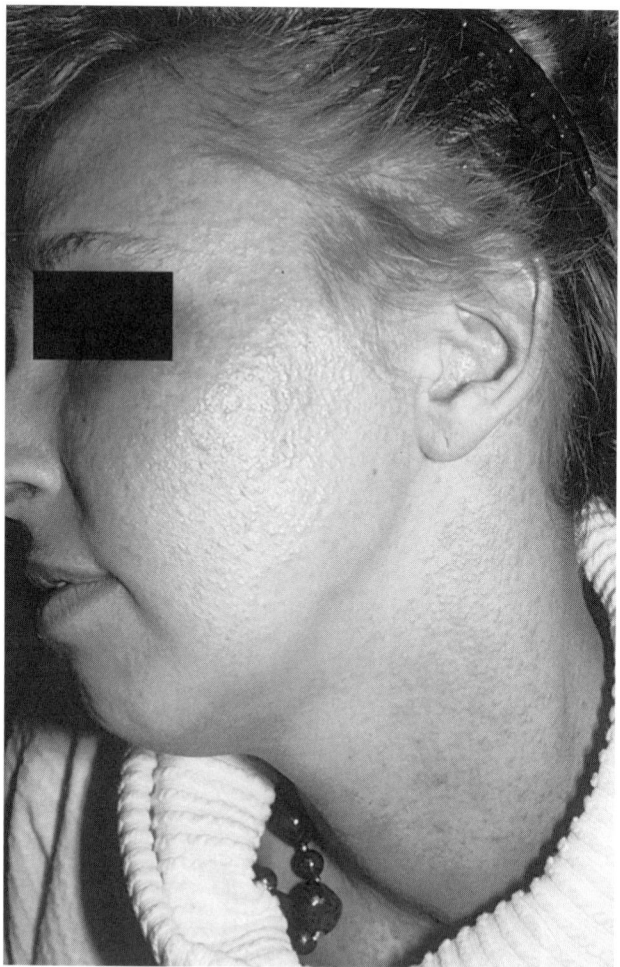

FIGURE 10.8 Photosensitivity versus phototoxic eruption due to Feldene (piroxicam). Two days after this patient began taking piroxicam, a nonsteroidal antiinflammatory drug, she went to the beach and developed an eruption in a photo distribution. Note the sparing under her sun-protected jaw (see color insert). (From Goodheart HP. Goodheart's Photoguide of Common Skin Disorders. 2nd ed. Philadelphia: Lippincott Williams & Wilkins, 2003.)

cancers are classified as either nonmelanoma (basal and squamous cell) or melanoma skin cancer. Most cases of skin cancer are nonmelanoma, but because they grow slowly and rarely spread, they have a high cure rate if detected and treated early. This is not the case for melanoma. Melanoma accounts for a small percentage of all skin cancers but makes up the majority of deaths from skin cancer.[87]

It is well established that UVR present in sunlight is a potent human carcinogen[88] and chronic sun exposure may lead to nonmelanoma skin cancers. Nonmelanoma cancers are found more often in sun-exposed areas and are enhanced by the cumulative exposure to UVR. Squamous cell cancers are most commonly shallow ulcers with a raised border that may present as red, raised, scaling lesions (Fig. 10.11). Basal cell carcinomas are more often nodules on the skin with a pearly, rolled border with prominent telangiectatic vessels on the surface, and they occasionally ulcerate (Fig. 10.12).

TABLE 10.4 | Common Photosensitizers

Oral Photosensitizers		Topical Photosensitizers

Oral Photosensitizers

Antidiabetics (sulfonylureas)
  Chlorpropamide
  Tolbutamide

Antihistamines
  Diphenhydramine
  Terfenadine

Diuretics
  Chlorothiazide
  Furosemide
  Hydrochlorothiazide

Phenothiazines
  Chlorpromazine
  Prochlorperazine
  Promethazine
  Thioridazine
  Trifluoperazine

Laxatives
  Bisacodyl

Sweetener
  Cyclamate

Antifungals
  Griseofulvin
  Voriconazole

Antimicrobials
  Demeclocycline
  Doxycycline
  Lomefloxacin

Antimicrobials *(continued)*
  Nalidixic acid
  Quinolones
  Sulfonamides
  Tetracycline

Furocoumarins (drugs)
  Methoxypsoralen
  Trimethylpsoralen

Antineoplastic
  Dacarbazine
  Vinblastine

Nonsteroidals
  Benoxaprofen
  Ibuprofen
  Ketoprofen
  Naproxen
  Piroxicam

Miscellaneous
  Amantadine
  Amiodarone
  Amlodipine
  Fenofibrate
  Isotretinoin
  Nifedipine
  Quinidine
  Quinine

Topical Photosensitizers

Antiseptics, deodorants, soaps
  Halogenated salicylanilides
  Hexachlorophene

Antifungals
  Buclosamide
  Fenticlor

Sunscreens
  Para-aminobenzoic acid

Fragrances
  Musk ambrette

Coal tar derivatives

Furocoumarins (plants)
  Lime, figs, celery, dill,
  lemon, bergamot, rye,
  anise, mustard, parsnip,
  carrot, cow parsley, fennel,
  masterwort, angelica,
  buttercup

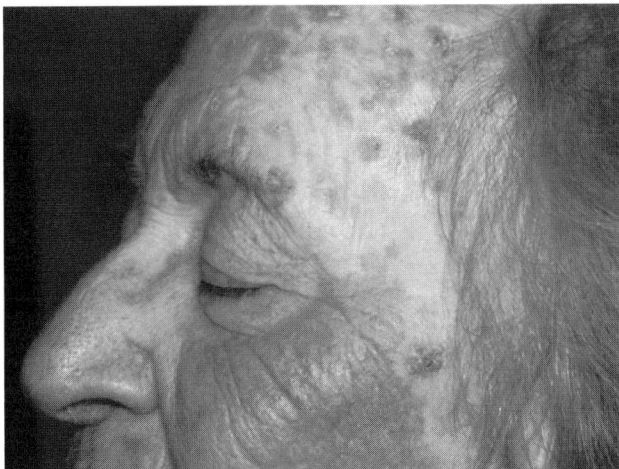

FIGURE 10.9 Actinic keratoses (*see color insert*). This elderly woman has vitiligo. The solar keratoses occur primarily in areas of unprotected, melanocyte-poor, vitiliginous skin. (From Goodheart HP. Goodheart's Photoguide of Common Skin Disorders. 2nd ed. Philadelphia: Lippincott Williams & Wilkins, 2003.)

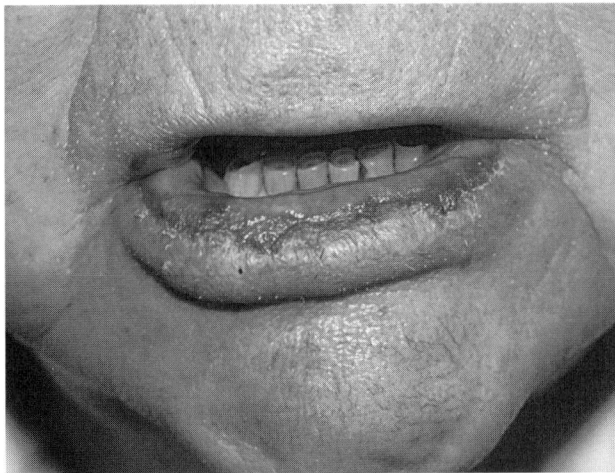

FIGURE 10.10 Actinic cheilitis (*see color insert*). This patient is undergoing treatment with topical 5-FU for multiple solar keratoses of the lower lip. (From Goodheart HP. Goodheart's photoguide of common skin disorders. 2nd ed. Philadelphia: Lippincott Williams & Wilkins, 2003.)

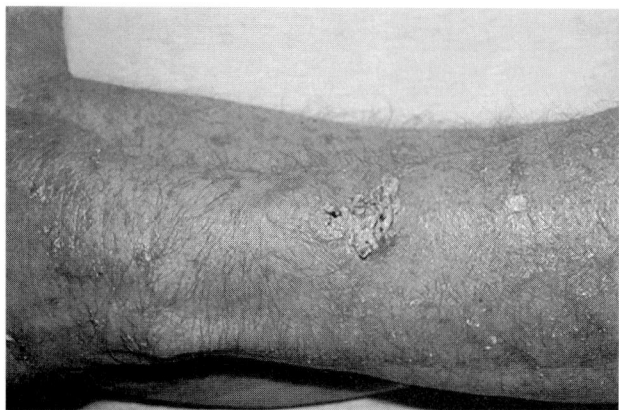

FIGURE 10.11 Nodular squamous cell carcinoma (*see color insert*). The surrounding, smaller lesions are actinic keratoses. (From Goodheart HP. Goodheart's photoguide of common skin disorders. 2nd ed. Philadelphia: Lippincott Williams & Wilkins, 2003.)

Melanoma is a cancer that originates in the melanocytes. It is considered the deadliest type of skin cancer, and the death rate is continuing to escalate.[89] When detected in its early stages and treated properly, melanoma is almost always curable. Therefore, early detection is essential. Malignant melanomas may have different clinical presentations; therefore, a dermatologist should evaluate any mole that appears to have differing shades of brown, black, or blue; irregular borders; asymmetry; or a rapid change in size.[87] These clinical characteristics can be summarized as the ABCDs of melanoma (Fig. 10.13). The risk of malignant melanoma appears to be increased in patients who have intermittent severe sunburn, especially if it occurred during childhood.[90] The individual risk also increases in people who burn easily, tan poorly, and have a large number of moles.[82] Malignant melanoma may have a grave prognosis if not treated adequately

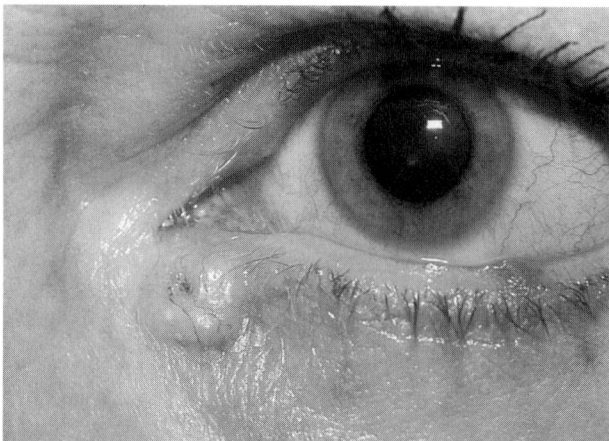

FIGURE 10.12 Basal cell carcinoma (*see color insert*). Well-circumscribed, pearly gray tumor of the epithelium, with raised, rolled edges and central ulceration. An independent vascular pattern is also visible. (From Tasman W, Jaeger E. The Wills Eye hospital atlas of clinical ophthalmology. 2nd ed. Lippincott Williams & Wilkins, 2001.)

and promptly. The best treatment for most skin cancers is surgical excision. Skin cancers can be cured in most cases if removed before they spread to the lymph nodes or distant organs.

THERAPEUTIC PLAN AND PREVENTION

There is strong evidence that sun exposure leads to photoaging and skin cancers. Sun protection should be stressed in the young, in people with fair skin, and in people prone to sun-sensitive disorders. One or more severe, blistering sunburns in childhood or adolescence can double the risk of skin cancer later in life.[91–93] The simplest and cheapest way to avoid sun exposure is to avoid outdoor exposure during hours of intense sunlight (10 AM to 4 PM), especially during the spring and summer, and to wear protective clothing and hats. If avoidance techniques are not feasible, sunscreens that provide maximum protection must be used.[94]

TREATMENT

PHARMACOTHERAPY

Sunscreens. Sunscreens are topical preparations that block the effect of UVR on the skin by absorbing, reflecting, or scattering UVR. They are divided into physical sunscreens (opaque products that reflect and scatter UVR) and chemical sunscreens (transparent products that absorb UVR) as shown in Table 10.5.

Physical Sunscreens. Physical sunscreens have traditionally been opaque and reflect, scatter, and absorb UVR.[78] They contain iron oxide, red petrolatum, titanium dioxide, talc, zinc oxide, ferric chloride, and/or ichthammol. These sunscreens are advantageous because they do not have to be absorbed into the skin and they reflect a broad spectrum of UVR, blocking both UVA and UVB. Because these chemically inert sunscreens are not absorbed, they do not cause allergic contact dermatitis. However, many people find these physical sunscreens to be cosmetically unacceptable, and therefore they are not used as often. Newer micronized formulations have better transparency and are much more cosmetically acceptable. Micronized zinc oxide and titanium oxide can also be found in several broad-spectrum, chemical sunscreens. Regardless of the formulation, physical sunscreens are not easily washed off, and they may melt with prolonged heat, necessitating repeated application.[94]

Chemical Sunscreens. Chemical sunscreens contain agents that absorb UVR. They may contain agents that absorb UVA or UVB. Newer sunscreens called broad-spectrum sunscreens will protect against both UVB and UVA. In general, sunscreens should be applied at least 20 minutes before going out into the sun to allow for adequate penetration into the dermis. It is also extremely important to reapply sun-

Asymmetry   Borders   Color   Diameter

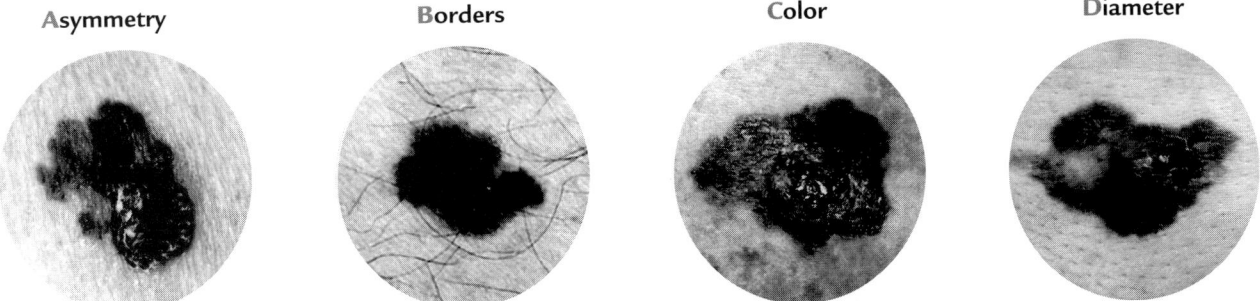

FIGURE 10.13 Skin cancer: the ABCDs of malignant melanoma (*see color insert*). A, asymmetry; B, borders; C, colors; D, diameter. (Provided by Anatomical Chart Co.)

screens frequently, especially if one is swimming or excessively sweating.

Ultraviolet B Absorbers. One of the most widely used chemical agents that absorb UVB used to be para-aminobenzoic acid (PABA) and its esters. PABA penetrates the stratum corneum of the skin, where it attaches to proteins, and thus it is not easily washed off after swimming or bathing. It should be applied at least 1 hour before sun exposure to allow adequate time for PABA binding to the skin. The high incidence of irritation and hypersensitivity reactions, however, caused PABA to fall out of favor. PABA esters have a lower potential for allergic or irritant reactions and staining and therefore are used instead of PABA in many products. Currently, the most commonly used esters are octyl-dimethyl-PABA, also known as padimate O and p-aminobenzoic acid.[95] Cross-reactivity between PABA and sulfonylureas, sulfonamides, thiazides, ''caine'' anesthetics such as lidocaine, and paraphenyldiamine has been described, and patients with sensitivity to these medications should avoid any sunscreens containing PABA or PABA derivatives.[96]

Cinnamates are increasingly being used in the United States for UVB absorption. They have a lower potential for hypersensitivity than the PABA agents and are non-staining. However, they do not bind to the stratum corneum and are easily removed with water. This class of agents includes cinoxate, ethylhexyl p-methoxycinnamate, octocrylene, and octyl methoxycinnamate.

Salicylates are UVB absorbers and have been ingredients in sunscreens since the 1920s. This class of salicylates includes triethanolamine salicylate, octyl salicylate, homosalate, and 2-ethylhexyl salicylate. They are the most common salicylates found in many sunscreens today.

Ultraviolet A Absorbers. The most widely used UVA absorbers are the benzophenone products such as oxybenzone and dioxybenzone. These two agents assist with both UVA and UVB protection, making them broad-spectrum sunscreens. A newer compound, butylmethoxydibenzoylmethane (Avobenzone, Parsol 1789), has been found to be a more effective UVA sunscreen than oxybenzone and has been approved for use in several sunscreens in the United States.[94] Physical sunscreens also protect against UVA, but with new micronized particles there are variations to the spectrum in which they cover. The smaller particles provide more UVB and less UVA protection.[97]

Sun Protection Factor (SPF). The concept of SPF was developed by Greiter of Austria and was adopted by the US Food and Drug Administration (FDA) in 1978.[98] Currently, manufacturers specify the SPF on sunscreen labels. The SPF is a quantitative measure of the product's ability to absorb UVB only. SPF is the ratio of the dose of UVB energy needed to produce minimal erythema on sunscreen-protected skin to the dose of energy needed to produce minimal erythema on skin without sunscreen protection.[99]

SPFs currently range from 2 to more than 50, with SPF 2 equaling a 50% block, SPF 15 a 93% block, and SPF 45 a 98% block. The FDA has proposed label changes to limit SPF values to 30. Sunscreens previously labeled with an SPF greater than 30 would be changed to SPF 30 plus. This

TABLE 10.5	Sunscreen Chemicals Used in the United States	
Chemical		**Physical (UVA and UVB)**
UVA Absorbers		Red petrolatum
Benzophenones (UVA and UVB)		Titanium oxide
Oxybenzone		Magnesium oxide
Dioxybenzone		Zinc oxide
Sulisobenzone		Magnesium salicylates
Avobenzone (Parsol 1789)		Ferric chloride
Anthranilates		
UVB Absorbers		
PABA		
PABA esters		
Padimate-O		
Glyceryl PABA		
Cinnamates		
Salicylates		

proposal is based upon the controversial issue of superpotent sunscreens being not only unnecessary, given the minimal increase in UVB protection above SPF 15, but also misleading.[100] SPFs are determined in a controlled environment with specific artificial lights and consistent, predetermined amounts of sunscreen (2 mg/cm^2), but studies have shown that most consumers still do not apply the correct amount of sunscreen to achieve the full benefit. Most apply only 0.5 to 1 mg per cm^2 of sunscreen before going into the sun, making a sunscreen labeled SPF 15 only a quarter to half its stated strength.[101] To evenly apply 2 mg per cm^2 of sunscreen to an average adult in a swimsuit, approximately 30 mL or 1 fluid ounce would be required, allowing only enough sunscreen for six applications from a regular-size bottle.[101,102] Furthermore, environmental factors such as sweating, swimming, rubbing off, and photodegradation diminish the sustainability of a sunscreen, further diminishing the claimed SPF on the label. Therefore, sunscreen should be applied at least every 2 hours and more often if swimming.

The sustainability of a sunscreen is a measure of its ability to adhere to the skin and remain effective despite swimming, bathing, or sweating. A sunscreen is considered water resistant if it maintains its SPF after two 20-minute immersions in a swimming pool.[103] Until recently, a sunscreen was classified as waterproof if it could withstand four 20-minute immersions.[100] The FDA has asked for a cessation of statements that are misleading, confusing, or absolute, such as waterproof, all-day protection, and sunblock.[100] Currently, there are no standardized guidelines for labeling the effectiveness of products for UVA protection.

Quick-Tanning Lotions. Sunless tanning lotions are becoming more popular to obtain color without sun exposure. These products contain 3% to 5% dihydroxyacetone (DHA) or 0.25% 1,4-dihydroxynaphthoquinone (lawsone). These compounds have no effect on melanocytes, do not stimulate melanin production, and do not provide photoprotection unless combined with a traditional sunscreen.[93] DHA becomes oxidized and polymerized to an orange-brown color that adheres to the skin and gives a tan appearance for 7 to 10 days.

Other Considerations. In older adults, it has been believed that the use of sunscreens is questionable because they block UV-induced vitamin D synthesis in the skin and may cause an older adult to be more prone to vitamin D deficiency and thus bone fractures. However, recent studies have shown this to be false. Sufficient sunlight is received, probably through the sunscreen itself and the lack of total skin coverage at all times, to allow for adequate vitamin D production.[104,105]

Systemic Photoprotective Agents. There is currently no effective, safe systemic photoprotective agent that would circumvent the shortcomings of topical sunscreens. Several agents have shown improvement in specific photosensitive diseases, but they are not as effective as general photoprotectors.

Antimalarials. Aminoquinolines (chloroquine, hydroxychloroquine, quinacrine) are occasionally used to treat several light-sensitive diseases, including systemic lupus erythematosus, polymorphous light eruption, solar urticaria, and porphyria cutanea tarda.

Chloroquine has been shown to have many diverse effects, including enzyme inhibition; protein, DNA, and melanin binding; and antihistaminic and anti-inflammatory effects. It is also an effective absorber of UVR. However, the exact mechanisms of action in photosensitive disorders are not known.[106] The toxicities of antimalarials are multiple, and they are not considered the first choice for treating photosensitive disorders. They should be used with close supervision and only after other therapies have failed.

Ocular toxicity is the greatest limitation of the aminoquinolines. They can cause an irreversible, dose-related retinopathy. To minimize the risk of ocular toxicity, the dose of chloroquine should not exceed 250 mg per day or hydroxychloroquine 400 mg per day (in a patient weighing more than 100 lb). An ophthalmologic examination should be performed before therapy and every 4 to 6 months during therapy. If any changes in vision occur, such as blurred vision or flashes of light, the drug should be stopped until an ophthalmologist can examine the patient.

Other reported side effects include headache, irritability, toxic psychosis, worsening of psoriasis, and leukopenia. They can cause a blue-black pigmentation of the skin, and quinacrine can give a yellow discoloration to the skin. Antimalarials are teratogenic and should be avoided during pregnancy.[107]

Carotenoids. Carotenoids can exert a photoprotective effect in humans and chlorophyll-containing organisms. β-Carotene has been found to absorb light in the visible spectrum (360 to 500 nm). However, some think its photoprotective effect results from its ability to quench single oxygen-derived photochemical reactions.[106] β-Carotene has been effective in treating erythropoietic protoporphyria, a rare hereditary photosensitivity disease caused by a defect in porphyrin metabolism. However, its usefulness in other photosensitivity diseases has been marginal. Oral ingestion should be regulated to keep a blood level between 600 and 800 mg per mL, which usually corresponds to an adult dosage of 150 mg.[106] The main side effect of β-carotene is a slight orange discoloration of the skin, most notable on the palms and soles. Results are not expected until 1 or 2 months of therapy.

Treatment of Photodamaged Skin. Although sunscreens and sun avoidance are important to prevent photodamage, once chronic photodamage has occurred, treatment that may obviate future surgical intervention may be needed. Several products have been used to treat photodamaged skin.

Topical Tretinoin. Two topical retinoids, tretinoin and tazarotene, are FDA approved for the palliation of fine wrinkles and irregular pigmentation of photoaging. Suspicion that topical tretinoin may reverse the seemingly irreversible (i.e., fine wrinkling, coarse wrinkling and hyperpigmented lesions) arose from clinical observations.[108] Clinical improvement is typically seen during the first 4 to 10 months of treatment. In photoaged skin, topical retinoids are thought to increase levels of collagen, the major structural protein of the skin. They may not only treat photoaging after it has occurred but also may retard or prevent photoaging before it occurs, although continued use seems to be necessary to maintain beneficial results. Experience with topical retinoids is limited and their long-term effects are unknown. The safety or efficacy of using topical retinoids for more than 52 weeks has not been established and therefore they should be used with caution. Whether their effects will persist past treatment is unknown. They should be used only in motivated patients who are committed to future sun protection and sun avoidance.

To treat photodamaged skin or precancerous lesions, topical retinoids usually are initiated at a low strength (0.02% or 0.05% cream) applied at bedtime to the entire face, including eyelids if desirable. The most significant side effect is irritation, which is readily treated by withholding treatment for 1 to 2 days and decreasing the dosage or changing to alternate-day therapy. A 30% increase in UVB penetration is noted when retinoids are used, requiring the patient to use sunscreen daily.[2] This treatment should be avoided during pregnancy because it is considered nonessential.

α-Hydroxyacids.
α-Hydroxyacids and α-keto acids, including glycolic, pyruvic, and lactic acids, are thought to be powerful keratolytic agents and have been used to treat photoaging with some success.[109] These agents may even increase the biosynthesis of collagen fibers, reversing the signs of aging skin.[109] Patients from two double-blind RCTs using a combination of 8% glycolic acid and L-lactic acid in one study and 5% glycolic acid daily in the other study reported a greater improvement in roughness, mottled pigmentation, and sallowness of their skin, although there was little success in the treatment of actinic keratoses and coarse wrinkles.[110,111] Twenty percent more UVB radiation is absorbed by skin treated with hydroxyacids than untreated skin.[112] Therefore, to maintain the benefits of these agents, they should be used with sunscreen daily. In addition, there are many different strengths and combinations of these acids on the market, producing varying degrees of effect on the skin. Low concentrations of α-hydroxyacids (less than 12%) are usually found in over-the-counter moisturizers and exfoliants, and high concentrations are used in chemical peels.

Newer generations of α-hydroxyacids called polyhydroxyacids have also been used to treat photoaged skin. Gluconolactone and lactobionic acid, types of polyhydroxyacids, have multiple hydroxyl groups that are considered moisturizing antioxidants and ultimately result in less sensitivity reactions than traditional α-hydroxyacids.[113] Because of their improved tolerability profile, polyhydroxyacids may now be used in combination with other types of antiaging products, which may result in improved outcomes.[114]

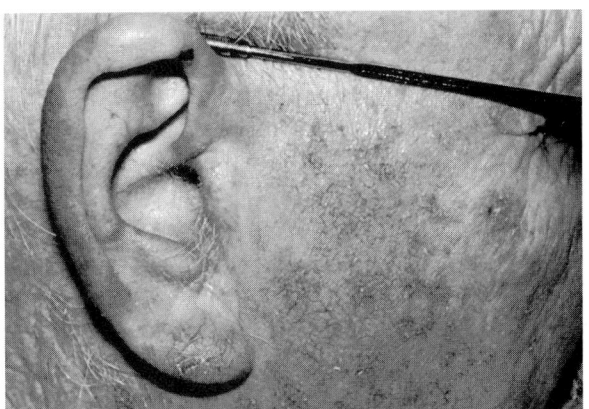

FIGURE 10.14 Actinic keratoses (*see color insert*). Before treatment, few lesions are clinically visible. (From Goodheart HP. Goodheart's photoguide of common skin disorders. 2nd ed. Philadelphia: Lippincott Williams & Wilkins, 2003.)

Topical Fluorouracil.
Topical 5-fluorouracil (5-FU) is an anticancer agent that has been used to treat many precancerous lesions and dermatoses. It is most often used to treat severe actinic keratoses but can also be used for superficial basal cell carcinomas at the highest strength. 5-FU is a structural analogue of uracil and blocks DNA synthesis. Cells that are rapidly growing, such as actinic keratoses, need more DNA and thus accumulate larger amounts of lethal 5-FU, resulting in their death. Normal skin is much less affected by 5-FU.[115]

5-FU is available as a 0.5%, 1%, or 5% cream and a 1%, 2%, or 5% solution. It is usually applied twice daily for 2 to 4 weeks, depending on the response. The response includes an inflammatory phase, followed by redness, burning, and oozing, followed by erosion or ulceration that occurs over 1 to 3 weeks, depending on the site and strength used (Figs.10.14 and 10.15). Treatment is stopped when ulcera-

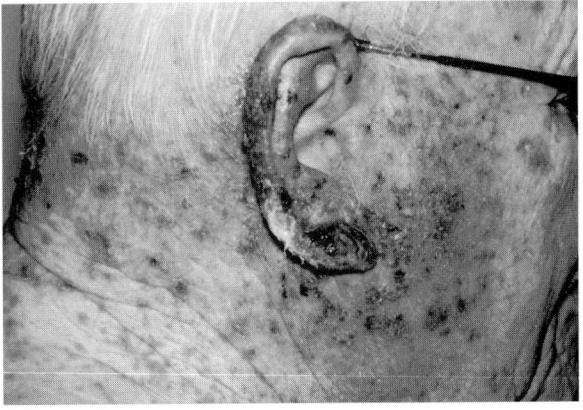

FIGURE 10.15 Actinic keratoses (*see color insert*). Two weeks after treatment with topical 5-FU, crusting and erythema are evident in areas that had lesions that were not initially apparent. (From Goodheart HP. Goodheart's photoguide of common skin disorders. 2nd ed. Philadelphia: Lippincott Williams & Wilkins, 2003.)

tion and crusting appear. The patient must be well informed of this expected response to avoid unnecessary or excessive worrying. Oozing and erosion are expected, and the patient should be given information pamphlets with pictures, which are provided by pharmaceutical companies. If 5-FU is applied with the fingers, the hands should be washed immediately afterward, or gloves can be used during application. 5-FU should not be applied too close to the eyes.

Topical 5-FU is a very effective treatment for actinic keratoses, reducing keratotic lesions by 70%. It has also been shown to give good cosmetic results and may eliminate the need for surgery. Side effects include an irritant dermatitis, which is difficult to distinguish from the desired effect of 5-FU. If severe, the treatment may have to be interrupted and lubricants or topical steroids used.

The most common local reactions are pain, pruritus, hyperpigmentation, and burning at the site of application. Rare side effects include photosensitivity, concealment of a cancer, nail changes, telangiectasias, and scarring.[115] Actinic keratoses that do not respond to treatment should be biopsied. Fluorouracil may cause fetal harm when administered to pregnant women and therefore should not be used during pregnancy.

Overall, when used with discretion and with consistent follow-up examinations, 5-FU is an effective and economical treatment for actinic keratoses and provides good cosmetic results.

Topical Diclofenac. Topical diclofenac sodium 3% gel is an NSAID approved by the FDA for the treatment of actinic keratoses.[116] The mechanism of action is related to diclofenac's ability to inhibit both cyclooxygenase and the upregulation of the arachidonic acid cascade. Inhibition of prostaglandin synthesis plays a role in preventing tumor progression in UVR-induced lesions.[117] Topical diclofenac was evaluated in a randomized, double-blind vehicle-controlled trial and was found to be an effective agent against actinic keratoses. In this study, diclofenac was applied twice daily for 90 days and resulted in complete disease clearance in 47% of the participants in the active treatment arm compared to 19% of participants treated with vehicle. Diclofenac was well tolerated, with pruritus, rash, and application-site reactions being the most common adverse reactions.[118]

Imiquimod. Imiquimod is an imidozoquinoline amine used for the treatment of external genital and perianal warts, actinic keratoses, and superficial basal cell carcinoma.[119] It is an immunomodulator that augments both innate and acquired cellular immunity through an increased production of the proinflammatory cytokines: interferon-alpha, interleukin-6, interleukin-8, and tumor necrosis factor alpha (TNF-α).[120] Although the exact mechanism of action is not fully understood, imiquimod has demonstrated significant efficacy over placebo in treating both actinic keratoses and superficial basal cell carcinoma. Imiquimod 5% cream is effective for the treatment of actinic keratoses. Imiquimod 5% cream applied twice a week for 16 weeks resulted in a 45% complete clearance rate.[121] Local skin reactions including erythema, itching, burning, and bleeding were the most common reported skin reactions.[121]

Masoprocol. Topical masoprocol cream comes in a 10% formulation that has antiproliferative activity against keratinocytes and is reported to be effective in treating actinic keratoses of the head and neck. It should be applied twice a day to the area of solar damage for 28 days. There is a high incidence (10%) of allergic contact dermatitis to this product.[122]

WARTS

DEFINITION

Warts, also known as verrucae, are caused by human papillomaviruses (HPVs). They are commonly classified by clinical appearance, histology, and location. The main classifications include common warts (verruca vulgaris), plantar warts (verruca plantaris), flat warts (verruca plana), and anogenital warts.[123] Nongenital warts in immunocompetent patients are generally harmless and resolve spontaneously within months to years. A policy of not treating these types of warts is often advised because of the probability of spontaneous remission and the absence of universally effective treatments. On the other hand, many patients seek and receive treatment for cosmetic and psychosocial discomfort.

EPIDEMIOLOGY

Cutaneous warts are most common in children and young adults. The main source of cutaneous HPV infection is through direct contact with affected individuals and via fomites. The peak incidence of warts occurs between the ages of 12 to 16, with the incidence estimated to be approximately 10%.[124,125] Spontaneous clearance was reported in 23% of patients at 2 months and 65 to 78% at 2 years.[126] The actual prevalence of warts in the general population is unknown, but both exposure and subclinical or latent infection are presumed to be common. The prevalence of warts in immunocompromised patients relates to the duration and intensity of immunosuppression.[127] The prevalence of warts in a small cohort of transplant patients was determined to be 16% at the time of transplant and increased to 54% at 7 years after the transplant.[128] Hand warts are also found in a high percentage of butchers and meat handlers, and plantar warts are frequently contracted in public baths and swimming pools.[129]

Anogenital warts are the most common sexually transmitted viral infection in the United States. The annual incidence of these warts is 10% to 20% in young adults, with the age of onset ranging from late teens to early 30s.[130] The lifetime risk for infection in sexually active young adults is estimated to be as high as 80%, and the transmission rate following a single sexual exposure is approximately 25%.[123,131] Most infections are asymptomatic, and the incubation period is variable and usually ranges from 1 to 6 months. Barrier contraceptive methods do not completely prevent the transmission of anogenital warts.[132]

PATHOPHYSIOLOGY

Warts are caused by various types of HPVs. The papillomaviruses belong to the Papillomaviridae family and are characterized by circular, double-stranded, supercoiled DNA approximately 8 kilobases in length. The virus particles are enclosed in an icosahedral capsid of 72 capsomers and are approximately 55 nm in diameter. The absence of a viral envelope confers resistance to drying, freezing, and solvents.[123] To date, nearly 100 different HPV types have been isolated with the use of DNA hybridization and polymerase chain reaction technology. The papillomaviruses are classified based upon DNA sequence homology. A variation by more than 10% in the L1 ORF gene distinguishes one type from another.[133]

HPV have a specific tropism for keratinocytes, and each HPV type tends to be associated with different clinical variants.[134] Table 10.6 lists the different HPV types correlated with common clinical lesions.[135,136] The potential for oncogenic transformation is associated with the high-risk subtypes, including HPV types 16, 18, 31, 33, 35, 45, and 56. HPV types 6 and 11 are found in 90% of anogenital warts, whereas HPV type 2 is most commonly associated with common warts.[131]

CLINICAL PRESENTATION

COMMON WART (VERRUCA VULGARIS)
Approximately 70% of warts are of the verruca vulgaris type. Initially the wart appears as a smooth, firm, circumscribed, flesh-colored papule. Common warts can develop into a grayish-brown, dome-shaped papule with an irregular scaly surface (Fig. 10.16). Although common warts can occur individually or grouped on any skin surface; they are usually located on the dorsal surface of the hands, particularly on the fingers and periungual region around the nail, and on the palms. Warts can also form at sites of trauma, a property known as the Koebner phenomenon. Although they are generally asymptomatic, periungual warts may become fissured, inflamed, and tender. Occasionally, warts consist of thread-

TABLE 10.6	HPV Types and Their Clinical Associations		
HPV Types	**Most Common Clinical Lesions**	**Less Common Lesions**	**Oncogenic Potential**
1, 2	Deep palmoplantar warts	Common warts	
2, 4, 7	Common warts	Superficial, mosaic-type palmoplantar warts, anogenital warts	
3, 10, 28, 41	Flat warts		
7	Common warts in butchers		
3, 5, 8–10, 12, 14, 15, 17, 19–29, 36–38, 47, 49	Epidermodysplasia verruciformis		Yes
6, 11, 42–44	Anogenital warts, cervical condyloma (acuminata)	Common warts	Low
16, 18, 31, 33, 35, 39, 42–45, 51, 52, 56, 58, 59, 66–68	Cervical condyloma (acuminata)	Anogenital warts	High

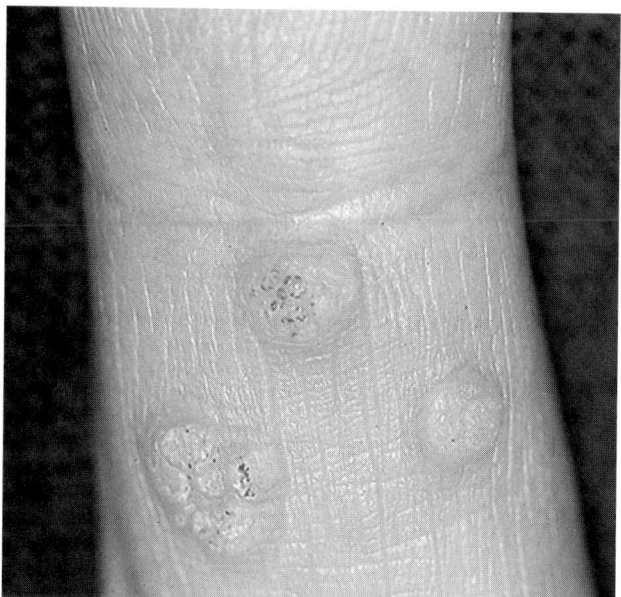

FIGURE 10.16 Common wart (verruca vulgaris) (*see color insert*). (From Goodheart HP. Goodheart's photoguide of common skin disorders. 2nd ed. Philadelphia: Lippincott Williams & Wilkins, 2003.)

like, thin, horny projections. This variant, called verruca filiformis, or filiform wart, occurs commonly on the face and scalp.[131,137]

PLANTAR WART (VERRUCA PLANTARIS)

Plantar warts occur most commonly on the palms and especially on pressure points on the soles of the feet. The surface of plantar warts is covered by a horny plate and surrounded by a horny ring. They are deep, grow endophytically, and are often painful (Fig. 10.17). Approximately one third of

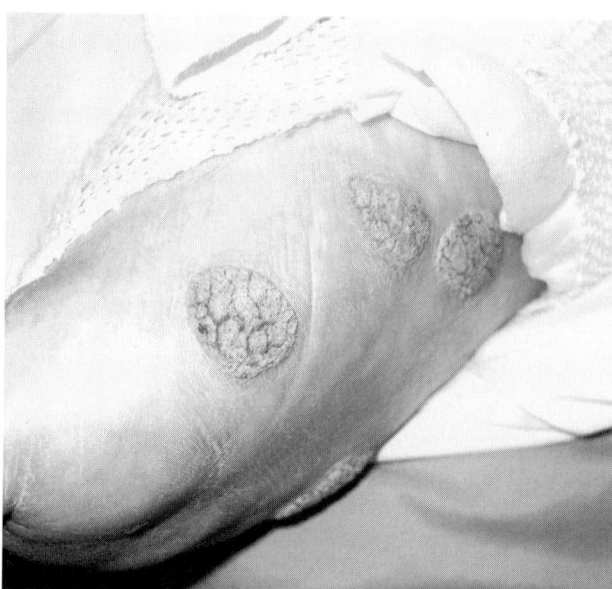

FIGURE 10.17 Plantar wart (verruca plantaris) (*see color insert*). (Image provided by Stedman's.)

patients with warts have the plantar type. Plantar warts can be difficult to distinguish from corns and calluses. Shaving off the keratotic surface aids in differentiating the two entities; warts have a soft central core with brown dots that are the result of thrombosed capillaries, whereas corns have a horny central core. Plantar warts are usually associated with inflammation and patients experience swelling, redness, pain, and considerable tenderness. Mosaic warts are multiple contiguous plantar warts that have coalesced to form one large plaque. The myrmecia type are deep, smooth-surfaced, dome-shaped papules that resemble anthills. This type of plantar wart is not usually painful but is more resistant to therapy.

FLAT WART (VERRUCA PLANA)

Flat warts are smooth, slightly elevated, flat-topped papules that usually range from 2 to 4 mm in diameter (Fig. 10.18). They may be flesh-colored, gray, or brown, and on darker skin they can be hyperpigmented. Numerous flat warts cluster on the face, neck, hands, and legs of children. The Koebner phenomenon is more common with this type of wart. Occasionally, men who shave their beards and women who shave their legs spread the condition to adjacent areas. Flat warts have the highest rate of spontaneous remission.[123]

ANOGENITAL WARTS (CONDYLOMATA ACUMINATA)

Anogenital warts, also known as venereal warts, can be acquired through sexual transmission and less frequently through vertical transmission from mother to newborn. Most infections are asymptomatic, subclinical, or unrecognized. Visible anogenital warts can occur with HPV types 6 or 11. High-risk HPV types 16 and 18 are strongly associated with cervical dysplasia. The vulva, vagina, penis, urethra, and

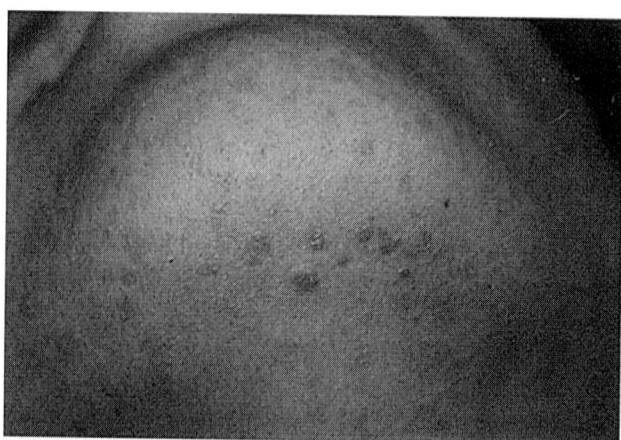

FIGURE 10.18 Flat warts (verruca plana) (*see color insert*). (From Goodheart H. A photoguide of common skin disorders. Baltimore: Williams & Wilkins, 1999.)

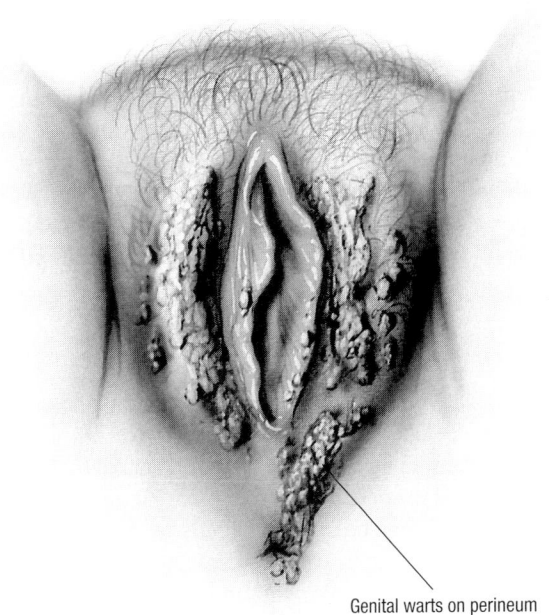

Genital warts on perineum

FIGURE 10.19 Vaginal warts (*see color insert*). (Provided by Anatomical Chart Co.)

perianal regions can also be affected (Fig. 10.19). Generally, anogenital wart infection appears to be transient and results in no sequelae. However, in a small subset of patients, the infection persists and can progress to cancer. Condylomata acuminata is a clinical variant that is associated with infection with the ''benign'' HPV types 6 and 11 (Fig. 10.20). Lesions consist of soft, lobulated, flesh-colored papules that can coalesce as cauliflower-like masses. Bowenoid papulosis is another clinical variant that is associated with the more ''malignant'' HPV type 16 infection. Lesions are typically flat, hyperpigmented papules that can progress to invasive squamous cell carcinoma.[123,131]

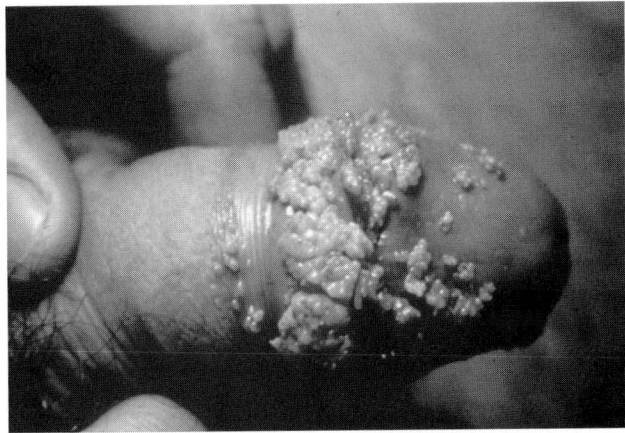

FIGURE 10.20 Condylomata acuminata (*see color insert*). (From Goodheart HP. Goodheart's photoguide of common skin disorders. 2nd ed. Philadelphia: Lippincott Williams & Wilkins, 2003.)

OTHER VARIANTS

Epidermodysplasia Verruciformis. Epidermodysplasia verruciformis is a rare, lifelong, HPV infection characterized by widespread flat warts with a tendency to coalesce into plaques and tinea versicolor-like lesions. Infection with these HPV types is considered harmless to the general population. However, infection in individuals with a genetic predisposition or compromised cell-mediated immunity can lead to the development of this condition. Although no specific gene has been found that predisposes patients to epidermodysplasia verruciformis, 90% of patients with the disorder have depressed cell-mediated immunity.[138] Defects in T-cell-mediated immunity may be related to disease susceptibility because of a decreased ability to eliminate HPV-infected cells. Epidermodysplasia verruciformis follows an autosomal recessive inheritance pattern, and parental consanguinity is approximately 10%.[131] The disorder begins in early childhood. Patients with this condition are predisposed to the development of squamous cell cancers, and approximately one third develop skin cancers in sun-exposed lesions approximately 20 to 30 years after the onset of the benign cutaneous lesions.[124,131]

THERAPEUTIC PLAN

The approach to treating warts depends on the patient's age, cooperation, immunologic status, and previous treatments. The location, number, size, duration, and type of lesions are also factors to consider. Although cutaneous warts commonly resolve spontaneously, the general indications for treatment include a patient's desire for treatment, painful, disfiguring warts, and a large number or size of warts. With genital warts, itching, burning, dyspareunia, and cervical dysplasia are indications for treatment. Warts rarely pose a serious health problem, but physical impairment and psychosocial discomfort often warrant clinical intervention. Although there are no data indicating that reinfection from untreated partners plays a role in recurrence, partners may benefit from routine examination to determine the presence of lesions and to get counseling on their own transmission potential.[139]

Therapeutic options can be divided into broad categories including chemical destructive therapy, physical destructive therapy, chemotherapeutic agents, immunotherapy, and new potential agents (Table 10.7). Topical salicylic acid and lactic acid paints are the usual first-line treatment for cutaneous warts. In general, most forms of wart treatment can be expected to have a 60% to 70% cure rate. Patients should be informed about the potential need for several treatments, often over a period of several weeks to months. In rare instances, a biopsy should be obtained to help distinguish benign warts from other verrucous-appearing lesions, such as squamous cell carcinoma, deep fungal infections, and verrucous carcinoma.[125,140]

TABLE 10.7	Treatment Modalities for Warts

Chemical Destruction	**Immunotherapy**
Acids	Imiquimod
Formaldehyde	Interferons
Glutaraldehyde	Contact sensitizers
Cantharidin	**Other Therapies**
Physical Destruction	Retinoids
Cryotherapy	Cidofovir
Electrosurgery	**Future Therapies**
Surgical excision	Vaccines
Carbon dioxide laser	
Chemotherapeutic Agents	
Podophyllotoxin	
Bleomycin	

TREATMENT

CHEMICAL DESTRUCTIVE THERAPY

Acids. Salicylic acid is a keratolytic agent available in concentrations ranging from 10% to 60% and can be used topically in paints, pastes, gels, or plasters. It is often used for common and palmoplantar warts, including periungual warts. Salicylic acid demonstrated treatment efficacy in 75% of patients compared to 48% of patients receiving placebo.[140] In 1991, the FDA issued a monograph mandating that all salicylic acid-based wart therapy products be changed to nonprescription status with a maximum concentration of 17% salicylic acid.[141] Preparations can be used on all skin sites except the face and anogenital areas. Other acids are also used in the treatment of various types of warts. Monochloroacetic acid crystals compounded with 60% salicylic acid are effective for plantar warts.[142] Weekly applications of 80% to 90% trichloroacetic acid, and less commonly, bichloroacetic acid are effective treatments for anogenital warts. These acids are applied in the physician's office, and although they do not need to be washed off, sodium bicarbonate or baking soda can be used to neutralize irritation and damage to adjacent tissue.[143] Trichloroacetic acid may be compounded with salicylic acid for treating common and palmoplantar warts. Lactic acid is no longer available as an active ingredient in over-the-counter products. However, pharmacists do compound these acids in higher concentrations as necessary for prescription use.

In general, acids act as keratolytic agents by physically destroying the keratin layer. Paints are most commonly used and are usually a collodion-based liquid. Treatment begins with soaking the wart in warm water for approximately 5 minutes, and then the wart is pared down as far as possible without causing bleeding. A pumice stone can be used if necessary. The acid solution is applied just to cover the wart and allowed to dry to a white film. The wart is then kept covered for 24 hours, and the procedure is repeated daily until the wart is gone. Salicylic acid plasters are especially suited for treating multiple mosaic plantar warts. A 40% salicylic acid adhesive plaster is a commonly used preparation. After the lesion is pared and moistened with warm water, the plaster is cut to the size of the wart and applied for 24 to 48 hours. Application should be repeated until the wart is gone.

Formaldehyde. Formaldehyde or formalin is a powerful disinfectant with desiccant properties. Following application, formaldehyde hardens the skin and disrupts the growth of epidermal cells.[144] It is especially effective in the treatment of plantar and mosaic warts. A 4% formaldehyde solution can be used to soak the pared wart for 30 minutes daily, or a 10% solution can be applied directly to the skin.[137] The surrounding normal skin can be protected with petroleum jelly. Cure rates for plantar warts in children are estimated to approach 80%. Potential complications of formaldehyde treatment include the development of allergic contact dermatitis, dryness, fissuring, and transient discoloration.

Glutaraldehyde. Glutaraldehyde is also a disinfectant that hardens the skin through the formation of polymers with keratin.[144] Topical application of 10% glutaraldehyde may be less irritating compared to formaldehyde preparations. A 20% aqueous solution of unbuffered glutaraldehyde was found to be effective in patients with resistant warts.[145] Daily application of glutaraldehyde over 12 weeks resulted in treatment efficacy in 72% of patients. Transient pigmentary changes were noted after application, but no evidence of scarring or permanent pigmentary change was noted.

Cantharidin. Cantharidin is an extract of the green blister beetle that destroys the epidermis by poisoning mitochondria and hindering oxidative metabolism. A solution containing 0.7% cantharidin in acetone or flexible collodion can be effective in treating common and plantar warts. The vehicle is applied to the pared wart and allowed to dry; the wart is then covered with adhesive tape for 24 hours. The process can be repeated weekly during physician office visits. It is not unusual for warts to recur in a doughnut-shaped ring around the original treated wart. Common side effects include postinflammatory hyperpigmentation and blistering.[137]

PHYSICAL DESTRUCTIVE THERAPY

Cryotherapy. Cryotherapy is an effective second-line treatment option for many types of common, palmoplantar, and genital warts.[123] Cryotherapy causes cell injury through intracellular ice formation, which leads to irreversible damage to the cell membrane and organelles.[146] Liquid nitrogen is the most commonly used vehicle, but solid carbon dioxide may also be effective. Before treatment, the wart is pared down, and a cotton-tipped applicator is used to apply liquid nitrogen to the wart, creating a white "ice ball" extending 1 to 2 mm beyond the visible wart. This process usually takes about 20 to 30 seconds. The lesion is allowed to thaw, and then the procedure is repeated several times, depending on the size and site of the wart. The lesion eventually dries and peels off with the wart. This regimen may involve multiple treatments at 1- to 3-week intervals over several months. Side effects mainly include pain, blistering, and the potential for hypopigmentation or hyperpigmentation.[137]

Several trials comparing the efficacy of cryotherapy with topical salicylic acid in the treatment of cutaneous warts found no difference between the treatments.[140] Cryotherapy offers patients a safe, inexpensive, and effective alternative to treatment with topical therapies. Although cure rates are slightly less than those reported with electrosurgery, cryotherapy is usually preferred because local anesthesia is not required and the potential for scarring is decreased. In the treatment of genital warts, cryotherapy is more effective than podophyllin and is safe to use during pregnancy.[123]

Electrosurgery. Electrosurgery is fairly common and involves the use of low-current electrodesiccation followed by gentle curettage of the wart to minimize scarring. Although the cure rates are slightly higher compared to cryotherapy, the disadvantages include the need for local anesthesia, pain, and greater risk of scarring and infection.[147] Electrosurgery should be used only on small warts.

Surgical Excision. Simple surgical excision of anogenital warts has been reported to be more effective than podophyllin application.[148] However, recurrence rates were reported to range from 20% to 30%.[146]

Carbon Dioxide Laser. Carbon dioxide lasers are distinguished by a favorable safety margin and precision in the ablation of cutaneous warts. Cure rates with the carbon dioxide laser may be as high as 90%, but the disadvantages include the high cost of the procedure, the possible need for general anesthesia, and the release of HPV in the laser smoke.[149] Carbon dioxide lasers are generally reserved for treating multiple, large, treatment-resistant anogenital, urethral, or vaginal condylomata.

CHEMOTHERAPY

Podophyllin. Podophyllin resin has been used to treat genital warts for many years. It is a nonhomogeneous, unstable extract obtained from the plants *Podophyllum peltatum* (found in North America) and *Podophyllum emodi* (found in India, Tibet, and Afghanistan). The resin has four active agents, or lignins: podophyllotoxin, 4-dimethylpodophyllotoxin, α-peltatin, and β-peltatin. The active lignin content of *P. emodi* is about 40% and consists primarily of podophyllotoxin and trace amounts of 4-dimethylpodophyllotoxin. *P. peltatum* has a lignin content of approximately 20% and consists of varying quantities of podophyllotoxin, α-peltatin, and β-peltatin. The primary active ingredient, podophyllotoxin, is cytotoxic and arrests cellular mitoses in metaphase by interfering with microtubule formation.[150] Podophyllin is compounded as a 10% to 25% solution in tincture of benzoin.

Podophyllin should be administered by physicians only and should not be dispensed directly to patients. It is applied sparingly to lesions weekly and then allowed to air dry. Contact with healthy tissue is avoided because podophyllin is caustic and very irritating. The resin is washed off with soap and water 4 hours after application. Because of a high percutaneous absorption and the potential for systemic toxicity, no more than 0.4 to 0.9 mL of the resin should be applied per week and the treatment area should not exceed 3 cm in diameter.[151,152] The typical treatment course ranges from 4 to 6 weeks and clearance rates range from 30% to 60%.[153]

Local irritation including erythema, burning, edema, pain, and ulceration are common side effects and occur in approximately 15% of patients.[150] Severe chemical burns, necrosis, scarring, and fistula formation have been reported with the improper use of podophyllin. Systemic toxicity has also been reported and is usually associated with the use of large volumes over extensive areas of the skin, or contact for extended periods of time. Systemic podophyllin toxicity affects multiple organ systems, but neurologic toxicity is the hallmark feature and may include mental status changes, peripheral neuropathy, seizures, psychosis, and coma. Other clinical symptoms include fever, nausea, vomiting, tachycardia, renal failure, ileus, bone marrow suppression, and death.[154] Podophyllin is contraindicated in pregnancy because of teratogenic effects. Furthermore, intrauterine deaths have been reported following topical application.[150] Podophyllin also contains two potential carcinogens, quercetin and kaempherol. Many clinicians avoid using podophyllin because of the significant toxicities, moderate efficacy, and availability of reliable alternatives.[152]

Podophyllotoxin (Podofilox). Podophyllotoxin is the purified and biologically active agent of podophyllin. It is indicated for the topical treatment of external genital warts and perianal warts, but it is not indicated for treatment of mucous membrane warts. The treatment area should be limited to 10 cm² or less and no more than 0.5 g of gel should be used per day. Standardized concentrations are commercially available in a 0.5% gel and solution.[155,156]

The efficacy of podophyllotoxin in the treatment of genital warts was reported in several clinical studies. A placebo-controlled trial compared twice-daily application of 0.5% podophyllotoxin gel for 3 days followed by a 4-day drug-free interval to vehicle in patients with anogenital warts.[157] After 8 weeks, the cure rate was 64% of warts in treated patients compared to 12% in the placebo group. Complete clearing occurred in 37% of patients in the treatment group compared to 2.3% of patients in the control group, and only 3% of patients discontinued therapy because of drug-related reactions. Studies in which the same preparation was applied twice daily for 4 and 5 days found no significant improvement in efficacy, but there was an increase in local irritation.[158] Patient application of a 0.5% podophyllotoxin preparation to penile warts for 3 consecutive days followed by a 4-day drug-free period was compared to a 20% podophyllin preparation applied by a physician. Patients who self-administered podophyllotoxin had an 88% cure rate compared to 63% who received podophyllin by a physician.[159] No systemic reactions were reported, and the incidence of local irritation was considerably less than commonly reported with podophyllin.

Podophyllotoxin is an attractive alternative to podophyllin resin because it is available in standardized formulations, is devoid of carcinogenic contaminants, has a lower potential for systemic toxicity, and has demonstrated increased treatment efficacy. Although podophyllotoxin is considerably more costly, the increased direct drug costs may be offset by a decrease in physician office visits because the patient may be able to apply this treatment at home.

5-Fluorouracil. 5-FU is a fluorinated pyrimidine antimetabolite that interferes with DNA synthesis and to a lesser degree inhibits RNA formation. This chemotherapeutic agent is not FDA indicated for the treatment of cutaneous or genital warts. The routine use of 5-FU is no longer recommended in the CDC guidelines for treatment of genital warts.[143] Although topical and intralesional administration of 5-FU has been used for cutaneous and genital warts, treatment is limited by evidence of modest efficacy and the development of moderate to severe irritation.[140,160]

Bleomycin. Bleomycin, an antibiotic produced by *Streptomyces verticillus*, has antiviral, antibacterial, and antitumor activity. It binds to DNA and prevents thymidine incorporation and single-stranded scission of DNA. Intralesional bleomycin has been reported to be effective as an alternative form of therapy, particularly for recalcitrant palmoplantar and periungual warts.[161] However, consistent evidence of the efficacy of bleomycin in the treatment of cutaneous warts is limited. The cure rates in five trials varied from 16% to 94%, and most trials used the number of warts rather than individuals as the unit of analysis.[140] Bleomycin has not been evaluated for the treatment of genital warts.

A 1 unit/mL solution of bleomycin in saline is injected intralesionally to blanch the entire wart. Tuberculin syringes are used to inject 0.1 to 1.0 mL, depending on the size of the wart. An alternative method in which topical bleomycin is ''pricked'' into the wart using a bifurcated needle usually requires topical anesthesia.[162,163] Local pain, erythema, and swelling may persist for 1 to 2 days after treatment. The wart usually blackens, thromboses, forms an eschar, and sloughs off several days after the injection.[161] Complications, usually from intralesional or perilesional infiltration of bleomycin, may include extensive necrosis, permanent nail dystrophy, sclerodermoid changes, joint destruction, and subcutaneous abscesses.[146]

IMMUNOMODULATORS

Imiquimod. Imiquimod is an imidazoquinoline amine used for the treatment of external genital and perianal warts, as well as actinic keratoses and superficial basal cell carcinoma.[119] Although the exact mechanism of action is not fully understood, imiquimod has demonstrated significant efficacy over placebo in clearing genital warts. A study in patients with external genital warts compared the effects of imiquimod 5% and 1% cream applied three times per week to vehicle. After 16 weeks of treatment, 50% of patients who received 5% imiquimod cream, 21% of patients who received 1% imiquimod cream, and 11% of patients who received vehicle experienced eradication of all treated warts. Patients who experienced total clearance were evaluated for symptom recurrence at 12 weeks after the end of the trial. Recurrences occurred in none of the patients who received imiquimod 1% cream, 13% of patients who received imiquimod 5% cream, and 10% of patients who received the vehicle.[164]

Imiquimod is commercially available in a 5% cream, and aside from podophyllotoxin, it is the only other agent available for patient-directed therapy of genital warts at home. Patient selection should be limited to responsible, compliant patients who can easily visualize and apply the cream to lesions. Imiquimod is applied to external lesions three times weekly before bedtime and should be washed off with soap and water 6 to 10 hours later. The cream may weaken condoms and vaginal diaphragms, so concurrent use is not advised. Furthermore, sexual contact should be avoided while the cream is on the skin.[119] Mild to moderate local inflammatory reactions and erythema were the most commonly reported side effects. Less frequently reported reactions included pruritus, burning, edema, and erosions. In clinical studies, approximately 1% to 2% of patients discontinued treatment because of adverse reactions.

Interferons. Interferons are endogenous glycoproteins with immunomodulatory and antiviral activity. Most of the published studies evaluating the efficacy of interferons were conducted in patients with genital warts. Limited success has been achieved with the use of intralesional interferon therapy in the treatment of cutaneous warts. Three types of interferons, α, β, and γ, administered intralesionally, subcutaneously, and intramuscularly have been evaluated. Although interferon-α is the only interferon that is FDA approved for the intralesional treatment of genital warts, interferons are no longer recommended in the CDC guidelines for the routine treatment of genital warts.[143,165]

Reported clearance rates range from 36% to 63%, but pooled data from three trials in patients with refractory warts found no significant advantage over placebo.[140,153] Side effects of interferons consist mainly of flu-like symptoms, including fatigue, malaise, fever, chills, nausea, vomiting, and headaches. Less commonly reported side effects include depression, liver dysfunction, and transient leukopenia. Intralesional interferon administration was generally associated with increased efficacy and less severe side effects. Relative contraindications include pregnancy, autoimmune disorders, renal disease, peripheral neuropathy, cardiovascular disease, and the use of other myelosuppressive medications. The use of interferons is not routinely recommended because of the modest efficacy, severe side effects, high cost of treatment, and availability of alternative treatments.[139]

Contact Sensitizers. The use of topical sensitizing agents such as dinitrochlorobenzene and diphencyprone is effective in the treatment of large, recalcitrant, nongenital warts. Dinitrochlorobenzene demonstrated mutagenic properties in the Ames test and is no longer recommended for clinical use. Diphencyprone immunotherapy involves initial sensitization, followed by applications of the same chemical in increasing concentrations to elicit a contact dermatitis at the base of the wart. The mechanism of contact immunotherapy may be related to the induction of type IV hypersensitivity or cell-mediated immunity, resulting in the destruction of wart-infected tissue.[166] A 0.1% diphencyprone solution in acetone may be used to sensitize the patient, followed by the application of a sequence of increasing strengths. This procedure is repeated at 1- to 3-week intervals, with the usual treatment duration of approximately 5 months. Controlled studies using diphencyprone therapy are limited. Based upon case studies, the cure rate varied from 8% to 88%.[167,168] A low rate of recurrence and a low incidence of scarring were noted in most studies. It is particularly effective for large, recurrent, recalcitrant periungual, plantar mosaic, and flat warts. Complications include localized or severe generalized dermatitis, urticaria, pruritus, blistering, and, rarely, secondary infection.

Cimetidine. Cimetidine may possess immunomodulatory activity and has been reported to be useful in treating warts in children. The mechanism of action may be related to an increase in antigen-induced lymphocyte proliferation and inhibition of T-suppressor cells. The most encouraging results were seen in several uncontrolled studies. However, three placebo-controlled trials and two open-label comparative trials failed to demonstrate efficacy.[169] The dose of cimetidine used in the treatment of warts ranged from 25 to 40 mg/kg/day, divided into three or four doses. Cimetidine is not specifically approved for use in children less than 16 years old; nevertheless, no untoward reactions have been observed.

OTHER THERAPIES

Retinoids. Retinoids are another treatment option for recalcitrant genital warts. Although the mechanism of action is unknown, the antiproliferative effects of vitamin A derivatives on epidermal cell growth and differentiation may be related to the observational benefit seen in the treatment of warts. Furthermore, retinoids have been associated with regression of cervical dysplasia, presumably by preventing malignant transformation. Oral isotretinoin, at doses ranging from 0.5 to 1 mg per kg daily, was effective in the treatment of genital warts in approximately 32% to 40% of men and women.[170,171] There are several anecdotal reports of topical and oral retinoids being effective in recalcitrant warts, partic-

ularly in immunosuppressed patients. Although no longer available in the United States, etretinate 1 mg/kg/day for 2 months improved epidermodysplasia verruciformis with widespread flat wart-like lesions and plaques.[172] Other reports state its effectiveness in recalcitrant plantar warts, but relapses are common and results are not consistent.[173] Topical retinoic acid has been used for flat warts, particularly on the face to minimize scarring.[174] Retinoids are associated with significant adverse effects, including teratogenicity, depression, and elevated liver function tests.[175] Therefore, the use of retinoids should be limited to patients with extensive disabling warts that fail to respond to other treatment options.

Cidofovir. Cidofovir is a nucleotide analogue used for the treatment of cytomegalovirus (CMV) retinitis.[176] Cidofovir suppresses CMV replication by selective inhibition of the viral DNA polymerase. It also has broad-spectrum anti-DNA virus activity, including activity against HPV.[177] The antiviral activity against HPV lesions was not expected because HPVs do not encode viral DNA polymerases but instead use the host cell's polymerases for DNA replication. The antiviral activity of cidofovir may be related to an accumulation of tumor suppressor proteins and subsequent apoptosis of HPV-infected cells.[177,178] Although cidofovir is marketed only as an intravenous formulation, the efficacy of a topical 1% gel for the treatment of cutaneous and genital warts was evaluated in several pilot studies. In a study of nonimmunocompromised patients with genital warts, 47% of patients in the treatment group had complete resolution compared to 0% in the placebo group.[179] Intravenous cidofovir is associated with significant toxicities, including acute renal failure, neutropenia, developmental abnormalities, and teratogenicity. However, the most frequently reported side effects with topical use were pain, pruritus, and rash at the application site. In animal studies of topical cidofovir, the bioavailability was 2.1% and 41% in intact and abraded skin, respectively.[178] Therefore, the use of topical cidofovir should be avoided in patients with contraindications and especially in infants and pregnant women.

FUTURE THERAPIES

VACCINES

The development of HPV vaccines based upon the viruslike-particle (VLP) technology is a remarkable breakthrough. VLPs mimic the true structure of the virion and induce a significant antibody response. VLPs of the oncogenic HPV types 16 and 18 were combined in a bivalent vaccine that has shown promise in protecting against infection by these viruses. A phase II trial of 1,113 women evaluated the efficacy of the vaccine over 2 years.[180] The vaccine was administered in three 0.5-mL doses at 0, 1, and 6 months and was generally safe and well tolerated. It was highly immunogenic and effective in preventing HPV infection in approximately 93% to 95% of study patients. However, consensus on the desirable efficacy endpoint has not been determined. In the absence of large-scale studies and long-term follow-up, it is essential to determine which surrogate endpoints will most accurately predict the preventive effect of the vaccine in the development of cervical cancer.[181]

SEBORRHEIC DERMATITIS

DEFINITION

Seborrheic dermatitis (SD) is a chronic, inflammatory, erythematous, and scaling eruption.

EPIDEMIOLOGY

SD is a common dermatologic disorder, affecting 1% to 3% of the immunocompetent population.[182] It is a recurrent, chronic inflammation of the skin that occurs predominately on sebum-rich areas of the face, scalp, and chest, and is characterized by greasy, red, scaly lesions. SD is most commonly seen in two distinct patient populations: infants and adolescents/young adults. It then generally follows a waxing/waning course throughout adulthood.[183] During infancy, it is commonly called ''cradle cap,'' with spontaneous remission tending to occur by 1 year of age. After this age, the disease is rare until puberty, most likely due to sebaceous gland activity, which is under hormonal influence.[184] In adults, seborrheic dermatitis has a predilection for men and African Americans, and tends to be more severe in the winter.[185] The disorder is often asymptomatic, but pruritus can be common and at times intense.

SD is also associated with immune deficiency, most evident in HIV-positive and AIDS patients.[185] The occurrence rate in these populations tends to be much higher than the general population, affecting 34% to 83% of patients.[186,187] The reason why infection with this virus predisposes this population to a rapid onset and atypical presentation is unknown.[183]

In addition to patients who are immunocompromised, patients with central nervous system disorders such as Parkinson's disease, cranial nerve palsies, and truncal paralysis also have a higher incidence of SD. Their form of SD is usually more severe and typically refractory to treatment. The residual pool of sebum caused by immobility may predispose the patient to an overgrowth of yeast, which may explain the frequent occurrence of SD in this population.[188]

PATHOPHYSIOLOGY

The etiology of SD is poorly understood. Clinicians initially believed that the development of SD was associated with increased sebum production because the condition is prevalent in areas of the body of high sebum production and almost absent in areas of low sebum production.[189] It is believed that increased sebaceous gland activity provides a good environment for colonization by the yeast *Malassezia* (previously *Pityrosporum ovale*).[190] *Malassezia* yeast is thought to play a role in triggering an inflammatory reaction leading to increased epidermal cell turnover and the development of SD.[191] Furthermore, this observation is consistent with the increased prevalence of SD in males who have more androgen activity and, therefore, increased sebum production. On the contrary, *Malassezia* yeast is also present on the skin of people without SD.[189] As a result of this finding, some clinicians believe that SD results from an inappropriate immunologic response by affected individuals to either the *Malassezia* yeast or the toxins it produces.[192,193] Regardless of the etiology, antifungal drugs are very effective in treating SD, supporting the theory that *Malassezia* plays some type of role in the development of SD.[189]

CLINICAL PRESENTATION AND DIAGNOSIS

SD dermatitis is characterized by the appearance of red, flaking, greasy areas on the skin (Fig. 10.21). It is also recognized by its characteristic distribution on skin areas that have a high frequency of sebaceous glands. Seborrheic areas in-

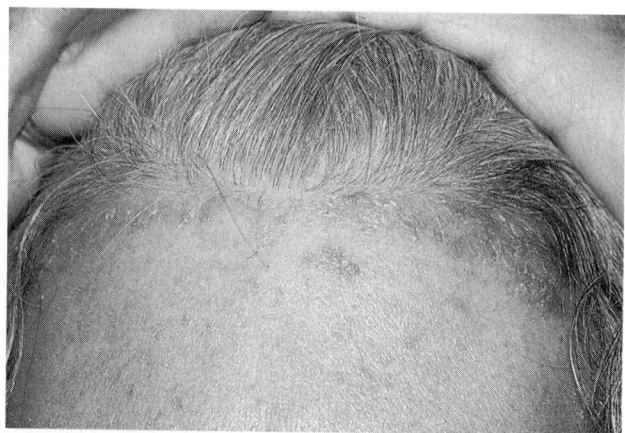

FIGURE 10.21 Seborrheic dermatitis (*see color insert*). Scale and erythema are evident along the frontal hairline. (From Goodheart HP. Goodheart's photoguide of common skin disorders. 2nd ed. Philadelphia: Lippincott Williams & Wilkins, 2003.)

clude the scalp, eyebrows, glabella, eyelid margins (often with marginal blepharitis and conjunctivitis), cheeks, paranasal areas, nasolabial folds, beard area, presternal area, central back, retroauricular creases, and the external ear canal.[185] Less commonly involved areas include the axillae, inframammary areas, naval, groin, and intergluteal cleft. SD in the intertriginous areas (areas where opposing skin surfaces touch or rub) may exist alone or in conjunction with other seborrheic areas. Similarly, psoriasis may occasionally have an intertriginous distribution, called inverse psoriasis, along with scalp involvement. In this form, it has been designated as seborrhiasis.

The severity of SD is varied. Some patients experience only a mild flaking dandruff, easily treated with over-the-counter medications, while others demonstrate more severe disease, with pruritic, red, flaky, inflamed scales covering a majority of their scalp, parts of the face, and trunk (Fig. 10.22). This severe form of the disease usually requires stronger prescription medications. The scales of seborrheic dermatitis vary from dry to thick powdery forms, with little to no erythema, to oily forms with greasy or oily scales and crusts on an inflamed erythematous base. The former manifestation is usually located on the scalp and is called simple dandruff. The greasier scales are found more commonly on the ears and central face such as the glabella,

eyebrows, and nasolabial folds but can occur on the scalp in more severe forms.

In infants, SD may become generalized to form an exfoliative erythroderma known as erythroderma desquamativum, or Leiner's disease. This syndrome is characterized not only by a generalized form of SD but also severe diarrhea, marked wasting, central nervous system deficiency, and failure to thrive. While rare, this condition can be fatal, primarily due to superimposed bacterial infections.[189]

Immunocompromised patients such as HIV-positive or AIDS patients typically present with a more severe form of the disease, commonly with lesions on the extremities, which is atypical in immunocompetent patients.[185,194] As these patients become more immunocompromised, their dermatitis usually worsens.[195]

TREATMENT

GENERAL TREATMENT OVERVIEW

The treatment of SD comprises three main categories: an antifungal, a corticosteroid, and a dandruff shampoo. The mainstay of treating seborrheic dermatitis of the scalp is medicated shampoos. The choice of shampoos depends on several factors, including physician and patient preference, cost, and cosmetic appeal to the patient. Depending on the severity of the disease, shampoos can be applied daily to twice weekly. Patients should be reminded that the scalp (not the hair) is being treated, so the patient should allow the shampoo to penetrate for at least 5 minutes, and preferably 10 minutes, before rinsing. It is also important to emphasize to patients that SD is a chronic condition and life-long intermittent treatment may be necessary to maintain control.

Some clinicians believe that removing the oils from the affected areas through frequent shampooing and cleansing may help control SD. Therefore, a commitment to good hygiene with bathing and shampooing hair daily is a requirement for treatment success. In some mild cases, this commitment may be all that is needed.[183]

Nonspecific Agents. Salicylic acid (Sebulex), coal tar (Denorex), 1% selenium sulfide (Selsun Blue), and 1% to 2% zinc pyrithione (Head & Shoulders) are the active ingredients in over-the-counter dandruff shampoos. They all have some degree of both antifungal and keratolytic action, but the most effective antifungal agents are 2.5% selenium sulfide and 2% ketoconazole, which can be obtained by prescription.[196] Using these shampoos daily may be necessary until the disease is under control; after that, only one to three times a week will usually be adequate to maintain remission.[183]

In more severe forms of the disease, predominately the scalp will be covered with thick yellow scales. For these diffused, dense, and scaly lesions, a mixture of liquid petrolatum, sodium chloride, and phenol can be applied overnight to soften scales and rinsed off in the morning using a deter-

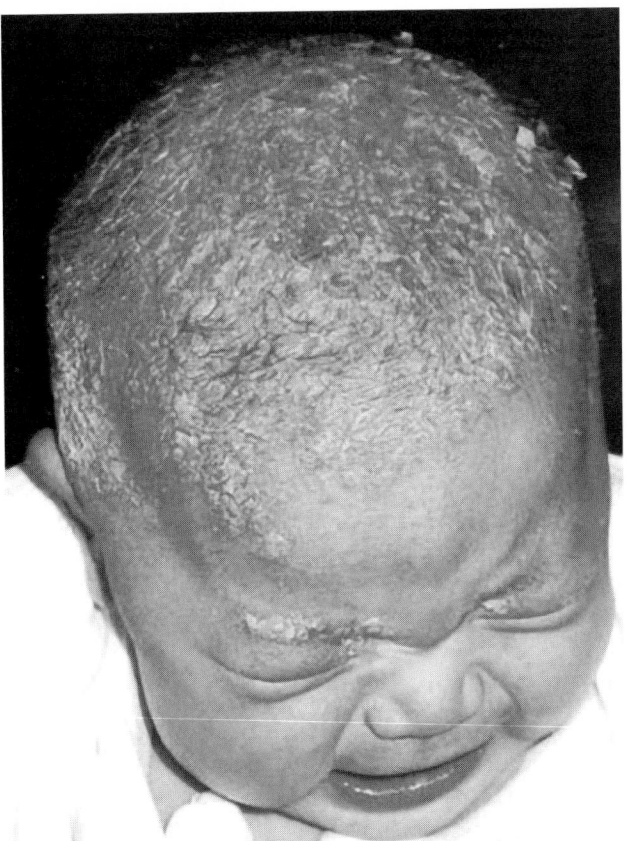

FIGURE 10.22 Infantile seborrheic dermatitis, also known as cradle cap (*see color insert*). (Image provided by Stedman's.)

gent such as dishwashing liquid or a coal tar preparation. Other preparations that use a similar application schedule include various concentrations of sulfur and salicylic acid in an ointment base.[183]

Corticosteroids. Topical corticosteroids are also common in the treatment of SD, especially if the scales are associated with inflammation and pruritus. A 1% hydrocortisone lotion, applied one or two times daily for 1 to 2 weeks, then discontinued when itching and erythema disappear, is usually safe and effective. Alternatives include 2.5% hydrocortisone cream or 0.5% desonide applied two or three times a day. More potent preparations, such as 0.025% triamcinolone lotion, 0.01% fluocinolone acetonide solution, 0.05% clobetasol solution, or 0.1% betamethasone valerate lotion, may be needed for more severe cases, but they should be used only for very short periods, no more than 2 weeks, due to the risk of skin atrophy and telangiectasia.[197]

If there is scaling in the auditory meatus, a polymyxin B-hydrocortisone suspension or 0.5% desonide and 2% acetic acid mixture may be effective by using four drops three or four times a day. The pruritus that sometimes accompanies the scaling is also relieved with this mixture. Topical steroids should not be used for seborrheic blepharitis (Fig. 10.23) because of the potential to induce glaucoma and cataracts. Hot compresses and gentle debridement using a cotton-tipped applicator with 2% ketoconazole shampoo one or more times daily are usually effective. If the lid margins are severely inflamed, topical antibiotic ointments may be added.

Topical Antifungal Medications. Unlike topical steroids, ketoconazole does not carry the same risks. Ketoconazole is available as a 2% cream or 1% to 2% shampoo. All these forms have been shown to be effective.[198] Other

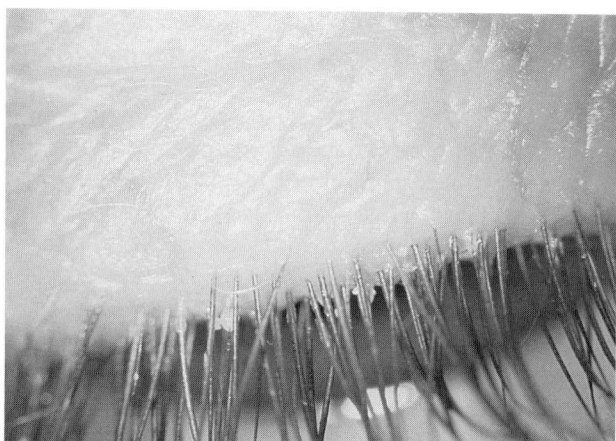

FIGURE 10.23 Seborrheic blepharitis is associated with crusting of the eyelids without meibomian gland inflammation and with seborrheic dermatitis of the eyebrows and scalp (*see color insert*). (From Tasman W, Jaeger E. The Wills Eye Hospital atlas of clinical ophthalmology. 2nd ed. Lippincott Williams & Wilkins, 2001.)

seborrheic areas of the body, including the scalp line, eyebrows, glabella, ears and nasolabial area, can be treated successfully with 2% ketoconazole cream applied twice a day. Other antifungals, such as terbinafine, have been shown to be effective both topically and orally.[193] A 1% solution of terbinafine used once daily for 4 weeks has been shown to reduce lesions and decrease the amount of *Malassezia* found on the skin.[193] Ciclopirox, with its broad-spectrum antifungal activity, has also been shown to be effective in treating SD and is available topically in a 1% shampoo and 0.77% cream, gel, and topical suspension.[199]

With the exception of accidental oral ingestion, systemic adverse reactions are minimal with topical medications. Local adverse reactions include skin irritation (usually from the vehicle), occasional reports of hair loss, and discoloration of hair (especially from selenium sulfide and coal tar). As with other shampoos, oiliness or dryness of the hair and scalp may occur.

Oral Antifungal Medications. If topical treatments are ineffective, oral agents might be necessary. Oral ketoconazole at a dose of 200 mg per day for 4 weeks is effective but may have significantly more side effects than the topical formulation. Ketoconazole and itraconazole are both very effective due to their activity against *Malassezia* yeasts in vitro.[200] Additionally, administration of itraconazole has been shown to result in high concentrations in the sebum after just 4 days of ingestion.[201] Oral terbinafine is also effective but has less in vitro activity against *Malassezia* than the azole antifungal drugs.[202] Oral terbinafine has been shown to improve clinical signs of SD when given for 4 weeks.[203]

SPECIAL PATIENT POPULATIONS

Special considerations must be made for infants with SD. Nonmedicated options should be attempted first. Applying mineral oil first to soften the scales before trying to remove them may decrease the chance of secondary infections. When treatment with drug therapy is necessary, it is important to keep in mind that an infant's scalp will absorb more drug compared to an adult's, especially if the infant has open lesions.[189] Therefore, special care should be taken to limit topical corticosteroids to 0.5% to 1% of hydrocortisone to avoid hypothalamic-pituitary-adrenal (HPA) axis suppression. Use of tar preparations should be avoided in infants because they may rub it into their eyes. However, 2% ketoconazole cream has been proven to be safe and should be the treatment of choice for infantile SD because of its minimal percutaneous absorption and lack of accumulation in the plasma.[204,205]

Patients who are immunocompromised or those with central nervous system disorders may find their SD very difficult to treat. Ketoconazole alone may not be enough to treat SD in these patients. Different combinations of an antifungal, a low-potency corticosteroid, and a dandruff shampoo may be necessary.[206]

PSORIASIS

DEFINITION

Psoriasis is an inflammatory skin disorder characterized by erythematous scaling plaques on virtually any area of the skin surface.[207]

EPIDEMIOLOGY

Psoriasis affects approximately 2% of the general population in the United States.[208] It ranks third, after acne and warts, as the most common reason for seeking the care of a dermatologist. It is a lifelong inflammatory disease with spontaneous remissions and exacerbations. Unlike other autoimmune disorders, psoriasis occurs with equal frequency in both sexes. Most patients develop the initial lesions of psoriasis in early adult life, around the third decade.[209] Approximately 30% of patients with psoriasis have a family history of the disease.[207]

Many factors have been associated with psoriasis exacerbations, including infections; winter weather; drugs such as lithium, β-blockers, terbinafine, antimalarials, NSAIDs, and corticosteroid withdrawal; stress; obesity; alcoholism; and skin trauma.[210] Conflicting data have been reported regarding the effect of these environmental factors on the development of flares. A true cause-and-effect relationship between these factors and the development of exacerbations has not been determined.[209]

PATHOPHYSIOLOGY

Localized areas of inflammation and unregulated epidermal cell growth and differentiation characterize the plaques typically seen in patients with psoriasis (Fig. 10.24).[211] Although the pathologic process that leads to the development of psoriasis is not fully understood, it is theorized that the clinical features of psoriasis develop as a secondary response triggered by T lymphocytes. The mechanism by which initial T-cell activation occurs is not known.

Sustained T-cell activation by antigen-presenting cells (APCs) in the psoriatic lesions is believed to activate a cytokine cascade, which leads to inflammation and the proliferation of keratinocytes.[212] TNF-α is a key component in the cytokine cascade and has become a molecular target in the treatment of psoriasis. The persistence of the plaques is mediated predominantly by a vicious cycle of further T-cell activation, cytokine release, and inflammation.

There is increasing support for the hypothesis that psoriasis is an autoimmune disease; however, the origin of the inciting antigen has not been elucidated.[213] Additionally, a genetic predisposition for the development of psoriasis may

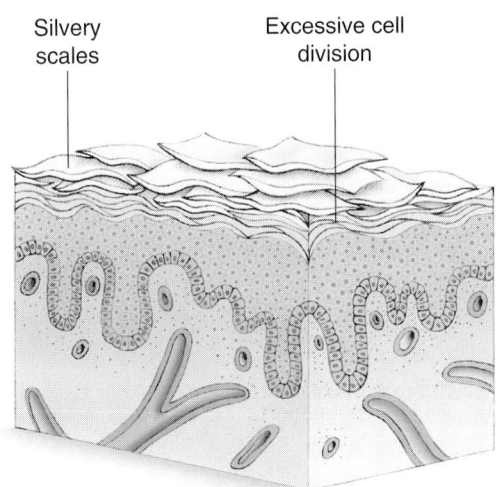

FIGURE 10.24 Psoriasis: silvery scales and excess cell division (*see color insert*). (From Goodheart HP. Goodheart's photoguide of common skin disorders. 2nd ed. Philadelphia: Lippincott Williams & Wilkins, 2003.)

exist.[214] The HLA-C gene on chromosome 6 encodes a family of antigen-presenting proteins that make up the major histocompatibility complexes on the surface of APCs. Scientists have found that approximately 60% of psoriasis patients carry the HLA-Cw6*0602 allele, compared to 10% to 15% of the general population.

CLINICAL PRESENTATION AND DIAGNOSIS

Most patients with psoriasis have symptoms of the disease throughout their lifetime. However, significant variability exists in both the severity of disease and the frequency of episodes of exacerbation and remission.[208] Patients who experience frequent relapses, occurring within months or even weeks, tend to develop more severe disease. The palm of one's hand, from the wrist to the fingertips, represents approximately 1% of the body surface area (BSA). Disease affecting less than 2% of the BSA is considered mild, moderate psoriasis involves 3% to 10%, and severe psoriasis involves more than 10% of the BSA. Several well-recognized clinical variants involve particular treatment modalities.

PSORIASIS VULGARIS OR PLAQUE PSORIASIS

Psoriasis vulgaris or plaque psoriasis, the most common form of the disease, affects approximately 80% of psoriasis

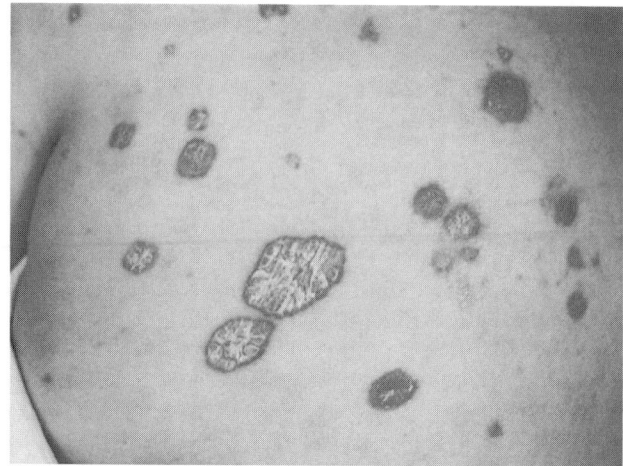

FIGURE 10.25 Typical lesions of plaque psoriasis on skin of the back (*see color insert*). (From Gold DH, Weingeist TA. Color atlas of the eye in systemic disease. Baltimore: Lippincott Williams & Wilkins, 2001.)

patients (Figs. 10.25 and 10.26). Lesions are usually distributed in a symmetrical pattern, typically located on the scalp, the lumbar region of the back, and the extensor surfaces of the elbows and knees. The well-demarcated erythematous plaques covered with silvery scales range in diameter from less than 1 cm to 10 cm. The lesions are associated with pain and pruritus and can occasionally crack and bleed. Scale removal may result in punctate bleeding, also called the Auspitz sign.[215]

GUTTATE PSORIASIS

Guttate psoriasis commonly affects children and young adults and is often associated with recent streptococcal infections (Fig. 10.27).[216] The lesions are usually small, scaly, and teardrop-shaped and typically are localized to the trunk, limbs, and scalp.

INVERSE PSORIASIS

Inverse psoriasis is a form of psoriasis that often exclusively involves the body folds (Fig. 10.28). Lesions usually present in the axillae, groin, inframammary folds, navel, intergluteal crease, and glans penis areas. Inverse psoriasis presents as a large, smooth, dry, and very erythematous lesion. This type of psoriasis is more common in obese patients.

PUSTULAR PSORIASIS

Pustular psoriasis is distinguished by the development of white pustules encircled by red skin (Fig. 10.29). The pustules contain noninfectious pus and are usually localized to the palms and soles. Generalized disease affecting the entire body often requires hospitalization and can be fatal.

ERYTHRODERMIC PSORIASIS

Erythrodermic psoriasis is an acute inflammatory, erythematous, scaling disorder involving the entire skin surface

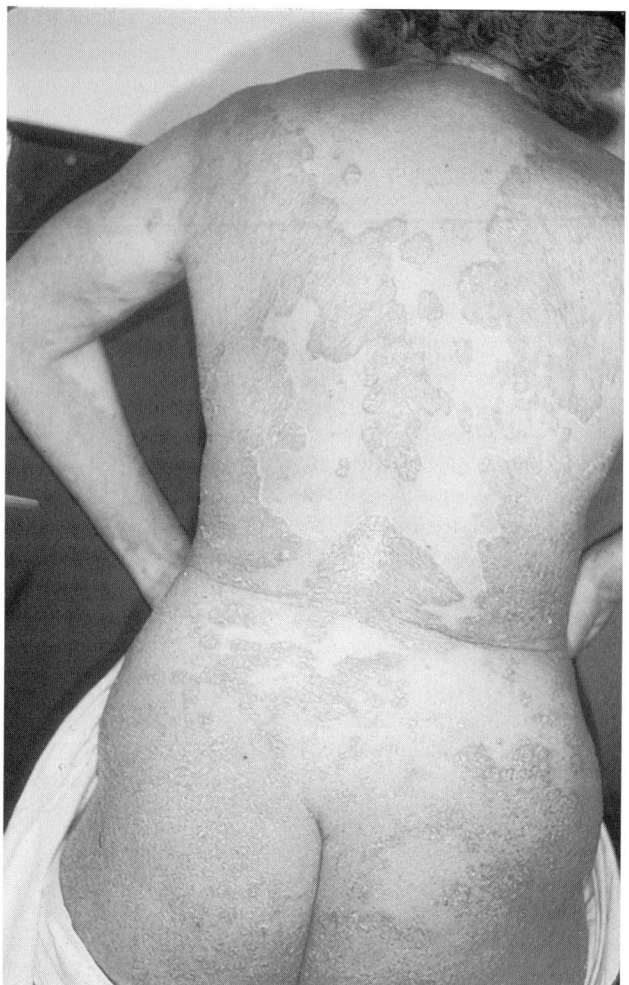

FIGURE 10.26 Psoriasis. Extensive, large plaques are evident on this patient (*see color insert*). (From Goodheart HP. Goodheart's photoguide of common skin disorders. 2nd ed. Philadelphia: Lippincott Williams & Wilkins, 2003.)

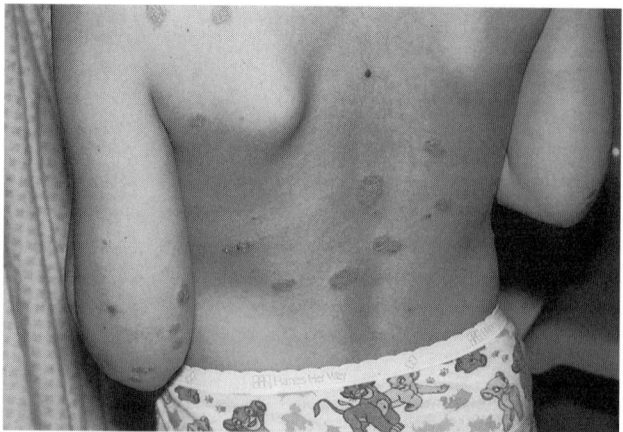

FIGURE 10.27 Guttate psoriasis (*see color insert*). (From Goodheart HP. Goodheart's photoguide of common skin disorders. 2nd ed. Philadelphia: Lippincott Williams & Wilkins, 2003.)

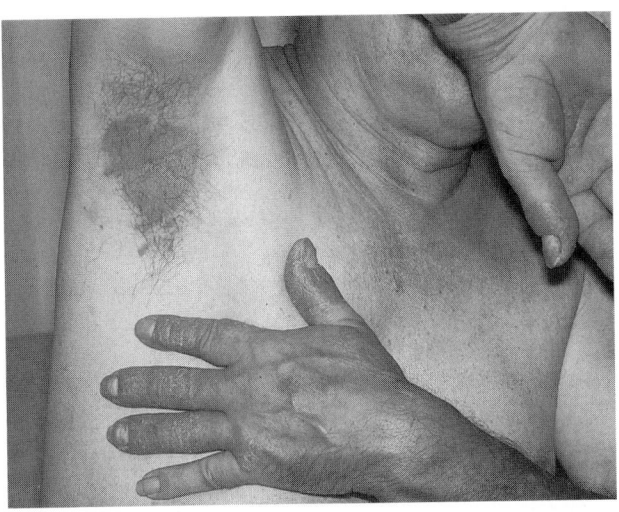

FIGURE 10.28 Inverse psoriasis (*see color insert*). (From Goodheart HP. Goodheart's photoguide of common skin disorders. 2nd ed. Philadelphia: Lippincott Williams & Wilkins, 2003.)

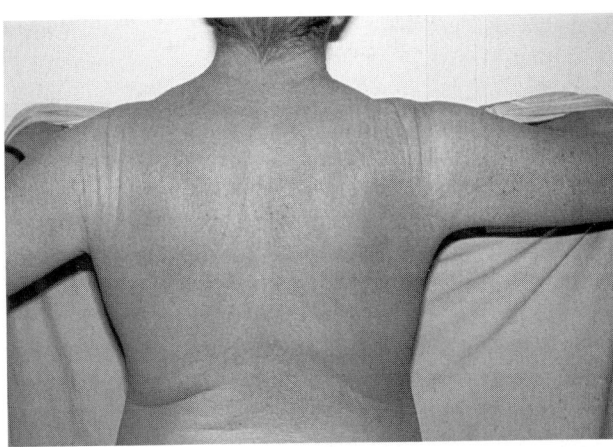

FIGURE 10.30 Erythrodermic psoriasis (*see color insert*). (From Goodheart HP. Goodheart's photoguide of common skin disorders. 2nd ed. Philadelphia: Lippincott Williams & Wilkins, 2003.)

(Fig. 10.30). Severe erythrodermic psoriasis and generalized pustular psoriasis are associated with the loss of the protective functions of the skin. These conditions are life-threatening because of the potential for systemic infections, loss of thermoregulation, and cardiovascular or pulmonary complications.

PSORIATIC ARTHRITIS

Psoriatic arthritis is a chronic, progressive, inflammatory arthritis that affects as many as about 30% of patients with psoriasis.[207,217] The arthritic symptoms are often associated with the development of skin lesions and include pain, swelling, and stiffness in the joints. Furthermore, approximately 5% to 10% of those patients may experience functional disability.

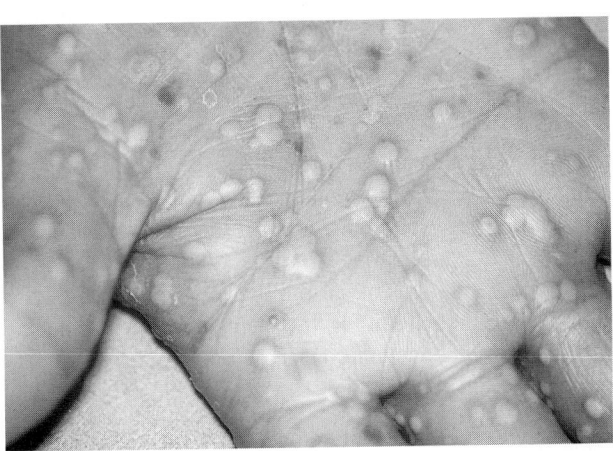

FIGURE 10.29 Pustular psoriasis (*see color insert*). (From Goodheart HP. Goodheart's photoguide of common skin disorders. 2nd ed. Philadelphia: Lippincott Williams & Wilkins, 2003.)

PSYCHOSOCIAL ASPECTS

Physical and psychological disability produced by the disease may range from minor to total. Severe psoriasis is associated with substantial morbidity and can cause functional impairment, skin disfigurement, and emotional distress. Approximately 30% of patients with psoriasis have moderate to severe disease.[218] The prevalence of depression and suicidal ideation among patients with psoriasis is consistent with figures seen in other populations with chronic illness and is estimated to be 44% to 51% and 2.5% to 5.5%, respectively.[219] Psoriasis directly affects the quality of life and may cause difficulty in work performance, problems with social rejection, sexual dysfunction, and depression.

THERAPEUTIC PLAN

The hyperproliferative and inflammatory components of the disease offer two different therapeutic approaches. Most pharmacologic interventions act by modifying one or both of these processes. Therapeutic consideration must also be given to the type of psoriasis, the extent and location of involvement, and the psychological impact of the disease. Clinical trials evaluating the efficacy of psoriasis treatment typically enroll patients with the more common plaque type of psoriasis. Therefore, the majority of clinical information available relates to this type of psoriasis. The therapeutic options for the treatment of the nonplaque type of psoriasis will also be discussed.

Topical therapy is the mainstay of treatment of mild psoriasis (Fig. 10.31). Agents are selected based upon efficacy, patient characteristics, and the potential for adverse drug reactions. Patients with moderate to severe disease representing approximately 10% BSA are candidates for phototherapy

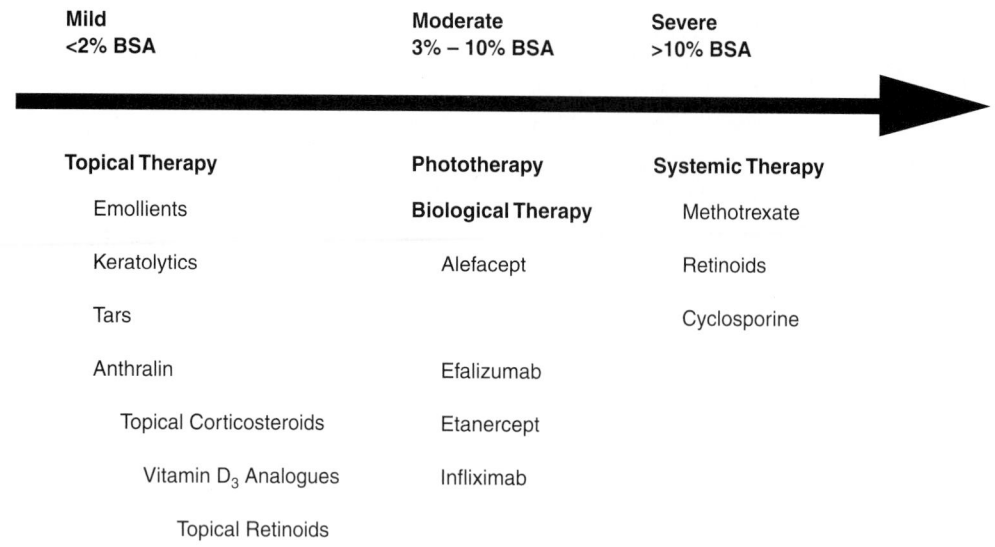

FIGURE 10.31 General approach to psoriasis treatment.

and/or systemic therapy in addition to topical therapy. The use of topical therapy alone in this case is not practical, given the tedious application to numerous lesions and restrictions on the total size of the application area associated with the use of topical steroids and calcipotriene.

New strategies in the treatment of moderate to severe psoriasis include sequential therapy, combination therapy, and rotational therapy. Sequential therapy involves of the use of several stronger and potentially more toxic agents in sequence to produce rapid disease remission, followed by a maintenance phase with an agent that has a low potential for toxicity. Combination therapy involves the simultaneous use of several synergistic agents, allowing the use of lower doses and decreasing the potential for toxicity with each agent. Rotational therapy involves alternating drug therapy every 1 to 2 years to minimize the risk of tachyphylaxis and long-term toxicity associated with many drugs.[220]

TREATMENT

TOPICAL PHARMACOTHERAPY

Emollients. Emollients are complex formulations of occlusive, humectant, and emollient ingredients. Most emollients are mineral oils and paraffins in an oil-in-water emulsion that hydrate the stratum corneum. Emulsifiers, stabilizers, and antimicrobial preservatives are common excipients added to the final product, which can cause allergic contact dermatitis in sensitive patients.

Occlusive ingredients are oily substances that form a film on the skin surface and prevent excessive transepidermal water loss. Petrolatum is the most effective occlusive moisturizer and is often blended with other ingredients to decrease the "greasy" feel. The use of lanolin is limited by its characteristic odor and the potential for allergic contact dermatitis. The silicone-based agents, which include dimeth-

icone and cyclomethicone, are popular because they are hypoallergenic and noncomedogenic. Furthermore, these products do not have a strong odor and are frequently found in "oil-free" products. Humectant ingredients enhance the hydrating properties of emollients by hygroscopically holding water in the stratum corneum. Common humectants include glycerin, urea, or pyrrolidone carboxylic acid. Emollient ingredients are esters and alcohols with both hydrophobic and hydrophilic properties. Unlike isopropyl alcohol, emollient alcohols do not have astringent properties and moisturize the skin by filling in the cracks and gaps between the desquamating corneocytes. Specialty ingredients are also added to emollients and include alpha hydroxy acids, urea, and retinoids.[221]

The preservation of skin pliability by maintaining skin hydration ultimately prevents fissuring and scaling in hyperkeratotic areas. Patients should be instructed to apply the emollients three or four times a day. Side effects from frequent application include acneiform folliculitis and exacerbation of existing acne. Occlusion of the sweat ducts may produce miliaria, especially in hot and humid climates.[222]

Keratolytics. Keratolytic agents promote the desquamation of scales. Salicylic acid, a beta hydroxy acid, is the most frequently used keratolytic agent. Concentrations ranging from 2% to 20% are formulated in a variety of ways. For smaller, thinner, scaling plaques, a 2% cream or a 3% ointment is used. A lotion base is excellent for scalp application. Higher concentrations of up to 6% have marked keratolytic activity and can be used for thicker, hyperkeratotic plaques. The use of salicylic acid concentrations up to 50% is currently limited to treatment of warts, corns, and calluses. Salicylic acid can also be used in combination with corticosteroids or tars.

Patients should be counseled to avoid the use of salicylic acid on the genitals, mucous membranes, unaffected skin, and around the eyes because of the irritant properties of the compound. Salicylic acid should be applied after phototherapy because it can block ultraviolet light. Prolonged use of salicylic acid over greater than 20% of the body area and use with occlusive dressings have been associated with the development of salicylism.[222,223] Side effects include allergic contact dermatitis and tenderness at the application site. Systemic side effects, which are more likely to occur when large areas of damaged skin are exposed to higher concentrations, include tinnitus, hyperventilation, and nausea.[222]

Lactic acid and glycolic acid are alpha hydroxy acids that can also be used to reduce scaling. Lactic acid is available in concentrations ranging from 5% to 10%. Urea-containing creams, gels, ointments, lotions, and shampoos also have keratolytic properties and are available in concentrations of 10% to 50%.[222]

Tars. Coal tar can be used in the treatment of psoriasis either as monotherapy or in combination with phototherapy and other topical agents. Use of coal tar products is limited because of poor patient acceptability and the availability of alternative topical agents. Crude coal tar is a byproduct of destructive carbonization and distillation of coal and is composed of approximately 10,000 compounds. Variations in the chemical composition of each batch depend on the type of coal used and the distillation process. Liquor carbonis detergens (LCD) is an extract of crude coal tar in a 10% concentration with alcohol. LCD is not considered a generic or pharmaceutical equivalent to standardized whole crude tar. Coal tar extracts and LCD are usually incorporated into various gel and cream-based vehicles and bath additives to facilitate application.[224]

The mechanism of action of coal tar is not known, but it is believed to have antimitotic effects. The initial application of coal tars to normal skin transiently increases epidermal proliferation during the first 2 weeks of treatment. If the coal tar is continued for up to 40 days, a cytostatic effect eventually produces epidermal thinning. Coal tars in combination with UVB light produce photo adducts that inhibit DNA synthesis.[225]

The Goeckerman regimen is used for moderate to severe psoriasis and involves the combination of daily ultraviolet light therapy followed by crude tar application for 8 hours per day for several weeks. This treatment regimen is typically administered in daily treatment centers. The average inpatient treatment course is approximately 18 days, and approximately 75% of patients remain disease-free after 12 months.[226,227]

Although coal tars typically require a longer treatment period to clear lesions, prolonged remission can be expected. Compliance is difficult because of odor, staining, and irritation. Coal tar should be applied in a downward motion in line with the growth of hair follicles to decrease the risk for developing folliculitis. When used as monotherapy, coal tar preparations are applied either once or twice daily, and the tar should be left on for at least 4 hours. Patients should be advised to avoid application to the groin and the anal, axillary, and periorbital regions because of the potential for irritation. Side effects include photosensitivity, acneiform eruptions, and folliculitis.[225] The incidence of skin carcinoma in patients treated with coal tar does not appear to be higher compared to the general population. However, further controlled studies and continued patient surveillance are necessary to determine the carcinogenic risk.[228]

Anthralin. Anthralin, or dithranol, is a topical treatment that is not commonly used in the United States. The compound 1,8-tri-hydroxy-anthracene has several modes of action, although inhibition of DNA synthesis and mitochondrial respiration may be the main mechanisms that confer the antiproliferative effect of anthralin on the epidermis.[225]

Commercial preparations of anthralin ointment and creams are available in concentrations of 0.1% to 1%. Short-contact anthralin therapy is effective for well-motivated, intelligent patients and can be used daily on an outpatient basis. Low concentrations of anthralin ointment (0.1% to 0.5%) are left on for 60 minutes or more, whereas higher concentrations (1%) may be left on for only 10 to 20 minutes. Anthralin is removed with mineral oil, followed by a shower with soap and water. Improvement can be expected to occur in approximately 8 to 16 weeks.[229] Application of a 10% triethanolamine aqueous cream can prevent inflammation and skin staining. This compound can be applied immediately after short-contact therapy without interfering with the therapeutic effect.[230]

Lassar's paste is used in the Ingram method for treating moderate to severe plaque-type psoriasis. It is a stiff paste that consists of 0.1% to 5% anthralin mixed into a zinc oxide paste containing paraffin and salicylic acid. The treatment program begins with a tar bath and UVB phototherapy, followed by the application of Lassar's paste to the plaques. The paste is left on for 4 to 12 hours and often can be left on overnight. It can be removed using a cloth with light mineral oil or baby oil. The excess is washed off in a shower or bath with soap. The advantages of short-contact therapy over the Ingram method are reductions in both irritation and staining of clothing.[225]

Patients should be instructed to use gloves when applying anthralin-containing products, to avoid smearing the product on unaffected areas, and to avoid leaving the product on the skin longer than the prescribed time. Although anthralin can permanently stain clothing and other fabrics, patients should be assured that skin staining will resolve several weeks after the discontinuation of therapy. Anthralin should not be used on the face because of the potential for eye irritation. Intertriginous areas, especially the antecubital and popliteal fossae, axillae, and inguinal folds, as well as the inner thighs should be avoided. Hair and nails may show discoloration, but low anthralin concentrations, short exposure time, and pretreatment with neutral henna to coat the hair prevent anthralin from penetrating into the hair shaft. Nail polish should be removed before treatment because it can prevent anthralin from penetrating the nail plate. No systemic toxic effects are associated with topical anthralin use.[224]

Topical Corticosteroids. Topical corticosteroids are the most frequently prescribed medications for psoriasis. They can be used alone or in combination with other agents. Several modes of action probably are important in explaining their antipsoriatic activity. Corticosteroids alter the hyperproliferative response seen in patients with psoriasis by reducing DNA synthesis and epidermal mitosis. The antiinflammatory activity of corticosteroids is mediated through a reduction in phospholipase A activity, which decreases arachidonic acid production and ultimately affects the production of inflammatory mediators such as prostaglandins, kinins, and histamine.[231]

Topical corticosteroids increase vascular smooth muscle tone. These vasoconstrictive properties correlate well with clinical efficacy and are used to rank preparations in order of antiinflammatory potency (Table 10.8).[232] The broad range of potency results in part from chemical modifications of hydrocortisone. Masking of the 16- or 17-hydroxyl groups with the addition of valerate, dipropionate, or acetonide groups dramatically enhances topical corticosteroid potency.[233]

The use of occlusive dressings and vehicle selection can also alter topical corticosteroid potency, and occlusive dressings can increase penetration by 10- to 100-fold.[234] Ointments generally are more effective than creams, and creams are usually more potent than lotions. Vehicle selection is usually based upon the location of the psoriatic lesion and patient preference. Ointments are best used on thick, scaly plaques; creams are a better option in the intertriginous areas. For the scalp and other hairy areas, gels, lotions, or sprays are preferable to ointments and creams.[231] Multiple formulations of an agent are often prescribed for versatility, and many patients may prefer a different vehicle depending on their attire, agenda, and the location of lesions.

Practitioners should use the lowest possible steroid strength to minimize the development of adverse drug reactions. Commonly used strengths include midpotency and high-potency agent. Less potent topical steroids have limited use in treating thick scaly lesions but can be used in steroid-sensitive areas. These areas are more prone to side effects and include the groin, face, and intertriginous areas. Potent topical corticosteroids are applied twice daily for approximately 2 weeks. Abrupt discontinuation can lead to rebound disease flares. Therefore, steroid holidays and ''weekend steroid pulse therapy'' in combination with an alternative topical agent during the week are tactics used to minimize the development of rebound disease, tachyphylaxis, and adverse drug reactions.[235]

The most common and concerning side effects associated with the use of topical corticosteroids include the development of cutaneous atrophy, striae, and telangiectasias. Cutaneous atrophy is characterized by thin, fragile skin and can lead to tearing of the dermal connective tissue, causing irreversible striae. Telangiectasias result from the dilation of epidermal blood vessels and become apparent through the thinned epidermis. These local cutaneous side effects are often the result of excessive application and extended treatment, particularly in steroid-sensitive areas. Although rare, systemic side effects, including HPA axis suppression, glucose intolerance, and Cushing syndrome, can occur with application to large areas or to patients with an increased BSA to mass ratio.[231]

Vitamin D₃. Calcitriol (1,25-dihydroxycholecalciferol) is the active form of vitamin D_3. When circulating calcitriol binds to receptors in the skin, keratinocyte proliferation is inhibited and basal skin cell differentiation is induced. In vitro, cultured cells from psoriatic skin exhibit a partial resistance to the effects of calcitriol, but increased concentrations can overcome this resistance.[236] Clinical studies confirm the effectiveness of topical calcitriol, and although well tolerated, topical calcitriol is rarely used because no commercial product is available in the United States.

Calcipotriol (calcipotriene in the United States) is a synthetic analogue of calcitriol. Like calcitriol, the effects of calcipotriol are mediated through the binding and activation of vitamin D receptors.[237] Calcipotriol demonstrated superior efficacy and appears to be at least 100 times less potent in its effects on calcium metabolism compared to calcitriol.[237,238] Calcipotriol is not associated with clinically significant effects on calcium homeostasis when used at recommended doses.[236] Rare cases of hypercalcemia have been reported with the use of more than 120 g per week.[239,240] Calcipotriol and potent topical corticosteroids are considered first-line therapy for the treatment of mild to moderate psoriasis. Meta-analyses of psoriasis trials suggest that calcipotriol is as effective as potent topical corticosteroids and is associated with increased efficacy compared to short-contact dithranol and coal tar.[241] Side effects are mild, and although irritation of the skin did occur in 10% to 15% of patients, treatment discontinuation is rarely required.

Calcipotriene is marketed under the brand name Dovonex and is available in a 0.005% cream, ointment, or solution. Although studies have demonstrated increased patient compliance with the cream formulation, the ointment demonstrated superior efficacy.[242] Therefore, substitution of one formulation for the other without careful consideration is not advised. Recommending the combination of calcipotriol cream in the morning and ointment in the evening may improve compliance.[243] Instruct patients to apply a liberal layer of the product to the affected areas twice daily. The onset of action is delayed, and signs of improvement usually manifest after 2 weeks of treatment. The average treatment duration to achieve disease remission is approximately 8 weeks. Approximately 60% of patients will relapse, with a mean relapse-free period of 43.3 days.[244] Educating patients about the delayed onset of action and expected treatment outcome

TABLE 10.8	Potency Ranking of Topical Corticosteroids
Super-potent	Augmented betamethasone dipropionate 0.05% ointment
	Clobetasol propionate 0.05% cream and ointment
	Diflorasone diacetate 0.05% ointment
	Halobetasol propionate 0.05% cream and ointment
Potent	Amcinonide 0.1% cream, ointment, and lotion
	Augmented betamethasone dipropionate 0.05% cream
	Betamethasone dipropionate 0.05% cream and ointment
	Betamethasone valerate 0.1% ointment
	Desoximetasone 0.25% cream, ointment, and 0.05% gel
	Diflorasone diacetate 0.05% cream and ointment
	Fluocinolone acetonide 0.2% cream
	Fluocinonide 0.05% cream, ointment, and gel
	Halcinonide 0.1% cream and ointment
	Triamcinolone acetonide 0.5% cream and ointment
Midstrength	Betamethasone benzoate 0.025% cream, gel, and lotion
	Betamethasone dipropionate 0.05% lotion
	Betamethasone valerate 0.1% cream
	Clocortolone pivalate 0.1% cream
	Desoximetasone 0.05% cream
	Fluocinolone acetonide 0.025% cream and ointment
	Flurandrenolide 0.05% cream, ointment, and lotion
	Flurandrenolide 0.025% cream and ointment
	Flurandrenolide 4 μg/cm^2 tape
	Fluticasone propionate 0.05% cream
	Fluticasone propionate 0.005% ointment
	Hydrocortisone butyrate 0.1% ointment, and solution
	Hydrocortisone valerate 0.2% cream and ointment
	Mometasone furoate 0.1% cream, ointment, and lotion
	Triamcinolone acetonide 0.1% cream, ointment, and lotion
	Triamcinolone acetonide 0.025% cream, ointment, and lotion
Low potency	Alclometasone dipropionate 0.05% cream and ointment
	Desonide 0.05% cream
	Dexamethasone sodium phosphate 0.1% cream
	Dexamethasone 0.04% aerosol
	Dexamethasone 0.01% aerosol
	Fluocinolone acetonide 0.01% cream and solution
	Hydrocortisone 2.5% cream, ointment, and lotion
	Hydrocortisone 1% cream, ointment, lotion, and solution
	Hydrocortisone 0.5% cream, ointment, lotion, and aerosol
	Hydrocortisone 0.25% lotion
	Hydrocortisone acetate 1% cream and ointment
	Hydrocortisone acetate 0.5% cream and ointment

(Facts & Comparisons, 2004)

is important to ensure compliance with the prescribed therapy.

Topical Retinoids. Tazarotene, a topical agent indicated for the treatment of psoriasis, belongs to a novel class of retinoids called acetylenic retinoids. Retinoids are useful in the treatment of psoriasis because they reduce inflammation and regulate keratinocyte differentiation and proliferation. These effects are mediated through the binding and activation of retinoid acid receptors (RARs) and retinoid X receptors (RXRs), which in turn modulate gene transcription and translation. In contrast to all-*trans* retinoic acid, which targets all three RARs with equal affinity and weakly targets the RXRs, tazarotene is specific for the RAR family of receptors. Furthermore, tazarotene preferentially binds RARs in the following rank order: RAR β > RAR γ > RAR α. The selective properties of tazarotene on RARs are associated with decreased topical and systemic toxicities compared to nonspecific retinoids.[245]

Tazarotene is a useful alternative to calcipotriene and topical corticosteroids for the treatment of mild to moderate psoriasis. Treatment is usually initiated with the 0.05% cream and increased to the 0.1% strength if tolerated and medically indicated. Plaques and scales tend to improve after 1 to 4 weeks of therapy, but redness may take longer to improve.[246] Treatment with tazarotene gel for up to 12 months has been studied in clinical trials for psoriasis. Use of tazarotene in combination with high-potency and midpotency topical corticosteroids was associated with increased efficacy, prolonged disease remission, and a decrease in both the irritation associated with tazarotene and the development of atrophy associated with topical steroid use.[247–249] Another study demonstrated increased efficacy with the combination therapy compared to calcipotriene 0.005% ointment alone; however, the combination was also associated with increased adverse effects.[250]

Tazarotene is available in a 0.05% or 0.1% cream or gel and marketed under the brand name Tazorac. Tazarotene should be applied to psoriatic lesions only once daily in the evenings and should not be used on more than 20% of the BSA. Tazarotene should be applied to dry skin after bathing; if emollients are used, they should be applied at least 1 hour before tazarotene. Unaffected skin may be more susceptible to irritation, so application to these areas should be avoided.[246]

Topical adverse effects, including pruritus, burning, irritation, and erythema, are the most common side effects, occurring in 10% to 30% of patients. Sun exposure should be avoided unless deemed medically necessary because of the potential for increased susceptibility to burning. Furthermore, patients should be encouraged to use protective clothing and sunscreen with an SPF of at least 15. The most concerning side effects are the embryotoxic and teratogenic effects in animal models and humans. The FDA classified tazarotene as pregnancy category X. Women of childbearing age must use contraception during therapy and should be

informed of the teratogenic risks associated with this medication.[246]

Novel Topical Treatment. Pimecrolimus and tacrolimus are macrolide immunosuppressants. The mechanism of action of these agents involves modulation of immune-cell function through the inhibition of calcineurin-dependent activation of nuclear factors, which ultimately results in the inhibition of T-cell activation and prevents the release of inflammatory cytokines from mast cells. Pimecrolimus and tacrolimus are available in topical formulations. The small molecular size of these agents produces good skin penetration with topical application. Although both agents have FDA indications for the topical treatment of mild to moderate atopic dermatitis, ongoing studies are evaluating the use of these agents in other inflammatory dermatologic conditions.[251] Currently neither agent holds a FDA indication for the treatment of psoriasis.

A public health advisory was issued by the FDA to inform healthcare providers and patients about a potential cancer risk with the use of topical pimecrolimus and tacrolimus. This concern was based on information from animal studies and case reports in a small number of patients, and on the mechanism of action. Calcineurin inhibitors suppress the body's normal immune defenses against cancer. Therefore, these agents should be used only as labeled and in patients who have failed to respond to treatment with other therapies where the potential benefits outweigh the risks.

Pimecrolimus. Pimecrolimus 1% cream may be an effective treatment option for patients with plaque-type psoriasis. Topical pimecrolimus 1% ointment applied once daily under occlusion was compared to clobetasol-17-propionate 0.05% ointment applied once daily under occlusion and placebo. After 2 weeks of treatment, total clinical scores decreased by 92% in the clobetasol group, 82% in the pimecrolimus group, and 18% in the placebo group. There was no significant difference in clinical scores between the clobetasol- and pimecrolimus-treated lesions at 2 weeks.[252] Topical pimecrolimus 1% cream applied twice daily without occlusion was also compared to calcipotriol 0.005% ointment, clobetasol-17-propionate 0.05% ointment, and placebo. Pimecrolimus was significantly more effective than placebo but less effective than clobetasol and calcipotriol.[252] Furthermore, topical pimecrolimus demonstrated increased efficacy compared to vehicle in the treatment of intertriginous psoriasis.[253]

The therapeutic potential of oral pimecrolimus for the treatment of psoriasis is being investigated. In animal models, pimecrolimus was highly active against skin inflammation. Unlike cyclosporine and tacrolimus, pimecrolimus demonstrated a low potential for systemic immunosuppression. Patients given oral pimecrolimus 30 mg twice daily for 12 weeks experienced a 75% reduction in the psoriasis area and severity index score compared to patients in the placebo group. Approximately 25% of patients given pimecrolimus reported a transient feeling of warmth on the upper chest occurring about 40 minutes after ingestion of the drug. No differences in skin and systemic infections were reported.[254]

Tacrolimus. Tacrolimus may be less promising than pimecrolimus in the treatment of psoriasis because of reduced penetration of the drug into psoriatic plaques. Topical tacrolimus 0.03% ointment once daily was compared to calcipotriol 0.005% ointment twice daily and placebo: a significant improvement was noted in the calcipotriol group compared to the tacrolimus and placebo groups. No statistically significant differences were observed between the tacrolimus and placebo groups after 6 weeks of treatment.[255] Topical tacrolimus did show increased efficacy compared to vehicle in the treatment of facial and intertriginous psoriasis.[256]

PHOTOTHERAPY

Phototherapy is a useful treatment option for moderate to severe psoriasis and involves the repeated exposure of affected skin to ultraviolet light. Although phototherapy is a good treatment option, poor reimbursement rates deter many physicians from using this therapy. Phototherapy was first used at the beginning of the 20th century in combination with crude coal tar. Today, phototherapy is used in combination with various topical and systemic therapies and is typically reserved for patients who have failed to respond to aggressive topical therapy or have widespread disease.[257] Several types of phototherapy are commonly used in the treatment of psoriasis, including broadband UVB and narrow-band UVB. Photochemotherapy is also effective and involves the use of light from the UVA spectrum in combination with a photoactive drug, psoralen. The efficacy of excimer laser therapy and heliotherapy has also been evaluated.

Broadband UVB. The broadband UVB spectrum ranges from 290 and 320 nm. The starting dose of UVB used in the treatment of psoriasis is usually based upon the minimal erythema dose (MED). The MED is determined by performing a test grid of varying wavelengths of light on the patient's back. The dose of ultraviolet light that results in a barely perceptible erythema 24 hours after exposure is the MED. This dose is associated with an optimal balance between treatment efficacy and minimizing side effects.[258] Although less accurate, the starting dose of UVB can also be estimated based on the Fitzpatrick skin type.[259] Modified protocols where the dose of UVB is varied are also used.

The most common outpatient protocol involves UVB exposure three times a week.[235] The application of a thin layer of clear emollients enhances the efficacy of UVB therapy. Although several small studies demonstrated treatment efficacy in 90% to 100% of patients with moderate to severe psoriasis, most practitioners expect two thirds of patients to experience disease clearing, and most patients clear after 20 to 30 treatments.[258] With disease remission, the treatment frequency can be tapered, but the use of maintenance UVB therapy once or twice weekly is associated with an extended remission time.[260]

UVB combined with crude coal tar is more effective than either agent alone. Although the mechanism behind the synergistic effects of crude coal tar and UVB is not known, the Goeckerman regimen is associated with a high treatment response and an extended duration of disease remission. It involves the combination of daily ultraviolet light therapy followed by crude tar application for 8 hours per day for several weeks. Because the tar layer prevents the UV light from reaching the skin, it is applied after UVB exposure. This treatment regimen is typically administered in daily treatment centers.[226,227] The combination of UVB with topical calcipotriene or tazarotene is also associated with accelerated efficacy. Furthermore, use with systemic methotrexate or acitretin reduces the total cumulative dose of either agent.[260]

The major side effects of UVB therapy are erythema and skin burning. Caution patients to avoid application of agents that may either sensitize them to phototherapy or block UVB therapy without the consent of their dermatologist. To prevent UV-induced conjunctival erosions, protective goggles are worn during treatment. It is generally advisable to minimize prolonged exposure to the face by using UVB-blocking face shields. In men, the genital skin is also routinely protected to decrease the theoretical potential for cutaneous cancers. Advise patients to avoid additional UVB exposure from sunbathing because of an increased risk for developing treatment complications. Although premature aging of the skin is dose-dependent, UVB used in the described manner is not associated with an increased risk for skin cancers.[261]

Narrowband UVB. Narrowband UVB is a newer technique that uses a narrower UV spectrum, ranging from 311 to 313 nm. By using longer wavelengths of light, it is hypothesized that narrowband UVB affords treatment efficacy and minimizes the burning and premature aging usually attributed to exposure to shorter wavelengths of light.[262] Although narrowband UVB demonstrated increased efficacy compared to broadband UVB, it was less effective than photochemotherapy.[263,264] The potential for photocarcinogenesis from narrowband UVB is unclear compared to the established safety of broadband UVB therapy. The use of narrowband UVB in the United States is becoming more popular largely due to the increased efficacy and good tolerability when used in sub-erythemogenic doses.

PUVA. Photochemotherapy, termed PUVA, is effective in the treatment of severe psoriasis and involves the use of light from the UVA spectrum in combination with psoralens, a class of photoactive drugs. The UVA spectrum ranges from 320 to 400 nm. Although UVA by itself is not effective, use in combination with psoralens is effective therapy for patients with disease that is resistant to other types of treatment or severe disability as a result of psoriasis, or for elderly patients.

Psoralens belong to the furocoumarin class of compounds and are thought to form photo adducts with DNA. The photochemically induced cross-linking of DNA strands is associated with inhibition of DNA synthesis and epidermal basal cell replication, ultimately resulting in antiproliferative effects. The two derivatives currently available in the United States are 8-methoxypsoralen (methoxsalen, 8-MOP) and 4,5′,8-trimethylpsoralen (trioxsalen, TMP). The third psoralen, 5-methoxypsoralen (bergapten, 5-MOP), is being investigated for clinical use in the United States but is available in Europe. The oral dose of the photoactive drug is administered 2 hours before UVA exposure.[265]

Methoxsalen is available in a hard gelatin capsule and a soft gelatin capsule and is marketed under the brand names Oxsoralen-Ultra and 8-MOP, respectively. These products should not be used interchangeably because the newer and more commonly used product, Oxsoralen-Ultra, has significantly greater bioavailability and earlier onset.[266] Methoxsalen is administered orally in a dose of 0.3 to 0.6 mg per kg. When Oxsoralen-Ultra is administered orally, blood levels peak at 2 hours, producing maximum sensitivity to UVA. Blood levels can be increased by a low-fat meal. Methoxsalen is metabolized through the liver by several pathways, including hydroxylation, glucuronide formation, epoxidation, and hydrolysis.[266]

The patient's skin type guides selection of the starting dosage of UVA. Treatment is usually administered two or three times per week because the erythema induced by PUVA may not be evident for up to 48 hours after exposure. In general, the dose of UVA is increased by 0.5 to 1.5 J per cm^2 with each consecutive treatment. The time to produce clearing with UVA is longer, usually after 10 to 20 treatments over 4 to 8 weeks. Once clearing has been achieved, the frequency of maintenance therapy is gradually decreased.[265]

Common side effects associated with PUVA therapy includes nausea, pruritus, and skin burning. Taking the psoralen with milk or food or dividing the dose in half and separating each dose by 30 minutes can reduce nausea. Pruritus occurs in approximately 10% of patients and can usually be alleviated with emollients. Transient mild erythema is expected 24 to 48 hours after PUVA therapy. Serious burns may occur from ultraviolet radiation or sunlight even if exposed through glass. Patients must avoid sun exposure for at least 8 hours after methoxsalen ingestion; if sun exposure cannot be avoided, shielding with protective clothing and use of sunscreens should be encouraged.

Methoxsalen has been associated with the development of cataracts in animal models. The concentration of methoxsalen in the lens of the eye is proportional to serum levels. The renal excretion of psoralens usually is completed within 8 hours, but elimination from the lens of the eye takes about 24 hours. Ocular UVA exposure from natural sunlight during the time methoxsalen is present may lead to irreversible DNA binding and can result in the formation of cataracts. Although the risk is small, this complication can be nearly eliminated by wearing UVA-blocking wraparound glasses for 12 to 24 hours after ingesting psoralen. More common and concerning chronic side effects of PUVA therapy in-

clude premature aging of the skin and a dose-dependent increased incidence of squamous cell carcinoma (SCC) and the development of PUVA lentigines. The association between the development of SCC and PUVA therapy is related to the cumulative dose. The results of a large prospective cohort study estimated an 11-fold increased risk of SCC in patients receiving more than 260 PUVA treatments compared to patients who received fewer than 160 treatments.[267] Furthermore, PUVA therapy may be associated with an increased risk of malignant melanoma, but more studies are necessary to determine whether a definite relationship exists.[266,268]

Topical psoralens in combination with UVA are a popular method for treating psoriasis in Scandinavia. This can be effective for both extensive plaque-type psoriasis and selected parts of the body. This method avoids the gastric side effects of oral psoralens and is ideal for patients with hepatic impairment. The patient applies topical psoralen before exposure to UVA. TMP usually is used because it has less percutaneous absorption than 8-MOP, but this method carries a greater risk of photosensitivity. To reduce the amount of UVA exposure and the number of treatments, oral retinoid agents, such as etretinate, can be used along with PUVA. Although the mechanism of synergism is not known, it does not seem to involve the increased photosensitivity seen with the retinoid agents.[265,266]

SYSTEMIC PHARMACOTHERAPY

Systemic therapy is reserved for patients with severe disabling psoriasis or psoriasis refractory to topical therapy and phototherapy. The most commonly used systemic agents for treatment of psoriasis include methotrexate, acitretin, and cyclosporine.

Methotrexate. Methotrexate (MTX) is a folic acid antagonist that inhibits dihydrofolate reductase, blocking key steps in DNA and RNA synthesis. Initially, MTX was thought to reduce the rapid keratinocyte proliferation that occurs in psoriasis, but it now appears that the primary effect of the drug is on cutaneous inflammation.[269] It is excreted by the kidneys almost unchanged; the clearance of MTX correlates with creatinine clearance. However, a small amount is excreted by active tubular secretion. MTX is 50% to 70% bound to albumin and may be displaced by acidic drugs such as phenylbutazone, sulfonamides, salicylates, and phenytoin. A potential for toxicity exists when MTX is used in combination with these drugs, especially in patients with impaired renal excretion. Weak organic acids such as salicylates, probenecid, ketoprofen, phenylbutazone, and sulfamethoxazole-trimethoprim can compete with MTX for active tubular secretion. Furthermore, direct renal toxicity occurs with the concomitant use of MTX and indomethacin. Therefore, both agents should be used cautiously in patients with psoriatic arthritis who have poor renal function.[270]

When initiating MTX therapy, one should consider the characteristics of the patient and disease and the contraindications to MTX therapy. Absolute contraindications to MTX therapy are pregnancy and lactation. As always, the benefits of therapy should be weighed against the potential risks. One relative contraindication that needs further elaboration is alcohol abuse. With chronic MTX administration, hepatotoxicity resulting in fibrosis and cirrhosis is a serious concern. Alcoholism significantly increases the risk of hepatotoxicity, and MTX should not be used in patients who abuse alcohol.

The usual oral dose of MTX is 10 to 20 mg in either a single weekly dose or divided into three doses given 12 hours apart once weekly. A test dose of 5 to 10 mg is given, and a complete blood count and liver function tests are done 7 days later. In general, 75% to 80% of patients with psoriasis respond within 4 weeks. If no response occurs, the dose is increased by 2.5 to 5 mg per week. Although the most common route of administration is by mouth, it may be given intramuscularly at doses of 10 to 25 mg per week. The total dose rarely exceeds 30 mg. Higher intramuscular doses are allowed because of the more rapid renal clearance. With remission, the dose of MTX may be tapered by 2.5 mg per week until the lowest possible dose that provides disease control is determined.[271]

Common acute side effects of MTX are nausea and gastrointestinal upset. MTX can also produce a phototoxic reaction similar to sunburn. If MTX is used with phototherapy, patients should omit their phototherapy treatments on the days MTX is administered. More serious long-term side effects include hepatotoxicity and bone marrow suppression. The hepatotoxicity seems to be related to the cumulative MTX dose. Liver function tests are an unreliable screening method for detecting MTX-induced hepatotoxicity. Liver biopsy is currently the only means of evaluating histologic changes attributed to MTX. A liver biopsy is recommended after the cumulative MTX dose exceeds 1.5 g, with subsequent biopsies being performed at regular intervals when therapy is continued beyond the 1.5-g cumulative dose. Specific guidelines for monitoring MTX toxicity are published elsewhere.[272] Folinic acid (leucovorin) is the treatment of choice for accidental overdose. Leucovorin rescue, as this is called, bypasses the step in folic acid reduction that is blocked by MTX.[270]

Retinoids. Two synthetic analogues of vitamin A, etretinate and acitretin, have been used to treat psoriasis. Etretinate, an aromatic retinoid, has been available for clinical use in the United States since 1986. Acitretin is an acid metabolite of etretinate with different pharmacokinetics. Acitretin has a shorter half-life, is less lipophilic, and does not distribute into subcutaneous fat as well as etretinate. The elimination half-lives of acitretin and etretinate are 2 and 100 days, respectively. Etretinate was withdrawn from the market following the FDA approval of acitretin because of the improved pharmacokinetics of acitretin.[273] Tazarotene is a topical retinoid approved for treatment of plaque psoriasis and acne in the United States, and the use of an oral form of tazarotene is under evaluation.[274]

The mechanism of action of retinoids in the treatment of psoriasis may be related to effects on cellular differentiation, resulting in the normalization of keratinization and proliferation. Retinoids also have an antiinflammatory effect associated with the reduction of leukotriene and hydroxyeicosatetraenoic acid (HETE) levels.[245] Retinoids should be reserved for psoriasis recalcitrant to topical therapy, UVB, and PUVA because of the increased potential for adverse side effects.

Acitretin is effective in the treatment of pustular, palmoplantar pustular, and exfoliative erythrodermic types of psoriasis. Rapid resolution of pustular psoriasis can usually be achieved within 10 days. The starting dosage of acitretin ranges from 25 to 50 mg per day. Plaque-type psoriasis responds more slowly, and acitretin is often used in combination with other treatment modalities to achieve disease remission. Dosages of acitretin ranging from 25 to 50 mg per day in combination with PUVA and UVB resulted in a faster onset and decreased total exposure to ultraviolet radiation.[275]

Side effects are similar to the clinical presentation of hypervitaminosis A syndrome. The major side effect of oral retinoid therapy is the teratogenic effect in humans. Women of childbearing age must use contraception for 3 years after the completion of acitretin treatment. Other side effects include diffuse hair loss, elevation of triglyceride or cholesterol levels, cheilitis, hepatotoxicity, and musculoskeletal changes. Pseudotumor cerebri is a rare but potentially devastating side effect of retinoid therapy.[273]

Cyclosporine. Cyclosporine is an 11-amino acid cyclic peptide commonly used as part of an immunosuppressive regimen in solid organ transplant recipients. Although the precise mechanism of action is not fully understood, the inhibition of lymphokine secretion by activated T cells plays a central role. The high potential for toxicity and expense limit the use of cyclosporine to patients with severe psoriasis that is unresponsive to more conventional therapies. Cyclosporine appears to be as effective as PUVA, UVB, MTX, or retinoid therapy in treating chronic severe plaque psoriasis but less effective in pustular psoriasis. Clearing with cyclosporine occurs more rapidly than with other systemic modalities. A good response is usually seen within 4 to 8 weeks, but relapse is common after therapy is withdrawn. The effective dose of cyclosporine for treatment of psoriasis ranges from 2.5 to 5 mg/kg/day, much lower than the doses used in solid organ transplant patients. Although a faster and more complete therapeutic response was observed with the use of higher doses, the potential for nephrotoxicity and hypertension are also dose-related. Most side effects were reversible following the discontinuation of treatment. Generally, the dose of cyclosporine should not exceed 5 mg/kg/day and the duration of treatment should not exceed 2 years.[273] Other side effects include hepatotoxicity, neurologic abnormalities, gingival hyperplasia, hypertrichosis, and an increased incidence of malignancies. Because of potentially life-threatening side effects, it has been recommended that patients with hypertension, evidence of compromised renal function, concurrent immunosuppression, or history of malignancy, pregnancy, or infection avoid cyclosporine. To date, little is known about the safety and efficacy of long-term maintenance therapy. Although systemic cyclosporine is efficacious in clearing psoriasis, several life-threatening side effects limit its use.[276,277]

Alternative Systemic Therapy

Hydroxyurea. Hydroxyurea (HU) is a hydroxylated molecule of urea that affects cell proliferation by inhibiting DNA synthesis. Although not approved by the FDA for treating psoriasis, it has been reported to be effective. HU is less effective than MTX, and the response is slower (6 to 8 weeks). A rapid response can be achieved with HU for the treatment of pustular psoriasis. Treatment efficacy ranges from a favorable response in 45% to 63% of patients to an excellent response in 18% to 38% of patients. This variation may be the result of different doses, varying time intervals, and different criteria for evaluating disease activity in studies. Although HU is not a first-line agent, it is an option for patients with contraindications to standard therapy. Major disadvantages associated with HU include the potential for bone marrow suppression and the development of lymphoproliferative disorders.[278]

BIOLOGIC AGENTS

Alefacept. Alefacept (Amevive) is a fusion protein consisting of portions of leukocyte function-associated antigen 3 (LFA3) bound to the Fc portion of IgG. LFA3 is a protein on the surface of APCs that facilitates the binding and activation of T cells via CD2 receptors on the T-cell surface. Alefacept binds to CD2 receptors on T-cells and targets that T-cell for apoptosis.[279] The FDA approved alefacept for the treatment of moderate to severe chronic plaque psoriasis in January 2003.

Alefacept is administered by either intravenous or subcutaneous injection. The recommended dose is 7.5 mg as an intravenous bolus over 30 seconds once weekly or 15 mg administered via an intramuscular (IM) injection once weekly for 3 months. Clinical signs of symptom improvement can be seen after 60 days, and a second course of therapy may be considered if necessary.[280] Approximately 33% of patients treated with alefacept 15 mg IM weekly achieved a 75% improvement in the psoriasis area and severity index at 12 weeks, compared to 28% of patients who received alefacept 10 mg IM weekly and 13% who received placebo.[281] In clinical trials, approximately 20% and 30% of patients achieved a "clear" or "almost clear" physician's global scale score after 12 and 24 weeks of treatment, respectively. The median duration of disease remission among studies ranged from 7 to 10 months in patients who responded to alefacept treatment.[282–284]

Alefacept is well tolerated, with the most common adverse events being headache, pruritus, infection, and injection site pain and inflammation. Injection site reactions are generally mild and do not lead to the discontinuation of ther-

apy. Infections were reported in approximately 15% of patients, with a majority of infections being attributed to the common cold. Less than 1% of patients treated with alefacept experienced a CD4+ T-cell count below 250/μL, and there was no association with an increased incidence of infection in these patients.[281] Nevertheless, treatment with alefacept is discouraged in patients with below-normal CD4+ T-cell counts. Weekly CD4+ T-cell counts should be monitored.[280] No clinically significant signs of immunosuppression, opportunistic infection, or increase in malignancy have been documented. A small percentage of patients tested positive for anti-alefacept antibodies, but the titers were not associated with any hypersensitivity reactions and were not considered clinically significant.[279,280,284] Strong evidence supports the use of alefacept in the treatment of moderate to severe psoriasis. It appears to be an effective and well-tolerated agent producing prolonged disease remission. Use of alefacept is currently limited by the lack of long-term safety data and its significant cost.

Efalizumab. Efalizumab (Raptiva) was approved by the FDA in 2003 for the treatment of moderate to severe chronic plaque psoriasis. Efalizumab is a humanized monoclonal antibody directed against CD11, a subunit of the leukocyte function-associated antigen 1 (LFA-1) on the surface of T cells. Binding to CD11 blocks the interaction between the LFA-1 and intercellular adhesion molecule 1 (ICAM-1) on the cell surface and inhibits T-cell activation trafficking into the epidermis and dermis.[285]

A conditioning dose of 0.7 mg per kg is initially administered by subcutaneous injection and followed by weekly injections of 1 mg per kg. The maximum single dose should not exceed 200 mg.[286] Approximately 27% of patients treated with efalizumab achieved a 75% improvement in the psoriasis area and severity index at 12 weeks, compared to 4% of patients in the placebo group. The proportion of patients with "clear" or minimal disease at week 12 was 26% and 3% in the efalizumab and placebo groups, respectively.[285] Following treatment discontinuation, patients experienced gradual recurrence of disease. A small proportion of patients (0.7%) developed serious worsening of disease, including the development of erythrodermic or pustular forms of psoriasis, requiring hospitalization.[286] As defined by the National Psoriasis Foundation, rebound disease occurs with a 25% increase over baseline disease severity or with the emergence of a new psoriasis morphology within 12 weeks of therapy discontinuation. According to this definition, it is estimated that approximately 14% of patients develop rebound disease with abrupt discontinuation of therapy.[287]

Efalizumab was well tolerated in clinical trials, and the most commonly reported adverse events reported at an incidence of at least 5% higher in efalizumab-treated groups were flu-like symptoms consisting of headache, chills, fever, myalgias, and pain.[285] These reactions tended to occur after the first one or two injections. Approximately 3% of patients discontinued study drug because of an adverse event. Infections were reported in approximately 27% of patients treated with efalizumab, with the majority of infections being attributed to the common cold. Serious infections occurred in 0.5% of patients in both treatment groups. No clinically significant laboratory changes or increase in incidence of malignancy were observed. A small percentage of patients tested positive for anti-efalizumab antibodies, but the titers were not associated with any hypersensitivity reactions and were not considered clinically significant.

Etanercept. Etanercept (Enbrel) is a TNF-α inhibitor currently approved by the FDA for the treatment of rheumatoid arthritis, ankylosing spondylitis, psoriatic arthritis, and chronic moderate to severe plaque psoriasis. Etanercept is a recombinant human fusion protein composed of two TNF receptor components bound to the Fc portion of IgG. Etanercept binds to TNF with greater affinity than natural TNF receptors and inactivates this proinflammatory cytokine.[288]

Etanercept is indicated for the treatment of moderate to severe plaque psoriasis in adults who are candidates for systemic therapy. Etanercept is administered by subcutaneous injection, and patients initially receive 50 mg twice weekly for 3 months, followed by a reduction to 50 mg per week for maintenance dosing.[288] Approximately 50% of patients treated with etanercept 50 mg twice weekly achieved a 75% improvement in the psoriasis area and severity index at 12 weeks, compared to 34% of patients receiving etanercept 25 mg twice weekly. Etanercept appears to be an effective and well-tolerated agent for the treatment of moderate to severe psoriasis.[289]

Treatment with etanercept should be discontinued in patients who develop a serious infection and should not be initiated in patients with active infections. Although there was no difference in the frequency of infections requiring hospitalization between the etanercept and placebo groups, etanercept may increase the risk for developing infections.[290] TNF antagonist therapy may increase the risk for reactivation of latent tuberculosis (TB) infections.[291] The CDC recommends postponing TNF antagonist therapy until patients complete treatment for latent TB and active TB infections.[292] In a small subset of patients, TNF antagonists were associated with the development of new-onset heart failure and exacerbation of preexisting disease. Data from the FDA's Medwatch program indicated that 38 patients developed new-onset heart failure during TNF antagonist therapy, and 50% of these patients did not have an identifiable risk factor for heart failure.[293] Large-scale epidemiologic studies are necessary to formally evaluate the risk for developing lymphomas following TNF antagonist therapy. Although rare, drug-induced lupuslike reactions, seizure disorder, pancytopenia, allergic reactions, and demyelinating disorders such as multiple sclerosis have also been observed. The most common side effects were injection site reactions, including erythema, pruritus, pain, and swelling. Patients should be informed about the recommended injection sites and the importance of rotating the site of injection.[288]

Infliximab. Infliximab (Remicade), a humanized murine monoclonal antibody directed against TNF-α, irreversibly binds soluble and transmembrane bound TNF-α with high affinity. In vitro evidence suggests that binding to soluble TNF-α inhibits initiation of the inflammatory cytokine cascade, and binding to membrane-bound TNF-α results in cell lysis via complement or antibody-dependent mechanisms. Although currently FDA approved only for the treatment of Crohn's disease and rheumatoid arthritis, infliximab has been used for the treatment of psoriasis.[294]

The use of infliximab in the treatment of adults with moderate to severe plaque psoriasis has been evaluated in several placebo-controlled trials. In a study of 33 patients, infliximab was administered by intravenous injection and patients initially received placebo or 5 or 10 mg per kg weekly on weeks 0, 2, and 6: approximately 82% of patients treated with infliximab 5 mg per kg achieved a 75% improvement in the psoriasis area and severity index at 10 weeks, compared to 73% of patients receiving infliximab 10 mg per kg and 18% in the placebo group.[295] In another study of 249 patients, infliximab doses of 3 and 5 mg per kg given on weeks 0, 2, and 6 were compared to placebo: approximately 88% of patients treated with infliximab 5 mg per kg achieved a 75% improvement in the psoriasis area and severity index at 10 weeks, compared to 72% of patients receiving infliximab 3 mg per kg and 6% in the placebo group.[296] Infliximab also appears to be an effective and well-tolerated agent for the treatment of moderate to severe psoriasis.

Treatment with infliximab should be discontinued in patients who develop a serious infection and should not be initiated in patients with an active infection. Data from pooled infliximab trials showed an increased incidence of infection in patients receiving infliximab compared to placebo. Approximately 21% of patients treated with infliximab developed an infection.[294] Infliximab may also be associated with an increased risk for reactivation of latent TB infections compared to etanercept.[291] Infliximab is associated with the potential for exacerbating heart failure, development of lymphomas, and rare demyelinating disorders.[292,293] Infusion-related reactions, usually including fever or chills, and occasionally including pain, hypotension, and dyspnea, can occur.[294]

Pharmacoeconomics. The new biologic agents are expected to raise the already considerable cost of managing psoriasis. Alefacept is the most expensive biologic agent for use in psoriasis. The added expense can be attributed to the favorable safety profile and length of remission. The average wholesale price for one course of therapy is approximately $8,400.[297] When weekly CD4+ monitoring is included, the cost could be as high as $16,000. Medicare reimburses for in-office administration of alefacept in patients with moderate to severe chronic plaque psoriasis who are candidates for phototherapy or systemic therapy and failed to respond to topical therapy. Infliximab, etanercept, and adalimumab are not currently reimbursed under Medicare guidelines.[298]

CLINICAL VARIANTS AND SPECIFIC TREATMENT MODALITIES

Several clinical variants of psoriasis have been recognized that will determine the type of treatment modality. The following discussion summarizes specific treatment modalities for these clinical variants.

Children and adults with guttate psoriasis usually are given systemic antimicrobial treatment, based on either cultures or antibody titers showing group A streptococcal infection. For both erythrodermic and generalized pustular psoriasis, MTX and etretinate have been successful in controlling these eruptions. Localized psoriasis of the palms and soles responds well to PUVA treatments concentrated in these areas, and adding etretinate to PUVA is reported to be more effective than PUVA alone. Inverse psoriasis of the body folds with associated group B streptococcus colonization has been reported to respond to 2% erythromycin ointment.

IMPROVING OUTCOMES

The choice of treatment for plaque-type psoriasis depends on the extent of body surface involvement. For more localized disease, topical corticosteroids, calcipotriene, or tazarotene may be used. If more than 10% of the body surface is involved, then phototherapy, photochemotherapy, or systemic therapy should be considered. Methotrexate and retinoids are the most commonly used systemic treatment for plaque-type psoriasis. However, retinoids are less effective and are usually used in combination with other treatments.[299] The biologics appear to be a safer alternative to traditional systemic and phototherapy therapy, but they lack long-term safety data, must be administered via intravenous or IM routes, and are associated with significant drug costs. Lastly, the use of combination, rotational, and sequential treatment strategies affords increased treatment efficacy and the potential for minimizing long-term and dose-related side effects.

ROSACEA

DEFINITION

Rosacea is a syndrome initially characterized by episodic central facial flushing. Progressive disease includes the development of erythema, papules, pustules, and facial edema and can lead to facial disfigurement.[300] Although no cure is available, treatment can prevent the progression of this chronic condition.

EPIDEMIOLOGY

Rosacea, also called middle-age acne or acne rosacea, is a chronic inflammatory disease that affects 13 to 14 million Americans each year.[301] It is most common after the age of 30 and more prevalent in people of Celtic and northern European heritage.[302] Women are two to three times more likely to be affected by rosacea compared to their male counterparts, but men experience more severe expressions of the disease.[302–304]

ETIOLOGY

Rosacea is thought to result from a vascular disorder; and although many factors have been associated with the condition, a definite cause is still unknown.[305] The microscopic mite *Demodex folliculorum* has been implicated as a cause

of rosacea. Although the mite is a normal inhabitant of human skin, it was found to be prevalent in higher numbers in patients with rosacea. The authors concluded that the mite may have a role in aggravating rosacea, but it is an unlikely cause of rosacea.[304,306] Some studies previously suggested that *Helicobacter pylori* may play a role, but more recent investigations have produced conflicting results.[307,308]

PATHOPHYSIOLOGY

Pathologic findings of rosacea include erythema, telangiectasia, edema, connective tissue hypertrophy, and fibroplasias. Erythema is caused by dilation of blood vessels in the papillary dermis and increased blood flow in the superficial vasculature of the face. The increased blood flow can lead to an accumulation of extracellular fluid if the lymphatics cannot maintain homeostatic drainage, resulting in edema. Connective tissue hypertrophy and fibroplasias may be the result of an inflammatory response to chronic cutaneous edema.[304,309]

CLINICAL PRESENTATION AND DIAGNOSIS

Many patients with rosacea suffer emotionally from the disfiguring effects of the syndrome. A survey by the National

Rosacea Society reported nearly 70% of patients felt low self-esteem and believed that it adversely affected their professional interactions. Prerosacea begins with a gradual onset of transient flushing and erythema (Fig. 10.32). Patients may notice flares secondary to emotional stress, alcoholic or hot drinks, and hot or spicy foods. Sun damage is commonly associated with rosacea.

The National Rosacea Society's standard classification system describes the four subtypes and one variant of rosacea.[309] Progression from one subtype to another may or may not occur.

Erythematotelangiectatic rosacea is characterized by flushing and persistent central facial erythema. Papulopustular rosacea may develop over a period of months to years and is characterized by persistent erythema with telangiectasias and eventually erythematous papules and pustules, resembling acne. Unlike acne, open comedones are never seen in rosacea. Phymatous rosacea occurs in severe, chronic cases and includes thickening skin and irregular surface nodularities. Rhinophyma is the most common presentation (Fig. 10.33). This is the irreversible soft tissue hypertrophy of the nose, producing the "W.C. Fields nose," and is more common in men.[310] Ocular rosacea may occur in 30% to 50% of the patients; symptoms can include a foreign body sensation in the eye, burning, stinging, dry eyes, blepharitis, conjunctivitis, styes, and corneal ulceration.[302,308,311–313]

Granulomatous rosacea is a variant subtype and is characterized by hard yellow, brown, or red monomorphic cutaneous papules or nodules that may or may not be associated with phymas.

The excessive, regular use of topical fluorinated corticosteroids on the face can provoke a skin eruption clinically indistinguishable from rosacea and is termed steroid rosacea.[314]

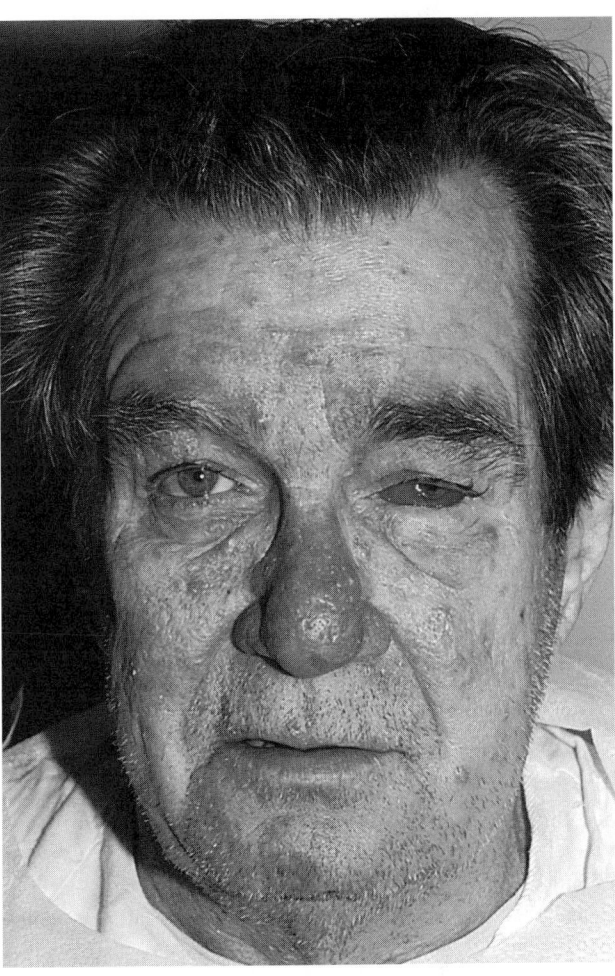

FIGURE 10.33 Rosacea is manifested by telangiectatic vessels on the skin—advanced case of rhinophyma. Blepharitis may also be associated (*see color insert*). (From Tasman W, Jaeger E. The Wills Eye Hospital atlas of clinical ophthalmology. 2nd ed. Lippincott Williams & Wilkins, 2001.)

TREATMENT

NONPHARMACOLOGIC THERAPY

Early rosacea, consisting primarily of vasodilation, is difficult to treat. Patients should be made aware of the stimuli commonly associated with the provocation of rosacea. The effects of these stimuli are variable and patient-specific. It is important to teach patients to evaluate the effect of these stimuli on their condition and to avoid the stimuli that aggravate their condition. Patients with rosacea who are sun sensitive should be counseled to use nonirritating sunblock. The presence of the protective ingredients dimethicone and cyclomethicone in sunblock preparations has been shown to decrease the irritation associated with PABA esters in patients with rosacea.[315]

PHARMACOTHERAPY

Topical metronidazole and oral tetracycline are the best-established treatment regimens for rosacea. Clinical improve-

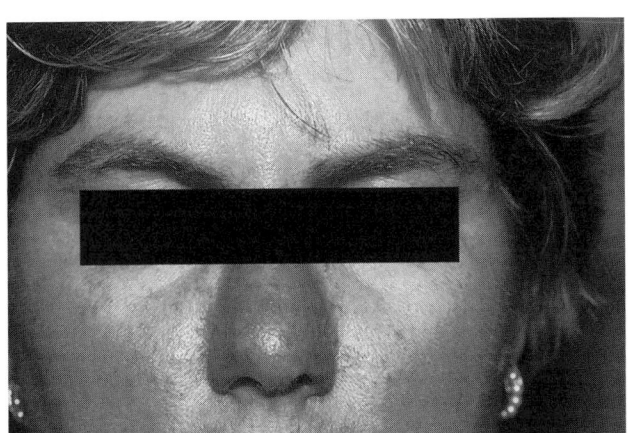

FIGURE 10.32 Prerosacea (*see color insert*). This woman has "rosy cheeks" and telangiectasias. (From Goodheart HP. Goodheart's photoguide of common skin disorders. 2nd ed. Philadelphia: Lippincott Williams & Wilkins, 2003.)

ment typically occurs between 1 to 3 months of therapy, and relapses often occur.[316] Prolonged treatment with topical metronidazole is often used to maintain remission.[317] Patients should be counseled on the expected treatment course to ensure a realistic understanding of the benefits of therapy and the importance of compliance.

Effective topical treatment includes metronidazole 0.75% gel, cream, or lotion twice daily, metronidazole 1% cream once daily, or clindamycin 1% lotion twice daily.[318–320] Sulfacetamide is available as 10% lotion or skin cleanser and may be effective for patients with rosacea but should be avoided in patients with sulfa allergies.[321] One study of 63 patients demonstrated that permethrin 5% cream applied twice daily was as effective as metronidazole 0.75% gel twice daily in the treatment of papulopustular rosacea.[322] Topical azelaic acid 20% cream applied twice daily has recently been shown to be as effective as topical metronidazole. Neither metronidazole or azelaic acid demonstrated any benefit in reducing telangiectasias or itching. In one study, azelaic acid 20% topical cream was associated with more stinging upon application but was preferred over metronidazole.[323] Patients should be instructed to apply a thin layer of topical medication uniformly over the entire affected areas rather than spotting inflammatory lesions.

The oral antibiotics are effective in the treatment of rosacea and include tetracycline 250 mg two to four times daily,[309] doxycycline 100 mg or 200 mg daily,[301] and minocycline 100 mg twice daily.[305,308,324] Metronidazole 200 mg twice daily, erythromycin 250 mg four times daily, and clarithromycin 250 mg to 500 mg twice daily have also demonstrated efficacy.[305,308,325] Oral and topical therapy is often initiated simultaneously; after inflammatory lesions clear, the oral therapy can be weaned.[309] Systemic isotretinoin, at a dosage of 0.5 to 1 mg per kg/day for 4 to 8 months, is a treatment option for severe disease.[326]

The treatment of ocular rosacea primarily consists of oral tetracycline and doxycycline. However, limited studies are available, and the optimal treatment dose or duration of therapy has not been established. Patients with severe disease should be referred to an ophthalmologist.[311,313]

Telangiectasias are often masked by erythema and become apparent after successful treatment of erythema.[309] Patients should be counseled about the appearance of telangiectasias to ensure that they do not attribute this condition to side effects from treatment of rosacea. Treatment of telangiectasias is limited to electrodestruction or laser techniques.[325] The only effective treatments for rhinophyma include cold steel, hot wire loop surgery, laser surgery, cryosurgery, and dermabrasion.[327]

Treatment of steroid-induced rosacea involves discontinuation of the topical steroid and administration of antihistamines, topical antibiotics, and oral tetracycline. Resolution can take several months. Steroid withdrawal leads to an intense rebound pustular reaction in 98% of patients. It is important to educate patients about this reaction to ensure that they do not attribute worsening symptoms to the discontinua-

tion of the steroid. Future therapy may include tacrolimus 0.075% ointment, as several case reports describe promising and rapid results.[314,328]

KEY POINTS

- Acne is a chronic condition and long-term therapy may be required.
- Acne treatment is directed at preventing new lesions, not treating existing lesions.
- Topical antibiotics are not useful in noninflammatory acne. They are most useful in mild to moderate inflammatory acne and as an adjunct in severe nodulocystic acne.
- Topical tretinoin is a superior agent for comedonal acne.
- Tetracycline and its derivatives and erythromycin are antibiotics of choice for moderate to severe inflammatory acne; however, therapy must be continued for at least 5 months and sometimes up to 2 years.
- Oral isotretinoin is the most effective agent for treating acne; however, potential teratogenicity and side effects warrant close patient monitoring.
- Blocking photodermatoses with protective clothing and sunscreens helps prevent chronic problems of photoaging and cancer. Treatment of these conditions is not as effective as prevention.
- Treatment options for warts are divided into chemical destructive therapy (acids, formalin, glutaraldehyde, cantharidin), physical destruction (cryotherapy, electrosurgery, surgical excision), chemotherapeutic agents (podophyllin, podophyllotoxin, 5-FU, bleomycin), immunotherapy (dinitrochlorobenzene, interferons, imiquimed), and retinoids.
- Therapies for seborrheic dermatitis include shampoos, topical antifungals, and corticosteroids.
- Psoriasis varies greatly in severity, and treatment must be based on a risk:benefit ratio.
- The selection of therapy for psoriasis depends on the location and clinical presentation.
- There is a wide range of therapies for psoriasis, and treatment must take into account the patient's quality of life.

SUGGESTED READINGS

Arnold HL, Odom RB, Berger TG. Warts. In: Andrews' Diseases of the Skin. 9th ed. Philadelphia: WB Saunders, 2000:509–520.

Callen JP, Krueger GG, Lebwohl M, et al. AAD consensus statement on psoriasis therapies. J Am Acad Dermatol 49:897–899, 2003.

Gollnick H, Cunliffe W, Berson D, et al. Management of acne: a report from a Global Alliance to Improve Outcomes in Acne. J Am Acad Dermatol 49:S1–37, 2003

Gupta AK, Bluhm R. Seborrheic dermatitis. J Eur Acad Dermatol Venereol 18:13–26, 2004.

REFERENCES

1. Gollnick H, Cunliffe W, Berson D, et al. Management of acne: a report from a Global Alliance to Improve Outcomes in Acne. J Am Acad Dermatol 49:S1–37, 2003.
2. Baur DA, Butler RC. Current concepts in the pathogenesis and treatment of acne. J Oral Maxillofac Surg 56:651–655, 1998.
3. Lucky AW. A review of infantile and pediatric acne. Dermatology 196:95–97, 1998.
4. Bataille V, Snieder H, MacGregor AJ, et al. The influence of genetics and environmental factors in the pathogenesis of acne: a twin study of acne in women. J Invest Dermatol 119:1317–1322, 2002.
5. Stewart ME, Downing DT, Cook JS, et al. Sebaceous gland activity and serum dehydroepiandrosterone sulfate levels in boys and girls. Arch Dermatol 128:1345–1348, 1992.
6. Beylot C, Doutre MS, Beylot-Barry M. Oral contraceptives and cyproterone acetate in female acne treatment. Dermatology 196:148–152, 1998.
7. Plewig G, Kligman AM. Acne and rosacea. 3rd ed. New York: Springer-Verlag, 2000.
8. Cunliffe WJ, Gollnick H. Acne: Diagnoses and management. London: Martin Dunitz, Ltd, 2001.
9. Nguyen QH, Kim YA, Schwartz RA. Management of acne vulgaris. Am Fam Physician 50:89–100, 1994.
10. Vowels BR, Yang S, Leyden JJ. Induction of proinflammatory cytokines by a soluble factor of Propionibacterium acnes: implications for chronic inflammatory acne. Infect Immun 63:3158–3165, 1995.
11. Eady EA. Bacterial resistance in acne. Dermatology 196:59–66, 1998.
12. Leyden JJ. A review of the use of combination therapies for the treatment of acne vulgaris. J Am Acad Dermatol 49:S200–210, 2003.
13. Shalita AR, Leyden JJ. New insights into pathogenesis of acne. 15 Symposium Digest 3:25–32, 1991.
14. Eady EA, Cove JH, Holland KT, et al. Superior antibacterial action and reduced incidence of bacterial resistance in minocycline compared to tetracycline-treated acne patients. Br J Dermatol 122:233–244, 1990.
15. Eady EA, Bojar RA, Jones CE, et al. The effects of acne treatment with a combination of benzoyl peroxide and erythromycin on skin carriage of erythromycin-resistant propionibacteria. Br J Dermatol 134:107–113, 1996.
16. Toyoda M, Morohashi M. An overview of topical antibiotics for acne treatment. Dermatology 196:130–134, 1998.
17. Leyden JJ, Hickman JG, Jarratt MT, et al. The efficacy and safety of a combination benzoyl peroxide/clindamycin topical gel compared with benzoyl peroxide alone and a benzoyl peroxide/erythromycin combination product. J Cutan Med Surg 5:37–42, 2001.
18. Cunliffe WJ, Holland KT, Bojar R, et al. A randomized, double-blind comparison of a clindamycin phosphate/benzoyl peroxide gel formulation and a matching clindamycin gel with respect to microbiologic activity and clinical efficacy in the topical treatment of acne vulgaris. Clin Ther 24:1117–1133, 2002.
19. Ellis CN, Leyden J, Katz HI, et al. Therapeutic studies with a new combination benzoyl peroxide/clindamycin topical gel in acne vulgaris. Cutis 67:13–20, 2001.
20. Eady EA, Farmery MR, Ross JI, et al. Effects of benzoyl peroxide and erythromycin alone and in combination against antibiotic-sensitive and -resistant skin bacteria from acne patients. Br J Dermatol 131:331–336, 1994.
21. Bojar RA, Cunliffe WJ, Holland KT. The short-term treatment of acne vulgaris with benzoyl peroxide: effects on the surface and follicular cutaneous microflora. Br J Dermatol 132:204–208, 1995.
22. Leyden JJ. Therapy for acne vulgaris. N Engl J Med 336:1156–1162, 1997.
23. Liden S, Lindelof B, Sparen P. Is benzoyl peroxide carcinogenic? Br J Dermatol 123:129–130, 1990.
24. Kraus AL, Munro IC, Orr JC, et al. Benzoyl peroxide: an integrated human safety assessment for carcinogenicity. Regul Toxicol Pharmacol 21:87–107, 1995.
25. Orfanos CE, Zouboulis CC. Oral retinoids in the treatment of seborrhoea and acne. Dermatology 196:140–147, 1998.
26. Leyden J, Grove G, Zerweck C. Facial tolerability of topical retinoid therapy. J Drugs Dermatol 3:641–651, 2004.
27. Leyden JJ. Meta-analysis of topical tazarotene in the treatment of mild to moderate acne. Cutis 74:9–15, 2004.
28. Haider A, Shaw JC. Treatment of acne vulgaris. JAMA 292:726–735, 2004.
29. Martinez-Frias ML, Rodriguez-Pinilla E. First-trimester exposure to topical tretinoin: its safety is not warranted. Teratology 60:5, 1999.
30. Jick SS, Terris BZ, Jick H. First-trimester topical tretinoin and congenital disorders. Lancet 341:1181–1182, 1993.
31. Lipson AH, Collins F, Webster WS. Multiple congenital defects associated with maternal use of topical tretinoin. Lancet 341:1352–1353, 1993.
32. Camera G, Pregliasco P. Ear malformation in baby born to mother using tretinoin cream. Lancet 339:687, 1992.
33. Shapiro L, Pastuszak A, Curto G, et al. Safety of first-trimester exposure to topical tretinoin: prospective cohort study. Lancet 350:1143–1144, 1997.
34. Navarre-Belhassen C, Blanchet P, Hillaire-Buys D, et al. Multiple congenital malformations associated with topical tretinoin. Ann Pharmacother 32:505–506, 1998.
35. Monga M. Vitamin A and its congeners. Semin Perinatol 21:135–142, 1997.
36. Leyden JJ. Antibiotic resistance in the topical treatment of acne vulgaris. Cutis 73:6–10, 2004.
37. Trexler MF, Fraser TG, Jones MP. Fulminant pseudomembranous colitis caused by clindamycin phosphate vaginal cream. Am J Gastroenterol 92:2112–2113, 1997.
38. Chu A, Huber FJ, Plott RT. The comparative efficacy of benzoyl peroxide 5%/erythromycin 3% gel and erythromycin 4%/zinc 1.2% solution in the treatment of acne vulgaris. Br J Dermatol 136:235–238, 1997.
39. Brown SK, Shalita AR. Acne vulgaris. Lancet 351:1871–1876, 1998.
40. Gibson JR. Azelaic acid 20% cream (AZELEX) and the medical management of acne vulgaris. Dermatol Nurs 9:339–344, 1997.
41. Hjorth N, Graupe K. Azelaic acid for the treatment of acne. A clinical comparison with oral tetracycline. Acta Derm Venereol (Stockh) 143(Suppl):45–48, 1989.
42. Gollnick HP, Graupe K, Zaumseil RP. Comparison of combined azelaic acid cream plus oral minocycline with oral isotretinoin in severe acne. Eur J Dermatol 11:538–544, 2001.
43. Graupe K, Cunliffe WJ, Gollnick HP, et al. Efficacy and safety of topical azelaic acid (20 percent cream): an overview of results from European clinical trials and experimental reports. Cutis 57:20–35, 1996.
44. Johnson BA, Nunley JR. Topical therapy for acne vulgaris. How do you choose the best drug for each patient? Postgrad Med 107:69–80, 2000.
45. Lookingbill DP, Abrams BB, Ellis CN, et al. Inocoterone and acne. The effect of a topical antiandrogen: results of a multicenter clinical trial. Arch Dermatol 128:1197–1200, 1992.
46. Burke B, Eady EA, Cunliffe WJ. Benzoyl peroxide versus topical erythromycin in the treatment of acne vulgaris. Br J Dermatol 108:199–204, 1983.
47. Battmann T, Bonfils A, Branche C, et al. RU 58841, a new specific topical antiandrogen: a candidate of choice for the treatment of acne, androgenetic alopecia and hirsutism. J Steroid Biochem Mol Biol 48:55–60, 1994.
48. Gottlieb A. Safety of minocycline for acne. Lancet 349:374, 1997.
49. Goulden V, Glass D, Cunliffe WJ. Safety of long-term high-dose minocycline in the treatment of acne. Br J Dermatol 134:693–695, 1996.
50. Driscoll MS, Rothe MJ, Abrahamian L, et al. Long-term oral antibiotics for acne: is laboratory monitoring necessary? J Am Acad Dermatol 28:595–602, 1993.
51. Hughes BR, Cunliffe WJ. Interactions between the oral contraceptive pill and antibiotics. Br J Dermatol 122:717–718, 1990.
52. Eady AE, Cove JH, Layton AM. Is antibiotic resistance in cutaneous propionibacteria clinically relevant? Implications of resistance for acne patients and prescribers. Am J Clin Dermatol 4:813–831, 2003.
53. Ross JI, Snelling AM, Carnegie E, et al. Antibiotic-resistant acne: lessons from Europe. Br J Dermatol 148:467–478, 2003.

54. Meigel WN. How safe is oral isotretinoin? Dermatology 195(Suppl 1):22–40, 1997.

55. Leyden JJ, McGinley KJ, Foglia AN. Qualitative and quantitative changes in cutaneous bacteria associated with systemic isotretinoin therapy for acne conglobata. J Invest Dermatol 86:390–393, 1986.

56. White GM, Chen W, Yao J, et al. Recurrence rates after the first course of isotretinoin. Arch Dermatol 134:376–378, 1998.

57. Stainforth JM, Layton AM, Taylor JP, et al. Isotretinoin for the treatment of acne vulgaris: which factors may predict the need for more than one course? Br J Dermatol 129:297–301, 1993.

58. Barth JH, Macdonald-Hull SP, Mark J, et al. Isotretinoin therapy for acne vulgaris: a re-evaluation of the need for measurements of plasma lipids and liver function tests. Br J Dermatol 129:704–707, 1993.

59. Goldsmith LA, Bolognia JL, Callen JP, et al. American Academy of Dermatology Consensus Conference on the safe and optimal use of isotretinoin: summary and recommendations. J Am Acad Dermatol 50:900–906, 2004.

60. Leachman SA, Insogna KL, Katz L, et al. Bone densities in patients receiving isotretinoin for cystic acne. Arch Dermatol 135:961–965, 1999.

61. Jacobs DG, Deutsch NL, Brewer M. Suicide, depression, and isotretinoin: is there a causal link? J Am Acad Dermatol 45:S168–175, 2001.

62. Strauss JS, Leyden JJ, Lucky AW, et al. Safety of a new micronized formulation of isotretinoin in patients with severe recalcitrant nodular acne: a randomized trial comparing micronized isotretinoin with standard isotretinoin. J Am Acad Dermatol 45:196–207, 2001.

63. Strauss JS, Leyden JJ, Lucky AW, et al. A randomized trial of the efficacy of a new micronized formulation versus a standard formulation of isotretinoin in patients with severe recalcitrant nodular acne. J Am Acad Dermatol 45:187–195, 2001.

64. Pochoi PE. The pathogenesis and treatment of acne. Ann Rev Med 41:187–198, 1990.

65. Lucky AW, Henderson TA, Olson WH, et al. Effectiveness of norgestimate and ethinyl estradiol in treating moderate acne vulgaris. J Am Acad Dermatol 37:746–754, 1997.

66. Redmond GP, Olson WH, Lippman JS, et al. Norgestimate and ethinyl estradiol in the treatment of acne vulgaris: a randomized, placebo-controlled trial. Obstet Gynecol 89:615–622, 1997.

67. Vessey M, Painter R, Yeates D. Mortality in relation to oral contraceptive use and cigarette smoking. Lancet 362:185–191, 2003.

68. Sciarra F, Toscano V, Concolino G, et al. Antiandrogens: clinical applications. J Steroid Biochem Mol Biol 37:349–362, 1990.

69. Sawaya ME, Hordinsky MK. The antiandrogens. When and how they should be used. Dermatol Clin 11:65–72, 1993.

70. van Wayjen RG, van den Ende A. Experience in the long-term treatment of patients with hirsutism and/or acne with cyproterone acetate-containing preparations: efficacy, metabolic and endocrine effects. Exp Clin Endocrinol Diabetes 103:241–251, 1995.

71. Muhlemann MF, Carter GD, Cream JJ, et al. Oral spironolactone: an effective treatment for acne vulgaris in women. Br J Dermatol 115:227–232, 1986.

72. Goodfellow A, Alaghband-Zadeh J, Carter G, et al. Oral spironolactone improves acne vulgaris and reduces sebum excretion. Br J Dermatol 111:209–214, 1984.

73. Pathak MA, Fitzpatrick TB, Greiter F, et al. Preventive treatment of sunburn, dermatoheliosis, and skin cancer with sun protective agents. In: Fitzpatrick TB, Eisen AZ, Wolff K, et al, eds. Dermatology in general medicine. 4th ed. New York: McGraw-Hill, 1993:1689–1717.

74. Braun-Falco O, Plewig G, Wolff HH, et al. Dermatology. 3rd ed. Berlin: Springer-Verlag, 1991.

75. Soter NA. Acute effects of ultraviolet radiation on the skin. Semin Dermatol 9:11–15, 1990.

76. Preston DS, Stern RS. Nonmelanoma cancers of the skin. N Engl J Med 327:1649–1662, 1992.

77. Burren R, Scaletta C, Frenk E, et al. Sunlight and carcinogenesis: expression of p53 and pyrimidine dimers in human skin following UVA I, UVA I + II and solar simulating radiations. Int J Cancer 76:201–206, 1998.

78. Chapman MS. Sunscreens: the importance of UVA protection. Medscape Website. Available at: http://www.medscape.com/viewprogram/1760_pnt. Accessed March 30, 2004.

79. Young AR. Cumulative effects of ultraviolet radiation on the skin: cancer and photoaging. Semin Dermatol 9:25–31, 1990.

80. Diffey BL. Human exposure to ultraviolet radiation. Semin Dermatol 9:2–10, 1990.

81. Scarlett WL. Ultraviolet radiation: sun exposure, tanning beds, and vitamin D levels. What you need to know and how to decrease the risk of skin cancer. J Am Osteopath Assoc 103:371–375, 2003.

82. Health issues of ultraviolet tanning appliances used for cosmetic purposes. Health Phys 84:119–127, 2003.

83. Eller MS, Ostrom K, Gilchrest BA. DNA damage enhances melanogenesis. Proc Natl Acad Sci USA 93:1087–1092, 1996.

84. Drake LA, Ceilley RI, Cornelison RL, et al. Guidelines of care for actinic keratoses. Committee on Guidelines of Care. J Am Acad Dermatol 32:95–98, 1995.

85. Foote JA, Harris RB, Giuliano AR, et al. Predictors for cutaneous basal- and squamous-cell carcinoma among actinically damaged adults. Int J Cancer 95:7–11, 2001.

86. Stern RS. Clinical practice. Treatment of photoaging. N Engl J Med 350:1526–1534, 2004.

87. Skin Cancer Facts. American Cancer Society Web site. Available at: http://www.cancer.org/docroot/PED/content/ped_7_1_What_You_Need_To_Know_About_Skin_Cancer.asp?sitearea = &level = . Accessed Feb. 28, 2005.

88. Matsumura Y, Ananthaswamy HN. Toxic effects of ultraviolet radiation on the skin. Toxicol Appl Pharmacol 195:298–308, 2004.

89. Greenlee RT, Hill-Harmon MB, Murray T, et al. Cancer statistics, 2001. CA Cancer J Clin 51:15–36, 2001.

90. Elwood JM, Jopson J. Melanoma and sun exposure: an overview of published studies. Int J Cancer 73:198–203, 1997.

91. Gallagher RP, Hill GB, Bajdik CD, et al. Sunlight exposure, pigmentation factors, and risk of nonmelanocytic skin cancer. II. Squamous cell carcinoma. Arch Dermatol 131:164–169, 1995.

92. Gallagher RP, Hill GB, Bajdik CD, et al. Sunlight exposure, pigmentary factors, and risk of nonmelanocytic skin cancer. I. Basal cell carcinoma. Arch Dermatol 131:157–163, 1995.

93. FDA/CFSAN Information about Suntan Products, Sunscreens, and Tanning. Food and Drug Administration Web site. Available at: http://www.cfsan.fda.gov/~dms/cos-sun.html.

94. Taylor CR, Stern RS, Leyden JJ, et al. Photoaging/photodamage and photoprotection. J Am Acad Dermatol 22:1–15, 1990.

95. Lowe NJ. Sunscreens and the prevention of skin aging. J Dermatol Surg Oncol 16:936–938, 1990.

96. Boger J, Araujo OE, Flowers F. Sunscreens: efficacy, use, and misuse. South Med J 77:1421–1427, 1984.

97. Herzog B, Katzenstein A, Quass K, et al. Physical properties of organic particulate UV-absorbers used in sunscreens. I. Determination of particle size with fiber-optic quasi-elastic light scattering (FOQELS), disc centrifugation, and laser diffractometry. J Colloid Interface Sci 271:136–144, 2004.

98. Pathak MA. Sunscreens: topical and systemic approaches for protection of human skin against harmful effects of solar radiation. J Am Acad Dermatol 7:285–312, 1982.

99. Federal Register. Sunscreen drug products for over-the-counter human drugs: proposed safety, effective, and labeling conditions. Washington, DC: Department of Health, Education and Welfare, Food and Drug Administration, Aug. 25, 1978;43:38206–38269.

100. Sunscreen Regulations Finalized. Food and Drug Administration Web site. Available at: http://www.fda.gov/bbs/topics/ANSWERS/ANS00955.html. Accessed Feb. 27, 2005.

101. Pinnell SR. Cutaneous photodamage, oxidative stress, and topical antioxidant protection. J Am Acad Dermatol 48:1–22, 2003.

102. Bech-Thomsen N, Wulf HC. Sunbathers' application of sunscreen is probably inadequate to obtain the sun protection factor assigned to the preparation. Photodermatol Photoimmunol Photomed 9:242–244, 1992.

103. Lowe NJ. Photoprotection. Semin Dermatol 9:78–83, 1990.

104. Naylor MF, Farmer KC. The case for sunscreens. A review of their use in preventing actinic damage and neoplasia. Arch Dermatol 133:1146–54, 1997.

105. Marks R, Foley PA, Jolley D, et al. The effect of regular sunscreen use on vitamin D levels in an Australian population. Results of a randomized controlled trial. Arch Dermatol 131:415–421, 1995.

106. Black HS. Systemic photoprotective agents. Photodermatology 4:187–195, 1987.

107. Swanbeck G. Aminoquinolones. In: Fitzpatrick TB, Eisen AZ, Wolff K, et al, eds. Dermatology in general medicine. 4th ed. New York: McGraw-Hill, 1993:2869–2871.
108. Kang S, Fisher GJ, Voorhees JJ. Photoaging and topical tretinoin: therapy, pathogenesis, and prevention. Arch Dermatol 133:1280–1284, 1997.
109. Van Scott EJ, Ditre CM, Yu RJ. Alpha-hydroxyacids in the treatment of signs of photoaging. Clin Dermatol 14:217–226, 1996.
110. Stiller MJ, Bartolone J, Stern R, et al. Topical 8% glycolic acid and 8% L-lactic acid creams for the treatment of photodamaged skin. A double-blind vehicle-controlled clinical trial. Arch Dermatol 132:631–636, 1996.
111. Thibault PK, Wlodarczyk J, Wenck A. A double-blind randomized clinical trial on the effectiveness of a daily glycolic acid 5% formulation in the treatment of photoaging. Dermatol Surg 24:573–578, 1998.
112. Center for Food Safety and Applied Nutrition. AHAs and UV sensitivity: results of new FDA-sponsored studies. Office of Cosmetics and Colors fact sheet. Rockville, MD: Food and Drug Administration, March 7, 2000.
113. Yu RJ, Van Scott EJ. Hydroxycarboxylic acids, N-acetylamino sugars, and N-acetylamino acids. Skinmed 1:117–126, 2002.
114. Grimes PE, Green BA, Wildnauer RH, et al.The use of polyhydroxy acids (PHAs) in photoaged skin. Cutis 73:3–13, 2004.
115. Goette DK. Topical chemotherapy with 5-fluorouracil. A review. J Am Acad Dermatol 4:633–649, 1981.
116. Tutrone WD, Saini R, Caglar S, et al. Topical therapy for actinic keratoses, II: Diclofenac, colchicine, and retinoids. Cutis 71:373–379, 2003.
117. An KP, Athar M, Tang X, et al. Cyclooxygenase-2 expression in murine and human nonmelanoma skin cancers: implications for therapeutic approaches. Photochem Photobiol 76:73–80, 2002.
118. Wolf JE, Jr., Taylor JR, Tschen E, et al. Topical 3.0% diclofenac in 2.5% hyaluronan gel in the treatment of actinic keratoses. Int J Dermatol 40:709–713, 2001.
119. Aldara [package insert]. Northridge, CA: 3M Pharmaceuticals; 2004.
120. Skinner RB, Jr. Imiquimod. Dermatol Clin 21:291–300, 2003.
121. Lebwohl M, Dinehart S, Whiting D, et al. Imiquimod 5% cream for the treatment of actinic keratosis: results from two phase III, randomized, double-blind, parallel group, vehicle-controlled trials. J Am Acad Dermatol 50:714–721, 2004.
122. Olsen EA, Abernethy ML, Kulp-Shorten C, et al. A double-blind, vehicle-controlled study evaluating masoprocol cream in the treatment of actinic keratoses on the head and neck. J Am Acad Dermatol 24:738–743, 1991.
123. Arnold HL, Odom RB, Berger TG. Warts. In: Andrews' diseases of the skin. 9th ed. Philadelphia: WB Saunders, 2000:509–520.
124. Cobb MW. Human papillomavirus infection. J Am Acad Dermatol 22:547–566, 1990.
125. Drake LA, Ceilley RI, Cornelison RL, et al. Guidelines of care for warts: human papillomavirus. Committee on Guidelines of Care. J Am Acad Dermatol 32:98–103, 1995.
126. Sterling JC, Handfield-Jones S, Hudson PM. Guidelines for the management of cutaneous warts. Br J Dermatol 144:4–11, 2001.
127. Bouwes Bavinck JN, Feltkamp M, Struijk L, et al. Human papillomavirus infection and skin cancer risk in organ transplant recipients. J Investig Dermatol Symp Proc 6:207–211, 2001.
128. Pruvost C, Penso-Assathiany D, Bachot N, et al. [Risk factors for cutaneous wart onset in transplant recipients]. Ann Dermatol Venereol 129:291–293, 2002.
129. Jablonska S, Majewski S, Obalek S, et al. Cutaneous warts. Clin Dermatol 15:309–319, 1997.
130. Koutsky L. Epidemiology of genital human papillomavirus infection. Am J Med 102:3–8, 1997.
131. Fazel N, Wilczynski S, Lowe L, et al. Clinical, histopathologic, and molecular aspects of cutaneous human papillomavirus infections. Dermatol Clin 17:521–536, viii, 1999.
132. Holmes KK, Levine R, Weaver M. Effectiveness of condoms in preventing sexually transmitted infections. Bull World Health Organ 82:454–461, 2004.
133. de Villiers EM, Fauquet C, Broker TR, et al. Classification of papillomaviruses. Virology 324:17–27, 2004.
134. Beutner KR, Tyring S. Human papillomavirus and human disease. Am J Med 102:9–15, 1997.
135. Penneys N. Diseases caused by viruses. In: Elder D, Elenitsas R, Jaworsky C, et al., eds. Lever's histopathology of the skin. 5th ed. Philadelphia: Lippincott-Raven, 1997:569–589.
136. Verdon ME. Issues in the management of human papillomavirus genital disease. Am Fam Physician 55:1813–1822, 1997.
137. Plasencia JM. Cutaneous warts: diagnosis and treatment. Primary Care 27:423–434, 2000.
138. Lowy DR, Androphy EJ. Warts. In: Fitzpatrick TB, ed. Dermatology in general medicine. 3rd ed. New York: McGraw-Hill, 1987:2355–2372.
139. Wiley DJ, Douglas J, Beutner K, et al. External genital warts: diagnosis, treatment, and prevention. Clin Infect Dis 35:S210–224, 2002.
140. Gibbs S, Harvey I, Sterling JC, et al. Local treatments for cutaneous warts. Cochrane Database Syst Rev 2003:CD001781.
141. Food and Drug Administration Health and Human Services. Wart removal drug products for over-the-counter human use: final monograph. 21 CFR, part 358, 1991.
142. Steele K, Shirodaria P, O'Hare M, et al. Monochloroacetic acid and 60% salicylic acid as a treatment for simple plantar warts: effectiveness and mode of action. Br J Dermatol 118:537–543, 1988.
143. 1998 guidelines for treatment of sexually transmitted diseases. Centers for Disease Control and Prevention. MMWR Recomm Rep 47:1–111, 1998.
144. Benton EC. Therapy of cutaneous warts. Clin Dermatol 15:449–455, 1997.
145. Hirose R, Hori M, Shukuwa T, et al. Topical treatment of resistant warts with glutaraldehyde. J Dermatol 21:248–253, 1994.
146. Mroczkowski TF, McEwen C. Warts and other human papillomavirus infections. Postgrad Med 78:91–98, 1985.
147. Stone KM, Becker TM, Hadgu A, et al. Treatment of external genital warts: a randomised clinical trial comparing podophyllin, cryotherapy, and electrodesiccation. Genitourinary Med 66:16–19, 1990.
148. Jensen SL. Comparison of podophyllin application with simple surgical excision in clearance and recurrence of perianal condylomata acuminata. Lancet 2:1146–1148, 1985.
149. Rapini RP. Venereal warts. Primary Care 17:127–144, 1990.
150. Miller RA. Podophyllin. Int J Dermatol 24:491–498, 1985.
151. Campbell BJ. The treatment of warts. Primary Care 13:465–476, 1986.
152. Longstaff E, von Krogh G. Condyloma eradication: self-therapy with 0.15–0.5% podophyllotoxin versus 20–25% podophyllin preparations: an integrated safety assessment. Regul Toxicol Pharmacol 33:117–137, 2001.
153. Rivera A, Tyring SK. Therapy of cutaneous human papillomavirus infections. Dermatol Ther 17:441–448, 2004.
154. Cassidy DE, Drewry J, Fanning JP. Podophyllum toxicity: a report of a fatal case and a review of the literature. J Toxicol Clin Toxicol 19:35–44, 1982.
155. Condylox solution [package insert]. San Rafael, CA: Oclassen Pharmaceuticals; 1997.
156. Condylox gel [package insert]. San Rafael, CA: Oclassen Pharmaceuticals; 1997.
157. Tyring S, Edwards L, Cherry LK, et al. Safety and efficacy of 0.5% podofilox gel in the treatment of anogenital warts. Arch Dermatol 134:33–38, 1998.
158. Beutner KR, von Krogh G. Current status of podophyllotoxin for the treatment of genital warts. Semin Dermatol 9:148–151, 1990.
159. Edwards A, Atma-Ram A, Thin RN. Podophyllotoxin 0.5% v podophyllin 20% to treat penile warts. Genitourinary Med 64:263–265, 1988.
160. Gibbs S, Harvey I, Sterling J, et al. Local treatments for cutaneous warts: systematic review. Br Med J 325:461, 2002.
161. Shumer SM, O'Keefe EJ. Bleomycin in the treatment of recalcitrant warts. J Am Acad Dermatol 9:91–96, 1983.
162. Shelley WB, Shelley ED. Intralesional bleomycin sulfate therapy for warts. A novel bifurcated needle puncture technique. Arch Dermatol 127:234–236, 1991.
163. Munn SE, Higgins E, Marshall M, et al. A new method of intralesional bleomycin therapy in the treatment of recalcitrant warts. Br J Dermatol 135:969–971, 1996.

164. Edwards L, Ferenczy A, Eron L, et al. Self-administered topical 5% imiquimod cream for external anogenital warts. HPV Study Group. Arch Dermatol 134:25–30, 1998.

165. Beutner KR, Ferenczy A. Therapeutic approaches to genital warts. Am J Med 102:28–37, 1997.

166. Naylor MF, Neldner KH, Yarbrough GK, et al. Contact immuno-therapy of resistant warts. J Am Acad Dermatol 19:679–683, 1988.

167. Higgins E, du Vivier A. Topical immunotherapy: unapproved uses, dosages, or indications. Clin Dermatol 20:515–521, 2002.

168. Buckley DA, Du Vivier AW. The therapeutic use of topical contact sensitizers in benign dermatoses. Br J Dermatol 145:385–405, 2001.

169. Rogers CJ, Gibney MD, Siegfried EC, et al. Cimetidine therapy for recalcitrant warts in adults: is it any better than placebo? J Am Acad Dermatol 41:123–127, 1999.

170. Tsambaos D, Georgiou S, Monastirli A, et al. Treatment of condy-lomata acuminata with oral isotretinoin. J Urol 158:1810–1812, 1997.

171. Georgala S, Katoulis AC, Georgala C, et al. Oral isotretinoin in the treatment of recalcitrant condylomata acuminata of the cervix: a randomised placebo controlled trial. Sexually Transmitted Infec-tions 80:216–218, 2004.

172. Lutzner MA, Blanchet-Bardon C. Oral retinoid treatment of human papillomavirus type 5-induced epidermodysplasia verruciformis. N Engl J Med 302:1091, 1980.

173. Gross G, Pfister H, Hagedorn M, et al. Effect of oral aromatic reti-noid (Ro 10–9359) on human papilloma virus-2-induced common warts. Dermatologica 166:48–53, 1983.

174. Bolton RA. Nongenital warts: classification and treatment options. Am Fam Physician 43:2049–2056, 1991.

175. Accutane [package insert]. Nutley, NJ: Roche Laboratories Inc; 2002.

176. Vistide [package insert]. Foster City, CA: Gilead Sciences, Inc; 2000.

177. Bernard HU. Established and potential strategies against papillo-mavirus infections. J Antimicrob Chemother 53:137–139, 2004.

178. Toro JR, Sanchez S, Turiansky G, et al. Topical cidofovir for the treatment of dermatologic conditions: verruca, condyloma, intraepi-thelial neoplasia, herpes simplex and its potential use in smallpox. Dermatol Clin 21:301–309, 2003.

179. Snoeck R, Bossens M, Parent D, et al. Phase II double-blind, placebo-controlled study of the safety and efficacy of cidofovir topi-cal gel for the treatment of patients with human papillomavirus in-fection. Clin Infect Dis 33:597–602, 2001.

180. Harper DM, Franco EL, Wheeler C, et al. Efficacy of a bivalent L1 virus-like particle vaccine in prevention of infection with human papillomavirus types 16 and 18 in young women: a ran-domised controlled trial. Lancet 364:1757–1765, 2004.

181. Pagliusi SR, Teresa Aguado M. Efficacy and other milestones for human papillomavirus vaccine introduction. Vaccine 23:569–578, 2004.

182. Erchiga VC, Martos OJ, Cassano AV, et al. Malassezia globosa as the causative agent of pityriasis versicolor. Br J Dermatol 143: 799–803, 2000.

183. Johnson BA, Nunley JR. Treatment of seborrheic dermatitis. Am Fam Physician 61:2703–2714, 2000.

184. Zouboulis CC, Xia L, Akamatsu H, et al. The human sebocyte cul-ture model provides new insights into development and manage-ment of seborrhoea and acne. Dermatology 196:21–31, 1998.

185. Gupta AK, Bluhm R. Seborrheic dermatitis. J Eur Acad Dermatol Venereol 18:13–26, 2004.

186. Berger RS, Stoner MF, Hobbs ER, et al. Cutaneous manifestations of early human immunodeficiency virus exposure. J Am Acad Der-matol 19:298–303, 1988.

187. Marino CT, McDonald E, Romano JF. Seborrheic dermatitis in ac-quired immunodeficiency syndrome. Cutis 48:217–218, 1991.

188. Cowley NC, Farr PM, Shuster S. The permissive effect of sebum in seborrhoeic dermatitis: an explanation of the rash in neurological disorders. Br J Dermatol 122:71–76, 1990.

189. Gupta AK, Bluhm R, Cooper EA, et al. Seborrheic dermatitis. Der-matol Clin 21:401–412, 2003.

190. Hay RJ, Graham-Brown RA. Dandruff and seborrhoeic dermatitis: causes and management. Clin Exp Dermatol 22:3–6, 1997.

191. Parry ME, Sharpe GR. Seborrhoeic dermatitis is not caused by an altered immune response to Malassezia yeast. Br J Dermatol 139: 254–263, 1998.

192. Shuster S. The aetiology of dandruff and the mode of action of therapeutic agents. Br J Dermatol 111:235–242, 1984.

193. Faergemann J, Jones JC, Hettler O, Loria Y. Pityrosporum ovale (Malassezia furfur) as the causative agent of seborrhoeic dermatitis: new treatment options. Br J Dermatol 134(Suppl 46):12–38, 1996.

194. Soeprono FF, Schinella RA, Cockerell CJ, et al. Seborrheic-like dermatitis of acquired immunodeficiency syndrome. A clinicopatho-logic study. J Am Acad Dermatol 14:242–248, 1986.

195. Matis WL, Triana A, Shapiro R, et al. Dermatologic findings asso-ciated with human immunodeficiency virus infection. J Am Acad Dermatol 17:746–751, 1987.

196. Brown M, Evans TW, Tooley PJH. The role of ketoconazole 2% shampoo in the treatment and prophylactic management of dan-druff. J Dermatol Treat 1:177–179, 1990.

197. Guin JD. Complications of topical hydrocortisone. J Am Acad Der-matol 4:417–422, 1981.

198. Green CA, Farr PM, Shuster S. Treatment of seborrhoeic derma-titis with ketoconazole: II. Response of seborrhoeic dermatitis of the face, scalp and trunk to topical ketoconazole. Br J Dermatol 116:217–221, 1987.

199. Aly R, Katz HI, Kempers SE, et al. Ciclopirox gel for seborrheic dermatitis of the scalp. Int J Dermatol 42(Suppl 1):19–22, 2003.

200. Faergemann J. Management of seborrheic dermatitis and pityriasis versicolor. Am J Clin Dermatol 1:75–80, 2000.

201. Cauwenbergh G, Degreef H, Heykants J, et al. Pharmacokinetic profile of orally administered itraconazole in human skin. J Am Acad Dermatol 18:263–268, 1988.

202. Leeming JP, Sansom JE, Burton JL. Susceptibility of Malassezia furfur subgroups to terbinafine. Br J Dermatol 137:764–67, 1997.

203. Scaparro E, Quadri G, Virno G, et al. Evaluation of the efficacy and tolerability of oral terbinafine (Daskil) in patients with sebor-hoeic dermatitis. A multicentre, randomized, investigator-blinded, placebo-controlled trial. Br J Dermatol 144:854–857, 2001.

204. Peter RU, Richarz-Barthauer U. Successful treatment and prophy-laxis of scalp seborrhoeic dermatitis and dandruff with 2% ketoco-nazole shampoo: results of a multicentre, double-blind, placebo-controlled trial. Br J Dermatol 132:441–445, 1995.

205. Taieb A, Legrain V, Palmier C, et al. Topical ketoconazole for in-fantile seborrhoeic dermatitis. Dermatologica 181:26–32, 1990.

206. Buchness MR. Treatment of skin diseases in HIV-infected patients. Dermatol Clin 13:231–238, 1995.

207. Guidelines of care for psoriasis. Committee on Guidelines of Care. Task Force on Psoriasis. J Am Acad Dermatol 28:632–637, 1993.

208. Christophers E. Psoriasis: epidemiology and clinical spectrum. Clin Exp Dermatol 26:314–320, 2001.

209. Naldi L. Epidemiology of psoriasis. Curr Drug Targets Inflamm Al-lergy 3:121–128, 2004.

210. Pardasani AG, Feldman SR, Clark AR. Treatment of psoriasis: an algorithm-based approach for primary care physicians. Am Fam Physician 61:725–736, 2000.

211. Nickoloff BJ, Nestle FO. Recent insights into the immunopathogen-esis of psoriasis provide new therapeutic opportunities. J Clin In-vest 113:1664–1675, 2004.

212. Robert C, Kupper TS. Inflammatory skin diseases, T cells, and im-mune surveillance. N Engl J Med 341:1817–1828, 1999.

213. Gudjonsson JE, Johnston A, Sigmundsdottir H, et al. Immunopatho-genic mechanisms in psoriasis. Clin Exp Immunol 135:1–8, 2004.

214. Capon F, Munro M, Barker J, et al. Searching for the major histo-compatibility complex psoriasis susceptibility gene. J Invest Der-matol 118:745–751, 2002.

215. Bernhard JD. Auspitz sign is not sensitive or specific for psoriasis. J Am Acad Dermatol 22:1079–1081, 1990.

216. Telfer NR, Chalmers RJ, Whale K, et al. The role of streptococcal infection in the initiation of guttate psoriasis. Arch Dermatol 128: 39–42, 1992.

217. Thumboo J, Uramoto K, Shbeeb MI, et al. Risk factors for the de-velopment of psoriatic arthritis: a population-based nested case con-trol study. J Rheumatol 29:757–762, 2002.

218. National Psoriasis Foundation. Statistics. Available at: http://www.psoriasis.org/resources/statistics/. Accessed Nov. 16, 2004.

219. Russo PA, Ilchef R, Cooper AJ. Psychiatric morbidity in psoriasis: a review. Australas J Dermatol 45:155–161, 2004.

220. Callen JP, Krueger GG, Lebwohl M, et al. AAD consensus statement on psoriasis therapies. J Am Acad Dermatol 49:897–899, 2003.

221. Draelos ZD. Therapeutic moisturizers. Dermatol Clin 18:597–607, 2000.

222. Marks R. Topical therapy for psoriasis: general principles. Dermatol Clin 2:383–388, 1984.

223. Lebwohl M. The role of salicylic acid in the treatment of psoriasis. Int J Dermatol 38:16–24, 1999.

224. Silverman A, Menter A, Hairston JL. Tars and anthralins. Dermatol Clin 13:817–833, 1995.

225. Lowe NJ, Ashton RE, Koudsi H, et al. Anthralin for psoriasis: short-contact anthralin therapy compared with topical steroid and conventional anthralin. J Am Acad Dermatol 10:69–72, 1984.

226. Gibson LE, Perry HO. Goeckerman therapy. In: Roenigk HH, Maibach HI, eds. Psoriasis. 3rd ed. New York: Marcel Dekker Inc; 1998:469–477.

227. Menter A, Cram DL. The Goeckerman regimen in two psoriasis day care centers. J Am Acad Dermatol 9:59–65, 1983.

228. Thami GP, Sarkar R. Coal tar: past, present and future. Clin Exp Dermatol 27:99–103, 2002.

229. van de Kerkhof PCM. Comparisons and combinations. In: van de Kerkhof PCM, ed. Textbook of psoriasis. Malden, MA: Blackwell Science Ltd; 1999:275–283.

230. Ramsay B, Lawrence CM, Bruce JM, Shuster S. The effect of triethanolamine application on anthralin-induced inflammation and therapeutic effect in psoriasis. J Am Acad Dermatol 23:73–76, 1990.

231. Miller JA, Munro DD. Topical corticosteroids: clinical pharmacology and therapeutic use. Drugs 19:119–134, 1980.

232. Drug Facts and Comparisons, 1998 ed. St. Louis: Facts and Comparisons, 1998:3136.

233. Katz HI. Topical corticosteroids. Dermatol Clin 13:805–815, 1995.

234. Hughes J, Rustin MHA. Corticosteroids. In: van de Kerkhof PCM, ed. Textbook of Psoriasis. Malden, MA: Blackwell Science Ltd, 1999:148–159.

235. Koo J, Kochavi G, Kwan JC. Contemporary Diagnosis and Management of Psoriasis. 1st ed. Newton, PA: Handbooks in Health Care Co., 2004:18–38.

236. Kragballe K, Wildfang IL. Calcipotriol (MC 903), a novel vitamin D3 analogue stimulates terminal differentiation and inhibits proliferation of cultured human keratinocytes. Arch Dermatol Res 282:164–167, 1990.

237. Kragballe K. Treatment of psoriasis by the topical application of the novel cholecalciferol analogue calcipotriol (MC 903). Arch Dermatol 125:1647–1652, 1989.

238. Bourke JF, Iqbal SJ, Hutchinson PE. A randomized double-blind comparison of the effects on systemic calcium homeostasis of topical calcitriol (3 micrograms/g) and calcipotriol (50 micrograms/g) in the treatment of chronic plaque psoriasis vulgaris. Acta Derm Venereol 77:228–230, 1997.

239. Bourke JF, Mumford R, Whittaker P, et al. The effects of topical calcipotriol on systemic calcium homeostasis in patients with chronic plaque psoriasis. J Am Acad Dermatol 37:929–934, 1997.

240. Guzzo C, Lazarus G, Goffe BS, et al. Topical calcipotriene has no short-term effect on calcium and bone metabolism of patients with psoriasis. J Am Acad Dermato; 34:429–433, 1996.

241. Ashcroft DM, Po AL, Williams HC, et al. Systematic review of comparative efficacy and tolerability of calcipotriol in treating chronic plaque psoriasis. Br Med J 320:963–967, 2000.

242. Duweb G, Aldebani S, Elzorghany A, et al. Calcipotriol ointment versus cream in psoriasis vulgaris. Int J Clin Pharmacol Res 23:47–51, 2003.

243. van de Kerkhof PC, Franssen M, de La Brassine M, et al. Calcipotriol cream in the morning and ointment in the evening: a novel regimen to improve compliance. J Dermatol Treat 12:75–79, 2001.

244. Giannotti B, Carli P, Varott C, et al. Treatment of psoriasis with calcipotriol: time onset and healing of relapses. Eur J Dermatol 7:275–278, 1997.

245. Chandraratna RA. Tazarotene: first of a new generation of receptor-selective retinoids. Br J Dermatol 135(Suppl 49):18–25, 1996.

246. Tazorac [package insert]. Irvine, CA: Allergan, Inc, 2004.

247. Koo JY, Martin D. Investigator-masked comparison of tazarotene gel q.d. plus mometasone furoate cream q.d. vs. mometasone furoate cream b.i.d. in the treatment of plaque psoriasis. Int J Dermatol 40:210–212, 2001.

248. Lebwohl M, Lombardi K, Tan MH. Duration of improvement in psoriasis after treatment with tazarotene 0.1% gel plus clobetasol propionate 0.05% ointment: comparison of maintenance treatments. Int J Dermatol 40:64–66, 2001.

249. Kaidbey K, Kopper SC, Sefton J, et al. A pilot study to determine the effect of tazarotene gel 0.1% on steroid-induced epidermal atrophy. Int J Dermatol 40:468–471, 2001.

250. Guenther LC, Poulin YP, Pariser DM. A comparison of tazarotene 0.1% gel once daily plus mometasone furoate 0.1% cream once daily versus calcipotriene 0.005% ointment twice daily in the treatment of plaque psoriasis. Clin Ther 22:1225–1238, 2000.

251. Marsland AM, Griffiths CE. The macrolide immunosuppressants in dermatology: mechanisms of action. Eur J Dermatol 12:618–622, 2002.

252. Mrowietz U, Graeber M, Brautigam M, et al. The novel ascomycin derivative SDZ ASM 981 is effective for psoriasis when used topically under occlusion. Br J Dermatol 139:992–996, 1998.

253. Gribetz C, Ling M, Lebwohl M, et al. Pimecrolimus cream 1% in the treatment of intertriginous psoriasis: a double-blind, randomized study. J Am Acad Dermatol 51:731–738, 2004.

254. Rappersberger K, Komar M, Ebelin ME, et al. Pimecrolimus identifies a common genomic anti-inflammatory profile, is clinically highly effective in psoriasis and is well tolerated. J Invest Dermatol 119:876–887, 2002.

255. Zonneveld IM, Rubins A, Jablonska S, et al. Topical tacrolimus is not effective in chronic plaque psoriasis. A pilot study. Arch Dermatol 134:1101–1102, 1998.

256. Lebwohl M, Freeman AK, Chapman MS, et al. Tacrolimus ointment is effective for facial and intertriginous psoriasis. J Am Acad Dermatol 51:723–730, 2004.

257. Abel EA. Phototherapy. Dermatol Clin 13:841–849, 1995.

258. Camisa C. Ultraviolet B phototherapy and coal tar. In: Camisa C. Handbook of Psoriasis. Malden, MA: Blackwell Science, 1998:144–165.

259. Rampen FH, Fleuren BA, de Boo TM, et al. Unreliability of self-reported burning tendency and tanning ability. Arch Dermatol 124:885–888, 1988.

260. Koo J, Lebwohl M. Duration of remission of psoriasis therapies. J Am Acad Dermatol 41:51–59, 1999.

261. Studniberg HM, Weller P. PUVA, UVB, psoriasis, and nonmelanoma skin cancer. J Am Acad Dermatol 29:1013–1022, 1993.

262. Krutmann J. Photo(chemo)therapy. In: van de Kerkhof PCM. Textbook of Psoriasis. Malden, MA: Blackwell Science, 1999:179–195.

263. Coven TR, Burack LH, Gilleaudeau R, et al. Narrowband UV-B produces superior clinical and histopathological resolution of moderate-to-severe psoriasis in patients compared with broadband UV-B. Arch Dermatol 133:1514–1522, 1997.

264. Tanew A, Radakovic-Fijan S, Schemper M, et al. Narrowband UV-B phototherapy vs photochemotherapy in the treatment of chronic plaque-type psoriasis: a paired comparison study. Arch Dermatol 135:519–524, 1999.

265. Helm TN, Camisa C. Psolarens and photochemotherapy (PUVA). In: Camisa C. Handbook of Psoriasis. Malden, MA: Blackwell Science, 1998:166–191.

266. Oxsoralen-Ultra Capsules [package insert]. Costa Mesa, CA: ICN Pharmaceuticals, Inc, 1998.

267. Stern RS, Lange R. Non-melanoma skin cancer occurring in patients treated with PUVA five to ten years after first treatment. J Invest Dermatol 91:120–124, 1988.

268. Wolff K. Side-effects of psoralen photochemotherapy (PUVA). Br J Dermatol 122(Suppl 36):117–125, 1990.

269. Zanolli MD, Sherertz EF, Hedberg AE. Methotrexate: anti-inflammatory or antiproliferative? J Am Acad Dermatol 22:523–524, 1990.

270. Olsen EA. The pharmacology of methotrexate. J Am Acad Dermatol 25:306–318, 1991.

271. Tung JP, Maibach HI. The practical use of methotrexate in psoriasis. Drugs 40:697–712, 1990.

272. Roenigk HH, Jr., Auerbach R, Maibach HI, et al. Methotrexate in psoriasis: revised guidelines. J Am Acad Dermatol 19:145–156, 1988.

273. McClure SL, Valentine J, Gordon KB. Comparative tolerability of systemic treatments for plaque-type psoriasis. Drug Safety 25: 913–927, 2002.

274. Singh F, Weinberg JM. Oral tazarotene and oral pimecrolimus: novel oral therapies in development for psoriasis. J Drugs Dermatol 3:141–143, 2004.

275. Yamauchi PS, Rizk D, Lowe NJ. Retinoid therapy for psoriasis. Dermatol Clin 22:467–476, x, 2004.

276. Griffiths CE. Systemic and local administration of cyclosporine in the treatment of psoriasis. J Am Acad Dermatol 23:1242–1247, 1990.

277. Guenther L. Cyclosporine. In: Wolverton SE, Wilkins JK. Systemic drugs for skin diseases. Philadelphia: WB Saunders, 1991: 167.

278. Boyd AS, Neldner KH. Hydroxyurea therapy. J Am Acad Dermatol 25:518–524, 1991.

279. Krueger GG. Current concepts and review of alefacept in the treatment of psoriasis. Dermatol Clin 22:407–426, viii, 2004.

280. Alefacept [package insert]. Cambridge, MA: Biogen, Inc, 2003.

281. Lebwohl M, Christophers E, Langley R, et al. An international, randomized, double-blind, placebo-controlled phase 3 trial of intramuscular alefacept in patients with chronic plaque psoriasis. Arch Dermatol 139:719–727, 2003.

282. Krueger GG, Ellis CN. Alefacept therapy produces remission for patients with chronic plaque psoriasis. Br J Dermatol 148:784–788, 2003.

283. Krueger GG, Papp KA, Stough DB, et al. A randomized, double-blind, placebo-controlled phase III study evaluating efficacy and tolerability of 2 courses of alefacept in patients with chronic plaque psoriasis. J Am Acad Dermatol 47:821–833, 2002.

284. Hodak E, David M. Alefacept: a review of the literature and practical guidelines for management. Dermatol Ther 17:383–392, 2004.

285. Gordon KB, Papp KA, Hamilton TK, et al. Efalizumab for patients with moderate to severe plaque psoriasis: a randomized controlled trial. JAMA 290:3073–3080, 2003.

286. Efalizumab [package insert]. South San Francisco, CA: Genentech, Inc, 2004.

287. Leonardi CL. Efalizumab in the treatment of psoriasis. Dermatol Ther 17:393–400, 2004.

288. Etanercept [package insert]. Thousand Oaks, CA: Immunex Corp, 2004.

289. Leonardi CL, Powers JL, Matheson RT, et al. Etanercept as monotherapy in patients with psoriasis. N Engl J Med 349:2014–2022, 2003.

290. Weinberg JM. An overview of infliximab, etanercept, efalizumab, and alefacept as biologic therapy for psoriasis. Clin Ther 25: 2487–2505, 2003.

291. Wallis RS, Broder MS, Wong JY, et al. Granulomatous infectious diseases associated with tumor necrosis factor antagonists. Clin Infect Dis 38:1261–1265, 2004.

292. Tuberculosis associated with blocking agents against tumor necrosis factor-alpha—California, 2002–2003. MMWR Morb Mortal Wkly Rep 53:683–686, 2004.

293. Kwon HJ, Cote TR, Cuffe MS, et al. Case reports of heart failure after therapy with a tumor necrosis factor antagonist. Ann Intern Med 138:807–811, 2003.

294. Winterfield L, Menter A. Psoriasis and its treatment with infliximab-mediated tumor necrosis factor alpha blockade. Dermatol Clin 22:437–447, ix, 2004.

295. Chaudhari U, Romano P, Mulcahy LD, et al. Efficacy and safety of infliximab monotherapy for plaque-type psoriasis: a randomised trial. Lancet 357:1842–1847, 2001.

296. Gottlieb AB, Evans R, Li S, et al. Infliximab induction therapy for patients with severe plaque-type psoriasis: a randomized, double-blind, placebo-controlled trial. J Am Acad Dermatol 51:534–542, 2004.

297. Redbook, 2004 edition; p. 196.

298. Centers for Medicare & Medicaid Services. Medicare Coverage Database. Available at: http://www.cms.hhs.gov/mcd/index_local_alpha.asp?from=alphalmrp&letter=A. Accessed April 29, 2005.

299. Matsunami E, Takashima A, Mizuno N, et al. Topical PUVA, etretinate, and combined PUVA and etretinate for palmoplantar pustulosis: comparison of therapeutic efficacy and the influences of tonsillar and dental focal infections. J Dermatol 17:92–96, 1990.

300. Wilkin J, Dahl M, Detmar M, et al. Standard classification of rosacea: report of the National Rosacea Society Expert Committee on the Classification and Staging of Rosacea. J Am Acad Dermatol 46:584–587, 2002.

301. Bikowski JB. Treatment of rosacea with doxycycline monohydrate. Cutis 66:149–152, 2000.

302. Berg M, Liden S. An epidemiological study of rosacea. Acta Derm Venereol 69:419–423, 1989.

303. Chalmers DA. Rosacea: recognition and management for the primary care provider. Nurse Pract 22:18–30, 1997.

304. Sibenge S, Gawkrodger DJ. Rosacea: a study of clinical patterns, blood flow, and the role of Demodex folliculorum. J Am Acad Dermatol 26:590–593, 1992.

305. Bleicher PA, Charles JH, Sober AJ. Topical metronidazole therapy for rosacea. Arch Dermatol 123:609–614, 1987.

306. Baima B, Sticherling M. Demodicidosis revisited. Acta Derm Venereol 82:3–6, 2002.

307. Bamford JT, Tilden RL, Blankush JL, et al. Effect of treatment of Helicobacter pylori infection on rosacea. Arch Dermatol 135: 659–663, 1999.

308. Webster GF. Acne and rosacea. Med Clin North Am 82: 1145–1154, vi, 1998.

309. Wilkin JK. Rosacea. Pathophysiology and treatment. Arch Dermatol 130:359–362, 1994.

310. Plewig G. Rosacea. In: Fitzpatrick T, Eisen A, Wolff K, et al, eds. Dermatology in general medicine. New York: McGraw-Hill, 1993: 727–735.

311. Stone DU, Chodosh J. Oral tetracyclines for ocular rosacea: an evidence-based review of the literature. Cornea 23:106–109, 2004.

312. Kligman AM. Ocular rosacea. Current concepts and therapy. Arch Dermatol 133:89–90, 1997.

313. Michel JL, Cabibel F. [Frequency, severity and treatment of ocular rosacea during cutaneous rosacea]. Ann Dermatol Venereol 130: 20–24, 2003.

314. Ljubojeviae S, Basta-Juzbasiae A, et al. Steroid dermatitis resembling rosacea: aetiopathogenesis and treatment. J Eur Acad Dermatol Venereol 16:121–126, 2002.

315. Nichols K, Desai N, Lebwohl MG. Effective sunscreen ingredients and cutaneous irritation in patients with rosacea. Cutis 61:344–346, 1998.

316. Schmadel LK, McEvoy GK. Topical metronidazole: a new therapy for rosacea. Clin Pharm 9:94–101, 1990.

317. Dahl MV, Katz HI, Krueger GG, et al. Topical metronidazole maintains remissions of rosacea. Arch Dermatol 134:679–683, 1998.

318. Blount BW, Pelletier AL. Rosacea: a common, yet commonly overlooked, condition. Am Fam Physician 66:435–440, 2002.

319. Wilkin JK, DeWitt S. Treatment of rosacea: topical clindamycin versus oral tetracycline. Int J Dermatol 32:65–67, 1993.

320. Thiboutot DM. Acne and rosacea. New and emerging therapies. Dermatol Clin 18:63–71, viii, 2000.

321. Plexion [package insert]. Scottsdale, AZ: The Dermatology Company, 2000.

322. Kocak M, Yagli S, Vahapoglu G, et al. Permethrin 5% cream versus metronidazole 0.75% gel for the treatment of papulopustular rosacea. A randomized double-blind placebo-controlled study. Dermatology 205:265–270, 2002.

323. Maddin S. A comparison of topical azelaic acid 20% cream and topical metronidazole 0.75% cream in the treatment of patients with papulopustular rosacea. J Am Acad Dermatol 40:961–965, 1999.

324. Quarterman MJ, Johnson DW, Abele DC, et al. Ocular rosacea. Signs, symptoms, and tear studies before and after treatment with doxycycline. Arch Dermatol 133:49–54, 1997.

325. Rebora A. The management of rosacea. Am J Clin Dermatol 3: 489–496, 2002.

326. Hoting E, Paul E, Plewig G. Treatment of rosacea with isotretinoin. Int J Dermatol 25:660–663, 1986.

327. Greenbaum SS, Krull EA, Watnick K. Comparison of CO$_2$ laser and electrosurgery in the treatment of rhinophyma. J Am Acad Dermatol 18:363–368, 1988.

328. Goldman D. Tacrolimus ointment for the treatment of steroid-induced rosacea: a preliminary report. J Am Acad Dermatol 44: 995–998, 2001.

Burns

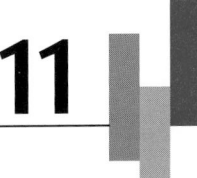

11

Ted L. Rice and Charles M. Karnack

TREATMENT GOALS

- Provide appropriate resuscitation.
- Preserve physical function.
- Promote wound healing and optimal cosmetic results.
- Minimize pain and anxiety.
- Provide adequate nutrition.
- Prevent or aggressively treat complications.

The clinical management of a severely burned patient is complex and frequently challenging. To get a general overview of the important issues, we recommend that clinicians read a recent publication in the "Case Records of the Massachusetts General Hospital" section of the *New England Journal of Medicine*.[1] The photographs and chronology of patient care provided by the authors provide an excellent presentation of patient management issues, treatment strategies employed in their resolution, and the long-term outcomes of a severely burned patient. Similarly, two recently published articles are of exceptional educational value in their description of burn patient management and the more global issues of public safety and the health care system response to disasters.[2,3]

The skin is the largest organ of the body, and it performs five major functions. It provides protection from the environment, sensory perception, vitamin production, excretion of water and some wastes, and regulation of body temperature. When the skin is damaged, bacteria are no longer prevented from invading, pain is produced (unless superficial sensory nerves are destroyed), and both fluid and heat are lost through the damaged area.

Extensive skin loss or damage requiring hospitalization can occur by many different mechanisms that produce similar effects, including thermal injury from hot liquids (scalds), flames, or extreme cold (frostbite), and injury from chemicals, radiation (sunburn), electricity, or trauma (abrasion). In addition, patients with extensive exfoliative dermatoses (e.g., Stevens-Johnson syndrome or toxic epidermal necrolysis) are often treated in burn centers. Because the presence of devitalized tissue increases the risk of tetanus, the patient's tetanus immunization status must be ascertained. In an audit of 269 trauma patients, 70 of whom had been burned, 15% of patients were not questioned about their tetanus status in the emergency room and 27% were incorrectly assessed.[4] Treatment with tetanus and diphtheria toxoids and tetanus immune globulin should be initiated according to promulgated guidelines.[5] In contrast to the rarity of tetanus, burn patients are at risk for the common adverse sequelae associated with intensive care unit admission, such as venous thromboembolism and sinusitis.[6,7]

Fire victims can suffer severe injury or death without significant body surface burning. A classic demonstration of this was the 1942 Coconut Grove Nightclub fire, in which 75 of the 114 deaths were caused by smoke inhalation. Carbon monoxide (CO) poisoning is a frequent cause of death. CO binds preferentially to hemoglobin, displacing oxygen and shifting the oxyhemoglobin dissociation curve to the left, resulting in tissue hypoxia. The smoke, which is a function of the burning material, contains toxins other than CO, such as cyanide, acrolein, benzene, and phosgene.[8,9]

TABLE 11.1	Burn Injury Severity Classification[a]					
	Percent of (TBSA) Affected[b]					
	Minor Injury		**Moderate Injury**		**Major Injury**	
Depth of Burn	Adult	Child	Adult	Child	Adult	Child
Partial Thickness						
First degree	<50	<10	50–75	10–20	>75	>20
Second degree	<15	<10	15–25	10–20	>25	>20
Full Thickness						
Third degree	<2	<2	2–10	2–10	>10	>10

[a] Irrespective of burn extent, injuries are classified as major when they involve areas of special importance, such as the eyes, ears, hands, feet, or genitals. Injuries are major when burns occur in conjunction with other major trauma (e.g., fractures) or inhalation injury.
[b] TBSA, total body surface area.

Outcome following thermal injury is determined by a combination of patient and burn factors. The very young, the very old, and those who were previously ill have a poorer prognosis than do healthy, young adults after a similar injury. Scoring systems for injury severity include the Thermal Injury Organ Failure Score, which correlates with outcome, and the Burn Specific Health Scale, which is used to accurately assess the impact of nonfatal burn injury.[10,11] One method for estimating the probability of death after burn injury found that the three risk factors with the strongest predictive value for death were age greater than 60 years, extent of burn, and level of inhalation injury.[12] The pathophysiology of inhalation injury is complex and incompletely understood; however, its impact on patient outcome is considerable, accounting for up to 77% of deaths in burn patients who also have inhalation injury.[13–15] Fiberoptic bronchoscopy is the preferred diagnostic strategy, although enthusiasm is growing among burn care clinicians for virtual bronchoscopy, because it is noninvasive and easy to perform in unstable patients.[16] Treatment of inhalation injury is mainly supportive (i.e., endotracheal intubation and mechanical ventilation).[17] High-frequency percussive ventilation is an innovative strategy that has been shown to benefit patients who do not respond to conventional ventilation.[18]

Burn factors that determine patient outcome include depth, extent, and body surface location.[19] A list of burn severity criteria is provided in Table 11.1. The important distinction regarding depth of burn is that partial-thickness injuries heal by cell regeneration, but full-thickness injuries, unless very small, require skin grafting. Small full-thickness burns heal by contraction and reepithelialization from progenitor cells at the edges of the wound.

WOUND ASSESSMENT

Traditionally, the depth of burns has been described according to degrees of injury, as listed in Figure 11.1. As the depth

of injury increases, the number representing degree of injury increases. A first-degree burn is very shallow and affects only the epidermis. A second-degree burn involves complete destruction of the epidermis and variable portions of the underlying dermis. When destruction to the dermis is limited to the upper third or less, the burn is called a *superficial second-degree burn*. Conversely, a deep second-degree burn appears as tissue destruction below the top one third, but not completely through the dermis. A third-degree, or full-thickness, burn reveals destruction of the entire epidermis and dermis. The terms *fourth-degree* and *fifth-degree burn* have been used to describe tissue destruction through subcutaneous fat and through muscle, respectively.[20]

The typical first-degree burn is easily identified. It is painful and erythematous, and it blanches to pressure. A superficial second-degree burn is painful, forms blisters, and blanches to pressure. A third-degree burn is usually not painful because superficial nerve endings are destroyed; may appear white, leatherlike, or black (charred); and contains thrombosed blood vessels. This dead tissue is called *eschar* (es'kar). Unfortunately, sometimes even the most experienced clinician cannot differentiate a partial-thickness from a full-thickness injury. In addition, flame injuries typically occur as a mixture of full- and partial-thickness injuries. This classic presentation, as depicted in Figure 11.2, was described as a target or bulls-eye, where the deepest injury is in the center, followed by increasingly superficial injury at increasing distance from the center. Early attempts to improve the accuracy of injury depth assessment included histologic staining, injection of radioactive compounds or dyes such as bromphenol blue, and fiberoptic perfusion fluorometry. These methods were disadvantageous in that they were invasive, cumbersome, labor intensive, and inaccurate. Although it is sensitive to variations in positioning and temperature, the laser Doppler has better than 90% accuracy when compared with histologic analysis of burn wound depth. The laser Doppler documents a reduction in red blood cell velocity in a burn wound, establishing the necessity for surgical

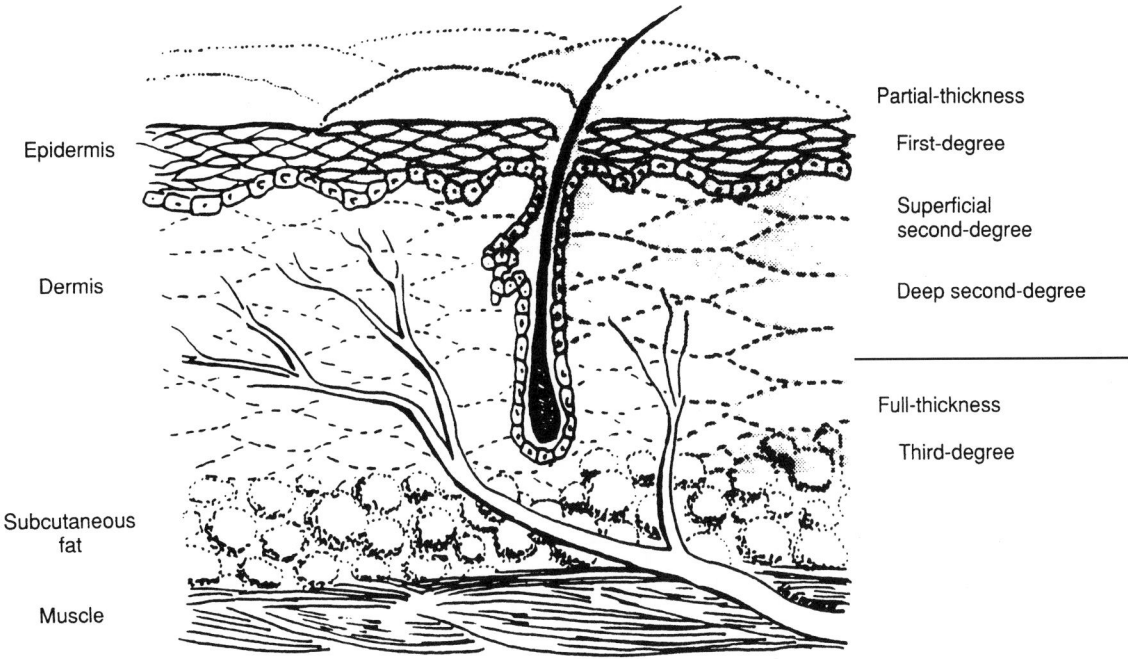

FIGURE 11.1 Diagram of burn depth in gross skin histology.

Epidermis

Dermis

Subcutaneous fat

Muscle

Partial-thickness

First-degree

Superficial second-degree

Deep second-degree

Full-thickness

Third-degree

removal and grafting.[21] Clinicians must remain cognizant of the need for confirmation of initial assessments of burn depth. Reassessment is necessary because of the changing nature of deep partial-thickness injuries, which may become full-thickness wounds because of infection or inadequate resuscitation.[22]

Several systems are used to calculate the relative percentage of total body surface area (TBSA) burned. The rule of nines is a simple system that can be used to estimate the extent of burn in adults. It represents regions of the body surface as 9% or multiples of 9%, for example, the head and arms each represent approximately 9% TBSA, the torso 36%, each leg 18%, and the perineum 1%. For burns with an uneven distribution, the patient's hand is a useful measuring tool. One side of the patient's complete hand (i.e., the palm and fingers) is about 1% TBSA.[23] In infants and children, the head represents a larger TBSA than that of adults; therefore, the rule of nines does not hold. A more accurate assessment of TBSA can be made with the Lund-Browder chart. The chart used at the University of Michigan Burn Center is reproduced in Figure 11.3. Favorable assessments of two computerized systems for estimating burn size and calculating fluid requirements [i.e., the Sage II (available at http://www.sagediagram.com) and the 3-D Burn Vision (CD-ROM from Electric Power Research Institute, Concord, CA, 1-800-313-3774)] have been reported.[24]

WOUND CLOSURE

Although some clinicians advocate the use of topical creams (i.e., papain-urea or the less painful collagenase) to enzymatically débride full-thickness injuries, the preferred surgical approach over the past decade has been staged eschar excision (débridement) with placement of autologous skin grafts.[25-28] Split-thickness skin grafts (STSGs) that are approximately 0.06 mm thick are harvested (with the use of a dermatome), expanded by a ratio of 1:1.5 (with the use of a meshing device), and applied to the wound after removal of devitalized tissue and achievement of hemostasis. An important detrimental problem during these operative procedures is coagulopathy, which is produced by hypothermia. To prevent or attenuate hypothermia, the ambient temperature of the operating room is maintained above 37°C, the amount of débridement is limited, and intravenous fluids are warmed to 40°C. Although it may appear hazardous, a pilot

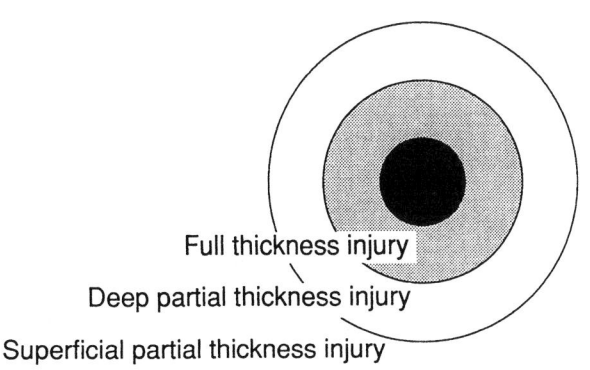

Full thickness injury

Deep partial thickness injury

Superficial partial thickness injury

Uninjured skin

FIGURE 11.2 Typical pattern of injury following flame burn.

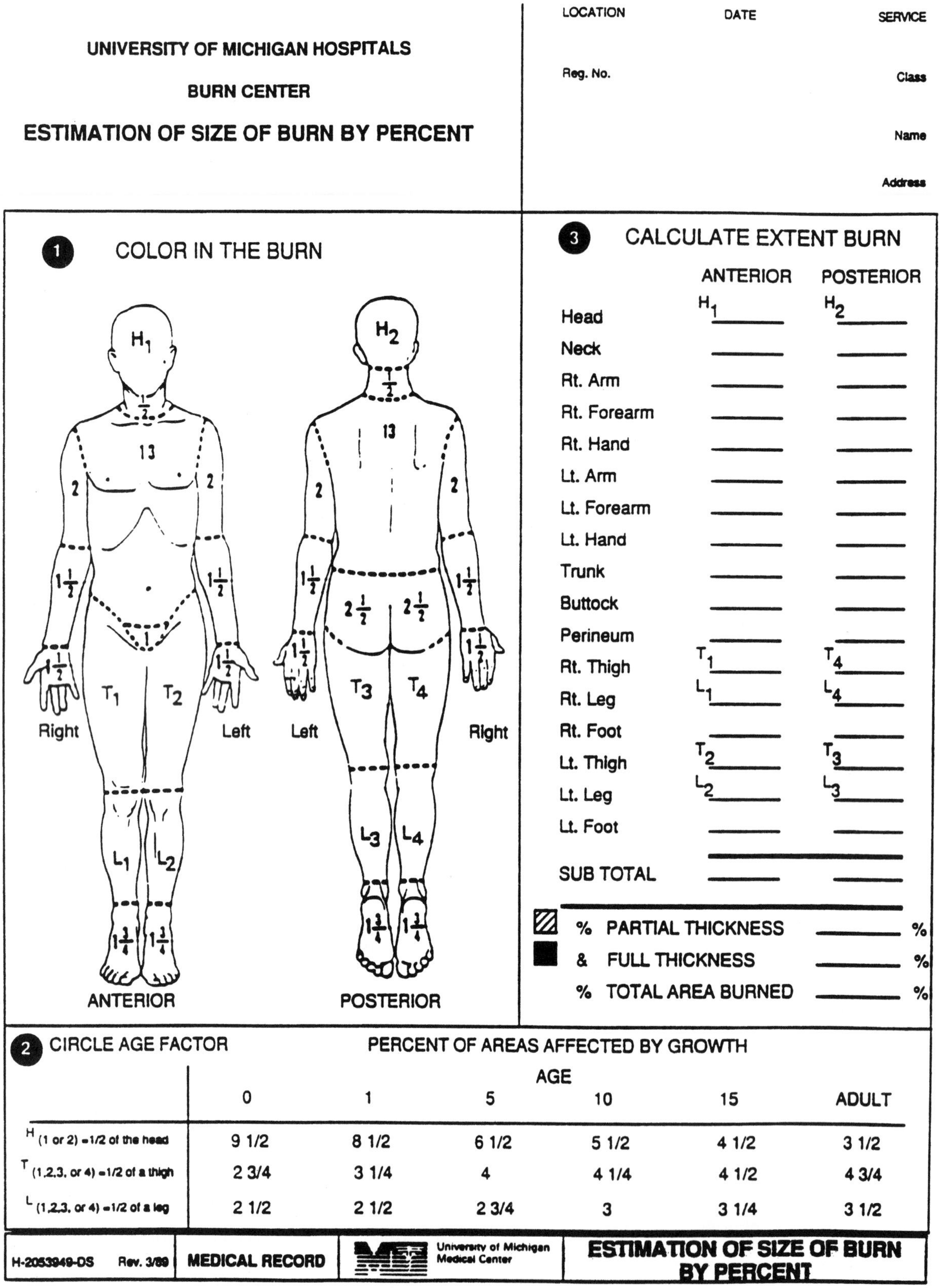

UNIVERSITY OF MICHIGAN HOSPITALS

BURN CENTER

ESTIMATION OF SIZE OF BURN BY PERCENT

LOCATION	DATE	SERVICE
Reg. No.		Class
		Name
		Address

1 COLOR IN THE BURN

Right Left   Left Right

ANTERIOR   POSTERIOR

3 CALCULATE EXTENT BURN

	ANTERIOR	POSTERIOR
Head	H_1 ____	H_2 ____
Neck	____	____
Rt. Arm	____	____
Rt. Forearm	____	____
Rt. Hand	____	____
Lt. Arm	____	____
Lt. Forearm	____	____
Lt. Hand	____	____
Trunk	____	____
Buttock	____	____
Perineum	____	____
Rt. Thigh	T_1 ____	T_4 ____
Rt. Leg	L_1 ____	L_4 ____
Rt. Foot	____	____
Lt. Thigh	T_2 ____	T_3 ____
Lt. Leg	L_2 ____	L_3 ____
Lt. Foot	____	____
SUB TOTAL	____	____

▨	%	PARTIAL THICKNESS	____ %
■	&	FULL THICKNESS	____ %
	%	TOTAL AREA BURNED	____ %

2 CIRCLE AGE FACTOR   PERCENT OF AREAS AFFECTED BY GROWTH

	AGE					
	0	1	5	10	15	ADULT
H (1 or 2) =1/2 of the head	9 1/2	8 1/2	6 1/2	5 1/2	4 1/2	3 1/2
T (1,2,3, or 4) =1/2 of a thigh	2 3/4	3 1/4	4	4 1/4	4 1/2	4 3/4
L (1,2,3, or 4) =1/2 of a leg	2 1/2	2 1/2	2 3/4	3	3 1/4	3 1/2

H-2053949-DS Rev. 3/89	MEDICAL RECORD	ME University of Michigan Medical Center	ESTIMATION OF SIZE OF BURN BY PERCENT

FIGURE 11.3 The University of Michigan Hospital Burn Center's estimation of size of burn by percentage.

study in eight patients demonstrated that intraoperative intravenous fluids could safely be heated to 60°C when administered through a central venous catheter.[29]

Once adherent and vascularized, the STSG from the patient's own noninjured skin (autograft or isograft) permanently closes the wound.[30] Unfortunately, the amount of noninjured skin available for STSGs often cannot completely cover the open wound. A number of skin substitutes can be used to temporarily cover the open wound while donor site healing and reharvesting of the autograft are awaited. A commonly used biologic skin substitute is cadaver skin (allograft or homograft). Less frequently used biologic skin substitutes include animal skin (xenograft or heterograft), amniotic membrane, and tissue-derived collagen. Synthetic skin substitutes include polyurethane film (e.g., Opsite) and petrolatum-impregnated fine mesh gauze (e.g., scarlet red and Xeroform). Biosynthetic skin substitutes have been developed that are combinations of biologic and synthetic materials, such as Biobrane and TransCyte, which combine collagen with a synthetic membrane.[31,32] Skin substitutes adhere to the wound, minimize pain, decrease protein, water, and electrolyte loss, and simulate many important skin functions, such as providing a barrier to bacteria. Although these skin substitutes perform important functions, they eventually must be replaced by autologous skin.

Advances in tissue bioengineering have focused on the development of a true dermal replacement or substitute. One approach is the in vitro production of new skin by culture of autologous epidermis. Since the first successful transplantation of cultured autologous epidermis in 1981, keratinocyte growth techniques have been so improved that current methods allow a several thousand–fold expansion of skin specimens within 3 to 4 weeks.[33] However, engraftment of cultured epidermis continues to be inconsistent and should be considered experimental.[34] Another strategy provides a dermal matrix attached to a silicon polymer membrane.[35] Finally, the availability of a ''living skin equivalent,'' such as Integra, Apligraf, and Alloderm, is an exciting, albeit costly, strategy for wound healing.[32,36,37]

Healing of burn wounds often results in scars that impair normal range of motion and are cosmetically unpleasant. Hypertrophic scars are associated with contractures, and they are raised, erythematous, and pruritic. Keloid scars extend beyond the original wound and rarely regress. Recently developed therapeutic strategies include the use of pressure, massage, physical therapy, silicone sheets and gels, glucocorticoids, and surgical procedures.[38,39] Another troublesome problem associated with a healing burn wound is pruritus. Attempts to control burn wound itch with the use of moisturizers and antihistamines have been disappointing. Increased success has been achieved by combining the histamine H_1 and H_2 receptor antagonists (H_1 and H_2RAs) cetirizine and cimetidine, through the use of a topical doxepin cream, with adjunct therapy that includes colloidal oatmeal baths, massage therapy, or analgesics.[40–43]

PAIN MANAGEMENT

Effective pain management in burn patients requires an understanding of physiologic responses to injury and the interrelationships between anxiety, depression, and pain. The extent of burn is a significant predictor of pain but only during the first week after injury. Pain varies greatly from patient to patient and undergoes wide fluctuations over time in each patient; the greatest pain is usually experienced during therapeutic procedures such as hydrotherapy with wound débridement and dressing changes.[44] Patients with high levels of anxiety or depression tend to report greater pain when at rest.

Historically, pain management practices for burn patients have not been optimal; some centers report that no analgesics or psychotropics were administered to children during wound débridement.[45] To the observant clinician, careful evaluation of signs such as heart rate, blood pressure, facial expression, and body movement and position, as well as the quality of an infant's cries, is sufficient to allow evaluation of pain intensity and to guide the need for and administration of analgesics. In addition, maintaining plasma analgesic concentrations within the range established for good analgesia may be beneficial in centers with rapid access to drug analysis laboratories.[46] Currently, a variety of pharmacotherapeutic agents are used in pain management, such as fentanyl, ketamine, propofol, and nitrous oxide. Indeed, a recent study applied the principle of patient-controlled opioid analgesia to the use of propofol for sedation during painful dressing changes.[47]

The amount of opioid necessary to achieve pain control in burn patients can be substantial, with reports of morphine sulfate self-administered at rates of 108 mg per hour.[48] This demonstrates that large doses of morphine sulfate can be administered safely without undue fear of hypoventilation—indeed a dose of 1,650 mg per hour has been reported.[49] Another important contribution to the enhanced usage of opioid analgesics is the allaying of unrealistic fears of narcotic addiction in hospitalized patients. The Boston Collaborative Drug Surveillance Program reported only four cases of reasonably well-documented addiction out of 11,882 patients who had received at least one narcotic preparation.[50]

Rather than conventional analgesic therapy, such as intermittent intravenous morphine injection, patient-controlled analgesia for both adult and pediatric burn patients is gaining popularity.[51,52] However, because of situations such as the need for neuromuscular blockade, many patients with acute burns are not suitable candidates for patient-controlled analgesia.[53] Another unconventional analgesic strategy that avoids opioid respiratory depression is the use of lidocaine as a continuous intravenous infusion.[54]

Nonpharmacologic methods or adjuncts to pain management include hypnotherapeutic intervention; distraction therapy, in which video programs of scenic beauty accompanied by music are used in combination with analgesics; and cognitive-behavioral therapies such as explanation, personal control, altering the meaning of pain, relaxation, imagery, distraction, and self-hypnosis.[55–59]

FLUID RESUSCITATION

Damaged skin loses the ability to serve as a barrier to percutaneous water loss. Evaporative water loss can be substantial.[60] In contrast to the normal vapor pressure of approximately 3 mm Hg, the vapor pressure of full-thickness burns is about 30 mm Hg. The amount of water loss in milliliters per hour can be estimated with the following formula:

Evaporative loss (mL/h) = (25 + TBSA % burn) × BSA
$$\text{(11-1)}$$

where *BSA* is body surface area in square meters and TBSA is total body surface area. In addition, injury to capillaries in the burn wound causes them to leak a protein-rich fluid into the interstitial space, producing edema and blisters. Blood vessels are generally thought of as solid-walled tubes like plumbing, when in fact, they are made up of individual cells. When injured or under the influence of cytokines or inflammatory mediators, these cells swell apart and produce small ''holes'' in the vessel wall. The problem resolves within 24 hours, but until then, large macromolecules (molecular weights up to 80,000) can leak out of the intravascular space. When the TBSA burned exceeds 25%, a generalized ''capillary leak'' is produced throughout the body, and fluid exudes from unburned vessels into tissue and organs. The exact pathophysiology of this phenomenon is not clear, but the effects of leukotrienes, prostaglandins, arachidonic acid, and oxygen-derived free radicals have been implicated.

FLUID REQUIREMENTS

Treatment or resuscitation of the burn patient who is in shock has been the subject of much interest, research, and controversy. Focused interest was generated in the 1940s because hypovolemic shock was the leading cause of death in burn patients who survived their initial injury. The goal of initial fluid resuscitation is to restore and maintain tissue perfusion while minimizing edema formation.[61,62] The success of fluid administration is judged primarily by urine production at a rate of 0.5 to 1.0 mL/kg/h. In addition, clinical observation of the adequately resuscitated patient should reveal a pulse rate less than 120 (adults) and a clear sensorium.[63] Use of a physiologic salt solution (crystalloid) such as Lactated Ringer's is recommended. A number of resuscitation strategies and adjunctive agents have been investigated with varying results; however, one intriguing report on 37 patients demonstrated a statistically significant reduction in resuscitation fluid volume when ascorbic acid was administered as a continuous intravenous infusion during the initial 24-hour period at a dose of 66 mg/kg/h.[64]

The primary controversy regarding fluid resuscitation of the burn victim involves the necessity of colloid infusion.[65–69] *Colloid* is a general descriptive term for nondiffusible, large-molecular-weight molecules that affect osmotic pressure. Available colloid suspensions include fresh frozen plasma, plasma protein fraction, albumin, dextrans, hetastarch, and pentastarch. Clinicians who routinely use colloids suggest that they are physiologic and can reduce nonburned tissue edema. Crystalloid proponents caution that administered colloids can escape from the intravascular space until the capillary leak is sealed. Although no definitive answer is available, it seems reasonable to exclude colloid infusion from resuscitation fluids for the first 12 hours. Representative resuscitation guidelines are listed in Table 11.2.

A second controversy regarding administration of colloid concerns the use of supplemental albumin to prevent or treat hypoalbuminemia in the postresuscitation phase. In two similar studies of pediatric patients, it was demonstrated that albumin administration did not improve pulmonary function, gastrointestinal tract function, wound healing, or out-

TABLE 11.2	Resuscitation Formulas for Postburn Fluid Requirements During the First 24 Hours Postburn[a]		
Formula	**Crystalloid**	**Colloid**	**Free Water**
Adults			
Parkland 1/2 in first 8 h 1/4 in next 8 h 1/4 in last 8 h	Lactated Ringer's 4 mL/kg/TBSA (%)	None	None
Evans	Lactated Ringer's 1 mL/kg/TBSA	1 mL/kg/TBSA	2,000 mL/m²
Brooke	Lactated Ringer's 1.5 mL/kg/TBSA	1 mL/kg/TBSA	2,000 mL/m²
Modified Brooke	Lactated Ringer's 2 mL/kg/TBSA	None	None
Children			
Graves	Lactated Ringer's 3 mL/kg/TBSA	None	Maintenance

[a] TBSA, total body surface area. Maintenance fluid requirements are 100 mL/kg/day for the first 10 kg body weight, 50 mL/kg/day for the second 10 kg body weight, 20 mL/kg/day for weight in excess of 20 kg.

come.[70,71] In addition, a recent meta-analysis of albumin administration in critically ill patients concluded that the risk of death was increased in the albumin-treated group.[72]

Fluid requirements after the first 24-hour postburn period are determined in the usual fashion, with consideration of fluids lost through the burn wound and nasogastric suction. The main benefit of published guidelines is to alert the clinician who is unfamiliar with burn care that unusually large volumes of fluids and rates of administration are required for severely injured patients.[73] Almost every author has acknowledged that patient variability prohibits development of a strictly calculated volume of resuscitative fluid and rate of administration.

In severe injuries, release of free hemoglobin from destroyed red cells and myoglobin from damaged muscle (especially following electrical injury) leads to destruction of renal tubules, acute renal failure, and possibly death.[74] Binding of free pigments to the renal tubules can be prevented by establishment of a brisk urine flow with the use of resuscitation fluids and diuretics such as furosemide or mannitol, and alkalinization of the urine (pH $\geq$6.5) with parenteral sodium bicarbonate. It is important to note that burn patients with rhabdomyolysis have estimated fluid requirements of 7 mL per kg/% TBSA—almost twice as large as the Parkland formula estimate.[74]

PHARMACOKINETIC CONSIDERATIONS IN BURN PATIENTS

The characteristic biphasic metabolic response to injury of an initial short ebb or shock phase (hypometabolic) followed by a flow phase (hypermetabolic) was described by Cuthbertson in 1930. A burn injury that exceeds 10% to 15% TBSA causes pathophysiologic alterations in the cardiovascular, gastrointestinal, renal, and hepatic systems. Plasma proteins responsible for drug binding either increase or decrease in concentration, resulting in decreased or increased unbound drug concentration, respectively. Finally, the movement of drugs into and out of the circulation is increased through the burn wound. The pharmacokinetics and pharmacodynamics of many drugs are changed after thermal trauma.[75]

CARDIOVASCULAR CHANGES

Cardiac output has been demonstrated to decrease by as much as 50% within 6 hours of severe thermal injury. This reduction in output has been attributed to hypovolemia, increased blood viscosity, increased peripheral vascular resistance, and the presence of a cardiotoxic protein called *myocardial depressant factor*.[76] Theoretically, intravenous drugs have a slower rate of distribution and elimination during this initial 48-hour period.

Following resuscitation, the hyperdynamic or recovery phase of injury is associated with increases of cardiac output of up to one and one half to three times normal. This may not occur in the patient with preexisting myocardial disease. This increase in tissue perfusion is associated with an increased rate of drug distribution and elimination following intravenous administration.[77]

GASTROINTESTINAL CONSIDERATIONS

Acute stress-related mucosal damage (SRMD) of the stomach and duodenum following severe burns is extremely common and is presumably related to increased acid secretion.[78] The first case of acute gastroduodenal ulcer associated with thermal injury was reported by Swan in 1823. Following the 1842 report on a series of 12 patients by Curling, the syndrome was established and named Curling ulcer. Prophylaxis and treatment of SRMD includes enteral feeding and administration of sucralfate, omeprazole, or H_2 receptor antagonists (H_2RAs).[79] Cimetidine appears to be unique among the H_2RAs in that after burns occur, it reduces resuscitative fluid requirements and has an increased elimination rate increased clearance. A study in burned children demonstrated a reduced cimetidine pharmacodynamic response, in addition to an altered pharmacokinetic profile. The absorption of orally administered drugs may be increased or decreased, depending on the drug pKa and whether intragastric pH has been modified by antacids or H_2RAs.

RENAL FUNCTION

Initial renal insults following a severe burn injury consist of general hypoxia and reduced perfusion. Following severe injury, liberation of free hemoglobin or myoglobin may result in acute renal failure. These problems can be reversed rapidly with resuscitative efforts and establishment of adequate urine flow. During the postburn hypermetabolic phase, renal blood flow and glomerular filtration rate (GFR) are increased, although tubular secretion may be impaired. This suggests that the elimination of freely filterable drugs such as the aminoglycosides and vancomycin will increase after burn injury. This effect was demonstrated in a study of 20 burn patients, which reported abnormal increases for both GFR and tobramycin elimination in 13 of 20 patients.[80] The need for increased dosage of gentamicin in burn patients has been demonstrated in numerous studies of both adults and children.[81–85] Similarly, application of the extended-interval dosing strategy for aminoglycosides, that is, the technically incorrect and confusingly named *once-daily aminoglycosides*, can be problematic.[86] Results are conflicting about increased renal elimination of vancomycin following burn injury, but the need for increased dosing is commonly observed.[87,88]

HEPATIC FUNCTION

The hepatocyte is the most important site for drug metabolism, and, in general, it produces a metabolite that is more water soluble (facilitates urinary excretion) and of greater molecular weight (facilitates biliary secretion) than metabolites produced at other sites. Chemical reactions are classified into phase I and phase II biotransformations, which may occur in series. Phase I reactions include the addition of a polar group (hydroxylation) or the deletion of a nonpolar group (N-demethylation). Phase II conjugation with endogenous compounds such as glucuronic acid may follow phase I reactions. The most important enzymes catalyzing these reactions make up the microsomal enzyme oxidation system and include cytochrome P-450 and cytochrome P-450 reductase.

Although the mechanism is not completely clear, burn injury is associated with a marked depression in phase I reactions, while phase II reactions are unaffected. Evidence indicates that decreased enzyme activity is due to oxygen-derived free radical damage to the hepatocyte. This discrepancy is evident in the postburn metabolism of diazepam and lorazepam.[76] The phase I metabolism of diazepam is impaired, while the phase II metabolism of lorazepam (glucuronidation) reveals no change in the normal pattern.[89]

PLASMA PROTEIN BINDING

Although problems associated with changes in unbound drug concentration associated with inverse changes in plasma protein concentration are theoretically possible, clinically important examples are few. The two proteins that account for the greatest quantity of drug serum protein binding are albumin and α_1-acid glycoprotein (AAG).[90]

Albumin is a large molecule (approximately 69,000 daltons) that is capable of binding acidic, neutral, and basic drugs. Despite its large molecular weight, albumin is not confined to the intravascular space; 30% of total exchangeable albumin is found in extravascular fluid. Postburn serum albumin concentration is commonly reduced by 50%, and it often reaches critical levels of 10 g per L (1 g/dL) (normal, 3.5 to 4.9 g/dL in adults). Free fractions of diazepam, phenytoin, and salicylic acid increase following burn injury, which has been attributed to decreased serum albumin concentration.

AAG is an acute-phase reactant that has a high affinity but low capacity for basic drugs; it may be saturated at therapeutic concentrations (e.g., lidocaine). The concentration of AAG may increase to as much as 300% of normal during the first postburn week and may not return to normal for 4 to 6 weeks. Free fractions of imipramine, lidocaine, meperidine, and propranolol decrease after the first postburn week, presumably in response to an increased AAG concentration.

The amount of drug that binds to serum protein becomes critically important when it approaches 90%. When binding involves less than 90%, the pharmacokinetic parameters change little following pathophysiologic changes in binding. Because of the first-pass effect, oral administration of drugs with a high hepatic extraction ratio (such as propranolol) is affected little by changes in plasma protein binding. Although the potential for problems is low, the clinician monitoring a patient who is receiving agents with low therapeutic indices or steep dose-response curves should consider the effects of altered protein binding when evaluating drug toxicity or suboptimal response.

The efficacies of the nondepolarizing neuromuscular blocking agents tubocurarine chloride, metocurine iodide, pancuronium bromide, and atracurium besylate are reduced after the first postburn week, which implies that increased plasma protein binding to AAG is responsible for this.[91,92] Although increased binding does occur, the relatively small increase cannot explain the sometimes dramatic decrease in response. Investigations of the mechanism for this resistance have ruled out changes in drug clearance or volume of distribution. The decreased potency of these agents may be due to an unidentified substance in the plasma of burn patients.

DRUG MOVEMENT THROUGH BURN WOUNDS

Destruction of normal barriers to percutaneous absorption occurs with burn injury. Diffusion resistance to water movement through injured skin can be less than one-tenth that of normal skin. Gentamicin is absorbed readily following topical application of a 0.1% cream, and it is absorbed to a smaller extent with a 0.1% ointment.[93] Eschar penetration has also been demonstrated in vitro for mafenide acetate, nitrofurazone, povidone-iodine, silver nitrate, and silver sulfadiazine.[94]

Drug penetration of the burn wound is not unidirectional. Historically, it has been assumed that eschar penetration by systemically administered drugs was prevented by the avascular nature of the wound. However, systemically administered gentamicin and tobramycin both penetrate burn eschar.[95] Drug loss through the burn wound may add substantially to total drug clearance.

INFECTION AND ANTIMICROBIALS

Despite therapeutic advances, infection in the burned patient remains the most important cause of death in those who survive initial resuscitation.[96–98] Colonization of the burn wound has been demonstrated, even when the patient is cared for in a laminar flow room. Explanations for this phenomenon are that endogenous bacteria translocate from the gastrointestinal tract, bacteria are iatrogenically transmitted, and normal skin flora proliferate.[99] In 15 patients with at least 20% TBSA evaluated within 24 hours of burn injury, the gastrointestinal barrier was compromised, as evidenced by increased absorption of lactulose and mannitol.[100] However, the potential consequences of bacterial translocation continue to be debated.[101]

BURN WOUND INFECTION

Methods and materials used in the treatment of burn wound infection have undergone significant changes.[102–104] Although the importance of bacteria in the burn wound has been recognized, the terminology describing the association between wound bacteria and systemic manifestations of infection is confusing. Moncrief and Teplitz suggested that the term *burn wound sepsis* be used to describe the events associated with bacterial proliferation to 100,000 colony-forming units (cfu) per gram of burn wound tissue and subsequent invasion of adjacent nonburned tissue.[105] Unfortunately, this number of bacteria per gram of tissue is not diagnostic of an invasive burn wound infection, and a complex classification scheme ranging from surface contamination to microvascular invasion (I, II, III, IV, V, VIa, VIb, VIc) has been suggested by Pruitt.[106]

Whether bacteria are localized to the burn or are disseminated, a rational method for selecting from available topical antimicrobials is necessary. Similar to the Kirby-Bauer method of determining bacterial susceptibility to systemic agents, Nathan et al first reported on the agar-well diffusion method for determining susceptibilities to topical antimicrobials.[107] Support for this method was supplied by Heggers et al, who demonstrated that the agar-well diffusion test was more reliable than minimum inhibitory concentration determination for predicting bacterial susceptibility.[108]

Topical Antimicrobials

Silver Nitrate. The "modern" use of silver nitrate began in the late 1800s with the prevention of ophthalmia neonatorum. Substantial improvement in the treatment of large burns through the use of continuously applied 0.5% silver nitrate solution was reported in 1965.[109] The characteristics that make 0.5% silver nitrate a useful topical antibacterial agent are its safety, water solubility, prolonged antibacterial action, lack of toxicity to viable skin, lack of antigenicity, and ease of preparation. Problems associated with its use include hypochloremia from formation of silver chloride salts, water intoxication because of the hypotonicity of the solution, and hyponatremia or hypokalemia from diffusion into the wet dressings. Other problems consist of a requirement for bulky dressings that restrict joint motion and ambulation, and black staining of everything that comes into contact with the solution.

Silver Sulfadiazine. The use of silver sulfadiazine (SSD) in burns was first reported in both a murine burn model and 16 patients.[110] SSD is unique among the usual topical antibacterial agents in effectively inhibiting *Candida albicans*. The exact antimicrobial mechanism of action of SSD has not been clearly elucidated, but its effect is attributed to silver inhibition of DNA replication or cell membrane modification. Two studies imply that the sulfadiazine component is not necessary for in vitro bacterial sensitivity. In addition, clinical efficacy may be associated with a reversal of injury-induced suppression of lymphocyte natural killer cell cytotoxicity rather than strict antibacterial effects.

SSD is the topical agent of choice worldwide because of its safety and efficacy.[111–113] Toxicity associated with SSD application is infrequent and is associated predominantly with the propylene glycol component of the cream base. The potential for allergic hypersensitivity is shown by circulating sulfadiazine antibodies [predominantly immunoglobulin (IgG)] in the serum of treated patients. Although SSD-associated leukopenia has been reported, it is probably an artifact of the physiologic response to burn injury of white blood cell margination or diapedesis (movement through vessels) from the intravascular space.[114] Clinicians should continue to apply SSD to patients who develop leukopenia.

Because of its demonstrated efficacy, SSD has been incorporated into a number of biologic and synthetic dressings or skin substitutes, to take advantage of its benefits and eliminate the inconvenience of dressing changes with reapplication of cream. Another method used to improve upon SSD is the addition of other agents such as nitrofurazone, gentamicin, fluoroquinolones, and cerium nitrate. The most successful combination is noted with chlorhexidine; Silvazine (Smith & Nephew, Clayton, Australia), a commercially available combination, has been used in Australia for over a decade.

Mafenide Acetate and Nitrofurazone. Although it causes pain upon application, mafenide acetate is a useful topical antimicrobial for the treatment of subeschar burn wound infection, because of its ability to penetrate the burn wound. Mafenide is often used on burned ears to prevent chondritis. Although the two are closely related chemically, mafenide is not a sulfonamide. The primary metabolite (p-carboxybenzene sulfonamide) is a sulfonamide, and it may cause allergic reactions in patients with sulfonamide hypersensitivity. When applied to large TBSA burns, mafenide can produce systemic metabolic acidosis secondary to carbonic anhydrase inhibition.[115] Another disadvantage of mafenide is its high cost—approximately four times that of SSD. The antimicrobial usefulness of nitrofurazone has been demonstrated since the mid-1940s.[116] Its primary use has been in prophylaxis of infection following skin grafting.

Miscellaneous Topical Agents. Topical nystatin may be useful in limiting candidal growth, even though fungal or yeast colonization in burn wounds has not been linked to increased mortality rates.[117] Although some reduced infection rates have been reported, there is little support for the use of unusual agents such as honey, gentian violet, or acetic acid. The use of polymyxin B and bacitracin ointments is limited to small wounds because of the potential for systemic toxicity when they are used over large areas. Mupirocin may be valuable in the treatment of methicillin-resistant staphylococci in burn wounds, but its use has been inadequately studied. The use of povidone-iodine solutions on burn wounds is considered inappropriate because its antibacterial activity is partially inactivated by wound exudates, and systemic absorption of iodine may cause renal dysfunction.

Systemic Antimicrobials. The use of prophylactic penicillin during the first postburn week was common during the 1950s and 1960s because of a justified concern about infection by *Streptococcus pyogenes*. This organism produced rapid conversion of partial-thickness to full-thickness wounds and fatalities. However, current laboratory methods for monitoring the burn wound and close clinical monitoring of patients allow the rapid recognition of infection. Recent prospective clinical trials have demonstrated no benefit for prophylactic penicillin. Indeed, subsequent wound cultures in penicillin-treated patients demonstrate a greater incidence of resistant organisms.

The choice of antibiotic for systemic infection in burn patients should be the same as for other patients.[118] However, because the pathophysiologic changes following burn trauma are dynamic, the dosing of systemic antimicrobials must be individualized when possible.[119] Increased requirements for aminoglycosides and vancomycin have been demonstrated in burn patients (as discussed in the pharmacokinetics section).

NUTRITIONAL SUPPORT

The intimate relationship between nutrition and wound healing has been described.[120] The injury-associated hypermetabolic response with altered nutritional requirements, including vitamins and micronutrients, is discussed.

METABOLIC RESPONSE TO TRAUMA

Hypermetabolism following trauma was initially explained as a physiologic response to increased heat loss. The rationale was that burned skin allows increased water loss that lowers the skin/wound temperature when the water evaporates. However, the precise relationship between evaporative water loss and postburn hypermetabolism is unclear, because conflicting results have been reported from similar investigations.

Similarly, it has been assumed that increased thermogenesis was necessary to compensate for heat loss in a cold environment, because damaged skin cannot respond with decreased perspiration and cutaneous vasoconstriction. However, postburn hypermetabolism is not attenuated, even when the environmental temperature is increased to above thermal neutrality. A resetting of the hypothalamic thermal regulatory setpoint is suggested by a study comparing burn patients with normal controls, in which burn patients selected a significantly higher environmental temperature when placed in a metabolic chamber.

Metabolic rate may be reduced following relief of pain, although the degree of reduction is not well defined.[121] Historically, pain management of hospitalized patients with opioids has been suboptimal because of unnecessary fears of addiction. Morphine requirements of burn patients can be substantial, exceeding 60 mg per hour before tolerance develops.[48]

Other contributors to postburn hypermetabolism are prostaglandins, interleukins, components of the complement cascade, and the catabolic neurohumoral milieu of elevated serum cortisol, growth hormone, catecholamines, and glucagon levels.[122,123] Initial insulin secretion inhibition is usually followed by normal or supernormal plasma insulin levels. Despite this insulin recovery, hyperglycemia persists, secondary to insulin resistance at the tissue insulin receptor.

Fuel stores that are mobilized to sustain postburn hypermetabolism include hepatic and muscle glycogen; visceral, plasma, and muscle protein; and fat. Because the major metabolic source of adenosine triphosphate (ATP) provided to the burn wound is anaerobic glycolysis, the obligatory glucose requirement is increased. Production of glucose from glycogenolysis is relatively short lived because stores only approximate 100 to 200 g and endogenous glucose production exceeds 400 g per day. Significant endogenous glucose is provided by efficient recycling of pyruvate and lactate via the Cori cycle and the glucose-alanine cycle. Catabolism of muscle protein and direct oxidation of amino acids provide approximately 15% to 20% of the total caloric expenditure in the fasting injured patient. The body adapts by using fat as its main energy source and can mobilize abundant energy from the typical fat stores of approximately 160,000 kilocalories.

Pharmacologic interventions that have been attempted to ameliorate the catabolic state following burn injury include anabolic steroids (testosterone and oxandrolone), insulin, insulinlike growth factor, and human growth hormone. A growing body of evidence supports the use of oxandrolone, with both short-term and long-term benefits demonstrated.[124–127] Although a number of studies have demonstrated clinical benefits from adjunctive growth hormone treatment, there is little enthusiasm for its use because it is expensive and must be administered parenterally, and there is some evidence that growth hormone administration is associated with premature mortality.[128,129]

The specific cause of postburn hypermetabolism is not clear, but it appears to be multifactorial. Complete arrest of postburn hypermetabolism is not currently possible. A reasonable approach is to provide the patient with a warm environment, adequate pain relief, early enteral nutrition, and aggressive wound coverage. In addition, an attempt should be made to minimize endogenous protein catabolism by providing exogenous protein and nonprotein calories.

METHOD OF NUTRIENT ADMINISTRATION

Patients with less than 20% TBSA burns can usually be maintained on a normal diet, unless there is an associated condition such as severe preburn malnutrition or an injury that prevents mastication. Patients with larger burns are often unwilling or unable to consume enough high-protein and caloric-dense food to fulfill requirements. For these patients, nutritional requirements can be met by insertion of a small-bore nasoenteric feeding tube and administration of commercially available enteral feeding formulations such as Osmolite-HN, TwoCal HN, Traumacal, and Replete. Enteral nutrition is preferred to parenteral nutrition because it is more physiologic and less costly, and it avoids the complications associated with parenteral nutrition, such as catheter-related sepsis.

In contrast to historical recommendations that focused on parenteral nutrition, current guidelines call for early enteral feeding.[130] Even in severely burned patients with absent bowel sounds, feeding into the small intestine through a nasoenteric tube is still possible, because postburn ileus is confined primarily to the stomach.[131] In these severely injured patients, a nasogastric tube is inserted and connected to suction for 2 to 3 days until gastric function returns. Experimental evidence favoring early enteral feeding demonstrated a reduction in catabolism and the hypermetabolic response in a guinea pig burn model. Another beneficial effect of early enteral feeding is the maintenance of gut mucosal mass. Improved gut wall integrity may prevent the increased intestinal permeability that allows translocation of enteric bacteria.

MACRONUTRIENT NEEDS

The metabolic demands of patients with severe burns exceed those of any other hospitalized patient. Postburn energy expenditure increases with increasing burn size. However, there is an upper limit to required calories. This upper limit is approximately twice the calculated basal energy expenditure (BEE), according to the Harris-Benedict equation. Numerous formulas have been developed to calculate a burn patient's daily energy requirement, and representative formulas are listed in Table 11.3. Unfortunately, an investigation into the bias and precision of 46 methods published from 1953 to 2000 demonstrated that none were precise.[132] Although mathematical calculation to estimate energy requirements is convenient, determination of the patient's specific caloric

TABLE 11.3	Various Formulas Used to Estimate Energy Requirements in Burn Patients[a]

Adults

1. Harris-Benedict equation [estimates basal energy expenditure (BEE)]

    Male : BEE (kcal) = 66 + (13.7 × W) + (5 × H) − (6.8 × A)

    Female : BEE (kcal) = 665 + (9.6 × W) + (1.7 × H) − 4.7 × A)

2. Burke and Wolfe

    Kilocalories per day = 2 × BEE

3. Curreri

    Kilocalories per day = 25 × W + (40 × TBSA)

4. Davies and Liljedahl

    Kilocalories per day = 20 × W + (70 × TBSA)

Children

1. Wolfe

    Kilocalories per day = 2 × BEE

2. Curreri Junior

    Kilocalories per day = {0–1 years} BEE + (15 × TBSA)

    {1–3 years} BEE + (25 × TBSA)

    {3–15 years} BEE + (40 × TBSA)

[a] W, weight in kilograms; H, height in centimeters; A, age in years; and TBSA, total body surface area burned (%).

needs is desirable.[133] A complex metabolic chamber is necessary to specifically measure energy expenditure, but a reasonably accurate estimation can be performed at the bedside with the use of indirect calorimetry.[134] Metabolic carts measure the respiratory gas exchange of oxygen (VO_2) and carbon dioxide (VCO_2), thereby indirectly measuring energy expenditure (via the reverse Fick equation). Refer to Chapters 29 and 30.

Carbohydrate Requirements. Energy liberated by oxidation of enterally administered carbohydrate is approximately 4 kilocalories per gram. The carbohydrate commonly administered parenterally is hydrous dextrose, which liberates 3.4 kilocalories per gram when completely oxidized. The optimal amount of administered carbohydrate will minimize gluconeogenesis without exceeding energy requirements and being stored as triglycerides.

The use of glucose for energy by burned patients has limits. When glucose is oxidized to liberate energy, equimolar concentrations of oxygen are consumed and carbon dioxide produced (respiratory quotient [RQ] = 1). The normal, fed RQ is approximately 0.84, and it rises when the rate of administered glucose exceeds the maximum rate of utilization. When glucose is converted into fat, more than eight times as much carbon dioxide is released for each mole of oxygen (RQ >1). Excretion of this extra carbon dioxide could be difficult for a burn patient with an associated inhalation injury. An additional negative aspect of lipogenesis is that it is an energy-consuming process. An elegant study of intravenous glucose, performed with isotopic tracers, demonstrated that the maximum rate of oxidation is approximately 5 mg/kg/min. At faster rates of glucose administration, the RQ rapidly increased above 1.0, suggesting lipogenesis. For a 70-kg patient, this maximum rate of glucose utilization translates into 2 liters of 25% dextrose–containing total parenteral nutrition solution (500 g) per day.[135]

Fat Requirements. Fat is an efficient provider of energy at 9 kilocalories per gram, but it is vital only for supplying essential fatty acids to prevent essential fatty acid deficiency syndrome. The amount of fat necessary in burn patients is not known, but fat should provide a minimum 20% of total calories. Fat is an essential component of cell membranes, functions as a carrier for fat-soluble vitamins, and is important for wound healing.

Patients with severe thermal injury may have reduced lipolytic capacity, especially following parenteral administration of fat emulsion. It appears that parenteral administration of long-chain triglycerides is associated with hepatomegaly, impaired clotting, and decreased resistance to infection. Another advantage of enteral administration is that medium-chain triglycerides are absorbed without the need for bile, and at the cellular level, these are transported into mitochondria without the need for carnitine.

Because of constraints on the rate of carbohydrate administration, fat must usually be provided in substantial quantities as an energy source. Although it is not often important clinically, fat has a specific advantage over glucose in patients with pulmonary dysfunction, for whom reduced carbon dioxide production for an equivalent amount of oxygen consumed is useful. The optimal fatty acid chain length and exact dietary fat requirements for burn patients remain to be determined.

Protein Requirements. Protein loss across burn wounds is considerable and is greatest during the first 3 postburn days. Although early protein loss across full-thickness burns is greater than that in partial-thickness burns, the rates become approximately the same after postburn day 3. The rate of protein loss is reduced by application of either antimicrobial creams or skin substitutes. With the use of average protein loss during the first postburn week ($0.5 \text{ mg/cm}^2/\text{h}$), a formula that estimates daily protein loss (grams) across the burn wound can be devised: $1.2 \times$ body surface area (m^2) $\times$ TBSA burned (%). Protein loss across the burn wound during the second postburn week occurs at approximately half this rate.

The recommended daily allowance of protein for healthy adults is 0.8 g per kg. The optimal amount of protein required by burn patients to prevent catabolism of protein stores and promote wound healing is not well defined. The importance of protein sparing attained by providing energy must be considered, but some clinicians advocate a high-protein diet aimed at achieving a 100:1 nonprotein calorie-to-nitrogen ratio, in contrast to the standard 150:1 ratio. In clinical practice, approximately 1.5 to 2 g/kg/day (according to lean body weight) of protein is provided initially. Nitrogen balance studies then determine the adequacy of this regimen. Although the nitrogen balance calculation appears simple:

$$\text{Nitrogen balance} = N\ (in) - N\ (out) \quad (11\text{-}2)$$

there is potential error in assessment of both $N\ (in)$ and $N\ (out)$. $N\ (in)$ is the number of grams of nitrogen ingested or infused; it is common practice to multiply the number of grams of protein or amino acid by 0.16 to estimate grams of nitrogen. This calculation assumes that the protein is made up of 16% nitrogen, but the percentage of nitrogen available in parenteral amino acid products varies from 11.1% to 16.9%.[136] The $N\ (out)$ is calculated by adding the urinary urea nitrogen (UUN) from a 24-hour urine collection to an estimate of nitrogen excretion other than that measured as urine urea. This estimate comprises nonurea urinary nitrogen (ammonia, uric acid, creatinine) and nonurinary nitrogen loss (fecal and skin). A commonly used estimate for non-UUN losses is 4 g per day. One group advocates the measurement of total urinary nitrogen rather than use of an inaccurate estimate.[137] As described previously, significant quantities of protein (nitrogen) are lost through open burn wounds and must be included when an estimate is used.

The branched-chain amino acids (BCAAs) leucine, isoleucine, and valine are unique in that skeletal muscle can oxidize them directly for energy. In contrast, the other amino acids are metabolized almost wholly by the liver. Under ordinary circumstances, only 6% to 7% of daily energy expenditure is provided through BCAA oxidation by skeletal muscle. The administration of supplemental BCAAs, especially leucine, to burn patients should theoretically reduce protein catabolism in skeletal muscle and increase protein synthesis. However, conclusive evidence of beneficial effects for BCAA-enriched solutions in burn patients has not been demonstrated, and further studies are needed.[138]

Another strategy for improving outcome in burn patients is the administration of beneficial nutrients, such as n-3 polyunsaturated fatty acids, arginine, glutamine, and nucleotides, in an attempt to reduce inflammation or enhance immunity. The hypothesis is that lipids high in linoleic acid (an omega-6 fatty acid in safflower or soybean oil) are potentially proinflammatory because linoleic acid gives rise to arachidonic acid, interleukins-1 and -6, and tumor necrosis factor-α. A number of clinical trials have been performed on several types of critically ill patients with the use of commercially available formulas such as Impact, Perative, and Crucial. Unfortunately, the results are conflicting, the benefits of these expensive diets have yet to be definitively demonstrated in burn patients, and much controversy exists.[139] Irrespective of these scientific limitations, some groups of experts advocate the use of these specialty diets.[140] The best evidence for a beneficial effect from these nutritional supplements appears to involve glutamine.[141,142]

Measurement of serum proteins such as albumin, prealbumin (transthyretin), transferrin, and retinol binding protein is often regarded as a reliable index of nutritional status. However, because of surgical excision and grafting of wounds, associated blood loss and transfusions, and administration of exogenous albumin, changes in serum protein concentrations as an indication of nutrition regimen adequacy must be viewed with caution. Nitrogen balance studies probably provide the best assessment of protein status, despite the limitations described previously.

MICRONUTRIENT NEEDS

In contrast to the extensive information that has been obtained about macronutrient requirements, little information is available about the micronutrient needs of burn patients. Evidence suggests that micronutrient needs are increased following burns, although the exact amounts have not been defined.[143,144]

Vitamins. At a minimum, burn patients should receive vitamin supplements based on the recommended dietary allowances (RDA) for enteral administration, or the American Medical Association (AMA) Nutrition Advisory Group recommendations for parenteral administration. With the exception of vitamin D, in the absence of preexisting deficiency, little information indicates that increased amounts of fat-soluble vitamins should be administered.[145] Vitamin C is often supplemented to $5 \times$ RDA because it has little inherent toxic potential and it plays an important role in collagen deposition and wound healing. Because of their role as cofactors in metabolism and the potential for increased losses through the wound and urine, the B vitamin group is supplemented to 2 × RDA.

Trace Elements. In the acute-phase reaction to trauma, plasma concentrations of zinc, iron, and copper are markedly decreased.[146] Similar to vitamin C, zinc is thought to promote wound healing, and it is supplemented to 2 × RDA. Aggressive iron supplementation must be undertaken with some caution because of the potential for increased bacterial growth due to plasma unbound iron. Deficiency syndromes of copper, selenium, chromium, iodine, manganese, and molybdenum occur in patients on long-term total parenteral nutrition, but no cases of deficiency appear to have been reported as a direct result of burn trauma. These trace elements are administered according to RDA or AMA guidelines.

CONCLUSION

The complex clinical management and rehabilitation of a severely burned patient require the efforts of a multidisciplinary team, including surgeons, nurses, a pharmacist, a dietitian, a psychotherapist, a physical therapist, an occupational therapist, a respiratory therapist, and a social worker. A large TBSA full-thickness burn requires surgical excision and split-thickness skin grafting. Fluid requirements during the initial postburn period are large, and guidelines for fluid resuscitation have been devised by experienced clinicians. The pharmacist must be aware that the postburn hyperdynamic and hypermetabolic phase produces multiple pharmacokinetic and pharmacodynamic changes. The nutritional requirements of burn patients can be substantial, with energy needs often approaching twice those of other hospitalized patients. A number of methods are available for estimating energy requirements through mathematical calculation, but determination of the patient's specific caloric needs by indirect calorimetry is desirable. The amount of dietary protein required by burn patients to promote wound healing, replace losses, and prevent catabolism of protein stores is not well defined. Usually, intravenous amino acids or enteral protein at 1.5 to 2 g/kg/day is provided, and nitrogen balance studies are performed. Current guidelines call for the preferential use of enteral (rather than parenteral) nutrition.

Prevention and treatment of infection in the burn patient are of paramount importance in that infection is the most common cause of death among patients who survive initial resuscitation. Treatment approaches for systemic infection in burn patients are similar to methods used for other patients, with dose individualization determined by antimicrobial serum concentration monitoring when possible. Microbial growth in the burn wound can be substantial following colonization by endogenous or exogenous organisms. The availability of topical antimicrobial agents has dramatically improved the control of burn wound infections.

KEY POINTS

- The complex clinical management and rehabilitation of a severely burned patient requires the efforts of a multidisciplinary team, including surgeons, nurses, a pharmacist, a dietitian, a physical therapist, an occupational therapist, a respiratory therapist, and a social worker.
- A large TBSA full-thickness burn requires surgical excision and split-thickness skin grafting.
- Fluid requirements during the initial postburn period are surprisingly large, and guidelines for fluid resuscitation have been devised by experienced clinicians.
- The pharmacist must be aware that the postburn hyperdynamic and hypermetabolic phase produces multiple pharmacokinetic and pharmacodynamic changes.
- The nutritional requirements of burn patients can be substantial, with energy needs often approaching twice those of other hospitalized patients. A number of methods are available for estimating energy requirements through mathematical calculation, but determination of the patient's specific caloric needs by indirect calorimetry is desirable.
- The amount of dietary protein required by burn patients to promote wound healing, replace losses, and prevent catabolism of protein stores is not well defined. Usually, intravenous amino acids or enteral protein at 1.5 to 2 g/kg/day is provided, and nitrogen balance studies are performed.
- Current guidelines call for the preferential use of enteral (rather than parenteral) nutrition.
- Prevention and treatment of infection in the burn patient are of paramount importance, because infection is the most common cause of death among patients who survive initial resuscitation. Treatment approaches for systemic infection in burn patients are similar to methods used for other patients, with dose individualization determined by antimicrobial serum concentration monitoring when possible.
- Microbial growth in the burn wound can be substantial following colonization by endogenous or exogenous organisms. The availability of topical antimicrobial agents has dramatically improved the control of burn wound infections.

SUGGESTED READINGS

1. Cassuto J, Tarnow P. The discotheque fire in Gothenburg 1998: a tragedy among teenagers. Burns 29:405–416, 2003.
2. Demling RH, DeSanti L, Orgill DP. Burn wound management: use of skin substitutes. [Module] [Online]. Available at: www.burnsurgery.org. Accessed April 2004.
3. National Guideline Clearinghouse—Burns (Revised November 2004). Available at: http://www.guideline.gov/summary/summary.aspx?ss=15&doc_id=5941&nbr=3910&string=burns. Accessed April 2004.

4. Sheridan RL, Schultz JT, Ryan CM, et al. Case 6-2004: a 35-year-old woman with extensive, deep burns from a nightclub fire. N Engl J Med 350:810–821, 2004.
5. Tarnow P, Gewalli F, Cassuto J. Fire disaster in Gothenburg 1998—surgical treatment of burns. Burns 29:417–421, 2003.

REFERENCES

1. Sheridan RL, Schultz JT, Ryan CM, et al. Case 6-2004: a 35-year-old woman with extensive, deep burns from a nightclub fire. N Engl J Med 350:810–821, 2004.
2. Tarnow P, Gewalli F, Cassuto J. Fire disaster in Gothenburg 1998—surgical treatment of burns. Burns 29:417–421, 2003.
3. Cassuto J, Tarnow P. The discotheque fire in Gothenburg 1998: a tragedy among teenagers. Burns 29:405–416, 2003.
4. Cassell OCS, Fiton AJ, Dickson WA, et al. An audit of the tetanus immunization status of plastic surgery trauma and burns patients. Br J Plast Surg 55:215–218, 2002.
5. Centers for Disease Control and Prevention. MMWR 40(RR12): 1–52, 1991.
6. Wibbenmeyer LA, Hoballah JJ, Amelon MJ, et al. The prevalence of venous thromboembolism of the lower extremity among thermally injured patients determined by duplex sonography. J Trauma 55:1162–1167, 2003.
7. McCormick JT, O'Mara MS, Wakefield W, et al. Effect of diagnosis and treatment of sinusitis in critically ill burn victims. Burns 29:79–81, 2003.
8. Arturson MG. The pathophysiology of severe thermal injury. J Burn Care Rehabil 6:129–146, 1985.
9. Silverman SH, Purdue GF, Hunt JL, et al. Cyanide toxicity in burned patients. J Trauma 28:171–176, 1988.
10. Blalock SJ, Bunker BJ, DeVellis RF. Measuring health status among survivors of burn injury: revisions of the burn specific health scale. J Trauma 36:508–515, 1994.
11. Saffle JR, Sullivan JJ, Tuohig GM, et al. Multiple organ failure in patients with thermal injury. Crit Care Med 21:1673–1683, 1993.
12. Ryan CM, Schoenfeld DA, Thorpe WP, et al. Objective estimates of the probability of death from burn injuries. N Engl J Med 338: 362–366, 1998.
13. Darling GE, Keresteci MA, Ibanez D, et al. Pulmonary complications in inhalation injuries with associated cutaneous burn. J Trauma 40:83–89, 1996.
14. Sheridan RL. Airway management and respiratory care of the burn patient. Int Anesthesiol Clin 38:129–145, 2000.
15. Fitzwater J, Purdue GF, Hunt JL, et al. The risk factors and time course of sepsis and organ dysfunction after burn trauma. J Trauma 54:959–966, 2003.
16. Gore MA, Anagha RJ, Ganesh N, et al. Virtual bronchoscopy for diagnosis of inhalation injury in burnt patients. Burns 30:165–168, 2004.
17. Sheridan RL. Specific therapies for inhalation injury. Crit Care Med 30:718–719, 2002.
18. Reper P, Van Bos R, Van Loey K, et al. High frequency percussive ventilation in burn patients: hemodynamics and gas exchange. Burns 29:603–608, 2003.
19. Punch JD, Smith DJ, Robson MC. Hospital care of major burns. Postgrad Med 85:205–215, 1989.
20. Wachtel TL. Major burns. Postgrad Med 85:178–196, 1989.
21. Schiller WR, Garren RL, Bay RC, et al. Laser doppler evaluation of burned hands predicts need for surgical grafting. J Trauma 43: 35–40, 1997.
22. Robson MC, Smith DJ, Heggers JP. Innovations in burn wound management. Adv Plast Reconstr Surg 4:149–176, 1987.
23. Perry RJ, Moore CA, Morgan BDG, et al. Determining the approximate area of a burn: an inconsistency investigated and re-evaluated. BMJ 312:1338, 1996.
24. Saffle JR. What's new in general surgery: burns and metabolism. J Am Coll Surg 196:267–289, 2003.
25. Wong L, Munster AM. New techniques in burn wound management. Surg Clin North Am 73:363–371, 1993.
26. Falanga V. Wound bed preparation and the role of enzymes: a case for multiple actions of therapeutic agents. Wound 14:47–57, 2002.
27. Barret JP, Herndon DN. Effects of burn wound excision on bacterial colonization and invasion. Plast Reconstr Surg 111:744–750, 2003.
28. Hart DW, Wolf SE, Chinkes DL, et al. Effects of early excision and aggressive enteral feeding on hypermetabolism, catabolism, and sepsis after severe burn. J Trauma 54:755–764, 2003.
29. Gore DC, Beaston J. Infusion of hot crystalloid during operative burn wound debridement. J Trauma 42:1112–1115, 1997.
30. Demling RH. Burns. N Engl J Med 313:1389–1398, 1985.
31. Nowicki CR, Sprenger CK. Temporary skin substitutes for burn patients: a nursing perspective. J Burn Care Rehabil 9:209–215, 1988.
32. Demling RH, DeSanti L, Orgill DP. Burn wound management: use of skin substitutes. [Module] [Online]. Available at: www.burnsurgery.org. Accessed April 2004.
33. Teepe RGC, Kreis RW, Koebrugge EJ, et al. The use of cultured autologous epidermis in the treatment of extensive burn wounds. J Trauma 30:269–275, 1990.
34. Williamson JS, Snelling CFT, Clugston P, et al. Cultured epithelial autograft: five years of clinical experience with twenty-eight patients. J Trauma 39:309–319, 1995.
35. Lorenz C, Petracic A, Hohl HP, et al. Early wound closure and early reconstruction. Experience with a dermal substitute in a child with 60 per cent total surface area burn. Burns 23:505–508, 1997.
36. Muhart M, McFalls S, Kirsner R, et al. Bioengineered skin. Lancet 350:1142, 1997.
37. Naughton G, Mansbridge J, Gentzkow G. A metabolically active human dermal replacement for the treatment of diabetic foot ulcers. Artif Organs 21:1203–1210, 1997.
38. Ahlering PA. Topical silastic gel sheeting for treating and controlling hypertrophic and keloid scars: case study. Derm Nursing 7: 259–267, 1995.
39. Mustoe TA, Cooter RD, Gold MH, et al. International advisory panel on scar management. International clinical recommendations on scar management. Plast Reconstr Surg 110:560–571, 2002.
40. Baker RAU, Zeller RA, Klein RL. Burn wound itch control using H_1 and H_2 antagonists. J Burn Care Rehabil 22:263–268, 2001.
41. Demling RH, DeSanti L. Topical doxepin cream is effective in relieving severe pruritis (sic) caused by burn injury: a preliminary study. Wounds 13:210–215, 2001.
42. Matheson JD, Clayton J, Muller MJ. The reduction of itch during burn wound healing. J Burn Care Rehabil 22:76–81, 2001.
43. Field T, Peck M, Hernandez-Reif M, et al. Postburn itching, pain, and psychological symptoms are reduced with massage therapy. J Burn Care Rehabil 21:189–193, 2000.
44. Choiniere M, Melzack R, Rondeau J, et al. The pain of burns: characteristics and correlates. J Trauma 29:1531–1539, 1989.
45. Perry S, Heidrich G. Management of pain during debridement: a survey of U.S. burn units. Pain 13:267–280, 1982.
46. Osgood PF, Szyfelbein SK. Management of burn pain in children. Pediatr Clin North Am:1001–1013, 1989.
47. Coimbra C, Choiniere M, Hemmerling TM. Patient-controlled sedation using propofol for dressing changes in burn patients: a dose-finding study. Anesth Analg 97:839–842, 2003.
48. Wermeling DP, Record KE, Foster TS. Patient-controlled high-dose morphine therapy in a patient with electrical burns. Clin Pharm 5:832–835, 1986.
49. Donahue SR. Morphine sulfate intravenous dose of 1650 mg per hour. Hosp Pharm 24:311, 1989.
50. Porter J, Jick H. Addiction rare in patients treated with narcotics. N Engl J Med 302:123, 1980.
51. Choiniere M, Grenier R, Paquette C. Patient-controlled analgesia: a double-blind study in burn patients. Anaesthesia 47:467–472, 1992.
52. Gaukroger PB, Chapman MJ, Davey RB. Pain control in paediatric burns—the use of patient-controlled analgesia. Burns 17:396–399, 1991.
53. Rovers J, Knighton J, Neligan P. Patient-controlled analgesia in burn patients: a critical review of the literature and case report. Hosp Pharm 29:106, 108–111, 1994.
54. Cassuto J, Tarnow P. Potent inhibition of burn pain without use of opiates. Burns 29:163–166, 2003.
55. Patterson DR, Questad KA, de Lateur BJ. Hypnotherapy as an adjunct to narcotic analgesia for the treatment of pain for burn debridement. Am J Clin Hypn 31:156–163, 1989.

56. Miller AC, Hickman LC, Lemasters GK. A distraction technique for control of burn pain. J Burn Care Rehabil 13:576–580, 1992.
57. Beyer JE, Levin CR. Issues and advances in pain control in children. Nurs Clin North Am 22:661–676, 1987.
58. Pal SK, Cortiella J, Herndon D. Adjunctive methods of pain control in burns. Burns 23:404–412, 1997.
59. Reilly M. Music distraction in burn patients: influencing postprocedure recall. Semin Periop Nurs 6:242–245, 1997.
60. Rubin WD, Mani MM, Hiebert JM. Fluid resuscitation of the thermally injured patient. Current concepts with definition of clinical subsets and their specialized treatment. Clin Plast Surg 13:9–20, 1986.
61. Demling RH. Fluid replacement in burned patients. Surg Clin North Am 67:15–30, 1987.
62. Graves TA, Cioffi WG, McManus WF, et al. Fluid resuscitation of infants and children with massive thermal injury. J Trauma 28:1656–1659, 1988.
63. Aikawa N, Ishibiki K, Naito C, et al. Individualized fluid resuscitation based on haemodynamic monitoring in the management of extensive burns. Burns 8:249–255, 1982.
64. Tanaka H, Matsuda T, Miyagantani Y, et al. Reduction of resuscitation fluid volumes in severely burned patients using ascorbic acid administration: a randomized, prospective study. Arch Surg 135:326–331, 2000.
65. Horton JW, White DJ, Baxter CR. Hypertonic saline dextran resuscitation of thermal injury. Ann Surg 211:301–311, 1990.
66. Gunn ML, Hansbrough JF, Davis JW, et al. Prospective, randomized trial of hypertonic sodium lactate versus lactated Ringer's solution for burn shock resuscitation. J Trauma 29:1261–1267, 1989.
67. Ross AD, Angaran DM. Colloids vs. crystalloids—a continuing controversy. DICP Ann Pharmacother 18:202–212, 1984.
68. Waters LM, Christensen MA, Sato RM. Hetastarch: an alternative colloid in burn shock management. J Burn Care Rehabil 10:11–16, 1989.
69. Bowser BH, Caldwell FT. The effects of resuscitation with hypertonic vs. hypotonic vs. colloid on wound and urine fluid and electrolyte losses in severely burned children. J Trauma 23:916–923, 1983.
70. Greenhalgh DG, Housinger TA, Kagan RJ, et al. Maintenance of serum albumin levels in pediatric burn patients: a prospective, randomized trial. J Trauma 39:67–74, 1995.
71. Sheridan RL, Prelack K, Cunningham JJ. Physiologic hypoalbuminemia is well tolerated by severely burned children. J Trauma 43:448–452, 1997.
72. Cochrane Injuries Group Albumin Reviewers. Human albumin administration in critically ill patients: systematic review of randomised controlled trials. BMJ 317:235–240, 1998.
73. Milner SM, Hodgetts TJ, Rylah LA. The burns calculator: a simple proposed guide for fluid resuscitation. Lancet 1993;342:1089–91.
74. Lazarus D. Hudson DA. Fatal rhabdomyolysis in a flame burn patient. Burns 23:446–450, 1997.
75. Murphy KD, Lee JO, Herndon DN. Current pharmacotherapy for the treatment of severe burns. Expert Opin Pharmacother 4:1–15, 2003.
76. Martyn J. Clinical pharmacology and drug therapy in the burned patient. Anesthesiology 65:67–75, 1986.
77. Bonate PL. Pathophysiology and pharmacokinetics following burn injury. Clin Pharmacokinet 18:118–130, 1990.
78. Czaja AJ, McAlhany JC, Pruitt BA. Acute duodenitis and duodenal ulceration after burns. Clinical and pathological characteristics. JAMA 232:621–624, 1975.
79. Cioffi WG, McManus AT, Rue LW, et al. Comparison of acid neutralizing and non-acid neutralizing stress ulcer prophylaxis in thermally injured patients. J Trauma 36:541–547, 1994.
80. Loirat P, Rohan J, Baillet A, et al. Increased glomerular filtration rate in patients with major burns and its effect on the pharmacokinetics of tobramycin. N Engl J Med 299:915–919, 1978.
81. Zaske DE, Sawchuk RJ, Gerding DN, et al. Increased dosage requirements of gentamicin in burn patients. J Trauma 16:824–828, 1976.
82. Glew RH, Moellering RC, Burke JF. Gentamicin dosage in children with extensive burns. J Trauma 16:819–823, 1976.
83. Zaske DE, Bootman JL, Solem LB, et al. Increased burn patient survival with individualized dosages of gentamicin. Surgery 91:142–149, 1982.
84. Zaske DE, Chin T, Kohls PR, et al. Initial dosage regimens of gentamicin in patients with burns. J Burn Care Rehabil 12:46–50, 1991.
85. Hollingsed TC, Harper DJ, Jennings JP. Aminoglycoside dosing in burn patients using first dose pharmacokinetics. J Trauma 35:394–398, 1993.
86. Hoey LL, Tschida SJ, Rotschafer JC, et al. Wide variation in single, daily-dose aminoglycoside pharmacokinetics in patients with burn injuries. J Burn Care Rehabil 18:116–124, 1997.
87. Garrelts JC, Peterie JD. Altered vancomycin dose vs. serum concentration relationship in burn patients. Clin Pharmacol Ther 44:9–13, 1988.
88. Brater DC, Bawdon RE, Anderson SA, et al. Vancomycin elimination in patients with burn injury. Clin Pharmacol Ther 39:631–634, 1986.
89. Martyn J, Greenblatt DJ. Lorazepam conjugation is unimpaired in burn trauma. Clin Pharmacol Ther 43:250–255, 1987.
90. Bloedow DC, Hansbrough JF, Hardin T, et al. Postburn serum drug binding and serum protein concentrations. J Clin Pharmacol 26:147–151, 1986.
91. Thompson DF. Neuromuscular blocking agents in burn patients. DICP Ann Pharmacother 23:1006–1008, 1989.
92. Dwersteg JF, Pavlin EG, Heimbach DM. Patients with burns are resistant to atracurium. Anesthesiology 65:517–520, 1986.
93. Stone HH, Kolb LD, Pettit J, et al. The systemic absorption of an antibiotic from the burn wound surface. Am Surg 34:639–643, 1968.
94. Stefanides MM, Copeland CE, Kominos SD, et al.: In vitro penetration of topical antiseptics through eschar of burn patients. Ann Surg 183:358–364, 1976.
95. Polk RE, Mayhall CG, Smith J, et al. Gentamicin and tobramycin penetration into burn eschar. Arch Surg 118:295–302, 1983.
96. McManus WF. Patterns of infection over the past ten years: historical patterns. J Burn Care Rehabil 8:32–35, 1987.
97. Gelfand JA. Infections in burn patients: a paradigm for cutaneous infection in the patient at risk. Am J Med 76 (Suppl 5A):158–165, 1984.
98. Luterman A, Dacso CC, Curreri PW. Infections in burn patients. Am J Med 81 (Suppl 1A):45–52, 1986.
99. Ziegler TR, Smith RJ, O'Dwyer RT, et al. Increased intestinal permeability associated with infection in burn patients. Arch Surg 123:1313–1319, 1988.
100. Deitch EA. Intestinal permeability is increased in burn patients shortly after injury. Surgery 107:411–416, 1990.
101. Barber A, Inner H, Shires GT. Bacterial translocation in burn injury. Semin Nephrol 13:416–419, 1993.
102. Ryan CM, Tompkins RG. Topical therapy II: burns. In: Chernow B, ed. The pharmacologic approach to the critically ill patient. 3rd ed. Baltimore: Williams & Wilkins, 1994:830–843.
103. Mayhall CG. The epidemiology of burn wound infections: then and now. Clin Infect Dis 37:543–550, 2003.
104. Edwards-Jones V, Greenwood JE. What's new in burn microbiology? James Laing Memorial Prize Essay 2000. Burns 29:15–24, 2003.
105. Moncrief JA, Teplitz C. Changing concepts in burn sepsis. J Trauma 4:233–245, 1964.
106. Pruitt BA. The diagnosis and treatment of infection in the burn patient. Burns Incl Therm Inj 11:79–91, 1984.
107. Nathan P, Law EJ, Murphy DF, et al. A laboratory method for selection of topical antimicrobial agents to treat infected burn wounds. Burns Incl Therm Inj 4:177–187, 1978.
108. Heggers JP, Velanovich V, Robson MC, et al. Control of burn wound sepsis: a comparison of in vitro topical antimicrobial assays. J Trauma 27:176–179, 1987.
109. Moyer CA, Brentano L, Gravens DL, et al. Treatment of large human burns with 0.5% silver nitrate solution. Arch Surg 90:812–867, 1965.
110. Fox CL. Silver sulfadiazine—a new topical therapy for *Pseudomonas* in burns. Arch Surg 96:184–188, 1968.
111. Monafo WW, West MA. Current treatment recommendations for topical burn therapy. Drugs 40:364–373, 1990.
112. Rice TL. Topical antibacterials. Hosp Pharm 27:1099–1108, 1992.
113. Sawhney CP, Sharma RK, Rao KR, et al. Long-term experience with 1 per cent topical silver sulphadiazine cream in the management of burn wounds. Burns Incl Therm Inj 15:403–406, 1989.

114. Thomson PD, Moore NP, Rice TL, et al. Leukopenia in acute thermal injury: evidence against silver sulfadiazine as the causative agent. J Burn Care Rehabil 10:418–420, 1989.
115. Liebman PR, Kennelly MM, Hirsch EF. Hypercarbia and acidosis associated with carbonic anhydrase inhibition: a hazard of topical mafenide acetate use in renal failure. Burns 8:395–398, 1982.
116. Hooper G, Covarrubias J. Clinical use and efficacy of furacin: a historical perspective. J Int Med Res 11:289–293, 1983.
117. Monafo WW, Bessey PQ. Wound care. In: Herndon DN, ed. Total burn care. London: WB Saunders Co. LTD, 1996.
118. Dacso CC, Luterman A, Curreri PW. Systemic antibiotic treatment in burned patients. Surg Clin North Am 67:57–68, 1987.
119. Mason AD, McManus AT, Pruitt BA. Association of burn mortality and bacteremia. A 25-year review. Arch Surg 121:1027–1031, 1986.
120. Meyer NA, Muller MJ, Herndon DN. Nutrient support of the healing wound. New Horizons 2:202–214, 1994.
121. Mackersie RC, Karagianes TG. Pain management following trauma and burns. Anesthesiol Clin North Am 7:211–227, 1989.
122. Drost AC, Burleson DG, Cioffi WG. Plasma cytokines following thermal injury and their relationship with patient mortality, burn size and time post burn. J Trauma 35:335–339, 1993.
123. DeBrandt JP, Chollet-Martin S, Hernvann A, et al. Cytokine response to burn injury: relationship with protein metabolism. J Trauma 36:624–628, 1994.
124. Andel H, Kamolzb L-P, Hörauf K, et al. Nutrition and anabolic agents in burned patients. Burns 29:592–595, 2003.
125. Wolf SE, Thomas SJ, Dasu MR, et al. Improved net protein balance, lean mass, and gene expression changes with oxandrolone treatment in the severely burned. Ann Surg 6:801–811, 2003.
126. Demling RH, DeSanti L. Oxandrolone induced lean mass gain during recovery from severe burns is maintained after discontinuation of the anabolic steroid. Burns 29:793–797, 2003.
127. Thomas S, Wolf SE, Murphy KD, et al. The long-term effect of oxandrolone on hepatic acute phase proteins in severely burned children. J Trauma 56:37–44, 2004.
128. Jenkins RC, Ross RJM. Growth hormone therapy for protein catabolism. QJM 89:813–819, 1996.
129. Maison P, Balkau B, Simon D, et al. Growth hormone as a risk for premature mortality in healthy subjects: data from the Paris prospective study. BMJ 316:1132–1133, 1998.
130. Enzi G, Casadei A, Sergi G, et al. Metabolic and hormonal effects of early nutritional supplementation after surgery in burn patients. Crit Care Med 18:719–721, 1990.
131. Garrel DR, Davignon I, Lopez D. Length of care in patients with severe burns with or without early enteral nutritional support. A retrospective study. J Burn Care Rehabil 12:85–90, 1991.
132. Dickerson RN, Gervasio JM, Riley ML, et al. Accuracy of predictive methods to estimate resting energy expenditure of thermally-injured patients. J Parent Enter Nutr 26:17–29, 2002.
133. Cunningham JJ, Hegarty MT, Meara PA, et al. Measured and predicted calorie requirements of adults during recovery from severe burn trauma. Am J Clin Nutr 49:404–408, 1989.
134. Saffle JR, Medina E, Raymond J, et al. Use of indirect calorimetry in the nutritional management of burned patients. J Trauma 25:32–39, 1985.
135. Bell SJ, Blackburn GL. Nutritional support of the burn patient. In: Martyn JAJ, ed. Acute management of the burned patient. Philadelphia: WB Saunders, 1990:138–158.
136. Miller SJ. The nitrogen balance revisited. Hosp Pharm 25:61–65, 1990.
137. Konstantinides FN, Radmer WJ, Becker WK, et al. Inaccuracy of nitrogen balance determinations in thermal injury with calculated total urinary nitrogen. J Burn Care Rehabil 13:254–260, 1992.
138. Oki JC, Cuddy PG. Branched-chain amino acid support of stressed patients. DICP Ann Pharmacother 23:399–408, 1989.
139. Saffle JR, Wiebke G, Jennings K, et al. Randomized trial of immune-enhancing enteral nutrition in burn patients. J Trauma 42:793–802, 1997.
140. Anonymous. Proceedings from summit on immune-enhancing enteral therapy, May 25–26, 2000, San Diego, California, USA. J Parent Enter Nutr 25:S1–S63, 2001.
141. Garrel D, Patenaude J, Nedelec B, et al. Decreased mortality and infectious morbidity in adult burn patients given enteral glutamine supplements: a prospective, controlled, randomized clinical trial. Crit Care Med 31:2444–2449, 2003.
142. Peng X, Yan H, You Z, et al. Effects of enteral supplementation with glutamine granules on intestinal mucosal barrier function in severe burned patients. Burns 30:135–139, 2004.
143. Pasulka PS, Wachtel TL. Nutritional considerations for the burned patient. Surg Clin North Am 67:109–131, 1987.
144. O'Neil CE, Hutsler D, Hildreth MA. Basic nutritional guidelines for pediatric burn patients. J Burn Care Rehabil 10:278–284, 1989.
145. Klein GL, Chen TC, Holick MF, et al. Synthesis of vitamin D in skin after burns. Lancet 363:291–292, 2004.
146. Shewmake KB, Talbert GE, Bowser-Wallace BH, et al. Alterations in plasma copper, zinc, and ceruloplasmin levels in patients with thermal trauma. J Burn Care Rehabil 9:13–17, 1988.

CASE STUDIES

CASE 3

TOPIC: Allergic and Drug-Induced Skin Diseases

THERAPEUTIC DIFFICULTY: Level 2
Kelly M. Smith

CHAPTER 9: Allergic and Drug-Induced Diseases

■ Scenario

Patient and Setting: JA, a 48-year-old white female; primary care provider's office

Chief Complaint: Pruritic, painful rash of palms, arms, and feet with fever, malaise, and weakness

■ History of Present Illness

Rash began 2 days prior with a spread from hands to arms and lower extremities, rash unresponsive to topical nonprescription medication; low-grade fever × 2 days

Medical History: Urinary tract infection (UTI) within past week; coronary artery disease (CAD) × 12 years; hypertension (HTN) × 10 years; generalized seizure disorder × 18 years; seasonal allergic rhinitis × 35 years

Surgical History: None

Family/Social History: Family History: Father died at age 53 of acute MI; mother positive for HTN and history of MI × 2 by age 45
Social History: JA works as an elementary school science teacher; has 28-pack per year cigarette history (1 pack per day); 1–2 glasses red wine per week

Medications:
Sulfamethoxazole, 800 mg/trimethoprim (SMX/ TMP) 160 mg PO BID × 3 days (completed 1 day prior)
Diphenhydramine/calamine lotion applied topically PRN
Lisinopril, 10 mg PO QD
Metoprolol, 100 mg PO BID
Simvastatin, 80 mg PO QD
Phenytoin, 300 mg PO QD
Cetirizine/pseudoephedrine, 1 tab PO BID

Allergies: Rash with unknown antibiotic (reaction as child)

■ Physical Examination

GEN: Well-developed, well-nourished woman
VS: BP 142/94, HR 68, RR 18, T 38.1°C, Wt 60 kg, Ht 150 cm
HEENT: Slight nystagmus
COR: WNL
CHEST: WNL
ABD: WNL
GU: Deferred
RECT: Deferred
EXT: Maculopapular, circular lesions with dark outer border on arms, hands, and feet; slightly erythematous
NEURO: Alert, 0 × 4; slightly ataxic

■ Results of Pertinent Laboratory Tests, Serum Drug Concentrations, and Diagnostic Tests

Na 136 (136)	Hct 0.37 (37)		T Bili 5.1 (0.3)
K 4.2 (4.2)	Hgb 130 (13)		
Cl 99 (99)	Lkcs 8.1 × 10⁹	AST 0.50 (30)	Glu 4.4 (80)
	(8.1 × 10³)		
HCO₃ 26 (26)		ALT 0.48 (29)	Ca 2.5 (9.8)
BUN 2.9 (8.2)	Plts (210 × 10⁹)	LDH 1.53 (92)	PO4 1.1 (3.3)
	(210 × 10³)		
CR 97.2 (1.1)		Alk Phos 1.5 (90)	Mg 0.8 (1.9)
	MCV 80 (80)	Alb 40 (4.0)	Uric Acid 249.8
			(4.2)

Total Chol 8.4 (323)
Triglycerides 1.7 (150)
HDL 0.8 (30)
LDL 6.2 (238)

Phenytoin serum concentration 100.3 μmol/L (25.3 mcg/ml)
ESR 18
Lkc differential: WNL
Urinalysis: WNL

■ Problem List

Identify principal problems from the scenario in priority order (see Answers in back of book for correct list of problems).

■ SOAP Note

To be completed by the student (see Answers in back of book for correct SOAP Note).

■ QUESTIONS

(See Answers in back of book for correct responses.)

1. The probable cause for JA's rash is: (EO-1)
   a. Erythema multiforme associated with sulfamethoxazole/trimethoprim
   b. Contact dermatitis reaction to poison ivy
   c. Stevens-Johnson syndrome secondary to sulfamethoxazole/trimethoprim
   d. Photoallergic response to lisinopril

2. _____ is another drug class that may result in JA's dermatologic condition. (EO-1)
   a. ACE inhibitors
   b. Fluoroquinolones
   c. Tetracyclines
   d. NSAIDs

3. Differentiate the dermatologic findings of Stevens-Johnson syndrome, erythema multiforme, and toxic epidermal necrolysis. (EO-2, 5)

4. In addition to the identified reaction (question 1), list other skin diseases that are known to be associated with the offending drug/drug class. (EO-1)

5. List additional clinical effects that may develop if JA's dermatologic condition progresses to a more severe form. (EO-5)

6. JA appears to have phenytoin toxicity. Which of the following is the most likely cause? (EO-5, 9)
   a. Drug interaction with simvastatin
   b. Hypoalbuminemia
   c. Lingering effects of drug interaction with sulfamethoxazole/trimethoprim
   d. Autoinduction of phenytoin metabolism

7. Identify the signs and symptoms of acute phenytoin toxicity. (EO-2, 5, 10)

8. Which one of the following of JA's medications is most likely to interact with phenytoin? (EO-9)
   a. Metoprolol
   b. Simvastatin
   c. Lisinopril
   d. Diphenhydramine/calamine

9. What is the nature of the above drug interaction with phenytoin? (EO-4, 9)
   a. Phenytoin-induced reduction in renal excretion of object drug
   b. Autoinduction of phenytoin metabolism
   c. Object drug's displacement of phenytoin from protein-binding sites
   d. Phenytoin induction of object drug's metabolism

10. Which medication is expected to contribute to JA's hypertension? (EO-7, 9, 10, 11)
    a. Simvastatin
    b. Diphenhydramine/calamine
    c. Pseudoephedrine
    d. Phenytoin

11. What intervention should be next to control JA's hypercholesterolemia? (EO-6, 8, 9, 12)
    a. Reduction of simvastatin to 10 mg PO QD and addition of cholestyramine powder
    b. Discontinuation of simvastatin and initiation of ezetimibe
    c. Continuation of simvastatin with dosage increase to 120 mg PO QD
    d. Discontinuation of simvastatin and initiation of atorvastatin

12. What is the goal for JA's LDL? (EO-12)
    a. <100 mg/dL
    b. <130 mg/dL
    c. <160 mg/dL
    d. <200 mg/dL

13. Summarize therapeutic, pathophysiologic, and disease management concepts for allergic and drug-induced diseases utilizing a key points format. (EO-18)

Common Eye Disorders

12

Andreas Katsuya Lauer and Ali J. Olyaei

TREATMENT GOALS

- Identify and differentiate vision-threatening from non–vision-threatening disorders.
- Differentiate periorbital disorders such as contact dermatitis from actual orbital disorders and orbital cellulitis.
- Recognize acute infectious and chronic inflammatory disorders of the eye.
- Identify and treat bacterial and viral conjunctivitis.
- Recognize vision-threatening disorders of the anterior segment, such as corneal ulcers and herpes keratitis.
- Recognize and treat corneal abrasions.
- Become familiar with the use of common topical ophthalmic medications, such as antibiotic drops and ointments, and educate the patient on use of these medications.

A number of conditions can affect the structures of the eye, with outcomes ranging from moderate discomfort to significant loss of vision. The healthcare provider should be familiar with the signs and symptoms of common eye disorders and should understand the decision-making process behind treatment. This chapter reviews common eye disorders by anatomic location and by medication classification. The clinical presentations of these disorders, principles of treatment, and a review of the mechanisms and profiles of commonly used ophthalmic medications are provided. Figure 12.1 depicts the anatomic structures of the eye.

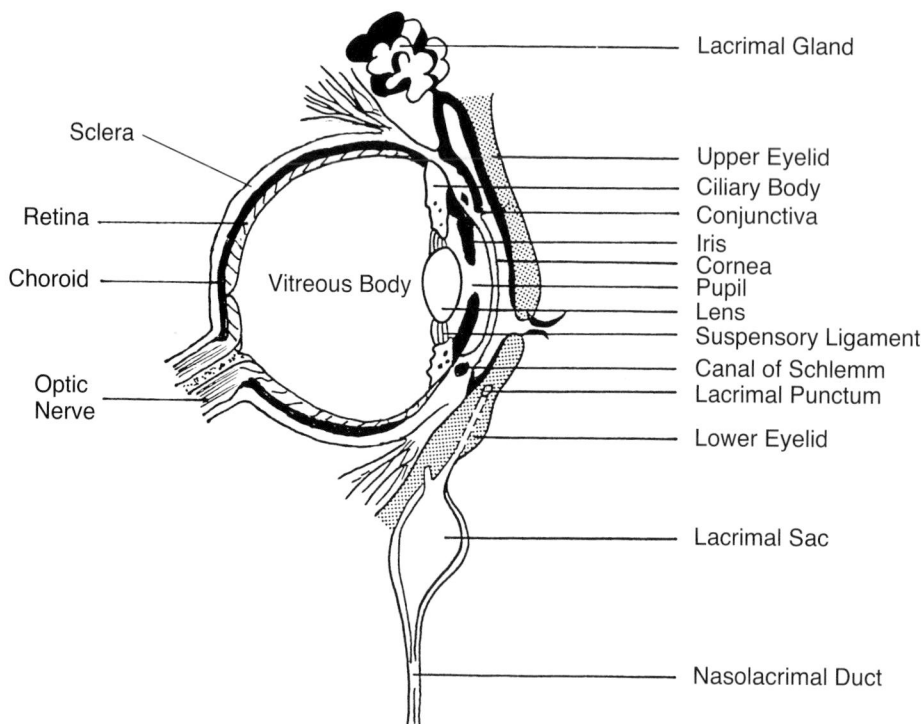

Sclera

Retina

Choroid

Vitreous Body

Optic
Nerve

Lacrimal Gland

Upper Eyelid
Ciliary Body
Conjunctiva
Iris
Cornea
Pupil
Lens
Suspensory Ligament
Canal of Schlemm
Lacrimal Punctum

Lower Eyelid

Lacrimal Sac

Nasolacrimal Duct

FIGURE 12.1 Cross-section of the eyeball and lacrimal passages.

DISORDERS OF THE EYELID AND LACRIMAL GLAND

The often nonspecific signs of eyelid swelling, diffuse tenderness to palpation, erythema, and increased tearing on presentation should elicit a differential diagnosis of causes ranging from chronic, benign disorders of the lid and lacrimal system to more acute conditions that warrant immediate intervention. The history and examination will aid in narrowing the differential diagnosis. The following are common, treatable conditions easily identified in an acute care setting.

HORDEOLUM AND CHALAZION

An external hordeolum, or stye, is a small abscess resulting from an acute infection of a lash follicle and its associated sebaceous gland (gland of Zeiss) or sweat gland (gland of Moll). Because *Staphylococcus* sp. are the most common pathogenic organisms, styes can also develop in patients with chronic, underlying staphylococcal blepharitis. On examination, visible or palpable discrete swelling in the lid margin may be appreciated. The patient may also report a history of previous episodes of stye formation.

An internal hordeolum is a small abscess caused by an acute staphylococcal infection of the glands on the conjunctival aspect of the lid, the meibomian glands. Everting the eyelid on examination may allow better visualization of the yellowish nodule.

Despite causing a moderate degree of discomfort to the patient, external and internal hordeola often resolve spontaneously. Application of warm compresses to the affected lid for 15-minute intervals four times a day often provides symptomatic relief. Coadministration of topical bacitracin or erythromycin ointment to the lid margin twice a day tends to result in more rapid resolution of the lesion. Patients should be advised that it may take up to 4 weeks before the lesion resolves completely.[1]

A chalazion is a focus of chronic granulomatous inflammation of the eyelid secondary to obstruction of the ducts of the sebaceous meibomian glands. These glands, located in the firm layer of the eyelid, the tarsal plate, produce the lipid layer of the tear film. When the gland is obstructed and its contents stagnate within the duct, a painless, round, firm nodule forms. During the acute, inflammatory phase of formation of this meibomian cyst, the treatment regimen is similar to that for hordeola. Warm compresses for 15 minutes four times a day, in addition to gentle massage over the lesion, may help to express the contents. Again, the patient should be informed that resolution occurs over weeks. If the chalazion persists for more than 4 weeks, the patient should be referred to an ophthalmologist for either steroid injection into the lesion or surgical incision and curettage of the lesion.[2] The latter is the more common method of treatment because it definitively decompresses the lesion and can be performed in an office setting under local anesthesia. Steroid injections of triamcinolone may need to be repeated for complete resolution of the lesion, and may lead to permanent depigmentation of the skin around the injection site.[2]

BLEPHARITIS AND MEIBOMITIS

Blepharitis is a chronic condition marked by red, crusty, thickened eyelids with engorged blood vessels at the margins. Patients often report itching, burning, and excessive tearing from a foreign-body sensation. Lid crusting waxes and wanes but is often worse in the morning. Infection with *Staphylococcus* at the base of the lashes is believed to have an important role in the genesis of this external eye disorder. Collarettes, hard scales at the lash bases, are associated with staphylococcal infection of the lid margins and contribute to epidermal ulceration. In longstanding cases, patients may suffer from loss of lashes (madarosis) and in-turning of lashes (trichiasis).

Proper lid hygiene is the mainstay for alleviating the symptoms of blepharitis. The patient should be advised to scrub the eyelid margins with a diluted baby shampoo twice a day, followed by a thin application of an antibiotic ointment, such as bacitracin or erythromycin, to the lid margin.[3] Frequent use of artificial tears relieves dry eye symptoms. Treatment is ongoing, with relief of symptoms occurring over 2 to 3 weeks, but the infection is seldom completely eradicated. Patients must resume a more intensive course of similar treatment when the symptoms recur.

Meibomitis, or posterior blepharitis, is characterized by inspissated oil glands at the eyelid margins. Patients often present with symptoms of burning and excessive tearing. About two thirds of patients have acne rosacea as an underlying disorder. Lid hygiene and cool compresses may help to alleviate symptoms, and the inflammation often is quieted with a course of systemic antibiotics. Oral tetracycline, 250 mg four times daily for 6 weeks, and doxycycline, 100 mg twice daily, have been shown to be efficacious in treating recurrent meibomitis.[1] Pregnant or lactating women and children younger than 12 years should receive oral erythromycin 250 mg four times daily instead, because tetracycline and doxycycline are contraindicated in these patients.[1]

CONTACT DERMATITIS

In a patient with the sudden onset of a periorbital rash with eyelid swelling and a mild, watery discharge who denies fever and tenderness to palpation, the diagnosis of contact dermatitis should be considered. A thorough history should be taken to elicit the recent use of a new ophthalmic drop or ointment, cosmetic, facial soap, or shampoo that could be the offending allergen. In some cases, patients may have used a particular ophthalmic drop for a significant length of time before developing a delayed hypersensitivity response to the drug. This is seen commonly in patients with glaucoma, who may receive a number of eye drops chronically. Treatment involves avoiding the offending agent, which can be identified by stopping one medication at a time. Cool compresses four times a day for 15-minute intervals offer symptomatic relief. For severe itching, an oral antihistamine, such as diphenhydramine 25 to 50 mg up to four times daily for several days, should be considered. In particularly severe cases, a mild steroid cream, such as dexamethasone 0.05%, applied to the affected area twice daily for several days may be used.[4]

PRESEPTAL CELLULITIS

Preseptal cellulitis must be considered in the patient presenting with mild fever, tightness of the eyelid skin, and bogginess (chemosis) of the conjunctiva of the eye, in addition to eyelid edema, erythema, and tenderness. This infection of the eyelid and periorbital structures anterior to the orbital septum usually is the result of inoculation from a puncture wound or laceration or from an adjacent area of infection, such as the sinuses. In adults, the most likely causative organisms are *S. aureus* and streptococci. *Haemophilus influenzae* should be considered in children under 5 years of age, who typically are affected by hematogenous spread from an otitis media or pneumonia.[5] A viral cause, such as herpes simplex virus, should be considered in patients with an associated skin rash. A severe, acute hordeolum may also predispose to a preseptal cellulitis.

To distinguish preseptal cellulitis from the more serious orbital cellulitis (discussed later), a thorough examination must be performed to assess ocular motility, visual acuity, and pupillary reactions, all of which should be normal. Even though the eyelids may be extremely edematous, the eye itself should not be proptotic. There is also generally no pain with eye movements.

Treatment entails systemic antibiotics and daily monitoring of the infection for regression. For a mild, preseptal cellulitis in a patient older than 5 years, amoxicillin-clavulanate or cefaclor provides good coverage and should be continued for a 10-day course.[6] For a moderate to severe preseptal cellulitis or in a patient less than 5 years old, hospital admission may be required for intravenous ceftriaxone and vancomycin.[5] An orbital computed tomography (CT) scan may also be obtained to rule out orbital cellulitis or subperiosteal abscesses.

DACRYOCYSTITIS AND DACRYOADENITIS

Dacryocystitis is an acute infection of the lacrimal sac resulting from blockage of the nasolacrimal duct. The obstruction prevents normal drainage of tears from the lacrimal sac into the nose and promotes stasis, predisposing the patient to secondary infection with bacteria. The patient presents with pain, redness, and swelling over most of the nasal aspect of the lower lid (medial canthus), where the lacrimal sac is located. In addition to tearing, there may be a mucopurulent discharge readily expressed from the punctum when pressure is applied to the lacrimal sac. These patients should be referred promptly to an ophthalmologist for an ocular examination assessing extraocular motility and proptosis, for Gram stain and culture of expressed discharge, and for systemic antibiotic treatment. Mild cases in both children and adults usually respond to amoxicillin-clavulanate in combination with topical antibiotics, such as trimethoprim-polymyxin.[7] Warm compresses with gentle massage over the lacrimal sac may help to relieve the obstruction. More severe cases of acute dacryocystitis may necessitate hospital admission for intravenous antibiotics and a CT scan to rule out orbital cellulitis.

Dacryoadenitis is an acute infection of the lacrimal gland. Patients often present with pain, redness, and swelling over the outer third of the upper eyelid. Gently lifting the upper lid may expose a prolapsed palpebral lobe of the lacrimal gland. The infecting bacteria tend to be *S aureus*, *Neisseria gonorrhoeae*, and streptococci.[1] Viruses such as mumps, infectious mononucleosis, and herpes zoster may also be the cause of the infection. For this reason, patients should also be referred promptly to an ophthalmologist for ocular examination, culture, and treatment with systemic antibiotics.

DISORDERS OF THE ORBIT

ORBITAL CELLULITIS

Orbital cellulitis is one of the few true ocular emergencies necessitating immediate medical attention. It is important to be aware of the signs and symptoms of this soft tissue infection, which extends behind the orbital septum. The patient may present with a red eye, blurred vision, fever, purulent discharge, and pain with eye movement. Critical signs include eyelid edema and conjunctival chemosis and injection. The eye may actually be proptotic, with restricted movement in the various directions of gaze.

The infection itself usually occurs secondarily, by direct extension from adjacent ethmoid sinuses (ethmoiditis).[8] However, it may also occur after a localized orbital infection, such as dacryoadenitis or dacryocystitis, after eye surgery, or after trauma to the eye. The most common causative organisms are *S. aureus*, *Streptococcus* sp., and *H. influenzae*.[6] A fungal cause, such as Mucormycosis, should be considered in diabetic or immunocompromised patients. Potential complications from orbital cellulitis include extension of the infection into the central nervous system, causing meningitis or brain abscess.

The patient should immediately undergo a complete ophthalmic examination to assess for afferent pupillary defects, proptosis, and restricted eye movements and should undergo a CT scan of the orbits and sinuses to confirm the diagnosis. Gram stain and cultures of any discharge should be collected before broad-spectrum intravenous antibiotics, usually ceftriaxone and vancomycin, are started.[1] In an uncomplicated case of orbital cellulitis that responds to treatment, a 14-day course of antibiotics usually is needed.

THYROID OPHTHALMOPATHY

Thyroid ophthalmopathy is the most common cause of unilateral or bilateral proptosis in adults.[9] Patients typically present with double vision, foreign-body sensation, and retraction of the eyelids, particularly on downgaze. The proptosis, if longstanding, may predispose the patient to corneal exposure with ulcer formation. The disorder commonly occurs in conjunction with Graves' disease, an autoimmune process marked by excessive secretion of thyroid hormones. Women are affected much more often than men. Although the majority of patients have a history of thyroid disease, approximately 16% of women and 34% of men have no evidence of an underlying thyroid disorder.[8] See Chapter 38 for further discussion.

These patients need medical management of their systemic thyroid disorder and referral to an ophthalmologist to screen for development of exposure keratopathy, restricted extraocular movement, and optic nerve compression.[1] Exposure keratopathy can be treated with a regimen of frequent artificial tears during the day (every 1 to 6 hours) and lubricating ointment at night. In thyroid ophthalmopathy, enlargement of the extraocular muscles may cause optic nerve compression at the orbital apex. When this is suspected, a color vision and formal visual field examinations should be performed.

DISORDERS OF THE CONJUNCTIVA AND SCLERA

Conjunctivitis is one of the most commonly treated disorders of the eye. Patients typically present with a red eye and discharge, which may range from mild to copious, clear to mucopurulent. Vision may be affected because of excessive tearing and irritation. The time of onset of symptoms, type of discharge, and laterality of the infection can aid in differentiating an acute from chronic bacterial or viral conjunctivitis.

BACTERIAL CONJUNCTIVITIS

Bacterial conjunctivitis is characterized by the acute onset of redness, foreign-body sensation, mucopurulent discharge, and excessive eyelid crusting upon waking. Typically, both eyes are involved, and the patient gives a history of symptoms in one eye preceding the other by a day or so. Examination is remarkable for conjunctival hyperemia, mucopurulent discharge, a papillary reaction at the palpebral conjunctiva, and the absence of preauricular lymphadenopathy. The most common causative organisms of a bacterial conjunctivitis are *S. aureus*, *S. epidermidis*, *S. pneumoniae*, and *H. influenzae*.[8]

Simple bacterial conjunctivitis is self-limiting; even without treatment, symptoms resolve in 10 to 14 days. However, it is common practice to treat the infection to alleviate the symptoms for patient comfort. A conjunctival swab on blood, chocolate, and mannitol media should be obtained for routine culture and sensitivities before treatment begins. The mainstay of therapy is 5 to 7 days of topical antibiotics, such as trimethoprim-polymyxin or ciprofloxacin four times daily, in combination with an antibiotic ointment (erythromycin or bacitracin) at bedtime.[1]

Gonococcal conjunctivitis should be high on the differential diagnosis in any patient presenting hyperacutely (onset within 12 hours) with extremely profuse mucopurulent discharge, marked conjunctival chemosis, and papillary conjunctival reaction. Examination may also reveal preauricular lymphadenopathy as well as pseudomembrane formation on the ocular and inner eyelid surfaces. Immediate Gram stain to detect intracellular Gram-negative diplococci and conjunctival scrapings for culture and sensitivity are essential. Treatment consists of ceftriaxone 1 g in a single intramuscular dose.[10] In particularly severe presentations with evidence of early peripheral corneal ulcer formation, the patient should be hospitalized for intravenous antibiotics (ceftriaxone 1 g every 12 to 24 hours) and close observation.[8] The eye should be irrigated frequently with sterile saline to clear the discharge, and topical erythromycin or bacitracin ointment should be applied four times daily. Concomitant infection with chlamydia should be suspected and the patient should also receive oral tetracycline 250 to 500 mg four times daily or doxycycline 100 mg twice daily for 2 to 3 weeks.[10]

VIRAL CONJUNCTIVITIS

Viral conjunctivitis usually presents acutely with the onset of a watery mucous discharge, conjunctival hyperemia, and lid edema. Examination often shows a palpebral follicular conjunctival response, preauricular lymphadenopathy, and, in severe cases, subconjunctival hemorrhages and pseudomembrane formation. Adenovirus is the most common causative organism.[11] In particular, serotypes 8 and 19 are implicated in epidemic keratoconjunctivitis (''pinkeye''), a severe and highly contagious form of viral conjunctivitis that causes a concomitant keratitis in up to 80% of cases.[8] Herpes simplex conjunctivitis should be considered in patients with a history of ocular herpes simplex or in whom herpetic vesicles are seen along the skin of the eyelid margin or in the distribution of the ophthalmic nerve (V_1).

In general, adenoviral conjunctivitis is a self-limited condition with spontaneous resolution over 2 to 3 weeks. Symptomatic discomfort may be treated with artificial tears every 3 to 4 hours during waking hours. Cool compresses at 15-minute intervals four times daily can help relieve lid swelling and itching. Although most patients have bilateral involvement by the time they present, they should be educated on the importance of handwashing, not sharing towels or linens, and modifying behavior likely to result in the spread of the infection.

Herpes simplex conjunctivitis, unlike adenovirus, tends to be unilateral. Patients should be referred to an ophthalmologist to rule out corneal involvement, which can be vision threatening. In an isolated conjunctivitis, topical antiviral therapy such as 1% trifluorothymidine (Viroptic) may be used 5 times a day for 7 to 10 days.[1] Cool compresses and artificial tears may also provide symptomatic relief.

CHRONIC CONJUNCTIVITIS

A chronic conjunctivitis is defined by the duration of symptoms, including discharge, conjunctival hyperemia, and generalized irritation for more than 4 weeks.[8] Adult inclusion conjunctivitis, or chlamydial conjunctivitis, is a chronic conjunctivitis typically affecting sexually active teenagers and young adults.[12] The patient presents with unilateral, mucopurulent discharge, a prominent palpebral and in some cases

bulbar follicular reaction, and preauricular lymphadenopathy. A history of a concomitant urethritis or cervicitis may be elicited.

Diagnosis is made from conjunctival smears with direct monoclonal fluorescent antibody microscopy. Treatment is directed at both the ocular and genital infection and consists of oral tetracycline 250 to 500 mg four times daily or oral doxycycline 100 mg twice daily for 3 weeks.[1] Both the patient and the asymptomatic sexual partner should be treated. Oral erythromycin 250 to 500 mg four times daily for 3 weeks should be administered instead of tetracycline in children younger than 12 years and in pregnant or lactating women.[1] A topical ointment, such as erythromycin or tetracycline, should be used three times daily for 3 weeks in combination with systemic treatment.

ALLERGIC CONJUNCTIVITIS

Hayfever, or seasonal allergic conjunctivitis, is a type I hypersensitivity immune response in which the binding of antigen-immunoglobulin E antibody complexes to mast cells causes the release of histamine and other inflammatory mediators.[13] The inciting antigen usually is airborne pollen, and the allergic response consists of a conjunctivitis marked by a watery discharge, pruritus, eyelid edema, conjunctival chemosis, and a palpebral conjunctival papillary reaction. The patient often has a history of allergies, and symptoms are worse during a particular season.

Treatment should involve avoiding the inciting agent. In addition, topical mast cell stabilizers, such as 4% cromolyn sodium, may be used four to six times per day to prevent degranulation of mast cells and release of histamine and leukotrienes, which would ultimately decrease the duration of most symptoms.[8] Though effective, cromolyn sodium must be used consistently for 7 to 10 days to achieve the desired effect. A topical antihistamine, such as levocabastine 0.05%, may be used four times daily, in combination with a mast cell stabilizer, to offer immediate relief of itching and burning.[1] Olopatadine (Patanol), a newly available combination topical mast cell stabilizer and antihistamine, is highly effective in relieving allergic symptoms and is used only twice daily. The antihistamine component provides immediate symptom relief, and the mast cell stabilizer provides long-term protection from the onset of symptoms.

KERATOCONJUNCTIVITIS SICCA

Keratoconjunctivitis sicca is one of the most common causes of dry eyes due to a decrease in production of tears. It presents insidiously, usually over a period of several years. Symptoms range in severity from dryness to a foreign-body sensation. Patients often describe a ''gritty'' or ''sandy'' feeling in their eyes, which is often worse in the evening. Keratoconjunctivitis sicca is one of the manifestations of Sjögren syndrome.

Artificial tears can be used for symptomatic relief. Cyclosporine ophthalmic emulsion 0.05% (Restasis) is an immunosuppressive drug that suppresses the ocular inflammation associated with keratoconjunctivitis sicca, resulting in increased tear production. The usual dose is one drop in each eye twice a day. It should not be used in patients with an active ocular infection. Most patients will notice an increase in tear production within 1 month of starting therapy.

SUBCONJUNCTIVAL HEMORRHAGE

A ruptured blood vessel in the subconjunctival layer can cause blood to collect beneath the conjunctiva in a sectoral or diffuse pattern. The patient may first notice the extremely red eye after coughing or straining, as during a Valsalva maneuver. The unsightly appearance of the eye usually is more disturbing to the patient or family member than any physical discomfort or irritation. Subconjunctival hemorrhages may also result from trauma, and a careful history should be taken to assess the possibility of more serious ocular damage, such as a ruptured globe or retrobulbar hemorrhage. In addition, underlying high blood pressure or a bleeding diathesis may rarely be the cause of a subconjunctival hemorrhage. A medication history should inquire about chronic use of medications such as warfarin (Coumadin). On examination, the presence of hemorrhage should be limited to the conjunctiva. The remainder of the examination should be normal.[1]

This condition usually clears spontaneously over 2 to 3 weeks, and no treatment is needed. Artificial tears can be prescribed as needed for mild irritation. A patient with a history of recurrent subconjunctival hemorrhage should be referred to an internist for a complete workup, including bleeding time, prothrombin and partial thromboplastin time, and complete blood count with platelets.[1]

EPISCLERITIS AND SCLERITIS

Episcleritis is a benign and self-limited disorder that often presents in young adults as an acutely red eye in a sectoral pattern. The patient may complain of mild discomfort in the affected eye, with some tenderness to palpation over the hyperemic area and excessive tearing, but vision is not affected. On examination, the small vessels beneath the conjunctiva, the episcleral vessels, appear prominent and engorged. Both eyes may be involved, and the pattern of hyperemia may also be diffuse. The patient may have a history of prior attacks.

Most cases of episcleritis are idiopathic and not associated with an underlying systemic disorder.[14] However, an attempt should be made to elicit a history of symptoms suggestive of rheumatoid arthritis, systemic lupus erythematosus, or other collagen-vascular diseases in a patient with recurrent bouts of episcleritis. Treatment is directed toward alleviating ocular irritation and decreasing redness of the eye. In mild cases, artificial tears used frequently during the day in combination with short-term use of a topical vasoconstrictor, such as 0.1% naphazoline twice daily, may be adequate therapy.[1] The patient should be warned against excessive or prolonged use of topical vasoconstrictors because they may result in rebound vasodilation and chronic redness.

In more severe cases of episcleritis, topical nonsteroidal anti-inflammatory drugs (NSAIDs), such as 0.5% ketorolac, or mild topical steroids, such as fluorometholone, may be used four times daily to provide relief.[8] In rare cases of unresponsiveness, oral NSAIDs, such as ibuprofen 200 to 600 mg three times daily, can be taken in combination with topical preparations. Patients should be advised to take their medication with meals.

Unlike episcleritis, where pain is absent or minimal, scleritis is a severe inflammatory condition of the sclera that typically presents with a severe, boring eye pain, sectoral or diffuse redness, tearing, and photophobia. Unlike the engorgement of preexisting vessels seen with episcleritis, dilated scleral vessels are formed with scleritis. These deeper, larger vessels do not blanch when topical phenylephrine is applied. The eye should be observed grossly under natural lighting conditions for the presence of scleral nodules or for the characteristic bluish hue of the uvea underlying thinned sclera.

Unlike episcleritis, scleritis often is associated with an underlying systemic disease; rheumatoid arthritis is the most common.[15] The disorder tends to be recurrent and may be associated with vision-threatening conditions such as anterior and posterior uveitis, keratitis, cataract, scleral or corneal thinning, risk of perforation with minor trauma, and exudative retinal detachments. In addition to care by an ophthalmologist, the patient should receive a rheumatologic workup to screen for other disorders such as Wegener's granulomatosis, ankylosing spondylitis, and systemic lupus erythematosus.

Treatment of the ocular disorder initially consists of oral NSAIDs, such as ibuprofen 400 to 600 mg four times daily or indomethacin 50 mg twice daily, for 1 to 2 weeks.[1] If there is no response to NSAIDs or if the presentation is particularly severe, systemic steroids, such as oral prednisone 60 to 100 mg daily for 2 to 3 days followed by a slow taper, may be needed to decrease the inflammation.[8] Steroid-resistant cases may respond to other immunosuppressive agents, such as cyclophosphamide or azathioprine, but such treatment should be prescribed in coordination with an internist or rheumatologist.

DISORDERS OF THE CORNEA AND ANTERIOR SEGMENT

CORNEAL INFILTRATE AND CORNEAL ULCER

Contact lens wear is the most common predisposing factor in the development of a corneal infiltrate and its progression to a corneal ulcer.[16] Typically, the patient presents with a red eye, tearing or discharge, a significant degree of ocular pain, photophobia, and foreign-body sensation, as well as decreased vision. Examination reveals an infiltrate, or localized, white opacification of the corneal stroma, that may or may not be associated with an overlying epithelial defect. The presence of an epithelial defect and evidence of decreased stromal thickness by slit-lamp examination is diagnostic of a corneal ulcer.[1] Anterior chamber inflammation ranging from mild cell and flare to frank hypopyon may also be seen on examination. A history of less-than-meticulous contact lens hygiene and overuse of extended-wear soft contact lenses may be elicited.

Bacterial keratitis is the most common form of corneal infection. *Pseudomonas aeruginosa*, *S. aureus*, and *S. pneumoniae* are common bacterial pathogens.[17,18] Fungal keratitis should be considered in patients who have sustained a traumatic corneal injury, especially involving vegetable matter, such as a scrape from a plant leaf.[8] These infiltrates appear suppurative, as in bacterial presentations, but tend to have feathery borders and may have small, adjacent satellite lesions. *Aspergillus* or *Fusarium* spp. are commonly the causative organisms after ocular trauma, whereas infection by *Candida* typically occurs in a baseline debilitated cornea.[8] Corneal infection by the protozoan *Acanthamoeba* should be suspected in soft contact lens wearers with a history of poor lens hygiene (i.e., swimming with contact lenses or using homemade instead of commercially processed cleaning solutions) who have negative bacterial, fungal, and viral cultures and are not responding to conventional treatment.[18] A ring-shaped infiltrate may be appreciated on examination in *Acanthamoeba* keratitis. Herpes simplex virus can also predispose to corneal infection and should be considered in any patient with a history of ocular herpes or in a patient presenting with eyelid vesicles or dendritic epithelial defects that stain with fluorescein.

Once a corneal infiltrate or ulcer is suspected, referral to an ophthalmologist is essential because this condition can be sight threatening. The ophthalmologist documents the dimensions of the infiltrate and the patient's visual acuity, intraocular pressure, and anterior chamber reaction daily to assess whether the condition is responding appropriately to therapy. Before antimicrobial therapy is started, cultures are taken on blood and chocolate agar for bacterial pathogens and Sabouraud's dextrose agar for fungal pathogens. If there is a high index of suspicion for *Acanthamoeba*, cultures can be sent on nonnutrient agar inoculated with *Escherichia coli*.[18] Confocal corneal microscopy may also assist in detecting *Acanthamoeba*. The contact lenses, cases, and cleaning solutions should be cultured as well. The patient should be warned of the serious complications that may arise, namely prolonged infection and risk of corneal perforation, if contact lens wear is resumed too early in the course of treatment.

If culture results are unavailable, treatment usually is directed toward broad-spectrum coverage of gram-negative and gram-positive bacteria, unless the history or examination is suspicious for a fungal, viral, or protozoan cause. In a patient with a small corneal infiltrate not associated with an overlying epithelial defect and with minimal discharge and anterior chamber reaction, fluoroquinolone eye drops every 2 hours while awake, supplemented with tobramycin ointment at bedtime, may be adequate therapy.[1] For larger infiltrates associated with an epithelial defect and moderate to severe anterior chamber inflammation, fortified tobramycin (15 mg/mL) and fortified cefazolin (50 mg/mL) or fortified vancomycin (50 mg/mL) should be used every hour around the clock until the infection begins to show signs of regression.[1] A cycloplegic, such as scopolamine 0.25% twice daily, can be used to prevent scarring of the iris during this acute phase of inflammation and to provide symptomatic pain relief from ciliary body spasm.

If the patient is not responding to fortified antibiotics or cultures are positive for fungus, natamycin 5% (50 mg/mL) drops may be used every waking hour and every 2 hours at night.[8] All topical or systemic steroid use should be tapered rapidly. It may be necessary to add amphotericin B 0.15% (1.5 mg/mL) drops every hour or oral fluconazole for a fungal keratitis slow to respond to treatment or for one involving the deep stroma and threatening corneal perforation.[1]

Culture-positive *Acanthamoeba* keratitis is treated with a combination of polymyxin, neomycin, and gramicidin (Neosporin) and propamidine isethionate 0.1% (Brolene) drops every hour.[1]

Hospitalization may be needed to ensure adequate treatment in patients who are noncompliant with the medical regimen or in whom topical therapy has failed and systemic treatment is needed. As a last resort, a corneal transplant may be needed to restore vision if medical therapy fails.[8]

HERPES SIMPLEX VIRUS: CORNEAL EPITHELIAL DISEASE AND KERATITIS

As in bacterial keratitis, the patient presenting with herpes simplex infection of the cornea has a red, painful eye with photophobia, tearing, and decreased vision. A periorbital rash may be present, and the patient often gives a history of previous episodes of a ''painful red eye.'' On examination, corneal sensitivity should be evaluated with a cotton-tipped applicator before topical anesthetic is instilled because corneal sensation may be decreased in the presence of a herpes infection of the cornea. A dendritic or branching epithelial defect usually is appreciated when the corneal surface is stained with fluorescein. A deeper infection of the corneal stroma may present with an intact epithelium but with a disc-shaped area of stromal edema that may later predispose the patient to postherpetic corneal scarring.[8]

Herpes simplex corneal epithelial disease is treated with trifluorothymidine 1% drops (Viroptic) nine times a day for 10 to 14 days.[1] If inflammation of the anterior chamber accompanies the epithelial disease, the patient should be given a cycloplegic agent such as scopolamine 0.25% twice daily. Any concomitant topical steroid use is contraindicated. Oral acyclovir at a dose of 2 g per day for 10 days or another oral antiviral in this class may be as effective as topical treatment for epithelial keratitis. This may be a better alternative for patients with preexisting ocular surface disease and those at high risk for toxicity from topical medications. The patient should be followed closely, every 2 to 3 days, to evaluate the size of the epithelial defect and the thickness of the corneal stroma. Once the lesion has healed, the topical antivirals should be tapered over the course of a week.

ANTERIOR UVEITIS

Uveitis is a term used to describe general inflammation of the structures that make up the uveal tract: the iris, ciliary body, and choroid. Anterior uveitis may consist simply of inflammation of the iris (iritis) or of inflammation of both the iris and ciliary body (iridocyclitis). Intermediate, posterior, and panuveitis are other categories in the anatomic classification of uveitis; however, because these types of inflammation occur in the deeper structures of the eye, where diagnostic optical lenses are needed for assessment, this discussion is limited to anterior uveitis, which can be assessed with slit-lamp examination.

The patient presenting with acute anterior uveitis reports photophobia, redness, and excessive tearing. Vision may be reduced to a variable extent. The hallmark finding on examination is the presence of white blood cells floating in the anterior chamber, ranging from scant to too numerous to count. Fine deposits of white cells may be appreciated on the inner aspect, or endothelial surface, of the cornea in the nongranulomatous type of uveitis (fine keratoprecipitates). In the granulomatous variety, larger ''mutton-fat'' keratoprecipitates and nodules on the iris surface may be appreciated.

There are many causes of anterior uveitis, including trauma, human lymphocyte antigen (HLA) B27 positivity (associated with ankylosing spondylitis and Reiter's syndrome, especially in young men), herpes simplex, sarcoidosis, syphilis, and tuberculosis.[19] The patient's history of underlying systemic conditions and previous episodes of iritis or uveitis is important in determining a course of treatment for the ocular manifestations. Regardless of the suspected cause of the uveitis, the patient should be referred promptly to an ophthalmologist for a complete eye examination to assess whether inflammation exists in the more posterior structures of the eye and to assess intraocular pressure. For a bilateral, granulomatous, or recurrent uveitis, an initial workup would include a complete blood count, a rapid plasma reagin (RPR) and a fluorescent treponemal antibody absorption test to rule out syphilis, a purified protein derivative test for tuberculosis, and an HLA-B27 test for Reiter's syndrome or ankylosing spondylitis.[19] If the history is suspicious for sarcoidosis, a chest radiograph should be ordered.

Despite the underlying cause of the uveitis, the initial treatment plan often consists of a topical steroid, such as 1% prednisolone acetate every 1 to 6 hours depending on the severity of the anterior chamber reaction, and a cycloplegic agent, such as homatropine 5% twice daily.[1] In addition, any detected systemic disorder should be treated. Initially, patients should be seen every 1 to 7 days until the anterior chamber reaction subsides and the intraocular pressure is stable. In addition, patients with chronic uveitis on long-term topical or systemic steroids should be seen periodically to monitor for elevated eye pressure (steroid-induced glaucoma) or steroid-induced cataract.

COMMON EYE DISORDERS SEEN IN THE EMERGENCY ROOM

CORNEAL ABRASION

A corneal abrasion should be suspected in any patient presenting with foreign-body sensation who gives a history of minor trauma such as a scratch to the eye or a history of contact lens wear. The patient reports pain and photophobia and has excessive tearing. The conjunctiva may be diffusely hyperemic. Vision is mildly to moderately diminished if the cornea becomes edematous or if the abrasion lies primarily over the visual axis. On slit-lamp examination, an epithelial staining defect is detected under cobalt blue light after a drop of fluorescein is instilled in the eye. The upper and lower eyelids should be everted to ensure that no retained foreign body exists that could cause recurrent mechanical trauma to the eye. While the epithelial defect is stained with fluorescein, its dimensions and location on the corneal surface should be recorded.

In a patient who does not wear contact lenses, treatment consists of applying an antibiotic ointment (erythromycin) to the eye prophylactically and then pressure patching the eye overnight to allow the epithelium to grow in over the defect. If the abrasion was caused by a contaminated object, such as a baby's fingernail or the leaf of a plant, or if the patient wears contact lenses, and the eye is at high risk for infection, pressure patching should be avoided.[8] Instead, topical antibiotics, such as a fluoroquinolone, should be administered every 2 to 6 hours, with erythromycin at bedtime.[8] In either case, the patient should be seen in 24 hours to check the vision and the size of the epithelial defect and to look for any evidence of anterior chamber inflammation or early evidence of corneal infiltrate. Topical antibiotics, with or without pressure patching, should be continued until the epithelium has regrown completely to cover the area of the previous defect. Contact lens wear should not be resumed for at least 1 week after the epithelial defect resolves.

RETAINED CORNEAL FOREIGN BODY OR RUST RING

Despite the similar presentation of painful foreign-body sensation, photophobia, tearing, and blurred vision, perhaps even with an epithelial defect visible on examination, any patient who gives a history of a foreign body forcibly striking the eye should be dilated and examined thoroughly. The nature of the trauma should be clear: Were glasses or safety glasses being worn? Was the foreign body generated from metal striking metal?[1] Was there an immediate change in the level of vision?

The vision should be documented before any attempt is made to retrieve a surface or intraocular retained foreign body. On examination, the upper and lower eyelids should be everted to rule out any remnant of a foreign body. The corneal surface should be stained with fluorescein to detect an epithelial defect where the foreign body may have entered. The anterior chamber should be examined carefully for signs of an intraocular retained body. The eye should then be dilated for a careful examination of the vitreous and retina.

A foreign body on the corneal surface can be removed in the office using a 25-gauge needle under magnification at the slit-lamp following instillation of topical anesthetic (proparacaine 0.5%). Often a rust ring remains on the corneal surface where a metal foreign body may have struck the eye and remained adherent to the cornea before being washed out of the eye by irrigation or tearing. The rust ring also can be removed with the use of a topical anesthetic and an ophthalmic drill bur. The eye should then be treated with topical antibiotics (fluoroquinolone every 2 to 6 hours) prophylactically and erythromycin at bedtime until the epithelial defect has healed.[1]

CHEMICAL BURN

Chemical injury to the eye is a true ocular emergency necessitating immediate and constant irrigation even before an examination is performed.[1] Normal saline solution or sterile water, rather than a neutralizing agent, should be used to flush the eye copiously for at least 30 minutes. During irrigation, the fornices and the undersurfaces of the lids should be swept with a cotton-tipped applicator to ensure that globules of the chemical are not being sequestered and continuing to damage ocular tissue. These areas should also be bathed in the irrigating solution. In general, irrigation is continued until the pH of the eye, as measured with litmus paper to the ocular surface, is neutral.

The patient should be seen by an ophthalmologist to assess the severity of the surface damage, including extent of corneal epithelial loss, degree of perilimbal ischemia, and intraocular pressure. Treatment ranges from a topical antibiotic (erythromycin) with pressure patching for an epithelial defect in mild cases to topical steroids, antiglaucoma medications, and/or corneal surgery or transplantation for moderate to severe cases.

COMMON OPHTHALMIC MEDICATIONS

Most ocular medications are solutions, suspensions, or ointments that are administered topically, reaching therapeutic levels in the anterior segment without usually causing systemic side effects. To ensure the delivery of an adequate concentration of topical drug to the anterior segment, patients can be instructed to perform maneuvers such as closing the eye after administration of a drop (to increase ocular absorption and decrease systemic absorption of the drug), waiting 5 minutes between drops (so that one medication doesn't simply wash out the other), and occluding the punctum after a drop (to decrease drainage of the medication with tears through the lacrimal system).[20] In addition, the traditional qualities of the drug itself, such as its lipid solubility, viscosity, and concentration, determine how much of the drug is absorbed from the ocular surface. Patients who wear contact lenses should remove them before administering topical medications, some of which may alter the clarity of the lenses.

To reduce the systemic absorption of eye drops, eyelid closure and punctual occlusion can be used as described earlier. In some instances, eye drops may enter the systemic circulation through the vasculature in the lacrimal apparatus and nasopharynx. When this occurs, the drug enters the venous system and bypasses the enterohepatic circulation. The avoidance of the first-pass effect may make certain individuals, such as infants or the elderly, more susceptible to the systemic side effects of eye drops.

ANTIMICROBIAL AGENTS

Topical ophthalmic antimicrobial agents (Tables 12.1 through 12.3) have the same mechanisms of action, coverage, and potential for side effects as their systemic counterparts. Therefore, a history of adverse reactions to these drug classes, ranging from local rash to anaphylaxis, should be elicited from the patient.

Bacitracin is an antibiotic that inhibits cell wall synthesis and is active against most gram-positive cocci, *Neisseria* sp, and *H. influenzae*. It is available as a single agent or in combination with neomycin and polymyxin B.

Chloramphenicol is a broad-spectrum bacteriostatic agent that inhibits bacterial protein synthesis. It provides good coverage against anaerobic bacteria, *H. influenzae*, and *Neisseria* sp. The topical form has been reported rarely to cause aplastic anemia in patients.

The fluoroquinolones, ciprofloxacin, ofloxacin, and norfloxacin, are highly effective antimicrobial agents with broad-spectrum activity against both gram-positive and gram-negative organisms. These agents interfere with the bacterial enzymes for replication and DNA repair. Ciprofloxacin in particular has a lower minimum inhibitory concentration than the aminoglycosides, gentamicin and tobramycin, and inhibits up to 90% of common bacterial pathogens infecting the cornea.[21] As a class, the fluoroquinolones are also less toxic to the corneal epithelium than the aminoglycosides.

Erythromycin belongs to the macrolide class of antibiotics and works by inhibiting bacterial protein synthesis. It is effective against gram-positive cocci and bacilli and *N. gonorrhoeae*.

Gentamicin and tobramycin belong to the class of aminoglycosides, which are bactericidal agents that interfere with the initiation of bacterial protein synthesis. These agents are effective against aerobic, gram-negative bacilli such as *P. aeruginosa*, a common corneal pathogen. They also provide coverage against gram-positive cocci such as *S. aureus* and *S. epidermidis*.

Sulfacetamide is a bacteriostatic drug that belongs to the sulfonamide class of inhibitors of bacterial folic acid synthesis. It is effective against *S. pneumoniae*, *Corynebacterium*

TABLE 12.1	Single-Agent Antibacterials		
Drug	**Dosage Form**	**Strength**	**Frequency of Dosing**
Bacitracin	Ointment	500 U/g	BID–QID
Chloramphenicol	Ointment	0.5%, 1.0%	BID–QID
Ciprofloxacin	Solution	0.3%	1 or 2 drops q1–6h
Erythromycin	Ointment	0.5%	BID–QID
Gentamicin	Ointment	0.3%	BID–QID
Ciprofloxacin	Ointment	0.3%	Half-inch ribbon BID or TID
Gatifloxacin	Solution	0.3%	1 drop q1–6h
Levofloxacin	Solution	0.3%	1 drop q1–6h
Moxifloxacin	Solution	0.3%	1 drop q1–6h
Norfloxacin	Solution	0.3%	1 drop q1–6h
Ofloxacin	Solution	0.3%	1 drop q1–6h
Sulfacetamide	Ointment	10%	BID–QID
	Solution	10%, 15%, 30%	1 drop q1–6h
Tobramycin	Ointment	0.3%	BID–QID
	Solution	0.3%	1 drop q1–6h

BID, twice a day; QID, four times a day; TID, three times a day.

diphtheriae, *H. influenzae*, and *Chlamydia trachomatis*. As with its systemic counterparts, the topical form has been implicated in cases of severe sensitivity reactions such as Stevens-Johnson syndrome.

Of the three topical antiviral agents for treating herpes simplex keratitis, trifluridine has the best corneal penetrance and the highest efficacy (Table 12.3). Natamycin is active against a range of filamentous fungi, such as *Aspergillus*, *Fusarium*, and the yeast *Candida albicans*.

ANTIINFLAMMATORY AND ANTIALLERGY AGENTS

The class of antiinflammatory agents (Tables 12.4 through 12.7) known as glucocorticoids or steroids works on the efferent limb of the immune response, decreasing the cellular response of macrophages and T lymphocytes at the site of inflammation.[22] Thus, these drugs are very effective in treating anterior and posterior segment inflammation as well as suppressing corneal graft rejection and preventing scarring. However, though useful for all the aforementioned reasons, topical steroids have potentially serious adverse effects. Ocular complications include steroid-induced glaucoma, posterior subcapsular cataracts, ptosis, and exacerbation of infection, especially when there is a herpetic cause.[8] In patients who respond to corticosteroids, the intraocular pressure spike rarely occurs before 2 weeks of chronic use of the medication. However, a pressure spike may occur any time during treatment, and even patients who have been taking topical steroids for months or years require periodic pressure checks.[22] Discontinuation of the steroid if it has been used for less than 1 year usually results in a return to baseline pressures. Dexamethasone, the most potent steroid agent, also tends to cause the greatest intraocular pressure spikes.[8]

TABLE 12.2	Combination Antibacterials	
Drug	**Dosage Form**	**Frequency of Dosing**
Neomycin/bacitracin/ polymyxin B (Neosporin)	Ointment Solution	BID–QID 1 drop q1–6h
Polymyxin B/bacitracin (Polysporin)	Ointment	BID–QID
Polymyxin B/trimethoprim (Polytrim)	Solution	1 drop q3h up to 6 drops/day

BID, twice a day; QID, four times a day.

TABLE 12.3	Antiviral and Antifungal Agents		
Drug	**Dosage Form**	**Strength**	**Frequency of Dosing**
Antiviral			
Idoxuridine	Solution	0.1%	1 drop q1h
Trifluridine	Solution	1%	1 drop 9 times/day
Vidarabine	Ointment	3%	0.5-inch ribbon 5 times/day
Antifungal			
Natamycin	Solution	5%	1 drop q1–6h

TABLE 12.4	Antibacterial and Corticosteroid Combinations		
Drug		**Dosage Form**	**Frequency of Dosing**
Neomycin/polymyxin/hydrocortisone 1% (Cortisporin)		Ointment	BID–QID
		Suspension	1 drop q3–4h
Dexamethasone/neomycin/polymyxin (Maxitrol)		Ointment	BID–QID
		Solution	1 drop q1–6h
Neomycin/dexamethasone (Neo-Decadron)		Ointment	TID or QID
		Solution	1 drop q1–6h
Tobramycin/dexamethasone (TobraDex)		Ointment	BID–QID
		Solution	1 drop q1–6h
10% Sulfacetamide/0.2% prednisolone acetate (Blephamide)		Ointment	BID
		Solution	1 drop q1–4h

BIB, twice a day; QID, four times a day; TID, three times a day.

TABLE 12.5	Corticosteroids		
Drug	**Dosage Form**	**Strength**	**Frequency of Dosing**
Dexamethasone	Ointment	0.05%	BID–QID
	Solution	0.1%	1 drop q1–6h
Fluorometholone	Solution	0.1%, 0.25%	1 drop q1–6h
Prednisolone acetate	Suspension	0.12%, 1%	1 drop q1–6h
Prednisolone sodium	Suspension	0.9%, 0.11%	1 drop q1–6h
Rimexolone	Suspension	1%	1 drop q1–6h
Loteprednol	Suspension	0.2%, 0.5%	1 drop q1–6h

BID, twice a day; QID, four times a day.

TABLE 12.6	Nonsteroidal Antiinflammatory Agents		
Drug	**Dosage Form**	**Strength**	**Frequency of Dosing**
Diclofenac	Solution	0.1%	1 drop QID
Ketorolac	Solution	0.4%, 0.5%	1 drop QID
Bromfenac	Solution	0.09%	1 drop BID
Nepafenac	Suspension	0.1%	1 drop QID

BID, twice a day; QID, four times a day.

TABLE 12.7	Antiallergy Agents		
Drug	**Dosage Form**	**Strength**	**Frequency of Dosing**
Cromolyn sodium	Solution	4%	1 drop 4–6 times/day
Levocabastine	Solution	0.05%	1 drop QID
Lodoxamide	Solution	0.1%	1 drop QID
Naphazoline	Solution	0.1%	1 drop BID–QID, PRN
Naphcon-A	Solution	Naphazoline 0.025%/ pheniramine 0.3%	1 drop BID–QID, PRN
Olopatadine	Solution	0.1%	1 drop BID

BIB, twice a day; PRN, as needed; QID, four times a day.

Combination antibacterial–steroid agents are available to treat mild conjunctival infections associated with inflammation, especially in the postoperative setting.

The NSAIDs work through the cyclooxygenase pathway to inhibit the production and inflammatory effects of prostaglandins.[23] Diclofenac is a topical NSAID used for the treatment of ocular inflammation. It is also effective in treating cystoid macular edema, a specific type of retinal inflammation that can occur after cataract surgery.[8]

The antihistamines and mast cell stabilizers work on the afferent limb of the immune response to decrease the cascade effect of histamines, prostaglandins, and leukotrienes in causing the itching and hyperemia of allergic and atopic conjunctivitis.[24] Cromolyn sodium blocks histamine release indirectly and must be used prophylactically for several weeks to alleviate symptom onset. Mast cell stabilizers, such as lodoxamide, also take several weeks to alleviate symptoms. The newer histamine receptor antagonists, such as levocabastine, have an onset of action within minutes and last for at least 4 hours.

MYDRIATICS AND CYCLOPLEGICS

This class of medications (Table 12.8) is used primarily in an office setting to perform a dilated fundus examination. In cases of moderate to severe postoperative inflammation or in cases of uveitis with significant anterior chamber inflammation, these agents are used to prevent permanent scar-ring of the pupil. The mydriatic agents dilate the pupil, and the cycloplegic agents paralyze the ciliary muscle to prevent painful spasm and to cause paralysis of accommodation. Atropine has the longest duration of any of these agents, causing dilation for as long as 2 weeks.

ARTIFICIAL TEARS

A wide range of agents are available to lubricate the eye and to prevent desiccation of the corneal surface (Table 12.9). These emollients vary in their viscosity; most are more viscous than water. The topical drops, which are up to seven times as viscous as water, are applied frequently during the day, every 30 minutes to 1 hour if necessary, and the lubricating ointments, such as Refresh PM, which is more than 20 times as viscous as water, are used before bedtime.

KEY POINTS

■ When treating a patient with a common eye disorder, elicit a thorough description of the symptoms, including decreased vision, pain with eye movement, discharge, and photophobia

■ Assess whether the patient has experienced an acute change from baseline vision or whether the symptoms have been chronic and progressive

TABLE 12.8	Mydriatics and Cycloplegics				
Drug	**Dosage Form**	**Strength**	**Frequency of Dosing**	**Duration**	**Effect**
Atropine	Solution	1%	1 drop QD–TID	Max 7–14 days	C, M
Cyclopentolate	Solution	0.5%, 1%, 2%	1 drop prior to exam	Max 2 days	C, M
Homatropine	Solution	2%, 5%	1 drop QD–TID	Max 3 days	C, M
Phenylephrine	Solution	2.5%, 10%	1 drop prior to exam	Max 5 h	M
Tropicamide	Solution	0.5%, 1%	1 or 2 drops prior to exam	Max 6 h	C, M
Scopolamine	Solution	0.25%	1 drop QD–QID	Max 6 h	C, M

C, cycloplegia; M, mydriasis; QD, once a day; QID, four times a day; TID, three times a day.

TABLE 12.9	Artificial Tears	
Drug	**Frequency**	**Viscosity (centistokes)[a]**
Dry Eye Therapy	1 drop PRN	0.7
HypoTears	1 drop PRN	1.2
Refresh Plus	1 drop PRN	2.0
Refresh	1 drop PRN	2.8
Tears Plus	1 drop PRN	2.8
Tears Naturale	1 drop PRN	3.7
Tears Naturale II	1 drop PRN	4.0
Tears Naturale Free	1 drop PRN	4.3
Bion Tears	1 drop PRN	4.5
OcuCoat PF	1 drop PRN	46
Celluvisc	1 drop PRN	170

When artificial tears are used more than 4 times a day, it is better to switch over to preservative-free types to avert ocular surface toxicity from the common preservative benzalkonium chloride.
[a] Water = 0.7 centistoke.

- Be systematic in the examination of the periorbital structures, such as the lid and lacrimal gland, as well as the structures of the eye, such as the conjunctiva, sclera, cornea, and anterior chamber
- If a vision-threatening disorder, such as orbital cellulitis or a corneal ulcer, is suspected, contact an ophthalmologist immediately
- Send routine cultures for suspected bacterial conjunctivitis before initiating treatment
- If gonococcal conjunctivitis is suspected, the patient should receive systemic as well as topical medication. An ophthalmologist should be consulted
- Consider a rheumatologic workup in patients with recurrent ocular inflammatory disorders, such as scleritis or uveitis
- The only instance where treatment should occur prior to eliciting symptoms and conducting a detailed examination is a chemical injury, where copious irrigation is of paramount importance and should occur at the location of the injury
- Know the indications and relative contraindications of the various topical antibiotic, antiviral, and anti-inflammatory agents

SUGGESTED READINGS

Lesar T. Proper use of ophthalmic products. J Am Pharm Assoc (Wash) NS36:704–706, 1996.

Ono SJ, Abelson MB. Allergic conjunctivitis: update on pathophysiology and prospects for future treatment. J Allergy Clin Immunol 11:118–122, 2005.

Raskin EM, Speaker MG, Laibson PR. Blepharitis. Infect Dis Clin North Am 6:777–787, 1992.

Syed NA, Hyndiuk RA. Infectious conjunctivitis. Infect Dis Clin North Am 6:789–805, 1992.

REFERENCES

1. Cullom RD Jr, Chang B. The Wills eye manual: office and emergency room diagnosis and treatment of eye disease, 2nd ed. Philadelphia: JB Lippincott, 1994.
2. Epstein GA, Putterman AM. Combined excision and drainage with intralesional corticosteroid injection in the treatment of chronic chalazion. Arch Ophthalmol 106:514–516, 1988.
3. McCulley JP, Dougherty JM, Deneau DG. Classification of chronic blepharitis. Ophthalmology 89:1173–1180, 1982.
4. Theodore FH, Bloomfield SE, Mondino BJ. Clinical allergy and immunology of the eye. Baltimore: Williams & Wilkins, 1983.
5. Weiss A, Friendly D, Eglin K, et al. Bacterial periorbital and orbital cellulitis in childhood. Ophthalmology 90:195–203, 1983.
6. Harris G. Subperiosteal inflammation of the orbit. A bacterial analysis of 17 cases. Arch Ophthalmol 106:947–952, 1988.
7. Berlin AJ, Rath R, Rich L. Lacrimal system dacryoliths. Ophthalmology 11:435–436, 1980.
8. Kanski JJ. Clinical ophthalmology, 3rd ed. Boston: Butterworth-Heinemann, 1994.
9. Sergott RC, Glaser JS. Graves' ophthalmopathy. A clinical and immunologic review. Surv Ophthalmol 26:1–21, 1981.
10. Haimovici R, Roussel TJ. Treatment of gonococcal conjunctivitis with single intramuscular ceftriaxone. Am J Ophthalmol 107:511–514, 1989.
11. Pettit TH, Holland GN. Chronic keratoconjunctivitis associated with ocular adenovirus infection. Am J Ophthalmol 88:748–751, 1979.
12. Schachter J. Chlamydiae. Am Rev Microbiol 34:285–309, 1980.
13. Butrus SI, Abelson MB. Laboratory evaluation of ocular allergy. Int Opthalmol Clin 28:324, 1988.
14. Watson PG. Diseases of the sclera and episclera. In: Tasman W, Jaeger EA, eds. Duane's clinical ophthalmology. Philadelphia: JB Lippincott, 1992:4.
15. Foster CS, Forstot SL, Wilson LA. Mortality rate and rheumatoid arthritis patients developing necrotizing scleritis or peripheral ulcerative keratitis: effects of systemic immunosuppression. Ophthalmology 91:1253–1263, 1984.
16. Poggio EC, Glynn RJ, Schein OD, et al. The incidence of ulcerative keratitis among users of daily-wear and extended-wear soft contact lenses. N Engl J Med 321:779–783, 1989.
17. Schein OD, Glynn RJ, Poggio EC, et al. The relative risk of ulcerative keratitis among users of daily-wear and extended-wear soft contact lenses. N Engl J Med 321:773–778, 1989.
18. Larkin DFP, Kilvington S, Dart JKT. Treatment of Acanthamoeba keratitis with polyhexamethylene biguanide. Ophthalmology 99:185–191, 1992.
19. Wakefield D, Montanaro A, McCluskey P. Acute anterior uveitis and HLA-B27. Surv Ophthalmol 36:223–232, 1991.
20. Zimmerman TJ, Kooner KS, Kandarakis AS, et al. Improving the therapeutic index of topically applied ocular drugs. Arch Ophthalmol 102:551–553, 1984.
21. Leibowitz HM. Antibacterial effectiveness of ciprofloxacin 0.3% ophthalmic solution in the treatment of bacterial conjunctivitis. Am J Ophthalmol 112:29S–33S, 1991.
22. Tripathi BJ, Millard CB, Tripathi RC. Corticosteroids induce a sialated glycoprotein (Cort-GP) in trabecular cells in vitro. Exp Eye Res 51:735–737, 1990.
23. Flach AJ. Nonsteroidal anti-inflammatory drugs. In: Zimmerman TJ, Kooner KS, eds. Ophthalmologic Clinics of North America. Philadelphia: WB Saunders, 1989.
24. Bito LZ. Prostaglandins: old concepts and new perspectives. Arch Ophthalmol 105:1036–1039, 1987.

Glaucoma

J. Douglas Wurtzbacher and Dick R. Gourley

13

TREATMENT GOALS

Current therapy remains targeted to reducing intraocular pressure (IOP), either medically or surgically. Studies have shown that reduction in IOP, even in patients with normal IOP (normal tension glaucoma), prevents progression of optic nerve damage and visual field loss.[1,2] Specific goals for the treatment of glaucoma include the following:

- Immediate medical attention to reduce IOP in cases of acute angle-closure glaucoma.
- Early diagnosis and management of glaucomatous changes to minimize chances of bilateral or unilateral blindness.
- Avoidance of medical therapy that may worsen the patient's glaucoma.
- Establishment of a target IOP to prevent initial or worsening ocular damage.
- Reduction of IOP with the use of topical medications with low systemic effects.
- Use of combination therapy only after monotherapy has proved unsuccessful.
- Provision of patient education to improve administration technique to reduce systemic adverse effects and improve compliance.
- Monitoring for effectiveness and adverse events.
- Surgical correction if medical therapy is not tolerated or is unsuccessful at maintaining the target IOP.

DEFINITION

Glaucoma is a group of diseases of the eye characterized by damage to the ganglion cells and the optic nerve. If left untreated, these effects may lead to various degrees of loss of vision and blindness. Increased intraocular pressure (IOP) remains the most important risk factor for the development of glaucoma, but it is no longer included as a part of the definition of disease. Glaucoma is typically classified as either open-angle or angle-closure (closed-angle), based upon causes of increased IOP.[3,4]

ETIOLOGY

Optic nerve damage that the different types of glaucoma cause is the result of a variety of initiating factors. Most commonly, genetic predisposition, physical changes, systemic diseases, or medications may increase an individual's risk of developing damage that may be broadly classified as IOP dependent (most commonly) or IOP independent.

Increased intraocular pressure remains the major causative risk factor for the development of glaucoma. Myopia may be an additional risk factor, especially in younger patients.[5,6] A summary of known risk factors associated with an increased risk of glaucoma is listed in Table 13.1.

The familial predisposition of glaucoma has been well established. A study by Wolfs et al[7] determined the prevalence of glaucoma in families of patients with glaucoma and in control patients. This population-based study found that 10.4% of siblings of patients and 1.1% of offspring of patients had glaucoma compared with 0.7% and 0% in families of control patients, respectively. At least three different genes have been identified that, when mutated, may be causally linked to the development of glaucoma.[8]

Glaucoma can occur as a secondary manifestation of systemic disorders or of trauma. A list of systemic diseases associated with increased IOP is shown in Table 13.2. In addition, the detection and recognition of drug-induced glaucoma as a potential cause of disease are important. Drugs that have autonomic effects produce several types of ocular changes. Of great significance is the effect of anticholinergic agents on angle-closure glaucoma. Several factors appear to be associated with drug-induced glaucoma (Table 13.3). Specific agents known to increase risk of glaucoma will be discussed in detail subsequently.

EPIDEMIOLOGY

Glaucoma, defined as damage to the optic nerve and ganglion cells, affects approximately 67 million individuals worldwide and 4 million Americans. There may be as many as 15 million Americans who have elevated IOP, or ocular hypertension, without clinical signs and symptoms of glaucoma who are at increased risk for development of disease and end-organ damage.[9]

Glaucoma usually manifests itself after age 35, but it can occur in younger people as well. The prevalence of glaucoma

TABLE 13.1	Risk Factors Associated with Glaucoma

Family history of glaucoma

High intraocular pressure

African or Asian descent

Diabetes mellitus

Myopia (nearsightedness)

Regular, long-term steroid/cortisone use

Previous eye injury

High blood pressure

TABLE 13.2	Systemic Conditions Associated with Secondary Glaucoma

Congenital rubella

Diabetes mellitus

Down's syndrome

Hallerman-Streiff syndrome

Homocystinuria

Hypertension

Idiopathic infantile hypoglycemia

Lowe's syndrome

Marfan's syndrome

Melanoma (intraocular tumor)

Neurofibromatosis (von Recklinghausen)

Turner syndrome

Uveitis (secondary)

(Modified from Scheie HG, Edwards DL, Yanoff MC. Clinical and experimental observations using alpha chymotrypsin. Am J Ophthalmol 59:469, 1965.)

increases with increasing age. Two percent of the population over 40 years of age and 5% to 9% of those over 65 years of age suffer from glaucoma. Although more men are diagnosed with open-angle glaucoma, sex predilections for the disease are not clinically apparent. Open-angle glaucoma is relatively more common in whites and blacks than in American Indians and Asians.

Glaucoma may be classified in a variety of ways (Table 13.4) according to causative factors, when known. Glaucoma is usually described as angle-closure or open-angle glaucoma. These terms are based on the mechanism of obstruction of outflow of aqueous humor, and they help clinicians develop treatment strategies. Open-angle glaucoma occurs in 80% to 90% of cases.[10] Angle-closure glaucoma is usually a more acute form of disease that occurs in 5% to 10% of

TABLE 13.3	Factors Implicated in Potential Drug Induction of Angle-Closure Glaucoma

Age—usually over 30

History—familial, genetic basis

Race—usually white

Sex—usually female

Anterior chamber angle—shallow and narrow

Vision—hyperopia, hypermetropia

Convexity of the iris—flattened

Dose and duration of the offending drug used

Duration of effect on the eye—longer duration

Route of administration—topical more than systemic

TABLE 13.4	Glaucoma Classified According to Etiology

A. Primary glaucoma

  1. Open-angle glaucoma

    a. Primary open-angle glaucoma (chronic open-angle glaucoma, chronic simple glaucoma)

    b. Normal-pressure glaucoma (low-pressure glaucoma)

  2. Angle-closure glaucoma

    a. Acute

    b. Subacute

    c. Chronic

    d. Plateau iris

B. Congenital glaucoma

  1. Primary congenital glaucoma

  2. Glaucoma associated with other developmental ocular abnormalities

    a. Anterior chamber cleavage syndromes

      Axenfeld's syndrome

      Sieger's syndrome

      Peter's anomaly

    b. Aniridia

  3. Glaucoma associated with extraocular developmental abnormalities

    a. Sturge-Weber syndrome

    b. Marfan's syndrome

    c. Neurofibromatosis

    d. Lowe's syndrome

    e. Congenital rubella

C. Secondary glaucoma

  1. Pigmentary glaucoma

  2. Exfoliation syndrome

  3. Due to lens changes (phacogenic)

    a. Dislocation

    b. Intumescence

    c. Phacolytic

  4. Due to uveal tract changes

    a. Uveitis

    b. Posterior synechiae (seclusio pupillae)

    c. Tumor

  5. Iridocorneoendothelial (ICE) syndrome

  6. Trauma

    a. Hyphema

    b. Angle contusion/recession

    c. Peripheral anterior synechiae

  7. Postoperative

    a. Ciliary block glaucoma (malignant glaucoma)

    b. Peripheral anterior synechiae

    c. Epithelial downgrowth

    d. After corneal graft surgery

    e. After retinal detachment surgery

  8. Neovascular glaucoma

    a. Diabetes mellitus

    b. Central retinal vein occlusion

    c. Intraocular tumor

  9. Raised episcleral venous pressure

    a. Carotid-cavernous fistula

    b. Sturge-Weber syndrome

  10. Steroid-induced

D. Absolute glaucoma: The end result of any uncontrolled glaucoma is a hard, sightless, and often painful eye.

Source: Reprinted with permission from Vaughan D, Asbury T, Riordan-Eva P. General ophthalmology. 14th ed. Norwalk, CT: Appleton & Lange, 1995.

all cases. A third type is congenital glaucoma, which results from developmental ocular abnormalities and occurs in less than 2% of cases. Finally, glaucoma may be secondary to other ocular disorders, systemic disorders, medications, or trauma, or it may occur after intraocular surgery is performed. This chapter discusses open- and closed-angle glaucoma and medication-related glaucoma and refers the reader to other sources[3,11] for a more detailed description.

Open-angle glaucoma can be further described as high tension or normal tension (also known as low tension) glaucoma. An estimated 25% to 30% of Americans and up to 70% of Asians with optic nerve damage characteristic of glaucoma have normal IOP, described as normal tension glaucoma. Long-term studies examining the effects of medi-

cal management of normal tension glaucoma have recently been completed[1,2] and are discussed later in this chapter.

Glaucoma is the second leading cause of irreversible blindness in the United States. Approximately 150,000 Americans have varying degrees of blindness caused by glaucoma.[10] However, medical treatment can decrease the risk of blindness secondary to glaucoma. Long-term surveillance studies of patients treated for glaucoma have demonstrated that 27% of patients are likely to become blind unilaterally and 9% bilaterally over a 20-year period. In patients who were not diagnosed or treated early in the disease, this estimate increased to 54% and 22%, respectively.[12] Therefore, early detection and control of IOP are important in the management of long-term outcomes of this disease.

PATHOPHYSIOLOGY

The pathogenesis of glaucoma occurs in five stages[3]: (1) a variety of initial events, causing (2) changes in aqueous outflow, resulting in (3) increased intraocular pressure, which leads to (4) optic nerve atrophy, and finally, (5) progressive loss of vision. This description highlights the importance of aqueous humor production and elimination in the progression of glaucoma and subsequent complications.

AQUEOUS HUMOR PRODUCTION AND ELIMINATION

The relative production and elimination of aqueous humor physiologically determines IOP. Increased IOP usually is the result of decreased elimination but may also be due to increased production of aqueous humor, or both.[13]

Aqueous humor is secreted by the ciliary processes into the posterior chamber of the eye (Fig. 13.1), where it flows to the trabecular meshwork and through the canal of Schlemm. Because of diurnal variability in aqueous humor production, IOP measurements vary according to the time of day. Many patients with open-angle glaucoma have the greatest IOP in the morning and the lowest IOP during the sleeping hours. Because a decrease in the outflow facility of aqueous humor is the primary mechanism causing an increase in IOP, anatomic changes associated with open-angle and angle-closure glaucoma are important.

OPEN-ANGLE GLAUCOMA

In open-angle glaucoma, a physical blockage occurs within the trabecular meshwork that retards elimination of aqueous humor. The obstruction is presumed to occur between the trabecular sheet and the episcleral veins into which the aqueous humor ultimately flows.

The impairment of aqueous drainage elevates the IOP to between 25 and 35 mm Hg (normal IOP is 10 to 20 mm Hg), indicating that the obstruction is usually partial. This increase in IOP is sufficient to cause progressive cupping of the optic disc and eventually visual field defects. As the trabecular spaces become more involved, detachment of the cornea and formation of bullae may occur. Because visual acuity remains largely unaffected until late in the disease process, areas of visual field disturbance or blind spots must be regarded as a major indication for medical therapy.

ANGLE-CLOSURE GLAUCOMA

In angle-closure glaucoma, increased IOP is caused by pupillary blockage of aqueous humor outflow and is typically severe. The basic requirements leading to an acute attack of angle-closure glaucoma consist of a pupillary block, a narrowed anterior chamber angle, and a convex iris. When a patient has a narrow anterior chamber or a pupil that dilates to a degree at which the iris comes into greater contact with the lens, interference with the flow of aqueous humor from the posterior to the anterior chamber is observed. Because aqueous humor is continually secreted, pressure from within the posterior chamber forces the iris to bulge forward, which may progress to complete blockage.

Pathologic complications of angle-closure and open-angle glaucoma include formation of cataracts, adhesion of the iris to the cornea, atrophy of the optic nerve and retina, complete blockage of aqueous outflow, and, ultimately, blindness.

CONGENITAL GLAUCOMA

Congenital glaucoma is a rare disorder in which IOP is increased as a result of developmental abnormalities of the ocular structures in the newborn or infant. It may occur in association with other congenital abnormalities and anomalies such as homocystinuria and Marfan's syndrome. Congenital glaucoma should be considered in newborns and infants who have sensitivity to light, or who exhibit excessive tearing or spasm of the eyelids.

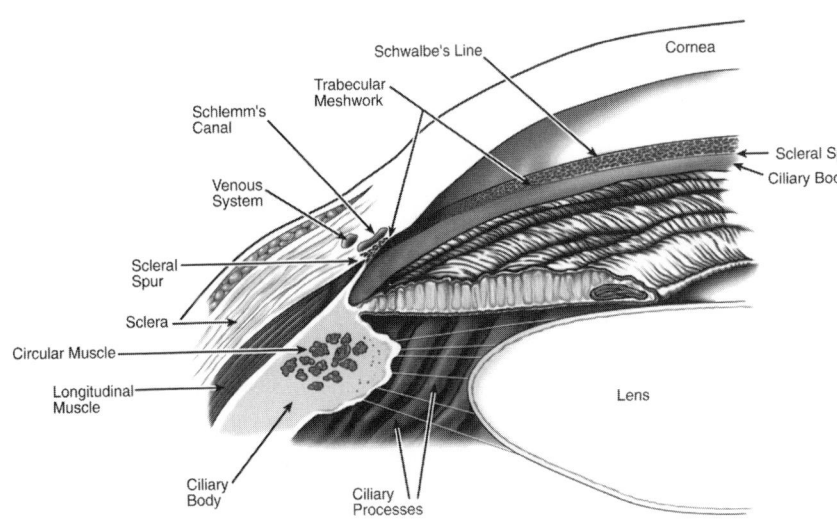

FIGURE 13.1 Aqueous humor is actively secreted by the ciliary epithelium into the posterior chamber; it flows through the pupil into the anterior chamber, and drains through Schlemm's canal and the trabecular meshwork. (From Tasman W, Jaeger E. The Wills Eye Hospital atlas of clinical ophthalmology. 2nd ed. Baltimore: Lippincott Williams & Wilkins, 2001, with permission.)

NORMAL-TENSION GLAUCOMA

The origin and pathogenesis of normal-tension glaucoma remain to be completely understood. Normal-tension glaucoma is believed to be related, at least in part, to decreased blood flow to the optic nerve. This may eventually cause neuronal damage. In addition, eyes appear to be more susceptible to pressure-related damage within the normal or high-normal range; therefore, a pressure lower than normal is often necessary to prevent further visual loss.[14]

DRUG-INDUCED GLAUCOMA

Several therapeutic classes of drugs, such as those with anticholinergic, adrenergic, or corticosteroid effects, have been implicated in the induction or worsening of glaucoma.

Medications affect open-angle and closed-angle glaucoma differently. Drugs that dilate the pupil, for instance, may precipitate an acute attack of angle-closure glaucoma but usually do not produce harmful effects in open-angle cases. Dilation of the pupil in angle-closure glaucoma may cause the peripheral iris to bulge forward, blocking the trabecular meshwork. The aqueous humor is prevented from reaching the outflow channels, which results in increased IOP. Because excessive resistance to outflow in open-angle glaucoma is caused primarily by changes within the trabecular outflow channels, dilation of the pupil usually does not exacerbate the IOP.

Topical administration of some drugs (Table 13.5) is known to elevate IOP in various patients with glaucoma,

TABLE 13.5	Ability of Drugs to Induce Glaucoma			
			Glaucoma Type	
Drug		Route	Open Angle	Angle Closure
Anticholinergics				
Atropine		Topical	Rare	Frequent
Scopolamine		Topical	Rare	Frequent
Belladonna		Topical	Rare	Frequent
Propantheline		Systemic	Rare	Rare
Adrenergics				
Phenylephrine 10%		Topical	Never	Occasional
Epinephrine		Systemic	Never	Rare
Miotics				
Pilocarpine 4%–8%		Topical	Never	Occasional
Echothiophate		Topical	Never	Occasional
Isoflurophate		Topical	Never	Occasional
Carbonic anhydrase inhibitors				
Acetazolamide		Systemic	Never	Rare
Antihypertensives		Systemic	Never	Never
β-Chymotrypsin		Topical	Rare	Occasional
Prochlorperazine		Systemic	Never	Never
Promethazine (high doses)		Systemic	Never	Rare
Ganglionic blocking agents		Systemic	Rare	Occasional
Amphetamines		Systemic	Rare	Occasional
Tricyclic antidepressants		Systemic	Rare	Occasional
Corticosteroids (at equipotent doses)				
Betamethasone		Topical	Frequent	Never
Dexamethasone		Topical	Frequent	Never
Hydrocortisone		Topical	Occasional	Never
Prednisolone		Topical	Occasional	Never
Triamcinolone		Topical	Occasional	Never
Dexamethasone		Systemic	Occasional	Never
Hydrocortisone		Systemic	Occasional	Never
Prednisolone		Systemic	Occasional	Never

and it has been assumed that systemic administration of such medications will have a similar effect. In patients with mild or controlled open-angle glaucoma, it is unwarranted to prohibit the use of systemic sympathomimetic, anticholinergic, and other atropine-like drugs because evidence that they exacerbate the condition is not well documented.[6,15]

Anticholinergics. In patients with normal eyes, topically instilled anticholinergics such as atropine, scopolamine, and cyclopentolate produce no significant elevation in IOP. However, in patients older than 30 years of age who have abnormally shallow anterior chambers, there is a risk that acute attacks of angle-closure glaucoma will be precipitated. The incidence has been estimated to be nearly 1 in 4,000.[16] Atropine and scopolamine have a profound effect on the eye because of their longer duration of action compared with other agents with anticholinergic effects, such as phenothiazines, tricyclic antidepressants, and antihistamines. These locally instilled agents cause mydriasis and cycloplegia that may persist for as long as 2 weeks. In some patients with open-angle glaucoma, they produce a slight rise in IOP (less than 6 mm Hg) when instilled into the eyes. Other mydriatics, however, do not appear to have this effect.[17]

Conventional doses of atropine systemically administered for preanesthesia have little ocular effect; in contrast, equivalent therapeutic doses of scopolamine can cause definite pupillary dilation.[18] Prolonged use of anticholinergics can exacerbate open-angle glaucoma to some extent, but studies have shown that oral atropine at a dose of 0.6 mg every 4 hours for 1 week produces only slight elevations of IOP.[19] In another study, the administration of proprietary cold remedies containing 0.2 mg of belladonna alkaloids (given twice daily for 4 days) caused no changes in IOP in 27 normal volunteers and 37 patients with glaucoma (including 18 patients with chronic angle-closure glaucoma).[20]

Propantheline, a commonly used anticholinergic, produces no significant elevation in IOP in normal patients or those with angle-closure glaucoma. Anticholinergics, in fact, can deepen the anterior chamber by inhibiting contraction of the ciliary body and can produce cycloplegia, which widens rather than narrows the anterior chamber angle, making angle-closure glaucoma less likely to occur. No recent reports of exacerbations of glaucoma with diazepam or amitriptyline have appeared in the literature, although the manufacturers of these drugs contraindicate their use in patients with this disorder. Very high doses of phenothiazines given for schizophrenia have produced slight elevations of IOP.[21] Treatment with miotics easily overcame the effect.

In summary, withholding systemic anticholinergics for fear of inducing open-angle glaucoma is not justified. This is true especially with parenteral atropine or scopolamine given before general anesthesia is administered. Sensitivity of the eye to systemic drugs is relatively low. Although these agents can induce angle-closure glaucoma in rare instances, the concomitant use of parasympathomimetic miotics will prevent any effects of IOP. However, ocularly instilled potent anticholinergics, such as atropine, scopolamine, cyclopentolate, and homatropine, should not be used in patients diagnosed with or predisposed to angle-closure glaucoma.

Sympathomimetics. Adrenergic agents commonly found in cough and cold preparations, appetite suppressants, bronchodilators, central nervous stimulants, and vasoconstrictors produce slight pupillary dilation. No adverse effects on open-angle glaucoma have been reported. After systemic administration of these agents, the frequency of deleterious effects on angle-closure glaucoma has been extremely small. Adrenergic agents such as epinephrine and phenylephrine have been used ocularly to treat open-angle-glaucoma. However, these agents elevate the IOP by narrowing the anterior chamber angle when instilled into the eyes of patients with angle-closure glaucoma.

General anesthetics producing parasympathetic and sympathetic imbalance may cause pupillary block. To prevent this complication, topical pilocarpine 1% may be instilled into the eye before anesthesia is induced.

Cardiovascular Drugs. Evidence is convincing that vasodilators significantly aggravate glaucoma, even though subconjunctival injection of strong vasodilators such as isoxsuprine and tolazoline can induce transient elevations in IOP, particularly in chronic open-angle glaucoma. Nitrates, nitrites, aminophylline, and cyclandelate can be used safely in glaucoma.[16,21] Antihypertensives decrease intraocular blood flow, which can lead to loss of small visual fields in patients with a high IOP. Therefore, it is best that blood pressure be decreased gradually in patients with angle-closure glaucoma. If it is necessary for blood pressure to be decreased rapidly, one should increase the patient's miotic medication or simultaneously lower the IOP rapidly with an agent such as acetazolamide.

Corticosteroid-Induced Glaucoma. Corticosteroid-induced glaucoma is well documented. This form of glaucoma usually occurs without pain, physical findings in the eye, or visual field defects. The lesion probably occurs in the trabecular meshwork and severely decreases the outflow facility. After topical therapy, glaucomatous change occurs in the eye instilled with the drug. This ocular hypertensive effect is usually fully reversible within 1 month after discontinuation of the medication.

The increase in IOP is approximately 10 mm Hg for patients with preglaucomatous anterior chambers and 5 mm Hg in normal persons. In some cases, irreversible eye damage occurs if ocular tension persists for 1 to 2 months or longer. In addition, cupping of the optic disc and defects of the visual field may develop a few months after topical administration of corticosteroids is begun. Patients on long-term topical steroid therapy should therefore have tonometric examinations every 2 months.

The degree of rise in pressure appears to be associated with the anti-inflammatory potency of the agents involved and is most marked with dexamethasone and betamethasone.[22] Equivalent doses of ophthalmic prednisolone and triamcinolone used four times daily resulted in elevations of IOP similar to those caused by betamethasone instilled only once daily. The duration of corticosteroid treatment and the age of the patient influence the degree of ocular hypertension experienced. In some instances, topical epinephrine or systemic carbonic anhydrase inhibitors can maintain ocular tension within normal limits. On other occasions, it may be necessary for clinicians to reduce the frequency of administration, substitute a less potent steroid, or withdraw therapy.

Ocular hypertension effect induced by topical steroids can be categorized into three groups of patients in the general population who do not have diagnosed glaucoma.[23] Two thirds of the general population (group 1) respond with an average increase in IOP of 1.6 mm Hg after 4 weeks of 0.1% dexamethasone given three times daily. A second group (29%) respond with an average rise of 10 mm Hg. Finally, a third group (5%) respond with a rise greater than 16 mm Hg. For each group, the rate of IOP increase differs significantly. The clinical implication is that patients who are receiving corticosteroid for at least 1 month and who have tonometric pressures below 21 mm Hg are unlikely to have glaucomatous complications. In addition, because approximately one third of the general population will have a group 2 or group 3 response to topical steroids, tonometric monitoring should be performed after the first month of therapy, then every 2 months while the patient is on therapy.

Miscellaneous Agents. Amphetamines, tricyclic antidepressants, monoamine oxidase inhibitors, indomethacin, and cocaine produce slight degrees of mydriasis, but the likelihood that angle-closure glaucoma can be induced with these drugs is very low. Strong miotics such as pilocarpine 4% to 8% and indirect-acting nonreversible cholinesterase inhibitors may lead to pupillary block and inhibition of aqueous humor outflow. This may result in vascular congestion of the peripheral part of the iris so that the swollen iris blocks the canal of Schlemm and prevents the outflow of aqueous humor.[21]

Polarizing neuromuscular blocking agents, such as succinylcholine, used as adjuvants to general anesthesia can cause a marked rise in IOP if the patient is not adequately anesthetized. These agents should not be used in glaucomatous patients. A nondepolarizing neuromuscular blocking agent, such as atracurium, does not increase the IOP.

Other medications, such as the serotonin-selective reuptake inhibitors (SSRIs) fluoxetine and paroxetine have also been implicated in case reports as causes of glaucoma.[24–27] Relative to the large number of patients who use these medications, the incidence of these problems is low, and there is no reason for clinicians to discourage therapy in patients with glaucoma. Rather, the clinician should closely monitor for potential drug-induced disease in patients who may benefit from either of these agents.

Summary of Drug-Induced Glaucoma. Table 13.5 lists drugs that can induce glaucoma. The following factors must be considered in assessment of the problem of drug-induced glaucoma: (a) topically administered drugs induce glaucoma more frequency than those given systemically; (b) conditions under which any drugs are contraindicated are specific about type of glaucoma and method of treatment for it; (c) seldom, if ever, does a warning against the use of a particular agent in glaucoma specify the type of glaucoma; and (d) patients with chronic open-angle glaucoma that is adequately controlled by therapy are not at risk when treated with systemic anticholinergics or sympathomimetics.

Finally, acute angle-closure glaucoma is an emergency, and any agent that might precipitate an attack must be used cautiously. Unfortunately, patients who are predisposed to angle-closure glaucoma are not accurately identified without a gonioscopic examination of the anterior angle. Additionally, patients with diagnosed angle-closure glaucoma who have had a corrective surgical procedure are not at risk for another episode of angle-closure glaucoma.[28]

CLINICAL PRESENTATION AND DIAGNOSIS

SIGNS AND SYMPTOMS

Glaucoma is insidious in onset and often produces no symptoms or only minor symptoms of discomfort, such as headache or "tired eyes." Many patients do not seek medical attention or do not adhere to medical therapy because of this lack of symptoms. Fortunately, optic nerve and retinal damage is a late finding of end-stage disease that can be minimized with effective medical treatment. Symptoms such as persistent headache and eye pain usually cause patients to seek medical assistance before these serious consequences develop.[15]

Open-Angle Glaucoma. Common findings of open-angle glaucoma may be minimal and do not appear immediately. As time progresses, the signs become more marked until they finally restrict vision. Common findings include increased IOP, visual field loss, optic disc changes, decreased outflow facility, and gonioscopically open angles.

An increased IOP can be interpreted in several ways. Most persons have pressures of 21 mm Hg or less. However, some patients may experience pressure-independent glaucomatous damage. This can occur with pressures under 20 mm Hg, called normal tension glaucoma. In general, pressure readings in the high 20s are suspicious, and those above 30 are cause for serious concern. Patients between the ages of 50 and 75 with pressures above 30 mm Hg as the only sign of glaucoma should be treated medically because decreased vascular perfusion in the elderly can damage the optic nerve. Younger patients with similar readings may require assessment for changes in the optic disc or visual fields at less frequent intervals. No cutoff IOP has been universally accepted for use in diagnosing glaucoma; the health care provider must judge whether to medically or surgically lower

IOP according to the patient's risk factors, diagnostic findings, and signs of existing optic nerve damage.[5,6,10,15]

Angle-Closure Glaucoma. Acute angle-closure glaucoma usually presents with signs and symptoms of blurred vision (often with colored halos around light), severe ocular pain, and nausea with occasional vomiting. Acute angle-closure glaucoma should be considered a medical emergency. The eye typically appears red, the cornea is cloudy, the pupil is halfway dilated, the anterior chamber is narrow, and the IOP is frequently above 50 mm Hg. Visual acuity is reduced by corneal changes or edema. Bullae may be present on the cornea if the acute attack is prolonged. Colored halos result from diffraction of light by the edematous cornea.[5,6,15] Ocular pain may vary from moderate to severe. The oculovagal reflex is thought to produce nausea, vomiting, bradycardia, and sweating that may accompany an acute attack. With very high IOPs, the pupil may become fixed in mid-dilation and may eventually be damaged. In severe cases, the pupil changes from a round to an oval shape and may resist constriction by topical parasympathomimetic agents.

Chronic angle-closure is a less severe form of glaucoma than acute angle-closure glaucoma; symptoms may range from none to intermittent and severe ocular pain, along with halo formation and ocular congestion. Synechiae do not form without ocular congestion, which may be evident only with a moderately high pressure reading.

Table 13.6 describes and differentiates clinical findings of patients with open-angle or angle-closure glaucoma.

DIAGNOSIS AND CLINICAL FINDINGS

Four common tests may be performed that allow diagnosis of glaucoma before visual loss occurs. Direct ophthalmoscopy, also known as slit-lamp examination, allows the physician to observe changes in the optic nerve head. Slit-lamp examination is a routine test performed by ophthalmologists to examine the cornea, anterior chamber (for depth), iris, and vitreous. Changes such as optic nerve cupping or hemorrhage may be evident upon examination. Photographs of the optic disc may be obtained that allow physicians to observe and compare changes over time with the use of repeat photographs. One problem with the use of direct ophthalmoscopy is that it requires a great amount of training, and considerable interobserver variability may occur. In addition, it is not easily available in most primary care settings.[10]

Tonometry measures IOP and may be useful as a screening test. Several different devices, such as the Goldmann tonometer, the Schiøtz indentation tonometer, or electrical strain gauges, measure how much force is required to flatten the central cornea (applanation of the cornea). As has been discussed, some patients with normal IOP may continue to develop glaucomatous damage. In addition, as many as 70% of patients with ocular hypertension will never develop visual problems due to glaucoma.[10] Therefore, many physicians use tonometry in combination with other diagnostic tests.

A third screening method is perimetry. Perimetry measures visual field defects by producing visual stimuli in various locations of the patient's field of vision. Because defects in the visual field and loss of vision are made apparent through perimetry, it is currently considered the ''gold standard'' diagnostic procedure. Unfortunately, perimetry is too time consuming and expensive to be a practical screening tool; it should be reserved for those patients who have optic nerve damage that is detected by other tests.[4,10]

Finally, gonioscopy is a procedure that allows quantitative measurement of the angle of the anterior chamber. Gonioscopy requires considerable training and is usually performed only by ophthalmologists.

TABLE 13.6	Clinical Findings and Symptoms of Primary Glaucoma		
Glaucoma	**Onset**	**Early Findings and Symptoms**	**Late Findings and Symptoms**
Open-angle	Insidious	Asymptomatic slight rise in IOP: decreased rate of aqueous humor outflow, optic disc changes (symptoms may be marginal or absent).	Gradual loss of peripheral vision (over months to years); persistent elevation of IOP; optic nerve degeneration; retinal nerve atrophy; edema of the cornea; cataracts; trabecular meshwork degeneration.
Angle-closure	Sudden	Blurred vision; severe ocular pain and congestion; conjunctival redness; cloudy cornea; moderately dilated pupil; poor pupil response to light; markedly elevated IOP; nausea and vomiting.	Complete blindness in 2–5 days if not treated.

TABLE 13.7	Recommended Initial Diagnostic Procedures for Open-Angle and Angle-Closure Glaucoma
Open-Angle Glaucoma	**Angle-Closure Glaucoma**
• Family history • Physical examination of the pupil • Measurement of intraocular pressure • Physical examination of the cornea and assessment of central and peripheral anterior chamber depth through the slit-lamp procedure • Measurement of angle with gonioscopy • Dilation of pupil and visualization of optic disc and nerve fiber layer • Photography or detailed drawing of optic nerve appearance • Examination of the fundus • Evaluation of the visual field	• Family history • Physical examination of the cornea and central and peripheral anterior chamber depth through the slit-lamp procedure • Measurement of angle with gonioscopy

(Adapted from the Medical Specialty Society, Primary Angle-Closure Glaucoma and Glaucoma Panel, Preferred Practice Patterns Committee. Primary open-angle glaucoma. San Francisco, CA: American Academy of Ophthalmology, 1996.)

Table 13.7 lists recommended initial diagnostic procedures for open-angle and angle-closure glaucoma while Table 13.8 describes these procedures in greater detail.

PSYCHOSOCIAL ASPECTS

It is estimated that 23% to 43% of patients whose condition has been diagnosed and is being treated do not adhere to drug therapy regimens.[29–31] It is important that clinicians recognize and appropriately assess several psychosocial factors when they are designing, implementing, and evaluating a therapeutic plan. First, as has been mentioned, most patients have few or no symptoms of disease. Second, open-angle glaucoma should be considered a chronic controllable disease. Finally, some patients may have difficulty with proper medication administration technique or may experience adverse effects from medications. All these aspects can lead to nonadherence to medication therapy. Finally, studies have shown that patients who have even mild visual field or visual acuity changes may have significantly impaired mobility.[29] Methods of educating the patient and minimizing psychosocial barriers that may affect management of the disease are discussed later throughout the chapter.

THERAPEUTIC PLAN

OPEN-ANGLE GLAUCOMA

Conservative medical treatment can successfully control most cases of chronic open-angle glaucoma. The stage or severity of disease as evidenced by the condition of the optic disc and the quality of the visual field should be the major factors assessed when treatment is selected. Mild elevation of IOP (<30 mm Hg) in the presence of a normal optic disc and visual field is not an absolute indication for therapy. Patients should have routine periodic examinations to detect optic changes because such changes can be detected long before permanent visual field impairment occurs. No absolute level of IOP that must be maintained to ensure therapeutic success. The IOP should be maintained at a level that prevents further deterioration of the optic disc and impairment of the visual field. If the disc is normal on gonioscopic examination, an IOP in the high 20s is not as important clinically as is one with concurrent disc involvement or abnormal visual field. The former situation may warrant only close periodic follow-up, whereas in the latter case, appropriate medical treatment should be started. If the slightest indication of disc pathology is noted, the IOP should be maintained at 20 mm Hg or even lower through medical management. In cases of considerable disc degeneration and visual field loss, vigorous treatment should be undertaken to attain a pressure of 15 mm Hg or lower. The target IOP reduction is therefore variable according to the patient's level of preexisting damage or risk of damage.

In situations where advanced cupping of the optic disc and visual loss are not apparent in the presence of high IOP (>30 mm Hg), medical therapy should be initiated. The aim of therapy is to lower the IOP sufficiently to interrupt the course of the disease. Problems common to antiglaucoma therapy must be considered before IOP is reduced with drugs. The expense and inconvenience of medications should be considered, as well as whether the adverse effects

TABLE 13.8	Diagnostic Studies for Glaucoma
Procedures	**Comments**
Tonometry	Measures intraocular tension; because of diurnal variation, repeated readings should be done before definitive diagnosis is made; between acute attacks of angle-closure glaucoma, intraocular tension may be normal; applanation tonometry measures the force applied per unit area, whereas indentation tonometry uses a plunger to produce a pit in the cornea, which serves as a measure of intraocular pressure.
Gonioscopy	Differentiates the type of glaucoma; gonioscopic appearance of narrowed anterior chamber angle is usually diagnostic of angle-closure glaucoma.
Tonography	May reveal impaired facility of aqueous humor outflow; early open-angle glaucoma can be detected by this technique; tonometer is applied to the eye and the resultant reduction in intraocular tension is measured as an indicator of outflow facility.
Water-drinking test	Rise in intraocular tension after rapid ingestion of a quart of water is significant indication of glaucoma; positive result occurs in 30% of open-angle glaucoma cases; negative result does not rule out glaucoma; tonography and water-drinking test reveal open-angle glaucoma with 90% reliability.
Ophthalmoscopy	Glaucomatous excavation or cupping of the optic disc is found in chronic primary open-angle and congenital glaucomas; glaucomatous changes of optic disc or occlusion of the central retinal vein in the absence of elevated intraocular tension should arouse suspicion of glaucoma in an early stage.
Visual field examination	Isolated areas of impaired vision surrounded by normal areas in a visual field is indicative of open-angle glaucoma; visual field changes are irreversible; parallel optic disc changes occur.
Corticosteroid instillation	Striking differences in ocular tension between patients with primary open-angle glaucoma and normal patients are produced by topically instilled corticosteroids; steroid provocative test is used to evaluate genetic predisposition of glaucoma; response of primary angle-closure glaucoma to corticosteroid instillation is similar to response in normal patients.
Dark room test	Intraocular tension is assessed in the patient before and after he or she is placed in a dark room; in chronic angle-closure glaucoma, a considerable rise in intraocular tension is observed after the patient has been in the dark.

and toxicities of the drugs constitute a greater risk to the patient than is posed by the increased level of IOP.

Trials of topical agents involving a single eye may be useful in determining the amount of IOP reduction attributable to medication. The effects of therapy on the IOP can be assessed within 1 week or longer. β-Blocker therapy remains the most widely prescribed drug therapy for the treatment of patients with glaucoma, although some clinicians now prefer newer agents that allow for less frequent dosing or greater reductions in IOP.[5,30] Well-designed cost-effectiveness studies and other pharmacoeconomic evaluations have not yet been completed for newer classes of antiglaucoma agents. Because of their higher costs, these agents should probably be reserved as second-line monotherapy for patients who do not tolerate or respond to less expensive topical therapy.

Refractoriness often occurs following prolonged use of cholinergic miotics. Rather than increasing the frequency of instillation or the strength used, the clinician should select an alternative agent. Responsiveness to the cholinergic miotics often is restored after their replacement for a brief period by an anticholinesterase miotic. Various combinations of glaucoma medications are often given together to potentiate their therapeutic effects. However, not all combinations produce an additive pharmacologic response.

The addition of an agent from another class of antiglaucoma drugs is preferred to substitution or addition of an agent from the same group. Deterioration of glaucoma should always be ruled out. The storage condition of the medication, the expiration date, and the method of administration (including observation of nasolacrimal occlusion) should be assessed when a patient experiences diminished effects from the eyedrops. Figure 13.2 summarizes an approach that may be useful in the treatment of open-angle glaucoma.

ANGLE-CLOSURE GLAUCOMA

Acute angle-closure glaucoma is a medical emergency that must be treated surgically. Before peripheral iridoplasty or laser iridotomy is performed, administration of one or more of the following agents may be used to eliminate pupillary block and decrease inflammation: hyperosmotic agents, carbonic acid inhibitors, miotics, or corticosteroids. Because therapy is largely surgical in nature, readers are referred to guidelines developed by the American Academy of Ophthalmology (www.aao.org) for the most current surgical treatment recommendations.

NORMAL-TENSION GLAUCOMA

The Collaborative Normal-tension Glaucoma Study found that when the IOP is lowered by 30%, the rate of visual field

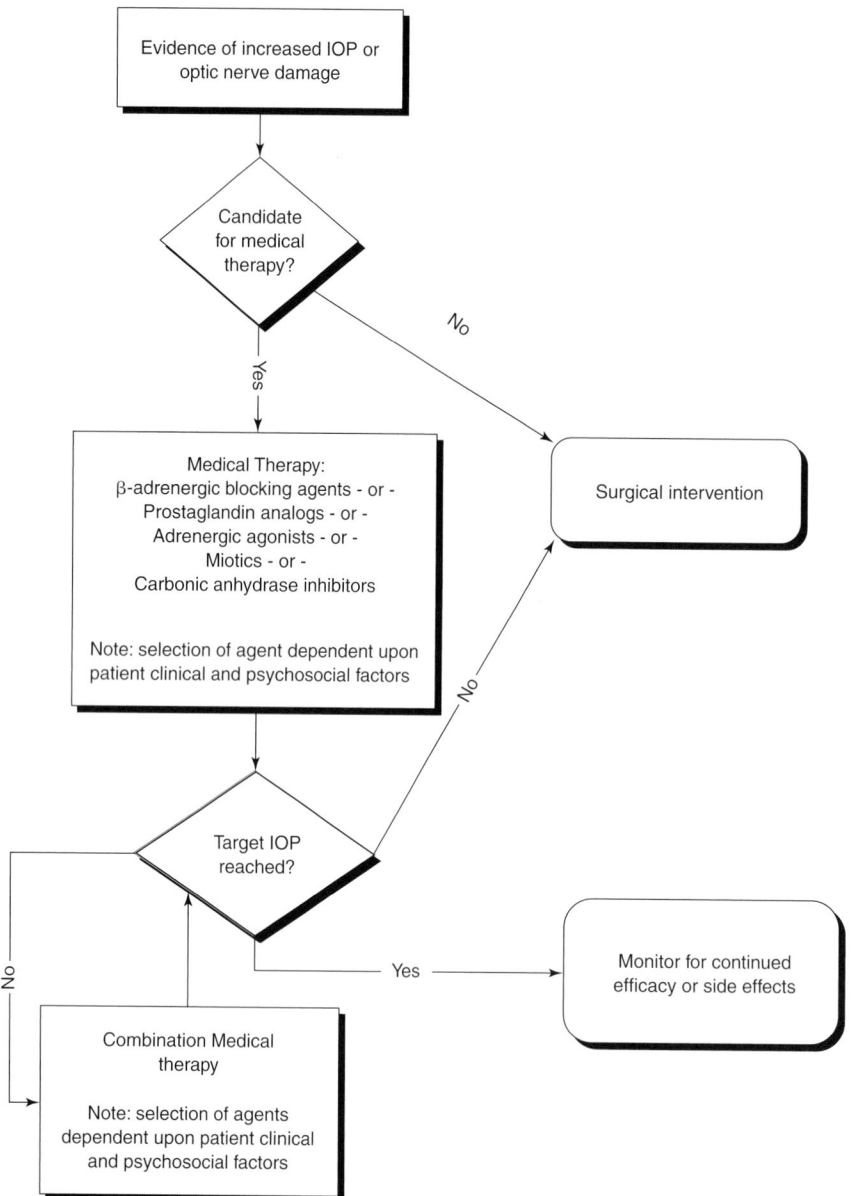

FIGURE 13.2 Algorithm for the medical management of open-angle glaucoma.

progression is lower.[1] On the basis of these results, it is now thought that patients with normal IOP who are at risk of progressing to optic nerve damage should be routinely examined for progression, and, if it is detected, they should be treated with drugs that effectively reduce baseline IOP by 25% to 30%.[31]

TREATMENT

PHARMACOTHERAPY

The goal of glaucoma therapy is the immediate and sustained reduction of IOP to prevent deterioration of the optic nerve and loss of vision. Medications used in the treatment of glaucoma may be classified as those that increase the elimination of aqueous humor and those that decrease its formation. The five major classes of medications used for the management of glaucoma include β-adrenergic blocking agents, miotics, adrenergic agonists, topical and oral carbonic anhydrase inhibitors, and prostaglandin analogs. Additionally, hyperosmotic agents are used for the short-term rapid decrease in IOP that is necessary in the management of acute angle-closure glaucoma. Table 13.9 summarizes the therapeutic classes of medications used in the treatment of patients with glaucoma; they are differentiated by their mechanisms of action.

β-Blocking Agents. β-blockers remain the most widely prescribed drugs for the treatment of glaucoma;[30] they may be used alone or in combination with other agents. The oc-

TABLE 13.9	Medications Used in the Treatment of Glaucoma		
Drug Class/Name	**Mechanism of IOP-Lowering Effect**	**Duration of Activity, h**	**Pregnancy Category**
β-blockers	Increase aqueous humor outflow		
Timolol		12–24	C
Levobunolol		12–24	C
Betaxolol		12	C
Metipranolol		12–24	C
Carteolol		12	C
Miotics (direct-acting)	Increase aqueous humor outflow		
Pilocarpine			C
Solution		4–8	
Gel		18–24	
Miotics (cholinesterase inhibitors)	Increase aqueous humor outflow		
Physostigmine		12–36	C
Demecarium		Days/weeks	X
Echothiophate		Days/weeks	C
Sympathomimetics	Decrease aqueous humor formation and increase aqueous humor outflow		
Apraclonidine		7–12	C
Epinephrine		12	C
Dipivefrin		12	B
Brimonidine		12	B
Carbonic anhydrase inhibitors	Decrease aqueous humor formation		
Acetazolamide			C
Tablets		8–12	C
ER capsules		18–24	C
Injectable		4–5	C
Dichlorphenamide		6–12	C
Methazolamide		10–18	C
Dorzolamide		8	C
Brinzolamide		8	C
Prostaglandin analogs	Increase aqueous humor outflow		
Latanoprost		12–24	C
Bimatoprost		24	C
Travoprost		24	C
Unoprostone		10–2	C

ER, extended-release.

ular hypotensive effect caused by β-blockers is probably due to suppression of aqueous humor formation by inhibition of the β-adrenoreceptors in the ciliary body.[30,32] β-blockers decrease aqueous humor production by approximately one third.[33] All agents are available as ophthalmic solutions that are usually administered one to two times daily.

Propranolol was used for the treatment of glaucoma as early as 1967.[34] However, because of adverse effects such as ocular anesthesia, the use of β-blockers was limited until timolol maleate became available.[35] β-Blockers that are commonly used for the treatment of open-angle glaucoma include timolol, betaxolol, levobunolol, carteolol, and metipranolol (Table 13.10). In addition, in 1995, timolol was approved by the US Food and Drug Administration (FDA) as a combination product with the carbonic anhydrase inhibitor

dorzolamide. The main clinical difference among the available topical β-blocking agents is their selectivity for the β-receptor. Betaxolol is the only currently available agent that is selective for the β_1-receptor.[36]

Timolol is a potent, short-acting, nonselective β-blocker. The usual starting dose is 1 drop of the 0.25% solution into the affected eye(s) once to twice a day. If this does not control the IOP, the dose may be increased to the 0.5% solution, one drop given twice a day.[37,38] When used alone, timolol can result in mean reductions in IOP of approximately 31% to 33%. Timolol may be used in combination with agents such as epinephrine, pilocarpine, carbachol, dorzolamide, acetazolamide, and prostaglandin agonists. The addition of timolol to these agents significantly reduces IOP farther than it is reduced by either agent alone.[33,37,39–42] A

TABLE 13.10	Selected Pharmacodynamic and Pharmacokinetic Properties of Ocular β-Adrenergic Blockers				
Property	**Timolol**	**Carteolol**	**Betaxolol**	**Levobunolol**	**Metipranolol**
Relative β-blockade potency (propranolol = 1)	6	10	4	6	2
β₁ selectivity	−	−	+ +	−	−
ISA	−	+ +	−	−	−
Local anesthetic effect	−	−	+	−	
Stinging, burning	+ +	+/−	+ + +	+ +	+
Heart rate decrease	+ +	+	+/−	+ +	+ +
Bronchoconstriction	+ +	+	+/−	+ +	+ +
Dyslipidemia	+	−	?	?	?
Ocular perfusion	+/−	+/−	+/−	?	?
Serum half-life, h	3–5	3–7	12–20	6	2

ISA, intrinsic sympathomimetic activity.
(Reprinted with permission from Zimmerman TJ. Topical ophthalmic β blockers: a comparative review. J Ocular Pharmacol 9 : 373–384, 1993.)

combination product that contains timolol maleate and dorzolamide may be useful in enhancing patient compliance to beyond the level of compliance seen with agents administered separately. A gel-forming product and a modified formulation of timolol are available for once-daily administration.

Stabilization of timolol therapy may take several weeks. A reevaluation should take place 2 and 4 weeks after therapy is begun. If the IOP is maintained, the schedule may be decreased to 1 drop once a day because of the daily variations in IOP. Tonometer readings should be performed at different times of the day.[35,43–45] Contraindications of timolol include use in patients with obstructive pulmonary disease and in those with congestive heart failure.[38]

Betaxolol, a β₁-selective adrenergic blocking agent, is available as a 0.5% solution and as a 0.25% suspension that is instilled into the eye every 12 hours. Betaxolol 0.5% and timolol 0.5% have been shown to have similar efficacy in reducing IOP.[46] The adverse effects reported most frequently were mild discomfort and tearing on administration, but adverse effects were not sufficient to cause discontinuation of therapy. Betaxolol, unlike timolol, offers the advantage of little or no effect[47] on pulmonary disease, but it should be used with caution in patients with preexisting disease.[30,48,49] Because of its selective β-adrenergic activity, betaxolol produces a greater additive effect than does timolol that is administered concomitantly with epinephrine. However, betaxolol, like other β-blockers, should not be administered to patients with heart failure.[50] Finally, betaxolol may cause more stinging and burning upon instillation than are caused by other available β-blocking agents.[36]

Levobunolol is available as a 0.25% and a 0.5% solution that can be given once or twice a day. Levobunolol is metabolized by the liver to an active metabolite, dihydrolevobunolol, which usually allows extended dosing intervals.[51] Levo-

bunolol 0.5% or 1% given once a day has been shown to have a greater effect on decreasing IOP than does timolol 0.5%.[52] If IOP is not controlled with a single dose of levobunolol, the frequency of administration should be increased to twice a day. In this case, levobunolol offers no advantage over timolol.[30,36]

Metipranolol is available as a 0.3% solution. Its relative β-blockage potency is the lowest of the β-blockers. Metipranolol may cause an increased risk of granulomatous anterior uveitis, resulting in iris nodules and precipitates.[36] Additionally, metipranolol has been reported to cause more stinging and burning upon administration than are caused by other agents.[36] Metipranolol has been discontinued in the United Kingdom because of these potential toxicities.

Carteolol is a nonselective β-adrenergic blocker that is available as a 1% solution. It is the most potent of the β-blockers and is the only agent with intrinsic sympathomimetic activity (ISA). Unfortunately, this has not been shown to decrease systemic cardiovascular or pulmonary adverse effects.[30,36,53]

Adverse effects of the topical β-blockers include burning or pain after instillation, blurring of vision, and dilated pupils (with epinephrine combination). Systemic adverse effects include cardiovascular problems (bradycardia, palpitations, hypertension, congestive heart failure), central nervous system disturbances (headaches, dizziness, drowsiness, anxiety, depression), and pulmonary system adverse effects, including deaths due to precipitation or exacerbation of existing bronchospasm.[30,43–45] Patients with diabetes should also use topical β-blockers with caution because of potential loss of symptoms of hypoglycemia.

Topical β-blockers cause only small changes in pupil size and accommodation. Additionally, blurred vision and night blindness associated with the use of miotic agents are less likely with β-blocking agents. β-Blockers should never be used in patients with angle-closure glaucoma without concomitant instillation of a topical miotic.

In summary, the available agents all typically reduce IOP by approximately 25% from baseline. Apparent advantages of one agent over another are limited to adverse effect profile, dosing schedule, and cost per effective dose. Levobunolol or timolol may allow for once-daily dosing. Betaxolol may be a safer alternative in patients with pulmonary disease. The ISA effect of carteolol has not been shown to reduce its adverse effect profile. Therefore, current recommendations usually consider timolol as the standard agent against which others must be judged.[36]

Miotics. Miotics act via direct cholinergic stimulation or as cholinesterase inhibitors. The resulting parasympathetic activity of either of these classes of medication facilitates the outflow of aqueous humor from the anterior chamber of the eye (Table 13.11). This is accomplished primarily by their action on the musculature of the iris and the ciliary body, which pulls the peripheral iris away from the trabecular meshwork. The trabecular meshwork and veins peripheral to the canal of Schlemm also may be dilated, thereby facilitating the outflow of aqueous humor. Miotics can lower IOP directly by stimulating the postfunctional effector cells innervated by cholinergic fibers. Structurally, these agents are similar to acetylcholine. Acetylcholine is used during surgery for rapid miosis, but it is not useful in the long-term treatment of glaucoma because it is rapidly hydrolyzed by acetylcholinesterase.[4]

Cholinergic miotics are therapeutically beneficial for treatment of open-angle glaucoma and for preoperative preparation for surgery in angle-closure glaucoma. Their disadvantage is their short duration of action, which requires frequent administration.

Direct-Acting Miotics. Pilocarpine is the cholinergic agent most commonly used for the treatment of glaucoma.[4–6,15,28] Dosage must be titrated to patient response; however, little additional benefit is derived from the use of solutions greater than 4% of pilocarpine.[54]

Pilocarpine penetrates the cornea after ocular instillation and decreases the IOP, reaching maximum levels in 30 to 40 minutes. The duration of IOP lowering is 4 to 8 hours. The usual frequency of instillation is two or three times daily, but pilocarpine may be given as often as every 2 hours.[6,55]

Pilocarpine gel is useful as an adjunct to the solution when given at bedtime. Because the patient is sleeping, typical adverse effects such as myopia and fixed pupils occur during the night. This may add to patient acceptance and compliance with medical therapy.[56] In general, however, newer agents have supplanted the use of pilocarpine by their relative dosing convenience.

Acetylcholine chloride is used only during surgical procedures. The solution is unstable, and it must be prepared immediately before the procedure. Additionally, pilocarpine or another miotic agent must be administered before the surgical dressing is placed if continued postoperative miosis is desired.

Patients who fail to control their IOP with direct-acting miotics may switch to more potent agents such as cholinesterase inhibitors.[4]

Cholinesterase Inhibitors. Cholinesterase inhibitors increase parasympathetic activity by inhibiting the enzyme

TABLE 13.11	Miotic Drugs Used in the Management of Glaucoma	
Drug	**Dose[a]**	**Comments**
Direct acting		
Pilocarpine hydrochloride, pilocarpine nitrate	0.25%–10%	Instill 1 or 2 drops in affected eye from q6–8h to as often as q4h. Onset of IOP-lowering effect is rapid with a 4- to 6-h duration; although strengths above 4% are available, little advantage is gained through the use of any strength above 4%.
Pilocarpine gel	4% gel	Apply to affected eye at bedtime. The gel dosage form is used as an adjunct to daytime medications.
Short-acting cholinesterase inhibitors		
Physostigmine sulfate	0.25%	Apply 0.25% ointment at bedtime. Onset of IOP-lowering effect similar to pilocarpine; considered to be stronger miotic than pilocarpine.
Long-acting cholinesterase inhibitors		
Demecarium bromide	0.125%–0.25%	This is rarely used clinically for the management of glaucoma.
Echothiophate iodide	0.03%–0.25%	This is rarely used clinically for the management of glaucoma.

[a] For open-angle glaucoma.

cholinesterase, thereby permitting the accumulation of ace-tylcholine and prolonging activity on the effector end organs of the eye. The key pharmacologic difference between avail-able compounds is the relative irreversibility or permanency of their parasympathomimetic activity. Physostigmine and neostigmine are reversible agents with short durations of effect. Organophosphate compounds such as demecarium, echothiophate, and isoflurophate are irreversible compounds that have long durations of action. Today, cholinesterase inhibitors are rarely used clinically in the United States for the treatment of glaucoma.

The adverse effect profiles of the parasympathetic miotic agents differ on the basis of pharmacologic activity. A direct and short-acting miotic such as pilocarpine can produce local conjunctival irritation as a result of frequent instillations. Allergic sensitivity or refractoriness to pilocarpine develops after prolonged use. Frequent instillation of the short-acting miotics can exacerbate chronic allergic conjunctivitis or blepharitis.

Miotics can produce additional annoying adverse effects such as transient headaches, ocular and periorbital pain, twitching of the eyelids, ciliary congestion, and spasms.[57] The long-acting agent echothiophate produces the most se-vere symptoms, including discomfort associated with bright lights and close-up work. The affected eye is extremely my-opic. This is particularly intense in younger patients who have active accommodation and are initially myopic. After intense and prolonged administration of the stronger miotics, pupillary cysts may occur.[58] These are seen more commonly in children, but the reason for this is not known.

Anticholinesterase miotics may produce vitreous hemor-rhaging, contact dermatitis, and allergic conjunctivitis. Reti-nal detachment and cataracts have been associated with the use of anticholinesterase miotics; however, these agents are probably only a contributing factor secondary to underlying retinal pathology.

Systemic absorption of antiglaucoma drugs after ocular instillation may result in undesirable effects.[59,60] These ef-fects are seen more commonly after administration of the indirect- and longer-acting anticholinesterase agents. Gas-trointestinal disturbances such as nausea, diarrhea, and ab-dominal pain, as well as muscle spasm and weakness, sweat-ing, lacrimation, salivation, hypotension, bradycardia, bronchial constriction, and respiratory failure, have been ob-served.[59,61] Most systemic effects reverse rapidly after the drug has been discontinued. In severe cholinergic toxicity, atropine sulfate 2 mg or pralidoxime chloride 25 mg per kilogram administered intravenously or subcutaneously can be given with no effect on the control of glaucoma.

Any potent long-acting miotic agent should be used with caution when a patient has asthma, Parkinson's disease, pep-tic ulcer disease, or other gastrointestinal disease, because anticholinesterase systemic effects can exacerbate their clin-ical course.

When known sensitivities to these agents exist, they should not be used. Considerable inhibition of plasma cho-linesterase can be produced by prolonged topical anticholin-esterase therapy.[62] A patient who receives these agents must be monitored closely for prolongation of apnea when succi-nylcholine chloride is given during surgery.[62]

Patients who may be exposed to organophosphate pesti-cides, such as professional gardeners, farmers, or workers in industries that produce these chemicals, should be made aware of the potential problems and risks associated with prolonged topical anticholinesterase exposure.[63] Additive and cumulative effects on the parasympathetic nervous sys-tem have been noted. Systemically administered cholinergic agents such as ambenonium, neostigmine, or physostigmine, which are used in disorders such as myasthenia gravis, can potentiate the action of the anticholinesterase miotics.

Glaucoma secondary to ocular inflammation may be ex-acerbated by these agents through further vascular disrup-tion. Lens opacities have been reported in patients treated with anticholinesterase miotics. Cataractogenic lens changes appear to be related to the drug, the concentration the patient is receiving, and the duration of treatment. Cataract forma-tion does not appear to be directly associated with glaucoma-tous eyes; patients treated with miotics other than the anti-cholinesterase miotics are less likely to develop lens opacity. Lens changes may be partially reversible when the drug is discontinued. Progressive worsening of the cataract may occur, however, necessitating surgical extraction.

If these agents are used clinically, undesirable adverse effects can be minimized through proper instillation of their lowest effective concentrations at reasonable intervals. Pa-tients should be instructed to tightly close their eyes or to occlude the nasolacrimal duct by pressing on the area be-tween the inside corner of the eye and the nose for approxi-mately 5 minutes after administration (see also the section on patient education).

Sympathomimetics. Reduction of IOP in open-angle glaucoma may be accomplished successfully by ocular in-stillation of sympathomimetics. These agents act as agonists at α- or β-adrenergic receptor sites, or both. Catecholamines, including epinephrine, norepinephrine, and dopamine, may act at many levels of aqueous humor production and elimina-tion. Sympathomimetic medications have a complex role in decreasing IOP; their mechanism of action includes both decreased production and increased outflow of aqueous humor.[64]

Epinephrine 1 to 2% solution instilled every 8 to 24 hours can reduce IOP in patients with open-angle glaucoma.[65] The rate of aqueous secretion is initially decreased, probably by adrenergic stimulation at receptor sites in the ciliary epithe-lium. Improved facility of outflow is not immediate but may be seen after several months of epinephrine therapy. The mechanism is believed to be α-adrenergic response to epi-nephrine at the trabecular meshwork. The pressure-lowering effect of epinephrine (3 to 15 mm Hg) occurs within 6 to 8 hours and lasts from several hours to days. Patient response appears to be highly variable. Epinephrine is seldom used alone for open-angle glaucoma but is usually used with miotics.[66,67] Epinephrine does not disturb accommodation and is especially beneficial in overcoming the disabling miosis induced by the parasympathomimetics. When used in combination, it should be given 5 to 10 minutes after the miotic has been instilled. Because of discomfort upon ocular administration, epinephrine use in the United States has declined as newer and better tolerated agents have become available.

Dipivefrin, a prodrug of epinephrine, is produced by the addition of two pivalyl side chains to epinephrine. Dipivefrin has greater lipid solubility than epinephrine, and thus better corneal penetration (approximately 17 times greater). The combination of dipivefrin 1% and epinephrine 2% has been shown to significantly lower IOP.[66,67] Dipivefrin was slightly less effective in lowering IOP than was epinephrine, but was also associated with fewer systemic adverse effects.[76] Dipivefrin has caused similar ocular adverse effects, however.

Apraclonidine was the first commercially available selective α$_2$-receptor agonist. It is structurally similar to the antihypertensive agent clonidine; the addition of an amide group causes apraclonidine to be a more polar molecule and allows for better ocular penetration. Its use was first limited to its role as an adjunctive agent during or immediately following surgical procedures.[64] Recent studies have shown that when it is used in this manner, apraclonidine is effective after procedures such as cataract removal[78,79] and argon laser trabeculoplasty.[80]

Apraclonidine may be used for long-term control of IOP. When given as a 0.5% solution three times a day, it has been shown to decrease IOP by approximately 3 to 5 mm Hg.[81] Apraclonidine may be added to other therapy as well.[82,83] Therapy with apraclonidine 0.5% or 1% added to timolol 0.5% results in additional benefit. When added to timolol, an additional 2.5- to 3.3-mm Hg (10.3% to13.6%) reduction was apparent at 8 AM, indicating improved control during sleeping hours. At 3 hours after apraclonidine administration, an additional reduction of 4.7 to 5.2 mm Hg (20.0% to 21.7%) was produced.[82] No significant difference was noted between 0.5% and 1% apraclonidine.

Apraclonidine 0.5% given three times a day to patients with inadequate IOP control despite the use of maximal pharmacotherapy has been shown to maintain adequate IOP and prevent the need for surgery. The adverse effect profile of apraclonidine limits its use as an initial agent for the treatment of glaucoma.[64] Most frequently, it causes follicular conjunctivitis. It may also cause dry nose and mouth. Because of ocular and nonocular adverse effects, 21% to 25% of patients may discontinue therapy.[82]

Apraclonidine is metabolized by the liver to an active metabolite, and its systemic effects may be increased in those patients with liver or kidney disease. Although apraclonidine is thought to cause minimal cardiovascular effects in normal persons, the manufacturer recommends close cardiovascular monitoring in patients with decreased liver or kidney function.[69] Finally, the IOP-lowering effect of apraclonidine ap-pears to persist for less than 4 weeks for some patients. Because of these limitations, apraclonidine is rarely used on a long-term basis for its IOP-lowering effects.

Brimonidine is a selective α$_2$-receptor agonist that has been approved for use in the United States. Brimonidine is available as a 0.2% solution, and its usual dose is 1 drop administered three times daily.

Brimonidine 0.2% and timolol 0.5% have been shown to significantly lower IOP.[70–72] Brimonidine was associated with more frequent dry mouth (33% vs. 19.4%), but burning and stinging were more common among patients treated with timolol (28.1% vs. 41.9%, respectively).[72] In addition, ocular allergy was reported in 9% of patients treated with brimonidine. Brimonidine has been shown to produce a greater peak effect but a lower mean decrease in IOP.[70,71]

Brimonidine does not cause significant decreases in heart rate compared with timolol. Brimonidine and apraclonidine are both contraindicated in patients taking monoamine oxidase inhibitors (MAOIs) because of a potential increase in the MAOI effect.

Appreciable local and systemic adverse effects are experienced by patients who use ocular sympathomimetics for long periods.[67] Local adverse effects include melanin deposits on the conjunctiva and cornea, hyperemia and corneal edema, and allergic blepharoconjunctivitis.[67] Headache, periorbital pain, and lacrimation with intermittent visual blurring and distortion are common complaints. Although the frequency is relatively low, cardiac irregularities and elevations of blood pressure after ocular administration of epinephrine have been reported.[73] Adverse effects, both local and systemic, are promptly relieved after the epinephrine has been discontinued. Closer supervision and caution should be exercised for patients who are receiving anesthetics in preparation for surgery because the reported rate of systemic adverse effects of the ocular sympathomimetic is higher in such cases. Gonioscopic examinations are advised before the ocular instillation of a sympathomimetic mydriatic, to rule out asymptomatic or subacute angle-closure glaucoma. Sympathomimetics are contraindicated in angle-closure glaucoma before peripheral iridectomy has been performed. After iridectomy takes place, sympathomimetics can be useful, especially if aqueous humor outflow is impaired. They should not be used if IOP can be adequately managed with the use of miotics alone.

Carbonic Anhydrase Inhibitors. The lowering of IOP can be achieved by topical or systemic administration of carbonic anhydrase inhibitors.[74] Of the systemic carbonic anhydrase inhibitors, acetazolamide is the most widely used for the treatment of glaucoma. Systemic agents are indicated when patients fail to respond to or cannot tolerate topical glaucoma therapy. The addition of topical agents such as dorzolamide and brinzolamide has largely replaced the use of systemic agents because they result in fewer adverse effects.[4]

Carbonic anhydrase catalyzes the reversible conversion of carbon dioxide to bicarbonate. In the eye, large concentrations of carbonic anhydrase are found in the ciliary process and retina. Bicarbonate flow into the posterior chamber is controlled by carbonic anhydrase and is decreased upon addition of carbonic anhydrase inhibitors. Bicarbonate decrease results in reduced sodium and water movement into the posterior chamber.[4,75,76]

Topical Agents. The early topical use of systemic agents was not effective because of the high concentrations that were necessary and the consequent changes in pH that caused irritation. The introduction of dorzolamide and brinzolamide sparked an interest in the use of carbonic anhydrase inhibitors as first-line therapy in selected patients.

Dorzolamide is available as a 2% solution (given alone or in combination with timolol maleate) and is indicated for monotherapy or in combination with other agents. When administered three times a day, dorzolamide lowers IOP by 4 to 6 mm Hg at peak, and by 3 to 4.5 mm Hg at trough (8 hours post dose). Dorzolamide 2% given three times daily as monotherapy lowers IOP by 22.8% compared with 31% to 36% lowering with add-on therapy with timolol or pilocarpine.[77] Therapy is generally well tolerated; the most common adverse effects are burning or stinging of the eyes, conjunctivitis, follicular conjunctivitis, and eyelid edema.[77]

When used as monotherapy, dorzolamide and latanoprost have been shown to significantly decrease IOP. The combination of these two agents, however, is more effective at lowering IOP than is either agent alone.[78]

Brinzolamide is available as a 1% suspension that is typically administered three times daily. When given two or three times a day, brinzolamide has similar efficacy to dorzolamide 2% in lowering IOP. Timolol 0.5% given twice a day has been shown to lower IOP to a greater extent than brinzolamide or dorzolamide.[79]

Brinzolamide is associated with fewer complaints of stinging and burning when compared with dorzolamide. Patients who receive brinzolamide should be reminded that the suspension must be shaken before administration to ensure proper dosing.

Systemic Agents. The systemic drug of choice is usually acetazolamide. Acetazolamide is available as 125-mg and 250-mg tablets and as 500-mg sustained-release capsules. Intravenous acetazolamide may also be useful in rapidly reducing IOP. A single dose of oral acetazolamide can reduce IOP for 8 to 12 hours. Maximum effect is seen about 2 hours after oral administration. Following intravenous administration, the maximum effect is attained within 15 minutes, and the duration of effect is approximately 4 to 5 hours.[74]

Acetazolamide can reduce aqueous inflow by approximately 40% to 60% and IOP by 25% to 40%. Dichlorphenamide and methazolamide have similar effects and only differ in their potency and adverse effects (Table 13.12).

TABLE 13.12	Carbonic Anhydrase Inhibitors Used to Manage Glaucoma			
Drug and Dosage Form	**Dose**	**Onset**	**Duration**	**Comment**
Acetazolamide Tablets 125 and 250 mg	125–250 mg qid	$\frac{1}{2}$–1 h	4–6 h	
Acetazolamide Sequels 500 mg	500 mg bid	1–2 h	10–18 h	May be better tolerated than immediate-release formulation.
Acetazolamide 500-mg vials	500 mg IV	1 min	4 h	Useful for attaining rapid decrease in IOP.
Methazolamide Tablets 25 and 50 mg	25–50 mg bid titrated to 50–100 mg bid to tid	1 h	10–14 h	50 mg is equivalent to 250 mg of acetazolamide; dose response for adverse effects and amount of IOP reduction.
Dichlorphenamide Tablets 50 mg	25–50 mg bid, tid, or qd	$\frac{1}{2}$ h	6–12 h	Metabolic acidosis occurs less frequently with dichlorphenamide than with other carbonic anhydrase inhibitors; used with patient intolerant of or refractory to acetazolamide; anorexia, nausea, paresthesias, dizziness, or ataxia and tremor should alert patients or clinicians of the possibility of toxicity.
Dorzolamide 2% Solution	1 drop to affected eye(s) tid		8 h	
Brinzolamide 1% Suspension	1 drop to affected eye(s) tid		8 h	Suspension must be shaken before administration.

IOP, intraocular pressure.
(Adapted from Flach AJ. Topical acetazolamide and other carbonic anhydrase inhibitors in the current medical therapy of the glaucomas. Glaucoma 8:20–27, 1986.)

These agents are more likely to cause adverse effects that lead to discontinuation of therapy and are rarely used.

Unfortunately, 50% of patients are unable to tolerate systemic carbonic anhydrase therapy.[74,80] Acetazolamide sustained-release capsules are somewhat better tolerated than are immediate-release tablets, but approximately 40% of patients cannot tolerate acetazolamide in this dosage form. A study of compliance with acetazolamide therapy in 87 patients demonstrated that 56% of patients either were not taking medication (30 patients) or were not taking medication as frequently as prescribed (19 patients).[81]

Older persons appear to be more intolerant of the carbonic anhydrase inhibitors than younger patients.[74,82] The most common adverse effects of the systemic carbonic anhydrase inhibitors are malaise, fatigue, weight loss, depression, and anorexia. Additional adverse effects, such as nausea, vomiting, intestinal colic, diarrhea, and paresthesia of the face and extremities, may also appear. Transient myopia is an unusual and rare occurrence.

Acetazolamide produces hyperglycemia in prediabetic and diabetic patients who are receiving oral hypoglycemic agents. Hyperuricemia has occurred after treatment with carbonic anhydrase inhibitors. Prolonged use of these drugs can lead to urinary and renal colic secondary to formation of calcium calculi.[83,84] Alkalinization of the urine by acetazolamide results in enhanced renal tubular reabsorption of drugs such as quinidine, amphetamine, and tricyclic antidepressants. Alkalinization of the urine can also decrease the acid-dependent antibacterial activity of methenamine. Carbonic anhydrase inhibitors are not recommended in patients with hemorrhagic glaucoma, hepatic or renal dysfunction, renocortical hypofunction, or a history of prior sensitivity to the drug.

The use of carbonic anhydrase inhibitors in chronic angle-closure glaucoma should be discouraged because symptoms of progressive angle narrowing can easily be obscured. Also, patients who are allergic to sulfa drugs should not take systemic or topical carbonic anhydrase inhibitors because these agents contain a sulfonamide group. Fatalities have occurred, although rarely, because of severe reactions to sulfonamides; these reactions include Stevens-Johnson syndrome, toxic epidermal necrolysis, fulminant hepatic necrosis, agranulocytosis, aplastic anemia, and other blood dyscrasias. A baseline complete blood count (CBC) should be obtained. For patients who are continuing on therapy, periodic monitoring should include CBCs and serum electrolytes. A summary of carbonic anhydrase inhibitors used to manage glaucoma is included in Table 13.12.

Prostaglandin Analogs. Prostaglandins are produced in the body by the action of the enzyme cyclooxygenase (COX) on arachidonic acid. Nonsteroidal anti-inflammatory agents (NSAIDs) block this activity, reducing the many known effects of prostaglandins throughout the body. Prostaglandins are known to cause increased IOP and inflammation when injected into animal models. Initial studies of the effects of prostaglandins on IOP demonstrated that, when given in high doses, IOP was increased upon administration.[85] When given in low concentrations, prostaglandin $F_{2\alpha}$ ($PGF_{2\alpha}$) effectively lowers IOP. The mechanism is thought to be the increased uveoscleral outflow of aqueous humor.[4,85] Currently, four different prostaglandin analogs are marketed in the United States for the treatment of glaucoma. Recent evidence suggests that clinicians in some countries, including the United States, have increasingly turned to prostaglandin analogs as first-line therapy.[86] In Italy, where medications are freely available to patients, DeNatale and colleagues found that their use had increased from 0% to 17% of all glaucoma prescriptions, while β-blockers had decreased from 79% to 55% of all glaucoma prescriptions.[87]

A number of trials have examined comparative efficacy of the available agents among other prostaglandin analogs or β-blockers or other agents.[88–91] Generally, the prostaglandin analogs are at least as effective as timolol and can be expected to decrease IOP from baseline by between 13% and 33%. Clinically, the agents appear to act very similarly. Unoprostone appears to have slightly fewer IOP-lowering effects compared with the other three marketed agents, and it requires twice-daily dosing. It is important to note that compliance and discontinuation of therapy with the prostaglandin analogs remain problematic. In a retrospective compliance study, patients who received bimatoprost or travoprost were approximately 30% more likely to discontinue therapy or switch therapy than were latanoprost users. The disparity in discontinuation rates may be due to differences in the adverse effect profiles of these drugs. Clinically, hyperemia occurs variably among the agents, with latanoprost typically described as causing fewer or less severe effects.[86]

Prostaglandin analogs may darken the iris by increasing the number of melanosomes (pigment granules) in melanocytes in about 7% of patients. Additionally, some patients may experience lengthened or darkened eyelashes. Patients who treat only a single eye may notice increased pigmentation only in the treated eye and may therefore experience heterochromia.[92,93] This effect may be permanent or may very slowly reverse. Clinical relevance and the possibility of histopathologic changes have been reviewed elsewhere.[93] This is not a reason to deny therapy when IOP lowering is deemed necessary.

It is important to note that the mechanisms of action of prostaglandin analogs and miotic agents are antagonistic. Therefore, patients should not receive these agents together, and any miotic agent should be discontinued before a prostaglandin analog is added.

The reader is directed elsewhere[94] for further comparative review of the agents, and a summary of available prostaglandin analogs is included in Table 13.9.

Hyperosmotic Agents. Hyperosmotic agents lower the IOP by creating an osmotic gradient between the plasma and the aqueous humor from the anterior chamber of the eye (Table 13.13). Given systemically, these agents draw fluid

TABLE 13.13	Hyperosmotic Agents Used in the Management of Glaucoma		
Drug	**Dosage, g/kg**	**Route**	**Comments**
Ascorbic acid	0.4–1	IV/oral	Gastric distress and diarrhea; oral administration; seldom used since more effective agents have become available.
Glycerin (50% solution)	1–1.5	Oral	Nausea, vomiting, hyperglycemia can occur; caution should be used in patients with diabetes.
Isosorbide	1–2	Oral	Can be given to patient with diabetes; tension comparable with that of intravenous hyperosmotics; diarrhea frequently experienced.
Mannitol (20% solution)	1–2	IV	Requires larger volumes than are required by other hyperosmotics; used in patients with diabetes; less irritating and free of tissue necrosis when solution extravasates; not contraindicated in patients with renal disease; patient should be monitored for cellular dehydration, hypokalemia, cardiac irregularities, urinary output, and chest pain; more effective for glaucoma with inflammation than urea or glycerol; avoid excessive use.
Urea (30% solution)	1–1.5	IV	Given IV over 30 min; unstable; adverse effects are sloughing, phlebitis, headache, nausea, vomiting, hemolysis "rebound diuresis"; contraindicated in nephrotic patients; caution required in patients with hepatic impairment; only freshly made solution should be used; maximal effect at 1 h.

from the anterior chamber of the eye into the intravascular space. Hyperosmotic agents are most useful in the preoperative management of primary acute angle-closure glaucoma. The degree of IOP lowering depends on the tension elevation and the osmotic gradient induced. The greatest effect of rapid changes in plasma osmolarity is noted on the eye, with profound pressure elevations. The most commonly used hyperosmotics are mannitol, urea, and glycerol.

Mannitol can effectively reduce acutely elevated IOP when given slowly by the intravenous route as a 20% solution to adults and a 10% solution to children.[95,96] The ocular hypotensive effect is produced in 30 to 60 minutes and lasts from 4 to 6 hours. The effectiveness of the hyperosmotic agents varies with the rate of administration. Mannitol is preferred in the management of secondary glaucoma accompanied by hyperemia or uveitis because it penetrates the eye less readily, which is an advantage when inflammation is present. Agents that enter the eye rapidly produce a lower osmotic gradient and a shorter duration of action than are produced by those that enter the eye slowly or not at all. Inflammation greatly increases the ocular permeability of agents such as urea. Therefore, it is less desirable under those circumstances. There is relatively less local tissue irritation, thrombophlebitis, and necrosis occurring with mannitol than with urea when given intravenously. Renal disease is not a contraindication to the use of mannitol.

Excessive thirst is a common sensation experienced by patients after hyperosmotic agents have been infused. However, these patients should not be given fluids during the period of osmotic dehydration. Secondary rises in IOP occur after administration of fluids, diminishing the therapeutic effects of the hyperosmotics. Headache is also a common complaint, but it can be minimized simply by bed rest. Symptoms of cellular dehydration and hypokalemia, and cardiac irregularities secondary to mannitol therapy should be monitored. On rare occasions, disorientation and severe agitation may be observed. Pulmonary edema and congestive heart failure may be precipitated in the elderly, especially with mannitol infusions. Potassium deficiency can accompany diuresis after hyperosmotic infusion. Patients with hepatic, renal, or cardiac disorders should be cautiously monitored. Mannitol is not absorbed and is ineffective when given orally.

Urea given by the intravenous route as a 30% solution reduces elevated IOP within 30 to 40 minutes. Miotics and carbonic anhydrase inhibitors are used concomitantly with urea before surgery in the management of acute glaucoma. Nausea, vomiting, confusion, disorientation, and anxiety may be seen. Severe headache, a common complaint, can begin soon after the initiation and continue for the duration of the intravenous infusion. The patient's head should not be elevated during this time.

Although urea produces less cellular dehydration because of its ease of penetrability into the cell, a "rebound phenomenon" can occur as the plasma level of the hyperosmotic agent drops to below that of the vitreous fluid. As urea is rapidly cleared from the circulation with diuresis, the osmolality of the blood declines. The hyperosmotic vitreous in turn draws fluid into the eye, resulting in increased IOP or pressure "rebound" effect.[97]

Ascorbic acid successfully reduces IOP in rabbits with glaucoma. In cases of refractoriness to acetazolamide and miotics, ascorbic acid given intravenously can lower the ocular hypertension. A 20% solution of sodium ascorbate at a pH of 7.2 to 7.4 can produce normal ocular tension in 60 to 90 minutes.

Oral hyperosmotic agents effectively reduce elevated IOP and are useful in situations where rapid-action infused preparations are not required. Glycerol is a convenient hyperosmotic agent when given as a 50% or a 75% solution.[98] The ocular penetration of glycerol is poor; therefore, a substantial osmotic gradient can be produced between the plasma and the aqueous humor. IOP reduction is as effective as with hyperosmotic agents given by intravenous infusion. IOPs normally return to pretreatment levels within 5 to 6 hours. Hyperglycemia and glycosuria can occur after glycerol is given and should be used with particular caution in labile diabetics.[98] Acute diabetic ketoacidosis has been reported after treatment with glycerol. Nausea, diarrhea, and headache are also common complaints after administration of oral glycerol.

The reduction of IOP with isosorbide is comparable with that associated with intravenous mannitol, urea, or oral glycerol. Given orally as a 50% solution, its absorption is rapid, and it is primarily excreted unchanged in the urine. Effective reduction in IOP occurs within 30 minutes after ingestion and remains for 1 to 2 hours or longer depending on the dose. Adverse effects include transient headaches and diarrhea. Other gastrointestinal disturbances such as nausea are usually less of a problem with isosorbide than with glycerol.[99]

NONPHARMACOLOGIC THERAPY

Surgical Management. Surgical management of open-angle glaucoma should be reserved for situations in which maximal efforts with single-drug and combination therapy are not tolerated or have been unsuccessful in maintaining an acceptable level of IOP and in preventing progressive changes of the optic disc or the visual field. The surgical procedure, peripheral iridectomy, involves creation of a collateral drainage from the anterior chamber.

Laser Therapies. Two differing laser therapies are available for patients, depending upon whether treatment is for open-angle or angle-closure glaucoma. Argon laser trabeculoplasty (ALT), an alternative to peripheral iridectomy, is the most often used nonpharmacologic means of treating chronic open-angle glaucoma. Laser surgery can reduce the IOP by 7 to 13 mm Hg in more than 80% of patients.[100]

Using the argon laser coupled with a high-magnification biomicroscope, the surgeon places approximately 50 to 100 lesions in an evenly spaced sequence on the inner surface of the trabecular meshwork. Histopathologic studies by scanning electron microscopy have shown that laser light energy produces fibrosis at the treatment site. It is theorized that these laser ''burns'' cause localized shrinkage, which in turn, produces tension on adjacent, untreated trabecular beams. The previously collapsed spaces between the beams are then pulled open, allowing aqueous humor to pass more easily and resulting in reduced IOP.

At least 1 hour before ALT, apraclonidine hydrochloride 1% is instilled into the operated eye for control of IOP.

Apraclonidine is used in conjunction with trabeculoplasty to prevent an acute elevation in IOP, which can occur after ALT. Its onset of action is within 1 hour of instillation, and maximal effect is seen within 3 to 5 hours. It is used 1 hour before ALT is undertaken, and a second drop is instilled immediately after completion of the laser surgical procedure.[101,102] Apraclonidine hydrochloride has replaced pilocarpine as the agent of choice before ALT. A topical anesthetic is instilled before the procedure is begun; then, the patient is seated at the slit-lamp laser photocoagulator.

Laser iridotomy is the treatment of choice for pupillary block or angle-closure glaucoma. In most cases, laser surgery is recommended over traditional surgery and is performed on an outpatient basis. One hour before laser iridotomy surgery, topical apraclonidine hydrochloride 1% is instilled in the eye, along with pilocarpine drops. The pilocarpine causes pupillary constriction, which thins the iris, making laser puncture easier. At the time of laser surgery, a topical anesthetic is instilled. An opening that measures approximately 50 to 100 microns in diameter is created in the peripheral iris for release of the pupillary block component of angle-closure glaucoma.[103]

Complications of laser treatment of glaucoma include intraocular inflammation in the form of uveitis, intraocular bleeding, elevated IOP, diplopia, pigment dissemination, and lens injury.[103]

ALTERNATIVE THERAPIES

The one alternative therapy that has received widespread attention is the use of marijuana to lower IOP. Historically, accounts of the use of marijuana to decrease IOP appeared as early as 1971.[104] The National Institutes of Health (NIH) in the United States sponsored studies from 1978 to 1984 that demonstrated that IOP decreased when marijuana was inhaled or was taken orally or intravenously. Unfortunately, topical administration was not shown to be effective, and serious adverse effects were noted with doses that were useful clinically. These included increased heart rate, decreased blood pressure, and dry eyes.[105]

Although the clinical usefulness of marijuana for the treatment of glaucoma has its limitations, research based on the active chemical component or components of marijuana (including tetrahydrocannabinol) may be valuable. Many unanswered questions remain regarding the safe and effective use of marijuana for glaucoma. The Institute of Medicine,[106] the American Academy of Ophthalmology,[107] and the National Eye Institute[105] of NIH all support continued research into the safety and effectiveness of various delivery systems for the use of marijuana in glaucoma.

IMPROVING OUTCOMES

The successful outcome of glaucoma treatment depends greatly on the patient's proper use of medications. Methods to improve the use of medication include patient education activities and assessment of patient compliance with therapy.

PATIENT EDUCATION

An asymptomatic patient who does not understand why expensive and inconvenient eyedrops are required will be less inclined to use them according to prescribed instructions. The blurring of vision and occasional discomfort or other adverse effects associated with the use of these medications further enhance noncompliance. The patient with glaucoma should understand the nature of the disorder and appropriate expectations for the drugs being used to control it.

Patients should be instructed regarding the proper technique for administration of eyedrops. This includes several steps such as: handwashing, checking the solution for discoloration or expiration date, shaking vials if medication is in suspension, not touching the dropper tip to the skin, tilting back the head, pulling down the lower lid, and administering the correct number of drops. It is important to stress (a) that the patient should close the eye or place an index finger over the tear duct for 3 to 5 minutes (called nasolacrimal occlusion) to minimize the amount of medication that reaches the systemic circulation, and (b) that drops of differing types of medication be spaced apart by at least 10 minutes. Ideally, the health care provider should also observe the patient after instruction to verify his or her understanding and manual dexterity.

Some authors[4] recommend that patients be taught to take their medications according to the colors of vial lids. This practice could lead to medication errors if vial lids are accidentally interchanged, or if the patient has other medications that appear similar. Pharmacists should remind patients to always check the instructions on the prescription label. If a patient cannot read the label because of loss of eyesight, or if the patient is not literate, large print instructions, the use of other caregivers, and other methods such as nontextual pictograms can help ensure proper medication technique.

METHODS TO IMPROVE PATIENT ADHERENCE TO DRUG THERAPY

Optimal therapeutic results can occur only in an environment of mutual cooperation and understanding between patients and the health care providers responsible for patient care. Physicians should assess compliance whenever IOP appears to be uncontrolled, before suggesting increases in medication strength or other changes in therapy.

Methods for improving medication compliance in patients with glaucoma should be attempted; these may include education about the importance of disease screening and the progression of disease, direct observation of administration technique, and modification of the therapeutic plan to simplify medication regimens or overcome adverse effects, whenever necessary.

Pharmacists are in a unique position to help clinicians monitor for compliance. If patients who are typically noncompliant take their medication before they make office vis-

its, their IOP may appear normal. A laboratory value that measures long-term IOP control is not available. Pharmacists, however, can monitor refill activity in patients who are receiving medications at one site. In addition, managed health plans that have prescription drug claims for payment purposes may be able to monitor for patients who do not receive refills within a certain time. Those patients may be targeted for educational interventions and resulting changes in their use of refills.

DISEASE MANAGEMENT STRATEGIES TO IMPROVE PATIENT OUTCOMES

The strategies to improve compliance with therapy that have already been discussed should be expected to improve IOP control, and ultimately, patient outcomes.

PHARMACOECONOMICS

Relatively few economic studies have been performed regarding the different agents available for the treatment of glaucoma. Part of this is due to the difficulty inherent in assigning an appropriate short-term treatment that reliably and accurately results in improved outcomes. The use of IOP as an end point may not be appropriate in all patients, in that no standard IOP target has been specified. Therefore, some patients will require a decrease of only 3 to 5 mm Hg, but others will require much more effect. A cost-effectiveness analysis that examines a cost per mm Hg lowering effect may therefore be misleading. Because of differing adverse effect profiles of the various classes of medications, a cost minimization analysis, which assumes equal outcomes, often is inappropriate. Finally, because of the chronic nature of glaucoma, cost utility analyses that examine blindness as an outcome will take many years to complete and may not be feasible.

Despite these problems, some economic evaluations have been completed.[108,109] A study by Stewart and colleagues examined the daily costs of therapy with six commercially available β blockers.[109] For study purposes, the authors assumed equal efficacy and safety among the available agents.

The protocol used 10 subjects to administer, per their normal techniques, 1 drop from each of 10 differing β-blocker preparations (differing pharmaceutical formulations and generic equivalents, when available, of timolol, levobunolol, carteolol, betaxolol, and metipranolol). The authors then calculated drop size and total bottle volume to determine amounts that would be wasted or used by patients. Sixty random pharmacies throughout the United States were then surveyed for the cost of the medications. With use of these data, the authors found a daily range of costs (based only on usable administered drops) of $0.55 to $1.35 (US). It is interesting to note that the amount wasted, as calculated from drop size, ranged from 27% to 54% of the stated dropper volume. This study was the first to highlight the importance of drop size through the use of volunteers to administer medication, as well as to examine the use of generic equivalent medications. Unfortunately, assumptions of equal efficacy and safety may not be valid for all patients.

A cost utility analysis comparing dorzolamide and pilocarpine was completed by Rocchi and Tingey.[108] The authors assumed a governmental payor perspective (Canadian provincial ministry of health) and assessed costs and consequences of alternatives over a 10-year period. A decision analysis model that used published and expert panel estimates of costs and probabilities of outcomes was completed. Quality adjusted life-years (QALYs) were calculated for adverse outcomes, and an incremental cost/QALY was calculated for the two alternatives. Results of the model demonstrated that patients who received dorzolamide had higher costs and higher QALYs. The incremental cost/QALY for a patient who received dorzolamide was $9,390 (CAN) over pilocarpine. The authors noted that a cost/QALY less than $20,000 (CAN) is usually regarded as worthwhile dollars spent in health care. Sensitivity analysis undertaken to change the adverse event rate and cost of medication did not change the overall calculated cost/QALY threshold of $20,000. The authors concluded that dorzolamide should be reimbursed by provincial formularies, on the basis of these results.

More economic studies of this type should help providers initiate medical therapy for glaucoma as efficiently as possible in selected patients and groups of patients.

FUTURE THERAPIES

Currently, several different agents in various clinical stages of development are being tested for the treatment of glaucoma.[110] Included are β-blocking agents (adaprolol), N-methyl-D-aspartate antagonists (dexanabinol), NSAIDs (diclofenac), and neuroprotective agents (memantine). Trials of agents designed to protect the retinal ganglion cells have begun recently and offer some hope based on positive animal studies.[111] Additionally, improved delivery systems that use submicron emulsions or other extended-release systems are being examined. Finally, agents that act through their effects on the ocular vasculature, such as verapamil, are being investigated as potential therapies to prevent the neuronal damage of glaucoma. It is hoped that these agents will progress to an ideal agent with improved safety, efficacy, and ease of administration that will effect improved clinical outcomes.

KEY POINTS

In summary, the following points should be remembered when one is treating a patient with glaucoma:

■ Increased IOP is the most important risk factor for progression of glaucomatous damage to the optic nerve.

■ Glaucoma is typically classified as open-angle (most common) or angle-closure glaucoma. Treatment strategies differ by glaucoma type.

■ Immediate medical attention is required to reduce IOP in cases of acute angle-closure glaucoma.

■ The patient's complete medical regimen should be evaluated to avoid medical therapy that may worsen the patient's glaucoma.

■ A target IOP is established on the basis of the patient's current IOP and risk factors for progression of end-organ damage, with the goal of preventing initial or worsening ocular damage.

■ Reduction of IOP should be attempted through the use of topical medications with low systemic effects. Typically, β-blocking agents are the agents first chosen, unless they are otherwise contraindicated.

■ Other medication classes, such as miotics, sympathomimetics, carbonic anhydrase inhibitors, and prostaglandin analogs, have all been useful in decreasing IOP. Each medication class has unique properties and adverse effect profiles that should be considered before therapy is initiated.

■ The patient should use combination therapy only after monotherapy proves unsuccessful or is not tolerated.

■ One of the most important factors in successful glaucoma therapy is compliance with medical regimens. Health care providers should educate the patient to improve administration technique, to reduce systemic adverse effects, and to improve compliance.

■ Health care providers should monitor for effectiveness and adverse events.

■ Surgical correction should be attempted only if medical therapy is not tolerated or is unsuccessful at maintaining the target IOP.

ACKNOWLEDGMENT

The authors acknowledge Constance McKenzie for her contributions to this chapter.

SUGGESTED READINGS

Alexander CL, Miller SJ, Abel SR. Prostaglandin analog treatment of glaucoma and ocular hypertension. Ann Pharmacother 36:504–511, 2002.

Alward WL. Medical management of glaucoma. N Engl J Med 339: 1298–1307, 1998.

American Optometric Association—Professional Association. Care of the patient with open angle glaucoma. 2nd ed. 1995 (revised August 17, 2002). Available at: http://www.guidelines.gov/summary/pdf.aspx-?doc_id=4599. Accessed June 22, 2005.

Chandler PA, Grant WM, Epstein DL, et al. Chandler and Grant's glaucoma. 4th ed. Baltimore: Williams & Wilkins, 1997.

Sorensen SJ, Abel SR. Comparison of the ocular beta-blockers. Ann Pharmacother 30:43–54, 1996.

REFERENCES

1. Collaborative Normal-Tension Glaucoma Study Group. Comparison of glaucomatous progression between untreated patients with normal-tension glaucoma and patients with therapeutically reduced intraocular pressures. Am J Ophthalmol 126:487–497, 1998.

2. Collaborative Normal-Tension Glaucoma Study Group. The effectiveness of intraocular pressure reduction in the treatment of normal-tension glaucoma. Am J Ophthalmol 126 :498–1505, 1998.

3. Shields MB, Ritch R, Krupin T. Classifications of the glaucomas. In: Ritch R, Sheilds MB, Krupin T, eds. The glaucomas: clinical science. 2nd ed. St. Louis: Mosby, 1996:717–725.

4. Alward WL. Medical management of glaucoma. N Engl J Med 339:1298–1307, 1998.

5. Danyluk AW, Paton D. Diagnosis and management of glaucoma. Clin Symp 43:2–32, 1991.

6. Vaughan D, Asbury T, Riordan-Eva P, et al. General ophthalmology. 13th ed. Norwalk, CT: Appleton & Lange, 1992.

7. Wolfs RC, Klaver CC, Ramrattan RS, et al. Genetic risk of primary open-angle glaucoma. Population-based familial aggregation study. Arch Ophthalmol 116:640–1645, 1998.

8. Alward WL, Fingert JH, Coote MA, et al. Clinical features associated with mutations in the chromosome 1 open-angle glaucoma gene (GLC1A). N Engl J Med 338:1022–1027, 1998.

9. The Glaucoma Foundation. Available at: http://www.glaucomafoundation. org. Accessed June 6, 2004.

10. Screening for Glaucoma. In: DiGuiseppi C, Atkins D, Woolf SH, et al, eds. Guide to clinical preventive services (CPS). 2nd ed. Alexandria, VA: National Library of Medicine, 1996.

11. Chandler PA, Grant WM, Epstein DL, et al. Chandler and Grant's glaucoma. 4th ed. Baltimore: Williams & Wilkins, 1997.

12. Hattenhauer MG, Johnson DH, Ing HH, et al. The probability of blindness from open-angle glaucoma. Ophthalmology 105: 2099–2104, 1998.

13. Epstein DL. Practical aqueous humor dynamics. In: Chandler PA, Grant WM, Epstein DL, et al, eds. Chandler and Grant's glaucoma. 4th ed. Baltimore: Williams & Wilkins, 1997:xvi, 670.

14. Doctor, I have a question: about glaucoma. Available at: http://www.glaucomafoundation.org/faqs_g.php?g = 2. Accessed July 1, 2004.

15. Newell FW. Ophthalmology : principles and concepts. 8th ed. St. Louis: Mosby, 1996.

16. Grant WM. Ocular complications of drugs. Glaucoma. JAMA 207: 2089–2091, 1969.

17. Harris LS. Cycloplegic-induced intraocular pressure elevations: a study of normal and open-angle glaucomatous eyes. Arch Ophthalmol 79:242–246, 1968.

18. Mehra KS, Chandra P, Khare BB. Ocular manifestations of parenteral administration of scopolamine (hyoscine). Br J Ophthalmol 49:557–558, 1965.

19. Lazenby GW, Reed JW, Grant WM. Anticholinergic medication in open-angle glaucoma. Long-term tests. Arch Ophthalmol 84: 719–723, 1970.

20. Mulberger RD. Effect of a common cold product containing belladonna on intraocular pressure. Eye Ear Nose Throat Mon 47: 61–64, 1968.

21. Fraunfelder FT, Meyer SM. Drug-induced ocular side effects and drug interactions. 2nd ed. Philadelphia: Lea & Febiger, 1982.

22. Smith CL. ''Corticosteroid glaucoma'': a summary and review of the literature. Am J Med Sci 252:239–244, 1966.

23. Pappa K. Corticosteroid drugs. In: Munger T, Craig E, eds. Havener's ocular pharmacology. 6th ed. St. Louis: CV Mosby, 364–428, 1994.

24. Eke T, Bates AK. Acute angle closure glaucoma associated with paroxetine. BMJ 314:1387, 1997.

25. Kirwan JF, Subak-Sharpe I, Teimory M. Bilateral acute angle closure glaucoma after administration of paroxetine [Letter] [See comments]. Br J Ophthalmol 81:252, 1997.

26. Lewis CF, DeQuardo JR, DuBose C, et al. Acute angle-closure glaucoma and paroxetine. J Clin Psychiatry 58:123–124, 1997.

27. Ahmad S. Fluoxetine and glaucoma. DICP 25:436, 1991.

28. Hiatt RL, Fuller IB, Smith L, et al. Systemically administered anticholinergic drugs and intraocular pressure. Arch Ophthalmol 84: 735–740, 1970.

29. Noe G, Ferraro J, Lamoureux E, et al. Associations between glaucomatous visual field loss and participation in activities of daily living. Clin Exp Ophthalmol 31:482–486, 2003.

30. Zimmerman TJ. Topical ophthalmic beta blockers: a comparative review. J Ocul Pharmacol 9:373–384, 1993.

31. Kamal D, Hitchings R. Normal tension glaucoma—a practical approach. Br J Ophthalmol 82:835–840, 1998.

32. Coakes RL, Brubaker RF. The mechanism of timolol in lowering intraocular pressure. In the normal eye. Arch Ophthalmol 96: 2045–2048, 1978.

33. Dailey RA, Brubaker RF, Bourne WM. The effects of timolol maleate and acetazolamide on the rate of aqueous formation in normal human subjects. Am J Ophthalmol 93 :232–237, 1982.

34. Phillips CI, Howitt G, Rowlands DJ. Propranolol as ocular hypotensive agent. Br J Ophthalmol 51:222–226, 1967.

35. Boger WP, Steinert RF, Puliafito CA, et al. Clinical trial comparing timolol ophthalmic solution to pilocarpine in open-angle glaucoma. Am J Ophthalmol 86:8–18, 1978.

36. Sorensen SJ, Abel SR. Comparison of the ocular beta-blockers. Ann Pharmacother 30:43–54, 1996.

37. Anon. timoptic in the management of chronic open-angle glaucoma. West Point, PA: Merck Sharp & Dohme Publishers, 1979.

38. Timolol maleate. In: Mosby's GenRx. 9th ed. (1999) Available at: http://www.mdconsult.com. Accessed March 15, 1999.

39. Kass MA. Efficacy of combining timolol with other antiglaucoma medications. Surv Ophthalmol 28 (Suppl):274–279, 1983.

40. Korey MS, Hodapp E, Kass MA, et al. Timolol and epinephrine: long-term evaluation of concurrent administration. Arch Ophthalmol 100:742–745, 1982.

41. Keates EU, Stone RA. Safety and effectiveness of concomitant administration of dipivefrin and timolol maleate. Am J Ophthalmol 91:243–248, 1981.

42. Cyrlin MN, Thomas JV, Epstein DL. Additive effect of epinephrine to timolol therapy in primary open angle glaucoma. Arch Ophthalmol 100:414–418, 1982.

43. Beta blockers for glaucoma [Editorial]. Lancet 1:1064–1065, 1979.

44. Phillips CI, Bartholomew RS, Kazi G, et al. Penetration of timolol eye drops into human aqueous humour. Br J Ophthalmol 65: 593–595, 1981.

45. LeBlanc RP, Krip G. Timolol. Canadian multicenter study. Ophthalmology 88:224–248, 1981.

46. Stewart RH, Kimbrough RL, Ward RL. Betaxolol vs timolol. A six-month double-blind comparison. Arch Ophthalmol 104:46–48, 1986.

47. Schoene RB, Abuan T, Ward RL, et al. Effects of topical betaxolol, timolol, and placebo on pulmonary function in asthmatic bronchitis. Am J Ophthalmol 97:86–92, 1984.

48. Lesar TS. Comparison of ophthalmic beta-blocking agents. Clin Pharm 6:451–463, 1987.

49. Allen RC, Hertzmark E, Walker AM, et al. A double-masked comparison of betaxolol vs timolol in the treatment of open-angle glaucoma. Am J Ophthalmol 101:535–541, 1986.

50. Betaxolol. Mosby's GenRx. 9th ed. (1999) Available at: http://www.md consult.com. Accessed March 15, 1999.

51. Levobunolol. Mosby's GenRx. 9th ed. (1999). Available at: http://www. mdconsult.com. Accessed March 15, 1999.

52. Wandel T, Charap AD, Lewis RA, et al. Glaucoma treatment with once-daily levobunolol. Am J Ophthalmol 101:298–304, 1986.

53. Diggory P, Cassels-Brown A, Fernandez C. Topical beta-blockade with intrinsic sympathomimetic activity offers no advantage for the respiratory and cardiovascular function of elderly people. Age Ageing 25:424–428, 1996.

54. Harris LS, Galin MA. Dose response analysis of pilocarpine-induced ocular hypotension. Arch Ophthalmol 84:605–608, 1970.

55. Pilocarpine. Mosby's GenRx. 9th ed. (1999). Available at: http://www.mdconsult.com. Accessed March 15, 1999.

56. Goldberg I, Ashburn FS Jr, Kass MA, et al. Efficacy and patient acceptance of pilocarpine gel. Am J Ophthalmol 88:843–846, 1979.

57. Taniguchi T, Kitazawa Y. A risk-benefit assessment of drugs used in the management of glaucoma. Drug Saf 11:68–74, 1994,.

58. Everitt DE, Avorn J. Systemic effects of medications used to treat glaucoma. Ann Intern Med 112:120–125, 1990.

59. Ellis PP. Systemic reactions to topical therapy. Int Ophthalmol Clin 11:1–11, 1971.

60. Ellis P. Systemic effects of locally applied anticholinesterase agents. Invest Ophthalmol 5:146, 1966.

61. Leopold IH. Cholinesterases and the effects and side-effects of drugs affecting cholinergic systems. Am J Ophthalmol 62: 771–777, 1966.

62. Eilderton TE, Farmati O, Zsigmond EK. Reduction in plasma cho-linesterase levels after prolonged administration of echothiophate io-dide eyedrops. Can Anaesth Soc J 15:291–296, 1968.
63. Echothiophate. Mosby's GenRx. 9th ed. (1999) Available at: http://www.mdconsult.com. Accessed March 18, 1999.
64. Gieser S, Juzych M, Robin A, et al. Clinical pharmacology of ad-renergic drugs. In: Ritch R, Shields M, Krupin T, eds. The glau-comas. 2nd ed. St. Louis: Mosby, 1996:1425–1448.
65. Obstbaum SA, Kolker AE, Phelps CD. Low-dose epinephrine. Arch Ophthalmol 92:118–120, 1974.
66. Kass MA, Mandell AI, Goldberg I, et al. Dipivefrin and epineph-rine treatment of elevated intraocular pressure: a comparative study. Arch Ophthalmol 97:1865–1866, 1979.
67. Kohn AN, Moss AP, Hargett NA, et al. Clinical comparison of dip-ivalyl epinephrine and epinephrine in the treatment of glaucoma. Am J Ophthalmol 87:196–201, 1979.
68. Package insert. Propine (dipivefrin). Markham, Ontario, Canada: Allergan, 1996.
69. Package insert. Iopidine (apraclonidine). Fort Worth: Alcon Labora-tories, 1998.
70. Katz LJ. Brimonidine tartrate 0.2% twice daily vs timolol 0.5% twice daily: 1-year results in glaucoma patients. Brimonidine Study Group. Am J Ophthalmol 127:20–26, 1999.
71. LeBlanc RP. Twelve-month results of an ongoing randomized trial comparing brimonidine tartrate 0.2% and timolol 0.5% given twice-daily in patients with glaucoma or ocular hypertension. Bri-monidine Study Group 2. Ophthalmology 105:1960–1967, 1998.
72. Schuman JS, Horwitz B, Choplin NT, et al. A 1-year study of bri-monidine twice daily in glaucoma and ocular hypertension. A con-trolled, randomized, multicenter clinical trial. Chronic Brimonidine Study Group. Arch Ophthalmol 115:847–852, 1997.
73. Carlstedt B, Stanaszek W. Glaucoma. US Pharmacist 12:7690, 1987.
74. Lippa E. Carbonic anhydrase inhibitors. In: Ritch R, Shields M, Krupin T, eds. The glaucomas. 2nd ed. St. Louis: Mosby, 1996:1463–1481.
75. Maren TH. The rates of movement of Na+, Cl−, and HCO-3 from plasma to posterior chamber: effect of acetazolamide and rela-tion to the treatment of glaucoma. Invest Ophthalmol 15:356–364, 1976.
76. Zimmerman TJ, Garg LC, Vogh BP, et al. The effect of acetazol-amide on the movement of sodium into the posterior chamber of the dog eye. J Pharmacol Exp Ther 199:510–517, 1976.
77. Adamsons IA, Polis A, Ostrov CS, et al. Two-year safety study of dorzolamide as monotherapy and with timolol and pilocarpine. Dor-zolamide Safety Study Group. J Glaucoma 7:395–401, 1998.
78. Kimal Arici M, Topalkara A, Guler C. Additive effect of latano-prost and dorzolamide in patients with elevated intraocular pres-sure. Int Ophthalmol 22:37–42, 1998.
79. Silver LH. Clinical efficacy and safety of brinzolamide (Azopt), a new topical carbonic anhydrase inhibitor for primary open-angle glaucoma and ocular hypertension. Brinzolamide Primary Therapy Study Group. Am J Ophthalmol 126:400–408, 1998.
80. Lichter PR. Reducing side effects of carbonic anhydrase inhibitors. Ophthalmology 88:266–269, 1981.
81. Alward PD, Wilensky JT. Determination of acetazolamide compli-ance in patients with glaucoma. Arch Ophthalmol 99:1973–1976, 1981.
82. Shrader CE, Thomas JV, Simmons RJ. Relationship of patient age and tolerance to carbonic anhydrase inhibitors. Am J Ophthalmol 96:730–733, 1983.
83. Pepys MB. Acetazolamide and renal stone formation. Lancet 1:837, 1970.
84. Parfitt AM. Acetazolamide and sodium bicarbonate induced nephro-calcinosis and nephrolithiasis: relationship to citrate and calcium ex-cretion. Arch Intern Med 124:736–740, 1969.
85. Camras C. Prostaglandins. In: Ritch R, Shields M, Krupin T, eds. The glaucomas. 2nd ed. St. Louis: Mosby, 1996:1449–1461.
86. Reardon G, Schwartz GF, Mozaffari E. Patient persistency with top-ical ocular hypotensive therapy in a managed care population. Am J Ophthalmol 137 (1 Suppl):S3–S12, 2004.
87. De Natale R, Draghi E, Dorigo MT. How prostaglandins have changed the medical approach to glaucoma and its costs: an obser-vational study of 2228 patients treated with glaucoma medications. Acta Ophthalmol Scand 82:393–396, 2004.
88. Fellman RL, Sullivan EK, Ratliff M, et al. Comparison of travo-prost 0.0015% and 0.004% with timolol 0.5% in patients with ele-vated intraocular pressure: a 6-month, masked, multicenter trial. Ophthalmology 109:998–1008, 2002.
89. Netland PA, Landry T, Sullivan EK, et al. Travoprost compared with latanoprost and timolol in patients with open-angle glaucoma or ocular hypertension. Am J Ophthalmol 132:472–484, 2001.
90. Haria M, Spencer CM. Unoprostone (isopropyl unoprostone). Drugs Aging 9:213–218; discussion 9–20, 1996.
91. Cardascia N, Vetrugno M, Trabucco T, et al. Effects of travoprost eye drops on intraocular pressure and pulsatile ocular blood flow: a 180-day, randomized, double-masked comparison with latanoprost eye drops in patients with open-angle glaucoma. Curr Ther Res Clin Exp 64:389–400, 2003.
92. Latanoprost. Mosby's GenRx. 9th ed. (1999) Available at: http://www.mdconsult.com. Accessed March 15, 1999.
93. Stjernschantz JW, Albert DM, Hu DN, et al. Mechanism and clini-cal significance of prostaglandin-induced iris pigmentation. Surv Ophthalmol 47(Suppl 1):S162–S175, 2002.
94. Alexander CL, Miller SJ, Abel SR. Prostaglandin analog treatment of glaucoma and ocular hypertension. Ann Pharmacother 36:504–511, 2002.
95. Weiss D, Shaffer R, Harrington D. Treatment of malignant glau-coma with intravenous mannitol infusion. Arch Ophthalmol 69:154, 1963.
96. Adams R. Ocular hypotensive effect of intravenously administered mannitol. Arch Ophthalmol 69:55, 1963.
97. Kolker AE. Hyperosmotic agents in glaucoma. Invest Ophthalmol 9:418–423, 1970.
98. McCurdy D, Schneider B, Scheic H. Oral glycerol: the mechanism of intraocular hypotension. Am J Ophthalmol 61:1244–124, 1966.
99. Krupin T, Kolker AE, Becker B. A comparison of isosorbide and glycerol for cataract surgery. Am J Ophthalmol 69:737–740, 1970.
100. Remis LL, Epstein DL. Treatment of glaucoma. Annu Rev Med 35:195–205, 1984.
101. Apraclonidine. Mosby's GenRx. 9th ed. (1999) Available at: http://www.mdconsult.com. Accessed January 19, 1999.
102. Pollack IP, Brown RH, Crandall AS, et al. Prevention of the rise in intraocular pressure following neodymium-YAG posterior capsulo-tomy using topical 1% apraclonidine. Arch Ophthalmol 106:754–757, 1988.
103. Reid F. Personal communication, 1991.
104. Hepler RS, Frank IR. Marijuana smoking and intraocular pressure. JAMA 217:1392, 1971.
105. NEI Statement. The use of marijuana for glaucoma. National Eye Institute, 1997. Available at: www.nei.nih.gov. Accessed April 28, 1999.
106. Marijuana and medicine: assessing the science base. Available at: http://bob.nap.edu/html/marimed/. Accessed May 1, 2004.
107. American Academy of Ophthalmology, 1997. The use of marijuana in the treatment of glaucoma. Available at: http://www.eyenet.org. Accessed April, 28, 1999.
108. Rocchi A, Tingey D. Economic evaluation of dorzolamide vs. pilo-carpine for primary open-angle glaucoma. Can J Ophthalmol 32:414–418, 1997.
109. Stewart WC, Sine C, Cate E, et al. Daily cost of beta-adrenergic blocker therapy. Arch Ophthalmol 115:853–856, 1997.
110. Carlson M, Goodfellow B, Frederick C, et al, eds. The NDA pipe-line—1998. Chevy Chase, MD: FDC Reports, 1999.
111. Levin LA. Retinal ganglion cells and neuroprotection for glau-coma. Surv Ophthalmol 48 (Suppl 1):S21–S24, 2003.

Common Ear Disorders

Michael A. Oszko

The ear is a complex structure that consists of bone and cartilage, nerve tissue, and mucous membranes and fluid. In addition to facilitating the sense of hearing, the structures of the ear are intimately involved in the maintenance of balance and equilib-rium. The ear is anatomically complex, and a wide range of conditions can alter normal ear function. This chapter describes two of the most common disease states that are likely to be encountered by the pharmacist: otitis media; and otitis externa.

OTITIS MEDIA

DEFINITION

The term *otitis media* commonly denotes an infection of the middle ear. It can be more precisely described by its duration, the presence or absence of infection, and the presence or absence of an effusion (a collection of fluid in the tympanic cavity).[1] Acute otitis media (AOM) refers to a clinically identifiable infection of the middle ear in which symptoms appear suddenly (over several hours) and resolve completely within 3 weeks. If the inflammatory state persists for longer than 3 weeks but less than 3 months, the condition is called *subacute*. A middle ear effusion or discharge that persists for longer than 3 months is called *chronic* otitis media. *Recurrent* otitis media denotes three distinct episodes of otitis media over the past 6 months, or four episodes in the past 12 months.

Acute otitis media is associated with abnormal collection of fluid in the tympanic cavity (known as middle ear effusion, or MEE). The effusion may be further characterized as sanguineous (bloody), serous (serumlike, thin), serosanguineous, mucoid (mucuslike, thick), or purulent (puslike). *Otitis media with effusion* (OME) is the term used if the effusion is located behind an intact tympanic membrane but is not infected. Otitis media with effusion is distinct from AOM.[2] A patient with OME may be symptomatic but is frequently asymptomatic.

Myringitis refers to an inflammation of the tympanic membrane and is not necessarily indicative of otitis media.

TREATMENT GOALS: OTITIS MEDIA

Because AOM is frequently a self-limiting condition with greater than 80% of cases resolving spontaneously without pharmacotherapy,[3] the clinician should consider careful observation of selected patients without the use of antimicrobial therapy (i.e., "watchful waiting").[4] When a decision is made to treat otitis media with drug therapy, the clinician should do the following:

- Treat the symptoms (primarily pain and fever) of acute otitis media with nonnarcotic analgesics and antipyretics.
- Render the middle ear effusion free from infection.
- Prevent complications (e.g., mastoiditis and impaired language development due to impaired hearing).
- Prevent recurrence of infection.
- Minimize or avoid adverse drug reactions.

EPIDEMIOLOGY

Otitis media is a common disease of early childhood, with the vast majority of children experiencing one or more episodes within the first 2 years of life.[5–7] It is one of the primary reasons that children see a physician, and it is estimated that this condition costs \$3.5 billion in direct and indirect health care costs.[8] Despite its high prevalence rate, a number of risk factors for the development of otitis media have been identified[1,5,7,9–11] (Table 14.1). On the other hand, breastfeeding has been shown to be protective against the development of otitis media, presumably because of the transfer of maternal immunoglobulins from the breast milk to the child.

PATHOPHYSIOLOGY

The ear can be divided anatomically into three sections: the outer (or external), middle, and inner (or internal) ear (Fig. 14.1).

The middle ear consists of the tympanic membrane (eardrum) and an air-filled tympanic cavity that houses three tiny bones known collectively as *ossicles* (Fig. 14.1). The middle ear is a relatively closed system, with a pressure approximately equal to atmospheric pressure. This pressure equivalency is maintained by the eustachian tube, which connects the tympanic cavity with the nasopharynx.

TABLE 14.1	Risk Factors for the Development of Otitis Media

First episode <18 months of age

Male sex

Positive family history of otitis media

Sibling history of recurrent otitis media

Exposure to secondhand smoke

Bottle-feeding

Use of a pacifier

Child care outside the home

Preceding upper respiratory infection

PATHOGENESIS

The pathogenesis of otitis media is not completely understood but is thought to be the result of two primary factors: eustachian tube dysfunction[10,12,13] and introduction of infectious material (viruses or bacteria) into the middle ear.

The eustachian tube equalizes the pressure between the tympanic cavity and the atmosphere. Cilia located in the eustachian tube continuously sweep mucus and debris toward the nasopharynx and away from the middle ear. Obstruction of the eustachian tube may result from mucous membrane edema (secondary to allergy or an upper respiratory tract infection) or from blockage by a foreign body, tumor, or lymphatic tissue (e.g., adenoid). In addition, developmental differences between children and adults with respect to anatomic positioning, length, and functional patency of the eustachian tube may predispose children, but not adults, to eustachian tube dysfunction.[11]

Once an obstruction occurs, a negative pressure (relative to the atmosphere) develops in the tympanic cavity. This pressure gradient is caused by the absorption of gases through the epithelial lining of the eustachian tube and tympanic cavity. In addition, normal drainage of the tympanic cavity is impeded. If the obstruction is suddenly relieved, nasopharyngeal mucus and viruses or bacteria may be insufflated (i.e., injected directly) into the tympanic cavity. Alternatively, a strong positive pressure originating in the nasopharynx (e.g., nose blowing) may force nasopharyngeal contents into the middle ear.

The role of viruses in the pathogenesis of otitis media is being increasingly recognized.[14] Viruses were identified in 6% to 42% of patients with otitis media,[15–17] with respiratory syncytial virus being the most commonly detected.[16,17] Whether viruses are directly involved in the development of otitis media is unclear, but they may predispose the patient to develop a secondary bacterial infection.

Other causative factors for otitis media include trauma, immunoglobulin deficiencies (particularly immunoglobulin [Ig]G-class antibodies against bacterial capsular polysaccharides),[18] human immunodeficiency virus (HIV) infection,[19] and, possibly, a genetic predisposition.[20]

MICROBIOLOGY

Although viruses appear to play a concomitant role in the development of otitis media, the major causative pathogens are bacteria. In acute otitis media, the bacteria most com-

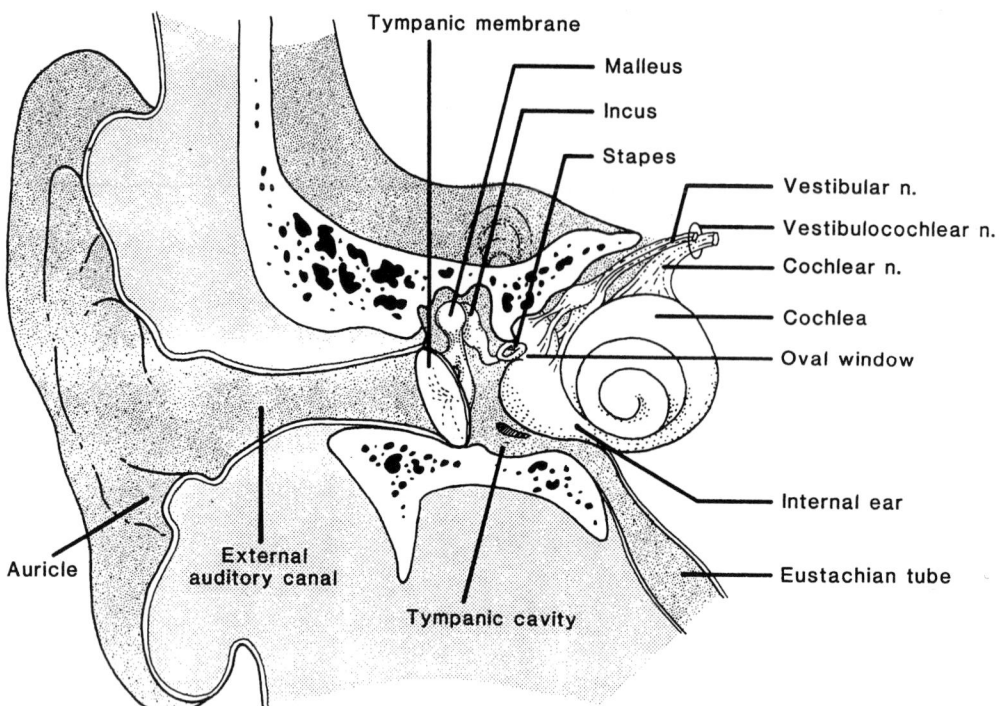

FIGURE 14.1 Anatomy of the ear.

monly isolated from the middle ear fluid are *Streptococcus pneumoniae, Haemophilus influenzae,* and *Moraxella catarrhalis.*[21] These organisms commonly colonize the nasopharynx of young children (<2 years) and are less frequently found in older children (<11 years).[22] In infants younger than 6 weeks of age, *Escherichia coli* and group B streptococci are common pathogens. Other less common organisms include staphylococci (both coagulase positive and negative), *Streptococcus pyogenes,* group A streptococci, other Gram-negative rods, *Chlamydia trachomatis,* and anaerobes. In chronic suppurative otitis media, the predominant organisms are *Staphylococcus aureus, Pseudomonas aeruginosa,* and *Klebsiella pneumoniae.*[23]

Up to 50% of *H. influenzae* and 100% of *M. catarrhalis* strains produce β-lactamases.[21] Resistant strains of *S. pneumoniae* (an organism that was once exquisitely sensitive to penicillins) are now appearing with increasing frequency in the United States.[24–26]

CLINICAL PRESENTATION AND DIAGNOSIS

SIGNS AND SYMPTOMS

The classical presentation of acute suppurative otitis media is that of an acute (within hours) onset of unilateral otalgia (ear pain), fever, and nasal discharge. Symptoms of otitis media displayed by neonates and small children include excessive fussiness, irritability, and tugging at the affected ear. Older children may complain of a sore throat or a sense of

''fullness'' or ''pressure'' in the ear. These symptoms may be associated with decreased hearing acuity. Less frequent symptoms include dizziness, lethargy, headache, anorexia (or reduced feeding in neonates), nausea, vomiting, diarrhea, and otorrhea (drainage from the ear). It is important to note that all these signs and symptoms are relatively nonspecific (i.e., many patients presenting with these signs or symptoms do not have otitis media),[27,28] and symptoms alone should not be used as the basis for establishing a diagnosis.[4]

DIAGNOSIS

To diagnose AOM, the clinician must establish the presence of an MEE, in addition to signs and symptoms of middle ear inflammation.[4] Otoscopic examination of the ear may reveal an erythematous tympanic membrane that is opaque or dull in appearance. The membrane is frequently bulging and, infrequently, it may become perforated and drain pus. The appearance of the tympanic membrane is highly variable, however, and otitis media is frequently overdiagnosed.[27,29] Evaluation of the compliance of the tympanic membrane is performed with either pneumatic otoscopy or tympanometry. The eardrum may exhibit reduced compliance, but its diagnostic usefulness is limited in that up to 25% of healthy children will have asymptomatic middle ear effusions.[30] Thus, the combination of patient symptoms, clinical signs, and information obtained through evaluation of the eardrum all must be used in making the diagnosis.

Otitis media is a usually a clinical diagnosis. However, isolation of the causative organism may be accomplished by aspirating fluid from the middle ear (tympanocentesis). This procedure is invasive and is performed only when the specific causative organism must be identified. Unfortunately, cultures may be negative in one third of patients with acute otitis media and in two thirds of those with recurrent or secretory otitis media.[31,32] Although colonization of the nasopharynx by the responsible bacteria appears to be a prerequisite for infection of the middle ear,[33] cultures of the nasopharynx are a poor predictor of the causative organism in AOM.[34]

PSYCHOSOCIAL ASPECTS

Although otitis media is obviously uncomfortable for the child, this condition takes its toll on parents and caregivers as well. The fussiness, inconsolability, and lack of appetite that many children experience during an episode of acute otitis media cause many parents to flee to the physician for ''something'' to alleviate the condition. Frequently, the result is the potentially inappropriate prescribing of antibiotics. Although antibiotic therapy has been shown to have only a modest effect on the overall course of the disease,[2] it may shorten the duration of symptoms.[35]

TREATMENT

PHARMACOTHERAPY

The treatment of otitis media with drug therapy can be divided into three categories: supportive therapy with analgesics and antipyretics; systemic antimicrobial therapy; and adjunctive therapy.

Analgesic and Antipyretic Therapy. Two of the most prominent symptoms of acute otitis media are pain and fever, both of which should be assessed and treated.[4] These symptoms can be effectively treated with acetaminophen (10 to 15 mg/kg q4–6h; maximum 60 mg/kg/day) or ibuprofen (5 to 10 mg/kg q6h; maximum 40 mg/kg/day). Aspirin should be avoided because of the potential risk of life-threatening Reye's syndrome.

A prescription-only otic solution containing antipyrine (an analgesic) and benzocaine (an anesthetic) has been shown to be effective in reducing ear pain associated with otitis media.[36]

Systemic Antimicrobial Therapy. Perhaps the most controversial aspect of the pharmacotherapy of acute otitis media is the use of systemic antimicrobial therapy. Despite the consensus that acute otitis media is primarily of bacterial origin, disagreement continues regarding three issues: whether or not this condition should be treated with oral antibiotics; the optimal duration of antibiotic therapy; and the end point by which antibiotic efficacy should be assessed.

In most patients, the symptoms of acute otitis media resolve spontaneously without treatment within 24 to 72 hours, with resolution of the effusion within 2 weeks. Moreover, meta-analyses[3,35,37] of clinical trials of antibiotic therapy in acute otitis media indicate that antibiotics produce only modest short-term improvement in the overall course of the disease. Thus, it has been suggested that antibiotic therapy should be reserved for those whose condition does not improve within 48 to 72 hours.[38] Unfortunately, it is impossible for clinicians to identify *a priori* patients whose otitis media will not resolve spontaneously, and antimicrobial therapy continues to be recommended in certain populations[4] to reduce the risk of suppurative complications, even though these complications are rare.

Because, in most cases, the causative organism is not isolated before treatment is initiated (and, in most cases, it is never identified), the choice of antibiotic is based on its efficacy against the most common pathogens reported in published studies in which microbiologic specimens were obtained. Table 14.2 lists antibiotics that are commonly used to treat otitis media.

Selection of an antibiotic to treat otitis media should take into account the drug's pharmacokinetic and pharmacodynamic profile with respect to efficacy and toxicity, as well as other factors (e.g., palatability, route of administration, cost). Ideally, an antibiotic that is used to treat otitis media should have several characteristics. It should (a) have excellent oral bioavailability; (b) readily distribute into the middle ear fluid in high concentrations for antibiotics that exhibit concentration-dependent killing or achieve concentrations that exceed the pathogen's minimum inhibitory concentration (MIC) for a significant portion (40% to 50%) of the dosing interval for antibiotics that exhibit time-dependent killing; (c) be bactericidal at low MICs; (d) have a long elimination half-life; (e) be devoid of drug-drug or drug-food interactions that are more common in children; and (f) have little or no toxicity at therapeutic doses.[39,40] Fortunately, all the antibiotics that are commonly used to treat otitis media reasonably satisfy these criteria.

Figure 14.2 presents an algorithm for treating acute otitis media. For most patients, high-dose (80 mg/kg/day) oral amoxicillin is an appropriate first choice. It is effective against the most likely causative organisms, relatively free of serious adverse effects (rash and diarrhea are the most common), and inexpensive. If a patient is allergic to penicillins, either trimethoprim/sulfamethoxazole or erythromycin/sulfisoxazole is an effective alternative. Both of these contain a sulfonamide, but the incidence of adverse effects is low (<5%) and hematologic toxicity is rare at the dose required to treat otitis media.

Because both *H. influenzae* and *M. catarrhalis* are capable of producing β-lactamases, an antibiotic that is stable against these enzymes should be considered if therapy with amoxicillin appears to be ineffective, or if the prevalence of these organisms in a particular geographic area is high. Amoxicillin combined with potassium clavulanate (a β-lactamase inhibitor), second- or third-generation cephalosporins, trimethoprim-sulfamethoxazole, clarithromycin, azithromycin, or erythromycin-sulfisoxazole is equally effective.[41] The initial empiric use of broad-spectrum, β-lactamase–stable antibiotics is unwarranted because they do not

TABLE 14.2	Antibiotics Used in the Treatment of Otitis Media	
Antibiotic	**Pediatric (<12 y) Dose**	**Comments**
Amoxicillin	40–45 mg/kg/day in 2–3 divided doses	80–90 mg/kg/day in high-risk patients, with penicillin-resistant pneumococci
Amoxicillin/potassium clavulanate	40 mg/kg/day in 3 divided doses, or 45 mg/kg/day in 2 divided doses, for 10 days	Dose based on amoxicillin content
Azithromycin	5 mg/kg/day	Day 1: 10 mg/kg ("loading dose")
Cefaclor	40 mg/kg/day in 3 divided doses	
Cefdinir	14 mg/kg/day in 1–2 divided doses for 5–10 days	
Cefpodoxime proxetil	10 mg/kg/day in 1–2 divided doses	
Cefprozil	30 mg/kg/day in 2 divided doses	
Ceftibuten	9 mg/kg/day	
Ceftriaxone	50 mg/kg	Administered intramuscularly; single dose
Cephalexin	75–100 mg/kg/day in 4 divided doses	
Cephradine	25–100 mg/kg/day in 2–4 divided doses	
Ciprofloxacin/ dexamethasone	4 drops instilled into the affected ear bid for 7 days	Otic solution
Clarithromycin	15 mg/kg/day in 2 divided doses	
Erythromycin/ sulfisoxazole	50 mg/kg/day in 3–4 divided doses	Dose based on erythromycin content
Loracarbef	30 mg/kg/day in 2 divided doses	
Ofloxacin	5 drops instilled into affected ear bid for 10 days	0.3% otic solution
Trimethoprim-sulfamethoxazole (TMP/SMX)	8 mg/kg/day in 2 divided doses	Dose based on trimethoprim content

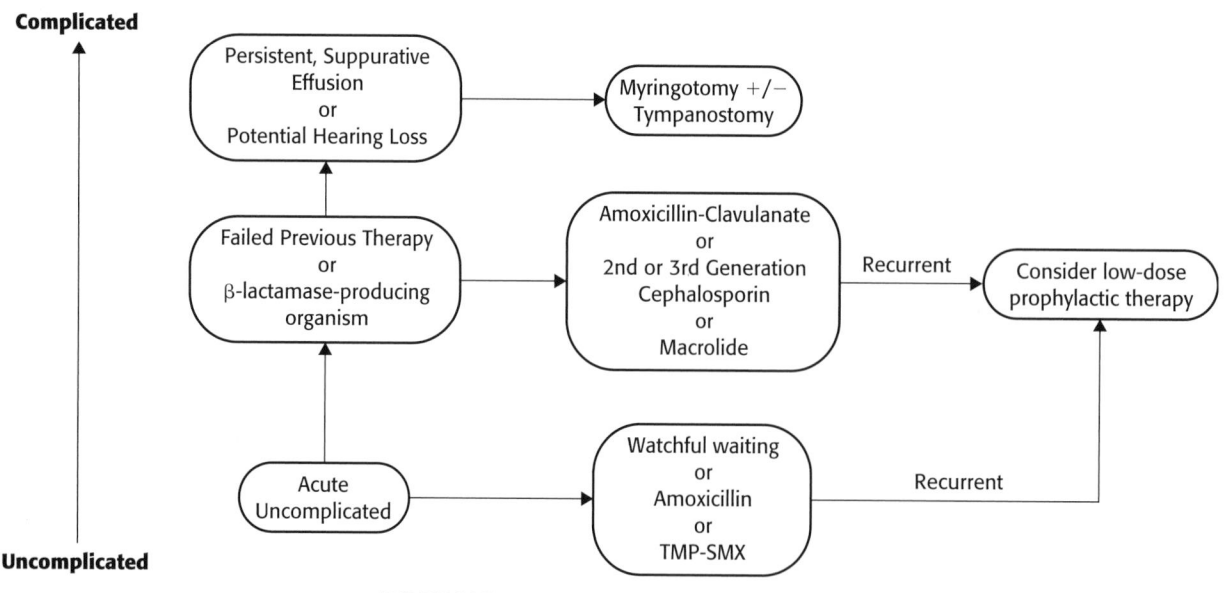

FIGURE 14.2 Algorithm for treating otitis media.

improve efficacy rates or reduce the incidence of suppurative complications. Furthermore, the newer agents are considerably more expensive than amoxicillin or trimethoprim-sulfamethoxazole, and their broad spectrum may contribute to the development of resistant strains of bacteria.

The traditional length of antibiotic therapy in acute otitis media has been 10 days. However, shorter courses of therapy (i.e., 5 days) have been shown to be equally effective.[42] In addition, a single intramuscular dose of ceftriaxone is as effective as 10 days of treatment with oral amoxicillin,[43] amoxicillin-clavulanate,[44] or trimethoprim-sulfamethoxazole[45] in uncomplicated acute otitis media in children. Similarly, a single oral dose of azithromycin is as effective as a 10-day course of amoxicillin/clavulanate or a single IM dose of ceftriaxone.[46] Although IM administration of ceftriaxone has drawbacks (e.g., it is painful, more expensive, may unnecessarily expose the patient to broad-spectrum therapy), it may be the appropriate treatment when a child is unable (or unwilling) to take oral medication, or when noncompliance is a documented problem. Moreover, parents prefer single-dose therapy because of its simplicity.[47] Longer-term therapy (i.e., 10 days) may still be appropriate for children younger than 2 years of age.[48]

If the patient's clinical response is unsatisfactory, an additional course of therapy with another antibiotic may be tried. This is unnecessary in most patients. Middle ear effusion will persist for several days to several months in a small number of patients, although in most children, the condition does not progress to chronic or recurrent otitis media.

Adjunctive Therapy. In addition to analgesics, antipyretics, and antibiotics, a number of other pharmacologic interventions have been tried. Decongestants, antihistamines, corticosteroids, mucolytics, and surfactants have been used to treat patients with otitis media. None of these agents has been shown to improve the outcome of otitis media. Influenza vaccine has been shown to be moderately effective in preventing episodes, and the conjugated pneumococcal vaccine has proved minimally effective. Intranasal beclomethasone may be a useful adjunct in the treatment of chronic otitis media when an allergic component is present.[49] Monthly administration of immune globulin to children with HIV infection was associated with a significant reduction in the frequency of bacterial infections, including otitis media.[50]

NONPHARMACOLOGIC THERAPY

In some children with complicated otitis media, it may be necessary to perform a bilateral myringotomy to place tympanostomy tubes. This allows the effusion to drain and the middle ear to be ventilated. This procedure is invasive (requiring general anesthesia) and is associated with a number of complications (e.g., otorrhea, granuloma formation, cholesteatoma, tube obstruction).[51] Despite these drawbacks, myringotomy with tympanostomy tube placement should be considered in children with recurrent otitis media or otitis media with effu-

sion lasting longer than 4 months, and in children with evidence of hearing loss or language delay.[2]

IMPROVING OUTCOMES

Although otitis media is a relatively benign process in most patients, a number of educational interventions can prevent future episodes, modify the course of an existing episode, and prevent complications from occurring.

PATIENT EDUCATION

Table 14.1 lists risk factors for otitis media, some of which can be modified by the parent or caregiver. Avoiding passive cigarette smoke, keeping the child out of day care centers, and limiting the child's exposure to others with upper respiratory infections may reduce the child's risk of developing otitis media. Minimizing these risk factors is particularly important for children who are prone to development of otitis media.

Parents should be made aware of the fact that antibiotic therapy has only a small impact on the overall course of acute otitis media, and their expectation of receiving a prescription for an antibiotic should be modified accordingly. When antibiotic therapy is prescribed, the importance of complying with treatment and recognizing potential treatment failure must be emphasized. Also, parents should be aware that adjunctive therapies commonly used in upper respiratory infections (e.g., antihistamines, decongestants, corticosteroids) are ineffective in otitis media but may nonetheless cause adverse effects.[52,53]

METHODS TO IMPROVE PATIENT ADHERENCE TO DRUG THERAPY

In general, the antibiotics listed in Table 14.2 are equally safe and effective for treating otitis media. With regard to compliance, three factors may distinguish these drugs from one another: cost, simplicity, and palatability.

With regard to cost, amoxicillin and trimethoprim-sulfamethoxazole are the least expensive antibiotics. Newer, more expensive antibiotics are not necessarily more effective or less toxic.

With regard to simplicity, the fewer the number of doses of a medication that must be given, the more likely it is that the regimen will be adhered to. Amoxicillin, although inexpensive, is frequently prescribed to be given three times daily. This may be problematic if the child is going to a day care facility, where someone other than the parent must be responsible for administering the midday dose. In this case, trimethoprim-sulfamethoxazole or another drug that can be administered in one to two daily doses (e.g., azithromycin) may be more appropriate.

Finally, the palatability of the antibiotic contributes to compliance as well. The use of oral syringes to deliver medication to the back of the mouth may be helpful in administering bad-tasting antibiotic suspensions.

PHARMACOECONOMICS

Although otitis media is responsible for an estimated $3.5 billion in health care costs annually, only a small percentage of this is attributable to pharmacotherapy.[54] Nonetheless, the fact that only a small, short-term improvement is seen with antimicrobial therapy calls into question the cost benefit of its use. Perhaps more important is the fact that the potential

development of bacterial resistance to antibiotics may, in the long run, prove to be far more costly from a public health standpoint. In addition, the financial impact of noncompliance and the adverse effects of drug therapy must be considered.[55] Pharmacists and other health care professionals must be cognizant of these issues when evaluating and selecting antibiotic therapy for the treatment of patients with otitis media.

OTITIS EXTERNA

DEFINITION

Otitis externa is an infectious condition of the external ear canal. Although it may be associated with chronic otitis media, it is more frequently an independent condition that

affects patients of all ages. One particularly severe form of this condition, malignant otitis externa, is characterized by extensive bacterial (predominantly *P. aeruginosa*) invasion into the surrounding bone, soft tissue, and nerve structures and is potentially life threatening.[56]

TREATMENT GOALS: OTITIS EXTERNA

- Facilitate an environment in the external ear canal that promotes healing of the inflamed, infected tissue.
- Dry the ear canal and treat the infection.

PATHOPHYSIOLOGY

The external ear consists of two structures: the auricle and the external auditory canal (Fig. 14.1). The purpose of these structures is to collect and transmit sound waves to the middle ear.

Two conditions produce an environment that is favorable for the development of otitis externa: the introduction of a sharp object (e.g., toothpick or hairpin) into the external auditory canal, which disrupts the integrity of the lining of the canal and permits the growth of bacteria or fungi; and the introduction and accumulation of moisture in the canal. Moisture not only softens the lining of the canal but also provides a medium for the growth of bacteria or fungi. Otitis externa commonly occurs when the ear is frequently exposed to water (e.g., swimming); for this reason, it is sometimes referred to as ''swimmer's ear.''

The two most common organisms that are isolated in otitis externa are *P. aeruginosa* and *S. aureus*.[57] Fungi, primarily *Aspergillus sp.* and *Candida sp.*, are found in about 10% of cases.

CLINICAL PRESENTATION AND DIAGNOSIS

SIGNS AND SYMPTOMS

Otitis externa is characterized by pain, swelling, maceration, and breakdown of the skin and subcutaneous tissues of the

external ear canal. Normally, the infection is limited to the external ear. However, it may spread to the surrounding soft tissue or bone.

DIAGNOSIS

The diagnosis of otitis externa is based on the clinical presentation of the patient. Additionally, culture and sensitivity data from the affected ear confirm the diagnosis and assist the clinician in the selection of antimicrobial therapy.[57] With malignant otitis externa, a number of diagnostic criteria have been proposed[56]; diagnostic imaging (e.g., computed tomography, magnetic resonance imaging) may be required for confirmation of the diagnosis.

TREATMENT

The goal of treatment of otitis externa is to produce an environment in the external ear canal that promotes healing of inflamed, infected tissue. This involves drying the ear canal and treating the infection. Table 14.3 lists those drugs commonly found in otic preparations used to treat otitis externa.

ANTIBIOTICS

Although antibiotics are found in many otic preparations, they may cause contact dermatitis, permit the overgrowth of

Drug Product	Antibiotic	Antibacterial/Antifungal	Corticosteroid	Analgesic	Local Anesthetic
TABLE 14.3	**Selected Topical Preparations for the Treatment of Otitis Externa**				
Auralgan Otic				Antipyrine	Benzocaine
Coly-Mycin S Otic	Neomycin SO$_4$, Colistin SO$_4$		Hydrocortisone		
Ciprodex	Ciprofloxacin		Dexamethasone		
Cortisporin Otic	Neomycin SO$_4$, Polymyxin B SO$_4$		Hydrocortisone		
Floxin Otic	Ofloxacin				
Otic Tridesilon		Acetic acid	Desonide		
Tympagesic[a]				Antipyrine	Benzocaine
Vosol HC Otic		Acetic acid	Hydrocortisone		Benzocaine

[a] Also contains phenylephrine.

resistant organisms (including fungi and viruses), and result in local (e.g., neomycin) or systemic (e.g., chloramphenicol) toxicities; therefore, they are generally not recommended. Ofloxacin is available as an otic solution and is as effective as bacitracin + polymyxin-B + hydrocortisone.[58] It remains to be seen whether this agent exhibits the same potential problems as have been noted with the older topical antibiotics. Otic preparations should be used with caution in patients with a perforated tympanic membrane. Oral antibiotics are indicated only when the infection has spread to surrounding soft tissue. For malignant otitis externa, a prolonged course of therapy with an antipseudomonal antibiotic, administered intravenously, is usually necessary.[56]

OTHER AGENTS
Corticosteroids possess anti-inflammatory, antipruritic, and vasoconstrictive activity and, when applied topically, may be useful in reducing swelling and inflammation in the external ear canal. Dexamethasone, in combination with acetic acid or an antibiotic, has been found to be more effective in treating otitis externa than either of these agents alone. A few drops of isopropyl alcohol 70% can serve as an excellent drying agent, but it should be used sparingly to prevent excessive drying and subsequent pruritus. Acetic acid may be combined in a 1:1 mixture with isopropyl alcohol to decrease the pH of the solution.

IMPROVING OUTCOMES

For topical therapy to be effective, the otic solution must be properly delivered to the site of infection. Proper technique is particularly important if the patient is going to self-administer the solution. This, along with proper attention to aural hygiene, will bring about resolution of the condition in most patients in 5 to 7 days.

In the treatment of otitis externa, 3 to 4 drops of the desired solution should be instilled into the ear canal four times daily. To prevent the solution from escaping from the ear canal, the otic drops may be placed on a cotton or gauze wick, which is then inserted into the ear canal and left in place. In addition to keeping the solution in contact with affected tissues, the wick prevents occlusion of the ear canal caused by swelling.

In a small number of patients, the condition becomes chronic and is characterized by dry, scaly, sometimes weeping skin that covers the auricle and external ear canal. Again, meticulous aural hygiene, combined with the application of a topical steroid cream (e.g., hydrocortisone) three to four times daily, will alleviate the patient's symptoms.

KEY POINTS

- Otitis media is a very common, yet relatively benign, condition of infancy and early childhood.
- Treatment is aimed at preventing acute (e.g., mastoiditis) or chronic complications (e.g., impaired language development secondary to hearing loss) resulting from chronic or recurrent infections.
- Because of the self-limited nature of the disease and its potential for inducing bacterial resistance, antimicrobial therapy should be reserved for acute episodes in children younger than 2 years of age, or in children with chronic or recurrent infections.
- Adjunctive therapies, such as antihistamines and decongestants, are of little value in the management of otitis media, but they are nonetheless capable of causing adverse effects.
- Education of the parent or caregiver and judicious selection and use of antimicrobial therapy will improve the outcome of otitis media.

- Otitis externa is an infection of the external auditory canal that affects both children and adults.
- Treatment of otitis externa involves meticulous aural hygiene, in addition to topical pharmacotherapy.
- Patient education on the administration of otic preparations is essential, especially if the patient is going to self-administer the medication.
- Malignant otitis externa is severe and potentially life threatening, and it requires aggressive, prolonged therapy with intravenous antibiotics.

REFERENCES

1. Klein JO, Tos M, Hussl B, et al. Recent advances in otitis media: definition and classification. Ann Otol Rhinol Laryngol 139(Suppl): 10, 1989.
2. American Academy of Pediatrics. Clinical practice guideline: otitis media with effusion. Pediatrics 113:1412–1429, 2004.
3. Rosenfeld RM, Vertrees JE, Carr J, et al. Clinical efficacy of antimicrobial drugs for acute otitis media: meta-analysis of 5400 children from thirty-three randomized trials. J Pediatr 124:355–356, 1994.
4. American Academy of Pediatrics and American Academy of Family Physicians Subcommittee on Management of Acute Otitis Media. Clinical practice guideline: diagnosis and management of acute otitis media. Pediatrics 113:1451–1465, 2004.
5. Teele DW, Klein JO, Rosner B, et al. Epidemiology of otitis media during the first seven years of life in children in greater Boston: a prospective cohort study. J Infect Dis 160:83–94, 1989.
6. Schappert SM. Office visits for otitis media: United States 1975–1990. Hyattsville, MD: US Public Health Service, 1992. DHHS publication PHS 92–1250.
7. Paradise JL, Rockette HE, Colborn DK. Otitis media in 2253 Pittsburgh-area infants: prevalence and risk factors during the first two years of life. Pediatrics 99:318–333, 1997.
8. Kaplan B, Wandstrat TL, Cunningham JR. Overall cost in the treatment of otitis media. Pediatr Infect Dis J 16 (Suppl):S9–S11, 1997.
9. Uhari M, Mantysaari K, Niemela M. A meta-analytic review of the risk factors for acute otitis media. Clin Infect Dis 22:1079–1083, 1996.
10. Fireman P. Otitis media and eustachian tube dysfunction: connection to allergic rhinitis. J Allergy Clin Immunol 99:S787–S797, 1997.
11. American Academy of Pediatrics Committee on Environmental Health. Environmental tobacco smoke: a hazard to children. Pediatrics 99:639–642, 1997.
12. Bluestone CD, Ostfeld EJ, Bakaletz LO, et al. Eustachian tube and middle ear physiology and pathophysiology. In: Recent advances in otitis media: report of the fifth research conference. Ann Otol Rhinol Laryngol 103 (Suppl 164):13–19, 1994.
13. Tücetürk AV, Ünlü HH, Okumuss M., et al. The evaluation of eustachian tube function in patients with chronic otitis media. Clin Otolaryngol 22:449–452, 1997.
14. Buchman CA, Brinson GM. Viral otitis media. Curr Allergy Asthma Rep 3:335–340, 2003.
15. Ruuskanen O, Arola M, Heikkinen T, et al. Viruses in acute otitis media: increasing evidence for clinical significance. Pediatr Infect Dis J 10:425–427, 1991.
16. Arola M, Ruuskanen O, Ziegler T, et al. Clinical role of respiratory virus infection in acute otitis media. Pediatrics 86:848–855, 1990.
17. Heikkenin H, Thint M, Chonmaitree T. Prevalence of various respiratory viruses in the middle ear during acute otitis media. N Engl J Med 340:260–264, 1999.
18. Yamakana N, Hotomi M, Shimada J, et al. Immunological deficiency in "otitis-prone" children. Ann NY Acad Sci 830:70–81, 1997.
19. Chen AY, Ohlms LA, Stewart MG, et al. Otolaryngologic disease progression in children with human immunodeficiency virus infection. Arch Otolaryngol Head Neck Surg 122:1360–1363, 1996.
20. Klein JO, Tos M, Casselbrant ML. Epidemiology and natural history. In: Recent advances in otitis media: report of the fifth research conference. Ann Otol Rhinol Laryngol 103 (Suppl 164):9–12, 1994.
21. Doern GV, Jones RN, Pfaller MA, et al. Haemophilus influenzae and Moraxella catarrhalis from patients with community-acquired respiratory tract infections: antimicrobial susceptibility patterns from the SENTRY Antimicrobial Surveillance Program (United States and Canada, 1997). Antimicrob Agents Chemother 43:385–389, 1999.
22. Stenfors LE, Räisänen S. Occurrence of middle ear pathogens in the nasopharynx of young individuals: a quantitative study in four age groups. Acta Otolaryngol 109:142–148, 1990.
23. Wintermeyer SM, Nahata MC. Chronic suppurative otitis media. Ann Pharmacother 28:1089–1099, 1994.
24. Roger G, Carles P, Thien HV, et al. Management of acute otitis media caused by resistant pneumococci in infants. Pediatr Infect Dis J 17:631–638, 1998.
25. Klein JO. Clinical implications of antibiotic resistance for management of acute otitis media. Pediatr Infect Dis J 17:1084–1089, 1998.
26. Dowell SF, Butler JC, Giebink GS, et al. Acute otitis media: management and surveillance in an era of pneumococcal resistance—a report from the drug resistant Streptococcus pneumoniae therapeutic working group. Pediatr Infect Dis J 18:1–9, 1999.
27. Weiss JC, Yates GR, Quinn LD. Acute otitis media: making an accurate diagnosis. Am Fam Physician 53:1200–1206, 1996.
28. Niemala M, Ukari M, Jounio-Ervasti K, et al. Lack of specific symptomatology in children with acute otitis media. Pediatr Infect Dis J 13:765–768, 1994.
29. Hendly JO. Otitis media. N Engl J Med 347:1169–1174, 2004.
30. Klein JO. Persistent middle ear effusions: natural history and morbidity. Pediatr Infect Dis J 1:S1–S11, 1982.
31. Qvarnberg Y, Kantola O, Valtonen H, et al. Bacterial findings in middle ear effusion in children. Otolaryngol Head Neck Surg 102:118–121, 1990.
32. Karma P. Secretory otitis media: infectious background and its implications for treatment. Acta Otolaryngol 449 (Suppl):47–48, 1988.
33. Ogra PL, Barenkamp SJ, Mogi G, et al. Microbiology, immunology, biochemistry, vaccination. In: Recent advances in otitis media: report of the fifth research conference. Ann Otol Rhinol Laryngol 103 (Suppl 164):27–43, 1994.
34. Groothuis JR, Thompson J, Wright PF. Correlation of nasopharyngeal and conjunctival cultures with middle ear fluid cultures in otitis media. Clin Pediatr 25:85–88, 1986.
35. Del Mar C, Glasziou P, Hayem M. Are antibiotics indicated as initial treatment for children with acute otitis media? A meta-analysis. Br Med J 314:1526–1529, 1997.
36. Hoberman A, Paradise JL, Reynolds EA, et al. Efficacy of Auralgan for treating ear pain in children with acute otitis media. Arch Pediatr Adolesc Med 151:675–678, 1997.
37. Williams RL, Chalmers TC, Stange KC, et al. Use of antibiotics in preventing recurrent otitis media and in treating otitis media with effusion: a meta-analytic attempt to resolve the brouhaha. JAMA 270:1344–1351, 1993.
38. Culpepper L, Froom J. Routine antimicrobial treatment of acute otitis media: is it necessary? JAMA 278:1643–1645, 1997.
39. Blumer JL. Implications of pharmacokinetics in making choices for the management of acute otitis media. Pediatr Infect Dis J 17:565–570, 1998.
40. Craig WA. Choosing an antibiotic on the basis of pharmacodynamics. Ear Nose Throat J 77 (6 Suppl):7–11, 1998.
41. Marcy M, Takata G, Shekelle P, et al. Management of acute otitis media. Evidence report/technology assessment no. 15. Rockville, MD: Agency for Healthcare Research and Quality, May 2001. AHRQ publication no. 01-E010.
42. Kozyrsky AL, Hildes-Ripstein GE, Longstaffe SE, et al. Treatment of acute otitis media with a shortened course of antibiotics: a meta-analysis. JAMA 279:1736–1742, 1998.
43. Green SM, Rothrock SG. Single-dose intramuscular ceftriaxone for acute otitis media in children. Pediatrics 91:23–30, 1993.
44. Varsano I, Volovitz B, Horev Z, et al. Intramuscular ceftriaxone compared with oral amoxicillin-clavulanate for the treatment of acute otitis media in children. Eur J Pediatr 156:858–863, 1997.
45. Barnett ED, Teele DW, Klein JO, et al. Comparison of ceftriaxone and trimethoprim-sulfamethoxazole for acute otitis media. Pediatrics 99:23–28, 1997.

46. Arguedas A, Loaiza C, Soley C. Single dose azithromycin for the treatment of uncomplicated otitis. Pediatr Infect Dis J 23 (Suppl): S108–S114, 2004.
47. Bauchner H, Adams W, Barnett E, et al. Therapy for acute otitis media: preference of parents for oral or parenteral antibiotic. Arch Pediatr Adolesc Med 150:396–399, 1996.
48. Paradise JL. Short-course antimicrobial treatment for acute otitis media: not best for infants and young children. JAMA 278: 1640–1642, 1997.
49. Tracy JM, Demain JG, Hoffman KM, et al. Intranasal beclomethasone as an adjunct to treatment of chronic middle ear effusion. Ann Allergy Asthma Immunol 80:198–206, 1998.
50. Olopoenia L, Young M., White D, et al. Intravenous immunoglobulin in symptomatic and asymptomatic children with perinatal HIV infection. J Natl Med Assoc 89:543–547, 1997.
51. Pizzuto MP, Volk MS, Kingston LM. Common topics in pediatric otolaryngology. Pediatr Clin North Am 45:973–991, 1998.
52. Mandel EM, Rockette HE, Bluestone CD, et al. Efficacy of amoxicillin with and without decongestant-antihistamine for otitis media in children. N Engl J Med 316:432–437, 1987.

53. Chonmaitree T, Saeed K, Uchida T, et al. A randomized, placebo-controlled trial of the effect of antihistamine or corticosteroid treatment in acute otitis media. J Pediatr 143:377–385, 2003.
54. Mainous AG, Hueston WJ. The cost of antibiotics in treating upper respiratory tract infections in a Medicaid population. Arch Fam Med 7:45–49, 1998.
55. Wandstrat TL, Kaplan B. Pharmacoeconomic impact of factors affecting compliance with antibiotic regimens in the treatment of acute otitis media. Pediatr Infect Dis J 16:S27–S29, 1997.
56. Amorosa L, Modugno GC, Pirodda A. Malignant external otitis: review and personal experience. Acta Otolaryngol 521(Suppl):3–16, 1996.
57. Bojrab DI, Bruderly T, Abdulrazzak Y. Otitis externa. Otolaryngol Clin North Am 29:761–782, 1996.
58. Jones RN, Milazzo J, Seidlin M. Ofloxacin otic solution for treatment of otitis externa in children and adults. Arch Otolaryngol Head Neck Surg 123:1193–1200, 1997.
59. van Balen FA, Smit WM, Zuithoff NP, et al. Clinical efficacy of three common treatments in acute otitis externa in primary care: randomised controlled trial. Br Med J 327:1201–1203, 2003.

CASE STUDIES

CASE 4

TOPIC: Glaucoma

THERAPEUTIC DIFFICULTY: Level 1
John Douglas Wurtzbacher

CHAPTER 13: Glaucoma

■ Scenario

Patient and Setting: ML, an 81-year-old female; community pharmacy

Chief Complaint: Excessive drowsiness and dizziness; fell at home this morning

■ History of Present Illness

ML presents to the pharmacy with prescriptions from her family physician after falling at home at approximately 8 AM this morning. She states, "I felt sleepy and dizzy, and then just went down." No loss of consciousness reported. Medications taken at approximately 6 AM include: tramadol 50 mg; acetaminophen 2 × 500 mg; conjugated estrogens 0.625 mg, and timolol eyedrops

Medical History: Remarkable only for open-angle glaucoma diagnosed 10 years ago; osteoarthritis × 12 years; and weight gain of 15 pounds over the past 2 years

Surgical History: Knee replacement: L knee, 2.5 years ago

Family History: Mother died at age 93 unknown cause; father Holocaust survivor, died age 89 unknown cause

Social History: No prior to bacco use; one glass of wine with dinner 3–4 times per week; unmarried and lives in assisted living facility; has skilled nursing provide weekly medication management via "pill boxes" filled with weekly medications separated into appropriate time of day dosing

Medications:
Acetaminophen, 500 mg; 2 PO Q 6 hours
Timolol maleate XL, 1–2 drops in both eyes at
  bedtime × 10 years
Tramadol, 50 mg PO q 4–6 hours PRN started 3
  weeks prior to visit

Conjugated estrogens, 0.625 mg PO QD 8 AM ×
  15–20 years
Presents to pharmacy with the following new prescriptions:
Ibuprofen, 400 mg PO TID × 10 days
Latanoprost, 1 drop in both eyes at bedtime

Allergies: Penicillins

■ Physical Examination

GEN: Well-developed, well-nourished woman, slightly distressed
VS: BP 130/70 (sitting) 125/65 (standing), HR 76, RR 20, T 37°C, Wt 54 kg, Ht 160 cm
HEENT: WNL; last IOP measurement noted from family physician as "good" 6 months ago
COR: WNL
CHEST: Clear to auscultation
ABD: WNL
GU: Deferred
RECT: Deferred
EXT: Surgical scar, L knee; contusions of obvious varying duration bilaterally on arms and legs; no visible open wounds; no noticeable swelling; noted mild tenderness bilateral lower legs
NEURO: Alert and oriented × 4
X-ray: Bilateral lower extremities normal; mild changes consistent with osteoarthritis present

■ Results of Pertinent Laboratory Tests, Serum Drug Concentrations, and Diagnostic Tests

Na 143 (143)	K 4.0 (4.0)	Cl 98 (98)
HCO$_3$ 26 (26)	BUN 6.4 (18)	CR 88 (1.0)
Hct 0.35 (35)	Hgb 120 (12)	Lkcs 6.0 × 10^9 (6.0 × 10^3)
MCV 80 (80)	Plts 156 × 10^9 (156 × 10^3)	Mg 1.2 (2.5)
AST 0.17 (10)	ALT 0.20 (12)	T Bili 3.4 (0.2)
Glu 6.1 (120)	Ca 2.2 (8.8)	PO4 0.92 (3.0)
Guaiac: negative		

■ Problem List

Identify principal problems from the scenario in priority order (see Answers in back of book for correct list of problems).

■ SOAP Note

To be completed by the student (see Answers in back of book for correct SOAP Note).

■ QUESTIONS

(See Answers in back of book for correct responses.)

1. The probable cause for ML's drowsiness and dizziness is: (EO-1)
   a. Atrial fibrillation
   b. Excessive intake of alcohol
   c. Secondary to timolol or tramadol
   d. New onset of depression

2. Which of the following signs and symptoms does ML report relative to her open-angle glaucoma? (EO-2)
   a. Pain in lower extremities
   b. Excessive tearing
   c. Extreme itching and redness of both eyes
   d. No signs or symptoms reported

3. List the common signs and symptoms of both open-angle and angle-closure glaucoma. (EO-2)

4. Which of the following might be related to ML's dizziness and drowsiness? (EO-3)
   a. Incorrect use of timolol eyedrops
   b. Excessive use of acetaminophen
   c. Weight gain of 15 pounds over 2 years
   d. Osteoarthritis

5. Which of the following findings might suggest systemic effects of timolol in ML? (EO-5)
   a. Na 143 (143)
   b. Guaiac: negative
   c. BP 130/70 (sitting), 125/65 (standing)
   d. T 37°C

6. Which of the following is considered the mechanism of both latanoprost and timolol in reducing the long-term consequences of untreated open-angle glaucoma? (EO-7)
   a. Decrease in serum sodium
   b. Decrease in intraocular pressure (IOP)
   c. Increase in serum potassium
   d. Increase in IOP

7. Describe how to properly administer eyedrops for treatment of glaucoma. (EO-14)

8. Which of the following methods might a community pharmacist best use to determine compliance with glaucoma therapy? (EO-16)
   a. Provide tonometry in the pharmacy to measure IOP
   b. Determine appropriateness of frequency of medication refills
   c. Question patient regarding use of OTC oxymetazoline for symptom relief
   d. Examine length of eyelashes in patients receiving latanoprost or other prostaglandin analogs

9. Which type of glaucoma is considered a medical emergency? (EO-8)
   a. Untreated open-angle glaucoma
   b. Congenital glaucoma
   c. Drug-induced glaucoma
   d. Untreated angle-closure glaucoma

10. Describe psychosocial factors that should be discussed when a patient presents to the pharmacy with therapy for newly diagnosed open-angle glaucoma. (EO-16)

11. Which of the following might result from untreated open-angle glaucoma? (EO-1)
    a. Darkening of the iris
    b. Reduction in effectiveness of ocular antibiotics
    c. Blindness due to changes of the optic nerve
    d. Increased risk of normal-tension glaucoma

12. Synthesize etiology, pathophysiology, epidemiology, therapeutic, and disease management concepts for open-angle glaucoma utilizing a key points format. (EO-18)

Pediatric and Neonatal Therapy

Sherry A. Luedtke

TREATMENT GOALS

- Explain the limitations of the research and drug approval processes for the pediatric population.
- Discuss the differences in drug absorption, distribution, metabolism, and excretion in infants and children, and describe the impact on drug therapy recommendations.
- Identify the drug additives and preservatives in commercially available drug formulations that may hinder their use in children.
- Recommend appropriate methods of drug administration for a given route in a pediatric patient.
- Identify the unique aspects of drug therapy in children that increase their risk for medication errors, and describe measures to limit the potential for medication errors.

GENERAL PRINCIPLES OF PEDIATRIC PHARMACOLOGY

Pediatric practitioners face many drug therapy challenges. In addition to employing medications for the management of diseases unique to the pediatric population, a pediatric practitioner may care for children as young and vulnerable as a 500-g premature infant who is struggling for life, or they may treat a 200-lb adolescent who is battling type 2 diabetes. Drug therapy challenges include age-related differences in the pharmacokinetics and pharmacodynamics of drugs, limited scientific evidence to support the use of most medications, and the lack of appropriate drug delivery systems/formulations for children—all of which can place a child at risk for adverse drug events.

The goal of this chapter is to provide the basis for an understanding of the important factors that the clinician must consider when providing pharmacotherapy to a pediatric patient. It is beyond the scope of this chapter to delve into individual diseases encountered in the clinical area of pediat-

rics or their pharmacologic management, as such an endeavor would require the devotion of an entire text.

LIMITATIONS OF DRUG THERAPY FOR CHILDREN

PEDIATRIC DRUG APPROVALS

Historical tragedies involving drugs and children have resulted in changes in the drug approval process; however, these changes have primarily affected and benefited adults. The tragedy involving sulfanilamide toxicity caused by the additive diethylene glycol resulted in the Food, Drug, and Cosmetic Act of 1938, which required the accumulation of safety data for marketed drugs.[1] The teratogenicity associated with thalidomide resulted in the Kefauver-Harris Drug Amendment, which mandated drug efficacy and improved drug safety data.[1] Until recently, the regulations of the US Food and Drug Administration (FDA) did little to require that manufacturers provide data regarding the use of their products in children. As a result, it is estimated that 75% of FDA-approved medications lack indications for use in children[2–5]; however, 30% are routinely used off-label to manage pediatric illnesses.[5] Pediatric practitioners essentially ''experiment'' each time they prescribe a drug, and it is a reality that off-label use of drugs in children is ''the cornerstone of pediatric practice.''[6] A practitioner may prescribe an off-label drug based on his or her judgment in an effort to provide appropriate treatment to a child, because the FDA does not regulate the use of medications in practice.[7,8] However, practitioners can be found negligent in civil court for inappropriate use of a drug, regardless of its FDA approval status.[7,8]

The lack of FDA indications for drugs in children leads to many other problems that affect their use. Information regarding appropriate dosing regimens, particularly for infants and young children, is lacking.[9] Most medications, such as oral solutions for infants and young children, lack appropriate formulations for administration to children, or the formulations are designed for adults and contain additives and preservatives that can be harmful to a young child.[10] Even parenteral formulations are marketed in concentrations that target adult dosing, and if those same products are to be used in a small child, 10- to 100-fold dilutions are required to allow measurement of small enough doses for an infant or young child. Finally, the off-label uses and lack of postmarketing monitoring have resulted in unfortunate and potentially preventable adverse events in children. Increased adverse event rates, such as gray baby syndrome with chloramphenicol in neonates, have been uncovered only after drugs were used in clinical practice in children.[11,12] Many unfortunate children have suffered and died because of lack of controlled study of a particular drug before it was granted approval.

Recent FDA regulations have pushed pediatrics to the forefront of the research and the drug approval process over the past decade. The first step taken by the FDA in 1994 was to request that all drug product labeling include pediatric dosing information when sufficient information was available to support its use and dosing.[13] Manufacturers were able to obtain a pediatric indication for their product with only pediatric pharmacokinetic and safety data if the disease state being treated was similar in children and adults. This first step resulted in FDA approval of a limited number of drugs for use in children. The greatest impact came when the Pediatric Exclusivity Provision of the FDA Modernization Act was passed in 1997; this provided an incentive to manufacturers of a 6-month patent extension in return for their implementation of pediatric studies on a respective product.[14] This act allowed manufacturers of patented drugs to extend their patents in exchange for clinical studies conducted in pursuit of pediatric indications. No such incentives existed for drugs already off-patent. By 2004, the FDA Modernization Act resulted in 73 agents with pediatric indications—this represented more pediatric indications than had ever been attained before.[15]

Because pediatric indications for off-patent drugs continued to be of concern, in 1998, the FDA developed the Pediatric Rule, which mandated that manufacturers must perform trials and provide safety and efficacy data for certain products.[16] The Pediatric Rule was implemented by the FDA in 1999, and shortly thereafter (2000), the FDA's authority to enforce the rule was contested and overturned in federal court. Much controversy and debate surrounded this action. However, no futile court battles were pursued; instead, new legislation was introduced to address the issue at hand. The Pediatric Research Equity Act of 2003 reiterated much of the content of the Pediatric Rule but clearly gave the FDA authority to enforce it.[17] In addition to the granting of enforcement authority to the FDA, a ''Pediatric Priority List'' of drugs was created, which lists drugs commonly used in children that lack indications.[18] By 2004, 54 agents that were seeking FDA approval sought pediatric indications under the Pediatric Rule, with 130 ongoing trials of additional agents.[19] Finally, under the Best Pharmaceuticals for Children Act of 2002, the Pediatric Exclusivity Provision was extended until the year 2007.[20] Thus, manufacturers who seek new approvals often do so under the exclusivity provision, and the FDA has a mechanism by which it can continue to require pediatric efficacy and safety data for off-patent medications under the Pediatric Research Equity Act.

As a result of the aforementioned legislation, by 1997, 38% of drugs that were seeking new drug approvals by the FDA had received pediatric indications, compared with only 20% before the legislative changes.[2] Not only have the legislative changes resulted in an increase in the number of drugs that have received FDA indications in children, they have also resulted in significant changes in the dosing recommendations or adverse effect profiles for 36% of those agents that had sought pediatric approval under the Pediatric Exclusivity Program.[21] This includes new dosing information on agents such as midazolam, gabapentin, and sotalol, as well as new safety information on agents such as betamethasone, propofol, and ribavarin.[21] It is clear that focused drug research, even for agents that have been used off-label for years, may reveal important information that will assist in the provision of safe and effective therapy for children.

RESEARCH ISSUES

Significant strides to enhance drug research in children have occurred over the past decade. In 1994, the National Institute of Child Health and Human Development created a network of Pediatric Pharmacology Research Units (PPRUs), which includes 13 academic institutions across the United States.[22] The PPRUs frequently partner with pharmaceutical companies to perform drug studies in children in an effort to obtain FDA approval. In 2001, the FDA strengthened its safeguards for children who participated in drug trials,[23] and the Best Pharmaceuticals for Children Act of 2002[20] established a program that provided public monies for pediatric studies funded through the National Institutes of Health (NIH). Collectively, these measures have increased the number and quality of pediatric drug trials while protecting the young patient.

Despite additional federal support and incentives for industry to perform drug studies in children, the actual launch of such studies remains a challenge. Children are considered a vulnerable population who require additional measures of protection while participating in clinical trials. Institutional review boards (IRBs) must carefully scrutinize all studies that involve children.[24] This increased scrutiny by IRBs often results in delays in the IRB approval process, or requirements of additional safety measures for pediatric enrollees. Although the American Academy of Pediatrics has developed guidelines for the ethical conduct of drug trials in children,[25] these are open to interpretation by individual IRBs. Controversies related to parental consent and assent of a child and remuneration of children/caregivers for a child's participation in trials are highly debated by pediatric researchers. One of the many challenges associated with pediatric research involves the design of trials that provide adequate protection for populations of children that are diverse and changing. For example, the dramatic physiologic changes that occur during infancy and childhood and that alter the pharmacokinetics and pharmacodynamics of drugs must be considered in the design of dosing schemes and the anticipation of responses during a trial. Altered or unique adverse effect profiles in children must also be anticipated and monitored closely. Knowledge and appreciation of all the unique aspects of the pediatric patient are essential if an investigator is to design a drug trial that ensures the validity of the research and the safety of his or her patients.

DEVELOPMENTAL PHARMACOLOGY

PHARMACOKINETIC DIFFERENCES

Because of ongoing changes that occur in the pediatric population, major changes in the disposition of drugs are noted. These changes significantly affect the dosing, monitoring, efficacy, and toxicity of drugs. Drugs that are safe and effective in one group of pediatric patients may be ineffective or toxic in another. Pharmacokinetic differences in children are described on the basis of age; therefore, it is important for the reader to review the accepted definitions of pediatric age groups. Table 15.1 provides a list of definitions for the various age categories of pediatric patients.[26]

Absorption. Gastric acid production is one factor that influences enteral drug absorption. The production of gastric acid has been reported to be low at birth. Although it has traditionally been believed that newborns are unable to produce gastric acid, increasing evidence indicates that this is not the case. It has been demonstrated that newborns have the ability to produce gastric acid by 24 hours of age.[27]

TABLE 15.1	Definitions of Age
Term	**Definition**
Gestational age	Weeks of gestation since conception
Postnatal age	Chronological age
Postconceptional age	Gestational age + postnatal age
Preterm	<36 weeks' gestation
Term	36–42 weeks' gestation
Post-term	>42 weeks' gestation
Neonate	≤1 month
Infant	1–12 months
Toddler	12–36 months
Child	3–12 years
Adolescent	12–18 years
Adult	>18 years

(From Milsap RL, Hill MR, Szefler SJ. Special pharmacokinetic considerations in children. In: Evans WE, Schentag JJ, Jusko WJ, eds. Applied pharmacokinetics, principles of therapeutic drug monitoring. Vancouver, British Columbia: Applied Therapeutics, 1992:1–32, with permission.)

Infants have been shown to have low baseline gastric acid production (pH of 6 to 7) until 20 months of age, at which time they reach a pH that is equivalent to that of adults.[28] However, a pH as low as 1 to 2 has been observed in premature infants under stress.[29] Because of their relatively low baseline gastric acidity, drugs that are weak bases (e.g., penicillin) may exhibit increases in absorption,[30] and drugs that are weak acids (e.g., phenobarbital) may exhibit reductions in enteral absorption.[31] Theoretically, drugs that require extensive acid hydrolysis for conversion to their active forms could lead to reductions in absorption as well.

The enzymatic activity and mucosal lining of the gastrointestinal tract are also immature in infants. Bile acid pools occur at approximately 50% of adult levels in term infants; this can lead to reduced absorption of lipophilic agents.[32] Reductions in levels of intestinal enzymes such as amylase and lipase, beta-glucuronidase, and glutathione peroxidase have all been reported and may lead to erratic absorption of oral agents in infants.[31] Reduced systemic levels of drugs that undergo significant enterohepatic recirculation may also be observed secondary to delayed bacterial colonization of the gastrointestinal tract.[31,33] Overall, all factors that are related to the immature development of the gastrointestinal tract may cause some reductions in absorption with most drugs that are used in children.

Gastric emptying times and intestinal motility also undergo physiologic changes in an infant that can influence the extent and timing of systemic drug absorption, but studies conducted to evaluate such changes are difficult to interpret because motility and drug absorption can be affected by numerous factors (e.g., type and volume of feedings, position).[33] Gastric emptying time is delayed in infants and reaches adult levels by 6 to 8 months of age.[31] Studies in older children to evaluate gastric emptying times have not been conducted. Intestinal transit time is delayed in infants and reaches adult levels by 4 to 6 months of age.[34] These changes in gastric and intestinal transit times are believed to slow the rate of drug absorption and delay the achievement of peak plasma concentrations, but they do not reduce the amount of drug that is absorbed in infants.[31] The impact of these delays in gastrointestinal transit on the newer sustained-release formulations of drugs has yet to be elucidated.

Absorption from the percutaneous and rectal routes of drug administration is altered in some pediatric age groups. Increased systemic absorption of drugs applied percutaneously in infants is believed to be related in part to a thin stratum corneum and increased skin hydration. However, to a larger extent, absorption is influenced by the larger body surface area relative to body weight (BSA:Wt) that is covered when agents are applied topically. Evidence of this is seen in reported toxicities to the use of topical agents such as hexachlorophene and povidone-iodine disinfectants, which have resulted in serious systemic toxicities.[33,35] In addition, recent studies have demonstrated significant hypothalamic-pituitary-adrenal (HPA) axis suppression secondary to topical betamethasone use.[21] Although practitioners are usually concerned about the systemic absorption of topical agents, some investigators have taken advantage of this increased absorption to employ an enhanced route of delivery of agents such as nitroglycerin and theophylline to preterm infants.[33] Rectal absorption of drugs may also be increased in infants because of reduced ''first-past'' hepatic metabolism.[35]

The intramuscular or subcutaneous route is a common route of administration for parenteral medications in children, particularly when intravenous access is problematic. Absorption of agents from these sites is dependent upon the relative muscle mass, fat stores, and blood flow to the respective area. Reductions in muscle mass or subcutaneous tissue and altered blood flow in a newborn may lead to erratic drug absorption.[33,35] Alterations in the absorption of intramuscular and subcutaneous drugs can be seen through the first month of life. Because of reductions in muscle size and subcutaneous tissue mass, volumes for drug administration by either route should be limited to 0.5 mL and 1 mL in infants and children, respectively.

Distribution. Distribution of a drug throughout the body once it reaches the circulation varies significantly with age. Neonatal body composition is 70% to 80% total body water and only 10% to 15% body fat. In contrast, at 1 year of age, total body water is 60% and total body fat is 20% to 25%.[31,33] Overall, decreases in body water occur with age, and total body water reaches 50% by adulthood. Clinically, this is seen by an enhanced volume of distribution and increased dosing requirements for water-soluble drugs (e.g., aminoglycosides) in infants. In contrast, drugs that are lipophilic (e.g., diazepam) may theoretically exhibit lower volumes of distribution.[31,33]

The tissue penetration and binding of drugs vary with age in pediatric patients. Tissue penetration of a drug is related to the mass of the target tissue and the transporter proteins within the tissue.[31] Historically, practitioners believed that adjustments in doses according to weight alone could account for these differences; however, it is clear that certain organ systems mature physiologically at different rates.[31] Thus, dosing for agents such as antiarrhythmics, which target the conduction system, should take into consideration the development of that tissue or system. For some agents, this may require higher serum concentrations to achieve the same effect; for others, increased toxicity may occur because of enhanced permeability, as is seen with increased permeability of drugs to the central nervous system (CNS).

The free or unbound potion of a drug in the body is the active portion, or the part that is available to bind to its site of action. Drugs bind to a variety of proteins in the body; primary drug-binding proteins consist of albumin and α_1 acid glycoprotein. Alterations in the concentration of these proteins or alterations in their binding affinity may result in higher free concentrations of the drug, leading to exaggerated responses. Lower concentrations of albumin and α_1 acid glycoprotein are found in infants and young children, and the affinity of many drugs to these proteins is reduced by 35% to 50% in neonates.[31,33,35] Neonates have a variety of fetal proteins that persist after birth and have reduced binding affinity for drugs.[33] Endogenous or exogenous substances may compete with drugs for binding proteins. Several highly protein-bound agents, such as sulfonamides, have been theorized to displace bilirubin from albumin-binding sites, warranting cautious use in infants at risk for kernicterus.[33] Although total serum concentrations of drugs may appear normal, if protein binding is reduced, one may see exaggerated or toxic responses. Thus, establishment of therapeutic concentration goals must take into account the level of protein binding.

Metabolism. Characterizing pediatric drug metabolism is extremely difficult because an ever-changing ''target'' is seen in the developing metabolic systems of infants and young children. Maturation of the metabolic systems of the liver in children has a huge impact on their ability to metabolize drugs, as well as on dosing requirements, potential for disease/drug interactions, and the ability of the body to use certain drug formulations that contain specific preservatives and additives.

The hepatic metabolic pathways by which drugs are metabolized are traditionally divided into phase 1 and phase 2 enzyme systems. Phase 1 enzyme systems are primarily responsible for the oxidation of drugs. The cytochrome (Cyp) P-450 enzymes are responsible for most phase 1 reactions, with Cyp1A2, Cyp2D6, Cyp2C9, and Cyp3A4 enzymes playing the major roles in drug metabolism. The extent of activity of the CypP450 enzymes at various stages of development varies by enzyme type (Table 15.2). Except for Cyp3A7, a fetal form of Cyp3A4, activity of most of the

TABLE 15.2	Hepatic Enzymes in Children[31,35,36,39]	
Enzyme	**Development**	**Common Pediatric Drugs Using the Pathway**
Cyp1A2	Negligible activity in utero; activity appears at 1–3 months; adult activity 6 months–2 years; exceeds adult activity in early childhood	Acetaminophen, caffeine, diazepam, theophylline, phenytoin, R-warfarin
Cyp2D6	Limited activity in utero; activity appears within hours of birth; 20% activity 1 month postnatal; adult activity reached by 1–3 years. Genetic polymorphisms in activity (5%–10%; white persons poor metabolizers)	Chlorpromazine, codeine, dextromethorphan, fluoxetine, hydrocodone, methadone, morphine, paroxetine, propranolol
Cyp2C9	Limited activity in utero; activity appears during 1st week of life; 50% activity by 1 month; adult activity reached by 6 months of age	Amitriptyline, diazepam, ibuprofen, omeprazole, phenytoin, topiramate, S-warfarin
Cyp3A4	Limited activity in utero; Cyp3A7 is fetal form of enzyme with high activity in utero. Activity appears during 1st week of life; 30%–40% of adult activity by 1 month; adult activity by 1 year; exceeds adult activity by 1–4 years of age	Carbamazepine, cyclosporine, dexamethasone, diltiazem, erythromycin, fluconazole, itraconazole, ketoconazole, lidocaine, midazolam, nifedipine, prednisone, sertraline, verapamil
Alchohol dehydrogenase	3%–4% of adult activity in infants; adult activity levels by 4–5 years	Benzyl alcohol, ethanol, steroids
Glucuronide conjugation	Low levels of activity in utero; 25% of adult activity by 3 months of age; adult activity by 3–30 months of age (dependent upon isoform)	Morphine, phenobarbital, acetaminophen, propofol, lorazepam, chloramphenicol, naloxone, zidovudine, propranolol
Acetylation	Low levels of activity in utero; adult activity by 1–3 years	Sulfonamides, hydralazine, procainamide, clonazepam
Sulfate conjugation	High levels of activity in utero (isoform and substrate dependent); exceeds adult activity in infancy	Acetaminophen, steroids
Methylation	30% adult activity in utero; exceeds adult levels of activity in newborns; insignificant activity in adults	Theophylline, acetaminophen

(Adapted from Kearns GL. Impact of developmental pharmacology on pediatric study design: overcoming the challenges. J Allergy Clin Immunol 106:S128–S138, 2000.)

CypP450 enzymes in utero is limited.[36] Each enzyme system matures at its own rate, generally reaching levels of adult activity by 1 to 3 years of age, and, in some circumstances (Cyp1A2, Cyp3A4), exceeding adult enzyme activity through adolescence.[31,33,35] For example, the Cyp1A2 enzyme, which is responsible for demethylation of theophylline, has minimal activity until 1 to 3 months of age, reaching adult levels by 6 months to 1 year.[31,36] Its activity in young children then exceeds that of adults, necessitating higher doses of theophylline on a weight-by-weight basis until early adolescence. Similarly, the Cyp3A4 enzyme is overexpressed in children and is thought to lead to increased metabolism of carbamazepine and overproduction of its metabolite carbamazepine epoxide.[31,35,36] This leads to increased dosing requirements of carbamazepine in children, and the increased carbamazepine epoxide may be responsible for some of the observed adverse drug reactions.

The activity of alcohol dehydrogenase, another phase 1 enzyme, is depressed in term infants at only 3% to 4% of

adult activity; it reaches adult activity levels by 4 to 5 years of age.[33] Benzyl alcohol, a bacteriostatic agent that is commonly used in parenteral drug formulations, is metabolized by alchohol dehydrogenase. The use of drugs that contain benzyl alcohol has led to numerous reports of kernicterus, metabolic acidosis, "gasping syndrome," and infant death, caused by its accumulation.[37] This tragedy resulted in the development of many of the preservative-free agents that are on the market today.

Phase 2 enzyme systems are primarily responsible for the conjugation of substances with a water-soluble molecule to enhance elimination. Four common phase 2 conjugation reactions that have been characterized in children include glucuronidation, acetylation, methylation, and sulfation. Probably the most well known of these systems is the glucuronidation pathway. Although significant maturation of this system occurs during the first week of life, as can be seen by the elimination of one of its major endogenous substrates, bilirubin, the activity of the glucuronidation system reaches only 25% of adult activity by 3 months of age.[36] Historically, the "gray baby syndrome" that was associated with chloramphenicol use in infants was due to its accumulation in infants with an immature glucuronidation system. Chloramphenicol undergoes extensive metabolism by the glucuronidation pathway; therefore, appropriate dose adjustments are required when it is used in infants and young children.

When a drug's primary route of metabolism is immature, it may be shunted through an alternate pathway. The sulfation pathway, another phase 2 enzyme, is active in fetal life, with activity in infancy exceeding that of adults.[36] Because of its relative overexpression, many drugs are preferentially shunted through the sulfation pathway during this time. Acetaminophen in adults undergoes glucuronidation; however, in infants, acetaminophen is primarily conjugated with sulfate because of this pathway's relatively high level of activity.[31,33] This is believed to result in lower rates of acetaminophen toxicity in infants because the toxic metabolite is produced through glucuronidation. Another similar shunting of metabolism can be seen with theophylline, which undergoes methylation in infants; in adults, it is primarily metabolized via the Cyp1A2 system. This occurs because the methylation pathway is overexpressed in infants relative to adults.

Clearly, an understanding of the extent of activity that occurs in the major metabolic pathways of infants and young children is important for clinicians to attain. Lack of awareness of enzyme activities can result in inappropriate extrapolations of doses from adults for use in children, or the use of agents with preservatives or additives that may be toxic. The study of a continuously changing or developing system to attempt to characterize drug metabolism in children is only one of many challenges for clinicians. Antenatal exposure to some substances can inhibit or induce fetal and postnatal enzymes.[33,36] Genetic polymorphisms for certain enzyme systems are known to exist and have been found to change during enzyme development in children.[35,36] Finally, changes that occur during puberty are believed to alter hepatic enzymatic activity.[33,35,36] It may be impossible to ever completely separate all of these factors and their influences on enzyme development in children.

Renal Elimination. The development of the kidney begins at 8 weeks' gestation, with all nephrons of the kidney developed and present by 36 weeks.[36] However, the functional capacity of a term infant is approximately 20% to 40% of that of an adult.[33] Dramatic increases in glomerular filtration occur within the first week of life as perfusion to the kidneys increases from the relatively low amounts of perfusion noted in intrauterine life. Glomerular filtration rates (GFRs) normalize after 4 to 5 weeks' postnatal age and reach maximum capacity by 6 to 12 months of age.[36] GFR at this time exceeds that observed in adults and gradually decreases with advancing age to reach adult rates at 1 year. Clinically, this can be seen with the aminoglycoside dosing requirements in neonates that vary

according to postnatal age. Neonates at less than 1 week of life require prolonged dosing intervals (24 to 48 hours, depending upon gestational age). After the first week of life, when GFR increases dramatically, shorter dosing intervals are required (8 to 12 hours). In addition to the changes in GFR that occur during the first year of life, tubular secretion and reabsorption of drugs undergo maturation during this time but at a slower pace, reaching maximal capacity at 1 year of age.[31,33,36] Dosing guidelines for infants and young children often require shorter intervals relative to adults so that serum concentrations can be maintained; this is so because of their increased GFRs and reduced tubular function.[36] Thus, more frequent serum concentration monitoring may be warranted for drugs that can be monitored.

In adults, GFR is frequently estimated with the use of creatinine clearance equations. Although similar equations exist and may be applied for a child with stable renal function (Table 15.3), their usefulness in many situations may be limited. Serum creatinine concentrations in infants and young children can be influenced by many factors, as is seen when newborn serum creatinine reflects maternal creatinine, muscle masses are reduced in children with chronic disease, or laboratory serum creatinine assays demonstrate limited sensitivity. Generally, in a healthy child, practitioners place great value in assessment of renal function performed by evaluating urinary output (normal 1 to 2 mL/kg/hour), although urine output can also be influenced by many factors. When concerns regarding acute changes in renal function arise, a 24-hour urine collection provides an accurate picture of renal function. Particularly in preterm infants, it is important that the clinician appreciate and empirically adjust dosing of renally eliminated drugs for factors that may indicate reduced renal perfusion and therefore development of GFR, such as neonatal asphyxia, presence of patent ductus arteriosus, or indomethacin use.[36] Because preterm infants are frequently on aminoglycosides for empiric therapy of neonatal sepsis, and because aminoglycoside clearance approximates GFR, calculation of aminoglycoside clearance may help guide the dosing of other renally eliminated drugs.

PHARMACODYNAMIC DIFFERENCES

As if the changes brought about by pharmacokinetic effects on drugs does not complicate matters enough, the pharmacodynamic response in children, or the body's response to a specific serum concentration, can also differ from that of adults. Limited research data are available regarding the pharmacodynamic responses of children to drugs. It is extremely difficult to separate the pharmacokinetic factors, such as protein binding or tissue penetration differences that may be contributing to an altered response to a drug concentration in the body, from the pharmacodynamic effects.[31,35] However, because the organ systems and receptor densities of the targets of our drug therapy are known to undergo major developmental changes during infancy and early childhood, it is

TABLE 15.3	Equations for Calculating Creatinine Clearance in Children

Infants and children >6 months of age:

$$CrCl = K \times L/Scr$$

Definitions	Age	K
CrCl = mL/min/1.73 m^2	Low birth wt ≤1 yr	0.33
K = constant of proportionality	Term infant <1 yr	0.45
L = length in centimeters	2–12 yr	0.55
Scr = serum creatinine in mg/dL	13–21 yr, female	0.55
	13–21 yr, male	0.70

Children 1–18 years of age:

$$CrCl = \frac{0.48 \times (Height)}{Scr}$$

Definitions

CrCl = mL/min/1.73 m^2

Scr = serum creatinine in mg/dL

Height = height in centimeters

(Adapted from Schwartz GJ, Brion LP, Spitzer A. The use of plasma creatinine concentration for estimating glomerular filtration rate in infants, children, and adolescents. Pediatr Clin North Am 34:571–590, 1987; Traub SL, Johnson CE. Comparison of methods of estimating creatinine clearance in children. Am J Hosp Pharm 37:195–201, 1980.)

theorized that the response of an organ or receptor to a given concentration of drug may be enhanced or reduced.

The infant response to β-agonists provides one such example. The pulmonary system is known to undergo significant growth and development within the first 2 to 5 years of life. Newborns are born with only 10% to 15% of the number of alveoli they will have in adulthood; adult values are not reached until they are 8 years of age.[38] Changes in responses to β-agonists may be due in part to differences in development of the pulmonary system and β-receptor density. Similarly, altered cardiovascular responses to α- and β-agonists, such as dopamine and dobutamine, may be related to changes in receptor densities on target organ systems.[40] Paradoxical CNS reactions of infants and young children to benzodiazepines or increased dystonic reactions to metoclopramide are theorized to be related to differences in neurotransmitter balance.[41] Until the maturation process of the targeted systems is clearly understood, differentiating pharmacokinetic from pharmacodynamic responses in children will continue to present a problem.

DRUG DOSING CONSIDERATIONS

Historically, pediatric dose adjustments from adult dosing have been performed based solely upon age, weight, or body surface area adjustments. Rules such as Clark's Rule and Young's Rule (Table 15.4) were commonly employed to approximate doses for young children. These rules made the assumption that an infant or child is just a "little adult," and did not take into consideration all the unique pharmacokinetic and pharmacodynamic differences that have been observed in children. Depending upon an infant's or child's age, adjustments based upon weight alone may result in significant overdosing of a young infant who cannot metabolize the drug, or significant underdosing of a child whose metabolism exceeds that of an adult. In addition, this has led and may lead to drug toxicity secondary to accumulation of drug or drug metabolites.

With the lack of pharmacokinetic and dosing studies in children, the practitioner is faced with a dosing dilemma. The easiest solution would be to avoid the use of any drug that lacks scientifically supported pediatric dosing; however, if pediatricians had taken this attitude in the past, much of the dosing information for drugs commonly used in children today would not exist. In practical terms, weight or body surface area adjustments may serve some role in a child over the age of 10 whose organ development and metabolism are similar to those of an adult. However, in an infant or young child, to ensure safety and efficacy, a practitioner must also apply his or her knowledge about a drug's pharmacokinetics and pharmacodynamics in adults, and must consider how those parameters may differ in an infant or young child. For example, if a practitioner chooses to employ a new drug in a newborn that lacks dosing information and undergoes significant glucuronidation, a dose reduction beyond that based on weight adjustment would be necessary.

| TABLE 15.4 | Useful Equations for Pediatric Drug Dosing |

Extrapolation of Adult Doses for Pediatrics[9,43,44,45]

Young's Rule (adjustment based on age)

$$\text{Pediatric Dose} = \frac{\text{Age} \times \text{Adult Dose}}{\text{Age} + 12}$$

Age = age in years

Clark's Rule (adjustment based on weight)

$$\text{Pediatric Dose} = \frac{\text{Wt} \times \text{Adult Dose}}{150}$$

Wt = weight in pounds

Fried's Rule (age adjustment for infants)

$$\text{Infant Dose} = \frac{\text{Age} \times \text{Adult Dose}}{150}$$

Age = age in months

Dose Adjustments for **Weight** or **BSA**

$$\text{Dose}_P = \text{Dose}_A \frac{(\text{Wt}_P)}{\text{Wt}_A}$$

$$\text{Dose}_P = \text{Dose}_A \frac{(\text{BSA}_P)}{\text{BSA}_A}$$

P = pediatric dose
A = adult dose

Body Surface Area Calculations

Body Surface Area

$$\text{BSA (m}^2) = \frac{\text{Ht (cm)} \times \text{Wt (kg)}}{3600}$$

Ht = height in cm
Wt = weight in kg

Body Surface Area (simplified)

$$\text{BSA (m}^2) = \frac{[4\,(\text{Wt}) + 7]}{90 + \text{Wt}}$$

Wt = weight in kg

Ideal Body Weight Calculations

Ideal Body Weight
Children 1–18 yr

$$\text{IBW} = \frac{(\text{Ht}^2 \times 1.65)}{1000}$$

IBW = ideal body weight in kg
Ht = height in cm

MEDICATION ADMINISTRATION ISSUES

FORMULATION ISSUES

An additional challenge of providing pharmacotherapy for children is the difficulty involved in obtaining dosage formulations appropriate for age. Many of the medications that are currently used are not available in dosage formulations for children.[10] Few medications on the market today have been developed primarily for pediatric use; therefore, most dosage formulations—tablet and capsule strengths—and concentrations of enteral and parenteral solutions are available in strengths for use in adults.[10] To administer small doses of an enterally administered drug to a young child, the practitioner often must resort to halving or quartering an adult-strength tablet. These must be further crushed and mixed with food, infant formula, or drink for delivery to an infant or young child. This requires that parents take additional steps to ad-

minister an appropriate dose to their child. It is important that the practitioner be aware of which medications can and cannot be crushed,[46] according to dosage formulation. In addition, it is important that parents and caregivers be educated about potential drug-food interactions that may occur.

An oral liquid drug formulation is preferred for children younger than 5 years of age who have difficulty swallowing capsules and tablets. It is also useful when agents cannot be crushed or mixed with foods. Although some medications have commercially available oral suspensions, solutions, or elixirs, many of these have been designed for adults. The concentrations of these liquids and the flavorings (e.g., mint flavoring) have been designed for adult use and adult tastes.[47] Without a pediatric FDA indication, manufacturers are unlikely to develop a "pediatric friendly" oral solution. This has led to significant effort from pediatric practitioners and independent researchers to develop oral solutions for use in children.[10] Many pharmacies devote most of their practice to compounding such formulations. Practitioners

TABLE 15.5	**Useful Pediatric Drug Information Resources**

Dosing References
Pediatric Dosing Handbook
Harriet Lane Handbook
Neofax
The Pediatric Drug Handbook

Pediatric Extemporaneous Formulations
Handbook of Extemporaneous Formulations
Pediatric Drug Formulations
Stability of Compounded Formulations
International Journal of Pharmaceutical Compounding

Compatibility References
Handbook on Injectable Drugs
King's Handbook of Intravenous Mixtures
Injectable Drug Reference
Micromedex DRUGDEX

Drug Administration References
The Teddy Bear Book: Pediatric Injectable Drugs
Handbook of Parenteral Drug Administration

Adverse Drug Events
Textbook of Adverse Drug Reactions
Vaccine Adverse Event Reporting System
(http://www.vaers.org)
Institute for Safe Medication Practices (http://www.ismp.org)
FDA Medwatch Program
(http://fda.gov/medwatch/safety.htm)
ClinAlert (www.nlm.nkh.gov/databases/clinical_alerts.html)
Mircomedex DRUGDEX

should be aware of and should recommend formulations with appropriate stability and sterility data.[10] Many useful references that provide formulation information have been compiled (Table 15.5).

The use of parenteral medications in children involves similar drug formulation problems. As with oral liquid formulations, most parenteral medications are packaged and formulated for adult dosing. Many single-use vials or ampules of medication are large, resulting in significant waste when only 1 mg of a 100-mg vial is used in a neonate. In addition, the accurate measuring of such small doses is problematic. Many parenteral medications require 10- or 100-fold dilutions of medications to allow for the accurate measurement of minute doses.[48,49] The large margin of error is a significant cause of many medication errors in children that are often life threatening. More concentrated parenteral solutions are needed for the delivery of small doses and for reduced dose volumes.

A common concern regarding the formulations of both enteral and parenteral drugs for use in children is the use of "inactive" drug additives in current formulations. Many commercially available drug formulations contain additives such as preservatives, sweeteners, dyes, or solubilizers. Although most of these agents do not pose a problem, particularly in adults, significant adverse reactions have been reported in children.[46,50] Traditionally, many of these additives were considered "inactive" by the FDA, and they were not required to be listed in the content labeling provided by the manufacturer. However, as individual agents have been linked to potential toxicities, the FDA has begun requiring labeling of the content of individual agents. A recent example of this is the requirement by the FDA to mandate labeling of aluminum content on small- and large-volume parenteral products used in total parenteral nutrition[52] because of potential CNS and bone marrow toxicity. A summary of common drug additives, their associated risks in children, and recommendations is provided in Table 15.6.

Drug additives are known to increase the osmolality of a drug formulation. Agents such as propylene glycol, alcohol, and sorbitol are known to significantly increase the osmolality of parenterally and enterally administered medications.[53–55] For enteral administration of drugs, an osmolality of less than 400 to 500 mOsm per liter is recommended, to limit the stress imposed on the gastrointestinal system; this stress could lead to pneumatosis intestinalis in preterm infants.[53,54] Many of the drugs commonly used in this population have osmolalities that exceed this amount, for example, acetaminophen drops have an osmolality of 10,000 to 16,000 mOsm per liter.[53] Selection of oral agents with low osmolalities is preferred; however, when this is not possible, enteral administration of parenteral agents with lower osmolalities may be considered.[53] Another way to reduce the osmolality of enteral agents is to administer doses along with an infant feeding to reduce the final osmolality exposure[53] (Table 15.7). Numerous reports of neonatal hypersomolality, hepatic necrosis, intestinal necrosis, and intraventricular hemorrhage with parenteral administration of hypersomolar drugs have been documented.[53,55,56] When such agents are employed, proper dilution to reduce the osmolality may prevent these toxicities. The recommended osmolarity limit for a peripheral infusion is 600 mOsm per liter,[54] when it is given to prevent pain, thrombophlebitis, and line infiltration. Many drugs such as phenytoin, phenobarbital, and digoxin have osmolarities that exceed 9000 mOsm per liter; these must be further diluted before they are administered.

PARENTERAL DRUG ADMINISTRATION

Once a drug has been selected for parenteral administration to a child, it is important that the clinician be cognizant of the intravenous (IV) access options for drug administration. Obtaining and maintaining peripheral IV access in an infant or young child is often problematic because of difficulty in cannulation and frailness of the veins. In newborns, the umbilical vein serves as a means of accessing the central circulation with the use of an umbilical vein catheter (UVC),[57] but its duration of use must be limited because of the risk of portal vein thrombosis. Other common sites for peripheral IV access for drug delivery in children include the dorsum of the hand or foot, the scalp, and the wrist or ankle, because of the size and ease of cannulation of veins, and the site can be immobilized to avoid decannulation.[57] Regardless of site, one must use extreme caution when administering drugs known to cause significant throm-

TABLE 15.6	Drug Additives of Concern in Children[46,50–52]		
Additive	**Role**	**Concern**	**Recommendation**
Alcohol	Solubilizer in tinctures and elixirs	Central nervous system (CNS) depression, gastrointestinal disturbances	Review drug labeling and avoid use of alcohol-containing products in children
Aluminum		Potential CNS and bone toxicity, microcytic anemia in infants and young children	Review drug labeling and limit exposure to <4–5 µg/kg/day.
Aspartame	Sweetener in enteral formulations	Use in children with phenylketonuria (PKU) contraindicated Headaches, neuropsychiatric reactions, seizures, and hypersensitivity reactions reported in children	Review drug labeling and avoid use of aspartame-containing products in children with PKU. Limit total ingestion amount in non-PKU children to 10 mg/kg/day aspartame
Benzyl alcohol	Preservative in parenteral agents	"Gasping syndrome," intraventricular hemorrhage, metabolic acidosis, kernicterus, cerebral palsy, death linked to exposure in preterm infants because of reduced metabolism Allergic reactions have also been reported	Review drug labeling and avoid use of benzyl alcohol–containing drugs, particularly in infants. When alternatives are not available, limit cumulative dose to <100 mg/kg/day
Benzalkonium chloride (BAK)	Preservative in nebulizer and nasal solutions	Dose-dependent and cumulative allergic reaction, including bronchoconstriction, pruritus, facial flushing	Review drug labeling and avoid use of agents that contain BAK in children who require frequent or long-term administration of such drugs
Dyes (various)	Coloring agent in enteral formulations	Cross-sensitivity reactions in aspirin-allergic children reported with many dyes Gastrointestinal intolerance, contact dermatitis, hyperactivity	Not required by FDA to be included in drug labeling Avoid use of dye-containing agents in aspirin-sensitive or -allergic children Avoid use of dye-containing agents in infants
Lactose	Diluent in tablets and capsules	Gastrointestinal distress in lactose-intolerant individuals Use in children with galactosemia contraindicated Allergic reactions reported	Review drug labeling and avoid use of agents that contain lactose in children with galactosemia and lactose-sensitive individuals
Propylene glycol	Solubilizer in parenteral, enteral, and topical agents	Serum hyperosmolality, lactic acidosis, hemolysis, CNS depression, seizures, and death reported in infants from use of topical, enteral, or parenteral agents because of increased absorption and decreased metabolism Cardiovascular reactions (hypotension, arrhythmias), respiratory depression, and seizures associated with rapid infusion rates of parenteral agents or large ingestions of enteral agents Local contact dermatitis and thrombophlebitis reported with topical and intravenous use, respectively	Review drug labeling and avoid use of propylene glycol–containing agents Limit exposure to propylene glycol via use of further dilutions of parenteral drug products. Reduce osmolarity of enterally administered agents by dilutions with infant formulas Limit rates of infusion of propylene glycol–containing products
Saccharin	Sweetener in enteral formulations	Sulfonamide derivative that leads to cross reactions in children with sulfa allergies Irritability, hypertonia, strabismus, and insomnia reported in infants Linked to bladder cancer in animal studies	Not required by FDA to be included in drug labeling Avoid use of such agents in children with sulfa allergies Limit intake of saccharine in infants and young children (<0.6–0.9 mg/kg/day)
Sulfites	Antioxidant in antiasthmatic and parenteral medications	Sulfite-allergic reactions in children with asthma	Review drug labeling and avoid use of agents that contain sulfites in children with underlying lung disease or history of sulfite allergy
Tartrazine (FD&C Yellow No. 5)	Coloring agent	Cross sensitivity in aspirin-allergic children	Review drug labeling and avoid use of agents that contain tartrazine in aspirin-sensitive or -allergic children
Thiomersal	Preservative that contains mercury	Neurotoxicity, behavioral disorders, and autism concerns in infants and young children Hypersensitivity reactions	Review drug labeling and avoid use of thiomersal- or mercury-containing agents Limit mercury exposure to 0.1 mg/kg/day

TABLE 15.7 | Calculating Final Osmolalities

$$OM = \frac{OD\,(VD) + OF(VF)}{VD + F}$$

OM = osmolality of mixture VD = volume of drug

OD = osmolality of drug VF = volume of formula

OF = osmolality of formula

Example of osmolality calculation:

Ferinsol drops (0.25-mL dose with osmolality of ~5010 mOsm/L

Premature Enfamil formula (24 cal/oz; 305 mOsm/L; 15 mL per feeding)

$$OM = \frac{(5010\ mOsm/L \times 0.00025\ L) + (305\ mOsm/L \times 0.015\ L)}{0.01525\ L}$$

$$= 382\ mOsm/L$$

bophlebitis or tissue ischemia upon extravasation (e.g., phenytoin). If available, central access is preferred for administering such drugs. Commonly used central access devices include peripherally inserted central catheters (PICCs) or traditional central lines (e.g., Broviac); selection depends upon the duration of access needed.[57,58] In emergency situations in infants and young children, the intraosseous route of administration serves as an excellent route of drug delivery to the central circulation; however, it is to be used only until alternative routes of access have been established.[57] Problems with limited IV access often complicate the drug delivery process, particularly in the critically ill child. Among the practitioner's most difficult problems is the delivery of numerous IV medications for which limited compatibility information is available. Resources for compatibility information (Table 15.5) are essential in such situations to help the clinician deal with this everyday dilemma.

Before advances were made in infusion technology, including syringe pumps and microbore tubing (which allow for precise delivery of medications at low infusion rates), numerous problems existed with the actual delivery of minute doses of medication to children.[59,60] Infants and children require low infusion rates of intravenous fluids relative to adults because of their reduced fluid requirements. With the use of adult infusion pumps and IV tubing, drugs were often "trapped" or lost in the deadspace of these lines, because of the low flow rates.[54,59,60] The use of microbore tubing and syringe pumps for infants and young children today has reduced the number of drug delivery problems; however, errors in drug administration are still more common with the intravenous route of drug delivery relative to other routes. A common method for individualizing drug therapy for infants that has been used by many neonatal and intensive care units—the "Rule of Sixes"—was designed as a simple calculation to accurately prepare concentrated

solutions for continuous infusion (Table 15.8).[61] Although it is still employed today, this method of drug preparation and infusion is falling out of favor in light of the new technology, which allows for more precise delivery of small volumes and concern for increased medication errors.[62] Several resources for pediatric intravenous drug administration have been developed to assist the practitioner (Table 15.5).

ENTERAL DRUG ADMINISTRATION

The oral delivery of medication to a young child brings on its own challenges. Numerous devices exist for measuring and delivering oral solutions to an infant or young child, such as oral syringes, medicine cups, medicine spoons, and droppers. Parents should be instructed to avoid the use of kitchen spoons that can vary in accuracy. Oral syringes are probably the most ideal method for delivery of oral solutions to young infants, as they allow for accurate and controlled delivery of medication. Caregivers should be instructed to squirt small amounts of solution from the oral syringe between the back gums of the mouth and cheek to avoid contact with the taste buds. Solutions should never be squirted di-

TABLE 15.8 | Rule of Sixes Calculation[61]

$$X\ mg/100\ mL = \frac{6 \times Wt\ (kg) \times dose\ (\mu g/kg/min)}{Rate\ (mL/hr)}$$

Normally make such that 1 mL/hr = 10 μg/kg/min

Example: 1.3-kg infant ordered to receive dopamine infusion such that 1 mL/hr = 10 μg/kg/min

$$X\ mg/100\ mL = \frac{6 \times 1.3\ (kg) \times 10\ (\mu g/kg/min)}{1\ (mL/hr)}$$

= 78 mg dopamine to put into 100 mL of D_5W

rectly to the back of the mouth; this precaution avoids choking or aspiration of drug. Many over-the-counter medications for children are packaged with medicine cups, medicine spoons, or droppers. Although these are all acceptable means of measuring and administering the respective medications, caregivers should be instructed to never interchange measuring devices from one product to another, to avoid serious dosing errors.

Children are generally able to swallow capsules and tablets by about 5 years of age. Until that time, oral solutions, chewable tablets, or crushed tablets or capsules are typically employed. Delivery of any oral medication can be a two-man job when an uncooperative child must be restrained. Additional strategies to improve cooperation in an uncooperative infant or child include administration of medication before infant feedings (when acceptance is higher and the child is less likely to vomit), use of chilled oral solutions to improve taste, and the mixing of medication with small amounts of food or formula. When medications are mixed into fluids, foods, or formula, the clinician must be aware of drug-food incompatibilities. The practitioner should avoid mixing in large amounts that may not be ingested entirely by the child; also, premixing in batches should be prevented because drug compatibility studies of these methods are non-existent.

ALTERNATIVE ROUTES OF DRUG ADMINISTRATION

Rectal administration serves as an excellent route of drug delivery, particularly for a young infant or child. Rectal absorption of medication is high in young infants but should be avoided in the presence of anal fissures and abnormalities of the rectum, as well as in the immunocompromised patient.[63] Additional modes of administration of pediatric medications include ophthalmic, otic, and nasal drops or ointments. Medications to be delivered rectally or via drops should be warmed before they are administered. To enhance delivery of drops or ointments to the targeted area, a child should be positioned such that his or her head is lower than the rest of the body. Because of the flat angle of the ear canal in infants, otic medications should be instilled by pulling the auricle down and out, rather than up and back, as is done with an adult.

The use of topical agents in infants and children requires a degree of caution. Application of topical products to large areas can result in systemic absorption of the medication or drug additive in infants, which is caused by their relatively large surface area relative to body mass.[63] This is of particular concern in preterm infants because of the immaturity of their skin. Generally, topical agents with the lowest concentrations of drug (e.g., steroids) should be employed in infants and young children. Occlusive dressings and barriers, such as petrolatum or infant diapers, have also been shown to enhance drug absorption from the site of application.

Numerous medications are available for inhalation to manage respiratory disorders in children. Many practitioners

feel more comfortable delivering inhaled medications to infants and young children with the use of a nebulizer rather than a metered-dose inhaler (MDI).[64] However, many drawbacks to nebulization of medications have been noted; these include significant drug loss in the nebulizer circuit or ambient air during nebulization of medication, cumbersome and expensive equipment, and the time-consuming nebulization process.[64] Also, many medications that are available in MDI form are not commercially available for nebulization; if they are, many contain preservatives and additives that themselves can be irritants to the respiratory tract. In contrast, MDIs or newer dry powder inhalers are frequently underused but equally effective means of inhaled drug delivery. The use of spacing devices with a face mask can be an effective and efficient method of delivery of MDI medications in an infant or young child.[65] Children as young as 5 can be taught to appropriately use an MDI, with or without a spacing device, or a dry powder inhaler. This allows them to quickly and effectively administer their own inhaled medication when a caregiver is unavailable. Guidelines for the selection of appropriate inhaler devices for children of various ages have been developed[64,66–67]; however, regardless of which inhaler device is chosen for a particular child, appropriate education is essential to ensure effective drug delivery.

MEDICATION COMPLIANCE ISSUES IN CHILDREN

Compliance with medication regimens among pediatric patients is similar to that reported for adults. Compliance rates ranging from 10% to 80% have been reported for both short-term and long-term drug therapy in children.[68] Numerous factors influence compliance in a pediatric patient; parental support and role modeling have been shown to be most influential in young children. For infants and young children, taste and palatability have a significant impact on their acceptance of a medication.[69] Palatability of drugs is influenced by smell, initial taste, flavor, texture, and aftertaste. Most efforts to improve the palatability of medications for children focus on improving the flavor through the use of homemade agents (e.g., peanut butter, honey, chocolate syrup) or commercially available flavoring systems. The use of ''chasers'' (Popsicle, lollipop, root beer soda) after a dose of medication can improve the aftertaste. In general, children prefer sweet flavors rather than the mint or citrus flavor favored by adults.

Additional factors that affect compliance in children include dosing frequency, adverse effects, education, school or day care policies, peer influences, and the adolescent need for autonomy.[68,69] As in adults, compliance in children is influenced by dosing frequency; however, this effect is compounded in children and adolescents who are faced with peer pressures and school or day care policies that may limit the use of medications. Drug regimens that avoid the need for drug administration during school or day care hours are preferred. The provision of two supplies of medication may help to improve compliance when mid-day doses are required for children who attend school or day care. Adolescents present a unique challenge for drug therapy compliance in that they are already struggling with their parents over issues of autonomy. Adolescents who are involved in and accountable for their own drug therapy have been shown to have improved compliance rates, as opposed to those for whom parents control drug therapy.[70–72] The practitioner must consider any barriers for medication compliance when prescribing drug therapy for children, as many may be out of the control of the patient or caregiver. Provision of written and verbal pediatric-specific drug information to the caregiver or child is key to success.[68] Children of all ages should be encouraged and praised for their medication compliance. Creative techniques for compliance through the use of reward systems, such as medication calendars, may be effective.[68]

MEDICATION ADVERSE EVENT POTENTIAL

By definition, adverse drug events include adverse drug reactions and medication errors. Adverse reactions are unwanted responses to a drug that may be predictable or unpredictable but are related to the pharmacologic properties of a drug.[73] In contrast, medication errors are preventable and result from human or system error.[73] As described earlier, pediatric patients are at risk for adverse drug reactions as a result of the limited research performed to date to support drug dosing regimens or altered adverse drug reaction profiles. Children also represent a population at significant risk for medication errors, with rates three times those reported in adults.[74] Unique aspects of drug therapy that may put children at higher risk for medication errors include the lack of appropriate dosing information or guidelines, the need to compound oral dosage forms or to dilute commercially available formulations, a child's inability to express his or her response to medication, the need for increased medication handling in preparation and dosage calculations, and the use of ambiguous dosing instructions for caregivers.[74] The medication errors that occur most commonly in children are dosing errors; however, errors may occur because of incorrect route of administration, inappropriate drug selection, insufficient drug monitoring, drug interactions, and inadequate communication.[73]

Medication errors occur more commonly with parenteral agents, placing pediatric patients in inpatient settings at highest risk for medication error. Analgesics (narcotics), antibiotics, fluid and electrolyte therapy, digoxin, and theophylline are the most common agents for which medication errors have been reported.[73,74] Many medication errors are system-related and can easily be prevented. The American Academy of Pediatrics has developed guidelines designed specifically to prevent medication errors in the pediatric inpatient setting[73]; similarly, the Institute for Safe Medication Practices (ISMP) and the Pediatric Pharmacy Advocacy Group

(PPAG) have developed guidelines for prevention of medication errors in all pediatric patients.[74] Both sets of guidelines emphasize the need for a multidisciplinary approach to preventing medication errors in children. Recommendations to reduce medication errors during the prescribing process include inclusion of patient age and weight on the prescription order, specification of drug strength or concentration, inclusion of calculations for double-checking (e.g., mg/kg/day dose), use of leading zeros (e.g., 0.1), avoidance of trailing zeros (e.g., 1.0), and use of metric units.[73,74] In addition, ISMP has created a list of ''error-prone'' abbreviations that should be avoided because they are commonly misinterpreted by health care professionals.[75] The use of these strategies, as well as the availability of pediatric-specific drug resources (Table 15.5), can assist in the prevention of medication-induced injuries.

KEY POINTS

- Lack of FDA indications and pediatric drug research has resulted in numerous tragedies in children.
- Recent regulatory changes by the FDA are anticipated to increase the quantity of safety and efficacy data regarding drug use in children.
- Despite additional funding and increased interest in pediatric drug therapy research, the process of conducting research in the pediatric population poses many unique challenges.
- Gastrointestinal tract acidity, enzymatic activity, and motility differences in infants and young children alter the absorption of oral drugs. Drugs that are weak bases increase drug absorption, and weak acids may reduce drug absorption in infants. Reduced gastric transit times may delay peak absorption times for infants and young children.
- Systemic absorption from the transcutaneous route of drug administration in infants may be enhanced, leading to the potential for increased adverse effects. Cautious use of topical agents should be employed in infants.
- The volume to which drugs distribute in an infant or young child is increased because of increased body water; this results in the need for increased drug doses for water-soluble drugs.
- Alterations in protein binding and tissue penetration of drugs may lead to reduced or exaggerated responses to drugs.
- In infants, the metabolism of most drugs is reduced and reaches adult levels by 1 to 3 years of age; then, it often exceeds adult levels until adolescence.
- Drugs may be shunted, or metabolized through alternate metabolic pathways, during infancy.
- Glomerular filtration is 20% to 40% of adult capacity at birth, increases dramatically after the first week of life, and reaches maximal levels by 6 to 12 months of age.

- Altered pharmacodynamic responses to drugs in children are believed to be related to the immature development of the target organ systems.
- Dose adjustments from adult doses for pediatric patients based upon weight alone should be applied only in children older than 10 years of age.
- Many drugs commonly used in children are not commercially available in appropriate dose formulations, resulting in problems with compliance and the potential for medication errors.
- ''Inactive'' drug additives in drug formulations can result in significant toxicities for pediatric patients.
- The osmolarity of a drug product should be considered during drug selection, and methods of reducing osmolarity should be used.
- Recommendations for parenteral drug delivery must take into consideration the available site of access, the IV line setup, the local toxicity potential of a particular drug, and the compatibility of the agent.
- Appropriate measuring devices should be employed when an oral liquid formulation is administered to an infant or young child.
- Parents should be provided with instructions for appropriate measurement and delivery of an oral agent to a child, along with strategies for enhancing child cooperation.
- Alternative routes of drug administration should be based on the age-related physiologic development of a child and the child's abilities.
- Strategies for improving medication palatability or reducing aftertaste should be recommended, to enhance medication compliance in a child.
- Practitioners should consider potential unique barriers to compliance in a pediatric patient.
- Children are at high risk for medication errors, the most common of which involve dosing errors.
- Prescribers should alter their prescribing process to eliminate practices that may place a child at risk for a medication error.

REFERENCES

1. Center for Drug Evaluation and Research. Timeline: chronology of drug regulation in the United States. Available at: http://www.fda.gov/cder/about/history/time.1.htm. Accessed May 13, 2004.
2. Steinbrook R. Testing medications in children. N Engl J Med 347:1462–1470, 2002.
3. Kauffman RE. Drug safety, testing, and availability for children. Child Legal Rights J 18:27–34, 1998.
4. Blumer JL. Off-label uses of drugs in children. Pediatrics 104 (Suppl):598–602, 1999.
5. Wilson JT. An update on the therapeutic orphan. Pediatrics 104:585–589, 1999.
6. Budetti PP. Ensuring safe and effective medications for children. JAMA 290:950–951, 2003.
7. Blumer JL. Off-label uses of drugs in children. Pediatrics 104:598–602, 1999.
8. American Academy of Pediatrics, Committee on Drugs. Uses of drugs not described in the package insert (off-label uses). Pediatrics 110:181–183, 2002.
9. Christensen ML, Helms RA, Chesney RW. Is pediatric labeling really necessary? Pediatrics 104:593–597, 2002.
10. Nahata MC. Lack of pediatric drug formulations. Pediatrics 104:607–609, 1999.
11. Burns LE, Hodgman JE, Cass AB. Fatal circulatory collapse in premature infants receiving chloramphenicol. N Engl J Med 261:1318–1321, 1959.
12. Sutherland JM. Fatal cardiovascular collapse of infants receiving large amounts of chloramphenicol. Am J Dis Child 97:761, 1959.
13. US Department of Health and Human Services, Food and Drug Administration. Specific requirements on content and format of labeling for human prescriptions: revision of ''pediatric use'' subsection in the labeling: final rule (21 C.F.R. part 201). Fed Regist 59:64240, 1994.
14. US Food and Drug Administration Modernization Act of 1997, Pub. L. 105–115, 105th Congress, November 21, 1997.
15. Center for Drug Evaluation and Research. Pediatric exclusivity statistics. Available at: http://www.fda.gov/cder/pediatric/wrstats.htm. Accessed May 13, 2004.
16. US Department of Health and Human Services, Food and Drug Administration. Regulations requiring manufacturers to assess the safety and effectiveness of new drugs and biological products in pediatric patients; final rule. Fed Regist 63:66632–66672, 1998.
17. Pediatric Research Equity Act of 2003, Pub. L. 108–155, 108th Congress, January 7, 2003.
18. US Department of Health and Human Services, National Institutes of Health. List of drugs for which pediatric studies are needed; final rule. Fed Regist 69:7243–7244, 2004.
19. Center for Drug Evaluation and Research. Pediatric rule statistics. Available at: http://www.fda.gov/cder/pediatric/wrstats.htm. Accessed May 13, 2004.
20. Best Pharmaceuticals for Children Act, Pub. L. 107–109, 107th Congress, January 4, 2002.
21. Roberts R, Rodriguez W, Murphy D, et al. Pediatric drug labeling: improving the safety and efficacy of pediatric therapies. JAMA 290:905–911, 2003.
22. National Institute of Child Health and Development Pediatric Pharmacology Research Network. A child is not just a miniature adult. Available at: http://www.nichd.nih.gov/about/crmc/eng/ped/ped2.htm. Accessed May 13, 2004.
23. US Department of Health and Human Services, Food and Drug Administration. Additional safeguards for children in clinical investigations of FDA-regulated products. Fed Regist 66:20589–20600, 2001.
24. National Commission for the Protection of Human Subjects of Biomedical and Behavioral Research. Research involving children. Washington, DC: Government Printing Office, 1977.
25. Committee on Drugs, American Academy of Pediatrics. Guidelines for the ethical conduct of studies to evaluate drugs in pediatric populations. Pediatrics 95:286–294, 1995.
26. Milsap RL, Hill MR, Szefler SJ. Special pharmacokinetic considerations in children. In: Evans WE, Schentag JJ, Jusko WJ, eds. Applied pharmacokinetics, principles of therapeutic drug monitoring. Vancouver, British Columbia: Applied Therapeutics, 1992:1–32.
27. Agunod M, Yamaguchi N, Lopez R, et al. Correlative study of hydrochloric acid, pepsin, and intrinsic factor secretion in newborns and infants. Am J Dig Dis 14:400–414, 1969.
28. Rodbro P, Krasilnikoff PA, Christiansen PM. Parietal cell secretory function in early childhood. Scand J Gastroenterol 2:209–213, 1967.
29. Hyman PE, Clarke DD, Everett SL, et al. Gastric acid secretory function in preterm infants. J Pediatr 106:467–471, 1985.
30. Huang NN, High RH. Comparison of serum levels following the administration of oral and parenteral preparations of penicillin to infants and children of various age groups. J Pediatr 42:657–668, 1953.
31. Kearns GL, Abdel-Rahman SM, Alander SW, et al. Drug therapy: developmental pharmacology—drug disposition, action, and therapy in infants and children. N Engl J Med 349:1157–1167, 2003.
32. DeBele RC, Vaupshas V, Bitullo BB, et al. Intestinal absorption of bile salts: immature development in the neonate. J Pediatr 94:472–476, 2979.

33. Stewart CF, Hampton EM. Effect of maturation on drug disposition in pediatric patients. Clin Pharm 6:548–564, 1987.
34. Berseth CL. Gestational evolution of small intestine motility in preterm and term infants. J Pediatr 115:646–651, 1989.
35. Kearns GL. Impact of developmental pharmacology on pediatric study design: overcoming the challenges. J Allergy Clin Immunol 106:S128–S138, 2000.
36. Alcorn J, McNamara PJ. Ontogeny of hepatic and renal systemic clearance pathways in infants. Clin Pharmacokinet 41:959–998, 2002.
37. Menon PA, Thach BT, Smith CH, et al. Benzyl alcohol toxicity in neonatal intensive care unit. Incidence, symptomatology and mortality. Am J Perinatol 1:288–292, 1984.
38. Merkus PJFM, Have-Opbroek AAW, Quanjer PH. Human lung growth: a review. Pediatr Pulmonol 21:383–397, 1996.
39. Michalets EL. Update: clinically significant cytrochrome P-450 drug interactions. Pharmacotherapy 18:84–112, 1998.
40. Bhatt-Mehta V, Nahata MC. Dopamine and dobutamine in pediatric therapy. Pharmacotherapy 9:303–314, 1989.
41. Robin C, Trieger N. Paradoxical reactions to benzodiazepines in intravenous sedation: a report of 2 cases and review of the literature. Anesth Prog 49:128–132, 2002.
42. Schwartz GJ, Brion LP, Spitzer A. The use of plasma creatinine concentration for estimating glomerular filtration rate in infants, children, and adolescents. Pediatr Clin North Am 34:571–590, 1987.
43. Traub SL, Johnson CE. Comparison of methods of estimating creatinine clearance in children. Am J Hosp Pharm 37:195–201, 1980.
44. Stoklosa MJ, Ansel HC, eds. Calculation of doses. In: Pharmaceutical calculations. 8th ed. Philadelphia: Lea & Febiger, 1986.
45. Monsteller RD. Simplified calculation of body surface area. N Engl J Med 317:1098, 1987.
46. Mitchell JF. Oral dosage forms that should not be crushed. Hosp Pharm 35:553–567, 2000.
47. Pawar S, Kumar A. Issues in the formulation of drugs for oral use in children, role of excipients. Pediatr Drugs 4:371–379, 2002.
48. Raju TN, Kecskes S, Thornton JP, et al. Medication errors in neonatal and paediatric intensive-care units. Lancet 2:374–376, 1989.
49. Perlstein PH, Callison C, White M, et al. Errors in drug computations during newborn intensive care. Am J Dis Child 133:376–379, 1979.
50. Committee on Drugs, American Academy of Pediatrics. ''Inactive'' ingredients in pharmaceutical products: update (subject review). Pediatrics 99:268–278, 1997.
51. US Food and Drug Administration Center for Biologics Evaluation and Research. Thiomersal in vaccines. Available at: http://www.fda.gov/cber/vaccine/thimerosal.htm#pres. Accessed May 18, 2004.
52. US Department of Health and Human Services, Food and Drug Administration. Aluminum in large and small volume parenterals used in total parenteral nutrition. Fed Regist 68:32981, 2003.
53. Ernst JA, Williams JM, Glick MR, Lemons JA. Osmolality of substances used in the intensive care nursery. Pediatrics 72:347–352, 1983.
54. Leff RD, Roberts RJ. Problems in pediatric drug therapy. Am J Hosp Pharm 44:865–870, 1987.
55. Doenicke A, Nebauer AE, Hoernecke R, et al. Osmolalities of propylene-glycol containing drug formulations for parenteral use.

56. Glascow AM, Boeckx RL, Miller MK, et al. Hyperosmolality in small infants due to propylene glycol. Pediatrics 72:353–355, 1983.
57. Gauderer MW. Vascular access techniques and devices in the pediatric patient. Surg Clin North Am 72:1267–1284, 1992.
58. Marcoux C, Fisher S, Wong D. Central venous access devices in children. Pediatr Nurs 16:123–133, 1990.
59. Roberts RJ. Intravenous administration of medication in pediatric patients: problems and solutions. Pediatr Clin North Am 28:23–34, 1981.
60. Gould T, Roberts RJ. Therapeutic problems arising from the use of the intravenous route for drug administration. J Pediatr 95:465–471, 1979.
61. McLeroy PA. The rule of six: calculating intravenous infusions in a pediatric crisis situation. Hosp Pharm 29:939–940, 1994.
62. Pinheiro JM, Mitchell AL, Lesar TS. Systematic steps to diminish multi-fold medication errors in neonates. J Pediatr Pharmacol Ther 8:266–273, 2003.
63. Committee on Drugs, American Academy of Pediatrics. Alternative routes of drug administration. Advantages and disadvantages (subject review). Pediatrics 100:143–152, 1997.
64. De Benedictis FM, Selvaggio D. Use of inhaler devices in pediatric asthma. Pediatr Drugs 5:629–638, 2003.
65. Delgado A, Chou KJ, Silver EJ, et al. Nebulizers vs metered-dose inhalers with spacers for bronchodilator therapy to treat wheezing in children aged 2–24 months in a pediatric emergency department. Arch Pediatr Adolesc Med 157:76–80, 2003.
66. O'Callaghan C, Barry PW. How to choose delivery devices for asthma. Arch Dis Child 82:185–187, 2000.
67. Everard ML. Guidelines for devices and choices. J Aerosol Med 14:S59–S64, 2001.
68. Matsui DM. Drug compliance in pediatrics. Clinical and research issues. Pediatr Clin North Am 44:2–14, 1997.
69. Ramgoolam A, Steele R. Formulations of antibiotics for children in primary care. Effects on compliance and efficacy. Pediatr Drugs 4:323–333, 2002.
70. Shemesh E, Shneider BL, Savitzky JK, et al. Medication adherence in pediatric and adolescent liver transplant patients. Pediatrics 113:825–832, 2004.
71. Rianthavorn P, Ettenger RB, Malekzadeh M, et al. Noncompliance with immunosuppressive medications in pediatric and adolescent patients receiving solid-organ transplants. Transplantation 77:778–782, 2004.
72. Hack S, Chow B. Pediatric psychotropic medication compliance: a literature review and research-based suggestions for improving treatment compliance. J Child Adolesc Psychopharmacol 11:59–67, 2001.
73. Committee on Drugs, American Academy of Pediatrics. Prevention of medication errors in the pediatric inpatient setting. Pediatrics 102:428–430, 1998.
74. Levine SR, Cohen MR, Blanchard NR, et al. Guidelines for preventing medication errors in pediatrics. J Pediatr Pharmacol Ther 6:246–262, 2001.
75. Institute for Safe Medication Practices. ISMP list of error prone abbreviations, symbols, and dose designations. Available at: http://www.ismp.org/PDF/ErrorProne.pdf. Accessed May 18, 2004.

Pediatric Nutrition Support

Emily B. Hak and Richard A. Helms

16

5

TREATMENT GOALS

- Provide nutrients for basal requirements, growth and development, wound healing, and recovery from acute illness.
- Use the gastrointestinal tract whenever possible.
- Provide nutrients in a safe and effective manner.
- Continually evaluate response and adjust nutrient intake according to growth and age, with consideration of underlying conditions.
- Engage patient, parents, and caregivers in nutrition management.
- Instill healthy eating habits in all people.

In addition to basal requirements, pediatric patients require nutrients to meet the demands of growth and development. Failure to obtain essential nutrients can result in growth retardation, immune system impairment, and neurologic deficits. The premature neonate presents a unique nutritional challenge because transition to the extrauterine environment occurs during a period of rapid lean body mass accretion, micronutrient accretion, and organ development. Thus, preterm neonates require early nutritional intervention, often with a combination of parenteral and enteral feedings.

Enteral formulas have been developed to meet the specialized nutrient needs of preterm and term infants who are not fed human milk. Commercially available enteral formulas have been designed to meet the nutritional requirements of older children who are unable to eat by mouth. Infants and children who cannot or should not be fed enterally can be provided adequate nutrition through the parenteral route. Standards have been developed to assist the clinician with appropriate nutrition therapies in children who require specialized nutrition support.[1]

Of significant importance is the recent dramatic increase in obesity in children that relates to an increase in sedentary lifestyle and the intake of large amounts of foods that are high in caloric and salt content. The impact of this change is directly related to the increased incidence in children of type 2 diabetes and polycystic ovarian syndrome and their associated morbidities.

ENTERAL NUTRITION IN HEALTHY INFANTS, CHILDREN, AND ADOLESCENTS

From 1941 until 1997, the Recommended Dietary Allowance (RDA) recommended nutrient intakes that would prevent disease caused by nutrient deficiency in most people.[2] In 1997, the Food and Nutrition Board of the Institute of Medicine reevaluated this approach and created a family of nutrient reference values with the broad heading of *Dietary Reference Intakes (DRI)*. DRI includes the RDA, the Estimated Average Requirement, the Adequate Intake (AI), the Tolerable Upper Intake Level, and others. The DRI for macronutrients in children is shown in Table 16.1. Energy required for growth is greatest during the newborn period, and, as infants grow, the overall caloric requirement increases, but the number of kilocalories required per kilogram de-

TABLE 16.1	Dietary Reference Intakes (DRI) of Macronutrients		
	Protein (g/kg)	Carbohydrate (g/d)	Total Fat (g/d)
0–6 months	1.5	60	31
6 months–1 year	1.5	95	30
>1–3 years	1.1	130	30–40[a]
4–13 years	0.95	130	25–35[a]
14–18 years	0.85	130	25–35[a]

[a] Acceptable Macronutrient Distribution Range associated with reduced risk of chronic disease and provides intakes of essential nutrients.

creases. From infancy to childhood, protein requirements decrease more rapidly than energy requirements. This reflects an increase in activity (requiring energy) and a decrease in growth rates (requiring protein). The DRIs for vitamins and minerals in infants and children are listed in Table 16.2. These recommendations are derived from population-based data; therefore, an individual patient may require more or less of a particular nutrient. For example, patients with cystic fibrosis require greater quantities of fat-soluble vitamins because they malabsorb fat.[3] Premature infants may require additional vitamin supplementation.[4]

INFANTS

Breast-feeding. The American Academy of Pediatrics recommends exclusive breast-feeding for the first 6 months of life.[5] When the child reaches 6 months of age, the diet can be supplemented with iron-rich foods; however, breast-feeding should continue until at least 12 months of age. Human milk is the most appropriate food for the vast majority of infants; it contains proteins of better biologic value (more whey than casein), more easily absorbed fat, immunoglobulins, lysozymes, antistreptococcal enzymes, complement, lactoferrin, and macrophages. In addition, the extra nutrient intake required by the mother costs about $400 less annually per child than the cost of infant formula.[5] Infants in the United States, Canada, Europe, and other developed countries who breast-feed have a lower incidence of gastrointestinal disease, including diarrhea and necrotizing enterocolitis, respiratory disease, bacteremia, meningitis, otitis media, and botulism.[5,6] Evidence is mounting that breast-feeding is somewhat protective against early-onset diabetes, Crohn's disease, ulcerative colitis, and allergy.[5,7] Breast-feeding also provides advantages for the mother; it enhances postpartum recovery, returns women to their prepartum weight more quickly, and enhances maternal-infant bonding.[5] Breast-feeding is usually supplemented with other types of iron-rich food in the child older than 6 months of age.

Difficulties can be encountered with breast-feeding. The mother must want to nurse if it is to be a satisfactory and rewarding experience for her and for her infant. Initially, the

TABLE 16.2	Dietary Reference Intakes for 14 Nutrients[a]							
	0–6 months	6–12 months	1–3 years	4–8 years	9–13 years, male	14–18 years, male	9–13 years, female	14–18 years, female
Thiamine (mg)	0.2	0.3	0.5	0.6	0.9	1.2	0.9	1
Riboflavin (mg)	0.3	0.4	0.5	0.6	0.9	1.3	0.9	1
Niacin (mg NE[b])	2[c]	4	6	8	12	16	12	14
Vitamin B$_6$ (mg)	0.1	0.3	0.5	0.6	1	1.3	1	1.2
Folate (µg DFE[d])	65	80	150	200	300	400	300	400
Vitamin B$_{12}$ (µg)	0.4	0.5	0.9	1.2	1.8	2.4	1.8	2.4
Phosphorus (mg)	100	275	460	500	1,250	1,250	1,250	1,250
Magnesium (mg)	30	75	80	130	240	410	240	360
Vitamin D (µg)	5	5	5	5	5	5	5	5
Pantothenic acid (mg)	1.7	1.8	2	3	4	5	4	5
Biotin (µg)	5	6	8	12	20	25	20	25
Choline (mg)	125	150	200	250	375	550	375	400
Calcium (mg)	210	270	500	800	1,300	1,300	1,300	1,300
Fluoride (mg)	0.01	0.5	0.7	1	2	3	2	3

[a] From the Food and Nutrition Board—National Academy of Sciences, 2004.
[b] Niacin equivalents.
[c] Milligrams of preformed niacin.
[d] Dietary folate equivalent.

nipples may be tender and breasts may become engorged and sore until the milk supply adapts to meet the demands of the infant. The breasts can be conditioned for nursing during the last trimester of pregnancy to minimize painful, sore nipples. The nursing mother should have a balanced diet and should ingest adequate nutrients and fluids to maintain her own health and promote adequate milk production.

Normal Composition of Human Milk. The composition of milk is determined by the mammary gland, with little or no external control.[8] Human milk occurs in three forms: colostrum, transitional milk, and mature milk. Colostrum, which serves as a precursor of milk, may be expressed from the breasts as early as the fourth month of pregnancy, but it usually appears after parturition. Colostrum production is low until the third or fourth day after delivery and usually continues for up to 5 days. It has, however, been reported to occur for as long as 10 days. Colostrum is a transudate that has undergone fatty degeneration and that consists primarily of serum albumin (3% to 5%) and cast-off epithelium (colostrum corpuscles). Compared with mature milk, the specific gravity is higher (1.030 to 1.060 vs. 1.026 to 1.036) and the average pH is higher (6.8 vs. 7.7). Colostrum is richer in vitamin A, sodium, potassium, and other minerals but lower in sugar and fat than mature milk.

Transitional milk is produced within the first week of breast-feeding and usually lasts for a few weeks, during which time fat and sugar content increase while protein and mineral concentrations decrease. Milk finally matures near the end of the first month of lactation. Mature milk comprises 0.9% to 1.6% protein, 2% to 6% fat, and 6.5% to 8% lactose. The composition of milk at the beginning of a feeding is highest in protein and lowest in fat. The hind milk composition, milk produced at the end of the feeding, is higher in fat and lower in protein. The effect of this on the excretion of drugs in breast milk is unknown.

Once established, mature milk changes little in composition.[8] If the mother has adequate nutritional intake, her diet can be varied with no effect on milk composition or volume. A deficiency in the maternal diet will at first cause a decrease in the quantity of milk but will not affect milk composition unless the mother's tissue stores are depleted. Decreased water intake causes maternal thirst before it affects milk production.

Control of Milk Production. Although the initiation and maintenance of human milk production have not been adequately studied, certain physiologic and endocrine factors that occur during lactation have been elucidated.[9,10] The inhibition of lactation during pregnancy is assumed to be the result of high estrogen or progesterone levels. Estrogen may work in part by affecting prolactin (lactogenic factor), which is secreted from the anterior pituitary. The effects of estrogen on milk secretion are dose dependent. At low endogenous levels, such as those that occur post partum, milk secretion occurs. High doses of estrogen (such as those that result from diethylstilbestrol given postpartum) inhibit lactation. In most women, low-dose oral contraceptives do not decrease lactation, even when given immediately post partum.[9]

During pregnancy, prolactin, estrogen, progesterone, and human growth hormone stimulate breast development. Prolactin concentrations are high during pregnancy and breast-feeding but decrease after birth in the absence of breast-feeding. If breast-feeding is successful and unrestricted, the increased prolactin concentration has been reported to be contraceptive in some societies in which breast-feeding is used almost exclusively.[9] This has not been observed in the United States, where infants are often supplemented with infant formula. The posterior pituitary, in addition to the anterior pituitary, is involved and stimulated when an infant breast-feeds. The release of oxytocin by the posterior pituitary initiates the "let-down" reflex—the expression or ejection of milk from the breast—whereas prolactin stimulates milk production. The let-down reflex is responsive to other internal and external factors. The actions and sounds associated with nursing, such as an infant crying, can stimulate this reflex.

The quantity of milk produced depends upon the demands of the infant. If the infant's demand increases, milk supply will adjust accordingly within 2 days, and vice versa. The actual secretion of milk is a discontinuous process. During feeding, milk secretion increases as a result of depleted milk stores. It is likely that drugs are excreted into milk in larger amounts when the milk is being actively secreted. See Chapter 19 for a discussion of drugs that are excreted in breast milk.

Factors That Interfere with Breast-feeding. Infants who are born prematurely are often unable to be breast-fed because of the need for ventilatory support or immaturity of the gastrointestinal tract. These infants can be fed human milk provided by their mothers via feeding tube. Most pediatric hospitals have lactation consultants to provide emotional support for these mothers and rooms where they can pump their breasts. The milk obtained can be refrigerated or frozen until the infant can be enterally fed. Pumping allows a mother to maintain lactation until her baby can be put to her breast. Although human milk is considered to be the ideal food for infants, supplements such as human milk fortifier may be added to human milk to enhance the nutrient content.

A mother should not breast-feed if she has active, untreated tuberculosis, breast cancer, or a serious infection. In the United States, women who are infected with the human immunodeficiency virus (HIV) should not breast-feed because of the risk of viral transmission to the baby. Many drugs are secreted in breast milk and may accumulate within or be harmful to the infant. As with women who are contemplating pregnancy, a mother who is taking medications daily should discuss this with her physician before making the decision to breast-feed. Nursing mothers should consult with their physicians about the appropriateness of any medication prescribed while nursing. See Chapter 19 on pregnancy and lactation for additional information.

Social factors may interfere with breast-feeding. Because it is impossible to know just how much milk the infant ingests, it is easy to believe that the infant is hungry shortly after having nursed just because he or she cries. First-time parents get a lot of well-intentioned advice about supplementing breast-feeding with infant formula. This practice can have a negative impact on milk production, especially if it is implemented early. In many cases, the active support and encouragement of health care personnel overcome most, if not all, maternal apprehension about breast-feeding.

Distractions such as fright, pain, and emotional distress can inhibit milk expression. It is hypothesized that the high concentrations of catecholamines, adrenaline, and norepinephrine that are produced in such circumstances cause vasoconstriction in the mammary circulation that prevents oxytocin from reaching the contractile cells.[7,10] Excessive doses of medications that also release endogenous catecholamines (e.g., amphetamines, most decongestants) may interfere with milk secretion.

Infants who are breast-fed may develop indirect hyperbilirubinemia or physiologic jaundice,[11] and it is speculated that a factor found in human milk may inhibit the conjugation of indirect bilirubin. The concern is that indirect bilirubin may cross the blood–brain barrier of neonates and cause kernicterus. This can be managed in several different ways. The infant can be bottle-fed for a time and when the bilirubin decreases, breast-feeding can resume. Phototherapy may be used. Some clinicians advocate continuing to breast-feed and monitor bilirubin concentrations closely to make sure they do not exceed some arbitrary concentration. Others advocate increasing the frequency of putting the infant to the breast for a feeding.

Standard Infant Formulas. The nutrient distribution in standard infant formulas that are available for infants younger than 1 year of age reflects their distribution in human milk. The composition of these products is similar (Table 16.3), and they contain 20 kcal per ounce when reconstituted according to the standard formula. Healthy young infants require from 85 to 120 kcal/kg/day to grow. This is equal to about 15 to 23 mL per kg of a standard infant formula given every 3 hours (or about 120 to 180 mL/kg/day).

Infant formulas have an osmotic load similar to that of human milk (277 to 303 mOsm/kg); this prevents diarrhea that may be induced by a high osmotic load. Cow's milk protein is commonly used as the protein source; it has less whey, the most easily digested protein, and more casein than human milk. Further, human milk contains very long chain omega-3 fatty acids. Infants are unable to conjugate long-chain fatty acids into very long chain products; therefore, infant formulas were developed that are supplemented with docosahexaenoic acid (DHA) and arachidonic acid (ARA). Studies have shown an improvement in visual and cognitive development in infants who received the supplemented product compared with those who did not receive DHA and ARA

supplements.[12,13] The protein and micronutrient content of cow's milk render it inappropriate for those younger than 12 months of age. Infants have developed an iron deficiency anemia from cow's milk ingestion.

Formula Reconstitution. Formulas are available as ready-to-feed products (usually 20 kcal per ounce), concentrated liquids, or dry powders. Before it is used, formula should be stored in a cool, dry place because temperature extremes can cause irreversible physical and chemical changes. Ready-to-feed formula should not be diluted unless a dilute formula has been prescribed. Of note, dry powder formulas, including human milk fortifier, are not sterile and may be intrinsically contaminated with *Enterobacter sakazakii*, as well as other bacteria that are usually nonpathogenic. In sick neonates, outbreaks of infection and at least one death have been reported.[14] Therefore, it is recommended that dry powder formulas not be used in sick neonates.

Concentrated liquid and dry powder formulas require dilution or reconstitution before feeding. Instructions for the amount of water to be added are provided on each container. Standard reconstitution results in a formula with 20 kcal per ounce. Regular tap water that meets federal drinking water standards is acceptable for reconstituting formula. However, in certain situations, sterilization of tap water before reconstitution, such as in the case of well water, may be necessary. Chemically softened water contains salts and should not be used to reconstitute infant formula. Commercially prepared sterile water is not necessary for formula preparation at home. Most city water supplies are fluoridated; however, sterile water and well water are not fluoridated, and supplementation may be required. Products can be reconstituted with less water so that they contain 24, 27, or 30 kcal per ounce. When formulas are concentrated in this manner, the protein, electrolyte, and mineral concentrations are also increased.

Formula preparation should take place in a clean area, with the use of clean utensils. The person who prepares the formula should have clean hands and should use good technique to avoid contaminating the formula during reconstitution. Immediately after concentrated formula is reconstituted or a ready-to-feed multiple-use container is opened, the portion required for an individual feeding should be put into an appropriate bottle for feeding, and the remainder should be stored in a clean container in the refrigerator. After the infant has begun feeding, any formula left in the bottle after 2 hours should be discarded. Reconstituted formula can be stored in the refrigerator for up to 24 hours.

After the initial opening, formula powder can be covered and stored in a cool, dry place for up to 4 weeks in the original container. Refrigeration is not necessary. However, opened liquid formula (ready-to-feed or concentrate) should be stored in the original container in the refrigerator and may be used only for up to 48 hours after opening. Reconstituted formula should be discarded if not used within 24 hours.

TABLE 16.3 | Composition of Human Milk and Infant Formulas[a]

	Kcal/oz	Carbohydrate Source	Protein Source	Fat Source	CHO[b] (g)	PRO (g)	Fat (g)	Na (mEq)	K (mEq)	mg Ca/mg P	Fe (mg)	mOsm/kg H₂O
Human milk (term)[c] Standard infant	20	Lactose			10.7	1.6	5.8	1.2	2	42/21	0.04	
Enfamil LIPIL with Iron	20	Lactose	Whey, nonfat milk	Palm olein, soy, coconut, sunflower oils, DHA[d], ARA[e]	10.9	2.1	5.3	1.2	2.8	78/53	1.8	
Similac Advance	20	Lactose	Nonfat milk, whey protein concentrate	Safflower, soy, coconut oils, 0.15% DHA, 0.4% ARA	10.8	2.07	5.4	1	2.7	73/42	1.8	300
Premature Transitional												
Enfamil Premature LIPIL	20	Corn syrup solids, lactose	Nonfat milk, whey protein	Soy, sunflower or safflower oil, MCT (40%) DHA, ARA	11	3	5.1	2.5	2.5	165/83	0.5	240
Similac Neosure Advance	22	Corn syrup solids, lactose	Nonfat milk, whey protein concentrate	Soy, coconut, MCT[f] (24.9%), 0.15% DHA, 0.4% ARA	10.3	2.6	5.5	1.4	3.6	105/62	1.8	250
Similac Special Care Advance with Iron 20	20	Corn syrup solids, lactose	Nonfat milk, whey protein concentrate	MCT (50%), soy and coconut oils, 0.25% DHA, 0.4% ARA	10.6	2.71	5.43	1.9	3.3	180/100	1.8	235

[a] Formula contents are reported for the ready-to-use product. Some specific nutrients may differ for powder formulas. Changes in formula contents are possible. The authors suggest referring to the most recent publication of product literature or consulting clinical dietetics for product information.
[b] Contents of CHO, PRO, fat, Na, K, Ca, P, and Fe are per 100 kcal.
[c] Composition may vary according to reference used.
[d] Docosahexanoic acid.
[e] Arachidonic acid.
[f] Medium-chain triglycerides.

Smaller infants should be fed formula that is not cooler than room temperature, and some infants prefer warmed formula. Older infants do not require warmed formula but may prefer it. The bottle with the required amount of formula for a single feeding can be warmed with warm, running tap water. If a bottle warmer is used, electric warmers are preferred over water-containing warmers because of the potential for bacterial contamination of the water contained in the warmer. Microwaves should never be used to warm infant formula because hot spots can develop and the infant may be burned. In addition, the excessive heat can physically alter the formula and degrade the nutrients.

Infant Formula Supplements. Some infants require more concentrated formula because of fluid considerations. In lieu of concentrating formulas, the caloric content can be enhanced by adding modular components such as carbohydrate (e.g., polycose) or fat (e.g., MCT Oil, Microlipid, Novartis Medical Nutrition, Minneapolis, Minnesota). The manufacturers recommend that medications not be added to infant formula because of potential drug-nutrient interactions. Because of the risk for botulism, neither honey nor corn syrup should be given to young infants.

Introduction of Solid Food. Solid food can be introduced at about 6 months of age. The foods used should be those with the least possible added salt, sugar, and monosodium glutamate. These substances are added to improve taste for increased adult acceptability. It has been speculated that increased sodium intake during infancy causes an increase in blood pressure later in life. However, when infants received low or high sodium from age 3 to 8 months, no difference in blood pressure was observed at 1 and 8 years.[15] Because increased sodium intake is associated with hypertension, it would seem prudent to choose low-salt prepared foods such as canned vegetables and to discourage the addition of salt to foods.

New foods should be added one at a time. Usually, plain rice cereal or applesauce is started. If the infant tolerates this, then another food can be tried. The daily intake of infant foods for the 8 to 12 month old should consist of two or more servings of meat, four or more servings of vegetables, one or more servings of citrus fruits, and four or more servings of bread or cereal. The size of each serving should increase as the child grows. Junior foods that contain small chunks of solid food are usually begun at 8 to 12 months of age. Cow's milk can be added to the diet at 12 months of age. Adult table food is usually begun at 1 year of age. Note that round foods such as hot dogs, sausage links, and hard candy can occlude the airway and result in asphyxiation, even in older children. These foods should be cut into a small size for young children or avoided. If the child receives a normal, varied diet that contains the required nutrients, no added supplements are needed. Vitamins and minerals should be used only if the diet is incomplete, such as with a vegan diet, or when nutritional deficiencies have been documented. If the water supply is deficient in fluoride (<0.3 ppm), the infant should be supplemented from 6 months to 3 years of age.[5]

TABLE 16.4	Suggested Portion Sizes for Children (those 2 to 3 years old should use smaller portions)
Milk	1 cup
1½ oz natural cheese	Two 9-volt batteries
2–3 oz lean meat, fish, poultry	Deck of cards
Raw vegetables	Baseball
Cooked vegetables	Small fist
1 slice bread	
Cooked cereal, rice, pasta	Small fist

Children 2 to 3 years old should use smaller portions.

CHILDREN AND ADOLESCENTS

Normal healthy children should follow the guidelines set out by the U.S. Department of Agriculture food pyramid, which can be accessed at http://www.usda.gov/cnpp/KidsPyra/. One problem for both children and adults involves determining an appropriate portion size. In general, portion sizes for those 4 years of age and older are shown in Table 16.4, and suggested numbers of portions per day are shown in Table 16.5. Note that active teenage boys require about 2,800 kilocalories per day, and girls require about 2,200 kilocalories per day.

A significant problem today is the increasing prevalence of excess weight and obesity among children.[16] Lifestyle factors that have been associated with this obesity epidemic include an increasing intake of carbonated beverages, the supersizing of meals, and a more sedentary lifestyle. The consumption of soft drinks provides significant carbohydrate calories, and these drinks often replace milk in the diet. The brown colas contain phosphoric acid that can bind calcium and prevent its absorption from the gastrointestinal tract. Thus, multiple dietary factors may adversely affect bone metabolism. A sedentary lifestyle has also been associated with obesity. One study found that not only was an increased body mass index associated with television and video games, but increased watching of television and use of video games were associated with greater intakes of soft drinks, fast foods, and snacks.[17]

SPECIALIZED NUTRITION SUPPORT

Those who are unable to select their food or orally ingest nutritional substrate may require specialized nutrition that is given enterally or parenterally.[1] In some cases, a combined approach that uses both enteral and parenteral nutrition is optimal.

TABLE 16.5	Suggested Number of Portions Per Day According to Age		
Food Group	Children 2–6 years, Women, Some Older Adults (~1,600 kcal)	Older Children, Teen Girls, Active Women, Most Men (~2,200 kcal)	Teen Boys, Active Men (~2,800 kcal)
Bread, cereal, rice, pasta (grains, especially whole grain)	6	9	11
Vegetable group	3	4	5
Fruit group	2	3	4
Milk, yogurt, cheese (preferably fat free or low fat)	2 or 3[a]	2 or 3[a]	2 or 3[a]
Meat, poultry, fish, dry beans, eggs, and nuts (preferably lean or low fat)	2 (5 oz)	2 (6 oz)	3 (7 oz)

[a]3 servings for women who are pregnant or breast-feeding, teenagers, and young adults under 24 years of age.

ENTERAL NUTRITION

The gastrointestinal tract should be used to provide nutrition whenever possible.

Premature Infant. Premature infant formulas are available to meet the needs of infants with immature gastrointestinal tracts (Table 16.3).[4] Protein, carbohydrate, and fat components of these products require less complex digestive processes. These formulas contain primarily whey protein, which forms smaller curds that are more easily digested than casein. In addition, whey protein has an amino acid composition that is high in cysteine and low in tyrosine, making it more desirable for the premature infant with immature enzymatic pathways (the Protein Requirements section provides a more detailed discussion). Lactose, a reducing sugar, is the carbohydrate found in human milk; however, low-lactase activity has been noted to occur in the intestinal mucosa of premature infants. Thus, the lactose content of preterm formulas has been limited to 40% to 50% of the available carbohydrate. The remaining carbohydrate is provided in the form of maltodextrins or "corn syrup," which is a mixture of monosaccharides, oligosaccharides, and polysaccharides that relies on multiple digestive and absorptive pathways, which results in enhanced usage.

Premature infants frequently have a decreased ability to digest long-chain triglycerides (LCTs) because of reduced bile acid pool size and limited pancreatic lipase activity. Up to 50% of fat in these formulas is provided as medium-chain triglycerides (MCTs) that do not require bile acids for solubilization or carnitine for transport into the mitochondria, where β-oxidation occurs. Linoleic acid, a long-chain fatty acid, prevents essential fatty acid deficiency; between 2% and 4% of caloric requirements must be supplied as linoleic acid to prevent deficiency. This is easily attained with the use of premature infant formulas because about half of the fat content occurs in the form of long-chain fatty acids.

Protein in the specialized infant formulas (Nutramigen, Pregestimil, Alimentum, and Neocate) takes the form of free amino acids or peptides that result from partial acid hydrolysis of cow's milk (Table 16.6). The protein in these formulas is easily digestible; thus, they may be appropriate for infants with intestinal resection, cow's milk allergy, or other protein allergies. The fat content of Pregestimil and Alimentum is similar, with about 50% MCTs; Nutramigen includes 100% of its fat as LCTs.

Lactose- and sucrose-free formulas (i.e., Isomil, Prosobee; Table 16.6) are also available for infants with disaccharidase deficiency or specific types of carbohydrate intolerance. Because all these formulas contain hypoallergenic soy protein, they may be indicated if cow's milk allergy is suspected.

Low–renal solute formulas (e.g., Similac PM 60/40) contain less sodium than is found in other specialized formulas; these are indicated when low sodium intake is desirable (Table 16.6). Although these formulas have a whey-to-casein protein concentration ratio of 60/40 (more like human milk), the carbohydrate content is lactose.

Formulas for Children between 1 and 10 Years of Age. Table 16.7 shows the nutrient content of several different enteral formulas designed for children. The protein concentration in these products is equal to or greater than that found in infant formulas; the percentage of carbohydrate is usually greater and fat is usually less compared with infant formulas. Unlike infant formulas, formulas for children contain equimolar amounts of calcium and phosphorus, and the renal solute load is greater. Vivonex Pediatric is designed for children who require a more elemental feeding solution. Portagen contains 87% of fat as MCTs. MCTs are not transported through the lymphatic system; Portagen has been used in patients with chylothorax because chyle production is minimized with this formula. Because of the low quantity of LCTs, children who receive Portagen may require supplemental LCTs if this product is used for extended periods.

TABLE 16.6 Specialized Infant Formulas[a,b]

	kcal/oz	Carbohydrate Source	Protein Source	Fat Source	CHO (g)	PRO (g)	Fat (g)	Na (mEq)	K (mEq)	mg Ca /mg P	Fe (mg)	mOsm/ kg H₂O
Hypoallergenic												
Enfamil Pregestimil	20	Corn syrup solids, modified corn starch, dextrose	Casein hydrolysates, amino acids	Soy, MCT (55%), safflower oils	10.2	2.8	5.6	2	2.8	115/75	1.88	280
Enfamil Nutramigen LIPIL	20	Corn syrup solids, modified corn starch	Casein hydrolysates, amino acids	Palm olein, soy, coconut, sunflower oil, DHA, ARA	10.3	2.8	5.3	2	2.8	94/63	1.8	
Similac Alimentum Advance	20	Sucrose, modified tapioca starch	Casein hydrolysates, amino acids	Safflower, MCT (33%), soy oils (0.15% DHA, 0.4% ARA)	10.2	2.75	5.54	1.9	3	105/75	1.8	370
SHS Neocate	20	Corn syrup solids	Amino acids	Safflower, coconut, soy oils	11.7	3.1	4.5	1.6	4	124/93.1	1.85	375
Soy formulas												
Similac Isomil	20	Corn syrup, sucrose	Soy protein isolate, L-methionine	Safflower, coconut, and soy oils	10.3	2.45	5.46	1.9	2.8	105/75	1.8	200
Enfamil ProSobee	20	Corn syrup solids	Soy protein isolate	Palm olein, soy, coconut, sunflower oils, DHA, ARA	10.6	2.5	5.3	1.6	3.1	105/83	1.8	
Infants with hypocalcemia												
Similac PM 60/40	20	Lactose	Whey (60%) protein concentrate, sodium caseinate (40%)	Corn, coconut, soy oils	10.2	2.2	5.59	1	2.2	56/28	0.7	280
Lactose free												
Enfamil Lactofree LIPIL®	20	Corn syrup solids	Milk protein	Palm olein, soy, coconut, sunflower oils, DHA, ARA	10.9	2.1	5.3	1.3	2.8	82/55	1.8	
Similac Lactose Free Advance	20	Maltodextrin, sucrose	Milk protein	Safflower, soy, coconut oils, DHA, ARA	10.7	2.14	5.4	1.3	2.7	84/56	1.8	200

a Formula contents are reported for the ready-to-use product. Some specific nutrients may differ for powder formulas. Changes in formula contents are possible. The authors suggest referring to the most recent publication of product literature or consulting clinical dietetics for product information.
b Contents of CHO, PRO, fat, Na, K, Ca, P, and Fe are per 100 kcal.

TABLE 16.7	Formulas for Children From 1 to 10 Years of Age[a]											
	kcal/oz	Carbohydrate Source	Protein Source	Fat Source	CHO (g)	PRO (g)	Fat (g)	Na (mEq)	K (mEq)	mg Ca/ mg P	Fe (mg)	mOsm/ kg H₂O
Enfamil Kindercal	31.8	Sugar and maltodextrin	Milk protein concentrate	Canola, corn, and sunflower oils, MCT	12.8	2.8	4.2	1.5	3.2	96/80	1	440
Pediasure	30	Sucrose and maltodextrin	Sodium caseinate and whey protein	Safflower and soy oils, MCT (20%)	11	3	4.98	1.7	3.3	97/80	1.4	430[c]
Peptamen Junior (unflavored)	30	Maltodextrin	Whey-based peptides	Soybean oil, canola oil, MCT (60%)	13.7	3	3.8	2	3.4	100/80	1.4	260[d]
Portagen	30	Corn syrup solids, sugar	Milk protein, sodium caseinate	MCT (87%), corn oil	11.48	3.5	4.68	2.4	3.2	94/70	1.9	350
Vivonex Pediatric	24	Maltodextrin, modified cornstarch	Free amino acids	MCT (68%), soybean oil	15.8	3	3	2.1	3.9	122/100	1.3	360

[a] Formula contents are reported for the ready-to-use product. Some specific nutrients may differ for powder formulas. Changes in formula contents are possible. The authors suggest referring to the most recent publication of product literature or consulting clinical dietetics for product information.
[b] Contents of CHO, PRO, fat, Na, K, Ca, P, and Fe are per 100 kcal.
[c] Chocolate flavored variety has 520 mOsm/kg H₂O.
[d] Vanilla flavored variety has 360 mOsm/kg H₂O.

TABLE 16.8	Kilocalories, Dextrose, Rice Syrup Solids, Electrolytes (mEq/L), and Osmolality (mOsm) of Infant Electrolyte Solutions							
	kcal	Dextrose (g)	Rice Syrup Solids (g)	Na$^+$	K$^+$	Cl$^-$	Citrate	mOsm
CeraLyte 50	160		40	50	20	40	30	220
CeraLyte 70	160		40	70	20	60	30	235
CeraLyte 90	160		40	90	20	80	30	260
Enfalyte	126		30	50	25	45	34	170
Pedialyte	100	25		45	20	35	30	250
Rehydralyte	100	25		75	20	65	30	300
ReVital	100	25		45	20	35	30	250
WHO/UNICEF	80	20		90	20	80	30	311
WHO/UNICEF reduced osmolarity	54	13.5[a]		75	20	65	10	245

[a] Anhydrous glucose.

Oral Rehydration during Disease. Oral electrolyte solutions are available for maintenance of fluid and electrolyte balance during mild to moderate diarrhea (Table 16.8). Rehydralyte contains more sodium and is better suited for use in infants with moderate to severe diarrhea than are products that contain less sodium. More recently developed oral rehydration solutions contain complex carbohydrate, rice syrup solids, instead of dextrose/glucose. Solutions with lower osmolality seem to be better tolerated; this has led to the reformulation of the World Health Organization (WHO)/United Nations Children's Fund (UNICEF) solution.

Routes of Enteral Feeding. The significance of the gastrointestinal tract in immune function has been recognized, and early enteral feedings are encouraged whenever possible, even in critically ill patients. Feeding tubes are placed soon after injury in patients with burns or after trauma, and, as with premature infants, continuous low-volume enteral feedings are started and advanced as tolerated. In many patients, parenteral nutrition can be avoided entirely. In those who cannot tolerate formula advancement, continuous low-volume trophic feeds should be continued if possible.

Maturation of the gastrointestinal tract is directly related to postconceptional age, thus premature neonates may be unable to be fed enterally immediately after birth.[18] In addition, the suck and swallow reflex develops at 34 to 36 weeks' gestation; therefore, even with a functionally mature gastrointestinal tract, these neonates may not be able to be fed orally. In these cases, a combination of parenteral and enteral feeding is used during the transition to full enteral and eventually oral feedings. To begin the transition to enteral feedings, a low volume of premature formula (or human milk) is infused continuously through an orogastric or nasogastric tube. Volumes are advanced very gradually as the infant tolerates the formula. Regularly during this process, gastric residuals are aspirated through the tube and volumes are measured to ensure that the formula is progressing through

the gastrointestinal tract. Abdominal distention and vomiting are indicative of too rapid advancement in feedings, or they may indicate outlet or intestinal obstruction. Stool consistency, volume, and frequency are monitored. During this rather slow process, parenteral nutrition is used as the primary source of substrate; however, the infant is encouraged to suck a pacifier for oral stimulation. As feedings progress, the parenteral nutrition solution is decreased, and the infant may be offered a small volume of formula by bottle. Close monitoring of weight gain is important to ensure adequate nutrient intake during the transition to full enteral feedings. In preterm neonates who develop abdominal distention and have evidence of intraluminal gas (pneumatosis intestinalis) on abdominal radiograph, enteral feedings should be discontinued and evaluation for necrotizing enterocolitis should be conducted. Initial therapy for this disease involves maintaining the patient's "nothing-by-mouth" status and providing parenteral nutrition and antibiotic coverage. Surgery is required for intestinal perforation.

Feeding routes for sick neonates, infants, and children are similar to those for adults and include orogastric, nasogastric, and transpyloric jejunal feeding routes and a gastrostomy tube. Type of illness and length of time the patient has continued without oral feedings should be considered when enteral feedings are reinstituted. Continuous low-volume feedings are often used initially; however, patients who are fed into the stomach may be given an appropriate formula at a specified volume for age as a bolus.

A significant problem in patients fed via a nasogastric or orogastric feeding tube is that the tube can be pulled out completely or may become dislodged from its intended position. Of concern is the possibility of reflux or vomiting and aspiration. In the past, blue coloring was added to enteral feedings for evaluation of reflux. Because of dye toxicity and lack of sensitivity in detecting reflux, the addition of blue dye to formula is not recommended.[19] Reflux precautions, including elevating the head of the bed and using low-volume and more frequent or continuous feedings, are helpful. Medications that promote gastrointestinal motility such as prokinetic agents (e.g., metoclopramide, bethanechol) and those that decrease gastric secretions (e.g., histamine 2 antagonists, proton pump inhibitors) may be beneficial. Erythromycin has been used as a promotility agent; however, neonates who receive erythromycin are at risk for developing pyloric stenosis.[20]

The primary manifestation of formula intolerance is diarrhea. Change to an age-appropriate elemental formula or a fiber-containing formula (e.g., Pediasure with fiber in those older than 1 year of age) or short-term therapy with an antiperistaltic agent such as loperamide may be indicated. Enteral feedings should be stopped in patients who manifest abdominal distention because they may have an ileus or a malpositioned feeding tube.

Gastrostomy tube (G-tube) placement is indicated in patients with upper gastrointestinal tract anomalies, esophageal injury, or tracheoesophageal fistula. Those who require prolonged tube feeding, such as patients with long-term coma or severe cardiac, neurologic, or respiratory disease, should be considered for G-tube placement. These can be placed percutaneously in older infants and children. Button-type G-tubes are available and are aesthetically more pleasing than standard G-tubes.

Jejunal feeding tubes may be used in infants and children with gastrointestinal anomalies or delayed gastric motility or after upper gastrointestinal surgery. With improved pediatric jejunal feeding tubes and refinement of surgical placement techniques, the use of jejunostomy feeding tubes in children is increasing. With jejunal feedings, continuous feedings are preferred because the small bowel cannot accommodate large volumes of fluid. Complications with jejunal feeding include malabsorption and bowel perforation.[21] In addition, the formula used in patients fed via jejunostomy may need to consist of less complex substrate, depending on the location of the feeding tube.

PARENTERAL NUTRITION

One of the most important advances in the nutritional care of the high-risk neonate was the development of parenteral nutrition. Successful use of total parenteral nutrition in an infant was first reported in the 1960s, but only since the mid 1970s has parenteral nutrition been routinely used in children with a variety of surgical or medical conditions. Knowledge of macronutrient and micronutrient metabolism and requirements has grown over time, and practitioners are able to individualize nutrients based on maturity, age, weight, nutritional status, and disease.

Venous Access. One problem with small infants and children is the limited number of peripheral intravenous access sites; thus, peripheral parenteral nutrition may be useful only for a few days. The dextrose concentration of parenteral nutrition infused peripherally is limited to 10% to 12.5%,

and the amino acid concentration is usually 2% to 3%. Coinfusion of fat emulsion with the dextrose and amino acid solution can provide 50 to 75 nonprotein kcal/kg/day. Peripheral parenteral nutrition may be used on a short-term basis, such as during the wait for a central venous line to be placed.[1] Different from plasma (295 mOsm/L), these solutions usually comprise 850 to 1,000 mOsm per L; they may cause phlebitis and tissue injury should infiltration or extravasation occur.[22] (This is discussed in greater detail in the Parenteral Nutrition Complications section.) Because of this, concentrations of calcium and potassium, two known tissue irritants, should be limited in peripherally infused solutions. Although each patient's need should be considered individually, limits of 10 mEq calcium and 40 mEq potassium per liter seem prudent for most infants and children who receive peripheral parenteral nutrition.

Percutaneous intravenous central (PIC) catheters are a good alternative in very small neonates and in infants who require parenteral nutrition but who have poor peripheral venous access. These catheters can be inserted into a peripheral vein and advanced into the central circulation with the use of sterile technique at the bedside. Placement must be validated by radiograph to ensure that the catheter tip is in the central circulation. PIC catheters have remained in place for an average of 24 days—significantly longer than the usual 2 to 3 days that a peripheral intravenous catheter typically lasts. For PIC catheters that are centrally placed, hypertonic solutions that contain more concentrated nutrients may be infused, and the risks associated with surgical central venous catheter placement are avoided as well.[23]

Children who require parenteral nutrition for an extended length of time should be given a tunneled catheter. PIC catheters can be placed in the central circulation by interventional radiology and tunneled. More commonly, Broviac and Hickman catheters are used for long-term parenteral nutrition. Usually, these are placed so that the catheter tip lies at the superior vena cava–right atrium junction (Fig. 16.1). Femoral insertion sites are also used, and the catheter is advanced to the inferior vena cava. The Dacron cuff is positioned subcutaneously near the exit site; this stimulates the formation of a fibrous adhesion that anchors the catheter, which prevents migration of microorganisms from the skin surface to the catheter tip and ultimately to the bloodstream. The location of the exit site should be decided according to cosmetic considerations because scars may remain after catheter removal. If placement is not performed with the use of fluoroscopy, a chest radiograph should be obtained after insertion to verify appropriate catheter placement before a more hypertonic parenteral nutrition solution is infused.

Totally implantable vascular access devices may be used in larger pediatric patients who require long-term central venous access; these are best suited for intermittent therapies that are most likely to be provided in the home. Compared with external catheters, implanted catheters require less maintenance, are less noticeable, impose fewer restrictions on patient activity, and have a lower infection rate.[24,25] In

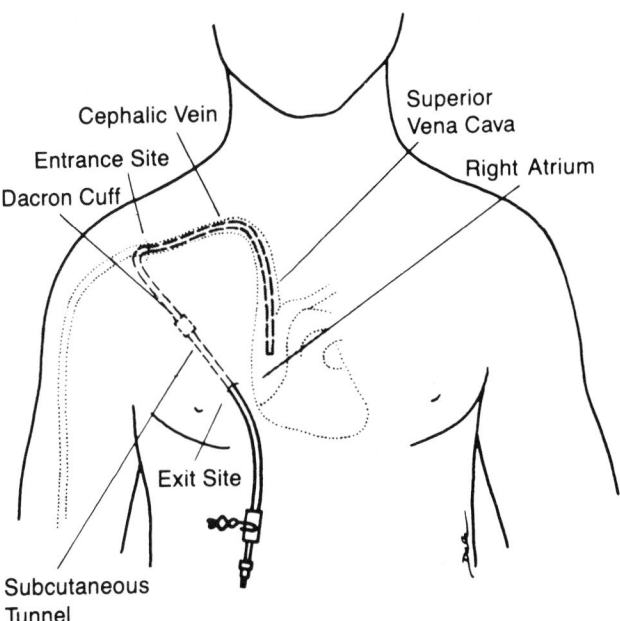

FIGURE 16.1 Placement of central venous catheter. The subclavian route as shown here is more commonly used in older children.

TABLE 16.9	Typical Peripheral (dextrose 10%) and Central (dextrose 25%) Line Solutions Used in Infants and Children (per L)			
	Peripheral	**Peripheral**	**Central**	**Central**
Solution name[a]	CPF 3%	IPF 2.4%	CCF 3%	ICF 2.4%
Amino acid (g)	30[b]	24[c]	30[b]	24[c]
Dextrose (g)	100	100	250	250
Electrolytes				
Sodium	51 mEq	38.5 mEq	51 mEq	38.5 mEq
Potassium	20 mEq	20 mEq	20 mEq	20 mEq
Chloride	51 mEq	38.5 mEq	51 mEq	38.5 mEq
Acetate	12 mEq	8.2 mEq	12 mEq	8.2 mEq
Phosphate	5.5 mmol	8 mmol	5.5 mmol	8 mmol
Calcium	6 mEq	10 mEq	8 mEq	24 mEq
Magnesium	3 mEq	4 mEq	3 mEq	4 mEq
Zinc[d]	1 mg	2 mg	1 mg	2 mg
Copper[e]	150 μg	200 μg	150 μg	200 μg
Selenium	20 μg	20 μg	20 μg	20 μg
Multivitamin[f]				

[a] CPF, child (≥12 kg) peripheral formula; IPF, infant (<12 kg) peripheral formula; CCF, child central formula; ICF, infant central formula.
[b] Standard crystalline amino acid formulation.
[c] Pediatric crystalline amino acid formulation (L-cysteine HCl at 40 mg/g protein admixed at dispensing).
[d,e] NR, none required for short-term administration.
[f] Pediatric multivitamin (see dosing recommendations in Vitamin section).

most cases, a Huber needle that is bent at a 90-degree angle is inserted through the skin into the port. This needle can be left in place up to 7 days before it is changed. According to product literature, the central silicone port can be punctured 1,000 to 2,000 times, depending on the brand. Extra care of the skin over the site is essential if infectious complications related to needle insertion are to be avoided.

Typical Parenteral Nutrition Solutions. Typical solution formulations for central venous infusion or peripheral venous infusion are shown in Table 16.9. The proportion of calories from each of the major nutrients should approach the percentages in the average enteral diet: 50% to 60% carbohydrate, 30% to 40% fat (higher percentage of fat in neonatal and infant diets), and 10% to 15% protein. Providing a balanced formula reduces the risks of toxicities or complications associated with excessive or inadequate administration of any single nutrient. Older children and adolescents may require solutions that contain up to 5% amino acids and lower dextrose concentrations, depending on the fluid volume available for infusion. Intravenous fat emulsions offer a concentrated source of calories and provide essential fatty acids.

In some institutions, the fat emulsion is added directly to the parenteral nutrition solution; this is referred to as a *total nutrient admixture (TNA)* or three-in-one admixture.[26] TNAs are not commonly used in infants because of several compositional limitations. First, parenteral nutrition solutions composed of pediatric amino acids have a lower pH that adversely affects TNA stability. Secondly, children require larger amounts of calcium (and phosphorus) to promote normal bone growth, and the increased amount of divalent cat-

ion (Ca, P) results in lipid particle instability. The ability to visualize particulates is lost in a TNA, and, finally, a 0.2-μm filter cannot be used because lipid particles range in size from 0.3 to 0.5 μm.

Fluid Requirements. Fluid needs are based on kilocaloric requirements; water losses from skin, respiration, and urine and stool output; water accumulation in newly formed tissues; and water produced from carbohydrate oxidation.[27] Because the body surface area per unit weight is greater in children than in adults, evaporative losses are increased, which results in greater fluid requirements per unit of weight in children. In general, fluid requirements are 90 to 100 mL per 100 kilocalories in those who weigh less than 10 kg,[27] decreasing to 45 mL per 100 calories in adults. Fluid needs are altered by prematurity, activity, environment, or pathology.[28,29] Maintenance kilocaloric (and fluid) requirements for term neonates and older children can be calculated from the equations described by Holliday and Segar (Table 16.10).[27]

Organ immaturity (primarily kidney and skin) in the preterm neonate results in increased sensible and insensible water losses. In preterm neonates, the skin and subcutaneous

TABLE 16.10	Daily Maintenance Caloric and Fluid Requirements for Term Infants and Children
Weight	**Fluid**
Up to 10 kg	100 mL/kg[a]
>10 to 20 kg	1,000 mL + 50 mL/kg for every kilogram >10 kg
>20 kg	1,500 mL + 20 mL/kg for every kilogram >20 kg

[a] Preterm infants may require 120 to 150 mL/kg.
(Adapted from Holliday MA, Segar WE: The maintenance need for water in parenteral fluid therapy. Pediatrics 19:823–832, 1957.)

tissue are thinner and more permeable, resulting in increased evaporative losses.[30] Infants who are under radiant warmers or who require ultraviolet light therapy for treatment of neonatal jaundice experience even greater evaporative water losses.[31] Preterm neonates are unable to concentrate urine because of renal immaturity; this results in an increased requirement for fluids.[32] Renal function matures with increasing postconceptional age; thus, the ability of neonates to regulate water and electrolyte metabolism improves with increasing age.[33] On the other hand, certain diseases common in preterm neonates have been associated with excessive fluid intake, including bronchopulmonary dysplasia,[34] intraventricular hemorrhage,[35] and patent ductus arteriosus.[36] Although the precise cause of necrotizing enterocolitis is unknown, it has been associated with aggressive fluid and enteral feeding practices.[37]

Children with congenital cardiac or renal anomalies, increased intracranial pressure, syndrome of inappropriate antidiuretic hormone (SIADH), or pulmonary edema may require varying degrees of fluid restriction. Conversely, patients with excessive fluid losses (e.g., gastric drainage, diarrhea, increased stool or ostomy output, vomiting, chest tube drainage, burn or wound exudate, fistula drainage) or those under radiant warmers, ultraviolet lights, or with fever may require additional fluids to compensate for these losses. These outputs should be replaced with fluids that are similar in volume and electrolyte composition (Table 16.11). In addition to electrolyte replacement, the albumin concentration can be measured in fluids that are expected to contain significant amounts of albumin, such as chest tube drainage or wound exudate. The addition of albumin to a replacement fluid may be the most appropriate method of compensating for estimated losses.

Macronutrient Requirements

Protein. Amino acid products comprise free-base amino acids or acetate salts (for those amino acids such as lysine that are not stable). The amino acid composition varies according to the specific product; therefore, the electrolyte content of amino acid solutions also varies (Table 16.12). Because of improved amino acid solutions, problems of hyperammonemia, compositional variability, occasional allergic reaction, poor nitrogen utilization, and acidosis seen with older formulations have been eliminated.[38] The graduation of amino acid doses over several days is rarely needed. Initial doses of 1 to 2 g per kg advanced to 3 to 3.5 g per kg in the preterm infant are well tolerated and are associated with increased growth, improved nitrogen balance, and enhanced catch-up growth.[39,40]

Because of increased tissue anabolism, protein requirements in children are greater on a per-kilogram basis than those in adults. Guidelines for protein doses are shown in Table 16.13. Because of immaturity, the preterm infant and neonate require qualitatively different amino acids for optimal growth and development.[41–43] Enzyme immaturity in the transsulfuration pathway prevents conversion of methionine to cysteine and cysteine to taurine, thereby rendering those two amino acids essential (Fig. 16.2). Similarly, phenylalanine hydroxylase insufficiency limits the conversion of phenylalanine to tyrosine. Thus, cysteine, taurine, and tyrosine are conditionally essential amino acids for preterm infants and neonates.

Target ranges for individual plasma amino acid concentrations were determined 2 to 3 hours after a human milk feeding in young infants.[44] It was not surprising that plasma amino acid patterns in neonates and infants infused with amino acid products designed for use in adults resulted in plasma amino acid concentrations that were different from the reference range.[41] Three pediatric-specific formulations (Aminosyn-PF, TrophAmine, PremaSol) were developed to address these metabolic differences (Table 16.14). These formulations require the addition of L-cysteine hydrochloride (pH 1.5) before infusion, and they contain reduced amounts of methionine, phenylalanine, and glycine and include the dicarboxylic amino acids (aspartate and glutamate) and taurine. They differ from each other in terms of the amounts of methionine, tyrosine (lower in Aminosyn-PF), and taurine (lower in TrophAmine and PremaSol) that are added. Because of solubility, tyrosine is added as *N*-acetyl L-tyrosine (NAT) in TrophAmine and PremaSol. NAT is not as efficiently converted to tyrosine in preterm neonates as it is in older infants and children; the clinical implications of this are not known. Unlike TrophAmine and Aminosyn-

TABLE 16.11	Range of Electrolyte Composition (mEq/L) of Gastrointestinal Secretions			
Secretion	**Na+**	**K+**	**Cl−**	**HCO3−**
Saliva	35–60	10–20	15–35	50
Gastric	10–115	5–35	10–150	0
Pancreatic	115–155	5–10	55–110	70–90
Bile	130–165	5–15	80–120	35–50
Midjejunum	70–125	5–30	70–135	10–20
Ileostomy	90–140	5–30	60–135	15–50
Diarrhea	25–50	35–60	0–40	35–45

TABLE 16.12	Electrolyte Content and pH of Commercially Available Amino Acid Products (mEq/L)					
	g/100 mL	OAc	Cl	Na	Phos[a]	pH
TrophAmine	6	56	<3	5		5–6
	10	97	<3	5		5–6
PremaSol	6	57	<3			5–6
	10	94	<3			5–6
Aminosyn-PF	7	32.5		3.4		5–6.5
	10	46		3.4		5–6.5
Aminosyn	7	105		5.4		4.5–6
	10	148		5.4		4.5–6
Aminosyn II	7	50.3		31.3		5–6.5
	10	71.8		45.3		5–6.5
Novamine	15	151				5.2–6
FreAmine III	8.5	72	<3	10	10	6–7
	10	89	<3	10	10	6–7
Travasol	8.5	73	34			6–8
	10	87	40			6–8
Cysteine HCl	5		5.7			1.5–2

[a] Units are mmol/L.

TABLE 16.13	Parenteral Protein Requirements (g/kg/day) in Stable Patients
Very Low Birth Weight	3–4
Preterm	2.5–3
Infant/neonate	2–2.5
Infant	1.5–2
Preschool/school age	1–1.5
Adolescent	0.8–1.5

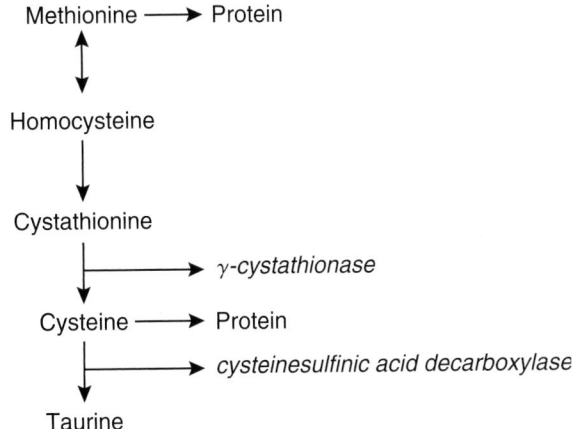

FIGURE 16.2 Metabolic pathway for the conversion of methionine to cysteine and taurine.

PF, PremaSol is sulfite-free and is packaged in a polyvinylchloride (PVC) bag; the other two products contain sulfites and are packaged in glass bottles.

The proposed benefits of using pediatric amino acid solutions with added L-cysteine hydrochloride include enhanced growth, improved nitrogen retention, better calcium and phosphorous solubility, and a potentially reduced risk for metabolic bone disease and cholestasis. Pediatric-specific amino acid formulations used in preterm postsurgical infants resulted in nitrogen balance and weight gain similar to those occurring during intrauterine growth.[41,42] Term neonates and older infants who received TrophAmine with L-cysteine supplementation had age-appropriate weight gain and nitrogen retention.[42] Infants given short-term peripheral parenteral nutrition with lower dosages of pediatric-specific amino acids and with caloric intakes that were below those described previously demonstrated weight gain and positive nitrogen balance.[45] This is likely the result of optimal plasma availability of amino acids for anabolism. As reported by Beck,[46] the lower incidence of cholestasis in very low birthweight neonates who received a pediatric amino acid formulation may be due in part to enhanced amino acid utilization. In addition, the lower solution pH allows more appropriate dosing of calcium and phosphorus, which may reduce the risk for metabolic bone disease.

Pediatric amino acid products should be supplemented with L-cysteine hydrochloride; however, this is not always done in practice because of the cost. The clinical implications of omitting L-cysteine have not been completely studied. One trial in a limited number of postsurgical adults who received a pediatric amino acid product found that those who

TABLE 16.14	Comparison of Amino Acid Composition (mole%) of Parenteral Amino Acid Products				
Amino Acid	Aminosyn-PF	TrophAmine	PremaSol	Aminosyn	FreAmine III
L-Isoleucine	7.4	8.2	8.2	6.4	6.3
L-Leucine	11.6	14.1	14.1	8.4	8.4
L-Lysine	5.9	7.3	7.3	5.7	6.0
L-Methionine	1.5	2.9	2.9	3.1	4.3
L-Phenylalanine	3.3	3.9	3.9	3.1	4.1
L-Tryptophan	1.1	1.3	1.3	0.9	0.9
L-Threonine	5.5	4.6	4.6	5.1	4.0
L-Valine	7.1	8.8	8.8	8.0	6.8
L-Arginine	9.1	9.2	9.2	6.6	6.6
L-Histidine	2.6	4.1	4.1	2.3	2.2
L-Alanine	10.1	7.9	7.9	16.8	9.6
L-Proline	9.1	7.8	7.8	8.7	11.7
Glycine	6.6	6.4	6.4	19.9	22.5
L-Serine	6.1	4.8	4.8	4.7	6.8
L-Tyrosine	0.4	0.5	0.5	0.3	0
N-Acetyl-L-tyrosine[a]	0	1.2	1.2	0	0
L-Glutamic acid	7.2	4.5	4.5	0	0
L-Aspartic acid	5.1	3.1	3.1	0	0
L-Cysteine[b]	0	0.4	0.4	0	0
Taurine	0.7	0.3	0.3	0	0
Total	100.4	101.3	101.3	100.0	100.2

[a] As tyrosine equivalents.

[b] Admixed to Aminosyn-PF, TrophAmine, PremaSol

received cysteine tended to have a more positive nitrogen balance than those who did not.[47] It is interesting to note that older children who received pediatric amino acids with different L-cysteine dosages demonstrated that plasma taurine, but not cysteine, concentrations were directly related to the L-cysteine dose.[48]

Protein requirements of the older child and adolescent can be met with the use of a standard amino acid formulation. Incremental increases in protein intake to above the requirements listed in Table 16.13 may be required for the severely catabolic patient.

Caloric Requirements. Children require calories for basal metabolic demands, activity, maintenance of body temperature, and, unlike adults, additional calories for growth and development. The most elegant work describing global and compartmental energy needs in preterm infants used indirect calorimetry.[49] Enterally fed low-birthweight infants had global energy requirements of 150 kcal/kg/day. Approximately 18 kcal/kg/day was lost in stool; thus, 132 kcal/kg/day was required for energy metabolism. Of this 132 kcal/kg/day, basal metabolism required 63 kcal/kg/day, activity required 4 kcal/kg/day, and the remaining 65 kcal/kg/day was used for growth.

Parenteral caloric requirements for optimal growth of the preterm infant and neonate range from 85 to 135 kcal/kg/day,[49,50] similar to fluid requirements. Caloric requirements (per kilogram body weight) decrease during the first year of life and continue to decrease until adult needs are approached (Table 16.10). As with protein, recommendations for caloric intake are merely guidelines for the practitioner. Assessment of clinical outcome, including weight gain, height or length, nitrogen balance, and visceral and somatic protein measurements, should be used to determine the adequacy of substrate intake.

Caloric requirements during critical illness may be decreased. Children who are pharmacologically paralyzed or mechanically ventilated, and whose thermal neutrality is controlled by cooling blankets or warming devices, have decreased caloric requirements because they do not expend calories for activity, breathing, or regulation of body temperature. To evaluate energy expenditure postoperatively, C-reactive protein (CRP), oxygen consumption, carbon dioxide production, measured energy expenditure, and nitrogen balance were measured in seven infants after abdominal or thoracic surgery was performed.[51] The quantity of calories provided (65 ± 18 kcal/kg/day) exceeded measured energy expenditure (43 ± 10 kcal/kg/day) by 50%. Investigators suggest providing no more calories than those equal to the measured energy expenditure until the CRP values are less than 2 mg per dL.[51]

Carbohydrate. Dextrose is used almost exclusively as the carbohydrate source. Premature neonates are less glucose tolerant and may spontaneously develop hypoglycemia or hyperglycemia. Because hyperglycemia increases the risk for development of hyperglycemia-induced hyperosmolar coma and intraventricular hemorrhage,[52] glucose should be advanced slowly by about 3 g/kg/day as serum glucose permits. Usually, older infants can be started on 10 g/kg/day (7 mg/kg/min) of dextrose, with doses increasing by 5 g per kg every 12 to 24 hours, to a maximum of 30 to 35 g/kg/day, if the patient has a central venous catheter and is glucose tolerant. Usually, dosages of 25 g/kg/day (17 mg/kg/min) when used with concomitant fat emulsion infusion are sufficient to achieve adequate weight gain in infants. With increasing age, maximum glucose oxidation rates decrease from approximately 12.5 mg/kg/min in infants to about 5 mg/kg/min in adults. Dextrose concentrations should be advanced slowly in all persons under severe stress and in those who are receiving corticosteroids because hyperglycemia may develop, even when dextrose intake is low.

Although higher dosages may not result in hyperglycemia, the maximum glucose oxidation rate may be exceeded and fat may accumulate, which can be desirable in an infant, particularly if he or she is undernourished. However, producing fat from carbohydrate is not energy efficient; it results in increased carbon dioxide (CO_2) production and may cause fatty infiltrations in the liver, all of which are undesirable. Glucose oxidation rates in children generally are higher than in adults; however, a study in burned children ages 1 to 11 years old who received parenteral nutrition during perioperative periods reported that the maximum glucose oxidation rate was 5 mg/kg/min, similar to adults.[53] Even when glucose oxidation rates were exceeded, these patients were euglycemic, suggesting that the excess glucose entered nonoxidative pathways.[53]

Insulin may be used to facilitate glucose metabolism for patients who are carbohydrate intolerant. Very low birthweight infants are started on 0.05 unit/kg/hour or less; older infants and children usually are started on dosages of 0.1 unit/kg/hour or less of insulin, with the dosage titrated to frequent (every 2 hours) assessments of serum glucose.[54] A concomitant insulin infusion will allow better glucose control than results from addition of insulin to the parenteral nutrition solution in infants with changing needs.

Fat. As in adults, fat emulsion infusion prevents or reverses essential fatty acid deficiency (EFAD), provides a concentrated and isotonic source of calories and a more physiologic "diet," and prolongs survival time of peripheral intravenous lines. The 20% fat emulsion products are compared in Table 16.15. Different from adults, biochemical evidence of EFAD (a triene [5,8,11-eicosatrienoic acid with 3 double bonds]-to-tetraene [arachidonic acid with 4 double bonds] ratio

TABLE 16.15	Composition of 20% Fat Emulsions[a]	
	Liposyn III	**Intralipid®**
Ingredient or Characteristic	Abbott Laboratories	Pharmacia & Upjohn
Source		
Soybean oil (%)	20	20
Safflower oil (%)	–	–
Fatty acid distribution		
Linoleic acid (%)	54.5	50
Oleic acid (%)	22.4	26
Palmitic acid (%)	10.5	10
Linolenic acid (%)	8.3	9
Stearic acid (%)	4.2	3.5
Egg yolk phospholipids (%)	1.2	1.2
Glycerin (%)	2.5	2.25
Calories (per mL)	2	2

[a] In 10% fat emulsions, the oil sources are the same for each product, but the amounts are halved, resulting in a higher phospholipid-to-triglyceride ratio and a 1.1-kcal/mL concentration.

above 0.4) may be evident after a few days of no fat intake in preterm neonates (Fig. 16.3). Linoleic acid reverses EFAD, but linolenic acid does not. However, evidence suggests that linolenic acid may also be essential.[55,56]

Carnitine acyltransferase is needed to transport free fatty acids across the mitochondria for β-oxidation and energy

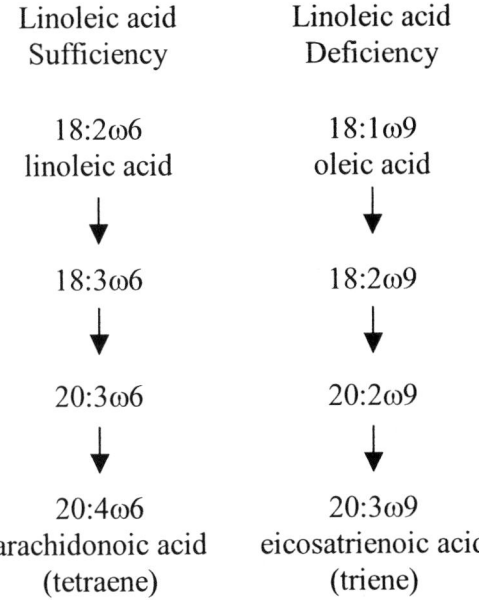

FIGURE 16.3 With adequate linoleic acid, the chain elongation pathway that results in arachidonic acid (a tetraene) predominates. With insufficient linoleic acid, the pathway that elongates oleic acid to eicosatrienoic acid (a triene) predominates. Thus, the ratio of the triene (eicosatrienoic acid) to the tetraene (arachidonic acid) is increased.

production. Neonates and infants may have a relative insufficiency of the hydroxylase enzyme required in the final step of carnitine synthesis in vivo. Consistent with this finding, plasma carnitine concentrations are low in preterm neonates[57] and in older infants who have received carnitine-free nutrition for longer than 1 month since birth.[58] The capacity for fatty acid oxidation can be enhanced by the provision of 10 to 20 mg/kg/day of carnitine.[58] Decreased carnitine concentrations have been associated with gastroesophageal reflux disease and apnea in low-birthweight infants; this has resolved with carnitine supplementation.[59]

Fat emulsion should be initiated at 0.5 g/kg/day in premature neonates; term infants and those older than 1 month of age can usually be started at 1 g/kg/day. If serum triglyceride concentrations are within acceptable limits (usually <150 mg/dL), the fat emulsion dose can be increased by 0.25 to 0.5 g/kg/day up to 3 g/kg/day in preterm neonates, or by 0.5 to 1 g/kg/day up to a maximum of 4 g/kg/day in term and older infants, respectively, as recommended by the American Academy of Pediatrics (AAP).[55] Ideally, fat emulsion is given continuously over 24 hours to promote clearance from the circulation. Those with increased triglyceride concentrations may not be clearing the exogenous chylomicron particles; others with increased values may be mobilizing endogenous fat stores because of low nutrient intake. The serum sample of those who are not clearing fat emulsion will be lipemic. Visual assessment of the serum sample can be helpful to the clinician in determining the most appropriate response to an elevated triglyceride concentration.

Neonates, particularly those who are premature, frequently develop physiologic (neonatal) jaundice or unconjugated (indirect) hyperbilirubinemia because they are not able to conjugate bilirubin. Because the blood–brain barrier is immature in neonates, indirect bilirubin can cross into the brain and cause a yellow staining known as *kernicterus*, which is associated with neurologic sequelae. Fatty acids and unconjugated bilirubin bind competitively to albumin; thus, unconjugated bilirubin can be displaced from high-affinity albumin-binding sites by free fatty acids. Hyperbilirubinemia alone should not be an absolute contraindication to the use of intravenous fat emulsion, and the provision of 2% to 4% of the total daily caloric requirement as fat emulsion to prevent EFAD should not present a problem.

The effects of fat emulsion on immune function are controversial, and study results are inconsistent. Both in vitro incubation of white blood cells with fat emulsion and in vivo infusion of fat emulsion inhibit leukocyte chemotaxis, phagocytosis, bactericidal capacity, and lymphoproliferation.[60–62] However, others report that fat has no effect, or that it restores and augments immune function.[63–65] These conflicting findings are probably secondary to the complexities (e.g., duration of exposure, lipid concentration and composition, responding cell type) of fatty acid and fatty acid metabolite interactions with immunoreactive cells. In practice, parenteral lipids are used conservatively in patients who are immunocompromised or who have sepsis, and serum triglycerides are monitored for assessment of tolerance.

Studies evaluating fat emulsion infusion and respiratory function are also inconsistent. Investigators found fat emboli in pulmonary capillaries during postmortem examinations of neonates who succumbed to respiratory compromise, and they attributed this finding to the infusion of fat emulsion. These findings were subsequently attributed to artifact, which occurred secondary to a delay in fixation of the lung after death.[66] Neonates younger than 1 week of age with respiratory distress syndrome who received 1 g per kg of fat emulsion (Intralipid) over 4 hours had lower partial pressure of oxygen (Po_2) values than did age-related neonates who received no Intralipid.[67] However, the changes in Po_2 did not correlate with elevations in serum triglyceride concentration.[67] Similarly, oxygen diffusion in the lungs of premature neonates was not affected by infusion of up to 4 g/kg/day of Intralipid over 24 hours.[68] Following AAP recommendations to infuse the daily fat dosage over 24 hours whenever possible helps avoid excessive fat concentrations in the circulation and minimizes potential changes in pulmonary microcirculation that may result in a lowering of Po_2.

The 10% and 20% concentrations of fat emulsion contain the same amount of phospholipid, resulting in a higher phospholipid-to-triglyceride ratio in the 10% (0.12) compared with the 20% (0.06) products. Infants who were randomly assigned to 7 days of continuous infusion of 10% had higher plasma concentrations of phospholipid and cholesterol than did those who received 20% fat emulsion.[69] In addition, the low-density lipoprotein (LDL) cholesterol had greater total cholesterol and phospholipid concentrations in those who received the 10% product. Two thirds of the phospholipid in 10% fat occurs in the form of liposomes, which may store cholesterol and apoproteins and potentially alter cholesterol regulation and triglyceride metabolism. Thus, the 20% product should be used whenever possible.

Micronutrients

Electrolyte and Mineral Requirements. The reader is referred to Chapter 28 for a discussion of electrolytes and minerals. As with adults, factors such as hydration, cardiovascular status, renal function, and concurrent medications should be considered when electrolyte requirements in children are determined.[70] In addition, age and organ maturity, in particular of the kidney, should be considered in premature infants.

Daily maintenance electrolyte requirements for neonates, infants, and children are listed in Table 16.16. As with adults, children with excessive gastrointestinal tract fluid losses should receive a replacement fluid composed of comparable electrolytes (Table 16.11). Replacement fluids are delivered most efficiently through a separate intravenous infusion.

Amino acid solutions also contain various amounts of anions (usually acetate) and cations, which should be considered when anion distribution is determined (Table 16.12). L-cysteine hydrochloride (HCl) provides additional chloride (5.7 mEq Cl/g L-cysteine) to parenteral nutrition solutions.

TABLE 16.16	Daily Electrolyte Doses (mEq/kg/day)[25,34,37–39,89,90]	
	Preterm Infants	Term Infants and Children
Sodium	2–8	2–5
Potassium	1.4–5[a]	2–3
Chloride	1.1–5	2–3
Magnesium	0.25–0.6	0.25–0.5
Calcium	2.5–3.5	1–2
Phosphate[b]	1.3–2	0.5–1

[a] Those receiving diuretics may require larger doses.

[b] Units are mmol/kg/day.

Sodium. Premature infants have functionally immature kidneys that may promote excessive urinary sodium losses.[71] Sodium requirements in these infants may be as high as 8 mEq/kg/day. When sodium needs are determined, other sources of sodium such as flushes, continuous infusion of normal saline through arterial lines, or antibiotics as sodium salts should be considered.

Frequent causes of hyponatremia or hypernatremia consist of vomiting and diarrhea. Patients who are receiving diuretics and those with certain renal disorders (e.g., renal tubular acidosis) have increased urinary sodium losses and often require additional sodium. Parenteral nutrition solutions that are high in sodium may be desirable in patients with closed head injury to increase serum osmolality and ultimately decrease intracranial pressure. Specific types of malignancies, pulmonary diseases, central nervous system disorders, and drugs (e.g., vincristine, carbamazepine, cyclophosphamide, barbiturates) may cause hyponatremia secondary to SIADH. Measurement of urine sodium concentration can be helpful in elucidating the cause of hyponatremia.

Potassium. Usual potassium dosages range from 2 to 4 mEq/kg/day; however, depending on organ maturity, presence of disease, and use of medications, much larger dosages may be needed in extreme cases. Vomiting, diarrhea, and draining fistulas are the primary causes of extrarenal potassium loss. Preterm infants may have increased potassium requirements because of increased urinary losses resulting from immature renal function. Metabolic acidosis may result in hyperkalemia because potassium shifts extracellularly as hydrogen ions are shifted into the cell. Diuretics (especially loop diuretics), amphotericin, and cisplatin are frequent causes of hypokalemia. Other drugs such as aminoglycosides and penicillins[72] promote renal potassium excretion.

Hypokalemia that is refractory to potassium supplementation may indicate concurrent hypomagnesemia, which must be addressed before serum potassium concentrations can be maintained. Because potassium is the principal intracellular cation, the extent of potassium depletion is difficult to estimate through the measurement of extracellular or serum po-

tassium concentrations; therefore, frequent serum concentration monitoring is necessary.

Peripheral infusion of potassium is irritating to vessels, may be painful to the patient, and should be limited to about 40 mEq per liter for peripherally infused solutions. Patients with central venous access can receive more concentrated solutions, but the maximum rate of potassium delivery should not exceed 0.5 to 1 mEq/kg/hour, when all sources are considered. Patients who receive more than 0.5 mEq/kg/hour should be monitored by electrocardiogram because cardiac dysrhythmias may develop when potassium is infused rapidly.[73] Potassium is most efficiently replaced by means of continuous infusions because the transient increase in potassium serum concentration attained with a 1-mEq/kg dose infused over 2 hours may stimulate aldosterone and promote potassium renal elimination.

Infant serum samples often are hemolyzed because they are obtained by heel puncture, which may require considerable squeezing to obtain an adequate blood volume. Hemolysis releases intracellular potassium, causing an apparent elevation in serum potassium concentration. When hyperkalemia is noted in an asymptomatic patient, the phlebotomy method should be determined and the serum evaluated for visual evidence of hemolysis. Validation of serum concentration by venipuncture may be desirable before aggressive treatment is undertaken.

Acetate. Amino acid products contain crystalline amino acids as acetate salts, and the amount of acetate varies widely among the commercially available products. For those who have an acidosis, it may be desirable to add ''base'' to the parenteral nutrition solution. Because bicarbonate is not compatible, acetate is added. Acetate is readily converted in vivo to bicarbonate (HCO_3). Older individuals may not require the addition of acetate unless they have significant stool losses or other types of metabolic acidosis. Acetate as either the potassium or the sodium salt can be added to the parenteral nutrition solution. Serum concentrations of HCO_3 should be monitored and doses adjusted accordingly. Premature infants often have increased requirements for ''base,'' and it is common to add about 1 to 2 mEq per kg of acetate as the sodium or potassium salt.

Minerals
Calcium. Calcium, the most abundant mineral in the body, is important for maintaining the functional integrity of cellular membranes and neuromuscular activity, and for regulating various endocrine and exocrine secretory activities, blood coagulation, and bone metabolism. In newborns, 98% of total body calcium is found in bone. Approximately 40% of total serum calcium is bound to serum proteins, and 80% to 90% of calcium is bound to albumin. Variations in the serum protein concentration and serum pH proportionately alter protein-bound and total serum calcium concentrations. Ionized calcium measurements may be more useful, especially during hypoalbuminemia.

Calcium homeostasis is regulated by parathyroid hormone (PTH), calcitonin, and vitamin D. PTH is stimulated by an increased need for available calcium, and calcitonin is stimulated in response to increased calcium concentrations. For example, an acute decrease in calcium concentration causes an increase in PTH concentration and a decrease in calcitonin, resulting in the mobilization of calcium from bone. Therefore, serum calcium concentration is neither a sensitive nor a specific measure of the adequacy of intake.

Calcium and phosphorous requirements are inversely related to postconceptional age. In utero, calcium accretion rates at 36 weeks' gestation are 5 to 7.5 mEq/kg/day of elemental calcium.[74] Because of limitations in solubility, it is impossible to provide this much calcium and phosphorus enterally or parenterally. It is interesting to note that adequate bone mineralization occurs with significantly less calcium as long as the appropriate amount of phosphate is provided. A physiologic ratio of calcium and phosphate (1.7 mg:1 mg) promotes retention of these minerals in premature infants and minimizes parenteral nutrition–related bone disease.[75,76] In addition to the inherently greater calcium requirement for normal bone mineralization, premature infants often have concurrent diseases that require aggressive diuretic therapy, which increases calcium urinary excretion,[77] or requires fluid restriction, which limits the amount of substrate that can be provided because of solubility. Thus, these infants are at increased risk for metabolic bone disease.

The solubility of calcium and phosphorus is enhanced by lower calcium and phosphorous concentrations, a lower pH, and colder temperature. Pediatric amino acid products have a lower pH, and the addition of L-cysteine further decreases the pH, thereby increasing calcium and phosphate solubility.[78–80] Therefore, the ability of pediatric amino acid–based formulations to provide more appropriate calcium and phosphate doses allows needs to be adequately addressed.

Calcium ionically bonds with phosphate to form monobasic, dibasic, or tribasic calcium phosphate, depending on pH. At low solution pH, monobasic calcium phosphate that is aqueously soluble predominates. As the pH increases, dibasic phosphate becomes available to bind with calcium, and precipitation occurs more easily.[78] Therefore, solutions compounded from amino acid products with a relatively high pH, such as FreAmine III with a pH of 6.5 to 6.8, have relatively low calcium phosphate solubility. In certain circumstances, L-cysteine HCl has been added to standard amino acid products to decrease solution pH and enhance calcium phosphate solubility. Another factor that influences calcium and phosphorous solubility is temperature. It is interesting to note that warmer temperatures result in decreased solubility because warmer temperatures increase calcium ionization. Radiant warmers used to maintain the infant's body temperature or phototherapy used to treat physiologic jaundice causes the temperatures near the infant to be increased. Under these conditions, solutions that are near solubility limits for calcium and phosphorus may precipitate. In some cases, precipitation has occurred within the catheter

as the infusing solution was warmed by the febrile patient's body temperature. Because calcium gluconate is less ionized in solution than is chloride salt, an equivalent calcium dose with gluconate salt results in less precipitation than occurs with chloride salt; thus, addition of calcium to parenteral nutrition solutions is generally provided with calcium gluconate.[81]

When the solution is compounded, phosphate is added early in the process because it is concentrated (3 mmol/mL) and consumes a small volume compared with calcium; therefore, it is more likely to remain in the injection port. The addition of other additives after phosphate helps clear the injection port. Calcium is more dilute (0.456 mEq/mL) than are phosphate salts and is added last.[82]

Phosphorus. Phosphate functions as a cofactor in multiple enzyme systems necessary for the metabolism of protein, carbohydrate, and fat, and it is required for the production of high-energy adenosine triphosphate (ATP) bonds. The refeeding syndrome occurs when a severely malnourished patient is fed without adequate provision of phosphate. The increased intracellular shifting of phosphate during refeeding has ultimately resulted in death.[83] Hypophosphatemia may also occur secondary to hyperparathyroidism (i.e., increased urinary phosphate excretion) or respiratory alkalosis (i.e., intracellular phosphate shifting). Similar to calcium, phosphorus is particularly important in bone growth. Phosphorous solubility in parenteral nutrition solutions is limited (for a more detailed discussion, see the previous section entitled Calcium).

Phosphate dosages provided to neonates and infants range from 1 to 2 mmol per kg. This amount can be provided to most patients who are not fluid restricted. Dosage requirements decrease to approximately 1 mmol per kg in older children and to 0.5 to 0.75 mmol per kg in adolescents and young adults. Because phosphate exists in three valence states that fluctuate with changing pH, phosphate requirements usually are described in millimoles (mmol) or milligrams (mg)—not milliequivalents (mEq). The use of milliequivalents does not reflect the concentration of phosphorus in solution and may lead to dosing errors. For example, 1 mmol phosphate is equal to 31 mg elemental phosphorus, and 3 mmol phosphate is contained in 4 mEq sodium phosphate or 4.4 mEq potassium phosphate. The different chemical states of phosphorus are listed in Table 16.17, and the

TABLE 16.17	Calcium Phosphate Solubility		
Salt	Formula	Molecular Weight	Parenteral Solubility
Monobasic	$Ca(H_2PO_4)_2$	234.06	Moderate
Dibasic	$CaHPO_4$	136.06	Insoluble
Tribasic	$Ca_3(PO_4)_2$	310.20	Insoluble

TABLE 16.18	Dissociation of Hydrogen Phosphate	
pKa_1	pH 2.12	$H_3PO_{4-} \leftrightharpoons H^+ + H_2PO_4^{(-1)}$
pKa_2	pH 7.21	$H_2PO_4^- \leftrightharpoons H^+ + HPO_4^{(-2)}$
pKa_3	pH 12.67	$HPO_4^- \leftrightharpoons H^+ + PO_4^{(-3)}$

dissociation constants of hydrogen phosphate are shown in Table 16.18.

Magnesium. Magnesium, the second most common intracellular cation, is necessary for numerous enzymatic reactions involving energy storage and use. Extracellular magnesium is used during neuromuscular transmission and is required for cardiovascular tone. Approximately 2% of the body's total magnesium is present in the extracellular compartment, whereas 98% is found intracellularly, primarily in bone.

Magnesium balance and serum magnesium concentration are largely determined by renal magnesium excretion, which is regulated primarily by glomerular filtration rate, tubular reabsorption, and PTH. When necessary, the kidney can conserve or increase urinary magnesium excretion, depending on body stores.[84]

As with hypocalcemia, hypomagnesemia often is present in infants with DiGeorge syndrome and those born to mothers with diabetes. Neonatal hepatitis and congenital biliary atresia are commonly associated with hypomagnesemia.[84] Because magnesium is absorbed in the proximal jejunum, patients who undergo intestinal resection are at risk for developing hypomagnesemia. Similarly, patients with extensive diarrheal or ileostomy fluid losses may have increased magnesium losses. Diuretics, amphotericin, cyclosporine, and cisplatin increase urinary magnesium losses and may contribute to hypomagnesemia. Magnesium depletion may precipitate refractory hypokalemia or hypocalcemia.[85] Because magnesium is an intracellular cation that equilibrates rather slowly, increases in magnesium content in parenteral nutrition solutions may not restore intracellular magnesium concentrations for days. Infusion of bolus doses of magnesium results in increased magnesium urinary concentrations, and, as with potassium, infusion of estimated deficits should be performed with continuous infusions.

Vitamins. A parenteral multivitamin product based on RDAs for oral vitamins was formulated in the 1980s according to recommendations of the Nutrition Advisory Group (NAG) of the American Medical Association (AMA). Twice during the 1990s, parenteral vitamin manufacturing was suspended, and at least two significant parenteral vitamin shortages resulted. During these vitamin shortages, several deaths were attributed to thiamine deficiency in adults.[86] Following resolution of the shortage, the FDA recommended that the adult parenteral vitamin products be reformulated. The newly formulated products contain 150 μg vitamin K and

increased amounts of thiamine, vitamin C, folic acid, and pyridoxine (vitamin B_6). Mayne Pharma continues to market an adult vitamin without vitamin K (M.V.I-12) that contains the increased amounts of thiamine, vitamin C, folic acid, and pyridoxine. The pediatric vitamins have not been reformulated. A 5-mL dose of the pediatric multivitamin contains 400 IU vitamin D (200 IU in the adult products), 200 μg vitamin K (150 μg in the adult products), and less of the other vitamins than is found in the adult products. The contents of these products are compared in Table 16.19.

Parenteral multivitamin preparations are sensitive to pH and temperature, and because they degrade in light, they are packaged in amber vials. In addition, vitamins may interact with one another or adsorb to the plastic matrix of administration sets, thereby decreasing bioavailability.[87]

Infants and children up to 11 years of age who weigh more than 2.5 kg should receive the full single-dose vial (5 mL) of a pediatric multivitamin product daily. Medically stable infants and children who receive parenteral nutrition with this dosage maintain acceptable vitamin serum concentrations.[87] During the AMA/NAG consensus meeting in 1987, it was recommended that preterm infants be dosed at 2 mL/kg/day, not to exceed 5 mL per day.[87] The retinol (vitamin A) contained in the pediatric products adsorbs to plastic tubing and bags, significantly reducing the amount of vitamin delivered. Vitamin A is important in retinal development, and supplementation of premature neonates with intramuscular injections of vitamin A has been recommended.[88] Of further concern in premature neonates is the possible decreased metabolism of the polysorbate emulsifiers because of immature hepatic metabolic pathways.[87]

Children older than 11 years of age should receive the adult multivitamin product at the recommended adult dosage. (For further discussion on this topic, see Chapter 29.)

Trace Elements. Trace elements constitute less than 0.01% of human body weight. Despite their low quantities in the body, trace elements have essential roles in biochemical processes, including growth and development. Pediatric trace element requirements have not been well defined; hence, RDAs and reports of deficiency currently guide intravenous dosage recommendations. Current recommendations for trace element dosing are shown in Table 16.20.

Because trace elements are stored during the last trimester of pregnancy, premature neonates have insufficient body stores, which put them at increased risk of developing deficiencies. Patients with persistent diarrhea or excessive ostomy outputs have increased zinc losses in these fluids and may require additional supplementation. Patients with exterior biliary drainage or jejunostomy may have increased copper losses because copper along with manganese is eliminated through the bile. Similarly, patients with cholestasis may accumulate copper and manganese, and it has been recommended that both of these elements be eliminated from parenteral nutrition solutions in patients with cholestasis.[87]

TABLE 16.19	Vitamin Content of Various Parenteral Vitamin Products			
Vitamin	**MVI Pediatric**[a]	**Infuvite Pediatric**[b]	**MVI-adult**[c]	**Infuvite Adult**[d]
Usual dose	5 mL	5 mL	10 mL	10 mL
Distributed by	Mayne Pharma	Baxter	Mayne Pharma	Baxter
A (retinol equivalents)	2300 IU	2300 IU	3300 IU	3300 IU
D (ergocalciferol)	400 IU	400 IU	200 IU	200 IU
E (l g tocopherol acetate)	7 IU	7 IU	10 IU	10 IU
K (phytonadione)	200 µg	200 µg	150 µg	150 µg
C (ascorbic acid)	80 mg	80 mg	200 mg	200 mg
B_1 (thiamine)	1.2 mg	1.2 mg	6 mg	6 mg
B_2 (riboflavin)	1.4 mg	1.4 mg	3.6 mg	3.6 mg
B_6 (pyridoxine)	1 mg	1 mg	6 mg	6 mg
Niacinamide	17 mg	17 mg	40 mg	40 mg
Dexpanthenol	5 mg	5 mg	15 mg	15 mg
Biotin	20 µg	20 µg	60 µg	60 µg
Folic acid	140 µg	140 µg	600 µg	600µg
B_{12} (cyanocobalamin)	1 µg	1 µg	5 µg	5 µg
Contaminant Al	≤43 µg/L	Vial 1: <800 µg/L Vial 2: <275 µg/L	<183 µg/L	Vial 1: <800 µg/L Vial 2: <275 µg/L

[a] MVI Pediatric contains 375 mg mannitol, sodium hydroxide, 50 mg polysorbate 80, 0.8 mg polysorbate 20, 58 mg butylated hyroxytoluene, and 14 mg butylated hydroxyanisole.

[b] Infuvite Pediatric: Vial 1 contains 50 mg polysorbate 80 and sodium hydroxide or hydrochloric acid to adjust pH; vial 2 contains 75 mg mannitol and citric acid or sodium citrate to adjust pH.

[c] MVI-12: Vial 1 contains contains 30% propylene glycol, 2% gentisic acid ethanolamide, sodium hydroxide to adjust pH, 1.6% polysorbate 80, 0.028% polysorbate 20, 0.002% butylated hydroxytoluene, 0.0005% butylated hydroxyanisole; vial 2 contains 30% propylene glycol and citric acid or sodium citrate to adjust pH.

[d] Infuvite Adult: Vial 1 contains 1.4% polysorbate 80 and sodium hydroxide or hydrochloric acid to adjust pH. Vial 2 contains 30% propylene glycol and citric acid or sodium citrate to adjust pH.

Selenium deficiency may result in cardiomyopathy and skeletal muscle myopathy.[87] Selenium, chromium, and molybdenum are excreted primarily by the kidneys; thus, doses should be adjusted in patients with renal insufficiency. Each trace element is available as a single-entity product for patients who require an individualized approach to supplementation. Because the most common multitrace products for use in term infants and children are no longer manufactured, individualization of trace elements is becoming a more common practice.

Complicating the use of trace element supplementation is the fact that parenteral products are contaminated with a variety of elements, and concerns about potential toxicity have been expressed.[89–95] Children on long-term parenteral

TABLE 16.20	Trace Element Daily Requirements for Zinc, Copper, Manganese, Chromium, Selenium, and Iodine				
Trace Element	**Preterm**[87]	**Term <3 months**[87]	**Term >3 months**[87]	**Children**[87]	**Adults**
Zn	400 µg/kg	250 µg/kg	100 µg/kg	50 µg/kg	2.5–6 mg
Cu µg	20 µg/kg	20 µg/kg	20 µg/kg	200 µg	300–500
Mn	1 µg/kg	1 µg/kg	2–10 µg/kg	50 µg	150 µg[95]
Cr	0.2 µg/kg	0.2 µg/kg	0.14–0.2 µg/kg	5 µg	10–20 µg
Se	2 µg/kg	2 µg/kg	2 µg/kg	20 µg	40–80 µg
I	1 µg/kg	1 µg/kg	1 µg/kg		

Zn, zinc; Cu, copper; Mn, manganese; Cr, chromium; Se, selenium; I, iodine.

nutrition who have received recommended dosages of chromium have plasma chromium concentrations that are five to ten times higher than normal.[91,92]

Manganese (Mn) is also a known contaminant of parenteral fluids.[89,93] Because Mn is eliminated through biliary secretions, it is not surprising that children with cholestasis who receive Mn supplements have increased plasma concentrations.[93] Even in children with normal liver function, both elevated Mn blood concentrations and Mn deposition in the basal ganglia have been reported.[94] In children, neurologic symptoms related to Mn deposition in the brain are reversible once the Mn has been discontinued. Recommendations are that Mn should be eliminated from parenteral nutrition solutions in those who have cholestasis[87,93] and, perhaps, in those without cholestasis.

Although measurable amounts of copper are found in many products used in compounding parenteral nutrition solutions, these amounts are relatively small. Copper is also eliminated through the bile, so patients with cholestasis may accumulate copper, and some clinicians suggest eliminating copper during cholestasis.[87] However, most infants on parenteral nutrition receive a pediatric amino acid product with cysteine that exists in equilibrium with cystine, the dimer, and contains a sulfhydryl bridge. This provides a binding site for copper and zinc. Therefore, as was demonstrated with zinc and cysteine infusion,[96] infants who receive cysteine may have increased urinary elimination of copper. In this case, the total elimination of copper may result in deficiency that includes anemia and neutropenia. Decreasing the dose by half, measuring serum concentrations monthly until they are stable, and observing for signs of deficiency or toxicity seem prudent in the care of cholestatic children who are on long-term parenteral nutrition.

Complications. During parenteral nutrition, the most basic forms of nutrients are delivered directly into the bloodstream, bypassing normal digestive and absorptive processes. Because of the nature of these solutions and catheters and the direct link to the bloodstream, a variety of technical, metabolic, and infectious complications can occur.

Technical. The intravenous catheter placed in a peripheral vein can back out of the vein or push through the other side, causing the infusate to accumulate in the tissues. The addition of 1 to 2 units of heparin per milliliter of dextrose/amino acid solution[97] and the concomitant infusion of fat emulsion with dextrose and amino acid solution[98] increase the length of time to extravasation in those receiving peripherally infused parenteral nutrition.

Patients who require parenteral nutrition for relatively long periods generally have central venous catheters placed for this purpose. In small infants and children with limited or difficult peripheral vascular access, a central venous catheter may be required, even if parenteral nutrition is required for a relatively short time.[99] Complications that may occur at the time of catheter placement include pneumothorax, vein or cardiac perforation, chylothorax,[100] and bleeding. Following catheter placement, the catheter hub or line may be punctured or may crack or break. Damage to the hub or proximal (exposed) portion of the catheter can be repaired in many cases, but catheter removal may be necessary.

The infusate may extravasate into the thoracic or pericardial cavity. These fluids will be resorbed, in time, after the infusion has been discontinued, but significant tissue injury may result. Furthermore, the abrupt discontinuation of a concentrated dextrose solution that is infusing into the central circulation may result in hypoglycemia. Extravasated or infiltrated solutions may accumulate in the pleural or pericardial region, resulting in respiratory or cardiac decompensation; this situation may require chest tube placement.

Central venous catheters can migrate out of position or may be accidentally removed.[101] This problem is more common with percutaneously placed central venous catheters than with Broviac or Hickman Silastic catheters that are tunneled and anchored by a Dacron cuff (Fig. 16.1).[102]

Catheters located in the right atrium may stimulate dysrhythmias by coming in contact with nodal tissue. These dysrhythmias may be resolved by pulling the catheter away from sensitive tissue.

Catheters may become occluded because of fibrin deposition,[103] precipitates,[104] or saponified material that accumulates within the lumen. In many instances, the catheter that is not completely occluded can be recannulated pharmacologically.[105–107] Fibrinolytic agents, primarily tissue plasminogen activator, are useful in dissolving fibrin that partially occludes a catheter. Precipitates such as calcium phosphate may be dissolved when the pH inside the catheter is decreased through the instillation of 0.1 N HCl into the catheter.[105] Other agents such as ethanol may be used to dissolve saponified material.[106] Depending on catheter volume, the appropriate agent is drawn into a 10-mL syringe and instilled into the lumen of the partially occluded catheter. After a defined period, usually 2 to 4 hours, the agent is withdrawn, along with an additional 5 mL of blood, and the catheter is flushed. This ensures that any loosened debris from the catheter lumen is removed and is not infused into the patient.

Metabolic. Most electrolyte and mineral abnormalities and acid-base complications can be avoided with adequate monitoring and appropriate forethought when solutions are formulated. Other metabolic complications include aberrant plasma amino acid patterns (see section entitled Protein Requirements), micronutrient deficiencies, hypersensitivity reactions, acid-base abnormalities, and alterations in pulmonary and immunologic function.[108]

Aluminum Contamination. Large-volume parenteral products are contaminated by aluminum that is present in raw materials, introduced during manufacturing, or leached from glass bottles during storage.[109,110] In premature infants, the elderly, and those with renal dysfunction, the renal elimination of aluminum is impaired. Aluminum accumulation can result in metabolic bone disease, cholestasis, and encephalopathy. In 2004, the US Food and Drug Administration (FDA) issued a rule mandating that parenteral products must contain less than 25 μg per L of contaminant aluminum. As a result, the amount of aluminum present in an individual parenteral nutrition solution is calculated, and if the aluminum content exceeds 5 μg/kg/day—the maximum amount the FDA considers to be safe—the physician must be notified.

Cholestasis. The cause of cholestasis is multifactorial and complex; it occurs most commonly in premature infants who are enterally fasted and receive long-term parenteral nutrition.[111] These infants are also at risk for infection, including hepatitis, and frequently receive medications, such as furosemide, that are associated with cholestasis; thus, it remains a diagnosis of exclusion. Proposed mechanisms include amino acid competition with bile salts for hepatocyte uptake, enhanced production of secondary bile salts,[112] accumulation of toxic trace elements, and provision of excessive calories and protein.[113] Increases in γ-glutamyltransferase (GGT) and direct bilirubin[114] are early indicators of cholestasis, but these are not seen until after at least 10 days of parenteral nutrition.

Initiation of small-volume enteral (trophic) feeding for gut stimulation is probably the most important intervention that should be initiated as soon as the patient is able to tolerate even minimal enteral feeding. Providing the patient a protein- and calorie-free period by cycling the parenteral nutrition solution off for a period of time during the day also may be beneficial. Young and small infants have difficulty maintaining euglycemia during the ''cycle-off'' and ''cycle-on'' periods, so it is imperative that blood glucose monitoring occur during this intervention. Phenobarbital, a choleretic agent, is not effective treatment for parenteral nutrition–associated cholestasis.[114] Cholecystokinin has been proposed as a useful agent for promoting bile flow and potentially treating cholestasis, but insufficient experience prevents recommendation of its use for this purpose.[115] Finally, the use of a pediatric-specific amino acid formulation should be considered. These solutions normalize plasma amino acid patterns; they should cause optimal substrate metabolism and should minimize the potential toxicity associated with amino acids. Cholestasis generally resolves when parenteral nutrition is discontinued.

Bone Disease. As with cholestasis, the cause of metabolic bone disease is multifactorial and may be related to inadequate calcium and phosphorous intake, end-organ resistance to vitamin D, increased calcium losses in the urine due to medications (in particular, loop diuretics), and aluminum intake as a contaminant. Adequate calcium and phosphorous dosing significantly decreases the occurrence of metabolic bone disease in infants. Because pediatric amino acid products have a lower pH, more appropriate amounts of calcium and phosphorus can be given, and, anecdotally, the occurrence of metabolic bone disease may be decreased. Aluminum is a significant contaminant in many parenteral fluids;

therefore, those who receive large-volume parenteral fluids may be at risk for aluminum accumulation not only in soft tissues such as the brain but also in bone, thereby resulting in osteomalacia.[109,110] Several amino acid manufacturers have set limits for aluminum content in individual amino acids included in their products; therefore, contaminant aluminum in these products is minimal. Patients suspected of having osteopenia and rachitic changes should be evaluated by roentgenography or radiographic densitometry.[116,117]

Other. Hypersensitivity reactions have been reported in patients receiving parenteral nutrition.[118–124] Anaphylaxis has been attributed to amino acid solutions,[118] vitamin preparations,[119,120] magnesium sulfate,[118] fat emulsion,[121] iron, and soybean oil.[122] In addition, bradycardia[123] and diarrhea[124] have been associated with fat emulsion infusions.

A variety of hematologic abnormalities have been reported in patients receiving parenteral nutrition. Thrombocytopenia has been related to fat emulsion infusion and appears to be dose related.[124] In contrast, an increased peripheral platelet count has been described in preterm neonates on parenteral nutrition.[125] Parenteral nutrition–associated eosinophilia[126] occurs with greater frequency in premature neonates and appears to be self-limiting. Hemolysis due to lipid peroxidation of red blood cell membranes may be associated with failure to provide sufficient antioxidant (vitamin E) or antioxidant cofactors such as selenium.[127] Intravascular hemolysis has been reported with rapid infusion of fat emulsion in adults.[128,129]

Impairment of immune function has been described with deficiency or insufficiency of a variety of micronutrients, including zinc[130]; selenium; pyridoxine and pantothenic acid[131,132]; vitamins E,[133,134] A, and D[133]; arginine[135]; and glutamine.[136]

Dextrose and amino acid solutions with added vitamins can generate free radicals because of interactions between amino acids and vitamins, especially in the presence of light.[137] Some neonatal institutions cover the solution and even the tubing with aluminum foil or an opaque plastic sleeve to minimize these degradations. Fat emulsion is also subject to generation of free radicals; in some cases, these bottles, syringes, or bags and tubing are covered to decrease these reactions.[138] It has been postulated that providing free radicals to premature neonates in particular may be detrimental. To effectively minimize these reactions, amino acids and fats must be kept out of the light during storage, compounding, and infusion to the patient.[137,138]

Di(2ethylhexyl)phthalate (DEHP), a plasticizer, is common in PVC plastic bags and tubing. DEHP is lipophilic and can leach into lipophilic substances that are infused through tubing that contains DEHP. Phthalates are teratogenic and are known carcinogens in animals. This has been proposed to also occur in humans but has not been proved. Because of concern about potential toxicity, DEHP has been removed from toys, infant bottle nipples, and other soft plastic objects that are likely to come into contact with young children.[139]

Concern continues over potential toxicity in those young infants who, through medical exposure, receive fat emulsion (including propofol) through PVC tubing that contains DEHP, or those who are on extracorporeal membrane oxygenation (ECMO)—an intervention that includes a setup similar to cardiopulmonary bypass, wherein the blood is oxygenated outside the body via an ECMO circuit that consists of a large amount of PVC tubing.[139] However, DEHP is metabolized via pancreatic lipase to monoethylhexyl phthalate, a toxic metabolite, and those younger than 6 months to 12 months of age who lack mature pancreatic lipase systems may have some protection from toxicity.

Infection. Infection, a serious complication associated with central venous catheters, may be blood-borne, or may manifest as exit site or tunnel tract infection. Mechanisms include introduction of organisms into the bloodstream through the catheter, hematogenous spread, and potentially, bacterial translocation, a process in which bacteria normally present in the bowel cross the intestinal lumen and enter the bloodstream. Because of problems with venous access in small children, central venous catheters are used for multiple purposes, thereby increasing the risk for infection. Young children often play with their catheters or infusion sets and may chew on lines or disconnect the infusion, which further increases the risk for infection. Infants who require parenteral nutrition often have bowel disease that results in frequent loose stools that are difficult to contain; it is not uncommon for fecal material to come into contact with tubing, also increasing the risk for accidental contamination of catheters or solutions. Furthermore, premature neonates have a greater risk for infection because of immune system immaturity. In some cases, infections are polymicrobial. The incidence of central venous line infections is inversely related to age and in pediatric patients ranges from 42% to 57%.[140] Organisms that commonly result in infection in pediatric patients on long-term parenteral nutrition are listed in Table 16.21.[141]

Solution contamination is often suspected to be the source of the infection. Dextrose amino acid solutions are very hypertonic and support bacterial growth poorly; however, yeast will grow in these solutions. On the other hand, lipid products facilitate bacterial and fungal growth; thus, repackaging of lipid products is discouraged. *Malassezia furfur* is a fungal infection that is found most often in children; it is almost exclusively associated with lipid infusion.

Ideally, infected catheters are removed. However, in children who require long-term central access, removal of an infected catheter and placement of a new catheter in a different site after the infection has cleared may not be feasible. Once a vein has been cannulated, collateral veins develop around the site so that blood flow to the area is not compromised. Collateral vessels are tortuous and narrow and can rarely be cannulated. In addition, veins may become thrombosed or scarred because of the presence of a catheter, rendering them unsuitable for subsequent line placement. Therefore, the decision to remove a central line in a child who depends on this route for hydration and nutrition must be made judiciously. Placement of a catheter directly into the right atrium has been performed in children without an alternative catheterization site. In patients with catheter-related infection who continued to require central venous access, 55% to 89% of catheter-related infections were successfully treated in situ by the administration of appropriate antibiotics through the catheter.[11,142] The appropriate dosage of an antimicrobial agent should be infused through the infected catheter. In addition, antibiotics or antifungals can be instilled and allowed to reside in the catheter for varying lengths of time, referred to as *dwell therapies*. Daily blood cultures are obtained through the catheter lumen and from a peripheral site to ensure that the microorganism is being eradicated.[11,142] Multiple-lumen catheters require careful evaluation because only one or all of the lumina may be infected. It is important that the infected lumina be effectively treated.

The body recognizes an indwelling central venous catheter as foreign; fibrin can accumulate outside and inside the lumen of the catheter, particularly if the line is used for blood withdrawal.[103] Microorganisms may be harbored within the fibrin, providing a nidus for infection. Even appropriate microbial therapy may not penetrate through the fibrin web to eradicate microorganisms residing inside. Although streptokinase, tissue plasminogen activator, and possibly HCl can dissolve the fibrin within the catheter lumen, it is less likely that fibrin around the outside of the catheter will be affected. Monthly treatment of central lines with a fibrinolytic has been suggested to decrease the number of central line infections. However, dissolution of a fibrin sheath that is harboring a large number of microorganisms has the potential to release the microorganisms into the bloodstream. The resultant bacteremia may cause an acute septic event or may seed distant sites.

The catheter exit site or tunnel tract may also become infected. Local antibiotic therapy may be used to treat certain exit site infections; however, both exit site and tunnel tract infections may require systemic antimicrobial therapy. In

TABLE 16.21	Microorganisms Cultured from Central Venous Catheters in Children on Home Parenteral Nutrition	
Staphylococcus epidermidis	25%	
Klebsiella	12%	
Staphylococcus aureus	10%	
Escherichia coli	6%	
Candida parapsilosis	5%	
Gram-positive organisms	43%	
Gram-negative organisms	36%	
Fungi	13%	
Polymicrobes	11%	

addition, more frequent central line dressing changes may be required.

NUTRITIONAL ASSESSMENT AND MONITORING

Similar nutritional assessment techniques are used in children and adults; however, children require special consideration for almost all parameters assessed.[143] Body composition in infants can be evaluated with the use of dual-energy x-ray absorptiometry (DEXA), total body electrical conductivity (TOBEC), and magnetic resonance imaging (MRI) techniques.[144,145] Because of the expense of equipment and personnel and the need for patients to remain motionless during the study, these procedures are not used in routine clinical pediatric practice.

WEIGHT, LENGTH, OR HEIGHT

Soon after birth, the extracellular fluid volume contracts, and a diuresis that results in weight loss occurs. The percentage of extracellular fluid increases with increasing prematurity; therefore, the percentage of total body weight loss after birth is increased in premature neonates.[27,28] When nutrient needs are met, infants should regain their birth weight by 7 to 10 days of age.

After fluid redistribution occurs shortly after birth, weight is the most important assessment tool used to evaluate nutritional outcome in infants and children. All infants who receive parenteral nutrition should have their weight measured daily, unless medically prohibited. Weights should be taken at the same time each day with the use of the same scale; assessments should be made by the same caregiver, and the infant should be nude. Wound dressings, arm boards used to stabilize an intravenous line, or other equipment can alter apparent weight, making interpretation of daily weight changes difficult. Because weight changes may relate to factors other than lean body mass accretion, assessment of weight changes should be averaged over several days. The younger the infant, the greater the expected gain per kilogram. Older children and adolescents may require less frequent weighing because growth occurs more slowly.

Length or height is measured less often than weight. Length should be measured at least monthly in small infants and semiannually in adolescents, unless a clinical condition or disease mandates more frequent measurement.

GROWTH CHARTS

The Third National Health and Nutrition Examination Survey (NHANES III) data collected between 1988 and 1994 were used to revise the pediatric growth charts in 2000. An individual child can be compared with population of the same age for length or height, weight, and head circumference[146]; these charts are available online at [http://www.cdc.gov/growthcharts]. In addition, a body mass index (BMI) chart that provides screening for overweight and for obesity was added for those older than 2 years of age.[146] Periodic weight and length/height plotting on growth charts provides an assessment of interindividual growth. In general, weight below the population standard indicates acute malnutrition; both weight and height below the population standard suggests a more chronic problem. When growth charts are interpreted, consideration must be given to gestational age and genetic factors (e.g., children whose parents are tall may be at greater than the 95th percentile for height). Head circumference is also plotted in infants and young children. This is not used as a nutritional index but is a way to screen for the development of hydrocephalus.

Estimates of desired average daily weight gains can be extrapolated from growth charts for better evaluation of changes over a relatively short period in younger, smaller infants whose growth velocity is greater in grams per kilogram per day. Growth charts for preterm infants ($\leq$37 weeks' gestational age) are available for low-birthweight (1,501 to 2,500 g) and very low birthweight ($\leq$1,500 g) infants at http://www.rosspediatrics.com under ''Practice Tools.'' A standard growth curve can be used if the postnatal age is adjusted for length of gestation (e.g., a 6-month-old infant born at 32 weeks' gestation, or 2 months early, should be plotted as a 4-month-old infant).

INTAKE AND OUTPUT

Intake consists of all substances delivered enterally and parenterally, including fluid used in the delivery of medications and flushes. Output includes urine, stool, nasogastric or gastrostomy tube drainage, chest tube outputs, emesis, blood loss, ventriculostomy drainage, and wound exudate. If possible, urine and stool volumes should be recorded separately. In infants, diapers can be weighed before they are put on the infant, and again after they are removed. The difference in weight approximates the volume of urine or stool contained in the diaper. Similarly, wound losses can be approximated when the bandage is weighed before and after it is placed. Measurement of total intake and output aids in the evaluation of fluid balance and the source of weight gain (e.g., lean body mass accretion vs. edema).

ANTHROPOMETRIC MEASUREMENTS

Age-related nomograms were developed for arm circumference and triceps skinfold thickness.[147] With the use of these nomograms, age-related percentiles can be calculated for arm muscle area, arm muscle diameter, and arm muscle circumference, and lean body mass can be assessed. Subscapular skinfold standards also have been compiled. To minimize variability, the same trained person and the same caliper type should be used to assess a given patient over time. These assessments are helpful for evaluation of interindividual progress.

VISCERAL PROTEINS

Serum albumin, transferrin, prealbumin (transthyretin), and retinol-binding protein are the visceral protein markers used in nutritional assessment.[148–152] Although the half-lives of these proteins in children are similar to those in adults, age-related normal serum concentrations may be lower in children. In healthy preterm infants and unhealthy term infants, prealbumin concentrations of 10.8 ± 3.9 and 9.7 ± 3.7 mg per dL, respectively, have been reported,[152] whereas concentrations in adults range from 23 to 41 mg per dL.[150] Prealbumin and retinol-binding protein concentrations increase following the provision of appropriate nutrients to otherwise healthy premature infants.[153,154] Likewise, concentrations increase in critically ill, malnourished infants who receive specialized nutrition support.[155] As in adults, these visceral protein markers are subject to concentration changes unrelated to nutrition status, including renal failure, iron status, liver disease, and acute illness.[156]

URINE STUDIES

Nitrogen balance measures the difference between nitrogen (protein) intake from parenteral and enteral nutrition and urinary urea nitrogen (UUN) lost during a 24-hour period. Although this is a relatively easy, noninvasive, reliable assessment of adequacy of intake in adults, it can be difficult to perform in infants. A common urine collection technique for an uncatheterized infant includes placing a urine collection bag around the genital area with an adhesive that remains affixed for the collection period. Problems include collection bags that do not fit well, adhesives that do not stick, skin breakdown under the adhesive, and stool contamination of the collected urine. These problems are avoided in catheterized infants.

Not only is it difficult to collect urine, but the total urine nitrogen (TUN) concentration relationship with UUN is unpredictable.[157] In adults, insensible nitrogen losses are estimated according to a set amount, and nonurea nitrogen losses are accounted for by multiplying the UUN measurement by 1.25. In young children, this factor can cause underestimation or overestimation of actual TUN losses. TUN can be measured through pyrochemiluminescence, although this is not available in many hospital clinical laboratories. A newer analytic method requires that all wet or soiled diapers be placed in a cooler after removal from the infant and collected over a 24-hour period. Soaking the diapers in a citrate buffer allows recovery of 90% to 95% of total urinary and stool nitrogen.[158]

IMMUNE FUNCTION

Assessment of immune function may not be helpful in determination of the nutritional status of infants and young children because lack of an immunologic response to a challenge may be due to lack of antigenic experience or to immaturity.[159,160] Also, as with visceral proteins, underlying disease can affect response to immunologic stimulation. On the other hand, improved lymphocyte function and enhanced expression of T-cell populations have been reported in malnourished infants who receive short-term parenteral nutrition.[161–163]

CONCLUSION

In this chapter, the reader has been apprised of the uniqueness of pediatric nutritional needs and the limitations of assessment techniques used in children. It is important to remember that children are not small adults; therefore, they should not be treated as such. Children (particularly neonates and infants) require quantitatively and qualitatively different nutrients than adults require. Failure to address these unique substrate requirements can result in abnormal physical and neurologic growth and development. However, through an understanding of the unique needs of children, the appropriate nutrients can be provided, normal growth can be achieved, and developmental milestones can be met.

KEY POINTS

- The ideal enteral feeding for infants is human milk.
- Infant formulas have been designed with the use of human milk as a template for nutrient composition.
- Whenever possible, the enteral route of feeding should be used.
- In general, fluid requirements (milliliters per kilogram) and caloric requirements (kilocalories per kilogram) are inversely related to patient age and weight.
- Parenteral amino acid products have been designed to address the unique amino acid needs of infants.
- Many metabolic complications associated with parenteral nutrition in neonates and infants can be avoided through an understanding of micronutrient needs and appropriate monitoring.
- Fat requirements are higher in pediatric patients to provide for normal growth and development.
- Normal growth and development can be achieved with parenteral nutrition.

REFERENCES

1. ASPEN Board of Directors and The Clinical Guidelines Task Force. Guidelines for the use of parenteral and enteral nutrition in adult and pediatric patients. JPEN J Parenter Enteral Nutr 26 (Suppl):1SA–138SA, 2002.
2. National Research Council. Recommended dietary allowances. 10th ed. Washington DC: National Academy Press, 1989:chapters 3–9.
3. Feranchak AP, Sontag MK, Wagener JS, et al. Prospective, long-term study of fat-soluble vitamin status in children with cystic fibrosis identified by newborn screen. J Pediatr 135:601–610, 1999.
4. Kennedy-Caldwell C, Caldwell MD, Zitarelli ME. Pediatric enteral nutrition. In: Rombeau JL, Caldwell MD, eds. Clinical nutrition—enteral and tube feeding. Philadelphia, Pa: WB Saunders, 1990:325–360.
5. American Academy of Pediatrics, Work Group on Breastfeeding. Breastfeeding and the use of human milk. Pediatrics 100: 1035–1039, 1997.
6. Chen Y, Yu S, Li WX. Artificial feeding and hospitalization in the first 18 months of life. Pediatrics 81:58–62, 1988.
7. Lawrence RA. Breastfeeding and medical disease. Med Clin North Am 72:583–603, 1989.

8. Riordan J. The biologic specificity of breastmilk. In: Riordan J, Auerback KG, eds. Breastfeeding and human lactation. 1st ed. Boston, Mass: Jones and Bartlett Publishers; 1993:105–134.

9. Rogers IS. Lactation and fertility. Early Human Dev 49 (Suppl): S185–S190, 1997.

10. Dewey KG. Maternal and fetal stress are associated with impaired lactogenesis in humans. J Nutr 131:3012S–3015S, 2001.

11. Martinez JC, Maisels MJ, Otheguy L, et al. Hyperbilirubinemia in the breast-fed newborn: a controlled trial of four interventions. Pediatrics 91:470–473, 1992.

12. Auestad N, Schoo DT, Janowsky JS, et al. Visual, cognitive and language assessments at 39 months: a follow-up study of children fed formulas containing long-chain polyunsaturated fatty acids to 1 year of age. Pediatrics 112:e177–e183, 2003.

13. Uauy R, Hoffman ER, Mena P, et al. Term infant studies of DHA and ARA supplementation on neurodevelopment: results of randomized controlled trials. J Pediatr 143:S17–S25, 2003.

14. Centers for Disease Control and Prevention. *Enterobacter sakazakii* infections associated with the use of powdered infant formula—Tennessee, 2001. MMWR 51:298–300, 2002.

15. American Academy of Pediatrics Committee on Nutrition. Sodium intake of infants in the United States. Pediatrics 68:444–445, 1981.

16. Helley AA, Ogden CL, Johnson CL, et al. Prevalence of overweight and obesity among US children, adolescents, and adults, 1999–2002. JAMA 291;2847–2850, 2004.

17. Utter J, Neumark-Sztainer D, Jeffery R, et al. Couch potatoes or French fries: are sedentary behaviors associated with body mass index, physical activity, and dietary behaviors among adolescents? J Am Diet Assoc 103:1298–3105, 2003.

18. Thureen PJ, Hay WW Jr. Early aggressive nutrition in preterm infants. Semin Neonatal 2001;6:403–415.

19. Maloney JP, Ryan TA, Brasel KJ, et al. Food dye use in enteral feedings: a review and a call for a moratorium. Nutr Clin Pract 17: 169–181, 2002.

20. Mahon BE, Rosenman MB, Kleiman MB. Maternal and infant use of erythromycin and other macrolide antibiotics as risk factors for infantile hypertrophic pyloric stenosis. J Pediatr 139:380–384, 2001.

21. American Academy of Pediatrics, Committee on Nutrition. Nutritional needs of low-birth-weight infants. Pediatrics 75:976–986, 1985.

22. Phelps SJ, Helms RA. Risk factors affecting infiltration of peripheral venous lines in infants. J Pediatr 111:384–389, 1987.

23. Oellrich RG, Murphy MR, Goldberg LA, et al. The percutaneous central venous catheter for small or ill infants. Maternal Child Nursing 16:92–96, 1991.

24. Wurzel CL, Halom K, Feldman JG, et al. Infection rates of Broviac-Hickman catheters and implantable venous devices. Am J Dis Child 142:536–540, 1988.

25. Mirro J, Rao B, Kuman M, et al. A comparison of placement techniques and complications of externalized catheters and implantable port use in children with cancer. J Pediatr Surg 25:120–124, 1990.

26. Rollins CJ, Elsberry VA, Pollack KA, et al. Three-in-one parenteral nutrition: a safe and economical method of nutritional support for infants. JPEN J Parenter Enteral Nutr 14:290–294, 1990.

27. Holliday MA, Segar WE. The maintenance need for water in parenteral fluid therapy. Pediatrics 19:823–832, 1957.

28. Costarino A, Baumgart S. Modern fluid and electrolyte management of the critically ill premature infant. Pediatr Clin North Am 33:153–178, 1986.

29. Bell EF, Oh W. Fluid and electrolyte balance in very low birth weight infants. Clin Perinatol 6:139–150, 1979.

30. Stuart HC, Sobel EH. The thickness of the skin and subcutaneous tissue by age and sex in childhood. J Pediatr 28:637–647, 1946.

31. Williams PR, Oh W. Effects of radiant warmer on insensible water loss in newborn infants. Am J Dis Child 128:511–514, 1974.

32. Leake RD, Zakuddin S, Trygstad CW, et al. The effects of large volume intravenous fluid infusion on neonatal renal function. J Pediatr 89:968–972, 1976.

33. Arant BS Jr. Developmental patterns of renal functional maturation compared in the human neonate. J Pediatr 92:705–712, 1978.

34. Van Marter LJ, Leviton A, Allred EN, et al. Hydration during the first days of life and the risk of bronchopulmonary dysplasia in low birth weight infants. J Pediatr 116:942–949, 1990.

35. Goldberg RN, Chung D, Goldman SL, et al. The association of rapid volume expansion and intraventricular hemorrhage in the preterm infant. J Pediatr 96:1060–1063, 1980.

36. Bell EF, Warburton D, Stonestreet BS, et al. Effect of fluid administration on the development of symptomatic patent ductus arteriosus and congestive heart failure in premature infants. N Engl J Med 302:598–604, 1980.

37. Uauy RD, Faranoff AA, Korones SB, et al. Necrotizing enterocolitis in very low birth weight infants: biodemographic and clinical correlates. National Institutes of Child Health and Human Development Neonatal Research Network. J Pediatr 119:630–638, 1991.

38. Stegink LD, Baker GL. Infusion of protein hydrolysates in the newborn infant: plasma amino acid concentrations. J Pediatr 78: 595–602, 1971.

39. Thureen PJ, Anderson AH, Baron KA, et al. Protein balance in the first week of life in ventilated neonates receiving parenteral nutrition. Am J Clin Nutr 68:1128–1135, 1998.

40. Van Goudoever JB, Colen T, Wattimena JLD, et al. Immediate commencement of amino acid supplementation in preterm infants: effect on serum amino acid concentrations and protein kinetics on the first day of life. J Pediatr 127:458–465, 1995.

41. Helms RA, Christensen ML, Mauer EC, et al. Comparison of pediatric versus standard amino acid formulation in preterm neonates requiring parenteral nutrition. J Pediatr 110:466–470, 1987.

42. Heird WC, Dell RB, Helms RA, et al. Amino acid mixture designed to maintain normal plasma amino acid patterns in infants and children requiring parenteral nutrition. Pediatrics 80:401–408, 1987.

43. Adamkin DH, McClead RE, Desai NS, et al. Comparison of two neonatal intravenous amino acid formulations in preterm infants: a multicenter study. J Perinatol 11:375–382, 1991.

44. Wu PY, Edwards N, Storm MC. Plasma amino acid pattern in term breast-fed neonates. J Pediatr 109:347–349, 1986.

45. Chessman K, Johnson M, Fernandes E, et al. Changing parenteral substrate requirements in neonates receiving a pediatric amino acid formulation. JPEN J Parenter Enteral Nutr 12:105, 1988. Abstract.

46. Beck R. Use of a pediatric parenteral amino acid mixture in a population of extremely low birth weight neonates: frequency and spectrum of direct bilirubinemia. Am J Perinatol 7:84–86, 1990.

47. Gazzaniga AB, Waxman K, Day AT, et al. Nitrogen balance in adult hospitalized patients with the use of a pediatric amino acid model. Arch Surg 123:1275–1279, 1988.

48. Helms RA, Storm MC, Christensen ML, et al. Cysteine supplementation results in normalization of plasma taurine concentrations in children receiving home parenteral nutrition. J Pediatr 134: 358–361, 1999.

49. Reichman BL, Chessex P, Putet G, et al. Partition of energy metabolism and energy cost of growth in the very low-birth-weight infant. Pediatrics 69:446–451, 1982.

50. Zlotkin SH, Bryan MH, Anderson GH. Intravenous nitrogen and energy intakes required to duplicate in utero nitrogen accretion in prematurely born human infants. J Pediatr 99:115–120, 1981.

51. Letton RW, Chwals WJ, Jamie A, et al. Early postoperative alterations in infant energy use increase the risk of overfeeding. J Pediatr Surg 30:988–992, 1995.

52. Thomas DB. Hyperosmolality and intraventricular haemorrhage in premature babies. Acta Paediatr Scand 65:429–432, 1976.

53. Sheridan RL, Yu Y, Prelack K, et al. Maximal parenteral glucose oxidation in hypermetabolic young children: a stable isotope study. JPEN J Parenter Enteral Nutr 22:212–216, 1998.

54. Collins JW Jr, Hoppe M, Brown K, et al. A controlled trial of insulin infusion and parenteral nutrition in extremely low birth weight infants with glucose intolerance. J Pediatr 118:921–927, 1991.

55. Committee on Nutrition, American Academy of Pediatrics. Commentary on parenteral nutrition. Pediatrics 71:547–552, 1983.

56. Bivins BA, Bell RM, Rapp RP, et al. Linoleic acid versus linolenic acid: what is essential. JPEN J Parenter Enteral Nutr 7:473–478, 1983.

57. Schiff D, Chan G, Seccombe D, et al. Plasma carnitine levels during intravenous feeding of the neonate. J Pediatr 95:1043–1046, 1979.

58. Helms RA, Whitington PF, Mauer EC, et al. Enhanced lipid utilization in infants receiving oral l-carnitine during long-term parenteral nutrition. J Pediatr 109:984–988, 1986.

59. Iofalla AK, Roe CR. Carnitine deficiency in apnea of prematurity. Pediatr Res 2:309A, 1995.
60. Nordenstrom J, Jarstrand C, Wienick A. Decreased chemotactic and random migration of leukocytes during Intralipid infusion. Am J Clin Nutr 32:2416–2422, 1979.
61. Jarstrand C, Berghem L, Lahnborg G. Human granulocyte and reticuloendothelial system function during Intralipid infusion. JPEN J Parenter Enteral Nutr 2:663–670, 1978.
62. Ladisch S, Poplark DG, Blaese RM. Inhibition of human lymphoproliferation by intravenous lipid emulsion. Clin Immunol Immunopathol 25:196–202, 1982.
63. Palmbald J, Brostrom O, Lahnborg G, et al. Neutrophil functions during total parenteral nutrition and Intralipid infusion. Am J Clin Nutr 35:1430–1436, 1982.
64. Strunk RC, Murrow BW, Thilo E, et al. Normal macrophage function in infants receiving Intralipid by low-dose intermittent administration. J Pediatr 106:640–645, 1985.
65. Escudier EF, Escudier BJ, Henry-Amar MC, et al. Effects of infused Intralipid on neutrophil chemotaxis during total parenteral nutrition. JPEN J Parenter Enteral Nutr 10:596–598, 1986.
66. Schroder H, Paust H, Schmidt R. Pulmonary fat embolism after Intralipid therapy—a postmortem artefact? Acta Paediatr Scand 73: 461–464, 1984.
67. Pereira GR, Fox WW, Stanley CA, et al. Decreased oxygenation and hyperlipemia during intravenous fat infusions in premature infants. Pediatrics 66:26–30, 1980.
68. Brans YW, Dutton EB, Andrew DS, et al. Fat emulsion tolerance in very low birth weight neonates: effect on diffusion of oxygen in the lungs and on blood pH. Pediatrics 78:79–84, 1986.
69. Haumont D, Deckelbaum RJ, Richelle M, et al. Plasma lipid concentrations in low birth weight infants given parenteral nutrition with twenty or ten percent lipid emulsion. J Pediatr 115:787–793, 1989.
70. Arnold WC. Parenteral nutrition, and fluid and electrolyte therapy. Pediatr Clin North Am 37:449–461, 1990.
71. Sulyok E, Varga F, Gyory E, et al. Postnatal development of renal sodium handling in premature infants. J Pediatr 95:787–792, 1979.
72. Stapleton FB, Nelson B, Vats TS, et al. Hypokalemia associated with antibiotic treatment. Am J Dis Child 130:1104–1108, 1976.
73. Schaber DE, Uden DL, Stone FM, et al. Intravenous KCl supplementation in pediatric cardiac surgical patients. Pediatr Cardiol 6: 25–28, 1985.
74. Knight PJ, Buchanan S, Clatworthy HW Jr. Calcium and phosphate requirements of preterm infants who require prolonged hyperalimentation. JAMA 243:1244–1246, 1980.
75. Pelegano JF, Rowe JC, Carey DE, et al. Simultaneous infusion of calcium and phosphorus in parenteral nutrition for premature infants: use of physiologic calcium/phosphorus ratio. J Pediatr 114: 115–119, 1989.
76. Koo WWK. Parenteral nutrition related bone disease. JPEN J Parenter Enteral Nutr 16:386–394, 1992.
77. Vileisis RA. Furosemide effect on mineral status of parenterally nourished premature neonates with chronic lung disease. Pediatrics 85:316–322, 1990.
78. Eggert LD, Rusho WJ, MacKay MW, et al. Calcium and phosphorus compatibility in parenteral nutrition solutions for neonates. Am J Hosp Pharm 39:49–53, 1982.
79. Lenz GT, Mikrut BA. Calcium and phosphate solubility in neonatal parenteral nutrient solutions containing Aminosyn-PF or TrophAmine. Am J Hosp Pharm 45:2367–2371, 1988.
80. Schmidt GL, Baumgartner TG, Fischlschweiger W, et al. Cost containment using cysteine HCl acidification to increase calcium/phosphate solubility in hyperalimentation solutions. JPEN J Parenter Enteral Nutr 10:203–207, 1986.
81. Henry RS, Jurgens RW Jr, Sturgeon R, et al. Compatibility of calcium chloride and calcium gluconate with sodium phosphate in a mixed TPN solution. Am J Hosp Pharm 37:673–674, 1980.
82. Niemiec PW Jr, Vanderveen TW. Compatibility considerations in parenteral nutrient solutions. Am J Hosp Pharm 41:893–911, 1984.
83. Solomon SM, Kirby DF. The refeeding syndrome: a review. JPEN J Parenter Enteral Nutr 14:90–97, 1990.
84. Tsang RC. Neonatal magnesium disturbances. Am J Dis Child 124: 282–293, 1972.
85. Whang R, Aikawa JK. Magnesium deficiency and refractoriness to potassium repletion. J Chron Dis 30:65–68, 1977.
86. Centers for Disease Control and Prevention. Lactic acidosis traced to thiamine deficiency related to nationwide shortage of multivitamins for total parenteral nutrition—United States, 1997. MMWR 46:523–528, 1997.
87. Greene HL, Hambidge KM, Schanler R, et al. Guidelines for the use of vitamins, trace elements, calcium, magnesium, and phosphorus in infants and children receiving total parenteral nutrition: report of the Subcommittee on Pediatric Parenteral Nutrient Requirements from the Committee on Clinical Practice Issues of The American Society for Clinical Nutrition. Am J Clin Nutr 48: 1324–1342, 1988.
88. Tyson JE, Wright LL, Oh W, et al. Vitamin A supplementation for extremely-low-birth-weight infants. N Engl J Med 340:1962–1968, 1999.
89. Pluhator-Murton MM, Fedorak RN, Audette RJ, et al. Trace element contamination of total parenteral nutrition. 1. Contribution of component solutions. JPEN J Parenter Enteral Nutr 23:222–227, 1999.
90. Hak EB, Storm MC, Helms RA. Chromium and zinc contaminant in components of parenteral nutrition solutions commonly used in infants and children. Am J Health-Syst Pharm 55:150–154, 1998.
91. Moukarzel AA, Song MK, Buchman AL, et al. Excessive chromium intake in children receiving total parenteral nutrition. Lancet 339:385–388, 1992.
92. Mouser JF, Hak EB, Helms RA, et al. Evaluation of zinc and chromium in infants and children receiving long-term parenteral nutrition. Am J Health-Syst Pharm 56:1950–1956, 1999.
93. Hambidge KM, Sokol RJ, Fidanza SJ, et al. Plasma manganese concentrations in infants and children receiving parenteral nutrition. JPEN J Parenter Enteral Nutr 13:168–171, 1989.
94. Masumota K, Suita S, Taguchi T, et al. Manganese intoxication during intermittent parenteral nutrition: report of two cases. JPEN J Parenter Enteral Nutr 25:95–99, 2001.
95. Fitzgerald K, Mikalunas V, Rubin H, et al. Hypermanganesemia in patients receiving total parenteral nutrition. JPEN J Parenter Enteral Nutr 23:333–336, 1999.
96. Zlotkin SH. Nutrient interactions with total parenteral nutrition: effect of histidine and cysteine intake on urinary zinc excretion. J Pediatr 114:859–864, 1989.
97. Alpan G, Eyal F, Springer C, et al. Heparinization of alimentation solutions administered through peripheral veins in premature infants: a controlled study. Pediatrics 74:375–378, 1984.
98. Phelps SJ, Cochran EB. Effect of the continuous administration of fat emulsion on the infiltration of intravenous lines in infants receiving peripheral parenteral nutrition solutions. JPEN J Parenter Enteral Nutr 13:628–632, 1989.
99. Eichelberger MR, Rous PG, Hoelzer D, et al. Percutaneous subclavian venous catheters in neonates and children. J Pediatr Surg 16: 547–552, 1981.
100. Ruggiero RP, Caruso G. Chylothorax—a complication of subclavian vein catheterization. JPEN J Parenter Enteral Nutr 9:750–753, 1985.
101. Gutcher G, Cutz E. Complications of parenteral nutrition. Semin Perinatol 10:196–207, 1986.
102. Welch GW, McKell DW, Silverstein P, et al. The role of catheter composition in the development of thrombophlebitis. Surg Gynecol Obstet 138:421–424, 1974.
103. Hoshal VL, Ause RG, Hoskins PA. Fibrin sleeve formation on indwelling subclavian central venous catheters. Arch Surg 102: 353–358, 1971.
104. Breaux CW Jr, Duke D, Georgeson KE, et al. Calcium phosphate crystal occlusion of central venous catheters used for total parenteral nutrition in infants and children: prevention and treatment. J Pediatr Surg 22:829–832, 1987.
105. Duffy LF, Kerzner B, Gebus V, et al. Treatment of central venous catheter occlusions with hydrochloric acid. J Pediatr 114:102–104, 1989.
106. Holcombe BJ, Forloines-Lynn S, Garmhausen LW. Restoring patency of long-term central venous access devices. J Intravenous Nursing 15:36–41, 1992.
107. Pennington CR, Pithie AD. Ethanol lock in the management of catheter occlusion. JPEN J Parenter Enteral Nutr 11:507–508, 1987.

108. Baker SS, Dwyer E, Queen P. Metabolic derangements in children requiring parenteral nutrition. JPEN J Parenter Enteral Nutr 10: 279–281, 1986.

109. Koo WWK, Kaplan LA, Horn J, et al. Aluminum in parenteral nutrition solution—sources and possible alternatives. JPEN J Parenter Enteral Nutr 10:591–595, 1986.

110. Klein GL, Alfey AC, Shike N, et al. Parenteral drug products containing aluminum as an ingredient or a contaminant; response to FDA notice of intent. Am J Clin Nutr 53:399–402, 1991.

111. Black DD, Suttle EA, Whitington PF, et al. The effect of short-term total parenteral nutrition on hepatic function in the human neonate: a prospective randomized study demonstrating alteration of the hepatic canalicular function. J Pediatr 99:445–449, 1981.

112. Farrell MK, Balistren WF, Sucky FY. Serum-sulfated lithocholate as an indicator of cholestasis during parenteral nutrition in infants and children. JPEN J Parenter Enteral Nutr 6:30–33, 1982.

113. Whitington PF. Cholestasis associated with total parenteral nutrition in infants. Hepatology 5:693–696, 1985.

114. Beale EF, Nelson RM, Bucciarelli RL, et al. Intrahepatic cholestasis associated with parenteral nutrition in premature infants. Pediatrics 64:342–347, 1979.

115. Gleghorn EE, Merritt RJ, Subramanian N, et al. Phenobarbital does not prevent total parenteral-associated cholestasis in noninfected infants. JPEN J Parenter Enteral Nutr 10:282–283, 1986.

116. Doty JE, Pitt HA, Porter-Fink V, et al. Cholecystokinin prophylaxis of parenteral nutrition–induced gallbladder disease. Ann Surg 201:76–80, 1985.

117. Lyon AJ, Hawkes DJ, Doran M, et al. Bone mineralization in preterm infants measured by dual energy radiographic densitometry. Arch Dis Child 64:919–923, 1989.

118. Pomeranz S, Gimmon Z, Zvi AB, et al. Parenteral-nutrition–induced anaphylaxis. JPEN J Parenter Enteral Nutr 11:314–315, 1987.

119. Bullock L, Etchason E, Fitzgerald JF, et al. Case report of an allergic reaction to parenteral nutrition in a pediatric patient. JPEN J Parenter Enteral Nutr 14:98–100, 1990.

120. Market AD, Lew DB, Schropp KP, et al. Anaphylactoid reaction associated with parenteral nutrition in a 4 year old. J Pediatr Gastroenterol Nutr 26:229–231, 1998.

121. Kamath KR, Berry A, Commins G. Acute hypersensitivity reaction to Intralipid. N Engl J Med 304:360, 1981.

122. Hiyama DT, Griggs B, Mittman RF, et al. Hypersensitivity following lipid emulsion infusion in an adult patient. JPEN J Parenter Enteral Nutr 13:318–320, 1989.

123. Sternberg A, Gruenevald T, Duetsch AA, et al. Intralipid-induced transient sinus bradycardia. N Engl J Med 304:422–423, 1981.

124. Connon JJ. Diarrhea possibly caused by total parenteral nutrition. N Engl J Med 301:273–274, 1979.

125. Campbell AN, Freedman MH, Pendarz PI, et al. Bleeding disorder from the ''fat overload'' syndrome. JPEN J Parenter Enteral Nutr 8:447–449, 1984.

126. Bhat AM, Scanlon JW. The pattern of eosinophilia in premature infants. J Pediatr 98:612–616, 1981.

127. Rotruck JT, Pope AL, Banther HE, et al. Selenium: biochemical role as a component of glutathione peroxidase. Science 179: 588–590, 1973.

128. Marks LM, Patel N, Kurtides ES. Hematologic abnormalities associated with intravenous lipid therapy. Am J Gastroenterol 73: 490–495, 1980.

129. McGrath KM, Zalcberg JR, Slonim J. Intralipid induced haemolysis. Br J Haematol 50:376–378, 1982.

130. Golden MHN, Harland PAEG, Golden BE, et al. Zinc and immunocompetence in protein-energy malnutrition. Lancet 1:1226–1227, 1978.

131. Hodges RE, Bean WB, Ohlson MA, et al. Factors affecting human antibody response V. Combined deficiencies of pantothenic acid and pyridoxine. Am J Clin Nutr 11:187–199, 1962.

132. Axelrod AE. Immune process in vitamin deficiency states. Am J Clin Nutr 24:265–271, 1971.

133. Kinsella JE, Lokesh B, Broughton S, et al. Dietary polyunsaturated fatty acids and eicosanoids: potential effects on the modulation of inflammatory and immune cells: an overview. Nutrition 6:24–44, 1990.

134. Meydani SN, Yogeeswaran G, Liu S, et al. Fish oil and tocopherol-induced changes in natural killer cell–mediated cytotoxicity and PGE_2 synthesis in young and old mice. J Nutr 118:1245–1252, 1988.

135. Barbul A, Sisto DA, Waserkurg HL, et al. Arginine stimulates lymphocyte immune response in healthy human beings. Surgery 90: 244–251, 1981.

136. Burke DJ, Alverdy JC, Aoys E, et al. Glutamine-supplemented total parenteral nutrition improves gut immune function. Arch Surg 124:1396–1399, 1989.

137. Laborie S, Lavoie JC, Pineault M, et al. Contribution of multivitamins, air and light in the generation of peroxides in adult and neonatal parenteral nutrition solutions. Ann Pharmacother 34:440–445, 2000.

138. Neuzil J, Darlow BA, Inder TE, et al. Oxidation of parenteral lipid emulsion by ambient and phototherapy lights: potential toxicity of routine parenteral feeding. J Pediatr 126:785–790, 1995.

139. American Academy of Pediatrics Technical Report. Pediatric exposure and potential toxicity of phthalate plasticizers. Pediatrics 111: 1467–1473, 2003.

140. Vargas JH, Ament ME, Berquist WE. Long-term home parenteral nutrition in pediatrics. Ten years of experience in 102 patients. J Pediatr Gastroenterol Nutr 6:24–37, 1987.

141. Buckman AL, Maukarzel A, Goodson B, et al. Catheter related infections associated with home parenteral nutrition and predictive factors for the need for catheter removal in their treatment. JPEN J Parenter Enteral Nutr 18:297–302, 1984.

142. Hartman GE, Shochat SJ. Management of septic complications associated with Silastic catheters in malignancy. Pediatr Infect Dis J 6:1042–1047, 1987.

143. Merritt RJ, Blackburn GL. Nutritional assessment and metabolic response to illness of the hospitalized child. In: Suskind RM, ed. Textbook of pediatric nutrition. New York: Raven Press, 1981:285.

144. Ponder SW. Clinical uses of bone densitometry in children: are we ready yet? Clin Pediatr 34:237, 1995.

145. Fiorotto ML, de Bruin NC, Brans YW, et al. Total body electrical conductivity measurements: an evaluation of current instrumentation for infants. Pediatr Res 37:94–100, 1995.

146. Olhager E, Thomas K, Wigstrom L, et al. Description and evaluation of a method based on magnetic resonance imaging to estimate adipose tissue volume and total body fat in infants. Pediatr Res 44: 572–577, 1998.

147. Kuczmarski RJ, Ogden CL, Grummer-Strawn LM, et al. CDC growth charts: United States. Advance data from vital and health statistics. Hyattsville, Md: National Center for Health Statistics; 2000. Report No. 314.

148. Wang J, Thornton JC, Kolesnik S, et al. Anthropometry in body composition. An overview. Ann NY Acad Sci 904:317–326, 2000.

149. Rothschild MA, Oratz M, Schreiber SS. Albumin synthesis. N Engl J Med 286:748–757, 1972.

150. Awai M, Brown EB. Studies of the metabolism of I131-labeled human transferrin. J Lab Clin Med 61:363–396, 1963.

151. Oppenheimer JH, Surks MI, Bernstein G, et al. Metabolism of I-131 labeled thyroxine binding prealbumin in man. Science 149: 748–751, 1965.

152. Peterson PA. Demonstration in serum of two physiological forms of the human retinol-binding protein. Eur J Clin Invest 1:437–444, 1971.

153. Thomas RM, Massoudi M, Byrne J, et al. Evaluation of transthyretin as a monitor of protein-energy intake in preterm and sick neonatal infants. JPEN J Parenter Enteral Nutr 12:162–166, 1988.

154. Giacoia GP, Watson S, West K. Rapid turnover transport proteins, plasma albumin, and growth in low birth weight infants. JPEN J Parenter Enteral Nutr 8:367–370, 1984.

155. Moskowitz SR, Pereira G, Spitzer A, et al. Prealbumin as a biochemical marker of nutritional adequacy in premature infants. Pediatrics 102:749–753, 1983.

156. Helms RA, Dickerson RN, Ebbert ML, et al. Retinol-binding protein and prealbumin: useful measures of protein repletion in critically ill, malnourished infants. J Pediatr Gastroenterol Nutr 5: 586–592, 1986.

157. Vehe KL, Brown RO, Kuhl DA, et al. The prognostic inflammatory and nutritional index in traumatized patients receiving enteral nutrition support. J Am Coll Nutr 10:355–363, 1991.

158. Boehm KA, Helms RA, Storm MC. Assessing the validity of adjusted urinary urea nitrogen as an estimate of total urinary nitrogen in three pediatric populations. JPEN J Parenter Enteral Nutr 18:172–176, 1994.
159. van Goudoever JB, Wattimena JDL, Carnielli VP, et al. Effect of dexamethasone on protein metabolism in infants with bronchopulmonary dysplasia. J Pediatr 124:112–118, 1994.
160. Lawton AR, Cooper MD. Ontogeny of immunity. In: Stiehm ER, Bulginiti VA, eds. Immunologic disorders in infants and children. Philadelphia, Pa: WB Saunders, 1980:36.
161. Shannon DC, Johnson G, Rosen FS, et al. Cellular reactivity to *Candida albicans* antigen. N Engl J Med 275:690–693, 1966.
162. Helms RA, Miller JL, Burckart FJ, et al. Clinical outcome as assessed by anthropometric parameters, albumin and cellular immune function in high-risk infants receiving total parenteral nutrition. J Pediatr Surg 18:564–569, 1983.
163. Helms RA, Herrod HG, Burckart GJ, et al. E-rosette formation, total T-cells and lymphocyte transformation in infants receiving intravenous safflower oil emulsion. JPEN J Parenter Enteral Nutr 7:541–545, 1983.

CASE STUDIES

CASE 5

TOPIC: Neonatal/Pediatric Nutrition

THERAPEUTIC DIFFICULTY: Level 3
Kathleen M. Gura

CHAPTER 15: Pediatric and Neonatal Therapy

■ Scenario

Patient and Setting: JL, a 45-day-old male infant; neonatal intensive care unit (NICU)

Chief Complaint: Abdominal distention, bilious emesis

■ History of Present Illness

Forty-five-day-old former 33-2/7 week Twin B delivered outside hospital via C/S for breech presentation with APGARS 9,9; transferred to NICU on day of life number 5 with medical necrotizing enterocolitis (NEC). On arrival, had KUB evidence of pneumatosis; was made NPO and started on triple antibiotics; resolution of pneumatosis occurred in 5 days; required a repogle (a type of suction catheter used for gastric decompression that runs from the mouth to the stomach) an additional 3 days; was transferred back to the community hospital where he was born after an 8-day NICU stay for further treatment of uncomplicated medical NEC.

While there, remained NPO until completed 14-day treatment course; prior to initiating feeds, received a KUB, which was reassuring, and a prefeed UGI, which was unremarkable, apart from evidence of reflux. Several days ago, small volume enteral feeds were restarted in combination with parenteral nutrition (PN) and was slowly advanced up to a maximum of 115 mL/kg/day of enteral feedings (TF = 150 mL/kg/day). Once reaching 115 mL/kg/day, PN was discontinued and he was maintained exclusively on enteral feedings. About 1 month later, developed abdominal distention, bilious emesis, and significant residuals; serial KUBs were significant for stacked, dilated bowel loops with stagnant air; positive evidence of intramural air; due to concerns for possible stricture, was transferred back to the NICU.

Medical History: H/O apnea of prematurity; treated with caffeine citrate (discontinued 10 days ago); H/O murmur s/p ECHO with structurally normal heart; H/O left knee swelling; hearing screen and hip ultrasound outstanding.

Surgical History: Broviac placement

Family/Social History: Intact parents; twin sister inpatient at local community hospital

Medication History: None at time of transfer; immunizations up to date
PN, 35 mL/kg/day current regimen at time of transfer:
Additives per day:
Dextrose, 18 g
Amino acids, 3.3 g (TrophAmine)
Sodium, 10 mEq
Potassium, 6 mEq
Calcium gluconate, 6 mEq
Magnesium, 1.6 mEq
Phosphorus, 5 mM
Minimum acetate
Pediatric trace elements, 2 mL/L
Pediatric MVI 5 mL/day
PN to run at 3.3 mL/hour × 24 hours
Intravenous fat emulsion (Intralipid) 20% 1.3 mL/hr × 24 hours, providing 62.4 calories, 6.3 g fat/day
EN: Enfamil 20 calories/oz 115 mL/kg/day, providing 241 calories/day, 362 mL fluid

Allergies: No known medication allergies

■ Physical Examination

GEN: Awake; alert; pale; irritable when examined
VS: T 38.3°C, HR 177, RR 40, Ht 43cm, Wt 3.15 kg, head circumference 33 cm, BP 64/30 MAP 43 O2SAT 100%
HEENT: Jaundiced sclera; normal ears; nares patent; palate intact, "wandering eyes"
NECK: Supple; stable clavicles
CV: RRR; no appreciable murmur; 2+ femoral pulses, hemodynamically stable
CHEST: Broviac dressing; clear to auscultation bilaterally, comfortable on RA
ABD: mildly distended; jaundiced; hypoactive BS; HSM noted
GU: NEMG; patent anus
EXT: right upper arm swollen, warm to touch
NEURO: Awake and alert; + palmer/plantar grasp; 2+ patellar reflexes

■ Results of Pertinent Laboratory Tests, Serum Drug Concentrations, and Diagnostic Tests

Na 137 (137)	Hct 0.26 (26)	ALT 4.1 (244)	Ca 3.9 (7.8)
K 3.2 (3.2)	Hgb 90 (9)	Alk Phos 12.3 (735)	Mg 1 (2)
Cl 104 (104)	Plts 60×10^9	GGT 4.43 (266)	PO4 1.3 (4)
HCO3 25 (25)	(60×10^3)	Alb 20 (2)	Tg 1.56 (138)
BUN 5.7 (16)	Lkcs 17×10^9	T bili 256 (15)	
CR 26.5 (0.3)	(17×10^3)	D bili 138 (8.1)	fecal fat 2+
Glu 9.9 (179)		CRP 1.2	reducing
			substances (−)

Radiology: KUB film: Stacked, dilated bowel loops, predominately in right upper abdomen; evidence of pneumatosis
Chest x-ray films: osteopenia, beading along ribs; CVC tip in brachiocephalic vein

■ Problem List

Identify principal problems from the scenario in priority order (see Answers in back of book for correct list of responses).

■ SOAP Note

To be completed by the student (see Answers in back of book for correct SOAP Note).

■ QUESTIONS

(See Answers in back of book for correct responses.)

1. List the complications that are associated with PN therapy. (EO-10)

2. What are the risk factors associated with PN liver disease? (EO-3)

3. What are the limitations associated with providing adequate calcium and phosphorus in neonatal parenteral nutrition solutions? (EO-6)

4. What is the optimal location for placement of a central venous catheter? How should tip placement be verified? (EO-5)

5. What risks are associated with aggressive enteral feedings in a child with pneumatosis intestinalis? (EO-3, 10)

6. JL's stool was positive for fecal fat. What changes to his trophic feedings should be considered? (EO-11, 12)

7. JL no longer has central access and now requires his PN to be infused via a peripheral line. How can his current solution best be adjusted to provide adequate calories? (EO-11, 12)

8. How does aluminum impact bone development? (EO-10)

9. In addition to metabolic bone disease, what other complications have been linked to aluminum toxicity? (EO-10)

10. Explain how intravenous fat emulsion can contribute to PN liver injury. (EO-7, 8)

11. What is the difference between pediatric and adult amino acid solutions? (EO-4)

12. How should growth be assessed in the PN-dependent infant? (EO-11)

13. JL's serum calcium is only 7.8 (normal 8–10.5). His serum albumin is 2 g/dL. Should the calcium in his PN be increased? (EO-4, 5)

14. List the factors that must be considered to avoid calcium phosphate precipitation. (EO-8)

15. Explain what is essential fatty acid deficiency (EFAD), including signs and symptoms and how to manage it. (EO-2, 11, 12)

16. Can 20% intravenous fat emulsion be infused through a peripheral line? Explain your reasoning. (EO-11, 12)

17. List the signs and symptoms associated with thiamine deficiency.

18. Summarize therapeutic, pathophysiologic, and disease management concepts for Pediatric and neonatal therapy/pediatric nutrition support utilizing a key points format. (EO-18)

Gynecologic Disorders

Linh Khanh Vuong

DYSMENORRHEA

TREATMENT GOALS

The goals of treating dysmenorrhea are to relieve the cramping pains associated with menstruation and to restore daily functions.

DEFINITION

Dysmenorrhea is defined as pelvic cramping pain occurring just before or during menstruation, and it can be categorized as primary or secondary. Primary dysmenorrhea, unlike secondary dysmenorrhea, lacks identifiable pelvic pathology such as endometriosis, uterine fibroids, and pelvic adhesions.[1]

EPIDEMIOLOGY

Primary dysmenorrhea is the most common gynecologic problem among menstruating women. The prevalence rate reported among adolescents and young women is usually >70% and up to 40% among adult women in the United States. Dysmenorrhea can be debilitating, causing an estimated 600 million lost school and working hours annually in the United States.[2]

ETIOLOGY AND PATHOPHYSIOLOGY

The cause of primary dysmenorrhea is unknown, but elevated levels of prostaglandins, leukotrienes, and possibly vasopressin released during endometrial sloughing appear to play a major role in the symptomatology.[3–5] Prostaglandins, particularly $PGF_{2\alpha}$ and PGE_2, are thought to increase myometrial contractions, leading to uterine ischemia and sensitization of nerve endings.[2] The severity of dysmenorrhea highly correlates with the duration of menstrual flow, amount of menstrual flow, and levels of prostaglandins released in menstrual fluid.

CLINICAL PRESENTATION AND DIAGNOSIS

SIGNS AND SYMPTOMS
Women with primary dysmenorrhea are diagnosed based on symptoms, presenting with cramping pains in the lower abdomen, which may be severe, and are often associated with symptoms of nausea, vomiting, diarrhea, headache, lower backache, fatigue, fever, or lightheadedness. Symptoms may present a few hours before or just after the onset of menses and can last for 48 to 72 hours.

TREATMENT

PHARMACOTHERAPY
Table 17.1 lists drug therapy regimens for primary dysmenorrhea. Nonsteroidal antiinflammatory drugs (NSAIDs), cyclooxygenase-2 (COX-2) inhibitors, and combined oral contraceptives (COCs) are mainstay treatment options. NSAID and COX-2 inhibitors relieve pain of dysmenorrhea via inhibition of cyclooxygenase (1 and 2), the enzyme that converts arachidonic acid to prostaglandins. NSAIDs are successful in 77% to 80% of patients with dysmenorrhea. Clinically, there is no way to predict if a certain NSAID will provide maximal benefit to any given patient based on current data in the literature. Few direct comparisons of one NSAID to another have been performed. Even though most studies show superiority of the active drug over placebo, no single NSAID has been found to be safer or superior.[6] However, one study of 1,649 women with dysmenorrhea found that the fenamates appeared to be more effective in providing pain relief than ibuprofen, indomethacin, or naproxen. The same study also showed a higher drop out rate with indomethacin due to gastrointestinal (GI) and central nervous system side effects.[7] The initial selection should be tried for at least two to four cycles. If therapy is unsuccessful, some patients may still respond to another NSAID class. Patients should be counseled to take NSAIDs at the onset of symptoms because the half-life of prostaglandins is only minutes. In patients with severe, monthly dysmenorrhea, NSAIDs can be taken the day before the expected day of menstruation, theoretically, to prevent the formation of prostaglandins. With the short-term use of NSAIDs for dysmenorrhea, side effects are infrequent and usually mild. GI irritation can best be avoided by taking the NSAIDs with food

TABLE 17.1	Pharmacotherapy for Primary Dysmenorrhea
Medication (NSAID)	**Usual Dose**
Acetic Acids	
Diclofenac	100 mg PO stat, then 50 mg tid
Indomethacin	25 mg PO tid
Tolmetin	400 mg PO tid
Sulindac	200 mg PO Q4–6H
Fenamates	
Mefenamic acid	500 mg PO stat, then 250 mg Q6H
Meclofenamate	100 mg PO stat, then 50–100 mg Q6H
Oxicams	
Piroxicam	20 mg PO daily
Propionic Acids	
Flurbiprofen	50 g PO qid
Ibuprofen	400–600 mg PO Q4–6H
Naproxen	500 mg PO bid
Naproxen sodium	550 mg PO bid
Ketoprofen	50 mg PO tid
Salicylic Acids	
Diflunisal	1000 mg PO stat, then 500 mg Q12H
Combination Oral Contraceptives	
Any 28-day cycle pack	1 table PO daily
COX-2 Inhibitors	
Celecoxib	400 mg PO stat, then 200 mg bid

NSAIDS, nonsteroidal anti-inflammatory drugs; PO, by mouth; tid, three times a day; qid, four times daily; bid, twice a day; COX-2, cyclooxygenase-2 inhibitors.
(From Ruggiero R. Gynecologic Disorders. In: Herfindal ET, Gourley D, eds. Textbook of therapeutics. 7th ed. Baltimore: Williams and Wilkins, 2003, with permission.)

or milk.[8] Aspirin should not be taken concurrently with NSAIDs because they can enhance side effects and toxic effects such as peptic ulceration, and liver and renal damage. NSAIDs are contraindicated in patients who have hypersensitivity, nasal polyps, angioedema, and bronchospasm to aspirin. In addition, these agents are also contraindicated in individuals with documented peptic ulceration and for those with preexisting chronic renal disease.

Recently, two COX-2 inhibitors, celecoxib and valdecoxib that have the potential benefit of fewer GI side effects, were approved for the treatment of dysmenorrhea. Selective inhibition of COX-2 versus COX-1 in the GI mucosa lends a better GI side effect profile. However, some clinicians have challenged the clinical significance of GI side effects in low-risk patients.[9] Valdecoxib 20 or 40 mg daily up to twice daily provided as effective pain relief as naproxen sodium 550 mg twice daily.[10] Second-generation COX-2 inhibitor lumiracoxib (400 mg daily) was comparable to rofecoxib (50 mg daily) and naproxen (500 mg twice daily) for moderate to severe dysmenorrhea.[11] Valdecoxib and celecoxib are con-

traindicated in patients with sulfonamide allergy. Valdecoxib was removed from the U.S. market in 2005 due to concerns about increased cardiovascular risk from its use.

COCs relieve dysmenorrhea in 90% of patients. The inhibition of ovulation, which suppresses proliferative endocrine activity and endometrial tissue growth, result in a concomitant reduction in the volume of menstrual fluid and in the levels of prostaglandins.[2] Evidence for the beneficial effects of COCs on dysmenorrhea is based on both higher dose and lower dose preparations. COC pills containing 20-μg ethinyl estradiol/150-μg desogestrel (Mircette) have been shown to decrease the incidence, duration, and severity of dysmenorrhea after three cycles of use.[2]

NONPHARMACOLOGIC THERAPY

Nonpharmacologic treatments of dysmenorrhea with some evidence include acupuncture, transcutaneous electrical nerve stimulation (TENS), psychotherapy, and a vegetarian diet low in fat.[12–15]

PHARMACOECONOMICS

The use of a generic NSAID as a first-line therapy is safe and effective short-term. Since treatment of dysmenorrhea is usually <5 days of the month, the risk of GI ulcer is low, especially in women <65 years of age, and the use of costly COX-2 inhibitors should be reserved as a last-line therapy. COCs can be used alone or added to a NSAID or COX-2 inhibitor if symptoms are not relieved by one treatment alone.

PREMENSTRUAL SYNDROME

DEFINITION

Premenstrual syndrome (PMS) is characterized by emotional and physical symptoms that consistently occur during the luteal phase, the period between ovulation and the onset of menses, but do not interfere with the patient's usual level of functioning. Typical symptoms include irritability, tension, dysphoria, mood lability, abdominal pain, breast tenderness, headache, and fatigue. In contrast to PMS, premenstrual dysphoric disorder (PMDD) consists of severe affective symptoms (depressed mood, anxiety, affective lability) that can substantially impair a patient's personal and social functioning.[16,17]

ETIOLOGY

PMDD, a severe form of PMS, is considered a multifactorial psychoendocrine disorder with altered regulation of neurohormones and neurotransmitters. Circulating sex steroid levels (progesterone, estrogen, and testosterone) are normal; however, the regulation of neurohormones may be severely affected in women afflicted with PMS. Because PMDD shares many affective clinical features with clinical depression, its etiology has been linked to serotonergic dysregulation. Trials with selective serotonin reuptake inhibitors (SSRIs) have yielded remarkable results in most women with severe PMS but not all, leading to the belief that other etiologic factors are probably involved. For example, levels of β-endorphin are found lower in PMS patients throughout the periovulatory phase, especially in postovulatory days 0 to 4, compared to controls.[18] Genetics may also play a role, as the concordance rate of PMS is twice as high among monozygotic twins as among dizygotic twins.[19]

EPIDEMIOLOGY

PMS usually begins when women are in their early 20s. Seventy-five percent of women of reproductive age report having PMS, whereas PMDD, the more severe form of PMS, accounts for only 3% to 8%.[17]

CLINICAL PRESENTATION AND DIAGNOSIS

SIGNS AND SYMPTOMS
PMS symptoms occur exclusively during the luteal phase of the menstrual cycle and generally disappear within 3 days after the onset of menses. A combination and variation of symptoms include mood swings, depressed mood, irritability, and anxiety. These can also be accompanied by physical symptoms such as headaches, breast tenderness, and bloating.

DIAGNOSIS AND CLINICAL FINDINGS
PMS or PMDD is diagnosed after other causes of physical and psychiatric disorders such as depressive disorders, panic disorder, generalized anxiety disorder, migraines, seizure disorders, irritable bowel syndrome, chronic fatigue syndrome, and thyroid and adrenal disorders are first ruled out.[16,19] The best way to diagnose is to have the patient document her symptoms using different diagnostic instruments, including the Calendar of Premenstrual Experiences, the Premenstrual Syndrome Diary, and the Daily Record of Severity of Problems for at least two menstrual cycles. Diagnosis is confirmed when three key factors are met: (a) symptoms are confined to the luteal phase of the menstrual cycle; (b) absence of symptoms during the follicular phase of the menstrual cycle; (c) symptoms cause a negative impact on function and lifestyle during the luteal phase. The American College of Obstetrics and Gynecology (ACOG) recommends the PMS diagnostic criteria developed by the University of California at San Diego and the National Institute of Mental Health (Table 17.2). In women with PMS who have more severe emotional symptoms, criteria from the *Diagnostic and Statistical Manual of Mental Disorders*, 4th edition can be used to diagnose PMDD (Table 17.3).

THERAPEUTIC PLAN

The goal of treatment is to improve the woman's daily function by targeting symptoms.

TABLE 17.2 | Diagnostic Criteria for Premenstrual Syndrome

National Institutes of Health

A 30% increase in the intensity of symptoms, measured instrumentally, from cycle days 5 to 10 as compared with the 6-day interval before the onset of menses

Documentation of these changes in a daily symptom diary for at least two consecutive cycles

University of California at San Diego

At least one of the following affective and somatic symptoms during the 5 days before menses in each of the three previous cycles (based on prospective self-reports):

- Affective symptoms: depression, angry outbursts, irritability, anxiety
- Confusion, social withdrawal
- Somatic symptoms: breast tenderness, abdominal bloating, headache
- Swelling of extremities

Symptoms must be relieved within 4 days of the onset of menses, without recurrence until at least cycle day 13

(From Dickerson LM, Mazyck PJ, Hunter MH. Premenstrual syndrome. Am Fam Physician 67:1743–1752, 2003, with permission.)

TABLE 17.3 | Research Criteria for Premenstrual Dysphoric Disorder

A. In most menstrual cycles during the past year, the following ≥5 symptoms must be present for most of the last week of the luteal phase, begin to remit at the onset of the follicular phase, and disappear during the week after menses. At least one of the first 4 symptoms must be present:

- markedly depressed mood, feelings of hopelessness, or self-deprecating thoughts
- marked anxiety, tension, feelings of being "keyed up" or "on edge"
- marked affective lability (e.g., feeling suddenly sad or tearful or having increased sensitivity to rejection)
- persistent and marked anger or irritability or increased interpersonal conflicts
- decreased interest in usual activities (e.g., work, school, friends, and hobbies)
- subjective sense of difficulty in concentrating
- lethargy, easy fatigability, or marked lack of energy
- marked change in appetite, overeating, or specific food cravings
- hypersomnia or insomnia
- subjective sense of being overwhelmed or out of control
- other physical symptoms, such as breast tenderness or swelling, headache, joint or muscle pain, a sensation of "bloating," weight gain

B. Marked interference with work or school or with usual social activities and relationships with others (e.g., avoidance of social activities or decreased productivity and efficiency at work or school)

C. Disturbance is not merely an exacerbation of the symptoms of another disorder, such as major depressive disorder, panic disorder, dysthymic disorder, or a personality disorder (although possibly superimposed on any of these disorders)

D. Criteria A, B, and C must be documented by prospective daily ratings during at least two consecutive symptomatic menstrual cycles (the diagnosis may be made provisionally before such confirmation)

Note: In menstruating women, the luteal phase corresponds to the time frame between ovulation and the onset of menses, and the follicular phase begins with menses. In nonmenstruating women (e.g., women who have had a hysterectomy), determination of the timing of the luteal and follicular phases may require measurement of circulating reproductive hormones.

(From the Diagnostic and Statistical Manual of Mental Disorders, 4th edition (DSM IV). Adapted from Dickerson LM, Mazyck PJ, Hunter MH. Premenstrual syndrome. Am Fam Physician 67:1743–1752, 2003, with permission.)

TREATMENT

NONPHARMACOLOGIC THERAPY

Although there are no medical sequelae if PMS is left untreated, the woman may seek treatment to improve her normal life functions. Treatment should be individualized based on the woman's symptoms and needs. Nonpharmacologic approaches should be tried first for at least two to three menstrual cycles, during which the woman should be documenting her symptoms using one of the approved diagnostic instruments. Patient education may help the woman understand her disorder and be in more control.

Supportive therapy such as relaxation therapy, getting adequate rest, aerobic exercise, and making dietary changes such as consuming carbohydrate-rich food or beverages and limiting caffeine intake may help.[19] Data supporting carbohydrate-rich foods need further support but it is thought that carbohydrates increase the levels of tryptophan, a precursor to serotonin.

ALTERNATIVE THERAPIES

Other ACOG recommendations, but with limited scientific evidence include calcium, vitamin E, vitamin B_6, magnesium, and primrose oil. Of these, calcium supplement is the only promising regimen. Few studies have found decreased levels of ionized and total calcium with a compensatory increase in the levels of parathyroid hormone (PTH) several days before ovulation, but that this cyclicity only occurs in a subset of premenstrual women.[20–22] It has been found that mid cycle elevations of PTH with a transient, secondary hyperparathyroidism only occurs in women with PMS.[23] Disturbances in intracellular calcium and PTH in patients with primary hyperparathyroidism have been linked to monoamine metabolism and serotonergic dysregulation. In a study involving 466 women with PMS, calcium carbonate (1,200 mg daily) reduced overall symptoms by 48% by the third treatment cycle compared with a 30% reduction in the placebo group.[24] Furthermore, all four symptom factors (negative affect, water retention, food cravings, and pain) were significantly reduced. Other trials using calcium supplements have also shown similar results.[25,26] Magnesium (200–400 mg/d), vitamin E (400 IU/d), and vitamin B_6 may have limited clinical benefit. Primrose oil and vitamin E may be useful in treating breast tenderness.

PHARMACOTHERAPY

If symptoms persist after three menstrual cycles of nonpharmacologic interventions, pharmacologic treatment should be considered (Table 17.4 lists pharmacotherapy options for PMDD). Treatment should be individualized and target the most troublesome symptoms.

Selective Serotonin Reuptake Inhibitors. SSRIs are the initial drugs of choice for severe PMS or PMDD. Several

double-blind, randomized, controlled clinical trials have shown the effectiveness of SSRIs in improving emotional and physical symptoms of PMDD within the first three menstrual cycles.[27–31] Fluoxetine (Sarafem) and sertraline (Zoloft) have been approved by the US Food and Drug Administration (FDA) for the treatment of PMDD and are the two most studied SSRIs in the treatment of PMDD. Other SSRIs with similar benefits are paroxetine,[29] citalopram,[30] and fluvoxamine.[31] In a study involving 277 patients with PMDD, fluoxetine (20 or 60 mg daily) reduced the severity of symptoms (tension, irritability, and dysphoria) by 50% from baseline in 52% of the patients compared with 22% of the patients receiving placebo within the first treatment cycle, and that benefit persisted throughout six treatment cycles.[27] The group receiving the 60-mg daily dose had more side effects leading to withdrawals, but not superior efficacy compared to the group receiving the 20-mg daily dose.[27] Other studies using fluoxetine (20 mg/day) show similar efficacy.[32–34] Similar efficacy has been shown with sertraline (50–150 mg daily) in multiple studies.[28,35–38]

SSRIs can be given continuously or intermittently during the symptomatic luteal phase. Intermittent therapy has been shown to be efficacious in several small, randomized, double-blind, placebo-controlled trials.[30,32,36–39] Women should be counseled to self-initiate treatment at onset of symptoms or 7 to 14 days before the next menstrual period with intermittent therapy. This method of administration is less expensive, reduces the overall rate of side effects, and is more acceptable to many women.[19] Common side effects of the SSRIs include insomnia, drowsiness, fatigue, nausea, headache, and decreased libido.

Other Pharmacologic Approaches. Alprazolam is the only anxiolytic studied for the treatment of PMS. Studies yielded mixed results. Coupled with the addictive and tolerance potential of alprazolam, this agent is only reserved for PMS patients with agitation and anxiety as primary symptoms. Other psychotropic agents with limited beneficial benefits include bupropion (Wellbutrin), tricyclic antidepressants, buspirone (BuSpar), lithium, and β-blockers such as atenolol and propranolol. However, their potential risks outweigh any benefit and use is not recommended.[16]

Another common PMS complaint is bloating or fluid retention that warrant diuretic therapy. Spironolactone, an aldosterone antagonist with antiandrogenic properties, 100 mg dosed in the morning during the 14-day luteal phase, in most studies, has been shown to significantly reduce somatic (including breast tenderness) and affective complaints.[40–44] Progesterone, in various forms, has been the most commonly prescribed therapy for PMS for several decades and yet is the most controversial. Uncontrolled clinical trials have consistently demonstrated that progesterone suppositories are an effective treatment for PMS, and they are the basis for the widespread use of progesterone in the United States.

TABLE 17.4	**Pharmacologic Treatment Options for PMS and PMDD**		
Medication	**Dosage**	**Therapeutic Use**	**Side Effects**
SSRIs Fluoxetine Sertraline Citalopram Paroxetine Fluvoxamine	10–20 mg daily 50–150 mg daily 20–40 mg daily 10–30 mg daily 50–100 mg daily	First-line treatment of PMDD. Intermittent dosing is given only during the luteal phase (14 days before menses).	Sexual dysfunction (anorgasmia, decreased libido) Sleep alterations (insomnia, sedation) Gastrointestinal distress (nausea, diarrhea)
Anxiolytic Alprazolam	0.25–0.75 mg three times daily	Second-line treatment. Use reserved for patients with predominant anxiety symptoms.	Drowsiness, sedation
GnRH agonists Leuprolide Goserelin	3.75 mg IM every month or 11.25 mg every 3 months 3.6 mg SC every month or 10.8 mg SC every 3 months	Third-line agent due to side effects, ease of use, and cost. Somewhat effective in alleviating physical and behavioral symptoms of PMS.	Hypoestrogenic side effects (atrophic vaginitis, hot flashes, osteoporosis with >6 months of use), night sweats, headache, nausea "add-back" therapy with estrogen and/or progesterone is necessary to prevent bone loss if use is >6 months
Diuretics Spironolactone	25–100 mg dosed in the morning during luteal phase	Effective in alleviating breast tenderness and bloating	Antiestrogenic effects, hyperkalemia
Oral contraceptives Any monophasic (preferred over triphasic) COCs	1 tablet daily	Third-line agent for hormonal suppression. Use is limited mostly to women with predominantly physical symptoms.	Although COCs improve physical symptoms, they can actually be exacerbated in the first 3 cycles: breast tenderness, nausea, mood alterations.

SSRIs, selective serotonin reuptake inhibitors; PMDD, premenstrual dysphoric disorder; GnRH, gonadotropin-releasing hormone; IM, intramuscularly; PMS, premenstrual syndrome; SC, subcutaneously; COCs, combined oral contraceptives.

(From the Diagnostic and statistical manual of mental disorders, 4th edition (DSM IV). Adapted from Dickerson LM, Mazyck PJ, Hunter MH. Premenstrual syndrome. Am Fam Physician 67:1743–1752, 2003; Grady-Weliky T. Premenstrual dysphoric disorder. N Engl J Med 348:433–438, 2003; Premenstrual syndrome. ACOG Practice Bulletin No 15, 2000, with permission.)

Unfortunately, most controlled clinical trials have failed to demonstrate the superiority of progesterone therapy whether administered as a vaginal suppository[45] or as oral micronized progesterone[46] over placebo. Progesterone may help with breast tenderness and bloating or specific psychological symptoms, such as worrying.[19]

If treatment with SSRIs and anxiolytics fail, hormonal suppression using combined COCs or gonadotropin-releasing hormone (GnRH) agonists may be tried. To date, there is only one controlled trial supporting the efficacy of an oral contraceptive combined with drospirenone (Yasmin) for mild-to-moderate symptoms.[47] Drospirenone is a chemical analogue of spironolactone and at a 3 mg per day dose (packaged in Yasmin) has antimineralocorticoid properties equivalent to spironolactone 25 mg. ACOG supports the use of any monophasic over triphasic COCs, citing less mood alterations with the monophasic formulations. Current evidence support COC use only in cases where physical symptoms dominate mood symptoms.

GnRH agonists are synthetic analogues of naturally occurring GnRH, and suppress ovulation by inhibiting the release of pituitary gonadotropins. GnRH agonists, including leuprolide and buserelin, were superior to placebo in the alleviation of premenstrual emotional symptoms (such as irritability and depression) and physical symptoms (such as bloating and breast tenderness) in four double-blind, controlled studies.[48–51] However, the routine use of GnRH is limited by their cost, parenteral route of administration (leuprolide), and hypoestrogenic side effects (hot flashes, vaginal dryness, bone loss). The risk of osteoporosis becomes a concern after 6 months of use. Bone loss may be prevented with "add-back" estrogen therapy, but this may be complicated by the return of symptoms. Thus, the GnRH agonists remain a third-line treatment option.

PHARMACOECONOMICS

ACOG recommends a stepwise approach to treating PMS by (a) using supportive therapy, complex carbohydrate diet, aerobic exercise, nutritional supplements (calcium, magne-sium, vitamin E), and spironolactone, (b) using the SSRI (fluoxetine or sertraline as the initial choice); for women who do not respond, consider an anxiolytic for specific symptoms, and (c) hormonal ovulation suppression using COCs or GnRH agonists.

ENDOMETRIOSIS

DEFINITION

Endometriosis is the presence and growth of glands and stroma of the lining of the uterus at an extrauterine site, usually in the peritoneal cavity.

ETIOLOGY

Many theories have arisen to explain the enigmatic nature of endometriosis. There are at least five different possible etiologies of endometriosis: (a) ectopic functioning endome-trium developing as a result of atypical development of ger-minal epithelium because various parts of the pelvic perito-neum are embryologically derived from totipotent coelomic epithelial cells; (b) metastases of normal endometrium spreading via uterine lymphatic vessels; (c) hematogenous spreading via blood vessels to distant sites; (d) cell rests of Müllerian epithelium developing into functioning ectopic endometrial implants; or (e) endometrial cells implanting themselves in the pelvic peritoneum via retrograde men-struation. Sampson's retrograde transplantation theory is widely accepted and supported by findings that (a) retro-grade menstruation is a common (90%) event in menstruat-ing women with patent fallopian tubes, (b) there is a high prevalence of pelvic endometriosis in girls with congenital menstrual outflow obstruction, and (c) endometriosis can be induced in animals by obstruction of antegrade menstrua-tion, thus forcing retrograde menstruation to take place. There is also ample evidence that endometriosis occurs in patients with altered cell-mediated immunity leading to im-paired mechanisms for the clearance of ectopic endometrial cells and that these cells thrive by acquiring a blood supply under the influence of local estrogens produced by the en-zyme aromatase.[52,53]

EPIDEMIOLOGY

The incidence and prevalence of endometriosis are only ap-proximations and vary depending on the criterion used to diagnose the disease. A conservative estimate of endometrio-sis in reproductive-age women is 5% to 15%. However, laparoscopic visualization of lesions approaches 45%. The average age at diagnosis is 28 years and 75% of women with endometriosis are between age 24 and 50 years.[8] Endometri-osis is recognized as the third leading cause for gynecologic hospitalization and a leading cause of hysterectomy.[54] It is estimated that endometriosis is present in 70% to 90% of women with chronic pelvic pain and in 30% to 45% of women with infertility.[55,56]

PATHOPHYSIOLOGY

Endometriosis is a disorder in which there is a presence of islands of endometrium in extrauterine locations that exhibit the histologic and hormonal responsiveness of native endo-metrium.[8] Physiologic levels of estrogen and progesterone produced by the ovaries stimulate the growth of ectopic en-dometrium. The principal manifestations of endometriosis are pelvic pain and infertility.[57]

The cyclic pelvic pain is related to the sequential swelling and the extravasation of blood and menstrual debris into the surrounding tissue. Chemical mediators responsible for inflammation and pain are prostaglandins and cytokines found in peritoneal fluid. Interestingly, the extent and sever-ity of pain are not always related to the extent of pelvic endometriosis. In fact, women with extensive endometriosis may be asymptomatic, whereas other patients with minimal implants may have incapacitating chronic pelvic pain. Rather, severe pelvic pain associated with endometriosis cor-relates with deep implants in highly innervated areas. Infer-tility secondary to endometriosis can result from the distor-tion of pelvic structures caused by fibrosis and the formation of adhesions or by chemical mediators produced by the endo-metriotic implants and/or the surrounding tissue, such as prostaglandins, cytokines, growth factors, and other em-bryotoxic factors.[58]

Endometriosis most commonly occurs within the pelvis, on or within the ovaries, on the peritoneum, or beneath the serosa of pelvic viscera. The most common site is the ovary, usually bilaterally and found in two of three women with endometriosis. Extrapelvic endometriosis, which occurs less often, involves locations outside the genital tract, such as

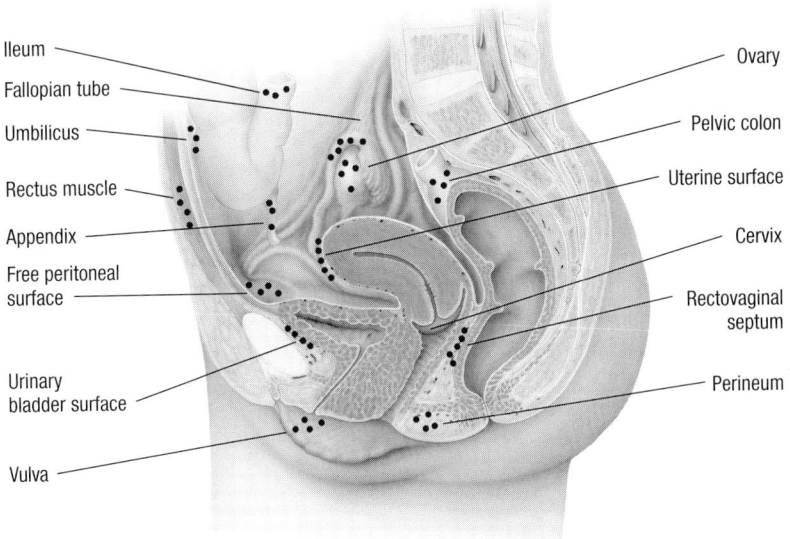

FIGURE 17.1 Common anatomic locations of endometriosis within the pelvic cavity (*see color insert*). (Asset provided by Anatomical Chart Co.)

the bowel, rectum, appendix, umbilicus, areas of previous surgical incisions of the anterior abdominal wall or perineum, the bladder, ureter, kidney, lung, arms, and legs (Fig. 17.1, *see color insert*).[59]

CLINICAL PRESENTATION AND DIAGNOSIS

SIGNS AND SYMPTOMS
Although up to one third of women with endometriotic implants are asymptomatic, other women with endometriosis usually present with chronic pelvic pain manifested as secondary dysmenorrhea and/or dyspareunia, cyclic pelvic pain, abnormal bleeding (premenstrual spotting and menorrhagia), and infertility.

DIAGNOSIS AND CLINICAL FINDINGS
When symptoms of pelvic pain, dysmenorrhea, dyspareunia, or infertility are present, endometriosis should be suspected.[53] Pelvic examination during the first or second day of menstrual flow, where maximum swelling and tenderness in the areas of endometriosis occurs, is most sensitive. Women with endometriosis may experience greater than normal tenderness during bimanual pelvic examinations. Diagnosis can be confirmed by direct laparoscopic visualization of endometriosis with its associated scarring and adhesion formation. Biopsy of selected implants confirms diagnosis.

THERAPEUTIC PLAN

Treatment of endometriosis aims at alleviating pain and restoring fertility. When medical therapy fails, surgical therapy should be considered.

TREATMENT

PHARMACOTHERAPY
Pharmacotherapy consists of NSAIDs, COCs, danazol, GnRH agonists, or progestins (Table 17.5 lists pharmacotherapy options for endometriosis). The goal of hormonal therapies is to interrupt the ovarian cycle and induce amenorrhea, since one of the main pathophysiologic symptoms of ectopic endometriotic implants is bleeding. Drugs used to treat endometriosis must, therefore, have the ability to induce anovulation, hypoestrogenism, and amenorrhea. Drug treatment with danazol or GnRH agonists is usually temporary, limited by their side effects. Symptomatic recurrences are common, occurring in up to 50% of patients shortly upon discontinuation of therapy. Thus, laparoscopic surgery is usually warranted.

Nonsteroidal Antiinflammatory Drugs. NSAIDs have consistently and conclusively been shown in many randomized-controlled trials (RCTs) to be safe and effective for the treatment of primary dysmenorrhea.[60–65] Their use in secondary dysmenorrhea or chronic pelvic pain associated with endometriosis has been extrapolated from these data. Although the COX-2 inhibitors have not been studied in chronic pelvic pain, they are expected to have comparable results for pain associated with endometriosis as well. NSAIDs and COX-2 inhibitors improve pain by reducing prostaglandins and possibly the amount of bleeding in endometriotic implants.

Combined Oral Contraceptives. Supraphysiologic doses of estrogen and progestin combinations are given to induce a ''pseudopregnant'' state. Only one RCT of cyclic COCs for chronic pelvic pain and endometriosis has been identified.[66] This was a 6-month study of 57 women given COCs cyclically or a GnRH agonist. Women on COCs had

TABLE 17.5	Pharmacotherapy Used in Endometriosis		
Medication	**Dose**	**Therapeutic Use**	**Side Effects**
NSAID (see options for dysmenorrhea)	Same as for dysmenorrhea	Empiric first-line agents used for secondary dysmenorrhea and/or CPP. May be combined with a COC.	Nausea, dizziness, gastric ulceration, renal dysfunction
Combined oral contraceptive pills Any (monophasic) pills	1 tablet daily (can be taken continuously, i.e., no placebo pills)	Empiric first-line agents used for secondary dysmenorrhea and/or CPP. May be combined with a NSAID.	Nausea, bloating, breast tenderness. These symptoms are temporary and usually resolve within three cycles of use.
Androgen Danazol (Danocrine)	Orally: 200 to 800 mg daily, dosed tid IUD: 400 mg inserted × 6 months	Considered "advanced medical therapy" but due to high drop out rates in studies, progestins and GnRH agonists are tried first.	Weight gain, acne, facial hair, decreased breast size, deepening of the voice, hot flashes, and vaginal atrophy. Monitor LFTs and lipid profiles
Progestins MPA (Provera) DMPA (Depo-Provera) Megestrol (Megace)	20–50 mg PO daily 150 mg IM every 3 months 20 mg PO bid	4 RCTs and 19 other studies have shown comparable efficacy to danazol and GnRH agonists for temporary relief of pelvic pain.	Uterine bleeding (spotting), bloating, weight gain
GnRH agonists Leuprolide (Lupron)	3.75 mg IM every month or 11.25 mg IM every 3 months	"Advanced medical therapy"; preferred over danazol. Induces a medical oophorectomy. Similar to progestins, danazol, GnRH agonists can be used before laparoscopic surgery or as adjunctive medical therapy postoperatively to prolong time to symptomatic recurrences.	Mostly *hypoestrogenic*: hot flashes, atrophic vaginitis, bone loss. "Add-back" therapy using estrogen, progestin, or both is essential when prolonged treatment (>6 months) is expected.
Goserelin (Zoladex)	3.6 mg SC every month or 10.8 mg SC every 3 months		
Nafarelin (Synarel)	200–400 mcg intranasally bid		

NSAID, nonsteroidal antiinflammatory drug; CPP, chronic pelvic pain; COC, combined oral contraceptive; tid, three times daily; IUD, intrauterine device; GnRH, gonadotropin releasing hormone; LFT, liver function test; MPA, medroxyprogesterone acetate; RCT = randomized controlled trial; PO, orally; DMPA, depot medroxyprogesterone acetate; IM, intramuscular; bid, twice daily; SC, subcutaneous.

less relief of dysmenorrhea compared to women on a GnRH agonist, but had similar relief of dyspareunia and nonmenstrual pain with less side effects. However, since COCs have been studied extensively in primary dysmenorrhea, their use as first-line agents with or without an NSAID in chronic pelvic pain associated with endometriosis is justified. In a recent ACOG publication and in another study where women have persistent dysmenorrhea despite cyclic COC, the use of continuous monophasic COCs in women with cyclic dysmenorrhea secondary to endometriosis is advocated.[53,67] In women whose symptoms are not relieved with an NSAID or COC, a full dose of GnRH agonist, a progestin, or danazol should be tried.

Androgen. Danazol was the first hormonal agent approved by the FDA in the 1970s for the treatment of endometriosis and has been the drug of choice for endometriosis since the 1980s. Danazol is a synthetic steroid that is a derivative of 17-alpha-ethinyltestosterone. Its complex mechanisms of action, though not fully elucidated, include inhibition of pituitary gonadotropin release with secondary suppression of ovarian steroidogenesis, and interaction with androgen and progesterone receptors. Danazol can be antagonistic or agonistic at different hormone-sensitive tissues. The relief of symptoms of endometriosis is directly related to the development of amenorrhea. Danazol has been shown to relieve pain and clinical improvement in 55% to 93% of women treated for 6 months.[53] Recommended therapy with danazol is 200 to 800 mg per day for 6 months. Lower doses of danazol have not been shown to be as effective in inducing amenorrhea. With a short half-life of 4 to 5 hours, danazol should be given three to four times a day to ensure adequate suppression of circulating sex steroids. Treatment is usually initiated within the first 5 days of menses to minimize spotting and to ensure that the woman is not currently pregnant. The manufacturer recommends a barrier method of contraception be used during the first month as the use of danazol during pregnancy could result in clitoral hypertrophy and labial fusion of the external genitalia in the female fetus.

Danazol binds to sex hormone-binding globulin, causing a threefold increase in endogenous-free testosterone levels, leading to androgenic side effects (e.g., deepening of the voice, weight gain of 8–10 pounds, facial hair, and acne). Hypoestrogenic side effects (hot flushes, uterine spotting, decrease in breast size, atrophic vaginitis) occur as a result of reduced circulating levels of ovarian steroids. Interestingly, bone loss has not been observed during therapy with danazol but in fact, several studies have shown no change or increased bone mass.[68–71] This may be attributed to the fact that levels of estrogen and progesterone during treatment with danazol remain in the follicular phase, unlike the state of estrogen deficiency seen with GnRH agonists. Side effects and metabolic changes with danazol are common, occurring in as much as 50% to 80% of women treated, especially when high doses (800 mg/day) are used. Changes in liver function tests and metabolic changes such as decrease in high-density lipoprotein (HDL) and increase in low-density lipoprotein (LDL) may be associated with danazol. Monitoring of liver function test is recommended if therapy continues for >6 months. Most side effects resolve on discontinuation of therapy except for deepening of the voice.[72] Recently, a novel danazol-loaded intrauterine device (IUD) was developed to minimize systemic absorption. A danazol-loaded IUD containing 400 mg was inserted into the uterine cavity of women in this prospective trial and maintained for 6 months. Symptoms of dysmenorrhea, dyspareunia, and pelvic pain were significantly decreased after the first month of therapy with spotting as the only local side effect seen during the first month.[73]

Progestational Agents. Various progestins have been studied for symptomatic endometriosis. Progestins may induce anovulation and hypoestrogenism according to their dosage, and they provoke marked decidualization and acyclicity of eutopic and ectopic endometria.[74] Progestins are effective, have a relatively good side effect profile, and are inexpensive. The most commonly used progestin in the United States is medroxyprogesterone acetate (MPA, Provera). Although utilization of MPA oral doses up to 50 mg per day has been studied, doses of 20 to 30 mg daily can induce endometrial atrophy and are equally efficacious. Depot medroxyprogesterone acetate (DMPA, Depo-Provera) at 150 mg given intramuscularly every 3 months has also been shown to be as effective as danazol and COC for endometriosis.[75] The most common complaint of unopposed progestational use (without estrogen) is abnormal uterine bleeding. Given the side effect profile of danazol, a progestational agent or GnRH agonist is a better alternative.

Gonadotropin-releasing Hormone Agonists. With the advent of the GnRH agonists, agents of comparable efficacy to danazol, but with more tolerable side effects, danazol

fell out of favor and GnRH agonists became the standard of treatment in the 1990s. Synthetic long-acting GnRH agonists create a temporary and readily reversible ''medical oophorectomy'' with dramatic reduction in levels of serum estradiol, testosterone, and androstenedione. Endogenous GnRH is normally released in a circadian pattern every 60 to 90 minutes in the follicular phase. Down-regulation of the pituitary-ovarian gonadal axis and diminution in levels of gonadotropins, follicle-stimulating hormone (FSH), and LH occur if the peptide is given continuously or as a long-acting synthetic agonist analogue. Treatment with a GnRH agonist usually reduces the level of serum estradiol to that seen in menopausal women and to 25% to 50% of the estradiol concentration observed in women taking danazol chronically. Oftentimes, these women have atrophic endometrium and as a result they become amenorrheic. In addition, chronic anovulatory amenorrhea leads to bone loss.

Although GnRH agonists can be administered intravenously, intramuscularly, subcutaneously, intranasally, intravaginally, or rectally, only subcutaneous 28-day implants or once-daily doses, intramuscular monthly doses of depot forms, or twice-daily nasal sprays are currently used in the United States. Goserelin acetate subcutaneous implants, depot leuprolide acetate, and intranasal nafarelin acetate have been FDA approved for the treatment of endometriosis (Table 17.5). The most commonly GnRH agonist used is leuprolide acetate 3.75 mg given intramuscularly monthly for 6 months. Improvements in symptoms can be expected in 85% to 100% of patients given GnRH agonist therapy. In several RCTs, treatment with a GnRH agonist has been shown to be more effective than placebo and comparable to danazol for secondary dysmenorrhea and/or chronic pelvic pain associated with endometriosis.[76–89] Danazol and GnRH agonists have similar effectiveness for improving pain during treatment and for maintenance of symptom relief (for at least 6–12 months) after the cessation of treatment.[53] Depot leuprolide 3.75 mg intramuscularly every month for 3 months has been shown to result in significant decreases in all pain measures including pelvic pain, dysmenorrhea, and pelvic tenderness compared to placebo.[90] It is not clear which of these hormonal therapies is the most efficacious for symptomatic endometriosis. Depot leuprolide, available in monthly or every 3-month dosage forms, and the goserelin implant that lasts for 28 days have the advantage of avoiding the compliance problems that occur with daily injections or twice-daily nasal spray with nafarelin. Initial treatment with GnRH agonists can actually exacerbate symptoms secondary due to a temporary surge in estradiol, FSH, or LH. The rise in estradiol and LH lasts for 1 week, and amenorrhea can be induced within 4 to 5 weeks if therapy is initiated during the luteal phase. However, if treatment is initiated during the follicular phase, the rise in estradiol and FSH can last up to 3 weeks and induction of amenorrhea is delayed for as long as 6 to 8 weeks.

Limitations to long-term use of GnRH agonists (>6–12 months) are hypoestrogenic side effects that include hot flashes, vaginal dryness, uterine spotting, and most importantly, bone loss. In contrast to all current medical therapies for endometriosis, GnRH agonist is the only therapy that has been shown to significantly decrease bone mineral content, necessitating treatment discontinuation or use of add-back therapy. A decrease in bone density has been observed at the trabecular bone of the lumbar spine, but not in the compact bone of the distal radius. A decrease in bone mass of 5% to 14% during a 6-month course of GnRH agonist therapy has been documented.[68–70] Bone loss has been documented as early as 3 months of therapy, and depot formulations produced more pronounced loss than daily intranasal sprays.[91] Most clinicians concur with the FDA's recommendation that a baseline bone mineral density (BMD) is not necessary before initiation of treatment with a GnRH agonist. The decision when to initiate add-back therapy varies among clinicians. Some will initiate add-back therapy simultaneously with the GnRH agonist to minimize hypoestrogenic side effects such as hot flashes and vaginal dryness. Others recommend add-back only for therapy >3 months to suppress bone loss. Several add-back options are available (Table 17.6); all have good evidence[92–99] supporting relief of hypoestrogenic symptoms and/or bone protection, with no return of symptoms during simultaneous treatment with GnRH agonists.

Although these hormonal therapies have been proven effective in relieving pain and combating the histologic manifestations of endometriosis, currently no clear evidence validates the efficacy of any medical approach in treating infertility.[8] Of concern, is a recent finding that hormonal suppressive therapy for endometriosis may actually increase the risk of malignant transformation in the endometriotic implants by causing a negative selection and increasing the rate of dyskaryosis and loss of heterozygosity.[100] In two other recent publications,[101,102] preliminary results have linked danazol to ovarian cancer.

Surgery can be conservative or nonconservative (bilateral salpingo-oophorectomy, with or without hysterectomy). According to an expert panel consensus[103] consideration for laparoscopically directed excision, ablation, or both should be offered to patients whose chronic pelvic pain or dysmenorrhea is not relieved by medical treatment, or in patients whose future fertility is important. Adjunctive medical therapy with danazol, GnRH agonist, or progestins should be provided to women after conservative surgical treatment since this method has been shown to provide a longer symptom-free period.

FUTURE THERAPIES

Currently, a phase II study[104] is being conducted using aromatase inhibitors in the treatment of endometriosis. These agents are thought to work by inhibiting conversion of peripheral estradiol. Other agents include modulators of the immune system, GnRH antagonist, pentoxifylline, levonorgestrel medicated intrauterine system (IUS) (Mirena), and possibly the antiprogestin, mifepristone.[105]

PHARMACOECONOMICS

From a pharmacoeconomic standpoint, 80% of women who are seen with chronic pelvic pain have endometriosis. The annual cost of chronic pelvic pain in the United States is

TABLE 17.6	Add-back Regimens Used with Gonadotropin Releasing Hormone Agonists*
CEE, 0.625 mg + MPA, 2.5 mg (Prempro) daily	
CEE, 0.625 mg + NE, 5 mg daily	
NE (Aygestin), 5 mg daily	
MPA (Provera), 20 mg daily	

CEE, conjugated equine estrogen; MPA, medroxyprogesterone acetate; NE, norethindrone acetate; GnRH, gonadotropin-releasing hormone; BMD, bone mineral density; COC, combined oral contraceptive.

* Any of these add-back regimens has been shown to be similarly effective in reducing hypoestrogenic symptoms including preserving bone loss. Add-back therapy may be used at the outset of GnRH agonist therapy or at 3 months. GnRH agonist therapy may be continued simultaneously with an add-back therapy for ≥12 months. A BMD is recommended every 2 years if therapy is >12 months. COCs should be avoided since the supraphysiologic dose of estrogen is likely to counteract the benefit of the GnRH agonist.

(From Winkel CA. Evaluation and management of women with endometriosis. Obstet Gynecol 102:397–408, 2003, with permission.)

estimated to be $2.8 billion, with another $600 million for indirect costs. These costs do not include the cost of diagnostic procedures such as ultrasonography or laparoscopy or costs associated with complications of laparoscopy. Chronic pelvic pain accounts for approximately 10% of all gynecologic outpatient visits. Therefore, there may be clinical and economic benefits when GnRH agonists are used to treat endometriosis without a surgical diagnosis.[8]

VAGINITIS

DEFINITION

Loosely defined, vaginitis is the inflammation of the vagina, usually manifested by a variety of vaginal complaints. Vulvovaginitis (VVC), bacterial vaginitis (BV), and trichomoniasis (TV) are three distinct infections that result in vaginitis (Fig. 17.2).

VULVOVAGINITIS

ETIOLOGY

Causative fungi of VVC are classified as *albicans* or non-*albicans*. *Candida albicans* account for about 80% to 90% of all VVC. *Candida tropicalis, Candida (Torulopsis) gla-*

brata, Candida parapsilosis, Candida krusei, and *Saccharomyces cerevisiae* comprise the group of non-albicans that are found in about 15% of VVC, and are usually causative organisms in recurrent VVC. Microscopic smears of vaginal secretions reveal hyphae, pseudohyphae, and budding yeast when *C. albicans* or *C. tropicalis* is present. In contrast, other non-*albicans* show only budding yeast and can usually be seen only under a higher power of magnification.[106]

EPIDEMIOLOGY

More than 50% of women age ≥25 years, and up to 75% of women by the time they reach menopause will have had at least an episode of VVC during their lifetime. About 5% of these women will develop recurrent VVC (RVVC), defined as having ≥4 episodes of VVC in a year. RVVC differs from persistent VVC in that it is separated by a symptom-free period. In 2002, women in the United States spent over half a billion dollars on drugs to treat VVC, with about half this amount spent on over-the-counter (OTC) yeast products. OTC antifungal therapies rank among the top ten selling OTC products in the United States.[107,108]

PATHOPHYSIOLOGY

In women of childbearing age, estrogen maintains a thick, protective epithelial cell layer of the vaginal mucosa. A pH <4.5 to 4.7 is maintained by the normal flora lactobacilli that break down epithelial cell carbohydrates, particularly glycogen, to lactic acid. The low pH encourages the growth of lactobacilli and inhibits the growth of other organisms. About 95% of the flora is made up of *Lactobacillus* species, with the remaining 5% of the flora comprising of facultative anaerobes (*Staphylococcus epidermidis*, corynebacteria, groups A and B streptococci, *Gardnerella vaginalis*, *Mobiluncus* species), anaerobes (*Peptostreptococcus* species, *Peptococcus* species, *Eubacterium* species, *Prevotella* species), aerobes (*Escherichia coli, Staphylococcus aureus*), *Mycoplasma hominis, Ureaplasma urealyticum,* and fungi (*Candida* species).[109] Factors that compromise the host's immunity, the normal flora makeup, or the integrity of the vaginal epithelium will lead to infectious vaginitis. Suppression of lactobacilli with antibiotics, altered immunity with

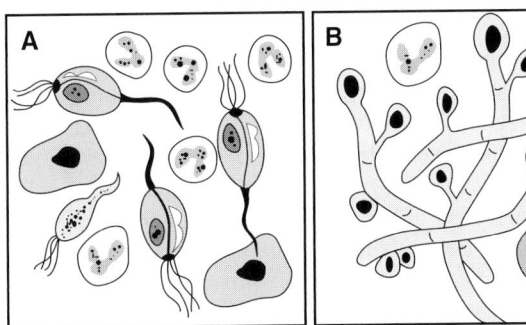
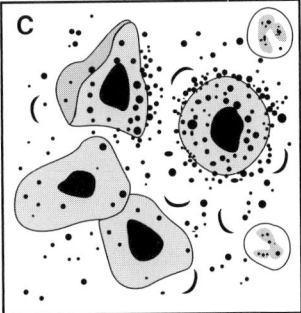

FIGURE 17.2 Microscopic findings of yeast in vulvovaginitis, clue cells in bacterial vaginosis, and trichomonads in trichomoniasis. **A.** flagellated protozoan *Trichomonas vaginalis*; **B.** pseudohyphae and spores in yeast candidiasis; **C.** epithelial cells dotted with adherent bacteria = clue cells in bacterial vaginosis. (From Beckmann CRB, Ling FW, Laube DW, et al. Obstetrics and gynecology. 4th ed. Baltimore: Lippincott Williams & Wilkins, 2002, with permission.)

local or systemic corticosteroids, diabetes, or menopause that leads to thinning of the vaginal epithelium can all contribute to VVC. Obese women or those who are incontinent also experience yeast infections more often because of the warm, moist environment and local maceration favorable to the growth of yeast.[110] Douches, vaginal cosmetic products, and spermicides containing nonoxynol-9 can negatively alter vaginal flora, elevating the risk of inhabitation of other pathogenic microorganisms by depleting lactobacilli.[111,112] Asymptomatic colonization of yeast organisms can be identified in 15% to 45% of nonpregnant women. A much higher number of yeast organisms and an inflammatory response to these fungi are present in symptomatic VVC requiring treatment. RVVC is usually caused by non-albicans, which are harder to treat and are often resistant to traditional treatment with azole antifungals. Vulvovaginal candidiasis is considered recurrent when at least four specific episodes occur in 1 year or at least three episodes unrelated to antibiotic therapy occur within 1 year.[113] Although antibiotic use has long been linked to an increase risk factor for developing VVC, a recent study of 316 women found no association between prior antibiotic use and incidence of VVC.[114] Similarly, a lack of association between antibiotic use and VVC has been seen in another study.[115] Perhaps, prolonged courses of broad-spectrum antibiotics are more culpable than short courses of narrow-spectrum ones.

CLINICAL PRESENTATION AND DIAGNOSIS

SIGNS AND SYMPTOMS

"Classic" signs and symptoms associated with *C. albicans* infection are intense vaginal itching with a white, curdy or cottage cheese-like discharge. Physical examination reveals redness at the introitus (vaginal entrance), generalized vulvar erythema, and/or skin-fold fissures. Characteristics of non-*albicans* infections (*C. glabrata*, *C. parapsilosis*, *C. krusei*, *S. cerevisiae*) are irritation and burning predominating pruritus, and an absence of discharge. The physical examination often shows no objective abnormalities.[110] Microscopy may show the presence of pseudohyphae or budding yeasts.

DIAGNOSIS AND CLINICAL FINDINGS

Although the majority of treatments for VVC are OTC, self-diagnosis of VVC is usually poor. In fact, even in a patient with a prior history of VVC, a second self-diagnosis is often incorrect. In a recent study published by ACOG, of the 95 symptomatic women who purchased an OTC antifungal product for treatment, only 34% actually had VVC while 19% had BV, 21% had mixed vaginitis, 14% had no infections, 2% had trichomoniasis, and 10% had other diagnoses.[116] The authors concluded that the availability of OTC antifungal products is associated with wasted financial expenditures, unfulfilled expectations, and a delay in correct diagnosis and treatment.

Pharmacists should encourage a woman to see a physician if the self-diagnosis made is the first one or if the woman is pregnant. Diagnosis of *C. albicans* VVC is confirmed if the pH of vaginal smear is normal and if microscopy of the sample in 10% potassium hydroxide (KOH) reveals hyphae or pseudohyphae. Detection of budding yeast in non-albicans VVC is easier if done on a saline versus KOH preparation. A culture is only considered in cases where therapy fails or in a patient with persistent and/or recurrent symptoms.

THERAPEUTIC PLAN

Treatment plans include restoring vaginal lactobacilli, achieving microbiologic cure, and preventing recurrence.

TREATMENT

PHARMACOTHERAPY

The goal of treatment is to rapidly alleviate symptoms by using a product that would enhance patient compliance. Treatment options available vary from 1-day oral, cream, or vaginal suppository to 3- to 7-day therapy. Oral and topical azole therapies listed in Table 17.7, including different duration of treatment, are equally effective for uncomplicated VVC in terms of mycologic cure. In patients with severe VVC, rated by intensity of pruritus and extent of vulvar involvement (erythema, edema, excoriation/fissure formation), a sequential dose of fluconazole separated by 3 days achieved superior clinical and mycologic eradication compared to the single dose.[117] The only FDA-approved oral therapy for VVC is fluconazole (150 mg taken once). Although oral ketoconazole and itraconazole have been shown to be effective for VVC, multiple dosing, multiple drug interactions, and risks of hepatotoxicity limit their use. Vaginal suppositories and oral therapies are less messy and are often preferred by patients. However, if vulvar involvement is extensive, the use of topical creams locally is recommended. Pregnant women should be treated with topical treatment to minimize systemic absorption and placental drug transfer. Most of the topical azole antifungal agents are available OTC with the exception of terconazole (Terazol).

Recurrent VVC is harder to treat and usually requires maintenance therapy. The intestinal reservoir theory, which suggests that recurrences are a result of persistence of the organism in the GI tract and later causing reinfection in the vagina, has been debunked and ongoing research focuses more on possible abnormalities of the local vaginal immune response to yeast and their role in laying the groundwork for the patient's next infection.[107] Behavioral factors associated with an increased risk in recurrent VVC include wearing panty liners or pantyhose and consuming cranberry juice or acidophilus-containing products.[115] It is thought that the high sugar content in cranberry juice or yogurt in this study contributed to recurrent VVC.

TABLE 17.7	Drug Therapy for Vulvovaginal Candidiasis	
Medication	**Dosage**	**Comments**
Miconazole (Monistat) Cream, suppository	Insert INV HS × 1, 3, or 7 days	Creams can be messy but useful for VVC with extensive vulvar involvement.
Clotrimazole (GyneLotrimin) Cream, suppository, tablet	Insert INV HS × 1, 3, or 7 days	
Butoconazole (Femstat, Gynazole) Ointment	Insert INV HS × 3 days (Femstat) Insert INV HS once (Gynazole)	Gynazole ointment is purported to coat vaginal epithelium evenly and stays coated longer and is less irritating due to similar pH of vagina.
Tioconazole (Vagistat) Suppository	Insert INV HS once	
Terconazole (Terazol 0.8%, 0.4%) Cream, suppository	Insert INV HS × 3 or 7 days	Although some studies[13] have suggested the use of terconazole and butoconazole × non-albicans VVC, other studies and experts have not agreed.[110,118]
Nystatin (Mycostatin) Tablet, ointment, cream	Insert INV HS × 14 days	Slightly less effective than newer azoles. Cream or ointment can be applied to vulva qid when significant vulvar disease is present.
Fluconazole (Diflucan) Tablet	150 mg PO once; give additional dose 3 days apart × severe VVC or frequently recurring *C. albicans* VVC	Convenient one-time dose, no irritation from ingredients in vehicles. Treats both vaginal and vulvar symptoms. Is as effective as topical azoles.[3] Headache is the most common side effect seen
Itraconazole (Sporanox) Capsule	Various dosing regimens: 200 mg bid once; 200 mg QD × 2 days; 200 mg qd × 3 days	Not FDA-approved for VVC, but shown to be very effective.
Ketoconazole (Nizoral) Tablet	200 mg bid × 5 days	Not FDA approved × VVC; also very effective. Drug interaction with multiple dosing. Idiosyncratic hepatotoxicity

Except for Terconazole and Nystatin, all listed topical azoles are available over-the-counter. INV, intravaginally; HS, at bedtime; VVC, vulvovaginal candidiasis; qid, four times daily; PO, orally; bid, twice daily; qd, every day; FDA, Food and Drug Administration.
(From Ringdahl E. Treatment of recurrent vulvovaginal candidiasis. Am Fam Physician 61 : 3306–3312, 2000; Edwards L. The diagnosis and treatment of infectious vaginitis. Dermatologic Ther 17 : 102–110, 2004; Sobel JD, Chaim W, Nagappan V, et al. Treatment of vaginitis caused by *candida glabrata*: use of topical boric acid and flucytosine. Am J Obstet Gynecol 189 : 1297–1300, 2003; Pharmacist's Letter, September 2003.)

Although *C. albicans* can also cause recurrent VVC, non-*albicans* species such as *C. glabrata*, *C. parapsilosis*, and *S. cerevisiae* are responsible for up to 33% of recurrent VVC. Treatment options depend on if infection is caused by *C. albicans* or *non-albicans*. When the infection is caused by *C. albicans*, recurrent VVC is best managed using an initial 14-day course of oral azole therapy to induce clinical remission and a negative fungal culture, followed by a 6-month maintenance regimen, which includes ketoconazole (100 mg daily), itraconazole (100 mg daily), or fluconazole (100–200 mg weekly).[107] A topical maintenance regimen using a clotrimazole vaginal suppository 500 mg weekly for 6 months has also been used with success. When azole therapy fails or if recurrent VVC is caused by non-*albicans* species, boric acid, nystatin, flucytosine, gentian violet, or amphotericin B can be used (Table 17.8). A boric acid capsule is com-

pounded by placing 600 mg of the powder into a gelatin capsule. Instruct the patient to insert one capsule intravaginally at bedtime for 14 days to 1 month. One author noted that failure is seen more commonly with the 2-week regimen in her vulvar clinic.[110] Nystatin is a polyene antifungal that is generally well tolerated when used intravaginally. Gentian violet is a fungicidal substance. Gauze soaked in a 1% solution can be applied to vaginal walls weekly for 4 to 6 weeks. This treatment is usually least favorable due to its messy application, staining of skin and clothing, and extremely irritating effects. Furthermore, concurrent therapy with nystatin or boric acid is required. Flucytosine cream is prepared by dissolving 14 capsules of 500-mg flucytosine (Ancobon) in 45 g of a hydrophilic ointment base or cold cream. Patients should be instructed to place cream in a 6.4-g vaginal applicator and insert in the vagina at bedtime for 2 weeks. This

TABLE 17.8	Drug Therapy for Resistant Non-*albicans* Vulvovaginal Candidiasis	
Medication	**Dosage**	**Comments**
Boric Acid	600-mg gelatin capsules inserted INV HS × 14 days to 1 month	Must be compounded. Locally irritating. More failure with 2-week course. Poisonous if ingested.
Nystatin Tablet or ointment	Insert INV bid × 1 month	Unrelated to azole. Generally well tolerated.
Gentian Violet 1% solution	Apply to vaginal walls with gauze swab weekly × 4–6 weeks.	Potent fungicidal agent. Very effective but therapy is used concurrently with nystatin or boric acid. Can produce erosive contact dermatitis, stains skin and clothing.
Flucytosine Compounded cream	5–6.4 g inserted INV HS × 1–2 weeks	Can be compounded using 14 of 500 mg flucytosine capsules (Ancobon) in 45 g of a hydrophilic cream or cold cream base. Well tolerated, fairly effective, but expensive. Resistance may quickly develop.
Amphotericin B Cream	Insert INV HS × 2–4 weeks	Available commercially, but is often intolerably irritating and expensive.

INV, intravaginally; HS, at bedtime; bid, twice daily.
(From Edwards L. The diagnosis and treatment of infectious vaginitis. Dermatologic Ther 17:102–110, 2004; Sobel JD, Chaim W, Nagappan V, et al. Treatment of vaginitis caused by *candida glabrata*: use of topical boric acid and flucytosine. Am J Obstet Gynecol 189:1297–1300, 2003.)

regimen has been demonstrated to be more effective against *C. glabrata* than boric acid in one study.[118] Although promising, this treatment has many limitations including rapid development of resistance and possible systemic toxicities (bone marrow toxicity) if extensive systemic absorption occurs. Finally, a combination of flucytosine and amphotericin B has been used but no comparative data in patients exist.[118] Before treatment failure to any of these therapies is declared, patient compliance and proper patient technique must be ruled out. It is important to counsel all patients on the use of intravaginal topical products and to emphasize the importance of completing therapy even after resolution of symptoms.

NONPHARMACOLOGIC THERAPY

Contrary to popular belief, eating yogurt does not seem to prevent VVC or recurrent VVC. Unpasteurized yogurt containing *Lactobacillus acidophilus* has been shown in small, unblinded studies to prevent VVC, but these results have not been replicated in other studies.[113] *Lactobacilli* species found in yogurt and other OTC products are derived from bovine sources and lack adherent properties found in human *lactobacilli* that allow them to attach to the vaginal epithelium and colonize.

PHARMACOECONOMICS

Generally, pricing of topical azoles for 1 day is more than 3 days and both are more than a 7-day therapy. Oral azoles and terconazole are available by prescription only and, thus,

require an office visit. Comparable efficacy has been shown among all topical azoles and oral azoles and for 1-day up to 7-day treatment in uncomplicated VVC. Therefore, patient preference usually dictates treatment option.

BACTERIAL VAGINOSIS

ETIOLOGY

Perturbations of the vaginal ecosystem leading to the overgrowth of mixed flora typically containing genital *Mycoplasma* spp., *Gardnerella vaginalis*, and anaerobic bacteria such as *Peptostreptococcus* spp., *Prevotella* spp., and *Mobiluncus* spp. contribute to the pathogenesis of BV. However, the cause of the microbial alteration is not fully understood.[119] Possible predisposing risk factors include lack of hydrogen peroxide producing lactobacilli, young sexual debut, low socioeconomic background, black ethnicity, multiple sex partners, recent change in sex partner, smoking, use of an IUD as contraception, lack of use of a barrier method of contraception, and douching.

EPIDEMIOLOGY

BV is seen in about 15% of private gynecologic patients,[120] 5% to 26% of pregnant women, and 24% to 37% of those attending sexually transmitted infection (STI) clinics.[121] BV in pregnant women seems to be more prevalent during second trimester screening. In the United States, the prevalence of BV among pregnant women ranges from 16% (23–26 weeks' gestation) to 42% (22–24 weeks' gestation). This is in concordance with several longitudinal cohort studies, which have shown that the prevalence of BV actually decreases in early pregnancy and in the third trimester.[122]

PATHOPHYSIOLOGY

The preponderance of *Lactobacillus* spp. in a normal, healthy vaginal ecosystem deters vaginal and cervical infection. Certain strains of lactobacilli produce hydrogen peroxide that interacts with host peroxidases to produce an oxidant, which in vitro has been shown to be cytotoxic to *G. vaginalis* and *Prevotella bivia*. Low vaginal pH (3.8–4.5) is attributed to the conversion of glycogen to lactic acid by lactobacilli. The adherence of lactobacilli to vaginal epithelium at low pH prevents the invasion of other pathogenic microorganisms. Lack of lactobacilli shifts the vaginal flora to that of predominantly anaerobes and facultative anaerobes, resulting in a degradation of mucins that form a natural gel barrier on the vaginal epithelium. It is thought that a symbiotic relationship exists between BV associated organisms and that the presence of one fuels the growth of another. For example, inoculation of *G. vaginalis* alone into a healthy vagina did not cause BV, but inoculation of vaginal secretions from women with BV caused disease. This suggests that the interrelation between the different groups of bacteria is important for overgrowth.[123] Production of amines including putrescine, cadaverine, and trimethylamine by the microbial flora contributes to the "fishy" odor detected in the vaginal fluid of women with BV.

BV increases a woman's risk of acquiring human immunodeficiency virus (HIV) and is a strong predictor of STIs including gonorrhea and chlamydia infections.[124] In addition, BV has been associated with endometritis, pelvic inflammatory disease (PID), and vaginal cuff cellulitis after invasive procedures such as endometrial biopsy, hysterectomy, hysterosalpingography, insertion of an IUD, cesarean section, and uterine curettage. The bacterial flora that characterize BV have been found in the endometria and salpinges (fallopian tubes) of women who have PID. Treatment with metronidazole substantially reduces postabortion PID.[119] In pregnant women, BV has been associated with premature rupture of the membranes, chorioamnionitis, preterm delivery (delivering before 37 weeks of gestation), postpartum endometritis, and postcesarean wound infection. Preterm delivery is one of the predominant causes of low birth weight and is the second leading cause of infant mortality in the United States.[122] Anaerobes and mycoplasma characteristic of BV have been isolated from sterile sites such as the amniotic fluid, the chorion, the placenta, and the uterus. It is thought that these bacteria travel through the ascending route, from the vagina through the cervix to the uterine cavity in pregnant and nonpregnant women. In pregnant women, the cause of preterm labor associated with BV may be related to the inflammation caused by the release of cervical cytokines.

It is not known whether BV is an independent risk factor for acquiring STIs, including HIV or simply that women who have BV tend to be more promiscuous and thus, are at high risk of being infected with other STIs. However, what is known is that women who are more susceptible to BV have a less healthy, altered vaginal ecosystem that would otherwise deter infections.

CLINICAL PRESENTATION AND DIAGNOSIS

SIGNS AND SYMPTOMS
The chief symptom of BV is vaginal discharge that has a characteristic foul "fish" odor that worsens after intercourse because of a shift to an alkaline pH in the vagina. This discharge is white and homogeneous and often coats the labia. Minimal vulvovaginal itching and burning may occur.[8]

DIAGNOSIS AND CLINICAL FINDINGS
There are four criteria used to diagnose BV: (a) thin, homogeneous, white vaginal discharge that smoothly coats the vaginal walls; (b) a vaginal fluid pH >4.5 or 4.7 depending on type of pH paper used; (c) the presence of clue cells (squamous epithelial cell whose border appears stippled with adherent *G. vaginalis*) on microscopic examination; and (d) a positive whiff test (a fishy odor from vaginal discharge before or after the addition of 10% KOH). Clue cells represent the best single criterion for the diagnosis of BV. Diagnosis of BV is made when three of the above signs and symptoms are found.

TREATMENT

PHARMACOTHERAPY
Treatment is aimed at relieving symptoms, achieving a clinical cure to prevent coinfection with other STIs, and restoring vaginal *Lactobacillus* spp. Currently, there are only two drugs used for BV, metronidazole and clindamycin. Clindamycin vaginal cream and metronidazole orally or intravaginally have been shown to be equally efficacious in achieving clinical cures with BV and preventing recurrences at follow-up in several randomized, double-blind, head-to-head comparison trials.[120,125–130] Clindamycin ovules are a relatively new formulation and like the vaginal suppositories used for VVC, they are less messy and generally preferred by patients.[131] Treatment with a one-time oral dose of metronidazole (2 g) was not shown to be as effective as the 1-week oral course.[132] In addition, single oral dose of metronidazole (2 g) and clindamycin ovules have relapse rates of 35% to 41% and 13%, respectively, after 2 to 3 weeks, and can reach as high as 50% for both after 1 month. Thus,

these regimens remain as ''alternative regimens.''[122] Short courses of treatment are a viable option for patients whose compliance may be problematic. Some patients may prefer metronidazole intravaginally over orally due to the frequent systemic side effects (nausea, abdominal cramping, taste perversion/metallic taste in 22% to 54% of patients) experienced with oral metronidazole. Although, the maximum serum concentration of metronidazole after a single dose of 0.75% vaginal gel is only approximately 2% of that obtained after a single 500-mg oral dose,[133] patients should be advised to abstain from alcohol consumption with either product formulation during treatment and for 24 hours after to avoid a disulfiram-like interaction.

Preference for clindamycin or metronidazole generally depends on the clinician's experience with one product over the other. However, most may prefer metronidazole due to its minimal effect on vaginal *lactobacillus*. In a classic widely cited study, treatment with intravaginal metronidazole normalized colonization of *lactobacillus* spp. by 83% after 1 week and 94% at ≥4 weeks after therapy, whereas treatment with clindamycin vaginal cream showed a recolonization rate of 25% at 1 week, but improved to 87% at ≥4 weeks.[134]

Symptomatic pregnant women should be tested and treated to prevent adverse pregnancy outcomes as previously mentioned. Systemic treatment using metronidazole or clindamycin is recommended. Oral metronidazole has been shown to reduce the risk of premature delivery by 25% to 75% in high-risk pregnant women (i.e., those who have delivered before term in the past)[122] and oral clindamycin, but not intravaginal clindamycin, has demonstrated a reduction in preterm birth and postpartum infectious complications. Lack of evidence with metronidazole vaginal gel and evidence of harm including preterm delivery and neonatal infections with clindamycin vaginal cream deter their use during pregnancy. Multiple studies and meta-analyses have not demonstrated a consistent association between metronidazole use during pregnancy and teratogenic or mutagenic effects in newborns, even with first trimester use.[119,122] It is not clear why a lower 3 times daily dose is chosen during pregnancy, but some clinicians also use the nonpregnant 500-mg twice daily dose.

Even though BV is associated with sexual activity, treatment of the sex partner has not been shown to improve clinical outcome or reduce the recurrence of BV.[119] Patients should be instructed to abstain from intercourse while being treated or to use condoms to optimize outcome. It is absolutely essential to complete the full course of therapy because symptoms may disappear before there is bacteriologic cure. Table 17.9 lists drug therapies for BV.

TABLE 17.9	**Drug Therapies for Bacterial Vaginosis**	
Medication	**Dosage**	**Comments**
Recommended Regimens		
Metronidazole tablet (Flagyl)	500 mg PO bid × 7 days	Common (22%–54%) systemic side effects with oral therapy: nausea, abdominal cramping, metallic taste. Cost of tablet is a lot less than Metrogel.
Metronidazole gel (MetroGel)	0.75%, one full applicator (5 g) INV HS × 5 days	
Clindamycin cream (Cleocin)	2%, one full applicator (5 g) INV HS × 7 days	Clindamycin cream is as effective as metronidazole. Clinical cure rate for both approaches 80%–90%. However, clindamycin is toxic against *lactobacilli*
Alternative Regimens		
Metronidazole tablet (Flagyl)	2 g PO in a single dose	Clindamycin ovules are less messy. These therapies are effective but recurrence of BV is common.
Clindamycin capsules (Cleocin)	300 mg PO bid × 7 days	
Clindamycin ovules (Cleocin ovules)	100 mg INV HS × 3 days	
Regimens in Pregnancy		
Metronidazole tablet (Flagyl)	250 mg PO tid × 7 days or 500 mg PO bid × 7 days	Both regimens have been shown to decrease the incidence of preterm birth and neonatal infections. Topical agents should not be used in pregnancy due to lack of evidence (MetroGel) and evidence of harm with clindamycin cream.
Clindamycin capsule (Cleocin)	300 mg PO bid × 7 days	

Note: Patients should be instructed to avoid consuming alcohol during treatment with metronidazole and for 24 hours thereafter. Clindamycin cream and ovules are oil-based and might weaken latex condoms and diaphragms.
PO, orally; bid, twice daily; INV, intravaginally; HS, at bedtime; BV, bacterial vaginosis; tid, 5 three times daily.
(From Centers for Disease Control and Prevention. Sexually transmitted diseases treatment guidelines 2002. MMWR 51 (No. RR-6):42–45, 2002, with permission.)

ALTERNATIVE THERAPIES

There is no other management of BV except to eradicate the offending organisms via antibiotics. However, ongoing research using hydrogen peroxide producing *Lactobacillus acidophilus* tablets to restore normal vaginal flora is being done. OTC lactobacilli products such as yogurt have not been shown to be beneficial in reconstituting the vaginal flora. This is due to the fact that strains of lactobacilli found in yogurt adhere poorly to vaginal epithelium compared to human-derived strains of *Lactobacillus*. Poor adherence leads to failure in recolonization.

TRICHOMONIASIS

ETIOLOGY

The flagellated protozoan *Trichomonas vaginalis* is transmitted almost exclusively by sexual intercourse. *T. vaginalis* is a parasite of the genitourinary tract and requires a warm (body temperature), moist, slightly alkaline pH (4.9–7.5) environment to thrive.

EPIDEMIOLOGY

Trichomoniasis is the most prevalent nonviral sexually transmitted infection in humans worldwide. Approximately 180 million women worldwide may be infected with *T. vaginalis*.[135] The highest rate of infection is reported among men and women who attend STI clinics. The recent estimate of 5 million new cases of trichomoniasis annually in the United States[136] far surpasses that for chlamydia or gonorrhea. Infection with *T. vaginalis* may not readily be recognized in men due to lack of symptoms and, thus, may be underreported.

PATHOPHYSIOLOGY

Sexual transmission of *T. vaginalis*, specifically, via direct genital contact is well established. Trichomonads can survive up to 45 minutes on toilet seats, washcloths, fomites (substances capable of absorbing and transmitting the contagium of disease), clothing, water, and rarely, be transmitted via objects. Transmission is greater from infected men (80% to 100%) to women compared to from infected women to men (70%).[136] Trichomonal infection in women is neither restricted to nor exclusive for the vagina,[135] with urinary tract infection and dysuria a common finding. Another disturbing finding is that women may harbor *T. vaginalis* for 3–5 years.[137] There are many sequelae to untreated trichomoniasis in women including: (a) an increased HIV transmission and infectivity, (b) a greater risk of tubal infertility and atypical PID, (c) an increased risk of cervical cancer, (d) an increased risk of postoperative infection, and (e) an association with preterm birth in pregnant women.[138–152]

STIs increase the likelihood of HIV transmission and trichomoniasis is no exception. Trichomoniasis is implicated as a cofactor in the transmission of HIV infection by increasing the susceptibility of an uninfected partner and infectivity of infected individuals.[136] Studies in HIV-positive men and women show that treatment of trichomoniasis significantly decreases HIV viral shedding in vaginal fluid and semen.[145,153] Studies evaluating infertility in women have shown an amplified risk of two- to sixfold in those with *T. vaginalis* infection.[141–143] Like BV, trichomoniasis is associated with postoperative infections. In fact, a recent study shows that *T. vaginalis* contributes to changes in vaginal flora and that this alteration may contribute to a coinfection with BV, a common finding in women with trichomoniasis.[154] Perhaps the most disconcerting news for women is that trichomoniasis may be a risk factor for the development of cervical neoplasia (benign or malignant changes of the squamous epithelium of the cervix). The result of a meta analysis of 22 cohort and two case-controlled studies show a doubling of risk of cervical neoplasia in women infected with *T. vaginalis*.[138] In a prospective, longitudinal cohort study of >19,000 Finnish women, the risk of developing cervical cancer in women infected with *T. vaginalis* was similar to that found in women infected with human papillomavirus (a known offender in the development of cervical cancer).[139] Strengthening these findings are results from two recent studies that showed the high prevalence of antibodies against *T. vaginalis* in women with invasive cervical cancer compared to controls.[150,151]

In pregnant women, *T. vaginalis* infection has also been shown to cause premature rupture of membranes, preterm delivery, and low-birth weight infants.[140,155] In addition, perinatal transmission from infected mothers via the birth canal occurs in about 5% of the time and can cause urinary tract infection, vaginitis, and severe respiratory distress in the neonates.[156–161] In female neonates, infection can also be localized to the vagina where the presence of maternal estrogen gives it an adult-like epithelium, making it favorable for the survival of *T. vaginalis*. Vaginal infection in female neonates is usually self-limiting once maternal estrogen is metabolized and the vaginal epithelium returns to the prepubescent state, at which time it becomes relatively resistant to *T. vaginalis* infection. Treatment of the woman and her sex partner(s) can potentially prevent premature delivery and infection in the neonates.

CLINICAL PRESENTATION AND DIAGNOSIS

SIGNS AND SYMPTOMS

In women, the chief symptoms of trichomoniasis are variable, ranging from a mild yellow-green or gray vaginal discharge, to a moderate malodorous discharge, to itching, burning discharge with odor, to intermenstrual or postcoital bleeding. Dysuria is present in at least 10% of patients. However, some women have minimal or no symptoms at all.[119]

DIAGNOSIS AND CLINICAL FINDINGS

Diagnosis can be made with different specimens including urine, vaginal fluid, and endocervical smear (via Papanicolaou). Microscopy of vaginal secretions has a sensitivity of 60% to 70%. Culture is the most sensitive diagnostic test available but because of the delay in results and consequently treatment, it is not usually performed. Flagellated motile trichomonads can be seen on a wet mount in normal saline. When present, a frothy green vaginal discharge with a pH >4.5 can be seen. Examination of the cervix may show colpitis macularis, or "strawberry cervix," cervical mucopurulence, erythema, and friability.[135]

TREATMENT

PHARMACOTHERAPY

In pregnant and nonpregnant women, the treatment of choice is metronidazole (2 g orally in a single dose). Treatment of partner is a must or reinfection will occur. Metronidazole vaginal gel (MetroGel) is not recommended since topical treatment does not achieve therapeutic levels in perivaginal glands. Tinidazole (Tindamax) is a second-generation nitroimidazole recently approved for the treatment of trichomoniasis. Tinidazole has greater potency against resistant *T. vaginalis* isolates than metronidazole in vitro. This has important implications in the treatment of this STI, since drug resistant *T. vaginalis* is on the rise. Tinidazole is dosed similar to metronidazole (2 g once), has the same GI side effects, and abstinence from alcohol during treatment is advised.

MENOPAUSE

DEFINITION

Menopause and climacteric are used interchangeably and are defined by the absence of menses in 12 consecutive months. Perimenopause is characterized by menstrual irregularities and is the period preceding menopause.

ETIOLOGY

Menopause results from the cessation of ovarian production of estrogen. Menopause can be induced by the removal of ovaries (oophorectomy), from premature ovarian failure, or from natural cause secondary to the physiologic depletion of ovarian follicles.

EPIDEMIOLOGY

The average age of women reaching menopause in the United States is 51 years, but ovarian production of estrogen and progestin begins to decrease years before the complete cessation of menses. Currently, it is estimated that more than 47 million women in the United States are over 50 years of age. The number will continue to rise, as the current average life expectancy of women is 79.5 years of age. As a result, women will spend more than one third of their lives in menopause. The probability of developing various chronic diseases is, thus, high in postmenopausal women. It is estimated that a postmenopausal woman has a 46% risk of developing coronary heart disease (CHD), 20% for stroke, 15% for hip fracture, 10% for breast cancer, and 2.6% for endometrial

cancer. In addition, postmenopausal women have a 1.4- to threefold higher risk for Alzheimer's disease than do men. The lifetime risk for developing colorectal cancer for a woman in the United States is 6%, with more than 90% of cases occurring after 50 years of age.[162]

PATHOPHYSIOLOGY

The number of ovarian follicles steadily decreases as a woman ages. When this number is depleted, ovarian production of estrogen ceases and menopause begins. Accompanying the decrease in gonadal estrogen secretion is the rise in pituitary FSH. The rise and fall of FSH is further controlled by inhibin, a glycoprotein made by the granulosa cells of developing follicles during the follicular phase of the cycle. Pituitary FSH and gonadal inhibin production are controlled in a closed-loop feedback system where FSH stimulates the production of inhibin, while inhibin suppresses the secretion of FSH. As the number of ovarian follicles decreases with increasing age, the level of inhibin also wanes with a concomitant rise in FSH. Initially, the rise in FSH contributes to an increased secretion of estradiol from the follicles. However, as the period of perimenopause progresses and more follicles are depleted, the elevated FSH levels will fail to stimulate sufficient estradiol production to maintain endometrial development. This eventually leads to the cessation of uterine bleeding or amenorrhea, clinically observed as menopause. It is important to note that during perimenopause, ovulatory cycles can still take place, and in a sexually active woman not using contraception, can result in a surprise pregnancy. Menopause is synonymously identified with an estrogen-deficient state with concomitant clinical sequelae such as vasomotor symptoms (hot flushes with or without night sweats), vaginal atrophy, and osteoporosis. However, the number one cause of death in women after reaching menopause is CHD.

THERAPEUTIC PLAN

GOALS OF TREATMENT

The goals of treatment with estrogen replacement are to prevent menopausal symptoms, vaginal atrophy, and osteoporosis. Patients should be instructed to perform monthly breast self-examinations and report any lumps or retractions discovered, and to report any irregular noncyclic bleeding that may indicate neoplastic changes in the genital tract. Postmenopausal patients on cyclic hormonal regimens should be told that withdrawal bleeding may occur.

VASOMOTOR SYMPTOMS

Approximately 75% of women in menopausal transition experience hot flushes and night sweats, classified as vasomotor symptoms of menopause. On average, vasomotor symptoms last for 3.8 years, with more than half of these women experiencing severe symptoms. Prevalence varies among different racial/ethnic groups, with the most frequently reported among African American women (45.6%), followed by Hispanics (35.4%), whites (31.2%), Chinese (20.5%), and Japanese (17.6%).[163] It is suggested that the change in estrogen levels leads to alterations in hypothalamic thermoregulation. The abrupt decline in estrogen as a result of oophorectomy or in early natural menopause produces the most pronounced vasomotor symptoms. Symptoms may last for at least 5 years for 70% of these women.[8] Homeostatic adjustments and abatement of symptoms eventually occur. The most likely explanation of why all women do not experience hot flushes or to different degrees seems to be varying amounts of endogenous estrogen produced in adipose tissue. The conversion of androstenedione (produced in adrenal glands and ovaries) to estrone (see estrogen pharmacology below) via aromatase in peripheral adipose tissues is higher in an obese postmenopausal woman than a slender woman, which may explain why obese women are less likely to develop hot flushes and other estrogen deficient symptoms and more likely to develop endometrial hyperplasia and adenocarcinoma of the endometrium. Slender women are at higher risk of developing osteoporosis and hot flushes.

CLINICAL PRESENTATION AND DIAGNOSIS

SIGNS AND SYMPTOMS

The chief vasomotor symptoms reported by patients are described as hot flushes or hot flashes occurring over the ante-rior part of the body, especially the chest, neck, and face. An episode lasts usually only a few minutes and is commonly precipitated by anxiety and excitement. The vasomotor symptoms vary considerably in duration, frequency, and severity. One variation, night sweats, is experienced by some patients who usually describe awakening at night, covered in perspiration, and throwing off the bed covers.[8]

It is estimated that following physiologic menopause, 15% of patients seek treatment for vasomotor symptoms; 50% of reproductive-age women undergoing castration request treatment.[8] Vasomotor symptoms do not pose any serious consequences, but they can be bothersome and affect a woman's quality of life and social functioning as a sudden onset of red flushing to the face or profuse sweating secondary to hot flushes can be embarrassing.

TREATMENT

PHARMACOTHERAPY

Hormonal therapy (HT) includes estrogen therapy (ET) or combination estrogen/progestin therapy (EPT) in woman with an intact uterus remains the treatment of choice for women with moderate-to-severe vasomotor symptoms. In controlled trials, estrogen consistently provides relief of hot flushes in 80% to 90% of women.[164] HT provides rapid relief of vasomotor symptoms, usually within 3 weeks and treats vaginal symptoms such as dryness and atrophy. In addition, HT provides benefits such as protection against fracture and colorectal cancer. Nonhormonal treatment options for hot flushes include clonidine, SSRIs (paroxetine, fluoxetine), serotonin-norepinephrine reuptake inhibitors (SNRIs) (venlafaxine), and gabapentin. For mild hot flushes, the North American Menopause Society (NAMS) recommends lifestyle-related strategies such as keeping the core body temperature cool, regular exercise, and using paced respiration.

All potential patients for HT should undergo a baseline evaluation, including pelvic examination, cytology, breast examination, blood pressure, and a thorough history, to rule out absolute and relative contraindications.[165]

Postmenopausal hormone therapy has been shown to cause exacerbation of asthma, epilepsy, and diabetes. However, women who are being treated for these conditions or are stable can safely use HT. In addition to treating vasomotor symptoms and vaginal atrophy, clinicians have long believed that HT also protects against CHD. Observational studies have suggested that postmenopausal HT confers a moderate degree of protection from CHD, with reductions in overall mortality rates for acute MI in comparison with nonestrogen users.[166] However, observational studies fail to control for other factors that can influence the outcomes such as baseline risks including genetic attributes, behaviors, and if patients were taking other medications. In contrast, clinical trials are designed to minimize confounding factors so that the results are that observed from the intervention(s). Furthermore, patients in control and intervention groups will be similar in age, education, and health at the time of entering the trial.

The first clinical trial to show positive markers for protection of CHD was the Postmenopausal Estrogen/Progestin Intervention (PEPI) Trial.[167] In all four hormone regimens [0.625 mg/day conjugated equine estrogens (CEE) alone; 0.625 mg/day CEE + 10 mg medroxyprogesterone (MPA) for the first 12 days of the cycle; 0.625 mg CEE + 2.5 mg MPA daily; 0.625 mg/d CEE + 200 mg micronized progesterone for the first 12 days of the cycle], there were reductions in LDL cholesterol, increases in HDL cholesterol, and decreases in levels of fibrinogen (high levels of fibrinogen allow blood clots to form more readily, thus increasing the risk of heart disease and stroke). The PEPI trial also showed that women with an intact uterus who took ET alone had a higher rate of endometrial hyperplasia, thus necessitating the need of adding a progestin.

The Heart and Estrogen/Progestin Replacement Therapy Study (HERS)[168] was the first clinical trial to specifically examine the effects of estrogen/progestin therapy (EPT) on diseases. This was a 4.1-year secondary prevention trial of 2,763 women with an intact uterus, average age of 67 years, using 0.625 mg CEE + 2.5 mg MPA daily as a treatment to protect against recurrent CHD events (nonfatal MI and CHD death). Additional patient risk factors for CHD included 18% of patients with diabetes, 55% of patients were overweight, and 13% were smokers. Hormone therapy in these postmenopausal women did not reduce the overall incidence of recurrent MI and CHD death compared with placebo [relative risk (RR)1.52; 95% confidence interval (CI) 1.01–2.29] in the first year. However, EPT resulted in fewer second events reducing linearly by the fourth and fifth years of treatment from 4.25 per 100 patients per year in the first year to 2.30 (RR 0.67; 95% CI 0.43–1.04). The rate of nonfatal heart attacks also reduced linearly from 3.13 during the first year to 1.39 by the fourth and fifth years. There were 13 venous thromboembolic events (VTEs) (in the legs and lungs) in the first year compared to 6 in the fourth and fifth year.[168] Recently, a follow-up to HERS (HERS II) was conducted in these women for an additional 2.7 years. The results for the total 6.8-year of EPT use did not differ in CHD events compared to placebo that is, the reduction in CHD events during the fourth and fifth years in HERS did not persist in HERS II.[169] Noncardiovascular events included an increase in venous thromboembolism and biliary tract surgery.[170]

In contrast to HERS, the Women's Health Initiative[171] (WHI), the largest clinical trial to date, was a primary prevention study that enrolled 16,608 healthy postmenopausal women (in EPT arm) age 50–79 years with an intact uterus to receive 0.625 mg CEE + 2.5 mg MPA or placebo, or 0.625 mg CEE unopposed (10,739 women in ET arm) for a planned duration of 8.5 years. The EPT arm of the study was halted early, after 5.2 years due to an ''unacceptable'' increased risk of invasive breast cancer and that, overall, risks from the use of EPT outweighed the benefits conferred.

The estimated risks and benefits after 5.2 years were as follows: CHD (RR 1.29; 95% CI 1.02–1.63); breast cancer (RR 1.26; 95% CI 1–1.59); stroke (RR 1.41; 95% CI 1.07–1.85); pulmonary embolism (PE) (RR 2.13, 95% CI 1.39–3.25); colorectal cancer (RR 0.63; 95% CI 0.43–0.92); and hip fracture (RR 0.66; 95% CI 0.45–0.98). RRs refer to the percentage change in a population that has been exposed to EPT to another that has not (placebo), which differs from absolute risks in that the latter is an estimate of the number of women who will (or will not) develop a disease when exposed to EPT. Absolute risks give a true picture of what will happen when a woman is exposed to the agent in question. For example, the results above showed that after 5 years, the women on EPT had a 29% greater chance of developing a CHD event than nonusers (RR 1.29), however, this translates to seven additional cases of CHD events per year in a group of 10,000 women in the EPT group, or an absolute excess risk of 0.07% per year. In the EPT arm of the WHI, the absolute excess risks per 10,000-person years (each year for every 10,000 women) were 7 more CHD events, 8 additional cases of invasive breast cancer, 8 more strokes, 8 more PEs, while the absolute risk reductions per 10,000 person-years were 6 fewer colorectal cancers and 5 fewer hip fractures. The increased risk of breast cancer appeared after 4 years, while that for MI and blood clots including PE appeared after the first year of use. Protection against colorectal cancer appeared after 3 years, while that for hip fracture was immediate.

The second arm of the WHI[172] consisted of 10,739 healthy postmenopausal women age 50 to 79 years, with prior hysterectomy, using unopposed CEE or placebo. This arm continued for an additional 2 years (6.8 years total) with somewhat better risk-to-benefit ratios. In contrast to the EPT arm of the WHI, there were only one or two adverse outcomes (increased strokes and perhaps PE) versus four (increased strokes, CHD, PE, and breast cancer) seen in the EPT arm of WHI. The incidence of CHD was not affected by the use of unopposed estrogen. It should be noted that this arm was also halted early due to an ''unacceptable'' elevated risk of strokes among healthy women in a study. There was an absolute excess risk of 12 additional strokes per 10,000 person-years and an absolute risk reduction of six fewer hip fractures per 10,000 person-years. Increased risk of stroke was the only outcome consistent among three trials, HERS, ET and EPT arms of the WHI. A consistent benefit was protection against hip fracture in both arms of the WHI. Surprisingly, an attenuated risk in breast cancer was seen in the WHI estrogen only arm, though, the result did not reach statistical significance (RR 0.77, 95% CI 0.59–1.01). These results implicated the role of progestin in breast cancer, and strengthened evidence from HERS and other large observational studies that MPA and other progestins increase risk for breast cancer above that associated with estrogen alone.[173–178] The levonorgestrel-releasing intrauterine device (Mirena) is currently being used to oppose the effects of estrogen on the endometrium. This device releases about 100 to 150 pg per milliliter of levonorgestrel into the bloodstream daily, a minimal exposure compared to other progestin therapy and thus, is expected to attenuate progestin-related events. Although both arms of the WHI have been halted, the women in the active phase of the studies are continued to be monitored to assess long-term effects of hormone use.

The WHI Memory Study (WHIMS)[179–182] evaluated the effects of ET or EPT on cognitive function in women between 65 and 79 years of age without signs of dementia on study entry. In both arms of the WHIMS, there was an increased incidence of dementia in women exposed to HT (estrogen alone or estrogen plus progestin), with Alzheimer as the most commonly diagnosed type of dementia compared to placebo. The absolute risk translates to 12 additional cases of dementia per 10,000 person-years in the ET group and 23 cases in EPT group. In addition, HT was not protective against cognitive decline, including memory, concentration, language, and abstract reasoning. In fact, global cognition was adversely affected with hormone use and that these effects were more pronounced among women who had relatively lower cognitive function at the start of therapy. Adverse findings in WHIMS occurred mostly in women >75 years of age. In contrast, the Cache County Memory Study, which followed 1,889 women (mean age 74.5 years) for 3 years, found that women who started HT at an earlier age had a decreased risk of Alzheimer's disease.[183]

After these compelling data and the ensuing media, it is difficult for any clinician to advise HT to a woman. However, as with all studies, the WHI is subjected to many criticisms and although may provide one view of the truth, it is by far, not gospel truth. Furthermore, all three trials mentioned (PEPI, HERS, WHI), used only CEE and MPA. Perhaps not all estrogens and progestins or routes of delivery are equal, a point of contention that has been shown in various studies. For example, in the PEPI trial, micronized progesterone was shown to preserve estrogen's benefits to lipid profiles, while MPA blunted these effects. In addition, transdermal estrogens have not been shown to increase C-reactive protein, sex hormone-binding globulin, cholesterol saturation of bile, or elevate the risk of venous thromboembolism to that of oral estrogens.[184] The largest criticism of the WHI is that, although it was designed as a primary prevention study, the average age of women enrolled in both arms was 63.3 years (an average of 13 years distant from menopause), 66% were age >60 years at study entry and 21% were age ≥70 years. Presumably, cardiovascular events may have already begun by this age and, thus, makes the study appear as a secondary prevention trial like HERS. Further, the use of statin drugs among patients in the WHI was not randomized, which can influence CHD outcomes. It is well documented that HT improves lipid profiles including lowering LDL and increasing HDL and intuitively, would be cardio-protective. It has been shown in a monkey model that early intervention with CEE significantly decreased plaque size compared to late intervention.[185]

With regards to breast cancer, age, and not HT is the greatest risk factor. Women >50 years of age have a six times elevated risk compared to that of younger women.[186] In the WHI, the excess risk of breast cancer associated with HT did not reach statistical significance until the fifth year. In addition, there were more cases of invasive breast cancer in the placebo group in the first 2 years than that seen in the HT group during the first 4 years. There was no difference in mortality rates from breast cancer between the placebo and HT group. In general, the absolute risk for many diseases approximately doubles with each decade of age.[168] On closer look at the WHI, women in the age group between 50 and 59 years of age appeared to respond more favorably to estrogen than older women. The high drop out rate of approximately 50% in the WHI can affect the statistical power of the study to accurately measure small differences between study groups. In addition, the lead statistician noted that the Global Index (the overall measurement of harm versus benefits) used in the WHI was for the purpose of decision-making by the Data Safety and Monitoring Board members (the group that halted the study prematurely) has no relevance to clinical practice.[187]

Although estrogen use has declined over the years, especially in light of the WHI, HT is still the gold standard for treatment of vasomotor symptoms. Compared to all the agents studied, HT remains the single therapy that consistently decreases hot flushes in frequency and severity with relief within the first few weeks of initiation. It is important to put data into perspective for patients, that results from the WHI do not apply to symptomatic, younger postmenopausal women, that the risks are small on an individual basis (since data were extrapolated per 10,000 woman-years), and that statistics are not fate but that other factors such as genetics, lifestyle, and personal medical history also play a role. Taken together, and in concordance with recommendations from major organizations (NAMS, FDA, ACOG), HT may be instituted in women with moderate-to-severe vasomotor symptoms at the lowest effective dose and for the shortest duration. Dose increase may be made if symptoms do not improve in 3 to 4 weeks. However, HT is not recommended for the prevention of chronic conditions in postmenopausal women.[162]

Estrogen Pharmacology[188]. The major circulating estrogen during the reproductive years is 17-β estradiol (E_2). Estradiol (E_2) in the premenopausal woman is produced by the ovaries. Other endogenous sources of estrogen come from the conversion of androstenedione into estrone (E_1), which primarily occurs in adipose tissues via aromatase. In postmenopausal women, the majority of estrogen is estrone, which has approximately one third the estrogenic potency of (E_2). Estradiol (E_2) is the most potent form of endogenous estrogen. It is produced in the ovaries, secreted into the bloodstream, and subsequently converted by hepatic enzymes into various metabolites with little or no estrogenic activities (Fig. 17.3).

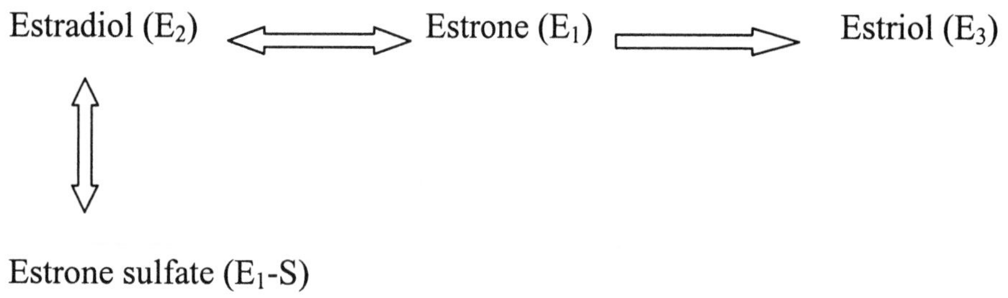

Estradiol (E$_2$) $\Longleftrightarrow$ Estrone (E$_1$) $\Longrightarrow$ Estriol (E$_3$)

$\Updownarrow$

Estrone sulfate (E$_1$-S)

FIGURE 17.3 At the cellular level, estrogenic potency is highest for E$_2$ > E$_1$ > E$_3$.

Estrogen and progestin can be ''natural'' or ''synthetic.'' The natural estrogen mimics the actions of (E$_2$), while that of progestin mimics the actions of progesterone. Progesterone is secreted by the ovaries, mainly from the corpus luteum during the luteal phase of the menstrual cycle. Drug marketing may be misleading, claiming that their products are natural when, in fact, naturally occurring compounds lack biological activity. The only natural estrogens are CEE, produced in the urine of pregnant mares. In contrast, the synthetic estrogens and progestins are derived from plant sources such as soybeans and White Mexican Yams must be chemically altered to achieve biological activities. The group of synthetic estrogens includes esterified, conjugated, micronized estradiol, and piperazine estrone sulfate.

HT for vasomotor symptoms can be administered orally or transdermally and most recently, vaginally (Femring). Transdermal formulations bypass first-pass hepatic metabolism and may attenuate the elevated levels of triglycerides and clotting factors seen with oral formulations.[184] Current oral ET users had approximately a fourfold increased risk of VTE, including PE and deep venous thrombosis (DVT) compared to current users of transdermal ET in a recent multicenter case control study.[189] These findings parallel biological evidence, which shows elevated levels of prothrombin fragments, decreased level of antithrombin, resistance to activated protein C, and elevated C-reactive protein, all markers of increased thrombotic risk.[190] In addition, transdermal formulations deliver a more physiologic steady serum levels of hormone. In several studies, transdermal HT improves hot flash scores (decreased frequency and severity) to a greater extent than oral formulations.[191] Two new transdermal formulations have recently been approved for the treatment of vasomotor symptoms and vulvovaginal atrophy. The topical emulsion, Estrasorb is packaged in individual pouches of 1.74 g of lotion that can be rubbed onto the skin. Two pouches a day deliver the equivalent dose of estradiol as a 0.05 mg per day patch. The emulsion is formulated and delivered via the micellar nanoparticle technology, which exploits the small-size particle to facilitate quick and complete absorption through the skin. EstroGel is dispensed from a metered dose pump to deliver 1.25 g per day containing 0.75 mg per day of estradiol. Since significant estradiol absorption occurs through the skin, the use of a progestin is needed to prevent endometrial hyperplasia. Refer to Table 17.10 for a list of HT options.

Nonhormonal Therapies. SSRIs (fluoxetine and paroxetine) and SNRI (venlafaxine) are the only antidepressants studied for the treatment of hot flushes. It is not fully understood how these agents work to alleviate vasomotor symptoms, but reduced serum serotonin (5-HT) levels, possibly secondary to estrogen withdrawal in women with spontaneous or surgical menopause[192] led to their interest. Furthermore, it has been suggested that 5-HT, specifically the subtypes 5-HT$_{1a}$ and 5-HT$_{2a}$ may play a role in thermoregulation in mammals and that these subtypes must be in balance to maintain optimal thermoregulation. The studies using these antidepressants were conducted in breast cancer survivors and the number of participants is usually small (≤220) and the duration short (≤13 weeks). Nevertheless, these studies achieve as much as 50% and 67% mean reduction in frequency and severity of hot flushes using doses lower than that used to treat depression, but they are often complicated by the high placebo effects (up to 40% in some studies).[192] Side effects were minimal and well tolerated thus, making these antidepressants favorable alternatives for the treatment of vasomotor symptoms. Gabapentin (300 mg three times daily) has been shown to decrease hot flash frequency by 45% in postmenopausal women with minimal side effects.[193] It is speculated that gabapentin's effect on hot flashes is mediated by mitigation of the hypothalamic tachykinin neurotransmitter.[193] There is a case report of a woman with severe hot flashes refractory to treatments with estrogen and SSRIs who was successfully managed with gabapentin (1,200–1,500 mg daily).[194] Gabapentin relieves hot flashes within days of therapy, in contrast to weeks with SSRIs and HT. These drugs are relatively safe and well tolerated and thus, have replaced the older nonhormonal substitutes for hot flashes such as clonidine and Bellergal (Table 17.10).

ALTERNATIVE THERAPIES

Data are inconsistent for phytoestrogens as treatment for vasomotor symptoms. Phytoestrogens are plant-derived compounds that exhibit estrogenic activity, are found in legumes, soybeans, vegetables, fruits, nuts, and grains.[164, 195] Other sources of phytoestrogens include herbs such as black cohosh, wild yam, dong quai, and valerian root. The three main classes of phytoestrogens are isoflavones, lignins, and coumestans. The most abundant soy isoflavones, genistein,

TABLE 17.10 | Hormonal and Nonhormonal Treatment Options for Vasomotor Symptoms

Types of Hormone Therapy	Trade Names and Usual Dosages (mg daily)	Comments
Oral Estrogen Therapy		CEE is the only type of estrogen used in HERS, WHI, PEPI trials. Unopposed use only in women without a uterus. A dose of 0.625 mg qd can prevent fractures. The most common side effects with initial therapy are breast tenderness and irregular vaginal bleeding or spotting. CEE (primarily sodium estrone sulfate and sodium equilin sulfate) are derived from the urine of pregnant mares, while synthetic estrogens (all others) are plant derived and chemically altered to yield desired biologic activities.
CEEs	Premarin: 0.3–1.25	
Synthetic conjugated estrogens	Cenestin: 0.3–1.25	
ESTs	Menest, Estratab: 0.3–1.25	
Estropipate (piperazine estrone sulfate)	Ogen, Ortho-Est: 0.625–5	
Micronized 17β-estradiol (E$_2$)	Estrace, Estradiol, Gynodiol: 0.5–2	
Injectable Estrogen Therapy		
Estrone	Estrone 5, EstraGyn 5: 0.1–1 mg IM q week	
Estradiol cypionate	Depo-Estradiol: 1–5 mg IM q 3–4 weeks	
Estradiol valerate	Delestrogen: 10–20 mg IM q 4 weeks	
Oral Progestin Therapy		Similar to the estrogens, progestins can be "natural" or synthetic. The only "natural" progestin is progesterone found in the Mexican yam. MP has neutral lipid effects.[167] Progestins are added to estrogen therapy to prevent endometrial hyperplasia in women with an intact uterus. The addition of a progestin usually increases initial side effects of HT such as mood changes and bloating. Higher doses of progesterone are needed to achieve similar endometrial protection (MP 100 mg ~2.5 mg MPA).
MPA	Provera, Amen, Cycrin: 10 mg for 10–12 days/month (cyclic dosing); or 2.5–5 mg qd	
NETA	Aygestin: 5 mg	
MP (Formulation is suspended in peanut oil and is contraindicated in patients allergic to peanuts)	Prometrium: 200 mg for 10–12 days/month (cyclic dosing); or 100 mg qd	
Megestrol acetate (Used for hot flushes, not for endometrial protection)	Megace: 20–40 mg qd	
Oral Estrogen + Progestin Therapy		Withdrawal bleeding (menses) is seen with cyclic progestin therapy such as Premphase and Prefest, where the progestin is given in a cyclic manner. With continuous dosing, where progestin is given daily, spotting may occasionally occur, but amenorrhea achieved by the majority of patients is reached by cycle 13. Spotting and/or bleeding with HT is a major factor for noncompliance. Increasing the dose of progestin usually eliminates spotting and/or bleeding. NETA 1 mg lowers HDL cholesterol level considerably, with no beneficial effects on triglyceride level, while at 0.5 mg in combination with E$_2$, has been shown to lower triglyceride levels below baseline in addition to reducing LDL cholesterol and apoB concentrations.[2]
CEE + MPA	Prempro: 0.625/2.5, 5 mg Prempro Lo: 0.45, 0.3/1.5 mg Premphase: 0.625/5 mg (for 14 days of the month)	
EE + NETA	Femhrt: 5 µg EE/1 mg NETA	
Estradiol (E$_2$) + norgestimate	Prefest: 1 mg (E$_2$)/0.09 mg norgestimate alternating q 3 days sequentially monthly	
Estradiol (E$_2$) + NETA	Activella: 1 mg (E$_2$)/0.5 mg NETA	
Other		Combination HT containing TES is thought to increase libido.[3] A progestin is required in a woman with an intact uterus. Therapy with TES requires periodic monitoring of liver enzymes. Androgenic side effects such as acne and facial hair are common.
EST + TES	Estratest, Syntest D.S.: 1.25 mg EST/2.5 mg TES Estratest HS, Syntest HS: 0.625 mg EST/1.25 mg TES	
Levonorgestrel IUD	Mirena IUD: releases 20 µg levonorgestrel daily in uterine cavity. Lasts 5 years	Plasma level of 100–150 pg/mL is minimal compared to other progestin options. Effective in preventing endometrial hyperplasia associated with ET use.

(continued)

TABLE 17.10	continued

Types of Hormone Therapy	Trade Names and Usual Dosages (mg daily)	Comments
Transdermal Hormone Therapy Patches Estradiol (E₂)	Alora, Esclim, Vivelle, Vivelle Dot, Estraderm: 0.025 mg to 0.1 mg BIW Climara, FemPatch, Estradiol: 0.025 mg q week Menostar: 14 μg q week	Transdermal route bypasses hepatic first-pass metabolism and has been shown to have many benefits over oral route including lack of effect on hemostasis, lipoproteins, and C-reactive protein. Irritation at site of application is common, occurring in up to 40% of patients. Due to the extremely low level of estradiol released, only 14 days of progestin is needed every 6–12 months with Menostar.
Estradiol (E₂) + NETA	CombiPatch: 0.05 mg (E₂)/0.14 mg, 0.25 mg NETA BIW	CombiPatch must be refrigerated before dispensing.
Estradiol (E₂) + Levonorgestrel	ClimaraPro: (0.045/0.015 mg/day) q week	
Percutaneous Estradiol (E₂)	Estrasorb (1.74 g/3.3 mL) EstraGel (1.25 g/dose)	Estrasorb is a topical emulsion that delivers the equivalent daily dose of E₂ as a 0.05-mg patch. Estragel dispenses 0.75 mg/day of E₂. The use of a progestin is needed to oppose their hyperplastic effects on the endometrium.
Vaginal Ring Estradiol (E₂) acetate	Femring (0.05–0.1 mg/day)	See comments in Table 17.11.
SSRIs Fluoxetine Paroxetine	Prozac: 20 mg qd Paxil, CR: 10–20 mg qd or 12.5 mg Paxil CR	Good alternatives to HT for treatment of hot flushes. Most studies have been done in breast cancer survivors, with small numbers and short duration, complicated by high placebo effect.
SNRI Venlafaxine	Effexor, XR: 37.5–75 mg	More data compared to SSRIs. High dose (≥150 mg qd) affects norepinephrine receptors, causing elevated diastolic blood pressure.
Anticonvulsant Gabapentin	Neurontin: 300 mg tid	Used for the treatment of vasomotor symptoms. Some anecdotal evidence for hot flashes resistant to treatment with HT and SSRI. Well-tolerated, with somnolence as most common side effect.

CEE, conjugated equine estrogens; HERS, Heart and Estrogen/Progestin Replacement Therapy Study; WHI, Women's Health Initiative; PEPI, Postmenopausal Estrogen/Progestin Intervention Trial; qd, daily; EST, esterified estrogen; IM, intramuscularly; q, every; MPA, medroxyprogesterone acetate; MP, micronized progesterone; NETA, norethindrone acetate; HT, hormonal therapy; EE, ethinyl estradiol; HDL, high-density lipoprotein; TES, methyltestosterone; LDL, low-density lipoprotein; HS, at bedtime; IUD, intrauterine device; ET, estrogen therapy; BIW, twice weekly; SSRI, selective serotonin receptor reuptake inhibitor; SNRI, serotonin-norepinephrine reuptake inhibitor; tid, three times daily.
(From The Writing Group for the PEPI Trial. Effects of estrogen or estrogen/progestin regimens on heart disease risk factors in postmenopausal women. JAMA 273:199–208, 1995; Speroff L, Rowan J, Symons, et al.The comparative effect on bone density, endometrium, and lipids of continuous hormones as replacement therapy (CHART study). A randomized controlled trial. JAMA 276:1397–1403, 1996; Lobo RA, Rosen RC, Yang HM, et al. Comparative effects of oral esterified estrogens with and without methyltestosterone on endocrine profiles and dimensions of sexual function in postmenopausal women with hypoactive sexual desire. Fertil Steril 79:1341–1352, 2003.)

and daidzein, have received the most attention as alternative treatments for hot flushes.[164] Soy isoflavones are believed to act as selective estrogen receptor modulators (SERMs), by acting as an agonist in certain estrogen-sensitive tissues and as an antagonist at others. For this reason, soy isoflavones may decrease hot flushes while having no effect on endometrial thickness. The preponderance of data indicate that phytoestrogens are no more effective than placebo in relieving hot flushes[164] and at least, in one recent study,

soy isoflavones have no effects on cognitive function, bone mineral density, or plasma lipids in postmenopausal women.[195] The existence of SSRIs, venlafaxine and gabapentin as alternatives to estrogen for the treatment of hot flushes has placed questions on supplemental phytoestrogen products (including black cohosh) as part of the armamentarium. Long-term safety data of phytoestrogens are lacking, making recommendations for their use difficult. However, this does not mean that postmenopausal women should be discouraged from consuming foods rich in phytoestrogens but simply to not use ''natural products'' containing excessive concentrated amounts.

VAGINAL ATROPHY

ETIOLOGY

Postmenopausal estrogen deficiency inevitably leads to a thinning and atrophy of the vaginal mucosa, an increase in vaginal pH, which can lead to vaginitis, dyspareunia, vaginismus, and infections of the vagina and urinary tract. In contrast to vasomotor hot flushes, vaginal atrophy, if left untreated, progressively worsens over time. A decrease in collagen content, elasticity, and vascularity as a consequence of estrogen loss contributes to vaginal atrophy.

CLINICAL PRESENTATION AND DIAGNOSIS

The chief symptoms are vaginal discharge secondary to infection (due to an increase in vaginal pH, favoring harboring of pathogenic organisms), complaints of painful intercourse (dyspareunia) due to dryness, and dysuria. Estrogens increase the vascularity and epithelial proliferation of the vagina, allowing greater lubrication, increased protection from vaginitis, and reduced vaginal trauma from coitus. The increased vascularity resulting from estrogen therapy is associated with increased blood flow through the periurethral venous plexus, leading to small increases in periurethral pressure occasionally sufficient to correct urinary stress incontinence.[8]

TREATMENT

PHARMACOTHERAPY

The atrophy and dysuria can be treated with equal effectiveness by systemic or vaginally applied estrogen. Estrogen therapy decreases vaginal pH, thickens and revascularizes the vaginal epithelium, increases the number of superficial cells, and reverses vaginal atrophy.[196] Improvements are usually seen within 1 to 3 months of treatment. Evaluation of effectiveness is done using the Vaginal Maturation Index, which measures the proportion of superficial cells, intermediate, and parabasal cells present in the vaginal epithelium. Postmenopausal vaginal cytology, in contrast to that seen in premenopause, mostly comprises of parabasal cells, not superficial and intermediate cells. Treatment with ET reverses this ratio.

Treatment options include oral HT, at the lowest dose, or vaginal estrogens. See Table 17.11 for a complete list. When local symptoms are the only concern, systemic oral HT should not be used. Vaginal estrogen creams containing CEE or estradiol are available in calibrated applicators in 0.625 and 0.1 mg per gram, respectively, for proper dose delivery. Estradiol

vaginal rings and tablets available are less messy than creams and the rings have an added convenience of remaining in place for 3 months. Initial starting dose is generally higher than maintenance dose. The duration of treatment for vaginal atrophy and urogenital symptoms (dysuria, urinary tract infections) is generally 6 to 12 months. Systemic absorption of local estrogens occurs, but there is insufficient data to recommend annual endometrial surveillance in asymptomatic women using local estrogens.[197] Vaginal ring containing 2 mg of estradiol (Estring) releases approximately 7.5 µg of estradiol daily for 3 months. This level of estradiol is comparable to that observed in a postmenopausal woman.[198] A new vaginal ring (Femring) (releasing 0.05 or 0.1 mg daily) has been found to treat urogenital and vasomotor symptoms. Femring showed comparable relief of hot flushes (84% vs. 73% at 12 weeks) compared to oral estradiol (1 mg daily), in a multicenter, double-blind, double dummy, placebo-controlled study of 159 women.[199] Unlike Estring, Femring may have significant systemic absorption, and therefore, it has the same potential risks of estrogen therapy as with other systemic methods. In several studies, vaginal tablets containing 25 µg of estradiol improve urogenital symptoms without raising serum estrogen level.[200,201] Another study suggested placing the vaginal tablet in the outer one third of the vagina to minimize the risk of endometrial hyperplasia and optimizing the local effect.[202] If withdrawal bleeding (spotting or actual menses) occurs with vaginal estrogen creams, then significant systemic absorption may be occurring, requiring the use of progestin after 3 to 6 months of therapy.

In addition to local estrogens, a nonhormonal vaginal moisturizer (Replens) has been shown to have similar benefits on vaginal cytology.[203–205] Replens is a polycarbophil-based vaginal moisturizer and should not be confused with an inert vaginal moisturizer. It is a bioadhesive polymer that is water insoluble but swells in the presence of water. The gel binds to vaginal epithelium and releases purified water to hydrate the epithelial cells, lubricating the vaginal wall and reduces the incidence of vaginal itching, irritation, and dyspareunia.[203] Postmenopausal women should be encouraged to have regular sexual activity to maintain vaginal health and to use vaginal moisturizers on a regular basis to prevent local urogenital symptoms such as vaginal itching, irritation, and dyspareunia. In women who experience frequent urinary tract infections, increase in consumption of pure cranberry-lingonberry juice rather than the high sugar content cranberry drink should be tried.[197]

OSTEOPOROSIS

DEFINITION

Osteoporosis is a systemic skeletal disease characterized by microarchitectural deterioration of bone tissue with a resultant increase in fragility.[206] The World Health Organization (WHO) defines osteopenia as a BMD between 1 and 2.5

TABLE 17.11	Treatment Options for Urogenital Symptoms	
Drug Therapy	**Usual Dosages**	**Comments**
Vaginal Creams		
Premarin Cream (CEE) 0.625 mg/g in 42.5-g tube	Applicator is in increments of 0.5 g. starting dose 1–2 g INV qd then decrease to 0.5g TIW then q weekly for 6–12 months	Significant systemic absorption may occur with prolonged use, requiring challenge with progestin therapy.
Estrace Cream (estradiol) 0.1 mg/g in 42.5-g tube	Initial dose is 2–4 g INV qd for 2 weeks then decrease	
Vaginal Rings		
Estring (estradiol) 2-mg ring	One ring INV for 90 days (delivers 7.5 μg estradiol/day)	Estring delivers minimal estradiol systemically and can be used safely in women who are not candidates for oral ET.
Femring (estradiol acetate)	One ring INV for 90 days (delivers 0.05–0.1 mg estradiol/day)	The only vaginal estrogen to relieve vasomotor and vaginal symptoms. Not recommended for women who only need local relief.
Vaginal Tablet		
Vagifem (estradiol) 25-μg tablet (in disposable single use applicator)	1 tablet INV qd for 2 weeks then 1 tablet INV TIW for maintenance	Studies have shown efficacy without endometrial hyperplasia or significant systemic absorption. Less messy to use than creams.
Vaginal Moisturizer		
Replens (polycarbophil bioadhesive polymer)	1 applicatorful INV TIW	Positive improvements in vaginal cytology, vaginal dryness, itching, irritation, and dyspareunia have been shown in numerous studies. Good alternative to ET for urogenital symptoms.

CEE, conjugated equine estrogen; INV, intravaginally; qd, daily; TIW, three times weekly; ET, estrogen therapy.
(From Simunic V, Banovic I, Ciglar S, et al. Local estrogen treatment in patients with urogenital symptoms. Int J Gynaecol Obstet 82:187–97, 2003; Notelovitz M, Funk S, Nanavati N, et al. Estradiol absorption from vaginal tablets in postmenopausal women. Obstet Gynecol 99:556–562, 2002; Cicinelli E, Di Naro E, De Ziegler D, et al. Placement of the vaginal 17 beta-estradiol tablets in the inner or outer one-third of the vagina affects the preferential delivery of 17 beta-estradiol toward the uterus or periurethral areas, thereby modifying efficacy and endometrial safety. Am J Obstet Gynecol 189:55–58, 2003; van der Laak JA, de Bie LM, de Leeuw H, et al. The effect of Replens on vaginal cytology in the treatment of postmenopausal atrophy: cytomorphology versus computerized cytometry. J Clin Pathol 55:446–451, 2002; Nachtigall LE. Comparative study: Replens versus local estrogen in menopausal women. Fertil Steril 61:178–180, 1994; Bygdeman M, Swahn ML. Replens versus dienoestrol cream in the symptomatic treatment of vaginal atrophy in postmenopausal women. Maturitas 23:259–263, 1996.)

standard deviations below the young adult peak mean (T score) and osteoporosis as a BMD 2.5 standard deviations or more below the young adult peak mean measured at the spine and hip. A decrease of 1 standard deviation in bone mass at either site is associated with approximately a twofold increase in fracture risk.

EPIDEMIOLOGY

Osteoporosis is more common in women than men because the loss of estrogen during menopause accelerates bone loss. Approximately 13% to 18% of U.S. women age ≥50 years have osteoporosis while another 37% to 50% has low bone mass (osteopenia).[206] Low BMD is the best indicator of increased fracture risk in postmenopausal women,[207] with hip fracture causing the highest morbidity and mortality (15% to 20%). Spinal fracture is more common and contributes to significant morbidity, including pain, deformity, loss of independence, and reduced cardiovascular, respiratory, and even digestive function. White and Asian women are at in-

creased risk for osteoporosis compared to African-American and Mexican-American women.

PATHOPHYSIOLOGY

Bone is considered a living organ with ongoing processes of bone remodeling that involves simultaneous resorption of old bone by osteoclasts and replacement of resorbed bone with new bone by osteoblasts. In young adults who have adequate nutrition and exercise, a homeostatic balance exists between formation and resorption. Peak bone mass is achieved by age 30 in men and women, with subsequent bone loss of 0.4% each year thereafter. Bone is made up of two major parts, cortical and trabecular. Cortical bone forms the outer shell of all bones and accounts for 75% of total bone mass. Trabecular bone is the spongy, interlacing network that forms the internal support within the cortical bone and accounts for 25% of total bone mass. Women lose approximately 2% of cortical bone and 5% of trabecular bone per year for the first 5 to 8 years after menopause,[208] followed by an annual loss of 1% for the rest of a woman's life. Excessive osteoclast-mediated resorption and suppressed osteoblast activity account for the resultant bone loss. In addition, the decline in estrogens enhances calcium efflux from bone mineral stores and increases the serum concentrations of ionized calcium. This suppresses secretion of PTH, which in turn reduces the synthesis of 1, 25-dihydroxyvitamin D_3 by the renal tubular cells.[8] The lowered concentration of 1, 25-dihydroxyvitamin D_3 causes a decrease in the intestinal absorption of calcium. Calcitonin inhibits bone resorption, but the level declines as a result of estrogen loss. Therefore, estrogen may play many roles in preventing bone loss. The management of osteoporosis and osteopenia is also discussed in Chapter 69.

TREATMENT

PHARMACOTHERAPY

Refer to Table 17.12 for a list of pharmacotherapy options. Treatment is aimed at preserving bone mass and preventing consequent fractures. Screening for osteoporosis should be initiated in all postmenopausal women age 65 years or older and younger if one or more risk factors for osteoporosis are

TABLE 17.12	United States FDA-Approved Treatment Options for Osteoporosis	
Drug Therapy	**Usual Doses**	**Comments**
Bisphosphonates Alendronate (Fosamax) Risedronate (Actonel)	Treatment: 10 mg qd, 70 mg weekly Prevention: 5 mg qd, 35 mg weekly Treatment/prevention: 5 mg qd, 35 mg weekly	Strong evidence for improving BMD and reducing incidences of vertebral (50% for alendronate, 40% for risedronate) and nonvertebral fracture (50% for alendronate, 40% for risedronate). Patient counseling including taking it with 8 oz of water, staying upright, and refrain from eating or drinking other meds, beverages for ≥30 minutes is important in improving bioavailability and decreasing incidence of esophagitis.
SERM Raloxifene (Evista)	Treatment/prevention: 60 mg qd	Strong evidence for improving BMD and reducing incidences of vertebral (30% reduction) but not nonvertebral fracture. Also reduces incidence of estrogen receptor positive breast cancer. Can precipitate hot flushes and has same risk of thromboembolism as estrogens.
Hormone Therapy Estrogens/Progestins, (various)	Various doses, depending on types and regimens used	WHI was the first clinical trial showing fracture reduction in addition to beneficial effects on BMD. A 34% reduction in vertebral and nonvertebral fractures was seen with Prempro 2.5 mg. Major organizations (FDA, ACOG, NIH, NAMS) recommend alternative to estrogens if prevention of osteoporosis is the sole indication for use.
Calcitonin Salmon nasal calcitonin (Miacalcin)	Treatment: 200 IU intranasally qd	Inconsistent results for fracture reduction despite increases in BMD. Reserved for use in patients with pain associated fractures or in patients who are not candidates for bisphosphonates, hormones.
Parathyroid Hormone PTH (1–34) (Forteo)	Treatment: 20 µg SQ daily	PTH is limited to patients who have failed other therapies or who have severe osteoporosis. PTH reduces vertebral fracture by 65% and nonvertebral fracture by 53%. A potential complication such as osteosarcoma has not been replicated in monkeys or seen in clinical trials with humans but safety has not been demonstrated beyond 2 years. The NOF cautions use in patients with Paget's disease, radiation of skeleton, bone malignancy, bone metastases, or hypercalcemia.

FDA, Food and Drug Administration; qd, daily; BMD, bone mineral density; SERM, selective estrogen receptor modulator; WHI, Women's Health Initiative; ACOG, American College of Obstetrics and Gynecology; NIH, National Institutes of Health; NAMS, North American Menopause Society; PTH, parathyroid hormone; NOF, National Osteoporosis Foundation.

(From National Osteoporosis Foundation. Physician's Guide to Prevention and Treatment of Osteoporosis, 2003. Available at http://www.nof.org with permission.)

TABLE 17.13	Risk Factors for Osteoporotic Fracture in Postmenopausal Women

- Old Age: Age ≥65 years
- Estrogen loss
  - Early menopause: physiological (ovarian failure) or induced (bilateral oophorectomy)
  - Prolonged premenopausal amenorrhea (>1 year)
- History of prior fracture or fragility fracture after 40 years of age
- Family history of osteoporosis or osteoporotic fracture (especially hip fracture in mother)
- White or Asian race
- Small frame: low weight (<58 kg) and body mass index
- Poor nutrition including long-term low calcium intake
- Sedentary lifestyle
- Propensity to fall
- Poor eyesight (usually leading to falls)
- Current smoking
- Excessive alcohol intake (>2 drinks/day)
- Dementia
- Prolonged systemic glucocorticoid therapy (≥3 months)

(From Osteoporosis. ACOG Practice Bulletin No 50, 2004; National Osteoporosis Foundation. Physician's guide to prevention and treatment of osteoporosis, 2003. Available at http://www.nof.org with permission.)

present (Table 17.13). In the absence of new risk factors, screening is recommended at 2-year intervals. Dual-energy x-ray absorptiometry (DXA) is the standard method for measuring BMD at the hip or spine. BMD testing should be performed on all postmenopausal women with fractures to confirm the diagnosis of osteoporosis and determine disease severity.[206] When the decision to treat is made, treatment should continue indefinitely unless a contraindication to the agent arises. The National Osteoporosis Foundation (NOF) recommends initiation of treatment in postmenopausal women with BMD T scores below −2 by hip DXA in the absence of risk factors and in women with T scores less than −1.5 by hip DXA in the presence of one or more risk factors.[208] Women with prior history of vertebral (spinal) or nonvertebral (hip) fracture should be treated irrespective of BMD scores. Regardless of treatment, all postmenopausal women should consume 1,000 to 1,500 mg of elemental calcium daily with or without vitamin D.

Estrogen with or without Progestin. Estrogen prevents bone loss by inhibition of bone resorption, generally, resulting in a 5% to 10% increase in BMD over 1 to 3 years. Estrogen or HT is best initiated in the first 5 to 10 years after menopause. However, even if started long after menopause, estrogen or HT still produces significant increases in bone mass. As demonstrated by the WHI, HT (0.625 mg CEE alone or + 2.5 mg MPA daily) initiated in women on aver-

age of 13 years from menopause reduced overall rates of fracture by 24% and reduced the risk of hip and clinical vertebral fractures by 34%. Lower dose of CEE (0.3–0.45 mg/day) with or without MPA (1.5 mg/day) has also been shown to increase BMD in postmenopausal women with low bone mass.[209–212] Although CEE and MPA are the two most studied formulations, other forms of estrogen and progestin such as 17 β-estradiol, esterified estrogen, norethindrone acetate, or micronized progesterone have also been shown to yield positive effects on bone mass.[206–213] Bone turnover increases and bone loss tends to accelerate initially when HT is discontinued. However, long-term treatment with HT carries untoward risks and should be reserved as treatment of osteoporosis only in an early menopausal woman needing treatment for vasomotor symptoms as well.

Selective Estrogen Receptor Modulators. SERMs are estrogen agonists in certain tissues and estrogen antagonists at others. Raloxifene, tamoxifen, and tibolone fall in this class. Raloxifene is currently the only SERM used for the treatment of osteoporosis in the United States. Tamoxifen has long been used as an adjuvant in the treatment of estrogen receptor positive breast cancer and for chemo-prevention of breast cancer in women at high risk of disease since it exhibits estrogen antagonistic activities in breast tissue. It is a partial agonist in bone and the endometrium. Its usefulness in the treatment of osteoporosis is limited by its ability to cause hyperplasia of the endometrium, leading to an increase risk of endometrial cancer. Furthermore, tamoxifen often causes abnormal uterine bleeding in menopausal women, prompting clinicians to perform endometrial biopsies. Other side effects include triggering or increasing vasomotor hot flashes and increasing venous thromboembolism.

Tibolone is a unique SERM with estrogenic, antiestrogenic, androgenic and progestogenic properties. It is indicated for the treatment of vasomotor symptoms and the prevention of osteoporosis in postmenopausal women in Europe but still awaits U.S. FDA approval. Tibolone improves vasomotor hot flashes without effects on breast tissue or the endometrium. In several studies, tibolone (2.5 mg) has been shown to prevent postmenopausal bone loss,[214–216] bone loss associated with GnRH therapy,[217] and at least as effective as HT in preventing bone loss in postmenopausal women.[218] A recent longitudinal study showed that tibolone increased BMD by 4.1% at the spine and 1.6% at the hip after 8 years of uninterrupted treatment.[219] However, fracture data for both spine and hip are lacking. Tibolone's androgenic effects on sexual function and progestational protective effect on the endometrium are the subjects of ongoing research.

Raloxifene is a benzothiophene that inhibits the action of estrogen on the breast and the endometrium and acts as an estrogen agonist on bone and lipid metabolism.[213] Although, raloxifene does not increase BMD as much as estrogen does, results from the Multiple Outcomes of Raloxifene Evaluation (MORE) study[220] found a 30% reduction in incidence of vertebral fracture (RR 0.7; 95% CI 0.4–0.7), but no differences in the incidence of nonvertebral fracture, despite a BMD increase of 2.1% at the femoral neck. The MORE study was a 3-year, multicenter, randomized, blinded, placebo-controlled trial evaluating the effects of raloxifene in 6,828 postmenopausal women with osteoporosis. Raloxifene (60 mg daily) produced an improvement in BMD of 2.1% at the femoral neck and 2.6% at the spine after 2 to 3 years. In addition, raloxifene reduces the risk of positive estrogen-receptor breast cancer by 65% (RR 0.35; 95% CI 0.21–0.58).[221] There were no increases in endometrial hyperplasia. Raloxifene was well tolerated but side effects include hot flushes and risks of therapy include venous thromboembolism similar to those of estrogens and tamoxifen.

Bisphosphonates. Bisphosphonates prevent bone resorption by inhibiting osteoclast activity and increasing osteoclast cell death.[222] Substantial fracture reductions at vertebral and nonvertebral sites have been demonstrated for risedronate and alendronate in patients with osteoporosis. In the Fracture Intervention Trial (FIT) study[223] for alendronate and the Vertebral Efficacy with Risedronate Therapy North America (VERT) study[224] for risedronate, clinical significant reductions in incidence of vertebral and nonvertebral fractures only occurred in women who met the WHO criteria for osteoporosis at study entry (T score < -2.5).[223–225] Alendronate (10 mg daily) reduced the risk of new vertebral and nonvertebral fractures by about 50%. Risedronate (5 mg daily) attenuated new vertebral fractures by 41% and nonvertebral fractures by 39%. Benefits with these agents are seen early in therapy, within 1 year of treatment, making them ideal for patients with high short-term fracture risk. Approximately 50% of ingested bisphosphonates is deposited in bones, with retention up to several years. Thus, accelerated bone loss associated with discontinuation of therapy is not as dramatic as that observed with estrogen or raloxifene and lack of fracture prevention may not be a problem in patients whose compliance is erratic. Similarly, the prolonged bone retention of alendronate (half-life 10 years), but relatively shorter in risedronate (half-life 484 hours) may have some unknown effects on bone. Due to the high cost, side effects, and prolonged bone half-life, the bisphosphonates should be reserved for women with documented osteoporosis and not in younger postmenopausal women with low bone mass who are not at great risk of sustaining a fracture.

Calcitonin. Calcitonin is a naturally occurring peptide secreted by thyroid C cells and reduces bone resorption by direct inhibition of osteoclast activity. Salmon calcitonin given intranasally is the preferred route of administration compared to subcutaneous injection, which causes many side effects such as nausea, facial flushes, and diarrhea. In the Prevent Recurrence Of Osteoporotic Fractures (PROOF)[226] study, a 5-year randomized, double-blind, placebo-controlled study of 1,255 postmenopausal women with osteoporosis, intranasal salmon calcitonin 200 international units (IU) daily reduced the rate of vertebral fractures by 33% (RR 0.67; 95% CI 0.47–0.97), but not hip fracture. The results in this study

were inconsistent, showing significant fracture reduction during years 1 and 2 in the group receiving 200 IU, with a small increase in BMD of 1.5% at the lumbar spine, but no reduction in fractures with the groups receiving 100 or 400 IU daily, despite positive changes in BMD in these groups. Calcitonin has demonstrated efficacy in relieving pain associated with osteoporotic vertebral compression fractures[227,228] and thus, may be a good option for bedridden patients who cannot take bisphosphonates due to the risk of esophageal insults or estrogen due to the risk of venous thromboembolism.

Parathyroid Hormone. Recombinant human PTH is the only anabolic agent in the armamentarium of treatment of osteoporosis. PTH stimulates new bone formation at both periosteal (outer) and endosteal (inner) bone surfaces, thickening the cortices, and increasing trabecular density and connectivity in postmenopausal women with osteoporosis.[206] In a randomized, double-blind, placebo-controlled prospective study of 1,637 postmenopausal women with prior vertebral fractures, PTH (20 or 40 μg) administered subcutaneously daily for 19 months reduced the incidence of new vertebral fractures by 65% and 69% respectively (RR 0.35 and 0.31; 95% CI 0.22–0.55 and 0.19–0.5) and new nonvertebral fractures by 53% and 54%, respectively (RR 0.47 and 0.46; 95% CI 0.25–0.88 and 0.25–0.86). Compared to placebo, PTH (20 or 40 μg) increased BMD by 9% and 13%, respectively, in the lumbar spine and by 3% and 6%, respectively, in the femoral neck.[229] Side effects were more pronounced in the PTH 40-μg group and include nausea and headache.

Combination Therapy. Approximately 10% to 20% of women continue to lose bone density while receiving HT alone and may need additional therapy for osteoporosis.[222] Studies of combination antiresorptive therapy with estrogen and a bisphosphonate or a bisphosphonate and raloxifene have shown small additional increases in BMD (approximately 1% to 3% in 2 years).[233–236] However, it is not known if the increases in BMD observed with combination therapies are sufficient to provide additional fracture protection.

NONPHARMACOLOGIC THERAPY

Physical activities including walking, weight training, and high impact exercises have shown a small increase in BMD but that this effect is not sustained once the exercise program stops. However, weight bearing exercise and muscle strengthening exercises are more effective at increasing bone mass. These types of exercise improve muscle tone and indirectly prevent fracture by reducing the risk of falls.[213]

Monitoring. Central bone densitometry is recommended to monitor a patient's response to therapy. Generally, it is recommended to wait 12 to 18 months after starting therapy to obtain a meaningful BMD change.[222] A decrease in vertebral BMD greater than 4% to 5% indicates a need to evaluate the patient's compliance and to search for secondary causes of bone loss.[206] ACOG recommends a repeat DXA testing in untreated postmenopausal women after 3 to 5 years have past.

KEY POINTS

DYSMENORRHEA
- Dysmenorrhea is the most common gynecologic problem in menstruating women.
- It is the single greatest cause of women's absenteeism from work or school.
- In contrast to primary dysmenorrhea, which can be managed with NSAID, COX-2 inhibitors, or COCs, the etiology of secondary dysmenorrhea must be ruled out before proper treatment ensues.

PREMENSTRUAL SYNDROME
- PMS is a common disorder affecting up to 75% of women during their reproductive years.
- Symptoms typically begin when women are in their early 20s.
- PMS with severe affective symptoms is considered PMDD. Both are difficult to diagnose and is usually made with the patient's documentation of her symptoms during the luteal cycle and when other psychological or physical disorders have been ruled out.
- When nonpharmacologic interventions fail, first-line pharmacotherapy with the SSRIs should be used.

ENDOMETRIOSIS
- Endometriosis may be asymptomatic, but is found in 70% to 90% of women with chronic pelvic pain, and in 30% to 45% of women with infertility.
- It is a benign, yet sometimes progressive disease that often recurs after cessation of treatment.
- Growth of endometriotic implants is spurred by estrogen, produced locally by the enzyme aromatase or by the ovaries and thus, usually regresses after menopause.
- First-line medical therapy includes COCs or NSAID for dysmenorrhea or cyclic or noncyclic pelvic pain. Advanced medical therapy includes hormonal suppression using danazol, GnRH agonists, or progestins.
- Diagnostic laparoscopy and conservative surgery are reserved for patients whose symptoms are not relieved by medical therapies alone.

VULVOVAGINAL CANDIDIASIS
- Vulvovaginal candidiasis is the most common vaginitis, affecting up to 75% of women.
- Self-diagnosis and treatment are common but accuracy in doing so has been challenged in a recent study published by ACOG. Thus, women are encouraged to seek a clinical diagnosis in a doctor's office with the first episode.
- Classic signs and symptoms include white, curdy discharge accompanied by itching.
- *C. albicans* is the cause in up to 90% of VVC.

- Non-*albicans*, especially *C. glabrata* is on the rise and contributes to azole-resistant recurrent VVC.
- Behavioral modifications to reduce the incidence of recurrent VVC include avoidance of tight pantyhose or pantyliner and decreasing consumption of cranberry juice.

BACTERIAL VAGINOSIS
- BV accounts for 35% of vaginitis.
- It is not known what leads to low or lack of lactobacilli in women with BV, but this seems to be an important predisposing factor, among sexual activity and douching.
- BV in nonpregnant and pregnant women have been shown to increase the risk of having PID and acquiring STIs such as HIV, gonorrhea, and chlamydia.
- In pregnant women, BV can cause preterm birth and postpartum infections.
- Although BV is rarely found in women who are not sexually active, it is not considered a sexually transmitted infection, since treatment of the sex partner has not altered outcomes.

MENOPAUSE
- Most women in the United States will spend at least one third of their lives in menopause.
- Menopause marks the time when ovarian function ceases, causing a drastic decrease in estrogen production.
- Estrogen deficiency results in vasomotor symptoms (hot flushes, night sweats), urogenital symptoms (vaginal atrophy, dyspareunia, vaginitis, incontinence), cardiovascular disease, osteoporosis, and decrease in cognitive function possibly leading to Alzheimer's disease.
- Vasomotor symptoms, although may be intense and extremely bothersome in the first few years after menopause, do abate over time; in contrast to urogenital symptoms which seem to worsen if left untreated.
- Estrogen therapy or hormone therapy (estrogen and progestin) for women with an intact uterus is usually initiated to prevent consequences of estrogen deficiency and still remain the gold standard for treatment of vasomotor symptoms.
- The hallmark prospective clinical trial, the WHI has shed much light on the risks and benefits of postmenopausal hormone therapy, specifically, the study showed a decrease in risk of fracture and colon cancer, but an increase in risk of strokes, cardiovascular events, and invasive breast cancer after 5 years of use and an increase in mild cognitive impairment.
- As with all studies, the WHI was subjected to many criticisms and although may provide one view of the truth, it is not gospel truth.
- Results from the WHI may not apply to an individual woman (absolute risk is low on an individual basis) but instead, to a large population.

- Therefore, the decision to initiate hormone therapy should be individualized to each woman, taking into account the presence of vasomotor and urogenital symptoms and the risks of osteoporosis and breast cancer.
- Most adverse events have been demonstrated with the oral formulations of hormone therapy, leading to investigations of alternate routes of administration.
- Transdermal hormone therapy bypasses hepatic first-pass metabolism, avoiding many untoward consequences including increases in clotting factors, triglycerides, and C-reactive protein.
- Local estrogens such as creams, vaginal tablets or rings, and a nonhormone vaginal cream, Replens, are used to relieve local urogenital symptoms.
- Hormone therapy is no longer recommended to prevent chronic diseases.
- Osteoporosis is another significant consequence of estrogen loss and is a leading cause of hospitalization, morbidity, and mortality in older women.
- Bisphosphonates, hormone therapy, raloxifene, and PTH have consistently shown reduction in fracture rates. The selection of agent should be individualized, based on age, degree of bone loss, and presence of other risk factors.
- BMD increases do not always correlate with fracture reduction. Significant fracture reduction may be seen with modest BMD improvements.
- BMD testing should be performed by DXA at central sites (spine, hip) to all postmenopausal women age ≥65 years.
- Given that reduction in fractures is greatest with established osteoporosis and the low incidence of fracture in younger postmenopausal women, initiation of treatment should be reserved in women who meet the WHO's definition of osteoporosis in the absence of other risk factors.
- Treatment should be offered to all women who have sustained a fracture at the spine or hip.
- In addition to treatment, all patients should be counseled to take adequate calcium and vitamin D supplementation and to incorporate a regular routine of weight bearing and muscle-strengthening exercises.

SUGGESTED READINGS

Centers for Disease Control and Prevention. Sexually transmitted diseases treatment guidelines, 2002. MMWR 51(RR-6), 2002.

Centers for Disease Control and Prevention. Sexually transmitted diseases treatment guidelines, 2002. MMWR 51(RR-6):42–45, 2002.

Stenchever M, Droegemueller W, Herbst A, et al, eds. Comprehensive Gynecology. 4th ed. St. Louis: Mosby, 2001.

REFERENCES

1. Sahin I, Saracoglu F, Kurban Y, et al. Dysmenorrhea treatment with a single daily dose of rofecoxib. Int J Gynecol and Obstet 83: 285–291, 2003.
2. Callejo J, Diaz J, Ruiz A, et al. Effect of a low-dose oral contraceptive containing 20 mcg ethinylestradiol and 150 mcg desogestrel on dysmenorrhea. Contraception 68:183–188, 2003.
3. Harel Z, Riggs S, Vaz R, et al. The use of the leukotriene receptor antagonist montelukast in the management of dysmenorrhea in adolescents. J Pediatr Adolesc Gynecol 17:183–186, 2004.
4. Coco AS. Primary dysmenorrhea. Am Fam Physician 60:489–496, 1999.
5. Dawood MY. Current concepts in the etiology and treatment of primary dysmenorrhea. Acta Obstet Gynecol Scand 138 (Suppl):7–10, 1986.
6. Marjoribanks J, Proctor ML, Farquhar C. Nonsteroidal anti-inflammatory drugs for primary dysmenorrhea. Cochrane Database Syst Rev 4: CD001751, 2003.
7. Owen PR. Prostaglandin synthetase inhibitors in the treatment of primary dysmenorrhea: outcome trials reviewed. Am J Obstet Gynecol 148:96–103, 1984.
8. Ruggiero R. Gynecologic disorders. In: Herfindal ET, Gourley D, eds. Textbook of therapeutics. 7th ed. Baltimore: Williams and Wilkins, 2003.
9. Laine L. Approaches to nonsteroidal anti-inflammatory drug use in the high risk patient. Gastroenterology 120:594–606, 2001.
10. Fenton C, Keating GM, Wagstaff AJ. Valdecoxib: a review of its use in the management of osteoarthritis, rheumatoid arthritis, dysmenorrhea and acute pain. Drugs 64:1231–1261, 2004.
11. Bitner M, Kattenhorn J, Hatfield C, et al. Efficacy and tolerability of lumiracoxib in the treatment of primary dysmenorrhea. Int J Clin Pract 58:340–345, 2004.
12. Helms JM. Acupuncture for the management of primary dysmenorrhea. Obstet Gynecol 69:51–53, 1987.
13. Dawood MY, Ramos J. Transcutaneous electrical nerve stimulation (TENS) for the treatment of primary dysmenorrhea: a randomized crossover comparison with placebo TENS and ibuprofen. Obstet Gynecol 75:656–661, 1990.
14. Barnard ND, Scialli AR, Hurlock D, et al. Diet and sex hormone binding globulin, dysmenorrhea and premenstrual syndrome. Obstet Gynecol 95:245–250, 2000.
15. Proctor ML, Smith CA, Farquhar CM, et al. Transcutaneous nerve stimulation and acupuncture for primary dysmenorrhea. Cochrane Database Syst Rev 1:CD002123, 2002.
16. Dickerson LM, Mazyck PJ, Hunter MH. Premenstrual Syndrome. Am Fam Physician 67:1743–1752, 2003.
17. Grady-Weliky T. Premenstrual dysphoric disorder. N Engl J Med 348:433–438, 2003.
18. Chuong CJ, His BP, Gibbons WE. Periovulatory beta-endorphin levels in premenstrual syndrome. Obstet Gynecol 83:755–760, 1994.
19. Premenstrual Syndrome. ACOG Practice Bulletin No 15, 2000.
20. Pitkin RM, Reynolds AR, Williams GA, et al. Calcium regulating hormones during the menstrual cycle. J Clin Endocrinol Metab 47: 626–632, 1978.
21. Gray TK, McAdoo T, Hatley L, et al. Fluctuation of serum concentration of 1,25 dihydroxyvitamin D_3 during the menstrual cycle. Am J Obstet Gynecol 144:880–884, 1982.
22. Tjellesen L, Christiansen C, Hummer L, et al. Unchanged biochemical indices of bone turnover despite fluctuations in 1,25 dihydroxyvitamin D_3 during the menstrual cycle. Acta Endocrinol 102: 476–480, 1983.
23. Thys-Jacobs S and Alvir MA. Calcium regulating hormones across the menstrual cycle: evidence of a secondary hyperparathyroidism in women with PMS. J Clin Endocrinol Metab 80:2227–2232, 1995.
24. Thys-Jacobs S, Starkey P, Bernstein D, et al. Calcium carbonate and the premenstrual syndrome: effects on premenstrual and menstrual symptoms. Am J Obstet Gynecol 179:444–452, 1998.
25. Thys-Jacobs S, Ceccarelli S, Bierman A, et al. Calcium supplementation in premenstrual syndrome. J Gen Intern Med 4:183–189, 1989.
26. Penland PG, Johnson PE. Dietary calcium and manganese effects on menstrual cycle symptoms. Am J Obstet Gynecol 168: 1417–1423, 1993.
27. Steiner M, Steinberg S, Stewart D, et al. Fluoxetine in the treatment of premenstrual dysphoria. N Engl J Med 332:1529–1534, 1995.

28. Yonkers KA, Halbreich U, Freeman E, et al. Symptomatic improvement of premenstrual dysphoric disorder with sertraline treatment: a randomized controlled trial. JAMA 278:983–988, 1997.

29. Eriksson E, Hedberg MA, Andersch B, et al. The serotonin reuptake inhibitor paroxetine is superior to the noradrenaline reuptake inhibitor maprotiline in the treatment of premenstrual syndrome. Neuropsychopharmacol 12:167–176, 1995.

30. Wikander I, Sundblad C, Andersch B, et al. Citalopram in premenstrual dysphoria: is intermittent treatment during luteal phases more effective than continuous medication throughout the menstrual cycle? J Clin Psychopharmacol 18:390–398, 1998.

31. Freeman EW, Rickels K, Sondheimer SJ. Fluvoxamine for premenstrual dysphoric disorder: a pilot study. J Clin Psychiatry 57 (Suppl):56–60, 1996.

32. Steiner M, Korzekwa M, Lamont J, et al. Intermittent fluoxetine dosing in the treatment of women with premenstrual dysphoria. Psychopharmacol Bull 33:771–774, 1997.

33. Pearlstein TB, Stone AB, Lund SA, et al. Comparison of fluoxetine, bupropion, and placebo in the treatment of premenstrual dysphoric disorder. J Clin Psychopharmacol 17:261–266, 1997.

34. Pearlstein TB, Stone AB. Long term fluoxetine treatment of late luteal phase dysphoric disorder. J Clin Psychiatry 55:332–335, 1994.

35. Pearlstein TB, Halbreich U, Batzar ED, et al. Psychosocial functioning in women with premenstrual dysphoric disorder before and after treatment with sertraline or placebo. J Clin Psychiatry 61: 101–109, 2000.

36. Halbreich U, Smoller JW. Intermittent luteal phase sertraline treatment of dysphoric premenstrual syndrome. J Clin Psychiatry 58: 399–402, 1997.

37. Young SA, Hurt PH, Benedek DM, et al. Treatment of premenstrual dysphoric disorder with sertraline during the luteal phase: a randomized, double blind, placebo controlled crossover trial. J Clin Psychiatry 59:76–80, 1998.

38. Jermain DM, Preece CK, Sykes FL, et al. Luteal phase sertraline treatment for premenstrual dysphoric disorder: results of a double blind, placebo controlled, crossover study. Arch Fam Med 8: 328–332, 1999.

39. Freeman EW, Rickels K, Arredondo F, et al. Full- or half-cycle treatment of severe premenstrual syndrome with a serotonergic antidepressant. J Clin Psychopharmacol 19:3–8, 1999.

40. O'Brien PM, Craven D, Selby C, et al. Treatment of premenstrual syndrome by spironolactone. Br J Obstet Gynaecol 86:142–147, 1979.

41. Vellacott ID, Shroff NE, Pearce MY, et al. A double blind, placebo controlled evaluation of spironolactone in the premenstrual syndrome. Curr Med Res Opin 10:450–456, 1987.

42. Wang M, Mammarback S, Lindhe BA, et al. Treatment of premenstrual syndrome by spironolactone: a double blind, placebo controlled study. Acta Obstet Gynecol Scand 74:803–808, 1995.

43. Burnet RB, Radden HS, Easterbrook EG, et al. Premenstrual syndrome and spironolactone. Aust N Z J Obstet Gynaecol 31: 366–368, 1991.

44. Hellberg D, Claesson B, Nilsson S. Premenstrual tension: a placebo controlled efficacy study with spironolactone and medroxyprogesterone acetate. Int J Gynaecol Obstet 34:243–248, 1991.

45. Freeman EW, Rickels K, Sondheimer SJ, et al. Ineffectiveness of progesterone suppository treatment for premenstrual syndrome. JAMA 264:349–353, 1990.

46. Freeman EW, Rickels K, Sondheimer SJ, et al. A double blind trial of oral progesterone, alprazolam, and placebo in treatment of severe premenstrual syndrome. JAMA 274:51–57, 1995.

47. Freeman EW, Kroll R, Rapkin A, et al. Evaluation of a unique oral contraceptive in the treatment of premenstrual dysphoric disorder. J Women's Health Gend Based Med 10:561–569, 2001.

48. Brown CS, Ling FW, Andersen RN, et al. Efficacy of depot leuprolide in premenstrual syndrome: effect of symptom severity and type in a controlled trial. Obstet Gynecol 84:779–786, 1994.

49. Freeman EW, Sondheimer SJ, Rickels K. Gonadotropin-releasing hormone agonist in the treatment of premenstrual symptoms with and without ongoing dysphoria: a controlled study. Psychopharmacol Bull 33:303–309, 1997.

50. Schmidt PJ, Nieman LK, Danaceau MA, et al. Differential behavioral effects of gonadal steroids in women with and in those without premenstrual syndrome. N Engl J Med 338:209–216, 1998.

51. Hammarback S, Backstrom T. Induced anovulation as treatment of premenstrual tension syndrome: a double blind, crossover study with GnRH agonist versus placebo. Acta Obstet Gynecol Scand 67: 159–166, 1988.

52. Nap AW, Groothuis PG, Demir AY, et al. Pathogenesis of endometriosis. Best Prac Res Clin Obstet Gynaecol 18:233–244, 2004.

53. Winkel C. Evaluation and management of women with endometriosis. Obstet Gynecol 102:397–408, 2003.

54. Eskenazi B, Warner ML. Epidemiology of endometriosis. Obstet Gynecol Clin 24:235–258, 1997.

55. Zhao SZ, Wong JM, Davis MB, et al. The cost of inpatient endometriosis treatment: an analysis based on the healthcare cost and utilization project nationwide inpatient sample. J Managed Care 4: 1127–1134, 1998.

56. Mathias S, Kupperman M. Chronic pelvic pain: prevalence, health related quality of life and economic correlates. Obstet Gynecol 87: 321–327, 1996.

57. Olive DL, Pritts EA. Treatment of endometriosis. N Engl J Med 345:266–273, 2001.

58. Burns WN, Schenken RS. Pathophysiology of endometriosis associated infertility. Clin Obstet Gynecol 42:586–610, 1999.

59. Markham SM, Carpenter SE, Rock JA. Extrapelvic endometriosis. Obstet Gynecol Clin North Am 16:193–219, 1989.

60. Hamann GO. Severe primary dysmenorrhea treated with naproxen. A prospective, double blind crossover investigation. Prostaglandins 19:651–657, 1980.

61. Hanson FW, Izu A, Henzl MR. Naproxen sodium, ibuprofen and a placebo in dysmenorrhea. Its influence in allowing continuation of work/school activities. Obstet Gynecol 52:583–587, 1978.

62. Henzl MR, Buttram V, Segre EJ, et al. The treatment of dysmenorrhea with naproxen sodium: a report on two independent double blind trials. Am J Obstet Gynecol 127:818–823, 1977.

63. Roy S. A double blind comparison of a propionic acid derivative (ibuprofen) and a fenamate (mefenamic acid) in the treatment of dysmenorrhea. Obstet Gynecol 61:628–632, 1983.

64. Jacobsen J. Naproxen in the treatment of OC-resistant primary dysmenorrhea. A double blind crossover study. Acta Obstet Gynecol Scand 113 (Suppl):87–89, 1983.

65. Arnold JD. Comparison of fenoprofen calcium, ibuprofen and placebo in primary dysmenorrhea. J Reprod Med 14:337–350, 1983.

66. Vercellini P, Trespidi L, Colombo A, et al. A gonadotrophin-releasing hormone agonist versus a low-dose oral contraceptive for pelvic pain associated with endometriosis. Fertil Steril 60:75–79, 1993.

67. Vercellini P, Frontino G, De Giorgi O, et al. Continuous use of an oral contraceptive for endometriosis associated recurrent dysmenorrhea that does not respond to a cyclic pill regimen. Fertil Steril 80: 560–563, 2003.

68. Dawood MY, Ramos J, Khan-Dawood FS. Depot leuprolide acetate versus danazol for treatment of pelvic endometriosis: changes in vertebral bone mass and serum estradiol and calcitonin. Fertil Steril 63:1177–1183, 1995.

69. Dodin S, Lemay A, Maheux R, et al. Bone mass in endometriosis patients treated with GnRH agonist implant or danazol. Obstet Gynecol 77:410–415, 1991.

70. Whitehouse RW, Adams JE, Bancroft K, et al. The effects of nafarelin and danazol on vertebral trabecular bone mass in patients with endometriosis. Clin Endocrinol 33:365–373, 1990.

71. Stevenson JC, Lees B, Gardner R, et al. A comparison of the skeletal effects of goserelin and danazol in premenopausal women with endometriosis. Horm Res 32 (Suppl 1):161–163, 1989.

72. Wong A and Tang L. An open and randomized study comparing the efficacy of standard danazol and modified triptorelin regimens for postoperative disease management of moderate to severe endometriosis. Fertil Steril 81:1522–1527, 2004.

73. Cobellis L, Razzi S, Fava A, et al. A danazol-loaded intrauterine device decreases dysmenorrhea, pelvic pain, and dyspareunia associated with endometriosis. Fertil Steril 82:239–240, 2004.

74. Vercellini P, Cortesi I, Crosignani P. Progestins for symptomatic endometriosis: a critical analysis of the evidence. Fertil Steril 68: 393–401, 1997.

75. Vercellini P, De Giorgi O, Oldani S, et al. Depot medroxyprogesterone acetate versus an oral contraceptive combined with very low

dose danazol for long term treatment of pelvic pain associated with endometriosis. Am J Obstet Gynecol 175:396–401, 1996.

76. Dlugi AM, Miller JD, Knittle J. Lupron depot in the treatment of endometriosis: a randomized, placebo controlled, double blind study. Fertil Steril 54:419–427, 1990.

77. Anonymous. Goserelin depot versus danazol in the treatment of endometriosis. Aus NZ J Obstet Gynaecol 31:55–60, 1996.

78. Chang SP, Ng HT. A randomized comparative study of the effect of leuprorelin acetate depot and danazol in the treatment of endometriosis. Chin Med J 57:431–437, 1996.

79. Cirkel U, Ochs H, Schneider HPG. A randomized, comparative trial of triptorelin depot and danazol in the treatment of endometriosis. Eur J Obstet Gynecol Reprod Biol 59:61–69, 1995.

80. Crosignani PG, Gastaldi A, Lombardi PL. Leuprorelin acetate depot versus danazol in the treatment of endometriosis: results of an open multicenter trial. Clin Ther 14 (Suppl A):29–36, 1992.

81. Dmowski WP, Radwanska E, Binor Z, et al. Ovarian suppression induced with buserelin or danazol in the management of endometriosis: a randomized, comparative study. Fertil Steril 51:395–400, 1989.

82. Fraser IS, Shearman RP, Jansen RP, et al. A comparative treatment trial of endometriosis using the gonadotrophin releasing hormone agonist, nafarelin, and the synthetic steroid, danazol. Aust NZ J Obstet Gynaecol 31:158–163, 1991.

83. Henzl MR, Corson SL, Moghissi K, et al. Administration of nasal nafarelin as compared with oral danazol for endometriosis. A multicenter double blind comparative clinical trial. N Engl J Med 318:485–489, 1988.

84. Wheeler JM, Knittle JD, Miller JD. Depot leuprolide versus danazol in treatment of women with symptomatic endometriosis. Am J Obstet Gynecol 167:1367–1371, 1992.

85. The Nafarelin European Endometriosis Trial Group (NEET). Nafarelin for endometriosis: a large scale, danazol-controlled trial of efficacy and safety, with 1 year follow up. Fertil Steril 57:514–522, 1992.

86. Rolland R and van der Heijden PF. Nafarelin versus danazol in the treatment of endometriosis. Am J Obstet Gynecol 162:586–588,1990.

87. Kennedy SH, Williams IA, Brodribb J, et al. A comparison of nafarelin acetate and danazol in the treatment of endometriosis. Fertil Steril 53:998–1003, 1990.

88. Rock JA. A multicenter comparison of GnRH agonist (Zoladex) and danazol in the treatment of endometriosis. Fertil Steril 56:S49, 1991.

89. Shaw RW. An open randomized comparative study of the effect of goserelin depot and danazol in the treatment of endometriosis. Fertil Steril 58:265–272, 1992.

90. Ling FW. Randomized controlled trial of depot leuprolide in patients with chronic pelvic pain and clinically suspected endometriosis. Obstet Gynecol 93:51–58, 1999.

91. Dawood MY. Hormonal therapies for endometriosis: implications for bone metabolism. Acta Obstet Gynecol Scand 159 (Suppl):22–34, 1994.

92. Surrey E and Judd H. Reduction of vasomotor symptoms and bone mineral density loss with combined norethindrone and long acting gonadotropin releasing hormone agonist therapy of symptomatic endometriosis: a prospective randomized trial. J Clin Endocrinol Metab 75:558–563, 1992.

93. Leather AT, Studd JW, Watson NR, et al. The prevention of bone loss in young women treated with GnRH analogues with ''add back'' estrogen therapy. Obstet Gynecol 81:104–107, 1993.

94. Makarainen L, Ronneberg L, Kauppila A. Medroxyprogesterone acetate supplementation diminishes the hypestrogenic side effects of gonadotropin releasing hormone agonists without changing its efficacy in endometriosis. Fertil Steril 65:29–34, 1996.

95. Kiiholma P, Korhonen M, Tuimala R, et al. Comparison of the gonadotropin releasing hormone agonist goserelin acetate alone versus goserelin combined with estrogen-progestogen add-back therapy in the treatment of endometriosis. Fertil Steril 64:903–908, 1995.

96. Moghissi KS, Schlaff WD, Olive DL, et al. Goserelin acetate with or without hormone replacement therapy for the treatment of endometriosis. Fertil Steril 69:1056–1062, 1998.

97. Surrey ES, Voigt B, Fournet N, et al. Prolonged gonadotropin releasing hormone agonist treatment of symptomatic endometriosis: the role of cyclic sodium etidronate and low dose norethindrone ''add back'' therapy. Fertil Steril 63:747–755, 1995.

98. Hornstein MD, Surrey ES, Weisberg GW, et al. Leuprolide acetate depot and hormonal add-back in endometriosis: a 12-month study. Obstet Gynecol 91:16–24, 1998.

99. Carr BR, Breslau NA, Peng N, et al. Effect of gonadotropin releasing hormone agoinst and medroxyprogesterone acetate on calcium metabolism: a prospective, randomized, double blind, placebo controlled, crossover trial. Fertil Steril 80:1216–1223, 2003.

100. Blumenfeld Z. Hormonal suppressive therapy for endometriosis may not improve patient health. Fertil Steril 81:487–492, 2004.

101. Weideman M. Danazol linked to ovarian cancer. Lancet Oncol 5:261, 2002.

102. Cottreau C, Ness R, Modugno F, et al. Endometriosis and its treatment with danazol or lupron in relation to ovarian cancer. Clin Cancer Res 9:5142–5144, 2003.

103. Gambone JC, Mittman BS, Munro MG, et al. Consensus statement for the management of chronic pelvic pain and endometriosis: proceedings of an expert-panel consensus process. Fertil Steril 78:961–972, 2002.

104. Ailawadi R, Jobanputra S, Kataria M, et al. Treatment of endometriosis and chronic pelvic pain with letrozole and norethindrone acetate: a pilot study. Fertil Steril 81:290–296, 2004.

105. Fedele L and Berlanda N. Emerging drugs for endometriosis. Expert Opin Emerg Drugs 9:167–177, 2004.

106. Spinillo A, Capuzzo E, Gulminetti R, et al. Prevalence of and risk factors for fungal vaginitis caused by non-albicans species. Am J Obstet Gynecol 176:138–141, 1997.

107. Nyirjesy P. Chronic vulvovaginal candidiasis. Am Fam Physician 63:697–702, 2001.

108. Rinkor L. Are OTC vaginal antifungals as effective as oral fluconazole? Pharmacist's Letter 19: No 190907, 2003.

109. Marrazzo J. Normal vaginal flora. A practical update on sexually transmitted infections. Ob Gyn News, 2003.

110. Edwards L. The diagnosis and treatment of infectious vaginitis. Dermatologic Ther 17:102–110, 2004.

111. Onderdonk AB, Delaney ML, Hinkson PL, et al. Quantitative and qualitative effects of douche preparations on vaginal microflora. Obstet Gynecol 80:333–338, 1992.

112. Richardson BA, Martin HL Jr, Stevens CE, et al. Use of nonoxynol-9 and changes in vaginal lactobacilli. J Infect Dis 178:441–445, 1998.

113. Ringdahl E. Treatment of recurrent vulvovaginal candidiasis. Am Fam Physician 61:3306–3312, 2000.

114. Glover D, Larsen B. Relationship of fungal vaginitis therapy to prior antibiotic exposure. Infect Dis Obstet Gynecol 11:157–160, 2003.

115. Patel D, Gillespie B, Sobel J, et al. Risk factors for recurrent vulvovaginal candidiasis in women receiving maintenance antifungal therapy: results of a prospective cohort study. Am J Obstet Gynecol 190:644–653, 2004.

116. Ferris D, Nyirjesy P, Sobel J, et al. Over-the-counter antifungal drug misuse associated with patient-diagnosed vulvovaginal candidiasis. Obstet Gynecol 99:419–425, 2002.

117. Sobel JD, Kapernick PS, Zervos M, et al. Treatment of complicated Candida vaginitis: comparison of single and sequential doses of fluconazole. Am J Obstet Gynecol 185:363–369, 2001.

118. Sobel JD, Chaim W, Nagappan V, et al. Treatment of vaginitis caused by *candida glabrata*: use of topical boric acid and flucytosine. Am J Obstet Gynecol 189:1297–1300, 2003.

119. Centers for Disease Control and Prevention. Sexually transmitted diseases treatment guidelines 2002. MMWR 51 (No. RR-6):42–45, 2002.

120. Paavonen J, Mangioni C, Martin M, et al. Vaginal clindamycin and oral metronidazole for bacterial vaginosis: a randomized trial. Obstet Gynecol 96:256–260, 2000.

121. Smart S, Singal A, Mindel A. Social and sexual risk factors for bacterial vaginosis. Sex Transm Infect 80:58–62, 2004.

122. Koumans EH, Markowitz LE, Hogan V, et al. Indications for therapy and treatment recommendations for bacterial vaginosis in nonpregnant and pregnant women: a synthesis of data. Clin Infect Dis 35 (Suppl 2):S152–72, 2002.

123. Wilson J. Managing recurrent bacterial vaginosis. Sex Transm Infect 80:8–11, 2004.
124. Wiesenfeld HC, Hillier SL, Krohn MA, et al. Bacterial vaginosis is a strong predictor of *Neisseria gonorrhea* and *Chlamydia trachomatis* infection. Clin Infect Dis 36:663–668, 2003.
125. Andres FJ, Parker R, Hosein I, et al. Clindamycin vaginal cream versus oral metronidazole in the treatment of bacterial vaginosis: a prospective double blind clinical trial. South Med J 85:1077–1080, 1992.
126. Fischbach F, Peterson EE, Weissenbacher ER, et al. Efficacy of clindamycin vaginal cream versus oral metronidazole in the treatment of bacterial vaginosis. Obstet Gynecol 82:405–409, 1993.
127. Schmitt C, Sobel JD, Meriwether C. Bacterial vaginosis: treatment with clindamycin cream versus oral metronidazole. Obstet Gynecol 79:1020–1023, 1992.
128. Arredondo JL, Higuera F, Hidalgo H, et al. Clindamycin vaginal cream vs oral metronidazole in the treatment of bacterial vaginosis. Arch AIDS Res 6:183–195, 1992.
129. Sobel JD, Schmitt C, Meriwether C. Long-term follow up of patients with bacterial vaginosis treated with oral metronidazole and topical clindamycin. J Infect Dis 167:783–784, 1993.
130. Ferris DG, Litaker MS, Woodward L, et al. Treatment of bacterial vaginosis: a comparison of oral metronidazole, metronidazole vaginal gel, and clindamycin vaginal cream. J Fam Pract 41:443–449, 1995.
131. Broumas AG, Basara LA. Potential patient preference for 3-day treatment of bacterial vaginosis: responses to new suppository form of clindamycin. Adv Ther 17:159–166, 2000.
132. Swedberg J, Steiner JF, Deiss F, et al. Comparison of single-dose versus one-week course of metronidazole for symptomatic bacterial vaginosis. JAMA 245:1046–1049, 1985.
133. Hanson JM, McGregor JA, Hillier SL, et al. Metronidazole for bacterial vaginosis. A comparison of vaginal gel vs. oral therapy. J Reprod Med 45:889–896, 2000.
134. Agnew KJ, Hillier SL. The effect of treatment regimens for vaginitis and cervicitis on vaginal colonization by lactobacilli. Sex Transm Dis 122:269–273, 1995.
135. Swygard H, Sena AC, Hobbs MM, et al. Trichomoniasis: clinical manifestations, diagnosis and management. Sex Transm Infect 80:91–95, 2004.
136. Soper D. Trichomoniasis: under control or undercontrolled? Am J Obstet Gynecol 190:281–290, 2004.
137. Bowden FJ, Garnett GP. *Trichomonas vaginalis* epidemiology: parameterising and analyzing a model of treatment interventions. Sex Transm Infect 76:248–256, 2000
138. Zhang Z, Begg C. Is *Trichomonas vaginalis* a cause of cervical neoplasia? Results from a combined analysis of 24 studies. Int J Epidemiol 23:682–690, 1994.
139. Viikki M, Pukkala E, Nieminen P, et al. Gynecological infections as risk determinants of subsequent cervical neoplasia. Acta Oncol 39:71–75, 2000.
140. Minkoff H, Grunebaum AN, Schwartz RH, et al. Risk factors for prematurity and premature rupture of membranes: a prospective study of the vaginal flora in pregnancy. Am J Obstet Gynecol 150:965–972, 1984.
141. Sherman KJ, Daling JR, Weiss N. Sexually transmitted disease and tubal infertility. Sex Transm Dis 14:12–16, 1987.
142. Sherman KJ, Chow W, Daling J, et al. Sexually transmitted diseases and the risk of tubal pregnancy. J Reprod Med 33:30–34, 1988.
143. Grodstein F, Goldman M, Cramer D. Relation of tubal infertility to history of sexually transmitted diseases. Am J Epidemiol 137:577–584, 1993.
144. Soper DE, Bump RC, Hurt WG. Bacterial vaginosis and Trichomonas vaginalis are risk factors for cuff cellulitis after abdominal hysterectomy. Am J Obstet Gynecol 163:1016–1021, 1990.
145. Wang C, McClelland S, Reilly M, et al. The effect of treatment of vaginal infections on shedding of HIV-type I. J Infect Dis 183:1017–1022, 2001.
146. Sorvillo F, Kerndt P. Trichomonas vaginalis and amplification of HIV-I transmission. Lancet 351:213–214, 1998.
147. Laga M, Monoka A, Kivuvu M, et al. Non ulcerative sexually transmitted diseases as risk factors for HIV-I transmission in women: results from a cohort study. AIDS 7:95–102, 1993.
148. Moodley P, Wilkinson D, Connolly C, et al. *Trichomonas vaginalis* is associated with pelvic inflammatory disease in women infected with HIV. Clin Infect Dis 34:519–522, 2002.
149. Sorvillo F, Smith C, Kerndt P, et al. *Trichomonas vaginalis*, HIV, and African Americans. Emerg Infect Dis 7:927–932, 2001.
150. Yap EH, Ho TH, Chan YC, et al. Serum antibodies to *T. vaginalis* in invasive cervical cancer patients. Genitourin Med 71:402–404, 1995.
151. Sayed SA, el-Wakil HS, Kamel WM, et al. A preliminary study on the relationship between *Trichomonas vaginalis* and cervical cancer in Egyptian women. J Egypt Soc Parasitol 32:167–178, 2002.
152. Paisarntantiwong R, Brockman S, Clarke L, et al. The relationship of vaginal trichomoniasis and pelvic inflammatory disease among women colonized with Chlamydia trachomatis. Sex Transm Dis 22:344–347, 1995.
153. Hobbs MM, Kzembe P, Reed AW, et al. *Trichomonas vaginalis* as a cause of urethritis in Malawian men. Sex Transm Dis 26:381–387, 1999.
154. Moodley P, Connolly C, Sturm W. Interrelationships among HIV type 1 infection, bacterial vaginosis, trichomoniasis and the presence of yeasts. J Infect Dis 185:69–73, 2002.
155. Cotch MF, Pastorek JG II, Nugent RP, et al. *Trichomonas vaginalis* associated with low birth weight and preterm delivery: the Vaginal Infections and Prematurity Group. Sex Transm Dis 24:353–360, 1997.
156. Hoffman DJ, Brown GD, Wirth FH, et al. Urinary tract infection with *Trichomonas vaginalis* in a premature newborn infant and the development of chronic lung disease. J Perinatol 23:59–61, 2003.
157. Temesvari P, Kerekes A, Tege A, et al. Demonstration of *Trichomonas vaginalis* in tracheal aspirates in infants with early respiratory failure. J Matern Fetal Neonatal Med 11:347–349, 2002.
158. Smith LM, Wang M, Zangwill K, et al. *Trichomonas vaginalis* infection in a premature newborn. J Perinatol 22:502–503, 2002.
159. Szarka K, Temesvari P, Kerekes A, et al. Neonatal pneumonia caused by *Trichomonas vaginalis*. Acta Microbiol Immunol Hung 49:15–19, 2002.
160. Danesh IS, Stephen JM, Gorbach J. Neonatal *Trichomonas vaginalis* infection. J Emerg Med 13:51–54, 1995.
161. McLaren LC, Davis LE, Healy GR, et al. Isolation of *Trichomonas vaginalis* from the respiratory tract of infants with respiratory disease. Pediatrics 71:888–890, 1983.
162. US Preventive Services Task Force. Postmenopausal hormone replacement therapy for primary prevention of chronic conditions: recommendations and rationale. Ann Intern Med 137:834–839, 2002.
163. North American Menopause Society. Treatment of menopause-associated vasomotor symptoms: position statement of the North American Menopause Society. Menopause 11:11–33, 2004.
164. Amato P, Marcus DM. Review of alternative therapies for treatment of menopausal symptoms. Climacteric 6:278–281, 2003.
165. Prempro [package insert]. Philadelphia, PA: Wyeth Pharmaceuticals, 2005.
166. Henderson BE, Ross RK, Paganini-Hill A, et al. Estrogen use and cardiovascular disease. Am J Obstet Gynecol 154:1181–1186, 1986.
167. The Writing Group for the PEPI Trial. Effects of estrogen or estrogen/progestin regimens on heart disease risk factors in postmenopausal women. JAMA 273:199–208, 1995.
168. Hulley S, Grady D, Bush T, et al. Randomized trial of estrogen plus progestin for secondary prevention of coronary heart disease in postmenopausal women: the heart and estrogen/progestin replacement study (HERS). JAMA 280:605–613, 1998.
169. Grady D, Herrington D, Bittner V, et al. Cardiovascular disease outcomes during 6.8 years of hormone therapy: heart and estrogen/progestin replacement study follow-up (HERS II). JAMA 288:49–57, 2002.
170. Hulley S, Furberg C, Barrett-Connor E, et al. Noncardiovascular disease outcomes during 6.8 years of hormone therapy: heart and estrogen/progestin replacement study follow-up (HERS II). JAMA 288:58–66, 2002.
171. Writing Group for the Women's Health Initiative Investigators. Risks and benefits of estrogen plus progestin in healthy postmenopausal women: principal results from the Women's Health Initiative (WHI) randomized controlled trial. JAMA 288:321–333, 2002.

172. The Women's Health Initiative Steering Committee. Effects of conjugated equine estrogen in postmenopausal women with hysterectomy: the Women's Health Initiative randomized controlled trial. JAMA 291:1701–1712, 2004.
173. Million Women Study Collaborators. Breast cancer and hormone replacement therapy in the Million Women Study. Lancet 362:419–427, 2003.
174. Berquist L, Adami H, Persson I, et al. The risk of breast cancer after estrogen and estrogen-progestin replacement. N Engl J Med 321:293–297, 1989.
175. Magnusson C, Baron JA, Correia N, et al. Breast cancer risk following long-term oestrogen and oestrogen-progestin replacement therapy. Int J Cancer 81:339–344, 1999.
176. Schairer C, Lubin J, Troisi R, et al. Menopausal estrogen and estrogen-progestin replacement therapy and breast cancer risk. JAMA 283:485–491, 2000.
177. Ross RK, Paganini-Hill A, Wan PC, et al. Effect of hormone replacement therapy on breast cancer risk: estrogen versus estrogen plus progestin. J Natl Cancer Inst 92:328–332, 2000.
178. Li CI, Malone KE, Porter PL, et al. Relationship between long durations and different regimens of hormone therapy and risk of breast cancer. JAMA 289:3254–3263, 2003.
179. Rapp SR, Espeland MA, Shumaker SA, et al. Effect of estrogen plus progestin on global cognitive function in postmenopausal women: the women's health initiative memory study (WHIMS), a randomized controlled trial. JAMA 289:2663–2672, 2003.
180. Shumaker SA, Legault C, Rapp SR, et al. Estrogen plus progestin and the incidence of dementia and mild cognitive impairment in postmenopausal women: WHIMS, a randomized trial. JAMA 289:2651–2662, 2003.
181. Shumaker SA, Legault C, Kuller L, et al. Conjugated equine estrogens and incidence of probable dementia and mild cognitive impairment in postmenopausal women: WHIMS. JAMA 291:2947–2958, 2004.
182. Espeland MA, Rapp SR, Shumaker SA, et al. Conjugated equine estrogens and global cognitive function in postmenopausal women: WHIMS. JAMA 291:2959–2968, 2004.
183. Zandi PP, Carlson MC, Plassman BL, et al. Hormone replacement therapy and the incidence of Alzheimer disease in older women: the Cache County Study. JAMA 288:2123–2129, 2002.
184. Lewis V. New hormone therapy formulations and routes of delivery: meeting the needs of your patients in the post-WHI world. OBG Management July(Suppl):11–18, 2004.
185. Clarkson TB, Anthony MS, Jerome CP. Lack of effect of raloxifene on coronary artery atherosclerosis of postmenopausal monkeys. J Clin Endocrinol Metab 83:721–726, 1998.
186. Ries et al., eds. SEER cancer statistics review, 1973–1996. National Cancer Institute, 1999.
187. Transcript of the FDA Endocrine and Bone Advisory Meeting, October 7, 2003. Available at: http://www.fda.gov/ohrms/dockets/ac/03/transcripts/3992T1.htm. Accessed October 5, 2005.
188. Vuong L. Estrogen and progestin options in hormone replacement therapy. Transcript from Embracing Menopause, an educational symposium at the University of California San Francisco, November 4, 2000.
189. Scarabin PY, Oger E, Plu-Bureau G, and the EStrogen and THromboEmbolism Risk (ESTHER) Study Group. Differential association of oral and transdermal oestrogen replacement therapy with venous thromboembolism risk. Lancet 362:428–432, 2003.
190. Minkin MJ. Considerations in the choice of oral vs. transdermal hormone therapy: a review. J Reprod Med 49:311–320, 2004.
191. Nelson H. Commonly used types of postmenopausal estrogen for treatment of hot flashes. JAMA 291:1610–1620, 2004.
192. Gonzales GF, Carrillo C. Blood serotonin levels in postmenopausal women: effects of age and serum oestradiol levels. Maturitas 17:23–29, 1993.
193. Gudelsky GA, Koenig JI, Meltzer HY. Thermoregulatory responses to serotonin (5-HT) receptor stimulation in the rat. Evidence for opposing roles of 5-HT2 and 5-HT1A receptors. Neuropharmacol 25:1307–1313, 1986.
194. Stearns V, Ullmer L, Lopez JF, et al. Hot flushes. Lancet 360:1851–1861, 2002.
195. Kockler DR, McCarthy MW. Antidepressants as a treatment for hot flashes in women. Am J Health-Syst Pharm 61:287–292, 2004.
196. Guttuso T Jr, Kurlan R, McDermott M, et al. Gabapentin's effects on hot flashes in postmenopausal women: a randomized controlled trial. Obstet Gynecol 101:337–345, 2003.
197. Guttuso T Jr. Hot flashes refractory to HRT and SSRI therapy but responsive to gabapentin therapy. J Pain Symptom Manage 27:274–276, 2004.
198. Kreijkamp-Kaspers S, Kok L, Grobbee DE, et al. Effect of soy protein containing isoflavones on cognitive function, bone mineral density, and plasma lipids in postmenopausal women: a randomized controlled trial. JAMA 292:65–74, 2004.
199. Marx P, Schade G, Wilbourn S, et al. Low-dose (0.3 mg) synthetic conjugated estrogens is effective for managing atrophic vaginitis. Maturitas 47:47–54, 2004.
200. Johnston SL, Farrell SA, Bouchard C, et al. The detection and management of vaginal atrophy. J Obstet Gynaecol Can 26:503–515, 2004.
201. Schmidt G, Anderson S, Nordle O, et al. Release of 17-beta-oestradiol from a vaginal ring in postmenopausal women: pharmacokinetic evaluation. Gynecol Obstet Invest 38:253–260, 1994.
202. Buckler H, Al-Azzawi F, UK VR Multicenter Trial Group. The effect of a novel vaginal ring delivering oestradiol acetate on climacteric symptoms in postmenopausal women. BJOG 110:753–9, 2003.
203. Simunic V, Banovic I, Ciglar S, et al. Local estrogen treatment in patients with urogenital symptoms. Int J Gynaecol Obstet 82:187–97, 2003.
204. Notelovitz M, Funk S, Nanavati N, et al. Estradiol absorption from vaginal tablets in postmenopausal women. Obstet Gynecol 99:556–562, 2002.
205. Cicinelli E, Di Naro E, De Ziegler D, et al. Placement of the vaginal 17 beta-estradiol tablets in the inner or outer one-third of the vagina affects the preferential delivery of 17 beta-estradiol toward the uterus or periurethral areas, thereby modifying efficacy and endometrial safety. Am J Obstet Gynecol 189:55–58, 2003.
206. van der Laak JA, de Bie LM, de Leeuw H, et al. The effect of Replens on vaginal cytology in the treatment of postmenopausal atrophy: cytomorphology versus computerized cytometry. J Clin Pathol 55:446–451, 2002.
207. Nachtigall LE. Comparative study: Replens versus local estrogen in menopausal women. Fertil Steril 61:178–180, 1994.
208. Bygdeman M, Swahn ML. Replens versus dienoestrol cream in the symptomatic treatment of vaginal atrophy in postmenopausal women. Maturitas 23:259–263, 1996.
209. Osteoporosis. ACOG Practice Bulletin No 50, 2004.
210. Siris ES, Miller PD, Barrett-Connor E, et al. Identification and fracture outcomes of undiagnosed low bone mineral density postmenopausal women: results from the National Osteoporosis Risk Assessment. JAMA 286:2815–2822, 2001.
211. National Osteoporosis Foundation. Physician's guide to prevention and treatment of osteoporosis, 2003. Available at: http://www.nof.org. Accessed October 5, 2005.
212. Lindsay R, Gallagher JC, Kleerekoper M, et al. Effect of lower doses of conjugated equine estrogens with and without medroxyprogesterone acetate on bone in early postmenopausal women. JAMA 287:2668–2676, 2002.
213. Recker RR, Davies KM, Dowd RM, et al. The effect of low dose continuous estrogen and progesterone therapy with calcium and vitamin D on bone in elderly women: a randomized controlled trial. Ann Intern Med 130:897–904, 1999.
214. Genant HK, Lucas J, Weiss S, et al. A low dose esterified estrogen therapy: effects on bone plasma estradiol concentrations, endometrium, and lipid levels. Estratab/Osteoporosis Study Group. Arch Intern Med 157:2609–2615, 1997.
215. Weiss SR, Ellman H, Dolder M. A randomized controlled trial of four doses of transdermal estradiol for preventing postmenopausal bone loss. Trandermal Estradiol Investigator Group. Obstet Gynecol 94:330–336, 1999.
216. Delmas P. Treatment of postmenopausal osteoporosis. Lancet 359:2018–2026, 2002.
217. Berning B, Kuijk C, Kuiper JW, et al. The effects of two doses of tibolone on trabecular and cortical bone loss in early postmenopausal women: a two-year randomized placebo controlled study. Bone 19:395–399, 1996.

218. Thiebaud D, Bigler JM, Renteria S, et al. A three year study of prevention of postmenopausal bone loss: conjugated equine estrogens plus medroxyprogesterone acetate versus tibolone. Climacteric 1: 202–210, 1998.

219. Rymer J, Robinson J, Fogelman I. Effects of eight years of treatment with tibolone 2.5mg daily on postmenopausal bone loss. Osteoporosis Int 12:478–483, 2001.

220. Linsay SP, Shaw RW, Coelingh HJ, et al. The effect of add back treatment with tibolone on patients treated with gonadotropin releasing hormone agonist triptorelin. Fertil Steril 6592:342–348, 1996.

221. Prelevic GM, Bartram C, Wood J, et al. Comparative effects on bone mineral density of tibolone, transdermal estrogen and oral estrogen/progestogen therapy in postmenopausal women. Gynecol Endocrinol 10:413–420, 1996.

222. Prelevic GM, Markou A, Arnold A, et al. The effect of tibolone on bone mineral density in postmenopausal women with osteopenia or osteoporosis—8 years follow up. Maturitas 47:229–234, 2004.

223. Ettinger B, Black DM, Mitlak BH, et al. Reduction of vertebral fracture risk in postmenopausal women with osteoporosis treated with raloxifene: results from a 3-year randomized clinical trial (MORE). JAMA 282:637–645, 1999.

224. Cummings SR, Eckert S, Krueger KA, et al. The effect of raloxifene on risk of breast cancer in postmenopausal women: results from the MORE randomized trial. JAMA 281:2189–2197, 1999.

225. Atkorn D, Vokes T. Treatment of postmenopausal osteoporosis. JAMA 285:1415–1418, 2001.

226. Cummings SR, Black DM, Thompson DE, et al. Effect of alendronate on risk of fracture in women with low bone density but without vertebral fractures: results from the Fracture Intervention Trial (FIT). JAMA 280:2077–2082, 1998.

227. Harris ST, Watts NB, Genant HK, et al. Effects of risedronate treatment on vertebral and nonverterbal fractures in women with postmenopausal osteoporosis: a randomized controlled trial (VERT). JAMA 282:1344–1352, 1999.

228. Black DM, Cummings SR, Karpf DB, et al. Randomized trial of effect of alendronate on risk of fracture in women with existing vertebral fractures (from the FIT trial). Lancet 348:1535–1541, 1996.

229. Chestnut CH, Silverman S, Andriano K, et al. A randomized trial of nasal spray salmon calcitonin in postmenopausal women with established osteoporosis: the prevent recurrence of osteoporotic fractures (PROOF) study. Am J Med 109:267–276, 2000.

230. Pun KK, Chan LW. Analgesic effect of intranasal salmon calcitonin in the treatment of osteoporotic vertebral fractures. Clin Ther 11:205–209, 1989.

231. Lyritis GP, Tsakalakos N, Magiasis B, et al. Analgesic effect of salmon calcitonin in osteoporotic fractures: a double blind placebo controlled clinical study. Calcif Tissue Int 49:369–372, 1991.

232. Neer RM, Arnaud CD, Zanchetta JR, et al. Effect of parathyroid hormone (1–34) on fractures and bone mineral density in postmenopausal women with osteoporosis. N Engl J Med 344:1434–1441, 2001.

233. Linsay R, Cosman F, Lobo RA, et al. Addition of alendronate to ongoing hormone replacement therapy in the treatment of osteoporosis: a randomized, controlled clinical trial. J Clin Endocrinol Metab 84:3076–3081, 1999.

234. Wimalawansa SJ. A four-year randomized controlled trial of hormone replacement and bisphosphonate, alone or in combination, in women with postmenopausal osteoporosis. Am J Med 104: 219–226, 1998.

235. Harris ST, Eriksen EF, Davidson M, et al. Effect of combined risedronate and hormone replacement therapies on bone mineral density in postmenopausal women. J Clin Endocrinol Metab 86: 1890–1897, 2001.

236. Bone HG, Greenspan SL, et al. Alendronate and estrogen effects in postmenopausal women with low bone mineral density. Alendronate/Estrogen Study Group. J Clin Endocrinol Metab 85: 720–726, 2000.

Contraception

Shareen El-Ibiary

DEFINITION

Contraception is defined as the prevention of conception, but generally it is understood to mean the intentional prevention of pregnancy. Contraceptives are pharmacologic agents or devices used to prevent pregnancy.

TREATMENT GOALS

- Prevent unintentional pregnancy.
- Help choose and recommend a patient-appropriate method that will reliably prevent pregnancy.
- Teach patients about the method and how to use it effectively and consistently.
- Avoid, manage, and recognize bothersome or potentially dangerous adverse effects of contraceptive methods.
- Reassess patient goals over time as contraceptive preferences may change.

EPIDEMIOLOGY

The control of fertility is a frequent concern of women and healthcare providers. In the United States alone, nearly half of all pregnancies each year are unintended.[1] The decisions of whether or not to use contraception and which method to use are not always easy to make. Significant advances in contraception have been made in the past several years, resulting in methods that are much safer, and highly effective when used properly. Unfortunately, there is still no 100% safe and effective contraceptive method available, besides complete abstinence. Healthcare providers, including pharmacists, can play a critical role in helping women and their partners choose a method that is consistent with their contraceptive goals.

PHYSIOLOGY

To understand the evolution of contraceptive methods, it is first necessary to review the physiology of the normal menstrual cycle.

The average menstrual cycle (Fig. 18.1) lasts 28 days, with a range of 23 to 35 days, and may vary with a woman's age. Several organ systems are involved in this cycle, including the hypothalamus, pituitary gland, uterus, and ovaries. The changes that occur in the ovaries during this 28-day cycle can be divided into three phases: the follicular phase, ovulation, and the luteal phase.

FOLLICULAR PHASE

The follicular phase lasts for approximately the first 14 days of the cycle. At the beginning of this phase, several follicles, each containing an oocyte, begin to enlarge, first independently and then in response to pituitary follicle-stimulating hormone (FSH). After 5 or 6 days, one of the follicles begins to develop more rapidly. The granulosa cells of this follicle multiply and, under the influence of FSH and pituitary luteinizing hormone (LH), synthesize and release estrogens from the ovary at an increasing rate. Peripheral levels of estradiol begin to rise significantly by cycle day 7. The estrogens appear to inhibit FSH before midcycle via negative feedback inhibition; however, the high level and rate of increase of estrogen stimulate a surge of LH at the end of this

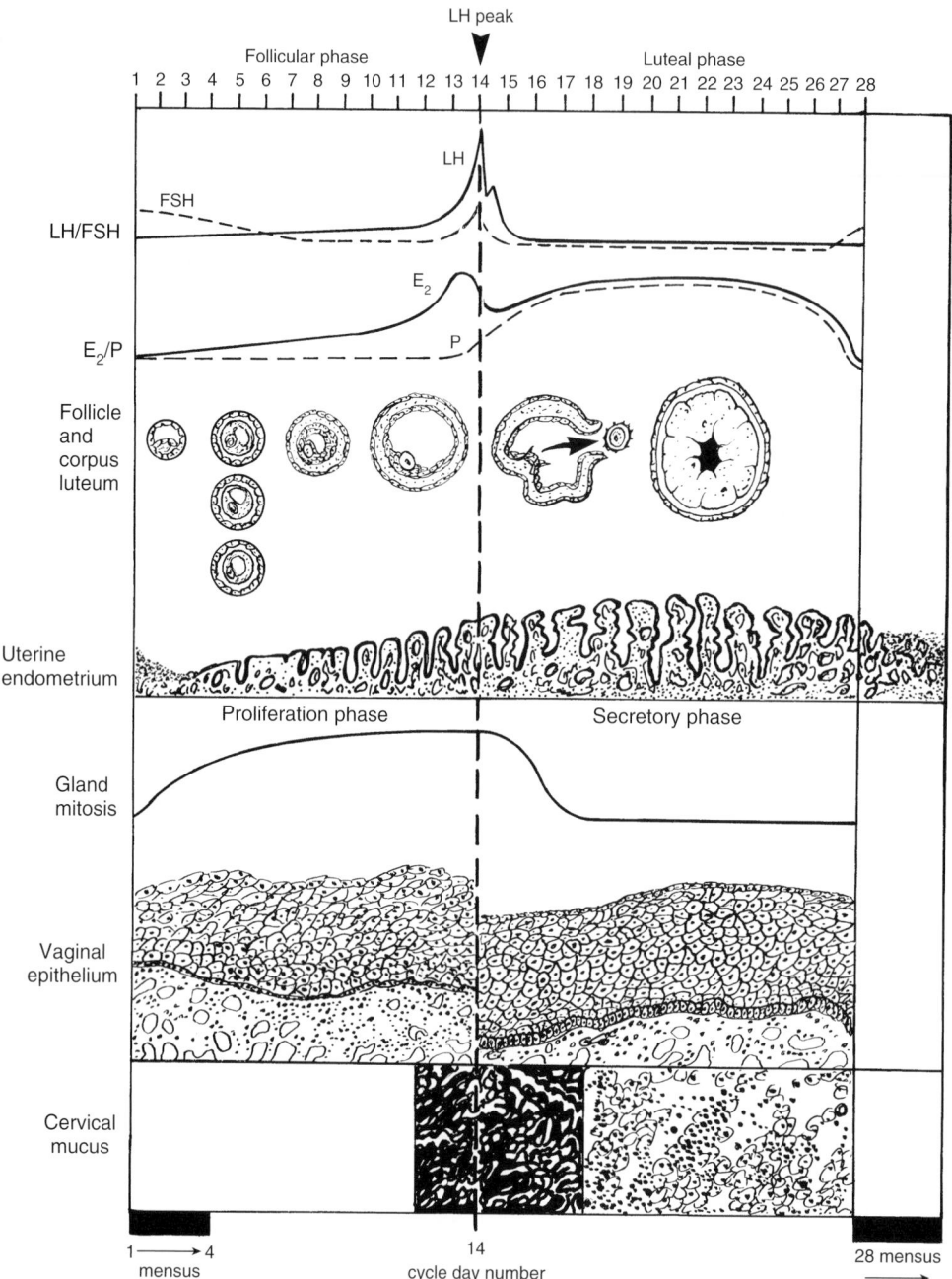

FIGURE 18.1 Composite changes in tissues and hormones during the reproductive cycle. E_2, estradiol; *FSH*, follicle-stimulating hormone; *LH*, luteinizing hormone; *P*, progesterone. (Reprinted with permission from Beckmann CRB, Ling FW, Herbert WNP, et al. Obstetrics and gynecology, 3rd ed. Baltimore: Williams & Wilkins, 1998.)

phase, which in turn causes final-stage growth and rupture of the ovum (ovulation).

OVULATION

Ovulation ordinarily occurs at midcycle, on day 14 or 15. As estrogen levels peak, a surge of LH occurs, leading to follicular maturation and ovulation. The onset of the LH surge appears to be the most reliable indicator of impending ovulation, occurring 34 to 36 hours before follicle rupture. At the time of ovulation, the granulosa cells of the follicle begin to secrete progesterone.

LUTEAL PHASE

The luteal phase follows ovulation and is dominated by progesterone effects. Under the influence of LH, the ruptured follicle fills with blood, and the surrounding theca and granulosa cells proliferate and replace the blood to form the corpus luteum. The cells of this structure produce estrogens and progesterone for the remainder of the cycle unless pregnancy occurs. If pregnancy does not occur during this cycle, the corpus luteum begins to degenerate and ceases hormone production. This drop in serum levels of estrogen and progesterone results in endometrial shedding (menstruation) and the beginning of a new cycle. If pregnancy does occur, the corpus luteum remains active because it is stimulated by human chorionic gonadotropin (hCG) derived from the developing placenta, thus maintaining the high levels of progesterone and estrogen necessary for pregnancy.

The changes that occur in the uterus over the 28-day cycle can also be divided into three phases: the menstrual phase, the proliferative phase, and the secretory phase. The menstrual phase starts on day 1 of the menstrual cycle with the sloughing of the old endometrium and the onset of vaginal bleeding. This phase lasts 3 to 6 days. The proliferative phase is a period of growth of the endometrial lining lasting from day 6 to day 14. Estrogen from the developing follicles is responsible for this growth as well as for the growth of uterine glands and the proliferation of uterine vessels. The secretory phase, which coincides with the luteal phase in the ovaries, is primarily under the influence of progesterone. During

this phase, the endometrium becomes thicker and is held in place, the uterine glands branch, and the secretory function of these glands begins, thus preparing the endometrium for implantation should fertilization of the ovum occur.

THERAPEUTIC PLAN

There are many methods of contraception available, including surgical, pharmacologic, and nonpharmacologic methods. Surgical options include tubal ligation for women and vasectomy for men. These are generally considered permanent options, although they may be reversible under certain rare circumstances. Other options that involve men include condoms and natural family planning. All other options are used by women. Figure 18.2 indicates the various methods available in a decision tree format. Table 18.1 compares the failure rates of these methods, both under "perfect use" conditions and "typical use" conditions. Perfect use is defined as the accidental pregnancy rate in the first year related to method failure (e.g., failure of the method itself). Typical use is defined as the accidental pregnancy rate in the first year related to user failure (e.g., failure of the couple to use the method properly). The decision to use a particular

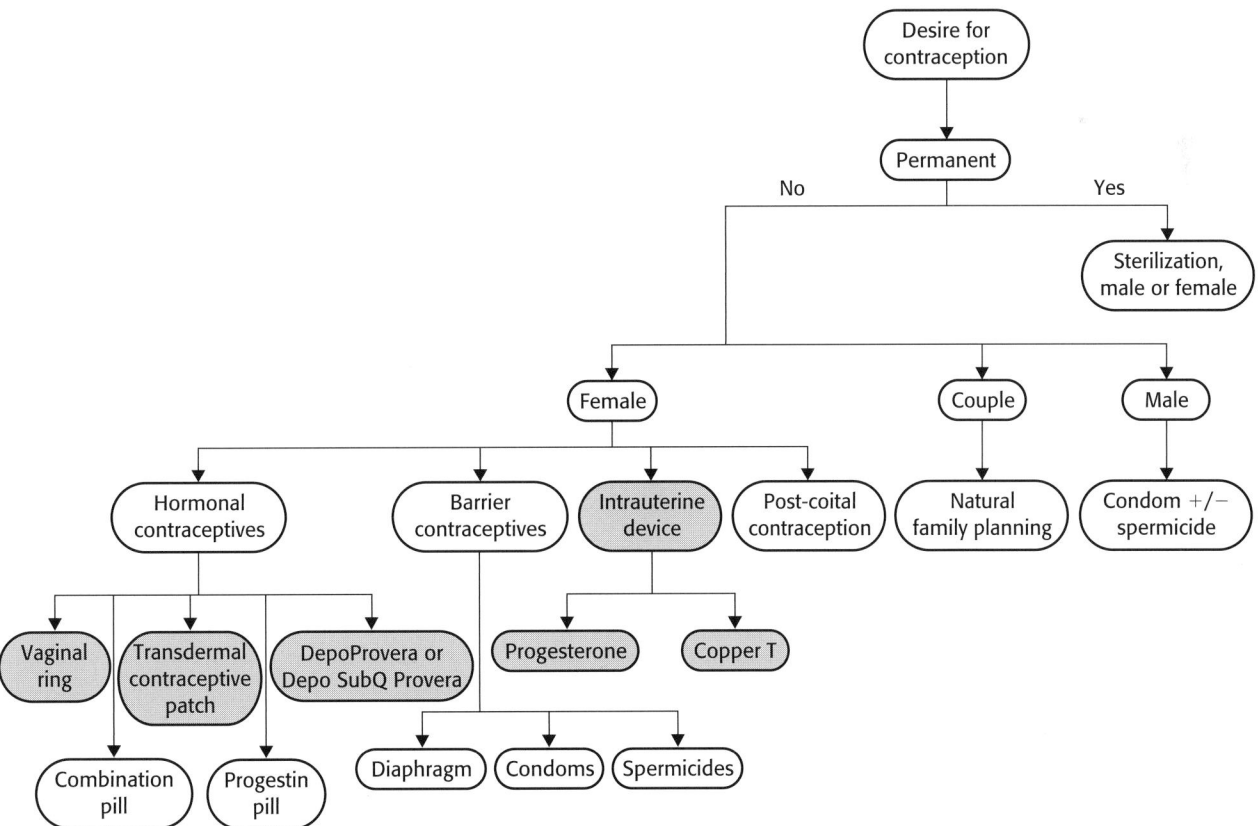

FIGURE 18.2 One of several possible algorithms to contraceptive choice. Shaded choices are less "use oriented"—that is, they require minimal action on the part of the couple to be effective. (Reprinted with permission from Beckmann CRB, Ling FW, Herbert WNP, et al. Obstetrics and gynecology, 3rd ed. Baltimore: Williams & Wilkins, 1998.)

| TABLE 18.1 | Success Rates of Various Contraceptive Methods: United States |

Method	% of Women Experiencing an Unintended Pregnancy Within the First Year of Use		% of Women Continuing Use at 1 Year[c]
	Typical Use[a]	Perfect Use[b]	
Chance[d]	85	85	
Spermicides[e]	26	6	40
Periodic abstinence	25		63
Calendar		9	
Ovulation method		3	
Symptothermal[f]		2	
Postovulation		1	
Cap[g]			
Parous women	40	26	42
Nulliparous women	20	9	56
Sponge			
Parous women	40	20	42
Nulliparous women	20	9	56
Diaphragm[g]	20	6	56
Withdrawal	19	4	
Condom[h]			
Female (Reality)	21	5	56
Male	14	3	61
Pill			
Progestin only	8	0.3	68
Combined	8	0.3	68
Ring		0.3	
Patch		0.3	
IUD			
Copper T 380A	0.8	0.6	78
LNg20	0.1	0.1	81
Depo-subQ Provera	3	0.3	70
Depo-Provera	3	0.3	
Norplant and Norplant-2	0.05	0.05	88
Female sterilization	0.5	0.5	100
Male sterilization	0.15	0.10	100

Emergency contraceptive pills: treatment initiated within 72 h after unprotected intercourse reduces risk of pregnancy by at least 75%[i]

Lactational amenorrhea method: a highly effective, *temporary* method of contraception[j]

[a]Among *typical* couples who initiate use of a method (not necessarily for the first time), the percentage who experience an accidental pregnancy during the first year if they do not stop use for any other reason.
[b]Among couples who initiate use of a method (not necessarily for the first time) and who use it *perfectly* (both consistently and correctly), the percentage who experience an accidental pregnancy during the first year if they do not stop use for any other reason.
[c]Among couples attempting to avoid pregnancy, the percentage who continue to use a method for 1 year.
[d]The percentages becoming pregnant in the "typical use" and "perfect use" columns are based on data from populations where contraception is not used and from women who cease using contraception to become pregnant. Among such populations, about 89% become pregnant within 1 year. This estimate was lowered slightly (to 85%) to represent the percentages who would become pregnant withint 1 year among women now relying on reversible methods of contraception if they abandoned contraception altogether.
[e]Foams, creams, gels, vaginal suppositories, and vaginal film.
[f]Cervical mucus (ovulation) method supplemented by calendar in the preovulatory and basal body temperature in the postovulatory phases.
[g]With spermicidal cream or jelly.
[h]Without spermicides.
[i]The treatment schedule is one dose within 72 hours after unprotected intercourse and a second dose 12 hours after the first dose. The Food and Drug Administration has declared the following brands of oral contraceptives to be safe and effective for emergency contraception: Ovral (1 dose is 2 white pills), Alesse (1 dose is 5 pink pills), Nordette or Levlen (1 dose is 4 light-orange pills), Lo/Ovral (1 dose is 4 white pills), Triphasil or Tri-Levlen (1 dose is 4 yellow pills).
[j]However, to maintain effective protection against pregnancy, another method of contraception must be used as soon as menstruation resumes, the frequency or duration of breastfeedng is reduced, bottle feeds are introduced, or the baby reaches 6 months of age.
(From Hatcher RA, Trussell J, Stewart F, et al. Contraceptive technology, 17th ed. New York: Ardent Media Inc, 1998, with permission.)

method is complex and dependent on individual factors, including the safety and efficacy of the method, the person's ability to use the method correctly, concurrent conditions, and the particular needs and desires of the couple, such as cost, side effect profile, reversibility of contraception, and access to healthcare.

METHODS OF CONTRACEPTION

HORMONAL CONTRACEPTION

Combination Oral Contraceptives. The use of female sex hormones to prevent the development of the ovum was suggested as early as 1931, but it was not until 1956, after the discovery of norethynodrel, that field trials were begun on what we now know as birth control pills.[2] In 1960, the U.S. Food and Drug Administration (FDA) first approved the use of Enovid 10, a combination pill containing 150 μg of mestranol and 9.85 mg of norethynodrel. Other products soon followed, containing varying amounts of estrogens and progestins.

All combination oral contraceptives (COCs) contain both an estrogen and a progestin component. Many products have been developed with lower doses of hormones to reduce the potential for adverse effects and to improve cycle control.

The major natural estrogens produced by women are estradiol (E2), estrone (E1), and estriol (E3). Estradiol is the major secretory product of the ovaries. Some estrone is also produced in the ovaries, although most estrone and estriol is formed in the liver from estradiol or converted in the peripheral tissues. To improve absorption and potency, synthetic estrogens were developed. Mestranol and ethinyl estradiol are the estrogens that have been used in the United States. Mestranol is an inactive synthetic estrogen that is demethylated in the liver to form the active ethinyl estradiol. Only one current COC contains mestranol in a dose of 50 μg, which is approximately equivalent to 35 μg ethinyl estradiol. All other COCs contain 50 μg or less of ethinyl estradiol. Pills containing 50 μg or greater ethinyl estradiol are considered "high dose." COCs are considered "low dose" if they contain 35 μg or less of ethinyl estradiol (e.g., 30 to 35 μg ethinyl estradiol). Pills containing less than 30 μg of ethinyl estradiol are considered "very low dose" (e.g., 20 to 25 μg ethinyl estradiol). However, most refer to COCs as just high or low dose.

Ethinyl estradiol undergoes extensive first-pass hepatic metabolism, which can result in considerable patient-to-patient variation in plasma and urine steroid concentrations. Circulating ethinyl estradiol is highly bound to albumin. It is metabolized primarily by the hepatic cytochrome P450 3A4 isoenzyme. Ethinyl estradiol also undergoes enterohepatic circulation and is excreted into the bile, deconjugated in the gastrointestinal (GI) system, and reabsorbed into the bloodstream. This may result in a rebound of blood levels of estrogen 10 to 14 hours after administration.

The role of estrogen in preventing pregnancy occurs through several mechanisms.[3,4] First, negative feedback inhibition by estrogen on the hypothalamus and pituitary gland suppresses the release of FSH and LH, preventing the selection of a dominant follicle and subsequent ovulation. Estrogen also may contribute by altering the endometrial lining, allowing changes in secretions, which results in alternating areas of edema and dense cellularity. In larger doses, estrogen stimulates the degeneration of the corpus luteum (luteolysis).

Progestin use in COCs has changed considerably. Progesterone itself is the most important natural progestin and also serves as a precursor to the estrogens, androgens, and adrenocortical steroids. Progesterone is rapidly absorbed after parenteral administration but is poorly absorbed when given orally. To overcome problems with absorption and high first-pass metabolism, synthetic progestins were developed. There are now nine different synthetic compounds in use in the United States: norethindrone, norethindrone acetate, ethynodiol diacetate, norgestrel, levonorgestrel, norethynodrel, desogestrel, norgestimate, and the spironolactone derivative drospirenone. Most synthetic progestins used in COCs are 19-nortestosterones derived from testosterone and differ from each other in terms of their biologic activities. Unlike the estrogens, progestins can exhibit not only progestin effects but also estrogenic and androgenic effects. This may result in subtle differences in side effects, but not in the ability to suppress ovulation. As a group, progestins exert their contraceptive effects by suppressing the release of LH (inhibiting ovulation), thickening the cervical mucus to hinder sperm transport, and producing an atrophic endometrial lining, which is inhospitable to implantation.

Progestins, like ethinyl estradiol, undergo first-pass metabolism.[3,5] Metabolism occurs in varying degrees in the intestinal wall and in the liver. Some of the older compounds (norethindrone acetate and ethynodrel diacetate) are converted to norethindrone, which exerts its activity and is then converted and excreted as sulfates and glucuronide. As first introduced, norgestrel was a mixture of d- and l-isomers. It has since been recognized that activity rests entirely with the levo form. Original products still contain the racemic norgestrel, but newer products contain half of the amount of levonorgestrel. There is enhanced potency of levonorgestrel and its derivatives of about 5-fold to 10-fold compared with norethindrone. Three derivatives of levonorgestrel represent one of the newest generation of orally active progestins: desogestrel, norgestimate, and gestodene (not currently available in the United States). It appears that neither desogestrel nor gestodene is converted to levonorgestrel, but norgestimate may undergo this transformation. However, one metabolite of norgestimate, 17-deacetylnorgestimate, is likely to also contribute to the pharmacologic response. Desogestrel is rapidly converted to 3-ketodesogestrel and is present in high circulating concentrations. Drospirenone, a derivative of spironolactone, is the newest progestin that has antimineralocorticoid and antiandrogenic effects.

Together, ethinyl estradiol and the progestin component work synergistically to produce very effective contraceptive effects. Compared to other methods of birth control, COCs remain one of the most effective forms. With perfect use (consistent and correct), only 3 of 1,000 women using COCs may accidentally become pregnant during the first year. With typical use (not always consistent and correct), approximately 8% of women may become pregnant.[4] Clearly, encouraging patients to strive for perfection with pill use will prevent many unintended pregnancies.

Risks. One reason why some women may be reluctant to take COCs consistently and correctly is a fear of possible adverse effects. It is important to discuss these fears and the potential risks as well as benefits before choosing this particular method. As stated earlier, older products contained higher doses of hormones and were associated with significant side effects. This reputation continues despite evidence to the contrary with more modern products. Also, with extensive study, many non-contraceptive health benefits from the use of COCs have been identified.

Cardiovascular Disease. Historically, COCs have been associated with increased risks for myocardial infarction (MI) and stroke. Much debate continues on the exact relationship of COC use and the risk of MI and stroke. Early data showed that dangers during therapy seem to increase substantially with age and the presence of risk factors such as smoking greater than 15 cigarettes daily, preexisting hypercholesterolemia, diabetes mellitus, or hypertension.[6,7] Overall, oral contraceptives were found to multiply the effects of age and other risk factors for MI and stroke rather than just add to them.[7] Because cigarette smoking is far more prevalent among women of reproductive age than any of these other risk factors, it becomes by far the most important factor.

While early epidemiologic studies of high-dose oral contraceptives found significantly increased risks of developing cardiovascular disease among users of COCs, several trends have led to a reassessment of that risk. First, studies have become more sophisticated and now take into account the potentially confounding effects of cigarette smoking. Second, in recent years women have been evaluated more carefully before they begin to take oral contraceptives, and women who have serious underlying medical problems and older women who smoke have been less likely to use oral contraceptives. Third, the formulations have changed dramatically; current formulations have a 3- to 4-fold decrease in estrogen dose and a 1-fold decrease in progestin dose compared with the formulations initially prescribed and studied. Hence, the findings of early epidemiologic studies are probably less important with today's products.[8]

Use of oral contraceptives by healthy women who do not smoke does not appear to be associated with an increased risk of either MI or stroke.[9–13] Data from the United States and the United Kingdom have documented no increase in the risk of death from cardiovascular disease among contemporary users of oral contraceptives. Data from the Oxford Family Planning Association study also support the hypothesis that oral contraceptives that contain less than 50 μg of estrogen are safer than high-dose formulations.[14]

Some evidence suggests that the pathophysiology of MI among women who used oral contraceptives in earlier studies was thrombosis and not atherosclerosis.[2] First, most studies, including the large Nurses' Health Study from the United States, have found no increased risk of MI among former users of COCs.[15,16] If atherosclerosis were the cause, then the risk should remain elevated after women discontinued COCs. Corroborating evidence comes from autopsy studies of women who died of MI. Second, there does not appear to be a duration-related effect between length of oral contraceptive use and risk of infarction. This also argues against deposition of plaque as the pathophysiologic mechanism.

Hypertension. As with the increased risks for MI and stroke, older formulations of COCs have been associated with significant elevations of blood pressure as well. The risk of hypertension appears to be much lower when estrogen and progestin doses are lowered. Although some studies have shown no clinically significant changes in blood pressure in low-dose COC users versus nonusers,[17,18] others have shown mildly increased systolic and diastolic blood pressures,[19] and rarely, individual patients have experienced idiosyncratic reactions and have developed hypertension after they begin taking the pill. A large epidemiologic study reported a relative risk of 1.8 in current users versus never-users, after adjustment for other risk factors for hypertension.[20] This relative risk appeared to decrease in past users. The mechanism for contraceptive-induced changes in blood pressure is still unclear, with alterations in plasma angiotensinogen and increases in sodium and water retention being noted. Although these are primarily estrogenic effects, progestins may have a synergistic effect, as significant elevations in blood pressure have been apparent only in the combination products and not with either hormone alone.

Hypertension associated with COCs is reversible on discontinuation of the pill, but it may take up to 3 to 4 months to return to normal. It is prudent to monitor patients at the initiation of combined hormonal contraception and periodically (e.g., 3 months later) thereafter. If the blood pressure rises significantly, the method may have to be discontinued, although some women may tolerate a lower-dose product with careful monitoring.

Thrombosis. Users of high-dose COCs have an increased risk of developing venous thrombosis and stroke with increasing doses of estrogen.[9,21] As doses of estrogen were lowered to less than 50 μg, a marked drop in the incidence of fatal and nonfatal pulmonary embolism was noted, thus implying an estrogen dose-related effect.[2] A large number of changes in the blood coagulation process have been attributed to estrogen, including an increase in platelet aggregation, increases in several clotting factors, and a decrease in antithrombin III activity.[22–24] The role of progestins is also unclear. It was generally accepted that the progestin component did not have a significant impact on clotting parameters, but several observational studies seemed to refute this belief.[25–28] In these reports, women using low-dose COCs containing either gestodene or desogestrel seemed to have an increased risk of thromboembolism compared to users of low-dose pills with the older progestins. This caused a great amount of concern about the safety of the newer agents. Further review and reanalysis of the data did not confirm the findings, but instead showed possible confounding and bias in the original studies.[13,29] Part of the problem may have been with patient selection, in that physicians may have prescribed these newer agents preferentially in patients who already had a higher risk for thromboembolism.[30] Also, duration of use may have been a confounding factor, in that it appears the risk for venous thromboembolism is greatest in the first year of use regardless of the formulation used.[31] Several recent studies have not been able to show significant differences between the older and newer progestins, but questions remain.[32,33] An explanation may involve differential effects of the different progestins on sensitivity to activated protein C, which acts as an endogenous anticoagulant.[34] Also, some women may have a newly identified genetic mutation called factor V Leiden, which also causes resistance to activated protein C and increases risk for deep vein thrombosis. The combination of the genetic mutation and a progestin that increases resistance to activated protein C may help explain the epidemiologic observations, but more study is needed.

As with the other concerns for MI, stroke, and hypertension, patient-appropriate product selection remains the most important method of reducing the incidence of these adverse effects. Women who are already at high risk for cardiovascular problems (hypertension, smoking, and older than 35 years, or diabetic with vascular complications) or have already had a cardiovascular or thromboembolic event should not use COCs.

Cancer. The data supporting the protective effects of COCs on the development of uterine and ovarian cancers are clear, but the effect of COCs on the risk of breast cancer is complex. Previous studies have found increased, decreased, or no change in risk in COC users. More recent studies have shed some light on the risk in various subgroups of women. The Collaborative Group on Hormonal Factors in Breast Cancer published an extensive study that reanalyzed the results of 54 studies.[35] This report indicated a small increase in relative risk of breast cancer in current users, which continues (although at an increasingly lower rate) in previous users up to 10 years after discontinuation. Thereafter, there was no increased risk in ever-users versus never-users. Also, it appeared that if breast cancer was diagnosed in a current or former user of COCs, the cancer was more likely to be less advanced, which may affect survival rates. It still remains to be shown whether estrogen use initiates the cancer or merely promotes its growth. In a population-based case-controlled study of women aged 35 to 64, there was no increased risk of breast cancer in current or former oral contraceptive users.[36]

Even more conflicting than the data on breast cancer are the studies evaluating the risk of cervical cancer. Several studies have shown a slightly increased risk, but it has been difficult to sort out the confounding risk factors such as multiple partners, coitus at an early age, and the role of human papillomavirus (HPV).[37,38] HPV seems to be a large factor in cervical cancer.[39] Those who are sexually active have a higher risk of contracting HPV. Consequently, those who are sexually active may also be likely to use COCs to prevent pregnancy. The exact role of COCs in cervical cancer is unknown. It may be a co-factor in conjunction with HPV, or it may act alone. There are some data that suggest the risk of cervical cancer increases with length of COC use.[40] Annual Pap smears are recommended for sexually active women taking COCs.

Hepatomas may occur in women taking oral contraceptives. A wide array of benign liver tumors has been reported, the most common of which are focal nodular hyperplasia and hepatic adenomas. Even though these tumors may rupture and bleed, since the advent of low-dose contraceptives this complication has been quite rare. Hepatocellular cancer was also thought to be associated with COC use, but interestingly enough there has not been an increase in death rates from liver cancer in the time since this method was introduced.[2]

Gallbladder Disease. Use of oral contraceptives was originally thought to increase the incidence of gallstones and cholecystitis. Estrogens alter the composition of bile, possibly by increasing cholesterol saturation of bile. With the decrease in estrogen content in newer products, this effect may be less common. One large prospective study showed the relative risk for symptomatic gallstones in ever-users of COCs to be 1.2, in long-term users 1.5, and in current users 1.6.[41] Overall, the incidence is quite low.

Benefits. Using controlled, cyclic doses of hormones, a woman's menstrual cycle can be more regulated and predictable. Menorrhagia (excessive blood loss during menstruation) can lead to iron deficiency anemia. For most women, with continued use of COCs, the endometrial lining becomes thinner, resulting in less menstrual blood loss and reduced anemia, as well as reduced menstrual cramping or dysmenorrhea. Reducing the frequency or even eliminating menstruation can have a significant impact on menorrhagia. In such cases, an extended-cycle regimen may be beneficial. Premenstrual symptoms such as depression, anxiety, and fluid retention may be lessened by the use of COCs, but in some women these symptoms worsen.[42] Chapter 17 offers further discussion on premenstrual syndrome.

Besides these benefits on the menstrual cycle itself, COCs offer other advantages. They convey protective effects against ovarian, endometrial, and perhaps colorectal cancer. Oral contraceptive use decreases the risk of endometrial cancer by approximately 50%, and its protective effects persist for at least 15 to 20 years after use is stopped.[43,44] Also, because of the inhibition of FSH and LH, ovarian stimulation is suppressed, and the incidence of functional ovarian cysts is reduced.[45] This appears to be somewhat dependent on dose, with older, higher-potency COCs offering the most benefit. With the inhibition of ovulation, the chances for an ectopic pregnancy are also markedly reduced.[46] In addition, the risk of ovarian cancer decreases with increased duration of COC use.[47] According to one study, after 4 years of use the incidence of ovarian cancer decreases by 41%, by 54% at 8 years, and 61% at 12 years.[47] Protective effects can be seen as early as 3 months and may continue up to 20 years after use.[47] After 10 years of COC use, one study found that COC use decreased the risk of those with a family history of ovarian cancer to similar risk of women without a family history.[48] The same study also found that COC use for 5 years lowered the risk of ovarian cancer in nulliparous women comparable to that of parous women who had not used COCs.[48] Benign breast diseases such as fibroadenomas and cysts are also less likely to develop in COC users.[49]

Acne and hirsutism may be either adversely affected or markedly improved by COCs, depending on the particular product. Combinations that are ''estrogen-dominant'' in their activity profile are useful in suppressing sebum production and reducing the production of androgenic hormones by the ovaries. Estrogens also increase sex hormone binding globulin levels by 3-fold to 4-fold, allowing increased binding of testosterone and a decrease in free testosterone. These effects result in reduced androgenic activity and improvement in acne and hirsutism. Progestins may have the opposite effects on sebum production and testosterone levels. If acne or hirsutism is a problem, it is advantageous to choose a COC that is estrogen dominant and/or contains a progestin with low androgenic activity (e.g., desogestrel, drospirenone, or norgestimate).[2,50] There are two COCs (Ortho Tri-Cyclen, Estrostep) that are FDA approved for the treatment of acne in women, although most COCs may help to clear acne regardless of FDA approval. Chapter 10 offers a further discussion on the management of acne.

Precautions. Table 18.2 indicates which women should not use combination oral contraceptives.

Types of Combination Oral Contraceptives. Table 18.3 lists the various formulations of COCs currently available, and their relative activities. Although products containing 50 μg ethinyl estradiol are still available, the vast majority of women use products containing less than 35 μg. All come in either 21- or 28-day pill packs, with active pills being taken for the first 21 days of each cycle, and either no pills or inactive pills for the last 7 days. Menstruation usually occurs 1 to 4 days after the last active pill, and a new pack must always be started 7 days after the last active pill. Monophasic pills contain the same amount of ethinyl estradiol and progestin in each pill. Biphasic formulations, which are seldom used, vary the amount of progestin between the first 10 days and last 11 days. Triphasic pills were

developed in an attempt to further lower total progestin doses over the 21-day cycle. In these formulations, both the estrogen and progestin doses may change throughout the cycle. Two new formulations are of note. Estrostep is the only multiphasic COC in which the progestin dose (1 mg norethindrone acetate) is fixed and the estrogen dose is gradually increased from 20 μg to 35 μg. Mircette, approved in 1998, is a monophasic pill containing low doses of estrogen (20 μg) and desogestrel (0.15 mg) and a shortened inactive pill interval. After 21 days of active pills, there are 2 days of inactive pills are followed by 5 days of pills containing 10 μg ethinyl estradiol. This differs from other formulations that contain 7 days of inactive pills. This formulation works well for women who suffer migraines due to withdrawal of estrogen in COCs because there are fewer inactive pills.

Initiation, Selection, and Monitoring. As shown in Table 18.3, there are many products from which to choose. Providing there are no reasons not to prescribe COCs and after obtaining a medical history, weight, blood pressure, and a Pap smear, any product containing 35 μg or less ethinyl estradiol may be recommended for the majority of women. Individual considerations will be discussed in the following sections.

All COCs can be initiated in one of three ways: (a) the first pill is taken on the first day of the menstrual period (''day 1 start''); (b) the first pill is taken on the Sunday after the onset of menses (''Sunday start''); or (c) anytime, if the woman is definitely not pregnant. The Sunday start will result in future periods occurring during the week instead of on the weekend, which may be preferable for some women. The day 1 start provides immediate protection, so backup contraception is probably not necessary with this method.[4] With the other two methods, a backup method is recommended until seven active consecutive pills have been taken.[4] Some clinicians recommend backup protection for the entire first month if patients may be inexperienced with daily pill taking and may miss pills. Patients should be advised to take the pill consistently every day at roughly the same time. Patients should also be informed what to do in the event of a missed pill. This is somewhat dependent on the type of pill being taken and at what point in the cycle the pill is missed. With low-dose pills, especially those containing 20 to 30 μg ethinyl estradiol, one missed pill could be enough to allow ovulation. Modest fluctuations in the levels of FSH and LH among pill users have been observed. This might indicate that follicular development may proceed to a greater extent in some women, resulting in breakthrough ovulation.

At times, patients may miss taking pills. There are a few different suggestions regarding how to handle a missed pill. The most conservative recommendation is as follows: 1) If one pill in the first 3 weeks is missed, it should be taken as soon as possible. If the missed pill is not remembered until the next day, the two pills should be taken together. To be on the safe side, backup protection or abstinence may be recommended for the next 7 days. 2) If two consecutive pills

TABLE 18.2	Precautions in the Use of Combined Oral Contraceptives (COCs)

Refrain from providing COCs for women with the following diagnoses (World Health Organization category 4):

Precautions	Rationale/Discussion
Deep vein thrombosis or pulmonary embolism, or embolism, or a history thereof	Estrogens promote blood clotting. Thromboembolic events related to known trauma or an IV needle are not necessarily a reason to avoid use of pills.
Cerebrovascular accident (stroke), coronary artery or ischemic heart disease, or a history thereof	Estrogens promote blood clotting.
Structural heart disease, complicated by pulmonary hypertension, atrial fibrillation, or history of subacute bacterial endocarditis	Estrogens promote blood clotting.
Diabetes with nephropathy, retinopathy, neuropathy, or other vascular disease; diabetes of more than 20 years' duration	Estrogens promote blood clotting.
Breast cancer	Breast cancer is a hormonally sensitive tumor. In theory, the hormones in COCs might cause some masses to grow.
Pregnancy	Current data do not show that hormonal contraceptives taken during pregnancy cause any significant risk of birth defects. However, hormonal contraceptives should not be given to pregnant women.
Lactation (<6 wk postpartum)	There is some theoretical concern that the neonate may be at risk due to exposure to steroid hormones during the first 6 weeks post-partum.
Liver problems: benign hepatic adenoma or liver cancer, or a history thereof; active viral hepatitis; severe cirrhosis	COCs are metabolized by the liver and their use may adversely affect prognosis of existing disease.
Headaches, including migraine, with focal neurologic symptoms	Focal neurologic symptoms such as blurred vision, seeing flashing lights or zigzag lines, or trouble speaking or moving may be an indication of an increased risk of stroke.
Major surgery with prolonged immobilization or any surgery on the legs	Increasesd risk for deep vein thrombosis and pulmonary embolism is seen.
Older than 35 years and currently a heavy smoker (15 or more cigarettes a day)	Smoking increases the risk of cardiovascular disease.
Hypertension, >160/100 mm Hg or with vascular disease	Hypertension is an important risk factor for cardiovascular disease.

(From Hatcher RA, Trussell J, Stewart F, et al. Contraceptive technology, 17th ed. New York: Ardent Media Inc, 1998, with permission.)
IV, intravenous.

are missed during the first 2 weeks, then two should be taken daily for 2 days, followed by resumption of the regular dosing. Backup contraception should be used for the remainder of the cycle. If unprotected intercourse occurred in the past 5 days, the woman may consider taking emergency contraception (EC) and then starting a new pill pack. 3) If two pills are missed during the third week, the woman should finish taking one active pill daily to the end of the active pills while using a backup birth control method for 7 days and then immediately start using a new pack without a pill-free interval in between. If unprotected intercourse occurred within 5 days of the missed doses, EC may be used and a new pill pack started. 4) If three pills are missed anytime, then the patient should stop the old pack and start over with a new pack. If a woman is a ''day 1'' starter, she may begin her new pill pack that day. If she is a ''Sunday'' starter, she

should take one active pill daily from her old pack until Sunday and then begin her new pack. A backup method of contraception should be used until seven active pills have been taken. Manufacturers of individual products may suggest different approaches; it is prudent to consult the package insert as well. Patients should also be advised about the availability of EC (see subsequent section).

Side Effects. In the first one or two cycles, as the body adjusts to new hormone levels, some women experience side effects such as nausea and irregular bleeding or spotting. It is generally recommended for women to continue with one COC product for at least 3 months to give the body time to adjust. ''Breakthrough bleeding'' is the term used for irregular bleeding that requires a tampon or maxi-pad; ''spotting'' is the term for a few droplets of blood that does not require

TABLE 18.3 | Estimated Relative Oral Contraceptive Progestin/Estrogen/Androgen Activity

Ingredients		Brand-Name Examples	Progestin Activity	Estrogen Activity	Androgen Activity
Monophasic	0.1 mg levonorgestrel/20 μg EE	Alesse, Aviane, Lessina, Levlite	Low	Low	Low
	0.25 mg norgestimate/35 μg EE	Ortho-Cyclen, Sprintec		Intermediate	
	0.5 mg norethindrone/35 μg EE	Brevicon, Modicon Necon 0.5/35, Nortrel 0.5/35		High	
	0.4 mg norethindrone/35 μg EE	Ovcon-35			
	0.15 mg levonorgestrel/30 μg EE	Levlen, Levora Nordette, Portia	Intermediate	Low	Intermediate
	0.3 mg norgestrel/30 μg EE	Cryselle, Lo-Ovral, Low-Ogestrel			
	1 mg norethindrone/50 μg mestranol	Necon 1/50, Norinyl 1 + 50, Ortho-Novum 1/50		Intermediate	
	1 mg norethindrone/35 μg EE	Necon 1/35, Norinyl 1 + 35, Nortrel 1/35, Ortho-Novum 1/35		High	
	1 mg norethindrone/50 μg EE	Ovcon-50			
	1 mg norethindrone acetate/ 20 μg EE	Loestrin 21 1/20, Loestrin Fe 1/20, Microgestin Fe 1/20	High	Low	
	1.5 mg norethindrone acetate/ 30 μg EE	Loestrin 21 1.5/30, Loestrin Fe 1.5/30, Microgestin Fe 1.5/30			High
	1 mg ethynodiol diacetate/ 35 μg EE	Demulen 1/35, Zovia 1/35E			Low
	Desogestrel/EE 0.15 mg-20 μg and EE 10 μg	Kariva, Mircette			
	0.15 mg desogestrel/30 μg EE	Apri, Desogen Ortho-Cept	High	Intermediate	
	1 mg ethynodiol diacetate/ 50 μg EE	Demulen 1/50, Zovia 1/50E			
	0.5 mg norgestrel/50 μg EE	Ovral, Ogestrel		High	High
	3 mg drospirenone/30 μg EE	Yasmin	No data	Intermediate[a]	None[a]
Biphasic	Norethindrone/EE 0.5–35/1-35 mg-μg	Necon 10/11 Ortho-Novum 10/11	Intermediate	High	Low
Triphasic	Norgestimate/EE 0.18-25/ 0.215-25/0.25-25 mg-μg	Ortho Tri-Cyclen Lo	Low	Low	
	Levonorgestrel/EE 0.05-30/ 0.075-40/0.125-30 mg-μg	Enpresse, Tri-Levlen, Triphasil, Trivora		Intermediate	
	Norgestimate/EE 0.18-35/ 0.215-35/0.25-35 mg-μg	Ortho Tri-Cyclen			
	Norethindrone/EE 0.5-35/ 1-35/0.5-35 mg-μg	Tri-Norinyl		High	
	Norethindrone/EE 0.5-35/ 0.75-35/1-35 mg-μg	Necon 7/7/7, Ortho-Novum 7/7/7	Intermediate		
	Norethindrone/EE 1-20/1-30/1-35 mg-μg	Estrostep 21, Estrostep Fe	High	Low	Intermediate
	Desogestrel/EE 0.1-25/ 0.125-25/0.15-25 mg-μg	Cyclessa			Low

EE, ethinyl estradiol.

[a]Preclinical studies have shown that drospirenone has no androgenic, estrogenic, glucocorticoid, antiglucocorticoid, or antiandrogenic activity.

(From Wickersham RM, Novak KK, eds. Drug facts and comparisons. St. Louis, MO: Wolters Kluwer Health, Inc, 2005, with permission.)

use of a feminine product. For most women, these problems tend to decrease substantially by the third cycle of pills, although for some women it may continue. If spotting or breakthrough bleeding continues after three cycles, the dose of estrogen or progestin can be adjusted based on the timing of breakthrough bleeding (e.g., early in cycle or late in cycle). Generally, if breakthrough bleeding occurs in the early part of the cycle, it may indicate either too high a progestin dose or too low an estrogen dose, and adjustments can be made (e.g., increasing the estrogenic potency or endometrial activity of the pill). If breakthrough bleeding occurs late in the cycle, it may likely be attributed to insufficient progestin support of the endometrial lining. Estrogen is involved in endometrial proliferation early on in the cycle and progestin is involved in endometrial atrophy and support later in the cycle. Both must be in the right combination to avoid breakthrough bleeding. If a patient reports breakthrough bleeding, nonadherence, drug–drug interactions, and infection should be ruled out first, as they may play a role.[4]

Many side effects can be attributed to the estrogen or progestin component, either because of an excess effect or a deficiency. Table 18.4 lists various hormone-related effects. With the wide variety of products available with differing hormonal activities, it is possible to manipulate the levels in an attempt to reduce a particular effect. For example, if a woman reports continued acne, she could switch to a product with less androgenic activity. Several guides are available that give detailed information on the evaluation of side effects and their management.[2,4,51]

Clearly, it is important to first rule out the possibility of serious adverse effects before continuing or changing the pill. Patients should be counseled to watch for warning signs that may indicate a serious problem and to report them immediately (Table 18.5).

An increase in the frequency of headache (both tension and migraine) has been noted to occur in women taking oral contraceptives. Approximately half of the women who develop vascular headaches with COCs report preexisting migraine attacks. There is evidence that falling estrogen levels may incite the cerebrovascular system to respond by producing cyclic migraine headaches.[52] Formulations that shorten the pill-free interval and provide very low doses of estrogen for the last several days (such as Mircette) may be useful for those women who have these menstruation-related migraines. Extended-use regimens may also be helpful. Patients with new-onset migraines or worsening headaches after initiation of a COC should see a physician and discontinue this method.

Increased corneal sensitivity, particularly contact lens discomfort, has been noted in about one of five women who take oral contraceptives.[53] Changes in corneal curvature and decreased tear secretion have been attributed to this side effect in oral contraceptive users. A variety of ocular changes have been attributed to the pill, ranging from retinal vascular accidents to decreases in visual acuity and color changes.[54]

TABLE 18.4 | Relation of Side Effects to Hormone Content

Estrogen Excess	Progestin Excess	Androgen Excess
Breast cystic changes	Cervicitis	Acne
Dysmenorrhea	Flow length decrease	Cholestatic jaundice
Heavy flow	Moniliasis	Hirsutism
Cervical exstrophy	Increased appetite	Libido increase
Uterine fibroid growth	Depression	Oily skin and scalp
Chloasma	Fatigue	Rash/pruritus
Telangiectasias	Noncyclic weight gain	Edema
	Libido decrease	

Estrogen Deficiency	Progestin Deficiency	Estrogen Excess or Progestin Deficiency
Absence of withdrawal bleeding	Breakthrough bleeding days 10–21	Bloating
Breakthrough bleeding days 1–9	Delayed withdrawal bleeding	Dizziness
Continuous bleeding and spotting	Dysmenorrhea	Edema
Flow decrease	Heavy flow	Cyclic headache
Atrophic vaginitis		Irritability
Vasomotor symptoms		Leg cramps
		Nausea/vomiting
		Cyclic visual changes
		Cyclic weight gain

Adapted with permission from Dickey RP. Managing contraceptive pill patients, 9th ed. Durant, OK: Essential Medical Information Systems, Inc., 1998.

TABLE 18.5 | Combination Oral Contraceptive Warning Signs

Symptom	Possible Significance
A: Abdominal pain	Hepatic tumor, gallbladder disease, thrombosis
C: Chest pain (severe cough or shortness of breath)	Myocardial infarction or pulmonary embolism
H: Headaches (severe dizziness or weakness)	Hypertension, migraines, or stroke
E: Eye problems (loss or blurring, speech problems)	Stroke or hypertension
S: Severe leg pain (calf or thigh)	Thrombosis

Repeated prospective and retrospective studies failed to find a correlation between the use of birth control pills and many of these abnormalities, which are found normally in a population of women of reproductive age. However, caution should be exercised in prescribing oral contraceptives to women with known ophthalmologic disorders.

Depression has been noted occasionally in COC users. Because of the lack of well-controlled trials and underlying prevalence of depression in this patient population, much controversy exists as to the cause. Depending on the severity and whether there is a temporal relationship, one could try altering the hormonal potency by switching to a lower-dose pill. Some women also seem to develop low pyridoxine levels while taking COCs and may respond to supplementation with 50 mg of vitamin B_6.[55] Careful monitoring of the depressed patient is recommended.

Drug Interactions. Evidence indicates that certain drugs may interfere with the efficacy of COCs. The converse is also true: COCs may modify the action of other drugs. Mechanisms thought to be responsible for these interactions include (a) interference with steroid absorption or reabsorption via enterohepatic circulation; (b) stimulation or inhibition of hepatic metabolism; (c) displacement of steroids from their receptor sites; and (d) opposing steroid action by some physiologic effect.

Gastroenteritis has long been associated with decreased GI transit time and steroid absorption. Because ethinyl estradiol conjugates are excreted in the bile, broken down by gut bacteria to active hormone, and then reabsorbed, anything that increases GI motility (e.g., diarrhea or stimulant laxatives) could reduce circulating concentrations of oral contraceptives and lead to contraceptive failure. Likewise, broad-spectrum antibiotics such as ampicillin or tetracycline may eliminate the gut microflora that is necessary for this enterohepatic circulation. Numerous well-documented clinical reports have appeared of pregnancies in women who have not missed COC doses but were also taking an antibiotic. However, no well-designed clinical studies have been able to prove an increased failure rate or even lower plasma hormone levels in patients taking antibiotics.[56]

The most clinically significant drug interactions occur with drugs that affect the hepatic metabolic enzymes through either induction or inhibition. Induction of microsomal enzymes results in increased clearance of the substrate, which in this case could lead to contraceptive failure and unintended pregnancy. Estrogens, including ethinyl estradiol, are substrates for the cytochrome P450 3A4 isoenzyme and thus may be affected primarily by drugs that induce this particular enzyme. These include rifampin, rifabutin, carbamazepine, felbamate, phenobarbital, phenytoin, primidone, and troglitazone.[57] Topiramate has also been reported to decrease estrogen levels through an unknown mechanism.[58] Options for patients requiring these medications include increasing the estrogenic strength of the pill to 50 μg (which may increase side effects) or, when possible, choosing another medication.

Of the class of antiepileptic drugs, valproic acid, ethosuximide, vigabatrin, and lamotrigine do not appear to interfere with the metabolism of estrogen. Griseofulvin use has also been reported to result in reduced serum hormone levels in several case reports.[59]

COCs may increase the clearance of benzodiazepines that undergo glucuronidation (e.g., lorazepam, oxazepam, temazepam). However, benzodiazepines that undergo oxidation (e.g., alprazolam, diazepam, chlordiazepoxide, triazolam), appear to compete with COCs for these enzymes; this could result in reduced effectiveness of the contraceptive or increased effects of the benzodiazepine.[4,5] Reduced clearance has also been suggested for corticosteroids, theophylline, aspirin, and acetaminophen. Patients taking these drugs should be monitored, with possible dose reduction if increased effects are seen. Chapter 3 offers a further discussion of potential drug–drug interactions.

Special Patient Groups

Patients With Diabetes. Historically, patients with established diabetes taking older, high-dose COCs showed a worsening of carbohydrate intolerance. It appears that these changes are caused by the progestin component because estrogens do not affect carbohydrate metabolism.[60] The newer progestins (desogestrel, gestodene [not available in the United States], and norgestimate), as well as low doses of COCs containing norethindrone, appear to have negligible effects on glucose tolerance.[61,62] Monophasic pills containing levonorgestrel have caused glucose intolerance in women who previously had gestational diabetes, but triphasic pills with levonorgestrel have not. A study evaluating the risk for development of type II diabetes in Latina women who previously had gestational diabetes found no increased risk for those using a low-dose COC containing ethinyl estradiol and norethindrone. Risk was significantly increased for those women using a contraceptive containing a progestin only.[63]

Generally, young women with a family history of diabetes or a personal history of gestational diabetes and some women with diabetes who do not have vascular complications can safely take low-dose COCs.

Women Older Than 35. Older women who are healthy and free of any contraindications can safely use low-dose COCs until menopause. The risk for MI seems to be increased primarily in women who are older than 35 years of age and who also smoke. Estrogen-containing contraceptives are not recommended in this population.

Postpartum Patients. Due to the hypercoagulable state of pregnancy, postpartum patients should avoid using estrogen-containing contraceptives at least 3 to 4 weeks after delivery. Right after pregnancy, women are at higher risk for developing blood clots. Progestin-only contraceptives may be used immediately postpartum if the patient does not intend to breastfeed.[4]

Breastfeeding Patients. The estrogen in COCs appears to reduce milk production in breastfeeding women.[4] Some constituents of COCs are found in breast milk as well, although adverse effects on infants have not been noted with the use of low-dose pills. Whereas some experts state that low-dose COCs can be used successfully in lactating women, others prefer progestin-only pills. If estrogen-containing pills are used, they should be delayed at least until 6 weeks postpartum, with 8 to 12 weeks being suggested by some, to allow milk production. Progestin-only pills, depot medroxyprogesterone acetate and medroxyprogesterone acetate injections, and the levonorgestrel intrauterine system do not appear to affect milk production and may be used while breastfeeding. Women should start progestin-only contraceptives approximately 6 weeks after delivery when breastfeeding, with the idea of preventing neonatal exposure to any steroids that may pass into the breast milk. In the first 6 weeks, infants still cannot metabolize or excrete drugs properly. Progestins probably do not harm lactation or nursing infants, but there are few data available on the subject because immediate postpartum use is not recommended.[4]

Unique Hormonal Combined Contraceptives

Transdermal Contraceptive Patch. In 2001, the FDA approved the transdermal contraceptive patch (Ortho Evra). The transdermal patch delivers the progestin norelgestromin 0.15 mg per day and the estrogen ethinyl estradiol 20 μg per day transdermally. The patch is a thin, matrix-like, pinkish-beige, adhesive square consisting of three layers. It is 1.75 inches long and has a surface area of 20 cm².[64] It contains a total of 6 mg of norelgestromin and 0.75 mg of ethinyl estradiol. Once absorbed into the body, norelgestromin is metabolized to the active progestin norgestimate.[64] The patch is very effective in preventing pregnancy. Unintended pregnancies in the first year of use with the patch were 1 per 100 women-years. In clinical trials, 5 out of the 15 pregnancies that occurred were in women who weighed 198 pounds (90 kg) or more.[64] Therefore, it has been concluded that the contraceptive patch is less effective in women who weigh more than 198 pounds (90 kg).

One patch is worn per week for 3 weeks. The fourth week is patch-free, and menses generally occurs at that time. The patch should be placed on a clean, dry, hairless skin area on the upper arm, shoulder, buttock, or abdomen. Application of the patch to the breasts should be avoided.[64] To remove the patch, users should peel the patch off the skin carefully and fold the adhesive sides together. The patch should be discarded in the trash away from the reach of children or pets. Patches should not be flushed down the toilet. Users should be instructed to rotate patch sites and apply the patch to a different area each week to avoid skin irritation. The patch may be worn while taking a shower, swimming, exercising, or sitting in a sauna.

Without prior use of a hormonal contraceptive, the patch should be applied either on the first day of menses or the Sunday following the start of menses.[64] A new patch is worn for 7 days and then changed on day 8, which is the "patch change day."[64] A backup birth control method should be used for the first 7 days of patch application. If switching from COCs to the patch, application of the patch should begin on the first day of withdrawal bleeding. If the patch is applied later than the first day of withdrawal bleeding, then a backup birth control method such as a condom, spermicide, or diaphragm should be used for 7 days. If more than 7 days go by after taking the last active COC pill, there is a chance that ovulation and conception may have occurred.[64] Patients should be advised to be using another nonhormonal birth control method until menses begins and the patch can be started at the appropriate time on the first day of menses.

From time to time, although rare, the patch may detach from the skin. If the patch falls off for less than 24 hours, it should be re-applied as soon as possible and no backup birth control method is necessary.[64] If the patch has been off for more than 24 hours, then a new patch should be applied. This will constitute a new cycle and a new "patch change day" for the user. A backup birth control method such as a condom and spermicide or diaphragm should be used for first 7 days of the "new cycle."[64] The user will experience a delayed menstrual period because she will be starting a new cycle of patches.

The most commonly reported side effects of the patch (9% to 20%) during clinical trials include breast symptoms, headache, application site reaction, nausea, upper respiratory infection, menstrual cramps, and abdominal pain.[64] Other possible side effects are similar to those of COCs.[64] Risks and benefits are similar to those of COCs. However, after a series of case reports involving blood clots with the use of the contraceptive patch, it was found that higher levels of ethinyl estradiol are absorbed from the patch. In late 2005, the FDA required label changes for Ortho Evra stating that "AUC and average concentration at steady state for ethinyl estradiol are approximately 60% higher in women using Ortho Eva compared to women using an oral contraceptive containing ethinyl estradiol 35μg." Precautions taken with COCs should also be taken with the contraceptive patch particularly those who might be at greater risk for blood clots, increased blood pressure, or stroke. Drug–drug interactions with the patch are not well studied and are thought to be similar to COCs.

Compliance and satisfaction with the contraceptive patch are high. According to one study, compliance with the patch was 88.7% versus 79.2% with the pill ($p < 0.001$) in women of reproductive age. In women less than 20 years old, the study showed a higher compliance rate of 87.8% with the patch versus 67.7% with the pill.[65] The contraceptive patch may be a good option in patients who have difficulty adhering to other contraceptive methods.[66] Women with skin sensitivity, those who have difficulty removing patches weekly, those sensitive to estrogen side effects or those who are self-conscious about the appearance of the patch on the skin are not good candidates for this method.

Contraceptive Vaginal Ring. In 2001, the FDA approved the use of a contraceptive vaginal ring (NuvaRing) that delivers the progestin etonogestrel 0.120 mg per day and the estrogen ethinyl estradiol 0.015 mg per day.[67] The ring is nonbiodegradable, flexible, transparent, and colorless. The ring's outer diameter is 54 mm and its cross-sectional diameter is 4 mm. It is made of ethylene vinylacetate copolymers and magnesium stearate and contains a total of 11.7 mg of etonogestrel and 2.7 mg of ethinyl estradiol.[67] The ring is highly effective in preventing pregnancy. During clinical trials, only one or two unintended pregnancies occurred in the first year per 100 women-years of use.[67]

The ring is inserted vaginally and left in place continuously for 3 weeks at a time. The fourth week, the ring is removed and withdrawal bleeding usually occurs. The ring may be worn during sexual intercourse, with a tampon, and with topical therapies such as antifungal creams or spermicides. Douching, however, is discouraged with vaginal ring use. In some instances, more commonly when removing a tampon, during bowel movements, or in cases of severe constipation and straining, the ring may be expelled from the vagina. If expelled, the ring should be rinsed with cool to lukewarm water (not hot) and re-inserted as soon as possible (within 3 hours). If the ring is left out of the vagina for longer than 3 hours, a backup birth control method such as condoms should be used until the ring has been in place for at least 7 days.[67] A diaphragm should not be used as a backup birth control method while using the vaginal ring, as the ring may interfere with proper placement of the diaphragm.

Without prior use of a hormonal contraceptive, use of the ring should be started within the first 5 days of the menstrual cycle, preferably the first day of menses. A backup birth control method should be used for at least 7 days after insertion of the ring. If switching from COCs to the ring, use of the ring should start within 7 days after taking the last active pill and no later than when the new cycle of active pills were to start.[67] Use of the ring can be started any day of the month when switching from progestin-only pills as long as no day has passed in between without taking a pill. Ring use may also be initiated on the scheduled day of the next progestin-only injection.[67]

Insertion of the vaginal ring may be done in various ways. The woman may insert the ring by standing with one leg up, by squatting, or while lying down. The ring should be squeezed so that the ends of the ring touch each other, and should be inserted into the vagina. The exact location of the ring is not important as long as it rests inside the vagina.[67] The ring is removed by hooking the index finger under the forward rim or grasping the ring between the index and middle finger and then pulling the ring out of the vagina.[67] The ring should be folded up in the foil packaging it came in and placed in the trash, out of the reach of children and pets. It should not be flushed down the toilet.

The most commonly reported side effects (5% to 14%) with the ring include vaginitis, headache, upper respiratory tract infection, leukorrhea, sinusitis, weight gain, and nausea.[67] Other possible side effects are similar to those of COCs.[67] Users have also reported feeling the ring. Sexual partners also reported sensing the ring during intercourse, but 90% of users did not cite this as a problem.[67] In one study of 1,950 women ages 18 to 41 who used the contraceptive ring for 13 cycles, 96% of users were satisfied with the ring and 97% said they would recommend it to a friend.[68] Users cited ''not having to remember anything'' and ''ease of use'' as top reasons for liking the ring.

The ring also has a good compliance profile. In another study of 247 women ages 18 to 40, a compliance rate of 92.4% was reported for ring users and 75.4% for pill users.[69] The contraceptive ring may be a suitable choice for women who have difficulty adhering to other methods. However, it may be not be suitable in women who are more susceptible to vaginal irritation or vaginal tears or who are uncomfortable with inserting the ring vaginally.

Risks and benefits are similar to those of COCs. Precautions taken with COCs should also be taken with the contraceptive vaginal ring. Drug–drug interactions with the ring are not well studied and are thought to be similar to COCs.[67]

Extended Use. More recently, extended-use regimens have become available. Extended-use contraception is described as using active hormonal contraception for longer than 1 month without a hormone-free interval—generally 3 months of active hormone and then a hormone-free week where menses occurs. In 2003, the FDA approved the first extended-use contraceptive regimen, Seasonale. This extended regimen of levonorgestrel 0.15 mg and ethinyl estradiol 30 μg is available in a 91-tablet pack containing 84 active tablets and 7 inert tablets.[70] The extended-cycle regimen effectively results in four menstrual periods a year, but it was associated with more breakthrough bleeding compared to the conventional 28-day cycle.[71]

Extended regimens can also be used with other monophasic COCs. The patient may take the active pills of one pack, skip the placebo pills, and begin a new pack of active COC pills. This should be done only under the supervision of a physician and only with monophasic pills. Other types of COCs, such as biphasic or triphasic packs, have varying amounts of estrogen and progestin, which may result in fluctuating hormone levels and unwanted side effects.

Extended regimens with the contraceptive patch and vaginal ring are also being studied. The patch regimen would entail wearing one patch a week for 12 weeks and then having one week patch-free for menses. One study found this regimen to decrease bleeding and spotting episodes.[72] Subjects in the study were also very satisfied with the extended regimen. The vaginal ring regimen would involve a new ring placed in the vagina every 3 weeks for 12 weeks and then a ring-free week when menses would occur. A recent study looked at 28-day, 49-day, 91-day, and 364-day extended regimens with the vaginal ring.[73] The study found that all regimens were well tolerated, but spotting and bleeding occurred more in the longer regimens.

The extended-use regimens may be ideal in women who prefer fewer menstrual cycles or who suffer from estrogen withdrawal side effects such as migraines or mood swings. Women using the extended regimens should be counseled about possible breakthrough bleeding and spotting. Other side effects are similar to regular-cycle COCs. Long-term side effects of the extended regimens are still being studied.

Progestin-Only Contraceptives

Oral Forms. The second type of oral contraceptive is sometimes called the "mini-pill." This form does not contain estrogen and provides low doses of either norethindrone or norgestrel taken daily without a pill-free interval. Progestins prevent pregnancy by inhibiting ovulation, thickening the cervical mucus, and causing a thin atrophic endometrium. In this case, though, ovulation is not inhibited with any predictability. Some women continue to ovulate regularly, some do not, and others ovulate sporadically.[4] The effectiveness of this method is thus less than that provided by COCs. Approximately 8% of women will become pregnant in the first year of typical use.[4]

Even though this method of birth control is slightly less effective, it does offer some advantages, particularly in women who should avoid estrogen-containing contraceptives. This includes those with estrogen-related adverse effects, smokers, and women who are breastfeeding, as well as those with a history of deep vein thrombosis or cardiovascular complications. The effectiveness in lactating women is nearly 100% because breastfeeding itself provides a contraceptive effect.[74] Progestin does not affect the quantity or quality of milk produced, making this an ideal form for this patient population, although many recommend initiating this method only after 6 weeks postpartum.[4] Other benefits include reduced menstrual blood loss and anemia, decreased dysmenorrhea, less risk of endometrial cancer, and possibly a lower risk for pelvic inflammatory disease (PID).

Because ovulation is not blocked consistently, and changes in cervical mucus can be affected by late pills, this is a method that requires absolute compliance: the pill must be taken every 24 hours. Other than the higher failure rate, risks are few with the mini-pill. As with all other forms of hormonal birth control, it should not be used in women with unexplained vaginal bleeding, breast cancer, or active liver disease. Women with cardiovascular conditions or diabetes who choose this method should be carefully monitored.

Mini-pills can have unpredictable effects on the menstrual cycle. Women who continue to ovulate will have regular periods, but others will experience irregular periods and spotting. Some will develop amenorrhea. Women considering the mini-pill should be informed about these effects and should accept the high probability of unpredictable bleeding. In some women, symptoms of depression, premenstrual syndrome, or breast tenderness worsen, rather than decrease, while taking progestin-only pills.

A missed pill with this method is more of a concern. Some experts recommend that a backup method of birth control be used at all times or at least for the first cycle while the routine is being established. If pill administration is delayed for more than 3 hours, it is considered a missed pill and should be taken as soon as possible. A backup contraception method should be used for the following 48 hours. Women who miss two pills should take two pills for 2 days, use backup contraception, or consider EC if intercourse has occurred.[4] Concurrent use with drugs that induce hepatic microsomal enzymes may result in unacceptably low levels of the progestin and contraceptive failure, and thus should be avoided.

Intramuscular Depot Medroxyprogesterone Acetate Injection. Depot medroxyprogesterone acetate (DMPA) has been used for many years in other countries as an injectable contraceptive and was approved for use in the United States in 1992. The drug suppresses the preovulatory surge of LH and reduces levels of LH and FSH, thus inhibiting ovulation; it also produces the cervical mucus changes and endometrial growth changes discussed earlier.[2] It provides effective contraception, resulting in a 0.3% pregnancy rate in the first year of use. DMPA is given as a deep intramuscular injection in a dose of 150 mg every 12 weeks. Plasma levels of contraceptive are reached within 24 hours, with peak concentrations in 20 days. The optimal time to initiate DMPA is within 5 days of the onset of menses. This ensures that the patient is not pregnant and prevents ovulation during the first month of use.

Along with providing the same benefits as the progestin-only pills, DMPA is also advantageous for women who have difficulty with daily compliance. Significant drug interactions are unlikely. Patients with sickle cell disease may experience improvements in their condition while receiving DMPA, possibly due to increased red blood cell stability and reduced painful crises.[75] Patients with seizures may experience a reduction in the frequency of seizures, which may be due to sedative effects of the hormone.[52,76]

Besides the general precautions with hormonal contraceptives, women considering DMPA should be aware that this is not a quickly reversible method. Because of the slow clearance of the drug from the body, it may take 6 to 12 months before fertility returns, which is a significant difference from other methods. Also allergic reactions are possible, although they are rare.

The most common side effect of DMPA is irregular bleeding. Rarely is the bleeding heavy; in most cases it results in prolonged light bleeding or spotting. Amenorrhea develops in at least 50% of women after 1 year of use, which may be seen as a benefit by some women. Weight gain (mean weight gain in clinical trials was 7.6 pounds after 2 years of use), headaches, abdominal discomfort, breast tenderness, and depression also may occur and if significant may require discontinuation of the injections.

Reduced bone density and reductions in high-density lipoprotein cholesterol levels have also been noted in DMPA users. In November 2004, the FDA issued a black box warning for DMPA stating that long-term use of the medication may result in significant bone density loss that may not be reversible after discontinuation of the drug. The black box warning reads, "Women who use Depo-Provera Contraceptive Injection may lose significant bone mineral density. Bone loss is greater with increasing duration of use and may not be completely reversible. It is unknown if use of Depo-Provera Contraceptive Injection during adolescence or early adulthood, a critical period of bone accretion, will reduce peak bone mass and increase the risk of osteoporotic fracture later in life. Depo-Provera Contraceptive Injection should be used as a long-term birth control method (e.g., longer than 2 years) only if other birth control methods are inadequate." Therefore, women using DMPA should take calcium supplements of 1,000 to 1,500 mg daily.

There was particular concern in women ages 15 to 20 years old and if DMPA exposure was increasing the risk of osteoporosis later in life.[77] In addition, 10% of female adolescents who use birth control use DMPA, compared to 3% of all women who use DMPA nationally. One study, however, found that lower bone density does appear to recover in adolescent females once DMPA use is discontinued.[78] Detailed guidelines on the management of adverse effects and delayed injections can be found in several references.[2,4,5,79]

Subcutaneous Medroxyprogesterone Acetate Injection.
In 2005, the FDA approved a subcutaneous form of medroxyprogesterone acetate (Depo-subQ Provera 104) to be administered every 12 to 14 weeks. Depo-subQ Provera 104 is available as prefilled syringes with a concentration of medroxyprogesterone acetate (MPA) of 160 mg per mL. Each syringe contains 0.65 mL (104 mg).[80] MPA works similarly to DMPA to prevent pregnancy. MPA is also FDA approved to treat endometriosis.

MPA is very effective in preventing pregnancy. In clinical trials, there were 0 pregnancies reported in the first year of use for 100 women-years. Side effects and precautions are similar to those of DMPA.[80] An advantage to MPA over DMPA is that patients can administer MPA to themselves and do not require a healthcare professional to administer the medication. This may help improve adherence and the timeliness of administration.

Initiation of MPA should be within the first 5 days after menses begins. If switching from COCs, the ring, or the patch, MPA should be administered no later than 7 days after the use of the hormonal contraceptive. Before use, women should make sure they are not pregnant. MPA should be injected in the upper thigh or abdomen every 12 to 14 weeks, preferably every 12 weeks. If the subsequent MPA injection is not administered within 14 weeks, a backup birth control method should be used and pregnancy should be ruled out before MPA is restarted.[80]

Subdermal Implants. Subdermal implants are an ideal choice for a woman who has difficulty complying with daily pill taking or regular injections and does not wish to become pregnant for several years. Currently, there are no subdermal implants available on the U.S. market. A few implants have been available in the past, but due to lack of efficacy have been removed. Among them was the progestin-only Norplant System. Norplant contained levonorgestrel (216 mg total) in six flexible silicone rods, each about 3.4 cm long. Under local anesthesia, a small incision was made in the upper arm, and the implants were inserted subdermally in a fan-like distribution. The hormone was released at a fairly constant rate, which slowly declined over time but provided very effective contraception for 5 years. The relatively low circulating levels of levonorgestrel were not sufficient to suppress the secretion of FSH and LH completely, but ovulation was suppressed at least 50% of the time.[5] Also, levonorgestrel in this form has the same impact on the endometrium and cervical mucus as with other forms. These effects and the lack of required compliance contributed to a low pregnancy rate of 0.05% in the first year and a cumulative rate of 3.9% after 5 years. Heavier women appeared to have a slightly higher failure rate.[5] Side effects included irregular bleeding that was heavy at times (but tended to decrease with time), headaches, nervousness, weight gain, acne, breast tenderness, and ovarian cysts. After Norplant was recalled due to lack of efficacy, it was found that many of the lots recalled did not lack efficacy, but Wyeth Pharmaceuticals decided not to market the drug again. A newer implant system containing two rods instead of six, Norplant II, is under review by the FDA and may be available in the future.

Levonorgestrel Intrauterine System. The levonorgestrel-releasing intrauterine system (Mirena) was FDA approved in 2000 for up to 5 years of use as a means of intrauterine contraception. The intrauterine system consists of a 32-mm T-shaped polyethylene frame with a total drug reservoir of 52 mg of levonorgestrel. The system releases 20 μg per day of levonorgestrel (LNg20) into the uterine cavity, which results in high endometrial tissue concentrations and low blood levels. The high local levels of levonorgestrel cause changes to the endometrium and cervical mucus that discourage sperm transport, implantation, and development of the blastocyst.

The levonorgestrel-releasing intrauterine system is extremely effective in preventing pregnancy: the unintended pregnancy rate in the first year of use was 0.1% for both perfect and typical use.[81] There is a fairly rapid return to fertility, with approximately 80% of women conceiving within 12 months of discontinuation.

The LNg20 system is inserted vaginally into the uterus by a healthcare professional such as a nurse practitioner or physician. Strings attached to the device hang down into the vagina to help ensure proper placement and to help patients know the device is inserted.

If a patient wants to start using a different hormonal contraceptive method, the device should be removed within the first 7 days of menses and the new method started at that time.[81]

While the copper intrauterine device (IUD; ParaGard) can increase menstrual flow, the levonorgestrel-releasing IUD can actually reduce menstrual flow (due to the progestin effects) and may be advantageous in women with menorrhagia, anemia, uterine myomas, and dysmenorrhea-related endometriosis.[82] Contraindications to the levonorgestrel device include pregnancy (or suspected pregnancy), uterine fibroids, acute PID or a history of PID, postpartum endometritis or infected abortion within the past 3 months, known or suspected uterine or cervical neoplasia or an abnormal Pap smear, genital bleeding of unknown etiology, untreated acute cervicitis or vaginitis, acute liver disease or liver tumor, multiple sexual partners (on the part of the patient or her partner), conditions associated with increased susceptibility to infections (e.g., leukemia, AIDS), genital actinomycosis, a previously inserted IUD that has not been removed, hypersensitivity to any component of this product, known or suspected breast cancer, or a history of ectopic pregnancy or condition that would predispose to ectopic pregnancy.[81] Irregular spotting is common following insertion of the device. Other adverse effects include menstrual changes, lower abdominal pain (cramps), back pain, headache, mood changes, and nausea. The section on intrauterine devices offers more information about serious side effects and reasons for discontinuation of IUDs.

NONHORMONAL CONTRACEPTION

A variety of nonhormonal contraceptive devices are available, including spermicidal agents, condoms, IUDs, and diaphragms. The efficacy of these products in theory and in use is shown in Table 18.1.

Spermicidal Agents. Spermicidal agents are available without a prescription in a wide variety of forms, including film, foam, jelly, cream, suppositories, or tablets. They may be used alone or in combination with other methods. Estimates of efficacy vary widely because of the difficulty in controlling all the variables with a method that is quite user-dependent. Pregnancy rates may range from as low as 3% to 6% to more than 40%.[83] These rates are improved when spermicides are combined with other methods.

The primary active ingredient used in the United States in nonoxynol-9, which kills sperm by disrupting the sperm cell membrane. For it to work properly, it must be applied on or near the cervix before intercourse. Products such as films, tablets, or suppositories must be inserted at least 15 minutes before intercourse to allow dissolution and dispersal of the product. When used alone, spermicides are effective for approximately 1 hour. More spermicide must be inserted for additional acts of intercourse.[83]

Benefits of using spermicidal agents include their wide availability in pharmacies and grocery stores, low cost, and reduced risk of some sexually transmitted infections (STIs) such as gonorrhea, chlamydia, and trichomoniasis.[4] Unfortunately, it does not appear that nonoxynol-9 provides adequate protection against human immunodeficiency virus (HIV).

Skin irritation or allergy may develop in either partner due to the spermicide or other ingredients. Switching to another form may be helpful. Women with abnormal vaginal anatomy may have difficulty using these products properly. Serious adverse effects have not been reported. Also, several well-designed recent studies have shown no increased risk of congenital malformations in newborns[84] or spontaneous abortions[85] of women who conceived while using spermicides.

With proper selection and appropriate use, these products can be successful. It is important to emphasize details such as timing and insertion techniques.

Condoms. Due to their ability to prevent STIs and pregnancy when used consistently and correctly, condoms are one of the most popular contraceptives. They are also accessible, inexpensive, and readily usable. During the 1980s, there was a dramatic increase in condom sales in the United States. Currently, condoms are made to be worn not only by men, but by women as well. Condoms for men are latex rubber or polyurethane sheaths that are worn over an erect penis during coitus. This forms a physical barrier that prevents the transmission of semen into the vagina. Although pregnancy rates are higher than for users of COCs, barrier methods are effective in preventing the transmission of STIs, including HIV, from either partner. Several in vitro and in vivo studies have demonstrated that latex condoms prevent the transmission of viruses, specifically herpes virus and HIV, when used for vaginal, orogenital, and anogenital intercourse.[86–88] In addition, *Chlamydia trachomatis* and gonorrheal infections can be prevented. There are also ''natural membrane'' condoms that are made of processed collagenous tissue from the intestinal cecum of lambs. This type of condom is thinner and more porous and conducts heat well, but it does not block the transmission of infectious organisms.[4,83] It still, however, may be used to prevent pregnancy in those sensitive to latex. Polyurethane condoms are also available for those who are sensitive to latex rubber. Polyurethane condoms are unique in that they can be used with a water-based or oil-based lubricant. They also conduct heat well but are more prone to breakage and slippage.[89,90]

More than 100 brands of condoms are available in different shapes, sizes, colors, and thicknesses. Some condoms have a small amount of spermicide applied to the inside and/or outside of the condom. Condoms are marketed rolled or unrolled, lubricated or unlubricated, and ribbed and may have reservoir ends to collect the semen. When the condom is put on, half an inch of empty space should be left at the tip if the condom does not have a reservoir end. To prevent spillage during withdrawal, the rim of the condom should be held against the base of the penis during withdrawal, promptly after ejaculation. A condom should be used only once.

Oil-based products (e.g., petroleum jelly, hand lotion, or vegetable oil) should never be used to lubricate a condom because they cause deterioration of the latex (except for polyurethane condoms, as noted earlier).[83]

K-Y jelly, contraceptive foams and gels, Astroglide, and saliva are examples of acceptable lubricants. Examples of unacceptable lubricants include rubbing alcohol, margarine or butter, edible oils, and petroleum jelly.[83] Trying to test a condom for holes by filling it up with water, as well as unrolling it and then sliding it over the penis, increases the probability of breakage.

A condom for women called the Reality condom has been available over-the-counter since 1993. It is a polyurethane sheath or pouch that is closed at one end and has two flexible polyurethane rings, one at each end. The female condom is approximately 17 cm in length and 7.8 cm in diameter. As with male condoms, the female condom will help prevent pregnancy and is believed to prevent the transmission of STIs, although this has not been proven.[5] The pouch is prelubricated on the inside with a silicone-based lubricant, with an additional bottle of lubricant included. The extrapolated unintended pregnancy rate for one year is 25% with typical use and 5% with perfect use.[83]

The open end with the outer ring remains outside the vagina to cover the perineum. The inner ring is needed for insertion and to hold the pouch in place. When inserting the pouch, the inner ring is held between the thumb and middle finger while the index finger is placed on the pouch between the other two fingers. While squeezing the inner ring, the pouch is inserted as far as possible into the vagina to cover the cervix. The pouch should not be twisted. The pouch should be removed before standing up by squeezing and twisting the outer ring and gently pulling. If the penis does not move freely in and out, if the outer ring is pushed inside, or if there is noise during intercourse, more lubricant can be applied. A new female condom should be inserted before each act of intercourse. The male condom and female condom should not be used together, as it may cause friction and displace the female condom and increase the risk of condom breakage.

There have been some problems with the acceptability of the female condom. The visibility of the outer ring, unpleasant noises during intercourse, and problems with the initial insertion are common complaints. However, with careful training and practice, it is a useful method of contraception and probably protects against STIs.

Intrauterine Devices. The idea of inserting a foreign body into the uterus to prevent pregnancy is not new. The use of intrauterine stones dates back to ancient times. Natural fibers such as silkworm gut were investigated in the early 1900s. After World War II, artificial fibers and various types of polyethylene became available and were molded in many ways to produce IUDs. The copper-containing IUD gained popularity in the 1960s, and an IUD that slowly releases progesterone was an innovative development of the 1970s.

Currently, IUDs are commonly used by women worldwide, but less than 1% of women in the United States choose them. Litigation concerning IUDs was responsible for many manufacturers voluntarily withdrawing their products, although at this point litigation has significantly dropped off, with an increased emphasis on patient selection, informed consent, and improved documentation.[4]

There are two products available now in the United States. The copper T 380A (ParaGard by FEI Women's Health) is a copper-containing IUD that can be left in place for up to 10 years, and the levonorgestrel-releasing intrauterine system (Mirena) can be left in place for up to 5 years.

The mechanism of action of the IUD depends on the type. Copper-containing IUDs appear to cause changes in uterine and tubal fluids that alter sperm and ova transport and prevent fertilization.[91] The copper ions inhibit acrosomal enzyme activation and sperm motility, thus inhibiting the sperm from reaching the fallopian tube and fertilizing the ovum.[4] The hormones in the Mirena system have the same types of effects on the uterus as other forms of progestin: thickening of cervical mucus, impairment of motility, and disruption of ovulation.

As long as the IUD is inserted correctly and remains in place, it is a highly effective method (Table 18.1). Users should be taught to check for the string extruding from the cervix to ensure that the IUD has not been expelled.

The IUD is a reasonable option for women who need reliable, reversible long-term contraception, who cannot take hormones (for the ParaGard Copper T 380A), and for whom compliance with other methods is a problem. Women in a mutually monogamous relationship who have already delivered at least one child may be better suited for this method, although with careful counseling others may consider it as well.

There is an increased risk of PID in women with IUDs who are subsequently exposed to STIs. The risk appears to be greatest in the first few weeks after insertion and could have ramifications for the woman's future fertility.[92] Also, should a pregnancy occur while the IUD is in place, there is a significantly increased chance of spontaneous abortion occurring, even if the IUD is removed early. Other problems with the IUD include dysmenorrhea and abnormal bleeding or spotting. The levonorgestrel-releasing device appears to decrease these types of side effects. Also, rarely an IUD gradually works its way through the uterine wall and may need to be removed from the abdominal cavity by laparoscopic procedures. In the first year, up to 10% of women may spontaneously expel the IUD.

Women should be informed about the following warning signs that require medical attention:[4]

P: period late (pregnancy); abnormal spotting or bleeding
A: abdominal pain or pain with intercourse
I: infection exposure (any STI) or abnormal discharge
N: not feeling well, fever, chills
S: string missing, shorter or longer

Diaphragm. The diaphragm is a flexible dome-shaped rubber cap that is available in several styles and diameters (50 to 95 mm). It is inserted into the vagina by the woman before intercourse and blocks the opening to the uterus by covering the cervix. The diaphragm must be fitted by a clinician and should be refitted at each annual examination or if the woman delivers a baby, has an abortion, or has a significant change in weight.

The most effective use of the diaphragm is in combination with spermicidal agents. The mechanical barrier is useful for holding the spermicide near the cervical os. Spermicides also aid insertion because of their lubricating properties. At least a teaspoonful of spermicidal jelly or cream should be placed into the dome and spread around the inside of the rim before insertion. The diaphragm must remain in place for at least 6 hours after intercourse. Oil-based lubricants (e.g., petroleum jelly or lotions) may cause deterioration of the diaphragm and are not recommended. If additional lubrication is needed, more spermicide or a water-soluble lubricant may be used. Another full applicator of spermicide should be inserted into the vagina, leaving the diaphragm in place, before each subsequent act of intercourse or if more than 6 hours has elapsed since insertion. There may be a risk of toxic shock syndrome if the diaphragm is left in place for more than 24 hours. After it has been removed, the diaphragm should be washed and stored carefully. The diaphragm may be used during menses.

The key to successful diaphragm use is motivation. Many clinicians fail to recognize the diaphragm as a viable contraceptive option. However, because of its mechanical action, it is a method of contraception practically devoid of side effects. The diaphragm is not advised for use in patients who have recurrent urinary tract infections or a history of toxic shock syndrome. Also, trained personnel are needed to fit the device and properly counsel the patient.

Cervical Cap. The cervical cap is a barrier method smaller than a diaphragm that fits over the cervix. It was removed from the U.S. market in March 2005 due to declining interest in the product.

Sponge. Another form of vaginal contraception is a nonprescription, disposable polyurethane foam sponge called the Today sponge. It is much smaller and thicker than a diaphragm, with a ribbon loop for removal. The sponge is impregnated with nonoxynol-9, which is activated by adding water shortly before insertion. The sponge can be left in place over the cervix for up to 24 hours. Contraceptive protection is provided for up to 24 hours regardless of the frequency of intercourse. It should be left in for at least 6 hours after intercourse. Its effectiveness is higher in nulliparous women: the failure rate was 18% to 20% in the first year versus 36% to 40% in parous women.[4] There is a risk of toxic shock syndrome with sponge use, so it should not be left in place for longer than 24 hours. Frequent use of the sponge may increase the risk of cervical and vaginal ulcerations.[4]

Production of the sponge was voluntarily halted by the manufacturer in 1995 because of an inability to comply with more stringent government-directed mandates at its manufacturing facility, but is now available again.

EMERGENCY CONTRACEPTION

EC is the use of a method after intercourse to prevent unintentional pregnancy. EC is well known and widely used in some countries, but few women in the United States have ever used EC, and many are unfamiliar with this method,[93,94] which is unfortunate given the high rate of unintended pregnancies. It has been known for years that a combination of high doses of estrogen and progestin is effective in preventing pregnancy, but it was not until 1997 that the FDA published an opinion supporting the use of the products as safe and effective postcoital contraception.[95] EC is sometimes referred to as the "morning-after pill," but the term "emergency contraception" is preferred because it does not give the impression that it is only to be taken the morning after sex. In the United States, EC is mainly known as hormonal emergency contraception, although there are other methods of EC.

The two methods that are widely used and best studied are the progestin-only and the combined estrogen and progestin (Yuzpe) regimens. Both regimens consist of two doses of oral contraceptive pills taken 12 hours apart after intercourse. Although to help improve adherence the two tablets may be taken at the same time, but this increases the risk of nausea particularly with the Yuzpe regimen. The progestin-only regimen consists of two doses of levonorgestrel 0.75 mg (Plan B). The combined estrogen and progestin regimen consists of two doses each of 100 μg of ethinyl estradiol plus 0.5 to 0.75 mg of levonorgestrel (or 1 mg of norgestrel). These two regimens can be made from a combination of the available oral contraceptive pills (Table 18.6).

At one time, both regimens (Plan B and Preven) were available as products specifically marketed for EC. Currently, the only product specifically marketed for EC is two doses of levonorgestrel 0.75 mg, known as Plan B. Preven (2 doses of levonorgestrel 0.5 mg and ethinyl estradiol 100 μg) was removed from the market in 2004.

EC is not an abortion; it works to prevent pregnancy. It was first thought that EC inhibited ovulation, prevented fertilization by changing the consistency of cervical mucus and altering the transport of sperm and egg, interfered with the maintenance of the corpus luteum, and reduced endometrial receptivity to implantation of the fertilized egg.[96–98] However, recent animal studies show that EC may not have a post-fertilization effect and affects only ovulation and sperm transport and prevents fertilization.[99,100] Clarification of this mechanism is important for those who consider fertilization to be conception.

EC is FDA approved for use with the first dose taken within 72 hours of unprotected intercourse. Indications for EC use include rape, exposure to a teratogen, unprotected intercourse, or a problem with a contraceptive (condom

TABLE 18.6	Oral Contraceptive Used for Emergency Contraception in the United States

Brand	Pills per Dose	Ethinyl Estradiol per Dose (μg)	Levonorgestrel per Dose (mg)[a]
Nordette	4 light-orange pills[b]	120	0.60
Levlen	4 light-orange pills[b]	120	0.60
Lo/Ovral	4 white pills[b]	120	0.60
Triphasil	4 yellow pills[b]	120	0.50
Tri-Levlen	4 yellow pills[b]	120	0.50
Ovral	2 white pills[b]	100	0.50
Alesse	5 pink pills[b]	100	0.50
Ovrette	20 yellow pills[c]	0	0.75

Reprinted with permission from Hatcher RA, Trussell J, Stewart F, et al. Contraceptive technology, 17th ed. New York: Ardent Media Inc., 1998.
[a] The progestin in Ovral, Lo/Ovral, and Ovrette is norgestrel, which contains two isomers, only one of which (levonorgestrel) is bioactive; the amount of norgestrel in each dose is twice the amount of levonorgestrel.
[b] The treatment schedule is one dose within 72 hours after unprotected intercourse and another dose 12 hours later.
[c] The treatment schedule in the only published prospective study of levonorgestrel was one 0.75 mg tablet (equivalent to 20 Ovrette pills) within 48 hours after unprotected intercourse and another tablet 12 hours later. However, interim data from a large World Health Organization study indicate that the regimen is effective when initiated up to 72 hours after unprotected intercourse.

breaks, contraceptive pills are missed, vaginal ring or IUD slips out, or contraceptive patch falls off).

While EC is more effective the sooner it is taken, it may provide protection up to 120 hours after unprotected intercourse.[101] When used within 72 hours after sex, the combined estrogen and progestin regimen prevents about 74% of expected pregnancies, the progestin-only regimen about 85%.[102,103]

Hormonal EC is very safe. The most frequent adverse events reported include nausea and vomiting, which are more common with the combined estrogen and progestin (Yuzpe) regimen. In some cases, particularly with the Yuzpe regimen, antiemetics such as meclizine may be given 1 hour prior to administration of EC.[104] If a woman vomits within 2 hours of taking her EC dose, she should take another dose. Other adverse effects include irregular bleeding, which should not be confused with onset of menses, dizziness, headache, abdominal pain, and breast tenderness.

There are no contraindications to using hormonal EC, but this method is not indicated for a woman with a confirmed or suspected pregnancy. This treatment will not work if the patient is already pregnant. However, if hormonal EC is given early in pregnancy, it is unlikely that the fetus will be harmed.[4,105]

There are other EC methods used, but they are not as well known to the lay public. Insertion of an IUD within 5 days of unprotected intercourse is a form of EC and very effective at preventing pregnancy.[106] The Copper-T IUD inhibits sperm motility, prevents fertilization, and stops implantation.[4] This method is not as easily accessible and requires a healthcare professional to insert the IUD. In some cases mifepristone (RU 486) can serve as a method of EC if used with 5 days of unprotected intercourse.[107] The timing of administration differentiates when mifepristone is considered an EC agent versus an abortive agent. Mifepristone is considered EC when given within 5 days of unprotected intercourse. It stops follicle maturation, prevents the LH surge, and disrupts endometrial support.[107] If mifepristone is given after pregnancy in confirmed, it is then being used as an abortive agent.

PREGNANCY TERMINATION

Despite the availability and effectiveness of contraceptive methods, unintended pregnancies still occur at a high rate. Women choosing to end a pregnancy are faced with several difficult decisions. Currently, women may opt for either surgical or pharmacologic methods for pregnancy termination.

Mifepristone (RU 486) has been available in a few European countries for several years and was FDA approved in 2000 for pregnancy termination. Mifepristone is a competitive progesterone antagonist and acts by causing decidual breakdown and detachment of the embryo. It also may increase responsiveness to uterine prostaglandins, resulting in increased uterine contractions and expulsion. It appears to be most effective when given in early pregnancy (i.e., before 7 weeks).[108] It is given orally, then two days later is followed by oral or vaginal misoprostol, a prostaglandin E_1 analogy, which improves efficacy by causing strong contractions, cervical ripening, and dialation of the cervix.[109] Most women will experience cramping and bleeding, sometimes up to 14 days after taking the medications. Most women will pass their pregnancy after the dose misoprostol, but some women may take up to four weeks to complete the process.

Misoprostol is also sometimes used with methotrexate, which acts by blocking folic acid in fetal cells, disrupting their division. This combination also appears to be highly effective but has not been extensively studied.[110,111] Most protocols use an intramuscular injection of methotrexate, followed several days later with misoprostol tablets inserted vaginally.

All pharmacologic options require close monitoring, follow-up, and support. In 2005, the FDA issued an alert for the mifepristone/misoprostol regimen after four women died of sepsis after their abortions. It is unknown if the regimen had any effect on the development of sepsis. Health care providers should educate patients electing to have an abortion on the signs and symptoms of sepsis.[112] Also it is important to note that women can quickly become pregnant again after abortion, and options for contraception should be thoroughly discussed.

IMPROVING OUTCOMES

Assisting women and men in choosing an appropriate contraceptive method and teaching them to use it consistently and correctly should help reduce the rate of unintended pregnancies. For women who choose oral contraceptives, it is important to stress the correct day to start the pills and how to avoid missing pills, such as choosing a time of day they will most likely remember, or connecting the pill administration with another daily routine such as brushing their teeth before bedtime. Patients should know what to do in the event of a missed pill and should be encouraged to refill their prescriptions before they finish a pack. Many failures occur because the next cycle of pills is not started on time.

With barrier methods, the appropriate techniques for insertion, removal, and lubricant use should be reviewed. Patients should be advised to keep adequate supplies on hand to encourage consistent use.

Regardless of the method chosen, patients should also choose a backup method to have on hand if their primary method fails or if doses are missed. Patients should also be aware of the availability of EC. They should be reminded that condoms provide protection against STIs, but most other contraceptive methods do not. Finally, every sexually active woman should be reminded of the need for regular physical examinations and screening for cervical cancer.

KEY POINTS

- The choice of a contraceptive method is dependent on individual factors, including the safety and efficacy of the method, the person's ability to use the method correctly, concurrent conditions, and the needs and desires of the couple, such as cost, side effect profile, reversibility of contraception, and access to healthcare
- Combined hormonal contraception can be used safely and effectively by many women if properly selected, counseled, and monitored
- Combined hormonal contraception provide many contraceptive and non-contraceptive health benefits, including significant reductions in ovarian and endometrial cancers
- Risks of combined hormonal contraception use increase in women who are already at risk for cardiovascular disease, including smokers, patients with hypertension or moderate to severe diabetes, and those who have already suffered a vascular event such as a MI, cerebrovascular accident, or deep vein thrombosis
- Many side effects of combined hormonal contraception may be managed by patient counseling an adequate

trial of three months, and careful manipulation of the hormonal content
- Progestin-only pills are not as effective as combined hormonal contraception but are good choices for women who are breastfeeding or who cannot take estrogen
- DMPA, MPA, and subdermal implants (if available) are highly effective forms of contraception and are good choices for those who have difficulty adhering to other methods or who cannot take estrogen. Women who choose this method should be adequately counseled on the likelihood of irregular bleeding and proper scheduling and timing of their next injection
- Barrier methods can be effective contraceptives with proper counseling in motivated users. Condoms provide the greatest protection against STIs
- IUDs and diaphragms can be used safely and effectively for long periods of time in properly selected patients
- Patients should be aware of the availability of EC

SUGGESTED READINGS

Dickey RP. Managing contraceptive pill patients, 12th ed. Durant, OK: Essential Medical Information Systems, 2004.
Hatcher RA, Trussell J, Stewart F, et al. Contraceptive technology, 18th ed. New York: Ardent Media Inc, 2004.
Hatcher RA, Zieman M, Cwiak C, et al. A pocket guide to managing contraception. Tiger, Georgia: Bridging the Gap, 2004.

REFERENCES

1. Brown SS. The best intentions: unintended pregnancy and the well-being of children and families. Washington DC: National Academy Press, 1995.
2. Speroff L. A clinical guide to contraception, 2nd ed. Baltimore: Lippincott Williams & Wilkins, 1997.
3. The pill and other hormones for contraception, 5th ed. Oxford, UK: Oxford University Press, 1997.
4. Hatcher RA, Trussell J, Stewart F, et al. Contraceptive technology, 18th ed. New York: Ardent Media Inc, 2004.
5. Hatcher RA, Trussell J, Stewart F, et al. Contraceptive technology, 17th ed. New York: Ardent Media, 1998.
6. Mann JI, Doll R, Thorogood M, et al. Risk factors for myocardial infarction in young women. Br J Prev Soc Med 30:94–100, 1976.
7. Oral contraceptives and stroke in young women. Associated risk factors. JAMA 231:718–722, 1975.
8. Grimes DA. The safety of oral contraceptives: epidemiologic insights from the first 30 years. Am J Obstet Gynecol 166: 1950–1954, 1992.
9. Mishell DR Jr. Cardiovascular risks: perception versus reality. Contraception 59 (1 Suppl):21S–24S, 1999.
10. Sidney S, Siscovick DS, Petitti DB, et al. Myocardial infarction and use of low-dose oral contraceptives: a pooled analysis of 2 US studies. Circulation 98:1058–1063, 1998.
11. Schwartz SM, Petitti DB, Siscovick DS, et al. Stroke and use of low-dose oral contraceptives in young women: a pooled analysis of two US studies. Stroke 29:2277–2284, 1998.
12. Lewis MA. Myocardial infarction and stroke in young women: what is the impact of oral contraceptives? Am J Obstet Gynecol 179:S68–77, 1998.
13. Farley TM, Meirik O, Collins J. Cardiovascular disease and combined oral contraceptives: reviewing the evidence and balancing the risks. Hum Reprod Update 5:721–735, 1999.

14. Mant D, Villard-Mackintosh L, Vessey MP, et al. Myocardial infarction and angina pectoris in young women. J Epidemiol Community Health 41:215–219, 1987.

15. Stampfer MJ, Willett WC, Colditz GA, et al. A prospective study of past use of oral contraceptive agents and risk of cardiovascular diseases. N Engl J Med 319:1313–1317, 1988.

16. Colditz GA. Oral contraceptive use and mortality during 12 years of follow-up: the Nurses' Health Study. Ann Intern Med 120:821–826, 1994.

17. Blumenstein BA, Douglas MB, Hall WD. Blood pressure changes and oral contraceptive use: a study of 2676 black women in the southeastern United States. Am J Epidemiol 112:539–552, 1980.

18. Tsai CC, Williamson HO, Kirkland BH, et al. Low-dose oral contraception and blood pressure in women with a past history of elevated blood pressure. Am J Obstet Gynecol 151:28–32, 1985.

19. Wilson ES, Cruickshank J, McMaster M, et al. A prospective controlled study of the effect on blood pressure of contraceptive preparations containing different types and dosages of progestogen. Br J Obstet Gynaecol 91:1254–1260, 1984.

20. Chasan-Taber L, Willett WC, Manson JE, et al. Prospective study of oral contraceptives and hypertension among women in the United States. Circulation 94:483–489, 1996.

21. Vandenbroucke JP, Rosing J, Bloemenkamp KW, et al. Oral contraceptives and the risk of venous thrombosis. N Engl J Med 344:1527–1535, 2001.

22. Dugdale M, Masi AT. Hormonal contraception and thromboembolic disease: effects of the oral contraceptives on hemostatic mechanisms. A review of the literature. J Chronic Dis 23:775–790, 1971.

23. Petersen C, Kelly R, Minard B, et al. Antithrombin III. Comparison of functional and immunologic assays. Am J Clin Pathol 69:500–504, 1978.

24. Howie PW, Mallinson AC, Prentice CR, et al. Effect of combined oestrogen-progestogen oral contraceptives, oestrogen, and progestogen on antiplasmin and antithrombin activity. Lancet 2:1329–1332, 1970.

25. Venous thromboembolic disease and combined oral contraceptives: results of international multicentre case-control study. World Health Organization Collaborative Study of Cardiovascular Disease and Steroid Hormone Contraception. Lancet 346:1575–1582, 1995.

26. Effect of different progestagens in low oestrogen oral contraceptives on venous thromboembolic disease. World Health Organization Collaborative Study of Cardiovascular Disease and Steroid Hormone Contraception. Lancet 346:1582–1588, 1995.

27. Jick H, Jick SS, Gurewich V, et al. Risk of idiopathic cardiovascular death and nonfatal venous thromboembolism in women using oral contraceptives with differing progestagen components. Lancet 346:1589–1593, 1995.

28. Spitzer WO, Lewis MA, Heinemann LA, et al. Third-generation oral contraceptives and risk of venous thromboembolic disorders: an international case-control study. Transnational Research Group on Oral Contraceptives and the Health of Young Women. Br Med J 312:83–88, 1996.

29. Lewis MA, Heinemann LA, MacRae KD, et al. The increased risk of venous thromboembolism and the use of third-generation progestagens: role of bias in observational research. The Transnational Research Group on Oral Contraceptives and the Health of Young Women. Contraception 54:5–13, 1996.

30. Westhoff CL. Oral contraceptives and venous thromboembolism: should epidemiologic associations drive clinical decision making? Contraception 54:1–3, 1996.

31. Lewis MA. The epidemiology of oral contraceptive use: a critical review of the studies on oral contraceptives and the health of young women. Am J Obstet Gynecol 179:1086–1097, 1998.

32. Farmer RD, Todd JC, Lewis MA, et al. The risks of venous thromboembolic disease among German women using oral contraceptives: a database study. Contraception 57:67–70, 1998.

33. Farmer RD, Lawrenson RA, Thompson CR, et al. Population-based study of risk of venous thromboembolism associated with various oral contraceptives. Lancet 349:83–88, 1997.

34. Rosing J, Tans G, Nicolaes GA, et al. Oral contraceptives and venous thrombosis: different sensitivities to activated protein C in women using second- and third-generation oral contraceptives. Br J Haematol 97:233–238, 1997.

35. Breast cancer and hormonal contraceptives: collaborative reanalysis of individual data on 53 297 women with breast cancer and 100 239 women without breast cancer from 54 epidemiological studies. Collaborative Group on Hormonal Factors in Breast Cancer. Lancet 347:1713–1727, 1996.

36. Marchbanks PA, McDonald JA, Wilson HG, et al. Oral contraceptives and the risk of breast cancer. N Engl J Med 346:2025–2032, 2002.

37. Thomas DB, Ray RM. Oral contraceptives and invasive adenocarcinomas and adenosquamous carcinomas of the uterine cervix. The World Health Organization Collaborative Study of Neoplasia and Steroid Contraceptives. Am J Epidemiol. 144:281–289, 1996.

38. Zondervan KT, Carpenter LM, Painter R, et al. Oral contraceptives and cervical cancer: further findings from the Oxford Family Planning Association contraceptive study. Br J Cancer 73:1291–1297, 1996.

39. Bosch FX, Lorincz A, Munoz N, et al. The causal relation between human papillomavirus and cervical cancer. J Clin Pathol 55:244–265, 2002.

40. Moreno V, Bosch FX, Munoz N, et al. Effect of oral contraceptives on risk of cervical cancer in women with human papillomavirus infection: the IARC multicentric case-control study. Lancet 359:1085–1092, 2002.

41. Grodstein F, Colditz GA, Hunter DJ, et al. A prospective study of symptomatic gallstones in women: relation with oral contraceptives and other risk factors. Obstet Gynecol 84:207–214, 1994.

42. Mortola JF. A risk-benefit appraisal of drugs used in the management of premenstrual syndrome. Drug Saf 10:160–169, 1994.

43. IARC. Monographs on the evaluation of carcinogenic risks to humans, 72: *Hormonal contraception and post-menopausal hormonal therapy*. Lyon: WHO, 1999.

44. La Vecchia C. Oral contraceptives, cancer and vascular disease. Eur J Cancer Prev 10:303–305, 2001.

45. Broome M, Clayton J, Fotherby K. Enlarged follicles in women using oral contraceptives. Contraception 52:13–16, 1995.

46. Franks AL, Beral V, Cates W, Jr., et al. Contraception and ectopic pregnancy risk. Am J Obstet Gynecol 163:1120–1123, 1990.

47. Hormonal contraception: recent advances and controversies. Fertil Steril 82(Suppl 1):S26–32, 2004.

48. Gross TP, Schlesselman JJ. The estimated effect of oral contraceptive use on the cumulative risk of epithelial ovarian cancer. Obstet Gynecol 83:419–424, 1994.

49. Oral contraceptives and neoplasia. WHO Scientific Group. World Health Organ Tech Rep Series 817:1–46, 1992.

50. Redmond GP, Olson WH, Lippman JS, et al. Norgestimate and ethinyl estradiol in the treatment of acne vulgaris: a randomized, placebo-controlled trial. Obstet Gynecol 89:615–622, 1997.

51. Dickey R. Managing contraceptive pill patients. 9th ed. Durant, OK: Essential Medical Information Systems, 1998.

52. Mattson RH, Rebar RW. Contraceptive methods for women with neurologic disorders. Am J Obstet Gynecol 168:2027–2032, 1993.

53. Smith M. Quantitative estimate of ocular iatrogenic disease in humans. J Am Optom Assoc 45:751–755, 1974.

54. Wood JR. Ocular complications of oral contraceptives. Ophthalmic Semin 2:371–402, 1977.

55. Adams PW, Rose DP, Folkard J, et al. Effect of pyridoxine hydrochloride (vitamin B 6) upon depression associated with oral contraception. Lancet 1:899–904, 1973.

56. Helms SE, Bredle DL, Zajic J, et al. Oral contraceptive failure rates and oral antibiotics. J Am Acad Dermatol 36:705–710, 1997.

57. Michalets EL. Update: clinically significant cytochrome P-450 drug interactions. Pharmacotherapy 18:84–112, 1998.

58. Rosenfeld WE, Doose DR, Walker SA, et al. Effect of topiramate on the pharmacokinetics of an oral contraceptive containing norethindrone and ethinyl estradiol in patients with epilepsy. Epilepsia 38:317–323, 1997.

59. McDaniel PA, Caldroney RD. Oral contraceptives and griseofulvin interactions. Drug Intell Clin Pharm 20:384, 1986.

60. Spellacy WN. Carbohydrate metabolism during treatment with estrogen, progestogen, and low-dose oral contraceptives. Am J Obstet Gynecol 142:732–734, 1982.

61. Mestman JH, Schmidt-Sarosi C. Diabetes mellitus and fertility control: contraception management issues. Am J Obstet Gynecol 168:2012–2020, 1993.

62. Baird DT, Glasier AF. Hormonal contraception. N Engl J Med 328:1543–1549, 1993.
63. Kjos SL, Peters RK, Xiang A, et al. Contraception and the risk of type 2 diabetes mellitus in Latina women with prior gestational diabetes mellitus. JAMA 280:533–538, 1998.
64. Ortho-McNeil. Ortho Evra Package Insert, 2001.
65. Archer DF, Bigrigg A, Smallwood GH, et al. Assessment of compliance with a weekly contraceptive patch (Ortho Evra/Evra) among North American women. Fertil Steril 77:S27–31, 2002.
66. Archer DF, Cullins V, Creasy GW, et al. The impact of improved compliance with a weekly contraceptive transdermal system (Ortho Evra) on contraceptive efficacy. Contraception 69:189–195, 2004.
67. Organon. NuvaRing Package Insert, 2004.
68. Novak A, de la Loge C, Abetz L, et al. The combined contraceptive vaginal ring, NuvaRing: an international study of user acceptability. Contraception 67:187–194, 2003.
69. Bjarnadottir RI, Tuppurainen M, Killick SR. Comparison of cycle control with a combined contraceptive vaginal ring and oral levonorgestrel/ethinyl estradiol. Am J Obstet Gynecol 186:389–395, 2002.
70. Seasonale prescribing information. Pomona, NY, 2003.
71. Anderson FD, Hait H. A multicenter, randomized study of an extended cycle oral contraceptive. Contraception 68:89–96, 2003.
72. Stewart FH, Kaunitz AM, Laguardia KD, et al. Extended use of transdermal norelgestromin/ethinyl estradiol: a randomized trial. Obstet Gynecol 105:1389–1396, 2005.
73. Miller L, Verhoeven CH, Hout J. Extended regimens of the contraceptive vaginal ring: a randomized trial. Obstet Gynecol 106:473–482, 2005.
74. Moggia AV, Harris GS, Dunson TR, et al. A comparative study of a progestin-only oral contraceptive versus non-hormonal methods in lactating women in Buenos Aires, Argentina. Contraception 44:31–43, 1991.
75. De Ceulaer K, Gruber C, Hayes R, et al. Medroxyprogesterone acetate and homozygous sickle-cell disease. Lancet 2:229–231, 1982.
76. Mattson RH, Cramer JA, Caldwell BV, et al. Treatment of seizures with medroxyprogesterone acetate: preliminary report. Neurology 34:1255–1258, 1984.
77. Scholes D, LaCroix AZ, Ichikawa LE, et al. The association between depot medroxyprogesterone acetate contraception and bone mineral density in adolescent women. Contraception 69:99–104, 2004.
78. Scholes D, LaCroix AZ, Ichikawa LE, et al. Change in bone mineral density among adolescent women using and discontinuing depot medroxyprogesterone acetate contraception. Arch Pediatr Adolesc Med 159:139–144, 2005.
79. Nelson AL. Counseling issues and management of side effects for women using depot medroxyprogesterone acetate contraception. J Reprod Med 41 (5 Suppl):391–400, 1996.
80. Pharmacia and Upjohn Co Depo-subQ Provera package information, 2005.
81. Berlex. Mirena package insert, 2004.
82. Jensen JT. Contraceptive and therapeutic effects of the levonorgestrel intrauterine system: an overview. Obstet Gynecol Surv 60:604–612, 2005.
83. Berardi RM, Newton GD. Handbook of nonprescription drugs, 14th ed. Washington DC: American Pharmacists Association, 2004.
84. Louik C, Mitchell AA, Werler MM, et al. Maternal exposure to spermicides in relation to certain birth defects. N Engl J Med 317:474–478, 1987.
85. Strobino B, Kline J, Lai A, et al. Vaginal spermicides and spontaneous abortion of known karyotype. Am J Epidemiol 123:431–443, 1986.
86. Carey RF, Herman WA, Retta SM, et al. Effectiveness of latex condoms as a barrier to human immunodeficiency virus-sized particles under conditions of simulated use. Sex Transm Dis 19:230–234, 1992.
87. Update: barrier protection against HIV infection and other sexually transmitted diseases. MMWR 42:589–591, 597, 1993.
88. Weller SC. A meta-analysis of condom effectiveness in reducing sexually transmitted HIV. Soc Sci Med 36:1635–1644, 1993.
89. Frezieres RG, Walsh TL, Nelson AL, et al. Breakage and acceptability of a polyurethane condom: a randomized, controlled study. Fam Plann Perspect 30:73–78, 1998.
90. Frezieres RG, Walsh TL, Nelson AL, et al. Evaluation of the efficacy of a polyurethane condom: results from a randomized, controlled clinical trial. Fam Plann Perspect 31:81–87, 1999.
91. Ortiz ME, Croxatto HB. The mode of action of IUDs. Contraception 36:37–53, 1987.
92. Farley TM, Rosenberg MJ, Rowe PJ, et al. Intrauterine devices and pelvic inflammatory disease: an international perspective. Lancet 339:785–788, 1992.
93. Delbanco SF, Mauldon J, Smith MD. Little knowledge and limited practice: emergency contraceptive pills, the public, and the obstetrician-gynecologist. Obstet Gynecol 89:1006–1011, 1997.
94. Ellertson C, Shochet T, Blanchard K, et al. Emergency contraception: a review of the programmatic and social science literature. Contraception 61:145–186, 2000.
95. FDA. Prescription drug products; certain combined oral contraceptives for use as postcoital emergency contraception. Federal Register 62:8610–8612, 1997.
96. Ling WY, Robichaud A, Zayid I, et al. Mode of action of DL-norgestrel and ethinylestradiol combination in postcoital contraception. Fertil Steril 32:297–302, 1979.
97. Kesseru E, Garmendia F, Westphal N, et al. The hormonal and peripheral effects of d-norgestrel in postcoital contraception. Contraception 10:411–424, 1974.
98. Croxatto HB, Devoto L, Durand M, et al. Mechanism of action of hormonal preparations used for emergency contraception: a review of the literature. Contraception 63:111–121, 2001.
99. Croxatto HB, Ortiz ME, Muller AL. Mechanisms of action of emergency contraception. Steroids 68:1095–1098, 2003.
100. Muller AL, Llados CM, Croxatto HB. Postcoital treatment with levonorgestrel does not disrupt postfertilization events in the rat. Contraception 67:415–419, 2003.
101. Rodrigues I, Grou F, Joly J. Effectiveness of emergency contraceptive pills between 72 and 120 hours after unprotected sexual intercourse. Am J Obstet Gynecol 184:531–537, 2001.
102. Trussell J, Rodriguez G, Ellertson C. Updated estimates of the effectiveness of the Yuzpe regimen of emergency contraception. Contraception 59:147–151, 1999.
103. Barr. Plan B package information, 2004.
104. Raymond EG, Creinin MD, Barnhart KT, et al. Meclizine for prevention of nausea associated with use of emergency contraceptive pills: a randomized trial. Obstet Gynecol 95:271–277, 2000.
105. De Santis M, Cavaliere AF, Straface G, et al. Failure of the emergency contraceptive levonorgestrel and the risk of adverse effects in pregnancy and on fetal development: an observational cohort study. Fertil Steril 84:296–299, 2005.
106. Fasoli M, Parazzini F, Cecchetti G, et al. Post-coital contraception: an overview of published studies. Contraception 39:459–468, 1989.
107. Glasier A, Thong KJ, Dewar M, et al. Mifepristone (RU 486) compared with high-dose estrogen and progestogen for emergency postcoital contraception. N Engl J Med 327:1041–1044, 1992.
108. Urquhart DR, Shinewi F. The efficacy and tolerance of mifepristone and prostaglandin in termination of pregnancy of less than 63 days gestation; UK Multicentre Study, final results. Contraception 55:1–5, 1997
109. el-Refaey H, Rajasekar D, Abdalla M, et al. Induction of abortion with mifepristone (RU 486) and oral or vaginal misoprostol. N Engl J Med 332:983–987, 1995.
110. Hausknecht RU. Methotrexate and misoprostol to terminate early pregnancy. N Engl J Med 333:537–540, 1995.
111. Wiebe ER. Abortion induced with methotrexate and misoprostol. Can Med Assoc J 154:165–170, 1996.
112. http:// www.fda.gov/cder/druginfopage/mifepristone/. Accessed January 16, 2006.

Drugs in Pregnancy and Lactation

Beth Logsdon Pangle

TREATMENT GOALS

- Utilize appropriate resources to determine the teratogenic risk of a drug and the amount excreted into breast milk.
- Assess the risk and benefits of pharmacotherapy to the mother and fetus.
- Utilize a drug regimen that is safe and effective for the mother and minimizes risk to the developing fetus.
- Use the lowest dose and for the shortest amount of time to minimize exposure to the fetus or neonate/infant.
- Minimize drug exposure to the neonate/infant during lactation.

EPIDEMIOLOGY

Despite limited or inconclusive information regarding medication effects on the fetus, exposure to drugs during pregnancy for treatment of such symptoms as pain, nausea and vomiting, gastrointestinal upset, edema, and the common cold remains a common occurrence. At least 35% of pregnant women have taken some sort of medication during pregnancy, and 40% of pregnant women have taken medications during their first trimester.[1–3] These figures are impressive when you consider that many medications are taken without medical supervision and without a clear indication, and may be taken immediately after conception before pregnancy is known. In 1991, the World Health Organization (WHO) completed an international survey of drug use in pregnancy involving nearly 15,000 pregnant women from 22 countries. Eighty-six percent of these women took a medication during pregnancy, receiving an average of 2.9 (range 1 to 15) prescriptions per pregnancy.[4] This survey did not take into account over-the-counter medications purchased without the advice of a physician. This extremely high drug utilization rate during pregnancy is then elevated by an increase in drug administration during the intrapartum period, when 79% of women in the WHO study received an average of 3.3 drugs. Little is known about the characteristics of the pregnant women who take medication, but one study identified non-white, unmarried, less educated women as less likely to use medication than other groups due to less prenatal care; medical care may be associated with increased use of medications.

In addition, surveys in Western countries indicate that 90% to 99% of women who are breast-feeding receive a medication during their first week postpartum, 17% to 25% at 4 months postpartum, and 5% of mothers receive chronic medications during breast-feeding.[5,6] With increasing information on the benefits of breast milk, which has nutritional and immunologic properties superior to those of infant formulas, the American Academy of Pediatrics (AAP) recommends breast-feeding for optimal nutrition during the first 12 months of life.[7] This increase in breast-feeding to more than 60% of American mothers today has led to questions regarding the safety and potential toxicity to neonates of drugs and chemicals that may be excreted in breast milk.

While heightened public awareness of medication use and concern for health of the fetus has reduced drug use in pregnancy, a great need for active patient counseling and education in the area continues to exist. It is the responsibility of all clinicians, including pharmacists, to counsel patients with complete, accurate, and current information on the risks and benefits of using medication while pregnant or breast-feeding. The fetus or nursing infant must always be kept in mind as a potential drug recipient. This chapter addresses challenges of treating pregnant or lactating women, suggests resources to refer, and discusses management approaches for commonly occurring conditions in this patient population.

TERATOGENS

The number of prescription and over-the-counter drugs available for human use is escalating each year. Attention should be paid to drugs that cause harm to the developing fetus. Of nearly 1,000 drugs evaluated for teratogenic potential, only about 30 are proven teratogens, and many of these are no longer used. A teratogen is an agent that is present during critical periods of development and is able to produce a congenital defect. The term ''congenital defect'' refers to major and minor malformations as well as functional abnormalities. Structural abnormalities that require major surgery or are incompatible with life occur at an incidence of 2% to 4% in the United States. Of approximately 10% of children with abnormal physical or mental development, only 2% to 3% of all abnormalities are believed to be chemical or drug-induced.[8] However, this figure may be an underestimate because many cases are not reported.

RESOURCES FOR INFORMATION

In reviewing the literature, the clinician should keep in mind that data on drugs in pregnancy and lactation are constantly being updated and may appear to be contradictory. Much of the data arises from case reports that may not be generalized to all women. Sound professional judgment based on clinical assessment of the patient and an understanding of the literature must be combined with direct patient counseling before medication is taken during pregnancy or lactation. Patient involvement in the decision-making process is important. This chapter provides a general review of common issues relating to drug use in pregnancy and lactation. Other references should be consulted because this chapter is not meant to include all issues necessary to making patient-specific therapeutic decisions.

In 1979, the Food and Drug Administration (FDA) devised a system that determines the teratogenic risk of drugs

TABLE 19.1	Food and Drug Administration Categories for Drug Use in Pregnancy
Category A:	Controlled studies in women fail to demonstrate a risk to the fetus in the first trimester, and the possibility of fetal harm appears remote.
Category B:	Either animal studies do not indicate a risk to the fetus and there are no controlled studies in pregnant women, or animal studies have indicated fetal risk but controlled studies in pregnant women failed to demonstrate a risk.
Category C:	Either animal studies indicate a fetal risk, and there are no controlled studies in women or there are no available studies in women or animals.
Category D:	There is positive evidence of fetal risk, but there may be certain situations where the benefit may outweigh the risk.
Category X:	There is a definite fetal risk based on studies in animals or humans, or a fetal risk based on human experience, and the risk clearly outweighs any benefit to pregnant women.

(From Food and Drug Administration labelling and prescription drug advertising: content and format for labeling for human prescription drugs. Federal Register 44:37434–37467, 1979.)

by considering the quality of data from animal and human studies[9] (Table 19.1). Benefits and risks of therapy are included for most drugs, providing therapeutic guidance for the clinician. Although category A is considered the safest category, some drugs with a B, C, or D rating are commonly used during pregnancy. Category X is the only rating that denotes a drug is absolutely contraindicated for use during pregnancy.

Drugs in Pregnancy and Lactation: a Reference Guide to Fetal and Neonatal Risk, by Briggs along with its quarterly updates, is an exhaustive reference that provides an up-to-date summary of available data on specific drugs.[10] An additional resource that may be useful is *Medication in Mothers Milk* by Hale.[11] Dr. Hale presents a lactation risk category to assess drug exposure to the nursing infant. Both of these references include recommendations by the American Academy of Pediatrics regarding use of medications in breast-feeding women.[12] Other potential sources for information include the drug manufacturer as well as medical journals. Most important, the data should be carefully evaluated before inferring results to an individual patient.

CHOOSING A DRUG FOR A PREGNANT OR NURSING MOTHER

Many drug and nondrug factors should be considered before prescribing medications for a pregnant or nursing mother. Principles of teratology have been identified and timing of exposure during fetal development is the most important factor to consider. Knowing the developmental stage when insult is applied can aid in predicting the possible defect. Exposure around the time of conception and implantation may kill the fetus, possibly without the woman knowing she was pregnant. However, if exposure occurs during the first 14 days after conception when the cells are still totipotential (i.e., if one cell is damaged, another can assume its function), the fetus may not be damaged.[13–15] The most sensitive period is from implantation to the end of organogenesis, days 18 to 60, during which damage to the developing organs may occur. From 8 weeks of gestation until birth, morphologic changes may occur as the developmental and growth phases continue, including brain maturation.[16]

Factors that influence teratogenicity of a drug include genotypes of the mother and the fetus, the embryonic stage at exposure, drug dose, duration of exposure, nature of the agent and the mechanism by which it causes a defect, simultaneous exposure to other drugs or environmental agents that may affect potential abnormalities, the maternal and fetal metabolism of the drug, and the extent to which the drug crosses the placenta.[16]

During breast-feeding, the amount of drug available to the nursing infant is influenced by maternal, drug, and infant factors (Table 19.2). A systematic approach has been proposed by the Drug Information Service of the University of California San Diego Medical Center to minimize infant exposure to drugs in breast milk with minimal disruption of nursing (Table 19.3).

TABLE 19.2	Factors Influencing Drug Concentration in Breastfed Infants
Maternal	Milk composition and pH Mammary blood flow Maternal drug metabolism
Drug	Molecular weight (<200) pKa Protein binding Lipid solubility Dose and dosing interval Formulation (i.e., immediate vs. sustained release)
Infant	Amount of breast milk consumed (i.e., fully vs. partially breastfed) Higher GI pH Altered GI flora Prolonged GI transit time Reduced amounts of bile salts and pancreatic enzymes Decreased affinity of neonatal proteins for drugs Greater percentage of body water and extracellular fluid volume Decreased hepatic and renal elimination

(From American Academy of Pediatrics Committee on Drugs. The transfer of drugs and other chemicals into human breast milk. Pediatrics 108:776–789, 2001; Anderson PO. Drug use during breast-feeding. Clin Pharm 10:594–624, 1991, with permission.)

TREATMENT OF SELECT CONDITIONS DURING PREGNANCY

ASTHMA

Asthma complicates up to 4% of pregnancies. The effect pregnancy has on asthma is variable: it may improve, go unaltered, or worsen. Women with severe asthma before pregnancy are more likely to have difficulty with the disease during pregnancy. Maternal and fetal morbidity and mortality increases when asthma is not adequately treated. Affected women are more likely to have hyperemesis gravidarum, uterine hemorrhage, preeclampsia, placenta previa, pregnancy-induced hypertension, and premature labor. Additionally, neonatal mortality, low birth weight, increased risk of transient tachypnea of the newborn, and increased risk of prematurity may be seen. If asthma is controlled, infants are born with no greater risk for congenital abnormalities than the general population. Complications may arise as a result of the disease or the drug therapy.[17–20]

The improved outcome of mother and child associated with treating pregnant asthmatic women supports administration of medications to these women.[21,22] Inhaled β2-agonists, such as albuterol (category C), have been used successfully in treating mild and infrequent asthmatic episodes. Systemic effects are lessened by using aerosolized therapy, the preferred route of administration for pregnant women. These agents may cause maternal tachycardia, hyperglycemia, hypotension, or neonatal hypoglycemia. Based on results of one surveillance study of 1,090 infants who were exposed in the first trimester, polydactyly may be associated with use in the first trimester.[10] Use of albuterol in the first trimester is limited, but use in the second and third trimester has not been linked to congenital defects. Terbutaline (category B) is another β-agonist that is commonly used as a tocolytic. There are no reports of adverse effects of albuterol use during lactation, and the β-agonists are considered compatible with breast-feeding.[10]

Theophylline (category C) in conjunction with inhalation therapy is considered safe in pregnancy and preferred in patients requiring long-term control.[23] Theophylline should be monitored throughout pregnancy to maintain nontoxic serum concentrations, particularly in the third trimester when a possible decrease in theophylline clearance and/or increase in volume of distribution occurs.[24] Theophylline crosses the placenta, and fetal concentrations are about equal to maternal concentrations. Adverse fetal or neonatal effects include jitteriness, cardiac arrhythmias, hypoglycemia, vomiting, tachycardia, and feeding difficulties. Theophylline does not appear to be associated with congenital defects. Theophylline is excreted in breast milk and may cause irritability and fretful sleep in infants.[25] Neonates may be more likely to be affected because of their slow elimination compared with older infants; therefore, extended-release preparations may be preferable.[10] This drug is considered compatible with lactation by the AAP with maternal plasma concentrations kept

| TABLE 19.3 | Stepwise Approach to Minimizing Infant Exposure |

1. *Withhold the drug.* Some medications such as headache or cold symptom medication is not essential and can be avoided with the mother's cooperation.

2. *Delay drug therapy.* If a mother is close to weaning her infant from breast-feeding, elective drug use or surgery can be postponed.

3. *Choose drugs that pass poorly into breast milk.* Within a class of drugs (i.e., β-blockers), there are large differences in the amount of drug distribution into milk among the different medications.

4. *Choose an alternative route of administration.* Minimizing maternal serum concentrations through the use of locally applied drugs will also minimize drug concentrations in milk and the infant's exposure to the medication. These include inhaled or topical corticosteroids, inhaled bronchodilators or decongestants, for example.

5. *Avoid nursing at times of peak drug concentrations in milk.* A general rule is that peak concentrations occur in milk approximately 1–3 hours after an oral dose. Nursing just before a dose may help avoid this peak effect on the infant. However, this may not always be successful, particularly in neonates who nurse irregularly and often. This strategy works best for medications with short half-lives in non-extended release dosage forms.

6. *Take medication before the infant's longest sleep period.* This is useful for long-acting drugs that may be given only once daily.

7. *Temporarily withhold breast-feeding when drug therapy is temporary.* If a dental or surgical procedure is undertaken with a short course of postoperative medication, mothers may be able to pump extra milk before the procedure to use while not nursing, or formula may be substituted. Pumping the breasts during the time of nursing abstinence is necessary to maintain milk flow and relieve engorgement. Breast-feeding may be resumed as early as one to two maternal half-lives (50%–75% elimination) after the last dose in drugs where the concern is that particularly toxic serum concentrations will accumulate in the infant with repeated dosing. For drugs with a high potential of toxicity that even a small dose may be harmful, a delay of four to five half-lives (94%–97% elimination) or longer may be advised.

8. *Discontinue nursing.* A small number of medications that may be necessary for the mother's health (i.e., cancer chemotherapy) are too toxic to allow nursing. In these cases, it is in the best interest of the child and mother to discontinue breast-feeding.

(From Anderson PO. Drug use during breast-feeding. Clin Pharm 10:594–624, 1991, with permission.)

as low as therapeutically possible and infant concentrations obtained if adverse effects occur.[12,25]

If corticosteroids are indicated, they should not be withheld.[20] Oral, intravenous (IV), or inhaled therapy may be used as necessary to control acute attacks. Two reports of infants exposed to prednisone throughout gestation resulted in one with congenital cataracts and the other immunosuppressed. Any association between these abnormalities and steroid therapy has not been supported by other studies. No evidence has confirmed that prednisone (category C) increases fetal morbidity and mortality and the risk to the newborn is considered to be low.[19] However, spontaneous abortion, prematurity, and cardiac malformations have been documented from experience with 40 women treated with inhaled beclomethasone.[26] Flunisolide or triamcinolone (category C) have been suggested as alternative anti-inflammatory agents for inhalation, but documentation on their use is sparse. Corticosteroids occur in small quantities in breast milk; therefore, at standard doses (<20 mg/day prednisone) or with single oral doses an infant is unlikely to receive significant amounts. With larger doses or long-term therapy, prednisolone is preferred, ideally with nursing delayed until 3 to 4 hours after a dose.[10,25] Depot injections and inhaled corticosteroids present little or no risk to the nursing infant.[25]

Cromolyn sodium (category B) by inhalation is indicated for the prevention of asthmatic attacks. Cromolyn does not have significant systemic absorption, and it is unknown if it crosses the placenta. Currently, there is no evidence of an association between cromolyn and fetal malformations. It has been used without maternal or fetal harm.[22,27]

COAGULATION DISORDERS

Despite pregnancy being a "hypercoagulable state" with increased risk of thromboembolism, the incidence is still low at 0.2% to 0.4%.[15,26] Current recommendations for a risk-adapted heparin prophylaxis and therapy during pregnancy and the puerperium are guided by the estimated thrombotic risk. This risk is predominantly based on the history of venous thromboembolism (especially with prior pregnancies) and the presence of hereditary risk factors. Although such therapy has risks, the reduction of antepartum mortality rates from 13% to 1% in women with thromboembolic disease receiving anticoagulants supports treatment of the pregnant patient.[15] Other pregnancy risk factors that increase the risk of venous thromboembolism in women without a prior history include age >35, operative delivery, and preeclampsia.[29]

The anticoagulant drug of choice in the pregnant patient is heparin. Heparin (category C) does not cross the placenta and has not been associated with congenital defects. Standard unfractionated heparin prophylaxis has been used with little risk to the mother or fetus, but may be inadequate during the second and third trimesters because of increasing heparin requirements in pregnancy.[30] Perinatal mortality rates are comparatively better for patients receiving heparin (3.6%) than with warfarin (26.1%).[31] Although advantageous in many respects, the use of heparin has risks for the mother such as bleeding, particularly during delivery, and heparin-induced thrombocytopenia (incidence up to 15%). Prolonged treatment with heparin is associated with a reversible dose-related osteopenia.[28] It appears that the use of low-molecular-weight heparin (LMWH) during pregnancy may be at least as safe and effective as unfractionated heparin with less frequent laboratory monitoring, less risk of bleeding, and less risk of osteoporosis, and it does not cross into the fetal circulation, and causes less osteoporosis.[32]

Exposure to warfarin (category D) during the sixth to ninth week of gestation may result in fetal warfarin syndrome; defects of the central nervous system and skeletal system and facial defects may occur with exposure throughout pregnancy. Stillbirths, spontaneous abortion, mental retardation, and impairment in physical growth may also occur. As a result of these risks, there is a contraindication to the use of warfarin in the first trimester and around the time of delivery. The use of warfarin in pregnancy should be restricted to situations in which heparin prophylaxis is contraindicated.

Heparin does not pass into breast milk because of its high molecular weight.[10] Warfarin therapy does not appear to cause significant risk to the breast-feeding neonate with little or no drug diffusing into the breast milk and is considered compatible with nursing by the AAP.[12] Also, because of the oral route of administration with warfarin and the significant risk of osteoporosis associated with protracted heparin therapy, warfarin is the ideal anticoagulant for use during the postpartum period for maintenance therapy. Despite lack of documentation, LMWHs still have a relatively high molecular weight and, as such, would not be expected to be excreted into human milk.[10]

COMMON COLD

The common cold often affects pregnant women whose resistance is weakened.[33] The viruses causing the common cold have not been found to be teratogenic. However, determining the risk associated with most cold medications is difficult because of confounding variables such as the underlying illness and polypharmacy. Because the short-lived symptoms such as watery eyes and nose, coughing, sneezing, and congestion are generally tolerable, medication therapy should be avoided if possible. If medication must be used, combination products should be avoided and single agents used to limit drug exposure.

If the patient's symptoms require an antihistamine, chlorpheniramine and triprolidine (both category B) have been commonly used during pregnancy. A significant increased risk of birth defects has been reported with brompheniramine (category C) use in the first trimester; therefore this drug is not recommended. Loratadine and cetirizine (both category B) should be considered alternatives after the first trimester if first-generation antihistamines cannot be tolerated. Anti-

histamine use in the last 2 weeks of pregnancy was found to increase the risk of retrolental fibroplasia in exposed premature infants.[10]

Antihistamines are excreted into breast milk. Brompheniramine and diphenhydramine have been classified by their manufacturers as contraindicated for use while nursing because of the increased sensitivity of newborn infants to antihistamines. The AAP recommends the use of clemastine with caution during breast-feeding.[12] Triprolidine, loratadine, and cetirizine are excreted in clinically insignificant amounts in human milk and can therefore be used.[10] Nasal cromolyn, beclomethasone, or flunisolide are useful alternatives.[12]

Minor malformations, including clubfoot and inguinal hernia, have been documented with first trimester use of decongestants. Of the decongestants, pseudoephedrine (category C) has not been associated with adverse outcomes and has been suggested as the drug of choice if an agent must be used.[33] Pseudoephedrine is excreted in breast milk, but the AAP considers the drug to be compatible with breast-feeding.[12] Phenylpropanolamine should be avoided because of possible significant physical deformations associated with early use; this drug has been withdrawn from the market. Phenylephrine and oxymetazoline (category C) may be used as topical nasal decongestants, which advantageously limits systemic absorption.[34]

Antitussives and/or expectorants, such as dextromethorphan and guaifenesin (both category C), have been used in pregnant women. Epidemiologic studies have not revealed an increase in congenital malformations after exposure to either of these agents.[10] Pregnant women should avoid those products containing alcohol, because of the risk of fetal alcohol syndrome, which has been documented in a woman who abused cough medication. The use of cough preparations that contain alcohol should also be discouraged during breast-feeding.

CONSTIPATION

Pregnant patients commonly complain of symptoms of constipation. Possible causes include increased pressure on the colon and rectum, decreased peristalsis, increased progesterone, decreased motilin, or increased colonic absorption of water.[35] Patients experiencing constipation should add fiber to their diet and increase water intake. Moderate exercise helps maintain regularity.

Bulk-forming laxatives appear to be safe in pregnancy and lactation and are the agents of choice. Because these agents are not absorbed systemically, they do not pose a threat to the fetus or neonate. Adequate fluid intake needs to be stressed when taking bulk laxatives to prevent intestinal obstruction. Surfactants, such as docusate sodium (category C), appear to be safe in pregnancy. Mineral oil (category C) should be avoided because of the risk of decreased absorption of fat-soluble vitamins. Use of senna (category C) in moderate doses is acceptable according to the AAP and may be used during lactation.[12] Also, bisacodyl is virtually non-absorbable and is considered safe to use during nursing.[11,12]

DEPRESSION

Overall, major depression is twice as prevalent in women as in men, and the childbearing years appear to be a time of increased vulnerability for the onset of mood disorders in women.[36] Despite this data, limited clinical investigation has been conducted with this population. Clinical data support the view that maternal depression has an adverse impact on mother-infant attachment and infant temperament.[37] Children of depressed mothers are more likely to suffer from adjustment disorders and childhood depression than children of nondepressed mothers.[38]

Postpartum depression is the most common complication of childbearing, occurring with 1 of every 8 births.[39] Several risk factors for depression during pregnancy have been identified, including personal history of depression, family history of depression, marital discord, recent adverse life events, and unwanted pregnancy.[40] There is no consistent evidence to suggest that any particular demographic factor places a woman at increased risk, including education level, the sex of her infant, whether or not she breast-feeds, or the mode of delivery.[41,42] Treatment of depression during pregnancy remains largely empirical, with little data to guide the clinician. Careful assessment of the risk/benefit ratio for the mother and fetus is essential. The risks of untreated depression include poor nutrition, disrupted sleep patterns, difficulty following medical and prenatal care recommendations, suicide, worsening of comorbid medical illness, and increased exposure to tobacco, alcohol, or drugs.

A recent meta-analysis failed to find any evidence for teratogenicity from any of the available classes of antidepressants [i.e., tricyclic antidepressants (TCAs), selective serotonin reuptake inhibitors (SSRIs), monoamine oxidase inhibitors (MAOIs), and bupropion during pregnancy.[43] Despite the fact that TCAs have been available for more than 30 years and data documenting their use during pregnancy is available, the majority of tricyclics are classified as pregnancy category C or D. Fetal abnormalities have been reported in patients taking TCAs; however, no clear association has been demonstrated.[10] If a TCA is used, the secondary amines [i.e., nortriptyline (category D), and desipramine (category C)] may be preferred because they generally are better tolerated than the other agents.[44]

Because of their favorable efficacy and side effect profile and relative safety in cases of overdose, the SSRIs have become the first-line agents for the treatment of depression during pregnancy.[45] Of the SSRIs, fluoxetine (category B) has been the most widely studied. While available animal and human experience indicate that it does not cause major congenital malformations (this is true for all of the SSRIs), animal data indicate that fluoxetine may produce potentially permanent changes to the brain. Also, a recent study showed that maternal use of high doses of fluoxetine may be associated with a risk for low birth weight.

A recent retrospective epidemiologic study found an increased risk of major congenital malformations for paroxetine when taken during the first trimester compared with other antidepressants [OR 2.2; 95% confedence interval, 1.34–3.63], as well as an increased risk of cardiovascular malformations [OR 2.08; 95% confidence interval, 1.03–4.23].[4]

Exposure to SSRIs late in the third trimester has been associated with such complications as prolonged hospitalization, respiratory support, and tube feeding. Also, symptoms of drug discontinuation such as respiratory distress, seizures, temperature instability, hypoglycemia, change in tone, jitteriness, and irritability have been noted.[46]

Eighty-five percent of known pregnancies will result in a live birth. Thirty-six percent of women who experience a miscarriage or stillbirth will experience severe depressive symptoms.[47] Evidence indicates that the length of gestation before pregnancy loss is proportional to the severity of depressive symptoms. Treatment of depression after miscarriage should be determined on an individual basis. Subsequent pregnancies in these women should be monitored closely, as there is an increased incidence of depression in women who previously experienced depression related to reproductive loss.

The event of childbirth is undeniably a time of biologic, psychologic, and economic adjustment. Despite historical knowledge of this apparent time of increased vulnerability, official recognition of postpartum-onset mental illness has occurred only recently. In addition to postpartum depression, two subtypes of postpartum mood disorders include maternity blues and postpartum psychosis.[48] Maternity blues (or ''baby blues'') is a relatively mild emotional disturbance characterized by mood lability, depression, increased sensitivity to criticism, and despondency during the first 2 weeks postpartum (peak between day 4 to 5 and resolution by day 10). This condition affects up to 85% of postpartum women. Symptoms are transient and require little intervention; however, approximately 20% of women with maternity blues go on to develop major depression in the first postpartum year. Postpartum psychosis refers to an acute onset of overt psychotic symptoms in the first 6 weeks postpartum. This condition is extremely rare, affecting 1 to 2 women per 1,000 deliveries, however, it is a psychiatric emergency requiring immediate intervention due to the risk of harm to the mother or her infant.[49]

Symptoms of major depression, as defined in the *Diagnostic and Statistical Manual of Mental Disorders IV* (DSM-IV) include: depressed mood, markedly diminished interest or pleasure in activities, sleep and/or appetite disturbance, fatigue, physical agitation, feelings of worthlessness or excessive guilt, decreased concentration or inability to make decisions, and/or recurrent thoughts of death or suicide.[50] Often many of the symptoms may be confused with normal sequelae of childbirth.

Hormonal theories have been postulated as triggers for postpartum emotional vulnerability, but the exact cause has yet to be pinpointed. The basis of the depressive thoughts may stem from inadequacy and insecurity in caring for the infant and can have significant functional impact. The social and psychologic insecurity in coping with the new role of parenthood may explain why first-time mothers are more likely to become depressed.

After women have been identified as suffering from postpartum depression, all treatment options should be evaluated. Psychosocial intervention has been effective in improving symptoms and disruptive interpersonal issues for postpartum women and is thought by some to be the first-line treatment. If treatment with antidepressants is deemed necessary, therapy should continue for 6 to 12 months postpartum to ensure complete recovery. Postpartum women may be more likely to respond to serotonergic agents, such as an SSRI or venlafaxine.[51] The treatment goals are the same as for other depressive episodes, but considerations for the risk versus benefit ratio to the baby and the mother complicate medication selection.[48]

Breast-feeding is an important consideration in treating women with postpartum depression. All antidepressants are excreted in human milk. While deleterious effects appear to be low, the effects of even trace amounts of medication on the developing brain are unknown. The use of antidepressants is not contraindicated during breast-feeding (the AAP classifies antidepressants as drugs whose effect on the nursing infant may be of concern) and should be considered in women with moderate to severe depression, suicidal thoughts or difficulty functioning, or those who have not responded to psychotherapy. In these women, the benefits of taking an antidepressant, particularly an SSRI, would most likely outweigh the risks to the infant. Because the FDA discourages use of fluoxetine by nursing mothers, sertraline, paroxetine, or citalopram would be preferable. Sertraline has been advocated as first-line treatment.[52] Newer antidepressants such as venlafaxine and nefazodone are excreted into human milk and caution has been urged with both of these agents in breast-feeding mothers. If the use of a tricyclic antidepressant is desired, nortriptyline appears not to accumulate in nursing infants. However, the AAP has expressed concerns about the effects of long-term exposure of tricyclic antidepressants on infants' neurobehavioral development; these concerns need to be considered.

DIABETES MELLITUS

The risk of congenital abnormalities is three times greater in pregnant overt diabetics than in the nondiabetic population.[53] Congenital anomalies occur in 3% to 22% of infants born to diabetic mothers and are associated with poor glucose control compared to 2% incidence in the normal population.[54] Blood glucose control is essential in decreasing the incidence of perinatal morbidity and mortality. When possible, pregnancy in the diabetic woman should be planned to prevent complications. It is important that the patient be normoglycemic before conception and during the first trimester because the congenital effects associated with dia-

betes are related to poor glucose control in the first 8 weeks of gestation.[55]

Patients at highest risk of complications during pregnancy include those with vasculopathy, poor glucose control, a previous stillbirth, and medication noncompliance. Diabetes during pregnancy is commonly categorized according to the White classification.[56] This system classifies patients based on presence of vascular disease, age of onset, and duration of diabetes mellitus in the patient. The potential effects on the infant include macrosomia, polyhydramnios, malformations, respiratory distress syndrome, and fetal behavior and intellectual impairment. With good prenatal management, diabetic patients now have a 96% chance of delivering a healthy child.

During pregnancy, diabetic patients have an increased risk of ketoacidosis, which may occur at lower glucose concentrations than in the nonpregnant diabetic woman. Ketoacidosis is associated with a 50% perinatal mortality rate and can be prevented with close monitoring at home by the patient. Glycosylated hemoglobin monitoring once each trimester is helpful in assessing control. Most women should be able to maintain glucose levels between 60 and 120 mg per dL (3.33 to 6.66 mmol/L).[57] About 70% of pregnant diabetic women have increased insulin requirements after the 24th week, and requirements usually double by the end of pregnancy. Insulin (category B) has a large molecular weight and crosses the placenta minimally with indirect effects on the fetus, making insulin the treatment of choice by the American College of Obstetricians and Gynecologists for patients with type I and II diabetes as well as gestational diabetes if diet alone fails. The use of insulin provides the best glucose control.[58] Breast-feeding significantly reduces blood sugars, allowing a reduced dose of insulin.[25] Diabetic mothers may breast-feed without insulin passing into breast milk.[11]

The use of the oral hypoglycemic agent, glyburide (category C), after the first trimester of pregnancy is considered an appropriate alternative to insulin in the control of glycemia in pregnancy not responsive to a reasonable trial of diet and exercise.[59] Glyburide offers the convenience to the patient of not having to use insulin and may improve patient compliance with no significant difference in adverse neonatal morbidity between the two treatment groups. Little information is available about the use of oral hypoglycemic agents during breast-feeding. Tolbutamide and chlorpropamide (both category C) are excreted in breast milk in small quantities, and tolbutamide is the recommended agent during nursing.[25] No reports describe the use of glipizide or glyburide during lactation, but an excretion pattern similar to that of chlorpropamide or tolbutamide should be expected.[10]

Gestational diabetes develops during the second half of pregnancy in 2% to 3% of patients.[54] Women with gestational diabetes have a lessened risk of congenital abnormalities compared to women with overt diabetes because gestational diabetes generally does not occur until the 24th week of gestation, after organogenesis is complete. The patient with gestational diabetes is initially placed on a diabetic diet and home glucose monitoring. If glucose control is not achieved with diet alone, insulin should be started.

Tight glucose control should be maintained during labor and delivery to reduce the risk of neonatal hypoglycemia. During delivery, the mother should receive regular insulin via IV infusion and glucose should be monitored every 1 to 2 hours with additional glucose or insulin given to maintain a glucose level of 100 mg per dL (5.55 mmol/L). Immediately after delivery, insulin requirements drop and remain low for 24 to 72 hours. The patient should be monitored closely to prevent hypoglycemic shock. If the mother chooses to breast-feed, lower insulin requirements are expected.

EPILEPSY

More than 1 million American women of childbearing age have epilepsy, but less than 1% of pregnancies are complicated by seizure disorders.[60] The primary goal in managing these patients is prevention of seizures with the fewest adverse effects on the fetus. Pregnancy has unpredictable effects on the frequency and severity of seizures. One third of patients reportedly have an increase in frequency of seizures; however, with increased attention to management of anticonvulsant therapy during pregnancy, this number is closer to 25%.[61] Women with epilepsy, both those taking medication and those not taking medication, have a higher incidence of delivering an infant with congenital malformations and mental retardation.[60,62] Although it is difficult to separate the effects of medication from the effects of disease, literature reviews indicate that anticonvulsants are associated with an increase in congenital defects. Although teratogenicity does occur with anticonvulsants, the benefits of treatment with appropriate anticonvulsants to prevent maternal seizures outweigh any risk to the infant.

The AAP recommends that a patient who is seizure-free for at least 2 years undergo a trial of medication withdrawal before becoming pregnant. Patient counseling should begin as soon as pregnancy is considered. The risk of delivering an infant with birth defects in the general population is 2% to 4% and increases to 4% to 6% in pregnant epileptic women receiving monotherapy. Pregnant epileptic women have a greater than 90% chance of having a normal child.[63]

Further research is needed to determine which anticonvulsant is safest for mother and child. Serious risks are inherent with each agent. Monotherapy is preferred, using the lowest effective dose possible to minimize risk. The clinician should be aware of the changes in anticonvulsant pharmacokinetics that occur during pregnancy, resulting in lower serum concentrations such as increased renal and hepatic clearance, decreased protein-binding capacity, and increased volume of distribution. Despite lower serum concentrations, seizure frequency may not increase because free drug concentrations do not decline proportionately with total drug concentration. Anticonvulsant serum concentrations should be monitored throughout pregnancy when appropriate and

dose adjustments made based on serum concentration, frequency of seizures, and adverse effects.

Serious and sometimes fatal hemorrhagic disease of the newborn may occur and be seen within 24 hours after delivery, particularly in infants exposed to anticonvulsants. This is caused by a deficiency in vitamin K-dependent clotting factors, and all infants should be treated prophylactically with vitamin K at birth.[62] Some physicians recommend administering oral vitamin K prophylactically to the mother during the last 2 to 4 weeks before expected delivery.[60] Prophylaxis is necessary because treatment may not be successful once there is clinical evidence of bleeding. Because folate deficiency occurs during anticonvulsant therapy, prophylactic administration of folic acid throughout gestation is recommended to prevent megaloblastic anemia and neural tube defects.[64]

Although the findings of fetal anticonvulsant syndrome have been described with virtually all of the antiepileptic agents, in some studies the use of certain agents was associated with a higher risk of specific malformations. Phenytoin (category D) causes fetal hydantoin syndrome, and effects may be evident in childhood. This syndrome includes school and learning problems, developmental problems, and physical abnormalities such as craniofacial abnormalities, growth retardation, limb defects, cardiac lesions, hernias, and distal digital and nail hypoplasias.[65] There is about a 10% risk for a fetus exposed to phenytoin to develop the full syndrome and about 30% risk for partial expression of the syndrome.[66]

Phenobarbital (category D) appears to be less teratogenic than phenytoin, but cleft lip and palate, and heart defects have been associated with its use in pregnancy.[62] Similar to phenytoin, coagulopathy and folate deficiency may occur with phenobarbital use. Unlike phenytoin, phenobarbital may cause neonatal addiction and withdrawal symptoms, such as hyperactivity, feeding disturbances, tremulousness, or diarrhea. Phenobarbital appears in milk in relatively large amounts, with drowsiness, potential feeding difficulties, infantile spasms after weaning, and one case of methemoglobinemia reported.[10,12,25] Phenobarbital may be used cautiously in low doses during breast-feeding with close monitoring of infant behavior, weight gain, and periodic infant serum concentrations.[12]

Carbamazepine (category D) has been used in pregnancy and was thought to be less teratogenic than other anticonvulsants. However, reports indicate that carbamazepine is teratogenic and has been associated with defects such as spina bifida (1%), craniofacial defects, nail hypoplasia, and developmental delay.[67,68] According to the AAP, carbamazepine may be used during lactation, but occasional monitoring of infant serum drug levels may be indicated.[12]

The fetal valproate syndrome is dose-related and has been described in case reports with associations of cleft palate, renal defects, and neural tube defects (1% to 2%).[69,70] Minor and major cardiovascular and craniofacial malformations, mental and physical developmental deficiencies, and meningomyelocele have also occurred with its use in pregnancy.

It appears that valproate (category D) is teratogenic and should be avoided during pregnancy.[71] However, low valproate concentrations are found in milk, and no adverse effects have been reported in breast-fed infants.[10]

The most recent results of the Lamotrigine Pregnancy Registry are encouraging that lamotrigine (category C) does not provide a major risk for congenital malformations or fetal loss following first trimester exposure compared with the older anticonvulsants.[72] The results of the Gabapentin Pregnancy Registry indicate that the numbers of malformations with gabapentin (category C) are similar to the other antiepileptics.[72] Oxcarbazepine (category C) has a more favorable teratogenic profile than carbamazepine due to its lack of a teratogenic epoxide metabolite. However, the available human data is too limited to assess the absolute risk to the fetus of exposure to oxcarbazepine. Data on the use of felbamate, levetiracetam, topiramate, and zonisamide during pregnancy are limited. The manufacturer of felbamate suggests that it be used with caution in breast-feeding mothers. Women receiving gabapentin, lamotrigine, topiramate, or tiagabine should breastfeed only if the benefits outweigh the risks. Because the AAP considers carbamazepine compatible with breast-feeding, oxcarbazepine probably can be similarly classified. [10]

HEARTBURN

Up to two thirds of pregnant women complain of heartburn, particularly during the third trimester.[73] A study conducted by Marrero et al. found that the prevalence of heartburn increased significantly in the first (22%), second (39%), and third (72%) trimesters, respectively.[74] Heartburn during pregnancy results from relaxation of the lower esophageal sphincter and increased pressure from the uterus onto the stomach, allowing regurgitation of stomach contents into the lower esophagus. Alternatively, it has been proposed that hormonal changes in pregnancy result in changes in gut motor function, which, among other effects, lead to abnormal gastroesophageal reflux.[74] Nonpharmacologic management should be tried initially and a low fat diet is recommended. Patients should also avoid caffeine, spicy foods, orange juice, tomato juice, or peppermint. Small, frequent meals and avoiding meals just before bedtime often help alleviate the symptoms. Elevating the head of the bed is sometimes effective as well. Antacids such as magnesium and/or aluminum hydroxides are usually effective and appear to be safe. Calcium carbonate may be used and has the added benefit of much needed calcium supplementation during pregnancy; however, its duration of action is very short. Although sucralfate is an aluminum salt, and aluminum has been associated with neurobehavioral and skeletal toxicity in animals, there is no evidence of absorption from the gastrointestinal tract and no reports of associated congenital defects when it is taken during pregnancy or adverse effects on breastfed infants.[73]

Drugs used in the nonpregnant patient to manipulate lower esophageal sphincter tone currently are not recommended during pregnancy. Antacids should be used rather than histamine-2 antagonists, bethanechol (category C), and metoclopramide (category B). Despite the antiandrogenic effects of cimetidine, this effect is not present with ranitidine. Data indicate no association of ranitidine and fetal or neonatal effects when used throughout pregnancy, and it would be the preferred agent if a histamine-2 antagonist is needed. Because famotidine has less excretion in breast milk, it is the histamine-2 antagonist of choice during lactation.[26] Although metoclopramide is used as a lactation stimulant for women with inadequate or decreased milk production, its use is classified by the AAP as a potential concern during breast-feeding because of the potent central nervous system effects. However, no adverse effects have been reported in nursing infants.[12]

HEMORRHOIDS

Hemorrhoids often develop or worsen during pregnancy owing to increased venous pressure below the uterus and constipation. Treating the constipation along with sitz baths are useful in reducing discomfort from hemorrhoids. Over-the-counter external medications are preferred over those inserted into the rectum because of possible systemic absorption across the rectal mucosa. Use of topical cleansing products containing witch hazel is also helpful in easing the discomfort. Nonprescription products containing topical anesthetics and prescription products containing corticosteroids should be avoided in pregnancy, except when recommended or prescribed by a physician, because of their potential for systemic absorption and effects on the fetus.

HYPERTENSION

Pregnancy-induced hypertension can be a serious and life-threatening obstetric complication. Gestational hypertension is diagnosed when the blood pressure exceeds 140/90 mm Hg in the absence of proteinuria or pathologic edema. Preeclampsia is divided into two forms, mild and severe. Mild preeclampsia is hypertension accompanied by proteinuria and/or pathologic edema. Preeclampsia is considered severe when proteinuria exceeds 4 g/24 hours or persistent values of 2+ are present by dipstick; blood pressure is 160/110 mm Hg; and/or severe headache, visual disturbances, or epigastric pain is noted. Eclampsia is the development of generalized seizures in a patient with pregnancy-induced hypertension. Pregnancy-aggravated hypertension is diagnosed in a patient with preexisting essential hypertension with diastolic increases of 15 mm Hg or systolic increases of 30 mm Hg after the 24th week of gestation. Preeclampsia is superimposed if proteinuria or pathologic edema is present.[1]

The incidence of preeclampsia is 5% to 8% in the United States.[1] Risk factors include first pregnancy (up to 85%), young or older maternal age, multiple gestation, family history, diabetes mellitus, essential hypertension, and molar pregnancies (i.e., tumor-like mass of cysts instead of embryo that grows from tissue of fertilized egg). Complications include intrauterine growth retardation (IUGR), placental insufficiency or abruption, and preterm labor and delivery. The incidence of complications increases in direct proportion to increased blood pressure.

Prevention of preeclampsia with low-dose aspirin has been suggested for patients who are at high risk of developing preeclampsia. Because of the potential imbalance of prostaglandins as a causative factor for preeclampsia, prophylactic aspirin has been studied. Low-dose aspirin (60 mg/day) has been shown to decrease thromboxane while sparing prostacyclin synthesis.[75,76] The usefulness of low-dose aspirin in preventing preeclampsia seemed promising in initial studies, but a meta-analysis found that aspirin failed to reduce the incidence of preeclampsia and did not improve maternal or fetal outcomes. A recent Cochrane review of the effectiveness and safety of aspirin concluded that despite small overall benefits, including a 15% reduction in preeclampsia, a number of questions remain. Therefore, there is insufficient evidence to make a clear recommendation for the use of low-dose aspirin for prevention of preeclampsia.[77]

The goal of treatment of preeclampsia is to decrease blood pressure, prevent or control seizures, and deliver a viable infant. Treatment for mild preeclampsia includes bed rest, daily urine protein measurements, and twice daily blood pressure monitoring. Diuresis usually begins within 48 hours with symptom regression within 5 days. Patients unable or unwilling to comply with these restrictions should be hospitalized. Women with severe preeclampsia must be hospitalized, IV or intramuscular (IM) magnesium sulfate given to prevent seizures, and plans for induction of labor or cesarean delivery made. IV administration may be preferred owing to the feasibility of rapid discontinuation if toxicity occurs. Monitoring for signs of magnesium toxicity is extremely important with maintenance of serum concentrations at 4 to 7 mEq per L (2–3.5 mmol/L). Patient patellar reflexes, respiratory rate, and urine output should also be followed. Neonates should be monitored for respiratory depression and hyporeflexia if exposed to magnesium sulfate for an extended period of time. Management of mild maternal magnesium toxicity may be treated with calcium, but this may not be effective for hypermagnesemia of the neonate. Maternal seizures not controlled by adequate serum concentrations of magnesium may respond to IV diazepam or phenytoin.

Antihypertensive medications have not been shown to improve perinatal outcomes in pregnancy-induced hypertension or mild to moderate preeclampsia (140–160/90–110 mm Hg) and should not be routinely prescribed.[77] Aggressive pharmacologic treatment of severe hypertension (>160 mm Hg systolic and/or >110 mm Hg diastolic) or rapidly rising blood pressure (>30 mm Hg) is warranted to decrease the risk of maternal eclampsia or stroke. IV hydralazine (category C) is most commonly used and has not been clearly associated with congenital defects; however, three cases of neonatal thrombocytopenia and bleeding have been documented with its use. Patients may experience tachycardia, headache, flushing, tremors, and palpitations. Propranolol (category C) may be useful for decreasing the cardiac effects

but should not be used alone for treatment of hypertension. Labetalol (category C) is an acceptable alternative to hydralazine for the treatment of hypertensive crisis of pregnancy. Labetalol has a faster onset with less tachycardia than hydralazine, but IV hydralazine tends to be more effective.[1,78] Neonatal bradycardia and mild transient hypotension have been reported rarely with labetalol. Nitroprusside (category C) has been used for life-threatening hypertensive emergencies, but should be avoided if possible because of the potential for neonatal cyanide toxicity.

Methyldopa (category B) remains the drug of choice for treating hypertension during pregnancy.[66] Data regarding long-term effects fail to document physical or mental abnormalities caused by the drug. Using methyldopa reportedly increases fetal survival rates and decreases midtrimester fetal loss. Clonidine (category C) is an alternative agent that has been effective for severe hypertension in late pregnancy with no associated reports of congenital abnormalities.[79] However, because clonidine offers no advantage over methyldopa and there is more experience with methyldopa, methyldopa is generally the preferred agent. Hydralazine has also been used in conjunction with methyldopa when needed for chronic hypertension.

β-Blockers, especially atenolol (category D), may be associated with fetal growth restriction and are not recommended for use in pregnancy unless methyldopa and/or hydralazine fail to control blood pressure. Because of the lower excretion of drug in milk, β-blockers labetalol, metoprolol, and propranolol would be preferred for use in breast-feeding mothers as supported by the AAP.[10,12,25]

Despite widespread use of calcium channel blockers (CCBs) in the treatment of hypertension in the nonpregnant population, there is limited information available on the use of calcium channel blockers in pregnancy.[80,81] However, one study of women with first-trimester exposure to CCBs found no increased risk of congenital malformations compared to controls. Nifedipine (category C) has been used effectively to treat acute hypertensive crises of pregnancy, however it has been associated with fatal and nonfatal cardiovascular events and is therefore not recommended for treatment of hypertensive crises. Although limited information is available, the AAP considers these agents safe for use in nursing mothers.[12]

Angiotensin-converting enzyme inhibitors (ACEIs) are contraindicated in pregnancy because they cause fetal and neonatal anuria, oligohydramnios, congenital malformations, and fetal death.[78,82] Angiotensin II receptor antagonists are believed to have similar effects as ACEIs and are not recommended for use in pregnancy. Mothers with exposure to ACEIs should receive counseling regarding potential adverse outcomes, and infants who were exposed should be monitored closely for renal failure and hypotension.[83] Captopril and enalapril are found in small quantities in breast milk with no adverse effects in infants and are considered compatible with breast-feeding according to the AAP.[12,25]

The use of diuretics in pregnancy is controversial. The main concern regarding diuretic use is their effect on the volume status of the patient by decreasing plasma and extracellular volume, decreasing cardiac output, and decreasing placental and uterine perfusion. This may accentuate problems in women with previously contracted fluid volumes and preeclampsia. Thiazides and loop diuretics have been used in late gestation for refractory hypertension. Adverse effects of thiazide diuretics include neonatal hypoglycemia resulting from maternal hyperglycemia, electrolyte imbalances, thrombocytopenia, decreased weight gain, and increased perinatal mortality. Therefore, these agents are not first-line therapy for treatment of hypertension in pregnancy. The AAP considers thiazide diuretics compatible with nursing, but thrombocytopenia, lactation suppression, and allergic reactions are potential adverse effects of sulfonamide diuretics.[12,25] Loop diuretics may suppress the volume of milk produced and should be avoided. Acetazolamide and spironolactone appear in negligible concentrations in milk and are compatible with breast-feeding.[12,25]

NAUSEA AND VOMITING

The nausea and/or vomiting of pregnancy is usually mild and often referred to as *morning sickness*. Up to 80% of pregnant women experience nausea and vomiting during pregnancy, most commonly during the first trimester. Nausea and vomiting of pregnancy is distinguished from hyperemesis gravidarum, which is intractable vomiting leading to electrolyte imbalance, maternal weight loss, altered nutritional status, and at times, end-organ or neurologic damage.[84] Hyperemesis gravidarum occurs in 1 in 1,000 births and generally requires hospitalization and treatment with IV fluids, electrolytes, antiemetics, and sedation. In very severe cases, parenteral nutrition may be necessary. Treatment with parenteral nutrition has been effective in providing the mother and fetus with adequate nutrition.[84]

Symptoms usually begin within a few weeks of conception and continue through the first 4 months. Nausea is often apparent on arising but abates as the day progresses. Some women report nausea and vomiting throughout the day and in some patients it persists throughout the pregnancy. Although symptoms are self-limiting, nearly 83% of women experiencing nausea and vomiting report taking medication for relief.[85,86]

The etiology of nausea and vomiting in pregnancy is unknown, but several possibilities are proposed, including increased concentrations of hormones during pregnancy, pyridoxine deficiency, and emotional and psychologic factors. Because the cause is unknown, treatment is focused on the symptoms. The goal of therapy is to eliminate the symptoms, improve the patient's quality of life, minimize harm to the fetus, and prevent hyperemesis gravidarum from occurring. Conservative nonpharmacologic measures should be tried first. Mild-to-moderate nausea and vomiting may be managed by efforts such as instructing the patient to eat small, frequent meals. High-carbohydrate meals, crackers, or high-protein snacks also may be helpful. Spicy foods and noxious odors should be avoided, and many patients find relief by lying down. Drinking ginger ale (made from real ginger) or salty liquids, such as sports beverages may be helpful. The use of elastic wristbands used to put pressure on the inner wrist (Seabands) has been advocated as safe and possibly effective. Two studies showed initial improvement and reduced symptom duration with this method, but the effect was not sustained.

When nondrug measures fail or if the nutritional and metabolic health of the mother is at risk, drug therapy may be required. Although teratogenic risk cannot be ruled out for any drug, the risk involved with the current agents used for nausea and vomiting in pregnancy appears to be minimal. The currently available over-the-counter products for nausea containing phosphorated carbohydrate appear to be benign and may be used. Meclizine (category B) is commonly used as the drug of choice; use in the first trimester has been associated with low teratogenic risk. Dimenhydrinate or doxylamine (both category B) have been used as an alternative with low risk of adverse outcomes.[87] When symptoms are not controlled and the health of the mother and fetus calls for drug therapy, phenothiazines (i.e., promethazine or prochlorperazine) may be used. Conflicting results have been reported regarding the safety of phenothiazines, therefore routine use is not recommended. Metoclopramide (category B) is the antiemetic of choice for treatment of nausea and vomiting of pregnancy in Europe.[88] A recent report indicated that metoclopramide during pregnancy is not associated with fetal malformations.[89] Other agents that appear safe in pregnancy include droperidol (category C) or trimethobenzamide (category C). Ondansetron (category B) recently has been given to women with nausea and vomiting of pregnancy and appears to be safe and effective.[90]

Pyridoxine deficiency has been hypothesized to cause nausea and vomiting of pregnancy. The demand for pyridoxine is increased during pregnancy, and women may develop a deficiency of this vitamin if supplementation is not given. However, the deficiency does not develop until the second or third trimester. Thus, this may not explain symptoms of nausea and vomiting that occur with normal pyridoxine levels or in the first trimester. One study confirmed previous reports that pyridoxine is useful for nausea and vomiting of pregnancy for the first 3 days of use, but the benefit decreases thereafter.[91]

OTHER COMMONLY USED DRUGS OF ABUSE

In addition to counseling pregnant women regarding various prescription and nonprescription medications during pregnancy and lactation, other substances that are commonly used should not be overlooked. Pregnant women should be informed of the risks of using any of the following substances.

ALCOHOL

The worldwide incidence of fetal alcohol syndrome (FAS) is estimated to be between 1:300 and 1:2,000 live births.[92,93] The syndrome is characterized by defects of the central nervous system, craniofacial abnormalities, and growth and mental difficulties. Affected infants can display a wide range of other abnormalities. Mental retardation is the most significant consequence. Nearly 30% to 40% of infants born to alcoholic women have complete FAS, and up to 70% may have partial expression of the syndrome, referred to as fetal alcohol effects (FAE). Additional maternal factors that may contribute to expression of the syndrome are poor nutrition, smoking, drug abuse, inadequate prenatal care, genetic disposition, and low socioeconomic status.

The effects are dose-related, but the amount of ethanol that may be ingested without causing abnormalities is unknown. Two drinks per day has been related to decreased birth weight, while binge drinking or more than six drinks per day are associated with adverse physical and intellectual outcomes and possibly stillbirth.[94,95] Pregnant women should be informed that a safe level of consumption and the phase of development of the fetus that is most susceptible to alcohol are not known. Women should thus avoid alcohol throughout pregnancy and when trying to conceive.

Although alcohol passes freely into breast milk, reaching concentrations of approximately maternal serum levels, the effects on infants have been considered insignificant except in rare cases or at very high concentrations. Potentiation of hypothrombinemic bleeding, a pseudo-Cushing syndrome, has been reported in nursing infants of alcoholic mothers.[10] Alcohol ingestion of 1 g/kg daily decreases the milk ejection reflex. Alcohol should be used in moderation during lactation and nursing should be withheld temporarily after alcohol consumption (i.e., 1 to 2 hours per drink).[25] Despite potential effects in infants such as drowsiness, diaphoresis, deep sleep, weakness, decrease in linear growth, and abnormal weight gain, the AAP considers maternal ethanol use compatible with breast-feeding.[12]

CAFFEINE

Caffeine (category B) is found in various quantities in many beverages, analgesics, diet aids, and stimulants. This makes caffeine the number one drug ingested by pregnant women. This potent central nervous system stimulant crosses the placenta, with fetal levels similar to maternal levels, but caffeine has not been shown to be a major teratogen in humans.[98] Numerous studies have been done to assess effects on the fetus, with results ranging from no effect to demonstration of complications. These studies are difficult to interpret because of confounding factors, such as cigarette and alcohol use. Long-term data through age 7 has shown no effects of perinatal caffeine exposure on intelligence, attention, or physical growth.[97] A positive correlation exists between heavy caffeine use and cigarette smoking. High doses of caffeine may cause fetal breathing movements and cardiac arrhythmias. Currently studies are looking at the risk of spontaneous abortion and intrauterine growth retardation because of conflicting results in prior studies.[98] In 1980 the FDA advised all women, based on animal toxicity data, to avoid caffeine use during pregnancy. However, no association with congenital malformations, spontaneous abortions, preterm birth, or low birth weight has been proven when caffeine is used in moderation.[10]

In breast-feeding, the concentrations of caffeine in breast milk after maternal ingestion is probably too small to be clinically important, and the AAP considers usual amounts of caffeine to be compatible with breast-feeding.[10] However, reports exist of infant jitteriness and difficulty sleeping with high maternal intake of caffeine (3–6 caffeinated drinks per day).[25]

NICOTINE

Maternal smoking is one of the few known preventable causes of perinatal morbidity and mortality. Despite documentation and information regarding the adverse effects on the fetus and the mother, young women continue to be a large consumer group of smokers.[99] Fetal, neonatal, and infant mortality is increased, birth weight and length are decreased, gestation is shortened, and the frequency of fetal breathing movements is reduced. Complications of pregnancy such as abruptio placentae, premature rupture of membranes, amnionitis, and placenta previa may also occur. Changes in uterine and placental oxygenation or blood flow may be the cause of infant death, prematurity, or spontaneous abortions. Complications in infancy and childhood may evolve into deficits in long-term physical growth or intellectual and behavioral performance.[100]

The effect of smoking is dose-related, including low birth weight and fetal death. According to the Surgeon General's report in 1990 on smoking cessation, women who quit smoking within the first trimester of pregnancy or before conception reduce the risk of having a low-birth-weight baby compared to those of women who never smoked.[101] Birth weight may not be improved if the woman simply reduces the number of cigarettes smoked per day. All women should be informed of the risk of smoking on the fetus and encouraged to quit during pregnancy. A recent study also suggests neurotoxic effects of prenatal tobacco exposure on newborn neurobehavior.[102]

Nicotine and its metabolite, cotinine, are concentrated in milk and excreted in amounts proportional to the number of cigarettes smoked by the mother.[25] Smoking is associated with infantile colic.[103] Nicotine shortens the period of breast-feeding by lowering maternal serum prolactin concentrations. The AAP considers smoking to be contraindicated during breast-feeding.[12] Some experts advise lactating women to stop or decrease smoking as much as possible, not to smoke before nursing, and not to smoke in the same room with the infant.[25]

TABLE 19.4	Over-the-Counter Drugs of Choice	
Drug Class	**During Pregnancy**	**During Lactation**
Analgesics	Acetaminophen	Acetaminophen
Antacids	Calcium carbonate	Calcium carbonate
Antihistamine	Chlorpheniramine	Chlorpheniramine
Decongestants	Oxymetazoline or phenylephrine nasal drops/spray	
Hemorrhoidal agents	Preparation H ointment	Preparation H ointment
Laxatives/stool softeners	Psyllium or docusate	Psyllium or docusate

(From Smith J, Taddio A, Koren G. Drugs of choice for pregnant women. In: Koren G, ed. Maternal-fetal toxicology: a clinician's guide 2nd ed. Rev. New York: Marcel Dekker, 1994; Koren G, Pastuszak A, Ito S. Drugs in pregnancy. N Engl J Med 338 : 1128–1137, 1998; Logsdon BA. Drugs in lactation. J Am Pharm Assoc 37 : 407–418, 1997, with permission.)

KEY POINTS

1. Medication use in pregnancy and lactation is a complex issue, and efforts must be made to provide the patient, as well as the fetus or neonate, with the most safe and effective medication(s). Over-the-counter agents that may be recommended as first-line treatment in pregnant or lactating mothers are summarized in Table 19.4.

2. Most medications taken by the mother reach the fetus to some extent, and effects on the fetus are often unknown. Patient education is imperative to insure optimal patient care with minimal risk of toxicity.

SUGGESTED READINGS

American Academy of Pediatrics Committee on Drugs. The transfer of drugs and other chemicals into human breast milk. *Pediatrics* 2001; 108:776–789.

Briggs GG, Freeman RK, Yaffe SJ. Drugs in pregnancy and lactation. 6th ed. Baltimore: Williams & Wilkins, 2002.

Hale T. Medications in mother's milk. 9th ed. Amarillo: Pharmasoft, 2000.

Koren G, Pastuszak A, Ito S. Drugs in pregnancy. New Engl J Med 338: 1128–1137, 1998.

REFERENCES

1. Cunningham FG, MacDonald PC, Grant NF, et al. Williams obstetrics. 19th ed. Norwalk: Appleton & Lange, 1993.
2. Bodendorfer TW, Briggs GG, Gunning JE. Obtaining drug exposure histories during pregnancy. Am J Obstet Gynecol 135: 490–494, 1979.
3. Bonati M, Bortolus R, Marchetti F, et al. Drug use in pregnancy: an overview of epidemiological (drug utilization) studies. Eur J Clin Pharmacol 38:325–328, 1990.
4. Collaboerative Group on Drug Use in Pregnancy. An international survey on drug utilization during pregnancy. Int J Risk Saf Med 1: 1, 1991.
5. Bennett PN, Matheson I, Dukes NMG, et al. Drugs and human lactation. Amsterdam: Elsevier, 1988.
6. Matheson I, Kristensen K, Lunde PKM. Drug utilization in breast feeding women. A survey in Oslo. Eur J Clin Pharmacol 38: 453–459, 1990.
7. American Academy of Pediatrics Work Group on Breastfeeding. Breastfeeding and the use of human milk. Pediatrics 100: 1035–1039, 1997.
8. Oakley GP. Frequency of human congenital malformations. Clin Perinatol 13:545–554, 1986.
9. Food and Drug Administration. Labeling and prescription drug advertising: content and format for labeling for human prescription drugs. Federal Register 44:37434–37467, 1979.
10. Briggs GG, Freeman RK, Yaffe SJ. Drugs in pregnancy and lactation. 6th ed. Baltimore: Williams & Wilkins, 2002.
11. Hale T. Medications in mothers' milk. 9th ed. Amarillo: Pharmasoft, 2000.
12. American Academy of Pediatrics Committee on Drugs. The transfer of drugs and other chemicals into human breast milk. Pediatrics 108:776–789, 2001.
13. Werler MM, Pober BR, Nelson K, et al. Reporting accuracy among mothers of malformed and nonmalformed infants. Am J Epidemiol 129:415–421, 1989.
14. Friedman JM. Teratogenic effects of drugs: a resource for clinicians. Baltimore: Johns Hopkins University Press, 1994.
15. Niebyl JR. Drug use in pregnancy. 2nd ed. Philadelphia: Lea & Febiger, 1988.
16. Dicke JM. Teratology: principles and practice. Med Clin North Am 73:567–582, 1989.
17. Perlow JH, Montgomery D, Morgan MA, et al. Severity of asthma and perinatal outcome. Am J Obstet Gynecol 167:963–967, 1992.
18. Clark SL. Asthma in pregnancy. Obstet Gynecol 82:1036–1040, 1993.
19. Demissie K, Marcella SW, Breckenridgee MB, et al. Maternal asthma and transient tachypnea of the newborn. Pediatrics 102: 84–90, 1998.
20. Tan KS, Thomson NC. Asthma in pregnancy. Am J Med 109: 727–733, 2000.
21. Schwartz DB. Medical disorders in pregnancy. Emerg Med Clin North Am 5:509–528, 1987.
22. Stenius-Aarniala B, Piirila P, Teramo K. Asthma and pregnancy: a prospective study of 198 pregnancies. Thorax 43:12–18, 1988.
23. Carter BL, Driscoll CE, Smith GD. Theophylline clearance during pregnancy. Obstet Gynecol 68:555–559, 1986.
24. Greenberger PA. Asthma in pregnancy. Clin Perinatol 12:571–584, 1985.
25. Anderson PO. Drug use during breast-feeding. Clin Pharm 10: 594–624, 1991.
26. Greenberger PA, Patterson R. Beclomethasone dipropionate for severe asthma during pregnancy. Ann Intern Med 98:478–480, 1983.
27. Wilson J. Use of sodium cromoglycate during pregnancy: results on 296 asthmatic women. J Pharm Med 8:45–51, 1982.
28. Rutherford SE, Phelan JP. Clinical management of thromboembolic disorders in pregnancy. Crit Care Clin 7:809–828, 1991.
29. Greer IA. Exploring the role of Low-molecular-weight heparins in pregnancy. SeminThromb Hemost 28:25–31, 2002.

30. Dahlman TC, Hellgreen MS, Blomback M. Thrombosis prophylaxis in pregnancy with use of subcutaneous heparin adjusted by monitoring heparin concentrations. Am J Obstet Gynecol 161: 420–425, 1989.

31. Ginsberg JS, Hirsh J, Turner DC, et al. Risks to the fetus of anticoagulant therapy during pregnancy. Thromb Haemost 61:197–203, 1989.

32. Wahlberg TB, Kher A. Low molecular weight heparin as thromboprophylaxis in pregnancy. Haemostasis 24:55–56, 1994.

33. Incaudo GA. Diagnosis and treatment of allergic rhinitis during pregnancy and lactation. Clin Rev Allergy 5:325–327, 1987.

34. Smith J, Taddio A, Koren G. Drugs of choice for pregnant women. In: Koren G, ed. Maternal-fetal toxicology: a clinician's guide. 2nd ed. Rev. New York: Marcel Dekker, 1994.

35. West L, Warren J, Cutis T. Diagnosis and management of irritable bowel syndrome, constipation, and diarrhea during pregnancy. Gastroenterol Clin North Am 21:793–802, 1992.

36. Weissman MM, Olfson M. Depression in women: implications for health care research. Science 269:799–801, 1995.

37. Campbell SB, Cohn JF, Meyers T. Depression in first-time mothers: mother-infant interaction and depression chronicity. Dev Psychol 31:349–357, 1995.

38. Gelfand DM, Teti DM. How does maternal depression affect children? Harvard Mental Health Letter November, 1995.

39. O'Hara MW, Swain AM. Rates and risk of postpartum depression: a meta-analysis. Int Rev Psychiatry 8:37–54, 1996.

40. O'Hara MW, Zeloski EM, Philipps LH, et al. Controlled prospective study of postpartum mood disorders: comparison of childbearing and nonchildbearing women. J Abnorm Psychol 99:3–15, 1990.

41. Nonacs R, Cohen LS. Postpartum mood disorders: diagnosis and treatment guidelines. J Clin Psychiatry 59 (Suppl 2):34–40, 1998.

42. Wisner KL, Peindl KS, Hanusa BH. Psychobiology of postpartum mood disorders. Semin Reprod Endocrinol 15:77–89, 1997.

43. Alshuler LL, Cohen L, Szuba MP, et al. Pharmacologic management of psychiatric illness in pregnancy: dilemmas and guidelines. Am J Psychiatry 153:592–606, 1996.

44. Potter WZ, Manji HK, Rudorfer MV. Tricyclics and tetracyclics. In: Schatzberg AF, Nemeroff CB, eds. Textbook of psychopharmacology. Washington DC: American Psychiatric Press, 1995.

45. Susman JL. Postpartum depressive disorders. J Fam Pract 43: S17–S24, 1996.

46. GlaxoSmithKline. Paxil package insert, 2004.

47. Neugebauer R, Kline J, O'Connor P, et al. Depressive symptoms in women in the six months after miscarriage. Am J Obstet Gynecol 166:104–109, 1992.

48. Llewellyn AM, Stowe ZN, Nemeroff CB. Depression during pregnancy and the puerperium. J Clin Psychiatry 58:26–32, 1997.

49. Kendall RE, Chalmers JC, Platz C. Epidemiology of puerperal psychoses. Br J Psychiatry 150:662–673, 1987.

50. American Psychiatric Association. Diagnostic and statistical manual of mental disorders. 4th ed. Washington, D.C.: American Psychiatric Association, 1994.

51. Wisner KL, Parry BL, Piontek CM. Postpartum depression. N Engl J Med 347:194–199, 2002.

52. Altshuler LL, Cohen LS, Moline ML, et al. The expert consensus guideline series: treatment of depression in women. Postgrad Med (special number):1–107, 2001.

53. Reece EA, Hobbins JC. Diabetic embryopathy: pathogenesis, prenatal diagnosis, and prevention. Obstet Gynecol Surv 41:325–335, 1986.

54. Barss VA. Diabetes and pregnancy. Med Clin North Am 73: 685–700, 1989.

55. Gabbe SG. Management of diabetes mellitus in pregnancy. Am J Obstet Gynecol 153:824–828, 1985.

56. White P. Classification of obstetric diabetes. Am J Obstet Gynecol 149:171–173, 1984.

57. Landon MB, Gabbe SG. Diabetes mellitus and pregnancy. Obstet Gynecol Clin North Am 19:633–654, 1992.

58. Committee on Technical Bulletins of the American College of Obstetricians and Gynecologists. ACOG Technical Bulletin, No. 200, December 1994.

59. Reece EA, Homko C, Miodovnik M, et al. A consensus report of the diabetes in pregnancy study group of north America conference. J Maternal Fetal Neonat Med 12:362–364, 2002.

60. Yerby MS, Devinsky O. Epilepsy and pregnancy. Adv Neurol 64: 53–63, 1994.

61. Devinsky O, Yerby MS. Women with epilepsy: reproduction and effects of pregnancy on epilepsy. Neurol Clin 12:479–495, 1994.

62. Dalessio DJ. Seizures and pregnancy. N Engl J Med 312:559–563, 1985.

63. American Academy of Pediatrics Committee on Drugs. Anticonvulsants and pregnancy. Pediatrics 63:331–333, 1979.

64. Delgado-Escueta AV, Janz D. Consensus guidelines: preconception counseling, management, and care of the pregnant woman with epilepsy. Neurology 42:149–160, 1992.

65. Buehler BA, Delimont D, Van Waes M, et al. Prenatal prediction of risk of the fetal hydantoin syndrome. N Engl J Med 322: 1567–1572, 1990.

66. Lewis DP, VanDyke DC, Shimbo PJ, et al. Drug and environmental factors associated with adverse pregnancy outcomes. Part I: Antiepileptic drugs, contraceptives, smoking, and folate. Ann Pharmacother 32:802–817, 1998.

67. Jones KL, Lacro RV, Johnson KA, et al. Pattern of malformations in the children of women treated with carbamazepine during pregnancy. N Engl J Med 320:1661–1666, 1989.

68. Roza FW. Spina bifida in infants of women treated with carbamazepine during pregnancy. N Engl J Med 324:674–675, 1991.

69. DiLiberti JH, Farndon PA, Dennis NR, et al. The fetal valproate syndrome. Am J Med Genet 19:473–481, 1984.

70. Omtzigt JG, Los FJ, Grobbee DE, et al. The risk of spina bifida after first trimester valproate exposure in a prenatal cohort. Neurology 42:119–125, 1992.

71. Nau H, Tzimas G, Mondry M, et al. Antiepileptic drugs after endogenous retinoid concentrations: a possible mechanism of teratogenesis of anticonvulsant therapy. Life Sci 57:53–60, 1995.

72. Pennell PB. The importance of monotherapy in pregnancy. Neurology 60:S31–8, 2003.

73. Baron TH, Ramirez B, Richter JE. Gastrointestinal motility disorders during pregnancy. Ann Intern Med 118:366–375, 1993.

74. Marrero JM, Goggin PM, Caestecker JS, et al. Determinants of pregnancy heartburn. Br J Obstet Gynecol 27:57–62, 1988.

75. Sibai BM, Caritis SN, Thom E, et al. Prevention of preeclampsia with low-dose aspirin in healthy, nulliparous pregnant women. N Engl J Med 329:1213–1218, 1993.

76. Hauth JC, Goldenberg RL, Parker CR, et al. Low-dose aspirin therapy to prevent preeclampsia. Am J Obstet Gynecol 168: 1083–1093, 1993.

77. Peters RM, Flack JM. Hypertensive disorders of pregnancy. J Obstet Gynecol Neonat Nurs 33:209–220, 2004.

78. Kyle PM, Redman CWG. Comparative risk-benefit assessment of drugs used in the management of hypertension in pregnancy. Drug Saf 7:223–234, 1992.

79. Horvath JS, Phippard A, Korda A. Clonidine hydrochloride—a safe and effective antihypertensive agent in pregnancy. Obstet Gynecol 66:634–638, 1985.

78. Goldberg CA, Schrier RW. Hypertension and pregnancy. Semin Nephrol 11:576–593, 1991.

79. Probst BD. Hypertensive disorders of pregnancy. Emerg Med Clin North Am 12:73–89, 1994.

80. Shotan A, Wilderhorn J, Hurst A, et al. Risks of angiotensin-converting enzyme inhibition during pregnancy: experimental and clinical evidence, potential mechanisms, and recommendations for use. Am J Med 96:451–456, 1994.

81. Rosa FW, Bosco LA, Graham CF, et al. Neonatal anuria with maternal angiotensin-converting enzyme inhibition. Obstet Gynecol 74:371–374, 1989.

82. Walters WAW. The management of nausea and vomiting during pregnancy. Med J Aust 147:290–291, 1987.

83. Vellacott ID, Cooke EJA, James CE. Nausea and vomiting in early pregnancy. Int J Gynecol Obstet 27:57–62, 1988.

84. Gadsby R, Barnie-Adshead AM, Jagger C. A prospective study of nausea and vomiting during pregnancy. Br J Gen Pract 43: 245–248, 1993.

85. Wernhoft E, Dykes AK. Effect of acupuncture on nausea and vomiting during pregnancy: a randomized placebo-controlled pilot study. J Reprod Med 46:835–839, 2001.

86. Norheim AJ, Pedersen EJ, Fonnebo V, et al. Accupressure treatment of morning sickness in pregnancy: a randomized, double-

blind, placebo-controlled study. Scand J Prim Health Care 19: 43–47, 2001.

87. Leathem AM. Safety and efficacy of antiemetics used to treat nausea and vomiting in pregnancy. Clin Pharm 5:660–668, 1986.

88. Einarson A, Koren G, Bergman U. Nausea and vomiting of pregnancy: a comparative European study. Eur J Obstet Gynecol Reprod Biol 76:1–3, 1998.

89. Berkovitch M, Elbirt D, Addis A, et al. Fetal effects of metoclopramide therapy for nausea and vomiting of pregnancy. N Engl J Med 2000 343:445–446.

90. World MJ. Ondansetron and hyperemesis gravidarum. Lancet 341: 185, 1993.

91. Vutyanovanich T, Wongha-Ngan S, Ruangsri R. Pyridoxine for nausea and vomiting of pregnancy: a randomized double-blind, placebo-controlled trial. Am J Obstet Gynecol 173:881–884, 1995.

92. Council on Scientific Affairs American Medical Association. Fetal effects of maternal alcohol use. JAMA 249:2517–2521, 1983.

93. Committee on substance abuse and committee on children with disabilities. Fetal alcohol syndrome and fetal alcohol effects. Pediatrics 91:1004–1006, 1993.

94. Frequent alcohol consumption among women of childbearing age-behavioral risk factor surveillance system, 1991. MMWR Morb Mortal Wkly Rep 42:328–335, 1994.

95. Streissguth AP, Barr HM, Sampson PD. Moderate prenatal alcohol exposure: effects on child IQ and learning problems at age 71/2 years. Alcohol Clin Exp Res 14:662–669, 1990.

96. Hill LM, Kleinberg F. Effects of drugs and chemicals on the fetus and newborn, part I. Mayo Clin Proc 59:707–716, 1984.

97. Barr HM, Streissguth AP. Caffeine use during pregnancy and child outcome: a 7-year prospective study. Neurotoxicol Teratol 13: 441–448, 1991.

98. Mills JL, Holmes LB, Aarons JH, et al. Moderate caffeine use and the risk of spontaneous abortion and intrauterine growth retardation. JAMA 269:593–597, 1993.

99. Cigarette smoking among women of reproductive age—United States, 1987–1992. MMWR-Morb Mortal Wkly Rep 43:789–797, 1994.

100. Olsen J, Pereira A, Olsen SF. Does maternal tobacco smoking modify the effect of alcohol on fetal growth? Am J Public Health 181: 69–73, 1991.

101. Centers for Disease Control. The Surgeon General's 1990 Report on the Health Benefits of Smoking Cessation [Executive Summary]. MMWR Morb Mortal Wkly Rep 39:RR12, 1990.

102. Law KL, Stroud LR, LaGasse LL, et al. Smoking during pregnancy and newborn neurobehavior. Pediatr 111:1318–1323, 2003.

103. Matheson I, Rivrud GN. The effect of smoking on lactation and infantile colic. JAMA 261:42–43, 1989.

CASE STUDIES

TOPIC: Drug Use in Pregnancy and Lactation

THERAPEUTIC DIFFICULTY: Level 3
Beth Logsdon Pangle

CHAPTER 19: Drug Use in Pregnancy and Lactation

■ Scenario

Patient and Setting CC, a 35-year-old MWF G3, P1, AB 1; presents to Ob/Gyn for her 24th week visit

Chief Complaint: "I have had headaches with nausea and vomiting."

■ History of Present Illness

CC presents to her Ob/Gyn with headaches without aura but with nausea and vomiting over the last 48 hours. She has a known history of hypertension (HTN) with BPs ranging from 125/85 to 130/90 at previous prenatal visits.

Medical History: HTN for 5 years; major depressive disorder for 5 years

Social History: Successful smoking cessation for 1 year but with previous 4-year pack history; admits to smoking (up to 4 cigarettes per day) and caffeine use to take edge off after discontinuation of Prozac, but denies alcohol or illicit drug use

Medications:
Diovan, HCT 80/12.5 mg QD
Prozac, 90 mg once a week
Both medications were stopped at initial Ob/Gyn visit approximately 8 weeks gestation; Tums PRN for Heartburn

Allergies: Penicillin (anaphylaxis noted), Sulfa

■ Physical Examination

Gen: WDWN female appearing stated gestational age
VS: BP 158/102, HR 100, RR 30, T 37°C, pre-pregnancy Wt 81 kg, current Wt 84 kg, Ht 163 cm

HEENT: PERRLA
CHEST: clear to auscultation
ABD: soft and nontender, no organomegaly noted, appropriate fundal height
GU: WNL
RECT: hemorrhoids noted
EXT: 2+ edema bilateral LE
NEURO: A/O × 3

■ Results of Pertinent Laboratory Tests, Serum Drug Concentrations, and Diagnostic Tests

Na 134 (134)	K 4.0 (4.0)	Cl 101 (101)
HCO_3 25 (25)	BUN 7.8 (22)	SCr 79.56 (0.9)
Glu 8.04 (145)		

Urinalysis: 1+ protein, 2+ glucose

■ Problem List

Identify principal problems from the scenario in priority order (see Answers in back of book for correct list of problems).

■ SOAP Note

To be completed by the student (see Answers in back of book for correct SOAP Note).

■ QUESTIONS

(See Answers in back of book for correct responses.)

1. List the physical assessment findings consistent with preeclampsia. (EO-5)

2. List the potential concerns to the mother for development of preeclampsia. (EO-1)

3. List the potential concerns to the baby for development of preeclampsia. (EO-1)

4. What is the greatest risk of smoking to the infant? (EO-2)
   a. Addiction to nicotine
   b. Addiction to other substances
   c. Lowered immunity
   d. Decreased birth weight

5. What psychosocial factors may affect CC's adherence to pharmacologic and nonpharmacologic therapy? (EO-15)

6. Which of the following would be the best choice of antidepressant for CC during her third trimester? (EO-14)
   a. Fluoxetine
   b. Amitriptyline
   c. Sertraline
   d. Buproprion

7. Which of the following would be the best choice of antidepressant for CC postpartum? (EO-14)
   a. Fluoxetine
   b. Amitriptyline
   c. Sertraline
   d. Buproprion

8. List CC's risk factors for development of hemorrhoids. (EO-8)

9. At 34 weeks, CC undergoes a group B strep screen that comes back positive. Which antibiotic would be the drug of choice for this patient during labor? (EO-10, 13)
   a. Ampicillin
   b. Penicillin G
   c. Clindamycin
   d. Cefazolin

10. Discuss the pros and cons of starting methyldopa in CC. (EO-8)

11. List CC's possible risk factors for postpartum depression. (EO-13)

12. Summarize therapeutic, pathophysiologic, and disease management concepts for drug use in pregnancy and lactation utilizing a key points format. (EO-18)

Hypertension

20

L. Brian Cross

TREATMENT GOALS: HYPERTENSION

- Use and maximize nonpharmacologic therapies in combination with pharmacotherapy.
- Individualize all therapies based on compelling indications and comorbid conditions.
- Treat systolic blood pressure to recommended goal as primary focus (especially in patients older than 50 years).
- Ultimate treatment goal is the reduction of cardiovascular and renal morbidity and mortality.

Hypertension continues to be one of the most significant risk factors for the development of stroke, congestive heart failure, coronary heart disease (CHD), and renal disease in the United States. Likewise, the appropriate treatment of hypertension has consistently proven to reduce both the morbidity and mortality associated with cardiovascular disease (CVD). The Seventh Joint National Committee on the Detection, Evaluation, and Treatment of High Blood Pressure (JNC-VII) sets forth recommendations to help healthcare providers improve the assessment and management of patients with hypertension.[1]

Though the trends are improving, still many patients are not aware of their condition, are not receiving therapy when needed, and when receiving therapy are not achieving recommended blood pressure (BP) goals. This represents a significant gap between recommended treatment goals and patients actually attaining those goals and is a clear opportunity for all healthcare providers to improve the outcomes of patients with hypertension.

DEFINITION

BP varies from minute to minute and is influenced by measurement technique, time of day, emotion, pain, discomfort, hydration, temperature, exercise, posture, and drugs. The dividing line between normal BP and hypertension is arbitrary.[1–3] Early insurance industry actuarial data showed a continuum—the higher the BP, the greater the risk of complications. Due to the design of earlier randomized controlled trials, diastolic blood pressure (DBP) served as the primary target for reduction of cardiovascular events until the 1990s. However, more recent evidence shows a clear and significant risk of cardiovascular events from elevated systolic blood pressure (SBP), especially in patients above the age of 50 years.[4] DBP is more predictive of cardiovascular risk before the age of 50 years, with SBP more predictive thereafter.[5] Some observational trials have shown a wide pulse pressure (SBP minus DBP) to be more predictive of negative cardiovascular outcomes than either SBP or DBP alone.[5,6]

TABLE 20.1	Classification of Blood Pressure for Adults					

					Management	
					Initial Drug Therapy	
Blood Pressure Classification	Systolic Blood Pressure (mm Hg)		Diastolic Blood Pressure (mm Hg)	Lifestyle Modification	Without Compelling Indication	With Compelling Indication
Normal	<120	and	<80	Encourage		
Prehypertension	120–139	or	80–89	Yes	No drug indicated	Drugs for compelling indications[b]
Stage 1 hypertension	140–159	or	90–99	Yes	Thiazide diuretic for most; may consider combination with other hypertension drugs[a]	Drugs for compelling indications; other hypertension drugs as needed
Stage 2 hypertension	≥ 160	or	≥ 100	Yes	2-drug combination for most (usually thiazide diuretic + other hypertension drugs[a])	Drugs for compelling indications; other hypertension drugs as needed

[a] Other hypertension drugs: angiotensin-converting enzyme inhibitor, angiotensin receptor blocker, β-blocker, calcium channel blocker, and thiazide-type diuretic (if not initial agent used for compelling indication)
[b] See Table 20.13 for compelling indications.

The JNC-VII defines hypertension as an SBP greater than 140 mm Hg or a DBP greater than 90 mm Hg. Measurements must be the average of two or more for a confirmed diagnosis of hypertension. JNC-VII classifies BPs as shown in Table 20.1. Single, casual measurements of BP may inaccurately classify patients as having hypertension and cause unnecessary emotional, social, and financial problems.[1]

ETIOLOGY

Hypertension is an extremely complex interplay of multiple influences from within and outside of the human body. Hypertension can be divided into two basic etiologic categories: unknown etiology (primary or essential hypertension) or a specific known etiology (secondary hypertension).

ESSENTIAL HYPERTENSION

More than 90% of patients with sustained elevation of arterial BP have essential hypertension with no identifiable cause. The term *essential hypertension* evolved from the mistaken belief that high BP was essential for adequate tissue perfusion.

SECONDARY HYPERTENSION

Remediable Hypertension. A few patients have potentially curable hypertension caused by renal disease, adrenal disease, coarctation of the aorta, or another rare condition.[1]

Renovascular hypertension, which is considered the most prevalent remediable cause of hypertension, is estimated to cause hypertension in less than 0.5% of the hypertensive population.[7]

Drug-Induced Hypertension. Hypertension occurs in up to 5% of patients who take oral contraceptives. However, most women show small but measurable BP increases (9/5 mm Hg) during the first 2 years on the pill.[8] Factors that may increase the likelihood of oral contraceptive hypertension include age greater than 35 years, smoking, obesity, and a family history of hypertension. Although the estrogen is the most important component, the amount and type of progestin may further influence the effect on BP. Proposed mechanisms for contraceptive-induced hypertension include stimulation of the renin-angiotensin-aldosterone system and sodium and fluid retention. Oral contraceptive-induced hypertension may develop gradually over 1 to 2 years and is usually reversible within 1 to 8 months after therapy is stopped. However, if BP does not normalize within 3 months, further evaluation and therapy are appropriate. Oral contraceptive-induced hypertension is best prevented by checking BP every 6 months and using the agent that has the lowest effective estrogen dosage (<30 μg) and a progestin content of 1 mg or less.[8] Women who are at higher risk or who actually develop hypertension may need to use an alternative form of contraception.

Other drugs may also significantly increase BP (see Table 20.19). A meta-analysis of the effect of nonsteroidal anti-inflammatory drugs (NSAIDs) on BP showed that they elevate supine mean BP by 5.0 mm Hg.[9] NSAIDs antagonized the antihypertensive effects of β-blockers (6.2-mm Hg increase) to a greater extent than they antagonized vasodilators or diuretics.[9] Recently, evidence suggested the cyclooxygenase-2 (COX-2)-specific inhibitor rofecoxib was associated with an increased risk of new-onset hypertension in patients aged 65 years or older.[10] This effect was not seen with celecoxib. Cyclosporine and tacrolimus cause vasoconstriction and sodium retention, inducing hypertension in a high percentage of patients. Recombinant human erythropoietin (rHuEPO) causes hypertension that is not responsive to antihypertensive therapy and must be managed by a dosage reduction or discontinuation of rHuEPO.[1] Also, corticosteroids, monoamine oxidase inhibitors, and products that contain large quantities of sodium, such as effervescent solutions, may increase BP.

EPIDEMIOLOGY

Some have estimated that as many as 1 billion people have hypertension worldwide. The World Health Organization has suggested that suboptimal treatment of hypertension represents the number-one risk for death in the world.[3] Most recent data suggest that at least 65 million Americans are hypertensive, defined as having a BP at least 140/90 mm Hg, taking an antihypertensive medication, or having been told at least twice by a healthcare professional they had high BP.[11] These results of the National Health and Nutrition Examination Survey (NHANES) IV from 1999–2000 showed a 30% increase in the prevalence of the disease compared with NHANES III from 1988–1994.

Older adults and non-Hispanic black adults are disproportionately affected by hypertension. Approximately 81% of Americans with hypertension are older than 45 years of age, but this age group represents only 46% of the population. In addition, recent data suggested that the lifetime risk of hypertension was 90% for those surviving to an age of 80 to 85 years.[12] Age-adjusted hypertension prevalence rates for non-Hispanic black men is 30.7% to 41.5% higher versus men of other races and 27% to 48.5% higher for non-Hispanic black women versus other races.[11]

Awareness of hypertension has improved from 50% during the period 1976–1980 to 70% during the period 1999–2000. Likewise, the percentage of hypertensive patients receiving therapy and the percentage of those receiving therapy actually reaching recommended BP goals have increased from 31% to 59% and 10% to 34%, respectively, during the same time period. Death from stroke and CHD has decreased by approximately 50% since 1972. These numbers represent significant improvements resulting from increased public and medical community awareness. However, 30% of patients are still unaware of their disease, 40% of hypertensive patients do not receive therapy, and 66% are not reaching recommended BP goals.

PATHOPHYSIOLOGY

BP is maintained within a fairly constant range, despite changes in posture and wide variations in the demand for blood supply. Although much is known about the complex system that regulates BP, the pathogenesis of essential hypertension remains unknown. The control of BP is done through a multifaceted interplay of neurohormonal, renal, vascular, adrenal, and genetic manipulations. Neurohormonal systems that play a significant role in BP regulation, both in healthy subjects and those with disease, include the sympathetic and parasympathetic systems, the renin-angiotensin-aldosterone system, the endothelin system, the natriuretic peptide system, and nitric oxide, in addition to adrenomedullin and leptin.[13] These systems, their relationships, and their contribution to endothelial dysfunction are the central focus of most theories of hypertension pathophysiology. Early theories suggested that renal sodium retention expanded vascular volume, increasing cardiac output. The increased cardiac output was believed to lead to increased vascular resistance. Further investigations suggested that natriuretic hormones may initiate sodium retention. Another theory suggests that inherited cellular defects cause increased intracellular sodium, leading to increases in ionic calcium and increased vascular tone and reactivity. A possible primary role of the sympathetic nervous system has also been suggested. It is likely that several interrelated mechanisms, rather than a single causative defect, control BP in essential hypertension. A relationship between hypertension and obesity, insulin resistance, hyperinsulinemia, glucose intolerance, and hypertriglyceridemia has been reported.[14]

The understanding of the role genetics plays in the development of hypertension has increased considerably. Genetic links have been identified for sodium transport, as well as nitric oxide, aldosterone, and angiotensinogen levels.[15] Though these findings may help to predict patient response to therapy in the future, essential hypertension remains a process that must be controlled rather than a curable disorder.

COMPLICATIONS

Target organ disease from arterial hypertension can be cardiac, cerebrovascular, peripheral vascular, renal, and ocular. The risk of complications and premature death is related to the degree of BP elevation. In fact, recent meta-analyses suggest death rates from both CHD and stroke increase linearly from BP levels as low as 115/75 mm Hg, and that there is a doubling of mortality for each increase of 20 mm Hg systolic or 10 mmHg diastolic beyond that level of 115/75 mm Hg.[16] A twofold increase in CVD was also shown in patients from the Framingham Heart Study with BP values in the 130 to 139/85 to 89 mm Hg range compared with

TABLE 20.2	Effect of Combined Risk Factors in Total Deaths per 1,000 in the Multiple Risk Factor Intervention Trial				
	Men Age 35–45 Years		**Men Age 46–57 Years**		
Risk Factor	**Deaths/1,000**	**Increase[a]**	**Deaths/1,000**	**Increase[a]**	
None	5.4		19.3		
Diastolic blood pressure >90	8.4	1.6	25.8	1.3	
Cholesterol >250 mg/dL	10.0	1.9	25.4	1.3	
Smoking	12.8	2.4	38.8	2.0	
Diastolic blood pressure + cholesterol	15.8	2.9	37.9	2.0	
Diastolic blood pressure + smoking	23.2	4.3	56.4	2.9	
Diastolic blood pressure, cholesterol, & smoking	33.2	6.1	70.7	3.7	

[a] Increased risk = deaths for men with risk factor vs. deaths for men with no risks.

those having BP values below 120/80 mm Hg.[17] Based on these data and the lifetime risk of developing hypertension data, JNC-VII created a new classification category called prehypertension that represents SBPs from 120 to 139 mm Hg and/or DBPs of 80 to 89 mm Hg (Table 20.1).

Hypertension is additive with other risk factors in the development of CHD and stroke.[18] Data from the Multiple Risk Factor Intervention Trial (MRFIT) study describe the combined effects of cardiovascular risk factors.[19] In men less than 46 years of age, a DBP greater than 90 mm Hg increased deaths to a rate 1.6 times the rate for men without risks, having two risk factors increased the rate 3 to 4 times, and having all three major risk factors increased the death rate 6 times (Table 20.2). The major correctable and noncorrectable risk factors are shown in Table 20.3.

CLINICAL PRESENTATION AND DIAGNOSIS

MEASUREMENT OF BLOOD PRESSURE

Because hypertension is usually an asymptomatic disease, it is usually detected during routine screening. The diagnosis of hypertension is made only after the average of two or more measurements, taken on separate occasions, determines the patient to be hypertensive based on the data in Table 20.1. Accurate and consistent technique in measuring BP is paramount, as many therapy decisions will be based on these results.[20] Table 20.4 describes the appropriate technique for the accurate measurement of BP.

Patient self-monitoring and ambulatory BP monitoring can both serve as important tools to assess BP outside the clinical setting, though self-monitoring may not be as reliable.[21] These techniques may be particularly helpful in the assessment of BP in smoking patients and patients with "white-coat hypertension." Ambulatory BP monitoring devices are worn for 24-hour periods with measurements taken

either at regular or random intervals throughout the entire day. Studies have suggested that readings from ambulatory monitoring may correlate better with target organ damage than measurements taken in the physician's office.[4] Though limited, Medicare reimbursement is available in defined situations for the use of ambulatory BP monitoring. Table 20.5

TABLE 20.3	Cardiovascular Risk Factors and Target Organ Damage
Major Risk Factors	**Target Organ Damage**
Hypertension	Heart
Age (>55 for men, >65 for women)[a]	Left ventricular hypertrophy
Diabetes mellitus[b]	Angina or prior myocardial infarction
	Prior coronary revascularization
Elevated LDL (or total) or low HDL cholesterol[b]	Heart failure
Microalbuminuria,	Brain
Estimated glomerular filtration rate <60 mL/min	Stroke or transient ischemic attack
Family history of premature cardiovascular disease	Dementia
(men aged <55 or women aged <65)	Chronic kidney disease
Cigarette smoking	Peripheral arterial disease
Physical inactivity	Retinopathy
Obesity (Body Mass Index ≥30 kg/m²)	

[a] Increased risk begins at approximately 55 and 65 for men and women, respectively. Adult Treatment Panel III used earlier cutpoints to suggest the need for earlier action.
[b] Components of the metabolic syndrome. Reduced HDL and elevated triglycerides are components of the metabolic syndrome. Abdominal obesity is also a component of metabolic syndrome.

TABLE 20.4	Appropriate Blood Pressure Measurement Technique

1. Patient should be resting for 5 minutes before blood pressure assessment.

2. Patient should avoid smoking, caffeine, or food for 30 minutes prior to blood pressure assessment.

3. Position arm (brachial artery) at heart level resting on a table or other support.

4. Uncover arm. Do not take blood pressure over clothes or allow rolled-up sleeve to serve as tourniquet.

5. Choose correct size cuff for patient. Cuff width should be 40% of limb circumference. With correct cuff length, the bladder should be at 80% of the limb's circumference. Use a large cuff or thigh cuff if the upper arm circumference is >34 cm. Use a forearm cuff (with radial palpation) if the upper arm circumference is >50 cm.

6. Position cuff 1 inch above antecubital crease.

7. Ask patient about previous blood pressure readings.[a]

8. Palpate the brachial artery and place the bell of the stethoscope over the brachial artery (location is medial to the center of the arm).

9. Place manometer with mercury column at examiner's eye level.

10. Inflate cuff rapidly to approximately 20 to 30 mm Hg above previous readings.

11. Deflate cuff slowly (approximately 2 mm/second).

    Note level of pressure at which first of repetitive audible sounds appear (phase I, systolic) and when they disappear (phase V, diastolic). Then continue to slowly deflate for at least another 10 mm Hg, checking for further Korotkoff sounds.

12. Remember to deflate the cuff completely when done.

13. Wait at least 2 minutes before repeating. Repeat again if second measurement varies by more than 5 mm Hg from first measurement.

14. On initial visit, take pressure in both arms.

15. If orthostatic hypotension is suspected, take measurements in sitting, standing, and supine positions.

[a] If previous readings are not available, inflate cuff while palpating radial pulse. The reading at which the pulse disappears and reappears with deflation represents a good estimation of the patient's systolic blood pressure. Subsequent auscultatory assessment uses this assessment, and the cuff should be inflated approximately 20 to 30 mm Hg beyond this number.

TABLE 20.5	Clinical Situations in Which Ambulatory Blood Pressure Monitoring May Be Helpful

Suspected "white-coat hypertension" in patients with hypertension and no target organ damage

Apparent drug resistance (office resistance)

Hypotensive symptoms with antihypertensive medication

Episodic hypertension

Autonomic dysfunction

lists clinical situations in which ambulatory monitoring may be indicated.

EVALUATION OF THE HYPERTENSIVE PATIENT

Evaluation of the patient newly diagnosed with hypertension has three purposes: (a) to assess the patient's lifestyle and cardiovascular risk factors and other significant diagnoses that will affect pharmacotherapy recommendations (Table 20.3); (b) to assess for secondary correctable causes of elevated BP (Table 20.6); and (c) to assess for preexisting target organ damage (Table 20.3) or cardiovascular or cerebrovascular disease. The initial evaluation visit of the hypertensive patient (Table 20.7) should include an interview for individual and family history issues, an appropriate physical examination to assess for target organ damage from preexisting hypertension as well as secondary causes of hypertension (Table 20.6), and appropriate laboratory testing to assess for secondary causes of hypertension as well as to control aspects of comorbid conditions (e.g., diabetes, hyperlipidemia, and chronic kidney disease).

TABLE 20.6	Identifiable Causes and Diagnostic Tests/Clinical Findings for Secondary Hypertension
Cause/Diagnosis	**Diagnostic Test (Clinical Finding)**
Chronic kidney disease	Estimated glomerular filtration rate (abdominal or flank mass for polycystic kidney disease)
Coarctation of the aorta	Computed tomographic angiography (delayed or absent femoral pulse)
Cushing syndrome and other glucocorticoid excess states, including chronic steroid therapy	History/dexamethasone suppression test (truncal obesity, "moonface," buffalo hump, abdominal striae, hirsutism)
Drug-induced or drug-related	History; drug screening (Table 20.19)
Pheochromocytoma	24-hour urinary metanephrine and normetanephrine (headache, palpitations, sweating)
Primary aldosteronism and other mineralocorticoid excess states	24-hour urinary aldosterone level or specific measurements of other mineralocorticoids (hypokalemia)
Renovascular hypertension	Doppler flow study; magnetic resonance angiography (abdominal bruit)
Sleep apnea	Sleep study with O_2 saturation (obesity, snoring, tired during daytime)
Thyroid/parathyroid disease	Thyroid-stimulating hormone; serum parathyroid hormone (goiter, hypercalcemia)

TABLE 20.7	Evaluation of Hypertensive Patients

A. Medical history

1. Family history of hypertension and hypertensive complications

2. History of cardiovascular, cerebrovascular, or renal disease or diabetes mellitus

3. Duration and level of blood pressure elevation

4. Effectiveness and side effects of previous drug treatment

5. Medication history of drugs that elevate blood pressure (Table 20.19)

6. Lifestyle and health habits

   a. Smoking

   b. Ethanol excess

   c. Sodium intake

   d. Caffeine

   e. Exercise

   f. Emotional stress

B. Physical examination

1. Two or more blood pressure measurements with patient supine or seated and standing

2. Verification of blood pressure in the contralateral arm

3. Height and weight (with calculation of Body Mass Index or measurement of waist circumference)

4. Funduscopic examination for arteriolar narrowing, arteriovenous compression, hemorrhages, exudates, and papilledema

5. Neck examination for carotid bruits, distended veins, and enlarged thyroid

6. Cardiac examination for increased rate, size, precordial heave, murmurs, arrhythmias, and S_3 and S_4 heart sounds

7. Abdominal examinations for bruits, enlarged kidneys, and aortic dilation

8. Extremity examination for edema, femoral bruits, and decreased or absent pulses

9. Neurologic assessment

C. Laboratory tests

1. Hemoglobin and hematocrit

2. Urinalysis—Urinary albumin/creatinine ratio optional

3. Serum potassium

4. Serum creatinine or estimated glomerular filtration rate (eGFR)

5. Serum uric acid

6. Serum calcium

7. Fasting lipid panel

8. Fasting plasma glucose

9. 12-lead electrocardiogram

In addition to the basic laboratory testing recommended in Table 20.7 during the initial assessment of the patient with hypertension, special consideration should be given to the assessment of renal function and newer emerging risk factors that may help in the further risk stratification of high-risk patients for CVD. Decreases in glomerular filtration rate (GFR) or the presence of albuminuria, including microalbuminuria, have been shown to increase cardiovascular risk.[22–24] The proper technique for GFR estimation has been debated, though results from the Modification of the Diet in Renal Disease (MDRD) study show an estimating tool for GFR that may better predict decreased renal function in some populations.[25] Though not recommended for all patients with hypertension, a quantitated assessment of urinary albumin excretion should be done in patients with diabetes or renal disease. Other risk factors that may provide improved cardiovascular risk assessment of patients in the future include elevated heart rate, high-sensitive C-reactive protein (hs-CRP), and homocysteine. Data from the Framingham Heart Study suggest that a resting heart rate greater than 83 beats per minute[26] or a reduction in heart rate variability[27] confers a significantly increased risk of cardiovascular death. hs-CRP levels, a marker of inflammation, have been suggested to predict independent higher risk for cardiovascular events,[28] especially in women.[29] However, recent evidence has suggested that the ability of hs-CRP to independently predict cardiovascular risk may not be as significant as originally thought.[30] Evidence suggesting a link between hyperhomocystinemia and atherothrombosis has been shown, although like hs-CRP, results have been conflicting.[31]

SECONDARY CAUSES OF HYPERTENSION

The initial laboratory tests and physical examination, in addition to patient age and BP severity, often provide clues suggestive of secondary causes of hypertension. Further consideration and possible workup for secondary hypertension is advised for patients who respond poorly to drug therapy, have increasing BPs after periods of good control, or have a sudden onset of hypertension. Table 20.6 describes secondary causes of hypertension and corresponding diagnostic tests and clinical findings.

TREATMENT

The treatment of hypertension requires a multimodal approach that encompasses the use of nonpharmacologic treatments such as weight reduction through appropriate physical activity and dietary habits, dietary sodium reduction, and moderation of alcohol consumption as well as individualized pharmacotherapy.

NONPHARMACOLOGIC THERAPY

Appropriate lifestyle modifications are important therapies in both the prevention and treatment of hypertension. The prevalence of hypertension is 50% greater in overweight adults than in normal-weight adults,[32] and weight loss of as little as 10 pounds has been shown to both reduce and prevent high BP.[33,34] The Dietary Approaches to Stop Hypertension (DASH) trial showed that eating a diet rich in fruits, vegetables, low-fat dairy products, potassium, and calcium with decreased dietary cholesterol and potassium can significantly improve BP.[35] This dietary modification was as effective as drug therapy with one agent in some patients. Patients with hypertension should take part in regular aerobic physical activity, after consultation with their physicians, 30 minutes a day on most days of the week.[36] Sixty to 90 minutes per week of walking has been shown to decrease cardiovascular mortality by approximately 50%.[37] Alcohol intake should be no more than two drinks (24 oz of beer, 10 oz of wine, or 3 oz of 80-proof liquor) per day in most men and one drink per day in women and lighter-weight people.[38] The lifestyle modifications recommended by JNC-VII (Table 20.8) not only help to lower BP, but also increase the effectiveness of pharmacotherapy regimens.

PHARMACOTHERAPY

The pharmacotherapy of hypertension comprises nine classes of medications: diuretics, aldosterone receptor blockers, β-blockers, angiotensin-converting enzyme (ACE) inhibitors, angiotensin II antagonists, calcium channel blockers, α_1-blockers, central α_2 agonists and other centrally acting drugs, and direct vasodilators (Tables 20.9 and 20.10). Therapy selection should be tailored to the patient, taking into consideration such issues as safety, cost, adverse event profile, presence of compelling indications for certain drug classes and risk factors for CVD, as well as clinical evidence of decreased morbidity and mortality secondary to their use.

Common adverse effects and special precautions for antihypertensive drugs are given in Table 20.11. Drug interactions are listed in Table 20.12.

With the most recent guidelines for the treatment of hypertension, the JNC-VII made several significant changes in an attempt to both simplify the treatment of hypertension and improve treatment rates of the disease.[1] SBP is now the recommended treatment focus for most patients, as it has been shown that if SBP is controlled, DBP will usually be controlled as well. A recent National High Blood Pressure Education Program (NHBPEP) advisory emphasizes this recommendation.[39] The JNC-VII guidelines also recommend thiazide diuretics as first-line therapy in patients with uncomplicated hypertension, and as the second agent to be added to other classes used for compelling indications if further BP reduction is required. Multiple clinical trials have shown that two out of every three patients will require at least two medications to lower their BP below 140/90 mmHg.[40–43] Therefore, the choice of which antihypertensive therapy should be used as initial therapy is much less significant. For patients whose BP is more than 20/10 mm Hg above their goal, JNC-VII now recommends that therapy be initiated with two agents.

Uncomplicated Hypertension. For 30 years thiazide-type diuretics have been the foundation of antihypertensive regimens used in placebo-controlled clinical trials showing reductions in major cardiovascular events, including myocardial infarction, stroke, and heart failure.[44] For patients without compelling indications that require specified antihypertensive therapies (Table 20.13), JNC-VII recommends that thiazide-type diuretics be considered as the initial agent

TABLE 20.8	Lifestyle Modifications to Manage Hypertension[a]	
Modification	**Recommendation**	**Approximate Reduction in Systolic Blood Pressure**
Weight reduction	Maintain normal body weight (Body Mass Index <25).	5–20 mm Hg per 10-kg weight loss
Adopt DASH (Dietary Approaches to Stop Hypertension) eating plan	Consume a diet rich in fruits, vegetables, and low-fat dairy products, with a reduced content of saturated and total fat.	8–14 mm Hg
Dietary sodium reduction	Reduce dietary sodium intake to no more than 100 mEq/L (2.4 g sodium or 6 g sodium chloride).	2–8 mm Hg
Physical activity	Engage in regular aerobic physical activity such as brisk walking at least 30 minutes per day, most days of the week.	4–9 mm Hg
Moderation of alcohol consumption	Limit consumption to no more than two drinks per day [1 oz or 30 mL ethanol (e.g., 24 oz beer, 10 oz wine, or 3 oz 80-proof whiskey)] in most men and no more than one drink in women and lighter-weight persons.	2–4 mm Hg

[a] Smoking cessation should be included in all lifestyle modification recommendations to reduce overall cardiovascular risk.

TABLE 20.9	Oral Antihypertensive Drugs		
Class	**Drug (Trade Name)**	**Usual Dose Range (mg/d)**	**Daily Frequency**
Thiazide diuretics	Chlorothiazide (Diuril)	125–500	1
	Chlorthalidone (Hygroton)	12.5–25	1
	Hydrochlorothiazide (Microzide, HydroDIURIL)	12.5–50	1
	Polythiazide (Renese)	2–4	1
	Indapamide (Lozol)	1.25–2.5	1
	Metolazone (Zaroxolyn)	2.5–5	1
Loop diuretics	Bumetanide (Bumex)	0.5–2	2
	Furosemide (Lasix)	20–80	2
	Torsemide (Demadex)	2.5–10	1
Potassium-sparing diuretics	Amiloride (Midamor)	5–10	1 or 2
	Triamterene (Dyrenium)	50–100	1 or 2
Aldosterone-receptor blockers	Eplerenone (Inspra)	50–100	1 or 2
	Spironolactone (Aldactone)	25–50	1 or 2
β-blockers	Atenolol (Tenormin)	25–100	1
	Betaxolol (Kerlone)	5–20	1
	Bisoprolol (Zebeta)	2.5–10	1
	Metoprolol (Lopressor)	50–100	1 or 2
	Metoprolol extended release (Toprol XL)	50–100	1
	Nadolol (Corgard)	40–120	1
	Propranolol (Inderal)	40–160	2
	Propranolol long-acting (Inderal LA)	60–180	1
	Timolol (Blocadren)	20–40	2
β-blockers with ISA	Acebutolol (Sectral)	200–800	2
	Penbutolol (Levatol)	10–40	1
	Pindolol (Visken)	10–40	2
Combined α- and β-blockers	Carvedilol (Coreg)	12.5–50	2
	Labetalol (Normodyne, Trandate)	200–800	2
Angiotensin-converting enzyme (ACE) inhibitors	Benazepril (Lotensin)	10–40	1 or 2
	Captopril (Capoten)	25–100	2
	Enalapril (Vasotec)	2.5–40	1 or 2
	Fosinopril (Monopril)	10–40	1
	Lisinopril (Prinivil, Zestril)	10–40	1
	Moexipril (Univasc)	7.5–30	1
	Perindopril (Aceon)	4–8	1 or 2
	Quinapril (Accupril)	10–40	1
	Ramipril (Altace)	2.5–40	1
	Trandolapril (Mavik)	1–4	1
Angiotensin II antagonists	Candesartan (Atacand)	8–32	1
	Eprosartan (Tevetan)	400–800	1 or 2
	Irbesartan (Avapro)	150–300	1
	Losartan (Cozaar)	25–100	1 or 2
	Olmesartan (Benicar)	20–40	1
	Telmisartan (Micardis)	20–80	1

(continued)

TABLE 20.9	continued			
Class	**Drug (Trade Name)**	**Usual Dose Range (mg/d)**	**Daily Frequency**
	Valsartan (Diovan)	80–320	1
Calcium channel blockers–nondihydropyridines	Diltiazem extended release (Cardizem CD, Dilacor XR, Tiazac)	180–240	1
	Diltiazem extended release (Cardizem LA)	120–540	1
	Verapamil immediate release (Calan, Isoptin)	80–320	2
	Verapamil long-acting (Calan SR, Isoptin SR)	120–360	1 or 2
	Verapamil-coer (Covera HS, Verelan PM)	120–360	1
Calcium channel blockers–dihydropyridines	Amlodipine (Norvasc)	2.5–10	1
	Felodipine (Plendil)	2.5–20	1
	Isradipine (Dynacirc)	2.5–10	2
	Nicardipine sustained release (Cardene SR)	60–120	2
	Nifedipine long-acting (Adalat CC, Procardia XL)	30–60	1
	Nisoldipine (Sular)	10–40	1
α_1-blockers	Doxazosin (Cardura)	1–16	1
	Prazosin (Minipress)	2–20	2 or 3
	Terazosin (Hytrin)	1–20	1 or 2
Central α_2-agonists	Clonidine (Catapres)	0.1–0.8	2
	Clonidine patch (Catapres TTS)	0.1–0.3	1 weekly
	Methyldopa (Aldomet)	250–1,000	2
	Reserpine (Serpasil)	0.05–0.25	1
	Guanfacine (Tenex)	0.5–2	1
Direct vasodilators	Hydralazine (Apresoline)	25–100	2
	Minoxidil (Loniten)	2.5–80	1 or 2

in most patients with stage 1 hypertension, and a two-drug combination that includes a thiazide-type diuretic in most patients with stage 2 hypertension. This is in contrast to most recent European guidelines, which encourage clinicians to choose initial therapy from the five major drug classes based on a more global cardiovascular risk assessment strategy.[2,3] Recent data from the Antihypertensive and Lipid-Lowering Treatment to Prevent Heart Attack Trial (ALLHAT),[45] as well as older data from the Systolic Hypertension in the Elderly Program (SHEP) trial,[46] confirm the ability of thiazide diuretics to consistently reduce cardiovascular morbidity and mortality. Figure 20.1 shows an algorithm for the treatment of hypertension as recommended by JNC-VII.

Diuretics. The initial mechanism by which thiazide diuretics lower BP is by direct diuresis. However, through compensatory mechanisms, plasma volume returns to predi-

uretic levels and long-term antihypertensive effects are maintained through a decrease in peripheral vascular resistance. The mechanism by which thiazide diuretics cause this is not clear, but it is thought to be by direct relaxation of the vascular smooth muscle.

In the ALLHAT trial, the largest hypertension trial to date, with nearly 40,000 patients enrolled, the thiazide diuretic chlorthalidone was compared to amlodipine, lisinopril, or doxazosin.[45] An increase in cardiovascular events, specifically heart failure, led to the early closing of the doxazosin arm in 2002.[47] In the remaining 33,357 patients, no difference was noted between the three treatment arms for the primary outcome of combined fatal CHD or nonfatal myocardial infarction. A significantly higher rate of heart failure was noted in the amlodipine group versus the chlorthalidone group, and the lisinopril group had higher rates of

TABLE 20.10	Combination Drugs for Hypertension	
Combination Type	**Fixed-Dose Combination (mg)**	**Trade Name**
Angiotensin-converting enzyme (ACE) inhibitors and calcium channel blockers	Amlodipine/benazepril (2.5/10, 5/10, 5/20, 10/20)	Lotrel
	Enalapril/felodipine (5/5)	Lexxel
	Trandolapril/verapamil (2/180, 1/240, 2/240, 4/240)	Tarka
ACE inhibitors and diuretics	Benazepril/hydrochlorothiazide (5/6.25, 10/12.5, 20/12.5, 20/25)	Lotensin HCT
	Captopril/hydrochlorothiazide (25/15, 25/25, 50/15, 50/25)	Capozide
	Enalapril/hydrochlorothiazide (5/12.5, 10/25)	Vaseretic
	Lisinopril/hydrochlorothiazide (10/12.5, 20/12.5, 20/25)	Prinizide
	Moexipril/hydrochlorothiazide (7.5/12.5, 15/25)	Uniretic
	Quinapril/hydrochlorothiazide (10/12.5, 20/12.5, 20/25)	Accuretic
Angiotensin receptor blockers and diuretics	Candesartan/hydrochlorothiazide (16/12.5, 32/12.5)	Atacand HCT
	Eprosartan/hydrochlorothiazide (600/12.5, 600/25)	Teveten HCT
	Irbesartan/hydrochlorothiazide (75/12.5, 150/12.5, 300/12.5)	Avalide
	Losartan/hydrochlorothiazide (50/12.5, 100/25)	Hyzaar
	Telmisartan/hydrochlorothiazide (40/12.5, 80/12.5)	Micardis HCT
	Valsartan/hydrochlorothiazide (80/12.5, 160/12.5)	Diovan HCT
β-blockers and diuretics	Atenolol/chlorthalidone (50/25, 100/25)	Tenoretic
	Bisoprolol/hydrochlorothiazide (2.5/6.25, 5/6.25, 10/6.25)	Ziac
	Propranolol LA/hydrochlorothiazide (40/25, 80/25)	Inderide
	Metoprolol/hydrochlorothiazide (50/25, 100,25)	Lopressor HCT
	Nadolol/bendroflumethiazide (40/5, 80/5)	Corzide
	Timolol/hydrochlorothiazide (10/25)	Timolide
Centrally acting drug and diuretic	Methyldopa/hydrochlorothiazide (250/15, 250/25, 500/30, 500/50)	Aldoril
	Reserpine/chlorothiazide (0.125/250, 0.25/500)	Diupres
	Reserpine/hydrochlorothiazide (0.125/25, 0.125/50)	Hydropres
Diuretic and diuretic	Amiloride/hydrochlorothiazide (5/50)	Moduretic
	Spironolactone/hydrochlorothiazide (25/25, 50/50)	Aldactone
	Triamterene/hydrochlorothiazide (37.5/25, 50/25, 75/50)	Dyazide, Maxzide

both heart failure and stroke compared to the chlorthalidone group. These differences in the lisinopril versus chlorthalidone groups were mostly seen in black patients, who had 4 mm Hg less BP lowering with the ACE inhibitor. These findings confirm previous results from the Captopril Prevention Project (CAPPP), which showed a 43% increase in stroke with captopril compared to diuretic and/or β-blocker therapy.[48] The differences in heart failure rates are also supported by previous data: the SHEP trial showed a 50% decrease in the risk of heart failure with diuretic therapy, and the Swedish Trial in Old Patients with Hypertension-2

(STOP-2)[49] showed an increase in heart failure in patients who received a calcium channel blocker. Finally, there was no difference in primary outcomes between the three groups in diabetic patients.

The Second Australian National BP (ANBP2) study was released shortly after ALLHAT and seemed to contradict the superior results of a thiazide-based regimen versus an ACE inhibitor-based regimen.[50] This trial of 6,000 patients actually found ACE inhibitors to be superior to hydrochlorothiazide. However, the ANBP2 study was done almost exclusively in white patients, and benefits were apparent only

TABLE 20.11	Adverse Effects of Antihypertensive Drugs	
Drug	**Adverse Effects**	**Special Precautions**
Thiazide diuretics	Hypokalemia, hyperuricemia, glucose intolerance, dyslipidemia, sexual dysfunction, dehydration, hyponatremia, hypomagnesemia, hypercalcemia, skin rash, photosensitivity	Gout, renal failure, digitalis, lithium
Loop diuretics	Similar to thiazide diuretics except hypocalcemia	Effective in patients with renal insufficiency
β-blockers	Fatigue, insomnia, nightmares, depression, sexual dysfunction, dyslipidemia, rash, gastrointestinal upset, worsening of psoriasis, withdrawal rebound coronary heart disease, bradycardia, decreased exercise tolerance, bronchospasm, Raynaud's phenomenon, masked symptoms of hypoglycemia	Asthma, chronic obstructive pulmonary disease, decompensated congestive heart failure, heart block, diabetes mellitus, peripheral vascular disease
β-blockers with intrinsic sympathomimetic activity	Less bradycardia and dyslipidemia, drug-induced lupus erythematosus	
α-β-blockers	Orthostatic hypotension, hepatotoxicity	No dyslipidemia
Angiotensin-converting enzyme (ACE) inhibitors	Hyperkalemia, cough, hypotension, angioedema, rash, loss of taste, proteinuria, renal failure, neutropenia, cholestasis, rash, blood dyscrasias, increased fetal mortality	Renal failure, pregnancy, renal artery stenosis
Angiotensin receptor blockers	Similar to ACE inhibitors but do not cause cough	
Calcium channel blockers	Headache, flushing, hypotension, dizziness, palpitations, nausea	Congestive heart failure, heart block
Dihydropyridines	Edema, tachycardia	
Diltiazem	Lupus-like rash	
Verapamil	Constipation, atrioventricular block, bradycardia	Digitalis
Central antiadrenergics	Sedation, dry mouth, fatigue, sexual dysfunction, postural hypotension, impaired mental concentration, withdrawal rebound hypertension, contact dermatitis from patch	Depression; taper dosage when discontinuing to avoid rebound
Methyldopa	Hepatitis, Coombs-positive hemolytic anemia, colitis, drug-induced lupus erythematosus	
Peripheral antiadrenergics	Sexual dysfunction, nasal congestion, orthostatic hypotension, dizziness, sodium and fluid retention	Asthma, congestive heart failure, advanced age
α-Adrenergic blockers	Syncope after first dose or dosage increase, orthostatic hypotension, headache, dizziness, drowsiness, tachycardia, sodium and fluid retention, priapism	Advanced age, first dose
Vasodilators	Headache, tachycardia, dizziness, sodium and fluid retention	Angina, congestive heart failure
Hydralazine	Positive antinuclear antibody (ANA), lupus-like syndrome, hepatitis, nasal congestion, gastrointestinal disturbances	
Minoxidil	Hypertrichosis, facial coarsening, pleural or pericardial effusion	

in male patients. This may explain much of the difference between the two trials. Finally, the thiazide therapy used in ANBP2 was hydrochlorothiazide; ALLHAT used chlorthalidone. Some have suggested there may be a difference between the two thiazide diuretics.[51] No studies have directly compared chlorthalidone and hydrochlorothiazide, but data from MRFIT suggested a reduction in nonfatal cardiovascular events when the diuretic treatment protocol was changed to replace hydrochlorothiazide with chlorthalidone.[52] Results of a recent observational study supported the superiority of chlorthalidone over hydrochlorothiazide.[53] However, the meta-analysis by Psaty et al predicted no significant

TABLE 20.12	Antihypertensive Drug Interactions		
Drug Class	**Increased Antihypertensive Effect**	**Decreased Antihypertensive Effect**	**Other Drug Interaction Effects**
Loop diuretics	ACEIs, antipsychotics, β-blockers, CCBs, ethanol, antiadrenergic agents	ASA/NSAIDs, anticonvulsants, bile acid resins, sympathomimetics	ACEI ↑ renal insufficiency Carbenoxolone ↓ K Corticosteroids ↓ K Digoxin ↑ toxicity from hypokalemia Fibric acids ↓ albumin binding ↑ Lithium toxicity SSRIs: severe hyponatremia
Thiazide diuretics	ACEIs, antipsychotics, β-blockers, CCBs, ethanol, antiadrenergic agents	ASA/NSAIDs, bsile acid resins, sympathomimetics	Calcium: milk alkali syndrome Carbenoxolone ↓ K ↑ Digoxin toxicity from hypokalemia ↑ Lithium toxicity ↓ Hypoglycemic agent effects from antagonism
β-blockers	α-blockers, antipsychotics, CCBs, ethanol, antiadrenergic agents, H₂ blockers, SSRIs, antiarrhythmics, quinolones (↑ β-blocker)	ASA/NSAIDs, antacids, sympathomimetics ↓ β-blocker levels: Barbiturate Carbamazepine Rifampin and rifabutin Sulfasalazine	α_1-blockers and α_2-agonists ↑ rebound hypertension Amiodarone: bradycardia, cardiac arrest Contrast media (intravenous): ↑ anaphylaxis ↓ Diazepam metabolism Digoxin: bradycardia, ↓ digoxin levels with carvedilol Ergot alkaloids: ↑ vasoconstriction Hypoglycemic agents: mask hypoglycemic symptoms ↓ Quinidine effect with hepatic metabolized β-blockers Sympathomimetics: ↑ blood pressure, ↑ terbutaline levels, ↑ theophylline levels
Calcium blockers	Antipsychotics, β-blockers, diuretics, ethanol (postural hypotension) ↑ Calcium blocker levels: α_1-blockers Cimetidine Erythromycin Grapefruit juice (↑ DHP) Proton pump inhibitors Quinidine Valproic acid	ASA/NSAIDs, sympathomimetics ↓ Calcium blocker levels: Carbamazepine Barbiturates Rifampin and rifabutin	8 ASA antiplatelet activity β-blockers: 8 cardiac depression ↑ Carbamazepine levels with diltiazem or verapamil ↑ Cyclosporine levels ↑ Digoxin levels except DHP ↑ Ethanol ↑ Lithium neurotoxicity ↑ Phenytoin levels with nifedipine ↑ Quinidine levels with nifedipine ↑ Quinidine bradycardia and hypotension with verapamil ↑ TCA levels

(continued)

TABLE 20.12	continued		
Drug Class	**Increased Antihypertensive Effect**	**Decreased Antihypertensive Effect**	**Other Drug Interaction Effects**
			↑ Theophylline levels with verapamil
			↑ HMG Co-A reductase inhibitor levels with diltiazem and verapamil
ACE inhibitors and ARBs	Antipsychotics, β-blockers, diuretics, ergot alkaloids	ASA/NSAIDs, sympathomimetics, antacids (captopril)	Azathioprine/6-MP toxicity
			↑ Lithium levels, hyperkalemia with K-sparing diuretics
$α_1$-blockers	ACE inhibitors, antipsychotics, β-blockers, calcium blockers, diuretics, ethanol	ASA/NSAIDs, sympathomimetics	↑ Orthostatic hypotension with diuretics
$α_2$-Agonists	Antipsychotics, diuretics, ethanol, nitrates	ASA/NSAIDs, MAOIs, TCAs, trazodone, phenothiazines, sympathomimetics	↑ Cyclosporine levels with clonidine TTS
			↓ Symptoms of hypoglycemia with clonidine
			↑ Rebound hypertension with β-blockers
			↑ Bradycardia with β-blockers
			↑ CNS depression with all CNS depressants
			↑ Lithium levels with methyldopa
Potassium- sparing diuretics	Antipsychotics, ethanol, nitrates	ASA/NSAIDs, sympathomimetics	↑ Amantadine levels with triamterene
			↑ Digoxin levels with spironolactone
			Acute renal failure with indomethacin and triamterene
			↑ Hyperkalemia with ACE/ARB
			↑ Quinidine toxicity with amiloride
Vasodilators	Antipsychotics, β-blockers, diuretics, ethanol	ASA/NSAIDs, sympathomimetics	
Peripheral adrenergic blockers	Diuretics, ethanol	ASA/NSAIDs, antipsychotics, MAOIs, sympathomimetics	

ACEIs, angiotensin converting enzyme inhibitors; ARB, angiotensin receptor blockers; ASA, aspirin; CCBs, calcium channel blockers; CNS, central nervous system; DHP, dihydropyridine; MAOIs, monoamine oxidase inhibitors; NSAIDs, nonsteroidal anti-inflammatory drugs; SSRIs, selective serotonin reuptake inhibitors; TCAs, tricyclic antidepressants.

differences between the two agents.[54] Therefore, when using thiazide diuretics, clinicians should try to titrate patients to the equipotent dose of chlorthalidone 25 mg, as tolerated, based on the results of ALLHAT.

Thiazide diuretics are generally well tolerated. Using lower dosages may reduce the incidence and severity of the metabolic abnormalities of hypokalemia, hyperuricemia, hypercalcemia, hypomagnesemia, and hyperglycemia. Hypokalemia is dose-related, and moderate hypokalemia (3.0 to 3.5 mEq/L) occurs in 2% of patients who are treated with hydrochlorothiazide 25 mg per day, compared to 11% of

patients treated with 50 mg per day.[55] Hypokalemia is worsened by high-sodium diets and can be minimized by using low-dose thiazide therapy, restricting sodium intake, using potassium supplements, and adding potassium-sparing drugs. The risk of primary cardiac arrest is increased by high-dose thiazide diuretic therapy.[56] For patients with a serum potassium level below 3.5 mmol per L in the SHEP trial, beneficial effects of the diuretic therapy were negated.[57] Thiazides increase the serum uric acid level by approximately 1 mg per dL, which is not associated with adverse effects on renal function and does not warrant uric

TABLE 20.13	Compelling Indications for Individual Drug Classes

High-Risk Conditions With Compelling Indication	Recommended Drugs					
	Diuretic	β-blocker	ACEI	ARB	CCB	AA
Heart failure	✓	✓	✓	✓		✓
Postmyocardial infarction		✓	✓			✓
High coronary heart disease risk	✓	✓	✓		✓	
Diabetes	✓	✓	✓	✓	✓	
Chronic kidney disease			✓	✓		
Recurrent stroke prevention	✓		✓			

ACEI, angiotensin-converting enzyme inhibitor; ARB, angiotensin receptor blocker; CCB, calcium channel blocker; AA, aldosterone antagonist.

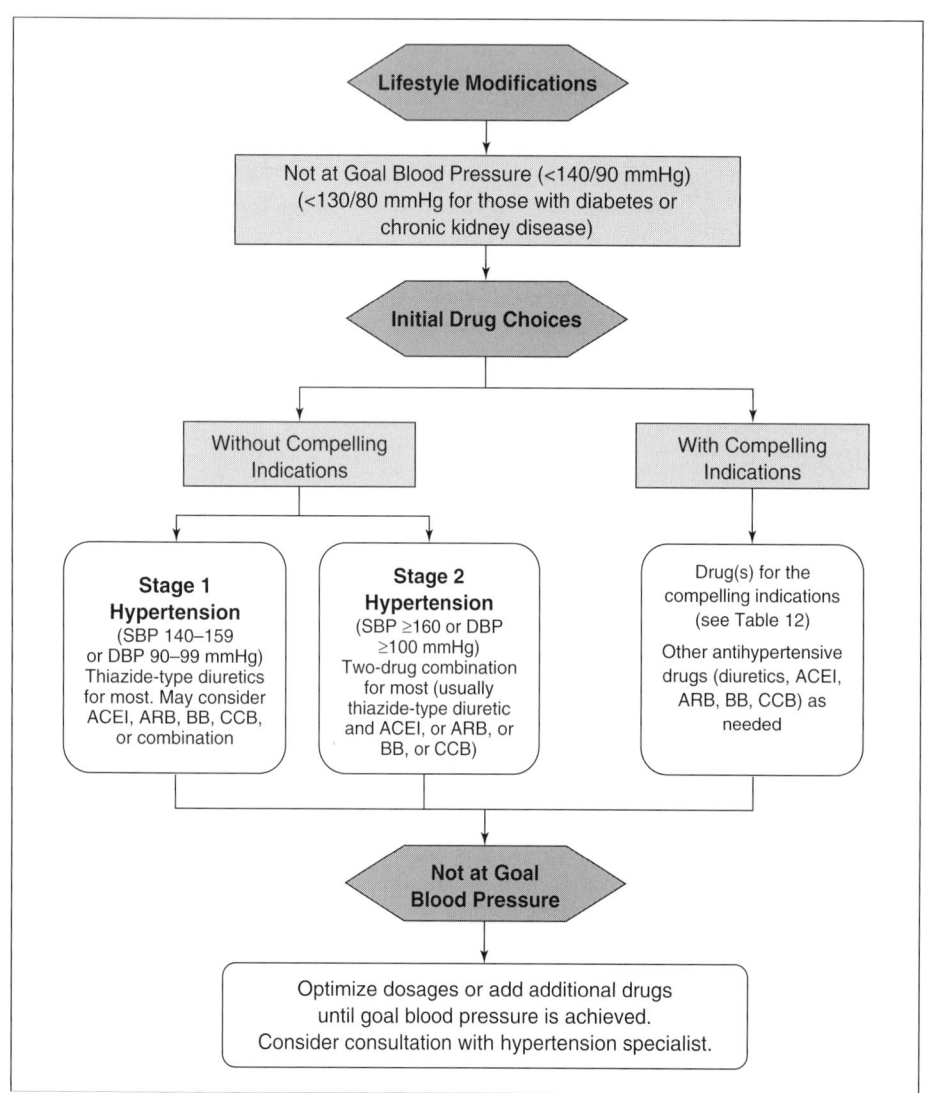

FIGURE 20.1 JNC-VII algorithm for treatment of hypertension. ACEI, angiotensin-converting enzyme inhibitor; ARB, angiotensin receptor blocker; BB, β-blocker; CCB, calcium channel blocker; DBP, diastolic blood pressure; SBP, systolic blood pressure.

acid-lowering drugs unless the patient has symptomatic gout.[39] Finally, significant changes in glucose metabolism did occur in patients receiving chlorthalidone versus those receiving amlodipine or lisinopril in ALLHAT. New diagnoses of diabetes were significantly greater for those receiving the diuretic therapy compared to the other groups. No significant changes in serum cholesterol levels occurred from baseline for patients receiving chlorthalidone, though levels decreased in both the calcium channel blocker and ACE inhibitor groups. The authors noted that despite these possible adverse metabolic effects, cardiovascular outcomes were not altered. The declining use of diuretics is not supported by the evidence.[58] Diuretic-induced metabolic effects and hypokalemia are minor with the smaller dosages of diuretics currently recommended, and cardiovascular mortality has been reduced even in patients with dyslipidemia and diabetes.[58] BP control in hypertensive patients will be improved with increased use of diuretic therapy.[58]

Metolazone is a thiazide-like diuretic that is effective for patients with renal impairment and is markedly effective in producing diuresis when combined with furosemide. Indapamide is a sulfonamide diuretic with antihypertensive effects that does not appear to elevate serum lipid levels. Recently, data have suggested that indapamide may have specific benefits in diabetic patients. In the PREMIER trial, the combination of perindopril and indapamide had a significantly better impact on microalbuminuria versus enalapril, independent of BP-lowering effects.[59] Indapamide monotherapy was shown to be equivalent to enalapril in the reduction of microalbuminuria of diabetes in the NESTOR trial.[60] Finally, the PROGRESS trial showed that when indapamide was added to the ACE inhibitor perindopril in patients with a previous stroke, recurrent cerebrovascular events were decreased by 43%.[61] No event reduction was noted in the perindopril monotherapy group. These data caused the JNC-VII to include recurrent stroke prevention in the compelling indications section of the guidelines (Table 20.13).

The potassium-sparing diuretics are used mainly to prevent or correct hypokalemia from other diuretics. Neither amiloride nor triamterene has a significant antihypertensive effect. There is a potential risk of hyperkalemia with these agents in patients with renal dysfunction or diabetes or those taking ACE inhibitors, angiotensin receptor blockers, NSAIDs, or potassium supplements. Combination products with thiazide diuretics may provide less hypokalemia and improved BP at a reasonable cost.

Though of significance in the symptomatic treatment of heart failure, loop diuretics for the treatment of hypertension should be used only in patients with impaired renal function (GFR <25 to 30 mL/min), who are not as responsive to normal thiazide-type diuretic therapy.[62]

β-Blockers. β-blockers competitively inhibit catecholamine neurotransmitters at both cardiac receptors (β_1) and noncardiac receptors (β_2).[63] Cardiac effects include reductions in heart rate, venous return, cardiac output, and cardiac

work. In addition, β-blockers reduce plasma renin activity, reduce norepinephrine release, and prevent the pressor response to exercise or stress catecholamine release. β-blockers are effective antihypertensive agents, particularly for young white patients, and have been proven to reduce mortality in randomized clinical trials.[64,65] β-blockers have additional favorable effects in patients with coexisting angina pectoris, atrial fibrillation or atrial tachycardia, essential tremor, hyperthyroidism, migraine headaches, or myocardial infarction. β-blockers should be avoided in patients with severe persistent asthma, and a risk-benefit assessment should be used to individualize β-blocker therapy in patients with mild intermittent or mild persistent asthma, perhaps well-controlled moderate persistent asthma, and probably chronic obstructive pulmonary disease.[66,67] In pulmonary patients for which the benefits of β-blocker therapy outweigh the potential risks, low-dose metoprolol XL or atenolol should be considered.[66,67] Individualization of β-blocker therapy should also be considered in patients with depression, diabetes, dyslipidemia, second- or third-degree heart block, and severe peripheral vascular disease.[1]

The use of β-blockers may be considered first line for hypertension in patients who also have a history of previous myocardial infarction, ischemic heart disease, arrhythmias or heart failure, or diabetes or high coronary disease risk. In earlier studies, β-blocker use in hypertension was associated with reductions in mortality,[68] stroke, and heart failure.[69] In the Swedish Trial in Old Patients with Hypertension (STOP-Hypertension trial), β-blocker use (metoprolol, pindolol, or atenolol) was associated with reductions in all-cause mortality and sudden death compared to placebo.[68] In the MAPHY study, β-blocker therapy (metoprolol) was associated with less mortality when compared with thiazide therapy.[70] However, in the Medical Research Council (MRC) trial, atenolol therapy was found to be no better than placebo or diuretics in reduction of cardiovascular events if patients did not also have a history of previous myocardial infarction, angina, or heart failure.[71] Again, these conflicting data were confirmed in a meta-analysis showing that β-blockers were superior to placebo but not diuretic therapy in preventing stroke and heart failure.[69]

Recent trials have shown β-blockers to be equal to calcium channel blockers[72] and ACE inhibitors.[48,49,72,73] However, results from the African American Study of Kidney Disease and Hypertension (AASK)[74] trial indicate that β-blocker therapy (metoprolol) may not be as effective as ramipril in protecting against the progression of renal impairment in black patients, and results from the Losartan Intervention For Endpoint reduction in hypertension (LIFE)[43] study suggest that β-blocker therapy (atenolol) may not prevent strokes as effectively as losartan in patients with hypertension with left ventricular hypertrophy (LVH) and no history of recent myocardial infarction, angina, or heart failure. Significant evidence to support the use of β-blockers in hypertensive patients with a history of myocardial infarction[75,76] or heart failure[77–79] supports these as compelling indications by JNC-VII.

Comparison of β-blockers. Although the available β-blockers are similar in efficacy and safety, there are two important differences in pharmacology. Cardioselective (β$_1$-selective) agents produce fewer negative effects on the heart in patients with congestive heart failure or conduction system disease, may be better tolerated by patients with chronic obstructive pulmonary disease and peripheral vascular disease, and produce less impairment in response to hypoglycemia in diabetic patients. Unfortunately, cardioselectivity is reduced or lost at higher dosages. Drugs with β-agonist activity or intrinsic sympathomimetic activity (ISA) may avoid the decrease in cardiac output and heart rate. β-blockers with ISA are preferred for patients who experience bradycardia with other β-blockers. β-blockers with ISA may also produce fewer problems for patients with peripheral vascular disease, lipid disorders, or diabetes mellitus, but they are not cardioprotective. A new β$_1$-selective agent, nebivolol, has been proposed to have a unique mechanism of peripheral vasodilation brought about by modulation of nitric oxide release. Preliminary data suggest it may be as effective as other accepted β-blockers in the treatment of heart failure.

β-blockers can also be classified into two groups on the basis of their pharmacokinetic properties. The β-blockers that are eliminated by hepatic metabolism are highly lipophilic, absorbed in the small intestine, undergo extensive first-pass metabolism, have variable bioavailability, have short plasma half-lives, and more readily penetrate the blood–brain barrier. β-blockers that are eliminated unchanged by the kidney are hydrophilic, are incompletely absorbed throughout the gut, have longer plasma half-lives, and are less able to penetrate the central nervous system. Because the antihypertensive effect of β-blockers appears to outlast the presence of the drug in plasma, all agents can be used on a twice-daily schedule, and the longer-acting drugs can be given once daily. The bioavailability of propranolol and metoprolol increases approximately 60% when the drugs are taken with food. Propranolol has a wide dosage range, and plasma concentrations from a fixed dosage may vary 20-fold between patients. The hydrophilic agents (atenolol and nadolol) have flat dose-response curves but accumulate in patients with renal failure.

Adverse Effects. Many adverse effects are related to β-adrenergic blockade in predisposed patients. Adverse effects from β$_1$-blockade include bradycardia, conduction abnormalities, and left ventricular failure. Adverse effects of β$_2$-blockade include bronchospasm, cold extremities, and worsening claudication. A meta-analysis concluded that β-blocker therapy did not worsen claudication in patients with mild to moderate peripheral vascular disease.[80] These adverse effects tend to occur early in therapy even at low dosages. Central nervous system effects may be most common with propranolol, and frank depression or vivid visual hallucinations can occur. However, a large case-control analysis did not show that β-blockers were causally related to depression.[81] β-blockers decrease HDL cholesterol, increase triglycerides, and blunt the effectiveness of dietary modification to lower cholesterol. Lipid changes are not associated with ISA β-blockers.

Withdrawing β-blockers may produce β-adrenergic supersensitivity. Both abrupt cessation and gradual withdrawal over 4 to 8 days have caused overshoot hypertension and cardiovascular complications within 48 to 72 hours after the last β-blocker dose.[82] Symptoms of the withdrawal syndrome are nervousness, restlessness, anxiety, malaise, fatigue, headaches, insomnia, vivid dreams, tachycardia, palpitations, tremors, diaphoresis, excessive salivation, abdominal cramps and pain, anorexia, nausea, and vomiting. Cardiovascular morbidity has included encephalopathy, cerebrovascular accidents, unstable angina, myocardial infarction, and sudden death. β-blocker withdrawal syndrome can be reversed by readministration of small dosages of the β-blocker. To prevent β-adrenergic supersensitivity, the β-blocker dosage should be reduced over 7 to 10 days to the equivalent of 30 mg per day of propranolol and then maintained at this low dosage for 2 additional weeks. The risk of β-blocker withdrawal is not only for patients with known ischemic heart disease: withdrawing β-blockers in patients who are free of CHD resulted in a fourfold increase in new onset of CHD.[82]

α–β-blockers. Labetalol is a nonselective β-blocker and an α$_1$-blocker that reduces the β$_2$-blockade increase in peripheral vascular resistance and sustains blood flow to the extremities and kidney. Labetalol does not reduce HDL cholesterol but may cause orthostatic hypotension and sexual dysfunction. Labetalol may be more effective than other β-blockers for older adults or black patients and has been used by patients with pulmonary disease. Carvedilol is also a nonselective β-blocker with α$_1$-blocker properties, but unlike labetalol it has been shown to have a significant impact in decreasing cardiovascular mortality in patients with a previous myocardial infarction or heart failure.

ACE Inhibitors. ACE inhibitors block the generation of angiotensin II, a potent vasoconstrictor and a stimulator of aldosterone and vasopressin secretion, as well as cause an increase in the levels of circulating bradykinin, which causes the release of nitric oxide and peripheral vasodilation. The antihypertensive efficacy of ACE inhibitors is comparable to that of diuretics and β-blockers as monotherapy for hypertension, but they are more effective in younger and white patients and somewhat less effective in black patients unless higher dosages are used or they are combined with diuretics.[83] ACE inhibitors are also synergistic with calcium entry blockers and additive with β-blockers. ACE inhibitors prolong the survival of patients with severe congestive heart failure and produce regression of LVH. ACE inhibitors also improve insulin sensitivity and have been associated with a decreased incidence of diabetes in several post-hoc analyses compared to other medications.[45,48,50,84,85] Another unique benefit of ACE inhibitors is the reduction of angiotensin II-mediated intraglomerular capillary pressure. This effect appears to retard the progression of diabetic renal disease, stabilize renal function, and decrease proteinuria.[83]

ACE inhibitors may be considered first-line treatment for hypertension in patients who also have a history of previous myocardial infarction, heart failure, diabetes, chronic kidney disease, stroke, or high coronary disease risk. The Appropriate Blood Pressure Control Diabetes (ABCD) trial suggested an advantage of enalapril compared to nisoldipine for fatal and nonfatal myocardial infarction, though total mortality was similar in both groups.[86] In an attempt to compare older agents (β-blockers or thiazides) with newer agents (ACE inhibitors or dihydropyridine calcium channel blockers), STOP-2 showed similar results in the combined primary endpoints of fatal stroke, fatal myocardial infarction, and other fatal cardiovascular disease between the groups with similar levels of BP reduction.[49] The CAPP trial found captopril to be equal to diuretics and β-blockers in preventing cardiovascular morbidity and mortality, though the incidence of stroke was higher in the captopril group.[48] The data concerning ACE inhibitors and stroke have continued to be conflicting. As discussed in the diuretic section, ALLHAT showed no difference among chlorthalidone, lisinopril, and amlodipine for the primary outcome of combined fatal CHD or nonfatal myocardial infarction, though the lisinopril group had higher 6-year rates of stroke as well as combined CVD, and heart failure.[45] ANBP2 seemed to contradict the findings of ALLHAT showing the ACE inhibitor, enalapril, was more effective than hydrochlorothiazide in cumulative rate of death and cardiovascular events. However, the difference between the groups was mainly due to a decrease in myocardial infarction, with no difference in stroke incidence. The effectiveness of ACE inhibitors in poststroke patients was addressed in the PROGRESS trial. Significant risk reduction of recurrent stroke in this high-risk group was seen only when the thiazide-like diuretic, indapamide, was added to perindopril versus ACE inhibitor monotherapy.

The use of ACE inhibitors in secondary prevention was addressed in the Heart Outcomes Prevention Evaluation (HOPE) trial[84] and the European Trial on Reduction of Cardiac Events with Perindopril in Stable Coronary Artery Disease (EUROPA).[87] The HOPE trial enrolled approximately 9,000 patients with either known atherosclerotic disease (coronary artery disease, peripheral arterial disease, stroke) or diabetes and one risk factor (hypertension, cigarette smoking, microalbuminuria, or dyslipidemia). Approximately 50% of the patients had hypertension and 40% had diabetes. For the patients who received ramipril, the primary endpoint of cardiovascular death, myocardial infarction, and stroke was significantly reduced compared to the control group. Secondary outcomes including all-cause mortality, revascularization need, new onset of diabetes, and worsening of angina or heart failure were all reduced from ramipril therapy. The mean difference in BP between the ramipril and control groups was 3.3 mm Hg. Based on this, the authors

concluded that the benefits derived the use of this ACE inhibitor was not attributed to BP reduction alone. However, a recent meta-regression analysis of 30 clinical trials found that the degree of cardiovascular event reduction in the HOPE trial was inconsistent with simply the BP-reduction effects of the drug.[88] Recent reports from the NHBPEP also support these findings in which a reduction of SBP should provide an 8% reduction in stroke and 5% reduction in CHD, numbers that are actually higher than those obtained in the HOPE trial.[89] Finally, the EUROPA trial showed results similar to the HOPE trial in patients slightly more stable than those in HOPE. However, in both these secondary prevention trials, ACE inhibitor therapy was compared to placebo and not other active drugs.

Initial ACE inhibitor therapy is an indirect means of classification of renin status and controls BP in about 50% of patients. Patients with a poor decrease in BP from ACE inhibitors are likely to have low-renin hypertension. For patients who do not respond to initial ACE inhibitor therapy, adding low dosages of a thiazide diuretic controls BP in up to 85% of patients by working synergistically with ACE inhibitor treatment.

Comparison of Ace Inhibitors. The available ACE inhibitors differ in pharmacokinetics. Captopril binds to ACE by a sulfhydryl group, and the other ACE inhibitors do not.[82] Benazepril, enalapril, fosinopril, perindopril, quinapril, and ramipril are administered as prodrugs; this delays their onset of action and prolongs the effect. Captopril should be taken without food and should be taken at least twice daily. Other agents are given once daily. The primary route of elimination is the kidney, and dosage should be reduced in renal insufficiency. Benazepril, trandolapril, and fosinopril are eliminated by both renal excretion and hepatic metabolism, and dosage reductions are not needed for patients with renal dysfunction. The ability of agents to inhibit ACE in different locations (vasculature, heart, kidneys, brain) of the body versus plasma ACE has seen much debate. However, the clinical significance of these proposed differences has not been proven.

Adverse Effects. ACE inhibitors avoid many of the adverse effects that were common to earlier antihypertensive drugs. They do not alter plasma lipids, glucose, or uric acid, nor do they aggravate bronchospastic disease or peripheral vascular disease. ACE inhibitors also do not cause central nervous system depression or sexual dysfunction. They may increase alertness and produce mood elevation, which may have contributed to the positive effect on the quality of life seen with captopril.[83] Adverse effects that are common to all ACE inhibitors are hypotension, hyperkalemia, cough, angioedema, and renal insufficiency.[83] Hypotension occurs when patients are sodium-depleted or have high renin and is more common with captopril because of its rapid onset of action. To reduce this risk, diuretics should be discontinued for 3 days before the initial ACE inhibitor dose. The risk of hyperkalemia is greater for patients with diabetes or renal insufficiency, if sodium intake is restricted, and if potassium-sparing diuretics, aldosterone antagonists, angiotensin receptor blockers, potassium supplements, or NSAIDs are given. Intractable, dry cough, warranting discontinuation of ACE inhibitor therapy, develops in more than 20% of patients. The mechanism of this is unclear, though it may be secondary to increased levels of bradykinin or substance P in the lungs. Other possible adverse effects include neutropenia, skin rash, proteinuria, and taste disturbances.[83] Finally, because of significant fetal abnormalities when given in the second or third trimester, ACE inhibitors are contraindicated during pregnancy.

Angiotensin II Receptor Antagonists. The newest pharmacologic class of drugs is the angiotensin II type 1 receptor (AT_1) antagonists (ARBs). The AT_1 antagonists displace angiotensin II from the type 1 receptor subtype, antagonizing smooth muscle contraction, sympathetic pressor response, and aldosterone release.[89] AT_1 antagonists lower BP and have cardiac and renal protective effects. Because they do not block the AT_2 receptor, the beneficial effects of angiotensin II that include vasodilation and tissue repair remain. Angiotensin II receptor antagonists also improve insulin sensitivity and have been associated with a decreased incidence of diabetes in several analyses compared to other medications.[43,85] Two significant large hypertension trials have compared ARBs with a calcium channel blocker [the Valsartan Antihypertensive Long-term Use Evaluation (VALUE) trial] and with a β-blocker (the LIFE trial).[85,90,91] The LIFE trial compared losartan with atenolol in 9,193 hypertensive patients with LVH. As discussed previously, the only primary end point that favored losartan was stroke. Fewer patients receiving losartan had new-onset diabetes or albuminuria. Though the results of LIFE indicate that an ARB had an impact on the composite endpoint of cardiovascular mortality, stroke, and myocardial infarction to the same degree as atenolol, many have questioned whether a β-blocker was the appropriate choice with which to compare losartan in this patient population, which contained 13% diabetic patients and had an average age of 67 years. As diuretic therapy has been shown to be more effective in elderly patients, it has been suggested that a diuretic may have been a better comparator. However, in a substudy of LIFE, the results in 1,195 diabetic patients showed a dramatic difference in cardiovascular and total mortality in favor of losartan versus atenolol as compared to the total study population, suggesting a possible patient population in which ARBs might be considered. This leads to a second criticism of the LIFE trial, which suggests that losartan should have been compared to an ACE inhibitor to give a better assessment of the medication's impact on clinical outcomes in diabetic patients. The VALUE trial was designed to test the hypothesis that for the same level of BP control, a valsartan-based regimen would offer better cardioprotection than would an amlodipine-based regimen.[85] In this trial 15,245 patients, aged 50 years or older with un-

treated hypertension and a high risk of cardiac events, were randomized to receive valsartan 80 mg or amlodipine 5 mg. For those not reaching BP goals, doses were titrated and hydrochlorothiazide 12.5 mg and other agents were added as needed. No significant differences were found between the two treatment groups for the primary composite endpoint of cardiac morbidity and mortality and for the secondary endpoint of all-cause mortality. However, patients receiving amlodipine had significantly lower BP levels early in the trial, which was the central reason for fewer myocardial infarctions and a favorable trend in stroke rates. There was no significant difference in the secondary endpoint of chronic congestive heart failure between the two treatment arms, but a trend favoring valsartan was apparent. Seventy-six percent of the entire observed excess of stroke occurred in the first 12 months of the study. Finally, the incidence of new-onset diabetes was significantly lower in the valsartan-based arm, which confirms the results from the LIFE trial with losartan and multiple trials with ACE inhibitors that suggest agents that antagonize the angiotensin system have beneficial effects on long-term glucose metabolism.

Trials have shown significant renal protective effects of ARBs in diabetic patients. The Reduction of End Points in NIDDM with the Angiotensin II Antagonist Losartan (RENAAL) was a placebo-controlled trial in patients with type 2 diabetes and nephropathy that assessed losartan's ability to reduce urinary protein excretion and the risk of end-stage renal disease.[92] Urinary protein excretion was reduced by 35% and the development of end-stage renal disease was reduced by 28% in the treatment group of losartan. Though these results showed significant clinical benefits with the use of an ARB in diabetic patients with nephropathy, the comparison with placebo has been questioned. Finally, the Irbesartan Diabetic Nephropathy Trial (IDNT) compared irbesartan to amlodipine in the combined endpoint of a doubling of the baseline serum creatinine level, the onset of end-stage renal disease, or death from any cause.[93] Significant reductions in the doubling of the serum creatinine concentration and relative risk of end-stage renal disease were seen in the irbesartan group versus the amlodipine group. The reduction could not be explained by differences in BP. However, similar to the results in the VALUE trial, there was a trend that favored amlodipine with regard to cardiovascular death, myocardial infarction, and stroke versus valsartan.

Comparison of Angiotensin II Receptor Antagonists. Though within the class there are kinetic differences, clinical trials have not revealed clinically relevant differences in efficacy among the ARBs at equipotent doses. The drugs differ in their metabolic pathways, with twice-daily dosing needed for losartan and possibly candesartan. Losartan is transformed to an active metabolite in the liver, which helps to prolong the antihypertensive effects of the drug. The drug is highly protein-bound (99%) and is cleared by both the hepatic and renal routes; therefore, it should be used with caution in patients with hepatic or renal dysfunction. Valsartan is also highly protein-bound (97%), reaches maximum antihypertensive effects in approximately 4 weeks, and is excreted as the parent compound 30% in the urine and 70% in the bile. Irbesartan has higher bioavailability than other agents in the class (80% vs. 20% to 30%) as well as having a high affinity for the AT_1 receptor. The drug does not require dosage adjustments for elderly patients and those with renal or hepatic insufficiency. Candesartan cilexetil is a prodrug that is rapidly hydrolyzed to the active compound, candesartan, in the gastrointestinal tract. Dosage adjustments are not required for patients with moderate renal or hepatic insufficiency.

Adverse Effects. The adverse effects that result from the blockade of angiotensin II are similar to those of the ACE inhibitors, which include orthostatic hypotension, especially in patients who are volume-depleted or with high renin levels, and hyperkalemia, especially in patients with renal insufficiency or diabetes and those with concomitant use of NSAIDs, potassium-sparing diuretics, ACE inhibitors, and potassium supplements. The unique difference between ACE inhibitors and ARBs with respect to adverse events is the lack of cough with ARBs, as they do not raise levels of bradykinin or substance P. Though it was thought that ARBs would not cause angioedema when originally released, case reports have confirmed the risk with this medication class as well.[94–96] AT_1 antagonists are contraindicated in pregnancy.

Calcium Channel Antagonists. Calcium antagonists may be the most controversial class of drugs considered to be effective monotherapy for initial hypertension treatment. Calcium antagonists impair the transport of calcium through the voltage-sensitive calcium channels in vascular smooth muscle cells; this decreases contractile force, vascular smooth muscle tone, and peripheral resistance. The calcium antagonists are particularly effective for patients with low-renin hypertension (i.e., hypertensive older adults and African Americans) and have greater antihypertensive efficacy in patients with higher pretreatment BPs. Calcium antagonists, especially dihydropyridines, are effective in treating isolated systolic hypertension. Calcium antagonists are also used to treat angina, variant angina, certain arrhythmias, and migraine headaches; this makes them attractive antihypertensive agents for patients with those conditions. Calcium antagonists also do not adversely affect asthma, gout, peripheral vascular disease, lipid levels, and diabetes mellitus.

The cardiovascular protective ability of calcium channel blockers, especially in diabetes, has been a subject of great debate. The ABCD trial[86] and the Fosinopril Versus Amlodipine Cardiovascular Events Randomized Trial (FACET)[97] raised the concern that dihydropyridine calcium antagonists may be dangerous in diabetic patients with hypertension, increasing the risk of myocardial infarction. However, in the HOT study, 1,500 diabetic patients with hypertension treated with felodipine had a significant reduction in cardiovascular mortality.[42] The Systolic Hypertension in Europe (Syst-Eur) trial found that nitrendipine reduced cardiovascular compli-

cations in older adults with isolated systolic hypertension.[98] Post-hoc analysis of the Syst-Eur trial in diabetic patients showed significant reductions in all cardiovascular endpoints as well.[99] The Intervention as a Goal in Hypertension Treatment (INSIGHT), another dihydropyridine outcomes trial, assessed the use of the long-acting version of nifedipine versus hydrochlorothiazide plus amiloride in 6,321 hypertensive patients.[100] No difference in overall cardiovascular outcomes was seen between the two treatment groups, but there was an increase in fatal myocardial infarctions and nonfatal heart failure in the nifedipine group. Finally, as discussed previously, the ALLHAT and VALUE trials both showed the dihydropyridine amlodipine to be at least as effective in preventing primary cardiovascular outcomes as a thiazide diuretic or an ACE inhibitor (ALLHAT) or an ARB (VALUE). Data from ALLHAT were consistent in the diabetic patients. As in previous trials, ALLHAT confirmed a significant 38% increased risk of heart failure in the calcium channel blocker group, but as shown in a recent meta-analysis, calcium channel blockers may be more effective in the prevention of stroke.[64,65] Though most recent data suggest improved cardiovascular outcomes for patients receiving dihydropyridines, results are still conflicting. Current recommendations are to avoid short-acting dihydropyridine calcium antagonists for the treatment of hypertension.[1] Some have proposed there may be a difference within the calcium channel blocker class, suggesting that dihydropyridines may increase adrenergic stimulation.[101] This was shown in the VAMPHYRE study in which the phenylalkylamine verapamil was associated with a 22% decrease in plasma norepinephrine as compared to amlodipine.[102] This increased adrenergic stimulation could explain poorer cardiovascular outcomes such as heart failure.

Two studies of nondihydropyridine calcium channel blockers (diltiazem and verapamil) suggest the non-dihydropyridine class of calcium channel blockers may be equivalent to diuretics, β-blockers, or ACE inhibitors on cardiovascular outcomes. The Nordic Diltiazem (NORDIL) trial compared the effects of diltiazem with those of diuretics, β-blockers, or both on cardiovascular morbidity and mortality in hypertensive patients.[103] This trial of 10,881 patients showed diltiazem to be equivalent to diuretics, β-blockers, or both in all outcomes, with stroke slightly better and heart attack slightly higher in the diltiazem group. The International Verapamil-Trandolapril Study (INVEST) was a comparison of antihypertensive treatment initiated with extended-release verapamil versus treatment initiated with atenolol in 22,576 high-risk patients aged 50 years or older with hypertension and coronary artery disease.[104] Trandolapril and/or hydrochlorothiazide, as well as other antihypertensive agents, could be added to either regimen to achieve the BP goals (<140/90 mm Hg or <130/85 mm Hg for patients with diabetes). Prevention of the primary outcome (all-cause mortality, nonfatal myocardial infarction, or nonfatal stroke) was equivalent between the two treatment regimens.

Comparison of Calcium Entry Blockers. There are three chemical classes of calcium antagonist. Verapamil is a phenylalkylamine, diltiazem is a benzothiazepine, and amlodipine, felodipine, isradipine, nicardipine, and nifedipine are dihydropyridines. All calcium antagonists that are used for hypertension have comparable efficacy, but they differ in their adverse effect profiles. The calcium antagonists have limited oral bioavailability because of first-pass hepatic metabolism. Only diltiazem (35%) has significant renal elimination. Because of short plasma half-lives, extended-release products are available for verapamil, diltiazem, and nifedipine, allowing once- or twice-daily administration. Extended-release products may also decrease dose-related adverse effects. Adding a diuretic to a calcium entry blocker usually has only minimal additive effect; this may be due in part to the natriuretic effect of the calcium entry blockers.

Adverse Effects. The adverse effects of the calcium antagonists are primarily extensions of their pharmacologic actions and can be categorized as vasodilation, negative inotropic effects, conduction disturbances, gastrointestinal effects, and metabolic effects. Vasodilatory side effects include headaches, flushing, palpitations, hypotension, and peripheral edema. Vasodilation is more common with dihydropyridine calcium antagonists. Negative inotropic effects are least with the dihydropyridines and greatest with verapamil. Although diltiazem has an intermediate negative inotropic effect, it can produce or worsen congestive heart failure in patients with preexisting left ventricular dysfunction. Conduction disturbances are greatest with verapamil, intermediate with diltiazem, and uncommon with dihydropyridines. Results from ALLHAT put to rest concerns of increased risk of gastrointestinal bleeding as well as cancer with calcium channel blockers. Verapamil often causes constipation, which may be relieved with stool softeners. Verapamil decreases digoxin elimination and can increase serum digoxin levels by 50% to 75%. A full list of drug interactions with calcium channel antagonists is given in Table 20.12. Other calcium antagonists may also interact with digoxin, but usually to a lesser degree. If a calcium antagonist is used in combination with a β-blocker, a dihydropyridine agent is preferred to reduce the additive negative chronotropic effects.

Aldosterone Receptor Antagonists. The ability of aldosterone to mediate water and electrolyte balance through mineralocorticoid receptors in the kidney is well established. Recent studies have revealed the presence of similar receptors in the brain, heart, and blood vessels.[105] These findings suggest that aldosterone may play a more significant role in cardiovascular disease, including LVH and heart failure, than originally thought. Because other therapies such as ACE inhibitors and ARBs may not have an impact on long-term suppression of aldosterone, there has been a renewed interest in effective receptor antagonists.

Spironolactone is a competitive aldosterone antagonist used in combination with thiazide diuretics to prevent or correct hypokalemia or in patients with mineralocorticoid-

influenced hypertension.[106] It has been suggested that primary aldosteronism may be present in up to 15% of patients with hypertension.[107] Food enhances the absorption of spironolactone, which is rapidly metabolized to pharmacologically active metabolites, including canrenone. Spironolactone may be superior to potassium supplements in correcting diuretic-induced hypokalemia and also corrects coexisting magnesium deficiency. In a trial of 1,663 heart failure patients with New York Heart Association (NYHA) functional class III or IV and an ejection fraction of less than 35%, spironolactone 25 mg was added to standard therapy for heart failure (ACE inhibitors and loop diuretics at the time) versus placebo.[108] The Randomized Aldactone Evaluation (RALES) study was stopped early after the spironolactone group showed a 30% decrease in mortality and a 35% reduction in hospitalization secondary to worsening heart failure. The side effects of spironolactone are secondary to its actions as an antagonist of androgen and progesterone (gynecomastia, menstrual irregularities, hirsutism, and impotence) as well as mineralocorticoid receptors (hyperkalemia). The risk of hyperkalemia is increased in patients taking ACE inhibitors or ARBs, NSAIDs, potassium-sparing diuretics, or potassium supplements, as well as patients with renal insufficiency or those who are volume-depleted. A recent Canadian study revealed that since the release of the RALES trial, the risk of hyperkalemia-related morbidity and mortality significantly increased, confirming the need for judicious monitoring when combining multiple agents that increase the risk of hyperkalemia.[109] Limiting spironolactone dosage to less than 100 mg per day appears to reduce the incidence of adverse effects.

Eplerenone, the first in a new class of agents, selective aldosterone receptor antagonists (SARAs), has significant less affinity for androgen and progesterone receptors. In controlled studies, eplerenone caused adverse effects related to androgen and progesterone antagonism no more than those seen with placebo.[110] The risk of hyperkalemia is dose-dependent and similar to that with spironolactone.[111] Eplerenone was as effective as spironolactone for lowering both SBP and DP.[111] The drug has also been shown to be effective as add-on therapy for patients with mild to moderate hypertension who were minimally responsive to ACE inhibitors or ARBs.[110] This suggested the drug might be effective in patients with low-renin hypertension, such as black patients. In one study, eplerenone was found to be equally effective in black patients and white patients for the treatment of hypertension, but more effective than losartan in black patients.[112] When compared to the ACE inhibitor enalapril, eplerenone was as effective as monotherapy in stage 1 or 2 hypertension, and more effective in reducing albuminuria in 12 months.[113] Eplerenone was shown to be equivalent to amlodipine in the reduction of BP in older patients with systolic hypertension and/or wide pulse pressures.[114] However, no pharmacoeconomic studies have suggested a compelling reason to use eplerenone versus spironolactone specifically for the treatment of hypertension.

Finally, the Eplerenone Post–Acute Myocardial Infarction Heart Failure Efficacy and Survival (EPHESUS) study assessed the addition of eplerenone 25 mg (titrated to a maximum of 50 mg) or placebo to optimal medical therapy in 6,642 patients with acute myocardial infarction complicated by left ventricular dysfunction (ejection fraction <40%) and heart failure.[115] The primary endpoints were death from any cause and death from cardiovascular causes or hospitalization for heart failure, acute myocardial infarction, stroke, or ventricular arrhythmia. All primary outcomes were significantly reduced by the addition of eplerenone. As seen in previous trials, the rate of hyperkalemia (>5.5 mmol/L) was significantly higher in the eplerenone group. Growing evidence suggests the appropriate antagonism of aldosterone may provide added benefits to patients at high risk for cardiovascular complications and hypertension. The JNC-VII lists heart failure and postmyocardial infarction as compelling indications to consider aldosterone antagonists in the pharmacotherapy plan for patients with those diagnoses and hypertension secondary to the RALES and EPHESUS trials. Until further long-term morbidity and mortality trials are available, aldosterone antagonists should be considered third- or fourth-line agents specifically for the treatment of hypertension.

Sympathetic Inhibitors. Many antihypertensive drugs interfere with the sympathetic nervous system. These agents may act in the central or peripheral nervous system.

α$_1$-Adrenergic Blocking Agents. These drugs produce a selective postsynaptic α$_1$-adrenoceptor inhibition, causing decreased peripheral resistance and vasodilation without reducing cardiac output or inducing a reflex tachycardia. These agents produce a slightly greater decrease in standing BP than in supine BP. They have additive effects with β-blockers and diuretics. Their advantages include a favorable lipid profile effect, equal efficacy in all age and race groups, and a favorable effect on plasma glucose levels.[1] Another group that may benefit from α$_1$-adrenergic inhibitors is patients with benign prostatic hypertrophy (BPH). α$_1$-Adrenergic inhibitors increase urine flow and decrease urinary frequency in patients with BPH by inhibiting norepinephrine-induced contraction of prostate smooth muscle. However, because the results of the ALLHAT arm containing the α$_1$-blocker doxazosin showed an increase in cardiovascular events, specifically heart failure, the use of this class for the treatment of hypertension should only be considered as third- or fourth-line therapy (usually in patients with concomitant BPH and hypertension) to be added to agents known to reduce cardiovascular events.[47]

Comparison of α$_1$-Adrenergic Blockers. The three α$_1$-adrenergic inhibitors appear to have similar antihypertensive effects and adverse effects. The α$_1$-adrenergic inhibitors undergo substantial hepatic first-pass metabolism. Doxazosin and terazosin have a longer duration of action than does prazosin and can be dosed once daily.

Adverse Effects. The most striking adverse effect of the α$_1$-adrenergic inhibitors is the first-dose syncope. Profound orthostatic hypotension with syncope can occur 1 to 3 hours after the first dose in patients with a low plasma volume from diuretic therapy or patients who are taking other antihypertensive drugs that blunt their response to the acute decrease in BP. To avoid this problem, the initial dose should be limited to the equivalent of 1 mg prazosin and should be taken at bedtime or when the patient can be observed.

Central α$_2$-Agonists. Central α$_2$-adrenergic agonists stimulate α$_2$-adrenergic receptors in the lower brain stem, which decreases sympathetic outflow to the cardiovascular system. Some agents also block peripheral α$_2$-adrenergic receptors. The combined sympatholytic effects cause a decrease in peripheral vascular resistance.[116] The central α$_2$-adrenergic agonists are equally effective in all age and race groups and can be used for patients with renal insufficiency, diabetes mellitus, bronchospastic disease, and ischemic heart disease. The efficacy of these drugs is similar to that of other antihypertensives. Unlike peripheral sympatholytics, the central α$_2$-adrenergic agonists do not cause significant sodium and fluid retention. The central α$_2$-adrenergic agonists do not adversely effect glucose metabolism and have neutral or favorable effects on plasma lipids.[116] These agents also produce a regression in LVH. In addition to its use in hypertension, clonidine has increased the success of smoking cessation, particularly for women, and decreasing craving as well as withdrawal symptoms.

Comparison of α$_2$-Adrenergic Agonists. Newer formulations of the central α$_2$-adrenergic agonists provide sustained antihypertensive efficacy with less frequent dosing and have reduced the occurrence of symptomatic side effects. Clonidine can be given twice daily. A clonidine suppression test has been used to assess the contribution of increased sympathetic outflow in patients with essential hypertension. Clonidine is also available as a transdermal therapeutic system that is applied once weekly. Transdermal clonidine controls BP in 60% to 80% of patients with mild hypertension.[117] Severe withdrawal rebound hypertension is less likely to occur with transdermal therapy than with oral clonidine.[117] The transdermal system is a convenient form of treatment with equal efficacy and fewer adverse effects than oral clonidine; the main adverse effect is contact dermatitis, which develops in 10% to 15% of patients.

Guanfacine is a long-acting central α$_2$-adrenergic agonist that is metabolized by the liver (70%) and excreted unchanged by the kidneys (30%), with a prolonged elimination half-life of 16 to 23 hours. The long duration of action allows once-daily dosing and reduces adverse effects. Guanfacine also has a flat dose-response curve, with little increase in antihypertensive effect from dosages greater than 1 mg.

Guanabenz is a guanidine derivative that blocks central sympathetic vasomotor impulses and produces a guanethidine-like postganglionic blockage. Guanabenz decreases cholesterol and triglycerides without changing HDL cholesterol. Guanabenz is used on a twice-daily dosing schedule.

Methyldopa, the first central α_2-adrenergic agonist, has largely been replaced by the newer agents. A methyldopa metabolite, α-methyl norepinephrine, is the active agonist that reduces central nervous system sympathetic outflow. Methyldopa has an orthostatic effect greater than that of clonidine, but both cardiac output and renal function usually are preserved. Because sodium and water retention can produce a pseudotolerance, methyldopa normally is combined with a diuretic. Methyldopa can be used on a twice-daily dosing schedule and has a long history of use in treating hypertension in pregnancy.

Adverse Effects. Sedation and dry mouth are the most common adverse effects of central α_2-adrenergic agonists. These symptoms often disappear after the first few weeks. Saliva substitutes or sugarless gum or candy can provide relief from dry mouth. Sedation is additive to the effects of other sedating drugs including alcohol; patients should be cautioned about these combinations and driving. Serious hypersensitivity reactions have occurred with methyldopa, including drug fever, colitis, hepatotoxicity, a positive Coombs test, and hemolytic anemia. The risks of serious toxicity and impaired mental function make alternative antihypertensive drugs preferable to methyldopa.

Abrupt discontinuation of clonidine has caused an acute withdrawal syndrome characterized by a rapid increase in BP, headaches, palpitations, tremor, restlessness, diaphoresis, and nausea. It appears to be rare with the use of transdermal clonidine and guanfacine. The risk of acute withdrawal syndrome is higher in younger patients with severe hypertension who are treated with high dosages and multiple antihypertensive agents. Combination with β-blockers increases the risk of a hypertensive episode on discontinuation of clonidine.[118] This combination should be avoided; if it is used, the β-blocker should be tapered and stopped before the clonidine is tapered. Avoiding excessive dosages, encouraging patient compliance, and tapering clonidine slowly may help to prevent the withdrawal syndrome. However, patients should be warned to seek immediate medical help if they develop signs and symptoms of the syndrome. Treatment by restarting medications usually is effective in reversing the withdrawal syndrome, and labetalol has been effective for combined central agonist-β-blocker acute withdrawal syndrome.[118,119]

Guanethidine is actively transported into the peripheral adrenergic neuron, where it depletes norepinephrine and produces a postural hypotension. Guanethidine decreases venous return to the heart, decreases cardiac output, and interferes with the sympathetic reflexes that control the resistance (arteriolar) and capacitance (venous) vessels. Because guanethidine depletes myocardial catecholamines, it can worsen congestive heart failure. Guanethidine is slowly and variably absorbed, undergoing partial first-pass hepatic metabolism. With chronic administration the half-life of guanethidine is

5 days, with 50% of the drug excreted unchanged in the urine. Because of the long half-life, guanethidine can be taken once daily, and dosage adjustments should be made only after 2 to 3 weeks. Prolonged standing, exercise, and heat increase postural hypotension. The guanethidine dosage should be adjusted on the basis of standing BP, and blocks can be used to elevate the head of the bed to sustain a nighttime postural effect. Guanadrel is an adrenergic blocking agent that also depletes norepinephrine from peripheral neurons. Guanadrel has a more rapid onset and a shorter duration of action than guanethidine. Because of the postural effect, standing BP must always be measured. These agents are reserved for treating resistant hypertension.

Adverse Effects. The major problem with both guanethidine and guanadrel is postural and exercise hypotension. Patients should be warned to rise slowly from supine or sitting positions, to flex their arms and legs before arising, and to avoid additive vasodilating factors such as prolonged standing, hot showers, and alcohol. Postural effects are most pronounced in the morning on arising. Other dose-related problems include sexual dysfunction and diarrhea, which may necessitate discontinuation of therapy. A pseudotolerance caused by fluid retention may develop unless diuretic therapy is adequate. Because guanethidine diffuses poorly into the central nervous system, sedation and depression are infrequent problems. Several drugs can interfere with the uptake of the sympatholytics into the adrenergic neuron and rapidly block the antihypertensive effects. Guanadrel may cause less sexual dysfunction and orthostasis than guanethidine. However, patients should be given similar precautions to minimize the risks of postural hypotension. Diuretics are needed to reduce sodium and water retention and weight gain.

Reserpine. Reserpine acts in both the central and peripheral sympathetic nervous systems, depleting norepinephrine and serotonin stores in the brain and peripheral adrenergic nerve endings. Reserpine also increases vagal tone; this contributes to the reduced heart rate and increased gastric acid secretions. The onset of action of reserpine may take several days; maximal hypotensive effects may take weeks. Adverse effects are common with high dosages and include nasal congestion from cholinergic stimulation. Central nervous system changes include drowsiness, sedation, dizziness, sleep disturbances, impaired concentration, poor memory, and depression. Other antihypertensive agents are preferred because they have greater efficacy and fewer adverse effects.

Vasodilators. Vasodilators directly relax arteriolar smooth muscle and decrease peripheral vascular resistance. They do not interfere with autonomic reflexes or produce postural hypotension. This stimulates carotid sinus baroreceptors, producing reflex increases in heart rate, renin release, and sodium and water retention. These drugs usually have been used in combination with a diuretic and a β-blocker or sympatholytic agent to prevent the reflex increases in cardiac output and fluid retention that blunt the effect of vasodilators when they are used alone. Older adults develop less reflex tachycardia.

Comparison of Vasodilators. Hydralazine is metabolized by hepatic acetylation with substantial first-pass elimination. Hydralazine is effective when taken twice daily; food increases bioavailability. The acetylation rate is genetically determined; slow acetylators experience greater hypotensive effects and usually should not receive more than 200 mg hydralazine daily.

Minoxidil is a potent vasodilator that markedly reduces peripheral vascular resistance and is reserved for severe hypertension. It can produce BP reductions of 30 to 40 mm Hg when combined with diuretics and β-blockers. Minoxidil is well absorbed and undergoes hepatic metabolism. Despite a short half-life, the antihypertensive effect persists for 12 to 24 hours, and minoxidil is dosed twice daily. Minoxidil produces marked sodium and water retention, and large dosages of loop diuretics often are needed to control the edema. Reflex tachycardia and increased cardiac output are prevented by adequate β-blocker therapy.

Diazoxide is a nondiuretic thiazide that dilates peripheral arterioles and is used to treat hypertensive emergencies.[119] Intravenous injection produces a profound decrease in both SBP and DBP that does not warrant continuous infusion and rarely causes hypotension. Diazoxide is metabolized in the liver and excreted in urine, with a duration of action of 2 to 24 hours. Diazoxide is administered as a minibolus (1 to 3 mg/kg) every 10 minutes, with a maximum of 150 mg, or as an infusion given at a rate of 15 mg per minute. Diazoxide produces sodium and water retention, and diuretic therapy is needed to maintain BP control. Hyperglycemia is a problem with prolonged use. Patients with renal failure or myocardial ischemia are predisposed to the adverse effects of diazoxide.

Nitroprusside is an instant-acting vasodilator that is useful in virtually all hypertensive emergencies. Nitroprusside relaxes both arteriolar and venous smooth muscles. Nitroprusside reacts with cysteine, forming nitrocysteine, which activates guanylate cyclase, leading to increased cyclic guanylic acid, which relaxes vascular smooth muscle. Controlled intravenous nitroprusside infusions are highly effective in treating hypertensive emergencies. The onset and cessation of the hypotensive action are immediate. Nitroprusside is unstable and must be protected from light. The nitroprusside metabolite thiocyanate may rapidly accumulate with impaired renal function, and plasma thiocyanate concentrations greater than 10 mg per dL are toxic. Nitroprusside decreases peripheral resistance and can improve left ventricular function in patients with congestive heart failure or with impaired cardiac output after a myocardial infarction.

Adverse Effects. Adverse effects from reflex sympathetic stimulation or direct vasodilation include headache, dizziness, postural hypotension, tachycardia, and palpitations.[120] The reflex tachycardia can precipitate or aggravate angina pectoris, and therefore hydralazine should always be given with concurrent β-blocker therapy. Hydralazine commonly causes throbbing headaches and also causes a pyridoxine deficiency-induced peripheral neuropathy. A positive antinuclear antibody (ANA) develops in 15% to 20% of hydralazine-treated patients, which can lead to a lupus-like syndrome, particularly if dosages greater than 200 mg per day are used. Symptoms can include arthralgia, arthritis, fever, malaise, rash, and weight loss. Symptoms can resolve rapidly and often disappear within 6 months; however, rheumatoid symptoms and a positive ANA can persist for years.

Minoxidil causes marked sodium and water retention, leading to weight gain, peripheral edema, cardiac enlargement, pulmonary hypertension, and pericardial effusion.[120] Like hydralazine, minoxidil therapy should only be given to patients already receiving diuretic and β-blocker therapy to minimize potential adverse effects. Minoxidil causes hypertrichosis in nearly all patients. This can be partly controlled with depilatories but limits its use by women. Coarsening of facial features can also occur.

Tailoring Antihypertensive Pharmacotherapy Regimens in Special Populations. As discussed previously, the JNC-VII recommends the use of thiazide-type diuretics for patients with uncomplicated hypertension (Fig. 20.1). However, many patients have concurrent diagnoses or are in high-risk groups that require proper selection of a pharmacotherapy regimen shown to specifically benefit patients with those diagnoses or high-risk groups (Table 20.13). As the evidence for individual agents for the treatment of hypertension with other disease states has been discussed in the agent class sections, this section will address specific population groups and the need for individualization of pharmacotherapy within them.

Diabetes. Greater than 70% of premature mortality in patients with type 2 diabetes is secondary to cardiovascular disease and stroke.[121,122] The interrelationship of the dual diagnoses of hypertension and diabetes is significant, with diabetes being diagnosed 2.5 times more often in hypertensive patients.[123] This combination of hypertension and diabetes has been shown to be a significant predictor of cardiovascular disease,[123,124] stroke,[41,45,84,122] and renal disease.[125] Because most diabetic patients require at least two medications to achieve the goal BP of less than 130/80 mm Hg,[41,45, 98,125] the initial medication chosen may not be as important as ultimately treating SBP aggressively. For diabetic patients without proteinuria, the most important issue may be aggressive reduction of SBP. However, in patients with either microalbuminuria (spot urinary microalbumin/creatinine ratio of 30 to 300 mg/g) or overt albuminuria (>300 mg/g), the JNC-VII[1] and the American Diabetes Association[126] both recommend the use of ACE inhibitors or ARBs preferentially due to their ability to slow nephropathy progression. The ability of thiazides to decrease fatal CHD and myocardial infarction was shown to be equal to that of lisinopril and amlodipine in the diabetic subpopulation of ALLHAT, even though these patients had worsening hyperglycemia and more new diagnoses of diabetes were seen in the total population compared to the other two treatment groups.[45] This concern of new diagnosis of diabetes in thiazide-based regimens is valid, as long-term outcomes of this impact may not be seen in the ALLHAT treatment groups for some time. Based on existing data, thiazide diuretics should be considered as add-on therapy for any diabetic patients with nephropathy whose hypertension is not controlled with an ACE inhibitor or ARB. Calcium channel blockers provide a useful addition to existing regimens of an ACE inhibitor or ARB plus a thiazide diuretic for further reduction of SBP, though their use as monotherapy is questionable secondary to conflicting data with nephropathy. β-blockers, like calcium channel blockers, may provide an option as add-on therapy to existing regimens of an ACE inhibitor or ARB plus a thiazide diuretic, though they are not recommended for monotherapy. They should still be used with caution secondary to their potential to mask epinephrine-based symptoms of hypoglycemia.

Chronic Kidney Disease. Normal renal function deterioration in GFR occurs with aging by 1 to 2 mL per minute per year. However, this deterioration is accelerated considerably by elevated SBP more so than DBP.[127] Chronic kidney disease, defined as either a decreased GFR of below 60 mL per minute or the presence of albuminuria, is a significant independent risk factor for CVD.[128] Recent research has suggested the possible need for replacing the reporting of serum creatinine by laboratories with eGFR, an index of renal function, which may better estimate current renal function.[25] Only 11% of patients with both hypertension and elevated creatinine were treated to a BP of below 130/80 mm Hg according to data from NHANES.[129] A recent meta-analysis identified reduced SBP (110 to 129 mm Hg) and albumin excretion rate (<1 g/d) as well as ACE inhibitor use as the factors most strongly correlated with improved outcomes in patients with chronic kidney disease and albuminuria.[130] The National Kidney Foundation recommends a BP of below 130/80 for all patients with chronic kidney disease and a medication regimen that includes an ACE inhibitor or an ARB in combination with a thiazide diuretic, though many will require a loop diuretic instead.[131] In patients with chronic kidney disease and proteinuria of 1 g per day or more, the National Kidney Foundation recommends a BP goal of below 125/75 mm Hg.

Left Ventricular Hypertrophy and Heart Failure. LVH, a risk factor for the development of dilated cardiomyopathy and heart failure, is seen in as many as 50% of patients with stage 1 and 2 hypertension, and contributes more attributable risk for all-cause mortality than does multivessel coronary artery disease or low ejection fraction.[132] LVH regression, which can be obtained with the use of most antihypertensive agents, is associated with a decreased overall CVD risk. A meta-analysis showed the best predictors of LVH regression were pretreatment left ventricular mass, greater SBP and DBP reductions, and longer treatment duration.[133] ACE in-

hibitor use was predictive of most consistent left ventricular regression, diuretic and calcium antagonist use was intermediate in left ventricular regression, and β-blocker use was associated with the least left ventricular regression. However, other studies suggested that diuretics may be most effective in LVH regression.[134,135] Recently, an antihypertensive regimen based on losartan was shown to be more effective at reducing LVH than an atenolol-based regimen.[43]

The diagnosis of hypertension confers a 2- to 3-fold increased risk for the development of heart failure, and 90% of those with heart failure will already have an existing diagnosis of hypertension.[136] The assessment and treatment of hypertension with heart failure is especially important in elderly and African American patients. As the average age of the American population continues to increase, it is expected that the prevalence of heart failure will also continue to increase. Heart failure is considered a compelling indication (Table 20.13) for the use of ACE inhibitors and β-blockers in patients with hypertension secondary to reductions in both morbidity and mortality in these patients. ARBs can be considered for patients who cannot tolerate an ACE inhibitor.

Minority Patients. African Americans have more severe hypertension, develop the disease earlier in life, have higher prevalence rates of hypertension, have lower rates of control when diagnosed with hypertension, and have more cardiovascular complications secondary to hypertension when compared to age-matched non-Hispanic white patients.[137] Likewise, though they have a lower prevalence rate as compared to African Americans, Mexican Americans have lower control rates than African Americans and non-Hispanic white patients.[138] There is a higher prevalence of stage 3 hypertension in African Americans, and hypertension is often poorly controlled in African American patients. Environmental factors, including dietary excess, high sodium consumption, and low dietary potassium, calcium, and magnesium, may contribute to these differences.[139] The greater prevalence of obesity and insulin resistance may be an important mechanism in hypertensive African Americans.[139] Many hypertensive African Americans show salt sensitivity, and hypertension often is associated with low plasma renin level and volume dependence.[137] In fact, African American patients had a more significant reduction in BP when following a low-sodium DASH diet compared to any other demographic subgroup.[35] When appropriately treated, cardiovascular events are reduced equally in hypertensive African American and non-Hispanic white patients.[137,139] However, monotherapy with ACE inhibitors, ARBs, and β-blockers was associated with lower control rates in hypertensive African Americans.[45,140–142] The use of the ACE inhibitor lisinopril in African American patients in ALLHAT was associated with a 40% increased risk of stroke, a 32% increased risk of heart failure, and a 19% increased risk of CVD compared to patients receiving the thiazide diuretic chlorthalidone. However, when combined with a diuretic, ACE inhibitors and β-blockers were equally effective in African American patients.[142,143] The AASK trial confirmed that the use of an ACE inhibitor was effective in preserving renal function in hypertensive African American patients with chronic kidney disease compared to a β-blocker or a calcium antagonist, though no difference in outcomes was noted between aggressive BP reduction (128/78 mm Hg) versus less aggressive reduction (141/85).[74] This trial showed that when treated aggressively, almost 80% of patients who would be considered "difficult to treat" could obtain a BP of below 140/90.[143]

In addition to differences in the efficacy of antihypertensive therapy in certain racial groups, differences in adverse effects may also exist. African Americans and Asians have been shown to have a significantly increased risk for both angioedema and cough from ACE inhibitors compared with non-Hispanic whites.

Older Patients. Patients over the age of 65 years are among the fastest-growing subset of the American population. Of the 34 million people aged 60 years or older, control rates are approximately 20%.[144] This low control percentage is due in large part to the significance of isolated systolic hypertension, defined as SBP above 160 mm Hg and DBP below 90 mm Hg, as the major contributor to hypertension in the older patient.[129] Isolated systolic hypertension is associated with an increased risk of stroke and CVD that is independent of other risk factors.[5] Two thirds of those aged 60 with hypertension have isolated systolic hypertension, and that number rises to greater than 75% by age 75.[129] Indeed, the lifetime risk of developing hypertension is greater than 90%, even for individuals who are normotensive at age 65.[12] In patients older than 60 years, SBP alone correctly classified their level of hypertension 94% of the time versus DBP alone, which correctly classified their hypertension level only 66% of the time.[129] Therefore, NBPEP issued a clinical advisory in 2000 emphasizing the need to use SBP as the primary target for both diagnosis and management in older patients with hypertension.[39]

Significant evidence exists supporting the need to appropriately treat elevated BP in older patients, even in those over 80 years old.[49,145] The SHEP trial demonstrated a 36% reduction in stroke, a 54% reduction in heart failure events, a 27% reduction in myocardial infarctions, and a 32% reduction in overall CVD events in patients age 60 years and older who were treated for isolated systolic hypertension.[97] Drug treatment in SHEP was low-dose chlorthalidone (12.5 to 25 mg) and atenolol 25 mg, with potassium supplements if needed. No evidence of increased risk was associated with more aggressive treatment (J-curve phenomenon) until DBP was below 55 mm Hg.[146] The Syst-Eur trial showed a 41% reduction in stroke and a 31% reduction in overall CVD events using a calcium antagonist-based treatment for older adults with isolated systolic hypertension.[98] A meta-analysis of hypertensive elderly patients showed a 23% reduction in coronary events, a 30% reduction in stroke, an 18% reduction in

cardiovascular deaths, and a 13% reduction in overall mortality in those receiving active therapy, especially in patients older than 70.[147] The Hypertensive Trialists group recently suggested that the overall reduction of BP was more important than the initial pharmacotherapy chosen for elderly patients, as most patients will require combination therapy.[65] Finally, nonpharmacologic therapy should be emphasized in elderly patients with hypertension. The Trial of Nonpharmacologic Interventions in the Elderly (TONE) study showed a significant impact of sodium restriction (less than 2 g/day) and weight loss on BP control rates in older patients, enabling 40% of patients to discontinue their antihypertensive medications.[148] Medication class selection for older patients should follow guidelines similar to the general population. However, due to more significant BP variations and a higher propensity for side effects in older patients, dosage titration should be approached with careful assessment.

Pregnant Patients. Hypertension complicates 10% of pregnancies and is more common in nulliparous women and women who have had multiple pregnancies.[149] Hypertension during pregnancy is classified into one of five categories (Table 20.14), and the use of this categorization system helps differentiate between preexisting chronic hypertension during pregnancy and new development of preeclampsia, a condition that increases the risk of mortality.[1] Chronic hypertension usually is well tolerated during pregnancy if SBP remains below 150 mm Hg and DBP below 100 mm Hg, and these patients are candidates for a trial of lifestyle modification therapy only. This approach puts the fetus at significantly less risk, with no exposure to medications in utero. A meta-analysis of the treatment of pregnant patients with stage 1 and 2 hypertension showed that an increase in small-for-gestational-age infants was directly related to the amount of reduction in mean arterial pressure and was independent of pharmacotherapy or stage of hypertension.[150] However, for pregnant patients with known target organ damage or previous BPs that required multiple medications for control, appropriate medications should be continued. Preeclampsia can be life-threatening to both the fetus and the mother and usually develops near term with pathophysiology of a marked increase in peripheral resistance.[149] Signs of preeclampsia include proteinuria, edema, hemoconcentration, hypoalbuminemia, increased urate, and hepatic or coagulation abnormalities.[149] Life-threatening complications are hemolytic anemia and marked hepatic dysfunction. Progression to seizures is called eclampsia, which is a major cause of maternal death.

Methyldopa has a long history of safe use in pregnancy, with normal follow-up evaluations in children up to 10 years after treatment.[151] β-blockers, labetalol, thiazide diuretics, and hydralazine have also been used to treat hypertension during pregnancy with apparent success. β-blockers are also considered to be safe when used later in pregnancy.[1] Limited information is available about the use of calcium entry blockers in pregnancy. ACE inhibitors and atenolol are avoided

TABLE 20.14	Classification of Hypertension in Pregnancy
Chronic hypertension	• Blood pressure ≥140/90 mm Hg prior to pregnancy or before 20 weeks' gestation
	• Persists 12 weeks postpartum
Preeclampsia	• Blood pressure ≥ 140/90 mm Hg with proteinuria (>300 mg/24 h) after 20 weeks' gestation
	• Can progress to eclampsia (seizures)
	• More common in nulliparous women, multiple gestation, women with hypertension ≥ 4 years, family history of preeclampsia, hypertension in a previous pregnancy, renal disease
Chronic hypertension with superimposed preeclampsia	• New-onset proteinuria after 20 weeks in a woman with hypertension
	• In a woman with hypertension and proteinuria prior to 20 weeks' gestation:
	• Sudden 2- to 3-fold increase in proteinuria
	• Sudden increase in blood pressure
	• Thrombocytopenia
	• Elevated alanine aminotransferase (ALT) or aspartate aminotransferase (AST)
Gestational hypertension	• Hypertension without proteinuria occurring after 20 weeks' gestation
	• Temporary diagnosis
	• May represent preproteinuric phase of preeclampsia or recurrence of chronic hypertension abated in midpregnancy
	• May evolve to preeclampsia
	• If severe, may result in higher rates of premature delivery and growth retardation than mild preeclampsia
Transient hypertension	• Retrospective diagnosis
	• Blood pressure normal by 12 weeks postpartum
	• May recur in subsequent pregnancies
	• Predictive of future primary hypertension

because they reduce uterine blood flow.[149,152] Intravenous hydralazine is commonly used to treat severe hypertension during pregnancy.[152] Diazoxide is used for refractory hypertension. Parenteral labetalol may become the second-choice agent. Calcium entry blockers are also effective, but concurrent magnesium sulfate may potentiate their effect and cause a precipitous fall in BP. Calcium entry blockers also reduce uterine blood flow.[152]

Children and Adolescents. Hypertension is defined in children and adolescents as a persistent elevation of BP at or above the 95th percentile for age, height, and gender (Tables 20.15 and 20.16). Likewise, the staging of hypertension in this population is defined with the comparison of the child to the 95th percentiles. This means that BP readings are ranked according to where they fall against the percentage of the reference population of all children, while taking into account variations in body weight, height, age, and other developmental parameters. Updated guidelines were recently released by the NHBPEP Working Group on High Blood Pressure in Children and Adolescents[153] and include the latest data from NHANES conducted in 1999 and 2000. The guidelines include a revised classification of BP, a guide

to the evaluation of hypertension in children, rationale and recommendations for identification and treatment of target organ damage, and updated recommendations for lifestyle changes and antihypertensive drug therapy. To conform to JNC-VII, a new category, prehypertension, was created. Prehypertension is defined as an average BP between the 90th and 95th percentiles (previously defined as "high normal"). It was noticed in the BP tables, however, that at age 12 years

TABLE 20.15	Classification of Blood Pressure in Children and Adolescents
Blood Pressure Category	**Definition**
Normal	<90th percentile
Prehypertension	90th to 95th percentile OR 120/80 mm Hg
Hypertension	
Stage 1	95th to 99th percentile + 5 mm Hg
Stage 2	>99th percentile + 5 mm Hg

TABLE 20.16	95th Percentile of Blood Pressure by Selected Ages, by the 50th and 75th Height Percentiles, by Gender in Children and Adolescents			
	Girls' SBP/DBP		Boys' SBP/DBP	
Age	50th Percentile for Height	75th Percentile for Height	50th Percentile for Height	75th Percentile for Height
1	104/58	105/59	103/56	104/57
6	111/74	113/74	114/74	115/75
12	123/80	124/81	123/81	125/82
17	129/84	130/85	136/87	138/87

in boys and 13 years in girls, the 95th percentile goes above SBP 120 mm Hg, so adolescents with BP of 120/80 mm Hg or higher should be considered hypertensive. The report recommends that if the BP obtained in the office is above the 90th percentile, a repeat measurement should be taken during the same office visit. The term ''white-coat hypertension'' has been included for the first time, and is said to exist when an individual's BP is above the 95th percentile in the physician's office or clinic but is normotensive outside this setting. Ambulatory BP monitoring is required to make this diagnosis. Children who are normotensive should be encouraged with regard to physical activity, a healthy diet, and sleep. Weight management and diet counseling for the overweight and introduction of physical activity should be ''instituted or strongly encouraged'' in children who are prehypertensive and as initial therapy in those who are hypertensive. Pharmacotherapy may be appropriate for prehypertension if there are compelling indications such as renal disease, diabetes, or signs of LVH. For stage 1 hypertension, pharmacotherapy should be initiated on the basis of indications; for stage 2, unless there is a dramatic response to lifestyle changes, pharmacotherapy should be given. Therapy should always begin with a single drug.

Hypertension is a significant health issue in children, with approximately 1% to 3% of children and adolescents having hypertension. An analysis of data from NHANES III (1988–1994) and NHANES IV (1999–2000) showed that BP in children and adolescents in the United States rose between the time of the two surveys.[154] The rise in DBP was particularly significant (an average of 2.2 mm Hg), and SBP rose by an average of 1.4 mm Hg. A strong association between Body Mass Index and SBP identified among children suggests that this increase in BP is at least in part attributable to an increased prevalence of overweight. The potential benefits of early recognition of hypertension and other cardiovascular risk factors in children and adolescents, and hence introduction of early interventions that may reduce premature cardiovascular morbidity and mortality, are therefore paramount.[155]

Resistant Hypertension. Patients with BP that is not controlled (160/100 mm Hg or higher) by a three-drug regimen that includes a diuretic are considered resistant. Table 20.17

lists the common causes of resistant hypertension that should be assessed in refractory patients. If after appropriate assessment and evaluation, causes of resistant hypertension are ruled out, the patient should be assessed for secondary causes of the hypertension (Table 20.6).

Hypertensive Crises: Emergencies and Urgencies. A hypertensive emergency is a clinical presentation in which BP is severely elevated (>180/120) and must be lowered immediately to limit progressive or impending target organ damage, including hypertensive encephalopathy, intracranial hemorrhage, acute myocardial infarction, acute left ventricular failure with pulmonary edema, unstable angina pectoris, dissecting aortic aneurysm, papilledema on funduscopic examination, acute renal failure, or eclampsia.[1,156,157] Hypertensive urgencies are categorized as severe elevations in BP with the absence of end-organ damage. Appropriate pharmacotherapy options for hypertensive urgencies are listed in Table 20.18. Hypertensive crises may involve an abrupt increase in vascular resistance secondary to increased circulating vasoconstrictor substances, leading to

TABLE 20.17	Causes of Resistant Hypertension

Improper blood pressure measurement
Volume overload
   Excess sodium intake
   Volume retention from kidney disease
   Inadequate diuretic therapy dose
Drug-induced or other causes
   Nonadherence
   Inadequate medication doses
   Inappropriate medication combinations
   Specific medications (Table 20.19)
Associated conditions
   Obesity
   Excess alcohol intake
   White-coat hypertension
Identifiable causes of hypertension (Table 20.6)

TABLE 20.18	Pharmacotherapy for Hypertensive Emergencies and Urgencies

Hypertensive Emergencies

Drug	Dose	Onset of Action	Duration of Action	Adverse Effects	Special Indications
Vasodilators					
Nitroprusside	0.25–10 µg/kg/min as IV infusion	Immediate	1–2 min	Nausea, vomiting, muscle twitching, sweating, thiocyanate & cyanide toxicity	Most hypertensive emergencies; caution with high intracranial pressure or azotemia
Nicardipine	5–15 mg/h IV	5–10 min	15–30 min, up to 4 hours	Tachycardia, headache, flushing, local phlebitis	Most hypertensive emergencies except acute heart failure; caution with coronary ischemia
Fenoldopam	0.1–0.3 µg/kg/min as IV infusion	<5 min	30 min	Tachycardia, headache, nausea, flushing	Most hypertensive emergencies; caution with glaucoma
Nitroglycerin	5–100 µg/kg/min as IV infusion	2–5 min	5–10 min	Headache, vomiting, methemoglobinemia, tolerance with prolonged use	Coronary ischemia
Enalaprilat	1.25–5 mg q6h IV	15–30 min	6–12 hours	Precipitous fall in pressure in high-renin states; variable response	Acute left ventricular failure; avoid in acute myocardial infarction
Hydralazine	10–20 mg IV	10–20 min	1–4 hours IV	Tachycardia, flushing, headache, vomiting, aggravation of angina	Eclampsia
	10–40 mg IM	20–30 min	4–6 hours IM		
Adrenergic Inhibitors					
Labetalol	20–80 mg IV bolus q10min	5–10 min	3–6 hours	Vomiting, scalp tingling, bronchoconstriction, dizziness, nausea, heart block, orthostatic hypotension	Most hypertensive emergencies; avoid in acute heart failure
	0.5–20 mg/min IV infusion				
Esmolol	250–500 µg/kg/min IV bolus, then 50–100 µg/kg/min by infusion; may repeat bolus after 5 min or increase infusion to 300 µg/kg/min	1–2 min	10–30 min	Hypotension, nausea, asthma, first-degree heart block, heart failure	Aortic dissection, perioperative
Phentolamine	5–15 mg IV bolus	1–2 min	10–30 min	Tachycardia, flushing, headache	Catecholamine excess

Hypertensive Urgencies

Captopril	25 mg, repeat in 1–2 hours as needed	5–15 minutes	4–6 hours	Hypotension, acute renal failure, angioedema	
Clonidine	0.1–0.2 mg, repeat in 1–2 hours as needed (up to 0.6 mg)	5–15 minutes	6–12 hours	Hypotension, drowsiness, sedation, dry mouth	

IV, intravenous; IM, intramuscular.

TABLE 20.19	Common Substances Associated With Hypertension in Humans

Prescription Medications	**Street Drugs and "Natural" Products**
Cortisone and other steroids (both cortico- and mineralo-), adrenocorticotropic hormone (ACTH)	Cocaine and cocaine withdrawal
	Ma huang, ephedra, bittersweet, "herbal Ecstasy," other phenylpropanolamine analogues
Estrogens	Nicotine and withdrawal
Nonsteroidal anti-inflammatory drugs	Anabolic steroids
Cyclooxygenase 2 inhibitors	Narcotic withdrawal
Phenylpropanolamines and analogues	Methylphenidate
Cyclosporine and tacrolimus	Phencyclidine
Erythropoietin	Ketamine
Sibutramine	Ergotamine and other ergot-containing herbal preparations
Ketamine	St. John's wort
Desflurane	**Food Substances**
Carbamazepine	Sodium chloride
Bromocryptine	Ethanol
Metoclopramide	Licorice
Antidepressants (especially venlafaxine and duloxetine)	Tyramine-containing foods (with monoamine oxidase inhibitors)
Buspirone	**Chemical Elements/Industrial Chemicals**
Clonidine/β-blocker combination	Lead
Pheochromocytoma: β-blocker without α-blocker first; glucagons	Mercury
Clozapine	Thallium and other heavy metals
	Lithium salts

ischemia, which triggers the further release of vasoconstrictors.[1,156,157] Therapy should interrupt this cycle and decrease BP to lower levels while avoiding an abrupt decrease to normotensive or hypotensive BPs, which may cause ischemia or infarction. For a hypertensive emergency the target usually is to lower BP by no more than 25% and then, if stable, to 160/100 mm Hg within the next 2 to 6 hours. Excessive falls in BP may precipitate renal, cerebral, or coronary ischemia and must be avoided.[1,156,157] Patients with hypertensive emergencies should be admitted to an intensive care unit and treated with the most appropriate parenteral antihypertensive pharmacotherapy for the given clinical situation (Table 20.18).[1,156] Sublingual or buccal fast-acting nifedipine has caused significant adverse effects and should not be used.[1]

FUTURE THERAPIES

Research into therapies for hypertension continues to focus on the systems that modulate and affect the ultimate structure that dictates BP, the endothelial lining of the vasculature.

The vasopeptidase inhibitors, a class of medication that inhibits both ACE and neutral endopeptidase (NEP), have shown great promise in the treatment of hypertension. Inhibition of NEP increases levels of vasodilator peptides such as natriuretic peptide, adrenomedullin, and bradykinin.[158] Omapatrilat, in a trial of 25,000 patients, was significantly better than enalapril by 3.6 mmHg in lowering BP.[159] However, the risk of angioedema was significantly higher with omapatrilat (2.17%) versus the ACE inhibitor (0.68%), and was significantly higher in smokers and African Americans. This problem with angioedema was also seen in a trial comparing omapatrilat to enalapril in congestive heart failure.[160] It has been suggested that this class of medication may be especially effective in patients with salt-sensitive hypertension.[161] US Food and Drug Administration approval was not given to omapatrilat due to the aforementioned safety concerns. Ongoing clinical trials will help to determine the clinical utility of this therapeutic class, which also includes fasidotril, sampatrilat, and gemopatrilat.

Important in regulating the body's balance of salt and water, aldosterone may play a larger role in pharmacotherapy regimens for hypertension in the future (see the section on aldosterone receptor antagonists for a complete discussion). Other compounds under investigation in the treatment of hypertension include the endothelin receptor antagonists sitaxsentan, tezosentan, ambrisentan and the oral renin inhibitor aliskiren, as well as an angiotensin vaccine.

At least one trial of "primary prevention" of hypertension has been described.[162] The TROPHY trial is a 4-year investigation assessing the ability of candesartan to decrease the number of patients with prehypertension who go on to develop clinical hypertension requiring treatment. Preliminary results are expected in 2007.

IMPROVING OUTCOMES

The single most important factor in successful hypertension treatment is patient compliance. Untreated and uncontrolled hypertension remains an important problem.[11] Public awareness programs have identified the majority of people with hypertension, but the problems of patient dropout and noncompliance with treatment still result in fewer than 50% of hypertensive patients having controlled BP. Continuous effort is needed to prevent patient dropout, encourage lifestyle changes, and improve medication compliance.

What has been described as clinical inertia of providers must also be overcome to improve control rates of hypertension. The use of decision support systems[163] and patient-centered behavioral interventions[164] as well as actions by nurse clinicians and pharmacists[165] have been shown to improve control in hypertensive patients.

METHODS TO IMPROVE THERAPEUTIC ADHERENCE

Nonadherence is a complex problem, and prediction of medication adherence by clinicians is poor. Factors affecting medication adherence include demographic characteristics, medication side effects, the complexity of the medication regimen (including cost issues), quality of life, patients' knowledge, beliefs, and attitudes, depression, and health system issues.[166] Adherence problems in hypertensive patients are multifactorial, and therefore solving these issues requires multiple, patient-specific interventions. Two recent meta-analyses confirmed the need for an individualized approach to the patient with adherence problems with antihypertensive medications.[167,168] Techniques to help overcome medication nonadherence include:

■ Simplify the drug regimen to once-daily, if possible.
■ Tailor medication times to coincide with existing daily habits.
■ Avoid side effects by starting with low dosages and individually selected drugs.
■ Label prescriptions with clear, explicit directions, and indicate the purpose of the drug.

■ Encourage the use of prompting cues such as stickers or calendars to remind patients to take medications.
■ Provide written schedules or pillbox organizers for patients who are taking multiple drugs.
■ Discuss potential problems such as drug costs, confusion with other drugs, and previous problems with drug therapy.
■ Involve the patient by providing feedback of BP response or self-monitoring of BP.
■ Encourage or reward patients for keeping appointments, taking medications, and reducing BP.
■ Screen for noncompliance by monitoring attendance, patient self-reports, BP response, and changes in biochemical or physical parameters (e.g., pulse or serum potassium).
■ Provide close professional supervision, and establish a positive relationship with patients.

In addition to patient nonadherence, the issue of clinician nonadherence to practice guidelines must also be addressed. As the National Committee for Quality Assurance's (NCQA) performance standards [Health Plan Employer Data and Information Set (HEDIS)] continue to be incorporated into the American healthcare system, clinicians will be held accountable for patients not treated by national standard guidelines. NCQA has now started monitoring patient charts for the percentage of patients with BP of 140/90 mm Hg or less.[169] In fact, hypertension control rates have approached 60% when clinicians' practices were monitored using this criteria.[1]

PATIENT EDUCATION

Education about the consequences of untreated hypertension and the role of drug and nondrug treatments serves as a foundation for compliance. The patient must understand and believe that hypertension is a serious condition that needs treatment (Table 20.19). With the release of the JNC-VII guidelines,[1] the NHBPEP has prepared a significant amount of patient education materials that can be ordered from the National Heart, Lung and Blood Institute. Important education points for the hypertensive patient include the following:

■ Assess the patient's understanding and acceptance of the diagnosis of hypertension.
■ Discuss the patient's concerns and clarify misunderstandings.
■ Tell the patient what his or her BP reading is and write it down for him or her.
■ Come to an agreement with the patient on a goal BP.
■ Ask the patient to rate his or her chance of staying on treatment.
■ Inform the patient about the recommended treatment and provide specific written information about the role of lifestyle, including diet, physical activity, dietary supplements, and alcohol intake. Use standard brochures when available.

- Elicit concerns and questions and provide opportunities for the patient to state specific behaviors to carry out treatment recommendations.
- Emphasize (a) the need to continue treatment; (b) that control does not mean cure; and (c) that the patient cannot tell if his or her BP is elevated merely by feelings or symptoms; BP must be measured.

DISEASE MANAGEMENT STRATEGIES TO IMPROVE PATIENT OUTCOMES

Involvement by the pharmacist in the care of patients with hypertension has been shown to have a consistently positive impact in both community pharmacy[170–172] and organized healthcare settings.[173–176] In these trials, involvement by pharmacists has been shown to bring about improved compliance, improved BP control, improved patient understanding of hypertension, and improved satisfaction with care. The JNC-VII guidelines strongly recommend the use of a multidisciplinary approach to the hypertensive patient, with a pharmacist as an integral part of the team of care. Though these data show positive trends, critical evaluation has found problems with study design.[177] Despite the tremendous increase in knowledge about hypertension and the explosion of drug therapy options, there remains a large gap between the JNC guidelines and the way that professionals implement them and, more importantly, the consistent control of BP in patients. Hypertension remains a largely untapped area for pharmacist participation in collaborative drug therapy management to optimize control of BP in a vast patient population.

PHARMACOECONOMICS

When tailoring an antihypertensive regimen for a patient, important concerns include the cost and clinical efficacy of treatment, as well as the adverse effects, likelihood of compliance with therapy, and impact on the quality of life. The cost efficacy of a given therapy for hypertension has been described as the net costs (therapy costs minus decreased costs of cardiovascular morbidity) divided by the increase in years of life gained.[178] The treatment of hypertension has been described as one of the most cost-effective methods of cardiovascular risk reduction,[179] though its undertreatment brings with it greater costs still.[180] Recent studies have suggested that medication persistence rates are influenced by the class of medication chosen, though the results are conflicting.[181,182] Secondary to low control rates of hypertension, some have done pharmacoeconomic evaluations of the role of combination therapy in the initial treatment plan.[183] Because more than two thirds of hypertensive patients will require at least two agents, this assessment, which showed a benefit to starting low-dose combinations earlier in therapy, may be very important. Finally, because no conclusive recommendations can be drawn from existing cost-effectiveness data favoring one drug class over another, the choice

of antihypertensive agent should be individualized based on patient characteristics, concomitant diseases, and cost.

KEY POINTS

- Hypertension continues to be a significant national health problem
- In most patients, SBP should be the primary target for therapeutic interventions
- Pharmacotherapy regimens for hypertension must be individualized to each patient based on other risk factors for cardiovascular disease, the presence of compelling indications for specific drug classes, and issues that may affect adherence
- Most patients will require combination pharmacotherapy to control hypertension, and that regimen should contain a diuretic

SUGGESTED READING

American College of Cardiology (http://www.acc.org)
American Heart Association (http://www.americanheart.org)
American Society of Hypertension (http://www.ash-us.org)
Hypertension Network (http://www.bloodpressure.com)
National Guideline Clearinghouse (http://www.guidelines.gov)
National Heart, Lung, and Blood Institute (http://www.nhlbi.nih.gov/guidelines/hypertension/index.htm)

REFERENCES

1. The Seventh Report of the Joint National Committee on Prevention, Detection, Evaluation, and Treatment of High Blood Pressure (JNC-VII). Hypertension 42:1206–1252, 2003.
2. 2003 World Health Organization (WHO)/International Society of Hypertension (ISH) statement on management of hypertension. J Hypertens 21:1983–1992, 2003.
3. 2003 European Society of Hypertension–European Society of Cardiology guidelines for the management of arterial hypertension. J Hypertens 21:1011–1053, 2003.
4. Franklin SS, Gustin W, Wong ND, et al. Hemodynamic patterns of age-related changes in blood pressure. The Framingham Heart Study. Circulation 96:308–315, 1997.
5. Franklin SS, Larson MG, Khan SA, et al. Does the relation of blood pressure to coronary heart disease risk change with aging? The Framingham Heart Study. Circulation 103:1245–1249, 2001.
6. Franklin SS, Khan SA, Wong DA, et al. Is pulse pressure useful in predicting risk for coronary heart disease? The Framingham Heart Study. Circulation 100:354–360, 1999.
7. Working Group on Renovascular Hypertension. Detection, evaluation, and treatment of renovascular hypertension. Arch Intern Med 147:820–829, 1987.
8. Woods JW. Oral contraceptives and hypertension. Hypertension 11 (Suppl I):11–14, 1988.
9. Johnson AG, Nguyen TV, Day RO. Do nonsteroidal anti-inflammatory drugs affect blood pressure? A meta-analysis. Ann Intern Med 121:289–300, 1994.
10. Solomon DH, Schneeweiss S, Levin R, et al. Relationship between COX-2 specific inhibitors and hypertension. Hypertension 44:140–145, 2004.
11. Fields LE, Burt VL, Cutler JA, et al. The burden of adult hypertension in the United States 1999 to 2000: a rising tide. Hypertension 44:1–7, 2004.

12. Vasan RS, Beiser A, Seshadri S, et al. Residual lifetime risk for developing hypertension in middle-aged women and men: the Framingham Heart Study. JAMA 287:1003–1010, 2002.

13. Savoia C, Schiffrin EL. Significance of recently identified peptides in hypertension: endothelin, natriuretic peptides, adrenomedullin, leptin. Med Clin North Am 88:39–62, 2004.

14. Ferrannini E, Buzzigoli G, Bonadonna R, et al. Insulin resistance in essential hypertension. N Engl J Med 317:350–357, 1987.

15. Luft FC. Present status of genetic mechanisms in hypertension. Med Clin North Am 88:1–18, 2004.

16. Lewington S, Clarke R, Qizilbash N, et al. Age-specific relevance of usual blood pressure to vascular mortality: a meta-analysis of individual data for one million adults in 61 prospective studies. Prospective Studies Collaboration. Lancet 360:1903–1913, 2002.

17. Vasan RS, Larson MG, Leip EP, et al. Impact of high-normal blood pressure on the risk of cardiovascular risk of cardiovascular disease. N Engl J Med 345:1291–1297, 2001.

18. Anderson KM, Wilson PWF, Odell PM, et al. Ten-year risk for CHD by SBP and presence of other risk factors. Circulation 83:356–362, 1991.

19. Kannel WB, Neaton JD, Wentworth D, et al. Overall and coronary heart disease mortality rates in relation to major risk factors in 325,348 men screened for MRFIT. Am Heart J 112:825–836, 1986.

20. Perloff D, Grim C, Flack J, et al. Human blood pressure determination by sphygmomanometry. Circulation 88:2460–2470, 1993.

21. Pickering TG, and American Society of Hypertension Ad Hoc Panel. Recommendations for the use of home (self) and ambulatory blood pressure monitoring. Am J Hypertens 9:1–11, 1996.

22. Beddhu S, Allen-Brady K, Cheung AK, et al. Impact of renal failure on the risk of myocardial infarction and death. Kidney Int 62:1776–1783, 2002.

23. Jensen JS, Feldt-Rasmussen B, Strandgaard S, et al. Arterial hypertension, microalbuminuria, and risk of ischemic heart disease. Hypertension 35:898–903, 2000.

24. Gerstein HC, Mann JF, Yi Q, et al. Albuminuria and risk of cardiovascular events, death, and heart failure in diabetic and nondiabetic individuals. JAMA 286:421–426, 2001.

25. Levey AS, Bosch JP, Lewis JB, et al. A more accurate method to estimate glomerular filtration rate from serum creatinine: a new prediction equation. Modification of Diet in Renal Disease Study Group. Ann Intern Med 130:461–470, 1999.

26. Gillman MW, Kannel WB, Belanger A, et al. Influence of heart rate on mortality among persons with hypertension: the Framingham Study. Am Heart J 125:1148–1154, 1993.

27. Tsuji H, Venditti FJ, Manders ES, et al. Reduced heart rate variability and mortality risk in an elderly cohort. The Framingham Heart Study. Circulation 90:878–883, 1994.

28. Ridker PM, Rifai N, Rose L, et al. Comparison of C-reactive protein and low-density lipoprotein cholesterol levels in the prediction of first cardiovascular events. N Engl J Med 347:1557–1565, 2002.

29. Ridker PM, Hennekens CH, Burning JE, et al. C-reactive protein and other markers of inflammation in the prediction of cardiovascular disease in women. N Engl J Med 342:836–843, 2000.

30. Danesh J, Wheeler JG, Hirschfield GM, et al. C-reactive protein and other circulating markers of inflammation in the prediction of coronary heart disease. N Engl J Med 350:1387–1397, 2004.

31. Stampfer MJ, Malinow MR, Willett WC, et al. A prospective study of plasma homocysteine and risk of myocardial infarction in US physicians. JAMA 268:877–881, 1992.

32. Schotte D, Stunkard AJ. The effect of weight reduction on blood pressure in 301 obese patients. Arch Intern Med 150:1701–1704, 1990.

33. The Trials of Hypertension Prevention Collaborative Research Group. Effects of weight loss and sodium reduction intervention on blood pressure incidence in overweight people with high-normal blood pressure. The Trials of Hypertension Prevention, phase II. Arch Intern Med 157:657–667, 1997.

34. He J, Whelton PK, Appel LJ, et al. Long-term effects of weight loss and dietary sodium reduction on incidence of hypertension. Hypertension 35:544–549, 2000.

35. Sacks FM, Svetkey LP, Vollmer WM, et al. Effects on blood pressure of reduced sodium and the Dietary Approaches to Stop Hypertension (DASH) diet. DASH-Sodium Collaborative Research Group. N Engl J Med 344:3–10, 2001.

36. Whelton SP, Chin A, Xin X, et al. Effect of aerobic exercise on blood pressure: a meta-analysis of randomized, controlled trials. Ann Intern Med 136:493–503, 2002.

37. Gregg EW, Cauley JA, Stone K, et al. Relationship of changes in physical activity and mortality among older women. JAMA 289:2379–2386, 2003.

38. Xin X, He J, Frontini MG, et al. Effects of alcohol reduction on blood pressure: a meta-analysis of randomized, controlled trials. Hypertension 38:1112–1117, 2001.

39. Izzo JL, Levy D, Black HR. Clinical advisory statement: importance of systolic blood pressure in older Americans. Hypertension 35:1021–1024, 2000.

40. Cushman WC, Ford CE, Cutler JA, et al. Success and predictors of blood pressure control in diverse North American settings: the Antihypertensive and Lipid-Lowering Treatment to Prevent Heart Attack Trial (ALLHAT). J Clin Hypertens 4:393–404, 2002.

41. Hansson L, Zanchetti A, Carruthers SG, et al. Effects of intensive blood-pressure lowering and low-dose aspirin in patients with hypertension: principal results of the Hypertension Optimal Treatment (HOT) randomized trial. HOT Study Group. Lancet 351:1755–1762, 1998.

42. Black HR, Elliott WJ, Grandits G, et al. Principal results of the Controlled Onset Verapamil Investigation of Cardiovascular Endpoints (CONVINCE) trial. JAMA 289:2073–2082, 2003.

43. Dahlöf B, Devereux RB, Kjeldesen SE, et al. Cardiovascular morbidity and mortality in the Losartan Intervention for Endpoint Reduction in Hypertension study (LIFE): a randomized trial against atenolol. Lancet 359:995–1003, 2002.

44. Psaty BM, Lumley T, Furberg CD, et al. Health outcomes associated with various antihypertensive therapies used as first-line agents: a network meta-analysis. JAMA 289:2534–2544, 2003.

45. The ALLHAT Officers and Coordinators for the ALLHAT Collaborative Research Group. Major outcomes in high-risk hypertensive patients randomized to angiotensin-converting enzyme inhibitor or calcium channel blocker vs. diuretic: the Antihypertensive and Lipid-Lowering Treatment to Prevent Heart Attack Trial (ALLHAT). JAMA 288:2981–2997, 2002.

46. SHEP Cooperative Research Group. Prevention of stroke by antihypertensive drug treatment in older persons with isolated systolic hypertension: final results of the Systolic Hypertension in the Elderly Program (SHEP). JAMA 265:3255–3264, 1991.

47. The ALLHAT Officers and Coordinators for the ALLHAT Collaborative Research Group. Major cardiovascular events in hypertensive patients randomized to doxazosin vs. chlorthalidone. The Antihypertensive and Lipid-Lowering Treatment to Prevent Heart Attack Trial (ALLHAT). JAMA 283:1967–1975, 2000.

48. Hansson L, Lindholm LH, Niskanen L, et al. The Captopril Prevention Project (CAPPP) study group: effect of angiotensin-converting-enzyme inhibition compared with conventional morbidity and mortality in hypertension: the Captopril Prevention Project (CAPPP) randomised trial. Lancet 353:611–616, 1999.

49. Hansonn L, Lindholm LH, Ekbom T, et al. Randomised trial of old and new antihypertensive drugs in elderly patients: cardiovascular mortality and morbidity the Swedish Trial in Old Patients with Hypertension-2 (STOP-2) study. Lancet 354:1751–1756, 1999.

50. Wing LM, Reid CM, Ryan P, et al. A comparison of outcomes with angiotensin-converting-enzyme inhibitors and diuretics for hypertension in the elderly. N Engl J Med 348:583–592, 2003.

51. Carter BL, Ernst ME, Cohen JD. Hydrochlorothiazide versus chlorthalidone: evidence supporting their interchangeability. Hypertension 43:4–9, 2004.

52. Mortality after 10-1/2 years for hypertensive participants in the Multiple Risk Factor Intervention Trial. Circulation. 82:1616–1628, 1990.

53. Khosla N, Chua D, Elliott WJ, et al. Greater efficacy of chlorthalidone over hydrochlorothiazide for achieving blood pressure goals. Am J Hypertens 17:114A, 2004.

54. Psaty BM, Lumley T, Furberg CD. Meta-analysis of health outcomes of chlorthalidone-based vs nonchlorthalidone-based low-dose diuretic therapies. JAMA 292:43–44, 2004.

55. Licht JH, Haley RJ, Pugh B, et al. Diuretic regimens in essential hypertension: a comparison of hypokalemic effects, BP control, and cost. Arch Intern Med 143:1694–1699, 1983.

56. Siscovick DS, Raghunathan TE, Psaty BM, et al. Diuretic therapy and the risk of primary cardiac arrest. N Engl J Med 330: 1852–1857, 1994.

57. Franse LV, Pahor M, Di Bari M, et al. Hypokalemia associated with diuretic use and cardiovascular events in the Systolic Hypertension in the Elderly Program. Hypertension 35:1025–1030, 2000.

58. Moser M. Why are more physicians not prescribing diuretics more frequently in the management of hypertension? JAMA 279: 1813–1816, 1998.

59. Mogensen, CE, Viberti G, Halimi S, et al. Effect of low-dose perindopril/indapamide on albuminuria in diabetes: preterax in albuminuria regression (PREMIER). Hypertension 41:1063–1071, 2003.

60. Marre M, Puig JG, Kokot F, et al. Equivalence of indapamide SR and enalapril on microalbuminuria reduction in hypertensive patients with type 2 diabetes: the NESTOR study. J Hypertens 22: 1613–1622, 2004.

61. PROGRESS Collaborative Group. Randomized trial of a perindopril-based blood-pressure regimen among 6,105 individuals with previous stroke or transient ischaemic attack. Lancet 358: 1033–1041, 2001.

62. Brater DC. Diuretic Therapy. N Engl J Med 339:387–395, 1998.

63. Tamargo JL, Delpón E. Optimisation of β-blockers pharmacology. J Cardiovasc Pharmacol 16 (Suppl 5):S8–S10, 1990.

64. Staessen JA, Wang JG, Thijs L. Cardiovascular prevention and blood pressure reduction: a quantitative overview updated until March 2003. J Hypertens 21:1055–1076, 2003.

65. Blood Pressure Lowering Treatment Trialists' Collaboration. Effects of different blood-pressure lowering regimens on major cardiovascular events: results of prospectively-designed overviews of randomized trials. Lancet 362:1527–1535, 2003.

66. Self TH, Soberman JE, Bubla JM, et al. Cardioselective beta-blockers in patients with asthma and concomitant heart failure or history of myocardial infarction: when do benefits outweigh risks? J Asthma 40:839–845, 2003.

67. Salpeter SR, Ormiston TM, Salpeter EE. Cardioselective β-blockers in patients with reactive airway disease: a meta-analysis. Ann Intern Med 137:715–725, 2002.

68. Dahlof B, Lindholm LH, Hansson L, et al. Morbidity and mortality in the Swedish Trial in Old Patients with Hypertension (STOP-Hypertension). Lancet 338:1281–1285, 1991.

69. Psaty BM, Smith NL, Siscovick DS, et al. Health outcomes associated with antihypertensive therapies used as first-line agents: a systematic review and meta-analysis. JAMA 277:739–745, 1997.

70. Olsson G, Tuomilehto J, Berglund G, et al. Primary prevention of sudden cardiovascular death in hypertensive patients. Mortality results from the MAPHY study. Am J Hypertens 4:151–158, 1991.

71. Medical Research Council Working Party. MRC trial of treatment of mild hypertension: principal results. Br Med J 291:97–104, 1985.

72. Blood Pressure Lowering Treatment Trialists' Collaboration. Effects of ACE inhibitors, calcium antagonists, and other blood pressure lowering drugs: results of prospectively designed overviews of randomized trials. Lancet 355:1955–1964, 2000.

73. UKPDS 39. Efficacy of atenolol and captopril in reducing risk of macrovascular and microvascular complications in type 2 diabetes: UKPDS 39. UK Prospective Diabetes Study Group. Br Med J 317: 713–720, 1998.

74. Wright JT Jr, Bakris G, Greene, et al. Effect of blood pressure lowering and antihypertensive drug class on progression of kidney disease: results from the AASK trial. JAMA 288:2421–2431, 2002.

75. β-blocker Heart Attack Trial Research Group. A randomized trial of propranolol in patients with acute myocardial infarction. I: Mortality results. JAMA 247:1707–1714, 1982.

76. The Capricorn Investigators. Effect of carvedilol on outcome after myocardial infarction in patients with left-ventricular dysfunction: the CAPRICORN randomized trial. Lancet 357:1385–1390, 2001.

77. MERIT-HF Study Group. Effect of metoprolol CR/XL in chronic heart failure: metoprolol CR/XL randomized intervention trial in congestive heart failure. Lancet 353:2001–2007, 1999.

78. Packer M, Bristow MR, Cohn JN, et al, for the US Carvedilol Heart Failure Study Group. The effect of carvedilol on morbidity and mortality in patients with chronic heart failure. N Engl J Med 334:1349–1355, 1996.

79. CIBIS Investigators and Committees. A randomized trial of beta-blockade in heart failure. The Cardiac Insufficiency Bisoprolol Study. Circulation 90:1765–1773, 1994.

80. Radack K, Deck C. β-adrenergic blocker therapy does not worsen intermittent claudication in subjects with peripheral arterial disease: a meta-analysis of randomized controlled trials. Arch Intern Med 151:1769–1776, 1991.

81. Bright RA, Everitt DE. β-blockers and depression: evidence against an association. JAMA 267:1783–1787, 1992.

82. Psaty BM, Koepsell TD, Wagner EH, et al. The relative risk of incident coronary heart disease associated with recently stopping the use of β-blockers. JAMA 263:1653–1657, 1990.

83. Williams GH. Converting-enzyme inhibitors in the treatment of hypertension. N Engl J Med 319:1517–1525, 1998.

84. Heart Outcomes Prevention Evaluation Study Investigators. Effects of an angiotensin-converting enzyme inhibitor, ramipril, on cardiovascular events in high-risk patients. N Engl J Med 342:145–153, 2000.

85. Julius S, Kjeldsen SE, Weber M, for the VALUE trial group. Outcomes in hypertensive patients at high cardiovascular risk treated with regimens based on valsartan or amlodipine: the VALUE randomized trial. Lancet 363:2022–2031, 2004.

86. Estacio R, Jeffers B, Hiatt W, et al. The effect of nisoldipine as compared with enalapril on outcomes in patients with non-insulin-dependent diabetes and hypertension. N Engl J Med 338:645–652, 1998.

87. The European Trial on Reduction of Cardiac Events with Perindopril in Stable Coronary Artery Disease Investigators. Efficacy of perindopril in reduction of cardiovascular events among patients with stable coronary artery disease; randomised, double-blind, placebo-controlled, multicentre trial (the EUROPA study). Lancet 362:782–788, 2003.

88. Wang JG, Staessen JA. Benefits of antihypertensive pharmacologic therapy and blood pressure reduction in outcome trials. J Clin Hypertens 5:66–75, 2003.

89. Whelton PK, He J, Appel LJ, et al. Primary prevention of hypertension: clinical and public health advisory from the National High Blood Pressure Education Program. JAMA 288:1882–1888, 2002.

90. Mimran A, Ribstein J. Angiotensin receptor blockers: pharmacology and clinical significance. J Am Soc Nephrol 10:273–277, 1999.

91. Lindholm LH, Ibsen H, Dahlöf B, et al. Cardiovascular morbidity and mortality in patients with diabetes in the Losartan Intervention for Endpoint Reduction in Hypertension study (LIFE): a randomised trial against atenolol. Lancet 359:1004–1010, 2002.

92. Brenner BM, Cooper ME, de Zeeuw D, et al. Effects of losartan on renal and cardiovascular outcomes in patients with type 2 diabetes and nephropathy. N Engl J Med 345:861–869, 2001.

93. Lewis EJ, Hunsicker LG, Clarke WR, et al. Renoprotective effect of the angiotensin receptor antagonist irbesartan in patients with nephropathy due to type 2 diabetes. N Engl J Med 345:851–860, 2001.

94. Irons BK, Kumar A. Valsartan-induced angioedema. Ann Pharmacother 37:1024–1027, 2003.

95. Warner KK, Visconti JA, Tschampel MM. Angiotensin II receptor blockers in patients with ACE inhibitor-induced angioedema. Ann Pharmacother 34:526–528, 2000.

96. Cha YJ, Pearson VE. Angioedema due to losartan. Ann Pharmacother 33:936–938, 1999.

97. Tatti P, Pahor M, Byington, et al. Outcome results of the Fosinopril versus Amlodipine Cardiovascular Events Randomized Trial (FACET) in patients with hypertension and NIDDM. Diabetes Care 21:597–603, 1998.

98. Staessen JA, Fagard R, Thijs L, et al. Randomized double-blind comparison of placebo and active treatment for older patients with isolated systolic hypertension: the Systolic Hypertension in Europe (Syst-Eur) trial. Lancet 350:757–764, 1997.

99. Tuomilehto J, Rastenyte D, Birkenhager WH, et al. Effects of effective calcium-channel blockade in older patients with diabetes and systolic hypertension. N Engl J Med 340:677–684, 1999.

100. Brown MJ, Palmer CR, Castaigne A, et al. Morbidity and mortality in patients randomized to double-blind treatment with a long-acting calcium-channel blocker or diuretic in the International Nifedipine

GITS study: Intervention as a Goal in Hypertension Treatment (IN-SIGHT). Lancet 356:366–372, 2000.

101. Grossman E, Messerli FH. Effect of calcium antagonists on plasma norepinephrine levels, heart rate and blood pressure. Am J Cardiol 80: 1453–58, 1997.

102. Lefrandt JD, Heitmann J, Sevre K, et al. The effects of dihydropyridine and phenylalkylamine calcium channel antagonist classes on autonomic function in hypertension: the VAMPHYRE study. Am J Hypertens 14:1083–1089, 2001.

103. Hansson L, Hedner T, Lund-Johansen P, et al, for the NORDIL Study Group. Randomised trial of effects of calcium antagonists compared with diuretics and beta-blockers on cardiovascular morbidity and mortality in hypertension: the Nordic Diltiazem (NOR-DIL) study. Lancet 356:359–365, 2000.

104. Pepine CJ, Hendberg EM, Cooper-DeHoff RM, for the INVEST Investigators. A calcium antagonist vs. a non-calcium antagonist hypertension treatment strategy for patients with coronary artery disease. The International Verapamil-Trandolapril Study (INVEST): a randomized controlled trial. JAMA 290:2805–2816, 2003.

105. Stier CT, Chandler PN, Rocha R, et al. Nonepithelial effects of aldosterone. Curr Opin Endocrinol Diabetes 5:211–216, 1998.

106. Gehr TWB, Sica DA, Frishman WH. Diuretic therapy in cardiovascular disease. In: Frishman WH, Sonnenblick EH, Sica D, eds: Cardiovascular pharmacotherapeutics, 2nd ed. New York: McGraw-Hill, 2003:157–176.

107. Lim PO, Rodgers P, Cardale K, et al. Potentially high prevalence of primary aldosteronism in a primary care population [letter]. Lancet 353:40, 1999.

108. Pitt B, Zannid F, Remme WJ, et al. The effect of spironolactone on morbidity and mortality in patients with severe heart failure. N Engl J Med 341:709–717, 1999

109. Juurlink DN, Mamdani MM, Lee DS, et al. Rates of hyperkalemia after publication of the Randomized Aldactone Evaluation Study. N Engl J Med 351:543–551, 2004.

110. Krum H, Nolly H, Workman D, et al. Efficacy of eplerenone added to renin-angiotensin blockade in hypertensive patients. Hypertension 40:117–123, 2002.

111. Weinberger MH, Roniker B, Krause SL, et al. Eplerenone, a selective aldosterone blocker, in mild-to-moderate hypertension. Am J Hypertension 15:709–716, 2002.

112. Flack JM, Oparil S, Pratt JH, et al. Efficacy and tolerability of eplerenone and losartan in hypertensive black and white patients J Am Coll Cardiol 41:1148–1155, 2003.

113. Williams GH, Burgess E, Kolloch RE, et al. Efficacy of eplerenone versus enalapril as monotherapy in systemic hypertension. Am J Cardiol 93:990–996, 2004.

114. White WB, Duprez D, St Hillaire R, et al. Effects of the selective aldosterone blocker eplerenone versus the calcium antagonist amlodipine in systolic hypertension. Hypertension 41:1021–1026, 2003.

115. Pitt B, Remme W, Zannad F, et al. For the Eplerenone Post–Acute Myocardial Infarction Heart Failure Efficacy and Survival Study Investigators. Eplerenone, a selective aldosterone blocker, in patients with left ventricular dysfunction after myocardial infarction. N Engl J Med 348:1309–1321, 2003.

116. Weber MA. Clinical pharmacology of centrally acting antihypertensive agents. J Clin Pharmacol 29:598–602, 1989.

117. Langley MS, Heel RC. Transdermal clonidine: a preliminary review of its pharmacodynamic properties and therapeutic efficacy. Drugs 35:123–142, 1988.

118. Mehta JL, Lopez LM. Rebound hypertension following abrupt cessation of clonidine and metoprolol: treatment with labetalol. Arch Intern Med 147:389–390, 1987.

119. Vaughan CJ, Delanty N. Hypertensive emergencies. Lancet 356:411–417, 2000.

120. Pettinger WA, Mitchell HC. Side effects of vasodilator therapy. Hypertension 11 (Suppl II):II34–36, 1988.

121. Haffner SM, Lehto S, Ronnemaa T, et al. Mortality from coronary heart disease in subject with type 2 diabetes and in nondiabetic subjects with and without prior myocardial infarction. N Engl J Med 339:229–234, 1998.

122. Davis M, Millns H, Stratton IM, et al. Risk factors for stroke in type 2 diabetes mellitus: United Kingdom Prospective Diabetes Study (UKPDS) 29. Arch Intern Med 159:1097–1103, 1999.

123. Gress TW, Nieto FJ, Shahar E, et al. Hypertension and antihypertensive therapy as risk factors for type 2 diabetes mellitus. Atherosclerosis Risk in Communities Study. N Engl J Med 342:905–912, 2000.

124. Fagan TC, Sowers J. Type 2 diabetes mellitus: greater cardiovascular risks and greater benefits of therapy. Arch Intern Med 159: 1033–1034, 1999.

125. UKPDS 38. Tight blood pressure control and risk of macrovascular and microvascular complications in type 2 diabetes: UKPDS 38. UK Prospective Diabetes Study Group. Br Med J 317:703–713, 1998.

126. American Diabetes Association. Nephropathy in diabetes. Diabetes Care 27: S79–83, 2004.

127. Maki DD, Ma JZ, Louis TA, et al. Long-term effects of antihypertensive agents on proteinuria and renal function. Arch Intern Med 155:1073–1080, 1995.

128. Hillege HL, Fidler V, Diercks GF, et al. Urinary albumin excretion predicts cardiovascular and noncardiovascular mortality in general population. Circulation 106:1777–1782, 2002.

129. Franklin SS, Jacobs MJ, Wong ND, et al. Predominance of isolated systolic hypertension among middle-aged and elderly US hypertensives: analysis based on National Health and Nutrition Examination Survey (NHANES) III. Hypertension 37:869–874, 2001.

130. Jafar TH, Stark PC, Schmid CH, et al. Progression of chronic kidney disease: the role of blood pressure control, proteinuria, and angiotensin-converting enzyme inhibition: a patient-level meta-analysis. Ann Intern Med 139:244–252, 2003.

131. National Kidney Foundation Guideline. K/DOQI clinical practice guidelines for chronic kidney disease: evaluation, classification, and stratification. Kidney Disease Outcome Quality Initiative. Am J Kidney Dis 39:S1–S266, 2002.

132. Levy D, Garrison RJ, Savage DD, et al. Prognostic implications of echocardiographically determine left ventricular mass in the Framingham Heart Study. N Engl J Med 322:161–165, 1990.

133. Schmieder RE, Schlaich MP, Klingbeil AU, et al. Update on reversal of left ventricular hypertrophy in essential hypertension (a meta-analysis of all randomized double-blind studies until December 1996). Nephrol Dial Transplant 13:564–569, 1998.

134. Liebson PR, Grandits GA, Dianzmba S, et al. Comparison of five antihypertensive monotherapies and placebo for change in left ventricular mass in patients receiving nutritional-hygenic therapy in the Treatment of Mild Hypertension Study (TOMHS). Circulation 91: 698–706,1995.

135. Gotdiener JS, Reda DJ, Massie BM, et al. Effect of single-drug therapy on reduction of left ventricular mass in mild to moderate hypertension: comparison of six antihypertensive agents. The Department of Veterans Affairs Cooperative Study Group on Antihypertensive Agents. Circulation 95:2007–2014, 1997.

136. Levy D, Kenchaiah S, Larson MG, et al. Long-term trends in the incidence of and survival in heart failure. N Engl J Med 247:1397–1402, 2002.

137. Cooper R, Rotimi C. Hypertension in blacks. Am J Hypertens 10: 804–812, 1997.

138. Crespro CJ, Loria CM, Burt VL. Hypertension and other cardiovascular disease risk factors among Mexican Americans, Cuban Americans, and Puerto Ricans from the Hispanic Health and Nutrition Examination Survey. Public Health Rep 111:7–10, 1996.

139. Douglas JG, Bakris GL, Epstein M, et al. Management of high blood pressure in African Americans: consensus statement from the Hypertension in African Americans Working Group of the International Society on Hypertension in Blacks. Arch Intern Med 163: 525–541, 2003.

140. Jamerson K, DeQuattro V. The impact of ethnicity on response to antihypertensive therapy. Am J Med 101:22S–32S, 1996.

141. Saunders E Weir MR, Kong BW, et al. A comparison of the efficacy and safety of a beta-blocker, a calcium channel blocker, and a converting enzyme inhibitor in hypertensive blacks. Arch Intern Med 150:1707–1713, 1990.

142. Cushman WC, Reda DJ, Perry HM, et al. Regional and racial differences in response to antihypertensive medication use in a randomized controlled trial of men with hypertension in the United States. Department of Veterans Affairs Cooperative Study Group on Antihypertensive Agents. Arch Intern Med 160:825–831, 2000.

143. Wright JT, Agodoa L, Contreras G, et al. Successful blood pressure control in African Americans Study of Kidney Disease and Hypertension. Arch Intern Med 162:1636–1643, 2002.
144. Burt VL, Cutler JA, Higgins M, et al. Trends in the prevalence, awareness, treatment, and control of hypertension in the adult US population: data from the health examination surveys, 1960 to 1991. Hypertension 26:60–69, 1995.
145. Gueyffier F, Bulpitt C, Boissel JP, et al. Antihypertensive drugs in very old people: a subgroup meta-analysis of randomized controlled trials. INDIANA Group. Lancet 353:793–796, 1999.
146. Somes GW, Pahor M, Shorr RI, et al. The role of diastolic blood pressure when treating isolated systolic hypertension. Arch Intern Med 159:2004–2009, 1999.
147. Staessen JA, Gasowski J, Wang JG, et al. Risks of untreated and treated isolated systolic hypertension in the elderly: meta-analysis of outcome trials. Lancet 355:85–872, 2000.
148. Appel LJ, Espeland MA, Easter L, et al. Effects of reduced sodium intake on hypertension control in older individuals: results from the Trial of Nonpharmacologic Interventions in the Elderly (TONE). Arch Intern Med 161:85–93, 2001.
149. National High Blood Pressure Education Program. Report of the National High Blood Pressure Education Program Working Group on High Blood Pressure in Pregnancy. Am J Obstet Gynecol 183:S1–S22, 2000.
150. von Dadelszen P, Ornstein MP, Bull SB, et al. Fall in mean arterial pressure and fetal growth restriction in pregnancy hypertension: a meta-analysis. Lancet 355:87–92, 2000.
151. ACOG Practice Bulletin. Chronic hypertension in pregnancy. ACOG Committee on Practice Bulletins. Obstet Gynecol 98:177–185, 2001.
152. Sibai BM. Treatment of hypertension in pregnant women. N Engl J Med 335:257–265, 1996.
153. National High Blood Pressure Education Program Working Group on High Blood Pressure in Children and Adolescents. The fourth report on the diagnosis, evaluation, and treatment of high blood pressure in children and adolescents. Pediatrics 114 (Suppl):555–576, 2004.
154. Hunter P, He J, Cutler JA, et al. Trends in blood pressure among children and adolescents. JAMA 291:2107–2113, 2004.
155. Ingelfinger JR. Pediatric antecedents of adult cardiovascular disease: awareness and intervention. N Engl J Med 350:2123–2126, 2004.
156. Cherney D, Straus S. Management of patients with hypertensive urgencies and emergencies. J Gen Intern Med 17:937–945, 2002.
157. Vaughan CJ, Delanty N. Hypertensive emergencies. Lancet 356:411–417, 2000.
158. Weber M. Vasopeptidase inhibitors. Lancet 358:1525–1532, 2001.
159. Kostis JB, Packer M, Black HR, et al. Omapatrilat and enalapril in patients with hypertension: the Omapatrialat Cardiovascular Treatment vs. Enalapril (OCTAVE) Trial. Am J Hypertens 17:103–111, 2004.
160. Packer M, Califf RM, Konstam MA, et al. Comparison of omapatrilat and enalapril in patients with chronic heart failure: the Omapatrilat versus Enalapril Randomized Trial of Utility in Reducing Events (OVERTURE). Circulation 106:920–926, 2002.
161. Ferrario CM, Smith RD, Brosnihen B, et al. Effects of omapatrilat on the renin-angiotensin system in salt-sensitive hypertension. Am J Hypertens 15:557–564, 2002.
162. Julius S, Nesbitt S, Egan B, et al for the TROPHY study group. Trial of preventing hypertension: design and 2-year progress report. Hypertension 44:146–151, 2004.
163. Balas EA, Weingarten S, Garb CT, et al. Improving preventive care by prompting physicians. Arch Intern Med 160:301–308, 2000.
164. Boulware LE, Daumit GL, Frick KD, et al. An evidence-based review of patient-centered behavioral interventions for hypertension. Am J Prev Med 21:221–232, 2001.
165. Hill MN, Miller NH. Compliance enhancement: a call for multidisciplinary team approaches. Circulation 93:4–6, 1996.
166. Neutel JM, Smith DHG. Improving patient compliance: a major goal in the management of hypertension. J Clin Hypertens 5:127–132, 2003.
167. Takiya LN, Peterson AM, Finley RS. Meta-analysis of interventions for medication adherence to antihypertensives. Ann Pharmacother 38:1617–1624, 2004.
168. Schroeder K, Fahey T, Ebrahim S. How can we improve adherence to blood pressure-lowering medication in ambulatory care? Systematic review of randomized controlled trials. Arch Intern Med 164:722–732, 2004.
169. Shih SC, Bost JE, Pawlson JG. Standardized health plan reporting in four areas of preventive health care. Am J Prev Med 24:293–300, 2003.
170. Carter BL, Billich AJ, Elliott WJ. How pharmacists can assist physicians with controlling blood pressure. J Clin Hypertens 5:31–37, 2003.
171. Carter BL, Barnett DJ, Chrischilles E, et al. Evaluation of hypertension patients after care provided by community pharmacists in a rural setting. Pharmacotherapy 17:1274–1285, 1997.
172. McKenney JM, Slining JM, Henderson HR, et al. The effect of clinical pharmacy services on patients with essential hypertension. Circulation 48:1104–1111, 1973.
173. Erickson SR, Slaughter R, Halapy H. Pharmacists' ability to influence outcomes of hypertension therapy. Pharmacotherapy 17:140–147, 1997.
174. Vivian EM. Improving blood pressure control in a pharmacist-managed hypertension clinic. Pharmacotherapy 22:1533–1540, 2002.
175. Borenstein JE, Graber G, Saltiel E, et al. Physician-pharmacist co-management of hypertension: a randomized, comparative trial. Pharmacotherapy 23:209–216, 2003.
176. Mehos BM, Saseen JJ, MacLaughlin EJ. Effect of pharmacist intervention and initiation of home blood pressure monitoring in patients with uncontrolled hypertension. Pharmacotherapy 20:1384–1389, 2000.
177. Kennie NR, Schuster BG, Einarson TR. Critical analysis of the pharmaceutical care research literature. Ann Pharmacother 32:17–26, 1998.
178. Johannesson M. The cost effectiveness of hypertension treatment in Sweden. Pharmacoeconomics 7:242–250, 1995.
179. Pardell H, Tressarras R, Armario P, et al. Pharmacoeconomic considerations in the management of hypertension. Drugs 59 (Suppl 2):13–20, 2000.
180. Esposti LD, Valpiani G. Pharmacoeconomic burden of undertreating hypertension. Pharmacoeconomics 22:907–928, 2004.
181. Marenette MA, Gerth WC, Billings DK, et al. Antihypertensive persistence and drug class. Can J Cardiol 18:649–656, 2002.
182. Conlin PR, Gerth WC, Fox J, et al. Four-year persistence patterns among patients initiating therapy with angiotensin II receptor antagonist losartan versus other antihypertensive drug classes. Clin Ther 23:1999–2010, 2001.
183. Ambrosioni E. Pharmacoeconomics of hypertension management: the place of combination therapy. Pharmacoeconomics 19:337–347, 2001.

Heart Failure

21

Wendy Gattis Stough, Paul E. Nolan Jr., and Dawn G. Zarembski

Although there is no precise definition of heart failure (HF), HF can be defined as a progressive, complex clinical syndrome characterized by dyspnea, fatigue, and fluid retention.[1,2] Patients move from asymptomatic left ventricular dysfunction to symptomatic heart failure. Over the course of the syndrome, patients will not always have symptoms of congestion. Therefore, the term ''congestive heart failure'' is beginning to fall out of favor; rather, ''chronic heart failure'' is being used to describe this population. Thus, for the remainder of this chapter, the abbreviation CHF will refer to ''chronic heart failure.'' These symptoms may arise from any cardiac disorder that causes left ventricular (LV) dysfunction and diminished cardiac output (CO). These disorders activate a number of cardiac and peripheral neurohormonal compensatory adaptive responses, which with continued stimulation become maladaptive and ultimately affect fluid retention, disease progression, and mortality. However, a subgroup of patients with LV dysfunction are asymptomatic.[2] This subgroup is considered to have HF but without symptoms. The primary cardiac mechanisms that underlie the clinical syndrome of CHF and asymptomatic HF are systolic (i.e., contracting) and diastolic (i.e., filling) dysfunction, usually in combination.

TREATMENT GOALS

- Relieve symptoms of central and peripheral circulatory congestion
- Improve quality of life
- Reduce neurohormonal activation
- Prevent CHF
- Minimize or prevent acute CHF exacerbations
- Slow progression of CHF
- Increase survival
- New therapies should neither worsen symptoms nor shorten life.

OVERVIEW

EPIDEMIOLOGY

ETIOLOGY

Some disparity exists in the reported frequencies of hypertension (HTN) and coronary artery disease (CAD) as causes of CHF. The Framingham Study, a community-based, longitudinal cohort investigation, reported an antecedent diagnosis of HTN, either alone or in conjunction with other causes, in 74% of the patients diagnosed with CHF.[3] In contrast, a summary of 13 multicenter CHF drug trials published over the past 10 years and involving more than 20,000 patients listed CAD as the primary cause for CHF in almost 70% of the patients.[4] One possible explanation for the discrepant findings is that in the Framingham Study, diastolic dysfunction was not distinguished from systolic dysfunction, whereas in the summary of the drug trials, CHF was caused principally by systolic dysfunction. Nonetheless, in the Framingham Study a majority of patients (54%) had CAD as an attributable cause of CHF, and CAD was found with accompanying HTN 31% of the time.[3] Two recent registries in patients hospitalized for HF report similar findings. In OPTIMIZE, 71% of the 48,681 patients enrolled had hypertension, 50% had CAD, and 46% were coded as having an ischemic etiology for heart failure.[5] In ADHERE, 73% of the 105,388 enrolled patients had hypertension, and 57% had CAD.[6] Additional causes of CHF include idiopathic dilated cardiomyopathy, valvular heart disease, viruses, genetic abnormalities that promote familial hypertrophic or dilated cardiomyopathies, congenital heart disease, anemia, thyrotoxicosis, and atrial fibrillation. Any of these causes ultimately can engender decreases in the contractile performance of the heart (i.e., systolic dysfunction) or the ability of the heart to fill adequately during diastole (i.e., diastolic dysfunction; Table 21.1).

DRUG-INDUCED DISEASE

Drugs are an uncommon cause of CHF (see Table 21.1).[7] Antineoplastic agents such as the anthracycline antineoplastic agents daunorubicin and doxorubicin are well-described causes of CHF. Other antineoplastic agents, some immunomodulating drugs, ethanol, and cocaine also may produce CHF. Thiazelinediones have also been associated with HF. These drugs appear to be associated with edema, weight gain, and volume expansion. It has not yet been determined whether they worsen symptoms in patients with existing HF or if they could be a cause of HF.[8]

PREVALENCE

Largely because of an aging population and the enhanced survival after acute myocardial infarction, CHF is becoming an increasingly prevalent healthcare problem, with notable socioeconomic consequences.[9] The 2002 prevalence was es-

TABLE 21.1	Causes of Heart Failure

A. Systolic dysfunction

  1. Echocardiographic and hemodynamic characteristics: ↓ LVEF, ↑ LVEDV, ↑ LVEDP

  2. Hypertension

  3. Coronary artery disease

  4. Idiopathic

  5. Valvular disease (e.g., mitral or aortic regurgitation)

  6. Viral

  7. Genetic abnormalities

  8. Drug-induced

    a. Anticancer drugs

      i. Anthracyclines

      ii. Cyclophosphamide

      iii. ?Paclitaxel

      iv. Mitoxantrone

      v. 5-Fluorouracil

      vi. ?Herceptin

    b. Ethanol

    c. Immunomodulating drugs

      i. Interferon-α

      ii. ?Interferons-β and -γ

      iii. Interleukin-2

    d. Cocaine

B. Diastolic dysfunction

  1. Echocardiographic and hemodynamic characteristics: normal or ↑ LVEF, ↑ LVEDP, normal or ↓ LVEDV

  2. Hypertension

  3. Advanced age

  4. Coronary artery disease

  5. Restrictive cardiomyopathies (e.g., amyloidosis)

  6. Valvular heart disease (e.g., aortic stenosis)

  7. Hypertrophic cardiomyopathy (e.g., idiopathic hypertrophic subaortic stenosis)

  8. Genetic abnormalities

LVEF, left ventricular ejection fraction; LVEDV, left ventricular end-diastolic volume; LVEDP, left ventricular end-diastolic pressure.

timated at 4.9 million Americans, with nearly equal numbers of men and women.[10] For Caucasian, African American, and Mexican American men and women age 20 and older, the percentages of people with CHF are 2.5%, 3.1%, and 2.7% (men) and 1.9%, 2.5%, and 1.6% (women), respectively.[10] The prevalence of CHF increases considerably with age. For the age ranges of 45 to 54 years, 55 to 64 years, 65 to 74 years, and 75 years and older, CHF is present in less than 2%, almost 5%, roughly 7%, and nearly 10%, respectively.[10] There are about 500,000 new cases of CHF per year.[10] The incidence of CHF, which also increases markedly with age, approaches 10 per 1,000 population after age 65 years.[10] Patients with CHF accounted for 970,000 hospital discharges in 2002, an increase of 157% since 1979.[10] For people 65 years and older, CHF is the most common cause of hospitalization.[10]

PATHOPHYSIOLOGY

Several generalized pathophysiologic conditions can lead to HF. These include pressure overload of the heart (e.g., HTN or aortic stenosis), volume overload (e.g., mitral or aortic valve regurgitation), loss of functional myocardial tissue (e.g., acute myocardial infarction), a generalized decrease

in myocardial contractility (e.g., several types of dilated cardiomyopathies), and restricted filling (e.g., constrictive pericarditis or amyloidosis). Clinically, these conditions manifest as a reduction in systolic emptying (i.e., systolic dysfunction) or diastolic relaxation and filling (i.e., diastolic dysfunction). Either systolic or diastolic dysfunction can lead to a decrease in stroke volume and CO. The decrease in CO is sensed as a decrease in end-organ perfusion pressure principally by arterial baroreceptors.

In response to decreased CO, a number of compensatory (i.e., adaptive) responses, many of which are neurohormonally mediated, become activated (Fig. 21.1). Within the heart, ventricular dilation and hypertrophy (i.e., ventricular remodeling) occur. Ventricular dilation develops in response to an elevated end-diastolic pressure, a consequence of either systolic or diastolic dysfunction. An elevated end-diastolic pressure produces mechanical stretch, which stimulates myocyte lengthening through replication of sarcomeres in series

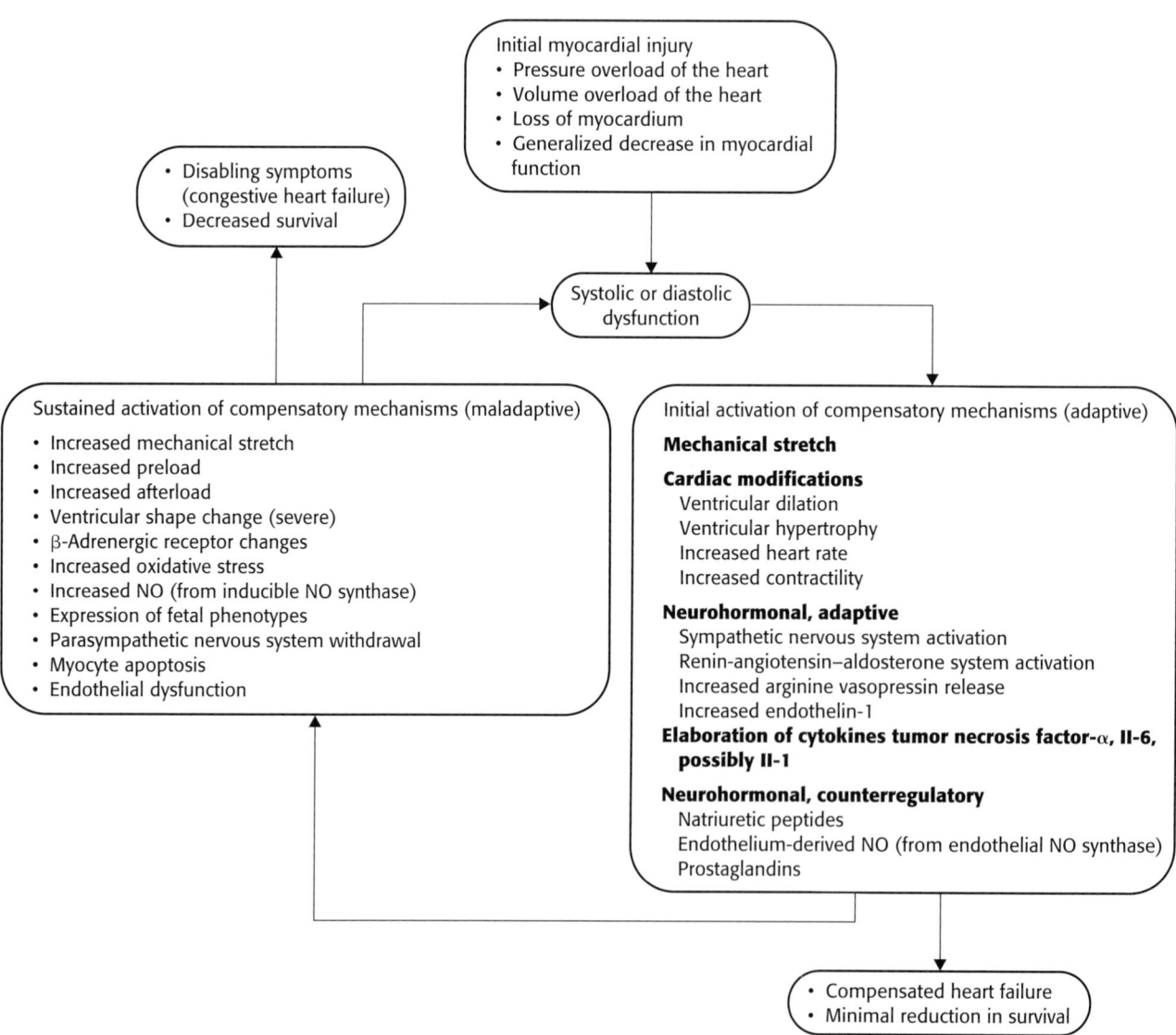

FIGURE 21.1 Pathogenesis of congestive heart failure. IL, interleukin.

(i.e., ventricular dilation or eccentric hypertrophy).[11] Ventricular dilation is an attempt to increase end-diastolic volume or preload to increase CO. As the ventricular chamber increases in size, it can fill to a greater extent during diastole, so stroke volume increases during systole. This response often is depicted by the Frank–Starling relationship between systolic performance and diastolic filling. Preload is determined largely by the extracellular fluid volume and venous return. However, an increase in preload may raise systolic wall tension or stress. According to the Laplace relationship, systolic wall tension equals the product of aortic pressure (P) and the internal radius of the ventricle (R) divided by the two times the wall thickness (2h): T = (PR)/2h. Preload is a component of wall tension in that it corresponds to the internal radius of the ventricular chamber. Therefore, increases in preload result in increases in wall tension.

Cardiac myocyte hypertrophy or an increase in wall thickness also occurs, especially in response to the pressure overload of HTN or aortic stenosis, and is the result of an increase in the diameter of myocytes through the parallel addition of new sarcomeres (i.e., concentric hypertrophy).[11] This response is analogous to a weightlifter's increase in skeletal muscle size in response to lifting heavier weights. According to the Laplace equation, the increase in wall thickness should result in a reduction in wall tension (or afterload) imposed on individual myocytes. Afterload is the hemodynamic load against which the ventricle must contract to deliver its stroke volume. Afterload corresponds to the systolic wall tension defined previously. A major peripheral component of afterload is the systemic arteriolar tone or systemic vascular resistance, which also is a component of blood pressure (i.e., P in the Laplace equation). In CHF it is common to see both parallel and series addition of sarcomeres.[11]

In addition to mechanical stretch, ventricular remodeling is mediated predominantly by initial activation of the sympathetic nervous system and secondary activation of the renin-angiotensin-aldosterone system (Fig. 21.1).[12,13] Norepinephrine and decreased renal perfusion pressure stimulate the release of renin by the kidney. Renin, both systemically and locally in the myocardium, first acts on angiotensinogen to convert it to angiotensin I. Angiotensin I is then converted to angiotensin II by angiotensin-converting enzyme (ACE). Angiotensin II also can be synthesized locally via chymase, an ACE-independent pathway.[13] Norepinephrine and angiotensin II act as mitogens for cardiac myocytes to increase the number of sarcomeres (i.e., cardiac hypertrophy).[11] Angiotensin II enhances sympathetic nervous system activity by facilitating presynaptic norepinephrine release.[13] Angiotensin II also stimulates the release of aldosterone from the adrenals and facilitates the secretion of arginine vasopressin. In turn, aldosterone and arginine vasopressin trigger renal sodium and water retention, respectively.[13] Blood volume is expanded, so preload is augmented. Angiotensin II also enhances the formation of preproendothelin by endothelial cells. Preproendothelin is cleaved by endothelin-converting enzyme to form endothelin-1, which stimulates further re-

lease of renin and aldosterone as well as further conversion of angiotensin I to angiotensin II in endothelial cells.[14] Therefore, endothelin-1 also promotes sodium retention. Furthermore, myocardial contractility is enhanced because norepinephrine, angiotensin II, and endothelin-1 are positive inotropic agents, the former via stimulation of β_1 receptors.[12–14] Norepinephrine also increases heart rate (HR) via β-receptor stimulation.[12] In addition, cytokines such as tumor necrosis factor-α (TNF-α) and interleukin-6, the former being secreted by cardiomyocytes, become elaborated and probably play a role in facilitating early ventricular dilation by stimulating increased activity of matrix metalloproteinases (MMPs).[15,16] MMPs are enzymes that degrade extracellular matrix, thereby augmenting LV remodeling. Thus, neurohormonally mediated increases in contractility, HR, preload, and myocardial hypertrophy, along with cytokine-mediated ventricular remodeling, maintain CO after initial myocardial injury.

In the peripheral circulation norepinephrine, angiotensin II, and endothelin-1 promote systemic vasoconstriction via stimulation of vascular α-receptors, angiotensin II type 1 receptor (AT_1), and endothelin-1 type A (ET_A) receptors, respectively, to maintain perfusion pressure.[12–14] However, systemic vasoconstriction causes an increase in afterload. Sustained increases in afterload can lead to a decreased stroke volume and CO, especially in advanced CHF. Nonetheless, the increase in afterload initially is compensated by release of atrial and brain natriuretic peptides (ANP and BNP) in response to atrial and ventricular stretch, respectively, which result from increased ventricular dilation.[17] ANP and presumably BNP decrease renin secretion, attenuate the stimulatory effects of angiotensin II on aldosterone release, inhibit the release of norepinephrine through stimulation of vagal afferents, inhibit the growth of vascular smooth muscle and endothelial cells, and produce vasodilatory and natriuretic effects to reduce the hemodynamic load on the heart.[17] A fourth natriuretic peptide, Dendraspis natriuretic peptide, has been identified in human atria and in the circulation of patients with CHF.[18] However, the role of Dendraspis natriuretic peptide in the neurohormonal activation characteristic of CHF has not been determined. In addition to ANP and BNP, vasodilation is also promoted by nitric oxide synthesized by endothelium-derived nitric oxide synthase (eNOS or NOS_3), which is expressed in cardiomyocytes and endothelial cells and upregulated by mechanical stress.[19] Prostaglandins prostacyclin (PGI_2) and prostaglandin E_2 also contribute to vasodilation. The increase in nitric oxide and prostaglandin synthesis may result from endothelin-1 stimulation of endothelial ET_B receptors.[14]

Thus, after the initial myocardial damage there appears to be a balance between vasoconstrictive and vasodilatory systems as well as sodium and fluid retaining and excreting systems. However, over time, the initial neurohormonal adaptive responses overshoot (i.e., become maladaptive), producing a progressive, vicious cycle in the disease process, leading to the signs and symptoms of CHF and ultimately death (Fig. 21.1). Within the heart there is norepinephrine-, angiotensin II-, and endothelin-1–mediated deposition of collagen and other components of the extracellular matrix among cardiomyocytes.[11] This increases chamber stiffness, decreases compliance, reduces delivery of nutrients to cardiomyocytes, and further elevates end-diastolic pressure and therefore mechanical stress. Conversely, continued eccentric ventricular remodeling may result from the dissolution of collagen and other extracellular matrix tethers by MMP, causing side-to-side slippage of myocytes, further ventricular dilation, and increased preload and wall stress.[11,16] Continued cardiomyocyte hypertrophy and extracellular matrix production also may result in cardiomyocyte energy starvation.[20] This can result from reductions in oxygen supply caused by a decreased capillary density; oxygen diffusion impairment caused by myocyte hypertrophy and adjacent fibrosis, both of which increase the distance between perfusing capillaries and the adenosine triphosphate (ATP)-consuming myofibrils; or impairments in mitochondrial ATP production. Each of these in turn may contribute to the development of cardiomyocyte apoptosis.

Continued activation of neurohormonal responses, although intended to maintain an effective CO, becomes deleterious. Diminished contractile response actually results from sustained, increased concentrations of norepinephrine caused by downregulation of principally myocardial β_1 receptors and uncoupling of β_1 and β_2 receptors. β-Receptor uncoupling is caused by phosphorylation of the β-receptor, which in effect inactivates the receptor; upregulation of inhibitory G-proteins; or sequestration of the receptors.[21] Impaired contractility may also result from alterations in other cardiac gene expressions, such as the downregulation of sarcoplasmic reticulum ATPase, a protein important in excitation–contraction coupling in the heart, and upregulation of β-myosin heavy chain (MyHC), a fetal form of MyHC that produces less energy for muscle contraction than adult α-MyHC.[12,21] In addition, elevated, persistent activation of the sympathetic nervous system promotes myocardial apoptosis[11] and impairs parasympathetic influence on the heart,[22] which diminishes the normal arterial baroreceptor response and increases the risk of proarrhythmia. Angiotensin II and endothelin-1 also promote myocyte apoptosis.[11] Peripheral vasoconstriction is further augmented and vasodilatory capacity impaired by norepinephrine, angiotensin II, and endothelin-1, along with increased sodium content of peripheral blood vessels. In addition, persistently increased levels of TNF-α and interleukin-6 diminish endothelium-mediated vasorelaxation and produce negative inotropic effects, largely by stimulating inducible nitric oxide synthase (iNOS or NOS₂) in cardiomyocytes.[19,23,24] This greatly increases myocardial concentrations of NO, which attenuates responsiveness to β-adrenergic stimulation and enhances myocyte apoptosis, perhaps by generating oxygen free radicals.[19,23,24] The counterregulatory vasodilator responses mediated by ANP, BNP, NO (produced by eNOS), and prostaglandins become overwhelmed. In addition, unrelenting

stimuli that trigger sodium and water retention override counterbalancing salt-excreting systems (natriuretic peptides and prostaglandins) and further expand intravascular volume and pressure, resulting in circulatory congestion and edema. Altered skeletal muscle structure and function combined with decreased perfusion produce fatigue and exercise intolerance.

In summary, HF begins when myocardial and peripheral adaptive responses are activated to maintain an effective perfusion pressure after initial myocardial damage. HF progresses when these compensatory, chiefly neurohormonally and cytokine-mediated responses persist. This leads to a series of deleterious effects on the heart, circulation, and end organs such as the kidney and liver, resulting in CHF, that are manifest by classic physical and laboratory signs, disabling symptoms, and ultimately death.

CLINICAL PRESENTATION AND DIAGNOSIS

With knowledge of the pathophysiology of CHF, it is easy to predict the expected signs, symptoms, and associated laboratory findings (Table 21.2).[25] However, many patients with impaired LV systolic function [i.e., LV ejection fraction (LVEF) <40%] may exhibit no signs or symptoms of CHF. Up to 20% of patients with LVEF less than 40% may not meet clinical criteria diagnostic for CHF.[26] Nonetheless, most patients with LVEF less than 40% exhibit signs and symptoms of CHF. An understanding of the essential elements of the cardiovascular physical examination is key to appropriate monitoring of HF therapy.

The underlying reduction in CO that occurs in CHF stimulates compensatory mechanisms, leading to sodium and water retention and increased sympathetic activity. Sodium and water retention produces an increase in preload, which the failing heart cannot manage. As is characteristic in most patients with CHF, systemic and pulmonary congestion ensues. Signs and symptoms of congestion relate to the failing ventricle. Pulmonary congestion develops secondary to failure of the LV, whereas systemic congestion occurs secondary to failure of the right ventricle. LV failure is more common, however, because the ventricles share a common wall, and given considerable interventricular dependence, most patients eventually develop biventricular failure and consequently exhibit both systemic and pulmonary congestion.

Pulmonary pressures are increased in CHF by the diminished ability of the LV to accept or eject the excess blood volume. Pulmonary congestion is manifest by varying degrees of breathlessness: dyspnea on exertion; orthopnea (dyspnea that occurs in the supine position); paroxysmal nocturnal dyspnea, an exaggerated form of orthopnea that occurs when the patient is awakened abruptly at night with a feeling of suffocation; dyspnea at rest; and pulmonary edema (fluid accumulation in the alveoli). Some patients complain of cough or asthma symptoms.

TABLE 21.2 Pathophysiologic Mechanisms Responsible for the Signs and Symptoms of Heart Failure

Left-Sided Sign or Symptom	Pathophysiologic Mechanism
Orthopnea Paroxysmal nocturnal dyspnea	Reintroduction of pooled blood from lower extremities after the patient assumes a supine position produces an abrupt increase in preload. The failing heart is unable to accommodate such abrupt increases in LVEDP, leading to pulmonary congestion and edema.
Pulmonary edema Bibasilar crackles	The failing heart is unable to accommodate increases in LVEDP, leading to pulmonary congestion, increased pulmonary vein hydrostatic pressure, and pulmonary edema.
Cough	Pulmonary congestion.
	Bradykinin accumulation secondary to the use of angiotensin-converting enzyme inhibitors.

Right-Sided Sign or Symptom	Pathophysiologic Mechanism
Peripheral edema Increased body weight	Sodium and water retention produces an increase in blood volume and venous hydrostatic pressure. Transudation of fluid into the subcutaneous tissue ensues. Albumin usually is decreased because of reduced hepatic synthesis and altered nutrition. Oncotic pressure is altered by the reduction in serum albumin.
Hepatomegaly Increased INR	Chronic venous congestion produces congestion of the liver. Synthesis of clotting factors can be reduced.
Jugular venous distention	Central blood volume is increased, leading to an increase in central venous pressure upon compression of the liver.

Nonspecific Sign or Symptom	Pathophysiologic Mechanism
Resting tachycardia Atrial fibrillation Ventricular arrhythmias	The reduction in cardiac output produces a compensatory increase in sympathetic nervous system activity, leading to an increase in heart rate and intracellular influx of calcium. The increase in norepinephrine along with parasympathetic withdrawal, myocardial architectural changes, and electrolyte disturbances predispose patients to arrhythmias.
Ventricular dilation and remodeling Enlarged heart (cardiac heave) Increased cardiothoracic ratio on chest roentgenograph	The ventricle dilates to accommodate increases in preload. Consequently, the natural elliptical shape of the ventricle is lost and the ventricle becomes spherical and baggy. Thus, the ratio of the size of the heart to thoracic cavity increases.
Fatigue and diminished exercise tolerance	Cardiac output is diminished, limiting oxygen delivery to brain and skeletal muscle. In addition, the ability to increase cardiac output in the face of exercise is reduced. Consequently, the skeletal muscles quickly become hypoxic. There are also defects in skeletal and respiratory musculature that contribute to fatigue and exercise limitations.
Altered mental status, confusion	Reduced cardiac output and oxygen delivery to central nervous system.
Hypotension	Blood pressure decreases secondary to a reduction in cardiac output (MAP ≈CO × SVR).
Nocturia	Reintroduction of pooled blood from lower extremities after the patient assumes a supine position produces an increase in venous return. An increase in blood flow to the kidney occurs.
Oliguria Increased blood urea nitrogen and serum creatinine Increased urine specific gravity Hyponatremia	Reductions in cardiac output and secondary increases in norepinephrine, angiotensin II, and other neurohormones reduce blood flow to the kidney, leading to a reduction in urine output. Urea and creatinine are not filtered normally. Effects of increased arginine vasopressin result in dilutional hyponatremia, a concentrated urine, and inability to excrete free water.

LVEDP, left ventricular end-diastolic pressure; MAP, mean arterial pressure; CO, cardiac output; SVR, systemic vascular resistance.

Typically, dyspnea on exertion is the first symptom of CHF.[27] As the disease progresses, the degree of physical activity that produces dyspnea decreases. The level of activity that produces dyspnea can be used to monitor disease severity. Patients with severe CHF complain of dyspnea at rest and may demonstrate Cheyne–Stokes breathing (alternating hyperventilation and apnea). Orthopnea occurs within minutes after the patient assumes a supine position. A supine position places the lower extremities on the same vertical plane as the heart. Venous pooling, which occurs while the patient is standing, is reduced and the fluid is reintroduced into the central circulatory system, leading to pulmonary congestion. Sitting upright relieves orthopnea. Increasing the number of pillows the patient uses to sleep on often circumvents orthopnea, and changes in the number of pillows used while sleeping can be used to monitor the patient's condition. Paroxysmal nocturnal dyspnea awakens the patient after 2 to 4 hours of sleep with the feeling of suffocation. Relief is obtained by maintaining an upright position and may take up to 30 minutes to occur. Severe pulmonary congestion, with accumulation of fluid in the alveoli, can occur, producing pulmonary edema. Patients may experience severe shortness of breath and anxiety as a result. Often patients with pulmonary edema expectorate a pink, frothy sputum. On physical examination, bibasilar rales (a crackling sound) may be heard on lung auscultation. Rales are consistent with fluid accumulation in the alveoli. Pulmonary congestion may also be observed in a chest roentgenogram. Findings consistent with pulmonary congestion include pleural effusions and Kerley lines. Careful interpretation of the physical examination is warranted in patients with CHF. For instance, because of a compensatory increase in lymphatic drainage, patients with chronic CHF can have very high LV filling pressures but no detectable rales. Therefore, the absence of rales does not preclude the existence of elevated pulmonary pressures.

Systemic venous congestion may manifest as weight gain, dependent peripheral edema, jugular venous distention, and congestive hepatomegaly. Hepatic edema may cause right upper quadrant pain. Generalized visceral edema may also occur and cause abdominal distention, anorexia, nausea, and constipation. The patient's weight should be assessed frequently because an increase in fluid retention is observed before the onset of peripheral edema. Short-term weight changes can be used to assess short-term fluctuations in fluid status. A gain of approximately 10 lb of extracellular fluid volume must occur before peripheral edema is noted. This edema usually develops in the gravity-dependent areas of the body such as the ankles and feet, or above the shinbone (i.e., pretibial) in ambulatory patients and in the sacral area when the patient is supine. Peripheral edema may be physically uncomfortable as well as cosmetically unattractive. Peripheral edema is specific for CHF in less than 30% of patients.[28] Additional populations at risk for peripheral edema include older adults, obese patients, and patients with peripheral vascular disease. In addition, the presence or absence of peripheral edema can be affected by the use of diuretics and vasodilators.

Central venous pressure is estimated by elevating the patient's head to a 45-degree angle and observing the peak of the maximal venous pulsation in the internal jugular vein. In this position, the central venous pressure normally does not exceed 2 cm of vertical distance above the sternal angle. Because the sternal angle usually lies about 5 cm above the right atrium, the central venous pressure can be estimated by noting the vertical distance and adding 5 cm to the value. The liver is also characteristically congested in CHF and is generally palpable several centimeters below the right costal margin. Pressure on the abdomen further increases the jugular venous pressure (because the right ventricle cannot accept the increased blood returned to the heart) and produces a positive hepatojugular reflex. Visual examination of the jugular veins remains a reliable way to noninvasively assess the overall fluid status of the patient, provided the assessment is performed appropriately.[29] In addition, a quick assessment of the jugular veins may be useful in determining which patients warrant further attention by a physician.[30] Again, it is important to remember that signs of systemic congestion may be affected by the use of diuretics and vasodilators. In addition, systemic signs of fluid overload reflect elevated right-sided pressures and can occur secondary to conditions other than CHF, such as mitral stenosis and pulmonary HTN.

Systemically, inadequate perfusion of the skeletal muscles often leads to easy fatigability and weakness. Exercise tolerance is diminished, and patients adjust their lifestyles accordingly, such as no longer walking up a flight of steps. Nocturia (increased urine formation at night), which results from redistribution of blood flow to the kidney during recumbency, often occurs early in the course of CHF. Oliguria may become manifest later as HF worsens. A host of cerebral symptoms may also be observed and can include memory impairment, confusion, and insomnia.

A number of cardiac and systemic physical findings are observed with varying frequencies. An early diastolic third heart sound, S_3 (i.e., "Ken-tuc-KY," where "Ken," "tuc," and "ky" represent S_1, S_2, and S_3 respectively) is believed to be related to impaired diastolic relaxation of the ventricle and suggests an elevated end-diastolic pressure. An S_3 is a hallmark of moderate to severe HF.[31] A resting sinus tachycardia is often present. Objective cardiac findings often include an enlarged heart (palpable as a cardiac heave) and an increased cardiothoracic ratio (>0.50) as determined by chest roentgenogram. LVEF is most commonly assessed via a two-dimensional echocardiogram.[1] Patients with an LVEF less than 40% are considered to have systolic dysfunction. In addition, echocardiography can be used to assess LV chamber size, geometry, wall thickness, and valve function. Segmental wall motion abnormalities, suggesting an ischemic cardiomyopathy, can be observed on echocardiography, but coronary angiography is needed to assess the presence and severity of atherosclerotic heart disease. Furthermore, an assessment of viability may be needed before revascularization is attempted. Coronary angiography and radionuclide ventriculography are alternatives to echocardiography that can be used to assess LVEF. LV function measurement may be indicated every 12 to 24 months in unstable patients.

Numerous laboratory abnormalities are observed in patients with CHF. Simple laboratory tests [i.e., body weight, serum electrolytes, serum creatinine (Scr) and blood urea nitrogen (BUN), and serum digoxin concentration], body weight, and chest roentgenograms are used most often in monitoring ambulatory patients with CHF.[32] At home, patients should monitor their weight daily. Serum electrolytes and markers of renal function can be checked every 1 to 3 months, depending on the patient's clinical status and provided there are no changes in therapy. Total body sodium (Na^+) often is increased. However, a dilutional hyponatremia is commonly seen because of a diminished ability to excrete free water. Hyponatremia may worsen with diuretic treatment. The presence of hyponatremia has been established as an important predictor of poor outcome.[33,34] Patients with CHF generally have deficits of both total body and intracellular potassium (K^+) and magnesium (Mg^{2+}), which may or may not be reflected in the serum concentrations of these cations.[35] These electrolyte deficiencies coupled with increased neurohormones may predispose patients to the development of potentially lethal ventricular arrhythmias. Impaired hepatic function may occur secondary to venous congestion and may be characterized by elevations in plasma concentrations of hepatic enzymes. Reductions in renal blood flow and glomerular filtration rate (GFR) are reflected by increases in both Scr and BUN levels. The urine usually is concentrated, with a high urine specific gravity, and there may be associated proteinuria.

A LVEF less than 40% indicates LV systolic dysfunction. CHF is a clinical diagnosis that can be observed in patients with either systolic or diastolic dysfunction. In the OPTIMIZE and ADHERE registries, HF symptoms in the setting of preserved systolic function were observed in 48% and 46% of the patients, respectively.[5,6] No one symptom can be considered the diagnostic gold standard of CHF. Rather, the presence of any single symptom warrants echocardiographic assessment of LV function with consideration of CHF as a possible cause. It is important to remember that symptoms alone are not indicative of CHF, and proper evaluation includes consideration of the clinical presentation and potential underlying causes. Past medical history is important to elicit the presence of prior myocardial infarction, HTN, and valvular disease and may aid in the diagnosis of CHF. Measurement of circulating BNP is a useful screening tool for LV systolic dysfunction.[36–39] In the Breathing Not Properly study, BNP values above 100 pg per mL had a diagnostic accuracy of 83.4%. The negative predictive value of BNP levels below 50 pg per mL was 96%.[36]

To evaluate both the severity of HF and the responses to therapy, two classification systems have been developed: the New York Heart Association (NYHA) Functional Classification[40] and the American College of Cardiology (ACC)/American Heart Association (AHA) stage classification for heart failure (Table 21.3).[41] The NYHA classification, despite its reliance on subjective findings during exertion, is commonly used to classify the severity of CHF.[40] Initially, patients may present with severe symptoms (NYHA class

TABLE 21.3	Classification Systems for Congestive Heart Failure	
Functional Capacity	**Objective Assessment**
New York Heart Association functional classification	
Class I. Patients with cardiac disease but without resulting limitation of physical activity. Ordinary physical activity does not cause undue fatigue, palpitation, dyspnea, or anginal pain.	A. No objective evidence of cardiovascular disease
Class II. Patients with cardiac disease resulting in slight limitation of physical activity. They are comfortable at rest. Ordinary physical activity results in fatigue, palpitation, dyspnea, or anginal pain.	B. Objective evidence of minimal cardiovascular disease
Class III. Patients with cardiac disease resulting in marked limitation of physical activity. They are comfortable at rest. Less than ordinary activity causes fatigue, palpitation, dyspnea, or anginal pain.	C. Objective evidence of moderately severe cardiovascular disease
Class IV. Patients with cardiac disease resulting in inability to carry out any physical activity without discomfort. Symptoms of heart failure or the anginal syndrome may be present even at rest. If any physical activity is undertaken, discomfort is increased.	D. Objective evidence of severe cardiovascular disease
Classification of heart failure based on maximal exercise tolerance	
Class A: No impairment: $Vo_{2max} \geq 20$ mL/min/kg	
Class B: Mild to moderate impairment: $Vo_{2max} = 16–20$ mL/min/kg	
Class C: Moderate to severe impairment: $Vo_{2max} = 10–15$ mL/min/kg	
Class D: Severe impairment: $Vo_{2max} < 10$ mL/min/kg	

Vo_{2max}, maximal oxygen (O_2) uptake. It is a function of the maximum cardiac output that the heart can generate and the maximum amount of oxygen that the exercising tissues can extract.

IV) despite well-preserved LV function. In addition, patients often downgrade their expectations for exercise tolerance as CHF progresses. Consequently, the NYHA classification system may not correlate accurately with disease severity. The NYHA classification probably will remain popular among practitioners because of its simplicity and convenience. In addition to NYHA classification, quality of life can be assessed via a variety of methods, including the Minnesota Living with Heart Failure Questionnaire, Kansas City Cardiomyopathy Questionnaire, the Chronic Heart Failure Questionnaire, the Specific Activity Scale, the Yale Scale, and the Quality of Life Questionnaire in Severe Heart Failure.[42]

The progression of CHF was recently incorporated in the AHA/ACC stage classification for heart failure.[41] Heart failure is now classified as stage A, B, C, or D, depending on risk factors, structural heart disease, and symptoms. This classification recognizes patients at risk for heart failure but who have not yet developed the syndrome.

The exercise tolerance classification system uses an incremental treadmill exercise protocol and noninvasive monitoring of respiratory gas exchange, HR, and blood pressure to grade the severity of chronic CHF.[43] Maximal oxygen uptake (Vo_{2max}, expressed in mL/minute/kg) is determined by maximal CO and by the maximal extraction of oxygen by the exercising muscles. Despite its relative objectivity and prognostic utility, it is a more complex, costly, and time-consuming method for evaluating CHF severity and responses to therapy. Furthermore, it is dependent on effort and may not be representative of the usual degree of physical activity for the typical patient. Its most appropriate uses may be to identify the patient's suitability for employment, rehabilitation programs, and cardiac transplantation.[1] An alternative measure of quantifying exercise capacity and its response to treatment is the 6-minute walk, which may better represent the patient's usual degree of physical activity.[44] The 6-minute walk distance is a significant predictor of mortality in patients with heart failure.[45]

THERAPEUTIC PLAN

Therapeutic goals are achieved using a combination of patient and family education and support, nonpharmacologic and pharmacologic therapies, surgical interventions, and device therapy (Table 21.4).[41,46–48] Nonpharmacologic treatment incorporates salt restriction, initial reduction of the heart's workload with abbreviated rest followed by exercise training upon recovery, lifestyle changes, and identification, treatment, and removal of precipitating causes.[46,47] Current pharmacologic therapy for CHF caused by systolic dysfunction consists of neurohormonal blockade with ACE inhibitors or angiotensin receptor blockers (ARBs) and β-adrenergic receptor blockers. Diuretics are prescribed as needed to manage fluid overload, but the dose should be the lowest that maintains euvolemia. Many patients can be managed

TABLE 21.4	General Nonpharmacologic and Pharmacologic Components in Treating the Patient with Heart Failure

Patient and family education

  Discussions and pamphlets on signs and symptoms of heart failure

  Discussions and pamphlets on medications

  Emphasis on compliance with complete treatment agenda

  Instructions on when to contact health care providers (see Table 40.5)

Diet

  Daily weight chart

  Individualized diet according to needs, preferences, and lifestyle

  Sodium restriction, mild (<3 g/day) or moderate (<2 g/day)

  Information about sodium content in foods

  Information about potassium content in foods

  Weight loss when appropriate

  Alcohol restriction

  Fluid restriction: ~2 L/day

  Nutritional supplements (e.g., vitamins)

  Emphasize importance of compliance

Other

  Smoking cessation

  Pharmacologic treatment of hyperlipidemia

  Pharmacologic treatment of diabetes

  Pharmacologic treatment of hypertension

  Pharmacologic treatment of coronary disease

Exercise

  Consultation and prescription

Psychosocial services

  Evaluate emotional needs and presence of depression

  Use individualized counseling or antidepressants

  Evaluate financial needs

  Support groups

  End-of-life issues

Intensive follow-up

  Telephone calls

  Home visits

  Outpatient clinic visits

with loop diuretics on an as-needed basis. Digoxin is recommended when patients are symptomatic despite ACE inhibitors and β-blockers. Aldosterone antagonists are indicated in patients with NYHA III/IV symptoms, who are treated with ACE inhibitors and β-blockers (Fig. 21.2).[41,47,48] Device therapies such as cardiac resynchronization and

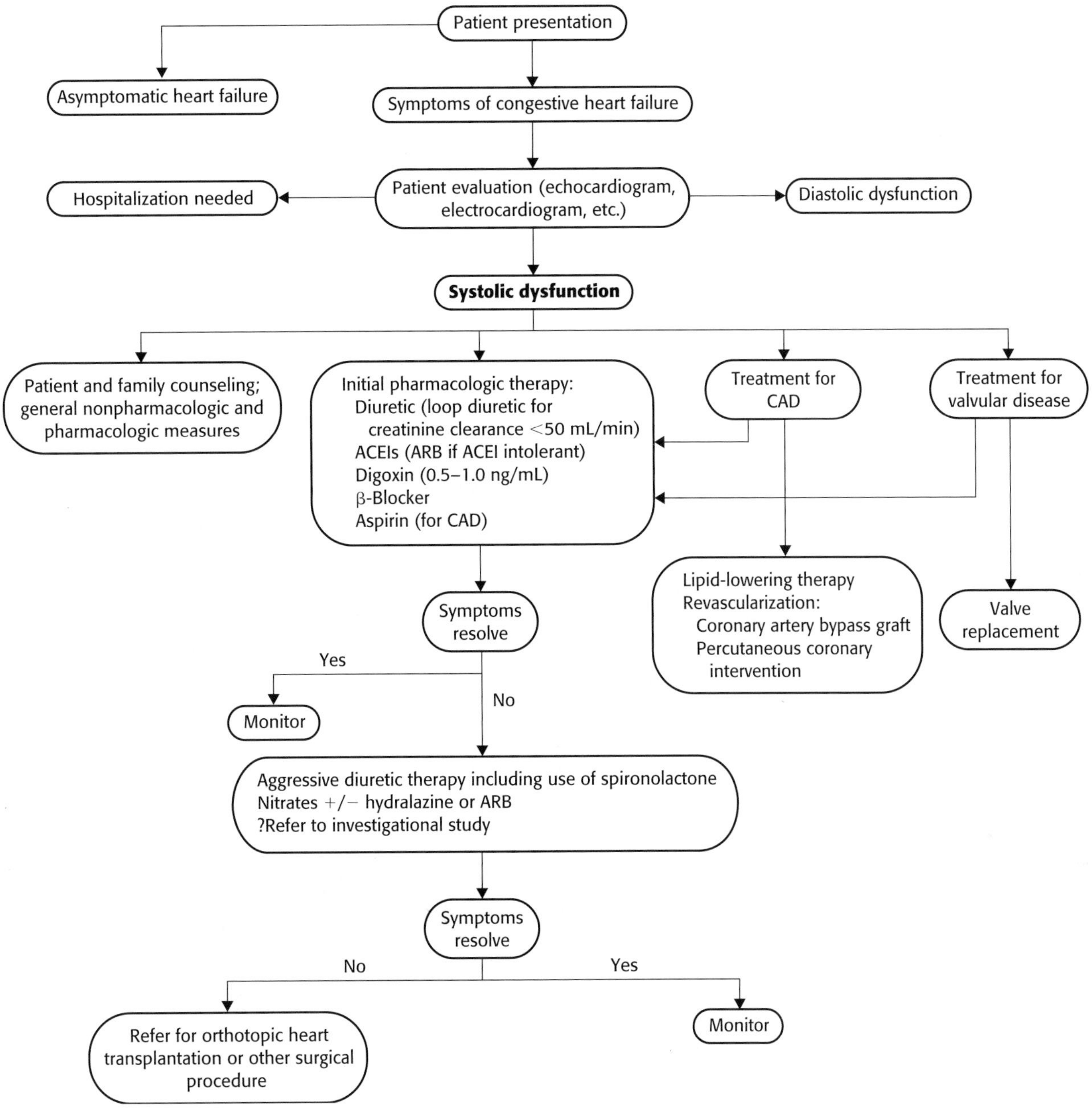

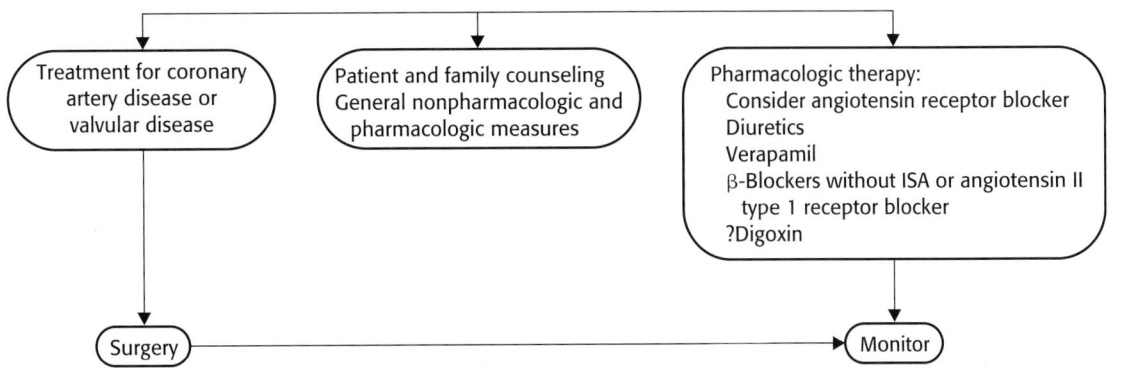

FIGURE 21.2 Treatment algorithm for symptomatic systolic dysfunction. ACE, angiotensin-converting enzyme; ARB, angiotensin II type 1 receptor blocker; CAD, coronary artery disease.

FIGURE 21.3 Treatment algorithm for symptomatic diastolic dysfunction.

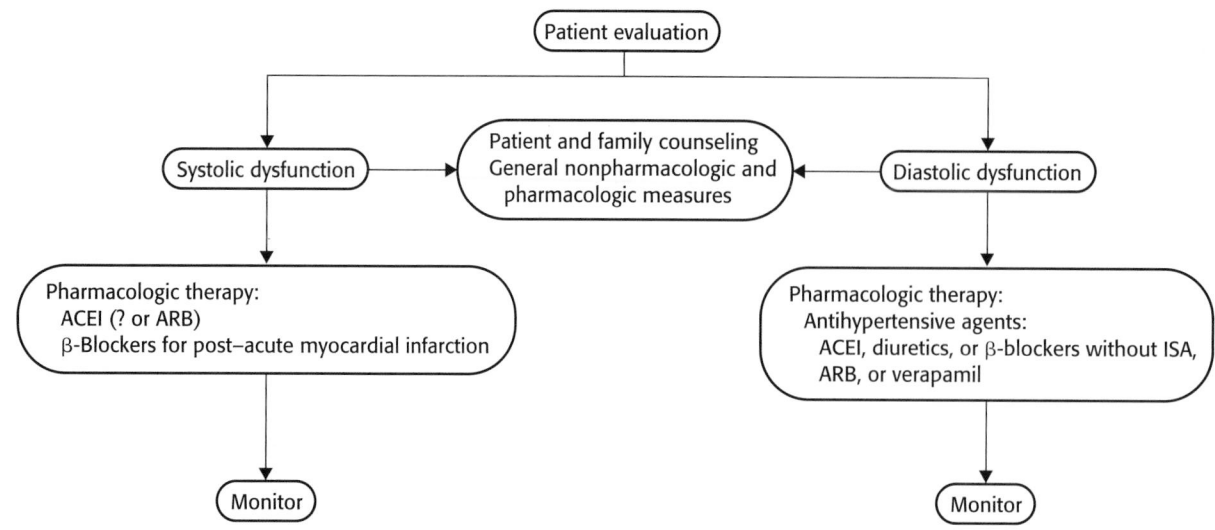

FIGURE 21.4 Treatment algorithm for asymptomatic heart failure. ACE, angiotensin-converting enzyme inhibitor; ARB, angiotensin II type 1 receptor blocker.

implantable cardioverter-defibrillators are standard treatment approaches for a subset of patients.[49,50] Surgical and related interventions include coronary artery bypass graft (CABG) surgery, LV assist devices, orthotopic heart transplantation, and the use of artificial ventricles as bridges to transplantation.[51]

The majority of this chapter is devoted to the treatment of symptomatic HF (i.e., CHF) caused by systolic dysfunction. HF secondary to diastolic dysfunction is treated very differently and is therefore discussed in a separate section (Fig. 21.3). A treatment algorithm for asymptomatic systolic dysfunction is shown in Figure 21.4.

CHRONIC CONGESTIVE HEART FAILURE SECONDARY TO SYSTOLIC DYSFUNCTION

TREATMENT

GENERAL NONPHARMACOLOGIC AND PHARMACOLOGIC MEASURES

Initial measures in CHF management (Table 21.4) should focus on preventing the disease.[52] For example, alteration of correctable risk factors for CAD, a major etiologic factor for CHF, should be attempted. Prevention should include attempts to normalize serum lipids, blood pressure, and body weight. Patient education should also emphasize the importance of smoking cessation and moderate exercise. As discussed earlier, the new "stage A" classification of patients with CHF in the AHA/ACC guidelines recognizes for the first time patients at high risk of developing heart failure. The guidelines now recommend consideration of the following interventions for stage A patients: treat HTN, encourage smoking cessation, treat lipid disorders, encourage regular exercise, discourage alcohol intake and illicit drug use, and prescribe ACE inhibition in appropriate patients.[41]

Proper CHF management includes attempts to modify or correct systemic diseases causing or precipitating CHF exacerbations.[52] CAD, if present, may impair ventricular function through ongoing myocardial ischemia. Attempts at revascularization in appropriate patients may enhance ventricular function and survival. Currently, there are no data from randomized, controlled clinical trials to determine the effect of revascularization on clinical outcomes in these patients. However, the Surgical Treatment for Ischemic Heart Failure Trial (STICH) is an NIH-funded randomized clinical trial that is studying surgical revascularization versus medical therapy on mortality and morbidity in patients with LV dysfunction and HF symptoms.[53] Patients with valvular disease may benefit from attempts to surgically repair or replace defective myocardial valves. In patients with symptomatic bradycardia, optimal CO can be ensured through the maintenance of sinus rhythm with pacemaker placement. Additional precipitating factors include systemic infection, pulmonary embolism, hypocalcemia, anemia, and endocrine disorders (e.g., hyperthyroidism). Acute CHF exacerbations may be prevented through judicious administration of pneumococcal and influenza vaccines.[52]

Initial restriction of physical activity to some degree is used to treat virtually every patient with CHF.[52] However, severe restrictions on physical activity may worsen a patient's exercise tolerance and lead to additional psychological problems. Many patients with CHF benefit from a carefully prescribed cardiac rehabilitation program. However, the actual minimum level of physical exertion needed to achieve improvements has not been defined. The actual type of physical activity that affords the greatest benefit to patients with CHF also is unknown. However, some form of regular aerobic exercise can enhance the cardiovascular system and improve exercise tolerance.[54,55] General improvement in physical condition can be accompanied by hemodynamic benefits, including reduction of the resting HR, reduction of exercise-associated peak systolic blood pressure, and an improvement in the tissue oxygen extraction. Long-term participation in exercise training may reduce mortality and improve quality of life for patients with CHF.[56] This concept is currently being tested in the NHLBI-sponsored Heart Failure A Controlled Trial Investigating Outcomes of Exercise Training (HF ACTION) study. HF ACTION is a randomized study of exercise training versus usual care in patients with HF and LV dysfunction. The primary endpoint of HF ACTION is a composite to determine the long-term safety and efficacy of exercise training, as well as the effects on quality of life.[57]

Exercise capacity varies widely. Patients with severe CHF may be unable to tolerate low-intensity exercise, and more strenuous physical activity may not be tolerated even in patients with compensated CHF. Therefore, each patient should receive individualized instruction. It is not possible to predict exercise tolerance from either LVEF or other clinical parameters. However, patients who cannot increase their CO with exercise probably will do poorly. These patients often experience a drop in systolic blood pressure while exercising, a finding that suggests that no cardiac reserve remains. Such patients may not tolerate any exercise program. Similarly, patients who have recently experienced a myocardial infarction should begin exercising only under the direction of a healthcare practitioner. Patients with HF should "begin low and go slow," thereby avoiding overexertion. Most cardiac rehabilitation programs include a combination of aerobic training and very light resistive exercises.[58] Many patients prefer walking programs. Such programs may improve mental health and combat some of the psychological problems typically seen in patients with CHF.

Patient education (Tables 21.4 and 21.5) should also focus on proper nutrition, with special attention to the potential harm of excess sodium intake,[46] because sodium overload is a leading cause of acute decompensation.[59] Limiting a patient's salt intake helps counteract the exaggerated renal retention of sodium. Higher or more frequent diuretic doses are needed to attenuate the effect of high sodium intake.

TABLE 21.5	Instructions on When to Contact a Healthcare Provider

UNIVERSITY MEDICAL CENTER
1501 N. Campbell Avenue
Tucson, Arizona 85724
Heart Failure Program
Signs and Symptoms of Heart Failure

Call your health care provider if you experience any of the following:

- Shortness of breath, especially if it does not go away with rest
- Difficulty breathing when lying down or waking up at night with shortness of breath
- Persistent cough or wheezing
- Fatigue or weakness with little or no energy for routine activities
- Weight gain of 2–3 lb in 2 days or 4–5 lb over 5–7 days, or if you do not achieve your desired weight after changing your diuretic dosage in response to the weight gain if you have been instructed to do so
- Swelling in your ankles, feet, legs, or abdomen
- Nausea or feeling full early with meals
- Abdominal pain or tenderness
- Confusion or difficulty with concentration

Also call your health care provider if you have

- Unusually prolonged or severe chest pain or angina
- Changes in the regularity of your heartbeat
- Dizziness or feeling faint when you stand up from a sitting position
- Any side effect from any of your medications

IN CASE OF A MEDICAL EMERGENCY, CALL 911 IMMEDIATELY.

Emergencies may include

- Chest pain or pressure not relieved with rest or after taking three nitroglycerin tablets 5 min apart
- Extreme shortness of breath
- Coughing up pink, frothy sputum
- Fainting spell, severe sweating, or passing out

Note: This is a sample list intended to serve as a guideline. It is not intended to include all potential medical problems for which a person with heart failure should seek urgent medical advice.

Source: Reference 222.

However, increasing diuretic dosages are not desirable given their ability to further activate the renin-angiotensin-aldosterone system, as well as retrospective data that suggest diuretics may be associated with poor outcomes.[60,61] Instead, dietary sodium restriction should be encouraged. Initial guidelines typically encourage that dietary intake be restricted to 3 g of sodium or less per day. Eliminating added salt and removing high-sodium foods (e.g., salted nuts, pretzels, salt-cured meats, potato chips, pickles, olives, processed meats, some canned vegetables and soups) will decrease daily sodium intake to about 1.5 to 3.0 g (3.75 to 7.5 g sodium chloride; 1.0 g Na = 2.5 g NaCl). The typical American diet usually contains twice this amount of sodium. Patients often find it difficult to keep track of daily sodium intake. Monitoring the sodium content per serving can be easier for patients. A general recommendation is for patients to avoid foods with more than 100 to 150 mg of sodium per serving. Patients must also be encouraged to read nutritional labels and to recognize the difference between a serving size on the label as compared to the portions they actually consume. Patients can use the Internet to obtain additional information about the sodium (www.ianr.unl.edu/pubs/FOODS/g916.htm) and potassium (www.consumermedhelp.com/HHPoCHrt.htm) content of foods. Excluding all salt from cooking further reduces the patient's sodium intake to 1.2 to 1.5 g. However, excessive sodium restriction may reduce the palatability of food and secondarily compromise adequate nutrition. Using spices for flavoring instead of salt should be encouraged and may enhance patient compliance with a low-sodium diet. Any family members involved in food preparation also should receive dietary education. In addition, over-the-counter medications may be a hidden source of sodium intake, and the patient can consult his or her pharmacist about appropriate selection.

Fluid restriction may also be recommended, particularly for patients with severe CHF. Fluid intake, when limited to 2 L per day or less, may reduce overall diuretic use.[62] Patients adhering to fluid restriction should be reminded to consider foods high in water, such as fruits and soup, in their total fluid intake. In addition, patients should be encouraged to abstain from alcohol. Ethanol and its metabolite acetaldehyde produce dose-related reductions in contractility via inhibition of actin and myosin coupling.[63] In addition, short-term alcohol intake can produce histologic alterations in the myocardium and is arrhythmogenic.[63] Chronic alcohol intake has been associated with the development of asymptomatic and symptomatic LV dysfunction, and abstinence has been associated with improvements in LV function and should therefore be encouraged.[64]

Patients should be informed about the use of herbal licorice, which is often advocated for gastrointestinal complaints but has mineralocorticoid properties that may antagonize the effects of the diuretic spironolactone.[65] The active component of licorice, glycyrrhizic acid, reduces 11-β-hydroxysteroid dehydrogenase activity, leading to excess mineralocorticoid effects. Consequently, sodium retention can occur, leading to an acute CHF exacerbation. In addition, hypokalemia may develop, increasing the patient's risk of arrhythmic complications. Patients with CHF should be advised to avoid using herbal licorice.

Patient noncompliance with prescribed medical and pharmacologic regimens often precipitates worsening of CHF. In a study of patients admitted to a Chicago hospital for HF treatment, 64% were noncompliant with their medical regimens.[66] Almost half of the patients in this study had uncontrolled HTN as a precipitating factor for HF. Hospital admissions may be reduced through proper attention to patient education.[46] Patient compliance improved in older adults with CHF enrolled in a 3-month patient education program provided by a pharmacist.[67] In addition, multidisciplinary interventions involving intensive patient education with detailed information about diet, medications, and instructions for calling healthcare providers (Table 21.5); increased patient monitoring through visits by pharmacists and nurses; and improved access to healthcare providers have been shown in randomized trials to reduce hospital readmissions, reduce length of stay, improve quality of life, enhance patient knowledge and medication compliance, improve functional capacity, and increase patient satisfaction.[68–72]

Some prescription medications may exacerbate CHF.[7] β-Adrenergic blocking therapy initiated at the usual antihypertensive dosages and first-generation calcium channel blocking agents (e.g., verapamil, diltiazem and nifedipine) are representative examples. Furthermore, adding antiarrhythmic agents with negative inotropic properties can worsen preexisting HF. Nonsteroidal anti-inflammatory drugs (NSAIDs) inhibit cyclooxygenase activity, leading to a reduction in vasodilatory prostaglandins, which oppose the renal and systemic effects of angiotensin II in patients with CHF.[7] Administering NSAIDs to patients with CHF produces a reduction in GFR and renal blood flow and an increase in sodium and water retention. Chronic use of NSAIDs in older adults with CHF is associated with increased hospitalization rates secondary to acute CHF decompensation.[73] NSAIDs are widely available and can be obtained without the knowledge or advice of a healthcare professional. Improved education about the possible detrimental effects of chronic NSAID use in patients with CHF is warranted.

Selective cyclooxygenase-2 (COX-2) inhibitors should also be avoided in patients with CHF. COX-2 is constitutively expressed in the kidney and is partially responsible for the synthesis of some renal prostaglandins.[74] Edema is also a reported adverse effect with COX-2 inhibitors.[75] Both NSAIDs and COX-2 inhibitors should be avoided in patients with HF.

Other medications can also be problematic in patients with HF. In general, sympathomimetic agents should be avoided because they increase sympathetic activity. Patients should be counseled to avoid using pseudoephedrine in over-the-counter or prescription cold medications; antihistamines or short-term topical decongestants are preferable in this setting. In addition, patients should be counseled to avoid over-the-counter "natural" or herbal products with sympathomimetic ingredients such as ephedrine or ma huang.

As discussed earlier, thiazelinediones have recently been associated with volume overload in patients with and without LV dysfunction. The exact mechanism is not known. Patients with HF who are started on thiazelinediones should be counseled to closely monitor their weight. The use of these drugs may require higher diuretic doses. The benefits of thiazelinedione therapy must be weighed against the risk of developing volume overload or requiring additional diuretic therapy to manage the patient. Thiazelinediones should be avoided in patients with unstable NYHA class IV heart failure.[8]

Pharmacist-conducted ''brown bag'' reviews may be of particular importance in patients with CHF because they can help identify drugs that may contribute to CHF exacerbations.[46] Stricter attention to these precipitating factors could significantly reduce the number of hospitalizations and ease the clinical and economic burden of CHF for patients and society.

PHARMACOTHERAPY

Vasodilators. Vasodilator therapy shows new promise in CHF treatment.[76] These agents, through varied mechanisms, have been shown to alter the capacitance (preload) and resis-

tance (afterload) of vessels, either directly or indirectly. The net result is that vasodilators enhance the physiologic performance of the diseased left ventricle, relieve symptoms of dyspnea, and improve exercise tolerance. Since the investigations of the early 1970s, vasodilator therapy has become an integral component of chronic CHF treatment. Most importantly, vasodilator therapy reduces mortality in patients with CHF.[77,78] However, not all vasodilators have been associated with a beneficial survival effect. It is now accepted that the mechanism of benefit of drugs such as ACE inhibitors is primarily due to the neurohormonal antagonist effects rather than hemodynamic properties. In general, the selection and dosing of a vasodilating agent for chronic CHF management should be based on studies that have evaluated the long-term beneficial and adverse effects of an agent (Table 21.6). The following section describes several classes of vasodilators used to treat CHF.

Angiotensin-Converting Enzyme Inhibitors. The ACE inhibitors, such as captopril, enalapril, fosinopril, lisinopril,

TABLE 21.6	Dosing Considerations for Vasodilators					
Drugs	Starting Dosage	Target Dosage (survival)	Maximum Dosage	Adverse Effects	Altered Kinetics	Monitoring Parameters
Angiotensin-converting enzyme inhibitors						
Captopril	3.125–6.25 mg TID	50 mg TID	100 mg TID	Hypotension	Renal dysfunction (dosage adjustments needed)	Blood pressure Renal function
Enalapril	1.25–2.5 mg BID	10 mg BID	20 mg BID	Renal dysfunction		Potassium
Lisinopril	2.5–5 mg QD	10 mg QD	40 mg QD	Angioedema		Cough
Ramipril	2.5 mg BID	5 mg BID	10 mg BID	Cough		Angioedema
Quinapril	2.5–5 mg BID	20 mg BID	20 mg BID			Volume status
Fosinopril	5–10 mg QD	20 mg QD	40 mg QD			CHF SS
Angiotensin II type I receptor blockers[a]						
Valsartan	40 mg BID	160 mg BID		Hypotension	Hepatic dysfunction	Blood pressure
Candisartan	4–8 mg QD	32 mg QD		Renal dysfunction		Renal function
Isosorbide dinitrate	10–20 mg TID	120 mg QD in 3 divided doses while ensuring a 12-hr nitrate-free interval		Hypotension Headache		Hepatic function CHF SS Blood pressure CHF SS
Hydralazine	25 mg TID	225 mg QD in 2 or 3 divided doses		Hypotension Headache Tachycardia Systemic lupus erythematosus	Renal dysfunction (dosage adjustments probably needed)	Blood pressure Heart rate CHF SS

CHF SS, signs and symptoms of congestive heart failure.
[a] Not approved by the U.S. Food and Drug Administration for treating heart failure

quinapril, and ramipril, competitively block the conversion of angiotensin I to angiotensin II. Angiotensin II is a potent peripheral arteriolar vasoconstrictor. It also stimulates the release of aldosterone and AVP and facilitates both central and peripheral activity of the sympathetic nervous system. In addition, the enzyme that converts angiotensin I to angiotensin II is identical to kinase II, the enzyme that degrades bradykinin, an endogenous vasodilator and smooth muscle relaxant.[79] Therefore, the vasorelaxant effects of these substances may be accentuated in the presence of ACE inhibitors. Thus, the reductions both in preload and afterload seen after an ACE inhibitor is administered may result from a number of different but interrelated mechanisms. Individual ACE inhibitors vary with respect to a number of different pharmacologic characteristics. Captopril contains a sulfhydryl group that binds directly to the zinc moiety of the enzyme. The remaining ACE inhibitors do not contain sulfhydryl groups and most, with the exception of fosinopril, bind via carboxyl groups. Fosinopril binds to ACE via a phosphoryl group. Captopril and lisinopril are active on administration, and the remaining ACE inhibitors are prodrugs that must be activated.

ACE inhibitors have emerged as the cornerstone in the medical management of CHF.[41,48,76] Currently captopril, enalapril, fosinopril, lisinopril, quinapril, and ramipril are approved by the U.S. Food and Drug Administration (FDA) for this indication.

Reductions in mortality and hospitalization rates have been found in patients with CHF receiving ACE inhibitor therapy regardless of the patient's NYHA functional class before treatment (Table 21.3).[77,78] Interestingly, in the patients with severe CHF (NYHA class IV) the reduction in total mortality was primarily a result of a reduction in progression of HF, whereas in the patients with mild to moderate CHF (NYHA class II to III) the mortality reduction was caused primarily by a reduction in sudden cardiac death. These findings have important implications for the mechanism through which ACE inhibitors exert their beneficial effects. Angiotensin II antagonism, reductions in sympathetic nerve activity and circulating norepinephrine,[80] and direct protective effects on the myocardium or coronary vasculature have been postulated as potential mechanisms through which ACE inhibitors affect mortality. In addition, the majority of healthcare costs attributed to CHF are direct costs of hospitalization. A 25% reduction in the hospitalization rate would lead to a $2 billion reduction in direct healthcare costs, or a net savings of more than $1 billion per year through the use of ACE inhibitors alone.[81]

ACE inhibitors also have important CHF-preventive effects when administered soon after acute myocardial infarction in patients with asymptomatic LV dysfunction (LVEF <40%; see Fig. 21.4).[82] These trials were based on the ability of ACE inhibitors to diminish the progressive ventricular remodeling observed soon after large myocardial infarctions. A meta-analysis of the trials in which ACE inhibitor therapy was initiated within 36 hours of myocardial infarction and

continued for 4 to 6 weeks showed a 7% reduction in mortality.[82] On average, approximately 5 lives would be saved per 1,000 patients treated with ACE inhibitor therapy. Approximately 85% of the mortality benefit occurs early, within the first week of therapy. Patients with large anterior infarcts and patients at high risk for post-acute myocardial infarction complications (Killip class 2 to 3, HR >100 bpm) derived the greatest benefit. A reduction in the frequency of CHF exacerbations also was observed. ACE inhibitor therapy was not associated with excess adverse effects in any subgroup, but hypotensive patients and patients in cardiogenic shock generally were excluded from analysis. In addition, a higher incidence of renal dysfunction and hypotension was observed in patients more than 75 years old.

ACE inhibitors appear to consistently improve the clinical status and longevity of patients with CHF. ACE inhibitor therapy should be initiated early, when signs and symptoms of CHF are absent or mild (i.e., NYHA class I and II). Current guidelines recommend the use of ACE inhibitors as first-line therapy before digoxin or diuretics in the absence of troubling symptoms and in combination with these agents and β-blockers (Fig. 21.2).[52] In addition, ACE inhibitors should be initiated early (days 1 and 2) after myocardial infarction if there is no evidence of cardiogenic shock or hypotension (systolic blood pressure <100 mm Hg).

Despite this extensive evidence of its beneficial effects, ACE inhibitors remain underused in patients with CHF. Analysis of prescribing patterns at an academic medical center in 1986 and 1994 indicated a significant but unsatisfactory increase in ACE inhibitor prescriptions among patients hospitalized for CHF (43% and 71%, respectively).[83] Additional analyses indicate that only 30% to 50% of patients with CHF receive ACE inhibitors.[84,85] Recent data suggest these numbers are improving. In ADHERE, 67.8% of eligible patients were treated with ACE inhibitors at hospital discharge.[86,87] In OPTIMIZE, 82.2% of eligible patients were treated with ACE inhibitors at discharge.[88] Similar evaluations in older adults with CHF have indicated underuse of ACE inhibitors, with an associated increase in adverse cardiovascular events in this population.[89,90]

ACE inhibitor dosages vary, but therapy generally should be initiated at low dosages (Table 21.6). Therapy initiation typically involves captopril dosages of 12.5 mg every 8 hours, enalapril maleate dosages of 5 mg twice daily, lisinopril 5 mg daily, or equivalent dosages of alternative ACE inhibitors. However, the actual dosage used depends on the patient's clinical status and risk of hypotension.[77] Risk factors associated with hypotension secondary to ACE inhibitor therapy include hyponatremia (serum sodium concentration <130 mEq/L), volume depletion after increased diuretic therapy or concurrent use of a potassium-sparing diuretic, and an elevated Scr concentration (>1.7 mg/dL).[91] The lowest possible starting dosage (e.g., captopril 3.125 mg, enalapril 1.25 mg, and lisinopril 2.5 mg) should be used in the aforementioned patients.

After therapy is initiated, current recommendations involve titrating the dosage upward at 3- to 7-day intervals to achieve the target dosages studied in the clinical trials.[77] Longer titration intervals may be indicated in patients at risk for adverse effects. Therefore, clinical observations such as systolic blood pressure, renal function, and the appearance of other adverse effects should be used to guide dosage adjustments until the target dosage is achieved. The beneficial effects of ACE inhibitor therapy appear to be dose-related, and every effort should be made to achieve the target dosage.[92,93] In support of this recommendation, results from the recent Assessment of Treatment with Lisinopril and Survival (ATLAS) trial indicated a trend toward lower mortality rates in patients receiving the higher lisinopril dosages (mean dosage difference 19 mg).[94] In addition, the higher dose was associated with greater improvements in the combined endpoint of mortality and progressive CHF. In contrast to the ATLAS study, the NETWORK trial did not find a significant dose-related reduction in mortality and morbidity for patients receiving 2.5 mg, 5 mg, and 10 mg twice daily.[95] However, the NETWORK trial was small, with relatively wide 95% confidence intervals. Despite data from the NETWORK trial, current recommendations suggest that ACE inhibitor dosages should be maximized to those used in clinical trials. Examples of target regimens used in clinical trials include captopril 50 mg every 8 hours, enalapril 10 mg twice daily, and lisinopril 10 mg daily (Table 21.6).[77] Patients unable to achieve target dosages should be maintained at the maximally tolerated dosage. Daily maintenance dosages probably can be reduced and the dosing interval extended (i.e., every 12 hours for captopril, every 24 hours for enalapril and quinapril, and every other day for lisinopril and ramipril) for patients with diminished renal function [i.e., estimated creatinine clearance (CL_{Cr}) <30 to 40 mL/minute; see Table 21.6].

The most common adverse effect of ACE inhibitors is hypotension. Peak hypotensive effects vary depending on the agent used. The peak hypotensive response to captopril generally occurs within 30 to 90 minutes of dosing, whereas this effect often occurs within 2 to 4 hours after enalapril and 7 hours after lisinopril. A single study showed that hypotension often was more severe and prolonged after enalapril than after captopril.[96] However, this investigation used large, fixed dosages of both drugs rather than optimizing the dosage of each agent to either hemodynamic or clinical effects. In patients at high risk of adverse events (NYHA class IV, baseline hypotension, baseline renal insufficiency) it may be advisable to administer the first dose under the watchful eye of a clinician so that first-dose syncope or presyncope can be treated appropriately. Blood pressure should be assessed before an ACE inhibitor is administered and closely monitored during the period of expected maximal hypotensive effects.[77] However, most HF patients tolerate ACE inhibitors without a problem and can be started on therapy without this close level of monitoring. An absolute blood pressure under which ACE inhibitor administration is contraindicated has not been identified.[77] Administration of an ACE inhibitor in patients with a systolic blood pressure below 90 mm Hg is left to the clinical judgment of the healthcare professional. Patients who are dehydrated or hyponatremic or have a low intravascular fluid volume are particularly susceptible to ACE inhibitor-induced orthostasis and syncope. Diuretics should be prescribed at the lowest dose that maintains euvolemia to avoid the potential pharmacodynamic drug interaction with ACE inhibitors. Patients who experience hypotension after ACE inhibitor initiation should have their drug regimen reviewed to evaluate whether diuretic doses can be decreased or unnecessary medications also affecting blood pressure can be discontinued.

Renal dysfunction is an adverse effect associated with ACE inhibitor therapy. Compensatory stimulation of angiotensin II production preserves renal blood flow in patients with CHF.[96] Therefore, after ACE inhibitor therapy is initiated, GFR is reduced and acute increases in BUN and Scr can occur, particularly during the first 6 weeks of therapy.[77] BUN and Scr may normalize with continued therapy or after decreases in the diuretic dosage in hypovolemic patients. Nonetheless, renal function may not improve, and some degree of renal insufficiency may persist in some patients. Use of an ACE inhibitor is not contraindicated in patients with underlying renal insufficiency because baseline renal function does not predict the development of subsequent renal dysfunction.[97] Interestingly, there is a strong association between long-term preservation of renal function and acute increases in Scr of less than 30% above baseline that stabilize within the first 2 months of ACE inhibitor therapy.[98] The relationship persists for patients with baseline Scr greater than 1.4 mg per dL. ACE inhibitor withdrawal should be considered only when Scr increases more than 30% above baseline within the first 2 months of ACE inhibitor therapy.[98] However, special attention is needed to detect patients who may have both CHF and bilateral renal artery stenosis (or single renal artery stenosis in patients with only one kidney). Because many patients with CHF have severe CAD, atherosclerosis of other arteries is expected. In a study of 89 patients referred to an HF unit, 6 (7%) had renal artery stenosis.[99] The suspicion of renal artery stenosis is raised when the Scr abruptly increases after ACE inhibitor therapy is initiated. Another clue to renal artery stenosis is late-onset (>50 years) HTN. When renal artery stenosis is confirmed (usually with digital subtraction angiography), angioplasty or surgery can correct the stenosis. The patient can then safely receive ACE inhibitor therapy for CHF. The ACE inhibitor must be discontinued if surgical or mechanical correction of the renal artery stenosis proves impossible.

ACE inhibitor-induced cough often contributes to the discontinuation of therapy.[77] The mechanism through which an ACE inhibitor produces cough is believed to involve the accumulation of bradykinin, a known mediator of bronchoconstriction.[100,101] The consequence is the development of a dry, nonproductive cough. However, cough in patients with CHF may also result from pulmonary edema. Consequently, the actual incidence of ACE inhibitor-induced cough is difficult to ascertain. In the Study of Patients Intolerant to Converting Enzyme Inhibitors (SPICE) registry, only 3.6% of patients were intolerant of ACE inhibitors due to cough.[102] The clinician should try to determine the cause of cough before discontinuing ACE inhibitor therapy. The ACE inhibitor should be discontinued or the dosage reduced only if the cough is believed to be related to the ACE inhibitor and is intolerable to the patient. Switching to an alternative ACE inhibitor[77] or to an ARB[103] may be helpful.

Urinary K^+ excretion is reduced and serum K^+ increased in patients receiving ACE inhibitor therapy. All diuretic and electrolyte therapy should be assessed before ACE inhibitor therapy is initiated. Discontinuation or dosage reductions of potassium supplements or minimizing intake of high-potassium foods (i.e., salt substitutes) may be necessary and should be considered in patients with high serum K^+ concentrations.

One week after ACE inhibitor therapy begins and after any dosage adjustments, BUN, Scr, and K^+ concentrations should be assessed.[77] Routine laboratory assessments should be obtained every 3 months. Maculopapular rashes, taste disturbances, leukopenia, and proteinuria have been observed during ACE inhibitor administration. Therefore, it is prudent to check a baseline complete blood cell count with differential and repeat it in 2 weeks and again every 6 months after ACE inhibitor therapy begins.

Pharmacodynamic drug interactions involving excessive hypotension can occur in patients receiving ACE inhibitors concurrently with other vasodilators. In addition, hyperkalemia can develop in patients receiving potassium supplements or potassium-sparing diuretics in combination with ACE inhibitor therapy.[77] NSAIDs, including aspirin, can attenuate the vasodilatory effects of ACE inhibitors in patients with CHF.[77] Chronic use of NSAIDs should be avoided, as previously discussed. The interaction between aspirin and ACE inhibitors has been evaluated in a limited number of clinical trials involving small numbers of patients. Single-dose aspirin administration has been associated with variable hemodynamic effects. Retrospective reviews indicate that the concurrent use of aspirin may reduce the mortality benefit produced by ACE inhibitors. However, a recent analysis of data from the Benzabrate Infarction Prevention (BIP) trial contradicts these findings.[104] In the BIP trial, mortality among patients with CAD and CHF was lower for patients receiving aspirin and ACE inhibitors than for those not taking aspirin (24% vs. 34%, respectively, $p < 0.001$). Consequently, concurrent use of ACE inhibitors and aspirin depends on the presence of additional indications for aspirin therapy and is warranted in patients with CAD. Although pharmacokinetic interactions with ACE inhibitors are rare, captopril has been shown to decrease digoxin clearance.

Angiotensin II Type 1 Receptor Blockers. Despite reductions in mortality, the use of ACE inhibitors in patients with CHF does not completely suppress angiotensin II formation.

In addition, angiotensin II formation can occur independently of ACE-mediated pathways.[13,105] Vasoconstriction, myocardial remodeling, and sodium and water retention result from binding of angiotensin II to the angiotensin II type 1 (AT_1) receptors. Recently, agents have been developed that bind to the AT_1 receptor, thereby blocking the deleterious effects of angiotensin II. Consequently, the ARBs may provide more complete suppression of angiotensin II activity than that achieved during ACE inhibitor therapy. However, ARBs, unlike ACE inhibitors, do not facilitate bradykinin accumulation. Given their different mechanisms of action, different clinical effects can be expected between the two classes.

ARBs produce dose-dependent inhibition of angiotensin II activity.[105] The individual ARBs vary in their pharmacokinetic profiles (Table 21.6). Losartan is metabolized to an active metabolite (E3174). Losartan and E3174 both antagonize the AT_1 receptor, but the metabolite is 10 times more potent and demonstrates noncompetitive receptor inhibition. Candesartan, also a prodrug, is converted in the gastrointestinal tract to the active compound (CV-11974). Valsartan, telmisartan, and irbesartan do not need activation after administration. All of the currently available agents selectively inhibit angiotensin II binding to the AT_1 receptor. Significant differences in clinical response to the agents remain to be determined.

The efficacy of AT_1 receptor blockade via administration of ARBs including losartan, irbesartan, valsartan, and candesartan has recently been evaluated in a number of small clinical trials. The Evaluation of Losartan in the Elderly (ELITE) trial randomized 722 patients with symptomatic HF (NYHA class II and III) older than 65 years of age to losartan (50 mg/day) or captopril (50 mg three times a day).[103] The trial was undertaken primarily to compare the safety of the two agents in patients with CHF. Patients enrolled were not previously receiving ACE inhibitor therapy. Duration of the trial was 48 weeks. Losartan administration was associated with a 32% lower mortality rate than that of the captopril group (4.8% vs. 8.7%, $p < 0.035$). However, the number of events was small and mortality was not a prespecified primary endpoint of the study. The difference in mortality resulted primarily from a difference in the rate of sudden death. Significant differences in renal function were not observed between the two agents. No difference in the incidence of hospital admission rates was observed between the two agents, and NYHA functional class improved equally in both treatment groups.

The results in the ELITE trial were not substantiated by the Randomized Evaluation of Strategies for Left Ventricular Dysfunction (RESOLVD) study, a dose-ranging trial comparing three different dosages of candesartan with enalapril alone or in combination with candesartan.[106] Data from the RESOLVD trial showed a 60% higher mortality associated with the use of candesartan than with enalapril. As with ELITE, RESOLVD was not powered to evaluate mortality (Fig. 21.2).

Several large trials evaluating AT_1 receptor blockers in heart failure have now been completed. ELITE II, Val-HeFT, the CHARM program, and VALIANT are recent trials that were adequately powered and prospectively defined mortality or a composite clinical outcome as a primary endpoint.

The ELITE II study was a randomized trial of losartan versus captopril in 3,152 patients with NYHA II to IV heart failure and systolic dysfunction. The primary endpoint of the study was all-cause mortality. Patients were titrated to a dose of captopril 50 mg three times daily or losartan 50 mg once daily. Patients were followed for a median of 1.5 years. There were 280 (17.7%) deaths in the losartan group compared with 250 (15.9%) deaths in the captopril group (hazard ratio 1.13, confidence interval 0.95 to 1.35, $p = 0.16$). Thus, no significant differences were detected between groups.[107]

The Val-HeFT trial was a randomized trial of valsartan versus standard therapy in 5,010 patients with NYHA II to IV clinical stable heart failure and systolic dysfunction. There were two primary endpoints of the study: mortality and the composite of mortality and morbidity (resuscitated cardiac arrest, hospitalization for HF, or HF symptoms requiring intravenous inotrope or vasodilator therapy). The majority of patients (93%) were receiving background ACE inhibitor therapy. Mortality was not different between the two treatment groups. The combined endpoint of mortality and morbidity was reduced in the valsartan group (28.8% vs. 32.1%, relative risk 0.87, confidence interval 0.77 to 0.97, $p = 0.009$).[108] The reduction in mortality and morbidity was largely driven by the subgroup of patients not on ACE inhibitor therapy or on suboptimal ACE inhibitor doses. Valsartan is FDA approved for heart failure. The specific indication as quoted from the product labeling reads, "Diovan is indicated for the treatment of heart failure (NYHA II-IV) in patients who are intolerant of angiotensin-converting enzyme inhibitors. In a controlled trial, Diovan significantly reduced hospitalizations for heart failure. There is no evidence that Diovan provides added benefits when it is used with an adequate dose of an ACE inhibitor."[109]

The CHARM program comprised three parallel, integrated, randomized, double-blind, placebo-controlled clinical trials comparing candesartan in three populations of patients with symptomatic HF. The CHARM added trial studied candesartan in addition to ACE inhibitor therapy, the CHARM alternative trial studied candesartan in patients with previous intolerance to ACE inhibitor therapy, and the CHARM preserved trial studied candesartan in patients with LVEF of more than 40%. The primary endpoint of the three studies combined was all-cause mortality. Each study independently evaluated the effect of candesartan on cardiovascular death or HF hospitalization. The study population consisted of 7,601 patients. For the overall study, there was a trend toward lower mortality in the patients treated with candesartan (23% vs. 25%, hazard ratio 0.91, confidence interval 0.83 to 1, $p = 0.055$). In the CHARM added trial,

a significant reduction in the composite endpoint was observed. In the CHARM intolerant trial, a reduction in the composite endpoint was also observed. A nonsignificant trend toward a lower risk of the composite endpoint was observed in the CHARM preserved trial.[110] The CHARM program resulted in an FDA-approved indication for candesartan for the treatment of NYHA II to IV heart failure and systolic dysfunction.

Finally, the VALIANT trial studied valsartan, captopril, or both in 14,808 patients 0.5 to 10 days after myocardial infarction with signs of HF. Thus, the study population in VALIANT differs from the other trials of AT_1 antagonists. There were two primary comparisons in VALIANT: valsartan versus captopril and valsartan plus captopril versus captopril alone. The primary endpoint was all-cause mortality. The mortality rate was 19.9% in the valsartan group, 19.3% in the valsartan plus captopril group, and 19.5% in the captopril group. There were no significant differences between treatment groups.[111]

Adverse effects associated with the ARBs are similar to those observed during ACE inhibitor therapy. The incidence of hypotension and renal dysfunction observed with ARB therapy appears equal to that observed during ACE inhibitor therapy. However, the incidence of cough is lower during ARB therapy, as would be expected given the absence of bradykinin accumulation.[103]

Nitrates. Nitrates were one of the initial groups of vasodilating agents used to manage CHF.[112] The beneficial effects of nitrates are believed to be mediated by nitric oxide formation. Nitric oxide, through cyclic guanosine monophosphate (cGMP) formation, reduces intracellular calcium concentrations, leading to vasodilation. Nitrates decrease preload predominantly through vasodilation of venous capacitance vessels. Nitrates may also decrease afterload via dilation of large arteries and arterioles when administered in high dosages. LV filling pressures, mean pulmonary artery pressure, systemic vascular resistance, severity of mitral regurgitation, and systolic blood pressure decrease but the cardiac index increases during exercise after nitrates are administered in patients with chronic CHF.[112] Improvements in treadmill exercise times, systolic function, CHF symptoms, and hospitalization rates have been observed after nitrates were added to ACE inhibitor therapy. Therefore, nitrates may be added to ACE inhibitors, but their impact on mortality is not known.[112]

The African American Heart Failure Trial (A-HeFT) demonstrated the effects of the combination of isosorbide dinitrate and hydralazine in African American patients with HF. All patients were African American, had NYHA III or IV symptoms of heart failure, had systolic dysfunction, and were treated with standard background therapy. The study enrolled 1,050 patients and randomized them to isosorbide dinitrate (titrated to 40 mg three times a day) plus hydralazine (titrated to 75 mg three times a day). The primary endpoint of the study was a clinical composite score calculated from weighted values for all-cause mortality, HF hospitalization, and change in quality of life. The trial was terminated early due to a significantly higher mortality rate in the placebo group compared to the hydralazine/nitrates group (10.2% vs. 6.2%, hazard ratio 0.57, $p = 0.01$). The primary composite score was also lower for the hydralazine/nitrates group.[113]

Nitrate tolerance has been found consistently when the vascular endothelium is constantly exposed to nitroglycerin.[112] Investigation into this issue has revealed that tolerance appears to be mediated by excessive free radical formation caused by continuous exposure of the vascular tissue to organic nitrates. Free radicals impair nitric oxide release, thereby preventing cGMP-mediated vasodilation. Inhibition of nitrate tolerance via antioxidant administration is under investigation. Currently, the most frequently used method of avoiding nitrate tolerance involves intermittent administration, which provides a daily "washout" period. Of the available nitrate formulations used to treat chronic CHF, isosorbide dinitrate (ISDN) is the most frequently prescribed and best-studied agent (Table 21.6). Although many large clinical trials have used a four-times-daily dosing strategy, 10 to 80 mg three times daily, administered at 7 AM, 12 noon, and 5 PM, for example, would retain a 12-hour nitrate-free dosing interval. Similarly, if nitroglycerin patches are prescribed, they should be applied for 12 hours and then removed for 12 hours. Isosorbide mononitrates, although not well studied, also are used in CHF. Because most patients experience dyspnea on exertion during the waking hours, the nitrate-free interval usually is at night. These intermittent dosing regimens do not preclude using short-acting sublingual tablets or lingual spray nitroglycerin for episodes of acute dyspnea or angina.

The most common adverse nitrate effect is headache, which often responds to mild analgesics such as acetaminophen (Table 21.6). Headaches usually disappear after several days of nitrate administration. Some patients continue to experience severe headaches with nitrates and may not tolerate any nitrate administration. Dizziness, flushing, postural hypotension, weakness, and occasionally skin rash have also been reported.

In summary, nitrates are safe and effective vasodilators useful as adjunctive therapy to ACE inhibitors or in combination with hydralazine in CHF treatment.

Hydralazine. Hydralazine is a direct-acting arteriolar dilator that principally reduces afterload. Reductions in afterload by hydralazine may also result in moderate reductions in preload because of the dependence of LV filling pressure on the resistance to ventricular emptying during systole. Hydralazine can markedly reduce LV filling pressure in patients with mitral or aortic valve regurgitation. Clinically, hydralazine is most commonly used in combination with other vasodilators with greater preload-reducing properties, such as nitrates.[114,115]

Studies using hydralazine monotherapy in patients with CHF (in dosages up to 225 mg per day) indicate that hydralazine, although improving quality of life, does not improve survival.[116,117] However, the combination of oral ISDN with hydralazine was the first pharmacologic therapy found to reduce mortality from CHF.[114] The Veterans Administrative Cooperative Study on Vasodilator Therapy of Heart Failure I (VHeFT-I) showed that the ISDN–hydralazine combination improved systolic function and reduced 2-year CHF mortality by 34%.[114] However, in VHeFT-II, enalapril conferred a greater survival benefit than the ISDN–hydralazine combination.[115] Consequently, combination ISDN–hydralazine therapy should be reserved for patients unable to tolerate ACE inhibitor therapy. However, the A-HeFT results, as reported earlier, suggest that the combination of hydralazine and nitrates may be particularly efficacious in the African American population. This may be due to the fact that African Americans have lower renin angiotensin system activity and a lower bioavailability of nitric oxide.[113]

Hydralazine dosages for treating patients with chronic CHF vary greatly, even though the placebo-controlled trials used fixed dosage regimens.[117] Baseline estimates of a patient's systolic blood pressure, resting HR, and renal function should be determined before therapy is initiated. Hydralazine and ISDN dosages for patients receiving both agents in the VHeFT trials were 270 and 136 mg per day, respectively.[114,115] The target dosage in A-HeFT was isosorbide 40 mg three times a day and hydralazine 75 mg three times a day; 68% of patients achieved this dosage. The total daily dosage can be divided into equal doses administered every 6, 8, or 12 hours, although the every-8-hours or three-times-daily schedule works best with current recommendations for prescribing ISDN (Table 21.6). Current data suggest that the dosage should be titrated to approximately 300 mg per day while systolic blood pressure ($\geq$95 mm Hg), HR (avoidance of a resting tachycardia), improvements in pulmonary and systemic symptoms, and the development of adverse effects are monitored. Patients with the highest elevations in central venous pressure have required dosages as high as 2,400 mg per day, and those with CL_{Cr} less than 35 mL per minute may exhibit the longest duration of action ($\geq$12 hours).

Unfortunately, side effects increase with increasing daily dosages (Table 21.6). Side effects forced discontinuation of therapy in 19% of patients receiving ISDN–hydralazine in the VHeFT-I trial.[114] The most common adverse effects include headache, palpitations, postural hypotension, nausea, vomiting, and systemic lupus erythematosus (seen particularly with dosages >200 mg/day). In A-HeFT, lupus was not reported as an adverse event in the main paper, but in a subsequent letter to the editor, the authors indicated that one patient in the entire study population (n = 1,050) reported a lupus-like syndrome.[118] In V-HeFT, antibody studies were performed and no excess of lupus was observed in the treatment group compared to the placebo group. However, previous studies in hypertension have reported an incidence of lupus of 10.4% with dosages over 200 mg per day.[119] Clinicians should be aware of the potential for this adverse effect and monitor patients accordingly. Salt and water retention may occur during long-term therapy with hydralazine. Mild to moderate increases in resting HR and myocardial ischemic events in patients with CHF also have been reported after hydralazine administration.

Prazosin. Prazosin is a specific, competitive antagonist of postsynaptic α_1-receptors located in the walls of precapillary arteriolar resistance vessels and postcapillary venous capacitance vessels. Therefore, prazosin is considered a balanced vasodilator in that it reduces both preload and afterload to approximately the same degree. Prazosin therapy was one of the treatment arms in the VHeFT-I trial.[114] However, prazosin therapy did not result in lower mortality rates than did placebo. Therefore, prazosin is not a component of the standard regimen for HF.

Calcium Channel Blockers. Several theoretical reasons exist for considering calcium channel blockers in CHF treatment: they are powerful arteriolar dilators and thus reduce LV afterload; they produce hemodynamic effects similar to those of hydralazine, which has improved survival in patients with mild to moderate CHF; they have anti-ischemic effects, making them an attractive therapeutic option for treating CHF caused by CAD; and they improve diastolic dysfunction, a significant cause of HF symptoms, through their beneficial effects on LV relaxation.[120] However, the first-generation calcium channel antagonists, verapamil, diltiazem, and nifedipine, have universally produced hemodynamic and clinical deterioration in patients with HF caused by systolic dysfunction. Possible explanations for these detrimental effects include direct negative inotropic properties, further activation of deleterious neurohormonal responses, and an increase in blood volume, which may increase afterload.

Two recent placebo-controlled trials evaluated the effects of second-generation dihydropyridines, amlodipine and felodipine, when added to ACE inhibitors, digoxin, and diuretics.[121–123]

In the Prospective Randomized Amlodipine Survival Evaluation (PRAISE) trial, amlodipine significantly reduced combined morbidity and mortality by 31% and all-cause mortality by 45% in patients with nonischemic CHF.[121] Reductions in both sudden cardiac death and death secondary to progressive HF were observed.[122] No beneficial effect was observed in patients with CHF secondary to ischemic cardiomyopathy. PRAISE II investigated the role of amlodipine in patients with nonischemic cardiomyopathy. The primary endpoint was all-cause mortality. No differences in outcome were observed for patients treated with amlodipine versus placebo. The results were presented at the American College of Cardiology 49th Scientific Sessions in Anaheim in March 2000 but have not yet been published in manuscript form.

VHeFT-III compared the addition of felodipine (5 mg twice daily) with placebo in 450 men (NYHA class II and

III) already receiving enalapril and a diuretic.[123] Felodipine did not significantly reduce mortality (13.8% vs. 12.8%) or hospitalization rates (43% vs. 42%) during an average follow-up of 18 months.

In summary, there is not currently a role for second-generation calcium channel blockers in CHF management. Amlodipine may be used in patients with HF to treat persistent hypertension or angina that is inadequately controlled by ACE inhibitors, AT_1 blockers, or β-blockers.

β-Adrenergic Blocking Agents. Until the late 1990s, β-blockers were not recommended for patients with HF. Today, however, β-blockers are a cornerstone of therapy for chronic HF patients. This transition is a result of several randomized trials showing improved survival and reduced need for hospitalizations for patients receiving β-blockers. Chronic activation of the sympathetic nervous system in patients with CHF is associated with alterations in the structure and function of the myocardium, particularly in β-receptor density and sensitivity. Interruption of sympathetic nervous system activity by β-adrenergic blockers counteracts the deleterious effects previously discussed. β-Adrenergic receptor blockers antagonize the adverse effects of excessive activation of the sympathetic nervous system, leading to a reduction in plasma norepinephrine and upregulation of myocardial β_1-receptors. β-Blockers also reverse the remodeling process that occurs in HF.

Three generations of β-blockers are available.[124] First-generation β-blockers nonspecifically block both β_1- and β_2-adrenergic receptors. Second-generation β-blockers include the β_1-specific antagonists, metoprolol and bisoprolol; the third-generation β-blockers, bucindolol and carvedilol, produce nonspecific β-blockade but have additional vasodilatory properties. Carvedilol produces vasodilation via α_1-blockade, inhibits vascular smooth muscle proliferation, and is an antioxidant. On the other hand, bucindolol produces vasodilation independent of α_1-blocking mechanisms. The efficacy of the different β-blockers has been examined in several large randomized trials.

Two different formulations of metoprolol have been studied in prospective, randomized, placebo-controlled trials.[125,126] The Metoprolol in Dilated Cardiomyopathy (MDC) trial evaluated the use of conventional-release metoprolol in 383 patients with dilated cardiomyopathy.[125] Metoprolol therapy was associated with improvements in exercise tolerance, quality of life, NYHA functional class, and the number of CHF exacerbations necessitating hospitalization. A significant difference in mortality (19 deaths in the metoprolol group and 23 in the placebo group, $p < 0.69$) was not observed. However, in a more recent study of nearly 4,000 patients with predominantly NYHA class II or III CHF, controlled-release/extended-release metoprolol conferred a 34% reduction in mortality.[126] Both sudden deaths and deaths caused by worsening CHF were significantly decreased.

The Cardiac Insufficiency Bisoprolol Study II (CIBIS-II) randomized 2,647 patients (NYHA class III and IV) to receive bisoprolol (maximum dose 10 mg) or placebo.[127] The trial was stopped early (mean follow-up, 1.3 years) upon observation of a 34% reduction in mortality, a 44% reduction in sudden death, and a 20% reduction in hospitalization rates in the group receiving bisoprolol.

The efficacy of carvedilol was assessed in the U.S. Carvedilol trial involving 1,094 patients with predominantly NYHA class II and III CHF.[128] The relative reductions in mortality and hospitalization for patients randomized to receive carvedilol were 65% and 36%, respectively. Reductions in mortality caused by progressive pump failure and sudden cardiac death were observed. Based on data extrapolated from the U.S. study, the cost per life-year saved for carvedilol ranges between $12,799 and $29,477, indicating that carvedilol therapy compares favorably with commonly used medical interventions.[129]

The U.S. Carvedilol Study provided interesting results, but it was not a mortality trial. To accurately evaluate the effect of carvedilol on mortality, the COPERNICUS trial was conducted. This trial randomized 2,289 patients to carvedilol or placebo. These patients had NYHA III or IV heart failure and systolic dysfunction. COPERNICUS randomized the most severely ill/symptomatic population to date in a β-blocker trial. All patients were treated with background standard therapy. In the placebo group, 190 patients died compared to 130 patients in the carvedilol group, a 35% decrease in the mortality risk ($p = 0.00013$).[130]

Given the reduction in mortality and hospitalization observed in these trials, the use of β-blockers is currently advocated in patients with stable CHF who lack contraindications to β-blockade. Patients should be clinically stable and on initial to medium ACE inhibitor doses before a β-blocker is added.[41,48,124]

However, despite these favorable effects, several questions remain with respect to β-blocker therapy. For instance, debate continues as to which generation of β-blockers affords the greatest clinical benefit. A meta-analysis that combined the results of 18 trials indicated a 49% reduction in mortality for patients receiving nonselective β-blockers (carvedilol, bucindolol), with a more modest 18% reduction in the group receiving β_1-selective agents (metoprolol, bisoprolol).[131] However, a small, prospective, randomized, open-label trial involving patients with predominantly mild to moderate HF (NYHA class II to III) directly compared the effects of carvedilol (n = 37) and metoprolol (n = 30).[132] After 6 months of therapy, no significantly different effects on mortality, quality of life, ejection fraction, exercise capacity, and incidence of adverse effects were observed between the two agents. Both drugs were well tolerated during initiation and upward titration of therapy, and no difference in the ability to achieve the target dosage was observed between the two groups. The Carvedilol or Metoprolol European Trial (COMET) compared the two β-blockers in patients with NYHA II to IV heart failure. The primary endpoint of the study was all-cause mortality and a composite of all-cause mortality and hospitalization. The study enrolled

1,511 patients. The target dose for carvedilol was 25 mg twice daily and 50 mg twice daily for metoprolol tartrate. Mortality was 17% lower for patients treated with carvedilol compared to metoprolol tartrate (hazard ratio 0.83, confidence interval 0.74 to 0.93, $P = 0.0017$).[133] The results of this study stimulated much controversy in the medical community.[134] Several criticisms of the trial were brought forth, including the dosing of metoprolol tartrate and the choice of metoprolol tartrate rather than the sustained-release succinate form studied in MERIT-HF. Despite the controversy, the practice of evidence-based medicine suggests that the only β-blockers that should be used in HF are carvedilol, metoprolol succinate (controlled release or extended release), or bisoprolol. The COMET results suggest that all β-blockers are not the same, and the clinical trial results cannot be equally applied to all β-blockers (i.e., atenolol). Atenolol is commonly used in patients with heart failure, yet no evidence exists supporting this approach. Carvedilol may be the preferred β-blocker in patients with severe HF, because the only study to specifically evaluate this population was COPERNICUS. Carvedilol is available in very low doses (3.125 mg, 6.25 mg, and 12.5 mg), and metoprolol succinate (controlled release or extended release) is also manufactured in doses appropriate for initiating in HF patients (25-mg scored tablet).

β-Blockers may also be prescribed in patients with severe CHF who are clinically stable. In a subgroup analysis of COPERNICUS, the most severely ill patients also benefitted from carvedilol therapy. The subgroup of severely ill patients in COPERNICUS were defined as patients with one of the following characteristics: pulmonary rales, ascites, or edema at randomization; three or more hospitalizations for HF within the previous 12 months; hospitalization at the time of randomization; need for intravenous inotropes or vasodilators within 14 days before randomization; or ejection fraction of 15% or less. These high-risk patients had fewer deaths and other clinical events both during the first 8 weeks and for the duration of the study compared to the subgroup of patients without the high-risk characteristics. There was no difference in adverse events for the high-risk versus non–high-risk patients.[135] Carvedilol has a FDA-approved indication for the treatment of mild to severe HF.

The Heart Failure Society of America Guidelines published in 1999 recommended that β-blockers be withheld until patients were clinically stable. It was recommended that β-blockers be withheld for a period of 2 to 4 weeks after a hospitalization for HF. Unfortunately, it became apparent that many patients were not receiving the life-saving benefits associated with β-blockade. Initiation of therapy in the hospital has previously been shown to be effective at ensuring that statins, aspirin, and other evidence-based therapies are prescribed after myocardial infarction. It was hypothesized that this would also be true for β-blockers in HF. The Initiation Management Predischarge Assessment of Carvedilol Therapy for Heart Failure (IMPACT-HF) study was performed to determine whether in-hospital initiation of carvedilol was a safe and effective method of ensuring that patients receive β-blockade. Patients hospitalized for HF who had been treated, were clinically stable, and were within 24 hours of discharge were randomized to receive in-hospital initiation of carvedilol or standard care. The study enrolled 363 patients. Slightly over 90% of patients randomized to in-hospital initiation of carvedilol remained on therapy at 60 days after the hospitalization. In-hospital initiation was not associated with worsening HF symptoms, hypotension, or bradycardia.[136] The revised Heart Failure Society of America Guidelines are expected to be published in 2005, and it is expected that these revisions will extend the recommendation to include all patients with mild to severe HF and will recommend that in-hospital initiation be considered.

Most studies of β-blockers for CHF have enrolled NYHA class II or III patients.[131] Retrospective analyses of the Survival and Ventricular Enlargement (SAVE) and Study of Left Ventricular Dysfunction (SOLVD) prevention trials revealed that the combination of β-blockers and ACE inhibitors significantly reduces mortality in patients with asymptomatic LV dysfunction but without CHF (Fig. 21.4).[137,138] Data from ongoing trials are needed to assess the impact of β-blockade in patients with regard to these issues. Additional data are needed about the use of β-blockers in older adults, because the majority of trials enrolled patients less than 80 years old.

As with ACE inhibitors, initiation of β-blocker therapy begins with low doses that are increased slowly and carefully (Table 21.7). The carvedilol dose begins at 3.125 mg twice daily and is doubled every 2 weeks to a maximum of 25 mg twice a day (weight <85 kg) or 50 mg twice a day (weight >85 kg). In the CIBIS trial, bisoprolol was initiated at 1.25 mg a day.[127] The dose was increased gradually at weekly intervals to 10 mg according to patient tolerance. The starting dosage for metoprolol (controlled release/extended release) was 12.5 mg and 25 mg once daily for 2 weeks for NYHA class III to IV and II, respectively.[126] Thereafter, the dosage was increased to 50 mg once daily for 2 weeks, then

100 mg daily for 2 weeks, and finally to the target dose of 200 mg per day. The titration can be very patient-specific, and the dose can be increased at biweekly intervals by 25% or 50%, rather than 100%, depending on the patient.

Patient monitoring is needed when initiating and titrating β-blocker therapy (Table 21.7). Blood pressure and HR should be assessed before initiation of therapy or dosage adjustment and after the first dose of the new dosing regimen is administered. Commonly observed adverse effects associated with β-blocker therapy include symptomatic and asymptomatic hypotension and bradycardia. Clinical decompensation of CHF can occur, and initiating β-blocker therapy in patients with CHF entails extensive patient education to ensure compliance with the medication regimen. Expected benefits are achieved after several months of continued drug use. Before therapy begins, patients should understand that although acutely their symptoms may worsen, long-term improvements in their CHF may be obtained with the use of β-blocker therapy. In addition, dosage adjustments of their other medications, especially diuretics and ACE inhibitors, may be needed to alleviate symptoms during the initial titration period. It may be necessary to reduce the β-blocker dosage during severe CHF exacerbations. It is generally recommended that a β-blocker be maintained during an HF exacerbation, unless the drug was recently started or if the patient is exhibiting signs of severe low-output failure.[48] These complications are rare, and the vast majority of patients tolerate β-blocker therapy without difficulty.

Many clinicians remain reluctant to use β-blockers in patients with pulmonary disease. Data support the use of these agents in patients with chronic obstructive pulmonary disease and in patients with mild intermittent or mild persistent asthma. The benefits of β-blockade outweigh the risks in these patients. In this setting, metoprolol succinate is preferred, because it is a β_1-selective agent. In addition, the sustained-release formulation minimizes the high peak concentrations that may be associated with blockade of the β_2 receptor. Selectivity may be lost at dosages of 150 to 200

TABLE 21.7	Dosing Considerations for β-Blockers				
Drugs	**Starting Dosage**	**Target Dosage**	**Adverse Effect**	**Altered Kinetics**	**Monitoring Parameters**
Carvedilol	3.125 mg BID	25 mg BID (wt <85 kg) 50 mg BID (wt >85 kg)	Hypotension Bradycardia CHF exacerbation	Hepatic dysfunction Concomitant administration of CYP2D6 inhibitors or substrates Poor metabolizers of CYP2D6	Blood pressure Heart rate CHF signs and symptoms Hepatic function Initiation of agents that inhibit CYP2D6
Metoprolol CR/XL	12.5–25 mg QD	200 QD	As for carvedilol	As for carvedilol	As for carvedilol

CHF, congestive heart failure; CR/XL, controlled release/extended release; CYP, cytochrome P-450.

mg per day, and patients taking doses above this threshold should be monitored for exacerbation of pulmonary disease. Carvedilol is a nonselective β-blocker and in general is not recommended in these patients.[139,140]

Diuretics. Diuretics continue to be an integral component of symptomatic CHF management; most patients are maintained on some diuretic regimen (Figs. 21.2 to 21.6). Principally through the excretion of excess sodium and water, the major beneficial effect of chronically administered diuretics is the relief of pulmonary and systemic congestive signs and symptoms.[141,142] Diuretics also may indirectly provide favorable hemodynamic effects by decreasing intraventricular wall tension. This occurs principally through a reduction in preload and secondary to venodilation. Thus, preload reduction may slightly improve systolic function. In addition to improving signs and symptoms, a home-based flexible diuretic regimen, adjusted by the patient according to changing dietary factors and weight, may enhance other quality-of-life aspects such as patient's control over this frustrating chronic condition and a decreased need for office visits or hospitalization. Diuretics as monotherapy do not prolong life. However, adding spironolactone (25 to 50 mg/day) to a regimen of an ACE inhibitor, loop diuretic, and digoxin in NYHA class III and IV patients resulted in a 30% reduction in the risk of mortality and a 35% decrease in the risk of hospitalization for worsening HF. There was also a 32% reduction in risk of death from cardiac causes. Spironolactone was well tolerated, with 10% of patients developing gynecomastia. The incidence of serious hyperkalemia was minimal.[143,144] A new aldosterone antagonist, eplerenone, has also shown a beneficial effect on survival for patients with HF after myocardial infarction. Eplerenone is a selective antagonist and has less hormone-related side effects such as gynecomastia.[145] Eplerenone is significantly more expensive than spironolactone. In general, eplerenone should be considered only for patients who have experienced gynecomastia with spironolactone.

ACE inhibitors do not completely suppress aldosterone production. Spironolactone antagonizes aldosterone, which mediates sodium retention, potassium loss, myocardial norepinephrine uptake, and myocardial fibrosis.[144,146] In addition, diuretics play an important preventive role by decreasing the occurrence of CHF in patients with HTN.[147] Further enhancement of neurohormonal activation is a negative aspect of the use of thiazides or loop diuretics in CHF.

Principles of Diuretic Use. Before diuretic therapy is initiated for a patient with symptomatic CHF, a number of general principles of diuretic usage should be considered[148,149]:

- Therapy to rid patients of all traces of peripheral edema often is unnecessary and may be harmful.
- Begin therapy with the smallest effective dose and titrate upward to minimize electrolyte imbalances and to keep weight loss at 0.5 to 1.0 kg per day, except in extreme cases of pulmonary edema.

- The more proximally a diuretic acts within the nephron, the greater the loss of fluid and electrolytes.
- Diuretics, which act proximally at the terminal distal tubule, where sodium is exchanged for both potassium and hydrogen, probably will produce both hypokalemia and metabolic alkalosis.
- Diuretics that induce hypokalemia often cause hypomagnesemia.
- Diuretics should be administered as frequently (or infrequently) as necessary.
- Combination diuretic therapy may be needed as CHF worsens.
- Osmotic diuretics generally are not useful in CHF management.
- Mild (<3 g/day) to moderate (<2 g/day) dietary Na^+ restriction is important for maintaining diuretic effectiveness.
- With the exception of spironolactone, all diuretics act at ionic luminal transport sites via access to renal tubular fluid.
- Potassium supplementation or a potassium-sparing diuretic generally is needed when large dosages of loop diuretics are prescribed, especially in combination with thiazide diuretics.

Classification of Diuretics

Thiazides. The major site of diuretic action of the thiazides is the early to mid-distal convoluted tubule, where they block the electroneutral sodium chloride transporter (Table 21.8).[148,149] This results in a maximal fractional excretion of sodium of approximately 3% to 6%.[148] Thus, these compounds are considered moderately potent diuretics. The effectiveness of thiazide diuretics depends on the proximal tubule organic acid secretory pathway and GFR for delivery to the site of action.[149] Because individual thiazide agents are essentially interchangeable in terms of diuretic effectiveness, hydrochlorothiazide (HCTZ) generally is prescribed because of its low cost. Unless the patient has impaired renal function (i.e., CL_{Cr} <50 mL/minute) or moderate to severe congestive symptoms, conditions when a loop diuretic is indicated, a thiazide is a rational initial diuretic choice.[149] Mild HF with preserved renal function (i.e., CL_{Cr} >50 mL/minute) may respond to daily dosages of HCTZ of 25 to 50 mg given once or twice daily (Table 21.8).[149] HCTZ dosages greater than 50 mg per day, generally in combination with a loop diuretic, are needed in instances of reduced renal function or worsening HF, at the risk of causing more severe electrolyte imbalances (Table 21.8).[149] Thiazide diuretic absorption may be delayed in CHF.[141] Adverse effects that may occur secondary to thiazide administration include hypokalemia, hyponatremia, hypomagnesemia, hyperuricemia, hyperlipoproteinemia (i.e., increases in total cholesterol, low-density lipoproteins, and triglycerides and decreases in high-density lipoproteins), and impaired carbohydrate tolerance (Table 21.8). NSAIDs and organic acids such as probenecid can diminish the response to thiazides (Table 21.8).[149] The for-

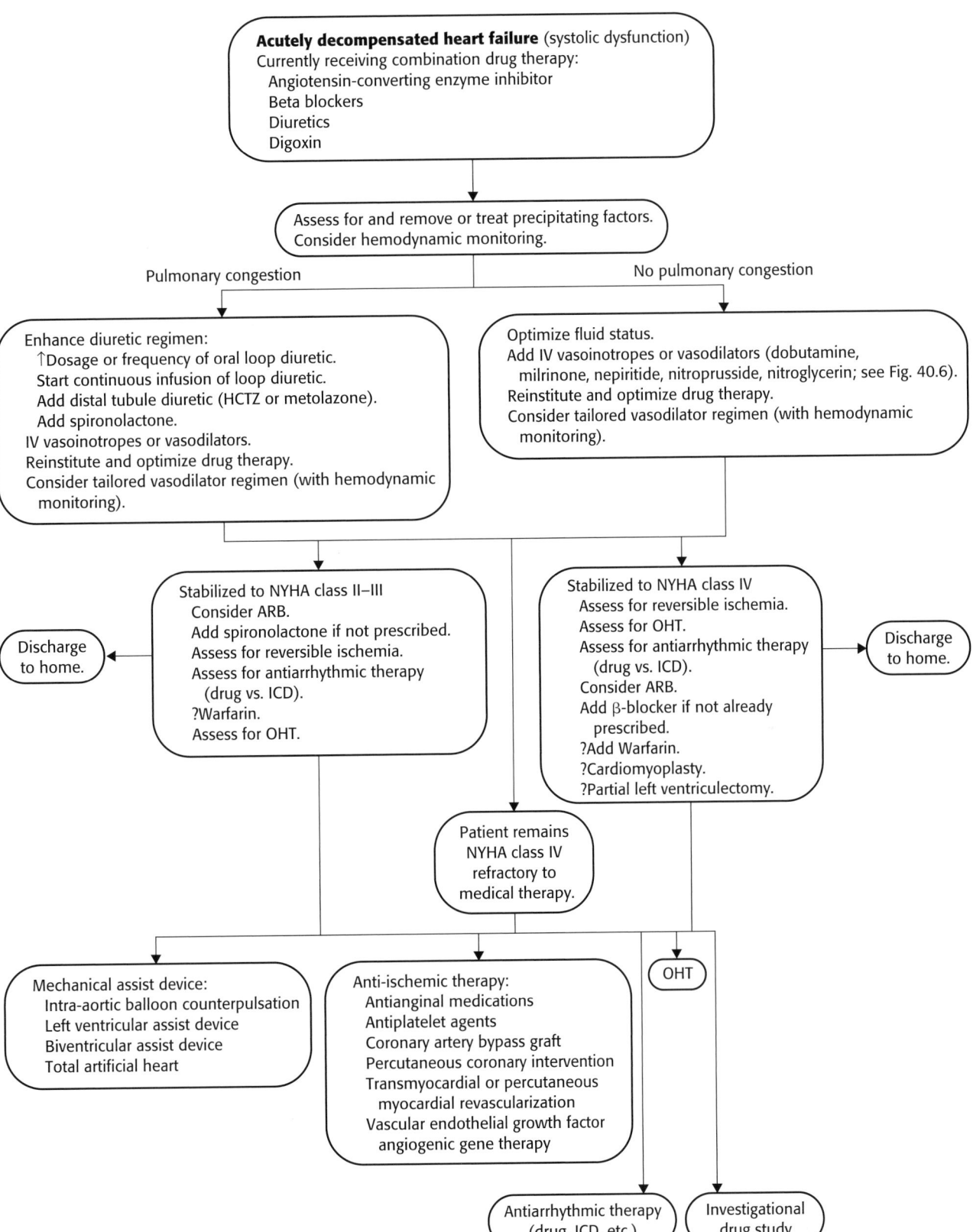

FIGURE 21.5 Algorithm for management of patient with acutely decompensated heart failure. ARB, angiotensin II type 1 receptor blocker; HCTZ, hydrochlorothiazide; ICD, implantable cardioverter–defibrillator; NYHA, New York Heart Association; OHT, orthotopic heart transplantation.

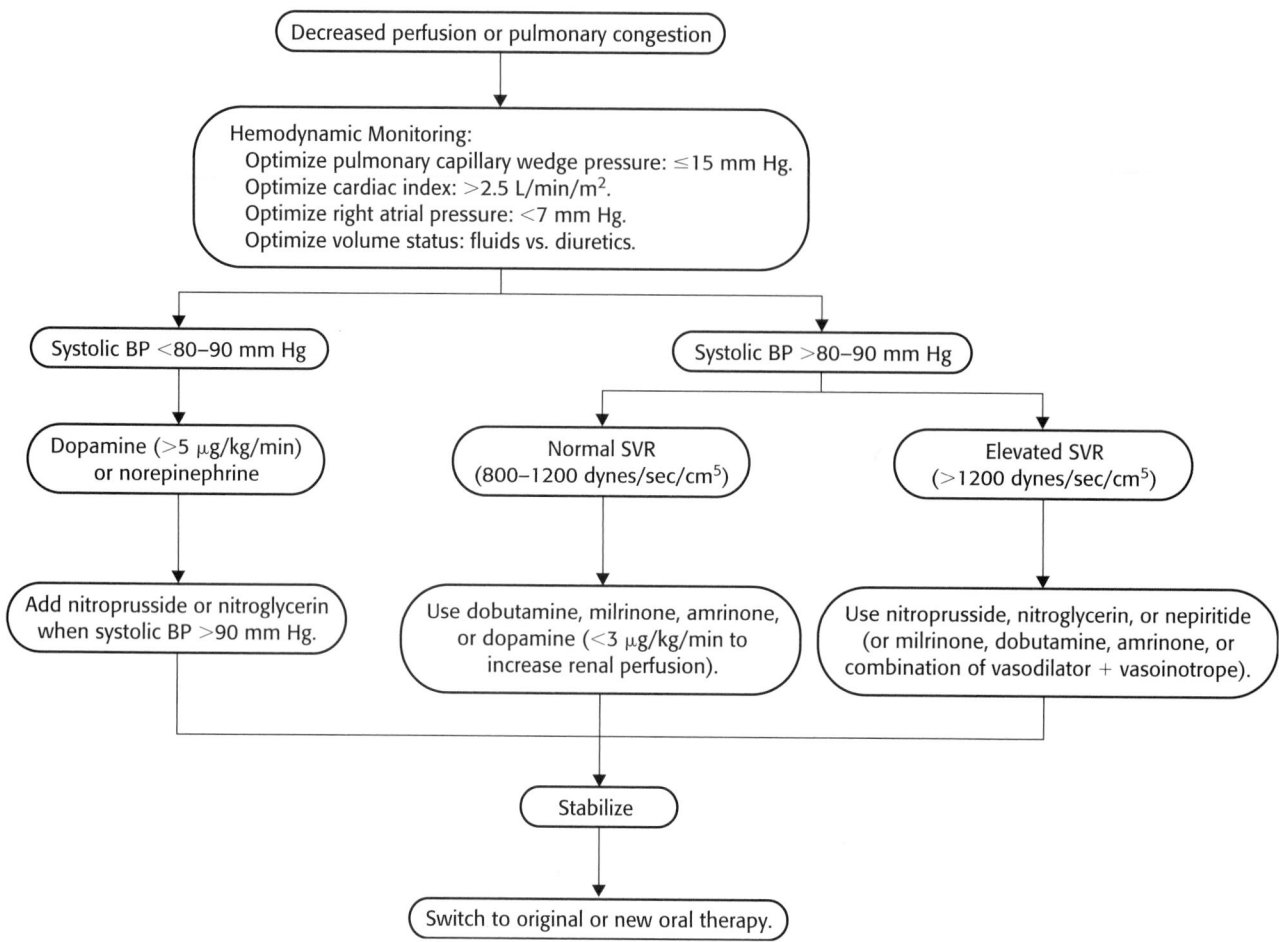

FIGURE 21.6 Algorithm for using vasoinotropes and vasodilators for patients hospitalized for congestive heart failure with acute decompensation. BP, blood pressure; SVR, systemic vascular resistance.

mer enhance sodium reabsorption in the thick ascending limb of the loop of Henle, and the latter impair proximal tubular secretion of the thiazide diuretic.

Metolazone. Metolazone is a thiazide-type drug that acts principally at the distal convoluted tubule (Table 21.8).[148] It also may have proximal tubular effects that further reduce sodium reabsorption. Major differences between metolazone and the thiazides are that metolazone retains its effectiveness even when renal function is markedly reduced and has a duration of action (elimination half-life of about 2 days) longer than that of most thiazides.[149] Metolazone and the thiazides produce similar adverse effects (Table 21.8). As a single diuretic, metolazone can be used in dosages starting at 2.5 mg daily. However, it is often used in combination with loop diuretics (i.e., sequential diuresis) and therefore may be prescribed as 2.5 mg every 1 to 4 days.[141–143,148–150] When metolazone is administered in conjunction with loop diuretics, it is advisable to administer metolazone (or any thiazide diuretic) about 1 hour before the loop diuretic to achieve maximal diuresis.[150]

Loop Diuretics. These drugs act principally at the thick ascending limb of the loop of Henle, where they block the sodium–potassium–chloride transporter and may increase the fractional excretion of sodium up to 25% (Table 21.8).[148] Like thiazides, loop diuretics depend on secretion into the proximal tubule via the organic acid pathway.[148,149] Loop diuretics also can increase renal blood flow by enhancing production of the renal vasodilatory prostaglandin. This effect contributes to the natriuretic effects of the loop diuretics. Loop diuretics remain effective despite reductions in GFR, although larger than usual dosages are needed in the setting of renal dysfunction (Table 21.8).

Furosemide, bumetanide, and torsemide are loop diuretics currently available in the United States. Furosemide is the most commonly prescribed agent in this subgroup because of cost. These agents differ predominantly with respect to milligram-to-milligram potency and pharmacokinetics (Table 21.8). Torsemide has a significantly longer half-life than the other two agents.[149] In addition, in CHF furosemide absorption is delayed and erratic, bumetanide absorption is delayed, and torsemide absorption is unaffected.[149] Adverse

TABLE 21.8 | Diuretics Used to Treat CHF

Class	Pharmacokinetics	Pharmacodynamics	Dosing Guidelines	Adverse Effects	Drug Interactions	Monitoring Parameters
Thiazides SOA: early to mid DCT HCTZ[a]	F: 65–75% $t_{1/2}$: RI: >2.5 hr CHF: ND	Onset: 2 hr Peak: 4–6 hr Duration: 6–12 hr	PO 25–50 mg/day (CL$_{cr}$ >50 ml/min) 50–100 mg/day (CL$_{cr}$ 20–50 mL/min) 100–200 mg/day (CL$_{cr}$ <20 mL/min)	Hypokalemia Hyponatremia Hypomagnesemia Azotemia Hyperlipoproteinemia Hyperglycemia Rash Pancreatitis Cholestatic jaundice	Loop diuretics (excessive hypokalemia) NSAIDs (antagonize diuretic effects) Probenecid (competes for secretion)	Body weight Serum electrolytes: K$^+$, Mg^{+2}, Na$^+$ Signs and symptoms of CHF Blood pressure BUN, Scr Drug interactions
Chlorothiazide[a]	F: 30–50% $t_{1/2}$: RI: 1.5 hr (N) ND CHF: ND	Onset: (IV): 15 min Peak (IV): 30 min Duration (IV): 2 hr	IV 250 mg q 12hr (CL$_{cr}$ >50 mL/min) 500 mg q 12 hr (CL$_{cr}$ 20–50 ml/min) 1 g q12 hr (CL$_{cr}$ <20 mL/min)	As above	As above	As above
Metolazone SOA: early to mid-DCT and possibly PCT	F: 40–65% $t_{1/2}$: 14 hr (N) RI: ND CHF: ND	Onset: 1 hr Peak: 2–8 hr Duration: 12–24 hr	PO: 2.5–20 mg/day or every other day	As for thiazides	As for thiazides	As for thiazides
Loop diuretics SOA: TAL Furosemide	F: 10–100% $t_{1/2}$: RI: ~ 3 hr CHF: ~ 3 hr	Onset PO: 30 min IV: 5 min Peak PO: 1–2 hr IV: 30 min Duration PO: 6–8 hr IV: 2 hr	PO: 40–80 mg × Scr IV infusion 40 mg LD, then 10 mg/hr (CL$_{cr}$ >75 mL/min) 40 mg LD, then 10–20 mg/hr (CL$_{cr}$ 25–75 mL/min) 40 mg LD, then 20–40 mg/hr (CL$_{cr}$ <25 mL/min)	As for thiazides except for hypocalcemia, transient tinnitus, or deafness	As for thiazides Thiazides or metolazone (excessive hypokalemia)	As for thiazides
Bumetanide	F: 80–100% $t_{1/2}$: RI: 1.6 hr CHF: 1.3 hr	Onset PO: 0.5–1 hr IV: 5 min Peak PO: 1–2 hr IV: 30–45 min Duration PO: 4–6 hr IV: 2 hr	PO: 1 mg × Scr IV infusion 1 mg LD, then 0.5 mg/hr (CL$_{cr}$ >75 mL/min) 1 mg LD, then 0.5–1 mg/hr (CL$_{cr}$ 25–75 mL/min) 1 mg LD, then 1–2 mg/hr (CL$_{cr}$ <25 mL/min)	As above	As above	As above

(continues)

TABLE 21.8	continued						
Class	**Pharmacokinetics**	**Pharmacodynamics**	**Dosing Guidelines**	**Adverse Effects**	**Drug Interactions**	**Monitoring Parameters**	
Torsemide	F: 80–100% $t_{1/2}$: RI: 4–5 hr CHF: 6 hr	Onset PO: 1 hr IV: 10 min Peak PO: 1–2 hr IV: 1 hr Duration PO: 8–12 hr IV: 6–8 hr	PO: 10 mg × Scr IV infusion 20 mg LD, then 5 mg/hr (CL$_{cr}$ >75 mL/min) 20 mg LD, then 5–10 mg/hr (CL$_{cr}$ 25–75 mL/min) 20 mg LD, then 10–20 mg/hr (CL$_{cr}$ <25 mL/min)	As above	As above	As above	
Potassium-sparing Spironolactone SOA: terminal DCT, aldosterone-dependent Na$^+$/K$^+$ exchange site	F: conflicting data $t_{1/2}$: >15 hr (N) (active metabolites) RI: ND CHF:ND	Onset: 3 days (active metabolites)	12.5–25 mg/day up to 200 mg/day	Hyperkalemia Gynecomastia	ACEIs, NSAIDs, or K$^+$ supplements (↑ risk of hyperkalemia) Digoxin (↓ SDC)	As for thiazides	
Triamaterene SOA: Na$^+$/K$^+$/H$^+$ exchange site, aldosterone-independent	F: >80% $t_{1/2}$: RI: > 5 hr CHF: ND	Onset: 2–4 hr Peak: 2–4 hr Duration: 7–9 hr	100 mg BID	Hyperkalemia Azotemia Renal stones	ACEIs, NSAIDs, or K$^+$ supplements (↑ risk of hyperkalemia) H$_2$-Antagonists and trimethoprim (compete for renal tubular secretion)	As for thiazides	
Amiloride SOA: same as triamterene	F: Conflicting data $t_{1/2}$: RI: 100 hr CHF: ND	Onset: 2 hr Peak: 3–4 hr Duration: 24 hr	5–10 mg/day up to 40 mg/day	Hyperkalemia Azotemia	As for triamterene	As for thiazides	

Source: Reference 149.

F, bioavailability; N, normals; ND, no data; RI, renal insufficiency; CL$_{cr}$ creatinine clearance; Scr, serum creatinine; ACEI, angiotensin-converting enzyme inhibitor; LD, loading dose; BUN, blood urea nitrogen; SDC, serum digoxin concentration; SOA, site of action within nephron; DCT, distal convoluted tubule; PCT, proximal convoluted tubules; TAL, thick ascending limb of the loop of Henle; HCTZ, hydrochlorothiazide.

^{a} Not effective as a single agent if CL$_{cr}$ < 50 mL/min.

effects of loop diuretics are similar to those of the thiazide diuretics (Table 21.8).[149] However, loop diuretics may produce hypocalcemia and transient ototoxicity, which are not shared with the thiazide compounds or metolazone. Initial dosages of furosemide (40 mg daily), bumetanide (1.0 mg daily), or torsemide (10 mg daily) can promote a prompt diuresis. However, as HF and secondary renal dysfunction progress, increasingly larger and more frequent doses are needed. Although dosages vary widely, patients with end-stage HF may need two or three oral daily doses of a loop diuretic (e.g., furosemide 160 to 400 mg).[149] A good rule for estimating the initial dosage of furosemide is 40 mg multiplied by the patient's Scr.[142]

Potassium-Sparing Diuretics. Spironolactone, triamterene, and amiloride exert their diuretic effects at the terminal portion of the distal convoluted tubule (Table 21.8).[148] Spironolactone, which is converted to the active metabolite canrenone, acts at an aldosterone-sensitive site, whereas triamterene and amiloride, which are secreted into the proximal tubule via the organic base pathway, block aldosterone-independent apical sodium channels. Potassium-sparing agents are considered weak diuretics because they induce a fractional excretion of sodium of only 1% to 2%.[148] Potassium-sparing diuretics are useful mainly as adjuncts with thiazides, metolazone, and loop diuretics to counteract the hypokalemia and hypomagnesemia often induced or exacerbated by these other drugs. Hypokalemia and hypomagnesemia are directly arrhythmogenic and may potentiate arrhythmias secondary to either digoxin or circulating catecholamines.[149] These combined electrolyte disturbances appear to be best prevented by potassium-sparing diuretics. However, therapy with potassium-sparing agents should be individualized.

In selecting a potassium-sparing diuretic, it should be noted that spironolactone is effective only in relative hyper-aldosteronemic states such as CHF (Table 21.8).[148,149] Triamterene and amiloride are effective even when aldosterone levels are not elevated. Both triamterene and amiloride attain steady-state effects in about 1 to 1.5 days. Spironolactone's effects do not peak for several days because it takes 3 to 4 days for active metabolites to attain steady-state concentrations. Likewise, the effects of spironolactone persist for several days after cessation of therapy because of the presence of the active metabolite. Adding single daily doses of spironolactone ranging from 12.5 to 75 mg to a regimen of digoxin, loop diuretic, and an ACE inhibitor significantly increases urinary excretion of aldosterone and serum potassium levels and decreases atrial natriuretic factor plasma concentrations.[151] As noted previously, spironolactone administration also is associated with almost a one-third reduction in 2-year mortality and hospitalization for HF.[143,144]

A potential consequence of prescribing any potassium-sparing diuretic is hyperkalemia. However, hyperkalemia appears to be dose-related[151] and is more likely to occur in patients with severe renal dysfunction or in patients receiving concomitant potassium supplements, salt substitutes (which contain potassium), NSAIDs, ACE inhibitors, or ARBs (Table 21.8). On the other hand, trimethoprim and H_2-receptor blockers, both of which are organic bases, may compete for the secretion of amiloride and triamterene.[149] Spironolactone can induce gynecomastia. Triamterene-containing renal stones have been reported.

Diuretic Resistance. To optimize diuretic therapy in patients with CHF, the clinician must be familiar with the physiologic and pharmacologic factors that mediate a diminished clinical response to diuretics (i.e., diuretic resistance).[141–143,149,150] Patient noncompliance with the prescribed diuretic regimen minimizes the effectiveness of the drug. Noncompliance can be minimized through patient education.[67] Also, an increased Na^+ intake can offset the natriuretic effects of the diuretic. Therefore, a reduction in Na^+ consumption usually must accompany diuretic therapy (Table 21.4).[46]

Uremia may diminish the response to loop diuretics, which chemically are highly protein-bound organic acids.[149] To reach their site of action within the nephron, loop diuretics depend largely on the proximal tubule organic acid secretory pump, which can be blocked by the increased circulating concentrations of endogenous organic acids seen in uremia and renal dysfunction. This example of diuretic resistance may be overcome either by using more frequent and much higher dosages of the loop diuretic or by combining the loop diuretic with another diuretic that has a different site of action within the nephron, such as a thiazide or metolazone.[142,143,149,150] A continuous infusion of a loop diuretic also may be useful in this clinical setting.[149]

NSAIDs significantly diminish the natriuretic effect of loop diuretics. NSAIDs block the renal hemodynamic effects of these agents by inhibiting prostaglandin synthesis.[73] The effect was initially reported with indomethacin and has subsequently been shown to occur with ibuprofen, sulindac, naproxen, and aspirin. The use of NSAIDs in patients with CHF taking diuretics is associated with a twofold higher need for hospitalization for CHF.[73] NSAID-induced diuretic resistance can be counteracted by discontinuing the offending agent, if possible, by using larger or more frequent doses of loop diuretics, or by combining the loop diuretic with a thiazide or metolazone.[141–143,149,150]

CHF also can partially attenuate the response to loop diuretics by a number of mechanisms.[141–143,149,150] In CHF, the natriuretic response is reduced secondary to neurohormonally mediated enhanced sodium reabsorption. In addition, in CHF the rate of gastrointestinal absorption of orally administered thiazide and some loop diuretics may decrease, slowing delivery of the diuretic to its site of action and thereby delaying or diminishing response.[149] A more effective diuresis can be achieved by administering more frequent doses of the oral loop diuretic, adding a thiazide diuretic or metolazone, or administering the loop diuretic intravenously, either as a single dose or via continuous infusion.[141–143,149,150] The coexistence of renal dysfunction also warrants higher dosages of the loop or thiazide diuretic.[149]

Patient-Adjusted Diuretic Therapy. After appropriate patient education, some patients may be able to assume responsibility for making minor adjustments in their diuretic regimen based on changes in weight, salt and fluid intake, symptoms of dyspnea, and increasing peripheral edema. A simple but useful monitoring tool is a daily log of the patient's weight.[46] Careful attention to clinical parameters at home with concomitant adjustments in the diuretic regimen may lead to reductions in the frequency of HF exacerbations and resultant hospital admissions.

Digoxin. Digitalis glycosides classically have been used as inotropic drugs to treat CHF. However, only recently have clinical studies better defined the actual value and role of these agents in CHF management.[152] In the discussion that follows, digoxin is the only cardiac glycoside extensively reviewed because of its predominant use in clinical medicine.

Mechanism of Action. The inotropic effects of digoxin are produced indirectly, through inhibition of the sarcolemmal transport enzyme sodium–potassium adenosine triphosphatase (Na^+–K^+ ATPase).[153] This enzyme complex catalyzes Na^+ efflux from the myocardial cell in exchange for K^+. When Na^+ efflux is inhibited by digoxin, high intracellular concentrations of Na^+ result. Sodium is subsequently exchanged for calcium (Ca^{2+}) via an Na^+-Ca^{2+} exchange carrier. The increased intracellular concentrations of Ca^{2+} ultimately enhance myocardial contractility through a complex series of intracellular Ca^{2+} movements. In the failing human myocardium there appears to be an increased sensitivity to the inotropic effects of digoxin, which is caused in part by decreased expression of Na^+-K^+ ATPase.[153]

Digoxin also has several neurohormonal effects. Digoxin increases parasympathomimetic activity, which slows both HR and atrioventricular conduction.[154] These effects may increase diastolic filling time and decrease myocardial oxygen consumption. Digoxin also decreases sympathetic activity, plasma renin, and aldosterone.[155] The combination of inotropic and neurohormonal-modulating effects may account for the recently observed beneficial outcomes in patients with CHF.[152]

Pharmacokinetics. A vast amount of literature describes the absorption, distribution, metabolism, and elimination of digoxin.[156] Digoxin is available parenterally and as a tablet, elixir, and capsule. For the oral preparations, the systemic availability is independent of the dosage administered and averages 70% to 80%, 75% to 85%, and 90% to 100%, respectively.

Digoxin is widely distributed into various tissues.[156] The highest concentrations of digoxin are found in the kidneys, heart, liver, adrenal glands, diaphragm, and intestinal tract. However, approximately 50% of the apparent total body stores of digoxin are found in the skeletal muscles. As a result of this extensive distribution to lean tissue, digoxin generally should be dosed using an estimate of the patient's ideal body weight. The plasma protein binding of digoxin is independent of concentration and averages 20% to 30%. Albumin is the principal binding protein. In patients with normal renal function, the volume of distribution at steady state (V_{ss}) averages 6 to 7 L/kg.

Digoxin undergoes metabolism primarily by two different pathways.[156] One of these pathways involves sequential hydrolysis of digitoxose sugar moieties, and the other route results in the formation of reduced metabolites. The reduced (i.e., dihydro) metabolites are inactive. In contrast, the hydrolysis products, digoxigenin bis- and mono-digitoxosides, have potencies that approach that of the parent compound. However, the contribution of these two metabolites to overall digoxin activity in humans is unknown. In adults with normal renal and hepatic function, the systemic clearance (CL_S) of digoxin averages approximately 180 mL/minute/1.73 m^2. Renal digoxin clearance (CL_R), which exceeds creatinine and inulin clearances, generally accounts for about 70% of the CL_S. The nonrenal clearance (CL_{NR}) of digoxin includes metabolism, biliary excretion, and possibly intestinal secretion and resultant fecal elimination. The CL_S of digoxin is linearly correlated, but the elimination half-life ($t_{1/2}$) is inversely correlated with creatinine clearance (CL_{Cr}). The $t_{1/2}$ of digoxin averages 36 hours in young adults with normal renal and hepatic function.

Numerous clinical conditions can alter digoxin pharmacokinetics (Table 21.9).[156–159] The bioavailability of digoxin tablets can be reduced by abdominal radiation, by various malabsorption syndromes such as hypermotility, diarrhea, and subtotal villus atrophy, and by several drugs.[157,158] In contrast, digoxin absorption may be enhanced by hypochlorhydria,[159] propantheline (and perhaps other anticholinergic drugs),[157] and oral antibiotics such as tetracycline and macrolides.[157,158] These antibiotics decrease the number of colonic bacteria that metabolize digoxin to inactive reduced metabolites. The V_{ss} of digoxin is reduced by chronic renal failure but increased by physical activity.[156] Chronic renal failure also increases the $t_{1/2}$ of digoxin. Drugs that consistently reduce the CL_S of digoxin include quinidine, verapamil, spironolactone, amiodarone, and propafenone.[157] Inhibition of the active drug transporter P-glycoprotein, for which digoxin acts as a substrate, is the likely mechanism for the reduced CL_S.[160] Captopril, hypothyroidism, and advanced CHF also decrease the CL_S of digoxin.[157] Hyperthyroidism, rifampin, and orally administered cholesterol-binding resins and activated charcoal increase the CL_S of digoxin.[156,157] Pharmacodynamic interactions may occur with β-adrenergic blocking drugs, amiodarone, verapamil, and diltiazem, all of which enhance the effects of digoxin on decreasing atrioventricular nodal conduction and sinoatrial nodal rate (Table 21.9).

Serum Digoxin Concentration–Response Relationships. Although many clinical laboratories and reference texts list the therapeutic range for digoxin as 0.5 or 0.8 to 2.0 ng per

TABLE 21.9	Conditions of Altered Digoxin Pharmacokinetics or Pharmacodynamics
Condition	**Clinical Management**

A. Reduced bioavailability

   1. Abdominal radiation   1. Consider administering digoxin as elixir or capsule.

   2. Malabsorption syndromes   2. Same as above.

      a. Hypermotility

      b. Diarrhea

      c. Subtotal villus atrophy

   3. Drugs   3. Consider administering digoxin 1–2 hr before or 2–3 hr after a, b, c, e, f, and g; consider administering digoxin as capsule or elixir for d.

      a. Cholesterol-binding resins

      b. Kaolin–pectin

      c. Large dosages (e.g., 30 mL) of antacid

      d. Metoclopramide (oral)

      e. Sulfasalazine

      f. Neomycin (oral)

      g. Sucralfate

B. Enhanced bioavailability

   1. Propantheline (and perhaps other anticholinergics)   1. Be alert for possible digoxin toxicity.

   2. Oral antibiotics   2. Thought to be a problem in 10% of population who extensively metabolize digoxin to inactive reduction products by colonic bacteria; avoid antibiotics if possible. If antibiotics must be administered, be alert for possible occurrence of digoxin toxicity.

      a. Erythromycin, clarithromycin, roxithromycin

      b. Tetracycline

   3. Hypochlorhydria, achlorhydria   3. Be alert for possible occurrence of digoxin toxicity.

C. Reduced systemic clearance

   1. Renal dysfunction   1. Adjust digoxin dosages to the reductions in creatinine clearance.

   2. Aging   2. As for C1: also monitor SDCs every few months.

   3. Drugs

      a. Quinidine   a. Reduce digoxin dosage by 50% upon start of quinidine; monitor SDCs.

      b. Verapamil   b. Consider reducing digoxin dosage by about 50% on initiation of verapamil, monitor SDCs, and look for additive effects on SA and AV nodes.

      c. Diltiazem   c. Monitor SDCs; be alert for additive effects on SA and AV nodes.

      d. Spironolactone   d. Consider reducing digoxin dosage by about 50%, monitor SDCs, and be alert for signs and symptoms of toxicity.

      e. Amiodarone   e. Consider reducing digoxin dosage by about 50%, monitor SDCs, and look for additive effects on SA and AV nodes.

      f. Captopril   f. Routine reduction of digoxin appears to be unnecessary; monitor SDCs and be alert for signs and symptoms of toxicity.

      g. Propafenone   g. Consider reducing digoxin dosage by about 25%, monitor SDCs, and be alert for signs and symptoms of toxicity.

D. Altered pharmacodynamics

   1. β-Blockers   1. Be alert for additive effects on SA and AV nodes.

   2. Other inotropic drugs   2. Try to avoid because they may increase risk of digoxin-induced arrhythmias.

   3. Diuretics   3. May produce hypokalemia or hypomagnesemia, which increase risk of digoxin-induced arrhythmias; replace depleted electrolytes.

SDCs, serum digoxin concentrations; SA, sinoatrial; AV, atrioventricular.

mL, relationships between the serum digoxin concentration and the intensity of its inotropic response, autonomic and neurohormonal effects, and the development of digoxin toxicity are not clearly defined. This lack of a definitive therapeutic range reflects digoxin's rather modest inotropic effects, the apparently flat dose–response curve with respect to digoxin's autonomic and neurohormonal modulating effects, and the overlap between therapeutic and toxic concentrations. In addition, many assay techniques used to quantify serum digoxin concentrations are nonspecific, failing to distinguish digoxin from active and inactive metabolites as well as endogenous digoxin-like immunoreactive substances. However, recent findings may lead to a better definition of the therapeutic range of digoxin.[161–163] For example, in patients with CHF caused by systolic dysfunction, serum concentrations ranging from 0.9 to 1.2 ng per mL were associated with significantly higher maximal treadmill exercise time than that of placebo.[161] This improvement was of the same magnitude as that observed at concentrations greater than 1.2 ng per mL but superior to that of concentrations ranging from 0.5 to 0.9 ng per mL. In another study, a near doubling of the serum concentration from 0.7 to 1.2 ng per mL resulted in a small increase in EF and a trend toward increased exercise time, but no further decrease in circulating neurohormones.[162] Other investigators reported no additional reductions in HR or sympathetic activity or improvements in ventricular performance after a near doubling of serum concentrations from 0.8 to 1.5 ng per mL.[163] Furthermore, at mean concentrations less than 1.0 ng per mL (and within a targeted range 0.5 to 2.0 ng/mL) the combined endpoint of death or hospitalization due to HF was significantly decreased by digoxin in the Digitalis Investigation Group (DIG) trial.[152] Last, despite considerable overlap between therapeutic and toxic concentrations, a review of data from more than 1,000 patients reported a mean serum concentration of 1.4 ng per mL in patients without toxicity, whereas concentrations two to three times greater were noted in patients with overt toxicity.[164] Collectively these observations suggest that serum digoxin concentrations between 0.7 and 1.2 ng per mL should maximize the hemodynamic, clinical, and neurohormonal benefits of digoxin and minimize the risk of digoxin toxicity.

Dosing Guidelines. Several pharmacokinetic equations provide prospective dosing guidelines for digoxin. However, most equations show a poor correlation between predicted and measured serum concentrations.[165] Nonetheless, because the equations generally overestimate the measured concentrations, they provide safe initial approximations of a patient's digoxin dosage. However, the method of Koup et al,[166] using a CL_{NR} of 20 mL/minute/1.73 m[2], best correlates the predicted and measured steady-state serum concentrations.[165]

To use this method, first estimate the patient's ideal body weight:

$$IBW_{male} = 50 \text{ kg} + 2.3 \text{ Height in inches above 5 ft}$$

$$IBW_{female} = 45 \text{ kg} + 2.3 \text{ Height in inches above 5 ft}$$

If the patient's actual weight is less than the estimated IBW, use the actual weight. Next estimate the patient's body surface area (BSA) in square meters:

$$BSA \text{ m}^2 = IBW \text{ (kg)}^{0.425} \text{ Height (cm)}^{0.725} \text{ } 0.007184$$

Then estimate the patient's CL_{Cr} using the Cockcroft and Gault equation[167]:

$$CL_{Cr} = (140 - \text{Age}) \text{ ABW72 Scr } 1.73 \text{ m}^2 \text{ BSA}$$

where Age is the patient's age in years, ABW is the patient's actual body weight in kg, and Scr is the patient's Scr in mg per dL. If the patient is female, multiply the result by 0.85. Then estimate the CL_S for digoxin:

$$CL_S = (1.303 \text{ } CL_{Cr}) + 20 \text{ mL/minute/1.73 m}^2$$

The initial estimate of the patient's daily digoxin dosage is computed using the steady-state equation and a target concentration (i.e., 1.0 ng/mL):

$$C_{SS} = F \text{ DCLS } \tau$$

where D = dosage (ng), C_{SS} = steady-state digoxin level (ng/mL), CL_S = systemic clearance (mL/minute/1.73 m[2]), τ = dosing interval (1,440 minutes/day), and F = fraction absorbed (0.75 for tablets).

These digoxin dosing guidelines for patients with CHF should result in a low probability of achieving a potentially toxic concentration. A trough concentration can be obtained either after a few days, to verify that a serious overprediction or underprediction of the measured concentration has not occurred, or at the attainment of steady state (usually 7 to 10 days for most adults). General indications for measuring serum concentrations include establishing an initial dose–concentration relationship, assessing known or suspected pharmacokinetic digoxin–drug interactions, evaluating the effect of a change in physiologic function known or suspected to alter the disposition of digoxin (e.g., renal dysfunction), monitoring after a change in the dosage form of digoxin, confirming suspected digoxin toxicity, evaluating a poor response to initial therapy or a decline in response after early therapeutic success, and assessing patient compliance. In addition, older adults may benefit from routine measurement of serum concentrations because of the difficulty of predicting digoxin dosages in this subgroup. Again, it must be emphasized that serum concentrations of digoxin do not predict efficacy or toxicity and should therefore be used only to complement good clinical judgment. Strict attention should be given to the timing of blood collection and its relationship to the time of last dose. Collecting blood during the distribution phase (lasting up to 12 hours after an oral dose) may cause the concentration to be falsely elevated and potentially useless in evaluating the possible risk of toxicity.

Digoxin Toxicity. Despite the objective means used to develop rational dosing guidelines for digoxin, digoxin toxicity remains a worrisome clinical problem. Previous estimates of the frequency of digitalis toxicity in hospitalized patients taking digoxin ranged from 4% to 35% and were accompanied by a high mortality rate of up to 41%.[164] However, today the incidence of definite or possible digoxin toxicity consistently approaches about 4%,[168,169] with hospitalization for digoxin toxicity needed for 1.5%[169] to 2%[152] of patients receiving digoxin.

The diagnosis of digoxin intoxication is challenging. It can be acute or chronic, and it generally results from excessive ingestion, a change in disposition, or an increased sensitivity to digoxin. Digoxin intoxication can manifest as a number of noncardiac symptoms (Table 21.10), the most common of which are anorexia, nausea, and vomiting.[170,171] In addition, virtually any cardiac arrhythmia or conduction disturbance can be associated with digoxin toxicity. These rhythm disturbances are common manifestations and may be the first sign of digoxin toxicity. Digoxin-induced arrhythmias are generally classified as decreases in impulse conduction, enhancement of automaticity, or a combination of both. In a recent study, the most commonly observed arrhythmias for patients with definite or probable digoxin toxicity were atrioventricular block and sinus bradycardia.[168] However, in the DIG trial, the most common arrhythmias in suspected digoxin toxicity were ventricular fibrillation or tachycardia, supraventricular arrhythmia, and second- or third-degree atrioventricular block.[152]

Digoxin toxicity is largely preventable[172] given the number of known risk factors, which usually can be modified and monitored. Digoxin toxicity occurs most commonly in older adults with impaired renal function (Table 21.11).[170] Older adults also may exhibit an increased sensitivity to the Na^+–K^+–ATPase inhibitory effects of digoxin. Renal dysfunction alone predisposes patients to digoxin toxicity because of decreases in the volume of distribution and elimination of digoxin. Hypokalemia and hypomagnesemia are associated with an increased incidence of digitalis-induced arrhythmias. Hypokalemia appears to increase myocardial uptake of digoxin. Magnesium (Mg^{2+}) acts as a cofactor for the enzyme Na^+–K^+ ATPase, so hypomagnesemia may decrease intracellular potassium. Alkalosis also decreases serum concentration and total body stores of K^+ and thereby increases the sensitivity to digitalis. Diuretic-induced alkalosis, even in the setting of a normal serum K^+, increases the frequency of digoxin-associated arrhythmias. Hypothyroidism and hypoxia, through unidentified mechanisms, increase a patient's sensitivity to digoxin. Finally, the development of digoxin toxicity may be enhanced by other inotropic drugs, drugs that produce electrolyte disturbances (e.g., diuretics), agents that slow atrioventricular nodal conduction or sinus rate (i.e., β-blockers), or drugs that decrease the CL_s of digoxin or increase its absorption (Table 21.9).

Treating Digoxin Toxicity. The severity of digoxin toxicity should be assessed before a treatment plan is initiated. In general, blood should be obtained for determination of serum K^+, Mg^{2+}, and digoxin levels. Efforts should be made to identify and remove predisposing factors. Discontinuation

TABLE 21.11	Factors That May Predispose Patients to Developing Digoxin Intoxication
Electrolyte abnormalities	Hypoxia
Hypokalemia	Renal dysfunction
Hypomagnesemia	Hypothyroidism
Hypercalcemia	Drug interactions
Advanced age	
Acid–base disturbances	
Alkalosis	

TABLE 21.10	Signs and Symptoms of Digoxin Intoxication
Noncardiac	Common cardiac arrhythmias[a]
Gastrointestinal: anorexia, nausea, vomiting	VPDs, including multifocal VPDs and bigeminy or trigeminy
Neurologic: fatigue, malaise, delirium, acute psychosis, neuralgic pain	First-degree AV block
	Mobitz type I AV block
Ocular: halo vision, green (chloropsia) or yellow (xanthopsia) vision	Nonparoxysmal junctional tachycardia
	Supraventricular tachycardia with block
Miscellaneous: gynecomastia and sexual dysfunction (men)	Ventricular tachycardia (including bidirectional ventricular tachycardia)

VPDs, ventricular premature depolarizations; AV, atrioventricular.
[a] Virtually every known cardiac arrhythmia has occurred secondary to digitalis intoxication.

of digoxin and supportive treatment may be sufficient to manage most noncardiac symptoms as well as asymptomatic cardiac manifestations such as first-degree atrioventricular block or Mobitz type I second-degree atrioventricular block.[171]

In the setting of an accidental or suicidal ingestion of large amounts of digoxin, syrup of ipecac can decrease absorption if administered within an hour of ingestion. Gastric lavage can be attempted if the patient presents within 2 hours of ingestion.[171] However, gastric lavage may provoke fatal arrhythmias. Orally administered activated charcoal, cholestyramine, or colestipol can also minimize absorption but may induce vomiting.

Altered potassium homeostasis often is observed in the setting of digoxin toxicity and can exacerbate digoxin-induced bradyarrhythmias or tachyarrhythmias.[170,171] Potassium should be administered if the potassium level is low or normal unless serum K^+ is 5.0 mEq per mL or higher, the patient is ingesting K^+-conserving drugs, severe renal insufficiency is present, markedly delayed atrioventricular conduction is observed (i.e., greater than first-degree atrioventricular block), or the patient has ingested a massive overdose of digoxin. Normal saline may be a better choice than 5% dextrose solution for diluting the potassium, avoiding the paradoxical worsening of the hypokalemia sometimes observed in the severely K^+-depleted patient. Hyperkalemia, which generally reflects extracellular distribution of K^+ secondary to inhibition of $Na^+–K^+$ ATPase, is best managed by administering digoxin-specific antibodies (Fab fragments, Digibind). Fab antibodies bind to tissue-bound, intravascular, and interstitial digoxin.[170,171]

Select digoxin-induced arrhythmias such as nonparoxysmal atrioventricular junctional tachycardia, atrial tachycardia with block, ventricular premature depolarizations, and ventricular tachycardia may be suppressed by potassium.[170] Magnesium also can suppress digitalis-induced ventricular arrhythmias even in the setting of mildly elevated Mg^{2+} levels.[171] The use of magnesium should be avoided in patients with severe renal insufficiency, a greater than first-degree atrioventricular block, or severe hypermagnesemia. The class IB antiarrhythmic drugs, lidocaine, and rarely phenytoin also may be useful in treating digitalis-induced ventricular arrhythmias. Other antiarrhythmics may be proarrhythmic in the setting of digoxin toxicity or may pharmacokinetically or pharmacodynamically interact with digoxin.[170,171] Cardioversion may produce severe arrhythmias or asystole in digoxin-intoxicated patients.[171]

Fab therapy is the most effective antiarrhythmic treatment for life-threatening ventricular arrhythmias secondary to digoxin toxicity.[170,171] An initial response, consisting of a 10- to 20-fold increase in total serum digoxin, a decrease in serum potassium, and a reversal of the adverse electrophysiologic effects of digoxin, often is observed less than 20 minutes after the Fab infusion. These digoxin-specific antibodies often completely reverse the toxic effects of digoxin within

a few hours. A treatment response is expected in at least 90% of patients with definitive life-threatening digoxin toxicity. Caution must be exercised in administering Fab fragments to patients with digoxin toxicity and concomitant severe renal impairment. However, plasmapheresis appears to be effective in removing the digoxin–antidigoxin antibody complexes in this setting.[173]

To reverse symptomatic digoxin-induced bradycardia or mild sinoatrial or atrioventricular conduction delays, atropine administered in intravenous dosages of 0.5 to 2.0 mg is indicated.[171] If the bradycardia or conduction delays are hemodynamically significant and refractory to atropine, Fab therapy should be administered.[170,171] Temporary pacing is associated with a high complication rate in digoxin-intoxicated patients.[171]

Use of Digoxin in Congestive Heart Failure. Digoxin offers several benefits for patients in normal sinus rhythm with CHF secondary to systolic dysfunction who are receiving concurrent treatment with diuretics and ACE inhibitors. Digoxin decreases symptoms, increases exercise performance, improves sympathetic/parasympathetic imbalances, reduces levels of harmful circulating neurohormones, and decreases hospital admissions secondary to HF. The latter effects especially may contribute to an estimated annual savings of $100 million.[174] Furthermore, in patients with coexistent atrial fibrillation, digoxin can offer the additional benefit of decreasing the ventricular rate response. The DIG trial also suggests that patients with CHF secondary to diastolic dysfunction may benefit from digoxin through a reduction in the need for hospitalization.[152] However, the currently limited information on the use of digoxin in these patients does not justify its routine use in this setting. The use of digoxin can result in digoxin toxicity, some of which is life-threatening. However, the incidence of digoxin toxicity is declining. Also, most cases of digoxin toxicity today are benign and can be prevented by targeting initial dosing to a lower serum concentration, monitoring the serum concentration, and monitoring for risk factors for digoxin toxicity and adjusting the dosage accordingly (Tables 21.9 to 21.11). Furthermore, all drugs used to treat CHF produce intolerable and difficult-to-manage adverse effects.

In summary, for patients with CHF secondary to systolic dysfunction, digoxin can be recommended as initial therapy in combination with diuretics, ACE inhibitors, and β-blockers (Fig. 21.2).[52] However, future post hoc analyses of β-blocker trials may suggest that little incremental benefit is associated with the use of digoxin with respect to hospitalization, sudden death, or HR response rates in patients with CHF treated with a β-blocker, ACE inhibitor, and diuretic.[155]

Additional Inotropic Drugs. A number of inotropic drugs have been investigated in chronic CHF management.[175] Each of these agents raises intracellular concentrations of calcium within myocardial cells, resulting in increases in contractility. Unfortunately, enthusiasm about positive inotropic agents has waned because of their tendency to increase mortality in patients with CHF. Recently, many clinicians have begun to advocate the use of intermittent intravenous milrinone and dobutamine in patients with CHF in an effort to improve quality of life, reduce hospitalization rates, and reduce healthcare costs. The use of these agents has been based on anecdotal data and small, nonrandomized trials. Typical regimens involve administering intermittent 4- to 6-hour infusions several days a week, 24-hour infusions several times a month, or continuous infusion of the drug.

Unfortunately, chronic use of intermittent intravenous inotropes has not been found to reduce mortality and may actually reduce survival.[176] Inotropic agents may precipitate ischemia and arrhythmias in patients with CHF. Consequently, intravenous inotropes should be reserved for temporary use in patients with acute CHF exacerbation or for hemodynamic support during diagnostic or surgical procedures.[177] In general, patients hospitalized for worsening heart failure with normal cardiac output (i.e., the volume-overloaded patient) do not benefit from inotropic therapy. Inotropes should be reserved for patients requiring inotropic support. Chronic, intermittent administration of intravenous inotropes either in a CHF clinic or at home is not routinely recommended by many cardiovascular specialists because of the lack of data demonstrating efficacy.[52] Rather, every effort should be made to maximize the patient's CHF medications. Intermittent or continuous inotropic infusions with dobutamine or milrinone or perhaps the combination of milrinone plus a β-blocker[178] should be reserved for patients with end-stage CHF who are awaiting cardiac transplantation or in whom alternatives do not exist.[177]

PREVENTING THROMBOEMBOLIC COMPLICATIONS

In the setting of LV dysfunction, abnormal, sometimes static flow through dilated cardiac chambers along with increases in platelet aggregability, coagulation activity, and neuroendocrine activation may predispose the patient to form an intraventricular thrombus and consequent emboli.[179] The incidence of arterial thromboembolism or stroke is approximately 1.9 per 100 patient-years.[179] Analysis of data from the SOLVD trial showed that the risk of embolic events was directly related to the severity of LV dysfunction.[180] Consequently, the use of oral anticoagulants has been proposed in an effort to reduce thromboembolic complications of LV dysfunction. Based on a number of small trials, the efficacy of oral anticoagulation in the prevention of thromboembolic events may be related to the cause of CHF. Early trials indicating a benefit secondary to oral anticoagulant therapy included primarily patients with idiopathic dilated cardiomyopathies.[179] However, recent studies, which included patients with ischemic heart disease, have not shown

a beneficial reduction in thromboembolic events in anticoagulated patients.[179]

Any beneficial reduction in thromboembolic events must be weighed against the risk of anticoagulant therapy. The annual risk of a major bleed for patients receiving oral anticoagulant therapy has been estimated at 2%, and the estimated risk of a fatal bleed is 0.8%.[179] Consequently, the risk of experiencing an adverse thromboembolic event is equivalent to and perhaps greater than the risk of experiencing a significant hemorrhagic adverse effect of anticoagulation. Anticoagulation management in patients with CHF is difficult because of a predilection to hepatic congestion and dysfunction, which can decrease warfarin metabolism. Results from CHF trials in which there was uncontrolled use of antiplatelet therapy also are contradictory with respect to favorable outcomes.[179] Thus, large randomized controlled trials that assess warfarin anticoagulation and antiplatelet therapy in patients with CHF and in normal sinus rhythm are needed before these treatments can be recommended routinely. However, for patients with coexisting atrial fibrillation, a history of thromboembolic events, or other known predisposing conditions, warfarin anticoagulation targeted to an international normalized ratio of 2.0 to 3.0 generally is indicated. Antiplatelet therapy probably is indicated for patients with CHF and concurrent CAD.

ARRHYTHMIAS IN CONGESTIVE HEART FAILURE

Patients with LV dysfunction are at high risk of ventricular arrhythmia and subsequent sudden cardiac death. The risks predisposing patients with HF to sudden death are multifactorial. Structural changes in the myocardium, such as enhanced protein deposition leading to fibrosis and stretching of tissues, may enhance arrhythmogenesis.[181] Also, neurohormonal activation with elevated circulating catecholamines[12] coupled with parasympathetic withdrawal[22] may stimulate arrhythmia development, as can hemodynamic derangements. Electrolyte disturbances, such as hypokalemia and hypomagnesemia, can occur secondary to diuretic therapy and further predispose patients to arrhythmias.[149] In addition, inotropic agents[176] and antiarrhythmic agents[182] can be proarrhythmic.

The use of antiarrhythmic agents to reduce sudden cardiac death has been evaluated in a number of clinical trials. Class Ic agents, such as flecainide, have negative inotropic, proarrhythmic effects and, as demonstrated in the Coronary Arrhythmia Suppression Trial, are associated with an increased mortality in patients with diminished LV function (LVEF <30%).[182] Surprisingly, mortality was increased despite suppression of ventricular premature complexes, thus demonstrating the proarrhythmic potential of antiarrhythmic agents. Consequently, the use of class IC antiarrhythmic agents for extended durations is contraindicated in patients with LV dysfunction. Conversely, class III antiarrhythmic agents, such as amiodarone and dofetilide, may have therapeutic benefit in patients with LV dysfunction.

Currently, amiodarone is the most commonly used antiarrhythmic agent in patients with LV dysfunction. The efficacy of prophylactic amiodarone administration in patients with LV dysfunction and asymptomatic, non–life-threatening ventricular arrhythmias has been evaluated in two clinical trials. In the Grupo de Estudia de la Sobrevida en la Insuficienca Cardiaca en Argentina trial, treatment with amiodarone (300 mg/day) was associated with a 30% reduction in mortality.[183] Reduction in both sudden cardiac death and progressive cardiac failure was observed. However, in the Congestive Heart Failure Survival Trial of Antiarrhythmic Therapy (CHF-STAT), amiodarone (300 mg/day) was associated with a trend of improved survival only in patients with CHF secondary to nonischemic causes.[184] Thus, amiodarone may be considered if antiarrhythmic therapy is used in patients with LV dysfunction and asymptomatic, non–life-threatening ventricular arrhythmias.

Dofetilide, a class III antiarrhythmic agent, was recently evaluated in patients with LV dysfunction in the Danish Investigations of Arrhythmia and Mortality on Dofetilide trial.[185] A 25% reduction in HF hospitalizations was observed. The role of dofetilide in patients with LV dysfunction must be elucidated, however.

A history of life-threatening ventricular arrhythmias warrants placement of an implantable cardioverter-defibrillator (ICD).[186] Since their development in the 1980s, ICDs have revolutionized the management of life-threatening ventricular arrhythmias in the setting of LV dysfunction. Technological improvements in the ICD now permit surgical insertion in a manner similar to pacemaker implantation. Current ICDs are capable of delivering a high-energy shock to patients with ventricular fibrillation and rapid ventricular tachycardia or providing antitachycardia pacing to patients with monomorphic ventricular tachycardia. Several trials have been conducted to compare the efficacy of antiarrhythmic therapy and ICD placement.[186] Based on the results of these trials, mild to moderate LV dysfunction and documented sustained or nonsustained ventricular tachycardia warrant placement of an ICD. In patients with severe CHF, the ICD may be used as a bridge to transplantation. In the absence of sustained, nonsustained, or inducible ventricular arrhythmias, sufficient data are currently lacking for empiric placement of an ICD in patients with LV dysfunction. Results from large, ongoing trials such as the Sudden Cardiac Death in Heart Failure trial are being awaited.

In addition to ventricular arrhythmias, atrial fibrillation occurs in 10% to 50% of patients with CHF, and its incidence increases with worsening CHF severity.[187] Elevated atrial pressures lead to hypertrophy and interstitial fibrosis, both of which in conjunction with increased concentrations of circulating norepinephrine and other neurohormones can alter the normal electrophysiologic properties of the atria, leading to multiple reentry circuits and atrial fibrillation. In CHF, atrial fibrillation can lead to systemic embolization, adverse hemodynamic effects, worsening symptoms, decreased exercise tolerance, and increased mortality.[187] Ret-

rospective analyses of the SOLVD trials also describe an association between atrial fibrillation and an increased risk of mortality and CHF progression.[188] If ventricular rate control is the goal of therapy, then digoxin, a β-blocker, or amiodarone can be tried.[187] If pharmacologic maintenance of normal sinus rhythm is the goal of therapy, then amiodarone is the drug of choice, and class I antiarrhythmics should be avoided.[187] Dofetilide may offer an alternative to amiodarone in the future. Warfarin anticoagulation, unless there are contraindications, is also indicated for patients with CHF and concomitant atrial fibrillation.[187]

SURGERY AND RELATED THERAPIES

Orthotopic Heart Transplantation. During the past three decades, orthotopic heart transplantation has emerged as the standard definitive therapy for patients with severe CHF refractory to medical therapy.[51] In the United States, the 1- and 5-year posttransplant survival rates are approximately 85% and 69%, respectively,[189] both of which far exceed corresponding survival rates for patients with severe CHF.[51] However, the number of patients needing transplants far outstrips the limited availability of donor hearts, thereby restricting the annual number of transplants to 2,300, with nearly 4,100 patients currently or soon to be listed for the procedure.[51] These figures do not begin to address the potential 40,000 patients in the United States who might benefit from transplantation.[189]

Given the shortage of available donor hearts, patients referred for cardiac transplantation undergo a specific evaluation to prioritize those most likely to benefit from the procedure. Most patients referred for transplantation are adults 50 to 64 years old with severe ventricular dysfunction (a resting LVEF <25%) secondary to advanced CAD or nonischemic cardiomyopathy.[51,189] The cause of CHF is determined for each patient; potentially reversible and precipitating factors are corrected; medical therapy, if possible, should be maximally tailored to delay the need for transplantation and to preserve end-organ function; and patients are evaluated with a measurement of exercise performance, Vo_{2max}.[51] Other comorbid conditions that may affect posttransplant morbidity or mortality (i.e., malignancy or a life-threatening infectious disease) should be identified.[51,189] These diagnostic and therapeutic efforts are used to stratify potential recipients as United Network for Organ Sharing (UNOS) status I or II patients. The former is the highest-priority status and specifies that potential recipients should be receiving inpatient parenteral pharmacologic (e.g., dobutamine or milrinone) or mechanical (e.g., intraaortic balloon pump or ventricular support device) support to maintain effective CO. All other patients are listed as UNOS status II patients.[51]

Proper selection and management of donor hearts and donor–recipient matching are essential to transplant success. Ideally, donors are under 40 years old and without cancer, cardiac disease, or active infection.[189] Potential donors also must meet both medical and legal criteria for brain death.[189] Donor hearts are allocated according to ABO blood type compatibility, accrued waiting time on the transplant list, body weight, and geographic region.[51,189] Recent data suggest that minimizing human lymphocyte antigen mismatches improves graft survival after transplantation.[51] Recipients are screened for preformed immunoglobulin G circulating antibodies against a panel of donor antigens (i.e., panel reactive antibodies) that are likely to trigger hyperacute rejection during the immediate posttransplant period.[51]

The impressive survival after cardiac transplantation can be traced largely to improved immunosuppression and perhaps most specifically to the introduction of cyclosporine. Cyclosporine is most commonly coprescribed with corticosteroids (usually prednisone) and mycophenolate mofetil (MMF) or azathioprine (i.e., triple-drug therapy) after a heart transplant.[51] A recent study comparing triple-drug therapy using MMF or azathioprine as the antiproliferative agent showed that MMF significantly reduced 1-year mortality and the need for antirejection treatment.[51] In addition, tacrolimus is replacing cyclosporine at some institutions. Immunosuppressive therapy must be tailored for each patient, with careful monitoring for potential adverse effects, cyclosporine or tacrolimus whole blood concentrations, drug interactions, signs and symptoms of rejection, and infectious complications. Induction therapy with antilymphocyte antibodies, usually rabbit or equine polyclonal antithymocyte globulin, may be used to facilitate earlier corticosteroid tapering or withdrawal and to hasten the development of immune tolerance, which should delay the mean time to initial allograft rejection. In addition, antilymphocyte antibodies are used to treat corticosteroid-resistant or hemodynamically severe allograft rejection.

Posttransplant complications may include a variety of bacterial, viral, fungal, or protozoal infections.[51] Perhaps the most worrisome is cytomegalovirus (CMV) infection because of its association with the development of coronary allograft vasculopathy.[51] Coronary allograft vasculopathy is a rapidly progressive, obliterative vasculopathy that leads to concentric myointimal hyperplasia in the coronary arteries of the donor heart and is the principal cause of death in long-term transplant survivors.[51] Preemptive treatment with intravenous ganciclovir may reduce the incidence of posttransplant CMV disease.[190] In addition, prophylactic intravenous ganciclovir administration may reduce coronary allograft vasculopathy.[191] Posttransplant HTN and renal dysfunction remain common complications, and the incidence of skin cancers and lymphoproliferative disorders increases after a cardiac transplant.[51]

Newer medical therapies are emerging for transplantation management. These include new immunosuppressive drugs such as sirolimus (previously known as rapamycin).[192] Calcium channel blockers such as diltiazem and HMG-CoA reductase inhibitors such as pravastatin may decrease the rate of development of coronary allograft vasculopathy.[192] In addition, coadministering ketoconazole, an inhibitor of cyclosporine metabolism, decreases the cost of cyclosporine therapy and may reduce the incidence of rejection.[192] In the future, agents such as soluble CTLA-4, which invokes T-cell anergy by inhibiting the binding of the CD28 receptor on the T cell to the B-7 receptor on the antigen-presenting cell and, therefore, T-cell activation and clonal expansion, may permit donor heart transplantation without concomitant immunosuppressive drug therapy.[193]

Coronary Artery Revascularization. Because of the prevalence of CAD as a cause for CHF and the growing waiting list for cardiac transplantation, coronary artery revascularization is an important therapeutic strategy and alternative for selected patients. It is clear that CABG confers an improved survival benefit in patients with moderate to severe LV systolic dysfunction and concurrent symptom-limiting angina pectoris.[51] In addition, CABG can be used in patients with ischemic cardiomyopathy without angina.[194] After CABG surgery for patients with severe LV dysfunction (LVEF <25%), 5-year survival rates range from 73% to 87%.[189] However, it is important to detect and quantify the amount of ischemic but viable myocardium with techniques such as thallium-201 scintigraphy, positron emission tomography, or dobutamine echocardiography to properly select patients with CHF for whom CABG surgery will improve clinical outcomes.[189]

With respect to alternatives to CABG surgery, prospective, comparative studies of percutaneous coronary interventions such as percutaneous transluminal coronary angioplasty (PTCA) and CABG surgery are lacking in patients with CHF. However, a clinical history of CHF in conjunction with a decreased LVEF in patients undergoing percutaneous coronary interventions (principally PTCA) is associated with significant increases in 6-month mortality.[195] Other emerging revascularization techniques for patients with ischemic cardiomyopathy and CHF include transmyocardial or percutaneous myocardial revascularization (TMR or PMR)[196] and intramyocardial angiogenic gene therapy.[197] With the former, channels from the LV cavity to the ischemic myocardium are created by a high-powered CO_2 laser applied either to the heart's epicardial surface (TMR) using an open chest procedure or to the endocardial surface of the heart (PMR) via standard femoral arterial access.[196] However, patency of these ventriculomyocardial channels is not maintained chronically, and the sustained improvement in anginal symptoms may occur secondary to the neovascularization that follows the thermal injury induced by the TMR or PMR procedure. PMR appears to be more suitable for patients with severely depressed LV dysfunction caused by CAD.[196] With intramyocardial angiogenic gene therapy, patients receive through a mini-thoracotomy an intramyocardial injection that contains DNA encoding vascular endothelial growth factor (VEGF).[197] VEGF induces neovascularization. A catheter-based system for percutaneous myocardial gene delivery is under investigation and, like PMR, it may hold promise for patients with CHF caused by ischemic cardiomyopathy.

Mechanical and Other Bridges or Alternatives to Orthotopic Heart Transplantation. In addition to cardiac transplantation and coronary revascularization procedures, other surgical approaches such as dynamic cardiomyoplasty, left ventriculectomy, and mechanical circulatory support devices are being investigated in advanced CHF management.[189,198] With dynamic cardiomyoplasty, the latissimus dorsi muscle, usually the left, while maintaining its blood supply is detached, moved into the chest, and wrapped around the heart. It is then electrically stimulated to convert it from a fast-twitch to slow-twitch muscle to reduce fatigability.[189,198] The electrically stimulated contractions of the latissimus dorsi muscle are intended to assist the systolic function of the heart. The Cardiac–Skeletal Muscle Assist Randomized Trial is under way to determine the role of dynamic cardiomyoplasty in CHF treatment.[198]

Left ventriculectomy, or the Batista procedure, is a direct attempt to surgically reduce ventricular dilation by removing a substantial segment of the LV free wall.[198] Therefore, according to the law of Laplace, ventricular wall stress is reduced. Mitral valve repair or modification is often performed at the time of ventriculectomy. Early single-center results with this procedure report an actuarial 11-month survival of nearly 90%, with a significant reduction in the need for cardiac transplantation.[198] However, better selection of the most suitable patients is needed before this procedure can be applied more widely.

Several mechanical circulatory support devices are available as transitions to myocardial recovery or as bridges to transplantation.[189] These include the intra-aortic balloon pump (IABP), HeartMate LV assist system (LVAS), the Novacor N100 LVAS, the Thoratec ventricular assist device (VAD), the Abiomed VAD, and the CardioWest total artificial heart (TAH).[189] The IABP is intended only for short-term support of acute HF. The LVAS and VAD systems are FDA-approved as bridges to transplantation, and the TAH is under investigation as a bridge to transplantation. In the future, it is highly likely that the LVAS and TAH systems will be used as alternatives to transplantation, given the mismatch between the number of donor hearts available and the number of patients needing a transplant.

ALTERNATIVE THERAPIES

In addition to the aforementioned conventional or investigational pharmacologic and surgical therapies, several alternative remedies have been studied in patients with CHF. Early open-label and placebo-controlled studies in which coenzyme Q_{10}, an endogenously synthesized provitamin with antioxidant properties that is also involved in mitochondrial ATP synthesis, was administered to patients with CHF showed improvements in LVEF, clinical symptoms, and NYHA status.[199] However, in a recent placebo-controlled crossover study, coenzyme Q_{10}, 100 mg per day for 3 months, did not improve resting LVEF or quality of life in patients with LV systolic dysfunction despite more than a doubling of coenzyme Q_{10} plasma levels.[200]

l-Carnitine is an essential endogenous cofactor that under ischemic conditions enhances carbohydrate metabolism by facilitating β-oxidation of lipids and reduces intracellular accumulation of the toxic metabolites long-chain acylcarnitine and long-chain acyl CoA.[201] Long-chain acylcarnitine can disrupt cell membranes, inhibit sarcolemmal Na^+–K^+–ATPase, impair normal cellular electrophysiology, and inhibit the release of endothelium-derived relaxing factor, whereas long-chain acyl CoA uncouples oxidative phosphorylation.[201] In CHF, serum l-carnitine levels are high, but myocardial levels are low.[201] Propionyl-l-carnitine (PLC), an analogue of l-carnitine that more rapidly enters into myocytes than l-carnitine and has additional antioxidant properties, when given in a randomized, placebo-controlled trial at dosages of 500 mg three times daily to patients with moderate CHF, significantly increased LVEF and exercise capacity.[201] However, the role of PLC in HF not secondary to carnitine deficiency syndromes remains to be determined.

Creatine and phosphocreatinine play important roles in ATP regeneration in exercising skeletal muscles.[202] In chronic CHF, resting skeletal muscle biopsies have shown reduced creatine concentrations, and magnetic resonance imaging studies have revealed a delay in the resynthesis of phosphocreatine after exercise.[202] In a recent study, patients with chronic CHF were randomized to receive creatine 5 g four times daily for 5 days, or placebo.[202] In the patients receiving creatine supplementation, there was a significant increase in forearm muscle contractions at 75% of maximal contraction and decreases in ammonia and lactate concentrations per contraction. However, sustained benefits and safety of creatine supplementation along with appropriate patient identification must be addressed before creatine can be routinely recommended for patients with CHF.

Other dietary supplements have been administered to patients with CHF. Thiamine deficiency may occur in patients as the result of long-term therapy with loop diuretics.[201] Although thiamine supplementation at dosages of 200 mg per day may significantly improve LVEF, other beneficial outcome measures have not been evaluated.[203] Vitamin C, in dosages of 1 g twice daily for 4 weeks, improved endothelial function by enhancing flow-dependent arterial dilation in patients with CHF via increased availability of nitric oxide.[204] However, as for thiamine, the long-term benefits of vitamin C supplementation remain to be determined. The administration of omega-3 fatty acids, 8 g per day for 18 weeks, to a patient with advanced CHF and cardiac cachexia resulted in a decrease in circulating TNF-α and increases in body weight, body fat percentage, and serum albumin.[205]

FUTURE THERAPIES

Several agents that influence a variety of pathophysiologic processes are under development. BNP, a hormone produced by the ventricles, is structurally similar to ANP and has been hypothesized to modulate fluid status in patients with CHF. Intravenous nesiritide, a recently developed synthetic form of BNP, was associated with reductions in pulmonary capillary wedge pressure (PCWP), systemic vascular resistance (SVR), and plasma norepinephrine and aldosterone levels.[206,207] A compensatory increase in the cardiac index also was observed. Nesiritide represents a new class of agents that may be used to manage acute CHF exacerbations. In addition, several endopeptidase inhibitors, which inhibit the degradation of natriuretic peptides, and combination endopeptidase and ACE inhibitors are under development.[208] An improvement in hemodynamics has occurred after both intravenous and oral administration of bosentan, an ET_A and ET_B antagonist.[209] Specific ET_A receptor antagonists and

ECE inhibitors also are under investigation. Administering the MMP inhibitor CP-471,474 has attenuated the early LV enlargement after experimental acute myocardial infarction.[210] Levosimendan, a calcium sensitizer, improves the response of myofilaments to calcium by binding troponin C, thereby stabilizing the troponin C conformation and augmenting calcium binding, which improves contractility.[211] Intravenous formulations are under investigation for management of acute CHF. Two agents have been studied that antagonize TNF-α.[212,213] Pentoxifylline, which suppresses TNF-α production, has improved NYHA functional class and LVEF.[212] Intravenous infusions of etanercept, a soluble TNF-α receptor two (TNF-R$_2$) fusion protein that binds TNF-α, has improved quality-of-life scores, 6-minute walk test, and LVEF.[213]

HEART FAILURE CAUSED BY DIASTOLIC DYSFUNCTION

Diastolic dysfunction, an inadequacy of ventricular relaxation and impaired LV filling, can present with the same signs and symptoms of CHF associated with systolic dysfunction or it can be asymptomatic.[2] Diastolic dysfunction is characterized by a normal or near-normal LVEF (i.e., >40% to >53%), abnormally elevated ventricular filling pressures, but normal or modestly increased ventricular volumes (Table 21.1).[214] The diagnosis of diastolic dysfunction is one of exclusion in which a patient exhibits clinical criteria for CHF but has preserved systolic function (i.e., normal LVEF) as determined by echocardiography.[214] In addition, radionuclide angiography can be used to evaluate ventricular filling, which is delayed in the setting of diastolic dysfunction.[214] Typical causes of diastolic dysfunction include HTN, aortic stenosis, hypertrophic cardiomyopathies, and CAD, which produce either significant LV hypertrophy, thereby altering the passive elastic properties of the ventricle, or myocardial ischemia, which impairs energy-dependent diastolic relaxation.[214] In some series of patients with CHF, diastolic dysfunction accounts for 14% to 51% of the cases.[214,215] In at least one series, women accounted for 65% of the group with CHF and normal LVEF.[215] Survival rates for patients with symptomatic diastolic dysfunction are about twice those of patients with symptomatic systolic dysfunction.[214,215] However, the mortality risk for patients with CHF and normal LVEF is four times greater than for controls without CHF.[215] Readmission rates for patients with CHF secondary to diastolic dysfunction are similar to those for patients with CHF caused by systolic dysfunction.[214]

The pharmacologic treatment of symptomatic or asymptomatic diastolic dysfunction is empiric because there have been no large-scale, prospective, controlled investigations.

Nonetheless, the goals of therapy should parallel those for treating systolic dysfunction, with special attention devoted to managing HTN aggressively to minimize or reverse LV hypertrophy and other remodeling responses, recognizing and treating CAD and myocardial ischemia to improve energy-dependent ventricular diastolic relaxation, relieving congestive symptoms related to increased ventricular filling pressures, and improving diastolic filling by slowing HR.[214] For symptomatic patients (Fig. 21.3), diuretics in conjunction with salt restriction are indicated initially to relieve congestive symptoms. Thereafter, β-adrenergic blockers, calcium channel blockers (e.g., verapamil), or ACE inhibitors, and by extension ARBs, may be beneficial. The former two are negative inotropic and negative chronotropic agents. In addition, both agents have anti-ischemic effects that would be beneficial for patients with symptomatic diastolic dysfunction secondary to CAD. All of these agents may promote regression of LV hypertrophy. ACE inhibitors, ARBs, and β-adrenergic blockers also have other benefits mediated via antagonism of neurohormonal maladaptive responses. Interestingly, in the DIG study, administering digoxin to a subgroup of patients with preserved systolic function resulted in a reduction in hospitalization for worsening CHF.[152] However, at this time routine digoxin use cannot be recommended. Nitrates plus hydralazine also can be beneficial.[214] Surgical therapy may be indicated for symptomatic diastolic dysfunction secondary to CAD or aortic stenosis.[214] For asymptomatic patients (Fig. 21.4), antihypertensive agents generally reduce LV hypertrophy.[216] The cost of treating CHF secondary to diastolic dysfunction is estimated to be one-fourth the cost of treating CHF caused by systolic dysfunction.[214]

Acute HF is a common medical emergency generally occurring in one of two clinical settings. Patients with chronic CHF may acutely decompensate. This condition may result from either a natural progression of CHF associated with a decline in cardiac function or some identifiable cardiovascular precipitating factors such as superimposed ischemia or new-onset atrial fibrillation. Alternatively, systemic or patient-related precipitating factors, including infection or medication or dietary noncompliance, may contribute to CHF decompensation. Acute, new-onset HF also may occur in association with acute myocardial infarction. Although similar agents are used to treat acutely decompensated chronic CHF and acute HF caused by acute myocardial infarction, selection of specific drugs may vary. The following discussion is limited to acute decompensation of chronic CHF.

PATHOPHYSIOLOGY

Acute decompensation of chronic severe CHF is characterized by failure of compensatory mechanisms to maintain adequate perfusion to the vital organs.[217] Most patients exhibit some or all of the following (Fig. 21.1): increased afterload or impedance to LV ejection, as evidenced by increased systemic vascular resistance; increased preload or elevated LV filling pressures and secondary pulmonary congestion; myocardial hypertrophy; sodium retention; peripheral edema; myocardial ischemia; and enhanced neurohormonal activation including the sympathetic nervous system, the renin-angiotensin-aldosterone system, and vasopressin antidiuretic hormone. Excessive activity of each of these mechanisms contributes to the vicious circle of CHF, ultimately leading to death.

Unlike the earlier stages of HF that may necessitate a multitude of tests for diagnosis, acute, severe decompensation is easily recognized.[217] Classically, hypotension occurs but blood pressure may be maintained by peripheral vasoconstriction. Compensatory tachycardia often is observed and is especially ominous if it persists. The patient's skin may appear cool and pale because of vasoconstriction. However, diaphoresis may be observed occasionally. Skin mottling and cyanosis indicate shunting of blood from the periphery in an effort to maintain perfusion to the heart and brain. Urine output decreases, and in severe failure states inadequate cerebral perfusion alters mental status. Dyspnea and tachycardia often are present. Systemic venous and pulmonary congestion may manifest as peripheral edema, elevated central venous pressure, and pulmonary edema.

Acute cardiogenic pulmonary edema is the most dramatic sign of LV failure.[217] The terrified patient is sitting bolt upright and expectorating pink, frothy sputum. The patient feels as if he or she is drowning. Diaphoresis may be accompanied by cool and ashen skin. Respiratory rate is rapid and accessory muscles are used for respiration. Pulmonary auscultation reveals rhonchi, wheezes, and rales. Although heart sounds may be difficult to hear, an S_3 usually is present. Overt signs of venous congestion usually are evident.

Therapy for patients with acutely depressed LV function is aimed at identifying and removing precipitating causes, reducing elevated LV filling pressure and systemic vascular resistance, and augmenting CO. Overall management depends on the severity of the acute exacerbation and the extent of compensatory mechanism activation. Some patients can be treated as outpatients with medication adjustment, but most patients need hospitalization for more intensive therapy, including parenterally administered diuretics, vasodilators, inotropic agents, and fluids. About 50% of hospitalized patients are admitted to an intensive care unit[218] for frequent patient assessment with the use of continuous ECG and hemodynamic monitoring. The latter is useful for distinguishing between cardiogenic and noncardiogenic causes of acute exacerbations and guiding therapeutic decisions. One-year survival for patients admitted with acute exacerbation of chronic CHF approaches 62%.[218]

HEMODYNAMIC MONITORING

The use of bedside hemodynamic monitoring with flow-directed pulmonary artery (i.e., Swan–Ganz) catheters and systemic arterial catheters remains a state-of-the art tool in critical care medicine. Although placing a pulmonary artery catheter is not risk-free and some experts contend that this procedure is overused, there is little disagreement over its value in treating patients with acutely decompensated chronic CHF.[219] However, because the hemodynamic parameters obtained are used to design patient-specific drug regimens, correct interpretation by skilled healthcare professionals is needed to optimize use of hemodynamic parameters and initiate appropriate therapeutic interventions. Recent data indicate that considerable variability exists in the ability of many healthcare professionals to assess patient data accurately. Erroneous interpretation and potential complications of right heart catheterization (pulmonary infarction, arrhythmias, thromboembolism, perforation, balloon rupture, and catheter knotting) usually are minimized by careful assessment of all hemodynamic data obtained and placement of the catheter by experienced physicians.

The pulmonary artery catheter is inserted at the bedside, often with the aid of fluoroscopy. A balloon is attached to the tip of the catheter and inserted into the central venous circulation, typically via the subclavian, internal jugular, or femoral vein. The catheter follows antegrade blood flow into the superior vena cava and the right atrium, across the tricuspid valve, and into the right ventricle (Fig. 21.7).[220] The

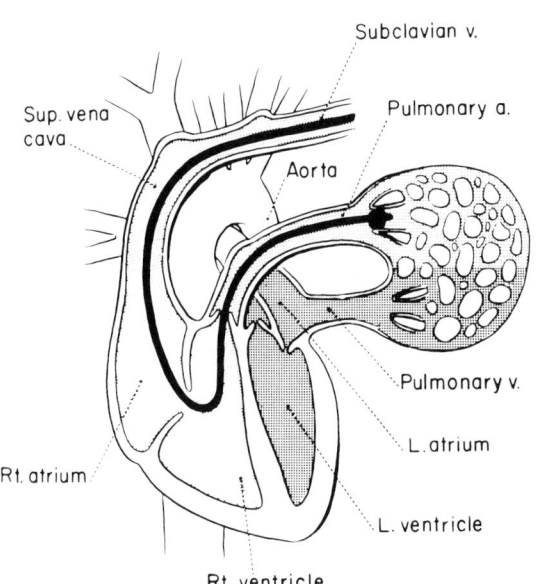

FIGURE 21.7 Final anatomic positioning of the Swan–Ganz Catheter, depicting balloon inflation in the pulmonary artery. (Reprinted with permission from Bollish SJ, Foster TJ. Swan–Ganz catheter: an important tool for monitoring drug therapy in the critically ill. Hosp Formul 16:99–103, 1980).

catheter is advanced into the pulmonary artery and is then inflated to obtain the pulmonary artery occlusion pressure (PAOP). The inflated catheter historically has been called a wedged catheter, so the PAOP is most often called the PCWP.

The systemic arterial pressure, obtained via an arterial line, is monitored continuously, but in severe HF states this is not a reliable indicator of tissue perfusion. The PCWP is extremely important because it indicates pulmonary venous pressure and correlates with signs of pulmonary congestion (Table 21.12). It also indirectly measures the filling pressure of the left ventricle or preload. The pulmonary artery diastolic pressure (PADP) is also a valuable index of LV filling pressure. The multilumen construction of the Swan–Ganz catheter also permits simultaneous measurements of right ventricular preload by measuring right atrial pressure, which is equal to the central venous pressure. SVR is a calculated parameter commonly used to estimate ventricular afterload. However, SVR does not accurately reflect the interaction of factors both internal and external to the myocardium. Stroke volume is the volume of blood ejected with each heartbeat. CO is the volume of blood ejected by the heart per unit time and usually is expressed in liters per minute. CO varies with body size and is therefore normalized by dividing the value by the patient's body surface area, yielding the cardiac index. Estimates of CO generally are obtained by the thermodilution technique. A thermal indicator (usually cooled sterile

TABLE 21.12	Normal Hemodynamic Values
Systemic arterial pressure (systolic/diastolic)	120/80 mm Hg
Mean arterial pressure	70–80 mm Hg
Pulmonary artery pressure (systolic/diastolic)	30/15 mm Hg
Pulmonary capillary wedge pressure	<12 mm Hg
Left atrial pressure	5–12 mm Hg (mean)
Left ventricular end-diastolic pressure	5–12 mm Hg (mean)
Pulmonary vascular resistance	150–250 dynes/sec/cm^5
Systemic vascular resistance	800–1200 dynes/sec/cm^5
Stroke volume	70–130 mL
Right ventricular stroke work	10–15 g·m
Left ventricular stroke work	60–80 g·m
Cardiac output	4–8 L/min
Cardiac index	2.2–4.0 L/min/m^2
Mixed venous oxygen content	13–16 mL/dL
Arterial oxygen content	18–20 mL/dL
Pulmonary capillary oxygen content	20 mL/dL
Arterial-mixed venous oxygen difference	5.0–5.5 mL/dL
Oxygen consumption	22 ± 40 mL/min

Source: Reference 219.

D_5W or normal saline) is injected into the right atrium. A thermistor at the end of the catheter measures the change in blood temperature downstream. The CO is then calculated by a computer using a modification of the Fick principle.

Even though it is not widely used, the arteriovenous oxygen difference is a better indicator of blood flow than is the cardiac index.[219] It is fairly constant and independent of body surface area, metabolic rate, or oxygen uptake. The arteriovenous oxygen difference assesses the adequacy of CO in relation to the metabolic needs of the tissues. It entails withdrawal of blood samples from the pulmonary and radial arteries. If the patient is not hypoxemic, the mixed venous oxygen content (or saturation) is a good predictor of clinical outcome. A mixed venous oxygen saturation of less than 40% is associated with a very poor prognosis.

TREATMENT

Nonspecific measures designed to decrease pulmonary congestion and improve oxygenation are indicated in all patients with acute failure (Figs. 21.5 and 21.6).[217] In addition, the patient should be evaluated for the presence of precipitating, potentially reversible factors. Supplemental oxygen, perhaps facilitated by mechanical ventilation, improves oxygen delivery. The patient should be seated to minimize respiratory distress. Morphine sulfate administration is beneficial because of its potent venodilatory effect and anxiolytic action. Small dosages (2 to 4 mg) are repeated often until acute pulmonary congestion is relieved or alternative parenteral vasodilator therapy is begun. Respiratory depression and systemic hypotension may limit morphine use. After the Swan–Ganz catheter and arterial line are inserted, patient-specific regimens may be tailored based on the hemodynamic profile and the clinical signs and symptoms.

DIURETICS

A mainstay of treatment for acute decompensation and pulmonary edema, intravenous furosemide or another loop diuretic, causes prompt venodilation and reduces PCWP and pulmonary artery pressure (Figs. 21.5 and 21.6).[221] The venodilatory action of intravenous furosemide is observed within several minutes of administration and precedes its natriuretic effect.[142] Intravenous furosemide administration should not be delayed due to the immediate unavailability of hemodynamic monitoring because dramatic relief of the signs and symptoms of pulmonary congestion may be obtained.[221,222] Either frequent intermittent intravenous injections or a continuous infusion of the drug can be used (Table 21.8). The latter is superior with respect to enhancing urinary output and avoiding potential ototoxic adverse effects. In either case, after the initial dose, hemodynamic data, urine output, and sustained relief of pulmonary congestion should guide the furosemide dosage. Oral furosemide generally does not exert an acute venodilatory effect. Bumetanide and torsemide are alternative loop diuretics, although furosemide usually is given first.

VASODILATORS

By blocking the positive feedback mechanisms of severe HF, parenteral vasodilators may abruptly improve CO and relieve pulmonary congestion.[217] The patient's hemodynamic profile guides selection of specific vasodilators according to their effects on preload and afterload (Fig. 21.6). Sodium nitroprusside often is the first vasodilator used because it acts on both preload and afterload. It has a fast onset of action and a short duration of action, so sodium nitroprusside is easily titrated. In many patients, it lowers pulmonary artery pressure, PCWP, and SVR, resulting in increased CO. The initial infusion rate is 0.25 to 0.5 μg/kg/minute and is titrated upward based on hemodynamic and clinical response. Generally blood pressure, pulmonary artery pressures, and urine output are monitored continuously. CO and SVR are assessed every 2 to 6 hours to aid in dosage adjustment. The most common hazard of nitroprusside in treating severe HF is hypotension.

Intravenous nitroglycerin is especially useful in acute decompensation because it is easily titrated. Because it predominantly increases venous capacitance (i.e., decreases preload), its effect is primarily to decrease PCWP and pulmonary artery pressures (Fig. 21.6).[217,221] Thus, it provides dramatic relief for patients with severe pulmonary congestion. It may also moderately decrease SVR and thus improve CO. Intravenous nitroglycerin dosages vary widely, but initial therapy may begin at 5 to 10 μg per minute. Dangers of nitroglycerin represent an extension of its pharmacologic action and usually are limited to hypotension and reflex tachycardia.

POSITIVE INOTROPIC AGENTS

Inotropic agents improve contractility by increasing intracellular calcium concentrations. In addition, calcium reuptake into the sarcoplasmic reticulum is improved during diastole. Agents used for inotropic support during acute CHF exacerbations include the β-adrenergic agonists and the phosphodiesterase inhibitors. Digoxin is of limited use in managing acute exacerbations. Because severe chronic congestive failure is complicated by overstimulation of the sympathetic nervous system and downregulation of β-receptors, exogenous catecholamine administration generally is reserved for acute exacerbations. Dopamine may be especially useful in patients with mild to moderate hypotension (Fig. 21.6).[175,217] The initial dosage is 0.5 to 1.0 μg/kg/minute and is titrated upward according to filling pressures, CO, and urine output. If hypotension is severe (i.e., ≤90 mm Hg), dopamine dosages in the range of 5 to 20 μg/kg/minute provide the α-adrenergic stimulation necessary to maintain perfusion to the vital organs and improve CO (Fig. 21.6). Dopamine side effects include tachycardia, ventricular arrhythmias, and excessive vasoconstriction, especially at higher dosages. Nevertheless, it remains a valuable agent, especially when used in combination with nitroprusside. Additionally, many clinicians advocate the use of dopamine at dosages of less than 2 μg/kg/minute to improve urine output in patients with renal dysfunction secondary to poor CO (Fig. 21.6).[177] However, objective data to support this indication are lacking.

Dobutamine is a synthetic catecholamine that is a selective β_1-agonist that augments cardiac contractility, HR, and cardiac output.[175,217] The improvement in CO may then cause a reflex decrease in both filling pressures and SVR (Fig. 21.6). Unfortunately, these improvements are achieved at the expense of increasing myocardial oxygen consumption. Careful dosage titration is needed to balance dobutamine's negative effects on myocardial oxygen consumption with the positive effects on CO and myocardial perfusion. Dobutamine infusions are begun at 1 to 2 μg/kg/minute and titrated upward every 10 to 30 minutes, with optimal maintenance infusions generally between 5 and 15 μg/kg/minute. Close monitoring of the patient's HR during the dosage titration is needed to achieve an optimal benefit:risk ratio between effects on CO and myocardial ischemia. Adverse effects usually are limited but may include tachycardia, arrhythmias, headaches, anxiety, and tremor. Combination therapy with dobutamine and either milrinone or amrinone therapy may provide greater improvement in LV performance than either agent alone.

Amrinone and milrinone inhibit phosphodiesterase III and subsequently increase intracellular cyclic adenosine monophosphate. Amrinone and milrinone have both positive inotropic actions and significant vasodilator activity.[175,217] Amrinone is associated with the development of a dose-dependent thrombocytopenia, so milrinone is used more often. In CHF associated with a low cardiac index, milrinone reduces pulmonary and systemic vascular resistances, right atrial pressure, and PCWP. The cardiac index increases as a consequence of these "unloading" properties and the positive inotropic effect of the drug. Therefore, their indications overlap those for the intravenous vasodilators, nitroglycerin and nitroprusside, and the parenteral sympathomimetics, dopamine and dobutamine (Fig. 21.6). In contrast to nitroglycerin and nitroprusside, milrinone has a long terminal $t_{1/2}$, so the time to peak pharmacodynamic effects is delayed, necessitating the use of a loading dose to achieve rapid hemodynamic effects. Milrinone dosing guidelines incorporate loading doses of 37.5 to 75 μg per kg, followed by maintenance infusions of 0.375 to 0.75 μg/kg/minute. Many clinicians prefer not to administer a loading dose, with the understanding that the peak pharmacologic effects will be delayed. Like other positive inotropic agents, milrinone can evoke tachycardia and precipitate myocardial ischemia. Additionally, milrinone may lead to hypotension through excessive vasodilation. Milrinone is renally cleared and may accumulate in renal failure, warranting close monitoring of renal function. Milrinone may be used as an alternative to dobutamine or in combination with dobutamine in patients who need intravenous inotropic support.

After hemodynamic and clinical stabilization with the use of intravenous diuretics, vasodilators, inotropes, and fluids, usually in combination, the patient is transitioned to an oral regimen.[222] The regimen should minimally consist of an ACE inhibitor titrated, if possible, to dosages shown to decrease mortality in clinical trials; loop diuretic dosages or loop diuretic–thiazide diuretic combinations adjusted for Scr (Table 21.8) and symptoms of fluid retention, especially pulmonary congestion; and digoxin dosed to the serum concentration as previously discussed. Dosages of diuretics and ACE inhibitors higher than those targeted in clinical trials may be administered, with titration guided by hemodynamic monitoring of PCWP, with a theoretical target of 15 to 16 mm Hg and right atrial pressure of 7 mm Hg or less in the absence of postural hypotension.[223] Normalizing the SVR (i.e., approximately 1,000 to 1,200 dynes/second/cm^{-5}), maintaining a systolic blood pressure of 80 mm Hg or higher, and maintaining a cardiac index adequate to support life (generally >2.0 L/minute/m^2 and possibly >2.5 L/minute/m^2) are other hemodynamic goals that can be achieved by tailoring vasodilator therapy with ACE inhibitors, either alone or in combination with other vasodilators such as nitrates, hydralazine, or perhaps ARBs.[223] When the patient is stabilized to a certain NYHA functional class with optimal, conventional medications, then decisions to add new drugs such as β-blockers or to evaluate the patient for additional nonpharmacologic therapies such as a heart transplant must be made (Fig. 21.5).

CONCLUSIONS

CHF remains a common clinical syndrome, the prevalence of which is increasing as the population ages. A sound working knowledge of the pathophysiology of CHF and how to implement, monitor, and integrate the various therapies is essential to preventing initiation and progression of CHF and improving the symptoms, quality of life, and longevity of patients with CHF. With the exception of diuretics, which are used to manage symptomatic complaints, current therapy is targeted largely at modifying maladaptive neurohormonal and cytokine-mediated mechanisms, which are initially activated in an attempt to maintain CO. ACE inhibitors remain the cornerstone of CHF therapy. In the future, however, ARBs may supplant ACE inhibitors, given the non-ACE pathways that can synthesize angiotensin II. Digoxin and especially β-blockers are additional agents that modulate maladaptive neurohormonal activation. The now-realized clinical importance of β-blockade introduces a new quadruple-drug therapy era in pharmacologic CHF management (Fig. 21.2). However, because clinician use of ACE inhibitors remains suboptimal and because patient compliance decreases as a function of the number of prescriptions, there will be difficulties in implementing this intricate quadruple-drug regimen. In the future, in addition to new pharmacologic treatments, the tailoring of existing pharmacotherapy to patient subsets to simplify treatment must be addressed.

PROGNOSIS

Despite the lack of published information describing the natural history of HF in the absence of treatment, studies in patients receiving some form of pharmacologic treatment have revealed that the overall prognosis is grim. In the Framingham study the 5-year survival after the diagnosis of CHF was 25% for men and 38% for women.[3] These survival statistics are worse than those reported for the placebo groups in several pharmacologic treatment trials.[224] However, the Framingham study covered a period before the more widespread use of ACE inhibitors and enrolled older patients. For hospitalized patients the 1-year mortality ranges from 30% to 50%, whereas for patients with less severe chronic stable CHF treated with appropriate therapy, the annual mortality is about 10%.[38] Between 1979 and 1996 deaths from CHF in the United States increased almost 120%.[10] The major causes of death from CHF are progression of disease or sudden death caused by lethal ventricular arrhythmias.

Several clinical variables have been shown to be predictive of prognosis in patients with CHF. Diminished LVEF, especially below 20%, or peak oxygen consumption (Vo_{2max}) during maximal exercise testing of 14 mL/minute/kg or less predicts a poor prognosis.[225] Increases in cardiothoracic ratio on chest roentgenogram, severity of symptoms (i.e., higher NYHA class), and a plasma norepinephrine level more than 600 pg per mL also predict a poor prognosis.[225] Elevated plasma levels of endothelin-1 and its inactive precursor, big ET-1,[226] and increased natriuretic peptide concentrations[38] appear to be of negative prognostic value as well. In some studies,[227] but not others,[228] nonsustained ventricular arrhythmias (i.e., couplets and triplets or nonsustained ventricular tachycardia) in patients with CHF are independent predictors of a diminished survival. Older patients also exhibit a worse prognosis than younger patients. Even patients who are treated with "life-saving" pharmacologic therapy have an unsatisfactory prognosis.[10,38] In VHeFT-II, for example, the 5-year survival in the enalapril group was approximately 55%. Thus, CHF remains a highly lethal clinical syndrome despite "effective" medical intervention.

PHARMACOECONOMICS

For 1999 the projected figure for healthcare expenditures for CHF in the United States was $21 billion.[10] This included $19.6 billion for direct costs (i.e., hospitalizations, professional fees, medications, and home health care) and $1.4 bil-lion for indirect costs, which consist of lost productivity from morbidity and mortality.[10] Of these costs, hospitalization and nursing home placement were the major component, accounting for $15 billion, or approximately 75% of the direct costs.[10]

Drug therapy costs for CHF for 1999 were estimated to be $1 billion, or about 5% of the direct costs.[10] However, for some drug therapies such as ACE inhibitors and β-adrenergic blockers, the cost per life gained ranges from a cost saving of $2,500 over 5 years.[174] These savings result principally from a decrease in hospitalization.[174] ACE inhibitors, β-blockers, and digoxin and perhaps diuretics appear to be cost-effective treatments for CHF.[174]

KEY POINTS

- CHF is a clinical syndrome that progresses to worsening symptoms and death largely as a consequence of maladaptive effects triggered by neurohormones and cytokines
- CHF can result from abnormalities in either systolic or diastolic dysfunction
- Participation in cardiac rehabilitation programs can improve exercise tolerance and quality of life and may reduce mortality in patients with CHF
- In CHF management, patient education is extremely important, especially with respect to facilitating compliance with dietary and medication treatment plans
- Based on their ability to consistently improve both clinical status and longevity, ACE inhibitors are considered first-line therapy for CHF
- ACE inhibitor therapy should begin with low dosages that are titrated slowly to target dosages
- Alternative vasodilator therapy such as ARBs or the combination of nitrates plus hydralazine should be reserved for patients intolerant of ACE inhibitors. β-Blockers are currently advocated for treating patients with stable NYHA class II or III CHF, based on their ability to reduce mortality and hospitalization rates.
- As with ACE inhibitors, the initiation of β-blocking therapy begins with low dosages that are increased slowly and carefully
- Diuretics are used to relieve CHF symptoms
- Digoxin can be used safely in most patients with CHF caused by systolic dysfunction, with target serum concentrations between 0.7 and 1.2 ng per mL
- The use of chronic, intermittent, or continuous inotrope infusions should be reserved for patients with severe, refractory CHF
- Anticoagulant therapy is indicated in patients with CHF and coexisting atrial fibrillation or other conditions that predispose them to thromboembolic conditions
- ICDs are indicated in patients with a history of sustained ventricular tachycardia

REFERENCES

1. Consensus Recommendations for the Management of Chronic Heart Failure. Part I. Evaluation of heart failure. Am J Cardiol 83 (Suppl A):2A–8A, 1999.
2. Gaasch WH. Diagnosis and treatment of heart failure based on left ventricular systolic or diastolic dysfunction. JAMA 271:1276–1280, 1994.
3. Ho KK, Anderson KM, Kannel WB, et al. Survival after onset of congestive heart failure in Framingham Heart Study subjects. Circulation 88:107–115, 1993.
4. Gheorghiade M, Bonow RO. Chronic heart failure in the United States. A manifestation of coronary artery disease. Circulation 97:282–289, 1998.
5. Fonarow GC, Abraham WT, Albert NM, et al. Organized Program to Initiate Lifesaving Treatment in Hospitalized Patients with Heart Failure (OPTIMIZE-HF): rationale and design. Am Heart J 148:43–51, 2004.
6. Adams, KF, Fonarow GC, Emerman CL, et al. Characteristics and outcomes of patients hospitalized for heart failure in the United States: rationale, design, and preliminary observations from the first 100,000 cases in the Acute Decompensated Heart Failure National Registry (ADHERE). Am Heart J 149:209–216, 2005
7. Feenstra J, Grobbee DE, Remme WJ, et al. Drug-induced heart failure. J Am Coll Cardiol 33:1152–1162, 1999.
8. Nesto RW, Bell D, Bonow RO, et al. American Heart Association, American Diabetes Association. Thiazolidinedione use, fluid retention, and congestive heart failure: a consensus statement from the American Heart Association and American Diabetes Association. Circulation 108:2941–2948, 2003.
9. Coats AJ. Is preventive medicine responsible for the increasing prevalence of heart failure? Lancet 352 (Suppl I):39–41, 1998.
10. American Heart Association. Heart Disease and Stroke Statistics, 2005 Update. Dallas, TX: American Heart Association, 2005.
11. Colucci WS. Molecular and cellular mechanisms of myocardial failure. Am J Cardiol 80 (Suppl L):15L–25L, 1997.
12. Jacob J, Gilbert EM. The sympathetic nervous system in chronic heart failure. Prog Cardiovasc Dis 41 (Suppl 1):9–16, 1998.
13. Schmermund A, Lerman Lo, Ritman EL, et al. Cardiac production of angiotensin II and its pharmacologic inhibition: effects on the coronary circulation. Mayo Clin Proc 74:503–513, 1999.
14. Love MP, McMurray JJ. Endothelin in chronic heart failure: current position and future prospects. Cardiovasc Res 31:665–674, 1996.
15. Rohde LE, Ducharme A, Arroyo LH, et al. Matrix metalloproteinase inhibition attenuates early left ventricular enlargement after experimental myocardial infarction in mice. Circulation 99:3063–3070, 1999.
16. Givertz MM, Colucci WS. New targets for heart-failure therapy: endothelin, inflammatory cytokines, and oxidative stress. Lancet 352 (Suppl I):34–38, 1998.
17. Stein BC, Levin RI. Natriuretic peptides: physiology, therapeutic potential, and risk stratification in ischemic heart disease. Am Heart J 135:914–923, 1998.
18. Schirger JA, Heublein DM, Chen HH, et al. Presence of Dendroaspis natriuretic peptide-like immunoreactivity in human plasma and its increase during human heart failure. Mayo Clin Proc 74:126–130, 1999.
19. Drexler H. Nitric oxide synthases in failing human heart. A double-edged sword? Circulation 99:2972–2975, 1999.
20. Katz AM. Is the failing heart energy depleted? Cardiol Clin 16:633–644, 1998.
21. Bristow MR. Why does the myocardium fail? Insights from basic science. Lancet 352 (Suppl I):8–14, 1998.
22. Floras JS. Clinical aspects of sympathetic activation and parasympathetic withdrawal in heart failure. J Am Coll Cardiol 22 (Suppl A):72A–84A, 1993.
23. Kapadia S, Dibbs Z, Kurrelmeyer K, et al. The role of cytokines in the failing human heart. Cardiol Clin 16:645–656, 1998.
24. Francis GS. TNF-α and heart failure. The difference between proof of principle and hypothesis testing. Circulation 99:3213–3214, 1999.
25. The Task Force on Heart Failure of the European Society of Cardiology. Guidelines for the diagnosis of heart failure. Eur Heart J 16:741–751, 1995.
26. Marantz PR, Tobin JN, Wassertheil-Smoller S, et al. The relationship between left-ventricular systolic function and congestive heart failure diagnosed by clinical criteria. Circulation 77:607–612, 1988.
27. Harlan WR, Oberman A, Grimm R, et al. Chronic congestive heart failure in coronary artery disease: clinical criteria. Ann Intern Med 86:133–138, 1977.
28. Economides E, Stevenson LW. The jugular veins: knowing enough to look. Am Heart J 136:6–7, 1998.
29. Butman SM, Ewy GA, Standen JR, et al. Bedside cardiovascular examination in patients with severe chronic heart failure: importance of rest or inducible jugular vein distension. J Am Coll Cardiol 22:968–974, 1993.
30. McGee SR. Physical examination of venous pressure: a critical review. Am Heart J 136:10–18, 1998.
31. Mattelman SJ, Hakki A, Iskandrian AS, et al. Reliability of bedside evaluation in determining left ventricular function and correlation with left-ventricular ejection fraction determined by radionuclide ventriculography. J Am Coll Cardiol 1:417–420, 1983.
32. Fleg JL, Hinton PC, Lakatta EG, et al. Physician utilization of laboratory procedures to monitor outpatients with congestive heart failure. Arch Intern Med 149:393–396, 1989.
33. Felker GM, Leimberger JD, Califf RM, et al. Risk stratification after hospitalization for decompensated heart failure. J Card Fail 10:460–466, 2004.
34. Klein L, O'Connor CM, Leimberger JD, et al. Lower serum sodium is associated with increased short-term mortality in hospitalized patients with worsening heart failure: results from the OPTIME-CHF Study. Circulation 111:2454–2460, 2005.
35. Packer M, Gottlieb SS, Kessler PD. Hormone-electrolyte interactions in the pathogenesis of lethal cardiac arrhythmias in patients with congestive heart failure. Am J Med 80 (Suppl 4A):23–29, 1986.
36. Maisel AJ, Krishnaswany P, Nowak RM, et al. Rapid measurement of B-type natriuretic peptide in the emergency diagnosis of heart failure. N Engl J Med 347:161–167, 2002.
37. Maisel A, Hollander JE, Guss D, et al. Primary results of the Rapid Emergency Department Heart Failure Outpatient Trial (REDHOT). A multicenter study of B-type natriuretic peptide levels, emergency department decision making, and outcomes in patients presenting with shortness of breath. J Am Coll Cardiol 44:1328–1333, 2004.
38. Sharpe N, Doughty R. Epidemiology of heart failure and ventricular dysfunction. Lancet 352 (Suppl I):3–7, 1998.
39. McDonagh TA, Robb SD, Murdoch DR, et al. Biochemical detection of left-ventricular systolic dysfunction. Lancet 351:9–13, 1998.
40. AHA Medical Scientific Statement. 1994 revisions to classification of functional capacity and objective assessment of patients with diseases of the heart. Circulation 90:644–645, 1994.
41. Hunt SA, Baker DW, Chin MH, et al. ACC/AHA guidelines for the evaluation and management of chronic heart failure in the adult: a report of the American College of Cardiology/American Heart Association Task Force on Practice Guidelines (Committee to Revise the 1995 Guidelines for the Evaluation and Management of Heart Failure). 2001. American College of Cardiology Web site. Available at: http://www.acc.org/clinical/guidelines/failure/hf_index.htm
42. Weber KT, Janicki JS. Cardiopulmonary exercise testing for evaluation of chronic cardiac failure. Am J Cardiol 55:22A–31A, 1985.
43. Guyatt GH. Measurement of health-related quality of life in heart failure. J Am Coll Cardiol 22 (Suppl A):185A–191A, 1993.
44. Guyatt GH, Sullivan MJ, Thompson PF, et al. The 6-minute walk: a measure of exercise capacity in patients with chronic heart failure. Can Med Assoc J 132:919–923, 1985.
45. Bittner V, Weiner DH, Yusuf S, et al. Prediction of mortality and morbidity with a 6-minute walk test in patients with left ventricular dysfunction. JAMA 270:1702–1707, 1993.
46. Uretsky BF, Pina I, Quigg RJ, et al. Beyond drug therapy: nonpharmacologic care of the patient with advanced heart failure. Am Heart J 135:S264–284, 1998.

47. O'Connor CM, Gattis WA, Swedberg K. Current and novel pharmacologic approaches in the management of advanced heart failure. Am Heart J 135:S250–263, 1998.
48. HFSA Guideline Committee. HFSA guidelines for management of patients with heart failure caused by left ventricular systolic dysfunction: pharmacological approaches. J Card Failure 4:357–382, 1999.
49. Abraham WT, Hayes DL. Cardiac resynchronization therapy for heart failure. Circulation 108:2596–2603, 2003.
50. Bardy GH, Lee KL, Mark DB, et al. Amiodarone or an implantable cardioverter-defibrillator for congestive heart failure. N Engl J Med 352:225–237, 2005.
51. Winkel E, DiSesa VJ, Costanzo MR. Advances in transplantation. Part 1: advances in heart transplantation. Dis Mon 45:63–87, 1999.
52. Consensus Recommendations for the Management of Heart Chronic Heart Failure. Part II: management of heart failure. Am J Cardiol 83 (Suppl A):9A–30A, 1999.
53. Joyce D, Loebe M, Noon GP, et al. Revascularization and ventricular restoration in patients with ischemic heart failure: the STICH trial. Curr Opinion Cardiol 18:454–457, 2003.
54. Sullivan MJ, Higginbotham M, Cobb FR. Exercise training in patients with chronic heart failure delays ventilation aerobic threshold and improves submaximal exercise performance. Circulation 79: 324–329, 1989.
55. Coats AJ, Adamopoulos S, Meyer TE, et al. Effects of physical training in chronic heart failure. Lancet 335:63–66, 1990.
56. Belardinelli R, Georgiou D, Cianci G, et al. Randomized, controlled trial of long-term moderate exercise training in chronic heart failure. Circulation 99:1173–1182, 1999.
57. Whellan DJ, O'Connor CM, Pina I. Training trials in heart failure: time to exercise restraint? Am Heart J 147:190–192, 2004.
58. Pina IL, Fitzpatrick JT. Exercise and heart failure: a review. Chest 110:1317–1327, 1996.
59. Bennett SJ, Huster GA, Baker SL, et al. Characterization of the precipitants of hospitalization for heart failure decompensation. Am J Crit Care 7:168–174, 1998.
60. Cooper HA, Dries DL, Davis CE, Shen YL, Domanski MJ. Diuretics and risk of arrhythmic death in patients with left ventricular dysfunction. Circulation 100:1311–1315, 1991.
61. Neuberg GW, Miller AB, O'Connor CM, et al. Diuretic resistance predicts mortality in patients with advanced heart failure. Am Heart J 144:31–38, 2002.
62. Silver MA. Conventional treatments for heart failure. In: Success with heart failure. Help and hope for those with congestive heart failure. New York: Plenum, 1994:25–34.
63. Regan TJ. Alcohol and the cardiovascular system. JAMA 264: 377–381, 1990.
64. Pavan D, Nicolosi GL, Lestuzzi C, et al. Normalization of variables of left ventricular function in patients with alcoholic cardiomyopathy after cessation of excessive alcohol intake: an echocardiographic study. Eur Heart J 8:535–540, 1987.
65. Miller LG. Herbal medicinals. Arch Intern Med 158:2200–2211, 1998.
66. Ghali JK, Kadakia S, Cooper R, et al. Precipitating factors leading to decompensation of heart failure: trait among urban blacks. Arch Intern Med 148:2013–2016, 1988.
67. Goodyer LJ, Miskelly F, Milligan P. Does encouraging good compliance improve patients' clinical condition in heart failure? Br J Clin Practice 49:173–176, 1995.
68. Stewart S, Pearson S, Horowitz JD. Effects of home-based intervention among patients with congestive heart failure discharged from acute hospital care. Arch Intern Med 158:1067–1072, 1998.
69. Shah NB, Der E, Ruggerio C, et al. Prevention of hospitalization for heart failure with an interactive home monitoring program. Am Heart J 135:373–378, 1998.
70. Rich MW, Brooks K, Luther P. Temporal trends in pharmacotherapy for congestive heart failure at an academic medical center: 1990–1995. Am Heart J 135:67–72, 1998.
71. Rich MW. Heart failure disease management: a critical review. J Card Fail 5:64–75, 1999.
72. Gattis WA, Hasselblad V, Whellan DJ, O'Connor CM. Reduction in heart failure events by the addition of a clinical pharmacist to the heart failure management team: results of the Pharmacist in Heart Failure Assessment Recommendation and Monitoring (PHARM) study. Arch Intern Med 159:1939–1945, 1999.
73. Heerdink ER, Leufkens HG, Herings RM, et al. NSAIDs associated with increased risk of congestive heart failure in elderly patients taking diuretics. Arch Intern Med 158:1108–1112, 1998.
74. Komhoff M, Grone HJ, Klein T, et al. Localization of cyclooxygenase-1 and 2 in adult and fetal human kidney: implication for renal function. Am J Physiol 272:F460–F468, 1997.
75. Feldman M, McMahon AT. Do cyclooxygenase-2 inhibitors provide benefits similar to those of traditional nonsteroidal anti-inflammatory drugs, with less gastrointestinal toxicity? Ann Intern Med 132:134–143, 2000.
76. Braunwald E. ACE inhibitors: a cornerstone of the treatment of heart failure. N Engl J Med 325:351–353, 1991.
77. American Society of Health-System Pharmacists. ASHP therapeutic guidelines for angiotensin-converting enzyme inhibitors in patients with left ventricular dysfunction. Am J Health Syst Pharm 54: 299–313, 1997.
78. Garg R, Yusuf S, for the Collaborative Group on ACE Inhibitor Trials. Overview of randomized trials of angiotensin-converting enzyme inhibitors on mortality and morbidity in patients with heart failure. JAMA 273:1450–1456, 1995.
79. Mason DT, Melmon KL. Effects of bradykinin on forearm venous tone and vascular resistance in man. Circ Res 17:106–113, 1965.
80. Grassi G, Cattaneo BM, Seravalle G, et al. Effects of chronic ACE inhibition on sympathetic nerve traffic and baroreflex control of the circulation in heart failure. Circulation 96:1173–1179, 1997.
81. Parmley WW. Cost-effective management of heart failure. Clin Cardiol 19:240–242, 1996.
82. ACE Inhibitor Myocardial Infarction Collaborative Group. Indications for ACE inhibitors in the early treatment of acute myocardial infarction. Circulation 97:2202–2212, 1998.
83. McGrae M, Feinglass J, Lee P, et al. Heart failure between 1986 and 1994: temporal trends in drug-prescribing practices, hospital readmissions, and survival at an academic medical center. Am Heart J 134:901–909, 1997.
84. Stafford RS, Saglam D, Blumenthal D. National patterns of angiotensin-converting enzyme inhibitor use in congestive heart failure. Arch Intern Med 157:2460–2466, 1997.
85. Philbin EF, Rocco RA. Use of angiotensin-converting enzyme inhibitors in heart failure with preserved left ventricular systolic function. Am Heart J 134:188–195, 1997.
86. Fonarow GC, Yancy CW, Chang SF. Variation in heart failure quality of care indicators among US hospitals: analysis of 230 hospitals in ADHERE. Circulation 108: 447, 2003.
87. Fonarow GC, et al. Adherence to heart failure quality-of-care indicators in US hospitals: analysis of the ADHERE Registry. Arch Intern Med 165(13):1455–6, 2005.
88. Fonarow GC. JACC 2005 abstract.
89. Havranck EP, Abrams F, Stevens E, et al. Determinants of mortality in elderly patients with heart failure. Arch Intern Med 158: 2024–2028, 1998.
90. Gattis WA, Larsen RL, Hasselblad V, et al. Is optimal angiotensin-converting enzyme inhibitor dosing neglected in elderly patients with heart failure? Am Heart J 136:43–48, 1998.
91. Packer M, Medina N, Yushak M. Relation between serum sodium concentration and the hemodynamic and clinical response to converting enzyme inhibition with captopril in severe heart failure. J Am Coll Cardiol 3:1035–1043, 1984.
92. Pacher R, Globits S, Bergler-Klein J, et al. Clinical and neurohumoral response of patients with severe congestive heart failure treated with two different captopril dosages. Eur Heart J 14: 273–278, 1993.
93. Reigger GA, Effects of quinapril on exercise tolerance in patients with mild to moderate heart failure. Eur Heart J 12:705–711, 1991.
94. Packer M, Poole-Wilson P, Armstrong P, et al. Comparative effects of low and high doses of angiotensin-converting enzyme inhibitor, lisinopril, on morbidity and mortality in chronic heart failure. ATLAS Study Group. Circulation 100:2312–2318, 1999.
95. NETWORK Investigators. Clinical outcome with enalapril in symptomatic chronic heart failure; a dose comparison. Eur Heart J 19: 481–489, 1998.
96. Packer M, Lee WH, Yushak M, et al. Comparison of captopril and enalapril in patients with severe heart failure. N Engl J Med 315: 847–853, 1986.

97. Levine TB. Effect of angiotensin converting enzyme inhibition on renal function in the treatment of heart failure. Clin Ther 11: 495–502, 1989.

98. Bakris GL, Weir MR. ACE inhibitor associated elevations in serum creatinine: is this a cause for concern? Arch Intern Med 160: 685–693, 2000.

99. Meissner MD, Wilson AR, Jessup M. Renal artery stenosis in heart failure. Am J Cardiol 62:1307–1308, 1988.

100. Adrejak M, Adrejak MT. Enalapril, captopril and cough. Arch Intern Med 148:249–251, 1988.

101. Varonier HS, Panzoni R. The effect of inhalations of bradykinin in healthy and atopic (asthmatic) children. Int Arch Allergy Appl Immunol 34:293–296, 1968.

102. Bart BA, Ertl G, Held P, et al. Contemporary management of patients with left ventricular systolic dysfunction: results from the Study of Patients Intolerant of Converting Enzyme Inhibitors (SPICE) Registry. Eur Heart J 20:1182–1190, 1999.

103. Pitt B, Segal R, Martinez FA, et al. Randomized trial of losartan versus captopril in patients over 65 with heart failure. Lancet 349: 747–752, 1997.

104. Leor J, Reicher-Reiss H, Goldbourt U, et al. Aspirin and mortality in patients treated with angiotensin-converting enzyme inhibitors: a cohort study of 11,575 patients with coronary artery disease. J Am Coll Cardiol 33:1920–1925, 1999.

105. Sander GE, McKinnie JJ, Greenberg SS, et al. Angiotensin-converting enzyme inhibitors and angiotensin II receptor antagonists in the treatment of heart failure caused by left ventricular systolic dysfunction. Prog Cardiovasc Dis 41:265–300, 1999.

106. McKelvie RS, Yusuf S, Pericak D, et al. Comparison of candesartan, enalapril, and their combination in congestive heart failure. Randomized Evaluation of Strategies for Left Ventricular Dysfunction (RESOLVD) Pilot Study. Circulation 100:1056–1064, 1999.

107. Pitt B, Poole-Wilson PA, Segal R, et al. Effect of losartan compared with captopril on mortality in patients with symptomatic heart failure: randomised trial—the Losartan Heart Failure Survival Study ELITE II. Lancet 355:1582–1587, 2000.

108. Cohn JN, Tognoni G. A randomized trial of the angiotensin receptor blocker valsartan in chronic heart failure. N Engl J Med 345: 1667–1675, 2001.

109. Diovan Product Labeling, Novartis, 2003.

110. Pfeffer MA, Swedberg K, Granger CB, et al. Effects of candesartan on mortality and morbidity in patients with chronic heart failure: the CHARM-Overall programme. Lancet 362:759–766, 2003.

111. Pfeffer MA, McMurray JJV, Velazquez EJ, et al. Valsartan, captopril, or both in myocardial infarction complicated by heart failure, left ventricular dysfunction, or both. N Engl J Med 349: 1892–1906, 2003.

112. Elkayam U, Karaalp IS, Wani OR, et al. The role of organic nitrates in the treatment of heart failure. Prog Cardiovasc Dis 41: 255–264, 1999.

113. Taylor AL, Ziesche S, Yancy C, et al. Combination of isosorbide dinitrate and hydralazine in blacks with heart failure. N Engl J Med 351:2049–2057, 2004.

114. Cohn JN, Archibald DG, Ziesche S, et al. Effect of vasodilator therapy on mortality in chronic congestive heart failure. N Engl J Med 314:1547–1552, 1986.

115. Cohn JN, Johnson G, Ziesche S, et al. A comparison of enalapril with hydralazine-isosorbide dinitrate in the treatment of congestive heart failure. N Engl J Med 325:303–310, 1991.

116. Franciosa JA, Weber KT, Levine TB, et al. Hydralazine in the long-term treatment of chronic failure: lack of a difference from placebo. Am Heart J 104:587–594, 1982.

117. Conradson TB, Ryden L, Ahlmark G, et al. Clinical efficacy of hydralazine dosage in refractory heart failure. Clin Pharmacol Ther 27:337–346, 1980.

118. Taylor AL, Cohn J. Isosorbide dinitrate and hydralazine in blacks with heart failure [letter to the editor]. N Engl J Med 352:1043, 2005.

119. Cameron HA, Ramsay LE. The lupus syndrome induced by hydralazine: a common complication with low dose treatment. Br Med J [Clin Res Ed] 289:410–412, 1984.

120. Elkayam U, Shotan A, Mehra A, et al. Calcium channel blockers in heart failure. J Am Coll Cardiol 122 (Suppl A):139A–144A, 1993.

121. Packer M, O'Connor CM, Ghali JK, et al. Effect of amlodipine on morbidity and mortality in severe chronic heart failure. Prospective randomized amlodipine survival evaluation study group. N Engl J Med 335:1107–1114, 1996.

122. O'Connor CM, Carson PE, Miller AB, et al. Effect of amlodipine on mode of death among patients with advanced heart failure in the PRAISE Trial. Am J Cardiol 82:881–887, 1998.

123. Cohn JN, Ziesche S, Smith R, et al. Effect of calcium antagonist felodipine as supplementary vasodilator therapy in patients with chronic heart failure treated with enalapril: VHeFT III. Vasodilator Heart Failure Trial (VHeFT) Study Group. Circulation 96: 856–863, 1997.

124. Bleske BE, Gilbert EM, Munger MA. Carvedilol: therapeutic application and practice guidelines. Pharmacotherapy 18:729–737, 1998.

125. Waagstein F, Bristow MR, Swedberg K, et al. Beneficial effects of metoprolol in idiopathic dilated cardiomyopathy: Metoprolol in Dilated Cardiomyopathy (MDC) Trial Study Group. Lancet 342: 1441–1446, 1993.

126. MERIT-HF Study Group. Effect of metoprolol CR/XL in chronic heart failure: metoprolol CR/XL randomized intervention trial in congestive heart failure (MERIT-HF). Lancet 353:2001–2007, 1999.

127. CIBIS-II Investigators. The cardiac insufficiency bisoprolol study II (CIBIS-II): a randomised trial. Lancet 353:9–13, 1999.

128. Packer M, Bristow MR, Cohn JN, et al. The effect of carvedilol on morbidity and mortality in patients with chronic heart failure. U.S. Carvedilol Heart Failure Study Group. N Engl J Med 334: 1349–1355, 1996.

129. Delea TE, Vera-Llonch M, Richner RE, et al. Cost effectiveness of carvedilol for heart failure. Am J Cardiol 83:890–896, 1999.

130. Packer M, Coats AJS, Fowler MB, et al. Effect of carvedilol on survival in severe chronic heart failure. N Engl J Med 344: 1651–1658, 2001.

131. Lechat P, Packer M, Chalon S, et al. Clinical effects of beta-adrenergic blockade in chronic heart failure. Circulation 98:1184–1191, 1998.

132. Kukin ML, Kalman J, Charney RH, et al. Prospective, randomized comparison of effect of long-term treatment with metoprolol or carvedilol on symptoms, exercise, ejection fraction, and oxidative stress in heart failure. Circulation 99:2645–2651, 1999.

133. Poole-Wilson PA, Swedberg K, Cleland JGF, et al. Comparison of carvedilol and metoprolol on clinical outcomes in patients with chronic heart failure in the Carvedilol Or Metoprolol European Trial (COMET): randomised controlled trial. Lancet 362:7–13, 2003.

134. Massie BM. A comment on COMET: how to interpret a positive trial? J Card Failure 9:425–428, 2003.

135. Krum H, Roecker EB, Mohacsi P, et al. Effects of initiating carvedilol in patients with severe chronic heart failure. JAMA 289: 712–718, 2003.

136. Gattis WA, O'Connor CM, Gallup DS, et al. Predischarge initiation of carvedilol in patients hospitalized for decompensated heart failure: results of the IMPACT-HF (Initiation Management Predischarge: Process for Assessment of Carvedilol Therapy in Heart Failure) trial. J Am Coll Cardiol 43:1534–1541, 2004.

137. Vantrimpont P, Rouleau JL, Wun CC, et al. Additive effects of beta-blockers to angiotensin-converting enzyme inhibitors in the Survival and Ventricular Enlargement (SAVE) Study. J Am Coll Cardiol 29:229–236, 1997.

138. Exner DV, Dries DL, Waclawiw MA, et al. Beta-adrenergic blocking agent use and mortality in patients with asymptomatic and symptomatic left ventricular systolic dysfunction: a post hoc analysis of the studies of left ventricular dysfunction. J Am Coll Cardiol 33:916–923, 1999.

139. Self T, Soberman JE, Bubla JM, Chafin CC. Cardioselective betablockers in patients with asthma and concomitant heart failure or history of myocardial infarction: when do benefits outweigh risks? J Asthma 2003;40:839–845, 2003.

140. Salpeter SR, Ormiston TM, Salpeter EE. Cardioselective beta blockers in patients with reactive airway disease: a meta-analysis. Ann Intern Med 137:715–725, 2002.

141. Cody RJ, Kubo SH, Pickworth KK. Diuretic treatment for the sodium retention of congestive heart failure. Arch Intern Med 154: 1905–1914, 1994.

142. Mokrzycki MH. Diuretic treatment of heart failure. Heart Fail 10: 181–191, 1994.
143. Kramer BK, Schweda F, Riegger GA. Diuretic treatment and diuretic resistance in heart failure. Am J Med 106:90–96, 1999.
144. Pitt B, Zannad F, Remme WJ et al. The effect of spironolactone on morbidity and mortality in patients with severe heart failure. N Engl J Med 341:709–717, 1999.
145. Pitt B, Remme W, Zannad F, et al. Eplerenone, a selective aldosterone blocker, in patients with left ventricular dysfunction after myocardial infarction. N Engl J Med 348:1309–1321, 2003.
146. Barr CS, Lang CC, Hanson J, et al. Effects of adding spironolactone to an angiotensin-converting enzyme inhibitor in chronic congestive heart failure secondary to coronary artery disease. Am J Cardiol 76:1259–1265, 1995.
147. Moser M, Herbert PR. Prevention of disease progression, left ventricular hypertrophy and congestive heart failure in hypertension treatment trials. J Am Coll Cardiol 27:1214–1218, 1996.
148. Antes LM, Fernandez PC. Principles of diuretic therapy. Dis Mon 44:254–268, 1998.
149. Brater DC. Diuretic therapy. N Engl J Med 339:387–395, 1998.
150. Ellison DH. The physiologic basis of diuretic synergism: its role in treating diuretic resistance. Ann Intern Med 114:886–894, 1991.
151. The RALES Investigators. Effectiveness of spironolactone added to an angiotensin-converting enzyme inhibitor and a loop diuretic for severe chronic congestive heart failure: the Randomized Aldactone Evaluation Study (RALES). Am J Cardiol 78:902–907, 1996.
152. The Digitalis Investigation Group. The effect of digoxin on mortality and morbidity in patients with heart failure. N Engl J Med 336: 525–533, 1997.
153. Schwinger RH, Wang J, Frank K, et al. Reduced sodium pump α_1, α_3, and β_1-isoform protein levels and Na$^+$, K$^+$-ATPase activity but unchanged Na$^+$–Ca^{2+} exchanger protein levels in human heart failure. Circulation 99:2105–2112, 1999.
154. Krum H, Bigger JT, Goldsmith RL, et al. Effect of long-term digoxin therapy on autonomic function in patients with chronic heart failure. J Am Coll Cardiol 25:289–294, 1995.
155. Hauptman PJ, Garg R, Kelly RA. Cardiac glycosides in the next millennium. Prog Cardiovasc Dis 41:247–254, 1999.
156. Reuning RH, Geraets DR, Rocci ML, et al. Digoxin. In: Evans WE, Shentag JJ, Jusko WJ. Applied pharmacokinetics: principles of therapeutic drug monitoring, 3rd ed. Vancouver, WA: Applied Therapeutics, Inc., 1992:20-1–20-28.
157. Magnani B, Malini PL. Cardiac glycosides. Drug interactions of clinical significance. Drug Saf 12:97–109, 1995.
158. Bizjak ED, Mauro VF. Digoxin-macrolide drug interaction. Ann Pharmacother 31:1077–1079, 1997.
159. Hui J, Geraets DR, Chandrasekaran A, et al. Digoxin disposition in elderly humans with hypochlorhydria. J Clin Pharmacol 34: 734–741, 1994.
160. Rodriquez I, Abernethy DR, Woosley RL. P-glycoprotein in clinical cardiology. Circulation 99:472–474, 1999.
161. Young JB, Gheorghiade M, Packer M, et al. Are low serum levels of digoxin effective in chronic heart failure? Evidence challenging the accepted guidelines for a therapeutic serum level of the drug. J Am Coll Cardiol 21:378A, 1993.
162. Gheorghiade M, Hall VB, Jacobsen G, et al. Effects of increasing maintenance dose of digoxin on left ventricular function and neurohormones in patients with chronic heart failure treated with diuretics and angiotensin-converting enzyme inhibitors. Circulation 92:1801–1807, 1995.
163. Slatton ML, Irani WN, Hall SA, et al. Does digoxin provide additional hemodynamic and autonomic benefit at higher doses in patients with mild to moderate heart failure and normal sinus rhythm? J Am Coll Cardiol 29:1206–1213, 1997.
164. Smith TW, Antman EM, Friedman PL, et al. Digitalis glycosides: mechanisms and manifestations of toxicity. Prog Cardiovasc Dis 26:413–458, 495–540; 27:21–56, 1984.
165. Jones WN, Perrier D, Trinca CE, et al. Evaluation of various methods of digoxin dosing. J Clin Pharmacol 22:543–550, 1982.
166. Koup JR, Jusko WJ, Elwood CM, et al. Digoxin pharmacokinetics: role of renal failure in dosage regimen design. Clin Pharmacol Ther 18:9–21, 1975.
167. Luke DR, Halstenson EC, Opsahl JA, et al. Validity of creatinine clearance estimates in the assessment of renal function. Clin Pharmacol Ther 48:503–508, 1990.
168. Williamson KM, Thrasher KA, Fulton KB, et al. Digoxin toxicity. An evaluation in current clinical practice. Arch Intern Med 158: 2444–2449, 1998.
169. Marik PE, Fromm L. A case series of hospitalized patients with elevated digoxin levels. Am J Med 105:110–115, 1998.
170. Kelly RA, Smith TW. Recognition and management of digitalis toxicity. Am J Cardiol 69:108G–119G, 1992.
171. Borron SW, Bismuth C, Muszynski J. Advances in the management of digoxin toxicity in the older patient. Drugs Aging 10: 18–33, 1997.
172. Gandhi AJ, Vlasses PH, Morton DJ, et al. Economic impact of digoxin toxicity. Pharmacoeconomics 12:175–181, 1997.
173. Rabetoy GM, Price CA, Findlay JW, et al. Treatment of digoxin intoxication in a renal failure patient with digoxin-specific antibody fragments and plasmapheresis. Am J Nephrol 10:518–521, 1990.
174. Cleland JG. Health economic consequences of the pharmacological treatment of heart failure. Eur Heart J 19 (Suppl P):P32–P39, 1998.
175. Chatterjee K, Wolfe CL, DeMarco T. Nonglycoside inotropes in congestive heart failure. Are they beneficial of harmful? Cardiol Clin 12:63–72, 1994.
176. Ewy GA. Inotropic infusions for chronic congestive heart failure. Medical miracles or misguided medicinals? J Am Coll Cardiol 33: 572–575, 1999.
177. Leier CV, Binkley PE. Parenteral inotropic support for advanced congestive heart failure. Prog Cardiovasc Dis 41:207–224, 1998.
178. Shakar SF, Abraham WT, Gilbert EM, et al. Combined oral positive inotropic and beta-blocker therapy for treatment of refractory class IV heart failure. J Am Coll Cardiol 31:1336–1340, 1998.
179. Garg RK, Gheorghiade M, Jafri SM. Antiplatelet and anticoagulant therapy in the prevention of thromboemboli in chronic heart failure. Prog Cardiovasc Dis 41:225–236, 1998.
180. Dries DL, Domanski MJ, Waclawiw MA, et al. Effect of antithrombotic therapy on risk of sudden coronary death in patients with congestive heart failure. Am J Cardiol 79:909–913, 1997.
181. Peters NS, Wit AL. Ventricular architecture and arrhythmogenesis. Circulation 97:1746–1754, 1997.
182. Echt DS, Liebson PR, Mitchell LB, et al. Mortality and morbidity in patients receiving encainide, flecainide, or placebo: the Cardiac Arrhythmia Suppression Trial. N Engl J Med 324:781–788, 1991.
183. Doval HC, Nul DR, Grancelli HO, et al. Randomised trial of low-dose amiodarone in severe congestive heart failure. Lancet 344: 493–498, 1994.
184. Singh SN, Fletcher RD, Fisher SG, et al. Amiodarone in patients with congestive heart failure and asymptomatic ventricular arrhythmias. N Engl J Med 333:77–82, 1996.
185. Torp-Pedersen C, Moller M, Bloch-Thomsen PE, et al. Dofetilide in patients with congestive heart failure and left ventricular dysfunction. N Engl J Med 341:857–865, 1999.
186. Pinski SL, Fahy GJ. Implantable cardioverter-defibrillators. Am J Med 106:446–458, 1999.
187. Stevenson WG, Ganz LI. Atrial fibrillation in heart failure. Heart Fail 13:22–29, 1997.
188. Dries DL, Exner DV, Gersh BJ, et al. Atrial fibrillation is associated with an increased risk for mortality and heart failure progression in patients with asymptomatic and symptomatic left ventricular systolic dysfunction: a retrospective analysis of the SOLVD trials. J Am Coll Cardiol 32:695–703, 1998.
189. Frazier OH, Myers TJ. Surgical therapy for severe heart failure. Curr Prob Cardiol 23:726–764, 1998.
190. Grossi P, Gasperina DD, Corona A, et al. Preemptive ganciclovir therapy as a strategy for prevention of human cytomegalovirus disease following thoracic organ transplantation: the experience of Pavia, Italy [abstract]. J Heart Lung Transplant 17:51, 1998.
191. Valantine HA, Gao SZ, Menon SG, et al. Impact of prophylactic immediate posttransplant ganciclovir on development of transplant atherosclerosis. A post hoc analysis of a randomized, placebo-controlled study. Circulation 100:61–66, 1999.
192. Valantine HA, Schroeder JS. Recent advances in cardiac transplantation. N Engl J Med 333:660–661, 1995.
193. Schwartz RS. The new immunology: the end of immunosuppressive drug therapy? N Engl J Med 340:1754–1756, 1999.
194. Townsend JN, Pagano D, Allen SM, et al. Results of surgical revascularization in ischaemic heart failure without angina. Eur J Cardiothorac Surg 9:507–510, 1995.

195. Anderson RD, Ohman EM, Holmes DR, et al. Prognostic value of congestive heart failure history in patients undergoing percutaneous coronary interventions. J Am Coll Cardiol 32:936–941, 1998.

196. Kantor B, McKenna CJ, Caccitolo JA, et al. Transmyocardial and percutaneous myocardial revascularization: current and future role in the treatment of coronary artery disease. Mayo Clin Proc 74: 585–592, 1999.

197. Losordo DW, Vale PR, Symes JF, et al. Gene therapy for myocardial angiogenesis. Initial clinical results with direct myocardial injection of phVEGF$_{165}$ as sole therapy for myocardial ischemia. Circulation 98:2800–2804, 1998.

198. Kass DA. Surgical approaches to arresting or reversing chronic remodeling of the failing heart. J Card Fail 4:57–66, 1998.

199. Pepping J. Coenzyme Q10. Am J Health Syst Pharm 56:519–521, 1999.

200. Watson PS, Scalia GM, Galbraith A, et al. Lack of effect of coenzyme Q on left ventricular function in patients with congestive heart failure. J Am Coll Cardiol 33:1549–1552, 1999.

201. Arsenian MA. Carnitine and its derivatives in cardiovascular disease. Prog Cardiovasc Dis 40:265–286, 1997.

202. Andrews R, Greenhaff P, Curtis S, et al. The effect of dietary creatine supplementation on skeletal muscle metabolism in congestive heart failure. Eur Heart J 19:617–622, 1998.

203. Leslie D, Gheorghiade M. Is there a role for thiamine supplementation in the management of heart failure? Am Heart J 131: 1248–1250, 1996.

204. Hornig B, Arakawa N, Kohler C, et al. Vitamin C improves endothelial function of conduit arteries in patients with chronic heart failure. Circulation 97:363–368, 1998.

205. Ventura HO, Mehra MR, Milani RV. Cardiac cachexia in advanced heart failure: suppression of tumor necrosis factor by omega-3 fatty acids. CHF 4:44–45, 1998.

206. Hobbs RE, Miller LW, Bott-Silverman C, et al. Hemodynamic effects of a single intravenous injection of synthetic brain natriuretic peptide in patients with heart failure secondary to ischemic or idiopathic dilated cardiomyopathy. Am J Cardiol 78:896–901, 1996.

207. Abraham WT, Lowes BD, Ferguson DA, et al. Systemic hemodynamic, neurohormonal, and renal effects of a steady-state infusion of human brain natriuretic peptide in patients with hemodynamically decompensated heart failure. J Card Fail 4:37–44, 1998.

208. Coleman SG, Duff R. Endopeptidase inhibitors. Drugs R&D 4: 339–340, 1999.

209. Sütsch G, Bertel O, Kiowski W. Acute and short-term effects of the nonpeptide endothelin-1 receptor antagonist bosentan in humans. Cardiovasc Drug Ther 10:717–725, 1996.

210. Rohde LE, Ducharme A, Arroyo LH, et al. Matrix metalloproteinase inhibition attenuates early left ventricular enlargement after experimental myocardial infarction in mice. Circulation 99: 3063–3070, 1999.

211. Hasenfuss G, Pieske B, Castell M, et al. Influence of the novel inotropic agent levosimendan on isometric tension and calcium cycling in failing human myocardium. Circulation 98:2141–2147, 1998.

212. Sliwa K, Skudicky D, Candy G, et al. Randomized investigation of effects of pentoxifylline on left-ventricular performance in idiopathic dilated cardiomyopathy. Lancet 351:1091–1093, 1998.

213. Deswal A, Bozkurt B, Seta Y, et al. Safety and efficacy of a soluble P75 tumor necrosis factor receptor (Enbrel, etanercept) in patients with advanced heart failure. Circulation 99:3224–3226, 1999.

214. Dauterman KW, Massie BM, Gheorghiade M. Heart failure associated with preserved systolic function: a common and costly clinical entity. Am Heart J 135:S310–S319, 1998.

215. Vasan RS, Larson MG, Benjamin EJ, et al. Congestive heart failure in subjects with normal versus reduced left ventricular ejection fraction. J Am Coll Cardiol 33:1948–1955, 1999.

216. Mosterd A, D'Agostino RB, Silbershatz H, et al. Trends in the prevalence of hypertension, antihypertensive therapy, and left ventricular hypertrophy from 1950 to 1989. N Engl J Med 340: 1221–1227, 1999.

217. Smith TW, Braunwald E, Kelly RA. The management of heart failure. In: Braunwald E, ed. Heart disease: a textbook of cardiovascular medicine, 4th ed. Philadelphia: WB Saunders, 1992:464–519.

218. Jaagosild P, Dawson NV, Thomas C, et al. Outcomes of acute exacerbation of severe congestive heart failure. Arch Intern Med 158: 1081–1089, 1998.

219. McGrath RB. Invasive bedside hemodynamic monitoring. Prog Cardiovasc Dis 29:129–144, 1986.

220. Bollish SJ, Foster TJ. Swan–Ganz catheter: an important tool for monitoring drug therapy in the critically ill. Formulary 16:99–103, 1980.

221. Nairns RG, Chusid P. Diuretic use in critical care. Am J Cardiol 10:139–145, 1984.

222. Stevenson LW, Massie BM, Francis GS. Optimizing therapy for complex or refractory heart failure: a management algorithm. Am Heart J 135:S293–S309, 1998.

223. Stevenson LW. Therapy tailored for symptomatic heart failure. Heart Fail 11:87–107, 1995.

224. Massie BM, Shah NB. Evolving trends in the epidemiologic factors of heart failure: rationale for preventive strategies and comprehensive disease management. Am Heart J 133:703–712, 1997.

225. Francis GS. Determinants of prognosis in patients with heart failure. J Heart Lung Transplant 13:S113–S116, 1994.

226. Pousset F, Isnard R, Lechat P, et al. Prognostic value of plasma endothelin-1 in patients with chronic heart failure. Eur Heart J 18: 254–258, 1997.

227. Doval HC, Nul DR, Grancelli HO, et al. Nonsustained ventricular tachycardia in severe heart failure. Circulation 94:3198–3203, 1996.

228. Singh SN, Fisher SG, Carson PE, et al. Prevalence and significance of nonsustained ventricular tachycardia in patients with premature ventricular contractions and heart failure treated with vasodilator therapy. J Am Coll Cardiol 32:942–947, 1998.

Cardiac Arrhythmias

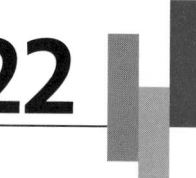

Tien M. H. Ng, J. Jason Sims, and Mark A. Gill

TREATMENT GOALS

- Prevent morbidity and mortality associated with cardiac arrhythmias
- Restore normal sinus rhythm in appropriate patients
- Balance therapeutic benefits of antiarrhythmic therapies with the potential for serious adverse effects

DEFINITION

An *arrhythmia* is any abnormality in the rate, regularity, or site of origin or a disturbance in conduction that disrupts the normal sequence of activation in the atria or ventricles. Arrhythmias can be due to a variety of reasons, such as electrolyte abnormalities, structural abnormalities, metabolic derangements, genetic mutations, and drug toxicity. Arrhythmias have varying degrees of severity and significance based on site of origin, symptoms, frequency, and duration. The aggressiveness of therapies is based on these factors.

CARDIAC ELECTROPHYSIOLOGY

NORMAL CELLULAR ELECTROPHYSIOLOGY

The majority of myocardial cells share the same basic cellular electrophysiologic properties that allow contraction when a transmembrane action potential develops. Fully polarized cells have a resting membrane potential of -90 mV. This resting membrane potential exists because of the electrical gradient created by differences in extracellular and intracellular ion concentrations. Specifically, sodium and potassium concentrations are controlled primarily by the sodium–potassium pump. This pump tries to maintain intracellular sodium concentrations at 5 to 15 mEq/L and intracellular potassium concentrations at 135 to 140 mEq/L. In comparison, the extracellular sodium concentration is normally 135 to 142 mEq/L and extracellular potassium 3 to 5 mEq/L.

Electrical stimulation of a myocardial cell results in depolarization. Depolarization is initiated by a slow inward leak of sodium. When the transmembrane potential reaches approximately -60 mV, the fast sodium channel opens, actively transporting sodium across the cell membrane and resulting in rapid cellular depolarization to approximately $+20$ mV. This is represented by phase 0 of the action potential and the QRS complex on a surface electrocardiogram (ECG). After the rapid membrane depolarization, the sodium channel closes and a complex exchange of sodium, calcium, and potassium occurs during the plateau phases 1 and 2 of the action potential. The dominant feature during the plateau phases of the action potential is movement of calcium ions into the intracellular space via L-type calcium channels. This feature differentiates myocardial cells from nerve tissue and starts the excitation–contraction cascade of the cell by initiating the release of intracellular calcium stores from the sarcoplasmic reticulum. Phase 3 of the action potential is dom-

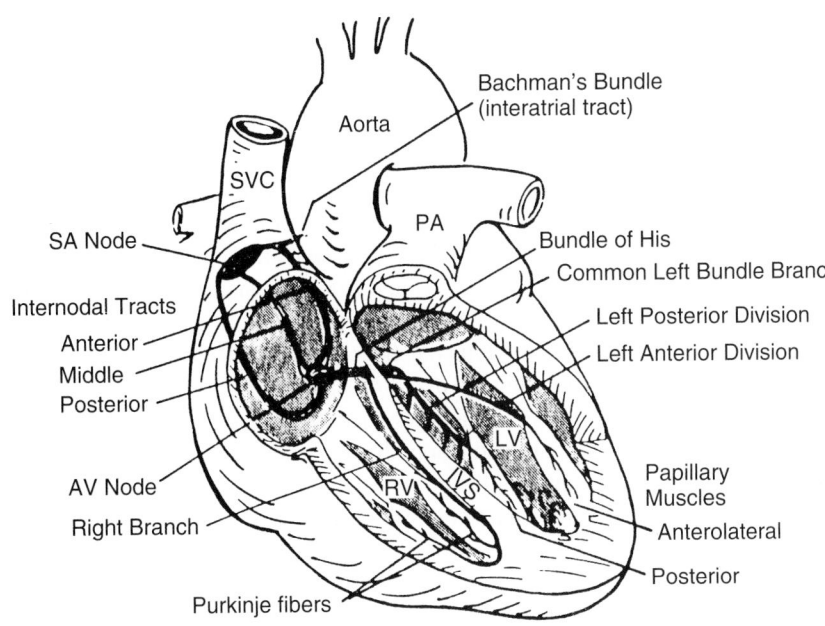

FIGURE 22.1 Anatomy of the electrical system of the heart. The impulse is generated by the sinoatrial (*SA*) node and is conducted through the atria to the atrioventricular node, which directs the current to the bundle of His, into the bundle branches, and finally to the Purkinje fibers. *PA*, pulmonary artery; *SVC*, superior vena cava.

inated by repolarization of the cell membrane by outward movement of potassium ions. The rate of fall of phase 3 and its depth determine membrane responsiveness to stimulation. Tissues may depolarize only after reaching a particular level of repolarization called the "threshold potential," at least -50 to -55 mV for normal Purkinje fibers. This level of repolarization therefore determines the absolute refractory period (ARP). The ARP varies in length depending primarily on the action potential duration (APD). Phase 4 is the resting membrane potential that results from a combination of ionic currents, primarily the slow inward sodium current.

NORMAL CARDIAC CONDUCTION

The electrical system of the heart consists of intrinsic pacemakers and conduction tissues. It is convenient to conceptualize the progression of normal cardiac rhythm in anatomic terms (Fig. 22.1). Figure 22.2 correlates the standard ECG with the normal electrical pathway.

The rate of electrical firing of the heart depends on the most rapid pacemaker. Spontaneous electrical firing or automaticity can occur anywhere in the heart under certain conditions. Normally, the sinoatrial (SA) node, located where the superior vena cava meets the right atrium, has the most rapid

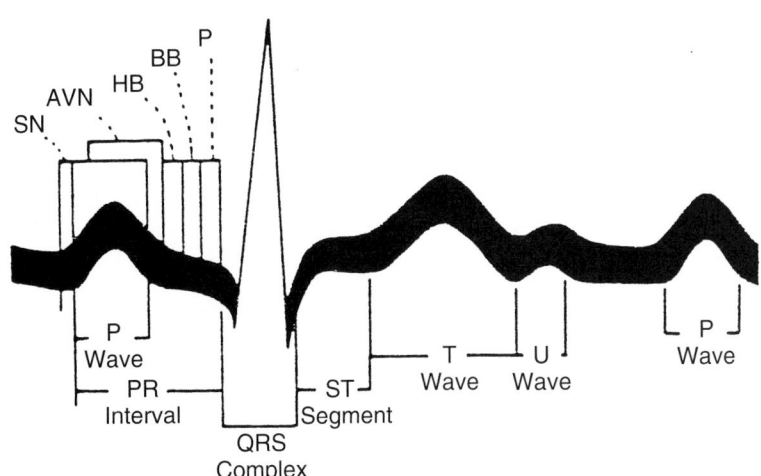

FIGURE 22.2 The normal electrocardiogram. The P wave is atrial depolarization. The P-R interval (0.12 to 0.20 seconds) is formed from the firing of the SA node (*SN*) and conduction through the AV node (*AVN*), bundle of His (*HB*), bundle branches (*BB*), and Purkinje fibers (*P*). The QRS complex (0.05 to 0.10 seconds) is ventricular depolarization. The ST segment is the refractory period. The T wave is ventricular repolarization. The Q-T interval is 0.35 to 0.44 seconds in duration.

intrinsic rate (60 to 100 bpm). Therefore, any electrical activity not initiated by the SA node is considered an arrhythmia. Consequently, most arrhythmias are labeled by the anatomic location and rate.

SA node firing initiates atrial contraction. The electrical impulse is conducted through the atria via the internodal tracts to the atrioventricular (AV) node near the coronary sinus, between the two atria. The AV node has pacemaker properties but normally coordinates atrial and ventricular contraction. The AV node normally limits excessively rapid atrial rates from activating the ventricles.

The conduction system in the ventricles is more elaborate than that in the atria because the muscle mass is larger. Rapid and effective excitation is critical because the ventricles contribute the most to cardiac output. Fibers leaving the AV node are called the bundle of His. They separate into the bundle branches, which traverse the septum between the ventricles. Conduction between the AV node and the bundle of His is measured by the P-R interval (Fig. 22.2). The final conducting components of the ventricles are the Purkinje fibers, which emanate from the bundle branches to stimulate the ventricular cardiac muscle to contract. The QRS complex measures depolarization of the ventricles. The Q-T interval reflects both ventricular depolarization and repolarization.

ARRHYTHMOGENESIS

In general, arrhythmia mechanisms have been described as abnormalities in electrical development, electrical conduction, or a combination of both. Abnormalities in electrical development arise from irregular automaticity or triggered activity from the SA node or other sites producing ectopic beats. Causes of irregular automaticity include hypoxia, electrolyte abnormalities, fiber stretch, catecholamine excess, ischemia, and edema. All of these factors increase the slope of phase 4 depolarization, resulting in heightened automaticity.

Triggered activity usually develops due to transient membrane depolarization during or immediately after repolarization. These early and delayed after-depolarizations can occur with oscillations in the plateau phase of the action potential, leading to a second depolarization before the first is completed. Hypoxia, fiber stretch, catecholamines, high P_{CO_2}, and digitalis overdose can lead to triggered activity.

Reentry and conduction block are the most common electrical conduction abnormalities associated with arrhythmogenesis. Reentry describes a concept of infinite impulse propagation by continued activation of previously refractory tissue. Reentry depends on different conduction velocities along adjacent myocardial fibers, with one fiber containing an area of unidirectional conduction block (Fig 22.3). This allows continued excitation in a repetitive manner. This circus rhythm may develop as areas of infarcted tissue block or delayed conduction. A single circuit of the fibers may induce a premature contraction, whereas continuous cycling of impulses might produce sustained tachycardia. This process may occur in both atrial and ventricular tissue. Conduction block occurs when the normal conduction pathway is blocked and the impulse either expires or conducts through an alternative inappropriate route to depolarize the myocardium.

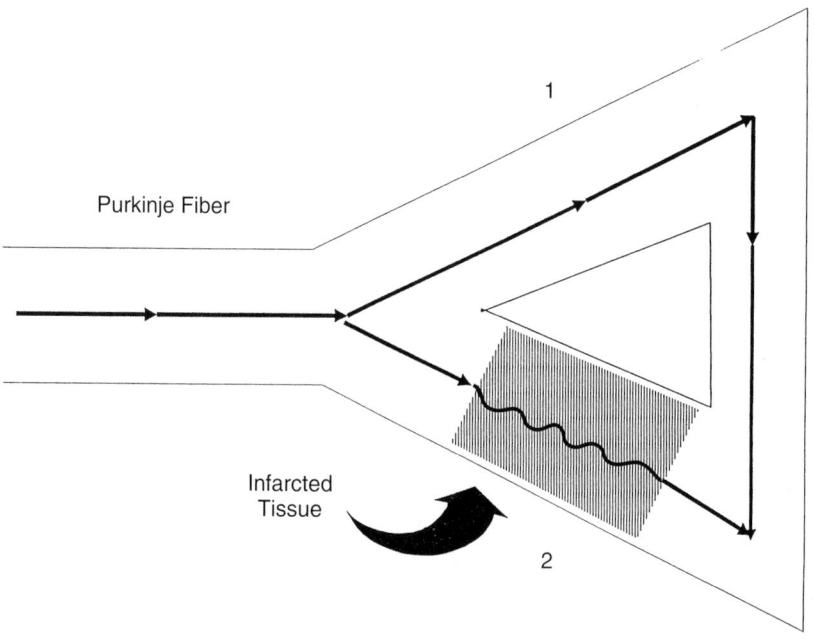

FIGURE 22.3 Reentry. A conduction fiber that bifurcates into fibers 1 and 2 to stimulate ventricular tissues. The normal pattern is for conduction through fibers 1 and 2 at similar rates. In this figure, fiber 2 is infarcted, which slows conduction until it is blocked by refractory cells. Fiber 2 is activated by the impulse crossing the ventricular muscle tissue. The retrograde impulse finds fiber 2 repolarized and initiates retrograde depolarization of fiber 2. This circuit may be repeated or may terminate if fiber 1 is depolarized.

ANTIARRHYTHMIC DRUGS BY VAUGHN-WILLIAMS CLASSIFICATION

CLASS I ANTIARRHYTHMICS

Class Ia. Quinidine, procainamide, and disopyramide represent this subclass of antiarrhythmics, which act by blocking the fast (sodium) channel for an intermediate duration of time (Table 22.1). The direct action is a generalized slowing of both automaticity and conduction velocity in the SA node, AV node, and His-Purkinje systems. In addition, all three agents are negative inotropes via their sodium channel blockade. As with most antiarrhythmics, each class Ia agent also exerts other pertinent pharmacologic effects. Quinidine exerts a vagolytic effect, which results in a physiologic override of the sodium channel slowing of conduction velocity in the SA and AV nodes. His-Purkinje conduction time remains delayed, reflecting the minimal autonomic influence in these tissues. The effects of quinidine are minimal in healthy, well-polarized tissues and most marked at rapid heart rates, in ectopic pacemakers, and in hypoxic or ischemic tissues. Pe-

ripheral α-adrenergic blockade and relaxation of vascular smooth muscle associated with intravenous administration may further influence cardiac action. Procainamide exerts additional class III effects (prolonging repolarization) through an active metabolite, N-acetylprocainamide (NAPA). NAPA is formed by acetylation of the parent compound in the liver. The rate of acetylation can vary between patients based on genetic predisposition for rapid acetylation or slow acetylation. Fast acetylators convert a higher percentage of procainamide to NAPA than slow acetylators. About 85% of NAPA is excreted unchanged by the kidneys; thus, NAPA accumulates more than procainamide as renal function deteriorates. It seems that procainamide and NAPA compete for renal tubular secretion. NAPA may thus prolong the procainamide elimination half-life.[1] Disopyramide exerts the strongest anticholinergic effects of any of the class Ia agents. Anticholinergic reactions may occur in as many as 45% of patients receiving disopyramide, and 25% may need to discontinue therapy.[2]

All three agents are used in the management of supraventricular tachyarrhythmias despite a paucity of controlled studies. Their efficacy in supraventricular tachycardias results from a decrease in atrial ectopy, which suppresses the inciting premature impulses, and a slowing of conduction in the retrograde fast path (Table 22.1). Quinidine is not useful after reentry has begun and may even be deleterious because of an increase in AV nodal conduction velocity. Patients should therefore have adequate AV node slowing before quinidine therapy is initiated for supraventricular tachyarrhythmias. In contrast, procainamide is commonly used to terminate supraventricular tachyarrhythmias caused by reentry. Procainamide is also approved for treating documented ventricular arrhythmias (e.g., sustained ventricular tachycardia) that are life-threatening.[3] Disopyramide currently is available for oral use (conventional or sustained-release) to treat ventricular arrhythmias. Disopyramide was approved in the United States in 1977. It also has antiarrhythmic efficacy in atrial fibrillation (AF).

Class Ia agents are generally used as second-line agents owing to new safer antiarrhythmic alternatives. They are limited by their negative inotropic effects, Q-T interval prolongation and proarrhythmia, drug interactions (especially quinidine), and extensive adverse effect profiles. Specific pharmacokinetic parameters, common or serious adverse effects, and monitoring parameters are listed in Tables 22.2 and 22.3.

Class Ib. Class Ib agents act by blocking the fast (sodium) channels, although they exhibit fast on-off binding characteristics as opposed to class Ia (intermediate) and class Ic (slow). Lidocaine, mexiletine, and tocainide are members of this category. These agents are effective only for ventricular tachyarrhythmias. Lidocaine, available as an intravenous preparation, used to be the drug of choice for rapid control of ventricular tachycardia until accumulating data suggested that amiodarone was generally safer in the acute setting.

TABLE 22.1	Electrophysiologic Effects of Antiarrhythmics			
Class	P-R Interval	QRS Duration	QTc Duration	Agent
Ia	0, +	+++	+++	Quinidine
				Procainamide[a]
				Disopyramide
				Moricizine[b]
Ib	0	0	0, !	Lidocaine
				Tocainide
				Phenytoin
				Mexiletine
Ic	+	+++	0, +	Flecainide
				Propafenone[c]
II	+++	0	0, !	β-blockers
III	+	+	+++	Bretylium
				Amiodarone[d]
				Sotalol[e]
				Ibutilide
				N-acetylprocainamide
IV	+++	0	0	Calcium channel blockers

0, no activity; *!*, slight shortening; *+*, slight prolongation; *+++*, significant prolongation.
[a] Procainamide is acetylated to active metabolite NAPA, which exerts properties of class III.
[b] Moricizine has been placed in various categories (e.g., Ia, Ib).
[c] Propafenone also has β-blocking properties of class II.
[d] Amiodarone also has properties of classes I, II, and IV.
[e] Sotalol also has β-blocking properties of class II.

TABLE 22.2	Pharmacokinetics of Antiarrhythmic Agents						
Agent	Dosage Forms	Bioavailability (%)	Protein Binding (%)	Volume of Distribution (L/kg)	Metabolism	CYP (substrate)	Half-Life (h)
Procainamide	PO, IV	83	14–23	2	R, H	–	2.5–4.7
Disopyramide	PO	80–90	50–65	0.8–2	R, H	(3A4)	4–10
Quinidine	PO	60–80	80–90	2.1–3.5	H, R	(3A4) −2D6,3A4	4–10
Lidocaine	IV	–	50	1–1.7	H	(1A2, 3A4)	1–2
Tocainide	PO	90	10–20	1.5–3.2	H, R	–	11–23
Mexiletine	PO, IV	90	50–70	5–9	H	(1A2, 2D6) −1A2	10–12
Phenytoin	PO, IV	50–90	88–93	0.5–1	H	(2C9/19) +2C9/19 +3A4	22–36
Flecainide	PO	70–95	40	5–10	H, R	(2D6)	12–27
Propafenone	PO	12	85–97	1.9–3	H	(2D6) −2D6	2–10 10–32
Metoprolol	PO, IV	40–50	12	5.6	H	(2D6)	3–7
Esmolol	IV	–	55	3.4	–	–	0.15
Amiodarone	PO, IV	20–80	96	60	H	(3A4) −2C9, 2D6 −3A4	60 d
Sotalol	PO	60–100	0	1.5× ABW	R	–	12
Ibutilide	IV	–	40	9–13	R	–	2–12
Dofetilide	PO	>90	60–70		R, H	(3A4)	7.5–10
Azimilide[a]	PO	100	94	12–14	H	–	96
Verapamil	PO, IV	20–35	83–92	2.4–6.8	H	−3A4	3–7
Diltiazem	PO, IV	40	77–93	5.3	H	(3A4) −3A4	3.5–6
Adenosine	IV	–	–	–	–	–	<10 s
Digoxin	PO, IV	60–80	20–25	4–7	R	–	30–40
Magnesium	PO, IV	33	33	–	R	–	–

[a] Azimilide is not yet FDA approved.
R, renal; H, hepatic.

Mexiletine is a class Ib agent with a structure and mechanism of action similar to those of lidocaine. At present, mexiletine is available in an oral dosage form only, with FDA approval for life-threatening ventricular arrhythmias such as sustained ventricular tachycardia. Tocainide, an amine analogue of lidocaine, is indicated for the suppression of life-threatening ventricular arrhythmias. It is especially useful if the arrhythmias responded first to lidocaine. It has very limited utility in atrial arrhythmias. Although tocainide may reduce the frequency of premature ventricular contractions (PVCs), it may not be as effective or as well tolerated as older drugs, such as quinidine.[4] Tocainide may be effective when class Ia drugs have failed.

Although similar in their mechanism of action, class Ib agents differ greatly in their tolerability. Lidocaine's adverse effects are largely limited to central nervous system toxicity when dosed too aggressively or in patients with hepatic impairment. Adverse effects often limit the mexiletine dosage and reduce the ability to suppress arrhythmias. The incidence of adverse effects may be as high as 54% of patients receiving chronic mexiletine, usually involving neurologic or gastrointestinal effects. When this occurs, it may be possible to add other drugs to a tolerated but ineffective dosage of mexiletine. The utility of tocainide chronically is limited by the high frequency of adverse reactions (up to 70%). Ataxia, tremor, dizziness, paresthesias, night sweats, nausea, and

| TABLE 22.3 | Common Adverse Effects and Monitoring Requirements for Antiarrhythmic Agents |

Agent	Adverse Effects	Routine Monitoring	Therapeutic Range
Procainamide	Lupus-like syndrome, hypersensitivity, torsades de pointes, blood dyscrasias, hepatitis, myopathy IV: hypotension, heart block	ECG, HR, CBC, LFTs, Scr	10–20 mg/L (total) 4–8 mg/L (parent compound)
Disopyramide	Anticholinergic effects, hypotension, heart failure, torsades de pointes, heart block, GI intolerance	ECG, HR, BP, urine output, Scr	2–8 mg/L
Quinidine	Diarrhea, GI intolerance, cinchonism, hepatic necrosis, thrombocytopenia, anemia, hypersensitivity, heart block, torsades de pointes, fever, lupus-like syndrome	ECG, HR, GI, LFTs, Scr, CBC	2–6 mg/L
Lidocaine	Drowsiness, confusion, coma, bradycardia, asystole	ECG, CNS, serum drug level	1.5–5 mg/L
Tocainide	GI upset, paresthesias, CNS side effects similar to lidocaine, nightmares, psychotic reactions, blood dyscrasias, hepatitis, interstitial pneumonitis	ECG, CNS, Scr, CBC	4–10 mg/L
Mexiletine	GI upset, fatigue, nervousness, dizziness, tremor, sleep disturbances, seizures, visual disturbances, psychosis, hepatitis, blood dyscrasias	ECG, CNS, LFTs, CBC	0.5–2 mg/L
Phenytoin	Nystagmus, ataxia, drowsiness, GI upset, rash, gingival hyperplasia, peripheral neuropathy	ECG, BP, serum drug level	10–20 mg/L
Flecainide	Bradycardia, heart block, sustained ventricular tachycardia, heart failure, GI upset, dizziness, blurred vision, neutropenia	ECG, HR, Scr	0.2–1 mg/L
Propafenone	Bradycardia, heart block, sustained ventricular tachycardia, heart failure, GI upset, dizziness, blurred vision, metallic taste, dry mouth, bronchospasm, hepatitis	ECG, HR, BP, LFTs	0.06–1 mg/L
Metoprolol	Fatigue, impotence, heart block, hypotension, heart failure, bronchospasm, depression	ECG, BP, HR, RR	–
Esmolol	Hypotension, heart block, heart failure, bronchospasm, pain at injection site	ECG, BP, HR, RR	0.15–2
Amiodarone	Ataxia, tremor, dizziness, pulmonary fibrosis, bradycardia, heart block, sustained ventricular tachycardia, GI upset, hepatitis, hypo– or hyperthyroidism, peripheral neuropathy, photosensitivity, blue-gray skin discoloration, corneal microdeposits	ECG, HR, BP CNS PFTs, CXR LFTs TSH Optic exams Skin	1–2.5+ mg/L
Sotalol	Heart block, hypotension, bronchospasm, bradycardia, torsades de pointes	ECG, BP, HR, RR, Scr	1–3.2
Ibutilide	AV block, torsades de pointes	ECG, HR, Scr	–
Dofetilide	AV block, torsades de pointes	ECG, HR, Scr	–
Azimilide[a]	Bradycardia, torsades de pointes, headache, diarrhea	ECG	–
Verapamil	Heart block, heart failure, hypotension, asystole, dizziness, headache, edema, constipation	ECG, BP, HR	–
Diltiazem	Heart block, hypotension, asystole, heart failure	ECG, BP, HR	–
Adenosine	Chest pain or discomfort, facial flushing, transient dyspnea, hypotension, bronchospasm in pts. with asthma	ECG, RR, BP	–
Digoxin	Bradycardia, AV block, arrhythmias, anorexia, nausea/vomiting, diarrhea, headache, confusion, abnormal vision	Serum digoxin level, serum potassium, ECG, HR	0.5–2.0 μg/L (0.5–1.0 μg/L in heart failure)
Magnesium	Areflexia	Serum Mg^{2+}	–

[a] Azimilide is not yet FDA approved in the United States.
ECG, electrocardiogram; HR, heart rate; CBC, complete blood count; LFTs, liver function tests; Scr, serum creatinine; GI, gastrointestinal; BP, blood pressure; CNS, central nervous system; RR, respiratory rate; PFTs, pulmonary function tests; CXR, chest x-ray; TSH, thyroid-stimulating hormone; AV, atrioventricular.

vomiting are common toxicities. There are case reports of an association between tocainide use and the development of pulmonary fibrosis and interstitial pneumonitis. The pulmonary toxicity may resolve after tocainide is discontinued.[5] Agranulocytosis has been reported with tocainide, and the mortality rate is high at 25%.[3]

Class Ic. Propafenone, flecainide, encainide, and moricizine are the classic Ic agents, but only propafenone and flecainide are still used. Encainide was removed from the U.S. market in 1991. These agents are characterized by their long binding to the fast (sodium) channels. Propafenone has the added ability to block β-adrenergic receptors.[6] Although the best tolerated of the class I antiarrhythmics, their use has been limited to patients without structural heart disease since the publication of the Cardiac Arrhythmia Suppression Trials (CAST I and II). These trials showed an increased mortality when encainide, flecainide, or moricizine was used after myocardial infarction (MI) to suppress PVCs.

Propafenone was approved in the United States in 1989. It is indicated for documented life-threatening ventricular arrhythmias (e.g., sustained ventricular tachycardia) and was approved in late 1997 for preventing recurrence of paroxysmal AF and paroxysmal supraventricular tachycardia associated with disabling symptoms.[3] Propafenone has shown efficacy in supraventricular arrhythmias, including AF and reentrant tachycardia, and is considered by some clinicians to be the antiarrhythmic of choice in Wolff-Parkinson-White (WPW) syndrome.[3,7] Efficacy has been comparable to sotalol and quinidine, and it is clearly more effective than placebo.[8–10] Because of the β-blocking properties of propafenone, the drug should be used cautiously in patients with chronic bronchitis or emphysema.[3] Drug interactions with propafenone are likely because of its extensive hepatic metabolism and high protein binding.

Flecainide is a fluorinated analogue of procainamide currently available in oral form only. Since the publication of CAST I, the FDA indications for flecainide have been limited to documented life-threatening arrhythmias, such as sustained ventricular tachycardia, and ventricular fibrillation. It is also indicated for paroxysmal AF and reentrant tachycardia associated with disabling symptoms. Flecainide should not be used for chronic AF because of an excess development of ventricular tachycardia and ventricular fibrillation. In addition, flecainide should not be used in patients with a recent MI or depressed left ventricular function. Unlike other class I drugs, flecainide does not frequently produce gastrointestinal toxicity.

Moricizine structurally resembles phenothiazines, but the antiarrhythmic does not have antidopaminergic effects. Moricizine has properties of all three subclasses of sodium channel blockers. Moricizine prolongs QRS duration (as class Ia drugs do), shortens APD (as class Ib agents do), and prolongs the P-R interval (as class Ic agents do). Moricizine has been described as a membrane stabilizer with anticholinergic properties and the ability to suppress both normal and abnor-

mal automaticity.[11] The current FDA-approved indication for moricizine is life-threatening, sustained ventricular tachycardia. It is recommended that therapy be initiated in the hospital.[3] Moricizine may be as effective as quinidine or disopyramide with fewer adverse effects in treating patients with ventricular arrhythmias.[12] In the Cardiac Arrhythmia Pilot Study (CAPS) trial, moricizine was less effective than encainide and flecainide in suppressing PVCs and nonsustained ventricular tachycardia.[13] In the CAST trial, where encainide and flecainide were withdrawn from randomization because of excessive mortality,[14] moricizine was also found to produce greater mortality than placebo.[15] Adverse effects of moricizine are infrequent and include dizziness, nausea, headache, and perioral paresthesia.

CLASS II ANTIARRHYTHMICS

β-adrenergic antagonists (β-blockers) are antiarrhythmic secondary to their ability to antagonize sympathetic influence over nodal tissues, resulting in reduced automaticity in the sinus node and conduction velocity through the AV node. β-blockers are most commonly used for rapid control of ventricular rate during supraventricular tachycardias such as AF and atrial flutter. They have also been shown to prevent the development of AF during states of adrenergic hyperstimulation, such as after cardiac surgery. In adrenergically mediated supraventricular tachycardias, β-blockers may actually terminate the arrhythmia. β-blockers have also been shown to reduce the incidence of ventricular tachycardia and sudden cardiac death. In clinical situations requiring rapid ventricular rate control, the intravenous β-blockers most commonly used are esmolol and metoprolol.

Esmolol is approved for rapid control of ventricular rate in patients with AF or atrial flutter when short-term control of ventricular rate is needed. It also is indicated for noncompensatory tachycardia when heart rate must be reversed. Esmolol demonstrates the typical effects of a cardioselective β-blocker without intrinsic sympathomimetic activity or membrane-stabilizing effects and has the additional unique property of an ultrashort duration of action. This permits its use to slow AV nodal conduction directly, with minimal concern for long-lasting adverse effects.[16,17] Clinical trials have shown esmolol to be comparable to propranolol in reducing the ventricular rate in supraventricular tachycardia, with an overall response rate of 64% to 72%, including 6% to 14% who converted to sinus rhythm.[16–18] Comparative studies with verapamil have shown similar reductions in ventricular rate, with a higher number of patients converting to sinus rhythm after esmolol.[19] Esmolol therefore allows the clinician to continually and rapidly titrate the dosage to the desired effect. Furthermore, there is an added element of safety if adverse effects occur because the effects subside soon after the infusion is discontinued.

The primary adverse effect is hypotension, occurring in 33% to 44% of patients.[16,18] The same studies support the safety of esmolol in patients with traditional contraindications to β-blockers such as diabetes mellitus or obstructive airway disease.

CLASS III ANTIARRHYTHMICS

Amiodarone. Amiodarone has become the most widely prescribed antiarrhythmic because of its wide spectrum of efficacy and relative safety in patients with structural heart disease. Amiodarone is a class III agent with properties of Vaughn-Williams classes I (sodium channel blocker), II (β-blocker), and IV (calcium channel blocker), and α-receptor antagonism as well. Amiodarone structurally resembles thyroxine. It is indicated for acute termination and maintenance of ventricular fibrillation, ventricular tachycardia (pulseless or with a pulse), AF, and atrial flutter. It is effective in the maintenance of sinus rhythm after direct current cardioversion in patients with AF[19] and in the termination of reentrant arrhythmias, including the WPW syndrome. Intravenous amiodarone also is effective in suppressing ventricular arrhythmias,[20–22] and oral amiodarone appears to decrease cardiac mortality after MI.[22–25] Low-dose amiodarone (200 mg/day) was compared with individualized antiarrhythmics or no therapy in patients with persisting asymptomatic complex arrhythmias after MI. During the first year after MI, amiodarone resulted in fewer deaths than in the other groups.[26] When amiodarone was used after MI in patients who could not take β-blockers, there were fewer deaths and a decreased frequency of ventricular arrhythmias.[24]

Pharmacokinetics. The bioavailability of oral amiodarone is poor and erratic, with 22% to 86% absorption.[27] The time to peak absorption is about 6 hours. After absorption, the drug is widely distributed to fat, lung, liver, muscle, and spleen, with a very large volume of distribution (approximately 5,000 L). The elimination half-life varies from 26 to 107 days and appears biphasic. Amiodarone is metabolized to its major active metabolite, desethylamiodarone (DEA). The utility of monitoring serum amiodarone concentrations is controversial because of the extensive distribution to tissues and the apparent role of DEA in arrhythmia suppression. There is evidence that arrhythmias may recur if concentrations fall below 1.0 mg per L. Toxicity may occur if serum concentrations exceed 2.5 mg per L. Variable correlations have been made with red cell concentrations of amiodarone. Various dosing schemes have been suggested to avoid the delay in reaching steady-state serum amiodarone concentrations. Up to 1,600 mg is given daily for a week, then 800 mg daily for 2 to 4 weeks, and finally the dosage is reduced to the minimally tolerable dosage, usually 200 to 600 mg daily in two divided doses. Intravenous amiodarone is given as a rapid infusion of 150 mg over 10 minutes, then a slow infusion of 1 mg per minute for 6 hours, followed by a maintenance infusion of 0.5 mg per minute.[3] In cardiac emergencies, such as pulseless ventricular tachycardia or ventricular fibrillation, amiodarone is given as a rapid 300-mg intravenous push. Although patients can be converted from parenteral to oral amiodarone, the products produce different cardiac effects. Intravenous amiodarone has more pronounced calcium channel-blocking effects and antiadrenergic effects than the oral form. Because of the high risk of phlebitis, intravenous infusions should be delivered via central lines. The surface tension of intravenous amiodarone makes drop counter infusions unreliable, necessitating the use of volumetric devices. Many of the dose-defining clinical trials used polyvinyl chloride tubing that adsorbs amiodarone. Glass or polyolefin should be used when infusions last longer than 2 hours.[3]

Toxicity. It is estimated that 80% of patients taking amiodarone will experience at least one adverse effect, most of which occur with chronic therapy. Corneal deposits are common, so annual eye examinations are recommended. In one series, 79% of patients developed microdeposits but no change in visual acuity.[28] Some cardiologists suggest observing only for visual symptoms such as photophobia or blurring, which develop less often than the microdeposits.[29] Abnormal liver enzymes may be encountered in 10% to 20% of patients.[30] The drug appears to concentrate in liver tissue. Although enzymes may rise, typically to two to three times normal, hepatic function may not change, and the drug may be continued with ultimate resolution of the problem. However, severe liver damage and death have been associated with amiodarone.[30] Dermatologic reactions to amiodarone occur in up to 11.6% of patients[29] and have been described as photosensitivity or blue-gray skin discoloration. Pulmonary abnormalities associated with amiodarone are considered to be a justification for discontinuing therapy. Pulmonary fibrosis, the most common reason for discontinuing therapy, is a dose- and time-dependent adverse effect.[30] The risk is greatest at high doses, but it can also occur with chronic use of low doses.[31] Pulmonary function tests are recommended at baseline and should be repeated if a subsequent chest radiograph indicates fibrosis. Chest radiographs are recommended if a patient develops unexplained or increasing dyspnea. A less common, but serious, pulmonary abnormality that can occur early and rapidly is interstitial pneumonitis, an autoimmune reaction that results in inflammation and acute lung damage. Treatment includes discontinuing amiodarone, intravenous corticosteroids, and other supportive therapy. Thyroid abnormalities are also common with amiodarone. The iodine content of amiodarone is 37%, which is thought to be responsible for the occurrence of hypothyroidism or hyperthyroidism. Amiodarone interferes with the metabolism of thyroxine (T_4) by the deiodinase enzyme, resulting in increased serum concentrations of T_4 and decreased serum concentrations of triiodothyronine (T_3). Patients typically do not display symptoms of hyperthyroidism; in fact, thyroid-stimulating hormone concentrations may be increased, which suggests insensitivity to thyroid hormone effect.[30] There is controversy over the predictability of antiarrhythmic response and toxicity with the use of the serum reverse T_3 (rT_3) concentrations. Very high rT_3 concentrations (greater than 130 ng/dL) have been associated with the development of pulmonary fibrosis, arrhythmogenicity, and sudden cardiac death.[32] Amiodarone-induced hyperthyroidism may warrant dosage reduction or withdrawal and antithyroid therapy. Amiodarone-induced hypothyroidism may present with signs of sinus bradycardia, which can reduce cardiac output or cause constipation. Hypothyroidism treatment includes amiodarone dosage reduction or withdrawal and thyroid hormone replacement therapy. Proarrhythmia associated with amiodarone is rare. A recent evaluation of pooled data from multiple trials of patients treated with amiodarone reported an overall proarrhythmia incidence of 2% and an incidence of less than 1% for torsades de pointes.[33]

Interactions. Amiodarone may produce drug interactions with warfarin, digoxin, procainamide, and quinidine.[34] It has been suggested that the dosage of these drugs be reduced empirically by 50% when amiodarone is added and that Q-T and QRS intervals be monitored for excessive prolongation.

Sotalol. Sotalol was approved by the FDA in 1992 for use in life-threatening ventricular arrhythmias. Sotalol is categorized as a class III agent that also has properties of class II (β-blockade). The marketed product is a racemic mixture of d- and l-sotalol, both with equal effect on lengthening the APD and refractory period. The main difference between the two compounds is the relative lack of β-blocking activity of d-sotalol.

The adverse effects of sotalol can be attributed to its β-blocking and Q-T prolongation properties. Fatigue, dyspnea, and bradycardia are the most common reasons for discontinuing sotalol.[35] Other adverse effects include dizziness, headache, bronchospasm, and congestive heart failure exacerbation. Proarrhythmia is the most serious adverse effect attributed to sotalol, with an overall occurrence of 4.3%.[35] The most common arrhythmias induced are torsades de pointes and sustained ventricular tachycardia or ventricular fibrillation. The incidence of proarrhythmia increases with increasing dosages of sotalol; most occur at dosages greater than 320 mg per day.[35] Proarrhythmias are most likely to occur within 7 days of sotalol initiation or dosage increase.

Initial sotalol dosing should begin with 40 to 80 mg twice a day, titrated every 2 to 3 days to the desired therapeutic effect. Most patients respond to dosages between 160 and 320 mg per day, but some patients need dosages up to 640 mg per day for arrhythmia suppression.[36] Dosages above 320 mg/day should be used only when the therapeutic benefit outweighs the risk. The class II and III properties of sotalol allow this drug to be effective in a variety of arrhythmias. Sotalol can suppress atrial and ventricular ectopy, depress reentrant conduction, and block the ventricular response to AF. A trial comparing sotalol with quinidine showed equal efficacy in maintaining sinus rhythm after direct current cardioversion for chronic AF, with better tolerance favoring sotalol.[37] In a study comparing seven drugs with antiarrhythmic properties (imipramine, mexiletine, pirmenol, procainamide, propafenone, quinidine, and sotalol) in patients with ventricular tachycardia, sotalol was more effective at sup-

pressing arrhythmias and had the least probability of discontinuation because of adverse effects.[38] Sotalol had a lower mortality rate and less proarrhythmic effect than class I agents in the Electrophysiologic Study Versus Electrocardiographic Monitoring (ESVEM) trial.[39] Enthusiasm for sotalol led to the Survival with Oral d-Sotalol (SWORD) trial that studied patients after MI with poor ejection fraction (i.e., less than 0.40). d-Sotalol resulted in a risk of death 20.7 times greater than that of placebo in the subgroup of remote MI and mildly impaired ejection fraction.[40] Women appeared to be at greater risk of mortality from sotalol than men. In no subgroup did d-sotalol perform better than placebo.

Ibutilide and Dofetilide. Ibutilide and dofetilide are indicated for the rapid conversion of AF or atrial flutter of recent onset. Ibutilide is an intravenous agent, whereas dofetilide is given orally. These compounds are structurally similar to sotalol. They are pure class III antiarrhythmics that prolong the action potential duration by a unique mechanism: activating the slow inward sodium current instead of slowing the potassium rectifier channel seen with other agents in its class.[41] An advantage is the lack of hypotensive or negative inotropic effects. However, they exert dose-related effects in prolonging Q-T intervals that are correlated with their antiarrhythmic activity.[3]

Ibutilide was compared with procainamide in patients with spontaneous, paroxysmal atrial flutter, or AF.[42] Ibutilide converted 64% of patients with atrial flutter, whereas procainamide did not convert any. Ibutilide converted 32% of patients with AF, procainamide only 5%. The low efficacy rates in this study may have been related to the long duration of the arrhythmia. Dofetilide was shown to be safe and effective in a randomized, double-blind study in patients with left ventricular systolic dysfunction.

The most common toxicity to ibutilide and dofetilide is QTc prolongation. Due to the risk of polymorphic ventricular tachycardia (torsades de pointes), continuous ECG monitoring is required even up to 4 hours after ibutilide is given or until the QTc has returned to baseline.[41] Dofetilide has strict restrictions on its use in the United States, with prescribing authority granted to specific physicians, mandatory initiation in the hospital setting, and specific dosing guidelines based on QTc and renal function. Serum potassium and magnesium concentrations should be measured and corrected before these agents are used.[43] They should not be used with other agents that prolong the QTc.

Azimilide. Azimilide (not yet FDA approved) is unique in that unlike other class III antiarrhythmics, it blocks both the rapidly (I_{Kr}) and slowly (I_{Ks}) activating components of the delayed rectifier potassium current.[44] Studies show that azimilide prolongs the refractory period in a dose-dependent manner.[45,46] The advantage of azimilide over conventional class III antiarrhythmics that block only the rapidly activating component is related to the increased importance of the slowly activating component at higher heart rates and conditions in increased sympathetic tone.[44] Therefore, it is hypothesized that azimilide will retain effectiveness (rate-independent) when tachycardia and adrenergic stimulation reduce the efficacy of other antiarrhythmics. Azimilide prolongs the Q-T interval but has no significant effect on the P-R interval or QRS duration. Studies have shown that azimilide is not associated with significant hemodynamic effects (heart rate or blood pressure) at doses adequate for antiarrhythmic efficacy.[44] Azimilide is capable of blocking inward sodium currents and L-type calcium channels at concentrations 5 to 10 times higher than required for blocking the delayed rectifier potassium channel. Azimilide also exerts β-adrenergic receptor blockade at approximately one-fourth the affinity as sotalol.

Azimilide was developed for use in prevention of recurrence of supraventricular arrhythmias. Studies have shown that azimilide 100 mg or 125 mg once daily is effective at prolonging the time to recurrence of symptomatic AF, atrial flutter, or paroxysmal supraventricular tachycardia.[44,46] Doses less than 100 mg once daily have not been shown to be effective. In addition, azimilide was studied in patients who had had an MI and had left ventricular dysfunction in the Azimilide Postinfarction Survival Evaluation (ALIVE) trial.[47] This randomized, double-blind study was designed to evaluate azimilide's efficacy in preventing sudden cardiac death in a high-risk population. Azimilide was associated with a neutral effect on all-cause mortality and a significant reduction in new-onset AF compared to placebo. This study showed that azimilide was safe for use in high-risk patients after MI and also effective for AF in this population.

Pharmacokinetics. Azimilide exerts linear pharmacokinetics.[44] After oral administration, peak concentrations are achieved in approximately 7 hours. The rate and extent of absorption are not affected by food. Azimilide is 94% protein bound. Clearance is mainly via metabolism, with renal elimination accounting for only 10% of total drug clearance. Only one metabolite has been found to be active, but its plasma concentrations represent less than 5% of the parent compound. The terminal elimination half-life of azimilide is approximately 4 days. Steady-state drug interaction studies have not shown any significant interactions with digoxin or warfarin. Based on its pharmacokinetic properties, azimilide is suitable for once-daily dosing, does not require dosage adjustments for age, gender, or renal function and can safely be administered in patients taking digoxin or warfarin.

CLASS IV ANTIARRHYTHMICS

Only the nondihydropyridine calcium channel blockers, verapamil and diltiazem, exert antiarrhythmic utility. Similar to β-blockers, these agents exert their antiarrhythmic efficacy by slowing AV nodal conduction and reducing ventricular rates during certain supraventricular tachyarrhythmias. These agents inhibit channel-mediated entry of calcium into the cell. Effects are most evident in the SA node, AV node, and cardiac and peripheral vascular smooth muscles because

these tissues depend on calcium flux for action potential generation. In contrast, atrial and ventricular myocardium and the His-Purkinje system normally are fast-channel (sodium flux dependent) tissues. This explains the lack of efficacy of verapamil or diltiazem in ventricular arrhythmias. Among the calcium channel-blocking agents, verapamil has the lowest degree of peripheral arterial dilation relative to its effects on the heart. This characteristic is advantageous in treating arrhythmias, but the prominent negative inotropic effect may be a limitation in patients with left ventricular dysfunction. Diltiazem has electrophysiologic and hemodynamic effects comparable to those of verapamil and has shown efficacy and safety in clinical trials.[48,49]

Verapamil and diltiazem are not thought to have a significant proarrhythmic effect but must be used cautiously in patients with preexisting conduction disorders. Premature atrial or ventricular impulses occasionally reactivate reentry. Atrial fibrillation and serious ventricular arrhythmias are uncommon. Bradycardia or heart block caused by excessive AV nodal effect may warrant treatment with isoproterenol, atropine, calcium, or pacemakers. Both agents are contraindicated in patients with preexisting SA nodal disease (sick sinus syndrome) because of the high risk of prolonged sinus arrest after termination of the arrhythmia.

An important drug interaction occurs between verapamil and β-blockers. Concomitant administration of these drugs results in AV blocking and negative inotropic effects by independent mechanisms. This increases the risk of serious cardiovascular effects such as congestive heart failure,[50] high-degree AV block, or hypotension. Serum concentrations of digoxin may be increased by verapamil[51] via an increase in half-life and reduction in the distribution volume and total clearance. Furthermore, verapamil should be used with caution in patients with suspected digoxin toxicity because of its additive effects on the AV node. Other significant drug interactions mediated through cytochrome P-450 3A4 inhibition with verapamil and diltiazem include pimozide, cyclosporine, tacrolimus, sirolimus, and ergotamine.

MISCELLANEOUS ANTIARRHYTHMICS

Digoxin. Digitalis has positive inotropic and negative chronotropic and dromotropic properties. The last effect accounts for its efficacy in AF, is seen only at higher dosages, and occurs via a variety of mechanisms. The predominant effect is indirect via vagal stimulation, with direct AV nodal action having a minor role. This vagotonic effect is largely attenuated by catecholamines, explaining the limited ability to control ventricular rates during exercise or stress.[52–54] Digoxin does not prevent recurrence of paroxysmal AF in patients in sinus rhythm. The effect of digitalis on accessory pathways differs from that on the AV node, and it should not be used in patients with AF and the WPW syndrome. Digoxin is no longer considered the drug of choice for ventricular rate control in AF; rather, verapamil, diltiazem, or a β-blocker should be used before digoxin unless hypotension or acute heart failure decompensation is present.[55]

Optimally, individual digoxin loading doses are determined based on the observed response to initial therapy. Dosages of 0.5 mg intravenously are followed by 0.125 to 0.25 mg intravenously or orally every 4 to 8 hours until the desired response is seen. The dosage and interval should take into account the time for tissue distribution of 6 to 8 hours. This regimen usually results in rate control in 12 to 24 hours. In a prospective observational study, the average total digoxin dosage needed for initial control of ventricular rate was 0.8 mg (range 0.125 to 6.125 mg), and the average time to initial ventricular rate control was 9.5 hours.[56] Intramuscular administration is not advised because of erratic absorption and excessive pain at the injection site. Infants, children, and patients with hyperthyroidism may need higher than estimated dosages, whereas those with coronary artery disease or obstructive airway disease may be especially sensitive to digitalis. Oral maintenance dosages for AF average 0.25 to 0.375 mg daily in adults with normal renal function. Calculated dosages may be used as a guideline, but the clinical response of the patient is a better criterion of efficacy.

Monitoring parameters for digoxin use in AF include ventricular rate (apical pulse) and the signs and symptoms of congestive heart failure. Renal function and serum electrolytes (especially potassium and magnesium) should also be monitored, along with observation for signs and symptoms of toxicity. Using serum concentrations as a guide to dosing is not advised in managing supraventricular tachycardias such as AV nodal reentry and AF. Correlation between therapeutic response (i.e., ventricular rate) and serum concentrations is poor.[57,58] This is probably because other factors (underlying autonomic tone, exogenous catecholamines, electrolyte concentrations) alter cardiac sensitivity to digitalis independently of serum concentrations. Despite this limitation, serum concentrations may be useful in evaluating patient compliance, suspected toxicity, or drug interactions. Concentrations should be measured at least 6 to 8 hours after administration to allow tissue distribution.

Three drug interactions of digoxin are relevant in supraventricular tachyarrhythmia management. An elevation of serum digoxin concentrations to two to three times baseline occurs in most patients taking digoxin and quinidine concomitantly. The mechanism is thought to be related to inhibition of p-glycoprotein.[59] Digoxin concentrations increase within hours of quinidine administration, reaching a new steady state in several days. This interaction depends on the serum concentration of quinidine but not that of digoxin and is caused by a decrease in the volume of distribution and renal and nonrenal clearance of digoxin by quinidine. A similar increase in digoxin concentration is also expected with coadministration of amiodarone or verapamil. Dosage reduction by 50% and careful serum concentration monitoring are advised.[51]

The subjective evaluation of patients for digoxin toxicity is difficult because of the nonspecific nature of the symptoms. Anorexia, nausea, vomiting, weakness, and lethargy are the most common symptoms. Vision changes, disorienta-

tion, and hallucinations are less common. Elevated serum concentrations may assist in the diagnosis, but there is overlap between toxic and therapeutic values. Moreover, electrolyte abnormalities (hypokalemia, metabolic alkalosis, hypomagnesemia, or hypercalcemia) or hypoxia may contribute to clinical toxicity even at "nontoxic" serum concentrations. Toxic cardiac effects result from enhanced automaticity, promotion of triggered activity, or a depression of AV nodal conduction. A useful monitoring tool for toxicity in patients with AF is the ECG. The excessive effects of digoxin result in an exaggerated AV nodal block, seen initially as occasional long equal pauses (intermittent junctional escape). Eventually, the ventricular rate becomes regular at 35 to 30 bpm, reflecting complete junctional escape. At higher concentrations, junctional pacemaker firing may accelerate, causing a junctional tachycardia. PVCs caused by enhanced firing of ectopic ventricular foci also are common. As toxicity progresses, essentially any arrhythmias can be seen. Toxicity is managed by discontinuation of the drug, potassium unless contraindicated, antiarrhythmics, or digoxin-immune Fab fragments.

Adenosine. Adenosine is a ubiquitous endogenous purine nucleoside. Its myriad biologic effects include regulating coronary, cerebral, renal, and skeletal blood flow, modulating neurotransmission and immune response, inhibiting platelet aggregation, stimulating gastrin secretion, inhibiting lipolysis, and inducing bronchoconstriction. The actions of adenosine on cardiac tissues include a very transient, powerful negative dromotropic effect on the AV node and a similar negative chronotropic effect in the sinus node, AV junction, and ventricles. On electrophysiologic studies the primary effects are a lengthening of sinus cycle and a prolongation of the A-H interval (i.e., the time from atrial excitation to the His bundle, which approximates the AV conduction time), followed by complete or partial AV nodal block.[60] Adenosine has no effect on the His-Purkinje interval. Cardiac activity is thought to occur secondary to activation of the A1 receptor, which leads to alterations in calcium and potassium ion currents, but the precise mechanisms are unclear.[61] Adenosine exerts minimal effect on vagal tone.

Adenosine (Adenocard) is an injectable product indicated for conversion of paroxysmal supraventricular tachycardia, including that associated with accessory bypass tracts (AV nodal reentry tachycardia or WPW). If vagal maneuvers are unsuccessful, adenosine is the drug of choice for terminating AV nodal reentrant rhythms.[62] Adenosine restores sinus rhythm within 10 to 20 seconds in 85% to 100% of adults and children with spontaneous or induced AV nodal reentrant tachycardias.[61,63–66] Despite the lack of FDA approval, adenosine is considered by some clinicians the drug of choice (after vagal maneuvers fail) for the acute management of AV nodal reentrant tachycardia in children.[67] Antegrade pathway conduction block occurs in the majority of patients.[61,63–66] In patients with sinus node or intraatrial reentry, AF or atrial flutter, ectopic atrial tachycardia, or ventricular tachycardia, adenosine induces a higher-grade AV block[61,68]; the transiently (less than 20 seconds) slower ventricular rate may allow visualization of P waves and therefore aid in diagnosis, but atrial activity is unchanged, and these arrhythmias are rarely terminated.

In randomized[63,66] and nonrandomized[65,69] comparative trials of adenosine and verapamil, conversion rates are comparable or favor adenosine for patients with AV nodal reentry or AV reentry involving an accessory pathway. Termination of the tachycardia generally is more rapid with adenosine than verapamil, but the clinical importance of this is unclear. Repetitive administration results in consistent conversion at a similar dosage each time or repeated failures.

Noncardiac adverse effects occur in 15% to 81% of patients.[60,63,65,66,70] The most common are flushing, dyspnea or a feeling of suffocation, and headache. Chest pain or pressure may mimic angina. Cough, malaise, and nausea have also been observed. Inhaled adenosine has been reported to induce bronchoconstriction in asthmatic patients.[60] The effect of intravenous adenosine in patients with preexisting obstructive airway disease is not known because most clinical trials have excluded asthmatics. Adenosine therefore should be used cautiously in these patients and avoided in patients with severe asthma. Adverse effects after intravenous adenosine abate within 1 to 2 minutes and are therefore limited in most patients.

Despite the action of adenosine to reduce systemic vascular resistance, intravenous boluses are well tolerated hemodynamically. Blood pressure remains unchanged or may even increase at the time of conversion to sinus rhythm. Masking of peripheral vasodilation in conscious subjects receiving bolus doses may be the result of autonomic reflexes. However, caution must be used when adenosine is administered to patients with underlying ischemic heart disease, as the vasodilation can precipitate angina. Postconversion arrhythmias or conduction disorders occur in up to 60% of patients receiving adenosine. Sinus bradycardia, sinus arrest, and various degrees of AV block last less than 1 to 2 minutes and do not warrant intervention in most patients. However, caution should be exercised in patients with sinus node disease because sinus arrest for up to 4 seconds has been observed.[63] Premature atrial or ventricular impulses after conversion to sinus rhythm occur in 33% to 60% of patients.[63,70] This may reinitiate reentry, an effect that is more common after adenosine than after verapamil. Self-limiting episodes of sinus tachycardia and AF are also relatively common.

Drug interactions with adenosine may involve alterations in extracellular and intracellular transport as well as receptor affinity. Although many drugs have in vitro or theoretical mechanisms for interaction, systematic clinical trials are lacking. Interactions with dipyridamole and theophylline have the strongest documentation. Dipyridamole blocks the cellular uptake of adenosine, thereby inhibiting its metabolism.[71] This may enhance the negative chronotropic and dromotropic effects of adenosine. Very limited evidence suggests a similar effect with diazepam. Aminophylline and theophylline bind to the extracellular adenosine receptor sites and therefore act as competitive antagonists.[60] Patients receiving these drugs (and possibly caffeine) may exhibit a blunted response to adenosine. Carbamazepine can suppress AV conduction at therapeutic or mildly elevated blood concentrations. In the presence of carbamazepine, conduction inhibition through the AV node by adenosine can be enhanced, producing a higher degree of heart block.[62,68] Adenosine should be used cautiously if combined with calcium channel blockers or β-blockers as it can potentiate both hypotensive and bradycardic effects. However, the ultrashort duration of action of adenosine usually minimizes the long-term effects of any drug interactions.

The ultrashort half-life of the drug necessitates careful attention to the site and rate of administration. The pharmacologic effect depends on the amount of drug delivered to the heart. A slow administration rate or slow rate of blood flow (e.g., heart failure) may result in significant metabolism before the drug reaches the heart, therefore attenuating the effect of the drug. Conversely, administration into central veins (e.g., femoral vein during electrophysiologic studies) may result in a more marked response. Reflex tachycardia caused by vasodilation has been reported after slow administration. Individual variation in underlying autonomic tone and the administration of other antiarrhythmics may enhance or attenuate adenosine's effect.

BRADYARRHYTHMIAS

SINUS BRADYCARDIA

Sinus bradycardia is defined in adults as a heart rate below 60 bpm, with each impulse originating in the SA node, followed by normal conduction through the AV node and His-Purkinje system. Although considered an arrhythmia, heart rates below 60 bpm are not uncommon in athletically active adults. However, sinus bradycardia may occur due to SA node dysfunction (sick sinus syndrome) due to underlying heart disease or the normal aging process. Acutely, sinus bradycardia may occur in patients with acute MI.

Sinus bradycardia usually reflects diminished SA node automaticity, although it may also be caused by improper impulse propagation out of the SA node. SA node automaticity is regulated by underlying autonomic tone (sympathetic and vagal) and is lower during sleep and in trained athletes. As long as the heart rate increases appropriately in response to elevations in sympathetic tone (e.g., exercise), many patients with resting sinus bradycardia remain asymptomatic. Asymptomatic sinus bradycardia is a benign condition that does not warrant treatment, aside from elimination of underlying factors that may worsen the bradycardia. These include drugs (e.g., β-blockers, digitalis, calcium channel blockers, or cholinergic agents), hypothyroidism, increased intracranial pressure, and certain electrolyte abnormalities.

Epidemiology. Sick sinus syndrome occurs in one of every 600 cardiac patients older than 65 years. Moreover, the syndrome may account for 50% of pacemaker implantations in the United States. Sinus bradycardia is seen in 10% to 41% of patients with acute MIs, especially the inferior type.[10] It is most often caused by increased vagal tone associated with inferior ischemia or infarction.

Clinical Presentation and Diagnosis.
Sick sinus syndrome is often asymptomatic or produces symptoms that are consistent with sinus bradycardia or AV block. Sinus bradycardia usually is seen in the early hours after infarction and is often asymptomatic. Ischemic sinus node dysfunction may also occur but is less common. Uncomplicated asymptomatic sinus bradycardia does not warrant treatment other than careful observation.

Treatment.
Therapy is indicated when hypotension, heart failure, chest pain, shortness of breath, ventricular irritability, or decreased level of consciousness is present.[11] Initial treatment should include lower extremity elevation and infusion of volume expanders. Drugs that may further worsen hypotension (e.g., morphine, nitroglycerin) or bradycardia (e.g., β-blockers, calcium channel blockers) should be used carefully. Severe bradycardia may increase ventricular irritability and result in arrhythmias such as PVCs. These often resolve after correction of the bradycardia and do not warrant treatment with conventional antiarrhythmics.

Pharmacotherapy
Atropine. The direct vagolytic action of atropine increases sinus node automaticity and accelerates conduction, usually producing a prompt increase in heart rate and blood pressure. The initial recommended dosage is 0.5 to 1 mg intravenously, repeated as needed to a maximum of 0.04 mg per kg or 3 mg.[11] Low dosages should be avoided because they may produce vagal stimulation with worsened bradycardia or a biphasic response of slowing followed by acceleration in 2 to 3 minutes. Total atropine dosages of 3 mg produce full vagal blockade and may induce unwanted effects.[11] Adverse cardiovascular effects include excessive tachycardia with increased myocardial oxygen consumption, ventricular irritability, and the potential for increasing infarct size.[12] This necessitates caution in patients with acute MI. Noncardiac effects include urinary retention, blurred vision, dry mouth, mydriasis, and toxic psychosis. Patients with sinus node disease may exhibit an inadequate response to atropine, whereas patients with denervated hearts after cardiac transplantation have no response to atropine; both need pacemakers.

Isoproterenol. Isoproterenol, a β-adrenergic agonist, is a second-line drug that should be used with extreme caution in a patient with acute MI because it increases heart rate, ventricular irritability, and myocardial oxygen consumption. Peripheral vasodilation may exacerbate hypotension, which further limits use. It may be temporarily useful for refractory torsades de pointes and hemodynamically unstable bradycardia until pacemaker therapy can be initiated.[11]

Nonpharmacologic Therapy
Pacemakers. Patients not responding to atropine or those with persistent symptoms need pacemakers. Either the transvenous or transcutaneous route may be used. Transvenous pacing is the most reliable, with ventricular pacing the traditional mode. Atrial pacing gives the best hemodynamic response, but intact and reliable AV conduction is needed. Dual-chamber pacemakers that sequentially pace the atrium and ventricle may be preferred in patients with severe heart failure. In transcutaneous cardiac pacing, a low-density current is passed between two self-adhesive pads located anteriorly and posteriorly over the apex of the heart. This results in a hemodynamic response comparable to that of transvenous pacing and has the advantages of faster, easier, and less invasive implementation.[13] Its primary limitation is a lower reliability, with successful pacing in 40% to 80% of patients.

Sinus bradycardia associated with acute MI usually is transient, so temporary pacemakers generally suffice. It is not associated with a higher incidence of complications or mortality. With proper management, this arrhythmia carries a good to excellent prognosis.

ATRIOVENTRICULAR BLOCK
Atrioventricular block occurs when the conduction of the atrial impulse to the ventricle is delayed or is not conducted at the time when the AV node is physiologically refractory. Abnormalities of AV conduction are classified into three types based on the extent of impulse transmission across the AV node. The anatomic location of the conduction block determines the clinical significance, prognosis, and therapy.

First-Degree Atrioventricular Block. First-degree AV occurs when every atrial impulse conducts to the ventricles and a regular ventricular rate is produced but the PR interval exceeds 0.20 seconds in adults. This is a common ECG finding, with an incidence of 0.5% to 10%. Conduction delay in the AV node is the most common cause. Both cardiac (AV nodal disease, AMI, myocarditis) and noncardiac (enhanced vagal tone) causes have been identified. Patients are rarely symptomatic, and treatment is not generally needed. Digitalis, β blockers, calcium channel blockers, and potassium may cause or worsen this pattern. First-degree AV block is not an absolute contraindication to these drugs, but close observation is necessary because they may produce higher-grade block.

Second-Degree Atrioventricular Block. In second-degree AV block, there is intermittent failure of AV impulse conduction. The nonconducted P wave can be intermittent or frequent, at regular or irregular intervals. The anatomic site of block may be the AV node, His bundle, or bundle branch system. This type of block is subdivided into Mobitz types I and II. Mobitz type I, or Wenckebach block, is characterized by a gradual prolongation of AV conduction (PR interval on ECG) until a P wave is not conducted to the ventricles. The cycle then begins anew with a short, followed by progressively longer, PR intervals and a nonconducted

P wave. EPS usually implicates a conduction abnormality in the AV node proximal to the bundle of His. The presence and extent of Mobitz type I AV block is influenced by underlying autonomic tone. It may be seen in normal subjects or may be caused by drugs (e.g., digitalis, β blockers, or verapamil), electrolyte abnormalities, or inflammation. This pattern is also seen in acute inferior myocardial infarction. It usually appears within the first 72 hours after infarction, is transient, and infrequently progresses to higher-grade block.

Many patients with Mobitz type I AV block are asymptomatic, in which case drugs or pacemakers are not needed.[71a] Close observation of patients with AMI or digitalis toxicity is warranted. Treatment is indicated when the patient exhibits symptoms (central nervous system or hemodynamic) or ventricular irritability or the ventricular rate persists at less than 40 bpm.[71a] Atropine facilitates AV nodal conduction by decreasing the effective and functional refractory periods of the AV node. It oftens restores 1:1 conduction in patients with Mobitz type I block and normal AV nodes and may be useful in managing digitalis toxicity. However, this effect is unpredictable in patients with AMI, and temporary pacemakers are therefore indicated.[71a] β-Blockers, verapamil, and digoxin should be used with caution in these patients.

Mobitz type II block is present when the PR interval of conducted beats remains constant, with unpredicted intermittent nonconduction of atrial impulses. It reflects a conduction abnormality distal to the bundle of His and is often associated with a wide QRS (bundle branch block) pattern on ECG. This type of block is seen in acute anterior or anteroseptal myocardial infarction, usually during the first 72 hours after infarction. It reflects extensive ischemia and necrosis of the septum, bundle branches, and Purkinje fibers. Almost all patients are symptomatic. Mobitz type II AV block with bundle branch block is an unstable rhythm with an ominous prognosis, often progressing abruptly to complete heart block, severe bradycardia, or asystole. Atropine is generally ineffective. Pacemakers are therefore mandatory and usually permanent.[71a] Most AV block rhythms are labeled according to the ratio of P waves to QRS complexers (e.g., 2:1 or 3:1). This information alone is of limited utility without the ventricular rate. A 3:1 block is not always more harmful than a 2:1 block. A 2:1 block is more dangerous if the atrial rate is 70 (leading to a ventricular rate of only 35) than a 3:1 block where the atrial rate is 150 (leading to a ventricular rate of 50).

Third-Degree Atrioventricular Block. Third-degree AV block occurs when no atrial activity is conducted to the ventricles; therefore, the atria and ventricles are controlled by independent pacemakers. Also known as complete heart block, it reflects a total absence of AV conduction. This results in an escape rhythm, with the AV junction, His bundle, or Purkinje cells acting as the pacemaker. The site of block is related to the symptoms, prognosis, and therapy. When conduction is blocked within the AV node (proximal conducting system), the AV junction or proximal His bundle cells function as the pacemaker. Normal-appearing QRS complexes are seen, reflecting normal ventricular impulse conduction. The physiologic escape rate for the AV junctional cells is 40 to 60 bpm, which increases in response to elevated sympathetic tone. Complete heart block with AV junctional escape may be a congenital rhythm, or it may be seen (usually transiently) in acute inferior myocardial infarction. This is a fairly stable rhythm. Normal ventricular conduction along with the ability to increase the rate with exercise allows some patients to remain asymptomatic. Infants and children with congenital proximal complete heart block may tolerate this rhythm well for long periods, needing close observation but no intervention.[9,15] Treatment is indicated in patients with symptoms such as hypotension, syncope, persistent chest pain, heart failure; inadequate chronotropic response to exercise; or ventricular arrhythmias. Atropine may be used in emergent situations but is of limited value and is not effective in the long term. Permanent pacemakers are the therapy of choice. Pacemakers are reliable and well tolerated in infants and children with the congenital form of this rhythm. The role of pacemakers in patients with myocardial infarction remains unclear.

Complete heart block in the distal His bundle or Purkinje system (distal conducting system) results in an idioventricular escape rhythm, with wide QRS complexes occurring at a rate of 30 to 40 bpm. This reflects abnormal impulse conduction through the ventricles and the slow intrinsic rate of ventricular pacemaker tissues. This pattern may be seen in AMI and other diseases such as myocarditis, cardiomyopathy, and sarcoidosis. The slow rate coupled with abnormal ventricular conduction usually causes hemodynamic or central nervous system symptoms. In patients with acute anterior or anteroseptal myocardial infarction, this is an unstable rhythm with abrupt progression to asystole or ventricular arrhythmias. Atropine is not effective. Patients with third-degree AV block and an idioventricular rhythm need permanent pacemakers regardless of symptoms.[71a] The abrupt occurrence of this type of block in the setting of an AMI carries an ominous prognosis and a high risk of sudden death.

SUPRAVENTRICULAR TACHYARRHYTHMIAS

SINUS TACHYARRHYTHMIAS

In the simplest terms, sinus tachyarrhythmias refer to heart rhythms originating in the SA node with normal conduction through the AV node and His-Purkinje system that generate a heart rate greater than 100 bpm. Sinus tachyarrhythmias can be subclassified as physiologic sinus tachycardia, inappropriate sinus tachycardia, and SA reentry tachycardia.[72] Sinus tachycardia refers to a sinus rate greater than 100 bpm that is proportional to a physiologic, pathologic, or pharmacologic stimulus. Inappropriate sinus tachycardia is characterized by a persistently elevated heart rate that is unrelated to a physiologic, pathologic, or pharmacologic stimulus, usually as a result of enhanced SA node automaticity or abnormal autonomic regulation of the SA node. SA reentry tachycardia is a result of reentry circuits within the SA node. Although there are subtle differences in electrophysiology, their respective clinical presentations and treatments are generally similar. Therefore, they will be discussed as a group, with pertinent differences highlighted.

Etiology and Pathophysiology. Automaticity of the SA node is normally between 60 and 100 bpm, but it is also under the influence of the autonomic nervous system and other stimuli. Sinus tachycardia most commonly results from an appropriate response to a physiologic stimulus, such as exercise or emotional stress, or a pathologic stimulus, such as hypoxia, acidosis, ischemia, pyrexia, atrial stretch, infection, hyperthyroidism, or pheochromocytoma. Pharmacologic stimuli can also contribute to an increase in SA node automaticity. These include stimulants such as sympathomimetics, catecholamines, β-adrenergic agonists, methylxanthines, and anticholinergic agents.

Clinical Presentation and Diagnosis. The majority of patients with sinus tachycardia are asymptomatic, except perhaps palpitations. Additional symptoms may also include shortness of breath, dizziness, and lightheadedness, with the rare possibility of severe symptoms such as chest pain and presyncope. In patients with underlying comorbid cardiovascular conditions, episodes of sinus tachycardia could precipitate ischemia or acute heart failure exacerbations.

Both physiologic and inappropriate sinus tachycardia are diagnosed based on the criteria of persistent heart rate greater than 100 bpm and the same P wave morphology as in sinus rhythm.[72] Sinus tachycardia is usually nonparoxysmal, characterized by gradual acceleration and deceleration. The exception is SA reentry tachycardia, which is paroxysmal in nature, usually triggered by a premature atrial beat. In all cases, workup for an underlying cause or stimulus is warranted.

Therapeutic Plan. Treatment is aimed at controlling the underlying etiology. Physiologic sinus tachycardia usually does not require treatment, and slowing the heart rate may be deleterious in situations where the increase in cardiac output is required for adequate tissue perfusion. However, if control of symptoms is desired, β-blockers or nondihydropyridine calcium channel blockers (verapamil and diltiazem) can be used to decrease the heart rate. In sympathetically driven rhythms, β-blockers may be particularly effective, in addition to providing secondary benefit for other cardiovascular diseases. Consideration of the usual contraindications to β-blocker and calcium channel blocker therapy remains prudent. In refractory cases of inappropriate sinus tachycardia, catheter ablation of the sinus node to modify or eliminate its function is an option.[73]

PAROXYSMAL SUPRAVENTRICULAR TACHYCARDIAS (AV NODAL RECIPROCATING TACHYCARDIA)

Paroxysmal supraventricular tachycardias (PSVTs) are a family of narrow QRS-complex tachycardias that share the common denominator of reentry (sometimes referred to as ''circus movement tachycardia'') as the primary underlying mechanism. The pathophysiology of reentry has been described in an early section of this chapter. The most common form of PSVT is AV nodal reciprocating tachycardia (AVNRT), where the reentry circuit is confined to the AV node or perhaps the perinodal atrial tissue. In most cases (90%), the anterograde pathway is the slow conducting pathway, while the retrograde pathway exhibits fast conduction. Less than 10% of the time is the reverse present.[74]

Epidemiology. Typically AVNRT occurs in healthy individuals and is not usually associated with structural heart disease. According to the American Heart Association statistics on arrhythmias, PSVT was directly linked to only 124 deaths and 29,000 hospital discharges in 2000.[75] These rhythms are also more common in females than males.

Clinical Presentation and Diagnosis. Reentry rhythms are characterized by sudden onset and termination, as opposed to sinus tachycardia, which follows a gradual acceleration and deceleration of heart rate. Symptoms depend on the ventricular response but are rarely life-threatening. Individuals with underlying heart disease, in whom an increase in ventricular rate can lead to hemodynamic compromise, are at the highest risk of severe symptoms. In general, patients may experience a sudden onset of palpitations, dizziness, lightheadedness, and neck pulsations. The heart rate is usually 140 to 250 bpm, with a regular rhythm. Patients may also experience polyuria secondary to atrial natriuretic peptide release in response to atrial stretch. In rare instances, patients may also experience syncope with the onset of AVNRT.[76]

Along with a history consistent with a sudden onset of symptoms, a 12-lead ECG is required for proper diagnosis of the rhythm.[77] Characteristic findings of AVNRT on an ECG include a narrow QRS complex (less than 120 ms), with no discernible P waves or P waves partially hidden in the QRS complex.[72] Since the retrograde pathway is fast in most instances, this results in a P wave remaining in close proximity to the QRS complex, with less than 70 ms in separation. A P wave located in the ST segment that is greater than 70 ms after the QRS complex is more indicative of atrioventricular reciprocating tachycardia (AVRT), a related supraventricular rhythm discussed in the following section. Termination of the rhythm by vagal maneuver is another clinical clue that the rhythm is secondary to a reentry circuit, and thus consistent with AVNRT or AVRT.

Other diagnostic tests may also be helpful in defining the rhythm but are not routinely ordered. Echocardiography may be useful in episodes of sustained supraventricular tachycardia to investigate possible structural heart disease, thus ruling out PSVT. For frequent and transient tachycardias,

24-hour ambulatory Holter monitoring may aid in detection of an aberrant rhythm.[78] Exercise testing is useful for detecting exercise-induced tachycardias. Other more invasive testing with more of a role in determining chronic management includes transesophageal atrial recordings and stimulation, and electrophysiologic testing.

Therapeutic Plan

Acute Management. If the rhythm has been confirmed as AVNRT and a wide QRS complex tachycardia has been ruled out, acute termination of the rhythm may be attempted. Termination of a reentry circuit is accomplished by interrupting the critically timed cyclical electrical impulses, either by slowing conduction or prolonging refractoriness in either the fast or slow conduction pathway. This increases the probability that an electrical impulse will encounter refractory tissue, leading to abrupt termination of the arrhythmia. In addition, correctable contributing factors such as fever, infection, hypoxia, anemia, or hyperthyroidism should be treated.

Acute rhythm termination can be achieved by direct current cardioversion or vagal maneuvers or with use of pharmacologic agents that slow AV nodal conduction. Globally, electrical cardioversion is more effective and quicker, but it is also associated with greater risks and discomfort to the patient. As such, the decision between electrical and vagal maneuvers/pharmacologic cardioversion is determined by the patient's hemodynamic stability and the severity of symptoms.

Direct Current Cardioversion. In patients with hemodynamic instability (severe hypotension or heart failure, pulmonary edema, myocardial ischemia, acute alteration in mental status), electrical cardioversion is the therapy of choice. Direct current cardioversion depolarizes a critical number of myocardial cells simultaneously, allowing the sinus node to reestablish dominance as the pacemaker. For conversion of SVTs, lower energies (10 to 50 joules, or 0.5 joules/kg) often are adequate. This is a uniformly effective, immediate method of termination with minimal adverse effects. The only major adverse effect is the potential for induction of ventricular arrhythmias, which can be avoided by synchronizing the electrical discharge to the QRS complex. Myocardial damage is rare with lower energies. Short-acting sedatives may be given before the procedure in older children and adults. Electroconversion is not advised in patients with stable cardiovascular status because other measures are considered less invasive and safer. Moreover, direct current cardioversion precludes a direct assessment of the efficacy of various other maneuvers and drugs on the arrhythmia. This information is useful in managing recurrent episodes.

Vagal Maneuvers. In hemodynamically stable patients, interventions to increase vagal tone are performed before antiarrhythmic agents are instituted. These maneuvers decrease conductivity, increase refractoriness in the AV node, and decrease automaticity in the SA node by increasing parasym-

pathetic tone. Used either alone or in conjunction with antiarrhythmic drugs, vagotonic maneuvers terminate 50% to 80% of cases of AVNRT.[79]

The most common vagal measures are carotid sinus massage (or pressure) and the Valsalva maneuver. Carotid sinus massage stimulates the baroreceptors of the carotid artery, which slows the sinus rate, prolongs AV conduction, lowers cardiac output, decreases venous return, and decreases peripheral vascular resistance.[80] Alteration in the critical balance between conduction and refractoriness disrupts the cycle and terminates the rhythm. The Valsalva maneuver (prolonged forced expiration against a closed glottis) may be induced by blowing into a blood pressure manometer tube to maintain a pressure of 30 to 60 mm Hg for 10 to 30 seconds. Conversion to sinus rhythm occurs during the relaxation phase, when a parasympathetic surge induces antegrade AV nodal block. Other vagotonic procedures include deep breathing, gagging, coughing, and squatting.

Carotid sinus massage and Valsalva maneuver may not be as successful in infants and young children. In these patients, the diving reflex may be initiated by immersing the face in a pan of ice water for 10 to 15 seconds or placing a washcloth soaked in ice water on the face. This causes an acute vagal surge that is more prominent and clinically effective in young patients. A slowing of the tachycardia rate is followed by abrupt conversion to sinus rhythm. The diving reflex may induce asystole and should be used only under monitored conditions.

Background increases in sympathetic tone may attenuate the effectiveness of vagal maneuvers.[79] This may explain the lower efficacy when standing, as compared with the supine position. These measures generally are more effective in young patients, probably because of a reduction in overall autonomic tone associated with aging. Vagal maneuvers should be performed as early as possible after arrhythmia initiation, before elevated sympathetic tone reduces efficacy.[79]

Vagotonic procedures should not be used in patients with a history of sinus node dysfunction because prolonged sinus node recovery time may cause sinus arrest after the reentry circuit is terminated. Carotid sinus massage or pressure may cause carotid artery ischemia in patients with preexisting atherosclerotic narrowing or (rarely) ventricular tachyarrhythmias.[80] Pressure to the carotid arteries should never be applied bilaterally. Both carotid arteries should be examined before the procedure, and it should not be attempted in patients with evidence of cerebrovascular insufficiency (e.g., carotid bruits). Because of the prevalence of sinus node and cerebrovascular disease in older adults, vagotonic stimuli should be avoided or used with great caution in this population.

Pharmacologic Agents. If vagal maneuvers fail, intravenous antiarrhythmic agents are instituted for termination of the rhythm as long as patients remain hemodynamically stable. The drug of choice is adenosine, which provides the fastest onset of action.[81] Nondihydropyridine calcium channel blockers and β-blockers are longer-acting alternatives if adenosine fails or is contraindicated, or if prevention of recurrences is warranted. Diltiazem inhibits antegrade AV nodal conduction with comparable effectiveness to verapamil.[49,82] Diltiazem is the more commonly used of the two calcium channel blockers due to the rapid titratability of the intravenous infusion, as opposed to the intermittent dosing of verapamil. Diltiazem also exerts a milder negative inotropic effect compared to verapamil,[83] which may allow its short-term use in patients with severe left ventricular impairment.[84] Propranolol prolongs antegrade AV conduction and refractoriness and also depresses automaticity at the SA node, AV junction, and His-Purkinje fibers. Propranolol is not a first-line drug because it is less efficacious than adenosine and verapamil, and it is contraindicated in patients who have received verapamil because of the additive effects on cardiac conduction and contractility. It is used primarily in infants and children who have not received verapamil and when digoxin is not desirable (e.g., accessory pathway conduction). Metoprolol and esmolol have the advantages of cardioselectivity and ultrashort half-life, respectively. Agents reserved for refractory patients include digoxin (preferable in patients with severe left ventricular function), amiodarone, sotalol, quinidine, procainamide, flecainide, and propafenone.

Nonpharmacologic Therapies. Patients who do not respond to pharmacologic treatment should receive electrical therapy, which may include direct current cardioversion (described earlier) or specialized pacing techniques. Pacing techniques include one or two critically timed extra stimuli or a rapid sequence of impulses (burst overdrive pacing).[85] As a rule, burst-pacing techniques are more effective. The goal of pacing is to create a strategically timed region of refractoriness. The paced impulse enters the circuit, collides with the advancing wavefront, blocks the succeeding wavefront, and stops the reentry circuit. Proximity of the pacing site to the anatomic origin of the arrhythmia enhances the likelihood of success. Though highly effective, pacing is an invasive technique that entails transvenous or transesophageal catheter placement and electrophysiologic studies for application. Complications include tachycardia acceleration and fibrillation of the paced chambers.

Chronic Management. The need for chronic prophylaxis is dictated by the frequency of episodes, the tachycardia rate, and its hemodynamic effects. In general, the presence and extent of symptoms are related to the rate and duration of the arrhythmia. Two approaches to chronic management are nonpharmacologic intervention by catheter ablation or pacing, or arrhythmia suppression with antiarrhythmics. The benefits of each modality must be balanced carefully against the risks and inconveniences of an invasive procedure or long-term antiarrhythmic therapy. In the absence of heart disease, most patients have infrequent attacks of short duration without cardiovascular compromise and do not require

chronic therapy. Patients with underlying heart disease, frequent attacks, or debilitating symptoms (syncope, angina, hypotension, heart failure) may benefit from either a nonpharmacologic or pharmacologic intervention. In addition, some patients who are candidates for a nonpharmacologic intervention may decline the procedure in favor of remaining on antiarrhythmic therapy.

The goal of chronic prophylaxis is to prevent or minimize the frequency of attacks and their hemodynamic consequences. Complete abolition is not necessary and may be worse than no therapy because of proarrhythmic or other adverse drug effects. Precipitating factors such as sympathomimetics, β-agonists, caffeine, tobacco, or ethanol should be limited or discontinued. Patients with arrhythmias responsive to physical maneuvers such as carotid sinus pressure should be instructed in their proper application. This may obviate pharmacologic prophylaxis.

Pharmacologic Agents. Strategies for the pharmacologic prophylaxis of AV nodal reentry are not as well established as those for managing acute episodes. Many therapeutic options exist, some or all of which may give a satisfactory outcome. As a rule, patient response is not as predictable and efficacy rates are lower than for acute episodes, with no single drug emerging as the treatment of choice. Initial selections are based on specific patient considerations, dosing intervals, adverse effect profile, cost of drugs and monitoring tests, and physician preference or experience. In the absence of large clinical trials dictating optimal therapy, agents targeting the AV node are usually initiated first. β-blockers, calcium channel blockers, and digoxin are common initial choices.[86,87] Unfortunately, successful termination with the intravenous formulation of any agents does not predict long-term efficacy with oral treatment. In patients who do not respond to AV nodal blocking agents, class I and III antiarrhythmics may be tried, although limited data support their use.[88–95] In general, class Ic agents are preferred in patients without structural heart disease and class III agents in patients with evidence of left ventricular dysfunction or left ventricular hypertrophy. Class Ia agents have fallen out of favor due to their numerous adverse effects and proarrhythmic potential.

For a subset of competent and compliant patients who experience infrequent and mild episodes of AVNRT, single-dose oral therapy may provide an alternative to the risks of chronic antiarrhythmic exposure.[96] A single oral dose of an antiarrhythmic is administered for acute termination of an arrhythmia after vagal maneuvers have been attempted. Limited data are available for flecainide (3 mg/kg) and the combination of diltiazem (120 mg) plus propranolol (80 mg).[96,97] These agents exhibit a relatively fast onset of action. For these agents to be used safely, left ventricular dysfunction, sinus bradycardia, or a preexcitation syndrome such as WPW syndrome must be ruled out.

Nonpharmacologic Therapies. Nonpharmacologic therapies for AV nodal reentry include percutaneous catheter ablation or modification and pacemakers. They are indicated when medical therapy is ineffective or not tolerated. Because these modalities allow patients to remain drug-free, non-compliant patients, younger patients unwilling to comply with lifelong drug treatment, older adults in whom symptoms of the arrhythmia or adverse effects of antiarrhythmic medication may be intolerable, or women desiring pregnancy may also be candidates. Extensive electrophysiologic studies and cardiac mapping studies are important in maximizing success.

Because the overall efficacy of chronic antiarrhythmic therapy is reported to be only 30% to 50%, *catheter ablation* has become the preferred therapeutic modality for patients with frequent episodes of recurrent AVNRT. According to the 2003 American College of Cardiology/American Heart Association/European Society of Cardiology guidelines for the management of supraventricular tachycardias, catheter ablation is a class I recommendation for patients with AVNRT accompanied by hemodynamic compromise, patients with recurrent symptomatic AVNRT, patients requesting complete control of a single episode or infrequent AVNRT, and even infrequent well-tolerated AVNRT.[72] However, the decision to pursue catheter ablation remains dependent on physician and patient preference, taking into account the frequency, severity, and duration of recurrent episodes, as well as the efficacy and safety of antiarrhythmic agents.

Antegrade pathway conduction modification is now preferred over retrograde conduction because of greater efficacy (more than 90% versus 50% to 90%, respectively) and minimal risk of AV block (less than 2% versus 2% to 8%, respectively).[98–100] The reported success rate of catheter ablation from the NAPSE Prospective Catheter Ablation Registry is approximately 96%. The main complication of this procedure is a low incidence of complete AV block, which would necessitate implantation of a permanent pacemaker.[101] Complications other than AV block include thromboembolism, arrhythmias (including inappropriate sinus tachycardia), and valvular damage. Intravenous heparin is infused during the procedure to prevent thromboemboli formation. Postmodification therapy may include 3 to 6 months of aspirin or warfarin therapy and β-blockers for the control of inappropriate sinus tachycardia if it occurs. The benefit of short-term antiplatelet or anticoagulation therapy after the modification procedure has not yet been determined.

Permanent pacemakers have been used in the chronic management of AV nodal reentry for many years. They either minimize arrhythmogenesis or terminate tachycardias after they occur. Overdrive pacing at a rate slightly faster than the sinus rate, or programmed atrial and ventricular stimulation, will alter refractoriness in the limbs of the reentrant circuit and therefore prevent the arrhythmia. Techniques for terminating the tachycardia are the same as those discussed under "Acute Management."[85] The most sophisticated devices are activated automatically by a sensing function, may be programmed both before and after insertion,

and have a memory function that remembers and delivers an algorithm of previously successful terminating sequences. Unfortunately, reliable termination of AV nodal reentry entails concomitant antiarrhythmic drug therapy in as many as 50% of patients receiving pacemakers.[85] Adverse effects include precipitation of tachyarrhythmias, syncope, and sudden death, especially in patients with accessory pathways. Additionally, pacemakers must be checked and reprogrammed regularly, may not eliminate symptoms, and are not curative. This last limitation has become more meaningful as surgical methods offering complete cure have evolved. Patients with sinus node disease are ideal candidates because the pacemaker can manage both tachycardic and bradycardic episodes. They are also useful in those who are not candidates for surgery or refuse surgery.

Additional nonpharmacologic strategies for treating AV nodal reentry and AV reentry associated with an accessory pathway are evolving rapidly. Their primary use at present is limited to patients who are resistant or intolerant to antiarrhythmic drug therapy. Their expeditious, cost-effective, and curative features are major attributes. As technologies are developed and refined, nonpharmacologic therapy is likely to be useful in a wide spectrum of patients.

WOLFF-PARKINSON-WHITE SYNDROME (AV RECIPROCATING TACHYCARDIA)

AV reciprocating tachycardias (commonly referred to as AV re-entry or AVRT) are reentrant arrhythmias characterized by the presence of an extranodal conduction pathway, which provides an electrical conduit between the atrium and ventricle. These pathways are called accessory pathways (or Kent bundle) because they provide an additional AV conduction pathway outside of the AV node. These pathways can be located anywhere in the heart but are usually located along the AV groove. Conduction through the accessory pathway can be antegrade (atrium to ventricle), retrograde (ventricle to atrium), or both.[102] Accessory pathways capable of only retrograde conduction are termed "concealed," whereas those capable of only antegrade conduction are known as "manifest." Conduction can also be intermittent or continuous. Because the accessory pathway can activate ventricular muscle directly (bypassing all or part of the AV node and His-Purkinje system), early or "preexcitation" of part of the ventricle occurs (Fig. 22.4). The most recognized presentation of AVRT with preexcitation is WPW syndrome. WPW syndrome is a congenital heart disease characterized by the presence of an anatomically distinct AV connection.[103] AVRTs account for the vast majority of all reentrant tachycardias with accessory pathways. Preexcitation tachycardias also occur with other supraventricular arrhythmias (such as AF, atrial flutter, atrial tachycardia, and AVNRT), where the accessory pathway is not critical to the reentry circuit. In these instances, the accessory pathway is termed a "bystander."

Epidemiology. WPW syndrome is often seen in otherwise healthy infants, children, and young adults. The clinical im-

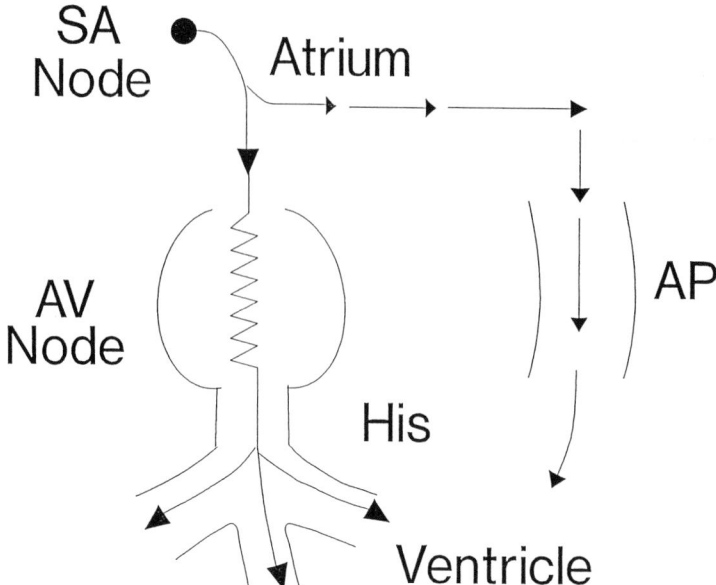

FIGURE 22.4 Wolff-Parkinson-White syndrome, sinus rhythm. The impulse reaches the ventricles via the atrioventricular (*AV*) node–His–Purkinje system with simultaneous pre-excitation via the accessory pathway (*AP*). *SA*, sinoatrial.

portance of the arrhythmias varies from benign to life-threatening, depending on the electrophysiologic properties of the accessory pathway and the AV node. Arrhythmias seen in infancy may persist, disappear, or disappear and then recur many years later.[7] This is thought to reflect a change in the conduction properties of the accessory pathway over time. The risk of sudden cardiac death is estimated to be 0.15% to 0.39% over a 3- to 10-year period. The risk is highest in patients with shorter preexcitation R-R′ intervals, a history of symptomatic tachycardias, multiple accessory pathways, or Ebstein's anomaly.

Etiology and Pathophysiology. Conduction in AVRT can be subclassified based on the direction impulses travel in the reentry circuit. Antegrade conduction over the AV node with retrograde conduction over the accessory pathway is termed ''orthodromic.'' The reverse situation is termed ''antidromic.'' Orthodromic reentry accounts for the majority of cases (90% to 95%), whereas antidromic reentry is less common (5% to 10%). Multiple accessory pathways are seen in 5% to 15% of patients, usually associated with antidromic reentry.

Patients are typically in sinus rhythm at baseline, with episodes of AVRT. Sinus rhythm is maintained as long as antegrade conduction is occurring over both the AV node and accessory pathway. Thus, ventricular activation is a fusion of the two impulses. However, if the accessory pathway and AV node form a reentry circuit, this results in the initiation of a supraventricular arrhythmia.[104] The trigger for reentry is usually a critically timed ectopic beat. AVRT is distinguished from AVNRT by the use of the accessory pathway as part of the circuit.

The most feared arrhythmia in patients with AVRT/WPW is AF with antegrade conduction down an accessory pathway

(antidromic), which exhibits a short refractory period. In this case, the protective effect of the AV node against very rapid ventricular rates is lost. Extremely rapid impulse transmission directly from the atrium to the ventricle may lead to ventricular flutter or fibrillation and sudden death.[105] Approximately one third of patients with WPW syndrome also have AF.

Clinical Presentation and Diagnosis

Signs and Symptoms. The clinical manifestations and hemodynamic consequences of AVRT are the same in patients with or without WPW syndrome, ranging from palpitations to syncope and sudden death.

Diagnosis and Clinical Findings. The most characteristic finding on an ECG for AVRT/WPW is the presence of δ waves, which indicate preexcitation of the ventricles.[106] The classic ECG in sinus rhythm includes a short P-R interval with a δ wave preceding the QRS complex. The QRS complex has abnormal morphology because of the fusion of normal conduction down the AV node–His bundle system and preexcitation of the left ventricular free wall.

In WPW patients experiencing AV reentry, ventricular rates average 100 to 280 bpm (higher in children). The direction of the reentry circuit (orthodromic or antidromic), variation in mode of ventricular activation, and different accessory pathway anatomies all contribute to marked interpatient and intrapatient ECG variation during SVTs. Detection of WPW syndrome and differentiation of its associated arrhythmias require an experienced ECG interpreter.

Therapeutic Plan. As for other tachyarrhythmias, acute management decisions are based on the clinical status of the patient. Acute management targets termination of the rhythm either by direct current cardioversion or pharmacologically with antiarrhythmics. As a rule, AV reentry associated with WPW syndrome is readily terminated using traditional maneuvers and drugs, as discussed in the AVNRT section. AV nodal blocking drugs are effective for some patients; however, if the reentry circuit involves multiple extranodal accessory pathways, they are ineffective. In addition, AV nodal blocking drugs must be used with caution as they may predispose to enhanced antegrade conduction through the accessory pathway, especially in patients with concomitant AF. This is a consideration in only a few patients (with a short antegrade accessory pathway refractory period), but it is not possible to identify susceptible patients on clinical grounds alone. In this sense, adenosine may be the safest AV node blocking alternative owing to its short duration of action. Since the characteristics of the reentry circuit are usually not known acutely, antiarrhythmics that target conduction of the accessory pathways are generally preferred. The most common agents used to terminate acute AVRT are ibutilide, flecainide, and procainamide.[72]

Chronic management involves identification of the most appropriate strategy for arrhythmia prevention. This is increasingly being accomplished by catheter ablation of the accessory pathway, or in some situations antiarrhythmics are used as prophylactic therapy. Unfortunately, there are no randomized, controlled trials of drug prophylaxis of AVRT. In addition, the small, nonrandomized trials that have been reported do not allow for comparison of the relative efficacy of the various antiarrhythmic agents. In general, AV nodal blocking drugs are safe in patients in whom electrophysiologic testing has determined that the accessory pathway is incapable of rapid antegrade conduction. Limited data are also available for various class Ic and III agents. These include propafenone, flecainide, sotalol, and amiodarone.[107-115] Data for the prophylactic efficacy of class Ia agents are lacking.

For either acute or chronic management, the choice of antiarrhythmic for AVRT poses some unique problems. It may be difficult to treat because the effect of the drug on the accessory pathway is not predicted by effect on the AV node. Moreover, drug action on antegrade conduction may differ from that on retrograde conduction. Underlying autonomic tone may alter conduction independently of drug effect. Therefore, a drug may be beneficial for one patient yet deleterious for another. Management should be individualized by electrophysiologic studies. These studies locate the accessory pathway, determine the conduction characteristics, identify the mechanism of the arrhythmia, and evaluate their effects on each anatomic component. Other termination techniques such as atrial pacing also may be evaluated. Electrophysiologic studies are also useful for risk-stratifying patients for sudden cardiac death, which may help in the determination of which therapy to use.

The role of extensive testing and treatment to prevent sudden death in asymptomatic patients remains controversial. Some may be entirely asymptomatic yet have electrophysiologic risk for sudden cardiac death. Moreover, the population at risk based on electrophysiologic risk stratification is much larger than that which will ultimately have a fatal arrhythmia. Little is known about the natural history of asymptomatic AVRT or WPW syndrome. In one study, one third of asymptomatic individuals eventually became symptomatic. The decision to ablate the accessory pathway in asymptomatic individuals is ultimately an individual one based on balancing perceived benefit with the risk of major complications with catheter ablation. Ablation may be of greater benefit to those with high-risk careers such as airline pilots and bus drivers.

Pharmacologic Therapy. After conversion to sinus rhythm, patients with recurrent symptomatic attacks may receive prophylactic therapy to minimize further episodes of SVT. Regimens commonly include class Ia or Ic drugs, sotalol, amiodarone, or β-blockers. Controlled comparative trials have not been performed, and no drug has demonstrated superiority. Drug treatment often is suboptimal because of limited efficacy and excessive toxicity. Preventive therapy is reserved for patients with recurrent disabling arrhythmias. Caution must be used with AV nodal blocking agents in patients in AF with documented or suspected preexcitation unless previous electrophysiologic studies have shown them to be safe. AV nodal blocking agents, which do not exert effects on the accessory pathways, are sometimes used with class I or III antiarrhythmics. There have been some reports of adenosine being effective for AVRT.[67,116]

Nonpharmacologic Therapy. Because of the unpredictable and often inadequate response to drugs, nonpharmacologic therapy is an important component of treating AVRT or WPW syndrome. Since pacing, surgery, and catheter ablation are curative, they may be considered the treatment of choice in patients unresponsive or intolerant to antiarrhythmics, those with arrhythmias associated with marked adverse hemodynamic effects, patients with AF with rapid antegrade accessory pathway conduction, young patients who would otherwise need lifelong drug therapy, or women desiring pregnancy.

Direct Current Cardioversion. Direct current cardioversion retains its near-uniform reliability and efficacy and is the treatment of choice in patients with hemodynamic instability.

Pacing. Atrial pacing may be used in AV reentry, although it may induce transient AF with rapid ventricular rate in patients with rapid antegrade accessory pathway conduction. Permanent ventricular pacing may be necessary in patients needing large dosages of antiarrhythmics or those with sinus node disease (pacing eliminates excessive bradycardia while the patient is in sinus rhythm).

Surgery. Surgical interruption of the accessory pathway is an effective and usually curative treatment. After detailed electrophysiologic and cardiac mapping studies, the accessory pathway is transected or ablated using an endocardial or epicardial approach.[7] AV nodal conduction is preserved. Surgical division of accessory pathways is 90% to 100% effective in experienced centers, with less than 1% mortality in uncomplicated cases and rare early or late recurrences.[98]

Percutaneous Catheter Ablation. A less invasive technique, percutaneous catheter ablation, uses direct current cardioversion, lasers, or radiofrequency to modify the AV node or destroy accessory pathways. Catheter ablation is performed in conjunction with an electrophysiologic study, which is used to confirm the presence and location of the accessory pathway and to determine its conduction characteristics. No prospective, randomized studies have formally evaluated the safety and efficacy of this technique for AVRT prevention, but smaller trials and multicenter registries have found an efficacy rate of approximately 95% after initial ablation.[117–121] There is a small recurrence rate of 5% once the inflammation and edema caused by the procedure have abated that requires a second ablation. The success rate and mortality of this procedure are similar to those of surgical ablation; however, this procedure does not entail an open chest or general anesthesia.

Although generally well tolerated, catheter ablation is associated with some risks. Intraprocedural mortality is reported to be up to 0.2%. Other complications result from establishing vascular access, manipulation of the catheter, and delivery of energy for ablation. These include hematomas, perforation of the peripheral or coronary artery, valvular damage, coronary artery spasm, embolic events, cardiac tamponade, and most commonly complete AV block. Complete AV block can occur if the ablation energy is delivered too close to the AV junction, and necessitates implantation of a permanent pacemaker.

FOCAL ATRIAL TACHYCARDIAS

Regular activation of ectopic foci from within atrial areas leads to the formation of focal atrial tachycardias. The electrical activity spawned from each ectopic focus spreads outward in a centrifugal pattern, eventually reaching the AV node.[122] Neither the SA nor the AV node is involved in the initiation or sustenance of the tachycardic rhythm. Focal atrial tachycardias can be nonsustained or sustained, and paroxysmal or permanent.

When three or more ectopic atrial foci are present, each with its own inherent rate of electrical discharge, the rhythm is known as multifocal atrial tachycardia.[123] This is a specific diagnosis that requires attention, as it is commonly mistaken for AF. Differentiation between the two rhythms is important since the approach to management is different.

Epidemiology. The prevalence of focal atrial tachycardias has been reported to be 0.34% in asymptomatic patients and 0.46% in symptomatic patients.[124] Patients experiencing focal atrial tachycardias usually follow a benign course, with the exception of those with incessant tachycardia, which can contribute to the development of a cardiomyopathy. Development of focal atrial tachycardias occurs in patients with

or without underlying heart disease. Multifocal atrial tachycardia has been reported to occur in 0.05% to 0.32% of hospitalized patients and is more common in adults than children.[123,125] In the hospitalized population multifocal atrial tachycardia is associated with a high in-hospital mortality rate (45%), but it is thought that this risk is attributable to the severity of underlying illnesses and not the atrial tachycardia itself.[125,126]

Etiology/Pathophysiology. The development of focal atrial tachycardias is largely linked to underlying disease states, metabolic derangements, or electrolyte abnormalities.[127] Multifocal atrial tachycardias are most commonly associated with pulmonary disease or hypoxemia. Specifically, a high percentage of patients with multifocal atrial tachycardias also present with chronic obstructive pulmonary disease (55%), hypoxemia (43%), pulmonary embolism (10% to 16%), and heart failure (28%).[128] Atrial tachycardias, in conjunction with AV block, are suspicious for digitalis (digoxin) toxicity. Other sympathomimetic agents, such as methylxanthines and β-agonists, can also predispose to the development of focal atrial tachycardias.

There are three distinct mechanisms proposed for the development of ectopic atrial foci. Enhanced focal activity most commonly results from abnormal automaticity, and less frequently from late after-depolarizations (triggered activity), or microreentry. Therefore, in contrast to abrupt-onset reentry tachycardias, focal atrial tachycardias usually initiate and terminate gradually. This "warming up" and "cooling down" phenomenon usually indicates some autonomic influence and is helpful in differentiating focal atrial tachycardias from reentry rhythms.[129] The distribution of ectopic foci is usually not random; instead, they tend to develop in specific areas of the left and right atria.[130,131] Right-sided atrial tachycardias are usually located in the crista terminalis of the SA node. Left-sided atrial tachycardias usually develop around the pulmonary veins, atrial septum, and mitral annulus.

Clinical Presentation and Diagnosis. Focal atrial tachycardias are characterized by atrial rates between 100 and 250 bpm, rarely achieving rates above 300. Signs and symptoms are consistent with those of other supraventricular tachyarrhythmias.

The diagnosis of focal atrial tachycardias is based on careful evaluation of the ECG, paying close attention to the timing and morphology of the P waves.[132] P waves are usually in the latter half of the tachycardia cycle and therefore are commonly masked by the T wave of the preceding QRS complex. The P-R interval varies proportionately with heart rate. In most cases, an isoelectric baseline is evident between P waves, and this can help in differentiation from atrial flutter or AF. If P waves are flattened or widened, focal atrial tachycardias can appear similar to the "sawtooth pattern" of atrial flutter. Multifocal atrial tachycardia is characterized by three or more distinct P wave morphologies, each with its own inherent rate. The ventricular rhythm is always irregular with an appearance similar to AF, although the ventricular rate is generally slower than in AF. Despite characteristic findings on an ECG, the only definitive method for diagnosing focal atrial tachycardias is an electrophysiologic study. This is usually performed with mapping and entrainment to determine the location of each ectopic focus.

Therapeutic Plan. Focal atrial tachycardias are generally difficult to terminate with conventional supraventricular antiarrhythmic interventions. Hence, acute therapy is largely targeted at the precipitating cause or contributory underlying disease states. Multifocal atrial tachycardia management usually involves treating the underlying pulmonary disease. Acute ventricular rate control with AV nodal blocking agents is only modestly effective for focal atrial tachycardias, even less so for multifocal atrial tachycardias. For chronic management, the decision to use antiarrhythmics for prophylaxis must be balanced against the risk of proarrhythmia and adverse effects. In patients with drug-refractory focal atrial tachycardia or those with incessant tachycardia (especially if tachycardia-induced cardiomyopathy has developed), the treatment of choice is catheter ablation. Catheter ablation is usually not an option for multifocal atrial tachycardia.

Pharmacologic Therapies. When antiarrhythmics are used for acute management of focal atrial tachycardia, a variety of outcomes are possible. AV nodal blocking agents such as adenosine, β-blockers, verapamil, and digoxin most commonly create AV block with persistence of the atrial rhythm. In a few instances where the underlying mechanism for focal activity is microreentry, termination of the arrhythmia may occur (adenosine-sensitive foci). Although these agents are usually ineffective at terminating the atrial arrhythmia, acute intravenous β-blockers and verapamil may reduce ventricular rates and aid in controlling symptoms of tachycardia.[133] Special care must be exercised in using digoxin because this drug may induce ectopic atrial tachycardia. In cases of suspected digitalis-induced arrhythmia, potassium is the agent of choice because it will counteract the action of digitalis at the cellular level. Phenytoin, lidocaine, propranolol, or digoxin-immune Fab fragments may also be used. Direct suppression of the ectopic foci may also be attempted with class Ia, Ic, and III antiarrhythmic agents.

The need for chronic prophylaxis of focal atrial tachycardias is controversial. The data for pharmacologic prevention are derived largely from observational studies. Before deciding on chronic therapy, the benefits and risk must be weighed accordingly. If the decision to treat is made, the usual approach is to begin by initiating a calcium channel blocker (verapamil) or β-blocker (metoprolol). Second-line therapy includes the addition of a class Ia or Ic agent, sotalol or amiodarone, for use in combination with verapamil or metoprolol.

Multifocal atrial tachycardias are often more difficult to manage than other focal atrial tachycardias. Pharmacologic attempts to block the AV node or decrease ectopic activity are rarely successful. Trials of digoxin, diltiazem, quinidine, procainamide, phenytoin, amiodarone, flecainide, and lidocaine have been disappointing. Treating the underlying disease is the only reliable therapy. Correcting predisposing factors terminates the arrhythmia in most patients, although recurrence is common. Verapamil[134] and metoprolol[135,136] have been reported to slow the ventricular rate, reduce atrial ectopy, or reduce abnormal atrial or AV junctional-triggered activity. In one trial, metoprolol was associated with a larger reduction in ventricular rate and a higher rate of conversion to sinus rhythm than verapamil.[136] However, the hypotensive and adverse pulmonary effects of β-blockers limit their utility. There are also limited data for intravenous magnesium in multifocal atrial tachycardia. Magnesium given as a 2-g bolus, followed by 2 g per hour for 5 hours, appeared to reduce heart rate and increase conversion rates in two small studies.[137,138] Antiarrhythmics have not been shown to reduce mortality.[139] Based on the available data, metoprolol, verapamil, or magnesium should be the first-line agent for multifocal atrial tachycardias.

Nonpharmacologic Therapies. Direct current cardioversion is highly ineffective for focal atrial tachycardias due to abnormal automaticity, but it may be effective in the small percentage of patients in whom triggered activity or microreentry is the driving force. Since the percentage of those without automatic atrial tachycardia is small, direct current cardioversion is usually not employed; it is also dangerous in digitalis toxicity because it may precipitate intractable ventricular arrhythmias. Multifocal atrial tachycardia has also been shown to be unresponsive to direct current cardioversion.

Although atrial pacing may temporarily slow the atrial rate, it has no demonstrable efficacy for rhythm termination and is not routinely used.

Catheter ablation targets the site of origin of the tachycardia. Mapping studies during electrophysiologic assessments are used to localize ectopic foci and determine which ones are responsible for the tachycardia. The success rate of the procedure is reported to be approximately 86%, with an 8% recurrence rate.[72] Complications of ablation largely depend on the location of the foci to be ablated. As stated above, ablation is the treatment of choice for refractory patients or those with tachycardia-induced cardiomyopathy.

ATRIAL FLUTTER AND ATRIAL FIBRILLATION

Atrial flutter is an organized rhythm characterized by an atrial rate usually between 250 and 350 bpm and a regular ventricular rhythm in patients with a functioning AV node. In contrast, AF is a disorganized rhythm with higher atrial rates of 350 to 600 bpm and an irregular ventricular rhythm but generally a slower ventricular rate.[140] The reported prevalence of AF in the general population is 0.4% and is directly related to age.[141] The prevalence is less than 1% in those under 60 years of age but greater than 6% in those over 80 years old.[140,142] Both rhythms are more common in males than in females, and in whites more than in blacks.[140,143]

There is no standard classification system for atrial flutter, but one has been proposed for AF to replace the previous conglomerate of terms (paroxysmal, acute, chronic, intermittent) used to describe it.[144] AF that spontaneously occurs, recurs, and terminates is termed paroxysmal. Sustained episodes of AF that do not terminate spontaneously are now termed persistent. If conversion to or maintenance of normal sinus rhythm cannot be achieved, this is known as permanent AF. Repeated episodes are termed recurrent AF. Finally, AF in patients less than 60 years of age without concomitant underlying cardiopulmonary disease is termed lone AF.[145,146] Lone AF accounts for approximately 12% of all cases.[147] AF is the most common sustained arrhythmia and the second most common overall. The long-term prognosis in patients with chronic AF is poor, with a yearly cardiovascular mortality (10%) twice that of age-matched controls (5%).[148] Mortality is related to age at onset and the presence and extent of coexisting heart disease.

Pathophysiology. Although a subset of 5% to 30% of atrial flutter or AF patients are without concomitant risk factors, the majority of these arrhythmias are associated with an acute or chronic disease process. Paroxysmal or single isolated episodes of AF are seen with cardiac surgery, fever, infection, pulmonary embolism, ethanol intoxication, or drug toxicity (sympathomimetics, β-agonists, and methylxanthines). Paroxysmal AF is also seen in 10% to 15% of patients with acute MI, with episodes usually lasting less than 24 hours.[149] Persistent or permanent AF is commonly associated with chronic heart failure, coronary artery disease, rheumatic heart disease, dilated or hypertrophic cardiomyopathy, hypertensive heart disease, hyperthyroidism, and certain congenital heart diseases. Heart failure is a strong risk factor for the development of atrial flutter or AF, with the incidence increasing in proportion to the severity of heart failure symptoms.[150–152] Other influencing factors include the autonomic nervous system, atrial ischemia or stretch, and older age. In addition, atrial flutter and AF can be isolated rhythms or they can present along with other arrhythmias such as atrial tachycardias. Atrial flutter is present in 25% to 35% of AF patients. Atrial flutter can degenerate into AF, while AF can precipitate atrial flutter. Other arrhythmias or premature beats may also trigger atrial flutter or AF.

Atrial flutter is also known as a macroreentrant tachycardia because the reentry circuit that is the underlying mechanism usually occupies a large portion of the atria. Abnormal automaticity is rarely a cause. AF can be caused by either enhanced automaticity, especially in the area of the pulmonary veins, or reentry.[153,154] Unlike atrial flutter, where usually only one or two reentry circuits are present, AF is characterized by multiple reentry circuits. This theory is called the multiple wavelet hypothesis.[155] Uneven refractoriness of adjacent atrial tissues allows the formation of multiple reentrant wavelets. These wavelets create self-perpetuating wavefronts of electrical activity that are completely disso-ciated from one another. These wavefronts are not organized and hence lead to the irregular nature of the rhythm.

Once a patient develops atrial flutter or AF, the risk of recurrent episodes is increased. In addition, the longer a patient remains in AF, the greater the difficulty in restoring normal sinus rhythm.[156] This phenomenon is known as atrial remodeling, a process of structural and electrical alterations that allow these rhythms to develop and persist.[157,158] Structural changes include fibrosis, fatty infiltrates, and atrial hypertrophy and dilation. Atrial electrical remodeling relates to progressive shortening of the effective refractory periods of atrial myocytes as the duration of AF increases. Atrial remodeling is purported to begin within the first 24 hours after onset of the arrhythmia and can impair atrial systolic function well beyond (2 to 4 weeks) the reestablishment of normal sinus rhythm. This has implications for prevention of thromboembolism, which will be discussed under treatment.

Apart from the atrial factors involved in the pathophysiology, the other key component ultimately affecting the clinical course is the AV node and its conduction characteristics. A properly functioning AV node regulates the number of impulses conducted from the atria to the ventricles.[159] In addition to the number of electrical impulses reaching the AV node from the atria, AV nodal conduction is also influenced by autonomic tone, intrinsic refractoriness, and concealed conduction.[160–162] Concealed conduction refers to electrical impulses that are only partially conducted across the AV node. These impulses modulate nodal refractoriness, effectively blocking other impulses from reaching the AV node. As a result, higher atrial rates usually translate into slower ventricular rates, while lower atrial rates may in fact generate faster ventricular rates, as seen in comparing atrial and ventricular rates of atrial flutter to AF. This concept is also clinically important when considering ventricular rate control, which will be discussed under treatment. Atrial flutter most commonly exhibits 2:1 conduction, meaning that for every two atrial impulses, only one is conducted to the ventricles. Higher AV conduction ratios (3:1 or 4:1) generally translate into more stable hemodynamics, whereas 1:1 conduction results in higher ventricular rates and a poorer prognosis. Conduction beyond the AV node is normal in the absence of a concomitant ventricular arrhythmia.

Clinical Presentation and Diagnosis
Signs and Symptoms. Patients with atrial flutter or AF may be asymptomatic to hemodynamically compromised. As many as 30% are asymptomatic at diagnosis.[163] However, most patients experience varying degrees of palpitations, dyspnea, lightheadedness, and dizziness. Palpitations may be especially troublesome in patients with paroxysmal AF. Additional symptoms tend to reflect underlying medical conditions. Patients with underlying ischemic heart disease, left ventricular dysfunction, or cerebrovascular disease may present with angina, heart failure exacerbation, or symptoms of cerebral insufficiency such as confusion, fatigue, or syncope. Older adults with AV nodal dysfunction may have

slow ventricular rates at rest but nonetheless have reduced cardiac reserve with exercise or stress.

Irregular apical and radial pulses result from random impulse transmission through the AV node and are the classic physical signs of AF, commonly noted as "irregularly irregular." Atrial flutter exhibits a more regular pulse upon palpitation. The principal hemodynamic effects of AF result from an elevated ventricular heart rate, irregularity of atrial and ventricular response, and loss of organized atrial contraction. An elevated irregular heart rate leads to a shortened diastolic filling time and decreased left ventricular end-diastolic volume and stroke volume. Loss of synchronized atrial contraction results in increased mean left atrial pressure.[164] Loss of atrial systole causes a 20% to 30% reduction in stroke volume in normal people, but it is proportionately increased in patients with heart disease (especially with left ventricular systolic dysfunction). The net effect is a decrease in cardiac reserve and cardiac output. Elevations in heart rate may partially compensate for the diminished cardiac output, but once a critical rate is exceeded, ventricular filling time becomes the limiting factor and further increases in heart rate result in reduced cardiac output.

The most important nonhemodynamic consequence of atrial flutter or AF is thromboembolism.[165–168] Embolic risk is highest in the first 2 to 4 weeks after the onset of AF and at any time the rhythm switches from AF to normal sinus rhythm or vice versa. In some patients, the embolic event is the presenting manifestation of previously undetected AF. Embolism to arteries in the cerebral circulation is most common and accounts for about 7% of all strokes.[148,169] Other locations include the extremities and the mesenteric, coronary, and renal circulations. Framingham study subjects with chronic AF caused by rheumatic mitral valve disease were found to have a 17.6-fold increase in stroke risk, with a 5.6-fold increase for AF of other causes.[170] The predisposition to embolic events is related to both AF and the presence of other risk factors. Studies have shown that AF is associated with all three components of Virchow's triad (stasis, endothelial dysfunction, hypercoagulable state). Left atrial appendage flow velocities are decreased in AF and to a lesser extent in atrial flutter compared to normal sinus rhythm.[171,172] Elevated levels of von Willebrand factor in AF indicate endothelial dysfunction.[173] Finally, markers of coagulation and platelet activity are elevated in AF, indicating a hypercoagulable state.[174,175] Other risk factors for embolism and stroke in chronic AF include a history of emboli, advanced age, congestive heart failure, hypertension, diabetes mellitus, thyrotoxicosis, and left atrial enlargement.[169,176] In patients with lone AF, stroke risk is low in young patients but probably higher in older patients and those with hypertension. Risk of thromboembolism is higher in AF than atrial flutter.

Diagnostic and Clinical Findings. Diagnostic workup for atrial flutter and AF should include a thorough clinical history, physical examination, and an ECG. The ECG is needed to confirm the diagnosis of the rhythm. ECG findings for AF include a lack of discrete atrial activity (no discernible P waves), variable R-R intervals, normal-appearing QRS complexes (unless aberrant conduction or bundle branch block is present), and an irregular baseline between QRS complexes (no isoelectric baseline is evident). Atrial flutter has a characteristic "sawtooth" pattern, especially in the inferior leads (II, III, aVF), and no obvious isoelectric baseline. In addition to confirming the arrhythmia diagnosis, an ECG can help identify evidence of preexcitation, ischemia, and left ventricular hypertrophy. The clinical history and physical examination are important for determining precipitating causes, identifying risk factors, assessing severity, and determining complications.

Once the diagnosis and initial workup are complete, other tests may be helpful in ruling out precipitating causes or guiding management. A chest radiograph may help identify a pulmonary disease. Blood tests should routinely include assessment of thyroid function. A transthoracic echo (TTE) is important for assessment of left ventricular function and left atrial and ventricular dimensions, parameters that affect therapy choices. A transesophageal echo (TEE) allows for better visualization of the supraventricular structures and may be used to rule out the presence of a thrombus prior to cardioversion.[168] In some instances, Holter monitoring may be required to confirm the diagnosis of paroxysmal AF or to assess the adequacy of ventricular rate control. Electrophysiologic studies confirm the mechanism for the arrhythmia and are required if ablation therapy is to be performed.

Therapeutic Plan

Acute Management. Acute management of AF or atrial flutter is largely determined by the clinical presentation of the patient. In patients with hemodynamic compromise, severe symptoms, or life-threatening complications, immediate direct current cardioversion would be performed.[62] Otherwise, a pharmacologic approach is used. The primary goals are correction of the hemodynamic manifestations, elimination of symptoms, prevention of complications (especially thromboembolism), and possible restoration of normal sinus rhythm. As stated above, the majority of clinical manifestations are a result of a reduction in cardiac output secondary to a rapid ventricular response. Therefore, stabilization of hemodynamics and elimination of symptoms are usually accomplished by pharmacologic slowing of the ventricular rate, which lengthens diastolic filling time and increases stroke volume.[177] Thromboembolic risk remains elevated in patients with AF or atrial flutter regardless of the ventricular rate; thus, anticoagulant therapy must also be considered acutely. After the patient is stabilized with ventricular rate control and the risk of thromboembolic complications is mitigated by anticoagulation, the focus moves to terminating the arrhythmia. In some patients, conversion is not attempted because the likelihood of sustained sinus rhythm is thought to be low. Others convert initially but revert to AF shortly thereafter. Therapy in these patients is directed at regulating

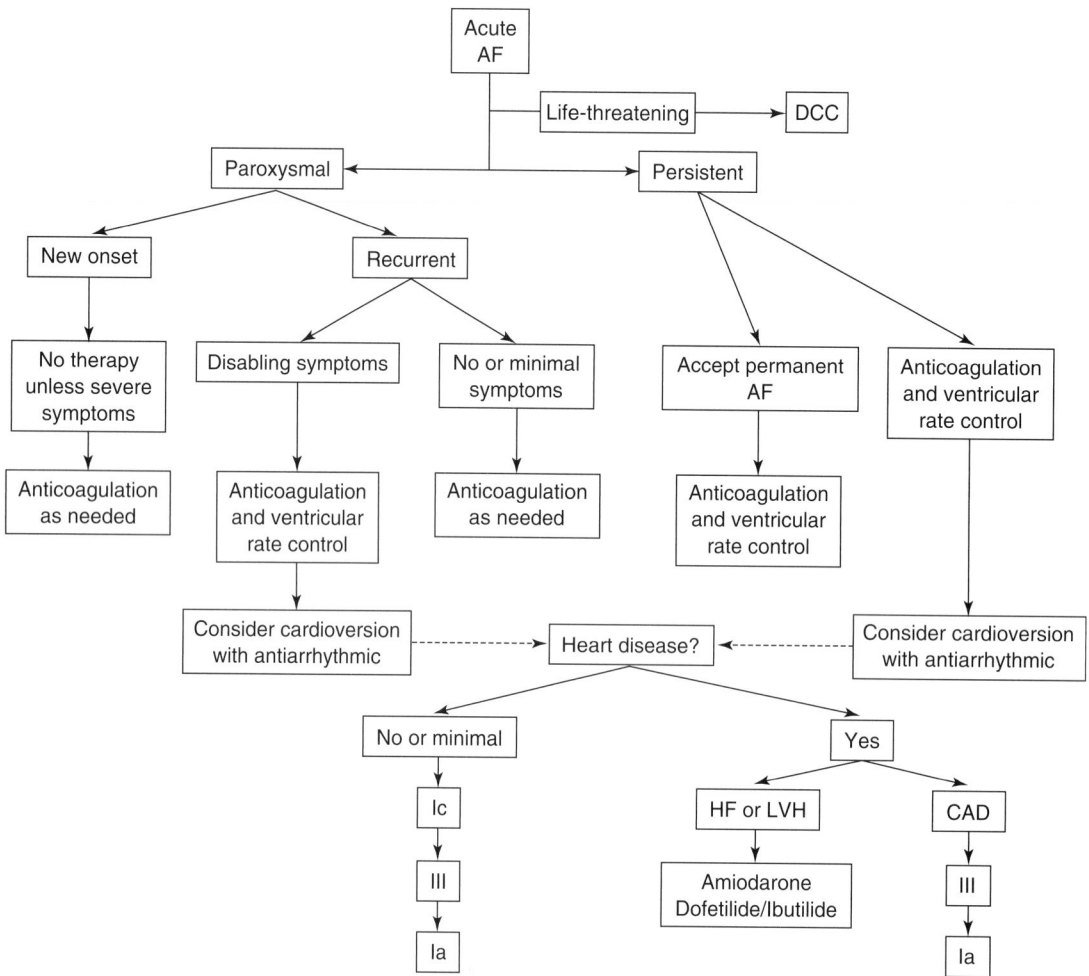

FIGURE 22.5 Treatment algorithm for acute atrial fibrillation and cardioversion.

the ventricular rate. An algorithm for acute management of AF or atrial flutter is depicted in Figure 22.5.

Ventricular Rate Control. A review of the role of the AV node in AF or atrial flutter is useful in understanding pharmacologic management of ventricular rate. The AV node is not involved in the initiation and perpetuation of these arrhythmias per se but plays a critical role as a filter of atrial impulses. The conduction characteristics of the AV node are the primary determinants of ventricular rate in AF. In contrast, the SA node determines the rate in sinus rhythm. The intrinsic conductivity of AV nodal tissues and extracardiac factors that may alter conduction (autonomic tone, drugs) have a critical influence on the number of atrial impulses that are conducted to the ventricles. Vagal stimulation results in less conduction across the AV node and increased filtering.[162] Increased sympathetic tone enhances AV nodal conduction and increases ventricular rate, as demonstrated with exercise or stress. Therefore, control of ventricular rate both at rest and during exercise is important in maintaining the stability and function of the patient. However, changes in AV nodal conductivity will not terminate these arrhythmias.

The optimal ventricular rate for maximizing cardiac output is unknown. An arbitrary ventricular rate of less than 80 bpm at rest and 100 bpm during moderate exercise is often chosen as a therapeutic goal, although they may vary with age.[178-180] In considering the adequacy of ventricular rate control, the following therapeutic aspects must be emphasized. Rate titration should consider the clinical appearance of the patient, as well as the anticipated rapidity of catecholamine correction. Underlying factors favoring tachycardia should be considered, especially excess catecholamine release as in infection, hyperthyroidism, or sympathomimetic drug overdose. In these patients, a rate of 100 to 120 bpm may be acceptable as long as the signs and symptoms are controlled. Aggressive treatment of coexisting conditions such as fever, infection, hypoxia, anemia, or hyperthyroidism is essential. In addition, strict adherence to a certain ventricular rate should not be at the expense of objective and symptomatic relief or of drug intoxication. Overly aggressive use of ventricular rate-controlling agents can result in bradycardia and heart block once the arrhythmia is terminated. The pharmacologic agents of choice for ventricular rate control are class II antiarrhythmics (β-blockers), class

IV antiarrhythmics (the nondihydropyridine calcium channel blockers verapamil and diltiazem), and digoxin. β-blockers are particularly useful in AF caused by high circulating catecholamine concentrations, including hyperthyroidism or sympathomimetic overdose, because they pharmacologically attenuate the underlying cause of the arrhythmia. Critically ill perioperative and cardiac patients should be treated with esmolol. β-blockers may be necessary for only a short time in these patients because correction of the precipitating cause may restore digoxin sensitivity or even allow conversion to sinus rhythm. A summary of the agents commonly used for ventricular rate control is provided in Table 22.4.

Preventing Thromboembolism. Several key concepts guide our decisions regarding the need for anticoagulation and how long it is required. First, after the onset of AF, generally several days (more than 48 hours) are needed for a thrombus to form.[181,182] Second, once a thrombus has formed, several weeks are needed to allow fibrotic organization and adherence to the atrial wall, thus forming a more stable clot. Third, in the presence of anticoagulant therapy, it also takes several weeks for an organized clot to dissolve secondary to the body's natural anticoagulant mechanisms.[183] Finally, upon restoration of normal sinus rhythm, normalization of atrial mechanical function (i.e., atrial systole) may be delayed for up to 4 weeks.[184] This delay in recovery of atrial mechanical function (systole) for several days or weeks after cardioversion occurs despite a return of normal electrical activity in certain patients.[184] This may account for the lack of improvement in exercise tolerance and cardiac output as well as the continued risk of embolism in the period immediately after

conversion. In a study of 52 patients who underwent cardioversion (electrical, pharmacologic, or spontaneous), 68% recovered effective mechanical atrial function by day 3 and 76% recovered by day 7.[185] Electrical conversion was more likely to cause a greater degree and longer duration of atrial dysfunction.

Hence, anticoagulation is not mandatory in patients with known AF or flutter duration for less than 24 to 48 hours if conversion to normal sinus rhythm is imminent. For patients with unknown duration or duration greater than 2 days, the American College of Chest Physicians (ACCP) recommends anticoagulation with warfarin to an international normalized ratio (INR) intensity of 2.0 to 3.0 for 3 weeks before and 4 weeks after cardioversion.[186] Anticoagulation with warfarin is also indicated in cases of AF or flutter of less than 2 days' duration if other risk factors for embolism are present. For patients needing emergent cardioversion, anticoagulation with intravenous heparin on the day of cardioversion is indicated if AF is of several days' duration, there is a high risk of recurrence, or other risk factors are present. Risk factors are previous transient ischemic attack or stroke, hypertension, diabetes, thyrotoxicosis, mitral stenosis, and other forms of heart disease.

In an ideal setting, all patients with AF or flutter episodes of known durations greater than 2 days could wait 3 weeks prior to attempting cardioversion. However, for symptomatic or logistical reasons (e.g., a return trip to the hospital for cardioversion is not feasible), it may be prudent to attempt cardioversion sooner despite a higher intrinsic thromboembolic risk. In these instances, TEE may be performed to rule

| TABLE 22.4 | Antiarrhythmics for Ventricular Rate Control and Rhythm Conversion in Atrial Fibrillation/Flutter |

Loading Dose, Maintenance Dose	IV	PO
Metoprolol	5 mg	50–200 mg/d
Esmolol	500 μg/kg over 1 minute, 25–200 μg/kg/min	–
Verapamil	5–10 mg over 2 min, 5 mg/h	120–480 mg/d
Diltiazem	0.15–0.25 mg/kg over 2 min, 5–15 mg/h infusion	120–540 mg/d
Digoxin	0.25–0.5 mg q6h ×2, 0.125–0.25 mg qd	0.25–0.5 mg q6h ×2, 0.125–0.25 mg qd
Procainamide	17 mg/kg at 20–30 mg/min, 1–4 mg/min	50 mg/kg/d in divided doses
Disopyramide	–	400–800 mg/d
Quinidine	<330 mg (gluconate)	200–600 mg q2–3h (max 4 g/d), 200–300 mg q6–8h (sulfate)
Flecainide	–	50–100 mg q12h
Propafenone	–	150–300 mg q8h OR 600 mg ×1
Amiodarone	150 mg over 10 min, 1 mg/min for 6 h, 0.5 mg/min for 18 h	800–1,600 mg/d, 400–800 mg/d, 100–400 mg/d
Sotalol	–	40–160 mg q12h
Ibutilide	1 mg over 10 minutes, repeat once in 10 minutes if necessary (0.01 μg/kg if <60 kg)	–
Dofetilide	–	125–500 μg q12h

out the presence of a thrombus to help decide whether the benefit of early cardioversion outweighs the risk of dislodging a thrombus during cardioversion.[187] Presence of a left atrial thrombus is a contraindication to cardioversion. However, absence of thrombus on TEE does not guarantee that a thromboembolic event will not occur if cardioversion is performed immediately.[188] Therefore, for patients undergoing immediate cardioversion, anticoagulation with intravenous heparin is still warranted. In support of using TEE as a risk-stratification tool, a recent prospective randomized study found similar outcomes between patients who underwent TEE-guided cardioversion compared to those following the conservative strategy of anticoagulation for 3 weeks prior to cardioversion.[189]

Cardioversion. The acuity of attempts to restore normal sinus rhythm is driven by the clinical status of the patient. Immediate cardioversion is indicated for patients in whom the AF or flutter results in hemodynamically instability, such as hypotension, acute heart failure, acute myocardial ischemia, or syncope. Patients with troublesome symptoms may require cardioversion during the hospitalization, while mildly symptomatic or asymptomatic patients with persistent AF or flutter may electively choose to undergo cardioversion. Patients with AF of recent onset may convert spontaneously, during initial drug treatment, or after the inciting stress is eliminated.

Unfortunately, not all patients remain in sinus rhythm. Although conversion to sinus rhythm is crucial for some patients, in others it may be neither practical nor useful. Ideally, an assessment of the likelihood of sustained sinus rhythm should be made before attempted conversion. Higher success rates are seen in patients with a corrected or controlled underlying cause and those with recent arrhythmia onset.[190,191] Once the decision to attempt cardioversion is made, a choice must be made between electrical or pharmacologic approaches. The risk of thromboembolism is similar regardless of the method used to convert the rhythm.

Pharmacologic conversion to sinus rhythm, though less invasive than direct current cardioversion, is also less successful (50% success rate). Digitalis, verapamil, and diltiazem rarely convert patients with AF to sinus rhythm, probably because of their minimal effects on atrial automaticity. β-blockers have been reported to facilitate conversion and may be helpful, especially if sympathetic stimulation is a contributing factor. However, the antiarrhythmics with proven efficacy at terminating AF or flutter are the class Ia, Ic, or III agents.[42,192–206] Few large comparative trials have been performed between agents. Therefore, much of the decision on which agent to select is governed by their safety in relation to both side effects and concomitant disease states. Antiarrhythmic therapy must be individualized to the patient. A summary of the most commonly used agents for cardioversion is provided in Table 22.4.

Electrical cardioversion is currently the only nonpharmacologic approach for acute rhythm management. In nonur-

gent cases, the patient should be fasting. Short-acting sedatives or anesthetics are given immediately before the procedure. Direct current cardioversion depolarizes a critical number of myocardial cells simultaneously, allowing the SA node to reestablish control as the pacemaker. The current should be synchronized with the QRS complex on the ECG to avoid delivery during the vulnerable period of ventricular recovery (could cause proarrhythmia). Lower initial energies are often used, although as much as 400 J may ultimately be needed. Atrial flutter generally responds to lower energies of 50 to 150 J, while AF usually requires 200 J or more.[207] An antiarrhythmic may be initiated a few days before attempted direct current cardioversion to facilitate termination of the arrhythmia and to help maintain sinus rhythm after conversion. Direct current cardioversion is initially successful in 80% to 95% of patients.[163,185,208,209] Any patient may be considered for direct current cardioversion, but the best candidates are those without mitral valve disease or significant atrial enlargement and those with recent-onset AF. Data compiled from 824 patients found a 2.4% incidence of complications, including emboli in 1.3%, ventricular arrhythmias in 0.4%, and miscellaneous complications in 0.6%.[208] Direct current cardioversion should be performed with caution in patients with digitalis toxicity because of the higher risk of ventricular arrhythmias. Generally it is not necessary to withhold digoxin immediately before cardioversion in patients without digitalis toxicity.[210] Patients with known or suspected sick sinus syndrome should be evaluated carefully for possible pacemaker insertion before attempted cardioversion, especially if receiving drugs that exacerbate bradycardia, such as calcium channel or β-blockers. Short-term anticoagulation is appropriate to decrease the embolic risk (see ''Preventing Thromboembolism'').

Chronic Management. Once conversion to sinus rhythm is achieved, the need for chronic maintenance therapy must be assessed. Maintenance of sinus rhythm is indicated for recurrent paroxysmal or persistent AF, especially in patients who experience severe or troublesome symptoms. Predictors of recurrence include underlying heart disease, hypertension, advanced age, duration of AF greater than 3 months, and atrial enlargement.[211,212] Patients experiencing their first episode of AF, lone AF, or AF secondary to a reversible cause probably do not require maintenance therapy if their symptoms were minor. The benefits of sinus rhythm maintenance are not entirely clear, but they include prevention of tachycardia-induced cardiomyopathy, potential improvement in cardiac function, and avoidance of the need for long-term anticoagulation. It does not appear that suppression of recurrent AF episodes translates into improved survival, a reduction in heart failure development, or a lower risk of thromboembolic events (see ''Rate Versus Rhythm Control'').[213–215]

Most patients receive pharmacologic maintenance therapy, with select patients being candidates for nonpharmacologic treatments. The approach to selection of an appropriate antiarrhythmic is shown in Figure 22.5. As for acute management, the decisions are largely based on safety considerations. In patients who were successfully converted to sinus rhythm pharmacologically, the same agent can be used for maintenance therapy in most cases.

Patients with chronic AF may also be candidates for long-term anticoagulation but usually receive antiplatelet therapy. The decision to anticoagulate an individual patient with AF is based on the presence of risk factors associated with stroke risk balanced against the risk of major bleeding. Cerebral embolism commonly results in large neurologic deficits with severe residual disability, occurs without warning symptoms, is recurrent in about 11% of patients, and carries a mortality of up to 25%.[216] Established risk factors for stroke are preexisting cardiovascular disease, prior thromboembolism, heart failure, hypertension, increasing age, diabetes mellitus, and thyrotoxicosis.[186] On the other hand, the incidence of major bleeding with anticoagulants at conventional intensities has been estimated at 2% to 5% yearly, with 1% per year suffering intracranial hemorrhage.[216] These values may be even higher in older adults, who make up the majority of patients with AF.

Currently, only two drugs are used for chronic thromboembolism prevention in AF, aspirin and warfarin.[186] There are ongoing studies with low-molecular-weight heparins and oral direct thrombin inhibitors, but they are not recommended at this time. An approach to selection of aspirin or warfarin is depicted in Figure 22.6. Assessment of embolic risk in patients with chronic AF remains an enigmatic clinical problem. Consensus exists about the high embolic risk in patients with documented recent embolism, AF associated with older mechanical heart valve prostheses, and mitral valve disease. Patients with a history of stroke, coronary disease, thyrotoxicosis, and modern mechanical valves are at a high but somewhat lower risk. The medium- to low-risk group comprises the largest number of patients, including those with mitral regurgitation, aortic valve disease, heart failure, hypertension, diabetes, advanced age, and bioprostheses. Risk/benefit data for anticoagulants in this group are limited. Several recent large placebo-controlled trials in patients with chronic nonvalvular AF[217-221] have found efficacy of warfarin therapy to an INR of 1.4 to 4.5. The overall risk reduction for stroke has been reported to be 68% from pooled data of five of these trials.[222] Aspirin 325 mg per day was also found to be beneficial for preventing stroke associated with AF[219] and is recommended by the ACCP in patients who are poor candidates for anticoagulation.[186] Compared with warfarin, aspirin is less effective but is asso-

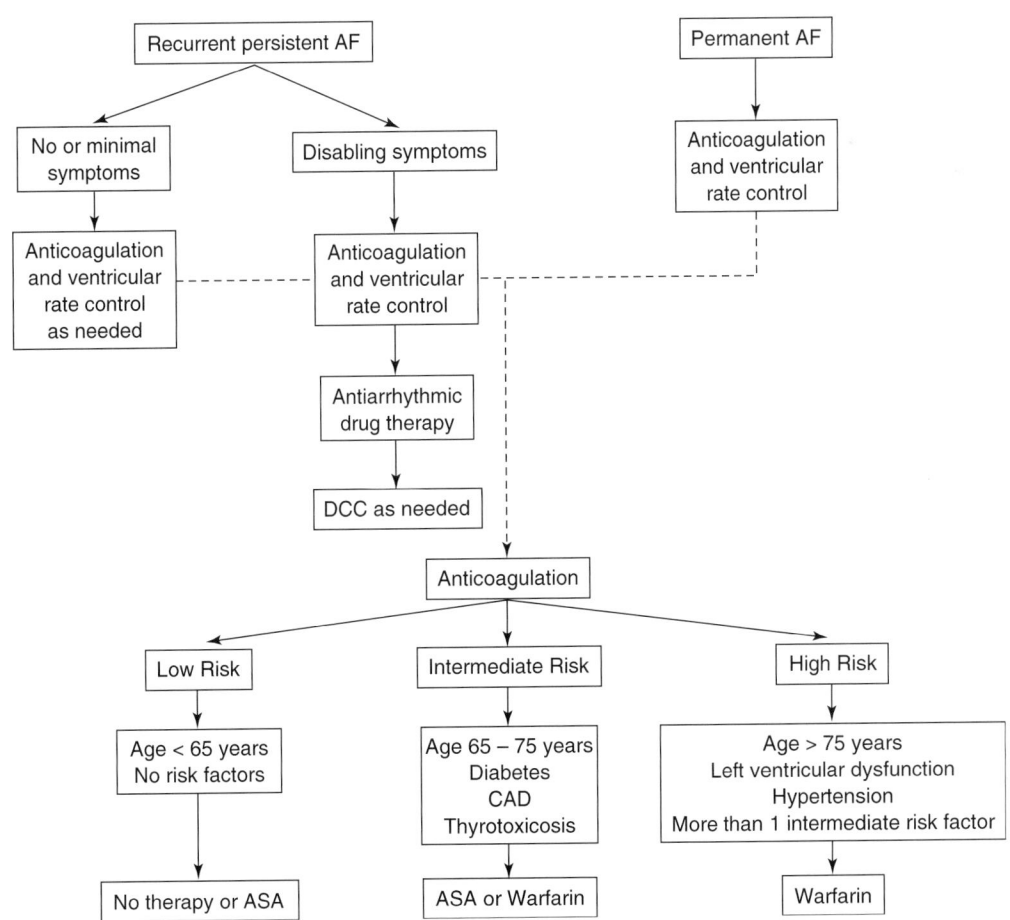

FIGURE 22.6 Treatment algorithm for recurrent persistent or permanent atrial fibrillation and anticoagulation.

ciated with less hemorrhagic complications.[219,223] Careful assessment of bleeding risk is a critical element in the decision for or against anticoagulant use in individual patients. Underlying risk factors for bleeding associated with warfarin therapy include age 65 years or older, history of gastrointestinal bleeding, stroke, cancer, recent surgery, and hypertension.[224] Patients unable to comply with medication regimens or laboratory follow-up, as well as those with dementia or alcohol abuse, may be poor candidates for anticoagulation regardless of embolic risk. Bleeding risk is also reduced by maintaining anticoagulants in the less intense range (INR 2.0 to 3.0) whenever possible.[224] Scrupulous monitoring is essential and can lower bleeding risk substantially. In the Stroke Prevention in Atrial Fibrillation trial, the annual rate of major hemorrhage for patients anticoagulated with warfarin to an INR of 2.0 to 3.5 was limited to 1.7% by meticulous supervision (compared with 0.9% for aspirin 325 mg orally daily and 1.2% for placebo).[219]

Rate Versus Rhythm Control. Until recently, there has been much controversy about the optimal approach to long-term management of patients with recurrent or persistent AF, and how aggressive therapy should be to maintain sinus rhythm. It was believed that maintaining normal sinus rhythm was tantamount to minimizing the risk of complications secondary to AF and improving prognosis. Only after failure to maintain sinus rhythm was ventricular rate control with concomitant anticoagulation considered. However, there has been increasing recognition of the inherent risks of chronic exposure to antiarrhythmic agents, especially proarrhythmia. In the last few years, several large, randomized, multicenter trials have been conducted to compare a ventricular rate control plus anticoagulation strategy to a rhythm control strategy. Three studies (PIAF, AFFIRM, and RACE) comprising just under 5,000 patients, most with recurrent persistent AF, consistently demonstrated no superiority of rhythm control over rate control in terms of mortality, symptomology, or incidence of ischemic stroke.[213,215,225,226] Moreover, there was a consistent increase in need for hospitalization in rhythm control patients. These studies enrolled "typical" AF patients, those over 60 years of age with risk factors for recurrent episodes or a history of recurrent episodes. The findings strongly suggest that achieving normal sinus rhythm at the expense of chronic exposure to antiarrhythmics is not imperative if the propensity for recurrence is high. In a large majority of patients with recurrent AF, especially if they are asymptomatic, rate control plus anticoagulation is appropriate. A rhythm control strategy is probably still appropriate for patients experiencing their first episode who have minimal or no (lone AF) risk factors for recurrence and in symptomatic patients in whom adequate rate control is difficult to achieve. The results also cast doubt on whether anticoagulation can safely be discontinued in patients who do convert to normal sinus rhythm, as no difference in ischemic stroke was found.

Nonpharmacologic Therapy. Nonpharmacologic therapy is reserved for patients with serious symptoms of AF that cannot be controlled by other methods. Patients with intolerable symptoms who are resistant to other therapies can be treated by surgical or catheter ablation of the AV node with permanent pacemaker placement. A surgical technique known as the maze procedure involves multiple small incisions in the atrium that disrupt the pathways that conduct the reentrant impulses.[227] This surgical technique terminates AF, restores AV synchrony, and preserves atrial transport function with a 93% success rate.[228] The intraoperative mortality rate of the maze procedure is less than 1%, but increases if combined with other cardiac surgery.

Catheter ablation techniques were devised after the success of surgical methods. Success rates of 60% to 70% have been reported for AF patients refractory to pharmacologic therapy, but recurrences may occur in up to 50% of cases.[229,230] Focal ablation appears to be more effective for atrial flutter.[230]

The effect of atrial pacing on the incidence of recurrent paroxysmal AF in patients with other indications for pacing has been studied to a limited extent. The incidence of AF is lower in patients undergoing atrial pacing compared to ventricular pacing. The incidence of AF is also lower with dual-site pacing than with single-site pacing. However, the utility of atrial pacing as a primary modality to prevent recurrent AF in patients not requiring a pacemaker for other indications has not been studied.

Atrial cardioverter-defibrillators have been in development for some time. Small studies have found efficacy with these devices in drug-refractory patients. However, current use of these devices is limited since the amount of energy for cardioversion (mean of 3 J in one study) results in intolerable discomfort without sedation, and most patients who would be candidates for these devices can also undergo catheter ablation. Research is continuing to develop new shock waveforms that are effective at lower energies.

Special Populations

Postoperative Atrial Fibrillation. Cardiac surgery is a direct stimulus for AF. The incidence of postoperative atrial arrhythmias is reported to be 20% to 50%, most commonly presenting within the first 5 days of surgery.[231,232] Advanced age, pericarditis, and increased sympathetic tone have been implicated as causative factors.[233,234] Most cases are self-limiting, and spontaneous conversion to sinus rhythm occurs in most patients within several weeks. Various antiarrhythmic agents have been studied for prevention of postoperative AF, with the most success being achieved by β-blockers, sotalol, and amiodarone.[232,235,236] Data with other agents such as diltiazem, verapamil, procainamide, and class Ic agents have been inconclusive. Treatment of postoperative AF should follow standard acute AF management. Direct current cardioversion is rarely indicated, as most cases are self-terminating. Ventricular rate control should normally involve a β-blocker, which has the advantage of antagonizing sympathetic tone. Anticoagulation should be instituted when the AF duration approaches 48 hours. Although several antiarrhythmics have been shown to be effective for conversion of postoperative AF, ibutilide and sotalol have shown the most promise.[237] In summary, patients undergoing cardiac surgery should receive an oral β-blocker to reduce the risk of postoperative AF. Sotalol and amiodarone can be administered prophylactically in patients at high risk for postoperative AF. If AF develops, ventricular rate control and anticoagulation should be instituted as indicated.

Pregnancy. Episodes of AF during pregnancy are usually associated with an underlying cardiac etiology or hyperthyroidism. Although the incidence is low, a rapid ventricular rate can be detrimental to both the mother and the fetus. Ventricular rate control can be achieved with all the standard rate-controlling agents. Heparin is the preferred anticoagulant as warfarin has been shown to be teratogenic during the first trimester and increases the risk of fetal hemorrhage as the pregnancy progresses. All antiarrhythmics have the potential to cross the placenta and be excreted in breast milk. There are more data with older antiarrhythmics than newer agents. Quinidine is the agent of choice for pharmacologic conversion.[144] In refractory or urgent cases, direct current cardioversion can be safely used without harming the fetus.

VENTRICULAR TACHYARRHYTHMIAS

PREMATURE VENTRICULAR CONTRACTIONS

A PVC is defined as an occurrence of a morphologically irregular QRS complex generated from electrical activity originating from ventricular muscle or below the bundle of HIS, not from a supraventricular focus. The QRS complex is usually greater than 120 ms in duration and not preceded by a P wave. They are also known as premature ventricular complexes or premature ventricular beats. PVCs are the most common arrhythmia found in both patients with underlying heart disease and apparently healthy individuals. The frequency of PVCs in otherwise healthy subjects is variable but was reported in one series of 50 male medical students to occur in one half of them over a 24-hour monitoring period.[238] The incidence and frequency of PVCs is highest in patients with underlying disease processes. The incidence is higher with increasing age and greater in males than females. Generally, PVCs follow a circadian pattern and are more frequent in the mornings. Exercise has been reported to increase the incidence, while sleep is associated with a lower incidence.

PVCs can be classified in several ways depending on their morphology and repetitiveness. Repetitive PVCs arising from a single focus will have similar QRS morphology and are classified as monomorphic or unimorphic. Multiple foci lead to multiple QRS morphologies and are known as polymorphic, multiform, or pleomorphic PVCs. A rhythm characterized by a single repetitive PVC that alternates with a normal QRS complex is called bigeminy. A single repetitive PVC alternating with two normal QRS complexes is known as trigeminy. Quadrigeminy is a repeating pattern of one PVC and three normal beats, and so on for similar patterns with four or more normal beats. Two and three consecutive PVCs are called a couplet and triplet, respectively. The spacing between PVCs and normal beats also lends itself to terminology. If the interval between the PVCs and normal beats remains stable, this is known as fixed coupling. If the interval changes, then the PVCs are said to exhibit variable coupling. Unifocal PVCs are usually seen in asymptomatic subjects with no cardiac disease. Multiform PVCs are uncommon in subjects with no cardiac disease but are common in patients with underlying heart disease.

PVCs can be precipitated by a variety of factors, mechanical, electrical, or chemical. Mechanical factors include ventricular stretch and surgery. Electrical factors include electrolyte abnormalities (especially hypokalemia), hypoxia, infection, and ischemia. Chemical factors include tobacco, caffeine, alcohol, and pharmacologic agents. Several classes of drugs are known inducers of PVCs: the sympathomimetic amines (epinephrine, pseudoephedrine, phenylephrine, phenylpropanolamine, amphetamine), the methylxanthines (caffeine, theophylline), digitalis, cocaine, and certain general anesthetics (cyclopropane and halothane). Type Ia antiarrhythmics, flecainide, and sotalol may also induce PVCs and ventricular tachycardias.

Clinical Presentation and Diagnosis. Patients with isolated PVCs generally do not present with remarkable findings on a physical examination, with the exception of a pause (the next ventricular beat is delayed) after a PVC has occurred. In most patients without an underlying disease process, this arrhythmia produces no symptoms and does not adversely affect prognosis. Some patients may experience palpitations and chest or neck discomfort. PVCs that are noninducible during an electrophysiologic study also appear to be associated with minimal risk for sudden cardiac death. However, when PVCs occur in relation to MI, they can contribute to hemodynamic compromise and have been shown to be independent predictors of sudden cardiac death.

Although PVCs are an independent risk factor for sudden death, it is not entirely clear whether they predispose to or trigger sudden death or are simply a marker for underlying heart disease. Previously there was an assumption that ''complex'' PVCs after MI were indicative of high risk for degeneration into ventricular fibrillation. These criteria included greater than five or six PVCs per minute, bigeminy, multiform PVCs, or R-on-T phenomenon (when the PVC occurs near or at the same time as repolarization of the previous beat). Their clinical utility has been called into question since ''complex'' arrhythmias occur in the majority of post-MI patients.

Treatment. Identification and removal of underlying causes or precipitating factors is paramount in many patients. PVCs can accompany both slow and fast heart rates. For

PVCs associated with bradycardia, suppression of PVCs can usually be accomplished with pharmacologic (atropine or isoproterenol) or pacing interventions to increase the heart rate. However, the general approach to treating PVCs has changed as a result of CAST I and CAST II.[15,239] These trials attempted to compare the use of encainide, flecainide, moricizine, and placebo in suppressing asymptomatic or mildly symptomatic PVCs on the premise that suppression of PVCs after MI would reduce sudden cardiac death and mortality. The trial with encainide and flecainide (CAST I) was suspended after a preliminary analysis revealed higher mortality with these agents than with placebo despite efficacy in suppressing PVCs.[15,239] The use of moricizine (CAST II) yielded similar results.[15,239,240] The results of the CAST trials indicate that suppression of asymptomatic PVCs after MI does not decrease sudden cardiac death, and use of antiarrhythmic therapy can contribute to a proarrhythmic effect that may paradoxically worsen outcomes. Therefore, in an otherwise healthy person, asymptomatic PVCs do not warrant suppression. Patients who experience intolerable palpitations can receive a β-blocker. Suppression of PVCs in the presence of other comorbid conditions to reduce sudden death must be balanced against the risk of increased mortality associated with antiarrhythmic therapy and is discussed in the "Sudden Cardiac Death" section below. If antiarrhythmic therapy is desired, a number of agents have shown efficacy in reducing or eliminating PVCs. These include amiodarone, sotalol, β-blockers, procainamide, lidocaine, and quinidine. The choice between agents should be largely based on safety and individualized for each patient.

Digitalis-Induced Premature Ventricular Contractions. PVCs are the most common arrhythmia produced by digitalis. Generally, this arrhythmia resolves when the digitalis is discontinued. For frequent or symptomatic PVCs, potassium replacement in hypokalemic or normokalemic patients may suppress the arrhythmia. For sustained digitalis-induced PVCs, lidocaine and phenytoin have been used successfully. Phenytoin is considered an ideal agent to treat digitalis-induced arrhythmias because it improves AV conduction while suppressing ventricular irritability. Unfortunately, phenytoin is not nearly as effective in PVCs of different causes. For refractory arrhythmias that are life-threatening, especially when an overdose of digitalis has produced hyperkalemia, digoxin-immune Fab (antigen-binding fragments to digoxin; Digibind) can be administered intravenously over 30 minutes or intravenous push if an arrest is imminent.[241] The use of digoxin-immune Fab is discussed in Chapter 4.

VENTRICULAR TACHYCARDIA

Ventricular tachycardia (VT) is defined as three or more consecutive PVCs, characterized by a QRS duration of more than 120 ms and a regular or irregular R-R interval resulting in a ventricular rate greater than 100 bpm. Contraction of the atria during VT can occur independent of the ventricular contractions (AV dissociation) or can occur after ventricular contraction secondary to retrograde conduction to the atria from the ventricles (VA association). Episodes of VT that spontaneously terminate and do not last greater than 30 seconds are termed nonsustained VT. Nonsustained VT usually does not lead to severe hemodynamic compromise. Ventricular tachycardia lasting greater than 30 seconds or requiring termination secondary to hemodynamic instability is called sustained VT. Based on the number of ventricular ectopic foci, VT can also be characterized based on the morphology of the QRS complexes. Single repeating QRS complex morphologies are monomorphic or unimorphic VT, whereas a rhythm consisting of multiple changing QRS morphologies is polymorphic, multiform, or pleomorphic VT. If electrical impulses from two ventricular foci depolarize the ventricle at a similar time point, the resulting QRS complex is sometimes referred to as a fusion beat. A specific VT usually associated with congenital long QT syndrome or drug-induced QT prolongation is torsades de pointes, a unique polymorphic VT that is discussed in the following section.

The onset of VT can be sudden (paroxysmal) or nonparoxysmal. Premature stimulation is usually required to trigger the onset of VT. The rhythm is then maintained as a result of either abnormal automaticity or reentry. Autonomic tone is also important is modulating the rate and sustenance of VT.

Clinical Presentation and Diagnosis. The clinical presentation of VT depends on the duration, the rapidity of the ventricular rate, and the extent of underlying heart disease. Ventricular rates are usually 70 to 250 bpm. Generally, short duration and slower heart rates result in asymptomatic and stable VT. Hemodynamic instability associated with prolonged rapid ventricular rates is more prone to degeneration into ventricular fibrillation, a life-threatening cardiac emergency discussed in the following section.

The most common risk factor associated with the development of VT is ischemic heart disease or coronary artery disease. VT tachycardia in the late hospital phase of an acute MI is often asymptomatic, but it is a highly important prognostic marker because patients who experience VT are five times more likely to die within 1 year than those remain arrhythmia free.[242] Other cardiac risk factors include dilated and hypertrophic cardiomyopathy, valvular heart disease, mitral valve prolapse, congenital heart disease, open heart surgery, and coronary reperfusion.

Studies have attempted to identify markers for risk of recurrence and sudden cardiac death. Clinical markers include left ventricular dysfunction, cardiac arrest at first presentation, and nonsustained VT after MI, while diagnostic markers include decreased baroreceptor sensitivity, increased Q-T interval dispersion, and inducible sustained VT during an electrophysiologic study. These markers, along with electrophysiologic testing, can be used to risk-stratify patients with a history of VT and guide therapeutic choices such as who requires an implantable cardioverter-defibrillator (ICD).

Treatment. The approach to treatment is largely dependent on symptoms. In the patient with VT and hemodynamic instability, the therapy of choice is electrical cardioversion. Pulseless VT should be treated as for ventricular fibrillation, where direct current cardioversion is mandatory (see ''Ventricular Fibrillation, Pulseless Ventricular Tachycardia, and Sudden Cardiac Death''). Treatment of asymptomatic VT should generally be avoided, since antiarrhythmic therapy has not been shown to improve outcomes. However, in asymptomatic patients with sustained VT that could lead to the development of a cardiomyopathy, treatment to terminate the rhythm and prevent recurrent episodes is warranted. In symptomatic but stable VT patients, a pharmacologic approach to management is justified.

Acute Ventricular Tachycardia Termination. VT with a pulse, accompanied by hemodynamic instability, may be cardioverted with synchronized shocks of 100 to 360 J.[62] An alternate, and much less effective, nonpharmacologic method for attempting to terminate VT is by administering a precordial thump or strike to the patient's chest. The mechanism of effect is thought to be generation of a PVC through mechanical stimulation of cardiac tissue that interrupts a reentry circuit. However, generation of a PVC can also trigger ventricular fibrillation.

In most instances of VT with a pulse, the patient can be managed pharmacologically. The approach to pharmacologic management follows the basic algorithm devised for Advanced Cardiac Life Support (ACLS). Intravenous amiodarone, given as a bolus and front-loaded infusion, is considered the first-line agent. Repeat boluses can be administered if breakthrough PVCs occur while on the infusion of amiodarone. The second- and third-line agents are intravenous procainamide and lidocaine, respectively. Both of these agents also require a bolus followed by an infusion. Quinidine and sotalol were also used historically but are not routinely used today. The agent that results in rhythm termination is continued as a maintenance infusion until it is deemed appropriate to discontinue antiarrhythmic therapy or the patient is switched to oral antiarrhythmics. If the VT is secondary to digitalis toxicity, a pharmacologic approach is desirable. In drug-refractory VT, options include competitive ventricular pacing and surgical or radiofrequency ablative techniques.[243,244]

Prevention of Recurrences. Preventing recurrent VT is more challenging and complex than terminating an acute episode. Elimination of reversible causes or precipitating factors is paramount to preventing recurrent VT. Some common reversible causes include ischemia, hypotension, and hypokalemia. Optimal control of other nonmodifiable risk factors, such as heart failure and ischemic heart disease, are also important. If ongoing ischemia is identified as a contributing factor, coronary revascularization may be successful in limiting the risk of recurrence.

Choosing an appropriate pharmacologic agent for chronic maintenance therapy can be a daunting task, since there are few outcome data for many antiarrhythmics, comparative efficacy has been poorly studied, and each antiarrhythmic has its own potential to induce arrhythmias and other severe adverse effects. As a consequence, the selection of an appropriate antiarrhythmic is largely based on safety and previously demonstrated clinical efficacy; in difficult cases, therapy is guided by electrophysiologic studies. Safety determination must include assessment of left ventricular function, Q-T interval, pharmacologic and adverse effect profile, and function of the eliminating organ. Refer to the sections on antiarrhythmic agents for a detailed discussion of the pharmacokinetics and potential adverse effects of each agent. For patients who have responded to a certain agent during the acute VT episode or during electrophysiologic testing, this agent is usually tried first if it meets all the safety requirements. Regardless of the choice, chronic maintenance therapy is initiated as single-drug therapy. If the patient continues to experience unacceptable ventricular ectopy, combination antiarrhythmic therapy is considered. Selecting an appropriate combination regimen requires an in-depth understanding of electrophysiologic principles and should be initiated only under the guidance of a cardiac electrophysiologist, since many combinations can enhance proarrhythmic potential. In patients refractory or intolerant to pharmacologic therapy, nonpharmacologic approaches may be instituted. These include ventricular or atrial pacing (with or without antiarrhythmic therapy), ICDs, and surgical ablation. Recent studies have suggested an expanded role for ICDs in patients with a history of VT (secondary prevention) or even those who have not experienced VT but have significant risk factors (primary prevention). The role of ICDs is discussed in more detail in the section ''Ventricular Fibrillation, Pulseless Ventricular Tachycardia, and Sudden Cardiac Death'' below.

TORSADES DE POINTES

Torsades de pointes is polymorphic VT characterized by variable-amplitude QRS complexes that appear to twist around an isoelectric point. This arrhythmia is usually associated with a Q-T interval of more than 500 ms secondary to delayed or prolonged ventricular repolarization, although this is not a prerequisite. Prominent U waves can also be distinctive for torsades de pointes. The electrophysiologic mechanisms have not been fully elucidated, but it may be triggered by early after-depolarizations and sustained by reentry in many cases. Some data support the notion that females are at greater risk of developing torsades de pointes. Torsades de pointes is frequently a proarrhythmia associated with pharmacologic agents that prolong the Q-T interval. Some of the most commonly implicated drugs are listed in

TABLE 22.5	Drugs Associated with Risk of Torsades de Pointes
Amiodarone	Arsenic trioxide
Bepridil	Chloroquine
Chlorpromazine	Cisapride
Clarithromycin	Disopyramide
Dofetilide	Domperidone
Droperidol	Erythromycin
Halofantrine	Haloperidol
Ibutilide	Levomethadyl
Mesoridazine	Methadone
Pentamidine	Pimozide
Procainamide	Quinidine
Sotalol	Sparfloxacin
Thioridazine	

Table 22.5. Other common etiologies are congenital Q-T prolongation (long Q-T syndrome), severe bradycardia, and hypokalemia and hypomagnesemia.

Clinical Presentation and Diagnosis. Similar to VT, the clinical presentation of a patient experiencing torsades de pointes depends on the ventricular rate, the duration of the arrhythmia, and underlying disease processes. However, unlike VT, which can be asymptomatic or associated with only mild symptoms, torsades de pointes is usually associated with faster ventricular rates (200 to 250 bpm) and more commonly results in significant symptomatic or clinical distress to the patient. Severe episodes can result in syncope and death.

Treatment. Vigilant monitoring is required to minimize the risk of developing torsades de pointes in patients receiving medications known to affect the Q-T interval. Many medications exhibit a dose-dependent effect on ventricular repolarization, an effect that can also be amplified by drug interactions and electrolyte abnormalities. Daily monitoring of the QTc interval (Q-T interval corrected for heart rate) should be mandatory for any medications known to prolong the Q-T interval. It is desirable to maintain the QTc below 500 ms at all times, and a reduction in dosage or discontinuation of therapy should be considered if the QTc increases by 60 ms above baseline. Increased attention should be paid to patients concomitantly receiving more than one Q-T–prolonging medication. In addition, since hypokalemia and hypomagnesemia can predispose to the development of torsades de pointes, serum potassium and magnesium levels should be monitored closely and they should be replaced as necessary.

For acquired torsades de pointes (not congenital long Q-T syndrome), elimination of the underlying etiology is critical. This usually means discontinuing an offending pharmaco-logic agent. If the patient is experiencing severe symptoms or hemodynamic compromise, direct current cardioversion may be attempted first. The drug of choice for acquired torsades de pointes is intravenous magnesium, given in 2-g boluses and repeated as needed up to 12 to 16 g total. Temporary pacing to overdrive the VT is an alternate effective approach. Overdrive pacing can also be accomplished with an infusion of isoproterenol. Agents not commonly used for torsades de pointes, but with reports of efficacy, include lidocaine, mexiletine, and phenytoin. Class Ia, Ic, and III antiarrhythmic agents should be avoided as they can worsen the QT prolongation. Episodes of torsades de pointes secondary to congenital causes are managed with β-blockers, surgery, and ICDs.

VENTRICULAR FIBRILLATION, PULSELESS VENTRICULAR TACHYCARDIA, AND SUDDEN CARDIAC DEATH

Sudden cardiac death due to pulseless VT or ventricular fibrillation accounts for 300,000 to 450,000 deaths in the United States each year.[245] This represents approximately 50% of all cardiac deaths.[246] There are numerous risk factors for sudden cardiac death, including coronary artery disease, left ventricular dysfunction, hypertrophic cardiomyopathy, congenital heart disease, and valvular heart disease. Coronary heart disease is present in approximately 80% of patients with sudden cardiac death, but sudden cardiac death is often the first manifestation of this underlying process.[245,247] Left ventricular function is an independent risk factor for sudden cardiac death, irrespective of underlying coronary heart disease. Unfortunately, resuscitation rates for out-of-hospital sudden cardiac death remain low, averaging 1% to 3% in most major cities.[246,248]

Most sudden cardiac deaths are attributable to VT that degenerates into ventricular fibrillation. The mechanism for these tachyarrhythmias is credited to reentry, a form of abnormal impulse conduction caused by reexcitation of an area of the heart previously activated. Reentrant arrhythmias can occur via anatomic pathways or functional pathways created by abnormalities such as ischemia, electrolyte imbalances, or proarrhythmic drugs. Regardless of the exact mechanism, the result is chaotic electrical activity that does not produce significant myocardial contraction and thus minimal cardiac output. Therefore, it is imperative to minimize the time from sudden cardiac event to medical evaluation and treatment.

Clinical Presentation and Diagnosis. Although some patients report antecedent palpitations for minutes before arrhythmia onset, sudden cardiac death often presents without any significant warning. This implies that the initial rhythm is likely VT. In most patients, as VT degrades to ventricular fibrillation, there is a sudden loss of consciousness with seizure-like activity. If left untreated, the arrhythmia uniformly results in death.

Successful resuscitation from sudden cardiac death implies a diagnosis of ventricular fibrillation. Due to the mixture of arrhythmia mechanisms, treatment goals, and varying prognosis based on the underlying coronary heart disease, a complete evaluation for heart disease should be performed. After the initial resuscitation, evaluation should include at least a 12-lead ECG, evaluation of left ventricular function, and coronary angiography. If warranted, more specific arrhythmia evaluation techniques may be used, such as ambulatory ECG (Holter) monitoring or electrophysiology studies.

Treatment. The key to treatment of sudden cardiac death regardless of etiology is time. Specifically, the survival rate from sudden cardiac death drops approximately 5% for every minute that resuscitation is delayed.[249] Thus, the American Heart Association has developed the Basic Cardiac Life Support survival chain that consists of immediate activation of emergency medical services, early cardiopulmonary resuscitation, early use of automatic external defibrillators, and quick transportation to emergency care centers.[250] Moreover, at emergency care centers, health care practitioners should use the American Heart Association's recommendations for ACLS.[251] The following section on acute treatment highlights these recommendations.

Acute Treatment. A patient with sudden cardiac death should be treated according to the American Heart Association's recommendations for ACLS.[251] The first step is assessment and appropriate treatment of the patient's airway (open the airway), breathing (provide positive-pressure ventilation), and circulation (give chest compressions). Since electrical defibrillation is the only effective treatment for sudden cardiac death, three attempts at external electrical defibrillation should be tried at 200 J, 300 J, and 360 J. If unsuccessful, then the health care team should resume cardiopulmonary resuscitation efforts via chest compressions and positive-pressure ventilation. Next, either epinephrine 1 mg via intravenous push every 3 to 5 minutes or a one-time dose of vasopressin 40 units intravenous push may be given. Vasopressin was added to the treatment algorithm in 2000 based on data showing it is as effective as epinephrine in return of spontaneous circulation.

Electrical defibrillation should be attempted again within 30 to 60 seconds after epinephrine or vasopressin. If electrical defibrillation is unsuccessful, then intravenous antiarrhythmic drug therapy with amiodarone or lidocaine should be considered. Furthermore, magnesium may be given if there is a known hypomagnesemic state. However, electrical defibrillation remains the most important intervention. Along with maintaining cardiopulmonary resuscitation efforts, electrical defibrillation should be attempted at least every 60 seconds.

Although continued arrhythmias are rare, it is important to continue the antiarrhythmic therapy that was given before successful defibrillation until the patient is stable. Once the patient is stable, the etiology for the arrhythmia needs to be determined. If the etiology of the arrhythmia is reversible, such as acute ischemia without heart failure, then no specific long-term antiarrhythmic therapies are warranted. However, if the etiology is not reversible or if there is significant left ventricular dysfunction, then further antiarrhythmic therapies are needed.

Secondary Prevention. Patients who have suffered a sudden cardiac death event and have been resuscitated need to be assessed for appropriate secondary prevention therapies. If the etiology for the sudden cardiac death event is not reversible or if significant left ventricular dysfunction is present after the event, the patient is at high risk for mortality due to ventricular arrhythmias. Based on current data, these patients should be evaluated for an ICD. Data from four studies showed an average reduction in all-cause mortality with ICD use of 9% over standard antiarrhythmic drug therapy, most often consisting of amiodarone.[252–255]

The largest of these studies was the Antiarrhythmics Versus Implantable Defibrillators (AVID) trial, published in 1997.[255] The AVID trial was a multicenter, randomized study that compared ICD to either empiric amiodarone or electrophysiology study/Holter-guided sotalol. The study was stopped early after 1,016 patients were enrolled due to the pronounced benefit in the ICD group. After a mean follow-up of 18 months, the overall death rates were 16% in the ICD group compared to 24% in the drug group. Based on AVID and the other secondary prevention studies, it is clear that patients with a reversible etiology for their sudden cardiac death event should be evaluated for implantation of an ICD.

For patients that refuse an ICD, amiodarone is the best pharmacologic alternative. There have been four large studies to assess the use of amiodarone to prevent death. Based on these studies, compared to placebo amiodarone may reduce mortality by approximately 5%.[256–259] Moreover, due to the high side effect profile, patients taking amiodarone need to be diligently monitored. The primary alternative to amiodarone is sotalol, but the data are not as conclusive.

Primary Prevention. Despite the multiple etiologies, certain groups of patients are at significant risk for sudden cardiac death: patients with coronary artery disease and impaired left ventricular dysfunction, heart failure, and hypertrophic cardiomyopathy. Therefore, primary prevention of ventricular arrhythmias should be considered. First and foremost, patients need to be aggressively treated for their underlying disease states with appropriate pharmacologic therapies. Specific treatment for arrhythmias has been studied for both drug and ICD therapies. Based on available data, implantation of an ICD appears to confer the most mortality benefit in patients at high risk for ventricular arrhythmias. Two patient populations have been studied. Patients with documented coronary artery disease and left ventricular dysfunction have been assessed in four large multicenter studies.[260–263] These studies indicate that the implantation of an ICD in this patient population should confer a 15% reduction in all-cause mortality. The second group of patients evaluated were patients with New York Heart

Association class II and III heart failure; the patients were studied in the Sudden Cardiac Death Heart Failure Trial (SCD-HeFT).[264] The SCD-HeFT study randomized 2,521 patients with heart failure to receive one of three therapies: an ICD, amiodarone, or placebo in addition to standard medical therapies. After a mean follow-up of 20 months, the mortality in the ICD group was 29% compared to 28% and 29% in the amiodarone and placebo groups, respectively. Based on the data from these studies, it is clear that patients with left ventricular ejection fractions of less than 35% with or without underlying coronary artery disease are at high risk for sudden cardiac death and derive significant mortality benefit from the implantation of an ICD. However, there is not significant evidence to recommend antiarrhythmic drug therapy in addition to standard medical care.

PHARMACOECONOMICS OF ARRHYTHMIAS

In the past, most cost-effectiveness studies of different strategies in the management of arrhythmias were derived from decision-analysis models. However, in recent years, cost-efficacy analyses are becoming a common part of prospective study designs. The most information on cost efficacy in arrhythmia treatment targets two main areas: AF and ICDs in ventricular tachycardia.

Cost-effectiveness studies in AF have evaluated the different therapeutic considerations of anticoagulation, the use of TEE screening, and rhythm conversion. Anticoagulation with warfarin and antithrombotic prophylaxis with aspirin have both been associated with a decrease in the risk of ischemic stroke in AF but an increased risk of bleeding. These assumptions have been used as the basis of decision-analysis models.[265] Overall, these analyses show that warfarin therapy is cost-effective ($4,500 to $98,300 per quality-adjusted year of life) in patients with at least a moderate to high risk of stroke when compared to aspirin or no therapy. There is concern that these numbers were derived from clinical trials that may not reflect true efficacy and bleeding rates in clinical practice.

The economic impact of TEE-guided cardioversion was also evaluated in the Assessment of Cardioversion Using Transesophageal Echocardiography (ACUTE) trial, which showed that a TEE-guided approach was safe.[266] The analysis concluded that in patients with AF for greater than 2 days, a TEE-guided strategy resulted in similar costs to a conventional strategy.

Comparisons of relative cost effectiveness of rate- versus rhythm-control strategies have been conducted as part of prospective, randomized trials evaluating these two treatment strategies for persistent AF. In both the RACE and AFFIRM studies (described in the "Atrial Fibrillation" section above), rate control was associated with a cost savings over rhythm control.[267,268] Rhythm control was associated with higher costs, largely secondary to a greater need for electrical cardioversions, hospital admissions, antiarrhythmic medications, and pacemaker procedures. Therefore, the rate-control strategy is considered a valid treatment approach not only from a patient outcome standpoint but also as a potentially more cost-effective approach.

Growing attention to arrhythmia cost efficacy has been directed at the expanding use of ICDs for ventricular arrhythmias. Results of recent studies are continuing to support wider indications for ICDs. Due to the inherent upfront costs of the device and implantation, there is concern that the health care system will not be able to sustain these new indications. Several ICD trials have included cost-efficacy analyses.[269] The cost-effectiveness ratios for ICDs compared to medically treated patients ranged from $27,000 to $139,000 per life-year saved. Initially, ICDs are expensive (for acquisition and implantation), but subsequently antiarrhythmics become more costly. Although the exact cost effectiveness can be debated, these analyses illustrate certain important facts. Cost efficacy decreases if the risk of death is very low or very high. In addition, ICD cost efficacy is affected by the mode of death, specifically being more effective in patients more likely to experience sudden death. Finally, cost effectiveness in different studies is largely influenced by the rate of efficacy of the ICD compared to standard therapy.[270] These studies can be applied only to patients with ventricular arrhythmias; extrapolations should not be made to supraventricular arrhythmias or the use of other devices such as pacemakers.

CONCLUSIONS

Cardiac arrhythmias are complex, exhibiting various predisposing etiologies and alterations in electrophysiology, and differing severity and prognosis. Management is complicated by treatment with potentially toxic drugs. Therefore, a thorough understanding of the pharmacology, pharmacodynamics, pharmacokinetics, and adverse reactions for each antiarrhythmic agent is needed for safe and effective treatment of patients with arrhythmias. No single drug is effective for all arrhythmias in all patients, although certain drugs are clearly first-line agents while others are contraindicated. Empiric dosing of many antiarrhythmics is based on using pharmacokinetic knowledge of the drug and the clinical status of the patient. Patients must be monitored carefully, which often involves drug concentration monitoring. In arrhythmia patients who are refractory to multiple antiarrhythmic agents, device or surgical options may also exist. The optimal or ideal methods for arrhythmia management remain elusive and an active area of research.

KEY POINTS

■ Cardiac arrhythmias can range from benign to lethal.
■ Arrhythmias can originate from almost any cardiac structure and arise from a variety of causes (e.g., elec-

trolyte disturbances, structural abnormalities, metabolic derangements, drug toxicity).

■ Correct identification of the arrhythmia is critical to deciding on a therapeutic strategy.

■ Antiarrhythmic drug therapy should be individualized to the patient's response and toxicity.

■ Many arrhythmias respond better to device or surgical therapies than drug therapy.

■ The risk/benefit ratio of treating each arrhythmia must be weighed when considering acute and chronic arrhythmia management.

REFERENCES

1. Funck-Brentano C, Light RT, Lineberry MD, et al. Pharmacokinetic and pharmacodynamic interaction of N-acetyl procainamide and procainamide in humans. J Cardiovasc Pharmacol 14(3): 364–373, 1989.
2. Teichman S. The anticholinergic side effects of disopyramide and controlled–release disopyramide. Angiology 36(11):767–771, 1985.
3. Drug Facts and Comparison CD-ROM. St. Louis: Kluwer, 1998.
4. Wasenmiller JE, Aronow WS. Effect of tocainide and quinidine on premature ventricular contractions. Clin Pharmacol Ther 28(4): 431–435, 1980.
5. Feinberg L, Travis WD, Ferrans V, et al. Pulmonary fibrosis associated with tocainide: report of a case with literature review. Am Rev Respir Dis 141(2):505–508, 1990.
6. Lee JT, Kroemer HK, Silberstein DJ, et al. The role of genetically determined polymorphic drug metabolism in the beta-blockade produced by propafenone. N Engl J Med 322(25):1764–1768, 1990.
7. Prystowsky EN. Diagnosis and management of the preexcitation syndromes. Curr Probl Cardiol 13(4):225–310, 1988.
8. Lee SH, Chen SA, Tai CT, et al. Comparisons of oral propafenone and sotalol as an initial treatment in patients with symptomatic paroxysmal atrial fibrillation. Am J Cardiol 79(7):905–908, 1997.
9. Capucci A. Quinidine versus propafenone for conversion of atrial fibrillation to sinus rhythm. Am J Cardiol 81(3):373–374, 1998.
10. A randomized, placebo-controlled trial of propafenone in the prophylaxis of paroxysmal supraventricular tachycardia and paroxysmal atrial fibrillation. UK Propafenone PSVT Study Group. Circulation 92(9):2550–2557, 1995.
11. Fitton A, Buckley MT. Moricizine. A review of its pharmacological properties, and therapeutic efficacy in cardiac arrhythmias. Drugs 40(1):138–167, 1990.
12. Mann HJ. Moricizine: a new class I antiarrhythmic. Clin Pharm 9(11):842–852, 1990.
13. Effects of encainide, flecainide, imipramine and moricizine on ventricular arrhythmias during the year after acute MI : the Cardiac Arrhythmia Pilot Study (CAPS) Investigators. Am J Cardiol 61(8): 501–509, 1988.
14. Bigger JT, Jr. The events surrounding the removal of encainide and flecainide from the Cardiac Arrhythmia Suppression Trial (CAST) and why CAST is continuing with moricizine. J Am Coll Cardiol 15(1):243–245, 1990.
15. Effect of the antiarrhythmic agent moricizine on survival after MI. The Cardiac Arrhythmia Suppression Trial II Investigators. N Engl J Med 327(4):227–233, 1992.
16. Abrams J, Allen J, Allin D, et al. Efficacy and safety of esmolol vs propranolol in the treatment of supraventricular tachyarrhythmias: a multicenter double-blind clinical trial. Am Heart J 110(5):913–922, 1985.
17. Anderson S, Blanski L, Byrd RC, et al. Comparison of the efficacy and safety of esmolol, a short-acting beta blocker, with placebo in the treatment of supraventricular tachyarrhythmias. The Esmolol vs Placebo Multicenter Study Group. Am Heart J 111(1):42–48, 1986.
18. Sung RJ, Blanski L, Kirshenbaum J, et al. Clinical experience with esmolol, a short-acting beta-adrenergic blocker in cardiac arrhythmias and myocardial ischemia. J Clin Pharmacol 26 Suppl A: A15–A26, 1986.
19. Platia EV, Michelson EL, Porterfield JK, et al. Esmolol versus verapamil in the acute treatment of atrial fibrillation or atrial flutter. Am J Cardiol 63(13):925–929, 1989.
20. Herre JM, Sauve MJ, Malone P, et al. Long-term results of amiodarone therapy in patients with recurrent sustained ventricular tachycardia or ventricular fibrillation. J Am Coll Cardiol 13(2): 442–449, 1989.
21. Weinberg BA, Miles WM, Klein LS, et al. Five-year follow-up of 589 patients treated with amiodarone. Am Heart J 125(1):109–120, 1993.
22. Randomized antiarrhythmic drug therapy in survivors of cardiac arrest (the CASCADE Study). Am J Cardiol 72(3):280–287, 1993.
23. Cairns JA, Connolly SJ, Gent M, et al. Post-MI mortality in patients with ventricular premature depolarizations. Canadian Amiodarone Myocardial Infarction Arrhythmia Trial Pilot Study. Circulation 84(2):550–557, 1991.
24. Ceremuzynski L, Kleczar E, Krzeminska-Pakula M, et al. Effect of amiodarone on mortality after MI: a double-blind, placebo-controlled, pilot study. J Am Coll Cardiol 20(5):1056–1062, 1992.
25. Pfisterer ME, Kiowski W, Brunner H, et al. Long-term benefit of 1-year amiodarone treatment for persistent complex ventricular arrhythmias after MI. Circulation 87(2):309–311, 1993.
26. Burkart F, Pfisterer M, Kiowski W, et al. Effect of antiarrhythmic therapy on mortality in survivors of MI with asymptomatic complex ventricular arrhythmias: Basel Antiarrhythmic Study of Infarct Survival (BASIS). J Am Coll Cardiol 16(7):1711–1718, 1990.
27. Naccarelli GV, Rinkenberger RL, Dougherty AH, et al. Amiodarone: pharmacology and antiarrhythmic and adverse effects. Pharmacotherapy 5(6):298–313, 1985.
28. Heger JJ, Prystowsky EN, Jackman WM, et al. Clinical efficacy and electrophysiology during long-term therapy for recurrent ventricular tachycardia or ventricular fibrillation. N Engl J Med 305(10):539–545, 1981.
29. Peter T, Hamer A, Mandel WJ, et al. Evaluation of amiodarone therapy in the treatment of drug-resistant cardiac arrhythmias: long-term follow-up. Am Heart J 106(4 Pt 2):943–950, 1983.
30. Gill J, Heel RC, Fitton A. Amiodarone. An overview of its pharmacological properties, and review of its therapeutic use in cardiac arrhythmias. Drugs 43(1):69–110, 1992.
31. Ott MC, Khoor A, Leventhal JP, et al. Pulmonary toxicity in patients receiving low-dose amiodarone. Chest 123(2):646–651, 2003.
32. Kerin NZ, Blevins RD, Benaderet D, et al. Relation of serum reverse T3 to amiodarone antiarrhythmic efficacy and toxicity. Am J Cardiol 57(1):128–130, 1986.
33. Hohnloser SH, Klingenheben T, Singh BN. Amiodarone-associated proarrhythmic effects. A review with special reference to torsades de pointes tachycardia. Ann Intern Med 121(7):529–535, 1994.
34. Saal AK, Werner JA, Greene HL, et al. Effect of amiodarone on serum quinidine and procainamide levels. Am J Cardiol 53(9): 1264–1267, 1984.
35. MacNeil DJ, Davies RO, Deitchman D. Clinical safety profile of sotalol in the treatment of arrhythmias. Am J Cardiol 72(4): 44A–50A, 1993.
36. Hohnloser SH, Woosley RL. Sotalol. N Engl J Med 331(1):31–38, 1994.
37. Juul-Moller S, Edvardsson N, Rehnqvist-Ahlberg N. Sotalol versus quinidine for the maintenance of sinus rhythm after direct current conversion of atrial fibrillation. Circulation 82(6):1932–1939, 1990.
38. Mason JW. A comparison of seven antiarrhythmic drugs in patients with ventricular tachyarrhythmias. Electrophysiologic Study versus Electrocardiographic Monitoring Investigators. N Engl J Med 329(7):452–458, 1993.
39. Reiffel JA, Hahn E, Hartz V, Reiter MJ. Sotalol for ventricular tachyarrhythmias: beta-blocking and class III contributions, and relative efficacy versus class I drugs after prior drug failure. ESVEM Investigators. Electrophysiologic Study Versus Electrocardiographic Monitoring. Am J Cardiol 79(8):1048–1053, 1997.

40. Pratt CM, Camm AJ, Cooper W, et al. Mortality in the Survival With ORal D–sotalol (SWORD) trial: why did patients die? Am J Cardiol 81(7):869–876, 1998.

41. Granberry MC. Ibutilide: a new class III antiarrhythmic agent. Am J Health Syst Pharm 55(3):255–260, 1998.

42. Stambler BS, Wood MA, Ellenbogen KA. Antiarrhythmic actions of intravenous ibutilide compared with procainamide during human atrial flutter and fibrillation: electrophysiological determinants of enhanced conversion efficacy. Circulation 96(12):4298–4306, 1997.

43. Murray KT. Ibutilide. Circulation 97(5):493–497, 1998.

44. Karam R, Marcello S, Brooks RR, et al. Azimilide dihydrochloride, a novel antiarrhythmic agent. Am J Cardiol 81(6A):40D–46D, 1998.

45. Connolly SJ, Schnell DJ, Page RL, et al. Dose–response relations of azimilide in the management of symptomatic, recurrent, atrial fibrillation. Am J Cardiol 88(9):974–979, 2001.

46. Pritchett EL, Page RL, Connolly SJ, et al. Antiarrhythmic effects of azimilide in atrial fibrillation: efficacy and dose–response. Azimilide Supraventricular Arrhythmia Program 3 (SVA–3) Investigators. J Am Coll Cardiol 36(3):794–802, 2000.

47. Pratt CM, Singh SN, Al-Khalidi HR, et al. The efficacy of azimilide in the treatment of atrial fibrillation in the presence of left ventricular systolic dysfunction: results from the Azimilide Postinfarct Survival Evaluation (ALIVE) trial. J Am Coll Cardiol 43(7):1211–1216, 2004.

48. Huycke EC, Sung RJ, Dias VC, et al. Intravenous diltiazem for termination of reentrant supraventricular tachycardia: a placebo-controlled, randomized, double-blind, multicenter study. J Am Coll Cardiol 13(3):538–544, 1989.

49. Dougherty AH, Jackman WM, Naccarelli GV, et al. Acute conversion of paroxysmal supraventricular tachycardia with intravenous diltiazem. IV Diltiazem Study Group. Am J Cardiol 70(6):587–592, 1992.

50. Packer M, Meller J, Medina N, et al. Hemodynamic consequences of combined beta-adrenergic and slow calcium channel blockade in man. Circulation 65(4):660–668, 1982.

51. Bussey HI. The influence of quinidine and other agents on digitalis glycosides. Am Heart J 104(2 Pt 1):289–302, 1982.

52. Lewis RV, Irvine N, McDevitt DG. Relationships between heart rate, exercise tolerance and cardiac output in atrial fibrillation: the effects of treatment with digoxin, verapamil and diltiazem. Eur Heart J 9(7):777–781, 1988.

53. Lewis RV, Laing E, Moreland TA, et al. A comparison of digoxin, diltiazem and their combination in the treatment of atrial fibrillation. Eur Heart J 9(3):279–283, 1988.

54. Lang R, Klein HO, Di Segni E, et al. Verapamil improves exercise capacity in chronic atrial fibrillation: double-blind crossover study. Am Heart J 105(5):820–825, 1983.

55. Drugs for cardiac arrhythmias. Med Lett Drugs Ther 38(982):75–82, 1996.

56. Roberts SA, Diaz C, Nolan PE, et al. Effectiveness and costs of digoxin treatment for atrial fibrillation and flutter. Am J Cardiol 72(7):567–573, 1993.

57. Beasley R, Smith DA, McHaffie DJ. Exercise heart rates at different serum digoxin concentrations in patients with atrial fibrillation. Br Med J (Clin Res Ed) 290(6461):9–11, 1985.

58. Goldman S, Probst P, Selzer A, et al. Inefficacy of "therapeutic" serum levels of digoxin in controlling the ventricular rate in atrial fibrillation. Am J Cardiol 35(5):651–655, 1975.

59. Fromm MF, Kim RB, Stein CM, et al. Inhibition of P-glycoprotein-mediated drug transport: a unifying mechanism to explain the interaction between digoxin and quinidine. Circulation 99(4):552–557, 1999.

60. Parker RB, McCollam PL. Adenosine in the episodic treatment of paroxysmal supraventricular tachycardia. Clin Pharm 9(4):261–271, 1990.

61. diMarco JP, Sellers TD, Lerman BB, et al. Diagnostic and therapeutic use of adenosine in patients with supraventricular tachyarrhythmias. J Am Coll Cardiol 6(2):417–425, 1985.

62. Guidelines for cardiopulmonary resuscitation and emergency cardiac care. Emergency Cardiac Care Committee and Subcommittees, American Heart Association. Part I. Introduction. JAMA 268(16):2171–2183, 1992.

63. DiMarco JP, Miles W, Akhtar M, et al. Adenosine for paroxysmal supraventricular tachycardia: dose ranging and comparison with verapamil. Assessment in placebo-controlled, multicenter trials. The Adenosine for PSVT Study Group. Ann Intern Med 113(2):104–110, 1990.

64. Till J, Shinebourne EA, Rigby ML, et al. Efficacy and safety of adenosine in the treatment of supraventricular tachycardia in infants and children. Br Heart J 62(3):204–211, 1989.

65. Rankin AC, Rae AP, Oldroyd KG, et al. Verapamil or adenosine for the immediate treatment of supraventricular tachycardia. Q J Med 74(274):203–208, 1990.

66. Hood MA, Smith WM. Adenosine versus verapamil in the treatment of supraventricular tachycardia: a randomized double-crossover trial. Am Heart J 123(6):1543–1549, 1992.

67. Till JA, Shinebourne EA. Supraventricular tachycardia: diagnosis and current acute management. Arch Dis Child 66(5):647–652, 1991.

68. Chronister C. Clinical management of supraventricular tachycardia with adenosine. Am J Crit Care 2(1):41–47, 1993.

69. Garratt C, Linker N, Griffith M, et al. Comparison of adenosine and verapamil for termination of paroxysmal junctional tachycardia. Am J Cardiol 64(19):1310–1316, 1989.

70. Rankin AC, Oldroyd KG, Chong E, et al. Adenosine or adenosine triphosphate for supraventricular tachycardias? Comparative double-blind randomized study in patients with spontaneous or inducible arrhythmias. Am Heart J 119(2 Pt 1):316–323, 1990.

71. Klabunde RE. Dipyridamole inhibition of adenosine metabolism in human blood. Eur J Pharmacol 93(1–2):21–26, 1983.

71a. Gregoratos G, Abrams J, Epstein AE, et al. ACC/AHA/NASPE 2002 Guideline update for implantation of cardiac pacemakers and antiarrhythmia devices: summary article: a report of the American College of Cardiology/American Heart Association Task Force on Practice Guidelines (ACC/AHA/NASPE Committee to Update the 1998 Pacemaker Guidelines). Circulation 106:2145–2161, 2002.

72. Blomstrom-Lundqvist C, Scheinman MM, Aliot EM, et al. ACC/AHA/ESC guidelines for the management of patients with supraventricular arrhythmias: executive summary. J Am Coll Cardiol 42(8):1493–1531, 2003.

73. Sato T, Mitamura H, Murata M, et al. Electrophysiologic findings of a patient with inappropriate sinus tachycardia cured by selective radiofrequency catheter ablation. J Electrocardiol 33(4):381–386, 2000.

74. Sung RJ, Styperek JL, Myerburg RJ, et al. Initiation of two distinct forms of atrioventricular nodal reentrant tachycardia during programmed ventricular stimulation in man. Am J Cardiol 42(3):404–415, 1978.

75. Heart disease and stroke statistics, 2004 update. 2004. (Accessed at www.americanheart.org).

76. Wood KA, Drew BJ, Scheinman MM. Frequency of disabling symptoms in supraventricular tachycardia. Am J Cardiol 79(2):145–149, 1997.

77. Josephson ME. Paroxysmal supraventricular tachycardia: an electrophysiologic approach. Am J Cardiol 41(6):1123–1126, 1978.

78. Crawford MH, Bernstein SJ, Deedwania PC, et al. ACC/AHA guidelines for ambulatory electrocardiography. J Am Coll Cardiol 34(3):912–948, 1999.

79. Mehta D, Wafa S, Ward DE, et al. Relative efficacy of various physical manoeuvres in the termination of junctional tachycardia. Lancet 1(8596):1181–1185, 1988.

80. Schweitzer P, Teichholz LE. Carotid sinus massage. Its diagnostic and therapeutic value in arrhythmias. Am J Med 78(4):645–654, 1985.

81. Glatter KA, Cheng J, Dorostkar P, et al. Electrophysiologic effects of adenosine in patients with supraventricular tachycardia. Circulation 99(8):1034–1040, 1999.

82. Buckley MM, Grant SM, Goa KL, et al. Diltiazem. A reappraisal of its pharmacological properties and therapeutic use. Drugs 39(5):757–806, 1990.

83. Bohm M, Schwinger RH, Erdmann E. Different cardiodepressant potency of various calcium antagonists in human myocardium. Am J Cardiol 65(15):1039–1041, 1990.

84. Heywood JT, Graham B, Marais GE, et al. Effects of intravenous diltiazem on rapid atrial fibrillation accompanied by congestive heart failure. Am J Cardiol 67(13):1150–1152, 1991.

85. De Belder MA, Malik M, Ward DE, et al. Pacing modalities for tachycardia termination. Pacing Clin Electrophysiol 13(2):231–248, 1990.

86. Winniford MD, Fulton KL, Hillis LD. Long-term therapy of paroxysmal supraventricular tachycardia: a randomized, double-blind comparison of digoxin, propranolol and verapamil. Am J Cardiol 54(8):1138–1139, 1984.

87. Rizos I, Seidl KH, Aidonidis I, et al. Intraindividual comparison of diltiazem and verapamil on induction of paroxysmal supraventricular tachycardia. Cardiology 85(6):388–396, 1994.

88. Anderson JL, Platt ML, Guarnieri T, et al. Flecainide acetate for paroxysmal supraventricular tachyarrhythmias. The Flecainide Supraventricular Tachycardia Study Group. Am J Cardiol 74(6):578–584, 1994.

89. Neuss H, Schlepper M. Long-term efficacy and safety of flecainide for supraventricular tachycardia. Am J Cardiol 62(6):56D–61D, 1988.

90. Pritchett EL, McCarthy EA, Wilkinson WE. Propafenone treatment of symptomatic paroxysmal supraventricular arrhythmias. A randomized, placebo-controlled, crossover trial in patients tolerating oral therapy. Ann Intern Med 114(7):539–544, 1991.

91. Tendera M, Wnuk-Wojnar AM, Kulakowski P, et al. Efficacy and safety of dofetilide in the prevention of symptomatic episodes of paroxysmal supraventricular tachycardia: a 6-month double-blind comparison with propafenone and placebo. Am Heart J 142(1):93–98, 2001.

92. Wanless RS, Anderson K, Joy M, et al. Multicenter comparative study of the efficacy and safety of sotalol in the prophylactic treatment of patients with paroxysmal supraventricular tachyarrhythmias. Am Heart J 133(4):441–446, 1997.

93. Wu D, Denes P, Bauernfeind R, et al. Effects of procainamide on atrioventricular nodal reentrant paroxysmal tachycardia. Circulation 57(6):1171–1179, 1978.

94. Wu D, Hung JS, Kuo CT, et al. Effects of quinidine on atrioventricular nodal reentrant paroxysmal tachycardia. Circulation 64(4):823–831, 1981.

95. Brugada P, Wellens HJ. Effects of intravenous and oral disopyramide on paroxysmal atrioventricular nodal tachycardia. Am J Cardiol 53(1):88–92, 1984.

96. Alboni P, Tomasi C, Menozzi C, et al. Efficacy and safety of out-of-hospital self-administered single-dose oral drug treatment in the management of infrequent, well-tolerated paroxysmal supraventricular tachycardia. J Am Coll Cardiol 37(2):548–553, 2001.

97. Musto B, Cavallaro C, Musto A, et al. Flecainide single oral dose for management of paroxysmal supraventricular tachycardia in children and young adults. Am Heart J 124(1):110–115, 1992.

98. Ferguson TB, Jr., Cox JL. Surgical therapy for patients with supraventricular tachycardia. Cardiol Clin 8(3):535–555, 1990.

99. Manolis AS, Wang PJ, Estes NA, 3rd. Radiofrequency catheter ablation for cardiac tachyarrhythmias. Ann Intern Med 121(6):452–461, 1994.

100. Akhtar M, Jazayeri MR, Sra J, et al. Atrioventricular nodal reentry. Clinical, electrophysiological, and therapeutic considerations. Circulation 88(1):282–295, 1993.

101. Hindricks G. Incidence of complete atrioventricular block following attempted radiofrequency catheter modification of the atrioventricular node in 880 patients. Eur Heart J 17(1):82–88, 1996.

102. Ross DL, Uther JB. Diagnosis of concealed accessory pathways in supraventricular tachycardia. Pacing Clin Electrophysiol 7(6 Pt 1):1069–1085, 1984.

103. Vidaillet HJ, Jr., Pressley JC, Henke E, et al. Familial occurrence of accessory atrioventricular pathways (preexcitation syndrome). N Engl J Med 317(2):65–69, 1987.

104. Berry V. WPW syndrome and the use of radiofrequency catheter ablation. Heart Lung 22:15–25, 1993.

105. Klein GJ, Bashore TM, Sellers TD, et al. Ventricular fibrillation in the Wolff-Parkinson-White syndrome. N Engl J Med 301(20):1080–1085, 1979.

106. Krahn AD, Manfreda J, Tate RB, et al. The natural history of electrocardiographic preexcitation in men. The Manitoba Follow-up Study. Ann Intern Med 116(6):456–460, 1992.

107. Janousek J, Paul T, Reimer A, Kallfelz HC. Usefulness of propafenone for supraventricular arrhythmias in infants and children. Am J Cardiol 72(3):294–300, 1993.

108. Musto B, D'Onofrio A, Cavallaro C, et al. Electrophysiological effects and clinical efficacy of propafenone in children with recurrent paroxysmal supraventricular tachycardia. Circulation 78(4):863–869, 1988.

109. Vassiliadis I, Papoutsakis P, Kallikazaros I, et al. Propafenone in the prevention of nonventricular arrhythmias associated with the Wolff-Parkinson-White syndrome. Int J Cardiol 27(1):63–70, 1990.

110. Kim SS, Lal R, Ruffy R. Treatment of paroxysmal reentrant supraventricular tachycardia with flecainide acetate. Am J Cardiol 58(1):80–85, 1986.

111. Cockrell JL, Scheinman MM, Titus C, et al. Safety and efficacy of oral flecainide therapy in patients with atrioventricular reentrant tachycardia. Ann Intern Med 114(3):189–194, 1991.

112. Hoff PI, Tronstad A, Oie B, et al. Electrophysiologic and clinical effects of flecainide for recurrent paroxysmal supraventricular tachycardia. Am J Cardiol 62(9):585–589, 1988.

113. Kunze KP, Schluter M, Kuck KH. Sotalol in patients with Wolff-Parkinson-White syndrome. Circulation 75(5):1050–1057, 1987.

114. Rosenbaum MB, Chiale PA, Ryba D, et al. Control of tachyarrhythmias associated with Wolff-Parkinson-White syndrome by amiodarone hydrochloride. Am J Cardiol 34(2):215–223, 1974.

115. Kappenberger LJ, Fromer MA, Steinbrunn W, et al. Efficacy of amiodarone in the Wolff-Parkinson-White syndrome with rapid ventricular response via accessory pathway during atrial fibrillation. Am J Cardiol 54(3):330–335, 1984.

116. Porter RS. Adenosine: supplementary considerations about activity and use. Clin Pharm 9(4):271–274, 1990.

117. Calkins H, Sousa J, el Atassi R, et al. Diagnosis and cure of the Wolff-Parkinson-White syndrome or paroxysmal supraventricular tachycardias during a single electrophysiologic test. N Engl J Med 324(23):1612–1618, 1991.

118. Jackman WM, Wang XZ, Friday KJ, et al. Catheter ablation of accessory atrioventricular pathways (Wolff-Parkinson-White syndrome) by radiofrequency current. N Engl J Med 324(23):1605–1611, 1991.

119. Calkins H, Langberg J, Sousa J, et al. Radiofrequency catheter ablation of accessory atrioventricular connections in 250 patients. Abbreviated therapeutic approach to Wolff-Parkinson-White syndrome. Circulation 85(4):1337–1346, 1992.

120. Scheinman MM. NASPE survey on catheter ablation. Pacing Clin Electrophysiol 18(8):1474–1478, 1995.

121. Hindricks G. The Multicentre European Radiofrequency Survey (MERFS): complications of radiofrequency catheter ablation of arrhythmias. Eur Heart J 14(12):1644–1553, 1993.

122. Saoudi N, Cosio F, Waldo A, et al. A classification of atrial flutter and regular atrial tachycardia according to electrophysiological mechanisms and anatomical bases. Eur Heart J 22(14):1162–1182, 2001.

123. Shine KI, Kastor JA, Yurchak PM. Multifocal atrial tachycardia. Clinical and electrocardiographic features in 32 patients. N Engl J Med 279(7):344–349, 1968.

124. Poutiainen AM, Koistinen MJ, Airaksinen KE, et al. Prevalence and natural course of ectopic atrial tachycardia. Eur Heart J 20(9):694–700, 1999.

125. Lipson MJ, Naimi S. Multifocal atrial tachycardia (chaotic atrial tachycardia). Clinical associations and significance. Circulation 42(3):397–407, 1970.

126. Wang K, Goldfarb BL, Gobel FL, et al. Multifocal atrial tachycardia. Arch Intern Med 137(2):161–164, 1977.

127. Chen SA, Chiang CE, Yang CJ, et al. Sustained atrial tachycardia in adult patients. Electrophysiological characteristics, pharmacological response, possible mechanisms, and effects of radiofrequency ablation. Circulation 90(3):1262–1278, 1994.

128. McCord J, Borzak S. Multifocal atrial tachycardia. Chest 113(1):203–209, 1998.

129. Goldreyer BN, Gallagher JJ, Damato AN. The electrophysiologic demonstration of atrial ectopic tachycardia in man. Am Heart J 85(2):205–215, 1973.

130. Kalman JM, Olgin JE, Karch MR, et al. "Cristal tachycardias": origin of right atrial tachycardias from the crista terminalis identified by intracardiac echocardiography. J Am Coll Cardiol 31(2):451–459, 1998.

131. Tada H, Nogami A, Naito S, et al. Simple electrocardiographic criteria for identifying the site of origin of focal right atrial tachycardia. Pacing Clin Electrophysiol 21(11 Pt 2):2431–2439, 1998.

132. Tang CW, Scheinman MM, Van Hare GF, et al. Use of P wave configuration during atrial tachycardia to predict site of origin. J Am Coll Cardiol 26(5):1315–1324, 1995.

133. Stock JP. Beta-adrenergic blocking drugs in the clinical management of cardiac arrhythmias. Am J Cardiol 18(3):444–449, 1966.

134. Salerno DM, Anderson B, Sharkey PJ, et al. Intravenous verapamil for treatment of multifocal atrial tachycardia with and without calcium pretreatment. Ann Intern Med 107(5):623–628, 1987.

135. Arsura EL, Solar M, Lefkin AS, et al. Metoprolol in the treatment of multifocal atrial tachycardia. Crit Care Med 15(6):591–594, 1987.

136. Arsura E, Lefkin AS, Scher DL, et al. A randomized, double-blind, placebo-controlled study of verapamil and metoprolol in treatment of multifocal atrial tachycardia. Am J Med 85(4):519–524, 1988.

137. Iseri LT, Fairshter RD, Hardemann JL, Brodsky MA. Magnesium and potassium therapy in multifocal atrial tachycardia. Am Heart J 110(4):789–794, 1985.

138. Cohen L, Kitzes R, Shnaider H. Multifocal atrial tachycardia responsive to parenteral magnesium. Magnes Res 1(3–4):239–242, 1988.

139. Scher DL, Arsura EL. Multifocal atrial tachycardia: mechanisms, clinical correlates, and treatment. Am Heart J 118(3):574–580, 1989.

140. Furberg CD, Psaty BM, Manolio TA, et al. Prevalence of atrial fibrillation in elderly subjects (the Cardiovascular Health Study). Am J Cardiol 74(3):236–241, 1994.

141. Ostrander LD, Jr., Brandt RL, Kjelsberg MO, et al. Electrocardiographic findings among the adult population of a total natural community, Tecumseh, Michigan. Circulation 31:888–898, 1965.

142. Wolf PA, Abbott RD, Kannel WB. Atrial fibrillation as an independent risk factor for stroke: the Framingham Study. Stroke 22(8):983–988, 1991.

143. Kannel WB, Abbott RD, Savage DD, et al. Coronary heart disease and atrial fibrillation: the Framingham Study. Am Heart J 106(2):389–396, 1983.

144. Fuster V, Ryden LE, Asinger RW, et al. ACC/AHA/ESC guidelines for the management of patients with atrial fibrillation: executive summary. Circulation 104(17):2118–2150, 2001.

145. Brand FN, Abbott RD, Kannel WB, et al. Characteristics and prognosis of lone atrial fibrillation. 30-year follow-up in the Framingham Study. JAMA 254(24):3449–3453, 1985.

146. Levy S, Maarek M, Coumel P, et al. Characterization of different subsets of atrial fibrillation in general practice in France: the ALFA study. The College of French Cardiologists. Circulation 99(23):3028–3035, 1999.

147. Evans W, Swann P. Lone auricular fibrillation. Br Heart J 16(2):189–194, 1954.

148. Stein B, Halperin JL, Fuster V. Should patients with atrial fibrillation be anticoagulated prior to and chronically following cardioversion? Cardiovasc Clin 21(1):231–249, 1990.

149. Hindman MC, Wagner GS. Arrhythmias during MI: mechanisms, significance, and therapy. Cardiovasc Clin 11(1):81–102, 1980.

150. Psaty BM, Manolio TA, Kuller LH, et al. Incidence of and risk factors for atrial fibrillation in older adults. Circulation 96(7):2455–2461, 1997.

151. Pedersen OD, Bagger H, Kober L, et al. The occurrence and prognostic significance of atrial fibrillation/–flutter following acute MI. TRACE Study group. TRAndolapril Cardiac Evalution. Eur Heart J 20(10):748–754, 1999.

152. Crijns HJ, Tjeersdma G, de Kam PJ, et al. Prognostic value of the presence and development of atrial fibrillation in patients with advanced chronic heart failure. Eur Heart J 21(15):1238–1245, 2000.

153. Moe GK, Abildskov JA. Atrial fibrillation as a self-sustaining arrhythmia independent of focal discharge. Am Heart J 58(1):59–70, 1959.

154. Rensma PL, Allessie MA, Lammers WJ, et al. Length of excitation wave and susceptibility to reentrant atrial arrhythmias in normal conscious dogs. Circ Res 62(2):395–410, 1988.

155. Moe GK, Abildskov JA. Observations on the ventricular dysrhythmia associated with atrial fibrillation in the dog heart. Circ Res 14:447–460, 1964.

156. Ricard P, Levy S, Trigano J, et al. Prospective assessment of the minimum energy needed for external electrical cardioversion of atrial fibrillation. Am J Cardiol 79(6):815–816, 1997.

157. Wijffels MC, Kirchhof CJ, Dorland R, Allessie MA. Atrial fibrillation begets atrial fibrillation. A study in awake chronically instrumented goats. Circulation 92(7):1954–1968, 1995.

158. Franz MR, Karasik PL, Li C, et al. Electrical remodeling of the human atrium: similar effects in patients with chronic atrial fibrillation and atrial flutter. J Am Coll Cardiol 30(7):1785–1792, 1997.

159. Prystowsky EN. Atrioventricular node reentry: physiology and radiofrequency ablation. Pacing Clin Electrophysiol 20(2 Pt 2):552–571, 1997.

160. Mazgalev T, Dreifus LS, Bianchi J, et al. Atrioventricular nodal conduction during atrial fibrillation in rabbit heart. Am J Physiol 243(5):H754–760, 1982.

161. Page RL, Wharton JM, Prystowsky EN. Effect of continuous vagal enhancement on concealed conduction and refractoriness within the atrioventricular node. Am J Cardiol 77(4):260–265, 1996.

162. Page RL, Tang AS, Prystowsky EN. Effect of continuous enhanced vagal tone on atrioventricular nodal and sinoatrial nodal function in humans. Circ Res 68(6):1614–1620, 1991.

163. Lundstrom T, Ryden L. Chronic atrial fibrillation. Long-term results of direct current conversion. Acta Med Scand 223(1):53–59, 1988.

164. Clark DM, Plumb VJ, Epstein AE, et al. Hemodynamic effects of an irregular sequence of ventricular cycle lengths during atrial fibrillation. J Am Coll Cardiol 30(4):1039–1045, 1997.

165. Halperin JL, Hart RG. Atrial fibrillation and stroke: new ideas, persisting dilemmas. Stroke 19(8):937–941, 1988.

166. Bogousslavsky J, Van Melle G, Regli F, et al. Pathogenesis of anterior circulation stroke in patients with nonvalvular atrial fibrillation: the Lausanne Stroke Registry. Neurology 40(7):1046–1050, 1990.

167. Kanter MC, Tegeler CH, Pearce LA, et al. Carotid stenosis in patients with atrial fibrillation. Prevalence, risk factors, and relationship to stroke in the Stroke Prevention in Atrial Fibrillation Study. Arch Intern Med 154(12):1372–1377, 1994.

168. Aschenberg W, Schluter M, Kremer P, et al. Transesophageal two-dimensional echocardiography for the detection of left atrial appendage thrombus. J Am Coll Cardiol 7(1):163–166, 1986.

169. Petersen P. Thromboembolic complications in atrial fibrillation. Stroke 21(1):4–13, 1990.

170. Wolf PA, Kannel WB, McGee DL, et al. Duration of atrial fibrillation and imminence of stroke: the Framingham study. Stroke 14(5):664–667, 1983.

171. Fatkin D, Kelly R, Feneley MP. Left atrial appendage blood velocity and thromboembolic risk in patients with atrial fibrillation. J Am Coll Cardiol 24(5):1429–1430, 1994.

172. Fatkin D, Herbert E, Feneley MP. Hematologic correlates of spontaneous echo contrast in patients with atrial fibrillation and implications for thromboembolic risk. Am J Cardiol 73(9):672–676, 1994.

173. Gustafsson C, Blomback M, Britton M, et al. Coagulation factors and the increased risk of stroke in nonvalvular atrial fibrillation. Stroke 21(1):47–51, 1990.

174. Heppell RM, Berkin KE, McLenachan JM, Davies JA. Haemostatic and haemodynamic abnormalities associated with left atrial thrombosis in nonrheumatic atrial fibrillation. Heart 77(5):407–411, 1997.

175. Oltrona L, Broccolino M, Merlini PA, et al. Activation of the hemostatic mechanism after pharmacological cardioversion of acute nonvalvular atrial fibrillation. Circulation 95(8):2003–2006, 1997.

176. Predictors of thromboembolism in atrial fibrillation: I. Clinical features of patients at risk. The Stroke Prevention in Atrial Fibrillation Investigators. Ann Intern Med 116(1):1–5, 1992.

177. Jung F, DiMarco JP. Treatment strategies for atrial fibrillation. Am J Med 104(3):272–286, 1998.

178. Rawles JM. What is meant by a "controlled" ventricular rate in atrial fibrillation? Br Heart J 63(3):157–161, 1990.

179. Resnekov L, McDonald L. Electroversion of lone atrial fibrillation and flutter including haemodynamic studies at rest and on exercise. Br Heart J 33(3):339–350, 1971.

180. Atwood JE, Myers J, Sandhu S, et al. Optimal sampling interval to estimate heart rate at rest and during exercise in atrial fibrillation. Am J Cardiol 63(1):45–48, 1989.

181. Stoddard MF, Dawkins PR, Prince CR, et al. Left atrial appendage thrombus is not uncommon in patients with acute atrial fibrillation and a recent embolic event: a transesophageal echocardiographic study. J Am Coll Cardiol 25(2):452–459, 1995.

182. Manning WJ, Silverman DI, Waksmonski CA, et al. Prevalence of residual left atrial thrombi among patients with acute thromboembolism and newly recognized atrial fibrillation. Arch Intern Med 155(20):2193–2198, 1995.

183. Collins LJ, Silverman DI, Douglas PS, et al. Cardioversion of non-rheumatic atrial fibrillation. Reduced thromboembolic complications with 4 weeks of precardioversion anticoagulation are related to atrial thrombus resolution. Circulation 92(2):160–163, 1995.

184. Harjai KJ, Mobarek SK, Cheirif J, et al. Clinical variables affecting recovery of left atrial mechanical function after cardioversion from atrial fibrillation. J Am Coll Cardiol 30(2):481–486, 1997.

185. Karlson BW, Herlitz J, Edvardsson N, et al. Prophylactic treatment after electroconversion of atrial fibrillation. Clin Cardiol 13(4):279–286, 1990.

186. Hirsh J, Guyatt G, Albers GW, et al. The Seventh ACCP Conference on Antithrombotic and Thrombolytic Therapy: evidence-based guidelines. Chest 126(3 Suppl):172S–173S, 2004.

187. Prystowsky EN, Benson DW, Jr., Fuster V, et al. Management of patients with atrial fibrillation. Circulation 93(6):1262–1277, 1996.

188. Black IW, Fatkin D, Sagar KB, et al. Exclusion of atrial thrombus by transesophageal echocardiography does not preclude embolism after cardioversion of atrial fibrillation. A multicenter study. Circulation 89(6):2509–2513, 1994.

189. Klein AL, Grimm RA, Murray RD, et al. Use of transesophageal echocardiography to guide cardioversion in patients with atrial fibrillation. N Engl J Med 344(19):1411–1420, 2001.

190. Capucci A, Lenzi T, Boriani G, et al. Effectiveness of loading oral flecainide for converting recent-onset atrial fibrillation to sinus rhythm in patients without organic heart disease or with only systemic hypertension. Am J Cardiol 70(1):69–72, 1992.

191. Capucci A, Boriani G, Rubino I, et al. A controlled study on oral propafenone versus digoxin plus quinidine in converting recent onset atrial fibrillation to sinus rhythm. Int J Cardiol 43(3):305–313, 1994.

192. Borgeat A, Goy JJ, Maendly R, et al. Flecainide versus quinidine for conversion of atrial fibrillation to sinus rhythm. Am J Cardiol 58(6):496–498, 1986.

193. Suttorp MJ, Kingma JH, Lie AHL, et al. Intravenous flecainide versus verapamil for acute conversion of paroxysmal atrial fibrillation or flutter to sinus rhythm. Am J Cardiol 63(11):693–696, 1989.

194. Suttorp MJ, Kingma JH, Jessurun ER, et al. The value of class IC antiarrhythmic drugs for acute conversion of paroxysmal atrial fibrillation or flutter to sinus rhythm. J Am Coll Cardiol 16(7):1722–1727, 1990.

195. Kochiadakis GE, Igoumenidis NE, Solomou MC, et al. Efficacy of amiodarone for the termination of persistent atrial fibrillation. Am J Cardiol 83(1):58–61, 1999.

196. Vardas PE, Kochiadakis GE, Igoumenidis NE, et al. Amiodarone as a first-choice drug for restoring sinus rhythm in patients with atrial fibrillation: a randomized, controlled study. Chest 117(6):1538–1545, 2000.

197. Galve E, Rius T, Ballester R, et al. Intravenous amiodarone in treatment of recent–onset atrial fibrillation: results of a randomized, controlled study. J Am Coll Cardiol 27(5):1079–1082, 1996.

198. Falk RH, Pollak A, Singh SN, et al. Intravenous dofetilide, a class III antiarrhythmic agent, for the termination of sustained atrial fibrillation or flutter. Intravenous Dofetilide Investigators. J Am Coll Cardiol 29(2):385–390, 1997.

199. Norgaard BL, Wachtell K, Christensen PD, et al. Efficacy and safety of intravenously administered dofetilide in acute termination of atrial fibrillation and flutter: a multicenter, randomized, double-blind, placebo-controlled trial. Danish Dofetilide in Atrial Fibrillation and Flutter Study Group. Am Heart J 137(6):1062–1069, 1999.

200. Peuhkurinen K, Niemela M, Ylitalo A, et al. Effectiveness of amiodarone as a single oral dose for recent-onset atrial fibrillation. Am J Cardiol 85(4):462–465, 2000.

201. Stambler BS, Wood MA, Ellenbogen KA. Comparative efficacy of intravenous ibutilide versus procainamide for enhancing termination of atrial flutter by atrial overdrive pacing. Am J Cardiol 77(11):960–966, 1996.

202. Stambler BS, Wood MA, Ellenbogen KA, et al. Efficacy and safety of repeated intravenous doses of ibutilide for rapid conversion of atrial flutter or fibrillation. Ibutilide Repeat Dose Study Investigators. Circulation 94(7):1613–1621, 1996.

203. Guo GB, Ellenbogen KA, Wood MA, et al. Conversion of atrial flutter by ibutilide is associated with increased atrial cycle length variability. J Am Coll Cardiol 27(5):1083–1089, 1996.

204. Boriani G, Capucci A, Lenzi T, et al. Propafenone for conversion of recent–onset atrial fibrillation. A controlled comparison between oral loading dose and intravenous administration. Chest 108(2):355–358, 1995.

205. Boriani G, Biffi M, Capucci A, et al. Oral propafenone to convert recent–onset atrial fibrillation in patients with and without underlying heart disease. A randomized, controlled trial. Ann Intern Med 126(8):621–625, 1997.

206. Boriani G, Diemberger I, Biffi M, et al. Pharmacological cardioversion of atrial fibrillation: current management and treatment options. Drugs 64(24):2741–2762, 2004.

207. Joglar JA, Hamdan MH, Ramaswamy K, et al. Initial energy for elective external cardioversion of persistent atrial fibrillation. Am J Cardiol 86(3):348–350, 2000.

208. Morris DC, Hurst JW. Atrial fibrillation. Curr Probl Cardiol 5(1):1–51, 1980.

209. Dalzell GW, Anderson J, Adgey AA. Factors determining success and energy requirements for cardioversion of atrial fibrillation: revised version. Q J Med 78(285):85–95, 1991.

210. Mann DL, Maisel AS, Atwood JE, et al. Absence of cardioversion-induced ventricular arrhythmias in patients with therapeutic digoxin levels. J Am Coll Cardiol 5(4):882–890, 1985.

211. Van Gelder IC, Crijns HJ, Tieleman RG, et al. Chronic atrial fibrillation. Success of serial cardioversion therapy and safety of oral anticoagulation. Arch Intern Med 156(22):2585–2592, 1996.

212. Suttorp MJ, Kingma JH, Koomen EM, et al. Recurrence of paroxysmal atrial fibrillation or flutter after successful cardioversion in patients with normal left ventricular function. Am J Cardiol 71(8):710–713, 1993.

213. Wyse DG, Waldo AL, DiMarco JP, et al. A comparison of rate control and rhythm control in patients with atrial fibrillation. N Engl J Med 347(23):1825–1833, 2002.

214. Blackshear JL, Safford RE. AFFIRM and RACE trials: implications for the management of atrial fibrillation. Card Electrophysiol Rev 7(4):366–369, 2003.

215. Van Gelder IC, Hagens VE, Bosker HA, et al. A comparison of rate control and rhythm control in patients with recurrent persistent atrial fibrillation. N Engl J Med 347(23):1834–1840, 2002.

216. Treatment of atrial fibrillation. Recommendations from a workshop arranged by the Medical Products Agency (Uppsala, Sweden) and the Swedish Society of Cardiology. Eur Heart J 14(10):1427–1433, 1993.

217. Petersen P, Boysen G, Godtfredsen J, et al. Placebo-controlled, randomised trial of warfarin and aspirin for prevention of thromboembolic complications in chronic atrial fibrillation. The Copenhagen AFASAK study. Lancet 1(8631):175–179, 1989.

218. The effect of low-dose warfarin on the risk of stroke in patients with nonrheumatic atrial fibrillation. N Engl J Med 325(2):129–132, 1991.

219. Stroke Prevention in Atrial Fibrillation Study. Final results. Circulation 84(2):527–539, 1991.

220. Connolly SJ, Laupacis A, Gent M, et al. Canadian Atrial Fibrillation Anticoagulation (CAFA) Study. J Am Coll Cardiol 18(2):349–355, 1991.

221. Ezekowitz MD, Bridgers SL, James KE, et al. Warfarin in the prevention of stroke associated with nonrheumatic atrial fibrillation. Veterans Affairs Stroke Prevention in Nonrheumatic Atrial Fibrillation Investigators. N Engl J Med 327(20):1406–1412, 1992.

222. Risk factors for stroke and efficacy of antithrombotic therapy in atrial fibrillation. Analysis of pooled data from five randomized controlled trials. Arch Intern Med 154(13):1449–1457, 1994.

223. Warfarin versus aspirin for prevention of thromboembolism in atrial fibrillation: Stroke Prevention in Atrial Fibrillation II Study. Lancet 343(8899):687–691, 1994.

224. Levine MN, Hirsh J, Landefeld S, Raskob G. Hemorrhagic complications of anticoagulant treatment. Chest 102(4 Suppl):352S–363S, 1992.

225. Gronefeld GC, Lilienthal J, Kuck KH, et al. Impact of rate versus rhythm control on quality of life in patients with persistent atrial fibrillation. Results from a prospective randomized study. Eur Heart J 24(15):1430–1436, 2003.

226. Hohnloser SH, Kuck KH. Randomized trial of rhythm or rate control in atrial fibrillation: the Pharmacological Intervention in Atrial Fibrillation Trial (PIAF). Eur Heart J 22(10):801–802, 2001.

227. Pritchett EL. Management of atrial fibrillation. N Engl J Med 326(19):1264–1271, 1992.

228. Cox JL, Boineau JP, Schuessler RB, et al. Five-year experience with the maze procedure for atrial fibrillation. Ann Thorac Surg 56(4):814–824, 1993.

229. Jais P, Shah DC, Takahashi A, et al. Long-term follow-up after right atrial radiofrequency catheter treatment of paroxysmal atrial fibrillation. Pacing Clin Electrophysiol 21(11 Pt 2):2533–2538, 1998.

230. Natale A, Newby KH, Pisano E, et al. Prospective randomized comparison of antiarrhythmic therapy versus first-line radiofrequency ablation in patients with atrial flutter. J Am Coll Cardiol 35(7):1898–1904, 2000.

231. Creswell LL, Schuessler RB, Rosenbloom M, et al. Hazards of postoperative atrial arrhythmias. Ann Thorac Surg 56(3):539–549, 1993.

232. Andrews TC, Reimold SC, Berlin JA, et al. Prevention of supraventricular arrhythmias after coronary artery bypass surgery. A meta-analysis of randomized control trials. Circulation 84(5 Suppl):III236–244, 1991.

233. Dixon FE, Genton E, Vacek JL, et al. Factors predisposing to supraventricular tachyarrhythmias after coronary artery bypass grafting. Am J Cardiol 58(6):476–478, 1986.

234. Aranki SF, Shaw DP, Adams DH, et al. Predictors of atrial fibrillation after coronary artery surgery. Current trends and impact on hospital resources. Circulation 94(3):390–397, 1996.

235. Parikka H, Toivonen L, Heikkila L, et al. Comparison of sotalol and metoprolol in the prevention of atrial fibrillation after coronary artery bypass surgery. J Cardiovasc Pharmacol 31(1):67–73, 1998.

236. Guarnieri T, Nolan S, Gottlieb SO, et al. Intravenous amiodarone for the prevention of atrial fibrillation after open heart surgery: the Amiodarone Reduction in Coronary Heart (ARCH) trial. J Am Coll Cardiol 34(2):343–347, 1999.

237. VanderLugt JT, Mattioni T, Denker S, et al. Efficacy and safety of ibutilide fumarate for the conversion of atrial arrhythmias after cardiac surgery. Circulation 100(4):369–375, 1999.

238. Brodsky M, Wu D, Denes P, et al. Arrhythmias documented by 24-hour continuous electrocardiographic monitoring in 50 male medical students without apparent heart disease. Am J Cardiol 39(3):390–395, 1977.

239. Echt DS, Liebson PR, Mitchell LB, et al. Mortality and morbidity in patients receiving encainide, flecainide, or placebo. The Cardiac Arrhythmia Suppression Trial. N Engl J Med 324(12):781–788, 1991.

240. Preliminary report: effect of encainide and flecainide on mortality in a randomized trial of arrhythmia suppression after MI. The Cardiac Arrhythmia Suppression Trial (CAST) Investigators. N Engl J Med 321(6):406–412, 1989.

241. Riddle K, Lee AJ. Digibind: emergency treatment for digitalis toxicity. J Emerg Nurs 15(3):266–268, 1989.

242. Bigger JT, Jr., Weld FM, Rolnitzky LM. Prevalence, characteristics and significance of ventricular tachycardia (three or more complexes) detected with ambulatory electrocardiographic recording in the late hospital phase of acute MI. Am J Cardiol 48(5):815–823, 1981.

243. Manolis AS, Linzer M, Salem D, et al. Syncope: current diagnostic evaluation and management. Ann Intern Med 112(11):850–863, 1990.

244. Blanck Z, Dhala A, Deshpande S, et al. Catheter ablation of ventricular tachycardia. Am Heart J 127(4 Pt 2):1126–1133, 1994.

245. Zheng ZJ, Croft JB, Giles WH, et al. Sudden cardiac death in the United States, 1989 to 1998. Circulation 104(18):2158–2163, 2001.

246. Myerburg RJ. Sudden cardiac death: exploring the limits of our knowledge. J Cardiovasc Electrophysiol 12(3):369–381, 2001.

247. Zipes DP, Wellens HJ. Sudden cardiac death. Circulation 98(21):2334–2351, 1998.

248. Cummins RO, Ornato JP, Thies WH, et al. Improving survival from sudden cardiac arrest: the "chain of survival" concept. Circulation 83(5):1832–1847, 1991.

249. Part 4: the automated external defibrillator: key link in the chain of survival. European Resuscitation Council. Resuscitation 46(1–3):73–91, 2000.

250. Part 1: Introduction to the International Guidelines 2000 for CPR and ECC: a consensus on science. Circulation 102(8 Suppl):I1–11, 2000.

251. Part 6: advanced cardiovascular life support. Section 1: introduction to ACLS 2000: overview of recommended changes in ACLS from the guidelines 2000 conference. European Resuscitation Council. Resuscitation 46(1–3):103–107, 2000.

252. Bocker D, Haverkamp W, Block M, et al. Comparison of d,l-sotalol and implantable defibrillators for treatment of sustained ventricular tachycardia or fibrillation in patients with coronary artery disease. Circulation 94(2):151–157, 1996.

253. Connolly SJ, Gent M, Roberts RS, et al. Canadian implantable defibrillator study (CIDS): a randomized trial of the implantable cardioverter defibrillator against amiodarone. Circulation 101(11):1297–1302, 2000.

254. Kuck KH, Cappato R, Siebels J, et al. Randomized comparison of antiarrhythmic drug therapy with implantable defibrillators in patients resuscitated from cardiac arrest: the Cardiac Arrest Study Hamburg (CASH). Circulation 102(7):748–754, 2000.

255. A comparison of antiarrhythmic drug therapy with implantable defibrillators in patients resuscitated from near-fatal ventricular arrhythmias. The Antiarrhythmics versus Implantable Defibrillators (AVID) Investigators. N Engl J Med 337(22):1576–1583, 1997.

256. Cairns JA, Connolly SJ, Roberts R, et al. Randomised trial of outcome after MI in patients with frequent or repetitive ventricular premature depolarisations: CAMIAT. Canadian Amiodarone Myocardial Infarction Arrhythmia Trial Investigators. Lancet 349(9053):675–682, 1997.

257. Doval HC, Nul DR, Grancelli HO, et al. Randomised trial of low-dose amiodarone in severe congestive heart failure. Grupo de Estudio de la Sobrevida en la Insuficiencia Cardiaca en Argentina (GESICA). Lancet 344(8921):493–498, 1994.

258. Julian DG, Camm AJ, Frangin G, et al. Randomised trial of effect of amiodarone on mortality in patients with left ventricular dysfunction after recent MI: EMIAT. European Myocardial Infarct Amiodarone Trial Investigators. Lancet 349(9053):667–674, 1997.

259. Massie BM, Fisher SG, Radford M, et al. Effect of amiodarone on clinical status and left ventricular function in patients with congestive heart failure. CHF-STAT Investigators. Circulation 93(12):2128–2134, 1996.

260. Bigger JT, Jr. Prophylactic use of implanted cardiac defibrillators in patients at high risk for ventricular arrhythmias after coronary artery bypass graft surgery. Coronary Artery Bypass Graft (CABG) Patch Trial Investigators. N Engl J Med 337(22):1569–1575, 1997.

261. Buxton AE, Lee KL, Fisher JD, et al. A randomized study of the prevention of sudden death in patients with coronary artery disease. Multicenter Unsustained Tachycardia Trial Investigators. N Engl J Med 341(25):1882–1890, 1999.

262. Moss AJ, Hall WJ, Cannom DS, et al. Improved survival with an implanted defibrillator in patients with coronary disease at high risk for ventricular arrhythmia. Multicenter Automatic Defibrillator Implantation Trial Investigators. N Engl J Med 335(26):1933–1940, 1996.

263. Moss AJ, Zareba W, Hall WJ, et al. Prophylactic implantation of a defibrillator in patients with MI and reduced ejection fraction. N Engl J Med 346(12):877–883, 2002.

264. Bardy GH, Lee KL, Mark DB, et al. Amiodarone or an implantable cardioverter–defibrillator for congestive heart failure. N Engl J Med 352(3):225–237, 2005.

265. Teng MP, Catherwood LE, Melby DP. Cost effectiveness of therapies for atrial fibrillation. A review. Pharmacoeconomics 18(4): 317–333, 2000.

266. Klein AL, Murray RD, Becker ER, et al. Economic analysis of a transesophageal echocardiography–guided approach to cardioversion of patients with atrial fibrillation: the ACUTE economic data at eight weeks. J Am Coll Cardiol 43(7):1217–1224, 2004.

267. Marshall DA, Levy AR, Vidaillet H, et al. Cost effectiveness of rhythm versus rate control in atrial fibrillation. Ann Intern Med 141(9):653–661, 2004.

268. Hagens VE, Vermeulen KM, TenVergert EM, et al. Rate control is more cost effective than rhythm control for patients with persistent atrial fibrillation—results from the RAte Control versus Electrical cardioversion (RACE) study. Eur Heart J 25(17):1542–1549, 2004.

269. Hlatky MA, Sanders GD, Owens DK. Cost effectiveness of the implantable cardioverter defibrillator. Card Electrophysiol Rev 7(4): 479–482, 2003.

270. Owens DK, Sanders GD, Heidenreich PA, et al. Effect of risk stratification on cost effectiveness of the implantable cardioverter defibrillator. Am Heart J 144(3):440–448, 2002.

Ischemic Heart Disease

23

Brian R. Overholser and Kevin M. Sowinski

TREATMENT GOALS

The goals of treatment for ischemic heart disease are twofold:

- Reduce cardiovascular morbidity and mortality.
- Minimize the frequency and severity of angina and increase functional capacity, while causing as few adverse effects as possible.

DEFINITION

Angina pectoris is a clinical syndrome of chest discomfort caused by reversible myocardial ischemia that produces disturbances in myocardial function without causing myocardial necrosis. Myocardial ischemia occurs secondary to increased myocardial demand and/or decreased myocardial oxygen supply. The specific causes of increased demand and decreased supply will be discussed. Myocardial ischemia causes several syndromes referred to collectively as ischemic heart disease including: stable angina, variant or Prinzmetal's angina, silent myocardial ischemia, and unstable angina. Unstable angina is discussed in detail in Chapter 24, and the goals of therapy for the remaining syndromes are discussed individually in this chapter.

EPIDEMIOLOGY

Chronic stable angina is initially present in approximately half of patients diagnosed with ischemic heart disease.[1] Ischemic heart disease, generally a manifestation of atherosclerotic coronary artery disease, is the leading cause of death in the United States. In 2001, coronary artery disease caused approximately 500,000 deaths (1 in every 5 deaths) in the United States.[2,3] The cost of treating coronary artery disease in 2004 is estimated at $133.2 billion.[3] It is difficult to estimate the prevalence of angina in the population as a whole, because its prevalence is affected by age, gender, and cardiovascular risk factor profile. Prevalence increases with age, is greater in males, and is dependent on the number of cardiovascular risk factors present. The average annual mortality rate from angina secondary to atherosclerosis is highly variable and is related to coronary artery anatomy, age, gender, other cardiovascular risk factors, anginal functional class, and the ischemic syndrome (i.e., stable angina, unstable angina, etc.) with which the patient presents.[4,5]

PATHOPHYSIOLOGY

Angina pectoris commonly is associated with large single- to multivessel atherosclerotic coronary artery disease, coronary artery vasospasm, or both. Significant coronary artery disease is generally defined as a 70% or greater atherosclerotic reduction of intraluminal area in one of the major epicardial coronary vessels or a 50% reduction of the left main coronary artery. Most patients presenting with angina have significant coronary disease although symptoms can manifest with less severe atherosclerotic stenosis.[6] The pathogenesis of atherosclerosis is discussed in detail in Chapter 41. The Third Report of the Expert Panel on Detection, Evaluation, and Treatment of High Blood Cholesterol in Adults[7] outlines the following as major risk factors for the development of atherosclerotic coronary artery disease: dyslipidemia [elevated low density lipoprotein (LDL) cholesterol or reduced high density lipoprotein (HDL) cholesterol], family history of premature myocardial infarction (MI) or sudden death, cigarette smoking, hypertension, diabetes mellitus, males >45 years of age, and females >55 years of age. The American Heart Association has additionally classified obesity as a major risk factor for the development of coronary artery disease.[8] In addition to these major risk factors, other clearly identified risk factors that may increase cardiovascular risk are: sedentary lifestyle, hypertriglyceridemia, small LDL particles, increased lipoprotein(a) concentrations, increased serum homocysteine concentrations, abnormalities in coagulation factors and markers of chronic infection or inflammation.[9,10]

Although most patients with ischemic heart disease have significant occlusions in one of the major epicardial coronary arteries, there is little correlation between the extent of atherosclerotic coronary artery disease and the severity of anginal symptoms.[11] Usually, the severity of anginal symptoms tends to be more significant in patients with multivessel coronary artery disease than in patients with single-vessel coronary artery disease, but, in any given patient, the extent of underlying atherosclerotic coronary artery disease cannot be predicted from the severity, nature, duration, or quality of discomfort. Two common examples of a lack of a correlation between clinical symptoms and underlying pathology are (a) a patient with advanced three-vessel coronary artery disease who does not experience angina but only silent myocardial ischemia or (b) a patient with Prinzmetal's (variant) angina with episodes of excruciating angina yet minimal or no coronary atherosclerosis.[11] In addition, the severity and duration of anginal symptoms is not necessarily related to prognosis. Prognosis is poorer in patients with left main coronary artery disease or three-vessel coronary artery disease and poor left ventricular systolic function.[4,11,12]

MYOCARDIAL OXYGEN SUPPLY AND DEMAND

Myocardial ischemia is caused by an imbalance between coronary blood flow (supply) and the metabolic needs of the myocardium (demand). Myocardial ischemia occurs when myocardial oxygen demand exceeds myocardial oxygen supply. It is useful to describe the determinants of myocardial oxygen supply and demand since drug therapy is designed to affect the balance between these variables (Fig. 23.1). The major determinants of myocardial oxygen demand are heart rate, contractility, and left ventricular systolic wall tension.[13] Of the three determinants, heart rate is the easiest to assess clinically with current drug therapies. Myocardial contractility refers to the rate of rise in the intraventricular pressure during isovolumetric contraction and is influenced by a number of variables including: the autonomic nervous system, heart rate, blood calcium concentration, and body temperature. Clinical assessment of the beneficial effects of drugs on myocardial contractility is difficult. The third determinant, systolic wall tension, is directly related to the ventricular systolic pressure and ventricular wall radius and is inversely related to wall thickness. Preload and afterload are important components of these factors. Reducing systolic blood pressure reduces afterload, which ultimately decreases oxygen demand. Reductions in preload reduce left ventricular dimension and ultimately reduce myocardial oxygen demand. One can clinically estimate myocardial oxygen demand by using the double-product (product of heart rate and systolic blood pressure). While the double-product provides a useful estimate of myocardial oxygen demand, it does not take contractility into consideration.

Myocardial oxygen supply is determined by two factors: coronary blood flow and the oxygen-carrying capacity of blood.[13] Although the oxygen-carrying capacity can be affected by certain conditions (e.g., anemia), the most important determinant of myocardial oxygen supply is coronary

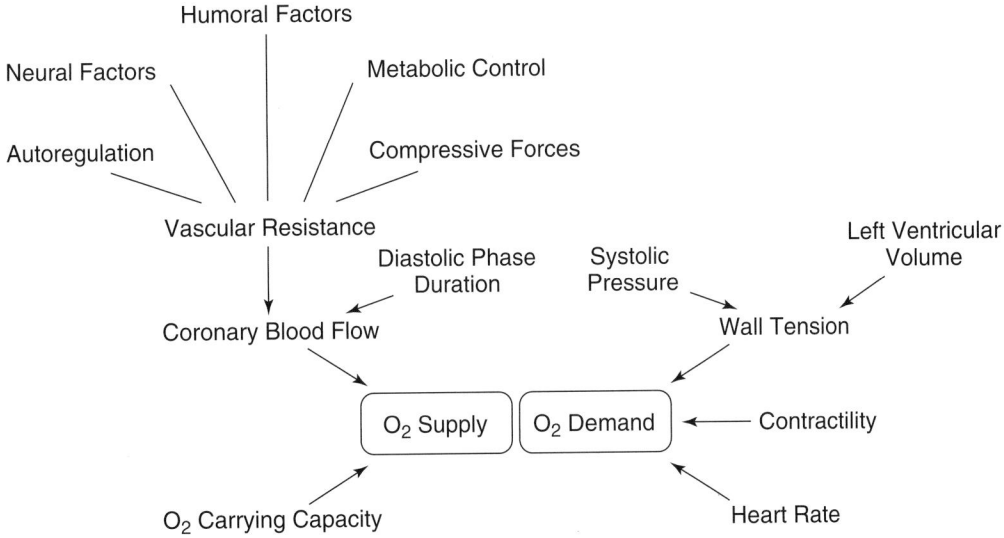

FIGURE 23.1 Factors affecting myocardial oxygen supply and demand. (Adapted from Ardehali A, Ports TA. Myocardial oxygen supply and demand. Chest 98:699–705, 1990, with permission.)

blood flow. Normally, the arteriolar resistance vessels are the most important regulators of coronary blood flow, whereas large epicardial arteries are low-resistance vessels. Myocardial ischemia develops when narrowing of the epicardial vessels by vasospasm or atherosclerosis results in high enough resistance to restrict coronary blood flow. Complex factors that determine coronary blood flow are the duration of diastole and coronary vascular resistance. Coronary vascular resistance is determined by metabolic control, autoregulation, extravascular compressive forces, and humoral and neural factors.

Drugs may precipitate ischemia or infarction by increasing myocardial oxygen demand and/or decreasing myocardial oxygen supply.[2] A few examples of these agents are cocaine (increased demand via increase heart rate and blood pressure and decreased supply via coronary vasoconstriction), ergot alkaloids (decreased supply via coronary vasoconstriction), β-agonists (increased demand via increase heart rate) oral contraceptives/estrogen replacement therapy (coronary artery thrombosis), and cytotoxic drugs.

CLINICAL PRESENTATION AND DIAGNOSIS

SIGNS AND SYMPTOMS

Chronic stable angina pectoris is termed stable because the characteristics of a given patient's anginal history (frequency, severity, duration of symptoms, time of day, etc.) is not changing with time.[11] Patients with stable angina are often classified as having mainly fixed-threshold angina or mainly variable-threshold angina. Anginal syndromes in patients with fixed-threshold angina or exertional angina are precipitated by increased myocardial oxygen demand and tend to occur at some reproducible level of myocardial work. This type of angina is caused by increased myocardial oxygen demand, associated with a fixed-obstruction of an epicardial coronary artery by an atherosclerotic plaque. During periods of increased metabolic demand (e.g., physical exertion), delivery of oxygen-carrying blood through the stenotic atherosclerotic coronary artery is insufficient to meet the myocardium's oxygen requirements, resulting in myocardial ischemia. Typically, an individual can predict what level of physical activity is likely to produce an anginal attack (e.g., walking up two flights of stairs, walking around the block, etc.). On any given day this is fairly reproducible. In contrast, patients with variable-threshold angina have difficulty predicting when or with what level of exertion they will experience an anginal attack. Daily anginal threshold is extremely variable causing these patients to have "good" and "bad" days. The reason for the somewhat variable threshold for causing angina is likely related to a predominance of a vasoconstrictive component leading to decreased oxygen supply and subsequent myocardial ischemia. Although individuals with variable-threshold angina have atherosclerosis, dynamic narrowing of the coronary vasculature by coronary vasoconstriction is important in the genesis of anginal symptoms. Finally, while it is easy to classify angina into the two

extremes of increased demand or decreased supply, most patients fall somewhere in between, often called mixed angina.[14]

Classically, angina presents as substernal, retrosternal, or transsternal discomfort that, usually radiates to the neck and left arm. Some patients may experience radiation to other areas of the body including the right arm. The quality of discomfort varies from patient to patient, which reflects wide variability in the way in which patients perceive pain and discomfort. The discomfort is usually a dull rather than a sharp or stabbing pain and patients may describe it as a strangling or constricting sensation. Patients often use the following descriptors to describe the discomfort: pressure, heaviness, fullness, squeezing, burning, aching, gas, "vise-like," or anxiety. It is important to realize that the severity of discomfort may range from slight discomfort to disabling pain. Anginal discomfort usually has a gradual onset and lasts only a few minutes if the precipitating factor is removed, and relief is usually afforded by rest and/or nitroglycerin. Longer durations of angina may imply severe ischemia, coronary vasospasm, unstable angina, and/or impending or ongoing MI. Symptoms lasting for several days are unlikely to be angina. The frequency of anginal attacks ranges from several per day to one per week or month. The New York Heart Association and Canadian Cardiovascular Society functional classifications (Table 23.1) for angina are the most widely used classification systems for assessing the frequency and patterns of angina. The classification systems can be used in documenting improvements or worsening in status but are not very useful for this purpose due to their broad classifications of the disease. In addition to the functional classifications, patient diaries documenting times and duration of anginal episodes and consumption of sublingual nitroglycerin should be used to classify anginal patterns and to monitor the effectiveness of prophylactic drug therapy and disease severity. Examples of activities that can be carried out by patients in each functional class are illustrated in Table 23.1. An increase in the consumption of sublingual nitroglycerin, number or duration of anginal episodes suggests worsening of the disease process and/or ineffectiveness of prophylactic drug therapy.

A partial list of the factors associated with the provocation of anginal episodes include: physical exertion, emotions (anger, excitation, frustration, anxiety), exposure to cold, heat, and humidity, meals, and sexual intercourse. Patients with variable-threshold angina tend to complain of angina evoked by changes in air temperature, emotion, and meals. Those factors that tend to increase myocardial oxygen demand (exertion, sexual intercourse, etc.) precipitate angina in those patients with fixed obstructions.

Certain patients may not experience typical symptoms of angina when experiencing myocardial ischemia, but rather have what are termed anginal equivalents.[2] Anginal equivalents are episodes of myocardial ischemia that may result in symptoms not necessarily associated with chest discomfort or other symptoms characteristic of anginal discomfort. Anginal equivalents are usually caused by exertion and are relieved by rest or nitroglycerin. Common symptoms of anginal equivalents include exertional dyspnea, fatigue, and exhaustion.

Table 23.1	Classification of Angina Pectoris		
Class	**New York Heart Association Functional Classification**	**Canadian Cardiovascular Society Functional Classification**	**Specific Activity Scale**
I	Symptoms occur with unusual activity, minimal or no functional impairment	*Angina does not occur with ordinary physical activity (walking, climbing stairs) but may occur with strenuous, rapid, or prolonged exertion (work, recreation).*	Patients can perform to completion any activity requiring ≤7 metabolic equivalents, e.g., can carry 24 lb up eight steps; carry objects that weigh 80 lb; do outdoor work (shovel snow, spade soil); do recreational activities (skiing, basketball, squash, handball, jog/walk 5 mph).
II	Symptoms occur with prolonged or slightly more than usual activity, mild functional impairment	*Slight limitation of ordinary activity.* Angina may occur with walking or climbing stairs rapidly, after meals, in the cold, in the wind or under emotional stress, walking uphill, walking more than two blocks on the level and climbing one flight of stairs at a normal pace under normal conditions.	Patients can perform to completion any activity requiring ≤5 metabolic equivalents—e.g., have sexual intercourse without stopping, garden (rake, weed), roller skate, dance fox trot, walk at 4 mph on level ground—but cannot and do not perform to completion any activity requiring ≥7 m Eq.
III	Symptoms occur with usual activities of daily living, moderate functional impairment	*Marked limitation of ordinary physical activity.* Angina may occur after walking one or two level blocks or climbing one flight of stairs in normal conditions at a normal pace.	Patients can perform to completion any activity requiring ≤2 mEq, e.g., shower without stopping, strip and make bed, clean windows, walk 2.5 mph, play golf, dress without stopping, but cannot and do not perform to completion any activity requiring ≥5 mEq.
IV	Symptoms occur at rest, severe functional impairment	*Inability to carry on any physical activity without discomfort.* Angina may be present at rest.	Patients cannot and do not perform to completion any activity requiring ≥2 mEq. Cannot carry out activities listed above.

(Adapted from: Goldman L, Hashimoto B, Loscalzo A. Comparative reproducibility and validity of systems for assessing cardiovascular functional class: advantages of a new specific activity scale. Circulation 64:1227, 1981. Copyright 1981, American Heart Association, with permission.)

In addition to symptomatic ischemia, many patients have myocardial ischemia in the absence of angina or anginal equivalents, termed silent myocardial ischemia. Silent myocardial ischemia is detected by exercise and pharmacologically induced stress electrocardiogram (ECG) testing (as asymptomatic ST-segment depression), by ambulatory ECG testing, or a combination of these tests.[15,16] Patients with silent myocardial ischemia are categorized into three types, patients with coronary artery disease who are totally asymptomatic (type 1), patients who are post-MI and have asymptomatic ischemia (type 2), and patients who experience symptomatic and asymptomatic ischemia (type 3). The incidence of silent myocardial ischemia is variable depending on the patient characteristics. In totally asymptomatic patients, the incidence is 2.5% to 3%, whereas in patients post-MI it is 30% to 43%.[15] Silent myocardial ischemia is present in approximately half of the patients with symptomatic ischemia. The prognostic value of silent myocardial ischemia can vary depending on the type of patient and the diagnostic procedure (i.e., stress testing vs. ambulatory ECG monitoring). Asymptomatic patients with coronary artery disease and a positive exercise ECG are at increased risk for coronary events, including MI, and death compared to the general population.[2] It is well established that the presence of is-

chemia manifesting as symptomatic, asymptomatic, or both is of prognostic importance. It is, however, less clear if silent myocardial ischemia contributes additional prognostic information to already symptomatic patients.[15]

Variant angina or Prinzmetal's angina is myocardial ischemia that is associated with coronary artery vasospasm and is not necessarily associated with atherosclerotic coronary artery disease. Imbalance between myocardial oxygen supply and demand is caused by reduced myocardial oxygen supply due to a critical narrowing of a large coronary vessel. The clinical manifestations of variant angina are similar to those seen with stable angina, although the pain may be somewhat more intense. The patient's history of angina is usually different than chronic stable angina because pain usually occurs at rest—most frequently between midnight and 8:00 AM.

Circadian rhythms are known to affect anginal occurrence. In fact, the incidence of MI, sudden cardiac death, Prinzmetal's angina, silent myocardial ischemia, and myocardial ischemia associated with stable angina is higher in the morning hours.[17] In addition, the threshold for precipitation of anginal attacks tends to be lower in the morning. This phenomenon may lead to patients experiencing anginal attacks in the morning at lower levels of exertion than would be necessary at other times of day. Patients should be instructed to perform morning activities at a somewhat slower pace to minimize the possibility of provoking myocardial ischemia.

DIAGNOSIS

Clinical Findings. While a detailed discussion of diagnostic procedures for chronic stable angina is beyond the scope of this text, the reader is directed to additional references.[1,2] The physical examination may be normal in patients with ischemic heart disease or it may reveal the presence of other risk factors for development of atherosclerotic coronary artery disease. The resting ECG is normal in approximately one half of patients with chronic stable angina.[18] Abnormal ECG findings include ST-segment depression, T wave inversion, and in patients with Prinzmetal's angina, ST-segment elevation.[19] Ambulatory ECG monitoring may be useful in detecting asymptomatic and symptomatic ischemic episodes as in patients with silent myocardial ischemia.

Exercise Testing. Treadmill or bicycle exercise testing provides a reproducible, objective method to study the relationship between myocardial oxygen supply and myocardial oxygen demand.[20,21] Testing usually is conducted by individualizing a specific protocol, such as the Bruce or Naughton protocols. These protocols allow incremental increases in workload of exercise in stages by increasing the speed and/or incline of the treadmill. Endpoints measured during exercise testing include duration of exercise, workload achieved, ECG changes, blood pressure, heart rate, and symptoms. The product of heart rate and systolic blood pressure (i.e., the *double product*) is used as an index of myocardial oxygen consumption. In patients with known ischemic heart disease (i.e., presence of angina symptoms, previous MI), exercise electrocardiography provides important prognostic information.[22] In addition, exercise testing with concomitant ECG monitoring may be useful in patients with an equivocal history of chest pain for risk stratification to determine whether medical or surgical treatment is appropriate and for assessment of drug efficacy. Short exercise duration with anginal symptoms, exercise-induced hypotension, and early onset of angina with ST-segment depression are all poor prognostic signs for development of cardiovascular events. Potential complications associated with exercise testing include MI, serious arrhythmias, and rarely death. It should be noted that exercise testing in the presence of drug therapy, notably β-blockers and calcium channel blockers, may complicate the interpretation of exercise testing by reducing the maximum heart rate achieved during exercise.

Radionuclide Imaging. Other techniques are also useful in the diagnosis and classification of ischemic heart disease both at rest and during exercise.[23,24] Thallium-201 myocardial perfusion scanning can be used in conjunction with exercise testing to provide additional information regarding reversible and irreversible defects in blood flow to the myocardium. Thallium is a potassium analog that is transported into normal cardiac cells. Thallium is injected at peak exercise and the patient undergoes a myocardial scanning procedure. Perfusion defects that are detected at this point can represent infarcted tissue or stress-induced ischemic tissues. Two to three hours later the patient undergoes repeat myocardial scanning and perfusion defects that are no longer present represent areas of reversible ischemia rather than infarction. Ischemic areas that on the first scan produced defects will now contain thallium. Thallium myocardial perfusion scanning in conjunction with exercise testing appears to be more sensitive and specific in the diagnosis of coronary artery disease, but is more expensive than exercise testing alone, cannot usually be performed in a physician's office, and requires the injection of a radionuclide. A combination test utilizing thallium-201 and the high-energy tracer, technetium-99m, is available that has the advantage of reducing the time of the procedure. Testing with radionucleotides should be reserved for special cases and a regular exercise test almost always should be used first.[2,23,24] In patients who are unable to exercise because of certain medical conditions or other factors (e.g., elderly age, patients with peripheral vascular disease), alternative tests are available that utilize pharmacologic agents to simulate the stress of exercise. Pharmacologic stress testing techniques[25] include dipyridamole- or adenosine-induced vasodilation and arbutamine or dobutamine stress echocardiography in conjunction with thallium myocardial scanning.

Other Diagnostic Techniques. Two-dimensional echocardiography may be useful in the detection of myocardial wall-motion abnormalities at rest and ischemic-induced wall-motion abnormalities during exercise. Echocardiography in conjunction with exercise testing may provide additional information about left ventricular function that would not be provided by exercise testing alone. Electron beam computed tomography is commonly used for the detection of coronary artery calcification, although its use in the diagnosis of coronary artery disease is controversial.[1]

Although each of the previously described tests yields important diagnostic and prognostic information in patients with coronary artery disease, definitive diagnosis and assessment of prognosis can only be attained invasively by cardiac catheterization, coronary arteriography, and left ventricular angiography.[26] These methods allow assessment of the severity of coronary anatomy obstruction and assessment of ventricular function. Left heart cardiac catheterization is accomplished by inserting a catheter into the brachial or femoral artery and advancing it into the left ventricle and coronary arteries. During coronary angiography, radiocontrast dye is injected into the coronary arteries and the coronary artery anatomy is visualized and the extent of coronary obstruction assessed. Due to the cost of this procedure and the risk associated with it, it has been suggested that coronary angiography only be considered under certain circumstances. Patients who may benefit from this procedure include: patients whose angina is unresponsive to maximal medical therapy and who are being considered for revascularization procedures (discussed later in the chapter) or patients in whom the definitive diagnosis of coronary artery disease cannot be made by less invasive means.

PSYCHOSOCIAL ASPECTS

Alterations in lifestyle are important in patients with angina because of certain factors that may provoke anginal episodes. Inclusion of the patient's family in discussions regarding lifestyle modifications may help patient compliance regarding these changes, but more importantly it fosters a family understanding of certain limitations that may be placed on the patient. Patients should be counseled to modify their participation in strenuous activities in an attempt to avoid excessive fatigue and exhaustion that may precipitate anginal attacks. An example of this would be the use of a golf cart rather than walking while playing golf. Another lifestyle modification would be the reduction or elimination of factors known to precipitate an anginal episode. Some patients may know exactly how much exertion they can tolerate before having an anginal attack, other patients may need to "learn" what their threshold is. In general, patients should perform morning activities at a slower pace and avoid sudden bursts of activity. Patients who are particularly susceptible to heat precipitating an anginal attack should have air conditioning. Patients who develop angina when going outside when it is very cold, should cover their mouth and face with a scarf. Eating small meals or napping after meals may help to avoid postprandial anginal attacks. Lastly, emotional outbursts (e.g., anger, anxiety, frustration) should be minimized.

THERAPEUTIC PLAN

The management of ischemic heart disease involves five areas: identification and treatment of concomitant conditions that may exacerbate or precipitate ischemia, correction of concomitant cardiovascular risk factors, lifestyle modifications, medical treatment, and revascularization techniques. Treatment strategies for ischemic heart disease syndromes have traditionally been targeted at symptom relief with nitrates, β-blockers, and calcium channel blockers. However, there is little evidence that these antianginal strategies alone reduce cardiovascular mortality in patients' naïve to an acute coronary event. β-blockers are the only class of drugs used for the symptomatic relief of angina that have been shown to reduce mortality in patients with a previous acute coronary event. There is considerable evidence that aspirin[27-29] and appropriate lipid-lowering therapy[7] reduce cardiovascular morbidity and mortality in primary and secondary prevention trials.

Because most patients with ischemic heart disease have underlying coronary artery disease, correction and treatment of all modifiable cardiovascular risk factors is essential in an effort to reduce the risk for future vascular events. Risk factor reduction should focus on hypertension management, smoking cessation, lipid-lowering therapy, antiplatelet therapy, cardiac rehabilitation, neurohormonal modulation, and weight loss. Although risk factor reductions may not reverse

existing coronary artery disease, they may aid in the secondary prevention of cardiovascular events. As with any disease or syndrome that increases cardiovascular risk (e.g., hypertension), the first goal of therapy is to decrease cardiovascular risk.

The ACC/AHA Practice Guidelines outline the following ABCDE mnemonic for the treatment of patients with chronic stable angina[1]:

A = Aspirin and Antianginal therapy
B = Beta-blocker and Blood pressure
C = Cigarette smoking and Cholesterol
D = Diet and Diabetes
E = Education and Exercise

The following section, "Treatment," discusses the components of the ABCDE treatment mnemonic by outlining strategies for coronary risk factor reduction, detailing the pharmacology of drugs used for the management of anginal symptoms, and combining these topics to discuss pharmacotherapy strategies for patients with chronic stable angina.

TREATMENT

CORONARY RISK FACTOR REDUCTION

Hypertension Management. Treatment of hypertension reduces cardiovascular morbidity and mortality and is the focus of Chapter 20. Blood pressure reduction also reduces myocardial oxygen demand and thus benefits patients with angina. The mortality associated with ischemic heart disease increases exponentially with increasing blood pressure.[30,31] The use of a single drug to treat multiple disease states is desirable and should always be taken into consideration. Antihypertensive agents that are beneficial for the management of anginal symptoms and decrease mortality and morbidity in patients with ischemic heart disease should be encouraged whenever possible.

Smoking Cessation. Intense efforts should be made to encourage smoking cessation to prevent the development or worsening of coronary artery disease. Smoking is associated with increased morbidity and mortality, silent ischemia, arrhythmias, and coronary vasospasm in patients with coronary artery disease.[32] Although controversial, the cessation of smoking has been reported to reduce the risk for sudden cardiac death in patients with overt coronary artery disease.[33] Pharmacologic and nonpharmacologic approaches are available and should be used to assist patients with smoking cessation. Chapter 60 details strategies for the implementation and execution of smoking cessation programs.

Dyslipidemia Management. American Heart Association (AHA)/American College of Cardiology (ACC) guidelines for the use of lipid-lowering therapy in patients with chronic stable angina have been adopted from the third report of the National Cholesterol Education Program Guidelines.[7] Bile acid sequestrants, fibric acid derivatives, 3-hydroxy-3-

methylglutaryl coenzyme A (HMG-CoA) reductase inhibitors, and niacin have beneficial lipid modification effects, including the lowering of total cholesterol. The reduction of total cholesterol with these agents along with diet and exercise have been reported to reduce coronary events.[7]

Drug therapy with HMG-CoA reductase inhibitors in patients with chronic stable angina and/or prior MI with average and elevated serum cholesterol concentrations have been reported in several trials to reduce cardiovascular morbidity and mortality. More recently the Heart Protection Study investigators reported a significant reduction in cardiovascular mortality in high-risk patients randomized to simvastatin irrespective of baseline cholesterol.[34] In addition to the established benefits on mortality, HMG-CoA reductase inhibitor treatment has stabilized vulnerable coronary plaques and hindered the natural progression of atherosclerotic disease.[35,36] These beneficial effects on morbidity have been particularly evident with intensive lipid-lowering treatment.[36,37] The differences in the baseline characteristics of LDL and total cholesterol in these clinical trials indicate that LDL-lowering therapy with HMG-CoA reductase inhibitors should be initiated in all patients with established coronary artery disease. This includes all patients presenting with chronic stable angina without absolute contraindications.

Modification of HDL concentrations may be beneficial in patients with low HDL despite acceptable triglyceride and LDL concentrations. It is well established that low HDL concentrations are associated with increased coronary risks.[7] Additionally, the raising of HDL concentrations with gemfibrozil in patients with normal LDL concentrations has been reported to significantly decrease major cardiovascular events.[38] A detailed discussion of lipid-modifying therapy is the focus of Chapter 41

Antiplatelet Therapy. Platelet aggregation is important in the pathogenesis of acute coronary syndromes, but less important in the pathogenesis of stable angina. Data from two studies in patients with chronic stable angina show that aspirin reduced the incidence of first MI.[27,28] Aspirin inhibits platelet aggregation and thrombus formation at the site of atherosclerotic plaque disruption. Although the lowest effective dose is controversial, it is recommended that all patients without contraindications that have angina or clinical or laboratory evidence of ischemic heart disease receive aspirin (75–325 mg/day) therapy indefinitely.[1]

Alternative pharmacologic approaches to antiplatelet therapy should be considered in patients with contraindications to aspirin therapy. Dipyridamole is an antithrombotic agent with vasodilatory effects that should not be used in patients with stable angina.[39] Ticlopidine and clopidogrel are thienopyridine derivatives that prevent adenosine diphosphate-mediated platelet activation. Ticlopidine has been associated with serious adverse events, including neutropenia that limits its use in clinical practice. Clopidogrel is therefore the agent of choice for patients with an absolute contraindication to aspirin therapy. Clopidogrel appears to be slightly more effective than aspirin in decreasing the composite endpoints of MI, vascular death, or ischemic stroke but more data are needed to confirm its benefits versus the relatively inexpensive aspirin alternative.[40] Antiplatelet therapy in patients with a previous MI will be discussed in Chapter 24.

Angiotensin-Converting Enzyme Inhibitor Therapy. Although angiotensin-converting enzyme (ACE) inhibitors do not have an indication for the symptomatic relief of ischemic heart disease, several large randomized trials have shown that they significantly lower mortality and morbidity rates when used in patients with different severities of coronary artery disease. ACE inhibitor therapy should be used in all patients with ischemic heart disease and left ventricular dysfunction or diabetes without absolute contraindications. The Survival and Ventricular Enlargement (SAVE) trial[41] and the Studies of Left Ventricular Dysfunction (SOLVD)[42] were the first to show that patients with left ventricular dysfunction and coronary artery disease significantly benefit from the addition of ACE inhibitor treatment. The Heart Outcomes Prevention Evaluation (HOPE) trial[43] reported significant mortality and morbidity benefits in high-risk patients with vascular disease or diabetes and no known left ventricular dysfunction that were randomized to ramipril versus placebo. This trial was the first to suggest that the role of ACE inhibitor therapy should be expanded outside of patients with left ventricular dysfunction or diabetes to almost all patients with chronic stable angina. The European Trial on Reduction of Cardiac Events with Perindopril in Stable Coronary Artery Disease (EUROPA) corroborated the findings from the HOPE study, although baseline differences in the patient population did exist.[44] Despite their dissimilarities, the HOPE and EUROPA trials provide convincing evidence that ACE inhibition may have benefits in most patients with chronic stable angina, especially those with additional coronary risk factors. The completion of the Prevention of Events with Angiotensin-Converting Enzyme inhibition (PEACE) trial[45] will add valuable insight into the role of ACE inhibitors in the management of chronic stable angina. Additionally, the angiotensin II receptor blockers (ARBs) promise to be the focus of future investigations in the treatment of coronary artery disease since a reduction in cardiovascular risk recently has been reported in patients receiving low-dose ARB.[46]

Cardiac Rehabilitation. Exercise training reduces cardiovascular mortality, improves functional capacity, and attenuates myocardial ischemia and thus is an important lifestyle modification. Exercise programs should adhere to accepted guidelines[47] for patients with heart disease. Exercise programs are also useful as adjuncts to reducing other coronary risk factors such as obesity, diabetes, and hypertension. Exercise has a beneficial conditioning effect on skeletal and cardiac muscle and may decrease oxygen demand for any level of exercise. Exercise also favorably affects fat and carbohydrate metabolism, which may aid in the reduction of cardiovascular risk.

PHARMACOLOGIC TREATMENT OF ANGINA AND ISCHEMIA

Nitrates

Mechanism of Action. Organic nitrates are prodrugs and must be converted to their active moiety before causing a therapeutic effect. The intracellular mechanism of action of organic nitrates is complex, although organic nitrates are known to be denitrated and liberate nitric oxide by multiple mechanisms. Nitric oxide reacts further with sulfhydryl groups to form S-nitrosothiols. The presence of sulfhydryl groups is necessary for the formation of nitric oxide and S-nitrosothiols and subsequent stimulation of guanylate cyclase.[48,49] Nitric oxide and/or S-nitrosothiols can activate smooth muscle guanylate cyclase, resulting in formation of intracellular cyclic guanosine monophosphate (cGMP). Cyclic guanosine monophosphate causes decreased intracellular calcium concentrations by increasing calcium extrusion from the cell.[48,49]

Nitrates act as vasodilators in virtually all vascular beds including veins, arteries, and arterioles. However, higher concentrations are required for vasodilatory effects in arteries and arterioles than in veins. This is especially true for arterioles, which require concentrations that may not be achieved clinically.[50] Hemodynamically, nitrates cause venodilation and thus reductions in venous tone leading to decreased venous return and decreased preload, ultimately resulting in reductions in myocardial oxygen demand. Additionally, at higher concentrations, nitrates may cause arterial vasodilation causing decreased systolic blood pressure and afterload, resulting in reductions in myocardial oxygen demand. However, because nitrates are such potent vasodilators, they may cause reflex sympathetic discharge, attenuating some of the beneficial effects of nitrates.[49,50]

Nitrates may also have several effects on the coronary circulation, including enhancement of coronary collateral blood flow, dilation of normal coronary arteries in patients with atherosclerosis, and dilation of stenotic coronary vessels.[2] Last, nitrates may reverse coronary vasospasm making them particularly useful in treatment of vasospastic angina. These effects may lead to increases in myocardial oxygen supply.

Nitrate Tolerance. A decreased pharmacologic response in the presence of continuously or frequently administered nitrates is well documented and is termed nitrate tolerance. Examples of regimens showing the development of tolerance are 24-hour ('round-the-clock) applications of transdermal nitroglycerin, continuous infusions of intravenous nitroglycerin, immediate-release isosorbide dinitrate (ISDN) administered four times daily, sustained-release isosorbide dinitrate (ISDN-SR) administered every 12 hours, and immediate-release isosorbide mononitrate (ISMN) administered every 12 hours. It is likely that all nitrates cause some degree of

tolerance and attenuation of pharmacologic effect if used continuously.[51] The hemodynamic and antianginal effects are attenuated with continuous administration.

The mechanism for nitrate tolerance appears to be multifactorial and is not well understood. Nitrates have a complex interaction with the endothelium and promote superoxide anion production that can lead to the scavenging of nitric oxide.[52-54] This interaction has been implicated as an underlying mechanism for the development of tolerance, but its relative importance has not been completely established.[55,56] Additional proposed mechanisms of nitrate tolerance include: (a) depletion of sulfhydryl donors impairing the intracellular formation of nitric oxide and S-nitrosothiols, resulting in decreased formation of cGMP; (b) sympathetic activation following vasodilation producing reflex vasoconstriction and sodium retention; (c) vascular production of endothelin-1; and (d) plasma volume expansion, minimizing the ability of nitrates to decrease left ventricular filling pressures.[49,51]

The prevention of nitrate tolerance via pharmacologic intervention based on proposed mechanisms of tolerance has been attempted with ACE inhibitors, thiazide diuretics, and sulfhydryl-donor compounds, although none have been effective clinically.[49,51] A recent investigation has shown benefits of an angiotensin II blocker to suppress the development of nitrate tolerance with transdermal nitroglycerin therapy, despite negative results from ACE inhibitor trials.[57] Additionally, L-arginine supplementation may decrease superoxide production and has been tested in a placebo-controlled, crossover study to patients with stable angina.[58,59] The administration of L-arginine increased treadmill walking time during continuous transdermal nitroglycerin therapy.[59] The results of these studies will need to be verified in large trials before the routine use of angiotensin II receptor blockers or L-arginine supplementation is implemented into clinical practice.

Currently, the best clinical method for the prevention of nitrate tolerance involves the provision of a daily nitrate-free interval. Nitrate-free intervals of at least 10 to 12 hours per day during chronic dosing have been shown to reduce occurrence of nitrate tolerance.[60-62] The time of day for provision of a nitrate-free interval is usually at night, however in patients who have nocturnal angina (i.e., most of their attacks at night), it would be prudent to move the nitrate-free interval to the daytime hours. Although nitrate-free intervals may benefit those who have angina that occurs predictably, those patients with severe or unpredictable (occurs day and night) angina would be left unprotected during the nitrate-free interval. In such patients, use of β-blockers (alone or in combination with nitrates) or calcium channel blockers (alone or in combination with nitrates) would be appropriate.

Nitrate Products. Table 23.2 lists the nitrates available for clinical use. Sublingual nitroglycerin is used in the management of acute episodes of angina and for prophylaxis against an expected anginal episode. It has been shown to be effec-

| Table 23.2 | Pharmacologic Characteristics of Currently Available Nitrates |

Indication Drug and Dosage Form	Route of Administration	Dose Range	Frequency of Administration (Dosing Interval)
Treatment of acute anginal attacks			
Nitroglycerin sublingual tablets	Sublingual	0.3–0.6 mg	As needed, repeat dose 1–3 times every 5 minutes
Nitroglycerin translingual spray	Sublingual	0.4–0.8 mg	As needed, repeat dose 1–3 times every 5 minutes
Nitroglycerin buccal tablets	Buccal	1–3 mg	Once
ISDN chewable tablets	Chewable	5–10 mg	Once
ISDN sublingual tablets	Sublingual	2.5–10 mg	Once
Prevention of anginal attacks			
Nitroglycerin tablets	Sublingual	0.15–0.6 mg	2–5 minutes before activity
Nitroglycerin spray	Sublingual	0.4–0.8 mg	2–5 minutes before activity
Nitroglycerin buccal tablets	Buccal	1–3 mg	2–5 minutes before activity or every 4–5 hours while awake
Isosorbide dinitrate tablets	Chewable	5–10 mg	5–10 minutes before activity
Isosorbide dinitrate tablets	Sublingual	2.5–10 mg	5–10 minutes before activity
Nitroglycerin SR tablets and capsules	Oral	2.5–26 mg	2–4 times per day; 12-hour dosage-free interval*
Nitroglycerin ointment	Transdermal	$^1/_2$–5 in.	3–4 times per day; 12-hour dosage-free interval*
Nitroglycerin patch	Transdermal	0.1–0.8 mg/hr	Once daily; 12-hour dosage-free interval
Isosorbide dinitrate tablets	Oral	5–40 mg	2–3 times per day; 14-hour dosage-free interval
Isosorbide dinitrate SR capsules and tablets	Oral	40–80 mg	1–2 times per day; 16-hour dosage-free interval*
Isosorbide mononitrate tablets	Oral	10–20 mg	2 times per day 7 hours apart, 17-hour dosage-free interval*
Isosorbide mononitrate SR tablets	Oral	30–240 mg	Once daily

SR sustained release.
* No data are available evaluating the long-term efficacy of these products. The nitrate dosage-free intervals are estimated and are not identical to the nitrate-free period (see text).

tive at increasing exercise time and relieving acute anginal symptoms and is available as sublingual tablets and aerosol spray. In the event of an acute attack, patients should be instructed to sit or lie down, place the dose (spray or tablet) under the tongue, and not swallow the tablet. Relief of pain should occur within 5 minutes. If the pain is not relieved within this time the process may be repeated until a total of three doses have been given (~15 minutes), after which time the patient should contact their physician, dial 911, or be transported to an emergency room. Failure of nitroglycerin to control the pain may be an indication of more serious ischemia or MI. Adverse effects seen with the sublingual form of nitroglycerin include lightheadedness, dizziness, tachycardia, and headache. Patients may or may not experience burning under the tongue after taking the sublingual dose. the absence of which is not necessarily an indication of a lack of dosage potency. Nitroglycerin is a labile com-

pound that requires special storage and handling. Sublingual tablets should be dispensed in the original, unopened, manufacturer's brown bottle. When the bottle is opened the patient should remove the cotton plug and discard it. The tablets should be stored in the manufacturer's brown bottle in a cool, dry place to avoid degradation of the tablets. Patients should be instructed to refill their prescriptions frequently (approximately every 6 months) to ensure adequate potency of the tablets. Because of the storage problems associated with sublingual nitroglycerin, the aerosol spray dosage form has some distinct advantages. Each canister has a shelf life of 2 years, has 200 metered doses, and does not require the same rigid storage conditions as the tablets. The adverse effects and efficacy of each product are similar.[63]

Buccal nitroglycerin tablets provide immediate and long-term delivery of nitroglycerin. The tablet is placed on the gum between the upper teeth and inner lip. A gel forms around the tablet, which contains nitroglycerin impregnated in a cellulose matrix. The tablet can stay in place for hours and provides immediate and sustained delivery of nitroglycerin as long as the tablet remains intact, which may be as long as 6 hours in some patients. This is advantageous in that the tablet can provide acute and prophylactic treatment of anginal episodes. Tolerance to the effects of buccal nitroglycerin is minimal, mainly because the tablet is not in place while the patient sleeps, allowing a nitrate-free interval.

Oral sustained-release formulations of nitroglycerin are available that are administered every 8 to 12 hours. However, there are no data suggesting maintenance of chronic efficacy throughout the duration of the dosing interval. Thus, no data are available to determine which dosing regimen would prevent tolerance (Table 23.2).

Nitroglycerin 2% ointment has documented efficacy in patients with angina.[64] It is easy to use, but rather inconvenient for patients because of the messiness that is involved with application of ointment. Patients should be instructed to apply the specified dose (from $\frac{1}{2}$–5 inches) of ointment to the chest, back, or upper limbs. Patients should rotate the application site daily in an attempt to reduce skin irritation. Family members or others applying the ointment to the patient should be instructed to use gloves during the application because of the chance for nitroglycerin absorption through their skin. The ointment can be easily removed by detaching the paper containing the ointment and wiping the skin clean of any residual ointment. There will be continued absorption of nitroglycerin for a short time because the skin acts as a reservoir for the drug.

Another form of topically available nitroglycerin, which has become enormously popular since their introduction in the early 1980s, is nitroglycerin transdermal patches. These patches deliver a constant amount of nitroglycerin per hour over a specific time period, maintaining constant nitroglycerin concentrations. Patients should be instructed to apply a new patch each day to a hairless area of the chest, back, or upper limbs. The site should be rotated on a daily basis to prevent local skin irritation. Various factors may increase the absorption of the drug, including physical exercise and high temperatures (e.g., saunas). The ease of administration compared to nitroglycerin ointment has made these agents very popular with patients. However, rapid development of nitrate tolerance[65,66] necessitates that patients wear the patch no more than 12 hours per day. Provision of a 12-hour nitrate-free period leads to effective exercise improvement in patients with angina.[60,67]

Two oral organic nitrates are available in the United States, isosorbide dinitrate (ISDN) and isosorbide 5-mononitrate (5-ISMN). Isosorbide 5-mononitrate is a metabolite of ISDN. Both ISDN and 5-ISMN are available as immediate-release and sustained-release preparations. Isosorbide dinitrate is also available as a sublingual and chewable tablet, which can be used for treatment and prophylaxis of acute anginal episodes. The sublingual tablet has a somewhat longer onset of action and a longer duration of action compared to sublingual nitroglycerin. The chewable tablet also has a longer duration of action versus sublingual nitroglycerin. When patients chew the tablet, particles remain in the mouth and continue to be absorbed.

Isosorbide dinitrate has widely variable bioavailability and a plasma half-life of 1 to 2 hours, whereas 5-ISMN has nearly complete bioavailability and a longer plasma half-life,[68] resulting in more predictable concentrations after oral dosing and allowing for once or twice daily dosing. Tolerance to the pharmacologic effects of ISDN and 5-ISMN have been described for both agents in the immediate-release and sustained-release preparations.[61,69] Avoidance of tolerance with ISDN is accomplished by administration of the immediate-release product three times daily at 7:00 AM, 12:00 Noon, and 5:00 PM.[62] This regimen provides a nitrate-free interval during the nighttime period. Twice daily dosing schedules of immediate release 5-ISMN, administered at 8:00 AM and 3:00 PM, enhanced exercise performance for 7 hours after the morning dose and for 5 hours after the afternoon dose.[62,70] Sustained-release 5-ISMN has been shown to be effective for up to 12 hours per day when administered once daily, thus it is recommended this agent be given once daily.[67]

Adverse Effects. Adverse effects caused by all nitrates are an extension of their pharmacologic actions. Headache occurs in most patients and may be described as a throbbing or pulsating sensation. Most patients can take over-the-counter analgesics (aspirin, acetaminophen, etc.) to alleviate this problem. Other adverse effects related to vasodilation include hypotension, dizziness, lightheadedness, and facial flushing. Patients may require lower doses if these adverse effects occur following sublingual doses of nitroglycerin. Reflex tachycardia may also occur due to the potent peripheral vasodilating effects of nitrates, which causes sympathetic nervous system activation. Patients should be instructed to vary the application site of nitroglycerin ointment and transdermal patches to avoid local skin irritation.

The use of the phosphodiesterase-5 inhibitors (sildenafil, vardenafil, and tadalafil) has gained widespread acceptance for the treatment of erectile dysfunction but these inhibitors possess vasodilatory properties similar to that of nitroglycerin. Severe and sometimes fatal hypotension has been reported following the co-administration of sildenafil with nitroglycerin. As a result of these isolated cases, the ACC and AHA have released a consensus statement recommending that phosphodiesterase-5 inhibitors not be used within 24 hours of nitroglycerin.[71] Participation in sexual activity is generally safe for patients with ischemic heart disease but can precipitate angina in some patients, which is termed coital angina. If coital angina is manifested during sexual activity with a phosphodiesterase-5 inhibitor, the patient should be instructed to seek immediate medical attention.

β-Blockers

Mechanism of Action. β-adrenergic receptor blockers competitively inhibit the binding of circulating and neurally released catecholamines to the β-adrenergic receptor.[72,73]

β-receptor blockade attenuates the cardiac responses to adrenergic stimulation by catecholamines. The beneficial effects provided by β-blockers in ischemic heart disease are severalfold. First, β-blockers reduce heart rate mainly during times of sympathetic stimulation that results in reduced cardiac work and thus reduced myocardial oxygen demand. In addition, by slowing heart rate, β-blockers increase diastolic filling time resulting in increased coronary perfusion and improved oxygen supply. Secondly, β-blockers reduce myocardial contractility and arterial blood pressure and as a result of each, reduce myocardial oxygen demand. A potential problem with β-blockers is the potential to promote coronary vasoconstriction. In the presence of blockade of β_2-receptors, which mediate vasodilation, there is unopposed α-receptor-mediated coronary vasoconstriction. This is a particular concern in patients with rest or variant angina where β-blockers could potentially precipitate an anginal episode.

Pharmacologic Characteristics. β-blockers differ in their pharmacologic characteristics, including receptor selectivity, pharmacokinetics, lipophilicity, and intrinsic sympathomimetic activity (Table 23.3).[72,73] β-adrenergic receptors are classified into two major subtypes (β_1-, and β_2-adrenoceptors) based on the physiologic responses they mediate. β_1-receptors predominately reside in the myocardium and their stimulation results in increased heart rate, myocardial contractility, and atrioventricular (AV) nodal conduction. β_2-receptors also reside in the heart but are the predominant receptors in pulmonary and vascular tissue where they are responsible for bronchodilation and vasodilation. β-blockers are classified as *nonselective* or *cardioselective* based on the selectivity at blocking β_1 receptors versus β_2 receptors. Cardioselective agents (atenolol, metoprolol, and acebutolol) are relatively more selective towards binding to β_1-receptors than β_2-receptors, whereas nonselective agents block β_1-receptors and β_2-receptors. Theoretically, β_1-selective agents would be more effective at antagonizing the effects of catecholamines at β_1-receptors, while causing minimal β_2-receptor blockade. β_1-selective antagonists have a theoretical advantage in patients with pulmonary disease (e.g., chronic obstructive pulmonary disease, asthma) or when blockade of β_2-receptor is undesirable, such as in patients with peripheral vascular disease or insulin-dependent diabetes mellitus. However, cardioselectivity is relative and achievement of high enough plasma concentrations, which can occur within the clinically used dosage range, will result in the diminishment of cardioselectivity.

β-blockers that possess intrinsic sympathomimetic activity (ISA) (Table 23.3) produce some degree of β-receptor stimulation at low states of sympathetic activation (e.g., at rest). However, at higher levels of sympathetic activation (e.g., during exercise), these agents act as antagonists. There are few data suggesting that drugs with ISA are more beneficial than agents without ISA in the prevention of angina or ischemia. Because these drugs tend not to lower resting heart rate or cardiac output, they may have theoretical advantages in a patient with already low resting heart rate and cardiac output. Finally, these agents may be detrimental in post-MI patients or those who experience resting angina.

Table 23.3	**Pharmacologic Characteristics of the Orally Available β-blockers**					
Agent	**Receptor Selectivity**	**ISA**	**Lipid Solubility**	**Primary Route of Elimination**	**Half-Life (hr)**	**Usual Maintenance Dose**
Acebutolol	β_1	+	Low–moderate	Renal/hepatic	3–4	200–600 mg BID
Atenolol*	β_1	0	Low	Renal	6–7	50–100 mg QD
Betaxolol	β_1	0	Low	Hepatic	14–22	10–20 mg QD
Bisoprolol	β_1	0	Low	Renal/hepatic	9–12	5–10 mg QD
Carteolol	$\beta_1\beta_2$	++	Low	Renal	5–6	2.5–10 mg QD
Carvedilol	$\beta_1\beta_2\alpha_1$	0	High	Hepatic	2–6	25–50 mg BID
Labetalol	$\beta_1\beta_2\alpha_1$	0	Moderate	Hepatic	6–8	200–400 mg BID
Metoprolol*	β_1	0	Moderate	Hepatic	3–7	50–100 mg BID
Metoprolol XL*						100–200 mg QD
Nadolol*	$\beta_1\beta_2$	0	Low	Renal	20–24	40–80 mg QD
Penbutolol	$\beta_1\beta_2$	+	High	Hepatic	5	20 mg QD
Pindolol	$\beta_1\beta_2$	+++	Low–moderate	Renal/hepatic	3–4	5–20 mg BID
Propranolol*	$\beta_1\beta_2$	0	High	Hepatic	3–5	Variable
Propranolol LA*						80–160 mg QD
Timolol	$\beta_1\beta_2$	0	Moderate	Hepatic	4	10–20 mg BID

ISA, intrinsic sympathomimetic activity; BID, twice daily; QD, once daily.
* Agents approved by the FDA for the treatment of chronic stable angina.

The pharmacokinetic properties of β-blockers are extremely variable and are related to the drug's lipophilicity or hydrophilicity.[74] In general, drugs that are highly lipid-soluble tend to be well absorbed from the gastrointestinal tract, hepatically metabolized, have highly variable oral bioavailability, undergo extensive hepatic first-pass metabolism, and have a short plasma terminal elimination half-life. Table 23.3 lists the lipid solubility of β-blockers ranging from low to high lipid solubility. β-blockers that are more water-soluble tend to be incompletely absorbed from the gastrointestinal tract, are eliminated mainly unchanged in the urine, and have a negligible first-pass hepatic metabolism and a longer plasma terminal elimination half-life. Although the pharmacokinetics of β-blockers are highly variable, most of these compounds can be dosed once or twice daily for the treatment of angina. The pharmacokinetic properties of a drug and individual patient characteristics should guide the selection of the appropriate agent. For example, if atenolol were to be used in a patient with angina and impaired renal function, a lengthening of the dosing interval may be necessary because atenolol is eliminated mainly by the kidneys, although response monitoring should always drive the dosing schedule.

Regardless of differences in pharmacologic characteristics described previously, it should be emphasized that all β-blockers are effective in preventing angina and ischemia.[75] The efficacy of β-blockers should be determined by effects on resting and exercise heart rate and the frequency and severity of anginal syndromes. The dose of β-blockers should be titrated to achieve a resting heart rate of 50 to 60 bpm and maximal exercise heart rate that remains less than 75% of the heart rate in which angina is manifested.

Adverse Effects. The adverse effects associated with β-blockers are an extension of their pharmacologic effects and include sinus bradycardia, sinus arrest, AV block, reduced left ventricular function, bronchoconstriction, fatigue, depression, nightmares, sexual dysfunction, and intensification of insulin-induced hypoglycemia.[72,73] Thus, β-blockers should be avoided or used with caution in patients with bradyarrhythmias (Table 23.4), AV conduction disturbances, asthma or chronic obstructive pulmonary disease, decompensated left ventricular systolic dysfunction, diabetes mellitus, and peripheral vascular disease. In selected patients (i.e., history of MI or heart failure) with mild-to-moderate asthma or chronic obstructive pulmonary disease, a low-dose β_1-selective blocker should be considered with close monitoring.[76]

A final issue of clinical importance is the β-blocker withdrawal syndrome. Prolonged therapy with β-receptor antagonists results in an increase in the number of β-receptors. Abrupt withdrawal of β-blockers in these patients may result in an increased number of receptors available for adrenergic stimulation and possible precipitation of anginal syndromes, unstable angina, and possibly MI. Because of this, when discontinuing the use of β-blockers it is prudent to decrease the dose gradually over a minimum of a 1- to 2-week time period or in some cases longer in patients receiving chronic, high-dose therapy.[77]

Calcium Channel Blockers

Mechanism of Action. Calcium channel blockers are a chemically heterogeneous group of agents that block the transmembrane flux of calcium into cardiac and vascular smooth muscle cells by noncompetitive blockade, thereby reducing the rate of calcium entry and intracellular calcium concentrations.[78–80] This reduction in intracellular calcium concentrations results in reduction in the excitation-contraction-coupling mechanism responsible for myocardial and smooth muscle contraction.

Pharmacologic Characteristics. Due to chemical heterogeneity of calcium channel blockers and the existence of three different binding sites (dihydropyridine site, phenylalkylamine site, and benzothiazepine site), these agents exert variable pharmacologic effects.[79] Based on these three binding sites calcium channel blockers are classified as dihydropyridines, phenylalkylamines, or benzothiazepines owing to the binding at each respective site. The prototype agents for these three sites are nifedipine, verapamil, and diltiazem, respectively. Table 23.5 illustrates the available calcium channel blockers and their pharmacologic effects. Due to the differential pharmacologic actions of these agents, they are collectively referred to as dihydropyridines or nondihydropyridines (Table 23.5).

Calcium channel blockers have five major physiologic effects: (1) decreased systemic vascular resistance (peripheral vasodilation), (2) decreased coronary vascular resistance (coronary vasodilation), (3) decreased myocardial contractility, (4) slowing of sinus nodal conduction (reduced heart rate), and (5) slowing of AV nodal conduction.[79–81] Reductions in systemic vascular resistance, heart rate, and myocardial contractility will result in decreased myocardial oxygen demand, whereas decreased coronary vascular resistance will increase myocardial oxygen supply. In general, the dihydropyridine agents exhibit greater vascular selectivity, and thus will preferentially cause peripheral and coronary vasodilation and have lesser or minimal effects on myocardial contractility and sinus and AV nodal conduction. However, due to their rapid and potent vasodilation, short-acting dihydropyridines (Table 23.5) may result in a reflex increase in heart rate leading to increased myocardial oxygen demand. As a result, short-acting dihydropyridines should be avoided in patients with angina. As shown in Table 23.5, the medium- and long-acting dihydropyridines have lessened effects on neurohormonal activation. However, the nondihydropyridines are neither vascular nor myocardial selective and thus exhibit all of the pharmacologic effects discussed previously. Given the pronounced differences in the clinical pharmacology of these agents, the selection of appropriate agent should be based on the characteristics of the drug and the characteristics of the patient being treated.

Table 23.4	Individualizing Anginal Therapy in Patients with Other Medical Conditions	
Indication		**Drug Therapy**
Compelling indication unless contraindicated		
Prior myocardial infarction		Non-ISA β-blockers
Isolated systolic hypertension		CCB (long-acting DHP)
Systemic hypertension		β-blockers
Left ventricular systolic dysfunction		Carvedilol, metoprolol XL, bisoprolol
May have favorable effects on co-morbid condition		
Sinus bradycardia, 2° or 3° trioventricular block		DHP CCB, nitrate
Sinus tachycardia; supraventricular tachycardia; atrial fibrillation		β-blockers, non-DHP CCB
Ventricular arrhythmias		β-blockers
Severe pre-existing headaches		β-blockers, non DHP-CCB
Hyperthyroidism		β-blockers
Diabetes mellitus		CCB
Essential tremor		β-blockers (noncardioselective)
Left ventricular systolic dysfunction		Isososorbide dinitrate
Systemic hypertension		CCB
May have unfavorable effects on co-morbid condition (*contraindicated)		
Sinus bradycardia, 2° or 3° atrioventricular block		β-blockers,* non-DHP CCB*
Sinus tachycardia, supraventricular tachycardia; atrial fibrillation		DHP CCB (short-acting), Nitrate
Left ventricular systolic dysfunction		CCB (except amlodipine and felodipine)
Prior myocardial infarction		ISA β-blockers, DHP CCB (short-acting)
Severe pre-existing headaches		Nitrates, DHP CCB
Bronchospastic disease (asthma/COPD)		β-blockers*
Peripheral vascular disease		β-blockers
Depression		β-blockers
Diabetes mellitus		β-blockers

Abbreviations COPD, chronic obstructive pulmonary disease; ISA, intrinsic sympathomimetic activity; CCB, calcium channel blockers; DHP, dihydropyridine.

Adverse Effects. Calcium channel blockers are relatively well tolerated. Most of the adverse effects associated with their use are related to their pharmacologic effects. However, both verapamil and diltiazem are inhibitors of the cytochrome P-450 3A enzymatic system and can cause clinically important drug interactions by inhibiting the metabolism of drugs that are metabolized by this pathway. Of particular importance with respect to this chapter, the concentrations of several HMG CoA reductase inhibitors (simvastatin, atorvastatin, and lovastatin) are significantly increased when used in combination with verapamil and diltiazem.[82,83] The major adverse effects are presented in Table 23.5. The degree or significance of each adverse effect depends on the individual agents. Flushing, headache, and dizziness are related to the vasodilatory effects of calcium channel blockers.[79–81] Dihydropyridines, which are the most potent peripheral vasodilators, tend to cause these adverse effects to the greatest extent. Use of long-acting or extended-release preparations

may lessen these adverse effects. Peripheral edema, likely related to arteriolar vasodilation, not sodium and water retention, is also most commonly seen in patients treated with dihydropyridines. Depression of myocardial contractility occurs most commonly in patients treated with verapamil and diltiazem, and to a lesser extent with dihydropyridines. The negative inotropic effects of dihydropyridines are typically masked by the peripheral vasodilation and resulting adrenergic activation. Calcium channel blockers should be used with caution in patients with left ventricular systolic dysfunction, with the exception of amlodipine and felodipine. Bradycardia and AV block can occur in patients receiving verapamil and diltiazem. These two adverse effects would occur most commonly in patients with baseline sinus bradycardia or AV nodal dysfunction or in patients receiving concomitant β-blockers. Calcium channel blockers also may cause gastrointestinal adverse effects such as nausea and constipation. The latter is caused most commonly by verapamil and may

Table 23–5	Pharmacologic Characteristics of Currently Available Calcium Channel Blockers		
	Major Adverse Effects	**Time to Peak Concentration (h)**	**Maintenance Dose**
Dihydropyridines	**Hypotension, headache, ankle edema**		
Short-acting	Reflex adrenergic and neurohormonal activation (tachycardia, flushing, dizziness)		
Nifedipine**		0.5	10–20 mg TID
Nicardipine*		0.5–2.0	20–40 mg TID
Medium-acting	Lessened incidence of but still significant reflex adrenergic and neurohormonal activation (tachycardia, flushing, dizziness)		
Nicardipine-SR		1–4	30–60 mg BID
Isradapine		1.5	5–10 mg BID
Long-acting	Subclinical reflex adrenergic and neurohormonal activation		
Amlodipine**		6–12	5–10 mg QD
Felodipine-ER		2.5–5	5–10 mg QD
Nifedipine-CC		6	30–60 mg QD
Nifedipine-XL**		6	30–60 mg QD
Nisoldipine-ER		6–12	20–40 mg QD
Nondihydropyridines	**Bradycardia, AV nodal conduction disturbances, heart failure, headache, dizziness, edema**		
Verapamil**	Constipation	1–2	60–90 mg TID-QID
Verapamil-SR		1–2	240 mg QD
Bepridil*	Proarrhythmia	5	300 mg QD
Diltiazem**		2–3	80–120 mg TID
Diltiazem-SR		6–11	60–120 mg BID
Diltiazem-CD**		10–14	180–360 mg QD
Diltiazem-XR*		4–6	180–540 mg QD
Diltiazem-ER			180–360 mg QD

* Approved by the FDA for the treatment of chronic stable angina.
** Approved by the FDA for the treatment of chronic stable angina and angina associated with coronary artery spasm.
Adapted from Frishman WH. Beta-adrenergic blockers. Med Clin North Am 72 : 37–81, 1988.[72]

be particularly problematic in the elderly. Finally, bepridil, a calcium channel blocker with type I antiarrhythmic effects, has the potential for causing proarrhythmia (ventricular tachycardia, ventricular fibrillation, etc.) and should not be used in patients with prolonged QT-intervals. Thus bepridil therapy should be reserved for those patients who do not respond adequately to other antianginal drugs.

PHARMACOTHERAPY

Chronic Stable Angina Pectoris. The highest priority in the pharmacotherapy of chronic stable angina should be given to pharmacologic agents that prevent MI and death. β-blockers and aspirin should be initiated in all patients without absolute contraindications. ACE inhibitor and antidyslipidemic therapy should also be strongly considered in most patients with coronary artery disease.[1] In addition, all pa-

tients with chronic stable angina require acute and in most cases chronic anti-ischemic therapy. Therefore, all patients should have access to sublingual nitroglycerin tablets or spray for the immediate relief of acute attacks (see Table 23.2 for treatment options). The specific dose administered depends upon the patient's hemodynamic response. Sublingual nitroglycerin tablets are available over a wide dosing range from 0.15 to 0.6 mg, whereas the spray delivers 0.4 mg with each dose. These products are also useful for the prevention of angina when taken just prior to the initiation of exertion or some other event that precipitates angina.

β-blockers, in addition to decreasing mortality, are effective in the management of anginal symptoms, although all are not approved by the Food and Drug Administration (FDA) for this purpose (see Table 23.3 for approved agents). The entire class, however, is effective in reducing ischemic episodes and may be selected as initial therapy for angina. Selection of an individual agent should be based on the pharmacologic characteristics of a given drug and patient characteristics (i.e., renal function, hepatic function, etc.). Those patients who would particularly benefit from β-blocker therapy are listed in Table 23.4.

Calcium channel blockers are also effective for the prevention of angina. They should be considered as second-line agents and used in patients with contraindications to β-blockers or patients with mainly variable threshold angina as well as with conditions listed in Table 23.4. All calcium channel blockers appear to be effective in the management of stable angina, although all are not approved by the FDA for this purpose (see Table 23.5, for approved agents). Selection of an individual agent should be based on the pharmacologic characteristics of a given drug and patient characteristics (i.e., renal function, hepatic function, etc.). The short-acting dihydropyridine calcium antagonists may increase the risk of MI in patients with coronary artery disease when used for preventing future cardiovascular events.[84,85] Thus, it is recommended that short-acting dihydropyridine agents such as the immediate-release formulations of nisoldipine, nifedipine, or nicardipine be avoided in patients with coronary artery disease.[1]

In addition to calcium antagonists, long-acting nitrate products may be used when β-blockers are contraindicated or not tolerated. These agents include: oral nitroglycerin capsules, transdermal nitroglycerin patches, nitroglycerin ointment, ISDN, and ISMN. The choice of one product over another should be based on patient preference and ease of administration. As illustrated in Table 23.4, patients with heart failure may benefit from the addition of a nitrate due to the reduction in preload and left ventricular filling pressures that accompany their use. However, there is no data indicating that nitrates alone decrease mortality in patients with left ventricular dysfunction. All patients treated with nitrates require a 10- to 12-hour nitrate-free period to avoid development of tolerance. Unfortunately, because a nitrate-free period is required, no nitrate product can provide 24-hour anti-ischemic coverage, thus necessitating additional therapy with β-blockers, calcium channel blockers, or combination therapy. Regardless of which nitrate is selected it should be started at a low dose to reduce the incidence of adverse effects early in therapy. Subsequent dosage adjustments can be based on incidence of adverse effects, headache, dizziness, and hypotension. Effectiveness can be assessed by decreased use of sublingual nitroglycerin for acute attacks, improvement in patient's quality of life (i.e., ability to have normal activities without experiencing angina), and objective assessment by exercise testing.

Combination drug therapy is indicated when monotherapy is unsuccessful or to treat concomitant disease states, such as hypertension or left ventricular dysfunction, in patients with infrequent anginal attacks. Selection of drug therapy based on concomitant disease states or conditions allows the treatment of two conditions with one drug. The addition of a calcium channel antagonist or long-acting nitrate to β-blocker therapy should be considered if angina persists (see Tables 23.2 and 23.5 for treatment options).[2] There are no data available to suggest that these second-line antianginal medications reduce mortality, thus treatment strategies are targeted at symptom relief and/or ischemia reduction. Drug selection for combination treatment of angina should be based on patient characteristics and concomitant conditions. The combination of β-blockers and nitrates is used commonly and has therapeutic rationale based on the pharmacology of each drug class. Nitrates offset the β-blockers' potential deleterious increase in left ventricular diastolic pressures and volumes by reducing preload, whereas the β-blockers inhibit the nitrate-induced sympathetically mediated reflex tachycardia.

Therapy with a β-blocker and calcium channel blocker should theoretically reduce myocardial oxygen demand further than could each agent alone. In addition, because β-blockers may increase coronary artery tone, the addition of a calcium channel blocker may attenuate this potentially detrimental effect.[86] The concern regarding the use of nondihydropyridines with β-blockers is the potential for additive adverse effects, specifically, slowing of AV and sinus nodal conduction, hypotension, and impairment of systolic function. These concerns may be minimized by selection of patients who are least likely to experience these adverse effects. Patients who are normotensive, have little or minimal systolic dysfunction, and have no conduction disturbances are the best candidates for this therapy. The combination of a β-blocker and verapamil should be reserved, if at all, for those patients failing combination therapy with other agents. Combination therapy with nondihydropyridine calcium channel blockers and nitrates also offer therapeutic benefit in patients who cannot tolerate β-blocker therapy. The combination of dihydropyridines and nitrates should be used cautiously due to the risk of excessive hypotension, rebound tachycardia, and headaches.

Triple combination antianginal therapy with β-blockers, calcium antagonists, and long-acting nitrates is warranted in patients with persistent angina on dual therapy or where it would be beneficial in the treatment of concomitant diseases. In those patients in whom medical therapy is not effective in reducing the number of anginal syndromes or where the underlying coronary artery disease is severe, revascularization therapy with percutaneous transluminal coronary angioplasty (PTCA) or coronary artery bypass graft (CABG) surgery are alternatives.

Silent Myocardial Ischemia. Therapy for all patients regardless of the type of silent myocardial ischemia should begin with coronary risk factor reduction. The drug therapies used for the treatment of silent myocardial ischemia, albeit controversial, are similar to those used to treat other types of chronic ischemia, namely nitrates, β-blockers, and calcium antagonists. Each of these agents, reduce the number of ischemic episodes,[15,87] but the impact on long-term prognosis is not clear. The treatment approach should be individualized depending on whether a patient has totally asymptomatic episodes of ischemia, postinfarction asymptomatic ischemia, or symptomatic and asymptomatic episodes. There is no consensus for therapy of totally asymptomatic individuals but ACE inhibitors should be administered to patients with left ventricular systolic dysfunction or diabetes and antidyslipidemics in patients with documented coronary artery disease and LDL greater than 130 mg per dL. In addition to beneficial lipid-lowering activity, HMG-CoA reductase inhibitors may reduce ambulatory ischemia.[88,89] In patients with postinfarction asymptomatic ischemia, therapy with β-blockers and aspirin is logical given the well-established benefits that these agents provide—preventing reinfarction and death in these patients.

Finally, the treatment of patients with asymptomatic and symptomatic ischemic episodes has received the largest attention as this group contains the largest number of patients. Several recent studies have increased the understanding of the correct therapy for these individuals. The placebo-controlled ASIST trial showed that atenolol was effective in asymptomatic and mildly symptomatic patients (with and without previous MI), at reducing ischemic episodes and reducing cardiovascular events.[90] A similar patient population was enrolled in a subsequent randomized trial[87,91] that was designed to investigate three approaches to treating these patients. The three approaches were revascularization with PTCA or CABG, drug therapy targeted at reducing ischemia, and drug therapy targeted at reducing angina. The drug therapies used in this trial were atenolol ± controlled-release nifedipine or sustained-release diltiazem ± sustained-release ISDN. Patients who were randomized to the revascularization group had improved 2-year survival and experienced fewer cardiac events than either of the medically managed groups. The outcome in the group of patients whose treatment was targeted at reducing ischemia did slightly better than the other medically managed group of patients. The question remains whether or not suppression of ischemic episodes will translate into reductions in long-term mortality. The results of these two studies suggest that β-blocker therapy with atenolol reduces ischemia and cardiovascular events, but that revascularization offers a significant advantage to this approach at improving prognosis. Future studies are required to address these issues further.

Variant Angina. Sublingual nitroglycerin therapy should be used for acute anginal episodes as was discussed for chronic stable angina. Calcium channel blockers are effective in the chronic prophylactic management of patients with variant angina. The selection of a particular drug depends mainly on patient characteristics. Nitrates are also effective in these patients, but the scheduling of a nitrate-free period may not necessarily be best during the sleeping hours. Because most episodes occur in the nighttime or morning hours, the nitrate-free interval should be scheduled during the day. Nitrate therapy should be reserved for patients with contin-

ued symptoms on maximized therapy with calcium channel blockers. Combination therapy with two calcium channel blockers (diltiazem and nifedipine) has reduced the frequency of anginal episodes in patients not receiving full benefit from either agent alone. However, this drug combination was associated with frequent adverse effects.[92] Finally, β-blockers should not be used in the treatment of variant angina as they may exacerbate coronary vasospasm.[93]

REVASCULARIZATION PROCEDURES

Two revascularization procedures, CABG and percutaneous coronary interventions (PCI), with or without coronary artery stent placement, are widely available for the treatment of ischemic heart disease. These procedures have become widely used in the United States. Because of the risk of morbidity and mortality associated with each procedure, each patient must be evaluated to determine whether the potential benefits of the procedure outweigh the risks. Extensive guidelines for each of these procedures have been published.[94–96] Additional, less established revascularization techniques may be useful in patients who are not candidates for CABG or PCI. These techniques include surgical laser transmyocardial revascularization, enhanced external counterpulsation, and spinal cord stimulation.[1,97]

Coronary Artery Bypass Grafting. CABG is a surgical procedure in which the affected stenosed coronary artery or arteries is bypassed in an attempt to reinstitute ''normal'' coronary blood flow. Two of the techniques are described here. The first technique involves removal of the saphenous vein from the leg, which is then used to bypass the affected vessel. The distal end of the vessel is connected to the aorta and the proximal end is connected to the coronary artery at a point distal to the obstruction. The second and most commonly used technique involves the connection of the distal end of the internal thoracic (mammary) artery beyond the narrowing of the coronary vessel. The following patients with stable angina should be recommended for CABG instead of medical therapy: patients with significant left main coronary artery disease, with stenosis of the proximal left anterior descending (LAD) and proximal left circumflex artery greater than 70%, patients with three-vessel coronary artery disease (or two-vessel with significant proximal LAD stenosis) and moderate to severe left ventricular dysfunction, patients with one- or two-vessel coronary artery disease that are high risk based on noninvasive testing but have a large area of viable myocardium, and patients who sustain disabling angina despite optimized medical treatment.[94] CABG generally is not recommended over medical therapy in patients with two-vessel (no LAD coronary artery involvement) or single-vessel disease with normal ventricular function. PCI may be a treatment option in these patients.[2]

In patients who have had CABG, stenosis of the bypass graft may occur. Coronary disease of the saphenous vein grafts are thought to occur in three stages: early (within 1 month), intermediate (within 1 year), and late (more than 1 year). Occlusion rates of 5% to15%, 15% to 25%, and up to 50 % have been reported for early, intermediate, and late phases, respectively.[98] The role of thrombosis in each of the phases has been documented. The use of lifelong antiplatelet therapy with aspirin or clopidogrel (if aspirin sensitive) may reduce the rate of occlusion. The late phase of vein graft occlusion is likely related to atherosclerosis of the graft. Prevention of late phase occlusion may be afforded by reducing risks for development of atherosclerosis with aggressive lipid-lowering therapy and lifestyle modifications.[99] Antiplatelet therapy should also be continued given its role in the management of ischemic heart disease.

Percutaneous Coronary Interventions. PTCA was the first PCI technique introduced in clinical practice in the early 1970s. PTCA is an extension of cardiac catheterization that involves passing a balloon-tipped catheter over a guidewire into the coronary artery that upon inflation dilates the stenosed vessel.[100] PCI has rapidly evolved in the past couple decades and now encompasses more advanced techniques than PTCA, including atherectomy, laser angioplasty, and intracoronary stent implantation. The advancement of PCI with these newer techniques along with advancements in balloon technology has been substantially beneficial in decreasing short-term complications following PCI including: abrupt coronary occlusion of the vessel, ischemia, emergency CABG, MI, and death. PCI is effective (defined as <20% obstruction after the intervention without acute complications) in approximately 96% to 99% of elective procedures.[96] In patients who have undergone successful PCI, the major concern remains to be long-term restenosis, which has been reported to be as high as 30% to 40% of patients—usually within 6 months of the procedure.

Currently, no interventions have convincingly been shown to reduce restenosis, but stent placement markedly reduces this risk. Coronary artery stents are stainless steel tubes that are inserted into coronary arteries at the site of atherosclerotic plaques to decrease the incidence of restenosis. The use of coronary artery stents is increasing rapidly and in some cardiac catheterization laboratories, more than 50% of patients undergoing angioplasty have coronary artery stents implanted. Due to the thrombogenic nature of a stent and the potential endothelial damage induced by the stent, antithrombotic drug therapy is needed to prevent thrombosis. Dual therapy should be used with pretreatment aspirin (80–325 mg) and clopidogrel (300 mg) initiated at least 2 hours prior to the procedure when possible. Clopidogrel increases the risk of bleeding when administered within 5 days prior to CABG. It should, therefore, be reserved for patients where this procedure is ruled out. A subgroup analysis of the Clopidogrel for the Reduction of Events During Observation trial suggests that clopidogrel administered at 3 hours prior to PCI did not significantly improve outcomes versus administration immediately following the procedure.[101] The optimal timing for the administration of antiplatelet therapy prior to a PCI has not been elucidated. Aspirin should be continued

indefinitely and clopidogrel (75 mg) continued for a minimum of 14 days and up to 1 year following stent placement.[101,102] Expert guidelines suggest that glycoprotein IIb/IIIa receptor inhibitors and/or unfractionated heparin should be considered in all patients undergoing PCI, especially those classified as high risk.[102] The initiation of lipid-lowering therapy with HMG-CoA reductase inhibitors may reduce mortality and also should be considered in patients requiring a PCI.[103] Anticoagulation for the prevention of restenosis in PCI is a rapidly expanding area in which the pharmacotherapy is constantly evolving. Future studies will better define the role of other agents in the management of these patients.

FUTURE THERAPIES

RANOLAZINE

Ranolazine is the first of a new class of antianginal drugs that is expected to gain FDA approval in the near future. It represents a new therapeutic option for the management of chronic stable angina by purportedly increasing myocardial energy production through the inhibition of fatty acid oxidation and subsequent increase in glucose oxidation leading to increased ATP generation. Two large clinical trials have reported that twice daily ranolazine therapy significantly increases exercise capacity in patients with symptomatic chronic angina, one as monotherapy and the other as an adjunct to standard therapy.[104,105] In the Combination Assessment of Ranolazine In Stable Angina (CARISA) trial,[105] ranolazine or placebo was administered twice daily to 823 patients with symptomatic chronic angina taking standard doses of atenolol, amlodipine, or diltiazem. In addition to increasing exercise capacity, both 750 and 1000 mg twice daily doses of ranolazine significantly reduced the number of anginal episodes per week. The most common adverse events reported for ranolazine in both clinical trials were constipation, dizziness, nausea, and asthenia. However, ranolazine was also reported to prolong QTc intervals in a dose-dependent manner in the CARISA trial. Although the increases in QTc intervals were relatively small, five patients receiving the larger dose reported experiencing syncope. This potential for serious adverse events will need to be investigated further before the widespread use of this agent. Ranolazine's role in the management of angina has not been determined but will most likely be introduced as adjunct or salvage therapy until long-term outcome data is obtained and its adverse event profile is better characterized.

ANTIMICROBIALS

The development of atherosclerosis contains an inflammatory component that may be partially derived from a bacteriologic origin in the arterial wall. Specifically, the roles of *Helicobacter pylori*, *Chlamydia pneumoniae*, and cytomegalovirus have been investigated as part of the etiology of coronary artery disease. Although there is an association between *C. pneumoniae* and coronary artery disease, current studies with prophylactic antibiotic therapy report conflicting evidence in the role of antimicrobial therapy.[106,107] Additional long-term investigations are being conducted to determine the potential prophylactic role of gatifloxacin, azithromycin, and clarithromycin in preventing cardiovascular events in patients with stable coronary artery disease. However, evidence is accumulating to suggest that azithromycin does not have clinical benefit for this purpose in this patient population.[107,108] Currently, there is not any convincing data to promote the use of antimicrobials in the treatment of ischemic heart disease and this treatment cannot be recommended.

IMPROVING OUTCOMES

PATIENT EDUCATION

Patient education in the management of chronic stable angina often can be overlooked by health care professionals. Proper education is critical to improve patient adherence to lifestyle modifications and pharmacologic treatment that improve clinical outcomes. The 2002 update of the ACC/AHA guidelines for the management of chronic stable angina outlines key principles to optimize patient education programs.[1] Education on ischemic heart disease therapy should begin by ensuring that the patient truly understands the etiology, pathogenesis, and progression of the disease along with the importance of risk factor reduction. This includes education on lifestyle changes that promote smoking cessation and weight loss through an appropriate exercise and diet program. All health care professionals should participate in patient education, but pharmacists are in a favorable position to ensure that patients fully understand their prescribed medication regimens. All patients with ischemic heart disease should have access to nitroglycerin, therefore, education on the appropriate use and storage of nitroglycerin tablets, ointment, and spray is critical to improve patient adherence and outcome. It must be reinforced that the inappropriate use of nitroglycerin or poor adherence to the treatment regimen will interfere with quality of life and increase mortality. Additionally, counseling on optimal dosing schedules to avoid the development of nitrate tolerance will help make certain that each patient has an adequate nitrate-free interval. Self-monitoring and the maintenance of patient log books should be encouraged for weekly nitroglycerin use, frequency of anginal attacks, resting and active heart rates, and daily blood pressures to optimize medical management of angina and concomitant diseases.

KEY POINTS

■ Ischemic heart disease is a manifestation of atherosclerotic coronary artery disease, the leading cause of death in the United States.

■ Myocardial ischemia causes several syndromes referred to collectively as ischemic heart disease including: stable angina, variant or Prinzmetal's angina, and silent myocardial ischemia.

■ The management of ischemic heart disease involves five areas: identification and treatment of concomitant conditions that may exacerbate or precipitate ischemia, correction of concomitant cardiovascular risk factors, lifestyle modifications, medical treatment, and revascularization techniques.

■ The goals of treatment for ischemic heart disease are to minimize the frequency and severity of angina and to reduce cardiovascular morbidity and mortality.

■ Drug therapy with nitrates, β-blockers, and calcium channel blockers, alone or in combination, are effective at reducing anginal episodes and reducing the frequency of anginal attacks.

■ Revascularization procedures are effective alternatives to medical therapy in certain patients.

SUGGESTED READING

Gibbons RJ, Abrams J, Chatterjee K, et al. ACC/AHA 2002 guideline update for the management of patients with chronic stable angina—summary article: a report of the American College of Cardiology/American Heart Association Task Force on practice guidelines (Committee on the Management of Patients With Chronic Stable Angina). J Am Coll Cardiol 41:159–168, 2003.

REFERENCES

1. Gibbons RJ, Abrams J, Chatterjee K, et al. ACC/AHA 2002 guideline update for the management of patients with chronic stable angina—summary article: a report of the American College of Cardiology/American Heart Association Task Force on practice guidelines (Committee on the Management of Patients With Chronic Stable Angina). J Am Coll Cardiol 41:59–168, 2003.
2. Gersh BJ, Braunwald E, Bonow RO. Chronic coronary artery disease. In: Braunwald E, Zipes DP, Libby P, eds. Heart disease. A textbook of cardiovascular medicine. Philadelphia: W.B. Saunders, 2001:1272–1363.
3. American Heart Association: Heart and Stroke Facts: 2004 Statistical Supplement. Dallas, TX, American Heart Association 2003.
4. Kannel WB, Feinleib M. Natural history of angina pectoris in the Framingham study. Prognosis and survival. Am J Cardiol 29:154–163, 1972.
5. Campeau L. Letter: Grading of angina pectoris. Circulation 54:522–523, 1976.
6. Lambert CR. Pathophysiology of stable angina pectoris. Cardiol Clin 9:1–10, 1991.
7. Third Report of the National Cholesterol Education Program (NCEP) Expert Panel on Detection, Evaluation, and Treatment of High Blood Cholesterol in Adults (Adult Treatment Panel III) final report. Circulation 106:3143–3421, 2002.
8. Eckel RH, Krauss RM. American Heart Association call to action: obesity as a major risk factor for coronary heart disease. AHA Nutrition Committee. Circulation 97:2099–2100, 1998.
9. Grundy SM, Balady GJ, Criqui MH, et al. Primary prevention of coronary heart disease: guidance from Framingham: a statement for healthcare professionals from the AHA Task Force on Risk Reduction. American Heart Association. Circulation 97:1876–1887, 1998.
10. Tousoulis D, Davies G, Stefanadis C, et al. Inflammatory and thrombotic mechanisms in coronary atherosclerosis. Heart 89:993–997, 2003.

11. Shub C. Stable angina pectoris: 1. Clinical patterns. Mayo Clin Proc 65:233–242, 1990.
12. Alderman EL, Bourassa MG, Cohen LS, et al. Ten-year follow-up of survival and myocardial infarction in the randomized Coronary Artery Surgery Study. Circulation 82:1629–1646, 1990.
13. Ardehali A, Ports TA. Myocardial oxygen supply and demand. Chest 98:699–705, 1990.
14. Maseri A, Chierchia S, Kaski JC. Mixed angina pectoris. Am J Cardiol 56:30E–33E, 1985.
15. Cohn PF, Fox KM, Daly C. Silent myocardial ischemia. Circulation 108:1263–1277, 2003.
16. Almeda FQ, Kason TT, Nathan S, et al. Silent myocardial ischemia: concepts and controversies. Am J Med 116:112–118, 2004.
17. Muller JE. Circadian variation in cardiovascular events. Am J Hypertens 12(2 Pt 2):35S–42S, 1999.
18. Connolly DC, Elveback LR, Oxman HA. Coronary heart disease in residents of Rochester, Minnesota. IV. Prognostic value of the resting electrocardiogram at the time of initial diagnosis of angina pectoris. Mayo Clin Proc 59:247–250, 1984.
19. Wang K, Asinger RW, Marriott HJ. ST-segment elevation in conditions other than acute myocardial infarction. N Engl J Med 349:2128–2135, 2003.
20. Chaitman BR. Exercise stress testing. In: Braunwald E, Zipes DP, Libby P, eds. Heart disease: a textbook of cardiovascular medicine. Philadelphia: W.B. Saunders, 2001:129–159.
21. Fletcher GF, Balady GJ, Amsterdam EA, et al. Exercise standards for testing and training: a statement for healthcare professionals from the American Heart Association. Circulation 104:1694–1740, 2001.
22. Goldman L, Cook EF, Mitchell N, et al. Incremental value of the exercise test for diagnosing the presence or absence of coronary artery disease. Circulation 66:945–953, 1982.
23. Klocke FJ, Baird MG, Lorell BH, et al. ACC/AHA/ASNC guidelines for the clinical use of cardiac radionuclide imaging—executive summary: a report of the American College of Cardiology/American Heart Association Task Force on Practice Guidelines (ACC/AHA/ASNC Committee to Revise the 1995 Guidelines for the Clinical Use of Cardiac Radionuclide Imaging). Circulation 108:1404–1418, 2003.
24. Wackers FJT, Soufer R, Zaret BL. Nuclear Cardiology. In: Braunwald E, Zipes DP, Libby P, eds. Heart disease: a textbook of cardiovascular medicine. Philadelphia: W.B. Saunders, 2001:273–323.
25. Navare SM, Kapetanopoulos A, Heller GV. Pharmacologic radionuclide myocardial perfusion imaging. Curr Cardiol Rep 5:16–24, 2003.
26. Scanlon PJ, Faxon DP, Audet AM, et al. ACC/AHA guidelines for coronary angiography. A report of the American College of Cardiology/American Heart Association Task Force on practice guidelines (Committee on Coronary Angiography). Developed in collaboration with the Society for Cardiac Angiography and Interventions. J Am Coll Cardiol 33:1756–1824, 1999.
27. Ridker PM, Manson JE, Gaziano JM, et al. Low-dose aspirin therapy for chronic stable angina. A randomized, placebo-controlled clinical trial. Ann Intern Med 114:835–839, 1991.
28. Juul-Moller S, Edvardsson N, Jahnmatz B, et al. Double-blind trial of aspirin in primary prevention of myocardial infarction in patients with stable chronic angina pectoris. The Swedish Angina Pectoris Aspirin Trial (APAT) Group. Lancet 340:1421–1425, 1992.
29. Eidelman RS, Hebert PR, Weisman SM, et al. An update on aspirin in the primary prevention of cardiovascular disease. Arch Intern Med 163:2006–2010, 2003.
30. Chobanian AV, Bakris GL, Black HR, et al. Seventh report of the Joint National Committee on Prevention, Detection, Evaluation, and Treatment of High Blood Pressure. Hypertension 42:1206–1252, 2003.
31. Lewington S, Clarke R, Qizilbash N, et al. Age-specific relevance of usual blood pressure to vascular mortality: a meta-analysis of individual data for one million adults in 61 prospective studies. Lancet 360:1903–1913, 2002.
32. Samet JM. The 1990 Report of the Surgeon General: The Health Benefits of Smoking Cessation. Am Rev Respir Dis 142:993–994, 1990.
33. Goldenberg I, Jonas M, Tenenbaum A, et al. Current smoking, smoking cessation, and the risk of sudden cardiac death in patients with coronary artery disease. Arch Intern Med 163:2301–2305, 2003.
34. MRC/BHF Heart Protection Study of cholesterol lowering with simvastatin in 20,536 high-risk individuals: a randomised placebo-controlled trial. Lancet 360:7–22, 2002.
35. Takano M, Mizuno K, Yokoyama S, et al. Changes in coronary plaque color and morphology by lipid-lowering therapy with atorvastatin: serial evaluation by coronary angioscopy. J Am Coll Cardiol 42:680–686, 2003.
36. Nissen SE, Tuzcu EM, Schoenhagen P, et al. Effect of intensive compared with moderate lipid-lowering therapy on progression of coronary atherosclerosis: a randomized controlled trial. JAMA 291:1071–1080, 2004.
37. Cannon CP, Braunwald E, McCabe CH, et al. Intensive versus moderate lipid lowering with statins after acute coronary syndromes. N Engl J Med 350:1495–1504, 2004.
38. Rubins HB, Robins SJ, Collins D, et al. Gemfibrozil for the secondary prevention of coronary heart disease in men with low levels of high-density lipoprotein cholesterol. Veterans Affairs High-Density Lipoprotein Cholesterol Intervention Trial Study Group. N Engl J Med 341:410–418, 1999.
39. Tsuya T, Okada M, Horie H, et al. Effect of dipyridamole at the usual oral dose on exercise-induced myocardial ischemia in stable angina pectoris. Am J Cardiol 66:275–278, 1990.
40. A randomised, blinded, trial of clopidogrel versus aspirin in patients at risk of ischaemic events (CAPRIE). CAPRIE Steering Committee. Lancet 348:1329–1339, 1996.
41. Pfeffer MA, Braunwald E, Moye LA, et al. Effect of captopril on mortality and morbidity in patients with left ventricular dysfunction after myocardial infarction. Results of the survival and ventricular enlargement trial. The SAVE Investigators. N Engl J Med 327:669–677, 1992.
42. Effect of enalapril on survival in patients with reduced left ventricular ejection fractions and congestive heart failure. The SOLVD Investigators. N Engl J Med 325:293–302, 1991.
43. Yusuf S, Sleight P, Pogue J, Bosch J, et al. Effects of an angiotensin-converting-enzyme inhibitor, ramipril, on cardiovascular events in high-risk patients. The Heart Outcomes Prevention Evaluation Study Investigators. N Engl J Med 342:145–153, 2000.
44. Fox KM. Efficacy of perindopril in reduction of cardiovascular events among patients with stable coronary artery disease: randomised, double-blind, placebo-controlled, multicentre trial (the EUROPA study). Lancet 362:782–788, 2003.
45. Pfeffer MA, Domanski M, Rosenberg Y, et al. Prevention of events with angiotensin-converting enzyme inhibition (the PEACE study design). Prevention of Events with Angiotensin-Converting Enzyme Inhibition. Am J Cardiol 82:25H–30H, 1998.
46. Kondo J, Sone T, Tsuboi H, Mukawa H, et al. Effects of low-dose angiotensin II receptor blocker candesartan on cardiovascular events in patients with coronary artery disease. Am Heart J 146:E20, 2003.
47. Thompson PD, Buchner D, Pina IL, et al. Exercise and physical activity in the prevention and treatment of atherosclerotic cardiovascular disease: a statement from the Council on Clinical Cardiology (Subcommittee on Exercise, Rehabilitation, and Prevention) and the Council on Nutrition, Physical Activity, and Metabolism (Subcommittee on Physical Activity). Circulation 107:3109–3116, 2003.
48. Ignarro LJ, Lippton H, Edwards JC, et al. Mechanism of vascular smooth muscle relaxation by organic nitrates, nitrites, nitroprusside and nitric oxide: evidence for the involvement of S-nitrosothiols as active intermediates. J Pharmacol Exp Ther 218:739–749, 1981.
49. Parker JD, Parker JO. Nitrate therapy for stable angina pectoris. N Engl J Med 338:520–531, 1998.
50. Abrams J. Beneficial actions of nitrates in cardiovascular disease. Am J Cardiol 77:31C–37C, 1996.
51. Elkayam U. Tolerance to organic nitrates: evidence, mechanisms, clinical relevance, and strategies for prevention. Ann Intern Med 114:667–677, 1991.
52. Skatchkov M, Larina LL, Larin AA, et al. Urinary NItrotyrosine Content as a Marker of Peroxynitrite-induced Tolerance to Organic NItrates. J Cardiovasc Pharmacol Ther 2:85–96, 1997.

53. Dikalov S, Fink B, Skatchkov M, et al. Formation of Reactive Oxygen Species in Various Vascular Cells During Glyceryltrinitrate Metabolism. J Cardiovasc Pharmacol Ther 3:51–62, 1998.

54. Mihm MJ, Coyle CM, Jing L, et al. Vascular peroxynitrite formation during organic nitrate tolerance. J Pharmacol Exp Ther 291: 194–198, 1999.

55. Gori T, Parker JD. Nitrate tolerance: a unifying hypothesis. Circulation 106:2510–2513, 2002.

56. Gori T, Parker JD. The puzzle of nitrate tolerance: pieces smaller than we thought? Circulation 106:2404–2408, 2002.

57. Hirai N, Kawano H, Yasue H, et al. Attenuation of nitrate tolerance and oxidative stress by an angiotensin II receptor blocker in patients with coronary spastic angina. Circulation 108:1446–1450, 2003.

58. Miner SE, Al Hesayen A, Kelly S, et al. L-arginine transport in the human coronary and peripheral circulation. Circulation 109: 1278–1283, 2004.

59. Parker JO, Parker JD, Caldwell RW, et al. The effect of supplemental L-arginine on tolerance development during continuous transdermal nitroglycerin therapy. J Am Coll Cardiol 39:1199–1203, 2002.

60. DeMots H, Glasser SP. Intermittent transdermal nitroglycerin therapy in the treatment of chronic stable angina. J Am Coll Cardiol 13:786–795, 1989.

61. Parker JO, Farrell B, Lahey KA, et al. Effect of intervals between doses on the development of tolerance to isosorbide dinitrate. N Engl J Med 316:440–1444, 1987.

62. Thadani U, Maranda CR, Amsterdam E, et al. Lack of pharmacologic tolerance and rebound angina pectoris during twice-daily therapy with isosorbide-5-mononitrate. Ann Intern Med 120:353–359, 1994.

63. Parker JO, Vankoughnett KA, Farrell B. Nitroglycerin lingual spray: clinical efficacy and dose-response relation. Am J Cardiol 57:1–5, 1986.

64. Reichek N, Goldstein RE, Redwood DR, et al. Sustained effects of nitroglycerin ointment in patients with angina pectoris. Circulation, 50:348–352 1974.

65. Reichek N, Priest C, Zimrin D, et al. Antianginal effects of nitroglycerin patches. Am J Cardiol 54:1–7.

66. Parker JO, Fung HL. Transdermal nitroglycerin in angina pectoris. Am J Cardiol 54:471–476, 1984.

67. Chrysant SG, Glasser SP, Bittar N, et al. Efficacy and safety of extended-release isosorbide mononitrate for stable effort angina pectoris. Am J Cardiol 72:1249–1256, 1993.

68. Fung HL. Pharmacokinetics and pharmacodynamics of organic nitrates. Am J Cardiol 60:4H–9H, 1987.

69. Thadani U, Prasad R, Hamilton SF, et al. Usefulness of twice-daily isosorbide-5-mononitrate in preventing development of tolerance in angina pectoris. Am J Cardiol 60:477–482, 1987.

70. Parker JO. Eccentric dosing with isosorbide-5-mononitrate in angina pectoris. Am J Cardiol 72:871–876, 1993.

71. Cheitlin MD, Hutter AM, Jr., Brindis RG, et al. ACC/AHA expert consensus document. Use of sildenafil (Viagra) in patients with cardiovascular disease. American College of Cardiology/American Heart Association. J Am Coll Cardiol 33:273–282, 1999.

72. Frishman WH. Beta-adrenergic blockers. Med Clin North Am 72: 37–81, 1988.

73. Sproat TT, Lopez LM. Around the beta-blockers, one more time. DICP 25:962–971, 1991.

74. Kazierad DJ, Schlanz KD, Bottoroff MB. β-Blockers. In: Evans WE, Schentag JJ, Jusko WJ, eds. Applied pharmacokinetics: principles of therapeutic drug monitoring. Vancouver: Applied Therapeutics, 1992.

75. Thadani U, Davidson C, Singleton W, et al. Comparison of the immediate effects of five beta-adrenoreceptor-blocking drugs with different ancillary properties in angina pectoris. N Engl J Med 300: 750–755, 1979.

76. Salpeter SR, Ormiston TM, Salpeter EE. Cardioselective beta-blockers in patients with reactive airway disease: a meta-analysis. Ann Intern Med 137:715–725, 2002.

77. Houston MC, Hodge R. Beta-adrenergic blocker withdrawal syndromes in hypertension and other cardiovascular diseases. Am Heart J 116(2 Pt 1):515–523, 1988.

78. Weiner DA. Calcium channel blockers. Med Clin North Am, 1988. 72:83–115.

79. Opie LH. Pharmacological differences between calcium antagonists. Eur Heart J 18 (Suppl A):A71–A79, 1997.

80. Opie LH. Calcium channel antagonists in the treatment of coronary artery disease: fundamental pharmacological properties relevant to clinical use. Prog Cardiovasc Dis 38:273–290, 1996.

81. Frishman WH, Sonnenblick EH. Calcium channel blockers. In: Schlant RC, Alexander RW, eds. The heart arteries and veins. New York: McGraw-Hill, Inc., 1994:1291–1308.

82. Kantola T, Kivisto KT, Neuvonen PJ. Erythromycin and verapamil considerably increase serum simvastatin and simvastatin acid concentrations. Clin Pharmacol Ther 64:177–182, 1998.

83. Azie NE, Brater DC, Becker PA, et al. The interaction of diltiazem with lovastatin and pravastatin. Clin Pharmacol Ther 64:369–377, 1998.

84. Furberg CD, Psaty BM, Meyer JV. Nifedipine. Dose-related increase in mortality in patients with coronary heart disease. Circulation 92:1326–1331, 1995.

85. Estacio RO, Jeffers BW, Hiatt WR, et al. The effect of nisoldipine as compared with enalapril on cardiovascular outcomes in patients with non-insulin-dependent diabetes and hypertension. N Engl J Med 338:645–652, 1998.

86. Strauss WE, Parisi AF. Combined use of calcium-channel and beta-adrenergic blockers for the treatment of chronic stable angina. Rationale, efficacy, and adverse effects. Ann Intern Med 109: 570–581, 1988.

87. Knatterud GL, Bourassa MG, Pepine CJ, et al. Effects of treatment strategies to suppress ischemia in patients with coronary artery disease: 12-week results of the Asymptomatic Cardiac Ischemia Pilot (ACIP) study. J Am Coll Cardiol 24:11–20, 1994.

88. van Boven AJ, Jukema JW, Zwinderman AH, et al. Reduction of transient myocardial ischemia with pravastatin in addition to the conventional treatment in patients with angina pectoris. REGRESS Study Group. Circulation 94:1503–1505, 1996.

89. Andrews TC, Raby K, Barry J, et al. Effect of cholesterol reduction on myocardial ischemia in patients with coronary disease. Circulation 95:324–328, 1997.

90. Pepine CJ, Cohn PF, Deedwania PC, et al. Effects of treatment on outcome in mildly symptomatic patients with ischemia during daily life. The Atenolol Silent Ischemia Study (ASIST). Circulation 90: 762–768, 1994.

91. Davies RF, Goldberg AD, Forman S, et al. Asymptomatic Cardiac Ischemia Pilot (ACIP) study two-year follow-up: outcomes of patients randomized to initial strategies of medical therapy versus revascularization. Circulation 95:2037–2043, 1997.

92. Prida XE, Gelman JS, Feldman RL, et al. Comparison of diltiazem and nifedipine alone and in combination in patients with coronary artery spasm. J Am Coll Cardiol, 1987. 9:412–419.

93. Robertson RM, Wood AJ, Vaughn WK, et al. Exacerbation of vasotonic angina pectoris by propranolol. Circulation 65:281–285, 1982.

94. Eagle KA, Guyton RA, Davidoff R, et al. ACC/AHA Guidelines for Coronary Artery Bypass Graft Surgery: A Report of the American College of Cardiology/American Heart Association Task Force on Practice Guidelines (Committee to Revise the 1991 Guidelines for Coronary Artery Bypass Graft Surgery). American College of Cardiology/American Heart Association. J Am Coll Cardiol 34: 1262–1347, 1999.

95. Pepine CJ, Holmes DR, Jr. Coronary artery stents. American College of Cardiology. J Am Coll Cardiol 28:782–794, 1996.

96. Smith SC, Jr., Dove JT, Jacobs AK, et al. ACC/AHA guidelines of percutaneous coronary interventions (revision of the 1993 PTCA guidelines)—executive summary. A report of the American College of Cardiology/American Heart Association Task Force on Practice Guidelines (committee to revise the 1993 guidelines for percutaneous transluminal coronary angioplasty). J Am Coll Cardiol 37:2215–2239, 2001.

97. Kleiman NS, Patel NC, Allen KB, et al. Evolving revascularization approaches for myocardial ischemia. Am J Cardiol 92:9N–17N, 2003.

98. Pearson T, Rapaport E, Criqui M, et al. Optimal risk factor management in the patient after coronary revascularization. A statement for healthcare professionals from an American Heart Association Writing Group. Circulation 90:3125–3133, 1994.

99. The effect of aggressive lowering of low-density lipoprotein cholesterol levels and low-dose anticoagulation on obstructive changes in saphenous-vein coronary-artery bypass grafts. The Post Coronary Artery Bypass Graft Trial Investigators. N Engl J Med 336: 153–162, 1997.

100. Landau C, Lange RA, Hillis LD. Percutaneous transluminal coronary angioplasty. N Engl J Med 330:981–993, 1994.

101. Steinhubl SR, Berger PB, Mann JT, III, et al. Early and sustained dual oral antiplatelet therapy following percutaneous coronary intervention: a randomized controlled trial. JAMA 288:2411–2420, 2002.

102. Popma JJ, Ohman EM, Weitz J, et al. Antithrombotic therapy in patients undergoing percutaneous coronary intervention. Chest 119 (Suppl):321S–336S, 2001.

103. Chan AW, Bhatt DL, Chew DP, et al. Early and sustained survival benefit associated with statin therapy at the time of percutaneous coronary intervention. Circulation 105:691–696, 2002.

104. Chaitman BR, Skettino SL, Parker JO, et al. Anti-ischemic effects and long-term survival during ranolazine monotherapy in patients with chronic severe angina. J Am Coll Cardiol 43:1375–1382, 2004.

105. Chaitman BR, Pepine CJ, Parker JO, et al. Effects of ranolazine with atenolol, amlodipine, or diltiazem on exercise tolerance and angina frequency in patients with severe chronic angina: a randomized controlled trial. JAMA 291:309–316, 2004.

106. Gupta S, Leatham EW, Carrington D, et al. Elevated Chlamydia pneumoniae antibodies, cardiovascular events, and azithromycin in male survivors of myocardial infarction. Circulation 96:404–407, 1997.

107. Anderson JL, Muhlestein JB, Carlquist J, et al. Randomized secondary prevention trial of azithromycin in patients with coronary artery disease and serological evidence for Chlamydia pneumoniae infection: The Azithromycin in Coronary Artery Disease: Elimination of Myocardial Infection with Chlamydia (ACADEMIC) study. Circulation 99:1540–1547, 1999.

108. O'Connor CM, Dunne MW, Pfeffer MA, et al. Azithromycin for the secondary prevention of coronary heart disease events: the WIZARD study: a randomized controlled trial. JAMA 290:1459–1466, 2003.

Acute Myocardial Infarction

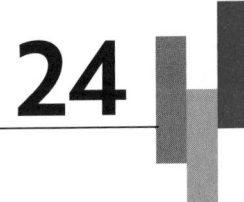

24

Edgar R. Gonzalez and Geneva C. Briggs

DEFINITION

Myocardial infarction (MI) is defined as death of myocardial tissue. The extent and location of the infarction depend on the degree of ischemic burden, the availability of coronary collateral blood flow, the rapidity of reperfusion, and the location of the afflicted coronary artery.

TREATMENT GOALS

- Abort the infarction.
- Salvage the area of jeopardized myocardium.
- Increase myocardial oxygen delivery.
- Decrease myocardial oxygen consumption.
- Provide symptomatic relief and reduce anxiety.
- Prevent complications and recurrences.
- Reduce mortality and improve quality of life.

EPIDEMIOLOGY

Every 20 seconds, someone in America has an acute myocardial infarction (AMI). Coronary artery disease (CAD), the primary predisposing factor for AMI, affects approximately 13 million Americans, 1.5 million of whom have an AMI each year.[1] In the United States, the magnitude of AMI as a public health concern is exemplified by the fact that 1 of 160 Americans has a heart attack. AMI is a frequent cause of emergency hospitalization in community hospitals and university medical centers and is the leading cause of death in the United States. Every hour, an American dies of a heart attack. In 1995, more than 400,000 Americans died of heart attacks; 50% of these patients suffered an out-of-hospital cardiac arrest within the first few hours from the onset of their cardiac symptoms.[2] Mortality among AMI victims ranges from 10% to 15% during the first year, decreasing to 3.5% per year thereafter.[2,3] Survival after AMI is determined partly by the extent of remaining viable myocardium and the occurrence of complications. Patients with anterior wall infarction, left ventricular dysfunction, and complex ventricular ectopy have the highest 1-year mortality rate after AMI (20%); patients with AMI without these risk factors have a 3% mortality rate.[4]

During the past decade, major improvements in the management of AMI patients have reduced AMI-related mortality by 50% in developed countries. Specifically, the introduction of intensive care units in the 1960s, improvement in pharmacologic reperfusion in the 1980s, and the widespread availability of percutaneous coronary intervention (PCI) in the 1990s have markedly reduced in-hospital mortality from AMI over the past 15 years.[5] Furthermore, the near-universal acceptance and prompt application of antiplatelet agents, β-adrenergic blockers, angiotensin-converting enzyme (ACE) inhibitors, and statins after an AMI have contributed to the improvement in long-term survival among AMI patients. Still, these great strides cannot diminish the impact of MI. First, the number of at-risk patients (e.g., genetic predisposition, smoking, poor dietary habits, or physical inactivity) is enormous and continues to increase, especially the population of diabetics, elderly patients, and other individuals with metabolic syndrome. Second, noncompliance with secondary preventive measures leads to a large population of post-MI patients at risk for recurrent events and death. Last, approximately 50% of AMI patients die before they can receive emergency prehospital care or acute interventions in the hospital.[5,6]

PATHOPHYSIOLOGY

An increase in myocardial oxygen demand relative to the available myocardial oxygen supply or an acute decrease in myocardial oxygen delivery can precipitate acute myocardial ischemic injury. Episodes of ischemia that last more than 30 minutes usually cause MI. The involved area can be divided into three zones: the zone of infarction, the zone of injury, and the zone of ischemia (Fig. 24.1). The infarction may be limited to the interior of the myocardium (subendocardial MI) or to a visceral layer of the pericardium (epicardial MI) or may extend through the full thickness of the myocardial wall (transmural MI). The most common cause of AMI is atherosclerosis of the coronary arteries, which narrows the coronary lumen and reduces myocardial blood supply. The terms *athero* and *sclerosis* are derived from the Greek words *gruel* and *hard*, respectively. The word *gruel* is similar to the rubbish located at the foundation of most formed plaques. *Hard* corresponds to the fibrotic cap of the lesion. The first noticeable sign of an atherosclerotic lesion is a fatty streak (yellow stripe) that runs parallel to the axis of the vessel.[7] The lesion progresses to form a necrotic core composed primarily of lipids and cellular debris. Fibrous caps composed of smooth muscle and collagen cover the fatty streaks, leading to ''vulnerable'' lesions[7] (Fig. 24.2). Ulceration of the vulnerable lesion or regional changes in blood flow trigger platelet aggregation, leading to thrombosis and coronary occlusion.[8,9]

Platelet involvement in thrombus formation begins with vessel wall injury, followed by platelet adhesion, activation, and aggregation.[7] After adhesion, platelets become activated through a cascade of steps that involve different agonists, including collagen, thrombin, serotonin, and epinephrine. These agonists trigger the release of agents that foster platelet aggregation [i.e., adenosine diphosphate (ADP) and thromboxane A_2 (TXA_2)]. Elevated shear force fosters the formation of atherosclerotic plaques within the intimal lumen. In the presence of disrupted blood flow or vascular insult, arterial thrombi or white clots form in these areas of high shear force.[2] Shear force-induced platelet aggregation is mediated by ADP. ADP and TXA_2 draw new platelets into areas of growing thrombi, leading to arterial thrombus formation. ADP and TXA_2 activate the glycoprotein IIb/IIIa

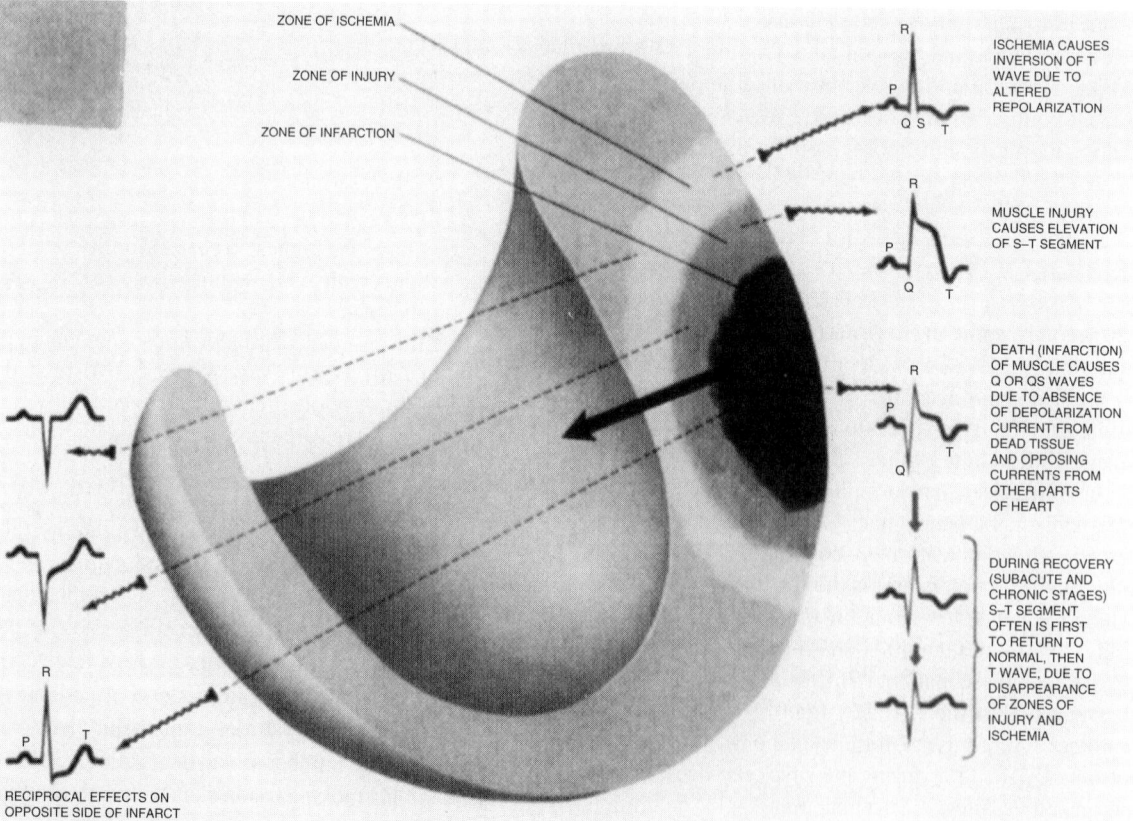

FIGURE 24.1 Effects of cardiac infarction, injury, and ischemia. (From Netter FH. The Netter Collection. In: Yonkmann FF, ed. The Ciba Collection of Medical Illustrations: Heart. New York: Ciba Pharmaceutical Company, 1969:62.)

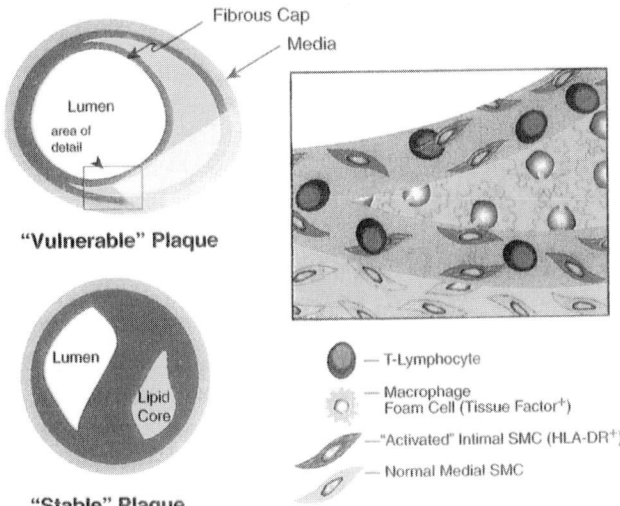

"Vulnerable" Plaque

"Stable" Plaque

— T-Lymphocyte
— Macrophage Foam Cell (Tissue Factor+)
— "Activated" Intimal SMC (HLA-DR+)
— Normal Medial SMC

FIGURE 24.2 Stable and vulnerable plaques. (From Libby P. Molecular bases of the acute coronary syndromes. Circulation 91:2844–2850, 1995.)

receptor complex to produce a transformational change that allows fibrinogen to bind and links the platelets together. Fibrin strands and erythrocytes coat the platelet-rich area and form thrombus (i.e., red plug).

Patients at highest risk for suffering an AMI are those with a prior history of AMI, CAD, or malignant arrhythmias.[10] Both modifiable and nonmodifiable risk factors increase the risk of AMI. Nonmodifiable risk factors such as increased age, male sex, and family history identify patients at risk for AMI. Common modifiable risk factors (i.e., cigarette smoking, diabetes mellitus, hyperlipidemia, hypertension, obesity, and physical inactivity) should be identified and, whenever possible, changed.

Diabetes mellitus, high levels of low-density lipoprotein (LDL) cholesterol, increased levels of catecholamines, or other factors affecting blood flow can contribute to the formation of an intravascular clot.[7] Less frequently, coronary vasospasm may precipitate clot formation and lead to complete coronary occlusion. Cocaine abuse has also been implicated as a possible cause of AMI due to complete coronary closure in the absence of coronary atherosclerosis. The morning hours are the peak times for suffering an AMI due to an increase in sympathetic activity that enhances platelet adhesiveness and coronary vasoconstriction. During the early morning hours, there is also an alteration in the plasminogen inhibitor and plasminogen ratio, making existing atherosclerotic plaques more vulnerable to rupture.[10] Antiplatelet agents and β-adrenergic blocking agents reduce the incidence of AMI by attenuating hyperaggregability of platelets and blunting the effects of circulating catecholamines, respectively. Precipitating factors for AMI include vasospasm, physical or emotional stress, hemorrhage, trauma, respiratory failure, hypoglycemia, exogenous sympathomimetics or other vasoactive substances, and hypersensitivity reactions.

Patients with >70% narrowing of the luminal diameter of one or more of the major coronary arteries [right coronary artery (RCA), left main, left anterior descending artery (LAD), or left circumflex artery (LCX)] are at greatest risk of ischemic injury (Fig. 24.3). The location of the coronary

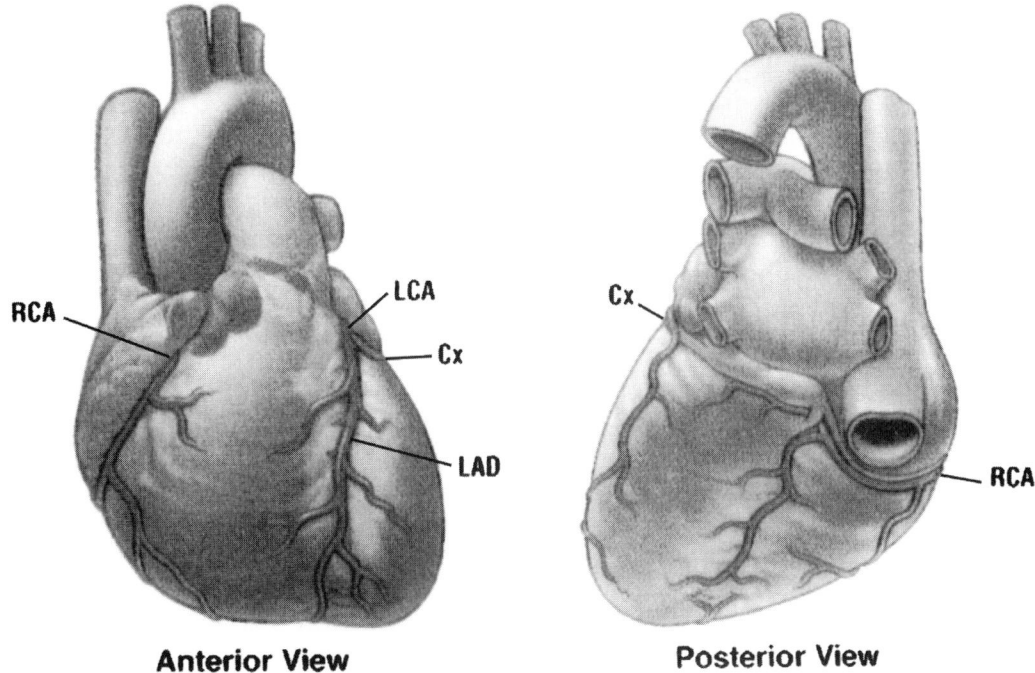

Anterior View

Posterior View

FIGURE 24.3 Common arteries of the heart: right coronary artery (RCA), left coronary artery (LCA), left circumflex artery (Cx). (Source: Advanced Cardiac Life Support. Dallas: American Heart Association, 1997–1999.)

thrombus determines the anatomic site of the AMI. Occlusion of the LAD usually causes an anterior wall infarction that may disrupt function of the left ventricle and may precipitate cardiogenic shock and sudden death. Occlusion of the RCA may produce an inferior wall infarction or a right ventricular (RV) infarction. RV infarction with bradycardia and hypotension may occur in patients with inferior wall MI.[11] Occlusion of the LCX usually results in a lateral wall infarction or a multiple-site infarction (e.g., anterolateral wall infarctions). A posterior wall infarction may also result from occlusion of the LCX, the RCA, or both.[10]

CLINICAL PRESENTATION AND DIAGNOSIS

SIGNS AND SYMPTOMS

The patient's chief complaint and medical history are invaluable in establishing a diagnosis of MI. Chest discomfort (i.e., oppressive, burning, squeezing, choking, or expanding sensation; tightness; or indigestion) is the most common presenting complaint. The discomfort is typically substernal; radiates to the neck, throat, jaw, shoulders, and arms; and may last from 30 minutes to several hours. Substernal chest pain associated with AMI does not subside with rest, is partially relieved by nitroglycerin, and produces a sense of ''impending doom.'' Most patients have prodromal symptoms (e.g., vague chest discomfort, weakness, fatigue, nausea, vomiting, and diaphoresis) before the acute attack.[12] Less commonly, an episode of light-headedness or syncope heralds the onset of AMI. However, approximately 15% to 20% of AMIs are asymptomatic (''silent MI''), and 33% of AMIs go undiagnosed, especially in women with preexisting hypertension, patients with diabetes, and elderly patients.

A detailed medical history may help to differentiate myocardial ischemic pain from noncardiac chest pain and may help uncover medication noncompliance. Review of systems may reveal a patient who is anxious, restless, cool, sweaty, and pale. Sinus tachycardia and mild fever are commonly observed. Sinus bradycardia is more common with inferior wall MI because occlusion of the RCA causes sinus node dysfunction. Blood pressure fluctuations are common during AMI. Hypertension may accompany pain and anxiety, whereas hypotension may result from drug-induced vasodilation, left ventricular dysfunction, or hypovolemia. Respirations are often rapid and shallow. Supplemental oxygen increases oxygen delivery and reduces the work of breathing. Heart sounds may be faint or normal, and an atrial gallop (S_4 sound) may be present.

Low-grade fever (i.e., <38°C) may be observed during the first 72 hours after AMI. Other physical findings include hypertensive retinopathy, diabetic nephropathy, and cholesterol-related xanthomas. Nonspecific laboratory abnormalities associated with AMI include polymorphonuclear leukocytosis (12,000 to 15,000/mm^3) that persists for 3 to 7 days and an elevated erythrocyte sedimentation rate, which peaks during the first week. Hypokalemia and hypomagnesemia may be present, especially in patients treated with diuretics, and may precipitate malignant ventricular arrhythmias.

A brief physical assessment by a pharmacist may promote rapid triage and rapid activation of the 911 system. A pharmacist's physical examination for AMI includes the following:

- Vital signs, general observation
- Pulmonary auscultation for rales
- Presence or absence of stroke
- Presence or absence of pulses
- Presence or absence of systemic hypoperfusion (cool, clammy, pale, and ashen extremities)

A more detailed physical examination aids in the differential diagnosis and is useful for assessing the extent, location, and presence of complications of the AMI and should be conducted only by appropriately trained personnel. Evidence of prior stroke or dementia may be suggested by the finding on examination of focal neurologic or cognitive deficits. A brief but focused examination can identify focal neurologic or cognitive deficits.

DIAGNOSIS

According to recent guidelines, patients must meet at least two of three criteria that define the presence of an AMI before a diagnosis can be established. The three criteria established by WHO are:

1. A clinical history of ischemic-type chest discomfort
2. Serial electrocardiographic (ECG) changes indicative of myocardial infarction, including the development of pathologic Q waves
3. A rise and fall in serum cardiac markers

A detailed history may help differentiate AMI from nonischemic chest pain syndromes (e.g., costochondritis, pericarditis, cardiac tamponade, or gastroesophageal reflux disease). The diagnosis of AMI is confirmed when any two of the following three clinical features are present: ischemic chest pain that lasts longer than 30 minutes and is unrelieved by nitroglycerin; new (ECG) changes that are consistent with AMI (i.e., ST-segment elevation in two contiguous precordial leads or more than 1- to 2-mm ST-segment elevation in two contiguous limb leads); or the presence of abnormally elevated levels of cardiac enzymes in the bloodstream.

Myocardial necrosis causes the release of intracellular enzymes [e.g., creatine kinase (CK), lactate dehydrogenase (LDH), and aspartate aminotransferase (AST)], myoglobin, and troponin into the systemic circulation. The temporal pattern of appearance in the systemic circulation after an AMI is of diagnostic importance (Table 24.1). Although the systemic release of CK is increased after skeletal muscle trauma related to surgery, exercise, or intramuscular injections, the MB fraction of CK is released only from heart muscle, and its concentration in blood may be used to determine the presence of an AMI. LDH increases more slowly than CK. When

TABLE 24.1	Myocardial Markers			
Parameter	Normal Range	Detectable (hr)	Time to Peak (hr)	Normalization (days)
Total CPK	Varies, 250–400 U/L	6–10	10–24	2–3
CK-MB mass	<8.0 ng/mL	3–6	10–24	3–4
Myoglobin	<76 ng/mL F	1–3	6–9	½–1
	<92 ng/mL M			
Troponin 1	<2.9 ng/mL	4–6	24	3–10

CPK, creatinine phosphokinase; CK-MB, MB fraction of creatinine kinase.

assessed within the second and third days after infarction, LDH has a relatively high specificity (94%) and good clinical sensitivity (85%) for AMI.[3,12] LDH_2 is the major LDH isoenzyme in blood; thus, the normal serum pattern shows more LDH_2 than LDH_1. A change in this relationship is seen after AMI, renal necrosis, and hemolysis. Within 48 hours after AMI, this serum pattern reverses in 80% of patients, who now show higher LDH_1 concentrations than LDH_2 concentrations. Because of poor sensitivity and specificity, the presence of AST is no longer used routinely to diagnose an AMI.

Serum myoglobin (S-Mgb) is an intracellular muscle protein that can serve as another marker for AMI. Because of the small size of S-Mgb compared with CK, S-Mgb can diffuse more quickly through injured cell membranes. S-Mgb appears at higher than normal levels as early as 1 to 3 hours after the onset of AMI, and the level peaks much more rapidly than either CK or LDH.[13] S-Mgb is of value in the early evaluation of patients with a potential AMI. A rapid rise in S-Mgb and a doubling of the S-Mgb concentration within the first 2 hours of treatment, even if the second level is within normal limits, is highly specific for AMI.[13] Because elevated S-Mgb levels usually return to normal

within 12 to 24 hours after the onset of symptoms, an isolated normal S-Mgb or a serial S-Mgb level that does not double does not necessarily rule out AMI.[13]

Studies now suggest that an assay based on monoclonal antibodies against troponin I is a better marker for AMI than CK-MB.[14] Troponin is part of the contractile apparatus of the myocardium. It is a regulatory subunit consisting of I, T, and C subunits.[15] Troponin I, or cardiac troponin, is used in the diagnosis of AMI because of its higher absolute cardiac specificity over the other troponin subunits.[15] Unlike CK and LDH, troponin I is highly specific to cardiac tissue and is not expressed in inflammatory and noninflammatory myopathies, skeletal muscle trauma, or chronic renal insufficiency.[15,16] Troponin I is undetectable in normal healthy adults.[16] The troponin I level peaks within 6 hours of the acute event and may remain elevated for as long as 7 to 10 days. Serial concentrations of troponin I should be measured at 3-hour intervals for the first 6 hours and then every 8 hours for the remaining 24 hours (Fig. 24.4). Once an elevated troponin I level is detected, the patient is likely to have myocardial injury. Many medical centers are now using troponin assays in the diagnosis of AMI. Recent studies show that an elevated cardiac troponin level on admission

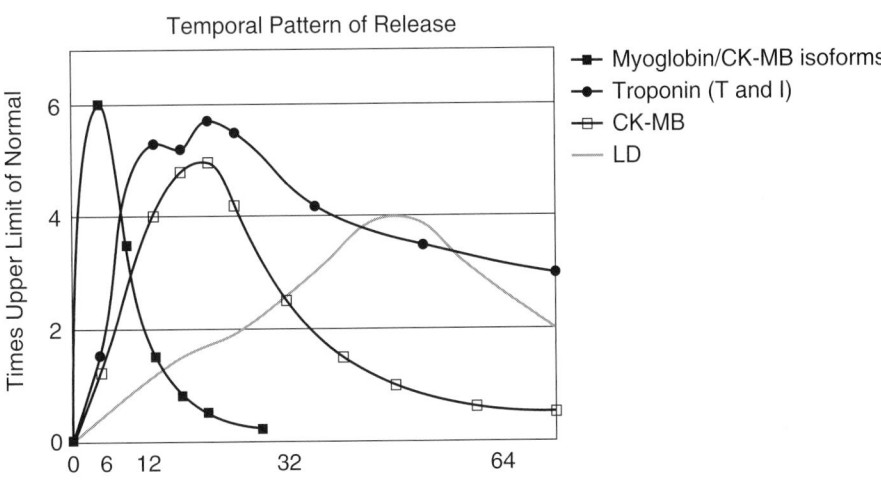

FIGURE 24.4 Temporal pattern of release of markers for myocardial necrosis. CK-MB, MB isoform of creatinine kinase; LD, lactate dehydrogenase.

is a predictor of subsequent cardiac events.[17] The recent changes to the definition of AMI reflect the increased emphasis on these specific biomarkers of myocardial injury.[17]

Recent research has evaluated the role of brain natriuretic peptide (BNP) in patients with AMI.[18] Unlike troponin, BNP is a counterregulatory hormone that plays an active role in the response to tissue injury. The levels of BNP may reflect the size and severity of myocardial ischemic injury. Ischemia may trigger the release of BNP via wall stress or directly from the myocytes. Additional studies are needed to define the role of BNP in AMI and acute coronary syndrome (ACS).

High-sensitivity C-reactive protein (CRP) is recognized as an independent predictor of short-term and long-term mortality in patients with ACS. However, there are limited data describing the time course of change for CRP in AMI. Yip et al evaluated the predictive value of CRP on 30-day outcomes in AMI patients when the CRP levels were measured within 6 hours of the onset of ischemia.[19] CRP levels were obtained in the cardiac catheterization laboratory before the onset of angiography. Patients were stratified as high CRP (>2.37 mg/L) and low CRP (≤ 2.37 mg/L). The 30-day composite for major adverse cardiac events was significantly higher ($p = 0.0008$) in the high CRP group (23%) than the low CRP group (4.1%). A recent study by Tanaka et al suggests that CRP levels correlate positively with the number of ruptured plaques during AMI.[20] In this study, patients with multiple plaque rupture had significantly higher CRP levels ($p = 0.01$) and a significantly worse prognosis ($p = 0.001$) after AMI. Additional studies will define the role of CRP as a prognosticator in AMI patients.

The ECG permits detection of the three pathophysiologic events occurring during an AMI: ischemia (T-wave inversion), injury (ST-segment elevation), and infarction (pathologic Q waves) (Fig. 24.1). The diagnostic feature of MI is a deep, wide Q wave or Q-S pattern (i.e., an initial slight upward deflection followed by a pronounced downward deflection) in the ECG leads corresponding to the area of injury. Although Q waves are seen more commonly in transmural than in nontransmural infarctions, both types may occur with or without Q waves. Therefore, it is more appropriate to use the terms *Q-wave* and *non–Q-wave* infarction.[21] Q waves do not diagnose an infarction; the presence of a Q wave will not be seen on an ECG until approximately 1 day after the event. If a patient is seen in the hospital with Q waves present on an ECG, this is evidence of a previous infarct. Non–Q-wave infarctions are associated with lower in-hospital mortality and complications but are also associated with an increased risk of subsequent events such as another infarction, a reinfarction, ischemia, or even death. Q-wave infarctions are associated with high rates of in-hospital death and complications, but the risk of reinfarction or subsequent events is lower.

An anterior wall MI is diagnosed by ST-segment elevations in leads V_1 and V_4 on an ECG strip. An inferior wall infarct results in ST-segment elevation in the inferior leads of an ECG, leads II, III, and aVF. RV infarctions usually cause ST-segment elevation in lead V4R and bradycardia because the RCA serves as the main blood supply to the sinoatrial node. If an inferior wall MI is identified on a left-sided ECG, a right-sided ECG should be done to exclude the possibility of a RV infarction in combination with inferior wall MI. A lateral infarction shows ST-segment elevation in leads I, aVL, V_5, and V_6. ECG changes seen with a posterior infarction are ST-segment depression in leads V_1 and V_2 with tall R waves.

However, patients with ischemic discomfort may present with or without ST-segment elevation on the ECG. Of patients with ST-segment elevation, most ultimately develop a Q-wave MI (QwMI), while a few develop a non–Q-wave MI (NQMI). Patients who present without ST-segment elevation are suffering from either unstable angina or a non–ST segment elevation MI (NSTEMI). Most patients presenting with NSTEMI ultimately develop a NQMI on the ECG; a few may develop a QwMI. The spectrum of clinical presentations ranging from unstable angina through NSTEMI and STEMI is referred to as the acute coronary syndromes.[17] Readers interested in learning more about the treatment of NSTEMI are referred to the excellent review by Gluckman.[22]

A conduction disturbance of the His bundle fibers (bundle branch block) may conceal the diagnosis of an AMI on an ECG. A bundle branch block distorts the ST segment on an ECG tracing. A left bundle branch block (LBBB) can shadow the diagnosis of an AMI more so than a right bundle branch block (RBBB). Blockage along the LAD can lead to LBBBs, whereas RCA occlusion can lead to RBBBs. A preexisting LBBB or RBBB will not interfere with ECG diagnosis of AMI. To determine if the conduction block is old or new requires previous ECG tracings. In the absence of an old ECG, the presence of either LBBB or RBBB makes the diagnosis of AMI difficult.

Pericarditis is inflammation of the pericardium, the fluid-filled sac that surrounds the heart. Pericarditis may produce chest pain and ECG changes and can confound the diagnosis of AMI. The ECG is useful in distinguishing pericarditis from an AMI based on the shape of the ST-segment elevation. The ST-segment elevation seen in AMI is rounded or concave, whereas pericarditis produces flat or convex ST-segment elevations.[23] In addition to ST-segment elevation seen with pericarditis, the T wave is often above the isoelectric line.

Radionuclide imaging techniques are valuable in assessing myocardial ischemic injury and confirming the suspicion of AMI in patients with atypical clinical presentations. Acute infarct scintigraphic (''hot spot'') imaging with infarct-avid Tc99m-pyrophosphatase aids in localizing and measuring the area of necrosis within 2 to 5 days after the AMI. Myocardial perfusion imaging with thallium-201, which is taken up and concentrated in viable myocardium, reveals a defect (''cold spot'') within 6 hours after AMI. Radionuclide ventriculography frequently reveals wall motion abnormalities and a reduced ventricular ejection fraction in patients with AMI.

PSYCHOSOCIAL ASPECTS

Time is a crucial factor in the treatment of AMI because thrombolytic therapy within the first hour after the onset of symptoms can salvage myocardial tissue and can abort an evolving AMI. Unfortunately, many patients fail to recognize the early signs of AMI and hesitate to seek prompt medical attention. The GISSI (Gruppo Italiano per lo Studio della Sopravvivenza nell'Infarto Miocardico) multicenter study compared 590 patients who were seen more than 12 hours after symptom onset with 600 patients treated within 2 hours and 603 patients treated between 6 and 12 hours.[24] Sixty percent of patients seen within 2 hours received thrombolytic therapy versus 18% of patients admitted more than 12 hours after the onset of symptoms. Factors associated with delayed hospital admission included age older than 65, living alone, diabetes mellitus, mild to moderate rather than severe pain, and onset of pain at night or at home.

Patients who are at risk for suffering an AMI as well as family members should be educated about the urgent need to seek help at the initial onset of symptoms; they should not wait to see if these symptoms abate with time. The classic symptoms as well as prodromal symptoms should be reinforced initially and again at each patient visit. National public awareness campaigns increase knowledge and awareness of the signs and symptoms associated with a heart attack.[25] Unfortunately, the results from these campaigns are disappointing because increased patient awareness appears to taper off several weeks after the end of the public awareness campaigns.[26] These observations suggest the need for patient education.

The American College of Cardiology/American Heart Association (ACC/AHA) guidelines for the treatment of AMI recommend that practitioners use the TIME method to help patients make a heart attack survival plan:[17]

- Talk with patients about:
  - The risks of a heart attack
  - Recognition of symptoms
  - Action steps to take and rationale for rapid action
  - Actions to take if symptoms develop
  - The importance of rapid activation of the 911 system
- Investigate:
  - The patient's thoughts and feelings about heart attacks
  - Potential barriers to symptom evaluation and response
  - Personal and family experiences with AMI and emergency medical treatment
- Make a plan:
  - For exactly what to do in case of heart attack symptoms, and make time for patients and their family members to rehearse the plan

- Evaluate:
  - The patient's understanding of risks in delaying the call to 911
  - The patient's understanding of your recommendations
  - The family's understanding of risks in delaying the call to 911

Pharmacists need to inform patients that death and disability from AMI can be reduced if artery-opening therapy is initiated within 1 hour of the onset of symptoms. Patients also need to be reminded that the most common barrier to initiation of treatment is their delay in seeking therapy. Patients need to know that unlike in the heart attacks commonly portrayed in movies, real heart attacks occur slowly with mild pain or discomfort. Therefore, a "wait-and-see attitude" is not in the patient's best interest. Patients should wait no more than 2 to 5 minutes at most to call 911.

THERAPEUTIC PLAN

After an AMI, sudden death is likely during the first 24 hours. If the infarction occurs outside the hospital setting, immediate transport to a hospital emergency department (ED) for management is essential. Activation of the 911 system reduces the time interval from ED arrival to definitive treatment and improves the likelihood of myocardial salvage (Fig. 24.5). Once acute therapy has been instituted and the patient's condition has been stabilized, he or she should be transferred to the coronary intensive care unit (CICU) for further observation and care.

Patients are triaged into risk and treatment categories for definitive diagnosis of AMI, for correction of underlying hematologic or electrolyte abnormalities, and for assessment of potential AMI-related complications. For example, a patient with ischemic chest pain who shows ECG changes consistent with an AMI will be rapidly evaluated for thrombolytic therapy. A complete history and physical examination, including rectal examination if not already obtained, should be completed. Routine clinical laboratory studies, including measurements of serum electrolytes and enzymatic markers of cardiac ischemia and injury, are performed. A 12-lead ECG and, if needed, a right-sided ECG should be obtained. Patients should receive oxygen, nitroglycerin, aspirin, and morphine. A chest radiograph with a portable x-ray machine should also be obtained soon after arrival at the ED.

Understanding the spectrum of acute coronary syndrome (i.e., unstable angina, NSTEMI, and STEMI) facilitates the tailoring of therapeutic strategies.[17] Because newly formed thrombus or impending thrombus may be present across the spectrum of acute coronary syndromes, antithrombin therapy and antiplatelet therapy should be administered to all patients with an acute coronary syndrome regardless of the presence or absence of ST-segment elevation.[17,27] Furthermore, because more than 90% of patients with STEMI have angiographic evidence of coronary thrombus formation, it is easy to justify the need for prompt initiation of reperfusion ther-

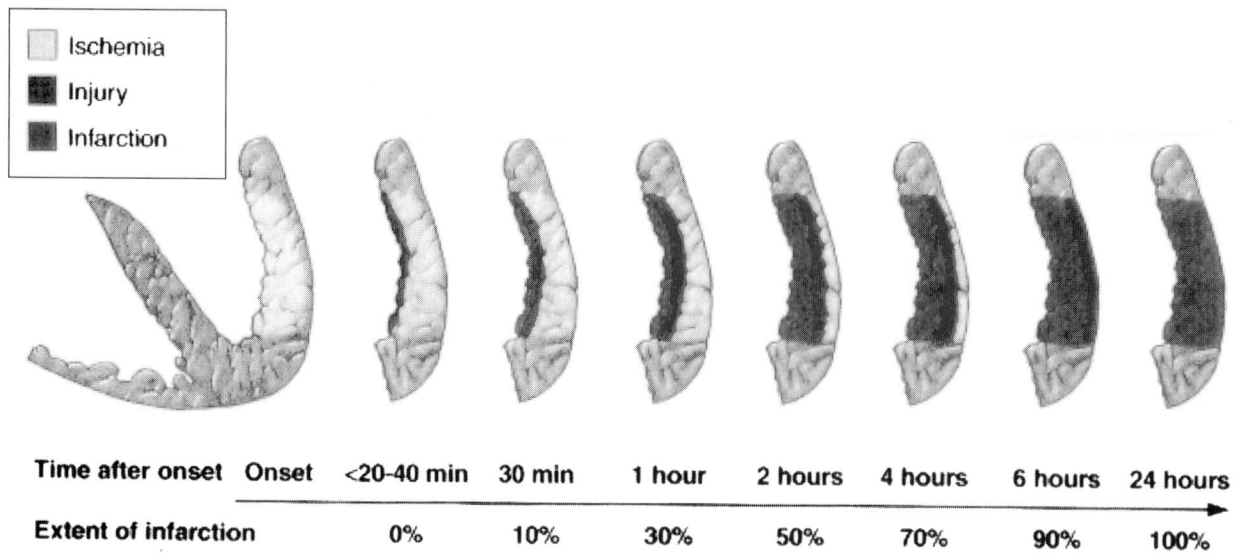

FIGURE 24.5 Time after onset—damage over time. (From Advanced Cardiac Life Support. Dallas: American Heart Association, 1997–1999.)

apy (either pharmacologic or catheter-based) to quickly restore flow in the occluded epicardial infarct-related artery in patients with STEMI.[17,27] Last, fresh thrombi are present in only 1% of patients with stable angina and in about 35% to 75% of patients with unstable angina or NSTEMI.[28] Therefore, patients presenting without ST-segment elevation are not candidates for immediate pharmacologic reperfusion but should receive anti-ischemic medical therapy; certain patients may benefit from catheter-based therapy.[28]

This chapter discusses only the acute treatment of STEMI. For a discussion on the treatment of NSTEMI and secondary preventive measures for long-term management of patients with myocardial ischemic disease, see the appropriate sections of this book.

TREATMENT

Treatments have been developed that reduce the morbidity and mortality of AMI, particularly when initiated early; it is therefore important to avoid delay in administering therapy. Although the greatest delay in treatment of AMI is usually the time it takes a patient to seek medical care, much of the emphasis on reducing delay has focused on the time between the patient's presentation to the ED and the administration of reperfusion therapy. A patient with symptoms suggestive of MI should be evaluated within 10 minutes after arrival to the ED. Early steps should include the following: hemodynamic stability should be assessed by measuring the patient's heart rate and blood pressure; a 12-lead ECG should be obtained; and oxygen should be given by nasal prongs and intravenous (IV) analgesia (most commonly morphine sulfate) should be administered, along with oral aspirin and sublingual nitroglycerin if the blood pressure is greater than

90 mm Hg. The challenge facing physicians who work in EDs is that more than 90% of patients who present to the ED with chest pain are not having an MI; many do not even have a cardiac etiology for their chest pain.

All patients with definite or suspected MI should be admitted to the hospital, undergo preparation for IV access, and be placed on continuous ECG monitoring. High-risk patients should be admitted to a coronary care unit. In many hospitals, patients at low risk for major complications are admitted to a telemetry unit, where emergency medical care can be quickly administered, rather than to a coronary care unit. Tachyarrhythmias and bradyarrhythmias may occur even in low-risk patients, particularly in the first 24 hours. Antiarrhythmic agents, an external or internal pacemaker, and a defibrillator should be readily available.

PHARMACOTHERAPY

Oxygen. Supplemental oxygen reduces the ischemic burden, but it is not known whether this therapy limits myocardial damage or reduces morbidity or mortality. Hypoxemia usually results from ventilation–perfusion abnormalities, commonly caused by left ventricular dysfunction and excessive lung water. Breathing oxygen may limit ischemic myocardial injury, and oxygen administration may reduce ST-segment elevation. Oxygen is administered at a rate of 4 L per minute by mask or nasal cannula for the first 24 to 48 hours. If oxygen saturation monitoring is used, therapy with supplemental oxygen is indicated if the saturation is less than 90%. Endotracheal intubation and positive airway pressure mechanical ventilation should be used if adequate oxygenation (oxygen saturation ≥90%) cannot be maintained by mask. High-level, continuous positive airway pressure improves tissue oxygenation and reduces the spontaneous respiratory effort without producing circulatory depression in patients with AMI and with left ventricular dysfunction.[29] Arterial blood gas determinations should be avoided shortly after the administration of thrombolytic therapy to minimize the risk of arterial bleeding. Continuous pulse oximetry assesses the adequacy of oxygenation and avoids the bleeding risk and discomfort produced by arterial punctures for blood gas monitoring.

For patients without complications, excess administration of oxygen can lead to systemic vasoconstriction, and high flow rates can be harmful to patients with chronic obstructive airway disease. In the absence of compelling evidence for established benefit in uncomplicated cases, and in view of its expense, there appears to be little justification for continuing its routine use beyond 6 hours.

Current 2004 ACC/AHA STEMI treatment guidelines recommend that supplemental oxygen therapy be continued beyond the first 6 hours in STEMI patients with Sa_{O_2} less than 90% or overt pulmonary congestion.[17]

Analgesics and Anxiolytics. Pain relief is an initial therapeutic objective. Prompt pain relief attenuates the sympathetic hyperactivity that increases myocardial oxygen demand and predisposes patients to tachyarrhythmias.[30] Numerous analgesic drugs (morphine, meperidine, and nalbuphine) have been used in AMI. Morphine is the agent of choice except in patients with a well-documented morphine hypersensitivity. In addition to relieving pain and anxiety, the hemodynamic effects of morphine are invaluable in patients with pulmonary edema. Morphine is a potent vasodilator. It increases venous capacitance and decreases systemic vascular resistance.[31] These effects are most pronounced in patients with heightened sympathetic tone. A dose of 2 to 4 mg should be administered intravenously over 1 to 2 minutes and repeated at 5- to 15-minute intervals until the pain is relieved or side effects occur (i.e., hypotension, respiratory depression, or vomiting) that preclude further administration. Adequate hydration and use of the recumbent position help reduce the risk of morphine-induced hypotension.

Concomitant administration of atropine 0.5 mg intravenously may help reverse the vagomimetic effects of morphine on blood pressure and heart rate. Meperidine 25 to 75 mg by slow intravenous injection every 2 to 3 hours as needed for pain control is a suitable alternative in morphine-intolerant patients. The anticholinergic effect of meperidine counteracts the heightened vagal tone in patients with AMI and either bradycardia or nausea. Tachycardia is a potential adverse effect of meperidine. Patients should be monitored for the respiratory-depressant effects of any narcotic analgesic.

Nalbuphine hydrochloride is a synthetic opioid analgesic with mixed narcotic agonist and antagonist effects. One study comparing the hemodynamic effects of nalbuphine and morphine in patients with AMI found that nalbuphine relieves pain and reduces myocardial oxygen demand without producing hypotension. Nalbuphine is a useful agent in patients with AMI because it produces less respiratory depres-

sion, less hypotension, and less vagal stimulation than morphine. Nalbuphine 10 mg is administered intravenously every 3 to 6 hours as needed for pain relief. Although butorphanol, a synthetic opioid agonist–antagonist, does not appear to significantly alter systemic hemodynamics, it should be avoided in patients with AMI because of concerns that it may increase systemic vascular resistance and myocardial oxygen demand.[32] Pentazocine and butorphanol should be used with caution in patients with AMI because they may increase systemic vascular resistance and myocardial oxygen demand.

Anxiolytics may be of value in patients with AMI for several reasons. First, the unfamiliar environment of the ICU and the stress and apprehension that accompany an acute illness may cause anxiety, restlessness, irritability, and delirium. These changes may cause tachycardia and increase the patient's myocardial oxygen demand. Second, anxiety, depression, irritability, and insomnia may develop in AMI patients who smoke and who experience symptoms of nicotine withdrawal during their hospitalization. Last, benzodiazepines decrease the outpouring of catecholamines from the brain, and this effect will decrease the workload of the heart. Therefore, short-term treatment with low-dose benzodiazepines may benefit AMI patients during their acute hospitalization and for a few days after hospital discharge. In patients with severe delirium, agitation, or reactive psychosis, intravenous haloperidol is a rapidly acting neuroleptic that can be given safely and effectively to patients with AMI. Haloperidol is extremely valuable since it is devoid of significant α-adrenergic blocking effects and anticholinergic effects and does not significantly alter respiratory drive or the ECG.

Current 2004 ACC/AHA STEMI treatment guidelines recommend morphine sulfate (2 to 4 mg IV with increments of 2 to 8 mg IV repeated at 5- to 15-minute intervals) as the analgesic of choice for the management of pain associated with STEMI.[17] Furthermore, it is reasonable to use anxiolytic medications (e.g., benzodiazepines) in STEMI patients to alleviate short-term anxiety or altered behavior related to hospitalization for STEMI, and to routinely assess the patient's anxiety level and manage it with behavioral interventions and referral for counseling as needed.

Nitrates. Organic nitrates, such as nitroglycerin and nitroprusside, reduce preload and afterload by their venodilatory and arteriodilatory effects, respectively.[33–39] Nitrates reduce myocardial oxygen demand and dilate the epicardial coronary vasculature. Nitroglycerin reduces intramyocardial wall tension, improves myocardial blood flow, and lowers systemic vascular resistance. Sublingual nitroglycerin is tried first unless the patient's systolic blood pressure is less than 90 mm Hg. In the presence of persistent ischemia and hypotension, nitroglycerin paste or IV nitroglycerin is preferred over sublingual nitroglycerin because the paste may be applied and removed promptly and the dose of IV nitroglycerin may be titrated to prevent further reductions in blood pressure.[33–39]

Nitroglycerin is generally well tolerated. Potential complications of IV nitroglycerin include reversible hypotension and bradycardia, hypoxemia due to increased pulmonary ventilation–perfusion mismatch, methemoglobinemia, and headache. Patients with nitroglycerin-induced hypotension usually respond to fluid resuscitation (e.g., 250 to 500 mL 0.9% saline solution) to maintain adequate cardiac output. Vasopressor agents are seldom required and should be avoided due to their propensity to worsen ischemia by increasing myocardial oxygen demand. Nitroglycerin may trigger a vasovagal reaction. In this situation, patients experience a paradoxical reduction in heart rate after nitroglycerin-induced hypotension.[33–36] These patients require fluid resuscitation and IV atropine (0.5 to 1.0 mg).

Nitroglycerin is contraindicated in patients who have an RV infarct or marked bradycardia (50 bpm or less). For patients with an RV infarction, the risk of precipitous hypotension with nitroglycerin is substantial because nitroglycerin increases venous capacitance and decreases venous return to the right atrium. These changes decrease the left ventricular filling volume and compromise cardiac output. Patients with nitroglycerin-induced hypotension usually respond to fluid resuscitation (e.g., 250 to 500 mL 0.9% saline solution) to maintain adequate cardiac output. Vasopressor agents are seldom required and should be avoided because of their propensity to worsen ischemia by increasing myocardial oxygen demand. Last, phosphodiesterase inhibitors potentiate the hypotensive effects of nitrates because of their mechanism of action in releasing nitric oxide and increasing cyclic guanosine monophosphate.[30] Practitioners need to ascertain whether such agents have been used, and nitrates should not be administered to patients who have received a phosphodiesterase inhibitor for erectile dysfunction in the prior 24 to 48 hours.[40]

The persistence of pain over several hours is a bad prognostic sign, usually indicative of continued myocardial ischemia and necrosis. Nitroglycerin relieves refractory angina in most patients. Patients with pulmonary edema derive great benefit from IV nitroglycerin because the venodilatory effects of nitroglycerin are directly proportional to preload (i.e., left ventricular end-diastolic pressure).[38] Prompt initiation of IV nitroglycerin therapy may reduce infarct size and decrease the incidence of congestive heart failure in patients with AMI.[38] Nitroglycerin infusion decreases both enzymatically assessed infarct size and hospital mortality in patients with AMI and left ventricular dysfunction.[33]

IV nitroglycerin is an effective adjunct in the management of heart failure associated with MI. It is administered by a continuous IV infusion at 10 to 20 μg per minute, increased by 5 to 10 μg per minute every 5 to 10 minutes until the desired hemodynamic or clinical response occurs. Low doses (30 to 40 μg/min) produce predominantly venodilation; high doses (250 μg/min) lead to arteriolar dilation as well.[34] In cardiogenic shock, the beneficial effects of ni-

troglycerin are due to systemic vasodilation, which increases cardiac output and lowers oxygen consumption, and to direct vasodilation of the coronary circulation, which increases the blood supply to ischemic areas more than nitroprusside.[34,35] The combination of nitroglycerin and an inotrope (dopamine and dobutamine), although not extensively studied, appears to produce marked hemodynamic improvements while reducing the risk of ischemic damage.[35] Overall, patients with the most severe degree of left ventricular failure have the most beneficial hemodynamic effects.

Studies show a difference between nitroglycerin and nitroprusside relative to their effect on myocardial blood flow.[36] Nitroglycerin has a greater vasodilatory effect on venous capacitance vessels than on arterial resistance vessels. In contrast, nitroprusside has a balanced vasodilatory effect on arteriolar resistance vessels and venous capacitance vessels. In patients with AMI, nitroglycerin is preferred over nitroprusside because nitroglycerin is less likely to produce ''coronary steal'' and worsen myocardial ischemia.[37,38] Coronary steal occurs either when blood is shunted away from the coronary arteries because of a fall in diastolic blood pressure or when blood is shunted away from the coronary collateral circulation because of a reduction in capillary resistance. Nitroglycerin is less likely to produce coronary steal than nitroprusside because nitroglycerin does not reduce coronary resistance, but facilitates blood flow along venous capacitance vessels in the coronary collateral circulation.

In summary, nitroglycerin does not readily relax resistance vessels and is less likely to reduce coronary perfusion pressure or shunt blood away from venous capacitance vessels (e.g., the collaterals) than nitroprusside.[37,38] The risk reduction in mortality in AMI trials with nitroglycerin is 45%, which is greater than the 23% reduction in mortality observed with nitroprusside.[38] These data suggest that IV nitroglycerin reduces mortality in AMI.

The 2004 ACC/AHA guidelines for STEMI offer the following recommendations for treatment with nitrates.[17] IV nitroglycerin is indicated in the first 48 hours after STEMI for treatment of persistent ischemia, congestive heart failure, or hypertension. The decision to administer IV nitroglycerin should not preclude therapy with other proven mortality-reducing interventions such as β-blockers or ACE inhibitors. IV, oral, or topical nitrates are useful beyond the first 48 hours after STEMI for treatment of recurrent angina or persistent congestive heart failure if their use does not preclude therapy with β-blockers or ACE inhibitors. The continued use of nitrate therapy beyond the first 24 to 48 hours in the absence of continued or recurrent angina or congestive heart failure may be helpful, although the benefit is likely to be small and is not well established in contemporary practice. Last, nitrates should not be administered to patients with systolic blood pressure less than 90 mm Hg or 30 mm Hg or more below baseline, severe bradycardia (<50 bpm), tachycardia (>100 bpm), or RV infarction.

Antiplatelet Agents. Aspirin inhibits platelet aggregation by irreversible acetylation of cyclooxygenase. Cyclooxygenase is an enzyme involved in the synthesis of TXA_2 and prostaglandin I_2 (PGI_2). TXA_2 is released by platelets, serving as a platelet aggregator as well as a vasodilator.[39] PGI_2 is produced by vascular endothelium and is an inhibitor of platelet aggregation and a vasodilator.[39] Aspirin shifts the balance in favor of PGI_2 because vascular endothelium synthesizes new cyclooxygenase within 6 hours, despite irreversible inactivation of platelet-derived cyclooxygenase.[39] Low-dose aspirin (i.e., 80 to 325 mg/day) inhibits TXA_2 for the lifetime of the platelet (i.e., 7 days).[39] High-dose aspirin (e.g., 1,000 mg/day) inhibits PGI_2 as well as TXA_2.[39,40]

Studies have been conducted using aspirin as well as other antiplatelet agents in the prevention of MI in patients with unstable angina.[41,42] Theroux et al[41] compared aspirin (325 mg twice daily) versus heparin (1,000 U/hr) or the combination of both in a double-blind, placebo-controlled trial of 479 patients with unstable angina pectoris. The incidence of MI was 3% with aspirin ($p = 0.01$), 0.8% with heparin ($p < 0.001$), and 1.6% with aspirin and heparin ($p = 0.003$) and 12% with placebo.[41] The mortality rate with active treatment was 0% compared to 1.7% with placebo. Theroux et al concluded that heparin decreased the incidence of MI; aspirin was also effective, but the combination of aspirin and heparin produced a greater number of complications and was no better than heparin alone.

The Second International Study of Infarct Survival Trial (ISIS-II) compared the relative efficacy of IV streptokinase (1.5 mU), oral aspirin (160 mg/day), both, or neither in patients with suspected MI.[42] Streptokinase reduced mortality at 5 weeks (9.2% with streptokinase vs. 12% with placebo ($p < 0.0001$). Similar results were observed with aspirin alone (9.4% with aspirin) versus placebo (11.8%) ($p < 0.00001$). The combination of aspirin and streptokinase was significantly more effective than either agent alone ($p < 0.0001$). Combination therapy had significantly fewer side effects than did either agent alone.

Aspirin was as effective as streptokinase in reducing the risk of death, but there was more benefit when the agents were used together.[42] Furthermore, aspirin reduced the rate of reinfarction.[42] Unless contraindicated, the administration of low doses (160 to 325 mg) of aspirin is advocated in all patients suspected of having an AMI. Upon arrival at the ED, patients with unstable angina or AMI should chew two baby aspirin tablets (160 mg total dose) irrespective of the need for thrombolytic therapy.[43] Patients should be maintained on aspirin indefinitely. Prolonged administration of aspirin in patients with a history of MI is associated with a 25% reduction in death, nonfatal reinfarction, and stroke.[44,45]

Although enteric-coated aspirin may be used in the AMI setting, chewing and swallowing regular aspirin is preferred since it produces more rapid peak serum aspirin concentrations, especially in the setting of opiate-induced decreased gastric motility such as that observed in morphine-treated patients.[17] Aspirin is contraindicated in those with a hypersensitivity to salicylate. Aspirin suppositories (300 mg) can be used safely, and this is the recommended route of administration for patients with severe nausea and vomiting or known upper gastrointestinal disorders. Clopidogrel or ticlopidine may be substituted in patients with true aspirin allergy (hives, nasal polyps, bronchospasm, or anaphylaxis).[44,45]

According to the 2004 ACC/AHA guidelines for STEMI,[17] a daily dose of aspirin (initial dose of 162 to 325 mg orally; maintenance dose of 75 to 162 mg) should be given indefinitely after STEMI to all patients without a true aspirin allergy.

Ticlopidine and clopidogrel are thienopyridine compounds that selectively bind adenylate cyclase-coupled ADP receptors and irreversibly inhibit platelet aggregation induced by epinephrine, collagen, thrombin, and platelet-activating factor.[46] Thienopyridine compounds reduce fibrinogen levels, platelet deposition on atheromatous plaque, and blood viscosity.[46,47] The antiplatelet effects of thienopyridines occur within 24 to 48 hours and peak after repeated administration around day 5 to 6.[46,47] The recommended dose of ticlopidine is 250 mg twice a day. The recommended dose for clopidogrel is 75 mg once a day.

Knudsen et al[48] compared ticlopidine (250 mg twice daily) with placebo on platelet function in patients with AMI treated within 12 hours of onset of precordial pain. Antiplatelet therapy was continued for 3 months after AMI.[47] Acute platelet survival was longer with ticlopidine (8 days) compared with placebo (5 days) ($p < 0.05$). Three months after the AMI there was no significant difference in platelet survival time between treatment groups. Knudsen et al concluded that ticlopidine decreased platelet activity and infarct size during AMI. The CAPRIE study was a randomized, blinded comparative trial of clopidogrel (75 mg once daily) and aspirin (325 mg once daily) in patients at risk for acute ischemia (i.e., stroke, AMI, or peripheral arterial disease).[49] For patients with AMI, the annual reduction in acute ischemic events did not differ between clopidogrel (5.03%) and aspirin (4.84%) ($p = 0.66$). The CAPRIE investigators concluded that clopidogrel and aspirin do not differ with respect to reduction of ischemic events in patients seen post-AMI.[49] The Antiplatelet Trialists' Collaboration reported a 2.4% incidence of neutropenia with ticlopidine.[50] In CAPRIE, the incidence of neutropenia with clopidogrel and aspirin was 0.1% and 0.17%, respectively.[49]

In patients with STEMI, clopidogrel combined with aspirin is recommended for patients who undergo coronary stent implantation.[17] There are no safety data available regarding the combination of fibrinolytic agents and clopidogrel. However, in patients with aspirin sensitivity, clopidogrel is probably useful as a substitute for aspirin to reduce the risk of occlusion.[17] There are no safety data comparing 300 and 600 mg as loading doses for clopidogrel in STEMI patients. The routine administration of clopidogrel as pretreatment in patients who have not yet undergone diagnostic cardiac catheterization and in whom coronary artery bypass surgery would be performed within 5 to 7 days is warranted.[17]

The 2004 ACC/AHA guidelines for STEMI provide the following recommendations regarding thienopyridines.[17] Clopidogrel is preferred because of fewer side effects, lack of need for laboratory monitoring, and once-daily dosing. In patients who have undergone diagnostic cardiac catheterization and for whom PCI is planned, clopidogrel should be started and continued for at least 1 month after bare-metal stent implantation, for several months after drug-eluting stent implantation (3 months for sirolimus, 6 months for paclitaxel), and up to 12 months in patients who are not at high risk for bleeding. In patients taking clopidogrel in whom coronary artery bypass surgery is planned, the drug should be withheld for at least 5 days, and preferably for 7 days, unless the urgency for revascularization outweighs the risks of excess bleeding. Clopidogrel is probably indicated in patients receiving fibrinolytic therapy who cannot take aspirin because of hypersensitivity or major gastrointestinal intolerance.

Unfractionated Heparin. Full-dose unfractionated heparin (UFH) is administered after thrombolytic therapy to prevent coronary artery reocclusion after successful thrombolysis in patients with AMI. The risk of reocclusion is high immediately after thrombolysis because blood flowing through the newly opened coronary artery is exposed to thrombin bound to fibrin on the residual thrombus. Clinical studies of patients with venous thrombosis and AMI indicate that there is a relation between the anticoagulant response to UFH and clinical efficacy.[51] Patients treated with streptokinase benefit from heparin therapy at relatively small doses (e.g., 12,500 U subcutaneously every 12 hours). Whereas this subcutaneous regimen of UFH failed to produce benefit in patients with AMI treated with tissue-type plasminogen activator (t-PA), full-dose heparin (e.g., 5,000-unit bolus followed by 30,000 U per 24 hours by continuous infusion) improves patency after coronary thrombolysis with t-PA. A plausible explanation for these apparently contradictory findings is that the lack of systemic lytic effect seen with t-PA requires heparin to be administered early and in high doses compared with UFH requirements after thrombolysis with streptokinase.

The Heparin-Aspirin Reperfusion Trial (HART) compared immediate administration of UFH (5,000-unit bolus), followed by a continuous infusion (106 patients), plus oral aspirin (99 patients) (80 mg) as adjunctive therapy, to recombinant t-PA (rt-PA) (100 mg over a 6-hour period).[52] Treatment was initiated within 6 hours of symptom onset. The three primary endpoints of the study were patency rates at 7 and 24 hours after rt-PA, ischemic or hemorrhagic complications during hospitalization, and angiography on day 7. Among patients treated with UFH plus aspirin, the infarct-related artery was patent in 82% of patients after the first angiogram compared with 52% in the aspirin group (*p* <0.0001). Of the vessels that were patent initially, 88% were still patent after 7 days in the heparin group, compared with 95% in the aspirin-treated group. This difference, however,

failed to reach statistical significance. There were 18 hemorrhagic complications in the heparin group compared with 15 in the aspirin-treated group. The number of recurrent events in both groups was similar. The authors concluded that UFH in combination with rt-PA produced a higher patency rate than rt-PA plus aspirin.[52]

The benefits of UFH are proven in unstable angina, but the role of UFH in AMI remained unproved until recently.[53] Current clinical practice is to use subcutaneous heparin for the prevention of venous thromboembolic events in patients with AMI. Heparin is recommended for patients receiving t-PA as well as for patients undergoing percutaneous transluminal coronary angioplasty (PTCA) or surgical revascularization, and those with severe left ventricular dysfunction, mural thrombi, or atrial fibrillation.[53]

The 2004 ACC/AHA guidelines for STEMI make the following recommendations regarding UFH.[17] Patients undergoing percutaneous or surgical revascularization should receive UFH. UFH should be given IV to patients undergoing reperfusion therapy with alteplase, reteplase, or tenecteplase. UFH should be given IV to patients treated with nonselective fibrinolytic agents (streptokinase, anistreplase, urokinase) who are at high risk for systemic emboli (large or anterior MI, atrial fibrillation, previous embolus, or known left ventricular thrombus). Platelet counts should be monitored daily. The dosing of UFH is as follows: bolus of 60 U per kg (maximum 4,000 U) followed by an infusion of 12 U/kg/hr (maximum 1,000 U) initially adjusted to maintain the activated partial thromboplastin time (aPTT) at 1.5 to 2.0 times control (approximately 50 to 70 seconds). The optimal duration of IV heparin therapy is unclear. Standard practice was to administer IV heparin for 3 to 5 days, although patients are now often discharged after only 3 days. Heparin should be discontinued more than 24 hours before the patient is discharged from the hospital because of the possibility of a rebound effect and recurrent thrombosis within 24 hours after cessation of heparin therapy.[17]

Side effects of UFH include hemorrhage (intracranial or gastrointestinal) and thrombocytopenia. Heparin is contraindicated in patients who have a history of hemorrhage, uncontrolled hypertension, vasculitis, blood dyscrasias, active bleeding, or a bleeding ulcer or who have recently had major surgery. Patients with AMI who do not have contraindications to heparin therapy should receive 5,000 U of heparin subcutaneously every 12 hours to decrease the risk of clot formation. Patients who are obese, who suffer from a ventricular aneurysm or cardiogenic shock, or who have a history of thrombophlebitis or arterial or venous embolism are predisposed to thrombus formation and should receive full anticoagulation. Patients with a transmural anterior MI have a 30% to 40% chance of developing left ventricular thrombi. Anticoagulation of these patients early in the course of therapy will prevent cerebrovascular accidents.

Low-Molecular-Weight Heparin. Compared with UFH, low-molecular-weight heparins (LMWHs, depolymerized

UFH with a mean molecular weight of approximately 5,000) have improved bioavailability, a longer duration of action, decreased binding to plasma proteins, decreased sensitivity to platelet factor 4, enhanced factor Xa activity, a more predictable anticoagulant response, and a decreased risk of bleeding and thrombocytopenia.[53,54] Gurfinkel et al[55] evaluated LMWH plus aspirin, UFH heparin plus aspirin, or aspirin alone in 219 patients with unstable angina. LMWH reduced the occurrence of recurrent angina compared with unfractionated heparin plus aspirin ($p = 0.002$) and of nonfatal AMI and urgent revascularization compared with aspirin alone ($p = 0.01$). Gurfinkel et al did not observe a difference in major bleeding episodes or death between treatment groups.

Klein et al[56] compared LMWH with UFH in 1,482 patients with unstable angina or non–Q-wave AMI. All patients received concurrent therapy with aspirin. Klein et al observed no significant difference with respect to recurrent angina, AMI, death, or adverse effects between LMWH and UFH.

LMWH is at least as effective in reducing ischemic events in patients with acute coronary syndromes.[54] Additional studies are needed to determine whether LMWHs are more cost-effective than UFH in patients with AMI. When coadministered with thrombolytics to patients with AMI, LMWH has the potential to reduce short-term mortality, in-hospital reinfarction, and in-hospital refractory ischemia, but the combined use of LMWH and thrombolytics carries a high risk of intracranial hemorrhage, especially in elderly patients.[17] Therefore, practitioners may need to reduce the dose of LMWH in elderly patients with AMI, especially if these patients are treated with thrombolytics.[54]

The 2004 ACC/AHA guidelines for STEMI make the following recommendations regarding LMWH.[17] LMWH might be considered an acceptable alternative to UFH as ancillary therapy for patients aged less than 75 years who are receiving fibrinolytic therapy, provided that significant renal dysfunction (serum creatinine >2.5 mg/dL in men or 2.0 mg/dL in women) is not present. Enoxaparin (30-mg IV bolus followed by 1.0 mg/kg given subcutaneously every 12 hours until hospital discharge) used in combination with full-dose tenecteplase is the most comprehensively studied regimen in patients less than 75 years of age. LMWH should not be used as an alternative to UFH as ancillary therapy in patients more than 75 years of age who are receiving fibrinolytic therapy. LMWH should not be used as an alternative to UFH as ancillary therapy in patients less than 75 years old who are receiving fibrinolytic therapy but have significant renal dysfunction (serum creatinine >2.5 mg/dL in men or 2.0 mg/dL in women).[17,57]

Direct Thrombin Inhibitors. The direct thrombin inhibitor bivalirudin may provide an alternative to UFH or LMWH because bivalirudin blocks both circulating and clot-bound thrombin.[57,58] In patients with unstable angina, bivalirudin provides a greater reduction in the rate of AMI and in the likelihood of dying from the acute coronary syndrome when compared with UFH.[58] Furthermore, bivalirudin produces a clinically relevant decrease in the rate of reinfarction but no change in mortality compared with UFH in patients with AMI. Unfortunately, bivalirudin may produce clinically relevant increases in the risk of major bleeding when compared with UFH in patients with AMI.[58]

The 2004 ACC/AHA guidelines for STEMI make the following recommendations regarding bivalirudin.[17] In patients with known heparin-induced thrombocytopenia, it is reasonable to consider bivalirudin as a useful alternative to heparin to be used in conjunction with streptokinase. The appropriate dose of bivalirudin in these patients is a bolus of 0.25 mg per kg followed by an IV infusion of 0.5 mg/kg/h for the first 12 hours and 0.25 mg/kg/h for the subsequent 36 hours, but with a reduction in the infusion rate if the partial thromboplastin time is above 75 seconds within the first 12 hours.[17,57]

Reperfusion Therapy. Important predictors of early clinical outcome in AMI (e.g., age of the patient, initial heart rate and blood pressure, initial Killip classification, and infarct location) are independent of treatment.[59] However, time to administration of reperfusion therapy is a critical determinant of long-term outcome and one of the few controllable determinants of early clinical outcome. Studies show that mortality and infarct size are directly proportional to the rapidity of reperfusion of the infarct-related artery.[59] The time between a patient's presentation to the ED and the administration of thrombolytic therapy should not exceed 60 minutes; ideally, it should be less than 30 minutes.[45] The critical interval is the time between symptom onset and reperfusion, not the time to the initiation of therapy. Therefore, a therapy that takes longer to initiate (e.g., PCI) may actually be superior if it achieves reperfusion more rapidly than one that can be initiated more rapidly (e.g., thrombolytic therapy).[44,59] Therefore, the best reperfusion therapy (coronary angioplasty or thrombolytic therapy) is not necessarily the one that can be most rapidly initiated; rather, it is the one that achieves coronary patency most rapidly.[44] Clinicians should have a working knowledge of their institution's elapsed time to successful PCI versus successful coronary thrombolysis. At institutions where a skilled catheterization team is on call 24 hours a day and can be rapidly assembled, coronary angioplasty would most likely be able to restore coronary blood flow in more patients more rapidly than thrombolytic therapy. Elsewhere, thrombolytic therapy may be preferable. However, transport of an AMI patient from one institution to another for the sake of obtaining primary PCI instead of thrombolytic therapy may be unwise if the patient is hemodynamically unstable or if the transport time is of such length that the time from symptom onset to initiation of PCI exceeds 90 minutes.[17]

Thrombolytic Agents. Thrombolytic therapy has been widely studied in prospective, randomized, controlled trials involving more than 50,000 patients and has been proved to reduce mortality 29% in patients with ST-segment elevation treated within 6 hours after the onset of chest pain. The survival benefit of thrombolytic therapy is maintained for 1 year.[45,59] The benefit of thrombolytic therapy is achieved through rapid restoration of blood flow in an occluded coronary artery. Thrombolytic therapy can save cardiac muscle in patients with AMI.[60,61] Sustained blood flow to the infarcted area reduces mortality and prevents electrical instability and left ventricular dysfunction. Thrombolytic agents activate both soluble plasminogen and surface-bound plasminogen to plasmin. Plasmin lyses fibrin and dissolves the clot. Fibrin selectivity is dose-dependent, and all agents activate circulating plasminogen to different degrees (streptokinase > reteplase = t-PA).[62] The activation of circulating plasminogen generates a systemic lytic response characterized by the conversion of fibrin to fibrin degradation products.[63] The fibrin degradation products have anticoagulant properties that prevent subacute vessel reclosure.

Many different thrombolytic regimens have been proved effective for the treatment of AMI, and many more are being studied. In principle, the preferred thrombolytic regimen would restore normal antegrade blood flow to an occluded coronary artery most rapidly and in the greatest number of patients, would have the lowest reocclusion rate, and would be associated with the lowest risk of severe hemorrhagic complications.[45] Table 24.2 compares the commercially available thrombolytic agents used in patients with AMI.[4]

Streptokinase binds plasminogen to form a complex that activates circulating plasminogen to plasmin. Streptokinase reduces blood viscosity and lowers systemic vascular resistance.[62] IV streptokinase is administered at a dose of 1.5 million U over 30 to 60 minutes. After the administration of streptokinase, patients should receive full-dose heparin for 24 to 72 hours. To reduce the risk of allergic reactions, patients may be given diphenhydramine 25 mg and hydrocortisone 100 mg IV before streptokinase infusion. Streptokinase therapy is contraindicated in patients who have recently received a dose of streptokinase because of antibodies that form against the drug; these antibodies limit the efficacy of repeat doses and increase the risk of allergic reactions. It has been suggested that the drug not be readministered for at least 2 years.

t-PA produces dose-dependent activation of fibrin-bound plasminogen.[62] Unlike streptokinase and APSAC, t-PA is not antigenic; hematoma and prolonged bleeding at the injection site are the most commonly reported adverse effects.[62] Because the speed of reperfusion is linked to the rate of administration of t-PA, accelerated (90-minute) infusions of t-PA produce more rapid reperfusion without compromising safety.[63,64] To prevent postlytic reocclusion, anticoagulation with full-dose IV unfractionated heparin is required for at least 24 hours. The dose of heparin is adjusted to maintain an activated partial thromboplastin time two times control for at least 24 hours.

Tenecteplase is a single-bolus formulation of t-PA. The single IV bolus is administered over 5 seconds and the dose is adjusted according to body weight (i.e., <60 kg, 30 mg; 60 to 69 kg, 35 mg; 70 to 79 kg, 40 mg; ≥80 kg, 50 mg).

Reteplase is a nonglycosylated deletion mutant of t-PA that is produced by expression of an appropriately constructed plasmid in *Escherichia coli*.[65] Reteplase lacks the kringle-1 domain, the finger domain, and the epidermal growth factor domain contained in t-PA.[66] These changes extend the half-life of reteplase (13 to 16 minutes) when compared to t-PA (5 to 6 minutes). The absence of the fibrin-specific finger region and the epidermal growth factor domain affects renal blood flow and fibrin specificity as well as affinity. In addition, reteplase has less affinity for binding fibrin when compared with t-PA. Reteplase is metabolized in the kidneys, liver, and blood. Renal failure produces a proportional decrease in the clearance of reteplase ($r = 0.713$; $p < 0.001$).[64,66] Renal dysfunction impairs the elimination of reteplase but not of t-PA.[66] The prolonged half-life and greater activity of reteplase, when compared with those of t-PA, have been demonstrated in animal studies.[65-68] Reteplase is 5.3 times more effective than t-PA in lysing jugular venous thrombus after single IV bolus administration.[68] The potential advantages of reteplase over t-PA include more rapid and more complete reperfusion and a longer half-life that allows bolus administration without a continuous infusion.[64,65] The recommended dose of reteplase is two 10-unit IV boluses given 30 minutes apart. This convenient regimen is especially valuable in a busy ED.[62]

Thrombolytics reduce morbidity and mortality if given within the first 6 hours after the onset of AMI symptoms.[67,69,70] The goals of thrombolytic therapy are to lyse coronary thrombi during the early phase of AMI, to limit

TABLE 24.2	Comparison of Thrombolytic Agents			
	Alteplase	**Reteplase**	**Streptokinase**	**Tenecteplase**
Dose	Up to 100 mg in 90 min according to body weight	10 U × 2 over 2 min via bolus injection	1.5 MU over 60 min	30–50 mg according to body weight via bolus injection
Antigenic/allergenic	No	No	Yes	No
Sytemic lytic effect	No	No	Yes	No
Expensive	Yes	Yes	No	Yes

TABLE 24.3	Eligibility Criteria for Thrombolytic Therapy

Clinical

Chest pain or chest pain-equivalent syndrome consistent with acute myocardial infarction ≤12 hours from symptom onset with

Electrocardiogram

≥1 mm ST-segment elevation in ≥2 contiguous limb leads

≥2 mm ST-segment elevation in ≥2 contiguous precordial leads

New bundle branch block

Cardiogenic shock

Emergency catheterization and revascularization if possible; consider thrombolysis if catheterization not immediately available.

infarct size by reperfusing jeopardized myocardium, and to reduce morbidity and mortality. Patients with recent onset of chest pain (usually <12 hours) or persistent ECG abnormalities indicating an evolving transmural AMI are candidates for thrombolytic therapy (Table 24.3).[69]

Treatment within the first hour after the onset of symptoms yields the maximal myocardial salvage in patients with AMI and ST-segment elevation.[71] Pooled data from mortality studies suggest that a 70% reduction in mortality can be achieved when thrombolytic therapy is initiated within 1 hour of symptom onset.[69,70] Afterward, the incremental benefit of thrombolytic treatment is less, and the degree of myocardial salvage is even further decreased after 3 hours. The Myocardial Infarction Triage and Intervention (MITI) trial showed a 1% mortality rate when thrombolytics are initiated within 70 minutes.[72] A delay in therapy beyond 70 minutes resulted in a 10% mortality rate.[73] Thrombolysis within the first hour of symptoms produces "an abortive effect on AMI" in approximately 40% of patients.[73] Data from the Global Utilization of Streptokinase and Tissue Plasminogen Activator for Occluded Coronary Arteries-I (GUSTO-I) investigators showed differences between clot-selective and non–clot-selective agents with respect to the open-artery principle.[74] Compared with streptokinase, t-PA opens occluded coronary arteries faster and improves survival if administered within 4 hours after symptom onset.[75]

In summary, controlled clinical trials demonstrate functional, clinical, and mortality benefits only if fibrinolytic therapy is given within 12 hours.[17,27,45] The reduction in mortality with fibrinolytic therapy is present regardless of sex, presence of diabetes, blood pressure (if <180 mm Hg systolic), heart rate, or history of previous MI. The mortality benefit is greater in the setting of anterior AMI, diabetes, low blood pressure (<100 mm Hg systolic), or high heart rate (>100 bpm). The earlier therapy begins, the better the outcome, with the greatest benefit decidedly occurring when therapy is given within the first 3 hours. Benefit occurs, however, up to at least 12 hours from the onset of symptoms.

The absolute benefit is less with inferior AMI, except for the subgroup with associated RV infarction or anterior ST-segment depression indicative of a greater territory at risk.[17]

Contraindications to the use of thrombolytic therapy are listed in Table 24.4. An absolute contraindication means that thrombolytic therapy is not to be given regardless of eligibility criteria. However, it is important to consider whether a contraindication is relative or absolute. A relative contraindication means that the clinician must weigh the benefits of giving the thrombolytic versus the risks to the patient. Hemorrhage is the most important risk of fibrinolytic therapy. Hemorrhagic complications of fibrinolytic therapy primarily include intracranial hemorrhage and other moderate or severe bleeding that may or may not require transfusion. The slight but definite excess risk of intracranial hemorrhage occurs predominantly within the first day of therapy; it may be fatal in half to two thirds of patients.[76] Typical presenting features include an acute change in level of consciousness, unifocal or multifocal neurologic signs, coma, headache, nausea, vomiting, and seizures, at times with acute hypertension. In many cases, onset is catastrophic and rapidly fatal. Therefore, practitioners should ascertain whether the patient has neurologic contraindications to fibrinolytic therapy, including any history of intracranial hemorrhage or significant closed head or facial trauma within the past 3 months, uncontrolled hypertension, or ischemic stroke within the past 3 months.[17,45]

TABLE 24.4	Contraindications to Thrombolytic Therapy

Intracranial neoplasms

Active internal bleeding

Previous history of hemorrhagic stroke

Previous allergic reaction to streptokinase

Suspected aortic dissection

A stroke or other cerebrovascular accident within the last year

Current use of anticoagulants (INR >2–3)

Prolonged and or potentially traumatic cardiopulmonary resuscitation (>10 min)

Severe uncontrolled hypertension upon presentation (blood pressure >180/110)

Recent internal bleeding episode (2–4 weeks)

Pregnancy

Active peptic ulcer

Noncompressible vascular punctures

Prior exposure to streptokinase within the past 2 years

Prior allergic reaction to streptokinase

Major surgery within the last 3 weeks

Menses is not a contraindication to thrombolytic therapy

INR, international normalized ratio.

Bleeding complications with thrombolytic agents are due to their general interference with hemostatic mechanisms. Thrombolytics do not differentiate between pathologic clots and hemostatic plugs. Lysis of hemostatic plugs can lead to bleeding complications after pharmacologic thrombolysis. Clinical studies show a 5% risk of major bleeding complications from thrombolytic therapy.[67,70] Bleeding complications are minimized by avoiding drugs that affect hemostasis and by avoiding excessive venipunctures. Compared with streptokinase, t-PA appears to be associated with a slightly higher risk of stroke in patients who have an AMI.[77] Any change in neurologic function, particularly in the first 24 hours after treatment, should be regarded as strongly indicative of intracranial hemorrhage.[17] Fibrinolytic, anticoagulant, antiplatelet, and combined therapies should be discontinued as soon as symptoms and signs are recognized. Immediate measures to reduce intracranial pressure are reasonable and include mannitol infusion, elevation of the head of the bed to 30 degrees, endotracheal intubation, and hyperventilation to achieve a p_{CO_2} of 25 to 30 mm Hg. If intracranial hemorrhage is documented, the patient should be given 10 U of cryoprecipitate, which will increase the fibrinogen level by approximately 0.70 grams per liter and the factor VIII level by approximately 30% in a 70-kg adult.[17] Fresh-frozen plasma can be used as a source of factors V and VIII and as a volume expander. In patients who are receiving UFH, 1 mg of protamine for every 100 U of UFH given in the preceding 4 hours may be administered. If the bleeding time is abnormal, infusion of 6 to 8 U of platelets is indicated. In rare cases, antifibrinolytic agents, such as ε-aminocaproic acid, may be necessary. Control of blood pressure and blood glucose levels may require a compromise between competing cardiologic and neurologic concerns. Mannitol and hyperventilation are reserved for patients with incipient brain herniation syndromes. After the patient is stabilized, catheter-based angiography may be necessary.

Data from the GISSI-2 trial suggest that there are four additional strokes per 1,000 patients treated with t-PA than with streptokinase. Logistic regression analysis on the data from the GISSI-2 trial revealed a significant association between the risk of stroke and older age, female sex, anterior infarction, and more extensive left ventricular dysfunction at the time of admission.[78] In the ISIS-3 study, streptokinase was associated with significantly fewer total strokes and noncerebral bleeding and intracranial bleeding episodes compared with either t-PA or APSAC.[79] When GISSI-2 and ISIS-3 data are combined, t-PA was associated with significantly higher total stroke rates (1.4% vs. 1%; 0.6% vs. 0.3%) compared with streptokinase.[80] The GUSTO trial showed that t-PA was associated with a significant excess in hemorrhagic strokes ($p = 0.03$) compared with streptokinase.[74]

Allergic reactions are more common with streptokinase and APSAC because these agents are derived from streptococci and act as haptens in the presence of antibodies to streptococci. Intravenous diphenhydramine and hydrocortisone may reduce the risk of anaphylaxis during administration of these two thrombolytics. Hypotension occurs in approximately 10% of patients treated with streptokinase or APSAC. Once the patient receives streptokinase, he or she then is sensitized to the drug and should not receive it again for at least 6 months.[33,81] Other side effects with thrombolytics include angina, flushing, dyspnea, mild febrile reactions, nausea and vomiting, and occasionally rash, all of which may be symptoms of mild allergic reactions. Allergic reactions and hypotension are rare in patients treated with t-PA.

Clinical trials show that streptokinase, APSAC, and t-PA improve left ventricular function.[63] Studies show that thrombolytics reduce AMI-related mortality compared with placebo. Streptokinase reduces in-hospital mortality by 3.7% to 10% and 1-year mortality by 13.9%. APSAC reduces 1-year mortality by 11.1%; t-PA produces a 3% to 7.2% reduction in prehospital mortality and a 5.9% to 7.3% reduction in 1-year mortality.[82] The International Joint Efficacy Comparison of Thrombolytics (INJECT) trial compared the 35-day mortality rates after treatment with reteplase (10 + 10 U in a bolus regimen) or streptokinase (1.5 mU over 60 minutes) in patients with AMI.[83] Mortality rates did not differ significantly between the reteplase group (9.02%) and the streptokinase group (9.53%; 95% confidence interval, −1.98% to 0.96%).[83]

ISIS-3,[79] GISSI-2,[78] the International Group, and GUSTO-1[74] confirmed the benefits of thrombolytic therapy on AMI-related mortality and morbidity. ISIS-3 assessed the relative efficacy of streptokinase, APSAC, and t-PA.[79] Mortality rates in all three groups were the same. GISSI-2 and the International Group compared streptokinase with t-PA and found no difference in mortality between treatment groups.[78,84] However, these trials were criticized because heparin was either withheld or given subcutaneously, a factor that would bias against clot-selective t-PA. The GUSTO-1 trial assessed the importance of IV and subcutaneous heparin after administration of streptokinase and t-PA.[74] The results showed one additional life saved per 100 treated patients with t-PA and IV heparin compared with streptokinase.[74]

Certain patients appear to benefit most from t-PA.[85] Patients with anterior wall MI have a lower mortality (8.6%) after treatment with t-PA versus streptokinase (10.5%).[74,75] Mortality rates for t-PA versus streptokinase in patients less than 75 years of age are 4.4% and 5.5%, respectively.[74,75] Neither age 75 years or more nor the presence of inferior wall MI affects the relative efficacy of the thrombolytics.[85] Mortality rates are lower with t-PA (5.5%) compared with streptokinase (6.7%) in patients treated within 2 to 4 hours after the onset of symptoms.[74,75] GUSTO-3 compared a 10-U double-bolus dose of reteplase with an accelerated dose of t-PA.[86] All patients received heparin and aspirin. There were no significant differences between the two treatment groups in mortality, stroke, or net clinical benefits.

A recent subanalysis of the MITI project compared in-hospital mortality, long-term mortality, and resource utilization among 3,145 patients with AMI; 1,050 patients were treated with acute angioplasty and 2,095 received thrombolytic therapy. After a 3-year follow-up period, the study showed no differences in acute mortality or long-term mortality rates between treatment groups.[72] However, after 3 years, the mean total cumulative inpatient costs were more than $3,000 higher for patients treated with angioplasty than those patients initially treated with thrombolytic therapy ($25,459 vs. $22,163, $p <0.001$).[72] As expected, the primary cost drivers were repeat angiograms and repeat angioplasties. The authors concluded that thrombolytic therapy may produce better short-term benefit when compared with angioplasty in patients with AMI.[72]

Successful thrombolytic therapy in AMI depends on more than just the ability to reperfuse the occluded coronary artery. Prevention of reocclusion and subsequent salvage of infarcted myocardium should reduce morbidity and mortality after thrombolytic therapy. Results of early studies that compared reperfusion rates achieved with t-PA and streptokinase suggested that t-PA was twice as effective as streptokinase in establishing reperfusion of acutely occluded coronary arteries.[87,88] In recent trials, myocardial salvage, mortality reduction, or bleeding complications have not differed in patients treated with t-PA versus streptokinase.[89] Clinical experience provides little evidence for the superiority of t-PA over other thrombolytic agents in AMI. The largest trials measuring myocardial function after thrombolytic therapy failed to show that t-PA is more effective than streptokinase[78,90] or APSAC.[91] Additionally, t-PA is no safer than other thrombolytics.[78,92] An international study of 20,749 patients with AMI showed no difference in mortality rates between t-PA (8.9%) and streptokinase (8.5%).[84] There was also no difference in the incidence of ventricular fibrillation (VF), reinfarction, or heart failure between treatment groups.

Not all patients suspected of having AMI receive thrombolytic therapy. This is unfortunate because mortality is substantially higher among patients who do not (18%) compared with those who do (2.5%).[85,93,94] Approximately 39% of patients with AMI are treated with thrombolytic therapy.[71] Clinical trials show a 30% to 40% reduction in acute mortality in patients with AMI who receive thrombolytic therapy.[74,95] The primary reason for not receiving thrombolytic therapy is too long a delay between symptom onset and arrival at a treatment facility.[71] Factors responsible for delay in the care of patients with AMI can be grouped into three phases: patient or bystander factors, prehospital factors, and hospital factors.

Because the benefit of fibrinolytic therapy is directly related to the time from symptom onset, treatment benefit is maximized by the earliest possible application of therapy. Thrombolytic treatment initiated within 60 to 90 minutes of symptom onset reduces the size of the AMI and its related mortality. Pharmacists can play a key role as healthcare team members to seek ways to ensure that "door-to-needle time" is reduced from the current 45 to 75 minutes to less than 30 minutes. Thrombolytic agents should be stocked in the ED

and the coronary care unit to avoid delays in administration. Pharmacists should help develop critical pathways and treatment guidelines for thrombolytic therapy in AMI.[96,97] Pharmacists can also collect patient outcome data and prescriber compliance information that may be used to make formulary decisions. Information obtained from these evaluations can also be used to implement procedural changes and educational efforts that can reduce hospital delays.[98]

Indications for Thrombolytics in Acute Myocardial Infarction. A constellation of clinical features must be present (although not necessarily at the same time) to serve as an indication for fibrinolysis. The 2004 ACC/AHA guidelines for STEMI make the following recommendations regarding thrombolytic agents.[17] In the absence of contraindications, fibrinolytic therapy should be administered to AMI patients with symptom onset within the prior 12 hours and ST elevation greater than 0.1 mV in at least two contiguous precordial leads or at least two adjacent limb leads. In the absence of contraindications, fibrinolytic therapy should also be administered to AMI patients with symptom onset within the prior 12 hours and new or presumably new LBBB. It is reasonable to administer fibrinolytic therapy to AMI patients with symptom onset within the prior 12 hours and 12-lead ECG findings consistent with a true posterior MI, or in patients with symptoms of AMI beginning within the prior 12 to 24 hours who have continuing ischemic symptoms and ST elevation greater than 0.1 mV in at least two contiguous precordial leads or at least two adjacent limb leads. In contrast, fibrinolytic therapy should not be administered to asymptomatic patients whose initial symptoms of AMI began more than 24 hours earlier, nor to patients whose 12-lead ECG shows only ST-segment depression, except if a true posterior MI is suspected.

Combination Therapy With Thrombolytics and Glycoprotein IIb/IIIa. Combination therapy with a thrombolytic agent and a glycoprotein IIb/IIIa inhibitor may offer an alternative to thrombolytic therapy for the primary treatment of AMI. However, controlled clinical trials do not support a decrease in mortality, and any benefits that may be observed with respect to secondary endpoints [e.g., nonfatal reinfarction, recurrent ischemia, VF, sustained ventricular tachycardia (VT), and atrioventricular block] were offset by an increased incidence of bleeding, especially among elderly patients.[17,27,45,99,100]

The 2004 ACC/AHA guidelines for STEMI make the following recommendations regarding the use of glycoprotein IIb/IIIa inhibitors in combination with thrombolytics.[17] Combination pharmacologic reperfusion with abciximab and half-dose reteplase or tenecteplase may be considered for prevention of reinfarction and other complications of STEMI in patients with an anterior MI, age less than 75 years, and no risk factors for bleeding in whom an early referral for angiography and PCI is planned. Combination pharmacologic reperfusion with abciximab and half-dose reteplase or tenecteplase should not be given to patients aged greater than 75 years because of an increased risk of intracranial hemorrhage.

Combination Glycoprotein IIb/IIIa Inhibitor Therapy and Primary Angioplasty for AMI.

The role of the platelet glycoprotein inhibitor abciximab in conjunction with primary coronary angioplasty has been examined in numerous trials.[99,100] Studies have found that abciximab is beneficial at reducing major adverse events, but the benefit appeared to be limited to patients undergoing balloon angioplasty without stent placement.[100] These data suggest that abciximab is beneficial in patients with AMI but that the benefit in patients undergoing balloon angioplasty alone may differ from that in patients who undergo balloon angioplasty with stent placement.[101] The combined use of stents and platelet glycoprotein inhibitors may maximize the frequency with which normal antegrade blood flow is achieved while reducing the need for repeat procedures in the following year. Last, when thrombolytic therapy plus abciximab is compared with primary angioplasty using both stents and abciximab, the reduction in infarct size is greater in the group undergoing primary angioplasty.

The 2004 ACC/AHA guidelines for STEMI make the following recommendations regarding the use of glycoprotein IIb/IIIa inhibitors in patients undergoing primary angioplasty.[17] It is reasonable to start treatment with abciximab as early as possible before primary PCI (with or without stenting) in patients with STEMI. Treatment with tirofiban or eptifibatide may be considered before primary PCI (with or without stenting) in patients with STEMI.

Percutaneous Coronary Interventions.

PCI provides a viable therapeutic alternative in patients who are seen at a hospital capable of performing PCI. In percutaneous balloon angioplasty (PCTA), a form of PCI, a balloon-tipped catheter is passed along the venous circulation into the coronary tree to the site of coronary occlusion. Once at the site, the balloon is inflated, causing the occlusive plaque to regress against the vessel wall. The balloon is deflated and reinflated several times until the plaque is reduced and approximately 70% of the arterial caliber has been restored. A major limitation of PTCA is that it requires a skilled team, a fully staffed catheterization laboratory, and a surgical team on standby. Potential complications of PTCA include catheter-induced occlusion caused by dissection, vasospasm, or subintimal hematoma and residual stenosis. Routine angioplasty performed within 24 hours of thrombolytic therapy offers no clinical benefit and is associated with an increased incidence of reocclusion and complications.[67] Angioplasty is recommended for patients with ongoing ischemia or pump failure. The use of emergency angioplasty for patients who have AMI may offer several advantages over thrombolytic therapy. PTCA is more effective than thrombolytic therapy in restoring patency and preventing reocclusion and in reducing the risk of death and reinfarction.[102] Angioplasty is associated with significantly less ($p = 0.05$) risk of hemorrhagic strokes than t-PA.[102] The benefits of angioplasty are especially apparent in patients who are of advanced age, have an anterior infarction, or have tachycardia.[103]

Primary Coronary Angioplasty With Stent Placement.

Primary coronary angioplasty, angioplasty without prior thrombolytic therapy, in AMI restores flow to the infarct-related artery with greater speed and frequency when compared with thrombolytic therapy and is considered preferable to thrombolytics when the procedure is done promptly by an experienced and skilled operator.[17] At institutions where a skilled catheterization team is on call 24 hours a day and can be rapidly assembled, coronary angioplasty would most likely be able to restore coronary blood flow in more patients more rapidly than thrombolytic therapy. Immediate transfer for primary angioplasty is an alternative treatment strategy for patients with AMI initially assessed at a hospital without on-site cardiac surgery facilities. Studies consistently show that long-distance transport from a community hospital to a facility with angioplasty facilities in the acute phase of AMI is safe and is associated with decreased mortality in patients who present more than 3 hours after symptom onset.

PCI with stent placement also improves the ability to achieve arterial patency early after thrombolytic therapy compared with balloon angioplasty alone. The administration of glycoprotein IIb/IIIa inhibitor may enhance the patency rate following PCI, but there appears to be an increase in the risk of bleeding when glycoprotein IIb/IIIa inhibitors are used early after full-dose thrombolytic therapy.[99–101] Data from several pilot studies suggest that the combination of a fibrin-specific thrombolytic agent, either t-PA or reteplase, combined with the glycoprotein IIb/IIIa inhibitor abciximab, may actually facilitate the performance of angioplasty with stent placement rather than reduce its safety and efficacy, as was seen when balloon angioplasty was performed after thrombolytic therapy.[17] When used correctly, half-dose thrombolytic therapy may facilitate the performance of PCI with stent after AMI.

According to the 2004 ACC/AHA STEMI guidelines, primary PCI, if immediately available, should be performed in patients with STEMI (including true posterior MI) or MI with new or presumably new LBBB who can undergo PCI of the infarct artery within 12 hours of symptom onset, if performed in a timely fashion (balloon inflation within 90 minutes of presentation) by persons skilled in the procedure (individuals who perform >75 PCI procedures per year).[17] The procedure should be supported by experienced personnel in an appropriate laboratory environment (a laboratory that performs >200 PCI procedures per year, of which at least 36 are primary PCI for STEMI, and has cardiac surgery capability). Primary PCI should be performed as quickly as possible with a goal of a medical contact-to-balloon or door-to-balloon interval of no more than 90 minutes. If the symptom duration is within 3 hours and the expected door-to-balloon time minus the expected door-to-needle time is within 1 hour, primary PCI is generally preferred; if it is greater than 1 hour, fibrinolytic therapy is generally preferred. If symptom duration is greater than 3 hours, primary PCI is generally preferred and should be performed with a medical contact-to-balloon or door-to-balloon interval as short as possible (goal ≤90 minutes).

Primary PCI should be performed in patients less than 75 years old with ST elevation or LBBB who develop shock within 36 hours of MI and are suitable for revascularization that can be performed within 18 hours of shock unless further support is futile because of the patient's wishes or contraindications/unsuitability for further invasive care.[17] Primary PCI should be performed in patients with severe CHF and/or pulmonary edema (Killip class 3) and onset of symptoms within 12 hours. The medical contact-to-balloon or door-to-balloon time should be as short as possible (goal ≤90 minutes).

Primary PCI should be performed in fibrinolytic-ineligible patients who present with STEMI within 12 hours of symptom onset.[17] It is reasonable to perform primary PCI for fibrinolytic-ineligible patients with onset of symptoms within the prior 12 to 24 hours and one or more of the following: severe congestive heart failure, hemodynamic or electrical instability, or persistent ischemic symptoms.

Primary PCI is reasonable for selected patients 75 years or older with ST elevation or LBBB or who develop shock within 36 hours of MI and are suitable for revascularization that can be performed within 18 hours of shock.[17] Patients with good prior functional status who are suitable for revascularization and agree to invasive care may be selected for such an invasive strategy. Furthermore, it is reasonable to perform primary PCI for patients with onset of symptoms within the prior 12 to 24 hours and one or more of the following: severe congestive heart failure, hemodynamic or electrical instability, or persistent ischemic symptoms.

The benefit of primary PCI for STEMI patients eligible for fibrinolysis is not well established when performed by an operator who performs fewer than 75 PCI procedures per year. PCI should not be performed in a noninfarct artery at the time of primary PCI in patients without hemodynamic compromise.[17] Primary PCI should not be performed in asymptomatic patients more than 12 hours after onset of STEMI if they are hemodynamically and electrically stable.

Facilitated PCI. Data from several pilot studies suggest that the combination of a fibrin-specific thrombolytic agent, either t-PA or reteplase, combined with the glycoprotein IIb/IIIa inhibitor abciximab, may actually facilitate the performance of angioplasty rather than reduce its safety and efficacy, as was seen when balloon angioplasty was performed after thrombolytic therapy.[17,59] Hence, the term *facilitated angioplasty* has been coined for the routine performance of angioplasty after the combination of half-dose thrombolytic therapy with a glycoprotein IIb/IIIa inhibitor.

Several studies have examined the role of the platelet glycoprotein inhibitor abciximab in conjunction with primary coronary angioplasty.[99–101] When evaluating these studies, practitioners should realize there were differences

in compliance with the protocol in some trials, and in part because of differences in the treatments used (balloon angioplasty alone vs. balloon angioplasty followed by stent placement). Collectively, these data show that stent placement in the setting of AMI slightly reduces the frequency with which normal antegrade blood flow in the infarct-related artery is achieved. This would suggest that glycoprotein IIb/IIIa inhibitors (e.g., abciximab) are beneficial in patients with AMI but that the benefit in patients undergoing balloon angioplasty alone may differ from that in patients who undergo balloon angioplasty with stent placement. Stents markedly reduce the frequency with which a repeat revascularization procedure is needed in the months after the angioplasty procedure.

The combined use of stents and platelet glycoprotein inhibitors may maximize the frequency with which normal antegrade blood flow is achieved while reducing the need for repeat procedures in the following year.[17] When thrombolytic therapy using t-PA is compared with primary angioplasty using both stents and abciximab, the reduction in infarct size is far greater in the group undergoing primary angioplasty; the clinical outcome was also better in the patients who underwent angioplasty.[44] Potential advantages include earlier time to reperfusion, improved patient stability, greater procedural success rates, higher TIMI flow rates, and improved survival rates. However, there are insufficient data to judge the value of facilitated PCI in high-risk patients when PCI is not immediately available.

According to the 2004 ACC/AHA STEMI guidelines, facilitated PCI might be performed as a reperfusion strategy in higher-risk patients when PCI is not immediately available and bleeding risk is low.[17]

Rescue Coronary Angioplasty. Rescue coronary angioplasty is used to re-establish antegrade flow in the infarct-related artery after failed thrombolytic therapy. When post-thrombolytic, conventional medical therapy (e.g., β-blockers, aspirin, and heparin) is compared with rescue coronary angioplasty, limited data suggest improved outcome with rescue angioplasty, although the benefits were not compelling.[17] Although the use of coronary stents and platelet glycoprotein inhibitors improves the results of percutaneous revascularization procedures and would be expected to further increase the benefit of angioplasty after failed thrombolytic therapy, this has not yet been proved. Based on available information, rescue coronary angioplasty is most likely to be beneficial in patients with a large MI in whom persistent pain, ST-segment elevation, or hemodynamic compromise is present more than 90 minutes after the administration of a thrombolytic agent. In contrast, rescue coronary angioplasty does not produce clinical benefits in other AMI patients with significant residual stenosis and should not be considered a potential treatment option in these patients.[17]

According to the 2004 ACC/AHA guidelines, rescue PCI should be performed in patients less than 75 years old with ST elevation or LBBB who develop shock within 36 hours of MI and are suitable for revascularization that can be performed within 18 hours of shock unless further support is futile because of the patient's wishes or contraindications/unsuitability for further invasive care.[17] Rescue PCI should be performed in patients with severe congestive heart failure and/or pulmonary edema (Killip class 3) and onset of symptoms within 12 hours. Rescue PCI is reasonable for selected patients 75 years or older with ST elevation or LBBB or who develop shock within 36 hours of MI and who are suitable for revascularization that can be performed within 18 hours of shock. Patients with good prior functional status who are suitable for revascularization and who agree to invasive care may be selected for such an invasive strategy. It is reasonable to perform rescue PCI for patients with one or more of the following: severe congestive heart failure, hemodynamic or electrical instability, or persistent ischemic symptoms.

Adjunctive Postreperfusion Management. After successful thrombolysis, the stenotic vessel may reocclude. The rate of reocclusion varies but may be as high as 30%.[69] The likelihood of reocclusion and recovery of regional ventricular function depends on the severity of residual stenosis. After successful thrombolysis, anticoagulation is advocated, although there is not consensus on the type, dosage, or duration of therapy. Most often, full-dose heparin is used for 24 to 72 hours. Aspirin (160 or 325 mg/day) is administered for 3 months or longer.[69] There is no role for dipyridamole as an adjunctive antiplatelet agent after thrombolytic therapy.[104,105]

β-Adrenergic Blocking Agents. β-Adrenergic blockade reduces myocardial oxygen consumption by reducing heart rate, contractility, and blood pressure. β-Adrenergic blockers can also reduce catecholamine levels in an ischemic heart and produce favorable redistribution of coronary blood flow.[106–108] Clinical trials with these agents can be divided into those in which treatment was begun early and endpoints such as cardiac enzyme levels, ECG changes, and reinfarction rates are investigated, and those in which treatment was begun later after resolution of the infarct, with mortality rate reduction as the endpoint. There is evidence that IV therapy followed by oral administration with atenolol, propranolol, metoprolol, sotalol, or timolol reduces serum CK concentrations.[43] Reduction in ECG abnormalities after AMI has been reported following acute intervention with propranolol, practolol, and metoprolol.[43] In AMI patients without known contraindications to β-blockers, these agents reduce the magnitude of infarction and incidence of associated complications in subjects not receiving concomitant fibrinolytic therapy; the rate of reinfarction in patients receiving fibrinolytic therapy; and the frequency of life-threatening ventricular tachyarrhythmias. In patients not receiving fibrinolytic therapy, IV β-blocking agents exert a modestly favorable influence on infarct size.

Studies show that β-blockers limit infarct size, reduce the incidence of malignant arrhythmias, and reduce mortality after acute administration in patients with AMI.[67] In the Met-

oprolol in Acute Myocardial Infarction (MIAMI) trial, a multicenter, double-blind, placebo-controlled randomized study, 2,877 patients with suspected or definite MI received 5 mg of metoprolol IV every 2 minutes for a total of 15 mg within 24 hours of onset of symptoms.[109] Patients were randomly assigned to the study after arrival to the coronary care unit. After IV dosing, patients received oral metoprolol 100 mg every 6 hours for the first 2 days beginning 15 minutes after the last IV injection. The dose was then decreased to 100 mg every 12 hours for the remaining 13 days of the study. The cumulative mortality for all patients at the conclusion of the 15-day trial was 123 (4.3%) deaths in the treatment groups compared with 142 (4.9%) deaths in the placebo group. This difference did not reach statistical significance. Mortality in patients with definite MI was 120 of 2,028 in the metoprolol group versus 137 of 2,099 in the placebo group. High-risk patients were found to benefit, whereas other subgroups did not benefit.

In ISIS-1, 16,207 patients were randomly assigned to receive 5 to 10 mg of atenolol, in 5-mg IV doses, or placebo within a mean of 5 hours of onset of suspected MI. Oral dosing in the treatment group followed with 100 mg of atenolol per day as either a single dose or every 12 hours for a total of 7 days. Vascular mortality occurred in 313 of 8,037 (3.89%) atenolol-treated patients and 365 of 7,990 (4.57%) control patients. The beneficial effect of atenolol in decreasing the incidence of mortality was statistically significant ($p < 0.04$).[110]

The Thrombolysis in Myocardial Infarction Phase II (TIMI II) study addressed the use of early and late β-adrenergic blocker therapy after t-PA administration.[111] Patients were randomly assigned to one of two groups: immediate β-adrenergic blocker administration (three doses of metoprolol 5 mg IV at 2-minute intervals followed by 50 mg orally twice a day for 24 hours, then 100 mg twice a day) or delayed administration (starting on day 6 after MI), consisting of metoprolol 50 mg twice a day for 24 hours, then 100 mg twice daily. The time of entry into the study was less than 4 hours since onset of AMI (mean 2.6 hours). Ejection fraction and early mortality were found to be similar between the two groups; however, at day 6, 16 patients in the immediate metoprolol intervention group and 31 patients in the delayed group had nonfatal reinfarctions ($p = 0.02$). Recurrent ischemic episodes occurred in 107 patients in the early metoprolol intervention group compared to 147 patients in the delayed intervention group ($p = 0.005$). Mortality at the end of the 6-week study was 5.0% in immediate metoprolol therapy versus 12.1% in the delayed intervention group ($p = 0.001$).

Based on TIMI II data, IV β-blocker therapy reduces the mortality and reinfarction rates when administered within 2 hours of the onset of symptoms in patients with AMI receiving thrombolytic therapy.[111] If IV β-blocker therapy is initiated within 4 hours of symptom onset, there is a reduction in nonfatal reinfarction and recurrent ischemia.[111] β-Blockers may also reduce the risk of intracranial bleeding in patients with AMI treated with thrombolytics. β-Adrenergic blockers are also valuable in patients with AMI and atrial tachyarrhythmias or rapid ventricular response rates in atrial fibrillation.[39] Well-designed trials with large numbers of patients show that timolol, metoprolol, and propranolol significantly reduce long-term mortality rates in AMI.[43] Because these agents were administered after reduction of MI, the decrease in mortality is probably a result of a drop in arrhythmias or reinfarction and is not related to infarct size reduction.[43]

Although β-adrenergic blockers are contraindicated in patients with serious myocardial dysfunction, cardiac conduction abnormalities, hypotension, peripheral hypoperfusion, or bronchospastic airway disease, it is reasonable to consider their use in all patients with AMI who have no contraindications, irrespective of concomitant thrombolytic therapy.[67] Recent studies suggest that esmolol infusions at a reduced dosage may be used safely and effectively in thrombolytic-treated patients with AMI who had relative contraindications to β-blocker therapy (e.g., congestive heart failure, pulmonary disease, peripheral vascular disease, bradycardia, or systolic blood pressure <100 mm Hg).[112]

There is overwhelming evidence for the benefits of early β-blockade in patients with STEMI and without contraindications to their use.[17] Benefits have been demonstrated for patients with and without concomitant fibrinolytic therapy, both early and late after STEMI. However, β-blockers should not be administered to patients with AMI precipitated by cocaine use because of the risk of exacerbating coronary spasm. Atrioventricular block, excessive bradycardia, or hypotension secondary to IV β-blocker administration is quickly reversed by infusion of dopamine (2.5 to 10 μg/kg/min). Patients with left ventricular dysfunction in the setting of AMI should not receive IV β-blockade until the heart failure has been compensated.[44] Nonetheless, these are the very patients who warrant post-MI oral β-blocker therapy before leaving the hospital, especially in the presence of sustained postinfarction left ventricular dysfunction. A reasonable general rule is to initiate β-blockade after 24 to 48 hours of freedom from a relative contraindication, such as bradycardia, mild to moderate heart failure, or first-degree heart block.

The 2004 ACC/AHA guidelines for the treatment of STEMI make the following recommendations regarding the use of β-blockers.[17] Patients receiving β-blockers within the first 24 hours of STEMI without adverse effects should continue to receive them during the early convalescent phase of STEMI. Patients without contraindications to β-blockers who did not receive them within the first 24 hours after STEMI should have them started in the early convalescent phase. Patients with early contraindications within the first 24 hours of STEMI should be re-evaluated for candidacy for β-blocker therapy.[17]

Calcium-Channel Blockers. Experimental data in animals suggest that calcium-channel blockers may prevent the progression of ischemia and subsequent necrosis by decreas-ing myocardial oxygen demand without comprising cardiac output.[12] Recent clinical trials indicate that these agents do not alter outcome in patients with AMI. Verapamil may reduce infarct size, but it does not alter acute mortality.[113] The Danish Multicenter Study Group randomly assigned 100 patients to receive verapamil 0.1 mg per kg IV followed by 120 mg orally three times a day or placebo for 6 months.[114] Patients were assigned within 4 hours of onset of symptoms of AMI. Verapamil failed to alter the acute mortality, long-term mortality, or reinfarction rate compared with placebo.[114]

Studies with nifedipine (20 mg orally every 4 hour for 14 days) failed to show a significant reduction in enzymatically assessed infarct size compared with placebo.[115] A slight trend for higher mortality was observed in the nifedipine group. The Nifedipine Angina Myocardial Infarction Study (NAMIS) was the first multicenter placebo-controlled trial to assess nifedipine (Procardia) 20 mg every 4 hours, starting 4.6 ± 0.1 hours after the onset of chest pain, for 14 days.[115] A total of 171 patients with either a threat of MI or early AMI were admitted into the study. No significant difference in size of infarction, as assessed by CK-MB serum levels, between the two groups was noted. A startling observation was that the nifedipine-treated group exhibited a higher incidence of mortality (7.9% vs. 0% in the control group) during the 2-week study period. Long-term mortality at the 6-month follow-up was not significantly different between the nifedipine and placebo groups.

In the Norwegian Nifedipine Multicenter Trial, 277 patients were randomly assigned to receive either nifedipine 10 mg five times a day or placebo.[116] Unlike the NAMIS trial, randomization occurred within 12 hours of onset of symptoms. Treatment was initiated within 5.5 ± 2.9 hours of symptom onset and was continued for 6 weeks. Results showed no difference in CK-MB release or 6-week mortality between the two groups.

A placebo-controlled trial of diltiazem in AMI reported a reduction in early recurrent infarction (one-tailed, $P = 0.03$; two-tailed, $P = 0.06$) in patients with non–Q-wave MI.[117] This multicenter, double-blind study consisted of 576 patients who were randomly assigned to receive either diltiazem or placebo within 24 to 72 hours of onset of infarction. Diltiazem 90 mg every 6 hours or placebo was continued for 14 days. Reinfarction, defined as a secondary increase in CK-MB during the study period, was observed in 15 of 287 (5.2%) diltiazem-treated patients compared with 27 of 289 (9.3%) control patients ($p = 0.0297$); however, 61% of the diltiazem patients and 64% of the placebo group were receiving concurrent β-adrenergic therapy and 80% were also receiving long-acting nitrates. Side effects such as heart block, bradycardia (heart rate ≤40 bpm), and hypotension (systolic blood pressure ≤90 mm Hg) were more pronounced in the diltiazem group compared with placebo. Although the study concluded that diltiazem was effective in preventing early reinfarction in non–Q-wave MI, no difference in mortality between the two groups was observed during the 14-day study period.[118]

The Multicenter Diltiazem Post-Infarction Trial (MDPIT) evaluated 2,466 patients with AMI.[119] Patients received either placebo or diltiazem 60 mg orally twice a day or four times a day. Therapy was initiated between 3 and 15 days after MI. There was no difference in mortality between groups; however, there were 11% fewer recurrent cardiac events (e.g., nonfatal reinfarction, death from a cardiac cause) in the diltiazem group. Further analysis of the MDPIT data indicates that diltiazem-treated patients with left ventricular dysfunction (ejection fraction <40%), pulmonary congestion, and acute anterolateral Q-wave MI at baseline had a predictably higher incidence of cardiac death and non-fatal reinfarction.[119] Long-term diltiazem therapy in patients with AMI failed to show any significant benefit and produced detrimental side effects in patients with left ventricular dysfunction.

Although there is laboratory evidence that calcium-channel blockers reduce infarct size, these results are not observed under clinical conditions.[107] Currently, there is no reason to recommend general treatment with calcium-channel blockers to reduce infarct size. However, patients with documented or suspected vasospastic angina and patients with AMI undergoing emergency angioplasty may benefit from the use of calcium-channel blockers as long as left ventricular function is relatively well preserved.[67]

According to the 2004 ACC/AHA STEMI guidelines, it is reasonable to give verapamil or diltiazem to patients in whom β-blockers are ineffective or contraindicated (e.g., bronchospastic disease) for relief of ongoing ischemia or control of a rapid ventricular response with atrial fibrillation or atrial flutter after STEMI in the absence of congestive heart failure, left ventricular dysfunction, or atrioventricular block.[17] Diltiazem and verapamil are contraindicated in patients with STEMI and associated systolic left ventricular dysfunction and congestive heart failure. Nifedipine (immediate-release form) is contraindicated in the treatment of STEMI because of the reflex sympathetic activation, tachycardia, and hypotension associated with its use.[17]

ACE Inhibitors. A key concept in the pathophysiology of STEMI is ventricular remodeling, a term that refers to changes in size, shape, and thickness of the left ventricle involving both the infarcted and noninfarcted segments of the ventricle.[52,53] Acute dilatation and thinning of the area of infarction that is not due to additional myocardial necrosis is referred to as infarct expansion.[55]

Recent studies by Pfeffer et al[120] show that early and continued use of captopril in patients with symptomatic left ventricular dysfunction after AMI improved survival and reduced morbidity and mortality due to major cardiovascular events.[120] Patients ($n = 2,231$) with ejection fractions 40% or less but without overt heart failure or recurrent ischemia were randomly assigned to receive either captopril 50 mg three times daily or placebo within 3 to 16 days after their

AMI. Patients were followed for an average of 42 months. Captopril reduced all-cause mortality by 19%, the risk of cardiovascular death was reduced by 21%, the risk of congestive heart failure requiring hospitalization was reduced by 22%, and the risk of recurrent MI was reduced by 25%. These benefits were seen in patients who received thrombolytic therapy, aspirin, and/or β-adrenergic blockers, and in those who did not.[120]

In contrast, the Second Cooperative New Scandinavian Enalapril Survival Study (CONSENSUS II) failed to show a benefit from the administration of enalapril (up to 20 mg/day) in patients in whom this therapy was initiated within 24 hours after their AMI.[121] A total of 6,090 patients were randomly assigned to receive either enalapril or placebo along with conventional therapy with thrombolytics, nitrates, aspirin, β-blockers, diuretics, analgesics, and calcium-channel blockers. The trial was prematurely stopped because of the high probability that enalapril was no more effective than placebo in improving 6-month survival.[121]

The Studies of Left Ventricular Dysfunction (SOLVD) Prevention Trial showed that long-term enalapril significantly reduced the incidence of heart failure and the need for hospitalization compared with placebo in patients with asymptomatic left ventricular dysfunction (ejection fraction ≤35%).[122] Approximately 80% of patients in the SOLVD Prevention Trial had suffered an AMI before enrollment in the study. The efficacy of enalapril in preventing the development of heart failure was evident as early as 3 months after the start of treatment.[122] Data produced by the SAVE and SOLVD trials suggest a possible benefit from the early administration of ACE inhibitors to patients with left ventricular dysfunction who are recovering from an AMI. The negative findings of the CONSENSUS II trial may have resulted from too early initiation of ACE inhibitor therapy or an inadequate follow-up period.[123] Patients with an anterior wall MI and reduced left ventricular function may benefit from therapy with an ACE inhibitor if it is initiated within the first 2 weeks after the AMI.[85] In patients with left ventricular dysfunction, the use of long-term ACE inhibitor therapy may reduce mortality. These agents attenuate the remodeling process that occurs after an AMI. As a result of the attenuation of remodeling, a reduction in ventricular dilation is observed. The effect of ACE inhibitors on remodeling is probably due to a suppression of endogenous catecholamines. ACE inhibitors prevent the degradation of bradykinin (a vasodilatory substance) that decreases systemic vascular resistance and reduce the workload of the heart. The initiation of ACE inhibitor therapy within the first 2 weeks after MI may save the lives of 5 patients for every 1,000 patients with left ventricular dysfunction.[85] Ideal candidates for ACE inhibitor therapy include patients with congestive heart failure or hypertension. For the patient to achieve the greatest benefit from the ACE inhibitor, therapy should be started during the first week after the AMI. However, ACE inhibitor therapy should not be instituted until blood pressure and renal function are assessed and stabilized. In patients with an evolving

AMI, ACE inhibitor therapy should be started shortly after hospitalization in the absence of hypotension or contraindications. If the patient has impaired left ventricular systolic function (ejection fraction ≤40%), ACE inhibitor therapy should be continued indefinitely and the dose should be titrated slowly upward to the maximum that can be tolerated. If the patient has no complications and no evidence of left ventricular dysfunction, the ACE inhibitor can be discontinued after 6 weeks of therapy.

The most common side effect associated with the administration of ACE inhibitor is a dry hacking cough. This cough may develop anytime from a few days up to a week after initiation of therapy or an increase in dose. If the patient can tolerate the cough, continuation of the drug is encouraged. If the cough becomes intolerable, therapy can be switched to an angiotensin II such as valsartan, irbesartan, or losartan. The only problem with the angiotensin II blockers is that they have not been shown to decrease mortality like the ACE inhibitors have.

Another side effect of ACE inhibitors is angioedema, an anaphylactic reaction that causes severe tongue swelling and can interfere with breathing. If this occurs, the ACE inhibitor should be discontinued and the patient should not be given this drug again. However, it is less likely to be a problem with angiotensin II blockers due to the lack of inhibition of bradykinin metabolism.

In summary, clinical studies suggests that ACE inhibitors should generally be started within the first 24 hours after AMI if the patient's blood pressure is stable and the systolic blood pressure is above 100 mm Hg or is no more than 30 mm Hg below baseline. ACE inhibitors should not be administered to patients with clinically relevant renal failure, bilateral renal artery stenosis, or a known allergy to ACE inhibitors.[17,45] ACE inhibitors produce the most benefit among post-AMI patients who are between 55 to 74 years of age, those with an anterior wall infarct, and those with a heart rate of 80 bpm or higher.[17] ACE inhibitor therapy should start with the lowest oral dose available as a test dose, and the oral regimen should be titrated to achieve a full-dose regimen within 24 to 48 hours. In contrast to oral regimens, IV ACE inhibitor therapy should be avoided in the immediate post-MI setting.[17] A possible exception may be patients with refractory hypertension for whom other more appropriate agents are contraindicated or not readily available. The potential interaction between aspirin and ACE inhibitors leading to an attenuation of the beneficial effects of the ACE inhibitor is unlikely, especially with aspirin regimens of 325 mg per day or less; this is not a reason to withhold either therapy.[44]

The 2004 ACC/AHA guidelines for STEMI make the following recommendations.[17] An ACE inhibitor should be administered orally within the first 24 hours of STEMI to patients with anterior infarction, pulmonary congestion, or a left ventricular ejection fraction less than 0.40 in the absence of hypotension (hypotension defined as systolic blood pressure <100 mm Hg or >30 mm Hg below baseline) or

known contraindications to that class of medications. An angiotensin receptor blocker should be administered to STEMI patients who are intolerant of ACE inhibitors and who have either clinical or radiologic signs of heart failure or a left ventricular ejection fraction less than 0.40. Valsartan and candesartan have established efficacy for this recommendation. An ACE inhibitor administered orally within the first 24 hours of STEMI can be useful in patients without anterior infarction, pulmonary congestion, or a left ventricular ejection fraction less than 0.40 in the absence of hypotension (hypotension defined as systolic blood pressure <100 mm Hg or >30 mm Hg below baseline) or known contraindications to that class of medications.[17] The expected treatment benefit in such patients is less (5 lives saved per 1,000 patients treated) than for patients with LV dysfunction. An IV ACE inhibitor should not be given to patients within the first 24 hours of STEMI because of the risk of hypotension.

Magnesium. The effect of hypomagnesemia in cardiac disease is well known.[124,125] Magnesium deficiency is associated with a high frequency of cardiac arrhythmias, symptoms of cardiac insufficiency, and sudden cardiac death.[124–127] Experimental and clinical studies show that magnesium and potassium metabolism are closely linked.[124,128] Diuretics[128,129] usually cause hypomagnesemia, often accompanied by hypokalemia. Transient hypomagnesemia not induced by renal magnesium loss has been observed in patients with AMI.[130] Because hypomagnesemia can precipitate refractory VF and can hinder the replenishment of intracellular potassium, it must be corrected if present. One or 2 g of magnesium sulfate (2 to 4 mL of a 50% solution) are diluted in 100 mL of dextrose 5% in water (D5W) and administered over 60 minutes.[131] A 24-hour magnesium infusion (8 g MgSO4 in 500 mL of D5W) started on admission to the CICU can significantly lower the incidence of VT.[130] Magnesium supplementation is a relatively safe method of reducing the incidence of postinfarction ventricular arrhythmias.[127,130] Magnesium toxicity is rare, but side effects from too-rapid administration include flushing, sweating, mild bradycardia, and hypotension. Hypermagnesemia may produce depressed reflexes, flaccid paralysis, circulatory collapse, respiratory paralysis, and diarrhea.

Clinical studies on the use of magnesium in AMI have yielded contradictory results. The Leicester Intravenous Magnesium Intervention Trial (LIMIT-2),[132] conducted before ISIS-4,[133] suggested that magnesium was highly effective in reducing the odds of death and capable of producing survival benefits comparable to those produced by aspirin and thrombolytic therapy in patients with AMI.[132] The ISIS-4 trial failed to show any benefit from magnesium with respect to mortality reduction after AMI.[133] Important differences in methodologic design between LIMIT-2 and ISIS-4 may explain the disparity in response produced by magnesium in patients with AMI. The primary difference is that although in the trials preceding ISIS-4, magnesium was usually administered before or at the time of reperfusion of the infarct-related artery, in ISIS-4 reperfusion was likely to occur in many patients before the administration of magnesium.[133] Considering the proposed mechanisms by which magnesium could improve survival in patients with AMI, administration before reperfusion seems to be of obvious importance. This applies to the postulated preservation of high-energy phosphates and reduction in mitochondrial calcium overload during acute ischemia as well as to a possible role in arrhythmia reduction and reduction in reperfusion injury and myocardial stunning.[134] Furthermore, the low mortality associated with the combined use of thrombolytics, anticoagulants, and antiplatelet drugs may mask the true benefit produced by magnesium.[135] Although further studies are needed to better define the role of early administration of magnesium in patients with AMI receiving thrombolytic therapy, magnesium improves left ventricular function and reduces mortality in patients after AMI, especially those who are not candidates for thrombolytic therapy.[135]

Magnesium should be reserved for use in patients with documented hypomagnesemia or hypokalemia. In the ISIS-4 trial[133] there was no decrease in mortality noted, but there was a slight possibility of harm due to drug-induced hypotension. However, one reason for this negative outcome could have been the administration of magnesium after the administration of the thrombolytic agent. When hypokalemia is present, magnesium should be replaced first, for magnesium is what drives the K⁺ pump.

The 2004 ACC/AHA guidelines for STEMI make the following recommendations regarding the use of magnesium.[17] It is reasonable that documented magnesium deficits be corrected, especially in patients receiving diuretics before the onset of STEMI. It is reasonable that episodes of torsades de pointes be treated with 1 to 2 g of magnesium administered as an IV bolus over 5 minutes. In the absence of documented electrolyte deficits or torsades de pointes, routine IV magnesium should not be administered to STEMI patients at any level of risk.

Potassium. Electrolyte abnormalities, most notably hypokalemia and hypomagnesemia, should be identified and corrected. These electrolyte abnormalities can precipitate malignant ventricular arrhythmias in patients with ischemia, hypertrophied or dilated hearts, or hypoxemia. Hypokalemia is the most common electrolyte abnormality encountered in clinical practice, occurring in 23% to 40% of patients treated with thiazide diuretics.[136] When loop and thiazide diuretics are used in combination, the incidence increases to approximately 100%.[126] Hypokalemia is present in 9% to 25% of patients with AMI and may predispose these patients to VF.[137] Ornato et al[138] found a 49% incidence of hypokalemia in their out-of-hospital cardiac arrest victims. Fifty-five percent of all hypokalemic sudden-death victims were receiving diuretics without potassium supplementation; hypokalemia occurred in 13% of victims receiving diuretics plus potassium supplementation. Fortunately, hypokalemia is significantly (*p* <0.001) less common in patients with uncompli-

cated AMI (11%) than in sudden-death victims (50%).[139] Nonetheless, hypokalemia should be identified and corrected in the AMI setting.

As with magnesium, potassium should not be given to every patient suspected of having an AMI; a documented potassium deficiency should be obtained first. A patient with an AMI should maintain a potassium level between 4 and 6 mEq per L. Replacement should be no faster than 10 mEq per hour. The most common side effect associated with the administration of potassium is a burning sensation. If this occurs, the infusion rate may be reduced.

Antiarrhythmics. The most common postinfarction complication is disturbance of the normal cardiac rhythm. Pharmacologic manipulation of the cardiac conduction system and the autonomic nervous system and correction of electrolyte abnormalities reduce the morbidity and mortality associated with cardiac arrhythmias in patients with AMI. Arrhythmias occurring in patients with AMI require vigorous treatment when they produce hemodynamic compromise or an increase in myocardial oxygen demand or predispose to malignant ventricular arrhythmias. Lidocaine hydrochloride is the prophylactic antiarrhythmic agent of choice in AMI. This agent decreases automaticity, blocks reentry pathways, and elevates the fibrillatory threshold. Lidocaine can reduce the incidence of malignant ventricular arrhythmias during the early phase of AMI, but mortality is unchanged.[140] Lidocaine may produce asystole and aggravate myocardial dysfunction, so it is not used very often. Prophylactic administration of lidocaine is no longer recommended after an AMI.[17]

Lidocaine is metabolized by the liver and has an elimination half-life of approximately 90 minutes. The metabolism of lidocaine is impaired in the presence of AMI, circulatory shock, hepatic failure, cimetidine, and β-adrenergic blockers. Accumulation of the metabolites of lidocaine may occur in elderly patients and in patients with hepatic or renal dysfunction. The dose of lidocaine should be reduced and individualized in such patients because excessive doses of lidocaine can produce central nervous system toxicity and possibly cardiovascular depression. The toxicity of lidocaine is directly related to its concentration in blood. Plasma lidocaine concentrations should be maintained between 1.5 and 5 μg per mL. Patients with AMI may tolerate higher plasma concentrations (8 μg/mL). This may be related to increased binding of lidocaine to α_1-acid glycoprotein, which is released into the systemic circulation in large concentrations after AMI. Lidocaine (1.0 mg/kg) is administered by IV injection over 2 minutes, followed immediately by an IV infusion of 1 to 4 mg per minute (20 to 50 μg/kg/min). Because of the short distribution half-life (6 to 8 minutes) of lidocaine, an additional bolus of 0.5 mg per kg should be given 10 minutes after the initial bolus to maintain adequate plasma lidocaine concentrations. If ventricular arrhythmias persist, 50-mg bolus injections can be repeated to a maximum of 250 mg of lidocaine over a 20-minute period.

Numerous studies support the use of amiodarone for malignant ventricular arrhythmias.[141] IV amiodarone was consistently effective in terminating these lethal arrhythmias in most patients.[141] Adverse events were usually characterized as hemodynamic events related to rapid administration or higher doses of IV amiodarone. Unlike many other antiarrhythmic agents, amiodarone does not exhibit significant arrhythmogenesis; the overall incidence of proarrhythmia is less than 2%.[141] Torsades de pointes has been reported in less than 1% of patients receiving amiodarone.[141] Amiodarone has been used safely as an alternative agent in patients who have developed torsades de pointes previously with class Ia agents.[141] Other manifestations of cardiovascular toxicity may include the overexpression of normal electrophysiologic actions of the drug, including sinus bradycardia, conduction abnormalities in the atrioventricular node, and heart block.[141] Caution should be exercised in administering amiodarone to patients with preexisting sinus node or conduction systems abnormalities. Amiodarone should not be administered to patients with profound sinus bradycardia or second- or third-degree atrioventricular block unless a functioning artificial ventricular pacemaker is available.[141] Amiodarone has a relatively mild negative inotropic effect, but it does not precipitate or exacerbate heart failure in most patients, even in those with left ventricular dysfunction.[141] Hypotension has also been observed in some patients receiving IV amiodarone.[141] Hypotension, when associated with IV amiodarone, is more dependent on the rate of drug administration than on the total amount of drug administered.[141] A decrease in the rate of infusion is usually all that is required to reverse amiodarone-induced hypotension. Although IV amiodarone is contraindicated in patients with cardiogenic shock or hypotension, the agent has been used safely in patients with cardiac arrest.[141]

Ventricular Fibrillation. VF is the most common cause of death in the early hours after MI and may occur without prior evidence of ventricular premature complexes.[142] VF occurs in approximately 11% of patients with AMI and carries a 46% mortality rate. Approximately 50% of episodes occur within 4 hours and 80% within 12 hours of symptom onset. Although there is no consensus regarding a reduction in morbidity and mortality, routine prophylactic antiarrhythmic therapy was once advocated during the initial 24 hours after MI.[140] Today, the routine use of prophylactic antiarrhythmics in patients with AMI is disputed. Treatment with antiarrhythmics is commonly instituted in patients with warning arrhythmias (i.e., couplets, multifocal premature ventricular contractions, or runs of three or more consecutive premature ventricular contractions).

According to the 2004 ACC/AHA guidelines for STEMI, VF or pulseless VT should be treated with an unsynchronized electric shock with an initial monophasic shock energy of 200 J; if unsuccessful, a second shock of 200 to 300 J should be given, and then, if necessary, a third shock of 360 J.[17] It is reasonable that VF or pulseless VT that is refractory

to electric shock be treated with amiodarone (300 mg or 5 mg/kg, IV bolus) followed by a repeat unsynchronized electric shock. It is reasonable to correct electrolyte and acid–base disturbances (potassium >4.0 mEq/L and magnesium >2.0 mg/dL) to prevent recurrent episodes of VF once an initial episode has been treated. It may be reasonable to treat VT or shock-refractory VF with boluses of IV procainamide.[17]

Ventricular Tachycardia. Electrical cardioversion is indicated for sustained VT, or whenever VT is accompanied by the absence of effective perfusion. Rapid, polymorphic-appearing VT should be considered similar to VF and managed with an unsynchronized discharge of 200 J, whereas monomorphic VT with rates greater than 150 bpm can usually be treated with a 100-J synchronized discharge. Immediate cardioversion is generally not needed for rates below 150 bpm unless hemodynamic compromise is present.

Hemodynamically stable sustained VT may respond to amiodarone or procainamide. Unfortunately, the data supporting the use of any specific antiarrhythmic therapy in this setting are scant. Therefore, knowledge of the pharmacokinetics of antiarrhythmic agents in patients with STEMI is important because dosing varies considerably, depending on age, weight, and hepatic and renal function. Prevention of drug toxicity is critical since efficacy remains unproved. Anecdotal evidence suggests that sustained VT, especially polymorphic VT, may be related to uncontrolled ischemia and increased sympathetic tone and is best treated by IV β-adrenoceptor blockade, IV amiodarone and/or IV magnesium, left stellate ganglion blockade, IABP, or emergency revascularization.

Nonsustained VT is rarely accompanied by hemodynamic compromise and usually does not require acute therapy. Nonetheless, nonsustained VT occurring more than 4 days after STEMI in patients with ejection fractions below 30% represents a risk factor for sudden cardiac death.

According to the 2004 ACC/AHA STEMI guidelines, sustained (>30 seconds or causing hemodynamic collapse) polymorphic VT should be treated with an unsynchronized electric shock with an initial monophasic shock energy of 200 J; if unsuccessful, a second shock of 200 to 300 J should be given, and, if necessary, a third shock of 360 J.[17] It is reasonable to manage refractory polymorphic VT by aggressive attempts to reduce myocardial ischemia, and adrenergic stimulation, including therapies such as β-adrenoceptor blockade, IABP use, and consideration of emergency PCI/coronary artery bypass surgery. Aggressive normalization of serum potassium to greater than 4.0 mEq per L and of magnesium to greater than 2.0 mg per dL is recommended.[17] If the patient has bradycardia to a rate less than 60 bpm or long QTc, temporary pacing at a higher rate may be instituted.

Episodes of sustained monomorphic VT associated with angina, pulmonary edema, or hypotension (blood pressure <90 mm Hg) should be treated with a synchronized electric shock of 100 J of initial monophasic shock energy.[17] Increasing energies may be used if not initially successful. Brief anesthesia is desirable if hemodynamically tolerable. Sustained monomorphic VT not associated with angina, pulmonary edema, or hypotension (blood pressure <90 mm Hg) should be treated with amiodarone [150 mg infused over 10 minutes (alternative dose 5 mg/kg); repeat 150 mg every 10 to 15 minutes as needed]. An alternative infusion is 360 mg over 6 hours (1 mg/min), then 540 mg over the next 18 hours (0.5 mg/min). The total cumulative dose, including additional doses given during cardiac arrest, must not exceed 2.2 g over 24 hours.

Sustained monomorphic VT not associated with angina, pulmonary edema, or hypotension (blood pressure <90 mm Hg) may be treated with a procainamide bolus and infusion.[17] The routine use of prophylactic antiarrhythmic drugs (i.e., lidocaine) is not indicated for suppression of isolated ventricular premature beats, couplets, runs of accelerated idioventricular rhythm, and nonsustained VT. The routine use of prophylactic antiarrhythmic therapy is not indicated when fibrinolytic agents are administered.[17] Treatment of isolated ventricular premature beats, couplets, and nonsustained VT is not recommended unless they lead to hemodynamic compromise.

Accelerated Idioventricular Rhythms. Accelerated idioventricular rhythms are characterized by a wide QRS complex, with a regular rate higher than the atrial rate and lower than 100 bpm. The appearance of an idioventricular rhythm is an inexact indicator of reperfusion. Treatment of idioventricular rhythm is not indicated, and suppression of the rhythm may lead to hemodynamic compromise. Accelerated junctional rhythms are characterized by a regular narrow QRS not preceded by atrial activity, with rates above 60 bpm. This rhythm may indicate digitalis intoxication and is more often seen in inferior STEMI than in anterior STEMI. In general, treatment of accelerated junctional rhythm is not indicated.[17]

Sinus bradycardia is a common finding in patients with inferior wall MI. Transient episodes of bradycardia are often observed during the initial hours after MI and may exert a protective function.[143] If the bradycardia is associated with hypotension or a ventricular arrhythmia, atropine 0.5 to 1 mg should be administered by rapid IV injection. Atropine may be repeated at 2- to 4-hour intervals as needed to maintain a heart rate greater than 60 bpm. Asymptomatic bradycardia should not be treated because the risk of increased myocardial oxygen demand outweighs any potential benefit from treatment. Atropine should not be administered in doses less than 0.5 mg because a paradoxical slowing of the heart rate may occur. Electrical pacing is used to manage atropine refractory bradycardia. IV isoproterenol (0.5 to 2.0 μg/min) should be used, if at all, only until a pacemaker can be placed because of the risks of tachyarrhythmias or hypotension.

Sinus tachycardia occurs in 30% of patients with AMI during the first few days postinfarction.[144] Anxiety, pain, fever, and ventricular dysfunction are common causes of this arrhythmia. Young patients with a first anterior wall MI may be seen in a hyperdynamic state with some tachycardia, hypertension, and ventricular ectopy. These patients may benefit from acute therapy with β-adrenergic blockers.[143,145–149] Atrial fibrillation or flutter occurs in up to 20% of patients with AMI and is often associated with left ventricular dysfunction.[144] Because of this association, these rhythms are seen more often with anterior wall MI and are associated with increased mortality. Therapy is indicated if the arrhythmia produces a rapid ventricular response and/or hemodynamic compromise. Restoration of normal sinus rhythm by electrical cardioversion is an immediate priority in the setting of acute hemodynamic instability.

Patients may develop hemodynamic instability from supraventricular tachycardia. IV verapamil 5 mg over 2 minutes and repeated in 30 minutes to a total of 20 mg may be used for conversion to normal sinus rhythm or for control of ventricular response rate. Verapamil should be used with caution, if at all, in patients with left ventricular dysfunction, hypotension, Wolff-Parkinson-White syndrome, or wide complex tachycardia. Adenosine has the advantage of a shorter half-life and is less likely to produce hypotension than verapamil. The usual dose of adenosine is 6 mg, followed by 12 mg in 3 to 5 minutes if a response is not observed. Total doses greater than 18 mg increase the risk of atrioventricular block, flushing, chest pain, and bronchospasm.

According to the 2004 ACC/AHA STEMI guidelines, sustained atrial fibrillation and atrial flutter in patients with hemodynamic compromise should be treated with one or more of the following: synchronized cardioversion with an initial monophasic shock of 200 J for atrial fibrillation and 50 J for flutter, preceded by brief general anesthesia or conscious sedation whenever possible; for episodes of atrial fibrillation that do not respond to electrical cardioversion or recur after a brief period of sinus rhythm, the use of antiarrhythmic therapy aimed at slowing the ventricular response is indicated.[17] One or more of these pharmacologic agents may be used: IV amiodarone or IV digoxin for rate control, principally for patients with severe left ventricular dysfunction and heart failure.[17]

According to the 2004 ACC/AHA STEMI guidelines, sustained atrial fibrillation and atrial flutter in patients with ongoing ischemia but without hemodynamic compromise should be treated with one or more of the following: β-adrenergic blockade is preferred, unless contraindicated; IV diltiazem or verapamil; synchronized cardioversion with an initial monophasic shock of 200 J for atrial fibrillation and 50 J for flutter, preceded by brief general anesthesia or conscious sedation whenever possible.[17]

For episodes of sustained atrial fibrillation or flutter without hemodynamic compromise or ischemia, rate control is indicated. In addition, patients with sustained atrial fibrillation or flutter should be given anticoagulants. Consideration should be given to conversion of sinus rhythm in patients without a history of atrial fibrillation or flutter prior to STEMI.

Reentrant paroxysmal supraventricular tachycardia, because of its rapid rate, should be treated with the following in this sequence:

Carotid sinus massage

IV adenosine (6 mg over 1 to 2 seconds; if no response, 12 mg IV after 1 to 2 minutes may be given; repeat 12-mg dose if needed)

IV β-adrenergic blockade with metoprolol (2.5 to 5.0 mg every 2 to 5 minutes to a total of 15 mg over 10 to 15 minutes) or atenolol (2.5 to 5.0 mg over 2 minutes to a total of 10 mg in 10 to 15 minutes) may facilitate rate control and convert the rhythm.

IV diltiazem [20 mg (0.25 mg/kg)] over 2 minutes followed by an infusion of 10 mg per hour may be used safely in patients with bronchospasm who cannot tolerate the hypotensive or negative inotropic effects of verapamil.

IV digoxin may be used to control the ventricular response rate, but there may be a delay of at least 1 hour before pharmacologic effects appear [8 to 15 μg/kg (0.6 to 1.0 mg in a person weighing 70 kg)].

Anticoagulants. All patients with MI should be considered for anticoagulant therapy. According to the Fourth American College of Chest Physicians Consensus Conference on Antithrombotic Therapy, if a patient receives warfarin, aspirin should be discontinued. Both warfarin and aspirin should be continued only if the patient experiences ischemic episodes with warfarin alone. In these patients, low-dose (81 mg) aspirin plus warfarin may be of benefit. Patients with contraindications to aspirin should receive warfarin for 1 to 2 years [international normalized ratio (INR) 2.5 to 3.5]. Although administration of anticoagulants to patients with AMI remains controversial, they may be used to prevent systemic and pulmonary embolism formation as well as to halt the progression of infarction. Most patients with uncomplicated AMI do not require full anticoagulation because the low incidence of deep venous thrombosis and pulmonary embolism outweighs the risks of anticoagulation.

Anticoagulation with warfarin for 3 months is recommended after an anterior wall transmural MI. Patients with AMI who are at increased risk for systemic thromboembolic events should be given warfarin for anticoagulation for at least 3 months. A prothrombin time of 1.5 to 2.5 times control (INR 2 to 3) should be the goal of oral anticoagulation.[140,149] Patients with inferior wall MI do not usually develop a left ventricular thrombus formation with resultant cerebrovascular accident. A two-dimensional echocardiogram can be used to assess the presence of a left ventricular thrombus.[140,149] Only patients with heart failure, atrial ar-

rhythmias, large AMI, old anterior wall MI, or apical dyskinesis or akinesis should receive anticoagulant therapy.

The Warfarin Re-Infarction Study Group[140] randomly assigned 1,214 AMI patients within 27 days from onset of symptoms to receive either warfarin to attain a prothrombin time of 1.5 to 2.0 times control or placebo for a mean duration of 37 months (range 24 to 63 months). Warfarin reduced mortality by 24%, the incidence of reinfarction fell by 34%, and there was a 55% decrease in the incidence of cerebrovascular accident. All differences reached statistical significance. The risk of a major bleeding episode was 0.6% per year. The authors concluded that warfarin therapy after AMI is safe and can significantly affect mortality and morbidity.

The incidence of hemorrhagic side effects from anticoagulation in patients with AMI ranges from 3% to 7%. The mortality rate as a result of hemorrhage is 2% to 4% in warfarin-treated patients and less than 1% in patients receiving heparin.[149] Cerebrovascular accidents occur in 2% to 3% and pulmonary embolus in 1% to 2% of patients after MI. On the basis of these observations, only patients at high risk (i.e., left ventricular hypokinesis or mural thrombus), as described earlier, should receive full anticoagulation.[149] The use of full-dose anticoagulation in patients with AMI must be based on the relative risk and potential benefit derived from anticoagulation. In patients with an absolute contraindication to anticoagulation (e.g., bleeding), the potential benefits of anticoagulation do not justify the risk. In patients with relative contraindications to anticoagulation (history of peptic ulcer disease or recent surgery), the risk of bleeding must be weighed against the risk of embolism. Warfarin is indicated for secondary prevention after MI in patients unable to take aspirin, patients with chronic atrial fibrillation, and patients with a left ventricular thrombus. Warfarin can be administered after MI in patients with extensive wall motion abnormalities and impaired ejection.

The 2004 ACC/AHA STEMI guidelines make the following recommendations regarding the role of anticoagulation.[17] Deep venous thrombosis or pulmonary embolism after STEMI should be treated with full-dose LMWH for a minimum of 5 days and until the patient is adequately anticoagulated with warfarin. Start warfarin concurrently with LMWH and titrate to an INR of 2 to 3. Patients with congestive heart failure after STEMI who are hospitalized for prolonged periods, who cannot walk, or who are considered to be at high risk for deep vein thrombosis and are not otherwise anticoagulated should receive low-dose heparin prophylaxis, preferably with LMWH. If true aspirin allergy is present, warfarin therapy with a target INR of 2.5 to 3.5 is a useful alternative to clopidogrel in patients less than 75 years of age who are at low risk for bleeding and who can be monitored adequately for dose adjustment to maintain a target INR range.

Strict Glucose Control During STEMI. Hyperglycemia on admission to the coronary care unit is associated with a poor outcome. It has now been reasonably well established that

IV insulin infusion during AMI has a protective role and reduces mortality.[150] In patients with AMI, hyperglycemia occurs in response to elevations in the circulating levels of catecholamines, cortisol, and glucagons and a deceased amount of circulating insulin. Reduction in insulin sensitivity contributes to impaired glucose utilization after AMI. Concentrations of free fatty acids and their metabolites rise after AMI. This rise potentiates ischemic injury by producing direct myocardial toxicity, by increasing oxygen demand, and by inhibiting glucose oxidation.

Agents that support glucose oxidation may reduce post-MI contractile dysfunction. Therefore, the administration of insulin may produce benefit during AMI because insulin promotes the oxidation of glucose, increases adenosine triphosphate levels, and may improve the fibrinolytic profile of patients with STEMI.[17] Insulin specifically enhances glucose, lactate, and pyruvate uptake and switches the reliance of the myocardium from fat to carbohydrate without a change in oxygen consumption. By reducing lipolysis and free fatty acid synthesis, insulin may produce beneficial effects on the myocardium, since free fatty acids increase myocardial oxygen demand without improving myocardial contractility.[17]

An insulin infusion to normalize blood glucose is recommended for patients with STEMI and complicated courses.[17] During the acute phase (first 24 to 48 hours) of the management of STEMI in patients with hyperglycemia, it is reasonable to administer an insulin infusion to normalize blood glucose even in patients with an uncomplicated course. After the acute phase of STEMI, it is reasonable to individualize treatment of diabetics, selecting from a combination of insulin, insulin analogs, and oral hypoglycemic agents that achieve the best glycemic control and are well tolerated.

Intensive insulin management of endogenous elevation of glucose in diabetics, supplemented by potassium as needed, has potential metabolic benefits similar to glucose-insulin-potassium (GIK) for nondiabetics. Short-term administration of insulin/glucose infusions followed by long-term subcutaneous insulin injections significantly improved glycemic control and produced strong trends toward reduced mortality rates at 30 days and 1 year of follow-up. These data, along with compelling evidence for tight glucose control in intensive care unit patients, support the importance of intensive insulin therapy to achieve a normal blood glucose level (80 to 110 mg/dL) in critically ill patients.[17]

Diabetic patients with STEMI should achieve the tightest glycemic control that is well tolerated and easy to comply with.[151] HbA1C levels should be less than 7%. Diabetics with STEMI should receive individualized therapy with insulin, insulin analogs, and oral hypoglycemic agents, alone or in combination.[17,151] A popular combination is metformin with insulin because it results in similar metabolic control, less weight gain, lower insulin doses, and fewer hyperglycemic episodes than insulin alone or insulin plus sulfonylurea therapy.[17] Metformin is contraindicated in the presence of

congestive heart failure and renal failure. It should be withheld for 48 hours after IV contrast injection.[17]

NONPHARMACOLOGIC THERAPY

Treatment for patients with suspected AMI in the intensive care or coronary care unit includes continuous monitoring and prompt response to emergencies. Intramuscular drug administration is avoided because of possible interference with cardiac enzyme determinations, unpredictable drug absorption during episodes of hypoperfusion, and bleeding during anticoagulation. Vital signs, pain relief, body weight, bowel habits, and diet are closely monitored.

Patients should limit their activities to bed rest during the first 24 hours after the acute event. This is done to decrease myocardial oxygen consumption and to prevent extension of the infarction during the healing process after an AMI. Activities over the next few days should begin gradually, starting with personal hygiene and in-bed range-of-motion exercises. A clear liquid diet is instituted for the first day during the convalescent period.[3,12] Upon discharge from the hospital after MI, a patient should be started on a Step II diet, which is low in saturated fat and cholesterol (<7% of total calories from saturated fat and <200 mg/day of cholesterol).

ALTERNATIVE THERAPIES

Anxiety may have deleterious effects on the cardiovascular system, especially in patients with AMI. The aim of treatment of anxiety should be to reduce not only the somatic complaints but also the adrenergic hyperactivity often present in MI patients. Three groups of medications can be used to treat cardiac symptoms and anxiety disorder. Antidepressant drugs lower anxiety but do not suppress adrenergic response and should be avoided in patients with AMI during acute recovery. In contrast, β-blockers blunt the adrenergic response but do not affect anxiety. Benzodiazepines can be used to relax the patient and theoretically decrease catecholamine release secondary to stress.[152,153] Alprazolam and diazepam have been shown to be effective in decreasing anxiety and catecholamine levels in patients with AMI. Once patients are consuming an appropriate diet, stool softeners are often used to decrease isometric stress associated with defecation. Either docusate sodium or docusate calcium, 240 mg once or twice daily, is satisfactory to soften the stool to avoid straining.

IMPROVING OUTCOMES

Approximately 50% of hospitalized MI patients develop complications.[154] Two general classes of complications have been defined: electrical (arrhythmias) and mechanical (heart failure). ECG monitoring and prompt recognition and treatment of arrhythmias have reduced the in-hospital mortality from MI. Unfortunately, a similarly favorable trend has not been observed with AMI-associated heart failure despite advances in hemodynamic monitoring and inotropic support. Left ventricular failure with subsequent pulmonary congestion is the primary cause of in-hospital death from MI.

Of the 500,000 patients hospitalized yearly for AMI, 400,000 survive to hospital discharge.[152] The major mortality risk is within the first 6 months of hospitalization; death is equally distributed between sudden and nonsudden cardiac events.[152,153] The major determinants of death after MI are the extent of jeopardized myocardium and the degree of electrical instability. Anterior infarction, early left ventricular failure, late significant arrhythmias, and poor left ventricular ejection fraction are major predictors of poor prognosis during the peri-infarction period.[152] Although Q-wave infarct patients have twice the initial mortality of patients with non–Q-wave infarction, their 1-year mortality rates are comparable.[155] Factors associated with late mortality after MI include advanced age,[155] history of prior infarction or chronic angina,[156] female sex,[157] hypertension,[158] diabetes mellitus,[158] and continued cigarette smoking.[15]

Considerable effort has been spent on the search for predictors of survival and factors determining the occurrence of reinfarction after AMI.[159] Most patients who survive AMI initially have an uncomplicated event; the pain subsides and there is no evidence of heart failure or arrhythmias. Mortality after MI in unselected groups of patients ranges from 4% to 6% per year.[159] Mortality is higher in patients with moderate impairment of left ventricular function and three-vessel coronary disease. These patients may benefit from elective coronary artery bypass graft after AMI.

Survival after AMI relates to the extent and location of the coronary obstructive lesion and to the adequacy of residual myocardial function. To prevent or retard the progression of atherosclerotic coronary heart disease, conventional coronary risk factor reduction is necessary.[160] Continued cigarette smoking after MI increases the likelihood of reinfarction and coronary death in men and women of all ages. Reduction of excess calorie and cholesterol intake is advisable. Control of systemic hypertension decreases both myocardial oxygen demand and the risk of stroke. Medical management with antianginal drugs reduces myocardial oxygen demand and decreases myocardial ischemia. By decreasing the ischemic burden, chronic therapy with β-adrenergic blockers reduces both the recurrence of MI and the incidence of sudden death for up to 2 years after AMI.[161] Exercise training improves physical work capacity and improves both weight control and psychological status.

LIPID-LOWERING THERAPY

Current clinical evidence strongly supports early, intensive treatment of patients with acute coronary syndromes to LDL-C goals substantially less than 100 mg per dL with statin therapy. Treatment with non-statin lipid-lowering therapy in the 1980s and early 1990s showed significant reductions of 25% in nonfatal MIs and 14% in fatal MIs. The landmark Scandinavian Simvastatin Survival Study reported results in

4,444 men and women with coronary heart disease (CHD) and moderate hypercholesterolemia observed over 5.4 years.[162] Coronary heart disease mortality was reduced by 42% and total mortality by 30% among those receiving simvastatin compared with placebo. The CARE trial was a similar study in a population of patients who had recovered from an earlier MI and whose total cholesterol (mean 209 mg/dL) and LDL-C (mean 139 mg/dL) levels were essentially the same as the average for the general U.S. population.[163] In this trial, 4,159 patients were randomly assigned to either 40 mg of pravastatin a day or placebo. After a median follow-up of 5 years, there was a significant reduction in the primary endpoint of fatal CHD and nonfatal confirmed MIs in the pravastatin cohort (24% RRR; $p = 0.003$).[163]

Approximately 25% of patients who have recovered from STEMI demonstrate desirable total cholesterol values but a low HDL-C fraction on a lipid profile. The Lipoprotein Cholesterol Intervention Trial (VA-HIT) revealed that modification of other lipid risk factors can reduce risk for CHD when LDL-C is in the range of 100 to 129 mg per dL.[164] In this trial, male patients with a relatively low LDL-C (mean 112 mg/dL) were treated with gemfibrozil for 5 years. Gemfibrozil therapy, which raised HDL-C and lowered triglycerides, reduced the primary endpoint of fatal and nonfatal MI (22% RRR) without significantly lowering LDL-C levels. There was no evidence of an increased risk of non-CHD mortality. This trial supports the concept that when LDL-C is in the range of 100 to 129 mg per dL, the use of other lipid-modifying drugs (e.g., fibrates) is a therapeutic option if the patient has a low HDL-C level (<40 mg/dL).

The benefits of lipid-lowering therapy after AMI are observed among all age, gender, and ethnic categories. A key to successful adherence to post-AMI lipid-lowering therapy is the initiation of pharmacotherapy while the patient is hospitalized. Patients hospitalized with AMI who start lipid-lowering therapy before discharge have been shown to be nearly three times as likely to be taking medication at 6 months as those starting therapy after discharge.[164]

PHARMACOECONOMICS

Advances in treatment have reduced the death rate from AMI by 30% since 1983; today, 13.5 million Americans have survived a heart attack or unstable angina pectoris.[2] Among those who survive their initial AMI, 31% of women and 23% of men will have another acute ischemic event (i.e., stroke, sudden death, or recurrent AMI) within 6 years.[2] The socioeconomic burden of AMI is substantial. Men with coronary artery disease have a 13-year reduction in life expectancy, whereas women have a 12-year reduction in life expectancy.[2,3] Direct costs from AMI (i.e., institutional care, medications, professional visits, home health care, and other medical goods) are $51.1 billion per year.[1] Indirect costs associated with AMI-related loss of income and productivity account for an additional $44.5 billion each year.[1]

Primary prevention measures aim to reduce the occurrence of AMI in disease-free, asymptomatic patients at risk for coronary artery disease. Smoking cessation, reduction in LDL cholesterol levels, control of hypertension, regular physical exercise, weight control, and estrogen replacement therapy in postmenopausal women are measures that may reduce the likelihood of AMI in high-risk patients. Secondary prevention attempts to avoid a second or repeat AMI. Because the number of Americans older than 65 years is expected to increase from 34.2 million in 1995 to 60.8 million in 2020 and AMI recurrence is directly proportional to age, secondary prevention is especially important in this age group. In these patients the administration of antiplatelet agents, ACE inhibitors, β-blockers, and HMG-CoA reductase inhibitors reduce the recurrence of AMI.

KEY POINTS

- MI is one of the most common reasons for hospitalization in the Western world
- Mortality in patients with MI results from both arrhythmias and heart failure
- The actual mortality rate is about 15%; approximately 10% of patients will die during the first year after their AMI
- Both short-term survival and long-term survival depend on the extent and location of the coronary obstructive lesions and the prompt correction of post-MI complications
- Appropriate medical and/or surgical treatment is based on the presence or absence of mechanical, electrical, ischemic, and vascular abnormalities
- MI evolves over a period of several hours. The extent of myocardial damage is related to the degree of reduction in myocardial tissue perfusion and level of myocardial oxygen consumption
- Reperfusion of the ischemic myocardium reduces infarct size and improves hemodynamics and functional recovery
- Thrombolytic therapy, percutaneous balloon angioplasty, and coronary artery bypass surgery are treatment modalities used to achieve prompt reperfusion
- Adjunctive therapy for MI includes aspirin, β-adrenergic blocking agents, and ACE inhibitors
- Primary prevention of MI includes smoking cessation, reduction in LDL cholesterol, management of systemic hypertension, exercise, weight control, and estrogen replacement therapy in postmenopausal women
- Secondary prevention of MI includes the use of antiplatelet agents, ACE inhibitors, β-adrenergic blocking agents, and HMG-CoA reductase inhibitors
- Advances in the treatment of MI have significantly reduced the death rate from MI

REFERENCES

1. American Heart Association. 1998 Heart and Stroke Statistical Update. Dallas: American Heart Association, 1998.
2. Overmyer RH. Treating atherosclerotic disease: current strategies. Formulary J Managed Care Hosp Decision Makers 33(Suppl 1): S3–S12, 1998.
3. Alpert JS, Braunwald E. Acute MI: Pathological, Pathophysiological, and Clinical manifestations. In: Braunwald E, ed. Heart Disease. 2nd ed. Philadelphia: WB Saunders, 1984:1262–1270.
4. Gonzalez ER. Thrombolytic therapy for acute myocardial infarction. Hosp Pharm 32:1498–1509, 1997.
5. Boersma E, Mercado N, Poldermans D, et al. Acute myocardial infarction. Lancet 2003;361:847–858.
6. Katritsis D, Karvouni E, Webb-Peploe MM. Reperfusion in acute myocardial infarction: current concepts. Prog Cardiovasc Dis 2003; 45:481–492.
7. Gonzalez ER, Kannewurf BS. Atherosclerosis: a unifying disorder with various manifestations. Am J Health Syst Pharm 55(Suppl 1): S4–S7, 1998.
8. Moseri A, L'Abbate A, Bardoldi G, et al. Coronary vasospasm as possible cause of myocardial infarction. A conclusion derived from the study of ''preinfarction'' angina. N Engl J Med 299: 1271–1277, 1978.
9. Epstein SE, Palmeri ST. Mechanisms contributing to precipitation of unstable angina and acute myocardial infarction: implications regarding therapy. Am J Cardiol 54:1245–1252, 1984.
10. Advanced cardiac life support. Dallas: American Heart Association, 1997–1999.
11. Kinch JW, Ryan TJ. Right ventricular infarction. N Engl J Med 330:1211–1217, 1994.
12. Zeller FP, Bauman JL. Current concepts in clinical therapeutics: acute myocardial infarction. Clin Pharm 5:553–572, 1986.
13. Tucker JF, Collins RA, Anderson AJ, et al. Value of serial myoglobin levels in the early diagnosis of patients admitted for acute myocardial infarction. Ann Emerg Med 24:704–708, 1994.
14. Adams JE III, Bodor GS, Davilla-Roman VG, et al. Cardiac troponin-1: a marker with high specificity for cardiac injury. Circulation 88:101–106, 1993.
15. Perviaz S, Anderson FP, Lohmann TP, et al. Comparative analysis of cardiac troponin I and creatine kinase-MB as markers of acute myocardial infarction. Clin Cardiol 20:269–271, 1997.
16. Antman EM, Tanasijevic MJ, Thompson B, et al. Cardiac-specific troponin I levels to predict the risk of mortality in patients with acute coronary syndromes. N Engl J Med 335:1342–1348, 1996.
17. Antman EM, Anbe DT, Armstrong PW, et al. ACC/AHA Guidelines for the Management of Patients With ST-Elevation Myocardial Infarction: A Report of the American College of Cardiology/ American Heart Association Task Force on Practice Guidelines (Committee to Revise the 1999 Guidelines for the Management of Patients With Acute Myocardial Infarction). 2004. Available at www.acc.org/clinical/guidelines/stemi/index.pdf.
18. Heeschen C, Hamm CW, Mitrovic V, et al. N-terminal pro-B-type natriuretic peptide levels for dynamic risk stratification of patients with acute coronary syndromes. Circulation 110:3206–3212, 2004.
19. Yip HK, Hang CL, Fang CY, et al. Level of high-sensitivity C-reactive protein is predictive of 30-day outcomes in patients with acute myocardial infarction undergoing primary coronary intervention. Chest 127:863–867, 2005.
20. Tanaka A, Shimada K, Sano T, et al. Multiple plaque rupture and C-reactive protein in acute myocardial infarction. J Am Coll Cardiol 45:1600–1602, 2005.
21. Zelma MJ. Q wave, S-T segment, and T wave myocardial infarction. Am J Med 78:391–398, 1985.
22. Gluckman TJ, Sachdev M, Schulman SP, et al. A simplified approach to the management of Non-ST-segment elevation acute coronary syndrome. JAMA 293:349–357, 2005.
23. Dubin D. Rapid interpretation of EKGs. 5th ed. Tampa: Cover Publishing, 1996.
24. GISSI–Avoidable Delay Study Group. Epidemiology; avoidable delay in the care of patients with acute myocardial infarction in Italy. Arch Intern Med 155:1481–1488, 1995.

25. Blohm MB, Herlitz J, Schroder U, et al. Reaction to a media campaign focusing on delay in acute myocardial infarction. Heart Lung 20:661–666, 1991.
26. Blohm MB, Hartfor M, Karlson BW, et al. An evaluation of the results of media and educational campaigns designed to shorten the time taken by patients with acute myocardial infarction to decide to go to hospital. Heart 76:430–434, 1996.
27. Cohen M, Arjomand H, Pollack CV. The evolution of thrombolytic therapy and adjunctive antithrombotic regimens in acute ST-segment elevation myocardial infarction. Am J Emerg Med 22:14–23, 2004.
28. Braunwald E, Antman EM, Beasley JW, et al. ACC/AHA 2002 Guideline Update for the management of Patients With Unstable Angina and Non–ST-Segment Elevation Myocardial Infarction: A Report of the American College of Cardiology/American Heart Association Task Force on Practice Guidelines (Committee on the Management of Patients With Unstable Angina). 2002. Available at: http://www.acc.org/clinical/guidelines/unstable/unstable.pdf.
29. Rasanen J, Vaisanen IT, Heikkila J, et al. Acute myocardial infarction complicated by left ventricular dysfunction and respiratory failure: the effects of continuous positive airway pressure. Chest 87:278–280, 1985.
30. Dole WP, O'Rourke RA. Pathophysiology and management of cardiogenic shock. Curr Probl Cardiol 8:1–72, 1983.
31. Lee G, DeMaria AN, Amsterdam EA, et al. Comparative effect of morphine, meperidine, and pentazocine on cardiopulmonary dynamics in patients with acute myocardial infarction. Am J Med 60:341–355, 1976.
32. Stadol. In: Physician's Desk Reference. Montvale, NJ: Medical Economics Publishing Co., 1995;49:739–742.
33. Mueller JE, Braunwald E. Can infarct size be limited in patients with acute myocardial infarction? Cardiovasc Clin 69:740–747, 1983.
34. Herling IM. Intravenous nitroglycerin: clinical pharmacology and therapeutic. Chest 73:441–445, 1981.
35. Roberts R. Intravenous nitroglycerin in acute myocardial infarction. Am J Med 74:45–52, 1983.
36. Swan NA, Evenson MK, Needham KE, et al. Effect of combined nitroglycerin and dobutamine infusion in left ventricular dysfunction. Am Heart J 106:35, 1983.
37. Chiarello M, Gold HK, Leinback RC, et al. Comparison between the effects of nitroprusside and nitroglycerin on ischemic injury during acute myocardial infarction. Circulation 54:766, 1976.
38. Flaherty JT. Comparison of intravenous nitroglycerin and sodium nitroprusside in acute myocardial infarction. Am J Med 74:53–60, 1983.
39. Pitt B, Shae MJ, Romson JL. Prostaglandins and prostaglandin inhibitors in ischemic heart disease. Ann Intern Med 99:83–92, 1983.
40. Hirsh J. The optimal antithrombotic dose of aspirin. Arch Intern Med 145:1582, 1985.
41. Theroux P, Quimet H, McCans J. Aspirin, heparin, or both to treat acute unstable angina. N Engl J Med 313:1369–1375, 1985.
42. ISIS-2 (Second International Study of Infarct Survival) Collaborative Group. Randomized trial of intravenous streptokinase, oral aspirin, both, or neither among 17,187 cases of suspected acute myocardial infarction: ISIS-2. Lancet 2:349–360, 1988.
43. American College of Cardiology/American Heart Association. Guidelines for the management of patients with acute myocardial infarction. Circulation 94:2341–2350, 1996.
44. Berger PB, Orford JL. Acute myocardial infarction. ACP Medicine 2004. Copyright 2004 WebMD.
45. Menon V, Harrington RA, Hochman JS, et al. Thrombolysis and adjunctive therapy in acute myocardial infarction: the Seventh ACCP Conference on Antithrombotic and Thrombolytic Therapy. Chest 126:549S–575S, 2004.
46. Gonzalez ER. Antiplatelet therapy in atherosclerotic cardiovascular disease. Clin Ther 20(Suppl B):B42–B53, 1998.
47. McTavish D, Faulds D, Gao KL. Ticlopidine: an updated review of its pharmacology and therapeutic use in platelet-dependent disorders. Drugs 40:239–259, 1990.
48. Knudsen JB, Kjoller E, Skagen K, et al. Randomized trial of prophylactic daily aspirin in British male doctors. Br Med J 296:313–316, 1988.
49. CAPRIE Steering Committee. A randomized, blinded trial of clopidogrel versus aspirin in patients at risk of ischemic events (CAPRIE). Lancet 348:1329–1339, 1996.
50. Antiplatelet Trialists Collaboration. Collaborative overview of randomized trials of antiplatelet therapy. I. Prevention of death, myocardial infarction, and stroke by prolonged antiplatelet therapy in various categories of patients. Br Med J 308:81–106, 1994.
51. Prins MH, Hirsh J. Heparin as an adjunctive treatment for thrombolytic therapy for acute myocardial infarction. N Engl J Med 323:147–152, 1990.
52. Hsia J, Hamilton WP, Kleiman N, et al. A comparison between heparin and low-dose aspirin as an adjunctive therapy with tissue plasminogen activator for acute myocardial infarction: Heparin-Aspirin Reperfusion Trial (HART) Investigators. N Engl J Med 323:1433–1437, 1990.
53. Trujillo TC, Nolan PE. Unfractionated heparin in acute coronary syndromes: has its time come and gone? Am J Health Syst Pharm 55:2402–2409, 1998.
54. Wong GC, Giugliano RP, Antman EM. Use of low-molecular-weight heparins in the management of acute coronary artery syndromes and percutaneous coronary intervention. JAMA 289:331–342, 2003.
55. Gurfinkel EP, Manos EJ, Mejail RI, et al. Low molecular weight heparin versus regular heparin or aspirin in the treatment of unstable angina and silent ischemia. J Am Coll Cardiol 26:313–318, 1995.
56. Klein W, Buchwald AB, Hillis SE, et al. Comparison of low molecular weight heparin with unfractionated heparin in the management of unstable coronary disease: Fragmin in Unstable Coronary Artery Disease Study. Circulation 96:61–68, 1997.
57. Haas S. The present and future of heparin, low molecular weight heparins, pentasaccharide, and hirudin for venous thromboembolism and acute coronary syndromes. Semin Vasc Med 3:139–146, 2003.
58. Eikelboom J, White H, Yusuf S. The evolving role of direct thrombin inhibitors in acute coronary syndromes. J Am Coll Cardiol 41(4 Suppl S):70S–78S, 2003.
59. Katritsis D, Karvouni E, Webb-Peploe MM. Reperfusion in acute myocardial infarction: current concepts. Prog Cardiovasc Dis 45:481–492, 2003.
60. Bahr RD. Reducing the time to therapy in AMI patients: the new paradigm. Am J Emerg Med 12:501–503, 1994.
61. Julian DG. Time as a factor in thrombolytic therapy. Int J Cardiol 49(Suppl):S17–S19, 1995.
62. Gonzalez ER, Sypniewski E. Acute myocardial infarction: diagnosis and treatment. In: DiPiro J, Talbert R, Hays M, et al, eds. Pharmacotherapy: A Pathophysiologic Approach. 2nd ed. New York: Elsevier, 1993:231–254.
63. Carney R. Randomized angiographic trial of recombinant tissue-type plasminogen activator in myocardial infarction. J Am Coll Cardiol 20:17–23, 1992.
64. Chen BP, Chow MS, Kluger J. Perspective on current, future thrombolytic therapy for acute myocardial infarction. Formulary 32:364–385, 1997.
65. Smalling RW, Bode C, Kalbfleisch J, et al. More rapid, complete, and stable coronary thrombolysis with bolus administration of reteplase compared with alteplase infusion in acute myocardial infarction. Circulation 91:2725–2732, 1995.
66. Martin U, Doerge L, Stegmeier K, et al. Influence of the degree of renal dysfunction on the pharmacokinetic properties of the novel recombinant plasminogen activator reteplase in rats. Drug Metab Dispos 24:288–292, 1996.
67. Gunnar RM, Bourdillon PD, Dixon DW, et al. Guidelines for the early management of patients with acute myocardial infarction: a report of the American College of Cardiology/American Heart Association Task Force on Assessment of Diagnostic and Therapeutic Cardiovascular Procedures. J Am Coll Cardiol 16:249–292, 1990.
68. Martin U, Kohnert U, Helerbrand K, et al. Effective thrombolysis by a recombinant *Escherichia coli*-produced protease domain of tissue-type plasminogen activator in rabbit model of jugular vein thrombosis. Fibrinolysis 10:87–92, 1996.
69. Gersh BJ. Role of thrombolytic therapy in evolving myocardial infarction. Mod Concepts Cardiovas Dis 54:13–17, 1985.

70. Schwartz DE, Yamago CC. Thombolysis for evolving myocardial infarction. Ann Intern Med 103;463–469, 1985.
71. National Heart Attack Alert Program Coordinating Committee. Emergency department: rapid identification and treatment of patients with acute myocardial infarction. Ann Emerg Med 23: 311–329, 1994.
72. Every NR, Spertus J, Fihn SD, et al. Length of hospital stay after acute myocardial infarction in the Myocardial Infarction Triage and Intervention (MITI) Project registry. J Am Coll Cardiol 28: 287–293, 1996.
73. Grines CL, DeMaria AN. Optimal utilization of thrombolytic therapy for acute myocardial infarction: concepts and controversies. J Am Coll Cardiol 16:223–231, 1990.
74. GUSTO-I Investigators. An international randomized trial comparing four thrombolytic strategies for acute myocardial infarction. N Engl J Med 329:673–682, 1993.
75. GUSTO Angiographic Investigators. The effects of tissue plasminogen activator, streptokinase, or both on coronary artery patency, ventricular function, and survival after acute myocardial infarction. N Engl J Med 329:1615–1622, 1993.
76. Schroeder WS, Gandhi PJ. Emergency management of hemorrhagic complications in the era of glycoprotein IIb/IIIa receptor antagonists, clopidogrel, low molecular weight heparin, and third-generation fibrinolytic agents. Curr Cardiol Rep 5:310–317, 2003.
77. Maggioni A. The risk of stroke in patients with acute myocardial infarction after thrombolytic and antithrombotic treatment. N Engl J Med 327:1–6, 1992.
78. Gruppo Italiano per lo Studio della Sopravvivenza nell'Infarto Miocardico. GISSI-2: A factorial randomised trial of alteplase versus streptokinase and heparin versus no heparin among 12,490 patients with acute myocardial infarction. Lancet 336:65–71, 1990.
79. ISIS-3 (Third International Study of Infarct Survival) Collaborative Group. ISIS-3: a randomised trial of streptokinase vs tissue plasminogen activator vs anistreplase and of aspirin plus heparin vs aspirin alone among 41,299 cases of suspected acute myocardial infarction. Lancet 339:753–770, 1992.
80. Ridker P. Large scale trials of thrombolytic therapy for acute myocardial infarction: GISSI-2, ISIS-3, and GUSTO-I. Ann Intern Med 119:530–532, 1993.
81. Sherry S. Appraisal of various thrombolytic agents in the management of acute myocardial infarction. Am J Med 83(Suppl 2A): 31–46, 1987.
82. Talley JD. Review of thrombolytic intervention for acute myocardial infarction: is it valuable? J Ark Med Soc 91:70–79, 1994.
83. International Joint Efficacy Comparison of Thrombolytics. Randomized, double-blind comparison of reteplase double-bolus administration with streptokinase in acute myocardial infarction (INJECT): trial to investigate equivalence. Lancet 346:329–336, 1995.
84. International Group. In-hospital mortality and clinical course of 20,891 patients with suspected acute myocardial infarction randomized between alteplase and streptokinase with or without heparin. Lancet 336:71–75, 1990.
85. Hochman J. Modern treatment of acute myocardial infarction. Cardiovasc Rev Rep 16:23–35, 1995.
86. GUSTO III. A comparison of reteplase with alteplase for acute myocardial infarction. N Engl J Med 337:1118–1123, 1997.
87. Crabbe SJ, Cloniger CC. Tissue plasminogen activator. A new thrombolytic agent. Clin Pharm 6:373–386, 1987.
88. Sherry S. Recombinant tissue activator (rt-PA): is it the thrombolytic agent of choice of an evolving myocardial infarction? Ann Intern Med 114:417–423, 1991.
89. Sherry S, Marder VJ. Streptokinase and recombinant tissue plasminogen activator (rt-PA) are equally effective in treating acute myocardial infarction. Ann Intern Med 114:417–423, 1991.
90. White HD, Rivers JT, Maslowski AH, et al. Effect of intravenous streptokinase as compared with that of tissue plasminogen activator on left ventricular function after first myocardial infarction. N Engl J Med 320:817–821, 1989.
91. Bassand JP, Cassagnes J, Machecourt T, et al. A multicenter trial of intravenous APSAC versus rt-PA in acute myocardial infarction: assessment of efficacy and safety [abstract]. J Am Coll Cardiol 13(Suppl A):214A, 1990.
92. Rao AK, Pratt C, Berke A, et al. Thrombolysis in Acute Myocardial Infarction (TIMI) Trial, phase I: hemorrhagic manifestations

and changes in plasma fibrinogen and the fibrinolytic system in patients treated with recombinant tissue plasminogen activator and streptokinase. J Am Coll Cardiol 11:1–11, 1988.
93. Gonzalez ER, Katz GM. Coronary thrombolysis: a comparison of intravenous streptokinase and intravenous tissue-type plasminogen activator. Fam Pract Recert 11:109–124, 1989.
94. McGovern PG, Pankow JS, Shaher E, et al. Recent trends in acute coronary heart disease: mortality, morbidity, medical care, and risk factors. N Engl J Med 334:884–890, 1996.
95. Granger CB. Data presented at the American College of Cardiology, 40th Annual Scientific Session. March 16–19, 1997.
96. Cragg DR, Bonemia JD, Jaiyesimi IA, et al. Ineligibility for intravenous therapy [abstract]. N Engl J Med 335:1253–1260, 1996.
97. Samama MM, Acar J. Thrombolytic therapy: future issues. Thromb Haemost 74:106–110, 1995.
98. Friedman BM. Early interventions in the management of acute myocardial infarction. West Med J 162:19–27, 1995.
99. Kandzari DE, Hasselblad V, Tcheng JE, et al. Improved clinical outcomes with abciximab therapy in acute myocardial infarction: a systematic overview of randomized clinical trials. Am Heart J 147: 457–462, 2004.
100. Moliterno DJ, Chan AW. Glycoprotein IIb/IIIa inhibition in early intent-to-stent treatment of acute coronary syndromes: EPISTENT, ADMIRAL, CADILLAC, and TARGET. J Am Coll Cardiol 41(4 Suppl S):49S–54S, 2003.
101. Ross AM. Glycoprotein IIb/IIIa receptor antagonists in the treatment of acute ST elevation MI: from hypotheses to unexpected recent observations. J Thromb Thrombolysis 15:85–89, 2003.
102. Gibbons R. Immediate angioplasty compared with the administration of a thrombolytic agent followed by conservative treatment for myocardial infarction. N Engl J Med 328:685–691, 1993.
103. Lange R, Hillis L. Immediate angioplasty for acute myocardial infarction [editorial]. N Engl J Med 328:685–691, 1993.
104. Klimt DR, Knatterud GL, Stamler J, et al. Persantine-aspirin reinfarction study. Part II. Secondary coronary prevention with persantine and aspirin. J Am Coll Cardiol 7:251–269, 1986.
105. Oates JA, Wood AJ. Dipyridamole. N Engl J Med 316:1247–1257, 1987.
106. May GS, Furbery CD, Eberlein KA, et al. Secondary prevention after myocardial infarction. A review of short-term acute phase trials. Prog Cardiovasc Dis 25:335–359, 1985.
107. Mueller HS, Ayres SM. Propranolol decreases sympathetic necrosis activity reflected by plasma catecholamines during evolution of myocardial infarction in man. J Clin Invest 65:338–346, 1980.
108. Pitt B, Crown P. Effect of propranolol in regional myocardial blood flow in acute ischemia. Cardiovasc Res 4:176–179, 1970.
109. MIAMI Trial Research Group. Metoprolol in acute myocardial infarction (MIAMI). A randomised placebo-controlled international trial. Eur Heart J 6:199–226, 1985.
110. ISIS-1 (First International Study of Infarct Survival) Collaborative Group. Randomized trial of intravenous atenolol among 16,027 cases of suspected acute myocardial infarction: ISIS-1. Lancet 2: 57–66, 1986.
111. TIMI Study Group. Comparison of invasive conservative strategies after treatment with intravenous tissue plasminogen activator in acute myocardial infarction: results of the Thrombolysis in Myocardial Infarction (TIMI) Phase II trial. N Engl J Med 320:618–627, 1989.
112. Moos AN, Hilleman DE, Mohiudin SM, et al. Safety of esmolol in patients with acute myocardial infarction treated with thrombolytic therapy who have relative contraindications to β-blocker therapy. Ann Pharmacother 28:701–703, 1994.
113. Bussman WD, Seher W, Gresengrus M. Reduction of creatine kinase and creatinine kinase-MB indexes of infarct size by intravenous verapamil. Am J Cardiol 54:1224–1230, 1984.
114. Danish Multicenter Study Group. Verapamil in acute myocardial infarction. Eur Heart J 5:516–528, 1984.
115. Mueller JE, Morrison J, Stone PH, et al. Nifedipine therapy for patients with threatened and acute myocardial infarction. A randomized double-blind, placebo-controlled comparison. Circulation 69: 740–747, 1984.
116. Sirnes PA, Overskeid K, Pedersen TR. Evolution of infarct size during the early use of nifedipine in patients with acute myocardial

infarction: The Norwegian Nifedipine Multicenter Trial. Circulation 70:638–644, 1984.

117. Gibson RS, Boden WE, Theroux P, et al. Diltiazem and reinfarction in patients with non-Q-wave myocardial infarction. N Engl J Med 315:423, 1986.

118. Gibson RS, Young OM, Boden WE, et al. Prognostic significance and beneficial effect of diltiazem on the incidence of early recurrent ischemia after non-Q wave myocardial infarction: Results from the Multicenter Diltiazem Reinfarction Study. Am J Cardiol 60: 203–209, 1987.

119. The Multicenter Diltiazem Postinfarction Trial Research Group. The effect of diltiazem on mortality and reinfarction after myocardial infarction. N Engl J Med 319:385, 1988.

120. Pfeffer M, Braunwald E, Moye LA, et al. Effect of captopril on mortality and morbidity in patients with left ventricular dysfunction after myocardial infarction. N Engl J Med 327:669–677, 1992.

121. Swedberg K, Held P, Kjekshus J, et al. Effects of early administration of enalapril on mortality in patients with acute myocardial infarction. N Engl J Med 327:678–684, 1992.

122. SOLVD Investigators. Effect of enalapril on mortality and the development of heart failure in asymptomatic patients with reduced left ventricular ejection fractions. N Engl J Med 327:685–691, 1992.

123. Cohn J. The prevention of heart failure: a new agenda [editorial]. N Engl J Med 327:725–727, 1992.

124. Dyckner T, Wester PO. Magnesium in cardiology. Acta Med Scand 666(Suppl):27–31, 1982.

125. Ebel H, Gunther T. Role of magnesium in cardiac disease. J Clin Chem Clin Biochem 21:249–265, 1983.

126. Hollifield JW. Potassium and magnesium abnormalities: diuretics and arrhythmias in hypertension. Am J Med 77:28–32, 1984.

127. Rasmussen HS, Norregard P, Lindeneg O, et al. Intravenous magnesium in acute myocardial infarction. Lancet 1:234–235, 1986.

128. Whang R, Flink EB, Dyckner T, et al. Magnesium depletion as a cause of refractory potassium repletion. Arch Intern Med 145: 1686–1689, 1985.

129. Whang R, Oei TO, Aikawa JK, et al. Predictors of clinical hypomagnesemia. Arch Intern Med 144:1794–1796, 1984.

130. Rasmussen HS, Aurup P, Hojberg S, et al. Magnesium and acute myocardial infarction. Arch Intern Med 146:872–874, 1986.

131. Ornato JP, Gonzalez ER. Refractory ventricular fibrillation. Emerg Decis 4:35–41, 1986.

132. Long-term outcome after intravenous magnesium sulphate in suspected acute myocardial infarction: the second Leicester Intravenous Magnesium Intervention Trial (LIMIT-2). Lancet 343: 816–819, 1994.

133. ISIS-4 (Fourth International Study of Infarct Survival) Collaborative Group. A randomized factorial trial assessing early oral captopril, oral mononitrate, and intravenous magnesium sulphate in 58,050 patients with suspected acute myocardial infarction. Lancet 345:669–685, 1995.

134. Heesch C, Eichhorn EJ. Magnesium in acute myocardial infarction. Ann Emerg Med 24:1154–1160, 1994.

135. Antman E. Randomized trials of magnesium in acute myocardial infarction: when big numbers do not tell the whole story [editorial]. Am J Cardiol 75:391–393, 1995.

136. Morgan DB, Davidson C. Hypokalemia and diuretics: an analysis of publications. Br Med J 280:905–909, 1980.

137. Kafka, S, Langevin L, Armstron PW. Serum magnesium and potassium in acute myocardial infarction. Arch Intern Med 147: 465–469, 1987.

138. Ornato JP, Gonzalez ER, Starke H, et al. Incidence and causes of hypokalemia association with cardiac resuscitation. Am J Emerg Med 3:503–506, 1985.

139. Salerno DM, Asinger RW, Elsperger J, et al. Frequency of hypokalemia after successfully resuscitated out-of-hospital cardiac arrest compared with that in transmural acute myocardial infarction. Am J Cardiol 59:84–88, 1987.

140. Smith P, Arnesen H, Holme I. The effect of warfarin on mortality and reinfarction after myocardial infarction. N Engl J Med 323: 147–152, 1990.

141. Gonzalez ER, Kannewurf BS, Ornato JP. Intravenous amiodarone for ventricular arrhythmias: overview and clinical use. Resuscitation 39:34–42, 1998.

142. Wyman MG, Gore S. Lidocaine prophylaxis in myocardial infarction: a concept whose time has come. Heart Lung 12:358–361, 1983.

143. Cristal N, Szwareberg J, Gueron M. Supraventricular arrhythmias in acute myocardial infarction: prognostic importance of clinical setting; mechanisms of production. Ann Intern Med 82:35–39, 1975.

144. Singh BN, Venkatesh N. Prevention of myocardial reinfarction and of sudden death in survivors of acute myocardial infarction: role of prophylactic beta-adrenoreceptor blockade. Am Heart J 108: 450–455, 1984.

145. Norris RM, Brown MA, Clarke ED, et al. Prevention of ventricular fibrillation during acute myocardial infarction by intravenous propranolol. Lancet 2: 883–886, 1984.

146. Ryden L, Arniego R, Arnman K, et al. A double-blind trial of metoprolol in acute myocardial infarction: effects on ventricular tachyarrhythmias. N Engl J Med 308:614–618, 1983.

147. Mueller H, Ayres SM, Religi A, et al. Propranolol in the treatment of acute myocardial infarction. Circulation 49:1078–1091, 1974.

148. Chadda K, Goldstein S, Byington R, et al. Effect of propranolol after acute myocardial infarction in patients with congestive heart failure. Circulation 73:503–510, 1986.

149. Kaplan K. Prophylactic anticoagulation following acute myocardial infarction. Arch Intern Med 146:595–597, 1986.

150. Imran SA, Malmberg K, Cox JL, et al. An overview of the role of insulin in the treatment of hyperglycemia during acute myocardial ischemia. Can J Cardiol 20:1361–1365, 2004.

151. Klein L, Gheorghiade M. Management of the patient with diabetes mellitus and myocardial infarction: clinical trials update. Am J Med 116(Suppl 5A):47S–63S, 2004.

152. Hoehn-Saric R, McLeod DR. Cardiac symptoms and anxiety disorders: contributing factors and pharmacologic. Am J Cardiol 60: 68j–73j, 1987.

153. Barker PH, Clanachan AS. Inhibition of adenosine accumulation into guinea pig ventricle by benzodiazepines. Eur J Pharmacol 78: 241–244, 1982.

154. Rude RE. Acute myocardial infarction and its complications. Cardiol Clin 2:163–171, 1984.

155. Forrester JS, Waters DD. Hospital treatment of congestive heart failure: management according to hemodynamic profile. Am J Med 65:173–180, 1978.

156. Herling IM. Intravenous nitroglycerin: clinical pharmacology and therapeutic considerations. Am Heart J 108:141–149, 1984.

157. Swan NA, Evenson MK, Needham KE, et al. Effect of continuous nitroglycerin and dobutamine infusion in left ventricular dysfunction. Am Heart J 106:35–41, 1983.

158. Parmley WW, Chatterjee K, Charuzi Y, et al. Hemodynamic effect of noninvasive systolic unloading (nitroprusside) and diastolic augmentation (external counterpulsation) in patients with acute myocardial infarction. Am J Cardiol 33:810, 1974.

159. Sanz G, Castaner A, Betrice A, et al. Determinants of prognosis in survivors of myocardial infarction. N Engl J Med 306:1065–1070, 1982.

160. Wenger NK. Uncomplicated acute myocardial infarction: long-term management. Am J Cardiol 52:658–660, 1983.

161. Turi ZG, Braunwald E. The use of beta blockers after myocardial infarction. JAMA 249:2512–2516, 1983.

162. Randomised trial of cholesterol lowering in 4444 patients with coronary heart disease: the Scandinavian Simvastatin Survival Study (4S). Lancet 344:1383–1389, 1994.

163. Sacks FM, Pfeffer MA, Moye LA, et al, for the Cholesterol and Recurrent Events Trial investigators. The effect of pravastatin on coronary events after myocardial infarction in patients with average cholesterol levels. N Engl J Med 335:1001–1009, 1996.

164. Rubins HB, Robins SJ, Collins D, et al, for the Veterans Affairs High-Density Lipoprotein Cholesterol Intervention Trial Study Group. Gemfibrozil for the secondary prevention of coronary heart disease in men with low levels of high-density lipoprotein cholesterol. N Engl J Med 341:410–418, 1999.

Thromboembolic Disease

25

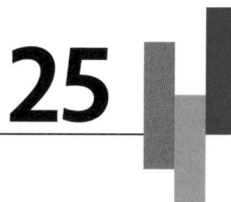

Christa M. George

TREATMENT GOALS

Objectives for the treatment of patients with deep vein thrombosis (DVT) and pulmonary embolism (PE) are to prevent thrombus extension, thrombus embolization, early and late recurrences of DVT and PE, and the development of postthrombotic syndrome (PTS) by restoring normal venous blood flow and maintaining normal venous valve function.[1,2] PTS is characterized by chronic posture-dependent swelling of the affected extremity and pain. It occurs in approximately 20% to 50% of patients with documented DVT.[2]

DEFINITION

Venous thromboembolism (VTE) is a disease that includes both DVT and PE. A deep vein thrombosis is a thrombus composed of cellular material and fibrin that can form in any vein in the body. Thrombi that occur in the larger leg veins pose a higher risk for pulmonary embolism than do those that occur in the smaller calf veins.[1] A pulmonary embolism is a thrombus that originates from any location in the systemic circulation and becomes lodged in the pulmonary artery, impeding blood flow to the lungs.[3,4]

ETIOLOGY

The pathogenesis of VTE involves three factors: venous stasis, hypercoagulability, and endothelial damage. These factors are collectively referred to as Virchow's triad. Many factors may contribute to the development of VTE (Table 25.1).[5,6]

Venous stasis inhibits the clearance and dilution of activated coagulation factors. Venous stasis may result from immobilization, major illness with hospitalization, obesity, or any obstruction of venous flow. Hypercoagulable states may be inherited or acquired. Activated protein C resistance (factor V Leiden mutation) is the most common of the heritable hypercoagulable disorders, with an incidence of 25%.[7] Other common inherited hypercoagulable disorders are protein C deficiency, protein S deficiency, prothrombin G20210A gene mutation, elevated factor VIII, antithrombin deficiency, and homocystinemia. Dysfibrinolysis manifests in five different forms and is relatively rare. The antiphospholipid antibody syndrome (APS) is an acquired hypercoagulable state that is divided into the lupus anticoagulant and the anticardiolipin antibody syndrome. APS is the most common hypercoagulable state, with an incidence of approximately 28%.[7] Cancer is the second most common acquired cause of hypercoagulability. In addition to producing a hypercoagulable state, tumors may cause endothelial injury and venous stasis.[7] The increased activity of clotting factors during pregnancy produces a hypercoagulable state. Oral contraceptives, hormone replacement therapy, and selective estrogen receptor modulators have also been associated with an increased risk of VTE. Acquired conditions that contribute to VTE through endothelial damage include major surgery or trauma. Increasing age may also contribute to the development of VTE.[7]

TABLE 25.1	Conditions Associated With Venous Thromboembolism
Inherited Conditions	**Acquired Conditions**
Antithrombin deficiency	Major surgery or trauma
Protein C deficiency	History of VTE
Protein S deficiency	Antiphospholipid antibodies (anticardiolipin antibodies, lupus anticoagulant)
Factor V Leiden mutation (activated protein C resistance)	Cancer
Prothrombin G20210A mutation	Increasing age
Homocystinemia	Pregnancy, OCs, HRT, SERMs
Elevated factor VIII	Obesity
Dysfibrinolysis	Major medical illness with hospitalization
	Immobility

VTE, venous thromboembolism; OCs, oral contraceptives; HRT, hormone replacement therapy; SERMs, selective estrogen-receptor modulators.
(Adapted from Bates SM, Ginsberg JS. Treatment of deep-vein thrombosis. N Engl J Med 351:268–277, 2004; Hyers TM, Agnelli G, Hull RD, et al. Antithrombotic therapy for venous thromboembolic disease. Chest 114:561S–578S, 1998.)

EPIDEMIOLOGY

The annual incidence of VTE is approximately 0.1%.[8,9] The incidence of VTE increases with age.[8–12] The rate of diagnosis of VTE was 4.9 per 100,000 children per year between 1979 and 2001.[13] The rate of diagnosis of DVT in elderly patients (≥70 years) was 655 per 100,000 population in 1999.[12] It is estimated that approximately 187,000 new cases of VTE are diagnosed each year in the United States.[14] VTE is a serious disorder that can often lead to death. Pulmonary embolism that stems from venous thrombosis is responsible for approximately 60,000 deaths each year.[1] Most patients who die of pulmonary embolism do so during the first hours after the event, making early detection and treatment essential in improving patient outcomes.[4]

PATHOPHYSIOLOGY

The coagulation system is activated in response to vascular endothelial injury. The system is composed of platelet-mediated primary hemostasis and the coagulation cascade. These two components work in concert to prevent hemorrhage secondary to the injury. Natural anticoagulant processes in the body closely regulate the coagulation system to avoid diffuse thrombosis. Any disturbance in the balance between the procoagulant and anticoagulant systems can lead to hemorrhage or thrombotic disease.[15]

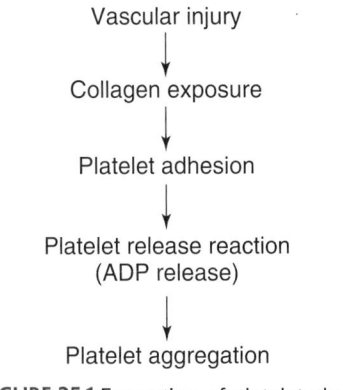

FIGURE 25.1 Formation of platelet plug.

Three steps are required for primary hemostasis to occur: platelet adhesion, granule release, and platelet aggregation. When injury occurs to the vascular endothelium, platelets adhere to exposed collagen fibers. This binding is facilitated by von Willebrand factor (vWF). Following platelet adhesion, numerous granules are released from platelets (adenosine diphosphate, platelet-derived growth factor, vWF, fibrinogen, heparinase, thromboxane A2, factor Va, thrombospondin, fibronectin), which stimulate platelet aggregation and aid in initiating the coagulation cascade (Fig. 25.1). Initiation of this cascade (Fig. 25.2) is necessary for the temporary platelet plug to be transformed into a permanent fibrin clot. The cascade may be initiated through intrinsic or extrinsic pathways.[15–17]

Clotting factors are proteins that circulate in an inactive form. Each factor must be converted to its active form for the clotting cascade to continue. The intrinsic pathway involves the formation of a complex between factor XII, high-

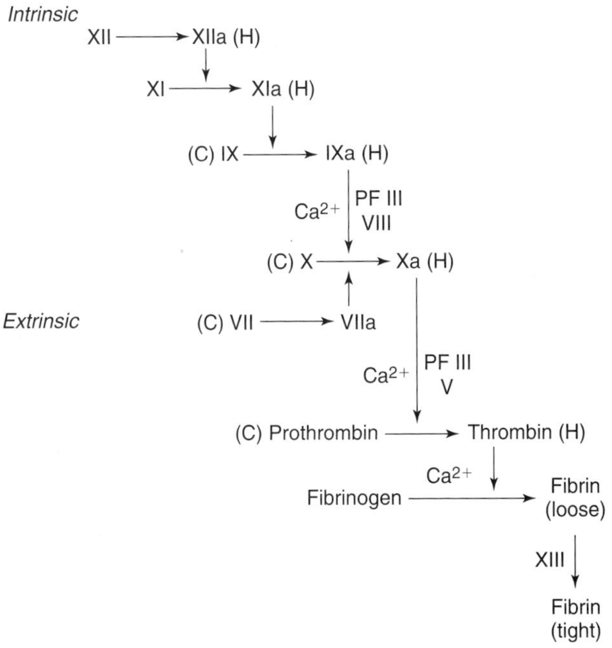

FIGURE 25.2 Soluble clotting cascade.

molecular-weight kininogen (HMWK) and prekalllikrein (PK), which binds to vascular subendothelial collagen. This results in the activation of factor XII. Factor XIIa then stimulates the conversion of factor XI to factor XIa. Factor XIa stimulates the conversion of factor IX to factor IXa. Factor IXa, in the presence of calcium, phospholipids, and factor VIII, stimulates the conversion of factor X to factor Xa. Factor Xa, in the presence of calcium, phospholipids, and factor V, stimulates the conversion of factor II (prothrombin) to factor IIa (thrombin).[15-17]

The extrinsic pathway is initiated when tissue factor, a membrane-bound protein that is exposed during endothelial injury, forms a complex with factor VIIa. This complex then stimulates the conversion of factor IX to factor IXa and factor X to factor Xa. Factor Xa then stimulates the conversion of factor II (prothrombin) to factor IIa (thrombin). Factor X thus occupies a central position at the junction of the extrinsic and intrinsic systems; the pathway at this point becomes the common pathway.[15-17]

Thrombin (factor IIa), which is generated by both pathways, stimulates the conversion of fibrinogen to fibrin in the presence of ionized calcium. The initial soluble fibrin clot is further converted to an insoluble fibrin polymer when factor XIII is converted to factor XIIIa by thrombin (factor IIa). Thrombin (factor IIa) also stimulates platelet aggregation and potentiates the activity of factors V, VIIa, VII, and Xa.[15-17]

Several natural anticoagulant systems regulate the activity of the clotting cascade. Antithrombin III neutralizes thrombin (factor IIa), factor Xa, and factor IXa. Protein C is activated when thrombin (factor IIa) binds to thrombomodulin (TM) on the surface of intact endothelial cells. With the aid of protein S, activated protein C (APC) then inhibits factors Va and VIIIa in the coagulation cascade. Tissue factor pathway inhibitor (TFPI) inhibits the activity of the tissue factor/factor VIIa complex in the coagulation cascade. The fibrinolytic system is activated upon formation of a soluble fibrin clot. When a clot is formed, tissue plasminogen activator (TPA) diffuses from endothelial cells and converts plasminogen to plasmin. Plasmin then degrades fibrin into soluble fibrin degradation products (Fig. 25.3).[15-17]

CLINICAL PRESENTATION AND DIAGNOSIS

DVT commonly originates in the deep venous sinuses of the calf muscles, but it can also form in the proximal veins

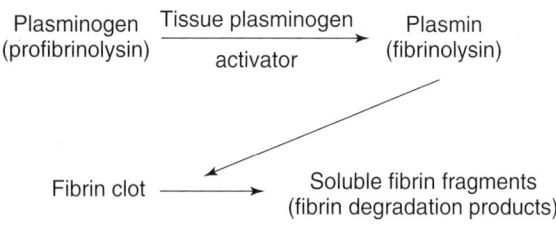

FIGURE 25.3 Fibrinolysis.

secondary to trauma or surgery. Symptoms of DVT result from venous outflow obstruction and inflammation of the vessel wall.[5]

SIGNS AND SYMPTOMS

Patients who experience VTE often manifest few specific symptoms, thereby making clinical diagnosis insensitive and unreliable.[18] Less than one third of patients with DVT who exhibit lower extremity symptoms present with the classic syndrome of calf pain/tenderness, lower extremity swelling, venous distention, and Homan's sign. Homan's sign is dorsiflexion of the foot that is associated with pain or incomplete dorsiflexion or flexion of the knee to prevent pain.[3,19,20]

The most common symptom of PE is dyspnea, and the most common sign is tachypnea.[21] Other frequent symptoms include sinus tachycardia and pleuritic pain. These symptoms are often inconsistent among patients and are nonspecific for the diagnosis of PE.[21,22] Syncope, cyanosis, cough, and hemoptysis may be present in some patients.[23]

DIAGNOSIS AND CLINICAL FINDINGS

For DVT to be accurately diagnosed, objective tests must be performed. Compression ultrasonography is the diagnostic test of choice when DVT is suspected. An ultrasound is considered positive for DVT when a proximal vein fails to flatten when compressed with an ultrasound probe. Historically, venography was considered the gold standard test in diagnosing DVT; however, its use has decreased secondary to its cost, invasiveness, technical demands, and risks (allergic reactions, renal dysfunction).[5]

Accurately diagnosing PE also requires objective testing; however, no single noninvasive diagnostic test is sufficiently sensitive or specific for the diagnosis in all patients.[22,24] Although pulmonary angiography is the gold standard test for diagnosing PE, it is reserved for those patients whose diagnosis cannot be established by less invasive tests. This is because of its cost, invasiveness, and associated risks. Specific diagnostic tests should be selected on the basis of the clinical probability of PE, according to the presence of specific risk factors (Table 25.2). For patients with a low probability of PE, a highly sensitive, standardized D-dimer assay may be used to rule out the diagnosis of PE. If the D-dimer result is positive, a helical computed tomography (CT) scan or ventilation-perfusion (VP) scan should be ordered to confirm the diagnosis. For patients with an intermediate probability of PE, CT or VP scanning is an appropriate initial test. If the CT scan is negative or VP scan indicates a low, intermediate, or high probability of PE, duplex ultrasonography (DUS) of the lower extremities should be performed. If the DUS is negative, pulmonary angiography should be performed for a definitive diagnosis. For patients with a high probability of PE, CT or VP scanning is the appropriate initial test. It the CT scan is negative or the VP scan indicates a low or intermediate probability of PE, then DUS should be performed. If DUS is negative, pulmonary angiography should be performed for a definitive diagnosis.[22,24]

TABLE 25.2	Criteria for Predicting the Probability of Embolism

Risk Factor	Number of Points
Clinical signs/symptoms of DVT	3
Alternative diagnosis less likely than PE	3
Heart rate >100 beats per minute	1.5
Immobilization or surgery in previous 4 weeks	1.5
Previous DVT or PE	1.5
Hemoptysis	1.0
Cancer (currently receiving treatment, treated in past 6 months, palliative care)	1.0

Clinical Probability	Score
Low	<2.0
Intermediate	2.0–6.0
High	>6.0

DVT, deep vein thrombosis; PE, pulmonary embolism.
(Adapted from Fedullo PF, Tapson VF. The evaluation of suspected pulmonary embolism. N Engl J Med 349:1247–1256, 2003; Wells PS, Anderson DR, Rodger M, et al. Derivation of a simple clinical model to categorize patients' probability of pulmonary embolism: increasing the model's utility with the SimpliRED D-dimer. Thromb Haemost 83:416–420, 2000.)

PSYCHOSOCIAL FACTORS

Many psychosocial factors can influence patient attitudes toward an understanding of anticoagulation therapy. These include educational levels, native language, literacy skills, cognitive function, diverse backgrounds, life experiences, family, employment, perceptions of their health status, and society. All of these issues must be addressed to enhance patient comprehension and improve outcomes.[25] Specific educational recommendations are discussed later in this chapter.

THERAPEUTIC PLAN

Patients diagnosed with VTE should be treated with anticoagulants as soon as possible. Patients diagnosed with DVT may be treated initially with body weight–adjusted low-molecular-weight heparin (LMWH), intravenous unfractionated heparin (UH), or subcutaneous UH with monitoring and subsequent dose adjustments. Therapy with warfarin should be initiated concurrently. Therapy with LMWH or UH should be continued until the patient's international normalized ratio (INR) is stable and greater than 2.0. Patients diagnosed with nonmassive PE may be treated initially with body weight–adjusted LMWH or intravenous UH. Therapy with

warfarin should be initiated concurrently. Therapy with LMWH or UH should be continued concurrently with warfarin for 4 to 5 days, until the patient's INR is stable and greater than 2.0. The target INR range for patients with VTE is 2 to 3. Duration of therapy with warfarin in the treatment of VTE depends upon several factors (Table 25.3). Patients with DVT should wear an elastic compression stocking to prevent PTS and should be encouraged to ambulate as tolerated. Systemic thrombolytic therapy should be reserved for those patients with massive ileofemoral DVT who are at risk for limb gangrene, and for patients with PE who are hemodynamically unstable. Catheter-directed thrombolysis should be reserved for patients with DVT who require limb salvage. Catheter extraction and pulmonary embolectomy should be reserved for patients with PE who are hemodynamically unstable and unable to receive thrombolytic therapy. An inferior vena cava filter should be placed in patients with VTE who have a contraindication for anticoagulant therapy, a complication of anticoagulant therapy, or recurrent VTE despite anticoagulant therapy.[2] Guidelines for the management of antithrombotic and thrombolytic therapy are published by the American College of Chest Physicians (ACCP) and are available at http://www.chestjournal.org/content/vol126/3_suppl/.[26]

TABLE 25.3	Duration of Therapy for Venous Thromboembolism

Indication for Therapy	Duration of Anticoagulation Therapy
First episode DVT with transient risk factor	3 months
First episode of idiopathic DVT	6–12 months; consider indefinite therapy
DVT and cancer	LMWH for 3–6 months; then warfarin until cancer has been resolved, or indefinitely
First episode DVT with antiphospholipid antibodies or two or more hypercoagulable states	12 months; consider indefinite therapy
First episode DVT with documented AT, protein C, or protein S deficiency; factor V Leiden or prothrombin gene mutation; homocystinemia; or high factor VIII levels	6–12 months; consider indefinite therapy
Two or more episodes of DVT	Indefinite

DVT, deep vein thrombosis; LMWH, low-molecular-weight heparin; AT, antithrombin.
(Adapted from Buller HR, Agnelli G, Hull RD, et al. Antithrombotic therapy for venous thromboembolic disease. Chest 126:401S–428S, 2004.)

TREATMENT

PHARMACOTHERAPY

Unfractionated Heparin. Heparin, a rapid-acting anticoagulant, exerts its antithrombotic effect by accelerating the action of antithrombin (formerly antithrombin III), a naturally occurring inhibitor of thrombin (factor IIa). Antithrombin (AT) inhibits activated clotting factors (Xa, IXa, XIa, XIIa) that have a reactive serine residue at their enzymatically active centers. Heparin, by binding at the lysine group of AT (Fig. 25.4), induces a conformational change in AT that allows increased access of the arginine residue to the serine group on the activated clotting factors.[27–29] Commercial heparin is obtained from hog mucosa or bovine lung. UH is a heterogeneous mixture of molecules with an average molecular weight of 12,000 to 15,000 daltons. Heparin must be administered parenterally and is effective following intravenous and subcutaneous administration. It should never be administered intramuscularly because of the risk of hematoma formation.

Standard UH is bound to a number of plasma proteins following administration. This binding leads to variation in patient response to heparin, and to heparin resistance. Heparin resistance occurs when a patient requires greater than 40,000 units of heparin in a 24-hour period to achieve a therapeutic activated partial thromboplastin time (aPTT). In these patients, heparin therapy should be adjusted to maintain anti-factor Xa heparin concentrations of 0.4 to 0.7 IU per mL. Heparin is metabolized primarily in the liver and reticuloendothelial system and is partly eliminated by excretion into the urine. The half-life of the anticoagulant effect of heparin in normal patients and in those with VTE, as measured by changes in the aPTT, is approximately 1.5 hours. The half-life, when plasma heparin activity is measured, depends on the dose and increases with an increased dose. Limited studies show that patients with PE have greater heparin clearance and a shorter half-life than do those with DVT. This may be the result of continuing thrombin formation on the surface of the embolus, leading to an increased rate of heparin clearance.[30–32]

Therapeutic Indications. Heparin is indicated for the prevention and treatment of VTE.[2,33] It is also indicated for use in early treatment of patients with unstable angina or acute myocardial infarction, during cardiac bypass surgery and vascular surgery, during and after coronary angioplasty, in patients with coronary stents, and in selected patients with disseminated intravascular coagulation.[32,34] These indications are discussed in detail in other chapters in this text.

Dosing and Administration. The starting dose of intravenous UH for the treatment of VTE is a bolus of 80 units per kg, followed by an infusion of 18 units/kg/hour. The dose should thereafter be adjusted to achieve and maintain a prolongation of the aPTT that corresponds to plasma heparin levels from 0.3 to 0.7 IU per mL anti-Xa activity by the amidolytic assay.[2,32] Heparin may also be given subcutaneously to treat patients with VTE. The initial bolus dose of 5,000 units is given intravenously and is followed by 17,500 units subcutaneously twice daily. The dose should thereafter be adjusted to achieve and maintain a prolongation of the aPTT that corresponds to plasma heparin levels from 0.3 to 0.7 IU per mL anti-Xa activity by the amidolytic assay.[2] Warfarin therapy should be initiated along with heparin therapy. Heparin therapy may be discontinued after 4 to 5 days, when the INR is stable and greater than 2.0. Heparin may also be used for the prevention of VTE in specific patient populations (Table 25.4).

Laboratory Assessment. Before the initiation of heparin, baseline clotting studies must be performed, including prothrombin time (PT), aPTT, platelet count, hemoglobin, and hematocrit. The aPTT is the standard test used to monitor heparin therapy. The aPTT is primarily a measure of the competence of the intrinsic and common clotting pathways. The aPTT is sensitive to the inhibitory effects of heparin on thrombin, factor Xa, and factor IXa. The aPTT is performed with platelet-poor plasma and so does not reflect the activity of platelets. Normal values for the aPTT are between 24 and 36 seconds. Historically, an aPTT of 1.5 to 2.5 times control was considered to be the therapeutic range for heparin; however, because of the numerous laboratory methods used to determine the aPTT, wide variation in the aPTT has been observed between different laboratories. The American College of Chest Physicians recommends that the aPTT therapeutic range be standardized for each laboratory by determining the aPTT values that correspond with therapeutic heparin levels. Therapeutic heparin levels are equivalent to 0.3 to 0.7 IU per mL anti-Xa activity by the amidolytic assay. The aPTT should be measured 6 hours after the first dose, and subsequent doses should be adjusted accordingly. An

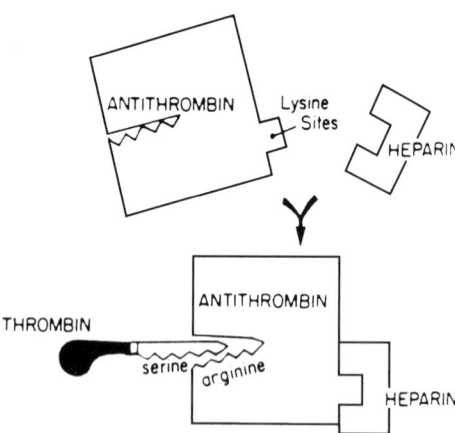

FIGURE 25.4 Model of heparin-induced confirmation change in antithrombin, resulting in rapid inhibition of thrombin. (Reprinted with permission from Rosenberg RD. Actions and interactions of antithrombin and heparin. N Engl J Med 292:146, 1975.)

TABLE 25.4	Prophylaxis of Venous Thromboembolism in Specific Patient Populations
Patient Type	**Recommendation**
General Surgery	
Low risk (minor surgery, <40 years of age, no additional risk factors for VTE[a])	Early and persistent ambulation
Moderate risk (minor surgery in patients with additional VTE risk factors; or surgery in patients aged 40–60 years without additional VTE risk factors)	LDUH 5,000 units SQ BID, or LMWH
High risk (patients >60 years of age; or patients age 40–60 years with additional VTE risk factors)	LDUH 5,000 units SQ TID, or LMWH
Highest risk (surgery in patients with multiple VTE risk factors, or hip or knee arthroplasty, hip replacement surgery; or major trauma or spinal cord injury)	Same as higher risk, combined with GCS and/or IPC
High risk of bleeding	GCS or IPC until bleeding risk decreases
Selected high risk (major CA surgery)	Discharge prophylaxis with LMWH
Vascular Surgery	
No additional VTE risk factors	No prophylaxis
Major procedures with additional VTE risk factors	LDUH or LMWH
Gynecologic Surgery	
Procedures ≤30 minutes for benign disease	Early and persistent ambulation
Laparoscopic procedures with additional VTE risk factors	One or more of LDUH, LMWH, IPC, or GCS
Major gynecologic surgery for benign disease; no additional VTE risk factors	LDUH 5,000 units SQ BID, or LMWH or IPC, until patient is ambulatory
Major gynecologic surgery for malignancy, with additional VTE risk factors	LDUH 5,000 units SQ TID, or LMWH or IPC alone until discharge, or IPC or GCS with LDUH or LMWH
Major gynecologic surgery for malignancy, age >60 years, previous VTE	Continue prophylaxis for 2–4 weeks after hospital discharge
Urologic Surgery	
Transurethral or low-risk procedures	Early and persistent ambulation
Major open procedures	LDUH 5,000 units BID or TID, or IPC and/or GCS
Actively bleeding or high risk of bleeding	GCS and/or IPC until bleeding risk decreases
Multiple VTE risk factors	LDUH or LMWH combined with GCS and/or IPC
Laparoscopic Surgery	
No additional VTE risk factors	Early and persistent ambulation
Additional VTE risk factors	One or more of LDUH, LMWH, GCS, or IPC
Orthopaedic Surgery	
Elective hip arthroplasty	LMWH started 12 hours before surgery or 12 to 24 hours after surgery; or fondaparinux 2.5 mg started 6 to 8 hours after surgery; or adjusted-dose warfarin started preoperatively or the evening after surgery. Target INR range 2–3. Give for at least 10 days; extended prophylaxis for 28–35 days recommended
Elective knee arthroplasty	LMWH, fondaparinux, or adjusted-dose warfarin at target INR range 2–3; or IPC alone. Give prophylaxis for at least 10 days
Knee arthroscopy	If no additional risk factors, early and persistent ambulation; if additional risk factors present, or prolonged, complicated procedure, use LMWH
Hip fracture surgery	Fondaparinux, LMWH, adjusted-dose warfarin at INR target 2–3, or LDUH. If surgery is delayed, use LMWH or LDUH from time of admission until time of surgery. If high risk of bleeding, use GCS and/or IPC instead of anticoagulation. Give for at least 10 days; extended prophylaxis for 28–35 days is recommended

(continued)

TABLE 25.4	continued	
Patient Type	**Recommendation**	
Elective Spine Surgery		
No additional VTE risk factors	Early and persistent ambulation	
Additional VTE risk factors (advanced age, known malignancy, neurologic deficit, previous VTE, anterior surgical approach)	Postoperative LDUH or LMWH alone; or perioperative IPC alone; or perioperative GCS alone; or perioperative GCS and IPC; in patients with multiple risk factors, LDUH or LMWH with GCS and/or IPC	
Isolated Lower Extremity Injuries	No routine prophylaxis recommended	
Neurosurgery		
Intracranial	IPC with or without GCS; or LDUH or LMWH	
High-risk patients	LDUH or LMWH with GCS and/or IPC	
Trauma		
All patients with one VTE risk factor	LMWH as soon as possible; IPC and/or GCS alone if high bleeding risk or LMWH delayed; continue prophylaxis until completely mobile (may use LMWH or adjusted-dose warfarin, target INR range 2–3)	
Acute Spinal Cord Injury	LMWH alone; or LMWH and IPC; or LDUH and IPC; if high risk for bleeding, IPC and/or GCS; continue LMWH or convert to adjusted-dose warfarin; target INR range 2–3 during rehabilitation	
Burns	Patients with additional risk factors—LMWH or LDUH as soon as possible	
Medical Conditions		
Acutely ill medical patients (CHF, respiratory disease)	LDUH or LMWH	
Confined to bed with one or more additional VTE risk factors	LDUH or LMWH	
Additional VTE risk factors and contraindication to anticoagulation	IPC or GCS	
Cancer		
Patients with long-term indwelling central venous catheters	No routine prophylaxis; do not use LMWH or fixed-dose warfarin	
Critical Care		
Moderate risk (medically ill, postoperative)	LDUH or LMWH	
High risk (major trauma, orthopaedic surgery)	LMWH	
High risk for bleeding	GCS and/or IPC until bleeding risk decreases	
Long Distance Travel		
Flights >6-hour duration	Avoid constrictive clothing around lower extremities or waist; avoid dehydration; frequent calf muscle stretching	
Patients with additional VTE risk factors	GCS providing 15–30 mm Hg pressure at the ankle; or single LMWH prophylactic dose injected before departure; aspirin not recommended	

[a] VTE risk factors: cancer, previous VTE, hypercoagulable states, age >40 years.
CHF, congestive heart failure; LDUH, low-dose unfractionated heparin; LMWH, low-molecular-weight heparin; GCS, graduated compression stockings; IPC, intermittent pneumatic compression; CA, cancer; INR, international normalized ratio; VTE, venous thromboembolism.
(Adapted from Geerts WH, Pineo GF, Heit JA, et al. Prevention of venous thromboembolism. Chest 126:338S–400S, 2004.)

example of a weight-based dosing nomogram is shown in Table 25.5.[2,32,35,36]

Adverse Reactions. The major adverse effect of heparin therapy is bleeding. The risk of bleeding increases with dose, concomitant thrombolytic therapy, recent surgery, trauma, invasive procedures, and concomitant hemostatic defects.[37] Other adverse effects include osteopenia and thrombocytopenia.[32] Osteopenia is due to the binding of heparin to osteoblasts, which then release factors that activate osteoclasts.[32] Reductions in bone density may occur in up to 30% of patients, and vertebral fractures occur in 2% to 3% of patients

TABLE 25.5	Body Weight–Based Dosing of Intravenous Heparin
aPTT	**Heparin Dose**
Initial dose	80 units/kg bolus, then 18 units/kg/hour
<35 seconds	80 units/kg bolus, then increase by 4 units/kg/hour
35–45 seconds	40 units/kg bolus, then increase by 2 units/kg/hour
46–70 seconds	No change
71–90 seconds	Decrease infusion rate by 2 units/kg/hour
>90 seconds	Hold infusion 1 hour, then decrease infusion rate by 3 units/kg/hour

(Adapted from Raschke RA, Gollihare B, Peirce JC. The effectiveness of implementing the weight-based heparin nomogram as a practice guideline. Arch Intern Med 156:1645–1649, 1996; Ansell J, Hirsh J, Poller L, et al. The pharmacology and management of the vitamin K antagonists. Chest 126:204S–233S, 2004.)

who take heparin for 1 month or longer.[37] Heparin-induced thrombocytopenia (HIT) is caused by an antibody to the heparin–platelet factor 4 complex. This antibody is produced by activated platelets. The frequency of HIT varies from 1% to 3%. It typically occurs 4 to 10 days after the initiation of heparin therapy in patients with no previous exposure to heparin; however, it may occur sooner (within hours of exposure) in patients with previous exposure to heparin. HIT is characterized by a 30% to 50% decrease in platelets from baseline, a platelet count of $50 \times 10^3/mm^3$ or less in patients with or without new VTE, and/or the development of new VTE in the presence of UH or LMWH. Management of HIT includes discontinuation of heparin, alternative anticoagulant therapy with lepirudin or argatroban, avoidance of primary anticoagulation with warfarin, and avoidance of platelet transfusions.[38]

Drug Interactions. A direct interaction between heparin and nitroglycerin has been proposed as a mechanism for increasing heparin requirements in some patients who receive both drugs concomitantly. This has not been a universal observation, however, and a controlled trial provides evidence that there is no interference with nitroglycerin at doses below 350 μg per minute. At doses of nitroglycerin greater than 350 μg per minute, a higher dose of heparin was required to achieve the same prolongation of the aPTT. The proposed mechanism is due to a qualitative antithrombin abnormality induced by nitroglycerin. Close patient monitoring is required, and resistance can usually be overcome with appropriate dose adjustments.[39] Heparin is physically incompatible with many other drugs, and appropriate sources should be consulted before heparin is mixed with other solutions. The concomitant administration of heparin and other antico-

agulant or antiplatelet agents must be done with caution to avoid bleeding complications.

Treatment of Patients Who Overdose. Protamine sulfate, a basic protein derived from fish sperm, combines with and inactivates heparin. If administered immediately after an intravenous bolus of heparin, 1 mg of protamine will neutralize approximately 100 units of heparin. For patients who receive a continuous infusion of heparin, only heparin received during the preceding few hours should be included in the dose calculation. Patients who have received heparin subcutaneously may require a prolonged infusion of protamine. The aPTT should be used to assess the effectiveness of protamine therapy. Protamine should be infused slowly over 1 to 3 minutes (maximum 50 mg in 10 minutes) to avoid hypotension and bradycardia. Patients with allergies to fish or previous exposure to protamine-containing insulin products may be at high risk for allergic reactions. These patients may be pretreated with antihistamines and corticosteroids.[32,40]

Low-Molecular-Weight Heparin. The LMWHs are glycosaminoglycans that are about one-third the molecular weight of UH. The average molecular weight is 4,000 to 5,000 daltons. Similar to UH, the LMWHs bind to AT, enhancing its activity against activated clotting factors, especially factor Xa. LMWHs have less affinity than UH for thrombin (factor IIa), plasma proteins, macrophages, endothelial cells, platelets, and osteoblasts. This characteristic gives LMWHs a more predictable anticoagulant response, making routine monitoring of the anticoagulant effect unnecessary. It also increases their plasma half-life and reduces the incidences of HIT and osteopenia when compared with UH.[32] The bioavailability of LMWHs approaches 100% after subcutaneous administration. The LMWHs are eliminated renally and have a half-life that ranges from 3 to 7 hours.[32]

Therapeutic Indications. Enoxaparin, dalteparin, and tinzaparin are the three LMWHs that are available in the United States. Enoxaparin and dalteparin are indicated for the prevention of VTE in patients undergoing abdominal surgery or hip replacement surgery, in medical patients at risk for VTE because of prolonged immobility, and for the prevention of ischemic complications due to unstable angina or non–Q-wave myocardial infarction in conjunction with aspirin therapy. Other indications for enoxaparin include the inpatient treatment of DVT with or without PE in conjunction with warfarin, the outpatient treatment of DVT without PE in conjunction with warfarin, and the prevention of VTE in patients undergoing knee replacement surgery.[41,42] Tinzaparin is indicated in the treatment of patients with DVT with or without PE in conjunction with warfarin.[43]

Dosing and Administration. LMWHs are administered subcutaneously every 12 to 24 hours, depending upon the indication for therapy. Table 25.4 lists indications and dosages for UH and LMWHs for the prevention of VTE. For the inpatient treatment of patients with acute DVT with or without PE, the dose of enoxaparin is 1 mg per kg of body weight given subcutaneously every 12 hours, or 1.5 mg per kg of body weight given subcutaneously every 24 hours. For the outpatient management of DVT without PE, the enoxaparin dose is 1 mg per kg of body weight given subcutaneously every 12 hours. The dose of tinzaparin for the treatment of DVT with or without PE is 175 anti-Xa units per kg of body weight given subcutaneously once daily. Warfarin therapy should be initiated concurrently and LMWHs should be continued for 4 to 5 days, until the INR is stable and greater than 2.0.[41–43]

Few data are available regarding the use of LMWHs in patients with a total body weight greater than 150 kg and a body mass index greater than 50 kg/m^2. The ACCP guidelines suggest anti-factor Xa testing in these patients with subsequent dose reduction if anti-factor Xa levels are elevated.[32] Clearance of the anti-factor Xa effect of LMWHs correlates strongly with creatinine clearance (CrCl).[32] Anti-factor Xa activity is prolonged in patients with renal dysfunction, which may predispose them to bleeding complications. The effect of renal dysfunction on clearance of the anti-factor Xa effect may also differ among LMWH preparations. There is no exact threshold for CrCl in terms of renal dysfunction; however, the ACCP guidelines suggest IV UH for anticoagulation therapy when CrCl is less than 30 mL per minute. If LMWH is used, anti-factor Xa activity should be monitored with subsequent dose adjustments made if anti-factor Xa levels are elevated.[32,44]

Laboratory Assessment. The aPTT and PT are not altered by the LMWHs. Anti-factor Xa activity may be monitored by a chromogenic assay; however, the predictable dose response of LMWHs negates the need for regular anti-factor Xa activity monitoring. Anti-factor Xa monitoring should be considered in patients with a total body weight greater than 150 kg and in patients with a CrCl of less than 30 mL per minute. The anti-factor Xa assay should be performed 4 hours after a subcutaneous dose of LMWH is administered. For twice-daily administration of LMWHs in the treatment of established VTE, the anti-factor Xa therapeutic range is 0.6 to 1.0 IU per mL. The therapeutic range for once-daily administration of LMWHs in the treatment of established VTE is estimated to be between 1.0 and 2.0 IU per mL. No therapeutic range has been established for LMWHs when used in prophylactic doses for the prevention of VTE.[2,32]

Adverse Reactions. Similar to UH, LMWHs may cause bleeding, HIT, and osteoporosis. However, the incidences of HIT and osteoporosis are lower with LMWHs because of less binding to plasma proteins.[32,45]

Drug Interactions. Similar to UH, the concomitant administration of LMWH and other anticoagulant or antiplatelet agents must be done with caution to avoid bleeding complications.

Treatment of Overdose. Currently, no proven method has been found for neutralizing the antithrombotic effects of LMWH.[32] Protamine neutralizes only 60% of the anti-factor Xa activity of LMWH.[32,46,47] ACCP guidelines recommend administration of protamine when LMWHs have been administered in the past 8 hours and reversal of the anticoagulant effect is required due to bleeding.[32] The recommended dose is 1 mg per 100 anti-factor Xa units of LMWH (1 mg of enoxaparin equals 100 anti-factor Xa units). A second dose of 0.5 mg of protamine per 100 anti-factor Xa units may be administered if necessary. Smaller doses of protamine may be used if the LMWH dose was administered more than 8 hours before the bleeding event.

Warfarin. Warfarin exerts its pharmacologic effect by interfering with the synthesis of the vitamin K-dependent clotting factors in the liver (factors II, VII, IX, and X). These clotting factors must undergo carboxylation to be converted into their active forms (IIa, VIIa, IXa, Xa). For carboxylation to occur, vitamin K undergoes cyclic interconversion to its epoxide form. Warfarin inhibits this interconversion of vitamin K, which then inhibits carboxylation, leading to production of inactivated clotting factors. Warfarin's effects can be overcome by the administration of vitamin K.[48,49]

Warfarin is the most commonly used coumarin. Among the coumarins, its pharmacokinetics have been the most extensively studied.[50] Warfarin is completely absorbed in the upper gastrointestinal tract, with peak blood levels occurring in 60 to 120 minutes. The volume of distribution of warfarin is 12.5% of body weight. The half-life of warfarin is independent of dose and ranges from 36 to 42 hours. Warfarin is 99.5% bound to albumin. Warfarin is metabolized in the hepatic microsomes by mixed-function oxidase enzymes. Warfarin is a racemic mixture of the two optically active isomers, R and S. The S isomer is approximately five times more potent than the R isomer. The half-life of the R isomer is 45 hours, and the half-life of the S isomer is 33 hours. It has been theorized that differences in permeability or affinity to the receptor site account for the differing potencies of the two isomers. Knowledge of these two isomers is important because drugs may stereoselectively interact with warfarin. For example, metronidazole inhibits the metabolism of the S isomer but has no effect on the R isomer.[51]

The response to a dose of warfarin may be modified by genetic and environmental factors. These factors may influence its absorption, pharmacokinetics, and pharmacodynamics.[52] Warfarin also inhibits the carboxylation of the vitamin K-dependent natural anticoagulants proteins C and S. This leads to decreased levels of proteins C and S, which induces a hypercoagulable state. Therefore, in patients with hereditary protein C and/or S deficiency, heparin therapy should be initiated with low-dose warfarin therapy to protect against this transient hypercoagulable state.[52]

Therapeutic Indications. Warfarin is effective in the primary and secondary prevention of venous thromboembolism, and in the prevention of systemic embolism in patients with artificial heart valves or atrial fibrillation. It is effective for the primary prevention of acute myocardial infarction in high-risk men, and for the prevention of stroke, recurrent infarction, or death in patients with acute myocardial infarction.[52]

Dosing and Administration. ACCP guidelines recommend an initial warfarin dose of 5 to 10 mg for the first 1 to 2 days for most patients. Loading doses are not recommended. Patients who are elderly, debilitated, malnourished, or have congestive heart failure or liver disease should be given an initial dose of less than 5 mg. Subsequent dose changes should be made on the basis of response of the INR.[52]

The onset of warfarin's effect depends not only upon its half-life, but also on the half-lives of the vitamin K–dependent clotting factors (II, VII, IX, and X). The half-life of factor VII is 6 hours. The half-lives of factors IX and X are 24 and 36 hours, respectively. The half-life of factor II is 60 to 72 hours.[52–54] Factor VII is responsible for the initial anticoagulant effect of warfarin and the subsequent rise of the INR. The antithrombotic response of warfarin is secondary to reduction of factor II, which takes about 3 to 4 days. Thus, heparin should be initiated with warfarin when a rapid antithrombotic response is needed. It should be continued for 4 to 5 days, until the INR is between 2 and 3 for at least 2 consecutive days.[52]

Optimal treatment duration with warfarin for VTE depends upon several factors, including risk of recurrent VTE, risk of bleeding during warfarin therapy, and number of episodes of previous VTE. Table 25.3 lists suggested treatment durations for VTE.[2]

Laboratory Monitoring. PT is the test that is used to monitor warfarin therapy. The PT reflects decreases in levels of factors II, VII, and X. A normal PT is approximately 11 seconds. Because of the variability in sensitivity of the thromboplastin reagent that is used in determination of PT, results from different laboratories may differ. The ratio of the patient's PT to the laboratory control PT will subsequently differ among laboratories. To standardize interpretation of the intensity of anticoagulation, the INR measurement was adopted in 1982.[55] A World Health Organization primary international reference preparation of thromboplastin is used to standardize the commercial source of thromboplastin that is used by a given laboratory. The INR is calculated by raising the calculated PT ratio (PT of the patient/PT control from the laboratory) to the power of the international sensitivity index (ISI) that is assigned to each batch of thromboplastin. For example, patient PT of 22 seconds and control PT of 11 seconds equals a PT ratio of 2; when raised to an ISI of 2, this equals an INR of 4 (i.e., 22/11 raised to the power of 2 = 4). Although several potential problems remain with measurement of the INR, overall, it allows for standardization of reporting.[52] Table 25.6 lists potential causes of erroneous INR measurements.[52] For hospitalized patients, the INR should be measured daily until the INR is within therapeutic range for 2 consecutive days. The INR may then be monitored two to three times per week for 1 or 2 weeks, depending on the stability of the INR. For outpa-

tients who begin warfarin therapy, the INR may be monitored every few days until stable. When the INR is stable, it should be monitored once every 4 weeks.[52] The INR should be monitored more frequently when dosing changes, dietary changes, or illnesses occur.

Determinants of Anticoagulant Response. Both genetic and environmental factors may alter the response to warfarin (Table 25.7). Genetic factors include a mutation in the cytochrome P-450 2C9 hepatic microsomal enzyme responsible for the metabolism of the S-isomer of warfarin, hereditary resistance to warfarin, and a mutation in factor IX, leading to a marked reduction in factor IX activity during warfarin therapy without an excessive prolongation of the INR.[52] Patients with one or more of the cytochrome P-450 2C9 muta-

TABLE 25.6	Potential Causes of Erroneous International Normalized Ratio Measurements
Sampling and blood collection problems	Instrument effects on INR at laboratory site
Incorrect normal PT value (nonuse of mean normal PT value)	Lupus anticoagulant effects on thromboplastin reagents
Unreliable ISI result from manufacturer of thromboplastin	Unreliable INR when measured at the onset of warfarin therapy or in patients with liver disease
Drift of ISI since original calibration	Unreliability of INR when >4.5 because these values are excluded from ISI calibrations

INR, international normalized ratio; PT, prothrombin time; ISI, International Sensitivity Index.
(Adapted from Ansell J, Hirsh J, Poller L, et al. The pharmacology and management of the vitamin K antagonists. Chest 126:204S–233S, 2004.)

TABLE 25.7	Factors That Alter Warfarin Response
Genetic Factors	Cytochrome P–450 2C9 polymorphism
	Hereditary warfarin resistance
	Factor IX propeptide mutation
Environmental Factors	Drugs (see Table 44.8)
	Diet (vitamin K–containing foods, enteral feeds, nutritional supplements)
	Diseases (gastrointestinal illnesses, CHF, hyperthyroidism/hypothyroidism, liver disease, fever)

CHF, congestive heart failure.
(Adapted from Ansell J, Hirsh J, Poller L, et al. The pharmacology and management of the vitamin K antagonists. Chest 126:204S–233S, 2004.)

tions have reduced warfarin requirements. These mutations have been associated with an increase in adverse outcomes.[56,57] Warfarin resistance is due to an altered affinity of the warfarin receptor. This leads to an increase in the amount of warfarin required to produce an anticoagulant effect.[52,58] The mutation in factor IX occurs in less than 1.5% of the population and has been associated with an increased risk of bleeding during warfarin therapy.[52,59,60]

Environmental factors that may alter the response to warfarin include diet, drugs, and various diseases.[52] Excessive intake of vitamin K–rich foods antagonizes the anticoagulant effect of warfarin, resulting in a decreased INR. Commonly consumed foods that contain vitamin K are spinach, cabbage, lettuce, broccoli, greens (turnip, mustard, collard), and mayonnaise. Reference 61 provides an extensive review of the vitamin K content of various foods. Liquid nutritional supplements, enteral nutrition formulas, and multivitamins are other potential dietary sources of vitamin K; however, their vitamin K content typically is low and may not be clinically significant. Conversely, poor nutrition may lead to an overall decrease in the intake of dietary vitamin K. This potentiates the anticoagulant effect of warfarin, resulting in an increased INR. Decreased dietary intake of vitamin K may result from recent illness (particularly gastrointestinal illnesses), antibiotic exposure, or chronic fat malabsorption.[52] Patients should be counseled on the importance of eating a consistent quantity of vitamin K–rich foods to avoid fluctuations in the INR. Drug interactions with warfarin are discussed in a subsequent section of this chapter. Disease states may also alter the anticoagulant effect of warfarin. Because vitamin K–dependent clotting factors are synthesized in the liver, any disruption of normal liver function may lead to an increased PT in the absence of warfarin therapy.[52] Hypermetabolic states such as fever or hyperthyroidism increase the catabolism of vitamin K–dependent clotting factors. This potentiates the anticoagulant effect of warfarin. Conversely, hypothyroidism decreases the catabolism of vitamin K–dependent clotting factors, thereby inhibiting the anticoagulant effect of warfarin.[62,63] Patients who experience congestive heart failure exacerbations may exhibit an exaggerated response to warfarin caused by plasma volume expansion and liver congestion.[64]

Adverse Reactions. Hemorrhage is the most common adverse effect of warfarin therapy. Estimates of the annual incidence of major hemorrhage (intracranial, retroperitoneal, requiring hospitalization and/or transfusion) during warfarin therapy vary according to patient populations, INR target ranges, patient characteristics, concomitant disease states, and concomitant drug therapy.[65] In five randomized trials in patients with atrial fibrillation, the annual incidence of bleeding was 1.3% for patients taking warfarin versus 1% for those taking placebo.[66] The risk of bleeding during warfarin therapy increases significantly when the INR is greater than 4.0 to 5.0. Patient characteristics associated with bleeding include increasing age, history of bleeding, hypertension,

cerebrovascular disease, ischemic stroke, serious heart disease, and renal insufficiency.[65] The concomitant use of aspirin and warfarin has been associated with an increased risk of bleeding; however, concomitant use is indicated in certain patient populations. These patients should be monitored closely for signs and symptoms of bleeding. Nonsteroidal anti-inflammatory agents (NSAIDs) have been shown to increase the risk of bleeding during warfarin therapy in some studies; however, these studies were not well-designed. Patients who use NSAIDs and warfarin should continue to be monitored for signs and symptoms of bleeding.[65] Any drug that potentiates the anticoagulant effect of warfarin may increase the risk of bleeding during warfarin therapy (Table 25.8).

Skin necrosis is a rare adverse effect of warfarin, the exact pathogenesis of which is poorly understood. It is caused by thrombosis of the venules and capillaries within subcutaneous fat. It typically occurs between the third and eighth days of warfarin therapy. A relationship between warfarin-induced skin necrosis and protein C deficiency has been reported; however, it also occurs in nondeficient individuals.[52]

Warfarin crosses the placenta and may cause fetal hemorrhage, nasal hypoplasia, and stippled epiphyses. The risk for these complications is highest when the fetus is exposed to warfarin at between 6 and 12 weeks' gestation. Warfarin has been used safely during the first 6 weeks of gestation.[67] It appears from limited studies that warfarin does not cross into breast milk.[68]

TABLE 25.8	Selected Drug Interactions With Warfarin
Drugs That Enhance Warfarin's Effect	**Drugs That Inhibit Warfarin's Effect**
Alcohol	Barbiturates
Amiodarone	Carbamazepine
Anabolic steroids	Cholestyramine
Cimetidine	Dicloxacillin
Ciprofloxacin	Phenytoin
Cotrimoxazole	Rifampin
Erythromycin	Sucralfate
Fluconazole, miconazole, itraconazole	
Isoniazid	
Metronidazole	
Omeprazole	
Propafenone	
Quinidine	
Simvastatin, lovastatin	
Tetracycline	

(Adapted from Ansell J, Hirsh J, Poller L, et al. The pharmacology and management of the vitamin K antagonists. Chest 126:204S–233S, 2004.)

Drug Interactions. Numerous drugs interact with warfarin to exacerbate or inhibit its anticoagulant effect. It is imperative that the clinician thoroughly assess for drug interactions with warfarin to avoid thromboembolic or hemorrhagic complications. Many drugs affect warfarin's pharmacokinetics and pharmacodynamics. For example, cholestyramine inhibits the anticoagulant effects of warfarin by reducing its absorption. Other drugs interact with warfarin by inducing or inhibiting its metabolism in the liver. For example, trimethoprim-sulfamethoxazole inhibits the metabolism of the S-isomer of warfarin, which potentiates its anticoagulant effect. Other drugs may interact with warfarin by inhibiting the synthesis of (third-generation cephalosporins) or increasing the clearance of (thyroxine) the vitamin K–dependent clotting factors. References 69 and 70 provide extensive reviews of warfarin drug interactions. Examples of drugs that significantly interact with warfarin are listed in Table 25.8.[52,69,70]

Treatment of Patients Who Overdose. The effects of excessive anticoagulation with warfarin may be reversed with the administration of vitamin K_1, fresh frozen plasma, prothrombin concentrates, or recombinant factor VIIa. Vitamin K_1 (phytonadione) is the vitamin K preparation of choice because of its rapid onset of action. It can be administered intravenously, subcutaneously, or orally. Intramuscular administration is contraindicated because of the risk of hematoma. Intravenous vitamin K_1 should be administered slowly to lower the risk of anaphylactic reactions. Patients who receive vitamin K_1 may exhibit resistance to subsequent warfarin therapy for 1 week or longer. For this reason, the lowest effective dose of vitamin K_1 should be used. Patients with INR measurements slightly above therapeutic range may be treated by omission of one or more warfarin doses or by reduction of the maintenance dose of warfarin.[52] Table 25.9 lists specific recommendations for treating patients with elevated INR measurements.[52]

Management of Surgical Procedures. Patients who are receiving anticoagulation therapy occasionally may require invasive procedures. The management of anticoagulation therapy during invasive procedures should be based upon the patient's risk for thromboembolism without anticoagulation, the risk of bleeding with continued anticoagulation, and the costs of various therapies. Table 25.10 lists recommendations for managing anticoagulation during invasive procedures.[52]

For most patients who require simple dental procedures, anticoagulation therapy need not be altered. Tranexamic acid or epsilon amino caproic acid mouthwash may be used to minimize local bleeding.[52,71]

Thrombolytic Agents. Thrombolytic agents dissolve venous thrombi, restoring blood flow through a previously obstructed vein. Three agents are currently available for use in the management of VTE: streptokinase, urokinase, and alteplase (rtPA). These agents activate plasminogen through

TABLE 25.9	Management of Elevated International Normalized Ratios and/or Bleeding in Patients Treated With Warfarin[a]
Condition	**Recommendation**
INR above target range but <5.0; no significant bleeding	Lower maintenance dose or omit dose, monitor more frequently, and resume at lower dose when INR in target range; if INR only slightly above range, no reduction may be necessary
INR >5.0 but ≤9.0; no significant bleeding	Omit next one or two doses, monitor more frequently, resume at lower dose when INR in target range; or omit dose and give vitamin K_1 ≤5 mg orally if at increased risk of bleeding. If rapid reversal required for an urgent invasive procedure, give vitamin K_1 2–4 mg orally. INR should decrease within 24 hours. If needed, additional vitamin K_1 (1 or 2 mg) may be given
INR ≥9.0; no significant bleeding	Hold warfarin and give vitamin K_1 5–10 mg orally. INR will be substantially reduced in 24–48 hours. Monitor more frequently and give additional vitamin K_1 if necessary. Resume warfarin at lower dose when INR in target range
Serious bleeding at any INR elevation	Hold warfarin and give vitamin K_1 10 mg by slow IV infusion, supplemented by fresh frozen plasma or prothrombin complex concentrate, depending on the urgency of the situation. Recombinant factor VIIa may be considered as an alternative to prothrombin complex concentrate. Repeat vitamin K_1 every 12 hours if needed
Life-threatening bleeding	Hold warfarin and give prothrombin complex concentrate supplemented with vitamin K_1 10 mg by slow IV infusion. Recombinant factor VIIa may be considered as an alternative to prothrombin complex concentrate. Repeat if necessary, on the basis of the INR measurement

INR, international normalized ratio.
(Adapted from Ansell J, Hirsh J, Poller L, et al. The pharmacology and management of the vitamin K antagonists. Chest 126:204S–233S, 2004.)

TABLE 25.10	Anticoagulation Management During Invasive Procedures
Condition	**Recommendation**
Low risk of VTE[a]	Stop warfarin 4 days before surgery, allow INR to return to near normal, briefly use postoperative prophylaxis with low-dose UH (5,000 units SQ) or prophylactic dose of LMWH, and begin warfarin therapy simultaneously. Or, use low-dose UH or prophylactic dose of LMWH preoperatively
Intermediate risk of VTE	Stop warfarin 4 days before surgery, allowing INR to decrease. Give low-dose UH or prophylactic dose of LMWH, beginning 2 days before surgery, and continue postoperatively with warfarin. Higher dose UH or full-dose LMWH may be used as an alternative
High risk of VTE[b]	Stop warfarin 4 days before surgery, allowing INR to return to normal. Give full-dose UH or full-dose LMWH, beginning 2 days before surgery. UH may be given SQ on an outpatient basis, then switched to continuous IV infusion upon admission. The infusion should be stopped 5 hours before surgery; or UH may be given SQ, with the last dose given 12–24 hours before surgery. The last dose of LMWH should be given 12–24 hours before surgery. UH or LMWH should be continued postoperatively, along with warfarin initiation
Low risk of bleeding	Continue warfarin at a lower dose, and operate with an INR of 1.3–1.5. The warfarin dose may be lowered 4–5 days before surgery. Restart warfarin therapy postoperatively. Supplemental low-dose UH or prophylactic dose LMWH may be given postoperatively if necessary

[a] Low risk of VTE—no recent (<3 months) VTE, atrial fibrillation with no history of stroke or other risk factors, bileaflet mechanical valve in the aortic position.
[b] High risk of VTE—recent (<3 months) history of VTE, mechanical cardiac valve in mitral position, old model cardiac valve (ball/cage).
VTE, venous thromboembolism; INR, international normalized ratio; UH, unfractionated heparin; LMWH, low-molecular-weight heparin; IV, intravenous; SQ, subcutaneous.
(Adapted from Ansell J, Hirsh J, Poller L, et al. The pharmacology and management of the vitamin K antagonists. Chest 126:204S–233S, 2004.)

various mechanisms. Plasminogen is then converted to plasmin, which degrades fibrin clots.[72–74]

Therapeutic Indications. Thrombolytic agents are not recommended for routine use in the treatment of patients with DVT. They should be reserved for patients with massive ileofemoral DVT who are at risk for limb gangrene because of severe venous occlusion. Thrombolytic agents are not recommended for routine use in the treatment of patients with PE. They should be reserved for patients with acute massive PE, or those who are hemodynamically unstable.[2] Thrombolytic agents are contraindicated in patients with active internal bleeding, recent stroke (within 2 months), recent intracranial or intraspinal surgery, recent trauma (including cardiopulmonary resuscitation), intracranial neoplasm, arteriovenous malformation, aneurysm, known bleeding diatheses, or severe uncontrolled arterial hypertension.[72–74] Catheter-directed thrombolysis is recommended only for selected patients with DVT, such as those who require limb salvage.[2] Catheter-directed thrombolysis is not recommended for the treatment of patients with PE because of increased bleeding risk at the catheter insertion site.[2]

Dosing and Administration. Treatment with streptokinase should be initiated with a loading dose of 250,000 IU, followed by an infusion of 100,000 IU per hour for 24 hours. Urokinase should be administered as a loading dose of 4,400 IU per kg of body weight, followed by an infusion of 2,200 IU per kg for 12 hours. rtPA should be administered as an infusion at a dosage of 100 mg over 2 hours.[2]

Laboratory Assessment. The aPTT, hematocrit, and platelets should be measured before thrombolytic agents are administered.[72–74]

Adverse Reactions. The most serious complication of thrombolytic therapy is bleeding. The incidences of bleeding following use of all agents are similar. Other adverse reactions include hypotension, allergic reactions, and fever.[72–74]

Drug Interactions. Anticoagulants and drugs that alter platelet function may increase the risk of bleeding if given concurrently with thrombolytic agents. UH or LMWHs should not be administered with thrombolytic agents; however, UH or LMWH therapy may be instituted near the end of an infusion of rtPA.[2,72–74]

Fondaparinux. Fondaparinux is a synthetic pentasaccharide. It is a selective inhibitor of activated factor X (Xa). It binds to a specific site on AT, forming a complex that accelerates AT's inactivation of factor Xa. This inhibits the formation of thrombin and thus, thrombus formation. It is currently the only drug in its class that has been approved by the US Food and Drug Administration (FDA).[75] Fondaparinux is completely absorbed from subcutaneous injections, exhibiting a bioavailability of 100%. Peak plasma concentrations are reached in 2 hours. The volume of distribution of fondaparinux is 7 to 11 L. It does not bind to plasma proteins, platelet factor 4, or red blood cells. Fondaparinux is eliminated renally and has a half-life of approximately 17 to 21 hours.[75,76] Clearance of fondaparinux may be increased by 20% during hemodialysis when given to patients who are undergoing long-term intermittent hemodialysis.[75]

Therapeutic Indications. Fondaparinux is indicated for the prevention of DVT/PE in patients undergoing hip fracture surgery, hip replacement surgery, or knee replacement surgery. Fondaparinux is indicated for the treatment of patients with acute DVT in conjunction with warfarin. It is indicated for the treatment of those with acute PE in conjunction with warfarin when therapy is initiated in the hospital. Fondaparinux is contraindicated in patients with CrCl less than 30 mL per minute. Prophylactic therapy in patients undergoing hip fracture, hip replacement, or knee replacement surgery is contraindicated in patients who weigh less than 50 kg, because of increased risk of bleeding. It is also contraindicated in patients with active bleeding, bacterial endocarditis, and thrombocytopenia associated with a positive in vitro test for antiplatelet antibody in the presence of fondaparinux.[75]

Dosing and Administration. For the prevention of DVT/PE in patients undergoing hip fracture surgery, hip replacement surgery, or knee replacement surgery, fondaparinux should be given subcutaneously in a dose of 2.5 mg once daily. The initial dose should be given 6 to 8 hours after surgery, when hemostasis has been established. The typical duration of therapy is 5 to 9 days; however, an extended course of an additional 24 days is recommended. Total therapy of up to 32 days has been tolerated in patients who are undergoing hip fracture surgery. The dose of fondaparinux for the treatment of patients with DVT/PE varies according to patient weight. For patients whose body weight is less than 50 kg, the dose is 5 mg. For patients whose body weight is 50 to 100 kg, the dose is 7.5 mg. For those whose body weight is greater than 100 kg, the dose is 10 mg. The dose should be given subcutaneously once daily. Treatment with warfarin should be initiated within 72 hours and should be continued for at least 4 to 5 days until an INR of 2.0 is obtained on 2 consecutive days. Fondaparinux should not be given intramuscularly.[75]

Laboratory Assessment. PT and aPTT measurements do not reflect the activity of fondaparinux and are not recommended during fondaparinux therapy. Complete blood counts should be measured at baseline and periodically during fondaparinux therapy. Fondaparinux should be discontinued if the platelet count falls to below 100,000 per mm³. Serum creatinine should be measured before fondaparinux therapy is initiated and periodically thereafter.[75] Periodic stool occult blood tests are recommended during fondaparinux therapy. The anti–factor Xa activity of fondaparinux may be measured using the anti-Xa assay calibrated to fondaparinux. Anti–factor Xa activity should be expressed in milligrams of fondaparinux, and is not comparable with the activities of heparin or the LMWHs.[75]

Adverse Reactions. The most common adverse effect of fondaparinux is bleeding. The incidences of major bleeding during premarketing clinical trials were 2.2%, 3.0%, and 2.1% during perioperative prophylaxis for hip fracture, hip replacement, and knee replacement surgery, respectively. The incidences of major bleeding increased to 3.8% and 4.8% for patients with CrCl of 30 to 50 mL per minute and less than 30 mL per minute, respectively, during prophylactic therapy. The incidence of major bleeding during treatment of patients with DVT or PE during premarketing trials was 1.2%.[75] The incidence of major bleeding increased to 2.2% or 7.8% for patients receiving treatment for DVT or PE with CrCl of 30 to 50 mL per minute or less than 30 mL per minute, respectively. Moderate thrombocytopenia (platelet counts between 100,000/mm³ and 50,000/mm³) occurred in 2.9% of patients receiving fondaparinux 2.5 mg daily for VTE prophylaxis during hip fracture, hip replacement, and knee replacement surgery in premarketing clinical trials. Severe thrombocytopenia (platelet counts less than 50,000/mm³) was reported in 0.2% of these patients.[75]

Drug Interactions. Any drug that may also increase the risk of bleeding should be discontinued before fondaparinux therapy is initiated. Patients should be monitored closely for signs and symptoms of bleeding when anticoagulants or antiplatelet agents are used concurrently with fondaparinux.[75]

Treatment of Patients Who Overdose. No antidote for fondaparinux is known; however, a study in 16 healthy male volunteers showed that recombinant factor VIIa reversed the effects of a single, subcutaneous 10-mg dose of fondaparinux.[75,77]

Argatroban. Argatroban is a synthetic direct thrombin inhibitor derived from L-arginine. It binds to the active site of thrombin, inhibiting thrombin-catalyzed and thrombin-induced reactions. Thus, it inhibits fibrin clot formation, the activation of factors V, VII, and XII, the activation of protein C, and platelet aggregation. It binds to both free and clot-associated thrombin.[78] Argatroban does not interact with heparin-induced antibodies, nor does it induce antibody formation to itself. Its volume of distribution is 174 mL/kg, and it is 54% bound to plasma proteins. Argatroban undergoes hydroxylation and aromatization in the liver. The cytochrome P-450 3A4/5 hepatic enzymes play a role in its metabolism; however, this is not a clinically important deactivation pathway in vivo. Argatroban has four metabolites, only one of which is active; however, it is three to five times weaker than argatroban. The total body clearance of argatroban decreased from 5.1 mL/kg/min to 1.9 mL/kg/min in patients with hepatic impairment. The half-life of argatroban is approximately 39 to 51 minutes. Steady state levels of argatroban are reached within 1 to 3 hours.[78]

Therapeutic Indications. Argatroban is indicated for the prevention and treatment of VTE in patients with HIT. It is also indicated as an anticoagulant in patients with or at risk for HIT who are undergoing percutaneous coronary intervention. Argatroban is contraindicated in patients with major bleeding or hypersensitivity to any of its components.[78,79]

Dosing and Administration. Each 2.5-mL vial of argatroban contains 250 mg of active drug. This must be diluted with 250 mL of 0.9% sodium chloride injection, 5% dextrose injection, or lactated Ringer's injection to a final concentration of 1 mg per mL. The solution should then be thoroughly mixed by repeated bag inversion for 1 minute. Argatroban should be given by continuous intravenous infusion at a dose of 2 μg/kg/min for patients with HIT. The dose should then be adjusted (maximum dose 10 μg/kg/min) according to subsequent aPTT measurements. The initial dosage of argatroban should be reduced to 0.5 μg/kg/min in patients with moderate hepatic impairment. For information on those who require subsequent warfarin therapy, please see the section on laboratory monitoring. All parenteral anticoagulants should be discontinued before therapy with argatroban is initiated.[78,79]

Laboratory Monitoring. Argatroban therapy is monitored through use of the aPTT. A baseline aPTT measurement should be obtained and repeated 2 hours after the infusion is begun. The desired aPTT is one and one half to three times the baseline level, not to exceed 100 seconds. Argatroban also increases the PT, INR, activated clotting time (ACT), and thrombin time (TT); however, therapeutic ranges for these tests have not been identified for argatroban. Argatroban produces an INR increase above that produced by warfarin therapy alone. When subsequent anticoagulation with warfarin is required, therapy with argatroban and warfarin should be overlapped. The expected maintenance dose of warfarin should be given, and the INR measured daily. For patients who are receiving argatroban doses up to 2 μg/kg/min, argatroban may be discontinued when the INR is greater than 4. The INR should be repeated 4 to 6 hours after argatroban is discontinued. If the INR is below therapeutic range, therapy with argatroban should be restarted at the previous dose. The procedure should be repeated daily until the INR on warfarin alone is within therapeutic range. For patients who are receiving argatroban doses greater than 2 μg/kg/min, the dose should be reduced to 2 μg/kg/min. The aforementioned procedure should then be followed for discontinuation of argatroban.[78]

Adverse Reactions. The most common adverse effect of argatroban is bleeding. Major bleeding occurred in 5.3% of patients with HIT who received argatroban in premarketing clinical trials. Dyspnea, hypotension, fever, and diarrhea have also been reported. Among 1,127 individuals who received argatroban during premarketing clinical trials, 156 allergic reactions were reported; however, 95% of those occurred in patients who had also received thrombolytic ther-

apy for acute myocardial infarction or intravenous contrast media for coronary angiography.[78] Argatroban is classified as pregnancy category B. Teratogenic effects have not been reported in animal studies; however, no well-controlled studies have been conducted in pregnant women.[78]

Drug Interactions. When argatroban is to be initiated after heparin therapy has been discontinued, adequate time for the anticoagulant effect of heparin to decrease should be allowed before argatroban therapy is initiated. The concomitant administration of argatroban and warfarin prolongs the INR to beyond that normally observed with warfarin therapy alone. Concomitant administration of thrombolytic and antiplatelet agents may increase the risk of bleeding.[78]

Treatment of Patients Who Overdose. No specific antidote has been identified for argatroban. Excessive anticoagulation may be reversed by discontinuing the argatroban infusion or decreasing the infusion rate. The INR should return to baseline 2 to 4 hours after discontinuation of the infusion. Reversal of the anticoagulant effect may be prolonged in patients with hepatic impairment. In the event of severe hemorrhage, the argatroban infusion should be discontinued and supportive care provided.[78]

Lepirudin. Lepirudin is a synthetic direct thrombin inhibitor. It is a recombinant hirudin that is derived from yeast cells. It binds directly to thrombin, directly inhibiting thrombin-catalyzed or thrombin-induced reactions. Lepirudin has a terminal half-life of 1.3 hours. Lepirudin is thought to undergo catabolic hydrolysis; however, 48% of the drug is excreted in the urine. Lepirudin has a volume of distribution of 12.2 L at steady state and a clearance of 164 mL per minute. The clearance of lepirudin is 25% lower in women than in men, and 20% lower in elderly patients than in young patients. Clearance of lepirudin decreased to 61 mL per minute in patients with a CrCl less than 80 mL per minute.[80] Lepirudin (antihirudin) antibodies were formed in 40% of patients with HIT who received lepirudin in premarketing clinical trials.[80]

Therapeutic Indications. Lepirudin is indicated for anticoagulation in patients with HIT and associated thromboembolic disease, to prevent further thromboembolic complications.[80]

Dosing and Administration. The initial dose is 0.4 mg per kg body weight (up to 110 kg) given slowly as an intravenous bolus over 10 to 20 seconds. This should be followed by 0.15 mg/kg/hour as a continuous intravenous infusion for 2 to 10 days, or longer as needed. The maximal initial bolus dose is 44 mg and the maximal initial infusion dose is 16.5 mg per hour. The dose is then modified according to the aPTT ratio. For patients who require long-term anticoagulation with warfarin, the lepirudin dose should be decreased to produce an aPTT ratio just above 1.5 before warfarin therapy is initiated. The expected maintenance dose of warfarin should be initiated. Loading doses of warfarin should not be used. Lepirudin should be continued for 4 to 5 days, until the INR is 2.0 on two consecutive days.[80]

Laboratory Monitoring. Lepirudin therapy is monitored by means of the aPTT ratio. The aPTT ratio is the ratio of the patient's aPTT to the aPTT reference value of the laboratory. The target range for the aPTT ratio is 1.5 to 2.5. A baseline aPTT ratio should be obtained and repeated 4 hours after the start of the lepirudin infusion. If the aPTT ratio is above or below therapeutic range, another aPTT ratio should be determined. If the confirmed aPTT ratio is above therapeutic range, the lepirudin infusion should be stopped for 2 hours. The infusion should then be restarted and the dose decreased by 50%. The aPTT ratio should be repeated 4 hours later and subsequent dose adjustments made. If the confirmed aPTT ratio is below therapeutic range, the dose should be increased by 20%. The aPTT ratio should be determined 4 hours later and subsequent dose adjustments made. The aPTT ratio should be determined at least once daily during lepirudin therapy. Lepirudin therapy should not be initiated in patients whose baseline aPTT ratio is 2.5 or greater. The initial bolus dose of lepirudin should be reduced to 0.2 mg per kg in all patients with renal insufficiency.

Adverse Reactions. The most common adverse effect of lepirudin is bleeding. Bleeding from puncture sites or wounds, anemia, other hematoma/unclassified bleeding, GI/rectal bleeding, epistaxis, hemothorax, and vaginal bleeding occurred in 14.1%, 13.1%, 11.1%, 6.6%, 5.1%, 3%, 3%, and 1.5% of patients, respectively, who received lepirudin during premarketing clinical trials.[80] Fever and abnormal liver function occurred in 6.1% of patients during premarketing clinical trials. Other nonhemorrhagic adverse events reported include pneumonia, sepsis, allergic skin reactions, and heart failure. These occurred in 4%, 4%, 3%, and 3% of patients, respectively.[80] Lepirudin is classified as pregnancy category B. No evidence of teratogenicity has been detected in rats; however, no well-controlled studies have been conducted in pregnant women. Lepirudin crosses the rat placenta. It is unknown whether lepirudin crosses the human placenta or is secreted into breast milk.[80]

Drug Interactions. Concomitant administration with thrombolytic, antiplatelet, or anticoagulant agents may increase the risk of bleeding and enhance lepirudin's effect on the aPTT.[80] Nine patients with HIT received lepirudin and thrombolytic therapy simultaneously during premarketing clinical trials. A 47% relative increase in risk of bleeding was noted for patients receiving lepirudin and thrombolytic agents simultaneously; however, no difference was seen in the rates of serious bleeding events between patients who received lepirudin and thrombolytics and those who received lepirudin alone.[80]

Treatment of Patients Who Overdose. No specific antidote for lepirudin has been identified. Lepirudin infusion should be stopped in the event of excessive aPTT prolongation or severe bleeding. The aPTT should be monitored, and supportive care should be administered.

NONPHARMACOLOGIC THERAPY

Surgical intervention in the treatment of patients with VTE is not routinely recommended. Venous thrombectomy should be reserved for patients with massive ileofemoral DVT who are at risk for limb gangrene because of venous occlusion.[2] Pulmonary embolectomy for the treatment of patients with PE is not routinely recommended. It should be reserved for patients who have massive PE, are hemodynamically unstable despite heparin therapy and proper resuscitation, or who fail thrombolytic therapy or have a contraindication to its use.[2] Catheter extraction techniques are not recommended for patients with DVT. Catheter extraction techniques should be reserved for selected patients with massive PE who are hemodynamically compromised and have contraindications to thrombolytic therapy.[2] Inferior vena cava filters are recommended for hospitalized patients with VTE who have a contraindication to or complication of anticoagulant therapy, and in patients with recurrent VTE despite adequate anticoagulation therapy.[2] Graduated compression stockings providing 30 to 40 mm Hg at the ankle should be worn by patients with DVT during the first 2 years after the event to decrease the incidence of PTS. They may also be used to treat patients with mild edema due to PTS. Intermittent pneumatic compression may be used to treat patients with severe edema due to PTS.[2] Patients with DVT should be encouraged to ambulate as tolerated to promote faster resolution of pain and swelling of the affected extremity.[2]

FUTURE THERAPIES

Several agents are under investigation for the prevention and treatment of patients with VTE. Idraparinux, a derivative of fondaparinux, binds to AT and inhibits factor Xa. It has a long half-life (130 hours) and is given once weekly. It is currently undergoing phase 3 clinical trials in the treatment of patients with VTE.[81,82] Soluble thrombomodulin is a recombinant analog of the extracellular domain of thrombomodulin. It binds to thrombin and induces a change in the enzyme that converts it into an activator of protein C. It is currently being evaluated in phase 2 dose-finding studies for the prevention of VTE in patients undergoing elective hip replacement.[82,83] Plasminogen activator inhibitor (PAI-1) inhibits the ability of tissue-type plasminogen activator to activate plasminogen and convert it to plasmin. This inhibits fibrinolysis. Several small-molecule PAI-1 inhibitors exhibit antithrombotic activity in rabbits.[82,84] Human studies are needed to further evaluate their role. Other investigational agents that may enhance fibrinolysis are targeted against activated thrombin–activatable fibrinolysis inhibitor (TAFIa) and factor XIIIa. These are still being studied in animals.[82] Ximelagatran is a prodrug of the direct thrombin inhibitor, melagatran. Potential advantages of ximelagatran over warfarin include fixed oral dosing, rapid onset/offset of effect, wide therapeutic index, predictable anticoagulant effect and patient response, no significant drug–food interactions, no risk of HIT, and no need for regular monitoring.[82] It has been studied in the prevention of stroke in patients with atrial fibrillation, treatment of and subsequent long-term prevention of VTE, VTE prophylaxis in patients undergoing orthopedic surgery, and secondary prevention of myocardial infarction.[82,85–93] Ximelagatran was found to be as effective as warfarin in the prevention of VTE in patients with atrial fibrillation, and as effective as enoxaparin and warfarin in the prevention of VTE in knee replacement surgery and in the treatment of VTE. On September 10, 2004, the FDA rejected ximelagatran, however, because of increased risk of hepatotoxicity during clinical trials.[94]

IMPROVING OUTCOMES

PATIENT EDUCATION

Patient education is essential to the success of anticoagulation therapy. Important educational topics include drug name and dose, indication for and duration of anticoagulant therapy, recognition and minimization of risk for adverse effects, risk of thrombosis without therapy, administration time and technique, drug–drug and drug–food interactions, importance of regular laboratory monitoring, management of adverse effects, and importance of regular follow-up with the health care provider.[95] Patient education has been positively associated with maintenance of the INR within therapeutic range.[96] Poor-quality patient education and lack of patient education have been associated with an increased risk of bleeding in elderly patients.[97]

METHODS FOR IMPROVING PATIENT ADHERENCE TO DRUG THERAPY

Adherence to anticoagulation therapy has been associated with maintenance of the INR within therapeutic range.[98] The length of time that the INR is within therapeutic range has been associated with decreased thromboembolic and hemorrhagic events in numerous studies.[52] Thus, strategies by which patient adherence to anticoagulation therapy can be improved are important. Generally, many factors have been associated with patient nonadherence to therapy, including psychiatric disorders, duration of treatment, number of medications prescribed, medication cost, frequency of dosing, patients' unresolved concerns, and poor communication between patient and provider.[99] A combination of educational and behavioral strategies should be employed to improve compliance.[99,100] Pill organizers, blister packs, calendars, and dosage counters may help to enhance compliance.[99] Access to culturally sensitive, appropriately written information, along with verbal reinforcement, may improve compliance. Additional strategies to be combined include involving the patient in establishing treatment goals, reducing the complexity of the medication regimen, tailoring the regimen to the patient's lifestyle, encouraging family support, informing the patient of possible adverse effects, monitoring adherence, and providing adequate feedback to the patient.[99]

DISEASE MANAGEMENT STRATEGIES FOR IMPROVING PATIENT OUTCOMES

Several studies have shown decreased incidences of bleeding and recurrent VTE when patients are managed by an anticoagulation management service (AMS) compared with usual care (typical care provided by a physician). However, these studies were not randomized. Although the benefits of an AMS are generally recognized, randomized, long-term, large-scale trials are needed to fully investigate these benefits.[52] Patient self-testing (PST) and patient self-management (PSM) of anticoagulation with the use of fingerstick measurements of the INR obtained with various machines have been compared with usual care (typical care provided by physicians). Several studies have shown that PST and PSM reduced the incidence of adverse events and increased times in the therapeutic range when compared with usual care.[52] PST and PSM have also been shown to increase times in the therapeutic range when compared with an AMS in several studies.[52] A recent study showed that PSM reduced the incidence of adverse events during anticoagulation therapy when compared with care provided by an AMS.[101] Various computer programs are available to assist with the management of warfarin dosing. In two studies, computerized dosing programs have been shown to be more effective at maintaining the INR within the therapeutic range when compared with manual dosing by health care providers.[52] Computerized dosing programs have yet to show a decreased incidence of adverse events when compared with manual dosing, however.[52]

PHARMACOECONOMICS

LMWHs have been shown to be more cost-effective than UH in the treatment of VTE in several studies.[102–106] This is attributed to ease of administration, fewer laboratory monitoring requirements, early hospital discharge, and outpatient management of VTE.[102] LMWHs are also more cost-effective than warfarin or UH in the prophylaxis of VTE.[102,107,108] Fondaparinux has been shown to be more cost-effective than LMWHs in the prophylaxis of VTE; it also demonstrates increased cost savings over time.[102,109]

KEY POINTS

■ Venous thromboembolism (VTE) is a disease that includes both DVT and PE. A deep vein thrombosis is a thrombus composed of cellular material and fibrin, which can form in any vein in the body. A pulmonary embolism is a thrombus that originates from any location in the systemic circulation and becomes lodged in

the pulmonary artery, impeding blood flow to the lungs
- Treatment goals for VTE are to prevent thrombus extension, thrombus embolization, early and late recurrences of DVT and PE, and the development of post-thrombotic syndrome (PTS) by restoring normal venous blood flow and maintaining normal venous valve function
- The pathogenesis of VTE involves three factors: venous stasis, hypercoagulability, and endothelial damage. These factors are collectively referred to as the Virchow triad
- The coagulation system is activated in response to vascular endothelial injury. The system is composed of platelet-mediated primary hemostasis and the coagulation cascade
- Patients who are experiencing VTE often manifest few specific symptoms, thereby making clinical diagnosis insensitive and unreliable. Compression ultrasonography is the diagnostic test of choice when DVT is suspected. Accurately diagnosing PE also requires objective testing; however, no single noninvasive diagnostic test is sufficiently sensitive or specific for the diagnosis in all patients
- Patients who are diagnosed with VTE may be treated initially with body weight–adjusted LMWH, intravenous UH, or subcutaneous UH, with monitoring and subsequent dose adjustments. Therapy with warfarin should be initiated concurrently. Therapy with LMWH or UH may be discontinued when the INR is within the target range of 2 to 3
- LMWHs have been shown to be more cost-effective than UH in the treatment of VTE. LMWHs are also more cost-effective than warfarin or UH in the prophylaxis of VTE. Fondaparinux has been shown to be more cost-effective than LMWHs in the prophylaxis of VTE
- Patients with DVT should wear an elastic compression stocking to prevent PTS and should be encouraged to ambulate as tolerated
- Surgical intervention and thrombolytic therapy are not routinely recommended and should be reserved for select patients
- Patient education is essential to the success of anticoagulation therapy. Important educational topics include drug name and dose, indication for and duration of anticoagulant therapy, recognition and minimization of risk for adverse effects, risk of thrombosis without therapy, administration time and technique, drug–drug and drug–food interactions, importance of regular laboratory monitoring, management of adverse effects, and importance of regular follow-up with the health care provider. A combination of educational and behavioral strategies should be employed to improve compliance
- Anticoagulation management services, patient self-testing, and patient self-management have been shown to decrease adverse events during anticoagulant therapy in several studies. Computerized warfarin dosing programs have been shown to increase the time that the INR spends within the therapeutic range
- Several agents are currently under investigation for the treatment of patients with VTE, including idraparinux, soluble thrombomodulin, PAI-1 inhibitors, TAFIa inhibitors, and factor XIII inhibitors

SUGGESTED READINGS

Ansell, J, Hirsh J, Poller L, et al. The pharmacology and management of the vitamin K antagonists. Chest 126:204S–233S, 2004.

Buller HR, Agnelli G, Hull RD, et al. Antithrombotic therapy for venous thromboembolic disease. Chest 126:401S–428S, 2004.

Geerts WH, Pineo GF, Heit JA, et al. Prevention of venous thromboembolism. Chest 126:338S–400S, 2004.

Hirsh J, Raschke R. Heparin and low-molecular-weight heparin. Chest 126:188S–203S, 2004.

REFERENCES

1. Hirsh J, Hoak J. Management of deep vein thrombosis and pulmonary embolism: a statement for healthcare professionals. Circulation 93:2212–2245, 1996.
2. Buller HR, Agnelli G, Hull RD, et al. Antithrombotic therapy for venous thromboembolic disease. Chest 126:401S–428S, 2004.
3. Weinmann EE, Salzman EW. Deep-vein thrombosis. N Engl J Med 331:1630–1641, 1994.
4. Stein PD. Acute pulmonary embolism. Dis Mon 40:467–523, 1994.
5. Bates SM, Ginsberg JS. Treatment of deep-vein thrombosis. N Engl J Med 351:268–277, 2004.
6. Hyers TM, Agnelli G, Hull RD, et al. Antithrombotic therapy for venous thromboembolic disease. Chest 114:561S–578S, 1998.
7. Thomas RH. Hypercoagulability syndromes. Arch Intern Med 161: 2433–2439, 2001.
8. Silverstein MD, Heit JA, Mohr DN, et al. Trends in the incidence of deep vein thrombosis and pulmonary embolism. Arch Intern Med 158:585–593, 1998.
9. Nordstom M, Lindblad B, Bergqvist D, et al. A prospective study of the incidence of deep-vein thrombosis within a defined urban population. J Intern Med 232:155–160, 1992.
10. Anderson FA Jr, Wheeler HB, Goldberg RJ, et al. A population-based perspective of the hospital incidence and case-fatality rates of deep vein thrombosis and pulmonary embolism: The Worcester DVT study. Arch Intern Med 151:933–938, 1991.
11. Gillum RF. Pulmonary embolism and thrombophlebitis in the United States, 1970-1985. Am Heart J 114:1262–1264, 1987.
12. Stein PD, Hull RD, Kayali F, et al. Venous thromboembolism according to age. Arch Intern Med 164:2260–2265, 2004.
13. Stein PD, Kayali F, Olson RE. Incidence of venous thromboembolism in infants and children: data from the national hospital discharge survey. J Pediatr 145:563–565, 2004.
14. Cushman M, Tsai AW, White RH, et al: Deep vein thrombosis and pulmonary embolism in two cohorts: the longitudinal investigation of thromboembolism etiology. Am J Med 117:19–25, 2004.
15. Dahlback B. Blood coagulation. Lancet 355:1627–1632, 2000.
16. Spronk HMH, Govers-Riemslag JWP, ten Cate H. The blood coagulation system as a molecular machine. BioEssays 25:1220–1228, 2003.
17. Furie B, Furie BC. Molecular and cellular biology of blood coagulation. N Engl J Med 326:800–806, 1992.
18. Geerts WH, Heit JA, Clagett GP, et al. Prevention of venous thromboembolism. Chest 119:132S–175S, 2001.
19. Gorman WP, Davis KR, Donnelly R. ABC of arterial and venous disease. Swollen lower limb: general assessment and deep vein thrombosis. BMJ 320:1453–1456, 2000.

SECTION VI ■ Cardiovascular Disorders appears in header.

20. Hirsh J. Diagnosis of venous thrombosis and pulmonary embolism. Am J Cardiol 65:45C–49C, 1990.
21. Stein PD, Terrin ML, Hales CA, et al. Clinical laboratory, roentgenographic, and electrocardiographic findings in patients with acute pulmonary embolism and no pre-existing cardiac or pulmonary disease. Chest 100:598–603, 1991.
22. Fedullo PF, Tapson VF. The evaluation of suspected pulmonary embolism. N Engl J Med 349:1247–1256, 2003.
23. Goldhaber SZ. Pulmonary embolism. N Engl J Med 339:93–104, 1998.
24. Wells PS, Anderson DR, Rodger M, et al. Derivation of a simple clinical model to categorize patients' probability of pulmonary embolism: increasing the model's utility with the SimpliRED D-dimer. Thromb Haemost 83:416–420, 2000.
25. Oertel LB. Education curriculum for patients and teaching methods. In: Ansell JE, Oertel LB, Wittkowsky AK, eds. Managing oral anticoagulation therapy: clinical and operational guidelines. Gaithersburg, Md: Aspen, 1999:6A–1, 1999.
26. The Seventh ACCP Conference on Antithrombotic and Thrombolytic Therapy: Evidence-based guidelines. Chest 126:163S–696S, 2004.
27. Hirsh J, Dalen JE, Deykin D, et al. Heparin: mechanism of action, pharmacokinetics, dosing considerations, monitoring, efficacy, and safety. Chest 102:337S–351S, 1992.
28. Hirsh J, Fuster V. Guide to anticoagulant therapy. Part 1: heparin. Circulation 89:1449–1468, 1994.
29. Hirsh J. Heparin. N Engl J Med 324:1565–1574, 1991.
30. Pineo GF, Hull RD. Classical anticoagulant therapy for venous thromboembolism. Prog Cardiovasc Dis 37:59–70, 1994.
31. Hirsch J, Van Aken WG, Gallus AS, et al. Heparin kinetics in venous thrombosis and pulmonary embolism. Circulation 53:691–695, 1976.
32. Hirsh J, Raschke R. Heparin and low-molecular-weight heparin. Chest 126:188S–203S, 2004.
33. Geerts WH, Pineo GF, Heit JA, et al. Prevention of venous thromboembolism. Chest 126:338S–400S, 2004.
34. Hirsh J, Warkentin TE, Raschke R, et al. Heparin and low-molecular-weight heparin: mechanisms of action, pharmacokinetics, dosing considerations, monitoring, efficacy, and safety. Chest 114:489S–510S, 1998.
35. Hirsh J, Anand SS, Halperin JL, et al. Guide to anticoagulant therapy: heparin. A statement for healthcare professionals from the American Heart Association. Circulation 103:2994–3018, 2001.
36. Raschke RA, Gollihare B, Peirce JC. The effectiveness of implementing the weight-based heparin nomogram as a practice guideline. Arch Intern Med 156:1645–1649, 1996.
37. Hirsh J, Warkentin TE, Shaughnessy SG, et al. Heparin and low-molecular-weight heparin: mechanisms of action, pharmacokinetics, dosing, monitoring, efficacy, and safety. Chest 119:64S–94S, 2001.
38. Niccolai CS, Hicks RW, Oertel L, et al. Unfractionated heparin: focus on a high-alert drug. Pharmacotherapy 24(8 Pt 2):146S–155S, 2004.
39. Becker RC, Corrao JM, Bovill EG, et al. Intravenous nitroglycerin-induced heparin resistance: a qualitative antithrombin III abnormality. Am Heart J 119:1254–1261, 1990.
40. Horrow JC. Protamine: a review of its toxicity. Anesth Analg 64:348–361, 1985.
41. Lovenox (enoxaparin) package insert. Bridgewater, NJ: Aventis, July 2004.
42. Fragmin (dalteparin) package insert. Kalamazoo, Mich: Pharmacia and Upjohn, March 2004.
43. Innohep (tinzeparin) package insert. Boulder, Colo: Pharmion, January 2003.
44. Nagge JN, Crowther M, Hirsh J. Is impaired renal function a contraindication to the use of low-molecular-weight heparin? Arch Intern Med 162:2605–2609, 2002.
45. Hirsh J, Levine MN. Low molecular weight heparin. Blood 79:1–17, 1992.
46. Racanelli A, Fareed J, Walenga JM, et al. Biochemical and pharmacologic studies on the protamine interactions with heparin, its fractions and fragments. Semin Thromb Hemost 11:176–189, 1985.
47. Woltz M, Weltermann A, Nieszpaur-Los M, et al. Studies on the neutralizing effects of protamine on unfractionated and low-molecular-weight heparin (Fragmin) at the site of activation of the coagulation system in man. Thromb Haemost 73:439–443, 1995.
48. Hirsh J. Oral anticoagulant drugs. N Engl J Med 324:1865–1875, 1991.
49. Sheareer MJ. Vitamin K. Lancet 345:229–234, 1995.
50. Hirsh J, Dalen JE, Deykin D, et al. Oral anticoagulants: mechanism of action, clinical effectiveness, and optimal therapeutic range. Chest 102:312S–326S, 1992.
51. Hirsh J, Fuster V. Guide to anticoagulant therapy. Part 2: oral anticoagulants. Circulation 89:1469–1479, 1994.
52. Ansell J, Hirsh J, Poller L, et al. The pharmacology and management of the vitamin K antagonists. Chest 126:204S–233S, 2004.
53. Hirsh J, Dalen JE, Anderson DR, et al. Oral anticoagulants: mechanism of action, clinical effectiveness, and optimal therapeutic range. Chest 119:8S–21S, 2001.
54. Zivelin A, Rao L, Viyaja M, et al. Mechanism of the anticoagulant effect of warfarin as evaluated in rabbits by selective depression of individual procoagulant vitamin K-dependent clotting factors. J Clin Invest 92:2131–2140, 1993.
55. Kirkwood TBL. Calibration of reference thromboplastins and standardization of the prothrombin time ratio. Thromb Haemost 49:238–244, 1983.
56. Wittkowsky AK. Pharmacology of warfarin and related anticoagulants. In: Ansell J, Oertel L, Wittkowsky A, eds. Managing oral anticoagulation therapy: clinical and operational guidelines (vol 1). St. Louis, MO: Facts and Comparisions, 2003:1–29.
57. Higashi M, Veenstra DL, Wittkowsky AK, et al. Influence of CYP2C9 genetic variants on the risk of overanticoagulation and of bleeding events during warfarin therapy. JAMA 287:1690–1698, 2002.
58. Alving BM, Strickler MP, Knight RD, et al. Hereditary warfarin resistance. Arch Intern Med 145:499–501, 1985.
59. Mannucci PM. Genetic control of anticoagulation. Lancet 353:688–689, 1999.
60. Oldenburg J, Quenzel E-M, Harbrecht V, et al. Missence mutations at ALA-10 in the factor IX neopeptide: an insignificant variant in normal life but a decisive cause of bleeding during oral anticoagulant therapy. Br J Haematol 98:240–244, 1997.
61. Sadowski JA, Booth SL, Mann KG, et al. Structure and mechanism of activation of vitamin K antagonists. In: Poller L, Hirsh J, eds. Oral anticoagulants. London, UK: Arnold, 1996:9–29.
62. Owens JC, Neely WB, Owen WR. Effect of sodium dextrothyroxine in patients receiving anticoagulants. N Engl J Med 266:76–79, 1962.
63. Richards RK. Influence of fever upon the action of 3,3-methylene bis-(4-hydroxycoumarin). Science 97:313–316, 1943.
64. Demirkan K, Stephens MA, Self TH. Response to warfarin and other oral anticoagulants: effects of disease states. Southern Med J 93:448–454, 2000.
65. Levine MN, Raskob G, Beyth RJ, et al. Hemorrhagic complications of anticoagulant treatment. Chest 126:287S–310S, 2004.
66. Atrial Fibrillation Investigators. Risk factors for stroke and efficacy of antithrombotic therapy in atrial fibrillation: analysis of pooled data from five randomized controlled trials. Arch Intern Med 154:1449–1457, 1994.
67. Bates SM, Greer IA, Hirsh J, et al. Use of antithrombotic agents during pregnancy. Chest 126:627S–644S, 2004.
68. Orme ML, Lewis PJ, DeSwiet MS, et al. May mothers given warfarin breast-feed their infants? Br Med J 1:1564–1565, 1977.
69. Wells PS, Holbrook AM, Crowther NR, et al. The interaction of warfarin with drugs and food: a critical review of the literature. Ann Intern Med 121:676–683, 1994.
70. Cropp JS, Bussey HI. A review of enzyme induction of warfarin metabolism with recommendations for patient management. Pharmacotherapy 17:917–928, 1997.
71. Wahl MJ. Dental surgery in anticoagulated patients. Arch Intern Med 158:1610–1616, 1998.
72. Streptase (streptokinase) prescribing information. Melbourne, Australia: ZLB Behring.
73. Abbokinase (urokinase) prescribing information. North Chicago, Ill: Abbott Laboratories, October 2002.
74. Activase (alteplase, recombinant) prescribing information. San Francisco, Calif: Genentech Inc, October 2002.

75. Arixtra (fondaparinux) prescribing information. Research Triangle Park, NC: GlaxoSmithKline, September 2004.

76. Alban S. From heparins to factor Xa inhibitors and beyond. Eur J Clin Invest 35 (Suppl 1):12–20, 2005.

77. Bijsterveld NR, Moons AH, Boekholdt SM, et al. Ability of recombinant factor VIIa to reverse the anticoagulant effect of the pentasaccharide fondaparinux in healthy volunteers. Circulation 106: 2550–2554, 2002.

78. Argatroban prescribing information. North Chicago, IL: Abbott Laboratories, April 2005.

79. Warkentin TE, Greinacher A. Heparin-induced thrombocytopenia: recognition, treatment, and prevention. Chest 126:311S–337S, 2004.

80. Refludan (lepirudin, recombinant) prescribing information. Montville, NJ: Berlex, October 2004.

81. Herbert JM, Herault JP, Bernat A, et al. Biochemical and pharmacological properties of SANORG 34006, a potent and long-acting synthetic pentasaccharide. Blood 91:4197–4205, 1998.

82. Weitz JI, Hirsh J, Samama MM. New anticoagulant drugs. Chest 126:265S–286S, 2004.

83. Kearon C, Comp C, Douketis D, et al. A dose-response study of a recombinant human soluble thrombomodulin (ART-123) for prevention of venous thromboembolism after unilateral total hip replacement (abstract). J Thromb Haemost 1(Suppl):OC330, 2003.

84. Friederich P, Levi M, Biemond B, et al. Low-molecular-weight inhibitor of PAI-1 (XR5118) promotes endogenous fibrinolysis and reduces postthrombolysis thrombus growth in rabbits. Circulation 96:916–921, 1997.

85. Executive Steering Committee on behalf of the SPORTIF III Investigators. Stroke prevention with the oral direct thrombin inhibitor ximelagatran compared with warfarin in patients with nonvalvular atrial fibrillation (SPORTIF III): a randomized trial. Lancet 362: 1691–1698, 2003.

86. Executive Steering Committee on behalf of the SPORTIF V Investigators. Ximelagatran versus warfarin for stroke prevention in patients with nonvalvular atrial fibrillation (SPORTIF V): a randomized trial. JAMA 293:690–698, 2005.

87. Eriksson BI, Agnell G, Cohen AT, et al. Direct thrombin inhibitor melagatran followed by oral ximelagatran in comparison with enoxaparin for prevention of venous thromboembolism after total hip or knee joint replacement. Thromb Haemost 89:288–296, 2003.

88. Francis CW, Berkowitz SD, Comp PC, et al. Comparison of ximelagatran with warfarin for the prevention of venous thromboembolism after total knee replacement. N Engl J Med 349:1703–1712, 2003.

89. Colwell CW, Berkowitz SD, Comp PC, et al. Randomized, double-blind comparison of ximelagatran, an oral direct thrombin inhibitor, and warfarin to prevent venous thromboembolism after total knee replacement: EXULT B. Abstract 39. Presented at: American Society of Hematology 45th Annual Meeting; December 6-9, 2003; San Diego, CA.

90. Eriksson BI, Agnelli G, Cohen AT, et al. The oral direct thrombin inhibitor ximelagatran, and its subcutaneous form melagatran, compared with enoxaparin for prophylaxis of venous thromboembolism in total hip or total knee replacement: the EXPRESS study (abstract). Blood 100:299, 2002.

91. Schulman S, Wahlander K, Lundstrom T, et al. Secondary prevention of venous thromboembolism with the oral direct thrombin inhibitor ximelagatran (THRIVE III). N Engl J Med 349:1713–1721, 2003.

92. Fiessinger JN, Huisman MV, Davidson BL, et al, on behalf of the THRIVE Investigators. Ximelagatran versus low-molecular-weight heparin and warfarin for the treatment of deep vein thrombosis: a randomized trial. JAMA 293:681–689, 2005.

93. Wallentin L, Wilcox RG, Weaver WD, et al, for the ESTEEM Investigators. Oral ximelagatran for secondary prophylaxis after myocardial infarction: the ESTEEM randomized controlled trial. Lancet 362:789–797, 2003.

94. Department of Health and Human Services, Food and Drug Administration, Center for Drug Evaluation and Research, Cardiovascular and Renal Drugs Advisory Committee Meeting transcript, September 10, 2004. Available at: http://www.fda.gov/ohrms/dockets/ac/04/transcripts/2004-4069T1.htm. Accessed May 20, 2005.

95. Oertel LB. Education curriculum for patients and teaching methods. In: Ansell JE, Oertel LB, Wittkowsky AK, eds. Managing oral anticoagulation therapy: clinical and operational guidelines. Gaithersburg, MD: Aspen, 1999:6A1.

96. Tang EOYL, Lai CSM, Lee KKC, et al. Relationship between patients' warfarin knowledge and anticoagulation control. Ann Pharmacother 37:34–39, 2003.

97. Kagansky N, Knobler H, Rimon E, et al. Safety of anticoagulation therapy in well-informed older patients. Arch Intern Med 164: 2044–2050, 2004.

98. Davis NJ, Billett HH, Cohen HW, et al. Impact of adherence, knowledge, and quality of life on anticoagulation control. Ann Pharmacother 39:632–636, 2005.

99. Vermeire E, Hearnshaw H, Royen PV, et al. Patient adherence to treatment: three decades of research. A comprehensive review. J Clin Pharm Ther 26:331–342, 2001.

100. Morris LS, Schulz RM. Patient compliance: an overview. J Clin Pharm Ther 17:183–195, 1992.

101. Menendez-Jandula B, Souto JC, Oliver A, et al. Comparing self-management of oral anticoagulant therapy with clinic management. A randomized trial. Ann Intern Med 142:1–10, 2005.

102. Hawkins D. Economic considerations in the prevention and treatment of venous thromboembolism. Am J Health Syst Pharm 61 (Suppl 7):S18–S21, 2004.

103. Lindmarker P, Hlmstrom M. Use of low molecular weight heparin (dalteparin) once daily, for the treatment of deep vein thrombosis. A feasibility and health economic study in an outpatient setting. Swedish Venous Thrombosis Dalteparin Trial Group. J Intern Med 240:395–401, 1996.

104. Gould MK, Dembitzer AD, Sanders GD, et al. Low-molecular-weight heparins compared with unfractionated heparin for treatment of acute deep venous thrombosis. A cost-effectiveness analysis. Ann Intern Med 130:789–799, 1999.

105. Lloyd AC, Aitken JA, Hoffmeyer UK, et al. Economic evaluation of the use of nadroparin in the treatment of deep-vein thrombosis in Switzerland. Ann Pharmacother 31:842–846, 1997.

106. Hull RD, Raskob GE, Rosenbloom D, et al. Treatment of proximal vein thrombosis with subcutaneous low-molecular-weight heparin vs intravenous heparin. An economic perspective. Arch Intern Med 157:289–294, 1997.

107. Menzin J, Colditz GA, Regan MM, et al. Cost-effectiveness of enoxaparin vs low-dose warfarin in the prevention of deep-vein thrombosis after total hip replacement surgery. Arch Intern Med 155:757–764, 1995.

108. Levine MN, Hirsh J, Gent M, et al. Prevention of deep vein thrombosis after elective hip surgery. A randomized trial comparing low molecular weight heparin with standard unfractionated heparin. Ann Intern Med 114:545–551, 1991.

109. Turpie AG, Bauer KA, Eriksson BI, et al. Fondaparinux vs enoxaparin for the prevention of venous thromboembolism in major orthopedic surgery: a meta-analysis of 4 randomized double-blind studies. Arch Intern Med 162:1833–1840, 2002.

CASE STUDIES

TOPIC: Hypertension and Congestive Heart Failure

THERAPEUTIC DIFFICULTY: Level 2
Sarah B. Karish and Joseph M. Calomo

Chapter 20: Hypertension
Chapter 21: Congestive Heart Failure

■ Scenario

Patient and Setting: WJ, a 59-year-old African American male; ambulatory care clinic

Chief Complaint: Increased shortness of breath (SOB) this past week; WJ attributes SOB to his "cold"

■ History of Present Illness

Requires two pillows to sleep, swollen legs, malaise, weakness, and weight gain; furosemide dose was decreased 2 weeks ago due to hypokalemia; increasing SOB; paroxysmal nocturnal dyspnea (PND); and ankle edema

Medical History: Heart failure (ejection fraction, 15%; New York Heart Association Class II); orthopnea; ventricular tachycardia (controlled with amiodarone); coronary artery disease (CAD); diabetes mellitus (DM) type 2 for 5 years; hypertension (HTN) for 30 years; chronic renal insufficiency

Surgical History: None

Family/Social History: Family History: Mother with heart failure (HR)
Social History: Prior cigarette smoker 3–4 packs/week; quit 30 years ago; 6 cans of beer/week

Medications:
Amiodarone, 200 mg PO QD
Furosemide, 80 mg PO QAM
Avandia, 8 mg PO QD
Spironolactone, 12.5 mg PO QD
Carvedilol, 25 mg PO QAM, 12.5 mg PO QPM
Coumadin, 6 mg PO QD
Digoxin, 0.125 mg PO QD initiated at today's visit

Allergies: No known drug allergies; ACEI-induced cough

■ Physical Examination

GEN: Well-developed, well-nourished man with noticeable SOB
VS: BP 153/91, HR 82, RR 25, T 37°C, Wt 78 kg (Wt 2 months earlier 71 kg), Ht 172 cm
HEENT: + jugular venous distension
COR: rrr, s1s2, no m/r/g
CHEST: Bibasilar rales
ABD: Hepatomegaly
GU: Deferred
RECT: Deferred
EXT: 2+ edema bilat LE
NEURO: Alert and 0 × 3

■ Results of Pertinent Laboratory Tests, Serum Drug Concentrations, and Diagnostic Tests

Fasting

Na 139 (139)	Hct 0.33 (33)	Lkcs 8.2 × 10^9
K 4.0 (4.0)	Hgb 140 (14)	(8.2 × 10^3)
Cl 103 (103)	AST 0.5 (30)	Plts 171 × 10^9
HCO$_3$ 25 (25)	ALT 0.5 (30)	(171 × 10^3)
BUN 11.4 (32)	Alb 20 (2.0)	MCV 80 (80)
Glu 11.6 (210)	SCr 168 (1.9)	Alk Phos 1.5 (90)
Uric Acid 190 (3.2)		T Bili 3.4 (0.2)
Ca 2.2 (8.8)		
HgA1C: 7.2 %		
PO4 0.92 (3.0)		
INR: 3.0		
Mg 1.2 (2.5)		

Lkc differential: WNL
Urinalysis: 2+ protein
Chest x-ray films: Enlarged cardiac silhouette

■ Problem List

Identify principal problems from the scenario in priority order (see Answers in back of book for correct list of problems).

■ SOAP Note

To be completed by the student (see Answers in back of book for correct SOAP Note).

■ QUESTIONS

(See Answers in back of book for correct responses.)

1. The most probable cause for WJ's heart failure exacerbation: (EO-1)
   a. Increased weight
   b. Decrease in furosemide dose

c. Poorly controlled blood pressure

d. Inability to take an ACE ihibitor due to cough

2. Which of the following is a sign and symptom of left-sided HF exacerbation currently present in WJ? (EO-2)
   a. Swollen legs
   b. Shortness of breath
   c. Altered mental status
   d. Increased body weight

3. Which of the following is a nonspecific symptom of HF noted in WJ: (EO-2)
   a. Swollen legs
   b. Shortness of breath
   c. Altered mental status
   d. Increased body weight

4. Which of the following is a contributing factor to WJ's heart failure? (EO-3)
   a. Gender
   b. Patient's age
   c. Hypertension
   d. Increased body weight

5. Which of the following disease processes is **LEAST** likely to be contributing to WJ's HF? (EO-1)
   a. Hypertension
   b. Increased age
   c. Atrial fibrillation
   d. Coronary artery disease

6. Which of the following is WJ's goal blood pressure based on JNC-VII guidelines? (EO-5)
   a. <120/80
   b. <130/80
   c. <140/80
   d. <140/90

7. Identify factors to consider when selecting current medication therapy for WJ. (EO-8)

8. WJ should be monitored for factors that predispose him to digoxin toxicity. Based on the information presented, which of the following is a current factor that would potentially predispose WJ to digoxin toxicity? (EO-4, 6, 8, 9)
   a. Increased age
   b. Hypokalemia
   c. Spironolactone
   d. Hypomagnesemia

9. Describe the mechanisms of action of the pharmacologic interventions in this case. (EO-7)

10. List the current pharmacological and nonpharmacological treatment problems with WJ's treatment plan. Explain your reasoning and provide solutions to therapy. (EO-11)

11. Describe what psychosocial factors may affect WJ's adherence to therapy. (EO-15)

12. Summarize therapeutic, pathophysiologic, and disease management concepts for hypertension utilizing a key points format. (EO-18)

CASE 8

TOPIC: Ischemic Heart Disease

THERAPEUTIC DIFFICULTY: Level 3
Kevin M. Sowinski and Brian R. Overholser

Chapter 21: Congestive Heart Failure
Chapter 23: Ischemic Heart Disease
Chapter 24: Acute Myocardial Infarction

■ Scenario

Patient and Setting: AD, a 60-year-old woman presents for follow-up at cardiology clinic

Chief Complaint: Follow-up appointment for coronary artery disease/post-myocardial infarction care; presents with increasing chest pain, shortness of breath, and leg swelling

■ History of Present Illness

Presents to cardiology clinic complaining of increased chest pain after climbing two flights of stairs or walking three blocks. All episodes of chest pain are relieved by sublingual nitroglycerin. AD reports that "they occur a bit more often" than before her myocardial infarction (MI); also complains of occasional shortness of breath, mainly when climbing stairs or walking, swelling in her ankles and lower legs, and having to get up several times during the night to go to the bathroom; she claims that the shortness of breath and leg swelling are new and have been occurring over the past several weeks.

Medical History: Came to the emergency department 6 months ago with an anterior-wall MI; received fibrinolytic therapy for the MI; has a long history of uncontrolled hypertension.

Surgical History: Tonsillectomy and adenoidectomy, age 9; appendectomy, age 22

Family/Social History: Family History: Mother died at age 55 of lung cancer; father died at age 61 of heart failure

Social History: Married with three children, all alive and well; active smoker, has smoked approximately one and a half packs of cigarettes per day for 40 years; drinks alcohol occasionally (~ 1–2 drinks per day, 5 × a week)

Medications:
Aspirin, 325 mg PO daily
Atenolol, 50 mg PO once daily
Nitroglycerin, 0.4 mg SL as needed for chest pain
Nifedipine XL, 30 mg PO daily
Hydrochlorothiazide (HCTZ), 50 mg PO twice daily
Potassium chloride, 10 mEq PO daily
Beclomethasone nasal inhaler
Conjugated estrogens, 0.625 mg PO daily
Medroxyprogesterone acetate, 2.5 mg PO daily

Allergies: PCN and "novocaine"

■ Physical Examination

GEN: Slightly obese female, in moderate distress, increased leg edema, nocturia, and SOB
VS: BP 145/105, HR 85, T 37.3, RR 24, Wt 80 kg, Ht 158 cm
HEENT: AV nicking and narrowing, retinal exudates
COR: Normal S_1, S_2, + S_3, and + S_4 with gallop, + JVD, − HJR
CHEST: Bilateral rales
ABD: Soft, nontender, hepatomegaly, abdominal striae
GU: Deferred
RECT: Heme (−)
EXT: 1+ ankle edema
NEURO: WNL

■ Results of Pertinent Laboratory Tests, Serum Drug Concentrations, and Diagnostic Tests

Na 137 (137)	Hct 0.37 (37)	AST 0.42 (25)
K 4.7 (4.7)	Hgb 123 (12.3)	ALT 0.32 (19)
Cl 103 (103)	Lkcs 4.8 x 10^9 (4.8 x 10^3)	LDH 1.30 (78)
HCO_3 23 (23)	Plts 220 x 10^9 (220 x 10^3)	Ca 2.27 (9.1)
BUN 8.57 (24)		PO_4 1.0 (3.2)
SCr 177 (2.0)	Cholesterol Panel (7 months ago)	Mg 0.9 (1.8)
Glu 7.05 (127)	TC: 249 mg/dL	
	LDL-C: 155 mg/dL	
	HDL-C: 38 mg/dL	
	TG: 280 mg/dL	

ECG: Old Q waves in leads V1–V4, voltage changes consistent with LVH, rate of 85 bpm with occasional premature ventricular contractions

■ Problem List

Identify principal problems from the scenario in priority order (see Answers in back of book for correct list of problems).

■ SOAP Note

To be completed by the student (see Answers in back of book for correct SOAP Note).

■ QUESTIONS

(See Answers in back of book for correct responses.)

1. Identify and list evidence of end-organ damage secondary to hypertension in AD. (EO-1, 2)

2. Which of the following is a sign or symptom of left-sided heart failure? (EO-2)
   a. Bilateral rales
   b. + JVD
   c. Hepatomegaly
   d. Splenomegaly

3. Which of the following is the most likely etiology of AD's heart failure? (EO-1, 3)
   a. Coronary artery disease
   b. Renal insufficiency
   c. Estrogen replacement therapy
   d. Hypertension

4. AD is to be started on ACE inhibitor therapy. Which of the following ACE inhibitor regimens will provide this patient with a dose shown to reduce mortality postmyocardial infarction in controlled clinical trials? (EO-8, 10, 12)
   a. Captopril 25 mg TID
   b. Enalapril 5 mg BID
   c. Lisinopril 20 mg daily
   d. Benazepril 10 mg daily

5. Six weeks after AD is initiated on enalapril therapy she develops a dry nonproductive cough that keeps her awake at night. Which of the following changes to her antihypertensive regimen is most appropriate for treating her hypertension, alleviating her cough, and reducing heart failure symptoms? (EO-10, 11, 12)
   a. Continue enalapril and add dextromethorphan at bedtime
   b. D/C enalapril and initiate lisinopril therapy
   c. D/C enalapril and initiate valsartan therapy
   d. D/C enalapril and initiate terazosin therapy

6. Which of the following physical assessment findings is most consistent with a prior myocardial infarction? (EO-2)
   a. ECG findings of old Q waves in leads V1–V4
   b. S_3 heart sound

c. ECG findings of voltage changes

d. Chest pain with exertion

7. Given AD's risk factors and previous myocardial infarction, which of the following is the *most* appropriate LDL goal in this patient? (EO-5, 12)

   a. <70 mg/dL
   b. <110 mg/dL
   c. <130 mg/dL
   d. <150 mg/dL

8. Which of the following anti-ischemic drugs have been shown to affect long-term outcome in patients who are postmyocardial infarction? (EO-8, 12)

   a. Carvedilol
   b. Amlodipine
   c. Isosorbide mononitrate
   d. Diltiazem

9. Your medical team wants to initiate digoxin therapy for this patient. What is an appropriate maintenance dose for AD? (EO-6, 8, 12)

   a. 0.125 mg PO every other day
   b. 0.125 mg PO daily
   c. 0.25 mg PO daily
   d. 0.375 mg PO daily

10. When communicating medication instructions to AD, which of the following is NOT a reason to immediately contact her health care provider? (EO-14, 15, 16)

    a. Shortness of breath that does not go away with rest
    b. Weight gain of 2 to 3 pounds in 1 week
    c. Swelling in ankles, feet, and/or legs
    d. Persistent cough and/or wheezing

11. To help AD stop smoking, she is started on nicotine gum. What should you tell AD about the proper use of nicotine gum? (EO-14, 16)

12. What patient education would you give AD about the proper use of her sublingual nitroglycerin tablets? (EO-12, 14, 15)

13. Summarize the risk-factor reduction therapies for this patient's ischemic heart disease. (EO-12, 14, 15)

14. Summarize the nonpharmacologic treatment options for this patient's heart failure.

15. Summarize therapeutic, pathophysiologic, and disease management concepts related to the treatment of heart failure/myocardial infarction in this patient utilizing a key points format. (EO-18)

CASE 9

TOPIC: Thromboembolic Disease

THERAPEUTIC DIFFICULTY: Level I
Laurie J. Schmitt

Chapter 25: Thromboembolic Disease

■ Scenario

Patient and Setting: GS, an 89-year-old Hispanic male, hospital

Chief Complaint: Hospitalized after 1 week of fever, vomiting, and mental status changes for empirical treatment of pneumonia. GS is not ambulating due to his illness and had one episode of vomiting in the past 24 hours. Renal function has improved since admission when BUN was 23 (65) and CR 186 (2.1); baseline CR 110 (1.2). GS is being given IV fluids for hydration and an albuterol inhaler PRN for shortness of breath (SOB).

■ History of Present Illness

GS has received 3 days of IV moxifloxacin 400 mg daily for treatment of pneumonia

Medical History: None

Surgical History: None

Family/Social History: Family History: Noncontributory
Social History: Lives alone at home, denies smoking or ETOH use

Medications:
MVI daily

Allergies: No known drug allergies

■ Physical Examination

GEN: Very pleasant, comfortable
VS: BP 138/76, HR 78, RR 18, T 37°C, Wt 62 kg, Ht 170 cm
HEENT: WNL
COR: RRR
CHEST: Diffuse rales present bilaterally, diminished breath sounds
ABD: WNL
GU: Deferred
RECT: Deferred

EXT: No edema
NEURO: Alert and oriented × 3

■ **Results of pertinent Laboratory Tests, Serum Drug Concentrations, and Diagnostic Tests**

Na 141 (141)	U/A: negative	T Bili 3.4 (0.2)
K 4.5 (4.5)	Hct 0.36 (36)	
Cl 105 (105)	Hgb 130 (13)	
HCO$_3$ 28 (28)	Lkcs 10 × 10^9 (10 × 10^3)	AST 0.50 (30)	Glu 6.1 (110)
BUN 14 (38)		ALT 0.50 (30)	Ca 2.2 (8.8)
CR 168 (1.9)	Plts 221 × 10^9 (221 × 10^3)	LDH 1.7 (100)	PO4 0.92 (3.0)
		Alk Phos 1.5 (90)	Mg 1.2 (2.5)
	MCV 93.8 (93.8)	Alb 3.5 (3.5)	Uric Acid 190 (3.2)

Chest x-ray–LLL infiltrate
Factor V Leiden–WNL
Protein C & S–WNL
Factor VIII–WNL
Urine culture: negative
ECG: normal

■ **Problem List**

Identify principal problems from the scenario in priority order (see Answers in back of book for correct list of problems).

■ **SOAP Note**

To be completed by the student (see Answers in back for book for correct SOAP Note).

■ **QUESTIONS**

(See Answers in back of book for correct responses.)

1. Which of the following is the likely etiology for the risk of developing VTE in GS? (EO-1)
   a. Venous stasis as a result of hospitalization
   b. Hypercoagulable state as a result of Factor V Leiden mutation
   c. Endothelial damage as a result of surgery
   d. Increased clearance of clotting factors as a result of renal disease

2. List 3 of the most common signs/symptoms to monitor that may indicate the presence of both DVT and PE in GS. (EO-2)

3. List the clinical risk factors that GS has for venous thromboembolic disease. (EO-3)

4. What is the diagnostic test that is preferred to diagnose both DVT and PE? (EO-5)

5. Which of the following statements is most accurate regarding the treatment options available to prevent VTE? (EO-6)
   a. The onset of UFH's antithrombotic effects may take up to 4 days.
   b. LMWHs do not require any laboratory monitoring.
   c. Warfarin is not associated with any drug-drug interactions.
   d. LMWHs are available in an oral formulation.

6. Which of the following represents the appropriate monitoring for each medication? (EO-5)
   a. Enoxaparin efficacy is monitored with an Aptt.
   b. Warfarin efficacy is monitored with an aPTT.
   c. Warfarin efficacy is monitored with an INR.
   d. UFH efficacy is monitored with an INR.

7. Which statement below is correct? (EO-7)
   a. LMWHs inhibit antithrombin III only.
   b. Unfractionated heparin inhibits thrombin and factor Xa.
   c. Warfarin interferes with clotting factors II, VII, IX, and X.
   d. Fibrinolytics inactivate plasminogen.

8. List two nonpharmacologic measures that can be used to help prevent VTE. (EO-7)

9. Which of the following is an adverse drug effect that should be monitored when using UFH and LMWHs? (EO-10)
   a. Hyperaldosteronism
   b. Hypercalcemia
   c. Thrombocytopenia
   d. Hypertension

10. What is an appropriate dose of enoxaparin (Lovenox) for the prevention of VTE? (EO-11)
    a. 1 mg/kg SQ q12 hrs
    b. 1.5 mg/kg SQ q24 hrs
    c. 5000 units SQ q12 hrs
    d. 40 mg SQ q24 hrs

11. Which of the following is the most appropriate agent to be used in a patient being administered UFH who becomes overanticoagulated? (EO-11)
    a. Protamine sulfate
    b. Danaparoid
    c. Vitamin K
    d. Alteplase

12. Summarize therapeutic, pathophysiologic, and disease management concepts for thromboembolic disease utilizing a key points format. (EO-18)

Critical Care Therapy

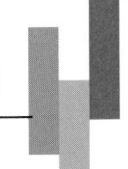

Bradley A. Boucher, G. Dennis Clifton, and Scott D. Hanes

Critical care medicine is a multidisciplinary subspecialty that has realized remarkable growth over the last 40 to 50 years, paralleling advances in life support technologies. Individuals requiring intensive care unit (ICU) management include general surgical, cardiothoracic, and neurosurgery patients; victims of major trauma and burns; medical patients with acute life-threatening single or multiple organ failure; and high-risk obstetric and neonatal patients. Common features among the majority of these patients are their acuity, complex pathophysiologic states, and the use of a large number of pharmacologic agents in their management. On average, these patients have six to nine drugs prescribed per day while being cared for in the ICU.[1] Table 26.1 lists categories of agents commonly administered to medical and surgical ICU patients. Recognition of the drug therapy selection, dosing,

and monitoring demands within the ICU by pioneering clinical pharmacists in the 1970s spawned the development of critical care as a specialty within the pharmacy profession.[1-3] Since that time, this practice area has grown immensely, with hundreds of pharmacists providing care to ICU patients on a full- or part-time basis in virtually all types of ICU settings (e.g., medical ICUs, coronary care units, surgical ICUs, trauma and burn centers, neonatal ICUs, neurology/neurosurgical ICUs). In addition, scores of aspiring practitioners and researchers continue to receive postgraduate critical care pharmacy training annually.[4] Further testimony to the maturation of critical care pharmacy practice was a landmark position paper endorsed jointly by the Society of Critical Care Medicine and the American College of Clinical Pharmacy published in 2000 outlining the scope of practice for critical care pharmacists.[5] This chapter intro-

TREATMENT GOALS

- Minimize patient mortality and morbidity through the use of invasive and noninvasive monitoring, extensive observation, and intensive care by health care providers specialized in critical care medicine.
- Restore curable patients to an independent state following acute injury or illness.
- Restore or improve the baseline state of chronically ill patients following an acute exacerbation or deterioration of their illness.
- Use pharmacologic and supportive therapies (e.g., mechanical ventilation, dialysis) to resuscitate unstable patients and restore them to physiologic stability.
- Use all pharmacotherapy in a rational and cost-effective manner.
- Individualize pharmacotherapy in patients with organ dysfunction through the application of relevant pharmacokinetic and pharmacodynamic principles.
- Maximize utilization of limited health care resources by appropriate selection and optimal management of patients receiving expensive or technically sophisticated therapies.
- Provide emotional and psychological support to patients and family members thrust into the typically overwhelming and unknown environment of the ICU.

Table 26.1	Medications Commonly Administered in Medical and Surgical Intensive Care Units
Analgesics	Anxiolytics/antipsychotics
Antianginals	Bronchodilators
Antiarrhythmics	Catecholamines
Antimicrobials	Corticosteroids
Anticoagulants	Diuretics
Anticonvulsants	Inotropes
Antiemetics	Insulin
Antihypertensives/vasodilators	Neuromuscular blocking drugs
Antipyretics (acetaminophen/aspirin)	Stress ulcer prophylaxis (H_2-receptor blockers, proton pump inhibitors, sucralfate)

duces the practice of critical care therapeutics by outlining several general principles relevant to the care of ICU patients and highlighting the management of medical problems frequently encountered in the critically ill patient population.

USE OF THE PROBLEM-ORIENTED METHOD

Developing a pharmacist-oriented problem list is an essential initial step in the process of formulating a monitoring and treatment plan for patients in general. Use of the problem-oriented approach is particularly important in the care of critically ill patients considering the relative complexities of their medical problems. Because these patients commonly have multiorgan system involvement, it is strongly recommended that the critical care pharmacy practitioner reflect on each respective organ system (e.g., central nervous system, pulmonary system, cardiovascular system) to determine whether a problem or potential problem amenable to initiation or modification of pharmacologic therapy exists. In so doing, the formidable challenge of evaluating critically ill patients is significantly simplified by breaking the medical problems down into more manageable pieces. Furthermore, the task of identifying appropriate monitoring parameters for treatment success or failure, including drug toxicity, is more easily accomplished. This latter task is aided substantially by the relative wealth of clinical and laboratory data available in critically ill patients for this purpose, compared to other hospitalized patients and the ambulatory patient care environment.

PHARMACOKINETIC AND PHARMACODYNAMIC CONSIDERATIONS

Critically ill patients undergo a number of physiologic changes during their acute stress that have the potential to dramatically affect drug disposition or response in these patients relative to more stable patients or healthy volunteers. Among these changes is a surge in catecholamines and other

vasoactive substances commonly observed in critically ill patients that can have significant effects on cardiac output (CO) and systemic vascular resistance (SVR). These effects may result in increases or decreases in drug delivery to the kidneys and liver by altering renal and hepatic blood flow, respectively. Mechanical ventilation (MV) settings, especially very high positive end-expiratory pressure (PEEP), may also reduce hepatic blood flow. Another important hemodynamic alteration often observed in critically ill patients is hypotension accompanying various shock states (e.g., cardiogenic, hemorrhagic, septic, neurogenic). Prolonged hypotension may not only result in acute pharmacokinetic alterations, but in end-organ damage as well [e.g., acute renal failure (ARF), hepatic dysfunction, gut ischemia]. In severe ARF cases, patients may require hemodialysis or other forms of renal replacement therapy to sustain homeostasis. Drug removal by the particular type of renal replacement therapy is another important factor to consider relative to design of dosing regimens.

A number of other factors may affect drug disposition in critically ill patients. One of these factors is the release of cytokines during the acute-phase response. Several in vitro and animal studies have provided evidence that many of the proinflammatory cytokines [e.g., interleukin-1 (IL-1), interleukin-6 (IL-6), and tumor necrosis factor (TNF)] decrease cytochrome P-450 enzyme concentrations or activity, which could affect many drugs used in the critical care setting that undergo hepatic oxidative metabolism.[6] Critically ill patients are also susceptible to protein binding changes as an indirect consequence of acute stress. For example, during the acute-phase response, patients typically become very catabolic, which can result in profound hypoalbuminemia. This may cause significant reductions in the protein binding of acidic drugs. Other patients receiving highly protein bound, basic drugs (e.g., lidocaine) may have significant increases in protein binding accompanying dramatic rises in α_1-acid glycoprotein (AAG) concentrations. The pharmacokinetic implications of these protein binding changes on the total and unbound drug concentrations are largely determined by the clearance properties of the drug in question

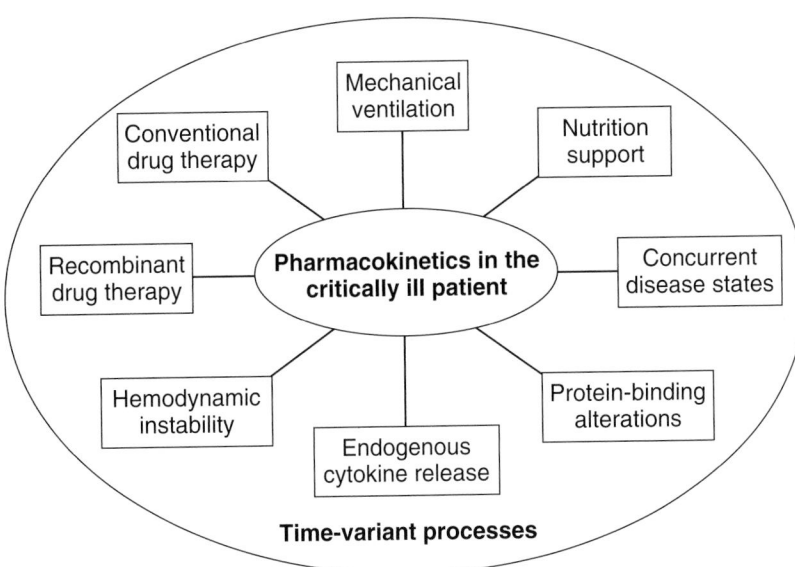

FIGURE 26.1 Potential factors affecting drug disposition in critically ill patients. The possibility of temporal changes in these factors must also be considered secondary to the dynamic nature of this patient subset.

(i.e., high extraction vs low extraction).[7] Finally, considering the large number of medications administered to critically ill patients, the potential for pharmacokinetic and pharmacodynamic drug interactions increases substantially. Although these interactions may be well tolerated in other patient populations, critically ill patients may be particularly susceptible to any associated adverse effects due to their unstable physiologic state.

Figure 26.1 summarizes the wide array of variables that may potentially affect drug disposition and response in critically ill patients. Superimposed on these many variables is the dynamic nature of the critically ill patient. For example, pharmacokinetic parameter estimates at one point in time may be dramatically different from those obtained only a short time later in the patient's hospital course. Thus, critical care pharmacy practitioners facing the daunting task of designing treatment regimens and monitoring therapy in these individuals need to have a keen appreciation of these many factors. In addition, surveillance of the primary literature for pharmacokinetic and pharmacodynamic investigations of specific drugs in various critically ill patient subsets is of utmost importance. Despite the difficulty in conducting these investigations because of numerous confounding variables, increasing numbers of studies are being published each year. Readers are directed to the textbook entitled *The Pharmacologic Approach to the Critically Ill Patient*, third edition, focusing on drug use in the critically ill for a more comprehensive treatment of this topic.[8]

DRUG ADMINISTRATION IN THE INTENSIVE CARE UNIT

Individual patient care plans in critically ill patients should always include assessment of the most appropriate and cost-effective route of drug administration. All routes of drug administration, including intravenous (IV), intramuscular (IM), intraarterial, epidural, intraventricular, intrathecal, subcutaneous (SC), oral, sublingual, rectal, inhalation, and topical, are used in the ICU setting. The route of drug administration depends on available dosage forms, intended use of the agent, functionality and availability of the gut, duration of action, urgency of treatment, and the hemodynamic stability of the patient. The duration of action of cardiovascular-acting agents is especially important when dealing with hemodynamically unstable patients. In these patients, IV administration of short-acting cardiovascular agents is generally preferred. The rapidity by which the desired effect takes place is also an important variable in deciding the type and route of drug administration. For example, the pharmacologic management of hyperkalemia may be performed over a period of hours by oral administration of sodium polystyrene sulfonate or more rapidly with the IV administration of insulin or sodium bicarbonate.

INTRAVASCULAR

Antimicrobials, inotropes, vasopressors, vasodilators, and analgesics administered to critically ill patients are most commonly administered intravenously. Additionally, the IV route is often used to administer nutrition, blood products, fluids, and electrolytes. Unfortunately, large numbers of concurrent drugs, limited sites of access, fluid restriction, and drug incompatibilities often complicate IV drug therapy in the ICU. These factors require critical care practitioners to be knowledgeable about many facets of IV therapy.

The number of IV medications that must be administered simultaneously often exceeds the available number of IV access sites. Consequently, it is essential that the chemical compatibility of agents mixed or infused together be known. In addition, a fluid-restricted patient may require that drugs be mixed in the minimum amount of fluid possible. Manufacturers' package inserts, along with a variety of published references and charts, are available to assist clinicians in determining the compatibility and stability of various drugs.[9] These publications provide useful guidelines but do not cover all possible combinations of specific drugs, their concentrations, routes, or conditions of administration. Pharmacists must be cautious, and generally should avoid mixing drugs together when no compatibility or stability data exist. The absence of visual changes when two drugs are admixed or when a single drug is highly concentrated does not ensure compatibility or stability. An additional consideration is the ability of the infusion device to be used to accurately deliver a highly concentrated solution.

Most IV solutions are administered to critically ill patients through peripheral veins. Central venous administration of agents is used when pharmacologic agents or electrolytes may be damaging to peripheral veins or when peripheral venous access is limited or nonexistent. Vasopressor agents (e.g., norepinephrine, dopamine) should always be administered via a central vein. Peripheral venous administration of these agents is associated with the risk of ischemic necrosis and sloughing of superficial tissues if extravasation occurs (i.e., infiltration of the catheter and solution out of the vein and into the surrounding tissues). If extravasation occurs, the medication should be discontinued and the tubing disconnected from the catheter. Highly concentrated solutions of certain agents (e.g., potassium chloride) may also be very irritating and damaging to the peripheral vein. A major concern for central venous catheters used for drug administration is the development of infection at the puncture site. This may lead to thrombophlebitis, venous thrombosis, embolism, or septicemia. Meticulous aseptic technique is essential for inserting and caring for the catheter. Other complications of central catheter placement include pneumothorax, systemic infection, arrhythmias (pulmonary artery catheter), pulmonary infarction, and air embolism.

Occasionally, drugs may be administered directly into an artery. The most common indication for this route is for local administration of a drug. For example, thrombolytic agents may be infused through a catheter whose tip is placed near an arterial thrombus. The high pressures encountered in the arterial circulation necessitate administration of such agents via an infusion pump capable of operating under these conditions. A catheter for monitoring arterial blood pressure and obtaining arterial blood gases is often placed in the radial or ulnar artery of critically ill patients. The patency of this catheter, or *art line*, is generally maintained with a slow-flowing heparinized solution.[10] These lines should not be used for drug administration.

EPIDURAL

Epidural administration of narcotics, particularly morphine, fentanyl, sufentanil, alfentanil, and hydromorphone alone or in combination with local anesthetics such as bupivacaine, is very effective for the relief of acute pain.[11] The analgesic

agent(s) may be administered by continuous infusion with or without intermittent bolus doses, or intermittent doses alone. Respiratory depression, however, is less common with continuous-infusion regimens. The incidence of pruritus, urinary retention, hypotension, vomiting, and sedation may be higher with this route of narcotic administration. Epidural analgesia is generally contraindicated in patients who have systemic infections, are receiving anticoagulant therapy, or have a coagulopathy. Only preservative-free medications should be administered directly into the epidural space.

INHALATIONAL

The pulmonary route for local and systemic drug administration is frequently used in critically ill patients. Inhalation of β-adrenergic and muscarinic bronchodilators, corticosteroids, mucolytics, surfactants, prostaglandin, and antibiotics is used to achieve local effects in the lower airways. These agents, if commercially available, may be administered via metered-dose inhalers (MDIs) or by nebulization. The choice of technique also depends on the ability of the patient to cooperate or assist with treatment. Nebulization treatments and MDIs can also be used in patients who are intubated and mechanically ventilated. Use of MDIs with or without a ventilator circuit has considerable advantages over nebulizers such as reduced personnel time, reduced use of specialized equipment, reduced cost, improved reliability of dosing, and lower risk of contamination.[12,13] Deposition of drug in the lung is highly variable when an aerosol is given through the ventilator circuit and is dependent on the technique of administration. Efficiency of the aerosol delivery to the lung approaches 30% to 35% of the administered dose when a spacer device is used, a value much higher than that reported for nebulizers.[13] Variables that may be modified to modify the quantity of drug deposited in the lower airways include the aerosol-generating characteristics of the delivery device, the delivery device's position in the ventilatory circuit, the mechanical ventilator settings, the characteristics of the ventilator circuitry and endotracheal tube, and the relative humidity of inspired air.[14]

Systemic administration of selective cardiovascular-acting agents via the endotracheal tube may be performed in emergency situations in which venous access has not been established. Agents in which endotracheal administration has proven to be effective include epinephrine, atropine, and lidocaine.[15] When administered by this route, a catheter for drug administration should be advanced beyond the tip of the endotracheal tube. Two to 2.5 times the normal dose should be administered followed by delivery of several quick breaths.[15]

OTHER ADMINISTRATION ROUTES

Although the IM, SC, and oral routes of drug administration frequently are used in the ICU, they cannot be used in every patient. IM, SC, and oral routes of administration require adequate blood flow to the site of administration for systemic absorption to occur. In patients with shock, the circulatory system redistributes blood flow away from the skeletal muscle, skin, and gastrointestinal system to preserve blood flow to vital organs. Thus both the extent and rate of systemic absorption may be severely affected in such conditions. Additionally, patients with thrombocytopenia, a coagulopathy, or those receiving anticoagulant medications should not receive IM injections due to the increased risk of bleeding and hematoma formation. Many drugs cannot be given IM due to limited solubility, pH of the solution, or the injection volume. For example, IM phenytoin is extremely painful due to the high pH required to manufacture a soluble formulation. When administering medications orally, the pharmacist should carefully monitor the gastrointestinal function of the patient. Significant changes in the extent or rate of absorption may occur in patients with gastroparesis, ileus, or diarrhea. Knowledge of food-drug interactions is also essential. For example, enteral feeds may significantly reduce the absorption of phenytoin, placing the patient at increased risk for seizure activity.[16]

SPECIAL PROBLEMS IN THE CRITICALLY ILL PATIENT

CENTRAL NERVOUS SYSTEM

Pain, Anxiety, Agitation, and Delirium. The most common central nervous system (CNS) problems encountered in critically ill patients are acute pain, anxiety, agitation, and delirium. Pain may be a consequence of direct trauma or invasive procedures, or it may accompany pre-existing medical problems.[3] Anxiety is the psychophysiologic response to the anticipation of real or imagined danger sensed by critically ill patients. The causes of anxiety are multifactorial including: inability to communicate, continuous noise and lighting within the ICU environment, sleep deprivation, and the circumstances leading to the ICU admission.[3] Agitation (i.e., excitement accompanied by motor restlessness) can result from excessive anxiety, delirium, and adverse drug effects and withdrawal in addition to pain.[3] Delirium is defined as an acute change or fluctuation in mental status, plus inattention, and either disorganized thinking or an altered level of consciousness.[3] Delirious patients may or may not have accompanying agitation.[3] Withdrawal in patients with a history of alcoholism is another common problem in critically ill patients, especially trauma victims. To minimize suffering and emotional stress in ICU patients, it is imperative that adequate attention be given to pain relief and sedative therapy.

In general, the goal of analgesic and sedation therapy is to provide an optimal level of comfort and safety for critically ill patients.[3] The Society of Critical Care Medicine has constructed an algorithm as a guide to critical care practitioners to assist in accomplishing this goal.[3] The most commonly used analgesics for acute pain within the ICU setting are parenteral opiate analgesics, most notably morphine, fentanyl, and hydromorphone.[3] The use of meperidine in this setting is not recommended.[3] In addition to a short duration of action, meperidine also has an active metabolite that can accumulate and result in CNS excitation.[3] Effective analgesic dosage requirements of these agents can vary tremendously, emphasizing the need for individualization of therapy while monitoring closely for adverse effects. *Adverse effect* is a relative term, however, because sedation associated with the use of opiates is often an added benefit in the ICU setting. Alternatives to systemic analgesic therapy include regional nerve blocks and epidural infusions. Advantages of these techniques are decreased risk of respiratory depression, hypotension, sedation, nausea, and hypomotility of the gastrointestinal tract.[3] Less potent analgesics such as acetaminophen and nonsteroidal anti-inflammatory drugs (e.g., ketorolac) should also be considered as the acute pain being experienced by the critically ill patient begins to subside. In the latter case, ketorolac use should be limited to 5 days or less to minimize adverse effects (e.g., gastrointestinal bleeding, ARF).[17,18] The benzodiazepines, midazolam and, lorazepam, and propofol are the most commonly used anxiolytics/sedatives in ICU patients. Midazolam is recommended for short-term use only (<48 to 72 hours) while proprofol is the preferred sedative when rapid wakening is important.[3] Lorazepam is recommended for most patients where intermittent or long-term use is anticipated.[3] Parenteral haloperidol is the preferred agent used to manage delirium in the critically ill patient because of its pharmacologic inhibition of dopaminergic activity in the CNS.[3,19] Use of individual treatment goals and objective assessment scales for pain, sedation, and delirium (Table 26.2) are recommended for ongoing monitoring critically ill patients.[3,20–22] Benzodiazepines are considered first-line therapy in the management of alcohol withdrawal.[23] Neuromuscular blocking agents such as pancuronium and vecuronium are important adjunctive agents in agitated patients requiring mechanical ventilation.[24] Regardless, use of these agents should be considered an option of last resort.[24] These agents should always be administered with sedative agents administered prior to the neuromuscular blocking agent to prevent further anxiety and emotional distress during the paralysis period.[24] The anxiety accompanying paralytic use relates to the feeling of helplessness and fear with loss of voluntary muscle control. Use of peripheral nerve stimulators for monitoring neuromuscular blockers is relatively commonplace in ICUs using continuous paralytic therapy. Specifically, the ''train-of-four'' response upon stimulation by the peripheral nerve stimulator is the most frequently used technique for monitoring neuromuscular blocking drugs.[24] Persistent paralysis after discontinuation is now appreciated as a significant risk associated with the use of neuromuscular blocking agents in ICU patients.[24] Hence, dosages and duration of therapy should be minimized as much as possible, with cessation of the paralytic therapy at least once daily to assess the need for continued paralysis.[24] Table 26.3 summarizes dosing regimens, typical onset of action, and duration of activity for the

Table 26.2	Sedation and Agitation Scales

Ramsay Scale

Awake levels:

1. Patient anxious and agitated or restless or both

2. Patient cooperative, oriented, and tranquil

3. Patient responds to commands only

Asleep levels, depends on response to a light glabellar tap or loud auditory stimulus:

4. Patient responds briskly

5. Patient responds sluggishly

6. Patient does not respond

Riker Sedation-Agitation Scale

Score	Description	Example
7	Immediate threat to safety	Pulling at endotracheal tube or catheters, trying to climb over bed rail, striking at staff
6	Dangerously agitated	Requiring physical restraints and frequent verbal reminding of limits, biting endotracheal tube, thrashing side-to-side
5	Agitated	Physically agitated, attempting to sit up, calms down to verbal instructions
4	Calm and cooperative	Calm, arousable, follows commands
3	Oversedated	Difficult to arouse or unable to attend to conversation or commands
2	Very oversedated	Awakens to noxious stimuli only
1	Unarousable	Does not awaken to any stimuli

(From Riker RR, Picard JT, Fraser GL. Prospective evaluation of the Sedation-Agitation Scale for adult critically ill patients. Crit Care Med 27:1325–1329, 1999; and Ramsay MA, Savege TM, Simpson BR, et al. Controlled sedation with alphaxalone-alphadolone. Br Med J 2:656–659, 1974.)

most commonly used analgesics, sedatives, and paralytics in the ICU setting.

Neurotrauma. In contrast to the symptomatic problems of pain and anxiety frequently encountered in critically ill patients, CNS disorders that may result in ICU admission include traumatic brain injury and spinal cord injury (SCI). Although not all patients with acute neurotrauma are admitted to an ICU, those with the most severe insults typically require supportive care and intensive monitoring. Patients suspected of having a brain injury or SCI should undergo a thorough physical and neurologic examination along with computed tomography. The Glasgow Coma Scale (GCS) is the most widely used system to grade the arousal and functional capacity of the cerebral cortex in these patients.[25] A GCS of 3–8, 9–12, and 13–14 is consistent with severe, moderate, and minor head injury, respectively (Table 26.4). The possibility that ethanol or drug intoxication, hypoglycemia, severe electrolyte disturbances, infection, hypoxia, hypotension, or spinal cord injury may alter the initial neurologic examination should always be considered. Thus initial laboratory tests for all patients with suspected neurologic injury should include a urine drug screen, blood ethanol concentration, complete blood count, electrolytes, glucose, blood urea nitrogen, and serum creatinine.

The initial management goal in these patients is to establish an adequate airway and maintain breathing and circulation during the initial period of evaluation (ABCs of resuscitation). Control of increased intracranial pressure (ICP) is also a priority in head injury patients, considering its potential to decrease cerebral blood flow (CBF) and thus cerebral delivery of oxygen (CDO_2). Nonpharmacologic and pharmacologic approaches in managing increased ICP (i.e., greater than 20 mm Hg) include mild hyperventilation ($PaCO_2$ 35–40 mm Hg); elevating the patient's head to 30 degrees; moderate, osmotic and loop diuretics; hypertonic saline and barbiturate coma in refractory patients.[26,27] See Boucher et al for a more extensive discussion of this topic.[28] In addition to close monitoring of ICP, cerebral perfusion pressure (CPP), which is the difference between MAP and ICP (i.e., CPP = MAP − ICP), should also be monitored. The CPP is essentially the pressure gradient driving CBF. It is recommended that the CCP be maintained greater than 60 mm Hg in patients with severe head injury.[29]

Neurotrauma patients should generally be kept euvolemic, with systemic blood pressure maintained in a normotensive range in an attempt to sustain CBF without exacerbating elevations in ICP. Patients with systemic hypertension should receive α-blockers, β-blockers, or angiotensin-converting enzyme inhibitors because they do not

Table 26.3	Clinical Use of Selected Analgesics, Sedatives, and Paralytics Commonly Used in Critically Ill Patients		
Agent	**Dose**	**Onset of Action**	**Duration of Activity**
Analgesics			
Morphine	0.01–0.15 mg/kg q 1–2 h IV	<1 min	4–5 h
	0.07–0.5 mg/kg/h IV infusion		
	5–10 mg q 4 h IM/SC	10–30 min	4–7 h
Fentanyl	0.7–10 µg/kg/h IV infusion	30 s	30–60 min
Hydromorphone	10–30 µg/kg q 1–2 h IV	5 min	3–4 h
	7–15 µg/kg/h IV infusion		
Ketorolac	15–30 mg q 6 h IV	10 min	6 h
Sedatives			
Lorazepam	0.02–0.06 mg/kg q 2–6 h IV	5–20 min	4 h
Midazolam	0.02–0.08 mg/kg q 0.5–2 h IV	2–5 min	15 min–6 h
	0.04–0.2 mg/kg/h IV infusion		
Haloperidol	0.03–0.15 mg/kg q 0.5–6 h IV	3–20 min	>24 h
Propofol	5–80 µg/kg/min IV infusion	1–2 min	8–10 min
Neuromuscular blocking drugs			
Pancuronium	0.06–0.1 mg/kg prn	2–5 min	90–100 min
	120–180 µg/kg/min IV infusion	3–6 min	
Vecuronium	0.08–0.1 mg/kg IV prn	3–5 min	35–45 min
	45–60 µg/kg/min IV infusion		

(From Hassan E, Fontaine DK, Nearman HS. Therapeutic considerations in the management of agitated or delirious critically ill patients. Pharmacotherapy 18 : 113–129, 1998; Murray MJ, Cowen J, DeBlock H, et al. Clinical practice guidelines for sustained neuromuscular blockade in the adult critically ill patient. Crit Care Med 30 : 142–156, 2002; Sedation, analgesia, and neuromuscular blockade of the critically ill adult: revised clinical practice guidelines for 2002. Am J Health Syst Pharm 59 : 147–149, 2002; and Jacobi J, Farrington EA. Supportive care of the critically ill patient. In: Carter B, L,, Lake KD, Raebel MA, et al, eds. Pharmacotherapy Self-Assessment Program, Critical Care, Module 2. Kansas City: American College of Clinical Pharmacy, 1998 : 129–159.)

typically affect ICP. Use of sedatives (e.g., benzodiazepines, barbiturates) and opiate analgesics may also be effective in lowering transiently increased blood pressure. Use of the venodilators, nitroprusside and nitroglycerin, and selected calcium channel blockers (e.g., nicardipine, diltiazem) should be avoided because they may have the undesirable effect of increasing cerebral blood volume, thereby increasing ICP.

By maintaining ventilation and CDO_2, further cerebral ischemia may be prevented or attenuated. This is of utmost importance because ischemia is thought to trigger extension of the primary insult into uninjured tissue (i.e., secondary neuronal injury) following acute head injury and SCI. In essence, cerebral ischemia results in cellular hypoxia and loss of cell membrane integrity. This can lead to major intracellular and extracellular ionic shifts, resulting in cytotoxic edema (with or without concurrent increased intracranial pressure), intracellular acidosis, electrical failure, and eventual generation of reactive oxygen species (e.g., oxygen-free radicals). The importance of understanding the pathophysiology of secondary neuronal injury is readily apparent in light of the many promising pharmacologic strategies available or under investigation that attempt to modulate this de-

structive cascade of events. These strategies include calcium channel blockers, glutamate antagonists, antioxidants, and nonsteroidal anti-inflammatory drugs.[27,28]

Despite several unsuccessful attempts at attenuating secondary neuronal injury, the results of two landmark investigations provide optimism for further breakthroughs in this arena. The first investigation was the second National Acute Spinal Cord Injury Study (NASCIS 2).[30] In this multicenter study, SCI patients randomized to receive methylprednisolone 30 mg per kg IV over 15 minutes followed by a 5.4 mg/kg/hour infusion for 23 hours had a significant increase in motor and sensory function at 6 weeks and 6 months compared to placebo patients in those patients receiving therapy within 8 hours after injury. Thus, all future SCI patients should receive methylprednisolone within this 8-hour treatment window because there is no alternative therapy of proven benefit at present to offer these patients. Results of the follow-up trial referred to as NASCIS 3 corroborated the findings of NASCIS 2 and suggested that patients receiving therapy between 3 and 8 hours after injury have improved outcomes when treated with methylprednisolone for 48 hours versus 24 hours (i.e., 5.4 mg/kg/hour).[31] Unfortunately, patients receiving the longer duration of therapy also

Table 26.4	Glasgow Coma Scale	
	Response	**Score**
Eyes	Open spontaneously	4
	To verbal command	3
	To pain	2
	No response	1
Best Motor Response		
To verbal command	Obeys	6
To painful stimulus (pressure to nail beds)	Localizes pain	5
	Flexion-withdrawal	4
	Flexion-abnormal (decorticate rigidity)	3
	Extension (decerebrate rigidity)	2
	No response	1
Best Verbal Response		
(Arouse patient with painful stimulus if necessary)	Oriented and converses	5
	Disoriented and converses	4
	Inappropriate words	3
	Incomprehensible sounds	2
	No response	1
	Total	3–15

(From Jennett B, Teasdale G. Aspects of coma after severe head injury. Lancet 1 : 878–881, 1977.)

had more severe sepsis and pneumonia compared with those receiving 24 hours of methylprednisolone.[31]

Seizure Treatment and Prophylaxis. Seizures are caused by a variety of conditions in ICU patients, including mechanical brain injury, cerebral hypoxia/ischemia, CNS infections, metabolic disorders, and chronic alcohol abuse. Of these conditions, seizures in patients with moderate to severe brain injury are of particular concern because the seizure activity can greatly increase cerebral metabolism. Patients experiencing status epilepticus (seizures lasting longer than 5 minutes or repetitive seizures without recovery of consciousness between events) should receive initial therapy consisting of incremental IV doses of lorazepam (0.1 mg/kg) followed by IV phenytoin or fosphenytoin if the seizures continue and/or prevent seizure recurrence.[32] In addition, prophylactic phenytoin or fosphenytoin should be considered in patients with mild to moderate brain injury based on a landmark study by Temkin and colleagues in 1990.[33] Data from this study do not support the use of phenytoin beyond 7 days unless seizures are observed. Aggressive phenytoin therapy is recommended during the treatment period to maintain total concentrations in the range of 10 to 20 mg per L (40 to 80 mmol/L). This can generally be achieved using an adult IV loading dose of 18 to 20 mg per kg followed by an initial adult daily maintenance dose of 2.5 to 3.0 mg per kg every 12 hours. The potential for phenytoin's metabolism to increase as a function of time should also be considered in severe brain injury patients.[34] See Chapter 63 for a thorough discussion of managing non–trauma-related seizures. The treatment of status epilepticus was reviewed by Lowenstein and Alldredge.[32]

PULMONARY SYSTEM

Mechanical Ventilation. A high percentage of critically ill patients are mechanically ventilated for all or a portion of their ICU stay. The objectives of mechanical ventilation (MV) include improvement of pulmonary gas exchange, relief of respiratory distress, alteration of pressure-volume relationships (e.g., atelectasis, decreased compliance), and allowance of lung and airway healing. Basic MV settings include the fraction of inspired oxygen (FiO_2) (i.e., the percent of oxygen contained in the inhaled gas), tidal volume (5 to 15 mL/kg), ventilation rate, and positive end-expiratory pressure (PEEP). Because of the toxic effects of oxygen to the lung, the lowest FiO_2 that will achieve satisfactory arterial oxygenation [arterial oxygen pressure (PaO_2) exceeding 60 mm Hg or arterial hemoglobin saturation (SaO_2) exceeding 90%] is used. Positive end-expiratory pressure is often used to prevent alveolar collapse at the end of expiration. The principal therapeutic effect of PEEP is to improve or maintain PaO_2 or SaO_2 while allowing a decrease in FiO_2. See recent review articles for a more thorough discussion of MV therapy.[35]

Several important factors and variables should be considered and monitored by pharmacists caring for patients who receive MV. Nosocomial pneumonia is a common complication of MV, occurring in up to 30% of patients and is associated with increased mortality.[36] If signs and symptoms of pneumonia appear, empiric antibiotic treatment aimed at the most likely pathogens should be promptly initiated. Infectious sinusitis also occurs frequently in mechanically ventilated patients, particularly those patients who have nasotracheal tubes.[37] The presence of infectious sinusitis also increases the likelihood of developing nosocomial pneumonia. Mechanical ventilation is an independent risk factor for the development of stress–related mucosal damage and gastrointestinal bleeding in critically ill patients.[38] Thus, patients at risk should receive appropriate acid-suppressive therapy or gut mucosal protection. Mechanical ventilation can also be an uncomfortable and frightening experience for patients. Although use of proper ventilatory settings and reassurance of the patient are the primary treatments for distress and agitation, analgesics, sedatives, and neuromuscular blocking agents are also frequently used to facilitate patient tolerance and delivery of optimal ventilation. The use of sedation scales is encouraged to prevent oversedation and potentially prolonged requirement for MV as previously noted. *Train of four* monitoring should be performed during neuromuscular blockade to minimize prolonged muscle paralysis. Finally, mechanical ventilation can have significant hemodynamic effects. Increased transmural pressure causes a decrease in ventricular distensibility and increases in peripheral vascular resistance. Consequently, cardiac output can be decreased secondary to decreased venous return and impaired contractility.

When weaning the patient from MV, a number of other factors should be considered to improve the patient's likelihood for successful extubation. These include the provision of adequate nutrition supplementation and correction of electrolyte disturbances, especially hypophosphatemia, which could impair oxygen delivery and respiratory muscle function.[39] Long-acting sedatives and narcotic analgesics should be used sparingly if at all when trying to wean patients from the ventilator. Optimization of bronchodilator therapy in patients with underlying obstructive or bronchospastic pulmonary disease may also aid in successful extubation of patients.

Acute Respiratory Distress Syndrome. The acute (formerly adult) respiratory distress syndrome (ARDS) is a condition defined by impaired oxygenation (P_aO_2/FiO_2 ratio 200) associated with bilateral pulmonary infiltrates on frontal chest radiograph and a pulmonary artery capillary wedge pressure (PCWP) of 18 mm Hg or less. Injury is characterized by diffuse alveolar damage, increased vascular permeability, and the development of noncardiogenic pulmonary edema. When damage is severe, the air spaces fill with fluid, resulting in deterioration in gas exchange and mechanical properties of the lung.[40] ARDS may result from direct lung injury such as pneumonia, aspiration of gastric contents, inhalation of toxins, or indirectly from conditions such as bacterial sepsis or pancreatitis. The mortality rate associated with ARDS approaches 50%, with most patients dying from the underlying predisposing illness, severe sepsis, or multiple organ dysfunction syndrome. The current clinical management of ARDS involves primarily supportive measures aimed at maintaining gas exchange and oxygen delivery. No specific measures currently exist to correct the abnormalities associated with ARDS. Mechanical ventilation with PEEP is typically required for at least 10 to 14 days in most patients. Although traditional tidal volumes were delivered at 10 to 15 mL per kg, the use of lower tidal volumes (6 mL/kg) has been shown to decrease patient mortality and ventilator days secondary to less mechanical stress on the lung tissue.[41] Fluid management is also important because intravascular hydrostatic pressures may contribute to pulmonary edema. Therapy should be aimed at achieving the lowest PCWP while maintaining an adequate CO. If sepsis is presumed to be the cause of ARDS, empiric antibiotic therapy should be instituted early. Evidence suggests that a trial of methylprednisolone, 2 mg/kg/day for 32 days, beginning 1 to 2 weeks following the onset of ARDS in patients with severe disease may attenuate the fibroproliferative phase of the disorder.[42]

CARDIOVASCULAR SYSTEM

Principles of Oxygen Delivery and Consumption. The primary goal of life support techniques used in modern critical care units is to achieve and maintain optimal tissue oxygenation. Although traditional hemodynamic monitoring of pressures and flow is important for providing measures of tissue perfusion, this monitoring does not allow assessment of oxygenation. Earlier studies have shown that oxygen transport monitoring is superior to hemodynamic monitoring alone, particularly in high-risk, critically ill patients.[43,44] Interventions designed to achieve supraphysiologic indices (cardiac index, oxygen delivery, oxygen consumption) are not universally accepted, secondary to equivocal evidence of efficacy[45] and possibly increased mortality rates.[46] A recent meta-analysis suggested that significantly decreased mortality rates may only occur in those who achieve early optimization prior to the onset of organ failure.[47] Nonetheless, ensuring adequate tissue oxygenation is still a cornerstone of medical therapy in the critically ill patient.

Oxygen demand is dependent on the overall rate of tissue metabolism rate and the intrinsic ability of tissues to extract oxygen. Generally, little can be done to alter oxygen demand. However, interventions aimed at reducing metabolic rate such as lowering body temperature, skeletal muscle paralysis, or sedation may modestly lower overall oxygen demand. Hence, most interventions are directed at improving the transportation of oxygen to tissues. The delivery of oxygen (DO_2) to tissues is the product of cardiac index (CI) and arterial oxygen content (CaO_2). The actual amount of oxygen consumed at the tissue level (VO_2) may be calculated as the product of CI and the difference between CaO_2 and mixed venous oxygen content (CvO_2). Arterial and venous oxygen content are dependent on the hemoglobin concentration, the percent oxygen saturation of arterial or mixed venous hemoglobin (SaO_2 or SvO_2), and, to a minor extent, the amount of oxygen dissolved in plasma. The percentage of oxygen extracted by the tissues (O_2 ER) is calculated as ($CaO_2 - CvO_2$)/CaO_2. Oxygen transport variables, their calculation, and normal values are listed in Table 26.5. In addition to SaO_2, SvO_2, CaO_2, CvO_2, DO_2, and VO_2, other clinical and laboratory parameters commonly used to monitor the adequacy of tissue oxygenation include arterial pH, total CO_2 content, lactic acid levels, blood pressure, heart rate, temperature, respiratory rate, urine output, and mental status.

Altering CI, CaO2, or both may increase oxygen delivery and result in improved tissue oxygenation. One approach to improving tissue oxygenation is outlined in Figure 26.2. Patients who are anemic, and subsequently have a low hemoglobin concentration, may benefit from transfusion of red blood cells. Commonly used methods to improve SaO_2 include increases in FiO_2 and PEEP. Improvements in CO can be achieved by ensuring appropriate heart rate and stroke volume. Stroke volume is dependent on preload, afterload, and contractility. Pharmacologic therapies aimed at correcting these hemodynamic variables are addressed in other chapters of this textbook and include the use of fluids, vasodilators (e.g., nitroprusside), inotropes (e.g., dobutamine), and antiarrhythmics (including atropine, β-blockers, and digoxin). The maneuver that yields the greatest improvement in DO_2 as determined by calculating its effect on oxygen transport variables is generally the one that should be used. This is usually determined by assessing the clinical status of the patient in conjunction with hemodynamic measurements

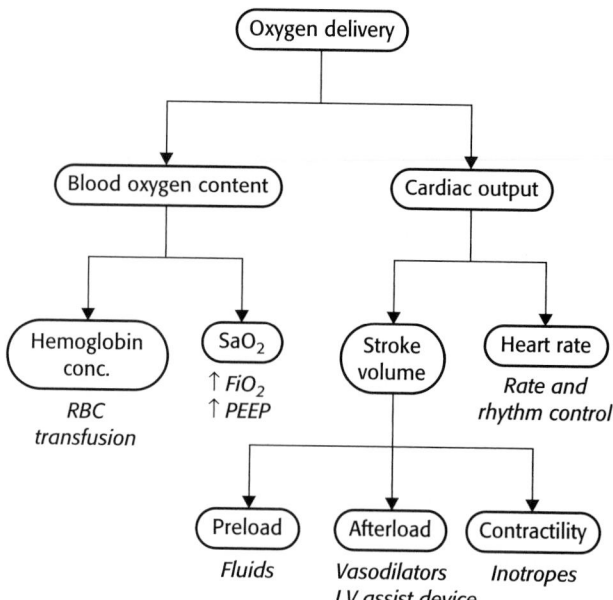

FIGURE 26.2 Factors influencing oxygen delivery to tissues. Means of altering each factor for improved oxygen delivery are provided in *italics*.

obtained from the pulmonary artery catheter. For instance, the volume status of the patient is estimated by analyzing the left ventricular end-diastolic pressure (LVEDP). Unfortunately, many factors, particularly increasing PEEP, can significantly affect the accuracy of correlating LVEDP with left ventricular end-diastolic volume. Recently, right ventricular end-diastolic volume has proven to be a more reliable indicator of volume status than LVEDP.[48] Thus assessing right rather than left ventricular function may more reliably optimize DO_2.

The drawback of oxygen transport monitoring as described is that it provides only an indication of global tissue

Table 26.5	Oxygen Transport Variables, Normal and Goal Values			
Parameter	**Abbreviation**	**Calculation**	**Normal Value**	**Goal**
Arterial Hgb saturation	SaO_2	Measured	95%–99%	>95%
Mixed venous oxygen saturation	SvO_2	Measured[a]	65%–75%	>60%
Arterial oxygen content	CaO_2	(Hgb × SaO_2 × 1.34[b]) 9 + (PaO_2 × 0.0031[c])	17–20mL O_2/dL	
Venous oxygen content	CvO_2	(Hgb × SvO_2 × 1.34) 9 + (PvO_2 × 0.0031)	12–15mL O_2/dL	
Oxygen delivery	DO_2	CI × CaO_2 × 10	529–720 mL/min/m²	
Oxygen consumption	VO_2	($CaO_2 - CvO_2$) × CI × 10	100–150 mL/min/m²	
Oxygen extraction ratio	O_2 ER	($CaO_2 - CvO_2$)/CaO_2	22%–30%	

Cardiac index (L/min/m²); Hgb, hemoglobin (g/dL); PaO_2, arterial pressure of oxygen in blood (mm Hg); PvO_2, venous pressure of oxygen in blood (mm Hg).
[a] Obtained from pulmonary artery blood.
[b] Milliliters of O_2/1 g Hgb.
[c] Solubility coefficient of O_2 in plasma.

oxygenation and may not detect regional or organ-specific mismatching of oxygen delivery and utilization. Tissue-specific markers of oxygen utilization such as gastric intra-mucosal pH (gastric tonometry) have been developed recently and are being used to obtain evidence of regional adequacy of tissue oxygenation.[49] Despite extensive experience with gastric tonometry, however, no trial has documented better outcomes with tonometry-directed therapy.

Acute Coronary Syndromes. Acute coronary syndromes encompass ST-segment elevated myocardial infarction, non–ST-segment myocardial infarction, and unstable angina. The medical management of uncomplicated ST-segment elevated acute myocardial infarction (AMI) is well established (see Chapter 24).[50] As an alternative to primary percutaneous coronary intervention (PCI) and in the absence of contraindications, pharmacologic treatment with thrombolytics and aspirin should be initiated within 30 minutes of patient presentation to the hospital. To achieve the greatest benefit, thrombolytics should be administered within 12 hours from the onset of symptoms. IV unfractionated or SC fractionated or unfractionated heparin should be initiated during alteplase, tenecteplase, and reteplase therapy and following streptokinase therapy when the APTT returns to <2 times control. In those patients not receiving thrombolytic therapy, standard heparin or low-molecular-weight heparin should be initiated. IV β-adrenergic blocking agents should be administered as early as possible in the course of therapy (i.e., within 12 hours), as should nitroglycerin. Chronic therapy with β-adrenergic blocking agents is also indicated, especially for patients at high risk for reinfarction. Oral angiotensin-converting enzyme inhibitors are indicated in patients with anterior myocardial infarctions, particularly those with ejection fractions below 40%. Therapy should be initiated as soon as the patient is hemodynamically stable, preferably within 24 hours after the infarction and continued indefinitely to reduce left ventricular remodeling and development of congestive heart failure. Additional consideration should be given as to providing adequate analgesia and correcting electrolyte disorders.

Treatment for patients suffering from non-ST elevated coronary syndromes is also well established.[51] Early use of aspirin, β-blockers, nitrates, and heparin parallel those therapies when used for ST segment elevated myocardial infarction. In addition, a platelet glycoprotein IIb/IIIa receptor antagonist such as eptifibatide or tirofiban should be considered in patients with continuing ischemia, other high-risk features (such as positive cardiac markers), or when PCI is planned.

Cardiogenic Shock. Cardiogenic shock can occur as a complication of AMI in 6% to 20% of survivors. However, the incidence and related mortality of cardiogenic shock after an AMI is decreasing because of advances in medical and invasive therapy. A variety of other conditions such as acute myocarditis, myocardial contusion, and decompensation in patients with end-stage heart failure may also result in car-

diogenic shock. Clinically, cardiogenic shock is defined as reduced cardiac index (<2.2 L/min/m^2) and evidence of tissue hypoxia (i.e., O$_2$ ER >31%, oliguria, cyanosis, cool extremities, altered mentation) in the presence of adequate intravascular volume.

Specific treatment of cardiogenic shock is preceded by correcting problems of hypoxia, fluid and electrolyte abnormalities, acidosis, and restoring sinus rhythm.[52] Restoration of adequate DO$_2$ to tissues occurs primarily through improving myocardial systolic function (Fig. 26.2). Inotropic agents such as dobutamine, amrinone, milrinone; and vasodilators such as sodium nitroprusside work to improve forward blood flow and reduce pulmonary edema. Dobutamine is preferred to dopamine and norepinephrine in cardiogenic shock; however, the latter two agents are useful in patients who are profoundly hypotensive. The phosphodiesterase inhibitors, amrinone and milrinone, have positive inotropic activity and vasodilatory action. The phosphodiesterase inhibitors can be used in conjunction with or substituted for dobutamine in cardiogenic shock because their mechanisms of action are different and thus additive. Sodium nitroprusside is particularly useful in reducing systemic vascular resistance (afterload), improving CI, and reducing myocardial VO$_2$. Sodium nitroprusside and nitroglycerin also lower left ventricular filling pressures (preload), which helps reduce oxygen consumption. Nesiritide (human B-type natriuretic peptide) has recently become available and may also be useful in lowering preload in selected patients. Venodilating agents such as nitroprusside, nitroglycerin, and nesiritide may also improve DO$_2$ by reducing pulmonary edema, improving gas exchange, and subsequently increasing blood oxygen content. Intra-aortic balloon counterpulsation, which increases diastolic coronary filling and decreases afterload, is used in cardiogenic shock, especially in patients with high systemic vascular resistance but low blood pressures (i.e., systolic <90 mm Hg.). Ventricular assist devices represent an even more aggressive approach to therapy, particularly when the cause of cardiogenic shock is potentially reversible.

Cardiogenic shock secondary to right ventricular failure occurs less frequently and is a challenge to manage. Adequate filling pressures must be maintained because these patients are particularly sensitive to volume depletion. Dobutamine is used to increase right ventricular contractility and reduce pulmonary vascular resistance.

Acute Cardiac Arrhythmias. Ventricular and supraventricular cardiac arrhythmias are frequently encountered in critically ill patients. The specific management of acute cardiac arrhythmias is covered in Chapter 22. When cardiac arrhythmias occur in critically ill patients, they are often precipitated by some other event or abnormality. Correctable causes of cardiac arrhythmias such as electrolyte abnormalities, hypoxia, acid-base disturbances, and drug toxicity should always be assessed and managed if present. Pharmacologic management of cardiac arrhythmias can generally be discontinued once the underlying abnormality is corrected or the precipitating factor removed. If the arrhythmia persists, the goals of therapy are to control the ventricular rate (atrial arrhythmias), convert to sinus rhythm, maintain sinus rhythm, and prevent complications (e.g., ischemic stroke).

Hypertensive Emergencies and Urgencies. *Hypertensive crisis* is a term used to refer to hypertensive emergencies and hypertensive urgencies. A *hypertensive emergency* is severe hypertension (i.e., systolic blood pressure 180 mm Hg or greater, diastolic blood pressure 110 mm Hg or greater) associated with symptoms of end-organ damage. Included in this definition are patients with hypertension associated with complications such as acute congestive heart failure, AMI, unstable angina, hypertensive encephalopathy, intracranial hemorrhage, dissecting aortic aneurysm, or eclampsia. These patients should be hospitalized with immediate lowering of their blood pressure. The initial goal of therapy is to reduce MAP by no more than 25% (within minutes to 2 hours) and then toward 160/100 mm Hg within 2 to 6 hours.[53]

Hypertensive urgency is a term used to describe asymptomatic patients with severe hypertension where lowering of the blood pressure over a period of hours is desirable. These individuals do not exhibit target organ damage and generally do not require hospitalization. Therapy should be initiated with a combination of oral antihypertensive therapy and close follow-up.

A variety of IV medications are available to treat hypertensive emergencies. Labetalol and sodium nitroprusside are especially effective and safe for lowering blood pressure in these situations. Alternative agents include nicardipine and fenoldopam.[53] Use of the once popular maneuver of administering sublingual nifedipine should be avoided due to serious adverse effects associated with its use and the inability to effectively control the fall in blood pressure. When hypertension is complicated by dissecting aortic aneurysm, sodium nitroprusside should be combined with IV β-adrenergic blockers (esmolol), or calcium antagonists (verapamil or diltiazem), or trimethaphan camsylate used. Oral medications agents used to treat hypertensive urgencies include loop diuretics, angiotensin-converting enzyme inhibitors, α_1-agonists, combination β-blocker/α_1-agonists, and calcium channel blockers.[53]

RENAL SYSTEM

Acute renal failure (ARF), defined as an abrupt decrease in the glomerular filtration rate (GFR), is a relatively common problem observed in critically ill patients. This is not surprising considering that shock, severe sepsis, and trauma are among the leading causes of ARF.[54] A smaller number of patients have exacerbation of their chronic renal failure (CRF) as the problem precipitating ICU admission or as a concurrent disease state accompanying an independent acute problem. Regardless of the circumstances, it is essential that the critical care practitioner be aware of the potential for renal insufficiency to be present or to develop in ICU patients and be adept at evaluating their level of renal impair-

ment. In essence, not only may specific treatment be warranted for reversing the ARF or managing the complications of CRF, but also major adjustments in drug-dosing regimens and fluid and electrolyte management may be necessary. In addition, because critically ill patients are particularly susceptible to developing ARF, drugs that may induce renal failure should be identified and used cautiously. The most noteworthy of these agents are the aminoglycosides, amphotericin B, radiocontrast dye, cyclosporine, and nonsteroidal anti-inflammatory drugs (e.g., ketorolac).[55]

Key laboratory tests and monitoring parameters in patients diagnosed or suspected of having acute renal insufficiency include serum creatinine, blood urea nitrogen, urine sodium, urine osmolality, urinalysis, urine creatinine, serum electrolytes, and urine output. After ruling out prerenal causes of ARF (e.g., dehydration, hemorrhage) and urinary obstruction, the primary goals of therapy should be to provide supportive care and avoid complications (e.g., fluid overload, electrolyte imbalances, etc.). An algorithm for management of ARF, including drug therapy can be found in Chapter 42. Restriction of fluids, dietary protein, and electrolytes, especially potassium, magnesium, and phosphorus, is important in oliguric patients to maintain homeostasis. Treating the underlying cause of ARF, such as the use of antibiotics for infected patients and discontinuation of nephrotoxic drugs when feasible, are additional considerations. Recommendations for dosage adjustments for renally eliminated drugs and active drug metabolites can be found in the manufacturer's package insert, selected secondary references sources, and/or the primary literature.[56] A caveat to consider in applying these guidelines is that most equations used to estimate creatinine clearance (e.g., Cockroft and Gault[57,58]) assume that the serum creatinine is at steady state. However, in patients with ARF, serum creatinine may be rising rapidly. Thus either special formulas that take this problem into account must be used,[59] or an acknowledgment must be made that the estimates obtained using the conventional formulas may be significantly overestimating the creatinine clearance.

In contrast to the diagnosis of ARF, the presence of CRF usually can be identified from the patient's history. When possible and appropriate, medications that the patient was receiving before admission should be continued as previously prescribed. Dosage adjustments for newly instituted medications should be made in a manner similar to adjustments in ARF patients, although in this instance, the problem of rapidly changing serum creatinine values usually is irrelevant. In ARF and CRF patients, renal replacement therapy (i.e., hemodialysis, peritoneal dialysis, continuous arteriovenous hemodialysis) may be needed to maintain a homeostatic state. The effects of intermittent hemodialysis and continuous renal replacement therapies on drug-dosing regimens and fluid and electrolyte supplementation are other important areas for the critical care practitioner to understand in order to optimize care in these patients. A thorough discussion of this topic can be found in Chapter 43.

GASTROINTESTINAL SYSTEM

Colonization of the Gastrointestinal Tract and Nosocomial Infections. It has been recognized since the early 1970s that critically ill patients are at risk to develop superficial gastroduodenal lesions (now termed stress-related mucosal damage) that can result in major gastric bleeding if untreated. Major risk factors for developing stress-induced gastrointestinal bleeding are presence of a coagulopathy, respiratory failure for more than 48 hours, and renal failure.[38,60] A thorough discussion of the pathophysiology and treatment alternatives can be found in Chapter 45. Because of the significant morbidity and mortality associated with major gastric hemorrhage, critically ill patients typically receive stress ulcer prophylaxis consisting of one of the following agents: H_2-receptor antagonists, proton-pump inhibitors, (PPIs) sucralfate, or antacids. Due to the frequency of administration required to maintain an elevated gastric pH with antacids, its use is not recommended. In the largest trial comparing prophylactic agents, Cook and colleagues found that ranitidine significantly decreased the incidence of clinically important gastric bleeding compared to sucralfate.[61] Despite the lack of large comparative clinical outcome trials, proton-pump inhibitors frequently are used to prevent stress-related gastrointestinal bleeding. Preliminary evidence from small trials appear to demonstrate that PPIs are at least as effective as H_2-receptor antagonists or sucralfate.[62,63] With the exception of sucralfate, these agents raise gastric pH thereby allowing gastric bacterial colonization. Theoretically, bacteria may migrate and colonize the nasopharynx area increasing the risk of pneumonia via microaspiration of the nasopharynx contents into the lungs. While some studies have found a higher rate of pneumonia with pH altering agents compared to sucralfate[64] a recent meta-analysis[65] found no major difference in pneumonia rates between ranitidine and sucralfate similar to the largest randomized, controlled trial for stress-related mucosal damage prophylaxis.[61] Stress-related mucosal damage prevention also has been questioned by some investigators arguing that many, if not the majority, of patients receive no benefit from these drugs.[38] More studies are needed in specific ICU patient subsets to discern which critically ill patients are at greatest risk for major gastrointestinal bleeding before the practice of no treatment can be advocated.

Liver Dysfunction. Liver dysfunction is a relatively common finding in critically ill patients. Some patients may have a history of severe chronic liver disease (e.g., alcoholic cirrhosis), whereas others may develop acute hepatic dysfunction secondary to direct trauma, infectious hepatitis, drug toxicity, or following an ischemic insult (e.g., hemorrhagic shock). From a therapeutic standpoint, one of the most important considerations in evaluating these patients is the potential for alterations in drug metabolism. Hepatic drug metabolism can be altered by changes in hepatic enzyme activity, blood flow, and protein binding.[6] Enzymatic activity is most commonly affected by drugs that inhibit or induce various cytochrome P-450 enzymes, however the potential for cytokine-induced changes in metabolism is appreciated. Changes in cardiac output (i.e., hyperdynamic sepsis, congestive heart failure, hypovolemic shock) produce significant changes in hepatic metabolism for drugs with a high-first pass effect. Protein binding can be dramatically decreased for acidic, highly protein-bound drugs secondary to hypoalbuminemia. Hyperbilirubinemia can result in protein-binding displacement as well. The pharmacodynamic profile of certain drugs such as anticoagulants may also be altered secondary to diminished clotting factor production and an increased sensitivity to CNS-active drugs.

Acknowledging the potential for pharmacokinetic and pharmacodynamic alterations in critically ill patients with suspected liver disease, several challenges face critical care practitioners in designing therapeutic drug regimens for an individual patient. One issue is that few, if any, hepatic processes are performed at 100% capacity. Therefore, even though liver dysfunction may be present, the effects of this impairment on drug metabolism may be insignificant. The liver also has reparative properties allowing function to return after an acute insult. Finally, unlike creatinine clearance, which is a good estimate of the glomerular filtration rate in patients with renal dysfunction, no analogous predictor of hepatic function is available for clinical use in patients with liver disease. Laboratory tests that are useful in identifying liver disease but not necessarily the extent of damage are: serum albumin; prothrombin time; bilirubin; and the liver enzymes, aspartate aminotransferase (AST), alanine aminotransferase (ALT), and alkaline phosphatase.[66] Thus, careful attention to signs and symptoms of severe liver impairment (e.g., hepatic encephalopathy, hepatomegaly, splenomegaly), in conjunction with these laboratory tests, remains the most viable approach for assessing the level of residual hepatic function in a given patient. After making this assessment, tables summarizing the pharmacokinetic literature relative to the normal disposition pathway for a particular drug or citing specific clinical drug trial findings from patients with liver disease can be used as general guides for drug usage in those individuals deemed to have significant impairment.[66] The use of potentially hepatotoxic drugs should also be carefully evaluated in those critically ill patients with evidence of hepatic dysfunction to avoid exacerbation of the condition.

HEMATOLOGIC SYSTEM

Coagulation and hematologic disorders are common in the ICU population. Routine laboratory monitoring should include a daily complete blood count with platelets, activated partial thromboplastin time (aPTT), and prothrombin time (PT). Commonly encountered hematologic problems include anemia, thrombocytopenia, and neutropenia. The recognition of various noncritical illness-related anemias and their treatment is discussed in Chapters 31 and 32. In the critical care setting, it is imperative that an adequate hematocrit and hemoglobin be maintained to ensure adequate tissue oxygenation. The majority of critically ill patients are anemic (hemoglobin <12 g/dL) on admission or during their ICU stay. The etiology of critical illness-related anemia is multifactorial and includes decreased erythropoiesis, alterations in iron metabolism, increased destruction of red blood cells, bleeding, and frequent phlebotomy.[67] Although transfusion of red blood cells in the form of whole blood or packed red blood cells is commonly used to correct anemia, recent evidence suggests that such transfusion may be harmful to critically ill patients.[68] Alternative treatments such as erythropoietin therapy have been shown to decrease the number of required transfusions while increasing hemoglobin concentrations but have not resulted in decreased mortality.[69]

Platelet Disorders. Thrombocytopenia is perhaps one of the most commonly encountered hematologic abnormalities in critically ill patients. As discussed in Chapter 33, a variety of factors may be responsible for the reduction in platelets seen in this population. Etiologies of thrombocytopenia commonly seen in critically ill patients include disseminated intravascular coagulation, liver disease, immune thrombocytopenic purpura, thrombotic thrombocytopenic purpura, splenic sequestration, physical destruction (cardiopulmonary bypass, intra-arterial balloon pump), massive blood loss or transfusion, and drug-induced causes.[70] The most common drug-related causes include cancer-related chemotherapy and heparin-induced thrombocytopenia (HIT). Immune-related HIT should be considered, particularly if platelet counts begin to fall precipitously following several days of therapy or if platelets fall immediately upon heparin re-exposure in patients recently treated with heparin. If suspected, heparin administration should be discontinued and removed from all flush solutions (e.g., arterial and pulmonary artery catheters). Treatment with direct thrombin inhibitors, argatroban or lepirudin, should be considered due to the high rate of thrombosis associated with HIT.[71]

Decreased platelet counts and/or platelet dysfunction (such as in renal failure) significantly increase the risk of a major bleeding episode. In addition to platelet transfusions, prolonged bleeding times caused by platelet dysfunction have empirically been treated with conjugated estrogens 0.6 mg/kg/day[72] and IV desmopressin at a dose of 0.3 mcg per kg.[73] Oprelviken, recombinant interleukin-11, stimulates platelet production via increased thrombopoietin concentrations and is approved for the prevention of chemotherapy-induced thrombocytopenia.

Disseminated Intravascular Coagulopathy. Disseminated intravascular coagulopathy (DIC), as discussed in Chapter 33, is a common occurrence in critically ill patients, especially those with viral, fungal, or bacterial sepsis, severe tissue injury or ischemia, and ARDS. Microvascular thrombosis associated with DIC may lead to further end-organ damage, including focal skin necrosis, ARF, seizures, and stroke. The management of DIC includes the treatment of the underlying disease while providing supportive measures to maintain circulation and oxygenation. Transfusion of blood products and coagulation factors frequently is administered in patients who demonstrate clinical manifestations of DIC. In addition, patients with DIC related to severe sepsis, should be considered for therapy with drotrecogin alfa activated (recombinant activated protein C).[74]

Deep Venous Thrombosis. Critically ill patients, particularly those suffering major trauma, are at significant risk for the development of deep venous thrombosis (DVT) and the catastrophic occurrence of pulmonary embolism.[75] Risk factors for the development of DVT include tissue injury secondary to trauma and surgery, immobilization, venous stasis, and cardiac dysfunction. Unless specific contraindications exist, all critically ill patients should receive DVT prophylaxis. Prophylaxis generally consists of subcutaneously administered low-dose unfractionated heparin or a low-molecular-weight heparin. Compression stockings and intermittent compression boots are alternatives for DVT prophylaxis in patients with contraindications to heparin-based treatment.[75]

Fluid and Electrolyte Disturbances. The homeostatic mechanisms that maintain normal electrolyte concentrations are often impaired in critically ill patients. In many instances, these abnormalities are a direct result of the patient's primary illness (e.g., hyperkalemia with diabetic ketoacidosis), whereas in others the disturbance may be the result of secondary disorders or a consequence of therapy (e.g., diuretics). Proper correction of the electrolyte disorder is dependent on identification of its cause, estimation of the degree of abnormality, and selection of the appropriate replacement source. Electrolyte abnormalities most commonly observed in critically ill patients include hypokalemia, hypophosphatemia, hypomagnesemia, hypocalcemia, and hyperkalemia. The etiology and manifestations of these electrolyte disorders and their treatment are discussed in Chapter 28.

Nutritional Support. Appropriate nutritional support enhances immune function, reduces length of ICU stay, and increases survival. Nutritional support of hospitalized patients is covered in Chapter 30. Enteral nutrition, particularly when administered distal to the pylorus, can be initiated early in most critically ill patients and should be considered as first-line therapy for those requiring nutritional support. Advantages of enteral nutrition in this population include a decreased rate of complications and mortality, lower cost, improved gastrointestinal protection, and a lower infectious risk profile. The latter advantages may largely be explained by attenuation of bacterial translocation from the gut by maintaining function integrity of the gastrointestinal tract with enteral nutrition.

The selection of the specific route and formulation of the nutritional product depends on the goals of nutritional support, caloric requirements, and the specific nutrients to be delivered. The determination and administration of caloric needs is paramount in critically ill patients. Underfeeding may result in impaired host defenses, delayed wound healing, muscle wasting, and prolonged weaning from MV. Overfeeding is associated with hepatic dysfunction, elevated blood urea nitrogen, hyperglycemia, fluid overload, and excessive carbon dioxide production. The commonly used Harris-Benedict equation is often inaccurate in critically ill patients, resulting in underprediction and overprediction of caloric needs. The measurement of resting energy expenditure by indirect calorimetry can be performed accurately in many critically ill patients and allows individualization of nutritional support. The use of a metabolic cart to measure resting energy expenditure may be particularly valuable in patients with multiple risk and stress factors. Patients who fail to respond adequately to estimated nutritional needs may also benefit from the use of indirect calorimetry.

SIRS, CARS, AND MODS

During periods of acute stress induced by sepsis, trauma, pancreatitis, and so on, critically ill patients undergo a number of metabolic changes secondary to activation of the sympathetic nervous system and the hypothalamic-pituitary-adrenal axis. Specific mediators involved in the acute-phase response include epinephrine, norepinephrine, cortisol, glucagon, and proinflammatory cytokines such as IL-1, IL-6, IL-8, and TNF.[76] The effect of this response is generally an acceleration of whole body metabolism proportional to the intensity of the initiating event or injury.[76] This can manifest itself as depletion of body stores of protein, fat, and carbohydrates or defects in intracellular energy metabolism that can ultimately contribute significantly to major organ dysfunction (e.g., lungs, heart, kidneys, gastrointestinal tract, CNS). Balancing the acute-phase response is an anti-inflammatory response mediated by substances such as IL-4, IL-10, transforming growth factor (TGF)-β, and soluble receptors to the proinflammatory mediators such as TNF and IL-1.[77,78] If the proinflammatory and anti-inflammatory mediators are balanced, homeostasis can be restored. When proinflammatory mediators dominate over anti-inflammatory mediators, an intense inflammatory response known as the systemic inflammatory response syndrome (SIRS) can occur.[79] Activation of polymorphonuclear neutrophils (PMNs), macrophages, endothelial cells, the complement pathway, coagulation factors, and fibrinolytic pathways are key secondary events in this process.[77] Relative tissue hypoxia and generation of reactive oxygen metabolites may be key events in the pathogenesis of organ failure in these patients. When these pathophysiologic processes affect two or more major organs it is referred to as the multiorgan dysfunction syndrome (MODS).[79,80] Regardless of the initiating event, MODS is a condition associated with significant morbidity and mortality in critically ill patients. If anti-inflammatory mediators dominate over proinflammatory mediators, a condition referred to as the compensatory anti-inflammatory response syndrome (CARS) can occur (Fig. 26.3).[81] This condition is characterized by anergy, an increased susceptibility to infection, or both.

Many different investigational therapeutic strategies have been employed that attempt to modulate the acute-phase response in critically ill patients. One such strategy is early and aggressive nutritional support. The goal of nutritional supplementation in this setting is to meet the increased energy and protein requirements typically present in these patients and thus diminish catabolism of body tissue. Another approach is intensive insulin therapy and strict blood glucose control. In a large, prospective randomized trial comparing conventional insulin treatment [i.e., administration if blood glucose >11.8 mmol/L (215 mg/dL)] with intensive insulin therapy [i.e., maintenance of blood glucose between 4.5–6.1 mmol/L (80–110 mg/dL)], a significant reduction in mortality and morbidity was observed in the latter study group.[82] The mechanism underlying the beneficial effects of intensive insulin therapy remain unknown although it could be a direct effect of insulin and/or the maintenance of normoglycemia.[83] Monoclonal antibodies directed against several of the proinflammatory cytokines or their receptors (e.g., anti-TNF antibody, IL-1 receptor antagonist) have also undergone clinical trials.[84] Another approach has been to develop antibodies to molecules responsible for binding PMNs to the endothelial cells during their migration following an inflammatory stimulus.[84] Other approaches include use of antioxidants, prostaglandin inhibitors, and mechanical removal of cytokines.[84,85] The first breakthrough was the use of recombinant activated protein C (drotrecogin alfa activated) in reducing mortality in severe sepsis patients compared to placebo from 31% to 24%.[74] While the success of drotecogin alfa activated in the treatment of severe sepsis is a landmark event, it remains clear that no single strategy will likely be successful in modulating sepsis, SIRS, and CARS in critically ill patients due to the overwhelming complexity of these syndromes. Nonetheless, improved understanding of the pathophysiology underlying the acute-phase response, SIRS, and CARS, and more sophisticated identification of patient subsets manifesting one or both of these latter syndromes offer some promise for affecting the devastating clinical course for these individuals in the future.

PHARMACOECONOMICS

Technologic advances in medical science, coupled with economic incentives, during the past three decades have led to a tremendous increase in the quantity and quality of critical care therapy provided to severely ill patients. This type of care is very expensive. An estimated $62 billion of the approximately $809 billion the United States spent on health care during 1992 was allocated to reimburse charges incurred in the ICU. Approximately 22% of deaths in America occur after ICU admission. The average length of stay for these individuals is 12.9 days at an average cost of $24,541.[86] Because of the high cost of ICU treatment, the aging of America, national debates over rising health care costs, and mechanisms for reimbursement, the cost-effectiveness of

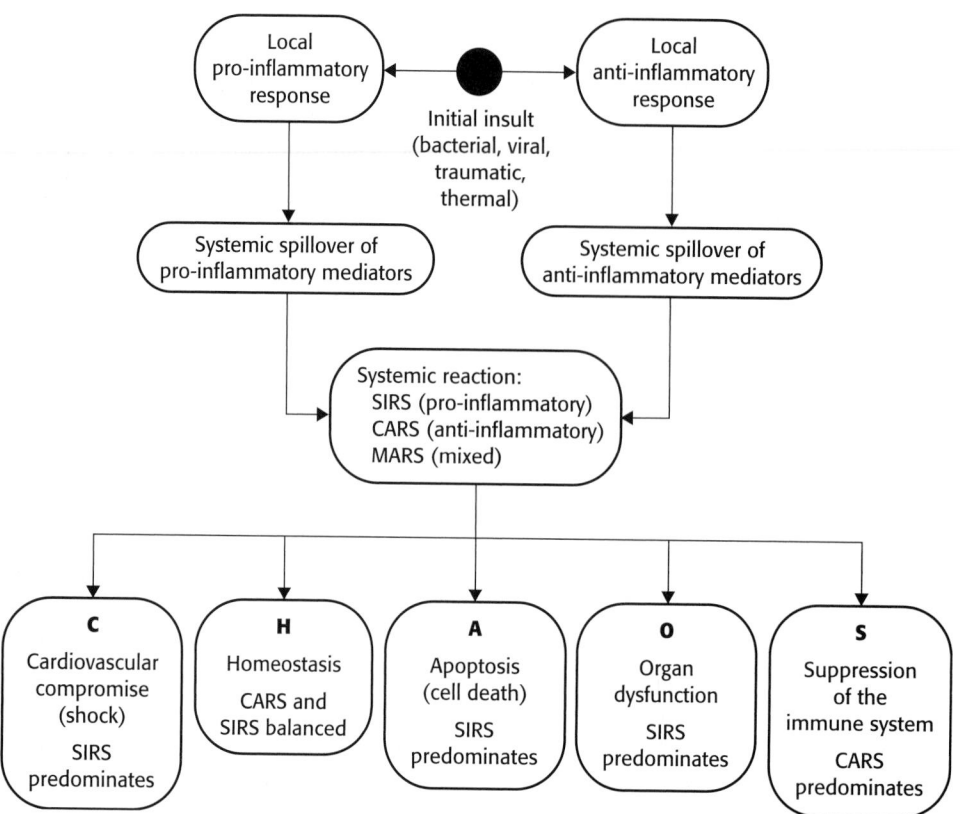

FIGURE 26.3 Clinical sequelae of the systemic inflammatory response syndrome (SIRS) and the compensatory anti-inflammatory response syndrome (CARS). MARS is the mixed antagonistic response syndrome. (Reprinted from Bone RC: Sir Isaac Newton, sepsis, SIRS, and CARS. Crit Care Med 24:1125–1128, 1996, with permission.)

health care provided in this setting is under increasing scrutiny.[87,88]

The introduction of new pharmacologic agents and an increased understanding of the properties and benefits of older agents have contributed significantly to the decrease in morbidity and mortality associated with critical illness. Considerable study has been devoted to determining the clinical benefit of various and competing pharmacologic therapies. Unfortunately, efficacy can no longer be the sole criterion that determines the use of a particular pharmacologic agent in caring for patients. This is particularly true in the critical care setting, where a patient's medication costs per day may reach into the thousands of dollars. A major question regarding the use of new and expensive agents, therefore, aside from their clinical efficacy, concerns their economic impact and added costs. If agents reduce morbidity and improve survival, any additional costs may be partially or completely obviated by reductions in other expenditures or improved quality of life. Rational use of new and expensive drugs involves proper patient selection, treatment guidelines, drug use evaluation techniques, and outcome indicators. The performance of pharmacoeconomic and outcomes research by critical care practitioners is of paramount importance in the development of treatment guidelines and the cost-effective use of drugs. Recent reviews highlight the im-

portance economic research in the critically ill patient, as well as the difficulties associated with this research.[89]

Nonetheless, pharmacists practicing in ICUs have a significant impact not only on the quality of pharmaceutical care but also on the cost of delivering that care. Pharmacotherapy of the critically ill patient typically involves administration of six to nine different drugs during a patient's ICU stay. Thus in-depth knowledge of potential pharmacokinetic and pharmacodynamic alterations, drug-drug interactions, preventable adverse reactions, and drug administration considerations allows the pharmacist to optimize drug therapy while minimizing or reducing costs. Pharmacist involvement in the drug therapy of critically ill patients has been estimated to reduce costs by $72,000 to more than $200,000 annually.[90,91]

CONCLUSION

Medical management of the critically ill patient can be an intimidating and daunting task for those individuals unfamiliar with the special needs of this patient population. Nonetheless, carefully delineating individual problems, identifying appropriate treatment regimens, and formulating a thoughtful monitoring plan can vastly simplify the complexity of caring for these patients. This chapter has attempted to high-light many of the problems frequently encountered in the ICU environment as a starting point in this effort. Although demanding and requiring a high level of commitment of those individuals accepting the challenge of providing care for the critically ill, the rewards can be personally and professionally gratifying. In addition, the demand for critical care pharmacy services is likely to be steadily increasing for the indefinite future.[92]

KEY POINTS

■ Developing a pharmacist-oriented problem list organized by organ system is a highly recommended strategy in monitoring complex, critically ill patients.

■ Critically ill patients undergo a number of physiologic changes and therapeutic maneuvers that can significantly alter pharmacokinetics and pharmacodynamics within the acute care setting.

■ The most appropriate route of drug administration should be individualized for each patient and should be based on available routes of administration, available dosage forms, the pharmacokinetics and pharmacodynamics of the drug, and the clinical situation

■ Provision of adequate analgesia and sedation is essential in the supportive care of virtually all critically ill patients.

■ Early use of high-dose methylprednisolone in the management of patients with spinal cord injury is among a very limited number of therapies demonstrated to be beneficial in attenuating CNS injuries in critically ill patients.

■ Mechanical ventilation frequently is required in critically ill patients and is associated with numerous complications requiring pharmacologic intervention.

■ Cardiac events occur frequently in critically ill patients and require numerous pharmacologic treatment strategies, the most important of which is to maximize tissue oxygen supply and minimize tissue oxygen demand.

■ ARF and hepatic dysfunction are common complications in critically ill patients that can have profound effects on drug product selection and dosing.

■ Use of prophylactic heparin and stress ulcer prophylaxis (e.g., H_2-receptor antagonists, proton pump inhibitors) should be considered in all critically ill patients deemed to be at risk to develop these complications.

■ Attempts to attenuate the acute-phase response and its sequelae (e.g., SIRS, MODS) have largely been unsuccessful to date, highlighting the immense complexity of these events.

REFERENCES

1. Dasta JF, Jacobi J, Armstrong DK. Role of the pharmacist in caring for the critically ill patient. In: Chernow B, ed. The pharmacologic approach to the critically ill patient. Baltimore: Williams & Wilkins,1994:156–166.
2. Majerus TC, Dasta. JF. Practice of critical care pharmacy. Rockville, MD: Aspen Systems, 1985.
3. Jacobi J, Fraser GL, Coursin DB, et al. Clinical practice guidelines for the sustained use of sedatives and analgesics in the critically ill adult. Crit Care Med 30:119–141, 2002.
4. Jacobi J. Critical care pharmacy practice. In: DiPiro JT, ed. Encyclopedia of clinical pharmacy. New York: Marcel Dekker, Inc., 2003: 233–239.
5. Position paper on critical care pharmacy services. Society of Critical Care Medicine and American College of Clinical Pharmacy. Pharmacotherapy 20:1400–1406, 2000.
6. McKindley DS, Hanes S, Boucher BA. Hepatic drug metabolism in critical illness. Pharmacotherapy 18:759–778, 1998.
7. Wilkinson GR, Shand DG. Commentary: a physiological approach to hepatic drug clearance. Clin Pharmacol Ther 18:377–390, 1975.
8. Todi SK, Hartmann RA. Pharmacologic principles. In: Civetta JM, Taylor RW, Kirby RR, ed. Critical care. New York: Lippincott-Raven, 1997:475–488.
9. Trissel LA. Handbook of injectable drugs. Bethesda, MD: American Society of Health-Systems Pharmacists, 2002.
10. Clifton GD, Branson P, Kelly HJ, et al. Comparison of normal saline and heparin solutions for maintenance of arterial catheter patency. Heart Lung 20:115–118, 1991.
11. Block BM, Liu SS, Rowlingson AJ, et al. Efficacy of postoperative epidural analgesia: a meta-analysis. JAMA 290:2455–2463, 2003.
12. Summer W, Elston R, Tharpe L, et al. Aerosol bronchodilator delivery methods. Relative impact on pulmonary function and cost of respiratory care. Arch Intern Med 149:618–623, 1989.
13. Georgopoulos D, Mouloudi E, Kondili E, et al. Bronchodilator delivery with metered-dose inhaler during mechanical ventilation. Crit Care 4:227–234, 2000.
14. Duarte AG, Fink JB, Dhand R. Inhalation therapy during mechanical ventilation. Respir Care Clin N Am 7:233–260, vi, 2001.
15. Guidelines 2000 for Cardiopulmonary Resuscitation and Emergency Cardiovascular Care. The American Heart Association in collaboration with the International Liaison Committee on Resuscitation. Circulation 102:II–384, 2000.
16. Fleisher D, Sheth N, Kou JH. Phenytoin interaction with enteral feedings administered through nasogastric tubes. J Parenter Enteral Nutr 14:513–516, 1990.
17. Feldman HI, Kinman JL, Berlin JA, et al. Parenteral ketorolac: the risk for acute renal failure. Ann Intern Med 126:193–199, 1997.
18. Strom BL, Berlin JA, Kinman JL, et al. Parenteral ketorolac and risk of gastrointestinal and operative site bleeding. A postmarketing surveillance study. JAMA 275:376–382, 1996.
19. Hassan E, Fontaine DK, Nearman HS. Therapeutic considerations in the management of agitated or delirious critically ill patients. Pharmacotherapy18:113–129, 1998.
20. Riker RR, Picard JT, Fraser GL. Prospective evaluation of the Sedation-Agitation Scale for adult critically ill patients. Crit Care Med 27:1325–1329, 1999.
21. Ramsay MA, Savege TM, Simpson BR, et al. Controlled sedation with alphaxalone-alphadolone. Br Med J 2:656–659, 1974.
22. Ely EW, Margolin R, Francis J, et al. Evaluation of delirium in critically ill patients: validation of the Confusion Assessment Method for the Intensive Care Unit (CAM-ICU). Crit Care Med 29: 1370–1379, 2001.
23. Mayo-Smith MF. Pharmacological management of alcohol withdrawal. A meta-analysis and evidence-based practice guideline. American Society of Addiction Medicine Working Group on Pharmacological Management of Alcohol Withdrawal. JAMA 278: 144–151, 1997.
24. Murray MJ, Cowen J, DeBlock H, et al. Clinical practice guidelines for sustained neuromuscular blockade in the adult critically ill patient. Crit Care Med 30:142–156, 2002.
25. Jennett B, Teasdale G. Aspects of coma after severe head injury. Lancet 1:878–881, 1977.
26. Marik PE, Varon J, Trask T. Management of head trauma. Chest 122:699–711, 2002.
27. Marshall LF. Head injury: recent past, present, and future. Neurosurgery 47:546–561, 2000.

28. Boucher BA, Phelps SJ, Timmons SD. Acute management of the brain injury patient. In: DiPiro JT TR, Yee GC, Matzke GR, et al, eds. Pharmacotherapy: a pathophysiologic approach. New York: McGraw-Hill Companies; 1061–1074, 2005.

29. Guidelines for the management of severe traumatic brain injury: cerebral perfusion pressure, March 14, 2003. Available at: www.braintrauma.org. Accessed September 29, 2005.

30. Bracken MB, Shepard MJ, Collins WF, et al. A randomized, controlled trial of methylprednisolone or naloxone in the treatment of acute spinal-cord injury. Results of the Second National Acute Spinal Cord Injury Study. N Engl J Med 322:1405–1411, 1990.

31. Bracken MB, Shepard MJ, Holford TR, et al. Administration of methylprednisolone for 24 or 48 hours or tirilazad mesylate for 48 hours in the treatment of acute spinal cord injury. Results of the Third National Acute Spinal Cord Injury Randomized Controlled Trial. National Acute Spinal Cord Injury Study. JAMA 277: 1597–1604, 1997.

32. Lowenstein DH, Alldredge BK. Status epilepticus. N Engl J Med 338:970–976, 1998.

33. Temkin NR, Dikmen SS, Wilensky AJ, et al. A randomized, double-blind study of phenytoin for the prevention of post-traumatic seizures. N Engl J Med 323:497–502, 1990.

34. Boucher BA, Hanes SD. Pharmacokinetic alterations after severe head injury. Clinical relevance. Clin Pharmacokinet 35:209–221, 1998.

35. Howman SF. Mechanical ventilation: a review and update for clinicians. Hosp Physc 12:26–36, 1999.

36. Chastre J, Fagon JY. Ventilator-associated pneumonia. Am J Respir Crit Care Med 165:867–903, 2002.

37. Rouby JJ, Laurent P, Gosnach M, et al. Risk factors and clinical relevance of nosocomial maxillary sinusitis in the critically ill. Am J Respir Crit Care Med 150:776–783, 1994.

38. Cook DJ, Fuller HD, Guyatt GH, et al. Risk factors for gastrointestinal bleeding in critically ill patients. Canadian Critical Care Trials Group. N Engl J Med 330:377–381, 1994.

39. Agusti AG, Torres A, Estopa R, et al. Hypophosphatemia as a cause of failed weaning: the importance of metabolic factors. Crit Care Med 12:142–143, 1984.

40. Brower RG, Ware LB, Berthiaume Y, et al. Treatment of ARDS. Chest 120:1347–1367, 2001.

41. The Acute Respiratory Distress Syndrome Network. Ventilation with lower tidal volumes as compared with traditional tidal volumes for acute lung injury and the acute respiratory distress syndrome. N Engl J Med 342:1301–1308, 2000.

42. Meduri GU, Headley AS, Golden E, et al. Effect of prolonged methylprednisolone therapy in unresolving acute respiratory distress syndrome: a randomized controlled trial. JAMA 280:159–165, 1998.

43. Teboul JL, Graini L, Boujdaria R, et al. Cardiac index vs oxygen-derived parameters for rational use of dobutamine in patients with congestive heart failure. Chest 103:81–85, 1993.

44. Shoemaker WC, Appel PL, Kram HB. Oxygen transport measurements to evaluate tissue perfusion and titrate therapy: dobutamine and dopamine effects. Crit Care Med 19:672–688, 1991.

45. Gattinoni L, Brazzi L, Pelosi P, et al. A trial of goal-oriented hemodynamic therapy in critically ill patients. SvO2 Collaborative Group. N Engl J Med 333:1025–1032, 1995.

46. Hayes MA, Timmins AC, Yau EH, et al. Elevation of systemic oxygen delivery in the treatment of critically ill patients. N Engl J Med 330:1717–1722, 1994.

47. Kern JW, Shoemaker WC. Meta-analysis of hemodynamic optimization in high-risk patients. Crit Care Med 30:1686–1692, 2002.

48. Leeper B. Monitoring right ventricular volumes: a paradigm shift. AACN Clin Issues 14:208–219, 2003.

49. Maynard N, Bihari D, Beale R, et al. Assessment of splanchnic oxygenation by gastric tonometry in patients with acute circulatory failure. JAMA 270:1203–1210, 1993.

50. Ryan TJ, Antman EM, Brooks NH, et al. 1999 update: ACC/AHA guidelines for the management of patients with acute myocardial infarction. A report of the American College of Cardiology/American Heart Association Task Force on Practice Guidelines (Committee on Management of Acute Myocardial Infarction). J Am Coll Cardiol 34:890–911, 1999.

51. Braunwald E, Antman EM, Beasley JW, et al. ACC/AHA guidelines for the management of patients with unstable angina and non-ST-segment elevation myocardial infarction. A report of the American College of Cardiology/American Heart Association Task Force on Practice Guidelines (Committee on the Management of Patients With Unstable Angina). J Am Coll Cardiol 36:970–1062, 2000.

52. Hollenberg SM, Kavinsky CJ, Parrillo JE. Cardiogenic shock. Ann Intern Med 131:47–59, 1999.

53. Chobanian AV, Bakris GL, Black HR, et al. Seventh report of the Joint National Committee on Prevention, Detection, Evaluation, and Treatment of High Blood Pressure. Hypertension 42:1206–1252, 2003.

54. Cole L, Bellomo R, Silvester W, et al. A prospective, multicenter study of the epidemiology, management, and outcome of severe acute renal failure in a "closed" ICU system. Am J Respir Crit Care Med 162:191–196, 2000.

55. Nolin TD, Abraham PA, Matzke GR. Drug-induced renal disease. In: DiPiro JT TR, Yee GC, Matzke GR, et al, eds. Pharmacotherapy: a pathophysiologic approach. New York: McGraw-Hill, 2002: 889–909.

56. St. Peter WL, Halstenson CE. Pharmacologic approach in patients with renal failure. In: Chernow B, ed. Pharmacologic approach to the critically ill patient. Baltimore: Williams & Wilkins, 1994: 41–79.

57. Cockcroft DW, Gault MH. Prediction of creatinine clearance from serum creatinine. Nephron 16:31–41, 1976.

58. Levey AS, Bosch JP, Lewis JB, et al. A more accurate method to estimate glomerular filtration rate from serum creatinine: a new prediction equation. Modification of Diet in Renal Disease Study Group. Ann Intern Med 130:461–470, 1999.

59. Lam YW, Banerji S, Hatfield C, et al. Principles of drug administration in renal insufficiency. Clin Pharmacokinet 32:30–57, 1997.

60. Cook D, Heyland D, Griffith L, et al. Risk factors for clinically important upper gastrointestinal bleeding in patients requiring mechanical ventilation. Canadian Critical Care Trials Group. Crit Care Med 27:2812–2817, 1999.

61. Cook D, Guyatt G, Marshall J, et al. A comparison of sucralfate and ranitidine for the prevention of upper gastrointestinal bleeding in patients requiring mechanical ventilation. Canadian Critical Care Trials Group. N Engl J Med 338:791–797, 1998.

62. Cohen H, Baldwin SN, Mukherji R, et al. A comparison of lansoprazole and sucralfate for the prophylaxis of stress-related mucosal damage in critically ill patients. Crit Care Med 28:A185, 2000.

63. Levy MJ, Seelig CB, Robinson NJ, et al. Comparison of omeprazole and ranitidine for stress ulcer prophylaxis. Dig Dis Sci 42: 1255–1259, 1997.

64. Driks MR, Craven DE, Celli BR, et al. Nosocomial pneumonia in intubated patients given sucralfate as compared with antacids or histamine type 2 blockers. The role of gastric colonization. N Engl J Med 317:1376–1382, 1987.

65. Messori A, Trippoli S, Vaiani M, et al. Bleeding and pneumonia in intensive care patients given ranitidine and sucralfate for prevention of stress ulcer: meta-analysis of randomised controlled trials. Br Med J 321:1103–1106, 2000.

66. Kubisty CA, Arns PA, Wedlund PJ. Adjustments of medications in liver failure. In: Chernow B, ed. The pharmacologic approach to the critically ill patient. Baltimore: Williams & Wilkins, 1994:95–113.

67. Scharte M, Fink MP. Red blood cell physiology in critical illness. Crit Care Med 31:S651–657, 2003.

68. Vincent JL, Baron JF, Reinhart K, et al. Anemia and blood transfusion in critically ill patients. JAMA 288:1499–1507, 2002.

69. Corwin HL, Gettinger A, Pearl RG, et al. Efficacy of recombinant human erythropoietin in critically ill patients: a randomized controlled trial. JAMA 288:2827–2835, 2002.

70. Drews RE, Weinberger SE. Thrombocytopenic disorders in critically ill patients. Am J Respir Crit Care Med 162:347–351, 2000.

71. Warkentin TE. Heparin-induced thrombocytopenia: pathogenesis and management. Br J Haematol 121:535–555, 2003.

72. Livio M, Mannucci PM, Vigano G, et al. Conjugated estrogens for the management of bleeding associated with renal failure. N Engl J Med 315:731–735, 1986.

73. Agnelli G, Parise P, Levi M, et al. Effects of desmopressin on hemostasis in patients with liver cirrhosis. Haemostasis 25:241–247, 1995.

74. Bernard GR, Vincent JL, Laterre PF, et al. Efficacy and safety of recombinant human activated protein C for severe sepsis. N Engl J Med 344:699–709, 2001.

75. Geerts WH, Heit JA, Clagett GP, et al. Prevention of venous thromboembolism. Chest 119:132S–175S, 2001.
76. Bessey PQ, Downey RS, Monafo WW. Metabolic response to injury and critical illness. In: Civetta JM, Taylor RW, Kirby RR, eds. Critical care. New York:Lippincott-Raven, 1997:325–335.
77. Pohlman TH, Boyle EM. The host response to injury and infection. In: Civetta JM, Taylor RW, Kirby RR, eds. Critical care. New York: Lippincott-Raven, 2000:291–301.
78. Shapiro L, Gelfand JA. Cytokines in disease. In: Shoemaker WC, Ayres SM, Grenvik A, et al, eds. Textbook of critical care. Philadelphia: W.B. Saunders, 2000:579–586.
79. Bone RC, Balk RA, Cerra FB, et al. Definitions for sepsis and organ failure and guidelines for the use of innovative therapies in sepsis. The ACCP/SCCM Consensus Conference Committee. American College of Chest Physicians/Society of Critical Care Medicine. 101:1644–1655, Chest 1992.
80. Levy MM, Fink MP, Marshall JC, et al. 2001 SCCM/ESICM/ ACCP/ATS/SIS International Sepsis Definitions Conference. Crit Care Med 31:1250–1256, 2003.
81. Bone RC. Sir Isaac Newton, sepsis, SIRS, and CARS. Crit Care Med 24:1125–1128, 1996.
82. van den Berghe G, Wouters P, Weekers F, et al. Intensive insulin therapy in the critically ill patients. N Engl J Med 345:1359–1367, 2001.
83. Mesotten D, Van den Berghe G. Clinical potential of insulin therapy in critically ill patients. Drugs 63:625–636, 2003.
84. Baumgartner JD, Calandra T. Treatment of sepsis: past and future avenues. Drugs 57:127–132, 1999.
85. Wheeler AP, Bernard GR. Treating patients with severe sepsis. N Engl J Med 340:207–214, 1999.
86. Angus DC, Black N. Improving care of the critically ill: institutional and health-care system approaches. Lancet 363:1314–1320, 2004.
87. Shorr AF. An update on cost-effectiveness analysis in critical care. Curr Opin Crit Care 8:337–343, 2002.
88. Angus DC, Barnato AE, Linde-Zwirble WT, et al. Use of intensive care at the end of life in the United States: an epidemiologic study. Crit Care Med 32:638–643, 2004.
89. Coughlin MT, Angus DC. Economic evaluation of new therapies in critical illness. Crit Care Med 31:S7–16, 2003.
90. Leape LL, Cullen DJ, Clapp MD, et al. Pharmacist participation on physician rounds and adverse drug events in the intensive care unit. JAMA 282:267–270, 1999.
91. Armstrong DK, Jacobi J, Dasta JF. Providing pharmaceutical services in critical care areas. In: Shoemaker WC, Ayres S, Grenvik A, et al, eds. Textbook of critical care. Philadelphia: WB Saunders, 1995:1151–1154.
92. Kelley MA, Angus D, Chalfin DB, et al. The critical care crisis in the United States: a report from the profession. Chest 125: 1514–1517, 2004.
93. Sedation, analgesia, and neuromuscular blockade of the critically ill adult: revised clinical practice guidelines for 2002. Am J Health Syst Pharm 59:147–149, 2002.
94. Jacobi J, Farrington EA. Supportive care of the critically ill patient. In: Carter BL, Lake KD, Raebel MA, et al, eds. Pharmacotherapy Self-Assessment Program, Critical Care, Module 2. Kansas City: American College of Clinical Pharmacy, 1998:129–159.

Transplantation

27

Heather J. Johnson

TREATMENT GOALS

The overall goal of solid organ transplantation is to return patients to a near-normal quality of life. The primary goal of immunosuppression is to prevent allograft rejection so that near-normal allograft function can be maintained. In addition, antirejection therapy must be balanced against the possibility of life-threatening infection and malignancy.

See important transplant definitions in Table 27.1.

Solid organ transplantation has become a widely accepted treatment for previously fatal end-organ failure. The success of transplantation has been a result of advances in immunology, immunopharmacology, and surgical technique. With the introduction of cyclosporine, 1-year graft survival rates improved dramatically for many types of transplants. Under cyclosporine-based immunosuppression, 1-year cardiac transplantation survival is 85%.[1] Cyclosporine (CSA) did not dramatically change the course of small-bowel transplantation, but recent success has been achieved with tacrolimus (TAC) therapy; 1-year graft survival of 75% has recently been reported, but morbidity and mortality still preclude the universal application of intestinal transplantation.[2]

The success of organ transplantation has led to an increasing demand for transplantation that is not currently met by the availability of donor organs. This discrepancy in supply and demand resulted in more than 83,000 patients awaiting transplantation in 2004. Living-donor transplantation has ex-

panded rapidly to relieve part of this shortage, accounting for almost 50% of renal transplantations in 2002. Living–related donor liver transplantation has also increased dramatically in adults and children. More than 500 living-donor liver transplantations were performed in 2001 (>10%) compared with just 33 in 1993.[1] In addition, successful living-donor pancreas and small bowel transplantations have been reported. Although still in the experimental stages, xenotransplantation and advancing cloning technology may provide alternative solutions for the current organ shortage. Research in the area of chimerism may one day yield clinical methods for inducing tolerance. Serious ethical issues and technological difficulties currently preclude the widespread use of xenografts.[3]

Very few absolute criteria for denial of organ transplantation have been delineated. Although strict age limits for kidney transplantation were once applied, patients older than 55 years of age represent the fastest growing group of kidney

Table 27.1	Important Transplant Definitions

Term	Definition
Allograft	A transplanted tissue or organ taken from a genetically different donor of the same species.
Autograft	A tissue or organ taken from the recipient and transplanted to a different location or at a different time.
Chimerism	The coexistence of genetic material from different individuals in one host.
Dual-therapy	Regimen containing two immunosuppressant agents (e.g., CSA or TAC + prednisone; CSA/AZA; TAC/MMF, AZA/prednisone).
Heterotopic transplant	Transplantation involving engraftment of the donor organ into an ectopic position, leaving the native organ intact.
Induction	The use of high-dose immunosuppression during the early post-transplantation period; often refers to the use of intravenous antibody immunosuppressive medications in quadruple therapy regimens.
Orthotopic transplant	Transplantation involving the removal of the recipient's native organ and the subsequent replacement with donor organ with normal or near-normal anatomic reconstruction.
Quadruple therapy	Regimen containing four immunosuppressant agents (e.g., ATG or OKT3 + CSA or TAC + AZA or MMF + prednisone).
Syngraft	A transplanted tissue or organ taken from an identical donor (monozygotic twins).
Tolerance	Indefinite unresponsiveness of a recipient to the allograft in the absence of long-term immunosuppression.
Triple therapy	Regimen containing three immunosuppressant agents (e.g., CSA or TAC + AZA or MMF + prednisone).
Xenograft	Transplanted tissue or organ taken from a donor of a different species.

CSA, cyclosporine; TAC, tacrolimus; AZA, azathioprine; MMF, mycophenolate mofetil; ATG, antithymocyte globulin.

transplant recipients. Metastatic malignancy is an absolute contraindication to transplantation. Many transplant programs do not perform transplantations on patients who are active substance abusers or who have demonstrated noncompliance. In addition, some patients have anatomic anomalies that preclude organ transplantation. The United Network for Organ Sharing (UNOS), which was established in 1977, maintains a registry of patients who are awaiting transplantation and coordinates the selection of donor and recipient. Selection is based on a multifactorial scoring system that includes blood type, human leukocyte antigen (HLA) typing, length of time on the waiting list, and degree of medical urgency. To optimize the use of donated organs, other strategies have been employed. These include the ''en bloc'' transplantation of pediatric kidneys into adult recipients, the use of two geriatric kidneys in adult recipients, split-liver transplantation, and the transplantation of ''expanded donor pool'' hearts that might normally be declined into ''older'' recipients who might otherwise wait longer for transplantation.

Kidney transplantation is the most commonly performed transplant procedure, with 1-year graft survival of almost 90% for cadaveric kidneys; more than 14,000 patients received kidneys in 2002.[1] Diabetes, hypertension, and chronic pyelonephritis are the most common diseases that lead to kidney transplantation. The allograft is generally placed retroperitoneally in the right iliac fossa. The renal artery and vein are anastomosed to the external iliac artery and vein, respectively. The donor ureter is connected directly to the bladder, and if the donor kidney has not undergone prolonged ischemia, the production of urine immediately follows revascularization. For the most part, native kidneys are not removed.[4] Residual function, therefore, should be taken into account when urine output is evaluated in the perioperative period.

Pancreas transplantation is usually performed in conjunction with kidney transplantation, but it can be performed after kidney transplantation or alone, before renal disease progresses. One-year graft survival is between 75% and 85%, depending on the nature of the transplant: pancreas after kidney, solitary pancreas, or kidney-pancreas transplant.[1] Although early pancreas transplantation might prevent long-term complications of insulin-dependent diabetes, such as gastropathy, nephropathy, neuropathy, peripheral vascular disease, and retinopathy, most insurance programs consider solitary pancreas transplantation an experimental procedure. Many potential candidates wait until renal failure ensues. As with kidney transplantation, the native pancreas is left in place. Either segmental (tail and body) or whole pancreas transplantation can be performed. Segmental grafts are usually placed intraperitoneally in the pelvis with vascular anastomosis to the iliac vessels. Whole organ grafts are obtained as a block that contains the pancreas, spleen, and long duodenal segment. Whole allografts are transplanted intraperitoneally, at a location where pancreatic secretions will be absorbed by the peritoneum. The exocrine duct is bladder-drained, which allows for urinary excretion of pancreatic enzymes. This technique is superior to intestinal drainage as it allows for monitoring of urinary amylase to detect rejection.[5] Transplantation of islet cells remains an important area of research.

Liver transplantation is the second most commonly performed transplant operation, with more than 5,000 liver transplantations performed in 2002.[1] Diseases that may lead to transplantation include hepatitis B and C, alcoholic cirrhosis, primary biliary cirrhosis, primary sclerosing cholangitis, and biliary atresia. In contrast to kidney and pancreas transplantation, the donor liver is placed orthotopically; the recipient's own liver must be removed. During the anhepatic phase, the patient is placed on venovenous bypass to preserve venous return from the kidney and lower extremities. Implantation of the donor liver begins with removal of the gallbladder. Vascular anastomoses are made with the suprahepatic vena cava, the infrahepatic vena cava, the hepatic artery, and the portal vein. The biliary tract is completed by connecting the donor and recipient common bile ducts over a drainage tube (T-tube). Although HLA matching is not as important for liver transplantation as it is for kidney transplantation, size may be a limiting factor. Donor and recipient are usually matched for size ($\pm 20\%$) to prevent splinting of the diaphragm and pulmonary complications that would result from transplantation of an excessively large liver.[6]

Heart transplantation is usually an orthotopic procedure. Transplants can be performed for ischemic, idiopathic, and viral cardiomyopathy, as well as for valvular heart disease or congenital anomalies. With most of the atria and septum of the recipient left in place, the patient is placed on cardiopulmonary bypass. The donor heart is implanted by anastomosis of the left atrium to the residual left atrial wall and by joining of the right atrial wall and septum. The main pulmonary artery is connected to the ascending aorta. The transplanted heart is denervated and relies on circulating catecholamines for normal function. In addition, it contains right atria with two sinus nodes. The native atrial impulse cannot cross the suture line, so it is the donor sinus node activity that is responsible for impulse generation. For this reason, cardiac transplant recipients do not experience symptoms of ischemia such as chest pain, and they may present with silent myocardial infarction or sudden cardiac death. Drugs such as digoxin and atropine that act primarily via the autonomic nervous system have no effect on the transplanted heart.[7]

Lung transplantation may involve one or two lungs, depending on the cause of the disease. Double-lung transplantation is generally performed in patients with cystic fibrosis because significant infectious risk would be associated with a remaining native lung. Patients with emphysema, however, are usually considered for a single-lung transplant. Other conditions that may lead to pulmonary transplantation include pulmonary hypertension, bronchiectasis, idiopathic pulmonary fibrosis, and sarcoidosis. After recipient pneumonectomy, the donor and recipient bronchi

are connected, followed by the pulmonary artery. A left atrial cuff is made from the recipient superior and inferior pulmonary veins and is anastomosed to the remnant donor left atria. Double-lung transplantation is generally performed as sequential single-lung transplants.[8] One-year graft survival rates approach 77%, but they fall dramatically to 43% by 5 years posttransplantation secondary to chronic rejection and infection.[1]

Most intestinal transplant recipients are younger than 20 years of age, and size matching is an important surgical consideration.[9] Intestinal transplantation is achieved by connecting the superior mesenteric artery and vein to the recipient aorta and inferior vena cava, respectively. The intestinal graft is anastomosed to the recipient intestine, and the distal portion is brought out as a stoma, which allows for periodic surveillance biopsies of the graft. The stoma is usually closed after 6 to 12 months.[10] Despite recent success, overall 3-year graft survival is 33%.[1] However, better results have been reported by single centers. A recent review of 10-year experience showed survival rates of 75% at 1 year, 54% at 5 years, and 42% at 10 years.[2] Recent advances in immunosuppression appear to have contributed to the success of intestinal transplantation. Intestinal transplantation is usually performed on patients with intestinal dysfunction who have failed long-term parenteral nutrition for various reasons, including liver dysfunction and recurrent line sepsis. Short-bowel syndrome is the primary indication that leads to intestinal transplantation. Other indications include severe intractable diarrhea and abdominal cancer.[9]

REJECTION

Allograft rejection is the immune system's natural response that protects the body from foreign substances (antigens) and ultimately destroys them. The general sequence of events that lead to graft loss includes (a) identification of donor histocompatibility differences by the recipient's immune system; (b) recruitment of activated lymphocytes; (c) initiation of immune effector mechanisms; and (d) graft destruction.

Three classes of antigens are coded for by the major histocompatibility complex (MHC): HLA classes I, II, and III. Classes I and II are important for histocompatibility in transplantation. Class I antigens are present on virtually all nucleated cells in the body, whereas class II molecules are primarily located on B-lymphocytes, antigen-presenting cells, and vascular endothelium.[11] Histocompatibility testing is used to minimize donor-specific immune responses to the allograft. In theory, the greater the number of antigens that match, the less likely rejection is to occur. Histocompatibility matching is significant only in kidney and pancreas transplantation. Secondary to limitations of organ availability, viability, and the critical condition of those awaiting transplantation, matching is not used in liver, heart, or lung transplantation. It is unclear whether HLA matching continues to affect graft survival since the introduction of potent immunosuppressants such as CSA and TAC.

The immune response is the result of a complex cascade of events that lead to the formation of antibodies (immunoglobulins) and sensitized cells (lymphocytes). Two lines of defense exist: humoral and cellular immunity. Humoral immunity is mediated by B-lymphocytes that develop into antibodies; cellular immunity is T-cell mediated. T-lymphocytes can further be differentiated based on their function. Helper T-cells secrete cytokines such as interleukins and interferons, which promote proliferation and differentiation of T-cells. For example, interleukin-2 (IL-2) is secreted by T-helper cells and stimulates the proliferation of other T-helper cells, as well as the differentiation of mature cytolytic T-cells. Cytolytic T-cells are responsible for the lysis of virus-infected cells, tumor cells, and allografts. Lymphocytes, the only cells in the body that can recognize specific antigens, are central to allograft rejection.[11]

When allograft histocompatibility antigens are recognized by the recipient's immune system, both B-lymphocytes and T-lymphocytes are activated, leading to a complex series of events that results in release of cytokines that aid in the overall rejection process (Figure 27.1). Recipient macrophages release IL-1, which in turn results in the stimulation of lymphocytic proliferation. In response, T-helper lymphocytes also produce IL-2 and interferon-gamma (IFN-γ). At the same time, cytotoxic T-lymphocytes express receptors for IL-2. Stimulation of these receptors by IL-2 leads to proliferation of cytotoxic T-lymphocytes, which can bind to the allograft and cause cell death. During this process,

helper T-lymphocytes can also acquire cytolytic activity and enhance this process. Following antigen recognition, helper T-lymphocyte–derived IL-2 promotes the release of B-lymphocyte growth factors, which results in the clonal expansion and differentiation of activated B-lymphocytes and antibody production. Antibodies target graft endothelium, whereas cell destruction is mediated by activation of the complement cascade or cell-mediated cytotoxicity.[11]

Despite advances in our understanding of immunology and improvements in immunosuppressive agents, rejection remains a major problem associated with transplantation. Approximately 30% to 75% of transplant patients experience rejection.[11] Allograft rejection is classified according to time posttransplantation and histologic findings. The types of rejection are summarized in Table 27.2. Hyperacute rejection occurs almost immediately after perfusion of the transplanted organ and is mediated by anti-HLA antibodies. Severe vascular damage occurs, including thrombosis, inflammation, and necrosis. It is believed that hyperacute rejection is caused by humoral presensitization to donor ABO blood and HLA antigens. Because hyperacute rejection is most frequent among renal and cardiac transplant recipients, a negative T-cell cross match (absence of donor-specific class I HLA antibodies) is generally required before transplantation is performed. Hyperacute rejection is less common in liver transplant recipients and generally occurs later—3 to 7 days after transplantation. In lung, pancreas, and small-bowel transplantation, the propensity for hyperacute rejection is unknown. Overall, hyperacute rejection occurs in about 1% of transplants. Because pharmacologic treatment is ineffective, the allograft must be removed.

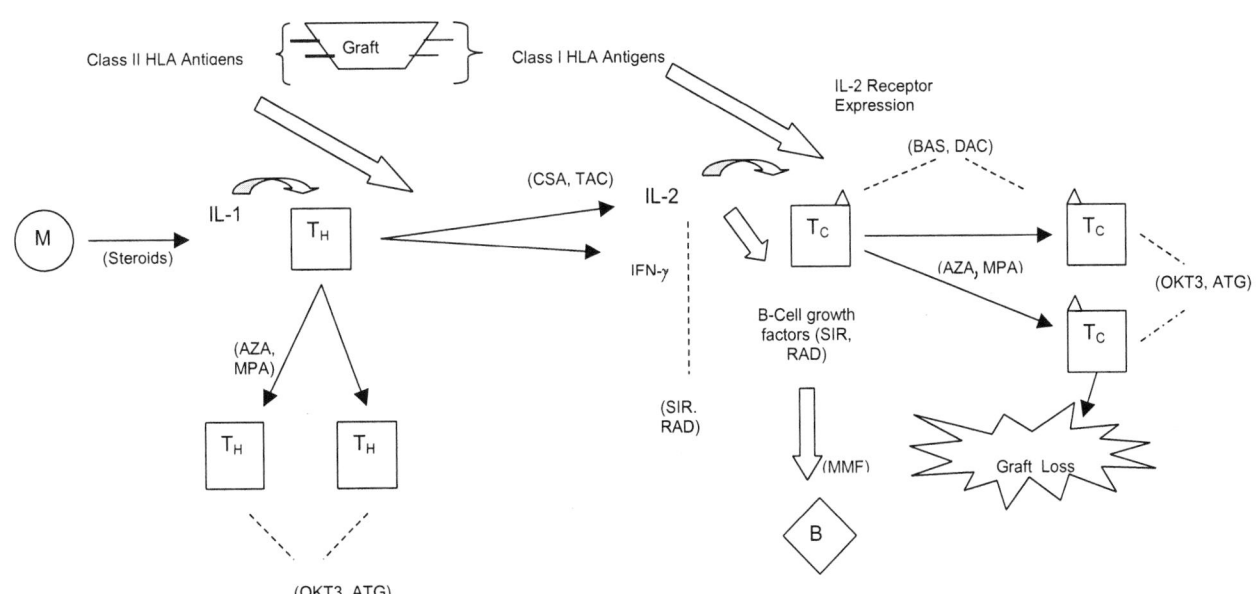

FIGURE 27.1 Summary of the cells responsible for transplant rejection and the sites of action of immunosuppressive medications. *M*, macrophage; *T*$_H$, helper T-lymphocyte; *T*$_C$, cytotoxic T-cell.

Table 27.2	Summary of Allograft Rejection		
Type	**Time Posttransplant**	**Probable Mechanism**	**Treatment**
Hyperacute	Immediate; 1–5 days	Presence of preformed donor-specific cytotoxic antibodies	Unresponsive to immunosuppressive therapy. Graft removal
Accelerated acute	7–10 days	Low levels of anti-class I antibodies; T-cell–mediated rejection in presensitized recipients	May be responsive to antibody therapy: OKT3, ATG
Acute	Weeks to 6 months, years	Newly developed antibodies, delayed-type hypersensitivity of helper and cytotoxic T-cells	Usually responsive to corticosteroids, OKT3, ATG
Chronic	Months to years	T-lymphocytes and donor-specific antibody directed to allograft vasculature	Unresponsive to immunosuppressive therapy

ATG, antithymocyte globulin.

Acute rejection can be subdivided according to onset. Accelerated acute rejection occurs within 3 to 10 days following renal transplantation and is a reflection of recipient antidonor presensitization. Patients who have received donor-specific transfusions or previous transplants, or who have had multiple pregnancies, are at highest risk for this type of rejection. Antirejection therapy may be effective in the short term, but an increased risk of graft failure remains over the long term.[11] Acute rejection is most common in the first few months following transplantation, but it can occur at any time during the life of the allograft. Acute rejection is generally reversible, especially if treated. Although most cases of acute rejection can be treated effectively, none of the currently available therapies prevents or changes the course of chronic rejection.

Chronic rejection is a major cause of late graft loss.[12] Although chronic rejection usually occurs months to years after transplantation, it may be evident within weeks of transplantation. Prevention and treatment of chronic rejection constitutes one of the most important problems to be addressed in transplantation. Although chronic rejection may simply be a slow and indolent form of cellular rejection, the involvement of the humoral immune system and of antibodies against the vascular endothelium appears to play a role. The clinical presentation of chronic rejection is organ dependent, but persistent perivascular and interstitial inflammation is common in kidney, liver, and heart transplants.[13] The pathogenesis of chronic rejection is difficult to determine because of prolonged exposure to multiple drugs, and because of the presence of other abnormalities that may predispose the patient to similar pathologic changes in organ function. For example, hypertension and hyperlipidemia are frequently associated with chronic renal allograft rejection. Chronic renal dysfunction, likewise, may lead to hypertension. Accelerated atherosclerosis and chronic cardiac rejection are also coexistent, but it is not always clear which is the primary event. In kidney transplantation, acute rejection is a strong predictor of chronic rejection, but it is unclear why reduction in the incidence of acute rejection associated with the widespread adoption of CSA and TAC has not affected the incidence of chronic rejection. The current tendency to decrease doses of CSA and TAC in the face of "good" graft function without dynamic measurement of immunologic factors may lead to subclinical rejection. In addition to increasing number and severity of acute rejection episodes, HLA mismatching, prolonged cold ischemia time, and the presence of cytomegalovirus are associated with the development of chronic rejection.

Chronic rejection is irreversible. Among lung transplant recipients, chronic rejection, manifested as bronchiolitis obliterans, is the leading cause of morbidity and mortality after the first year posttransplant, affecting up to 50% of patients.[13] Arteriosclerosis is the hallmark of chronic rejection in heart transplant patients, affecting up to 50% of patients 5 years after transplantation. Among liver transplant recipients, chronic rejection is characterized by the loss of bile ducts; thus, it is called *vanishing bile duct syndrome* and affects 10% to 15% of patients. In renal transplant recipients, chronic rejection is associated with proteinuria, hypercholesterolemia, and hypertension. Recent data indicate that the administration of low-dose aspirin (100 mg per day) may have an important role in renal allograft survival, in addition to its cardioprotective effects.[14] Chronic rejection accounts for about 10% of renal allograft loss.

CLINICAL PRESENTATION AND DIAGNOSIS

Several factors make the diagnosis of rejection in transplant patients difficult. Many symptoms of organ rejection, such as fever and malaise, are nonspecific. In addition, some symptoms may be blunted or "masked" by the antirejection agents themselves. In particular, CSA and TAC are both nephrotoxic and may cloud the diagnosis of rejection in kidney transplant patients. Because of the complexity of this situation, clinicians rely on clinical symptoms, laboratory values, imaging studies, and biopsy findings to make the diagnosis of rejection. Table 27.3 summarizes signs and symptoms of rejection by organ.

Table 27.3	Signs and Symptoms of Acute Allograft Rejection	
Organ	**Symptoms**	**Objective Findings**
Kidney	Fever, malaise, oliguria, edema, graft tenderness	SCr >120% of baseline; increased BUN; hypertension, weight gain
Pancreas	Graft swelling/tenderness	Elevated fasting blood sugar, leukocytosis, C peptide <0.7 ng/mL, urinary amylase <167 ukat/L (bladder-drained)
Liver	Fever, lethargy, graft tenderness or swelling, back pain, anorexia, ileus Severe: jaundice, ascites, encephalopathy	Elevated LFTs: rapid rise in γ-glutamyl transpeptidase; elevated serum bilirubin, alkaline phosphatase, transaminases, and prothrombin time
Heart	Fever, lethargy, weakness, dyspnea	Leukocytosis, tachycardia, arrhythmia, pericardial friction rub
Lung	Fever, malaise, shortness of breath, anxiety	Infiltrates on chest x-ray, decreased FEV_1, hypoxia
Intestine	Increased ostomy output; fever, abdominal pain, nausea, vomiting, diarrhea, ileus, and distention	Blood cultures positive for enteric organisms; acidosis

SCr, serum creatinine; BUN, blood urea nitrogen; LFT, liver function test; FEV_1, forced expiratory volume in 1 second.

KIDNEY

Approximately 50% of renal transplant recipients will experience at least one episode of acute rejection. Acute rejection occurs most commonly within the first 3 months following transplantation. Renal allograft rejection is characterized by an acute increase in serum creatinine over baseline, decreased urine output, and allograft swelling and tenderness. Patients may also report fever, malaise, edema, and hypertension. Increased serum creatinine may be the result of other disease. CSA or TAC concentrations may help rule out drug toxicity; ultrasound may be used to rule out stenosis of renal arteries or veins. In addition, dehydration, urinary tract infection, and cytomegalovirus infection may result in increased serum creatinine. Renal biopsy is the gold standard for diagnosing rejection and may allow clinicians to choose specific therapies. Lymphocytic infiltration and interstitial tissue damage are the most common findings; vascular damage revealed on biopsy may predict a rejection that will be unresponsive to high-dose corticosteroids.

PANCREAS

The diagnosis of pancreatic rejection is difficult because no reliable markers of rejection have been discerned. Pancreatic biopsy is technically difficult to perform and is associated with patient morbidity. In addition, pathologic findings are often difficult to interpret. In patients who have simultaneous kidney-pancreas transplants, kidney transplant rejection usually precedes pancreas rejection; rejection of the pancreas without kidney rejection is uncommon. Pancreas function can be monitored by measurement of changes in urinary amylase. Serum amylase and lipase have also been used. Elevated serum glucose may not occur until late in rejection.

LIVER

In liver transplant recipients, rejection most commonly occurs within the first 2 weeks following transplantation. Of the 70% of recipients who develop rejection, about 75%

will have complete resolution with antirejection therapy; the remainder will go on to develop chronic rejection. Signs and symptoms of rejection include abnormal liver function tests [γ-glutamyl transpeptidase (GGTP), alanine transaminase (ALT), aspartate transaminase (AST), bilirubin], fever, ileus, ascites, abdominal pain, and jaundice. Liver biopsy, which generally reveals a mixed inflammatory cell infiltrate of the portal tracts, bile duct damage, lymphocytic infiltration, and hepatic and portal venous endothelial inflammation, can confirm rejection.

HEART

The period of highest risk for rejection in heart transplant recipients is the first 3 months. The signs and symptoms of rejection are very nonspecific and are usually not present unless the rejection is prolonged or severe. These include fever, lethargy, weakness, elevated jugular venous pressure, a new S3 gallop, arrhythmia, shortness of breath, and hypotension. Because the transplanted heart is denervated, patients will not experience angina or chest pain. Because rejection is so common and difficult to diagnosis, routine surveillance endomyocardial biopsies are performed weekly during the early postoperative period. Histology consistent with acute rejection includes diffuse mononuclear infiltrates.

LUNG

Most lung transplant recipients experience an episode of acute rejection within the first few weeks; 60% to 70% experience biopsy-proven acute rejection within the first month. Diagnosis is usually based on symptoms such as elevated temperature, impaired gas exchange, decreased forced expiratory volume, and the appearance of infiltrates on chest x-ray. In addition, transbronchial biopsy and radionuclide perfusion studies are useful in aiding the diagnosis of rejection.

SMALL BOWEL

The incidence of rejection is especially high in intestinal transplantation, with more than 90% of patients requiring treatment. The high incidence of rejection and the lack of specific chemical markers warrant the use of surveillance biopsies. Clinical signs of rejection occur late in the course of rejection. The earliest clinical indication of rejection may be an increase in ostomy output, which is generally followed by fever and abdominal pain.[2]

TREATMENT OF ACUTE REJECTION

The treatment approach to acute rejection varies between transplant centers. The primary goals are to minimize the intensity of the immune response and to prevent irreversible injury to the allograft. An algorithm for the treatment of rejection is given as Figure 27.2. Common doses of immunosuppressants are summarized in Table 27.4.

THERAPEUTIC STRATEGIES TO PREVENT REJECTION

Immunosuppression must be balanced in terms of graft and patient survival. The ideal immunosuppressive agent would specifically inhibit the cells responsible for organ rejection while leaving intact the means to fight off infection. Until the ideal immunosuppressant becomes available, most transplant clinicians use a multidrug approach to prevent rejection. The rationale for this approach is twofold. Several immunosuppressants with different mechanisms of action and different adverse effect profiles are given simultaneously to maximize therapeutic benefit while minimizing adverse effects. The challenge is to maintain adequate immunosuppression to preserve allograft function while avoiding infec-

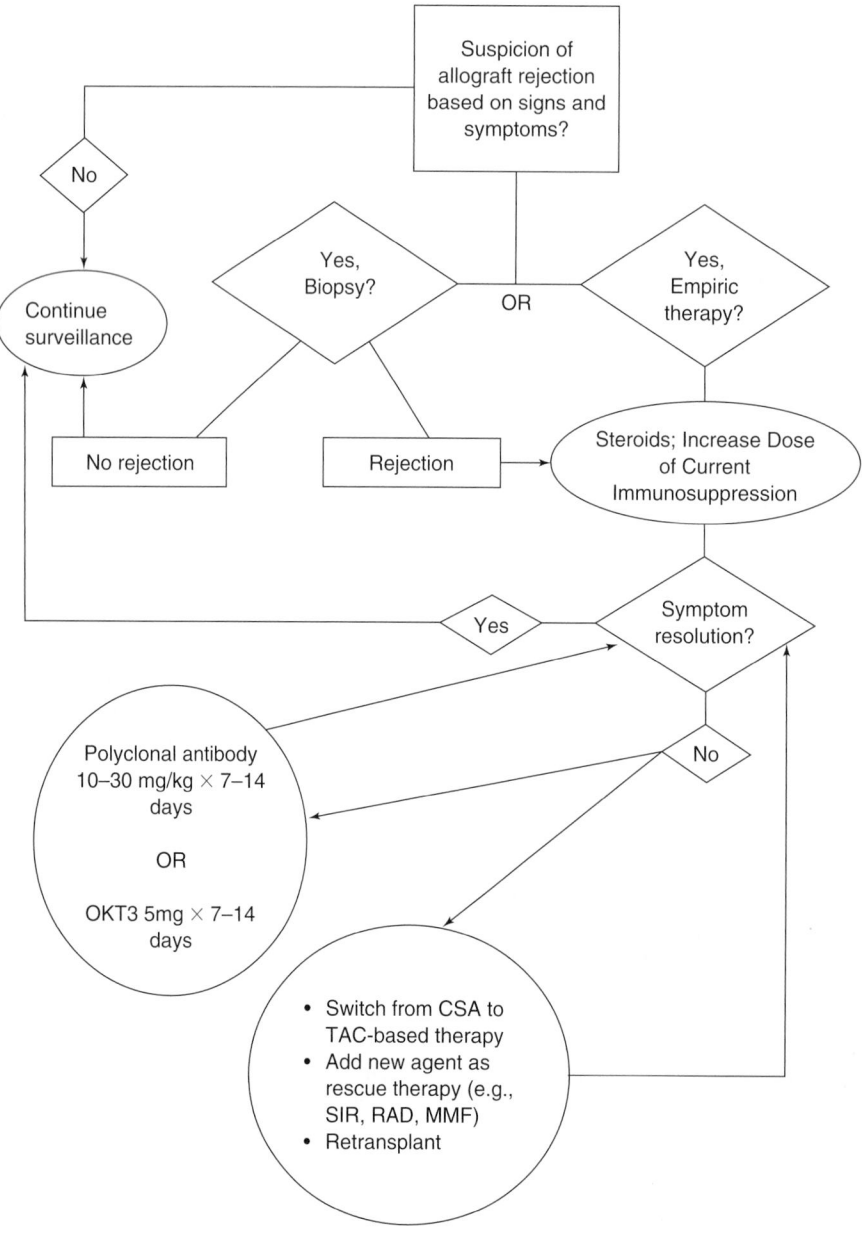

FIGURE 27.2 Algorithm for the treatment of rejection.

Table 27.4 | Summary of Immunosuppressive Agents

Agent	Induction	Maintenance	Rejection	Comments
Monoclonal Antibodies				
Basiliximab	20 mg IV day 0, day 4	–	–	
Daclizumab	1 mg/kg IV q14days × 5	–	–	
Muromonab	2.5–5 mg/day IV × 7–14 days	–	5–10 mg/day IV qd × 7–10	Check for antibodies if second course
Polyclonal Antibodies				
Antithymocyte globulin (ATGAM)	10–30 mg/kg/day IV × 7–14 days	–	15–30 mg/kg IV qd × 7–14	Dose-limiting thrombocytopenia
Antithymocyte globulin (rATG-thymoglobulin)	1–2 mg/kg/day IV × 10–14 days (renal)	1.5 mg/kg IV qd × 7–14		Dose-limiting thrombocytopenia
Corticosteroids				
Prednisone	Perioperative taper: 50 mg qid × 4 doses, 40 mg qid × 4 doses, 30 mg qid × 4 doses, 20 mg qid × 4 doses, 10 mg qid × 4 doses, then 20 mg/day	20–60 mg/day tapering by 2.5–5 mg q2–4 weeks OR 0.5–0.75 mg/kg/day, tapering to 0.15 mg/kg/day @ 6 months	5-day oral "recycle": 100 mg, 80 mg, 60 mg, 40 mg, 20 mg. Taper slowly from 20 mg	Protocols vary widely depending on institution and concomitant agents
Methylprednisolone	1,000 mg × 1 then pred OR 1,000 mg × 1, 500 mg × 1, 250 mg × 1, then pred OR 1,000 mg × 1, 50 mg qid × 4 doses, 40 mg qid × 4, 30 mg qid × 4, 20 mg qid × 4, 30 mg bid × 2, 20 mg × 1, then pred	–	IV "burst": 500 mg/day × 3 OR 1,000 mg × 2, 500 mg × 2, 250 mg × 2, then pred	Protocols vary widely depending on institution and concomitant agents
Antiproliferative Agents				
Azathioprine	3–5 mg/kg PO/IV qd	1–3 mg/kg IV PO qd	–	Monitor LFTs and WBC.
Mycophenolate mofetil	1–1.5 gm po bid	1–1.5 g PO bid	Conversion from AZA, doses up to 3.5 g/day	Monitor WBC
Calcineurin Inhibitors				
Cyclosporine	5–6 mg/kg/day IV until GI function resumes OR 6–20 mg/kg/day PO divided bid	5–15 mg/kg/day PO divided bid		Initial Neoral doses are usually lower than Sandimmune doses; adjust doses based on target concentrations.
Tacrolimus	0.05–0.1 mg/kg/d IV until GI function resumes	0.1–0.3 mg/kg/d divided bid	Conversion from CSA in refractory rejection	TAC levels may be as high as 40 ng/mL for intestinal transplant
Rapamycin Derivatives				
Sirolimus	6-mg loading dose (renal)	2 mg PO qd		Target levels with CSA therapy 12–24 ng/mL

AZA, azathioprine; LFT, liver function test; WBC, white blood cell count; GI, gastrointestinal; CSA, cyclosporine; TAC, tacrolimus.

tion and the nonimmunologic toxicities of the various immunosuppressive agents. Transplant immunosuppression is often divided into two phases: induction and maintenance. *Induction* refers to the period of immunosuppression immediately posttransplantation, when the level of immunosuppression is kept the highest. Immunosuppression during this period may include up to four immunosuppressive agents, that is, quadruple-therapy. Transplant protocols may include a monoclonal or polyclonal antibody until therapeutic concentrations of other immunosuppressive medications are demonstrated. Most protocols also include high-dose corticosteroids, a calcineurin inhibitor such as CSA or TAC, and an antiproliferative agent such as azathioprine (AZA) or mycophenolate mofetil (MMF). The decision to use triple or quadruple immunosuppression during the induction period varies according to transplant center, type of transplant, previous transplant or rejection history, race, and pregnancy history, as well as donor-specific factors such as cold ischemia time. Typically, doses of immunosuppressive agents are kept highest during the first 3 months posttransplantation, when the risk for rejection is the greatest. Doses are then slowly titrated downward in an attempt to minimize the long-term adverse effects of immunosuppression. This period of lower immunosuppressive doses is often referred to as the *maintenance phase*, and transplant protocols usually include between two and three immunosuppressant agents during this time, depending on the time posttransplant and the overall rejection history. Most combinations of immunosuppressants administered during the maintenance phase include CSA or TAC, AZA or MMF, and corticosteroids.

The number and variety of immunosuppressive agents available present opportunities and obstacles for transplant clinicians. Now, more than ever before, clinicians have the tools to individualize and optimize therapy for transplant patients. Evaluating the safety and efficacy data, as well as the pharmacoeconomic impact, of new immunosuppressive agents is important in choosing the most appropriate therapies for transplant recipients. Common doses of immunosuppressant agents are summarized in Table 27.4. A summary of their toxicity profiles can be found in Table 27.5.

CORTICOSTEROIDS

Because many recent advances have been made in immunosuppressive therapy, corticosteroids such as prednisone and methylprednisolone are being successful eliminated or reduced in many transplant centers. However, corticosteroids remain an important part of the treatment of acute rejection and are essential for some maintenance immunosuppressive regimens.

Corticosteroids inhibit the inductive phase of cytotoxic T-cells by decreasing the production of immunomodulatory proteins such as IL-1 and IL-2, resulting in a diminished T-cell proliferative response to alloantigens.[15] High-dose rejection or induction therapy can also decrease expression of HLA antigens and β_2-microglobulin on peripheral blood

lymphocytes, thus decreasing the immunogenicity of transplanted organs.

Doses of corticosteroids used in transplantation vary widely. Dose adjustments are based on therapeutic and toxic responses. Clinical monitoring of corticosteroid concentrations is not routinely done. The pharmacokinetics of corticosteroids is complex and varies with disease state, race, sex, and level of renal function. The introduction of CSA and TAC has allowed the reduction of prednisone doses from those used in earlier protocols. Most protocols use high-dose intravenous corticosteroids (e.g., 120 to 1,000 mg methylprednisolone) in the first several days, followed by oral prednisone at doses of 20 to 140 mg per day, tapered to 5 to 20 mg by 3 months posttransplantation. Maintenance doses at 12 to 18 months posttransplant range from 5 to 10 mg per day. Some centers attempt to completely withdraw steroids in rejection-free patients at this point. Other protocols use every other day administration to minimize long-term adverse effects. High-dose corticosteroids are also used for the treatment of acute rejection. A typical course may include 2 to 3 g of methylprednisolone over 5 to 7 days, or an oral "recycle" of 300 mg, which is tapered by 20 mg each day from 100 mg to 20 mg per day over 5 days.

AZATHIOPRINE

Azathioprine (AZA) was first used in organ transplantation in 1962. Today, it has largely been replaced by mycophenolic acid derivatives.[16] AZA is a prodrug of 6-mercaptopurine (6-MP), which is further converted to active 6-thioguanine nucleotides. These metabolites are incorporated into DNA, where they inhibit purine nucleotide synthesis.

AZA is readily absorbed after oral administration and undergoes extensive first-pass metabolism. AZA and 6-MP are rapidly metabolized to 6-thioguanine and 6-thiouric acid via xanthine oxidase. Renal dysfunction does not affect the overall elimination of AZA.[15]

Dose-related bone marrow suppression is the main toxicity of AZA. Leukopenia is the most common manifestation, although thrombocytopenia and megaloblastic anemia may occur. Gastrointestinal upset may be allayed by administration of the agent with food.

Concomitant treatment with allopurinol, a xanthine oxidase inhibitor, prevents the metabolism of 6-MP and markedly increases the toxicity of AZA. To prevent profound myelosuppression, AZA doses should be reduced by 25% to 50%, and complete blood count (CBC) should be monitored. Another effective strategy is to convert patients who require allopurinol from AZA to MMF.

AZA is clinically used in combination with other immunosuppressive agents from the time of transplant; common starting doses of 2 to 5 mg/kg/day are tapered to 1 to 3 mg/kg/day. Doses are adjusted on the basis of white blood cell count, which is monitored throughout therapy so that counts of 3,000 to 5,000 per cubic millimeter are maintained.

Table 27.5	Summary of Adverse Effects of Immunosuppressive Agents	
Adverse Effect	**Potential Causes**	**Special Notes/Management**
CNS		
Neurotoxicity (tremors, seizures, headache, paresthesia)	CSA, TAC, OKT3	Check CSA/TAC concentrations, usually responds to dose reduction; discontinue OKT3
Insomnia	Steroids, TAC	May be transient or may respond to dose reduction
Psychiatric	Steroids, OKT3	Provide patient counseling/support; may be transient and may respond to dose reduction
Cardiovascular		
Hyperlipidemia	Steroids, CSA, SIR	Impose dietary restrictions, pharmacotherapy; may respond to changes in immunosuppressants
Hypertension	Steroids, CSA, TAC	Restrict sodium, provide home blood pressure monitoring
Metabolic		
Hyperglycemia, Diabetes	Steroids, TAC>CSA	Monitor blood glucose; adjust or add hypoglycemic; may respond to changes in immunosuppressants
Hyperkalemia	CSA, TAC	Provide dietary counseling; consider fludrocortisone
Hypomagnesemia	CSA, TAC	Provide dietary counseling, electrolyte replacement
Hematologic		
Anemia	AZA, MMF	Reduce dose; ensure adequate iron stores
Leukopenia	ATG, AZA, MMF, SIR	Reduce dose or discontinue; titrate to WBC $>4,000/mm^3$
Thrombocytopenia	ATG, OKT3, SIR	Reduce dose or discontinue for platelet count $<70,000/mm^3$
Leukocytosis	Steroids	Usually present with high-dose intravenous therapy and corrects with dose reduction. Rule out infection
Dermatologic		
Acne	Steroids	Dose related; may consider topical retinoids (e.g., tretinoin)
Alopecia	AZA, TAC	Provide patient counseling, not usually permanent
Gingival hyperplasia	CSA	Promote oral hygiene; greater risk with concomitant calcium channel blockers
Hirsutism	CSA	Provide patient counseling; consider TAC
Rash	AZA, MMF, ATG	
Gastrointestinal		
Gastritis	MMF	Reduce dose; administer with food; H_2-blocker or proton pump inhibitor. Rule out CMV, gastritis
Nausea, vomiting, diarrhea, anorexia	AZA, MMF, TAC, CSA, ATG, OKT3, steroids	Administer oral steroids with food
Hepatotoxicity	AZA, CSA, TAC	Usually dose dependent and reversible upon discontinuation of offending agent
Nephrotoxicity	CSA, TAC	Monitor serum creatinine, immunosuppressant concentrations
Pulmonary edema	OKT3	Follow administration precautions; weight <103% of dry weight
Anaphylaxis	ATG, OKT3	ATG test dose. Provide close observation with first few doses

(continues)

Table 27.5	continued

Adverse Effect	Potential Causes	Special Notes/Management
Fever, chills	ATG, OKT3	Premedicate with acetaminophen
Edema	Steroids	Restrict sodium, provide furosemide
Cataracts/glaucoma	Steroids	Require annual eye exams
Osteoporosis/aseptic necrosis	Steroids	Promote weight-bearing exercise; adequate calcium intake; dose minimization
Weight gain	Steroids	Provide patient counseling; promote exercise
Malignancy	All	Provide patient counseling regarding sun exposure/ protection; routine follow-up

CNS, central nervous system; CSA, cyclosporine; TAC, tacrolimus; SIR, sirolimus; AZA, azathioprine; MMF, mycophenolate mofetil; ATG, antithymocyte globulin; WBC, white blood cell count; CMV, cytomegalovirus.

MYCOPHENOLIC ACID DERIVATIVES—MYCOPHENOLATE MOFETIL AND MYCOPHENOLATE SODIUM

Mycophenolate mofetil (MMF), the ester prodrug of mycophenolic acid, is currently available in the United States and is a component of many immunosuppression protocols. Mycophenolate sodium is the sodium salt of mycophenolic acid.

Mycophenolic acid (MPA), a potent noncompetitive inhibitor of inosine monophosphate dehydrogenase, causes the inhibition of de novo purine biosynthesis. The antiproliferative effects of MPA are specific to lymphocytes, which rely on the de novo pathway of purine synthesis; most other cell lines can proliferate via a salvage pathway. MPA also inhibits the proliferation of B-lymphocytes and reduces antibody formation and the generation of cytotoxic T-cells.[17] Although early animal reports suggested that MMF may prevent chronic rejection, this has not been borne out in human trials.

Pharmacokinetics and Metabolism. MMF is rapidly and completely converted to MPA, resulting in an oral bioavailablity of 94% in healthy subjects. Maximal concentration (C_{max}) occurs at about 1 hour, with a secondary peak at 6 to 12 hours caused by enterohepatic circulation. Mycophenolate sodium is enterically coated and allows MPA to be released directly into the small intestine, where it is absorbed. MPA is highly protein bound—97% in normal plasma.[17] MPA is eliminated primarily as an inactive glucuronide metabolite, referred to as MPAG. MPA area under the curve (AUC) is unchanged in patients with renal impairment. MPAG, however, is renally eliminated and accumulates in patients with renal dysfunction.[17] Pharmacokinetic studies with MMF in renal transplant recipients showed an increase in AUC and C_{max} in patients at least 3 months posttransplant when compared with those less than 40 days posttransplant.[17] The clinical significance of this finding remains to be determined. Dose reduction during the first year posttransplant, according to the pharmacokinetic and pharmacodynamic properties of MMF, has not been evaluated.

Drug Interactions. Few drug interactions with MMF have been documented. Concomitant administration of aluminum- or magnesium-containing antacids significantly decreases the C_{max} (37%) and AUC (15%) of MPA and should be avoided.[18] Whether or not other divalent cations such as calcium and iron cause the same effect has not been tested. Acyclovir competes with MPAG for renal tubular secretion. The AUCs for both entities are increased with concomitant acyclovir and MMF administration. Although no clinically significant interaction has been established, patients with severe renal insufficiency may be at increased risk of adverse effects associated with the accumulation of acyclovir, such as seizures and delirium. Single-dose pharmacokinetic assessment of intravenous ganciclovir in combination with MMF in renal transplant recipients produced no change in the disposition of ganciclovir, MPA, or MPAG.[19] This finding does not preclude the potential for additive pharmacodynamic effects, such as bone marrow suppression. CSA appears to have no effect on MPA disposition and elimination; whereas concomitant administration of TAC and MMF may result in increased MPA trough levels and AUC. MMF does not affect the pharmacokinetics of CSA or TAC.[20]

Toxicity. Gastrointestinal (GI) adverse effects such as nausea, vomiting, and diarrhea are the predominant toxicities of MMF. It is thought that mycophenolate sodium should be associated with less GI toxicity because it is released into the small intestine. Leukopenia and anemia may occur.[17] These adverse effects are generally responsive to dose reduction or cessation. Other strategies that have been used to improve the GI tolerance of MMF include dividing the total daily dose by three and administering it with food; the latter approach decreases the C_{max} of MPA but has no effect on the AUC.

Dosing and Monitoring. MMF is available as 250-mg capsules and 500-mg tablets, as well as in an injectable formulation. The recommended dose for the prevention of renal allograft rejection is 1,000 mg twice daily; doses up to 3.5

Table 27.6	Pharmacokinetic Summary of Maintenance Immunosuppressants				
Drug	**Pharmacokinetics**				
	CL (ml/min/kg)	**Vd (L/kg)**	**t1/2 (hr)**	**F (%)**	**Protein Binding (%)**
Azathioprine	0.81	0.8	0.2	60	Unknown
Cyclosporine	2–11.8	3.5	6–20	2–89	96
Everolimus			43		73.5
Mycophenolic acid	193 mL/min	3.6	17.9	94	97
Prednisone/prednisolone	1.6–2.8	0.3–0.7	2.2	85–99	70–95
Sirolimus	0.4	5.6–16.7	57–63	20	40
Tacrolimus	5.8–103	5–65	3.5–40.5	5–67	88

g per day have been evaluated for the treatment of rejection. Pediatric patients and those undergoing small-bowel transplantation may benefit from three-times-daily dosing to maintain therapeutic MPA concentrations. Mycophenolate sodium 1.44 g per day is considered equivalent to MMF 2 g per day.[21] In contrast to CSA and TAC, plasma appears to be the most appropriate medium for measuring MPA.[17] Although the measurement of MPA concentrations may be useful in pediatric patients and those with absorption anomalies, therapeutic drug monitoring is not routinely performed. Both therapeutic drug monitoring and pharmacodynamic monitoring are being evaluated for their usefulness in tailoring dosing regimens to achieve optimal immunosuppression.[17]

CALCINEURIN INHIBITORS—CYCLOSPORINE AND TACROLIMUS

CSA or TAC provides the cornerstone for most immunosuppressive regimens. These agents have similar mechanisms of action and similar toxicity profiles. CSA and TAC decrease cytotoxic T-cell activation by inhibiting the same intermediate signaling protein, calcineurin. Calcineurin in turn activates the promoter region for the gene that encodes for IL-2. CSA must bind to an intracellular receptor, cyclophilin.[22] This complex is responsible for disrupting calcineurin signaling, thus blocking the transcription of IL-2. The result is T-cells that are unable to release cytokines and induce an immune response.[22] CSA also appears to have effects on IL-1, IL-3, IL-5, B-cells, tumor necrosis factor-α (TNF-α) and IFN-γ. CSA spares suppressor T-cells and is inactive against mature cytotoxic T-cells; it is, therefore, ineffective in the treatment of ongoing rejection.

TAC also binds to an intracellular protein known as *FK binding protein (FKBP)* to cause inhibition of calcineurin. TAC ultimately inhibits the production of IL-2, IL-3, IL-4, TNF-α, and IFN-γ.[23] Unlike CSA, TAC appears to be able to reverse ongoing rejection and thus may be used as "rescue" therapy in patients who are receiving CSA-based immunosuppression.[24]

Pharmacokinetics. CSA and TAC both exhibit a high degree of pharmacokinetic variability. Variability of CSA

absorption has been identified as a risk factor for rejection.[25] The pharmacokinetic parameters of these and other immunosuppressant agents are summarized in Table 27.6. CSA is currently available in two distinct formulations: Sandimmune and Neoral (a microemulsion formulation of CSA). These two agents do not have the same pharmacokinetic profile and should not be interchanged.[26] Absorption of CSA is slow and incomplete. Bioavailability ranges from 2% to 89%, with a mean of 30%. The microemulsion formulation generally results in increased C_{max} and AUC, which often translates to lower milligram per kilogram dose requirements to yield concentrations comparable with those of Sandimmune. Bioavailability of CSA seems to increase with time posttransplantation. High-fat meals also improve the bioavailability of CSA.[27] To decrease variability, patients should be instructed to take each dose of CSA in a similar manner with respect to food. CSA requires bile for emulsification and ultimate absorption, but the microemulsion formulation of CSA does not depend on bile for absorption. Factors that influence bile flow, such as cholestasis and biliary diversion (T-tube), can decrease CSA absorption. Absorption may also be reduced in patients with liver disease, postoperative ileus, gastroparesis, or diarrhea. TAC has poor bioavailability, ranging from 5% to 67% (mean, 27%). Unlike CSA, TAC is not dependent on bile for absorption; thus, it is particularly useful in liver transplant recipients.[28] Food also causes a reduction in the rate and extent of TAC absorption. As with CSA, patients should take TAC in a consistent manner to avoid large fluctuations in drug exposure.

Both agents are widely distributed throughout the body. CSA has a volume of distribution that ranges from 0.9 to 4.8 L per kg (average, 3.5 L per kg).[26] Highest concentrations are found in fat and in the liver. Other sites where CSA may be found include the thymus, spleen, lymph nodes, bone marrow, pancreas, kidneys, lungs, and skin. About 60% of CSA in the blood is bound to red blood cells. In plasma, 85% to 90% is bound to lipoproteins, most often high-density lipoproteins (HDLs). It has been suggested that patients with very low cholesterol levels may be susceptible to CSA neurotoxicity.[29] Tacrolimus is highly lipophilic and is extensively distributed in red blood cells. In contrast to CSA, TAC is primarily bound to α_1-acid glycoprotein. Tacrolimus sequesters in the heart, lung, spleen, kidney, and pancreas. Both CSA and TAC distribution are influenced by hematocrit, concentration, and temperature.

CSA and TAC are metabolized predominantly in the liver and intestine by cytochrome P-450 3A4 (CYP3A4).[22] Because both are extensively metabolized, patients with hepatic dysfunction have markedly reduced clearance and usually require lower doses to achieve adequate blood concentrations. Renal dysfunction does not affect the elimination of CSA or TAC. Dosage adjustments in the presence of renal insufficiency are usually made to minimize nephrotoxicity.

Drug Interactions. Because these immunosuppressive agents are extensively metabolized by CYP3A4, which may be responsible for more than half the metabolism of all drugs, the potential for drug interactions is immense. The narrow therapeutic ranges of CSA and TAC underscore the importance of monitoring for drug interactions to prevent toxicity and to avoid subtherapeutic concentrations that may increase the risk of allograft rejection. Table 27.7 outlines important drug interactions with CSA and TAC. All new medications should be viewed as having the potential to alter CSA and TAC concentrations until data and experience dictate otherwise. Agents such a phenytoin, phenobarbital, carbamazepine, and rifampin induce P-450 enzymes and increase CSA and TAC metabolism, thereby markedly decreasing concentrations. On the other hand, ketoconazole, fluconazole, itraconazole, erythromycin, verapamil, and diltiazem result in increased CSA and TAC concentrations via inhibition of CYP3A4.[30–33] Tacrolimus is subject to pH-dependent degradation. Administration with antacids should be avoided.[32]

In addition to those drugs that cause pharmacokinetic interactions, drugs with potential nephrotoxicity should be used with caution. Drugs such as aminoglycosides, amphotericin B, trimethoprim/sulfamethoxazole, nonsteroidal anti-inflammatory drugs (NSAIDs), and angiotensin-converting enzyme (ACE) inhibitors can potentiate the nephrotoxicity of CSA and TAC.[30–33]

Toxicity. Dose-limiting nephrotoxicity is the most common adverse effect of CSA and TAC. Prolonged treatment with these agents may lead to end-stage renal failure in approximately 10% of cardiac transplant patients and 4% of liver transplant patients at 10 years following transplantation.[34,35] Such treatment often makes the diagnosis of rejection in renal transplant recipients especially difficult. CSA and TAC nephrotoxicity may present acutely and may be noted as an increase in serum creatinine over several days that is usually accompanied by increased drug concentrations and that reverses with dose reduction. Nephrotoxicity can also manifest in a more chronic manner that occurs slowly over time and is not readily reversible.

Dose-related neurotoxicity occurs with both agents but is more extensive and common with TAC than with CSA.[22] Common manifestations include tremor, headache, paresthe-

sia, and seizure. Concomitant administration of other seizurogenic medications should be approached with caution. Insomnia, nightmares, tingling sensations, myalgia, itching, and sensitivity to light and heat are reported by patients who are taking TAC.

Although both agents are associated with glucose intolerance, this condition has been reported more commonly with TAC than CSA.[22] Tacrolimus may cause alopecia, whereas CSA is associated with hirsutism, as well as gingival hyperplasia.

Monitoring. Drug level monitoring is an integral part of therapy with CSA or TAC. Because both agents exhibit wide interpatient and intrapatient variability in pharmacokinetics, and because both have narrow therapeutic ranges, it is often difficult for clinicians to tailor therapy to specific patients. Drug level monitoring is used to help guide therapy and dosage adjustment decisions in an attempt to optimize immunosuppressive effects while minimizing toxicity. In addition, concentration monitoring may be useful in monitoring compliance.

Three strategies have been employed to optimize CSA therapy: trough concentration monitoring, complete AUC monitoring, and abbreviated AUC monitoring. Although trough concentration monitoring is practical, a single concentration may not adequately characterize the average drug exposure. Alternatively, AUC has been suggested to correlate with outcome; however, complete pharmacokinetic profiles are cumbersome and costly to obtain, and a single profile may be of little use. Abbreviated AUC monitoring with a limited sampling strategy can be used in patients who are given Neoral secondary to a somewhat predictable pharmacokinetic profile.[36]

CSA levels can be measured by several means. Radioimmunoassay (RIA) and fluorescence polarization immunoassay are employed most frequently. High-performance liquid chromatography (HPLC) remains the gold standard but is infrequently used because it is costly and time consuming. Because different assays have variable specificity for CSA and its metabolites, accepted ranges vary widely between methodologies.[36]

RIAs and fluorescence polarization immunoassays can further be subdivided. One class uses a CSA-specific monoclonal antibody; the nonspecific monoclonal antibody measures CSA, as well as some metabolites. In general, specific RIA and HPLC are used to measure CSA concentrations in whole blood with target concentrations ranging from 150 to 400 ng per mL.

Trough level monitoring is used to optimize TAC therapy. As with CSA, whole blood is the preferred medium for analysis because concentrations are higher and analysis times faster with blood than with plasma. Two assays are available to measure TAC concentrations: an enzyme-linked immunosorbent assay (ELISA) and a microparticle enzyme immunoassay (MEIA). Each has its disadvantages: MEIA lacks sensitivity at low TAC concentrations, whereas ELISA has a

Table 27.7	**Potential Drug Interactions with Immunosuppressive Drugs**

Reported Effect on Immunosuppressant Concentration

	CSA	TAC	SIR	MMF
Amiodarone	↑			
Antacids		↓		↓
Allopurinol	↑			
Bromocriptine		↑		
Carbamazepine	↓			
Cimetidine	↑	↑		
Cisapride	↑			
Clarithromycin	↑	↑		
Clotrimazole	↑, ↔	↑		
Corticosteroids	↑, ↔	↑		
Cyclosporine		↑	↑	
Danazol	↑	↑		
Dexamethasone		↑		
Diltiazem	↑	↑	↑	
Ergotamine		↑		
Erythromycin	↑	↑		
Fluconazole	↑	↑		
Glipizide	↑			
Itraconazole	↑	↑		
Ketoconazole	↑	↑	↑	
Metoclopramide	↑			
Miconazole	↑			
Midazolam		↑		
Nafcillin	↓			
Nefazodone		↑		
Nicardipine	↑	↑		
Nifedipine		↑		
Octreotide	↓			
Omeprazole		↑		
Phenobarbital	↓	↓		
Phenytoin	↓			
Primidone	↓			
Rifampin	↓	↓	↓	
Sirolimus	↑, ↔	↔		
Sodium bicarbonate		↓		
Tacrolimus	↑			↑
Tamoxifen		↑		
Ticlopidine	↓			
Verapamil	↑	↑		

CSA, cyclosporine; TAC, tacrolimus; SIR, sirolimus; MMF, mycophenolate mofetil.

slower turnaround time. Therapeutic whole blood TAC concentrations range from 5 to 20 ng per mL, depending on the time posttransplantation and the organ that was transplanted.[36–38]

Dosing. CSA doses vary widely between transplant centers, depending on type of organ transplant, time posttransplantation, other immunosuppressive agents used, and targeted concentrations. Initial doses range from 6 to 20 mg/kg/day. Because of its improved bioavailability and decreased variability, Neora is becoming the most commonly used form of CSA for CSA-naive patients. The conversion from Sandimmune to Neoral in stable patients is a topic of controversy. With increased CSA exposure associated with Neoral, patients taking it may be at greater risk for toxicity. Conversion is usually made on a milligram per milligram basis, with frequent monitoring of blood levels and serum creatinine. Most patients ultimately require a lower dose of Neoral than of Sandimmune. Both Neoral and Sandimmune are available as 25- and 100-mg capsules and as an oral solution of 100 mg per mL. Parenteral CSA is available as a solution of 250 mg per 5 mL. CSA is usually dosed every 12 hours and should be administered in a consistent fashion with respect to time of day and meals. The oral solution is not very palatable and is best administered in chocolate milk. The oral solution may be flushed with water in patients receiving CSA via nasogastric tube. Parenteral CSA is usually administered over 2 to 24 hours in 5% dextrose or 0.9% sodium chloride in glass. Intravenous CSA is empirically started at one third the oral dose and is titrated according to concentration.

TAC may be administered intravenously in the early postoperative setting at doses ranging from 0.05 to 0.1 mg/kg/day over 4 to 24 hours. TAC in a final concentration of 4 to 20 µg per mL can be administered with 5% dextrose or with 0.9% sodium chloride in glass. TAC is available as a 5-mg per mL intravenous concentrate, and as 0.5-, 1-, and 5-mg capsules. Oral therapy may be initiated posttransplantation at a dose of 0.15 to 0.3 mg/kg/day, divided every 12 hours. When patients are converted from intravenous to oral therapy, the daily intravenous dose is generally tripled and administered divided in two equal doses at 12-hour intervals. Grapefruit juice inhibits gut CYP3A4 metabolism, resulting in increased immunosuppressant absorption. Patients should be advised against administration of CSA and TAC with grapefruit juice so that erratic CSA or TAC exposure and toxicity can be avoided.

SIROLIMUS

Sirolimus (SIR), formerly known as rapamycin, is a macrolide immunosuppressant that is structurally similar to TAC; it inhibits T-cell activation via suppression of proliferation driven by IL-2 and IL-4.[39] This mechanism is distinct from that of CSA and TAC. Whereas CSA and TAC inhibit cytokine production, SIR appears to inhibit response to these cytokines. The SIR-FKBP12 complex binds to the mammalian target of rapamycin (mTOR). IL-2 stimulates mTOR to activate kinases that ultimately advance the cell cycle from G_1 to S phase. Thus, the SIR-FKBP12 complex inhibits T-cell proliferation by inhibiting cellular response to IL-2 and progression of the cell cycle.[39]

Pharmacokinetics and Metabolism. SIR is a lipophilic compound with a high volume of distribution; it readily distributes into most tissues of the body. Bioavailability of the oral formula is poor at only 15%; peak concentrations are reached within 1 to 2 hours.[39] Metabolism occurs primarily by CYP3A4 and p-glycoprotein, both in the gut and in the liver. The average half-life is reported to be 60 hours but can range up to 110 hours in patients with liver dysfunction.[40]

Drug Interactions. As with CSA and TAC, CYP3A4 is the major metabolic pathway for SIR. Therefore, drug interactions mediated by induction or inhibition of the CYP3A4 enzyme system are similar with SIR. Although concomitant administration of CSA microemulsion with SIR significantly increases SIR AUC trough levels, the same is not seen with the standard formulation of CSA. Additionally, CSA concentrations and AUC are increased by SIR, probably because of competitive binding to CYP3A4 and p-glycoprotein. It is recommended that patients separate the doses of SIR and CSA by 4 hours to minimize interaction and prevent potential toxicities of the combination.[41] Concomitant administration of TAC does not affect SIR levels.[42]

Toxicity. SIR is associated with dose-related myelosuppression, which has been correlated with SIR trough levels greater than 15 ng per mL.[43] Thrombocytopenia usually manifests within the first 2 weeks of therapy but generally improves with continued treatment. Leukopenia and anemia are typically transient.[44] Hypercholesterolemia and hypertriglyceridemia are common with SIR. It is postulated that these adverse effects are mediated through overproduction of lipoproteins or inhibition of lipoprotein lipase. Peak cholesterol and triglyceride levels are seen within 3 months of initiation of SIR, but these usually decrease after 1 year of therapy and can be managed by dose reduction or discontinuation, or by the use of antihyperlipidemic agents such as hydroxymethyl glutaryl coenzyme A (HMG-CoA) reductase inhibitors or fibric acid derivatives. A recent study suggests that SIR-associated dyslipidemia is not a major risk factor for early cardiovascular complications following kidney transplant.[44,45] Delayed wound healing and wound dehiscence have been reported in patients receiving SIR therapy; these could be due to inhibition of smooth muscle proliferation and intimal thickening.[46] Mouth ulcers have also been reported with SIR, more commonly with the oral solution. This may be a direct effect of the drug itself or may result from activation of the herpes simplex virus.[47] Interstitial pneumonitis, which has been described in kidney, liver, and heart-lung transplant recipients, is reversible after discontinuation of SIR.[40] Other adverse effects reported with

SIR include increased liver enzymes, hypertension, rash, acne, diarrhea, and arthralgia.

Similar to CSA and TAC, grapefruit juice produces increases in SIR levels. Administration of SIR with a high-fat meal delays the rate of absorption and decreases the C_{max} when compared with the fasting state. However, the AUC increases, indicating increased drug exposure, while the half-life remains unchanged.[48] The clinical significance of this is unknown. Consistency should be maintained with administration of SIR with regard to meals and food.

Dosing and Monitoring. A fixed SIR dosing regimen has been approved for concomitant use with CSA; it includes a loading dose that is three times the maintenance dose (usually, a 6-mg or 15-mg loading dose), followed by 2 mg or 5 mg daily, respectively. Similar dosing strategies have been used in clinical trials that combined SIR with TAC. Similar to TAC, SIR binds extensively to erythrocytes because of the high FKBP12 concentration found in red blood cells (RBCs). Therapeutic monitoring of SIR with the use of whole blood concentrations is advocated to a target level of 10 to 15 ng per mL when used in combination with a calcineurin inhibitor, or to higher levels (12 to 24 ng/mL) when used in regimens that involve CSA withdrawal.[36]

ANTIBODY-BASED THERAPY

Both polyclonal and monoclonal antibody preparations have a role in immunosuppressant therapy. Polyclonal antibodies have been used for induction and for rejection treatment. Monoclonal antibodies are more specific in their targets. OKT3, the first available monoclonal antibody, has been used for induction and for rejection treatment, whereas the newest monoclonal antibodies, the IL-2 receptor antagonists, have a primary role in induction.

Antithymocyte Globulins. Two antithymocyte globulin (ATG) preparations are currently available: ATGAM is produced from horses, whereas thymoglobulin (rATG) is derived from rabbits. When used as part of induction protocols, ATG is given immediately after transplant to prevent or delay the first rejection, or to protect early kidney function from the nephrotoxicity of CSA or TAC. ATG is also effective in treating steroid-resistant rejection.[49] ATG causes complement-mediated lysis of lymphocytes, removal by the reticuloendothelial system, or alteration of T-cell function. One of the limitations of polyclonal antibody therapy is the high degree of immunosuppression that puts patients at risk for the development of malignancy and viral infection.[50] These products are associated with dose-related thrombocytopenia and leukopenia. In addition, patients may experience a serum sickness reaction that resembles a flulike syndrome, with fever, chills, malaise, arthralgia, nausea, vomiting, and lymphadenopathy. Acetaminophen, diphenhydramine, and corticosteroids may be administered as premedication to allay some of these effects. Doses should be reduced or held for platelet counts lower than 70,000 per cubic millimeter (or profound leukopenia). ATGAM is available as a 50-mg

per mL solution that must be diluted in 0.45% or 0.9% sodium chloride before it is administered. Thymoglobulin is compatible with 0.9% sodium chloride or 5% dextrose solutions. It should be diluted to a final concentration of 0.5 mg per mL before administration. Both products must be filtered and administered over 4 to 6 hours via a central venous catheter; this minimizes the risks of phlebitis and tissue necrosis.

MONOCLONAL ANTIBODIES

Muromonab (OKT3). OKT3 is a purified murine immunoglobulin G (IgG)2a monoclonal antibody to the CD3 receptor on the surface of mature human T-cells. OKT3 is thought to exert anti–T-cell proliferative effect by two mechanisms: T-cell depletion and T-cell receptor modulation. OKT3 may bind mature T-cells, causing opsonization and removal by the reticuloendothelial system. Minutes after intravenous injection of OKT3, CD3+ cells are rapidly cleared from the circulation. This process is complete within 1 hour. OKT3 can also remove CD3 molecules on the surface of T-cells, thus rendering T-lymphocytes unable to function properly.[15]

OKT3 is used for induction therapy and for the treatment of rejection. Because of several limitations, however, OKT3 is often reserved for steroid-resistant rejection, by which it is effective in 75% to 95% of patients. Significant T-cell suppression by OKT3 may result in increased lymphomas and viral infection, in particular, cytomegalovirus. In addition, neutralizing antibodies can develop against OKT3, preventing its further use. OKT3 is also associated with a severe ''first-dose reaction'' or ''cytokine release syndrome,'' which consists of flulike symptoms, dyspnea, tremor, chest pain, pulmonary edema, and possibly asepsis. Seizures have also been associated with its use. The reaction is thought to be due to the release of cytokines during initial T-cell depletion. Several strategies have been employed to lessen the severity and duration of this response. These include premedication with various combinations of corticosteroids, acetaminophen, indomethacin, diphenhydramine, and pentoxyfilline.[51] The first few doses of OKT3 are usually administered in a controlled setting, such as the intensive care unit.

The recommended dose of OKT3 is 5 mg given intravenously daily for 7 to 14 days. The dose can be given peripherally or centrally by intravenous (IV) push. Patients who weigh less than 30 kg should receive 2.5 mg per day. To decrease the risk of pulmonary edema, OKT3 should not be administered to patients who are more than 3% over their dry weight.

Immunologic monitoring has been used to determine the efficacy of OKT3 therapy. Three tactics have been employed, either alone or in combination.[15,51] First, CD3+ cells can be quantified. OKT3 administration results in rapid disappearance of CD3+ cells from the circulation. For optimal efficacy, CD3+ cells should remain undetectable. This method, however, measures only circulating CD3+ cells and does not quantify those infiltrating the allograft. With this approach, CD3 + cells are measured three times weekly. If CD3 + cells remain elevated, the dose of OKT3 may be increased. Second, serum OKT3 concentrations can be monitored. Two factors influence OKT3 concentrations: the number of available CD3 molecules and the gradual formation of anti-OKT3 antibodies. OKT3 concentrations should therefore provide information on the efficacy of OKT3 and should serve as an indirect measure of xenosensitization (formation of antibodies against OKT3 by the patient). This method remains controversial. Third, anti-OKT3 antibodies can be monitored to determine the level of recipient sensitization. Most centers measure anti-OKT3 antibodies if a patient is to receive a second course of OKT3. OKT3 may remain effective if the antibody titer is less than 1:100; OKT3 should not be given if the titer is greater than 1:1,000.

IL-2 Receptor Antagonists — Basiliximab and Daclizumab. The introduction of basiliximab and daclizumab has provided several opportunities in transplant immunosuppression. These agents are being used in steroid-limiting and calcineurin-limiting protocols, in addition to having replaced ATG and OKT3 in many induction protocols. These IL-2 receptor antagonists (IL-2-RAs) are monoclonal antibodies that exert their immunosuppressive effects by binding to and blocking the α-subunit of the IL-2 receptor on the surface of activated T-lymphocytes; they inhibit IL-2–mediated activation of lymphocytes, which is a necessary step for the clonal expansion of T-cells. Clinical trials in renal transplant patients using daclizumab or basiliximab versus placebo in combination with CSA-based immunosuppression have demonstrated significant reductions in the incidence of biopsy-proven rejection over the first 12 months posttransplantation.[52–55] These agents have not been associated with infusion-related adverse effects that are common with other antibody preparations. In addition, these agents are far easier to administer than are other monoclonal or polyclonal antilymphocyte preparations. The recommended dose of basiliximab is 20 mg in 50 mL of dextrose or normal saline infused over 20 to 30 minutes before transplantation, followed by 20 mg on the fourth day posttransplantation. Daclizumab is administered at a dose of 1 mg per kg in 50 mL of normal saline over 15 minutes every 14 days for 5 doses, starting on the day of transplant. Both agents can be administered via peripheral or central venous catheter. The adverse effects reported in clinical trials of these agents were comparable with those reported in the placebo arms. It is important to note that this greater degree of immunosuppression did not seem to confer an increased risk of infection. Although experience is extremely limited, no drug interactions with IL-2 receptor antagonists have been reported. Few patients have developed anti-idiotype antibodies to basiliximab and daclizumab. Anaphylaxis has been reported in a small number of patients with the second dose of basiliximab.

ALTERNATIVE IMMUNOSUPPRESSIVE OPTIONS

In addition to the aforementioned immunosuppressants, chemotherapeutic agents such as methotrexate and cyclophosphamide have been used in lung and heart transplant recipients for refractory rejection. Inhaled CSA has been used as rescue therapy in lung transplant recipients with some success. Other immunosuppressive strategies include total lymphoid irradiation as an adjuvant to pharmacologic immunosuppression, photopheresis for the treatment of heart and lung rejection, and donor-specific blood or bone marrow transfusion in patients with various types of transplants.[56]

INVESTIGATIONAL THERAPIES

ALEMTUZUMAB

Alemtuzumab is a humanized monoclonal antibody directed at cells that express the CD52 surface antigen, such as T-lymphocytes and B-lymphocytes, macrophages, monocytes, and natural killer cells. Binding of alemtuzumab to the CD52 surface antigen results in antibody-dependent lysis and subsequent T-cell depletion.[57]

Adverse effects of alemtuzumab include infusion-related reactions such as rigors, hypotension, fever, shortness of breath, bronchospasm, and chills; hematologic effects such as pancytopenia, neutropenia, thrombocytopenia, and lymphopenia; and infection. Infusion-related reactions may be attenuated by the administration of premedications such as steroids, diphenhydramine, and acetaminophen, or by gradual dose escalation from small starting doses. Dose modifications are recommended according to the degree of thrombocytopenia present.

Various dosing regimens of alemtuzumab have been tried in patients undergoing solid organ transplantation. For induction therapy, the most commonly reported doses in the literature are two 20-mg doses, given on day 0 and day 1, and a 0.3 mg/kg/dose. Early experience indicates that monotherapy with CSA, TAC, or SIR may be used following alemtuzumab induction.[57–59] For the treatment of rejection, doses of 5 to 10 mg for 6 to 10 days have been reported. In practice, increments of 30 or 60 mg are often used to minimize product waste.

EVEROLIMUS

Everolimus, also known as SDZ-RAD, is a rapamycin derivative with immunosuppressive activity similar to that of SIR. Everolimus exerts the same mechanism of action, binding to FKBP12 and inhibiting mTOR and the cellular response to IL-2, ultimately preventing progression of the cell cycle. It is a lipophilic compound that readily distributes into red blood cells because of the high concentration of FBKP12, as well as into tissues. The half-life of everolimus is shorter than that of SIR at 16 to 19 hours, resulting in twice-daily dosing as compared with once-daily dosing with SIR.[60,61] Severe hepatic impairment decreases everolimus clearance.[62] Additionally, preliminary experience with macrolides such as erythromycin and azithromycin and the azole antifungal itraconazole indicates that drug interactions via cytochrome P-450 3A4 influence everolimus elimination.[63]

As with SIR, thrombocytopenia and leukopenia are common within the first 2 months of everolimus therapy. Both total cholesterol and triglyceride levels increase with everolimus use and generally peak within the first month of therapy, but they usually plateau after 2 to 3 months of therapy, most likely because of initiation of antihyperlipidemic agents.[61] These hematologic and cholesterol adverse effects have been reported within the accepted therapeutic range of 7 to 15 ng per mL.[64]

Phase 3 clinical trials are currently evaluating doses of 0.75 mg twice daily and 1.5 mg twice daily in combination with CSA and steroids.

LEFLUNOMIDE, FK778

Leflunomide, currently approved for use in rheumatoid arthritis, has increasingly been used in patients with solid organ transplantation. Leflunomide is a prodrug for the active metabolite A77,1726, which inhibits de novo pyrimidine synthesis and tyrosine kinase activity in T-lymphocytes and B-lymphocytes. It is currently approved for use in patients with rheumatoid arthritis. Bioavailability is 80% after oral administration. Leflunomide is metabolized in the liver, and biliary recirculation of A77,1726 contributes to the long half-life of 15 to 18 days. Adverse effects noted with leflunomide in solid organ transplant studies include skin rash, anemia, and elevated liver enzymes.

In limited experience with leflunomide in the treatment of kidney and liver transplant recipients, loading doses of 1,400 mg over 7 days, followed by maintenance doses of 40 to 60 mg daily have been used to achieve target concentrations of 50 to 80 μg per mL. This has allowed administration of lower doses of steroids and calcineurin inhibitors.[65] A small, open-label pilot study also reported on the potential for leflunomide to reverse chronic renal allograft dysfunction.[66]

FK778, a synthetic derivative of A77,1726, is being evaluated in animal models of solid organ transplantation. It has a shorter half-life than the parent compound and is described as having equivalent or superior immunosuppressive effects.[67]

INFECTION

Infection is a common complication following transplantation. Multiple factors affect the incidence and severity of infectious complications. These factors include the type, intensity, and duration of immunosuppressive therapy, as well as the organisms encountered by the patient in the hospital and community.[68]

Bacterial infection related to the transplant surgery predominates in the first month posttransplantation. Renal transplant recipients, for example, are at risk for urinary tract infection; heart and lung transplant patients for intrathoracic infection and pneumonia; and liver and pancreas transplant patients for intra-abdominal infection. Bacterial infection

may also be transmitted from the donor. Should a donor culture become positive after the time of transplantation, organism-specific anti-infective prophylaxis should be initiated in the transplant recipient. As a result of high-dose steroids and antimicrobial pharmacotherapy, candidal infections are also common in the early posttransplant period. Routine prophylaxis with oral antifungal agents such as nystatin or clotrimazole troches four times daily greatly reduces the incidence of these infections.[68]

CYTOMEGALOVIRUS

Viral infection usually occurs at between 1 and 6 months after transplantation. Cytomegalovirus (CMV) is the most important viral pathogen in transplant patients, affecting up to 70%.[68–70] CMV infection commonly refers to the presence of serologic evidence of CMV, whereas CMV disease indicates symptomatic presentation.[70] CMV may be present as latent infection in the donor or the recipient or both. CMV-seronegative recipients (R–) of CMV-seropositive organs (D+) are at higher risk of symptomatic infection than are seropositive recipients (R+) of seropositive (D+) or seronegative (D–) organs. Administration of antilymphocyte antibodies and cytotoxic drugs heightens the risk for primary activation or reactivation of symptomatic CMV disease in seropositive patients. The direct effects of acute CMV disease include unexplained fever, malaise, myalgia, leukopenia, thrombocytopenia, and mild hepatitis. The immunomodulatory effects of CMV also render patients susceptible to opportunistic infection. It is not uncommon for patients with *Pneumocystis carinii* pneumonia (PCP) or aspergillosis to have concomitant (but previously undiagnosed) CMV disease. CMV has been associated with acute and chronic allograft rejection: bronchiolitis obliterans—lung; coronary atherosclerosis—heart; vanishing bile duct syndrome—liver.[71–73]

Because of the importance of CMV in transplantation, several strategies have been employed to minimize its effects. Prophylaxis remains controversial. Prophylactic measures include high-dose oral acyclovir, oral or intravenous ganciclovir, oral valganciclovir, and CMV hyperimmuoglobulin.[69,74] For the treatment of CMV disease, intravenous ganciclovir remains the standard 5 mg per kg every 12 hours, adjusted for renal insufficiency. Another strategy is to preemptively treat patients at high risk for the development of CMV disease, such as patients who are treated with antibody therapy or those who have antigenic evidence of the CMV virus in their blood, based on surveillance monitoring.[70] Table 27.8 reviews the pharmacologic approaches to management of CMV disease.

Other viral infections are also important. Patients may experience reactivation of viral infection, such as oral or genital herpes or varicella zoster virus, as shingles. Recurrence of these latent infections often reflects a state of overimmunosuppression; such infection usually responds to antiviral therapy with or without reduction in immunosuppression.

Table 27.8	Strategies for the Treatment of Cytomegalovirus Disease in Transplant Recipients	
Strategy	**Treatments Employed**	**Considerations**
Prophylactic		
Goal: prevention of CMV disease	IV ganciclovir 5 mg/kg/day × 3 months	Development of resistant organisms; unnecessary exposure to toxic drugs; cost of therapies; availability and variable potency of CMVIG
Treat all patients	PO ganciclovir 1 g tid × 3 months	
	PO valganciclovir 900 mg qd	
	PO acyclovir 800 mg qid × 12 weeks	
	CMVIG 150 mg/kg at transplant; 50–100 mg/kg every 2–4 weeks post-transplant for ~16 weeks	
Preemptive		
Goal: prevention of CMV disease	IV ganciclovir × 14 days (or until resolution of infection) based on positive surveillance monitoring during 0–6 months post-transplant	Sensitivity and specificity of surveillance to predict who would develop clinical disease
Treat patients with serologic evidence of infection or at high risk		Does surveillance marker become positive early enough to prevent clinical disease?
	IV ganciclovir prophylaxis for high-risk patients (i.e., antibody therapy)	
Treatment		
Goal: prevent morbidity and mortality of CMV disease	IV ganciclovir; minimize immunosuppression	May be too late to prevent serious complications of CMV disease

CMV, cytomegalovirus; CMVIG, cytomegalovirus immune globulin.

PNEUMOCYSTIS CARINII PNEUMONIA

PCP can be virtually eliminated through the use of prophylactic trimethoprim/sulfamethoxazole (TMP/SMX) (80/400 mg per day). In untreated patients, the incidence of PCP ranges from 2% to 12%.[75] Prophylaxis with TMP/SMX also reduces the risk of *Listeria monocytogenes*, *Nocardia*, and *Toxoplasma gondii* infections. This combination also decreases the rate of urinary tract infection in renal transplant recipients. For patients who are intolerant of TMP/SMX, monthly inhalation treatment with pentamidine 300 mg or daily oral dapsone provides protection against PCP.[76,77] Prophylaxis generally continues for 6 to 12 months; however, some centers employ lifelong prophylaxis.

CARDIOVASCULAR COMPLICATIONS

Cardiovascular disease is especially common among transplant patients and is a major cause of morbidity and mortality. In fact, cardiovascular disease is the most common cause of death after kidney transplantation.[78] It may lead to end-stage renal or cardiac disease. In addition, hypertension, hyperlipidemia, and diabetes may be exacerbated by immunosuppressant agents.

Hypertension is often present at the time of transplantation but may develop as a result of immunosuppressive medications, such as corticosteroids, CSA, and TAC. Impaired graft function may also result in hypertension after renal transplantation. With some special precautions, the treatment of hypertension in transplant patients can generally be approached according to the guidelines established by the Joint National Committee on the Detection, Evaluation, and Treatment of High Blood Pressure.[79] Calcium channel blockers are often considered first-line agents for the treatment of posttransplant hypertension in patients receiving CSA or TAC. Calcium channel blockers may also attenuate the nephrotoxic effects of the calcineurin inhibitors and may improve renal hemodynamics.[80] Calcium channel blockers are generally well tolerated, but gingival hyperplasia may be more common in patients who are also taking CSA.

Diltiazem, verapamil, and nicardipine inhibit CSA and TAC metabolism by inhibiting CYP3A4. This interaction, if unmonitored, may lead to CSA- or TAC-induced nephrotoxicity and neurotoxicity. With proper monitoring and CSA or TAC dosage adjustments, agents like diltiazem and verapamil can be used to decrease the daily dose of CSA or TAC. The end result is a decrease in overall medication costs.

ACE inhibitors and angiotensin II (AT2) blockers may be effective after transplantation. However, the combination of efferent arteriolar vasodilatation caused by the ACE inhibitor or AT2 blocker and afferent vasoconstriction caused by CSA or TAC may result in decreased glomerular filtration when these agents are used together. In addition, the hyperkalemia caused by CSA or TAC is frequently aggravated by concomitant therapy with an ACE inhibitor. If ACE inhibitor therapy is used in renal transplant patients, close monitoring of serum creatinine and potassium is required.

Therapy with CSA, corticosteroids, diuretics, and β-adrenergic blockers can have a detrimental effect on serum lipids. Traditionally, clinicians have started treatment according to the guidelines of the National Cholesterol Education Program (NCEP).[81] However, these may not adequately reflect the need for aggressive lipid-lowering therapy following solid organ transplantation. In addition, the National Kidney Foundation recently published guidelines for the treatment of renal transplant patients.[82] Effective lipid-lowering modalities may not only arrest the progress and prevent the complications of atherosclerosis but may promote renal and cardiac graft survival. Potential strategies for the treatment of hyperlipidemia in transplant patients include dietary intervention, reduced immunosuppression, and the use of lipid-lowering agents.[78]

HMG-CoA reductase inhibitors are highly effective in the treatment of patients with hyperlipidemia, specifically, increased low-density lipoprotein (LDL). They are generally well tolerated, especially when used as monotherapy. Studies in renal and cardiac transplant recipients treated with pravastatin and simvastatin have demonstrated a reduction in the incidence of rejection and improved survival.[78] This class of agents should be used with caution because of several reports of rhabdomyolysis resulting in renal failure when lovastatin was used in combination with CSA. Safety measures, including the use of low doses of an HMG-CoA reductase inhibitor and avoidance of inappropriately high CSA concentrations, should be used with all drugs in this class. The concurrent use of medications known to increase the risk of myopathy (e.g., gemfibrozil) should be avoided. Patients should be informed of the signs and symptoms of rhabdomyolysis. Baseline and follow-up creatine phosphokinase (CPK) measurements (every 6 months) have been used to identify patients who develop subclinical rhabdomyolysis when cholesterol-lowering therapy is used. In addition, because of the potential for hepatotoxicity from HMG-CoA reductase inhibitors, close monitoring of liver function is indicated, especially in liver transplant patients.

Several studies have examined the use of niacin in transplant patients. It is not recommended for routine use. In addition to the potential for liver toxicity, niacin may impair glucose control. Bile acid–binding resins may be used to lower cholesterol in transplant patients, although adequate doses are difficult to achieve without the development of GI adverse effects. Because the absorption of CSA is dependent on the presence of bile in the GI tract, patients should be instructed to separate dosing of bile acid–binding resins and CSA by 2 hours. Because the absorption of TAC is not dependent on bile, this interaction is not of significance in patients taking TAC. For those transplant patients who have hypertriglyceridemia and are refractory to dietary intervention, fish oil and fibric acid derivatives appear to be well tolerated and are effective alternatives. Gemfibrozil is most effective in lowering serum triglyceride concentrations. Doses of gemfibrozil must be reduced in patients with decreased renal function.[78]

Management of diabetes in the posttransplant period can be difficult. Immunosuppressive medications may cause glucose intolerance, occasionally leading to new-onset diabetes. New-onset diabetes in posttransplant patients is commonly referred to as posttransplant diabetes mellitus (PTDM) and is present in 4% to 20% of renal transplant patients.[83]

Immunosuppressive medications, including corticosteroids, CSA, and TAC, are known to be diabetogenic. AZA and MMF do not contribute to glucose intolerance. Corticosteroids seem to induce insulin resistance, but other mechanisms have been suggested, including decreased insulin receptor number and affinity; impaired peripheral glucose uptake; and impaired suppression of endogenous insulin production.[83] The contribution of CSA to PTDM appears to be mediated by inhibition of insulin production. Patient factors that may contribute to PTDM include African American race, advanced age, obesity, specific HLA subtypes, receipt of cadaveric kidney, and aspects of family history.

Regardless of therapy, frequent blood glucose monitoring is imperative in the early posttransplant period. Tapering of immunosuppressive medications may result in lower insulin requirements, whereas steroid pulses for the treatment of rejection may result in increased insulin requirements.

MALIGNANCY

Malignancy affects as many as 6% to 18% of patients following transplantation; the risk of tumor increases over time. Immunosuppressive therapy may allow for the development of malignant tumors because of depressed immunosurveillance. Immunosuppressive agents such as AZA and cyclophosphamide may damage DNA and potentiate the effects of other carcinogens such as sunlight.[84] The development of malignancy posttransplantation is related to the relative amount of immunosuppression as evidenced by a difference in rates of malignancy associated with quadruple versus triple versus dual immunosuppressant regimens.[85]

Posttransplant malignancies are often divided into three classes: de novo malignancy, recurrent disease, and disease that is directly transmitted from donor to recipient. Transplant patients do not seem to be at increased risk for cancers that are common in the general population (e.g., lung, breast; colon; and prostate cancers). The malignancies that are most commonly diagnosed in transplant patients are those that can be linked to viral origins: Kaposi sarcoma, squamous cell carcinoma, non-Hodgkin lymphoma, skin cancer, and cancer of the vulva and perineum.[84] Transplant patients should be counseled on the use of sunscreen and protective clothing. Regular self-examination of the skin and lymph nodes may also aid in early diagnosis of some malignancies. Attempts should be made to minimize the amount of immunosuppression patients receive and to prevent viral infection where possible. When cancer is diagnosed in a transplant patient, immunosuppressive medications should be reduced or discontinued. Treatment with appropriate antineoplastic, surgical, or radiologic intervention should then begin.

Lymphomas after transplantation are of particular interest. Compared with matched controls, relative risk for the development of lymphoma ranges from 11.8 to almost 240 for renal and heart-lung transplant recipients, respectively.[85] Lymphoma is related not only to the intensity of immunosuppression, but also to the type. OKT3 and ATG have been associated with higher risks of lymphoma. In pediatric patients, TAC may confer greater risk. Posttransplant lymphoproliferative disorder (PTLD), the presence of an abnormal proliferation of lymphoid cells, appears to have viral origins in Epstein-Barr virus (EBV) infection. PTLD results when immunosuppression limits T-cell responses that control proliferation of EBV-infected B-cells; it is most common in the first year after transplant, when the level of immunosuppression is highest. Incidence ranges from 0.2% of kidney transplant recipients to 15% of intestinal transplant patients.[85] Patients may present with persistent malaise, fever, and leukopenia. Serologic evidence of EBV infection may be present, but diagnosis relies on the demonstration of abnormal lymphoid proliferation. Reduction in immunosuppression is the cornerstone of treatment for PTLD. Because of the viral origins of PTLD, acyclovir and ganciclovir have been used to promote its regression.

Recurrence of a previous cancer is dependent on both the length of time since cancer treatment was provided and the type of cancer. More than half of cancers that recur do so in patients who are treated less than 2 years before transplantation. Malignancies that recur most frequently are renal carcinoma, malignant melanoma, sarcoma, and nonmelanoma skin cancer.[84] Most directly transplanted malignancies occurred in the early transplant era, before the risk of malignancy was fully appreciated.

ALTERNATIVE MEDICINE

Increasingly, patients are seeking information about and self-administering "natural" or "herbal" medicines. Transplant patients are no exception. Although information about alternative medicines is often sparse, data on these therapies in immunosuppressed and transplant recipients are even less common. Most transplant patients usually have a variety of other disease states that must be considered. Little information is available about the immunomodulatory effects of alternative medicines, or about their effects on the pharmacokinetics of immunosuppressive agents.

Echinacea, which is touted to aid wound healing and demonstrate antiviral activity, should not be used by transplant recipients. Echinacea has been shown to stimulate T-lymphocyte proliferation and interferon production, both of which could interfere with immunosuppressive medications and precipitate allograft rejection.[33] Oral aloe, ginseng, and cat's claw are among other herbal medications that might have immunomodulatory effects. These should be avoided as well. St. John's Wort has been shown to induce cytochrome P-450 3A4 and p-glycoprotein, thus resulting in significant reductions in trough levels of both CSA and TAC.[33] All medicines, herbal or otherwise, should always be used with caution in patients who take medications with narrow therapeutic windows.

PATIENT EDUCATION

Compliance with immunosuppressant medications is essential for long-term graft survival.[86] Unfortunately, the first clinical indication of gross noncompliance may be irreversible allograft rejection. Pharmacists can play a key role in teaching patients about the importance of immunosuppressant medications. Initially, transplant medication regimens are very complex. Patients may benefit from individualized schedules with administration times tied to daily triggers such as meals. It is important that the clinician try to minimize the number of medication administration times per day. Compliance with prophylactic medications is important; noncompliance may lead to life-threatening infection. Patients should be educated about the adverse effects of their medications, as well as the common symptoms of rejection.

CONCLUSIONS

Solid organ transplantation is an increasingly common therapeutic option for patients with life-threatening end-stage organ disease. Continued development of new immunosuppressive therapies and improvement in our understanding of the immune system have resulted in lower complication rates and improved graft survival. Improved survival means that clinicians will be caring for transplant patients well into the future and must be mindful of the many chronic conditions that may accompany transplantation. Transplantation continues to be associated with many challenges, including the shortage of donor organs compared with the growing need, economic barriers to transplantation and compliance, and chronic rejection. Pharmacists can play an important role in caring for transplant patients and promoting long-term well-being, medication compliance, and graft survival.

KEY POINTS

■ Organ transplantation is a life-saving treatment for many end-organ diseases.

- The primary goal of immunosuppressive therapy is the prevention of allograft rejection, which remains a major cause of graft loss and morbidity.
- The use of immunosuppressive drugs in the prevention of rejection must be balanced against the risks of infection, cardiovascular disease, and malignancy.
- Cytomegalovirus is the most important infection in transplant recipients and may predispose allografts to chronic rejection.
- Immunosuppressant medications have many toxicities. Many new chronic medical conditions such as diabetes, hypertension, hyperlipidemia, and osteoporosis may require treatment following transplantation.
- Immunosuppressive medications have narrow therapeutic indices. Patients must be monitored closely for signs and symptoms of efficacy and toxicity.
- Concomitant therapy with nephrotoxic agents or drugs that interfere with CYP3A4 metabolism should be approached with caution. Increased monitoring is warranted (e.g., serum creatinine [SCr], CSA, TAC, or SIR levels).
- Noncompliance is a treatable cause of late allograft loss. Pharmacists can play a key role in providing patient education and actively assessing transplant patients for noncompliance.

REFERENCES

1. 2003 OPTN/SRTR annual report. Available at: http://www.optn.org. Accessed July 12, 2004.
2. Abu-Elmagd K, Reyes J, Bond G, et al. Clinical intestinal transplantation: a decade of experience at a single center. Ann Surg 234: 404–417, 2001.
3. Dorling A, Riesbeck K, Warrens A, et al. Clinical xenotransplantation of solid organs. Lancet 349:867–871, 1997.
4. Merion RM, Magee JC. Renal transplantation. In: Greenfield LJ, ed. Surgery: scientific principles and practice. Philadelphia: Lippincott Williams & Wilkins, 2001:568–576.
5. Auchincloss H, Shaffer D. Pancreas transplantation. In: Ginns LC, Cosimi AB, Morris PJ, eds. Transplantation. Malden, Mass: Blackwell Science, 1999:395–412.
6. Campbell DA, Magee JC, Rudich SM, et al. Hepatic transplantation. In: Greenfield LJ, ed. Surgery: scientific principles and practice. Philadelphia: Lippincott Williams & Wilkins, 2001:577–597.
7. Pierson RN. Cardiac transplantation. In: Greenfield LJ, ed. Surgery: scientific principles and practice. Philadelphia: Lippincott Williams & Wilkins, 2001:597–608.
8. Kaiser LR. Pulmonary transplantation. In: Greenfield LJ, ed. Surgery: scientific principles and practice. Philadelphia: JB Lippincott, 1993:548–559.
9. Goulet O, Jan D, Brousse N, et al. Intestinal transplantation. J Pediatr Gastroenterol Nutr 25:1–11, 1997.
10. Soin AS, Friend PJ. Recent developments in transplantation of the small intestine. Br Med Bull 53:789–797, 1997.
11. LeMoine A, Goldman M, Abramowicz D. Multiple pathways to allograft rejection. Transplantation 73:1373–1381, 2002.
12. Massy ZA, Guijarro C, Wiederkehr MR, et al. Chronic renal allograft rejection. Immunologic and nonimmunologic risk factors. Kidney Int 49:518–524, 1996.
13. Reichenspurner H, Girgis RE, Robbins RC, et al. Stanford experience with obliterative bronchiolitis after lung and heart-lung transplantation. Ann Thorac Surg 62:1467–1473, 1996.
14. Grotz W, Siebig S, Olschewski M, et al. Low-dose aspirin therapy is associated with improved allograft function and prolonged allograft survival after kidney transplantation. Transplantation 77: 1848–1853, 2004.
15. Bush WW. Overview of transplantation immunology and the pharmacotherapy of adult solid organ transplant recipients: focus on immunosuppression. AACN Clin Issues 10:253–269, 1999.
16. Murray JE, Merrill JP, Harrison JH, et al. Prolonged survival of human kidney homografts by immunosuppressive therapy. N Engl J Med 268:1315–1323, 1963.
17. Cox VC, Ensom MHH. Mycophenolate mofetil for solid organ transplantation: does the evidence support the need for clinical pharmacokinetic monitoring? Ther Drug Monit 25:137–157, 2003.
18. Bullingham R, Shah J, Goldblum R, et al. Effects of food and antacid on the pharmacokinetics of single doses of mycophenolate mofetil in rheumatoid arthritis patients. Br J Clin Pharmacol 41: 513–516, 1996.
19. Wolfe EJ, Mathur V, Tomlanovich S, et al. Pharmacokinetics of mycophenolate mofetil and intravenous ganciclovir alone and in combination in renal transplant recipients. Pharmacotherapy 17:591–598, 1997.
20. Zucker K, Rosen A, Tsaroucha A, et al. Augmentation of mycophenolate mofetil pharmacokinetics in renal transplant patients receiving Prograf and Cellcept in combination therapy. Transplant Proc 29: 334–336, 1997.
21. Granger DK. Enteric-coated mycophenolate sodium: results of two pivotal global multicenter trials. Transplant Proc 33:3241–3244, 2001.
22. Tanabe K. Calcineurin inhibitors in renal transplantation: what is the best option? Drugs 63:1535–1548, 2003.
23. Peters DH, Fitton A, Plosker GL, et al. Tacrolimus: a review of its pharmacology, and therapeutic potential in hepatic and renal transplantation. Drugs 46:746–794, 1993.
24. Jordan ML, Naraghi R, Shapiro R, et al. Tacrolimus rescue therapy for renal allograft rejection—five year experience. Transplantation 63:223–228, 1997.
25. Kahan BD, Welsh M, Schoenberg L, et al. Variable oral absorption of cyclosporine: a biopharmaceutical risk factor for chronic renal allograft rejection. Transplantation 62:599–606, 1996.
26. Wahlberg J, Wilczek HE, Fauchald P, et al. Consistent absorption of cyclosporine from a microemulsion formulation assessed in stable renal transplant recipients over a one-year study period. Transplantation 60:648–652, 1995.
27. Gupta SK, Manfro RC, Tomlanovich SJ, et al. Effect of food on the pharmacokinetics of cyclosporine in healthy subjects following oral and intravenous administration. J Clin Pharmacol 30:643–653, 1990.
28. Kelly PA, Burckart GJ, Venkataramanan R. Tacrolimus: a new immunosuppressive agent. Am J Health-Syst Pharm 52:1521–1535, 1995.
29. Hauben M. Cyclosporine neurotoxicity. Pharmacotherapy 16:576–583, 1996.
30. Campana C, Regazzi MB, Buggia I, et al. Clinically significant drug interactions with cyclosporine: an update. Clin Pharmacokinet 30: 141–179, 1996.
31. Mignat C. Clinically significant drug interactions with new immunosuppressive agents. Drug Saf 16:267–278, 1997.
32. Van Gelder T. Drug interactions with tacrolimus. Drug Saf 25: 707–712, 2002.
33. Christians U, Jacobsen W, Benet LZ, et al. Mechanisms of clinically relevant drug interactions associated with tacrolimus. Clin Pharmacokinet 41:813–851, 2002.
34. Woolfson RG, Neild GH. Cyclosporine nephrotoxicity following cardiac transplantation. Nephrol Dial Transplant 12:2054–2056, 1997.
35. Fisher NC, Nightingale PG, Gunson BK, et al. Chronic renal failure following liver transplantation: a retrospective analysis. Transplantation 66:59–66, 1998.
36. Kahan BD, Keown P, Levy G, et al. Therapeutic drug monitoring of immunosuppressant drugs in clinical practice. Clin Ther 24: 330–350, 2002.
37. Jusko WJ, Thomson AW, Fung J, et al. Consensus document: therapeutic monitoring of tacrolimus (FK-506). Ther Drug Monit 17: 606–614, 1995.
38. Laskow DA, Vincenti F, Neylan JF, et al. An open-label, concentration-ranging trial of FK506 in primary kidney transplantation. Transplantation 62:900–905, 1996.

39. Ingle GR, Sievers TM, Hold CD. Sirolimus: continuing the evolution of transplant immunosuppression. Ann Pharmacother 34: 1044–1055, 2000.

40. Kahan BD, Camardo JS. Rapamycin. Clinical results and future opportunities. Transplantation 72:1181–1193, 2001.

41. Kaplan B, Meier-Kriesche HU, Napoli KL, et al. The effects of relative timing of sirolimus and cyclosporine microemulsion formulation coadministration on the pharmacokinetics of each agent. Clin Pharmacol Ther 63:48–53, 1998.

42. McAlister VC, Mahalati K, Peltekian KM, et al. A clinical pharmacokinetic study of tacrolimus and sirolimus combination immunosuppression comparing simultaneous to separated administration. Therap Drug Monit 23:346–350, 2002.

43. Kahan BD, Napoli KL, Kelly PA, et al. Therapeutic drug monitoring of sirolimus: correlations with efficacy and toxicity. Clin Transplant 14:97–109, 2000.

44. Saunders RN, Metcalfe MS, Nicholson ML. Rapamycin in transplantation: a review of the evidence. Kidney Int 59:3–16, 2001.

45. Chueh SCJ, Kahan BD. Dyslipidemia in renal transplant recipients treated with a sirolimus and cyclosporine-based immunosuppressive regimen: incidence, risk factors, progression, and prognosis. Transplantation 76:375–382, 2003.

46. Guilbeau JM. Delayed wound healing with sirolimus after liver transplant. Ann Pharmacother 36:1391–1395, 2002.

47. van Gelder T, ter Meulen CG, Hené R, et al. Oral ulcers in kidney transplant recipients treated with sirolimus and mycophenolate mofetil. Transplantation 75:788–791, 2003.

48. Zimmerman JJ, Ferron GM, Lim HK, et al. The effect of a high-fat meal on the oral bioavailability of the immunosuppressant sirolimus (rapamycin). J Clin Pharmacol 39:1155–1161, 1999.

49. Gaber AO, First MR, Tesi RJ, et al. Results of the double-blind, randomized, multicenter, phase III clinical trial of thymoglobulin versus ATGAM in the treatment of acute graft rejection episodes after renal transplantation. Transplantation 66:29–37, 1998.

50. Suthanthiran M, Morris RE, Strom TB. Immunosuppressants: cellular and molecular mechanisms of action. Am J Kidney Dis 28: 159–172, 1996.

51. Wilde MI, Goa KL. Muromonab CD3: a reappraisal of its pharmacology and use as prophylaxis in solid organ transplant rejection. Drugs 51:865–894, 1996.

52. Cibrik DM, Kaplan B, Meier-Kriesche H. Role of anti-interleukin-2 receptor antibodies in kidney transplantation. BioDrugs 15:655–666, 2001.

53. Carswell CI, Plosker GL, Wagstaff AJ. Daclizumab: a review of its use in the management of organ transplantation. BioDrugs 15: 745–773, 2001.

54. Adu D, Cockwell P, Ives NJ, et al. Interleukin-2 receptor monoclonal antibodies in renal transplantation: meta-analysis of randomized trials. BMJ 326:789–794, 2003.

55. Bumgardner GL, Hardie I, Johnson RWG, et al. Results of 3-year phase III clinical trials with daclizumab prophylaxis for prevention of acute rejection after renal transplanation. Transplantation 72: 839–845, 2001.

56. Hausen B, Morris RE. Review of immunosuppression for lung transplantation: novel drugs, new uses for conventional immunosuppressants, and alternative strategies. Clin Chest Med 18:353–366, 1997.

57. Tzakis AG, Kato T, Nishida S, et al. Preliminary experience with Campath 1H (C1H) in intestinal and liver transplantation. Transplantation 75:1227–1231, 2003.

58. Kirk AD, Hale DA, Mannon RB, et al. Results from a human renal allograft tolerance trial evaluating the humanized CD52-specific monoclonal antibody alemtuzumab (Campath-1H). Transplantation 76:120–129, 2003.

59. Calne R, Moffatt SD, Friend PJ, et al. Campath IH allows low-dose cyclosporine monotherapy in 31 cadaveric renal allograft recipients. Transplantation 68:1613–1616, 1999.

60. Kahan BD, Wong RL, Carter C, et al. A phase I study of a 4-week course of SDZ-RAD (RAD) quiescent cyclosporine-prednisone-treated renal transplant recipients. Transplantation 68:1100–1106, 1999.

61. Kovarik JM, Kahan BD, Kaplan B, et al. Longitudinal assessment of everolimus in de novo renal transplant recipients over the first posttransplant year: pharmacokinetics, exposure-response relationships, and influence on cyclosporine. Clin Pharmacol Ther 69:48–56, 2001.

62. Nashan B. Early clinical experience with a novel rapamycin derivative. Ther Drug Monit 24:53–58, 2002.

63. Kovarik JM, Hsu C-H, McMahon L, et al. Population pharmacokinetics of everolimus in de novo renal transplant patients: impact of ethnicity and comedications. Clin Pharmacol Ther 70:247–254, 2001.

64. Kovarik JM, Sabia HD, Figueiredo JL, et al. Influence of hepatic impairment on everolimus pharmacokinetics: implications for dose adjustment. Clin Pharmacol Ther 70:425–430, 2001.

65. Williams JW, Mital D, Chong A, et al. Experiences with leflunomide in solid organ transplantation. Transplantation 73:358–366, 2002.

66. Hardinger KL, Wang CD, Schnitzler MA, et al. Prospective, pilot, open-label, short-term study of conversion to leflunomide reverses chronic renal allograft dysfunction. Am J Transplant 2:867–871, 2002.

67. Jin MB, Nakayama N, Ogata T, et al. A novel leflunomide derivative, FK778, for immunosuppression after kidney transplantation in dogs. Surgery 132:72–79, 2002.

68. Fishman JA, Rubin RH. Infection in organ-transplant recipients. N Engl J Med 338:1741–1751, 1998.

69. Hebart H, Kanz L, Jahn G, et al. Management of cytomegalovirus infection after solid-organ or stem-cell transplantation. Drugs 55: 59–72, 1998.

70. Schnitzler MA. Costs and consequences of cytomegalovirus disease. Am J Health-Syst Pharm 60:S5–S8, 2003.

71. Pouria S, State OI, Wong W, et al. CMV infection is associated with transplant renal artery stenosis. Q J Med 91:185–189, 1998.

72. Koskinen P, Lemstrom K, Mattila S, et al. Cytomegalovirus infection associated accelerated heart allograft arteriosclerosis may impair the late function of the graft. Clin Transplant 10:487–493, 1996.

73. Lautenschlager I, Hockerstedt K, Jalanko K, et al. Persistent cytomegalovirus in liver allografts with chronic rejection. Hepatology 25:190–194, 1997.

74. Pescovitz MD. Formulary considerations for drugs used to prevent cytomegalovirus disease. Am J Health-Syst Pharm 60:S17–S21, 2003.

75. Higgins RM, Bloom SL, Hopkin JM, et al. The risks and benefits of low-dose cotrimoxazole prophylaxis for *Pneumocystis* pneumonia in renal transplantation. Transplantation 47:558–560, 1989.

76. Saukkonen K, Garland R, Koziel H. Aerosolized pentamidine as alternative primary prophylaxis against *Pneumocystis carinii* pneumonia in adult hepatic and renal transplant recipients. Chest 109: 1250–1255, 1996.

77. Kemper CA, Tucker RM, Lang OS, et al. Low-dose dapsone prophylaxis of *Pneumocystis carinii* pneumonia in AIDS and AIDS-related complex. AIDS 4:1145–1148, 1990.

78. Mathis AS, Dave N, Knipp GT, et al. Drug-related dyslipidemia after renal transplantation. Am J Health-Syst Pharm 61:565–587, 2004.

79. Chobanian AV, Bakris GL, Black HR, et al. The seventh report of the Joint National Committee on Prevention, Detection, Evaluation, and Treatment of High Blood Pressure: the JNC 7 report. JAMA 289:2560–2572, 2003.

80. Weir MR. Calcium channel blockers in organ transplantation: important new therapeutic modalities. J Am Soc Nephrol 1:S28–S30, 1990.

81. Expert Panel on Detection, Evaluation, and Treatment of High Blood Cholesterol in Adults (Adult Treatment Panel III). Executive Summary of the Third Report of the National Cholesterol Education Program (NCEP). JAMA 285:2486–2497, 2001.

82. National Kidney Foundation. Introduction, assessment of dyslipidemias, treating dyslipidemias, and research recommendations. Am J Kidney Dis 41 (Suppl 3):S11–S91, 2003.

83. Jindal RM, Sidner RA, Milgrom ML. Posttransplant diabetes mellitus: the role of immunosuppression. Drug Saf 16:242–257, 1997.

84. Penn I. Posttransplant malignancy: the role of immunosuppression. Drug Saf 23:101–113, 2000.

85. Opelz G, Dohler B. Lymphomas after solid organ transplantation: a collaborative transplant study report. Am J Transplant 4:222–230, 2004.

86. Schweizer R, Rovelli M, Palmieri D, et al. Noncompliance in organ transplant recipients. Transplantation 49:374–377, 1990.

CASE STUDIES

CASE 10

TOPIC: Critical Care Therapy

THERAPEUTIC DIFFICULTY: Level 3
Joseph Swanson and Bradley A. Boucher

Chapter 26: Critical Care Therapy

■ Scenario

Patient and Setting: JS, a 32-year-old male admitted 10 days ago to the trauma intensive care unit (TICU) status post all-terrain vehicle (ATV) accident. He was not wearing a helmet and had positive loss of consciousness.

Chief Complaint: ATV accident

■ History of Present Illness

Small subdural hematoma; fractured ribs, right 2–8; fractured ribs, left 8–10; grade II spleen laceration; fractured vertebra: cervical 5th and 6th

Medical History: Asthma (mild intermittent)

Surgical History: None

Family/Social History: Family History: Noncontributory
Social History: Occasional alcohol (2–3 beers or mixed drinks on weekends); no tobacco, no recreational drugs

Medications:
Albuterol inhaler, 2 puffs q4h PRN
Ibuprofen, 400 mg PO PRN for occasional headaches

Allergies: No known drug allergies

Hospital Course: On admission JS's Glasgow Coma Scale (GCS) was nine. Prior to arrival in TICU, the patient was intubated and mechanical ventilation was provided; day 2 of hospitalization, underwent fixation of cervical spine fractures; day seven, mental status began to improve; day 8, developed a new right lower lobe infiltrate on chest roentogram, had a temperature spike of 38.9°C (102°F), and WBC count of 15,000; nurse reports copious purulent respiratory secretions. Within 15 minutes of JS's fever, blood and urine cultures were obtained. As a result of listed signs, bronchoscopy with bronchoalveolar lavage (BAL) was

performed based on suspicion of ventilator associated pneumonia (VAP). Immediately following BAL, empiric antibiotics were started; day 10, nurse notices an acute decline in JS's mental status. Soon after, JS experiences a drop in mean arterial pressure (MAP) to 50 mm Hg, which only increased to 57 mm Hg several hours later despite 6 liters of normal saline.

■ Physical Examination

GEN: Well-developed, well-nourished intubated male
VS: BP 70/50, MAP 57, HR 115, RR 18, T 39°C (102.2°F), Ht 69″, Wt 85 kg
HEENT: Minor facial lacerations, Miami J cervical collar
NEURO: GCS of 8 intubated (E 2, M 5, V 1 intubated) down from 11 intubated on day 9, SAS of 2
COR: Tachycardia, nl S1, S2, grade II/VI SEM
CHEST: Bibasilar rhonchi
ABD: Soft, nontender, nondistended, positive bowel sounds
GU: Foley catheter
RECT: Deferred
EXT: Slightly cool

■ Results of Pertinent Laboratory Tests, Serum Drug Concentrations, and Diagnostic Tests Results (Day 10)

Na 142 (142)	Ca 4 (8)	Lkcs 22 × 10^9 (22 × 10^3)
K 3 (3)	PO$_4$ 0.7 (2.2)	Hgb 103 (10.3)
Cl 110 (110)	Mg 0.75 (1.5)	Hct 0.31 (31)
CO$_2$ 15 (15)	Alb 25 (2.5)	Plt 300 × 10^9 (300 × 10^3)
BUN 10.7 (30)	Phenytoin level 5 mg/L	Bands 0.05 (5)
CR 132.6 (1.5)	Glu 10.3 (185)	

pH 7.16, PCO$_2$ 41.2, PO$_2$ 91.5, HCO$_3$ 14.2 (14.2), BE: −13.8 mmol/L, FiO$_2$: 40%

Imaging Results: Computed tomography of head: stable, small subdural hematoma
Chest roentogram: right lower lobe infiltrate

Microbiologic Laboratory Results: BAL:
Acinetobacter baumanii 150,000 CFU/mL
Staphylococcus aureus 100,000 CFU/mL
Blood: No growth to date (NGTD)
Urine: NGTD

Medications:

Acetaminophen, 650 mg per tube q4h PRN temp >38.6°C (101.5°F)

Albuterol, 0.083% via nebulization q4h PRN for wheezing

Morphine, 2 mg IV q2h

Midazolam, 1 mg IV q2h PRN to maintain a SAS of 4

Phenytoin, 100 mg IV q8h

Enoxaparin, 30 mg SQ q12h (started 48 hours after admission)

Ranitidine, 50 mg IV q8h

Vancomycin, 1250 mg IV q12h

Piperacillin/tazobactam, 4.5 g IV q6h

Tobramycin, 560 mg IV q24h

IV Fluids: 0.9% NaCl (normal saline) IV infusing at 150 mL/hr

Nutrition: 1 kcal/mL standard formula to provide 2,500 kcal/day and 170 g/day protein via orogastric flexiflo tube

■ Problem List

Identify principal problems from the scenario in priority order (see Answers in back of book for correct list of problems).

■ SOAP Note

To be completed by the student (see Answers in back of book for correct SOAP Note).

■ QUESTIONS

(See Answers in back of book for correct responses.)

1. If JS were to develop delirium, which of the following medications would be the preferred agent? (EO-8, 12)
   a. Meperidine
   b. Propofol
   c. Haloperidol
   d. Lorazepam

2. The incidence of pneumonia in mechanically ventilated patients has been reported to be: (EO-3)
   a. 61%–70%
   b. 75%–80%
   c. 40%–60%
   d. 9%–30%

3. The drug of choice for JS's pneumonia caused by *Acinetobacter baumannii* is: (EO-8)
   a. Sulfamethoxazole/trimethoprim
   b. Imipenem/cilistatin
   c. Ciprofloxacin
   d. Piperacillin/tazobactam

4. Based on JS's shock state, what medication should be recommended to improve JS's MAP? (EO-5, 8)
   a. Dobutamine
   b. Phenylephrine
   c. Vasopressin
   d. Norepinephrine

5. Which of the following electrolyte disturbances is most common in critically ill patients? (EO-3)
   a. Hypomagnesemia
   b. Hypernatremia
   c. Hypercalcemia
   d. Hyponatremia

6. Which of the following therapy goals has been shown to improve mortality in patients like JS? (EO-3, 5, 8)
   a. Maintain MAP >100
   b. Maintain blood glucose between 80–110 mg/dL (4.5–6.1 mmol/L)
   c. Maintain serum magnesium between 1.8–2
   d. Maintain gastric pH <4

7. Which of the following is a true statement pertaining to the selection of a proton pump inhibitor (PPI) versus a histamine-2 receptor (H-2) antagonist for the prevention of stress ulcer prophylaxis? (EO-8)
   a. PPIs have superior efficacy compared to an H-2 antagonist.
   b. Patients generally develop tolerance to a PPI.
   c. PPIs have more dosage forms than an H-2 antagonist.
   d. PPIs have equal or better pH control compared to H-2 antagonists.

8. How does sucralfate prevent stress ulcers? (EO-7)
   a. Inhibits histamine-provoked acid secretion
   b. Binds hydrogen ion to reduce stomach acid
   c. Inhibits hydrogen-potassium-ATPase
   d. Binds and covers damaged gastric mucosa

9. What is JS's phenytoin level when adjusted for hypoalbuminemia? (EO-5, 6)
   a. 5 mg/L
   b. 12 mg/L
   c. 8 mg/L
   d. 18 mg/L

10. What two ways could JS's hypophosphatemia contribute to difficulty in weaning him from the ventilator? (EO-1)

11. What criteria for severe sepsis does JS have that would make him a possible candidate for drotrecogin alfa? What contraindication does JS have for receiving drotrecogin alfa? (EO-2, 8)

12. What risk factors for deep vein thrombosis does JS have that would put him at particularly high risk for deep vein thrombosis? (EO-8)

13. Describe one pharmacologic and two nonpharmacologic therapies that could improve DO_2 in JS. (EO-1, 12)

14. JS's vancomycin trough was drawn 30 minutes prior to the third dose and the peak was drawn 1 hour after the end of the third dose infusion. The peak was 20 μg/mL and the trough was 6 μg/mL. What is your recommendation pertaining to the vancomycin dosing? Include pertinent pharmacokinetic information. (EO-4, 5, 6, 8)

15. JS develops acute renal failure as a result of septic shock with an estimated creatinine clearance of approximately 15 mL/min. Using this and all other clinical information provide recommendations pertaining to JS's medication regimen. (EO-4, 5, 8, 10, 11, 12)

16. Summarize therapeutic, pathophysiologic, and disease management concepts for critical care therapy utilizing a key points format. (EO-18)

Fluid and Electrolyte Therapy and Acid-Base Balance

28

Jane M. Gervasio

The body maintains its internal fluid environment by balancing the amounts, volume, and composition of water, electrolytes, proteins, acids, and bases. The most abundant constituent of the body is water, which accounts for 60% of body mass. Within this water are dissolved or suspended elements and formed substances needed to generate energy, maintain and manufacture body components, metabolize nutrients and drugs, and eliminate waste. Changes in body water, salts, and pH are deviations from the environmental conditions within which the body can function normally and protect and repair itself. Metabolic processes can continue only within very narrow limits of size, composition, and pH of body fluid. Efforts to normalize the amount, composition, distribution, and pH of body fluids, whether by internal homeostatic processes or by externally applied therapeutic measures, are aimed at restoring and maintaining an environment in which body functions can proceed normally.

PHYSIOLOGY OF BODY WATER BALANCE

Body water is divided into two main compartments: intracellular fluid (ICF) and extracellular fluid (ECF). The ECF is further divided into the interstitial and vascular compartments.[1-3] In the nonobese, well-conditioned 70-kg man, ICF (water inside the cells) makes up 40% to 45% (30 L) of body weight. Interstitial fluid (water between the cells) accounts for 11% to 15% (10 L), and vascular water (that inside the walls of the blood vessels) is approximately 5% (3.5 L). The actual amount of body water varies slightly according to age, sex, body muscle, and fat content. When body water in a patient is estimated, the contribution of these factors must be taken into consideration. At maturity, men usually have a water content of 60%. Women tend to have lower water content per body mass, estimated to be about 5% less, because of their smaller amount of muscle mass. At birth, a newborn is made up of approximately 75% water because of small amounts of adipose tissue. The slight weight loss seen after birth is actually water loss from evaporation as the infant adjusts to an air environment. By the end of the first year of life, the infant's total body water (TBW) is about 60%. The TBW of older adults usually is below 60% because of their lower muscle mass, resulting from lower levels of exercise and endogenous anabolic hormones. Obese people are less than 60% water by weight because fat includes negligible intracellular water; the absolute decrease in percentage of TBW is a function of the degree of obesity. For practical purposes, TBW in obese patients is estimated according to ideal rather than actual body weight, and without factoring in the negligible amount of water contained in fat.

Body water is constantly being circulated between the three body compartments. Under stable conditions, the volume of each compartment remains constant, but a continuous interchange of individual molecules occurs across the water-permeable cell membranes. This exchange is regulated by the differences in hydrostatic and oncotic (protein) pressure on the arteriole and the venule side of the capillaries. At the heart, cardiac output and arterial tone determine the intravascular or blood hydrostatic pressure. At the arteriole side of the capillary, this hydrostatic pressure is approximately 17 mm Hg, and solute-free water is pushed out into the interstitial or third space. Proteins, primarily albumin, and negative hydrostatic pressure in the third space simultaneously pull water from the vascular space into the third space. The combined effect of these two processes accounts for the movement of water out of the vascular space. On the venule side

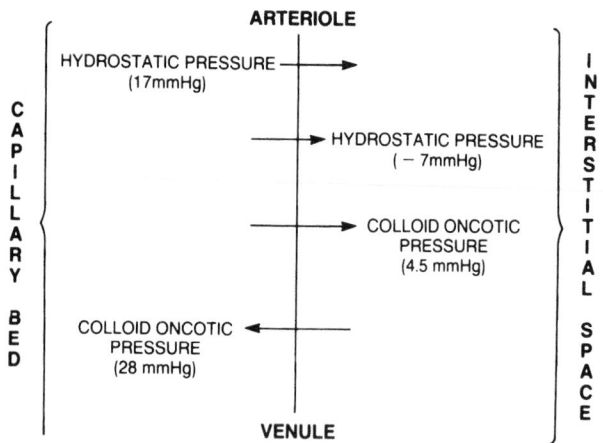

FIGURE 28.1 Forces regulating water movement in extracellular fluid.

of the capillary bed, intravascular oncotic pressure pulls 95% of the extruded water back into the vascular space, with the remaining 5% returned by the action of the lymphatic collecting system (Fig. 28.1).

The volumes of the three compartments remain standard only as long as the described hydrostatic and oncotic forces remain constant relative to each other. In assessment of the appropriateness of body water content, evaluation of not only the total volume but also its distribution among the three body compartments must be determined. Dehydration is the state in which the volume of fluid is low in all three compartments. Hypovolemia is a condition in which the intravascular volume is low, but the volumes of the interstitial and intracellular spaces are not described or quantified. TBW overload means only that TBW is greater than 60%, but this does not describe specifically the volume of any individual compartment. When the phrase *TBW overload* is used, the actual distribution of volume in each compartment must be known before an appropriate therapeutic intervention can be determined. For example, fluid accumulates in the interstitial space if blood (hydrostatic) pressure is normal but oncotic pressure is low; the resulting clinical condition is called *edema*. With low albumin concentrations, the vol-

ume of the third space gradually expands at the expense of the vascular space. In the most severe cases, death results from too low circulating blood volume (hypovolemia) in the presence of interstitial space overload (edema) and TBW greater than 60%. In this situation, more fluid must be given to support the circulating vascular volume, even though the edema will worsen and the TBW will continue to rise. Only correction of the underlying disequilibrium between the hydrostatic and oncotic pressures, brought about by raising the low albumin or lowering the blood pressure, will normalize the volumes of the three fluid compartments.

PHYSIOLOGY OF BODY SOLUTE BALANCE

Osmotic pressure keeps the volume of the three body fluid compartments constant, and only solute-free water moves freely across cell membranes. The concentration of dissolved ions (electrolytes) in each compartment creates the osmotic pressure responsible for containing the water in each space. These ions and their distribution are listed in Table 28.1. The normal serum osmolality (osmotic concentration) is 280 to 300 mmol per kg (280 to 300 mOsm/L). Sodium and chloride are the main ions in the ECF, and potassium and phosphate are those of the ICF. Other ions are present but occur at concentrations too low to contribute significantly to the osmotic gradient. Other important osmotically active substances are glucose, urea, phospholipids, cholesterol, and neutral fats. A molecule of glucose has one-eighteenth and urea has one-third the osmotic strength of an atom of an electrolyte. Osmolality is determined by all the particles mentioned, but the nonelectrolytes contribute little unless their values are abnormally high (Table 28.1).

The equation used to determine osmolality is as follows:

$$\text{Osmolality (mmol/kg)} = 2 \times \text{Sodium (mmol/L)} + \text{Glucose (mmol/L)}/18 + \text{BUN (mmol/L)}/2.8$$

Body processes function best within a serum osmolality of 280 to 300 mmol per kg; therefore, the kidneys will attempt to maintain this value by increasing glucose and urea

Table 28.1	Approximate Composition of Body Fluid (mmol/L)		
	Plasma (total = 300)	**Interstitium (total = 304)**	**Cell (total = 300)**
Na	141	144	16
K	4	4	150
Ca	2.5	2.5	–
Mg	2	2	34
Cl	100	114	–
HCO$_3$	25	30	10
PO$_4$/SO$_4$	1	1.5	50
Protein/acid	25	6	40

excretion when their concentrations rise above normal. When this is not possible or sufficient, the kidneys will increase sodium excretion. In the physiologic sense, the biologic priority to maintain a normal osmolality is greater than the need to maintain a normal body sodium concentration.

When the concentration of ions in any compartment changes, water migrates across cell membranes to reestablish osmotic equilibrium. If the serum sodium rises, the osmolality of the vascular space is momentarily higher than that of the interstitial and intracellular spaces. Water moves from these two areas to dilute the vascular space until the correct relative osmolalities of all three compartments are reestablished. The result is a decrease in the size of the interstitial and intracellular spaces and an increase in the volume of the vascular space. If the serum sodium falls, the opposite happens, and the size of the interstitial and intracellular compartments increases.

MAINTENANCE FLUID AND ELECTROLYTE NEEDS

Salt and water balance in the body is maintained by the equilibrium between intake of fluid and electrolytes, evaporation of solute-free water across the skin and lungs, and controlled renal excretion of water and electrolytes. The amount of water that evaporates (insensible loss) is a function of body surface area and respiratory rate. In a 70-kg man, the amount is approximately 1 L per day and remains constant. The kidneys increase or decrease their fluid and electrolyte output by the action of antidiuretic hormone (ADH) and aldosterone. This activity compensates for daily variations in fluid and electrolyte intake. ADH, also called *vasopressin*, regulates the amount of water reabsorbed in the distal tubule of the kidney by assessing the volume and osmolality of the ECF. If the osmolality of the ECF is higher than normal or the blood volume low, ADH is released and water is reabsorbed in the renal tubules. If the osmolality is low or blood volume high, the converse is true. Aldosterone increases sodium reabsorption, and release of this hormone is stimulated by low total body sodium. These two hormones, along with stimulation of thirst centers in the brain, enable the body to maintain TBW and sodium within 1% of normal over wide variations in daily intake.

The amount of water and electrolytes needed to replace insensible loss, maintain adequate perfusion of body cell mass, and cause urine output sufficient to excrete metabolic waste varies according to body size in a nonlinear way. This is because the change in body surface area relative to body mass as size increases is not linear. The first 10 kg of body weight needs 100 mL per kg, the next 10 kg needs 50 mL per kg, and each kilogram beyond 20 needs 20 mL per kg. A 50-kg man has a water need of 2,100 mL per day; this is derived from 1,000 mL for his first 10 kg of weight, 500 mL for the next 10 kg, and 600 mL for the remaining 30 kg. Calculation of water needs in children follows the same

rule. Insensible loss of free water increases in febrile patients. A patient needs an extra 10% of the calculated need for water for each 1°C elevation in body temperature.

Electrolyte quantities needed to maintain normal total body concentration vary because the kidneys increase or decrease sodium excretion to maintain a normal circulating vascular volume and composition. When necessary, the kidney can prevent sodium loss by increasing potassium and hydrogen excretion (Fig. 28.2). For practical purposes, the amounts of electrolytes needed to maintain homeostasis without stimulating inordinate amounts of ADH and aldosterone release are linearly related to the water needs. The values used to determine daily maintenance fluid and electrolyte needs are listed in Table 28.2. Oral or intravenous replacement of maintenance needs should always include sodium and potassium. Deficiencies of the other electrolytes develop more slowly, and they are not always given during short-term therapy.

Cations must be given with an equal number of anions to maintain electrical neutrality, but giving excess chloride ions almost never causes hyperchloremia in patients with adequate renal function. Acetate salts of sodium and potassium are available and can be used if chloride anions must be avoided. Acetate is converted to bicarbonate in the body. Bicarbonate salts can be added directly to intravenous solutions, but they raise the pH of the product and may cause precipitation of electrolytes or drugs.

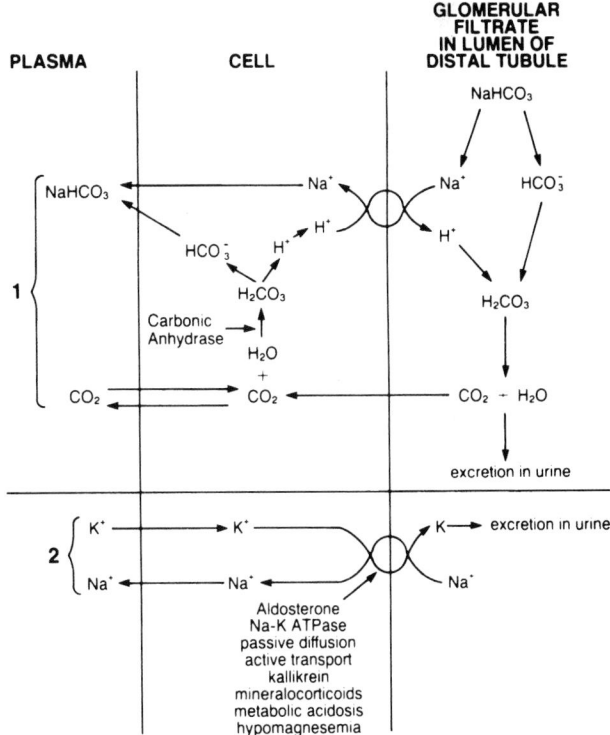

FIGURE 28.2 Mechanisms of Na-K exchange in the distal renal tubule.

Table 28.2	Maintenance Needs per 24 Hours
Water	
0–10 kg	100 mL/kg
10–20 kg	50 mL/kg
>20 kg	20 mL/kg
Electrolytes	
Na	3 mmol (3 mEq)/100 mL H_2O need
K	2 mmol (2 mEq)/100 mL H_2O need
Cl	2 mmol (2 mEq)/100 mL H_2O need
Ca	0.05–0.1 mmol (0.1–0.2 mEq)/kg
Mg	0.05 mmol (0.1 mEq)/kg
PO_4	0.1 mmol (2.8 mg)/kg

Use ideal body weight in obese patients.

DISORDERS OF BODY WATER AND SOLUTE

SODIUM

Serum sodium is the major determinant of intravascular volume because it is the osmotically active substance that occurs in greatest concentration.[4–12] Abnormalities in salt and water intake or excretion alter sodium concentration. This affects the interstitial volume because its major osmotic substance is also sodium, and the two compartments are in equilibrium with each other.

The usual serum sodium concentration is 135 to 145 mmol per L (135 to 145 mEq /L). Concentrations above or below this are called *hypernatremia* or *hyponatremia*, respectively. The terms refer only to concentration and do not indicate whether the abnormality is the result of increases or decreases in the total amounts of sodium, water, or both in the body.

Hypernatremia. Hypernatremia usually results from a free water deficit with sodium loss (hypovolemic hypernatremia) or without sodium loss (isovolemic hypernatremia). Elevated total body sodium can result from excessive intake of water and salt (hypervolemic hypernatremia), but this is usually iatrogenic. Clinically, complications of hypernatremia generally do not appear until the serum concentration is greater than 160 mmol per L, and they are the result of central nervous system (CNS) dehydration (Table 28.3). Hypernatremia is always hypertonic, and hyperosmolar states result in stimulation of the thirst response. Therefore, patients at risk for hypernatremia are those with an impaired thirst response, those not able to access water, and those who have not been adequately hydrated, such as infants, the elderly, or disabled individuals.

Treatment of Hypernatremia. The treatment for hypernatremia depends on whether the cause is too little water or too much sodium. Hypernatremia from water loss indicates

a decrease in TBW, not just in intravascular volume. Because the concentration of osmotically active substances across the three compartments is always in equilibrium, the interstitial sodium concentration and the intracellular potassium concentration are as elevated as the intravascular sodium. Calculating the amount of free water needed to correct the concentrations of all electrolyte values and return the volumes of all three compartments to normal involves the use of the following equation:

Water deficit (L) = [(Measured serum sodium (mmol/L) − 140) − 1] × Body weight (kg) × 0.6

If sodium loss accompanies the water deficit, normal saline (0.9% saline; NS) is administered to correct the ECF. When the volume status is correct, electrolyte-free or hypotonic solutions, such as 5% dextrose in water (D_5W) or 0.45% saline, may be given. If sodium loss does not accompany free water loss, hypotonic solutions are the treatment of choice.

Aggressive treatment to correct an altered serum or total body sodium concentration is not indicated because it may create or further complicate central nervous system (CNS) problems. Equilibration across the blood–brain barrier is slower than across other semipermeable membranes in the body, and rapid changes may cause seizures. If hypernatremia has developed rapidly over a few hours, treatment to decrease sodium concentrations should not exceed 1 mEq/L/hour. If hypernatremia has developed slowly, correction of sodium concentration should be no greater than 0.5 mEq/L/hour.

If hypernatremia is the result of an actual increase in the amount of sodium in the body, treatment is directed at removal of sodium from the body and may involve the use of diuretics and D_5W to increase renal elimination while maintaining a normal TBW.

Hyponatremia. Hyponatremia is characterized by a serum sodium concentration less than 135 mmol per L, but clinically, symptoms usually do not appear until the concentration is below 125 mmol per L and are the result of CNS water intoxication (Table 28.3). Although hypernatremia is always hypertonic, hyponatremia may be hypotonic, isotonic, or hypertonic. Hyponatremia can result from dilution or depletion or may be translocational. As with hypernatremia, the cause must be determined before treatment begins.

Hypertonic Hyponatremia: Clinical Presentation and Treatment. Hypertonic (translocational) hyponatremia manifests when a gain of impermeable solutes other than sodium occurs in the vascular compartment. The most common solute responsible for this disorder is glucose, although mannitol and glycine have also been identified. In hypertonic hyponatremia, solutes shift water from the ICF compartment into the ECF compartment. Glucose, as well as mannitol and glycine, contributes to the osmolality of the serum, thereby creating a hypertonic hyponatremia. An increase of 100 mg per dL (5.6 mmol/L) of serum glucose concentration de-

Table 28.3	Symptoms and Causes of Hypernatremia and Hyponatremia
Hypernatremia	**Hyponatremia**
Serum concentration >145 mmol/L (145 mEq/L)	Serum concentration <135 mmol/L (135 mEq/L)
Causes	
Decreased water intake	Low-sodium diet with diuretics
Excessive water loss	Diuretics
Diabetes insipidus	Congestive heart failure
Excessive salt intake	Cirrhosis
Iatrogenic causes	Replacement of body secretion loss with electrolyte-free solutions
Fever	Adrenal insufficiency
Hyperventilation	Osmotic diuresis
	Syndrome of inappropriate secretion of antidiuretic hormone
Signs and Symptoms	
Thirst	Apathy or agitation
Dry mucous membranes	Fatigue
Decreased skin turgor	Anorexia or nausea
Acute weight loss	Headache
Confusion	Muscle cramps
Hallucinations	Tachycardia
Intracranial hemorrhage	Oliguria or anuria
Coma	Confusion
	Seizures
	Coma
	Shock

creases serum sodium concentrations by approximately 1.7 mmol per L, although some data has demonstrated decreases of 2.4 mmol per L. Treatment for hypertonic hyponatremia involves correcting the elevated blood glucose concentrations or eliminating the mannitol or glycine.

Hypotonic Hypervolemic Hyponatremia: Clinical Presentation and Treatment. Hypotonic hypervolemic (dilutional) hyponatremia is a condition in which the total body sodium is actually high, but TBW is increased to a greater degree. The result is a low serum sodium concentration. It occurs in conditions such as cirrhosis and congestive heart failure, when effective cardiac output reaching the kidneys is diminished. This, along with the low sodium concentration, is a stimulus for ADH and aldosterone secretion. The result is further salt and water retention, and affected patients usually are edematous because of the attendant increase in interstitial fluid compartment size. Salt and water restriction, bed rest (to increase venous return to the heart), and correction of the primary disorder are the initial treatments. These measures must not be so aggressive as to compromise intravascular volume or further decrease renal blood flow. Diuretics may be necessary but should be used judiciously to

prevent exacerbation of the hyponatremia by causing sodium excretion that exceeds water elimination.

Hypotonic Euvolemic Hyponatremia: Clinical Presentation and Treatment. Hypotonic euvolemic hyponatremia occurs when both the ECF and the ICF compartments expand because of water retention, but the body sodium stores are normal or slightly decreased. Increases in the ECF are usually not sufficient to cause edema. Hypotonic euvolemic hyponatremia is commonly associated with syndrome of inappropriate antidiuretic hormone (SIADH), but other disorders such as adrenal insufficiency, hypothyroidism, and primary and psychogenic polydipsia may cause euvolemic hyponatremia. The underlying cause must be identified and treated. Medications reported to cause SIADH are listed in Table 28.4. Fluid restriction is often the first-line treatment for SIADH. Demeclocycline 900 to 1,200 mg per day may also be initiated in patients with chronic complications, but it is not indicated for acute situations because of its long half-life.

Hypotonic Hypovolemic Hyponatremia: Clinical Presentation and Treatment. Hypotonic hypovolemic hyponatremia is characterized by a decrease in TBW, along with a

Table 28.4	**Medications Causing SIADH**
Azithromycin	Melphalan
Bromperidol	Methyldopa
Bupropion	Metrizamide
Chlorpromazine	Miconazole
Chlorpropamide	Oxytocin
Cilazapril	Paroxetine
Citalopram	Perphenazine/amitriptyline
Clomipramine	Phenoxybenzamine
Cyclophosphamide	Piroxicam
Cyclothiazide	Propafenone
Dyphylline	Reboxetine
Enalapril	Rifabutin
Fentanyl	Sertraline
Fluoxetine	Thioridazine
Fluphenazine	Thiothixene
Fluvoxamine	Tolazamide
Glipizide	Tolbutamide
Haloperidol	Tranylcypromine
Hydrochlorothiazide	Trazodone
Ifosfamide	Triamterene/hydrochlorothiazide
Imipramine	Valproic acid
Interferon alfa-2A	Venlafaxine
Levodopa/carbidopa	Vinblastine
Lofepramine	Vincristine
Lorcainide	Vinorelbine

(From Chan TY. Drug-induced syndrome of inappropriate secretion of antidiuretic hormone. Causes, diagnosis and treatment. Drugs Aging 11:27–44, 1997, with permission.)

greater decrease in sodium. It most commonly results from gastrointestinal (GI) losses caused by vomiting, excessive diuretic therapy, or replacement of losses with electrolyte-fluid. Patients show signs of dehydration (e.g., dry mucous membranes, skin tenting, lethargy) and, in extreme cases, hypovolemia. Volume replacement with NS is usually the first-line treatment.

Treatment of Severe Hyponatremia. Patients with symptomatic hyponatremia or serum sodium concentrations below 120 mmol per L (associated with ~50% mortality) require administration of intravenous sodium. The amount of sodium needed to replace the total body deficit is calculated with the use of the following equation:

$$\text{Sodium deficit (mmol)} = [140 - \text{Measured serum sodium}$$
$$\text{(mmol/L)}] \times \text{Body weight (kg)} \times 0.6$$

Appropriate solutions to replace the sodium deficit are 0.9% saline (154 mmol sodium and chloride/L) or 3% hypertonic saline (513 mmol sodium and chloride/L). Approximately 50% of an amount equal to the deficit should be administered over a 12-hour period at a rate that increases the serum sodium concentration by no more than 2 mEq/L/hour, or a maximum of 12 mEq/L/24 hour. Rapid infusions of 3% hypertonic saline at 1 to 2 mL/kg/hour over 2 to 3 hours should be used only in patients with seizures or coma. Severe chronic hyponatremia should be corrected more slowly at a rate not to exceed 0.5 mEq/L/hour. Because hyponatremia usually does not occur acutely, the deficit may be replaced over several days to avoid intravascular volume overload, seizures, pulmonary edema, or congestive heart failure.

ALTERATIONS IN FLUID COMPARTMENT INTEGRITY

Trauma, tissue ischemia, endotoxemia, hypoalbuminemia, and decreased cardiac output cause hypovolemia by damaging capillary membranes or disrupting the hydrostatic and oncotic forces governing fluid movement across them.[13–15] Symptoms of hypovolemia include tachycardia, low central venous pressure (CVP), low pulmonary capillary wedge pressure, and decreased urine output. Blood pressure is not a good measure of this condition because increases in sympathetic tone can maintain the blood pressure at near-normal levels in the presence of a greatly decreased circulating volume.

In cases of trauma, ischemia, and endotoxemia, capillary pore size increases (capillary leak syndrome); in addition, water, solute, and plasma proteins, primarily albumin, flow into the interstitial space. This leak may be localized to an area of injury or ischemia (surgery, trauma) or generalized throughout the body (endotoxemic shock from Gram-negative sepsis). The amount of fluid lost from the intravascular space varies with the degree of injury but can result in hypovolemia severe enough to cause cardiovascular collapse and death if the circulating volume is not maintained.

Treatment for Hypovolemia. Treatment consists of correcting the underlying disorder to normalize capillary permeability while replacing the lost intravascular fluid with a solution of the same composition. Blood has no role in this therapy because the formed elements of the intravascular fluid are not lost to the third space. The two categories of replacement solutions are crystalloid and colloid. *Crystalloid* is a general term for an aqueous solution that contains electrolytes. NS and lactated Ringer (LR) solutions are most commonly used for treating hypovolemia because they are isotonic with the ECF and are most effective in maintaining the circulating volume. *Colloid* is a general term for a solution that contains plasma proteins or other colloidal molecules. Three colloid solutions are available. Plasma protein fraction (PPF) is approximately 85% albumin and 15% globulin and is available as a 5% solution. Albumin is available as a 5% or 25% solution, and hetastarch as a 6% solution. Hetastarch is a mixture of ethoxylated amylopectin molecules that exerts the same hemodynamic effect as albumin. Hetastarch is not extracted from pooled human plasma and is much less expensive than PPF or albumin, but severe bleeding complications have been reported with hetastarch. All three products also contain 130 to 160 mmol sodium and chloride per L.

The use of colloid infusions remains controversial. Although some albumin does move into the third space when capillary pore size increases, it is much less than the amount of salt and water that leaks out. Colloids act by temporarily decreasing the rate at which fluid migrates into the third space, but hypovolemia may be exacerbated 24 to 36 hours later as colloids move into the interstitial space and begin to draw fluid there. Unless the actual serum albumin concentration is below the concentration needed to maintain the capillary venule oncotic pressure gradient (20 to 25 g/L) or aggressive crystalloid therapy is not restoring intravascular volume, the routine use of colloid solutions is not recommended.

During treatment of patients with hypovolemia, the rate of fluid administration into the vascular space must meet or exceed the rate of loss if tissue perfusion is to be maintained.

In extreme cases, this may exceed 1 L per hour. Urine output should be kept at a minimum of 0.5 mL/kg/hour, the concentration at which the circulating volume is sufficient to perfuse body tissues. Normalized heart rate and CVP also are indicators of normal intravascular volume that can be monitored along with urine output. During resuscitation, the rate of fluid administration is adjusted hourly to maintain adequate intravascular volume. It is important to remember that although edema may appear in some patients during this process, it is the capillary leak that causes the edema, not the resuscitation process. When healing begins, this extra fluid and solute are returned to the vascular compartment and excreted.

Hypoalbuminemia without concurrent capillary leak can result in hypovolemia with edema. Capillary venule oncotic pressure is low, and fluid that moved into the interstitial space on the arterial side of the capillary bed is not returned to the vascular system. Treatment for this condition consists of intravenous albumin in sufficient amounts to normalize arteriovenous capillary oncotic pressure. Edema resolves only when this can be accomplished.

Hypovolemia caused by decreased cardiac output (e.g., congestive heart failure, cardiomyopathy, myocardial infarction) cannot be corrected by administration of fluids. In these conditions, hypovolemia exists on the arterial side of the heart because of pump failure. The venous side of the circulatory system may be overloaded and the patient may be edematous. Treatment options are confined to agents that improve cardiac output, such as inotropes.

If hypovolemia is the result of blood loss, then whole blood or packed red blood cells with NS or LR are indicated to reestablish the hematocrit at above 0.25 g per L (25%) with a normal circulating volume.

LOSSES OF BODY WATER AND SOLUTE AND TREATMENT

With prolonged vomiting, diarrhea, or losses through perforations in organs or the GI tract leading to the skin (fistulas), water and solute are lost from the body. The compositions of these fluids vary according to the area affected and are listed in Table 28.5. When the exact origin of the fluid is not

Table 28.5	Approximate Concentrations of Body Secretions (mmol/L and mEq/L)			
	Na	**K**	**Cl**	**HCO$_3$**
Saliva	60	20	15	50
Stomach	60	10	130	–
Bile	150	5	100	40
Pancreas	140	5	80	120
Small bowel	140	5	105	30
Terminal ileum	120	5	105	–
Sweat	45	5	60	–
Cerebrospinal fluid	140	3	130	–

known, laboratory analysis helps in selecting an appropriate replacement solution. This analysis often is necessary in the case of enterocutaneous fistula (communication between the GI tract and the skin). Because such fistulas can make circuitous tracts through the body before reaching the skin, the organ nearest the exit site is not necessarily the one from which the fluid is draining. Diarrhea is most often of distal small-bowel or colonic origin, but in cases of secretory diarrhea, such as in giardiasis or acquired immunodeficiency syndrome, the fluid may arise from the duodenum or jejunum. In all cases of abnormal loss, the fluid composition should be determined. Appropriate replacement solutions, in addition to maintenance quantities, are given at a rate designed to restore and maintain normal body water and solute.

ACID-BASE BALANCE

For physiologic processes to occur at a normal rate, body pH must remain within a narrow range.[1-3,16-24] Although it varies slightly among body compartments (the ICF has a pH of approximately 6.9, and some subcellular components, such as the mitochondria, have even lower usual concentrations), normal total body acid-base balance is assumed to be present when the arterial pH is between 7.35 and 7.45.

Cellular metabolism, energy generation, and protein metabolism add large amounts of acid to the body daily. This occurs predominantly in the form of carbon dioxide (CO_2), but some hydrogen ions and weak organic and inorganic nonvolatile acids also are generated. Almost no alkaline substances result from metabolic processes, so body acid-base homeostatic mechanisms exclusively buffer or eliminate acids. Hemoglobin, proteins, and phosphate buffer only nonvolatile acids, and their concentrations are fixed in the body; therefore, their buffering capacity does not change. Additionally, hemoglobin, proteins, and phosphate contribute little to the total buffering capacity of the body.

The bicarbonate–carbonic acid system buffers CO_2 and can adjust quickly to changes in the daily acid load. It keeps body pH in the normal range by maintaining the correct ratio between concentrations of bicarbonate (HCO_3) and carbonic acid (H_2CO_3) in the blood. This relationship is described by the Henderson-Hasselbalch equation:

$$pH = pK_{carbonic\ acid} + \log (HCO_3/H_2CO_3)$$

When the HCO_3/H_2CO_3 (24 mmol per 1.2 mmol) concentrations are at a ratio of 20:1, the pH is 7.4 because the pK of carbonic acid is 6.1 and the log of 24/1.2 is 1.3. Carbonic acid concentrations are not obtained in the patient care setting. The value reported by clinical laboratories is the partial pressure of CO_2 (pCO_2). A 40-mm Hg pCO_2 corresponds to a H_2CO_3 concentration of 1.2 mmol. The pCO_2 is maintained within the normal range because CO_2 generated by cellular metabolism is continuously diffused and eliminated across the lungs. The capacity of the lungs to excrete CO_2 is so

great that they are saturated only in cases of severe pulmonary disease.

The kidneys are responsible for maintaining serum HCO_3 within the normal range by reabsorbing bicarbonate ions from the glomerular filtrate and by generating new HCO_3 ions in renal tubular cells. This generation is accomplished by carbonic anhydrase action on CO_2 and water to form carbonic acid. Carbonic acid quickly dissociates into H and HCO_3. The hydrogen ion is secreted into the urine and the bicarbonate transported from the renal tubular cells into the vascular system. The capacity of this reaction to generate new HCO_3 is not saturated unless renal function is severely compromised (Fig. 28.2).

Acid-base disturbances are attributed to CO_2 or bicarbonate serum concentration changes. If the problem originates with CO_2, the resultant change in pH is said to be of respiratory origin. If it begins with bicarbonate, the change is said to be of metabolic origin. A plasma pH below 7.35 is called *acidosis* and can be of respiratory or metabolic origin; a plasma pH above 7.45 is called *alkalosis* and is also of respiratory or metabolic origin. When plasma pH goes outside the normal range, the lungs and the kidneys begin processes that act to compensate and normalize the pH value. Therefore, it is the ratio between CO_2 and HCO_3, not the absolute numbers, that determines the pH. The body has a greater physiologic need (biologic priority) to have a plasma pH between 7.35 and 7.45 than it does to have ''normal'' concentrations of pCO_2 and HCO_3. When the respiratory center in the medulla oblongata perceives a change in pH, it causes the lungs to adjust the pCO_2 by increasing or decreasing the respiratory rate. Although it occurs quickly, this process can completely correct the pH only when the change in HCO_3 concentration is minor; it is limited by how quickly or slowly a person can breathe in and out, and by the capacity of the intracellular hemoglobin and phosphate buffering systems. The kidneys, by increasing or decreasing the plasma HCO_3, may take several days to fully compensate and normalize a pH that is altered by a change in CO_2 concentration, but they have a much greater total buffering capacity.

PRIMARY ACID-BASE DISTURBANCES

METABOLIC ACIDOSIS

Metabolic acidosis is the condition in which the plasma pH is below 7.35 as a result of a low HCO_3 concentration in the blood. A low serum HCO_3 concentration results from losses from the body, decreased renal regeneration of HCO_3, or increased amounts of acid added to the body by ingestion or metabolic processes. As the HCO_3 concentration declines, the lungs attempt to lower the pCO_2 and maintain a normal pH by increasing the depth and rate of respiration (Kussmaul breathing). The symptoms of metabolic acidosis occur in the cardiopulmonary system or CNS but usually are not clinically important at a pH greater than 7.1 (Table 28.6).

Table 28.6	Metabolic Acidosis [pH <7.35, HCO₃ <22 mmol (22 mEq)/L]
Causes	**Signs and Symptoms**
Ketoacidosis	Kussmaul breathing
Renal failure	Hyperkalemia
Hypoxia or anoxia	Ventricular arrhythmias
Diarrhea	Lethargy
Salicylates	Stupor
Methanol	Coma
Chloride loading	

The number of positively charged ions in the body must always equal the number negatively charged. In the plasma, this electrical neutrality is achieved by dissolved electrolytes and proteins in the following relationship:

$$Sodium = Cl + HCO_3 + Unmeasured\ anions$$

Unmeasured anions consist of plasma proteins and small amounts of other negatively charged substances, such as sulfate and phosphate, that are not measured by the tests usually done in clinical laboratories. The usual amounts of these anions in the blood have a combined ionic strength of 8 to 16 mmol per L (8 to 16 mEq/L). This value is called the *anion gap*, and it rarely changes. Assuming that sodium remains constant, a change in the number of any one of the anions necessitates a change in one or both of the others to maintain electrical neutrality. Because the number of unmeasured anions is fixed, the chloride (Cl) and HCO_3 are alterable. With the addition of acid, the fall in HCO_3 actually is an appropriate compensatory response to maintain the electrical neutrality of the blood (a condition with an even higher biologic priority than maintenance of a normal pH). Metabolic acidosis occurs when the HCO_3 declines and the HCO_3/CO_2 ratio becomes abnormal. Metabolic acidosis is divided into nonanion gap and anion gap.

Nonanion Gap Metabolic Acidosis. In nonanion gap acidosis, the number of unmeasured anions is the same as usual, so the decreased serum HCO_3 concentration is secondary to Cl loading, an actual loss of HCO_3 from the body, or decreased HCO_3 generation. In anion gap acidosis, the number of unmeasured anions has increased and the HCO_3 has dropped to maintain electrical neutrality. The cause of an anion gap acidosis is the contribution of nonvolatile acids to the blood. This can result from abnormal metabolic processes, such as diabetic ketoacidosis and hypoxia, or from poisonings by substances that dissociate at physiologic plasma pH. Salicylate and methanol overdoses commonly cause this particular type of metabolic acidosis. It is important for the clinician to determine which type of metabolic acidosis is occurring before any treatment regimen is begun.

Treatment of Nonanion Gap Metabolic Acidosis. Nonanion gap metabolic acidosis may occur from loss of HCO_3 (prolonged diarrhea, upper GI fistulas), inability to generate HCO_3 (renal failure), or Cl loading (NS infusions, NaCl overdoses). Treatment consists of correcting the underlying cause and replacing the HCO_3 deficit. Except in cases of renal failure or profound and continuing GI losses, the kidneys generate sufficient HCO_3 and normalize pH when the cause of the acidosis has been corrected. Acute HCO_3 replacement is provided only when the plasma pH is at or below 7.1, or the patient is exhibiting life-threatening symptoms of acidosis. The amount of bicarbonate deficit can be determined with the following equation:

$$HCO_3\ deficit\ (mmol) = [24 - Measured\ HCO_3\ (mmol/L)] \times Body\ weight\ (kg) \times 0.5$$

The volume of distribution of HCO_3 is estimated to be 10% less than the TBW, so the factor used is 0.5 rather than 0.6. One half of the calculated dosage is given (this amount usually changes the pH by 0.2). The goal of emergency bicarbonate replacement therapy is to correct existing cardiac or CNS disturbances by achieving a plasma pH at or above 7.2. Because the onset of acidosis usually is gradual, the CNS has slowly equilibrated to a low pH. Rapid change in the plasma pH relative to the CNS pH may cause seizures and death because CNS pH normalization lags behind. As plasma pH normalizes over hours or days by renal HCO_3 generation, CNS pH equilibrates at a rate tolerable to the patient, and complications are avoided. The additional risks of inducing alkalosis or hypernatremia by administering sodium bicarbonate often outweigh any benefit derived from quick normalization of the pH.

Nonanion gap acidosis in renal failure is the result of the reduced ability of damaged kidneys to generate HCO_3. The condition is usually chronic and mild, and most patients are asymptomatic. Renal failure severe enough to cause significant acidosis almost always necessitates hemodialysis. The composition of the dialysate is modified to improve serum HCO_3 concentrations and pH.

In cases of diarrheal losses or fistula outputs that exceed the ability of the kidneys to generate HCO_3, bicarbonate must be given. This usually is done with sodium or potassium acetate rather than bicarbonate salts, for reasons stated previously, but sodium bicarbonate can be used. The composition of the fluid that is being lost should be determined by laboratory analysis. The amount of base given should be enough to correct the initial deficit with maintenance therapy in quantities sufficient to match daily losses.

Anion Gap Metabolic Acidosis. Anion gap acidosis is the result of a rise in the number of unmeasured anions (nonvolatile acids) in the plasma with a resultant drop in HCO_3 concentration. These acids may be the byproducts of metabolic processes seen in diabetes and prolonged starvation (ketosis), or they may result from anaerobic carbohydrate metabolism and accumulation of ingested acids (salicylate and methanol poisoning) or acids normally produced in the body that cannot be eliminated, as is the case in renal failure.

During intracellular hypoglycemia, fat becomes the sole substrate for energy generation. This quickly results in the production of ketone bodies. In diabetes, the cause of low intracellular glucose is lack of insulin, which prevents glucose transport from the blood into cells. In starvation, a total absence of glucose from the body forces a change to fat metabolism. Ketone bodies dissociate and contribute hydrogen ions and the anion β-hydroxybutyrate. In cases of tissue hypoxia, insufficient oxygen to support the action of the Krebs cycle results in the activation of an alternative pathway for energy generation—the Cori cycle. Its metabolic byproduct is lactic acid. An accumulation of hydrogen ions and lactate results in acidosis.

Treatment of Anion Gap Metabolic Acidosis. The treatment for anion gap acidosis always is correction of the underlying problem. Intravenous insulin is given in the case of diabetes. In lactic acidosis, restoration of an appropriate circulating volume or plasma oxygen–carrying capacity is indicated. Patients suffering from anion gap acidosis from poisoning may need hemodialysis or gastric lavage to remove the toxic substances from the body. HCO_3 treatment is reserved for patients with a pH at or below 7.1, or for those with severe adverse symptoms of acidosis.

METABOLIC ALKALOSIS

Metabolic alkalosis is defined as a plasma pH above 7.45 caused by a high HCO_3 concentration in the blood. The anion gap is never affected by this condition. As the HCO_3 rises, the lungs compensate by lowering the depth and rate of respiration (Cheyne-Stokes breathing) in an effort to increase the pCO_2, thereby normalizing the plasma pH. Important symptoms associated with alkalosis generally do not appear at a pH below 7.6 (Table 28.7).

The most common causes of metabolic alkalosis are loss of Cl ion (nasogastric suction, loop diuretics, mineralocorticoid excess), ECF depletion, and hepatic failure. Diuretics and mineralocorticoids stimulate exchange of hydrogen and potassium ions for sodium in the renal tubules; this may result in both hypokalemia and alkalosis (Fig. 28.2). Diuretics cause volume depletion and hyponatremia, which further results in hydrogen and potassium losses. Volume depletion itself leads to alkalosis because of the increased concentration of HCO_3 in a reduced plasma space. This condition is referred to as *contraction alkalosis*. Because the body generates almost no basic substances during metabolism and base ingestion is uncommon, alkalosis from other causes is rare.

Treatment of Metabolic Alkalosis. Metabolic alkalosis as the result of sodium and Cl loss accompanying volume contraction is called *saline responsive*. Replacing sodium stops aldosterone-stimulated exchange of hydrogen for sodium in the renal tubules, and replacing Cl ions stops the generation of HCO_3 needed to maintain electrical neutrality. Volume expansion reduces the HCO_3 concentration in the vascular space. NS is the treatment of choice in this condition because it is slightly higher in sodium (154 mmol/L) and much higher in chloride (154 mmol/L) compared with the ECF. The quantity of NS required to restore the TBW deficit should normalize body sodium and chloride. Some patients with metabolic alkalosis present with TBW overload and may not be able to tolerate a sodium load. This alkalosis can be treated with an infusion of hydrochloric acid (HCl) or arginine hydrochloride. HCl is preferred because severe hepatic dysfunction usually is the cause of alkalosis in these patients, and administering arginine can precipitate hepatic coma. The dosage of HCl needed to replace hydrogen and Cl deficits can be determined by the use of the following equation:

$$HCl \ (mmol) = [103 - \text{Measured Cl (mmol/L)}] \times \text{Body weight (kg)} \times 0.2$$

The volume of distribution of chloride is 33% of TBW, so the multiplication factor is 0.2. Giving one-half the HCl deficit over 12 to 24 hours should lower plasma pH by 0.2 and should not cause a significant CNS pH gradient. Hydrochloric acid solutions for intravenous use are commercially available, or extemporaneous compounding of a 0.1- to 0.2-N solution (10 to 20 mmol HCl/L) can be prepared. Infusion into a central venous catheter rather than a peripheral intravenous line is recommended to reduce the risk of phlebitis.

Metabolic alkalosis may be the result of hypokalemia secondary to ICF/ECF exchange of hydrogen for potassium ions and mineralocorticoid excess. These types of alkalosis are saline resistant, and treatment consists of potassium replacement. Alkalosis caused by decreased aldosterone degradation (secondary hyperaldosteronism) seen in severe hepatic disease may respond to the aldosterone antagonist spironolactone. Patients with mineralocorticoid-producing tumors of the adrenal or pituitary gland require therapy with aminoglutethimide or surgery.

RESPIRATORY ACIDOSIS

Respiratory acidosis is characterized by a plasma pH lower than 7.35, which occurs as the result of a pCO_2 higher than

Table 28.7	Metabolic Alkalosis [pH >7.45, HCO_3 >28 mmol (28 mEq]/L)]
Causes	**Signs and Symptoms**
Liver failure	Cheyne-Stokes breathing
Diuretics	Hypokalemia
Nasogastric suction	Muscle cramping
Hyponatremia	Seizures
Hyperaldosteronism	
Corticosteroids	

40 mm Hg. The hemoglobin buffering system is activated in acute respiratory acidosis and sequesters hydrogen ions inside red blood cells. However, it is a weak system and can raise the HCO_3 by only 1 mmol per L for every 10-mm Hg rise in pCO_2. To completely correct the plasma pH, a 5-mmol/L rise in HCO_3 is needed for every 10-mm Hg rise in pCO_2. It is the slow generation of HCO_3 in the kidney that eventually raises the plasma HCO_3 enough to compensate for respiratory acidosis and normalize the pH. Because the CO_2 excretion capacity of normal lungs is always greater than the metabolic production, respiratory acidosis occurs only as a result of severe pulmonary disease (Table 28.8).

Treatment of Respiratory Acidosis. Treatment, which involves correcting the underlying pulmonary disorder, may include antibiotics, bronchodilators, and steroids. Intubation and mechanical ventilation may be needed if respiratory depression accompanies the acidosis. Rapid correction of pH should be avoided, and bicarbonate is indicated only if plasma pH is at or below 7.1. Chronic respiratory acidosis with emphysema and chronic obstructive pulmonary disease develops slowly and is rarely severe enough to necessitate treatment. The stimulus for respiration in these patients may still be an elevated CO_2, but many have adapted to hypoxia as the respiratory drive. Attempts to lower the pCO_2 and raise the pO_2 acutely are not recommended because apnea can result.

RESPIRATORY ALKALOSIS

Respiratory alkalosis occurs with a pCO_2 lower than 40 mm Hg that causes a plasma pH higher than 7.45. The defense against this type of alkalosis is the movement of hydrogen ions (intracellular H_2PO_4 goes to HPO_4) to the vascular space. The phosphate buffering system, as for hemoglobin, is small in capacity and cannot normalize the pH in severe respiratory alkalosis; it can lower the HCO_3 only by 3.5 mmol per L for every 10-mm Hg drop in pCO_2 (Table 28.9).

Treatment of Respiratory Alkalosis. Voluntary hyperventilation, mechanical ventilation, and rapid breathing caused by hypoxemia lower the pCO_2. Correcting this disorder involves normalizing the pCO_2 by raising the CO_2 concentration of inspired air. This can be done by increasing the concentration of inspired CO_2 delivered by a ventilator,

Table 28.9	Respiratory Alkalosis (pH >7.45, pCO_2 <40 mm Hg)
Causes	**Signs and Symptoms**
Hyperventilation	Confusion
Respiratory stimulants	Tetany
Hypoxemia	Syncope

or by having the patient rebreathe his or her own expired air (bag placed loosely over the nose and mouth).

COMPENSATORY RESPONSES TO ACID-BASE DISTURBANCES

All primary acid-base disturbances engender a compensatory response. It may be difficult to determine the primary disturbance if the plasma pH is within normal limits. It is also possible for two primary acid-base problems to occur together. The only exception is that respiratory acidosis and respiratory alkalosis cannot occur simultaneously. Correctly diagnosing the patient's diseases and obtaining a medication history are essential for establishing the causes of an acid-base disorder and initiating treatment. No simple calculation using the arterial blood gases and serum electrolyte concentrations will suffice, given the complexity of the body's buffering and compensatory mechanisms. Nomograms (Fig. 28.3) exist to help the clinician determine the constituents of an acid-base disturbance. This determination, combined with the patient history, should be used to guide appropriate treatment decisions.

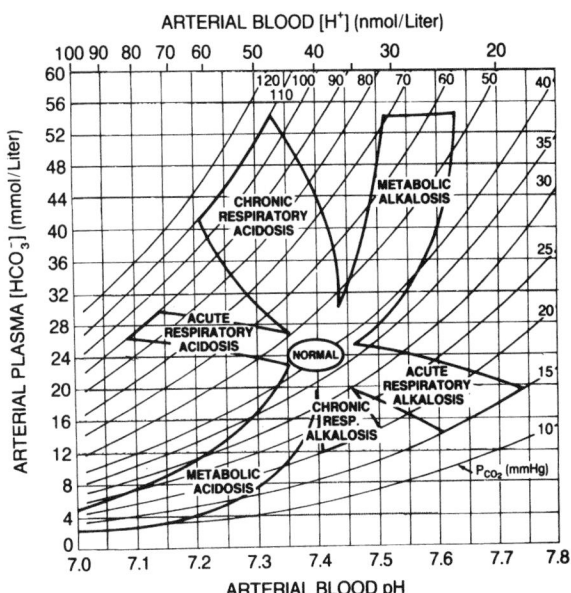

FIGURE 28.3. Acid-base nomogram. (Reprinted from Cogan MG, Rector FC. Acid-base disorders. In: Brenner BM, Rector FC, eds. The kidney. 3rd ed. Philadelphia: WB Saunders, 1986: 457–518, with permission.)

Table 28.8	Respiratory Acidosis (pH <7.35, pCO_2 >40 mm Hg)
Causes	**Signs and Symptoms**
Emphysema	Anxiety
Airway obstruction	Disorientation
Bronchoconstriction	Vasodilation
Pneumonia	Increased cardiac output
Respiratory depression	Coma

ELECTROLYTES

The major electrolytes in the body consist of sodium, Cl, HCO_3, potassium, calcium, magnesium, and phosphorus. Normal serum concentrations are listed in Table 28.1. Sodium is linked to TBW, and maintenance of normal concentrations and correction of abnormalities were discussed earlier. The role of Cl in the body is as an osmotic substance and the major anion in the ECF. Cl has no innate physiologic function. HCO_3 is linked to the acid-base homeostatic system and was also discussed earlier. The physiologic functions of the remaining electrolytes are to maintain membrane potentials for nerve conduction and muscle contraction (potassium, calcium, and magnesium), to generate the energy needed to maintain these potentials and to do the work of body functions and movement (phosphorus), and to maintain the strength of bone mass (calcium and phosphorus). The main reservoirs of these ions are the intracellular space and bone. Serum concentrations fall slowly when intake goes down because numerous hormonal and homeostatic mechanisms exist to keep serum concentrations within the normal range. The serum concentrations of these electrolytes are low relative to sodium and to their own intracellular concentrations, but it is their intravascular concentrations that control physiologic activities. Serum concentrations must be kept within a narrow range, or serious complications such as arrhythmias, seizures, and tetany may result.

POTASSIUM

The amount of potassium in the vascular space accounts for only 0.4% of the total amount in the body.[25–30] Normal serum concentrations range from 3.5 to 5.0 mmol per L (3.5 to 5 mEq/L), and the major functions of potassium include impulse transmission, cardiac contractility, and aldosterone secretion. The major route of potassium excretion is the kidney. Elimination can increase when intake is high, but the kidneys have no mechanism with which to conserve potassium. A deficiency develops rapidly when potassium intake is inadequate. Hyponatremia also causes potassium loss via renal exchange processes that are discussed in the Sodium section (Fig. 28.2).

Serum concentrations of potassium do not completely depend on the relationship between intake and output and sodium homeostasis. The large intracellular pool of potassium can be a source of ions to support the intravascular concentration when a low serum concentration develops. Because of this process, depletion of potassium usually represents not just a low circulating amount of potassium but also an acquired intracellular deficit that can approach several hundred millimoles. Changes in acid-base status alter the distribution of potassium ions in the body. In acidosis, potassium is exchanged across cell membranes with hydrogen ions as the body attempts to buffer protons (acid) in the intracellular space to help maintain a normal pH. The converse is true in alkalosis. The serum potassium concentration increases (acidosis) or decreases (alkalosis) by 0.6 mmol per L for every 0.1 change in pH from the value of 7.4.

Hyperkalemia. Elevated serum potassium concentrations may represent a medical emergency and almost always manifest as the sudden appearance of cardiac arrhythmias. This usually occurs at serum concentrations above 6 mmol per L. The symptoms and causes of hyperkalemia are listed in Table 28.10. Actual total body potassium can be high, normal, or (occasionally) low, and it is the intravascular concentration that effects physiologic activities and causes cardiac disorders. The life-threatening potential of the cardiac abnormality determines the type, complexity, and sequence of treatment given. Any exogenous sources of potassium such as IV fluids or drugs that contain potassium should be discontinued immediately.

Treatment of Hyperkalemia. Measures used to correct hyperkalemia act by normalizing neuromuscular membrane potential, shifting ions back into the intracellular space, or removing potassium from the body. Membrane potential and, therefore, the strength of muscular contraction are determined by the relative concentrations of potassium, calcium, and magnesium at the cell membrane. If the potassium-induced arrhythmia is life threatening, 2.5 to 5 mmol (5 to 10 mEq) calcium is given over several minutes to temporarily correct the potassium-to-calcium ratio and eliminate the cardiac problem. A constant infusion of intravenous calcium at a rate determined by simultaneous electrocardiographic (ECG) monitoring may be necessary to maintain cardiac function until measures that permanently normalize serum potassium concentrations take effect. Calcium gluconate (2.3 mmol/g) or calcium chloride (6.8 mmol/g) is used, but therapy cannot be continued for long periods because complications of hypercalcemia may occur.

Potassium ions may be shifted from the vascular space to the intracellular space through the administration of glucose and insulin. Potassium ions move with glucose across cell membranes in the presence of insulin. A ratio of 2 to 3 g glucose per unit of insulin is needed to maintain a normal blood glucose concentration during this process. Commonly administered solutions include 25 to 30 units of regular insulin per L 10% dextrose solution and 10 units in 50 mL 50% dextrose.

β_2-agonists may also be used to cause a transcellular shift of potassium. A total of 10 to 20 mg of albuterol may be administered by nebulizer, in combination with glucose and insulin.

Sodium bicarbonate is another treatment option used to shift potassium intracellularly. A temporary alkalosis is caused, thereby lowering serum potassium concentrations by 0.6 mmol per L for every 0.1 elevation in pH. Sodium bicarbonate is recommended in combination with insulin and glucose because of its poor efficacy when used as a solo agent for the treatment of hyperkalemia. Additionally, this pharmaceutical therapy, similar to calcium infusion, cannot be continued for long periods because sodium overload and

Table 28.10	Symptoms and Causes of Hyperkalemia and Hypokalemia
Hyperkalemia	**Hypokalemia**
Serum concentration >5 mmol/L (5 mEq/L)	Serum concentration <3.5 mmol/L (3.5 mEq/L)
Causes	
Renal failure	Amphotericin B
Acidosis	Diuretics
Crush injury	Diarrhea
Red cell hemolysis	Decreased intake
Potassium-sparing diuretics	Corticosteroids
Excess ingestion of potassium (salt substitutes)	Renal tubular acidosis
Adrenal insufficiency	Alkalosis
Hypoaldosteronism	Vomiting
	Fanconi syndrome
	Hyperaldosteronism
	Licorice
Signs and Symptoms	
Electrocardiographic findings	Electrocardiographic findings
Peaked T waves	Flat or inverted T waves
Depressed ST segment	Depressed ST segment
Disappearance of P wave	Muscle weakness
Widened QRS complex	Diminished reflexes
Muscle weakness	Paralysis
Paresthesias	Weak pulse
Gastrointestinal hypermotility	Ileus
Flaccid paralysis	Depression
	Confusion
	Hypotension

metabolic alkalosis may result. Fifty-mL vials and preloaded syringes of 8.4% (1 mmol/mL) and 500-mL containers of 5% (0.6 mmol/mL) sodium bicarbonate are commercially available; 4.2% (0.5 mmol/mL) preloaded syringes are available for pediatric or neonatal use. These treatments are a temporary solution because potassium ions are not removed from the body. However, they do allow treatment to continue for long periods without significant complications.

Three different treatments may be used to *remove* potassium from the body. Although these should be initiated as soon as possible, they may not correct cardiac arrhythmias in a timely fashion and cannot be considered acute treatment for hyperkalemia. The cationic-anionic exchange resin sodium polystyrene sulfonate (SPS), given orally or rectally, binds potassium to itself through exchange with sodium in the GI tract. One gram of SPS removes approximately 1 mmol potassium and adds 2 to 3 mmol sodium. The resin is very constipating, so it is given with sorbitol, an osmotic cathartic, and water to prevent fecal impaction. The oral route is preferred over rectal administration because contact time with the GI mucosa is longer. The initial dosage is 30 to 60 g resin in 20% sorbitol (commercial preparations are available) and can be repeated every 1 to 2 hours if the serum potassium concentration remains high. Sodium overload may occur, so monitoring for congestive heart failure, edema, and pulmonary edema is necessary in patients at risk of developing these complications.

Loop diuretics, specifically furosemide, have been used as treatment for patients with hyperkalemia because of the renal wasting of potassium caused by the drug. Hemodialysis can be used to remove potassium from the body. Although its onset is immediate and potassium is removed from the plasma, the procedure is very invasive and should be used only when the patient's condition is life threatening and other treatment methods have failed.

Hypokalemia. Hypokalemia can also be a cardiac medical emergency, with rhythm disturbances appearing at serum concentrations below 3 mmol per L. Patients may exhibit muscle weakness and malaise before ECG changes appear. Symptoms and causes of hypokalemia are listed in Table 28.10. Correction of underlying disease or discontinuation of drug therapy that contributes to hypokalemia is a basic part of the initial treatment.

Hypokalemia secondary to hyponatremia is almost always accompanied by hypochloremic alkalosis as the renal conservation of sodium causes secretion of potassium and hydrogen ions (Fig. 28.2). For every 3 mmol sodium reabsorbed, 2 mmol potassium and 1 mmol hydrogen are lost in the urine. The hydrogen ion needed for exchange with sodium is generated from the action of carbonic anhydrase on water and CO_2. Carbonic acid in renal tubular cells dissociates into hydrogen and HCO_3. The hydrogen ion is secreted into the urine, and HCO_3 is resorbed into the blood. When enough HCO_3 ions accumulate in serum, alkalosis results. Any concomitant hyponatremia and alkalosis must be corrected for hypokalemia treatment to be successful. The Cl salt of potassium is the treatment of choice because alkalosis must be corrected. As Cl loading proceeds, HCO_3 excretion by the kidneys increases, generation decreases, and alkalosis resolves. If a nonchloride salt of potassium is given, renal excretion and intracellular shifting of potassium will continue, and hypokalemia will not be corrected (Fig. 28.2).

Treatment of Hypokalemia. An intracellular deficit of potassium almost always precedes and accompanies an intravascular deficit, thereby requiring large amounts of potassium to restore total body deficits and normalize serum concentrations. Orally or intravenously administered potassium shifts slowly into the ICF to correct that deficit, so the rate of potassium chloride infusion must not be so rapid as to cause interim hyperkalemia. Under most conditions, intravenous potassium chloride at 10 mmol per hour will not cause hyperkalemia in a patient with a serum concentration below 3.5 mmol per L, and 30 to 40 mmol given over 3 to 4 hours in D_5W or NS is a common rate of potassium replacement. Serum potassium concentration should be reassessed and potassium administered until normal serum concentrations are obtained (3.8 to 4.0 mmol/L). In patients with profound hypokalemia and continued potassium wasting, such as those with renal tubular acidosis from amphotericin B therapy, replacing the potassium deficit may entail very large dosages. In these instances, 20 to 40 mmol per hour may be needed, and a central line is always necessary because infusion into a peripheral vein at a rate greater than 10 mmol per hour almost always causes intolerable pain and phlebitis at the infusion site.

Oral administration of potassium chloride can correct hypokalemia, but many patients experience considerable GI irritation and vomiting when given more than 20 mmol per dose or 60 mmol per day. Wax matrix tablets have greater patient acceptance than does liquid potassium because of the unpleasant taste of the oral solutions. The problem of gastric irritation is the same for both tablets and solution. Attempts to replace large potassium deficits by mouth often are unsuccessful, and simultaneous IV replacement may be needed.

CHLORIDE

Chloride is the major anion in the ECF, but it has no inherent physiologic function.[2,4,14] It usually increases or decreases in synchronous fashion with total body sodium, but a change in Cl concentration causes an acid-base disturbance. Because electrical neutrality must be maintained and the concentration of unmeasured ions is fixed, an immediate change in the serum HCO_3 concentration will be noted. The effect will occur as metabolic acidosis or alkalosis, depending on the resultant increase or decrease in the HCO_3:pCO_2 ratio.

Disorders of body Cl result from its loss from the body (vomiting, diuretics), hypernatremia, Cl loading (saline infusion), or changes in acid-base balance. In acidosis and alkalosis, the change in serum Cl concentration is almost always a compensatory response to an initial change in the HCO_3 value. In this instance, the serum Cl will not normalize, nor should an effort be made to correct the concentration by giving or withholding Cl until the cause of the acid-base abnormality is identified and corrected. When this occurs, the Cl concentration normalizes naturally via renal homeostatic mechanisms.

Hyperchloremia. Hyperchloremia, defined as a serum concentration greater than 105 mmol per L, results from metabolic acidosis, respiratory alkalosis, hypernatremia, or Cl loading. Treatment is aimed at correcting the underlying disorder. If the cause of the hyperchloremia is metabolic acidosis or respiratory alkalosis, correcting these disturbances is the only treatment. The composition of oral or intravenous fluids should be determined and adjustments made if they appear to be the cause of the problem. Changing a NS infusion to 0.45% saline infusion or replacing sodium chloride with sodium acetate may resolve the problem. When hyperchloremia is caused by overingestion of sodium chloride, treatment consists of free water replacement and diuresis. In hypernatremia caused by water loss, the treatment is TBW fluid replacement (see Sodium).

Hypochloremia. A serum chloride below 95 mmol per L is considered hypochloremia. Because ECF chloride changes with ECF sodium, hyponatremia causes hypochloremia. This is an appropriate compensatory mechanism for maintaining electrical neutrality; chloride normalizes with correction of the ECF sodium concentration.

The most common causes of hypochloremia are nasogastric suction, vomiting, and diuretic therapy. Large amounts of chloride and acid are lost along with stomach fluid, so therapy consists of replacing the volume of the nasogastric aspirate or vomiting with high-chloride solutions such as NS or LR. Diuretics cause hypochloremia through mechanisms discussed in the Hyponatremia section. Therapy consists of liberalizing sodium chloride intake, reducing the diuretic dosage, and correcting symptomatic hyponatremia and hypokalemia with saline and potassium chloride solutions.

CALCIUM

The major repository of calcium in the body is bone, with only 1% of the total amount of calcium in the body found in the fluid spaces.[31–39] Normal serum concentration is 2.2 to 2.6 mmol per L (8.8 to 10.3 mg/dL). Only 50% is available to exert its physiologic effect; the other 50% is bound to albumin and other proteins. Serum calcium concentration does not fluctuate as a direct result of daily intake and excretion of the ion. The synchronous activity of parathyroid hormone, vitamin D, and calcitonin regulates GI absorption, renal excretion, and skeletal deposition or resorption of calcium and determines the serum calcium concentration. An inverse relationship occurs between serum calcium and phosphate; an increase or decrease in one mineral necessitates a change in the opposite direction of the other mineral to maintain equilibrium.

Calcium has a variety of specific physiologic functions in the body. It is essential to neuromuscular conduction because it stabilizes cell membrane permeability and excitability; it inhibits some enzymes in the Krebs cycle, stimulates gastrin, reduces renal blood flow, and is active in the blood coagulation cascade as factor IV. The normal serum range is narrow, and many laboratories measure only total serum calcium, not just the active ionized 50%. This presents a problem for determination of the physiologically active amount of ion in the serum. Because 50% is protein bound, primarily to albumin, low serum albumin results in low total serum calcium concentration. Low serum calcium concentration in the presence of low albumin does not necessarily indicate a low ionized concentration. Corrected, measured total serum calcium can be calculated by accounting for a patient's decreased albumin on the basis of a normal value of 4 g per dL. It can be assumed from this correction that the free calcium is normal and physiologic hypocalcemia is not present. The formula for this calculation is as follows:

$$\text{Corrected serum calcium} = [4 \text{ g/dL} - \text{Measured albumin} \\ (\text{g/dL})] \times 0.8 + \text{Serum calcium measured}$$

When the ionized calcium is reported, this correction need not be made. Acid-base disturbances affect the ionized: bound calcium ratio but not the total serum calcium. Some hydrogen ions circulate in the blood while bound to albumin. In acidosis, more hydrogen ions are bound to albumin as the body attempts to buffer acid and normalize the plasma pH. This action displaces calcium ions from their binding sites, and the amount of free calcium in the blood rises. The converse is true in alkalosis. For each 0.1 change in pH, the ionized calcium changes by 0.42 mmol per L in the opposite direction.

Hypercalcemia. Hypercalcemia is defined as corrected total serum calcium above 2.6 mmol per L (10.3 mg/dL) or an ionized value above 1.15 mmol per L. The symptoms and causes are listed in Table 28.11. Any sources of exogenous calcium should be discontinued immediately. It is important to note that mental aberrations seen with hypercalcemia may be profound and are not always related in a linear fashion to the degree of hypercalcemia. Any evaluation of mental status changes or of a comatose patient should include serum calcium concentration.

Treatment of Hypercalcemia. Therapies for hypercalcemia involve shifting calcium ions into the bone or eliminating calcium from the body. Therapies administered to remove calcium from the body are given first because they work faster and are generally more effective in an acute situation. Loop diuretics, such as furosemide and bumetanide, increase renal calcium excretion. The initial furosemide dosage is 1 mg per kg and is given with an amount of NS that will maintain normal body water and sodium concentration when a urine output of 200 to 500 mL per hour is achieved. Electrolytes must be carefully monitored and potassium and magnesium administration may need to be implemented to prevent hypokalemia and hypomagnesemia caused by the action of the loop diuretic. This washout therapy may need to be continued for extended periods if the cause of the hypercalcemia is severe or if abnormally large amounts of calcium continue to appear in the vascular compartment.

Treatments that shift calcium back into bone are slow and may become ineffective because of tachyphylaxis. Parenteral calcitonin is used because it rapidly increases bone uptake of calcium; although the effect is rapid, it is of short duration, and tachyphylaxis develops within days. The initial parenteral dosage for treating hypercalcemia is 4 IU per kg salmon calcitonin given every 12 hours by subcutaneous or intramuscular injection. After 2 days, this can be increased to a maximum dosage of 8 IU per kg given every 6 hours, but additional hypocalcemic effect usually does not result. Intranasal calcitonin is not useful in managing acute or chronic hypercalcemia. Etidronate disodium is a bisphosphonate that inhibits osteoclastic bone resorption by binding hydroxyapatite. Initial treatment consists of 7.5 mg/kg/day given intravenously once daily for 3 days. The infusion time must be at least 2 hours to avoid proximal renal tubular damage (seen in patients with preexisting renal disease) and the theoretical risk of transient hypocalcemia. Once serum calcium has been normalized, oral therapy with 20 mg/kg/day can be given if the hypercalcemia is expected to recur (e.g., bone metastases in patients with cancer). Pamidronate disodium appears to be more effective than etidronate in treating hypercalcemia and offers the advantages of quicker onset and longer duration of action without the disadvantage of inhibiting bone mineralization at high dosages. It is dosed at 60 to 90 mg given intravenously over at least 2 hours. The treatment may be repeated as often as every 7 days if necessary. Calcitonin in combination with bisphosphonates is used in the acute management of hypercalcemia.

Steroids such as prednisone are useful in managing chronic mild hypercalcemia. The initial prednisone dosage varies between 15 and 100 mg per day, with an onset of action of 3 to 10 days. Steroids work by antagonizing the activation of vitamin D in the liver and reducing bone resorption. For these reasons, steroids are not effective in hypercal-

Table 28.11	Symptoms and Causes of Hypercalcemia and Hypocalcemia
Hypercalcemia	**Hypocalcemia**
Serum concentration >2.6 mmol/L (10.3 mg/dL)	Serum concentration <2.2 mmol/L (8.8 mg/dL)
Ionized >1.2 mmol/L (2.3 mEq/L)	Ionized 1.0 mmol/L (2.0 mEq/L)
Causes	
Bone neoplasms	Renal failure
Hyperparathyroidism	Hypoparathyroidism
Hypervitaminosis D	Vitamin D deficiency
Prolonged immobilization	Diuretics
Sarcoidosis	Mithramycin
Paget disease	Transfusion with citrated blood
Acidosis	Lithium
Idiopathic hypercalcemia	Adrenal insufficiency
Alkalosis of infancy	Pancreatitis
Hypervitaminosis A	Hyperphosphatemia
Aluminum osteodystrophy	Colchicine
Thiazide diuretics	Hypomagnesemia
	Fluoride poisoning
	Loop diuretics
Signs and Symptoms	
Muscle weakness	Numbness or tingling of fingertips or around mouth
Anorexia	Fatigue
Lethargy	Nausea
Depression	Hyperactive reflexes
Psychosis	Chvostek sign
Stupor	Trousseau sign
Coma	Tetany
	Lethargy
	Depression
	Psychosis
	Stupor
	Coma

cemia secondary to hyperparathyroidism. Oral phosphate is not a treatment option in this type of hypercalcemia. Because the ordinarily reciprocal relationship between serum calcium and phosphorous concentrations has not been sustained, the amount by which the serum calcium falls when phosphorous concentration rises usually is small. The risk of soft tissue calcification by calcium-phosphate complexes often exceeds the benefit of this therapy. If raising the serum phosphorus results in a calcium-phosphate product [serum calcium (mg/dL) multiplied by phosphate (mg/dL)] above 60, precipitation can occur. In the rare instances when hypophosphatemia is the cause of hypercalcemia, administering 30 to 100 mmol per day (1 to 3 g) of phosphorus should resolve the problem.

Sodium phosphate replacement products are available; Phospho-Soda solution contains 25 mmol (800 mg) phosphate per 5 mL, Neutra-Phos capsules contain 8 mmol (250 mg) phosphate, and the solution contains 32 mmol (1 g) phosphate per 300 mL. These products also contain considerable amounts of sodium as the obligate cation, so they must be used with caution.

An effective but potentially toxic therapy for hypercalcemia is mithramycin, which is indicated only when other therapies fail. Mithramycin is a cancer chemotherapeutic agent that acts by inhibiting DNA-dependent bone osteoclast RNA synthesis. This slows or stops bone resorption. The initial dosage is 25 Φg per kg daily up to a weekly maximum of

150 Φg per kg. The onset of action is 12 to 48 hours, and the duration 3 to 7 days. Although these dosages are considerably smaller than those used in cancer treatment, the risk of hematologic and GI toxicity remains.

Hypocalcemia. Hypocalcemia is defined as a corrected serum concentration below 2.20 mmol per L (8.8 mg per dL) or an ionized concentration below 1 mmol per L. Symptoms and causes are listed in Table 28.11. Acute treatment involves intravenous calcium. The chloride salt contains 6.8 mmol per gram (13.5 mEq calcium per gram), and the gluconate and gluceptate salts 2.3 mmol per gram (4.6 mEq calcium per gram). The initial dosage is 2.5 to 5 mmol calcium followed by an infusion of 0.075 to 0.1 mmol calcium/kg/hour. Calcium concentration, blood pressure, and ECG should be monitored during this process for evaluation of cardiac function and avoidance of hypercalcemia. Patients whose symptoms of hypocalcemia do not resolve with calcium replacement should be evaluated for hypomagnesemia because the abnormalities can mimic each other and often appear together.

Treatment of Hypocalcemia. Treatment of chronic hypocalcemia is directed at correcting the underlying cause. Most often, the cause of chronic hypocalcemia is a low concentration of biologically active vitamin D. This appears in advanced hepatic or renal disease because of decreased transformation of cholecalciferol (D_3) by these organs to the active form, 1,25-dihydroxycholecalciferol (1,25-DHC). The serum concentration of calcium will not normalize until the concentration of 1,25-DHC is normal. Therapy usually involves calcium and vitamin D supplementation. Ergocalciferol (D_2) in a dosage of 1.25 to 5 mg (50,000 to 200,000 IU per day) or dihydrotachysterol (DHT) in a dosage of 0.25 to 1 mg per day (equivalent to 30,000 to 120,000 IU of D_2) is used. The onset of action can take several weeks and the effect may be prolonged because of the long half-life of vitamin D. Activated forms of vitamin D must be given when renal or hepatic transformation of ergocalciferol and dihydrotachysterol is absent or unreliable. 25-Hydroxycholecalciferol (calcifediol) in dosages of 50 to 100 Φg per day or 1,25-DHC (calcitriol) in dosages of 0.25 to 1 Φg per day is available. Active forms of vitamin D have an onset of action of 3 to 7 days and are preferred because their shorter half-lives reduce the risk of prolonged hypercalcemia. Calcium supplementation with 25 to 100 mmol per day (1 to 4 g) elemental calcium is begun simultaneously. Several salts of calcium are available for oral therapy, but calcium carbonate contains the highest amount of elemental calcium—10.2 mmol (400 mg) per 1,000 mg calcium carbonate. Calcium lactate contains 1.5 mmol (60 mg) per 300 mg, calcium gluceptate 2.2 mmol (80 mg) per 1,000 mg, and calcium gluconate 2.3 mmol (90 mg) per 1,000 mg. Calcium carbonate is the preferred preparation because the number of tablets the patient must take is lower than with the other salts. Liquid calcium carbonate and calcium gluceptate are available for use in patients with achlorhydria or those receiving H_2-an-

tagonist therapy because tablet dissolution in the GI tract may be incomplete without gastric acid. When hypocalcemia is caused by hypoparathyroidism, parathyroid hormone replacement is indicated and is the only therapy that raises the serum calcium.

MAGNESIUM

The average adult body contains approximately 1,000 mmol (2000 mEq) magnesium, 99% of which is in bone and the intracellular compartment.[40–43] Of the 1% remaining in the vascular space, 25% is bound to proteins. It is the ionized 75% that exerts the physiologic effect. Serum magnesium is maintained in the normal range of 0.8 to 1.2 mmol per L (1.6 to 2.4 mEq/L) through efficient renal conservation and excretion mechanisms and the ability to draw on the intracellular space for replacement ions when intake falls. In conjunction with calcium and potassium, magnesium regulates neuromuscular excitability and conduction on the cell membrane. Magnesium also has a role in parathyroid hormone release. Deviations from normal serum magnesium rarely appear as an isolated problem. Most often, calcium, potassium, and phosphate concentrations also are abnormal, indicating a generalized abnormality in the solute concentration of the intracellular compartment. This pattern of electrolyte disturbances is most commonly seen in prolonged starvation or malnutrition.

Hypermagnesemia. Hypermagnesemia is defined as a serum concentration above 1.2 mmol per L (2.4 mEq/L), but serious symptoms usually do not occur until the concentration is above 2.4 mmol per L (4.8 mEq/L). Symptoms and causes of hypermagnesemia are listed in Table 28.12. Because the kidneys can easily excrete large amounts of magnesium, hypermagnesemia is rarely seen without attendant severe renal dysfunction. Magnesium-containing antacids are often a contributing factor in this situation. All sources of exogenous magnesium should be discontinued.

Treatment of Hypermagnesemia. Treatments for an elevated magnesium concentration involve resolving the adverse symptoms, shifting the magnesium intracellularly, and eliminating it from the body. Patients with neuromuscular or cardiovascular symptoms of hypermagnesemia may be administered intravenous calcium in dosages of 100 to 200 mg elemental calcium. This therapy can be used hourly until the magnesium concentration is normalized or the symptoms subside. Glucose and insulin can be used for brief periods, as occurs in the treatment of hyperkalemia, to mobilize the magnesium intracellularly. Forced diuresis with saline boluses and looped diuretics may be given to eliminate the magnesium in patients with adequate renal function. Potassium may have to be replaced in patients because of possible depletion from loop diuretics. In patients with chronic renal insufficiency, loop diuretics may be employed on a long-term basis. Hemodialysis may be necessary in patients who are unresponsive to the previously described therapies, or in those with end-stage renal disease.

Table 28.12	Symptoms and Causes of Hypermagnesemia and Hypomagnesemia
Hypermagnesemia	**Hypomagnesemia**
Serum concentration >1.2 mmol/L (2.4 mEq/L)	Serum concentration <0.8 mmol/L (1.6 mEq/L)
Causes	
Renal failure	Amphotericin B
Hyperparathyroidism	Cis-platinum
Hypoaldosteronism	Diuretics
Adrenal insufficiency	Diarrhea
Lithium	Hypervitaminosis D
	Vitamin D deficiency
	Vomiting
	Hyperaldosteronism
	Aminoglycosides
Signs and Symptoms	
Weakness	Tremor
Nausea or vomiting	Hyperactive reflexes
Hypotension	Confusion
Respiratory depression	Seizures
Coma	

Hypomagnesemia. Hypomagnesemia is defined as a serum concentration below 0.8 mmol per L (1.6 mEq/L), and symptoms may appear at concentrations below 0.6 per L (1.2 mEq/L). Symptoms and causes of hypomagnesemia are found in Table 28.12. Hypomagnesemia usually appears with hypokalemia, hypocalcemia, and hypophosphatemia. Concentrations of these electrolytes should be measured when a low magnesium concentration is identified.

Treatment of Hypomagnesemia. A large magnesium deficit is usually present when serum magnesium concentrations decline, making exact replacement dosages of magnesium difficult to determine from the serum concentrations alone. Therapy consists of intravenous magnesium sulfate or oral magnesium oxide or gluconate salts. Intravenous magnesium sulfate is administered at a dosage of 1 mEq/kg/day if the serum concentration is less than 0.6 mmol per L, and 0.5 mEq/kg/day if it is between 0.7 and 1.2 mmol per L. Intravenous magnesium sulfate is administered slowly at 0.5 to 1 g per hour. Serum magnesium concentrations may take up to 48 hours to equilibrate with intracellular shifting. The oral replacement of large deficits can be difficult. Magnesium is a saline cathartic, and the large dosages required for replacement may cause diarrhea. When this route of administration is chosen, up to 20 mmol per day given in divided doses is usually tolerated. Magnesium oxide capsules are most commonly given (6.2 mmol per 250 mg MgO) because of convenience for the patient, but solutions of magnesium sulfate and gluconate are also available.

PHOSPHORUS

Of the total body phosphate, 99.99% is contained in bone and the intracellular space.[43–46] The normal serum concentration is 0.8 to 1.6 mmol per L (2.5 to 5 mg/dL). The equilibrium between serum calcium (reciprocal with phosphate), intracellular stores, parathyroid hormone, vitamin D, renal conservation and excretion mechanisms, and oral intake maintains a normal serum concentration. The specific physiologic function of phosphate in the body is the formation of high-energy phosphate bonds of adenosine diphosphate and triphosphate in glycolysis (anaerobic metabolism) and in the Krebs cycle. Another important function of phosphate, as 2,3-diphosphoglycerate, is facilitation of the release of oxygen from hemoglobin.

Hyperphosphatemia. Hyperphosphatemia, defined as a serum concentration above 1.6 mmol per L (5 mg/dL), almost always results from decreased excretion in the presence of severe renal dysfunction. Symptoms and causes of hyperphosphatemia are listed in Table 28.13. The major risk of hyperphosphatemia, and the reason it is most commonly corrected, is the hypocalcemia it reciprocally causes. A high phosphorous concentration alone does not have significant negative physiologic consequences. Serum calcium concentration should be evaluated in a patient with an elevated phosphate concentration because the physiologic disturbances caused by an abnormal calcium concentration are serious.

Treatment of Hyperphosphatemia. Available treatments for hyperphosphatemia involve reducing phosphorous intake

Table 28.13	Symptoms and Causes of Hyperphosphatemia and Hypophosphatemia
Hyperphosphatemia	**Hypophosphatemia**
Serum concentration >1.6 mmol/L (5.0 mg/dL)	Serum concentration <0.8 mmol/L (2.5 mg/dL)
Causes	
Renal failure	Aluminum antacids
Hypoparathyroidism	Prolonged starvation
	Nutritional depletion
	Diuretics
	Vitamin D deficiency
	Hyperaldosteronism
	Corticosteroids
	Alkalosis
	Renal tubular defects
	Syndrome of inappropriate secretion of antidiuretic hormone
Signs and Symptoms	
Renal osteodystrophy	Muscle weakness
Ca-PO₄ complex deposition in soft tissue	Bone pain
	Paresthesias
	Irritability
	Respiratory insufficiency
	Hemolytic anemia
	Rhabdomyolysis
	Proximal muscle atrophy
	Cardiomyopathy
	Seizures
	Coma

and decreasing its absorption from the GI tract by precipitating it with aluminum-containing antacids, calcium salts, or sevelamer, a polymeric compound. Care must be used in patients with renal dysfunction. Calcium and aluminum accumulation may result from aggressive treatment with aluminum-containing antacids or calcium salt. Short-term treatment (<48 hours) with antacids or calcium salt or sevelamer may be necessary.

Hypophosphatemia. Hypophosphatemia is defined as a serum concentration below 0.8 mmol per L (2.5 mg/dL). Abnormality usually is the result of starvation and appears with simultaneous deficits in other intracellular ions. Symptoms and causes are listed in Table 28.13.

Treatment of Hypophosphatemia. Therapy consists of replacement with the sodium or potassium salts of phosphate. Repletion must be slow because calcium-phosphate precipitation in soft tissue can result from aggressive therapy. The initial phosphate dosage is 0.64 mmol/kg/day if the serum concentration is below 0.5 mmol per L (1.5 mg/dL), and 0.32 mmol/kg/day if it is between 0.5 mmol per L (1.6 mg/dL) and 0.7 mmol per L (2.2 mg/dL). Therapy should be given over at least 6 hours to allow for equilibration into the intracellular space, where the majority of the body deficit occurs. Oral sodium and potassium phosphate replacement may be given as capsules, packets, or solution, but because of the high propensity to cause GI upset and diarrhea, large dosages are not recommended. Dosages of 8 to 16 mmol phosphate (250 to 500 mg) four times a day after meals and at bedtime are usually tolerated may be used to help correct hypophosphatemia.

KEY POINTS

■ Identifying and correcting disorders of fluids, electrolytes, and acid-base balance can be difficult. The body's internal environment is constantly changing, adjusting to and correcting for internal and external forces that disturb homeostasis. Normal serum concentrations of electrolytes do not always reflect normal body water or pH status. Values outside the normal range may represent appropriate compensatory responses to maintain homeostasis, and treatment consists of finding and correcting the primary disturbance. Normal body functions continue only within narrow ranges of ionic composition, pH, and intravascular volume and pressure

- When any patient is evaluated, establishing and maintaining hemodynamic status sufficient to perfuse and oxygenate cells is the first priority and must be done quickly

- With the exception of exsanguination (acute, massive blood loss), changes in fluids, electrolytes, and pH usually occur slowly, and some compensatory mechanisms operate

- Correcting an isolated abnormal laboratory value without regard to its cause and contribution to overall patient status will further complicate the patient's condition with no derived benefit

- Therapy chosen must be administered to reestablish and support homeostasis without causing treatment-induced (iatrogenic) complications

REFERENCES

1. Brenner BM, Levine SA, eds. The kidney. 5th ed. Philadelphia: WB Saunders, 1995.
2. Halperin ML, Goldstein MB, eds. Fluid, electrolyte, and acid-base physiology: a problem-based approach. 3rd ed. Philadelphia: WB Saunders, 1999.
3. Hill LL. Body composition, normal electrolyte concentrations, and the maintenance of normal volume, tonicity and acid-base metabolism. Pediatr Clin North Am 37:241–256, 1990.
4. Adrogue HJ, Madias NE. Hypernatremia. N Engl J Med 342:1493–1499, 2000.
5. Adrogue HJ, Madias NE. Hyponatremia. N Engl J Med 342:1581–1589, 2000.
6. Zarinetchi F, Berl T. Evaluation and management of severe hyponatremia. Adv Intern Med 41:251–283, 1996.
7. Hillier TA, Abbott RD, Barrett EJ. Hyponatremia: evaluating the correction factor for hyperglycemia. Am J Med 106:399–403, 1999
8. Kovacs L, Robertson GL. Syndrome of inappropriate anti-diuresis. Endocrinol Metab Clin North Am 21:859–875, 1992.
9. Chan TY. Drug-induced syndrome of inappropriate secretion of anti-diuretic hormone. Causes, diagnosis and treatment. Drugs Aging 11:27–44, 1997.
10. Faber MD, Kupin WL, Heilig CW, et al. Common fluid and electrolyte and acid-base problems in the intensive care unit: selected problems. Semin Nephrol 14:8–22, 1994.
11. Field M, Rao M. Intestinal electrolyte transport and diarrheal disease, part 1. N Engl J Med 321:800–806, 1989.
12. Field M, Rao M. Intestinal electrolyte transport and diarrheal disease, part 2. N Engl J Med 321:879–883, 1989.
13. Harris BH, Gelfand JA. The immune response to trauma. Semin Pediatr Surg 4:77–82, 1995.
14. Choi PT, Yip G, Quinonez LG, et al. Colloids vs crystalloids in fluid resuscitation: a systematic review. Crit Care Med 27:200–210, 1999.
15. Roberts JS, Bratton SL. Colloid volume expanders. Problems, pitfalls and possibilities. Drugs 55:621–630, 1998.
16. Gluck SL. Acid-base. Lancet 352:474–479, 1998.
17. Rutecki GW, Whittier FC. An approach to clinical acid-base problem solving. Compr Ther 24:553–559, 1998.
18. McLaughlin M, Kassirer J. Rational treatment of acid-base disorders. Drugs 39:841–855, 1990.
19. Fulop M. Flow diagrams for the diagnosis of acid-base disorders. J Emerg Med 16:97–109, 1998.
20. Adrogue HJ, Madias NE. Changes in plasma potassium concentration during acute acid-base disturbances. Am J Med 71:456–469, 1981.
21. Khanna A, Kurtzman NA. Metabolic alkalosis. Respir Care 46:354–365, 2001.
22. Adrogue HJ, Madias NE. Management of life-threatening acid-base disorders. First of two parts. N Engl J Med 338:26–34, 1998.
23. Adrogue HJ, Madias NE. Management of life-threatening acid-base disorders. Second of two parts. N Engl J Med 338:107–111, 1998.
24. Franch HA, Mitch WE. Catabolism in uremia: the impact of metabolic acidosis. J Am Soc Nephrol 9:S78–S81, 1998.
25. Brater DC. Serum electrolyte abnormalities caused by drugs. Prog Drug Res 30:9–69, 1986.
26. Paltiel O, Salakhov E, Ronen I, et al. Management of severe hypokalemia in hospitalized patients. Arch Intern Med 161:1089–1095, 2001.
27. Clark BA, Brown BS. Potassium homeostasis and hyperkalemic syndromes. Endocrinol Metab Clin North Am 24:573–591, 1995.
28. Halperin ML, Kamel KS. Potassium. Lancet 352:135–140, 1998.
29. Perazella MA, Mahnansmith RL. Hyperkalemia in the elderly: drugs exacerbate impaired potassium homeostasis. J Gen Intern Med 12:646–656, 1997.
30. Gennari FJ. Hypokalemia. N Engl J Med 339:451–458, 1997.
31. Bushinsky DA, Monk RD. Calcium. Lancet 352:306–311, 1998.
32. Tohme JF, Bilezikian JP. Hypocalcemic emergencies. Endocrinol Metab Clin North Am 22:363–375, 1993.
33. Gucalp R, Ritch P, Wiernik PH, et al. Comparative study of pamidronate disodium and etidronate disodium in the treatment of cancer-related hypercalcemia. J Clin Oncol 10:134–142, 1992.
34. Boden SD, Kaplan FS. Calcium homeostasis. Orthop Clin North Am 21:31–42, 1990.
35. Wu-Wong JR, Tian J, Goltzman D. Vitamin D analogs as therapeutic agents: a clinical study update. Curr Opin Investig Drugs 5:320–326, 2004.
36. Kanis J. Vitamin D metabolism and its clinical application. J Bone Joint Surg 64B:542–557, 1982.
37. Siminoski K, Josse RG. Prevention and management of osteoporosis: consensus statements of the Scientific Advisory Board of the Osteoporosis Society of Canada. Calcitonin in the treatment of osteoporosis. CMAJ 155:962–965, 1996.
38. Pun KK, Chan LWL. Analgesic effect of intranasal salmon calcitonin in the treatment of osteoporotic vertebral fractures. Clin Ther 2:205–208, 1989.
39. Sekima M, Takami H. Combination of calcitonin and pamidronate for emergency treatment of malignant hypercalcemia. Oncol Rep 5:197–199, 1998.
40. Abbott LG, Rude RK. Clinical manifestations of magnesium deficiency. Miner Electrolyte Metab 19:314–322, 1993.
41. Rude RK. Magnesium metabolism and deficiency. Endocrinol Metab Clin North Am 22:377–395, 1993.
42. Whang R, Hampton EM, Whang DD. Magnesium homeostasis and clinical disorders of magnesium deficiency. Ann Pharmacother 28:220–225, 1994.
43. Weisinger JR, Bellorin-Font E. Magnesium and phosphorus. Lancet 352:391–396, 1998.
44. Malluche HH, Monier-Faugere MC. Hyperphosphatemia: pharmacologic intervention yesterday, today and tomorrow. Clin Nephrol 54:309–317, 2000.
45. Daily WH, Tonnesen AS, Allen SJ. Hypophosphatemia—incidence, etiology, and prevention in the trauma patient. Crit Care Med 18:1210–1214, 1990.
46. Clark CL, Sacks GS, Dickerson RN, et al. Treatment of hypophosphatemia in patients receiving specialized nutrition support using a graduated dosing scheme: results from a prospective clinical trial. Crit Care Med 23:1504–1511, 1995.

General Nutrition and Vitamins/Minerals

29

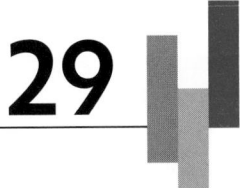

Diane Nykamp McCarter and Leisa L. Marshall

Researchers have discovered a relationship between the maintenance of an optimal state of health and good nutritional practices. Nutrition, including dietary intake and vitamin/mineral supplementation, is a topic of interest to the United States public. Obesity in American adults and children has increased over the last several decades with a disturbing increase in the incidence of diabetes. Nutrition is also critical to the prevention and management of other diseases such as heart disease and hypertension. Health care practitioners, in particular pharmacists, have an ideal opportunity to provide nutritional and health promotion advice to the public on a daily basis. This chapter begins with a discussion of general nutritional guidelines and population-specific nutrition considerations and concludes with a detailed discussion of vitamin and minerals. Nutrition and vitamin/mineral supplementation important in select patient populations is discussed, but the reader is referred to specific chapters pertaining to particular disease state for additional information.

TREATMENT GOALS: GENERAL NUTRITION AND VITAMINS AND MINERALS

- Understand the components of a healthful diet based on the food guide pyramid.
- Recognize the importance of regular exercise.
- Encourage patients to develop good nutritional practices that will promote wellness and prevent disease.
- Enhance the patient's ability to recognize and treat nutrient deficiencies or toxicity.
- Maintain an optimal state of health in patients with special needs caused by medical conditions or use of medications, which alter nutritional status.
- Foster awareness that optimal nutritional intake, not supplements, is the most appropriate and cost-effective way to obtain vitamins and minerals.

GENERAL NUTRITION GUIDELINES

The following section describes the current recommendations for healthful eating and general dietary guidelines. Appropriate use of vitamin and mineral supplements, including a description of the dietary reference intakes (DRIs), which vary with age, gender, and other factors, are discussed later in the vitamin and mineral section of the chapter.

Dietary guidelines and health policy recommendations are designed to educate consumers to promote the selection of foods to achieve a nutritionally adequate diet.[1] They include recommendations on daily food choices, portion size, and advice regarding sodium, saturated and unsaturated fat, and cholesterol intake. Advice on health promoting lifestyle modifications, including regular exercise, maintaining ideal body weight (IBW), limiting alcohol ingestion, and smoking cessation are often included.[1,2] The *Dietary Guidelines for Americans*, from the U.S. Departments of Agriculture (USDA) and Health and Human Services (USHHS), is a well-known general dietary guideline to promote health and prevent disease that is updated every 5 years. The current guidelines are the *Year 2000 Dietary Guidelines for Americans*. The complete guidelines, available at www.health/gov/dietaryguidelines, include the 13-page summary *Dietary Guidelines for Americans*, a brochure *Using the Dietary Guidelines for Americans*, a 1-page summary of the guidelines, and the complete *Report of the Dietary Guidelines Advisory Committee on the Dietary Guidelines for Americans, 2000*.[3] The 2000 guidelines were revised extensively from the 1995 version with increased emphasis on maintaining a healthy weight and the importance of physical activity. The 2000 guidelines include ten goals in an ABC format: Aim for fitness, Build a healthy base, and choose sensibly (Table 29.1).[3] The guidelines emphasize balance, moderation, and eating a variety of foods. They also recommend eating whole grains, fruits, and vegetables, and limiting sugar, salt, saturated and total fat, and cholesterol intake.

Section A of the Dietary Guidelines, ''Aim for Fitness,'' includes the goals of aiming for a healthy weight and being physically active each day.[3] Individuals should calculate their body mass index (BMI) to evaluate their weight. The BMI is the ratio of weight in kilograms to height in meters squared.[4] According to the Dietary Guidelines, a BMI of 18.5 to 25 is considered a healthy weight, 25 to 30 is considered overweight, and over 30 is considered obese.[3] Other references use the BMI to determine a person's heath risks. A person with a BMI of 25 to 29.9 is considered to have relatively low risk, BMI of 30 to 40 to have a moderate risk, and BMI over 40 to have high health risks.[4] A person with a BMI of over 40 is considered morbidly obese and is approximately 30% overweight.[5] People who are obese, especially those with central adiposity, are at high risk for the development of co-morbid conditions such as diabetes mellitus and cardiovascular disease. However, in some cases a

TABLE 29.1	Dietary Guidelines for Americans

Aim for Fitness

Aim for a healthy weight

Be physically active each day

Build a healthy base

Let the Pyramid guide your food choices

Choose a variety of grains daily, especially whole grains

Choose a variety of fruits and vegetables daily

Keep food safe to eat

Choose sensibly

Choose a diet that is low in saturated fat and cholesterol and moderate in total fat

Choose beverages and food to moderate your intake of sugars

Choose and prepare foods with less salt

If you drink alcoholic beverages, do so in moderation

(From U.S. Department of Agriculture and U.S. Department of Health and Human Services (2000) Year 2000 Dietary Guidelines for Americans. U.S. Government Printing Office, Washington, D.C., available at www.health.gov/dietaryguidelines. Accessed November 11, 2005.)

person's BMI may appear in the healthy range, despite their being overweight, if they have decreased muscle mass and increased fat. Males with a waist measurement greater than 40 inches and women with a waist measurement greater than 35 inches are at increased risk of health problems, even with an acceptable BMI.[3] Occasionally an athlete with increased muscle mass may not be overweight but may appear so based on the BMI.[3,4]

According to the Dietary Guidelines, most adults should exercise at a moderate level at least 30 minutes most days of the week to promote physical fitness and decrease health risks.[3] Regular physical activity decreases the risk of developing hypertension, cardiovascular disease, type 2 diabetes, and colon cancer.[3] However, to maintain weight loss most adults need to exercise 45 minutes or more per day. The Institute of Medicine guidelines recommend 60 minutes a day of moderate to vigorous physical activity to prevent weight gain, promote weight loss, and achieve the health benefits of physical activity.[6] Although 30 minutes of physical activity most days of the week results in health benefits, according to the Institute of Medicine report, most adults are not able to maintain weight in a BMI of 18.5 to 25 kg per m[2] with 30 minutes and should spend 60 minutes a day in moderate intensity physical activity, such as walking or jogging 4 to 5 miles per hour.[6] Even so, as little as 30 minutes a day of physical activity may be sufficient to prevent weight gain and promote weight loss in most overweight sedentary adults.[6-8]

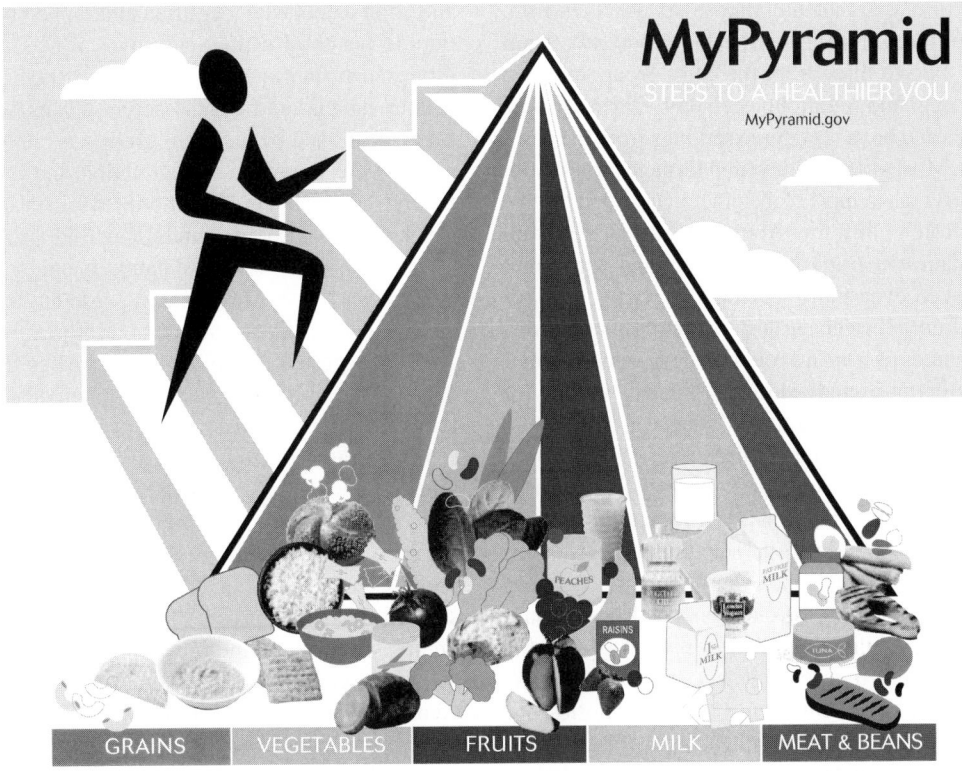

FIGURE 29.1 The USDA Food Guide Pyramid, My Pyramid, updated in April 2005. (available at www.mypyramid.gov)

The American public can use the current U.S. Department of Agriculture and Health and Human Services Food Guide Pyramid, My Pyramid, (Fig. 29.1 *see color insert*), helps in selecting food choices to achieve a healthy diet.[3,9,10] The food guide pyramid contains suggestions for daily servings in each of the major food groups. Grains, especially whole grains, vegetables, and fruits form the basis of a diet based on the food pyramid.[10] Choosing a variety of foods from the food groups of the pyramid should provide needed nutrients and appropriate carbohydrate, protein, and fat.[2,9,10] Each food group contains a range for the suggested number of servings, as this varies by age, gender, and activity level. Active men and women and older children and teenagers will need to choose more servings in each food group (with the exception of dairy) than children 2 to 8 years old, nonactive women, and some older adults.[3,9] Most adults should choose a diet low in cholesterol and saturated fat and moderate in total fat.[3] Normal healthy adults require between 25 to 30 kcal/kg/day, with a maximum of 30% of these calories from fat.[9] Intake of saturated and polyunsaturated fat should not exceed 10% of kilocalories.[11] Daily cholesterol intake should not exceed 300 mg per day, and protein intake should be approximately 0.8 g per kg body weight.[3,9,11] Ingestion of food or beverages high in added sugars should be limited to avoid weight gain.[3] Individuals who are gaining weight despite using the food pyramid to guide food choices may need to increase their physical activity and decrease the number of servings or size of servings to achieve a modest reduction in caloric intake.[8,9,12]

Besides these general nutrition recommendations, several patient populations have more specific concerns and recommendations. A discussion of nutritional considerations for children and adolescents, pregnant patients, obese patients, patients with diabetes or hypertension, and geriatric patients follows.

POPULATION-SPECIFIC NUTRITIONAL CONSIDERATIONS

CHILDHOOD AND ADOLESCENCE

Appropriate nutrition and physical activity during childhood and adolescence is imperative to maintain healthy growth. The Dietary Guidelines suggest a minimum of 60 minutes of physical activity each day for children and adolescents to promote health and maintain appropriate weight.[3] Several reports indicate that children and adolescents in the United States are spending less time in physical activity at school and outside of school, and more time involved in sedentary activities such as using computers.[8,13,14]

Along with encouraging an appropriate amount of physical activity each day, parents of children and adolescents are encouraged to use the food guide pyramid to select food choices to achieve adequate nutrition.[3,9,10] In general, children age 2 to 6 years should choose six servings from the grain group, three from the vegetable group, two from the fruit group, two to three from the dairy group, and two from the meat, egg, and nut group each day. Older children and teenage girls and boys need three servings from the dairy group each day. Most older children and teenage girls should increase their servings in most of the other major food groups as well to nine from grains, four from vegetables, three from fruit, and maintain two from the meat, egg, and nut group. Teenage boys need even more servings.[3]

Young children and teenage girls should choose foods that are good sources of iron to avoid iron deficiency anemia. Good sources of iron include enriched breads, cereal with added iron, cooked dry beans and peas, shellfish, lean meats, and spinach.[3] Adolescents and children over age 2 should also adhere to the Dietary Guidelines suggestions for limiting saturated fat and cholesterol as described in the general nutrition section above.[3] The American Heart Association (AHA) also now recommends their Step I diet as a safe and healthy diet for the majority of children.[15] For some time the AHA has advocated the adoption of the Step I diet for most adults to prevent the development of cardiovascular disease. The Step I diet recommends that fat calories not exceed 30% of total calories, saturated fat not exceed 8% to 10% of total calories, and total cholesterol intake be below 300 mg per day. These are the same percentages as recommended by the general dietary guidelines. In 1997 an AHA nutrition committee concluded that this diet could be safely recommended for most children over the age of 2, as long as dietary fat intake remained above 20%.[15] Adopting a heart healthy diet in youth reduces the incidence of obesity, hypertension, and elevated cholesterol common in adults and does not impair normal growth and development.[15]

Despite widespread knowledge of appropriate diet and the need for physical activity in childhood and adolescence, the prevalence of childhood and adolescent obesity has increased significantly since the 1960s. The increasing incidence of childhood and adolescent obesity in the United States has alarmed health care professionals concerned about the long-term health risks associated with obesity early in life.[8,16,17] Because it is difficult for overweight children and adolescents to lose weight and maintain that weight loss, greater attention needs to be focused on prevention.[17,18] Being overweight or obese as a child or adolescent increases health risks later throughout life, including increased incidence of cardiovascular disease and insulin resistance.[19,20] Increasingly, children who are obese are developing type 2 diabetes and hypertension as children, chronic medical conditions that were once rare in childhood.[17] Children who are obese are also developing myocardial changes and coronary and carotid artery pathology.[17] Behavioral therapy to alter dietary intake and increase physical activity is modestly successful.

More information is needed on motivation and barriers to good diet and exercise in children and adolescents. One recently published study involved focus groups of children and adolescents who identified and ranked benefits and barriers to healthful eating and physical activity.[21] The focus groups also suggested strategies for overcoming barriers to healthy eating and physical activity. The five themes most often mentioned by the focus groups as benefits of healthful eating were improved concentration and mental alertness, feeling good physically, improved physical performance, psychological benefits, and increased production of energy.[21] Barriers to healthful eating included convenience of alternatives that are less healthy, taste and cravings for less healthful alternatives, and social reinforcement.[21] The focus groups suggested the following strategies to overcome the barriers to healthful eating habits: parental support, planning ahead, reducing the availability of junk food at home and at school, using self-motivation, and increased education. The three most common perceived benefits of physical activity were social benefits, psychological enhancement, and feeling good physically. Major barriers to physical activity were preference for indoor activities, low energy level, time constraints, social factors, and lack of motivation.[21] The focus groups suggested numerous strategies to increase physical activity, including planning and organization, such as becoming involved in a team, increasing the variety of sports available at school, increased parental involvement and support, and time management.[21] Children and adolescents expect and need parents and schoolteachers to encourage healthful eating and increased physical activity.[21] Obesity in children should be seen as a chronic medical condition that needs to be prevented and treated if it occurs.

PREGNANT WOMEN

Proper nutrition during pregnancy is vital because the mother needs nourishment for herself and the unborn child. Pregnant women need to increase servings per day in all of the major food groups, with the exception of fats, oils, and sweets, to provide the appropriate amount of calories, nutrients, and vitamins.[22] All pregnant women should take a prenatal vitamin as several minerals and vitamins should be supplemented during pregnancy. A discussion of all the mineral and vitamin supplements recommended in pregnancy is beyond the scope of this chapter, but a mention of folic acid supplementation is in order. Folic acid deficiency can cause neural tube defects, preterm labor, and low birth weight infants.[22] When used for prevention of neural tube defects, folate levels must be adequate in the first 4 weeks after conception, before neural tube closure.[23] Because many women do not realize they are pregnant until after this time, difficulties arise in establishing the most appropriate method of supplementation. Therefore, women of childbearing age are encouraged to have a daily folic acid intake of at least 400 μg as pregnant women need 600 μg per day.[24]

OBESE ADULTS

The prevalence of overweight and obese adults in the United States has increased over the last three decades. Disturbingly, the percentage of obese adults, those with a BMI more than or equal to 30, has increased greatly. According to the National Health and Nutrition Examination Survey (NHANES) of 1999 to 2000 and the 2001 Behavioral Risk Factor Surveillance System (BRFSS), the percentage of U.S. adults classified as obese is estimated to be approximately 30%.[25,26] Health problems associated with being overweight and obese include insulin resistance, dyslipidemia, glucose intolerance, elevated blood pressure, diabetes, and pain in weight-bearing joints. Complications that develop include diabetes, hypertension, cardiovascular disease, and osteoarthritis.[7,8,25] The term *metabolic syndrome* is used to describe individuals who have three or more conditions that greatly increase their risk of hypertension and cardiovascular disease, one of which is normally obesity. The specific conditions are abdominal obesity, glucose intolerance, elevated triglycerides, or low high-density lipoprotein.[27–29] These individuals are at increased risk for complications associated with hypertension and cardiovascular disease, and should begin lifestyle modification, including appropriate diet and exercise, as well as being treated with appropriate drug therapy.[27,29]

For the majority of overweight and obese adults, an appropriate diet with calorie reduction and increased physical activity are the mainstay of any weight loss program.[8] Goals are to prevent further weight gain, reduce body weight, and maintain a lower body weight over time. Reducing calorie intake by 500 to 1,000 kcal per day with a moderate increase in physical activity should result in a weight loss of 1 or 2 pounds per week.[12] A reasonable goal for overweight and obese adults is a 10% weight loss over 6 months.[12] Total fat intake should be 30% or less of the daily energy intake.

As well as reducing calorie intake, overweight and obese adults should be encouraged to increase physical activity after consulting with their physician. Patients with chronic medical conditions will need to increase exercise time and intensity gradually. Mild to moderate activities, such as walking or swimming at a slow pace, are good starting points for most adults. A reasonable goal would be to increase exercise time and intensity to a level of moderate intensity for at least 45 minutes per day most days of the week. However, mild to moderate exercise is still beneficial. For example, in the Studies of Targeted Risk Reduction Interventions Through Defined Exercise (STRRIDE) trial, sedentary, middle-aged, overweight adults were randomized into four groups: no exercise, low-dose moderate intensity exercise (e.g., walking 12 miles per week), low-dose vigorous intensity exercise (e.g., jogging 12 miles per week), or higher dose vigorous intensity exercise (e.g., jogging 20 miles per week).[7] Participants were to maintain their usual diet during the 8-month study. The majority of the participants in the three exercise groups lost weight, while most (73%) of the control group gained weight. Not surprisingly, the higher dose vigorous intensity exercise group experienced greater benefits than the other two exercise groups in weight loss, body fat mass decrease, and lean body mass increase. Even

so, 75% of the participants of the low-dose moderate intensity group lost weight.[7]

Eating disorders as a psychiatric disorder are discussed in Chapter 57.

ADULTS WITH DIABETES MELLITUS

The current American Diabetes Association (ADA) nutrition principles and recommendations for diabetic patients are similar to health promotion recommendations for the general population.[30,31] ADA nutrition goals are to maintain appropriate metabolic outcomes, prevent and treat diabetes complications, improve health, and address individual considerations in designing an appropriate diet.[31] Individuals at risk of developing type 2 diabetes are encouraged to avoid weight gain and hopefully lose a moderate amount of weight. Patients treated with insulin should try to avoid weight gain that often accompanies increased glycemic control if at all possible.[31]

For most individuals with diabetes, carbohydrates and monounsaturated fat should provide 60% to 70% of energy intake.[30,31] Intake of carbohydrates, with an appropriate amount of fiber, from whole grains, fruits, vegetables, and low-fat milk are encouraged. Sucrose and sucrose-containing foods do not have to be avoided altogether, but should be incorporated into the meal plan. Diabetics should limit saturated fat to less than 10% of energy intake and those with elevated LDL levels are advised to further limit intake to less than 7%. Limiting saturated fat should promote weight maintenance and weight loss.[30,31] For diabetics where weight loss is not needed, monosaturated fat or carbohydrate should replace saturated fat. In general, diabetics should consume no more than 300 mg of dietary cholesterol each day, and those with elevated low density lipoprotein (LDL) levels should limit dietary cholesterol intake to less than 200 mg each day. Protein intake should be between 15% to 20% of energy intake each day, but may need to be lowered with reduced renal function. Although protein does not increase glucose concentrations and high-protein low-carbohydrate diets may promote weight loss and improved glucose control, the long-term effects of these diets on diabetes and plasma cholesterol levels are not conclusive at this time.[30,31]

Adults with type 2 diabetes are often overweight, and many have hypertension and dyslipidemia. For these individuals the nutrition guidelines described previously in this chapter are especially important. Advice on appropriate nutrition and lifestyle modifications should focus on a realistic plan to increase physical activity and modify dietary intake to decrease intake of saturated fat, cholesterol, and sodium. Even modest weight loss in overweight type 2 diabetics leads to increased glycemic control and decreased insulin resistance, a more favorable lipid profile, and a reduction in blood pressure.[30,31]

Strict dietary restrictions in geriatric diabetics is not appropriate in most cases, especially for geriatric diabetics who live in assisted living or nursing facilities.[30,31] Underweight older diabetics are at increased risk of morbidity and mortality, as are all underweight geriatric patients. Adjusting the diabetic medication regimen, rather than adopting strict dietary restrictions, is normally recommended.[30,31]

ADULTS WITH HIGH BLOOD PRESSURE

Adults with high blood pressure are at risk of numerous cardiovascular, renal, and neurologic complications that increase their morbidity and mortality. A healthy lifestyle, including appropriate diet and exercise, helps prevent hypertension and is an essential component of managing existing hypertension.[27] The Joint National Committee made several recommendations regarding lifestyle changes and dietary modification in the Seventh Report on the Prevention, Detection, Evaluation and Treatment of High Blood Pressure (JNC7).[27] JNC 7 recommendations are consistent with advice for a general healthful diet and lifestyle in normal healthy people. They include maintaining a normal weight, adopting the DASH eating plan, restricting sodium intake, engaging in regular physical activity, and limiting alcohol intake to no more than two drinks per day in males and one per day in women.[27] The DASH diet is the Dietary Approaches to Stop Hypertension eating plan. The DASH diet contains similar recommendations as the *Dietary Guidelines for Americans*, and recommends consuming a diet with a decreased intake of saturated and total fat, and increased consumption of fruits, vegetables, and dairy products, which are rich in calcium and potassium.[32] Sodium from the diet should be 2.4 g per day at the most. JNC 7 also recommends routine aerobic physical activity for at least 30 minutes almost every day.[27] Adults with elevated blood pressure can reduce their blood pressure and increase the effectiveness of their medication by adopting the recommended lifestyle modifications.[27]

GERIATRIC POPULATION

The geriatric population of the United States continues to increase. By 2050 approximately one in five Americans will be older than 65 years of age.[33] Recommended intake of protein, carbohydrate, and fat for older individuals follows the recommendations for U.S. adults.[33] Suggested daily vitamin intake for older individuals is discussed later in the chapter. Protein intake may need to be increased when an older adult is injured or the body is under stress, for example with acute or chronic infection.[33] Obese older individuals may need to modify intake, as described previously in the section on obesity. Older individuals should be encouraged to drink plenty of fluid as dehydration is more common than in younger adults. Risk factors for dehydration in geriatric individuals include a decreased thirst response, use of diuretics or laxatives, cognitive or physical impairment, and acute infection or fever.[33]

Although the incidence of obesity in geriatric individuals is rising, unplanned or involuntary weight loss leading to malnutrition remains a common problem, especially among the frail elderly living in the community or nursing facilities.[34–36] Malnutrition in older adults is associated with increased morbidity and mortality.[34,35,37] Specific complications include muscle weakness and wasting, anemia, decubitus ulcers, increased infections, loss of independence and failure to thrive.[34,36] Unplanned weight loss and malnutrition in this population is often the result of multiple causes. Common causes are listed in Table 29.2.[38–42] Acute and chronic illness, cognitive decline, depression, physiologic changes with aging, and psychosocial and environmental factors increase the risk of malnutrition in the geriatric patient.[41] An example of a nutritional assessment instrument recommended for use in assessing nutritional status of geriatric patients is the Mini-Nutritional Assessment.[42] Another assessment instrument was recently developed by the Coun-

TABLE 29.2	Possible Causes of Malnutrition in Older Adults

Changes in taste and smell
Swallowing disorders
Poor dentition
Lack of mobility
Living alone
Poverty
Acute or chronic infection
Depression or other emotional problems
Dementia
Numerous chronic medical conditions:
    Cancer
    Diabetes
    Hyperthyroidism
    Arthritis
    Congestive heart failure
    Chronic obstructive lung disease
    Parkinson's disease
Decreased absorption from:
    Bowel surgery
    Malabsorption syndromes
Catabolic illness:
    Infection
    Inflammation
    Trauma
Adverse effects from medications:
    Drug–nutrient interactions
    Gastrointestinal side effects
    Altered taste
    Dry mouth
    Sedation or confusion

cil for Nutritional Strategies in Long-term Care. Their ''Clinical guide to prevent and manage malnutrition in long-term care for physicians, pharmacists, and dieticians,'' is available at www.LTCnutrition.org.[40] Due to the multi-faceted nature of weight loss and malnutrition in the frail elderly, a multidisciplinary team is often needed to determine the causes of weight loss and design a plan to address the problem.

VITAMINS

Vitamins are non–energy-producing organic substances that are essential in small amounts for the maintenance of normal metabolic functions. They are categorized into two groups: the fat-soluble vitamins (A, D, E, and K) and the water-soluble vitamins (B complex and C). All vitamins, with the exception of D, K, and biotin, must be supplied completely from dietary sources.[43,44] The majority of vitamins are obtained from plant and animal sources, with the exceptions of vitamin K and biotin, which are produced by microorganisms in the intestinal tract, and vitamin D, which is synthesized from cholesterol in the skin. The amount of vitamin K synthesized is sufficient to meet the body's needs, but some dietary supplementation of biotin usually is required. The amount of vitamin D produced in the skin may or may not be sufficient to meet the body's needs because its synthesis depends on exposure to ultraviolet light.

VITAMIN REQUIREMENTS—DIETARY REFERENCE INTAKES

Reference values for nutrient requirements for the American population have changed. The Recommended Dietary Allowances (RDAs) of 1989 have been replaced with the Dietary Reference Intakes (DRIs). The RDAs were developed for groups of the population rather than for individuals. The Food and Nutrition Board of the Institute of Medicine has redefined the recommendations for individuals as well as groups. The RDAs were associated with nutrient values designed to prevent deficiencies such as scurvy or beriberi. The DRIs are an estimate of nutrient intakes designed to assist healthy individuals meet dietary intake requirements to prevent chronic diseases such as diabetes, heart disease, hypertension, and osteoporosis. The DRIs also provide tolerable upper values. DRIs are an umbrella term and are based on four categories:

■ Estimated Average Requirement (EAR): The intake value estimated to meet the requirement defined by a specified indicator of adequacy in 50% of an age- and gender-specific group. The EAR for a nutrient is used primarily as a basis for establishing a RDA and for evaluating the diet of a population.
■ Recommended Dietary Allowance (RDA): The average dietary intake level of a nutrient that prevents a deficiency in 98% of the population.
■ Adequate Intake (AI): Values used when sufficient evidence is not available to estimate an average intake re-

quirement or RDA. AIs indicate an average intake that appears to sustain a desired indicator of health, such as calcium in bone.
■ Tolerable Upper Intake Level (UL): The highest level of a nutrient that is likely to pose no risk of adverse health effects to 98% of the population. As the intake increases above the UL, the potential for adverse reactions increases. Table 29.3 lists the published 2003 DRIs for vitamins. Table 29.4 lists the upper limits for vitamins.[45–49]

VITAMIN STABILITY

In general, fat-soluble vitamins are not destroyed during cooking. However, water-soluble vitamins are easily dissolved in cooking water and may be destroyed through heating. Ascorbic acid (vitamin C) suffers the greatest loss in nutritive value through cooking. Riboflavin is only sparingly water-soluble and is not removed as quickly (when cooked in water) as the other water-soluble vitamins. When meats are broiled or roasted, thiamine losses are 25% or less. Constant low-temperature cooking improves palatability of meat but decreases the nutritive value. Wilting of vegetables or dehydration of most foods results in considerable nutrient loss. Improper storage or dicing and cutting of fruits and vegetables before cooking in water can also result in vitamin loss. Fruits and vegetables should be consumed raw or cooked in a minimum amount of liquid to help retain their maximum vitamin content. Other vitamin-conserving cooking methods include steaming, microwaving, and stir frying.[50] Steaming or microwaving is especially beneficial for vegetables containing thiamine, riboflavin, pyridoxine, folic acid, and ascorbic acid. Microwave cooking requires a shorter cooking time and less water and generally results in greater retention of heat-labile nutrients.[51]

FAT-SOLUBLE VITAMINS

Vitamins A, D, E, and K are classified as fat-soluble vitamins. Their absorption is facilitated by bile salts or dietary fat, and they are stored in moderate amounts in the body. Vitamins A and D function like hormones, interacting with specific intracellular receptors in their target tissues. Toxicity associated with the fat-soluble vitamins can occur

(text continues on page 10)

TABLE 29.3 | Dietary Reference Intakes (DRIs): Recommended Intakes for Individuals, Vitamins Food and Nutrition Board, Institute of Medicine, The National Academies

Life Stage Group	Vitamin A (μg/d)[a]	Vitamin C (mg/d)	Vitamin D (μg/d)[b,c]	Vitamin E (mg/d)[d]	Vitamin K (μg/d)	Thiamin (mg/d)	Riboflavin (mg/d)	Niacin (mg/d)[e]	Vitamin B6 (mg/d)[e]	Folate (μg/d)[f]	Vitamin B12 (μg/d)	Pantothenic Acid (mg/d)	Biotin (μg/d)	Choline (mg/d)[g]
Infants														
0–6 mo	400*	40*	5*	4*	2.0*	0.2*	0.3*	2*	0.1*	65*	0.4*	1.7*	5*	125*
7–12 mo	500*	50*	5*	5*	2.5*	0.3*	0.4*	4*	0.3*	80*	0.5*	1.8*	6*	150*
Children														
1–3 y	300	15	5*	6	30*	0.5	0.5	6	0.5	150	0.9	2*	8*	200*
4–8 y	400	25	5*	7	55*	0.6	0.6	8	0.6	200	1.2	3*	12*	250*
Males														
9–13 y	600	45	5*	11	60*	0.9	0.9	12	1.0	300	1.8	4*	20*	375*
14–18 y	900	75	5*	15	75*	1.2	1.3	16	1.3	400	2.4	5*	25*	550*
19–30 y	900	90	5*	15	120*	1.2	1.3	16	1.3	400	2.4	5*	30*	550*
31–50 y	900	90	5*	15	120*	1.2	1.3	16	1.3	400	2.4	5*	30*	550*
51–70 y	900	90	10*	15	120*	1.2	1.3	16	1.7	400	2.4[h]	5*	30*	550*
>70 y	900	90	15*	15	120*	1.2	1.3	16	1.7	400	2.4[h]	5*	30*	550*
Females														
9–13 y	600	45	5*	11	60*	0.9	0.9	12	1.0	300	1.8	4*	20*	375*
14–18 y	700	65	5*	15	75*	1.0	1.0	14	1.2	400[i]	2.4	5*	25*	400*
19–30 y	700	75	5*	15	90*	1.1	1.1	14	1.3	400[i]	2.4	5*	30*	425*
31–50 y	700	75	5*	15	90*	1.1	1.1	14	1.3	400[i]	2.4	5*	30*	425*
51–70 y	700	75	10*	15	90*	1.1	1.1	14	1.5	400	2.4[h]	5*	30*	425*
>70 y	700	75	15*	15	90*	1.1	1.1	14	1.5	400	2.4[h]	5*	30*	425*
Pregnancy														
≤18 y	750	80	5*	15	75*	1.4	1.4	18	1.9	600[j]	2.6	6*	30*	450*
19–30 y	770	85	5*	15	90*	1.4	1.4	18	1.9	600[j]	2.6	6*	30*	450*
31–50 y	776	85	5*	15	90*	1.4	1.4	18	1.9	600[j]	2.6	6*	30*	450*
Lactation														
≤18 y	1,200	115	5*	19	75*	1.4	1.6	17	2.0	500	2.8	7*	35*	550*
19–30 y	1,300	120	5*	19	90*	1.4	1.6	17	2.0	500	2.8	7*	35*	550*
31–50 y	1,300	120	5*	19	90*	1.4	1.6	17	2.0	500	2.8	7*	35*	550*

NOTE: This table (taken from the DRI reports, see www.nap.edu) presents Recommended Dietary Allowances (RDAs) in **bold type** and Adequate Intakes (AIs) in ordinary type followed by an asterisk (*). RDAs and AIs may both be used as goals for individual intake. RDAs are set to meet the needs of almost all (97% to 98%) individuals in a group. For healthy breastfed infants, the AI is the mean intake. The AI for other life stage and gender groups is believed to cover needs of all individuals in the group, but lack of data or uncertainty in the data prevent being able to specify with confidence the percentage of individuals covered by this intake.

[a] As retinol activity equivalents (RAEs). 1 RAE = 1 μg retinol, 12 μg β-carotene, 24 μg α-carotene, or 24 μg β-cryptoxanthin. To calculate RAEs from REs of provitamin A carotenoids in foods, divide the REs by 2. For preformed vitamin A in foods or supplements and for provitamin A carotenoids in supplements, 1 RE = 1 RAE.

[b] cholecalciferol. 1 μg cholecalciferol = 40 IU vitamin D.

[c] In the absence of adequate exposure to sunlight.

[d] As α-Tocopherol. α-Tocopherol includes RRR-α-tocopherol, the only form of α-tocopherol that occurs naturally in foods, and the 2R-stereoisomeric forms of α-tocopherol (RRR-, RSR-, RRS-, and RSS-α-tocopherol) that occur in fortified foods and supplements. It does not include the 2S-stereoisomeric forms of α-tocopherol (SRR-,SSR-, SRS-, and SSS-α-tocopherol), also found in fortified foods and supplements.

[e] As niacin equivalents (NE). 1 mg of niacin = 60 mg of tryptophan; 0–6 months = preformed niacin (not NE).

[f] As dietary folate equivalents (DFE). 1 DFE = 1 μg food folate = 0.6 μg of folic acid from fortified food or as a supplement consumed with food = 0.5 μg of a supplement taken on an empty stomach.

[g] Although AIs have been set for choline, there are few data to assess whether a dietary supply of choline is needed at all stages of the life cycle, and it may be that the choline requirement can be met by endogenous synthesis at some of these stages.

[h] Because 10% to 30% of older people may malabsorb food-bound B12, it is advisable for those older than 50 years to meet their RDA mainly by consuming foods fortified with B12 or a supplement containing B12.

[i] In view of evidence linking folate intake with neural tube defects in the fetus, it is recommended that all women capable of becoming pregnant consume 400 μg from supplements or fortified foods in addition to intake of food folate from a varied diet.

[j] It is assumed that women will continue consuming 400 μg from supplements or fortified food until their pregnancy is confirmed and they enter prenatal care, which ordinarily occurs after the end of the periconceptional period—the critical time for formation of the neural tube.

TABLE 29.4 | Dietary Reference Intakes (DRIs): Tolerable Upper Intake Levels (UL^a), Vitamins Food and Nutrition Board, Institute of Medicine, National Academies

Life Stage Group	Vitamin A (μg/d)^b	Vitamin C (mg/d)	Vitamin D (μg/d)	Vitamin E (mg/d)^{c,d}	Vitamin K	Thiamin	Riboflavin	Niacin (mg/d)^d	Vitamin B$_6$ (mg/d)	Folate (μg/d)^d	Vitamin B$_{12}$	Pantothenic Acid	Biotin	Choline (g/d)	Carotenoids^e
Infants															
0–6 mo	600	ND^f	25	ND	ND	ND	ND	ND	ND	ND	ND	ND	ND	ND	ND
7–12 mo	600	ND	25	ND	ND	ND	ND	ND	ND	ND	ND	ND	ND	ND	ND
Children															
1–3 y	600	400	50	200	ND	ND	ND	10	30	300	ND	ND	ND	1.0	ND
4–8 y	900	650	50	300	ND	ND	ND	15	40	400	ND	ND	ND	1.0	ND
Males, Females															
9–13 y	1,700	1,200	50	600	ND	ND	ND	20	60	600	ND	ND	ND	2.0	ND
14–18 y	2,800	1,800	50	800	ND	ND	ND	30	80	800	ND	ND	ND	3.0	ND
19–70 y	3,000	2,000	50	1,000	ND	ND	ND	35	100	1,000	ND	ND	ND	3.5	ND
> 70 y	3,000	2,000	50	1,000	ND	ND	ND	35	100	1,000	ND	ND	ND	3.5	ND
Pregnancy															
≤ 18 y	2,800	1,800	50	800	ND	ND	ND	30	80	800	ND	ND	ND	3.0	ND
19–50 y	3,000	2,000	50	1,000	ND	ND	ND	35	100	1,000	ND	ND	ND	3.5	ND
Lactation															
≤ 18 y	2,800	1,800	50	800	ND	ND	ND	30	80	800	ND	ND	ND	3.0	ND
19–50 y	3,000	2,000	50	1,000	ND	ND	ND	35	100	1,000	ND	ND	ND	3.5	ND

^{a} UL = The maximum level of daily nutrient intake that is likely to pose no risk of adverse effects. Unless otherwise specified, the UL represents total intake from food, water, and supplements. Due to lack of suitable data, ULs could not be established for vitamin K, thiamin, riboflavin, vitamin B$_{12}$, pantothenic acid, biotin, or carotenoids. In the absence of ULs, extra caution may be warranted in consuming levels above recommended intakes.

^{b} As preformed vitamin A only.

^{c} As α-tocopherol; applies to any form of supplemental α-tocopherol.

^{d} The ULs for vitamin E, niacin, and folate apply to synthetic forms obtained from supplements, fortified foods, or a combination of the two.

^{e} β-Carotene supplements are advised only to serve as a provitamin. A source for individuals at risk of vitamin A deficiency.

^{f} ND = Not determinable due to lack of data of adverse effects in this age group and concern with regard to lack of ability to handle excess amounts. Source of intake should be from food only to prevent high levels of intake.

Reprinted with permission from (**Dietary Reference Intakes: Guiding Principles for Nutrition Labeling and Fortification**) © (**2003**) by the National Academy of Sciences, courtesy of the National Academies Press, Washington, D.C.)

because fat-soluble vitamins can be stored with other lipids in fatty tissues and can accumulate. The characteristics of fat-soluble vitamins are listed in Table 29.5.

VITAMIN A

Functions of Vitamin A. Vitamin A is essential for vision, dental development, growth, and reproduction. Vitamin A is also necessary for the synthesis of hydrocortisone and the regulation and differentiation of epithelial tissue. The integrity of the mucous membranes of the eyes, skin, mouth, gastrointestinal tract, and genitourinary tract is maintained by this vitamin, which is required for the production of mucus.[52]

Properties of Vitamin A. Vitamin A includes three natural compounds found in animal sources (retinol, retinal, and retinoic acid) and three provitamins found in plants (α-, β-, and γ-carotene). Retinol apparently is responsible for the actions of the vitamin in the reproductive process and retinal is the functional compound of the visual cycle. Retinoic acid, the active form of vitamin A, is associated with growth and cell differentiation. Retinoic acid cannot replace retinal in the visual cycle and is not able to support reproduction.[53] β-carotene, the most abundant plant source, does not possess inherent vitamin A activity but yields retinol after absorption and metabolism. One international unit (IU) of vitamin A is equal to 0.3 Φg retinol or 0.6 Φg β-carotene. Large amounts of β-carotene can be ingested over a long period of time without development of toxic effects (other than skin pigmentation) because only 20% to 30% of a dose is absorbed from the gastrointestinal tract, and it is metabolized at a rate of approximately 50% to 60% of normal dietary intake.[54] When the dietary intake of retinol is in the range of the recommended dietary allowance, the majority is absorbed but excess amounts ingested in the diet are excreted. The recommended daily intake of vitamins is 3,000 IU (900 μg).

Vitamin A Deficiency. There is now evidence that β-carotene has important functions other than being the precursor of vitamin A and therefore should be ingested in amounts greater than needed to meet the vitamin A requirements. Vitamin A deficiency usually is caused by fat malabsorption syndromes or malnutrition. Deficiency produces a variety of symptoms that include nyctalopia (night blindness), diminished production of corticosteroids, xerophthalmia (drying of the cornea), keratinization of the skin, growth failure, and fetal malformations. Vitamin A deficiency can impair resistance to infections by breaking down mucous membranes.[55]

Vitamin A Toxicity. Acute and chronic vitamin A toxicity are well-recognized conditions in adults. Acute poisoning may occur after a single dose greater than 1,000,000 IU. Chronic toxicity is determined mainly by the dosage and duration of therapy. Usually a dosage of more than 10,000 IU (3,000 μg) daily for several months causes hypervitaminosis

A.[56] Prolonged daily use of vitamin A in dosages of 25,000 IU or more may result in hypervitaminosis resembling a cirrhosis-like liver syndrome. Symptoms of chronic use of vitamin A include fatigue, vomiting, cheilosis, dizziness, nausea, and irritability, followed by generalized skin desquamation. Pruritus, dry, scaly skin, bone pain, changes in hair and nail texture, increased cerebrospinal fluid pressure, and hypercalcemia may also occur. Concern about an excess intake of vitamin A during pregnancy has increased in recent years because of its structural and metabolic relationship to other vitamin A analogs (retinoids), especially 13-cis-retinoic acid (isotretinoin), which is teratogenic. A daily dosage lower than 10,000 IU is not thought to be teratogenic.[57]

Therapeutic Uses of Vitamin A. Vitamin A analogs (retinoids) have been developed to improve the therapeutic index of vitamin A. Isotretinoin, etretinate, and acitretin were developed as less toxic and more effective agents. However, they have caused embryopathy.[57] Retinoids have had a major impact on the practice of dermatology[58] and are under investigation for the possible effect of decreasing the risk of cancer[59–61] and reducing the rate of infections.[62] There remains controversy about the relationship between an above-average β-carotene intake and a lowered incidence of cancer and cardiovascular disease, especially when β-carotene is used in combination with vitamins E and C.[63–65]

Until further research is conducted, advice to vitamin A users is understandably conservative. Dosages higher than 10,000 IU should not be recommended and consumers should rely on dietary intake of foods containing β-carotene.[66,67] Excess use of retinol supplements may cause serious adverse reactions however, increasing the dietary intake of retinol by eating more green and yellow vegetables may be beneficial and avoid toxicity. No definitive statement can be made at this time about the use of vitamin A in wound healing, although recent studies have reported that vitamin A promotes wound healing.

VITAMIN D

Functions of Vitamin D. Vitamin D is considered a hormone rather than a vitamin, although it is not a natural hormone. Vitamin D, in conjunction with parathyroid hormone (PTH) and calcitonin, is needed for calcium and phosphate metabolism. This in turn supports normal mineralization of bone and neuromuscular activity.

Properties of Vitamin D. Vitamin D refers to D_2 (calciferol, ergocalciferol) and D_3 (cholecalciferol). D_2 and D_3 occur naturally and are equipotent. Either may supply the body's daily requirements. These forms have an onset of action time of 10 to 24 hours and may be stored in the body for prolonged periods.

Ninety percent of dietary vitamin D is absorbed from the small intestine. Vitamin D_3 may be absorbed more rapidly and completely than vitamin D_2.

The supply of vitamin D depends on ultraviolet light radiation for conversion of plant ergosterol to vitamin D_2 or

TABLE 29.5 | Summary of Fat-Soluble Vitamins

Vitamin	Function	Deficiency	Large Dosages	Therapeutic Uses	Sources
Vitamin A Retinol Retinal Retinoic acid β-carotene	Growth Vision Dental development Reproduction Hydrocortisone synthesis Epithelial tissue differentiation Mucous membrane maintenance	Nyctalopia Xerophthalmia Faulty bone and tooth development Keratinization Fetal malformation Decreased production of cortical steroids Impaired resistance to infection	Acute Fatigue Cheilitis Dizziness Nausea and vomiting Irritability Desquamation Chronic Hypercalcemia Dry, scaly skin Bone pain Changes in hair and nail texture Increased cerebrospinal pressure Pruritus	Dermatology Oncology	Liver Milk Butter and margarine Dark-green, leafy vegetables Carrots Sweet potatoes
Vitamin D Ergocalciferol (D₂) Cholecalciferol (D₃)	Bone mineralization Maintenance of normal neuromuscular activity Maintenance of serum calcium and phosphorus levels	Associated with inadequate calcium and phosphorus Rickets (children) Osteomalacia (adults) Secondary hyperparathyroidism	Hypercalcemia (weakness anorexia, vomiting, diarrhea, polydipsia, polyuria, and mental changes) Constipation Proteinuria Vague aches Metallic or bad taste Renal failure Hypertension	Renal osteodystrophy Hypoparathyroidism	Sunlight Butter Egg yolk Fatty fish Liver Fortified milk and bread
Vitamin E dl-α-tocopherol (1 mg = (1.49 IU)	Antioxidant: maintains integrity of cell membrane Enhances vitamin A uptake Inhibition of prostaglandin production Cofactor in steroid metabolism Related to action of selenium	Neurologic syndrome (ataxia, muscle weakness, nystagmus, loss of touch or pain) Anemia in premature infants Hemolysis of red blood	Increase the effects of oral anticoagulants	Intermittent claudication Retrolental fibroplasia	Wheat germ oil Nuts Green, leafy vegetables
Vitamin K Phylloquinone (K₁) Menaquinone (K₂) Analog: Menadione (K₃)	Coagulation Formulation of prothrombin and other clotting proteins	Prolonged clotting time Deficiency symptoms can be produced by coumarin anticoagulants and antibiotic therapy	Vomiting Toxicity can be induced by water-soluble analog Neonatal jaundice Dietary supplements can block effect of oral anticoagulant	Coagulation disorders Anticoagulant-induced prothrombin deficiency	Green leaves (spinach, cabbage) Liver Synthesis in intestine by bacteria Cheese, egg yolk

(From Williams SR, ed. Nutrition and diet therapy. St. Louis: Mosby, 1997; Sizer FS, Whitney EN, eds. Hamilton & Whitney's nutrition: concepts and controversies, 6th ed. St. Paul: West Publishing, 1994; Weigley ES, Mueller DH, Robinson CH, eds. Robinson's basic nutrition and diet therapy, 8th ed. Columbus, OH: Merrill, 1997.)

for conversion of skin 7-dehydrocholesterol to vitamin D_3. Dietary intake of vitamin D is unnecessary in people who spend adequate amounts of time in sun (5 to 15 minutes exposure of face, neck, and arms per day). However, factors thought to predispose adults to inadequate amount of vitamin D include long hours spent working indoors or consistent use of sunscreens.[68] The recommended daily intake of 600 IU (15 μg) of vitamin D is estimated to provide enough vitamin D even for people with limited sun exposure. Vitamins D_2 and D_3 require activation (hydroxylation) by the liver and the kidney. Vitamin D_3 is absorbed into the circulation and converted by hepatic microsomal enzymes to 25-hydroxycholecalciferol, which is hydroxylated in the kidney to its active metabolite, 1,25-dihydroxycholecalciferol (calcitriol). Calcitriol has pharmacologic activity that lasts from 3 to 5 days. The production rate of calcitriol is closely regulated by plasma calcium and PTH. PTH mobilizes calcium from bone to maintain normal calcium concentrations, whereas vitamin D promotes bone mineralization.

Dihydrotachysterol (DHT) is a synthetic vitamin D analog activated in the liver that does not require renal hydroxylation. DHT has a rapid onset of action (2 hours), a shorter half-life, and a greater effect on mineralization of bone salts than does vitamin D.

Vitamin D Deficiency. Vitamin D deficiency may be induced by renal and hepatic disease, malabsorption syndromes, short bowel syndrome, hypoparathyroidism, and long-term anticonvulsant therapy. Vitamin D deficiency results in inadequate absorption of calcium and phosphorus from the intestinal tract. A deficiency of these minerals leads to faulty mineralization of bone and teeth, resulting in rickets in children and osteomalacia in adults. The clinical symptoms of vitamin D deficiency in adults can include bone pain, and muscle weakness and pain. Also, increased PTH secretion is caused by a decreased serum calcium level, resulting in secondary hyperparathyroidism.

Vitamin D Toxicity. The dosages of vitamin D (50,000 IU or more per day) may result in toxicity, although tolerance to vitamin D varies widely. Initial manifestations of toxicity result from hypercalcemia and include weakness, anorexia, vomiting, diarrhea, polydipsia, polyuria, mental changes, and proteinuria. Prolonged hypercalcemia may result in calcification of soft tissue, including the heart, blood vessels, renal tubules, and lungs. Death can result from cardiovascular or renal failure.

Therapeutic Uses of Vitamin D. A vitamin D–resistant state exists in chronic renal failure. Renal osteodystrophy is characterized by a decreased ability of the kidney to convert 25-hydroxycholecalciferol to 1,25-dihydroxycholecalciferol. Active vitamin D (calcitriol) or dihydrotachysterol must be supplemented to lower the concentrations of PTH and raise the plasma calcium concentration to allow bone formation. Vitamin D supplementation is also needed in hypoparathyroidism, which is characterized by hypocalcemia and

hyperphosphatemia. Generally, if a patient has an inadequate diet and little exposure to sunlight, a vitamin D supplement may be appropriate.

An anticonvulsant-induced hypocalcemia is thought to be caused by induction of the hepatic microsomal P-450 enzyme system and is treated with vitamin D, 25-hydroxycholecalciferol, and possibly calcium. Combination therapy is required because vitamin D obtained from the diet, supplements, or sun exposure is converted to inactive metabolites with prolonged anticonvulsant use.

VITAMIN E

Functions of Vitamin E. Many of the actions of vitamin E are related to its antioxidant properties. Vitamin E stabilizes the lipid portion of the cell membrane by preventing oxidation of polyunsaturated phospholipids, thereby maintaining the integrity of the cell membrane. Other functions of vitamin E include enhancement of vitamin A use, inhibition of prostaglandin production, and stimulation of an essential cofactor in steroid metabolism.

Properties of Vitamin E. α-Tocopherol is the most active and abundant form of vitamin E, occurring naturally in substances such as wheat germ oil. Vitamin E is 20% to 40% absorbed from the gastrointestinal tract and is distributed to all tissues via the lymphatic system. Natural vitamin E is commonly referred to as d-alpha tocopherol and synthetic vitamin E as d,l-alpha tocopherol. The recommended daily allowance of vitamin E is 15 mg (equivalent to 22 IU of natural vitamin E or 33 IU of synthetic vitamin E).

Vitamin E Deficiency. Vitamin E deficiency occurs primarily in premature infants and in patients with severe malabsorptive disease, such as cystic fibrosis. The neurologic syndrome of ataxia, muscle weakness, nystagmus, and loss of the senses of touch and pain have been attributed to vitamin E deficiency.[69,70]

Vitamin E Toxicity. The upper limit of vitamin E is 1,000 mg per day (1,500 IU of natural and 1,100 IU of synthetic vitamin E). The most commonly recurring complaint with large dosages (300 to 3,200 IU per day) is gastrointestinal upset (nausea, flatulence, or diarrhea), weakness, or fatigue.[71] Large dosages of vitamin E may increase the risk of hemorrhagic stroke, and intravenous use has been associated with infant death.[72] Although vitamin E has been reported to increase the effects of oral anticoagulants, this interaction remains controversial.[73,74]

Therapeutic Uses of Vitamin E. In the past, vitamin E was thought to protect or decrease the risk of cardiovascular disease and decrease the incidence of cancer. These theories are no longer thought to be valid. Vitamin E does not appear to have a direct association with protection from cancer or cardiovascular disease.[63,75–78] Vitamin E is being investigated in its role of slowing the cognitive decline in Alzheimer's disease.[79–81]

Parenteral administration of vitamin E appears to be effective in preventing retrolental fibroplasia, hemolysis, and pulmonary oxygen toxicity in premature infants.[82]

Scientists now believe that vitamin E acts with selenium as a cellular antioxidant, protecting cell membranes from peroxidase damage. However, there is no scientific basis for vitamin E supplementation in a host of conditions, including infertility, arthritis, angina, muscular dystrophy, diabetes, premenstrual syndrome, nocturnal leg cramps, and in the enhancement of athletic performance.

VITAMIN K

Functions of Vitamin K. The only rational use of vitamin K is for the correction of bleeding tendencies caused by its deficiency. Such a deficiency is unlikely to occur because of intestinal bacterial synthesis of the vitamin. For this reason, there are no dietary recommended allowances.

Properties of Vitamin K. Vitamin K is essential for the hepatic synthesis of prothrombin and other clotting proteins. Vitamin K compounds are chemically called *quinones* and include phylloquinone (K_1) and menaquinone (K_2), which are synthesized by intestinal flora, and menadione (K_3), the water-soluble analog.

Vitamin K Deficiency. Vitamin K deficiency, clinically resulting in hemorrhage, may result from destruction of intestinal flora associated with antibiotic use and especially with prolonged poor dietary intake, as may be seen during hospitalization. The role of antibiotics, especially select second- and third-generation cephalosporins, in producing hypoprothrombinemia is thought to result from a common structural side chain that inhibits a vitamin K–dependent step in the synthesis of prothrombin in the liver. When these antibiotics are used, prothrombin time should be monitored, and in many instances a prophylactic dose of vitamin K is given.[83] Aspirin and other salicylates can also induce hypoprothrombinemia. Also, large amounts of vitamins A and E, mineral oil, and bile acid sequestrants interfere with absorption of vitamin K.[84] Advanced liver damage, when caused by cancer and cirrhosis, results in a deficiency of clotting factors that cannot be alleviated by administering vitamin K. However, increased prothrombin time as a result of vitamin K deficiency responds to supplementation.

Infants are unable to synthesize vitamin K because they have a sterile intestinal tract at birth. A single prophylactic dose of vitamin K (0.5 to 1 mg intramuscularly or subcutaneously) should be given to infants to protect them until synthesis begins and to supplement dietary intake. Phylloquinone (phytonadione) is the agent of choice to prevent bleeding tendencies,[85] but caution must be exercised with intravenous use.

Vitamin K Toxicity. Vitamin K is nontoxic, even in massive dosages. Too rapid an intravenous injection of phylloquinone may result in flushing and cause a sense of constriction in the chest. Menadione in dosages of more than 10 mg parenterally may produce hemolysis, hyperbilirubinemia, and kernicterus in premature newborns.

WATER-SOLUBLE VITAMINS

The B complex vitamins and vitamin C are the water-soluble vitamins. The B complex includes thiamine, riboflavin, nicotinic acid, pyridoxine, pantothenic acid, biotin, folic acid, and cyanocobalamin.

Water-soluble vitamins act as co-factors for specific enzyme systems in the body. Many water-soluble vitamins are not active until phosphorylation occurs after ingestion (thiamine, riboflavin, niacin, and pyridoxine) or until coupled to specific nucleotides (riboflavin, niacin).

Water-soluble vitamins are stored only to a limited extent, so a daily supply is desirable. When excessive amounts are ingested, the unneeded portion generally is excreted. However, even water-soluble vitamins can be toxic, especially when large amounts are ingested for prolonged periods.

Certain conditions or situations may cause depletion of water-soluble vitamins and result in the appearance of deficiency symptoms. These include fever (which may accelerate vitamin metabolism), the stress of injury or surgery, and hyperthyroidism. Deficiencies of water-soluble vitamins may begin as a depletion of body stores without evidence of clinical symptoms such as abnormal laboratory indices. Initial clinical symptoms include loss of appetite, weight loss, headache, apathy, insomnia, or excitability. In severe deficiency states, specific clinical syndromes such as beriberi or pellagra occur. Characteristics of the water-soluble vitamins are listed in Table 29.6.

THIAMINE

The principal role of thiamine (B_1) is as a coenzyme in the form of thiamine pyrophosphate, which plays a vital role in the intermediate metabolism of carbohydrates in decarboxylation (removal of carbon dioxide) and transketolation (transfer of carbon units), such as the conversion of pyruvic acid into acetyl-coA and the synthesis of acetylcholine. Individual requirements for thiamine are related to metabolic rate and are greatest when carbohydrates are the primary source of calories. Thiamine is also necessary for the transmission of nerve impulses.

Thiamine deficiency results in beriberi, characterized by peripheral neuritis. The symptoms of peripheral neuritis include sensory disturbances in the extremities, loss of muscle strength, muscle wasting (dry beriberi), edema (wet beriberi), tachycardia, and an enlarged heart.

In the United States, the most common cause of thiamine deficiency is excessive alcohol intake, which is often associated with poor dietary habits, decreased absorption of nutrients, and decreased activation of thiamine pyrophosphate. The Wernicke–Korsakoff syndrome, characterized by paralysis of eye muscles and nystagmus and associated with

TABLE 29.6	Water-Soluble Vitamins

Vitamin	Function	Deficiency	Large Dosages	Sources
Thiamine Vitamin B$_1$	Carbohydrate metabolism Normal growth Nervous system function Acetylcholine synthesis	Beriberi Peripheral neuritis Loss of memory Depression Muscle wasting Edema Tachycardia Enlarged heart	Nontoxic even in very large dosages of 100–500 mg parenterally	Milk Pork Liver Nuts Whole grains Enriched flour and cereals
Riboflavin Vitamin B$_2$ Flavin mono-nucleotide Flavin adenine dinucleotide	Building and maintaining body tissues	Cheilosis Glossitis Seborrheic dermatitis Burning and itching eyes Achlorhydria	No toxicity	Milk Eggs Meat Liver Green, leafy vegetables
Niacin Nicotinic acid Nicotinamide	Conversion of food to energy Tissue respiration Fat synthesis Growth Healthy skin	Pellagra Erythematous eruptions Dermatitis Diarrhea Dementia	Transient flushing of skin and tingling sensation (vasodilation) Dizziness Nausea Gastrointestinal upset Peptic ulcer disease Liver toxicity Hyperuricemia Glucose intolerance Lower serum lipids with 3–6 g cholesterol and triglycerides	Lean meats Fish Whole grains Green vegetables
Pyridoxine Vitamin B$_4$ Pyridones: Pyridoxine Pyridoxamine Pyridoxal	Amino acid transformation Metabolism of tryptophan to serotonin Modify action of steroid hormones	Seborrheic-like skin Glossitis Stomatitis Peripheral neuropathy Anemia Drugs: hydralazine, penicillamine, isoniazid, cycloserine, and estrogen	Peripheral sensory neuropathy Ataxia	Wheat Corn Meat Potatoes
Ascorbic acid (Vitamin C)	Synthesis of collagen, important for wound healing and reducing stress of injury and infection Synthesis of epinephrine from adrenal glands Conversion of folic acid to folinic acid Iron absorption	Defect in collagen formation: poor wound healing, aching joints, increased susceptibility to infection, weakened cartilage and capillary walls Scurvy	Possible kidney stones Diarrhea with 4–15 g/day Gout Lower serum cholesterol Rebound scurvy Increased absorption of iron Interference with oral anticoagulants Treatment of pressure sores Impaired bacterial activity	Citrus fruits Tomatoes Leafy vegetables Melons
Pantothenic acid	Carbohydrate metabolism Gluconeogenesis Synthesis and degradation of fatty acids Sterol synthesis Steroid hormone synthesis Porphyrin synthesis	Usually seen only with severe, multiple B-complex deficits	Essentially nontoxic in humans	Meat Poultry Fish Cereals Fruits and vegetables Milk
Biotin	Carbohydrate metabolism Fat metabolism	Seborrheic dermatitis Algesia	Essentially nontoxic in humans	Liver Egg yolk Synthesized by intestinal bacteria
Folic acid	Red blood cell maturation Interrelated with B$_{12}$	Megaloblastic anemia In pregnancy, neural tube defects in offspring	Essentially nontoxic in humans	Liver Green, leafy vegetables
Cobalamin B$_{12}$	DNA synthesis Red blood cell formation	Pernicious anemia Peripheral neuropathy Macrocytic anemia	Essentially nontoxic in humans	Liver, meat, milk, eggs, cheese

Source: Marcus R, Coulston AM. Water-soluble vitamins. In Hardman JG, Limbird LE, Molinoff PB, et al., eds. Goodman & Gilman's the pharmacological basis of therapeutics. 9th ed. New York: McGraw-Hill, 1996; Cataldo CB, DeBruyne LK, Whitney EN, eds. Nutrition and diet therapy. 3rd ed. St. Paul: West Publishing, 1992; Siaer FS, Whitney EN, eds. Hamilton & Whitney's nutrition: concepts and controversies. 6th ed. St. Paul: West Publishing, 1994, Weigley ES, Mueller DH, Robinson CH, eds. Robinson's basic nutrition and diet therapy. 8th ed. Columbus, OH: Merrill, 1997.

excess alcohol intake, is caused primarily by a thiamine deficiency.[86]

RIBOFLAVIN

Riboflavin (vitamin B_2) is converted to two coenzymes, flavin mononucleotide (FMN) and flavin adenine dinucleotide (FAD), which are required for normal tissue respiration. Riboflavin is also required for activation of pyridoxine. Under normal conditions, riboflavin, like all B vitamins, is readily absorbed from the gastrointestinal tract, specifically the duodenum. Dietary sources of riboflavin include dairy products, meats, and green, leafy vegetables. Large dosages may cause yellow discoloration of urine.

A deficiency of riboflavin, as with inadequate dietary intake, malabsorption syndromes, or high alcohol consumption, leads to stomatitis, cheilosis, corneal vascularization, or dermatoses.

NIACIN

Niacin (vitamin B_3) is a component of the coenzymes nicotinamide adenine dinucleotide (NAD) and nicotinamide adenine dinucleotide phosphate (NADP). These two coenzymes are important in the oxidation-reduction reactions essential for tissue respiration. Niacin (nicotinic acid) is essential for conversion of food to energy, fat synthesis, growth, and healthy skin. Niacin may be converted in the body to niacinamide (nicotinamide), but either form can be used by the body.

Both excessive intake of alcohol and protein-calorie malnutrition may lead to the niacin deficiency state known as pellagra, with initial symptoms of an erythematous eruption resembling sunburn. Later, the three Ds of dermatitis, diarrhea, and dementia occur, followed by death if the deficiency is not corrected.

Niacin (but not niacinamide) affects lipid levels by causing a decrease in total cholesterol, triglycerides, LDLs, and an increase in high density lipoproteins (HDLs). Niacin produces a prostaglandin D2-mediated vasodilation, resulting in a transient flushing of the skin (especially the face and upper trunk) and a tingling sensation, dizziness, nausea, gastrointestinal upset, and activation of peptic ulcer disease. The flushing sensation is common and occurs in approximately 70% of those who take niacin. Generally the flushing begins 30 minutes after ingestion and lasts 30 to 60 minutes.[87,88] After 3 to 6 weeks of therapy, the flushing side effect usually decreases markedly if the patient remains compliant with drug therapy.[88,89] The adverse effects of niacin may be diminished by increasing the dosage slowly, administering with food or milk, or administering 60 minutes after a 325-mg dose of aspirin or 200 mg of ibuprofen. Niacin should not be taken in conjunction with alcohol or hot drinks. Consumption of alcohol or hot beverages increases the amount of flushing. Niacin is available at a low cost, but is not free of serious side effects.

Three formulations of niacin are available: Immediate release (IR) is absorbed over 1–2 hours, extended release (ER) is absorbed over 8 to 12 hours and sustained release (SR) is absorbed over 12 or more hours. The immediate release formulation is associated with the greatest incidence of flushing. The extended release formulation (Niaspan) is dosed at bedtime, has a lower incidence of flushing compared to the IR formulation and is not associated with increased hepatic toxicity.[90,91] The SR formulation has been associated with hepatoxicity and liver failure due to its metabolism. The SR formulation is metabolized through two pathways, nonconjugated and conjugated. The SR formulation is absorbed over a period of 12 or more hours and metabolized by the nonconjugated pathway with metabolites associated with hepatoxicity.[92]

Laboratory monitoring is required with niacin therapy. Niacin therapy for treating dyslipidemias requires baseline lipid levels (then at 4–6 weeks, and whenever the dose is increased), blood glucose, serum uric acid, and liver function tests (ALT and AST). Niacin may cause hyperglycemia, increase in uric acid, and hepatoxicity. The IR formulation is initially dosed from 50–100 mg three times daily. The dose is slowly increased at weekly intervals to a dose of 100 mg three times daily. Daily doses greater than 3,000 mg are generally not tolerated.[93] Extended release niacin is initially dosed at bedtime from 500 mg to 2,000 mg for a period of 8 weeks. The dose of the ER formulation should be limited to an increase of 500 mg at a time and at 4-week intervals to a maximum dose of 2,000 mg.[94] The SR formulation should not be substituted for equal doses of the IR niacin.[88] The maximum dose of SR that should be used daily is 2,000 mg.[93]

Niacin is also available in a no-flush formulation. The no-flush formulation generally contains a small concentration of niacin or does not contain any free nicotinic acid.[95]

PYRIDOXINE

Vitamin B_6 consists of a group of related compounds known as the pyridines, which include pyridoxine, pyridoxamine, and pyridoxal. The pyridines are converted to the active form of vitamin B_6, pyridoxal phosphate, in the gastrointestinal tract.

Pyridoxal phosphate is a coenzyme involved in the metabolism of protein, carbohydrates, and fat. In protein metabolism, vitamin B_6 participates in the decarboxylation of amino acids and the conversion of tryptophan to niacin or serotonin.

Vitamin B_6 deficiency caused by dietary restrictions is seldom seen in adults, although a deficiency in the alcoholic population may be as high as 30%. Symptoms of pyridoxine deficiency include seborrhea like skin lesions on the face, glossitis, stomatitis, peripheral neuropathy, and anemia. Drug-induced deficiencies have been observed with vitamin B_6 antagonists such as hydralazine, penicillamine, isoniazid, cycloserine, and estrogen. Pyridoxine has been reported to decrease phenobarbital and phenytoin serum levels when daily doses of 200 mg are administered for 4 weeks. Pyridoxine antagonizes the therapeutic action of levodopa by facilitating the conversion of levodopa to dopamine outside the central nervous system. Patients treated with levodopa should avoid supplemental B_6. Concurrent B_6 use does not adversely affect the levodopa–carbidopa combination because carbidopa is a peripheral dopa decarboxylase inhibitor.

Large dosages of 0.2 to 6 g per day for 2 months to 3 years may result in toxic symptoms of peripheral sensory neuropathies, with associated ataxia and numbness and clumsiness of the hands and feet.[96,97]

Pyridoxine supplementation has been reported to be beneficial in decreasing nausea and vomiting associated with pregnancy,[98] reducing carpal tunnel syndrome pain, and alleviating premenstrual syndrome (PMS) symptoms. Although clinical trials do not support pyridoxine therapy for PMS, it is used and should be limited to a dosage of 100 mg daily to prevent sensory neuropathies.[99] Low levels of vitamin B_6, vitamin B_{12}, and folic acid are associated with high levels of homocysteine. Homocysteine, and amino acid, may contribute to plaque formation and an elevated level of homocysteine is a risk factor in cardiovascular disease.[63,100–102] Under investigation is if the combination should be used by patients after percutaneous coronary angioplasty with or without stent placement.[103–105]

VITAMIN C (ASCORBIC ACID)

Ascorbic acid is involved in a variety of metabolic functions, including direct stimulation of peptide synthesis and hydroxylation of proline and lysine in collagen formation, epinephrine synthesis, and conversion of folic acid to folinic acid. Vitamin C also facilitates the gastrointestinal absorption of iron. The adrenal cortex, leukocytes, and platelets contain high concentrations of vitamin C. The amount found in the leukocytes is less susceptible to depletion than that present in plasma.[106] Ascorbic acid deficiency results in defective collagen synthesis, joint pain, anemia, poor wound healing, and increased susceptibility to infection. The severe form of vitamin C deficiency is called scurvy. The clinical findings in patients with scurvy include ecchymoses, petechial hemorrhages, easy bruising, loosening of the teeth secondary to gum inflammation, muscle weakness, and joint pains. Plasma levels of vitamin C may be low in cigarette smokers and women taking oral contraceptives.[107,108]

Large daily doses of 1 to 3 g ascorbic acid may result in formation of kidney stones because of excessive excretion of oxalate produced by the metabolism of ascorbic acid.[109] Severe diarrhea and precipitation of gout as the result of excretion of uric acid in predisposed people may also occur.[110]

Rebound scurvy may be seen in both infants and adults after cessation of the use of megadoses of vitamin C.[111] An infant born to a mother taking large amounts of vitamin C can metabolize the vitamin at a more rapid rate than normal. Adults who abruptly stop high-dose therapy experience loosened teeth and bleeding gums. In both instances, an increased rate of vitamin C elimination results in a relative deficiency when large quantities are no longer available. Therefore, patients should be advised to taper the dosage of vitamin C instead of suddenly discontinuing therapy.

Other adverse effects that have been reported with intake of megadoses of vitamin C include absorption of excessive amounts of iron, uricosuria with resultant stone formation, gastrointestinal disturbances, interference with anticoagulants, cell damage, and impaired bactericidal activity of leukocytes.

Ingestion of 1 to 3 g vitamin C has been advocated by Linus Pauling as a protective factor against the common cold.[112] Some studies show a decrease in frequency and severity of symptoms of the common cold[113,114] or an enhanced resistance to upper respiratory infections.[115,116] Others have found this not to be true.[117–119] The value of vitamin C in prevention of the common cold or as a cure for cancer remains unsubstantiated by randomized, well-designed, double-blind clinical studies.[120,121]

Vitamin C and other antioxidants have been associated with protection against cataract formation and macular degeneration.[122,123]

PANTOTHENIC ACID

Pantothenic acid, a constituent of coenzyme A, is needed for enzyme-catalyzed reactions such as the metabolism of carbohydrates, gluconeogenesis, synthesis and metabolism of fatty acids, and synthesis of sterols, steroid hormones, and porphyrins. Because pantothenic acid is widely distributed in the diet, a deficiency is rare and would be expected to occur only in a malnourished person.

BIOTIN

Biotin is important in carbohydrate and fat metabolism. Biotin is available from a wide variety of foods and is also synthesized by bacteria in the intestinal tract. A deficiency is rare but may result from inadequate synthesis. Exfoliative dermatitis is the primary deficiency symptom. Infants who are deficient in biotin because of malabsorption syndromes exhibit the symptoms of Leiner's disease. These infants should be treated with an intravenous form of biotin that is available as an investigational drug.

VITAMIN B_{12}

Vitamin B_{12} participates as a coenzyme in DNA synthesis, cell reproduction, red blood cell (RBC) formation, and nerve maintenance. It may also be needed for the incorporation of folic acid into cells.

Vitamin B_{12} also occurs in several forms designated as cobalamins. Commercially available cyanocobalamin is the most stable form.

Intrinsic factor is secreted by parietal cells in the stomach and regulates the amount of vitamin B_{12} absorbed in the terminal ileum. Because vitamin B_{12} is so well conserved by the body through enterohepatic recycling, signs of deficiency may not be seen for 3 to 4 years after absorption has ceased.[124] Because cyanocobalamin is important in cell production, the signs and symptoms of deficiency are manifested in organ systems with rapidly replicating cells. A deficiency results in megaloblastic anemia, characterized by mature red blood cells that lack oxygen-carrying capacity. Megaloblastic anemia may also occur after surgical removal of the body or fundus of the stomach, which contains parietal cells that secrete intrinsic factor, or removal of part of the ileum, where absorption of the vitamin occurs. Pernicious anemia, a genetic disorder, occurs when intrinsic factor is not produced and, consequently, vitamin B_{12} is not absorbed. In pernicious anemia, mature RBCs are not produced because of a lack of DNA synthesis. The characteristic symptoms of the disorder include pallor, anorexia, dyspnea, prolonged bleeding time, weight loss, glossitis, and neurologic disturbances including depression and unsteady gait.

A vitamin B_{12} deficiency may exist in older adults without the classic laboratory, hematologic, or clinical manifestations. This vitamin B_{12} deficiency appears to be caused by an inability to absorb protein-bound vitamin B_{12}. It is manifested in neurologic and psychiatric abnormalities without the classic hematologic abnormalities. Older adults with a serum B_{12} level of less than 200 pg per mL should be treated initially with 1 µg per day B_{12} until serum B_{12} exceeds 300 pg per mL or with B_{12} intramuscularly (100 µg/ day for 2 weeks, then 1,000 µg per month for life) if serum B_{12} does not exceed 300 pg per mL.[125] Vitamin B_{12} is available as a tablet, a solution for intramuscular injection, and an intranasal gel. The gel is reported by the manufacturer to have greater bioavailability than oral tablets and is easier to administer than an intramuscular injection.

Cyanocobalamin has no therapeutic value beyond that of correcting deficiencies. The use of vitamin B_{12} to boost energy is not supported by the literature.

FOLIC ACID

Folic acid is functionally related to cyanocobalamin because both are essential for DNA synthesis. Folic acid is also important in cell reproduction, including RBC formation and protein synthesis.

Folacin or folate are the terms for folic acid (pteroylglutamic acid). Approximately 25% of the folacin found in food is in the active (tetrahydrofolic acid) form and is readily absorbed and stored in the liver. Ascorbic acid prevents its oxidation.

The usual causes of folic acid deficiency are similar to those previously discussed with other B vitamins. In addition, a deficiency may occur during pregnancy, causing birth defects such as neural tube defects (spina bifida and anencephaly). Women of childbearing age should have an intake of at least 0.4-mg folic acid daily to reduce the risk of fetal neural tube defects.[126,127] As of January 1998, the FDA has required all cereal and grain products to be fortified with folic acid at a concentration that on average provides an additional 0.1-mg folic acid.[128-130] Fortification of food products with folic acid is also being investigated as a way to reduce the risk of heart disease by reducing blood levels of homocysteine.[63,131]

Deficiencies can also occur with oral contraceptive use, in older adults as the result of a poor diet, and in infants whose formulas lack folic acid or vitamin C. A folic acid deficiency can also occur with anticonvulsants such as phenytoin or primidone. These agents lower serum folate by inhibiting deconjugase enzymes in the gastrointestinal tract. The anemia that results from folic acid is characterized by a reduction in the number of RBCs, the release of large nucleated cells (macrocytic, megaloblastic), low hemoglobin levels with a high color content in RBCs, and lowered leukocyte and platelet counts.

Folic acid therapy corrects the anemia associated with vitamin B_{12} deficiency, but it does not prevent or correct neurologic disturbances associated with vitamin B_{12} deficiency. Folic acid in combination with vitamin B_6 and vitamin B_{12} are being investigated for the role in decreasing cardiovascular disease. See section on vitamin B_6.

MINERALS

Minerals are inorganic substances that are classified as either macronutrients or micronutrients. Macronutrients are required in daily amounts of 100 mg or more, whereas micronutrients are required in amounts of less than 100 mg daily. A summary of essential minerals is included in Table 29.7. Other minerals are found widely in nature and in the human body, but their functions are uncertain, and many are considered contaminants. With all minerals, a narrow therapeutic index exists between general requirements and toxic levels.

Sources of minerals vary according to the composition of the soil in which they are found. In regions where the soil has been depleted of minerals, the population may experience deficiencies. Deficiencies may result from chronic ingestion of highly refined foods (flour and cereals) unless they have been fortified with the minerals lost during processing. Whole-grain foods are preferred to refined foods because of their higher content of zinc, copper, iron, pyridoxine, pantothenic acid, biotin, folic acid, and vitamin E.

In this section, emphasis is placed on a discussion of calcium, iron, and zinc because of their well-understood functions. Table 29.8 lists the DRIs for minerals that are labeled elements. Table 29.9 lists the upper limits of the

TABLE 29.7	Summary of Minerals

Mineral	Physiologic Functions	Deficiency	Clinical Applications
Chlorine (chloride), major anion of extracellular fluid	Required for fluid–electrolyte balance, acid–base balance, gastric acidity	Deficiency of chloride alone rare	Losses in GI disorders, vomiting, diarrhea, and GI tube damage
Chromium	Favors normal glucose tolerance	Impaired glucose clearance, peripheral neuropathy, ataxia	Required for normal glucose use, role in management of diabetes controversial, required for carbohydrate and lipid metabolism, lowers serum cholesterol and LDL, increases HDL
Cobalt	Integral part of B_{12}	Pernicious anemia	Excess leads to polycythemia
Copper 30% absorbed from diet inversely related to zinc, essential for proper iron use	Synthesis of melanin, collagen, hemoglobin, and connective tissue	Decreased red blood cell production and poor wound healing	Menke's kinky hair syndrome, absorption disorder, toxicity, Wilson's disease
Fluoride	Contributes to structure of teeth and soft tissues	Dental caries	May be useful in osteoporosis, toxicity, fluorosis, mottled enamel
Iodine	Thyroxine and tri-iodothyronine synthesis	Cretinism, goiter, myxedema	Regulation of basal metabolic rate growth, reproduction, cellular metabolism
Magnesium 25%–65% absorbed primarily in small intestine. Efficiently absorbed and highly conserved. A person on a high-magnesium diet absorbs only about 1/4 of the intake but on a low magnesium diet more than 3/4 of the intake is absorbed.	Nerve cell function enzyme activator, skeleton synthesis	Occurs in alcoholics, diabetics, and with malabsorption syndrome (symptoms: tremor, spasm, irritability, lack of coordination, convulsions) Excretion enhanced by mineralocorticoids, hypercalcemia, phosphate depletion, and alcohol ingestion	Uses in therapy include intravenous magnesium sulfate as anticonvulsant, electrolyte replenisher, uterine relaxant magnesium gluconate for oral supplementation, magnesium citrate or sulfate as laxative magnesium carbonate, oxide hydroxide, or trisilicate as antacid Hypermagnesemia rare except in renal failure excess may cause diarrhea
Manganese Substitute for magnesium in some reactions	Cofactor for enzyme systems involved in bone formation required for formation of mucopolysaccharides	Not observed in humans	
Molybedenum	Cofactor for xanthine oxidase	Not observed in humans	
Phosphorus 70% absorbed by jejunum, maintained by renal resorption, normal plasma concentration, 30 mg/dL to 4.5 mg/dL	Skeletal synthesis, component of vitamins and essential for coenzyme formation, contributes to structure of teeth and soft tissue	Occurs with prolonged excessive use of alcohol or nonabsorbable antacids, prolonged vomiting, liver disease, hyperparathyroidism	Dibasic calcium phosphate used orally, hyperphosphatemia associated with chronic renal disease, hypoparathyroidism, tetany
Potassium Major cation of intracellular fluid normal range, 3.5–5.0 mEq/L, 3–4.5 mg/dL	Required for fluid–electrolyte balance, acid–base balance, muscle activity, carbohydrate metabolism, protein synthesis	Produces sore, weak, or painful muscles	Losses occur in GI disorders and diarrhea, used in treatment of diabetic acidosis, required for fluid balance

(continues)

TABLE 29.7 | **continued**

Mineral	Physiologic Functions	Deficiency	Clinical Applications
Selenium 90% absorbed	Acts synergistically with vitamin E to protect cell membranes from oxidative damage	Thigh tenderness, deficiency due to total parenteral nutrition, malnutrition	Incidence of cancer may result from low intake of selenium, marginal deficiency when soil content is low
Sodium Major cation of extracellular fluid normal range, 136–145 mEq/L, under hormonal control of aldosterone	Required for fluid balance, acid–base balance, cell permeability, normal muscle irritability	Losses occur in GI disorders and diarrhea weakness, mental confusion, nausea, lethargy, and muscle cramping may result	Fluid balance, blood pressure, membrane permeability, neuromuscular function may be altered by depletion or retention
Sulfur Obtained from protein	Structure of skin and cartilage, component of vitamins, important coenzyme formation		

GI, gastrointestinal; LDL, low-density lipoprotein; HDL, high-density lipoprotein.
(Adapted from Williams SR, ed. Nutrition and diet therapy, 8th ed. St. Louis: Mosby, 1997: 223–224; Weigley ES, Mueller DH, Robinson CH, eds. Robinson's basic nutrition and diet therapy. 8th ed. Columbus, OH: Merrill, 1997: 208–209.)

elements. Table 29.10 lists the interactions that involve minerals.

CALCIUM

Calcium is essential for the functional integrity of the nervous and muscular systems, for normal cardiac function, for conversion of prothrombin into thrombin, and as the major mineral component of bone.

Of total body calcium, 99% is found in bone and 1% is present in serum. Of the calcium found in serum, 45% is bound to plasma proteins. The calcium in bone serves as a reservoir to maintain normal plasma calcium levels.[132] The interaction of PTH, vitamin D, and calcitonin is responsible for maintaining a normal calcium level of 2.12 to 2.62 mmol per L (8.5 to 10.5 mg/dL).

Calcium absorption occurs in the small intestine at a steady rate of 30% of intake, increasing to approximately 50% during growth periods, pregnancy, and lactation.

Hypocalcemia usually occurs when the plasma calcium level falls below 8 mg per dL. An exception occurs when plasma protein concentration is low. In this case, calcium is reported as less than normal. Chronic, excessive intake of calcium causes adverse effects that range from minor to life threatening and are clearly dose related. In a healthy person, 1 to 2 g calcium per day is unlikely to cause problems. However, possible adverse effects include nausea, bloating, constipation (which may be prevented by increased fiber and water consumption), and flatulence (especially with oral intake of calcium carbonate).[133] Symptoms of hypercalcemia generally occur with ingestion of more than 4 to 5 g per day.[134] Signs and symptoms of hypercalcemia include nausea, vomiting, anorexia, headache, muscle weakness,

depression, apathy, fatigue, hypertension, nervousness, insomnia, and urolithiasis.[135,136]

Calcium supplements are suggested for prevention or control of osteoporosis,[137,138] hypertension,[139,140] colon cancer,[141] and weight control[142] but the only confirmed use is for correction of dietary deficiency. Of commercially available supplements, calcium carbonate (oyster shell) provides the greatest amount of elemental calcium (40%). Taking calcium carbonate with food increases its absorption. Calcium absorption is impaired in patients with achlorhydria (especially geriatric patients). Calcium citrate (21% elemental calcium) has been shown to have better solubility and absorption, particularly in patients with impaired acid secretion. Absorption of calcium decreases with age.[143]

Three natural sources of calcium, bone meal, dolomite, and coral should be avoided because of the risk of lead contamination. The risk of contamination is especially great for pregnant or lactating women, infants, children, and possibly older adults.[144]

IRON

Iron is essential in the functioning of all biologic systems. It is essential for oxygen transport as a constituent of hemoglobin and myoglobin and is also found in a number of enzymes such as cytochromes, catalases, and oxidases.

Iron in the body is either functional or stored. Functional iron is found in hemoglobin and myoglobin, whereas stored iron is found in association with transferrin, ferritin, and hemosiderin. The storage sites of ferritin and hemosiderin are the liver, spleen, and bone marrow.

(text continues on page 23)

TABLE 29.8 Dietary Reference Intakes (DRIs): Recommended Intakes for Individuals, Elements Food and Nutrition Board, Institute of Medicine, National Academies

Life Stage Group	Calcium (mg/d)	Chromium (µg/d)	Copper (µg/d)	Fluoride (mg/d)	Iodine (µg/d)	Iron (mg/d)	Magnesium (mg/d)	Manganese (mg/d)	Molybdenum (µg/d)	Phosphorus (mg/d)	Selenium (µg/d)	Zinc (mg/d)
Infants												
0–6 mo	210*	0.2*	200*	0.01*	110*	0.27*	30*	0.003*	2*	100*	15*	2*
7–12 mo	270*	5.5*	220*	0.5*	130*	11	75*	0.6*	3*	275*	20*	3
Children												
1–3 y	500*	11*	340*	0.7*	90	7	80	1.2*	17	460	20	3
4–8 y	800*	15*	440	1*	90	10	130	1.5*	22	500	30	5
Males												
9–13 y	1,300*	25*	700	2*	120	8	240	1.9*	34	1,250	40	8
14–18 y	1,300*	35*	890	3*	150	11	410	2.2*	43	1,250	55	11
19–30 y	1,000*	35*	900	4*	150	8	400	2.3*	45	700	55	11
31–50 y	1,000*	35*	900	4*	150	8	420	2.3*	45	700	55	11
51–70 y	1,200*	30*	900	4*	150	8	420	2.3*	45	700	55	11
>70 y	1,200*	30*	900	4*	150	8	420	2.3*	45	700	55	11
Females												
9–13 y	1,300*	21*	700	2*	120	8	240	1.6*	34	1,250	40	8
14–18 y	1,300*	24*	890	3*	150	15	360	1.6*	43	1,250	55	9
19–30 y	1,000*	25*	900	3*	150	18	310	1.8*	45	700	55	8
31–50 y	1,000*	25*	900	3*	150	18	320	1.8*	45	700	55	8
51–70 y	1,200*	20*	900	3*	150	8	320	1.8*	45	700	55	8
>70 y	1,200*	20*	900	3*	150	8	320	1.8*	45	700	55	8
Pregnancy												
≤18 y	1,300*	29*	1,000	3*	220	27	400	2.0*	50	1,250	60	13
19–30 y	1,000*	30*	1,000	3*	220	27	350	2.0*	50	700	60	11
31–50 y	1,000*	30*	1,000	3*	220	27	360	2.0*	50	700	60	11
Lactation												
≤18 y	1,300*	44*	1,300	3*	290	10	360	2.6*	50	1,250	70	14
19–30 y	1,000*	45*	1,300	3*	290	9	310	2.6*	50	700	70	12
31–50 y	1,000*	45*	1,300	3*	290	9	320	2.6*	50	700	70	12

NOTE: This table presents Recommended Dietary Allowances (RDAs) in bold type and Adequate Intakes (AIs) in ordinary type followed by an asterisk (*). RDAs and AIs may both be used as goals for individual intake. RDAs are set to meet the needs of almost all (97 to 98 percent) individuals in a group. For healthy breastfed infants, the AI is the mean intake. The AI for other life stage and gender groups is believed to cover needs of all individuals in the group, but lack of data or uncertainty in the data prevent being able to specify with confidence the percentage of individuals covered by this intake.

(Reprinted with permission from (**Dietary Reference Intakes: Guiding Principles for Nutrition Labeling and Fortification**) © (**2003**) by the National Academy of Sciences, courtesy of the National Academies Press, Washington, D.C.)

TABLE 29.9 | Dietary Reference Intakes (DRIs): Tolerable Upper Intake Levels (UL[a]), Elements Food and Nutrition Board, Institute of Medicine, National Academies

Life Stage Group	Arsenic[b]	Boron (mg/d)	Calcium (g/d)	Chromium	Copper (μg/d)	Fluoride (mg/d)	Iodine (μg/d)	Iron (mg/d)	Magnesium (mg/d)[c]	Manganese (mg/d)	Molybdenum (μg/d)	Nickel (mg/d)	Phosphorus (g/d)	Selenium (μg/d)	Silicon[d]	Vanadium (mg/d)[e]	Zinc (mg/d)
Infants																	
0–6 mo	ND	ND	ND	ND	ND	0.7	ND	40	ND	ND	ND	ND	ND	45	ND	ND	4
7–12 mo	ND	ND	ND	ND	ND	0.9	ND	40	ND	ND	ND	ND	ND	60	ND	ND	5
Children																	
1–3 y	ND	3	2.5	ND	1,000	1.3	200	40	65	2	300	0.2	3	90	ND	ND	7
4–8 y	ND	6	2.5	ND	3,000	2.2	300	40	110	3	600	0.3	3	150	ND	ND	12
Males, Females																	
9–13 y	ND	11	2.5	ND	5,000	10	600	40	350	6	1,100	0.6	4	280	ND	ND	23
14–18 y	ND	17	2.5	ND	8,000	10	900	45	350	9	1,700	1.0	4	400	ND	ND	34
19–70 y	ND	20	2.5	ND	10,000	10	1,100	45	350	11	2,000	1.0	4	400	ND	1.8	40
>70 y	ND	20	2.5	ND	10,000	10	1,100	45	350	11	2,000	1.0	3	400	ND	1.8	40
Pregnancy																	
≤18 y	ND	17	2.5	ND	8,000	10	900	45	350	9	1,700	1.0	3.5	400	ND	ND	34
19–50 y	ND	20	2.5	ND	10,000	10	1,100	45	350	11	2,000	1.0	3.5	400	ND	ND	40
Lactation																	
≤18 y	ND	17	2.5	ND	8,000	10	900	45	350	9	1,700	1.0	4	400	ND	ND	34
19–50 y	ND	20	2.5	ND	10,000	10	1,100	45	350	11	2,000	1.0	4	400	ND	ND	40

[a] UL = The maximum level of daily nutrient intake that is likely to pose no risk of adverse effects. Unless otherwise specified, the UL represents total intake from food, water, and supplements. Due to lack of suitable data, ULs could not be established for arsenic, chromium, and silicon. In the absence of ULs, extra caution may be warranted in consuming levels above recommended intakes.

[b] Although the UL was not determined for arsenic, there is no justification for adding arsenic to food or supplements.

[c] The ULs for magnesium represent intake from a pharmacological agent only and do not include intake from food and water.

[d] Although silicon has not been shown to cause adverse effects in humans, there is no justification for adding silicon to supplements.

[e] Although vanadium in food has not been shown to cause adverse effects in humans, there is no justification for adding vanadium to food and vanadium supplements should be used with caution. The UL is based on adverse effects in laboratory animals and this data could be used to set a UL for adults but not children and adolescents.

[f] ND = Not determinable due to lack of data of adverse effects in this age group and concern with regard to lack of ability to handle excess amounts. Source of intake should be from food only to prevent high levels of intake.

(Reprinted with permission from **(Dietary Reference Intakes: Guiding Principles for Nutrition Labeling and Fortification)** © **(2003)** by the National Academy of Sciences, courtesy of the National Academies Press, Washington, D.C.)

TABLE 29.10	Mineral Interactions	
Mineral	**Drug or Agent**	**Interaction or Effect**
Calcium	β-blockers	Decreased β-blocker absorption
	Calcium channel blockers	Possible reduction in efficacy of calcium channel blocker
	Corticosteroids	Decreased calcium absorption
	Fiber	Decreased calcium absorption
	Iron	Decreased iron absorption
	Oxalic acid (found in rhubarb and spinach)	Decreased calcium absorption
	Phenytoin	Decreased phenytoin absorption
	Phosphorus (found in dairy products)	Decreased calcium absorption
	Phytic acid (found in bran and cereals)	Decreased calcium absorption
	Quinidine	Decreased quinidine renal excretion and increased pharmacologic effects
	Salicylates	Increased salicylic acid renal excretion and decreased pharmacologic effects
	Tetracycline	Decreased serum tetracycline levels
	Thiazide diuretics	Increased calcium absorption
	Vitamin D	Increased calcium absorption
Copper	Penicillamine	Copper deficiency
Iodine	Lithium	Additive or synergistic effect in inhibiting thyroid function
Iron	Antacids	Decreased iron absorption
	Ascorbic acid	200-mg ascorbic acid per 30-mg iron increases iron absorption
	Caffeine	Decreased iron absorption
	Dairy products	Decreased iron absorption
	Oxalic acid (found in rhubarb and spinach)	Decreased iron absorption
	Phosphorus (found in dairy products)	Decreased iron absorption
	Phytic acid (found in bran and cereals)	Decreased iron absorption
Magnesium	Alcohol	Decreased magnesium absorption
	Calcium	Decreased magnesium absorption
	Diuretics	Increased magnesium absorption
	Phosphorus	Decreased magnesium absorption
Phosphorus	Antacids (Al or Mg)	Decreased phosphorus absorption
	Calcium	Decreased phosphorus absorption
	Iron	Decreased phosphorus absorption
Zinc	Alcohol	Decreased serum zinc levels
	Bran or dairy products	Decreased zinc absorption
	Copper	An excess of either may cause decreased absorption of the other
	Diuretics	Increased zinc excretion
	Penicillamine	Zinc deficiency
	Phytic acid	Decreased zinc absorption
	Phosphorus	Decreased zinc absorption
	Tetracycline	Decreased tetracycline absorption

Dietary iron absorption is highly variable, ranging from 2% to 40% depending on the type and source. Heme iron and nonheme iron are the two forms of dietary iron. Heme iron is obtained from animal protein sources and is 15% to 35% absorbed.[145] Meat may facilitate the absorption of heme iron by stimulating production of gastric acid. Nonheme iron constitutes most dietary iron found in grain products, vegetables, and dairy products and has an absorption rate of 2% to 20%. A healthy person absorbs approximately 10% of dietary iron. Iron absorption may increase to 20% if iron stores are low or iron requirements are high, as in menstruation, pregnancy, or growth stages. In the presence of iron deficiency anemia, absorption becomes more efficient to help meet the body's needs. Absorption of nonheme iron is influenced by the levels of iron stores and by concomitantly consumed dietary components. A factor such as availability of ascorbic acid may increase the bioavailability of nonheme iron.

Iron supplementation with 256 mg per day has been used to suppress the cough associated with angiotensin converting enzyme inhibitors. The theory is iron may reduce the amount of nitric oxide that is increased with use of these drugs.[146]

Iron deficiency is a recognized nutritional deficiency in the United States. Iron deficiency usually occurs in high-risk groups that include infants, children, adolescents, women of childbearing age, frequent blood donors, and chronic aspirin users. Iron deficiency in these groups usually is treated or prevented with supplements.

Iron preparations are available in three salt formulations: fumarate (33% iron), sulfate (20% iron), and gluconate (12% iron). The fumarate salt may cause a greater incidence of gastrointestinal irritation due to the higher concentration of the fumarate salt. Iron is also available in a time-released preparation which is promoted to cause less incidence of gastrointestinal upset. The preparation may cause less stomach upset since iron absorption occurs in the upper part of the small intestine and the time released preparation permits iron to be released past the site of iron absorption.

ZINC

Zinc is important in the growth and maintenance of healthy skin and in the development and continued functioning of the male sex organs. It is also necessary for the synthesis of DNA, RNA,[147] and connective tissue and bone. It is necessary for normal sense of taste, increased oxygen-carrying capacity in normal and sickle RBCs, spermatogenesis, ova formation, and the mobilization and transport of vitamin A from the liver. Zinc supplementation may affect behavior.[148]

Ten to 40% of dietary zinc is absorbed from the small intestine. The absorption of zinc appears to be associated with nutritional status and may also be influenced by a zinc-binding ligand secreted by the pancreas. Zinc absorption is inhibited by the formation of insoluble complexes with other nutrients such as phytate (found in cereals), calcium, vitamin D, protein, and fiber. Excessive copper or iron intake competes with zinc to interfere with absorption. Zinc salts (acetate and sulfate) appear to have the highest degree of bioavailability.[147] Zinc sulfate can be irritating to the gastrointestinal tract.

Zinc deficiency related to increased urinary excretion may be associated with surgery, diabetes, fever, alcohol consumption, and therapy with corticosteroids, estrogens, and thiazide diuretics. Clinical manifestations of zinc deficiency include loss of taste (hypogeusia) or smell, dermatitis, macular degeneration, and poor wound healing.[147,149,150] Acrodermatitis enteropathica is the deficiency syndrome resulting from human genetic deficiency.

Zinc therapy in dosages of 220 mg two or three times daily may be of value in facilitating wound healing and treating hypogeusia in zinc-deficient patients. Zinc gluconate lozenges may reduce the duration of cold symptoms.[151,152] Reported signs of zinc toxicity in humans include anorexia, nausea, lethargy, dizziness, and diarrhea. Vomiting may occur after ingestion of more than a 2-g dose.

CHROMIUM

Chromium is a trace mineral needed for appropriate glucose use, lipid metabolism, and insulin receptor sensitivity.[152] Chromium has been reported to be beneficial in the treatment of type II diabetes but studies and reports remain inconclusive regarding chromium supplementation to control type II diabetes or glucose and insulin responses.[152,153]

The adequate intake for chromium is 25 to 35 Φg. It is found in nature as a component of glucose tolerance factor in whole grain products, mushrooms, liver, brewer's yeast, raw sugar, beets, honey, grapes, raisins, and clams. Chromium found in dietary supplements (chromium picolinate) may be absorbed differently from dietary chromium. Chromium picolinate is incorporated into cells unchanged and generates hydroxyl radicals.[152] Chromium deficiency symptoms include hyperglycemia, glucosuria, peripheral neuropathy, and ataxia, some of the same symptoms associated with diabetes.

Chromium supplementation has been used to treat certain types of depression[154,155] and as an adjunct to obesity treatment because of its ability to increase insulin sensitivity, lower plasma glucose levels, and improve lean body mass. However, some concerns have been raised about the potential for accumulation and toxicity.

SELENIUM

Selenium, an antioxidant, is a component of the enzyme glutathione peroxidase, thought to deactivate lipid peroxidases, which are strong oxidizing agents that cause cell injury. The relationship between dietary selenium intake and cancer incidence is being investigated. Limited epidemiologic evidence suggests that the risk of certain types of cancer and stroke[63,94,156,157] are inversely related to selenium intake. Because of the potential for toxicity, unsupervised use of selenium for cancer prevention should be discouraged. Selenium is being used (although claims remain unfounded) in heart disease, arthritis, heavy metal poisoning, sexual dysfunction, and aging. Selenium toxicity includes loss of hair, brittle fingernails, fatigue, irritability, and garlic odor or breath. Selenium deficiency rarely occurs in humans and supplementation generally is not recommended.

PSYCHOSOCIAL ISSUES

Several psychosocial issues are important, especially as they relate to socioeconomic status, cultural beliefs, and consumer fads.

■ Vitamins are not energy sources. They function as coenzymes or enzymes in biochemical processes in which energy is produced during the metabolism of carbohydrates, lipids, and protein.

■ Vitamin and mineral supplements can never be considered substitutes for adequate dietary intake.

■ There is little or no advantage to using vitamins from natural sources rather than those produced synthetically. The primary difference between natural and synthetic vitamins is their cost.

■ Vitamin deficiencies are most common in older adults because of inadequate dietary intake and physiologic changes associated with aging.

■ Use of vitamin or mineral supplements does not enhance one's ability to cope with stress unless one is deficient in B complex vitamins.

■ No current research shows definitively that vitamin or mineral supplements improve athletic skill, enhance sexual performance, or prevent aging except when a deficiency is present.

■ Vitamins are not cure-alls. They are capable only of preventing diseases caused by deficiency.

CONCLUSIONS

Vitamins are organic compounds that are essential for the body's biochemical processes. Vitamins, or their precursors, must be obtained through the diet because they generally are not manufactured by the body or under certain circumstances are produced in insufficient amounts. A positive relationship exists between the maintenance of optimal health and an optimal diet. Vitamin supplementation should not be a substitute for a well-balanced diet. For the normal population, the recommended number of daily servings from the five basic food groups (meats, vegetables, fruits, dairy products, and grains) provide the needed recommended dietary allowances. However, certain groups in the general population with high metabolic requirements, malabsorption syndromes, inadequate dietary intake, or stress require additional nutrients.

The fat-soluble vitamins A, D, E, and K are stored in the body for months. Therefore, fat-soluble vitamin toxicity is related to accumulation of vitamins in fatty tissues. The water-soluble vitamins, vitamin B complex and C, have very small reserves maintained in the body, and a daily supply is desired. Water-soluble vitamins usually are nontoxic but can cause adverse effects when they are ingested for prolonged periods in excessive quantities.

Minerals are inorganic substances. Several of these elements, particularly calcium, iron, and zinc, are important catalysts in various enzymatic activities or play a role in hormonal metabolism. The importance of these elements must not be overlooked while investigators attempt to understand the nutritional importance of other minerals.

Consumers often have questions about compounds that are not considered "true" or "real" vitamins. To protect the consumer's health and finances, health care practitioners must be knowledgeable and provide the necessary information about vitamin like substances.

KEY POINTS

■ Advocate the principles of a healthful diet rich in fruits and vegetables and low in saturated fat

■ Encourage achievement and maintenance of an appropriate body weight through dietary modification and exercise

■ Ensure women of childbearing age have a folic acid intake of at least 400 μg per day

■ Pay attention to the special nutritional needs of high-risk groups, including patients with diabetes mellitus and hypertension and older adults

■ Daily Reference Intakes have replaced the 1989 Recommended Dietary Allowances

■ Niacin remains a successful treatment for the management of hypercholesterolemia as long as ongoing supervision and instructions are provided by a qualified health care provider

■ Minerals are important to good health, but the consumer must be cautioned that with all minerals, the therapeutic index between general requirements and toxic levels is narrow

REFERENCES

1. Dwyer JT. Nutrition guidelines and education of the public. J Nutr 131(11S): S3074–S3077, 2001.

2. Peckenpaugh NJ. Guides for good food choices in a family meal environment. In: Peckenpaugh NJ. Nutrition essentials and diet therapy, 9th ed. St. Louis: WB Saunders, 20033–20035.

3. U.S. Department of Agriculture and U.S. Department of Health and Human Services (2000) Year 2000 Dietary Guidelines for Americans. U.S. Government Printing Office, Washington, DC. Available at www.health.gov/dietaryguidelines. Accessed November 11, 2005.

4. Sardesai VM. Obesity and eating disorders. In: Sardesai VM. Introduction to clinical nutrition, 2nd ed. New York: Marcel Dekker, Inc., 2003:317–337.

5. Peckenpaugh NJ. Obesity and healthy weight management. In: Peckenpaugh NJ. Nutrition essentials and diet therapy, 9th ed. St. Louis: WB Saunders, 2003:201–224.

6. Institute of Medicine Food and Nutrition Board. Dietary reference intakes for energy, carbohydrate, fiber, fat, fatty acids, cholesterol, protein, and amino acids (macronutrients). Institute of Medicine of the National Academies. Washington, DC: National Academy Press, 2005. Available at http://books.nap.edu/catalog/10490.html. Accessed November 11, 2005.

7. Slentz CA, Dusch BD, Johnson JL, et al. Effects of the amount of exercise on body weight, body composition, and measures of central obesity: STRRIDE–a randomized controlled study. Arch Intern Med 164:31–39, 2004.

8. Manson JE, Skerrett PJ, Greenland P, et al. The escalating pandemics of obesity and sedentary lifestyle. Arch Intern Med 164: 249–258, 2004.

9. U.S. Department of Agriculture. My Pyramid, 2005. Available at www.mypyramid.gov/downloads.miniposter.pdf. Accessed November 11, 2005.

10. Food and Nutrition Information Center. Food Guide Pyramid. Available at www.nal.usda.gov/fnic/Fpyr/pyramid.html. Accessed November 11, 2005.

11. Peckenpaugh NJ. Carbohydrate, protein, and fat: the energy macronutrients of balanced meals. In: Peckenpaugh NJ. Nutrition essentials and diet therapy, 9th ed. St. Louis: WB Saunders, 2003:33–55.

12. American Pharmaceutical Association. Concepts in comprehensive weight management: managing obesity as a chronic disease. Srnka QA, Early JL, Maddox RW, Ploehn LC as advisory board. American Pharmaceutical Association. Washington, DC, 2001:1–20.

13. Lowry R, Wechsler H, Kann L, et al. Recent trends in participation in physical education among U.S. high school students. J Sch Health 71:145–152, 2001.

14. National Institute of Child Health and Human Development Study of Early Child Care and Youth Development Network. Frequency and intensity of physical activity of third grade children in physical education. Arch Pediatric Adolesc Med 157:186–190, 2003.

15. Fisher EA, Van Horn L, McGill HC. Nutrition and children: a statement for healthcare professional from the nutrition committee, American Heart Association. Circulation 95:2332–2333, 1997.

16. Ogden CL, Flegal KM, Carroll MD, et al. Prevalence and trends in overweight among US children and adolescents, 1999–2000. JAMA 288:728–1732, 2002.

17. Sorof D, Daniels S. Obesity hypertension in children: a problem of epidemic proportions. Hypertension 40:441–447, 2002.

18. Jackson Y, Dietz WH, Saunders C, et al. Summary of the 2000 Surgeon General's listening session: toward a national action plan on overweight and obesity. Obesity Res 10:1299–1305, 2002.

19. Yanovski JA, Yanovski SZ. Treatment of pediatric and adolescent obesity. JAMA 289:1851–1853, 2003.

20. Deitz WH. Childhood weight affects adult morbidity and mortality. J Nutr128:S411–S414, 1998.

21. O'Dea JA. Why do kids eat healthful food? Perceived benefits of and barriers to healthful eating and physical activity among children and adolescents. J Am Diet Assoc103:497–501, 2003.

22. Zavod RM. Essentials of nutrition. In: Wolinsky I, Williams L, eds. Nutrition in pharmacy practice. Washington, DC: American Pharmaceutical Association, 2002:1–54.

23. Czeizel AE, Dudas I. Prevention of the first occurrence of neural tube defects by periconceptional vitamin supplementation. N Engl J Med 327:1832–1835, 1992.

24. Sardesai VM. Water soluble vitamins II. In: Introduction to clinical nutrition, 2nd ed. New York: Marcel Dekker, Inc., 2003:211–240.

25. Flegal KM, Carroll MD, Ogden CL, et al. Prevalence and trends in obesity among US adults, 1999–2000. JAMA288:1723–1727, 2002.

26. Mokdad AH, Ford ES, Bowman BA, et al. Prevalence of obesity, diabetes, and obesity–related health risk factors, 2001. JAMA 289: 76–79, 2003.

27. Chobanian AV, Bakris GL, Black HR, et al. The seventh report of the joint national committee on prevention, detection, evaluation, and treatment of high blood pressure. JAMA 289:2560–2572, 2003.

28. Expert Panel on Detection, Evaluation, and Treatment of High Blood Cholesterol in Adults. Executive summary of the third report of the National Cholesterol Education Program (NCEP) expert panel on detection, evaluation, and treatment of high blood cholesterol in adults (Adult Treatment Panel III). JAMA 285:2486–2497, 2001.

29. National Cholesterol Education Program. Third report of the National Cholesterol Education Program (NCEP) Expert Panel on Detection, Evaluation, and Treatment of High Blood Cholesterol in Adults (Adult Treatment Panel III) final report. Circulation 106: 3143–3421, 2002.

30. Franz MJ, Bantle JP, Beebe CA, et al. Evidence-based nutrition principles and recommendations for the treatment and prevention of diabetes and related complications (Technical Review). Diabetes Care, 2002 25:148–198.

31. American Diabetes Association. Nutrition principles and recommendations in diabetes. Diabetes Care 27:S36–S46, 2004.

32. Sacks FM, Svetkey LP, Vollmer WM, et al, for the DASH-Sodium Collaborative Research Group. Effects on blood pressure of reduced dietary sodium and the Dietary Approach to Stop Hypertension (DASH) diet. N Engl J Med 344:3–10, 2001.

33. McGee M, Jensen GL. Nutrition in the elderly. J Clin Gastr 2000 30:372–380.

34. Huffman GB. Evaluating and treating unintentional weight loss in the elderly. Am Fam Physician 65:640–650, 2002.

35. Miller LJ, Kwan RC. Pharmacologic treatment of undernutrition in the geriatric patient. Cons Pharm17:739–747, 2002.

36. Demling RH, Walaszek P, Collins N. Involuntary weight loss: causes and consequences in the elderly long-term care facility resident. Cons Pharm 17 (Suppl A):3–10, 2002.

37. Wedick NM, Barrett-Conner E, Knoke JD, et al. The relationship between weight loss and all-cause mortality in older men and women with and without diabetes mellitus: the Rancho Bernardo study. JAGS 50:1810–1815, 2002.

38. Malone M. General nutrition. In: Herfindal ET, Gourley DR, eds. Textbook of therapeutics: drug and disease management, 7th ed. Baltimore: Lippincott Williams and Wilkins, 2000:163–174.

39. Morley JE, Silver AJ. Nutritional issues in nursing home care. Ann Intern Med 123:850–859, 1995.

40. Thomas DR, Ashmen W, Morley JE, et al. Nutritional management strategies in long-term care: development of a clinical guideline. Council for Nutritional Strategies in Long-Term Care. Journals of Gerontology Series A-Biological Science and Medical Sciences 55A:M725–M734, 2000.

41. Walaszek P, Collins N, Demling RH. Involuntary weight loss: treatment issues in long-term care. Cons Pharm17 (Suppl A):1–21, 2002.

42. Guigoz Y, Vellas B, Garry PJ. Assessing the nutritional status of the elderly: the Mini Nutritional Assessment as part of the geriatric evaluation. Nutr Rev 54:S59–S65, 1996.

43. Rulemaking History for OTC Vitamins and Minerals. Federal Register 44:16139, 1979. Available at www.fda.gov/cder/otcmonographs/vitamin&mineral/new_vitamin&mineral.htm/.

44. American Dietetic Association. Position paper: vitamin and mineral supplementation. J Am Diet Assoc 96:73–77, 1996.

45. Dietary Reference Intakes: Applications in dietary planning. Washington DC: National Academies Press Publications 2003:229–237.

46. Dietary Reference Intakes: Guiding Principles for Nutrition Labeling and Fortification. Washington, DC: National Academic Press; 2003:179–193.

47. Dietary References Intakes: an update. International Food Information Council Foundation. August 2002. www.ific.org/publications/other/driupdateom.cfm. Accessed November 11, 2005.
48. Barr SI, Murphy SP, Poos MI. Interpreting and using the Dietary Reference Intakes in dietary assessment of individuals and groups. J Am Diet Assoc 102:780–788, 2002.
49. Anonymous. Dietary reference intakes. Nutr Rev 55:319–326, 1997.
50. Sizer FS, Whitney EN, eds. Hamilton & Whitney's nutrition: concepts and controversies. 6th ed. St Paul: West Publishing, 1994: 550–553.
51. Boyle MA, Zyla G. Personal nutrition. 3rd ed. New York: West Publishing, 1996:213–215.
52. Marcus, Coulston AM. Fat soluble vitamins. In Hardman JG, Limbird LE, eds. Goodman and Gilman's the pharmacological basis of therapeutics. 10th ed. New York: McGraw-Hill, 2001:1773–1783.
53. Hathack JN, Hattan DG, Jenkins MY, et al. Evaluation of vitamin A toxicity. Am J Clin Nutr 52:183–202, 1990.
54. Sirling HF, Laing SC, Barr DG. Hypercarotenemia and vitamin A overdosage from proprietary baby food. Lancet 1:1089, 1986.
55. Sommer A, Djunaedi E, Loeden AA, et al. Impact of vitamin A supplementation on childhood mortality. Lancet 1:1169–1173, 1986.
56. Rothman KJ, Moore LL, Singer MR, et al. Teratogenicity of high vitamin A intake. N Engl J Med 333:1369–1373, 1995.
57. Lammer EJ, Chen DT, Hoar RM, et al. Retinoic acid embryopathy. N Engl J Med 313:837–841, 1985.
58. Orfanos CE, Zouboulis CC. Current use and future potential role of retinoids in dermatology. Drugs 53:358–388, 1997.
59. deKlerk NH, Musk AW, Ambrosini GL, et al. Vitamin A and cancer prevention II: comparison of the effects of retinol and beta-carotene. Int J Cancer 75:362–367, 1998.
60. Fairfield KM, Hankinson SE, Rosner BA, et al. Risk of ovarian carcinoma and consumption of vitamins A, C, and E and specific carotenoids: a prospective analysis. Cancer 92:2318–2326, 2001
61. Zhang S, Hunter DJ, Forman MR, et al. Dietary carotenoids and vitamins A, C, and E and risk of breast cancer. J Natl Cancer Institute 91:547–56, 1999.
62. Fawzi WW, Msamanga G, Hunter D, et al. Randomized trial of vitamin supplements in relation to vertical transmission of HIV-1 in Tanzania. J Acquir Immune Defic Syndrome 23:246–254, 2000.
63. Morris CD, Carson S. Routine vitamin supplementation to prevent cardiovascular disease: a summary of the evidence for the U.S. Preventive Services Task Force. Ann Inter Med 139:56–70, 2003.
64. Greenberg ER, Baron JA, Karagas ME, et al. Mortality associated with low plasma concentration of beta carotene and the effect of oral supplementation. JAMA 275:699–703, 1996.
65. Todd S, Woodward M, Tunstall-Pedoe H, et al. Dietary antioxidant vitamins and fiber in the etiology of cardiovascular disease and all-causes mortality: results from the Scottish heart health study. Am J Epidemiol 150:1073–1080, 1999.
66. Institute of Medicine. Dietary reference intakes for vitamin A, vitamin K, arsenic, boron, chromium, copper, iodine, iron, manganese, molybdenum, nickel, silicon, vanadium, and zinc. Washington, DC: Academy Press, 2001.
67. Koo LC. Diet and lung cancer 20+ years later: more questions than answers? Int J Cancer 10(Suppl):22–29, 1997
68. Plotinikoff GA, Quigley JM. Prevalence of severe hypovitaminosis D in patients with persistent, unspecific musculoskeletal pain. Mayo Clin Proc 78:1463–1470, 2003.
69. Cavalier L, Ouahchi K, Kayden HJ, et al. Ataxia with isolated vitamin E: heterogeneity of mutations and phenotypic variability in a large number of families. Am J Hum Genet 62:301–310, 1998.
70. Sokol RJ, Butler-Simon N, Conner C, et al. Multicenter trial of d-alpha-tocopheryl polyethylene glycol 1000 succinate for treatment of vitamin E in children with chronic cholestasis. Gastroenterology 104:1727–1735, 1993.
71. Bendich A, Machlin LJ. Safety of oral intake of vitamin E. Am J Clin Nutr 48:612–619, 1988.
72. Mino M. Clinical uses and abuses of vitamin E in children. Proc Soc Exp Biol Med 200:266–270, 1992.
73. Food and Nutrition Board, Institute of Medicine. Dietary Reference Intakes for vitamin C, vitamin E, selenium and carotenoids. Washington, DC: National Academy Press 2000. Available at http://

www.nap.edu/books/0309069351/htm/. Accessed November 11, 2005.
74. Liu M, Wallmon A, Olsson Morlock C, et al. Mixed tocopherols inhibit platelet aggregation in humans: potential mechanism. Am J Clin Nutr 77:700–706, 2003.
75. Office of Dietary Supplements. Vitamin and Minerals Fact Sheets, Vitamin E. Available at www.ods.od.nih.gov/Health_Information/Vitamin_and_Mineral_Supplement_Fact_Sheets.aspx. Accessed November 11, 2005.
76. Brown BC, Cheung MC, Lee AC, et al. Antioxidant vitamins and lipid therapy: end of a long romance. J Am Heart Assoc 22: 1535–1546, 2002.
77. The Heart Outcomes Prevention Evaluation Study Investigators. Vitamin E supplementation and cardiovascular events in high-risk patients. N Engl J Med 342:154–160, 2000.
78. GISS-Prevenzione Investigators. Dietary supplementation with n-3 polyunsaturated fatty acids and vitamin E after myocardial infarction: results of the GISSI-Prevenzione trial. Lancet 354:447–455, 1999.
79. Sano M, Ernesto C, Thomas RG, et al. A controlled trial of selegiline, apha-tocopherol, or both as treatment for Alzheimer's disease. The Alzheimer's Disease Cooperative Study. N Engl J Med 336: 1216–1222, 1997.
80. Carlsson CM, Papcke-Benson K, Caenes M, et al. Health-related quality of life and long-term therapy with pravastatin and tocopherol (vitamin E) in older adults. Drugs and Aging 19:793–805, 2002.
81. Dekosky ST. Pathology and pathways of Alzheimer's disease with an update on new developments in treatment. J Am Geriatr Soc 51: 5314–5320, 2003.
82. Bell EF. History of vitamin E in infant nutrition. Am J Clin Nutr 46:183–186, 1987.
83. Breen GP, St Peter WL. Hypoprothrombinemia associated with cefmetazole. Ann Pharmacother 31:180–184, 1997.
84. Weigley ES, Mueller DH, Robinson CH, eds. Robinson's basic nutrition and diet therapy. 8th ed. Columbus, OH: Merrill, 1997:175.
85. Marcus R, Coulston AM. Fat soluble vitamins. In: Hardman JG, Limbird LE, eds. Goodman & Gilman's the pharmacological basis of therapeutics, 10th ed. New York: McGraw-Hill, 2001:1785.
86. Hoyumpa AM. Mechanisms of thiamine in chronic alcoholism. Am J Clin Nutr 33:2750, 1980.
87. Food and Nutrition Board, Institute of Medicine. Dietary Reference Intakes for Thiamin, Riboflavin, Niacin, Vitamin B6, Folate, Vitamin B12, Pantothenic Acid, Biotin, and Choline. Washington, DC: National Academy Press, 2000. Available at http://books.nap.edu/books/0309065542/html/. Accessed November 11. 2005
88. Anonymous. ASHP therapeutic position statement on the safe use of niacin in the management of dyslipidemia. Am J Health Syst Pharm 54:2816–2819, 1997.
89. Marcus R, Coulston AM. Water-soluble vitamins. The vitamin B complex and ascorbic acid. In: Hardman JG, Limbird LE, Molinoff PB, et al, eds. Goodman & Gilman's the pharmacological basis of therapeutics, 10th ed. New York: McGraw-Hill, 2001:991–992.
90. Knopp RH, Alagona P, Davidson M, et al. Equivalent efficacy of a time-release form of niacin (Niaspan) given once-a-night versus plain niacin in the management of hyperlipidemia. Metabolism 47: 1097–1104, 1998.
91. Knopp RH. Evaluating niacin in its various forms. Am J Cardiol 86(Suppl 12A):51L–56L, 2000.
92. Piepho RW. The pharmacokinetics and pharmacodynamics of agents proven to raise high-density lipoprotein cholesterol. Am J Cardiol 86 (Suppl 12A):35–40L, 2002.
93. Daily JH, Gray DR, Bradberry JC, et al. Lipid-modifying drugs. In: McKenny JM, Hawkins D, eds. Handbook of the management of lipid disorders, 2nd ed. St. Louis: National Pharmacy Cardiovascular Council c/o Health Tech Solutions 124–166, 2001.
94. Brown BG, Zhao XQ, Chait A, et al. Simvastatin and niacin, antioxidant vitamins or the combination for the prevention of coronary disease. N Engl J Med 345:1583–1592, 2001.
95. Meyers CD, Carr MC, Parks S. Varying cost and free nicotinic acid content in over-the-counter niacin preparations for dyslipidemia. Ann Intern Med 139:996–1002, 2003.
96. Schaumburg H, Kaplan J, Windebank A, et al. Sensory neuropathy with low dose pyridoxine abuse. A new megavitamin syndrome. N Engl J Med 310:445–448, 1983.

97. Girman A, Lee R, Kliger B. An integrative medicine approach to premenstrual syndrome. Clin J Womens's Health 2:116–127, 2002.
98. Quinlan JD. Nausea and vomiting of pregnancy. Am Fam Physician 68:121–128, 2002.
99. Wyatt KM, Dimmock PW, Jones PW, et al. Efficacy of vitamin B6 in the treatment of premenstrual syndrome. BMJ 318:1375–1381, 1999.
100. Nallamothu BF, Fendrick AM, Omenn GS. Homocysteine and coronary heart disease: pharmacoeconomic support interventions to lower hyperhomocysteinaemia. Pharmacoeconomics 20:429–442, 2002.
101. McKinley MC, McNulty H, McPartlin J, et al. Low–dose vitamin B-6 effectively lowers fasting plasma homocysteine in healthy elderly persons who are folate and riboflavin replete. Am J Clin Nutr 73:759–764, 2001.
102. Rodrigo R, Passalacqua W, Araya J, et al. Homocysteine and essential hypertension. J Clin Pharm. 43:1299–1306, 2003.
103. Schnyder G, Roffi M, Pin R, et al. Decreased rate of coronary restenosis after lowering of plasma homocysteine levels. N Engl J Med 345:1593–1600, 2001.
104. Schnyder G, Roffi M, Flammer Y, et al. Effect of homocysteine-lowering therapy with folic acid, vitamin B12, and vitamin B6 on clinical outcome after percutaneous coronary intervention. The Swiss Heart Study: A randomized controlled trial. JAMA 288:973–979, 2002.
105. Lange HW, Dambrink JH, Pasalary M, et al. Folate therapy increases instant restenosis: results from the folate after coronary intervention trial (FACIT). American College of Cardiology 52nd Annual Scientific Session. Chicago March 30–April 4, Abstract 31–37.
106. Levine M, Cantilena CC, Dhariwal KR. In situ kinetics and ascorbic acid requirements. World Rev Nutr Diet 72:114–127, 1993.
107. Kallner AB, Hartmann D, Hornig DH. On the requirements of ascorbic acid in man: steady-state turnover and body pool in smokers. Am J Clin Nutr 34:1347–1355, 1981.
108. Rivers JM. Oral contraceptives and ascorbic acid. Am J Clin Nutr 28:550–554, 1975.
109. Schmidt KH, Hagmaier V, Horning DH, et al. Urinary oxalate excretion after large intakes of ascorbic acid in man. Am J Clin Nutr 34:305–311, 1981.
110. Stein HB, Hasan A, Fox IH. Ascorbic acid-induced uricosuria: a consequence of megavitamin therapy. Ann Intern Med 84:385–388, 1976.
111. Marcus R, Coulston AM. Water-soluble vitamins. In: Hardman JG, Limbird LE, eds. Goodman & Gilman's the pharmacological basis of therapeutics, 10th ed. New York: McGraw-Hill, 2001:1770.
112. Pauling L. Vitamin C and the common cold. San Francisco: WH Freeman, 1970:39–52, 83–88.
113. Baird IM, Hughes RE, Wilson HK, et al. The effects of ascorbic acid and flavonoids on the occurrence of symptoms normally associated with a common cold. Am J Clin Nutr 32:1686–1690, 1979.
114. Schwartz J, Weiss ST. Dietary factors and chronic respiratory symptoms. Am J Epidemiol 132:67–76, 1990.
115. Peters EM, Goetzsche JM, Grobbelaar B, et al. Vitamin C supplementation reduces the incidence of postrace symptoms of upper-respiratory-tract infection in ultramarathon runners. Am J Clin Nutr 57:170–174, 1993.
116. Hemila H. Vitamin C supplementation and the common cold: was Linus Pauling right or wrong? Int J Vitam Nutr Res 67:329–335, 1997.
117. Hemila H. Vitamin C intake and susceptibility to the common cold. Br J Nutr 77:59–72, 1997.
118. Levine M, Rumsey Sc, Daruwala R, et al. Criteria and recommendations for vitamin C intake. JAMA 281:1415–1423, 1999.
119. Audera C, Patulny RV, Sander BH, et al. Mega-dose vitamin C in treatment of the common cold: a randomized controlled trail. Med J Aust 175:359–362, 2001.
120. Loria CM, Klag MJ, Caulfield LE, et al. Vitamin C status and mortality in US adults. Am J Clin Nutr 72:139–145, 2000.
121. Michels KB, Holmberg L, Bergkvist L, et al. Dietary antioxidant vitamins, retinal, and breast cancer incidence (United States). Cancer Causes Control 11:279–283, 2000.
122. Age-Related Eye Disease Study Research Group. A randomized, placebo controlled, clinical trial of high-dose supplementation with vitamins C and E, beta carotene, and zinc for age-related macular degeneration and vision loss. AREDS report no. 8 Arch Ophthalmol 119:1417–1436, 2001.
123. Age-Related Eye Disease Study Research Group. Potential public heath impact of age-related eye disease study results: AREDS report no. 11. Arch Ophthalmol 121:1621–1624, 2003.
124. Hillman R. Hematopoietic agents. In Hardman JG, Limbird Le, eds. Goodman and Gilman's the pharmacological basis of therapeutics. 10th ed. New York: McGraw Hill, 2001:105–110.
125. McRae TD, Freedman ML. Why vitamin B_{12} deficiency should be treated aggressively. Geriatrics 44:70–79, 1989.
126. Willett WC. Folic acid and neural tube defect: can't we come to a closure? Am J Public Health 82:666–668, 1992.
127. Anonymous. Use of folic acid–containing supplements among women of childbearing ages: United States, 1997. MMWR Morb Mortal Wkly Rep 47:131–435, 1998.
128. Anonymous. Food standards: amendment of the standards of identity for enriched grain products to require addition of folic acid (21 CFR 136, 137, and 139). Federal Register 58:5305–5312, 1993.
129. Anonymous. Recommendations for the use of folic acid to reduce the number of cases of spinal bifida and other neural tube defects. MMWR Morb Mortal Wkly Rep 41(RR–14):1–7, 1992.
130. Anonymous. Food labeling health claims and label statements: folate and neural tube defects. Federal Register 58(197):53254–53295, 1993.
131. Milinow MR, Duell PB, Hess DL, et al. Reduction of plasma homocysteine levels by breakfast cereal fortified with folic acid in patients with coronary heart disease. N Engl J Med 338:1009–1015, 1998.
132. Marcus R. Agents affecting calcification: calcium parathyroid hormone, calcitonin, vitamin D, and other compounds. In: Hardman JG, Limbird LE, eds. Goodman & Gilman's the pharmacological basis of therapeutics, 10th ed. New York: McGraw-Hill, 2001:1520–1521.
133. Leverson DI, Bockman RS. A review of calcium preparations. Nutr Rev 52:221–232, 1994.
134. Beall DP, Scofield RH. Milk-alkali syndrome associated with calcium carbonate consumption. Report of 7 patients with parathyroid hormone levels and an estimate of prevalence among patients hospitalized with hypercalcemia. Medicine 74:89–96, 1995.
135. Bullimore DW, Miloszewski KJ. Raised parathyroid hormone levels in the milk alkali syndrome: an appropriate response? Postgrad Med 63:789–792, 1987.
136. French JK, Holdaway, IM Williams LC. Milk alkali syndrome following over-the-counter antacid self-medication. NZ Med J 99:322–323, 1986.
137. Heaney RP. Calcium, dairy products and osteoporosis. J Am Coll Nutr 19:83S–99S, 2000.
138. McGarry KA, Kiel DP. Postmenopausal osteoporosis. Strategies for preventing bone loss, avoiding bone fracture. Postgrad Med. 108:79–82, 85–91, 2000.
139. Jorde R, Bonaa KH. Calcium from dietary products, vitamin D intake, and blood pressure: the Tromso study. Am J Clin Nutr 71:1530–1535, 2000.
140. McCarron DA, Resser ME. Are low intakes of calcium and potassium important causes of cardiovascular disease? Am J Hypertension 14:2065–2125, 2000.
141. Terry P, Baron JA, Bergkvist L, et al. Dietary calcium and vitamin D intake and risk of colorectal cancer: a prospective cohort study in women. Nutr and Cancer 43:39–46, 2002.
142. Zemel MB. Regulation of adiposity and obesity by dietary calcium: mechanisms and implications. J Am Coll Nutr 21:145S–151S, 2002.
143. Heller HJ, Greer LG, Haynes SD, et al. Pharmacokinetics and pharmacodynamic comparison of two calcium supplements in postmenopausal women. J Clin Pharmacol 40:1237–1244, 2000.
144. Ross EA, Szabo NJ, Tebbett IR. Lead content of calcium supplements. JAMA 284:1425–1429, 2000.
145. Monsen ER. Iron nutrition and absorption: dietary factors which impact iron bioavailability. J Am Diet Assoc 88:786–790, 1990.
146. Lee SC, Park SW, Kim DK, et al. Iron supplementation inhibits cough associated with ACE inhibitors. Hypertension 38:166–170, 2001.

147. Peckenpaugh NJ. Nutritional Essentials and Diet Therapy 9th ed. WB Saunders St. Louis 2003, 119.

148. Billici M, Yildirim F, Kandil S, et al. Double-blind, placebo-controlled study of zinc sulfate in treatment of attention deficit hyperactivity disorder. Pro Neuropsychopharmacol Biol Psychiatry 28:181–190, 2004

149. Bressler NM, Bressler SB, Congdon NG, et al. Potential public health impact of age-related eye disease study results: AREDS report no. 11. Arch Ophthalmol 121:1621–1624, 2003.

150. Mossad SB, Mackin ML, Medendork SV, et al. Zinc gluconate lozenges for treating the common cold: a randomized, placebo-controlled, double-blind study. Ann Intern Med 125:81–88, 1996.

151. Jackson JL, Lesho E, Peterson C. Zinc and the common cold: a meta-analysis revisited. J Nutr 130:1512S–1515S, 2000.

152. Vincent JB. The biochemistry of chromium. J Nutr 130:715–718, 2002.

153. Althius MD, Jordon NE, Ludington EA, et al. Glucose and insulin responses to dietary chromium supplements: a meta-analysis. Am J Clin Nutr 78:148–155, 2002.

154. Davidson JR, Abraham K, Connor KM, et al. Effectiveness of chromium in atypical depression: a placebo-control trial. Biol Psychiatry 53:261–264, 2003.

155. Attenburrow MJ, Odontiadis J, Murray BJ, et al. Chromium treatment decreases the sensitivity of 5-HT2A receptors. Psychopharmacology 159:432–436, 2002.

156. Clark LC, Dalkin B, Krongrad A, et al. Decreased incidence of prostate cancer with selenium supplementation: results of a double-blind cancer prevention trial. Br J Urol 81:730–734, 1998.

157. Helzlsouer KJ, Huang HY, Alberg AJ, et al. Association between alpha-tocopherol, gamma-tocopherol, selenium, and subsequent prostate cancer. J Natl Cancer Inst. 92:2018–2023, 2000.

Parenteral and Enteral Nutrition in Adult Patients

30

Rex O. Brown

TREATMENT GOALS

Specialized nutrition support includes parenteral nutrition (PN) and enteral nutrition (EN). In 1968, Dudrick et al reported that growth and development could be sustained with long-term PN in an infant who could not be fed via the gastrointestinal tract.[1] Most practitioners consider this the beginning of modern clinical nutrition. EN has been used for many years but did not become a safe and efficacious method of nutrient delivery until the 1970s. During the past 40 years, many advances have been made to improve safe and efficacious delivery of PN and EN. The following are general treatment goals for patients receiving PN and/or EN:

- Repletion of patients with undernutrition.
- Maintenance of nutritional status in patients who have adequate nutritional stores and require parenteral or enteral nutrition.
- Achievement of appropriate fluid, electrolyte, trace element, and vitamin balance in patients requiring parenteral or enteral nutrition.
- Adequate wound healing in patients who have undergone major gastrointestinal surgery or have suffered thermal injury.
- Improve the quality of life in patients who require parenteral or enteral nutrition.

Since the original report by Dudrick et al,[1] the prevalence of complications of malnutrition has become more appreciated. A practical way to assess malnutrition in patients is to include components of weight change, dietary intake, gastrointestinal (GI) symptoms, muscle and fat loss, and functional capacity as part of a history and physical examination.[2] Despite this increased awareness of malnutrition and an appreciation for its negative effects on patient outcomes, in many patients undernutrition goes undetected or is undertreated.[3]

PN and EN can be effective medical therapies, but they are not without complications. This has led to the development of nutrition support teams or nutrition support committees that assist in making specialized nutrition support safe and efficacious. Traditionally, the nutrition support team has consisted of multidisciplinary health care practitioners including a physician, pharmacist, nurse, and dietitian. The physician has usually been the director of the nutrition support team. Surgeons, gastroenterologists, and intensivists most commonly serve as nutrition support team physicians. The pharmacist's role has ranged from ensuring provision of a properly compounded PN formulation to being the director of the team. Most commonly, the pharmacist provides assistance in prescribing the nutrient formulation, monitors the patient for metabolic or mechanical complications, educates other practitioners about compatibilities and drug–nutrient interactions, and assists the health care system in developing a cost-effective formulary of nutrition products. In some health care systems, the pharmacist is the director or coordinator of the nutrition support team, with complete or nearly complete responsibility for PN and EN prescribing, compounding, and delivery. Nurses have also directed nutrition support teams, but traditionally their role has been involved with intravenous (IV) catheter insertion and site care, nasogastric enteral tube placement, and selection of nutrition support products. These products include central line insertion kits, dressing trays, parenteral and enteral pumps, and multilumen catheters. Nurses also monitor patients receiving PN or EN for mechanical, infectious, GI, and metabolic complications. Registered dietitians perform nutritional or metabolic assessments, establish caloric and protein goals, monitor patients, and document calorie counts from PN, EN, and oral intake. The roles of the disciplines will invariably overlap depending on staffing and the training and experience of each member. Many practitioners serve on the nutrition support team on a part-time basis.

NUTRITIONAL ASSESSMENT

Nutritional assessment evaluates a patient's nutritional status and can be used to detect and quantitate malnutrition in a variety of diseases. The ideal nutritional assessment would include a measurement of body cell mass. Body cell mass includes fat-free tissue such as skeletal muscle, smooth muscle, and solid organs. Malnutrition appears to be prevalent in ambulatory care patients,[3] subacute care patients,[4] and critically ill hospitalized patients.[5] It is also not surprising that malnutrition is more prevalent in the elderly.[6] There has been considerable interest recently in assessing body mass index (BMI) and patient outcome with various diseases. In seriously ill hospitalized adults, a depressed body mass index (below the 15th percentile) has been associated with a significant increase in hospital mortality.[6] A 7-year study of 18,316 patients reported that the lowest mortality rate among men and women was in those with BMIs from 25 to 27.4 kg/m^2.[7] These type of studies usually report a U-shaped graph for mortality. Those with clear undernutrition (below 20 kg/m^2) and those with obesity (>30 kg/m^2) have increased rates of death compared to patients with BMIs in the mid-20s.[7] A study of 3,975 men and women with hypertension found that treated patients showed a U-shaped mortality curve for both men and women; the lowest mortality

rates were for BMI = 26 for men and BMI = 29.6 for women.[8] Patients with BMIs below 24 had a marked increase in strokes.[8] A large U.S. trial that included over 1 million adults reported that the lowest mortality rate for nonsmokers was a BMI of 23.5 to 24.9 kg/m^2 for men and 22 to 23.4 kg/m^2 for women.[9] Smoking clearly increased mortality for all BMI groups. Mortality increased significantly at higher BMIs, especially in whites.[9] Interestingly, a slightly depressed body weight in healthy, middle-aged women showed an improvement in mortality compared to heavier females.[10] In this 16-year longitudinal study of female registered nurses, all-cause mortality increased substantially as BMI increased. Women who maintained their weight as least 15% less than the U.S. average did not show an increase in mortality.[10]

Nutritional assessment has traditionally been divided into four parts: history and physical examination, anthropometric measurement, biochemical assessment of serum proteins, and evaluation of immune status. The reader is referred to a comprehensive review of nutritional assessment that addresses this topic in more depth.[11]

HISTORY AND PHYSICAL EXAMINATION

The history and physical examination should be used as a screening mechanism to identify patients who require a more thorough assessment. A history of unintentional weight loss, either chronic or acute, is usually a sign of suboptimal nutritional intake or altered metabolism. Chronic disease, GI disease, certain social factors, or an abnormal metabolic state all may be risk factors for developing malnutrition (Table 30.1). Physical signs suggestive of malnutrition include edema, decubitus ulcers, muscle wasting, poor wound healing, and glossitis. Patients with documented unintentional weight loss, chronic disease, or physical signs as described can be categorized after a comprehensive history and physical examination. This alternative to a complete nutritional assessment is to use clinical judgment during the patient history and physical. Detsky et al[2] have suggested asking a short series of questions that include information about weight loss over the previous 6 months, recent dietary intake in relation to usual patterns, presence of significant GI symptoms, and the patient's functional capacity. This technique, called *subjective global assessment*, is easier and less expensive than a comprehensive nutritional assessment.[12]

ANTHROPOMETRIC MEASUREMENTS

Anthropometric measurements are used to assess fat and somatic protein stores. The somatic protein stores include skeletal muscle and the visceral organs. Subcutaneous fat is often assessed by a series of measurements with a skinfold caliper. The most popular sites for skinfold measurement are the triceps, subscapular, and calf areas. The sum of the triceps and calf skinfolds (in mm) can be used to determine the percentage of body fat:

Table 30.1	Risk Factors for Undernutrition That Can Be Detected in a Patient History and Physical Examination
Chronic diseases	
	Renal failure
	Liver failure
	Pulmonary disease
	Congestive heart failure
	Diabetes mellitus
Gastrointestinal diseases	
	Peptic ulcer disease
	Inflammatory bowel disease
	Pancreatitis
	Short-bowel syndrome
Social factors	
	Alcohol abuse
	Drug abuse
Abnormal metabolic state	
	Cancer
	Sepsis or pneumonia
	Trauma or thermal injury

$$\text{Males (\% body fat)} = 0.735 \text{ (triceps skinfold + calf skinfold)} + 1$$
$$\text{Females (\% body fat)} = 0.610 \text{ (triceps skinfold + calf skinfold)} + 5.1 \quad (30.1)$$

This method is attractive because it is relatively noninvasive and inexpensive. The assessment of skinfold measurements can be erroneous if a patient has edema, if the equipment is not standardized, or if multiple observers are used. Also, some individuals may have very little subcutaneous fat and yet be in excellent physical condition (e.g., trained athletes such as runners or body builders).

The somatic protein compartment may be assessed indirectly by using the BMI. Arm muscle area and mid-arm muscle circumference have been used in the past to assess somatic protein but are rarely used now.

BIOCHEMICAL ASSESSMENT OF SERUM PROTEINS

Serum concentrations of several constitutive proteins have been used initially and serially during specialized nutrition support intervention. Unfortunately, other factors such as metabolic stress, hydration status, and hepatic function influence these serum concentration measurements. Although these serum markers lack sensitivity and specificity, some of them serve as good prognostic indicators of patient outcome and therefore continue to be the subject of intense study. Albumin, transferrin, and prealbumin are the constitu-

tive proteins used most frequently. Other serum proteins are being studied, but their role in nutritional assessment has not yet been determined.

Albumin is a protein with a half-life of 21 days and a large body pool compared with other secretory proteins. The normal serum concentration of albumin is 3.5 to 5 g per dL (35 to 50 g/L) in adults. A decrease in the serum concentration of albumin suggests inadequate protein intake, especially when the serum concentration is chronically depressed. Bed rest, overhydration, and transcapillary escape secondary to metabolic stress such as sepsis can all depress the serum concentration of albumin. Regardless of the cause, a depressed serum albumin concentration is associated with increased hospital morbidity and mortality. Because factors other than nutrition can lower the serum concentration of albumin, it must be interpreted cautiously when used as a nutritional marker. Its use as a prognostic indicator, however, cannot be ignored.

Transferrin, a secretory protein with a half-life of 8 days, serves as a carrier for iron. It has a much smaller body pool than albumin, and its normal serum concentration is 200 to 350 mg per dL (2 to 3.5 g/L). Because transferrin has a smaller body pool and shorter half-life than albumin, it is much more sensitive to protein–calorie deprivation or nutritional repletion. Therefore, it is used frequently in serial monitoring of patients receiving specialized nutrition support. Serum transferrin concentrations are attractive because they respond to nutritional repletion rather quickly (e.g., with weekly monitoring), are easy to measure, and are available in many institutions. Iron-deficiency anemia increases the transferrin serum concentration, while injury and sepsis depress it.[13] The normal serum concentration of prealbumin, also called thyroxine-binding prealbumin and transthyretin, is 15 to 40 mg per dL (0.15 to 0.4 g/L). It is the major carrier protein for thyroxine and retinol-binding protein and has a half-life of 2 days. Because of its short half-life and relatively small body pool, prealbumin is quite sensitive to nutritional deprivation and repletion. Many health care systems have added this laboratory test because it is inexpensive and relatively easy to perform.

The serum concentration of prealbumin rises during nutrition support, even when the nitrogen balance remains negative. The correlation between improvement in nitrogen balance and increase in serum prealbumin concentration is highly significant. Acutely stressful events such as trauma or sepsis are known to depress the serum prealbumin concentration, and chronic renal failure elevates it.

Retinol-binding protein, fibronectin, and insulin-like growth factor I have all been studied for their role in documenting nutritional repletion. Retinol-binding protein serum concentration is influenced by vitamin A status and the glomerular filtration rate. Its short half-life of 12 hours may make it too sensitive to nutritional deprivation or intake.[13] Fibronectin is a glycoprotein that is a nonspecific opsonin. It has a half-life of about 24 hours and is synthesized by the liver. Although fibronectin appears to respond positively during nutrition support, many other factors can alter its serum concentration (e.g., sepsis, trauma, shock). Insulin-like growth factor I is a growth hormone-dependent protein that possesses broad anabolic activity. The concentration correlates very well with nitrogen balance and increases during nutritional repletion.[13,14] Recent work has suggested that mitochondrial complex I activity has potential as a biochemical marker of repletion in malnourished patients.[15]

EVALUATION OF IMMUNE STATUS

The relationship between malnutrition, depressed immune status, and infection has been appreciated for years. Immune stores (total lymphocyte count) and immune function (cell-mediated immunity) are sometimes assessed in patients who require specialized nutrition support.

Immune stores are usually assessed by determining the total lymphocyte count (TLC), which includes predominantly thymus-derived lymphocytes (T-cells). The TLC is calculated from the product of the peripheral white blood cell count (WBC) and the percentage of lymphocytes:

$$\begin{aligned} \text{TLC (cells/mm}^3\text{) (10}^6 \text{ cells/L)} \\ = \text{WBC (cells/mm}^3\text{) (10}^6 \text{ cells/L)} \\ \times \text{ \% lymphocytes/100} \end{aligned} \quad (30.2)$$

A TLC above 2,000/mm³ (2,000 × 10⁶ cells/L) suggests adequate immune stores in adult patients. Immune function can be assessed by measuring the response to common antigens through skin testing. Antigens that have been used in this procedure include *Candida albicans,* mumps, streptokinase/streptodornase, tetanus, and *Trichophyton.* Most patients who have intact immune function will respond to both *Candida* and mumps skin tests, so these are the most commonly used. A positive test results in skin induration of more than 5 mm at the site of application within 24 to 48 hours.

Geriatric patients may react slowly and not demonstrate a positive response until 72 hours after application. Many other factors, such as drug therapy (e.g., steroids, histamine antagonists, anesthetic agents) and certain disease states (e.g., cancer), can interfere with the body's cell-mediated immunity, severely limiting the usefulness of these tests in the clinical setting.

BIOELECTRICAL IMPEDANCE

A promising method for assessment of lean body mass or body cell mass is bioelectric impedance analysis (BIA).[16] This noninvasive technique is based on the premise that lean tissue is an excellent electrical conductor due to its high water and electrolyte composition. When a high-frequency alternating current is passed through the human body, electrical impedance can be measured with electrodes positioned on the subject's wrist and ankle. Impedance measurements are translated into electrical reactance and resistance values, which can be used to derive body composition parameters such as lean body mass, body cell mass, body fat, and total body water.

Although further validation of this technique is needed before widespread use can be recommended, BIA does offer a safe, inexpensive, and reproducible method for evaluating body composition, especially in the outpatient setting.

TYPES OF MALNUTRITION

Marasmus is a form of undernutrition that results from chronic deprivation of protein and calories. Patients with this disorder are relatively easy to identify, as they have considerable wasting of somatic protein and fat. Their serum protein concentrations and immune status are often normal. This disorder is seen in patients who suffer from chronic disease and ingest a suboptimal amount of nutrition over a relatively long period of time. Table 30.2 contrasts the various types of malnutrition.

Kwashiorkor is traditionally classified as protein deficiency. Patients with kwashiorkor typically have adequate or excess caloric stores, as evidenced by sufficient body fat (see Table 30.2). They have depressed serum concentrations of constitutive proteins and often have depressed immune function. The most common cause of this disorder is severe metabolic stress (e.g., trauma, sepsis, thermal injury). Kwashiorkor is often difficult to diagnose at the bedside because these patients appear to be well nourished or even overnourished.

A kwashiorkor/marasmus mix results when a patient with marasmus is subjected to metabolic stress. These patients have deficits in all categories of the nutritional assessment and have the highest risk for hospital morbidity and mortality (see Table 30.2).

Table 30.2	Types of Malnutrition			
Characteristic	**Marasmus**	**Kwashiorkor**	**Kwashiorkor–Marasmus Mix**	**Obesity**
Weight for height	Decreased	Normal or increased	Decreased	Increased
Fat stores	Decreased	Increased	Decreased	Increased
Somatic protein stores	Decreased	Normal or increased	Decreased	Increased
Serum protein concentrations	Normal	Decreased	Decreased	Normal
Immune function	Normal	Decreased	Decreased	Normal

Patients with excess body weight secondary to fat are classified as obese if they are more than 20% above their ideal body weight. *Obesity* is a type of malnutrition that usually results from a prolonged increase in calories over what is needed or used. If subjected to metabolic stress, these patients can quickly develop kwashiorkor.

Because no one nutritional assessment marker effectively identifies all patients at nutritional risk and because many nonnutritional factors alter the currently used tests, investigators continue to evaluate new methods of nutritional assessment. Some of the methods that have been investigated include underwater weighing, muscle-strength testing, magnetic resonance imaging, neutron activation analysis, and radioisotope analysis. Some of these methods will be too expensive or invasive for general clinical use; however, BIA shows particular promise.

TOTAL CALORIE AND PROTEIN REQUIREMENTS

After completion of the nutritional assessment in a patient who is going to receive specialized nutrition support, the total calorie and protein goals must be determined. There continues to be controversy among nutritional support practitioners on whether nonprotein calories and protein should be separated when determining calorie goals.[17] More recently, practitioners have been dosing nutritional support using total calories, which includes the protein component. All EN products are marketed in total calories (i.e., 1 kcal/mL), so total calorie dosing is the only practical method using this nutrition intervention. By using total calories with PN, the practitioner would be using a similar method of dosing both PN and EN. The nutritional goals will be different for each patient, based on the nutritional assessment results, the purpose for initiating specialized nutrition support, and the size of the patient.

TOTAL CALORIES

The total caloric requirement for an individual patient may be predicted by several different methods. The degree of metabolic stress and any chronic disease afflicting the patient also help determine energy requirements. The most widely used method is the calculation of the basal energy expenditure (BEE) using the Harris-Benedict equations developed in 1919.[18] The BEE was developed by measuring oxygen consumption using direct calorimetry in 239 healthy male and female subjects. The two equations use the patient's gender, weight, height, and age:

$$\text{Males: BEE (kcal/day)} = 66.4730 + 13.7516\,\text{Wt} + 5.0033\,\text{Ht} - 6.7550\,\text{Age}$$
$$\text{Females: BEE (kcal/day)} = 655.0950 + 9.5630\,\text{Wt} + 1.8496\,\text{Ht} - 4.6756\,\text{Age} \quad (30.3)$$

Weight is in kilograms, height in centimeters, and age in years. BEE reflects the number of kilocalories expended during a 24-hour period in a subject at bed rest in a fasted state in a semidark room. There are several nomograms and stress factor calculations that can be used to estimate the actual resting energy expenditure (REE) of a patient with certain clinical conditions (e.g., injury). Unfortunately, when patients have multiple conditions, the estimates far exceed the actual REE in most patients. Therefore, use of these nomograms and stress factors should be abandoned. As more knowledge of the effects of disease states on caloric needs has been gained, there has been a gradual reduction in total calorie estimates to sustain health and support patients with stressful conditions.[19] A total calorie dose of 10% to 20% above the BEE should be adequate for most patients. Patients with severe trauma, major burns, or sepsis may require up to 50% more calories than the calculated BEE. Some investigators have even challenged the use of the BEE equations, since other calculated equations, like the WHO equations, have proved superior across some patient populations.[20] These equations were developed after measuring approximately 11,000 people.

$$\text{Men (18 to 30 years old): EE} = 64.4 \times \text{weight (kg)} - 113 \times \text{height (m)} + 3,000$$
$$\text{Men (30 to 60 years old): EE} = 19.2 \times \text{weight (kg)} + 66.9 \times \text{height (m)} + 3,769$$
$$\text{Women (18 to 30 years old): EE} = 55.6 \times \text{weight (kg)} + 1397.4 \times \text{height (m)} + 146$$
$$\text{Women (30 to 60 years old): EE} = 36.4 \times \text{weight (kg)} - 104.6 \times \text{height (m)} + 3,619 \quad (30.4)$$

Energy expenditure (EE) using the WHO equations above is calculated in kilojoules per day. By dividing kilojoules by 4.1, one can calculate kilocalories per day. In certain circumstances, not all the information required to calculate caloric needs using the BEE or WHO equations may be available, so an alternative method is used to determine the total calorie requirements. If the patient's weight is known, an estimated total calorie goal may be calculated. A range of 25 to 35 kcal/kg/day is generally accepted for most patients. A total caloric goal of 25 kcal/kg/day would be used for an elective surgical patient who is otherwise healthy, whereas a septic or trauma patient would require up to 35 kcal/kg/day. A severely burned patient may require as much as 40 kcal/kg/day initially.

Patients who are older or have an abnormal body size create a particular dilemma when dosing total calories by body weight. For example, infusing calories to an obese patient at 35 kcal/kg/day will result in overfeeding and potential exacerbation of the obesity. Most practitioners would use an adjusted weight (e.g., ideal body weight + 0.25 [actual body weight − ideal body weight]) for total calorie and protein dosing. Barak et al[21] have reported reasonable data in obese patients using 50% of the difference between ideal body weight and actual body weight to set caloric goals.

This would, of course, result in a higher BEE in obesity, resulting in more calories administered. Undernourished patients should always be dosed on actual body weight, never ideal body weight. Dosing of energy in pediatrics and neonates is discussed in Chapter 16. Because of gradual loss of body cell mass over time, geriatric patients require a lower dose of energy based on body weight (e.g., 25 kcal/kg/day). It may be most prudent to determine energy doses in the elderly using the BEE formulas because age is a factor in the equations.

When available, indirect calorimetry is an ideal way to measure a patient's REE. This involves using a metabolic cart and measuring the amount of oxygen consumed (V_{O_2}) and carbon dioxide produced (V_{CO_2}) over time.[22] After measuring V_{O_2} and V_{CO_2} and collecting a 24-hour urine sample for urine urea nitrogen (UUN), the complete Weir formula can be used to calculate the patient's REE:[23]

$$REE = (3.941\ V_{O_2} + 1.106\ V_{CO_2})\ 1.44 - 2.14\ UUN \quad (30.5)$$

REE is in kilocalories per day, V_{O_2} is in milliliters per minute, V_{CO_2} is in milliliters per minute, and UUN is in grams per 24 hours. If a 24-hour urine sample is obtained the same day indirect calorimetry is performed, the nitrogen data are used in the calculation. The difference between the REE obtained from the complete Weir formula and the abbreviated Weir equation (without the UUN term) is less than 2%.[23] Thus, a 24-hour urine specimen is not required for each REE determination by indirect calorimetry. Many practitioners add 10% to 30% to the measured REE to allow for movement and patient interventions during the day. This presumably provides enough energy to maintain body weight. Use of BIA for calculation of REE has been proposed and appeared to be a reasonable alternative to calculation of BEE in a small patient sample.[24]

PROTEIN

Protein requirements for an individual depend on many factors. In health, the recommended dietary allowance (RDA) for protein for an adult is 0.8 g/kg/day. In a hospital environment patients are generally stressed and thus may require higher doses of protein. Depending on the clinical status of the patient, the protein requirement may range from 0.6 to 2.2 g/kg/day. As metabolic stress increases, the protein dose required to maintain adequate protein stores increases. An elective operative procedure such as cholecystectomy results in mild stress and a modest increase in protein requirements. Patients with infections have a moderate degree of stress, while those who experience a traumatic injury or sepsis may be severely stressed.[25] Severe thermal injury may require protein doses of more than 2 g/kg/day in selected situations.

Each patient should be monitored closely to determine whether the desired response is achieved (e.g., nutritional repletion, wound healing). During periods of metabolic stress, protein turnover is markedly increased and urinary excretion of urea nitrogen is elevated, which can lead to

Table 30.3	**Nitrogen Balance Calculation**

Nitrogen balance (g/d) = Nitrogen intake (g/d) – Nitrogen output (g/d)

Nitrogen intake = protein intake (g)/6.25

Nitrogen output = [urine urea nitrogen concentration (g/L) × 24-h urine volume (L)] + 4 g

rapid erosion of the body cell mass if adequate protein is not administered. The gold standard to measure protein nutriture is nitrogen balance, with the obvious goal of achieving nitrogen equilibrium or a positive balance. This measurement is obtained by subtracting nitrogen output from nitrogen input during a 24-hour period (Table 30.3). Nitrogen input is calculated by dividing protein intake for 24 hours by 6.25 (protein is approximately 16% nitrogen). Nitrogen output is calculated by adding 4 g to the grams of urea nitrogen excreted in the urine during a 24-hour period. The 4 g represent nonmeasurable nitrogen losses such as stool losses, skin losses, and nonurea nitrogen losses in the urine. A nitrogen balance of 2 to 6 g per day suggests adequate intake of total calories and protein. A nitrogen balance between -2 and 2 g per day suggests that nitrogen equilibrium has been attained. A nitrogen balance below -2 g per day suggests that more protein or more total calories are needed.

PARENTERAL NUTRITION

Parenteral nutrition should be reserved for patients who require specialized nutrition support and who do not have a functional or accessible GI tract. With the multitude of available PN products, the practitioner needs sound guidelines so patients may receive this therapy in a safe and efficacious manner. Practice guidelines and standards have been developed by the American Society for Parenteral and Enteral Nutrition[26] and the American Gastroenterology Association.[27] The guidelines are summarized in Table 30.4. The American Society for Parenteral and Enteral Nutrition has prepared guidelines for the use of PN and EN in adult patients with cancer, acquired immune deficiency syndrome (AIDS), liver failure, renal failure, pancreatitis, respiratory failure, inflammatory bowel disease, short-bowel syndrome, intestinal pseudoobstruction, critical illness, pregnancy, neurologic impairment, and old age.[26] Pediatric nutritional needs for EN and PN are also addressed in this document.

TYPES OF PARENTERAL NUTRITION

PN may be given via a central or peripheral vein. Although central PN is more commonly used, peripheral PN is used by some institutions in certain patients.[28]

Peripheral PN can be used as a sole source of nutrition or as an adjunct to an oral or enteral diet. Generally, 900 mOsm/L is the maximum osmolality tolerated by peripheral

Table 30.4	**Parenteral Nutrition Practice Guidelines**

Patients who do not have access to the GI tract or a functioning GI tract should be considered for parenteral nutrition. This includes patients with diffuse peritonitis, paralytic ileus, intestinal obstruction, GI ischemia, or intractable vomiting or diarrhea.

Peripheral PN generally can be used for only 1 week secondary to frequent vein rotation.

Central PN should be used when PN support will be needed for more than 1 week. It is also required when nutritional requirements are elevated or fluid restriction is necessary.

Patients should be monitored by health care professionals trained to detect and treat mechanical, metabolic, and infectious complications.

The indications for home PN should be the same as for patients in the hospital requiring this method of nutrition support.

Patients receiving home PN should be reevaluated periodically for potential benefits of this therapy.

PN, parenteral nutrition; GI, gastrointestinal.
(From Guidelines for the use of parenteral and enteral nutrition in adult and pediatric patients. J Parenteral Enteral Nutr 26 : 1SA–138SA, 2002, with permission.)

veins. Actually, a solution of 600 mOsm/L is better tolerated and may lower the risk of phlebitis. The electrolytes added to PN formulations contribute substantially to the osmolality of the PN solution (e.g., NaCl 50 mEq/L contributes 100 mOsm to each liter of solution). Subtherapeutic doses of heparin or hydrocortisone or concurrent infusions of fat emulsion with peripheral PN have been used in attempts to decrease the risk of phlebitis. Peripheral PN is intended to be used for short periods of time (e.g., 5 to 7 days) as adjunctive therapy. A formulation with a final protein concentration of 3% to 5% and a dextrose concentration of 5% to 10% is commonly used for this type of therapy. It is extremely difficult to meet a patient's nutritional requirements because of the large volumes of fluid required. Also, the administration of peripheral PN has not demonstrated a significant benefit over the infusion of crystalloid, which makes this therapy questionable.[29]

Most patients receive PN via a central vein. The superior vena cava is used most often after percutaneous catheterization of the subclavian, internal, or external jugular vein. The catheter may be placed in the operating room or at the patient's bedside using sterile technique and radiographic verification. A double- or triple-lumen catheter is used most often because patients who require PN often receive other IV medications or blood products. This provides access for the additional IV infusions without interrupting the administration of the PN. By having the catheter tip placed into the superior vena cava, concentrated substrates may be infused because of the high rate of blood flow in this vein. Thus, required nutrients may be delivered in relatively small volumes without causing thrombophlebitis. This method is par-

ticularly effective in patients who have large energy and protein requirements or who require fluid restriction. If the catheter is properly cared for, it can be used indefinitely.

PARENTERAL NUTRITION FORMULATION COMPONENTS

Protein. The initial protein products used in PN formulations were hydrolysates of naturally occurring proteins (fibrin, casein). Today, commercially available forms of parenteral protein are provided as crystalline amino acids. If protein is oxidized for energy, it will yield 4 kcal/g. Patients undergoing severe metabolic stress may require large doses of protein and actually use it as a preferential calorie source. Currently marketed amino acid products in the United States are provided as standard or modified amino acids. Standard amino acid products are used for patients with normal organ function and relatively normal nutritional needs. The modified amino acid formulations are marketed for patients with hepatic failure, renal failure, fluid restriction, or metabolic stress. Currently available amino acid products for adult parenteral nutrition are listed in Table 30.5. The standard amino acid formulas are composed of physiologic mixtures of essential and nonessential amino acids. Although these products are commercially available in several concentrations, many institutions are now stocking only the 15% or 20% concentrations because lower concentrations can easily be made by adding sterile water via an automated compounder. These products are marketed with or without maintenance electrolytes.

Patients with severe liver failure develop many metabolic abnormalities, including disturbances in electrolyte and amino acid homeostasis. Some of these patients develop hepatic encephalopathy associated with decreased concentrations of branched-chain amino acids (BCAA) and elevated concentrations of aromatic amino acids (AAA) and methionine. The BCAAs include leucine, isoleucine, and valine, and the AAAs are phenylalanine, tyrosine, and tryptophan. In the absence of encephalopathy, liver failure patients who require PN may be maintained on standard amino acids. However, when hepatic encephalopathy is severe (grade 3 or 4), the modified amino acid formula for hepatic failure

Table 30.5	**Parenteral Amino Acid Categories and Products**
Patient Category	**Product Examples**
Standard	Aminosyn II, Travasol, FreAmine III
Fluid-restricted	Aminosyn II 15%, Clinasol 15%, Prosol 20%
Liver failure	HepatAmine, Hepatasol
Renal failure	Aminosyn RF, NephrAmine, RenAmin, Aminess
Metabolic stress	BranchAmin, Aminosyn-HBC, FreAmine HBC

may be used. Generally, patients should meet one of the following criteria to receive the modified amino acid: hepatic encephalopathy above grade 2 or hepatic encephalopathy associated with PN formulations containing standard amino acid solutions in doses needed for nutritional support. The modified amino acid formula contains high concentration of BCAAs and low concentrations of AAAs and methionine. Although normalization of the amino acid profile has been shown with this product, an improvement in overall patient outcome has not been uniformly demonstrated in clinical trials. One randomized clinical trial[30] found a decrease in hepatic encephalopathy scores and a lower prevalence of mortality in patients receiving this formulation, while another study failed to show any difference in encephalopathy scores and mortality with this product.[31]

Patients with severe renal failure also have several metabolic changes, including electrolyte alterations and protein intolerance. Those who are not undergoing dialysis should have their daily protein dose restricted to 0.6 to 0.8 g/kg/day. Acute renal failure patients undergoing hemodialysis may be given 1.2 to 1.4 g protein/kg/day, while peritoneal dialysis patients may receive 1.2 to 1.5 g protein/kg/day. Patients receiving continuous renal replacement therapy (e.g., continuous venovenous hemodialysis) may receive protein doses in the range of 1.2 to 2 g/kg/day if clinically indicated. Modified amino acids for renal failure, which contain primarily essential amino acids, are more expensive than standard amino acids and have not demonstrated clinical benefit over standard amino acids.[32] Thus, patients with severe renal failure should be given standard amino acids as part of PN.

Some critically ill patients who require PN are markedly fluid-overloaded. In these patients, it is usually beneficial to use the smallest possible volume to deliver PN. Commercially available 15% and 20% amino acid products can be used to concentrate the PN formula in patients with overhydration or edema.

Patients who are highly stressed have altered energy and protein metabolism. These patients take up BCAAs into skeletal muscle for energy. This has led to the development of modified amino acid products with enhanced concentrations of the BCAAs. These products have been proposed to stimulate protein synthesis, decrease protein catabolism, and serve as a preferential fuel source. The many clinical trials using amino acids with an enhanced BCAA content have produced equivocal results. Some suggest that patients receiving these modified amino acids have decreased skeletal muscle catabolism and enhanced protein synthesis.[33] In contrast, other studies have found a lack of clinical benefit when BCAA-enriched solutions were compared with standard amino acids.[34] Given the expense of the products and the equivocal results of clinical trials, careful evaluation is needed before using these products.

Carbohydrate. The nonprotein energy source in PN solutions may be carbohydrate only or a combination of carbohydrate and fat. The carbohydrate component of the nutrient solutions is usually dextrose. Other carbohydrates such as xylitol, fructose, or sorbitol have been studied but have not gained wide acceptance in the United States. Each gram of hydrated dextrose provides 3.4 kcal. Dextrose stock solutions of 5% to 70% are available for use in PN solutions. Many institutions purchase only the 70% dextrose solution because dilutions can be made using an automated compounder and sterile water. Generally, dextrose infusions should not exceed 5 mg/kg/min (25 kcal/kg/day) during PN.[35] This appears to be the maximum rate of glucose oxidation by the human body. Rates above 5 mg/kg/min can be associated with lipogenesis, increased carbon dioxide production, and hepatic steatosis. Many clinicians use dosages of dextrose of 3 to 4 mg/kg/minute (15 to 20 kcal/kg/day) in PN formulations, especially in glucose-intolerant patients.

An advisory group of nutrition support pharmacists have prepared an excellent report on the safe practices for prescribing, labeling, and compounding PN formulations.[36] Information regarding PN stability, compatibility, and filtration is also included in this report. Dosage ranges for dextrose and total calories in adults, children, and neonates receiving PN are included in this report.

Overfeeding patients with dextrose via PN continues to be a problem in acute care institutions, especially academic medical centers where there are multiple inexperienced prescribers.[37] In one study of PN patients, hyperglycemia was noted in 49% of patients given dextrose at a rate of more than 5 mg/kg/minute, compared to 11% and 0% in patients given dextrose at rates of 4 to 5 mg/kg/minute and less than 4 mg/kg/minute, respectively.[38] Van Den Berghe et al[39] have provided data in a large clinical trial that support aggressive control of hyperglycemia in critically ill patients receiving nutrition support: mortality and the incidence of acute renal failure and bacteremia were significantly lower in the group receiving intensive regular insulin therapy.

Fat. The first IV fat emulsion product introduced into the United States contained cottonseed oil, but it was removed from the U.S. market in 1965 because of severe adverse reactions. Today, commercially available fat emulsions contain soybean oil or combinations of soybean and safflower oils. Fat emulsions should be given as part of a patient's PN regimen to prevent essential fatty acid deficiency or to serve as a calorie source. Essential fatty acid deficiency has both biochemical and clinical signs. Biochemical evidence usually becomes apparent within 1 to 3 weeks after fat-free parenteral nutrition is started. Biochemical evidence includes increased serum concentrations of saturated fatty acids, decreased concentrations of essential fatty acids, and a triene:tetraene ratio greater than 0.4. Clinical evidence of essential fatty acid deficiency does not usually appear until several weeks of fat-free PN has been given. Manifestations of essential fatty acid deficiency include thrombocytopenia, delayed wound healing, fatty liver, alopecia, and dry, thick, desquamating skin.

IV fat emulsions provide a concentrated source of calories (9 kcal/g of fat) and can correct or prevent essential fatty acid deficiency. Absolute contraindications to the administration of fat emulsions include pathologic hyperlipidemia, lipoid nephrosis, severe egg allergy, and acute pancreatitis associated with hyperlipidemia. Patients with acute pancreatitis who do not have hyperlipidemia may receive IV fat emulsions safely. Fat emulsions should be used cautiously in patients with severe liver disease, acute respiratory distress syndrome, or blood coagulation disorders. Most clinicians recommend administration of about 30% of the total calories as fat, with the remainder being carbohydrate and protein. The usual adult daily dose of fat is 0.5 to 1 g/kg/day, with the maximum dose being 2.5 g/kg/day; however, the maximum dose is rarely used in clinical practice. Table 30.6 lists commercially available fat emulsions, which are composed of mainly long-chain triglycerides. Fat emulsion products are marketed in concentrations of 10% (1.1 kcal/mL), 20% (2 kcal/mL), and 30% (3 kcal/mL). The 30% product is not approved for direct infusion into patients in the United States, but only for preparation of total nutrient admixtures. The 10% and 20% products can be infused at a maximum rate of 125 mL per hour and 60 mL per hour, respectively, but they are rarely given that fast. The 20% product is favored because of the lower phospholipid/triglyceride ratio. Currently, most clinicians infuse the daily dose of fat over a 12-hour period as a continuous infusion or as a component of a total nutrient admixture. The lipid emulsions contain varying amounts of the essential fatty acids, egg yolk phospholipid as an emulsifying agent, and glycerin, which makes the products isotonic.

If administered in the recommended doses, IV fat emulsions are very safe. Most side effects are due to the administration of excessive doses of fat emulsions or excessive rates of infusion. Adverse reactions include nausea and vomiting, headache, fever, chills, chest or back pain, and irritation at the infusion site. Reactions that may be associated with long-term use include hepatomegaly, jaundice, splenomegaly, and thrombocytopenia. Considerable controversy exists surrounding the ability of IV fat emulsions to modify immune function. Because of the complexity associated with induction and control of the immune system, fat emulsions may alter different components of the immune response. Some studies suggested that IV fat emulsions impair the bactericidal and migratory functions of polymorphonuclear cells and decrease bacterial clearance by the mononuclear phagocyte system. Biochemical mediators derived from the omega-6 family of fatty acids may induce inflammation and immunosuppression, while metabolic end products from the omega-3 fatty acids may produce the opposite effects. One clinical study in trauma patients receiving PN suggested an increase in morbidity, mechanical ventilation, and hospital stay in patients receiving IV fat emulsions as part of PN compared to a similar group receiving PN without fat.[40] It is not clear whether the fat in the control group or the higher calorie dose was responsible for the difference in clinical outcome. This type of study needs to be confirmed. Other types of fats can also have unique and potent effects on the immune system. Medium-chain triglycerides may have less immunosuppressive properties and serve as more rapidly available and high-energy lipid fuel sources than traditional IV fat emulsions.[41] Currently, fat emulsion products are being developed that contain different fatty acid profiles, designed for better utilization of fat. Fat emulsions containing medium-chain triglycerides, omega-3 fatty acids, short-chain triglycerides, or carnitine may become available after clinical trials are completed. Most likely, these new products will be marketed as a physical mixture of the different triglycerides (e.g., long-chain triglyceride 25%, medium-chain triglyceride 75%) or as a structured triglyceride. A structured triglyceride has different fatty acids attached to the glycerol backbone in distinct proportions (e.g., two medium-chain fatty acids and one long-chain fatty acid on each glycerol).

Electrolytes. Electrolytes in maintenance or therapeutic doses must be added to the PN daily to maintain electrolyte homeostasis (Table 30.7). Requirements for individual electrolytes vary, depending on many factors in a patient's clinical course.[36] Electrolyte imbalance may arise from insufficient intake, extraordinary losses, or a combination of both. Patients receiving PN may have large renal or extrarenal losses of electrolytes and fluid. Extrarenal electrolyte losses may include losses from diarrhea, vomiting, ostomies, fistulas, or nasogastric suctioning. In addition, various pharmacotherapeutic interventions may decrease or increase individual electrolyte requirements. For example, sodium ticarcillin administration delivers a substantial amount of sodium to the patient and causes renal potassium wasting. Amphotericin B therapy increases magnesium and potassium renal losses. Relative electrolyte deficiencies may develop as a result of intracellular shifts of electrolytes from the extracellular fluid compartments. For instance, intracellular

Table 30.6 | IV Fat Emulsion Products

Product	Strength (%)	Kcal/mL[a]	Source
Intralipid	10	1.1	Soybean oil
Intralipid	20	2	Soybean oil
Intralipid[b]	30	3	Soybean oil
Liposyn-II	10	1.1	Soybean oil 50%, safflower oil 50%
Liposyn-II	20	2	Soybean oil 50%, safflower oil 50%
Liposyn-III	10	1.1	Soybean oil
Liposyn-III	20	2	Soybean oil

[a] Glycerol is added to all IV fat emulsions and contributes some calories to the respective products.
[b] The 30% lipid product can be used only for the preparation of total nutrient admixtures in the United States.

Table 30.7	Electrolytes Available for Additives to Parenteral Nutrition Formulations	
Salt	**Preparation**	**Concentration**
Sodium	Phosphate	3 mmol/mL
		4 mEq Na/mL
Sodium	Chloride	2 mEq/mL
Sodium	Acetate	2 mEq/mL
Potassium	Phosphate	3 mmol/mL
		4.4 mEq K/mL
Potassium	Chloride	2 mEq/mL
Potassium	Acetate	2 mEq/mL
Calcium	Gluconate	4.6 mEq/10 mL
Magnesium	Sulfate	4 mEq/mL

shifts of potassium occur during metabolic alkalosis because intracellular hydrogen ions are exchanged for extracellular potassium ions. Also, refeeding chronically starved patients results in an intracellular shift of potassium, phosphorus, and magnesium.[42]

Electrolytes are available as single- or multiple-entity products. Once the phosphorus dose has been determined and added, the remaining anions are given as chloride or acetate salts. Patients with metabolic acidosis should have the majority of electrolytes added as acetate salts, while patients with metabolic alkalosis should have most salts added as chloride.

Vitamins/Trace Elements. Vitamins are an essential component of a patient's daily PN regimen, as they are necessary for normal metabolism and cellular function. There are four fat-soluble and nine water-soluble vitamins recognized as essential. The American Medical Association Nutrition Advisory Group established guidelines for daily parenteral administration of vitamins during PN in 1975.[43] The revised recommendations emanated from a workshop in 1985 but were not published until 2000 in the Federal Register.[44] Several modifications were recommended and a daily dose of vitamin K was added. The suggested amounts for daily administration have been summarized recently[45] and appear in Table 30.8. There currently are two commercial manufacturers of multiple-entity vitamin products that are used for daily administration in PN formulations. Patients not receiving anticoagulants may receive vitamin K as phytonadione 250 μg per day during PN if the 12-vitamin product is used. Many of the vitamins are available as single-entity products that can be used for patients with documented vitamin deficiencies. The United States experienced two prolonged periods of parenteral multivitamin shortage during the 1990s that required rationing of these products.

Trace elements are also a necessary part of a daily PN solution. Trace elements are metabolic cofactors essential to the proper functioning of several enzyme systems in the body. Suggested amounts for zinc, copper, chromium, manganese, and selenium appear in Table 30.9.[36] Zinc requirements are increased in metabolic stress or with large GI losses. Zinc, chromium, and selenium are excreted by the kidneys, while manganese and copper are excreted through the biliary tract. Therefore, patients with cholestatic liver disease should have copper and manganese restricted or withheld from the PN solution. There is evidence that manganese can accumulate in the brain with chronic administration of standard doses of this trace element in home PN patients.[46] This has led to a lower recommended dose of 80 μg per day in patients receiving long-term PN.[36] The trace

Table 30.8	Recommended Adult IV Dosages of Vitamins and Commercially Available Products			
Vitamin	**Recommendations of 1975 Conference**	**MVI-12**	**Recommendations of 1985 Conference**	**Infuvite Adult MVI-Adult**
Vitamin A (IU)	3,300	3,300	3,300	3,300
Vitamin D (IU)	200	200	200	200
Vitamin E (IU)	10	10	10	10
Vitamin K (μg)	–	–	150	150
Thiamine (mg)	3	3	6	6
Riboflavin (mg)	3.6	3.6	3.6	3.6
Niacin (mg)	40	40	40	40
Pantothenic acid (mg)	15	15	15	15
Pyridoxine (mg)	4	4	6	6
Cyanocobalamin (μg)	5	5	5	5
Folic acid (μg)	400	400	600	600
Biotin (μg)	60	60	60	60
Ascorbic acid (mg)	100	100	200	200

Table 30.9	Recommended Adult IV Dosages of Trace Elements
Trace Element	**Daily IV Dosage**
Zinc	2.5–5 mg
Copper	0.3–0.5 mg
Chromium	10–15 μg
Manganese	60–100 μg
Selenium	20–60 μg

(From ASPEN Board of Directors and the Clinical Guidelines Task Force. Guidelines for the use of parenteral and enteral nutrition in adult and pediatric patients. J Parenteral Enteral Nutr 26:1SA–138SA, 2002, with permission.)

elements are available as single- or multiple-entity products for admixture into PN formulations. Parenteral guidelines for molybdenum and iodine have not been established; however, these trace elements are available commercially.

TOTAL NUTRIENT ADMIXTURES

In the past, PN formulations consisted of an admixture of dextrose and protein (two-in-one); however, IV fat is being added to these solutions at some health system pharmacies. The IV admixture of dextrose, amino acids, and fat emulsion is known as a total nutrient admixture (TNA). IV fat is a water-in-oil emulsion stabilized by the anionic emulsifier egg yolk phospholipid. When properly prepared, the TNA is stable for at least 48 hours. The use of TNAs has several advantages over two-in-one formulations. It may decrease the risk of infection because fewer central-line manipulations are involved. It also decreases the time spent by the nursing staff in PN administration. In addition, lipids mixed with dextrose and amino acids do not support bacterial growth as well as the fat emulsion alone. By giving the fat emulsion slowly and continuously over a 24-hour period (as a component of the TNA), there is improved oxidation of the lipids and less potential for immunosuppression from the long-chain triglycerides.

Despite these advantages, there are some concerns about TNAs. It is not possible to detect particulate matter in a TNA. Also, because the fat particles are fairly large, the TNA cannot be filtered with a 0.22-micron filter (but they can be filtered with a 1.2-micron filter). Also, it is difficult knowing the particle size before the emulsion actually cracks. Furthermore, only a few medications are known to be compatible with and can be added to the TNAs. Drugs known to be compatible include cimetidine, ranitidine, famotidine, heparin, and insulin. There is also potential for increased waste using this method of PN administration because most pharmacies prepare one bag for each 24-hour period.

The method of preparation of a TNA is important to ensure stability.[36] Creaming and coalescence of the fat emulsion results when electrolytes are added directly to it. The anionic emulsifier in the fat emulsion may be adversely affected by divalent cations and acidifying agents. Therefore, limitations exist on the doses of divalent cations that may be added to the TNA. Adding these electrolytes beyond the recommended amounts will neutralize the negative potential at the surface of the emulsion and cause the admixture to coalesce.

PRESCRIBING AND LABELING

The National Advisory Group on Standards and Practice Guidelines for Parenteral Nutrition also addressed the prescribing and labeling of PN formulations.[36] It is suggested that all PN formulation labels be standardized by showing the amounts of macronutrients, electrolytes, micronutrients, and medications given per day. For health care systems that prescribe by amounts per liter, the daily amount should be listed first, followed by an amount per liter in parentheses. When IV fat emulsion is infused as a separate entity, a label listing product, strength, volume, g/kg, and g is proposed. This proposed standardization should be particularly useful as patients move across health care environments (i.e., hospital, extended care facility, clinic, home).

COMPLICATIONS

The complications of PN support may be divided into three broad categories: infectious, technical, and metabolic. Catheter-related sepsis, the most common infectious complication, may occur as a result of contamination during line placement or poor catheter care. Catheter sepsis can be minimized by following a strict protocol for line insertion and catheter care. Many institutions have nutrition support nurses who assist in line placement and perform the central catheter dressing changes.

Technical complications, such as pneumothorax, hydrothorax, and arterial puncture, may occur during placement of the catheter. Proper training and careful technique minimize the chance of these technical complications. Several metabolic complications may occur. Fluid overload may occur because patients receiving PN often require several other IV fluids. Metabolic acidosis and metabolic alkalosis occur with relative frequency in critically ill patients who receive PN. Metabolic complications related to the carbohydrate component of PN include hyperglycemia, hyperosmolar coma, and adverse effects of overfeeding. Hyperglycemia is usually identified by frequent monitoring of serum glucose concentrations. This complication may be managed by adding insulin to the PN formulation, by decreasing the dextrose concentration in the PN, or by decreasing the infusion rate. As discussed earlier in this chapter, normal or near-normal glucose concentrations during PN should be a goal.[39] This has resulted in increased use of regular insulin infusions to maintain glucose homeostasis. Carbohydrate overfeeding may cause excess carbon dioxide production, leading to respira-

Table 30.10	Guidelines for Monitoring Patients Receiving Parenteral Nutrition

Fingersticks for glucose q6h initially. Patients who are glucose-intolerant and/or receiving an insulin infusion should be monitored more frequently.

Use sliding scale or insulin infusions with regular human insulin.

Measure total fluid intake and output daily.

Weigh patient at least once per week if possible.

Draw serum for serum concentrations of prealbumin or transferrin once per week.

Draw serum for comprehensive metabolic panel at least once per week, basic metabolic panel daily in the ICU.

Draw serum for magnesium and phosphorus at least two times per week.

Collect a 24-hour urine sample for nitrogen balance determination once per week in the ICU.

tory acidosis, elevations of liver function test results, and hepatic steatosis. These problems can usually be avoided with a dextrose infusion rate of 5 mg/kg/min or less (25 kcal/kg/day).[35] Disorders may occur with virtually all of the electrolytes. Malnourished patients who begin PN often experience hypokalemia and hypophosphatemia secondary to the intracellular shift of those ions, induced by dextrose. Vitamin and trace element disorders may also occur (e.g., vitamin A toxicity during PN in patients with renal failure and decreased serum zinc concentrations in severe metabolic stress). The doses of these micronutrients may be increased or decreased as necessary to alleviate metabolic complications.

MONITORING

Because many metabolic complications may occur in patients receiving PN support, patients should be monitored daily. Table 30.10 lists guidelines for monitoring patients receiving PN.

DRUG COMPATIBILITY

By using the PN formulation as a drug vehicle, the overall amount of fluid administered and the number of IV line manipulations are decreased. Patients who are fluid-restricted, receive home PN, or have limited venous access may benefit from receiving their medications in the PN formulation.

Drugs that are added to the PN formulation must be physically and chemically stable in it. It is not wise to add a drug to these formulations when frequent dosage changes are anticipated. When no dosage changes are anticipated, pharmacodynamic actions are consistent with continuous delivery, and the drug is physically compatible, addition to the PN formulation is reasonable. The amino acid concentration, the pH of the solution, and the ambient room temperature all may affect the stability of the drug added to PN formulations. Also, drugs added to the PN formulation may have an adverse effect on selected nutrients. Heparin, regular human insulin, and most histamine-2 receptor antagonists are compatible in TNAs. Iron dextran, metoclopramide, human albu-

min, theophylline, heparin, regular human insulin, and histamine-2 receptor antagonists are compatible in two-in-one PN formulations.

Numerous studies have been conducted on calcium and phosphorus compatibility in PN formulations. A number of factors may contribute to calcium/phosphate precipitation, such as the respective amounts of calcium and phosphorus additives, the pH of the PN formulations, the concentration of the amino acid solution, and the order of mixing the minerals used for preparation of PN admixtures. An FDA safety alert cautioned that improper preparation of TNAs with automated compounding systems may result in calcium phosphate precipitates.[47] Life-threatening hazards such as microvascular pulmonary emboli and subacute interstitial pneumonitis have been linked to calcium/phosphate precipitates from improperly prepared PN formulations. Recommendations for proper compounding of TNAs have been suggested by the National Advisory Group on Standards and Practice Guidelines for Parenteral Nutrition (Table 30.11). Generally, solutions with amino acid concentrations of more than 2.5% and a pH of less than 6 favor solubility of calcium and phosphorous. Some studies have reported incompatibilities between therapeutic doses of iron and fat. Human albumin is reported to be compatible in most two-in-one solutions and TNAs by some manufacturers (e.g., Abbott). There is a lack of data on albumin compatibility with TNAs by other manufacturers.

Table 30.11	Summary of Recommendations for Extemporaneous Compounding and Filtration of Parenteral Nutrition Admixtures

Optimize additive sequence and validate as safe and efficacious.

Review manual methods of compounding regularly and when contracts with macronutrient manufacturers change.

Manufacturers of automated compounders should provide an additive sequence that ensures safety.

Whenever a question of compatibility arises, it is best to obtain information from a recent text on IV admixtures. If no data exist on a particular combination, the safest approach is not to add the medication to the PN formulation, but to administer it separately.

ENTERAL NUTRITION

The use of EN dates back to the ancient Egyptians, who used nutritional enemas to preserve health. Enteral nutrition by tube has been mentioned and used over the subsequent centuries; however, only during the past 35 years has it been used safely and effectively in acute and chronic care settings.

Most practitioners believe that if the GI tract is functional and accessible, it should be used for the delivery of specialized nutrition support. The development of new feeding tubes, modern equipment for administration, surgically placed enterostomies, and sophisticated enteral formulas have greatly improved this method of administering nutrients. Enteral feeding by tube is thought to preserve the GI mass and possibly maintain the immune status of this organ. When compared to EN, PN has been associated with sepsis and multiple organ dysfunction syndrome in critically ill patients. Consequently, practitioners in specialized nutrition support are making extraordinary efforts to deliver enteral nutrients to critically ill patients.

Practice guidelines published by the American Society for Parenteral and Enteral Nutrition address the rational use of EN too.[26] A summary of these recommendations appears in Table 30.12. EN should not be used when the GI tract is not functional (e.g., postoperative ileus) or when enteral nutrients are undesirable (e.g., severe acute pancreatitis).

Table 30.12	EN Practice Guidelines

Requires a functioning and accessible GI tract

Can be administered into the stomach, duodenum, or jejunum

Full EN support can usually be attained in 2 to 3 days

EN administration maintains the mucosal structure and function of the GI tract

EN is more cost effective than parenteral nutrition

EN administration is associated with pulmonary, GI, mechanical, and metabolic complications

Metabolic complications of EN can be reduced when patients are managed by a multidisciplinary team

EN should be initiated within 7 to 14 days in a patient with inadequate oral intake

EN, enteral nutrition.
(From ASPEN Board of Directors and the Clinical Guidelines Task Force. Guidelines for the use of parenteral and enteral nutrition in adult and pediatric patients. J Parenteral Enteral Nutr 26:1SA–138SA, 2002, with permission.)

TYPES OF ENTERAL FEEDING DELIVERY

There are many ways to deliver enteral nutrients into the GI tract, and EN can be delivered safely and efficaciously in most patients, as either short- or long-term therapy (Fig. 30.1). Nasogastric or nasoduodenal feeding tubes are used for patients who need enteral access for a short-term period (e.g., a few weeks). These soft, small-bore tubes have virtually replaced the large nasogastric tube, which is now only used for nasogastric suction. These tubes, made of polyurethane or silicone, have several advantages over the large nasogastric tubes. Most of them have a weighted tip, which facilitates transpyloric passage of the tube into the small bowel. Irritation to the nose, pharynx, and esophagus is decreased when these smaller tubes are used compared to larger, more rigid nasogastric tubes. Also, patients may eat food and swallow without difficulty when these softer tubes are used. These tubes are usually packaged with a stylet, which aids in proper placement during intubation.

A surgical gastrostomy provides enteral access for long-term EN therapy (months to years). The nutrients are infused directly into the stomach via the gastrostomy tube, bypassing the mouth, pharynx, and esophagus. The Stamm gastrostomy and percutaneous endoscopic gastrostomy (PEG) are the two most common types of gastrostomies for long-term use. The Stamm gastrostomy is usually done by a general surgeon in the operating room, using general anesthesia. PEGs are done by general surgeons or gastroenterologists in a surgical suite or at the bedside, using local anesthesia. Jejunostomies for enteral feeding administration are done for both short-term and long-term access.[48] A tube jejunostomy is placed during laparotomy and can be used for long-term enteral access. This type of jejunostomy is particularly effective in a patient who has severe, chronic gastroparesis (e.g., some diabetics). When supplemental enteral feedings are no longer needed and the patient is taking adequate nutrients by mouth, the jejunostomy can be removed at the bedside without surgical intervention.

ENTERAL NUTRITION PRODUCTS

Currently, more than 200 enteral products are marketed in the United States. Most health care systems that are involved in the administration of these products develop formularies by creating several categories and stocking one product in each one. Table 30.13 lists 14 categories of enteral formulas and gives examples in each category. Patients with normal fluid requirements, normal nutritional needs, and normal electrolyte status can usually be treated with isotonic, nutritionally complete formulas. Several institutions use products with added dietary fiber as their standard enteral formula in the conditions above, presumably for improved GI tolerance. Patients who are eating part of their diet orally can often be supplemented through ingestion of 8 to 32 ounces of an oral enteral supplement. This obviates placement of an enteral feeding tube. Fluid-restricted enteral formulas are reserved for patients who have a problem with overhydration and edema (e.g., congestive heart failure). These products are

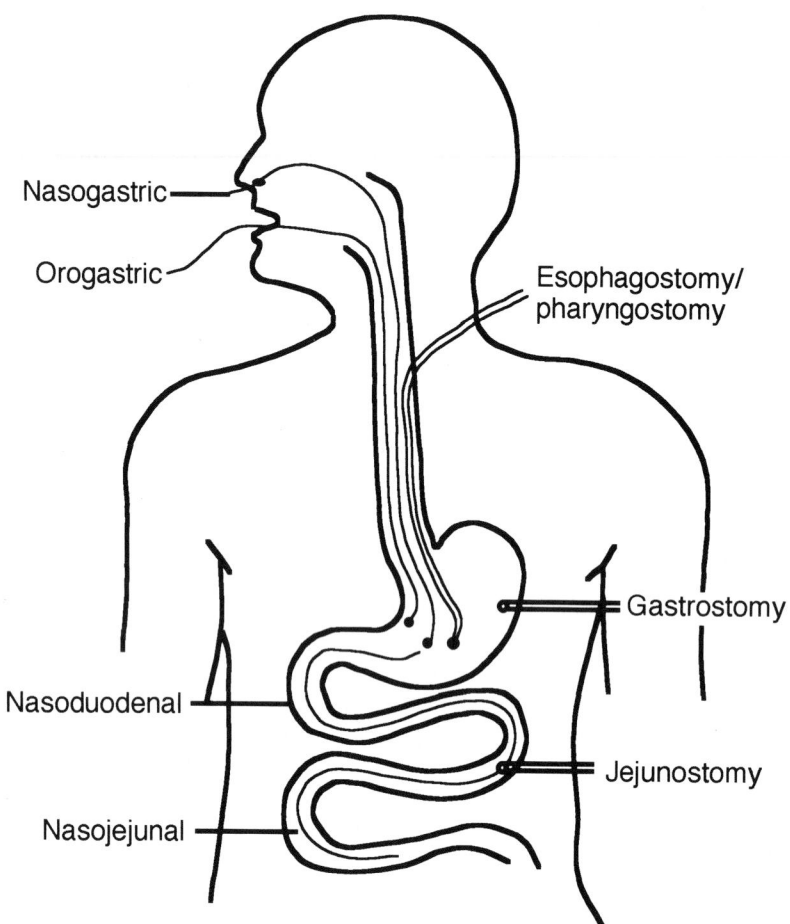

FIGURE 30.1 Enteral nutrition access sites. Enteral access can be obtained at the bedside or in a surgical suite. Nasogastric and orogastric feeding tubes are usually placed at the bedside. Placement of nasoduodenal or nasojejunal tubes usually requires fluoroscopy or esophagogastroduodenoscopy. Percutaneous endoscopic gastrostomy tubes may be placed under local anesthesia at the bedside or in an endoscopy suite. Open gastrostomy or jejunostomy requires an operative procedure.

Table 30.13	Categories of Enteral Formulations with Examples	
Isotonic tube feeding	Isocal, Osmolite
Standard tube feeding with fiber	Jevity, Ultracal, Fibersource
Oral supplements	Ensure, Boost
Fluid-restricted tube feeding	Novasource 2, Two-Cal-HN
Chemically defined tube feeding (elemental)	Vivonex TEN, Vital-HN
Low-protein, low-electrolyte or electrolyte-free tube feeding (acute renal failure)	RenalCal, Suplena
Regular-protein, low-electrolyte tube feeding (renal failure with dialysis)	Nepro, Novasource Renal
Modified protein for hepatic failure with encephalopathy	Hepatic-Aid, Nutrihep
Low-carbohydrate, high-fat tube feeding (diabetes)	Resource Diabetic, Choice-DM, Glucerna, Pulmocare
High-protein tube feeding	Promote, TraumaCal
High-protein with fiber tube feeding	Promote with fiber, Isosource-VHN, Fibersource-HN
Immune-enhancing tube feeding	Immun-Aid, Perative, Impact-Glutamine
High-fat with omega-3 fatty acids and antioxidants tube feeding	Oxepa
Protein supplement	ProMod, Proteinex

extremely low in free water and are potentially dangerous in a patient who does not need severe fluid restriction. When GI digestive capabilities are compromised, a chemically defined or elemental enteral formula is often used because most of the nutrients are in elemental or predigested form. Elemental formulations are generally reserved for patients with chronic pancreatitis or early short-bowel syndrome. Several products are marketed for patients with renal failure, liver failure, respiratory failure, diabetes, compromised immune function, and severe metabolic stress (see Table 30.13). These products are more expensive than standard enteral formulas. When a patient's specific needs cannot be met with commercially available enteral formulations, specific macronutrients (carbohydrate, fat, protein) can be added to these formulas to meet special needs.

ADMINISTRATION OF ENTERAL FEEDINGS

There are essentially three ways to administer enteral feeding to institutionalized or home-bound patients: continuous, intermittent, and bolus. Continuous feeding, used preferentially in the institutionalized patient, involves an enteral pump so that the formula can be infused at a constant rate. The advantages of this method are less risk of aspiration, less nursing time, decreased GI distention, and decreased diarrhea. Continuous feeding is more sophisticated and more expensive than the other methods. Intermittent feeding is used in the home setting and in some extended-care facilities. The desired volume of formula (usually 240 to 480 mL) is infused over a short period of time (e.g., 1 hour), several times each day. Bolus feeding consists of rapid administration of the desired volume of formula into the patient's ostomy tube. This method is most often used in the home-bound patient who has a gastrostomy tube in place. When bolus feedings are administered into the stomach, the risk of aspiration, gastric distention, and diarrhea is higher. The bolus method is, however, the simplest method of administering enteral nutrients, making it attractive in the home setting. In general, bolus feedings should not be given via jejunostomy.

EN is usually started at a slow rate that is increased gradually over time to the desired goal. Most adult patients can tolerate an initial rate of 25 to 50 mL per hour. The isotonic formulas can often be started at 50 mL per hour, while the more concentrated formulas (2 kcal/mL) are started at 25 mL per hour. Patients who are slowly regaining bowel function should be started at a more conservative rate (e.g., 25 mL/hour or less). Many institutions advance the infusion rate of the enteral nutrition formula by 25 mL/hour/day when GI tolerance and fluid/electrolyte status are acceptable. This enables most patients to achieve the desired rate within 3 to 4 days. There is little evidence supporting dilution of hyperosmolar formulas to enhance GI tolerance. In fact, in one study patients who received an undiluted hyperosmolar enteral formula received more calories and protein without any increase in GI side effects than groups receiving diluted hyperosmolar formulas or isotonic formulas.[49] Therefore, the use of diluted enteral formulas (e.g., half-strength) should be abandoned.

COMPLICATIONS

The complications of EN support can be divided into four categories: pulmonary, GI, mechanical, and metabolic.[50] Aspiration of EN formula into the lungs is a serious complication of this type of therapy. It occurs in the patient who has developed vomiting or impaired gastric emptying. This serious complication often results in pneumonia, requiring mechanical ventilation in an intensive care unit. Frequent examination of the abdomen and meticulous checking of gastric residuals aspirated through the feeding tube may help to identify patients at risk for aspiration. Prokinetic drugs such as metoclopramide and erythromycin have been used with some success in patients who have poor gastric emptying of EN formulas. Diabetics and patients who have sepsis are particularly prone to delayed gastric emptying.

GI complications include vomiting, diarrhea, and constipation. Vomiting can usually be prevented by advancing the enteral feeding rate slowly, as described earlier, and checking the patient's abdomen often. Most institutions elevate the head of the patient's bed at least 30 degrees in gastric-fed patients. Diarrhea is a frequent problem in patients who receive EN support, but its cause is often elusive. Patients who have their enteral nutrient rate decreased by half often demonstrate decreased diarrhea.[51] The rate may then be gradually increased to the desired goal, as tolerated.

Suggested causes of diarrhea in association with enteral tube feeding include antibiotic administration, hypoalbuminemia, hyperosmolar formulas, lactase deficiency, and lack of a nutrition support team. The authors of an excellent report carefully examined diarrhea in tube-fed patients and found hyperosmolar drug solutions containing sorbitol to be the most likely cause.[52] Therefore, all drugs administered via the GI tract should be inspected in patients who have diarrhea associated with EN. Some patients demonstrate decreased stool volume and frequency when they are switched from a standard enteral formula to a chemically defined formula. Pharmacologic agents such as kaolin pectin may be helpful as first-line pharmacotherapy. Loperamide and diphenoxylate should be used as a last resort in treating diarrhea.

A severe GI complication of EN via jejunostomy is pneumatosis intestinalis with bowel infarction/necrosis. This has been reported to occur in up to 5% of patients receiving EN by this route. It appears that this is a complication of critically ill patients who are hemodynamically unstable (e.g., patients with hypotension and tachycardia who are receiving IV pressor agents) and fed via jejunostomy.[53] Regular abdominal examinations of patients receiving feedings by this route and stopping EN during periods of instability are prudent approaches to help prevent this complication.

Constipation is often a complication of long-term EN. It is often managed effectively by keeping the patient well hydrated and administering regular doses of fiber. Regular laxative use is sometimes required for the patient to have regular bowel movements.

Mechanical complications occur in a feeding tube that has become kinked or occluded. A kinked tube can be made functional by slowly withdrawing the tube until it straightens out. This should be done without the enteral formula infusing. Slow irrigation of the tube lumen with warm water administered by a 30-mL syringe will open some occluded feeding tubes. Cranberry juice, cola syrup, and pancreatic enzymes in water have also been used with some success. Some practitioners have found a decrease in tube occlusion by using a pancreatic enzyme flush prophylactically.[54] Occasionally, an occluded tube can be saved by passing the stylet back into the lumen of the tube. This may remove or break up any concretion formed within the lumen. This should be done by a physician and only in tubes that do not let the stylet exit through a side port.

Virtually all of the metabolic complications that happen with PN can occur with EN. Hyperglycemia is usually not as severe with EN support because the nutrients are being infused into the GI tract rather than into a large vein. It is not uncommon, though, to use regular insulin infusions in patients receiving EN who have profound glucose intolerance. Some institutions where the pharmacy department prepares and dispenses the enteral formulas have programs that allow the addition of electrolytes (e.g., KCl, Fleet Phosphosoda) to help treat or prevent metabolic complications.

MONITORING

Patients who receive EN should be monitored frequently to ensure safety and efficacy. Many of the complications described above can be averted with meticulous patient monitoring. Enteral tube feeding guidelines for monitoring are listed in Table 30.14.

DRUG COMPATIBILITY

In many patients receiving EN, the feeding tube may be the only way to administer drugs.[55] Therefore, any incompatibil-

Table 30.14	Monitoring Guidelines for Patients Receiving Enteral Nutrition

Raise head of bed to at least 30 degrees at all times.

Check gastric residuals every 6 hours. If more than 150 mL, replace residual and hold feedings for 4 hours and recheck. If less than 150 mL, restart. If still more than 150 mL, continue to hold feedings.

Fingerstick glucose assessment every 6 hours with regular insulin to scale.

Draw blood for a comprehensive metabolic panel, phosphorus, and magnesium at least weekly and as needed.

Draw blood for a basic metabolic panel daily in the ICU.

Draw blood for a prealbumin or transferrin each week.

Collect a 24-hour urine sample for nitrogen balance weekly until positive.

ities between drugs and the enteral formula or tube are of paramount importance. The actions of phenytoin and warfarin have been reported to be altered during EN administration. Patients who received both phenytoin (300 mg/day as the suspension) and EN were reported to have subtherapeutic serum concentrations of the drug compared with patients who received the drug without EN.[56] Interestingly, there does not appear to be a problem with this drug administered to normal subjects who receive concomitant oral enteral supplements or nasogastric tube feedings.[57] It is unclear what effect the difference in subjects (patients versus normal subjects) has on this interaction. Difficulty has been reported in attaining a therapeutic INR with warfarin administration during concurrent EN. Initially this was thought to be caused by the large vitamin K content of some commercially available enteral formulas. The manufacturers have decreased the vitamin K content of most enteral formulas, but the problem with warfarin and enteral formulas still exists. One study found reduced recovery of warfarin mixed with an enteral formula compared to when it was mixed with distilled water.[58]

HOME CARE

HOME NUTRITION THERAPY

Although most hospitalized patients receiving PN or EN can be changed to an oral diet before discharge, some require continued specialized nutrition support at home. The hospital nutrition support team members usually work with an assigned home health care company. The team devises a specialized nutrition support prescription that will meet the patient's fluid and nutritional requirements with an administration schedule that will be compatible with the patient's lifestyle. PN and EN are often given as a nocturnal continuous infusion over an 8- to 18-hour period. This allows patients to hold employment or participate in other activities during the day. Some patients receiving EN, however, prefer periodic bolus feedings during the day. The home health pharmacy will compound the EN or PN formulation and provide the patient with the necessary equipment for its administration. Approximately 2 to 5 days prior to hospital discharge, clinicians from the home health agency or nutrition support team will begin training the patient and family to administer the nutrition regimen. The patient and family are also trained to detect adverse effects that may occur during administration. In addition, the home health agency works with the patient's physician, nurse, and pharmacist to ensure that the patient is monitored between office visits. Provision of specialized nutrition support in the home setting is costly but is much more economical than keeping the patient hospitalized for extended periods. Examples of patients who may require home PN are those with extensive small bowel resection (short-bowel syndrome), chronic enteritis from radiation therapy, or severe Crohn's disease. These patients receive PN via a permanent, centrally placed catheter [e.g., Hickman catheters, peripherally inserted central catheters (PICC lines), and implanted ports]. Patients who receive home EN can absorb nutrients via the GI tract but cannot consume adequate nutrients by mouth; examples of those who receive home EN include patients with severe ulcerative colitis, colon cancer, cerebral trauma, or head and neck cancer. The administration route chosen for enteral feeding will depend on the patient's diagnosis and the estimated duration of EN. Surgical gastrostomy or jejunostomy is often used in these patients.

Home nutrition programs have increased the quality of life for many patients who require these therapies and have allowed many to return to nearly normal lifestyles.

PHARMACOKINETIC AND PHARMACODYNAMIC CONSIDERATIONS

Altered disposition of drugs has been shown with both malnutrition and changes in macronutrient intake.[59] In general, the systemic clearance of many drugs is decreased significantly in patients in an undernourished state compared with well-nourished patients. Some drugs show increased clearance when they are given concurrently with aggressive doses of macronutrients (e.g., protein). Clearance of theophylline in children[60] and gentamicin in normal adults[61] increased significantly when they were given relatively high-protein diets. This may be clinically important, as there is a trend to give higher doses of protein to patients who require specialized nutrition support, especially in the critical care setting.

CONCLUSION

There are still questions in specialized nutrition support that need to be answered through basic and clinical research.[62] Nutrition support team members should now be as involved in EN as PN. Many patients, especially those hospitalized in the intensive care unit, are now receiving EN as a sole source of nutrition support or in combination with PN. If the nutrition support team member focuses only on the PN component, he or she will miss an enormous opportunity to affect patient care. EN is associated with pulmonary, mechanical, GI, and metabolic complications that all can be prevented or treated efficiently if patients are monitored closely. There is an association between the use of EN in critical illness and the development of morbidity. Clearly, patients receiving EN have a significantly lower incidence of pneumonia and abdominal abscesses compared to patients receiving PN. Most of this work has been done in trauma patients. It will be unfortunate if nutrition support team members are not involved with this therapy as more data become available; most likely, an increased number of patients will receive EN and fewer PN over the next few years.

KEY POINTS

- Nutritional assessment is used to detect and quantitate malnutrition. The ideal measure for nutritional assessment is body cell mass. Marasmus, Kwashiorkor, Kwashiorkor-Marasmus Mix, and obesity are the major types of malnutrition.
- Basal energy expenditure equations and World Health Organization equations are reasonable to use to estimate total calorie needs of stable patients. Indirect calorimetry is the best method to determine calorie needs of hospitalized patients.
- Peripheral vein parenteral nutrition should only be used for about 1 week because of the need for frequent vein rotation.
- Central vein parenteral nutrition should be used for patients who have high calorie and protein needs, who need fluid restriction, and who will need parenteral nutrition for an extended amount of time.
- The maximum amount of dextrose provided to adults receiving parenteral nutrition should not exceed 5 mg/kg/minute.
- The newer formulations of parenteral vitamins contain all 13 vitamins.
- Enteral nutrition can be provided via the nasogastric, nasoduodenal, nasojejunal, orogastric, gastrostomy, or jejunostomy route.
- Initial treatment of enteral tube feeding-related diarrhea includes elimination of sorbitol in drug vehicles and administration of dietary fiber via the formulation.

REFERENCES

1. Dudrick SJ, Wilmore DW, Vars HM, et al. Long-term parenteral nutrition with growth, development, and positive nitrogen balance. Surgery 64:134–142, 1968.
2. Detsky AS, Smalley PS, Chana J. Is this patient malnourished? JAMA 271:54–58, 1994.
3. Wilson MM, Vaswani S, Liu D, et al. Prevalence and causes of undernutrition in medical outpatients. Am J Med 104:56–63, 1998.
4. Thomas DR, Zdrowski CD, Wilson MM, et al. Malnutrition in subacute care. Am J Clin Nutr 75:308–313, 2002.
5. Galanos AN, Pieper CF, Kussin PS, et al. Relationships of body mass index to subsequent mortality among seriously ill hospitalized patients. Crit Care Med 25:1962–1968, 1997.
6. Kyle UG, Unger P, Mensi N, et al. Nutrition status in patients younger and older than 60 y at hospital admission: a controlled population study in 995 subjects. Nutrition 18:463–469, 2002.
7. Landi F, Onder G, Gambassi G, et al. Body mass index and mortality among hospitalized patients. Arch Intern Med 160:2641–2644, 2000.
8. Wassertheil-Smoller S, Fann C, Allman RM, et al. Relation of low body mass to death and stroke in the systolic hypertension in the elderly program. Arch Intern Med 160:494–500, 2000.
9. Calle EE, Thun MJ, Petrelli JM, et al. Body-mass index and mortality in a prospective cohort of U.S. adults. N Engl J Med 19;341:1097–1105, 1999.
10. Manson JE, Willett WC, Stampfer MJ, et al. Body weight and mortality among women. N Engl J Med 333 677–685, 1995.

11. Hensrud DD. Nutrition screening and assessment. Med Clin North Am 19;83:1525–1546, 1999.
12. Baker, JP, Detsky AS, Wesson DE, et al. Nutritional assessment: a comparison of clinical judgment and objective measurements. N Engl J Med 306:969–972, 1992.
13. Lopez-Hellin J, Baena-Fustegueras JA, Schwartz-Riera S, et al. Usefulness of shortlived proteins as nutritional indicators in surgical patients. Clin Nutr 21:119–125, 2002.
14. Donahue SP, Phillips LS. Response of IGF-1 to nutritional support in malnourished hospital patients: a possible indicator of short-term changes in nutritional status. Am J Clin Nutr 50:962–969, 1989.
15. Briet F, Twomey C, Jeejeebhoy KN. Effect of feeding malnourished patients for 1 mo on mitochondrial complex I activity and nutritional assessment measurements. Am J Clin Nutr 79:787–794, 2004.
16. Brodie D, Moscrip V, Hutcheon R. Body composition measurement: a review of hydrodensitometry, anthropometry, and impedance methods. Nutrition 14:296–310, 1998.
17. Miles JM. Should protein be included in calorie calculations for a TPN prescription? Yes, protein should be included. Nutr Clin Prac 11:204–205, 1996.
18. Harris JA, Benedict FC. A Biometric Study of Basal Metabolism. Carnegie Institute of Washington, publication no. 279. Washington DC: 1919.
19. Elia M. Changing concepts of nutrient requirements in disease: implications for artificial nutritional support. Lancet 345:1279–1284, 1995.
20. Garrel DR, Jobin N, Dejonge LH. Should we still use the Harris and Benedict equations? Nutr Clin Prac 11:99–103, 1996.
21. Barak N, Wall-Alonso E, Sitrin MD. Evaluation of stress factors and body weight adjustments currently used to estimate energy expenditure in hospitalized patients. J Parenter Enteral Nutr 26:231–238, 2002.
22. McClave SA, Snider HL. Use of indirect calorimetry in clinical nutrition. Nutr Clin Prac 7:207–221, 1992.
23. Weir JB. New methods for calculating metabolic rate with special reference to protein metabolism. J Physiol (London) 109:1–9, 1949.
24. Barak N, Wall-Alonso E, Cheng A, et al. Use of bioelectrical impedance analysis to predict energy expenditure of hospitalized patients receiving nutritional support. J Parenter Enteral Nutr 27:43–46, 2003.
25. Shaw JHF, Wildbore M, Wolfe RR. Whole body protein kinetics in severely septic patients: the response to glucose infusion and total parenteral nutrition. Ann Surg 205:288–294, 1987.
26. ASPEN Board of Directors and the Clinical Guidelines Task Force. Guidelines for the use of parenteral and enteral nutrition in adult and pediatric patients. J Parenteral Enteral Nutr 26:1SA–138SA, 2002.
27. AGA technical review on parenteral nutrition. Gastroenterology 121:970–1001, 2001.
28. Everitt NJ, McMahon MJ. Peripheral venous nutrition. Nutrition 10:49–57, 1994.
29. Doglietto GB, Gallitelli L, Pacelli F, et al. Protein-sparing therapy after major abdominal surgery. Lack of clinical effects. Ann Surg 223:357–362, 1996.
30. Cerra FB, Cheung NK, Fischer JF, et al. Disease-specific amino acid infusion (F080) in hepatic encephalopathy: a prospective, mixed double-blind, controlled trial. J Parenter Enteral Nutr 9:288–295, 1985.
31. Michel H, Bories P, Aubin JP, et al. Treatment of acute hepatic encephalopathy in cirrhotics with a branched-chain amino acids versus a conventional amino acids mixture. Liver 5:282–289, 1985.
32. Mirtallo JM, Schneider PS, Marko, et al. A comparison of essential and general amino acid infusions in the nutritional support of patients with compromised renal function. J Parenter Enteral Nutr 6:109–113, 1982.
33. Garcia-de-Lorenzo A, Ortiz-Leyba C, Palnas M, et al. Parenteral administration of different amounts of branched-chain amino acids in septic patients: Clinical and metabolic aspects. Crit Care Med 25:418–424, 1997.
34. von Meyenfeldt MF, Soeters PB, Vente JP, et al. Effect of branched chain amino acid enrichment of total parenteral nutrition on nitrogen sparing and clinical outcome of sepsis and trauma. A prospective randomized double-blind trial. Br J Surg 19;77:924–929, 1990.
35. Burke JF, Wolfe RR, MuDancy CJ, et al. Glucose requirements following burn injury: parameters of optimal glucose infusion and possible hepatic and respiratory abnormalities following excessive glucose intake. Ann Surg 190:275–285, 1979.
36. Task Force for the Revision of Safe Practices for Parenteral Nutrition. Safe practices for parenteral nutrition. J Parents Enteral Nutr 28:S39–S70, 2004.
37. Schloerb PR, Henning JF. Patterns and problems of adult total parenteral nutrition use in U.S. academic medical centers. Arch Surg 133:7–12, 1998.
38. Rosmarin DK, Wardlaw GM, Mirtallo J. Hyperglycemia associated with high, continuous infusion rates of total parenteral nutrition dextrose. Nutr Clin Prac 11:151–156, 1996.
39. Van Den Berghe G, Wouters P, Weekers, F, et al. Intensive insulin therapy in critically ill patients. N Engl J Med 345:1359–1367, 2001.
40. Battistella FD, Wildergren JT, Anderson JT, et al. A prospective, randomized trial of IV fat emulsion administration in trauma victims requiring total parenteral nutrition. J Trauma 43:52–58, 1997.
41. Hyltander A, Sandstrom R, Lundholm K. Metabolic effects of structured triglycerides in humans. Nutr Clin Prac 10:91–97, 1995.
42. Solomon SM, Kirby DF. The refeeding syndrome: a review. J Parenter Enteral Nutr 19;14:90–97, 1990.
43. Multivitamin preparations for parenteral use: a statement by the Nutrition Advisory Group. J Parenter Enteral Nutr 3:253–262, 1979.
44. Department of Health and Human Services. Parenteral multivitamin products. Federal Register 65:21,200–21,201, 2000.
45. Helpingstine CJ, Bistrian BR. New food and drug administration requirements for inclusion of vitamin K in adult parenteral multivitamins. J Parenter Enteral Nutr 27:220–224, 2003.
46. Bertinet DB, Tinivella M, Balzola FA, et al. Brain manganese deposition and blood levels in patients undergoing home parenteral nutrition. J Parenter Enteral Nutr 24:223–227, 2000.
47. McKinnon BT. FDA safety alert: Hazards of precipitation associated with parenteral nutrition. Nutr Clin Prac 11:59–65, 1996.
48. Sarr MG, Mayo S. Needle catheter jejunostomy: an unappreciated and misunderstood advance in the care of patients after major abdominal operations. Mayo Clin Proc 63:565–572, 1988.
49. Keohane PP, Attrill H, Love M, et al. Relation between osmolality of diet and gastrointestinal side effects in enteral nutrition. Br Med J 288:678–680, 1984.
50. Cabre E, Gassull MA. Complications of enteral feeding. Nutrition 9:1–9, 1993.
51. Heimburger DC, Sockwell DG, Geels WI. Diarrhea with enteral feeding: prospective reappraisal of putative causes. Nutrition 10:392–396, 1994.
52. Edes TE, Walk BE, Austin JL. Diarrhea in tube-fed patients: feeding formula not necessarily the cause. Am J Med 19;88:91–93, 1990.
53. Delany HM, Lindine P. The pros and cons of needle catheter jejunostomy. Nutrition 4:119–124, 1988.
54. Sriram K, Jayanthi V, Lakshimi RG, et al. Prophylactic locking of enteral feeding tubes with pancreatic enzymes. J Parenter Enteral Nutr 21:353–356, 1997.
55. Beckwith MC, Barton RG, Graves C. A guide to drug therapy in patients with enteral feeding tubes: dosage form selection and administration methods. Hosp Pharm 32:57–64, 1997.
56. Bauer LA. Interference of oral phenytoin absorption by continuous nasogastric feedings. Neurology 32:570–572, 1982.
57. Doak KK, Haas CE, Dunningan KJ, et al. Bioavailability of phenytoin acid and phenytoin sodium with enteral feedings. Pharmacotherapy 18:637–645, 1998.
58. Kuhn TA, Garnett WR, Wells BK, et al. Recovery of warfarin from an enteral nutrient formula. Am J Hosp Pharm 46:1395–1399, 1989.
59. Anderson KE. Influences of diet and nutrition on clinical pharmacokinetics. Clin Pharmacokinet 14:325–346, 1988.
60. Feldman CH, Hutchinson VE, Sher TH, et al. Interaction between nutrition and theophylline metabolism in children. Ther Drug Monit 4:69–76, 1982.
61. Dickson CJ, Schwartzman MS, Bertino JS. Factors affecting aminoglycoside disposition: effects of circadian rhythm and dietary protein intake on gentamicin pharmacokinetics. Clin Pharmacol Ther 39:325–328, 1986.
62. Klein S, Kinney J, Jeejeebhoy K, et al. Nutrition support in clinical practice: review of data and published recommendations for future research directions. Am J Clin Nutr 66:683–706, 1997.

CASE 11

TOPIC: Fluid and Electrolyte Therapy and Acid-Base Balance

THERAPEUTIC DIFFICULTY: Level 2
Lisa M. McDevitt and Mark E. Klee

Chapter 28: Fluid and Electrolyte Therapy and Acid–Base Balance

■ Scenario

Patient and Setting: MH is a 46-year-old male admitted yesterday to the surgical intensive care unit

Chief Complaint: Status postorthotopic liver transplant (OLT)

■ History of Present Illness

MH was on the liver transplant waiting list (MELD score = 39) and was called in yesterday to receive a deceased donor liver transplant.

Medical History: End-stage liver disease secondary to chronic active hepatitis C complicated by ascites, portal hypertension, esophageal varices, and hepatic encephalopathy

Surgical History: Variceal band ligation for esophageal varices 2 years ago

Family/Social History: Family History: Noncontributory
Social History: MH has a history of intravenous drug use and alcoholism. He is married with no children and lives at home. He is not working (on disability).

Medications:
Prior to transplant:
Pantoprazole, 40 mg PO QD
Nadolol, 20 mg PO QD
Spironolactone, 100 mg PO QD
Furosemide, 40 mg PO QD
Lactulose, 20 mg PO QID
Today:
Tacrolimus, 2 mg NG BID

Methylprednisolone, 40 mg IV q6h × 4 doses (part of a steroid taper)
Valganciclovir, 900 mg NG QD
Sulfamethoxazole/trimethoprim, 800/160 mg NG QD
Nystatin, 500,000 units to oral cavity QID
Lansoprazole, 30 mg NG QD
Ursodiol, 300 mg NG TID
Hydromorphone, IV continuous infusion
Regular insulin, IV continuous infusion

Allergies: No known medication allergies

■ Physical Examination

GEN: Jaundiced, awake, alert
VS: T 37.3°C, BP 116/55, HR 76, RR 12 (on vent at 50% FiO2), Wt 75 kg, Ht 168 cm
HEENT: Intubated, NPO except medications; NG tube to suction
COR: RRR
CHEST: CTA
ABD: Soft, nontender, mildly distended
GU: Foley in
EXT: 3+ bilateral edema of LE, + radial pulses, + DP pulses
NEURO: Awake and alert
WOUND: Clean, dry, and intact

■ Results of Pertinent Laboratory Tests, Serum Drug Concentrations, and Diagnostic Tests

Na 144 (144)	Lkcs 4.4 × 10^9 (4.4 × 10^3)	Tbili 143.6 (8.4)
K 3.4 (3.4)	Hgb 107 (10.7)	AST, SGOT 7.32 (439)
Cl 99 (99)	Hct 0.322 (32.2)	ALT, SGPT 6.03 (362)
HCO$_3$ 35 (35)	Plt 156 × 10^9 (156 × 10^3)	Alk Phos 0.8 (50)
BUN 7.5 (21)	Ca 1.85 (7.4)	LDH 665 (665)
CR 106.1 (1.2)	Mg 1 (2)	
Glu 9.1 (164)	Phos 1.19 (3.7)	
Lactate 2.1 (2.1)	Alb 24 (2.4)	
pH 7.51 (7.51)		
pO2 37.8 kPa (284 mmHg)		
pCO2 5.3 kPa (40 mmHg)		
Tacrolimus <3 (goal: 8–10 ng/ mL)		

■ Problem List

Identify principal problems from the scenario in priority order (see Answers in back of book for correct list of problems).

■ SOAP Note

To be completed by the student (see Answers in back of book for correct SOAP Note).

■ QUESTIONS

(See Answers in back of book for correct responses.)

1. Diarrhea is a possible side effect of mycophenolate mofetil. Which of the following most accurately describes the electrolyte disturbances associated with diarrhea? (EO-2)
   a. Dehydration, hypokalemia, metabolic acidosis
   b. Dehydration, hypokalemia, metabolic alkalosis
   c. Dehydration, hyperkalemia, metabolic acidosis
   d. Dehydration, hyperkalemia, metabolic alkalosis

2. Calcineurin inhibitor (cyclosporine or tacrolimus) use is frequently associated with hypomagnesemia and hypophosphatemia. Give an appropriate threshold for initiating therapy and suggest a management strategy for magnesium and phosphorus replacement. (EO-8, 11)

3. Which of the following adverse effects are associated with oral magnesium replacement? (EO-10)
   a. Diarrhea
   b. Tachycardia
   c. Seizures
   d. Tetany

4. Which of the following is the best way to manage MH's calcium? (EO-5, 6, 8)
   a. Administer intravenous calcium chloride
   b. Administer oral calcium carbonate
   c. Administer oral vitamin D
   d. No treatment is necessary.

5. List the pertinent lab values needed to correctly identify an acid-base disorder. (EO-8)

6. Which of the following best describe MH's compensatory response to his metabolic alkalosis? (EO-1, 5)
   a. He has a compensatory respiratory acidosis from hyperventilating.
   b. He has a compensatory respiratory acidosis from hypoventilating.
   c. There is no respiratory compensation because his mechanical ventilation does not allow him to hyperventilate.
   d. There is no respiratory compensation because the mechanical ventilation does not allow him to hypoventilate.

7. Identify MH's total body water status and describe the etiology behind it. (EO-1)

8. Which of the following best describes why 0.9% NaCl is not a good choice to treat MH's metabolic alkalosis? (EO-9)
   a. He is hypernatremic and could not tolerate the additional sodium load.
   b. He is hyperchloremic and could not tolerate the additional chloride load.
   c. He has a total body water overload, and 0.9% NaCl would exacerbate it.
   d. He has a total body water deficit, and 0.9% NaCl would correct it too quickly.

9. Which of the following statements is true regarding potassium replacement? (EO-6, 8)
   a. The wax matrix tablet offers a more rapid onset of action than the oral liquid.
   b. Patients with symptomatic hypokalemia should receive intravenous rather than oral potassium replacement.
   c. The maximum rate of peripheral infusion is 40 mmol/hr.
   d. Potassium can be administered via IV push.

10. Which of the following statements is correct regarding management of hyperkalemia? (EO-7)
    a. Albuterol can be used to stabilize cellular membranes.
    b. Calcium chloride can be used to drive potassium into the cells.
    c. Kayexalate can be used to increase potassium excretion.
    d. Dextrose can be used to drive potassium into the cells.

11. Which of the following most accurately describes MH's daily fluid requirements? (EO-6)
    a. 50 mL/hr
    b. 100 mL/hr
    c. 200 mL/hr
    d. 300 mL/hr

12. Compare and contrast crystalloids and colloids. Give two examples of each. (EO-7)

13. Analyze pharmacoeconomic factors associated with management of MH's metabolic alkalosis. (EO-17)

14. Summarize pathophysiologic, pharmacotherapeutic, and disease management concepts for management of acid/base and electrolyte disorders utilizing the key points format. (EO-18)

CASE 12

TOPIC: Parenteral and Enteral Nutrition in Adult Patients

THERAPEUTIC DIFFICULTY: Level 1

Paul J. Kiritsy

Chapter 30: Parenteral and Enteral Nutrition in Adult Patients

■ Scenario

Patient and Setting: JN, a 49-year-old Caucasian male; community hospital ER

Chief Complaint: Weight loss, fatigue, depression

■ History of Present Illness

Presents in ER with general weakness, slightly withdrawn with inappropriate feelings of worthlessness and worry; states that he usually eats 2–3 meals day but admits to having at best one meal a day for the past couple of months; states he is always tired and has not left his apartment in days; admits that he has stopped taking his Zoloft prescription when it ran out about 2 months ago

Medical History: One episode of depression following divorce 2 years ago (controlled on sertraline) with weight loss >20% (requiring short course of nutritional support); fractured collarbone in hockey game as teen.

Surgical History: Nephrolithiasis with ureteroscopic removal 8 years ago

Family/Social History: Family History: Father died at age 67 with liver disease secondary to alcoholism; mother retired clerk in generally good health, lives out of state
Social History: Divorced with two adult children; laid-off computer programmer (11 weeks ago); collecting unemployment

Medication History:
Acetaminophen (APAP), 650 mg PO q4–6h PRN
Sertraline, 50 mg PO QD

Allergies: No known drug allergies

■ Physical Examination

GEN: Slightly withdrawn, weak male, apparent fatigue

VS: T 37°C, BP 118/72, HR 72, RR 18, O2 sat 99% RA, Wt 55 kg, Ht 175 cm
HEENT: PERRLA, EOMI, appreciate dry mouth
NECK: Supple
COR: RRR, normal S1, S2, no M/R/G
CHEST: WNL
ABD: Soft, NT/ND, no BS
GU: WNL
RECTAL: WNL
EXT: Cold to touch, decreased turgor
NEURO: A and O $\times$ 3

■ Results of Pertinent Laboratory Tests, Serum Drug Concentrations, and Diagnostic Tests

Lkcs 6.0 $\times$ 10^9	Na 148 (148)	Ca 2.25 (4.5)
(6.0 $\times$ 10^3)	K 3.5 (3.5)	Mg 1.1 (2.2)
Hct 0.48 (48)	Cl 110 (110)	Alb 34 (3.4)
Hgb 160 (16)	HCO$_3$ 22 (22)	PO$_4$ 0.65 (2.0)
Plts 200 $\times$ 10^9	BUN 8.5 (24)	
(200 $\times$ 10^3)	SCr 97.2 (1.1)	
	Glucose 3.9 (70)	

■ Problem List

Identify principal problems from the scenario in priority order (see Answers in back of book for correct list of problems).

■ SOAP Note

To be completed by the student (see Answers in back of book for correct SOAP Note).

■ QUESTIONS

(See Answers in back of book for correct responses.)

1. JN is most likely suffering from which type of malnutrition? (EO-2, 5)
   a. Marasmus
   b. Kwashiorkor
   c. Kwashiorkor-Marasmus
   d. Obesity

2. Using the Harris-Benedict equation, calculate JN's BEE. (EO-5, 13)
   a. 1,275
   b. 1,367
   c. 1,641
   d. 1,955

3. Describe how JN's daily volume and total calorie requirement is determined. (EO-12)

4. Compare and contrast the risks and benefits of the two primary ways to administer PN solu-

tions and recommend the best choice for JN. (EO-8)

5. The serum protein that best indicates acute nutrition status is: (EO-4, 5)
   a. Albumin
   b. Transferrin
   c. Prealbumin
   d. Retinol-binding protein

6. The carbohydrate component to JN's solution is formulated using a 70% solution of dextrose. At a starting rate of 15 kcal/kg/day, how many mL of dextrose solution should be used to compound JN's PN? (EO-13)
   a. 55
   b. 242
   c. 350
   d. 825

7. The protein component to JN's solution is formulated using a 15% solution of Aminosyn. At a starting rate of 1 g/kg/day, how many mL of amino acid solution should be used to compound JN's PN? (EO-13)
   a. 366
   b. 167
   c. 55
   d. 42

8. After reviewing the pertinent labs, identify the electrolytes that require adjusting and recommend a daily amount to achieve optimal therapeutic control. (EO-11, 12)

9. A 24-hour urine collection reveals that JN excreted 6.5 g of nitrogen. Based on the above PN formulation and taking into account nonmeasurable nitrogen loss, calculate JN's daily nitrogen balance (g/day).

10. Describe the role of the pharmacist with the nutrition support team in assisting with JD's plan of care. (EO-16)

11. The combined osmolarity of JN's PN is 803 mOsm/L (includes carbohydrate, protein, electrolytes, trace elements). His daily intravenous fat emulsion (1 g/kg/day) requires 275 mL of 20% solution (total 71 mOsm). What is the best recommendation for JN's intravenous fat emulsion administration? (EO-5, 8, 11, 12)
    a. Prepare as separate solutions and administer peripherally
    b. Prepare as separate solutions that must be administered centrally
    c. Prepare as a TNA (3-1) solution and administer peripherally
    d. Prepare as a TNA (3-1) solution that must be administered centrally

12. Summarize therapeutic, pathophysiologic, and disease management concepts for the utilization of parenteral and enteral nutrition utilizing the key points format. (EO-18)

Iron Deficiency and Megaloblastic Anemias

31

David J. Quan

OVERVIEW

DEFINITION

Anemia is a hematologic condition in which there is quantitative deficiency of circulating hemoglobin (Hb), often accompanied by a reduced number of red blood cells (erythrocytes). Causes of anemia are blood loss, impaired erythropoiesis, and abnormal erythrocyte destruction. Nutritional deficiencies [iron, cobalamin (B$_{12}$), folate] are the most common cause of anemia throughout the world.[1,2]

Erythropoiesis is a controlled physiologic process. In response to changes in tissue oxygen availability, the kidney regulates production and release of erythropoietin that stimulates the bone marrow to produce and release red blood cells. Erythrocytes originate from pluripotent stem cells in the bone marrow and undergo multiple steps of differentiation and maturation. Early stages of red cell production consist of large cells with immature nuclei (pronormoblasts and basophilic normoblasts). As cells mature, Hb is incorporated, the nucleus is extruded, and cell size decreases. Various nutrients are needed for normal erythropoiesis. Lack of B$_{12}$ or folate can interfere with cell maturation, resulting in the release of megaloblasts (erythroid precursors with immature nuclei). Iron deficiency interferes with Hb production and incorporation into the maturing cells, which continue to divide, resulting in the release of smaller cells (microcytosis).

TREATMENT GOALS: ANEMIAS

- Identify patients at risk for developing nutritional anemias.
- Prevent nutritional deficiencies and anemia.
- Treat nutritional deficiency and/or anemia by providing the appropriate nutrient.
- Document and confirm the deficiency state as the cause of the anemia.
- Identify and, when possible, rectify the pathologic state responsible for the deficiency.
- Develop therapeutic monitoring plans.
- Optimize patient compliance with treatment plan by minimizing treatment side effects, costs, and inconvenience.
- Prevent long-term sequelae.

PATHOPHYSIOLOGY

Anemia, which has many causes, is not a single disease entity but a sign of disease. Regardless of the cause, anemia is associated with a reduction in circulating Hb because of reduced numbers of erythrocytes or less Hb per erythrocyte.

The number of erythrocytes in normal people varies with age, sex, and atmospheric pressure. People who live at high altitudes have more erythrocytes to compensate for the reduced oxygen in the air. At sea level, the average man has 5.5×10^{12} erythrocytes/L ($5.5 \times 10^6/mm^3$). The erythrocytes occupy approximately 47% of the blood and are often referred to as the packed cell volume or hematocrit (Hct). The normal ranges for red blood cell measurements (Hb, Hct) vary with age and laboratory, but in general, values that are more than two standard deviations (SD) below the mean warrant further investigation.[1] Blood from healthy men contains approximately 9.9 mmol/L (16 g/dL) Hb. All these parameters are lower for healthy women. Values for neonates, which show no sex differences, are higher at birth, but after several weeks they decrease to below those of women. Thereafter the values rise gradually, and at puberty sex differences appear (Table 31.1). The physiologic result of low circulating Hb is the reduced capacity for blood to carry oxygen. Consequently, less oxygen is available to tissues, including those of the heart, brain, and muscles, leading to the clinical manifestations of anemia.

CLINICAL PRESENTATION AND DIAGNOSIS

Regardless of the cause of anemia, the clinical features depend on the rate of development and the compensatory ability of the cardiovascular and pulmonary system to adjust to tissue hypoxia. Lower Hb levels often are tolerated with minimal symptoms if the anemia develops slowly and the body is able to compensate.

SIGNS AND SYMPTOMS

Overt signs of anemia are listed in Table 31.2. Cardiomegaly and high-output heart failure also are possible in severe cases. Although the symptoms of anemia are distinctive, they can also be manifestations of other disorders, such as cancer or an inflammatory process. A comprehensive history and physical examination are important in the assessment of the

TABLE 31.1	Normal Hematologic Values by Age			
	Mean Hb (−2 SD)		**Mean Hct (−2 SD)**	
Age	Conventional (g/dL)	SI (mmol/L)	Conventional (g/dL)	SI (mmol/L)
1–3 days	18 (14)	11.2 (8.7)	54 (42)	0.54 (0.42)
6 months–2 years	12 (10.5)	7.4 (6.5)	36 (32)	0.36 (0.32)
12–18 years				
Male	14.5 (13)	9 (8.1)	43 (38)	0.43 (0.38)
Female	14 (12)	8.7 (7.5)	41 (36)	0.41 (0.36)
Adult				
Male	15.5 (13.5)	9.6 (8.4)	47 (40)	0.47 (0.40)
Female	14 (12)	8.7 (7.5)	41 (36)	0.41 (0.36)

TABLE 31.2	Signs and Symptoms of Anemia and Vitamin Deficiency	
Anemia in General	**Iron Deficiency**	**Vitamin B$_{12}$ Deficiency**
Fatigue	Development delays	Peripheral neuropathy
Pallor		"Strange" feeling in extremities
Dyspnea	Behavioral disturbances	
Light-headedness	Altered central nervous system development	Loss of hand coordination
Dizziness		Deterioration in handwriting
Palpitations		
Increased heart rate	Impaired work capacity	Tingling of extremities
		Loss of proprioception
Chest pain	Preterm delivery	Depression
Loss of concentration	Delivery of low-birthweight baby	Psychosis
		Spinal cord degeneration
		Sore tongue or mouth

From references 1–5, 18, 27, and 69.

TABLE 31.3	High-Risk Populations for Development of Nutritional Anemias	
Population	**Predisposing Factors**	**Type of Anemia**
Children[3,16]	Growth, poor diet	Iron deficiency
Teenagers[3]	Growth, diet, menstruation	Iron deficiency
Women[3,16]	Menstruation, diet	Iron deficiency
Pregnant women[3,16]	Fetal needs, diet	Iron, folate deficiency
Older adults[4,91,92]	Achlorhydria	Iron, B$_{12}$ deficiency
	Diet	Iron, B$_{12}$, folate deficiency
	Underlying disease	Iron, B$_{12}$, folate deficiency
	Organ function	Iron, B$_{12}$, folate deficiency
	Drug-induced	Iron, B$_{12}$, folate defiency
Alcoholics[69]	Diet	Iron, folate deficiency
	Liver or gastrointestinal disease	Iron, B$_{12}$, folate deficiency
Patients with human immunodeficiency virus[4,93,94]	Achlorhydria	Iron, B$_{12}$ deficiency
	Diet	Iron, B$_{12}$, folate deficiency
	Drug-induced	B$_{12}$, folate deficiency

anemic patient. More specifically, dietary habits, drug histories, surgical procedures, and occupation should be documented. Careful questioning about blood loss, menses, gastrointestinal symptoms, and history of pregnancy may provide useful information.

In addition, vitamin deficiencies may cause other symptoms before overt anemia develops. As noted in Table 31.2, neurologic or oral changes may occur with B$_{12}$ deficiency and may precede anemia.

DIAGNOSIS

A detailed medical and medication history along with hematologic and biochemical tests, including a full blood screen, are essential for identifying the type of anemia and in many cases directing the treatment. As the nutritional anemias progress in stages (normal, negative nutrient balance, nutrient depletion, nutrient deficiency, anemia), monitoring early indicators of depletion may prevent the progression to overt anemia. Risk factors for certain vitamin deficiencies (Table 31.3) and reported symptoms (Table 31.2) often suggest the possible cause of anemia or alert the physician to the potential for anemia.

Hematologic Tests. Hematologic tests (Table 31.4) are less expensive and more available than biochemical tests and provide information on the characteristics of the red blood cells. A full blood screen provides information on Hb and Hct levels as well as cell size and color. Many aspects of the cellular elements of blood can be quantified by automated blood analyzers, including blood Hb concentration, cell counts, and the mean corpuscular volume (MCV). From these primary measurements, the Hct, mean corpuscular hemoglobin (MCH), and the mean corpuscular hemoglobin

concentration (MCHC) are calculated automatically. MCV, MCH, and MCHC are collectively known as the erythrocyte indices. The MCV correlates with cell size (smaller cells take up less volume) and is particularly valuable in differentiating microcytic anemias, which have a reduced MCV (<80 fL), from macrocytic anemias, which have a greater than normal MCV (>100 fL). However, the MCV may appear normal in mixed anemias, where the microcytic cells of iron deficiency are counterbalanced by the macrocytic cells of B$_{12}$ or folate deficiency. In this instance, a peripheral blood smear can aid in identifying the existence of a mixed anemia. The MCH and MCHC provide information on cell color [lower Hb, less color (hypochromia)]. Hypochromic anemias, such as iron deficiency anemia, have a low MCHC indicating lower-than-normal Hb concentrations. Another parameter, the red blood cell distribution width (RDW), is an index of the variation in cell volume of the erythrocyte population. With iron deficiency anemia, there is an increased RDW, reflecting the anisocytosis (cells of unequal size) seen in blood smears.

Other hematologic investigations include reticulocyte counts, differential white cell count, platelet count, and microscopic examination of peripheral blood smears and bone marrow aspirates. The normal life span of an erythrocyte is 120 days. As old erythrocytes are removed from the circulation by the reticuloendothelial system, they are replaced by young erythrocytes from the bone marrow. These immature cells, called reticulocytes, make up 1% to 1.5% of the total erythrocyte population in a normal person. Because reticulo-

| TABLE 31.4 | Selected Hematologic and Biochemical Parameters |

Component	Specimen		Representative Reference Range Conventional	Representative Reference Range SI
Hematocrit	B	M	45%–52%	0.45–0.52
		F	37%–48%	0.37–0.48
Hemoglobin	B	M	13%–18% g/dL	130–180 g/L
		F	12%–16% g/dL	120–160 g/L
Erythrocyte count	B		$4.2\%–5.9\% \times 10^6/mm$	$4.2–5.9 \times 10^6/mm$
Reticulocyte count	B		0.5%–1.5% erythrocytes	
Mean corpuscular volume	Ery			80–94 fmol
Mean corpuscular hemoglobin	Ery		27–32 pg	1.7–2.0 fmol
Mean corpuscular hemoglobin concentration	Ery		32–36 g/dL	19–22.8 mmol/L
Red cell distribution width	Ery		11.5%–14.5%	
Iron	S	M	80–200 µg/dL	14–35 µmol/L
		F	60–190 µg/dL	11–29 µmol/L
Transferrin	S		170–370 mg/dL	1.7–3.7 g/L
Total iron-binding capacity	S		250–410 g/mL	45–72 µmol/L
Transferrin saturation	S		20%–55%	
Transferrin receptors	S			2.8–8.5 mg/L
Ferritin	S	M>F	1.5–30 µg/dL	15–300 µg/L
Zinc protoporphyrin			<70 µg/dL red cell	<80 µmol/mol heme
Folate (as pteroglutamic acid)				
Normal	S		2–10 ng/mL	4–22 nmol/L
Borderline	S		1–1.9 ng/mL	2.5–4 nmol/L
	Ery		150–800 ng/mL	
Vitamin B_{12}	S		200–1,000 pg/mL	150–750 pmol/L
Methylmalonic acid (mean ± 3 SD)	S			53–376 nmol/L
Homocysteine (mean ± 3 SD)	S			4.1–21.3 µmol/L
Holo-transcobalamin II	P			Mean for control group +2 SD

B, whole blood; M, male; F, female, Ery, erythrocyte; S, serum. (From references 1, 6, 7, and 9.)

cytes are a young population of red blood cells, they are an important marker of bone marrow activity. Reticulocytosis, an increase in reticulocyte numbers, indicates increased bone marrow activity. Transient reticulocytosis often occurs in response to iron, B_{12}, or folic acid therapy for the respective deficiency states.

Biochemical Tests. Biochemical tests (Table 31.4) for assessing anemias include measurement of serum iron vitamin concentrations (B_{12}, folate), transport proteins (transferrin, transcobalamin II [TCII]), saturation of protein-binding sites (transferrin saturation), and storage amounts (ferritin). More specific tests also can be used: serum transferrin receptors (TfR), erythrocyte zinc protoporphyrin (ZPP) concentration (iron deficiency), homocysteine (Hcy) and methylmalonic acid (MMA) serum concentrations (B_{12} and folate deficiencies), and antibodies to intrinsic factor (IF) or parietal cells (B_{12}).[3–12]

Selected laboratory characteristics of iron deficiency anemia and megaloblastic anemias are summarized in Table 31.5. In general, the diagnosis of a nutritional anemia depends on an accurate and complete medical, drug, and symptom history and assessment of multiple laboratory and biochemical tests rather than a single result.

TREATMENT

Treating nutritional anemia involves identifying and correcting the cause if possible, replenishing deficient nutrients, and alleviating symptoms. This may involve restoring missing nutrients, restoring blood volume by transfusions, or treating the cause by medical or surgical methods. Inadequate dietary intake of nutrients often is a cause of nutritional deficiencies that may lead to anemia. Dietary counseling and follow-up

TABLE 31.5	Selected Laboratory Characteristics of the Nutritional Anemias			
Type	Mean Corpuscular Volume	Red Blood Cell Distribution Width	Peripheral Smear	Additional Investigations
Iron deficiency	L[a]	H	Hypochromic, microcytic	↓ Iron, ↓ ferritin, ↑ transferrin, ↑ zinc protoporphyrin, ↑ TfR
Vitamin B$_{12}$ deficiency[b]	H	H	Macrocytic	↓ S-vitamin B$_{12}$, ↑ methylmalonic acid, ↑ homocysteine, ↑ intrinsic factor antibodies
Folate deficiency	H	H	Macrocytic	↓ S-folate[c], ↓ erythrocyte folate
Chronic disease	L	H	Hypochromic, normocytic	↓ Iron, ↓ transferin, nl TfR
	N	N	Normochromic, normocytic	nl TfR
Blood loss	N	N	Normochromic, normocytic	Clinical evidence, occult blood loss

[a]Normal in early iron deficiency.
[b]Includes pernicious anemia.
[c]Varies with diet.
L, low; H, high; TfR, transferrin receptors; nl, normal; s, serum.

may be sufficient for some patients, but many need supplementation. Careful assessment of the patient's drug history may help identify possible pharmacotherapeutic agents that affect nutrient status or red blood cells directly. Some deficiencies may necessitate long-term or lifelong therapy, and patients must be counseled and monitored appropriately.

IRON DEFICIENCY ANEMIA

Iron deficiency occurs when the body's iron stores are insufficient for the normal formation of Hb, iron-containing enzymes, and other functional iron compounds such as myoglobin and those of the cytochrome system. Iron deficiency can be classified according to its severity (Table 31.6): normal stores; negative iron balance; iron store depletion (low serum ferritin); decreased serum iron [low serum iron, increased total iron-binding capacity (TIBC)]; and anemia (reduced Hb with microcytic, hypochromic erythrocytes).[3] Erythrocytes of patients with mild, early-stage iron deficiency often appear to be normal in color and size (i.e., normochromic, normocytic).

Other conditions with low MCV and MCHC, such as thalassemia and anemia of chronic disease, generally can be

TABLE 31.6	Laboratory Values in Various Stages of Iron Deficiency						
Stage	Serum Ferritin (μg/L)	Serum Iron	Total Iron-binding Capacity	Zinc Protoporphyrin	Transferrin Saturation (%)	Transferrin Receptors	Hemoglobin
Normal	>15	nl	nl	nl	>16	nl	nl
Negative balance	>15	nl	nl	nl	>16	nl	nl
Iron store depletion	<15	nl	nl	nl	>16	nl	nl
Iron deficiency	<15	↓	nl	↑	<16	↑	nl
Iron deficiency anemia	<15	↓	↑	↑	<16	↑	↓
Anemia of chronic desease	↓, ↑, or nl	nl	nl or ↓	↑	nl or ↓	nl	↓
Thalassemia	nl or ↑	nl	nl	nl	nl	nl	↓

nl, normal.
(From references 1, 3, 10, and 18.)

differentiated from iron deficiency anemia by assessment of various laboratory values (Table 31.6).

PHYSIOLOGIC IMPORTANCE OF IRON

Iron is an essential element for many physiologic processes, including erythropoiesis, tissue respiration, and several enzyme-catalyzed reactions.[1] The average adult body contains 3 to 5 g elemental iron, distributed into two major components: functional iron and storage.[1,3] Functional iron exists predominantly as Hb (1.5–3 g) in circulating erythrocytes, with lesser amounts in iron containing proteins such as myoglobin and cytochromes (0.4 g), 3 to 7 mg bound to transferrin in plasma, and the remainder in storage iron in the form of ferritin or hemosiderin.

Hb is the oxygen-binding protein in erythrocytes that transports oxygen absorbed from the lungs to the tissues. Each Hb molecule consists of a globin surrounded by four heme groups that contain all the iron. Globin consists of linked pairs of polypeptide chains. Fetal Hb has two α- and two γ-globin chains. In normal erythrocyte development, the γ-chains are replaced by β-chains, and a normal human adult has two α- and two β-chains. The composition of these chains differs in patients with genetically determined disorders such as thalassemia and sickle cell anemia (Chapter 32).

Hb forms an unstable, reversible bond with oxygen, allowing oxygen release at a lower oxygen tension that is encountered in the tissues. In iron deficiency anemia and other chronic anemias, Hb has a reduced affinity for oxygen. This allows oxygen to transfer more readily from the erythrocytes to the tissues. Myoglobin, a hemoprotein in muscle, accepts oxygen from Hb and acts as an oxygen store in muscle. If oxygen supply is limited, myoglobin releases its oxygen to cytochrome oxidase, the terminal enzyme in the mitochondrial respiratory chain, which has a higher affinity for oxygen than myoglobin, allowing oxidative phosphorylation to occur.

Transferrin, a β-globulin synthesized by the liver, is a specific iron-binding protein in blood that transports iron through the plasma and extravascular space. Each molecule of transferrin can bind two molecules of iron in the ferric state (Fe^{3+}). In normal circumstances, it is only about 30% to 50% saturated. The ability of transferrin to bind iron is called the iron-binding capacity. The total iron binding capacity (TIBC), which reflects serum transferrin concentrations, is a well-recognized value in the investigation of anemias. It represents the amount of iron that can bind to transferrin to give 100% saturation of the binding sites. The TIBC is high in iron deficiency and low in iron overload. Most cells obtain their iron from transferrin. In the case of reticulocytes and developing erythrocytes in the bone marrow, most of the iron taken up is used for Hb synthesis.

Storage iron (0.3–1.5 g), in the form of ferritin and hemosiderin, is located mainly in the parenchymal cells of the liver, the reticuloendothelial cells of the spleen, and bone marrow, and it replenishes functional iron. Iron stores account for one third of body iron in healthy men. Iron stores are more variable and are generally lower in children and women of childbearing potential. Low iron stores are an early sign of iron deficiency and may help differentiate between iron deficiency anemia and other causes of anemia (Table 31.6).

IRON NEEDS

Body iron usually is kept constant by a delicate balance between the amount lost and absorbed. There is no physiologic mechanism for excreting iron in humans. Consequently, there is only a limited ability to compensate for excessive loss or absorption of iron. Iron balance is a conservative system, and in the normal adult, even if iron intake is negligible, it takes at least 2 to 3 years to develop iron deficiency.

Iron needs are determined by total losses from the body. Daily iron needs vary according to age and sex (Table 31.7). Total daily iron loss amounts to 1 mg daily in men. Iron losses in women of childbearing potential are higher than those in men because of menstruation and pregnancy. Iron is lost from the gastrointestinal tract by sloughing of iron-containing mucosal cells and extravasation of erythrocytes, by skin exfoliation, and by shedding of urinary tract epithelial cells. Iron loss through sweat is minimal.

Blood loss in menstruating women varies, but if it exceeds 80 mL, it can lead to iron deficiency. Average iron losses through menstruation are about 0.3 to 0.5 mg daily. Menstrual iron losses are lower in women taking oral contraceptives and higher in those using an intrauterine device.[1,3]

Iron needs increase to 3 to 4 mg daily during pregnancy to account for obligatory losses, the expanded maternal erythrocyte mass that occurs in pregnancy and in the placenta and fetus. Iron needs are greatest in the second and third trimester when the highest fetal erythrocyte needs occur. Some of the iron incorporated in the expanded maternal erythrocyte mass returns to the iron pool after pregnancy, but peripartum blood loss partly nullifies this contribution. Because menstruation does not start until several weeks after delivery, iron losses are reduced. However, breast-feeding offsets some of the gain.[1,3]

The need for iron is high in the first year of life and throughout childhood because of rapid growth and erythropoiesis during this period. Normal full-term infants need to absorb a minimum of 0.3 mg of iron daily in the first year of life. Premature infants can need up to 1 mg daily. Children's iron needs increase with age (Table 31.7).

IRON ABSORPTION

Iron absorption is regulated by iron needs and body stores. When iron stores are low or depleted, a higher proportion of available iron is absorbed. Absorption decreases when the

Age	Iron (mg/day)	Folic Acid (μg/day)	Vitamin B$_{12}$ (μg/day)
Infants			
0–6 months	0.27	65	0.4
7–12 months	11	80	0.5
Children			
1–3 years	7	150	0.9
4–8 years	10	200	1.2
Males			
9–13 years	8	300	1.8
14–18 years	11	400	2.4
19–30 years	8	400	2.4
31–50 years	8	400	2.4
50–70 years	8	400	2.4
>70 years	8	400	2.4
Females			
9–13 years	8	300	1.8
14–18 years	15	400	2.4
19–30 years	18	400	2.4
31–50 years	18	400	2.4
50–70 years	8	400	2.4
>70 years	8	400	2.4
Pregnancy			
≤18 years	27	600	2.6
19–30 years	27	600	2.6
31–50 years	27	600	2.6
Lactation			
≤18 years	10	500	2.8
19–30 years	9	500	2.8
31–50 years	9	500	2.8

(From http://www.nal.usda.gov/fnic/etext/000105.html. Accessed 11/29/2005.)

stores are replete. The serum ferritin concentration, which reflects body iron stores, is inversely related to iron absorption. However, this feedback process can be overwhelmed when large amounts of iron are presented for absorption (e.g., in iron overdose or toxicity cases).[1] In some clinical states, such as primary hemochromatosis, thalassemia, and sideroblastic anemia, iron absorption remains normal and even elevated despite increased iron stores.

The iron content of food and its bioavailability determine if the diet can meet physiologic needs. Dietary iron is present as two major pools: heme iron and nonheme iron. Heme iron, found only in meats, is two to three times more absorbable than nonheme iron, found in plant-based and iron-fortified foods. Ingested heme compounds and organic non-

heme iron complexes are broken down in the acid environment of the stomach to ferric ions (Fe^{3+}) and heme molecules, respectively. The stomach's acidity promotes reduction of iron from the ferric state to the ferrous state (Fe^{2+}), which is better absorbed. Patients with achlorhydria secondary to age or gastrectomy tend to absorb nonheme iron poorly.[1,3,13–15]

Iron is absorbed primarily in the upper duodenum (Fig. 31.1; color insert). The iron-absorptive capacity is limited by the rate at which iron is transferred from the intestinal lumen to the plasma. The reduced (ferrous) iron binds to specific sites on the lumen and is actively carried across the intestinal membrane. Iron absorbed by these cells is incorporated into an iron carrier pool, most of which is deposited

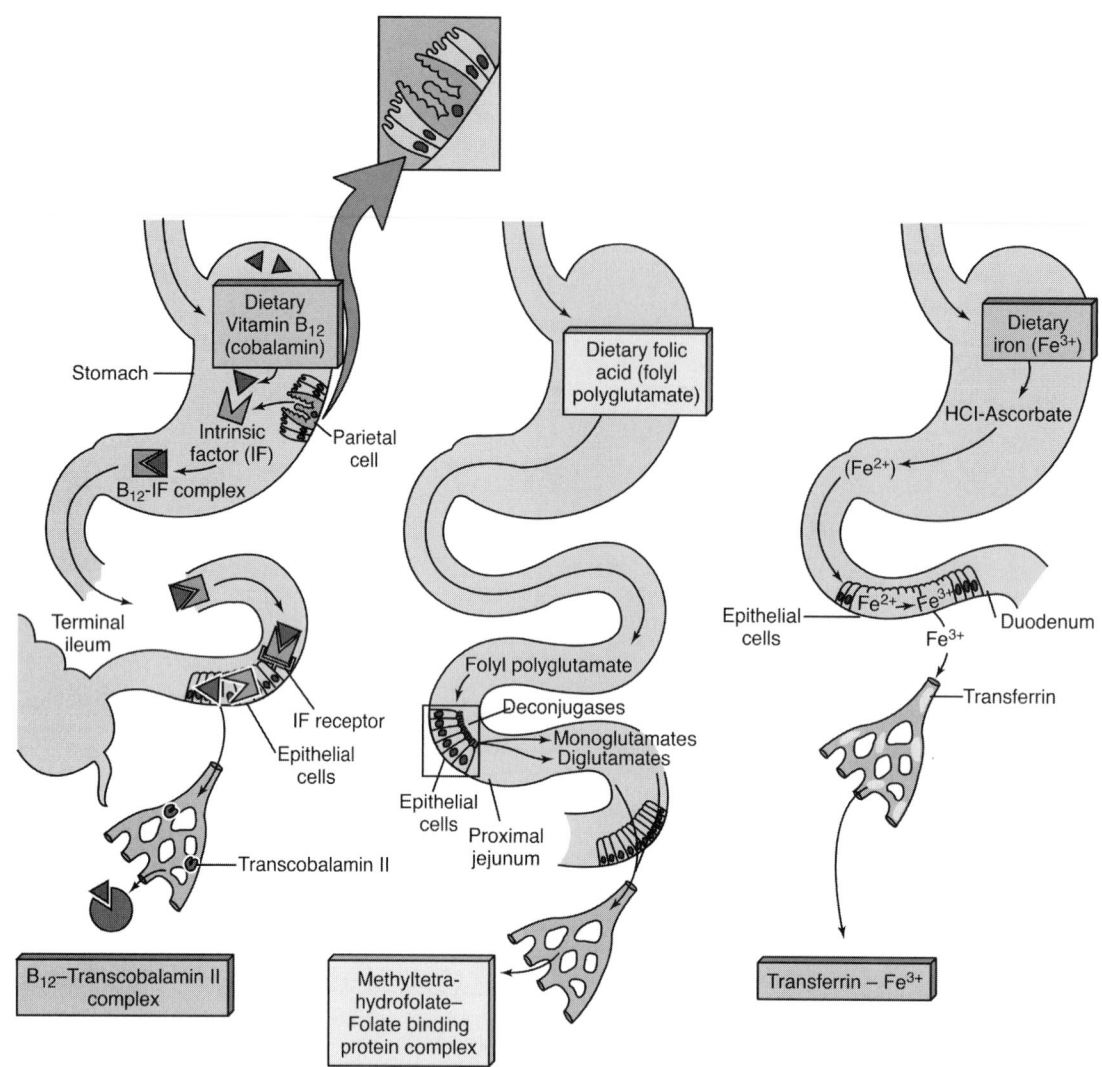

FIGURE 31.1 Absorption of vitamin B12, folic acid, and iron (*color insert*). Absorption of vitamin B12 requires initial complexing with intrinsic factor (IF), which is produced by the parietal cells of the gastric mucosa. Absorption then occurs in the terminal ileum, where there are receptors for the IF-B12 complex. Dietary folic acid is conjugated by conjugase enzymes to polyglutamate. Absorption occurs in the jejunum following deconjugation in the intestinal lumen. Reduction and methylation result in the generation of methyl tetrahydrofolate, which is then transported by folate binding protein. Dietary ferric iron is reduced to ferrous iron in the stomach and absorbed principally in the duodenum. Iron is transported by transferrin in the circulation. (Image from Rubin E MD and Farber JL MD. Pathology. 3rd ed. Philadelphia: Lippincott Williams & Wilkins, 1999, with permission.)

as ferritin or used by the mitochondria for enzyme synthesis. A small amount of iron is lost through the normal sloughing of the mucosal cells in the gastrointestinal tract. A smaller proportion of the iron from the carrier pool is transferred to the plasma, where the ferric form binds tightly to transferrin.

A number of factors can inhibit or promote iron absorption (Table 31.8). Foods that can reduce iron absorption by forming less soluble complexes include coffee, tea, milk and milk products, eggs, whole grain breads and cereals, and any food containing bicarbonates, carbonates, oxalates, or phosphates. Commercial processing or enhancers can im-

prove absorption from food in some cases. Enhancers of nonheme iron absorption are food acids such as citric, lactic, or ascorbic acids, and meats.[3,13–15] Ascorbic acid, the most powerful promoter, has a dose-related effect on nonheme iron absorption. In its presence, ferric iron is converted to the ferrous state, maintaining iron solubility in the alkaline environment of the duodenum and upper jejunum. Ascorbic acid also forms an alkaline-stable chelate with ferric chloride in the stomach. Meat, itself a rich source of iron, also promotes absorption of nonheme iron. Approximately 1 g of meat enhances nonheme iron absorption to about the same

TABLE 31.8	Factors Associated With Iron Absorption
Factor	**Associations**
Promoting absorption	
Inorganic iron	Ionic iron, particularly in the ferrous form, is better absorbed than ferric iron and organically bound iron.
Ascorbic acid	Ascorbic acid helps to convert ferric iron to ferrous iron.
Acid	Gastric hydrochloric acid promotes the release and conversion of dietary iron to the ferrous form.
Chelates	Iron chelated to low-molecular-weight substances such as sugars (fructose and sucrose), amino acids, and succinate facilitates iron binding to the intestinal mucosa.
Clinical states	Iron deficiency, increased erythropoiesis, pregnancy, anoxia, and pyridoxine deficiency promote absorption.
Reducing absorption	
Alkaline	Alkaline pancreatic secretions containing phosphate probably convert iron to insoluble ferric hydroxide; antacids.
Dietary	Dietary phosphates and phytates in cereals and tannins in tea probably complex iron.
Clinical states	Chronic diarrhea, steatorrhea, adequate iron stores, decreased erythropoiesis, and acute or chronic inflammation reduce absorption.
Medications	Anatacids, tetracycline

extent as 1 mg of ascorbic acid. Citric acid, a common food additive and a less powerful promoter of iron absorption, has an additive effect to ascorbic acid.

EPIDEMIOLOGY

OCCURRENCE

Iron deficiency, estimated to occur in more than 2.5 billion people throughout the world, is the most common cause of nutritional anemia.[3,16–18] Data from the third Nutritional Health and Nutrition Examination Survey (NHANES III) in the United States indicated that the incidence of iron deficiency was highest for toddlers aged 1 to 2 years (9%), adolescent girls (9%), and women of childbearing potential (11%), with iron deficiency anemia occurring in 3%, 2%, and 5%, respectively. This corresponds to approximately 240,000 toddlers and 3.3 million women having iron deficiency anemia. For women of childbearing potential, iron deficiency was more common in minorities, people with lower incomes, and multiparous women. Iron deficiency occurred in less than 1% of men and adolescent boys between 12 and 50 years of age and in 4% of men 70 years and older.[19]

ETIOLOGY

The primary causes of iron deficiency are listed in Table 31.9. Blood loss is the major cause of iron deficiency in men and nonmenstruating women and girls. Bleeding may be overt or occult. A common site of blood loss is the gastrointestinal tract. If bleeding is not obvious, a test for occult blood in the stool may give the first indication of blood loss. Common sources of blood loss in the gastrointestinal tract are peptic ulcers, esophageal varices, and colon cancer. Nonsteroidal anti-inflammatory agents, such as aspirin and indomethacin, can cause gastrointestinal bleeding, especially if taken with warfarin. In the absence of upper gastrointestinal symptoms, investigations should be directed to the lower gastrointestinal tract. Bleeding hemorrhoids rarely result in anemia, but neoplasms are a common cause of bleeding, particularly in older adults. The incidence of colon cancer, which can cause bleeding, increases 40-fold between ages 40 and 80. Other causes of gastrointestinal blood loss include hookworm infestation, Meckel's diverticulum, and ulcerative colitis. Hookworm is a major cause of iron deficiency anemia in tropical areas.

Iron deficiency has also been noted in athletes, particularly adolescent girls, marathon runners, and other endurance athletes. Up to 50% of adolescent female athletes demonstrate some degree of iron depletion, but anemia is uncommon. Blood loss is believed to result from ischemia of the gastrointestinal tract because blood is shunted to muscles

TABLE 31.9	Factors Associated With Iron Deficiency	
Factor	**Association**	
Dietary	Starvation, poverty, vegetarianism, religious practice, food fads	
Blood loss		
Women and girls	Menstruation, postmenopausal bleeding, pregnancy	
General	Esophageal varices, peptic ulcer, drug-induced gastritis, carcinomas of stomach and colon, ulcerative colitis, hemorrhoids, renal or bladder lesions (hematuria), hookworm infestation, other organ bleeding (hemoptysis), frequent blood donation, athletic training, widespread bleeding disorders	
Malabsorption	Celiac disease (gluten-induced enteropathy), partial and total gastrectomy, chronic inflammation	
Increased requirements	Rapid growth (as in childhood and adolescence), pregnancy; erythropoiesis	

during prolonged exercise. Marathon runners can lose at least 3 mg of iron daily for several days after a marathon race. Another short-term anemia related to sports is the dilutional anemia that can result from plasma volume expansion in the early weeks of conditioning.[20,21]

Poor nutrition, defective intake, and decreased assimilation of iron rarely cause iron deficiency in people living in Western countries. Iron deficiency caused by inadequate dietary iron intake is predominantly a problem of infants, children, and pregnant women, whose daily needs are higher. In some populations, where the diet is mainly of vegetable origin with little meat, women are more likely to suffer from nutritional iron deficiency. Iron malabsorption may occasionally cause iron deficiency, although it is rarely an important cause unless iron stores are low or there are other contributing factors such as blood loss, pregnancy, or poor nutrition. The two most common conditions in which iron absorption is a problem are gluten enteropathy (celiac disease) and gastrectomy. Other conditions associated with iron deficiency anemia include pernicious anemia,[22,23] pica syndrome,[24] and chronic inflammatory disease such as rheumatoid arthritis.[1,2]

CLINICAL PRESENTATION AND DIAGNOSIS

SIGNS AND SYMPTOMS

Iron deficiency precedes the manifestations of anemia. Most people with iron deficiency have minimal anemia and are asymptomatic.[25] Progression to iron deficiency anemia is often insidious, although mildly lowered Hb concentrations generally decrease work capacity. The development of symptoms depends on the rate of iron loss and the body's ability to compensate. Symptoms generally become evident when the blood Hb concentration falls below 6.2 mmol per liter (10 g/dL), although some patients remain asymptomatic even with Hb concentrations of 4.3 mmol per liter (7 g/dL).

The usual signs and symptoms of iron deficiency anemia are often present (Table 31.2). Other problems caused by the gross epithelial changes associated with chronic iron deficiency include brittle or spoon-shaped nails, angular stomatitis, atrophic tongue, pharyngeal and esophageal webs causing dysphagia, and atrophic gastric mucosa. Iron deficiency, in addition to its hematologic effects, may also be associated with diverse problems such as impaired work performance[2,3]; low birthweight, prematurity, and increased perinatal mortality;[2,3] and impaired psychomotor behavior, cognitive function, and central nervous system development in infants and young children.[18,26,27]

A common symptom of iron deficiency anemia is pica, a condition in which the person craves unusual substances that generally have no nutritional value, such as clay (geophagia), paper products, or starch (amylophagia). Pagophagia (pica for ice), or habitual ice eating, is a common form of pica in some communities. Other people consume earth and particles of clay cooking pots. Such ingestions have led to metabolic problems, including heavy metal poisoning.[24]

DIAGNOSIS

Most cases of iron deficiency anemia are identified on the basis of a medical history, complete blood count, and peripheral smears.[1–3,9] In iron deficiency anemia, hematologic changes are evident only after all body iron stores have been depleted and there is insufficient iron to maintain normal erythrocyte morphology and mass (Table 31.6). Blood Hb concentrations and erythrocyte numbers are normal in mild cases. Serum ferritin is the first parameter to change with iron deficiency. As the deficiency worsens, the MCV and erythrocyte count decrease markedly, the RDW increases, and eventually, the Hb decreases. When Hb concentrations are 4.4 mmol per liter (7 g/dL) or less for women or 5.6 mmol per liter (9 g/dL) or less for men, microscopic examination of peripheral blood smears shows hypochromia (Fig. 31.2; *color insert*) and poikilocytosis.

Although the ultimate proof of iron deficiency is the absence of stainable iron in bone marrow aspirates, this procedure is not routinely performed because it is painful and expensive. The proportion of reticulocytes usually is normal, but transient increases may follow acute hemorrhage or treatment with iron. The white cell and platelet count generally are normal.

Serum ferritin concentration is an early and specific indicator of body iron stores and is very useful in distinguishing iron deficiency from other causes of microcytic anemia. Ferritin concentrations fall in iron deficiency states but increase abnormally in iron storage conditions. Serum ferritin concentrations of less than 15 μg per liter (normal, 15–300 μg/L) generally are diagnostic for iron deficiency in adults (Table 31.6). However, interpretation of ferritin levels entails consideration of other patient factors, such as coexisting inflammatory processes, liver disease, or malignancy. Ferritin is an acute phase reactant to inflammatory diseases such as rheumatoid arthritis or acute infection. In these conditions, serum ferritin concentrations increase, with the lower level

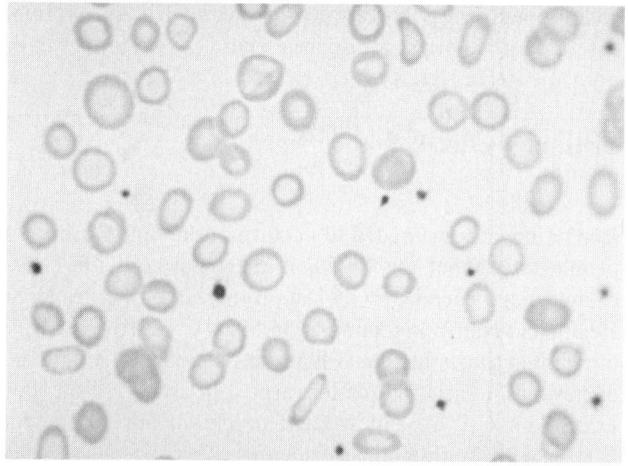

FIGURE 31.2 Iron deficient erythrocytes (hypochromic/microcyte; *see color insert*). Pink central pallor greater than one third of cell. (From Anderson's Atlas of Hematology; Anderson, Shauna C., PhD. © 2003. Phildelphia: Wolters Kluwer Health/Lippincott Williams & Wilkins, with permission.)

of normal increasing to 50 μg per liter. Patients with levels between 12 μg per liter and 50 μg per liter should be investigated further for iron deficiency anemia. An abnormal release of ferritin from hepatocytes can also occur with acute hepatic necrosis or inflammation. To rule out iron deficiency anemia in patients with an inflammatory disease or liver disease, especially hepatitis, other tests, such as ZPP or serum TfR concentration, which are not affected by these underlying processes, should be used.

Final heme synthesis involves the incorporation of iron into the protoporphyrin ring. When there is insufficient iron to support heme production, zinc is incorporated into the protoporphyrin and ZPP is produced instead of heme. Serum concentrations of ZPP, which measure the amount of protoporphyrin not incorporated into heme, increase when insufficient iron is available for Hb synthesis. A concentration of more than 80 μmol per mole heme indicates iron deficiency. This measurement has less daily variability than serum iron concentration or transferrin saturation and is an earlier indicator of iron-deficient erythropoiesis than anemia. However, it is not as early an indicator of deficiency as serum ferritin. Some advocate its use before or concurrently with serum ferritin because it correlates with deficiency at the tissue level.[3,9,18] In assessing ZPP values, one must be aware that other conditions in which iron support for erythropoiesis is insufficient (lead poisoning, myelodysplastic syndromes, anemia of chronic disease) also result in increased ZPP concentrations.

Serum TfR measurement reflects the number of transferrin receptors on immature red cells and is an indication of bone marrow erythropoiesis. While ferritin is an early indicator of iron deficiency, TfR measurement provides information on the later stages of iron deficiency, increasing only after iron stores are depleted. It is not affected by inflammatory processes, and is useful in differentiating iron deficiency from anemia caused by chronic disease, infection, or inflammation.[9,10,25,28,29] Use of the TfR to serum ferritin ratio has been advocated for earlier and more sensitive detection of iron deficiency.[28,29]

Serum iron levels and the TIBC are other traditional measures for evaluating iron deficiency. However, these are less sensitive and more variable than ferritin determination and often are normal in the early stages of iron deficiency. A low serum iron with a high TIBC level generally is characteristic of iron deficiency. Normal to low serum iron levels with a normal or low TIBC is associated with anemias of chronic disease. In thalassemia, hemoglobinopathies, and sideroblastic anemia, serum iron levels are normal or high. Transferrin saturation, another indicator of body iron stores, is below 16% in most cases of iron deficiency anemia. Transferrin saturation levels below 5% are found only in iron deficiency. However, there is considerable overlap with anemias of chronic disease.

Assessment of the predictive values of some of these tests in patients without evidence of inflammatory disease showed that bone marrow examination and serum ferritin were 100% predictive in patients with iron depletion, iron deficiency (insufficient for erythropoiesis), and iron deficiency anemia. The ZPP values were normal (0% predictive value) with iron depletion but 100% predictive in patients with iron deficiency or iron deficiency anemia. Transferrin saturation had 0% predictive value for iron depletion, 71% for iron deficiency, 78% for mild iron deficiency anemia, and 96% for severe iron deficiency anemia. Hb concentrations were not predictive until anemia developed (100% for mild or severe anemia), and MCV was 22% predictive for mild and 100% predictive for severe anemia.[25]

Which tests are used to assess iron status depends on the patient's history and condition, the goal of the evaluation (early detection of iron depletion versus assessment of the existence or cause of an anemia), and laboratory equipment available. To check for anemia, Hb or Hct may be assessed, with other tests ordered if anemia is found. Monitoring iron depletion to prevent anemia includes using tests with sensitivity for the earlier stages of iron deficiency. Many clinicians use the ferritin test as the first-line test of iron status because it is an early indicator of iron store depletion. However, concurrent inflammatory or infectious processes or neoplasms reduce its reliability. Therefore, multiple tests often are used to assess iron status.

In the absence of a specialized hematology facility, a tentative diagnosis of iron deficiency can be made by giving a trial of iron therapy, and monitoring Hb concentrations and reticulocyte counts. Significant reticulocytosis occurs 7 to 10 days after the start of treatment, and the Hb concentrations increase over 3 to 4 weeks. Inflammatory disease may retard reticulocytosis.

PREVENTION

Prevention is accomplished by identifying high-risk patients (Table 31.3) and correcting iron deficiencies before anemia develops. Management is directed toward identifying and treating the underlying cause of the iron deficiency and correcting the iron deficiency with diet or supplementation.

DIETARY MANIPULATION

The primary prevention of iron deficiency, and hence anemia, should occur using dietary manipulation. For overall prevention of iron deficiency, food fortification has been recommended, especially in developing countries where diets do not contain iron-rich foods such as red meat.[30,31] Targeted fortification for infants through formula and commercial cereals and for schoolchildren through meal programs has been successful in developed countries. Widespread fortification of foods in the United States may account for the lower incidence of iron deficiency anemia in women of childbearing potential. However, even with fortification, iron deficiency and iron deficiency anemia can still occur.[19,31] When dietary iron supplementation is not possible or adequate, oral supplementation should be initiated.

The U.S. Centers for Disease Control (CDC) published guidelines for preventing iron deficiency in high-risk groups.[3] In infants, the CDC recommends the following:

- Breast-feeding for 4 to 6 months after birth
- Use of 1 mg/kg/day of iron from supplemental foods or iron drops when breast-feeding is stopped
- Use of only iron-fortified infant formula as a substitute for breast milk
- Use of 2- to 4-mg/kg/day of iron drops (max 15 mg/day) for preterm or low-birthweight infants starting at 1 month and continuing until 12 months after birth
- Introduction of iron-fortified infant cereal at age 4 to 6 months (two or more servings should meet iron needs)

For adolescent girls and nonpregnant women of childbearing potential, iron-rich foods and foods that enhance iron absorption should be encouraged. For pregnant women, the CDC recommends starting oral low-dose (30 mg/day) iron supplementation at the first prenatal visit.[3]

Generally, iron stores become depleted by 4 months of age in term infants unless an adequate exogenous supply of iron is provided. Although breast milk is thought to provide enough iron to prevent deficiency, a study performed in Argentina demonstrated a 27.8% incidence of iron deficiency anemia in children breast-fed for 6 months and a 7.1% incidence in children who received formula.[32] This indicates the need for caution in relying solely on breast milk to meet iron needs through 6 months of age in all children. Maternal diet and amount of breast milk consumed may affect the amount of iron provided to the infant.

The iron content of infant formulas continues to be evaluated to ascertain the optimal amount of iron to prevent iron deficiency anemia. Lower iron concentrations (2.3 mg/L vs. 12.7 mg/L and 3 mg/L vs. 5 mg/L) in healthy, noniron-deficient, term infants were as efficacious as higher concentrations in preventing iron deficiency anemia.[33,34] However, in a high-risk group of infants, an iron concentration of 12.8 mg per liter was found to be superior to 1.1 mg per liter in maintaining iron status (preventing iron deficiency) and psychomotor development.[35] This enforces the need to monitor therapy to ensure appropriate response and dosing.

Providing supplemental iron to other high-risk groups, such as children with inadequate dietary intake, women of childbearing potential, and pregnant women, continues to be recommended, but the optimal dose and schedule are debated.[3,16,17,36,37] Anemic and nonanemic children 3 to 6 years of age who received 6 mg per kilogram elemental iron daily, twice weekly, or weekly had similar hematologic response after 3 months of therapy. In the children with anemia, all three regimens reversed the anemia and replenished ferritin levels. The incidence of side effects was dramatically different between the dosing groups: 35.4%, 7.4%, and 0% for daily, twice weekly, and weekly administration, respectively, in children with anemia at the start of the study and 39.7%, 6.6%, and 5.7%, respectively, in the nonanemic children. The major complaints were anorexia, nausea, abdominal discomfort, constipation, and diarrhea.[38] This study, and other clinical trials in preschool-age children, adolescent girls, and pregnant women, have demonstrated that weekly iron supplementation provides similar efficacy with fewer side effects than daily iron therapy for the prevention and possible treatment of iron deficiency.[16,17,36] However, the design limitations of many of these studies have lessened the value of the results.[37]

Iron supplementation during pregnancy is controversial. Treatment can be geared toward prevention of iron deficiency anemia, prevention of iron store depletion, or avoidance of a negative iron balance. The CDC recommends universal treatment with 30 mg iron daily during pregnancy to prevent iron deficiency.[3] This can be done using a prescribed multivitamin and iron preparation or over-the-counter iron preparations. However, because iron can cause side effects and potentially affect absorption of other nutrients, selective supplementation only for women at risk of iron deficiency anemia also has been advocated.[16] The recommended dosages and schedules of iron supplements also vary from 30 to 240 mg daily to 60 mg once a week.[3,16] The higher doses may be needed in populations in which the prepregnancy anemia rate is high because the women are more likely to have depleted iron stores before becoming pregnant. Patient tolerance and compliance with the iron regimen must be assessed. If patients are not able to tolerate daily supplementation, reducing the daily dosage or dosing on a weekly schedule are other options.

SCREENING FOR IRON DEFICIENCY

The CDC recommends assessing infants for risk of iron deficiency and screening (Hb and/or Hct) those who are at risk (preterm, low birthweight, low-iron diet) at 9 to 12 months and at 15 to 18 months of age. In addition, the CDC recommends screening all nonpregnant girls starting in adolescence and continuing every 5 to 10 years throughout their childbearing years. Women with high risk factors (poor diet, excessive menstrual bleeding, chronic blood loss) should be screened annually. In pregnant women, Hb should be measured at the first prenatal visit to assess the need for iron replacement therapy or prophylaxis.[3]

TREATMENT

Although dietary improvements may reduce the risk of iron deficiency, the poor absorption of iron from foods limits the usefulness of dietary therapy in correcting an existing deficiency. Therefore, iron deficiency generally is corrected with oral or parenteral iron. A workup should be completed before therapy is initiated because indiscriminate iron administration can delay the diagnosis of underlying causes. Most iron therapy is given by the oral route, with few situations justifying the use of parenteral iron. With appropriate therapy, the Hb levels improve within a few weeks, and the patient feels better. Adequate iron must be supplied in the early stages of treatment to optimize the response.

PHARMACOTHERAPY

Oral Iron Therapy. Oral iron supplementation is safer, more convenient, and less expensive than parenteral therapy. Oral iron preparations are salt forms, which vary in elemental iron content, cost, and effectiveness. Iron absorption from ferrous salts is considered better than that from ferric salts.

The dosage of the iron product is based on the elemental iron content. In general, 30 to 40 mg daily elemental iron is used to treat iron deficiency states. These numbers are derived from calculating the maximum rate of Hb regeneration:

$$\begin{aligned} &0.25 \text{ g Hb}/100 \text{ mL blood/day} \\ &\times 5000 \text{ mL blood} \quad\quad (31\text{-}1) \\ &\times 3.4 \text{ mg iron}/1 \text{ g Hb} \approx 40 \text{ mg iron/day} \end{aligned}$$

Since only 10% to 20% of iron is absorbed, 200 to 400 mg of iron would result in absorption of approximately 40 mg elemental iron. Ferrous sulfate tablets contain 20% elemental iron (60 mg iron per 300-mg tablet). The standard dosing of ferrous sulfate is 300 mg three times a day, which provides 180 mg of elemental iron per day. Assuming 20% absorption, only about 40mg of elemental iron will be absorbed. When switching from one form of iron to another, care must be taken in calculating the dosages of different salts needed to provide equivalent elemental iron quantities (Table 31.10). Maximum absorption occurs if iron is taken before or between meals.

The most common side effects of oral iron therapy are epigastric distress, abdominal cramping, nausea, diarrhea, and constipation caused by gastric irritation. The reported incidence of these side effects ranges from 15% to 46% with daily dosing.[1,16,39] These side effects appear to be dose related. Options for minimizing these side effects include reducing the daily dose, taking the iron with food (at the expense of lower absorption), or changing to once-a-week dosing.[16,39] Use of enteric-coated products to minimize gastrointestinal effects is not recommended because the coating prevents dissolution in the stomach, thus minimizing iron absorption.[1,14] Iron therapy can cause the stools to appear black. Patients should be educated about differences between stool changes from iron and those associated with gastrointestinal bleeding.

Iron absorption may be reduced in patients with reduced gastric acid production or prior gastrointestinal surgeries. When an inability to absorb iron is suspected, an oral iron absorption test should be administered. This consists of administering an oral bolus dose of 325 mg ferrous sulfate (65 mg elemental iron) and measuring the serum iron level 2 and 4 hours later. The serum iron level should rise by 21 to 23 μmol per liter (115–128 μg/dL). Failure to attain this response generally indicates decreased absorption.[14] Antacids, histamine-2 blockers, and proton pump inhibitors may also decrease iron absorption (Table 31.8). A careful medication history should be obtained to check for potential drug interactions before an absorption test or parenteral therapy is initiated.

Parenteral Iron Therapy. Oral iron replacement therapy is usually sufficient for most patients. Oral iron may be inadequate in patients who are intolerant to oral iron, noncompliant, have abnormal absorption due to surgery or gastrointestinal conditions, or significant blood loss. Parenteral iron may be necessary in these patients.[14,15] Iron deficiency anemia in patients with chronic kidney disease and hemodialysis patients receiving erythropoietin or darbepoetin supplementation is discussed in further detail in Chapter 43.

The amount of parenteral iron needed to replenish iron stores and restore Hb levels in patients with iron deficiency anemia can be approximated using the following formula:[14,15]

$$\text{Dose (mg)} = 0.3 \times \text{Body weight (lb)} \quad (31\text{-}2a)$$
$$\times \left[100 - \frac{\text{Hb (g/dL)} \times 100}{14.8} \right]$$

The formula can be modified to use kilograms instead of pounds:

$$\text{Dose (mg)} = 0.66 \times \text{Body weight (kg)} \quad (31\text{-}2b)$$
$$\times \left[100 - \frac{\text{Hb (g/dL)} \times 100}{14.8} \right]$$

For example, a 65 kg man with a Hb of 10 g/dL would require approximately 1,400 mg of iron.

$$= 0.66 \times 65 \text{ (kg)} \times \left[100 - \frac{10 \text{ (g/dL)} \times 100}{14.8} \right]$$
$$= 1391 \text{ mg} \approx 1400 \text{ mg}$$

For children weighing less than 15 kg, the normal mean Hb of 12 g/dL is used in place of 14.8 g/dL in the equation.[15]

These formulas do not take into account active blood loss. To determine the iron replacement dose in these patients, it is assumed that 1 mL of normochromic, normocytic erythrocytes contains 1 mg of elemental iron:

$$\text{Dose (mg)} = 1 \text{ mg iron/mL blood} \quad (31\text{-}3)$$
$$\times \text{ blood loss (mL)} \times \text{Hct}$$

For example, a patient with a blood loss of 250 mL and a Hct of 23% would need approximately 58 mg of iron.

$$58 \text{ mg} = 1 \text{ mg iron/mL} \times 250 \text{ mL} \times 0.23$$

Iron Dextran. Iron dextran is a complex of ferric hydroxide and dextran. Following administration, the iron dextran complex is separated by the reticuloendothelial system. The iron that is released then binds to transferrin for transport to the liver, spleen, and bone marrow.

Iron dextran can be given as an intravenous infusion, slow intravenous injection, or by intramuscular injection. Regardless of the route, a test dose of 0.5 mL (25 mg) should be given before therapy is initiated. The test dose should be given by the same route as the intended therapy. Patients should be observed for at least 1 hour for any reactions. Most adverse reactions occur during or shortly after the test dose and range from mild transient reactions to life-threatening anaphylactic reactions. Mild reactions are generally transient and include dyspnea, headache, nausea, vomiting,

TABLE 31.10	Common Oral Iron Preparations	
Iron Salt	**Dosage Form (Brand)**	**Strength (elemental iron)**
Ferrous fumarate	Capsules (Neo-Fer)	300 mg (100 mg)
	Extended release capsules (Span-FF)	325 mg (106 mg)
	Oral solution (Feostat)	100 mg (33 mg)/5 mL
	Tablets	
	Femiron	63 mg (20 mg)
	Fumerin	195 mg (64 mg)
	Fumasorb, Ircon	200 mg (66 mg)
	Generic	300 mg (99 mg)
	Ferretts, Hemocyte, generic	325 mg (106 mg)
	Nephro-Fer	350 mg (116 mg)
	Chew tabs (Feostat)	100 mg (33 mg)
Ferrous gluconate	Capsules (Simron)	86 mg (10 mg)
	Elixir (Fergon)	300 mg (34 mg)/5 mL
	Tablets	
	Generic	300 mg (34 mg)
	Fergon	320 mg (37 mg)
	Generic	325 mg (38 mg)
	Extended release tablets (Ferralet slow release)	320 mg (37 mg)
Ferrous sulfate	Capsules (Ferrospace, generic)	250 mg (50 mg)
	Capsules (dried) (Fer-In-Sol)	190 mg (60 mg)
	Extended release capsules (dried)	
	Feosol	159 mg (50 mg)
	Ferralyn, Lanacaps, Ferra-TD	250 mg (50 mg)
	Elixir (Feosol)	220 mg (44 mg)/5 mL
	Oral solution	
	Fer-In-Sol drops	75 mg (15 mg)/0.6 mL
	Fer-Iron drops, generic	125 mg (25 mg)/mL
	Tablets	
	Mol-Iron	195 mg (39 mg)
	Ferratab	300 mg (160 mg)
	Generic	325 mg (65 mg)
	Enteric coated tablets (generic)	325 mg (65 mg)
	Extended release tablets (generic)	325 mg (65 mg)
	Tablets (dried) (Feosol)	200 mg (65 mg)
	Extended release tablets (dried) (Slow Fe)	160 mg (50 mg)

(From United States Pharmacopeia Drug Information: Drug Information for the Health Care Professional. Vol 1.21st ed. Greenwood Village, CO: Thomson Micromedex, 1774–1785, 2001, with permission.)

flushing, itching, urticaria, fever, hives, and chest, abdominal, or back pain. Anaphylactic reactions are characterized sudden onset of respiratory difficulty or cardiovascular collapse. Emergency medications such as epinephrine, diphenhydramine, and corticosteroids to treat the anaphylactic reaction should be readily available. Severe reactions can still occur during therapeutic administration even though the test dose was uneventful. Systemic reactions may also occur 1 to 2 days after iron dextran therapy. These delayed reactions may include myalgias, arthralgias, and back pain.[14,15] Adverse events are more frequent in patients with rheumatoid arthritis (flare in symptoms or severe anaphylactic reaction), other collagen vascular disease, or infection, and in patients receiving large doses.[14,15] There are two iron dextran products available, which differ in their molecular weight (Dexferrum, molecular weight = 265,000; INFeD, molecular weight = 96,000).[40,41] There does not appear to be any therapeutic advantage with using a higher molecular weight iron dextran preparation, however, the incidence of adverse events appears to be greater compared to the lower molecular weight iron dextran product.[42]

If the intramuscular route is selected, a Z-track method technique is recommended for administration. This technique involves moving the subcutaneous tissue over the injection site laterally before inserting the needle. After the iron dextran is administered, the tissue is slowly released as the needle is removed, covering the needle track. This technique minimizes leakage through the needle track and skin staining. This technique is painful, and may result in necrotic skin ulcerations after multiple injections.[15] Another limitation of the intramuscular route is that only 100 mg (2 mL) can be delivered per injection, with a total daily dose not to exceed 100 mg. Iron dextran should be injected only into the muscle mass of the upper outer quadrant of the buttock.[41]

One advantage of iron dextran is the ability to infuse to the patient's total iron requirement in one dose [total dose infusion (TDI)], thus, minimizing patient discomfort and increasing convenience and compliance. Although TDI is not approved by the Food and Drug Administration (FDA), it is commonly used in clinical practice.[1,14,15] For TDI, the total dose of iron dextran is diluted in 250 to 1,000 mL of normal saline or 5% dextrose and administered over 4 to 6 hours. Local phlebitis is less likely to occur if normal saline is used; slower infusion rates may also minimize irritation.

Iron Sucrose. Iron sucrose is a complex of ferric hydroxide and sucrose. Like iron dextran, iron sucrose is dissociated into iron and sucrose in the reticuloendothelial system. Iron sucrose (Venofer) was approved by the FDA in November of 2000 for treatment of iron deficiency anemia in nondialysis and dialysis-dependent chronic kidney disease patients receiving erythropoietin. The recommended dose of iron sucrose in hemodialysis-dependent patients is 100 mg (5 mL) undiluted as a slow intravenous injection over 2 to 5 minutes or diluted in 100 mL of 0.9% normal saline given as an intravenous infusion over 15 minutes on consecutive dialysis sessions to a cumulative dose of 1,000 mg. In nondi-

alysis patients with chronic kidney disease, the recommended dose is 200 mg, given as a slow intravenous injection over 2 to 5 minutes on five different occasions in a 14-day period to a cumulative dose of 1,000 mg. Doses of 500 mg diluted in 250 mL of 0.9% normal saline given over 3.5 to 4 hours on days 1 and 14 have been administered. For peritoneal dialysis patients, a cumulative dose of 1,000 mg is given in three divided doses within a 28-day period, with two infusions of 300 mg each given over 1.5 hours 14 days apart followed by one 400-mg infusion over 2.5 hours 14 days later.[43] Iron sucrose is more readily available for erythropoiesis than iron dextran, with increases in hemoglobin noted after 1 week of administration.[44,45] Iron sucrose has been used in patients with documented iron dextran sensitivity.[46]

Ferric Gluconate. Sodium ferric gluconate complex in sucrose was approved by the FDA in February 1999 for the treatment of patients with iron deficiency anemia undergoing chronic hemodialysis who are receiving erythropoietin therapy. The recommended dose is 125 mg (10 mL) diluted in 100 mL of 0.9% normal saline given as an intravenous infusion over 1 hour. It can also be given undiluted as a slow intravenous injection (not to exceed 12.5 mg/min). Most patients will require a cumulative dose of 1,000 mg given over eight sequential dialysis sessions to achieve the desired hemoglobin or hematocrit response. Doses exceeding 125 mg and/or infusion rates exceeding the recommended rate have been associated with a higher incidence of adverse reactions.[47] Ferric gluconate has been safely administered to iron dextran-sensitive patients.[48]

Parenteral Iron Toxicities. Adverse reactions to iron dextran, iron sucrose, and ferric gluconate have been reported in 50%, 36%, and 35% of patients, respectively. The most common adverse events include hypotension, hypertension, nausea, vomiting, diarrhea, abdominal pain, bradycardia, chest pain, headache, fever, pruritus, malaise, arthralgias, myalgias, back pain, and allergic reactions.[43,49]

The parenteral administration of iron dextran is associated with significant morbidity and anaphylactic reactions. Anaphylactic reactions are believed to be due to the dextran moiety rather than iron. The incidence of serious life-threatening anaphylactic reactions with dextran has been reported to be 0.6% to 0.7%,[50,51] and 0.002% and 0.05% for iron sucrose and ferric gluconate respectively.[52]

Iron dextran has been available in the United States for over 40 years. Despite the extensive medical experience with its efficacy and the ability to deliver the total dose in a single infusion, many clinicians are reluctant to use iron dextran because of the greater potential for severe allergic reactions. As a result, iron sucrose and ferric gluconate have become the predominant parenteral iron preparations used.[53]

Contraindications to Iron Therapy. Iron preparations should not be used in conditions, such as hemochromatosis and hemosiderosis, that already signify iron overload. In thalassemia and anemic conditions with chronic inflammatory disease, such as rheumatoid arthritis, iron is contraindicated because these conditions have normal to high iron stores because of impaired use of iron. Care must be exercised in giving iron to alcoholic patients because of elevated iron stores. Patients with alcoholic liver disease, such as cirrhosis, generally do not suffer from hemochromatosis, but those with marked increases in iron deposition and body stores may have genetically determined hemochromatosis. Iron should be used carefully in enteritis, diverticulitis, colitis, and ulcerative colitis because of local effects. Patients receiving repeated blood transfusions generally become iron overloaded because of the high erythrocyte iron content.

Iron Toxicity. Iron toxicity can be acute, such as in overdose and accidental poisoning, or chronic, as in overload that occurs in hemochromatosis, hemosiderosis, and thalassemia. A person with iron overload usually has more than 4 g body iron. Iron, which is ordinarily stored in reticuloendothelial cells, is deposited as ferritin and hemosiderin into hepatocytes of the liver and eventually other tissues and organs. Hemochromatosis is associated with severe iron overload, and may lead to liver and heart failure. Recently, noninvasive methods, such as computed tomography and magnetic resonance imaging, have been used to determine hepatic iron content.

The pathogenesis of iron overload is associated with increased mucosal iron absorption, the iron load associated with blood transfusions, or injections of therapeutic iron preparations. Diet is unlikely to cause iron overload unless other factors or problems are present. Normal people absorb the usual amounts of iron, even when the dietary iron load is increased 5 to 10 times. Amounts of 300 to 500 mg per day can be tolerated, although there are some exceptions. Alcohol consumption can contribute to the development of iron overload. Another potential cause of iron overload is the controversial practice in some developed countries of fortifying food with iron. Although this addition may be useful for women, it may lead to a grossly excessive iron intake by men. The prevalence of hemochromatosis is 0.5%, which is higher than that of iron deficiency in men. Indiscriminate use of iron supplements can be harmful. Intrinsic metabolic abnormalities may account for increased iron ab-

sorption from the small intestine. Such abnormalities occur in primary idiopathic hemochromatosis (hereditary hemochromatosis) and in some anemias.

Iron overload secondary to anemias can be divided into two classes: that in patients with hypoplastic bone marrow, where the main source of iron is blood transfusion (e.g., aplastic anemia, sickle cell disease) and that in patients with hyperplastic bone marrow, where the iron excess results from increased iron absorption secondary to ineffective erythropoiesis (e.g., thalassemia major, sideroblastic anemia, and some hemolytic anemias). Treatment of transfusional iron overload generally consists of chelation therapy, such as deferoxamine.[54]

Monitoring Iron Deficiency Therapy. The primary objective is to reverse the anemia. Response to iron therapy generally is evident within the first week by reticulocytosis. Hb should also increase, although the rate of increase depends on the severity of the anemia, whether the cause of iron depletion (blood loss, increased needs) has resolved, and the usual range for an individual. The rate of increase for a man with a usual blood Hb of 10 mmol per liter (16 g/dL) is faster than that for a pregnant woman who would normally have a blood Hb of about 6.5 mmol/L (10.5 g/dL). Serial blood hemoglobin measurements generally indicate an increase of 0.02 to 0.9 mmol per liter per day (0.03–0.14 g/dL/day). However, for practical purposes, most patients are not reevaluated until after 3 or 4 weeks of oral therapy. Anemia is corrected within about 6 weeks. A rapid recovery generally indicates that the cause of iron loss is no longer present. Poor responders should be evaluated to ensure adequacy of the dosage to meet the patient's iron needs, patient compliance, potential sources of iron loss (bleeding), and potential drug interactions.

A second objective in instituting iron therapy is to replenish iron stores. Generally this is a nonurgent phase of treatment that takes about 4 to 6 months to accomplish. Serum ferritin concentration and iron saturation can be used as guides for this stage of therapy. Some patients need long-term iron therapy because of blood loss or malabsorption problems. Iron dosages for these patients should be adjusted for the losses. Periodic serum ferritin determinations should be used as a guide to the patient's iron status.

MEGALOBLASTIC ANEMIAS

Megaloblastic anemia is a subclass of the macrocytic anemias. Megaloblastic anemia is characterized by a lowered blood Hb mass because of reduced erythropoiesis secondary to defective DNA synthesis in the developing erythroid cells of the bone marrow. Nonmegaloblastic macrocytic anemias (those not resulting from disorders of DNA synthesis) are caused primarily by alcoholism, liver disease, and hypothyroidism. Deficiencies of vitamin B_{12} or folate are the major

causes of megaloblastic anemia, followed by drug-induced interference, direct or indirect, with DNA synthesis or nutritional status.

Reduced availability or absence of one-carbon-unit coenzymes, such as methylcobalamin (active B_{12}) or formyltetrahydrofolic acid (active folic acid), results in impaired DNA synthesis in developing erythroid cells. These cells do not divide normally, and fewer large but well-hemoglobinated cells (megaloblasts) form in the bone marrow. The resulting megaloblasts are characterized by an abnormal nucleus because of greater cytoplasmic (rather than nuclear) maturity. Cells released into the circulation are larger than normal (macrocytic) and are generally normochromic. Morphologic changes observed in the peripheral smear include macro-ovalocyte erythrocytes and multilobed neutrophilic granulocytes. These erythrocytes have a reduced life span.

In addition to the erythroid changes, similar effects on other hemopoietic cell lines in the bone marrow can lead to leukopenia, thrombocytopenia, or pancytopenia. Other rapidly dividing tissue can also be affected, particularly the mucosal epithelium of the gastrointestinal tract.[5,55,56]

It is important to distinguish anemia caused by B_{12} from folate deficiency to optimize treatment. A positive response (correction of anemia) to folate therapy does not confirm that folate deficiency was the cause of the anemia because folate supplementation can correct anemia caused by B_{12} deficiency. If this situation occurs, the B_{12} deficiency continues and the neurologic and gastrointestinal effects of B_{12} deficiency may develop.[5,57,58]

VITAMIN B_{12} DEFICIENCY ANEMIA

Like iron deficiency, B_{12} deficiency anemia is preceded by various stages of B_{12} depletion (Table 31.11).[59,60] Because the liver B_{12} stores are large (2–5 mg), B_{12} deficiency develops over many years, and the onset of symptoms tends to be gradual. In addition to affecting erythropoiesis, B_{12} deficiency results in neurologic and gastrointestinal manifestations (Table 31.2).

These symptoms do not appear to correlate with the development of anemia and often occur without evidence of hematologic effects of B_{12} deficiency. More importantly, the neurologic damage is progressive and, if untreated, can be permanent.

PHYSIOLOGIC IMPORTANCE OF VITAMIN B_{12}

Vitamin B_{12}, also known as cobalamin (Cbl), occurs in synthetic and biologically active forms. It is a cobalt-containing vitamin that cannot be synthesized by mammalian tissue. Therefore, it must be obtained via dietary intake or supplementation. Some bacterial synthesis of B_{12} occurs in the large bowel and the cecum, but there is no absorption at these sites.

B_{12} is an essential cofactor for three known enzymatic reactions: conversion of methylmalonyl-Co A to succinyl-Co A, a critical step in propionate metabolism; methylation of Hcy to methionine by methionine synthetase; and interconversion of leucine and β-leucine by leucine 2,3-aminomutase.[4] B_{12} deficiency inhibits the activity of these enzymes, resulting in increases in metabolites such as MMA and Hcy. Some speculate that excess of 2-MMA (part of the conversion of methylmalonyl-Co A to succinyl-Co A) may be associated with the neurologic symptoms of B_{12} deficiency.[61]

VITAMIN B_{12} NEEDS

The daily requirement for humans is 0.4 to 2.4 µg, and higher in pregnant and lactating mothers. The average diet in the United States supplies 5 to 15 µg/day, but there is a wide variation. Some diets, such as vegan, macrobiotic, or weight-reduction diets that drastically restrict food selection, may not meet the minimum daily needs. The total body stores amount to 2 to 5 mg, mainly in the liver. Thus, B_{12} deficiency takes years to develop.[56,59]

VITAMIN B_{12} ABSORPTION AND METABOLISM

Vitamin B_{12}, particularly at the usual low levels in foods, is well absorbed from the gastrointestinal tract by an orderly sequence of events involving three different binding proteins: R-proteins, IF, and TCII (Fig. 31.1).[4,62,63] The R-proteins, a group of high-affinity, B_{12}-binding glycoproteins, are produced predominantly by leukocytes and are present in a variety of biologic secretions, including gastric fluid, plasma, saliva, tears, milk, and bile. Their function is not fully understood. Extravascular R-proteins, also known as cobalophilins, are the first binding proteins encountered as B_{12} and is released from food in saliva and gastric juices. Although cobalamin can bind to R-proteins or IF, at the low gastric pH, binding to gastric R-proteins is favored. The relative binding of B_{12} also depends on the dosage and the amounts of R-protein and IF secreted. The cobalamin re-

TABLE 31.11	Stages of Vitamin B_{12} Deficiency			
Stage	**B_{12} Concentration**	**Mean Corpuscular Volume**	**Hemoglobin**	**Signs and Symptoms**
Normal	Normal	Normal	Normal	None
Negative balance	Normal	Normal	Normal	None
Depletion of stores	Slight decrease	Normal	Normal	Possible
B_{12} deficient erythropoiesis	Moderate decrease	Increased	Normal	Possible
B_{12} deficiency anemia	Severe decrease	Increased	Decreased	Probable

(Modified from Goodman KI, Salt WV. Vitamin deficiency: important new concepts in recognition. Postgrad Med 88:147–158,1990, with permission.)

mains bound to R-proteins in the upper small intestine until pancreatic proteases, such as trypsin, partially degrade the complex, releasing B_{12}, which then binds to IF. IF, a specific B_{12}-binding glycoprotein, is synthesized and secreted by the parietal cells of the stomach. Its secretion parallels hydrochloric acid secretion. IF functions as a chaperone for B_{12} once it is liberated from the cobalophilins. The IF-B_{12} complex, which is highly resistant to proteolysis, passes down the small intestine to the distal ileum, where it attaches to specific receptors on the luminal side of the mucosal cells (enterocytes). The attachment is not energy dependent, but extracellular calcium and a pH higher than 5.4 are needed. IF is released at the cell surface, and the vitamin is taken up by the enterocyte. Approximately 4 hours later, B_{12} exits the cells bound to transcobalamin. The majority (approximately 80%) of B_{12} in the circulation is bound to transcobalamin I (TCI), an intravascular R-protein (also called haptocorrin). However, haptocorrins are not responsible for delivering B_{12} to peripheral tissues. TCII is the functional binding protein that delivers B_{12} to the tissues. Patients with TCII deficiency may have normal serum B_{12} concentrations because binding to TCI compensates for lowered TCII levels. However, features of severe B_{12} deficiency occur because the TCI-B_{12} complex does not deliver the vitamin to the tissues.

Another mechanism for B_{12} absorption involves diffusion and not IF. This mechanism is biologically important only when large amounts are ingested and generally provides only small quantities of the vitamin. This mechanism is being explored as a potential method of providing oral B_{12} therapy to people with low levels of IF (pernicious anemia).

The daily cellular needs for B_{12} are low, and much of what is ingested is stored in the liver. Vitamin B_{12} is conserved in the body by enterohepatic recycling. Biliary excretion of B_{12} is much higher than excretion in urine or feces. Vitamin B_{12} and its analogs in bile are excreted bound to biliary R-protein. When the complex comes into contact with pancreatic enzymes in the upper small intestine, B_{12} and its analogs are released because of biliary R-protein degradation. Only B_{12} binds to fresh IF; the analogs are excreted in the feces. In addition to being the major route of B_{12} analog excretion, bile may play a role in enhancing B_{12} absorption. When the diet contains little or no B_{12}, as may be the case for strict vegans, biliary cobalamin is conserved to the extent that clinical deficiency may take up to 20 years to develop. When malabsorption occurs, as in pernicious anemia, endogenous and dietary B_{12} are lost and deficiency develops within 3 to 6 years. This accounts for the slow and insidious course of pernicious anemia.

EPIDEMIOLOGY

OCCURRENCE

B_{12} deficiency becomes increasingly prevalent with advancing age. In people over age 65, the incidence ranges from 5% to 40.5% depending on the criteria used to define deficiency.[11,60,62,64,65] African-Americans tend to have higher B_{12} concentrations than do whites, and it is unclear if using standard normal range values to assess B_{12} status underrecognizes mild B_{12} deficiency in this population.[48] Metabolic evidence (deoxyuridine suppression, MMA, and Hcy tests) of B_{12} deficiency is present in approximately 50% to 75% of people with low B_{12} concentrations, despite the absence of clinical signs or symptoms of deficiency.[62] This means that B_{12} is deficient at the cellular (bone marrow and other tissues) level. Anemia is a later finding of B_{12} deficiency, so the deficiency often is diagnosed and treated before anemia develops.

ETIOLOGY

Populations at high risk for B_{12} deficiency are listed in Table 31.3. Causes of B_{12} deficiency include inadequate intake, malabsorption, B_{12} degradation, and inadequate B_{12} use (Table 31.12). In developed countries, dietary causes are rare and may be important only in vegans (strict vegetarians who do not consume foods of animal origin, including milk, cheese, and eggs), breast-fed babies of vegan mothers, and people living in countries where poor nutrition is widespread. Most cases of deficiency are secondary to malabsorption associated with pernicious anemia, gastric lesions, gastrectomy, achlorhydria, and a number of small bowel disorders.[4,17,56,65,66] Inadequate B_{12} use results from drug interactions, congenital or acquired enzyme deficiencies, and abnormal B_{12} binding proteins.

Pernicious Anemia. Pernicious anemia, defined as B_{12} malabsorption caused by the loss of gastric IF secretion, is thought to be the most common cause of B_{12} deficiency. The term ''pernicious'' is used because the anemia is insidious and progressive (Table 31.11). Current evidence suggests that pernicious anemia is caused by an autoimmune reaction against gastric parietal cells. Most patients have

TABLE 31.12	Causes of Vitamin B_{12} and Folic Acid Deficiencies
Vitamin B_{12} deficiency	
Dietary	Inadequate intake
Malabsorption	Inadequate production of intrinsic factor, competition for B_{12}, disorders of terminal ileum, drugs
Impaired transport	Transcobalamin II deficiency
Folic acid deficiency	
Dietary	Inadequate intake, unbalanced diet, excessive cooking
Malabsorption	Intestinal mucosal changes
Increased requirements	Pregnancy, infancy, malignancy, increased hematopoiesis
Impaired metabolism	Drugs, enzyme deficiencies

increased levels of circulating antibodies, particularly those directed against parietal cells and IF.[4,8]

The incidence of pernicious anemia is about 1% in the general population, with most cases occurring in people over 60 years of age. There is a distinctive racial and geographic distribution, with pernicious anemia more common in temperate regions such as North America and northern Europe than in tropical countries. Juvenile pernicious anemia is less common. These patients often develop clinical features of B_{12} deficiency during the second decade of life. Inherited conditions leading to pernicious anemia in infancy or early childhood may be caused by a lack of IF or the production of abnormal IF by an otherwise normal stomach.[26,60,62,65]

Gastric Disorders. Gastric disorders, most commonly gastrectomy, are the second most common cause of vitamin B_{12} malabsorption. Complete gastrectomy results in an absolute deficiency of IF, and megaloblastic anemia develops 3 to 6 years after surgery unless supplementation is given. Partial gastrectomy is a variable cause of B_{12} deficiency. Deficiency is also possible if sufficient gastric mucosa has been destroyed by ingestion of corrosive chemicals, by tumors, or by chronic gastritis.

Even when the diet is adequate, some stomach abnormalities prevent the release of the vitamin from foods. These include atrophic gastritis, achlorhydria, vagotomy, partial gastrectomy, and the use of H_2-receptor antagonists and proton pump inhibitors.

Intestinal Problems. Small intestine disorders are the third most common cause of B_{12} deficiency. Abnormal situations leading to malabsorption range from impaired transfer of the vitamin from R-protein to competition for luminal B_{12} or a low pH in the ileum.

B_{12} malabsorption also occurs with Zollinger-Ellison syndrome if the associated hypersecretion of gastric acid is left uncontrolled. The associated lowering of pH in the duodenum inactivates pancreatic proteolytic enzymes.

Surgical resection or bypass of the ileum also increases the likelihood of malabsorption. Most patients who have lost more than 5 cm of distal ileum have abnormal Schilling test results. Even in the presence of IF, B_{12} malabsorption occurs in conditions, such as tropical sprue, Crohn's disease, celiac disease, lymphomas, and Whipple's disease, in which alteration or destruction of the ileal absorptive surface occurs. In the recessive disorder, Imerslund-Grasbeck's disease, selective B_{12} malabsorption through a poorly understood mechanism occurs in association with proteinuria.

Bacterial overgrowth, particularly by *Bacteroides* sp. and coliforms in blind loops or diverticula, results in B_{12} malabsorption. Absorption returns to normal when patients are given tetracycline, lincomycin, or metronidazole. The mechanism of B_{12} uptake by bacteria is unclear. Most intestinal bacteria avidly absorb the unbound vitamin, but only small amounts are taken up when it is bound to IF. Parasitic infections, such as tapeworm *Diphyllobothrium latum* (from eat-

ing undercooked freshwater fish) or *Giardia lamblia*, also cause B_{12} deficiency.

Drug-Induced Vitamin B_{12} Deficiency. Drug-induced B_{12} deficiency has been associated with a number of pharmacotherapeutic agents. Colchicine, *p*-aminosalicylic acid, neomycin, H_2-receptor blockers, proton pump inhibitors, and biguanide hypoglycemic agents decrease absorption of B_{12}.[4,60,66–68] Agents that reduce B_{12} absorption in the ileum include ethanol and cholestyramine. Nitrous oxide oxidizes the central cobalt atom, which inhibits its ability to function as a cofactor in the methionine synthase reaction,[4] thus affecting cells of the bone marrow, nervous system, and other tissues. Use of nitrous oxide in patients over 60 years of age or with other potential risk factors for B_{12} deficiency should be avoided.[4,5,66]

CLINICAL PRESENTATION AND DIAGNOSIS

SIGNS AND SYMPTOMS

Clinical manifestations reflect abnormalities of the blood, gastrointestinal tract, and nervous system (Table 31.2). In severe cases the peripheral blood smear exhibits severe macrocytic anemia, leukopenia with hypersegmentation of the polymorphonuclear cells, and thrombocytopenia (Fig. 31.3; *color insert*). Nonspecific symptoms related to anemia include apathy, weakness, fatigue, palpitations, and breathlessness. The mucous membranes usually are pale, and in Caucasians the skin is pale and yellow-tinted because of the anemia and the mild jaundice of ineffective erythropoiesis.

Gastrointestinal tract or neurologic changes may occur in the absence of hematologic changes. Sore tongue is the most common oral complaint. Glossitis, burning of the mouth,

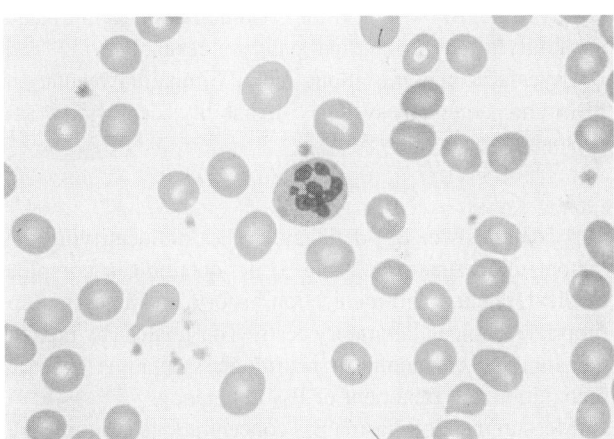

FIGURE 31.3 Vitamin B_{12} deficiency (*see color insert*). Macrocytic, normochromic anemia, thrombocytopenia with large platelets and hypersegmented neutrophils. (From Anderson's Atlas of Hematology; Anderson, Shauna C., PhD. Copyright 2003. Phildelphia: Wolters Kluwer Health/Lippincott Williams & Wilkins, with permission.)

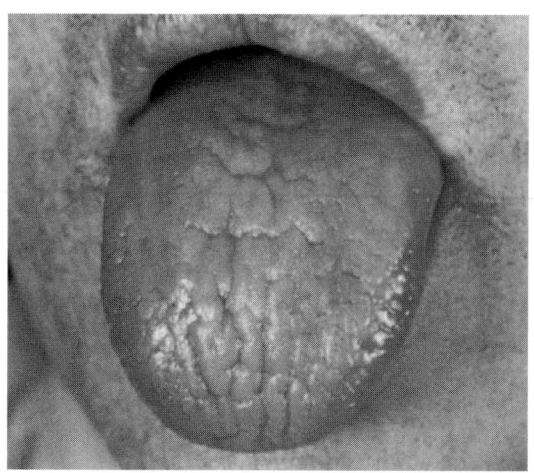

FIGURE 31.4 Smooth, reddish, shiny tongue without papillae due to vitamin B_{12} deficiency (*see color insert*). (From Weber J, Kelley J. Health Assessment in Nursing. 2nd ed. Philadelphia: Lippincott Williams & Wilkins, 2003, with permission.)

and a beefy red tongue are other manifestations (Fig. 31.4; *color insert*). Other gastrointestinal symptoms include diarrhea, gas, heartburn, nausea, and vague abdominal pain.[4,5,56,69]

Neurologic manifestations include peripheral neuropathies, degeneration of the spinal cord, and altered mental states.[4,5,56,57,60,65,69] B_{12} deficiency results in distinct changes in the nervous system, beginning with demyelination of nerves. These changes often are progressive, and if the deficiency is not corrected, they can be irreversible. Peripheral nerve damage results in symmetric paresthesias (numbness and tingling of the extremities) and reduction of pain and temperature sensation. The most serious problem, subacute degeneration of the spinal cord, is associated with loss of position and vibration sense, resulting in ataxia and weakness. Lateral column disruption leads to weakness and spasticity, exemplified by myoclonus, hyperreflexia, and a positive Babinski's sign. If the condition remains untreated, instability of gait and virtual paralysis result.

Psychiatric manifestations include impaired mentation, delirium, paranoia, psychosis, irritability, depression, and personality changes.[4,5,56,57,60,65,69]

DIAGNOSIS

Early diagnosis of B_{12} deficiency relies on identifying risk factors for deficiency (Table 31.3), obtaining a complete medical, dietary, and medication history, and assessing appropriate clinical laboratory tests. The goal is to prevent development of anemia or neurologic symptoms by early recognition and treatment of B_{12} deficiency.

Measurement of plasma B_{12} concentrations is simple and inexpensive and is considered the standard test for diagnosing B_{12} deficiency.[4,55,62,63,70] Limitations of the test include the inability to distinguish total from metabolically active B_{12} (bound to TCII, or holo-TC), discrepancies between concentrations and symptoms, and reference ranges that may

not be applicable to all patients, such as African-Americans and older adults.[4,60,62,63] For example, people with TCII deficiency could have a normal B_{12} concentration but be B_{12} deficient at the tissue level because of a lack of the transport protein. Measurement of holo-TC would overcome this problem and be a better measure of actual B_{12} available to the tissues. However, limited assay availability has hindered clinical use of this test. Another alternative is measurement of TCII saturation, which decreases early in B_{12} deficiency. However, because only small amounts of B_{12} are bound to TCII, low levels of detection are needed that results in increased variability, thus limiting its clinical usefulness.

''Normal'' B_{12} concentrations also occur despite an actual B_{12} deficiency in liver disease, myeloproliferative disorders, and nitrous oxide anesthesia.[4,55,70] Cutoff points for normal B_{12} concentrations also vary, and symptoms do not always occur with low values. Recent studies have documented that asymptomatic patients with low B_{12} concentrations have metabolic abnormalities strongly suggestive of B_{12} deficiency at the cellular level, which reverse with B_{12} treatment.[4,6,11,64,65] Therefore, in patients with B_{12} concentrations in the low normal range (whether they are symptomatic or not), additional tests, such as biochemical assessment of metabolite production (MMA and Hcy), should be conducted.

Functional deficiency of B_{12} inhibits reactions converting MMA to succinyl-Co A and Hcy to methionine, resulting in accumulation of MMA and Hcy (Fig. 31.5). Marked elevation of these serum metabolites (more than 3 SDs increase from the mean) occurs in more than 95% of patients with B_{12} deficiency.[7] MMA is considered more specific for B_{12} deficiency because folate deficiency can also result in accumulation of Hcy. However, MMA also increases in renal disease, so renal function should be assessed when MMA is measured. Disadvantages of using metabolite concentrations are cost and availability, which have limited their clinical use.[4,6,7,61,63,65,70]

Once B_{12} deficiency is determined, assessment of the cause (malabsorption vs. other) guides treatment selection. Antigastric parietal cell or anti-IF antibodies (IFAs) can be measured to provide information about a patient's ability to absorb B_{12}. Antigastric parietal cell antibodies often are found in patients with gastritis not affecting B_{12} absorption and, thus, are not sensitive or specific for assessing B_{12} absorption.[8,70] However, IFAs rarely occur without B_{12} malabsorption and are found in 50% to 75% of patients with pernicious anemia.[8,55,70] The British Committee for Standards in Haematology guidelines state that detection of IFAs eliminates the need for absorption tests (e.g., Schilling test) in most patients.[70]

A Schilling test (with or without IF) is an alternative method of assessing B_{12} malabsorption.[4,55,59,62,63,70] Several types of Schilling tests are available. The standard test is divided into three stages. In stage I, an oral dose (1 μg for adults, 0.5–1 μg for children) of ^{57}Co-labeled B_{12} is given, followed by a 1-mg intramuscular dose of unlabeled B_{12}.

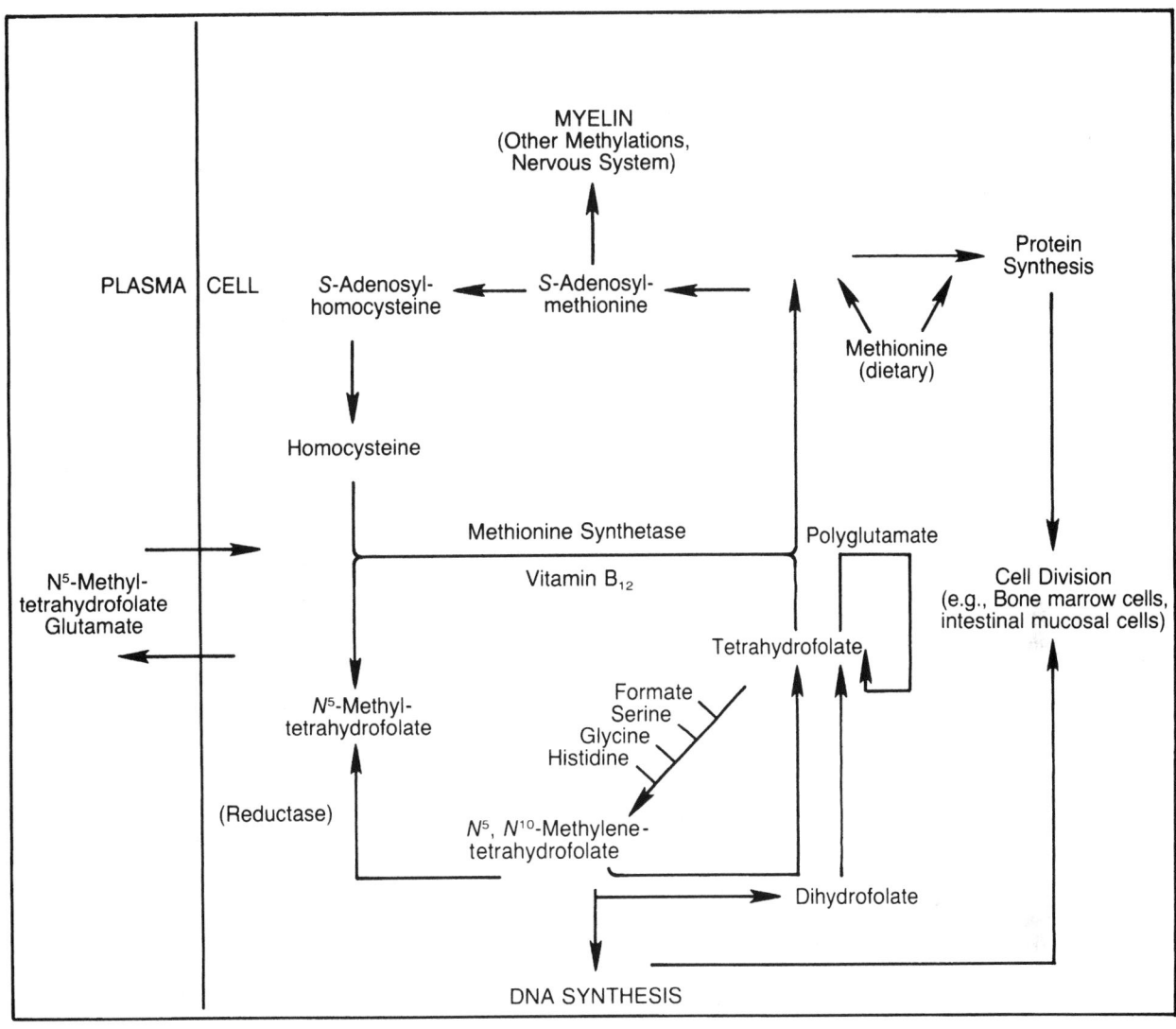

FIGURE 31.5 Normal vitamin B_{12} and folate metabolism in mammalian cells.

The large intramuscular dose saturates B_{12}-binding proteins in the blood. Consequently, there are fewer binding sites for ^{57}Co-labeled B_{12}, and a substantial proportion is excreted in the urine. Urine is collected over 24 hours and the amount of labeled B_{12} measured. B_{12} absorption is considered to be impaired if less than 10% of the label is excreted in the urine. If less than 5% is excreted, the diagnosis is consistent with pernicious anemia.

Stage II of the test distinguishes between the possible causes of the malabsorption (e.g., pernicious anemia, lack of ileal absorptive sites, or bacterial overgrowth proximal to the terminal ileum). The same procedure is followed as in stage I except that IF is given with the radiolabeled B_{12}. If the B_{12} deficiency is caused by lack of IF (pernicious anemia), stage I should be abnormal and stage II should be normal. If both stages are abnormal, an ileal disorder, bacterial overgrowth, pancreatic disorders, or fish tapeworm infestation may be causing B_{12} malabsorption. Stage III of the

test, which involves giving the patient an antibiotic (usually tetracycline 250 mg orally four times a day for 10–14 days) and then repeating the stage I test, checks for possible bacterial overgrowth (Table 31.13). The Schilling test depends on renal function and a complete 24-hour urine collection.

TABLE 31.13	Summary of Schilling Test Results in Vitamin B_{12} Deficiency		
Condition	**Stage I**	**Stage II**	**Stage III**
Normal	Normal		
Inadequate diet	Normal		
Pernicious anemia	Low	Normal	
Bacterial overgrowth	Low	Low	Normal
Ileal defect	Low	Low	Low

Decreased renal function and incomplete urine collection lead to inaccurate results. In addition, H_2-antagonists and proton pump inhibitors may cause falsely abnormal results by preventing the degradation of R-protein and decreasing the secretion of endogenous IF. Conditions that reduce hydrochloric acid production (H_2-antagonists and proton pump inhibitors) and other situations in which acid and IF secretion are reduced (achlorhydria, complete or partial gastrectomy) can give falsely normal Schilling test results. The problem is that the aqueous, crystalline B_{12} used in the test differs in bioavailability from the usually food-bound vitamin that must be released to participate in the uptake process. A modified Schilling test [protein bound absorption test (PBAT)] using protein-bound B_{12} more closely resembles the physiologic state.[4]

Use of the Schilling test may decrease as other tests become available to assess B_{12} absorption that are less expensive, do not expose patients to radiation, and do not entail 24 hours of sample collection.[4,62,63,70]

Anemia is a late presentation of B_{12} deficiency (Table 31.11) that may be avoided with early detection and correction of B_{12} depletion. Hematologic tests, such as a blood smear and the red cell indices, help differentiate the cause of anemia. Macrocytosis (MCV >100 fL) often occurs with B_{12} deficiency, but it also occurs with other conditions, such as liver disease, myxedema, acute myelogenous leukemia, acquired sideroblastic anemia, aplastic anemia, hemolytic anemia, posthemorrhagic states, splenectomy, and certain medications (e.g., zidovudine). Evaluating the smear for megaloblastic changes, such as neutrophil hypersegmentation and oval-shaped erythrocytes, generally differentiates a B_{12} or folate deficiency from other causes. If iron deficiency occurs along with B_{12} deficiency, the MCV may appear normal, but the blood smear should show megaloblastic and microcytic cells.[21,55,56,60,70]

Less commonly used tests include thymidine uptake [deoxyuridine suppression test (dUST)] by bone marrow cells, food cobalamin absorption, erythropoietin measurement, and gastrin and pepsinogen analysis.[4,63,70] Folate concentrations also are generally assessed to rule out a concurrent folate deficiency.

TREATMENT

Management includes identifying B_{12} deficiency early (before anemia or neurologic symptoms develop), correcting the cause of the deficiency if possible, replenishing depleted stores, and if necessary, administering maintenance B_{12} therapy. Once anemia or other symptoms develop, the aim of treatment is to reverse the symptoms (achieve hematologic remission, reverse or retard nervous system complications, and eliminate gastrointestinal symptoms) and replenish B_{12} stores.

Treatment options include dietary changes and supplemental B_{12} given orally, intranasally, or parenterally.

Dietary adjustments may be warranted in patients with poor or restricted diets. Dietary sources of B_{12} include fresh liver (the richest source), eggs, meat, kidney, milk, dairy products, fish, and shellfish. However, dietary changes provide little benefit for patients with malabsorption states such as pernicious anemia.

PHARMACOTHERAPY

Oral Vitamin B_{12} Therapy. When B_{12} absorption is normal but there is dietary deficiency (e.g., strict vegetarian or restricted diets), oral B_{12} therapy is the preferred route. In the presence of adequate absorption, the usual oral dose of B_{12} supplementation is 1 to 10 μg daily. Oral B_{12} therapy may also be used to treat some drug-induced B_{12} deficiencies (e.g., nitrous oxide).[5] Oral cyanocobalamin is well absorbed with peak serum concentrations being reached 8 to 12 hours after ingestion.

A debated area is use of oral B_{12} therapy in patients with impaired absorption (e.g., pernicious anemia, complete or partial gastrectomy).[4,60] Because approximately 1% of an oral dose of B_{12} can be absorbed by a nonspecific, non–IF-dependent process, large oral dosages may provide sufficient B_{12} to correct the deficiency, replenish stores, and resolve symptoms. In a randomized, controlled trial in 33 patients with B_{12} deficiency, 2 mg oral cyanocobalamin taken daily for 120 days was compared with 1 mg given intramuscularly on days 1, 3, 7, 10, 14, 21, 30, 60, and 90. The oral therapy resulted in significantly higher serum B_{12} concentrations and lower serum MMA concentrations than intramuscular therapy.[71] Symptoms of B_{12} deficiency resolved in both groups, but the incidence of anemia at baseline was low. In another study, eight patients with megaloblastic anemia were treated with daily oral dosages of 1.5 mg of cyanocobalamin (n = 3), hydroxy-cobalamin (n = 4), or methyl-cobalamin (n = 1) for 1 year. After 3 or 4 days of therapy, patients reported increased appetite, alertness, and well-being. Reticulocytosis occurred after a few days with peak effect by the end of the first week of therapy. B_{12} concentrations returned to normal range in a median of 14.5 days, and Hb rose to above 6.2 mmol per liter (10 g/dL; normal range 7.5–11.2 mmol/L, or 12–18 g/dL) in a median of 34.4 days. The responses were similar to those reported after intramuscular administration, although the hematologic response appeared to be slightly slower.[72] Other reports also support the use of oral therapy.[73,74] The dosing of the oral product is important. Dosages of less than 150 μg generally do not restore B_{12} and Hb concentrations, and dosages between 250 and 500 μg may be affected by variable absorption, resulting in erratic responses. Therefore, in patients with malabsorption, B_{12} dosages should be 1,000 μg or higher to produce favorable long-term results.[75] Concerns with oral therapy are the potential for erratic absorption, poor compliance, and subsequent development of neurologic symptoms. Patient evaluation and monitoring for compliance and therapeutic response should determine if long-term oral therapy is optimal for each patient.

TABLE 31.14	**Summary of Various Parenteral B$_{12}$ Regimens**	
Dosage	**Frequency**	**References**
100 μg	Daily for 1 week, then every other day for 7 doses, then every month for life	95
100 μg	Every week, then	92
1,000 μg	Every 1–3 months for life	
500–1,000 μg	Daily for 1 week, then weekly for 1 month, then monthly for life	56,59
1,000 μg	Every week ×4, then every month for life	60
1,000 μg	On days 1, 3, 7, 10, 14, 21, 30 then monthly for life	5,71

Parenteral Vitamin B$_{12}$ Therapy.A number of different parenteral B$_{12}$ treatment plans exist (Table 31.14), but no controlled treatment studies were found in the literature to support the regimens.[62] Because of the safety of these agents, dosages of 100 to 1,000 μg of B$_{12}$ can be given. Dosages under 15 μg generally are insufficient to completely correct the later stages of B$_{12}$ deficiency. All regimens use more frequent dosing initially to correct the deficiency, followed by injections every 1 to 3 months, based on the patient's response, for life.

Proponents for the higher (>1,000 μg) dosage argue that lower (<300 μg) dosages sometimes are insufficient to maintain serum concentrations within the normal range because B$_{12}$ needs vary (1.5–10 μg/day) and there is a wide intrasubject response to replacement dosages.[60] In addition, few problems have been reported with parenteral B$_{12}$, with any extra B$_{12}$ (beyond the daily needs) being excreted, largely unchanged, in the urine. The excess B$_{12}$ that is eliminated is an argument for use of the lower dose; it is less wasteful and should meet the needs of most patients. B$_{12}$ generally is administered intramuscularly, although subcutaneous injection also can be used. Peak serum concentrations after intramuscular injection are reached in about 1 hour. The half-life of the parenteral B$_{12}$ is about 6 days; its half-life in the liver is 400 days. With impaired liver or kidney function, more frequent dosing is necessary.

Two synthetic forms of B$_{12}$ are available: cyanocobalamin and hydroxocobalamin. After intramuscular administration, cyanocobalamin appears to be excreted more rapidly than hydroxocobalamin, which is more highly protein bound. Therefore, hydroxocobalamin may allow less frequent dosing (every 3 months) during maintenance therapy.[4] Indications for both of these agents are similar, although hydroxocobalamin may be preferred for treating B$_{12}$ deficiencies because optic neuropathies may worsen with cyanocobalamin administration.

The synthetic B$_{12}$ products are well tolerated, and allergic reactions are rare. Medical attention should be sought if a rash or wheezing develops. Although anaphylactic reactions can occur after parenteral administration, they are rare. An intradermal test dose is recommended for patients with a history of suspected allergic reactions to B$_{12}$. No adverse effects have been documented when the normal daily needs for these agents are administered during pregnancy. B$_{12}$ crosses the placenta, and at birth the neonatal level can be two to five times that of the mother. Injections containing benzyl alcohol should not be used in neonates or immature infants because of possible toxicity from the preservative. B$_{12}$ is excreted in breast milk, and no problems have been reported for humans taking the normal daily allowances. No problems in the geriatric population have been reported.[60]

Intranasal Vitamin B$_{12}$ Therapy.A more recent development in B$_{12}$ therapy is intranasal administration.[60] Currently, an intranasal gel (cyanocobalamin 500 μg/actuation) is available in the United States, with recommended dosing of three times a week.[76] Because the experience with the gel is limited, it is generally used in patients who refuse or cannot tolerate parenteral therapy and do not respond to oral treatment. A recent report documents the efficacy of a metered-dose nasal spray of hydroxocobalamin (750 μg per puff) in treating six patients with documented B$_{12}$ deficiency.[77] One puff was administered in each nostril on days 0, 14, and 21. B$_{12}$ concentrations increased significantly 1 hour after the dose. However, most of the concentrations fell below the normal range before the next dose. The spray was well tolerated, with no reports of nasal irritation or sensitivity. This study supports further investigation into the dosing and efficacy of this product.

MONITORING VITAMIN B$_{12}$ DEFICIENCY THERAPY
Response varies depending on the stage (Table 31.11) of B$_{12}$ deficiency being treated. In the later stages, reticulocytosis occurs rapidly, with a maximum reticulocyte count seen 4 to 7 days after treatment starts. The neutrophil count also increases by this time, although the hypersegmented polymorphonuclear neutrophils persist for several weeks. Hb concentrations gradually increase over the first 2 months of therapy. Macrocytosis may persist for several months after treatment is started because of the long lifespan of erythrocytes.[56,73] Serum iron concentrations may decrease because the accelerated erythropoiesis requires more Hb production. Some patients may need supplemental iron. If iron stores become depleted, the hematologic response to B$_{12}$ therapy could be diminished.[22,23] The rapid erythropoiesis may also cause hypokalemia. Serum potassium concentrations should be monitored during the first 48 hours of treatment in patients who have cardiac disease (especially those on potassium-depleting diuretics) or other risk factors for significant potassium depletion.

Oral and gastrointestinal symptoms generally resolve within the first 3 days of therapy, and patients report an overall feeling of well-being.[5,69] Reversal of neurologic manifestations and dementia may take several weeks. Most resolve by 6 months of B_{12} therapy, although maximum benefit may take as long as 1.5 years. However, some patients have incomplete responses, which is thought to depend on the duration of the neurologic problem before treatment.[5,56] Serum B_{12} concentrations increase to within the normal range, and metabolite concentrations (MMA and Hcy) decrease to within the normal range, generally within the first month of therapy.[71] Patients not responding to therapy may need a dosage adjustment (higher dose), a change in dosage form (oral to intramuscular), and evaluation for drug interactions, drug-induced bone marrow effects, and other medical problems.

FOLATE DEFICIENCY

Like B_{12} deficiency, folate deficiency occurs in stages, with depletion of stores leading to deficiency that can result in megaloblastic anemia and other hematologic abnormalities (thrombocytopenia, leukopenia).[78] Treating a B_{12} deficiency megaloblastic anemia with folic acid may correct the anemia, but does not correct the B_{12} deficiency or prevent the development of neurologic changes. Therefore, it is important to determine the cause of a megaloblastic anemia before initiating therapy. Folate also is critical in early pregnancy for fetal neural tube development.[79] To reduce the incidence of neural tube defects, since January 1998 the FDA has required enriched grains to be fortified with folic acid at a concentration that provides, on average, 100 µg per day.[80]

A high plasma Hcy concentration is a risk factor for the development of atherosclerosis, coronary artery disease, stroke, and peripheral vascular disease.[81,82] Hyperhomocystinemia is related to low levels of folate and B vitamins. A folate-rich diet as well as folic acid supplementation has been shown to decrease plasma Hcy concentrations.[83,84] It has been speculated that folate replenishment may have an important role in the prevention and treatment of cardiovascular disease.[78,85–88]

PHYSIOLOGIC IMPORTANCE OF FOLATE

Reduced forms of folate (tetrahydrofolate) are cofactors for transformylation reactions in the biosynthesis of purines and thymidylates of nucleic acids. In folate deficiency, reduced thymidylate synthesis leads to defective DNA synthesis, resulting in megaloblast formation and bone marrow suppression. Folate is also involved in the methylation cycle and is essential in providing methyl groups for a wide range of cellular methyltransferases. In particular, folate is needed in Hcy metabolism (Fig. 31.5), which accumulates in folate deficiency.[7,78,79,86]

FOLATE NEEDS

Folate needs depend on metabolic and cell turnover rates. In general, the minimum daily requirement is 65 to 400 µg daily.[56,78] In pregnancy, 600 µg daily is recommended, and 500 µg daily for lactating mothers (Table 31.7).[57,80] More than 2% is degraded daily, so a continuous dietary supply is essential. The average amount stored in the body is 5 to 10 mg, one half of which is found in the liver. With folate depletion, deficiency leading to anemia generally occurs within 6 months.

FOLATE ABSORPTION AND METABOLISM

Folate is a water-soluble vitamin found in many plant and animal foods. Dietary sources are primarily polyglutamates, which must be converted to the monoglutamate form for absorption. This process often is impaired in malabsorption syndromes, such as sprue. The percentage of dietary folate absorbed depends on the source, with liver, yeast, and egg yolk having high absorption; only 10% of most other dietary sources are absorbed. Active absorption of dietary folate occurs mainly in the proximal part of the small intestine (Fig. 31.1). Synthetic folate (folic acid) is already in the monoglutamate form and has greater stability and better absorption (almost twice the bioavailability) than dietary folate.[78,79] Folic acid from pharmaceutical products is almost completely absorbed in the upper duodenum, even in the presence of malabsorption.

The principal circulating form of folic acid, *N*-5- methyltetrahydrofolate, is extensively bound to plasma proteins. There is no specific transport protein. Some enterohepatic cycling of folic acid occurs, although significant amounts are not reabsorbed from the bile.

Amounts of folic acid beyond the daily needs are excreted almost entirely as metabolites by the kidney.

EPIDEMIOLOGY

Inadequate diet, alcoholism, and pregnancy are the most common causes of folate deficiency. Other causes include increased requirements, malabsorption, enhanced metabolism, and interference in the metabolism or clearance by other pharmacotherapeutic agents.

Malnutrition is often a significant cause of folate deficiency. Folate-rich foods include raw spinach, broccoli, cauliflower, peanuts, and peas. Folate is highly susceptible to cooking or processing. Heating foods (microwaving or boiling) decreases the amount of folate available by up to 50%. People at risk of inadequate folate intake include alcoholics whose main caloric intake is in the form of ethanol, narcotic addicts who have a poor diet, older adults who often do not feel like eating or who eat commercially prepared foods, institutionalized people who have no control over their diet, adolescents who may skip meals and eat junk foods, and pregnant women who have increased needs, that often are not met by dietary intake.[56,57,70,78]

In alcoholics, the incidence of folate deficiency has been reported to be as high as 60%.[89] Poor diet and altered absorption are the primary causes.

During pregnancy, a large increase in nucleic acid synthesis is associated with growth of the fetus, placenta, and uterus and with the increased maternal erythrocyte mass. Folate needs may triple during pregnancy, and if supplements are not taken, particularly in the last trimester, megaloblastic anemia may develop in the mother. In addition, folate is essential for fetal neural tube development, and supplementation in the periconceptional period has been shown to reduce the occurrence of neural tube defects.[57,79] Worldwide, folate deficiency occurs in up to one third of pregnancies. In the United States, the incidence is about 4%, but it increases up to eight fold with multiple gestations, teenage pregnancies, and closely spaced pregnancies.[64]

Folate needs increase during malignancy, increased erythropoiesis, and conditions causing rapid cell turnover. Folate deficiency is very common in myeloproliferative disorders, such as chronic myeloid leukemia and myelofibrosis, often leading to thrombocytopenia or anemia. The increased folate needs in chronic hemolytic anemia, exfoliative dermatitis, generalized psoriasis, or extensive burns can also lead to folate deficiency. In these cases, adequate supplementation is needed. Anemia is more likely to occur if several contributing factors are present.

Various drugs can affect folate absorption, metabolism, and use (Table 31.15). Folate supplementation generally is not necessary during short courses of these drugs (e.g., oral sulfonamide antibiotics). However, chronic or high-dose therapy may necessitate folate supplementation to prevent deficiency. Methotrexate, a folate antagonist, binds to dihydrofolate reductase and prevents reduction of folate to its active intracellular form. When high dosages of methotrexate are given (e.g., in cancer treatment protocols), bone marrow suppression and mucositis generally occur unless leucovorin, a reduced form of folate, is coadministered. It should be noted that supplemental folate may alter the central nervous system effect of phenytoin, and patients may need an increase in phenytoin dosage to maintain efficacy.

CLINICAL PRESENTATION AND DIAGNOSIS

SIGNS AND SYMPTOMS

Signs and symptoms of folate deficiency are similar to those of other anemias (Table 31.2). In addition, megaloblastosis, glossitis, diarrhea, and weight loss may occur.

DIAGNOSIS

As with B_{12} deficiency, early diagnosis and prevention of anemia depend on identification and treatment of high-risk patients (Table 31.3). Serum or erythrocyte folate concentrations may be determined to assess folate status (Table 31.4). Within 5 weeks of inadequate folate intake, the serum folate concentration declines to the subnormal range, whereas the erythrocyte folate concentration does not decline until about 3 months.[55] However, serum folate measurement has the disadvantage of being sensitive to dynamic changes in folate metabolism, such as reflecting folate absorbed from a recent meal. Therefore, serum folate concentrations fluctuate from day to day, closely reflecting dietary intake. Falsely normal values can be obtained if folate-rich foods are consumed within a few days before evaluation. Erythrocyte folate concentration reflects tissue status and is felt to be a better indicator of depletion.[55,70]

Increased plasma Hcy concentration with normal MMA levels is another indicator of folate deficiency.[7] Elevated Hcy levels may also be increased by B_{12} deficiency and with decreased renal function. Both of these conditions should be concurrently evaluated when this test is used to determine the exact nature of the anemia.

In the later stages of folate deficiency, a blood smear and hematologic evaluation often show macrocytosis with megaloblastosis (Fig. 31.6; *color insert*). Megaloblastosis must be interpreted in light of B_{12} status because of similar findings in B_{12} deficiency. Erythrocyte folate and serum B_{12} concentrations should be measured.[78] Anemia occurs only when tissue levels are depleted, so a normal serum folate concentration does not exclude deficiency. The diagnosis of megaloblastic anemia caused by folate deficiency entails a demonstration of reduced folate tissue levels, as reflected by erythrocyte folate concentrations.

TREATMENT

The primary prevention of folate deficiency, and hence anemia, should occur through dietary manipulation or oral supplementation.

TABLE 31.15	Drug-Induced Folate Deficiency

Reduced absorption

Ethanol

Metformin

Cholestyramine

Sulfasalazine

Sulfamethoxazole

Oral contraceptives

Some anticonvulsants

Altered metabolism

Some anticonvulsants

Methotrexate

Trimethoprim

Triamterene

Pentamidine

Alcohol

(From references 55 and 78.)

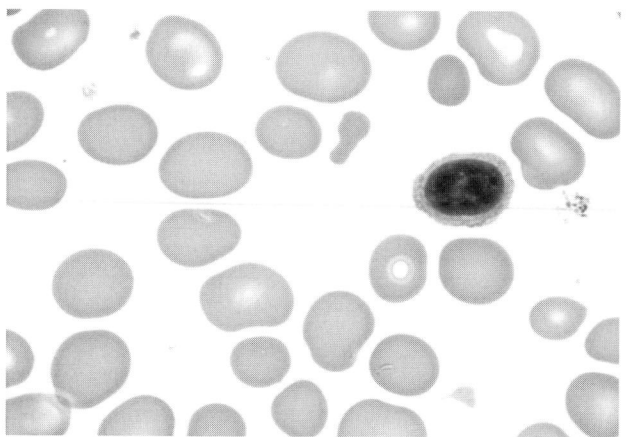

FIGURE 31.6 Folate deficiency (*see color insert*). Peripheral blood smear showing macrocytic, normochromic anemia. (From Anderson's Atlas of Hematology; Anderson, Shauna C., PhD. Copyright 2003. Phildelphia: Wolters Kluwer Health/Lippincott Williams & Wilkins, with permission.)

PHARMACOTHERAPY

Women planning to become pregnant should take at least 400 μg daily to prevent fetal neural tube defects. Because many pregnancies are not planned, the FDA has mandated food fortification to enhance the daily folate intake in all women by 100 μg daily.[80] There are two concerns with this approach. One is that the increase in folate intake could mask a B_{12} deficiency by "correcting" the anemia.[88] However, one would hope to detect a B_{12} deficiency before anemia develops. Also, folate dosages of 1 mg or more generally are needed to produce and maintain a remission in a B_{12} deficiency anemia.[57] The other concern is that the folate amount is too low and does not provide enough to prevent neural tube defects.[80] Therefore, 400 μg folic acid daily is still recommended for pregnant women and women who are trying to become pregnant.[78,80] This dosage will also minimize the chance of the women developing folate-deficiency anemia during the latter part of the pregnancy, when folate needs increase. Dosages less than 1 mg are available in numerous over-the-counter preparations.

Folate deficiency usually is treated with oral folic acid 1 mg daily.[90] This dose is available only by prescription. Parenteral administration is indicated when oral administration is unacceptable (preoperatively, postoperatively, or if nausea or vomiting is a problem) or not possible (malabsorption syndromes or after gastric resection). Available parenteral formulations contain 5 mg per milliliter and may be given intramuscularly, subcutaneously, or intravenously.[90]

The duration of therapy depends on the underlying cause. Replacement therapy should be continued until the underlying problem has been corrected. If this is impossible, lifelong therapy is needed. B_{12} studies should also be undertaken in people requiring long-term folate supplementation. Long-term therapy may be needed in chronic hemolytic states, myelofibrosis, and refractory malabsorption. Postgastrec-

tomy states, prolonged stress or infection, chronic fever, and persistent diarrhea may also increase needs.

MONITORING FOLATE DEFICIENCY THERAPY

In anemic patients, treatment response can be monitored by following the reticulocyte count, which peaks 5 to 8 days after treatment begins. Hematologic findings (Hb, MCV) should be normal in about 2 months. Measuring erythrocyte folate levels for several months during the treatment can confirm replenishment of tissue stores. For patients with deficiency without anemia, folate stores are replenished in about 3 weeks.[56]

KEY POINTS

- Nutritional anemias may be prevented by early identification of at-risk patients, monitoring for vitamin deficiency, and providing supplementation or replacement therapy
- Pregnant women, young children, and older adults are prone to nutritional anemias and should be monitored for potential deficiencies of iron, B_{12}, and folate
- Nutritional deficiencies develop in stages, with anemia occurring at the final stage. Other hematologic and biochemical changes occur earlier in the deficiency, allowing diagnosis to be made before anemia develops
- If anemia does result, it usually can be treated simply and effectively, although determining and correcting the primary cause of anemia can be difficult
- Where possible, dietary manipulation should be used as a maintenance strategy. In some cases, particularly with pernicious anemia, lifelong therapy is necessary
- Iron deficiency is common during pregnancy and early childhood. The CDC recommends supplementation in both groups
- Based on elemental iron content and absorption, the usual dosage of ferrous sulfate to treat iron deficiency is 300 mg taken three times a day
- Oral B_{12} therapy (dosages >1 mg/day) may be used to treat B_{12} deficiencies, even those caused by malabsorption (pernicious anemia)
- Maintenance B_{12} therapy generally is 1 mg intramuscularly every 1 to 3 months or 1 mg orally daily
- Gastrointestinal and neurologic symptoms of B_{12} deficiency can develop before anemia
- Pregnant women and women planning to become pregnant should take supplemental folic acid (400 μg/day)
- Because 1 mg folic acid per day can reverse the anemia associated with B_{12} deficiency but does not prevent the neurologic symptoms, the cause of a megaloblastic anemia should be determined before therapy is initiated
- For patients who need long-term vitamin supplementation, compliance should be monitored because patients may discontinue use once symptoms improve

■ Response to therapy generally occurs within the first week (reticulocytosis), although correction of the anemia may take 2 to 3 months

SUGGESTED READINGS

Little DR. Ambulatory management of common forms of anemia. Am Fam Physician 15:1598–1604, 1999.

Oh R, Brown DL. Vitamin B12 deficiency. Am Fam Physician 67: 979–986, 2003.

Anonymous. Recommendations to prevent and control iron deficiency in the United States. Centers for Disease Control and Prevention. MMWR Recomm Rep 47(RR-3):1–29, 1998.

REFERENCES

1. Massey AC. Microcytic anemia. Differential diagnosis and management of iron deficiency anemia. Med Clin North Am 76:549–566, 1992.
2. Brown RG. Determining the cause of anemia. General approach, with emphasis on microcytic hypochromic anemias. Postgrad Med 89:161–170, 1991.
3. Anonymous. Recommendations to prevent and control iron deficiency in the United States. Centers for Disease Control and Prevention. MMWR Morb Mortal Wkly Rep 47(RR-3):1–29, 1998.
4. Markle HV. Cobalamin. Crit Rev Clin Lab Sci 33:247–356, 1996.
5. Schilling RF. Vitamin B_{12} deficiency: underdiagnosed, overtreated? Hosp Pract 30:47–54, 1995.
6. Metz J, Bell AH, Flicker L, et al. The significance of subnormal serum B_{12} concentration in older people: a case control study. J Am Geriatr Soc 44:1355–1361, 1996.
7. Savage DG, Lindenbaum J, Stabler SP, et al. Sensitivity of serum methylmalonic acid and total homocysteine determinations for diagnosing cobalamin and folate deficiencies. Am J Med 96:239–246, 1994.
8. Carmel R. Reassessment of the relative prevalences of antibodies to gastric parietal cell and to intrinsic factor in patients with pernicious anemia: influence of patient age and race. Clin Exp Immunol 89: 74–77, 1992.
9. Worwood M. The laboratory assessment of iron status: an update. Clin Chim Acta 259:3–23, 1997.
10. Ahluwalia N. Diagnostic utility of serum transferrin receptors measurement in assessing iron status. Nutr Rev 56:133–141, 1998.
11. Lindenbaum J, Rosenberg IH, Wilson PWF, et al. Prevalence of cobalamin deficiency in the Framingham elderly population. Am J Clin Nutr 60:2–11, 1994.
12. Phekoo K, Williams Y, Schey SA, et al. Folate assays: Serum or red cell? J R Coll Physicians Lond 31:291–295, 1997.
13. Layrisse M, Garcia-Casal MN. Strategies for the prevention of iron deficiency through foods in the household. Nutr Rev 55:223–239, 1997.
14. Swain RA, Kaplan B, Montgomery E. Iron deficiency anemia. When is parental therapy warranted? Postgrad Med 100:181–193, 1996.
15. Kumph VJ. Parenteral iron supplementation. Nutr Clin Pract 11: 139–146, 1996.
16. Viteri FE. Iron supplementation for the control of iron deficiency in populations at risk. Nutr Rev 55:195–209, 1997.
17. Stephenson LS. Possible new developments in community control of iron-deficiency anemia. Nutr Rev 53:23–30, 1995.
18. de Andraco I, Castillo M, Walter T. Psychomotor development and behavior in iron-deficient anemic infants. Nutr Rev 55:125–132, 1997.
19. Looker AC, Dallman PR, Carroll MD, et al. Prevalence of iron deficiency in the United States. JAMA 277:973–976, 1997.
20. Beddall A. Anemias. Practitioner 234:714–715, 1992.
21. Rowland TW. Iron deficiency in the young athlete. Pediatr Clin North Am 37:1153–1163, 1990.
22. Demiroglu H, Dundar S. Pernicious anemia patients should be screened for iron deficiency during follow-up. N Z Med J 110: 147–148, 1997.
23. Hash RB, Sargent MA, Katner H. Anemia secondary to combined deficiencies of iron and cobalamin. Arch Fam Med 5:585–588, 1996.
24. Sayetta RB. Pica: an overview. Am Fam Physician 33:181–185, 1986.
25. Hastka J, Lasserre J-J, Schwarzbeck A, et al. Laboratory tests of iron status: Correlation or common sense? Clin Chem 42:718–724, 1996.
26. Roncagliolo M, Garrido M, Walter T, et al. Evidence of altered central nervous system development in infants with iron deficiency anemia at 6 mo: delayed maturation of auditory brainstem responses. Am J Clin Nutr 68:683–690, 1998.
27. Lozoff B, Jimenez E, Wolf AW. Long-term developmental outcome of infants with iron deficiency. N Engl J Med 325:687–694, 1991.
28. Punnonen K, Irjala K, Rajamaki A. Serum transferrin receptor and its ratio to serum ferritin in the diagnosis of iron deficiency. Blood 89:1052–1057, 1997.
29. Skikne BS. Circulating transferrin receptor assay: coming of age. Clin Chem 44:7–9, 1998.
30. Hurrell RF. Preventing iron deficiency through food fortification. Nutr Rev 55:210–222, 1997.
31. Hallberg L, Hulten L, Gramatkovski E. Iron absorption from the whole diet in men: how effective is the regulation of iron absorption? Am J Clin Nutr 66:347–356, 1997.
32. Calvo EB, Galindo AC, Aspres NB. Iron status in exclusively breast-fed infants. Pediatrics 90:375–379, 1992.
33. Walter T, Pino P, Pizarro F, et al. Prevention of iron deficiency anemia: Comparison of high- and low-iron formulas in term healthy infants after six months of life. J Pediatr 132:635–640, 1998.
34. Haschke F, Vanura H, Male C, et al. Iron nutrition and growth of breast- and formula-fed infants during the first 9 months of life. J Pediatr Gastroenterol Nutr 16:151–156, 1993.
35. Moffatt MEK, Longstaffe S, Besant J, et al. Prevention of iron deficiency and psychomotor decline in high-risk infants through use of iron-fortified infant formula: a randomized clinical trial. J Pediatr 125:527–534, 1994.
36. Beard JL. Weekly iron intervention: the case for intermittent iron supplementation. Am J Clin Nutr 68:209–212, 1998.
37. Hallberg L. Combating iron deficiency: daily administration of iron is far superior to weekly administration. Am J Clin Nutr 68: 213–217, 1998.
38. Lui XN, Kang J, Zhao L, et al. Intermittent iron supplementation in Chinese preschool children is efficient and safe. Food Nutr Bull 16: 139–146, 1995.
39. Harju E. Clinical pharmacokinetics of iron preparations. Clin Pharmacokinet 17:69–89, 1989.
40. Dexferrum [package insert]. Shirley, NY: American Reagent Laboratories Inc.; 2001
41. INFed [package insert]. Morristown, NJ: Watson Pharmaceuticals Inc.; 2001.
42. Chertow G, Mason PD, Vaage-Nilsen O, et al. Update on adverse drug events associated with parenteral iron. Nephrol Dial Transplant 2005.
43. Venofer [package insert]. Shirley, NY: American Reagent Laboratories Inc.; 2005.
44. Yee J, Besarab A. Iron sucrose: the oldest iron therapy becomes new. Am J Kidney Dis 40:1111–1121, 2002.
45. Charytan C, Leven N, Al-Saloum M, et al. Efficacy and safety of iron sucrose for iron deficiency in patients with dialysis-associated anemia. North American Clinical Trial. Am J Kid Dis 37:300–307, 2001.
46. Van Wyck DB, Cavalllo G, Spinowitz BS, et al. Safety and efficacy of iron sucrose in patients sensitive to iron dextran. North American Clinical Trial. Am J Kidney Dis 36:88–97, 2000.
47. Ferrlecit [package insert]. Morristown, NJ: Watson Pharmaceuticals Inc.; 2004.
48. Coyne DW, Adkinson NF, Nissenson AR. Sodium ferric gluconate complex in hemodialysis patients. II. Adverse reactions in iron dextran-sensitive and dextran-tolerant patients. Kidney Int 63: 217–224.

49. Ifudu O. Parenteral iron: pharmacology and clinical use. Nephron 80:249–256, 1998.

50. Bastani B, Rahman S, Gellens M. Lack of reaction to ferric gluconate in hemodialysis patients with a severe reaction to iron dextran. ASAIO J 48:404–406, 2002.

51. Hamstra RD. Block MH, Shocket AL. Intravenous Iron dextran in clinical medicine. 243:1726–1731, 1980.

52. Silverstein SB, Rodgers GM. Parenteral iron therapy options. Am J Hematol 76:74–78, 2004.

53. St Peter LW, Obrador GT, Roberts TL, et al. Trends in intravenous iron use among dialysis patients in the United States (1994–2002). Am J Kid Dis 46:650–660, 2005.

54. Cohen A. Treatment of transfusional iron overload. Am J Pediatr Hematol Oncol 12:4–8, 1990.

55. Colon-Otero G, Menke D, Hook CC. A practical approach to the differential diagnosis and evaluation of the adult patient with macrocytic anemia. Med Clin North Am 76:581–597, 1992.

56. Davenport J. Macrocytic anemia. Am Fam Physician 53:155–162, 1996.

57. Bower C, Wald NJ. Vitamin B_{12} deficiency and the fortification of food with folic acid. Eur J Clin Nutr 49:787–793, 1995.

58. Dickinson CJ. Does folic acid harm people with vitamin B_{12} deficiency? Q J Med 88:357–364, 1995.

59. Goodman KI, Salt WB. Vitamin B_{12} deficiency. Important new concepts in recognition. Postgrad Med 88:147–158, 1990.

60. Swain R. An update of vitamin B_{12} metabolism and deficiency states. J Fam Pract 41:595–600, 1995.

61. Allen RH, Stabler SP, Savage DG, et al. Elevation of 2-methylcitric acid I and II levels in serum, urine, and cerebrospinal fluid of patients with cobalamin deficiency. Metabolism 42:978–988, 1993.

62. Delva MD. Vitamin B_{12} replacement. To B_{12} or not to B_{12}? Can Fam Physician 43:917–922, 1997.

63. Nexo E, Hansen M, Rasmussen K, et al. How to diagnose cobalamin deficiency. Scand J Clin Lab Invest 54 (Suppl 219):61–76, 1994.

64. Stott DJ, Langhorne P, Hendry A, et al. Prevalence and haemopoietic effects of low serum vitamin B_{12} levels in geriatric medical patients. Br J Nutr 78:57–63, 1997.

65. Carmel R. Cobalamin, the stomach, and aging. Am J Clin Nutr 66:750–759, 1997.

66. Brigden ML. A systematic approach to macrocytosis. Sorting out the causes. Postgrad Med 97:171–186, 1995.

67. Marcuard SP, Albernaz L, Khazanie PG. Omeprazole therapy causes malabsorption of cyanocobalamin (vitamin B_{12}). Ann Intern Med 120:211–215, 1994.

68. Termanini B, Gibril F, Sutliff VE, et al. Effect of long-term gastric acid suppressive therapy on serum vitamin B_{12} levels in patients with Zollinger-Ellison syndrome. Am J Med 104:422–430, 1998.

69. Field EA, Speechley JA, Rugman FR, et al. Oral signs and symptoms in patients with undiagnosed vitamin B_{12} deficiency. J Oral Pathol Med 24:468–470, 1995.

70. Amos RJ, Dawson DW, Fish DI, et al. Guidelines on the investigation and diagnosis of cobalamin and folate deficiencies. A publication of the British Committee for Standards in Haematology. Clin Lab Haematol 16:101–115, 1994.

71. Kuzminski AM, Del Giacco EJ, Allen RH, et al. Effective treatment of cobalamin deficiency with oral cobalamin. Blood 92:1191–1198, 1998.

72. Kondo H. Haematological effects of oral cobalamin preparations on patients with megaloblastic anemia. Acta Haematol 99:200–205, 1998.

73. Altay C, Cetin M. Oral treatment in selective vitamin B_{12} malabsorption. J Pediatr Hematol Oncol 19:245–246, 1997.

74. Lederle FA. Oral cobalamin for pernicious anemia: medicine's best kept secret? JAMA 265:94–95, 1991.

75. Elia M. Oral or parenteral therapy for B_{12} deficiency. Lancet 352:1721–1722, 1998.

76. Romeo VD, Sileno A, Wenig DN. Intranasal cyanocobalamin [letter]. JAMA 268:1268–1269, 1992.

77. Slot WB, Merkus FWHM, Van Deventer SJH, et al. Normalization of plasma vitamin B_{12} concentration by intranasal hydroxocobalamin in vitamin B_{12}-deficient patients. Gastroenterology 113:430–433, 1997.

78. Swain RA, St Clair L. The role of folic acid in deficiency states and prevention of disease. J Fam Pract 44:138–144, 1997.

79. Eskes TKAB. Folates and the fetus. Eur J Obstet Gynecol Reprod Biol 71:105–111, 1997.

80. Oakley GP. Eat right and take a multivitamin. N Engl J Med 338:1060–1061, 1998.

81. Robinson K, Arheart K, Refsum H, et al. Low circulating folate and vitamin B6 concentrations: risk factors for stroke, peripheral vascular disease, and coronary artery disease. European COMAC Group. Circulation 97:437–443, 1998.

82. Chasan-Taber L, Selhub J, Rosenberg IH, et al. A prospective study of folate and vitamin B6 and risk of myocardial infarction. J Am Coll Nutr 15:136–143, 1996.

83. Pinto X, Vilaseca MA, Balcells S, et al. A folate-rich diet is as effective as folic acid from supplements in decreasing plasma homocysteine concentrations. Int J Med Sci 2:58–63, 2005.

84. Homocysteine Lowering Trialists' Collaboration. Dose-dependent effects of folic acid on blood concentrations of homocysteine: a meta-analysis of the randomized trials. Am J Clin Nutr 82:806–812, 2005.

85. Rimm EB, Willett WC, Hu FB, et al. Folate and vitamin B6 from diet and supplements in relation to risk of coronary artery disease among women. JAMA 279:359–364, 1998.

86. Folsom AR, Nieto J, McGovern PG, et al. Prospective study of coronary heart disease incidence in relation to fasting total homocysteine, related genetic polymorphisms, and B vitamins. The Atherosclerosis Risk in Communities (ARIC) Study. Circulation 98:204–210, 1998.

87. Malinow MR, Duell PB, Hess DL, et al. Reduction of plasma homocyst(e)ine levels by breakfast cereal fortified with folic acid in patients with coronary heart disease. N Engl J Med 338:1009–1015, 1998.

88. Tucker KL, Mahnken B, Wilson PWF, et al. Folic acid fortification of the food supply. Potential benefits and risks for the elderly population. JAMA 276:1879–1885, 1996.

89. Gloria L, Cravo M, Camilo ME, et al. Nutritional deficiencies in chronic alcoholics: relationship to dietary intake and alcohol consumption. Am J Gastroenterol 92:485–489, 1997.

90. United States Pharmacopeia Drug Information: Drug Information for the Health Care Professional. Vol 1. 21 ed. Greenwood Village, CO: Thomson Micromedex, 2001:1561–1563.

91. Quinn K, Basu TK. Folate and vitamin B_{12} status of the elderly. Eur J Clin Nutr 50:340–342, 1996.

92. Mansouri A, Lipschitz DA. Anemia in the elderly patient. Med Clin North Am 76:619–630, 1992.

93. Rule SAJ, Hooker M, Costello C, et al. Serum vitamin B_{12} and transcobalamin levels in early HIV disease. Am J Hematol 47:167–171, 1994.

94. Paltiel O, Falutz J, Veilleux M, et al. Clinical correlates of subnormal vitamin B_{12} levels in patients with the human immunodeficiency virus. Am J Hematol 49:318–22, 1995.

95. United States Pharmacopeia Drug Information: Drug Information for the Health Care Professional. Vol 1. 21 ed. Greenwood Village, CO: Thomson Micromedex, 2001:3012–3016.

Other Anemias

32

Janice L. Stumpf and Kevin A. Townsend

TREATMENT GOALS

- Improve the anemia of chronic disease by treating the underlying infectious, inflammatory, or neoplastic condition and administering erythropoiesis-stimulating agents, when appropriate.
- Increase hemoglobin concentrations toward normal values in patients with anemia of chronic kidney disease by administering erythropoiesis-stimulating agents while maintaining iron stores.

- Remove the causative agent in patients who develop aplastic anemia and provide supportive care with transfusions and antibiotic therapy as well as definitive therapy with immunosuppressive agents or bone marrow transplantation.
- Prevent the adverse consequences of sickle cell anemia by providing transfusions, vaccinations, and prophylactic antibiotics as indicated; provide effective treatment for painful vaso-occlusive crises, infections, and other complications; and treat the disorder itself with hydroxyurea or bone marrow transplantation.
- Correct the anemia and suppress the ineffective erythropoiesis of β-thalassemia major by providing regular blood transfusions.
- Avoid blood transfusion-associated iron overload by administering concomitant iron chelation therapy.
- Manage hemolytic anemia by identifying and controlling etiologic factors and providing appropriate supportive care.

Although the clinical features of anemias resulting from many causes are often similar, treatment modalities and prognosis are quite distinct. In this chapter, a variety of anemias are discussed, including the anemias of chronic disease and kidney disease, aplastic anemia, sickle cell anemia, thalassemia, and hemolytic anemia.

ANEMIA OF CHRONIC DISEASE

The anemia of chronic disease is a mild, often asymptomatic condition that occurs in conjunction with a variety of infectious, inflammatory, and neoplastic disorders. The anemia develops 1 to 2 months after the onset of diseases such as chronic osteomyelitis, tuberculosis, rheumatoid arthritis, systemic lupus erythematosus, vasculitides, and carcinomas, including Hodgkin's disease and solid tumors. Although renal insufficiency also is a chronic disease, the associated anemia manifests differently and therefore is discussed separately.

PATHOPHYSIOLOGY

The pathology of anemia of chronic disease is multifactorial, but it appears to be a defense mechanism to hinder the progression of the underlying disease.[1,2] Inflammatory cytokines mediate a disruption of iron homeostasis. The cytokines tumor necrosis factor (TNF-α) and interleukin-1 induce the synthesis of ferritin, increasing iron storage in the reticuloendothelial system (RES) and restricting the amount of iron available to the bone marrow. The supply of iron that may promote the growth of rapidly proliferating malignant cells or infectious pathogens is thereby diminished. Interferon may also directly suppress erythropoiesis by inhibiting proliferation and differentiation of erythroid progenitor cells. In addition, a moderate shortening of the red blood cell (RBC) life span may be noted that is unaccompanied by increased erythrocyte production. In fact, erythropoietin concentrations may be low relative to the measured hematocrit.

CLINICAL PRESENTATION AND DIAGNOSIS

Because it is associated with many diseases and a unifying pathogenesis has not been elucidated, the anemia of chronic disease remains a diagnosis of exclusion. The erythrocytes typically are normochromic and normocytic, but they may be microcytic. The hematocrit concentration rarely falls below 30%; if it does, other causes of anemia should be investigated thoroughly. The reticulocyte count is low or within normal limits and serum iron levels and iron binding protein saturation are low. However, in contrast to the picture of iron deficiency anemia, ferritin levels are elevated in the anemia of chronic disease. Anemia caused by iron deficiency as a sole diagnosis or in conjunction with the anemia of chronic disease is unlikely if the serum ferritin concentration exceeds 50 ng/mL (112.35 pmol/L). The serum transferrin receptor assay may assist in differentiation between functional and true iron deficiency in patients with anemia of chronic disease.[1,2] These and other manifestations, including elevations in haptoglobin and fibrinogen levels and erythrocyte sedimentation rate, are known collectively as the acute phase reaction, a response to inflammation that may persist with chronic conditions.

TREATMENT

Because the anemia of chronic disease generally is mild, no specific therapy is necessary in most cases. The degree of anemia correlates well with the severity of the associated disease state, and reversal of the underlying disorder corrects the anemia. However, if the patient becomes symptomatic, blood transfusions may be beneficial. Iron replacement regimens have been attempted but have been uniformly ineffective and may place the patient at risk by providing iron to proliferating micro-organisms or malignant cells.[1] Administration of recombinant human erythropoietin (epoetin) may reduce the need for blood transfusions and improve quality-of-life indices. Epoetin has improved anemia of chronic disease in patients with underlying malignancies, chronic infections, and autoimmune disorders, with response dependent on the availability of iron (i.e., serum ferritin levels) and the degree of inflammation.

ANEMIA OF CHRONIC KIDNEY DISEASE

The anemia that complicates chronic kidney disease generally is more severe than that associated with other chronic diseases. The severity of the anemia appears to correlate with the extent of the uremia, but not with the cause of the underlying renal disease. Anemia is typically apparent in patients with glomerular filtration rates of less than 30 mL per min or serum creatinine concentrations greater than 2.3 to 5.7 mg/dL (200 to 500 μmol/L).[3] Over 85% of patients have hemoglobin concentrations less than 12 g/dL (120 g/L) when therapy for end-stage renal disease is initiated.[4]

PATHOPHYSIOLOGY

The anemia of renal failure is primarily the result of reduced secretion of erythropoietin by the diseased kidneys. This hormone stimulates the proliferation and maturation of erythrocytes and is released when the availability of oxygen to the organs is diminished. Although to some extent the hormone is synthesized extrarenally in the liver, serum erythropoietin concentrations in uremic patients are markedly lower than those in patients with similar degrees of anemia and normal renal function.

Other factors that contribute to the anemia are the accumulation of inhibitors of erythropoiesis, reduced RBC life span, and chronic blood loss.[5,6] In support of the presence of suppressive substances, erythropoietin-induced stimulation of erythroid progenitors is blunted in vitro by uremic serum. In addition, while erythropoietin levels remain stable, the anemia improves after dialysis, perhaps indicating removal of these substances. Parathyroid hormone and the polyamine spermine have been implicated in reducing marrow responsiveness to erythropoietin; however, data are conflicting and the identity of the inhibitory substances remains unknown.

Erythrocyte survival also decreases to an average of one half of normal in uremia due to a mild, chronic hemolysis. The cause of the RBC destruction is unclear; however, hypersplenism or increases in erythrocyte fragility induced by parathyroid hormone may contribute. This abnormality may not be corrected by dialysis, yet it also does not appear to be a defect in the red cells. A similar reduction in erythrocyte life span is noted after transfusion of blood products from nonuremic donors to patients with renal failure.

Chronic blood loss both from a gastrointestinal source and during hemodialysis may also contribute to the anemia. Because of defects in platelet function, uremic patients have an elevated risk of bleeding; occult blood loss is reported in >20% of patients receiving dialysis. An estimated 2 g of iron is lost annually during hemodialysis, increasing the likelihood of a concurrent iron deficiency anemia. In addition, the intestinal absorption of iron may be compromised by the chronic use of iron-chelating antacids. Other factors that may aggravate the anemia of chronic kidney disease include folic acid deficiency caused by losses to the dialysate, the accumulation of the fat-soluble vitamin A, aluminum toxicity caused by long-term hemodialysis and the use of aluminum-containing phosphate binders, and osteitis fibrosa, a complication of hyperparathyroidism in which myelofibrosis reduces viable erythroid cellular mass.

CLINICAL PRESENTATION AND DIAGNOSIS

The RBCs in the anemia of chronic kidney disease are normochromic and normocytic but often are irregular in shape. Although hematocrit levels may fall to 30% or less, not all patients become symptomatic. This tolerance of such low hematocrit concentrations may be explained by the compensatory reduction in oxygen–hemoglobin affinity, allowing improved delivery of oxygen to the tissues. Despite this adaptation, an estimated 25% of patients receiving dialysis needed treatment with blood transfusions before the widespread use of recombinant erythropoietin.[5] In addition to improving common symptoms of anemia (e.g., fatigue, angina, shortness of breath), adequate therapy also improves vague complaints of generalized coldness, anorexia, insomnia, and depression and increases survival and quality of life.

TREATMENT

Before initiating therapy aimed at the primary abnormality, other potential causes of anemia should be identified and addressed. Iron and folate supplementation should be provided as necessary, and blood loss and the use of aluminum-containing antacids should be minimized whenever possible. The treatment for acute symptoms of hypoxia consists of the transfusion of RBCs. However, although transfusions may readily correct the anemia, they carry the risk of hypersensitivity reactions and the transmission of viral hepatitis. In addition, bone marrow suppression and iron overload necessitating deferoxamine therapy may occur after multiple, chronic transfusions.

ANDROGENS

In the past, androgens such as parenteral nandrolone decanoate and testosterone enanthate or oral fluoxymesterone were recommended for treating the anemia of chronic kidney disease. These agents stimulate the synthesis of erythropoietin, the production of RBCs in the bone marrow, or both. However, they are not universally effective and rarely fully correct the anemia. In addition, the use of androgens is limited by virilizing effects as well as the association of the oral agents with liver dysfunction.

ERYTHROPOIESIS-STIMULATING AGENTS

The availability of recombinant human erythropoietin, a peptide whose 166-amino acid structure is identical to that of the native hormone, has revolutionized the therapy of anemia associated with chronic kidney disease and essentially eliminated therapy with androgens. Administration of epoetin intravenously (IV) three times weekly after hemodialysis resulted in target hematocrit concentrations of 35% or 6% increases from baseline in >97% of patients within 12 weeks.[7] The need for routine RBC transfusions was eliminated and quality of life was enhanced. Darbepoetin alfa, a long-acting analogue of epoetin, is the second erythropoiesis-stimulating agent to gain approval from the U.S. Food and Drug Administration (FDA) and is similar in safety and efficacy.

Although epoetin was once commonly administered as IV bolus doses three times weekly after hemodialysis, subcutaneous administration is more cost-effective and is preferred.[6] Subcutaneous epoetin produces equivalent efficacy with doses 15% to 50% lower than those required by the IV route. Subcutaneous epoetin has also been used successfully in predialysis and peritoneal dialysis populations. The bioavailability of epoetin and darbepoetin after subcutaneous injection is 20% and 37%, respectively; however, lower, more sustained plasma concentrations are achieved through slow release from the subcutaneous depot. The elimination half-lives of both agents are prolonged after subcutaneous injection compared to IV administration. An initial epoetin regimen of 80 to 120 units/kg/week divided into two or three subcutaneous doses per week is currently recommended.[6]

The chief advantage of darbepoetin over epoetin is the convenience afforded by its long half-life and subsequent need for less frequent administration. Following subcutaneous administration, darbepoetin has an elimination half-life of 49 hours (range 27 to 89 hours), approximately three times that of epoetin.[8] Darbepoetin should be initiated with IV or subcutaneous doses of 0.45 µg/kg once weekly; dosage requirements are not affected by route of administration. Predialysis patients may require lower maintenance doses, and some patients can be maintained within the target hemoglobin range of 11 to 12 g/dL (110 to 120 g/L) with IV or subcutaneous injections every 2 to 4 weeks.[3] The dose of epoetin or darbepoetin should be increased no more often than monthly.

Monitoring Parameters. Dose-dependent increases in hemoglobin concentrations and reticulocyte counts are seen after 2 to 6 weeks of therapy. In general, hemoglobin increases of 0.3 g per dL (3 g/L) per week are expected. Hemoglobin concentrations should be determined weekly, and the dose of the erythropoiesis-stimulating agent reduced by 25% if the concentration increases by more than 1 to 1.5 g/dL (10 to 15 g/L) within a 2-week period. In addition, the dose should be decreased if the hemoglobin continues to rise, approaching the target range. Once a stable hemoglobin concentration and dose are achieved, the hemoglobin should be reassessed every 2 to 4 weeks.

Adverse Effects. Adverse effects associated with erythropoiesis-stimulating agents include myalgias, headache, flank pain, hypertension, and seizures. In addition, local reactions, such as burning, pain, and irritation, have been reported after subcutaneous injection. Increases in blood pressure appear to be a hemodynamic consequence of the rising hematocrit, although the exact mechanism of this effect remains to be elucidated. Blood pressure elevations necessitate the institution or upward titration of antihypertensive medications in 30% to 40% of patients early in the course of epoetin or darbepoetin therapy.[8,9] Seizures may accompany uncontrolled hypertension. Therefore, close monitoring and control of blood pressure levels are essential.

Increases in predialysis concentrations of serum creatinine, potassium, and phosphate have also been documented. The reduced effectiveness of dialysis noted with higher hematocrit levels and increased dietary intake may account for these changes. In addition, clotting of arteriovenous access sites, venous thrombosis, and pulmonary emboli have been associated with erythropoiesis-stimulating agents.

Lack of Response. Iron deficiency is the most common reason for resistance to erythropoiesis-stimulating agents. During the acute erythroid response, iron may be used more rapidly than it is released to transferrin from the RES. A functional and an absolute iron deficiency may therefore develop, which may compromise further response to epoetin. Patients with pretreatment iron overload have experienced beneficial 39% reductions in serum ferritin levels within 6 months. Ferritin levels and transferrin saturation should be determined at baseline and monthly until the goal hemoglobin is achieved; iron stores should be measured at 3-month intervals thereafter. If the ferritin concentration or transferrin saturation falls below 100 ng/mL (224.7 pmol/L) or 20%, respectively, IV iron supplementation should be initiated.[6] There is some evidence that therapy with angiotensin-converting enzyme inhibitors may reduce the efficacy of the erythropoietic agents; however, data are conflicting at present. Rarely, loss of response to epoetin has been associated with the presence of neutralizing antibodies to native and recombinant erythropoietins, leading to pure red cell aplasia.[10]

The erythropoiesis-stimulating proteins epoetin and darbepoetin allow clinicians to correct the anemia of chronic kidney disease on a long-term basis in both dialysis and predialysis patients. The high response rate indicates that the predominant cause of the anemia is erythropoietin deficiency. Other pathogenetic mechanisms, such as the presence of inhibitors of erythropoiesis, may also be operative yet may be overwhelmed clinically by excessive exogenous erythropoietin. The high cost of these agents should be considered in the context of savings resulting from reductions in other interventions (e.g., blood transfusions). In addition, improvements in quality-of-life parameters may lead to greater rehabilitation potential and a return to productive lives for more patients with chronic kidney disease.

APLASTIC ANEMIA

Aplastic anemia is distinguished by hypocellularity of the bone marrow and subsequent pancytopenia that is unrelated to malignancy or myeloproliferative disease. The characteristic anemia, neutropenia, and thrombocytopenia result from failure of the pluripotential stem cell due to congenital or acquired processes. Although the causative mechanisms remain unknown, advances in therapy have greatly improved the overall prognosis.

ETIOLOGY

Although many causes have been identified, the majority of cases of aplastic anemia are classified as idiopathic. Myelosuppression is a component of several congenital diseases but is more commonly acquired after exposure to drugs, chemicals, ionizing radiation, or viruses (Table 32.1). Aplastic anemia and paroxysmal nocturnal hemoglobinuria are closely associated; aplastic anemia may precede or progress to paroxysmal nocturnal hemoglobinuria.

Bone marrow suppression resulting from drugs or chemicals is often dose and duration dependent and may result from direct or immune-mediated stem cell toxicity. Chloramphenicol is the best-documented cause of drug-induced aplastic anemia. Reversible erythroid suppression is noted in approximately 50% of those receiving more than 1 week of high-dose systemic therapy. In contrast, rare idiosyncratic marrow suppression manifesting weeks to months after exposure is also associated with chloramphenicol. Before the availability of bone marrow transplantation (BMT) and alternative treatments, this reaction was fatal in 90% of cases, often within 1 year of clinical presentation.

Aplastic anemia may also arise concurrently with or after viral infection. Hepatitis, most often non-A, non-B (including hepatitis C), precedes up to 5% of cases of aplastic anemia; however, the severity of the infection does not predict the subsequent development of bone marrow suppression. Myelosuppression usually is noted within 6 months of the onset of hepatitis.

EPIDEMIOLOGY

The annual incidence of aplastic anemia in the West is estimated to be two to five cases per million population.[11] The prevalence of disease is higher in developing countries, perhaps reflecting increased exposure to viral hepatitis and environmental toxins. Two peaks are evident in the distribution of ages of onset: approximately 25% of those affected are under 20 years of age, and one third are over 60 years of age.

PATHOPHYSIOLOGY

In normal hematopoiesis, three cell lines originate from the pluripotential stem cell, producing erythrocytes, granulocytes, and platelets. Both cellular and humoral factors regulate the stem cells to maintain a balance between self-replication and differentiation into particular cell types. Aplastic anemia develops when hematopoiesis is interrupted because of deficient or defective stem cells. In addition to reduced numbers of progenitor cells, suggested pathophysiologic mechanisms include immune-mediated suppression of stem cell function, disturbances in the bone marrow microenvironment, and alterations in the cellular or humoral interactions that normally sustain hematopoiesis.[12] Research with a variety of treatment modalities supports T-cell–mediated destruction of marrow cells as the most likely cause of the majority of cases of acquired aplastic anemia.

CLINICAL PRESENTATION AND DIAGNOSIS

Stem cell dysfunction may be incomplete and result in unequal effects on each cell type. Therefore, the earliest clinical signs are determined by the cell line affected to the greatest degree. Often, features of a mild anemia, such as pallor and

TABLE 32.1	Causes of Aplastic Anemia

Acquired
  Drugs and chemicals
    Acetazolamide
    Allopurinol
    Antibiotics
      Chloramphenicol
      Quinacrine
      Sulfonamides
    Anticonvulsants
      Carbamazepine
      Felbamate
      Phenytoin
      Primidone
    Arsenic
    Benzene
    Cancer chemotherapy
    Ethanol
    Gold salts
    Insecticides
    Methylene dioxymethamphetamine (MDMA, Ecstasy)
    Nonsteroidal anti-inflammatory drugs
      Diclofenac
      Indomethacin
      Naproxen
      Phenylbutazone
      Piroxicam
    Penicillamine
    Phenothiazines

    Thiouracil
    Ticlopidine
  Viral
    Cytomegalovirus
    Epstein-Barr virus
    Hepatitis
    Herpes varicella zoster
    Human immunodeficiency virus
    Influenza
    Parvovirus
    Rubella
  Other
    Anorexia nervosa
    Eosinophilic fasciitis
    Ionizing radiation
    Mycobacterial infection
    Paroxysmal nocturnal hemoglobinuria
    Pregnancy
    Thymoma
    Transfusional graft versus host disease
Congenital
    Amegakaryocytic thrombocytopenia
    Dubowitz syndrome
    Dyskeratosis congenita
    Familial aplastic anemia
    Fanconi's anemia
    Shwachman-Diamond syndrome

fatigue, are reported initially and may be more pronounced if accompanied by bleeding due to thrombocytopenia. Ecchymoses and petechiae also indicate a low platelet count. Less commonly, infection caused by the underlying neutropenia is the presenting manifestation of aplastic anemia. Signs of infection such as fever should be monitored closely as the neutropenia progresses because inflammation may not be apparent.

Decreased numbers of morphologically normal cells are observed in the peripheral blood. The erythrocytes are normochromic and normocytic or slightly macrocytic. The corrected reticulocyte count is markedly reduced, as is the absolute granulocyte count. Bone marrow biopsy reveals extensive areas of hypocellularity in which the marrow is replaced by fat, interspersed with small patches of hematopoietic cells (Fig. 32.1; *see color insert*).

DIAGNOSIS

Diagnosis of aplastic anemia depends on the presence of at least two of the following measurements in the peripheral

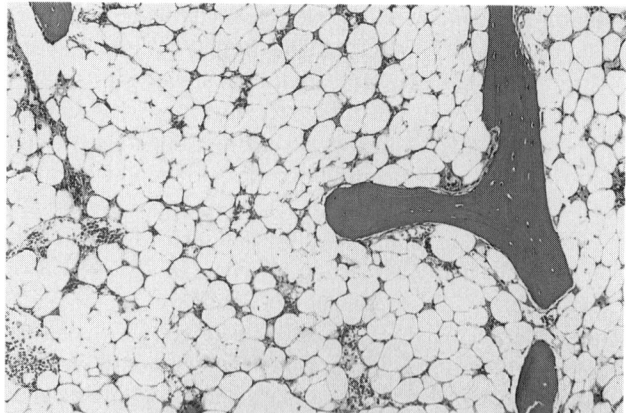

FIGURE 32.1 Aplastic anemia. The bone marrow consists largely of fat cells and lacks normal hemopoietic activity (*see color insert*). (From Rubin E, Farber JL. Pathology, 3rd ed. Philadelphia: Lippincott Williams & Wilkins, 1999.)

TABLE 32.2	Criteria for the Diagnosis of Severe Aplastic Anemia

Peripheral blood counts must reveal at least two of the following:

Neutrophils $<0.5 \times 10^9/L^a$

Platelets $<20 \times 10^9/L$

Reticulocytes $<1\%$

Bone marrow biopsy must reveal either:

Severe hypocellularity ($<25\%$ of normal)

or

Moderate hypocellularity (25% to 50% of normal), with $<30\%$ of residual cells being hematopoietic

---

^{a} A neutrophil count of $<0.2 \times 10^9/L$ with other criteria for severe aplastic anemia is defined as very severe aplastic anemia.

blood: hemoglobin less than 10 g/dL (<100 g/L), platelet count less than 50,000/mL ($<50 \times 10^9/L$), and neutrophil count $<1.5 \times 10^9/L$.[12,13] Severe aplastic anemia is further defined as even lower neutrophil, platelet, and reticulocyte counts, with marked bone marrow hypocellularity (Table 32.2). Differentiation of aplastic anemia from other syndromes accompanied by hypocellularity, such as hypoplastic myelodysplasia, may be difficult.

TREATMENT

Treating patients with aplastic anemia includes removal of potential causative agents, supportive care, and the restoration of normal hematopoiesis with pharmacologic therapy or BMT.[12–14] In mild cases, supportive care should be provided in anticipation of spontaneous recovery. Blood transfusions, preferably leukocyte-depleted products, should be reserved for patients with symptomatic anemia to delay sensitization to alloantigens. Blood products from family members should not be used in candidates for marrow transplantation because of the development of antibodies to histocompatibility antigens of the donor, increasing the risk of graft rejection. Overall, nontransfused patients fare better after BMT than their transfused counterparts.

Antiplatelet antibodies that reduce platelet function and life span also develop after 1 to 2 months of repeated transfusions. Patients often become refractory to subsequent transfusions, although a dose–response relationship has not been established. Platelets should be administered to treat active bleeding or to maintain a platelet count greater than 10,000/mL ($10 \times 10^9/L$), or greater than 20,000/mL ($20 \times 10^9/L$) if febrile. Because of the risk of hematoma, intramuscular injections should be avoided whenever possible in patients with thrombocytopenia, as should aspirin, nonsteroidal anti-inflammatory drugs, and other agents with antiplatelet prop-

erties. Menses should be suppressed hormonally to prevent menorrhagia in female patients with aplastic anemia.

Prompt recognition and treatment of infection are vital in the patient with aplastic anemia and severe neutropenia. Broad-spectrum antibiotics should be initiated in any patient with fever of unknown origin. If a pathogen is not identified and the patient continues to be febrile after 48 to 72 hours of treatment, empiric antifungal therapy with amphotericin B should be considered.

BONE MARROW TRANSPLANTATION

BMT has become the treatment of choice for younger patients (<40 to 45 years) with severe acquired aplastic anemia, with greatest success achieved in those undergoing the procedure soon after diagnosis.[13,14] Initially, a donor who is human lymphocyte antigen (HLA) compatible must be identified. There is a 25% chance that a sibling will be HLA identical. Graft rejection may develop because of minor antigenic differences between donor and recipient marrow and previous sensitization by blood transfusions. Therefore, a course of immunosuppressive therapy is administered before transplantation. This conditioning regimen consists of IV cyclophosphamide (50 mg/kg daily for 4 days) with or without antithymocyte globulin (ATG); methylprednisolone and fludarabine have also been added in some protocols. A 12-month course of cyclosporine is administered posttransplantation to prevent late graft failure. These regimens have reduced the rate of graft rejection to 5% to 10%.[13,14] Two to 6 weeks after IV infusion of marrow cells, the donor cells have engrafted, and blood cells begin to be produced.

The interval between transplantation and the return of hematopoiesis and normal immune function poses the greatest threat to the patient. Supportive care should include isolation in a sterile environment, transfusions of blood products as needed, and close monitoring for signs of infection. Prophylactic antifungal therapy and bowel sterilization with nonabsorbable oral antibiotics may be undertaken in attempts to reduce the incidence of systemic infections. Interstitial pneumonitis may complicate transplantation within the first 3 months; it occurs in approximately 18% of patients with aplastic anemia. In $>39\%$ of cases, cytomegalovirus is implicated, and it is associated with a mortality rate of $>70\%$.[15] Infection with *Aspergillus, Candida, Pneumocystis carinii*, herpes simplex virus, and herpes varicella zoster virus has also been reported. Acyclovir and trimethoprim–sulfamethoxazole prophylaxis may be administered to inhibit activation of herpes viruses and *Pneumocystis*, respectively. In addition, the use of immune globulin to prevent cytomegalovirus activation is advocated at some centers.

Acute graft-versus-host disease (GVHD), in which donor lymphocytes attack the host tissue, occurs in approximately 20% of patients within 2 months after transplantation despite prophylactic immunosuppression with cyclosporine alone or in combination with methotrexate.[14] Initial presenting signs of acute GVHD include skin rash and diarrhea. Elevations in liver function tests and severe immunodeficiency may also develop. Once established, GVHD may be managed with ATG, prednisone, or cyclosporine, with response rates of 30% to 50%.

Chronic GVHD manifests as a serious complication more than 3 months after transplantation in approximately 25% of surviving patients.[13,14] The reaction is similar to that of a systemic autoimmune disease (e.g., systemic lupus erythematosus) with skin, gastrointestinal, hepatic, lymphoid, lung, and ophthalmic involvement. After treatment with prednisone and cyclosporine or azathioprine, 80% of afflicted patients recover. The risk of acquiring GVHD and the severity of GVHD are directly correlated to patient age. Therefore, most transplantations are performed in patients <40 years of age.

IMMUNOSUPPRESSION

Immunosuppressive therapy generally is reserved for older patients with aplastic anemia and those without an HLA-matched sibling marrow donor. A variety of agents, both alone and in combination, have been used to treat the disease, including ATG, antilymphocyte globulin (ALG), corticosteroids, and cyclosporine.[12–14] High doses of corticosteroids have not improved responses and are therefore no longer recommended. A regimen of ATG with cyclosporine appears to be most efficacious, with survival rates of 70% to 87% at 5 years.

ATG is prepared in animals and reacts against human thymocytes. Although the exact mechanism is unknown, ATG presumably inactivates cytotoxic lymphocytes responsible for the suppression of hematopoiesis. In addition, proliferation and differentiation of hematopoietic progenitors may be stimulated. In a typical treatment protocol, a test dose is administered, followed, in the absence of anaphylaxis, by a total ATG (equine) dose of 40 mg per kg IV daily for 4 days. Positive effects are observed in 90% of responders within 3 months. A second course may be effective in those in whom initial therapy fails and in the 25% to 30% of patients who relapse.

Adverse effects of ATG include fever, chills, rash, headache, and hypotension. Serum sickness, manifesting with fever, rash, and arthralgias, may be evident 1 to 2 weeks after therapy; symptoms may be alleviated by corticosteroid therapy. Transient reductions in white blood cell and platelet counts are also reported.

Adding cyclosporine to the immunosuppressive regimen increases the hematologic response rate to 70% to 80% compared to 40% to 50% with ATG alone.[12,13] Therapy with cyclosporine for 6 to 12 months is often needed, increasing the risk of renal toxicity and other adverse effects. A slow tapering of the cyclosporine dose may reduce the rate of relapse; however, many patients require continued low doses to maintain a response. Because clonal disorders subsequently develop in 5% to 15%, patients should be closely monitored for myelodysplasia, leukemia, and paroxysmal nocturnal hemoglobinuria.[14]

ALTERNATIVE THERAPIES

CYCLOPHOSPHAMIDE

High doses of cyclophosphamide have produced complete remissions without relapses or induction of clonal disorders, although hematologic recovery is 2 to 3 weeks slower than conventional immunosuppressive therapy.[16] Responses to cyclophosphamide have also been reported in patients refractory to standard immunosuppression. However, a trial comparing the combination of cyclophosphamide and ATG/cyclosporine with ATG/cyclosporine alone was terminated prematurely when increased toxicity, severe fungal infections, and early deaths were noted in cyclophosphamide recipients.[17] In light of these results, more studies are required before high-dose cyclophosphamide can be recommended as an alternative to immunosuppression or BMT.

ANDROGENS

Androgens once were widely used to treat aplastic anemia because of their stimulatory effects on hematopoiesis (predominantly RBC production). However, in patients with severe disease, oral oxymetholone and intramuscular nandrolone decanoate produced responses similar to those produced by supportive care alone. Although androgens have no apparent role in the management of severe forms of the disease, those with mild aplastic anemia or Fanconi's anemia not amenable to BMT may benefit from treatment.

HEMATOPOIETIC GROWTH FACTORS

Hematopoietic growth factors stimulate the proliferation of progenitor cells and thus may have applications in many hypoplastic disorders.[14] Although recombinant human granulocyte colony-stimulating factor (G-CSF, filgrastim) and granulocyte-macrophage colony-stimulating factor (GM-CSF, sargramostim) have been the most extensively studied, interleukins (IL-1, IL-3, IL-6) and epoetin have also been used with some success in refractory aplastic anemia. Both G-CSF and GM-CSF have produced marked elevations in leukocyte counts, primarily through increases in neutrophils. In general, response is inversely related to the severity of disease, and the effects do not persist after G-CSF or GM-CSF discontinuation. Because growth factors do not correct the underlying stem cell disorder, these agents should be used only in conjunction with definitive therapies for aplastic anemia (i.e., immunosuppression or BMT). Administration of G-CSF as supportive therapy may reduce mortality caused by infection; however, improvements in response and survival were not found when G-CSF was added to ATG/cyclosporine immunosuppression in a prospective, randomized trial.[18] Routine therapy with granulocyte-stimulating factors is therefore not currently recommended.

PROGNOSIS

The prognosis of aplastic anemia is related to blood cell counts, especially the degree of neutropenia.[12–14] Bacterial sepsis and fungal infections are the most common causes of death. With supportive care alone, 80% to 90% of patients with severe aplastic anemia die within 1 to 2 years.[11] Advances in BMT and immunosuppressive protocols have dramatically improved this outcome. The rate of long-term disease-free survival after transplantation ranges from 75% to 90%.[12–14] Survival rates following immunosuppressive therapy are comparable to those of transplantation, with best outcomes in patients >20 years of age with absolute neutrophil counts >200 per mL.

SICKLE CELL ANEMIA

The term *sickle cell disease* encompasses a variety of hemoglobinopathies, including sickle cell anemia, sickle hemoglobin C (SC) disease, and sickle cell thalassemia. Although the clinical presentation of these disorders is often similar, the manifestations of sickle cell anemia are more severe and are therefore the focus of the following discussion.

EPIDEMIOLOGY

The Hb S gene confers protection against *Plasmodium falciparum* infection in infancy. Therefore, populations residing in or originating from areas where malaria is endemic have the highest frequency of the AS and SS genotypes. The distribution of sickle disease is no longer restricted to Africa, the Middle East, and India, but areas of concentration remain. Up to 25% of people in West Africa possess the Hb S gene. Among African Americans in the United States, 1 in 600 have sickle cell anemia, whereas 1 in 12 have the sickle trait.[19]

PATHOPHYSIOLOGY

The hemoglobin molecule is a tetramer composed of four polypeptides linked to iron-carrying heme groups. More than 600 different types of hemoglobin have been distinguished, including hemoglobins A_1, A_2, C, F, and S. Only three variants are considered to be normal: hemoglobin A_1 (Hb A_1), hemoglobin A_2 (Hb A_2), and fetal hemoglobin (Hb F). Hb F accounts for 70% to 80% of the hemoglobin in the red cells of newborns. A gradual conversion occurs over the first year until the normal adult pattern of 97% Hb A_1, less than 3% Hb A_2, and less than 1% Hb F is represented.

The Hb A_1 tetramer consists of two pairs of globin chains, α and β, which have distinct primary structures. Sickle cell anemia is a homozygous condition that results from the substitution of valine for glutamic acid in both of the β-chains. Because each parent contributes a single β-chain gene, the heterozygous genotype AS is also possible and is expressed as the sickle cell trait phenotype.

Deoxygenation in the capillaries induces rapid polymerization of the sickling hemoglobin, Hb S, and results in formation of helical strands of parallel fibers.[20] The elongated, crescent-shaped cells characteristic of sickle cell anemia are thereby produced (Fig. 32.2). The erythrocytes adhere to the endothelia of the postcapillary venules, and then aggregates of white blood cells and sickled cells are formed. Inflammation, abnormalities in vasomotor tone, and increased rates of Hb S polymerization due to local hypoxia and other factors lead to vaso-occlusion, with subsequent painful ischemia and chronic organ damage. In general, the sickling is reversible upon re-exposure to oxygen; however, repeated sickling episodes eventually damage the cell membrane. The sickled conformation is sustained and the cells are subject to hemolysis and removal by the liver or spleen.

The rate of Hb S polymerization depends on its concentration in the erythrocyte. The copolymerization of Hb S with

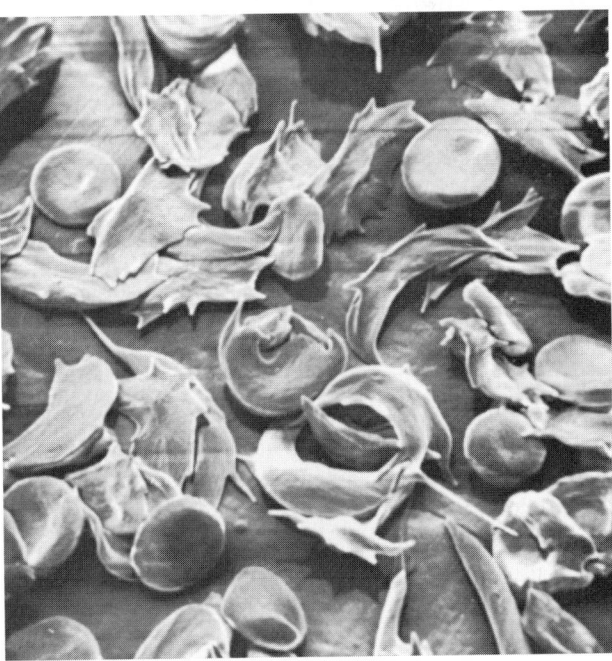

FIGURE 32.2 Sickle cell anemia. (Reprinted with permission from McKenzie SB. Textbook of Hematology, 2nd ed. Baltimore: Williams & Wilkins; 1996:155, Fig. D.)

Hb F inhibits further polymer growth; intracellular Hb F concentrations are inversely correlated with disease severity.

CLINICAL PRESENTATION AND DIAGNOSIS

SIGNS AND SYMPTOMS

Sickle cell anemia presents with constitutional, hematologic, and vaso-occlusive manifestations (Table 32.3) late in the first postnatal year, after levels of the protective Hb F have diminished. Skeletal growth and sexual maturation are impaired, although catch-up growth is apparent by adulthood.

Because of recurrent microinfarcts, the spleen is initially enlarged and then completely fibrosed by 6 years of age. This functional autosplenectomy and defects in other host defenses greatly increase the likelihood of infection, especially with *Streptococcus pneumoniae* and *Haemophilus influenzae.*

Hemolysis accompanied by inadequate erythropoiesis results in a normochromic, normocytic anemia, with hematocrit levels ranging from 18% to 30%. The chronic anemia leads to a hyperdynamic circulatory system and subsequent cardiac hypertrophy and systolic ejection murmurs. The anemia is aggravated during aplastic crises, when erythropoiesis is further suppressed by acute infection or folate deficiency.

Painful vaso-occlusive crises produced by aggregates of sickled cells in the microcirculation are the most common reason for hospitalization. The frequency and severity of painful crises vary greatly between individuals. In one review of more than 12,200 pain episodes, approximately 5% of patients with sickle cell anemia had 3 to 10 pain episodes each year, whereas another 39% did not experience pain.[21] The episodes are sudden and last an average of 4 to 6 days. Pain is most often reported in the long bones, spine, pelvis, chest, and abdomen and must be differentiated from infection and other acute processes. Factors that may precipitate vaso-occlusive crises include acidosis, heat or exercise (dehydration), cold (vasoconstriction), infection, stress, menses, and high altitudes.

Recurrent sickling and subsequent infarction produce chronic damage to many organ systems. Hematuria and an inability to concentrate urine progress in some patients to renal failure. Neurologic complications such as cerebrovascular accidents and seizures develop in 25% of patients, with a recurrence rate of >60% in children with cerebral infarction.[22] Acute chest syndrome, manifesting with pleuritic chest pain, dyspnea, and pulmonary infiltrates, may eventually result in pulmonary fibrosis and chronic obstructive disease. Intrahepatic fibrosis is also reported. Impotence may occur, usually after multiple episodes of priapism.

In addition to indices of anemia, laboratory abnormalities include elevations in platelet count and leukocytosis caused by demargination of granulocytes from vessel walls into the circulation. Irreversibly sickled cells are seen in the blood smear.

TABLE 32.3	**Complications of Sickle Cell Anemia**

Constitutional
  Impaired growth and development
  Increased risk of infection
    Meningitis
    Osteomyelitis
    Pneumonia
    Pyelonephritis
    Septicemia
Hematologic
  Hemolytic anemia
  Aplastic crises
  Splenic sequestration crises
Vaso-occlusive
  Cardiovascular
    Cardiac enlargement
    Systolic murmur
  Gastrointestinal
    Autosplenectomy
    Gallstones/cholecystitis
    Hepatic crises/right upper quadrant syndrome
    Hepatic insufficiency
    Intrahepatic cholelithiasis
  Genitourinary
    Hematuria
    Impotence
    Priapism
    Renal insufficiency
  Neurologic
    Cerebral thrombosis
    Intracerebral hemorrhage
    Seizures
    Subarachnoid hemorrhage
  Ocular
    Retinopathy
    Secondary glaucoma
Painful crises
Pulmonary
  Acute chest syndrome
  Chronic obstructive disease
  Infarction
  Pulmonary hypertension
Skin and skeletal
  Arthropathy
  Aseptic necrosis
  Dactylitis
  Leg ulcers

Individuals with sickle cell trait generally are asymptomatic, although sickling manifestations may occur at extreme levels of hypoxia, acidosis, or other physiologic stress. Hematuria associated with renal papillary necrosis and splenic infarction have been rarely associated with the AS phenotype. The ability to maximally concentrate the urine is lost in most adults with sickle cell trait, due to infarction of the renal medulla. Life expectancy is normal in those with the sickle trait. In contrast, although 85% to 90% of patients with sickle cell anemia may now survive to the age of 20 years, median ages at death for men and women are 42 and 48 years, respectively.[23] Increased mortality has been correlated with increased disease symptoms, elevated white blood cell counts and Hb less than 7.1 g/dL (<71 g/L), whereas higher Hb F levels have been found to reduce mortality risk. Preliminary data suggest that the severity of the clinical course of the disease may be predicted by the presence of dactylitis (pain or tenderness in hands or feet), anemia with Hb less than 7 g/dL (<70 g/L), and leukocytosis by age 2 years.[24]

DIAGNOSIS

Universal neonatal screening for sickle cell disease is currently conducted in 44 states, identifying approximately 2,000 infants with the disease annually.[19] Sickle cell diseases are diagnosed by hemoglobin electrophoresis, which reveals the types and proportion of hemoglobins present. Once the patient's genotype is established, appropriate genetic counseling and education may be provided. If both parents have the AS genotype, there is a 1 in 4 chance that their child will have homozygous SS disease. Prenatal diagnosis is also possible. Genotyping may be performed in the first trimester of pregnancy using fetal cells obtained by amniocentesis or chorionic villus sampling.

TREATMENT

MANAGEMENT OF MAJOR COMPLICATIONS

Anemia. Physiologic adaptations such as low Hb S–oxygen affinity allow patients with sickle cell anemia to tolerate relatively low hematocrit levels. Therefore, therapy is supportive, with blood transfusions reserved for acute, symptomatic exacerbations in the anemia. High folate utilization arising from continuously elevated RBC production may lead to folate deficiency; folate supplementation (1 mg orally daily) is recommended to maintain adequate stores. Transient RBC aplasia (aplastic crises) may be caused by viral (most commonly, human parvovirus B19) infections. Prompt diagnosis and administration of IV immune globulin (IVIG) and RBC transfusions are necessary to treat the viral infection and correct the severe anemia, respectively.[19] Recovery of erythropoiesis generally occurs within 5 to 10 days, as the underlying infection resolves. Acute splenic sequestration, in which the spleen traps erythrocytes, may cause a rapid reduction in hemoglobin and is a leading cause

of death in children with sickle cell disease. RBCs should be transfused immediately. Prevention of recurrence relies on splenectomy or chronic transfusion to maintain Hb S levels <30%.

Infection. Bacterial infection is the leading cause of death in patients with sickle cell anemia. Therefore, a thorough search for an infectious source should be undertaken in any patient with a painful crisis and fever. Pneumonia may be treated empirically with parenteral antibiotics such as cefuroxime or ceftriaxone that cover the most likely pathogens, *S. pneumoniae* and *H. influenzae*. If a clinical response is not apparent after 24 to 48 hours, infection with *Mycoplasma pneumoniae* should be suspected and erythromycin or azithromycin added to the antibiotic regimen. Meningitis occurs 200 to 300 times more frequently in children with sickle cell anemia, with *S. pneumoniae* isolated in approximately 80% of cases.

A series of four doses of pneumococcal-conjugated vaccine (Prevnar) is recommended for children with sickle cell disease. In addition, children ≥2 years old should be immunized with pneumococcal polysaccharide vaccine, and a booster dose should be given after 3 to 5 years. Although a 50% reduction in the incidence of pneumococcal infection has been found after immunization, these vaccines protect against a limited number of pneumococcal serotypes. Prophylactic oral penicillin for patients with sickle cell disease reduces the incidence of pneumococcal septicemia by 84%.[25] Therefore, oral penicillin VK 125 mg should be given twice daily beginning at the age of 2 months. The dosage should be increased to 250 mg twice daily at 3 years of age and therapy continued at least to age 5 years. Continued penicillin prophylaxis beyond 5 years of age is no longer recommended because the incidence of pneumococcal meningitis or sepsis is not reduced.[26] Other routine immunizations and annual influenza vaccination should also be provided.

Salmonella species are isolated in up to 80% of patients with sickle cell disease and osteomyelitis. A 4- to 6-week course of treatment with ampicillin or a cephalosporin is needed. Leg ulcers should receive local care and should be monitored closely for potential progression to osteomyelitis.

Painful Crises. The goals of therapy for painful vaso-occlusive crises are to provide supportive care and effective analgesia while eliminating potential precipitating factors. Vigorous enteral or parenteral hydration should be initiated and oxygen administered if hypoxia from pulmonary involvement is evident. Both nonnarcotic and narcotic analgesics are used, depending on the severity of pain.

Those with mild to moderately painful crises should be treated as outpatients. Oral hydration with 3 to 4 L (150 mL/kg for children) of fluid daily should be encouraged, and pain should be treated with acetaminophen or nonsteroidal anti-inflammatory drugs.[19] Pain unresponsive to these agents may be controlled by codeine or oxycodone, as single agents or in combination with acetaminophen.

Inpatient treatment with parenteral hydration and narcotic analgesics is necessary for severe painful crises. Scheduled, around-the-clock narcotic administration is preferred over as-needed regimens. The pain–anxiety cycle is thereby diminished and relief often is achieved with lower total dosages. Oral narcotic protocols have been used but are not universally accepted by patients, especially if nausea and vomiting are present. Frequent intramuscular or subcutaneous injections cause local pain and promote abscesses and subsequent infection. In addition, drug absorption may be erratic. Peak effects associated with IV bolus administration may lead to excessive central nervous system depression. Continuous IV infusions are ideal for initial therapy because a dosage range may be specified, allowing safe titration to pain control. Success with patient-controlled analgesia (PCA) has also been reported.

Because narcotics have similar effects at equianalgesic dosages, various regimens alleviate symptoms. Agents with mixed agonist–antagonist properties (e.g., pentazocine, butorphanol) are not recommended for those using narcotics chronically because withdrawal may be precipitated in these physically dependent patients. Although once widely used, meperidine should be avoided because its metabolite, normeperidine, accumulates after repeated high doses and may induce seizures, especially in the presence of renal insufficiency or underlying neurologic disease. The short duration of action of meperidine (2 to 4 hours) also makes administration less practical. Morphine sulfate is the narcotic of choice. In patients unable to tolerate morphine because of nausea, vomiting, or pruritus, hydromorphone may be substituted. Adjuvant therapy with promethazine or hydroxyzine may promote analgesia and reduce narcotic requirements; however, adverse effects also may be potentiated.

Analgesic dosages must be individualized and based on the intensity of pain, degree of outpatient narcotic use, and previous inpatient needs. Tolerance to narcotic analgesic effects after chronic administration may dramatically increase parenteral needs. Although patients may appear manipulative and exhibit drug-seeking behavior, this may be a response to the reluctance of health care professionals to provide the high doses of opiates frequently required to relieve pain. Adequate analgesia should be administered; placebos should not be given.

A continuous IV infusion of morphine (100 mg/100 mL 5% dextrose) at a rate of 0.05 to 0.10 mg/kg/hour may be used for the first 24 to 48 hours. Alternatively, 5 to 10 mg morphine may be administered to adult patients as an IV bolus every 2 to 4 hours. In one protocol, a morphine loading dose is followed by PCA pump delivery of two thirds of the estimated 24-hour morphine requirements as divided doses per hour on demand, with lock-out intervals initially set at every 5 minutes and then adjusted to every 15 to 30 minutes once pain is controlled. In addition, the pump is programmed to infuse another one third of the 24-hour morphine requirements IV.[19] Adverse effects such as respiratory depression,

oversedation, and blood pressure reductions should be monitored and the dosage decreased if indicated.

As the pain subsides, the continuous infusion should be discontinued and the total daily morphine dosage divided into four to six IV bolus doses. The dosage should be tapered by 20% to 30% daily while the interval is maintained. Once the daily IV dosage is 50% of that initially needed, conversion to an equianalgesic dosage of an oral narcotic can be made.

Some patients have chronic pain that may be debilitating and that may require long-term oral narcotic use. Unfortunately, psychological dependence (i.e., addiction) may develop, although this is generally not noted in patients using narcotics appropriately for pain relief. Continuity of care and communication between health care providers are essential to eliminate the possibility of multiple sources of narcotic prescriptions. Psychosocial support and nonpharmacologic coping techniques, such as relaxation therapy, behavior modification, and self-hypnosis, should be explored thoroughly.

MANAGEMENT OF THE SICKLE CELL DISEASE

Transfusion Therapy. Partial exchange transfusions, in which more than 50% of the patient's erythrocytes are replaced by donor RBCs, prevent vaso-occlusive crises. Hypertransfusion until the hematocrit level has doubled temporarily halts erythroid Hb S production and also inhibits sickling. Because of the inherent risks of hepatitis transmission and iron overload, however, transfusions generally are reserved for the management of acute complications and, chronically, for indications such as prevention of cerebral infarctions or hemorrhages in children at high risk (Table 32.4).[22,27] A randomized trial in children to determine

TABLE 32.4	Indications for Transfusion in Patients with Sickle Cell Anemia

Management of acute complications
   Acute chest syndrome
   Anemia exacerbation
   Aplastic crises
   Cerebrovascular accidents
   Multiple organ failure syndrome
   Priapism
   Splenic sequestration
Prophylaxis
   Preoperative
Chronic transfusion therapy
   Prevention of recurrent splenic sequestration
   Prevention of stroke in high-risk patients
   Pulmonary hypertension
   Refractory pain
   Recurrent acute chest syndrome

whether RBCs transfused at 3- to 4-week intervals must be continued indefinitely was terminated early when an increase in the risk and incidence of stroke was documented.[27]

Pharmacologic Management. Many pharmacologic modalities have been directed against the sickling abnormality (Table 32.5), but most have yielded minimal clinical benefit, in part because of limiting adverse effects. Inhibitors of Hb S polymerization, such as sodium cyanate and urea, are not dependably effective; in addition, sodium cyanate is associated with neurologic toxicity. Cetiedil, desmopressin, and clotrimazole alter fluid and electrolyte transport across the RBC membrane. These agents functionally decrease intracellular Hb S concentrations and thereby reduce the polymerization rate. Pentoxifylline may prevent vaso-occlusive crises by increasing RBC deformability and decreasing blood viscosity. These effects improve blood flow through the microvasculature in peripheral vascular occlusive diseases; however, further studies are needed to establish the role of pentoxifylline in sickle cell anemia.

Increasing production of the protective Hb F is another approach to therapy. The antineoplastics 5-azacitidine and cytarabine enhance Hb F production; however, bone marrow suppression produced by these agents is problematic and long-term efficacy is uncertain. Treatment with hydroxyurea increases the proportion of Hb F and the number of cells containing Hb F, resulting in prolonged RBC survival.[28,29] In addition, reductions in neutrophil counts, increases in RBC water content and the deformability of sickled cells, and alterations in erythrocyte–endothelial adhesiveness may contribute to its efficacy. Clinical response, including a 50% reduction in the frequency of painful crises and hospitalizations for sickling complications, was shown in 299 patients enrolled in a multicenter placebo-controlled, double-blind study.[29] In a follow-up observational study,[30] the cumulative mortality rate at 9 years was 15% in those whose Hb F was ≥0.5 g per dL compared to 28% in those with Hb F levels <0.5 g/dL (5 g/L) ($p = 0.03$). Use of hydroxyurea was associated with a 40% reduction in the mortality rate.

Hydroxyurea is approved by the FDA for adults with recurrent moderate or severe painful crises (i.e., three or more episodes per year). Experience with hydroxyurea in infants and children is limited but encouraging. Initial adult dosages of 10 to 15 mg/kg once daily may be increased every 6 to 8 weeks until Hb F increases to 15% to 20%.[19] The maximum daily dosage is 35 mg/kg. Reversible, dose-dependent myelosuppression and the potential for carcinogenic effects of long-term therapy underscore the importance of close monitoring. Complete blood counts should be performed every 2 weeks initially and then at 1- to 2-month intervals once a stable dosage is reached. Discontinuation of the drug should be considered if Hb F levels fail to increase after 6 to 12 months of therapy. Data regarding the benefit of epoetin in conjunction with hydroxyurea are conflicting; however, studies of hydroxyurea with other agents with differing mechanisms of action are under way.

Bone Marrow Transplantation. BMT can cure sickle cell anemia, and those with successful engraftment have had no progression of organ damage or other sickle cell-related events.[31,32] Over 90% of patients survive after BMT, with 85% free of sickle cell disease after up to 11 years. Recurrence of sickle cell anemia has been reported in 10% of patients, and the transplant-related mortality rate is approximately 5%. Optimal candidates for BMT are younger (<16 years) patients with an HLA-matched sibling and a high risk of severe morbidity (e.g., history of cerebrovascular accident, recurrent acute chest syndrome, debilitating pain) who have been minimally transfused and have no significant disease-associated organ damage. The clinical course of sickle cell anemia is quite variable and symptoms may not be apparent for months to years after birth. Studies to identify factors that predict poor outcome and thereby allow selection of patients who would benefit most from BMT are essential. The risks of transplantation must be carefully considered in light of the reduced morbidity noted with improved management of complications and advances in antisickling drug therapy.

FUTURE THERAPIES

Therapeutic modalities that hold promise for the future include agents that reduce the erythrocyte–endothelium adhesiveness that leads to vaso-occlusion; the use of nonmyeloablative regimens prior to BMT, allowing a mixed chimerism of normal and sickle cell populations to coexist; umbilical cord blood transplantation; stem cell transplantation from unrelated donors; and gene therapy in which normal hemoglobin genes are transferred into patients with sickle cell anemia.[20]

TABLE 32.5	Agents Studied for the Treatment of Sickle Cell Anemia
5-Azacytidine	Medroxyprogesterone
Butyrate	Nifedipine
Cetiedil	Nitric oxide
Clotrimazole	Papaverine
Cytarabine	Pentoxifylline
Desmopressin	Piracetam
Dextran	Sodium cyanate
Epoetin alfa	Ticlopidine
Hydergine	Urea
Hydroxyurea	Valproic acid
Isoxsuprine	Zinc sulfate

THALASSEMIAS

The thalassemias are a group of hereditary disorders of hemoglobin synthesis characterized by impaired production of one or more of the normal polypeptide chains of globin. Any of the four polypeptides that occur in normal hemoglobin may be involved (α, β, γ, δ). However, the most prevalent thalassemia syndromes are those that involve diminished or absent synthesis of either the alpha (α-thalassemia) or beta (β-thalassemia) globin chains of Hb A_1.[33-36]

ETIOLOGY

The imbalance in polypeptide chain production secondary to impaired synthesis of either the α chain or the β chain of globin is the underlying factor that accounts for the pathogenesis of all the clinically severe thalassemia syndromes. Reduced production of the normal $\alpha_2\beta_2$ tetramer of Hb A_1 (also known as Hb A) results in the production of smaller erythrocytes with a low hemoglobin content.[33] The synthesis and accumulation of excess normal globin chains within the RBC leads to the formation of unstable aggregates, which may precipitate and cause cell membrane damage. These deformed cells undergo premature destruction either in the bone marrow (extravascular hemolysis) or the peripheral circulation (intravascular hemolysis).[34,37] Chronic hemolysis is a primary complication of the clinically significant α- and β-thalassemia syndromes (e.g., Hb H disease and β-thalassemia major). The "ineffective erythropoiesis" and microcytic, hypochromic anemia described previously is associated with a compensatory increase in the absorption of dietary iron. This may contribute to the iron overload that can result in patients receiving therapy with blood transfusions. There is also an increase in erythropoietic activity in the bone marrow and in extramedullary sites (i.e., liver, spleen, and lymph nodes). In severe forms of thalassemia (e.g., β-thalassemia major), excessive erythropoiesis causes significant bone marrow hypertrophy, growth retardation, lymphadenopathy, and hepatosplenomegaly.[34,37] Bone marrow expansion in untreated patients leads to skeletal deformities and fragility.

EPIDEMIOLOGY

The thalassemia syndromes are collectively one of the most common genetic disorders in humans. Approximately 200 million people throughout the world carry a hemoglobinopathy gene, and greater than half of these are thalassemia genes.[38] Populations that are most affected include Asian, African, Eastern Indian, and Mediterranean cultures.[33,35,39] Since the geographic distribution of this disorder is similar to that of malaria, it is thought that certain types of thalassemia may offer protection from *Plasmodium falciparum* infection.[34,36] The incidence of α-thalassemia is higher in Southeast Asia, China, and certain areas of Africa, while β-thalassemia syndromes are more common in Mediterranean countries such as Greece and Italy. In North America, β-thalassemia is found primarily in people of Greek, Italian, and African ancestry. Genetic analysis studies indicate that approximately 30% of black Americans are "silent carriers" of α-thalassemia.[35]

Because of their similar geographic distributions, coinheritance of sickle cell anemia with thalassemia is not uncommon. Detailed discussion of various sickle cell–thalassemia syndromes can be found elsewhere.[35]

α-THALASSEMIA

There are four genes involved in the production of α globin chains, with one pair occurring on each DNA strand ($\alpha\alpha/\alpha\alpha$). The most common forms of α-thalassemia result from deletion of one or more of these genes. Excess production of β and γ chains results in the formation of unstable and nonfunctional γ_4 (hemoglobin Bart's) and β_4 (hemoglobin H) tetramers.[34] Four α-thalassemia syndromes have been identified (Table 32.6).

TABLE 32.6	Comparison of α-Thalassemia Syndromes			
Syndrome	**Genotypes**	**Hb**[a]	**RBC Morphology**	**Clinical Manifestations**
Silent carrier	-α/$\alpha\alpha$	150 (15)	Normal	None
α-thalassemia trait	-α/-α or -/$\alpha\alpha$	120–130 (12–13)	Microcytic	Mild anemia
Hb H disease	-/-α	60–100 (6–10)	Microcytic; deformed	Chronic hemolysis; splenomegaly
Hydrops fetalis	-/-	-	Nucleated red blood cells	Intrauterine or neonatal death

[a] Typical hemoglobin concentrations in untreated patients are expressed as g/L (g/dL).

The deletion of a single α gene is classified as a "silent carrier state" and is the most common single gene abnormality in the world. Up to 2% Hb Bart's can be isolated in cord blood of these individuals at birth. Hb Bart's disappears within the first year of life. Fortunately, there are virtually no clinical manifestations of the silent carrier state, and laboratory values such as hemoglobin concentration and mean corpuscular volume (MCV) are usually within normal limits.[40,41] These individuals do not require treatment.

The deletion of two α genes is classified as "α-thalassemia trait" or "α-thalassemia minor." The most common genotype for this disorder is a homozygous α gene deletion $(-\alpha/-\alpha)$. Individuals with α-thalassemia trait experience a mild microcytic, hypochromic anemia without hemolysis.[40,41] In Southeast Asians, however, both α gene deletions frequently occur on the same chromosome $(--/\alpha\alpha)$. This genotype is associated with a more pronounced microcytosis [MCV 70–80 fL (70 to 80 μm^3)] and mild hemolysis. In α-thalassemia trait, Hb Bart's (γ_4) makes up 2% to 10% of hemoglobin in cord blood and disappears within the first year of life.[35] Hemoglobin concentrations of adults with α-thalassemia trait are usually normal or only slightly decreased.[40,41] Not surprisingly, this disorder is often identified in patients by chance during routine laboratory blood tests. Because most patients are asymptomatic, treatment is seldom warranted.

Another α-thalassemia syndrome, more common in Asian populations, is Hb H disease. This disorder is associated with the deletion of three of the four α genes $(--/-\alpha)$. As mentioned, Hb H is an unstable tetramer of β globin chains (β_4) that is formed when there is a marked reduction of α globin production, yielding a substantial surplus of β globin chains. This hemoglobin variant constitutes 5% to 30% of total circulating hemoglobin in affected adults. In patients with Hb H disease, Hb Bart's represents 10% to 40% of the hemoglobin pool at birth and is found in trace amounts during adulthood.[35] The unstable β_4 containing Hb H gradually undergoes oxidation and precipitates within the cell. These deformed cells are removed and hemolyzed primarily by the spleen.

Clinical manifestations associated with Hb H disease include microcytosis, mild to moderate chronic hemolytic anemia, mild jaundice, and splenomegaly.[41] Enlargement of the spleen results from both the trapping of deformed red cells and from extramedullary erythropoiesis in that organ. In most patients, Hb H disease is not severe enough to impair routine activities, interfere with reproductive function, or reduce longevity.[41] However, circumstances such as infection, pregnancy, or exposure to oxidant drugs can precipitate severe exacerbations of the hemolytic anemia. Treatment usually involves supplementation with daily folic acid, monitoring of spleen size, and monitoring of hemoglobin levels.[33] Patients should also be advised to avoid drugs or substances associated with increased oxidative stress to RBCs and, therefore, increased risk of hemolysis (see "Hemolytic Anemia").

In certain patients with Hb H disease, especially those with severe splenomegaly, splenectomy is often beneficial in reducing symptoms and slowing the rate of hemolysis. In rare instances, patients with severe forms of Hb H disease are dependent on blood transfusions.[41]

Deletion of all four α genes is classified as "Hb Bart's hydrops fetalis" and is incompatible with life.[34,41] An affected fetus will either be prematurely stillborn in the second or third trimester or will die within hours after birth. Hemoglobin in an affected fetus will be >80% Hb Bart's. Physical findings include massive edema (hydrops), ascites, and hepatomegaly; peripheral blood examination reveals immature nucleated erythrocytes (erythroblasts), target cells, reticulocytosis, and hypochromia.

Diagnosis of severe forms of α-thalassemia can be done by demonstrating the presence of Hb Bart's or Hb H. After treatment with an oxidant dye such as brilliant cresyl blue, microscopic evaluation of erythrocytes of affected patients will reveal precipitated globin aggregates ("inclusions").[40] Diagnosis of milder forms may be done through DNA electrophoretic analysis.[40,41] Since most α-thalassemia syndromes are associated with a relatively benign clinical course, prenatal diagnosis is usually not critical. An exception to this would be situations where couples are at risk of a hydrops pregnancy (e.g., Southeast Asians, Chinese, or a prior hydrops fetalis pregnancy). Prenatal diagnosis of the fetus involves gene mapping of DNA acquired by chorionic villus sampling (first trimester) or by amniocentesis (second trimester).[41] A diagnosis of Hb Bart's hydrops fetalis allows the option of early termination of the pregnancy, which may protect the health of the mother by avoiding such problems as toxemia and peripartum hemorrhage.[34]

β-THALASSEMIA

In contrast to α-thalassemia, where gene deletion is the mechanism, β-thalassemia syndromes usually result from faulty mRNA transcription of the β gene.[35] Excess α chains accumulate and cause membrane damage in RBC precursors. This process leads to the premature destruction of the cells in the bone marrow or peripheral blood.[34,40] Since α and δ chain production is usually unaffected, increased levels of Hb A_2 $(\alpha_2\delta_2)$ are common to most of the β-thalassemias. More than 200 different genetic mutations associated with β-thalassemia have been described.[33] However, patients can be classified as either heterozygous or homozygous for the β gene. Further distinction is then made based on clinical manifestations and severity (i.e., phenotype) of the syndrome (Table 32.7).

Heterozygous β-thalassemia is much less severe than homozygous forms of the disease. Patients either have a clinically undetectable disorder ("β-thalassemia minima") or one that results in only mild anemia ("β-thalassemia minor" or "β-thalassemia trait"). In general, patients with β-thalassemia minima are asymptomatic, have laboratory

TABLE 32.7	Comparison of β-Thalassemia Syndromes			
Syndrome	**Hb**[a]	**Clinical Manifestations**	**Conventional Treatment**	
Heterozygous				
Minima	Normal	None	None	
Minor (trait)	>100 (>10)	Mild anemia	Genetic/medical counseling	
Homozygous				
Intermedia	70–100 (7–10)	Moderate–severe anemia; impaired growth and splenomegaly in severe cases	Intermittent blood transfusion and chelation therapy	
Major	20–70 (2–7)	Severe anemia; abnormal skeletal growth; splenomegaly; iron overload complications	Chronic blood transfusion and chelation therapy	

[a] Typical hemoglobin concentrations in untreated patients expressed as g/L (g/dL).

blood values (i.e., hemoglobin concentration and MCV) within normal limits, and require no treatment. Definitive diagnosis can be made by measuring the relative synthetic rates of β and α chains.[35,40]

Patients with β-thalassemia minor usually have a mild hypochromic, microcytic anemia. Hemoglobin concentration in these individuals is generally greater than or equal to 100 g/L (10 g/dL). Microcytosis is more pronounced, with MCV values of approximately 60 fL (60 μm^3). Clinical manifestations such as splenomegaly and hyperplastic marrow are usually absent. Nutritional deficiencies, infection, and pregnancy may exacerbate anemia in patients with β-thalassemia minor. However, since these individuals are predisposed to iron overload due to enhanced absorption of dietary iron, long-term iron supplementation and routine blood transfusions during pregnancy should be avoided, if possible. Medical care for these individuals should also involve genetic counseling.[35] Screening patients for β-thalassemia minor is often done through quantification of Hb A$_2$. Ranges of Hb A$_2$ levels are 2% to 3% in normal patients and 3.5% to 8% in those with β-thalassemia minor.[35]

Homozygous forms of β-thalassemia can be classified as either ''β-thalassemia intermedia'' or ''β-thalassemia major.'' The intermedia form is associated with moderate anemia and may require intermittent treatment with blood transfusions. Hemoglobin concentrations in patients with β-thalassemia intermedia usually range from 70 to 100 g/L (7 to 10 g/dL). In contrast, β-thalassemia major (Cooley's anemia) is associated with severe anemia and requires intensive chronic treatment. Hemoglobin concentration and MCV in these patients usually range from 20 to 70 g/L (2 to 7 g/dL) and 50 to 60 fL (50 to 60 μm^3), respectively.[35,42]

CLINICAL PRESENTATION OF β-THALASSEMIA MAJOR

Excessive erythropoiesis (secondary to severe anemia) in the bone marrow and extramedullary sites is a primary compli-

cation of untreated patients with β-thalassemia major. Bone marrow hypertrophy with subsequent abnormal skeletal growth usually develops in children from the second year of life through 10 years of age. Skeletal manifestations before age 6 to 24 months are less common due to the presence of Hb F through early infancy.[43] Abnormal skeletal changes are most apparent in the craniofacial bones due to maxillary overgrowth, protrusion of teeth, and separation of orbits. Cortical thinning of weight-bearing bones may lead to recurrent fractures in these patients. Fortunately, skeletal abnormalities are almost completely prevented if adequate blood transfusion therapy is initiated early in life. Excessive extramedullary erythropoiesis leads to significant lymphadenopathy and hepatosplenomegaly.[37]

RBC damage and the subsequent chronic hemolysis that occur in β-thalassemia major are due to precipitated intracellular aggregates of excess α chains. Removal of these deformed RBCs by the spleen contributes to splenomegaly; if uncorrected by splenectomy, this can significantly increase blood transfusion requirements of patients. Chronic hemolysis is also associated with gallstone formation, which is present in 70% of children with thalassemia >15 years of age.[37,42]

TREATMENT

Conventional treatment for most patients with β-thalassemia major continues to be supportive therapy with chronic blood transfusion and iron chelation regimens. The main goal of this approach is to avoid or reduce major complications of the disease. Experience with BMT in patients with thalassemia has progressed substantially, and this approach offers a curative treatment for a few patients. Research in gene therapy is ongoing and may eventually provide a more widely available cure of clinically significant thalassemias.

Transfusion and Chelation. The primary approach to treatment for patients with β-thalassemia major is chronic blood transfusions in conjunction with intensive iron chelation therapy. The goals of transfusion and chelation therapy are to suppress excessive erythropoiesis, prevent anemia, and minimize or prevent the accumulation of toxic amounts of excess iron.

An appropriate transfusion regimen is critical in accomplishing these goals.[44] Current approaches focus on transfusion protocols designed to achieve pretransfusion hemoglobin concentrations of 95 to 105 g/L (9.5 to 10.5 g/dL) and posttransfusion hemoglobin concentrations of 130 to 135 g/L (13.0 to 13.5 g/dL). These have been shown to result in a reduced transfusion requirement and optimal control of total body iron accumulation compared to more aggressive ("supertransfusion") regimens designed to maintain higher pretransfusion hemoglobin concentrations.[33,44] Variations in transfusion protocols exist between institutions and different types of patients will have different requirements. However, typical transfusion programs involve transfusing patients every 3 to 4 weeks on an outpatient basis. Longer intervals between transfusions (i.e., every 5 to 6 weeks) have been shown to increase iron accumulation and therefore should be avoided. Packed red blood cells (PRBCs), rather than whole blood, are used for all thalassemia transfusion protocols. The adequacy of a given transfusion regimen is best evaluated by monitoring a patient's growth rate and serum hemoglobin concentrations.[33,37,42,45,46]

Important complications associated with chronic blood transfusions include sensitization reactions, transmission of viral infection, and iron overload. Febrile and urticarial reactions to PRBCs caused by sensitization to leukocyte surface antigens may occur. However, the incidence of these reactions has been greatly reduced through improved typing and matching techniques and the use of leukocyte-depleted RBC products.[37,42,46] A more hazardous problem of chronic blood transfusions is the transmission of viral infections. Careful screening of donors and donated blood products has reduced the risk of human immunodeficiency virus (HIV) transmission to less than 1 per 150,000 units transfused. Hepatitis B may be prevented through proper vaccination of uninfected patients with thalassemia who are starting or being maintained on chronic transfusion programs. Hepatitis C transmission remains a relatively common threat to transfused patients, with an incidence of about 5%.[37,42] The screening for donors infected with hepatitis C has reduced the risk of transmission of this disease. Patients who become infected with hepatitis C are at risk for liver failure and hepatocellular carcinoma.[44] The use of alpha interferon is a treatment option for patients with hepatitis C. In patients with thalassemia infected with the virus, the effectiveness of antiviral therapy is improved in patients with lower total body iron accumulations. Therefore, optimal iron chelation takes on increased importance in this population.[44]

The primary cause of morbidity and mortality in patients with β-thalassemia major who receive adequate transfusion therapy is iron overload associated with the intensive administration of blood products. Each unit of PRBCs (450 mL) contains 200 to 250 mg of elemental iron. By 12 years of age, a properly transfused patient with thalassemia has likely received over 50 g of iron. The normal iron content of the body is 2 g, and there is no natural mechanism by which excess amounts may be excreted. Iron overload and subsequent toxicity occur when the capacity of the storage proteins (ferritin and hemosiderin) and the transport protein (transferrin) is exceeded. The molecular mechanism of toxicity is thought to be due to excess unbound iron that accumulates both intracellularly and in the circulation acting as a catalyst in Haber-Weiss and Fenton reactions. This produces reactive oxygen radicals that subsequently oxidize membrane lipids and damage cellular components.[37,42,46]

The clinical effects of iron overload are most pronounced on normal growth, the liver, endocrine function, and the heart. The impairment of normal growth in children with β-thalassemia major is most likely multifactorial and may involve hypogonadism, impaired growth hormone system, hyposecretion of adrenal androgen, and impaired cartilage growth.[44] With respect to effects on the liver, hepatic fibrosis often develops in transfused children with thalassemia during the first decade of life, and older patients often have histologic evidence of cirrhosis. Hepatic iron accumulation may occur after only 2 years of transfusion therapy and can lead to the rapid development of portal fibrosis. Mild prolongations of clotting time are often observed. Liver disease remains a relatively common cause of death in patients with β-thalassemia major.[44] Diabetes mellitus secondary to the effects of hemochromatosis on the pancreas may occur and can be managed by standard insulin replacement therapy. The manifestations of iron overload on the heart include pericarditis, atrial and ventricular arrhythmias, and congestive heart failure. Cardiomegaly secondary to hypoxia is usually not significant in adequately transfused patients. In underchelated patients, cardiac dysfunction is the primary cause of death.[37,42,44] For all of these reasons, chronic iron chelation therapy must accompany standard blood transfusion regimens.

Deferoxamine, a trihydroxamic acid produced by *Streptomyces pilosus*, remains the primary option for chelating and removing excess iron.[33,44] Following parenteral administration, deferoxamine penetrates cell membranes and combines with free intracellular iron to form the complex ferrioxamine. Liver parenchymal cells serve as a large source of chelatable iron. Ferrioxamine is then transported extracellularly and is readily excreted in the urine and the bile. The general goal of treatment with deferoxamine is to control total body iron and, if possible, create a "negative iron balance" where the amount of iron removed exceeds the amount of iron administered during transfusions.[37,42,44,46] Adequate chelation therapy with deferoxamine in patients with thalassemia major has been shown to decrease the risks of iron overload, such as diabetes and cardiac disease, and improve survival.[45,47]

One component of iron chelation therapy that plays an important role in making initiation and dose-adjustment decisions is the assessment of total body iron. No single, preferred method for this assessment exists.[33] Measurement of hepatic iron concentration may be the most quantitative indicator of total body iron.[44] Several methods to accomplish this have been described. The indirect assessment of body iron burden has been performed by measuring serum ferritin, 24-hour deferoxamine-induced urinary iron excretion, computed tomography (CT) imaging, and magnetic resonance imaging (MRI). Of these methods, the measurement of serum ferritin is the most commonly used technique to assess body iron. However, because serum ferritin is an acute phase reactant, its concentrations may fluctuate independently of total body iron due to conditions such as fever, acute infection, chronic inflammation, and hepatic damage. Because of this, the use of serum ferritin alone may provide an inaccurate assessment of body iron in certain patients.[33,44] Measurement of urinary iron excretion induced by deferoxamine is of limited value due to the poor correlation between urinary iron concentration and hepatic iron concentration. The amount of iron excreted in the urine is dependent on several factors, including the degree of body iron load, the dose of deferoxamine, and the rate of erythropoiesis. The use of magnetic resonance imaging (MRI) may play a role in detecting the presence of iron within cardiac tissue. However, this approach is limited in terms of making quantitative estimates of iron load.

The direct assessment of total body iron may be performed through liver biopsy and the subsequent measurement of hepatic tissue iron concentration. This method, though invasive, is the most sensitive and specific approach for determining total body iron in patients with thalassemia.[44]

In clinical practice, the initiation of chelation therapy is often based on the serial measurement of serum ferritin concentrations during regular blood transfusions. Alternatively, liver biopsy to determine hepatic iron concentrations may provide a more accurate indicator for the initiation of deferoxamine. In general, chelation therapy is started after approximately 1 year of regular blood transfusions.[44] Chelation therapy is usually initiated in transfusion-dependent patients by 3 to 4 years of age. Due to poor oral absorption, deferoxamine must be given parenterally. The subcutaneous route is generally considered to achieve the best balance between safety and efficacy for promoting iron removal in patients with thalassemia. Because of its short half-life (5 to 10 minutes), deferoxamine is usually administered by continuous infusion to maximize exposure time between the drug and excess iron. Typical deferoxamine dosing regimens are 30 to 50 mg/kg/day infused subcutaneously over 8 to 12 hours, 5 or 6 days a week. In children <5 years of age, lower dosages (25 mg/kg/day 3 to 5 days a week) have been used to avoid potential growth disturbances.[33] Treatment is usually administered with a portable infusion pump, infusing the drug at night while the patient is sleeping. One approach toward the management of deferoxamine iron chelation therapy is summarized in Table 32.8. The clinical benefits of regular transfusion and chelation therapy initiated at an early age include a reduced risk of complications from iron-induced organ damage (e.g., cardiac disease and impaired glucose tolerance) and a reduced risk of early death.[45,47]

Intravenous deferoxamine dosing regimens (50 to 80 mg/kg/day) have also been shown to be safe and efficacious.[48] Continuous IV ambulatory deferoxamine therapy may be appropriate for patients with greatly elevated hepatic iron concentrations who are at increased risk for complications and early death from iron overload. Because rapid IV infu-

| TABLE 32.8 | **Example Guidelines for Iron Chelation Management With Deferoxamine (DFO)** |

Time Course	Assessment Interval	HIC[a] (mg/g)	DFO Regimen
Baseline[b]	Yearly	<3.2	No DFO; recheck in 6 months
		≥3.2	25 mg/kg/night × 5 nights/week
Before age 5	Yearly	<3.2	Stop DFO; recheck in 6 months
		3.2–6.9	25 mg/kg/night × 5 nights/week
		≥7	35 mg/kg/night × 6 or 7 nights/week
Age 5–10	Every 18 months	<3.2	Stop DFO; recheck in 6 months
		3.2–6.9	40 mg/kg/night × 5 nights/week
		7–14.9	40 mg/kg/night × 6 or 7 nights/week
		≥15	40–50 mg/kg/night × 7 nights/week
After age 10	Every 18 months	<3.2	Stop DFO; recheck in 6 months
		3.2–6.9	40 mg/kg/night × 5 nights/week
		7–14.9	40 mg/kg/night × 6 or 7 nights/week
		≥15	50 mg/kg/night × 7 nights/week

[a] Hepatic iron concentration from liver biopsy expressed as mg iron per gram of dry weight of liver biopsy
[b] After 1 year of regular transfusions
(From Fosburg MT, Nathan DG. Treatment of Cooley's anemia. Blood 76:435–444, 1990.)

sion may cause hypotension, the rate of administration should not exceed 15 mg/kg/hr.[46,49]

Monitoring total body iron burden and chelation therapy efficacy should include the measurement of hepatic iron concentrations, serum ferritin concentrations [normal: 18 to 300 μg/L (18 to 300 ng/mL)], and possibly urinary iron excretion. Chelation therapy with deferoxamine designed to maintain hepatic iron concentrations of 0.2 to 1.6 mg of iron per gram of liver tissue (dry weight) has been shown to reduce the risk of complications from iron overload. However, this approach has also been associated with an increased risk of adverse drug effects. In contrast, maintaining hepatic iron concentrations of more than 15 mg of iron per gram of liver (dry weight) results in a lower risk of drug toxicity but an increased risk of cardiac disease and early mortality secondary to iron overload.[44] Therefore, some authors have suggested a target reference range of 3.2 to 7 mg of iron per gram of liver (dry weight). Maintaining a serum ferritin value less than 2,500 ng/mL has been correlated with an excellent prognosis for prolonged survival without cardiac disease.[47] As previously discussed, urinary iron excretion is dependent on many factors and may not reliably correlate with the efficacy of iron chelation therapy.[37,46,50]

In most patients, deferoxamine used in typical chelation regimen doses is a relatively safe drug. Common side effects during subcutaneous infusion programs include local irritation and urticaria at the injection site, diarrhea, leg cramps, tachycardia, and abdominal discomfort. Some reports have associated deferoxamine with a variety of adverse visual and auditory effects. The mechanism of this toxicity is not well understood. Patients taking deferoxamine should have regular vision and hearing evaluations. Other serious adverse effects that have been reported with deferoxamine include changes in renal function and pulmonary toxicity.[44] Patients with lower iron burdens and patients receiving high doses of deferoxamine (>50 mg/kg) are likely to be at greater risk for toxicity.[42,44,49]

Because of the inconvenience, high cost, and frequent noncompliance with parenteral deferoxamine therapy, research efforts have focused on the development of a safe, effective, and inexpensive oral medication for iron chelation. One orally active agent that has shown efficacy similar to that of subcutaneous deferoxamine is deferiprone, an α-keto-hydroxypyridone.[51–53] Doses of this agent ranging from 50 to 120 mg/kg/day are associated with iron removal and negative iron balance.[54] The combined use of deferiprone and deferoxamine has been reported to have additive and synergistic effects on iron removal.[33,51,55,56] Adverse effects that have been associated with deferiprone include agranulocytosis, neutropenia, musculoskeletal pain, gastrointestinal complaints, and hepatotoxicity. Due to a relative lack of controlled studies and conflicting results with respect to safety and efficacy, additional evaluation of this agent may be necessary to better understand its role in the management of thalassemia in the United States.[33,57] Deferiprone is currently designated as an orphan drug under the FDA's Office

of Orphan Products Development. Clinical data regarding another oral iron chelating agent, deferasirox, is currently under priority review by the FDA for the treatment of chronic iron overload due to blood transfusions.

Patients with β-thalassemia intermedia are often not dependent on blood transfusions. However, in severe forms of this syndrome, ineffective erythropoiesis and anemia are sometimes significant enough to inhibit growth and development and lead to skeletal fragility and injury. In these cases, patients with β-thalassemia intermedia should be treated with intermittent courses of transfusion and chelation therapy, as described above.[42,44]

Ascorbic Acid. Ascorbic acid (vitamin C) supplementation may enhance iron removal during chelation therapy in some patients with thalassemia by increasing the iron pool with which deferoxamine is available to bind.[33,44] However, some evidence exists that this process may also increase iron-induced formation of cytotoxic oxygen free radicals. One approach recommended is to check tissue ascorbic acid concentrations in patients with diminished response to deferoxamine. Patients with reduced levels may be supplemented with 100 mg of ascorbic acid 30 minutes to 1 hour prior to receiving their deferoxamine.[44]

Splenectomy. Due to increased erythropoietic activity and trapping of red cells by the spleen, patients with β-thalassemia major develop splenomegaly. Proper transfusion therapy may slow the process, but gradual enlargement of the spleen usually occurs. In patients who receive chronic transfusion therapy, enlargement of the spleen is associated with increased transfusion requirements to maintain an adequate hemoglobin concentration. The administration of greater volumes of blood products increases the amount of iron a patient receives and makes successful chelation therapy more difficult. Therefore, when blood transfusion requirements exceed 200 mL/kg/year, splenectomy may be indicated. Following spleen removal, transfusion requirements will decrease substantially. However, the benefits and risks of splenectomy should be carefully considered.[33] Since splenectomized patients, especially young children, are predisposed to certain bacterial infections, removal of the spleen should be avoided until the age of 4 or 5 years. Furthermore, all splenectomized patients should be vaccinated against pneumococcus, meningococcus, and *H. influenzae* at the earliest appropriate age.[37,42,46] Postsplenectomy initiation of oral penicillin for prophylaxis against pneumococcus is recommended.[33]

Bone Marrow Transplantation. BMT from an HLA-identical donor is currently the only cure for thalassemia.[33,58] Since the initial successful case in 1982, considerable experience has been gained with BMT in patients with β-thalassemia major. Survival and disease-free survival rates in a group of 139 patients receiving BMT for thalassemia were 73% and 58%, respectively.[59] A later report of a series of 89 patients ages 1 to 15 years found survival and rejection-free survival rates of 92% and 85%, respectively.[60] Therefore, assuming an HLA-compatible donor exists, BMT offers patients with thalassemia a reasonable chance for cure. The risk of graft failure and mortality associated with BMT varies among different institutions and different patients and must be weighed against the high rate of survival and the good quality of life that is associated with conventional transfusion and chelation therapy for at least the first two decades. Patients with thalassemia who have the highest chances for rejection-free survival after BMT are those who are young, well chelated, and in good clinical condition.[59,60]

FUTURE THERAPIES

Another technique that has shown some success in treating patients with β-thalassemia major is to reduce transfusion requirements by increasing Hb F synthesis.[61–64] Agents currently available that have been investigated as clinical stimulators of Hb F synthesis include hydroxyurea, butyrate, and azacitidine. The adverse effects (i.e., bone marrow suppression and mutagenicity) and unknown long-term efficacy of these agents may limit their widespread use in the treatment of thalassemia. However, this approach may be a cost-effective and viable alternative when safe transfusion and chelation therapy is not available.[33]

Gene therapy is another treatment approach that holds great potential for providing a definitive cure of patients with severe forms of thalassemia.[65] Current limitations in the use of this therapy for the treatment of thalassemia include inefficient gene expression and regulation.

PREVENTION

Prevention is another effective approach in dealing with β-thalassemia major. Multifaceted programs involving education, genetic counseling, and prenatal diagnosis have led to a significant reduction in the incidence of this disease in certain areas.[33,34] In Sardinia, for example, implementation of such a program was associated with a 95% reduction in the incidence of thalassemia major over a 16-year period.[66] Inexpensive and simple DNA analysis techniques can provide a safe and accurate diagnosis at 8 to 14 weeks' gestation.[42]

PROGNOSIS

Prior to the implementation of adequate transfusion and chelation programs, children with β-thalassemia major suffered from skeletal deformities, growth and development retardation, progressive enlargement of the liver and spleen, congestive heart failure, and recurrent infections. More than 80% of these patients died within the first 5 years of life. The introduction and widespread use of regular transfusion programs, along with effective chelation therapy, has led to a significant improvement in the quality and duration of life for patients with thalassemia who have such therapy available. BMT provides a chance for a cure in a few patients.

HEMOLYTIC ANEMIA

Hemolytic anemias are due to an increased rate of RBC destruction. The anemia is of greatest clinical concern when the rate of RBC destruction exceeds that of erythropoiesis. The hemolytic process may occur chronically or manifest as an acute episode, depending on the etiologic mechanism. Acute hemolysis is generally a more clinically threatening event. Many anemias have a hemolytic component due to the production of defective or damaged RBCs (e.g., megaloblastic anemias, thalassemias, sickle cell anemia).[67,68] As there are a multitude of causes of hemolytic anemia, this section will focus on those amenable to specific medical treatment and those that are drug-induced.

ETIOLOGY AND CLASSIFICATION

Hemolytic anemias can be categorized as either inherited or acquired disorders. Inherited hemolytic anemias include defective globin synthesis, erythrocyte membrane defects, and erythrocyte enzyme deficiencies. Acquired hemolytic disorders are those caused by some extrinsic event and do not involve a genetic component. Typically, the acquired hemolytic anemias are either immune-mediated, due to physical stress on the RBC, or are induced by certain infections (Table 32.9).

EPIDEMIOLOGY

The prevalence and distribution of sickle cell anemia and thalassemia have been discussed previously. With respect to other inherited hemolytic disorders, the incidence of hereditary spherocytosis and hereditary elliptocytosis in the United States is approximately 220 and 400 per million, respectively. Glucose-6-phosphate dehydrogenase (G6PD) deficiency is the most common inherited erythrocyte enzyme

| TABLE 32.9 | Classification of Common Hemolytic Anemias |

I. Inherited

  Globin synthesis defect

    Sickle cell anemia

    Thalassemia

    Unstable hemoglobin disease

  Erythrocyte membrane defect

    Hereditary spherocytosis

    Hereditary elliptocytosis

    Hereditary stomatocytosis

  Erythrocyte enzyme defect

    Hexose-monophosphate shunt defect (e.g., glucose-6-phosphate dehydrogenase)

    Glycolytic (Embden-Meyerhof) enzyme defect (e.g., pyruvate kinase)

    Other enzyme defect (e.g., adenylate kinase)

II. Acquired

  Immune-mediated

    Warm reacting antibody (IgG)

      Primary (Idiopathic)

      Secondary (e.g., collagen vascular disease, lymphoproliferative disorders)

    Drug-induced

    Cold agglutinin disease (IgM)

      Acute (e.g., *Mycoplasma* pneumonia, infectious mononucleosis)

      Chronic (e.g., lymphoid neoplasms, idiopathic)

    Paroxysmal nocturnal hemoglobinuria

    Transfusion reactions

    Hemolytic disease of newborns

  Microangiopathic and traumatic

    Disseminated intravascular coagulation

    Hemolytic-uremic syndrome

    Thrombotic thrombocytopenic purpura

    Prosthetic or diseased heart valves

  Infection

  Exogenous substances

  Other

    Liver disease

    Hypophosphatemia

disorder worldwide, affecting close to 200 million people, but not all patients with G6PD deficiency are significantly predisposed to oxidative hemolysis.[35,67,69]

The majority of acquired hemolytic anemias are idiopathic. Many are due to immune reactions, collagen vascular disease, or malignancy. Drugs are the causative agents in 10% of cases.

PATHOPHYSIOLOGY

The average RBC life span is 120 days, but during severe hemolytic episodes this can be reduced to as low as 5 to 20 days. RBCs are hemolyzed either within the circulation (intravascular hemolysis) or taken up by the RES and destroyed (extravascular hemolysis). Intravascular hemolysis may be caused by trauma to the RBC, complement fixation to the RBC (immune-mediated), or exposure to exogenous substances. Under normal circumstances, however, most RBC catabolism occurs extravascularly by the RES in the liver and spleen. Specific drug-induced mechanisms of RBC hemolysis are discussed later in the context of G6PD deficiency and immune-mediated hemolysis.

Following lysis of the RBC, hemoglobin is released into the blood, where it is bound by the plasma protein haptoglobin. Free heme molecules are bound by the plasma protein hemopexin. The hemoglobin–haptoglobin complex is rapidly cleared from the circulation by the RES, and the heme component is metabolized to unconjugated (indirect) bilirubin. In the liver, this is linked with glucuronic acid, forming conjugated (direct) bilirubin, which passes from the bile duct into the intestine. Fecal bacteria then metabolize conjugated bilirubin to urobilinogen, which is primarily excreted in the feces. Iron from heme catabolism is stored as ferritin or hemosiderin.[68,70]

During hemolysis, if the haptoglobin binding capacity is exceeded, unbound hemoglobin levels increase, resulting in hemoglobinemia. In this case, free hemoglobin is filtered through the glomerulus and is usually reabsorbed by the proximal tubules. In severe intravascular hemolysis, the reabsorptive capacity is exceeded, causing hemoglobinuria. Also during severe intravascular hemolysis, some heme molecules in the circulation are transferred from hemopexin to albumin, forming methemalbumin. When the liver's conjugating capacity is exceeded during moderate or severe hemolysis, unconjugated (indirect) bilirubin serum levels increase.[67,68]

CLINICAL PRESENTATION AND DIAGNOSIS

The primary diagnostic features of hemolytic anemia are a marked reticulocytosis and jaundice (including scleral icterus) due to hyperbilirubinemia. A corrected reticulocyte count >0.025 (2.5%) is a typical response to hemolysis. The severity of the anemia may also be judged by the extent to which the hematocrit is decreased. The enzyme lactate dehydrogenase (LDH) is released from the RBC during hemolysis, and plasma levels may be elevated. RBC membranes may sustain incomplete damage, resulting in the formation of spherocytic-shaped erythrocytes. These cells have an increased susceptibility to splenic removal.[70] Splenomegaly is usually present in cases of chronic hemolysis. A sum-

TABLE 32.10	Common Diagnostic Features of Hemolytic Anemia	
	Moderate Hemolysis	**Severe Hemolysis**
Physical findings		
Jaundice	+	+
Hemoglobinuria	0	+
Laboratory indices plasma/serum:		
Reticulocytosis	+	++
Plasma hemoglobin	+	++
Red cell hemoglobin	Decreased	Decreased
Hematocrit	Decreased	Decreased
Bilirubin (unconjugated)	+	++
Haptoglobin	Decreased	Decreased or absent
Hemopexin	Normal or decreased	Decreased or absent
Methemalbumin	0	+
Lactate dehydrogenase	+ (variable)	++ (variable)
Laboratory indices: urine		
Hemoglobin	0	+
Hemosiderin	0	+

mary of important findings in hemolytic anemia is presented in Table 32.10.

With respect to immune-mediated hemolysis, diagnostic evaluation includes the direct antiglobulin test (DAT or Coombs' test), which detects the presence of IgG or C3 (complement) on the surface of RBCs.[67] Patients may have positive DAT results without hemolysis (up to 15% of hospitalized patients). Therefore, this must be correlated with other clinical evidence of a hemolytic process. The indirect antiglobulin test (IAT or indirect Coombs' test) detects the presence of antibodies against RBCs in the serum rather than on the surface of the RBC itself. This test is most commonly used in blood banks for antibody screening and cross-matching blood for transfusion.[70] During oxidative hemolytic anemias, denatured hemoglobin precipitates within the RBC, forming Heinz bodies, which are visible during microscopic examination. Heinz bodies are rapidly removed by the spleen, creating "bite" cells, which are erythrocytes that appear to have a bite of cytoplasm removed.[69]

INHERITED HEMOLYTIC ANEMIAS: G6PD DEFICIENCY

Hereditary spherocytosis, elliptocytosis, and stomatocytosis are all genetic disorders inherited in an autosomal dominant fashion and are associated with altered RBC morphology. Hemolysis and clinical sequelae tend to be more pronounced with hereditary spherocytosis than with the other two. Sple-

nectomy usually corrects anemia in these individuals. Supplemental folic acid therapy (1 mg daily) is also recommended.[68] Sickle cell anemia and thalassemia may also be considered inherited hemolytic anemias.

The most prevalent inherited RBC enzyme defect is G6PD deficiency, a sex-linked (X-chromosome) disorder. Affected females are predominantly heterozygous and have both normal and G6PD-deficient RBCs. They are fairly resistant to RBC hemolysis. Men and homozygous women, however, have predominantly G6PD-deficient RBCs and are predisposed to more severe hemolytic episodes. Cultural distribution of this disorder is similar to that of thalassemia, occurring frequently in blacks and people of Mediterranean cultures. The "A−" variant of G6PD is found primarily in blacks. Enzyme activity in these individuals is 8% to 20% of normal. In the United States, approximately 13% of black males and 3% of black females are affected. The Mediterranean-type variant of G6PD has 0% to 4% of normal enzyme activity. Consequently, these individuals are generally at greater risk of developing hemolytic anemia, and the associated clinical manifestations are more pronounced.[69]

HEMOLYTIC MECHANISM

The G6PD enzyme, in conjunction with glutathione and nicotinamide adenine dinucleotide phosphate (NADPH), serves as a protective antioxidant for RBCs against external oxidative stresses (Fig. 32.3). In the presence of G6PD deficiency, oxidative stresses on the RBC such as drugs, infection, or acidosis can lead to denaturation of the globin chains. Dena-

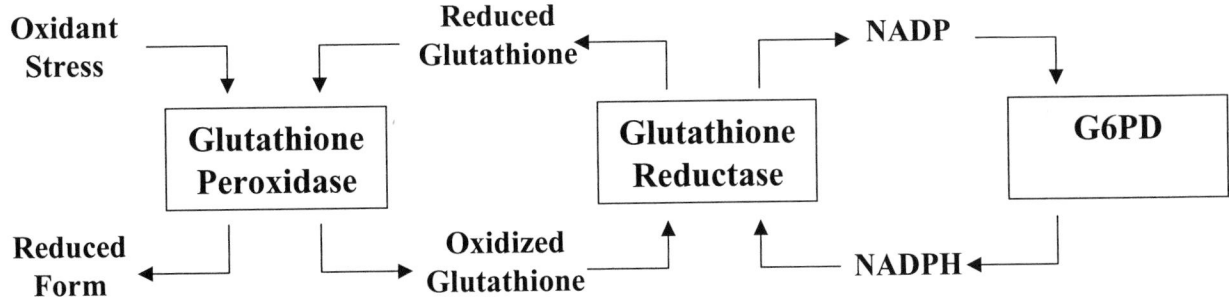

FIGURE 32.3 Antioxidant mechanism of G6PD. NADP, nicotinamide adenine dinucleotide phosphate.

tured globin precipitates intracellularly onto the cell membrane as Heinz bodies, and premature hemolysis occurs.[67,69,71] This type of disorder is frequently referred to as oxidative hemolysis.

Many drugs and substances have been associated with hemolytic anemia in G6PD-deficient individuals. However, the list of agents for which there is strong evidence of an association is relatively small (Table 32.11).[69,71] A patient's susceptibility to oxidative stress of a particular drug varies according to several factors. The type of G6PD genetic variant present (i.e., type A- or Mediterranean-type) is a major determinant. Other factors include patient age, other sources of oxidant stress, dose of an offending drug, patient metabolism of an offending drug, and patient elimination of an offending drug. During hemolytic episodes in susceptible patients, signs and symptoms usually develop within 2 to 3 days of drug initiation. The hemolysis is primarily intravascular and generally results in pronounced hemoglobinuria.

TREATMENT

Withdrawal or avoidance of any potentially oxidant drugs or other substances is the most important component of treatment. In patients with A- variant G6PD deficiency, hemolysis is usually mild and self-limited and therapy is seldom required. In patients with Mediterranean-type deficiency experiencing severe hemolysis, blood transfusions are occa-

TABLE 32.11	Drugs and Substances Associated with Hemolytic Anemia in Glucose-6-Phosphate Dehydrogenase (G6PD) Deficiency
Primaquine	Sulfapyridine
Nalidixic acid	Phenazopyridine
Ciprofloxacin	Dapsone
Nitrofurantoin	Methylene blue
Sulfacetamide	Naphthalene (mothballs)
Sulfamethoxazole	Fava beans

sionally warranted in symptomatic patients. Folic acid supplementation should be given for 2 to 3 weeks following an acute hemolytic episode and may be necessary for extended periods in patients with chronic hemolysis. In patients who develop severe hemolytic anemia with hemoglobinuria, IV hydration to maintain adequate urine output may be necessary to prevent acute renal failure.[69,71]

The primary approach when caring for patients who have documented G6PD deficiency or those who may be at risk (e.g., family history, ethnic background) is prevention. Several factors should be considered prior to starting a potentially hemolyzing drug in such patients, including patient age, renal function, type of G6PD variant that may be present, availability of alternative drugs, and severity of primary illness. A specific quantitative assay of G6PD is available for screening patients who may be deficient.[71]

ACQUIRED HEMOLYTIC ANEMIAS: AUTOIMMUNE HEMOLYSIS

Acquired hemolytic anemias are made up of a diverse group of disorders (Table 32.9). Microangiopathic hemolytic anemias, including disseminated intravascular coagulation, hemolytic-uremic syndrome, and thrombotic thrombocytopenic purpura, are generally caused by alterations such as fibrin deposition or narrowing of the microvasculature. Therapy for these disorders involves treatment of the underlying disease. Acquired hemolytic anemias secondary to RBC trauma occur in up to 10% of patients with prosthetic or diseased heart valves due to pressure gradient stresses placed on the RBC membrane. Treatment in these patients includes correcting iron deficiency and limiting exertional activity. Valve replacement may be necessary when less invasive measures fail.

Autoimmune hemolytic anemia results from the binding of complement or anti-RBC antibodies to the RBC membrane in affected individuals. These disorders may be classified according to the temperature at which the antibodies have the greatest affinity for and interaction with red cells.

COLD AGGLUTININ HEMOLYTIC ANEMIA

Cold agglutinin disorders involve the binding of IgM antibodies to RBCs at low temperatures (4°C). This agglutination process is quickly reversed during warming. Most cold agglutinins do not appreciably shorten RBC survival. Acute cold agglutinin disease is frequently associated with *Mycoplasma* pneumonia or infectious mononucleosis. Hemolysis typically begins 5 to 10 days after recovery from the infection and is mild and self-limited. Chronic cold agglutinin disease often occurs spontaneously in elderly patients, especially those with lymphoproliferative disorders, and results in poor peripheral circulation. Treatment of cold agglutinin disease involves preventing exposure to cold environments, folic acid supplementation, blood transfusions (if necessary), and treatment of any underlying diseases. Occasionally patients respond to plasmapheresis or cytotoxic agents such as cyclophosphamide or chlorambucil. Splenectomy and corticosteroids are of questionable value.[68,70]

WARM AUTOIMMUNE HEMOLYTIC ANEMIA

Warm reacting antibodies have the greatest affinity for RBCs at room temperature (37°C) and are usually of the IgG or, occasionally, IgA type. The mechanism of hemolysis involves the attachment, and subsequent destruction, of IgG-coated erythrocytes to receptors on macrophages in the RES. This process occurs primarily in the spleen. This type of immunohemolytic anemia may be idiopathic, secondary to an underlying disease that affects the immune system (e.g., chronic lymphocytic leukemia, non-Hodgkin's lymphoma, or systemic lupus erythematosus), or secondary to certain drugs. Many of these patients have a chronic mild anemia and splenomegaly, but the clinical presentation varies widely. This disorder is more common in adults and in women. The presence of IgG autoantibodies is detected by a positive DAT.[68,70]

TREATMENT OF WARM AUTOIMMUNE HEMOLYTIC ANEMIA

Prior to treating patients with immunohemolytic anemia, drugs that have been associated with this condition (discussed later) should be excluded as the cause. Therapy should be guided by the severity of the anemia. Patients with mild hemolysis usually do not require therapy. When hemolysis is clinically significant, corticosteroid therapy is usually effective and blood transfusions may be required. The mechanism of steroid action in immunohemolytic anemia is thought to involve a reduction in the clearance of IgG-coated RBCs from the circulation by interfering with macrophage receptor function or phagocytosis. Typically, prednisone is administered in a dosage of 1 to 2 mg/kg/day and continued until hemoglobin levels have normalized. Hemoglobin concentration usually begins to increase within 3 to 4 days after prednisone is initiated. Once hemoglobin has returned to baseline, prednisone therapy is tapered slowly over a period of several months. Approximately 60% to 70% of patients treated in this manner will have a sustained suppression of hemolysis. However, more than 80% of these patients will relapse as steroids are tapered or after they are withdrawn. IVIG is less effective in treating warm autoimmune hemolytic anemia, producing transient remission in only 40% of patients. Splenectomy is indicated in patients who relapse or fail to respond to corticosteroids and will benefit 50% to 60% of these individuals. In patients who are refractory to steroids and splenectomy (about 10% of cases), alternative therapies include immunosuppressive agents (e.g., cyclophosphamide or azathioprine), danazol, IVIG, and cyclosporine. Corticosteroids may also be reinstituted and maintained indefinitely at the lowest effective dose. Patients who undergo splenectomy should receive vaccination against pneumococcus, meningococcus, and *H. influenzae* approximately 2 weeks prior to surgery. Cross-matching patients with immunohemolytic anemia for blood transfusions is difficult because the antibody that is present will often react with all normal donor cells.[68,70]

DRUG-INDUCED IMMUNOHEMOLYTIC ANEMIAS

Drugs that have been associated with immunohemolytic anemias are listed in Table 32.12. There are three proposed mechanisms by which drugs may initiate this condition.

AUTOIMMUNE (METHYLDOPA TYPE)
Up to 10% of patients receiving methyldopa in daily doses of 2 g develop a positive DAT. This usually occurs after 6 to 12 months of therapy. Only a few of these patients (≤1%) will develop an extravascular hemolysis. The patient's RBCs are coated with IgG but not complement. The mechanism of this condition is not well understood but may involve the inhibition of suppressor T cells. If hemolysis occurs, it gradually subsides over a period of weeks after drug discontinuation, but the DAT may remain positive for more than 1 year.[68,70]

DRUG ADSORPTION (HAPTEN TYPE)
In patients receiving large dosages of penicillins (e.g., 15 to 20 million units/day) or cephalosporins, the drug nonspecifically adsorbs to the RBC membrane, forming a hapten complex. Antibodies are then formed against this complex, resulting in extravascular hemolysis within 7 to 14 days following initiation of the drug. The DAT is positive for IgG

TABLE 32.12	Examples of Drugs Associated with Immunohemolytic Anemia	
Autoimmune (Methyldopa Type)	**Drug Adsorption (Hapten Type)**	**Immune Complex Adsorption (Innocent Bystander Type)**
Methyldopa	Penicillins	Quinidine
Levodopa	Cephalosporins	Quinine
Mefenamic acid	Tetracycline	Phenacetin
Cimetidine		Acetaminophen
Procainamide		

during therapy. Hemolysis subsides quickly after the drug is withdrawn.[68,70]

IMMUNE COMPLEX ADSORPTION (INNOCENT BYSTANDER TYPE)

In this rare type of drug-induced immunohemolytic anemia, the offending agent binds to plasma proteins and induces the production of IgM antibodies. A drug–antibody complex forms and then adheres nonspecifically to the RBC membrane. Complement (C3) is activated and irreversibly fixes to the membrane surface. The drug–antibody complex dissociates from the RBC, and only C3 is detected by a DAT. The hemolytic process usually occurs intravascularly and may be associated with hemoglobinemia, hemoglobinuria, and acute renal failure.[68,70]

A fourth type of process may occur secondary to the administration of high-dose cephalosporins. In this case, the drug binds to the RBC membrane, causing it to be modified, which results in the nonspecific adsorption of serum proteins. This process is not immune-mediated, nor does hemolysis occur.

CONCLUSION

Anemia is a reduction in the concentration of viable erythrocytes or hemoglobin in the circulation, resulting in a reduced oxygen-carrying capacity of blood. There are several basic mechanisms discussed in this chapter by which anemia may occur, including impaired or absent erythropoiesis (e.g., anemia of chronic disease, aplastic anemia, anemia of chronic kidney disease), impaired hemoglobin synthesis (e.g., sickle cell anemia, thalassemia), and premature RBC destruction (e.g., hemolytic anemia). These mechanisms may coexist. Diseases or conditions that are frequently the primary cause of anemia include chronic infection or inflammation, neoplastic diseases, renal disease, exposure to certain pathogens or chemicals, exposure to certain drugs, inherited abnormalities, and autoimmune processes.

Anemia has many potential etiologies and is actually a symptom of an underlying condition. The treatment of patients should focus not only on correcting the anemia and its associated symptoms but also on identifying and correcting underlying causes, when possible.

KEY POINTS

- Anemia is a reduction in the concentration of viable erythrocytes or hemoglobin in the circulation, resulting in a reduced oxygen-carrying capacity of blood.
- There are several basic mechanisms by which anemia may occur, including impaired or absent erythropoiesis (e.g., anemia of chronic disease, aplastic anemia, anemia of chronic kidney disease), impaired hemoglobin synthesis (e.g., sickle cell anemia, thalassemia), and premature RBC destruction (e.g., hemolytic anemia). These mechanisms may coexist.
- Diseases or conditions that are often the primary cause of anemia include chronic infection or inflammation, neoplastic diseases, renal disease, exposure to pathogens or chemicals, exposure to certain drugs, inherited abnormalities, and autoimmune processes.
- Anemia has many potential causes and is actually a symptom of an underlying condition. Treatment should focus not only on correcting the anemia and its associated symptoms but also on identifying and correcting underlying causes, when possible.
- Anemia of chronic disease generally is mild and associated with infectious, inflammatory, and neoplastic disorders.
- Anemia of chronic disease remits with successful management of the underlying condition. Therapy with recombinant erythropoietin may reduce the need for blood transfusions and improve quality of life.
- Although there are many potential pathogenetic mechanisms, the anemia of chronic kidney disease is primarily caused by deficiency of the hormone erythropoietin.
- Definitive management of the anemia of chronic kidney disease consists of supplementation with an erythropoiesis-stimulating agent to increase hemoglobin concentrations to 110 to 120 g/dL while maintaining iron stores.

■ Aplastic anemia is caused by a defect or deficiency of the pluripotential stem cell, resulting in anemia, agranulocytosis, and thrombocytopenia.

■ Management of aplastic anemia includes removal of the causative agent when possible, supportive care with transfusions and antibiotic therapy, and, depending on patient-specific factors, immunosuppressive therapy or BMT.

■ Sickle cell anemia is a genetic disorder whose manifestations are highly variable but may include vaso-occlusive crises, cerebrovascular accidents, aplastic crises, splenic dysfunction and associated infectious complications, and recurrent, debilitating pain.

■ In addition to managing complications, definitive therapy for sickle cell anemia may now include hydroxyurea or BMT. Hydroxyurea is associated with a 40% reduction in mortality.

■ The thalassemias are a group of hereditary disorders of hemoglobin synthesis characterized by impaired production of one or more of the normal polypeptide chains of globin.

■ Chronic hemolysis is a primary complication of the clinically significant α- and β-thalassemia syndromes.

■ Clinical manifestations of untreated β-thalassemia major include bone marrow hypertrophy, skeletal deformities and fragility, growth retardation, lymphadenopathy, and hepatosplenomegaly.

■ Standard therapy of β-thalassemia major includes regular blood transfusions to correct anemia and suppress ineffective erythropoiesis, along with iron chelation therapy to avoid the systemic toxicities of iron overload associated with transfusions.

■ Other potential therapies for treating patients with β-thalassemia major include hemoglobin switching (i.e., stimulation of Hb F production) and BMT.

■ Hemolytic anemias, which may occur as an acute episode or chronic condition and may take place intravascularly or extravascularly, have many different etiologies but generally occur when the rate of RBC destruction is increased and exceeds that of erythropoiesis.

■ Many types of anemias have a hemolytic component (e.g., megaloblastic anemias, thalassemias, sickle cell anemia) due to the production of defective or damaged RBCs.

■ Management of hemolytic anemia should focus on controlling etiologic factors.

SUGGESTED READINGS

Dhaliwal G, Cornett PA, Tierney LM. Hemolytic anemia. Am Family Phys 69:2599–2606, 2004.

Louise L, Singer LT. Thalassemia: current approach to an old disease. Pediatr Clin North Am 49:1165–1191, 2002.

National Institutes of Health National Heart, Lung, and Blood Institute. Management and therapy of sickle cell disease. National Institute of Health publication no. 02-2117, 2002.

National Kidney Foundation. K/DOQI clinical practice guidelines for anemia of chronic kidney disease, 2000. Am J Kidney Dis 37 (Suppl 1):S182–238, 2001.

Shah A. Thalassemia syndromes. Indian J Med Sci 58:445–449, 2004.

Weiss G. Pathogenesis and treatment of anaemia of chronic disease. Blood Rev 16:87–96, 2002.

Young NS. Acquired aplastic anemia. Ann Intern Med 136:534–546, 2002.

REFERENCES

1. Weiss G. Pathogenesis and treatment of anaemia of chronic disease. Blood Rev 16:87–96, 2002.
2. Spivak JL. Iron and the anemia of chronic disease. Oncology 16 (Suppl 10):25–33, 2002.
3. European Best Practice Guidelines II Working Group. Revised European best practice guidelines for the management of anaemia in patients with chronic renal failure. Nephrology Dialysis Transplant 19 (Suppl 2):ii1–47, 2004.
4. U.S. Renal Data System. USRDS 2004. Annual data report: atlas of end-stage renal disease in the United States, National Institutes of Health, National Institute of Diabetes and Digestive and Kidney Disease, Bethesda, MD, 2004.
5. Erslev AJ, Besarab A. Erythropoietin in the pathogenesis and treatment of the anemia of chronic renal failure. Kidney Int 51:622–630, 1997.
6. National Kidney Foundation. K/DOQI clinical practice guidelines for anemia of chronic kidney disease, 2000. Am J Kidney Dis 37 (Suppl 1):S182–238, 2001.
7. Eschbach JW, Abdulhadi MH, Browne JK, et al. Recombinant human erythropoietin in anemic patients with end-stage renal disease. Ann Intern Med 111:992–1000, 1989.
8. Darbepoetin alfa (Aranesp) package insert. Amgen, Inc. Thousand Oaks, CA: December 2004.
9. Maschio G. Erythropoietin and systemic hypertension. Nephrology Dialysis Transplant 10 (Suppl 2):4–79, 1995.
10. Casadevall N, Nataf J, Viron B, et al. Pure red-cell aplasia and anti-erythropoietin antibodies in patients treated with recombinant erythropoietin. N Engl J Med 346:469–475, 2002.
11. Gale RP. Aplastic anemia: biology and treatment. Ann Intern Med 95:477–494, 1981.
12. Young NS. Acquired aplastic anemia. Ann Intern Med 136: 534–546, 2002.
13. Killick SB, Marsh JCW. Aplastic anaemia: management. Blood Rev 14:157–171, 2000.
14. Marsh JCW, Ball SE, Darbyshire P, et al. Guidelines for the diagnosis and management of acquired aplastic anaemia. Br J Haematol 123:782–801, 2003.
15. Weiner RS, Dicke KA. Risk factors for interstitial pneumonitis following allogeneic bone marrow transplantation for severe aplastic anemia: a preliminary report. Transplant Proc 19:2639–2642, 1987.
16. Brodsky R. Acquired severe aplastic anemia in children: is there a standard of care? Pediatr Blood Cancer 43:711–712, 2004.
17. Tisdale JF, Dunn DE, Geller N, et al. High-dose cyclophosphamide in severe aplastic anaemia: a randomized trial. Lancet 356: 1554–1559, 2000.
18. Gluckman E, Rokicka-Milewska R, Hann I, et al. Results and follow-up of a phase III randomised study of recombinant human-granulocyte stimulating factor as support for immunosuppressive therapy in patients with severe aplastic anaemia. Br J Haematol 119: 1075–1082, 2003.
19. National Institutes of Health National Heart, Lung, and Blood Institute. Management and therapy of sickle cell disease. National Institute of Health publication no. 02-2117, 2002.
20. Stuart MJ, Nagel RL. Sickle-cell disease. Lancet 364:1343–1360, 2004.
21. Platt OS, Thorington BD, Brambilla DJ, et al. Pain in sickle cell disease: rates and risk factors. N Engl J Med 325:11–16, 1991.
22. Ballas SK. Sickle cell anaemia. Progress in pathogenesis and treatment. Drugs 62:1143–1172, 2002.

23. Platt OS, Brambilla DJ, Rosse WF, et al. Mortality in sickle cell disease. Life expectancy and risk factors for early death. N Engl J Med 330:1639–1644, 1994.
24. Miller ST, Sleeper LA, Pegelow CH, et al. Prediction of adverse outcomes in children with sickle cell disease. N Engl J Med 342:83–89, 2000.
25. Gaston MH, Verter JI, Woods G, et al. Prophylaxis with oral penicillin in children with sickle cell anemia. N Engl J Med 314:1593–1599, 1986.
26. Falletta JM, Woods GM, Verter JI, et al. Discontinuing penicillin prophylaxis in children with sickle cell anemia. Prophylactic Penicillin Study II. J Pediatr 27:685–690, 1995.
27. National Heart, Lung, and Blood Institute. Clinical alert: results of the Stroke Prevention in Sickle Cell Anemia II (STOP II) Trial. National Institutes of Health, Dec. 5, 2004.
28. Rodgers GP, Dover GJ, Noguchi CT, et al. Hematologic responses of patients with sickle cell disease to treatment with hydroxyurea. N Engl J Med 322:1037–1045, 1990.
29. Charache S, Terrin ML, Moore RD, et al. Effect of hydroxyurea on the frequency of painful crises in sickle cell anemia. N Engl J Med 332:1315–1322, 1995.
30. Steinberg MH, Barton F, Castro O, et al. Effect of hydroxyurea on mortality and morbidity in adult sickle cell anemia. JAMA 289:1645–1651, 2003.
31. Vermylen C, Cornu G, Ferster A, et al. Haematopoietic stem cell transplantation for sickle cell anaemia: the first 50 patients transplanted in Belgium. Bone Marrow Transplant 22:1–6, 1998.
32. Walters MC, Storb R, Patience M, et al. Impact of bone marrow transplantation for symptomatic sickle cell disease: an interim report. Blood 95:1918–1924, 2000.
33. Louise L, Singer LT. Thalassemia: current approach to an old disease. Pediatr Clin North Am 49:1165–1191, 2002.
34. Weatherall DJ. The thalassemias. Br Med J 314:1675–1678, 1997.
35. Jandl JH. Blood: textbook of hematology. Boston: Little, Brown & Co, 1987.
36. Steinberg MH. Thalassemia: molecular pathology and management. Am J Med Sci 296:308–321, 1988.
37. Festa RS. Modern management of thalassemia. Pediatr Ann 14:597–606, 1985.
38. Wonke B. Prospects of β-thalassemia major. Indian Pediatr 24:969–975, 1987.
39. Huisman TH. Frequencies of common β-thalassemia alleles among different populations: variability in clinical severity. Br J Haematol 75:454–457, 1990.
40. Beutler E. Disorders of hemoglobin. In Fauci AS, Braunwald E, Isselbacher KJ, et al, eds. Harrison's principles of internal medicine, 14th ed. New York: McGraw-Hill, 1998:650–652.
41. Liebhaber SA. α-Thalassemia. Hemoglobin 13:685–721, 1989.
42. Fosburg MT, Nathan DG. Treatment of Cooley's anemia. Blood 76:435–444, 1990.
43. Shah A. Thalassemia syndromes. Indian J Med Sci 58:445–449, 2004.
44. Oliveri NF, Brittenham GM. Iron-chelating therapy and the treatment of thalassemia. Blood 89:739–761, 1997.
45. Brittenham GM, Griffith PM, Nienhuis AW, et al. Efficacy of deferoxamine in preventing complications of iron overload in patients with thalassemia major. N Engl J Med 331:567–573, 1994.
46. Lerner N. Medical management of β-thalassemia. Progr Clin Biol Res 309:14–22, 1989.
47. Olivieri NF, Nathan DG, MacMillan JH, et al. Survival in medically treated patients with homozygous β-thalassemia. N Engl J Med 331:574–578, 1994.
48. Olivieri NF, Berriman AM, Tyler BJ, et al. Reduction in tissue iron stores with a new regimen of continuous ambulatory intravenous deferoxamine. Am J Hematol 41:61–63, 1992.
49. Cohen A. Current status of iron chelation therapy with deferoxamine. Semin Hematol 27:86–90, 1990.
50. Pippard MJ. Iron overload and iron chelation therapy in thalassemia and sickle cell haemoglobinopathies. Acta Haematol 78:206–211, 1987.
51. Maggio A, D'Amico G, Morabito A, et al. Deferiprone versus deferoxamine in patients with thalassemia major: a randomized clinical trial. Blood Cells Mol Dis 28:196–208, 2002.
52. Richardson DR. The controversial role of deferiprone in the treatment of thalassemia. J Lab Clin Med 137:324–329, 2001.
53. Olivieri NF, Koren G, Matsui D, et al. Reduction of tissue iron stores and normalization of serrum ferritin during treatment with the oral iron chelator L1 in thalassemia intermedia. Blood 79:2741–2748, 1992.
54. Kontoghiorghes GJ, Neocleous K, Kolnagou A. Benefits and risks of deferiprone in iron overload in thalassemia and other conditions: comparison of epidemiological and therapeutic aspects with deferoxamine. Drug Safety 26:553–584, 2003.
55. Wu KH, Chang JS, Tsai CH, et al. Combined therapy with deferiprone and desferrioxamine successfully regresses severe heart failure in patients with β-thalassemia major. Ann Hematol 83:471–473, 2004.
56. Tsironi M, Deftereos S, Andriopoulos P, et al. Reversal of heart failure in thalassemia major by combined chelation therapy: a case report. Eur J Haematol 74:84–85, 2005.
57. Oliveri NF, Brittenham GM, McLaren CE, et al. Long-term safety and effectiveness of iron-chelation therapy with deferiprone for thalassemia major. N Engl J Med 339:417–423, 1998.
58. Lucarelli G, Andreani M, Angelucci E. The cure of thalassemia by bone marrow transplantation. Blood Rev 16:81–85, 2002.
59. Barrett AJ, Lucarelli G, Gale RP, et al. Bone marrow transplantation for thalassemia: a preliminary report from the International Bone Marrow Transplant Registry. Progr Clin Biol Res 309:173–185, 1989.
60. Lucarelli G, Galimberti M, Polchi P, et al. Marrow transplantation in patients with thalassemia responsive to iron chelation therapy. N Engl J Med 329:840–844, 1993.
61. Stamatoyannopoulos JA, Nienhuis AW. Therapeutic approaches to hemoglobin switching in treatment of hemoglobinopathies. Ann Rev Med 43:497–521, 1992.
62. Lowrey CH, Nienhuis AW. Treatment with azacitidine of patients with end-stage β-thalassemia. N Engl J Med 329:845–848, 1993.
63. Dover GJ. Hemoglobin switching protocols in thalassemia: experience with sodium phenylbutyrate and hydoxyurea. Ann NY Acad Sci 850:80–86, 1998.
64. Loukopoulos D, Voskaridou E, Stamoulakatou A, et al. Hydroxyurea therapy in thalassemia. Ann NY Acad Sci 850:120–128, 1998.
65. Steinberg MH. Prospects of gene therapy for hemoglobinopathies. Am J Med Sci 302:298–303, 1991.
66. Higgs DR. The thalassemia syndromes. Q J Med 86:559–564, 1993.
67. Dhaliwal G, Cornett PA, Tierney LM. Hemolytic anemia. Am Fam Phys 69:2599–2606, 2004.
68. Tabbara IA. Hemolytic anemias: diagnosis and management. Med Clin North Am 76:649–668, 1992.
69. Beutler E. G6PD deficiency. Blood 84:3613–3636, 1994.
70. Winkelstein A, Kiss JE. Immunohematologic disorders. JAMA 278:1982–1992, 1997.
71. Mehta AB. Glucose-6-phosphate dehydrogenase deficiency. Postgrad Med J 70:871–877, 1994.

Coagulation Disorders

33

Joan M. Stachnik and Michael P. Gabay

TREATMENT GOALS

- Identify and correct underlying medical or surgical conditions where possible.
- Discontinue known drug therapies that cause thrombocytopenia.
- Initiate drug therapies that ameliorate or arrest thrombocytopenia.
- Administer coagulation factors and platelets where indicated.
- Offer supportive care for the associated signs and symptoms.

HEMOSTASIS

Hemostasis is the body's ability to maintain blood in its fluid state while it is within the vasculature and minimize blood loss by promoting clotting when the blood is outside of the vasculature. For this to occur there must be coordination of blood vessels, platelets, coagulation factors, natural inhibitors, and the fibrinolytic proteins existing in an overlapping system of checks and balances.[1] Normal hemostasis requires three responses: the vascular response, formation of a platelet plug, and formation of a fibrin clot. At the same time, naturally occurring anticoagulant proteins inhibit the action of clotting factors in an attempt to control thrombosis, fibrinolysis, and inflammation. The fibrinolytic system also dissolves and removes excess fibrin deposits to preserve vascular patency.

THE VASCULATURE

The main role of the vasculature is to prevent bleeding. Normal intact vascular endothelium repels platelets and red blood cells (RBCs) and secretes substances to inhibit clotting. The initial vascular response to trauma is vasoconstriction, which shunts blood away from the damaged area. Traumatic disruption of the vessel endothelial lining triggers formation, binding, and/or activation of various substances. Trauma also exposes substrates that facilitate attachment and formation of the platelet plug, which is the primary hemostatic mechanism. The secondary hemostatic mechanism controls the formation of a fibrin clot via the ordered interaction of a series of tissue and blood components or factors. Primary and secondary hemostasis operates simultaneously. During this time, inhibitor systems also operate to prevent propagation of the clot, and fibrinolysis is activated for eventual removal of the clot.

PLATELET PATHOPHYSIOLOGY

Platelets play a dominant role in the spontaneous prevention of blood loss from damaged blood vessels. Immediately after tissue injury, platelets clump together to form a primary he-

mostatic plug through a series of overlapping phases, which stops blood flow while maintaining vascular integrity. These phases include adhesion, aggregation, secretion, and elaboration of procoagulant activity. This series of steps ultimately results in the formation of a permanent insoluble fibrin clot that is essential for long-term hemostasis.

Platelets are fragments of megakaryocytes, which are large stem cells that are formed in the bone marrow. A normal platelet concentration is 150,000 to 450,000/mm³ of blood, and production appears to be directly proportional to demand. This allows for the repair of minor ruptures that occur routinely in everyday life. The bone marrow contains a limited quantity of ''reserve'' platelets. This reserve can be readily exhausted after a noxious intervention resulting in platelet destruction. Platelet cells mature over a 4- to 5-day period and have a typical life span of approximately 9 to 10 days.[1] After formation and release from the bone marrow, approximately 25% to 35% of platelets are found in the spleen and the remainder in the circulation. Younger platelets are more physiologically active than older ones.[2]

COAGULATION AND FIBRINOLYSIS

The nomenclature and characteristics of the factors involved in the coagulation cascade are summarized in Table 33.1. The Roman numeral designations for clotting factors generally correspond to their order of discovery. Many clotting factors fall into one of two major groups, based on their biochemical properties. Factors XI, XII, prekallikrein, and high-molecular-weight kininogen are known as contact activation factors because they initiate the contact phase of the coagulation pathway. Factors II, VII, IX, and X are vitamin K-dependent coagulation factors synthesized by the liver. Vitamin K is an essential cofactor for hepatic carboxylation of glutamic acid residues. The t-carboxyglutamic acid residues allow the calcium binding that is essential for normal clotting activity. Vitamin K-deficient persons continue to produce factors II, VII, IX, and X, but in inactive forms. Factor III (tissue factor) is found in many tissues; factor IV (calcium) comes from diet and bone. No factor VI exists.

TABLE 33.1	Characteristics of Coagulation				
Factor	Synonyms	Plasma Half-Life (h)	Plasma Concentration (mg/dL)	Coagulation Pathway (E, I, C)	Biochemical Group
Procoagulants					
I	Fibrinogen	100–150	200–400	C	
II	Prothrombin, prethrombin	50–80	10	C	Vitamin K-dependent
III	Tissue factor, tissue thromboplastin	0		E	
IV	Calcium ion		9–10	E, I, C	
V	Proaccelerin, labile factor	24	1	C	
VII	Proconvertin, SPCA, stable factor	6	0.05	E	Vitamin K-dependent
VIII	Antihemophilic factor (AHF)	12	0.01	I	
	Antihemophilic globulin				
	Antihemophilic factor A				
	Platelet cofactor I				
vWF	von Willebrand factor	24	1		
IX	Christmas factor	24	0.3	I	Vitamin K-dependent
	Antihemophilic factor B				
	Plasma thromboplastin component				
	Platelet cofactor II				
X	Stuart-Prower factor	25–60	1	C	Vitamin K-dependent
XI	Plasma thromboplastin antecedent	40–80	0.5	I	Contact factor
	Antihemophilic factor C				
XII	Hageman factor	50–70	3	I	Contact factor
XIII	Fibrin stabilizing factor	150	1–2	C	
Prekallikrein	Fletcher factor	35	5	I	Contact factor
High-molecular-weight kininogen	Contact activation factor	150	6	I	Contact factor
Inhibitors/fibrinolysis					
Antithrombin		24–36	18–30	I	Vitamin K-dependent
Protein C		16	0.4	I, C	Vitamin K-dependent
Protein S		42	2.3	I, C	Vitamin K-dependent
Plasminogen		48	20–40	C	

E, Extrinsic; I, intrinsic; C, common; SPCA, serum prothrombin conversion accelerator.
(From Goodnight SH, Hathaway WE. Disorders of hemostasis & thrombosis, 2nd ed. New York: McGraw-Hill; 2001, and Comp PC. Production of plasma coagulation factors. In: Williams WJ, Beutler E, Erslev AJ, et al., eds. Hematology, 4th ed. New York: McGraw-Hill, 1990:1285–1294.)

Hepatic biosynthesis provides the other factors listed in Table 33.1.[3]

The traditional model of coagulation cascade comprises reaction complexes, each including an enzyme, a substrate, and a reaction accelerator. The numerous steps amplify the activation process, which ensures a rapid response at sites of injury. The product of these reactions is the potent enzyme thrombin, which is formed by the catalytic action of factor Xa (activated factor X) on prothrombin (Fig. 33.1). Historically, there have been two classic independent pathways that lead to the generation of factor Xa and subsequently give rise to the common pathway: the extrinsic and intrinsic pathways. More recently, these two independent pathways have been merged into one in order to account for clinical observations not explained by the traditional coagulation cascade, such as why patients with hemophilia, who lack either factor VIII or IX, continue to bleed when neither of these deficiencies affects the extrinsic pathway.[1] Even though this new model of coagulation has been developed, the fundamental principles behind clot formation remain the same.

After the fibrin clot is formed, fibrinolysis is initiated to remove the clot and restore blood flow. Fibrinolysis is mediated by the enzyme plasmin. Plasmin circulates in the inactive form of plasminogen. Tissue plasminogen activators (t-PAs) that are present in endothelial cells and other tissues activate plasminogen to form plasmin, which in turn cleaves fibrin into fibrin degradation products (FDPs) (Fig. 33.2).

The intact vessel endothelium and natural anticoagulants continuously maintain normal blood flow. Disruption of endothelial integrity or release of tissue factor after injury activates both the platelet and coagulation systems, resulting in an insoluble fibrin clot that limits further bleeding. Fibrinolysis is then activated, which results in vascular patency by breaking down the fibrin clot. Abnormalities in these systems may occur at virtually any step and may result in bleeding or coagulation disorders.

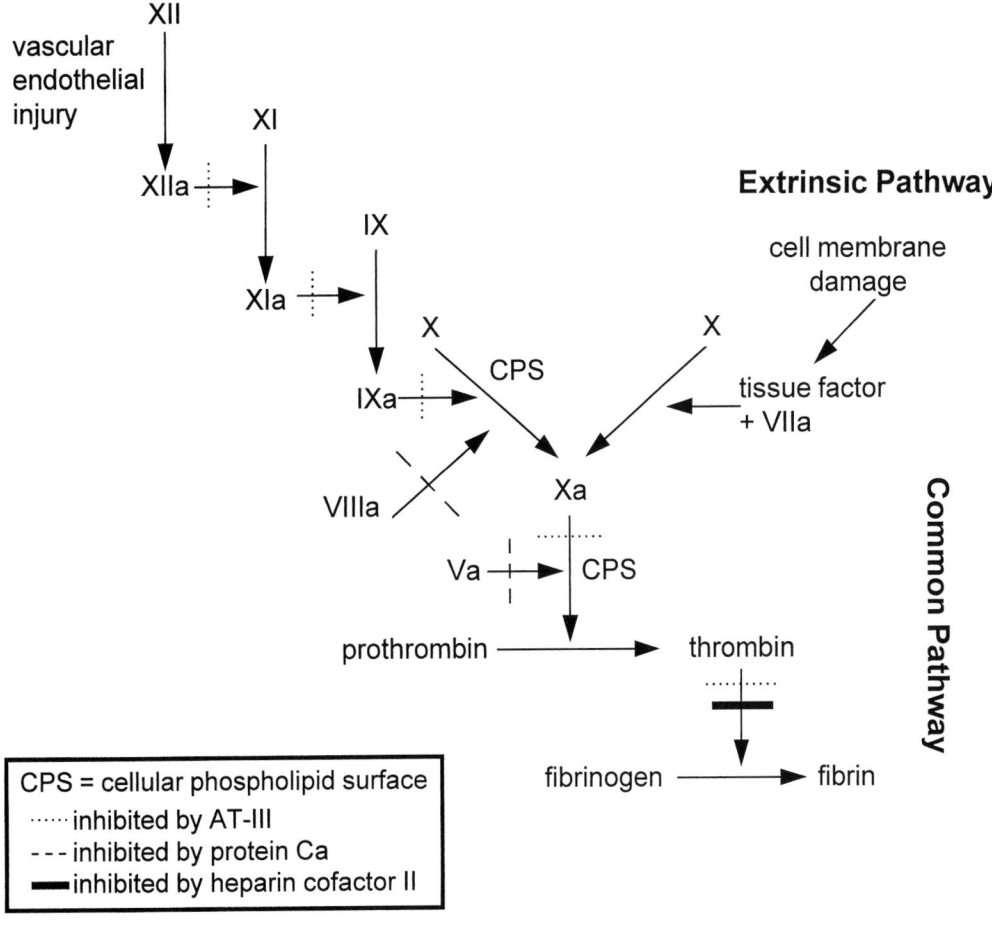

FIGURE 33.1 Components and inhibitors of the intrinsic, extrinsic, and common coagulation pathways.

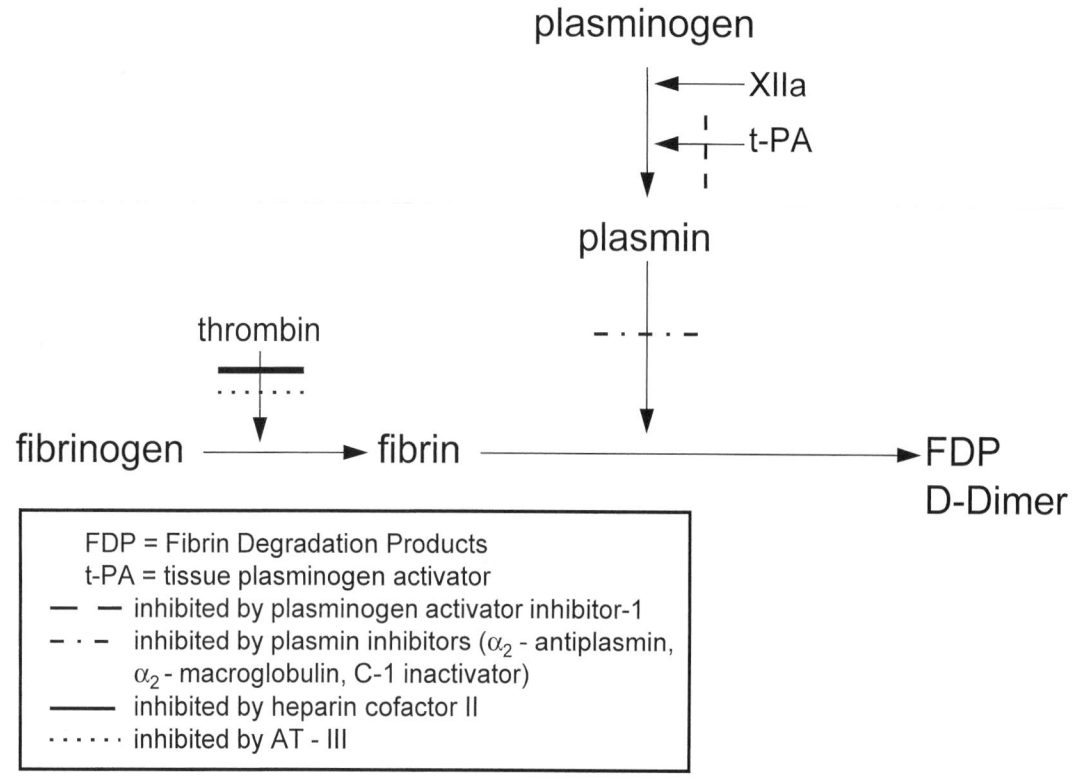

FIGURE 33.2 Components of fibrin formation and degradation.

PLATELET DISORDERS

THROMBOCYTOPENIA

A normal platelet count ranges from 150,000 to 450,000/mm³. Thrombocytopenia, defined as a decrease in the normal number of blood platelets, is one of the most common causes of abnormal bleeding. A platelet count less than 150,000 per mm³ generally indicates the presence of thrombocytopenia; however, clinical trials evaluating the existence of a reduced platelet count use a variety of values to define thrombocytopenia.[1] Mild thrombocytopenia (50,000 to 150,000/mm³) is associated with few symptoms. Counts less than 50,000/mm³ constitute moderate thrombocytopenia and are associated with some bleeding potential. In severe thrombocytopenia (<10,000 to 20,000/mm³), spontaneous life-threatening bleeding can occur. At platelet counts less than 100,000/mm³ bleeding time becomes progressively longer. However, the actual risk for bleeding depends on both the number of platelets available and how well they function.

Thrombocytopenia has many causes, which may vary with both age and development.[1] The causes of thrombocytopenia should be distinguished to optimize the therapeutic approach. A decrease in the platelet count may occur from a decrease in production of platelets, altered distribution (sequestration) of platelets, or increased destruction of platelets.

A decrease in platelet production may occur from conditions that either alter normal formation of platelets (thrombopoiesis) or decrease the number of marrow megakaryocytes. Examples include marrow injury (e.g., myelosuppressive drugs, chemicals, radiation, or viral infections such as rubella, cytomegalovirus, Epstein-Barr virus, and human immunodeficiency virus), marrow failure (e.g., aplastic anemia and hereditary disorders), or marrow replacement (e.g., leukemia, tumor metastases, and fibrosis). Ineffective thrombopoiesis caused by severe vitamin B_{12} or folate deficiency is characterized by a normal or increased number of megakaryocytes in the bone marrow associated with inadequate availability of platelets in the circulation.

Altered distribution of platelets can result from any disorder that causes splenomegaly (e.g., alcoholic liver disease, congestive heart failure, lymphomas, sickle cell disease, and myeloproliferative diseases). In this situation the actual number of total body platelets is normal, but their distribution in the body is altered.

Increased destruction of platelets can result from increased platelet utilization and from immunologic and nonimmunologic mechanisms. Disseminated intravascular coagulation (DIC) is an example of a nonimmunologic condition that causes increased platelet consumption. Immunologic causes of thrombocytopenia include drug-induced immune thrombocytopenia (e.g., quinidine, quinine, gold, and heparin), autoimmune disorders [e.g., systemic lupus erythematosus (SLE) and autoimmune thrombocytopenic purpura], and autoantibody-produced thrombocytopenia (e.g., placental transfer and history of multiple transfusions).

Massive blood loss may result in dilutional thrombocytopenia when treated with large amounts of fluids having few or no platelets. Other miscellaneous causes of thrombocytopenia are thrombotic thrombocytopenic purpura (TTP), prosthetic heart valves, extracorporeal perfusion, hemodialysis, and snake envenomation.

The symptoms of thrombocytopenia include symmetric petechiae and purpura on the extremities and trunk, mild to moderate bleeding of mucosal surfaces (oropharynx, nose, and the gastrointestinal, pulmonary, and genitourinary systems), and easy or spontaneous bleeding.

IMMUNE THROMBOCYTOPENIC PURPURA

Immune thrombocytopenic purpura (ITP; also known as idiopathic thrombocytopenic purpura), an autoimmune disorder, is characterized by decreased numbers of circulating platelets, normal or increased numbers of megakaryocytes in the bone marrow, and clinical signs and symptoms related to the low platelet count. Most cases of ITP involve shortened platelet survival due to immune-mediated platelet destruction by antiplatelet autoantibodies of the immunoglobulin (Ig) G or IgM subtypes.[4,5]

EPIDEMIOLOGY

Clinically, ITP is classified as acute (lasting 6 months or less) or chronic. The acute form most commonly occurs in young, previously healthy children 2 to 8 years of age and affects both sexes equally. The onset in most pediatric patients is seen within days to several weeks after an acute viral infection, most often an upper respiratory infection but also varicella, rubeola, or rubella. The syndrome has also been seen after immunizations. Approximately 80% of pediatric patients will have a complete remission within several weeks to months, regardless of therapy. The annual incidence of the acute form is approximately 4 to 5.3 per 100,000 children; however, many times ITP remains undiagnosed because of its transient and self-limiting nature. About 15% to 20% of children with acute ITP will develop chronic ITP.[4,5]

The chronic form occurs more often in adults, usually women between 20 and 40 years of age, with a female:male ratio of 3:1.[4–9] Chronic ITP has an insidious onset and a lower rate of acute bleeding. Often, the chronic form is an incidental finding. It is sometimes a secondary disorder, associated with another underlying disease (e.g., SLE, other autoimmune disorders, chronic lymphocytic leukemia, or lymphoma) and is not usually preceded by a viral infection. Chronic ITP undergoes remissions and exacerbations, persisting for more than 6 months and often for years. Only about 20% of patients with chronic ITP will have a spontaneous remission, regardless of therapy. The incidence of chronic ITP in adults has been reported to be 5.8 to 6.6 per 100,000.

CLINICAL PRESENTATION AND DIAGNOSIS

SIGNS AND SYMPTOMS
Acute ITP is characterized by an abrupt onset.[4–6] The platelet count is frequently low, between 10,000 and 20,000/mm^3. In most patients the physical examination is remarkable only for the hemorrhagic abnormalities associated with the low platelet count. Small punctate red macules (petechiae) and a dark red-purple discoloration of the skin reflecting larger areas of hemorrhage (purpura) are the classic signs of ITP. These can occur anywhere on the external surface of the skin as well as internally, the gastrointestinal tract being the most common internal site. Bleeding of the nasal, oropharyngeal, and vaginal mucosa; easy bruising with ecchymoses; conjunctival hemorrhage; epistaxis; and menorrhagia are common. Hematuria, retinal hemorrhage, and joint bleeding are less common. Splenomegaly is absent. Central nervous system (CNS) bleeding is seen in approximately 1% of patients. Intracranial hemorrhage occurs early in the acute form of ITP and is most common in patients with platelet counts less than 20,000/mm^3. It is considered the most serious risk with ITP, owing to its associated high morbidity and mortality. Manifestations include altered mental status and headache.

Patients with chronic ITP usually have a higher platelet count compared to those with the acute form.[4,6] Minor skin and mucous membrane bleeding may be the sole manifestations, and some patients are asymptomatic. However, serious bleeding, such as intracranial hemorrhage, can occur in patients with chronic ITP and a low platelet count.

DIAGNOSIS
The diagnosis is usually a process of eliminating other disorders that also cause thrombocytopenia.[4,6] This is especially true for children with signs and symptoms of acute ITP. The differential diagnosis of ITP includes a wide array of hematologic diseases, including leukemia, marrow hypoplasia, DIC, aplastic anemia, TTP, and lymphoma. Nonhematologic causes of thrombocytopenia include systemic infection, thyroid disease, tuberculosis, and autoimmune diseases such as SLE. Human immunodeficiency virus (HIV) infection should be considered as a possible diagnosis for patients who fit into high-risk categories. Drug-induced thrombocytopenia should also be excluded, and any drug that is capable of causing thrombocytopenia should be discontinued (Table

TABLE 33.2	Drugs That Cause Thrombocytopenia

Amrinone (8)	Ethanol (7)
Anti-inflammatory agents (1, 2, 3)	Estrogens (7)
Aspirin	Furosemide (1, 5)
Fenoprofen	Gold salts (2)
Indomethacin	Heparin (2)
Phenylbutazone	Histamine h2
Piroxicam	antagonists (8)
Tolmetin	Cimetidine
β-Blockers (3, 4, 8)	Ranitidine
Alprenolol	Methyldopa (2)
Oxprenolol	Penicillins (3, 5, 8)
Propranolol	Ampicillin
Carbamazepine (2, 8)	Carbenicillin
Clofibrate (3)	Methicillin
Cytotoxic agents (7)	Penicillin G
Busulfan	Ticarcillin
Cytarabine	Penicillamine (2, 8)
Daunorubicin	Phenytoin (2)
Flucytosine	Quinidine (2)
Fluorouracil	Quinine (2)
Mechlorethamine	Rifampin (8)
Mercaptopurine	Sulfinpyrazone (1, 4)
Methotrexate	Thiazide diuretics (8)
Mithramycin	Chlorothiazide
Mitomycin	Hydrochlorothiazide
Dextran (4, 8)	Tocainide (8)
Digitoxin (2)	Trimethoprim (8)
Dipyridamole (3, 5, 6)	Valproic acid (2)

Numbers in parentheses indicate confirmed and suspected mechanisms of thrombocytopenia: 1, Inhibits cyclooxygenase; 2, Drug-induced immune; 3, Inhibits aggregation; 4, Inhibits adhesion; 5, Inhibits release reaction; 6, Inhibits phosphodiesterase; 7, Myelosuppression; 8, Mechanism not documented.

33.2). Splenomegaly, adenopathy, fever, and malaise are uncommon in acute ITP and may suggest other disorders when present.

Laboratory testing reveals isolated thrombocytopenia, unless bleeding has been sufficient to cause anemia. A complete blood examination shows a decreased number of platelets with an elevated mean platelet volume and platelet distribution width. On peripheral smear, the platelets are larger and appear to be less mature than normal. Thrombocytopenia in acute ITP may be severe (platelet count 10,000 to 20,000/mm^3), whereas patients with chronic ITP generally have higher counts (30,000 to 75,000/mm^3). Bleeding time is prolonged in proportion to the degree of thrombocytopenia. The bleeding time for a given platelet count is shorter than that

for thrombocytopenia caused by decreased platelet production, because the circulating platelets are young and "superactive."

This accounts for the lack of bleeding symptoms in some patients despite severe thrombocytopenia. The prothrombin time (PT), activated partial thromboplastin time (aPTT), and erythrocyte sedimentation rate usually remain normal. Almost all patients have normal hemoglobin, hematocrit, and RBC indices, although chronic gastrointestinal hemorrhage or menorrhagia occasionally causes iron deficiency anemia. Bone marrow examination shows normal or increased numbers of immature megakaryocytes.[4,5]

TREATMENT

The major goals in the treatment of ITP are to decrease the risk of hemorrhage and to obtain complete remission of the disease. Traditionally, these goals are met either by suppressing the production of antiplatelet antibodies or by inhibiting platelet phagocytosis. Supportive measures to reduce the risk of bleeding include restriction of physical activity and avoidance of drugs that alter platelet activity; these should be implemented for all patients. For patients with chronic ITP secondary to another disorder, treatment of the underlying disease will benefit the ITP.

ACUTE IMMUNE THROMBOCYTOPENIC PURPURA

The initial course of treatment in children with acute ITP is controversial.[5] Part of this controversy is due to the fact that more than 80% of patients with acute ITP will have a complete spontaneous recovery within a few weeks to months of the disease onset, irrespective of the treatment given.[2,4,5,9] Intracranial hemorrhage is the primary concern of clinicians who prefer early treatment. The risk of intracranial hemorrhage, however, is low (incidence of 0.2% to 1%). Others choose not to treat because of adverse effects, cost, the low frequency of CNS bleeding, and the self-limiting nature of the disease. Some clinicians base the decision to treat on the platelet count, electing to treat when the count is less than 20,000/mm^3. Recent surveys, however, have shown that the majority of children with acute ITP do not have serious bleeding episodes even with low platelet counts.[4] A "watch and wait" approach is frequently used for initial management of children with acute ITP and mild to moderate symptoms. Platelet counts should be repeated within 7 to 10 days after diagnosis to rule out the development of serious bone marrow disorders.

If treatment is initiated, the goal is to rapidly increase the platelet count to a hemostatically safe level.[4,5,10] Prednisone has been considered the drug of choice for treating acute ITP. Dosages range from 1 to 4 mg per kg daily for a maximum of 2 to 3 weeks.[11] Lower doses of prednisone (1 to 2 mg/kg) are effective in raising platelet counts but may not be faster than no treatment.[12] Higher dosages (4 mg/kg) may produce a more rapid rise in platelet count, with a reported median of 4 days to reach a platelet count of greater than 50,000/mm³. Short-term therapy (4 days) at this higher dosage may also be effective. Higher-dose prednisone may be preferred for children with mucous membrane bleeding and more severe cutaneous symptoms.[4,10,13,14] However, the optimal corticosteroid dosage and route of administration have not been established. Adverse effects are minimal at low doses, whereas higher doses have been associated with weight gain, epigastric discomfort, glycosuria, and behavioral changes.[14,15] High-dose methylprednisolone (30 mg/kg daily for 2 to 3 days) has been used for urgent treatment (e.g., neurologic symptoms, evidence of internal bleeding, or when surgery is needed).[5]

Intravenous high-dose immune globulins (IVIGs) have been shown to shorten the duration of platelet counts less than 20,000/mm³. IVIG has many simultaneous effects on platelet function, which occur through inhibition of Fc receptor-mediated platelet binding in the reticuloendothelial system. IVIG alters T- and B-cell numbers and function. It also produces a reduction in platelet-associated immunoglobulins, which is seen within 3 days. The total dose of IVIG to be administered is 2 g/kg, given as either 0.4 g/kg/day for 5 days or 1 g/kg/day for 2 days. This usually results in a response in 1 to 3 days, with about 80% of patients showing a platelet count greater than 50,000/mm³ at 72 hours after treatment. If the effect is not sustained, repeat doses may be given. Adverse effects of IVIG include nausea, vomiting, headache, and fever, which seem to occur more often (50% to 60%) in patients who receive the total dose over 2 days.[9,10] However, these symptoms usually abate after about 1 day and are readily managed with acetaminophen. The long-term response to IVIG, assessed as maintenance of a platelet count greater than 20,000/mm³ with no subsequent bleeding, is about 62%.[16] IVIG may be used with methylprednisolone when urgent therapy is needed.[5] This combination has been shown to increase the platelet count more rapidly than either drug alone.[8,15,16]

The decision whether to use prednisone or IVIG as initial therapy requires consideration of many factors. IVIG may be preferable because it has a more rapid onset of action compared to traditional doses of prednisone; however, higher prednisone doses may yield a comparable onset of action. Some investigators prefer IVIG, with the belief that it may have a disease-modifying role.[15] Some practitioners consider prednisone to be the gold standard and favor its use because of familiarity with the drug. Much lower cost and concern regarding administration of blood products also favor prednisone, although a shortened hospital stay with IVIG may offset some of the cost. Additional studies are clearly necessary to clarify this clinical decision.[5]

Anti-D immunoglobulin (WinRho) is an Rh_o (D) immune globulin made from freeze-dried γ-globulin (IgG) fraction and contains antibodies to Rh_o (D). It has been successfully used in the treatment of ITP in nonsplenectomized, Rh_o (D)-positive children and adults. When given at a dosage of 25 μg/kg/d for 2 days, the platelet response is slower compared to IVIG.[5] However, higher doses (40 to 75 μg/kg) result in increases in platelet counts similar to those seen with IVIG.[4,5] It has some advantages over IVIG, such as cost and method of administration. Anti-D may, however, cause reductions in hemoglobin and, rarely, renal failure.

Splenectomy is generally avoided as a treatment for children with ITP because of the high rate of spontaneous remission of the disorder and the risks associated with the surgery (e.g., postsplenectomy sepsis).[4,5] If splenectomy is contemplated, pneumococcal and *Haemophilus influenzae* immunizations should be given before the surgery; prophylaxis with penicillin is needed after surgery, and some clinicians recommend lifetime prophylaxis.

CHRONIC IMMUNE THROMBOCYTOPENIC PURPURA

Chronic ITP is primarily a disease of adults, but approximately 10% to 20% of children with acute ITP have a poor response to treatment, and their ITP will evolve into the chronic form. The decision to treat patients with chronic ITP depends on a number of factors, including severity of the disorder, platelet count, lifestyle, and adverse effects of treatment. Studies have suggested that the risk for clinically significant bleeding is low when platelet counts are greater than 10,000/mm³. For patients with nonactive lifestyles, a platelet count greater than 30,000/mm³ is thought to be acceptable. For more active patients, higher platelet counts (>50,000/mm³) are needed. However, bleeding can still occur despite higher platelet counts; other factors (i.e., age, uremia, chronic liver disease) must be considered when assessing the risk of bleeding in patients with chronic ITP. In addition, there are no strict recommendations as to what a "safe" platelet count is for patients with chronic ITP.[4–6] Therapy for chronic ITP is usually begun with 1 to 2 mg/kg/day of prednisone. A positive response should be seen in 3 to 7 days, although 2 to 4 weeks may be needed for maximal response.[15] If a response is not seen within 4 weeks, the corticosteroid should be tapered and discontinued. An alternative therapy should be considered in patients who fail to respond to corticosteroids or who cannot be maintained on low-dose or alternate-day therapy. The initial response rate to steroid therapy may be as high as 50% to 80%, but less than 20% of patients will be able to receive long-term corticosteroid therapy, owing to relapse or adverse reactions.[15,17] IVIG has been used for chronic ITP, but its effect is transient, with return to pretreatment levels 3 to 4 weeks after therapy.[4]

In patients with refractory disease, splenectomy is usually considered next. Nearly 70% of patients who undergo splenectomy respond with a normal platelet count.[4] Postulated mechanisms for efficacy of splenectomy in chronic ITP include a reduction in the phagocytosis of antibody-coated platelets and a reduction of platelet-associated antibody production. It is important that the operative procedure include a search for and removal of all accessory splenic tissues.

The presence of accessory splenic tissues has been associated with relapse following splenectomy. Corticosteroids or IVIG are often given before surgery to boost the platelet count ($>30,000/mm^3$) and reduce the risk of perioperative bleeding. Oral dexamethasone (40 mg/d for 4 days) has also been used preoperatively. Polyvalent pneumococcal vaccine should be administered preoperatively. Some clinicians also advocate daily oral penicillin therapy for several years after surgery.[2] A complete remission of ITP has been reported in up to 80% of patients after splenectomy.[2,17,18] Platelet kinetic studies may be performed to assess the degree of splenic sequestration; this may assist in the decision to perform splenectomy. In one study, a platelet count greater than $120,000/mm^3$ at the time of discharge, age less than 30 years, preoperative corticosteroid dependence, and splenic sequestration (measured preoperatively) were associated with a more favorable response to splenectomy.[17]

A number of second-line agents have been used to treat patients who are refractory to corticosteroids and splenectomy. Immunosuppressive therapy is usually considered next. Azathioprine, cyclophosphamide, and the vinca alkaloids (vincristine and vinblastine) are the most commonly used agents.[6] Azathioprine is believed to interfere with the response of T cells to antigenic challenge, with an additional more generalized reduction in T-helper activity. About 20% of patients given azathioprine respond with a normal platelet count, which may be sustained for several years. Between 30% and 40% have a partial response. The dosage of azathioprine used is 1 to 4 mg/kg/day (or 100 to 200 mg/day); the dose is reduced if the patient becomes leukopenic.[12] It is usually given in conjunction with steroids and may have a steroid-sparing effect for some patients.[15] Side effects are usually less serious than with cyclophosphamide, bone marrow suppression being the most important. Azathioprine is considered the safest agent for long-term therapy.

Cyclophosphamide is given in an oral dosage of 1 to 2 mg/kg/d or as an intermittent intravenous dose (1 to 1.5 g/m^2 intravenously every 3 to 4 weeks).[6,15] Improvement is usually seen in 2 to 10 weeks, with a maximum response in platelet count seen in 8 weeks. Treatment is continued for 4 to 6 weeks after an adequate platelet count is achieved. Studies showing complete remission in 30% to 40% of patients are an advantage with cyclophosphamide. Unfortunately, side effects, including bone marrow suppression, hemorrhagic cystitis, and bladder fibrosis, may limit its use.

Vinca alkaloids have been reported to be beneficial in more than 50% of patients who are refractory to steroids and splenectomy. Vincristine (0.25 mg/kg to a maximum dose of 2 mg) and vinblastine (0.125 mg/kg to a maximum dose of 10 mg) are given intravenously every 2 to 6 weeks.[6,15,19] Response occurs more rapidly than with azathioprine or cyclophosphamide, but relapses usually occur in 3 to 4 weeks. These agents are believed to decrease the rate of destruction of platelets by inhibiting phagocytosis and decreasing antibody levels.[7] Vincristine may also bind selectively to platelet tubulin, such that when the antibody-coated platelet is phagocytosed, the macrophages are poisoned. Vincristine and vinblastine have been loaded onto platelets in an attempt to deliver them selectively to macrophages that are responsible for platelet destruction, but this is not commonly done because of its impracticality and lack of advantage over conventional administration. The incidence of side effects is relatively high with the vinca alkaloids. Vincristine may cause transient malaise, fever after injection, temporary jaw pain, alopecia, and a variety of neuropathies. Leukopenia, abdominal pain, and headache are associated with vinblastine.

Danazol, an anabolic steroid, is thought to decrease phagocytosis of platelets by decreasing the number of phagocytic cell IgG Fc-receptors.[7] Dosage is usually 400 to 800 mg per day initially, then tapered to 50 to 200 mg daily. Clinical response is normally seen within 8 weeks, however, treatment should be continued for up to 6 months since response may be slow. Between 30% and 40% of patients have a sustained increase in platelets.[6,19] Side effect frequency is low; side effects include virilization, fibrinolysis, and hepatic dysfunction. Danazol is contraindicated during pregnancy.

High-dose corticosteroids have also shown some efficacy in patients with refractory disease. Dexamethasone 40 mg per day (oral or intravenous) for 4 days given every 4 weeks for up to six cycles has been reported to result in a complete and sustained response.[6,19] However, results have not been consistent. Methylprednisolone given at a dosage of 30 mg/kg/d for 3 days tapered to 1 mg per kg increased platelet counts within 3 to 4 days, but the response was transient in some patients.

Rituximab, an anti-CD20 monoclonal antibody, has been successful in some patients with refractory ITP.[20–22] In one small pilot study, rituximab at a dosage of 375 mg per m^2 once weekly for 4 weeks resulted in a complete response (defined as normalization of platelet counts for $\geq$30 days) in 5 of 12 patients, with a partial response (platelet count $>30,000/mm^3$) in 2 of 12 patients. However, relapse after discontinuation of rituximab has occurred.[22]

Other therapies that have been studied in limited numbers of patients include colchicine, dapsone, cyclosporine, and interferon-α.[19,23] However, no clear consensus exists as to optimal treatment for patients with refractory ITP. A meta-analysis conducted by Vesely et al found azathioprine, cyclophosphamide, and rituximab to be associated with the highest rates of complete response, but these rates were still low, ranging from 17% to 27% of patients.

Although spontaneous complete remission of chronic ITP is unusual, the long-term prognosis is usually favorable. Most patients will have stable, mild to moderate thrombocytopenia. The objective of therapy in chronic ITP is to keep the patient hemostatically safe (i.e., platelet counts $>30,000$ to $50,000/mm^3$), not necessarily to obtain a complete remission. A review of the literature on patients with refractory disease showed a median death rate of 5.1%, caused either by uncontrolled bleeding or by complications of therapy.

High-risk groups included patients with a history of bleeding, those with the concomitant presence of other bleeding disorders, and those more than 60 years of age.[17]

THROMBOTIC THROMBOCYTOPENIC PURPURA

TTP is an uncommon but potentially devastating disorder of multiorgan involvement. The clinical manifestations are often described as a pentad of signs and symptoms: thrombocytopenia, microangiopathic hemolytic anemia, neurologic abnormalities, renal failure, and fever.[24–27] A patient with TTP may also have abdominal and chest pain and sometimes cardiac arrhythmias.[25] The hallmark of TTP is widespread formation of platelet microthrombi, which results in end-organ damage and intravascular hemolysis as fragmented RBCs flow through partially occluded arterioles and capillaries.[26] In the past, TTP was associated with a mortality rate greater than 90%; however, with the introduction of plasma exchange therapy, survival has increased markedly.[26–28]

EPIDEMIOLOGY

TTP is a rare disorder, occurring at a reported rate of 3.7 per million adults.[25] Women are more frequently affected by the disease than men (3:2).[27] Pregnant or postpartum women represent 10% to 25% of patients with TTP.[29] TTP may be familial or acquired. Familial TTP is rare and usually manifests in infancy or childhood; however, some patients with a familial disposition to TTP may not exhibit symptoms of the disease for years. Acquired TTP is observed more frequently in older children and adults and is usually associated with a single acute episode. However, 11% to 36% of patients experience intermittent recurrence of disease. Although TTP may occur at any age from infancy onward, the peak incidence is observed during the fourth decade of life, with a median age at diagnosis of 35.[27]

Precipitating factors may be found in as many as 70% of patients.[30] Bacterial or viral infection is the most common (including HIV infection at any stage), occurring in up to 40% of patients. Other precipitating conditions include pregnancy, postoperative status, transplantation, myocardial infarction, lymphoma, carcinoma, autoimmune disorders, bee stings, and dog bites.[27,31] Drugs such as penicillins, sulfonamides, cyclosporine, penicillamine, oral contraceptives, iodine, ticlopidine, clopidogrel, mitomycin, cisplatinum, and bleomycin have also been implicated.[32,33]

PATHOPHYSIOLOGY

Historically, the pathogenesis of TTP has been unknown; however, recent advances in the understanding of the pathophysiology of TTP have begun to paint a clearer picture of the disease. The microvascular thrombi observed in TTP consist of aggregations of platelets with small amounts of fibrin.[24] These thrombi, which result in organ damage, actually contain significant amounts of von Willebrand factor (vWF).

Endothelial cells produce multimers of vWF, which are typically larger than those observed in normal plasma.[24] These unusually large multimers bind to glycoprotein Ibα and subsequently to glycoprotein IIb/IIIa complexes. This binding induces platelet aggregation. In a normal individual, the presence of such unusually large vWF multimers results in the activation of an enzyme known as ADAMTS13. ADAMTS13 is a metalloprotease that cleaves the vWF multimers into smaller subunits.[34,35] In most patients with TTP, the plasma activity level of ADAMTS13 is less than 5% of the normal value.[24] In this situation, the large multimers of vWF are not cleaved, and passing platelets begin to adhere to these molecules. As additional platelets bind to the complex, large occlusive thrombi are formed, which may result in an episode of TTP.

Although the above pathophysiologic mechanism explains the development of TTP in most patients, some with acquired TTP have large multimers of vWF in the plasma without a corresponding reduction in ADAMTS13 activity.[24] These patients may produce autoantibodies that prevent ADAMTS13 from cleaving the large vWF multimers.

CLINICAL PRESENTATION AND DIAGNOSIS

SIGNS AND SYMPTOMS

Although a classic pentad of signs and symptoms of TTP has been described, a patient may present with variable and nonspecific manifestations of disease, including malaise, weakness, fatigue, abdominal pain, nausea and vomiting, arthralgia, and hemorrhage.[27] Neurologic symptoms include headache, syncope, vertigo, ataxia, aphasia, behavioral or mental status changes, and seizures. Signs of hemorrhage, including petechiae and purpura, are common. Target organ dysfunction may also be observed in the eyes, heart, and lungs. Not all patients have symptoms in each of these categories.

DIAGNOSIS

TTP should be suspected in patients who have these symptoms. The workup for TTP includes an evaluation for sepsis, hemolysis, elevated liver function tests, and low platelets (HELLP) syndrome, autoimmune disorders, and potentially an underlying malignancy.[27] In clinical practice, a triad of signs and symptoms—thrombocytopenia, schistocytosis, and an elevated lactate dehydrogenase (LDH) level—is usually all that is required to suggest a diagnosis of TTP.[24] Even if a firm diagnosis of TTP cannot be made, the clinician may initiate treatment as soon as possible due to the increased mortality observed if appropriate therapy is delayed.

The key component in the diagnosis of TTP is an evaluation of a peripheral blood smear.[27] The smear should contain fragmented RBCs (i.e., schistocytes) suggestive of microangiopathic hemolysis.[26] Bilirubin and LDH levels are markedly elevated owing to RBC hemolysis. The hemoglobin concentration averages 8 to 9 g per dL. Thrombocytopenia is invariably present, with platelet counts usually less than 30,000 to 50,000 per mm[3] and bone marrow biopsies showing large numbers of megakaryocytes. The coagulation screen is normal except for mild elevations in fibrin degradation products in up to 70% of patients[30]; this is a useful parameter for distinguishing TTP from DIC. Renal involvement is present in 40% of patients,[7] with laboratory tests showing proteinuria, microscopic hematuria, and elevated blood urea nitrogen (BUN) and serum creatinine levels. Obtaining an ADAMTS13 activity level is not currently recommended for most patients.[34]

TREATMENT

In the past, TTP was almost uniformly fatal, but with the introduction of successful treatment strategies, survival rates have increased.[27] Therapies include plasma infusion or exchange, corticosteroids, splenectomy, and antiplatelet, immunosuppressive, and cytotoxic agents. Success with therapy varies from individual to individual, each approach showing some benefit in certain patients but little benefit in others. The individual effectiveness of each modality is not known, because several or all are commonly administered simultaneously.

Plasmapheresis [exchange transfusion with fresh-frozen plasma (FFP) or cryosupernatant] is the treatment of choice for TTP, producing a response rate near 80%.[2] The therapeutic rationale for plasmapheresis has been more fully explained with the recent discovery of ADAMTS13 deficiency in patients with TTP.[24,27] Plasmapheresis results in the removal of the large vWF multimers and autoantibodies against ADAMTS13 while also replenishing the missing enzyme itself through the infusion of FFP or cryosupernatant. Plasmapheresis has been associated with a higher response rate and lower mortality than plasma infusion, although it is technically more difficult and expensive. It should be initiated as soon as possible, with a single plasma volume exchange daily (40 mL/kg of body mass) and continued for several days after clinical manifestations improve and platelet count, hemoglobin level, and LDH values have normalized.[27] The standard replacement fluid for plasma exchange is FFP; use of albumin or plasma protein fraction is not recommended. Patients with a poor response to plasmapheresis with FFP may benefit from the substitution of cryosupernatant as the replacement solution. Patients who do not respond favorably to once-daily exchange therapy may be administered plasmapheresis on a twice-daily regimen. Once

a successful response is observed, plasma exchange should be slowly tapered over 1 to 2 weeks. Relapse of TTP can occur, typically within 1 week to 1 month after discontinuation of therapy. Adverse effects of plasma therapy include hypersensitivity reactions, paresthesias, twitching, muscle cramps, or tetany related to citrate toxicity, infusion-related reactions, catheter-related complications, potential for blood-borne infections, and volume overload.[26,27,30,36]

Infants or young children with familial TTP may respond favorably to treatment with infusions of FFP, cryosupernatant, or solvent/detergent-treated plasma approximately every 3 weeks.[24] Plasmapheresis is not recommended for this patient population. All of these infusion solutions contain the metalloprotease enzyme ADAMTS13, which is deficient in patients with familial TTP.

Corticosteroids have a variable benefit but are almost universally used as an adjunctive therapy, in part because of the theoretical autoimmune hypothesis for the pathogenesis of TTP.[25,26] Although randomized studies evaluating the effectiveness of corticosteroids in TTP are nonexistent, dosages of prednisone of 1 to 2 mg/kg/day (or its equivalent) have been used.[7,26,30,36] The dosage is then slowly tapered. Corticosteroids alone are not generally effective in treating the acute disease. They are also used (alone or in combination) to reduce the remission rate and treat relapses.

Antiplatelet agents such as aspirin and dipyridamole may be administered in the acute phase. However, in some patients they worsen bleeding without providing a beneficial effect.[2,7] After remission is achieved, maintenance doses of aspirin and dipyridamole may be given to prevent relapse. The antiplatelet agents ticlopidine and clopidogrel should not be used, because they have been implicated as causative factors in some cases of TTP.[25] Infusions of prostacyclin have been administered because deficiencies of this vasodilator and platelet aggregation inhibitor have been observed in patients with TTP. The effectiveness of this modality has been questionable, and its use is restricted to patients whose disease is unresponsive to other treatments. Sulfinpyrazone and dextran are also reserved for patients with refractory disease.

Splenectomy is reserved for patients who show no response to other therapies and those who cannot be weaned off plasma therapy. It has also been shown to reduce the relapse rate. Vincristine may be given in severe cases at a dosage of 2 mg weekly.[30,36] Other immunosuppressives reported to produce anecdotal benefit in refractory TTP include azathioprine, cyclophosphamide, and cyclosporin.[25] Rituximab, a monoclonal antibody, has also recently been investigated for use in chronic recurring TTP.[37] IVIG has shown a variable effect and is used only in patients with refractory disease.

Platelet transfusions have been shown to worsen the microvascular occlusion and are therefore not given.[2,30,36] Because TTP is a disease of the platelets, heparin has no beneficial effect and can even be harmful by increasing the risk of bleeding.

Supportive care for the associated symptoms should be provided. Hemodialysis may be necessary for patients with severe renal failure. Anticonvulsants may be indicated in patients who develop seizures.[27]

PROGNOSIS

Before 1965, TTP was considered an infrequent, complicated, progressive, and nearly always fatal disease. Without treatment, TTP remains a fatal disorder in 80% to 90% of patients. Fortunately, with advances in the understanding and treatment of the disease, up to 70% to 80% of patients can now be expected to survive with appropriate treatment, most with few or no sequelae.[30,36] Early intervention minimizes the risk of long-term neurologic or renal sequelae.

The improved survival rate has resulted in larger numbers of patients with relapsed or chronic disease. Approximately 15% to 50% of patients who survive after TTP will have a relapse.[2,30] Relapses are usually milder than the initial disease. They occur at intervals of months or years, and the patient is relatively healthy in the interim periods.

PLATELET FUNCTION DISORDERS

Disorders of platelet function may cause bleeding or thrombosis independent of the platelet count.[38,39] Congenital disorders of platelet function are rare and encompass defects in any of the four previously described actions. Acquired platelet function disorders are common, are often associated with clinically significant bleeding, and may be caused by medical conditions as well as by a variety of drugs.

Uremia is a commonly encountered medical condition that is associated with a variety of platelet function defects. Almost all uremic patients have prolonged bleeding times and abnormal in vitro platelet function,[40] with a correlation between the bleeding time prolongation and the degree of renal insufficiency. The abnormalities are thought to be caused by unknown substances that are present in uremic plasma, because most defects abate with dialysis or improved renal function. Most patients experience bleeding, but this is rarely a cause of serious morbidity.

Cardiac bypass induces a platelet function disorder that is caused by factors related to the bypass procedure itself. Most defects correct spontaneously after completion of the bypass. Other conditions that are associated with abnormalities in platelet function include liver disease, dysproteinemias (e.g., multiple myeloma or macroglobulinemia), and myeloproliferative disorders.

The management of patients with platelet function disorders consists of both supportive care and administration of specific agents to improve platelet function. Supportive measures include avoiding situations associated with a high risk of bleeding and medications that alter platelet function or

numbers (Table 33.2). The underlying disorder should be corrected or treated when possible. Platelet transfusions are useful for patients after bypass surgery but are otherwise avoided unless bleeding is life-threatening. For uremic patients with bleeding, desmopressin or conjugated estrogens will correct the bleeding time and slow clinical bleeding.[40] Oral contraceptives may be given to reduce menorrhagia.

DRUG-INDUCED PLATELET DISORDERS

The healthcare professional must recognize drugs that adversely affect platelets. Avoidance of their use entirely or close monitoring of platelet counts and function may be necessary for certain patients. Familiarity with these agents also facilitates assessment of drugs as potential causative factors in patients with platelet abnormalities. Although many drugs affect platelet activity adversely, the literature must be evaluated carefully before an ''antiplatelet'' label is placed on a therapeutic agent that only rarely produces clinically significant manifestations.

Drug-induced platelet disorders include those that alter platelet function and those that cause thrombocytopenia. Drug-induced disorders of platelet function are further subdivided (in descending order of prevalence) into drug interference with (a) platelet membranes or membrane receptor sites, (b) prostaglandin biosynthetic pathways, (c) phosphodiesterase activity, and (d) unknown mechanisms.[41] Either decreased production or increased destruction of platelets may cause drug-induced thrombocytopenia. Table 33.2 lists commonly implicated drugs and their proposed mechanisms of action.

Aspirin is by far the most common and well-documented cause of drug-induced platelet dysfunction. This is mediated by aspirin-induced abnormalities on both platelets and endothelial cells. At the platelet level, aspirin irreversibly acetylates cyclooxygenase. This reduces platelet synthesis of cyclic endoperoxides and thromboxane A_2, resulting in loss of thromboxane A_2-mediated platelet stimulation and vasoconstriction. Platelets cannot regenerate cyclooxygenase; therefore, the effect of aspirin on thromboxane A_2 is irreversible. In contrast, endothelial cells can synthesize new cyclooxygenase; therefore, prostacyclin synthesis resumes after the aspirin is metabolized. The net effect of aspirin reflects its action on the platelets and endothelial cells. The irreversible loss of platelet cyclooxygenase often dominates, with a reduction in platelet stimulation. The peak effect of a single dose occurs in 2 to 4 hours, but because aspirin's effect on platelets is irreversible, its pharmacodynamic activity may last up to 10 days or the life span of the platelet. When aspirin is administered to a normal person, bleeding time is prolonged by a factor of 1.5 to 2,[40] but significant bleeding is uncommon. Aspirin may be associated with clinically significant hemorrhage when the hemostatic system is stressed (e.g., surgery or other invasive procedure), such as in older adults, patients with hemophilia, patients with coexisting thrombocytopenia or other bleeding risk (e.g., peptic ulcer disease), patients taking other drugs with antiplatelet effect, or patients undergoing neurologic or ophthalmic surgery. It should also be avoided late in pregnancy.

Other nonsteroidal anti-inflammatory agents such as indomethacin, ibuprofen, naproxen, piroxicam, and ketorolac also prevent thromboxane A_2 generation by inhibiting platelet cyclooxygenase.[40,41] With these drugs the platelet effect is reversible, occurring only while the drug is present in the circulation. The bleeding time is only slightly prolonged, and the effects abate as the drug is cleared from the plasma.

Dipyridamole is sometimes used therapeutically for its antithrombotic activity, usually in combination with aspirin. The mode of action is believed to be prevention of cyclic adenosine monophosphate (AMP) breakdown by inhibition of phosphodiesterase activity. Increased platelet cyclic AMP levels inhibit platelet aggregation and release. Unlike aspirin, dipyridamole does not alter bleeding time or platelet survival.

Ticlopidine-induced antiplatelet effects occur via a mechanism that is not well established. Ticlopidine induces a thrombasthenic-like state without altering the expression of platelet membrane receptors. This may occur via inhibition of common signal transduction pathways in platelets. The drug prolongs bleeding time; however, severe hemorrhage is not a prominent side effect.[40]

Penicillin and related compounds prolong bleeding time and occasionally have clinically important effects on platelet function. These effects are mediated by an interaction with platelet membrane receptors that reduces responsiveness to stimulation by adenosine diphosphate (ADP) and epinephrine and decreases platelet aggregation.[40] Platelet dysfunction begins several days after initiation and abates several days after discontinuation of the drug. High-dose carbenicillin is the prototype example of a drug that produces this effect. Similar effects have been seen with penicillin G, ampicillin, ticarcillin, piperacillin, methicillin, and nafcillin. Cephalosporins may also alter platelet function, although this effect is not as well documented, and the clinical relevance is not well established. Significant bleeding is uncommon unless the patient has other risk factors such as renal failure or ulcer disease.

Dextran, a partially hydrolyzed polymer of glucose, is used as a plasma volume expander in patients with certain types of shock, impaired renal function, and other conditions in which improved circulation is desirable. It also prolongs bleeding time, impairs fibrin polymerization, decreases blood viscosity, and alters platelet function. For these reasons, dextran is sometimes used in the prophylaxis of venous thrombosis and pulmonary thromboembolism. The mechanism of the antiplatelet activity is not known but may involve inhibition of platelet aggregation and reduced platelet agonist activity. Dextran should be used with caution in treating patients with coexisting thrombocytopenia.

Alcohol impairs platelet function and primary hemostasis. Large quantities of ethanol can inhibit prostaglandin endoperoxide synthesis and decrease thromboxane A_2 production, thereby causing a decrease in platelet aggregation and release. Alcohol ingestion may also directly suppress bone marrow thrombocyte production. Alcoholism can decrease ADP storage pools and platelet agonist (ADP and epinephrine) activity. Moreover, alcoholism is associated with other factors that may cause platelet dysfunction. Alcohol-mediated platelet dysfunction can occur in the absence of liver disease and is reversible; the platelet count returns to baseline 7 to 21 days after discontinuation.[7]

Drug-induced immune thrombocytopenia is a relatively uncommon platelet disorder that is caused by a number of drugs.[42] A variety of mechanisms have been postulated to explain drug-induced immune thrombocytopenia.

Drug-induced immune thrombocytopenia is more common in adults, is not dose-related, and is associated with antibody persistence for many years. The clinical presentation of petechiae, purpura, and mucous membrane bleeding is similar to that for the chronic form of autoimmune thrombocytopenia. However, its rapid onset (6 to 12 hours after re-exposure), the severity of both symptoms and thrombocytopenia (commonly <10,000/mm^3), and the rapid sustained recovery after the drug is terminated are distinguishing features of the drug-induced form.[2,43] The primary management is discontinuation of the drug. Platelet destruction generally abates in 3 to 7 days but may persist for weeks to months after drug discontinuation in some patients. High-dose IVIG or a short course of corticosteroids may be given to shorten the recovery period.[23] Plasmapheresis may be used for critically ill patients. Drug-induced immune thrombocytopenia has been best documented with heparin, gold, quinidine, and quinine (which may be used therapeutically or found in soft drinks and street drugs). Other common drugs that cause this syndrome are listed in Table 33.2.

Heparin is the most common cause of drug-induced thrombocytopenia, with an overall incidence of 3% to 5% with intravenous therapy[44–46] and with less than 3% of patients developing platelet counts less than 100,000/mm^3. The incidence is much lower with subcutaneous administration, yet this syndrome has been seen after the use of the small doses used in heparin flushes or even in patients with heparin-coated intravenous catheters. Thrombocytopenia is more common with bovine-derived heparin (versus porcine). Heparin causes two types of platelet disorders, type I and type II.

In type I, a mild gradual thrombocytopenia develops over the first few days of treatment. Platelet counts rarely fall to less than 100,000/mm^3. The thrombocytopenia usually resolves spontaneously, even with continued heparin therapy. It is not dose-dependent and is thought to be caused by an induced platelet proaggregant effect that results in enhanced sequestration and destruction.[47] Most patients are asymptomatic, and treatment is not indicated.

Type II is much less common, appearing after 5 to 14 days of therapy (unless the patient has been previously exposed). Characteristics include platelet counts of 60,000 to 100,000/mm^3 that remain low until the drug is discontinued. After heparin is stopped, platelet counts return to normal values in 5 to 7 days. The development of type II involves a complex interaction between heparin, platelet factor 4 (PF4), platelet Fc receptors, and heparin-like molecules on the endothelial cell surface, ultimately resulting in an increased risk of thrombosis. The resultant ''paradoxical'' thrombosis may be arterial (more common) or venous, may occur at multiple sites, and in some cases is devastating. Concomitant with the onset of thrombocytopenia, extensive arterial or venous thrombosis with limb ischemia or gangrene, myocardial infarction, stroke, recurrent pulmonary embolism (PE), and skin necrosis has been observed.

Treatment of type I consists of monitoring the platelet count every 2 to 3 days. In type II, heparin should be immediately discontinued and alternative anticoagulants such as dextran, aspirin, argatroban, lepirudin, thrombolytics, and/or warfarin should be initiated. Platelet counts should return to normal a few days after discontinuation.[43] Unfortunately, thrombectomy or limb amputation may be necessary in some patients with type II disease, and mortality may be as high as 30%. A high in vitro cross-reaction rate has been reported with various low-molecular-weight heparins (LMWHs).[47] These should therefore also be avoided unless a lack of cross-reactivity has been shown. In addition, therapy with warfarin in patients with heparin-induced thrombocytopenia (HIT) must be approached cautiously.[48,49] Several case reports have described warfarin-induced skin necrosis and venous limb gangrene in patients with HIT given unopposed warfarin therapy. One retrospective study found that 12% of patients with HIT-associated deep venous thrombosis (DVT) given warfarin developed venous limb gangrene. HIT produces a hypercoagulable state; when given alone, the early procoagulant effects of warfarin (due to inhibition of protein C) can worsen thromboses in these patients, resulting in progression to venous limb gangrene. Warfarin-induced skin necrosis (due to microthrombotic lesions) has also occurred. In some cases, this complication might have been due to initial use of high-dose warfarin or concurrent use of ancrod. The risk of these complications may be reduced if warfarin therapy is initiated after normalization of platelet levels, use of low doses of warfarin (<5 mg daily), or use of alternative anticoagulants that reduce thrombin formation during early warfarin therapy (e.g., lepirudin or argatroban) until platelet counts have normalized.

Lepirudin is a treatment option for HIT. It inactivates fibrin clot-bound and soluble thrombin. Because its chemical structure is different from that of the heparins, no platelet aggregation cross-reactivity occurs between the agents. Lepirudin has been found to trigger the formation of IgG antihirudin antibodies in approximately 50% of patients with HIT who receive it for >5 days. Also, in patients with renal failure, there is a high risk associated with bleeding due to drug accumulation because it is renally metabolized and excreted.[50] One advantage for using lepirudin is the ability to monitor its effect through aPTTs. The loading dose is an intravenous bolus of 0.4 mg/kg, followed by a maintenance intravenous dose of 0.15 mg/kg/hour. Adjustments should be made to the maintenance dose to maintain an aPTT of 1.5 to 3.0 times normal.[51]

Argatroban, another agent useful for the management of HIT,[44] is a synthetic, L-arginine derivative that does not cross-react with heparin. Although published efficacy data for argatroban in HIT are limited, the recommended dose is 2 μg/kg/min as a continuous infusion. The infusion should be adjusted to maintain an aPTT of 1.5 to 3 times control.

Cytotoxic agents can cause thrombocytopenia because of their myelosuppressive action on the hematopoietic system. In contrast to other forms of drug-induced thrombocytopenia, which affect mature platelets in the circulation, antineoplastic agents cause a dose-dependent reduction in bone marrow platelet precursors. Precursors of all three cell lines [white blood cells (WBCs), RBCs, and thrombocytes] are suppressed, the onset and severity being related to the life span of existing cells. In this regard, thrombocytopenia is intermediate, occurring gradually over 7 to 10 days.[52] Host factors such as age, nutritional status, and preexisting bone marrow compromise affect the severity and symptoms. Drugs that may cause significant bone marrow suppression include cytarabine, the nitrosoureas, busulfan, methotrexate, cyclophosphamide, and mercaptopurine.[7,43] Busulfan may cause a severe prolonged thrombocytopenia due to an irreversible reduction in the number of marrow stem cells. Vincristine is an exception and may even stimulate thrombopoiesis.[43,53] The primary management consists of prophylactic platelet transfusions when the counts fall to less than 10,000 to 20,000/mm^3, single-donor platelets being preferable because of a lower incidence of alloimmunization.[52] When possible, chemotherapeutic regimens should be tailored to avoid the simultaneous administration of drugs that are known to cause this effect. A new therapeutic approach is the administration of interleukins; several have megakaryocyte-stimulating properties. One of these is interleukin-11 (IL-11), which causes the proliferation of hematopoietic stem cells and megakaryocyte progenitors. It also can induce megakaryocytic maturation. Dosages of 25 to 75 μg/kg/day have been found to ameliorate chemotherapy-induced thrombocytopenia in women who have stage 3 or 4 breast cancer. IL-11 was also found to decrease the number of platelet transfusions in patients with various cancer diagnoses undergoing chemotherapy with different regimens.[54]

Cocaine may also have a toxic effect on megakaryocytes, causing oropharyngeal and mucous membrane bleeding with platelet counts less than 10,000/mm^3.[7] This effect is unrelated to the route of administration. Bone marrow aspiration shows a reduced number of megakaryocytes, without involvement of the WBC and RBC cell lines. The platelet count generally increases over 2 to 3 weeks after discontinuation of the drug.

DISSEMINATED INTRAVASCULAR COAGULATION

DIC is an acquired syndrome, secondary to some underlying cause.[55–57] Conditions resulting in DIC are varied, with septicemia the most common precipitating disease. Nearly 50% of patients with gram-negative sepsis exhibit clinical signs of DIC; it is also common among patients with gram-positive sepsis. Other clinical conditions associated with DIC are given in Table 33.3. Regardless of the underlying cause of DIC, the end result is a breakdown of the intricate balance between coagulation and fibrinolysis, the systems that maintain blood in a fluid state within the vasculature. In DIC, simultaneous in vivo activation of the coagulation and fibrinolytic systems results in both thrombosis and hemorrhage. The clinical manifestations of DIC are highly variable and depend on the underlying disease process and the relative balance between coagulation and fibrinolysis in the individual patient.

Once initiated, DIC results in (a) in vivo activation of the coagulation system, resulting in intravascular thrombin generation, (b) intravascular fibrin clot formation with end-organ ischemia, (c) activation of the fibrinolytic systems, and (d) depletion of blood coagulation proteins and platelets.

The severity of DIC and the degree of morbidity and mortality depend in part on the severity of the underlying triggering clinical condition. The stronger the triggering process and the longer the process continues, the more severe the associated DIC.

PATHOPHYSIOLOGY

IN VIVO ACTIVATION OF THE COAGULATION SYSTEM

Two major pathways have been identified as a cause of DIC: (a) the release of procoagulant materials—such as thromboplastin-like materials, enzymes, fat, and phospholipids—into the circulation due to either vascular endothelial or tissue injury that initiates the coagulation system, and (b) a systemic inflammatory response, resulting in cytokine release.[55,56] This inflammatory response may be induced by exposure to bacterial cell membrane components (i.e., lipopolysaccharides or endotoxins) or bacterial exotoxins. Endothelial damage may result in the activation of coagulation, with platelet aggregation and activation of clotting factors.[55,57,58] Activation of either the intrinsic or extrinsic pathway results in intravascular thrombin generation. The smooth layer lining the vascular endothelium normally repels clotting factors and platelets.

TABLE 33.3	Conditions Associated with Disseminated Intravascular Coagulation (DIC)

Acute (Fulminant)

Septicemia	Tissue injury	Acute liver disease
Bacterial	Burns	Obstructive jaundice
Gram-negative (endotoxin)	Crush injuries and tissue necrosis	Acute hepatic failure
Gram-positive (mucopolysaccharides)	Multiple trauma	Prosthetic devices
Viremia	Head trauma	LeVeen or Denver shunt
Cytomegalovirus	Extensive surgery	Aortic balloon assist device
Hepatitis	Malignancy	Cardiovascular
Varicella	Leukemia	Postcardiac arrest
Human immunodeficiency virus (HIV)	Acute promyelocytic (M-3)	Aortic aneurysm
Rickettsial	Acute myelomonocytic (M-4)	Giant hemangiomas
Rocky mountain spotted fever	Most metastatic solid tumors	Acute myocardial infarctio
		Peripheral vascular disorders

Chronic (Low Grade)

Malignancy	Collagen vascular disorders	Hematologic disorders
Leukemia	Systemic lupus erythematosus	Polycythemia rubra vera
Most metastatic solid tumors	Rheumatoid arthritis	Inflammatory disorders
Cardiovascular disease	Sjögren's syndrome	Crohn's disease
Aortic aneurysm	Dermatomyositis	Ulcerative colitis
Giant hemangioma	Renal vascular disorders	Sarcoidosis
		Eclampsia

(From Gilbert JA, Scalzi RP. Disseminated intravascular coagulation. Emerg Med Clin North Am 11:465–480, 1993, and Bick RL. Disseminated intravascular coagulation: objective criteria for diagnosis and management. Med Clin North Am 78:511–543, 1994.)

INTRAVASCULAR FIBRIN CLOT FORMATION WITH END-ORGAN DAMAGE

In the presence of thrombin, fibrinogen is cleaved into fibrinopeptides A and B and fibrin monomer (Fig. 33.3, left path).[57] Fibrin monomer is then polymerized to form a fibrin clot. This results in micro- and macrovascular thrombosis, impeding blood flow and causing peripheral ischemia and end-organ damage, which can be extensive. As polymerized fibrin is deposited in the microvascular circulation, platelets are trapped, resulting in thrombocytopenia.

ACTIVATION OF THE FIBRINOLYTIC SYSTEMS

Fibrin clot activates the fibrinolytic system, beginning with plasminogen conversion to plasmin by t-PA (Fig. 33.4). Systemic plasmin cleaves fibrinogen into FDPs, with formation of fragments X, Y, D, and E. The FDPs also complex with fibrin monomers, solubilizing the monomer—called a soluble-fibrin monomer. All of these events act to further impair hemostasis and promote hemorrhage.[57]

DEPLETION OF BLOOD COAGULATION PROTEINS AND PLATELETS

The ongoing processes of fibrin formation and breakdown result in consumptive depletion of coagulation factors, natural anticoagulants, and platelets. The intensity and duration of the DIC determine the degree of depletion.

PATHOPHYSIOLOGY SUMMARY

The simultaneous presence of thrombin and plasmin in the systemic circulation generates a paradox of concurrent clotting and bleeding. Polymerized fibrin clot and microthrombi result in thrombosis and ischemia. At the same time, fibrinolysis, depletion of coagulation factors, natural anticoagulant proteins, and platelets, coupled with the platelet function disorder, cause hemorrhage. Depending on the balance between coagulation and fibrinolysis, both processes may be clinically evident in DIC, although sometimes one dominates. In infection, thrombosis usually predominates. In acute leukemia, bleeding is the primary manifestation.[58]

CLINICAL PRESENTATION AND DIAGNOSIS

The diagnosis of DIC is established when all four processes previously noted occur in a patient who also has a condition that is known to be a precipitating cause of DIC. Prompt diagnosis requires a high index of suspicion and aggressive laboratory testing. Signs and symptoms are variable and confusing because of the wide spectrum of manifestations contributed by the coagulopathy and the underlying disease. In some patients the diagnosis is obvious (e.g., gangrene of the extremities, bleeding, and multiorgan failure in a patient with

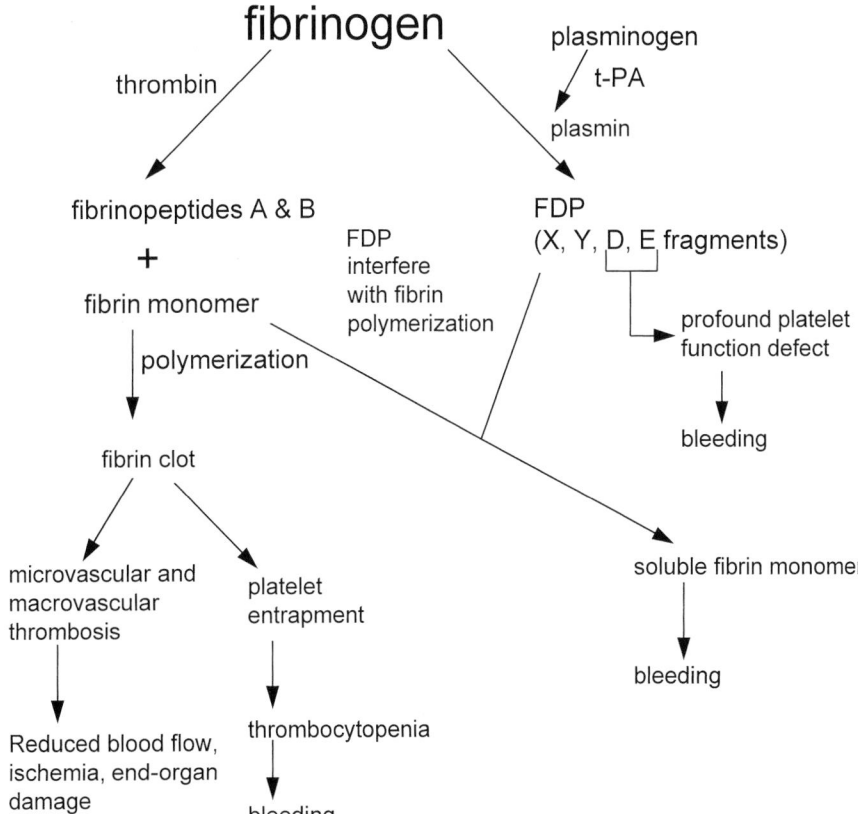

FIGURE 33.3 Pathogenesis of disseminated intravascular coagulation. *FDP,* fibrin degradation product; *t-PA,* tissue plasminogen activator.

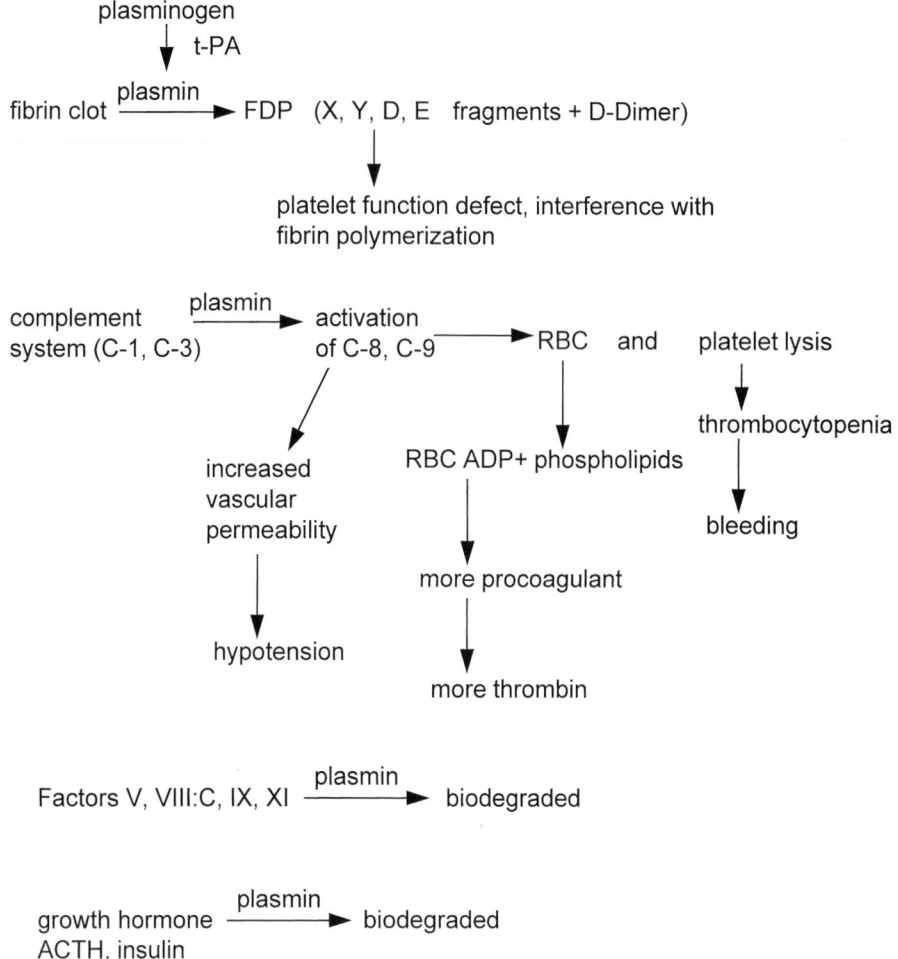

FIGURE 33.4 Additional actions of plasmin. *ACTH,* adrenocorticotropic hormone; *FDP,* fibrin degradation product; *RBC,* red blood cell; *t-PA,* tissue plasminogen activator.

meningococcemia). In others there may be mild or no bleeding at all, clinically silent microvascular thrombosis, and only subtle laboratory abnormalities. A single patient may manifest one or more of these findings alone, simultaneously, or serially at different times in the disease process.[59] The signs and symptoms of the underlying disorder further complicate the clinical presentation. The total picture for an individual patient therefore reflects both the DIC and the underlying disorder and depends on the tissues and organs that are involved and the severity of the DIC and disease processes. Vigilant correlation of physical examination and laboratory results is essential in the diagnosis, management, and evaluation of DIC.

In general, there are two modes of presentation of DIC: acute and chronic (also called low-grade or compensated DIC). In chronic DIC, subacute bleeding and diffuse thromboses may be present in place of massive hemorrhage.[57,60] This is generally the result of a decrease in production and an increase in the turnover of factors associated with hemostasis. Acute (''fulminant'') DIC is more common than the chronic form. In acute DIC the clinical and laboratory features develop rapidly (over a few hours to days), often with catastrophic consequences. The patient is critically ill from the underlying disease as well as from the DIC. Acute DIC

usually presents with both bleeding and thrombosis, bleeding being more clinically evident in most patients. Hemorrhage can range from low-grade oozing to massive bleeding. Bleeding from unrelated, multiple sites (at least three) is usually seen, because even small wounds lack normal hemostasis (Table 33.4). Areas of trauma, sites of surgical or other invasive procedures (including venipuncture sites or intra-arterial lines), or other area with pathologic manifestations are common sources of bleeding. In the skin, microvascular thrombosis of end-arterioles with concurrent bleeding results in petechiae and purpura, hemorrhagic bullae, and even gangrene.[57] End-organ dysfunction secondary to microvascular and macrovascular thrombosis is also common, although organ failure may also be caused by the underlying disease. End-organ malfunction is often less evident clinically but requires early identification and treatment to avoid irreversible damage. The organ systems affected most often (respiratory, renal, central nervous, cardiovascular, and hepatic) exhibit progressive organ failure (see Table 33.4). Fluid and electrolyte disorders, hypotension, and fever are also common. Pallor and jaundice secondary to microangiopathic hemolytic anemia are less common. The intermingling of these findings with those of the underlying disease

TABLE 33.4	Signs and Symptoms of Acute Disseminated Intravascular Coagulation

Hemorrhage	Thrombosis
Surgical or trauma sites	Skin and soft tissue
Wound bleeding	Cyanosis of hands, feet, nose, cheeks
Internal bleeding	Acral cyanosis
Skin and soft tissue	Cold, mottled fingers, toes, hands, feet
Oozing at venipuncture, IV catheter insertion, and arterial-line sites	Purpura
	Infarction, necrosis or gangrene of digits, hands, feet, nose, earlobes
Petechiae, purpura	Venous thromboembolism
Ecchymoses	End-organ dysfunction
Spreading hematomas	Lung (hypoxia, acidosis, respiratory failure, ARDS)
Hemorrhagic bullae	Kidney (elevated BUN, creatinine, oliguria, proteinuria, hematuria, acute renal failure)
Ear, nose, throat	
Gingival or oral mucosal bleeding	Central nervous system (altered mental status, seizures, coma)
Epistaxis	
Respiratory	Cardiovascular (hypotension, shock, hemodynamic instability or failure)
Blood-tinged respiratory secretions	Liver (elevated ALT, AST)
Gastrointestinal	Gastrointestinal (vomiting, diarrhea, abdominal distress, ileus)
Hematemesis	
Blood in nasogastric secretions (occult or gross)	
Fecal blood (occult or gross)	
Urinary	
Hematuria	

ARDS, adult respiratory distress syndrome; BUN, blood urea nitrogen; ALT, alanine aminotransferase; AST, aspartate aminotransferase.
(From Gilbert JA, Scalzi RP. Disseminated intravascular coagulation. Emerg Med Clin North Am 11:465–480, 1993, and Rubin RN, Coleman RW. Disseminated intravascular coagulation: approach to treatment. Drugs 44:963–971, 1992.)

make the diagnosis of DIC impossible without coagulation studies.

Currently, there is no one single laboratory test that can accurately diagnose DIC.[55] In practice, many clinicians use a combination of laboratory tests—platelet count, clotting times (aPTT and PT), protamine sulfate measurement of clotting factors and inhibitors, and FDP measurements—to aid in the diagnosis of DIC. However, abnormal findings in some of these measures may be due to other disorders.[56,57] A number of other laboratory tests have been shown to have a reliability of 75% or greater—prothrombin fragment (PF) 1 + 2, fibrinopeptides A and B, and antithrombin—but these are generally not widely available[55–57,59] (Table 33.5). FDP levels are elevated in almost all patients with DIC; FDP levels are considered a sensitive but not specific test for DIC, because they do not distinguish between fibrin versus fibrinogen degradation. D-dimer is a specific biochemical marker for fibrin breakdown; assays are therefore more use-

ful, although they are not always available.[57,58] Thrombocytopenia is a cardinal finding. The platelet count is less than 50,000 to 60,000/mm^3 in about 50% of patients (range 2,000 to 100,000/mm^3). Results of platelet function tests such as template bleeding time or platelet aggregation studies are abnormal in almost all patients as well.[57,58] The plasma fibrinogen level is less than 150 mg/dL in 70% to 80% of patients; levels less than 50 mg/dL are often associated with severe bleeding. A normal fibrinogen level may be observed in DIC associated with pregnancy, sepsis, or malignancy, because the baseline fibrinogen level may be elevated in these conditions.[33–35] Conversely, liver disease is associated with low baseline fibrinogen levels. The protamine sulfate test measures the presence of circulating soluble fibrin monomer. It is usually positive in patients with DIC, although it is not specific for this disease process. The PT is prolonged in 50% to 75% of patients with DIC, owing to factor consumption.[58] However, because the PT is normal

TABLE 33.5	Laboratory Findings in Acute Disseminated Intravascular Coagulation	
	Reference Range	**Findings in DIC**
Fibrin degradation products	<10 µg/mL	Increased
D-dimer	<500 ng/mL	Increased
Platelet count	150,000–400,000/mm^3	Decreased
Fibrinogen	200–400 mg/dL	Decreased
Protamine sulfate	Negative	Positive
Prothrombin time	0.88–1.12 INR	Increased

INR, international normalized ratio.
(From Nachman RL, Silverstein R. Hypercoagulable states. Ann Intern Med 119:819–827, 1993; Levi M. Current understanding of disseminated intravascular coagulation. Br J Haematol 124:567–576, 2004; Rick R. Disseminated intravascular coagulation: current concepts of etiology, pathophysiology, diagnosis, and treatment. Hematol Oncol Clin North Am 17:115–147, 2003; Alving BM. The hypercoagulable states. Hosp Pract 28:109–121, 1993; Eby CS. A review of the hypercoagulable state. Hematol Oncol Clin North Am 7:1121–1142, 1993.)

or even shorter than the control time in as many as 50% of patients, this test is less useful for diagnosing DIC.

Other laboratory tests are commonly performed in the screening and evaluation of patients with suspected acute DIC but have limited value. These include the aPTT, thrombin clotting time (TT), euglobulin clot lysis time, coagulation factor assays, and peripheral blood smear examination. The aPTT is prolonged in 50% to 60% of patients with acute DIC, but it may also be normal or short[57,58] and is therefore unreliable for patient assessment. Likewise, the TT may be prolonged, the euglobulin clot lysis time may be shortened, and blood coagulation factor levels are often low, but these findings are not reliable and do not add meaningful information. Examination of a peripheral blood smear provides evidence of RBC fragmentation, mild reticulocytosis, mild leukocytosis with a mild to moderate shift to immature neutrophil forms (''left shift''), and thrombocytopenia with large young platelets. Unfortunately, these findings also lack specificity and sensitivity.

Chronic DIC is characterized by abnormal low-grade coagulation and fibrinolysis accompanying an array of less acute conditions (Table 33.4). Chronic DIC is thought to be less common than the acute form. However, the subtle manifestations of this form may contribute to underdiagnosis. Many believe that acute and chronic DIC are simply different phases in the continuum of a single disease. Chronic DIC is not generally considered an emergency. Clinical findings are less florid, and laboratory abnormalities are more subtle. Enhanced turnover with increased production of platelets, fibrinogen, and coagulation proteins may yield normal or near-normal levels. If the rate of fibrinolysis is sufficient to balance the rate of fibrin formation, there may be no obvious clinical symptoms. Patients with chronic DIC uniformly have elevated D-dimer levels. Measurement

of D-dimer (or FDP) levels is therefore very useful in establishing the diagnosis.

Over time patients with chronic DIC may develop overt problems, especially thrombotic complications such as thrombophlebitis, PE, or stroke.[59,61] Patients with metastatic malignancies often manifest DIC as a ''hypercoagulable syndrome'' with recurrent local or diffuse thrombotic events. Trousseau's syndrome, a recurrent migratory venous thrombosis, is a variant of this condition.[61] Subacute or ''bothersome'' bleeding may also be seen. Patients with chronic DIC may develop the acute form with hemostatic stress, such as surgery or invasive procedures.

In summary, no single physical finding or laboratory test is diagnostic for acute or chronic DIC. Careful physical examination and laboratory assessment, combined with vigilance and good judgment, are essential in establishing the diagnosis. Normal D-dimer (or FDP) levels make DIC unlikely. A combination of elevated D-dimer (or FDP) level, thrombocytopenia, low or falling fibrinogen (in the absence of liver disease), a positive protamine sulfate test, and a prolonged PT in a patient with a disease known to cause DIC will establish the diagnosis in most patients, with the degree of abnormality roughly correlating with disease acuity. These tests are also the most useful in monitoring the response to therapy.

MANAGEMENT

The cornerstone of DIC management is treatment of the underlying disease and supportive therapy for the signs and symptoms.[55,56] For some patients, aggressive control of the underlying disease may result in resolution of bleeding. Antibiotic therapy for sepsis and evacuation of the uterus for an obstetric accident are examples in which successful treatment of the underlying disorder alone may resolve the DIC. In addition, vigorous supportive therapy for control of acid–base, fluid and electrolyte, hemodynamic, respiratory, and renal disturbances may be needed. Intramuscular medications and venipunctures should be minimized to avoid additional sites of bleeding and hematoma formation. Frequent clinical and laboratory monitoring is essential. With aggressive therapy and improvement in laboratory parameters, additional treatment should be needed only transiently or may even be unnecessary. Careful observation and follow-up may be the only additional measures required.[56,62] In other situations, efforts to treat the precipitating disease are unsuccessful or inadequate, or the manifestations fail to resolve. Patients with acute leukemia may even experience an initial worsening of the DIC after administration of chemotherapy, owing to massive blast cell lysis with subsequent generation of large amounts of procoagulant.

Specific treatment modalities for acute DIC beyond supportive care and treatment of the underlying diseases are highly controversial, are poorly documented, and lack consensus. A general lack of prospective randomized clinical trials exists, largely because of the complex spectrum of underlying diseases and clinical manifestations. Published trials are difficult to compare because of differences in diagnostic and outcome criteria. Moreover, patient outcomes are often dependent more on the underlying disease than on the DIC. Individualization of therapy is essential. Treatment may involve measures to (a) interrupt the coagulation process, (b) replace depleted coagulation factors and platelets, and (c) interrupt fibrinolysis.

Measures to interrupt the coagulation process include administration of anticoagulants and replacement of natural anticoagulant proteins. Although bleeding is often more obvious and alarming, thrombosis is more dangerous and has a greater impact on morbidity and mortality because of its potential to cause irreversible ischemic end-organ damage.[58] Heparin has been used in the treatment of DIC for nearly 50 years, although data from controlled studies are lacking.[56,63] Anecdotal evidence suggests that some patients benefit in terms of hemorrhage control and survival.[59,64] Because bleeding in acute DIC is caused by massive coagulation cascade activation with subsequent depletion of clotting factors and platelets, it seems reasonable to interrupt this process with heparin. Heparin will also inhibit growth of existing thrombi, thereby stabilizing the coagulation system while the underlying disease is treated.[57,59,61] However, some clinicians do not advocate the routine use of heparin for all patients with DIC, in part because the safety of heparin in patients prone to bleeding is unknown.[56,62,63] Heparin is clearly indicated for patients with clinically evident thromboembolism or fibrin deposits (e.g., those with purpura fulminans or acral ischemia).[61] Dosages of 5 to 8 U/kg/hour or 300 to 500 units per hour have been recommended, possibly in combination with plasma and platelet replacement if appropriate.[55,63] All patients should be carefully monitored

for evidence of microvascular and macrovascular thrombosis, including progressive organ failure (Table 33.4). Immediate heparin therapy is required if necrosis, gangrene, and irreversible end-organ damage are to be prevented.

The timing of heparin administration relative to blood component replacement in patients with hemorrhage but no clinical evidence of thrombosis is debatable. Many clinicians recommend anticoagulants before blood component replacement therapy. This is based on the theory that administration of more coagulation factors and platelets will only increase coagulation unless the thrombosis has been interrupted; moreover, the exogenous blood components will be rapidly depleted and therefore will not be effective for stopping the hemorrhage.[57,59] Others disagree on the premise that early administration of heparin may worsen bleeding. These clinicians base the initial treatment on the dominant abnormality (i.e., anticoagulants for thrombosis, replacement therapy for hemorrhage).[58]

LMWHs have also been used in the treatment of DIC, due to their lower risk of bleeding compared to unfractionated heparin (UFH).[63,65] The anticoagulant effect of UFH occurs via complexation with antithrombin III, which inhibits activated coagulation factors, principally thrombin and factor Xa. LMWHs possess selective antifactor Xa properties and do not inhibit thrombin. They do not markedly prolong the aPTT and have less effect on platelet activation and aggregation than UFH does; these attributes have translated into a lower incidence of bleeding with LMWHs. This offers attractive possibilities in treating patients with DIC, because LMWHs may therefore abort thrombus formation without exacerbating bleeding. A double-blind randomized study of intravenous dalteparin versus UFH in 126 patients suggested a more favorable profile for dalteparin with respect to improvement of clinical symptoms and safety, although there was no difference in overall efficacy.[66] A dose-finding trial of dalteparin[37] and case studies using enoxaparin[67] have been reported with promising results.

Contraindications to heparin in any form include CNS bleeding (e.g., intracranial or subarachnoid hemorrhage or subdural hematoma), bleeding into other closed spaces where vital functions might be compromised (e.g., intraspinal, pericardial, or peritracheal hemorrhage), and DIC associated with fulminant liver failure.[56,61] Caution should also be used when treating patients with a high risk of heparin-induced bleeding (e.g., those with intracranial metastases, severe hypertension, or a recent history of peptic ulcer disease).

Depletion of natural anticoagulant proteins (antithrombin and proteins C and S) is another important contributor to clotting in patients with acute DIC. Antithrombin depletion may be particularly significant, because it is an anticoagulant (Fig. 33.1) and is also required for the in vivo activity of heparin. Restoration and maintenance of adequate antithrombin levels may therefore ameliorate the coagulopathy via both direct and indirect mechanisms. Antithrombin administration may be especially useful in treating patients with acute DIC with bleeding, because it does not exacerbate hemorrhage. Patients with apparent heparin resistance or those with severe bleeding may benefit from antithrombin replacement via transfusion with FFP or antithrombin concentrate. FFP has the advantages of containing multiple coagulation proteins and derivation from a single donor, but the large volumes that are required may be a limitation.

Antithrombin concentrate (Thrombate-III, Talecris Biotherapeutics) is a plasma-derived heat-treated preparation of purified human antithrombin, the major plasma inhibitor of thrombin. It has been studied alone and in combination with heparin in treating acute DIC, primarily in patients with sepsis, septic shock, or both.[56,63] Overall, antithrombin concentrate has provided some beneficial effect in patients with DIC, shortening the duration of the disorder, with improvements in laboratory parameters or organ function.[68–70] An important finding in one study[70] was a significantly higher RBC transfusion requirement in the group receiving both antithrombin and heparin, yielding the conclusion that antithrombin alone was effective and had a more favorable safety profile. Clinical improvement has also been shown in a cohort of children[71] and in a patient with recurrent multisite arterial thrombosis refractory to heparin.[72] Limited data also support efficacy in DIC associated with pregnancy or acute fatty liver of pregnancy. However, a significant effect on mortality was not observed, even when antithrombin concentrate was administered at high doses.[56,69,73] In a double-blind, placebo-controlled trial, 2,314 adult patients with severe sepsis were randomly assigned to treatment with antithrombin concentrate (6,000 units as a loading dose followed by 6,000 units daily given as a continuous infusion) or placebo.[73] Heparin (UFH or LMWH) at a dose of 10,000 units or less per day could also be administered. No difference was seen between the two groups in 28-day mortality, the primary outcome (38.7% vs. 38.9% for placebo). In addition, 28-day mortality was increased when antithrombin concentrate was used in combination with any heparin, including heparin flushes for catheter patency compared to antithrombin concentrate without heparin, as was the risk of bleeding. Based on available data, the role of antithrombin concentrates in patients with sepsis and DIC is unclear.[60]

Two important considerations specific to the use of antithrombin concentrate in treating acute DIC are a shorter half-life, which necessitates twice-daily initial administration,[40] and the interaction between antithrombin and heparin. Some clinicians administer heparin only after antithrombin functional levels >70% have been established,[67,70] because the efficacy of heparin depends on the presence of antithrombin. Patients who are already receiving heparin before antithrombin may demonstrate a markedly enhanced heparin effect after antithrombin is added. Careful monitoring of heparin dosing is therefore important in this scenario.

Protein C is another natural anticoagulant (Fig. 33.1) that is commonly depleted in acute DIC. In one study, a recombinant protein C (drotrecogin alfa) was investigated for its effects on organ dysfunction in patients with severe sepsis.

A total of 1,690 adult patients with severe sepsis received recombinant protein C (24 μg/kg/hour) or placebo as a 96-hour infusion. Significant reductions in organ dysfunction (cardiovascular and respiratory) were seen with recombinant protein C compared to placebo.[56,74] In addition, recombinant protein C was associated with resolution of coagulation abnormalities compared to placebo. An independent, unpublished analysis of the outcomes of this study found a greater benefit from recombinant protein C among patients with overt DIC at study entry, with a relative risk reduction in mortality of 38% with recombinant protein C compared to 18% for patients without DIC.[56]

TREATMENT

REPLACEMENT OF DEPLETED COAGULATION FACTORS AND PLATELETS

Blood component replacement therapy is indicated when the patient continues to have active bleeding after initial supportive measures or when an invasive procedure or surgery is required.[56,60,62,63] Although clinical trial data are unavailable, the use of blood components is still recommended as rational therapy. If depletion of coagulation factors and platelets is believed to be a major cause of bleeding, replenishment may slow hemorrhage. It is unnecessary in most patients with chronic DIC (factors are not usually depleted) and may even be harmful for patients with gross thrombosis (may cause thrombus extension).

Replacement therapy includes platelets, FFP, and cryoprecipitate.[55,62] If bleeding is severe, administration of packed RBCs may also be necessary. Platelet transfusions are indicated for marked thrombocytopenia (platelet count <50,000/mm^3 in patients with bleeding or undergoing invasive procedures or <20,000/mm^3 if no bleeding is present) or for ongoing hemorrhage.[60,62] At least 5 to 10 units of platelet concentrate (or 0.1 units/kg) should be given.[58] One or two units of FFP (or 10 to 15 mL/kg) or 15 units of cryoprecipitate (or 0.2 bag/kg) usually improve factor deficiencies.[58] Use of FFP requires administration of larger volumes but is advantageous because it contains clotting factors plus antithrombin and proteins C and S. However, because of the differences in the half-life of the various coagulation factors contained in FFP, an imbalance of the factors may occur with repeated administration of FFP.[60] Cryoprecipitate contains 10 times more fibrinogen per unit than FFP. It is indicated for patients with very low fibrinogen levels (<50 mg/dL) or those with fibrinogen levels less than 100 mg/dL who are bleeding.

Use of coagulation factor concentrates, such as factor IX complexes (also known as prothrombin complex concentrate), may avoid the need for large volumes of plasma. Factor IX complexes may be useful for patients with sepsis and vitamin K deficiency or in combination with FFP.[60] Doses of 20 to 30 units per kg have been recommended. However, some essential factors may be missing in factor IX complexes if used alone, and there is still concern that the trace amounts of activated factors present may worsen the coagulation disorder.[55,56] Factor VIII concentrates are not appropriate, because DIC depletes multiple coagulation factors. However, several case reports have described the successful use of recombinant factor VIIa in the treatment of DIC bleeding refractory to other therapies. Bolus doses of 60 to 120 μg/kg have been used, repeated every 2 to 6 hours if needed. Administration of platelets may be needed if platelet counts are less than 20,000/mm^3.[60,75,76]

The timing of blood component administration in the management of acute DIC is controversial. If given while clotting is still ongoing, exogenous coagulation factors will simply be integrated into the coagulation process; this will not elevate factor levels and may even worsen the thrombosis. Although this "fuel-the-fire" scenario is theoretically possible and may rarely occur, it has not been substantiated with clinical trials.[56,60,61,64] Nonetheless, many believe that factor replacement should be withheld until intravascular clotting has been suspended with heparin, especially when using components containing fibrinogen.[58,59] After intravascular clotting has been interrupted, any depleted component can be given; this should raise factor levels and reduce bleeding. If heparin is contraindicated, products with high fibrinogen content (e.g., FFP and cryoprecipitate) should be avoided.

Vitamin K deficiency may occur in patients with acute DIC, depending on the degree and duration of DIC, whether factor replacement is given, the type of nutritional support given, and other issues such as administration of broad-spectrum antibiotics. In patients with vitamin K deficiency, supplementation will facilitate production of vitamin K-dependent clotting factors.

INTERRUPTION OF FIBRINOLYSIS

Fibrinolytic (or fibrinogenolytic) inhibitors such as ε-amino-caproic acid or tranexamic acid are generally not recommended in patients with DIC. Although successful use of tranexamic acid in patients with DIC refractory to heparin, antithrombin III, and FFP has been reported, antifibrinolytics are thought to block the already compromised fibrinolytic system, allowing for increased deposition of fibrin.[55,63,77] If intravascular clotting has not been suspended before use, antifibrinolytics may cause catastrophic widespread fibrin deposition in the microcirculation, leading to irreversible ischemic multiorgan damage, which is sometimes fatal.[61] These agents should be used with extreme caution and always with concurrent heparin therapy. They should be restricted to last-recourse situations with life-threatening bleeding or evidence of extensive secondary fibrinolysis and after failure of other therapies.[58,61] An exception to this is the patient with acute promyelocytic leukemia, who may have primary activation of both the coagulation and fibrinolytic systems caused by the malignancy. When antifibrinolytics are used in conjunction with other modalities, the benefits may outweigh the risks for these patients.

OTHER THERAPIES

Exchange transfusions are sometimes used in the treatment of DIC. Plasma exchange, plasmapheresis, leukapheresis, and whole blood exchange have been used. The efficacy of exchange or pheresis procedures is thought to be related to removal of FDPs, activated clotting factors, and toxins from the patient's plasma, all of which aggravate bleeding.[64,78] Replacement of antithrombin, proteins C and S, and other proteins in the exchanged plasma may also contribute to a successful outcome by re-establishing the normal balance of circulating coagulation factors and natural anticoagulants.[79] Exchange transfusion is not considered part of the routine management of DIC because of its associated risks and the need for specialized equipment and trained personnel. In one published report, 76 patients with DIC and sepsis underwent plasma exchange in addition to standard therapies (UFH or LMWH, corticosteroids, antibiotics, fluids, inotropes). Plasma exchange was performed until improvements in coagulation were seen, with a median of two exchanges reported (range 1 to 14). A beneficial effect was seen, with a reported survival rate of 82%.[78]

A number of drugs for the management of acute DIC are being clinically investigated or have been reported as successful in case reports.[55,63] These include gabexate mesilate (FOY), a synthetic inhibitor of serine proteases in the coagulation, fibrinolysis, and other systems (complement, kinins, prostaglandins, superoxide). Gabexate has antithrombin and antiplasmin effects that are independent of antithrombin and account for its efficacy in acute DIC.[80–82] Recombinant nematode anticoagulant protein c2 is an antithrombotic agent that exerts its effect through inhibition of tissue factor/factor VIIa after initially binding with activated factor X.[83,84] This protein was originally isolated from the hematophagous hookworm *Ancylostoma caninum*. Additional agents that are under research include recombinant human soluble thrombomodulin (rhs-TM), recombinant hirudin (including lepirudin, as well as other direct antithrombotic agents such as argatroban), and an inhibitor of factor Xa (DX-9065).[85,86]

MONITORING PARAMETERS FOR ACUTE DIC

All patients with acute DIC should have regular monitoring of fibrinogen levels, D-dimer (or FDP) levels, protamine sulfate test results, and platelet counts. Measurements of antithrombin levels and other biochemical markers (PF 1 + 2, fibrinopeptides A and B) are also useful if available. Attainment and maintenance of adequate fibrinogen levels and platelet counts, with falling D-dimer (or FDP) levels, normal protamine sulfate test results, and stable hematocrit are indicators of successful interruption of the coagulopathy. Initial monitoring every 6 to 12 hours is appropriate, with once-daily assessment after the patient's condition is stable. Changes in the balance between fibrinogen synthesis and consumption can be seen within hours, whereas it may take 1 to 2 days for platelet and D-dimer (or FDP) levels to show meaningful trends.[64] In patients with certain conditions, such as acute leukemia, D-dimer levels will increase initially, then decline. Clinical response begins shortly after improvement in laboratory parameters,[57] with stabilization of bleeding, thrombosis, and end-organ dysfunction. Blood pressure, cardiac output, systemic vascular resistance, the Glasgow Coma Scale score, and urine output may be measured, as well as arterial blood gases, serum BUN, creatinine, alanine aminotransferase, and aspartate aminotransferase. A reduction in the need for continued use of pressor agents, ventilators, dialysis, and transfusion of coagulation factors, platelets, and packed RBCs also indicates improvement. Of course, improvement or worsening of the underlying disease will also influence the patient's clinical status.

Patients who are receiving heparin require additional monitoring. aPTT, TT, PT, and hematocrit are measured 4 to 6 hours after initiation of heparin and every 12 to 24 hours thereafter. Although the aPTT is a primary tool for monitoring and adjusting heparin therapy in other situations, most patients with acute DIC have an abnormal baseline aPTT. The aPTT therefore provides limited guidance, as do plasma heparin levels. The inability to ameliorate the general manifestations of acute DIC as described earlier (e.g., D-dimer, fibrinogen) can indicate a need to increase the heparin dose. In general, heparin should be continued until the fibrinogen level is greater than 100 mg/dL and the platelet count is greater than 100,000/mm³. The hematocrit should also be monitored frequently to assess both beneficial and adverse effects of heparin.

Patients who are receiving antithrombin (either via FFP or antithrombin concentrate) should have plasma antithrombin levels measured every 12 hours until their condition is stable and then daily. Clinical improvement should occur in 1 to 3 days.

Objective measures of successful management in patients who are receiving coagulation factor or platelet transfusions include an increase in platelet count and plasma fibrinogen concentration, as well as the criteria reviewed earlier for the general monitoring of acute DIC. Platelet and fibrinogen levels should be determined 30 to 60 minutes after a transfusion and every 6 to 12 hours thereafter until they are stable. With effective therapy, the fibrinogen concentration and platelet count should stabilize and then increase. Similarly, clinical improvement, measured as a slowing and then cessation of bleeding, occurs over several days. A subsequent need for transfusion will depend on clinical response, treatment of the underlying disorder, and the half-life of the platelets and clotting factors. Once consumption is interrupted, the bone marrow and liver usually take several days to replenish endogenous platelet and fibrinogen levels.

Treatment of the precipitating disorder and supportive therapy for clinical manifestations should be the first steps for chronic DIC. For some patients, especially those who are asymptomatic and have a correctable underlying disease,

these alone are adequate. Careful observation and follow-up are essential, because these patients can develop acute florid DIC when they are subjected to stressors such as surgery, invasive procedures, infection, or disease progression.[61,64]

Patients who have DVT should be managed with intravenous heparin at standard therapeutic doses (20,000 to 30,000 U/day via constant intravenous infusion). LMWH has also been used.[65] Special care should be exercised when treating patients with intracranial metastases or other risk factors for bleeding. Oral anticoagulants are only rarely successful in treating patients with thrombotic complications of chronic DIC. DIC associated with neoplastic disease is caused by direct activation of the extrinsic pathway via release of procoagulant material from the malignant cells. Warfarin and other coumarin derivatives are not effective in this situation because they simply reduce the amounts of activated vitamin K-dependent clotting factors but will not otherwise affect coagulation and fibrinolysis. Patients who require long-term secondary prophylaxis of thrombotic events in these situations should receive chronic subcutaneous heparin.[59] Patients with untreatable malignancies and other persistent symptoms of DIC should also be managed with subcutaneous heparin. The use of antiplatelet agents (e.g., aspirin, dipyridamole) and pentoxifylline is controversial. Some advocates believe that they may correct coagulation parameters and reduce bleeding or thrombosis[58]; others find no documented clinical benefit.[61] Replacement therapy with blood components or antifibrinolytic drugs is rarely necessary for patients with chronic DIC.

Monitoring parameters for chronic DIC include routine assessment of signs and symptoms. If treatment is given, D-dimer (or FDP) and fibrinogen levels, protamine sulfate test results, and platelet counts should be monitored. Patients receiving long-term heparin therapy should be monitored and counseled.

PROGNOSIS

Much remains to be investigated regarding the pathophysiology and management of DIC. Randomized controlled large-scale trials have been difficult to perform because of the broad spectra of underlying diseases, diagnostic criteria, and outcome measurements. Most clinicians therefore base their treatment decisions on clinical judgment and prior experience.

Acute DIC may be an incidental preterminal event occurring in a variety of acute catastrophic illnesses. It may be brief and end promptly with effective treatment of the underlying disorder. Alternatively, patients may die of hemorrhage and progression of the underlying disorder. Mortality rates for patients with acute DIC are reported to be 50% to 85%. However, this may be more reflective of the mortality rates of the precipitating disorders rather than DIC. Morbidity and mortality are reduced with early recognition and aggressive treatment of DIC; however, the prognosis may not improve until better methods of prevention and treatment of the underlying disorders become available.

Some patients with chronic DIC may be asymptomatic, with only laboratory evidence of the disorder. Others may have recurrent episodes of thromboembolism requiring long-term therapy with subcutaneous heparin for prophylaxis. In most cases the prognosis for chronic DIC is related to that of the precipitating disease rather than the treatment strategy.

HYPERCOAGULABLE STATES

Hypercoagulable states involve a number of conditions that share the common endpoint of inappropriate thrombus formation.[87] Patients with these disorders are at higher risk for both venous and arterial thromboembolic disease. Disruption of coagulation may occur on an inherited (primary) or acquired (secondary) basis. Inherited hypercoagulable disorders are abnormalities in the synthesis or function of various proteins in the coagulation and fibrinolytic systems. Exaggerated formation or impaired breakdown of fibrin results in clotting, which may occur in the microvasculature or in large vessels such as the iliac veins. Acquired disorders include a wide spectrum of conditions associated with an enhanced risk of thromboembolism. Acquired risk factors for venous thromboembolism (Table 33.6) are varied, including production of abnormal proteins, diseases, drugs, or clinical situations. This discussion will focus on the venous manifestations of hypercoagulable states.

INHERITED HYPERCOAGULABLE STATES

As previously discussed, hemostasis is regulated by two major physiologic systems, the coagulation and fibrinolytic systems. Under normal conditions, they are intricately balanced to maintain the blood in a fluid state within the vessels while at the same time minimizing blood loss from the vasculature at sites of injury. Disruption of this intrinsic balance may result in either bleeding or thrombosis. Thrombosis occurs when large amounts of thrombin are produced via the coagulation cascade. Thrombin catalyzes the conversion of fibrinogen to fibrin, which then polymerizes to form an insoluble clot (Fig. 33.1). The fibrin clot is degraded by another endogenous cascade called the fibrinolytic system (Fig. 33.2). Physiologic inhibitors of coagulation act to either inhibit thrombin formation or enhance fibrinolysis. In this manner, almost every protein in the coagulation and fibrinolytic systems has a natural inhibitor or lytic mechanism.

A number of endogenous proteins act as major deterrents to thrombin formation and are sometimes called ''natural'' or ''physiologic'' anticoagulants. The best-understood include antithrombin, protein C, and protein S. Each has a critical role in preventing the formation of pathologic amounts of thrombin (Fig. 33.1). Patterns of inheritance, prevalence, and site(s) of endogenous production are summarized in Table 33.7.

TABLE 33.6	Acquired Risk Factors for Venous Thromboembolism

Abnormal function of the coagulation cascade or fibrinolyti system

  Surgery (especially orthopedic surgery of the lower limb)

  Trauma

  Pregnancy

  Oral contraceptives

  Infection (associated with disseminated intravascular coagulation)

  Nephrotic syndrome

  Antiphospholipid syndrome

  Hepatic insufficiency

Abnormal platelet number or function

  Myeloproliferative disorder (e.g., essential thrombocytosis)

  Paroxysmal nocturnal hemoglobinuria

Abnormal vessel endothelial cell function or blood rheology

  Stasis (prolonged sitting or bed rest, acute hemiplegia or paraplegia, congestive heart failure, varicose veins)

  Trauma

  Abnormal blood rheology (previous venous thrombosis, extrinsic compression)

  Hyperviscosity syndromes (including myeloproliferative syndromes such as polycythemia vera)

  Artificial surfaces (heart valves, vascular patches)

  Vasculitis

Miscellaneous

  Malignancy

  Obesity

  Drugs (heparin-associated thrombocytopenia, warfarin skin necrosis, antineoplastic agents)

(From Nachman RL, Silverstein R. Hypercoagulable states. Ann Intern Med 119:819–827, 1993; Alving BM. The hypercoagulable states. Hosp Pract 28:109–121, 1993; Eby CS. A review of the hypercoagulable state. Hematol Oncol Clin North Am 7:1121–1142, 1993.)

ANTITHROMBIN DEFICIENCY

In the past, a deficiency of the plasma cofactor, antithrombin, was referred to as antithrombin III deficiency, based upon an erroneous coagulation classification system.[88] Today, this blood coagulation disorder is simply referred to as antithrombin deficiency. The presence of a deficiency in antithrombin results in a markedly (5- to 50-fold) increased risk of thrombosis.[88,89] Antithrombin is a serine protease inhibitor that irreversibly complexes with factors IXa, Xa, XIa, XIIa, and thrombin[88] (Fig. 33.1). Antithrombin is considered a crucial component in limiting ongoing activation of the

| TABLE 33.7 | Natural Inhibitors of Coagulation |

			Prevalence		
	Half-Life	Inheritance	General Population	8 Reports of Unselected Patients With Thrombosis[a]	Site of Synthesis
Antithrombin III	2.5 days	Autosomal dominant	1/2,000 to 1/5,000	0.5–8%, mean 4%	Hepatocyte; vitamin K-independent
Protein C	6–8 h	Autosomal dominant	1/15,000	1.5–11.5%, mean 5.4%	Hepatocyte; vitamin K-dependent
		Autosomal recessive	1/200 to 1/300		
Protein S	Unknown	Autosomal dominant	Unknown	1.5–13.2%, mean 5.9%	Hepatocyte; vitamin K-dependent; α-Platelet granules; Endothelial cells; Megakaryocytes

[a] Data from Bick RL. Hypercoagulability and thrombosis. Med Clin North Am 78:635– 665, 1994.
(From Nachman RL, Silverstein R. Hypercoagulable states. Ann Intern Med 119:819–827, 1993; Menache D. Antithrombin III concentrates. Hematol Oncol Clin North Am 6:1115–1120, 1992; Bick RL. Hypercoagulability and thrombosis. Med Clin North Am 78:635– 665, 1994; and Marlar RA, Sills RH, Groncy PK, et al. Protein C survival during replacement therapy in homozygous protein C deficiency. Am J Hematol 41:24–31, 1992.)

coagulation pathway; it is sometimes called the primary physiologic inhibitor of in vivo coagulation. The antithrombin molecule contains not only a site responsible for inactivation of procoagulant factors, but also a heparin-binding site.[88] When heparin is administered, the ability of antithrombin to inactivate the aforementioned procoagulant factors is significantly enhanced. A deficiency of antithrombin in the blood, or a decreased ability to interact with the antithrombin molecule, may ultimately result in procoagulant effects and the eventual development of a thrombus. Assays for both the quantity (antigen) and function of antithrombin are reported as a percentage compared to normal pooled plasma; normal values for both assays range from 70% to 120% of control. Antithrombin levels in 20-week fetuses and term babies are about 25% and 50% of control, respectively; adult levels are achieved at about 6 months of age. In utero or neonatal clotting is uncommon because of a concurrent physiologic reduction in procoagulant factor levels. Antithrombin plasma levels may be measured in patients taking warfarin but should be avoided during heparin therapy and during acute thromboembolic events.

A deficiency of antithrombin may be either inherited or acquired.[90] Inherited antithrombin deficiency occurs more commonly and is an autosomal dominant trait, the effects of which are observed equally among males and females.[88] Acquired antithrombin deficiency may occur as a result of a variety of disease states affecting antithrombin serum levels, including DIC, chronic liver disease, and nephrotic syndrome.[89,90]

The estimated prevalence of antithrombin deficiency in the general population is approximately 0.02%.[88] For pa-

tients who present with a first-time thrombus, the estimated prevalence of antithrombin deficiency is 1% to 3%. Inherited antithrombin deficiency typically presents as a heterozygous state.[88–90] A homozygous state occurs rarely and results in death in utero or during infancy in most patients. In the antithrombin-deficient population, two subtypes are seen. Type I deficiency is more common and is characterized by decreased synthesis of a functionally normal antithrombin molecule (i.e., a quantitative defect). In these persons, functional and antigenic assays yield similar values; most have approximately 35% to 70% of control levels.[53,89,91–93] Formation of a biologically dysfunctional form of antithrombin (qualitative, or type II, deficiency) is less common. These persons have normal antigenic levels but abnormal antithrombin activity as measured in functional assays. Type II antithrombin deficiency has been further broken down into subtypes IIa, IIb, and IIc based on the nature of the genetic defect.[89] These subtypes typically are linked to genetic mutations at different sites within the antithrombin molecule.

The wide array of clinical manifestations of inherited antithrombin deficiency reflects an inheritance pattern with variable expression. Only moderate reductions (50% to 70% of normal) of antithrombin levels may induce thrombophilia.[79] Some patients remain asymptomatic, although many clinically asymptomatic patients have laboratory evidence of a procoagulant state.[51] In families with antithrombin deficiency, the prevalence of venous thromboembolism in heterozygotes is about 50%.[89,94] The cumulative incidence of thrombosis increases with age, with most patients having their first event in adolescence or young adulthood (10 to 35 years).[89,90] By age 50, approximately 85% of individuals with antithrombin deficiency will have experienced a thrombotic event.[89] Typically, the initial event is a DVT of a lower extremity, PE, or both. Thrombosis may also occur at unusual sites such as the upper extremity (axillary or brachial vein), viscera (mesenteric, renal, or retinal vein), cerebrum (the cerebral sinuses), or vena cava. Superficial thrombophlebitis and arterial thrombosis are relatively uncommon with antithrombin deficiency. The initial event in antithrombin deficiency usually occurs in the presence of a known thrombogenic risk factor (most commonly pregnancy or surgery/trauma but also during prolonged immobilization or exposure to other factors or drugs, as listed in Table 33.6). Recurrence of thrombosis is a common event. Apparent heparin resistance may occur with antithrombin deficiency and occasionally is a clue to its presence.

Antithrombin deficiency is also associated with a high risk of maternal and fetal complications due to the natural hypercoagulable state present during pregnancy.[95] The risk of a thromboembolic event occurring in a pregnant woman with antithrombin deficiency has been estimated to range between 44% and 70%. Of women diagnosed with a thrombotic event during pregnancy, approximately 12% are antithrombin deficient.[92,95] A significantly increased incidence of fetal morbidity and mortality is observed among pregnant women with antithrombin deficiency, manifested as spontaneous abortions, intrauterine growth retardation, and preterm delivery. Widespread microvascular thrombosis with subsequent fibrosis of the placenta has been observed and is presumed to cause placental insufficiency.[96,97] In pregnant women with antithrombin deficiency, prophylactic therapy against the formation of thromboembolism is a critical component of overall care.[95]

TREATMENT

The management of acute thromboembolism in most antithrombin-deficient patients is the same as that for the general population.[98] Unfractionated heparin, the dose being titrated according to aPTT, or LMWH should initially be administered. Treatment with warfarin should be initiated within the first 24 hours of either heparin or LMWH therapy. Heparin or LMWH administration should be continued for at least 5 days or until an international normalized ratio (INR) for warfarin of between 2 and 3 is maintained. The dose of heparin required to attain a therapeutic aPTT is not related to the degree of antithrombin deficiency. Some patients with antithrombin deficiency are resistant to treatment with heparin. This resistance occurs in part due to the ability of heparin itself to reduce antithrombin levels by approximately 30% over several days. For patients experiencing severe thrombosis, those with difficulty maintaining adequate anticoagulation, and those with recurrent thrombosis despite appropriate anticoagulation, therapy with antithrombin concentrate is recommended.

Antithrombin concentrate (Thrombate-III, Talecris Biotherapeutics) is a purified, lyophilized preparation of human antithrombin.[99–101] This pooled plasma product is currently indicated for the treatment of acute venous thromboembolism in patients with inherited antithrombin deficiency. In addition, antithrombin concentrate may be administered to patients with inherited antithrombin deficiency undergoing surgical or obstetric procedures as a preventive indication. Antithrombin concentrate is not indicated for the long-term prophylaxis of antithrombin-deficient patients.

Dosing of antithrombin concentrate should be determined on an individual basis.[99,100] A determination of a patient's baseline antithrombin level is required to calculate the appropriate amount of units of antithrombin needed. The following formula may be used to calculate the initial units required of antithrombin concentrate:

$$\text{Units required (IU)} = \frac{[\text{desired} - \text{baseline antithrombin level}] \times \text{weight (kg)}}{1.4} \quad (33.1)$$

A common initial "desired" antithrombin level is 120% of normal. The formula is based upon an expected increase above baseline antithrombin levels of 1.4% per IU per kilogram administered.[99,100] The antithrombin concentrate dosing formula is intended only as a guide for clinicians. Improvements in recovery of antithrombin levels above baseline may vary from patient to patient; therefore, antithrombin levels should be drawn not only at baseline but also 20 minutes after infusion. The observed recovery with the initial dose of antithrombin concentrate can be used to determine subsequent dosing.

The goal of therapy is to maintain a plasma antithrombin level of 80% to 120%. Normally, goal plasma levels may be preserved by administering maintenance doses that are 60% of the initial loading dose every 24 hours. After administration of the initial antithrombin concentrate dose, antithrombin plasma levels should be obtained at least every 12 hours and also prior to the next dose.[100] More frequent monitoring of antithrombin levels may be needed in situations where the half-life (normal biologic half-life of 2.8 to 4.8 days) of antithrombin is reduced, such as after surgery, during acute thrombosis, and when heparin therapy is administered.[98,100] Antithrombin levels should be maintained at goal for 2 to 8 days, depending on the indication, type of surgery, past medical history of the patient, and the clinical judgment of the physician. Concurrent heparin therapy may also be administered if deemed necessary by the clinician.

Adverse drug reactions reported with antithrombin concentrate have been minimal. Rarely chest tightness, dizziness, and fever have occurred.[93,102] Other rarely reported effects in clinical trials included nausea, foul taste in the mouth, chills, cramps, lightheadedness, and hives.[99,100] An interesting finding in patients with DIC who received antithrombin concentrate plus heparin was a greater need for RBC transfusion compared with that with either drug alone.[70] A higher incidence of wound hematoma and bleeding was also noted after joint replacement surgery compared to dextran 40.[103] Conversion of hepatitis B antigen and antibody has been reported; however, these patients also received other blood products.[102] Transmission of hepatitis C and HIV-1 has not been reported.

In administering antithrombin concentrate and heparin concurrently, it is important to consider their interaction. Replenishment of antithrombin to a deficient patient may result in a significantly lower dosage requirement for heparin. Empiric dosage reduction, frequent laboratory monitoring, or both would be appropriate when antithrombin concentrate is added to heparin therapy.

Monitoring parameters for antithrombin concentrate include hemoglobin and hematocrit every 12 hours until stable, then every 24 hours. Antithrombin plasma levels should be monitored as described previously. Care should be exercised during monitoring to ensure that antithrombin functional rather than antigenic or immunologic levels are determined. Patients receiving heparin and warfarin should also have regular monitoring of aPTT, PT, and TT. Other laboratory indicators of ongoing thrombin formation such as fibrinopeptide A, prothrombin fragment $1+2$, and thrombin–antithrombin complex levels should be assessed if available. The patient should be examined regularly for the signs and symptoms of thromboembolism, such as lower extremity pain, swelling, and warmth; shortness of breath; pleuritic chest pain; and hypoxemia. Appropriate monitoring of nasogastric aspirate, stools, and urine should be performed for the presence of occult blood.

LONG-TERM MANAGEMENT

Once a thrombotic event has occurred, the antithrombin-deficient patient will have a significant lifelong risk of recurrence, which can happen spontaneously or in the presence of thrombosis risk factors. In a retrospective analysis of 238 patients from 73 families with inherited deficiency of antithrombin, protein C, or protein S, the incidence of an initial episode of venous thromboembolism was 1.3 per 100 patient-years; in contrast, the incidence of recurrent events was 4.8 per 100 patient-years.[94] In another retrospective cohort study involving individuals with antithrombin, protein C, or protein S deficiency, the 1- and 5-year cumulative incidences of recurrent venous thromboembolism were 10% and 23%, respectively.[104] These findings emphasize the importance of long-term secondary prophylaxis; however, guidelines for prophylaxis are lacking. Lifelong replacement therapy with antithrombin concentrate is neither indicated nor practical; therefore, most clinicians advise lifelong therapy with oral anticoagulants for patients with antithrombin deficiency after a single thrombotic event, adjusted to a target INR of 2.0 to 3.0.[53,92,98,105,106] Some clinicians take a more conservative approach, advising lifelong therapy only for patients with recurrent DVT, or a single episode that was life-threatening or spontaneous.[94] The decision about long-term anticoagulant therapy should be made for each individual patient. Patients with dementia, peptic ulcer disease, or chronic bleeding or who have a history of frequent falls or trauma, poor or unreliable compliance with drug therapy, or alcohol abuse may not be suitable candidates for lifelong treatment.

The management of pregnant women (or those desiring pregnancy) merits special discussion. The risk of maternal thrombosis during pregnancy is higher among women with a past or family history of venous thromboembolism.[98] Antithrombin deficiency, whether inherited or acquired, is associated with both maternal and fetal complications.[95,101] For women with antithrombin deficiency, prophylactic anticoagulant therapy is recommended throughout the pregnancy.[98,107,108] Patients receiving warfarin before becoming pregnant should discontinue use in advance, if possible, because of its known teratogenic effects.[108] The preferred anticoagulant therapy for antithrombin-deficient pregnant women (i.e., a situation with high risk of thrombosis) is either subcutaneous adjusted-dose unfractionated heparin or LWMH. A typical adjusted-dose heparin prophylactic regimen is $\geq$10,000 U subcutaneously two or three times daily to maintain an aPTT of 1.5 to 2.5 times control.[107] LWMH may be preferred over unfractionated heparin in this setting due to its increased bioavailability, prolonged half-life, and ease of administration. No clinical studies have been performed to definitively determine the appropriate dose and duration of LWMH in pregnancy; however, dalteparin 5,000 to 10,000 U and enoxaparin 30 to 80 mg every 12 hours are two frequently used regimens. Both unfractionated heparin and LWMH regimens should be administered throughout pregnancy and for approximately 6 weeks postpartum in antithrombin-deficient patients. Firm monitoring guidelines for LWMH therapy during pregnancy have not been established; however, antifactor Xa levels may be drawn every 4 to 6 weeks beginning in the second trimester. A goal antifactor Xa level of 0.5 to 1 U per mL 2 to 3 hours after injection is recommended.[98,107] Patients with difficulty managing subcutaneous injections should receive heparin or LMWH at least during the first trimester and the last 1 to 2 months of pregnancy and oral anticoagulants during the remainder of the pregnancy.[94,108] This recommendation is supported by the American College of Obstetricians and Gynecologists, who stated that administration of warfarin during pregnancy should be restricted to the second and early third trimesters only in patients for whom heparin therapy is contraindicated.[107] Twice-weekly antithrombin concentrate infusions plus subcutaneous heparin have been successfully used in treating two women with congenital antithrombin deficiency and heparin resistance.[93] For most patients, however, antithrombin concentrate is withheld until the peripartum period, when it is given at the time of delivery and for several days thereafter.[97,102] Additionally, warfarin therapy (usually with 5 to 7 days of concurrent heparin) should be promptly reinitiated postpartum. Warfarin is considered safe for an infant whose mother is breastfeeding[109]; however, this assessment of safety does not extend to other coumarin derivatives.

All antithrombin-deficient patients who undergo surgery, incur trauma, or are exposed to other high-risk situations should receive prophylaxis with heparin, LMWH, warfarin, or antithrombin concentrate, whether or not they are receiving long-term oral anticoagulant therapy. Short-term prophylaxis should be given before, during, and for a few days after exposure to thrombosis risk factors.[94]

The use of long-term oral anticoagulant prophylaxis in patients with antithrombin deficiency who have not experienced a thrombotic event (e.g., a person detected in family screening) is controversial. Short-term prophylaxis as described earlier during exposure to high-risk situations (including pregnancy) is appropriate. However, there are no studies showing a definite benefit of long-term anticoagulant therapy for these patients.[106,109] The decision to initiate such treatment should therefore be individualized on the basis of the family history and after patient consultation regarding the risks and benefits of treatment. If the patient and clinician elect to treat with warfarin, it may be initiated on an outpatient basis without concomitant heparin.

The value of a management strategy that incorporates short-term prophylaxis for all patients and long-term anticoagulants for symptomatic patients with inherited deficiencies of antithrombin, protein C, or protein S was evaluated in a retrospective study of 238 patients from 73 families.[94] At the time of diagnosis, the incidence of recurrent venous thrombosis was 4.8 per 100 patient-years. This was reduced to 1.4 per 100 patient-years with the described treatment strategy; if those who complied poorly with the drug regimen were excluded, the incidence was further reduced to 0.3 per 100 patient-years. Specific analysis of antithrombin-deficient patients yielded a reduction in the overall incidence (single event or recurrent, long-term prophylaxis or not) of major thrombotic events from 2.5 to 1.3 per 100 patient-years after implementation of the strategy (0.5 if those who complied poorly were excluded). Four antithrombin-deficient women (two with and two without a prior history of thrombosis) became pregnant and were managed with heparin, with or without oral anticoagulants and antithrombin concentrate; none had a thrombotic event. Six antithrombin-deficient patients were given perioperative prophylaxis with heparin, antithrombin concentrate, or both, with no thrombotic events. During follow-up of 42 asymptomatic antithrombin-deficient patients over a mean of 5.3 years, 2 developed major thrombotic manifestations. This last finding may argue for long-term prophylaxis for asymptomatic patients, although confirmation with larger patient populations is desirable.

IMPROVING OUTCOMES

Counseling for all patients with inherited antithrombin deficiency should include a review of thrombosis risk settings and the importance of avoiding such situations. All patients should be informed of the symptoms of DVT and PE and the need for prompt medical evaluation should they occur. All patients should consider short-term prophylaxis with heparin, warfarin, or antithrombin concentrate when risk factors are present. The following information should be given to patients who are receiving long-term warfarin therapy: rationale for treatment, symptoms of bleeding, need to avoid contact sports or activities, importance of consistent dietary intake of vitamin K, abundance of drug interactions, and the need for regular coagulation studies and dosage adjustment. Women of childbearing age who are receiving long-term anticoagulant therapy must be counseled regarding the teratogenic effects of coumarin derivatives and the need for effective contraception. Women who are not receiving long-term anticoagulant therapy should be informed of the maternal and fetal risks during pregnancy and the advisability of prophylaxis during pregnancy and shortly thereafter.

ACQUIRED ANTITHROMBIN DEFICIENCY

In addition to congenital aberrations of the physiologic anticoagulant and fibrinolytic proteins, certain diseases may alter their levels or function, resulting in acquired deficiencies. This may occur in patients with increased antithrombin consumption (DIC, preeclampsia, major surgery, extensive acute DVT, or PE), decreased production (liver failure, fatty liver of pregnancy, malnutrition, or preterm infants), or increased plasma loss (nephrotic syndrome or inflammatory bowel disease).[96,101,110] Patients with malignancy may develop antithrombin deficiency via an uncertain mechanism. Most patients with acquired antithrombin deficiency do not develop thrombosis. Although nephrotic syndrome is associated with a high risk of thromboembolism, a causative relationship with antithrombin deficiency remains unclear.[110] Prophylaxis for acquired antithrombin deficiency is therefore not generally necessary. For patients with acute thromboembolism with known low plasma antithrombin levels, DIC, fatty liver of pregnancy with DIC, or fulminant hepatic failure, the usefulness of antithrombin concentrate has been demonstrated.[40,50,55] Patient counseling regarding avoidance of high-risk situations is appropriate.

Two randomized double-blind trials of antithrombin concentrate, either alone or in combination with heparin, that involved patients with DIC have been reported. When compared with heparin[79] or placebo,[69] a significantly shorter duration of DIC in groups receiving antithrombin concentrate was observed. One trial found a trend toward a reduction in mortality in patients receiving antithrombin concentrate, but it was not statistically significant.[69] The need for RBC transfusion in patients receiving antithrombin concentrate was higher in one study[70] than in the other.[69] Uncontrolled trials or case reports have been published on patients with fatty liver of pregnancy and DIC,[97] children with DIC,[71] and patients with DIC and arterial thrombosis that was unresponsive to heparin alone.[72] Whereas antithrombin concentrate has been found to improve the clinical and laboratory markers for patients with DIC, the ultimate outcome as measured by mortality is primarily related to the underlying disease.

A third randomized trial of antithrombin concentrate was performed in normal patients after total hip or knee replacement surgery.[103] Patients in the group receiving antithrombin concentrate plus heparin (treated for 5 days) had a significantly lower incidence of venous thrombosis compared to those who received dextran 40. An interesting finding was the occurrence of venous thrombosis in 100% of patients with antithrombin plasma levels <65%, suggesting that this value may represent an important threshold.

Drug-induced antithrombin deficiency has been reported with L-asparaginase, oral contraceptives, and heparin.[101]

L-Asparaginase is thought to cause thrombosis via reduced endogenous synthesis of the coagulation and fibrinolytic proteins, via drug-induced endothelial damage, or both. Thrombosis during or immediately after L-asparaginase administration is well documented, occurring in 3% to 5% of patients.[111] Antithrombin concentrate has been evaluated in a small cohort of patients undergoing induction therapy for acute lymphoblastic leukemia, yielding a reduction in laboratory test abnormalities and clinical thrombosis.

Oral contraceptives are the triggering event for the initial episode of venous thrombosis in 5% to 10% of antithrombin-deficient patients and are generally avoided in this population.[94,96] To assess the additional risk of oral contraceptives in 48 patients with hereditary thrombophilia, a retrospective study of antithrombin-deficient women compared those who had taken oral contraceptives at least once with age-matched control subjects.[112] The antithrombin-deficient patients who had taken oral contraceptives had a significantly higher probability for thrombosis (48% and 77% after 12 and 60 months, respectively), with a yearly incidence of 27.5% compared to 3.4% of control subjects. It was concluded that oral contraceptives were contraindicated in patients with antithrombin deficiency and that relatives of those with known antithrombin deficiencies should be screened before initiation of oral contraception. A limitation of this study was the very small sample size of 15 antithrombin-deficient patients.

PROTEIN C DEFICIENCY

Protein C is a vitamin K-dependent proenzyme that circulates as an inactive zymogen.[113–115] Activation of protein C occurs when thrombomodulin, a vascular endothelial cell receptor, binds to thrombin; conformational changes in the thrombomodulin–thrombin complex allow for the binding of protein C to endothelial cell protein C receptors.[113,114] Activated protein C is released from the complex and, along

with protein S as a cofactor, inhibits thrombin formation by proteolytic inactivation of factors Va and VIIIa (Fig. 33.1). Activated protein C also enhances fibrinolysis by inactivating tissue plasminogen activator inhibitor (PAI-1). In this capacity, activated protein C is a major physiologic modulator of blood fluidity and hemostasis.

Protein C in plasma can be measured quantitatively [using an immunologic or antigenic assay, such as enzyme-linked immunosorbent assay (ELISA)] or functionally [using amidolytic (fluorescent) or anticoagulation detection methods].[114,116,117] These two different assays reflect the different types of protein C deficiencies that are found—a type I deficiency and a type II deficiency. Type I deficiency is a quantitative deficiency resulting from reduced synthesis of the protein. In type II deficiency, the quantity of protein synthesized is normal, but the protein itself is dysfunctional. Most individuals with protein C deficiency (about 76%) have a type I deficiency.[114] Findings for assays of protein C can be expressed as a percentage of normal (considered to be 100%), with 95% of values found between 70% and 140% of a normal plasma pool. Individuals with assay results below the lower end of this range may have a hereditary protein C deficiency. Standard deviations (SD) have also been used as a reference range for protein C assay results; individuals with protein C levels less than 3 SD below the mean of the reference range are likely to have hereditary protein C deficiency. The diagnosis is less clear when the results are between 3 and 2 SD below the mean. Protein C levels are not affected by heparin; however, warfarin will decrease protein C levels, since it is a vitamin K-dependent protein.[87,114,115] Protein C levels should be assayed 10 to 30 days after discontinuation of warfarin. If discontinuation of warfarin is not possible, the magnitude of protein C reduction may be compared with that of another vitamin K-dependent protein such as factor X, but this has less precision in identifying deficient patients. Assays that measure the anticoagulant activity of protein C are recommended to screen for deficiencies; quantitative immunologic assays can be used to confirm the deficiency and to differentiate between type I and type II deficiencies.[117]

Protein C deficiency is described as an inherited autosomal dominant trait,[87] reported to occur at a prevalence of 1:200 to 1:300.[113] However, a higher number of individuals (1:60) may have protein C levels similar to those with a heterozygous deficiency. It is thought, therefore, that additional risk factors for thrombosis may be present in heterozygous individuals.[118–120] The occurrence of thrombotic events usually begins in adolescence in heterozygous individuals.[87] Nearly 50% experience some type of thrombosis by age 45, compared to about 10% of normal-related individuals.[114,119,120] Homozygous protein C deficiency (or a compound or double heterozygous state) is relatively rare, occurring in 1 out of every 500,000 to 1,000,000 births.[113,114,121,122] With severe homozygous mutations, thrombosis is often seen in the neonatal period, with the development of purpura fulminans neonatorum. This syndrome manifests with necrotic dermal lesions, CNS and retinal thrombosis, and ecchymosis occurring hours to days after birth. Protein C levels may be low (<1%) or undetectable.[113] About 200 different mutations in protein C deficiency have been identified.[122,123]

Another type of congenital protein C abnormality has been described in the literature.[124] Activated protein C resistance (APCR) is an autosomal-dominant inherited single-point genetic mutation on the coagulation factor V gene that results in resistance by factor Va to the proteolytic actions of activated protein C.[118,125] The procoagulant activity of factor Va is retained, increasing the risk of thrombosis in affected individuals. With APCR, protein C levels (measured by immunologic and functional assays) are normal; resistance can be detected with a dual measurement of aPTT, performed in the absence and presence of activated protein C.[124] The prevalence of heterozygotes for APCR in the general population is high, ranging from 2% to 15%. Most are asymptomatic, which suggests that APCR alone is not a major risk factor for thrombosis. However, a high risk for thrombosis exists when APCR occurs concomitantly with a second abnormality such as antithrombin, protein C or S deficiency, the lupus anticoagulant, or homozygous APCR. APCR is found in as many as 50% of patients with hereditary thrombophilia, compared with 3% to 7% of healthy control subjects. APCR is, therefore, the most common hereditary abnormality identified to date.[118]

CLINICAL PRESENTATION AND DIAGNOSIS

In neonatal purpura fulminans, homozygotes with severe mutations develop symptoms within hours after birth. Microvascular thrombosis with DIC is seen clinically as ecchymoses, purpura, and hemorrhagic bullae, followed by necrosis and gangrene, usually on the extremities, trunk, scalp, and pressure points (also occasionally in other organs). In some individuals with homozygous protein C deficiency, the type of mutation present still allows for limited protein C synthesis, delaying manifestations of the disorder.[122] Laboratory findings resemble those of DIC, except for nondetectable protein C immunologic and functional levels. Skin biopsies reveal extensive thrombosis of the arterioles and venules. CNS and vitreous or retinal thrombosis with hemorrhage may occur in utero, resulting in mental retardation, developmental delay, and blindness.[64] Most reported infants with neonatal purpura fulminans have been the offspring of consanguineous parents.[123]

Individuals with heterozygous protein C deficiency may develop a wide spectrum of thrombotic diseases.[87,113,114,117] DVT and PE are the most frequent manifestations. Arterial events such as myocardial infarction, transient ischemic attacks, and ischemic stroke are uncommon overall, but the prevalence is higher with proteins C or S deficiency (8.4%) than with antithrombin (1%) deficiency.[94] Superficial throm-

bophlebitis is also relatively more common with protein C deficiency. Events begin in adolescence or young adulthood, with 80% of instances occurring before age 40 years.[94,110,126] About 50% of events occur during periods of thrombosis risk such as pregnancy or surgery. The risk is intensified in patients <40 years old; the incidence of thromboembolism before age 40 is 120-fold and 14-fold higher in protein C-deficient males and females, respectively, than in the general population.[94] Thrombosis in unusual sites such as the upper extremities, viscera (renal, mesenteric veins), or brain (cerebral sinuses) occurs with a prevalence similar to that of other inherited deficiencies. Some patients have only a single thrombotic episode, but about 50% have recurrent events.

Although warfarin is used for treatment of protein C deficiency, a syndrome of warfarin-induced skin necrosis may occur infrequently.[113] The syndrome is characterized by the sudden onset of painful edematous erythema followed by hemorrhagic bullae, gangrene, and necrosis of the skin and subcutaneous tissues of the extremities, trunk, breasts, buttocks, or penis.[127,128] These symptoms typically occur 2 to 3 days after initiation of warfarin therapy. Laboratory findings in severe cases resemble those of DIC. Histologic examination reveals microvascular thrombosis, a finding that was previously considered paradoxical, since the reaction was caused by an anticoagulant. It is now believed that warfarin-induced skin necrosis is caused by a transient hypercoagulable state that occurs because of the short half-life of protein C (6 to 8 hours) compared with that of the other vitamin K-dependent clotting factors, especially factors II, IX, and X (24 to 80 hours). When warfarin is begun, rapid depletion of protein C to homozygous levels (0% to 30%) may be seen, while levels of factors II, IX, and X are near normal.[110,113,114,127,128] This exaggerated imbalance causes the thrombosis. Replacement of protein C is needed, using FFP, or protein C concentrate, if available. The occurrence of warfarin-induced skin necrosis is generally considered a contraindication to future warfarin use, although some patients have been successfully treated when FFP was infused at the time of initiation of warfarin therapy.[113]

TREATMENT

For severe protein C deficiency, presenting as neonatal purpura fulminans, prompt recognition and treatment are essential for survival. Protein C may be replaced by infusion of FFP (8 to 12 mL/kg every 12 hours) or with factor IX complex. This has been reported to halt the formation of new lesions and to induce regression of evolving lesions.[119] However, the large volumes of FFP needed by be problematic in some situations, and the amount of clotting factors present in prothrombin complex concentrates may vary, making consistent replacement difficult. In addition, the presence of procoagulants in prothrombin complex concentrates may worsen the coagulopathy. Coadministration of heparin with prothrombin complex concentrates may reduce this risk.[116,124] An alternative source of protein C is protein C concentrate (plasma-derived or recombinant).[129–132] In one published report, plasma-derived protein C concentrate (Ceprotin, Baxter AG) was successfully used to treat patients with severe congenital protein C deficiency (homozygous or double heterozygous).[132] A total of 22 patients received protein C concentrate under an open-label compassionate-use protocol. All patients responded to treatment, with resolution or improvement in lesions due to purpura fulminans or warfarin-induced skin necrosis. However, blindness secondary to retinal thrombosis or hemorrhage was not prevented in five of seven patients. Protein C concentrate was used for long-term prophylaxis (up to 7 years) in nine patients, with good outcomes reported; no patients developed inhibitory antibodies to protein C. One available case report described the use of recombinant activated protein C (drotrecogin) for treatment of purpura fulminans in a 14-year-old with severe inherited protein C deficiency: a dose of 20 μg/kg/hour was infused over a 5-hour period, with some resolution of symptoms.[121] Replacement of protein C is followed by UFH or LMWH.[129] Supportive care for the dermatologic, neurologic, and ophthalmic manifestations should be provided. Replacement therapy should be continued until all lesions are healed. If the patient survives, healing occurs over 4 to 8 weeks, often with residual scarring and sometimes requiring plastic surgery or amputation.

Plasma-derived human protein C concentrate (Ceprotin, Baxter AG) is available in the United States on a compassionate-use basis.[116,132,133] It is prepared as a monoclonal antibody-purified concentrate that undergoes vapor (steam) heating and detergent treatment for additional viral safety. The initial recommended dose of protein C concentrate is 60 to 80 IU per kg, with subsequent doses based on protein C activity, recovery, and half-life.[133] Both activity and half-life of protein C are variable and are influenced by the severity of the thrombotic event. A recombinant activated protein C (drotrecogin alfa; Xigris, Eli Lilly) is available in the United States for treatment of patients with severe sepsis.[134]

In patients with moderate protein C deficiency, acute thromboembolism (acute DVT and PE) is the most common clinical symptom. Most patients can be managed with UFH or LMWH and warfarin in doses to produce the same target laboratory values as in the general population. Oral anticoagulants are continued for 3 to 6 months after the initial thrombotic episode.[116] An important precaution in protein C-deficient patients is to ensure that therapeutic doses of UFH or LMWH are being administered at the time of initial warfarin therapy and until a therapeutic prothrombin time INR is achieved. Warfarin must be started at low doses in conjunction with UFH or LMWH. This reduces the risk of warfarin-induced skin necrosis. Resistance to heparin may occur rarely in protein C-deficient patients. This was managed in a homozygous patient with acute DVT by infusion of protein C concentrate during the warfarin titration period.[126]

For warfarin skin necrosis, prompt diagnosis and management are required to avoid ischemic necrosis of the subcuta-

neous tissues. It is managed with heparin (to stop the clotting process), FFP or cryoprecipitate (to replace protein C), and vitamin K (to facilitate endogenous protein C production). Protein C concentrate with intravenous heparin administration has also been reported to induce a rapid improvement in laboratory abnormalities and clinical manifestations over 24 hours, with complete healing over 15 days.[135] Appropriate supportive therapy to minimize complications such as infection is essential. Reconstructive surgery may be necessary in severe cases.

LONG-TERM MANAGEMENT

Until recently, neonatal purpura fulminans was considered a uniformly and rapidly fatal disorder.[121,131] Advances in its diagnosis and management have improved short-term survival and allowed development of long-term treatment strategies. With intensive anticoagulation, some children with homozygous protein C deficiency have remained asymptomatic for long periods of time, with occasional episodes of purpura fulminans. When symptomatic, protein C replacement—as FFP or protein C concentrate—has been successfully used. In some cases, however, patients require regular replacement of protein C with protein C concentrate.[119,123,136]

Problems with long-term use of protein C-containing products include risk of viral transmission, fluid overload (with FFP use), cost, need for venous access, and variable and unpredictable protein C content, with the possibility of drug-induced thromboembolism with factor IX complex. Oral warfarin carefully titrated to a prothrombin INR that is adequate to maintain an asymptomatic state (3.0 to 3.5 or higher) is the most common long-term treatment.[114,119,121] Special considerations in the use of warfarin in protein C-deficient patients include delaying treatment until all lesions of purpura fulminans have healed and the need for 5 to 7 days of overlapping heparin or FFP when initiating therapy. The latter precaution is recommended to reduce the likelihood of warfarin skin necrosis. If the symptoms of purpura fulminans recur, prompt replacement of protein C with FFP or protein C concentrate is indicated (prothrombin complex concentrate may be harmful in this situation). Liver transplantation was reported to cure protein C deficiency in a single case.[113]

Patients with protein C deficiency or APCR associated with recurrent thrombosis should be managed with lifelong warfarin therapy to a prothrombin INR goal of 3.0 to 3.5 (or sometimes higher).[115,116] Symptomatic patients with APCR and a second inherited deficiency (antithrombin, protein C, or protein S) should be similarly treated. LMWH has also been successfully used as long-term secondary prophylaxis in treating patients who have a history of warfarin skin necrosis.[115,120] Patients who refuse or are not suitable candidates for long-term anticoagulant therapy should be counseled regarding avoidance of thrombosis risk situations and the advisability of short-term prophylaxis.

Management of asymptomatic persons and those with a single thrombotic event is controversial because of variable and unpredictable clinical expression of the deficiency. The decision to maintain lifelong treatment is made only after individualized consultation regarding its potential risks and benefits. Many practitioners advise long-term prophylaxis after only one event if it is life-threatening or spontaneous. The value of this strategy was assessed in 141 protein C- or S-deficient patients who were followed for 598 patient-years.[94] The overall incidence (initial or recurrent events, with or without long-term prophylaxis) was reduced from 1.4 (protein C) to 2.0 (protein S) per 100 patient-years before the strategy was initiated to 0.8 (combined) per 100 patient-years after implementation. If oral anticoagulants were given and patients who complied poorly were excluded, this was further reduced to 0.5 per 100 patient-years. The reduction in recurrent thromboembolism was even more striking, from 4.8 per 100 patient-years (baseline incidence) to 1.4 after the strategy was initiated and 0.3 if patients who complied poorly were excluded. A disturbing finding in this report was the occurrence of major thrombosis in 2 of 51 protein C-deficient patients and 2 of 16 protein S-deficient patients who were asymptomatic at presentation and therefore did not receive long-term prophylaxis. Although this finding may support prophylaxis in all patients, the risk of treatment must also be considered for each patient. Patients who are unreliable, those who are subject to trauma, and those with a condition that has a risk of bleeding, such as peptic ulcer disease, should be carefully evaluated before long-term anticoagulant therapy is given. An important therapeutic distinction in protein C-deficient patients is the need for either intravenous or subcutaneous heparin in doses to achieve a therapeutic aPTT before the first dose of warfarin and until a therapeutic prothrombin INR is achieved. Alternatively, FFP or protein C concentrate may be given during warfarin titration.[126]

Approximately 50% of major thrombotic events occur in association with a risk situation. Short-term prophylaxis should be given to all patients during exposure to high-risk situations such as surgery, trauma, or prolonged immobilization, regardless of the history of thrombosis. Heparin, warfarin, FFP, and/or protein C concentrate may be used. Limited evidence favors the use of replacement therapy, either alone or with heparin. Prophylaxis should be given before, during, and immediately after risk exposure and is especially important in patients less than 40 years of age.[94]

The risk of maternal and fetal complications during pregnancy in protein C-deficient women is not as high as that seen with antithrombin deficiency but is nonetheless higher than that of the general population. All patients should therefore receive prophylaxis, regardless of history of thrombosis. Pregnancy is managed as previously described in the discussion of antithrombin deficiency, with the elimination of antithrombin concentrate. FFP or protein C concentrate may be considered in the peripartum period.[137] Warfarin should be initiated promptly after delivery, with overlapping heparin therapy.

MONITORING PARAMETERS

Frequent clinical assessment of the affected areas should be performed.[115,116] Relevant laboratory studies in patients with purpura fulminans include markers of DIC (see Table 33.5). If available, levels of fibrinopeptide A, PF 1 + 2, thrombin–antithrombin complex, and protein C are also useful in assessing response. Patients who receive FFP should be regularly assessed for fluid overload and hypertension, with periodic evaluation of cardiac, renal, and hepatic function. Indwelling intravenous catheters should be evaluated for function, patency, and infection. Patients who are receiving long-term warfarin therapy should have regular monitoring of prothrombin INR, hematocrit, and signs of bleeding. All patients should receive longitudinal assessment for recurrence of the thrombotic manifestations. Childhood growth and development should also be followed.

IMPROVING OUTCOMES

Counseling for patients with protein C deficiency is similar to that described in the discussion of antithrombin deficiency. Patients should be apprised of both the potential for reduction in subsequent events with treatment and the lack of effect if compliance with treatment is poor. Family screening should be performed to identify other family members with this deficiency. Females who desire to take oral contraceptives should be advised of the potential for drug-induced thromboembolism. Although the incremental risk in protein C-deficient females who have taken oral contraceptives appears to be less than that for antithrombin deficiency,[112] in one study oral contraceptives were the precipitating factor for five initial thrombotic events in 57 protein C-deficient patients.[94] Therefore, these patients should be advised to use other forms of contraception.

ACQUIRED PROTEIN C DEFICIENCY

Protein C levels may be reduced in severe liver disease, DIC, acute respiratory distress syndrome, malignancy, acute thromboembolic disease, and pregnancy and after surgery.[113–115] Patients with previously normal protein C levels may have reduced levels during extensive DVT or PE due to consumption. Drugs that may alter levels include oral anticoagulants and L-asparaginase. Treatment includes control of the underlying disease state and anticoagulation in patients with acquired protein C deficiency. As with inherited protein C deficiency, there is a risk of warfarin-induced skin necrosis. Use of heparin (UFH or LMWH) during initiation of anticoagulation and maintenance of INR between 3.0 and 3.5 will reduce this risk.[115] Long-term heparin therapy or use of protein C concentrates may be necessary.

PROTEIN S DEFICIENCY

Protein S is a vitamin K-dependent entity synthesized in the liver.[113,115,117,138] It differs from protein C in that it does not require activation and is not itself an anticoagulant but rather a cofactor for the actions of other proteins. Binding of activated protein C to protein S markedly augments the proteolytic activity of activated protein C on factors Va and VIIIa. Protein S may also be a cofactor for the profibrinolytic actions of protein C. Protein S is present in the plasma in two different forms. Approximately 30% to 50% of body stores circulate in the free (active) form.[118] The remainder exists in an inactive membrane-bound complex with C4b binding protein, a regulator of the complement system. Protein S levels are altered by warfarin but not by heparin.

Protein S deficiency in the general population is now known to be common. Among patients <45 years of age with DVT, the incidence of protein S deficiency has been reported to be up to 10%.[115] In other populations, the incidence has ranged from 1.5% to 7%. The inheritance of protein S deficiency is autosomal dominant; heterozygous patients have a strong tendency to develop DVT.[106,109,118] The prevalence in patients with venous thromboembolism is at least as high as that of antithrombin and protein C deficiency.[118] Three types of protein S deficiency have been described[113,138,139]:

■ Type I (quantitative) is the most common and is characterized by a reduction in both total and free protein S antigen. The protein S produced has normal or moderately reduced activity. C4b binding protein levels are also reduced.

■ Type II is rare, with normal levels of free protein S and reduced cofactor activity.

■ In type III, total protein S antigen and C4b binding protein levels are normal, but the levels of free protein S are reduced.[63,72] In general, the functional protein S levels in type III patients are higher than in type I patients.[72]

Normal levels of protein S are generally considered to be 60% to 130% of protein S levels found in pooled normal plasma.[113,138] However, certain groups, such as women <45 years of age may have a lower normal range, with a lower limit of about 55%.[117]

CLINICAL PRESENTATION AND DIAGNOSIS

Like the other deficiency syndromes, protein S deficiency has a variable clinical and biologic expression. Homozygous protein S deficiency manifests as death in utero or a syndrome similar to neonatal purpura fulminans seen in protein C deficiency. Some heterozygotes are completely asymptomatic (even during exposure to risk factors). DVT and pulmonary thrombosis account for 64% of initial events,[139] which typically begin in young adulthood. Superficial thrombophlebitis (30% of events) occurs at a rate greater than that in antithrombin deficiency and comparable to that in protein C deficiency. Venous thrombosis in unusual sites (e.g., axillary, cerebral sinuses, mesenteric, portal, or jugular) is seen with a prevalence comparable to that of other deficiencies. Arterial thrombosis (primarily in the cerebrum or coronary arteries) occurs in 5% to 8% of patients.[102,139–141] Approximately half of initial events are spontaneous. Pregnancy is a common predisposing condition, especially for patients with combined protein S deficiency and APCR.[140,142] Recurrence is common, with some patients reported to have as many as 15 thrombotic episodes. Warfarin-induced skin necrosis has also been reported in protein S deficiency.

Thrombotic events appear to be more common in isolated protein S deficiency than in protein C deficiency,[102] although some have suggested that the high incidence may be due to selection of severely affected families[140] or misdiagnosis in patients who actually have APCR.[118] At least 50% to 70% have their first episode before the age of 40.[94,139,141] Some investigators have suggested that with prolonged follow-up, all persons with heterozygous protein S deficiency will eventually develop thrombosis.[57,73] There is no relationship between the type of deficiency, the levels of immunologic or functional protein S, and the incidence of thrombosis,[139,141] a finding that suggests that factors other than the antigenic or functional concentration regulate the degree of clinical expression. Evidence suggests that patients with both protein S deficiency and APCR have a significantly greater incidence of thrombosis than do patients with either disorder alone.[141,142]

TREATMENT

The acute and long-term management of patients with protein S deficiency is similar to that for protein C deficiency.[113,115] Heparin (UFH or LMWH) is used for acute thrombosis; maintenance therapy is long-term, low-dose UFH, LMWH, or warfarin. Because of the higher incidence of thrombotic events, however, there is a greater tendency to give lifelong oral anticoagulants to patients with protein S deficiency after even one event. Some practitioners maintain a conservative approach, treating with long-term warfarin only patients with recurrent thrombosis.[110] When given in doses titrated to the standard desired prothrombin INR, warfarin has been found to be effective in preventing subsequent events[139,141]; detailed documentation of value is discussed in the section of this chapter titled "Protein C Deficiency."[94] Moreover, temporary discontinuation of warfarin resulted in recurrent thrombosis.[73] Asymptomatic patients are generally not treated with long-term warfarin. The occurrence of initial thrombotic events in 2 of 16 previously asymptomatic patients who were followed for a mean of 5.3 years, coupled with the severity of these events (stroke in a 23-year-old and myocardial infarction in a 42-year-old),[94] suggests that further studies should be performed to assess the value of long-term warfarin therapy in asymptomatic protein S-deficient patients. Replacement therapy with either FFP or prothrombin complex concentrate (factor IX concentrate) has been used both therapeutically and prophylactically.[106] The use of FFP requires larger volumes; however, it may otherwise be advantageous, since it exposes the patient to fewer infectious complications and does not have the potential to enhance thrombosis risk by providing other coagulant factors.

On the basis of available data, all protein S-deficient individuals should receive short-term prophylaxis before, during, and immediately after exposure to risk situations such as surgery or trauma, regardless of the history of thrombosis. Pregnant women with isolated protein S deficiency have a lower risk of thrombosis than those with antithrombin or protein C deficiency.[112] Most clinicians nonetheless prefer to give prophylaxis to pregnant patients in the same fashion as for patients with protein C deficiency.[94]

Liver disease, DIC, nephrotic syndrome, and pregnancy have all been associated with low protein S levels and are all seen in patients with acquired protein S deficiency.[113,115] Drug-induced reductions in protein S levels may occur during treatment with oral anticoagulants, oral contraceptives,[141,142] estrogens, and L-asparaginase. The C4b binding protein that complexes with protein S is an acute phase reactant; therefore, levels will increase in acute inflammatory processes (e.g., postoperative states or infection). This may reduce levels of free (active) protein S, thereby partially explaining the high risk of thrombosis associated with these conditions.[53,106]

As with other inherited thrombotic disorders, effective management includes familial studies to identify those at risk for thrombosis. Counseling for affected patients is important so that risk factors, such as obesity, oral contraceptive use, and comorbidities, can be avoided and prophylactic use of anticoagulants can be started in clinical situations such as pregnancy and delivery and after surgery.

OTHER INHERITED HYPERCOAGULABLE STATES

The miscellaneous causes of hypercoagulable states may be broadly grouped into impaired fibrinolysis, abnormal fibrinogen, or heparin cofactor II deficiency. Fibrinolysis is a complex process that is regulated by numerous proteins (Fig. 33.2). Abnormalities in the fibrinolytic system are common in patients with acute thrombosis but in this context are probably due to the disease and are unlikely to be the cause of the thrombosis. Inherited deficiency, dysfunction, and impaired release of plasminogen, t-PA, PAI-1, or factor XII have been reported[53,106,110] and occur in an autosomal-dominant pattern. Acute ethanol ingestion, drugs (e.g., oral contraceptives), other conditions (e.g., acute myocardial infarction, malignancy, or infection), or surgery may also alter fibrinolysis. The clinical presentation of thrombosis is similar to that of antithrombin or protein C or S deficiency.[53,110] However, abnormalities in fibrinolysis appear to be much less important, since associated thrombosis is rare. An important therapeutic consideration in these patients is that abnormal plasminogen function or activation may preclude the use of thrombolytic agents.[87,143]

Abnormal inherited fibrinogen defects may result in inadequate quantity or function, the latter condition being more common. Congenital fibrinogen disorders are clinically asymptomatic in most patients and more commonly cause bleeding rather than thrombosis when symptoms are seen.[106,110] Thrombosis is rare; when present, it is caused by the production of abnormal fibrinogen that is resistant to lysis by plasmin. Acquired quantitative abnormalities are more common than the inherited form. A low fibrinogen level is one of the hallmark signs of DIC and contributes to its associated bleeding. Accelerated fibrinogen consumption by thrombolytic drugs and decreased production in liver disease are other causes of fibrinogenemia.

Heparin cofactor II has a specific antithrombin effect (Fig. 33.1) that is accelerated by heparin, dermatan sulfate, and dextran. Inherited deficiency may manifest clinically as arterial or venous thrombosis; however, the vast majority of heparin cofactor II-deficient patients are asymptomatic. Low levels are also seen in DIC, but not in nephrotic syndrome or acute venous thrombosis.

HEMOPHILIA

The hemophilias are a variety of inherited bleeding disorders that involve a deficiency of one or more coagulation factors.[144,145] The most common hemophilias are hemophilia A and hemophilia B, resulting from a deficiency in coagulation factors VIII and IX, respectively. Both of these hemophilias are X-linked recessive traits, with bleeding tendencies manifesting in male offspring. Hemophilia A is the more common of the disorders, with an incidence of 1 in 5,000 male live births; in the general population, the incidence is 1 in 10,000. Hemophilia B occurs in 1 in 30,000 male live births, or 1 in 60,000 in the general population. Deficiencies in other coagulation factors may also occur but are rare.

Hemophilia A and B affect secondary hemostasis. Factors VIII and IX are necessary for activation of factor X, followed by generation of thrombin; thrombin in turn leads to formation of fibrin. When injury occurs in an individual with hemophilia, platelet function (part of primary hemostasis) is normal, with the formation of a platelet plug. However, stabilization of the formed platelet plug by fibrin does not occur (since thrombin formation is inadequate to generate fibrin), leading to a failure in secondary hemostasis and continued bleeding.

Factor deficiency is not absolute in hemophilia; factor VIII and factor IX procoagulant levels remain relatively constant in a patient and correspond to hemorrhagic frequency and severity. Bleeding can occur spontaneously in patients with severe deficiency or only after trauma in patients with some factor activity.[144,145] The most common sites for bleeding are muscles and large joints.

Factor VIII or factor IX levels of 100% correspond to factor VIII or factor IX activity of 1.0 U/mL. Factor VIII and factor IX levels in a normal person range from 50% to 200% (0.5 to 2.0 U/mL). Although hemostasis occurs at 25% to 30% of normal factor VIII activity, most symptomatic patients with hemophilia A have factor VIII levels less than 5%. The severity of the deficiency is categorized as mild, moderate, and severe. Patients with factor levels less than 1% (0.01 U/mL) are classified as having severe hemophilia. Hemorrhagic episodes are more frequent in these patients (20 to 30 or more annually) and often occur without evidence of trauma. Patients with factor levels greater than 5% are considered to have mild hemophilia. These patients usually hemorrhage only after trauma or surgery. Patients with factor levels between 1% and 5% are considered to have moderate hemophilia, with manifestations between the two extremes. Most patients with hemophilia have moderate to severe disease.[144,145]

CLINICAL PRESENTATION AND DIAGNOSIS

The clinical hallmarks of hemophilia A and B are identical and include: (a) lack of excessive hemorrhage from minor cuts or abrasions, owing to the normalcy of platelet function; (b) joint and muscle hemorrhages; (c) easy bruising; and (d) prolonged and potentially fatal postoperative hemorrhage.[144–146]

The diagnosis of hemophilia is made based on family history (which may not be present in up to 30% of individuals) or bleeding episodes.[144] With severe hemophilia, neonates have a 1% to 4% risk of intracranial hemorrhage. Bleeding tendencies usually become evident in the toddler stage, when the child is learning to crawl or walk. Most children with severe hemophilia have a first bleeding episode prior to age 4. Moderate hemophilia is usually diagnosed slightly later in childhood, whereas mild hemophilia may not be recognized until after some type of trauma.

Bleeding into joints results in hemarthrosis, the most common and often the most disabling manifestation of hemophilia. Repeated exposure of the synovium to blood results in swelling and hypertrophy; blood leukocytes in the joint space erode both the cartilage and bone, with narrowing of the joint space. Continued damage causes loss of joint motion and contracture, leading to disability in target joints (joints with recurrent bleeding). The joints that are most often involved include the knees, elbows, ankles, shoulders, hips, and wrists. The spine and hands are rarely involved.[147]

An aura consisting of joint warmth and tingling often signals the onset of hemorrhage. Mild discomfort gives way to pain, swelling, erythema, and decreased range of motion over the next several hours. Young children often display guarding, irritability, and decreased movement in an affected joint. Classic symptoms in a reliable patient are a sufficient basis for immediate treatment.

There is no cure for hemophilia, and treatment is directed at increasing concentrations of the deficient factor.[144,148] Joint hemorrhage should be treated when the earliest symptoms appear to limit acute effects and prevent long-term sequelae. Within 8 to 12 hours of treatment, symptoms of hemarthrosis begin to resolve. Initial treatment with factor VIII or factor IX concentrate requires that levels be increased to 30% to 50%.[149] The duration of therapy depends on the severity of bleeding. Once bleeding has stopped, blood is resorbed, and the joint returns to normal over several days to weeks. Use of nonsteroidal anti-inflammatory agents for joint pain should be avoided because of their disruptive effects on platelet function.

Microscopic and macroscopic hematuria is a common problem among hemophiliac patients.[148,150,151] Treatment with factor concentrate to elevate levels to 40% to 50% for 2 to 4 days is necessary if conservative treatment, such as bed rest and increased fluid intake, is unsuccessful. The use of ε-aminocaproic acid should be avoided, since decreasing clot lysis may prevent removal of a clot occluding the ureter.

Spontaneous and posttraumatic hematomas are frequent complications of hemophilia. Although most are small and resolve spontaneously, large soft tissue bleeding episodes may cause anemia and compartment syndromes with ischemic and neurologic complications. Large hematomas require treatment with factor concentrates to increase levels to 50% to 60% or more. Maintenance therapy for several days may be required to reduce rebleeding. Aggressive therapy can reduce the incidence of long-term complications, including pseudocysts, calcifications, and fibrosis.[148,149,151]

Spontaneous or posttraumatic intracranial bleeding is an infrequent but serious complication of hemophilia.[152] The annual incidence of intracranial bleeding has been reported to be 54 to 200 per 10,000 individuals with hemophilia. Even with prompt treatment, patients who experience intracranial bleeding are at risk for reduced quality of life due to functional disability. Treatment of intracranial bleeding should be immediate and aggressive. Any patient with a history of head trauma and signs of head injury, including abrasions, lacerations, or scalp hematoma, should be treated. Factor VIII or factor IX concentrates should be given to increase and maintain the level near 100%.[148,151]

Mucosal bleeding is not uncommon among patients with hemophilia.[148,151] Factor replacement to a level greater than or equal to 30% is often indicated. Supplementation with ε-aminocaproic acid or tranexamic acid may be advantageous to stabilize clot formation. Temporary restriction of oral intake and repeated treatment may be required if clot dislodgment is a problem.

TREATMENT

Care of patients with hemophilia and related bleeding disorders has improved dramatically over the past several decades, resulting in lower morbidity, increased life expectancy, and significantly better quality of life.[153] Hemophilia treatment centers, established in the mid-1970s, not only provide comprehensive medical care to patients with bleeding disorders, but also provide patients and families with educational and social services to help cope with this lifelong disorder.[144,154] These centers, along with wider availability of coagulation factor products and early and accurate diagnoses, have substantially reduced mortality among patients with hemophilia.

Treatment of hemophilia consists primarily of administration of products that increase the concentration of deficient clotting factors [e.g., factor concentrates, FFP, cryoprecipitate, or desmopressin (DDAVP)] and inhibiting fibrinolysis with antifibrinolytics, such as ε-aminocaproic acid and tranexamic acid.[148,151,155] Various organizations, including individual hemophilia treatment centers, have developed comprehensive protocols and guidelines for the treatment of patients with hemophilia and related bleeding disorders. Two organizations are well-recognized: the National Hemophilia Foundation (www.hemophilia.org) and the World Federation of Hemophilia (www.wfh.org). The Medical and Scientific Advisory Committee (MASAC) of the National Hemophilia Foundation has developed an extensive list of treatment guidelines for all aspects of hemophilia care, both therapeutic and social issues. Similar guidelines are available from the World Federation of Hemophilia.

FRESH-FROZEN PLASMA

FFP is the fluid portion of 1 unit of whole blood, taken from a single donor. It contains about 1 U of factor VIII and 1 U of factor IX per mL of plasma (some factor activity may be lost during frozen storage of the plasma).[151,155] However, because of the large amount of fluid that would be required, FFP is not the optimal means of factor replacement. Several guidelines on the treatment of hemophilia and bleeding disorders recommend the use of FFP for coagulation factor deficiencies for which there is no coagulation factor concentrate available.[156,157] For patients with hemophilia B, FFP has been recommended for use only in life-threatening emergencies, when factor IX concentrates are not available.[151] Factor IX levels may be increased by up to 15% with FFP, if the volume needed can be tolerated by the patient (up to 18 mL/kg).

CRYOPRECIPITATE

Cryoprecipitate is prepared by thawing FFP and removing the cell-free fluid remaining after centrifugation, leaving factor VIII, vWF, and fibrinogen. The amount of factor VIII in cryoprecipitate varies; on average a 10- to 20-mL bag contains about 80 units of factor VIII.[155] Cryoprecipitate contains no factor IX. Because of the risk of viral transmission, availability of factor concentrates, and variability in factor VIII content, cryoprecipitate is not recommended for treatment of hemophilia A.[156,158]

FACTOR VIII REPLACEMENT

Two types of factor VIII concentrate are available: plasma-derived and recombinant (Table 33.8).[148] Plasma-derived factor VIII concentrate is produced from factor VIII isolated from pooled plasma generated from thousands of donors. Although plasma-derived concentrates are considered safe, a large percentage of hemophilia patients were infected with hepatitis C or HIV in the mid-1980s, before the risk of transmission of these viruses through human plasma products was recognized, resulting in significant mortality.[158] Today, the safety of plasma-derived concentrates is ensured through strict plasma-donor screening and testing. Factor concentrates also undergo viral removal and inactivation methods to reduce the risk of viral transmission; these include solvent/detergent, heat treatment, pasteurization, vapor heating, and filtration. Chromatographic methods (e.g., immunoaffinity with monoclonal antibodies) are used to purify the concentrate, removing any nonfactor proteins and contaminants.[148]

Recombinant factor VIII concentrates are produced by recombinant technology, using hamster cell lines (kidney or ovary cells) transfected with the human gene for factor VIII.[156,159–161] Three generations of recombinant products are currently available. First-generation recombinant factor concentrates use animal and/or human plasma-derived proteins (e.g., albumin) in the cell culture medium and as a stabilizer in the final formulation. With second-generation agents, animal and/or human plasma-derived proteins are used in the cell culture medium but not in the final product. These agents use a sugar (e.g., mannitol or sucrose) as a stabilizer in the final product. No animal or human plasma-derived proteins are used in third-generation recombinant products. The development of third-generation recombinant products is in keeping with the MASAC recommendation of removing all animal or human protein sources from recombinant products to eliminate the risk of transmission of known or unknown pathogens from human or animal proteins.

Although the viral inactivation and removal methods used during the manufacture of plasma-derived coagulation factor concentrates have made these products safe in regard to

TABLE 33.8	Factor VIII Concentrates	
Product	**Viral Inactivation**	**Manufacturer**
Third-Generation Recombinant		
Advate	Immunoaffinity chromatography; solvent detergent	Baxter
Second-Generation Recombinant		
Helixate FS	Immunoaffinity chromatography; solvent detergent	ZLB Behring
Kogenate FS	Immunoaffinity chromatography; solvent detergent	Bayer
ReFacto	Immunoaffinity chromatography; solvent detergent	Wyeth
First-Generation Recombinant		
Recombinate		Baxter
Plasma-Derived		
Monoclate-P	Immunoaffinity chromatography; pasteurization	ZLB Behring
Hemofil M	Immunoaffinity chromatography; solvent detergent	Baxter
Monarc-M	Immunoaffinity chromatography; solvent detergent	Baxter/American Red Cross
Humate-P	Pasteurization	ZLB Behring
Alphanate	Affinity chromatography; solvent-detergent; dry heat	Grifols
Koate-DVI	Solvent detergent; Dry heat	Talecris Biotherapeutics

(From MASAC recommendations concerning the treatment of hemophilia and other bleeding disorders. MASAC Document #151.)

transmission of HIV or hepatitis, there is still concern about other potential pathogens, such as new variant Creutzfeldt-Jakob disease and parvovirus.[161,162] Recombinant factor products have been shown to be safe, with no reports of disease transmission. Whenever possible, recombinant factor concentrates are generally preferred over plasma-derived products for the treatment of hemophilia.

The goal of factor replacement therapy is to achieve hemostasis by maintaining adequate levels of deficient factor. The level of clotting factor to achieve this goal depends on the indication for treatment. Volume of distribution or recovery (ratio of observed peak factor concentration to predicted peak concentration), baseline factor concentration, factor half-life, and the presence of inhibitors can all influence the dose of factor replacement required.

Factor VIII distributes into plasma volume and initially to extravascular space. The volume of distribution is approximately 50 mL per kg. A simple dose calculation based on volume of distribution is that each unit of factor VIII infused per kilogram of body weight yields a 2% increase in plasma level (0.02 U/mL or 2 U/dL).[148] With an average elimination half-life of 12 hours, factor VIII may be dosed every 12 hours, with 50% of the initial dose used as a maintenance dose, every 12 hours. Factor VIII concentrate has also been given as a continuous infusion.[148,163] This method of administration may reduce the amount of factor needed and maintain a more constant factor concentration to reduce the risk of bleeding from trough concentrations that are too low.

FACTOR IX REPLACEMENT

Bleeding in patients with hemophilia B (deficiency of factor IX) can be treated with factor IX concentrates. As for factor VIII, factor IX is available as a plasma-derived product and as a recombinant product (Table 33.9).

Factor IX complexes (prothrombin complex concentrates) have been used for patients with hemophilia B. These concentrates contain not only factor IX, but also significant quantities of the other vitamin K-dependent clotting factors II, VII, and X. Although these agents are effective, they increase the risk of thrombosis, especially when used at high doses.[164]

TABLE 33.9	Factor IX Concentrates	
Product	**Viral Inactivation**	**Manufacturer**
Factor IX complex plasma-derived		
Bebulin VH	Vapor-heated	Baxter
Profilnine SD	Solvent detergent	Grifols
ProPlex T	Dry heat	Baxter
Factor IX concentrates Plasma-derived		
AlphaNine SD	Dual-affinity chromatography; solvent detergent; nanofiltration	Grifols
Mononine	Immunoaffinity chromatography; sodium thiocyanate; ultrafiltration	ZLB Behring
Second-generation recombinant		
BeneFIX	Affinity chromatography; ultrafiltration	Wyeth

(From MASAC recommendations concerning the treatment of hemophilia and other bleeding disorders. MASAC Document #151.)

Because the molecular size of factor IX is one-fifth that of factor VIII, the volume of distribution of factor IX is twice that of factor VIII. A simple dose calculation based on volume of distribution is that each unit of factor IX infused per kg of body weight yields a 1% increase in plasma level (0.01 U/mL or 1 U/dL).[148] The longer half-life of factor IX allows for every-24-hours dosing, with 50% of the initial dose used as a maintenance dose every 24 hours.

TREATMENT COMPLICATIONS

One of the major complications of treatment of hemophilia is the development of inhibitors. As many as 50% of patients with hemophilia A and 3% of patients with hemophilia B have been reported to develop inhibitors to the respective factors with repeated administration of the concentrate.[144,148,165,166] Inhibitors are IgG antibodies that bind to and inactivate the coagulation factor, reducing the efficacy of the factor concentrate and therefore the response to treatment. Inhibitors to factor VIII (the more commonly occurring) are expressed as titers called Bethesda units (BU). Low responders (3 to 5 BU) have low inhibitor titers that do not rise after further exposure to factor VIII. High responders (the majority of patients with inhibitors) may have low inhibitor titers initially, but they rise markedly (>1,000 BU) with further exposure to factor VIII (called an anamnestic response).[167] Inhibitor titers usually rise 2 to 3 days after exposure, peak in 7 to 21 days, then decline slowly.

Patients with inhibitors do not bleed more often than patients without inhibitors, but treatment of bleeding is more difficult for these patients and the use of prophylactic therapy is not possible.[166,168] Options for treatment of patients with inhibitors are to (a) administer sufficient quantities of factor concentrate to overwhelm antibodies that are present with an excess of factor to produce hemostasis, (b) restore hemostasis with factors other than factor VIII (called bypassing agents), and (c) remove antibodies by use of immune tolerance induction therapy. Patients who are low responders can sometimes be successfully treated with higher doses of factor concentrate. However, for most patients with inhibitors, use of bypassing agents or immune tolerance induction (ITI) is often necessary.

Human factor VIII can be used to treat hemorrhages in patients with low or high responses with inhibitor levels <5 BU and in patients with inhibitor levels between 5 and 30 BU after inhibitor removal. To neutralize inhibitors and achieve therapeutic hemostatic concentrations of 30% to 50%, an adult patient can be given an initial factor VIII bolus of 70 to 140 U/kg, followed by an infusion of 4 to 14 U/kg/hour.[169] Factor VIII levels should be monitored regularly to ensure that therapeutic concentrations are maintained. Porcine-derived factor VIII concentrate is another option for patients with inhibitors (titers to human factor VIII <50 or <15 BU to porcine factor VIII). There is a risk of cross-reactivity to porcine factor VIII (averaging 25%), and inhibitors to the porcine factor should be measured prior to therapy.[148] The recommended dose of porcine factor VIII for patients with low titers to human factor VIII (<5 BU) is 20 to 50 U/kg; for patients with titers 5 to 50 BU, porcine factor VIII can be dosed at 50 to 100 U per kg. Infusion reactions to porcine factor VIII (chills, fever, rash) occur in about 10% of patients; pretreatment with corticosteroids or antihistamines may be beneficial. Thrombocytopenia and an anamnestic response may also occur with porcine factor VIII. However, as of this writing, porcine factor VIII (Hyate:C, Ipsen) has been discontinued; it is available in limited quantities from the manufacturer while existing supplies last. A recombinant B-domain deleted porcine factor VIII (OBI-1) is currently under investigation by Octagen and is in phase II trials.

When factor VIII inhibitor levels are too high (>30 to 50 BU), bypassing agents may be needed to control bleeding. Anti-inhibitor coagulant complexes [AICC; also known as activated prothrombin complex concentrates (aPCC)] and factor IX complexes [also known as prothrombin complex concentrates (PCC)] have been successfully used to treat bleeding in patients with inhibitors to factor VIII. However, the clinical response with these agents is variable, and there may be a risk of thromboembolic complications and anamnestic response.[148,166,169]

Another bypassing agent that has been shown to be effective in patients with inhibitors to factor VIII or factor IX is recombinant factor VIIa.[165,166] It does not appear to be associated with an anamnestic response and has a low risk for thromboembolic events. However, the response rate is variable and it has a short half-life, requiring frequent dosing (every 2 to 4 hours). Bleeding has been reported to be controlled with a dose of 35 μg/kg; a greater effect was seen with doses of 70 to 90 μg/kg.

The third option for treatment of inhibitors in patients with hemophilia is ITI.[165] Some clinicians have recommended ITI for most patients with hemophilia as a means to eradicate inhibitors. ITI regimens include long-term, regular infusion of factor concentrates with or without immunosuppressive or immunoadsorptive therapies.[144] This approach is most successful when initiated during periods of low inhibitor titers, shortly after the development of inhibitors (i.e., in childhood), and when therapy is uninterrupted. Although costly, the life-long consequences of poorly controlled bleeding episodes in children with hemophilia must be considered. ITI is more effective in patients with inhibitors to hemophilia A (about 85% response); about 50% of patients with inhibitors to hemophilia B respond to ITI. Use of recombinant factor VIIa may be a more effective approach to treatment of patients with inhibitors to hemophilia B.[144]

DESMOPRESSIN

Desmopressin (DDAVP) is a synthetic analog of the hormone vasopressin.[170] Although its mechanism is unknown, DDAVP produces up to a five-fold increase in factor VIII concentrations in most patients with mild hemophilia.[171] DDAVP does not increase production of factor VIII but stimulates the release of stored factor VIII. DDAVP does not increase the concentration of factor IX, so patients with severe hemophilia A or with hemophilia B do not benefit from this therapy.

To determine whether patients will respond to DDAVP, a plasma factor concentration is obtained after an infusion. Testing for responsiveness should be conducted when a patient is asymptomatic. This prevents a delay in the decision to use more aggressive forms of therapy while the DDAVP response is being assessed during a bleeding episode. Most patients with mild hemophilia A and factor VIII levels >10% respond to DDAVP.

For patients who are known to respond and who do not have life-threatening bleeding or who are not undergoing major surgery, DDAVP is the treatment of choice.[149,170] The recommended intravenous dosage of DDAVP is 0.3 μg per kg, given over 30 minutes. For patients weighing more than 10 kg, the dose should be diluted in 50 mL and in 10 mL for patients less than 10 kg. DDAVP should result in an increase in factor VIII concentrations of three to five times baseline within 1 hour of the infusion. DDAVP may be administered daily for 2 to 3 days, after which tachyphylaxis may develop.[172] If therapy is needed for longer periods, factor VIII concentrate should be considered instead. DDAVP may also be given subcutaneously, but the maximal response is delayed. A dose of 250 μg can be used intranasally, resulting in a 2.5-fold increase in factor VIII levels. Blood pressure, fluids, electrolytes, and heart rate should be monitored in patients receiving DDAVP, because it may cause a slight pressor response and fluid retention. Seizures secondary to hyponatremia have also been reported.[89]

ANTIFIBRINOLYTIC AGENTS

ε-Aminocaproic acid and tranexamic acid are lysine-derived antifibrinolytic agents that bind to plasminogen at the lysine binding site, inhibiting fibrinolysis and stabilizing a formed fibrin clot.[151,170] The primary role of these antifibrinolytic agents is as a single-dose prophylactic agent after dental procedures.

ε-Aminocaproic acid is administered orally as a loading dose of 200 mg/kg (maximum 10 g) followed by maintenance doses of 50 to 100 mg/kg every 6 hours (maximum 24 g over 24 hours) for 5 to 7 days. Tranexamic acid is administered orally at 25 mg/kg every 6 to 8 hours for 5 to 7 days. The two agents are generally well tolerated, gastrointestinal complaints being the most reported complication.

PROPHYLAXIS

In addition to "on demand" therapy (i.e., use of factor concentrates for control of active bleeding), factor concentrates have been used for prophylaxis of bleeding.[173–176] When initiated early, prophylactic factor VIII or factor IX infusions can eliminate or minimize disabling arthropathies. Prophylaxis has been described as primary (initiation of therapy prior to the age of 2 years or before any significant joint bleeding occurs) or secondary (treatment started after the age of 2 years or after two or more joint bleeds have occurred).[176] Both types of prophylaxis are effective in improving joint function and quality of life, although more data are available for primary prophylaxis. The optimal duration of prophylaxis is unknown.

Current MASAC guidelines recommend the use of prophylactic factor concentrates for patients with severe hemophilia A or B (factor concentrations <1%). The goal of regular administration is to keep factor VIII or factor IX trough concentrations >1% between dosing.[175] Dosages of factor VIII concentrate of 25 to 40 U/kg three times weekly or every other day and 40 to 100 U/kg of factor IX concentrate twice weekly have been suggested. Although prophylactic therapy is nearly 100% effective in preventing bleeding, considerations in its use include cost, need for venous access, availability of factor concentrates, and patient and family acceptability.

FUTURE THERAPIES

No cure for hemophilia currently exists. Liver transplantation has been reported to be successful in returning factor production to normal in a few patients with hemophilia A and end-stage liver disease.[177]

The most promising therapy under investigation is likely to be gene therapy. One feature of hemophilia that makes gene therapy or gene transfer a viable approach is the need to raise factor concentrates by a very small amount (1% to 5% of normal) for a clinical effect to be seen.[144,178,179] Beneficial effects of gene therapy have been seen in early phase I trials; however, the potential risks of gene therapy must also be considered.

ANTIPHOSPHOLIPID SYNDROME

The antiphospholipid syndrome (APS) is the most commonly observed cause of acquired thrombophilia. The syndrome is characterized by the presence of antiphospholipid antibodies, recurrent thrombosis of veins and arteries, spontaneous abortions, and thrombocytopenia.[180] In healthy subjects, an incidence of antiphospholipid antibodies of 1% to 5% is observed. Patients with APS have an increased risk of thrombosis of approximately 0.5% to 30%. APS may be primary (occurring separately from any disease process) or secondary (occurring within the context of a concurrent, usually autoimmune, disease process). An example of an autoimmune disease with an associated high prevalence of antiphospholipid antibodies is SLE. Patients with SLE and antiphospholipid antibodies have a significantly increased chance of developing APS. The syndrome occurs more frequently in young to middle-aged adults and has a higher prevalence among females.

APS is an autoimmune process, but the exact mechanism behind the formation of antiphospholipid antibodies is unknown.[180] What is known is that these formed antibodies react with endothelial cell membranes and platelets, resulting in disruptions to the coagulation system and the formation of thrombi. Research is ongoing to determine the exact role of antiphospholipid antibodies in the development of coagulation abnormalities.

CLINICAL PRESENTATION AND DIAGNOSIS

The clinical manifestations of APS are varied and include thrombotic, neurologic, and obstetric complications. APS is associated with many types of venous thrombosis, including DVT of the upper extremities, intracranial veins, inferior vena cava, hepatic veins (Budd-Chiari syndrome), portal vein, renal vein, and retinal veins, and PE.[180–184] Arterial thrombotic sites associated with APS include the coronary arteries, carotid arteries, cerebral arteries, retinal arteries, subclavian or axillary arteries, brachial arteries, mesenteric arteries, peripheral (extremity) arteries, renal arteries, and both the proximal and distal aorta.[182,183] APS has been associated with premature or precocious coronary artery disease, early angioplasty (percutaneous transluminal coronary angioplasty) failure, and early and late coronary artery bypass graft occlusion.[185]

The neurologic syndromes associated with APS have included transient ischemic attacks, small stroke syndrome, arterial and venous retinal occlusive disease, cerebral arterial and venous thrombosis, migraine headache, Degos disease, Sneddon syndrome, Guillain-Barré syndrome, chorea, seizures, and optic neuritis.[186–190]

APS is associated with a high chance of fetal wastage; the characteristics of this syndrome are frequent abortion,

particularly in the first trimester; recurrent fetal wastage in the second and third trimesters; placental vasculitis; and, less commonly, maternal thrombocytopenia. Successful anticoagulant therapy can increase the chances of normal term delivery to about 80%.[191–193]

Patients with APS usually experience recurrent single thrombotic events; however, in rare situations, catastrophic APS can occur.[180,194,195] Catastrophic APS involves multiple organ failure due to the formation of widespread microthrombi. Approximately 50% of all patients with catastrophic APS die despite treatment.

In 1998, an international consensus statement was developed that included criteria for a diagnosis of definite APS.[196] Prior to development of this consensus statement, no uniform diagnostic criteria existed across the multiple medical disciplines involved in the care of patients with APS. The criteria for classification of APS include two broad sections: clinical criteria and laboratory criteria. The clinical criteria include an evaluation of vascular thrombosis and pregnancy morbidity. An examination of the presence of anticardiolipin antibody and lupus anticoagulant is the main laboratory criteria. If at least one clinical criterion and one laboratory criterion are present, a definitive diagnosis of APS is established.

When testing for the anticardiolipin antibody, the laboratory test to be performed is the ELISA. The clinician should look for the levels of IgG and/or IgM isotypes on two or more occasions at least 6 weeks apart.[180,196,197] These isotypes should be present in the blood in medium or high titers. Tests to order when looking for lupus anticoagulant are aPTT, kaolin clotting time, and dilute Russell's viper venom time (dRVVT).[198] Again, the presence of lupus anticoagulant in plasma should be confirmed on two or more occasions at least 6 weeks apart.

TREATMENT

Disagreement continues over the optimal management of patients with APS due to the lack of prospective clinical trials in this area.[180] Generally, clinicians agree that patients who experience recurrent thrombotic episodes require lifelong anticoagulation. In addition, patients with APS who have recurrent spontaneous abortions should receive anticoagulant therapy throughout gestation. Less agreement regarding the management of APS is observed when discussing patients who have never experienced a spontaneous thrombotic event or asymptomatic pregnant women with antiphospholipid antibodies.

Some clinicians consider the administration of anticoagulant therapy to a patient with antiphospholipid antibodies, but no history of thrombotic events, to be unjustified.[180]

Others state that current data support the use of low-dose aspirin as a prophylactic measure in these patients.[199] Hydroxychloroquine may also be used as a prophylactic agent for patients who have not experienced a thrombosis.[180,199,200]

For secondary prophylaxis, debate continues to rage regarding the benefits of aspirin, warfarin, or a combination of the two. Until more clinical trials are performed to address this issue, lifelong secondary prophylaxis should be given with warfarin, with a goal INR of 3.[180] A goal INR of 3 to 4 has traditionally been warranted in the setting of APS and may still be useful, particularly in patients who have experienced an arterial thromboembolism.

The treatment of pregnant patients with APS who have experienced a prior thrombosis is another area where differences in approach to therapy exist.[180,191,192] However, most clinicians agree that pregnant women with APS should receive combination therapy with low-dose aspirin and heparin. Administration of LMWH is preferred over UFH despite the limited data involving the LMWHs in pregnancy.[192] Commonly used dosages of LMWHs in pregnant patients with APS include enoxaparin 1 mg per kg or dalteparin 5,000 IU twice daily subcutaneously. The combination of low-dose aspirin and heparin is also recommended for pregnant women with a history of pregnancy losses or complications due to APS; however, many clinicians administer a lower dosage of LMWH to these patients (i.e., enoxaparin 1 mg/kg or dalteparin 5,000 IU once daily). Therapy should be initiated as soon as pregnancy is diagnosed and continued until delivery.

ANTIPHOSPHOLIPID SYNDROME AND THROMBOCYTOPENIA

Thrombocytopenia is associated with both primary and secondary forms of APS. Moderate to severe thrombocytopenia is common and occurs in 50% of patients with secondary APS; however, it occurs in <10% of those with primary APS.[182,183,201,202]

PATHOPHYSIOLOGY

The autoimmune pathophysiology is thought to be platelet sensitization by antibodies attached to surface phospholipids. A high correlation between IgA anticardiolipin antibodies and thrombocytopenia exists, although thrombocytopenia may accompany IgG and IgM antibodies as well. Regardless of the severity of the thrombocytopenia, thrombosis, not bleeding, remains the major clinical consequence.

TREATMENT

IVIG or plasma exchange may be beneficial as additive therapy to the standard management of APS in patients with severe thrombocytopenia and thrombosis.[182,183,201,202]

SUMMARY

This chapter discusses the common hereditary and acquired coagulation disorders associated with thrombosis and hypercoagulability. The most common of the hereditary defects appear to be deficiencies in antithrombin and proteins C and S, and the most commonly observed acquired defect is the presence of antiphospholipid antibodies. Therefore, these are the coagulation abnormalities that should initially be suspected in a patient with unexplained thrombosis.

The importance of determining the presence of these coagulation abnormalities has significant implications for therapy of the individual patient and for institution of familial studies to identify, inform, and possibly treat others at risk.

Finally, a diagnosis of thrombosis is only generic and partial; the cause must be clearly defined. Only in this manner can cost-effective and appropriate therapy for both primary treatment and secondary prevention be initiated. Treatment options are summarized in Table 33.10.

KEY POINTS

■ Normal hemostasis requires three responses: the vascular response (vasoconstriction), formation of a platelet plug (primary hemostatic mechanism), and the formation of a fibrin clot (secondary hemostatic mechanism).

■ Immediately after tissue injury, platelets clump together to form a primary hemostatic plug through a series of the following overlapping phases: adhesion, aggregation, secretion, and elaboration of procoagulant activity.

■ The extrinsic, intrinsic, and common pathways are components of the traditional coagulation cascade, which results in the formation of thrombin. Thrombin and platelets form a clot, which acts as a plug to minimize further blood loss. More recently, this traditional model has evolved into a model that merges the extrinsic and intrinsic pathways into one.

■ Naturally occurring anticoagulation proteins inhibit the action of clotting factors in an attempt to control thrombosis, fibrinolysis, and inflammation.

■ The fibrinolytic system dissolves and removes excess fibrin deposits to preserve vascular patency and restore blood flow. Fibrinolysis is mediated by the enzyme plasmin.

■ Platelets are formed in the bone marrow. They have an average life span of 9 to 10 days, and younger platelets are more physiologically active than older ones.

■ Thrombocytopenia, defined as a decrease in the number of blood platelets, is one of the most common causes of abnormal bleeding. A decrease in platelets may occur from (a) a decrease in production, (b)

TABLE 33.10	Treatment Options for Coagulation Disorders
Coagulation Disorder	**Treatment**
Thrombocytopenia	Correct underlying conditions.
	Discontinue drug therapies known to cause thrombocytopenia.
	Administer coagulation factors and platelets if indicated.
	Offer supportive care of associated signs and symptoms.
Acute immune thrombocytopenic purpura	Treatment is controversial:
	No treatment due to self-limiting nature and low incidence of side effects, or
	Treat when platelet count <20,000/mm^3 with:
	Prednisone
	High-dose IVIG
	Anti-Rh(D) (WinRho)
Chronic immune thrombocytopenic purpura	Corticosteroids
	Splenectomy
	For refractory chronic ITP:
	Azathioprine
	Cyclophosphamide
	Vinca alkaloids
	Danazol
	High-dose corticosteroids
	Rituximab
Thrombotic thrombocytopenic purpura	Give simultaneously:
	Plasma infusion or exchange
	Splenectomy
	Corticosteroids
	Antiplatelet agents (aspirin, dipyridamole)
	IVIG
	Other options:
	Cytotoxic agents (vincristine)
	Other antiplatelet agents (prostacyclin, sulfinpyrazone, dextran)
Platelet function disorders	Avoid situations associated with a high risk of bleeding.
	Avoid medications that alter platelet function or numbers.
	Treat underlying disorder.
	Decrease in platelets after bypass surgery:
	Platelet transfusion
	Uremia-associated decrease in platelets:
	Desmopressin, conjugated estrogens
Drug-induced immune thrombocytopenia	Type I heparin-induced thrombocytopenia:
	Monitor platelet counts every 2–3 days.
	Type 2 heparin-induced thrombocytopenia:
	Discontinue heparin immediately.

(continues)

TABLE 33.10	continued	
Coagulation Disorder	**Treatment**	
Acute disseminated intravascularr coagulation	Give alternative anticoagulants:	
	Dextran	
	Aspirin	
	Warfarin	
	Lepirudin	
	Argatroban	
	Thrombolytics (if needed)	
	Treat underlying disease.	
	Give supportive therapy for signs and symptoms.	
	Interrupt the coagulation process:	
	Heparin	
	LMWH	
	Replacement of depleted coagulation factors and platelets:	
	FFP	
	Protein C concentrate	
	Antithrombin concentrate	
	Platelets	
	Cryoprecipitate	
	Factor IX complex	
	Interruption of fibrinolysis:	
	Fibrinolytic inhibitors: ϵ-aminocaproic acid or tranexamic acid	
	Other therapies:	
	Recombinant hirudin	
	Argatroban	
	Exchange transfusions (plasma exchange, plasmapheresis, leukapheresis, whole blood exchange)	
Chronic disseminated intravascular coagulation	Treat underlying disease.	
	Give supportive therapy for clinical manifestations.	
	Treatment: heparin or LMWH	
Antithrombin deficiency	Acute thromboembolism, prevention of thromboembolism during high-risk situations, and long-term prophylaxis after first thrombotic event:	
	Heparin or LMWH + warfarin	
	Antithrombin concentrate	
	Warfarin (long-term management only)	
Protein C deficiency	Neonatal purpura fulminans treatment and long-term management:	
	FFP	
	Factor VIII concentrate	
	Protein C concentrate	
	Warfarin (long-term management only)	
	Acute thromboembolism, prevention of thromboembolism during high-risk situations, and long-term prophylaxis after first thrombotic event:	

(continues)

Coagulation Disorder	Treatment

TABLE 33.10	continued

Coagulation Disorder	Treatment
	Heparin or LMWH + warfarin (must have therapy with heparin or LMWH before starting warfarin)
	FFP, protein C concentrate (prevention in high-risk situations only)
	Warfarin skin necrosis:
	Stop warfarin
	Heparin
	FFP
	Cryoprecipitate
	Vitamin K
	Protein C concentrate + heparin
Protein S deficiency	Acute thromboembolism, prevention of thromboembolism during high-risk situations, and long-term prophylaxis after first thrombotic event:
	Heparin
	LMWH
	FFP
	Factor IX concentrate
	Factor VIII concentrate
	Warfarin (long-term prophylaxis only)
Hemophilia	Products that increase clotting factors:
	Desmopressin
	Factor VIII concentrate
	Factor IX concentrate
	Bypassing agents (for patients with inhibitors)
	Antifibrinolytic agents:
	ε-Aminocaproic acid
	Tranexamic acid
Antiphospholipid syndrome	Acute thromboembolism, prevention of thromboembolism during high-risk situations, and long-term prophylaxis after first thrombotic event:
	Heparin
	LMWH
	Warfarin (long-term prophylaxis only)

IVIG, immune globulin; LMWH, low-molecular-weight heparin; FFP, fresh frozen plasma; AT-III, antithrombin III.

altered distribution (sequestration), or (c) increased destruction of platelets.
- ITP causes shortened platelet survival due to immune-mediated platelet destruction by antiplatelet autoantibodies of the IgG or IgM subtypes. There are two forms of ITP: acute, affecting previously healthy children, and chronic, affecting mainly women from 20 to 40 years of age.
- TTP is an uncommon disorder that causes widespread occlusion by platelets and hyaline material in the capillaries and arterioles (but not the venules) of nearly all organs, resulting in high mortality. The treatment of choice is plasma infusion or exchange.
- Platelet function disorders may cause bleeding or thrombosis independent of the platelet count and are commonly associated with uremia, cardiac bypass,

liver disease, dysproteinemias, and myeloproliferative disorders. The underlying disorder should be corrected or treated when possible.

■ Drug-induced platelet disorders include those that alter platelet function and those that cause thrombocytopenia by decreased production or increased destruction of platelets.

■ Drug-induced immune thrombocytopenia can be caused by the formation of an immunoglobulin–drug immune complex that attaches to and destroys the platelet or the binding of the drug to the platelet membrane, creating a hapten that ultimately results in the formation of antiplatelet antibodies.

■ Heparin causes two types of drug-induced thrombocytopenia. Type I is a mild, gradual thrombocytopenia that develops over the first few days of treatment and usually resolves spontaneously even with continued heparin treatment. Type II generally appears 5 to 14 days after therapy, or sooner if the patient has been previously exposed, and is thought to be caused by a complex interaction between heparin, platelet factor 4 (PF4), platelet Fc receptors, and heparin-like molecules on the endothelial cell surface.

■ DIC is an intermediary syndrome caused by an underlying disorder, which results in the simultaneous in vivo activation of the coagulation and fibrinolytic systems, causing both thrombosis and hemorrhage. The cornerstone of DIC management is treatment of the causative disease and supportive care for the signs and symptoms associated with the syndrome. Other treatments include interruption of the coagulation process, replacement of depleted coagulation factors and platelets, and interruption of fibrinolysis.

■ Hypercoagulable states include a number of conditions (antithrombin deficiency, protein C deficiency, protein S deficiency, and antiphospholipid syndrome) that share the common endpoint of inappropriate thrombus formation. Patients with these disorders are at higher risk for both venous and arterial thromboembolic disease. Disruption of coagulation may occur on an inherited (primary) or acquired (secondary) basis.

■ Treatments for acute thromboembolism for patients with antithrombin deficiency, protein C deficiency, protein S deficiency, or APS are heparin or LMWH with or without warfarin. Patients with protein C deficiency should be given heparin or LMWH before warfarin is initiated.

■ All patients with antithrombin deficiency, protein C deficiency, protein S deficiency, or APS should receive short-term prophylaxis before, during, and immediately after exposure to situations with a high risk of thrombosis, such as surgery, pregnancy, delivery, major trauma, and prolonged bed rest, with heparin or LMWH with or without warfarin, regardless of thromboembolic history.

■ Because of the high risk of recurrence after the first episode of thromboembolism, prophylaxis against future events should be considered in patients with inherited antithrombin deficiency, protein C deficiency, protein S deficiency, or APS, especially after a life-threatening or spontaneous thrombotic event. Patients should be advised about the risks and benefits of treatment. Warfarin is generally the drug of choice.

■ Pregnancy increases the risk of thromboembolism in patients with inherited antithrombin deficiency, protein C deficiency, protein S deficiency, or APS. Therefore, patients who become pregnant should receive anticoagulation prophylaxis therapy with heparin or LMWH, regardless of thrombotic history.

■ Oral contraceptives can increase the risk of thrombosis in patients with antithrombin deficiency, protein C deficiency, or protein S deficiency and should be avoided.

■ Warfarin-induced skin necrosis can occur in patients who have inherited protein C deficiency when large warfarin loading doses are given. It is caused by a transient hypercoagulable state that occurs because of the short half-life of protein C compared to that of the other vitamin K-dependent clotting factors. Other acute complications of protein C deficiency include neonatal purpura fulminans and acute thromboembolism.

■ Miscellaneous causes of hypercoagulable states may be broadly grouped into impaired fibrinolysis, abnormal fibrinogen, or heparin cofactor II deficiency.

■ Hemophilia results in spontaneous or posttraumatic bleeding into muscles, joints, and body cavities. There is generally a lack of excessive hemorrhage from minor cuts or abrasions, owing to normal platelet function. A defect in or absence of the procoagulant portion of factor VIII or factor IX causes hemophilia A and B, respectively. Joint hemorrhage is the most common and often most disabling manifestation of hemophilia and should be treated at the earliest manifestation of symptoms to limit acute and prevent long-term sequelae.

REFERENCES

1. Goodnight SH, Hathaway WE. Disorders of hemostasis & thrombosis, 2nd ed. New York: McGraw-Hill, 2001.
2. Goebel RA. Thrombocytopenia. Emerg Med Clin North Am 11: 445–464, 1993.
3. Comp PC. Production of plasma coagulation factors. In: Williams WJ, Beutler E, Erslev AJ, et al, eds. Hematology, 4th ed. New York: McGraw-Hill, 1990:1285–1294.
4. British Committee for Standards in Haematology, General Haematology Task Force. Guidelines for the investigation and management of idiopathic thrombocytopenic purpura in adults, children and in pregnancy. Br J Haematol 120:574–596, 2003.
5. Cines D, Blanchette V. Immune thrombocytopenic purpura. N Engl J Med 346:995–1008, 2002.
6. Stasi R, Provan D. Management of immune thrombocytopenic purpura in adults. Mayo Clin Proc 79:504–522, 2004.
7. Rutherford CJ, Frenkel EP. Thrombocytopenia: issues in diagnosis and therapy. Med Clin North Am 78:555–575, 1994.

8. Waters AH. Autoimmune thrombocytopenia: clinical aspects. Semin Hematol 29:18–25, 1992.
9. Blanchette VS, Kirby MA, Turner C. Role of intravenous immunoglobulin G in autoimmune hematologic disorders. Semin Hematol 29 (Suppl 2):72–82, 1992.
10. Blanchette V, Imbach P, Andrew M, et al. Randomised trial of intravenous immunoglobulin G, intravenous anti-D, and oral prednisone in childhood acute immune thrombocytopenic purpura. Lancet 344:703–707, 1994.
11. Yetman R. Evaluation and management of childhood idiopathic immune thrombocytopenia. J Pediatr Health Care 17:261–263, 2003.
12. Warkentin TE, Kelton JG. Current concepts in the treatment of immune thrombocytopenia. Drugs 40:531–542, 1990.
13. Blanchette VS, Luke B, Andrew M, et al. A prospective, randomized trial of high-dose intravenous immune globulin G therapy, oral prednisone therapy, and no therapy in childhood acute immune thrombocytopenic purpura. J Pediatr 123:989–995, 1993.
14. Albayrak D, Islek I, Kalayci G, et al. Acute immune thrombocytopenic purpura: a comparative study of very high oral doses of methylprednisolone and intravenously administered immune globulin. J Pediatr 125 (Part 1):1004–1007, 1994.
15. Collins PW, Newland AC. Treatment modalities of autoimmune blood disorders. Semin Hematol 29:64–74, 1992.
16. Imbach P. Immune thrombocytopenic purpura and intravenous immunoglobulin. Cancer 68 (Suppl):1422–1425, 1991.
17. Naouri A, Feghali B, Chabal J, et al. Results of splenectomy for idiopathic thrombocytopenic purpura. Acta Haematol 89:200–203, 1993.
18. Schattner E, Bussel J. Mortality in immune thrombocytopenic purpura: report of seven cases and consideration of prognostic indicators. Am J Hematol 46:120–126, 1994.
19. McMillan R. Classical management of refractory adult immune (idiopathic) thrombocytopenic purpura. Blood Rev 16:51–55, 2002.
20. Giagounidis A, Schneider A, Germing U, et al. Treatment of relapsed idiopathic thrombocytopenic purpura with anti-CD20 monoclonal antibody rituximab: a pilot study. Eur J Haematol 69:95–100, 2002.
21. Bengtson K, Skinner M, Ware R. Successful use of anti-CD20 (rituximab) in severe, life-threatening childhood immune thrombocytopenic purpura. J Pediatr 143:670–673, 2003.
22. Thude H, Gruhn B, Werner U, et al. Treatment of a patient with chronic immune thrombocytopenic purpura with rituximab and monitoring by flow cytometric analysis. Acta Haematol 111:221–224, 2004.
23. Vesely S, Perdue J, Rizvi M, et al. Management of adult patients with persistent idiopathic thrombocytopenic purpura following splenectomy. Ann Intern Med 140:112–120, 2004.
24. Moake JL. Thrombotic microangiopathies. N Engl J Med 347:589–600, 2002.
25. Yarranton H, Machin SJ. An update on the pathogenesis and management of acquired thrombotic thrombocytopenic purpura. Curr Opin Neurol 16:367–73, 2003.
26. Elliott MA, Nichols WL. Thrombotic thrombocytopenic purpura and hemolytic uremic syndrome. Mayo Clin Proc 76:1154–1162, 2001.
27. Nabhan C, Kwaan HC. Current concepts in the diagnosis and management of thrombotic thrombocytopenic purpura. Hematol Oncol Clin North Am 17:177–199, 2003.
28. Tsai HM. Advances in the pathogenesis, diagnosis, and treatment of thrombotic thrombocytopenic purpura. J Am Soc Nephrol 14:1072–1081, 2003.
29. Proia A, Paesano R, Torcia F, et al. Thrombotic thrombocytopenic purpura and pregnancy: a case report and a review of the literature. Ann Hematol 81:210–214, 2002.
30. Rose M, Rowe JM, Eldor A. The changing course of thrombotic thrombocytopenic purpura and modern therapy. Blood Rev 7:94–103, 1993.
31. Naqvi TA, Baumann MA, Chang JC. Post-operative thrombotic thrombocytopenic purpura: a review. Int J Clin Pract 58:169–172, 2004.
32. Majhail NS, Lichtin AE. Clopidogrel and thrombotic thrombocytopenic purpura: no clear case for causality. Cleve Clin J Med 70:466–470, 2003.
33. Medina P, Sipols J, George J. Drug-associated thrombotic thrombocytopenic purpura-hemolytic uremic syndrome. Curr Opin Hematol 8:286–293, 2001.
34. Zheng X, Majerus EM, Sadler JE. ADAMTS13 and TTP. Curr Opin Hematol 9:389–394, 2002.
35. Tsai HM. Deficiency of ADAMTS13 causes thrombotic thrombocytopenic purpura. Arterioscler Thromb Vasc Biol 23:388–396, 2003.
36. Dabrow MB, Wilkins JC. Hematologic emergencies. Postgrad Med 93:193–202, 1993.
37. Yomtovian R, Niklinski W, Silver B, et al. Rituximab for chronic recurring thrombotic thrombocytopenic purpura: a case report and review of the literature. Br J Haematol 124:787–795, 2004.
38. Shapiro AD. Platelet function disorders. Haemophilia 6 (Suppl 1):120–127, 2000.
39. Fausett B, Silver RM. Congenital disorders of platelet function. Clin Obstet Gynecol 42:390–405, 1999.
40. Bennett JS, Kolodziej MA. Disorders of platelet function. Dis Mon 38:579–631, 1992.
41. Bick RL. Platelet function defects associated with hemorrhage or thrombosis. Med Clin North Am 78:577–607, 1994.
42. Aster RH. Drug-induced immune thrombocytopenia: an overview of pathogenesis. Semin Hematol 36 (Suppl 1):2–6, 1999.
43. Salama A, Mueller-Eckhardt C. Immune-mediated blood cell dyscrasias related to drugs. Semin Hematol 29:54–63, 1992.
44. Deitcher SR. Heparin-induced thrombocytopenia: pathogenesis, management, and prevention. Formulary 36:26–41, 2001.
45. Brieger DB, Kottke-Marchant K, Topol EJ. Heparin-induced thrombocytopenia. J Am Coll Cardiol 31:1449–459, 1998.
46. Fabris F, Luzzato G, Stefani PM, et al. Heparin-induced thrombocytopenia. Haematologica 85:72–81, 2000.
47. Chong BH. Heparin-induced thrombocytopenia. Aust NZ J Med 22:145–152, 1992.
48. Srinivasan A, Rice L, Bartholomew J, et al. Warfarin-induced skin necrosis and venous limb gangrene in the setting of heparin-induced thrombocytopenia. Arch Intern Med 164:66–70, 2004.
49. Hirsch J, Warkenti T, Shaughnessy S, et al. Heparin and low-molecular-weight heparin. Chest 119 (Suppl):64S–94S, 2001.
50. Kelton JG. The clinical management of heparin-induced thrombocytopenia. Semin Hematol 36 (Suppl 1):17–21, 1999.
51. Warkentin TE, Chong BH, Greinacher A. Heparin-induced thrombocytopenia: towards consensus. Thromb Haemost 19:1–7, 1998.
52. Bodensteiner DC, Doolittle GC. Adverse haematological complications of anticancer drugs. Drug Saf 8:213–224, 1993.
53. Nachman RL, Silverstein R. Hypercoagulable states. Ann Intern Med 119:819–827, 1993.
54. Isaacs C, Robert NJ, Bailey FA, et al. Randomized placebo-controlled study of recombinant human interleukin-11 to prevent chemotherapy-induced thrombocytopenia in patients with breast cancer receiving dose-intensive cyclophosphamide and doxorubicin. J Clin Oncol 15:3368–3377, 1997.
55. Levi M, ten Cate H. Disseminated intravascular coagulation. N Engl J Med 341:586–592, 1999.
56. Levi M. Current understanding of disseminated intravascular coagulation. Br J Haematol 124:567–576, 2004.
57. Bick R. Disseminated intravascular coagulation: current concepts of etiology, pathophysiology, diagnosis, and treatment. Hematol Oncol Clin North Am 17:115–147, 2003.
58. Gilbert JA, Scalzi RP. Disseminated intravascular coagulation. Emerg Med Clin North Am 11:465–480, 1993.
59. Rubin RN, Coleman RW. Disseminated intravascular coagulation: approach to treatment. Drugs 44:963–971, 1992.
60. Dempfle C. Coagulopathy of sepsis. Thromb Haemost 91:213–224, 2004.
61. Feinstein DI. Treatment of disseminated intravascular coagulation. Semin Thromb Hemost 14:351–362, 1988.
62. Toh C, Dennis M. Disseminated intravascular coagulation: old disease, new hope. Br Med J 327:974–977, 2003.
63. deJonge E, Levi M, Stoutenbeek C, et al. Current drug treatment strategies for disseminated intravascular coagulation. Drugs 55:767–777, 1998.
64. Colman RW, Rubin RN. Disseminated intravascular coagulation due to malignancy. Semin Oncol 17:172–186, 1990.
65. Cummins D, Segal H, Hunt B, et al. Chronic disseminated intravascular coagulation after surgery for abdominal aortic aneurysm: clini-

cal and haemostatic response to dalteparin. Br J Haematol 113: 658–660, 2001.

66. Sakuragawa N, Hasegawa H, Maki M, et al. Clinical evaluation of low-molecular-weight heparin (FR-860) on disseminated intravascular coagulation (DIC): a multicenter co-operative double-blind trial in comparison with heparin. Thromb Res 72:475–500, 1993.

67. Oguma Y, Sakuragawa N, Maki M, et al. Treatment of disseminated intravascular coagulation with low molecular weight heparin. Semin Thromb Hemost 16 (Suppl):34–40, 1990.

68. Gillis S, Dann E, Eldor A. Low molecular weight heparin in the prophylaxis and treatment of disseminated intravascular coagulation in acute promyelocytic leukemia. Eur J Haematol 54:59–60, 1995.

69. Fourrier F, Chopin C, Huart JJ, et al. Double-blind, placebo-controlled trial of antithrombin III concentrates in septic shock with disseminated intravascular coagulation. Chest 104:882–888, 1993.

70. Vinazzer H. Therapeutic use of antithrombin III in shock and disseminated intravascular coagulation. Semin Thromb Hemost 15: 347–352, 1989.

71. Hanada T, Abe T, Takita H. Antithrombin III concentrates for treatment of disseminated intravascular coagulation in children. Am J Pediatr Hematol Oncol 7:3–8, 1985.

72. Wisecarver JL, Haire WD. Disseminated intravascular coagulation with multiple arterial thromboses responding to antithrombin-III concentrate infusion. Thromb Res 54:709–717, 1989.

73. Warren B, Eid A, Singer P, et al. High-dose antithrombin III in severe sepsis. JAMA 286:1869–1878, 2001.

74. Vincent J, Angus D, Artigas A, et al. Effects of drotrecogin alfa (activated protein C) on organ dysfunction in the PROWESS trial. Crit Care Med 31:834–840, 2003.

75. Moscardo F, Perez F, de la Rubia J, et al. Successful treatment of severe intra-abdominal bleeding associated with disseminated intravascular coagulation using recombinant activated factor VII. Br J Haematol 114:174–176, 2001.

76. Chuansumrit A, Chantarojanasiri T, Isarangkura P, et al. Recombinant activated factor VII in children with acute bleeding resulting from liver failure and disseminated intravascular coagulation. Blood Coagul Fibrinolysis 11 (Suppl 1):S101–S105, 2000.

77. Takada A, Takada Y, Mori T, et al. Prevention of severe bleeding by tranexamic acid in a patient with disseminated intravascular coagulation. Thromb Res 58:101–108, 1990.

78. Stegmayr B, Banga R, Berggren L, et al. Plasma exchange as rescue therapy in multiple organ failure including acute renal failure. Crit Care Med 31:1730–1736, 2003.

79. Baker B, Keeling D, Murphy M. Plasma exchange as a source of protein C for acute-onset protein C pathway failure. Br J Haematol 120:166–171, 2003.

80. Yokota T, Yamada Y, Takahashi M, et al. Successful treatment of DIC with a serine proteinase inhibitor. Am J Emerg Med 19: 334–335, 2001.

81. Tamaki S, Hiyoyama K, Minamikawa K, et al. Treatment of disseminated intravascular coagulation with gabexate mesilate. Clin Ther 15:1076–1084, 1993.

82. Okamura T, Niho Y, Itoga T, et al. Treatment of disseminated intravascular coagulation and its prodromal stage with gabaxate mesilate (FOY): a multi-center trial. Acta Haematol 90:120–124, 1993.

83. DePont A, Moons A, DeJonge E, et al. Recombinant nematode anticoagulant protein c2, an inhibitor of tissue factor/factor VIIa, attenuated coagulation and the interleukin-10 response in human endotoxemia. J Thromb Haemost 2:65–70, 2004.

84. Lee A, Vlasuk G. Recombinant nematode anticoagulant protein c2 and other inhibitors targeting blood coagulation factor VIIa/tissue factor. J Intern Med 254:313–321, 2003.

85. Pernerstorfer T, Hollenstein U, Hansen J, et al. Lepirudin blunts endotoxin-induced coagulation activation. Blood 95:1729–1734, 2000.

86. Mukundan S, Zeigler Z. Direct antithrombin agents ameliorate disseminated intravascular coagulation in suspected heparin-induced thrombocytopenia thrombosis syndrome. Clin Appl Thrombosis/Hemostasis 8:287–289, 2002.

87. Thomas R. Hypercoagulability syndrome. Arch Intern Med 161: 2433–2439, 2001.

88. Buchanan GS, Rodgers GM, Branch DW. The inherited thrombophilias: genetics, epidemiology, and laboratory evaluation. Best Pract Res Clin Obstet Gynaecol 17:397–411, 2003.

89. Kottke-Marchant K, Duncan A. Antithrombin deficiency: issues in laboratory diagnosis. Arch Pathol Lab Med 126:1326–1336, 2002.

90. Baker WR, Bick RL. Treatment of hereditary and acquired thrombophilic disorders. Semin Thromb Hemost 25:387–406, 1999.

91. Hassouna HI. Laboratory evaluation of hemostatic disorders. Hematol Oncol Clin North Am 7:1161–1249, 1993.

92. Menache D. Antithrombin III concentrates. Hematol Oncol Clin North Am 6:1115–1120, 1992.

93. Schwartz RS, Bauer KA, Rosenberg RD, et al. Clinical experience with antithrombin III concentrate in treatment of congenital and acquired deficiency of antithrombin. Am J Med 87 (Suppl 3B): 53S–60S, 1989.

94. De Stefano V, Leone G, Mastrangelo S, et al. Clinical manifestations and management of inherited thrombophilia: retrospective analysis and follow-up after diagnosis of 238 patients with congenital deficiency of antithrombin III, protein C, protein S. Thromb Haemost 72:352–358, 1994.

95. Yamada T, Yamada H, Morikawa M, et al. Management of pregnancy with congenital antithrombin III deficiency: two case reports and a review of the literature. J Obstet Gynaecol Res 27:189–197, 2001.

96. Hathaway WE. Clinical aspects of antithrombin III deficiency. Semin Hematol 28:19–23, 1991.

97. Owen J. Antithrombin III replacement therapy in pregnancy. Semin Hematol 28:46–52, 1991.

98. Bauer KA. Management of thrombophilia. J Thromb Haemost 1: 1429–1434, 2003.

99. Cada DJ, ed. Drug facts and comparisons. St. Louis: Wolters Kluwer Health, Inc., 2004.

100. Thrombate III [package insert]. Elkhart, IN: Bayer Corp., 2001.

101. Bucur SZ, Levy JH, Despotis GJ, et al. Uses of antithrombin III concentrate in congenital and acquired deficiency states. Transfusion 38:481–498, 1998.

102. Menache D, O'Malley JP, Schorr JB, et al. Evaluation of the safety, recovery, half-life, and clinical efficacy of antithrombin III (human) in patients with hereditary antithrombin III deficiency. Blood 75:33–39, 1990.

103. Francis CW, Pellegrini VD Jr, Harris CM, et al. Prophylaxis of venous thrombosis following total hip and total knee replacement using antithrombin III and heparin. Semin Hematol 28:39–45, 1991.

104. van den Belt AGM, Sanson BJ, Simioni P, et al. Recurrence of venous thromboembolism in patients with familial thrombophilia. Arch Intern Med 157:2227–2232, 1997.

105. Couturaud F, Kearon C. Long-term treatment for venous thromboembolism. Curr Opin Hematol 7:302–308, 2000.

106. Bick RL. Hypercoagulability and thrombosis. Med Clin North Am 78:635–665, 1994.

108. Briggs GG, Freeman RK, Yaffe SJ. Drugs in pregnancy and lactation. Baltimore: Williams & Wilkins, 1994:223c–229c.

107. American College of Obstetricians and Gynecologists. ACOG Practice Bulletin. Thromboembolism in pregnancy. Int J Gynaecol Obstet 75:203–212, 2001.

108. Ginsberg J, Greer I, Hirsch J. Use of antithrombotic agents during pregnancy. Chest 119 (Suppl 1):122S–131S, 2001.

109. Alving BM. The hypercoagulable states. Hosp Pract 28:109–121, 1993.

110. Eby CS. A review of the hypercoagulable state. Hematol Oncol Clin North Am 7:1121–1142, 1993.

111. Pogliani EM, Parma M, Baragetti I, et al. l-Asparaginase in acute lymphoblastic leukemia treatment: the role of human antithrombin III concentrates in regulating the prothrombotic state induced by therapy. Acta Haematol 93:5–8, 1995.

112. Pabinger I, Schneider B, GTH Study Group on Natural Inhibitors. Thrombotic risk of women with hereditary antithrombin III-, protein C- and protein S-deficiency taking oral contraceptive medication. Thromb Haemost 71:548–552, 1994.

113. Nizzi F, Kaplan H. Protein C and S deficiency. Semin Thromb Hemost 25:265–272, 1999.

114. Kottke-Marchant K, Comp P. Laboratory issues in diagnosing abnormalities of protein C, thrombomodulin, and endothelial cell protein C receptor. Arch Pathol Lab Med 126:1337–1348, 2002.

115. Bick R. Prothrombin G20210A mutation, antithrombin, heparin co-factor II, protein C, and protein S defects. Hematol Oncol Clin North Am 17:9–36, 2003.

116. Pescatore S. Clinical management of protein C deficiency. Exp Opin Pharmacother 2:431–439, 2001.

117. Aiach M, Borgel D, Gaussem P, et al. Protein C and protein S deficiencies. Sem Hematol 34:205–216, 1997.

118. Dahlback B. Molecular genetics of venous thromboembolism. Ann Med 27:187–192, 1995.

119. Marlar RA, Montgomery RR, Broekmans AW, Working Party. Diagnosis and treatment of homozygous protein C deficiency. J Pediatr 114 (Pt 1):528–534, 1989.

120. Pescatore P, Horellou HM, Conard J, et al. Problems of oral anticoagulation in an adult with homozygous protein C deficiency and late onset of thrombosis. Thromb Haemost 69:311–315, 1993.

121. Manco-Johnson M, Knapp-Clevenger R. Activated protein C concentrate reverses purpura fulminans in severe genetic protein C deficiency. J Pediatr Hematol Oncol 26:25–27, 2004.

122. Reitsma P. Genetic heterogeneity in hereditary thrombophilia. Haemostasis 30(Suppl 2):1–10, 2000.

123. Abu-Amero K, Al-Hamed M, Al-Batniji F. Homozygous protein C deficiency with purpura fulminans: report of a new case and a description of a novel mutation. Blood Coagul Fibrinolysis 14:303–306, 2003.

124. Nicolaes G, Dahlbäck B. Activated protein C resistance (FV_{Leiden}) and thrombosis: factor V mutations causing hypercoagulable states. Hematol Oncol Clin North Am 17:37–61, 2003.

125. Dahlbäck B. The discovery of activated protein C resistance. J Thromb Haemostas 1:3–9, 2003.

126. De Stefano V, Mastrangelo S, Schwarz HP, et al. Replacement therapy with a purified protein C concentrate during initiation of oral anticoagulation in severe protein C congenital deficiency. Thromb Haemost 70:247–249, 1993.

127. Broekmans AW, Bertina RM, Loeliger EA, et al. Protein C and the development of skin necrosis during anticoagulant therapy [letter]. Thromb Haemost 49:251, 1983.

128. McGehee WG, Klotz TA, Epstein DJ, et al. Coumarin necrosis associated with hereditary protein C deficiency. Ann Intern Med 101:59–60, 1984.

129. Segel G, Francis C. Anticoagulant proteins in childhood venous and arterial thrombosis: a review. Blood Cells Mol Dis 26:540–560, 2000.

130. Nakayama T, Matsushita T, Hidno H, et al. A case of purpura fulminans is caused by homozygous $\Delta 8857$ mutation (protein C-Nagoya) and successfully treated with activated protein C concentrate. Br J Haematol 110:727–730, 2000.

131. Gatti L, Carnelli V, Rusconi R, et al. Heparin-induced thrombocytopenia and warfarin-induced skin necrosis in a child with severe protein C deficiency: successful treatment with dermatan sulfate and protein C concentrate. J Thromb Haemost 1:387–388, 2003.

132. Moritz B, Rogy S, Tonette S, Efficacy and safety of a high purity protein C concentrate in the management of patients with severe congenital protein C deficiency. 31st Hemophilia Symposium Hamburg 2000; 101–109.

133. Ceprotin [package insert]. Vienna, Austria: Baxter AG, 2002.

134. Xigris [package insert]. Indianapolis: Eli Lilly, 2003.

135. Schramm W, Spannagl M, Bauer KA, et al. Treatment of coumarin-induced skin necrosis with a monoclonal antibody purified protein C concentrate. Arch Dermatol 129:753–756, 1993.

136. Marlar RA, Sills RH, Groncy PK, et al. Protein C survival during replacement therapy in homozygous protein C deficiency. Am J Hematol 41:24–31, 1992.

137. Sekiyama K, Itoh H, Sagawa N, et al. Successful management of a pregnant woman with heterozygous protein C deficiency using activated protein C concentrate. J Obstet Gynaecol Res 29:412–415, 2003.

138. Bogel D, Gandrille S, Aiach M. Protein S deficiency. Thromb Haemost 78:351–356, 1997.

139. Gouault-Heilmann M, Leroy-Matheron C, Levent M. Inherited protein S deficiency: clinical manifestations and laboratory findings in 63 patients. Thromb Res 76:269–279, 1994.

140. Zoller B, Berntsdotter A, Garcia de Frutos P, et al. Resistance to activated protein C as an additional genetic risk factor in hereditary deficiency of protein S. Blood 85:3518–3523, 1995.

141. Heistinger M, Rumpl E, Illiasch H, et al. Cerebral sinus thrombosis in a patient with hereditary protein S deficiency: case report and review of the literature. Ann Hematol 64:105–109, 1992.

142. Hellgren M, Svensson PJ, Dahlback B. Resistance to activated protein C as a basis for venous thromboembolism associated with pregnancy and oral contraceptives. Am J Obstet Gynecol 173:210–213, 1995.

143. Mazza J. Hypercoagulability and venous thromboembolism: a review. WMJ 103:41–49, 2004.

144. Bolton-Maggs P, Pasi K. Haemophilia A and B. Lancet 361:1801–1809, 2003.

145. Mannucci P, Tuddenham E. The hemophilias—from royal genes to gene therapy. N Engl J Med 344:1773–1779, 2001.

146. Brettler DB, Forsberg AD, Levine PH, et al. The use of porcine factor VIII concentrate (hyate:C) in the treatment of patients with inhibitor antibodies to factor VIII. Arch Intern Med 149:1381–1385, 1989.

147. Hilgartner M. Current treatment of hemophilia arthropathy. Curr Opin Pediatr 14:46–49, 2002.

148. Shord S, Lindley C. Coagulation products and their uses. Am J Health-Syst Pharm 57:1403–1420, 2000.

149. Furie B, Limentani SA, Rosenfield CG. A practical guide to the evaluation and treatment of hemophilia. Blood 84:3–9, 1994.

150. Kulkarni R, Soucie JM, Evatt B. Renal disease among males with haemophilia. Haemophilia 9:703–710, 2003.

151. Hemophilia of Georgia. Protocols for the treatment of hemophilia and von Willebrand disease. World Federation of Hemophilia. www.wfh.org. (accessed June 2004).

152. Revel-Volk S, Golomb M, Achonu C, et al. Effect of intracranial bleeds on the health and quality of life of boys with hemophilia. J Pediatr 144:490–495, 2004.

153. Jones P. The early history of haemophilia treatment: a personal perspective. Br J Haematol 111:719–725, 2000.

154. Soucie J, Nuss R, Abdelhak A, et al. Mortality among males with hemophilia: relations with source of medical care. Blood 96:437–442, 2000.

155. Kasper C. Hereditary plasma clotting factor disorders and their management. 1999. Treatment of Hemophilia Monograph Series. World Federation of Hemophilia. www.wfh.org (accessed June 2004).

156. The Medical and Scientific Advisory Council (MASAC). MASAC recommendations concerning the treatment of hemophilia and other bleeding disorders (document #151). The National Hemophilia Foundation. www.hemophilia.org (accessed June 2004).

157. British Committee for Standards in Haematology, Blood Transfusion Take Force. Guidelines for the use of fresh-frozen plasma, cryoprecipitate and cryosupernatant. Br J Haematol 126:11–28, 2004.

158. The Medical and Scientific Advisory Council (MASAC). Guidelines for emergency department management of individuals with hemophilia. (document #155). The National Hemophilia Foundation. www.hemophilia.org (accessed June 2004).

159. Luban N. The spectrum of safety: a review of the safety of current haemophilia products. Semin Hematol 40 (Suppl 3):10–15, 2003.

160. Manno C. The promise of third-generation recombinant therapy and gene therapy. Semin Hematol 40 (Suppl 3):23–28, 2003.

161. Mannucci P, Giangrande P. Choice of replacement therapy for hemophilia: recombinant products only? Hematol J 1:72–76, 2000.

162. The Medical and Scientific Advisory Council (MASAC). MASAC recommendations regarding the use of recombinant clotting factor replacement therapies. (document #106). The National Hemophilia Foundation. www.hemophilia.org (accessed June 2004).

163. Stachnik J, Gabay M. Continuous infusion of coagulation of factor products. Ann Pharmacother 36:882–891, 2002.

164. Abildgaard CF. Hazards of prothrombin complex concentrates in the treatment of hemophilia. N Engl J Med 304:670–671, 1981.

165. Paisley S, Wight J, Currie E, et al. The management of inhibitors in haemophilia A: introduction and systematic review of current practice. Haemophilia 9:405–417, 2003.

166. Jones M, Wight J, Paisley S, et al. Control of bleeding in patients with hemophilia A with inhibitors: a systematic review. Haemophilia 9:464–520, 2003.

167. Feinstein DI. Acquired disorders of hemostasis. In: Coleman RW, Hirsch J, Marder VJ, et al, eds. Hemostasis and thrombosis, 3rd ed. Philadelphia: JB Lippincott, 1994:881.

168. Blatt PM, White GC, McMillan CW, et al. Treatment of antifactor VIII antibodies. Thromb Haemost 38:514–523, 1977.
169. Kasper CK. The therapy of factor VIII inhibitors. Prog Hemost Thromb 9:57–86, 1989.
170. Villar A, Jimenez-Yuste V, Quintana M, et al. The use of haemostatic drugs in haemophilia: desmopressin and antifibrinolytic agents. Haemophilia 8:189–193, 2002.
171. Mannucci PM, Ruggeri ZM, Pareti FI, et al. 1-Deamino-8-*d*-arginine vasopressin: a new pharmacologic approach to the management of hemophilia and von Willebrand's disease. Lancet 8: 869–872, 1977.
172. Mannucci PM, Bettega D, Cattaneo M. Patterns of development of tachyphylaxis in patients with haemophilia and von Willebrand's disease after repeated doses of desmopressin (DDAVP). Br J Heamatol 82:87–93, 1992.
173. Weinstein RE, Bona RD, Altman AJ, et al. Severe hyponatremia after repeated intravenous administration of desmopressin. Am J Hematol 32:258–261, 1989.
174. Manco-Johnson M. Update on treatment regimens: prophylaxis versus on-demand therapy. Semin Hematol 40 (Suppl 3):3–9, 2003.
175. The Medical and Scientific Advisory Council (MASAC). MASAC recommendations concerning prophylaxis (prophylactic administration of clotting factor concentrate to prevent bleeding). (document #117). The National Hemophilia Foundation. www.hemophilia.org (accessed June 2004).
176. Valentino L. Secondary prophylaxis therapy: what are the benefits, limitations and unknowns? Haemophilia 10:147–157, 2004.
177. Bontempo F, Lewis J, Gorenc T, et al. Liver transplantation in hemophilia A. Blood 69:1721–1724, 1987.
178. Monahan P, White G. Hemophilia gene therapy: update. Curr Opin Hematol 9:430–436, 2002.
179. Walsh C. Gene therapy for the hemophilias. Curr Opin Pediatr 14: 12–16, 2002.
180. Gezer S. Antiphospholipid syndrome. Dis Mon 2003;49:696–741.
181. Meroni PL, Moia M, Derksen RHWM, et al. Venous thromboembolism in the antiphospholipid syndrome: management guidelines for secondary prophylaxis. Lupus 12:504–507, 2003.
182. Bick RL. The antiphospholipid thrombosis syndromes: lupus anticoagulants and anticardiolipin antibodies. Adv Pathol Lab Med 8: 391, 1995.
183. Bick RL. Antiphospholipid thrombosis syndromes: etiology, pathophysiology, diagnosis and management. Int J Hematol 65:193–213, 1997.
184. Oppenheimer S, Hoffbrand B. Optic neuritis and myelopathy in systemic lupus erythematosus. Can J Neurol Sci 13:129–132, 1986.
185. Bick RL, Ismail Y, Baker WF. Coagulation abnormalities in patients with precocious coronary artery thrombosis and patients with failing coronary artery bypass grafting and percutaneous transcoronary angioplasty. Semin Thromb Hemost 19:412–417, 1993.
186. Katzau A, Chapman J, Shoenfield Y. CNS dysfunction in the antiphospholipid syndrome. Lupus 12:903–907, 2003.
187. Englert H, Hawkes C, Boey M. Dagos' disease: association with anticardiolipin antibodies and the lupus anticoagulant. Br Med J 289:576, 1984.
188. Frampton G, Winer JB, Cameron JS. Severe Guillain-Barré syndrome: an association with IgA anti-cardiolipin antibody in a series of 92 patients. J Neuroimmunol 19:133–139, 1988.
189. Hinton RC. Neurological syndromes associated with antiphospholipid antibodies. Semin Thromb Hemost 20:46–54, 1994.
190. Levine SR, Welch K. The spectrum of neurologic disease associated anticardiolipin antibodies. Arch Neurol 44:876–883, 1987.
191. Derksen RHWM, Khamashta MA, Branch DW. Management of the obstetric antiphospholipid syndrome. Arthritis Rheum 50: 1028–1039, 2004.
192. Tincani A, Branch W, Levy RA. Treatment of pregnant patients with antiphospholipid syndrome. Lupus 12:524–529, 2003.
193. Khamashta MA, Cuadrado MJ, Mujic F, et al. The management of thrombosis in the antiphospholipid-antibody syndrome. N Engl J Med 332: 993–997, 1995.
194. Erkan D, Cervera R, Asherson RA. Catastrophic antiphospholipid syndrome. Where do we stand? Arthritis Rheum 48:3320–3327, 2003.
195. Asherson RA, Cervera R, de Groot PG, et al. Catastrophic antiphospholipid syndrome: international consensus statement on classification criteria and treatment guidelines. Lupus 12:530–534, 2003.
196. Wilson WA, Gharavi AE, Koike T, et al. International consensus statement on preliminary classification criteria for definite antiphospholipid syndrome. Arthritis Rheum 42:1309–1311, 1999.
197. Sibilia J. Antiphospholipid syndrome: why and how should we make the diagnosis? Joint Bone Spine 70:97–102, 2003.
198. Devine DV, Brigden ML. The anti-phospholipid syndrome. When does the presence of antiphospholipid antibodies require therapy? Postgrad Med 99:105–122, 1996.
199. Alarcón-Seovia D, Boffa MC, Branch W, et al. Prophylaxis of the antiphospholipid syndrome: a consensus report. Lupus 12:499–503, 2003.
200. Petri M. Evidence-based management of thrombosis in the antiphospholipid antibody syndrome. Curr Rheumatol Rep 5:370–373, 2003.
201. Bick RL, Baker WF. The antiphospholipid and thrombosis syndromes. Med Clin North Am 78:667–684, 1994.
202. Bick RL. Disseminated intravascular coagulation: objective criteria for diagnosis and management. Med Clin North Am 78:511–543, 1994.

CASE STUDIES

CASE 13

TOPIC: Megaloblastic Anemia

THERAPEUTIC DIFFICULTY: Level 2
Erica Murrell

Chapter 31: Iron Deficiency and Megaloblastic Anemias

■ Scenario

Patient and Setting: EC, an 83-year-old female; home visit by nurse to perform dressing change for bedsore

Chief Complaint: Pain and tingling in her lower extremities, shortness of breath, fatigue, increased anxiety, difficulty sleeping, and constipation

■ History of Present Illness

Recent bedsore due to failure to thrive after a recent hip replacement. Visiting nurse performing dressing changes discovered the patient was non-adherent with her medication regimen and had a 5% loss in weight over the last 30 days. Pharmacy consult for review of patient medications requested.

Medical History: Hypertension (20 years), chronic obstructive pulmonary disease (COPD), depression, osteoporosis, gout, GERD

Surgical History: Hip replacement s/p fall 1 year ago

Family/Social History: Family History: Noncontributory
Social History: Patient denies smoking tobacco but admits to drinking two shots of bourbon at bedtime to help with recent sleeping problems; lives alone with no family members in the area; only financial resources are her retirement check and Medicare

Medications:
HCTZ, 25 mg PO daily
Lisinopril, 40 mg PO daily
Fosamax, 70 mg PO qweek
Colchicine, 0.6 mg PO QOD
Pepcid, 20 mg PO BID
Klonopin, 0.5 mg PO BID
Zoloft, 50 mg PO daily
Combivent, 2 puffs QID
Ambien, 5 mg PO QHS PRN

Allergies: No known drug allergies

■ Physical Examination

GEN: Frail and pale, moderate distress
VS: 126/80, HR 75, RR 14, T 37.8°C, Wt 50 kg
HEENT: Pale conjunctiva, pale and dry mucous membranes
COR: RRR
CHEST: Bilateral wheezes
ABD: Soft, slightly tender, decreased bowel sounds
GU: Deferred
RECT: Guaiac negative stool
EXT: Slow capillary refilling with slightly pale nail beds and palms of hands, dry and flaky skin, level 2 bedsore noted slightly below the lower back area
NEURO: Alert, oriented to person, place, and time

■ Results of Pertinent Laboratory Tests, Serum Drug Concentrations, and Diagnostic Tests

Na	147 (147)	Hgb	100 (10)	Albumin	31 (3.1)
K	4.0 (4.0)	MCV	110 (110)	Uric acid	428 (7.2)
Cl	97 (97)	MCH	1.8 (29)	Glucose	5.8 (105)
HCO3	26 (26)	RDW	0.16 (16)	Serum B$_{12}$	98.1 (133)
BUN	8.9 (25)	Ca	2.1 (8.4)	Serum Folate	20 (8.8)
Cr	97.2 (1.1)	PO4	0.94 (2.9)		
Hct	0.30 (30)	Mg	1.0 (2.0)		

Peripheral blood smear: normochromic, macrocytic RBCs

■ Problem List

Identify principal problems from the scenario in priority order (see Answers in back of book for correct list of problems).

■ SOAP Note

To be completed by the student (see Answers in back of book for correct SOAP Note).

■ QUESTIONS

(See Answers in back of book for correct responses.)

1. What predisposing factor places EC at a greater risk for developing vitamin B_{12} deficiency? (E-03)
   a. GERD
   b. Bedsore
   c. Elderly
   d. Postmenopausal status

2. What lab finding coupled with a decreased vitamin B_{12} level would suggest vitamin B_{12} deficiency? (E0-05)
   a. Decreased iron level
   b. Increased folate level
   c. Decreased homocysteine level
   d. Increased MCV level

3. List the potential causes of vitamin B_{12} deficiency to consider in EC. (EO-01)

4. A physical assessment finding of ECs that is consistent with anemia is: (EO-05)
   a. T 37.8°C
   b. Wt 50 kg
   c. Slow capillary refilling
   d. Pale nail beds

5. List the signs and symptoms of anemia. (EO-02)

6. Which of the following medications is the most likely contributor to EC's B_{12} deficiency? (EO-09)
   a. Colchicine
   b. HCTZ
   c. Zoloft
   d. Lisinopril

7. Vitamin B_{12} must be obtained through dietary intake or supplementation because it contains which of the following elements?
   a. Zinc
   b. Iron
   c. Cobalt
   d. Selenium

8. Vitamin B_{12} is stored primarily in which of the following organs?
   a. Kidney
   b. Spleen
   c. Gallbladder
   d. Liver

9. List pros and cons of oral, parental, and intranasal forms of B_{12} supplementation. (EO-11)

10. Develop an education plan for EC regarding the treatment option you would select for EC and why that is the best option for her. (EO-14)

11. What psychosocial factors may affect EC's adherence to both pharmacologic and nonpharmacologic therapy? (EO-15)

12. Describe the health care provider's role in managing EC's vitamin B_{12} deficiency. (EO-16)

13. Evaluate the pharmacoeconomic considerations relative to EC's plan of care. (EO-17)

14. Summarize the therapeutic, pathophysiologic, and disease management concepts for megaloblastic anemias utilizing a key points format. (EO-18)

Asthma

Kathryn Blake and H. William Kelly

DEFINITION

The National Asthma Education and Prevention Program (NAEPP) of the Heart, Lung, and Blood Institute and the Global Initiative for Asthma (GINA) have published guidelines on the diagnosis, management, and prevention of asthma.[1,2] These guidelines can be downloaded from the Internet at http://www.nhlbi.nih.gov/guidelines/asthma/asthgdln.pdf or at http://www.ginasthma.com/workshop.pdf. An update on the NAEPP report on selected topics was published in 2002 and can be downloaded from http://www.nhlbi.nih.gov/guidelines/asthma/asthmafullrpt.pdf. According to these guidelines, asthma is defined largely as a chronic inflammatory disorder of the airways, which emphasizes that asthma is not simply a disease of smooth muscle bronchoconstriction, as was once thought.

Focus on the genetic origins of asthma is increasing, and descriptions of asthma subtypes in the future may be defined by genetic loci. Genetic studies have yielded susceptibility loci for asthma, and several may be major gene effects for asthma. Many of these studies have focused on portions of the genome that contain genes responsible for immune function. Because asthma is a complex disease, the physiologic definition as described by NAEPP and GINA is broad. However, results of genetic studies may allow for precise identification of asthma phenotypes. Chromosome locations of interest for asthma genes include 2p, 4q, 5q23–q33, 6p21–24, 11q13–21, 13q12–14, 16q21–23, and 19q.[3] In addition, five novel asthma genes have been identified over the past few years.[3] Genetic information on asthma can be searched on databases found at http://www.cdc.gov/genomics/info/database.htm.

ETIOLOGY

It is well recognized that expression of the disease is the result of a complex interrelationship between the presence and absence of genetic susceptibility and environmental influences. The difficulty in defining asthma relates to the multiple factors that trigger bronchospasm; these include allergens, environment (weather changes, perfumes, smoke), emotions, exercise, and respiratory infection. Family and twin studies support the heritable basis of the disease.[3]

EPIDEMIOLOGY

According to data compiled by the American Lung Association, an estimated 20.3 million persons (7.2% of persons) in the United States have self-reported asthma, as of 2001.[4] The incidence of asthma has risen from 6.8 million persons in 1980, to 14.6 million persons in 1994, to 20.3 million persons in 2001, which represents a threefold increase over approximately 20 years. Twenty-five percent of asthmatics are 5 to 17 years old, and 38% are between 18 and 44 years of age. Thus, nearly two thirds of persons affected by asthma are children and young adults. Children with asthma younger than 15 years of age accounted for 35% of hospital admissions in 2000, with asthmatic females (children and adults) accounting for 57% of admissions. African-Americans, who accounted for 25% of all hospitalizations for asthma in 2000, have a death rate of 3.9 per 100,000 compared with a rate of 1.3 for whites (2000 data). A total of 4,487 deaths resulted from asthma in 2000—a decrease from a peak of 5,667

TABLE 34.1	Risk Factors for Death from Asthma

Past history of sudden severe exacerbations

Previous intubation for asthma

Previous admission for asthma to an intensive care unit

Two or more hospitalizations for asthma in the past year

Three or more emergency care visits for asthma in the past year

Hospitalization or an emergency care visit for asthma within the past month

Use of >2 canisters per month of an inhaled short-acting β_2-agonist

Current use of systemic corticosteroids or recent withdrawal from systemic corticosteroids

Difficulty perceiving airflow obstruction or its severity

Co-morbidity, as from cardiovascular disease or chronic obstructive pulmonary disease

Serious psychiatric disease or psychosocial problems

Low socioeconomic status and urban residence

Illicit drug use

Sensitivity to *Alternaria*

(From National Asthma Education and Prevention Program. Expert panel report 2: guidelines for the diagnosis and management of asthma. Bethesda, MD: US Department of Health and Human Services, Public Health Service, National Institutes of Health, National Heart, Lung, and Blood Institute, April 1997; Publication no 97–4051.)

deaths in 1996. The risk factors for death from asthma are shown in Table 34.1.[1]

PATHOPHYSIOLOGY

The pathophysiology of asthma is characterized by a variable degree of airflow obstruction secondary to bronchial smooth muscle constriction, airway wall inflammation and edema, epithelial desquamation, mucous hypersecretion, bronchial hyperresponsiveness, and, in some but not all, airways remodeling (Fig. 34.1 *see color insert*).[2,5] Airway wall inflammation is characterized by an influx of eosinophils, neutrophils, lymphocytes, and degranulated mast cells. Airway inflammation is considered to be the primary pathologic event in asthma.[1,2,5,6] Initially, it was described in postmortem observations of patients with asthma who died from an attack of asthma or from other causes; however, both bronchial biopsy and bronchoalveolar lavage (BAL) studies have consistently demonstrated most if not all the above components of inflammation in all patients with asthma, regardless of the variant of asthma, the disease severity, or the principal triggering event (allergy, virus, or occupational trigger).

More recently, remodeling of the airways thought to be secondary to persistent inflammation has been described in a number of patients with asthma. Airway remodeling refers to structural changes that consist of collagen deposition in the subbasement membrane, airway smooth muscle hypertrophy and hyperplasia, increased numbers of mucous glands, and enhanced vasculature of the airway walls.[5] These changes may lead to irreversible narrowing of the airway lumen. It has been hypothesized that airway remodeling is the cause of the increased loss in lung function over time reported in adults with asthma compared with normal adults without asthma.[5,6] However, certain aspects of airway remodeling have been noted in airway tissues from children and adults with asthma and those with normal lung function.[5]

The precise pathologic mechanism for the development and persistence of airway inflammation in asthma has yet to be elucidated. However, a large body of research has described the cells and mediators that are involved in the inflammatory process; these are briefly described here. It appears that there are two predominant forms of asthma: extrinsic or allergic (atopic) asthma, and intrinsic or nonallergic asthma.[6] Atopy is associated with 40% to 50% of patients with asthma, but not all allergic patients develop asthma.[6] However, much of our understanding of the patho-

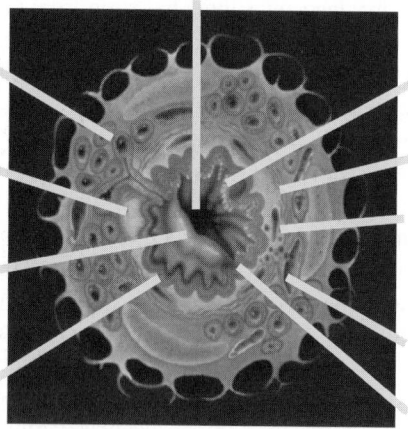

Airway lumen narrowing

Mucous gland hypertrophy and hyperplasia

Edema

Mucus hypersecretion

Thickening of basement membrane

Epithelial damage

Airway smooth-muscle hypertrophy, hyperplasia, and bronchoconstriction

Inflammatory cell infiltration

Vascular dilation

Goblet cell hyperplasia

FIGURE 34.1 Diagram illustrating the changes present in a fully contracted small airway (*see color insert*).

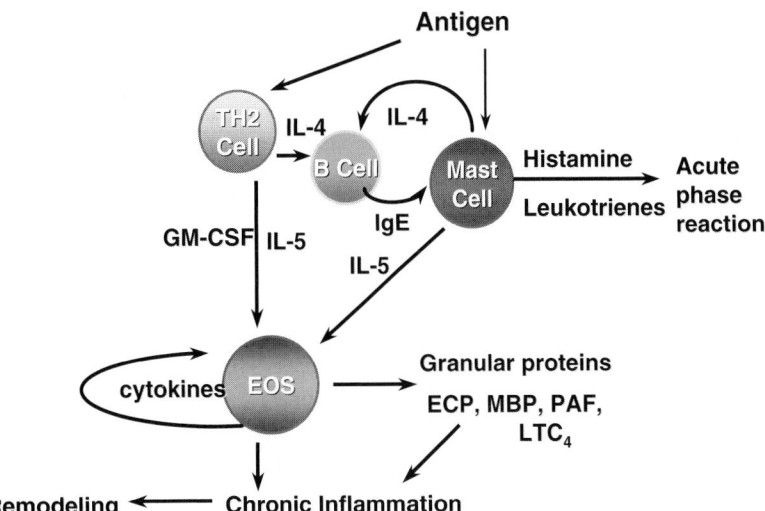

FIGURE 34.2 Pathophysiologic findings in the asthmatic airway. (Adapted from National Asthma Education and Prevention Program. Expert panel report. Guidelines for the diagnosis and management of asthma (*see color insert*).)

physiology of asthma comes from studies of patients with this phenotype. Intrinsic asthma commonly follows respiratory viral infection; it is not associated with specific immunoglobulin E (IgE) antibodies, is associated with aspirin sensitivity, and may be more severe than extrinsic asthma.[6] Although intrinsic asthma is clinically different from extrinsic asthma and is not associated with high serum IgE concentrations, it is not necessarily immunopathologically distinct, as patients with intrinsic asthma also have shown a Th2 cytokine profile in biopsy studies.[6,7] Figure 34.2 (*see color insert*) provides a simplistic schematic of the interaction of inflammatory cells, cytokines, and mediators in asthma. However, it should be remembered that well over 20 cytokines alone have been described that could be involved in regulating the inflammation of asthma, and that the cytokine system is a highly duplicative process with more than one cytokine performing specific functions.[6] Thus, it is no wonder that therapies that reduce the presence of one cytokine have not been successful in treating asthma.

INFLAMMATORY CELLS

Lymphocytes. Two types of lymphocyte responses are mediated by T-helper CD4+ cells. Type 1 T-helper (Th1) cells produce interleukin (IL)-2 and interferon-γ, both essential in cellular defense mechanisms for fighting infection.[7] Th2 cells produce cytokines (IL-4, -5, -6, -9, and -13) that mediate allergic inflammation.[7] Asthmatic inflammation is thought to result from a Th2-mediated mechanism (an imbalance between Th1 and Th2 cells).[6,7] The Th1/Th2 imbalance also provides the immunologic basis for the *hygiene hypothesis*, which attempts to explain the increasing prevalence of asthma in westernized urban environments. The T-cell population in the cord blood of newborn infants is skewed toward a Th2 phenotype.[6] The newborn's immune system then requires timely and appropriate environmental stimuli to create a balanced immune response. Factors that enhance Th1-mediated response include infection with *Mycobacte-*

rium tuberculosis and numerous viruses, as well as endotoxin exposure.[2] Th2-lymphocyte cytokines direct undifferentiated B-lymphocytes to make specific IgE antibodies following allergen presentation.[2,7] Th2 cytokines also promote the production and influx of mast cells and eosinophils into the airways. Lastly, lymphocytes provide the memory that likely promotes the chronicity of the inflammation. Selective retention of airway T-cells occurs, along with the release of selected proinflammatory mediators and cytokines involved in the recruitment and activation of inflammatory cells.[8,9] The activation of T-cells after allergen challenge leads to the release of Th2-like cytokines that may be key in the mechanism of the late-phase response.[2]

Mast Cells. Following the release of IgE into the circulation, these cytokines bind to the high-affinity IgE receptors (FcεRI) in tissue mast cells and circulating basophils.[2] Mast cells are found throughout the walls of the respiratory tract, and threefold to fivefold increases have been described in the airways of atopic patients with asthma. Once binding and cross-linking of allergen to cell-bound IgE occur, mediators such as histamine, eosinophil and neutrophil chemotactic factors, leukotrienes (LT) B_4, C_4, and D_4, prostaglandins, platelet-activating factor, and others are released from mast cells (Fig. 34.2). Histologic examination has revealed degranulated mast cells in the airways of patients who have died from acute asthma attacks. Mast cell degranulation is believed to be the primary event that produces decreased lung function and symptoms immediately following inhalation of an allergen.[5,6] In addition, infiltration of mast cells into the airway smooth muscle may be responsible for ongoing airway hyperresponsiveness in asthma.[5,7]

Inhaled allergen challenge in atopic patients leads to an early-phase allergic reaction that, in some cases, may be followed by a late-phase reaction. The early asthmatic response is characterized by a rapid drop in lung function secondary to the release of preformed inflammatory mediators such as histamine, eicosanoids, and reactive oxygen species that induce contraction of airway smooth muscle, mucous secretion, and vasodilatation.[2,5] Spontaneous recovery occurs within an hour. However, these inflammatory mediators also induce microvascular leakage with exudation of plasma in the airways, inducing a thickened, engorged, and edematous airway wall and consequent narrowing of the airway lumen. This may contribute to the influx of inflammatory cells that produces the late-phase allergic reaction (see section on Eosinophils). Plasma proteins also may promote the formation of exudative plugs mixed with mucus and inflammatory and epithelial cells. Mast cell degranulation is felt to be an important mechanism for exercise-induced bronchospasm (EIB).[7] In this case, the degranulation appears to be secondary to cooling or increased osmolarity of the bronchial fluids, or both.

Eosinophils. Eosinophils appear to be the primary effector cells in asthma inflammation because they release cytotoxic mediators (oxygen free radicals, eicosanoids, and major basic protein) and cytokines.[2,5] The late-phase inflammatory reaction or late asthmatic response occurs 4 to 8 hours after allergen inhalation and involves the recruitment and activation of eosinophils.[5] It is characterized by a prolonged drop in lung function that is difficult to reverse. Nonspecific bronchial hyperresponsiveness is increased after the late-phase reaction, but not after the early-phase reaction, following allergen or occupational challenge.[5]

Eosinophilopoiesis is regulated by IL-5 and granulocyte-macrophage colony-stimulating factor (GM-CSF). Circulating eosinophils migrate to the airways through cell rolling or interactions with selectins, and they eventually adhere to the endothelium through the binding of integrins to adhesion proteins (vascular cell adhesion molecule-1 (VCAM-1) and intercellular adhesion molecule-1 (ICAM-1)). Once at the site of airways inflammation, the survival of eosinophils as activated cells is increased as a consequence of reduced apoptosis (normal programmed cell death) and increased expression of adhesion molecules on epithelial cells. Several cytokines and chemokines, including GM-CSF, IL-3, IL-5, and regulated upon activation, normal T-cell expressed and secreted (RANTES; a member of the interleukin-8 superfamily), may promote cell survival.[6]

Alveolar Macrophages and Neutrophils. Alveolar macrophages and neutrophils are also found in the airways of patients with asthma. Their role in asthma remains to be elucidated.[6] Alveolar macrophages serve as ''scavengers,'' engulfing and digesting bacteria and other foreign materials. They are found in large and small airways and may be capable of amplifying the inflammatory response through the release of the following mediators: platelet-activating factor, LTB_4, LTC_4, LTD_4, neutrophil chemotactic factor, and eosinophil chemotactic factor.[5]

Neutrophils may be present normally in the airways and usually do not infiltrate tissues with chronic allergic inflammation. However, high numbers of neutrophils have been reported to be present in the airways of patients who died from sudden-onset fatal asthma.[1,5] They are also increased in the airways following exacerbation during viral respiratory infection and have been present in adults with severe corticosteroid-dependent asthma, which suggests that neutrophils may play a role in the disease process.[6] Neutrophilic inflammation is more prominent in inflammation secondary to smoking (chronic obstructive pulmonary disease (COPD)). The neutrophil may be a source for a variety of mediators, including platelet-activating factor, prostaglandins, thromboxanes, and leukotrienes.[5]

Epithelial Cells. Bronchial epithelial cells traditionally have been considered to act as a barrier that participates in mucociliary clearance and removal of noxious agents. In asthma, especially fatal asthma, epithelial shedding occurs. However, epithelial cells also participate in inflammation through the release of eicosanoids, peptidases, matrix proteins, cytokines, and nitric oxide (NO).[5] Epithelial cells can be activated by IgE-dependent mechanisms, viruses, pollutants, or histamine. Epithelial cells appear to be important in the repair process and may contribute to airway remodeling through the release of fibrogenic growth factors.[5] Epithelial shedding may be caused by plasma exudation, toxic inflammatory mediators, oxygen free radicals, tumor necrosis factor-alpha (TNF-α), mast cell proteolytic enzymes, and metalloproteases from epithelial cells or macrophages.[5] The functional consequences of epithelial shedding may include heightened airways responsiveness through increased penetration of various provocative stimuli, depletion of epithelial-derived relaxant factors, and loss of enzymes responsible for degrading proinflammatory neuropeptides.

Fibroblasts and Myofibroblasts. Fibroblasts are found frequently in connective tissue and act as precursors for various cell types. In asthma, myofibroblasts are increased in numbers beneath the reticular basement membrane, and they increase in number following the late asthmatic response. Their numbers are positively associated with the thickness of the reticular basement membrane.[5]

MEDIATORS

As with specific cytokines, no single mediator is responsible for the pathogenesis of asthma. Histamine is capable of inducing smooth muscle constriction, mucosal edema, and mucous secretion.[2] Lung mast cells are an important source of histamine.[5,6] Histamine is involved in acute bronchospasm following allergen exposure; however, other mediators such as leukotrienes and prostaglandins are also involved. Antihistamines are not effective in the treatment of patients with asthma. Several classes of important mediators, including arachidonic acid and its metabolites (i.e., prostaglandins, leukotrienes, thromboxane A_2, and platelet-activating factor), are derived from cell membrane phospholipids.

The 5-lipoxygenase pathway of arachidonic acid breakdown is responsible for production of the class of compounds called *cysteinyl leukotrienes* (LTs).[10] Leukotrienes C_4, D_4, and E_4 (cysteinyl LTs) share a common receptor (the LTD_4 receptor) that, when stimulated, produces bronchospasm, mucous secretion, microvascular permeability, and airway edema. The only specific mediator inhibitors that demonstrate efficacy in asthma are those that inhibit leukotriene synthesis or act as leukotriene receptor antagonists, and these have only a modest effect.

BRONCHIAL HYPERRESPONSIVENESS

Hyperresponsiveness of the airways to physical, chemical, and pharmacologic stimuli is a hallmark of asthma.[2,5] Although it is found in other respiratory diseases, the degree of responsiveness is quantitatively greater in patients with asthma. The degree of responsiveness correlates with the clinical course of asthma and the medication necessary to control symptoms.[2] Patients with mild symptoms or who are in remission demonstrate lower levels of responsiveness, although still greater than the normal population; some patients in remission have normal responsiveness. The increased responsiveness seen in asthma is at least in part caused by an inflammatory response within the airways.[2,5] Investigators have found correlations between inflammatory cells in BAL fluids and degree of hyperresponsiveness.[2] Newer evidence suggests that airways remodeling correlates with bronchial hyperresponsiveness.[2,5,6] Although the precise link is not known, bronchial hyperresponsiveness is in part related to the extent of inflammation in the airways; it worsens upon exposure to inflammatory triggers and lessens when effective anti-inflammatory therapy is provided.[2]

MUCOUS PRODUCTION

The mucociliary system is the lung's primary defense mechanism against irritants and infectious agents. Mucus, composed of 95% water and 5% glycoproteins, is produced by bronchial epithelial glands and goblet cells.[2,5] Normal mucociliary clearance is dependent upon maintenance of a continuous aqueous layer controlled by active ion transport across the epithelium and the viscoelastic properties of the mucus. Mucus that is too watery or too viscous will not be transported optimally. The inflammatory process of asthma impairs mucociliary transport. In addition, the remodeling process produces an increase in size and number of goblet cells in the airways. Mucous plugs found in the airways of patients who died from severe asthma exacerbations are highly viscous and tend to be connected by mucous strands to the goblet cells.[2] There have also been reports of airways being plugged with casts that consisted of sloughed epithelial cells and inflammatory cells.[2] Autopsies of patients with asthma who died from other causes also have revealed mucous plugging.

AIRWAY SMOOTH MUSCLE

Smooth muscle is wrapped around the airways in a spiral arrangement.[2] A threefold to fourfold increased muscle volume has been reported in the airways of patients with asthma, although significant heterogeneity has been noted.[5] Airway

smooth muscle contraction displays a sphincteric action that is capable of completely occluding the airway lumen. The airway smooth muscle extends from the trachea through the respiratory bronchioles. When expressed as percentage of wall thickness, the smooth muscle represents 5% of the large central airways and up to 20% of the wall thickness in the bronchioles. In patients with asthma, smooth muscle may account for 11% to 20% of wall thickness.[5] The precise cause of the increased smooth muscle mass in asthma is not known, but it is important in magnifying and maintaining bronchial hyperresponsiveness in chronic asthma.[5]

NEURAL MECHANISMS

Parasympathetic, sympathetic, and nonadrenergic inhibitory nerves innervate the airways.[2] The normal resting tone of human airway smooth muscle is maintained by parasympathetic efferent activity via the vagus nerve.[11] Numerous chemical and physical irritants produce bronchoconstriction through stimulation of nonmyelinated C-fibers of the afferent system that lie immediately beneath the tight junctions between epithelial cells that line the airway lumen.[2] In contrast, the sympathetic innervation of the airway smooth muscle is sparse and does not directly control airway smooth muscle tone.[2] However, airway smooth muscle contains an abundance of noninnervated β_2-adrenergic receptors that produce bronchodilation.[11] Thus, circulating catecholamines play an important role in regulating bronchial tone.

The nonadrenergic, noncholinergic nervous system releases the excitatory neuropeptides substance P and neurokinin A following stimulation of C-fiber nerve endings. Vasoactive intestinal peptide is an inhibitory neurotransmitter within the system, but inflammatory cells in asthma can release peptidases that may degrade it, thereby amplifying bronchoconstriction.[2] The nonadrenergic, noncholinergic nervous system also amplifies inflammation in asthma by releasing NO, a potent smooth muscle relaxant that produces vasodilation and bronchodilation.[2] Endogenous NO is generated from the amino acid L-arginine by the enzyme NO synthase.[12] One of the three isoforms of NO synthase is induced in response to cytokines from airway epithelial cells and inflammatory cells of asthmatic airways; thus, NO is upregulated in asthma and correlates with the degree of airways inflammation.[12] The fraction of exhaled NO (FeNO) in expired air appears to be a useful measure of ongoing lower airways inflammation in patients with asthma, and it is helpful for measuring effectiveness of therapy.[12]

CLINICAL PRESENTATION AND DIAGNOSIS

SIGNS AND SYMPTOMS

Chronic Asthma. Symptoms of chronic asthma include shortness of breath or dyspnea, wheezing, cough, and sputum production. Chest "tightness" is a common complaint among patients with asthma; symptoms may occur continuously or may be episodic. On the basis of symptoms and objective measures, the NAEPP guidelines provide treatment recommendations on the classification of asthma as mild intermittent, mild persistent, moderate persistent, or severe persistent.[1]

Acute Asthma. Symptoms of acute asthma are similar to those of chronic asthma and are characterized by shortness of breath, wheezing, cough, and chest tightness. Tachypnea, tachycardia, retractions, cyanosis, and hypoxemia may also be present. Asthma of sudden onset may be referred to as acute asthma, asthma exacerbation, or status asthmaticus. Patients with these symptoms may present to the emergency department or may be appropriate for home self-management under the supervision of health care professionals. Acute asthma that results from progressive inflammatory processes may progress over many hours, days, or even weeks before functional deterioration is reached. Eighty percent to 90% of adults with acute asthma who present to an emergency department have asthma progression of this type, which has often been triggered by upper respiratory tract infection.[13] Eosinophils may be present in the airways, indicating an allergic component, and patients are often slow (days or weeks) to respond to treatment.[13] Conversely, in a minority of patients, symptoms are of sudden onset, and bronchospasm is the primary pathologic process. Airway obstruction typically occurs quickly (over less than 6 hours) after onset; typical triggers include allergens (such as exposure to a cat), exercise, and psychosocial stress.[13] Patients respond to treatment more quickly and completely. They may have a preponderance of neutrophils in their airways, which is also a finding in patients with fatal asthma.

Exercise-Induced Bronchospasm. EIB, also called exercise-induced asthma or thermally induced asthma, is defined as "transient narrowing of the airway that follows vigorous exercise."[14] It is present in 30% to 90% of patients with asthma, although when exercise is sufficiently vigorous, EIB is present in nearly all patients with asthma.[15] EIB can be further provoked when the patient breathes in cold, dry air. Symptoms of EIB are similar to those of asthma that are provoked by other stimuli; they include wheezing, chest tightness, cough, and possibly, hypoxemia. When exercise occurs, airways bronchodilate and when exercise ceases, airways bronchoconstrict. However, when exercise is sufficiently prolonged, or if other triggers are present (such as pollens on a soccer or football field), bronchoconstriction may occur during exercise. The peak fall in lung function typically occurs within 5 to 10 minutes after activity ceases; function returns to normal within 20 to 30 minutes.[1] Clinically, EIB is defined as a fall in forced expiratory volume in 1 second (FEV_1) of at least 15% following exercise.[1] Only rarely are delayed (hours later) bronchoconstrictor effects noted after the initial bronchostriction has resolved.

Nocturnal Asthma. Nocturnal asthma may represent a manifestation of more severe disease or a discrete disease process. In some patients, increased inflammatory markers are present that do not demonstrate circadian variability, whereas in others, diurnal variation in cytokine levels, oxygen radicals, and alveolar inflammation may occur.[16] Nocturnal asthma is defined as an increase of greater than 15% in normal diurnal variation in lung function that occurs with peak lung function at 4:00 PM and minimal lung function at 4:00 AM.[16] Symptoms include dyspnea and cough that may awaken the patient and result in bronchodilator treatment. Gastroesophageal reflux disease, obesity, and increasing age (middle age and older) are associated with nocturnal asthma.[16] Evaluation of nocturnal symptoms is essential to the classification of asthma and may influence treatment provided according to the NAEPP guidelines.[1,17]

Premenstrual Asthma. Premenstrual asthma is characterized by an increase in asthma symptoms in the days before and during menstruation. The incidence of premenstrual asthma is estimated at 8% to 40% among women; it tends to occur in women who are older and who have had long-standing asthma.[18,19] Sex steroid hormones have an effect on premenstrual asthma, although the exact mechanisms are unclear. In addition, evidence suggests that the usual increase in β_2-receptor density that occurs during the luteal phase of the menstrual cycle in nonasthmatic women is absent in women with premenstrual asthma.[18,19] Treatment includes hormonal therapies, leukotriene antagonists, and inhaled corticosteroids plus long-acting inhaled β_2-agonists.[18,19]

DIAGNOSIS AND CLINICAL FINDINGS

History. The diagnosis of asthma is usually made on the basis of clinical history and objective measures of pulmonary function. It can be elusive in that a number of other conditions, including foreign body aspiration, laryngotracheomalacia, bronchiolitis, and cystic fibrosis, may manifest as wheezing (Table 34.2).[1] Recurrent exacerbations, which may provoke factors such as allergens, irritants, exercise, or viral respiratory infection, and a history of nocturnal symptoms are particularly characteristic of asthma. Although the history is of great importance and is helpful in narrowing the diagnosis of the disease, it is not diagnostic. Of note, the physical examination may be normal when no symptoms are present. Rhinitis, sinusitis, eczema, blood eosinophilia, and nasal secretion and sputum eosinophilia may also be present.[1,20]

A number of factors, such as allergens (pollens, moulds, mites, animal danders), viral respiratory tract infections, environmental irritants (smoke, strong odors, cold dry air), exercise, food additives (sulfites, tartrazine), and medications (aspirin, nonsteroidal anti-inflammatory drugs (NSAIDs), β-blockers), may trigger asthma symptoms or exacerbations. Although the psychological effects of emotions do not induce asthma, the physiologic response to certain emotions (hard laughter, crying) may precipitate asthma symptoms. Following exposure to a relevant allergen, an immediate

TABLE 34.2	Differential Diagnosis of Asthma
Infants and Children	**Adults**
Allergic rhinitis and sinusitis	Chronic obstructive pulmonary disease (chronic bronchitis or emphysema)
Foreign body in trachea or bronchus	Congestive heart failure
Vocal cord dysfunction	Pulmonary embolism
Vascular rings or laryngeal webs	Laryngeal dysfunction
Laryngotracheomalacia, tracheal stenosis, or bronchostenosis	Mechanical obstruction of the airways (tumors)
Enlarged lymph nodes or tumor	Pulmonary infiltration with eosinophilia
Viral bronchiolitis or obliterative bronchiolitis	Cough secondary to drugs
Cystic fibrosis	Vocal cord dysfunction
Bronchopulmonary dysplasia	
Heart disease	
Aspiration from dysfunction of swallowing	
Recurrent cough not due to asthma	
Mechanism dysfunction or gastroesophageal reflux	

(From National Asthma Education and Prevention Program. Expert panel report 2: guidelines for the diagnosis and management of asthma. Bethesda, MD: US Department of Health and Human Services, Public Health Service, National Institutes of Health, National Heart, Lung, and Blood Institute, April 1997; Publication no 97–4051.)

asthmatic response (IAR)—a drop in pulmonary function within minutes—and a late asthmatic response (LAR)—a second drop in pulmonary function after several hours of exposure—may be observed (Fig. 34.3C) (see also section on mast cells and eosinophils). It is believed that many symptoms of persistent asthma are due to unrelenting inflammatory responses that are triggered by continued exposure to allergens or other provocateurs.

Spirometry. Airflow is easily measured, and although reduced airflow is a characteristic feature of asthma, other diseases may manifest with similar obstruction. Airflow is typically measured by spirometry or peak expiratory flow (Fig. 34.3A,B), and normal (predicted) values based on height, age, sex, and race are established. FEV_1, the most commonly used spirometric evaluation of pulmonary function, consists of the volume of air expelled within the first second of forced expiration after maximal inhalation. It is normally >70% of the total volume of expired air (forced vital capacity (FVC)); however, in obstructive processes such as asthma, FEV_1 is reduced, as is FVC (although to a lesser extent); therefore, the FEV_1/FVC ratio is also reduced. Peak expiratory flow (PEF) is the maximal rate at which air is exhaled from the lungs with a forced expiratory maneuver; it correlates fairly well with FEV_1, although for some patients, it does not correlate well with symptoms. Peak flowmeters are simple, portable, and relatively inexpensive devices that facilitate accurate and objective self-monitoring of pulmonary function. Patients should be encouraged to use the same brand of peak flow device during monitoring as

they usually use, as different brands can give clinically significant different measurements. A disadvantage of both FEV_1 and PEF is their dependence on patient effort.[1]

Bronchial Challenge. Demonstration of bronchial hyperresponsiveness by inhalation challenge testing with histamine, methacholine, or exercise can also be helpful to clinicians in making the diagnosis; however, these tests can pose some danger and require sufficient precautions. Because of safety concerns, provocation with specific allergens is rarely recommended.[20]

Bronchial hyperresponsiveness is the exaggerated bronchoconstrictor response that may follow exposure to physical and chemical stimuli; it may persist for weeks to months following exposure to stimuli such as viral respiratory infections. Bronchial hyperresponsiveness can be measured by inhalation challenge testing, with patients inhaling increasing doses of histamine or methacholine; the end point is the dose required to elicit a ≥20% fall in pulmonary function, typically FEV_1. The provocative concentration or dose required for a 20% fall in FEV_1 (PC_{20} or PD_{20}) is inversely proportionate to bronchial hyperresponsiveness; thus, a lower PD_{20} is indicative of greater reactivity (Fig. 34.3D). Not only can measures of bronchial hyperresponsiveness be used for the diagnosis of asthma, but changes in PD_{20} over time may be useful for guiding therapy and gauging response to therapy.

Assessment of Allergy. It is estimated that 60% to 78% of adult patients with asthma[21] and up to 93% of children

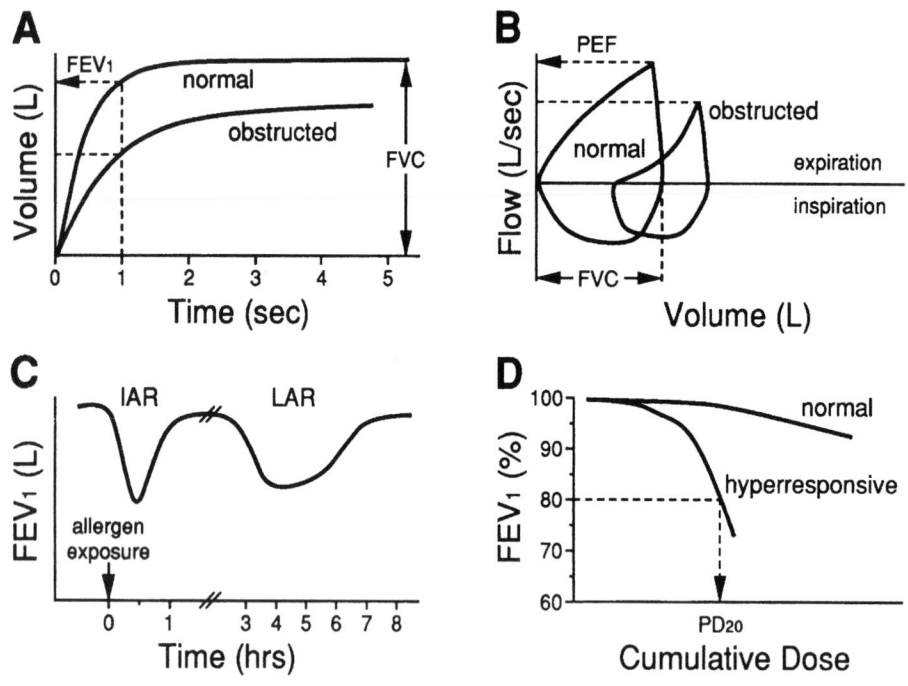

FIGURE 34.3 A. Typical spirometry of normal and obstructed patients. Note the lower forced expiratory volume at 1 second (FEV₁), forced vital capacity (FVC), and FEV₁/FVC ratio in the obstructed patient. **B.** Typical flow-volume loops of a normal and obstructed patient. Note the lower peak expiratory flow, increased lung volume, and typical "scooped out" expiratory curve in the obstructed patient. **C.** Typical immediate and late asthmatic responses seen following exposure to relevant allergen. Immediate asthmatic response (IAR) occurs within minutes, and late asthmatic response (LAR) occurs several hours after exposure. Patients may demonstrate an isolated IAR, an isolated LAR, or dual responses. **D.** Typical pulmonary function seen with histamine or methacholine challenge testing in normal and hyperresponsive patients. The provocative concentration or dose of histamine or methacholine required to elicit a drop in FEV₁ of 20% (PC₂₀ or PD₂₀) is inversely proportionate to bronchial hyperresponsiveness.

and adolescents with asthma have an allergic component to their disease.[22] Inhalation of allergens directly into the lungs or exacerbations of allergic rhinitis can evoke symptoms of asthma.

Allergen prick skin testing is the most commonly used diagnostic test for atopy. The skin is first cleansed with alcohol, then a drop of allergen extract is placed onto the skin. With the use of a sterile lancet, a small prick is made through the drop; this allows a small amount of allergen to enter the skin. If sensitivity is present, a wheal and flare response will occur within 20 minutes. Skin testing can be performed on infants as young as 3 months of age. If the patient is unable to withhold oral antihistamines before skin testing is performed, or is otherwise not a candidate for skin testing, a radioallergosorbent test can be performed. IgE antibody testing may also be used to assess the allergic component of a patient's asthma and, more recently, to determine the appropriateness of treatment with anti-IgE monoclonal antibody therapy.

Chest X-Ray. Chest radiographs (posterior-anterior) may be normal in mild disease; however, signs of air trapping (hyperinflation) are more often present with severe, chronic asthma. Radiographs may be more useful in younger children, particularly infants, to exclude alternative conditions that may be causing symptoms of reduced airflow such as pneumonia, cystic fibrosis, recurrent milk inhalation, congenital heart disease, or other congenital malformations.[1,2] Chest radiographs taken in the emergency department for

patients with acute asthma add little to the medical management of these patients, except possibly for those with other complicating findings.[23]

PSYCHOSOCIAL ASPECTS

Patients with asthma may also suffer from psychosocial problems that affect their ability to care for themselves, thus adversely affecting their overall health and quality of life. Depression and anxiety appear to be relatively common disorders in patients with asthma, and in children, these are positively correlated with severity of asthma.[24,25] In a small study, 25% of patients with moderate to severe asthma had major depression, 16% had anxiety disorder, and 13% had a social phobia (28% had a specific phobia).[25] Because it is difficult to control asthma symptoms in patients with high levels of depression, co-management of psychiatric and asthma symptoms is often needed.[25]

Panic disorder appears to occur with greater prevalence in patients with asthma (approximately 10% compared with 3% of the general population), and these patients tend to have more frequent emergency department visits and greater asthma morbidity.[24,26] Asthma tends to precede the development of a panic disorder in 20% of patients, suggesting that treatment of asthma should be maximized before drug therapy for an anxiety disorder is added.[25] Additionally, chronic respiratory disorders are three times more common in patients with panic disorders than in those with other psychiatric diseases.[24] It is interesting to note that mild asthma tends to provoke greater symptoms of anxiety, whereas more severe symptoms are better recognized as being related to asthma and thus generate asthma coping behaviors.[24] Confusion between asthma and panic symptoms can lead patients to overmedicate with asthma medications.[24,25] Hyperventilation in asthma can invoke bronchoconstriction, which may also precipitate a panic response.

Patients with brittle asthma (i.e., asthma characterized by frequent and significant fluctuations in daily peak flow readings, or sudden, severe exacerbations in relatively stable disease) or those who have nearly died from asthma or have ultimately died from asthma frequently have (had) psychosocial problems (Table 34.3).[27] Most patients with near-fatal asthma are women; exacerbations occur frequently on Sundays, asthma is characterized as severe persistent and has an adverse effect on work or school, visits to the emergency department or intensive care unit are frequent, and routine asthma care is considered suboptimal. In addition to these characteristics, patients who have died from asthma are often from a lower socioeconomic group. In patients with near-fatal asthma or fatal asthma, psychosocial issues are believed to have contributed to the event in more than 80% of cases.[27]

Factors that have been identified as being associated with asthma death include (a) an underestimation of the severity of disease caused by lack of objective measures of lung function (such as peak expiratory flow) in evaluating disease, (b) failure of the patient and family to appreciate the severity of episodes because the patient is used to having a suboptimal level of health, and (c) underuse of oral and inhaled corticosteroids for long-term treatment.[27] It is interesting to note that since the introduction of more effective treatment for asthma such as inhaled corticosteroid therapy in the 1970s, interest in the psychological and psychosocial aspects of the disease has diminished.[27] In fact, recent asthma guidelines fail to include specific discussion of these issues,[1,2] although guidelines stress the need to involve the patient (and family) with all members of the health care team to optimize care. This partnership encourages joint development of treatment goals, review of these goals and outcomes on a regular basis, open communication, and teaching and reinforcing of self-management techniques. Through these processes, improvements in the psychosocial well-being of the patient are to be expected.

Poor adherence with prescribed medications has been associated with increased mortality from asthma. Patients who are nonadherent with their medications tend to be younger; to have higher scores for depression on certain scales; to feel ashamed, embarrassed, or angry about their disease; and to be concerned about adverse effects of corticosteroids and the possibility of becoming addicted to their medications.[27]

TABLE 34.3 Adverse Psychosocial Factors in Near-Fatal (NFA) and Fatal Asthma

	NFA	Fatal Asthma
Depression or other psychiatric illness, currently or previously	+	+
Denial	+	+
Personality disorder		+
Psychiatric case-ness	+	+
Current or recent use of major tranquilizers or sedatives	+	+
Deliberate self-harm		+
Learning disability or mental retardation	+	+
Psychiatric history in a first-degree relative	+	+
Alcohol or drug abuse	+	+
Recent bereavement		+
Severe domestic stress	+	+
Social isolation, living alone, homelessness	+	+
Unemployment, self-employment, threatened redundancy	+	+
Marital problems		+
Marital separation or single parenthood	+	+
Extreme poverty		+
Childhood abuse		+
Smoking or passive smoking	+	+
Legal problems		+

Many patients had more than one adverse factor.
(From Harrison BD. Psychosocial aspects of asthma in adults. Thorax 53:519–525, 1998.)

Adolescents, in particular, are poorly adherent with their medications because of denial, peer pressure, lack of perception of disease, reluctance to seek medical advice, ignorance, and desire for a simpler medication regimen.[28] However, once adolescents realize that asthma does not have to be disabling, and that participation in sports is encouraged, medication adherence improves because of their desire to be normal.[28]

THERAPEUTIC PLAN

TREATMENT GUIDELINES

The National Asthma Education and Prevention Program (NAEPP) of the National Institutes of Health (NIH) and the Global Initiative for Asthma (GINA) of the World Health Organization (WHO) have provided evidence-based national and international guidelines for the diagnosis and management of asthma.[1,2] The overriding goal of these guidelines is to improve the quality of care of patients with asthma by improving outcomes. The main precepts of the NAEPP and GINA guidelines, as well as of guidelines developed by other countries, are similar. The four major components of asthma management are as follows: (a) use of objective measures to assess and monitor, (b) control of factors that contribute to asthma severity, (c) use of optimal pharmacologic therapy, and (d) provision of patient education with the goal of developing a partnership in asthma care.[1] Attention to each of these components is essential if optimal care is to be provided. The goals of asthma management put forth by the NAEPP and GINA are listed here[1,2]:

1. Maintain normal activity levels (including exercise and other physical activity).
2. Maintain (near) normal pulmonary functions.
3. Prevent chronic and troublesome symptoms (e.g., coughing or breathlessness in the night, in the early morning, or after exertion).
4. Prevent recurrent exacerbations of asthma and minimize the need for emergency department visits or hospitalizations.
5. Provide optimal pharmacotherapy with minimal or no adverse effects.
6. Meet patients' and families' expectations of satisfaction with asthma care.

The NAEPP recommends spirometry at the time of diagnosis in patients old enough to produce accurate results (i.e., those older than 5 years of age) for the purpose of assessing airflow obstruction and reversibility.[1] Spirometry is then recommended following initiation of therapy after signs and symptoms stabilize, and at least every 1 to 2 years to monitor for progression of the disease.[1] Ongoing periodic assessment of the signs and symptoms of asthma, patient functional status or quality of life, the history of asthma exacerbations, the amount of pharmacotherapy required, and patient satisfaction with the health care provider is also recommended.[1]

Ongoing PEF monitoring with home peak flowmeters is no longer recommended for all patients.[17] However, it is recommended that patients with persistent asthma be taught how to use a peak flowmeter, and that patients with more severe asthma and those who might have difficulty perceiving symptoms of airflow obstruction monitor their morning PEF on a regular basis. Peak flow monitoring can be used as part of patient education to help the patient recognize symptoms of airflow obstruction and determine specific triggers that induce bronchoconstriction.

Long-Term Treatment. The NAEPP and GINA guidelines recommend therapy that is based on the persistence and severity of symptoms. Figure 34.4 provides the stepwise approach to therapy for adults and children older than 5 years, as recommended by the 2002 update of the NAEPP guidelines.[17] Only mild intermittent asthma (Step 1) does not require long-term control therapy. All patients should be prescribed a short-acting inhaled β_2-agonist for the treatment of acute symptoms. The dosage can be found in Table 34.4[17] and varies with the severity of symptoms and the response to initial therapy (Fig. 34.5).[1] It is recommended that all patients receive a written action plan for their daily long-term medications and for what to do for acute exacerbations of asthma.[17] This should be part of the patient education process.

Drugs with anti-inflammatory activity, specifically, the inhaled corticosteroids, are the cornerstone of long-term daily therapy for persistent asthma. As monotherapy, the inhaled corticosteroids are more effective than cromolyn, leukotriene modifiers, nedocromil, and theophylline.[17] The alternative long-term controllers are listed alphabetically because review of the evidence did not find any to be more effective than the other. In addition, inhaled corticosteroids are the only long-term controller therapy that has been associated with a reduced risk of dying from asthma.[29] Patients with persistent asthma should not use regular administration of short- or long-acting inhaled β_2-agonists as long-term controller monotherapy.

In moderate persistent asthma, the preferred therapy (Step 3) is the addition of a long-acting inhaled β_2-agonist to inhaled corticosteroids in the low to medium dose range.[29] The evidence clearly demonstrated that this combination was more effective at improving lung function and reducing asthma exacerbations than was doubling the dose of inhaled corticosteroids.[29] In patients with a history of frequent or severe exacerbations, it is recommended that the inhaled corticosteroid dose be increased, and that a long-acting inhaled β_2-agonist be added to the treatment. However, current evidence suggests that a fourfold increase in inhaled corticosteroid dosage is required to produce a significant reduction in asthma exacerbations.[30–32] The addition of sustained-release theophylline or a leukotriene modifier is as effective as doubling the dose of inhaled corticosteroids and could provide an alternative for patients who do not tolerate long-acting inhaled β_2-agonists. No evidence supports the use

Classify Severity: Clinical Features Before Treatment or Adequate Control			Medications Required To Maintain Long-Term Control
	Symptoms/Day Symptoms/Night	PEF or FEV$_1$ PEF Variability	Daily Medications

Step 4
Severe Persistent
	Continual
	Frequent
		≤60%
		>30%
			■ Preferred treatment:
			  – High-dose inhaled corticosteroids
			  AND
			  – Long-acting inhaled beta$_2$-agonists
			  AND, if needed,
			  – Corticosteroid tablets or syrup long term (2 mg/kg/day, generally do not exceed 60 mg per day). (Make repeat attempts to reduce systemic corticosteroids and maintain control with high-dose inhaled corticosteroids.)

Step 3
Moderate Persistent
	Daily
	>1 night/week
		>60% – <80%
		>30%
			■ Preferred treatment:
			  – Low-to-medium dose inhaled corticosteroids and long-acting inhaled beta$_2$-agonists.
			■ Alternative treatment (listed alphabetically):
			  – Increase inhaled corticosteroids within medium-dose range
			  OR
			  – Low-to-medium dose inhaled corticosteroids and either leukotriene modifier or theophylline.
			
			If needed (particularly in patients with recurring severe exacerbations):
			■ Preferred treatment:
			  – Increase inhaled corticosteroids within medium-dose range and add long-acting inhaled beta$_2$-agonists.
			■ Alternative treatment:
			  – Increase inhaled corticosteroids within medium-dose range and add either leukotriene modifier or theophylline.

Step 2 Mild Persistent	>2/week but < 1x/day >2 nights/month	≥80% 20–30%	■ Preferred treatment: – Low-dose inhaled corticosteroids. ■ Alternative treatment (listed alphabetically): cromolyn, leukotriene modifier, nedocromil, OR sustained release theophylline to serum concentration of 5–15 mcg/mL.
Step 1 Mild Intermittent	≤2 days/week ≤2 nights/month	≥80% <20%	■ No daily medication needed. ■ Severe exacerbations may occur, separated by long periods of normal lung function and no symptoms. A course of systemic corticosteroids is recommended.

Quick Relief **All Patients**	■ Short-acting bronchodilator: 2–4 puffs short-acting inhaled beta$_2$-agonists as needed for symptoms. ■ Intensity of treatment will depend on severity of exacerbation; up to 3 treatments at 20-minute intervals or a single nebulizer treatment as needed. Course of systemic corticosteroids may be needed. ■ Use of short-acting beta$_2$-agonists >2 times a week in intermittent asthma (daily, or increasing use in persistent asthma) may indicate the need to initiate (increase) long-term-control therapy.

 Step down
Review treatment every 1 to 6 months; a gradual stepwise reduction in treatment may be possible.

 Step up
If control is not maintained, consider step up. First, review patient medication technique, adherence, and environmental control.

Goals of Therapy: Asthma Control

- Minimal or no chronic symptoms day or night
- Minimal or no exacerbations
- No limitations on activities; no school/work missed
- Maintain (near) normal pulmonary function
- Minimal use of short-acting inhaled beta$_2$-agonist
- Minimal or no adverse effects from medications

Note
- The stepwise approach is meant to assist, not replace, the clinical decisionmaking required to meet individual patient needs.
- Classify severity: assign patient to most severe step in which any feature occurs (PEF is % of personal best; FEV$_1$ is % predicted).
- Gain control as quickly as possible (consider a short course of systemic corticosteroids); then step down to the least medication necessary to maintain control.
- Minimize use of short-acting inhaled beta$_2$-agonists. Overreliance on short-acting inhaled beta$_2$-agonists (e.g., use of short-acting inhaled beta$_2$-agonist every day, increasing use or lack of expected effect, or use of approximately one canister a month even if not using it every day) indicates inadequate control of asthma and the need to initiate or intensify long-term-control therapy.
- Provide education on self-management and controlling environmental factors that make asthma worse (e.g., allergens and irritants).
- Refer to an asthma specialist if there are difficulties controlling asthma or if step 4 care is required. Referral may be considered if step 3 care is required.

FIGURE 34.4 Stepwise approach to asthma therapy for older children and adults, from the NAEPP update on the management of asthma. (From the National Asthma Education and Prevention Program. Expert panel report: guidelines for the diagnosis and management of asthma update on selected topics—2002. J Allergy Clin Immunol 110 (5 Suppl):S141–S219, 2002. Reproduced with permission.)

TABLE 34.4 Dosages of Drugs for Acute Severe Exacerbations of Asthma in the Emergency Department or Hospital

Medications	Dosages		Comments
Inhaled β2 agonists	**>6 years old**	**≤ 6 years old**	
Albuterol Nebulizer Soln (5 mg/mL)	2.5–5 mg every 20 min for 3 doses, then 2.5–10 every 1–4 h as needed, or 10–15 mg/hr continuously.	0.15 mg/kg (minimum dose 2.5 mg) every 20 min for 3 doses, then 0.15–0.3 mg/kg up to 10 mg every 1–4 h as needed, or 0.5 mg/kg/hour by continuous nebulization	Only selective β2 agonists are recommended. For optimal delivery dilute aerosols to minimum of 4 mL at gas flow of 6–8 L/min.
MDI 90 μg/puff	4–8 puffs every 30 min up to 4 hours then every 1–4 hours as needed.	4–8 puffs every 20 min for 3 doses, then every 1–4 hours as needed.	In patients in severe distress nebulization is preferred, use holding-chamber type spacer.
Levalbuterol Nebulizer Soln	Give at one-half the mcg dose of albuterol above	Give at one half the mcg dose of albuterol above	The single isomer of albuterol is likely to be twice as potent
Bitolterol Nebulizer Soln (2mg/ml)	See albuterol dose	See albuterol dose, thought to be as potent to one-half as potent as albuterol on a μg basis.	Has not been studied in acute severe asthma. Do not mix with other drugs.
Pirbuterol MDI 200 μg/puff	See albuterol dose	See albuterol dose, one-half as potent as albuterol on a μg basis.	Has not been studied in acute severe asthma.
Systemic β agonists			
Epinephrine 1:1000 (1 mg/mL)	0.3–0.5 mg every 20 min for 3 doses SQ	0.01 mg/kg up to 0.5 mg every 20 min for 3 doses SQ	No proven advantage of systemic therapy over aerosol.
Terbutaline (1 mg/ml)	0.25 mg every 20 min for 3 doses SQ	0.01 mg/kg every 20 min for 3 doses then every 2–6 h as needed SQ	Not recommended.
Anticholinergics			
Ipratropium Br-Nebulizer Soln (.25mg/ml)	500 μg every 30 min for 3 doses then every 2 to 4 hours as needed	250 μg every 20 min for 3 doses, then 250 μg every 2 to 4 hours.	May mix in same nebulizer with albuterol. Do not use as first-line therapy, only add to β2 agonist therapy.
MDI 18 μg/puff	4–8 puffs as needed every 2 to 4 hours	4–8 puffs as needed every 2 to 4 hours	Not recommended as dose in inhaler is low and has not been studied in acute asthma.
Corticosteroids			
Prednisone Methylprednisolone Prednisolone	60–80mg in 3 or 4 divided doses for 48 hours, then 30–40 mg/d until PEF reaches 70% of personal best.	1 mg/kg every 6 hours for 48 hours then 1–2 mg/kg/day in 2 divided doses until PEF 70% of normal predicted	For outpatient "burst" use 1–2 mg/kg/day max 60 mg for 3–7 days. It is unnecessary to taper course.

No advantage has been found for very high dose corticosteroids in acute severe asthma, nor is there any advantage for intravenous administration over oral therapy. The usual regimen is to continue the frequent multiple daily dosing until the patient achieves an FEV$_1$ or PEF of 50% of personal best or normal predicted value and then lower the dose to twice daily dosing. This usually occurs within 48 hours. The final duration of therapy following a hospitalization or emergency department visit may be from 7 to 14 days. If patients are then started on inhaled corticosteroids, studies indicate there is no need to taper the systemic steroid dose. If the follow-up therapy is to be given once daily, studies indicate there may be an advantage to giving the single daily dose in the afternoon at around 3:00pm. (From National Asthma Education and Prevention Program. Expert panel report: guidelines for the diagnosis and management of asthma update on selected topics—2002. J Allergy Clin Immunol 110 (5 Suppl):S141–S219, 2002.)

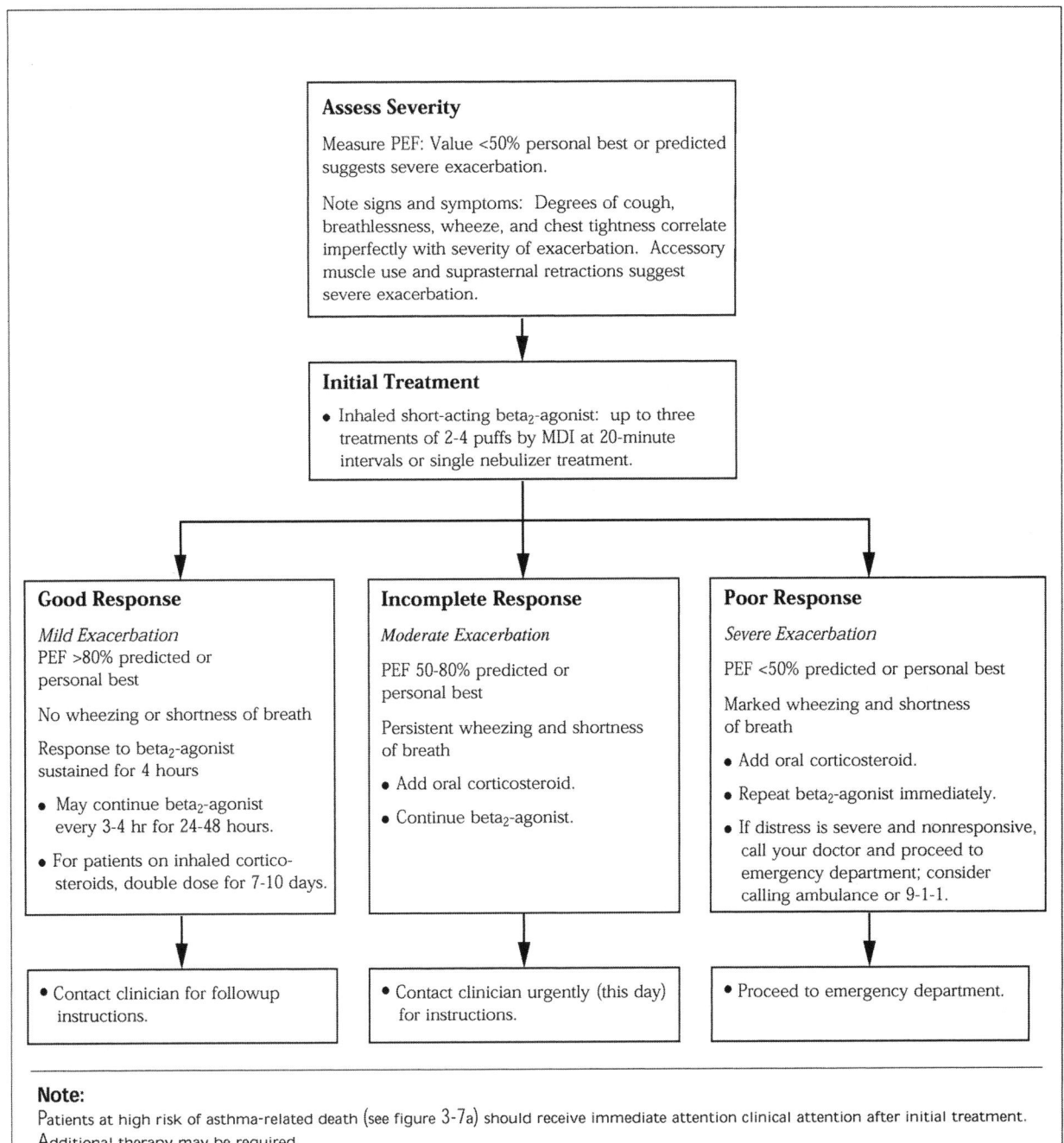

Assess Severity

Measure PEF: Value <50% personal best or predicted suggests severe exacerbation.

Note signs and symptoms: Degrees of cough, breathlessness, wheeze, and chest tightness correlate imperfectly with severity of exacerbation. Accessory muscle use and suprasternal retractions suggest severe exacerbation.

Initial Treatment

- Inhaled short-acting beta$_2$-agonist: up to three treatments of 2-4 puffs by MDI at 20-minute intervals or single nebulizer treatment.

Good Response

Mild Exacerbation
PEF >80% predicted or personal best

No wheezing or shortness of breath

Response to beta$_2$-agonist sustained for 4 hours

- May continue beta$_2$-agonist every 3-4 hr for 24-48 hours.
- For patients on inhaled corticosteroids, double dose for 7-10 days.

Incomplete Response

Moderate Exacerbation

PEF 50-80% predicted or personal best

Persistent wheezing and shortness of breath

- Add oral corticosteroid.
- Continue beta$_2$-agonist.

Poor Response

Severe Exacerbation

PEF <50% predicted or personal best

Marked wheezing and shortness of breath

- Add oral corticosteroid.
- Repeat beta$_2$-agonist immediately.
- If distress is severe and nonresponsive, call your doctor and proceed to emergency department; consider calling ambulance or 9-1-1.

- Contact clinician for followup instructions.

- Contact clinician urgently (this day) for instructions.

- Proceed to emergency department.

Note:
Patients at high risk of asthma-related death (see figure 3-7a) should receive immediate attention clinical attention after initial treatment. Additional therapy may be required.

FIGURE 34.5 Home therapy of acute asthma exacerbations from the NAEPP Expert Panel Report 2 on the management of asthma. (From National Asthma Education and Prevention Program. Expert panel report 2: guidelines for the diagnosis and management of asthma. Bethesda, MD: US Department of Health and Human Services, Public Health Service, National Institutes of Health, National Heart, Lung, and Blood Institute, April 1997; Publication no 97-4051.)

of cromolyn, nedocromil, or oral long-acting β_2-agonists as adjunctive therapy. The goal in both mild persistent and moderate persistent asthma is to convert patients to the mild intermittent category (normal lung function and the use of as-needed short-acting inhaled β_2-agonists for symptoms that occur less often than 3 days per week).

The recommended therapy for patients with severe persistent asthma is high-dose inhaled corticosteroids plus long-acting inhaled β_2-agonists.[17] Increasing the dose of the long-acting inhaled β_2-agonists over the standard dose has not been shown to be beneficial.[2,17] Many clinicians and asthma specialists may prescribe a third long-term controller (i.e., leukotriene modifiers or sustained-release theophylline) for these patients before placing them on oral corticosteroids to avoid the toxicities associated with long-term systemic corticosteroid exposure (see later discussion). However, current evidence does not support additional efficacy obtained by addition of a third or a fourth long-term controller.[17] All these patients should be referred to a specialist for investigation into factors that may be interfering with response to therapy such as chronic sinusitis, psychological factors that are affecting compliance, workplace exposures, and gastroesophageal reflux.[1,2] Patients with atopy with severe asthma and high IgE concentrations have been able to discontinue oral corticosteroid therapy following omalizumab therapy.[2] Other therapies for severe persistent asthma that have been used to lower the need for systemic corticosteroids include cyclosporine, methotrexate, gold, intravenous immunoglobulin, and hydroxychloroquine.[1] Although some small studies show benefit, the evidence is far from conclusive; therefore, it is recommended that these agents be used only by specialists in asthma care.

Acute Treatment. Patients at all levels of severity are at risk for acute exacerbations of asthma. Even those patients whose persistent symptoms are well controlled on long-term therapy may experience acute exacerbations when exposed to specific triggers such as allergens, smoke, air pollution, or upper respiratory tract viral infections.[1,2] Although patients with more severe disease may be at greater risk for severe exacerbation, patients considered to have mild disease are also at risk for life-threatening asthma exacerbations.[33] Thus, all patients should be instructed on what to do for asthma exacerbations, and they should be given a written action plan. Action plans based on symptoms have been shown to be as effective as action plans based on PEF monitoring.[17] Sample action plans can be found at the NAEPP and GINA Web sites. Figure 34.5 is an algorithm for home management of acute exacerbations.[1] Whether or not to provide a patient with oral prednisone to be initiated at home is an individual decision made according to the comfort level of the physician and the patient. Regardless, it is recommended that the clinician be contacted if oral corticosteroids are to be started.[1,2] Figure 34.6 provides the algorithm for treating acute exacerbations in the physician's office, urgent care center, emergency department, and hospital.[1]

Recommended dosages of drugs for severe acute exacerbations are provided in Table 35.4.[17] The short-acting inhaled β_2 agonists are the most effective quick relief medications.[33] There does not appear to be any advantage for using nebulized therapy over metered-dose inhaler (MDI) plus a valved holding chamber (VHC) spacer device for delivering the aerosol, so the choice is left to the treating clinician.[34,35] The short-acting inhaled anticholinergic ipratropium bromide should be used only for those patients who are intolerant to short-acting inhaled β_2-agonists (a very rare phenomenon) as it can reverse only bronchospasm mediated by cholinergic stimulation. However, in those patients who are not completely responding to the usual doses of short-acting inhaled β_2-agonists in the emergency department, the addition of ipratropium bromide has been shown to reduce the risk of hospitalization.[10,36]

Most patients who seek care for an asthma exacerbation at an urgent care center or an emergency department will respond adequately to the first three doses of short-acting inhaled β_2-agonists and can be discharged home.[37] Most of the research in severe acute asthma therapy involves those patients with an inadequate response to the first three doses. It is recommended that patients with an inadequate response to the initial bronchodilators be started on systemic corticosteroids to treat the inflammatory component of the exacerbation.[1,2] These corticosteroids may be administered orally or parenterally, although there is no advantage in efficacy for either mode of administration.[8,33] Other therapies shown to enhance outcomes and reduce the risk of hospitalization in patients in the emergency department include the addition of frequent doses of ipratropium bromide and the use of very frequent or continuous delivery of aerosolized short-acting inhaled β_2-agonists.[9,10,35,36]

Therapies for which numerous studies have been conducted with inconclusive or no evidence for greater efficacy than the standard therapy include the parenteral administration of short-acting β_2-agonists, the addition of theophylline (parenterally or orally), the parenteral administration of magnesium sulfate, the use of high-dose inhaled corticosteroids, and the administration of heliox.[1,33,38] The parenteral use of β_2-agonists increases the risk of adverse effects without enhancing efficacy.[39] Theophylline, particularly in its parenteral form aminophylline, was a mainstay of therapy for severe acute asthma in the 1970s and 1980s; however, it has since been shown that it does not add to the efficacy of the inhaled β_2-agonists.[38,40] In some studies, the use of theophylline has been associated with an increase in adverse effects.[40,41] Although inhaled corticosteroids are not as effective as systemic corticosteroids in the treatment of severe acute asthma, the introduction of inhaled corticosteroids to the usual short course of systemic corticosteroids appears to prevent relapse following discharge from the emergency department.[8,42]

Two therapies that are still considered experimental by the NAEPP are magnesium sulfate and heliox. Magnesium sulfate is a smooth muscle relaxant used for preeclampsia.

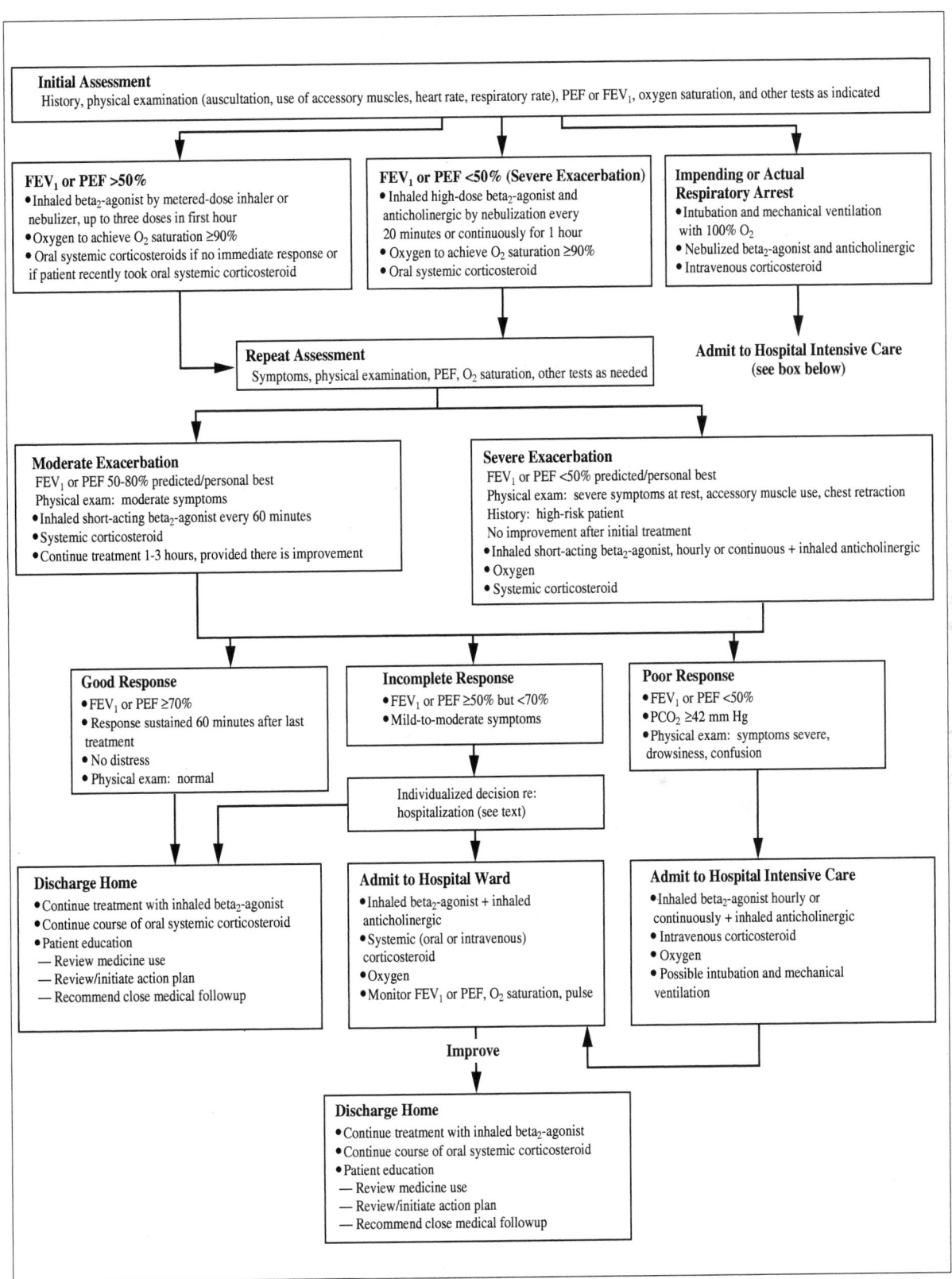

Initial Assessment
History, physical examination (auscultation, use of accessory muscles, heart rate, respiratory rate), PEF or FEV_1, oxygen saturation, and other tests as indicated

FEV_1 or PEF >50%
• Inhaled beta₂-agonist by metered-dose inhaler or nebulizer, up to three doses in first hour
• Oxygen to achieve O_2 saturation ≥90%
• Oral systemic corticosteroids if no immediate response or if patient recently took oral systemic corticosteroid

FEV_1 or PEF <50% (Severe Exacerbation)
• Inhaled high-dose beta₂-agonist and anticholinergic by nebulization every 20 minutes or continuously for 1 hour
• Oxygen to achieve O_2 saturation ≥90%
• Oral systemic corticosteroid

Impending or Actual Respiratory Arrest
• Intubation and mechanical ventilation with 100% O_2
• Nebulized beta₂-agonist and anticholinergic
• Intravenous corticosteroid

Repeat Assessment
Symptoms, physical examination, PEF, O_2 saturation, other tests as needed

Admit to Hospital Intensive Care
(see box below)

Moderate Exacerbation
FEV_1 or PEF 50-80% predicted/personal best
Physical exam: moderate symptoms
• Inhaled short-acting beta₂-agonist every 60 minutes
• Systemic corticosteroid
• Continue treatment 1-3 hours, provided there is improvement

Severe Exacerbation
FEV_1 or PEF <50% predicted/personal best
Physical exam: severe symptoms at rest, accessory muscle use, chest retraction
History: high-risk patient
No improvement after initial treatment
• Inhaled short-acting beta₂-agonist, hourly or continuous + inhaled anticholinergic
• Oxygen
• Systemic corticosteroid

Good Response
• FEV_1 or PEF ≥70%
• Response sustained 60 minutes after last treatment
• No distress
• Physical exam: normal

Incomplete Response
• FEV_1 or PEF ≥50% but <70%
• Mild-to-moderate symptoms

Poor Response
• FEV_1 or PEF <50%
• PCO_2 ≥42 mm Hg
• Physical exam: symptoms severe, drowsiness, confusion

Individualized decision re: hospitalization (see text)

Discharge Home
• Continue treatment with inhaled beta₂-agonist
• Continue course of oral systemic corticosteroid
• Patient education
— Review medicine use
— Review/initiate action plan
— Recommend close medical followup

Admit to Hospital Ward
• Inhaled beta₂-agonist + inhaled anticholinergic
• Systemic (oral or intravenous) corticosteroid
• Oxygen
• Monitor FEV_1 or PEF, O_2 saturation, pulse

Admit to Hospital Intensive Care
• Inhaled beta₂-agonist hourly or continuously + inhaled anticholinergic
• Intravenous corticosteroid
• Oxygen
• Possible intubation and mechanical ventilation

Improve

Discharge Home
• Continue treatment with inhaled beta₂-agonist
• Continue course of oral systemic corticosteroid
• Patient education
— Review medicine use
— Review/initiate action plan
— Recommend close medical followup

FIGURE 34.6 Emergency department and hospital treatment of a patient with acute asthma exacerbation, as recommended by the NAEPP Expert Panel Report. (From National Asthma Education and Prevention Program. Expert panel report 2: guidelines for the diagnosis and management of asthma. Bethesda, MD: US Department of Health and Human Services, Public Health Service, National Institutes of Health, National Heart, Lung, and Blood Institute, April 1997; Publication no 97-4051.)

Early, small open trials suggested benefit, but larger, randomized clinical trials have failed to confirm improved outcomes with the exception of post hoc analysis of a small subset of patients.[43] Thus, its efficacy is still in question. Heliox is a mixture of helium and oxygen, usually in an 80:20 ratio.[38] It is used with a mixture of oxygen so that the final helium concentration is 60% to 70%. Because helium is lighter than nitrogen, it has been proposed that it be used as a means of improving airflow in obstructed airways, thereby enhancing oxygenation.[38] However, clinical trials have proved to be inconclusive.[44] Heliox has also been used as the driving gas for nebulizing β_2-agonists. Improved delivery was seen in one but not all studies.[45,46]

Nondrug management of severe acute asthma includes low-flow oxygen therapy, usually by nasal cannulae, to prevent hypoxemia.[1,2,38] Routine monitoring of oxygenation by pulse oximetry is warranted in all patients who do not respond to initial bronchodilator therapy. The oxygen flow should be adjusted to maintain oxygen saturations above 90%. In very severe cases, blood gases are used to monitor the arterial pressure of CO_2 ($PaCO_2$). A $PaCO_2$ that is normal or elevated following intensive therapy indicates risk of respiratory failure. All patients who are physically capable should have their PEFs measured.[1,2] This can take place following initial β_2-agonist therapy, if necessary. Patients should be adequately hydrated but not overhydrated. If high-dose or continuously inhaled β_2-agonists are used, monitoring of serum electrolytes, particularly potassium and glucose, is indicated.[38] Mucolytics, sedation, and routine use of antibiotics are not indicated, nor are chest radiographs routinely indicated without symptoms indicating pneumonia or pneumothoraces.[1,2]

Pediatric Treatment. The NAEPP guidelines for the management of asthma provide separate long-term treatment guidelines for children 5 years of age and younger (Fig. 34.7).[17] This separation is necessary primarily because children younger than 6 years have difficulty performing spirometric measurements; therefore, lung function often cannot be used to assess the severity of asthma or response to therapy. In addition, drugs approved by the US Food and Drug Administration (FDA) for use in pediatric patients are often divided into various age ranges according to differences in metabolic capabilities, as well as in outcome measures to be attained.[47] For asthma, the age ranges 6 to 12 years, 3 to 5 years, and 2 years of age and younger are often used as cutoffs by the pharmaceutical industry for the testing of asthma drugs. Many asthma drugs that are used in children may not be FDA approved for all ages of children. Most long-term control medications, including all the older inhaled corticosteroids in chlorofluorocarbon (CFC)-propelled MDIs (beclomethasone dipropionate, flunisolide, and triamcinolone acetonide), are approved for children down to 6 years of age. The following medications have been FDA approved for various age ranges of children younger than 6 years old: nebulizer suspension of budesonide for children

1 to 8 years old, dry-powder inhaler (DPI; Diskhaler) of fluticasone propionate for children 4 to 11 years old, DPI combination of fluticasone propionate 100 μg/salmeterol xinafoate 50 μg for children 4 to 11 years old (Diskus), DPI of salmeterol xinafoate 50 μg for children 4 to 11 years old (Diskus), DPI of formoterol fumarate 12 μg for children 5 to 12 years old (Aerolizer), hydrofluoroalkane (HFA)-propelled MDI of beclomethasone dipropionate for children 5 to 12 years old, cromolyn nebulizer solution 20 mg for patients age 2 years and older, montelukast for those 1 year of age and older, and zafirlukast for children 5 to 11 years old.[17]

According to the new pediatric initiative of the FDA, drugs may be approved for young children following safety and pharmacokinetic studies and extrapolation of data from efficacy studies in older children with the same disease.[47] As an example, montelukast was approved in this manner for children younger than 6 years old. However, this is more difficult for aerosolized drugs in that systemic pharmacokinetics is not a reliable predictor of efficacy. Aerosol deposition in young children is complicated by their inability to coordinate the steps necessary for MDI administration, requiring the addition of a valved holding chamber–type spacer device with a mask or the generation of adequate inspiratory flows for the use of DPIs. Thus, currently, the only FDA-approved aerosol medications for very young children are those administered by nebulizer.[17] Although a number of studies have demonstrated the efficacy of MDI plus VHC as an effective delivery device for inhaled corticosteroids and β_2-agonists in young children, none has been approved as yet.[48–50]

Much of the 2002 update of the NAEPP guidelines was targeted to issues concerning pediatrics, particularly the safety of long-term inhaled corticosteroid use. This led to new recommendations for children 5 years of age and younger (Fig. 34.7).[17] The inhaled corticosteroids are now considered to be the preferred therapy for long-term control for children of all ages with asthma. The leukotriene receptor antagonists (montelukast and zafirlukast), chromones (cromolyn and nedocromil), and theophyllines are considered alternative therapies; no advantage of one over the other for efficacy has been noted, although the leukotriene receptor antagonists and chromones have significantly better safety profiles than does theophylline.[17] The inhaled corticosteroids can be administered by nebulizer or MDI plus VHC with face masks in children younger than 4 years of age, or with DPIs down to 4 years of age. There is no need to reduce the dosage of drugs administered to infants via face mask with a nebulizer or an MDI plus VHC, given that the low tidal volume of infants lowers the total dose delivered to the lungs.[51] Dosages for children are given in Tables 34.4 and 34.5.[17]

In young children with moderate persistent asthma, the guidelines provide two alternatives for Step 3 therapy: medium doses of inhaled corticosteroids or the addition of a long-acting inhaled β_2-agonist.[17] Currently, the latter choice is not an option in children younger than 4 years, as no

Classify Severity: Clinical Features Before Treatment or Adequate Control		Medications Required To Maintain Long-Term Control
	Symptoms/Day ──── Symptoms/Night	Daily Medications
Step 4 Severe Persistent	Continual ──── Frequent	■ Preferred treatment: – High-dose inhaled corticosteroids **AND** – Long-acting inhaled beta$_2$-agonists **AND**, if needed, – Corticosteroid tablets or syrup long term (2 mg/kg/day, generally do not exceed 60 mg per day). (Make repeat attempts to reduce systemic corticosteroids and maintain control with high-dose inhaled corticosteroids.)
Step 3 Moderate Persistent	Daily ──── >1 night/week	■ Preferred treatments: – Low-dose inhaled corticosteroids and long-acting inhaled beta$_2$-agonists **OR** – Medium-dose inhaled corticosteroids. ■ Alternative treatment: – Low-dose inhaled corticosteroids and either leukotriene receptor antagonist or theophylline. ·········· If needed (particularly in patients with recurring severe exacerbations): ■ Preferred treatment: – Medium-dose inhaled corticosteroids and long-acting beta$_2$-agonists. ■ Alternative treatment: – Medium-dose inhaled corticosteroids and either leukotriene receptor antagonist or theophylline.
Step 2 Mild Persistent	>2/week but <1x/day ──── >2 nights/month	■ Preferred treatment: – Low-dose inhaled corticosteroids (with nebulizer or MDI with holding chamber with or without face mask or DPI). ■ Alternative treatment (listed alphabetically): – Cromolyn (nebulizer is preferred or MDI with holding chamber) OR leukotriene receptor antagonist.
Step 1 Mild Intermittent	≤2 days/week ──── ≤2 nights/month	■ No daily medication needed.

Quick Relief All Patients	■ Bronchodilator as needed for symptoms. Intensity of treatment will depend upon severity of exacerbation.
	   – Preferred treatment: **Short-acting inhaled beta$_2$-agonists** by nebulizer or face mask and space/holding chamber
	   – Alternative treatment: Oral beta$_2$-agonists
	 ■ With viral respiratory infection
	   – Bronchodilator q 4–6 hours up to 24 hours (longer with physician consult); in general, repeat no more than once every 6 weeks
	   – Consider systemic corticosteroid if exacerbation is severe or patient has history of previous severe exacerbations
	 ■ Use of short-acting beta$_2$-agonists >2 times a week in intermittent asthma (daily, or increasing use in persistent asthma) may indicate the need to initiate (increase) long-term-control therapy.

 Step down
Review treatment every 1 to 6 months; a gradual stepwise reduction in treatment may be possible.

 Step up
If control is not maintained, consider step up. First, review patient medication technique, adherence, and environmental control.

Goals of Therapy: Asthma Control
- Minimal or no chronic symptoms day or night
- Minimal or no exacerbations
- No limitations on activities; no school/parent's work missed
- Minimal use of short-acting inhaled beta$_2$-agonist
- Minimal or no adverse effects from medications

Note
- The stepwise approach is intended to assist, not replace, the clinical decision-making required to meet individual patient needs.
- Classify severity: assign patient to most severe step in which any feature occurs.
- There are very few studies on asthma therapy for infants.
- Gain control as quickly as possible (a course of short systemic corticosteroids may be required); then step down to the least medication necessary to maintain control.
- Minimize use of short-acting inhaled beta$_2$-agonists. Overreliance on short-acting inhaled beta$_2$-agonists (e.g., use of short-acting inhaled beta$_2$-agonist every day, increasing use or lack of expected effect, or use of approximately one canister a month even if not using it every day) indicates inadequate control of asthma and the need to initiate or intensify long-term-control therapy.
- Provide parent education on asthma management and controlling environmental factors that make asthma worse (e.g., allergens and irritants).
- Consultation with an asthma specialist is recommended for patients with moderate or severe persistent asthma. Consider consultation for patients with mild persistent asthma.

FIGURE 34.7 Stepwise approach to asthma therapy for children 5 years old and younger, from the NAEPP update on the management of asthma. (From the National Asthma Education and Prevention Program. Expert panel report: guidelines for the diagnosis and management of asthma update on selected topics—2002. J Allergy Clin Immunol 110 (5 Suppl):S141–S219, 2002. Reproduced with permission.)

TABLE 34.5	Comparable Daily Doses in Micrograms for Children Younger than 12 years and Adults		
	Low Dose **Child/Adult**	**Medium Dose** **Child/Adult**	**High Dose** **Child/Adult**
Beclomethasone dipropionate			
CFC-MDI (42 & 84 μg/actuation)	84–336/168–504	336–672/504–840	>672/>840
HFA-MDI (40 & 80 μg/actuation)	80–160/80–240	160–320/240–480	>320/>480
Budesonide			
DPI (200 μg/inhalation)	200–400/200–600	400–800/600–1,200	>800/>1,200
Nebules (200 & 500 μg/ampule)	250–500/Unknown	500–1,000/Unknown	>1,000/Unknown
Flunisolide			
CFC-MDI (250 μg/actuation)	500–750/500–1,000	750–1,250/1,000–2,000	>1,250/>2,000
Fluticasone propionate			
CFC-MDI (44, 110, 220 μg/actuation)	88–176/88–264	176–440/264–660	>440/>660
DPIs (50, 100, 250 μg/inhalation)	100–200/100–300	200–400/300–600	>400/>600
Mometasone furoate[a]			
DPI (200 & 400 μg/inhalation)	Unknown/200–400	Unknown/400–800	Unknown/>800
Triamcinolone acetonide			
CFC-MDI (100 μg/actuation)	400–800/400–1,000	800–1,200/1,000–2,000	>1,200/>2,000

[a] Comparative doses based upon National Asthma Education and Prevention Program. Expert panel report: guidelines for the diagnosis and management of asthma update on selected topics—2002. J Allergy Clin Immunol 110 (5 Suppl):S141–S219, 2002.

long-acting inhaled β$_2$-agonist given by MDI or nebulizer is commercially available. Alternative therapies include the addition of a leukotriene receptor antagonist or theophylline. It must be pointed out that none of the preferred treatments or alternatives has been adequately studied in younger children. Combination therapy with an inhaled corticosteroid and a long-acting inhaled β$_2$-agonist has been approved down to 4 years of age. Combination therapy with an inhaled corticosteroid and leukotriene receptor antagonist has been studied only down to 6 years of age. Few dose-response studies of the inhaled corticosteroids have been performed, and these provide conflicting results.

Many infants have virally induced wheezing and are otherwise normal between upper respiratory tract viral infections. Clinicians are sometimes reluctant to diagnose these patients with asthma or to treat them with long-term medications. It has been common practice to treat virally induced exacerbations with oral corticosteroids, usually with oral prednisone or prednisolone and short-acting inhaled β$_2$-agonists, without the use of long-term control therapy. The new guidelines recommend that long-term control medication be started in infants and young children who had more than three episodes of wheezing in the past year that lasted longer than 1 day and affected sleep, and who have risk factors for developing persistent asthma.[17] The risk factors for developing persistent asthma include the following: (a) parental history of asthma and/or (b) physician-diagnosed atopic dermatitis; or two or more of (c) physician-diagnosed allergic rhinitis, (d) blood eosinophilia greater than 4%, and (e)

wheezing apart from viral infection (colds). Therapy in infants and young children should be monitored carefully, and if no clear benefit is discerned in 4 to 6 weeks, alternative therapies or diagnoses should be considered.

Therapy for severe acute asthma in infants and young children is not different from that for older children and adults (Figs. 34.5 and 34.6), with the exception of differing dosages for various drugs (Table 34.4).[1,17] Although many of the aerosolized drug doses are listed on a weight basis in milligrams per kilogram, they can be given as safely as standard fixed doses for age, such as a nebulized albuterol dose of 2.5 mg every 20 minutes for patients 5 years of age or older, and 1.25 mg for those younger than 5 years old.[51] Following initial dosing, the doses may be adjusted according to response.

PHARMACOTHERAPY

As outlined by the NAEPP guidelines,[1] treatment includes *providing optimal pharmacotherapy with minimal or no adverse effects.* Maintaining an affordable cost of care and reasonable medication regimens (facilitating better adherence) could also be included in this list of treatment goals. Because asthma is a chronic condition with periodic exacerbations, therapy requires continuous attention, along with efforts at preventing or minimizing acute symptoms.

The medications used to treat asthma can be divided into the general categories of bronchodilators and anti-inflammatory agents. The NAEPP guidelines categorize medications into "quick-relief agents," which include short-acting inhaled β_2-agonists, anticholinergics, and short-term systemic corticosteroids, and "long-term control agents," which include inhaled and systemic corticosteroids, cromolyn and nedocromil, long-acting β_2-agonists, methylxanthines, and leukotriene modifiers.

Bronchodilators

β_2-Adrenergic Agonists. β_2-adrenergic agonists are the safest and most effective bronchodilators. Adrenergic receptors belong to the superfamily of G-protein–coupled receptors. Activation of the receptor by a β_2-adrenergic agonist results in coupling of the β_2-adrenergic receptor complex with G_s binding protein. Guanosine diphosphate is released from G-protein, which is a membrane-associated heterotrimer. This enables guanosine triphosphate to bind to the β-receptor, which activates adenylyl cyclase, thereby catalyzing formation of cyclic 3', 5'-adenosine monophosphate (cAMP).[52] A reduction in cytosolic calcium ion concentration occurs, and smooth muscle relaxation ensues.[53] Other mechanisms of smooth muscle relaxation include shifting of myosin light-chain kinase to a less active form, cAMP inhibition of phos-

pholipase C and reduction of 1,4,5-triphosphate formation (reducing intracellular calcium), stimulation of a calcium-activated potassium channel, and inhibition of acetylcholine release from cholinergic neurons.[53,54] This ultimately leads to smooth muscle relaxation and bronchodilation.

Currently available β-adrenergic agonists stimulate the α-, β_1-, and β_2-receptors, but it is the action on the β_2-receptors that produces the therapeutic response in asthma. Table 34.6 compares the β-agonists for route of administration, relative potency, duration of effect, and receptor selectivity. β_2-agonists can be divided into two classes—clinically short-acting (albuterol, bitolterol, metaproterenol, pirbuterol, terbutaline) and long-acting (salmeterol, formoterol)—which have different roles in the treatment of asthma. The long duration of effect of salmeterol is believed to be due to the binding to an exocite, which may permit nearly continuous stimulation of the β-receptor; the long action of formoterol is believed to be due to its extreme lipophilicity and high affinity at the β_2-agonist receptor.[55,56]

β_2-agonists produce the same degree of bronchodilation at equipotent doses, with differences in the duration of bron-

TABLE 34.6 | Adrenergic Stimulants Used in the Treatment of Obstructive Airways Disease[a]

Agent	Route of Administration[a]			Relative Potency	Duration (hr)		Receptor Stimulation		
	Injected	Inhaled	Oral	(Scale of 4)	Bronchodilation	Bronchoprotection	β_2	β_1	α
Catecholamines									
Ephedrine	−	−	+	1	2–3		+	+	+
Epinephrine	+	+	−	3 (injected [d])	1–2	0.5–1.0	+	+	+
Isoproterenol	+	+	−	4	1–2	0.5–1.0	+	+	−
Isoetharine	+	+	−	2+	2–3	0.5–1.0	+ +	+	−
Rimiterol[b]	+	+	−	2+	2–3		+ +	+	−
Hexoprenaline[b]	+	+	+	2+	2–3		+ +	+	−
Bitolterol[c]	−	+	−	3+	4–6	2–4	+ + +	±	−
Resorcinols									
Metaproterenol	+[b]	+	+	3	3–4	1–2	+ +	+	−
Terbutaline	+	+	+	4	4	2–4	+ + +	±	−
Fenoterol[b]	+	+	+	4	4–6	2–4	+ + +	±	−
Saligenins									
Albuterol	+[b]	+	+	4	4–6	2–4	+ + +	±	−
Salmeterol	−	+	−	4	8–12	8–12	+ + +	±	−
Other									
Pirbuterol	−	+	+	4	4–6	2–4	+ + +	±	−
Procaterol	−	+	+	4	4–6	2–4	+ + +	±	−
Carbuterol[b]	−	+	+	3	4	2–4	+ + +	±	−
Formoterol	−	+	+	4	8–12	8–12	+ + +	±	−

[a] Not all dosage forms are marketed in the U.S.

[b] Drug not available in U.S.

[c] Active moiety is colterol.

[d] By the inhaled route, epinephrine is the least potent β-agonist, with the shortest duration of action. Available O.T.C. (Primatene-Mist, others).

chodilation and bronchoprotection against an asthma trigger such as exercise. Acute adverse effects are common when β_2-agonists are administered orally, and they are significantly reduced when administration occurs by the inhaled route. The most common adverse effects are palpitations, sinus tachycardia, tremor, and increased blood pressure. Other adverse effects include nausea and vomiting, throat irritation, insomnia, headache, decreased serum potassium levels, and nightmares. Tolerance to these adverse effects generally occurs within several weeks of regular use.

β_2-agonists have anti-inflammatory effects that are demonstrated in vitro but are not apparent clinically as they do not inhibit the late-phase inflammatory response following allergen inhalation, nor do they prevent a subsequent increase in bronchial hyperreactivity (an indicator of airway inflammation).[1,57] Even with long-term administration, β_2-agonists do not reduce airway hyperreactivity.[57] In addition, neither short-acting nor long-acting β_2-agonists affect inflammation when evaluated by lung biopsy.[58,59] Combined administration of long-acting β_2-agonists with inhaled corticosteroids provides better asthma control than is provided by doubling the dose of inhaled corticosteroids.[60–66] This is not the result of additive inflammatory effects but rather likely occurs because β_2-agonists and inhaled corticosteroids treat different components of airway narrowing; long-acting β_2-agonists relax airway smooth muscle bronchospasm, and inhaled corticosteroids reduce the inflammatory processes of asthma. β_2-agonists may, however, enhance the function of inhaled corticosteroids at the molecular level.[67]

Concern has been expressed in recent years regarding the potential for β_2-agonists to cause worsening asthma, near death, or death with regular or excessive use. The package insert for short-acting β_2-agonists states the maximum daily dose as two inhalations four to six times daily. Early clinical and epidemiologic studies demonstrated that frequent β_2-agonist use was associated with worsening asthma control and death or near death due to asthma.[68] However, these studies were confounded by disease severity, and subsequent studies demonstrated that the risk of death or near death from asthma was increased with excessive use of short-acting inhaled β_2-agonists during the 2 months before the event[29] (i.e., with use that exceeded approximately two canisters per month).[69,70] In addition, several carefully designed short-term studies have now shown that asthma control is not worsened in most patients with regular administration of short-acting inhaled β_2-agonists,[71,72] although a subset of patients with selected β_2-adrenergic receptor polymorphisms may be at increased risk of adverse effects from regularly scheduled short-acting β_2-agonist use.[73] In summary, these data suggest that the increased use of short-acting β_2-agonist therapy can be a marker of worsening asthma control, rather than a direct cause of increased morbidity or mortality.

In the Salmeterol Multicenter Asthma Research Trial (SMART), the use of salmeterol was directly associated with an increased risk of adverse asthma outcomes with long-

term use.[74] In this study, greater morbidity and mortality were observed in the salmeterol group compared with the placebo group. In a subgroup analysis, African-Americans, but not whites, had a statistically significantly increased occurrence of death when treated with salmeterol compared with placebo. However, African-Americans were less likely to be on inhaled corticosteroids and had more severe asthma, which could have contributed to these findings. As a result of this study, in 2003, the FDA required that a black box warning be placed on the labeling for products that contain salmeterol, and in 2005, an FDA advisory panel recommended a similar black box warning for products containing salmeterol or formoterol.

The synthetic production of β_2-agonists results in a racemic mixture of (R)- and (S)-enantiomers.[75] The pharmacologic activity is caused by the (R)-enantiomer, and it was originally thought that the (S)-enantiomer was essentially inactive because of the 1,000-fold potency difference between the (R)- and (S)-enantiomers.[76,77] Animal and in vitro studies suggest that the (S)-enantiomer could be proinflammatory and could increase bronchial hyperreactivity,[77] although no supporting clinical studies have been conducted in patients with asthma. Several outpatient studies with levalbuterol (the (R)-enantiomer of albuterol) have suggested greater potency compared with racemic albuterol,[78–81] although these studies have been criticized for poor study design and statistical analysis.[15,82] A carefully controlled pediatric study found that children treated with levalbuterol versus albuterol in the emergency department had a reduced hospital admission rate, but that no differences in clinical indices nor in duration of hospital stay were observed between levalbuterol and albuterol.[83] Additional studies are needed to confirm this finding. Thus, levalbuterol may have some therapeutic benefit over albuterol in the short-term management of pediatric asthma in the emergency department, but current studies do not support its use over albuterol in the outpatient setting in children or adults, particularly given the approximately five times greater cost over albuterol.

Thirteen polymorphisms of the β_2-receptor have been identified; these are organized into five common (frequency greater than 5%) haplotypes (single nucleotide polymorphisms in tight linkage disequilibrium).[84] Numerous studies have found associations between polymorphisms at positions 16 and 27 and asthma severity, response to β_2-agonist therapy, and adverse effects, but findings have been inconsistent and conflicting.[85] In a prospective, carefully designed study,[73] patients homozygous for Arg-16 had lower peak expiratory flow, and patients homozygous for Gly-16 had higher peak expiratory flow, when treated with regularly scheduled albuterol compared with placebo. The authors suggest that a pharmacogenetic approach to treatment may be warranted and propose that patients who are homozygous for Arg-16 may be better treated with nonalbuterol (possibly ipratropium bromide) bronchodilator treatments.[86]

The NAEPP and GINA guidelines recommend that short-acting β_2-agonists be used as needed to treat intermittent symptoms of bronchoconstriction and as first-line therapy for severe acute asthma.[1,2] In the treatment of severe acute asthma, short-acting β_2-agonists can be administered by MDI plus spacer, intermittent nebulization, or continuous nebulization. Intravenous administration of short-acting β_2-agonists is not recommended because no benefit over other delivery methods has been proved, even in patients with more severe asthma.[39] Delivery by MDI plus spacer or intermittent nebulization provides no difference in efficacy outcomes, with perhaps only a small advantage of the MDI plus spacer seen in children treated in the emergency department.[34] In addition, no difference in outcome is seen in adults when continuous delivery is provided in the emergency department[36] compared with intermittent delivery, but children treated in the intensive care unit demonstrate greater improvement with continuous nebulized albuterol.[87] Short-acting β_2-agonists are also the treatment of choice for the prevention of exercise-induced asthma; they have a 4-hour duration of effect.[88] Because short-acting β_2-agonists are prescribed to be used only as needed for symptom relief, the number of inhalations used per day can provide a measure of asthma control. Increased use or daily use is an indicator of poorly controlled asthma that requires added or intensified therapy with inhaled corticosteroids.[1,2] Similarly, a reduction in immediate symptom relief or duration of effect indicates worsening asthma that requires medical attention and possible treatment with systemic corticosteroids.[1,2]

Long-acting β_2-agonists, which are recommended for use in persistent asthma, are to be used only in combination with an inhaled corticosteroid.[1,2] Salmeterol should not be used for relief of intermittent symptoms of bronchospasm because bronchodilation (defined as at least a 15% improvement in FEV_1) may not occur for 20 minutes, and maximum effect occurs after 1 to 4 hours.[89] Formoterol has an onset of effect within 4 minutes but is currently not indicated for relief of acute asthma symptoms.[90] Both salmeterol and formoterol are indicated for the prevention of exercise-induced asthma when used at least 30 minutes and 15 minutes before exercise, respectively. When used in combination with an inhaled corticosteroid, long-acting β_2-agonists can provide control of exercise-induced asthma for up to 12 hours[88]; however, the duration of protection tends to decrease after several weeks of use.[91]

Theophylline. Methylxanthines, of which theophylline is the primary drug, have been used in the treatment of acute and chronic asthma for more than 50 years. Dyphylline, caffeine, and theobromine (found in chocolate) are methylxanthines with much weaker bronchodilator properties than theophylline, and enprofylline, although more potent, has unacceptable cardiovascular effects. Salts of theophylline have been developed to improve solubility and absorption. Because theophylline absorption is related to lipophilic characteristics rather than water solubility, only the ethylenedi-amine salt (aminophylline) that is used for intravenous administration is of clinical importance. Oral salt formulations (choline, calcium salicylate, sodium glycinate) simply contain less anhydrous theophylline by weight; thus, it is the fraction of theophylline in these dosage forms that determines the prescribed dose.

Evidence suggests that theophylline exerts its bronchodilator effects via inhibition of phosphodiesterase (PDE).[92] PDE III and IV, as well as PDE V, catalyze the breakdown of intracellular cAMP and cyclic 3′,5′ guanosine monophosphate (cGMP), respectively. PDE isoenzymes may have differential expression depending on the cell type studied; PDE III and PDE IV, and possibly PDE V, are present in smooth airway muscle, whereas PDE IV is the predominant isoenzyme in inflammatory cells. Inhibition of PDE III and IV increases cAMP, which opens maxi-K$^+$ channels. These channels assist in recovery and stabilization of excitable cells following activation; opening these channels contributes to smooth muscle relaxation. It has been suggested that PDE expression may be activated in asthmatic airways, thus enhancing the effects of theophylline. The fact that theophylline demonstrates bronchodilator activity in patients with asthma but not in nonasthmatic patients provides a foundation for this hypothesis. In addition, theophylline may inhibit isoenzymes of phosphodiesterase at clinically relevant therapeutic concentrations.

Theophylline is now believed to have modest anti-inflammatory or immunomodulatory effects, which occur at low serum concentrations of 27.5 to 55 μmol per liter (5 to 10 μg/mL). Theophylline inhibits adenosine-stimulated release of mediators from mast cells at therapeutic serum concentrations, modulates T-cell trafficking within the airways, inhibits eosinophil activation and degranulation, decreases the total number of eosinophils beneath the basement membrane, and attenuates eosinophil cationic protein release from eosinophils following allergen challenge.[92] Recently, a molecular mechanism for theophylline has been proposed to explain these effects.[93] Acetylation of core histones by acetyltransferase activates inflammatory genes. Inhaled corticosteroids and theophylline reverse acetylation by activating histone deacetylase (HDAC); inhaled corticosteroids bind and activate glucocorticoid receptors to increase HDAC activity, whereas theophylline appears to activate HDAC directly.[93] These parallel mechanisms suggest that theophylline would have relatively weak anti-inflammatory effects when used as monotherapy but would potentiate the effects of inhaled corticosteroids when used concurrently. Several clinical trials have confirmed the beneficial effect on asthma symptoms when theophylline and inhaled corticosteroids are used in combination.[94–96]

Other related pharmacologic actions of theophylline include increased right and left ventricular ejection fraction, reduced fatigue of the diaphragmatic muscles, which may decrease the work of breathing, decreased vascular permeability, and enhanced mucociliary clearance, although some of these effects have not been consistently observed in all studies.[97]

Theophylline is a relatively weak bronchodilator compared with inhaled β_2-adrenergic agonists. However, similar to the β_2-adrenergic agonists, theophylline is a functional antagonist that can inhibit bronchospasm induced by various stimuli, including histamine, methacholine, exercise, and distilled water, in a serum concentration–related manner.[97] Protection has been noted at serum concentrations less than 55 μmol per liter (10 μg/mL) for exercise- and methacholine-induced bronchoconstriction. However, studies examining the long-term effects of theophylline in reducing bronchial hyperresponsiveness measured by bronchoprovocation with histamine or methacholine have been conflicting.[97] It appears that theophylline is effective in preventing a fall in airway function during IAR and LAR after an allergen is inhaled, and in inhibiting the subsequent increase in airway responsiveness to histamine.[98] The effect seen with theophylline is similar to that noted after cromolyn is inhaled from an MDI.[98]

Theophylline is administered orally, intravenously, and rectally, although the latter method is rarely used because of unpredictable absorption. Theophylline has no antiasthma effects when given by the inhaled route. Familiarity with the pharmacokinetics of theophylline is essential for the safe and effective use of this drug. In addition, recognition that differences in the formulations of slow-release products can result in significant differences in the rate and extent of absorption is also important. Inappropriate use that leads to toxicity can have dire consequences for the patient.

The therapeutic range for theophylline is 27.5 to 82.5 μmol per liter (5 to 15 μg/mL).[1] Theophylline pharmacokinetics is largely dependent on factors that influence hepatic metabolism after 1 year of age, when approximately 90% of a dose is metabolized in the liver. At younger than 1 year of age, nearly half a dose is excreted as unchanged theophylline in the urine. N-demethylation and hydroxylation are the major metabolic pathways; they are regulated by several P-450 enzymes, including 1A2, 2E1, and 3A3. Both pathways are saturable within the therapeutic range, and persons with high initial clearance rates may be at greatest risk. Factors that may influence hepatic metabolism of theophylline include age, concurrent diseases, and drug interactions. Hyperthyroidism, cystic fibrosis, smoking, and ingestion of a high-protein/low-carbohydrate diet are common conditions known to increase theophylline clearance, whereas age younger than 1 year or older than 60 years, congestive heart failure, prolonged fever (greater than 102°F), hypothyroidism, and liver disease are some of the conditions known to decrease theophylline clearance. Ninety drugs have been evaluated with respect to their effect on theophylline clearance, and approximately half have clinically important interactions (Tables 34.7 and 34.8).[99] Theophylline rarely affects the pharmacokinetics of other drugs.

Dosing schemes and monitoring guidelines for theophylline administration in persistent asthma are presented in Table 34.9.[100] However, the dosages listed are merely guidelines for attaining serum concentrations within the therapeutic range and should be confirmed with serum concentration measurement. Intravenous administration and monitoring should be provided by persons who are experienced in theophylline pharmacokinetics.

Adverse effects of theophylline, which are generally mild and temporary when serum concentrations are less than 110 μmol per liter (20 μg/mL), include caffeine-like effects such as nausea and vomiting, headache, and insomnia. The severity of adverse effects worsens as the serum concentration exceeds 110 μmol per liter (20 μg/mL).[101] However, minor symptoms of toxicity such as nausea and vomiting may not precede more severe toxicity (seizures and arrhythmias) and cannot be relied upon as a dosing end point. Only serum concentration measurement can reliably predict the potential for severe or life-threatening toxicity. Non–serum concentration–related effects are uncommon. Controlled studies and meta-analyses have failed to show an adverse effect of theophylline on behavior and school performance.[92]

Until inhaled β_2-adrenergic agonists were introduced in the early 1970s and 1980s, theophylline had a well-established role in the treatment of acute asthma in the emergency department or in the inpatient setting. Many well-designed studies have been published that demonstrate that the addition of theophylline to optimal inhaled β_2-adrenergic agonists plus systemic corticosteroids in both the emergency department and the inpatient setting provides no added benefit in acute severe asthma over optimal treatment with inhaled β_2-adrenergic agonists plus systemic corticosteroids alone.[92] Therefore, intravenous theophylline should be reserved for those patients who fail to respond to high-dose inhaled β_2-adrenergic agonists and systemic corticosteroids.[92,102]

Similarly, the role of theophylline in the treatment of chronic asthma has also lessened with the introduction of potent inhaled corticosteroids, long-acting inhaled β_2-agonists, and leukotriene modifiers. With the addition of theophylline, some patients, despite the regular use of inhaled corticosteroids, have fewer symptoms, less inhaled β-adrenergic agonist use, and fewer exacerbations that require systemic corticosteroids.[97] The addition of theophylline to low-dose inhaled corticosteroids provides benefit similar to that attained by increasing the dose of inhaled corticosteroids.[94] The NAEPP guidelines reserve theophylline as second-line add-on therapy in the treatment of persistent asthma.[1]

Anticholinergics. Anticholinergic drugs have been used in the treatment of asthma-like symptoms for more than 400 years. Until the introduction of quaternary ammonium derivatives such as ipratropium bromide, glycopyrrolate, atropine methonitrate, oxitropium bromide, and tiotropium bromide, central nervous systemic adverse effects limited their use.

The parasympathetic (vs. the sympathetic) nervous system is largely responsible for the control of baseline airway caliber. Therefore, anticholinergic drugs, which are competi-

TABLE 34.7	Clinically Significant Drug Interactions with Theophylline	
Drug	**Type of Interaction**	**Effect**[a]
Adenosine	Theophylline blocks adenosine receptors	Higher doses of adenosine may be required to achieve desired effect
Alcohol	A single large dose of alcohol (3 mL/kg of whiskey) decreases theophylline clearance for up to 24 h	30% increase
Allopurinol	Decreases theophylline clearance at allopurinol doses ≥600 mg/day	25% increase
Aminoglutethimide	Increases theophylline clearance by induction of microsomal enzyme activity	25% decrease
Carbamazepine	Similar to aminoglutethimide	30% decrease
Cimetidine	Decreases theophylline clearance by inhibiting cytochrome P450 1A2	70% increase
Ciprofloxacin	Similar to cimetidine	40% increase
Clarithromycin	Similar to erythromycin	25% increase
Diazepam	Benzodiazepines increase central nervous system (CNS) concentrations of adenosine, a potent CNS depressant, while theophylline blocks adenosine receptors	Larger benzodiazepine doses may be required to produce desired level of sedation; discontinuation of theophylline without reduction in diazepam dose may result in respiratory depression
Disulfiram	Decreases theophylline clearance by inhibiting hydroxylation and demethylation	50% increase
Enoxacin	Similar to cimetidine	300% increase
Ephedrine	Synergistic CNS effects	Increased frequency of nausea, nervousness, and insomnia
Erythromycin	Erythromycin metabolite decreases theophylline clearance by inhibiting cytochrome P450 3A3	35% increase; erythromycin steady-state serum concentrations decrease by a similar amount
Estrogen	Estrogens that contain oral contraceptives decrease theophylline clearance in a dose-dependent fashion. The effect of progesterone on theophylline clearance is unknown	30% increase
Flurazepam	Similar to diazepam	Similar to diazepam
Fluvoxamine	Similar to cimetidine	Similar to cimetidine
Halothane	Halothane sensitizes the myocardium to endogenous catecholamines; theophylline increases the release of endogenous catecholamines	Increased risk of ventricular arrhythmias
Interferon, human recombinant alpha-A	Decreases theophylline clearance	100% increase
Isoproterenol (IV)	Increases theophylline clearance	20% decrease
Ketamine	Pharmacologic	May lower theophylline seizure threshold
Lithium	Theophylline increases lithium renal clearance	Lithium dose required to achieve a therapeutic serum concentration increased an average of 60%
Lorazepam	Similar to diazepam	Similar to diazepam
Methotrexate (MTX)	Decreases theophylline clearance	20% increase after low-dose MTX; higher-dose MTX may have a greater effect
Mexiletine	Similar to disulfiram	80% increase
Midazolam	Similar to diazepam	Similar to diazepam
Moricizine	Increases theophylline clearance	25% decrease
Pancuronium	Theophylline may antagonize nondepolarizing neuromuscular blocking effects, possibly because of phosphodiesterase inhibition	Larger dose of pancuronium may be required to achieve neuromuscular blockade

(continued)

TABLE 34.7	continued		
Drug	**Type of Interaction**	**Effect[a]**
Pentoxifylline	Decreases theophylline clearance	30% increase
Phenobarbital (PB)	Similar to aminoglutethimide	25% decrease after 2 weeks of concurrent PB
Phenytoin	Phenytoin increases theophylline clearance by increasing microsomal enzyme activity. Theophylline decreases phenytoin absorption	Serum theophylline *and* phenytoin concentrations decrease about 40%
Propafenone	Decreases theophylline clearance and pharmacologic interaction	40% increase. β_2-blocking effect may decrease the efficacy of theophylline
Propranolol	Similar to cimetidine in clearance and pharmacologic interaction	100% increase; β_2-blocking effect may decrease efficacy of theophylline
Rifampin	Increases theophylline clearance by increasing cytochrome P450, 1A2, and 3A3 activity	20% to 40% decrease
Sulfinpyrazone	Increases theophylline clearance by increasing demethylation and hydroxylation. Decreases renal clearance of theophylline	20% decrease
Tacrine	Similar to cimetidine, also increases renal clearance of theophylline	90% increase
Thiabendazole	Decreases theophylline clearance	190% increase
Ticlopidine	Decreases theophylline clearance	60% increase
Troleandomycin	Similar to erythromycin	33% to 100% increase, depending on troleandomycin dose
Verapamil	Similar to disulfiram	20% increase
Zafirlukast	Decreases theophylline clearance	120% increase
Zileuton	Decreases theophylline clearance	73% increase

[a] Average effect on steady state theophylline concentration or other clinical effect for pharmacologic interactions. Individual patients may experience larger changes in serum theophylline concentration than the value listed.
(Updated from Hendeles L, Harman E, Huang D, et al. Theophylline attenuation of airway responses to allergen: comparison with cromolyn metered-dose inhaler. J Allergy Clin Immunol 95:505–514, 1995.)

tive antagonists rather than functional antagonists, will be most useful in those patients whose symptoms are caused by excessive cholinergic stimulation. However, it is not possible to predict who those patients are. Because most mediators, such as histamine, allergens, and exercise, cause bronchoconstriction only partially through cholinergic stimulation, anticholinergics will be less effective than β_2-adrenergic agonists and theophylline, which are functional antagonists.

Five muscarinic receptor subtypes have been discovered; three receptors have been characterized pharmacologically.[103] Acetylcholine stimulation of the muscarinic receptor may activate an inhibitory G-protein and decrease the activity of adenylate cyclase, resulting in decreased cAMP and causing smooth muscle contraction. Two other mechanisms include activation of phospholipase C via a different G-protein, which releases stores of intracellular calcium and produces smooth muscle contraction and formation of a second messenger, diacylglycerol, which activates protein kinase C and causes a slow and prolonged contraction.[104] Stimulation of M_1 receptors on the terminal of parasympathetic preganglionic neurons facilitates cholinergic transmission. M_2 receptors, located on the postganglionic terminal,

inhibit acetylcholine release and stimulate uptake, thus functioning as inhibitory feedback receptors. It is believed that abnormal functioning or absence of the M_2 receptors occurs in asthma.[104] M_3 receptors located on airway smooth muscle also facilitate cholinergic transmission. Therefore, selective blockers at the M_1 and M_3 receptors would likely have enhanced benefit over nonselective muscarinic receptor blockers. Antagonism of M_3 receptors, also located on mucous glands, causes drying of secretions; therefore, drugs must be developed for inhalation use to avoid unwanted systemic adverse effects.[103]

Currently available short-acting (duration of effect less than 12 hours) anticholinergics (ipratropium bromide, glycopyrrolate, and oxitropium bromide) are nonselective competitive antagonists at the muscarinic receptor. Tiotropium bromide, approved in 2004 for patients with COPD, is a selective M_1/M_3 receptor antagonist with a bronchodilator effect that lasts up to 24 hours.

With the availability of ipratropium bromide for nebulization, no reason remains for the use of nebulized atropine sulfate. Atropine sulfate is rapidly absorbed when given by the inhaled route, resulting in dose-related peripheral and central nervous system adverse effects. Ipratropium is re-

TABLE 34.8	Drugs That Have Been Documented to Not Interact with Theophylline or Drugs That Produce No Clinically Significant Interaction with Theophylline

Albuterol, systemic and inhaled	Medroxyprogesterone
Alosetron	Methylprednisolone
Amoxicillin	Metoprolol
Ampicillin, with or without sulbactam	Metronidazole
Atenolol	Montelukast
Azithromycin	Moxifloxacin
Caffeine, dietary ingestion	Nadolol
Cefaclor	Nifedipine
Clopidogrel	Nizatidine
Co-trimoxazole (trimethoprim and sulfamethoxazole)	Norfloxacin
	Ofloxacin
Diltiazem	Omeprazole
Dirithromycin	Pantoprazole
Donepezil	Prednisone, prednisolone
Enflurane	Ranitidine
Famotidine	Rifabutin
Felodipine	Ropinirole
Finasteride	Roxithromycin
Gemifloxacin	Sorbitol
Hydrocortisone	(purgative doses do not inhibit theophylline absorption)
Indinavir	
Influenza vaccine	Sucralfate
Isoflurane	Tamsulosin
Isoniazid	Tegaserod
Isradipine	Terbinafine
Ketoconazole	Terbutaline, systemic
Lansoprazole	Terfenadine
Levofloxacin	Tetracycline
Lomefloxacin	Tocainide
Mebendazole	Trovafloxacin

(Updated from Hendeles L, Harman E, Huang D, et al. Theophylline attenuation of airway responses to allergen: comparison with cromolyn metered-dose inhaler. J Allergy Clin Immunol 95:505–514, 1995.)

markably free of unwanted adverse effects because of its minimal systemic absorption. Adverse effects may include dry mouth, irritated throat, and bitter taste.

Anticholinergics do not produce maximal bronchodilation when compared with β_2-adrenergic agonists in patients with asthma, but they do have a longer duration of effect. Maximum bronchodilation occurs in 1.5 to 2 hours; however, 50% of the eventual maximum occurs within 3 to 5 minutes, and 80% within 30 minutes,[105] which is comparable clinically to the time of peak effect (30 minutes) with inhaled β_2-adrenergic agonists. Ipratropium bromide has a bronchodilator effect for 4 to 8 hours. Both intensity and duration of effect are dose dependent. The NAEPP guidelines recommend the use of nebulized anticholinergic therapy in combination with β_2-agonist therapy for the treatment of acute severe asthma in patients who fail to respond to initial treatment with inhaled β_2-agonists.[1] The addition of several doses (vs. a single dose) of an anticholinergic decreases the risk of hospital admission by approximately 30%.[10,36] In patients who are hospitalized, the combination of anticholinergic and β_2-agonist therapy should be continued for at least 36 hours for an effect such as reduced length of hospitalization to be seen.[106] The NAEPP guidelines do not include therapy with anticholinergics in the management of chronic asthma, as other more effective drugs are available.[1,107] Limited data indicate that anticholinergics may be effective in psychogenic asthma.

Anti-inflammatory Agents

Cromolyn Sodium/Nedocromil Sodium. Cromolyn sodium has been a long-standing treatment for asthma, and nedocromil sodium has been available since 1992. Although they are structurally and possibly pharmacologically distinct, these two drugs are often discussed together. Neither drug has acute bronchodilator effects. The exact mechanism of action for each is largely unknown, but both are capable of inhibiting the IgE-mediated release of mediators from mast cells. However, this effect seems to vary depending on the species and the cell type tested; other drugs with greater mast cell–stabilizing activity do not have therapeutic efficacy.[51] Cromolyn is also effective in preventing mast cell degranulation induced by nonimmunologic stimuli such as phospholipase A, dextran, and polymyxin B. The mechanism by which cromolyn and nedocromil inhibit mediator release at the cellular level is unclear but likely involves regulation of intracellular calcium, probably by phosphorylation of a specific membrane protein, which inhibits calcium influx into the cell. Cromolyn and nedocromil also inhibit the release of mediators from eosinophils, alveolar macrophages, neutrophils, and monocytes.[108] Other effects regulated by cromolyn include inhibition of phosphodiesterase, modification of the vagal reflex, and inhibition of irritant receptors. Cromolyn and nedocromil also inhibit chemotaxis of inflammatory mediators and may inhibit release of inflammatory neuropeptides that induce bronchoconstriction through efferent cholinergic pathways.[51]

Neither cromolyn nor nedocromil is effective orally or intravenously. Cromolyn or nedocromil which is systemically absorbed is excreted largely unchanged in the urine or the bile. The half-life for clinical effectiveness is short (less than 4 hours); thus, these drugs require dosing three to four times daily.[51] Adverse effects of cromolyn and nedocromil are rare and most often include transient bronchospasm,

	TABLE 34.9	Dosage Guidelines for Theophylline in Children Older Than 6 Months and Adults Who Have No Risk Factors for Decreased Theophylline Clearance[a]		
Variable	**Weight-Adjusted and Maximal Dose**	**Comments**	**Adjustment to Dose**
Initial dose	~10 mg/kg of body weight/day; maximum, 300 mg/day	If initial dose is tolerated, increase the dose no sooner than 3 days later to the first increment	
First increment	~13 mg/kg/day; maximum, 450 mg/day	If the first incremental increase is tolerated, increase the dose no sooner than 3 days later to the second increment	
Second increment	~16 mg/kg/day; maximum, 600 mg/day	Measure the peak serum concentration after at least 3 days at the highest tolerated dose[b]	
Serum theophylline concentration (μg/mL)			
<10			Increase by approximately 25%
10–15			Maintain dose, if tolerated
15.1–19.9			Consider a reduction of approximately 10%[c]
20–25			Withhold next dose, then resume treatment with next lower dose increment
>25			Withhold next 2 doses, then resume treatment with initial dose or lower dose

[a] For infants 6 weeks to 6 months of age, the initial daily dose is calculated according to the following regression equation: dose (in milligrams per kilogram per day) = (0.2)(age in weeks) + 5.0. Subsequent increases in the dose in this age group should be based on peak serum concentrations measured no sooner than 3 days after the start of therapy. The guidelines listed use doses that are lower than those used in previous guidelines to account for the most recent assessment of population dose requirements and to minimize the risk of even minor adverse effects. With the use of these guidelines, one to two measurements of serum theophylline are usually sufficient to determine the dose requirement, with annual checks thereafter unless clinical indications suggest the need for more frequent assessment.
[b] The length of time to the peak serum concentration depends on the rate of absorption, the rate of elimination, and the dosing interval.
[c] This decreases the likelihood of adverse effects due to fluctuations in the absorption or elimination rate that may result in serum concentrations above 20 μg per milliliter and is especially important for patients who require doses higher than those used in the second increment.
(From Weinberger M, Hendeles L. Theophylline in asthma. N Engl J Med 334: 1380–1388, 1996.)

cough, and dry throat. Bronchospasm is quickly relieved with administration of an inhaled β_2-agonist. Infrequent adverse effects include anaphylaxis, generalized or facial dermatitis, myositis, gastroenteritis, and immunologic reactions in the lung. Because of the lack of systemic effects, cromolyn is often regarded as the safest anti-inflammatory therapy for asthma for use in children and during pregnancy.

Both cromolyn and nedocromil inhibit the IAR and LAR to inhaled allergens after a single dose, in contrast to inhaled corticosteroids, which inhibit only the LAR after a single dose. They also prevent exercise-induced asthma (although to a much lesser extent than inhaled β_2-agonists). Protection against exercise is dose dependent, with higher doses providing more complete and prolonged effects.[51] Despite the variety of effects, cromolyn and nedocromil are most valued for their ability to decrease airway hyperresponsiveness measured by histamine- or methacholine-induced bronchoconstriction when given for at least 12 weeks. There appears to be no advantage to theophylline versus cromolyn,[109] and no well-controlled studies have compared cromolyn and nedocromil with leukotriene modifiers. Cromolyn and nedocromil have effects on airway reactivity similar in magnitude to those of low-dose inhaled corticosteroids (<400 μg/day beclomethasone equivalent), although their effects have not been found to be uniformly consistent. There appears to be no benefit to adding cromolyn or nedocromil to high-dose inhaled corticosteroids (>1,000 μg/day beclomethasone equivalent) or oral corticosteroids or theophylline. However, some patients on moderate doses of inhaled corticosteroids may achieve a reduction in corticosteroid dose with added cromolyn or nedocromil.[51]

Cromolyn and nedocromil are not indicated for the relief of acute symptoms of asthma, as neither has bronchodilator effects. Results of studies using allergen challenge suggest that cromolyn and nedocromil may be useful for preventing symptoms due to a one-time exposure (such as exposure to a cat or vacuuming). In this case, use of cromolyn or nedocromil 15 to 30 minutes before anticipated exposure may prevent symptoms.[110] Although clinical effects may be noted within 1 week of initiation of therapy, 4 weeks is generally required for clinicians to determine whether an individual is responding to therapy. Guidelines from the NAEPP[1] and from the American Academy of Allergy, Asthma, and Immunology[111] recommend cromolyn or nedocromil as second-line therapy only in mild persistent asthma in children and adults. However, a Cochrane Library review of the efficacy of cromolyn in children concluded that no evidence demonstrates that cromolyn is more effective than placebo, even in children with mild asthma.[112] Thus, there appears to be only a minor role for cromolyn and nedocromil in the management of persistent asthma.

Leukotriene Modifiers. The leukotriene modifiers (zileuton, zafirlukast, and montelukast) constitute the newest pharmacologic class of drugs for the treatment of asthma. Leukotrienes are released from inflammatory cells in the airway and interact with specific receptors to cause bronchoconstriction, airway hyperresponsiveness, increased microvascular permeability leading to edema, leukocyte activation, eosinophilia, and enhanced mucous secretion. Leukotrienes are formed when the enzyme 5-lipoxygenase (5-LO), in conjunction with the cofactor 5-lipoxygenase–activating protein (FLAP), metabolizes arachidonic acid. An unstable intermediate product (LTA_4) is initially formed. Further conversion occurs to derive the cysteinyl leukotrienes (CysLTs) LTC_4, LTD_4, and LTE_4, or, via a separate pathway, to form LTB_4. The bronchoconstriction produced by LTD_4 has been estimated at 1,000 to 10,000 times greater than the activity of histamine and methacholine. LTC_4, LTD_4, and LTE_4 are highly potent inducers of airway smooth muscle contraction and bronchoconstriction, with an approximate equal potency between LTC_4 and LTD_4; however LTE_4 is approximately only 10% as potent.[113] LTC_4 is rapidly (minutes) converted to LTD_4, which is then converted to LTE_4 over approximately 30 minutes.[114] LTC_4, LTD_4, and LTE_4 act by binding to a common receptor, $CysLT_1$; however, because LTD_4 is extremely potent and has the longest half-life of the leukotrienes, it has been the focus of antimediator drug development. Leukotriene modifiers block leukotriene-mediated effects, either by preventing the enzymatic conversion of arachidonic acid to LTA_4 by blocking the 5-lipoxygenase enzyme (zileuton) or by blocking the binding of leukotrienes to the $CysLT_1$ receptor site (zafirlukast and montelukast).

Several polymorphisms within the leukotriene pathway have been identified.[115,116] Preliminary studies have shown an association between certain polymorphisms and response to leukotriene modifiers, but polymorphisms occur with a low frequency within the population and are unlikely to explain the significant variability that occurs with response to these drugs.[115] Pharmacogenetic studies will serve as an area of active research in which investigators will try to identify patients who are most likely to respond to leukotriene modifiers.

Leukotriene modifiers are administered orally and do not have clinically significant effects when inhaled. The pharmacokinetics and adverse effects differ significantly between zileuton, zafirlukast, and montelukast. Zileuton is dosed four times daily, zafirlukast twice daily, and montelukast once daily. Montelukast should be dosed at bedtime so that the highest serum concentrations of montelukast are provided during the night and early morning hours when asthma symptoms tend to be worse. Only montelukast is approved for use in children as young as 1 year of age. Zafirlukast bioavailability is significantly reduced by concomitant food ingestion; therefore, it must be dosed 1 hour before or 2 hours after a meal. Drug interactions occur with zileuton and zafirlukast, but to date, these have not been found with montelukast. Zileuton decreases the clearance of warfarin and theophylline, and zafirlukast decreases the clearance of warfarin, corticosteroids, theophylline (rare cases reported), and possibly other drugs metabolized by the cytochrome

P-450 2C9 isoenzyme, such as tolbutamide, phenytoin, and carbamazepine.[117]

Zileuton can cause liver dysfunction, and liver function monitoring is currently recommended before therapy is begun and every month for the first 3 months and every 3 months for the next 9 months. Reports of Churg-Strauss syndrome, which is characterized by eosinophilia, pulmonary infiltrates, and myocardial dysfunction, have occurred in patients treated with leukotriene modifiers who were being weaned from oral or high-dose inhaled corticosteroid therapy. It is believed that this syndrome is unmasked by the withdrawal of corticosteroid therapy rather than caused by the leukotriene modifier, as the syndrome also has been observed when oral corticosteroids are withdrawn from patients receiving maintenance therapy with inhaled corticosteroids.[117] Given the convenience of once-daily dosing, the lack of food and drug interactions, and the fact that it has been approved for use in children, montelukast is the preferred leukotriene modifier for patients with persistent asthma.

The leukotriene modifiers are effective in attenuating induced asthma, and all have similar clinical efficacy in asthma treatment. After allergen inhalation, these drugs attenuate the IAR and LAR by approximately 50% after a single dose but are not effective in inhibiting the increased airway hyperresponsiveness that occurs 24 hours later. Similarly, these drugs attenuate the fall in pulmonary function after exercise by 50% to 80% after a single dose, but significant bronchospasm can still occur at the end of the dosing interval.[113] In many but not all asthmatic patients with aspirin sensitivity, leukotriene modifiers are effective in preventing bronchoconstriction, which can occur after ingestion of aspirin or nonsteroidal anti-inflammatory drugs.[113,118] However, selective cyclooxygenase-2 inhibitors have not been shown to have cross-reactivity with aspirin or NSAIDs, and they appear to be safe when used in asthmatic patients with aspirin sensitivity.[119]

Clinical trials indicate that therapy with leukotriene modifiers can improve pulmonary function by approximately 10% to 12%, can reduce inhaled β_2-agonist use by 30%, and can decrease nocturnal awakenings due to asthma by 30%.[113] However, in these studies, significant asthma symptoms remained when leukotriene modifiers were used as monotherapy. Most published clinical trials, however, evaluated these drugs in patients with moderate to severe persistent asthma; therefore, it is not surprising that these drugs did not provide complete control of asthma symptoms.

Results of studies comparing low-dose inhaled corticosteroid therapy versus montelukast as monotherapy in patients with mild to moderate asthma are conflicting, depending upon the sponsor of the study.[6,120–123] Montelukast combined with inhaled fluticasone appears to be less effective than salmeterol combined with inhaled fluticasone in short-term (12-week) studies but is similarly effective in preventing asthma exacerbations when evaluated over 1 year or longer.[124–127] Montelukast combined with an inhaled corti-

costeroid is similarly effective to a doubled dose of inhaled corticosteroid.[128] Single doses of intravenous montelukast rapidly improve FEV_1, suggesting a possible role in the treatment of asthma in the emergency department in the future.[129,130]

The NAEPP guidelines currently recommend leukotriene modifiers as single-drug therapy for the treatment of patients with mild persistent asthma as an alternative *after* therapy with inhaled corticosteroids has been considered. In moderate persistent asthma, they are considered second-line therapy after a long-acting β_2-agonist as add-on therapy to inhaled corticosteroids. Probably the greatest advantage of leukotriene modifier therapy is that it is available in oral dosage forms. Studies indicate that patients prefer, and are more adherent with, oral versus inhaled therapy for asthma.[131–133]

Corticosteroids.

Inhaled Corticosteroids. The corticosteroids are the most potent anti-inflammatory drugs used for the treatment of asthma, and the inhaled corticosteroids are the most effective long-term control therapy for persistent asthma.[2,17] The use of inhaled corticosteroids is associated with a reduced risk of asthma exacerbations and hospitalizations for patients with asthma (up to 80%), and they offer the only long-term control therapy associated with a decreased risk of dying from asthma.[134] Despite this, numerous studies have reported that inhaled corticosteroids are underused in the treatment of persistent asthma, particularly in children and underrepresented minorities and socioeconomically deprived patient populations, who are at highest risk for adverse outcomes from asthma.[11,135,136] The underuse of inhaled corticosteroids is multifactorial, but concern for adverse effects by both clinicians and patients undoubtedly contributes.

Corticosteroids work by forming a complex with the glucocorticoid receptor that exists in the cytoplasm of most cells.[137] The corticosteroid-glucocorticoid receptor complex is a transcription factor that modulates gene activation and suppression. Thus, corticosteroids have a broad anti-inflammatory action, suppressing the action of several inflammatory cytokines (i.e., IL-1, GM-CSF, IL-3, IL-4, IL-6, and IL-8). In addition, corticosteroids can reduce cell inflammatory activation, improve cell apoptosis, and decrease vascular permeability and cell recruitment and activation.[137] It is interesting to note that corticosteroids do not influence degranulation of mast cells or inhibit the activity of histamine and leukotrienes once released, so they do not inhibit the IAR or EIB.[5,137] However, long-term administration results in an overall reduction in the number of lung tissue mast cells, so that acute responsiveness to allergens and exercise is markedly reduced over time.[137] Corticosteroids produce significant suppression of the late-phase inflammatory response to allergens and reduce markers of chronic inflammation and bronchial hyperresponsiveness.[2,5,137] However, their effects on airway remodeling and long-term progression of irreversible airways obstruction in asthma have not been established.[5,17] Cessation of corticosteroid therapy even after a number of years of therapy results in the return of markers of airway inflammation, along with worsening airflow obstruction and increased bronchial hyperresponsiveness.[5,17,138]

Chemical modification of endogenous cortisol has produced synthetic corticosteroids that are more selective for the glucocorticoid receptor (anti-inflammatory activity) with minimal to no mineralocorticoid (sodium retention) effects. However, glucocorticoid receptors, which are ubiquitous throughout the body, modulate the numerous effects that are listed in Table 34.10.[139] Further modifications have been made to enhance potency and systemic metabolism and to decrease oral absorption of the exogenous corticosteroids to increase their activity when administered topically and reduce their potential for systemic activity.[140,141] The inhaled corticosteroids are far more lipophilic than are the systemic corticosteroids, which enhances glucocorticoid receptor binding affinity (potency), metabolic clearance, and first-pass liver metabolism and decreases oral absorption.[141] These latter effects reduce systemic activity. More lipophilic

TABLE 34.10	Potential Adverse Effects from the Use of Corticosteroids
Short-term effects	Cough
	Dysphonia
	Thrush
	Suppression of basal cortisol secretion
	Suppression of ACTH and CRH secretion
	Suppression of lower leg growth
	Suppression of bone formation
	Sex hormone suppression
Intermediate effects	HPA axis suppression
	Linear growth velocity reduction
	Bone mineral density reduction
	Weight gain
	Cushing syndrome
	Mood swings, psychosis
	Hypokalemia
	Hyperglycemia
	Dermal thinning and skin bruising
	Glaucoma
Long-term effects	Adrenal insufficiency and crisis
	Growth suppression
	Failure to attain expected adult height
	Osteoporosis and fractures
	Cataracts

ACTH, adrenocorticotropic hormone; CRH, corticotropin-releasing hormone; HPA, hypothalamic-adrenal.

compounds may also be retained in the lung tissue for a longer time, which improves the topical-to-systemic activity ratio (therapeutic index).[140] Some inhaled corticosteroids are esterified intracellularly (budesonide and ciclesonide), and this may contribute to longer lung tissue retention.[141]

Although the inhaled corticosteroids have a significantly greater therapeutic index than do systemically administered corticosteroids, if given in large enough dosages, they all produce the same adverse effects.[139] Systemic activity is caused by the portion of drug that is absorbed orally plus that portion that is deposited in the lung. Table 34.11 lists the various pharmacodynamic/pharmacokinetic properties of inhaled corticosteroids. Decreased oral bioavailability and prolonged lung retention enhance the therapeutic index, whereas increased potency merely alters the dose required to produce a specific effect. Relative potency can also be affected by the delivery device, which determines the amount of initial dose that is deposited in the lung (see later discussion).[139] It has been estimated that at least a fourfold difference in potency or dose delivered is required for a significant difference in clinical efficacy to be demonstrated.[137,141] For those compounds with significant oral absorption, use of a VHC with an MDI significantly reduces the systemic load, as the large particles that are normally deposited in the oropharynx and swallowed (70% to 80% of the dose) are deposited instead in the VHC.[139] However, the addition of a VHC to an MDI may also enhance the systemic activity of inhaled corticosteroids with poor oral absorption by increasing lung delivery compared with the MDI alone.[139] Gargling with water and spitting immediately after taking an inhaled corticosteroid by DPI may reduce the gastrointestinal load.[140] Both gargling and the use of a VHC with MDI have been shown to be effective in reducing local adverse effects, including oropharyngeal thrush and hoarseness. The NAEPP has provided a comparative dosing table for the inhaled corticosteroids (Table 34.5), as they differ significantly in potency and lung delivery from various devices.[17] When they are administered in comparable doses, one should expect similar clinical efficacy. However, there is evidence that they differ in their systemic activity at comparable efficacy.[139,142] Most patients should be treated with low to medium doses.[17] At high doses, the potential for systemic effects is significant, warranting periodic monitoring of the patient. It is recommended that patients who require high-dose inhaled corticosteroids be referred to an asthma specialist.[17]

Although most of the systemic effects listed in Table 34.10 occur at high doses of inhaled corticosteroids, growth suppression or growth retardation has been reported in children at low to medium doses of inhaled corticosteroids. Most studies suggest that this is a small effect of 1 to 2 cm over 1 year that occurs in the first 3 to 6 months and is not cumulative.[17,139] Retrospective cohort studies also suggest that final predicted adult height is not affected; however, long-term, longitudinal studies have not been completed, so it is not absolutely certain whether final adult height is affected.[17]

| TABLE 34.11 | Pharmacodynamic/Pharmacokinetic Comparison of Corticosteroids |

Systemic	Anti-inflammatory Potency	Mineralocorticoid Potency	Duration of Biologic Activity (h)	Elimination Half-life (h)
Hydrocortisone	1	1.0	8–12	1.5–2.0
Prednisone	4	0.8	12–36	2.5–3.5
Methylprednisolone	5	0.5	12–36	3.3
Dexamethasone	25	0	36–54	3.4–4.0

ICS	Receptor Binding Affinity[a]	Lung Delivery[b] (% dose/device)	Oral Bioavailability (%)	Systemic Clearance (L/h)	Half-life (h) IV/inhaled
Beclomethasone dipropionate/monopropionate	0.4/13.5	4%–10%/CFC-MDI 55%–60%/HFA-MDI	15–20	UK	0.5/1.5–6.5
Budesonide	9.4	32% (16%–59%)/DPI 6%/Nebulizer ampules	11	55–84	2.8/2.0
Flunisolide	1.8	32%	20	58	1.6/1.6
Fluticasone propionate	18	26%–30%/CFC-MDI 15%/DPI	≤1	66	7.8/14.4
Mometasone furoate	27	Unknown	≤1	53	5.8/Unknown
Triamcinolone acetonide	3.6	22%/CFC-MDI	23	45–69	2.0/3.6

[a] Receptor binding affinities are relative to dexamethasone equal to 1.
[b] Based on in vivo scintigraphy or pharmacokinetic studies.

There may be a difference between the inhaled corticosteroids and their delivery devices, as studies with fluticasone propionate by DPI and ciclesonide have not detected growth suppression at low to medium doses, whereas studies with beclomethasone dipropionate by MDI and DPI and budesonide by DPI have consistently shown an effect at low to medium doses.[139]

However, higher doses of any of the inhaled corticosteroids are likely to produce an effect on height, so the risks and benefits of this therapy should be evaluated for all patients. It should be noted that severe uncontrolled persistent asthma also is associated with growth retardation in children.[2,17] It is recommended that children on inhaled corticosteroids have their height monitored routinely, which should be done anyway as part of routine pediatric care.[17]

The inhaled corticosteroids have been associated with decreased bone mineral density and increased risk of fracture in groups of patients already predisposed to these problems (elderly and postmenopausal females).[139] These effects are dose dependent, and the increased risk is associated with high-dose inhaled corticosteroids. Clinically significant hypothalamic-adrenal axis (HPA) suppression is rare and occurs at high doses; however, severe adrenal crisis has been reported in patients on excessive doses.[139] Currently, only those patients who are receiving high doses of inhaled corticosteroids must have their bone mineral density and HPA axis monitored.[17,139] Patients at high risk for lower bone mineral density should take normal prophylactic measures (see Chapter 69 for discussion of osteoporosis).

The dosing of inhaled corticosteroids is initially based on severity (Table 34.5; Figs. 34.4 and 34.7).[17] The usual recommendation is to administer inhaled corticosteroids twice daily; however, a number of studies have shown that once control is achieved, many patients with mild disease can be controlled on once-daily administration in the late afternoon or evening.[140,143] One method of reducing the dose of inhaled corticosteroid is to administer it in combination with a long-acting inhaled β$_2$-agonist, such as salmeterol or formoterol. Combination therapy is more effective at improving lung function and decreasing acute exacerbations of asthma than is doubling the dose of inhaled corticosteroids.[17] By contrast, the addition of leukotriene receptor antagonists or theophylline results in the same improvement as is caused by doubling the inhaled corticosteroid dose.[17] Although the addition of long-acting inhaled β$_2$-agonists allows a reduction in inhaled corticosteroid dose, such agonists cannot replace inhaled corticosteroids because of the associated lack of anti-inflammatory activity.

Systemic Corticosteroids. Systemic corticosteroids are used primarily as rescue medication for acute asthma exacerbations.[1,2] Oral prednisone and prednisolone are the most commonly used preparations. These drugs have minimal mineralocorticoid effects and a relatively short biological half-life; they therefore produce less adrenal suppression than is caused by agents with longer biological half-lives such as dexamethasone. Evidence from clinical trials does not support an advantage for parenteral administration in onset or in overall efficacy.[8,33] Higher doses over those recommended also do not produce a greater effect but may produce a greater number of adverse effects (central nervous system and electrolyte disturbances). Case reports have documented severe muscle myopathy associated with excessively high doses of systemic corticosteroids.[2] Although it has been suggested that early initiation of systemic corticosteroids in the emergency department may decrease the rate of hospitalization, this is an inconsistent finding across studies.[8,33] Thus, the use of corticosteroids is recommended only for those patients who do not respond to the initial three doses of inhaled β_2-agonists.[1,2] The use of systemic corticosteroids for an additional 7 to 10 days following discharge from the emergency department to home may reduce the number of relapses (patients returning within 2 weeks of discharge).[33] The addition of inhaled corticosteroids at this time may produce additional benefits.

In children with virally induced exacerbations of such severity that they result in hospitalization, it has been proposed that prednisone be available at home to be initiated at the first signs of deterioration following upper respiratory tract infection.[144] However, this recommendation is based primarily on the results of a single study. Outpatient management of acute exacerbations of asthma with systemic corticosteroids in children is common practice, yet studies supporting this practice are somewhat equivocal.[144] Most studies used dosage regimens that ranged from 3 to 10 days. The current recommendation is found in Table 34.4.[17] One of the issues involving systemic corticosteroids is the potential for long-term adverse effects such as growth suppression, adrenal suppression, and osteoporosis when frequent short courses are used. Although any dose of corticosteroid that exceeds normal physiologic cortisol excretion for longer than 5 days produces some suppression of the HPA axis, this is relatively short-lived (1 to 3 days) at the usual dose of 1 to 2 mg per kg daily of prednisone equivalent for up to 21 days.[38] Patients who receive three to four ''short bursts'' of prednisone (10 or fewer days) do not show evidence of long-term corticosteroid toxicity.[144] However, patients who receive at least eight bursts (at least 10 days each) demonstrate a similar reduction in bone mineral density as those receiving daily or alternate-day corticosteroids.[38] Patients who require more than three to four courses of prednisone should be placed on appropriate long-term control therapy with inhaled corticosteroids.

Another common practice is to use tapering doses of systemic corticosteroids to prevent relapse of the disease and to allow recovery of the HPA axis. No evidence proves that tapering the dose improves either outcome. Prolonging dosing by tapering prolongs the duration of supra-physiologic

doses of corticosteroid, thus increasing the risk of HPA suppression. However, if a patient has been receiving long-term daily therapy for longer than 2 weeks, appropriate tests of adrenal function should be performed and the dose tapered slowly with appropriate monitoring. Studies in patients in the emergency department and in hospitalized patients have shown tapering to be unnecessary for preventing relapse if patients are started on inhaled corticosteroids.[33,38,144]

Anti-IgE Monoclonal Antibodies. Omalizumab, an anti-IgE monoclonal antibody, is the first monoclonal drug developed for asthma; it was approved by the FDA in June of 2003 for patients 12 years of age and older. IgE plays a critical role in the inflammatory process of allergic asthma. High-affinity receptors for circulating IgE (FcεR1) are found on mast cells and basophils. When allergen is inhaled into the lungs, the allergen molecules cross-link IgE bound to mast cells and basophils, which causes the mast cells and basophils to degranulate and release preformed mediators (histamine, tryptase) and rapidly synthesized mediators (bradykinin, prostaglandin E2, prostaglandin F2, and leukotrienes). Omalizumab binds to the Cε3 domain of free IgE in the serum and forms a complex that prevents IgE from binding to the FcεR1 on mast cells and basophils. Omalizumab does not bind to IgE that is already bound to mast cells. Thus, although a single dose of omalizumab can reduce free IgE serum levels by more than 99% within the first hour, the clinical effects takes several weeks to manifest, presumably because of continued degranulation of mast cells with bound IgE molecules.[145] Serum IgE levels are not to be measured for monitoring purposes, as most clinical assays measure both free and bound IgE in the serum; serum IgE levels actually rise after treatment is begun, as the IgE-omalizumab complex has a slower clearance than does free IgE.[146]

The dose of omalizumab is determined by actual body weight and total serum IgE concentration and is administered subcutaneously. Current recommended dosing guidelines allow for omalizumab administration to patients who weigh less than 150 kg and who have a baseline IgE between 30 and 700 IU per mL. Patients outside these ranges have not been studied in clinical trials; therefore, no dosing recommendations are available. Calculated doses that exceed 300 mg are to be divided and administered every 2 weeks. In addition, any single dose that exceeds 150 mg must be divided and administered at two or three injection sites. Therefore, large patients with high baseline serum IgE levels could receive three subcutaneous injections every 2 weeks; such a regimen could certainly hinder adherence, particularly in children.

Immune complex reactions have not occurred with omalizumab, presumably because of the relatively small size of the IgE-omalizumab complex.[146] Anaphylaxis is a potential adverse effect; thus, patients should be observed after dosing. Risk of malignancy is included in the labeling, although many patients with reported cancers have had a history of cancers, premalignant conditions, or other risk factors.[146]

Antibody formation to omalizumab has not been observed.[147]

A Cochrane Database Review indicated that omalizumab is effective in reducing asthma exacerbations and steroid dose in patients with moderate to severe asthma and in improving quality of life.[147] It is not clear whether differences in response occur between patients with moderate and severe asthma, and further study is needed to define patients who are most likely to respond.[147] Long-term studies are needed to determine whether patients with more severe asthma require a prolonged period to slowly reduce steroid doses while receiving omalizumab, and also to confirm safety.

Depending on the dose required, the per annum cost of omalizumab ranges from approximately $6,500 to $40,000 per year.[146] Clearly, patients must be carefully chosen for a favorable cost-to-benefit ratio. Omalizumab is not currently included in the NAEPP or GINA guidelines,[2,17] and comparative studies with regimens that have been shown to reduce asthma exacerbations and steroid dose are needed.

Inhaled Drug Delivery. Administration of medications by the inhaled route offers the advantage of delivery directly to the site of action. Inhaled delivery allows for reduced dosage and results in less risk of systemic adverse effects and the potential for improved efficacy and a faster onset of action compared with oral administration. However, inhaled drug delivery can be affected by a number of factors, including aerosol particle size, inhalation technique, propellants, and delivery device used for administration.

Deposition of inhaled aerosol particles occurs primarily by inertial impaction, sedimentation, and diffusion. Inertial impaction is the means by which larger particles, those unable to flow in the airstream with changes in direction, are deposited. This typically occurs with particles >6 μm in aerodynamic diameter and results in oropharyngeal deposition, as well as deposition into the bifurcations of the larger airways.[35] Particles between 2 and 6 μm flow in the slower airstream in central airways (the target for drug delivery in asthma) and are deposited by gravitational sedimentation, especially with breathholding maneuvers. Particles <2 μm deposit in the peripheral airways, and those <1 μm in diameter are deposited by random Brownian diffusion in bronchioles or alveoli or are exhaled.[35] Thus, the ideal or "respirable range" of aerosol particles for deposition in the lower respiratory tract is 1 to 6 μm aerodynamic diameter.[35]

Generation of therapeutic aerosols is caused by nebulizers, MDIs, and DPI devices. Each type of delivery device, nebulizer, MDI, and DPI has distinct advantages and disadvantages (Table 34.12).

Nebulizers. Two types of nebulizers are available—those driven by compressed air ("jet") and ultrasonic nebulizers. Jet nebulizers produce an aerosol when compressed gas is delivered up through the bottom of the nebulizer, creating a region of negative pressure that entrains the solution of drug. The air and solution strike a baffle and break into droplets to be inhaled.[35] Larger droplets adhere to the sides

of the nebulizer and drip back into the nebulizer base to be renebulized. Jet nebulizers require a gas flow of approximately 8 L per minute for particles to be generated within the respirable range,[35] and tidal breathing and deep inhalation with breathholding are acceptable methods of delivery. Aerosols from ultrasonic nebulizers are produced by a piezoelectric transducer that vibrates at a high frequency (1 to 3 MHz). Ultrasonic nebulizers are not effective for delivery of suspensions and viscous solutions, as most of what is nebulized is water and not drug.[148] Only about 10% of the dose placed in the nebulizer reaches the patient's lungs, with 60% to 80% retained in the nebulizer, 20% exhaled, and 2% deposited into the mouth.[140] A face mask is typically needed for young children, but holding the face mask only 2 cm from the face can reduce delivery by 80%.[149] A nebulizer is not indicated for routine use and should be reserved as second-line therapy after MDI or DPI.[148] A Cochrane Database Review found similar outcomes for β2-agonist treatment of acute asthma with the use of an MDI plus holding chambers versus nebulizers.[34]

Metered-Dose Inhalers and Spacers/Holding Chambers. Metered-dose inhalers are the standard for aerosolized delivery because of their convenience and efficacy; however, they can be difficult to use correctly. MDIs deliver suspensions or solutions of drug mixed with propellants and other chemicals via a pressurized canister with a metering valve. The CFC propellants are being phased out of production, and hydrofluoroalkane propellant alternatives (non-CFC) and powder delivery devices are available.

Technique is extremely important for the proper use of MDIs, as significant hand-lung coordination is required (Table 34.13). Most patients and health care professionals (more than 60%) do not use an MDI correctly, and frequent reinstruction is needed because correct use declines over periods as short as 6 to 10 weeks.[35,150] With appropriate technique, approximately 10% to 25% of drug is delivered to the lungs,[35] but drugs with HFA propellant may demonstrate different lung delivery. Breath-actuated devices have further simplified the use of MDIs by significantly lessening the degree of coordination needed; however, these provide no advantage in patients with good inhaler technique and cannot be used with spacer and holding chambers, which have advantages of their own.

Spacers and valved holding chambers (Fig. 34.8)[151] increase pulmonary drug deposition in patients with poor MDI technique, reduce oropharyngeal deposition of drug (thus decreasing the risks for topical as well as systemic adverse effects), lessen bad taste and the cold freon effect, and minimize the amount of coordination required for proper use of MDIs.[35] A spacer is a simple device that is an open-ended tube or bag that creates a space for the aerosol to expand to allow the propellant to evaporate.[35] Spacers must be at least 100 mL in volume and 10 to 13 cm in length; smaller spacers reduce drug delivery.[35] Valved holding chambers are larger and allow the aerosol to expand; however, drug remains in the device until

TABLE 34.12	Advantages and Disadvantages of Various Inhalation Delivery Systems	
Device	**Advantages**	**Disadvantages**
Nebulizer	Simple to use (requires minimal coordination) Can be used in mechanically ventilated patients	Requires water-soluble drug Inefficient delivery Significant drug wasted (residual volume) Numerous factors can affect delivery Device variability (brand to brand, lot to lot) Inconvenient, bulky, costly, and time consuming Requires electrical power source Nebulizer must be kept clean (potential for infection) Potential for breakdown of drug (ultrasonic) Costly
Metered-dose inhaler	Requires minimal time for treatments Small, portable Can be used in mechanically ventilated patients	Requires significant coordination Chorofluorocarbon propellants to be phased out Difficulty in determining number of doses remaining Numerous excipients
MDI with spacer	Significantly reduces coordination required Improves pulmonary drug deposition Reduces risk for adverse effects	Bulky, costly Overall cost of drug treatment may decrease with increased delivery of drug to the lung (greater efficacy) and less oropharyngeal deposition (fewer systemic effects)
Breath-actuated MDI	Requires minimal coordination Potential for improved pulmonary drug deposition	No additional benefit if good inhaler technique used Cannot be used with spacer (potential for adverse effects) Difficulty in determining number of doses remaining Cannot be used in mechanically ventilated patients Chorofluorocarbon propellants to be phased out
Dry-powder inhaler	Breath-actuated, requires minimal coordination Improves pulmonary drug deposition Lactose excipients Some are single-dose units that require assembly	Young children and acutely obstructed patients may not generate adequate inspiratory flow to actuate Requires change in inhalation technique Increased oropharyngeal drug deposition and systemic absorption increase risk for systemic adverse effects Potential for drug to aggregate Potential to provoke cough (not widely reported) Cannot be used in mechanically ventilated patients

inhaled, and exhaled air does not return to the chamber; thus, multiple inhalations can be used to completely empty the aerosol from the chamber.[35] The latter is particularly important for children with tidal volumes that do not exceed the volume of the holding chamber. The advantages of spacer devices and VHC are often worth the extra cost and bulkiness.

Dry Powder Inhalers. Dry-powder inhalers consist of a varied group of inhalers from which patients inhale a micronized dry powder of drug or drug plus excipient such as lactose.[35] They do not contain a pressurized propellant, the patient must inspire deeply and forcefully to empty a small holding chamber or capsule of the powder following activa-tion. Activation of a DPI consists of shaving off a dose from solid depot (Turbuhaler), releasing the micronized powder from a blister pack (Diskus), or puncturing a single-dose capsule (Aerolizer and HandiHaler). Once it has been activated, the patient should not exhale into the device, as the moisture will prevent dispersion of the powder or will tip the device upside down, causing the powder to fall out. Inspiratory flow is important for dispersal of the micronized powder with an optimal flow of about 60 L per minute.[35,51] This is about twice the rate of the lower flows used for optimal MDI inhalation technique. Advantages of DPIs are that they do not require significant hand-lung coordination, and the

TABLE 34.13	Recommended Technique for the Proper Use of a Metered-Dose Inhaler

1. Remove cap

2. Shake canister

3. Exhale (to functional residual capacity or fully, if *slow* exhalation)

4. Hold MDI upright and:

   a. Place lips around mouthpiece, or

   b. Place mouthpiece ~2 inches or 2 fingerwidths from mouth, or

   c. Place lips around spacer mouthpiece (if using a spacer device)

5. Start to inhale slowly (≤30 L/min) immediately before actuation

6. Actuate MDI while continuing to inhale

7. Inhale completely and hold breath for 10 seconds (or at least 4 to 5 seconds)

8. Wait 1 minute

9. Repeat treatment (Steps 2–7), if more than one inhalation prescribed

10. For inhaled steroids, rinse mouth with water or mouthwash and expel contents

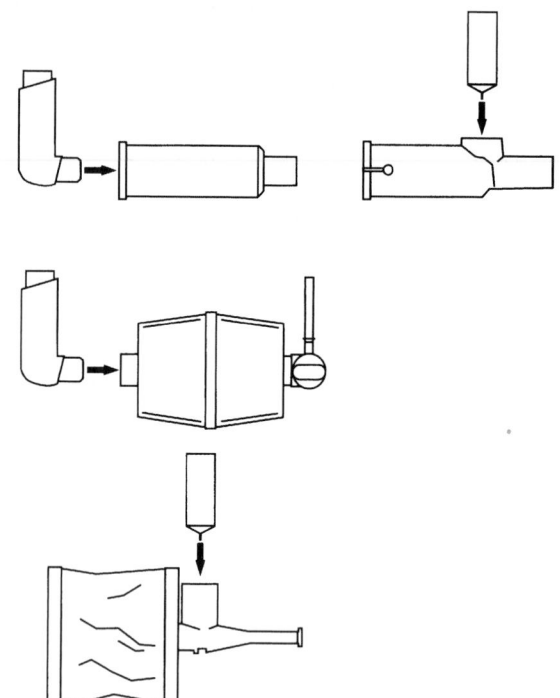

FIGURE 34.8 Diagram of various spacer devices. (From the National Asthma Education and Prevention Program. Practical guide for the diagnosis and management of asthma. Based on the expert panel report 2: guidelines for the diagnosis and management of asthma. Bethesda, MD: US Department of Health and Human Services, Public Health Service, National Institutes of Health, National Heart, Lung, and Blood Institute, October 1997; Publication no 97-4053.)

deep, forceful inhalation technique is easier to teach.[51] The primary disadvantage is the requirement of a higher inspiratory flow for optimal delivery. Some differences among DPIs have been noted in that high-resistance DPIs (such as the Turbuhaler) exhibit significant differences in delivery at low flows (30 L/min) compared with low-resistance DPIs (such as Diskus and Aerolizer).[35] The Turbuhaler delivers one-half the dose at 30 L per minute than is delivered at 60 L per minute, whereas the Diskus and Aerolizer deliver approximately the same dose at 30 and 60 L per minute.[35,51] Children younger than 4 years of age generally cannot consistently generate an inspiratory flow greater than 30 L per minute, so DPIs are not indicated in infants and toddlers.[51]

NONPHARMACOLOGIC THERAPY

Environmental control measures, along with pharmacotherapy, are an integral component of successful asthma therapy. Environmental controls include allergen and trigger avoidance measures (Table 34.14). Patients must be counseled that environmental controls must be adhered to consistently if any beneficial effect is to be achieved. However, a Cochrane Database Review[152] on house dust mite control measures in patients with asthma did not find an effect of these interventions and concluded that chemical and physical methods to reduce house dust mite exposure cannot be recommended. Many trials had methodologic flaws, and it is likely that elimination of a single allergen would have little effect in persons with sensitivities to multiple allergens. A large, carefully controlled trial is under way with controls for problems in other studies may provide further clarification.[152]

Immunotherapy, provided by subcutaneous administration of standardized allergen extracts, is generally reserved for patients who have incomplete symptom control with drug therapy despite adherence with the regimen, have intolerable adverse effects from drug therapy, or are unable to avoid exposure to the allergen. Only allergens to which the patient has demonstrated IgE-mediated sensitivity and positive clinical history should be included in an immunotherapy plan. A single subcutaneous injection often contains multiple allergens to which the patient is sensitive. Physician visits are frequent (once or twice a week, initially), and it may take as long as 6 months for symptom relief to be obtained. Because treatment can continue for up to 5 years or longer, it is imperative that a patient's commitment be assessed before treatment is begun. Patients often have misconceptions and a lack of knowledge about the safety and efficacy of immunotherapy, suggesting that health care providers must provide regular education to patients throughout the duration of treatment.[153] Immunotherapy should be continued for at least 3 years because relapse is common when therapy is discontinued sooner. Approximately 80% to 85% of patients obtain

| TABLE 34.14 | **Strategies to Reduce Allergen Exposure** |

Indoor Allergen Control

Dust mite	Encase mattresses and pillows in mite-proof coverings
	Remove carpeting entirely from home, if possible, or at least from bedrooms
	Replace upholstered furniture with vinyl or leather
	Wipe down surfaces of dressers, window sills, blinds weekly
	Wash bedding (sheets, mattress covers, blankets) weekly in water in temperatures of at least 130°F
	Remove stuffed animals and toys from the bedroom
	Place stuffed animals and toys in dryer at 140°F for 1 h, or place in freezer overnight
	Vacuum wearing a face mask or use high-efficiency particulate air (HEPA) filter on vacuum to avoid inhalation of mite fecal balls
	Apply acaricides[a] to carpet and upholstered furniture
	Keep relative humidity in home below 45% and temperature below 70°F by using refrigerated air conditioning
	Vacuum baseboard and wall heaters weekly
Cats[b]	Remove cat from household or at least from bedroom; keep outdoors if possible
	Wash and wipe walls weekly
	Use HEPA filters or electrostatic filters on forced air central heating/cooling units to remove cat allergen from air.[c] For room air filtration, use HEPA filters; do not use electrostatic room air filters, which release ozone
	Encourage children to play in homes that are cat-free
	Keep clothing in closet with door closed
Moulds	Use 5% bleach solution to clean bathrooms and kitchens to kill mould
	Remove stacks of old newspapers and books
	Use a dehumidifier
	Change air filters monthly
	If building a home, create airspace between cement floor and carpeting, or use vinyl tile
	Keep plants outdoors
Cockroaches	Use professional extermination services

Outdoor Allergen Control

Pollens	Keep windows in car and home closed during pollen season and use air conditioning
	Shower and wash hair nightly to remove pollen
Moulds	Avoid mowing grass, which releases mould spores into the air

[a] Benzyl benzoate products are acaricidal; tannic acid–containing products denature the allergenic protein but are not acaricidal and thus are not recommended. Do not use if there is a toddler present in the household. Products may need to be applied more frequently than is stated in instructions.
[b] Products applied directly to the cat's fur are not effective in reducing cat allergen load.
[c] Filters can also remove dust mite fecal balls when they are airborne (i.e., after vacuuming).

significant relief when they continue therapy.[154] Patients should be much improved or symptom free for at least 1 to 2 years before treatment is discontinued. If no improvement is noted after 1 year, a reassessment of clinical allergen sensitivities and of the method of immunotherapy used should be conducted. For example, if too many allergens are included in each injection, none may be provided at a sufficient concentration to stimulate an immune response. Patients with coronary artery disease, severe hypertension, severe asthma, or severe atopic dermatitis should not receive immunotherapy because anaphylaxis to the allergen injection would increase the risk of life-threatening consequences. Immunotherapy may be continued in women who become pregnant but should not be initiated in pregnant patients. In addition, patients who require β-blockers or monoamine oxidase inhibitors should not receive immunotherapy because these drugs hamper treatment of anaphylaxis with adrenergic agonist drugs. Immunotherapy has proved effective for grass, ragweed, birch, and mountain cedar pollens, dust mites, and cat allergen; the efficacy of mould immunotherapy is still being evaluated.

The efficacy of immunotherapy may involve several mechanisms, including generation of a rise in serum IgG antibodies that bind but do not cross-link allergens, suppression of IgE antibody levels, and reduction of basophil and lymphocyte responsiveness to allergens.

ALTERNATIVE THERAPIES

Because of the many toxicities and adverse effects associated with long-term oral corticosteroid use, several other asthma therapies have been investigated for patients with severe persistent asthma. These include methotrexate, troleandomycin (TAO), gold, intravenous gamma globulin (IVIG), and cyclosporine. Consideration and institution of alternative treatments are reserved for steroid-dependent patients with severe asthma. Although the goal of therapy is usually to reduce systemic corticosteroid doses, some studies have demonstrated improvements in pulmonary function (although no corticosteroids are bronchodilators in the traditional sense) and bronchial hyperresponsiveness.[155] With alternative treatments, it is particularly important that the goal of therapy be defined, as improving pulmonary function may not be realistic in the patient with severe asthma who is undergoing concomitant corticosteroid dose reductions.

Patients with asthma are increasingly using alternative and complementary therapies such as herbs, vitamins, massage, acupuncture, prayer, healing touch, and homeopathy.[156–158] Up to 41% of persons with asthma in the United States have used complementary therapies.[159] A thorough review of herbal therapies in asthma is presented by Bielory and Lupoli.[156] However, common complementary therapies, including herbal, acupuncture, homeopathy, breathing exercises, and dietary therapies, have not shown benefit in patients with asthma.[159] Many studies have been poorly de-

signed, and access to and interpretation of literature from other cultures is nearly impossible.[159] The FDA maintains a list of harmful dietary supplements at http://www.cfsan.fda.gov/~dms/ds-warn.html.

FUTURE THERAPIES

With increased research and improved knowledge of the pathophysiology of asthma, many novel treatment modalities are being developed,[160] in addition to improvements in inhaled corticosteroids and long-acting β₂-agonists. Mediator antagonists (NO inhibitors, interleukin antagonists), cytokines, chemokine receptor inhibitors, PDE-4 inhibitors, transcription factor inhibitors, kinase inhibitors, and cell adhesion blockers are being investigated for their potential in asthma therapeutics.[160] Other modalities include immunostimulation, vaccinations to induce the Th1 response, and antisense and gene therapy.[160]

IMPROVING OUTCOMES

Outcome studies comparing the effects of different interventions, including improving medication adherence, teaching self-management strategies, and providing intensive follow-up, on the morbidity, mortality, and quality of life of patients with asthma have recently been the subject of renewed interest. Such studies have become important in guiding the treatment of patients covered by health maintenance organizations (HMOs) and other health insurers, and as part of the FDA drug approval process. Many insurers are developing asthma management programs for their enrollees in an attempt to better control expensive asthma outcomes such as emergency department visits and hospitalizations. The NAEPP guidelines provide extensive information on how to educate patients about asthma and self-management.[1]

PATIENT EDUCATION

Patient education strategies are well described in the NAEPP guidelines.[1] The emphasis in these guidelines is on developing a partnership between the patient (and family) and the caregivers. This partnership serves to provide both patient and family members with the education and skills needed for appropriate self-management, with regular feedback and reinforcement provided by caregivers. Areas that should be covered in patient education sessions include the following:

- Basic facts about asthma
- Roles of medications (especially the distinction between quick-relief and long-term-control medications)
- Skills for proper inhaler use with or without a VHC/spacer and for peak flow meter monitoring and self-assessment
- Environmental control measures
- Appropriate use of rescue plans and medications

Educational materials and forms for self-monitoring are available in these guidelines for photocopying, or they can be downloaded from the Internet at the address provided in the opening paragraphs of this chapter.

METHODS TO IMPROVE PATIENT ADHERENCE TO DRUG THERAPY

Patients with asthma, similar to others with chronic diseases, are poorly adherent to drug therapy. Rates of medication nonadherence among patients with asthma range from 30% to 70%.[161] Adherence does seem to improve as disease severity worsens from mild to moderate asthma, but it declines in patients with severe asthma, and as expected, adherence declines with an increase in the number of times per day a medication is prescribed; adherence is better with oral than with inhaled medications.[161] Unfortunately, no common characteristics appear to be predictive of medication nonadherence, except that barriers can be divided into (a) treatment-related, (b) clinician-related, and (c) patient-related factors.[161] Steps that can be taken to improve adherence include simplifying treatments, ensuring patient understanding of the disease and its treatment, gaining the confidence of the patient, addressing psychological disorders, and assessing the motivation of the patient for self-management.[161]

The NAEPP guidelines stress a partnership between the patient and the caregiver. A satisfying relationship between patient and caregiver is the most important factor required for changing health care behavior, including medication adherence.[162] Skills that the health care provider should use include the following:

- Making direct eye contact
- Transmitting genuine interest
- Explaining all recommendations thoroughly and in language the patient can understand
- Praising good medication adherence
- Expressing a willingness to modify the treatment plan in accord with concerns expressed by the patient[162]

Once a positive relationship has been established, other changes that can be negotiated, which may lead to improved adherence, include the following:

- Prescribing less costly medications
- Prescribing medications with fewer adverse effects that are of concern to the patient
- Working with the patient to determine appropriate reminders to help with taking medications on schedule
- Changing dosing schedules to accommodate work or school
- Reducing the number of medications taken[162]

Adolescents are predictably nonadherent with medication regimens. Suggestions given by adolescents for improving communication between the adolescent patient and the health care provider include the following:

- Provide practical information on how to prevent symptoms

- Explain how medications work and discuss the purpose of each medication (especially important when multiple medications are taken)
- Provide information in person and not as written material
- Use language understood by adolescents
- Use drawings, pictures, or videos to illustrate information (this could include demonstration on use of MDIs, DPIs, or peak flowmeters)
- Keep drawings childlike (simple) to facilitate remembering[163]

DISEASE MANAGEMENT STRATEGIES TO IMPROVE PATIENT OUTCOMES

The NAEPP guidelines provide the methods needed for establishing a comprehensive asthma management program.[1] These guidelines, initially published in 1991,[164] have been implemented communitywide in several metropolitan areas, and have been found to reduce emergency department visits and hospitalizations.[165,166]

PHARMACOECONOMICS

Morbidity from asthma, in particular, acute exacerbation, is the driving force for the estimated $14.5 billion cost of asthma recorded in the United States in the year 2000.[167] Direct medical costs account for 50% of total societal costs, with about 50% of that spent on the treatment of acute exacerbations. In comparison, indirect societal costs are exclusively due to lost work, schooldays lost, and mortality secondary to exacerbation. For example, it is estimated that at least $1 billion is lost annually by parents who must care for their children secondary to asthma exacerbations.[167] Thus, therapies that reduce the risk of exacerbation, particularly of severe exacerbations that lead to emergency department visits and hospitalizations, can have a significant impact on the overall cost of asthma. Finally, low-income, minority, and other underserved populations disproportionately share the burden of asthma morbidity and mortality.[168] In addition, numerous studies have documented the undertreatment of these populations, so that programs directed to these populations represent a public health priority.[168]

Pharmacoeconomic studies in asthma consist of prospective cost-effectiveness trials attached to randomized clinical trials, retrospective cost analysis from large integrated medical and pharmaceutical claims databases, and retrospective mathematical model assessments that use outcomes data from various randomized clinical trials and cohort studies. These economic studies reflect the findings of randomized clinical trials and meta-analyses of asthma management. Educational interventions that teach asthma self-management, particularly to high users of health care resources, reduce both direct and indirect costs over the short term, but the effects begin to wane over the long term, emphasizing the need for continued reinforcement of patient education.[169–172] In addition, the introduction of clinical pathway protocols in the emergency department reduces hospital admissions and relapses, producing considerable cost savings.[33,38]

By significantly reducing severe asthma exacerbations, corticosteroids have clearly demonstrated cost-effectiveness, even in newly diagnosed patients with mild asthma and in small infants and young children.[173–175] Compared with leukotriene modifiers as monotherapy, inhaled corticosteroids significantly reduce the cost of asthma care.[176,177] The addition of a long-acting inhaled β_2-agonist to an inhaled corticosteroid reduces health care use, offsetting the increased cost of medication in patients with moderate persistent asthma.[178] The combination of long-acting inhaled β_2-agonists with inhaled corticosteroids is significantly more cost-effective than is the combination of a leukotriene modifier with an inhaled corticosteroid.[179,180] The relative cost-effectiveness of omalizumab was recently evaluated because of its modest efficacy and high annual cost.[181] Its incremental cost-effectiveness ratio suggested that it should be reserved for those patients hospitalized at least five times a year despite maximal asthma therapy. For the treatment of children with severe acute asthma, the addition of ipratropium bromide has been shown to be cost-effective in that it reduces hospitalization.[10,38] Continuous nebulization of albuterol reduces the overall cost of care of children admitted to an intensive care unit.[38] On the other hand, although the use of an MDI plus a spacer device in the emergency department has been promoted as more cost-effective than the use of nebulized bronchodilators, accurate economic analyses have not been performed to support this conclusion.[35] In conclusion, pharmacoeconomic analyses support the current clinical guideline recommendations for asthma therapy.[2,17]

KEY POINTS

Asthma is now recognized as constituting much more than bronchoconstriction, and it may well represent a number of defects with similar clinical presentations. Therapy must target not only the symptoms that result from bronchospasm, but also the underlying inflammation and characteristic bronchial hyperresponsiveness. As new therapies and delivery systems are developed, choices between potentially equally efficacious regimens will become more complex. It is extremely important that treatment goals be developed in a collaborative effort between health care providers and patients. To reiterate, the NAEPP goals of asthma management include the following[1]:

■ Prevent chronic and troublesome symptoms (e.g., coughing or breathlessness in the night, in the early morning, or after exertion)
■ Maintain (near) ''normal'' pulmonary function
■ Maintain normal activity levels (including exercise and other physical activity)
■ Prevent recurrent exacerbations of asthma and minimize the need for emergency department visits or hospitalizations

■ Provide optimal pharmacotherapy with the lowest number of adverse effects
■ Meet patients' and families' expectations of and satisfaction with asthma care

With implementation of an individualized asthma management plan that includes appropriate medications and informative asthma education, both of which can be provided by pharmacists, patients with asthma should have a realistic probability of reaching these goals.

SUGGESTED READINGS

National Asthma Education and Prevention Program. Expert panel report: guidelines for the diagnosis and management of asthma update on selected topics—2002. J Allergy Clin Immunol 110 (5 Suppl): S141–S219, 2002.
National Asthma Education and Prevention Program. Expert panel report 2: guidelines for the diagnosis and management of asthma. Bethesda, MD: US Department of Health and Human Services, Public Health Service, National Institutes of Health, National Heart, Lung, and Blood Institute, April 1997; Publication no 97-4051.
National Asthma Education and Prevention Program. Practical guide for the diagnosis and management of asthma. Based on the expert panel report 2: guidelines for the diagnosis and management of asthma. Bethesda, Md: US Department of Health and Human Services, Public Health Service, National Institutes of Health, National Heart, Lung, and Blood Institute, October 1997; Publication no 97-4053.

REFERENCES

1. National Asthma Education and Prevention Program. Expert panel report 2: guidelines for the diagnosis and management of asthma. Bethesda, Md: US Department of Health and Human Services, Public Health Service, National Institutes of Health, National Heart, Lung, and Blood Institute, April 1997; Publication no 97-4051.
2. Global Initiative for Asthma (GINA). Global strategy for asthma management and prevention. NHLBI/WHO workshop report. Bethesda, Md: National Institutes of Health, 2002; NIH Publication no 02-3659.
3. Wills-Karp M, Ewart SL. Time to draw breath: asthma-susceptibility genes are identified. Nat Rev Genet 5:376–387, 2004.
4. American Lung Association Epidemiology and Statistics Unit Research and Scientific Affairs. Trends in asthma morbidity and mortality. Available at: www.lungusa.org/data. Accessed March 12, 2004.
5. Bousquet J, Jeffery PK, Busse WW, et al. Asthma. From bronchoconstriction to airways inflammation and remodeling. Am J Respir Crit Care Med 161:1720–1745, 2000.
6. Busse WW, Lemanske RF Jr. Asthma. N Engl J Med 344:350–362, 2001.
7. Larche M, Robinson DS, Kay AB. The role of T lymphocytes in the pathogenesis of asthma. J Allergy Clin Immunol 111:450–463, 2003.
8. Rowe BH, Edmonds ML, Spooner CH, et al. Corticosteroid therapy for acute asthma. Respir Med 98:275–284, 2004.
9. Camargo CA Jr, Spooner CH, Rowe BH. Continuous versus intermittent beta-agonists in the treatment of acute asthma (Cochrane Review). Cochrane Review 4, 2003.
10. Plotnick LH, Ducharme FM. Should inhaled anticholinergics be added to beta2 agonists for treating acute childhood and adolescent asthma? A systematic review. BMJ 317:971–977, 1998.
11. Boudreaux ED, Emond SD, Clark S, et al. Race/ethnicity and asthma among children presenting to the emergency department: differences in disease severity and management. Pediatrics 111: e615–e621, 2003.
12. Kharitonov SA, Barnes PJ. Exhaled markers of pulmonary disease. Am J Respir Crit Care Med 163:1693–1722, 2001.

13. Rodrigo GJ, Rodrigo C, Hall JB. Acute asthma in adults: a review. Chest 125:1081–1102, 2004.
14. Anderson SD, Daviskas E. The mechanism of exercise-induced asthma is. . . . J Allergy Clin Immunol 106:453–459, 2000.
15. Hendeles L, Asmus MJ, Chesrown S. Management of exercise-induced bronchospasm in children. J Pediatr Pharmacol Ther 8:13–21. 2003.
16. Calhoun WJ. Nocturnal asthma. Chest 123 (3 Suppl):399S–405S, 2003.
17. National Asthma Education and Prevention Program. Expert panel report: guidelines for the diagnosis and management of asthma update on selected topics—2002. J Allergy Clin Immunol 110 (5 Suppl):S141–S219, 2002.
18. Redmond AM, James AW, Nolan SH, et al. Premenstrual asthma: emphasis on drug therapy options. J Asthma 41:687–693, 2004.
19. Tan KS. Premenstrual asthma: epidemiology, pathogenesis and treatment. Drugs 61:2079–2086, 2001.
20. Fabbri LM, Caramori G, Maestrelli P. Definition, clinical features, investigations and differential diagnosis of asthma. In: Kay AB, ed. Allergy and allergic diseases. Oxford: Blackwell Science Ltd, 1997:1347–1359.
21. Nayak AS. The asthma and allergic rhinitis link. Allergy Asthma Proc 24:395–402, 2003.
22. Corren J. The association between allergic rhinitis and asthma in children and adolescents: epidemiologic considerations. Pediatr Ann 29:400–402, 2000.
23. Gentile NT, Ufberg J, Barnum M, et al. Guidelines reduce x-ray and blood gas utilization in acute asthma. Am J Emerg Med 21:451–453, 2003.
24. Lehrer P, Feldman J, Giardino N, et al. Psychological aspects of asthma. J Consult Clin Psychol 70:691–711, 2002.
25. Rietveld S, Creer TL. Psychiatric factors in asthma: implications for diagnosis and therapy. Am J Respir Med 2:1–10, 2003.
26. Harvmedlet. Panic disorder. Cambridge, Mass: Harvard Health Publications, 2001:1–5.
27. Harrison BD. Psychosocial aspects of asthma in adults. Thorax 53:519–525, 1998.
28. Randolph C, Fraser B. Stressors and concerns in teen asthma. Curr Probl Pediatr 29:82–93, 1999.
29. Suissa S, Ernst P, Benayoun S, et al. Low-dose inhaled corticosteroids and the prevention of death from asthma. N Engl J Med 343:332–336, 2000.
30. O'Byrne PM, Barnes PJ, Rodriguez-Roisin R, et al. Low dose inhaled budesonide and formoterol in mild persistent asthma: the OPTIMA randomized trial. Am J Respir Crit Care Med 164:1392–1397, 2001.
31. Sont JK, Willems LN, Bel EH, et al. Clinical control and histopathologic outcome of asthma when using airway hyperresponsiveness as an additional guide to long-term treatment. The AMPUL Study Group. Am J Respir Crit Care Med 159:1043–1051, 1999.
32. Pauwels RA, Lofdahl CG, Postma DS, et al. Effect of inhaled formoterol and budesonide on exacerbations of asthma. Formoterol and Corticosteroids Establishing Therapy (FACET) International Study Group. N Engl J Med 337:1405–1411, 1997.
33. McFadden ER Jr. Acute severe asthma. Am J Respir Crit Care Med 168:740–759, 2003.
34. Cates C, Rowe BH, Bara A. Holding chambers versus nebulisers for beta-agonist treatment of acute asthma (Cochrane Review). Cochrane Review 2, 2002.
35. Dolovich MA, MacIntyre NR, Anderson PJ, et al. Consensus statement: aerosols and delivery devices. American Association for Respiratory Care. Respir Care 45:589–596, 2000.
36. Rodrigo GJ, Rodrigo C. The role of anticholinergics in acute asthma treatment: an evidence-based evaluation. Chest 121:1977–1987, 2002.
37. Strauss L, Hejal R, Galan G, et al. Observations on the effects of aerosolized albuterol in acute asthma. Am J Respir Crit Care Med 155:454–458, 1997.
38. Kelly HW, Murphy SJ. The management of acute severe asthma in children. Asthma and rhinitis. Boston, Mass: Blackwell Science, 2001:1944–1960.
39. Travers A, Jones AP, Kelly K, et al. Intravenous beta2-agonists for acute asthma in the emergency department. Cochrane Database Syst Rev 2:CD002988, 2001.
40. Goodman DC, Littenberg B, O'Connor GT, et al. Theophylline in acute childhood asthma: a meta-analysis of its efficacy. Pediatr Pulmonol 21:211–218, 1996.
41. Rodrigo C, Rodrigo G. Treatment of acute asthma. Lack of therapeutic benefit and increase of the toxicity from aminophylline given in addition to high doses of salbutamol delivered by metered-dose inhaler with a spacer. Chest 106:1071–1076, 1994.
42. Rowe BH, Bota GW, Fabris L, et al. Inhaled budesonide in addition to oral corticosteroids to prevent asthma relapse following discharge from the emergency department: a randomized controlled trial. JAMA 281:2119–2126, 1999.
43. Rowe BH, Bretzlaff JA, Bourdon C, et al. Intravenous magnesium sulfate treatment for acute asthma in the emergency department: a systematic review of the literature. Ann Emerg Med 36:181–190, 2000.
44. Rodrigo G, Rodrigo C, Pollack C, et al. Helium-oxygen mixture for nonintubated acute asthma patients. Cochrane Database Syst Rev 1:CD002884, 2001.
45. Kress JP, Noth I, Gehlbach BK, et al. The utility of albuterol nebulized with heliox during acute asthma exacerbations. Am J Respir Crit Care Med 165:1317–1321, 2002.
46. Rose JS, Panacek EA, Miller P. Prospective randomized trial of heliox-driven continuous nebulizers in the treatment of asthma in the emergency department. J Emerg Med 22:133–137, 2002.
47. US Food and Drug Administration (FDA). Guidance for industry: E11 clinical investigation of medicinal products in the pediatric population. Washington, DC: US Food and Drug Administration, 2004.
48. Bisgaard H, Gillies J, Groenewald M, et al. The effect of inhaled fluticasone propionate in the treatment of young asthmatic children: a dose comparison study. Am J Respir Crit Care Med 160:126–131, 1999.
49. Bisgaard H, Munck SL, Nielsen JP, et al. Inhaled budesonide for treatment of recurrent wheezing in early childhood. Lancet 336:649–651, 1990.
50. Castro-Rodriguez JA, Rodrigo GJ. Beta-agonists through metered-dose inhaler with valved holding chamber versus nebulizer for acute exacerbation of wheezing or asthma in children under 5 years of age: a systematic review with meta-analysis. J Pediatr 145:172–177, 2004.
51. Kelly HW. Aerosol delivery. New York: Marcel Dekker, 1999:463–487.
52. Johnson JA, Lima JJ. Drug receptor/effector polymorphisms and pharmacogenetics: current status and challenges. Pharmacogenetics 13:525–534, 2003.
53. Bai TR. Adrenergic agonists and antagonists. In: Kay AB, ed. Allergy and allergic diseases. Oxford: Blackwell Science Ltd, 1997:568–583.
54. Hakonarson H, Grunstein MM. Regulation of second messengers associated with airway smooth muscle contraction and relaxation. Am J Respir Crit Care Med 158:S115–S122, 1998.
55. Anderson GP. Formoterol: pharmacology, molecular basis of agonism, and mechanism of long duration of a highly potent and selective beta 2-adrenoceptor agonist bronchodilator. Life Sci 52:2145–2160, 1993.
56. Rong Y, Arbabian M, Thiriot DS, et al. Probing the salmeterol binding site on the beta 2-adrenergic receptor using a novel photoaffinity ligand, ((125)I)iodoazidosalmeterol. Biochemistry 38:11278–11286, 1999.
57. Nelson HS. Beta-adrenergic bronchodilators. N Engl J Med 333:499–506, 1995.
58. Laitinen LA, Laitinen A, Haahtela T. A comparative study of the effects of an inhaled corticosteroid, budesonide, and of a β_2-agonist, terbutaline, on airway inflammation in newly diagnosed asthma. J Allergy Clin Immunol 90:32–42, 1992.
59. Roberts JA, Bradding P, Britten KM, et al. The long-acting beta2-agonist salmeterol xinafoate: effects on airway inflammation in asthma. Eur Respir J 14:275–282, 1999.
60. Condemi JJ, Goldstein S, Kalberg C, et al. The addition of salmeterol to fluticasone propionate versus increasing the dose of fluticasone propionate in patients with persistent asthma. Salmeterol Study Group. Ann Allergy Asthma Immunol 82:383–389, 1999.
61. Faurschou P, Steffensen I, Jacques L. Effect of addition of inhaled salmeterol to the treatment of moderate-to-severe asthmatics uncon-

trolled on high-dose inhaled steroids. European Respiratory Study Group. Eur Respir J 9:1885–1890, 1996.

62. Greening AP, Ind PW, Northfield M, et al. Added salmeterol versus higher-dose corticosteroid in asthma patients with symptoms on existing inhaled corticosteroid. Lancet 344:219–224, 1994.

63. Pauwels R. Physiological aspects of airway, pulmonary and respiratory muscle function in asthma. In: Kay AB, ed. Allergy and allergic diseases. Oxford: Blackwell Science Ltd, 1997:682–691.

64. van Noord JA, Schreurs AJ, Mol SJ, et al. Addition of salmeterol versus doubling the dose of fluticasone propionate in patients with mild to moderate asthma. Thorax 54:207–212, 1999.

65. Woolcock A, Lundback B, Ringdal N, et al. Comparison of addition of salmeterol to inhaled steroids with doubling of the dose of inhaled steroids. Am J Respir Crit Care Med 153:1481–1488, 1996.

66. Verberne AA, Frost C, Duiverman EJ, et al. Addition of salmeterol versus doubling the dose of beclomethasone in children with asthma. The Dutch Asthma Study Group. Am J Respir Crit Care Med 158:213–219, 1998.

67. Barnes PJ. Scientific rationale for inhaled combination therapy with long-acting beta2-agonists and corticosteroids. Eur Respir J 19:182–191, 2002.

68. Sears MR. Adverse effects of beta-agonists. J Allergy Clin Immunol 110 (6 Suppl):S322–S328, 2002.

69. Suissa S, Ernst P, Boivin JF, et al. A cohort analysis of excess mortality in asthma and the use of inhaled beta-agonists. Am J Respir Crit Care Med 149:604–610, 1994.

70. Spitzer WO, Suissa S, Ernst P, et al. The use of beta-agonists and the risk of death and near death from asthma. N Engl J Med 326:501–506, 1992.

71. Drazen JM, Israel E, Boushey HA, et al. Comparison of regularly scheduled with as-needed use of albuterol in mild asthma. Asthma Clinical Research Network. N Engl J Med 335:841–847, 1996.

72. Dennis SM, Sharp SJ, Vickers MR, et al. Regular inhaled salbutamol and asthma control: the TRUST randomised trial. Therapy Working Group of the National Asthma Task Force and the MRC General Practice Research Framework. Lancet 355:1675–1679, 2000.

73. Israel E, Chinchilli VM, Ford JG, et al. Use of regularly scheduled albuterol treatment in asthma: genotype-stratified, randomised, placebo-controlled cross-over trial. Lancet 364:1505–1512, 2004.

74. Knobil K, Yancey S, Kral K, et al. Salmeterol multi-center asthma research trial (SMART): results from an interim analysis. Chest 124 (4 Suppl):335S, 2003.

75. Waldeck B. Beta-adrenoceptor agonists and asthma—100 years of development. Eur J Pharmacol 445:1–12, 2002.

76. Lotvall J, Palmqvist M, Arvidsson P, et al. The therapeutic ratio of R-albuterol is comparable with that of RS-albuterol in asthmatic patients. J Allergy Clin Immunol 108:726–731, 2001.

77. Waldeck B. Enantiomers of bronchodilating beta2-adrenoceptor agonists: is there a cause for concern? J Allergy Clin Immunol 103:742–748, 1999.

78. Nelson JA, Strauss L, Skowronski M, et al. Effect of long-term salmeterol treatment on exercise-induced asthma (see comments). N Engl J Med 339:141–146, 1998.

79. Gawchik SM, Saccar CL, Noonan M, et al. The safety and efficacy of nebulized levalbuterol compared with racemic albuterol and placebo in the treatment of asthma in pediatric patients. J Allergy Clin Immunol 103:615–621, 1999.

80. Milgrom H, Berger W, Nayak A, et al. Treatment of childhood asthma with anti-immunoglobulin e antibody (omalizumab). Pediatrics 108:E36, 2001.

81. Nowak RM, Emerman CL, Schaefer K, et al. Levalbuterol compared with racemic albuterol in the treatment of acute asthma: results of a pilot study. Am J Emerg Med 22:29–36, 2004.

82. Asmus MJ, Hendeles L, Weinberger M, et al. Levalbuterol has not been established to have therapeutic advantage over racemic albuterol. J Allergy Clin Immunol 110:325–328, 2002.

83. Carl JC, Myers TR, Kirchner HL, et al. Comparison of racemic albuterol and levalbuterol for treatment of acute asthma. J Pediatr 143:731–736, 2003.

84. Drysdale CM, McGraw DW, Stack CB, et al. Complex promoter and coding region beta 2-adrenergic receptor haplotypes alter receptor expression and predict in vivo responsiveness. Proc Natl Acad Sci U S A 97:10483–10488, 2000.

85. Palmer LJ, Silverman ES, Weiss ST, et al. Pharmacogenetics of asthma. Am J Respir Crit Care Med 165:861–866, 2002.

86. Israel E, Drazen JM, Liggett SB, et al. The effect of polymorphisms of the beta(2)-adrenergic receptor on the response to regular use of albuterol in asthma. Am J Respir Crit Care Med 162:75–80, 2000.

87. Papo MC, Frank J, Thompson AE. A prospective, randomized study of continuous versus intermittent nebulized albuterol for severe status asthmaticus in children. Crit Care Med 21:1479–1486, 1993.

88. Shapiro GS, Yegen U, Xiang J, et al. A randomized, double-blind, single-dose, crossover clinical trial of the onset and duration of protection from exercise-induced bronchoconstriction by formoterol and albuterol. Clin Ther 24:2077–2087, 2002.

89. van Noord JA, Smeets JJ, Raaijmakers JA, et al. Salmeterol versus formoterol in patients with moderately severe asthma: onset and duration of action. Eur Respir J 9:1684–1688, 1996.

90. Palmqvist M, Persson G, Lazer L, et al. Inhaled dry-powder formoterol and salmeterol in asthmatic patients: onset of action, duration of effect and potency. Eur Respir J 10:2484–2489, 1997.

91. Jackson CM, Lipworth B. Benefit-risk assessment of long-acting beta2-agonists in asthma. Drug Saf 27:243–270, 2004.

92. Blake K. Theophylline. In: Murphy S, Kelly HW, eds. Pediatric asthma. New York: Marcel Dekker, 1999:363–431.

93. Barnes PJ. Theophylline: new perspectives for an old drug. Am J Respir Crit Care Med 167:813–818, 2003.

94. Evans DJ, Taylor DA, Zetterstrom O, et al. A comparison of low-dose inhaled budesonide plus theophylline and high-dose inhaled budesonide for moderate asthma. N Engl J Med 337:1412–1418, 1997.

95. Ukena D, Harnest U, Sakalauskas R, et al. Comparison of addition of theophylline to inhaled steroid with doubling of the dose of inhaled steroid in asthma. Eur Respir J 10:2754–2760, 1997.

96. Youngchaiyud P, Permpikul C, Suthamsmai T, et al. A double-blind comparison of inhaled budesonide, long-acting theophylline, and their combination in treatment of nocturnal asthma. Allergy 50:28–33, 1995.

97. Barnes PJ, Pauwels RA. Theophylline in the management of asthma: time for reappraisal? Eur Resp J 7:579–591, 1994.

98. Hendeles L, Harman E, Huang D, et al. Theophylline attenuation of airway responses to allergen: comparison with cromolyn metered-dose inhaler. J Allergy Clin Immunol 95:505–514, 1995.

99. Hendeles L, Jenkins J, Temple R. Revised FDA labeling guideline for theophylline oral dosage forms (see comments). Pharmacotherapy 15:409–427, 1995.

100. Weinberger M, Hendeles L. Theophylline in asthma. N Engl J Med 334:1380–1388, 1996.

101. Hendeles L, Bighley L, Richardson RH, et al. Frequent toxicity from IV aminophylline infusions in critically ill patients. Drug Intell Clin Pharm 11:12–17, 1977.

102. Self TH, Redmond AM, Nguyen WT. Reassessment of theophylline use for severe asthma exacerbation: is it justified in critically ill hospitalized patients? J Asthma 39:677–686, 2002.

103. Barnes PJ. New drugs for asthma. Eur Respir J 5:1126–1136, 1992.

104. Fryer AD, Jacoby DB. Muscarinic receptors and control of airway smooth muscle. Am J Respir Crit Care Med 158:S154–S160, 1998.

105. Pakes GE, Brogden RN, Heel RC, et al. Ipratropium bromide: a review of its pharmacological properties and therapeutic efficacy in asthma and chronic bronchitis. Drugs 20:237–266, 1980.

106. Brophy C, Ahmed B, Bayston S, et al. How long should Atrovent be given in acute asthma? Thorax 53:363–367, 1998.

107. McDonald NJ, Bara AI. Anticholinergic therapy for chronic asthma in children over two years of age. Cochrane Database Syst Rev 3: CD003535, 2003.

108. Brogden RN, Sorkin EM. Nedocromil sodium: an updated review of its pharmacological properties and therapeutic efficacy in asthma. Drugs 45:693–715, 1993.

109. Sorkness CA. Cromolyn, nedocromil, leukotriene modifiers, and alternative anti-inflammatory agents in the treatment of pediatric asthma. In: Murphy S, Kelly HW, eds. Pediatric asthma. New York: Marcel Dekker, 1999:433–462.

110. Cockcroft DW, Murdock KY. Comparative effects of inhaled salbutamol, sodium cromoglycate, and beclomethasone dipropionate on allergen-induced early asthmatic responses, late asthmatic responses, and increased bronchial responsiveness to histamine. J Allergy Clin Immunol 79:734–740, 1987.

111. AAAAI. Pediatric asthma: promoting best practice. guide for managing asthma in children. Milwaukee, Wis: American Academy of Allergy, Asthma and Immunology, Inc, 1999.

112. van der Wouden JC, Tasche MJ, Bernsen RM, et al. Inhaled sodium cromoglycate for asthma in children. Cochrane Database Syst Rev 3:CD002173, 2003.

113. Drazen JM, Israel E, O'Byrne PM. Treatment of asthma with drugs modifying the leukotriene pathway. N Engl J Med 340:197–206, 1999.

114. Dahlen SE, Kumlin M, Bjorck T, et al. Airway smooth muscle and disease workshop: leukotrienes and related eicosanoids. Am Rev Respir Dis 136:S24–S28, 1987.

115. Wechsler ME, Israel E. Pharmacogenetics of treatment with leukotriene modifiers. Curr Opin Allergy Clin Immunol 2:395–401, 2002.

116. Pillai SG, Cousens DJ, Barnes AA, et al. A coding polymorphism in the CYSLT2 receptor with reduced affinity to LTD4 is associated with asthma. Pharmacogenetics 4:627–633, 2004.

117. Deykin A, Israel E. Newer therapeutic agents for asthma. Dis Mon 45:117–144, 1999.

118. Pauls JD, Simon RA, Daffern PJ, et al. Lack of effect of the 5-lipoxygenase inhibitor zileuton in blocking oral aspirin challenges in aspirin-sensitive asthmatics. Ann Allergy Asthma Immunol 85:40–45, 2000.

119. Szczeklik A, Stevenson DD. Aspirin-induced asthma: advances in pathogenesis, diagnosis, and management. J Allergy Clin Immunol 111:913–921, 2003.

120. Meltzer EO, Lockey RF, Friedman BF, et al. Efficacy and safety of low-dose fluticasone propionate compared with montelukast for maintenance treatment of persistent asthma. Mayo Clin Proc 77:437–445, 2002.

121. Maspero JF, Duenas-Meza E, Volovitz B, et al. Oral montelukast versus inhaled beclomethasone in 6- to 11-year-old children with asthma: results of an open-label extension study evaluating long-term safety, satisfaction, and adherence with therapy. Curr Med Res Opin 17:96–104, 2001.

122. Williams B, Noonan G, Reiss TF, et al. Long-term asthma control with oral montelukast and inhaled beclomethasone for adults and children 6 years and older. Clin Exp Allergy 31:845–854, 2001.

123. Malmstrom K, Rodriguez-Gomez G, Guerra J, et al. Oral montelukast, inhaled beclomethasone, and placebo for chronic asthma. A randomized, controlled trial. Montelukast/Beclomethasone Study Group (see comments). Ann Intern Med 130:487–495, 1999.

124. Bjermer L, Bisgaard H, Bousquet J, et al. Montelukast and fluticasone compared with salmeterol and fluticasone in protecting against asthma exacerbation in adults: one year, double blind, randomised, comparative trial. Br Med J 327:891, 2003.

125. Ilowite J, Webb R, Friedman B, et al. Addition of montelukast or salmeterol to fluticasone for protection against asthma attacks: a randomized, double-blind, multicenter study. Ann Allergy Asthma Immunol 92:641–648, 2004.

126. Nelson HS, Busse WW, Kerwin E, et al. Fluticasone propionate/salmeterol combination provides more effective asthma control than low-dose inhaled corticosteroid plus montelukast. J Allergy Clin Immunol 106:1088–1095, 2000.

127. Ringdal N, Eliraz A, Pruzinec R, et al. The salmeterol/fluticasone combination is more effective than fluticasone plus oral montelukast in asthma. Respir Med 97:234–241, 2003.

128. Price DB, Hernandez D, Magyar P, et al. Randomised controlled trial of montelukast plus inhaled budesonide versus double dose inhaled budesonide in adult patients with asthma. Thorax 58:211–216, 2003.

129. Dockhorn RJ, Baumgartner RA, Leff JA, et al. Comparison of the effects of intravenous and oral montelukast on airway function: a double blind, placebo controlled, three period, crossover study in asthmatic patients (see comments). Thorax 55:260–265, 2000.

130. Camargo CA Jr, Smithline HA, Malice MP, et al. A randomized controlled trial of intravenous montelukast in acute asthma. Am J Respir Crit Care Med 167:528–533, 2003.

131. Kelloway JS, Wyatt RA, Adlis SA. Comparison of patients' compliance with prescribed oral and inhaled asthma medications. Arch Intern Med 154:1349–1352, 1994.

132. Ringdal N, Whitney JG, Summerton L. Problems with inhaler technique and patient preference for oral therapy—tablet zafirlukast vs inhaled beclomethasone. Am J Respir Crit Care Med 157:A416, 1998.

133. Sherman J, Patel P, Hutson A, et al. Adherence to oral montelukast and inhaled fluticasone in children with persistent asthma. Pharmacotherapy 21:1464–1467, 2001.

134. Suissa S, Ernst P. Inhaled corticosteroids: impact on asthma morbidity and mortality. J Allergy Clin Immunol 107:937–944, 2001.

135. Halterman JS, Aligne CA, Auinger P, et al. Inadequate therapy for asthma among children in the United States. Pediatrics 105:272–276, 2000.

136. Finkelstein JA, Lozano P, Farber HJ, et al. Underuse of controller medications among Medicaid-insured children with asthma. Arch Pediatr Adolesc Med 156:562–567, 2002.

137. Barnes PJ. Efficacy of inhaled corticosteroids in asthma. J Allergy Clin Immunol 102:531–538, 1998.

138. Covar RA, Szefler SJ, Martin RJ, et al. Relations between exhaled nitric oxide and measures of disease activity among children with mild-to-moderate asthma. J Pediatr 142:469–475, 2003.

139. Kelly HW, Nelson HS. Potential adverse effects of the inhaled corticosteroids. J Allergy Clin Immunol 112:469–478, 2003.

140. Kelly HW. Pharmacology of inhaled glucocorticoids: comparative properties. Immunol Allergy Clin North Am 19:725–738, 1999.

141. Kelly HW. Pharmaceutical characteristics that influence the clinical efficacy of inhaled corticosteroids. Ann Allergy Asthma Immunol 91:326–334, 2003.

142. Martin RJ, Szefler SJ, Chinchilli VM, et al. Systemic effect comparisons of six inhaled corticosteroid preparations. Am J Respir Crit Care Med 165:1377–1383, 2002.

143. Pauwels RA, Pedersen S, Busse WW, et al. Early intervention with budesonide in mild persistent asthma: a randomised, double-blind trial. Lancet 361:1071–1076, 2003.

144. Rachelefsky G. Treating exacerbations of asthma in children: the role of systemic corticosteroids. Pediatrics 112:382–397, 2003.

145. Milgrom H, Fick RB Jr, Su JQ, et al. Treatment of allergic asthma with monoclonal anti-IgE antibody. rhuMAb-E25 Study Group (see comments). N Engl J Med 341:1966–1973, 1999.

146. Ruffin CG, Busch BE. Omalizumab: a recombinant humanized anti-IgE antibody for allergic asthma. Am J Health-Syst Pharm 61:1449–1459, 2004.

147. Walker S, Monteil M, Phelan K, et al. Anti-IgE for chronic asthma in adults and children. Cochrane Database Syst Rev 3:CD003559, 2004.

148. De Benedictis FM, Selvaggio D. Use of inhaler devices in pediatric asthma. Paediatr Drugs 5:629–638, 2003.

149. Everard ML, Clark AR, Milner AD. Drug delivery from jet nebulisers. Arch Dis Child 67:586–591, 1992.

150. De Blaquiere P, Christensen DB, Carter WB, et al. Use and misuse of metered-dose inhalers by patients with chronic lung disease. A controlled, randomized trial of two instruction methods (see comments). Am Rev Respir Dis 140:910–916, 1989.

151. National Asthma Education and Prevention Program. Practical guide for the diagnosis and management of asthma. Based on the expert panel report 2: guidelines for the diagnosis and management of asthma. Bethesda, Md: US Department of Health and Human Services, Public Health Service, National Institutes of Health, National Heart, Lung, and Blood Institute, October 1997; Publication no 97-4053.

152. Gotzsche P, Johansen H, Schmidt L, et al. House dust mite control measures for asthma. Cochrane Database Syst Rev 4:CD001187, 2004.

153. Sade K, Berkun Y, Dolev Z, et al. Knowledge and expectations of patients receiving aeroallergen immunotherapy. Ann Allergy Asthma Immunol 91:444–448, 2003.

154. Druce HM. Allergic and nonallergic rhinitis. In: Middleton E Jr, Reed CE, Ellis EF, et al, eds. Allergy principles and practice. St. Louis: Mosby-Year Book, 1993:1433–1453.

155. Szefler SJ. Alternative therapy in severe asthma: rationale and guidelines for applications. In: Middleton E Jr, Reed CE, Ellis EF, et al, eds. Principles and practice. St. Louis: Mosby, 1991:1–14.

156. Bielory L, Lupoli K. Herbal interventions in asthma and allergy. J Asthma 36:1–65, 1999.

157. Ernst E. Complementary therapies for asthma: what patients use. J Asthma 35:667–671, 1998.

158. Kemper KJ, Lester MR. Alternative asthma therapies: an evidence-based review. Contemp Pediatr 16:162–195, 1999.

159. Gyorik SA, Brutsche MH. Complementary and alternative medicine for bronchial asthma: is there new evidence? Curr Opin Pulm Med 10:37–43, 2004.

160. Barnes PJ. New drugs for asthma. Nat Rev Drug Discov 3: 831–844, 2004.

161. Bender B. A simple scoring system predicted clinical progression in HIV patients receiving highly active antiretroviral therapy. ACP J Club 137:37, 2002.

162. Bender B, Milgrom H, Rand C. Nonadherence in asthmatic patients: is there a solution to the problem? Ann Allergy Asthma Immunol 79:177–185, 1997.

163. van Es SM, le Coq EM, Brouwer AI, et al. Adherence-related behavior in adolescents with asthma: results from focus group interviews. J Asthma 35:637–646, 1998.

164. National Asthma Education and Prevention Program. Expert panel report: guidelines for the diagnosis and management of asthma. Bethesda, Md: US Department of Health and Human Services, Public Health Service, National Institutes of Health, National Heart, Lung, and Blood Institute, August 1991; Publication no 91-3042.

165. Wilson SR, Scamagas P, Grado J, et al. The Fresno Asthma Project: a model intervention to control asthma in multiethnic, low-income, inner-city communities. Health Educ Behav 25:79–98, 1998.

166. Greineder DK, Loane KC, Parks P. A randomized controlled trial of a pediatric asthma outreach program. J Allergy Clin Immunol 103:436–440, 1999.

167. Weiss KB, Sullivan SD. The health economics of asthma and rhinitis. I. Assessing the economic impact. J Allergy Clin Immunol 107: 3–8, 2001.

168. Lara M, Rosenbaum S, Rachelefsky G, et al. Improving childhood asthma outcomes in the United States: a blueprint for policy action. Pediatrics 109:919–930, 2002.

169. Schermer TR, Thoonen BP, van den BG, et al. Randomized controlled economic evaluation of asthma self-management in primary health care. Am J Respir Crit Care Med 166:1062–1072, 2002.

170. Sullivan SD, Weiss KB, Lynn H, et al. The cost-effectiveness of an inner-city asthma intervention for children. J Allergy Clin Immunol 110:576–581, 2002.

171. Castro M, Zimmermann NA, Crocker S, et al. Asthma intervention program prevents readmissions in high healthcare users. Am J Respir Crit Care Med 168:1095–1099, 2003.

172. Kauppinen R, Vilkka V, Sintonen H, et al. Long-term economic evaluation of intensive patient education during the first treatment year in newly diagnosed adult asthma. Respir Med 95:56–63, 2001.

173. Paltiel AD, Fuhlbrigge AL, Kitch BT, et al. Cost-effectiveness of inhaled corticosteroids in adults with mild-to-moderate asthma: results from the asthma policy model. J Allergy Clin Immunol 108: 39–46, 2001.

174. Bisgaard H, Price MJ, Maden C, et al. Cost-effectiveness of fluticasone propionate administered via metered-dose inhaler plus babyhaler spacer in the treatment of asthma in preschool-aged children. Chest 120:1835–1842, 2001.

175. Sullivan SD, Buxton M, Andersson LF, et al. Cost-effectiveness analysis of early intervention with budesonide in mild persistent asthma. J Allergy Clin Immunol 112:1229–1236, 2003.

176. Stempel DA, Meyer JW, Stanford RH, et al. One-year claims analysis comparing inhaled fluticasone propionate with zafirlukast for the treatment of asthma. J Allergy Clin Immunol 107:94–98, 2001.

177. Orsini L, Limpa-Amara S, Crown WH, et al. Asthma hospitalization risk and costs for patients treated with fluticasone propionate vs montelukast. Ann Allergy Asthma Immunol 92:523–529, 2004.

178. Andersson F, Stahl E, Barnes PJ, et al. Adding formoterol to budesonide in moderate asthma—health economic results from the FACET study. Respir Med 95:505–512, 2001.

179. Stempel DA, O'Donnell JC, Meyer JW. Inhaled corticosteroids plus salmeterol or montelukast: effects on resource utilization and costs. J Allergy Clin Immunol 109:433–439, 2002.

180. O'Connor RD, O'Donnell JC, Pinto LA, et al. Two-year retrospective economic evaluation of three dual-controller therapies used in the treatment of asthma. Chest 121:1028–1035, 2002.

181. Oba Y, Salzman GA. Cost-effectiveness analysis of omalizumab in adults and adolescents with moderate-to-severe allergic asthma. J Allergy Clin Immunol 114:265–269, 2004.

Chronic Obstructive Pulmonary Disease

35

Dennis M. Williams

TREATMENT GOALS

- To halt or slow the progression of pathologic changes
- To improve the patient's quality of life
- To prevent acute exacerbations of the disease

Chronic obstructive pulmonary disease (COPD) is characterized by chronic airflow obstruction and accelerated loss of lung function. The loss of lung function is progressive and the patient develops chronic symptoms and disabilities as the disease worsens. The primary goals of COPD treatment are described in Table 35.1.

DEFINITION

Chronic obstructive pulmonary disease (COPD) is a chronic condition of the airways characterized by airflow obstruction that is progressive and not fully reversible. The disease process is associated with an abnormal response to noxious chemicals or gases. Patients with COPD experience chronic symptoms such as productive cough and dyspnea. The most common risk factor for COPD is a history of cigarette smoking. COPD is both preventable and treatable.

Airflow obstruction in COPD does not change markedly over time. It is characterized as fixed or irreversible, although individual patients may demonstrate varying degrees of reversibility. During the past two decades, there has been a dearth of research and exploration concerning potential treatment strategies due to the chronic and progressive nature of the disease. More recently, two international guidelines[1,2] have focused on an evidence-based approach to management and have identified areas where further research is warranted. International guidelines are available from the American Thoracic Society (ATS) and European Respiratory Society as well as the National Heart Lung and Blood Institute and the World Health Organization. The latter document is referred to as the "Global Initiative for Chronic Obstructive Pulmonary Diseases" (GOLD) guidelines. In addition, the introduction of new therapies has sparked a renewed interest in this disease.

The major obstructive pulmonary diseases are asthma, chronic bronchitis, and emphysema. Obstruction to expiratory airflow is the common element in these conditions, in contrast to restrictive lung disease, in which the defect is reduced lung expansion capability due to fibrosis of the lung parenchyma. Asthma is characterized by narrowing of the airways as a result of bronchial hyperreactivity, excessive bronchial secretions, and airway inflammatory changes. Airflow obstruction in asthma is usually reversible.

TABLE 35.1	General Goals of Management for Chronic Obstructive Pulmonary Disease

- Prevent or slow disease progression
- Relieve symptoms
- Improve exercise tolerance
- Improve overall health status
- Prevent and treat complications
- Prevent and treat exacerbations
- Reduce mortality

TABLE 35.2	Asthma Versus Chronic Obstructive Pulmonary Disease	
Feature	Asthma	COPD
Past or current history of cigarette smoking	Maybe	Usually
Symptoms present before age 40 years	Common	Rare
Spirometry improvement after bronchodilator	≥12%	Minimal
Chronic productive cough present	Uncommon	Common
Breathlessness	Intermittent	Persistent
Night-time awakening with dyspnea/wheeze	Common	Uncommon
Significant intra- and inter-day variability in symptoms	Common	Uncommon

In contrast, COPD describes the presentation of chronic cough that is typically productive, varying degrees of exertional dyspnea, and a significant and progressive reduction in expiratory airflow.[1] COPD airflow obstruction is largely fixed or irreversible, but it is now apparent that there is variability in the degree of airflow reversibility among patients in response to treatment.

The two major forms of COPD are chronic bronchitis and emphysema. Chronic bronchitis is defined clinically as chronic excessive mucus secretion into the bronchial tree that occurs on most days during a period of at least 3 months of the year for at least 2 consecutive years. Emphysema is defined anatomically by abnormal permanent enlargement of the airspaces distal to the terminal bronchioles, accompanied by destruction of their walls, but without obvious fibrosis. Chronic bronchitis and emphysema are often indistinguishable on clinical examination, and many patients have components of both diseases. Chronic bronchitis and emphysema share similar risk factors and management strategies are also similar; therefore, the type of presentation is often not relevant.

Asthma is also a disease characterized by airflow obstruction, but the pathophysiologic features and response to treatment differ significantly from COPD, as described in Table 35.2. Therapeutic principles for asthma and COPD are quite different. However, some patients with asthma exhibit poorly reversible obstruction, and the relationship between longstanding asthma and COPD is not clear.

ETIOLOGY

The major risk factor for COPD development is a history of cigarette smoking. It is unique that a common chronic disease is attributed to a single risk factor. Nearly 80% to 90% of COPD patients have a current or past history of cigarette smoking, although only 15% to 20% of smokers go on to develop obstruction.[3] The latter fact suggests that other factors, including genetics, influence the subsequent development of the disease. Passive smoking has been identified as a possible factor in COPD development, and other environmental factors such as pollution and occupational

exposures and serious or recurrent pulmonary infections during childhood have also been implicated.

Like other chronic diseases, COPD develops as the result of the interaction between the host and environmental exposures. Host factors include a genetic basis, gender, and the presence of airway hyperresponsiveness, but the basis for these host risks is not clear. Beyond the purely inherited disorder of α_1-antitrypsin deficiency, which is rare, the genetic predisposition that results in COPD development is not known. Disease is more common in men than women, although the contribution of environmental exposures on these data is unclear, since men historically have a higher smoking prevalence. Recent evidence suggests that women may be more susceptible to developing smoking-related COPD; thus, the role of gender is less clear.[4] The presence of airway hyperresponsiveness appears to confer an increased risk for COPD, although the progression from asthma to COPD is not well defined.

The inherited deficiency of α_1-antitrypsin is a rare cause of emphysema (less than 1%), and these patients typically present with significant symptoms at an earlier age (in their 30s or 40s). A deficiency of α_1-antitrypsin (or α-proteinase inhibitor), an elastase inhibitor, is the genetic basis for alveolar wall destruction in the inherited form of emphysema. In this case, the lack of α_1-antitrypsin, an important inhibitor of serum proteases, allows the action of proteases (e.g., elastase, an enzyme that degrades elastin in the lung parenchyma) to go unchecked and results in alveolar destruction.

Environmental exposures other than cigarette smoking that play an important role in COPD development include occupational exposures, air pollution, serious respiratory disease during childhood, and recurrent bronchopulmonary infections. Occupational exposures include inhalation of dust from grains, coal, and other minerals, as well as fumes from adhesives and welding materials.[5]

EPIDEMIOLOGY

The reported physician-diagnosed COPD prevalence is approximately 10 million people in the United States,[6] but this figure may be low due to underreporting: in self-report surveys, nearly 24 million persons indicate that they have COPD. Some estimates suggest that less than 50% of patients with COPD may have a physician's diagnosis.[7] Among the 10 million people with a COPD diagnosis, most have features of chronic bronchitis. Compared to other common chronic diseases, the prevalence of COPD has steadily increased during the past 30 years.

Morbidity data include physician visits and visits to emergency departments or hospitalization. Morbidity is significant in COPD, increases with disease severity, and is higher in patients with lower socioeconomic status.[8] In 2000, COPD was the second leading cause of disability after heart disease.[6] This disease accounted for 8 million medical outpatient visits, 1.5 million visits to emergency departments, and over 700,000 hospitalizations in 2000.[9] Based on the advancing age of the U.S. population in general, the prevalence, severity, and morbidity of COPD will likely increase.[10]

COPD is the fourth leading cause of death in the United States, accounting for 120,816 deaths in 2002.[11] The mortality rate from COPD is increasing, particularly among older patients. This rising mortality rate occurs at a time when deaths from heart disease and strokes are decreasing. By 2020, it is anticipated that COPD will be the third leading cause of death for both men and women.[12] Mortality rates for women has doubled over the past two decades; however, it remains higher in whites than blacks and in men than women. This latter trend is changing, however, with predictions that within 10 to 20 years there will be an equal number of deaths between men and women related to cigarette consumption.

In 2004, the economic impact of COPD was estimated at $37.2 billion, including over $16 billion in indirect morbidity and mortality costs.[13] This is significantly higher than the cost of asthma, although a similar number of individuals are affected. Direct costs reflect diagnosis and care; indirect costs include the consequences of disability, reduced productivity in the workplace, and early mortality. Much of the direct cost is attributed to treatment of acute exacerbations either in ambulatory or hospitalized patients.

PHYSIOLOGY, PATHOLOGY, AND PATHOPHYSIOLOGY

NORMAL PHYSIOLOGIC FUNCTION

The respiratory apparatus refers to the lungs and surrounding tissues, muscles, and nervous system. The respiratory system is responsible for gas exchange and acid–base homeostasis, in addition to providing physical and immunologic protection against foreign material. The process of respiration is the exchange of oxygen (O_2) and carbon dioxide (CO_2) so that oxygen is delivered to and carbon dioxide is removed from the blood. Inhaled air moves through the upper airway (nose, pharynx, larynx, trachea, and bronchi) and the lower respiratory tract (bronchioles, alveolar ducts, alveolar sacs, and alveoli). Gas exchange occurs in the alveoli of the lung through a process of simple diffusion based on concentration gradients. Oxygen moves from the alveoli to the pulmonary capillaries, and carbon dioxide is removed from the vascular supply to the alveoli for subsequent exhalation. Normal airway integrity is maintained through the relationship of pressures in and around the airway and the elasticity of the airway.

The respiratory system plays a role in maintaining acid–base balance by retaining or excreting carbon dioxide through exhalation. The primary stimulus to breathe in humans is the carbon dioxide concentrations in the central nervous system. This occurs in the respiratory center in the medulla of the brain. When carbon dioxide concentrations are elevated, the rate and depth of ventilation is increased. Peripheral chemoreceptors that are sensitive to lower oxygen concentrations provide a secondary drive to ventilation.

The respiratory system also serves an important role in protecting the body from foreign bodies, including microorganisms. This defense is provided through physical and immunologic mechanisms. The upper and lower respiratory tract includes mucous glands and ciliated epithelial surfaces that trap inhaled particles and remove them from the respiratory tract. Immunologic activity is attributed to immunoglobulins, enzymes, and other mediators that destroy or inactivate inhaled foreign materials. A delicate balance exists between the aggressive and protective enzyme systems in the airways, and disruption of this balance is the basis for COPD development.

PATHOLOGIC FEATURES AND PATHOGENESIS

Our understanding of the disease process of COPD has improved significantly over the past decade. Four areas of the lung are affected: the central airways, peripheral airways, lung parenchyma, and pulmonary vasculature. Pathologic changes in these areas lead to the pathophysiologic characteristics of COPD.

Chemicals and gases from noxious exposures (e.g., tobacco smoke) cause increased bronchial reactivity and inflammation. In patients with COPD, inflammatory cells have been found throughout the airways, including the epithelium of the trachea, bronchi, and bronchioles. Macrophage function is also inhibited, and release of lysosomal enzymes destroys the connective tissue in the lung. Chronic inflammation leads to remodeling and narrowing of the airway lumen, resulting in fixed or irreversible airflow obstruction. Prominent cells participating in inflammation are $CD8^+$ lymphocytes, macrophages, and neutrophils. Inflammatory mediators involved in COPD include tumor necrosis factor α, interleukin-8, and leukotriene-B4. Inflammation results in chronic or recurrent excessive mucus secretion. Although inflammation is an important feature of COPD, the process is distinct from that seen in asthma, where eosinophils are prominent.

In the central airways, bronchial glands and mucus-producing cells are increased in size and number, resulting in increased mucus production. Airway cilia are destroyed and ciliary function is compromised, resulting in decreased clearance of mucus and particles. There is also evidence of smooth muscle proliferation and fibrosis.[14] In smaller peripheral airways, there is also evidence of inflammatory changes, proliferation of goblet cells, and fibrosis.

In the lung parenchyma of COPD patients, airspaces are enlarged and attachments are lost, leading to alveolar collapse. Inflammatory cells and mediators present in other areas of the lung are also active in the parenchyma. There are differences in parenchymal involvement depending on the risk factor. Tobacco-related COPD is described as centrolobular, with primary effects on respiratory bronchioles, and α_1-antitrypsin–associated disease affects the entire parenchyma, including the lower lung zones (panlobular).

Pathologic changes are also present in the pulmonary vasculature. Inflammatory cells, including lymphocytes and macrophages, are present, and there is thickening and fibrosis of vascular walls. These changes, as well as the loss of vasculature associated with destruction of alveoli, contribute to the later development of pulmonary hypertension and cor pulmonale.[15]

The presence of chronic inflammation leads to numerous changes associated with the development and progression of COPD. Current theories suggest that a combination of inflammation, imbalances between proteinases and antiproteases, and increased oxidative stress leads to lung damage.

Normally, there is a balance between protective and aggressive enzyme activity (antiproteases and proteases) in the lungs; this balance is perturbed in COPD. Aggressive factors (proteases) may be increased in number and have greater activity, triggered by components of cigarette smoke or other environmental exposures. Protective factors (antiproteases) may have reduced production and activity. The resultant imbalance contributes to injury and damage to normal lung tissue.[1,2]

Noxious chemicals and gases increase oxidative stress in the airways and stimulate inflammatory cells to release additional proteases. Various markers of oxidative stress have been found in the airways of COPD patients, including nitric oxide and hydrogen peroxide.[16] Oxidative stress also inhibits antioxidant activity.

PATHOPHYSIOLOGY

The pathologic changes in COPD are exhibited as airflow limitation; a reduced ratio of forced expiratory volume in 1 second (FEV_1) to forced vital capacity (FVC) is the hallmark of obstructive lung disease. Another spirometric change is an increased functional residual capacity (FRC) due to air trapping, especially during exercise, and thoracic hyperinflation. The changes contribute to airflow limitation in several ways. Airway integrity is compromised through smooth muscle contraction, inflammation, edema, and peribronchiolar fibrosis.

The various pathologic changes in the lungs of COPD patients are manifested as the pathophysiologic features of the disease. These include chronic mucus hypersecretion with impaired removal due to ciliary dysfunction, chronic airflow limitation, and thoracic hyperinflation, which disturbs normal ventilatory dynamics. Consequences of advanced disease include abnormalities of gas exchange, changes in pulmonary vasculature as a result of hypoxia, pulmonary hypertension, with elevated mean pulmonary artery pressures and pulmonary vascular resistance, hypertrophy of the right ventricle, and development of cor pulmonale.

Mucus hypersecretion and decreased ciliary function occur early in the course of COPD. The result is mucus plugging, primarily in the small peripheral airways. In the presence of increased mucus production and reduced clearance of airway secretions, airways that are typically sterile may become colonized with bacteria. This constant presence of bacteria contributes further to the chronic inflammation associated with COPD.

Numerous factors contribute to airflow obstruction, including increased mucus, airway wall fibrosis, and loss of alveolar support leading to collapse. Airflow limitation is also worsened by a loss of the normal elastic recoil of the lung during exhalation. As a result, the patient is required to use abdominal and chest wall muscles to force air out of the lung, resulting in further collapse of airways and air trapping, which leads to thoracic hyperinflation. Hyperinflation of the lungs due to excess air trapping inhibits normal diaphragm contraction and reduces the efficiency of this primary muscle of ventilation, especially during exercise.[17] As COPD advances, gas exchange worsens, resulting in significant hypoxemia, which may require chronic supplemental oxygen. Some patients with severe disease develop hypercapnia, which affects the primary drive to breathe. In these patients, respiratory drive becomes less responsive to changes in arterial pH and $Paco_2$ and hypoxic drive begins to play a larger role. Patients with chronic carbon dioxide retention tolerate the increased carbon dioxide concentrations and do not exhibit the signs of acute hypercapnia, including somnolence and altered mental status. Supplemental oxygen in these patients can result in an acute worsening of hypercapnia and acidosis, so it should be administered cautiously. However, concerns about oxygen supplementation causing narcosis should not prohibit its administration.[18]

In addition to the significant pathophysiologic effects of COPD in the lung, the disease also has consequences outside the lung. The cardiovascular consequences of advanced COPD have been discussed. Significant reductions in skeletal muscle mass can occur and can limit exercise capacity and worsen the overall prognosis.[19]

Pathophysiology of Exacerbations. COPD is characterized by periodic episodes of worsening lung function and symptoms called *exacerbations*. Exacerbations have a significant impact on the morbidity and mortality of COPD. The inflammatory mediators that contribute to COPD play a role in exacerbations, although it appears that eosinophils are more prominent during exacerbations.

Exacerbations of COPD typically have an infectious etiology, either viral or bacterial. Some estimates suggest that at least 50% of episodes are viral. Some patients' airways are chronically colonized with bacteria, which reduces the utility of sputum cultures in identifying a cause. *Haemophilus influenzae*, *Streptococcus pneumoniae*, and *Moraxella catarrhalis*, common colonizers of the upper airway, cause most of the bacterial respiratory infections.[20] Mucus hypersecretion predisposes patients to repeated infections. Decreased removal of bronchial secretions physically impairs the defenses of the lungs against infection, and the mucus provides a good growth medium for bacteria. The bacteria, together with the host's immune responses, contribute to further lung tissue damage.[20,21]

During an exacerbation, there are increased symptoms, increased mucus production, and worsening of gas exchange and airflow obstruction. Spirometry may not be markedly decreased because airflow limitation is fixed and does not change substantially. The increased work of breathing required during periods of increased symptoms can result in respiratory muscle fatigue and an increased risk of respiratory failure.

CLINICAL PRESENTATION AND DIAGNOSIS

Clinical assessment of the patient with COPD includes medical history and physical examination. A diagnosis of COPD should be considered in any patient with complaints of chronic cough, dyspnea, and sputum production, especially if there is a positive history of exposure to risk factors. In COPD, the cough is typically productive of sputum and may be intermittent progressing to chronic. Sputum production should be characterized in terms of quantity and appearance. Dyspnea is also progressive as disease severity worsens. Initially it occurs with exertion, but it can progress to being always present, including at rest.

The medical history also includes a review of pertinent exposures, including a current or past history of tobacco use. Smoking history is quantified into pack-years by multiplying the number of packs per day smoked times the number of years smoked. The pack-year smoking history provides insight into the general level of risk for COPD and other smoking-related diseases. Pertinent data to gather in a medical history are listed in Table 35.3.

SIGNS AND SYMPTOMS

By the time the patient seeks medical attention, the disease is usually far advanced, with symptoms of airway obstruction. This delay in medical intervention occurs because the

TABLE 35.3	Components of Medical History for Patients with Chronic Obstructive Pulmonary Disease (COPD)

Evaluate the presence of symptoms:
- Cough
- Sputum production
- Dyspnea

Collect past medical history and review of systems:
- History of asthma, allergies, or childhood respiratory infections
- Episodes of wheezing, chest pain, or morning headache
- Past history of COPD exacerbations
- Comorbidities related to cigarette smoking
- Unexplained weight loss
- History of depression or anxiety
- Family history of COPD

Collect risk exposure history:
- Cigarette smoking (past or present)
- Passive cigarette smoke exposure
- Occupational or environmental exposures

pathologic changes have been progressing for years, but overt clinical symptoms occur later. Screening programs to identify patients at risk for COPD, or in the earliest stages of the disease, are not as common as programs for detection of heart disease or cancer, but recently there has been an increased awareness about early detection.[22] Much of this effort is directed toward primary care providers to assist in the early identification and intervention in COPD and related disorders. This initiative aims at preventing or forestalling premature morbidity and mortality from COPD and related disorders.

There is significant overlap between the clinical presentations of chronic bronchitis and emphysema. The usual presentation of chronic bronchitis begins with morning cough productive of sputum. Cough and increased sputum production are not generally present in emphysema. The patient may report a decline in exercise tolerance, although he or she may not appreciate this decline until questioned. Fatigue also correlates with worsening pulmonary function.[23] Weight loss (sometimes profound) may be reported by the patient with primary emphysema, but the patient with chronic bronchitis is typically obese. Dyspnea occurs later in the course of COPD and may be worsened by exposure to cold, dampness, pollution, or acute infection. Considerable interpatient variation exists in the subjective perception of dyspnea, but there is a close intrapatient correlation between dyspnea and worsening degree of airway obstruction in patients with advancing COPD.

DIAGNOSIS AND CLINICAL FINDINGS

All patients being evaluated for COPD should undergo spirometry testing with bronchodilator reversibility and should receive a chest radiograph. The gold standard for COPD diagnosis is spirometry, which provides objective evidence of airflow limitation. Spirometry should be performed by a qualified person and according to ATS criteria.[2] By definition, obstruction to air outflow is present when the FEV_1/FVC ratio is less than 70%. Spirometry provides the best information on the degree of airway obstruction and also is useful to assess the efficacy of drug therapy. In spirometry testing, the patient exhales as rapidly and forcefully as possible for a minimum of 6 seconds through a device that measures airflow.

Commonly reported parameters of spirometry include FEV_1, FVC, and the FEV_1/FVC ratio. Normal values are determined based on age, gender, race, and height among people without lung disease. Results are often reported as absolute numbers or the percentage of predicted values based on the normal values.

FEV_1 is decreased in patients with an obstruction to outflow, and the extent to which it is decreased is associated with disease severity in COPD. FEV_1 above 2 L is usually not associated with dyspnea with normal activity. With a 50% decrease in FEV_1, dyspnea on exertion is present. A 75% decrease is associated with dyspnea at rest. There can be considerable day-to-day variability in FEV_1, with most stable COPD patients showing up to 20% fluctuation.[12]

FVC denotes the volume of gas expelled from the lungs during rapid and complete exhalation and is also reduced in COPD. In a patient without lung disease, the FEV_1/FVC ratio is normally 0.8 or greater. Therefore, a patient with chronic or acute airway obstruction would have an FEV_1/FVC ratio less than 0.8.

When appropriately performed and interpreted, spirometry testing serves as an early screening tool for identifying patients at risk for COPD, identifies patients with COPD and other disorders, provides positive reinforcement to patients attempting smoking cessation, and assesses response to drug therapy. It also allows staging of COPD based on the FEV_1 result.

Bronchodilator reversibility testing should be performed at least initially to establish a baseline, rule out other causes, and estimate prognosis.[24] A short-acting bronchodilator (e.g., albuterol) is administered and spirometry is repeated in 15 to 30 minutes. COPD is typically characterized by less than a 12% improvement in FEV_1 after the bronchodilator administration, or less than 200 mL in patients with very low lung volumes. However, COPD patients can exhibit varying degrees of improvement. A large increase in the FEV_1 is more consistent with a diagnosis of asthma. The absence of a significant increase after a single dose does not justify withholding bronchodilator therapy.

Chest radiography is not often useful in assessing and managing COPD; however, it can be used initially to exclude other diseases, including pneumonia, congestive heart failure, pleural effusion, or pneumothorax. Characteristic findings on radiographs in patients with COPD include diffuse scarring, a flattened diaphragm, thoracic overinflation, and diminished pulmonary vasculature.

Additional testing can be helpful in some patients, such as more extensive assessments of lung volumes through body plethysmography, carbon dioxide diffusion capacity, measurement of arterial blood gases for acid–base status, exercise testing, computed tomography, and tests of respiratory muscle strength. These evaluations may be warranted if the diagnosis is uncertain or difficult.

Patients who have evidence of airflow limitation of COPD at a relatively early age (third to fourth decade of life) should undergo serologic testing for an α_1-antitrypsin deficiency. This testing is also warranted in patients who have COPD symptoms in the absence of a significant smoking history or in patients with a family history of an α_1-antitrypsin deficiency. The diagnosis is made by serum protein electrophoresis testing. α_1-Antitrypsin deficiency presents as emphysema. If serum concentrations of α_1-antitrypsin are 15% to 20% of normal, genotype testing is warranted.

Findings on the physical examination may be unremarkable in patients with early or mild disease. Major components of the physical examination are listed in Table 35.4. A prolonged expiratory effort may be seen as a sign of airway obstruction in primary emphysema. These patients may also exhale through pursed lips in an attempt to control the rate of expiration. Grunting may be heard on inspiration. Patients with predominant emphysema may prefer an upright, forward-leaning posture. The patient may be using the accessory respiratory muscles to aid in breathing. An overall increase in respiratory rate is common. Wheezes may be heard

TABLE 35.4	Components of Physical Examination for Patients with Chronic Obstructive Pulmonary Disease

Respiratory rate

Body mass index calculation based on weight and height

Chest examination
- Inspect for barrel chest, pursed-lip breathing, paradoxical movement of respiratory and abdominal muscles.
- Percuss for diaphragm movement and evidence of hyperinflation or bullae.
- Auscultate for normal or absent lung sounds, as well as abnormal (added) sounds.

Cardiac examination for findings associated with lung disease

Other areas for focused examination
- Distention for neck veins
- Liver size
- Peripheral edema
- Muscle wasting and weakness
- Cyanosis of extremities or mucous membranes

during bouts of airway obstruction in both chronic bronchitis and emphysema. An increase in the anteroposterior diameter of the chest and the classic ''barrel chest'' may occur in both diseases. These signs and symptoms do not correlate well with the severity of illness.

As COPD progresses, other acute and chronic complications may develop. Some patients may develop cor pulmonale and right-sided congestive heart failure; the term ''blue bloater'' has been used to describe this presentation. Hypoxemia and respiratory acidosis are common findings. The other common presentation is a patient with predominantly emphysematous changes. These patients are termed ''pink puffers'' because alveolar ventilation is maintained until the terminal stages of the disease.

CLASSIFICATION OF SEVERITY

The international guidelines can be used to classify COPD severity. Although there are minor differences between the two international documents, the severity classification from the GOLD guidelines is summarized in Table 35.5. As disease severity worsens, patients experience worsening health and more frequent exacerbations, utilize more healthcare resources, and are at greater risk for death.

Although spirometry represents the gold standard in diagnosing and classifying COPD severity, other factors affect the patient's overall health status, as well as morbidity and mortality risks. Two important parameters are nutritional status, as reflected by body mass index (BMI), and dyspnea, assessed according to a standardized scale. Patients with COPD who have a BMI less than 21 are at risk for increased mortality. BMI is determined by the following formula: BMI (kg/m^2) = body weight (kg)/ height (m^2). Dyspnea is a subjective symptom, but a scale is available from the Medical Research Council (Table 35.6). These assessments have been shown to be of prognostic value.[25,26]

TABLE 35.5 Severity Classification for Chronic Obstructive Pulmonary Disease

Severity Stage	Classification	Predicted FEV_1[a]
0	At risk[b]	≥80%
1	Mild	≥80%
2	Moderate	≥50% and <80%
3	Severe	≥30% and <50%
4	Very Severe	<30% (or <50% with respiratory failure)

Based on the Global Initiative for Chronic Obstructive Pulmonary Diseases (GOLD Guidelines). Available at www.goldcopd.com
[a]FEV_1, forced expiratory volume in 1 second; results should be obtained after bronchodilator administration.
[b]''At risk'' indicates a positive history of risk factor exposure, family history of respiratory disease, and the presence of symptoms. At-risk patients have a normal FEV_1/FVC ratio (>70%); patients with stage 1 to 4 COPD have an FEV_1/FVC ratio of 70% or less.

TABLE 35.6 Dyspnea Assessment (Based on the Medical Research Council Dyspnea Scale)

Level	Description
0	Shortness of breath occurs only with strenuous exercise
1	Shortness of breath occurs when hurrying or walking up a slight hill
2	Walks more slowly than people of same age due to shortness of breath, or has to stop for breath when walking at own pace on a level surface
3	Stops for breath after walking 100 m or a few minutes on a level surface
4	Too breathless to leave the house, or develops shortness of breath with normal activities (e.g., dressing or undressing)

NATURAL COURSE

COPD is characterized by a steady progressive decline in lung function, although the rate of loss varies among patients. This variation is often attributed to genetic factors, combinations of environmental risks, continued exposure, and the extent of exposure. In the third decade of life, lung function begins a decline of approximately 10 to 20 mL of FEV_1 annually. Some patients with COPD are at risk for an accelerated decline of up to 120 mL annually. Removing the exposure can slow the subsequent loss of function within a few years.[27]

The best indicators of prognosis are the degree of obstruction and age. Complications such as cor pulmonale and hypoxia are negative indicators for survival. FEV_1 obtained after bronchodilator administration is a good predictor of survival. Once FEV_1 decreases below 0.75 L, severe airway obstruction is present; this is associated with an increased 5-year mortality rate. When patients have dyspnea, the mortality rate increases; up to 50% of patients die within 5 years. The course will probably be characterized by multiple exacerbations, hospitalizations, and multiple-drug therapies to treat symptoms or prevent progression. Poor nutrition and exercise intolerance commonly develop, and patients with severe disease face significant alterations in lifestyle.

PSYCHOSOCIAL ASPECTS

Depression and anxiety are common in patients with COPD. Studies are lacking, but psychosocial interventions are believed by patients and physicians to be an important part of a pulmonary rehabilitation program. This may include smoking cessation efforts for patients who have not already quit smoking. Quitting can be very difficult for patients who are feeling anxious or depressed. Adherence to other treatment interventions can also be improved.

Discussion of end-of-life decisions is difficult for patients, families, and health care providers; COPD is no exception. Therapy of COPD is not currently curative, and progression of disease is inevitable. However, COPD patients are no more likely than other patients to have expressed their wishes about end-of-life decisions to their physicians or families. The crucial decision usually centers around mechanical ventilation: Does the patient want to be placed on mechanical ventilation for respiratory failure? If mechanical ventilation is initiated and the patient does not improve, does the patient wish to be removed from mechanical support? Physicians may be reluctant to remove a patient from mechanical ventilation, particularly in light of family objections. However, the patient's right of self-determination in these cases should outweigh concerns about legal liability or personal beliefs. Open discussion, before the point of medical crisis, should occur between caregivers, the patient, and family members. Decisions not to implement mechanical support or to withdraw mechanical support once begun are both ethically appropriate but are only made harder when the patient has not expressed his or her wishes.

THERAPEUTIC PLAN

The therapy of COPD is discussed in this section, with areas of particular benefit in primary chronic bronchitis or primary emphysema highlighted. Evidence supporting management strategies has improved during the past decade. The primary goals of therapy should be to halt or slow the progression of the pathologic changes, improve the patient's quality of life, and prevent acute exacerbations of the disease. An individualized approach to therapy is appropriate and should be based on the severity classification of the disease and the patient's risk factors. COPD is a complex disease, and patients will have varying health-related needs depending on the severity of their disease. A comprehensive model of care that uses the skills of a multidisciplinary team of clinicians and others is useful.

For most patients, an important initial intervention is to reduce or eliminate exposure to risk factors. Smoking cessation is the only treatment strategy proven to slow the chronic progressive loss of lung function. The majority of cases of COPD are attributed to cigarette smoking, and strategies for stopping and continued cessation are the most important intervention for all patients, independent of their current stage of disease.

APPROACHES TO TREATMENT

PHARMACOTHERAPY

The goals of pharmacotherapy for COPD are listed in Table 35.7. None of the currently available therapies has been shown to prevent or slow the progressive loss of lung function. As a result, the primary role of drug therapy has been for

TABLE 35.7	Goals of Pharmacotherapy for Chronic Obstructive Pulmonary Disease

- Reduce, control, or abolish symptoms
- Improve lung function if reversibility is present
- Improve exercise capacity
- Reduce the frequency and severity of exacerbations
- Improve general health status

symptomatic relief of symptoms, and the primary strategy is the use of bronchodilator therapy. The response to medications varies among patients with COPD. The clinician should periodically assess the patient for improvement in symptoms and for side effects (Table 35.8).

Some patients demonstrate reversibility of airflow limitation as measured through spirometry, but many patients do not exhibit improvement in this objective measure. Recently there has been increased interest in evaluating the benefit of various therapies on reducing exacerbation frequency and in decreasing symptoms of dyspnea. Exacerbations have a significant impact on morbidity and prognosis, and dyspnea is a major debilitating symptom for patients with advanced disease.

When pharmacotherapy is used, the inhaled route of administration is preferred because it is more efficacious and safer than available oral therapies. Inhaled bronchodilators are preferred over systemic treatment. Inhaled therapy can be delivered by a metered-dose inhaler (MDI), a dry powder

TABLE 35.8	Assessment of Benefits and Side Effects From Pharmacotherapy for Chronic Obstructive Pulmonary Disease

During periodic evaluations, the clinician should evaluate whether the patient has improved with medications or if any side effects are present. The following questions can be useful:

Do you feel improved since the medication was started? If so, what is improved?

- Shortness of breath
- Exercise tolerance
- Cough or wheezing
- Sputum production
- General health
- Sleep

Is there anything that you can do or do more easily than before? If so, what?

Have you experienced any side effects that you attribute to your medication?

Do you have any difficulty using your medication?

Do you have any questions about your medication?

inhaler (DPI), or a nebulizer. The patient should be instructed about proper use and care of the inhalation device to obtain optimal benefit from therapy. In general, these routes for inhalation therapy are equally effective, especially for chronic management. The device used to deliver inhaled medication appears less important, although MDIs and DPIs are more convenient than jet nebulizers. Nebulization therapy is used in the initial treatment of exacerbations. If the patient is able to use all of the devices, the choice is based on costs, reimbursement considerations, and patient preference. A comprehensive review has identified several factors that should be considered in selecting a specific inhalation delivery system for an individual patient; these are listed in Table 35.9.[28]

Among the agents currently used in COPD treatment, no medication has been effective in slowing the progressive decline in lung function that characterizes the disease. Often, drug therapy does not result in substantial improvements in spirometry results; therefore, appropriate outcome measures are to control or reduce symptoms, improve exercise tolerance, reduce the frequency and severity of exacerbations, and improve overall health status. The focus of treatment recommendations currently is on bronchodilators. Within this class, inhaled therapy is generally preferred, and combinations are often used for additive benefits and to reduce side effects.[29]

Bronchodilators. Bronchodilators typically provide minimal improvement in objective measures of lung function due to the irreversible nature of COPD. However, relaxing airway smooth muscle can help empty the lungs during breathing at rest (FRC) and reduce the amount of trapped air in the lung after maximal exhalation (residual volume). These changes are associated with improvements in symptoms of dyspnea.[30]

Several options exist, including short- and long-acting inhaled β-agonists, short- and long-acting inhaled anticholinergics, and methylxanthines. Each agent is effective in reducing symptoms. Inhaled therapy is preferred over systemic therapy due to improved efficacy and a more favorable

TABLE 35.9	Factors to Consider When Selecting an Inhalation Device

Availability of desired medication in the delivery device

Clinical setting for inhalation therapy use

Patient's age and skill to use device optimally

Device availability with multiple medications

Cost and reimbursement issues

Convenience of use in multiple settings

Prescriber and patient preference

Adapted from Dolovich MB, Ahrens RC, Hess DR, et al. Device selection and outcomes of aerosol therapy: evidence-based guidelines. Chest 127:335–371, 2005.

safety margin. Although spirometry improvements with bronchodilator therapy may be small, reductions in obstruction can reduce hyperinflation and air trapping, which helps reduce symptoms of dyspnea.[30]

For patients with more frequent or chronic symptoms, long-acting bronchodilators are more effective at improving lung function, exercise tolerance, and quality of life. The long-acting therapies also can reduce the frequency of exacerbations.

β_2-Agonists. β_2-Agonists are in the broader class of sympathomimetic agents, which include agents that stimulate α-, β_1-, and β_2-receptors. β_2-Receptors are located primarily in airways. Currently available β_2-selective therapies include albuterol, levalbuterol, pirbuterol, and terbutaline as short-acting agents and formoterol and salmeterol as long-acting agents. β_2-Agonists stimulate β_2-receptors that increase adenyl cyclase, an enzyme that increases cyclic AMP (cAMP) and results in smooth muscle relaxation and bronchodilation. The most commonly used β-agonists are inhaled β_2-agonists are administered via inhalation, although oral and parenteral products are available. Systemic therapy is associated with more frequent adverse effects and lower efficacy and has limited clinical utility. Rapid airway response is seen with inhaled β_2-agonists, whereas the onset of action with oral therapy is delayed in acute airway obstruction.

Albuterol is the most commonly used inhaled, short-acting β_2-agonist. It has a rapid onset of action (less than 5 minutes) and a relatively short duration of action (approximately 4 hours) with chronic use. Other short-acting β_2-agonists exhibit similar effects. In patients with COPD, treatment relieves symptoms and improves exercise tolerance without a significant effect on lung function.

As inhaled therapy, short-acting β_2-agonists are relatively well tolerated. Side effects of inhaled β_2-agonists are dose-related and occur less commonly when given by the inhalation route compared to orally or parenterally. Tachycardia and palpitations can occur from stimulation of β_1-receptors in cardiac tissue. Patients may initially experience a fine skeletal muscle tremor that improves with continued use. High-dose therapy during exacerbations can precipitate hypokalemia in some patients.

Levalbuterol, the R isomer of albuterol, is available in an MDI and nebulized dosage form. There are some small studies and retrospective evaluations suggesting that levalbuterol offers clinical benefits over albuterol based on the theory that the S isomer of albuterol is not inert and exerts contradictory or antagonistic activity to the R isomer at the β_2-receptor. Comparisons of levalbuterol to albuterol for COPD have included small numbers of patients or have been retrospective evaluations.[31]

Although some studies suggest a benefit of levalbuterol therapy compared to albuterol in selected clinical or economic outcomes, there is not sufficient evidence to support its routine use over albuterol. The acquisition cost of levalbuterol is currently much higher than that of albuterol.

Long-acting inhaled β_2-agonists include formoterol and salmeterol. Clinical studies conducted during the past few years suggest a significant advantage of these long-acting bronchodilators over short-acting therapies. In addition to improving symptoms and exercise tolerance, they reduce the frequency of exacerbations and improve quality of life. They should be considered for patients whose symptoms are not controlled with short-acting therapies.

Both salmeterol and formoterol have been compared with ipratropium in patients with COPD. Salmeterol was superior to ipratropium and placebo in improving spirometric measures and in reducing time to the first exacerbation, but both treatments were similar in relieving dyspnea and reducing rescue inhaler use.[32] In another study, formoterol was significantly better than ipratropium in improving spirometry and reducing symptoms and rescue inhaler use, but there was no difference in reducing exacerbation rates.[33]

Although the two long-acting inhaled β_2-agonists have similar profiles in terms of duration of effect (approximately 12 hours), formoterol has a faster onset (5 minutes), with peak effect on FEV_1 in 30 minutes. Salmeterol has an onset of 15 minutes and peak effect in 1 to 2 hours. Based on the proposed role of these long-acting agents in providing long-term control of symptoms, this difference may not be clinically important.

Anticholinergics. Cholinergic tone predominates in the airways and has a major influence on airway diameter. COPD patients exhibit an increased cholinergic tone in the airway, although the basis for this is unclear. An increased tone is associated with smaller airway diameter due to bronchoconstriction. This feature is the basis for inhaled anticholinergic therapy in COPD management.

Cholinergic stimulation increases the activity of guanyl cyclase, the enzyme responsible for catalyzing the formation of cyclic guanosine $3',5'$-monophosphate (GMP). Cyclic GMP stimulates bronchoconstriction; therefore, administration of an anticholinergic agent prevents the formation of cyclic GMP. The result is inhibition of bronchoconstriction. Two anticholinergic therapies are used commonly as inhalation therapy: ipratropium, a short-acting anticholinergic, and tiotropium, a long-acting agent.

Ipratropium bromide, an analogue of atropine, acts as a bronchodilator by the same mechanism as atropine; however, because it is a quaternary compound, little systemic absorption occurs. Studies comparing ipratropium to β-agonists in stable COPD patients show that ipratropium bromide produces equal or greater bronchodilation at usual doses.[34,35] At maximal doses, the bronchodilation produced by β-agonists probably equals that of ipratropium in COPD,[36] but adverse effects are more common. Ipratropium bromide produces a response within 15 minutes when inhaled, with effects seen for 4 to 6 hours.[34] Because of its slower onset compared with β_2-agonists, patients may prefer to use β_2-agonists for acute bronchospasm, with ipratropium being used on a scheduled basis. Ipratropium bromide is adminis-

tered as two inhalations four times a day, increasing to six inhalations if needed. Adverse effects are uncommon and consist of dry mouth and throat, bitter taste, cough, and nausea.

Tiotropium, a long-acting inhaled anticholinergic therapy, has been available for use in the United States since 2004. Tiotropium is an inhaled anticholinergic agent that blocks cholinergic (or muscarinic) receptors in bronchial smooth muscle (M1, M2, and M3), resulting in smooth muscle relaxation. However, tiotropium disassociates from M2 receptors more rapidly than the M1 and M3. Physiologically, activation of M2 receptors is associated with reduced acetylcholine release. Tiotropium's prolonged action in blocking the M1 and M3 receptors results in prolonged and sustained bronchodilation. A major advantage of tiotropium is the once-a-day dosing regimen. Like ipratropium, tiotropium has an excellent safety profile. The most common complaint with this therapy is dry mouth due to its anticholinergic properties, although this is well tolerated by most patients.

Tiotropium has been compared with other therapies, including ipratropium and long-acting β_2-agonists. In a comparison of once-daily tiotropium with four-times-daily ipratropium in COPD patients, the tiotropium group had significantly higher improvements in FEV_1,[37] the percentage of patients experiencing multiple exacerbations was significantly lower with tiotropium compared to ipratropium, and the time to first exacerbation was significantly longer. For most outcome measures, tiotropium is more effective than the short-acting ipratropium, but it is more expensive.

Tiotropium has also been compared with long-acting β_2-agonists. In a study comparing tiotropium with salmeterol, both active treatments improved FVC, but tiotropium improved FEV_1 and reduced symptoms of dyspnea more than salmeterol at 6 months.[38] Supplemental albuterol use was similar between treatments. In another trial, tiotropium and salmeterol reduced exacerbation and improved dyspnea symptoms to a similar extent.[39]

Combination of Short-Acting β_2-Agonist/Anticholinergic. Data have been conflicting regarding the effects of using an anticholinergic medication with a β_2-agonist. The overall weight of the evidence favors an additive effect with chronic use but not acute use. Additive effects during chronic use have been recently supported by a large multicenter trial, although it is not clear whether the combination is superior to maximal doses of either agent alone.[40] The study found 20% to 40% additional bronchodilation for the combination over single agents, but clinical COPD symptom scores were not significantly different. The increased effectiveness of the combination is not surprising because the two classes of drugs have different mechanisms and sites of action. Anticholinergic drugs appear to act primarily in the central airways where cholinergic receptors are abundant; the β_2-agonists' site of action includes peripheral as well as central airways.[41] Despite the paucity of data supporting the use of short-acting combination bronchodilators, this practice is supported by treatment guidelines and is commonly used in the management of mild to moderate COPD.

Combinations of Long-Acting Bronchodilators. To date, there are limited data about combination therapy with long-acting β_2-agonists and tiotropium in the chronic management of COPD. Single dose studies with both formoterol and salmeterol combined with tiotropium have been performed but have not shown any benefit from the combination. It is likely that combinations of long-acting agents are used for patients with severe COPD. Further research is warranted to evaluate the benefit of these combinations. In addition, data about the benefit of combination bronchodilator therapy compared with bronchodilator and inhaled corticosteroid combinations would be useful.

Methylxanthines. Methylxanthines, including theophylline, have been used as bronchodilator therapy for over 50 years. Until 20 years ago, these agents were the mainstay of bronchodilator therapy in COPD, but with more effective bronchodilators now available, theophylline's role in COPD has diminished substantially. However, theophylline may still be beneficial in the management of chronic COPD, especially if a reversible component is present.

Theophylline, when added to regimens of inhaled anticholinergics or β_2-agonists, produces additive bronchodilation.[42–44] Once therapy is maximized with inhaled bronchodilators with suboptimal response, patients may be given a trial of theophylline followed by pulmonary function testing to assess response to therapy. Outcome measures that should be evaluated include FEV_1, dyspnea scores, and quality of life measures. Theophylline may also reduce overnight declines in FEV_1 and resultant morning respiratory symptoms when administered as an evening dose, and it may still have an important role in this setting.[45]

Although there is evidence that theophylline may provide benefit by improving symptoms for patients with COPD, it currently is considered a third-line agent due to the availability of safer and more potent therapies and its risk of toxicity.

The mechanism of action for methylxanthines in COPD is not well understood. Proposed effects on the cardiac and respiratory systems include bronchodilation, improved respiratory muscle contractility and reserve, stimulation of central ventilatory drive, increased mucociliary clearance, decreased mean pulmonary artery pressure and pulmonary vascular resistance, increased collateral ventilation, and improved biventricular cardiac performance, but the significance of these effects has not been fully examined in COPD patients.

Theophylline has been proposed to exert various mechanisms of actions, including inhibition of phosphodiesterase, alteration in calcium movement, blockade of adenosine receptors, prostaglandin antagonism, and alteration of cAMP binding to the binding protein. Although phosphodiesterase inhibition has traditionally been accepted as the mechanism of action of theophylline, it is questionable whether this accounts for its effects at clinically used doses. The other effects have been noted at clinically useful levels and thus may be responsible for the efficacy of the drug.

When a decision is made to use theophylline, several issues must be considered. Various dosage forms and salts of theophylline are available, although the most appropriate therapy to select is a sustained-release theophylline product that can be taken once or twice daily. There is significant variability in bioavailability among available products as well as intrapatient and interpatient variability in pharmacokinetics. Clinicians planning to use theophylline for chronic COPD treatment should consult a pharmacokinetics resource to guide dosing and monitoring.

Theophylline exhibits a dose–response relationship. Clinically, the recommended therapeutic range for COPD is 8 to 12 μg per mL. When used in COPD, theophylline therapy should be monitored closely to assess the degree of benefit the patient is receiving (primarily symptomatic control). Careful monitoring is also warranted to prevent or limit adverse effects that may be more common in these patients (e.g., they may be particularly sensitive to the arrhythmogenic effects of theophylline). Many COPD patients continue to smoke, thereby increasing theophylline clearance. The clearance of theophylline may be reduced in advanced stages of COPD or in the presence of cor pulmonale with or without heart failure, and careful monitoring of serum concentrations is essential.

Primary reasons that theophylline use has declined over the past 20 years are the greater efficacy of other therapies and the risk of side effects, toxicities, and drug interactions with its use. Theophylline's adverse effect profile affects the gastrointestinal, cardiac, and central nervous systems. The drug is poorly tolerated by some patients, and there is significant overlap between side effects at therapeutic versus toxic concentrations. Common side effects include nausea, vomiting, diarrhea, tachycardia, palpitations, cardiac arrhythmias, headaches, and convulsions.

Given the adverse effect profile of theophylline, evidence of significant benefit should be obtained before subjecting the patient to long-term therapy. The clinician must be able to monitor the patient for side effects and toxicity such as nausea, vomiting, tremors, headaches, confusion, arrhythmias, and seizures.

Summary of Bronchodilator Therapy. Bronchodilators are the mainstay of therapy for chronic COPD management. Although several options exist, inhaled therapy is preferred over systemic agents in most cases. Short-acting agents can be used initially, but if the patient continues to have symptoms, long-acting agents are more effective and convenient. In various clinical trials, long-acting bronchodilators (β-agonists and anticholinergics) have provided greater benefit in terms of improving various outcome measures compared to short-acting agents.[37,46] Combinations of bronchodilators are commonly used to take advantage of the different mechanisms of other agents and to reduce side effects from higher doses of a single agent. Combinations have provided additional benefit for various outcome measures in COPD patients.[47–49] Oral theophylline is an option that is usually reserved for patients who are not responding to inhaled regimens or who refuse to use inhalation therapies.

Corticosteroids. Although inflammation plays a major role in the development and progression of COPD, corticosteroid therapy has not resulted in a dramatic response. This lack of benefit may be related to the neutrophilic nature of inflammation in COPD: although corticosteroids have widespread anti-inflammatory effects, their activity against activated neutrophils is minimal.

Historical data suggest that only 20% of COPD patients benefit from systemic corticosteroid therapy, and these patients appear to have characteristics more consistent with asthma. Systemic corticosteroid therapy should be avoided in the chronic management of COPD due to lack of benefit and the potential for serious toxicity, including immunosuppression, muscle wasting, and accelerated bone loss leading to osteoporosis and fractures.

Inhaled corticosteroids exhibit a superior safety profile compared to systemic corticosteroids. Therefore, if clinical benefit is apparent with inhaled corticosteroid therapy, these agents could play an important role in chronic COPD management. Several trials have evaluated moderate to high doses of inhaled corticosteroids in the long-term management of COPD.[50–53] Results from four long-term prospective clinical trials failed to show any benefit from inhaled corticosteroid therapy in slowing the progressive decline in FEV_1. However, a subset of patients with more severe disease (FEV_1 less than 50% predicted) who experienced frequent exacerbations showed improvements in quality-of-life scores and had a reduced frequency of exacerbations.[50] A meta-analysis of several published studies suggested that regular treatment with inhaled corticosteroids reduced exacerbation rates in COPD, especially for patients with an FEV_1 less than 50% predicted.[54] As a result, current guidelines suggest that a trial of inhaled corticosteroid therapy is warranted in patients who have an FEV_1 less than 50% and who experience frequent exacerbations of COPD.[1,2] An in-depth discussion of inhaled corticosteroid products is available in Chapter 34.

If inhaled corticosteroid therapy is used, patients should be monitored for local problems such as thrush and dysphonia, and periodic monitoring of bone mineral density is recommended. Inhaled corticosteroids have an improved safety profile compared to systemic corticosteroids, but there is some evidence of reduced bone mineral density.[51] Newer agents such as budesonide, fluticasone, and mometasone may have less of a risk, but periodic monitoring of bone mineral density is still warranted with long-term treatment.

Combination of Long-Acting β_2-Agonists and Inhaled Corticosteroids. A combination product containing a long-acting β_2-agonist and inhaled corticosteroid is available in the United States and has been evaluated in several clinical trials comparing the combination to individual agents.[55,56]

The FEV_1 response was greatest with the combination, although there was no difference in exacerbation rates among the treatments. The combination product offers advantages in convenience and ease of use compared to separate inhalers.

Mucolytic/Expectorant Agents. Although they have been used for many years, no clinical benefit of mucolytic or expectorant agents has been established in COPD patients. Acetylcysteine thins secretions in chronic bronchitics but does not improve airflow in COPD patients. Acetylcysteine is not well tolerated and can induce airway irritation and bronchospasm, requiring bronchodilator use.

Respiratory Stimulants. Chronic hypercapnia in the COPD patient is usually well tolerated and may be compensatory to reduce respiratory muscle fatigue.[57] It is best managed by proper muscle conditioning and bronchodilators. Although respiratory stimulants such as doxapram, medroxyprogesterone, and acetazolamide are available, any beneficial effect is short-lived. The potential risks of therapy are also significant concerns. Further respiratory fatigue from overstimulation of respiratory muscles may worsen respiratory failure. At this time, their use cannot be recommended. Almitrine bismesylate is a peripheral chemoreceptor stimulant shown to improve P_{O_2} concentrations in COPD patients, but its benefit is limited, it has significant toxicity, and it is unavailable in the United States.

α_1-Proteinase Inhibitors. In the rare inherited form of emphysema, patients have a deficiency of α_1-antitrypsin. This deficiency leads to progressive destruction of elastin tissues and alveolar destruction caused by unopposed neutrophil elastase activity. Three replacement therapy products are available in the United States. α_1-Antitrypsin replacement therapy requires weekly or twice-weekly infusions to maintain circulating concentrations at acceptable levels (approximately 60% of normal). The usual weekly dose is 60 mg per kg. This treatment is not indicated for patients who have not developed signs and symptoms of emphysema, patients with other forms of emphysema, or patients with an FEV_1 less than 20% of predicted.

α_1-Antitrypsin replacement therapy was approved as an orphan drug based on the concept that a minimum concentration of circulating protein was necessary to prevent disease progression. There are limited data from a national registry showing that replacement therapy is associated with a slower decline in lung function. Therapy is expensive, averaging $500 to $1,500 per week, depending on the patient's weight. Although α_1-antitrypsin from pooled human plasma is found to be nonreactive for the human immunodeficiency virus (HIV) antibody and hepatitis B surface antigen, hepatitis B immunization is still recommended.

NONPHARMACOLOGIC APPROACHES

Tobacco Cessation Strategies. The most important intervention in the treatment or prevention of COPD is smoking cessation. Cigarette smoking results in an addiction to nicotine, so cessation is difficult to achieve and maintain. Smoking cessation guidelines are available and provide comprehensive information about the risks of cigarette smoking and proven cessation strategies.[58]

Smoking cessation slows the rate of loss of lung function.[59] The Lung Health Study, conducted in the late 1980s, showed that cessation was associated with a slower decline in FEV_1. After a few years without smoking, the decline in FEV_1 usually returns to that of a nonsmoker. In the Lung Health Study, patients in the early stages of COPD were randomized to three groups: usual care with no specific smoking intervention, smoking intervention and the use of ipratropium bromide, or smoking intervention and a placebo inhalation.[59] Rates of decline in FEV_1 were followed over 5 years. This study provided strong evidence that smoking cessation results in substantial benefit to lung function, with FEV_1 improving over the first year. During the second year after smoking cessation, FEV_1 continued unchanged and thereafter exhibited a similar rate of decline as nonsmokers. Smoking cessation is therefore the most important and beneficial intervention and is associated with immediate and sustained health benefits.

All clinicians should take an active role in identifying individuals who smoke, encouraging them to consider stopping, and offering assistance with quit attempts. A key to success is the interest and willingness of the patient to quit. Smokers have varying interest in cessation, and an effective approach is to encourage patients to reach the phase when they are actively interested in quitting. Attempts to initiate smoking cessation in a patient who is not interested or who is in the ''precontemplation stage'' are inappropriate and likely to fail.

A common system to evaluate and assist patients who smoke is described as the ''5 A's'' (Table 35.10). Brief interventions are effective when used consistently and provided by multiple clinicians during encounters. Patients benefit

---

TABLE 35.10	Strategies for Assisting Patients in Smoking Cessation: "The 5 A's"

Ask: Collect and document smoking histories among all patients encountered. For current smokers, inquire about interest in smoking cessation.

Advise: Strongly encourage smoking cessation among current smokers with a clear, concise, and personal message.

Assess: Determine the patient's interest and willingness in smoking cessation now.

Assist: Provide education, advice, and support to the patient in making a cessation attempt. Use proven methods of counseling, social support, and smoking cessation pharmacotherapies (nicotine replacement or bupropion).

Arrange: Schedule follow-up contacts to monitor success, failed attempts, relapses, and continued cessation.

---

from continued encouragement and support. Failed attempts and relapses are not uncommon, and patients should be encouraged to try again. A comprehensive discussion regarding smoking cessation is found in Chapter 60.

Other occupational or environmental exposures, including air pollution, can contribute to disease progression in some patients. Identification of potential exposures is important, and patients can be given advice about minimizing continued exposure. Recommendations can include removing the patient from certain environments at home or work, or avoiding prolonged periods of exposure to poor air quality.

Pulmonary Rehabilitation. The value of pulmonary rehabilitation programs in the management of COPD has been proven in well-controlled studies.[60] Rehabilitation programs include a variety of interventions such as education, exercise, and psychosocial counseling. Pulmonary rehabilitation programs for COPD patients should be multidisciplinary and individually tailored in an effort to optimize the patient's physical and social performance and autonomy.

There is convincing evidence about the value of pulmonary rehabilitation programs in relieving symptoms, improving exercise tolerance, and improving overall health status.[61] Pulmonary rehabilitation is less beneficial in preventing complications and exacerbations (as measured by healthcare utilization) and has no effect on reducing mortality or slowing disease progression.[62]

A comprehensive pulmonary rehabilitation program includes patient education, exercise training, psychosocial support and intervention, and nutritional therapy, with assessments for each area. Endurance training of both the lower and upper extremities can be helpful. Improved lower extremity muscle training improves ambulation and therefore the ability to do routine daily tasks. Upper extremity training can be important because arm activities can produce shortness of breath due to competition with accessory respiratory muscles. Even though these exercises may not improve pulmonary function, they improve motivation and quality of life by enhancing the patient's ability to carry out daily activities. Strength training is supplemental to endurance training and often focuses on ventilatory muscle training, although this is of questionable benefit alone.

Among the educational components in the program are information about the disease and its course, techniques to improve adherence, and improving coping and self-management skills. Psychosocial interventions are targeted to address anxiety and depression if present.

Nutritional Status. Severe COPD can be associated with significant loss of weight and muscle mass. Decreased caloric intake, increased energy expenditure due to the increased work of breathing, and declining pulmonary function measures are possible explanations. Nutritional status is often addressed as part of pulmonary rehabilitation programs; poor nutrition has a significant impact on COPD survival. Weight loss may be the result of inflammation manifesting as a systemic feature of the disease. Reduction in fat-free mass, a marker of weight loss, is present in 20% of COPD patients with moderate to severe disease and in 35% of patients who are candidates for pulmonary rehabilitation.[63] Although depleted fat-free, mass is associated with weight loss, muscle wasting can be present in COPD patients with stable weights.

BMI should be calculated in COPD patients so they can be classified as underweight (BMI less than 21), normal weight (BMI 21 to 25), overweight (BMI 25 to 30), or obese (BMI 30 or more). Nutritional interventions should be considered in underweight patients or those reporting involuntary weight loss of more than 10% over 6 months or more than 5% within 1 month.

Nutritional interventions may consist of adjusting the patient's dietary intake toward a caloric goal as well as the use of energy-dense supplements. However, in patients with advanced disease, it is difficult to meet the nutritional goals of patients as a result of poor compliance, decreased appetite, and ongoing muscle wasting and weight loss.[64] It is likely that nutritional interventions would be more successful if used earlier in the course of disease or if greater efforts at prevention were made.

Keeping Immunizations Current. Risk reduction and immunizations should be used consistently in management, independent of disease severity. Immunization against the influenza virus has been shown to reduce serious illness and death in patients with COPD.[65] The intramuscular inactivated influenza vaccine should be used. Vaccination with pneumococcal vaccine is also recommended in high-risk patients. Pneumococcal vaccine is formulated to provide prophylaxis against the most common strains of *S pneumoniae*. Clear evidence that COPD patients are at an increased risk of infection by *S pneumoniae* and thus increased risk of death has not been presented.[66] Antibody titers to the organisms may be elevated in COPD, probably as a result of chronic upper airway colonization. When given the vaccine, these patients respond by further increasing their antibody titers. Therefore, many clinicians recommend giving the vaccine to individuals with COPD. The most current dosing recommendation for adults is 0.5 mL by subcutaneous or intramuscular injection.

Supplemental Oxygen Therapy. Supplemental oxygen therapy, termed long-term oxygen therapy, improves survival in some COPD patients with chronic hypoxemia. This benefit is present in patients with a Pa_{O_2} of less than 55 mm Hg or less than 60 mm Hg with evidence of end-organ effects of COPD, including cor pulmonale, polycythemia, or cognitive impairment.[67,68] The number of hours per day the patient uses oxygen continuously seems to relate to the effectiveness of this therapy: patients who use oxygen for at least 15 hours per day show the greatest benefit. Some patients who experience desaturation with exertion or during the night can be prescribed intermittent or nocturnal oxygen therapy, but there is no evidence that it improves life expectancy.

The primary methods of determining oxygen saturation in arterial blood are through arterial blood gas measurements and pulse oximetry. Arterial blood gas measurements provide information about acid–base status and P_{CO_2} in addition to P_{O_2} and are recommended when long-term oxygen therapy is initiated to identify COPD patients who are CO_2 retainers and at risk for depressed ventilatory drive from oxygen therapy. Pulse oximetry is noninvasive; a small device is placed on the finger or earlobe, beams of light are transmitted through the blood vessels, and an estimate of oxygen saturation is computed. This method is generally reliable and convenient for periodic monitoring of oxygen saturation.[69]

Oxygen can be administered by devices that allow for ambulation or by fixed devices. The former are preferable. Oxygen use in combination with a structured exercise program may improve exercise tolerance. The most common and convenient method of supplementation is from an oxygen supply delivered through a nasal cannula that does not interfere with talking or eating. The goal of therapy is to maintain oxygen saturation at or above 90%. Most patients are managed at flow rates of 1 to 4 L per minute.

The main risks of long-term oxygen therapy relate to reducing ventilatory drive in patients with carbon dioxide retention and the physical hazards of oxygen gas. Oxygen therapy is generally well tolerated even in CO_2 retainers; however, these patients should be cautioned about the risks of adjusting oxygen flow rates without monitoring. Oxygen is combustible, and the most common injuries occur if the patient smokes while using oxygen and if the oxygen containers are knocked over and explode.

SURGICAL MANAGEMENT

Surgical options—bullectomy, lung volume reduction surgery (LVRS), and lung transplantation—are available for patients whose disease cannot be managed medically. However, patients with advanced COPD may be a poor surgical risk. Depending on the severity of underlying disease as well as comorbid conditions, patients with COPD are at increased risk for postoperative complications, including venous thromboembolism and ventilation difficulties.

Lung surgery is an option to relieve symptoms and improve the well-being of patients with COPD. Bullectomy involves removing bullae (large airless spaces) in the lung. These areas are not participating in gas exchange, and their presence increases the risk of pneumothoraces and can limit gas exchange in adjacent lung through compression. Removing large bullae can reduce obstruction and improve functional lung volumes, hypoxemia, and hypercapnia. Other benefits include improved exercise tolerance and reduced dyspnea.

In recent years, LVRS procedures have become more common. Compared to bullectomy, LVRS is a more comprehensive procedure in removing nonfunctional segments of lung tissue. Before surgery, patients undergo a series of evaluations to estimate the extent to which various portions of the lung are participating in gas exchange. The goal of LVRS is to change dynamics and allow remaining functional areas of the lung to be ventilated. LVRS procedures have been shown to improve compliance of the lung and reduce the work of breathing by allowing the diaphragm and other respiratory muscles to function more efficiently. LVRS also improves short-term spirometric parameters, exercise tolerance, dyspnea, and quality of life.

A large national trial concluded that patients with primarily upper lobe emphysema and low exercise capacity receive the most benefit from LVRS.[70] This surgery is associated with improvements in spirometry in some patients, but the range varies significantly and up to 50% of patients have minimal improvement. There is a reduction in total lung capacity and residual volume. Similarly, improvements in dyspnea, quality of life, and exercise tolerance are quite variable among patients. In many patients, spirometry, symptoms, and exercise tolerance returned to preoperative baselines. These results suggest that LVRS will provide benefit for a subset of COPD patients but that patient selection is important to identify the patients who will receive the greatest benefit.

In advanced COPD, lung transplantation is an option. COPD is the most common indication for lung transplantation consideration, but data are lacking concerning the relative value of either single-lung or double-lung transplant. Surrogate outcomes are often improved (spirometry, symptoms, exercise tolerance, quality of life), but the survival benefit of lung transplantation is uncertain, and numerous transplant-related problems may develop.

MANAGING EXACERBATIONS

COPD exacerbations occur periodically in the natural course of the disease and are described as an acute worsening in the patient's baseline, including worsening dyspnea, increased cough, and change in the volume and appearance of sputum beyond the usual day-to-day variation. The change in symptoms is sufficient to warrant a change in treatment. Determining the presence of an exacerbation is based on a variety of subjective assessments. Airflow limitation may be slightly reduced. Due to increased inflammation and an increase in the work of breathing, gas exchange is worsened and respiratory muscle fatigue more prominent. These factors can contribute to more problems with hypoxemia, hypercapnia, respiratory acidosis, and respiratory failure.

Exacerbations can be classified according to severity from level 1 to level 3. Level 1 exacerbations can be managed on an outpatient basis, level 2 typically requires hospitalization, and level 3 is complicated by respiratory failure. The underlying COPD severity and the presence of comorbidities also influence the classification.

General management of exacerbations includes supplemental oxygen if warranted, intensification of bronchodilator regimens, systemic corticosteroid therapies, antimicrobial therapy in most cases, and ventilatory support if respiratory failure is present.

Acute exacerbations of COPD are associated with increased morbidity and mortality.[71,72] In addition to the increased symptoms and reduced health status, exacerbations have a significant economic impact, and patients are at increased risk of death after an exacerbation. Nearly one third of patients treated in the emergency department for an acute exacerbation had a relapse within 2 weeks.[73] Reducing exacerbation frequency is an important outcome parameter in chronic management of COPD.

Level 1 exacerbations are commonly treated with intensification of bronchodilator therapy. The dosage of short-acting bronchodilators is typically increased, usually with a combination of a short-acting, inhaled β_2-agonist and ipratropium.[74] These agents are chosen because of their relatively faster onset of action and the ability to titrate doses. Therapy can be administered either by MDI or nebulizer, although patients with severe symptoms may have difficulty using the MDI.[75] There is less evidence to support the role of long-acting bronchodilators during acute exacerbations; however, expert guidelines recommend that they be continued or added to therapy if the patient's condition warrants.

Level 1 treatment also involves the use of systemic corticosteroids. A short course of systemic corticosteroids improves lung function and reduces relapse rates. Prednisone 0.5 to 1 mg per kg for 10 to 14 days is adequate; tapering is not required, although it is frequently used.[76] There are insufficient data to support the use of inhaled corticosteroids for COPD exacerbations.

Frequent isolation of *S. pneumoniae*, *H. influenzae*, and *M. catarrhalis*, both in patients with stable COPD and exacerbations, poses a dilemma for the clinician. This finding may represent colonization of the airway, not infection. The presence of two of three findings (increased dyspnea, increased sputum volume, and sputum purulence) has been recommended as an indicator for antibiotic treatment.[77] Improved clinical outcomes, fewer therapeutic failures, and quicker recovery of lung function were noted in antibiotic-treated patients. This finding is reinforced by a meta-analysis of antibiotic trials in COPD patients that also identified a statistical improvement in patients treated with antibiotics versus placebo.[78]

Despite the lack of consensus on the value of antibiotic use and the prevalence of viral infections in these patients, the fact remains that antibiotics are commonly prescribed in COPD patients. This practice results in increased drug therapy expense and almost certainly contributes to the widespread problem of antibiotic resistance. Common antibiotics prescribed include doxycycline, ampicillin or amoxicillin, cephalosporins, and cotrimoxazole. However, newer and broader-spectrum antibiotics continue to be introduced to the market and are commonly prescribed as well. Quinolones, clarithromycin or azithromycin, and β-lactamase inhibitor combination drugs are also commonly used.

Antimicrobial therapy is commonly used for level 1 COPD exacerbations if there is a worsening in at least two chronic symptoms. They provide a small but significant benefit. Traditional agents (e.g., cotrimoxazole or doxycycline) are as effective as newer therapies. Local resistance patterns should be considered when selecting the antimicrobial agent. A course of 7 to 10 days is usually sufficient for treatment.

Level 2 exacerbations are frequently treated on an inpatient basis, although the approach to treatment is similar to level 1 exacerbations. If the patient can take corticosteroids and antibiotics orally, this route is as effective as parenteral therapy. Consideration should be given to using extended-spectrum antimicrobial therapy especially if *Pseudomonas aeruginosa* is suspected as a potential pathogen.

Level 3 exacerbations may require ventilatory support using invasive or noninvasive methods. Aggressive bronchodilator therapy is used; corticosteroid therapy and broad-spectrum antimicrobial therapy may be warranted initially. Noninvasive ventilation using bilevel positive airway pressure (BiPAP) has become popular in recent years because it can reduce the need for intubation and reduce mortality.

Noninvasive ventilation provides ventilatory support through a nasal or face mask. Its use is associated with reduced mortality, improved gas exchange, and shorter hospital stay. It is considered when hypercapnia persists despite aggressive treatment. If noninvasive ventilation does not improve objective and subjective parameters, invasive ventilation must be considered.

For patients hospitalized for a COPD exacerbation, discharge can be considered once the reasons for hospitalization have been treated or controlled. Patients should be stable and close to their pre-exacerbation baseline in terms of their general health. Symptoms should be improving daily and adequate support at home should be available. After hospitalization for an exacerbation, a follow-up evaluation should be scheduled within 1 month.

Some therapies have no proven benefit and should not be used to treat COPD exacerbations or to reduce exacerbation frequency. Oral or intravenous methylxanthines provide minimal benefit during acute exacerbations and should be avoided due to the risk of toxicity and the potential for drug interactions. The use of prophylactic antibiotics to reduce repeated exacerbations has also not proven to be effective. This practice should be avoided because of the potential problems of increasing antimicrobial resistance.

ALTERNATIVE THERAPIES

There is no proven role for the use of alternative therapies in the management of COPD. There is a paucity of data about these therapies, and little is known about the potential for drug interactions. The use of alternative therapies should be avoided.

FUTURE THERAPIES

One class of new therapies that may emerge for the future is phosphodiesterase 4 (PDE4) inhibitors. There is evidence that PDE4 plays an important role in airway inflammation associated with COPD. At least two agents that are selective inhibitors of phosphodiesterase enzyme have been investigated in human studies, cilomilast and roflumilast.

PDE4 inhibitors relax airway smooth muscle and suppress inflammatory mediators that are active in COPD. However, clinical benefits of PDE4 inhibitors have been modest in improving FEV_1 in COPD patients. Another limitation may be the side effect profile: these agents are associated with significant gastrointestinal side effects in nearly 20% of patients.

IMPROVING OUTCOMES

PATIENT EDUCATION

Patient education is an important component of COPD management. Counseling and education can help the patient develop self-management skills, improve coping abilities, and improve overall health status.[79] Important educational topics include risk reduction through smoking cessation strategies, advanced care planning and end-of-life discussions, and early recognition of exacerbations. For inhalation therapies, the patient must understand how to use the various delivery devices correctly. Administering medications for the treatment of lung disease can be difficult, and COPD patients may have specific problems due to comorbidities and advancing age.

METHODS TO IMPROVE ADHERENCE TO DRUG THERAPY

When therapy with ipratropium or another inhaled aerosol is prescribed, the patient should be instructed on the proper administration technique. MDIs are a convenient way to deliver aerosolized drugs, but many patients find it difficult to actuate the inhaler properly and to synchronize inhalation and exhalation for maximum drug deposition. Patients who have difficulty using these delivery devices may experience decreased aerosol deposition within the airways. Patients have also been known to exhale during actuation of the inhaler, preventing any drug from being deposited in the airways. Pharmacologic activity occurs only when sufficient drug is deposited at the bronchial receptors.

Many authorities have made recommendations on the optimal use of MDIs. Actuation of the MDI between tightly closed lips and actuation up to 2 inches in front of widely opened lips are both recommended, and study results disagree on the optimal technique. However, a properly performed closed-mouth technique is as efficacious as using an add-on auxiliary device (spacer). Therefore, either open- or closed-mouth technique is acceptable.

Thorough, repeated instructions, involving observation of the patient's technique whenever possible, should be given during each patient visit. Instructions to the patient for appropriate use of MDIs should include the following:

1. Use the inhaler only at the frequency and dose prescribed. If symptoms worsen, seek medical attention before routinely increasing the dose.
2. Shake the MDI canister thoroughly immediately before use.
3. Exhale slowly and completely.
4. Depress the MDI canister at the beginning of a slow deep inhalation and continue to inhale for 3 to 4 seconds.
5. Hold your breath for 10 seconds (or as long as possible, if not able to do so for 10 seconds).
6. Wait at least 30 seconds between administration of multiple doses.
7. Clean the MDI case and cap thoroughly with water once per day.

Many experts prefer to have patients use spacers routinely. Spacers decrease particle size, resulting in decreased particle deposition in the upper airway and greater delivery of drug to the more distal airways. In doing so, these devices prevent aerosols from being deposited in the oral mucosa and systemic absorption. These auxiliary systems may be useful in patients who fail to properly use MDIs despite education, although many patients may benefit equally from proper explanation and reinforcement of correct MDI use.

Currently, several medications are available as DPIs. These are sometimes called breath-activated inhalers. Technique is just as important when using DPIs as when using MDIs, but the technique for use varies among the devices. Generic instructions for DPI use are as follows:

1. Open the mouthpiece of the device.
2. Load a dose of medication into the device as instructed by the manufacturer.
3. Hold the device upright or horizontal after loading a dose.
4. Exhale fully with your mouth away from the device.
5. Place your lips firmly around the mouthpiece.
6. Begin a steady forceful inhalation from the device, inhaling for 3 to 4 seconds.
7. Remove the device from your mouth and hold your breath for 10 seconds.
8. Exhale and use a second dose if prescribed.
9. Close the mouthpiece on the device.

DISEASE MANAGEMENT STRATEGIES TO IMPROVE PATIENT OUTCOMES

The natural course of COPD is chronic progressive loss of lung function and increasing disability, especially if there is continuing exposure to noxious chemicals and gases. Awareness about screening for COPD has increased in recent years. Identifying patients with risk factors based on exposures or their past medical history, and performing spirometry on these patients, allows early detection and intervention, which can be helpful in slowing disease progression.

A comprehensive approach to disease management for the patient with COPD offers the advantage of addressing diverse issues and needs that are present at various points in the natural course of the disease. Prevention strategies can be directed toward the population at risk for COPD development. The primary focus of prevention is tobacco cessation. For patients with evidence of airflow limitation, prevention also includes providing appropriate immunizations to protect against vaccine-preventable diseases (influenza and pneumococcal infections).

For patients with chronic disease, providing advice about risk factor reduction and pharmacotherapy to relieve symptoms, improve exercise tolerance, and prevent exacerbations and complications can be effective in maintaining overall health status. Early recognition and treatment of exacerbations can reduce the morbidity and mortality associated with these periodic worsenings of disease activity.

Ongoing monitoring of lung function and general health status is an important component to determine the need for additional management strategies. The management goals are the appropriate outcome measures. The effectiveness of various treatments in meeting the goals of COPD management should be evaluated periodically.

Response to pharmacotherapy varies among COPD patients. After therapy is initiated, the clinician should perform periodic assessments of benefit and side effects. The general principles of chronic management are summarized in Table 35.11. Many therapies for chronic management of COPD should be initiated as therapeutic trials; if no benefit is apparent, the therapy should be discontinued. A stepwise approach outlining primary options and alternatives is given in Table 35.12.

TABLE 35.11	General Principles for Pharmacotherapy for Chronic Obstructive Pulmonary Disease (COPD)

- Pharmacotherapy for COPD is used to prevent and control symptoms, improve exercise tolerance and overall health status, and reduce or prevent complications and exacerbations.
- For patients with mild or intermittent symptoms, treatment with short-acting bronchodilators should be initiated on a scheduled or PRN basis.
- For patients who have symptoms despite short-acting bronchodilators, long-acting bronchodilator therapy can improve symptom control and is more convenient.
- Inhaled bronchodilator therapy is preferred. Theophylline is an alternative for patients who cannot or will not use inhaled therapy. However, periodic monitoring of serum concentrations is required due to significant variability in metabolism and the risk for toxicity.
- A trial of inhaled corticosteroid therapy should be considered for patients who continue to have COPD exacerbations despite treatment with one or more long-acting bronchodilators.

TABLE 35.12	Stepwise Approach for Management of Chronic Obstructive Pulmonary Disease (COPD)

Normal Spirometry

Provide education and advice about risk reduction.

For Intermittent Symptoms

Primary Options

SABA for PRN use

Alternative Options

Ipratropium for PRN use

For Mild COPD or Patients With Symptoms Less Than Twice Daily

Primary Options

Ipratropium four times daily + SABA PRN

OR

Ipratropium/SABA combination four times daily

For Moderate COPD or Patients With Symptoms More Than Three Times Daily or Chronic

Primary Options

LABA twice daily + SABA PRN

OR

Tiotropium once daily + SABA PRN

Alternative Options

LABA twice daily + ipratropium PRN

LABA twice daily + ipratropium four times daily + SABA PRN

ICS + LABA twice daily + SABA PRN

ICS twice daily + tiotropium daily + SBA PRN

Theophylline titrated to 8 to 12 μg per mL + SABA PRN

LABA twice daily + tiotropium daily + SABA PRN

LABA twice daily or tiotropium daily + theophylline titrated to 8 to 12 μg per mL + SABA PRN

Patient education and advice about risk reduction (e.g., tobacco cessation) and immunizations should be provided at each level. All therapies above refer to inhaled route of administration, except for theophylline.
SABA, short-acting β-agonist; LABA, long-lasting β-agonist; ICS, inhaled corticosteroid.

PHARMACOECONOMICS

There is a paucity of data concerning pharmacoeconomic assessments of various management strategies. However, it is clear that smoking cessation strategies and administering appropriate immunizations to high-risk patients are two of the most cost-effective interventions in modern medicine. Those strategies should be used in COPD patients independent of disease severity.

According to COPD management guidelines, pharmacotherapy for patients with mild disease and intermittent symptoms should be initiated with short-acting, inhaled bronchodilators (e.g., short-acting inhaled β-agonists or ipratropium). This is based on the efficacy of these treatments in relieving intermittent symptoms and the favorable cost compared to newer long-acting therapies.

A pharmacoeconomic assessment of two clinical trials totaling over 1,000 patients was conducted to compare the cost savings of combining albuterol and ipratropium compared with either treatment alone for COPD management.[80] The combination therapy and the ipratropium treatment group experienced one-third fewer exacerbations compared to the albuterol treatment group, and this translated to a 24% lower overall cost of care.

There is a need for similar data concerning other interventions. Pulmonary rehabilitation programs require significant resources, and the cost/benefit ratio of instituting and maintaining these efforts would be useful information. Similarly, long-acting bronchodilator therapies and inhaled corticosteroids are significantly more expensive than short-acting bronchodilators. However, assessments of overall cost savings due to fewer exacerbations and reduced morbidity and mortality would provide insight into the best candidates for these therapies.

ETHICAL AND ADVANCED CARE PLANNING

The natural course of COPD is a chronic progressive decline in lung function. Recurrent exacerbations of COPD increase the risk of respiratory failure and mortality. Respiratory failure is characterized by worsening hypoxemia and hypercapnia that may require assisted ventilatory support. Advanced care planning enables the patient, family, and clinician to determine the patient's wishes in the event of an acute event. Most patients with advanced COPD have not participated in advanced care planning.[81]

Patients with severe COPD are more likely to experience severe exacerbations accompanied by respiratory failure requiring ventilatory support. The use of ventilatory support is associated with a poor prognosis. In addition, treatment may not result in substantial improvement of this chronic progressive disease. Advanced care planning, including end-of-life directives, allows for patients to be transitioned to palliative care, which can provide relief of symptoms and address emotional and spiritual issues.

The use of advanced care planning and end-of-life directives allows patients and their families to carefully consider their wishes before decisions are required emergently. These approaches allow for flexibility in integrating palliative care with routine care. When used appropriately, advanced care planning can relieve much of the discomfort and anxiety associated with progression of COPD as a terminal illness.

KEY POINTS

- COPD is a potentially preventable disease. Because smoking contributes to the majority of COPD cases, smoking cessation would dramatically decrease its incidence. Public education about the hazards of smoking should continue. Health care professionals should model wellness by not smoking, and they should make concerted efforts to have patients stop smoking
- Increased awareness about risk factors for COPD may improve early identification and intervention of COPD
- Smoking cessation is the most important and most effective strategy to slow the progressive loss of lung function that characterizes COPD
- For patients with mild disease or intermittent symptoms, short-acting bronchodilator therapy is recommended based on safety, efficacy, and cost-effectiveness
- Long-acting inhaled bronchodilators (β-agonists or tiotropium) are effective in controlling symptoms and improving exercise capacity in patients who continue to have symptoms despite the use of short-acting agents
- Inhaled corticosteroids can be added to long-acting bronchodilator therapies for patients with moderate to severe disease who continue to experience two or more exacerbations annually
- Greater attention should be focused on the use of comprehensive pulmonary rehabilitation programs and advanced care planning to address the needs of patients with more severe forms of COPD

SUGGESTED READINGS

Celli BR, MacNee W. Standards for the diagnosis and treatment of patients with COPD: a summary of the ATS/ERS position paper. Eur Respir J 23:932–946, 2004; full report available at www.thoracic.org/copd/

Chronic obstructive pulmonary disease: management of chronic obstructive pulmonary disease in adults in primary and secondary care. Clinical Guideline 12. National Collaborating Centre for Chronic Conditions. National Institute for Clinical Excellence. London, February 2004. Available at: www.nice.org.uk/CG012NICEguideline.

Sin DD, McAlister FA, Man SFP, et al. Contemporary management of chronic obstructive pulmonary disease. JAMA 290:2301–2312, 2003.

REFERENCES

1. Celli BR, MacNee W. Standards for the diagnosis and treatment of patients with COPD: a summary of the ATS/ERS position paper. Eur Respir J 23: 932–946, 2004. Full report available at www.thoracic.org/copd/
2. Global Initiative for Chronic Obstructive Pulmonary Diseases (GOLD Guidelines). Available at www.goldcopd.com.
3. Fletcher C, Peto R, Tinker C, et al. The Natural History of Chronic Bronchitis and Emphysema. New York: Oxford University Press, 1976:82–84.
4. Prescott E. Tobacco-related diseases: the role of gender. Dan Med Bull 47:115–131, 2000.
5. Rahman Q, Nettesheim P, Smith K, et al. International conference on environmental and occupational lung diseases. Environ Health Perspect 109:425–443, 2001.
6. Clancy C. Improving Health Care for Americans With Disabilities. Bethesda, MD: Agency for Healthcare Research and Quality: U.S. Department of Health and Human Services, 2002. AHRQ Publication No. 02–M016.
7. Mannino DM, Gangon RC, Petty TL, et al. Obstructive lung disease and low lung function in adults in the United States: data from the National Health and Nutrition Examination Survey, 1988–1994. Arch Intern Med 160:1683–1689, 2000.
8. Prescott E, Vestbo J. Socioeconomic status and chronic obstructive pulmonary disease. Thorax 54:737–741, 1999.
9. Mannino DM, Homa DM, Akinbami LJ, et al. Chronic obstructive pulmonary disease surveillance, United States, 1971–2000. MMWR Surveill Summ 51:1–16, 2002.
10. Feenstra TL, van Genugten MLL, Hoogenveen RT, et al. The impact of aging and smoking on the future burden of chronic obstructive pulmonary disease. Am J Respir Crit Care Med 164:590–596, 2001.
11. National Center for Health Statistics. FASTATS for COPD. Available at awww.cdc.gov/nchs/fastats/copd.htm.
12. Calverley PMA, Walker P. Chronic obstructive pulmonary disease. Lancet 362:1053–1061, 2003.
13. National Heart Lung and Blood Institute. Morbidity and Mortality Chartbook, 2004. Available at www.nhlbi.nih.gov/resources/docs/cht-book.htm.
14. Mullen JB, Wright JL, Wiggs BR, et al. Reassessment of inflammation of airways in chronic bronchitis. Br Med J 291:1235–1239, 1985.
15. MacNee W. Pathophysiology of cor pulmonale in chronic obstructive pulmonary disease. Part 2. Am J Respir Crit Care Med 150:1158–1168, 1994.
16. Repine JE, Bast A, Lankhorst I. Oxidative stress in chronic obstructive pulmonary disease. Oxidative Stress Study Group. Am J Respir Crit Care Med 156:341–357, 1997.
17. O'Donnell DE, Revill SM, Webb KA. Dynamic hyperinflation and exercise intolerance in chronic obstructive pulmonary disease. Am J Respir Crit Care Med 164:770–777, 2001.
18. Carroll GC, Rothenberg DM. Carbon dioxide narcosis. Chest 102:986, 1992.
19. Schols AM, Slangen J, Volovics L, et al. Weight loss is a reversible factor in the prognosis of chronic obstructive pulmonary disease. Am J Respir Crit Care Med 157:1791–1797, 1998.
20. Murphy TF, Sethi S. Bacterial infection in chronic obstructive pulmonary disease. Am Rev Respir Dis 146:1067–1083, 1992.
21. Wilson R, Dowling R, Jackson A. The biology of bacterial colonization and invasion of the respiratory mucosa. Eur Respir J 9:1523–1530, 1996.
22. National Lung Health Education Program (NLHEP) Committee. Strategies in preserving lung health and preventing COPD and associated diseases—The National Lung Health Education Program (NLHEP). Chest 113:2 (Feb Suppl):123–163, 1998.
23. Breslin E, van der Schens C, Breukink S, et al. Perception of fatigue and quality of life in patients with COPD. Chest 114:958–964, 1998.
24. Gibson GJ, MacNee W. Chronic obstructive pulmonary disease: investigations and assessment of severity. In: Postma DS, Siafakas NM, eds. Management of Chronic Obstructive Pulmonary Disease. Eur Respir Mon 7:25–40, 1998.
25. Landbo C, Prescott E, Lange P, et al. Prognostic value of nutritional status in chronic obstructive pulmonary disease. Am J Respir Crit Care Med 160:1856–1861, 1999.
26. Nishimura K, Izumi T, Tsukino M, et al. Dyspnea is a better indicator of 5-year survival than airway obstruction in patients with COPD. Chest 121:1434–1440, 2002.
27. Anthonisen NR, Connett JE, Murray RP, et al. Smoking and lung function of Lung Health Study participants after 11 years. Am J Respir Crit Care Med 166:675–679, 2002.
28. Dolovich MB, Ahrens RC, Hess DR, et al. Device selection and outcomes of aerosol therapy: evidence-based guidelines. Chest 127:335–371, 2005.
29. Gross N, Tashkin D, Miller R, et al. Inhalation by nebulization of albuterol-ipratropium combination (Dey combination) is superior to

either agent alone in the treatment of chronic obstructive pulmonary disease. Respiration 65:354–362, 1998.

30. O'Donnell DE, Lam M, Webb KA. Spirometric correlates of improvement in exercise performance after anticholinergic therapy in chronic obstructive pulmonary disease. Am J Respir Crit Care Med 160:542–549, 1999.

31. Truitt T, Witko J, Halpern M. Levalbuterol compared to racemic albuterol: a retrospective evaluation in hospitalized patients with COPD or asthma. Chest 123:128–138, 2003.

32. Rennard, SI, Anderson W, ZuWallack R, et al. Use of a long-acting inhaled beta-2 adrenergic agonist, salmeterol xinafoate, in patients with chronic obstructive pulmonary disease. Am J Respir Crit Care Med 163:1087–1092, 2001.

33. Dahl R, Greefhorst LAPM, Nowak D, et al. Inhaled formoterol dry powder versus ipratropium bromide in chronic obstructive pulmonary disease. Am J Respir Crit Care Med 164:778–784, 2001.

34. Braun SR, Keim NL, Dixon RM, et al. The prevalence and determinants of nutritional changes in chronic obstructive pulmonary disease. Chest 86:558–563, 1984.

35. Braun SR, Levy SF. Comparison of ipratropium bromide and albuterol in chronic obstructive pulmonary disease: a three-center study. Am J Med 91:28S–32S, 1991.

36. Tashkin DP, Ashutosh K, Bleecker ER, et al. Comparison of the anticholinergic bronchodilator ipratropium bromide with metaproterenol in chronic obstructive pulmonary disease. Am J Med 81:81–90, 1986.

37. Vincken W, van Noord JA, Greefhorst APM, et al. Improved health outcomes in patients with COPD during one year's treatment with tiotropium. Eur Respir J 19:209–216, 2002.

38. Donohue JF, van Noord JA, Bateman ED, et al. A six-month, placebo-controlled study comparing lung function and health status changes in COPD patients treated with tiotropium or salmeterol. Chest 122:47–55, 2002.

39. Brusasco V, Hodder R, Miravittles M, et al. Health outcomes following treatment for six months with once-daily tiotropium compared with twice-daily salmeterol in patients with COPD. Thorax 58:399–404, 2003.

40. Combivent Inhalation Aerosol Study Group. In chronic obstructive pulmonary disease, a combination of ipratropium and albuterol is more effective than either agent alone: an 85-day multicenter trial. Chest 105:1411–1419, 1994.

41. Ohrui T, Yanai M. Sekizawa K, et al. Effective site of bronchodilation by beta-adrenergic and anti-cholinergic agents in patients with chronic obstructive pulmonary disease: direct measurement of intrabronchial pressure with a new catheter. Am Rev Respir Dis 146:88–91, 1992.

42. Bleecker ER. Acute bronchodilating effects of ipratropium bromide and theophylline in chronic obstructive pulmonary disease. Am J Med 91:24S–27S, 1991.

43. Filuk RB, Easton PA, Anthonisen NR. Responses to large doses of salbutamol and theophylline in patients with chronic obstructive pulmonary disease. Am Rev Respir Dis 132:871–874, 1985.

44. Guyatt GH, Townsend M, Pugsley SO, et al. Bronchodilators in chronic air-flow limitation: effects on airway function, exercise capacity, and quality of life. Am Rev Respir Dis 135:1069–1074, 1987.

45. Martin RJ, Park J, Overnight theophylline concentrations and effects on sleep and lung function in chronic obstructive pulmonary disease. Am Rev Respir Dis 145:540–544, 1992.

46. Jones PW, Bosh TK. Quality of life changes in COPD patients treated with salmeterol. Am J Respir Crit Care Med 155:1283–1289, 1997.

47. Gross N, Tashkin D, Miller R, et al. Inhalation by nebulization of albuterol-ipratropium combination (Dey combination) is superior to either agent alone in the treatment of chronic obstructive pulmonary disease. Respiration 65:354–362, 1998.

48. Van Noord JA, de Munck DR, Bantje TA, et al. Long-term treatment of chronic obstructive pulmonary disease with salmeterol and the additive effect of ipratropium. Eur Respir J 15:878–885, 2000.

49. Zuwallack RL, Mahler DA, Reilly D, et al. Salmeterol plus theophylline combination therapy in the treatment of COPD. Chest 119:1661–1670, 2001.

50. Burge PS, Calverley PM, Jones PW, et al. Randomized, double-blind placebo-controlled study of fluticasone propionate in patients with moderate to severe chronic obstructive pulmonary disease. Br Med J 320:1297–1303, 2000.

51. Lung Health Study Research Group. Effect of inhaled triamcinolone on the decline in pulmonary function in chronic obstructive pulmonary disease. N Engl J Med 343:1902–1909, 2000.

52. Vestbo J, Sorensen T, Lange P, et al. Long-term effect of inhaled budesonide in mild and moderate chronic obstructive pulmonary disease: a randomized controlled trial. Lancet 353:1819–1823, 1999.

53. Pauwels RA, Lofdahl CG, Laitinen LA, et al. Long-term treatment with inhaled budesonide in persons with mild chronic obstructive pulmonary disease who continue smoking: European Respiratory Society Study on Chronic Obstructive Pulmonary Disease. N Engl J Med 340:1948–1953, 1999.

54. Alsaeedi A, Sinn DD, McAlister FA. The effects of inhaled corticosteroids in chronic obstructive pulmonary disease: a systematic review of randomized placebo-controlled trials. Am J Med 113:59–65, 2002.

55. Calverley PM, Boonsawat W, Cseke Z, et al. Maintenance therapy with budesonide and formoterol in chronic obstructive pulmonary disease. Eur Respir J 22:912–919, 2003.

56. Calverley P, Pauwels R, Vestbo J, et al. Combined salmeterol and fluticasone in the treatment of chronic obstructive pulmonary disease: a randomized controlled trial. Lancet 361:449–456, 2003.

57. Begin P, Grassino A. Inspiratory muscle dysfunction and chronic hypercapnia in chronic obstructive pulmonary disease. Am Rev Respir Dis 143:905–912, 1991.

58. Clinical Practice Guideline. Treating tobacco use and dependence. Available at www.surgeongeneral.gov/tobacco/default.htm.

59. Anthonisen NR, Connett JE, Kiley JP, et al. Effects of smoking intervention and the use of an inhaled anticholinergic bronchodilator on the rate of decline of FEV1. JAMA 272:1497–1505, 1994.

60. Pulmonary rehabilitation: official statement of the American Thoracic Society. Am J Respir Crit Care Med 159:1666–1682, 1999.

61. Ries AL, Kaplan RM, Limberg TM, et al. Effects of pulmonary rehabilitation on physiologic and psychosocial outcomes in patients with chronic obstructive pulmonary disease. Ann Intern Med 122:823–832, 1995.

62. Trooster T, Gosselink R, Decramer M. Short and long-term effects of outpatient rehabilitation in patients with chronic obstructive pulmonary disease: a randomized trial. Am J Med 109:207–212, 2000.

63. Schols AMWJ, Soeters PB, Dingemans AMC, et al. Prevalence and characteristics of nutritional depletion in patients with stable COPD eligible for pulmonary rehabilitation. Am Rev Resp Dis 147:1151–1156, 1993.

64. Creutzberg EC, Schols AM, Weling Scheepers CA, et al. Characterization of nonresponse to high caloric oral nutritional therapy in depleted patients with chronic obstructive pulmonary disease. Am J Respir Crit Care Med 161:745–752, 2000.

65. Nichol KL, Baken L, Nelson A. Relation between influenza vaccination and outpatient visits, hospitalization, and mortality in elderly patients with chronic lung disease. Ann Intern Med 130:397–403, 1999.

66. Williams JH, Moser KM. Pneumococcal vaccine and patients with chronic lung disease. Ann Intern Med 104:106–109, 1986.

67. Nocturnal Oxygen Therapy Trial Group. Continuous or nocturnal oxygen therapy in hypoxemic chronic obstructive lung disease. Ann Intern Med 93:391–398, 1980.

68. Report of the Medical Research Council Working Party. Long-term oxygen therapy in chronic hypoxic cor pulmonale complicating chronic bronchitis and emphysema. Lancet 1:681–686, 1981.

69. Carter R. Oxygen and acid–base status: measurement, interpretation, and rationale for oxygen therapy. Chapter 5. In: Tiep BL, ed. Portable Oxygen Therapy: Including Oxygen-Conserving Methodology. Mt Kisco, NY: Futura Publishing Co, 1991:136–138.

70. National Emphysema Treatment Trial Research Group. A randomized trial comparing lung volume reduction surgery with medical therapy for severe emphysema. N Engl J Med 348:2059–2073, 2003.

71. Connors AF Jr, Dawson NV, Tomas C, et al. Outcomes following acute exacerbation of severe chronic obstructive lung disease. Am J Respir Crit Care Med 154:959–967, 1996.

72. Fuso L, Incalzi RA, Pistrelli R, et al. Predicting mortality of patients hospitalized for acute exacerbated chronic obstructive pulmonary disease. Am J Med 98:272–277, 1995.

73. Emerman CL, Effron D, Lukens TW. Spirometric criteria for hospital admission of patients with acute exacerbations of COPD. Chest 99:595–599, 1991.

74. Karpel JP, Pesin J, Greenberg D, et al. A comparison of the effects of ipratropium bromide and metaproterenol sulfate in acute exacerbations of COPD. Chest 98:835–839, 1990.

75. Turner MO, Patel A, Ginsburg S, et al. Bronchodilator delivery in acute airflow obstruction: a meta-analysis. Arch Intern Med 157:1736–1744, 1997.

76. Thompson WH, Nielson CP, Carvalho P, et al. Controlled trial of oral prednisone in outpatients with acute COPD exacerbations. Am J Respir Crit Care Med 154:407–412, 1996.

77. Anthonisen NR, Manfreda J, Warren CPW, et al. Antibiotic therapy in exacerbations of chronic obstructive pulmonary disease. Ann Intern Med 106:196–204, 1987.

78. Saint S, Bent S, Vittinghoff E, et al. Antibiotics in chronic obstructive pulmonary disease exacerbations: a meta-analysis. JAMA 273:957–960, 1995.

79. Celli BR. Pulmonary rehabilitation in patients with COPD. Am J Repir Crit Care Med 152:861–864, 1995.

80. Friedman M, Serby CW, Menjoge SS, et al. Pharmacoeconomic evaluation of a combination of ipratropium bromide plus albuterol compared with ipratropium alone and albuterol alone in COPD. Chest 115:635–641, 1999.

81. Heffner JE, Fahy B, Hilling L, et al. Attitudes regarding advance directives among patients in pulmonary rehabilitation. Am J Respir Crit Care Med 154:1735–1740, 1996.

Cystic Fibrosis

Paul Beringer and Emily Han

TREATMENT GOALS

- Slow progressive deterioration in pulmonary function and maintain normal growth and maturation.
- Treat infection and inflammation and reduce airway obstruction to improve or maintain pulmonary function.
- Replace pancreatic enzymes and ensure adequate caloric intake to achieve normal growth.

Cystic fibrosis (CF) is one of the most common lethal genetic disease in the United States today, affecting nearly 30,000 children and young adults.[1] It is caused by a single gene mutation on the long arm of chromosome 7, whose protein product is the cystic fibrosis transmembrane regulator (CFTR). According to current theory, CFTR regulates sodium and chloride transport across the apical membrane of epithelial cells. CFTR is present in many organs throughout the body, including sweat glands, respiratory tract, pancreas, and gastrointestinal, hepatobiliary, and reproductive organs. The primary clinical characteristics of CF are malabsorption and malnutrition caused by pancreatic insufficiency (PI, 80% to 90%), chronic sinopulmonary infection, and male infertility. The major causes of morbidity and mortality are bronchiectasis and obstructive pulmonary disease, which account for more than 90% of deaths.

Improvements in airway clearance techniques, pancreatic enzyme replacement, and treatment of pulmonary infection provided at CF care centers have greatly improved longevity, increasing median survival from 16 years in 1970 to 32.5 years in 2000 (Fig. 36.1). The percentage of adult patients has also increased: adults represented 29.5% of the population with CF in 1988, and this increased to 40.2% in 2002. The rapid pace of research into the pathophysiology of the disease promises to bring new treatment strategies that will contribute to even greater improvements.

EPIDEMIOLOGY

CF is an autosomal recessive trait that affects 1 of every 3,300 live births.[1] To inherit CF, an individual must receive a defective copy of the CF gene from each parent. If both parents are carriers, there is a 25% chance of inheriting CF, a 50% chance of becoming a carrier, and a 25% chance of being unaffected. Currently, 1 in 29 Americans (nearly 10 million) is an asymptomatic carrier of this disease.

Because of the great degree of variability in the clinical course of CF, much work is being conducted to identify specific mutations of CFTR. Since the discovery of the gene responsible for CF, more than 1,300 different mutations have been identified (http://www.genet.sickkids.on.ca/cftr/). A classification scheme for mutations based on CFTR protein alterations has been proposed.[2] The six classes include class I, defective synthesis; class II, block in processing and trafficking; class III, defective regulation; class IV, decreased conductance; class V, reduced synthesis; and class VI, decreased stability. The most common mutation (accounting for 70% among whites) is a processing defect (class II mutation) that arises from a 3-bp deletion, resulting in the loss of the amino acid phenylalanine at position 508 in the CFTR protein (ΔF508). Patients who are homozygous for ΔF508

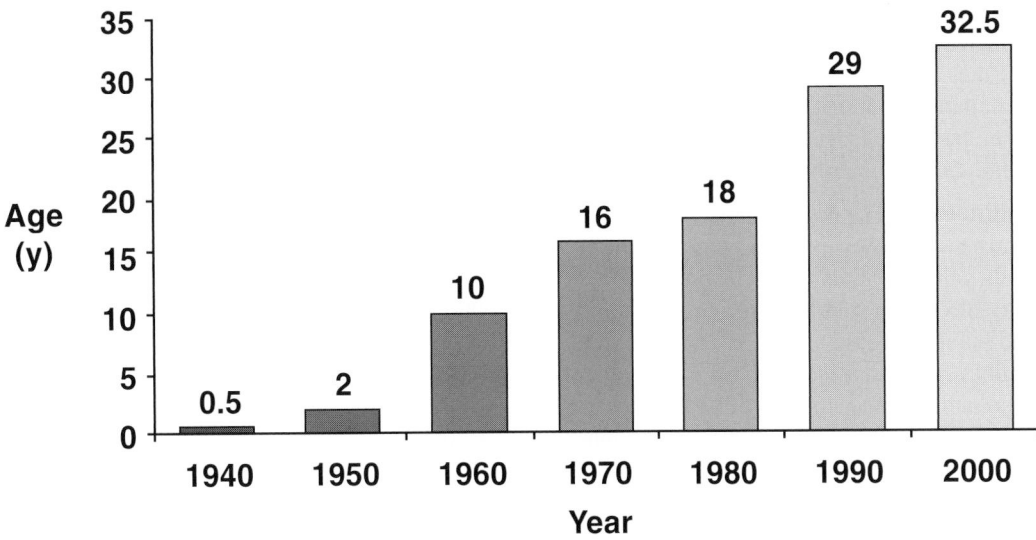

Data from Cytstic Fibrosis Foundation, Bethesda, Md.

FIGURE 36.1 Median survival age for patients with cystic fibrosis in the United States.

(both genes carry the mutant allele) are pancreatic insufficient. Patients who are pancreatic sufficient tend to have a better overall prognosis than their pancreatic-insufficient counterparts. In some cases, therefore, knowledge of a patient's genotype provides information about the phenotype. This type of classification scheme may serve as a prognostic indicator and provide a framework for specific treatments based on the class of mutation involved.

PATHOPHYSIOLOGY

The present theory holds that the basic defect in CF is decreased chloride transport. Reduced chloride transport is accompanied by alterations in sodium and water transport, leading to dehydrated, thickened secretions. These thickened secretions are associated with obstruction and eventual destruction of exocrine glands. The primary systems affected include the sweat gland, the respiratory system, the pancreas, the gastrointestinal and hepatobiliary systems, and the reproductive organs.

SWEAT GLAND

In the sweat duct, CFTR reabsorbs chloride from sweat. Dysfunctional CFTR therefore inhibits reabsorption of chloride, resulting in a nearly fivefold elevation in sweat chloride concentrations. This aberration is the principal laboratory criterion for diagnosis of CF. Sweat chloride concentrations lower than 40 mmol per L are normal (person does not have CF); values between 40 and 60 mmol per L are borderline, and sweat chloride concentrations greater than 60 mmol per L are consistent with the diagnosis of CF. The sweat chloride defect predisposes patients with CF to heat prostration. Ade-

quate attention to dietary salt and fluid intake, especially during the summer, is necessary.

REPRODUCTIVE SYSTEM

Infertility among men and women is common. More than 95% of men with CF have congenital bilateral absence of the vas deferens (CBAVD) and are therefore sterile. In women with CF, cervical mucus is dehydrated and fails to increase during midcycle, which can reduce fertility.[3] Pregnancy was of concern in the past because it was thought to result in increased health risk to the mother. However, results of a study of 258 women with CF indicate that pregnancy does not alter the rate of deterioration in pulmonary function.[4]

GASTROINTESTINAL TRACT

Pancreas. One of the primary functions of the pancreas is secretion of lipase and colipase, which are responsible for hydrolyzing a large proportion of dietary triglycerides. PI results in malabsorption principally of fat through incomplete digestion. In addition, secretion of bicarbonate by the pancreas is reduced in both pancreatic-sufficient and -insufficient patients. This impairs digestion because an alkaline environment is necessary for optimal activity of both endogenous and exogenous pancreatic enzymes. Although the exact function of CFTR in the pancreatic duct cells has not been identified, it is presumed that its dysfunction results in reduced chloride and water secretion, leading to protein precipitation and ductule plugging.[5] Progression of pancreatic disease is associated with the onset of cystic fibrosis–related diabetes mellitus (CFRD). Evidence suggests that CFRD results from insulin resistance and decreased insulin secretion and is associated with worsened clinical status.[6] The prevalence of CFRD is 12%.

Stomach and Esophagus. Gastroesophageal reflux results from an increased number of inappropriate transient relaxations of the lower esophageal sphincter (LES).[7] Cough, forced expirations during chest physiotherapy, and hyperinflation of the lung increase the abdominothoracic pressure gradient, thereby contributing to reflux.[8]

Liver and Gallbladder. The pathogenesis of liver disease in CF is currently unclear; however, the presence of CFTR in epithelial cells lining the biliary ductules suggests a deficiency in biliary electrolyte and fluid secretion, leading to obstruction and biliary cirrhosis if severe.[9,10] The development of cholelithiasis (gallstones) increases with age (15% of young adults) and is associated with PI.[11] Fecal loss of bile acids, resulting in diminished reserves, is thought to be the predisposing factor in the formation of gallstones in patients with CF.[12]

LUNG

Respiratory disease is of major importance in patients with CF because it is the primary factor responsible for repeated hospitalizations, pulmonary function decline, and more than 90% of mortality. Chronic bronchitis that progresses to bronchiectasis and eventual respiratory failure characterizes this process. The pathogenesis of CF airway disease is depicted in Figure 36.2. (a) In normal individuals, a thin mucous layer resides on top of the periciliary liquid, which facilitates mucociliary clearance. Mucociliary clearance is a part of the innate host defense mechanisms designed to clear the airways of unwanted substances to which an individual may have been exposed (bacteria, allergens). (b) In patients with CF, the CFTR defect reduces the periciliary liquid layer, resulting in markedly thickened mucus and impaired mucociliary clearance.[13] (c) Continued mucous hypersecretion

Pathophysiological Cascade

Treatment

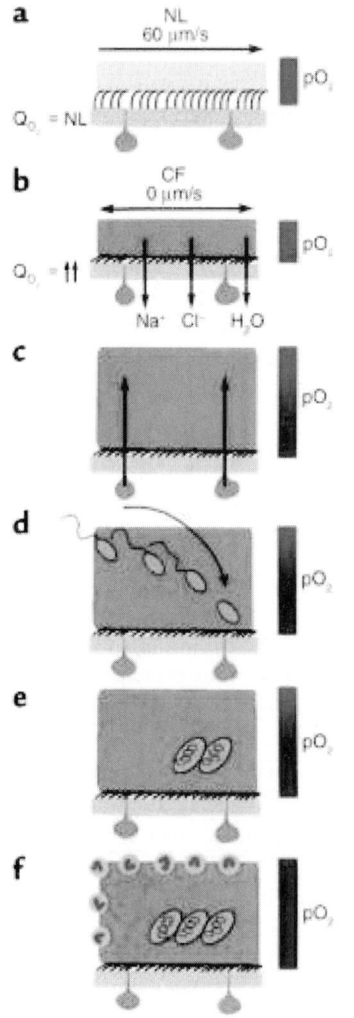

Excessive CF volume depletion
INS 37217 (activate alternate CL- channel)
SPI-8811 (activate alternate CL- channel)
AAV (gene therapy)

Persistent mucus hypersecretion
DNase
Talniflumate

Initial Infection
Inhaled tobramycin

Chronic Infection
Azithromycin
Inhaled tobramycin
Corus 1020 (inhaled aztreonam)

Chronic Inflammation
DNase
Ibuprofen
Azithromycin
DHA (correct fatty acid imbalance)
BIIL-284 (LTB4 Antagonist)

FIGURE 36.2 Proposed pathophysiologic cascade for cystic fibrosis (*CF*) lung disease and the therapeutic interventions targeted at each step. (Reproduced with permission from Worlitzsch D, Tarran R, Ulrich M. Effects of reduced mucus oxygen concentration in airway *Pseudomonas* infections of cystic fibrosis patients. J Clin Invest 109(3):317–325, 2002.)

leads to mucous plugging and airway obstruction. Accelerated ion transport increases oxygen consumption, leading to hypoxic gradients within the mucus. (d) The local environment is suitable for bacteria, resulting in initial/intermittent infection caused by *Pseudomonas aeruginosa*. In addition, reduced host defense proteins (nitric oxide synthase) in the airway epithelial cells of patients with CF[14] and the finding that CFTR acts as a receptor for ingestion of bacteria (e.g., *P. aeruginosa*) also contribute to the predisposition of patients with CF to airway infection.[15] (e) *P. aeruginosa* adapts to the anaerobic environment by increasing alginate production and the formation of biofilms. (f) These biofilms resist secondary defenses, including neutrophils, leading to a chronic cycle of infection and inflammation.

Neutrophil elastase plays a central role in perpetuating the chronic cycle of infection, inflammation, and tissue damage (Fig. 36.3). In the normal host, proteases (e.g., neutrophil elastase), which are released in response to an infectious insult, digest the bacteria, and lung tissue is protected by the presence of antiproteases. However, an exaggerated response occurs in patients with CF because the persistence of bacteria in the lungs overwhelms the antiproteases. Free elastase impairs phagocytosis, causes direct and indirect (through release of free radicals) tissue damage, contributes to airway plugging, and increases neutrophil migration, resulting in further increases in elastase.

Occasionally, infections involve atypical organisms, including *Stenotrophomonas maltophilia* (9.4%) or *Burkholderia cepacia* (3.1%). Infections involving *B. cepacia* are of particular concern because it is typically multidrug resistant, can be transmitted from patient to patient, and may result in deterioration in pulmonary function.[16,17] *Aspergillus* species present a unique challenge in patients with CF. The presence of these organisms ignites an immunologic response characterized by an increase in serum IgE and wheezing in some patients called allergic bronchopulmonary aspergillosis (ABPA).[18] The disease is not invasive; however, damage to the airways as a result of eosinophilic infiltration occurs.[19] The drug of choice for treating ABPA is corticosteroids. Antifungals have also been used as adjunctive therapy, resulting in a reduced corticosteroid requirement.

CLINICAL PRESENTATION AND DIAGNOSIS

SIGNS AND SYMPTOMS

Pancreatic Insufficiency. Pancreatic dysfunction is one of the principal abnormalities in patients with CF. According to the Cystic Fibrosis Foundation (CFF), more than 90% of patients with CF in the United States currently receive pancreatic supplements. In most patients, PI manifests at

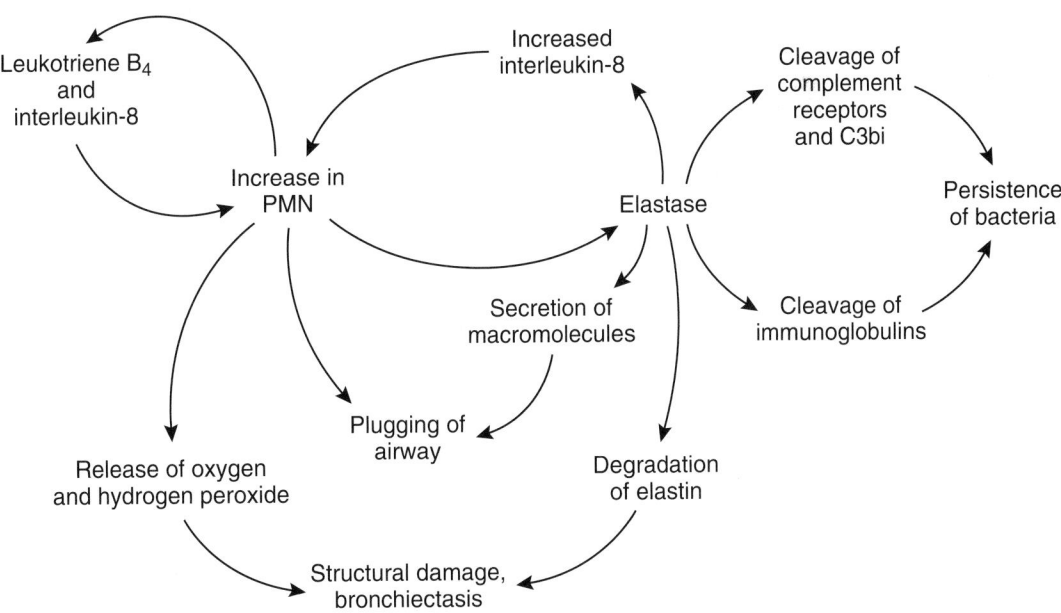

FIGURE 36.3 Products derived from polymorphonuclear leukocytes and their secondary effects on inflammation in the airways of patients with lung disease caused by cystic fibrosis. Leukotriene B$_4$ and interleukin-8 are chemoattractant substances that elicit an increased influx of polymorphonuclear leukocytes (PMNs), which release large quantities of elastase and other proteolytic enzymes as they die. These enzymes degrade structural proteins such as elastin and stimulate the hypersecretion of mucus. Elastase can inhibit phagocytosis of bacteria by cleaving immunoglobulins, complement receptors, and proteins of the complement cascade (C3bi). (Reprinted with permission from Ramsey BW. Drug therapy: management of pulmonary disease in patients with cystic fibrosis. N Engl J Med 335:179–188, 1996. Copyright © 1996 Massachusetts Medical Society. All rights reserved.)

birth or shortly thereafter as failure to grow or gain weight despite adequate oral intake. Additional symptoms include crampy abdominal pain after high-fat meals and frequent bulky, foul-smelling stools. Fifteen percent of patients with CF are pancreatic sufficient.[20] However, PI eventually develops in 10% to 20% of these patients.[21] Pancreatitis is a potential complication that occurs in both pancreatic-sufficient and -insufficient patients. A number of different direct and indirect methods of diagnosing PI have been described. The most widely used is the 72-hour fecal fat analysis, which provides a quantitative measurement of fecal fat losses caused by malabsorption. Recently, measurement of fecal elastase-1 has proved to be a sensitive and specific measure of pancreatic function in patients with moderate to severe PI.[22] These tools can also be used to determine adequacy of the pancreatic enzyme replacement regimen.

Diabetes Mellitus. A period of glucose intolerance usually precedes CFRD onset. The association of the occurrence of CFRD with advancing age suggests that this problem will become more prevalent as further improvements in survival are made. The cumulative incidences identified in a recent prospective evaluation were 1%, 12.5%, and 25% at ages 6 to 10, 18 to 24, and 35 to 44, respectively. A casual or random glucose determination should be performed annually in all patients with CF older then 13 years of age.[23] The incidence of diabetic complications, including retinopathy, nephropathy, and neuropathy, is similar in diabetic patients with and without CF.[24] In addition, the presence of CFRD may increase mortality.[25] Pharmacologic management is similar to that associated with type 1 diabetes. However, dietary considerations differ significantly. A low-fat, low-carbohydrate diet typically is recommended for patients with diabetes. In contrast, in patients with CF, a high-fat high-calorie diet is recommended to prevent malnutrition.

Gastroesophogeal Reflux. Gastroesophogeal reflux is a common symptom of CF. Heartburn and regurgitation are reported in 20% of patients.[26] Progression to esophagitis as evidenced by endoscopy occurs in more than 50% of patients with prominent respiratory symptoms.[27] Treatment is similar to that provided to patients without CF and includes both nonpharmacologic and pharmacologic approaches. Special attention is necessary to avoid possible drug interactions (antacid-quinolones, cimetidine-theophylline) and medications that can decrease LES pressure (theophylline, α-adrenergic agents).

Meconium Ileus and Distal Intestinal Obstruction Syndrome. In the neonate, reduced chloride and water secretion in the intestine is responsible for the presence of meconium ileus (intestinal obstruction) in 10% to 15% of patients.[28] With rare exception, meconium ileus occurs in patients with PI. Pancreatic replacement therapy, therefore, should be considered in affected patients. Treatment typically involves a therapeutic enema or surgical removal as a last resort. Distal intestinal obstruction syndrome (DIOS) is

an analogous complication that is present in 15% of adolescents and adults.[26] This syndrome typically manifests with abdominal pain, nausea and vomiting, and a palpable mass in the right lower quadrant. The use of oral polyethylene glycol electrolyte solution is the preferred treatment. Because of its recurrent nature, maintenance therapy with a high-fiber diet and laxatives is recommended. Prokinetic agents (e.g., metoclopramide) or stimulant laxatives can be used in patients with persistent symptoms.[20]

Cirrhosis and Cholelithiasis. Liver disease is the second leading cause of death among patients with CF (2% annual mortality).[1] The prevalence increases with age, so the overall incidence is expected to increase as further improvements in lung disease treatment are made. Liver disease is more common in patients with PI.[20] Most patients with mild disease are asymptomatic, with the only clinical sign being the presence of a firm, enlarged, or tender liver. Further progression in some patients is evidenced by the clinical manifestations of portal hypertension, variceal bleeding, and liver failure. Laboratory data typically are unremarkable. Elevations in γ-glutamyltranspeptidase are the only significant evidence of cirrhosis.[11] The primary determinant of morbidity and mortality is the presence of portal hypertension and variceal hemorrhaging.[20]

The clinical presentation of cholelithiasis is similar to that of other disorders, with intermittent right upper quadrant pain, nausea, vomiting, jaundice, and dietary fat intolerance. Cholecystectomy is the treatment of choice that is considered for patients who are symptomatic.

Malnutrition. Nutritional deficits can significantly affect the growth and survival of patients with CF.[29] The causes of malnutrition are multifactorial and are influenced by energy intake, losses, and use. Recurrent vomiting caused by coughing or gastroesophageal reflux, chronic respiratory infections, and psychosocial stresses have been implicated in reduced energy intake. PI and reduced bile acid secretion result in malabsorption and loss of fat, protein, and carbohydrates. Increased resting energy expenditure correlates with severity of pulmonary disease.[30]

Deficiencies of fat-soluble vitamins (A, D, E, and K) can occur in patients with CF as a result of PI. Clinical symptoms that result from these deficiencies are uncommon but have been reported.[20] Vitamin D deficiency is found predominantly in patients with inadequate sunlight exposure or cholestatic liver disease. Rickets is extremely rare among patients with CF; however, bone demineralization is a significant problem that occurs in 10% to 15% of adults.[31] Vitamin K production by intestinal flora is reduced during antibiotic use and therefore warrants replacement, particularly in patients with frequent pulmonary exacerbations. Hemorrhagic diathesis resulting from inadequate vitamin K levels is a serious complication that can be prevented by the administration of supplements to patients at greatest risk.

The CFF recommends routine nutritional status assessment, including quarterly anthropometric measurements (e.g., height, weight, triceps skinfold thickness), annual dietary intake and 3-day fat balance, and laboratory studies (e.g., complete blood count, vitamins A and E), to facilitate early intervention. Pancreatic replacement therapy, a high-fat and high-calorie diet, and aggressive pulmonary therapy are essential to improving nutritional status.

Respiratory Disease. The presentation of pulmonary disease is unique, which accounts for its importance in establishing the diagnosis of CF. Chronic cough and sputum production are almost universally present. The frequency of cough and the quantity and appearance of sputum are useful in monitoring for acute exacerbations. Patients also commonly experience wheezing, shortness of breath, and chest tightness as a result of airway obstruction. Hemoptysis is seen occasionally, particularly during exacerbations. Episodes of hemoptysis typically resolve spontaneously after a few days, but medications that may exacerbate bleeding (e.g., nonsteroidal anti-inflammatory drugs (NSAIDs)) should be avoided. Pneumothorax, which occurs in 5% to 8% of patients, occurs with simultaneous onset of dyspnea and unilateral chest pain.[19] Impaired gas exchange, leading to respiratory failure, is observed in patients with severe lung disease or during a severe pulmonary exacerbation in patients with moderate pulmonary disease. In severe cases, respiratory failure can result in pulmonary hypertension and cor pulmonale. Aggressive therapy to treat infection and inflammation is necessary to improve gas exchange. Supplemental oxygen and mechanical ventilation may also be necessary.

CF also affects the upper respiratory tract, manifesting as chronic sinusitis. In addition to the pain, pressure, and congestion it causes, infection can be transmitted to the lower respiratory tract. Sinus surgery is needed in 10% to 20% of patients with recurrent disease and is beneficial in reducing pulmonary exacerbations. Long-term antibiotic lavage has been recommended in patients who need repeated surgical treatment.[32]

Acute pulmonary exacerbations of chronic infection are an inevitable consequence of pulmonary disease in most patients with CF. Pulmonary exacerbations are characterized by increased cough and sputum production, decreased exercise tolerance, weight loss, new findings on chest examination, and fever.[26] Approximately one third of patients experience at least one pulmonary exacerbation annually. Although the exact inciting event is not known, improvement in signs and symptoms is highly correlated with a reduction in sputum bacterial density.[33] *Staphylococcus aureus, Haemophilus influenzae,* and particularly *P. aeruginosa* are commonly cultured pathogens. The goals of therapy in acute pulmonary exacerbation are to reduce bacterial density and improve pulmonary function and nutritional status.

Pulmonary function tests are useful tools for assessing respiratory status. They are typically used periodically to assess disease progression or to determine the effect of a therapeutic intervention (e.g., bronchodilators, a course of antibiotics). The benefit of such interventions is determined by comparison of pulmonary function test results after the intervention with baseline measurements. The two most commonly used measures are forced expiratory volume in 1 second (FEV_1) and forced vital capacity (FVC); the latter represents the total volume of air expelled through the mouth during forced maximal expiration after maximal inspiration. A classification scheme for stratifying patients according to severity of pulmonary disease has been developed. Mild disease is defined as an FEV_1 greater than 70%, moderate as FEV_1 of 40% to 69%, and severe as FEV_1 less than 40% of predicted value for a person of same age and weight with normal lung function.[34] Pulmonary function as measured by FEV_1 declines steadily throughout childhood, adolescence, and early adulthood (Fig. 36.4).

DIAGNOSIS

CF is most commonly diagnosed on the basis of typical signs and symptoms (Table 36.1) and is confirmed by laboratory evidence of CFTR dysfunction. Because of its sensitivity, an abnormal sweat chloride concentration (>60 mEq/L) is the recommended method of identifying CFTR dysfunction. Additional diagnostic methods include abnormal nasal potential differences and genetic mutational analysis, which may be useful in patients with atypical presentations.

Identification of the genetic defect responsible for CF has opened the door for genetic testing. Potential benefits of genetic testing consist of the identification of carriers of a single gene with a mutation and the early diagnosis of CF. However, because more than 1,300 mutations are known, many of which are currently not tested for, a negative result on genetic analysis does not exclude the possibility that the patient has CF or is a carrier of the defective gene. For this reason, a 1997 consensus panel of experts did not recommend routine genetic screening for the entire population.[35] The rapid evolution in technology (i.e., gene chip technology) has resulted in the recommendation for routine newborn screening of the population.

TREATMENT

REPRODUCTIVE DYSFUNCTION

Treatment for infertility in both men and women is available. In men, sperm can be removed from the testes and used for artificial insemination of the partner. In women, infertility has been overcome by artificial insemination beyond the obstructing cervical mucus. However, this raises a number of psychosocial issues, including increased risk of CF in the fetus, perpetuation of an abnormal gene, and increased risk of early parental loss.

LIVER DISEASE

The beneficial effects of ursodeoxycholic acid (UDCA) in treating liver disease in patients with CF have been demon-

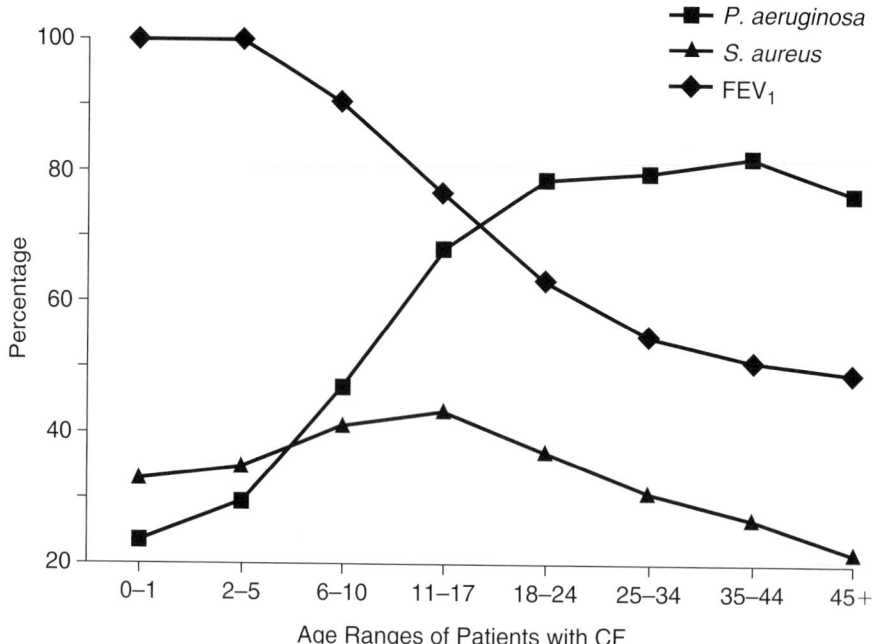

FIGURE 36.4 Age-related changes in microbiology and pulmonary function in patients with cystic fibrosis.

TABLE 36.1	Clinical Features Consistent with a Diagnosis of Cystic Fibrosis

Chronic sinopulmonary disease manifested by the following:

Persistent colonization with typical cystic fibrosis pathogens, including *Staphylococcus aureus,* nontypable *Haemophilus influenzae,* mucoid and nonmucoid *Pseudomonas aeruginosa,* and *Burkholderia cepacia*

Chronic cough and sputum production

Persistent chest radiograph abnormalities (e.g., bronchiectasis, atelectasis, infiltrates, hyperinflation)

Airway obstruction manifested by wheezing and air trapping

Nasal polyps, radiographic or computed tomographic abnormalities of the paranasal sinuses

Digital clubbing

Gastrointestinal and nutritional abnormalities, including the following:

Intestinal: meconium ileus, distal intestinal obstruction syndrome, rectal prolapse

Pancreatic: pancreatic insufficiency, recurrent pancreatitis

Hepatic: chronic hepatic disease manifested by clinical or histologic evidence of focal biliary cirrhosis or multilobular cirrhosis

Nutritional: failure to thrive (protein/calorie malnutrition), hypoproteinemia and edema, complications secondary to the following:

Fat-soluble vitamin deficiency

Salt loss syndromes: acute salt depletion, chronic metabolic alkalosis

Male urogenital abnormalities resulting in obstructive azoospermia

(Reprinted with permission from Cystic Fibrosis Foundation. Clinical practice guidelines for cystic fibrosis. Bethesda, MD; Cystic Fibrosis Foundation, 1997.)

strated in a number of studies. UDCA improves liver function by reducing bile viscosity and preventing obstruction. UDCA is thought to increase clearance and inhibit intestinal absorption of toxic bile acids.[20] Treatment for a 1-year period was associated with significant improvement in clinical score (Shwachman) and liver function tests when compared with placebo in the largest controlled trial conducted to date.[36] However, the biochemical parameters have been shown to reverse to pretreatment values upon discontinuation of UDCA.[20] A prospective study that used liver biopsy testing demonstrated a significant improvement in liver morphology (based on a subjective scoring system that reflected inflammation, bile duct proliferation, and fibrosis) over a 2-year treatment period with UDCA. In addition, UDCA has been shown to improve lipoprotein metabolism, resulting in improvement in essential fatty acid deficiency and correction of vitamin A levels.[37] The long-term benefit in terms of slower progression to portal hypertension is unknown. On the basis of published studies to date, patients with biochemical evidence of liver disease and abnormal morphology on liver biopsy or ultrasound are good candidates for a trial of UDCA. The dosages used were 15 to 20 mg/kg/day and were well tolerated.

PANCREATIC DISEASE

PI is treated with supplementation of exogenous pancreatic enzymes derived from bovine or porcine sources. The available products contain varying quantities of pancreatin or pancrelipase, protease, and amylase formulated as powders, tablets, enteric-coated tablets, and enteric-coated microencapsulated tablets or spheres. The microencapsulated formulations are the most widely used because they provide the greatest protection against inactivation of enzymes by the acidic gastric environment. However, reduced bicarbonate secretion within the CF pancreas fails to provide the optimal pH for dissolution in the intestine. In addition, lipase is inactivated at pH values below 4, which may further reduce the activity of pancreatic enzyme supplements[38]; therefore, normal absorption characteristics are not typically achieved in patients with CF. Treatment usually is sufficient to control symptoms and promote adequate nutrition for most patients. In patients in whom enzyme supplementation is inadequate (symptomatic at dosages of 1,000 to 2,000 units lipase/kg/meal), the use of histamine (H_2) receptor blockers has been shown to increase body weight and reduce stool fat and nitrogen.[38] In addition, alternative factors that contribute to an inadequate response such as poor adherence, alterations in diet, and "generic substitutions" should be considered. Because pancreatic enzymes were available before the Food, Drug, and Cosmetic Act was passed, they have not been subjected to the same scrutiny as other drug products. However, the FDA has recently announced that manufacturers have 4 years within which they must submit a new drug application (NDA) for each of their products to receive marketing approval. Products not receiving approval must be taken off the market by April 28, 2008. This announcement was made in response to numerous reports claiming that these drug products do not have the expected therapeutic effect (http://www.fda.gov/cder/drug/infopage/pancreatic_drugs/pancreatic_QA.htm).

Dosing of pancreatic enzymes is based on lipase content. Ideally, dosing should be based on the quantity of fat grams ingested to mimic the normal physiologic response. It has been estimated that patients need an average of 1,800 lipase U per g of fat per day.[26] A more practical method is to base the dosage on weight. The recommended initial dosage for children younger than age 4 is 1,000 lipase U/kg/meal, and 500 U/kg/meal for patients older than 4, to account for the reduced fat intake per kg of body weight.[26] Dosages can be increased after several days if symptoms persist; however, dosages should not exceed 2,500 lipase U/kg/meal unless they are determined to be effective based on 72-hour fecal fat measurements. Dosages exceeding 6,000 U/kg/meal have been associated with colonic strictures and should be avoided.[39,40]

NUTRITION

In addition to pancreatic enzyme supplements, an adequate caloric intake is necessary to achieve normal nutritional status. A high-fat diet in combination with pancreatic enzymes is recommended because fat is a dense source of energy. A study in children (mean age, 12 years) with CF found that a target of 100 fat g per day provided more than 110% of the recommended daily intake for energy.[41] A common method for assessing nutritional status is to determine the patient's weight-to-height ratio. In patients who are unable to maintain adequate nutrition (weight-to-height ratio less than 90% of ideal) despite appropriate pancreatic supplementation and dietary modifications, oral nutritional supplements are indicated. More aggressive nutritional management (enteral or parenteral support) is necessary for patients in whom significant improvements have not been made within 3 months, or whose weight-to-height ratio declines to less than 85% of ideal. The nutritional status of patients with CF is closely related to pulmonary status, so aggressive pulmonary therapy also improves nutritional status.

Fat-soluble vitamins (A, D, E, and K) are replaced by administration of one or two multivitamins daily. In addition, supplementation with water-miscible forms of vitamin A (5,000 IU) and vitamin E (100 to 400 IU) is needed to normalize the vitamin levels. Alternatively, a higher dosage of the fat-soluble form of vitamin E (200 to 800 IU) may be more cost efficient. Additional vitamin D supplementation typically is not necessary unless the patient has little sunlight exposure. Similarly, vitamin K supplementation above that provided by the standard multivitamin preparation is not necessary unless the patient receives frequent antibiotic exposures or has liver disease. Supplemental dosages are individualized on the basis of measured levels (vitamins A, D, and E) or clinical response (prothrombin time). Multivitamin preparations containing water-miscible preparations of vitamins A, D, E, and K are available and may be helpful in improving patient adherence.

LUNG DISEASE

Reducing Airway Obstruction. The primary way to mobilize thickened pulmonary secretions is through chest physiotherapy. The basic components of chest physiotherapy have been chest percussion and vibration to loosen the mucus, combined with postural drainage to facilitate mobilization and removal via cough. Although effective, this method is time consuming, and a partner is needed. Recently, newer techniques such as airway oscillation (flutter device) and high-frequency chest oscillation (ThAIRapy Vest) have been shown to provide similar or greater improvement in pulmonary function and sputum production with greater independence.[42] The choice of method is determined on an individual basis after effectiveness and compliance have been considered.

Bronchodilators. Response to bronchodilators in patients with CF is variable; patients may demonstrate improvement, no change, or even deterioration in pulmonary function. One method of determining whether a patient may exhibit a positive response to bronchodilators is by bronchoprovocation studies with the use of methacholine and histamine to evaluate patients for airway hyperreactivity. The degree of hyperresponsiveness correlates with airflow limitation severity.[43] In the clinical setting, bronchodilator therapy is considered in patients who demonstrate an increase of 10% or more in FEV_1 after use of an inhaled bronchodilator. However, response within an individual patient may vary over time.[44] Inhaled adrenergic agonists (e.g., albuterol) and parasympatholytic agents (e.g., ipratropium) used alone and in combination have been shown to improve pulmonary function in clinical trials. In addition, β_2-agonists may assist in airway clearance and are often used before chest physiotherapy is performed.[45] The recommended dosages of agents used are similar to those recommended for asthma treatment. The long-acting β_2-agonist salmeterol provides greater improvement in pulmonary function and symptoms than do short acting β_2-agonists.[46]

Mucolytics. The viscoelasticity of airway secretions in patients with CF results primarily from the accumulation of DNA from neutrophil turnover. The abnormal viscosity makes it difficult for patients with CF to expectorate sputum and serves as a medium for bacterial growth. Recombinant human DNase digests extracellular DNA and has been shown to reduce the viscoelasticity of sputum in vitro.[47] Treatment with recombinant human DNase has been associated with significant improvement in pulmonary function and a reduction in the risk of pulmonary exacerbations for which intravenous antibiotics are required.[48] Recombinant human DNase has been recommended for use in patients with chronic endobronchial infection with mucopurulent secretions and an obstructive pattern on pulmonary function testing. Recent evidence demonstrates that DNase also re-

duces airway inflammation and may therefore be an integral early treatment modality in patients with mild pulmonary disease.[49] The emphasis on early treatment in patients with mild pulmonary disease is based on the observation that these patients are at greatest risk for reduction in pulmonary function. Therefore, intensive early treatment may preserve pulmonary function, resulting in improved quality of life. Of note, recombinant human DNase has been shown to form a precipitate when combined with tobramycin solution,[50] and its activity is inhibited when it is combined with macrolides.[51] Recombinant human DNase is available as Pulmozyme in 2.5-mg vials and is administered once daily via jet nebulizer.

Managing Infection. Treatment of pulmonary infection has been integral in the management of CF and has significantly improved survival of this population. Several approaches to the use of antibiotics in CF have been proposed. Intermittent courses of intravenous antibiotics given during acute exacerbations have been the primary mode of administration at CF care centers for a number of years. More recently, maintenance therapy with oral or inhaled antibiotics has been instituted to control the bacterial burden with the intention of extending the time between pulmonary exacerbations. In addition, prophylactic antibiotic therapy has been shown to prevent chronic infection in a few preliminary reports.

Pulmonary Exacerbations. The value of antibiotic therapy in treating pulmonary exacerbations has been demonstrated in a placebo-controlled study that compared the addition of antibiotic therapy with a regimen of chest physiotherapy and bronchodilators alone. A moderate improvement in pulmonary function as measured by FEV_1 (6.6%) was demonstrated in patients treated with chest physiotherapy and bronchodilators alone. The addition of intravenous antibiotics resulted in further improvement in FEV_1 (16%). This improvement was highly correlated with a decline in the density of *P. aeruginosa* in sputum.[33]

Selection of Antibiotic. Antibiotic selection is based on sputum culture and susceptibility data. In the absence of these data, empiric therapy directed at the most commonly occurring organisms (*P. aeruginosa, S. aureus,* and *H. influenzae*) is recommended. Patients may be treated with oral antibiotics in the outpatient setting when respiratory symptoms are mild to moderate.[52] In cases of severe pulmonary exacerbation, or when no improvement is seen with oral antibiotic treatment, intravenous antibiotic therapy is warranted.

P. aeruginosa. Two antibiotics with different mechanisms of action often are used when *P. aeruginosa* is suspected or known to be involved, to prevent the development of resistance and provide potential synergistic activity. For these reasons, the combination of an antipseudomonal β-lactam and an aminoglycoside is the recommended treatment regimen. If recent culture results are available, then the antibiotic therapy should be directed against the identified organisms. Recent studies demonstrate that organisms isolated during exacerbations are of the same strains as those isolated during the asymptomatic period.[53] Therefore, it is not necessary to wait for the culture and susceptibility data from a new sputum culture specimen. It is now known that chronic airway infection with *P. aeruginosa* in patients with CF exists as freely motile or planktonic forms in microcolonies encased within a layer of alginate (biofilms). These biofilms create a significant therapeutic challenge in that they impair local defense mechanisms, are slow growing, and can sequester β-lactamase.[54] Susceptibility results performed with planktonic and biofilm forms of *P. aeruginosa* demonstrate significant discordance, particularly with the β-lactam agents. Because β-lactam agents work by disrupting bacterial cell wall formation, it is not surprising that they demonstrate poor activity against the slowly growing biofilm forms.[55] Clinical trials undertaken to evaluate the outcomes of patients treated according to biofilm susceptibility versus conventional planktonic forms are ongoing. Until these data become available, combination therapy that includes agents active against both planktonic and biofilm forms of *P. aeruginosa* is recommended.

Multidrug-resistant *P. aeruginosa* isolates (defined as resistance to all agents in two of the following classes of antibiotics: β-lactams, aminoglycosides, or quinolones) are frequently isolated among patients who have received frequent courses of antibiotic treatment. Synergy testing may be useful under these conditions to identify combinations of antibiotics with activity that would not be identifiable through standard susceptibility testing of individual compounds. The CF Referral Center for Susceptibility and Synergy Studies (http://syngergy.columbia.edu) performs synergy testing, specifically for isolates obtained from the sputum of patients with CF. Data obtained from synergy testing have not been correlated with clinical efficacy; however, they do provide more susceptibility information than is provided by standard testing performed at most institutions, and they are a good guide for antimicrobial treatment. The combinations of a β-lactam (e.g., ticarcillin, piperacillin, or aztreonam) with tobramycin and of ciprofloxacin with piperacillin have been shown to consistently provide synergistic activity against multidrug-resistant *P. aeruginosa* isolates.[56] Intravenous colistin is another viable option that is being used increasingly in patients with CF because of the lack of new effective agents against multidrug-resistant *P. aeruginosa*. Colistin is a member of the polymixin family, which exerts its action through disruption of the permeability barrier of the outer membrane of gram-negative organisms. It exhibits potent concentration-dependent bactericidal activity and reportedly a low rate of resistance. Primary adverse effects include nephrotoxicity and neurotoxicity, which must be monitored carefully in patients who receive this agent.[57]

B. cepacia. *Burkholderia cepacia*, formally known as *Pseudomonas cepacia*, was first reported in 1980 in patients with CF.[54] *B. cepacia* is a complex that consists of several distinct species or genomovars. Genomovar III (*B. cenocepacia*) is the most frequently isolated and most clinically relevant species in patients with CF.[58] *B. cepacia* is easily transmitted via inhalation or contact with a reservoir of *B. cepacia*, including other patients with CF, health care professionals, or contaminated medical instruments.[59] Colonization with *B. cepacia* can manifest as chronic asymptomatic carriage, progressive deterioration of lung function over a time,[60] or fatal deterioration (known as ''*B. cepacia* syndrome''), ultimately leading to a 50% reduction in life expectancy.[61,62] Chronic infection with *B. cenocepacia* can exclude patients from lung transplant, emphasizing the importance of preventing acquisition of this organism through active infection control measures. When potential outbreak situations arise, isolates can be genotyped via field gel electrophoresis (PFGE) (National Lab of *Burkholderia cepecia*, www.cff.org) to determine whether patients are infected by the same strain. *B. cepacia* is intrinsically resistant to many antibiotics, including aminoglycosides and β-lactams, and quickly acquires resistance to other agents that may have possessed initial activity.[59] Similar to multidrug-resistant *P. aeruginosa*, synergy testing (CF Referral Center for Susceptibility and Synergy Studies) can be useful for identification of combination therapy regimens.

Dosage. The antibiotics most commonly used to treat acute pulmonary exacerbations and their dosage ranges are listed in Table 36.2. Typical dosage regimens used in other populations may be inadequate in patients with CF because of altered pharmacokinetics, reduced lung penetration, decreased activity in sputum, presence of biofilm with *Pseudomonas* isolates, heavy bacterial inocula, and more resistant isolates. Oral antibiotics are used to treat patients with mild to moderate exacerbations, and parenteral administration is reserved for patients with severe exacerbations or those who do not respond to oral therapy.

Antimicrobial Pharmacokinetics and Pharmacodynamics. The pharmacokinetics of a number of compounds appears to be altered in patients with CF. Currently, no unifying mechanism linking the altered pharmacokinetics to a specific alteration in patients with CF exists.[63, 64] Therefore, the appropriate dosage should be determined on the basis of data derived from controlled pharmacokinetic studies or by individualization using measured serum concentrations if possible. In general, higher dosages or more frequent dosing is needed in patients with CF in order to achieve similar peak and trough serum antibiotic concentrations as are achieved in non-CF patients. This approach maximizes lung penetration and antibiotic concentrations at the site of infection.

Aminoglycosides. Results of controlled trials of aminoglycoside (amikacin, gentamicin, and tobramycin) pharmacokinetics indicate that the total body clearance and volume of distribution are greater for patients with CF than for age-matched controls.[65–67] The increased clearance of tobra-

TABLE 36.2	Intravenous Antibiotic Dosage Recommendations for Treating Pulmonary Exacerbations in Patients with Cystic Fibrosis

Antibiotic	Dosage (mg/kg/day)	Doses per Day	Maximum Daily Dosage (g) or Desired Serum Concentration
Amikacin	30	2 or 3	Peak 25–30
		1[a]	Trough <5
Ampicillin-sulbactam	100–150	4	12
Aztreonam	150–200	3 or 4	8
	>100	CI	8
Cefepime	150–200	3 or 4	8
Ceftazidime	150–200	3 or 4	8
	>100	CI	8
Cefuroxime	100–150	3	4.5
Ciprofloxacin	20–30	2 or 3	1.2
Ciprofloxacin (PO)	40	2 or 3	2.25
Colistin	5–8	2–3	0.3
Gentamicin	10	1	Peak 20–30
			Trough <0.5
Imipenem-cilastatin	50–100	4	4
Meropenem	50–100	3–4	6
Nafcillin	100–200	4	12
Piperacillin, ± tazobactam	400[b]	4	24
Ticarcillin, ± clavulanate	400[b]	4	24
Tobramycin	10	1	Peak 20–30
			Trough <0.5
Trimethoprim-sulfamethoxazole	10–20	2	20 mg/kg/day (trimethoprim)

CI, continuous infusion.
[a] Efficacy data with once-daily amikacin administration are limited; a large randomized, multicenter clinical trial with tobramycin demonstrated similar efficacy and reduced nephrotoxicity when compared with multiple daily dosing.
[b] Refers to dosing of piperacillin and ticarcillin components.
(From Mouton JW, Kerrebyn KR. Antibacterial therapy in cystic fibrosis. Med Clin North Am 74:837–850, 1990; Ramsey BW. Management of pulmonary disease in patients with cystic fibrosis. N Engl J Med 335:179–188, 1996; Turpin SU, Knowles MR. Treatment of pulmonary disease in patients with cystic fibrosis. In: Davis PB, ed. Cystic fibrosis. Lung biology in health and disease. New York: Marcel Dekker, 1993:277–234.)

mycin has been attributed to increased nonrenal clearance (e.g., biliary),[67] whereas an increased renal clearance was identified with amikacin.[64] The increased volume of distribution may result from reduced adipose tissue in patients with CF. Because aminoglycosides distribute poorly into adipose tissue, the volume of distribution when expressed per kg of body weight appears elevated.[68]

The pharmacodynamics of the aminoglycoside antibiotics, which is characterized by concentration-dependent bactericidal activity, demonstrates postantibiotic effects (PAEs) against gram-negative organisms, including *P. aeruginosa*. The goal of therapy with these agents is to maximize the peak concentrations relative to the minimal inhibitory concentration (MIC) of the infecting organism, preferably to a ratio of 8 or greater.[69] Because the median MIC for *P. aeruginosa* isolates obtained from patients with CF is 1 μg per mL, peak concentrations in the range of 8 to 12 mg per L are desirable. However, because of the risks of potential nephrotoxicity and ototoxicity with excessive tissue accumulation, serum trough concentrations greater than 2 mg per L for gentamicin or tobramycin should be avoided.[70] Recently, studies evaluating once-daily aminoglycoside dosing have been performed.[71] The goal of these dosage regimens is to administer higher dosages of aminoglycosides at prolonged intervals to maximize the peak concentration (and bactericidal activity) while minimizing accumulation (and risk of toxicity). In theory, the presence of the PAE provides some protection against bacterial regrowth between doses. Currently, data on efficacy with this dosing modality in treating pulmonary exacerbations in patients with CF are limited.[72,73] A randomized, multicenter clinical trial conducted in the UK demonstrated equivalent efficacy between once-daily and multiple daily dosing regimens of tobramycin. It is important to note that the safety data indicate that once-daily administration reduces the incidence of nephrotoxicity in children.[74]

Routine monitoring of serum aminoglycoside concentrations is recommended to maximize efficacy and minimize the risk of toxicity. Because many patients with CF receive multiple courses of aminoglycosides (average, one pulmonary exacerbation per year), sometimes for extended durations (longer than 2 weeks), they are particularly predisposed to developing nephrotoxicity and ototoxicity. Despite this concern, the incidence of renal failure among patients with CF is low (0.2%). However, when the potential for concurrent use of other nephrotoxic agents (e.g., ibuprofen) is considered, vigilant monitoring is an appropriate measure. Auditory toxicity affects high-frequency hearing; appropriate audiometric testing is needed for early detection. Thus, audiometric testing may be appropriate in patients with frequent exacerbations and in those who receive a prolonged course of treatment (longer than 21 days).

β-Lactams. Results of controlled pharmacokinetic studies indicate that the clearances of several commonly prescribed intravenous β-lactams are higher (ticarcillin,[75] ceftazidime[76,77]) or unchanged (cefepime)[78,79] compared with those in matched controls. Similarly, the volume of distribution is shown to be greater (ceftazidime)[76,77] or unchanged (ticarcillin, cefepime) compared with that in matched controls. One possible explanation for the disparity in the clearance of these agents may be related to their specificity for renal transporters. P-glycoprotein is a luminal efflux transporter that, if upregulated in patients with CF, could account for the altered renal clearance of several antibiotics that are substrates for this transporter.[80] Clinical trials undertaken to further investigate this hypothesis are ongoing. In contrast to the aminoglycosides, β-lactams do not demonstrate any appreciable PAE against gram-negative organisms. In addition, they do not exhibit concentration-dependent bactericidal activity, if serum concentrations of at least four times the MIC are achieved. The goal of therapy with this class of antibiotics is therefore to maintain concentrations above this threshold for the entire dosing interval. Because higher concentrations (those exceeding four times the MIC) offer no advantages, some have suggested administering β-lactams as a continuous infusion.[81] Studies with continuous infusion ceftazidime have demonstrated that this method of administration more consistently maintains concentrations above the MIC of *P. aeruginosa* in patients with CF than

does intermittent dosing. In addition, continuous infusion appears to be more efficient: One-third less drug per day is needed to maintain therapeutic concentrations (100 mg/kg/day compared with 150 mg/kg/day for continuous and intermittent dosing, respectively).[82] A recent randomized, crossover study in 70 patients demonstrated significantly greater improvements in pulmonary function in those receiving continuous infusion ceftazidime (200 mg/kg).[83]

Fluoroquinolones. The pharmacokinetics of the fluoroquinolones, particularly ciprofloxacin, has been extensively evaluated in patients with CF. Conflicting results have been demonstrated with respect to differences in pharmacokinetics when compared with age-matched controls.[84–87]

The pharmacodynamic characteristics of the fluoroquinolones are similar to those of the aminoglycosides, demonstrating concentration-dependent bactericidal activity and PAEs against gram-negative organisms, including *P. aeruginosa*. Data about ciprofloxacin pharmacodynamics in CF are limited.

Monitoring Antibiotic Therapy. The typical treatment duration of an acute exacerbation is 10 to 14 days but can extend to 21 days or longer if the signs and symptoms have not improved significantly. Research studies conducted to evaluate new antibiotics have often used improvements in sputum bacterial density or formal measures of pulmonary function (e.g., FEV_1) to assess treatment outcomes. In the clinical setting, improvement in subjective signs and symptoms (decreased cough and sputum production), a return to baseline in spirometric measurements (FEV_1), and an increase in weight are indicative of treatment success. Although slight elevations in temperature and white blood cell counts occur with acute exacerbations, they do not correlate closely with the clinical status of the exacerbation. Elevations in erythrocyte sedimentation rate (ESR) can also occur during exacerbations, reflecting an increase in inflammation. However, ESR is a nonspecific marker of inflammation and therefore may be elevated secondary to other processes (e.g., arthritis).

The availability of home infusion services has enabled patients to be treated at home for pulmonary exacerbations. The advantages of home intravenous antibiotic therapy are that it is less disruptive to normal daily activities and it is substantially less expensive than is hospitalization. Home therapy should be considered for patients with mild to moderate exacerbations for whom the home environment supports this therapy.

Long-term Maintenance Antibiotic Therapy. Recognition of progressive decline in pulmonary function despite aggressive treatment of acute exacerbations and the availability of oral and inhaled therapies with activity against typical CF pathogens have led to increased use of long-term maintenance antibiotic therapy. The goals are to suppress the bacterial infection with the hope of reducing the frequency and severity of pulmonary exacerbations and to slow the progressive deterioration in lung function. Results of controlled clinical trials have established the benefit of long-term inhaled tobramycin and oral azithromycin in improving these outcomes. Currently, the fluoroquinolones are the only oral antibiotics with significant activity against *P. aeruginosa*; however, because of the rapid emergence of resistance during therapy, some clinicians suggest that these agents be reserved for acute exacerbations. Antibiotics and dosage recommendations are listed in Table 36.3. Other approaches such as prophylactic administration of oral or inhaled antibiotics to prevent or delay the onset of chronic infection are being evaluated.

Administering antibiotics via inhalation has the advantage of achieving high concentrations at the site of infection while minimizing systemic exposure and resultant toxicity. A number of different trials performed to evaluate various antibiotics (aminoglycosides, β-lactams, and polymyxins) have demonstrated clinical benefit in long-term maintenance with this route of administration. The most widely studied drug is tobramycin, which is available as TOBI Solution for inhalation. The recommended dose of TOBI is 300 mg twice daily in cycles of 28 days on and 28 off. Therapy with inhaled tobramycin significantly improves pulmonary function (improvement in FEV_1 of 9% to 14%), reduces the risk of hospitalization (37%), and lessens the need for intravenous antipseudomonal antibiotics (32%).[88] These benefits must be weighed against the high cost of aerosolized tobramycin solution (average wholesale price, $18,000/year).

The macrolide antibiotics do not exhibit significant antibacterial activity against *P. aeruginosa* when conventional susceptibility testing methods are used; however, they do inhibit production of alginate, the principal component of biofilms. Biofilm susceptibility testing has demonstrated that the MIC is well within clinically achievable concentrations in sputum.[55] In addition, the macrolides exhibit potent anti-inflammatory activities. Results of a recent randomized controlled trial demonstrated that patients who were treated with azithromycin had significant improvements in FEV_1 and nutritional status, as well as reduced hospitalizations for acute pulmonary exasperation.[89] The recommended doses for azithromycin in patients with CF are 250 mg (weight <40 kg) or 500 mg (weight >40 kg) given three times a week. Subgroup analysis indicates that the beneficial effect of azithromycin on pulmonary function is additive with other long-term therapies such as TOBI and recombinant human DNase.[89]

Early Antibiotic Treatment (Initial Acquisition/Intermittent Infection). The difficulty of eradicating *P. aeruginosa* from the airways once it has been established has led to investigations into early intervention at the time of initial acquisition or during the time of intermittent infection. Early treatment of *P. aeruginosa* in asymptomatic patients with CF can reduce or prolong the time to chronic infection.[90] The goal of this therapy is to prevent or slow the rate of decline in pulmonary function in patients with CF by eradicating the organism from the airways before chronic infection is established. Several therapeutic options have been used for this purpose, including intravenous (IV) antibiotics, oral fluoroquinolones, aerosolized antibiotics, and

TABLE 36.3	Oral and Inhaled Antibiotic Dosage Recommendations for Long-term Suppressive Therapy in Patients with Cystic Fibrosis		
Antibiotic	**Dosage (mg/kg/day)**	**Doses per Day**	**Maximum Daily Dosage (g)**
Oral			
Amoxicillin, ± clavulanate	50[a]	4	2
Cefuroxime	50	2	2
Cephalexin	100	4	4
Ciprofloxacin	40	2 or 3	2.25
Doxycycline	4	2	
Trimethoprim-sulfamethoxazole	10[b]	2	0.32 (trimethoprim)
Inhaled			
Colistin	300 mg/day	2	
Tobramycin	600 mg/day	2	

[a] Based on amoxicillin component.
[b] Based on trimethoprim component.
(From Mouton JW, Kerrebyn KR. Antibacterial therapy in cystic fibrosis. Med Clin North Am 74:837–850, 1990; Ramsey BW. Management of pulmonary disease in patients with cystic fibrosis. N Engl J Med 335:179–188, 1996; Turpin SU, Knowles MR. Treatment of pulmonary disease in patients with cystic fibrosis. In: Davis PB, ed. Cystic fibrosis. Lung biology in health and disease. New York: Marcel Dekker, 1993:277–234.)

combinations of these. Administering antibiotics via inhalation is a convenient method of achieving high concentrations at the site of infection while minimizing systemic exposure and resultant toxicities. Higher rates of *P. aeruginosa* eradication from the airways have been demonstrated in patients receiving aerosolized tobramycin compared with patients receiving placebo. Longer-term studies with larger numbers of subjects are currently under way to more clearly establish the outcomes associated with this treatment.[90]

Managing Inflammation. Recognition of the potent inflammatory response to chronic infection in the airways and its destruction of the lung has led to investigations of various anti-inflammatory agents. The goal of such therapies is to interrupt the infection-inflammation cycle with the intent of slowing deterioration in pulmonary function. As was previously mentioned, the course of lung disease progresses rapidly throughout childhood and adolescence, so early therapy is desirable to slow the deterioration (Fig. 36.4). Therapeutic agents that have been evaluated include oral and inhaled corticosteroids and oral NSAIDs. Because of an increased incidence of growth retardation, cataracts, and glucose intolerance in children, prolonged therapy (longer than 2 years) is not recommended.[91]

Inhaled corticosteroids are an attractive treatment option because in theory they could provide efficacy similar to that of oral corticosteroids without the systemic toxicities. Several short-term trials of inhaled corticosteroids have been reported, demonstrating marginal benefit in pulmonary function. Larger trials evaluating longer-term uses are necessary to determine the role of inhaled corticosteroids in managing chronic inflammation.

NSAIDs are also beneficial in controlling airway inflammation. Ibuprofen is the most widely used and studied agent for treatment of airway inflammation in patients with CF. NSAIDs as a class do not interfere with the lipoxygenase pathway that releases potent neutrophil chemoattractants such as leukotriene B_4 (LTB_4).[92] Ibuprofen is unique in that it is believed to inhibit this lipoxygenase pathway at high doses (serum concentrations of 50 to 100 µg/mL), which ultimately inhibits neutrophil migration and activation. Ibuprofen has been shown to be beneficial in children aged 5 to 13 with mild lung disease.[93] Typical starting dose is 20 to 30 mg per kg given twice daily, but dosage individualization is recommended because of the high dosages needed to achieve therapeutic concentrations and the large interpatient variability in pharmacokinetic parameters. Although results of this trial indicate that ibuprofen therapy is well tolerated, concern about adverse effects (e.g., bleeding, renal failure) has limited the widespread use of this agent. Concern about renal failure is relevant because concurrent aminoglycoside therapy for pulmonary exacerbations may increase the nephrotoxic potential of these agents.[94]

Lung Transplantation. Lung transplantation has been a treatment option for patients with end-stage lung disease since the mid-1980s. Bilateral lung transplantation is the most common operative procedure; however, living-donor lobar transplantation is an alternative that is becoming more common because of a shortage of available organs. The current 5-year survival rate for patients with CF is 48% and appears comparable between the two transplant procedures (bilateral lung versus living-donor lobar). A patient should be considered for transplantation if his or her survival is expected to just exceed the expected waiting period for donor lung availability (currently 6 to 24 months). Specific criteria for lung transplantation include progressive pulmonary function impairment (i.e., FEV_1 less than 30% predicted, severe hypoxemia and hypercarbia), increased frequency and duration of hospitalization for pulmonary exacerbations, the presence of life-threatening pulmonary complications (e.g., massive hemoptysis), and increasing antibiotic resistance of bacteria infecting the lungs.[95] Contraindications to lung transplantation include inability to adhere to the complex treatment plan, major complications affecting other organ systems (e.g., hepatic or renal insufficiency, diabetes with end-organ damage, malignancy), and active infection (human immunodeficiency virus, hepatitis B, *Mycobacterium tuberculosis*). Currently, the lack of sufficient organ donors limits the availability of this treatment for many patients who meet these criteria.

FUTURE THERAPIES

Advances in understanding of the pathophysiology of lung disease have led to investigations of new therapies that act against infection and inflammation and correct the basic defect (impaired chloride conductance). Agents in clinical trials include new inhaled antibiotics for infection, docosahexaenoic acid and LTB_4 antagonists for inflammation, and stimulation of alternative chloride channels and gene therapy for correcting the basic defect (http://www.cff.org/research/clinical__trials.cfm).

INFECTION

The emergence of multidrug-resistant isolates of *P. aeruginosa*[96,97] and *B. cepacia* pose a difficult challenge for clinicians who manage infection in patients with CF. Corus 1020 is an inhaled version of the monobactam antibiotic aztreonam, which is currently in phase 3 testing. When the high levels of antibiotic achieved locally within the airways are considered, it is expected that this agent will provide a new therapy for patients chronically infected with *B. cepacia*. In addition, it will be a useful agent to add for those individuals who experience significant declines in pulmonary function during the TOBI off-cycle month. Of potential concern is the potential collateral damage to susceptibility patterns of other β-lactam agents, which are the primary therapies used in the treatment of patients with acute pulmonary exacerbation.

INFLAMMATION

Recognition of the significant contribution of chronic inflammation to lung destruction has led to investigation of a number of new agents. A recent study shows that people with the CF gene have increased levels of a fatty acid that causes inflammation, and decreased levels of another that reduces inflammation. The two fatty acids in question, arachidonic acid (AA) and docosahexaenoic acid (DHA), are involved in many biological functions, including inflammation. This understanding offers the potential to correct this imbalance through pharmacologic supplementation with DHA. Clinical trials in infants with CF are currently being initiated.

BIIL-284 is an LTB_4 antagonist that is being developed to improve airway inflammation in CF by reducing neutrophil accumulation (Fig. 36.3). Phase 2 trials are currently underway.

The effect of these agents on reducing inflammation and the associated decline in pulmonary function await longer-term evaluation in larger numbers of patients.

CORRECTING THE BASIC DEFECT

Three strategies directed at correcting the basic defect include activation of mutant CFTR, modulation of electrolyte (sodium and chloride) transport, and gene therapy. The advantage of these approaches is that they are directed at the primary defect of CF and therefore are potentially curative. INS 37217 is an agonist for the P2Y2 receptor in airway epithelial cells. Stimulation of this receptor leads to secretion of chloride/water via non-CFTR chloride channels, mucin secretion via goblet cells, and more rapid ciliary beating. The combination of these effects results in increased mucociliary clearance in patients with CF. Phase 2 trials have recently been completed and demonstrated significant improvement in pulmonary function over placebo. SPI-8811 promotes chloride transport through activation of the ClC-2 chloride channel, which is also distinct from the CFTR channel. Restoration of chloride transport should improve airway volume depletion, resulting in improved mucociliary clearance. Phase 2 studies are currently under way. Much recent attention has been placed on curcumin, which has been shown in CFTR knockout mice to correct the intracellular trafficking defect of the ΔF508 CFTR protein. Administration of large doses of curcumin to CFTR ΔF508 mice results in correction of nasal potential difference defect. Currently, phase 1 studies have been initiated in patients with CF who are homozygous for the CFTR ΔF508 defect.[98]

AAV (GENE THERAPY)

The most promising area of research is gene replacement therapy. A number of clinical trials are evaluating the safety and effectiveness of gene therapies mediated by viral and liposomal vectors. The current obstacle is a lack of an efficient delivery system to provide sufficient expression of the gene.[84] When an effective gene transfer strategy is developed, there is hope that this therapy may be curative. A phase 2b study with an adeno-associated virus (tgAAVCF) to deliver a normal copy of the gene into CF airways is ongoing.

KEY POINTS

- CF is a genetic disorder that results from impairment of chloride transport across epithelial cells, causing obstruction of exocrine glands, including sweat glands, respiratory tract, pancreas, and gastrointestinal, hepatobiliary, and reproductive organs.
- Respiratory disease characterized by chronic endobronchial infection and inflammation that results in tissue damage is the primary cause of morbidity and mortality, accounting for more than 90% of deaths.
- Nonpharmacologic therapies (chest physiotherapy) and pharmacologic therapies (bronchodilators, mucolytics) are used to reduce airway obstruction.
- Intermittent courses of antibiotics are used to treat patients with acute pulmonary exacerbation and to decrease bacterial burden.
- Patients with CF exhibit altered pharmacokinetics of many antibiotics and other drugs, necessitating the use of CF-specific dosage guidelines or individualization based on measured concentrations.
- Long-term administration of inhaled antibiotics is used to suppress infection and disrupt the cycle of infection and inflammation that leads to tissue destruction.
- Pancreatic enzyme replacement and a high-fat, high-calorie diet are needed to ensure adequate absorption of food and nutrients necessary to achieve and maintain normal growth.
- As lung disease treatment improves, the incidence of complications involving other organs (e.g., cirrhosis, diabetes mellitus) is likely to increase.
- The most promising area of clinical research is gene replacement therapy. There is hope that this treatment may be curative. However, until it is further developed, conventional therapies directed at maintaining pulmonary function and nutritional status remain the best treatment strategies.

REFERENCES

1. Cystic Fibrosis Foundation. Patient registry 1996 annual data report. Bethesda, MD: Cystic Fibrosis Foundation, August 1997.
2. Zielenski J. Genotype and phenotype in cystic fibrosis. Respiration 67:117–133, 2000.
3. Kotloff RM. Reproductive issues in patients with cystic fibrosis. Semin Respir Crit Care Med 15:402–413, 1994.
4. Fiel SB. Pulmonary function during pregnancy in cystic fibrosis: implications for counseling. Curr Opin Pulm Med 2:462–465, 1996.
5. Kopelman H, Durie P, Gaskin K, et al. Pancreatic fluid secretion and protein hyperconcentration in cystic fibrosis. N Engl J Med 312:329–334, 1985.
6. Hardin DS, LeBlanc A, Lukenbaugh S, et al. Insulin resistance is associated with decreased clinical status in cystic fibrosis. J Pediatr 130:948–956, 1997.
7. Cucchiara S, Santamaria F, Andreotti MR, et al. Mechanisms of gastroesophageal reflux in cystic fibrosis. Arch Dis Child 66:617–622, 1991.

8. Stern RC. Cystic fibrosis and the gastrointestinal tract. In: Davis PB, ed. Cystic fibrosis. Lung biology in health and disease. New York: Marcel Dekker, 1993:401–434.

9. Cohn JA, Strong TV, Picciotto MR, et al. Localization of the cystic fibrosis transmembrane conductance regulator in human bile duct epithelial cells. Gastroenterology 105:1857–1864, 1993.

10. Columbo C, Battezzati PM, Podda M. Hepatobiliary disease in cystic fibrosis. Semin Liver Dis 14:259–269, 1994.

11. Roy CC, Weber AM, Morin CL, et al. Hepatobiliary disease in cystic fibrosis: a survey of current issues and concepts. J Pediatr Gastroenterol Nutr 1:469–478, 1982.

12. Watkins JB, Tercyak AM, Szczepanik P, et al. Bile salt kinetics in cystic fibrosis: influence of pancreatic enzyme replacement. Gastroenterology 72:1023–1028, 1977.

13. Smith A. Pathogenesis of bacterial bronchitis in cystic fibrosis. Pediatr Infect Dis J 16:91–96, 1997.

14. Kelley TJ, Drumm ML. Inducible nitric oxide synthase expression is reduced in cystic fibrosis murine and human airway epithelial cells. J Clin Invest 102:1200–1207, 1998.

15. Pier GB, Grout M, Zaidi TS. Cystic fibrosis transmembrane conductance regulator is an epithelial cell receptor for clearance of *Pseudomonas aeruginosa* from the lung. Proc Natl Acad Sci U S A 94: 12088–12093, 1997.

16. Muhdi K, Edenborough FP, Gumery L, et al. Outcome for patients colonised with *Burkholderia cepacia* in a Birmingham adult cystic fibrosis clinic and the end of an epidemic. Thorax 51:374–377, 1996.

17. Smith DL, Gumery LB, Smith EG, et al. Epidemic of *Pseudomonas cepacia* in an adult cystic fibrosis unit: evidence of person-to-person transmission. J Clin Microbiol 31:3017–3022, 1993.

18. Greenberger PA. Immunologic aspects of lung diseases and cystic fibrosis. JAMA 278:1924–1930, 1997.

19. Stern RC. Pulmonary complications. In: Davis PB, ed. Cystic fibrosis. Lung biology in health and disease. New York: Marcel Dekker, 1993:345–373.

20. Shalon LB, Adelson JW. Cystic fibrosis: gastrointestinal complications and gene therapy. Pediatr Clin North Am 43:157–196, 1996.

21. Waters DL, Dorney SA, Gaskin KJ, et al. Pancreatic function in infants identified as having cystic fibrosis in a neonatal screening program. N Engl J Med 322:303–308, 1990.

22. Walkowiak J, Cichy WK, Herzig KH. Comparison of fecal elastase-1 determination with the secretin-cholecystokinin test in patients with cystic fibrosis. Scand J Gastroenterol 34:202–207, 1999.

23. Moran A, Hardin D, Rodman D, et al. Diagnosis, screening and management of cystic fibrosis related diabetes mellitus: a consensus conference report. Diabetes Res Clin Pract 45:61–73, 1999.

24. Lanng S, Thorsteinsson B, Lund-Andersen C, et al. Diabetes mellitus in Danish cystic fibrosis patients: prevalence and late diabetic complications. Acta Paediatr 83:72–77, 1994.

25. Finkelstein SM, Wielinski CL, Elliott GR, et al. Diabetes mellitus associated with cystic fibrosis. J Pediatr 112:373–377, 1988.

26. Cystic Fibrosis Foundation. Clinical practice guidelines for cystic fibrosis. Bethesda, MD: Cystic Fibrosis Foundation, 1997.

27. Feigelson J, Girault F, Pecau Y. Gastroesophageal reflux and esophagitis in cystic fibrosis. Acta Paediatr Scand 76:989–990, 1987.

28. Kerem E, Cory M, Kerem B, et al. Clinical and genetic comparisons of patients with cystic fibrosis, with or without meconium ileus. J Pediatr 114:767–773, 1989.

29. Corey M, McLaughlin FJ, Williams M, et al. A comparison of survival, growth, and pulmonary function in patients with cystic fibrosis in Boston and Toronto. J Clin Epidemiol 41:583–563, 1988.

30. Vaisman N, Pencharz PB, Corey M, et al. Energy expenditure of patients with cystic fibrosis. J Pediatr 111:496–500, 1987.

31. Reiter EO, Brugman SM, Pike JW, et al. Vitamin D metabolites in adolescents and young adults with cystic fibrosis: effects of sun and season. J Pediatr 106:21–26, 1985.

32. Moss RB, King VV. Management of sinusitis in cystic fibrosis by endoscopic surgery and serial antimicrobial lavage: reduction in recurrence requiring surgery. Arch Otolaryngol Head Neck Surg 121:566–572, 1995.

33. Regelmann WE, Elliott GR, Warwick WJ, et al. Reduction of sputum *Pseudomonas aeruginosa* density by antibiotics improves lung function in cystic fibrosis more than do bronchodilators and chest physiotherapy alone. Am Rev Respir Dis 141:914–921, 1990.

34. Fiel SB, FitzSimmons S, Schidlow D. Evolving demographics of cystic fibrosis. Semin Respir Care 15:349–355, 1994.

35. Centers for Disease Control and Prevention. Newborn screening for cystic fibrosis: a paradigm for public health genetics policy development. Proceedings of a 1997 workshop. MMWR 46:1–24, 1997.

36. Colombo C, Battezzati PM, Podda M, et al. Ursodeoxycholic acid for liver disease associated with cystic fibrosis: a double-blind multicenter trial. Hepatology 23:1484–1490, 1996.

37. Lepage G, Paradis K, Lacaille F, et al. Ursodeoxycholic acid improves the hepatic metabolism of essential fatty acids and retinol in children with cystic fibrosis. J Pediatr 130:52–58, 1997.

38. Cotton CU, Davis PB. The pancreas in cystic fibrosis. In: Davis PB, ed. Cystic fibrosis. New York: Marcel Dekker, 1993:161–192.

39. Fitzsimmons SC, Burkhart GA, Borowitz D, et al. High-dose pancreatic-enzyme supplements and fibrosing colonopathy in children with cystic fibrosis. N Engl J Med 336:1283–1289, 1997.

40. Stevens JC, Maguiness KM, Hollingsworth J, et al. Pancreatic enzyme supplementation in cystic fibrosis patients before and after fibrosing colonopathy. J Pediatr Gastroenterol Nutr 26:80–84, 1998.

41. Collins CE, O'Loughlin EV, Henry RL. Fat gram target to achieve high energy intake in cystic fibrosis. J Paediatr Child Health 33: 142–147, 1997.

42. Hardy KA. A review of airway clearance: new techniques, indications, and recommendations. Respir Care 39:440–445, 1994.

43. Mitchell I, Corey M, Woenne R, et al. Bronchial hyperreactivity in cystic fibrosis and asthma. J Pediatr 93:744–748, 1978.

44. Pattishall EN. Longitudinal response of pulmonary function to bronchodilators in cystic fibrosis. Pediatr Pulmonol 9:80–85, 1990.

45. Cropp GJ. Effectiveness of bronchodilators in cystic fibrosis. Am J Med 100 (Suppl 1A):19S–29S, 1996.

46. Bargon J, Viel K, Dauletbaev N, et al. Short-term effects of regular salmeterol treatment on adult cystic fibrosis patients. Eur Respir J 10:2307–2311, 1997.

47. Shak S, Capon DJ, Hellmiss R, et al. Recombinant human DNase I reduces the viscosity of cystic fibrosis sputum. Proc Natl Acad Sci U S A 87:9188–9192, 1990.

48. Fuchs HJ, Borowitz DS, Christiansen DH, et al. Effect of aerosolized recombinant human DNase on exacerbations of respiratory symptoms and on pulmonary function in patients with cystic fibrosis. N Engl J Med 331:637–642, 1994.

49. Paul K, Rietschel E, Ballmann M, et al. Bronchoalveolar lavage for the evaluation of antiinflammatory treatment study group. Effect of treatment with dornase alpha on airway inflammation in patients with cystic fibrosis. Am J Respir Crit Care Med 169:719–725, 2004.

50. Cipolla D, Clark A, Pearlman R, et al. Pulmozyme rhDNase should not be mixed with other nebulizer medications (abstract 236). Presented at: Eighth Annual North American Cystic Fibrosis Conference; October 20–23, 1994; Orlando, Fla.

51. Ripoll L, Reinert P, Pepin LF, et al. Interaction of macrolides with alpha dornase during DNA hydrolysis. J Antimicrob Chemother 37: 987–991, 1996.

52. Gibson RL, Burns JL, Ramsey BW. Pathophysiology and management of pulmonary infections in cystic fibrosis: state of the art. Am J Respir Crit Care Med 168:918–951, 2003.

53. Aaron SD, Ramotar K, Ferris W, et al. Adult cystic fibrosis exacerbations and new strains of *Pseudomonas aeruginosa*. Am J Respir Crit Care Med 169:811–815, 2004.

54. Lyczak JB, Cannon CL, Pier GB. Lung infections associated with cystic fibrosis. Clin Microbiol Rev 15:194–222, 2002.

55. Moskowitz SM, Foster JM, Emerson J, et al. Clinically feasible biofilm susceptibility assay for isolates of *Pseudomonas aeruginosa* from patients with cystic fibrosis. J Clin Microbiol 42:1915–1922, 2004.

56. Saiman L, Mehar F, Niu WW, et al. Antibiotic susceptibility of multiply resistant *Pseudomonas aeruginosa* isolated from patients with cystic fibrosis, including candidates for transplantation. Clin Infect Dis 23:532–537, 1996.

57. Beringer P. The clinical use of colistin in patients with cystic fibrosis. Curr Opin Pulm Med 7:434–440, 2001.

58. Chen JS, Witzmann KA, Spilker T, et al. Endemicity and inter-city spread of *Burkholderia cepacia* genomovar III in cystic fibrosis. J. Pediatr 139:643–649, 2001

59. Knowles MR, Gilligan PH, Boucher RC. Cystic fibrosis. In: Mandell GL, Bennett JE, Dolin R, eds. Principles and practice of infectious diseases. 5th ed. Philadelphia: Churchill Livingstone, 2002: 767–772.

60. Mc Manus TE, Moore JE, Crowe M, et al. A comparison of pulmonary exacerbations with single and multiple organisms in patients with cystic fibrosis and chronic *Burkholderia cepacia* infection. J Infect 46:56–59, 2003.

61. Hutchison M, Govan JRW. Pathogenicity of microbes associated with cystic fibrosis. Microbes Infect 1:1005–1014, 1999.

62. Vartivarian S, Anaissie E. *Stenotrophomonas maltophilia* and *Burkholderia cepacia*. In: Mandell GL, Bennett JE, Dolin R, eds. Principles and practice of infectious diseases. 5th ed. Philadelphia: Churchill Livingstone, 2002:2335–2339.

63. De Groot R, Smith AL. Antibiotic pharmacokinetics in cystic fibrosis: differences and clinical significance. Clin Pharmacokinet 13: 228–253, 1987.

64. Spino M. Pharmacokinetics of drugs in cystic fibrosis. Clin Rev Allergy 9:169–210, 1991.

65. Vogelstein B, Kowarski AA, Lietman PS. The pharmacokinetics of amikacin in children. J Pediatr 91:333–339, 1977.

66. Kearns GL, Hilman BC, Wilson JT. Dosing implications of altered gentamicin disposition in patients with cystic fibrosis. J Pediatr 100: 312–318, 1982.

67. Levy J, Smith AL, Koup JR, et al. Disposition of tobramycin in patients with cystic fibrosis: a prospective controlled study. J Pediatr 105:117–124, 1984.

68. Kavanagh RE, Unadkat JD, Smith AL. Drug disposition in cystic fibrosis. In: Davis PB, ed. Cystic fibrosis. New York: Marcel Dekker, 1993:91–136.

69. Moore RD, Lietman PS, Smith CR. Clinical response to aminoglycoside therapy: importance of the ratio of peak concentration to minimal inhibitory concentration. J Infect Dis 155:93–99, 1987.

70. Dahlgren JG, Anderson ET, Hewitt WL, et al. Gentamicin blood levels: a guide to nephrotoxicity. Antimicrob Agents Chemother 8: 58–62, 1975.

71. Bates RD, Nahata MC, Jones JW, et al. Pharmacokinetics and safety of tobramycin after once-daily administration in patients with cystic fibrosis. Chest 112:1208–1213, 1997.

72. Vic P, Ategbo S, Turck D, et al. Efficacy, tolerance, and pharmacokinetics of once daily tobramycin for *Pseudomonas* exacerbations in cystic fibrosis. Arch Dis Child 78:536–539, 1998.

73. Powell SH, Thompson WL, Luthe MA, et al. Once-daily vs. continuous aminoglycoside dosing: efficacy and toxicity in animal and clinical studies of gentamicin, netilmicin and tobramycin. J Infect Dis 147:918–932, 1983.

74. Smyth A, Tan K, Hyman-Taylor P, et al. A randomized controlled trial of once vs three times daily tobramycin for pulmonary exacerbations of cystic fibrosis (The Topic Study) (abstract). Ped Pulm 36: 292, 2003.

75. de Groot R, Hack BD, Weber A, et al. Pharmacokinetics of ticarcillin in patients with cystic fibrosis: a controlled prospective study. Clin Pharmacol Ther 47:73–78, 1990.

76. Leeder JS, Spino M, Isles AF, et al. Ceftazidime disposition in acute and stable cystic fibrosis. Clin Pharmacol Ther 36:355–362, 1984.

77. Hedman A, Adan-Abdi Y, Alvan G, et al. Influence of the glomerular filtration rate on renal clearance of ceftazidime in cystic fibrosis. Clin Pharmacokinet 15:57–65, 1988.

78. Huls CE, Prince RA, Seilheimer DK, et al. Pharmacokinetics of cefepime in cystic fibrosis patients. Antimicrob Agents Chemother 37: 1414–1416, 1993.

79. Hamelin BA, Moore N, Knupp CA, et al. Cefepime pharmacokinetics in cystic fibrosis. Pharmacotherapy 13:465–470, 1993.

80. Susanto M, Benet LZ. Can the enhanced renal clearance of antibiotics in cystic fibrosis patients be explained by P-glycoprotein transport. Pharm Res 19:457–462, 2002.

81. Mouton JW, Vinks AA. Is continuous infusion of β-lactam antibiotics worthwhile? Efficacy and pharmacokinetic considerations. J Antimicrob Chemother 38:5–15, 1996.

82. Vinks AA, Touw DJ, Heijerman GH, et al. Pharmacokinetics of ceftazidime in adult cystic fibrosis patients during continuous infusion and ambulatory treatment at home. Ther Drug Monitor 16:341–348, 1994.

83. Hubert D, Wallaert B, Scheid P, et al. Continuous infusion versus intermittent administration of ceftazidime in cystic fibrosis patients. Pediatr Pulmonol 36:294, 2003.

84. Lebel M, Bergeron MG, Vallee F, et al. Pharmacokinetics and pharmacodynamics of ciprofloxacin in cystic fibrosis patients. Antimicrob Agents Chemother 30:260–266, 1986.

85. Davis RL, Koup JR, Williams-Warren J, et al. Pharmacokinetics of ciprofloxacin in cystic fibrosis. Antimicrob Agents Chemother 31: 915–919, 1987.

86. Reed MD, Stern RC, Myers CM, et al. Lack of unique ciprofloxacin pharmacokinetic characteristics in patients with cystic fibrosis. J Clin Pharmacol 28:691–699, 1988.

87. Christensson BA, Nilsson-Ehle I, Ljungberg B, et al. Increased oral bioavailability of ciprofloxacin in cystic fibrosis patients. Antimicrob Agents Chemother 36:2512–2517, 1992.

88. Ramsey B, Burns JL, Smith AL. Safety and efficacy of tobramycin solution for inhalation in patients with cystic fibrosis: the results of two phase III placebo controlled clinical trials. Presented at: Eleventh Annual North American Cystic Fibrosis Conference; October 23–26, 1997; Nashville, Tenn. Abstract S10.4.

89. Saiman L, Marshall BC, Mayer-Hamblett N, et al. Azithromycin in patients with cystic fibrosis chronically infected with *Pseudomonas aeruginosa*; a randomized controlled trial. JAMA 290:1749–1756, 2003.

90. Marchetti F, Giglio L, Candusso M, et al. Early antibiotic treatment of *Pseudomonas aeruginosa* colonisation in cystic fibrosis: a critical review of the literature. Eur J Clin Pharmacol 60:67–74, 2004.

91. Rosenstein BJ, Eigen H. Risks of alternate-day prednisone in patients with cystic fibrosis. Pediatrics 87:245–246, 1991.

92. Voter KZ. Adjunctive therapy in cystic fibrosis (CF). Pediatr Infect Dis J 17:341–342, 1998.

93. Konstan MW, Byard PJ, Hoppel CL, et al. Effect of high-dose ibuprofen in patients with cystic fibrosis. N Engl J Med 332:848–854, 1995.

94. Kovesi TA, Swartz R, MacDonald N. Transient renal failure due to simultaneous ibuprofen and aminoglycoside therapy in children with cystic fibrosis (letter). N Engl J Med 338:65–66, 1998.

95. Yankaskas JR, Mallory GB. Lung transplantation in cystic fibrosis: consensus conference statement. Chest 113:217–226, 1998.

96. Lambert L, Mitchell C, Scannon P. Recombinant bactericidal/permeability-increasing protein (rBPI21) is bactericidal in vitro against *Pseudomonas aeruginosa* strains isolated from cystic fibrosis patients (abstract E-149:140). Proceedings of the 37th Conference on Antimicrobial Agents and Chemotherapy, September 28-October 1, 1997; Toronto, Ontario, Canada.

97. Pier GB. *Pseudomonas aeruginosa:* a key problem in cystic fibrosis. ASM News 64:339–347, 1998.

98. Egan ME, Pearson M, Weiner SA, et al. Curcumin, a major constituent of turmeric, corrects cystic fibrosis defects. Science 304: 600–602, 2004.

CASE STUDIES

CASE 14

TOPIC: Asthma

THERAPEUTIC DIFFICULTY: Level 3

Kathryn Blake

Chapter 34: Asthma

■ Scenario

Patient and Setting: RP, a 51-year-old female; urgent clinic visit

Chief Complaint: Severe wheezing, shortness of breath, coughing, and painful sinuses

■ History of Present Illness

Frequent asthma attacks for the past 2 months (April and May); frequent sinus headaches over the last 6 weeks, worse in the last week

Medical History: History of periodic asthma attacks since childhood and worsening during adolescence and early adulthood; placed on inhaled corticosteroids in her 30s and prednisone when she was 45 years old; severe osteoporosis diagnosed 2 years ago; wrist fracture 2 years ago; placed on alendronate; severe menopausal symptoms; placed on ERT 2 years ago for menopausal symptoms and osteoporosis management; stage II hypertension diagnosed 3 years ago; placed on hydrochlorothiazide and enalapril; hypertension intermittently controlled for the past year

Surgical History: None

Family/Social History: Family History: Father died age 59 of kidney failure secondary to hypertension; mother died age 62 from a stroke
Social History: Nonsmoker; no alcohol intake; caffeine use: 4 cups of coffee and 4 diet colas per day

Medications:
Prednisone, 10 mg PO QD (since she was 45 years old)
Serevent Diskus inhaler 500/50 (fluticasone propionate 500 μg and salmeterol 50 μg per inhalation), 1 inhalation BID

Albuterol inhaler, PRN
Alendronate; 5mg QD
Hydrocholorothiazide tablets, 25 mg PO BID
Enalapril tablets, 5 mg PO BID
Conjugated estrogens (Premarin); 0.625 mg PO QD and medroxyprogesterone acetate, 2.5mg PO QD

Allergies: No known drug allergies

■ Physical Examination

GEN: Pale, well-developed, anxious-appearing woman
VS: BP 150/92, HR 92, RR 24, T 38.5°C, Wt 61 kg, Ht 161 cm
HEENT: PERRLA, oral cavity without lesions, TM without signs of inflammation; sinuses tender to palpation
COR: RRR, normal S_1 and S_2
CHEST: Bilateral inspiratory and expiratory wheezes
ABD: Nontender, nondistended, no masses
GU: Unremarkable
ECT: Guaiac negative
EXT: Unremarkable
NEURO: Oriented to time, place, and person; cranial nerves intact

■ Results of Pertinent Laboratory Tests, Serum Drug Concentrations, and Diagnostic Tests

Na 134 (134)	Ca 2.23 (8.9)	PT 12 sec
K 4.9 (4.9)	Cl 100 (100)	INR 1.0
HCO_3 30 (30)	BUN 7.5 (21)	AST 0.45 (27)
Mg 0.65 (1.3)	Cr 106.1 (1.2)	ALT 0.4 (24)
PO_4 0.872 (2.7)	Glu 6.1 (110)	Alb 38 (3.8)
T Bili 3.4 (0.2)	Hct 0.37 (37)	Alk Phos 1.32 (79)
LDH 2.5 (150)	Hgb 130 (13)	
WBC 10.4×10^9	Plts 201×10^9	
(10.4×10^3)	(201×10^3)	

Spirometry: <u>Prebronchodilator</u> [last dose of albuterol (2 inhalations) 3 hours previously]
FVC 2.26L (60% of predicted)
FEV_1 1.34L (45% of predicted)
FEF_{25-75} 0.71L/s (25% of predicted)
FEV_1/FVC 59% [last dose of albuterol (2 inhalations) 3 hours previously]
Spirometry: <u>Post 2.5 mg albuterol</u>
FVC 2.50L (66% of predicted)
FEV_1 1.44L (48% of predicted)
FEF_{25-75} 0.92L/s (32% of predicted)
BMD: −3.1 SD below mean

■ Problem List

Identify principal problems from the scenario in priority order (see Answers in back of book for correct list of problems).

■ SOAP Note

To be completed by the student (see Answers in back of book for correct SOAP Note).

■ QUESTIONS

(See Answers in back of book for correct responses.)

1. List the intermediate and long-term adverse effects seen with corticosteroid use. (EO-10)

2. List advantages of using a spacer device with a MDI. (EO-8)

3. Describe the mechanisms of action of each of the pharmacologic interventions in this case. (EO-7)

4. List the specific steps that you would include when educating RP about appropriate administration of the albuterol inhaler. (EO-14)

5. What are the advantages of inhaled versus oral administration route of β_2-agonists? (EO-8)

6. List common adverse effects of alendronate. (EO-10)

7. Omalizumab is recommended for asthmatics who are/have: (EO-8)
   a. Diagnosed with mild to moderate asthma
   b. Currently being managed with prednisone and/or high-dose inhaled corticosteroids
   c. No prior hospitalizations or visits to the emergency department for asthma
   d. Negative skin prick tests to allergens

8. To correctly use the Advair Diskus inhaler, patients should do which of the following? (EO-8)
   a. Exhale into the device before inhaling
   b. Forceful and deep inhalation
   c. Shake the device before using
   d. Rinse the device in warm water after each use

9. RP was admitted to the emergency department with signs and symptoms of acute asthma attack. List these signs and symptoms. (EO-2)

10. What psychosocial factors may affect RP's adherence to both pharmacologic and nonpharmacologic therapy? (EO-15)

11. List common adverse effects seen with amoxicillin/clavulanate when used in the treatment of acute sinusitis. (EO-8, 10)

12. Evaluate the pharmacoeconomic considerations relative to RP's plan of care. (EO-17)

13. Summarize therapeutic, pathophysiologic, and disease management concepts for asthma utilizing a key points format. (EO-18)

Adrenocortical Dysfunction and Clinical Use of Steroids

37

Karen J. Tietze

OVERVIEW OF THE ADRENAL GLANDS

ANATOMY AND PHYSIOLOGY

Each of the two adrenal glands is located at the superior pole of the kidney (Fig. 37.1, *see color insert*). The adult adrenal is a pyramidal structure approximately 2 to 3 cm wide, 4 to 6 cm long, and 1 cm thick. The adrenals are supplied with blood from the abdominal aorta and renal and phrenic arteries. Drainage of the adrenal gland occurs via the renal vein on the left and the inferior vena cava on the right.

The adrenal gland is composed of two physiologically distinct glands: the adrenal cortex and the adrenal medulla (85%–90% and 10%–15% of the total adrenal gland, respectively). Histologically, the adrenal cortex is differentiated into three separate zones: (a) zona glomerulosa, (b) zona

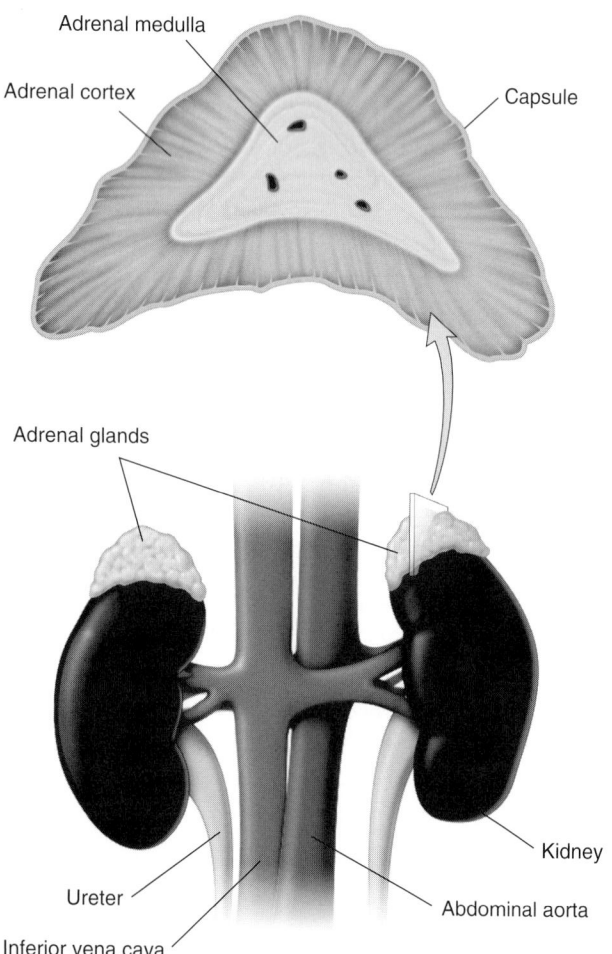

Adrenal medulla

Adrenal cortex

Capsule

Adrenal glands

Kidney

Ureter

Abdominal aorta

Inferior vena cava

FIGURE 37.1 Location and structure of the adrenal glands (*see color insert*). (From Premkumar K. The Massage Connection Anatomy and Physiology. Baltimore: Lippincott Williams & Wilkins, 2004, with permission.)

fasciculata, and (c) zona reticularis. The outer zone (glomerulosa) produces mineralocorticoids (aldosterone). The inner zones (fasciculata/reticularis) produce androgens [dehydroepiandrosterone (DHEA), androstenedione] and glucocorticoids (cortisol). The adrenal medulla secretes catecholamines (epinephrine). Adrenocortical steroids are derived from endogenous and exogenous cholesterol (Fig. 37.2, *see color insert*). Hepatic cytochrome P-450 enzymes (cholesterol side chain cleavage, 3β-hydroxysteroid dehydrogenase, 17α-hydroxylase, 21-hydroxylase, and 11β-hydroxylase) are primarily responsible for adrenal steroid conversion.

ADRENAL HORMONES

Glucocorticoids. The principal glucocorticoid, cortisol, is secreted at a rate of 5 to 10 mg/m^2 per day (equivalent to 20–30 mg/day hydrocortisone or 5–7 mg/day prednisone),[1,2] but can increase five- to tenfold to a maximum of approximately 100 mg/m^2 per day.[3] Cortisol is produced via two cytochrome P-450-mediated hydroxylations at the 21-position, yielding cortisol.

Cortisol is converted in the kidneys, colon, sweat glands, and salivary glands to the inactive form, cortisone, by the enzyme 11 β-hydroxysteroid dehydrogenase type 2 (11β-HSD2).[4] Cortisone is converted in the liver, adipose, and central nervous system to the active form, cortisol, by the enzyme 11β-hydroxysteroid dehydrogenase type 1 (11β-HSD1).[4] When high levels of circulating cortisol overwhelm the 11β-HSD2 and 11βHSD1 pathways, cortisol binds to and activates mineralocorticoid receptors, resulting in typical mineralocorticoid effects (e.g., expanded plasma volume, elevated blood pressure, and hypokalemia). The half-life of cortisol is 70 to 120 minutes, with less than 1% of unchanged cortisol excreted by the kidneys over 24 hours. Mineralocorticoid and glucocorticoid equivalencies are listed in Table 37.1.[5,6]

Although the name ''glucocorticoid'' is derived from the carbohydrate effects of the hormone, glucocorticoids have multiple physiologic actions.[7] Glucocorticoid receptors are found in the anterior pituitary, hypothalamus, hippocampus, brain, muscle, adipose tissue, and liver.[4] Glucocorticoids affect vascular tone, vascular permeability, and distribution of total body water. Glucocorticoids stimulate lipolysis, gluconeogenesis, glycogen secretion, and conversion of lactic acid to glycogen. In addition, they increase the responsiveness of β-adrenergic receptors and mobilize amino acids from muscle. Glucocorticoids inhibit protein synthesis and insulin secretion, impair leukocyte migration, and inhibit nuclear factor-kappa B (NF-κB), a nuclear transcription factor that regulates the production of proinflammatory proteins (cytokines, interleukins, interferons, chemokines, colony stimulating factors, endothelial-leukocyte adhesion molecules, and enzymes).[8]

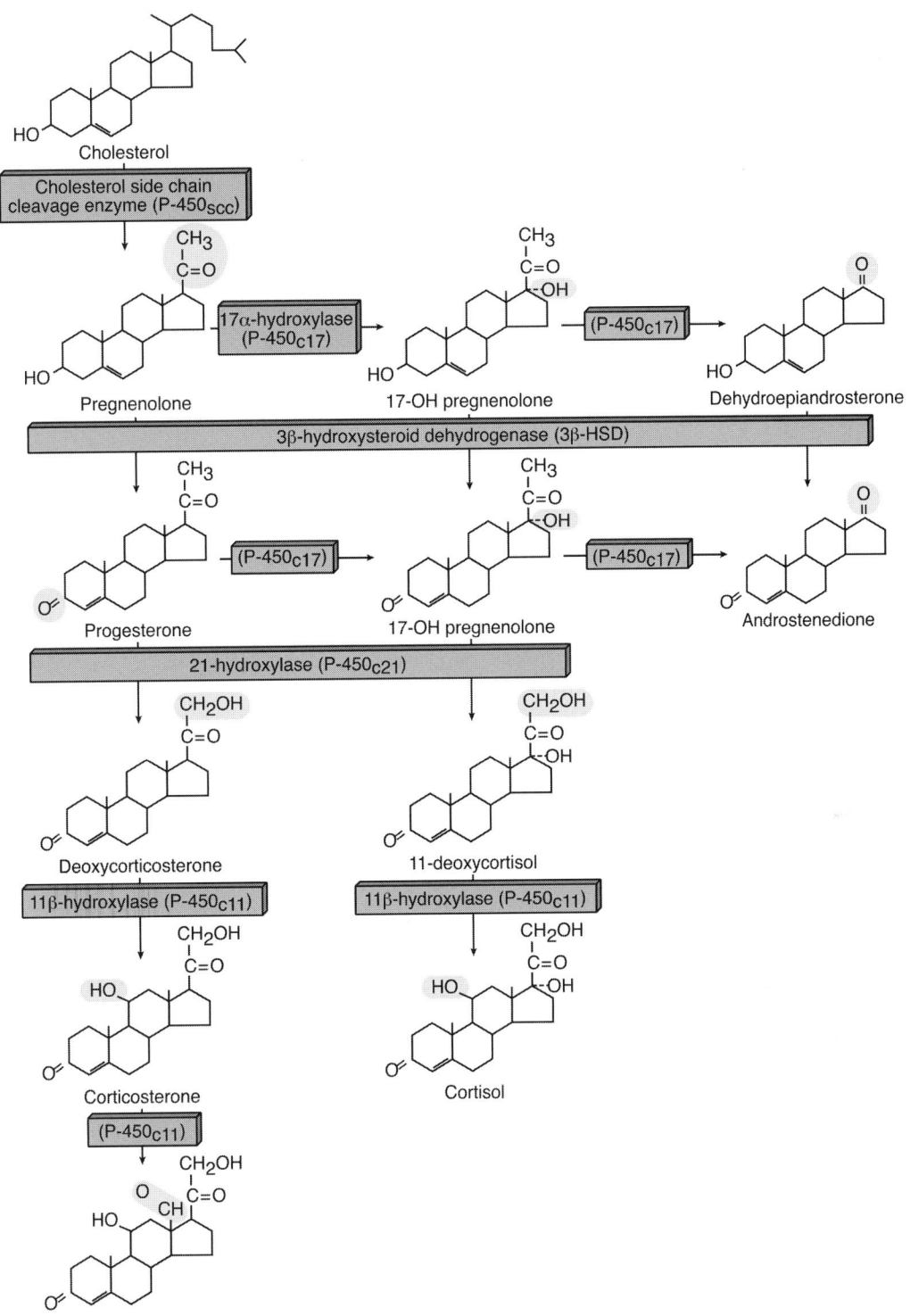

FIGURE 37.2 Biosynthetic pathways in the synthesis of adrenal corticosteroids (*see color insert*). (From Rubin E, Farber JL. Pathology. 3rd ed. Philadelphia: Lippincott Williams & Wilkins, 1999, with permission.)

TABLE 37.1	Glucocorticoid and Mineralocorticoid Equivalencies				
	Equivalent Dose	Anti-inflammatory Potency	Sodium-retaining Potency	Plasma t½ (min)	Biologic t½ (h)
Glucocorticoids					
Short acting					
Cortisone	25	0.8	2	30	8–12
Hydrocortisone	20	1	2	80–118	8–12
Intermediate-acting					
Prednisone	5	4	1	60	12–36
Prednisolone	5	4	1	115–212	12–36
Triamcinolone	4	5	0	200+	12–36
Methylprednisolone	4	5	0	78–188	12–36
Long-acting					
Dexamethasone	0.75	20–30	0	110–210	36–72
Betamethasone	0.6–0.75	20–30	0	300+	36–72
Mineralocorticoids					
Fludrocortisone	2	10	250	200	18–36

(From Drug Facts and Comparisons. Available at: http://www.efactsweb.com. Accessed March 31, 2004; Schimmer BP, Parker KL. Adrenocorticotrophic hormone; adrenocortical steroids and their synthetic analogs; inhibitors of the synthesis and action of adrenocortical hormones. In: Hardman JG, Limbird LE, eds. Goodman and Gilman's the pharmacological basis of therapeutics. 10th ed. New York: McGraw-Hill, 2001:1649–1679; with permission.)

Glucocorticoids inhibit or induce the secretion of end-effector proteins by regulating cellular transcription. Free glucocorticoid diffuses through plasma membranes and binds with specific cytoplasmic receptors to form ligand-receptor complexes. The ligand-receptor complex undergoes a conformational change, translocates into the nucleus, and binds to specific elements within the DNA. The bound complex modulates the transcription of specific genes, resulting in the production of end-effector proteins or the inhibition of specific proteins.

Glucocorticoids circulate in the blood free or bound to proteins [cortisol-binding globulin (CBG; transcortin) and albumin]. In physiologic concentrations, approximately 95% of circulating cortisol is protein bound. Unbound cortisol, about 5% of circulating cortisol, is the biologically active hormone. The reservoir of protein-bound hormone prevents rapid fluctuations in a free steroid concentration that would otherwise occur given the episodic cortisol secretion and may ensure more uniform distribution to target tissues.

Mineralocorticoids. The principal mineralocorticoid, aldosterone, is secreted at a rate of 100 to 150 μg per day.[2] Sodium depletion or hyperreninism increase the production rate tenfold or more. Mineralocorticoids regulate intravascular blood volume and sodium and potassium balance by enhancing renal sodium and water reabsorption at the distal tubule and increasing urinary potassium and hydrogen ion

excretion. The net result is expanded plasma volume, elevated blood pressure, and hypokalemia. Other adrenal steroids with some mineralocorticoid activity include cortisol, corticosterone, and deoxycorticosterone.

Androgens. The principal androgen, DHEA, is secreted at a rate of about 4 mg per day.[2] Adrenal androgens are the precursors for the peripheral synthesis of androgen and estrogen.[9] Adrenal androgens are an important source of androgens for women but not for men since most androgens are produced in the testes. Androgens regulate sexual differentiation, gonadotropin secretion, spermatogenesis, and sex drive, and they may have positive influences on cognition, memory, and mood.[9]

HYPOTHALAMUS-PITUITARY-ADRENAL AXIS

The three major components of the hypothalamus-pituitary-adrenal (HPA) axis (hypothalamus, anterior pituitary, adrenals) function as an integrated system. Corticotropin-releasing hormone (CRH) is released from the hypothalamus in response to a variety of stimulants, including neurotransmitters, arginine vasopressin, and catecholamines. Adrenocorticotropic hormone (ACTH), the anterior pituitary hormone, is released into the systemic circulation in response to stimulation by the CRH. ACTH stimulates the adrenal cortex to produce cortisol. ACTH also binds to melanocortin-2 receptors, increasing pigment deposition. As serum cortisol levels increase, the biosynthesis and secretion of CRH and ACTH decrease in a classic negative feedback mechanism.

CIRCADIAN RHYTHM

CRH, free cortisol plasma concentration, and the sleep-wake cycle control ACTH release.[10,11] ACTH, secreted in brief episodic bursts, causes sharp increases in the plasma concentrations of ACTH and cortisol. The ACTH plasma concentration peaks early in the morning, decreases throughout the morning, and nadirs at about midnight.[2] The cortisol plasma concentration peaks at awakening at about 10 to 20 μg/dL, declines throughout the late afternoon and evening, and nadirs an hour or two after falling asleep to less than 5 μg/dL.[2,12] Stress (pyrogens, injury, pain, hypoglycemia, hypovolemia, exercise, severe emotional trauma) enhances ACTH release and abolishes ACTH circadian rhythmicity. High-dose glucocorticoid administration suppresses stress-related ACTH release.

CUSHING'S SYNDROME

TREATMENT GOALS: Cushing's Syndrome

The treatment goals for Cushing's syndrome are to:

- Restore HPA axis function by eliminating glucocorticoid and mineralocorticoid excess
- Eradicate tumors (pituitary, adrenal, ectopic) that directly or indirectly increase cortisol secretion
- Reduce long-term need for medications

DEFINITION

Cushing syndrome is a disorder caused by persistent glucocorticoid excess.

ETIOLOGY

Cushing's syndrome is caused by ACTH-dependent or ACTH-independent disorders that increase serum cortisol (Table 37.2).[2,13] Cushing's disease is a specific type of Cushing's syndrome caused by ACTH-secreting pituitary tumors. Described first by William Osler in 1899, Harvey W. Cushing postulated 20 years later that the "polyglandular syndrome" (Cushing's disease) was caused by primary pituitary dysfunction.[14] Pseudo-Cushing's syndrome, a nonendocrine disorder characterized by some of the clinical and biochemical manifestations of Cushing's syndrome, is associated with major depressive disorders and alcoholism.

EPIDEMIOLOGY

A recent population-based study estimated the overall incidence of new cases of Cushing's syndrome to be approximately 2 to 2.6 cases per million per year with more than half the new cases caused by Cushing's disease.[15,16] Other estimates of the incidence of Cushing's syndrome and Cushing's disease are higher (5–25 cases per million per year and 660 cases per million per year, respectively).[17]

TABLE 37.2	Cushing Syndrome Etiology
ACTH-dependent Disorders	**Etiology**
Cushing's disease[a]	Pituitary ACTH hypersecretion
Ectopic ACTH syndrome	Ectopic (nonpituitary) ACTH secretion
Ectopic CRH syndrome	Ectopic (nonhypothalamic) CRH secretion causing pituitary ACTH hypersecretion
Iatrogenic/Factitious	Exogenous ACTH administration
ACTH-independent Disorders	**Etiology**
Iatrogenic[b]	Exogenous glucocorticoid administration
Factitious	Exogenous glucocorticoid administration
Adrenal adenomas and carcinomas	HPA-axis independent cortisol production
Micronodular and macronodular adrenal hyperplasia	Increased cortisol secretion

[a] Most common ACTH-dependent disorder.
[b] Most common ACTH-independent disorder.
ACTH, adrenocorticotropic hormone; CRH, corticotropin-releasing hormone; HPA, hypothalamus-pituitary-adrenal.
(From Stewart PM. The adrenal cortex. In: Larsen PR, Kronenberg HM, et al, eds. Williams textbook of endocrinology. 10th ed. Philadelphia: WB Saunders, 2003:491–551; Nieman LK, Orth DN. Causes and pathophysiology of Cushing's syndrome. In: UpToDate Online Release 11.3. Available at: http://www.uptodate.com. Accessed February 11, 2004; with permission.)

Cushing's disease causes about 70% of all cases of ACTH-dependent Cushing's syndrome.[2] Ectopic secretion of ACTH or CRH by nonpituitary and nonhypothalamic tumors (e.g., small cell lung carcinoma) are a less common cause of ACTH-dependent Cushing's syndrome. The most common cause of ACTH-independent Cushing syndrome is exogenously administered glucocorticosteroids.[13,18,19] Less commonly, ACTH-independent Cushing's syndrome is caused by adrenal adenomas and carcinomas.

Women are three to eight times more likely than men to develop Cushing's disease and four to five times more likely to have adrenal tumor-associated Cushing's syndrome.[20] Men present with Cushing's disease at a younger age and with a more severe clinical presentation than women.[21] Ectopic ACTH secretion-associated Cushing's syndrome is more common in men, most likely reflecting the increased incidence of lung cancer in men.[22]

PATHOPHYSIOLOGY

Cushing's syndrome is the result of prolonged exposure to excessive glucocorticoids. Patients with Cushing's disease have pituitary micro- or macroadenomas or corticotroph hyperplasia, resulting in increased ACTH secretion that is relatively resistant to glucocorticoid negative feedback. Ectopic tumors secrete ACTH or CRH, resulting in adrenocortical hyperplasia and hyperfunction. Exogenously administered glucocorticoids increase serum cortisol, which inhibits CRH and ACTH secretion, resulting in bilateral adrenocortical atrophy.

CLINICAL PRESENTATION AND DIAGNOSIS

SIGNS AND SYMPTOMS

The clinical manifestations of Cushing's syndrome are insidious in onset and include multiple organ systems; none is pathognomonic (Fig. 37.3, *see color insert*). Signs and symptoms depend on the degree and duration of hypercortisolism, the presence or absence of androgen excess, and other tumor-related effects (adrenal carcinoma or ectopic ACTH syndrome) (Table 37.3).[2,17,22]

General. Progressive obesity, the most common sign of Cushing's syndrome, usually is central, involving the face, neck, trunk, and abdomen; the extremities are spared. Facial fat accumulation in the cheeks produces moon facies, often accompanied by facial plethora. Fat pads fill and bulge above the supraclavicular fossae and the dorsocervical fat pad enlarges creating the characteristic "buffalo hump." Exophthalmos, caused by increased retroorbital fat, may be present. Weakness, usually associated with proximal muscle wasting,

is caused by the catabolic effects of cortisol on muscle tissue.[23] Patients with severe disease may be unable to climb stairs, get up from a deep chair, or raise their arms.

Cardiovascular. Moderate hypertension (diastolic blood pressure >100 mmHg) is common. The elevated blood pressure is caused by increased peripheral vascular sensitivity to adrenergic agonists and mineralocorticoid excess. Dependent edema is another sign of mineralocorticoid excess. Congestive heart failure has been reported in almost half of patients more than 40 years of age.[24]

Dermatologic. The skin is atrophic and fragile with a loss of subcutaneous fat making the subcutaneous blood vessels visible. Loss of connective tissue results in easy bruisability. Striae, caused by stretched skin, appear purplish or reddish because the thin, transparent skin reveals the color of venous blood in the dermis. Striae, often more than 1 cm wide, appear most often on the breasts, hips, buttocks, upper abdomen, shoulders, and upper thighs and in the axillae. Thinning scalp hair is common. Chronic ACTH elevation (e.g., ectopic ACTH syndrome) is associated with hyperpigmentation of light-exposed skin (e.g., face, neck, arms) and scars.

Endocrine and Metabolic. Osteopenia and osteoporosis are caused by cortisol osteoblast inhibition, resulting in back pain, vertebral compression fractures, pathologic rib fractures, and, less commonly, long bone fractures. Hypercalciuria and renal caliculi may be present. Glucose intolerance and hyperinsulinemia are common. True diabetes mellitus occurs in less than 20% of patents, probably in those with a familial predisposition; ketoacidosis is rare. Oligomenorrhea in women, impotence in men, and decreased libido in both sexes are common. Androgen excess is manifested by oily facial skin, acne, mild facial hirsutism, and virilization (deep voice, temporal balding, clitoral hypertrophy).

Psychological. More than half of patients with Cushing's syndrome experience psychological complications including emotional lability, agitated depression, loss of energy, irritability, anxiety, panic attacks, and mild paranoia.[25–27] Most patients have increased appetite and weight gain. Insomnia is a common early symptom.

Other. Patients are at an increased risk of phlebothrombosis and thromboembolic events.[28] Glucocorticoids suppress immune function and inflammatory and febrile responses, but infection occurs only with severe hypercortisolemia. Intraocular pressure is reversibly increased.

DIAGNOSIS AND CLINICAL FINDINGS

The diagnosis of Cushing's syndrome is based on recognizing the signs and symptoms, establishing the presence of hypercortisolism, and testing of the HPA axis. The first step is to rule out iatrogenic (prescribed glucocorticoids), surreptitious (nonprescribed glucocorticoids used without intent of self-harm), or factitious (nonprescribed glucocorticoids used

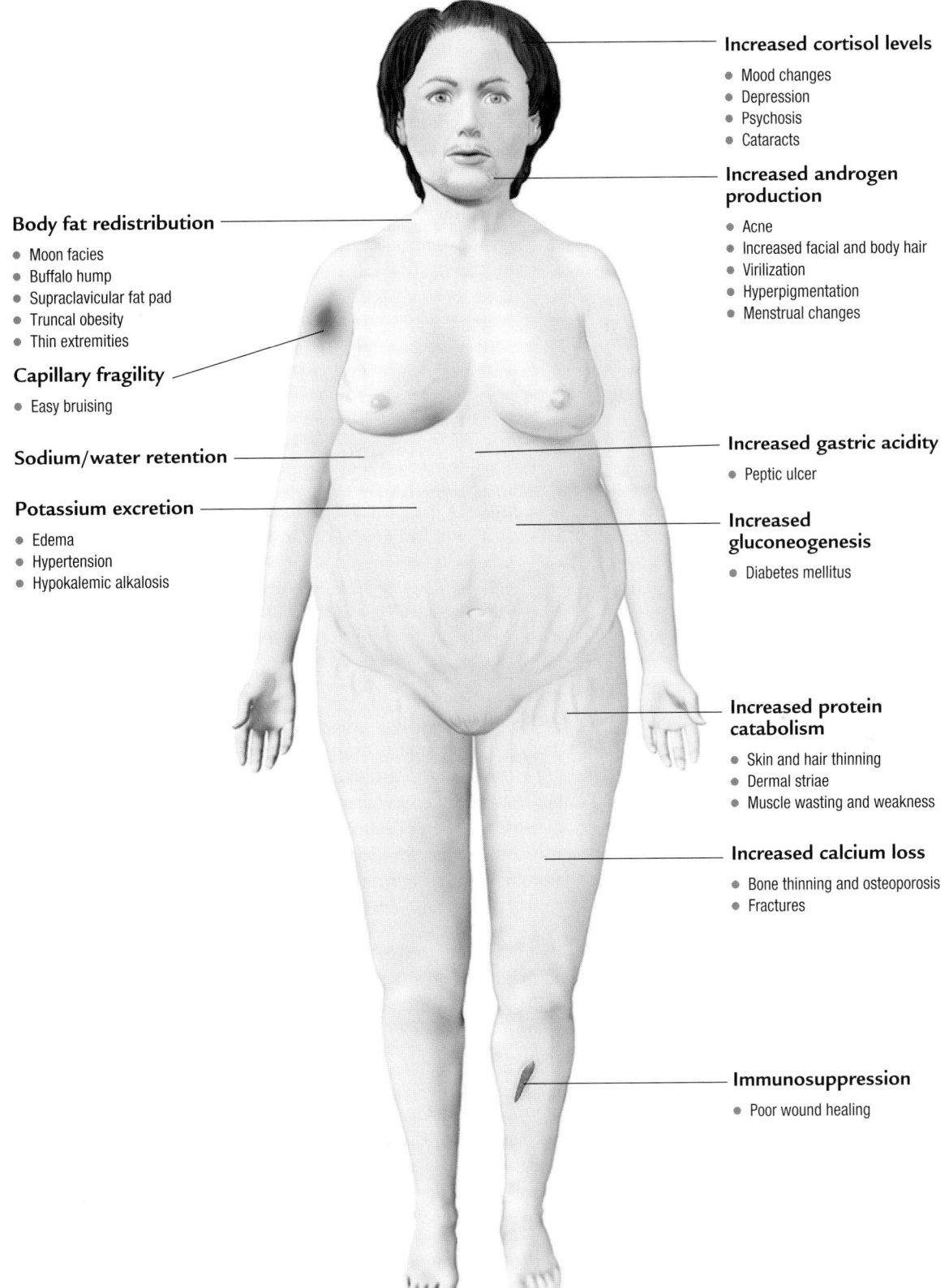

Increased cortisol levels

- Mood changes
- Depression
- Psychosis
- Cataracts

Increased androgen production

- Acne
- Increased facial and body hair
- Virilization
- Hyperpigmentation
- Menstrual changes

Body fat redistribution

- Moon facies
- Buffalo hump
- Supraclavicular fat pad
- Truncal obesity
- Thin extremities

Capillary fragility

- Easy bruising

Sodium/water retention

Potassium excretion

- Edema
- Hypertension
- Hypokalemic alkalosis

Increased gastric acidity

- Peptic ulcer

Increased gluconeogenesis

- Diabetes mellitus

Increased protein catabolism

- Skin and hair thinning
- Dermal striae
- Muscle wasting and weakness

Increased calcium loss

- Bone thinning and osteoporosis
- Fractures

Immunosuppression

- Poor wound healing

FIGURE 37.3 Manifestations of Cushing's syndrome (*see color insert*). (Asset provided by Anatomical Chart Co.)

TABLE 37.3	**Cushing's Syndrome Signs and Symptoms**		
General	**Cardiovascular**	**Skin**	**Endocrine and Metabolic**
Centripetal obesity	Edema (ankle)	Acne	Decreased libido
Elevated intraocular pressure	Heart failure	Ecchymoses	Delayed bone growth (children)
Headache	Hypertension	Facial plethora	Glucose intolerance
Insomnia		Fungal skin infections	Hypercalciuria
Proximal muscle weakness		Hirsutism	Hypokalemic alkalosis
Psychiatric (emotional lability, depression, irritability, anxiety, mild paranoia)		Hyperpigmentation	Impotence
		Skin atrophy	Leukocytosis
		Wide (>1 cm) purple striae	Menstrual irregularities
			Osteopenia, osteoporosis
			Polyuria
			Renal calculi

(From Stewart PM. The adrenal cortex. In: Larsen PR, Kronenberg HM, et al, eds. Williams textbook of endocrinology. 10th ed. Philadelphia: WB Saunders, 2003:491–551; Nieman LK, Orth DN. Clinical manifestations of Cushing's syndrome. In: UpToDate Online Release 11.3. Available at: http://www. uptodate.com. Accessed February 12, 2004; Meier CA, Biller BMK. Clinical and biochemical evaluation of Cushing's syndrome. Endocrinol Metab Clin North Am 26:741–762, 1997; with permission.)

with intent of causing harm) hypercortisolism; the most definitive test for factitious or surreptitious hypercortisolism is high-performance liquid chromatography (HPLC) analysis of urine for synthetic corticosteroids.[29,30] The next step is to establish the presence of hypercortisolism. Further testing of the HPA axis is required to determine the exact cause of the hypercortisolism. There is no current consensus on how best to confirm the diagnosis of Cushing's syndrome and define the cause.

Associated Laboratory Abnormalities. Packed red blood cell volume and hemoglobin concentration tend to be high normal. The total leukocyte count usually is normal but may be elevated. Half of all patients have a relative or absolute lymphopenia and one third have eosinopenia. Hypercalciuria occurs in almost half of patients despite normal serum calcium and phosphorus levels. Electrolyte levels are normal except in extreme hypercortisolism. Serum cholesterol and triglyceride concentrations often are elevated secondary to increased levels of very low-density lipoprotein, low-density lipoprotein, and high-density lipoprotein. Clotting factors V and VIII and prothrombin may be elevated.[31]

Establishing Hypercortisolism
Urinary Free Cortisol. The 24-hour urinary free cortisol (UFC) excretion test is the best screening test for endogenous hypercortisolism.[4] At least two, preferably three consecutive 24-hour urine specimens are collected to minimize collection errors and hormonal secretion variability. Patients are in-

structed to void at 8 AM, discard the specimen, and then collect all urine until 8 AM the next morning; creatinine excretion is measured to assess adequacy of the urine collection. Steroids, ACTH, CRH adrenal enzyme inhibitors, and all other unnecessary medications should be avoided during the collection periods. The cortisol reference range is less than 80 to 120 μg per 24 hours (220–330 nmol/24 hours); free cortisol less than 10 μg per 24 hours (<28 nmol/24 hours) excludes Cushing's syndrome.[2,4]

Late Night Serum and Salivary Cortisol. The late night cortisol nadir is not preserved in patients with Cushing's syndrome. An elevated midnight serum cortisol is a useful diagnostic test, but it is difficult to obtain an unstressed blood sample. The nighttime salivary cortisol concentration is easier to obtain and appears to be a sensitive and specific test.[32] The reference range for late night salivary cortisol (using an enzyme-linked immunosorbent assay) is less than 0.11 to 0.15 μg per dL (<3–4 nmol/L); salivary cortisol levels more than 0.25 μg per dL (>7 nmol/L) are diagnostic of Cushing syndrome.[4]

Low-Dose Dexamethasone Suppression Test. Patients with Cushing's syndrome lack normal negative feedback cortisol regulation.[33] Dexamethasone, used to test for negative feedback control, does not cross-react in most radioimmunoassays for serum cortisol or UFC.[33,34] Suppression tests include the overnight (1 mg dexamethasone at 11 PM) and the 2-day (0.5 mg dexamethasone every 6 hours for eight doses) low-dose dexamethasone suppression tests.[35] In the overnight test, a single blood sample is drawn at 8 AM. Cushing's syndrome is excluded if the plasma cortisol concentration is less than 1.8 μg per dL (<50 nmol/L).[4,34] The 2-day test includes at least one 24-hour urine collection for cortisol metabolites and UFC, but is no longer recommended because of poor sensitivity and specificity.

Dexamethasone-CRH Test. Used to test patients with equivocal results from standard tests for cortisol hypersecretion, the dexamethasone-CRH test combines tests for HPA axis sensitivity to endogenous glucocorticoid and pituitary sensitivity to stimulation with CRH. Dexamethasone, 0.5 mg, is given every 6 hours for eight doses starting at 12 noon day 1. CRH (1 μg/kg) is given intravenously at 8 AM on day 2. Plasma cortisol and ACTH are measured every 15 minutes for 1 hour. Cushing's syndrome is identified by an elevated 15-minute plasma cortisol [>1.4 μg/dL (>39 nmol/L)] and ACTH [>15 pg/mL (>3.3 pmol/L)].[4]

Differential Diagnosis. Defining the precise cause of the Cushing's syndrome is essential to appropriate surgical management. Additional diagnostic procedures are indicated when biochemical testing suggests the presence of specific lesions.

Plasma ACTH. Plasma ACTH concentrations are elevated in patients with ACTH-dependent Cushing's syndrome and low in patients with ACTH-independent Cushing's syndrome. The ACTH nadir is assessed with a midnight blood sample. A plasma ACTH less than 5 pg per mL (<1.1 pmol/ L) indicates ACTH-independent Cushing's syndrome.[4] A plasma ACTH more than 20 pg per mL (>4.4 pmol/L) indicates ACTH-dependent Cushing's syndrome.[4] Intermediate plasma ACTH concentrations [5–20 pg/mL (1.2–4.4 pmol/ L)] are indeterminant and require a follow-up CRH test (see below).[4]

Corticotropin-Releasing Hormone Stimulation Test. CRH stimulates ACTH secretion in patients with Cushing's disease but not ectopic ACTH-secreting tumors. An intravenous bolus dose (1 μg/kg body weight) of synthetic ovine CRH is injected. Blood samples for plasma ACTH and cortisol are obtained before and after CRH injection. A subnormal response to CRH [ACTH <30 pg/mL (<6.6 pmol/L)] establishes ACTH-independent Cushing syndrome; an elevated ACTH establishes ACTH-dependent Cushing syndrome.

Inferior Petrosal Sinus Catheterization. Inferior petrosal sinus catheterization (IPSC) determines the origin (pituitary vs. ectopic) and lateralization (left vs. right side of the pituitary) of ACTH-secreting lesions. Catheters are placed into the left and right inferior petrosal venous system draining the pituitary gland; blood is sampled simultaneously from both sides and the peripheral circulation. With a pituitary source, the petrosal-peripheral gradient for ACTH is greater than 2 or 3.[4] CRH administration (1 μg/kg) during the procedure enhances the diagnostic accuracy.

Metyrapone Test. The metyrapone test differentiates between Cushing's disease and ectopic ACTH-secreting tumors. Though nearly replaced by the plasma ACTH test and adrenal CT, the metyrapone test is sometimes performed when other tests are equivocal. Metyrapone blocks the synthesis of 11-deoxycortisol to cortisol at the level of the adrenal enzyme, 11β-hydroxylase, resulting in decreased circulating cortisol. Plasma 11-deoxycortisol increases in response to increased pituitary ACTH secretion. Patients with Cushing's disease have a supranormal increase in plasma 11-deoxycortisol, whereas patients with ectopic ACTH-secreting tumors show little or no response.[33]

Radiologic Imaging. Computed tomography (CT) and magnetic resonance imaging (MRI) are the standard imaging techniques for evaluating Cushing's syndrome. CT is used to determine the location and size of tumors and to differentiate between adrenal adenomas and carcinomas (small, rounded, well-circumscribed unilateral masses vs. large, irregular infiltrated masses, respectively).[33,36] CT of the adrenals of patients with ACTH-dependent Cushing's syndrome generally shows bilateral hyperplastic glands though the adrenals may be normal or atrophic.[33] MRI has greater sensitivity for detecting ACTH-producing pituitary microadenomas than CT scans.[37]

PSYCHOSOCIAL ASPECTS

Cushing's syndrome is a serious but potentially curable disease. Major depressive disorder is a severe and life-threatening complication of Cushing's syndrome; other psychiatric symptoms, including anxiety disorders, mania, and cognitive dysfunction, may be present, though to a lesser degree. Depression may have a profound impact on the patient's quality of life. Correction of the hypercortisolism is more effective than antidepressant medication, though patients may benefit from cognitive-behavioral therapies, antidepressants, or anxiolytics after the hypercortisolism is corrected.[38]

THERAPEUTIC PLAN

The treatment of Cushing's syndrome depends on the etiology. With appropriate treatment, the signs and symptoms of hypercortisolism resolve over several weeks to months. Iatrogenic Cushing's syndrome is treated by slowly tapering the steroid over several weeks as tolerated and managing the adverse physiologic consequences of excessive chronic glucocorticoid administration (e.g., control hyperglycemia with diet and hypoglycemic medications; control the elevated blood pressure with antihypertensive medications; monitor for and treat infections; replace potassium; give supplemental calcium; supplement the glucocorticoid dosage when the patient has an acute illness, injury, or surgery). Cushing's disease is treated by selective surgical removal of the pituitary microadenomas (transsphenoidal adenectomy).[39] ACTH production temporarily drops after surgery; patients typically require glucocorticoid replacement therapy for 3 to 12 months until the HPA axis function recovers.[39] Pituitary irradiation is indicated for those who failed or are unable to tolerate pituitary surgery. Ectopic ACTH-secreting tumors, adrenal adenomas, and adrenalomas are surgically removed or treated with radiation or standard chemotherapy; adrenocorticolytic drugs control cortisol production during treatment.

TREATMENT

PHARMACOTHERAPY

Pharmacotherapy of Cushing's syndrome is indicated to reduce cortisol production before surgery, to maintain normal plasma cortisol levels while awaiting the results of surgical or radiation therapy, to treat patients with severe physical or psychiatric symptoms of hypercortisolism, and to reduce cortisol effects in patients with nonresectable tumors.

The three categories of medications used to treat Cushing's syndrome include the (a) steroidogenic inhibitors, (b) neuromodulators of ACTH secretion, and (c) glucocorticoid receptor antagonists (Table 37.4).[2,40,41] Steroidogenic inhibitors, used almost exclusively to treat ACTH-dependent syn-

TABLE 37.4	Medications for the treatment of Cushing's Syndrome		
Medication	**Dosage**	**Mechanism of Action**	**Major Side Effects**
Ketoconazole[a,b] (Nizoral)	Initial: 200 mg tid MD: 300–400 mg tid	Inhibits cortisol synthesis	Nausea, vomiting, abdominal pain, headache, sedation, gynecomastia, pruritus, decreased libido, impotence, edema, rash
Metyrapone[a] (Metopirone)	Initial: 250 mg daily MD: 500–750 mg tid-qid	Inhibits cortisol synthesis	Dizziness, sedation, hirsutism, nausea, ataxia, edema
Aminoglutethimide[c] (Cytodren)	250 mg bid-tid	Inhibits cortisol synthesis	Transient generalized pruritic rash, headache, sedation, nausea, vomiting, anorexia, blurred vision, lethargy, dyscrasias
Mitotane[b] (Lysodren)	Initial: 500 mg at bedtime MD: 2–4 g/d (one-half at bedtime)	Inhibits cortisol synthesis; Adrenocorticolytic	Nausea, vomiting, diarrhea, anorexia, rash, lethargy, dizziness, ataxia, leukopenia, hypercholesterolemia, hepatotoxicity
Etomidate[a,b,d] (Amidate)	0.3 mg/kg/h IV	Inhibits cortisol synthesis	Sedation
Bromocriptine[a,e] (Parlodel)	3.75–30 mg daily	Inhibits ACTH release	Nausea, dry mouth, headache, nasal congestion, postural hypotension
Cyproheptadine[a,f] (Periactin)	Initial: 8 mg daily MD: Up to 24 mg daily	Inhibits ACTH release	Sedation, hyperphagia, weight gain
Valproate[a,c] (Depakene)	200–400 mg tid	Inhibits ACTH release	Nausea, vomiting, abdominal pain, sedation, thrombocytopenia, hepatotoxicity, rash
Mifepristone[a,g] (Mifeprex)	400 mg daily	Blocks glucocorticoid receptors	Headache, fatigue, nausea, vomiting, diarrhea, abdominal pain

[a] Not an FDA-approved indication; [b] Pregnancy Category C; [c] Pregnancy Category D; [d] Contains 0.1813 g propylene glycol/g of etomidate; [e] Pregnancy category not determined; [f] Pregnancy Category B; [g] Indicated to terminate pregnancy. tid, three times daily; MD, maintenance dose; qid, four times daily; bid, twice a day; IV, intravenous; ACTH, adrenocorticotropic hormone.
(From Stewart PM. The adrenal cortex. In: Larsen PR, Kronenberg HM, Melmed S, et al, eds. Williams textbook of endocrinology. 10th ed. Philadelphia: WB Saunders, 2003:491–551; Miller JW, Crapo L. The medical treatment of Cushing's syndrome. Endocrin Rev 14:443–458, 1993; Nieman LK, Orth DN. Treatment of Cushing's syndrome: diminishing adrenal cortisol synthesis. Release 11.3. 2003. Available at: http://www.uptodate.com. Accessed April 1, 2004; with permission.)

dromes, are the most effective agents available for treating Cushing's syndrome. Results with neuromodulator agents have been disappointing,[42–45] and clinical experience with the glucocorticoid receptor antagonist mifepristone is limited.[46,47]

Therapy is often initiated with ketoconazole.[41] Metyrapone may be added as a second steroidogenic inhibitor and aminoglutethimide, a third steroidogenic inhibitor may be added if the combination of ketoconazole and metyrapone is ineffective. The steroidogenic inhibitors act synergistically; side effects are reduced when used in combination at less than maximal doses of each agent.

Dexamethasone (0.25–0.5 mg daily) is added as cortisol serum concentrations approach normal (10 μg/dL; 28 nmol/L); the dosage is adjusted to alleviate the symptoms of hypocortisolism. Dexamethasone has the advantage over other glucocorticoids of not interfering with the serum cortisol assay and has a long half-life, allowing for once daily dosing. Depending on the specific treatment, mineralocorticoid replacement therapy with fludrocortisone may be indicated. The fludrocortisone dose is adjusted to alleviate signs and symptoms of volume depletion and normalize serum electrolytes and plasma renin.

Coexisting ovulatory disorders make pregnancy rare in patients with Cushing's syndrome. The general treatment approach is the same with no significant maternal or perinatal complications reported in one series of patients.[48] The potential benefits and risks of each medication must be considered.

Steroidogenic Inhibitors

Ketoconazole. Ketoconazole inhibits the first step in cortisol synthesis (side-chain cleavage), inhibits the conversion of 11-deoxycortisol to cortisol, and inhibits ACTH secretion. Ketoconazole is very effective in lowering cortisol in patients with Cushing's syndrome.[40] Treatment is initiated with 200 mg orally every day and increased at 4- to 7-day intervals until UFC concentrations decrease to the upper limits of normal. Treatment typically requires a daily dose of 600 to 800 mg. Antacids, histamine$_2$ antagonists, antisecretory agents, and sucralfate decrease the absorption of ketoconazole. Isoniazid and rifampin decrease ketoconazole levels and should be avoided. Ketoconazole can inhibit the metabolism of many drugs. Careful clinical monitoring, including serum drug levels when appropriate, is indicated when ketoconazole is given concomitantly with drugs that are metabolized in the liver, such as warfarin, cyclosporine, and phenytoin. See Chapter 3 for a further discussion on drug interactions.

Metyrapone. Metyrapone blocks the final step in cortisol synthesis by inhibiting the enzyme 11β-hydroxylase. Metyrapone is used to treat Cushing's syndrome when dose-limiting side effects occur with ketoconazole or as part of combination therapy with other steroidogenic inhibi-

tors.[19,40,42] The initial dose of metyrapone is 250 mg daily; doses up to 2,000 mg per day are well tolerated. Metyrapone induces hepatic mixed-function oxidases; concurrent use of phenytoin or phenobarbital requires careful clinical monitoring.

Aminoglutethimide. Aminoglutethimide inhibits cortisol synthesis, but the effects are short-lived due to a compensatory rise in ACTH. The duration of effect is longer in patients with cortisol-secreting adenocarcinomas or when aminoglutethimide is used in combination with metyrapone or pituitary irradiation.[42,49] Treatment is initiated with 250 mg four times daily and increased as required to normalize UFC concentrations; doses less than 1 g per day usually are well tolerated.[50] Aminoglutethimide induces the metabolism of dexamethasone, but has no effect on the metabolism of cortisone.[51]

Mitotane. The mitotane acylchloride metabolite binds to adrenocortical cellular mitochondria, destroying the cells (sometimes called a "medical adrenalectomy"). Mitotane also inhibits cortisol synthesis by inhibiting 11β-hydroxylase and cholesterol side chain cleavage enzyme. Used most commonly with pituitary irradiation, mitotane may be used in combination with other steroidogenic inhibitors. Most patients (80%–90%) respond to pituitary irradiation and do not require chronic mitotane therapy.[19] Treatment is initiated with 500 mg once daily at bedtime and increased as required to normalize UFC concentration. Concomitant glucocorticoid replacement therapy is required during and after mitotane therapy. Mitotane accumulates in fatty tissues and persists in plasma for several months after discontinuation[52]; patients may require glucocorticoid replacement therapy for weeks after mitotane is discontinued. Mitotane induces a state of mineralocorticoid deficiency. Replacement therapy with fludrocortisone is guided by signs and symptoms of volume depletion or excess.

Etomidate. Etomidate, a hypnotic parenteral anesthetic medication, inhibits cortisol synthesis at low doses by inhibiting 11β-hydroxylase; high doses also inhibit the side-chain cleavage enzyme.[53] Data regarding the use of etomidate for the short-term or long-term treatment of Cushing's disease are quite limited.[54,55]

Neuromodulators. Bromocriptine, a dopamine receptor agonist and prolactin inhibitor, cyproheptadine, a sedating antihistamine, and valproate sodium, an antiepileptic, have all been used experimentally in the treatment of Cushing's syndrome. All three are thought to inhibit ACTH secretion but data are extremely limited.[43,45,56–58]

Glucocorticoid Receptor Antagonists. Mifepristone competitively binds to glucocorticoid and progestin receptors, blocking agonist-induced activation.[59] Data regarding the use of mifepristone to treat Cushing's syndrome are limited.[60] Serum cortisol concentrations are unaffected. Concomitant administration of spironolactone, a mineralocorticoid receptor antagonist, may be required to control hypokalemia secondary to cortisol activation of mineralocorticoid receptors.[61]

NONPHARMACOLOGIC THERAPY

Surgery. Transsphenoidal microadenomectomy is the surgery of choice for circumscribed microadenomas.[62,63] With a cure rate of approximately 95%, the surgery preserves normal anterior pituitary function.[63] Resection of nonpituitary ACTH- and CRH-secreting tumors is curative, however, most tumors are nonresectable.[62] Bilateral total surgical adrenalectomy is indicated for bilateral micronodular or macronodular adrenal hyperplasia and nonresectable ectopic tumors, when rapid hypercortisolism reduction is needed, or when all other therapies have failed.[62]

Irradiation. Pituitary irradiation is indicated for treating Cushing's disease not cured by transsphenoidal surgery. Newer forms of radiotherapy, including computer-assisted linear accelerator (photon knife) or cobalt-60 (gamma knife) may be more effective, but experience is limited. In one series, 83% of patients treated with a total dose of 48 to 54 Gy administered in fractions of 1.8 to 2 Gy per day for 5 days a week, achieved remission during the first 2 years.[64] Until remission, hypercortisolism is controlled with adrenal enzyme inhibitors (e.g., ketoconazole).

ALTERNATIVE THERAPIES

Numerous alternative therapies, including KH3, DHEA, vitamin C, phosphatidylserine, and melatonin, are mentioned in the lay literature, but little data are available regarding the efficacy or toxicity of these therapies in the treatment of Cushing's syndrome or Cushing's disease. KH3, a European drug, not approved by the U.S. Food and Drug Administration (FDA), that contains some form of procaine HCL, purportedly protects against cortisol toxicity. DHEA supposedly protects against overproduction of cortisol by the adrenal gland. Vitamin C and phosphatidylserine are used to suppress stress-induced cortisol release. Conflicting data are available regarding whether the circadian profile of serum melatonin secretion is abnormal in patients with Cushing's syndrome.[65,66] There are no data regarding the efficacy or safety of supplemental melatonin therapy in Cushing's syndrome.

FUTURE THERAPIES

Current Cushing's syndrome-related research is focused on improved diagnostic and surgical techniques. Positron emission tomography (PET) scans may improve the detection of ectopic ACTH-secreting tumors. Synthetic ovine CRH can also be used for the diagnosis of Cushing's syndrome. Genetic and molecular research may provide the foundation for new therapeutic strategies.

IMPROVING OUTCOMES

PATIENT EDUCATION

Patients with Cushing's syndrome or disease should wear a medical alert bracelet or other form of identification and carry written documentation identifying their current medications and prescriber contact information. Counsel patients to follow corticosteroid tapering instructions carefully, to not discontinue the corticosteroid (or any other medication used to treat the disorder) without prescriber permission and guidance, and to ask about potential drug interactions with any coprescribed medication or self-selected nonprescription drug. Advise patients to eat a high protein, low carbohydrate, low calorie, and low sodium diet; a high potassium diet may be recommended depending on the specific treatment. Instruct patients to contact their doctor if they have any signs or symptoms of infection (fever or chills) or steroid deficiency (dizziness, muscle pain, headache).

METHODS TO IMPROVE ADHERENCE TO DRUG THERAPY

Though not specifically evaluated in patients with Cushing's disease, strategies to improve patient adherence to chronic drug therapy include patient education, refill reminders, enlisting the aid of a family member or friend, and participation in patient support groups. Some patients respond best to a paternalistic approach; other patients respond best to a shared decision-making approach.

DISEASE MANAGEMENT STRATEGIES TO IMPROVE PATIENT OUTCOMES

Cushing's syndrome patients require long-term follow-up and monitoring during and after treatment for the hypercortisolism. The signs and symptoms of hypercortisolism resolve slowly over several months, though hypertension and diabetes may persist.[2] Markers of reduced bone mass persist for several years after resolution of hypercortisolism[67] and patients remain at a high risk for adverse cardiovascular events.[68] After surgical cure, patients may feel worse with increased mood changes, lethargy, postural hypotension, and arthropathy; these symptoms may respond to temporary increases in the glucocorticoid dose.

PHARMACOECONOMICS

There are no pharmacoeconomic data for Cushing's syndrome or Cushing's disease. Unanswered questions include cost-effective diagnostic, surgical, and treatment strategies. Given the rarity of Cushing's syndrome, these questions will be difficult to answer.

ADDISON'S DISEASE

TREATMENT GOALS: Addison's Disease

The treatment goals for Addison's disease are to:

■ Restore HPA hormonal balance by replacing glucocorticoids and mineralocorticoids.
■ Manage hormonal needs during intercurrent illnesses.

DEFINITION

Addison's disease, also known as primary adrenal insufficiency, was first described in 1855 by Thomas Addison.[69] A rare disease most often caused by autoimmune-mediated destruction of the adrenal cortex, the signs and symptoms of Addison's disease result from decreased production of glucocorticoids, mineralocorticoids, and androgens.

ETIOLOGY

Adrenal insufficiency is classified as primary or secondary adrenal insufficiency. Primary adrenal insufficiency (Addison's disease), caused by adrenal gland disease, is associated with glucocorticoid, mineralocorticoid, and androgen deficiencies. More than 90% of patients with primary adrenal insufficiency have autoimmune-associated Addison's disease.[70] Other causes of primary adrenal insufficiency include infections (e.g., bacterial infections, granulomatous infections), infiltrating diseases (e.g., sarcoidosis, amyloidosis), hemorrhage or infarction, and tumors.[2,71,72]

Secondary adrenal insufficiency caused by ACTH deficiency is associated with glucocorticoid deficiency; the renin-angiotensin-aldosterone axis is intact. The most common cause of secondary adrenal insufficiency is the sudden withdrawal of chronically administered exogenous glucocorticoids.[2] Other causes of secondary adrenal insufficiency include hypothalamic or pituitary tumors or lesions, surgical removal of the pituitary, pituitary irradiation, aneurysm of the internal carotid artery, and proopiomelanocortin (POMC) gene mutation.[2,71,72]

EPIDEMIOLOGY

The prevalence of Addison's disease is estimated to be approximately 110 per million population with an incidence of 5 to 6 per million per year.[73,74] Addison's disease occurs as an isolated disorder or as one component of multiple coexisting endocrinopathies known as polyglandular autoimmune (PGA) syndromes.[75] As an isolated endocrine disorder, autoimmune adrenal insufficiency most commonly is first diagnosed in women in their third or fourth decade.

PATHOPHYSIOLOGY

In Addison's disease, all three zones of the adrenal glands are progressively destroyed and replaced by fibrotic tissue; the medulla is spared but may be atrophic. Adrenal dysfunction may be gradual or abrupt; clinical signs and symptoms of adrenal insufficiency appear when ≥90% of the adrenal cortex is destroyed.[76] The zona glomerulosa is affected first, followed by zona fasciculata dysfunction months to years later. Acute adrenal gland hemorrhage or infection is associated with sudden and complete loss of adrenal function.

Autoimmune Addison's disease is characterized by the presence of autoantibodies directed against adrenal cortex steroid-producing cells. Antibodies to at least three of the cytochrome P-450 enzymes involved in steroidogenesis, including 17α-hydroxylase, 21α-hydroxylase, and side-chain cleavage enzyme, have been identified.[77,78]

The adrenal cortex may be destroyed by disseminated infection with *Mycobacterium tuberculosis*, histoplasmosis, and paracoccidioidomycosis; metastatic tumor (e.g., disseminated breast or lung cancer); and acute hemorrhage associated with anticoagulation or meningococcemia. Patients infected with the human immunodeficiency virus are at risk of Addison's disease on the basis of infection with cytomegalovirus, *Mycobacterium avium intracellulare,* cryptococcus, and metastatic Kaposi's sarcoma.[79] Drugs that interfere reversibly with steroidogeneis (aminoglutethimide, etomidate, ketoconazole, metyrapone, and mitotane[71] or competitively inhibit glucocorticoid and progestogens (mifepristone) can cause Addison's disease.

CLINICAL PRESENTATION AND DIAGNOSIS

SIGNS AND SYMPTOMS

Addison's disease has been called the "unforgiving master of non-specificity and disguise."[80] Addison's disease is considered when patients complain of persistent vague symptoms, especially in the presence of other autoimmune disease, and when critically ill patients remain hypotensive despite maximal vasopressor therapy. The signs and symptoms range from vague feelings of unwellness to acute syncope and mental status changes (Table 37.5).[2,71,72,80,81] Addison's disease patients crave salt and have characteristic

TABLE 37.5	Addison's Disease Signs and Symptoms

Glucocorticoid Deficiency	Mineralocorticoid Deficiency	Other	Electrocardiographic	Radiologic
Fatigue	Dehydration	Hyperpigmentation	Changes secondary to hyperkalemia	Abdominal computed tomography: small, normal, enlarged adrenals (depending on the cause)
Lassitude, malaise	Hypotension	Salt craving		
Weight loss	Orthostatic hypotension	Amenorrhea		
Anorexia	↓ Cardiac output	↓ Libido		Skull radiograph: enlarged sella turcica (chronic untreated or undertreated disease)
Nausea, vomiting, abdominal pain	↓ Catecholamine response	↓ Axillary and pubic hair		
Diarrhea		Premature menopause		Head computed tomography: enlarged pituitary
Steatorrhea		Multiple dental caries		
Hypotension		Splenomegaly		
Weakness		Lymphoid hyperplasia		
Myalgias, arthralgias				
Depression				
Organic brain syndrome				
Psychosis				
Perceptual disturbances				

(From Stewart PM. The adrenal cortex. In: Larsen PR, Kronenberg HM, Melmed S, et al, eds. Williams textbook of endocrinology. 10th ed. Philadelphia: WB Saunders, 2003:491–551; Chin R Jr, Zekan JM. Adrenal insufficiency. Prob Crit Care 4:312–324, 1990; Loriaux DL. Syndromes of adrenal insufficiency. In: Becker KL, ed. Principles and practice of endocrinology and metabolism. 3rd ed. Philadelphia: Lippincott Williams & Wilkins, 2001:739–743; Brosnan CM, Gowing NFC. Lesson the week: Addison's disease. BMJ 312:1085–1087, 1996; Oelkers W. Current concepts: adrenal insufficiency. N Engl J Med 335:1206–1212, 1996; with permission.)

hyperpigmentation of the sun-exposed skin, the skin over areas of pressure or irritation (e.g., knuckles, knees), and mucosal membranes. Vitiligo and alopecia may be observed in patients with autoimmune disease.

More than 90% of patients with Addison's disease present with biochemical abnormalities including hyponatremia, hyperkalemia, hypoglycemia, mild normocytic normochromic anemia, neutropenia, lymphocytosis, eosinophilia, hypercalcemia, mild hyperchloremic metabolic acidosis, elevated plasma creatinine, elevated aspartate transaminase, and elevated erythrocyte sedimentation rate.[2,72,81,82]

An adrenal crisis typically occurs in the setting of undiagnosed adrenal insufficiency and untreated stress. The signs and symptoms mimic septic shock and include profound anorexia and nausea and vomiting, severe dehydration, hypotension, shock unresponsive to vasopressors and inotropic agents, tachycardia, fever, hypoglycemia, progressively deteriorating mental status, and biochemical changes.

Acute Addison's disease may occur in the setting of previously normal adrenal function or may be superimposed on chronic adrenal insufficiency. When acute Addison's disease occurs in isolation, serum sodium and potassium are within normal limits and patients are not hyperpigmented. When an acute Addisonian crisis is superimposed on chronic adrenal insufficiency, dehydration, hyperpigmentation, hyponatremia, hyperkalemia, weight loss, and azotemia are typically present.

DIAGNOSIS AND CLINICAL FINDINGS

Diagnosis begins with a high degree of clinical suspicion but depends on provocative testing of the HPA axis. Screening tests include complete blood count with differential, chest radiograph, serum biochemistries, renal function, urinalysis, and skin testing. Tests for suspected pituitary dysfunction include thyroid stimulating hormone, follicle stimulating hormone, leuteinizing hormone, growth hormone, thyroxine, and testosterone levels.

Establishing Adrenal Insufficiency

Basal Serum Cortisol. Basal morning cortisol may be decreased or, if partial adrenal function is preserved, nearly normal, limiting the diagnostic usefulness of the test. A very low basal serum cortisol concentration [<3 μg/dL (<80 nmol/L)] or salivary cortisol [<1.8 ng/mL (<5 nmol/L)] suggests adrenal dysfunction. A high basal cortisol serum concentration [>15 μg/dL (>400 nmol/L)] suggests an intact HPA axis.[2]

Short ACTH Stimulation Test. Synthetic ACTH (cosyntropin; Cortrosyn) is used for the short ACTH stimulation test instead of human ACTH, which is allergenic. The short ACTH stimulation test can be conducted any time of the day and does not require fasting. Serum cortisol is measured before and 30 to 60 minutes after intramuscular or intravenous administration of 250 μg of cosyntropin. Depending on the assay, Addison's disease is ruled out if the peak serum cortisol concentration is greater than or equal to 19 μg per dL (525 nmol/L).[2,83] The short cosyntropin test does not exclude mild primary or secondary adrenal insufficiency, does not distinguish between primary and secondary adrenal insufficiency, and does not always predict the response to surgery, hypoglycemia, or other forms of stress.

Differential Diagnosis

Basal Plasma ACTH. The morning basal plasma ACTH is used to differentiate between primary and secondary adrenal insufficiency. Plasma ACTH follows a circadian rhythm with the highest concentration at about 8 AM and the lowest concentration at about midnight.[84] The 8 AM plasma ACTH is normally 20 to 80 pg per mL (4.5–10 pmol/L).[84] A high 8 AM plasma ACTH [>4,000 pg/mL (880 pmol/L)] establishes primary adrenal insufficiency; a low or low normal basal plasma ACTH establishes secondary adrenal insufficiency. Since ACTH secretion is episodic, the test may need to be repeated on several consecutive days to establish a consistent basal concentration. Exogenous glucocorticoid administration suppresses ACTH secretion. When possible, the test should be performed before glucocorticoid therapy is initiated. Patients taking glucocorticoids should be switched to hydrocortisone, a short-acting glucocorticoid, for several days before the test is performed and the test performed 24 hours after the last hydrocortisone dose.

2-Day ACTH Stimulation Test. The 2-day ACTH stimulation test may distinguish Addison's disease from secondary adrenal insufficiency. In Addison's disease, the adrenal glands are destroyed and cannot secrete cortisol. In secondary adrenal insufficiency, the atrophic adrenal glands will secrete cortisol when chronically exposed to ACTH. ACTH (250 μg) is infused over 8 hours on 2 consecutive days. Serum cortisol and 24-hour UFC are collected daily. In Addison's disease, serum cortisol remains low [<18–20 μg/dL (500–550 nmol/L)]; urinary 17-OHCS (hydroxycorticosteroid) is low and does not increase with time.[2] In secondary and tertiary adrenal insufficiency, serum cortisol and urinary 17-OHCS are increased at 24 and 48 hours.

Short Metyrapone Test. Metyrapone blocks the synthesis of cortisol at the level of the adrenal enzyme 11β-hydroxylase, the final step in cortisol synthesis. The blockade causes a decrease in circulating cortisol and an increase in 11-deoxycortisol. Metyrapone (30 mg/kg) is administered at midnight. Plasma 11-deoxycortisol and cortisol are measured at 8 AM the next morning. Adrenal insufficiency is established if the plasma cortisol is less than 8 μg per dL (<230 nmol/L) and the plasma 11-deoxycortisol is less than 7 μg per dL (200 nmol/L).[81]

Insulin-Induced Hypoglycemia. The insulin-induced hypoglycemia test is the most sensitive and accurate test of HPA axis function. However, the test is physiologically stressful and contraindicated in patients with seizure disorders, cerebrovascular disease, and cardiovascular disease. Insulin-induced symptomatic (sweating, tachycardia, tremor) hypoglycemia [plasma glucose <40 mg/dL (<2.2 mmol/L)] stimulates the HPA axis. Regular insulin (0.1–0.15 U/kg) is administered by intravenous injection. Plasma glucose and cortisol are measured at baseline and then every 15 minutes for 90 minutes. Adrenal insufficiency is suggested if the plasma cortisol concentration is less than 18 to 20 μg per dL (497–552 nmol/L) at 60 to 90 minutes.[81]

Other Diagnostic Tests. Adrenal CT is used to identify adrenal atrophy, hemorrhage, or enlargement caused by tumors and disseminated mycobacterial and fungal infections.[81] MRI is used to image the hypothalamic-pituitary region. Autoantibodies against 17α-hydroxylase, 21α-hydroxylase, and side-chain cleavage enzyme may be detected by the indirect immunofluorescence technique or radiobinding assay.[85,86] The corticotropin-releasing hormone test differentiates between corticotropin-releasing hormone and corticotropin deficiencies.[84] Plasma renin is increased and plasma aldosterone is decreased in primary adrenal insufficiency, but it is normal in secondary adrenal insufficiency.[2]

PSYCHOSOCIAL ASPECTS

Addison's disease is an incurable and potentially life-threatening disease. With appropriate medical therapy, patients can live fairly normal lives. Patients with Addison's disease may present with or develop psychiatric symptoms making it difficult to recognize secondary psychiatric complications such as reactive depression. Neuropsychiatric symptoms, including fatigue and depression, may occur if corticosteroid replacement therapy is tapered too quickly.

THERAPEUTIC PLAN

The treatment of Addison's disease consists of hormone replacement therapy and supplemental glucocorticoid therapy during periods of stress (Table 37.6).[2,72,77,87] Replacement glucocorticoid and mineralocorticoid drug therapy is continued indefinitely, though some cases of subclinical autoimmune adrenal insufficiency may be self-limiting.[88] Androgen replacement therapy, though not routinely recommended, may be considered.[2,72,87]

TREATMENT

PHARMACOTHERAPY

Chronic Replacement Therapy. Chronic replacement therapy consists of daily glucocorticoid and mineralocorticoid replacement therapy; androgen replacement therapy may be considered. The target cortisol replacement therapy is slightly higher than the physiologic cortisol production rate of approximately 12 to 15 mg per m² per day.[89–91] In the past, a short-acting glucocorticoid (cortisone acetate or hydrocortisone) was given twice daily to simulate normal

TABLE 37.6 | Treatment of Addison's Disease

Acute Adrenal Crisis

- Establish IV access with a large-gauge needle.
- Obtain blood for stat serum electrolytes, glucose, plasma cortisol, and ACTH.
- Rapidly infuse 2–3 L 0.9% sodium chloride or 5% dextrose/normal saline; subsequent rate depends on patient response.
- Inject hydrocortisone 100 mg IV every 6 hours.
- Taper the glucocorticoid over the next 2–3 days to standard replacement therapy if physiologic stress resolving.
- Initiate mineralocorticoid replacement therapy with fludrocortisone 0.1 mg daily when patient is able to eat and drink.

Chronic Replacement Therapy

- Dexamethasone 0.5 mg (0.25–0.75 mg) or prednisone 5 mg daily at bedtime. May add hydrocortisone 5–10 mg mid-afternoon if needed.
- Fludrocortisone 0.1 mg (0.05–0.2 mg) daily.

Self-care

Minor febrile illnesses or stress: Double or triple the glucocorticoid dose for 2–3 days. Continue usual mineralocorticoid dose. Contact physician if condition worsens or persists more than 3 days.

Emergency self-treatment of severe stress or trauma: Inject dexamethasone 4 mg IM. Get to a physician as soon as possible.

Pregnancy

Continue usual glucocorticoid and mineralocorticoid replacement doses; some women may need slightly higher doses during the third trimester. For women unable to take oral medications, give dexamethasone 1 mg IM daily plus 1–2 mg deoxycorticosterone acetate in oil daily. Give 25 mg IV hydrocortisone every 6 hours and adequate saline hydration during labor; increase the dose to 100 mg every 6 hours if labor is prolonged. Rapidly taper the doses to the patient's usual maintenance doses within 3 days of delivery.

Steroid Coverage for Hospitalized Patients

- Moderately stressful outpatient and inpatient procedures (barium enema, arteriogram, endoscopy): Give 100 mg IV hydrocortisone immediately prior to the procedure.
- Moderate illness: Give 50 mg IV or oral hydrocortisone twice daily. Rapidly taper to the patient's maintenance dose as the illness resolves.
- Major surgery: Give 100 mg IV hydrocortisone immediately before induction of anesthesia. Give 100 mg IV hydrocortisone every 8 hours for 24 hours following the surgery. Taper to the patient's maintenance dose by reducing the dose by 50% daily; adjust the taper based on clinical course.
- Severe illness: Give 100 mg IV hydrocortisone every 8 hours. Taper to the patient's maintenance dose by reducing the dose by 50% daily; adjust the taper based on clinical course.

IV, intravenous; ACTH, adrenocorticotropic hormone; IM, intramuscular.
(From Stewart PM. The adrenal cortex. In: Larsen PR, Kronenberg HM, Melmed S, Polonsky KS, eds. Williams textbook of endocrinology. 10th ed. Philadelphia: WB Saunders, 2003:491–551; Loriaux DL. Syndromes of adrenal insufficiency. In: Becker KL, ed. Principles and practice of endocrinology and metabolism. 3rd ed. Philadelphia: Lippincott Williams & Wilkins, 2001:739–743; Ten S, New M, Maclaren N. Addison's disease 2001. J Clin Endocrinol Metab 86:2909–2922, 2001; Nieman LK, Orth DN. Treatment of adrenal insufficiency. In: UpToDate Online Release 11.3, 2003. Available at: http:www.uptodate.com. Accessed December 3, 2003; with permission.)

circadian rhythm. However, this regimen caused fluctuating serum concentrations and periods of transient adrenal insufficiency.[92] Currently, dexamethasone is the glucocorticoid of choice for chronic replacement therapy, patient-initiated rescue therapy, and initial treatment of an adrenal crisis before the diagnosis is confirmed. The glucocorticoid dosage is titrated to a sense of well-being, blood pressure, and weight.[2] Dexamethasone does not interfere with serum cortisol measurements and has the advantage of prolonged ACTH suppression. Fludrocortisone is the mineralocorticoid of choice for chronic replacement therapy. Fludrocortisone is approximately equipotent with aldosterone but is only available as an oral dosage form. The mineralocorticoid dosage is titrated to relieve postural hypotension symptoms, normalize standing and sitting blood pressure, and normalize serum potassium and plasma renin activity.

The current recommended regimen is dexamethasone 0.5 mg (0.25–0.75 mg) plus fludrocortisone 0.1 mg (0.05–0.2 mg) daily at bedtime; doses are individualized to clinical response. Patients who have drug-associated insomnia can take the glucocorticoid when arising in the morning. Some patients need a small (5–10 mg) mid-afternoon supplemental hydrocortisone dose. For women, whose primary source of androgens are the adrenals, androgen replacement therapy with dehydroepiandrosterone (DHEA) (25–50 mg daily), though not well-established, may improve mood, sense of well-being, and sexual function, but with a high incidence of side effects such as increased sweat odor, scalp itching, acne, and hirsutism.[9,93,94]

Acute Adrenal Crisis. Acute adrenal insufficiency is life threatening. Empiric glucocorticoid replacement therapy and supportive therapy must be initiated before the diagnosis is confirmed (Table 37.6).[2,72,77,87] Hydrocortisone is the drug of choice for the acute treatment of an Addisonian crisis or for short-term parenteral use; dexamethasone may be substituted to avoid confounding the results of an anticipated ACTH stimulation test. Hydrocortisone has about 1% of the mineralocorticoid activity of aldosterone; concomitant mineralocorticoid replacement therapy is not necessary when large hydrocortisone doses are administered.[95] The glucocorticoid dose is titrated to relieve clinical signs and symptoms and normalize the morning plasma ACTH. Hydrocortisone is tapered to maintenance doses over 1 to 3 days as the precipitating illness resolves. Mineralocorticoid deficiency is treated with saline and fluid loading; specific aldosterone replacement therapy is not effective since it takes several days for the sodium-retaining effects to be apparent. Once the patient is stabilized, intravenous fluids are continued at a lower rate for another 1 to 2 days. Mineralocorticoid replacement therapy with fludrocortisone is started when the patient is stable and able to take oral medications.

Supplemental Stress-Dose Steroids. Patients with Addison disease who are physiologically stressed by acute medical illnesses or other trauma need supplemental steroids. Steroid supplementation is not needed for routine un-

complicated dental procedures, minor procedures performed with local anesthesia, or most radiology procedures. Adrenal reserve can be assessed if adrenal status is uncertain and time permits. For treatment of special situations, including short-term minor stress or febrile illnesses, pregnancy, emergency treatment of stress or trauma, and severe stress or febrile illness, refer to Table 37.6.

NONPHARMACOLOGIC THERAPY

Nondrug therapy for normotensive patients consists of liberalizing the dietary salt intake and avoidance of sodium-wasting diuretics and spironolactone. However, hypertensive patients should be maintained on salt-restricted diets.

ALTERNATIVE THERAPIES

Although numerous alternative therapies, including minerals (sea salt, magnesium, zinc), vitamins (pantothenic acid, ascorbic acid), nutrients (trimethylglycine, phosphatidylserine), botanicals (licorice root, ginseng), and adrenal cortical extract are mentioned in the lay literature, few data are available regarding the efficacy or toxicity of these therapies in the treatment of Addison's disease. However, two of these therapies, licorice and adrenal cortical extract, may be quite harmful. Licorice (*Glycyrrhiza glabra*) has mineralocorticoid effects. Taken in excess or in combination with prescribed mineralocorticoid therapy, licorice can cause signs and symptoms of mineralocorticoid excess (sodium retention, hypokalemia, suppression of the renin-angiotensin-aldosterone system, increased blood pressure, and edema).[96] Adrenal cortex extract (ACE), an unlicensed parenteral product derived from the adrenal cortex of domestic food animals, was withdrawn from the market in 1978[97] but is available through the internet. There is a risk of infection (new variant Creutzfeldt-Jakob disease) if the product is derived from a cow infected with bovine spongiform encephalopathy. Patients are at risk of other infections from contaminated products. Recently, the largest outbreak of *Mycobacterium abscessus* infections in the United States was linked to contaminated adrenal cortex extract.[98]

FUTURE THERAPIES

Current Addison's disease-related research is focused on improved diagnostic techniques. Genetic and molecular research may provide the foundation for new therapeutic strategies.

IMPROVING OUTCOMES

PATIENT EDUCATION

Patients with Addison's disease should wear a medical alert bracelet or other form of medical identification and carry written documentation identifying their current medications and physician contact information. Patients should be counseled to follow corticosteroid taper instructions carefully, to not change the dose or discontinue any medication without prescriber permission and guidance, and to ask about potential drug interactions with any coprescribed or self-selected nonprescription drug. Patients should have prefilled syringes containing 4 mg dexamethasone with them at all times and should know when and how to administer the drug. Patients should also be instructed to contact their doctor if they are scheduled for surgery or medical procedures or if they have an illness with symptoms of nausea, vomiting, or diarrhea.

METHODS TO IMPROVE ADHERENCE TO DRUG THERAPY

Though not specifically evaluated in patients with Addison's disease, strategies to improve patient adherence to chronic drug therapy may include patient education, refill reminders, enlisting the aid of a family member or friend, and participation in patient support groups. Some patients respond best to a paternalistic approach; other patients respond best to a shared decision-making approach.

DISEASE MANAGEMENT STRATEGIES TO IMPROVE PATIENT OUTCOMES

Addison's disease patients require long-term monitoring and follow-up. Drug therapy requires careful titration of the corticosteroid and mineralocorticoid replacement therapy. The corticosteroid dose is adjusted to relieve signs and symptoms and normalize the morning ACTH and avoid signs and symptoms of hypercortisolism. The mineralocorticoid dose is adjusted to relieve postural hypotension symptoms, normalize standing and sitting blood pressures, serum potassium, and plasma renin activity. Appropriate anticipation and treatment with supplemental corticosteroids during physiologically stressful situations should improve patient outcomes.

PHARMACOECONOMICS

There are no pharmacoeconomic data for Addison's disease. Unanswered questions include cost-effective diagnostic, surgical, and treatment strategies. Given the rarity of Addison's disease, these questions will be difficult to answer.

CLINICAL USE OF STEROIDS

Corticosteroids, introduced into clinical practice in the late 1940s, are indicated for treating endocrine insufficiency disease and virtually all immunologically mediated diseases. Marketed in numerous dosage forms, including oral, parenteral, topical, compartmental (i.e., intraarticular), inhalational, and intranasal, corticosteroids have multiple effects on almost all cells involved in the inflammatory process.

CORTICOSTEROID PHARMACOKINETICS

Corticosteroid pharmacokinetics are complex and drug specific.[99] Oral bioavailability is high, ranging from nearly 100% with prednisone and methylprednisolone to about 70% with cortisol. The volume of distribution ranges from 0.5 L per kg with cortisol to 1.2 L per kg with dexamethasone and methylprednisolone. Corticosteroids are hepatically metabolized; prednisone and cortisone are inactive until hepatically converted to prednisolone and cortisol, respectively. Prednisone, cortisol, methylprednisolone, and dexamethasone undergo extensive interconversion between active and inactive forms, reducing serum fluctuations and prolonging the half-life.

Corticosteroid receptor pharmacokinetics greatly influence the clinical response to corticosteroids.[100] Biologic activity depends on the corticosteroid-receptor interactions and

activity of newly produced proteins. Corticosteroid-receptor interactions are influenced by receptor-binding affinity, corticosteroid-receptor association and disassociation rates, and corticosteroid-receptor complex half-life.[101] Limited corticosteroid-receptor pharmacokinetic data are available. Although lung-receptor studies demonstrate clear differences among the corticosteroids, the clinical relevance is not known.

CORTICOSTEROID DOSING

Corticosteroid dosing depends on indication, route of administration, and acuity of disease. Physiologic or replacement doses are indicated for deficiency disease. Pharmacologic doses are indicated for treating acute and chronic immune-mediated disease such as acute organ transplant rejection. Corticosteroid doses applied directly to a target tissue (skin, eyes, lungs, joints) are small compared to systemic doses. To minimize toxicity, corticosteroids are used in the lowest effective dose for the shortest period of time. Topical corticosteroids, usually associated with the least risk, may cause systemic side effects at high doses. The benefit to risk ratio must be weighed when deciding whether to use corticosteroids during pregnancy. The fluorinated corticosteroids (fludrocortisone, triamcinolone, betamethasone, dexamethasone) readily cross the placenta and should be used with caution during pregnancy. Newborns exposed to high-dose fluorinated corticosteroids in utero must be evaluated for adrenal insufficiency.

TOPICAL CORTICOSTEROIDS

Cutaneous penetration depends on potency, concentration, formulation, application technique, skin condition, and site of application.[102] Systemic absorption is higher with potent drugs (betamethasone dipropionate, clobetasol dipropionate, diflorasone diacetate, and halobetasol propionate), higher drug concentration, ointments, excipient use (urea or difluoromethylornithine), drug application to damaged or thin skin, increased skin hydration, occlusive dressing use, and continuous application. Creams are indicated for acute or weeping lesions, ointments for dry or chronic lesions, and lotions, creams, and gels for hairy areas.

SYSTEMIC THERAPY

High initial systemic doses suppress immune-mediated processes and reduce subsequent tissue damage. Initial systemic doses (0.6–1 mg/kg/day prednisone or equivalent) are given as single-morning or twice-daily regimens; twice-daily regimens generally are preferred. Once the acute illness resolves, the dose is changed to once daily and rapidly tapered off. Tapering is individualized according to the clinical response. Too rapid a taper may exacerbate the precipitating disease; too slow a taper increases the risk of corticosteroid side effects.

PULSE THERAPY

Large daily intravenous doses (methylprednisolone sodium succinate 1 g/m^2) for short durations (<10 days) are indicated for the initial treatment of progressive immune-mediated diseases. Pulse therapy suppresses disease activity with minimal risk of HPA axis suppression.

STRESS-DOSE THERAPY

Stress-dose therapy is indicated for patients who have received pharmacologic doses of corticosteroids (>7.5 mg/day prednisone or equivalent) for more than 2 or 3 weeks and during the first 6 months after discontinuation of long-term corticosteroid therapy. Hydrocortisone 100 mg daily in two to three divided doses is indicated for minor stress or surgery; higher doses are required for more severe stress. Physiologic replacement doses are continued for 4 weeks after resolution of the acute stress.

SEPSIS-ASSOCIATED FUNCTIONAL ADRENAL INSUFFICIENCY THERAPY

The term "functional adrenal insufficiency" is used to describe subnormal adrenal corticosteroid production during acute severe illness[103,104]; supplemental corticosteroid therapy improves survival in critically ill septic patients.[103] Functional adrenal insufficiency is suspected in septic patients who are hemodynamically unstable despite adequate fluid resuscitation and vasopressors.[105] Corticosteroids are

indicated if a random serum cortisol level less than 15 μg per dL (<400 nmol/L) or if the random cortisol level is 15 to 34 μg per dL (400–940 nmol/L) and the increase in serum cortisol in response to the short 250-mg ACTH stimulation test is less than 9 μg per dL (<240 nmol/L).[103] Treatment consists of hydrocortisone 50 mg intravenously (IV) every 6 hours for 7 days; one group of investigators also administered fludrocortisone 50 μg per day, though the mineralocorticoid status of the patients was not assessed.[106]

TAPERING AND CHRONIC ALTERNATE DAY THERAPY

Corticosteroids can be rapidly tapered and discontinued abruptly if used for less than 2 to 3 weeks. If tapered too quickly and the patient is adrenally suppressed, the patient may experience corticosteroid withdrawal symptoms (anorexia, fatigue, nausea, vomiting, fever, orthostatic hypotension, dizziness, syncope, hypoglycemia, and exacerbation of immune-mediated disease).

Chronic alternate day therapy reduces the risk of corticosteroid toxicity, allows recovery of HPA axis function, and minimizes the risk of infection and delayed growth in children. There is no single rule for changing therapy from daily to an alternate day corticosteroid regimen except to slowly decrease one day's dose and increase the alternate day's dose while monitoring the patient closely. The goal is to place the patient on a regimen consisting of the lowest effective corticosteroid dose on one day, alternating with no corticosteroid the next day. Each dose is given as a single morning dose. Some patients tolerate only very small dose decreases (e.g., 1-mg decreases monthly). Underlying disease states masked by the corticosteroid therapy may be unmasked as the dose is decreased. Patients should wear medical identification and have instructions on how to manage stress.

ADVERSE REACTIONS OF CORTICOSTEROIDS

Corticosteroids are associated with significant morbidity (Table 37.7).[107–109] Some side effects are apparent within days of initiation (e.g., euphoria, insomnia, leukocytosis); some side effects are associated with long-term therapy (e.g., osteoporosis, cataracts, delayed growth). Strategies to limit systemic corticosteroid toxicity include use of the lowest effective dose for the shortest period of time, single morning regimens, alternate day regimens, exercise, low-fat diet, smoking cessation, adequate dietary calcium (1,000 mg/day), and limited alcohol intake.

CARDIOVASCULAR

Mineralocorticosteroids are associated with systemic hypertension and vascular disease. Retained sodium and water increases circulating volume and elevates systemic blood pressure. Multiple steroid-associated factors (hypertension, obesity, hypercholesterolemia, hypertriglyceridemia, insulin resistance, hyperinsulinemia, electrolyte disturbances,

TABLE 37.7	Corticosteroid Side Effects
Target Organ/System	**Side Effects**
Cardiovascular and Renal	Hypercalciuria[a], hypertension[a], hypokalemic metabolic alkalosis[a], sodium and water retention[a]
Central Nervous System	Insomnia[a], mood disorders[a], psychosis[a], pseudotumor cerebri
Endocrine and Metabolic	Acne[a], adrenal suppression, amenorrhea[a], delayed growth in children, carbohydrate intolerance, hyperinsulinemia, insulin resistance, diabetes mellitus, Cushingoid features, impotence, ↓ thyroid-stimulating hormone and T_3, hypokalemia, hirsutism, hypercholesterolemia[a], hyperosmolar nonketotic coma[a], hypertriglyceridemia, negative nitrogen balance[a], impaired wound healing, subcutaneous tissue atrophy, ↑ appetite[a]
Gastrointestinal	Negative calcium balance[a], pancreatitis[a], fatty infiltration of liver
Hematopoietic	Leukocytosis[a], monocytopenia, lymphopenia, eosinopenia
Immune System	Immunosuppression, infections, impaired wound healing
Musculoskeletal	Osteoporosis, aseptic necrosis, myopathy

[a] May be evident within days of starting therapy.
(From Rossi SJ, Schroeder TJ, Hartharan S, et al. Prevention and management of the adverse effects associated with immunosuppressive therapy. Drug Saf 9 : 104–131, 1993; Truhan AP, Ahmed AR. Corticosteroids: a review with emphasis on complications of prolonged systemic therapy. Ann Allergy 62 : 375–390, 1989; Magiakou MA, Chrousos GP. Corticosteroid therapy, nonendocrine disease, and corticosteroid withdrawal. Curr Ther Endocrinol Metab 6 : 138–142, 1997; with permission.)

endothelial cell damage, hypercoagulability, catecholamine potentiation, and altered monocyte and macrophage function) contribute to the development of thrombi and premature atherosclerosis.[110]

GASTROINTESTINAL

Historically, corticosteroids were thought to increase the risk of peptic ulceration. However, a meta analysis of 93 studies concluded that peptic ulceration is a rare complication of corticosteroid use.[111] Risk factors for corticosteroid-associated peptic ulceration include concomitant nonsteroidal anti-inflammatory agents, cumulative corticosteroid dose, duration of corticosteroid usage, and a prior history of peptic ulcers.[112,113] Pancreatitis also is a rare complication of corticosteroid use.

GROWTH

Corticosteroids delay linear bone growth and closure of bone epiphyses. Although the mechanism is unclear, corticosteroids decrease growth hormone secretion and competitively inhibit insulin and somatostatin receptors. Growth resumes and catches up if corticosteroids are discontinued before puberty.

HYPOTHALAMUS-PITUITARY-ADRENAL AXIS SUPPRESSION

HPA axis suppression depends on the type of corticosteroid, dose, dosing interval, time of administration, route of administration, and duration of corticosteroid therapy.[114,115] Recovery of function is slow and may take several months; patients are considered adrenally suppressed for as long as 6 to 12 months after discontinuation of chronic corticosteroid therapy.[116]

METABOLIC

Corticosteroids alter fat, glucose, and protein metabolism. Fat redistribution from the periphery to the trunk causes centripetal obesity, characterized by moon facies, buffalo hump, and protuberant abdomen. Easy bruisability occurs in 50% of patients and is the most common side effect associated with inhaled corticosteroids.[117] Hyperglycemia usually is mild but may persist for several months after the corticosteroid is discontinued. The risk of corticosteroid-induced hyperglycemia is dose related; the greater the dose, the greater the risk. Corticosteroids are more likely to uncover latent diabetes mellitus and to increase the insulin requirement in known diabetics than to cause new cases of diabetes mellitus.

MUSCLE

Corticosteroid-associated myopathy may be acute or chronic. In the acute form, proximal and distal muscle weakness develops acutely in association with significant serum creatine phosphokinase elevations and type IIB muscle fiber atrophy; recovery takes weeks to months after the corticosteroids are discontinued.[112] In the chronic form, proximal muscle weakness develops slowly and the serum creatine phosphokinase and type IIB muscle fibers usually are normal.[112,118] Corticosteroid-associated myopathy is more commonly associated with prolonged courses of high-dose corticosteroids.

OPHTHALMIC

Systemic and topical corticosteroids are associated with an increased risk of posterior subcapsular cataracts.[119,120] Risk factors may include daily dose, cumulative dose, duration of corticosteroid use, age, and ethnicity.[119–121] The cataracts develop slowly, are bilateral, and occur more often in children than in adults. Glaucoma, less predictable and not necessarily reversible, is more likely in patients with diabetes mellitus, myopia, or a family history of glaucoma.

PSYCHOLOGICAL

Corticosteroids cause numerous emotional disturbances, including euphoria, depression, mania, and psychotic reactions.[122] Corticosteroids generally make people feel well, although severe depression with suicidal ideation may occur. These effects usually are dose related, occur within a few days of initiation, and resolve spontaneously within a few weeks of discontinuation.[123] High-dose alternate day regimens may cause mood swings resembling manic-depressive states. A psychiatric history does not predispose patients to corticosteroid-associated psychological side effects. If an acute psychotic reaction occurs, the corticosteroid should be tapered off over a period of several days to avoid rebound depression and increased anxiety.

SKELETAL

Osteoporosis, one of the most serious corticosteroid-associated side effects, is caused by the combination of multiple factors including protein catabolism, osteoblast inhibition, growth hormone inhibition, decreased calcium absorption, decreased renal calcium reabsorption, and mild secondary hyperparathyroidism.[124] Skeletal decalcification occurs quickly; bone fractures are commonly reported during the first year of treatment. All bones are affected, however, lumbar spine compression and rib fractures are more common. Biochemical markers of bone turnover are not sensitive or specific predictors.

A combination of nondrug and drug therapy is recommended to preserve bone.[125] Lifestyle modification includes smoking cessation, avoidance of excessive alcohol intake, and adequate weight-bearing and resistive exercise (30–60 minutes/day). Drug therapy includes calcium (approximately 1,500 mg/day) unless contraindicated, vitamin D (400 IU/day), or calcitriol (0.5 μg/day), bisphosphonates, and low-dose thiazide diuretic if hypercalcuria is detected.

DRUG INTERACTIONS OF CORTICOSTEROIDS

Numerous drug interactions have been reported with corticosteroids (Table 37.8).[126] Glycyrrhizin, the saponin of licorice root, increases the steroid effect. The effectiveness of glucocorticoids is greatly impaired by rifampin administration through induction of hepatic steroid-metabolizing enzymes. The steroid dose may need to be doubled or tripled to maintain adequate replacement therapy when rifampin is added to a chronic steroid regimen.[127] In addition to these typical pharmacokinetic drug interactions, corticosteroids have numerous pharmacodynamic drug interactions. The hypokalemic effect of corticosteroids may exaggerate the hypokalemic effects of amphotericin B, potassium-depleting diuretics, and digitalis glycosides. Corticosteroids may inhibit the growth-promoting effect of growth hormone. The expected immune response to vaccines may be impaired in the presence of corticosteroids. The risk of duodenal ulcer is greatly increased when corticosteroids and nonsteroidal anti-inflammatory drugs are administered concomitantly.[113] Patients must be monitored closely and drug doses adjusted to achieve the desired clinical effect.

KEY POINTS

CUSHING'S SYNDROME

- The goal of therapy is to restore HPA hormonal balance by eliminating excess glucocorticoids and mineralocorticoids.
- Most cases of Cushing's syndrome are caused by iatrogenic administration of glucocorticoids.
- Other causes of Cushing's syndrome are rare, but are important to identify because many are curable.
- Signs and symptoms of Cushing's syndrome are nonspecific and usually insidious in onset.
- Diagnosis depends on documenting hypercortisolism and identifying the precise cause.
- Treatment of exogenous Cushing's syndrome consists of minimizing glucocorticoid or ACTH exposure.
- Treatment of endogenous Cushing's syndrome consists of reducing cortisol production.
- Three types of drugs are used to treat Cushing's syndrome: steroidogenic inhibitors, neuromodulators of ACTH release, and glucocorticoid receptor antagonists.
- Nonpharmacologic therapy for Cushing's syndrome includes surgery for resectable tumors and pituitary irradiation for Cushing's disease not cured by surgery.

ADDISON'S DISEASE

- The goal of therapy is to restore HPA hormonal balance by replacing glucocorticoids and mineralocorticoids.
- Addison's disease, also known as primary adrenal insufficiency, is a chronic, incurable disease.
- Most cases of Addison's disease are caused by autoantibodies directed against steroid-producing cells.
- Although the signs and symptoms of Addison's disease are nonspecific, nearly all patients present with biochemical abnormalities.
- The presenting signs and symptoms and biochemical findings depend on the acuity of presentation.
- Diagnosis depends on provocative tests of the HPA axis.
- An acute adrenal crisis is life threatening; drug treatment should be delayed for diagnostic testing or blood chemistry results.

TABLE 37.8	Corticosteroid Drug Interactions
Drug	**Effect**
Aminoglutethinide[a]	Decreased steroid effect
Antacids (aluminum hydroxide, aluminum-magnesium hydroxide, magnesium hydroxide)	Decreased steroid effect
Anticholinesterases (edrophonium, neostigmine, pyridostigmine)[b]	Refractory muscle depression
Anticoagulants (warfarin sodium)	Variable
Azole antifungals (fluconazole, itraconazole, ketoconazole, miconazole, voriconazole)	Increased steroid effect
Barbiturates (amobarbital, butabarbital, butalbital, mephobarbital, pentobarbital, phenobarbital, primidone, secobarbital)	Decreased steroid effect
Bile acid sequestrants[c] (cholestyramine, colestipol)	Decreased steroid effect
Contraceptives, oral (see estrogens, below)	Increased steroid effect
Cyclosporine[a]	Increased steroid and cyclosporine effects
Diltiazem	Increased steroid effect
Ephedrine[a]	Decreased steroid effect
Estrogens (conjugated estrogens, esterified estrogens, estradiol, estropipate, ethinyl estradiol)	Increased steroid effect
Hydantoins (fosphenytoin sodium, phenytoin)	Decreased steroid effect
Interferon alfa	Decreased interferon alfa effect
Isoniazid	Decreased isoniazid effect
Macrolide antibiotics (clarithromycin, erythromycin, troleandomycin)	Increased steroid effect
Nondepolarizing muscle relaxants (pancuronium bromide, tubocurarine chloride, vecuronium bromide)	Decreased nondepolarizing muscle relaxant effects
Rifamycins (rifabutin, rifampin, rifapentine)[b]	Decreased steroid effect
Salicylates (aspirin, bismuth subsalicylate, choline salicylate, magnesium salicylate, salsalate, sodium salicylate, sodium thiosalicylate)	Decreased salicylate effect
Theophyllines (aminophylline, oxtriphylline, theophylline)	Variable

[a] Dexamethasone only; [b]Potentially severe or life-threatening interaction; [c]Hydrocortisone only.
(From Drug Interactions Facts. Available at: http://www.efactsweb.com.. Accessed March 8, 2004, with permission.)

■ The current recommended chronic replacement regimen is dexamethasone (0.5 mg) plus fludrocortisone (0.1 mg daily at bedtime).
■ Nondrug therapy for normotensive patients consists of liberalizing the dietary salt intake.

SUGGESTED READINGS

Burchard K. A review of the adrenal cortex and severe inflammation: question of the "eucorticoid" state. J Trauma 51:800–814, 2001.
Ernst E. Harmless herbs? A review of the recent literature. Am J Med 104:170–178, 1998.
Ulick S. Cortisol as mineralocorticoid [editorial]. J Clin Endocrinol Metab 81:1307–1308, 1996.

REFERENCES

1. Coursin DB, Wood KE. Corticosteroid supplementation for adrenal insufficiency. JAMA 287:236–240, 2002.
2. Stewart PM. The adrenal cortex. In: Larsen PR, Kronenberg HM, Melmed S, et al, eds. Williams textbook of endocrinology. 10th ed. Philadelphia: WB Saunders, 2003:491–551.
3. Lamberts SWJ, Bruining HA, de Jong FH. Drug therapy: corticosteroid therapy in severe illness. N Engl J Med 337:1285–1292, 1997.
4. Raff H, Findling JW. A physiologic approach to diagnosis of the Cushing syndrome. Ann Intern Med 138:980–991, 2003.
5. Drug Facts and Comparisons. Available at: http://efactsweb.com. Accessed March 31, 2004.
6. Schimmer BP, Parker KL. Adrenocorticotrophic hormone; adrenocortical steroids and their synthetic analogs; inhibitors of the synthesis and action of adrenocortical hormones. In: Hardman JG, Limbird LE, eds. Goodman and Gilman's the pharmacological basis of therapeutics. 10th ed. New York: McGraw-Hill, 2001:1649–1679.

7. Riad M, Mogos M, Thangathurai D, et al. Steroids. Curr Opin Crit Care 8:281–284, 2002.
8. van Leeuwen HJ, van der Bruggen T, van Asbeck BS, et al. Effect of corticosteroids on nuclear factor-κB activation and hemodynamics in late septic shock. Crit Care Med 29:1074–1077, 2001.
9. Hunt PJ, Gurnell EM, Huppert FA, et al. Improvement in mood and fatigue after dehydroepiandrosterone replacement in Addison's disease in a randomized, double blind trial. J Clin Endocrinol Metab 85:4650–4656, 2000.
10. Moore-Ede MC, Czeisler CA, Richardson GS. Circadian timekeeping in health and disease. N Engl J Med 309:469–476, 1983.
11. Czeisler CA, Chiasera AJ, Duffy JF. Research on sleep, circadian rhythms and aging: applications to manned space flight. Exp Gerontol 26:217–232, 1991.
12. Pincus G, Nakao T, Tait JF, eds. Symposium on the dynamics of steroid hormones. New York: Academic Press, 1965:387.
13. Nieman LK, Orth DN. Causes and pathophysiology of Cushing's syndrome. In: UpToDate Online Release 11.3. Available at: http://www.uptodate.com. Accessed February 11, 2004.
14. Cushing H. The basophil adenomas of the pituitary body and their clinical manifestations (pituitary basophilism). Bull Johns Hopkins Hosp 50:137–195, 1932.
15. Ross NS. Epidemiology of Cushing's syndrome and subclinical disease. Endocrinol Metab Clin North Am 23:539–546, 1994.
16. Lindholm J, Juul S, Jørgensen JO, et al. Incidence and late prognosis of Cushing's syndrome: a population-based study. J Clin Endocrinol Metab 86:117–123, 2001.
17. Nieman LK, Orth DN. Clinical manifestations of Cushing's syndrome. In: UpToDate Online Release 11.3. Available at: http://www.uptodate.com. Accessed February 12, 2004.
18. Becker M, Aron DC. Ectopic ACTH syndrome and CRH-mediated Cushing's syndrome. Endocrinol Metab Clin North Am 23:585–606, 1994.
19. Tsigos C, Chrousos GP. Differential diagnosis and management of Cushing's syndrome. Annu Rev Med 47:443–461, 1996.
20. Carpenter PC. Diagnostic evaluation of Cushing's syndrome. Endocrinol Metab Clin North Am 17:445–472, 1988.
21. Giraldi FP, Moro M, Cavagnini F. Gender-related differences in the presentation and course of Cushing's disease. J Clin Endocrinol Metab 88:1554–1558, 2003.
22. Meier CA, Biller BMK. Clinical and biochemical evaluation of Cushing's syndrome. Endocrinol Metab Clin North Am 26:741–762, 1997.
23. Wajchenberg BL, Bosco A, Marone MM, et al. Estimation of body fat and lean tissue distribution by dual energy X-ray absorptiometry and abdominal body fat evaluation by computed tomography in Cushing's disease. J Clin Endocrinol Metab 80:2791–2794, 1995.
24. Ross EJ, Marshall-Jones P, Friedman M. Cushing's syndrome: diagnostic criteria. Q J Med 35:149–192, 1966.
25. Jeffcoate WJ, Silverstone JT, Edwards CRW, et al. Psychiatric manifestations of Cushing's syndrome: response to lowering of plasma cortisol. Q J Med 48:465–472, 1979.
26. Loosen PT, Chambliss B, DeBold CR, et al. Psychiatric phenomenology in Cushing's disease. Pharmacopsychiat 25:192–198, 1992.
27. Dorn LD, Burgess ES, Dubbert B, et al. Psychopathology in patients with endogenous Cushing's syndrome: 'atypical' or melancholic features. Clin Endocrinol 43:433–442, 1995.
28. Ross EJ, Linch DC. Cushing's syndrome—killing disease: discriminatory value of signs and symptoms aiding early diagnosis. Lancet 2:646–649, 1982.
29. Quddusi S, Browne P, Toivola B, et al. Cushing syndrome due to surreptitious glucocorticoid administration. Arch Intern Med 158:294–296, 1998.
30. Cizza G, Nieman LK, Doppman JL, et al. Factitious Cushing syndrome. J Clin Endocrinol Metab 81:3573–3577, 1996.
31. Sjoberg HE, Blomback M, Granberg PO. Thromboembolic complications, heparin treatment in increase in coagulation factors in Cushing's syndrome. Acta Med Scan 199:95–98, 1976.
32. Papanicolaou DA, Mullen N, Kyrou I, et al. Nighttime salivary cortisol: a useful test for the diagnosis of Cushing's syndrome. J Clin Endocrinol Metab 87:4515–4521, 2002.
33. Perry LA, Grossman AB. The role of the laboratory in the diagnosis of Cushing's syndrome. Ann Clin Biochem 34:345–359, 1997.
34. Wood PJ, Barth JH, Freedman DB, et al. Evidence for the low dose dexamethasone suppression test to screen for Cushing's syndrome – recommendations for a protocol for biochemistry laboratories. Ann Clin Biochem 34:222–229, 1997.
35. Liddle GW. Tests of pituitary adrenal suppressibility in the diagnosis of Cushing's syndrome. J Clin Endocrinol Metab 20:1539–1560, 1960.
36. Lumachi F, Zucchetta P, Marzola MC, et al. Usefulness of CT scan, MRI and radiocholesterol scintigraphy for adrenal imaging in Cushing's syndrome. Nucl Med Commun 23:469–473, 2002.
37. Kaye TB, Crapo L. The Cushing syndrome: an update on diagnostic tests. Ann Intern Med 112:434–444, 1990.
38. Sonino N, Fava GA. Psychiatric disorders associated with Cushing's syndrome. CNS Drugs 15:361–373, 2001.
39. Freda PU, Wardlaw SL. Diagnosis and treatment of pituitary tumors. J Clin Endocrinol Metab 84:3859–3866, 1999.
40. Miller JW, Crapo L. The medical treatment of Cushing's syndrome. Endocrin Rev 14:443–458, 1993.
41. Nieman LK, Orth DN. Treatment of Cushing's syndrome: diminishing adrenal cortisol synthesis. Release 11.3. 2003. Available at: http://www.uptodate.com. Accessed April 1, 2004.
42. Atkinson AB. The treatment of Cushing's syndrome. Clin Endocrinol 34:507–513, 1991.
43. Koppeschaar HPF, Croughs RJM, Thijssen JHH, et al. Response to neurotransmitter modulating drugs in patients with Cushing's disease. Clin Endocrinol 25:661–667, 1986.
44. Lamberts SWJ, Klijn JGM, de Quijada M, et al. The mechanism of the suppressive action of bromocriptine on adrenocorticotropin secretion in patients with Cushing's disease and Nelson's syndrome. J Clin Endocrinol Metab 51:307–311, 1980.
45. Colao A, Pivonello R, Tripodi FS, et al. Failure of long-term therapy with sodium valproate in Cushing's disease. J Endocrinol Invest 20:387–392, 1997.
46. Bertagna X, Bertagna C, Laudat MH, et al. Pituitary-adrenal response to the antiglucocorticoid action of RU 486 in Cushing's syndrome. J Clin Endocrinol Metab 63:639–643, 1986.
47. Chu JW, Matthias DF, Belanoff J, et al. Successful long-term treatment of refractory Cushing's disease with high-dose mifepristone (RU486). J Clin Endocrinol Metab 86:3568–3573, 2001.
48. Buescher MA, McClamrock HD, Adashi EY. Cushing syndrome in pregnancy. Obstet Gynecol 79:130–137, 1992.
49. Thorén M, Adamson U, Sjöberg HE. Aminoglutethimide and metyrapone in the management of Cushing's syndrome. Acta Endocrinol 109:451–457, 1985.
50. Misbin RI, Canary J, Willard D. Aminoglutethimide in the treatment of Cushing's syndrome. J Clin Pharmacol 16:645–651, 1976.
51. Santen RJ, Wells SA, Runic S, et al. Adrenal suppression with aminoglutethimide. I. Differential effects of aminoglutethimide on glucocorticoid metabolism as a rationale for use of hydrocortisone. J Clin Endocrinol Metab 45:469–479, 1977.
52. Child DF, Burke CW, Burley DM, et al. Drug control of Cushing's syndrome. Acta Endocrinol 82:330–341, 1976.
53. Lamberts SW, Bons EG, Bruining HA, et al. Differential effects of the imidazole derivatives etomidate, ketoconazole and miconazole and of metyrapone on the secretion of cortisol and its precursors by human adrenocortical cells. J Pharmcol Exp Ther 240:259–264, 1987.
54. Schulte HM, Benker G, Reinwein D, et al. Infusion of low dose etomidate: correction of hypercortisolemia in patients with Cushing's syndrome and dose-response relationship in normal subjects. J Clin Endocrinol Metab 70:1426–1430, 1990.
55. Krakoff J, Koch CA, Calis KA, et al. Use of a parenteral propylene glycol-containing etomidate preparation for the long-term management of ectopic Cushing's syndrome. J Clin Endocrinol Metab 86:4104–4108, 2001.
56. McKenna MJ, Linares M, Mellinger RC. Prolonged remission of Cushing's disease following bromocriptine therapy. Henry Ford Hosp Med J 35:188–191, 1987.
57. Jeffcoate WJ. Treating Cushing's disease. Br Med J 296:227–228, 1988.
58. Krieger DT. Cyproheptadine for pituitary disorders. N Engl J Med 295:394–395, 1976.
59. Bamberger CM, Chrousos GP. The glucocorticoid receptor and RU 486 in man. Ann N Y Acad Sci 761:296–310, 1995.

60. Sartor O, Cutler GB Jr. Mifepristone: treatment of Cushing's syndrome. Clin Obstet Gynecol 39:506–510, 1996.
61. Chu JW, Matthias DF, Belanoff J et al. Successful long-term treatment of refractory Cushing's disease with high-dose mifepristone (RU 486). J Clin Endocrinol Metab 86:3568–3573, 2001.
62. Orth DN. Medical progress: Cushing's syndrome. N Engl J Med 332:791–803, 1995.
63. Mampalam TJ, Tyrrell JB, Wilson CB. Transsphenoidal microsurgery for Cushing's disease. Ann Intern Med 109:487–493, 1988.
64. Estrada J, Boronat M, Mielgo M, et al. The long-term outcome of pituitary irradiation after unsuccessful transsphenoidal surgery in Cushing's disease. N Engl J Med 336:172–177, 1997.
65. Soszynski P, Stowinska-Srzednicka J, Kasperlik-Zatuska A, et al. Decreased melatonin concentration in Cushing's syndrome. Hormone Met Res 21:673–674, 1989.
66. Terzolo M, Piovesan A, Ali A, et al. Circadian profile of serum melatonin in patients with Cushing's syndrome or acromegaly. J Endocrinol Invest 18:17–24, 1995.
67. Di Somma C, Pivonello R, Loche S, et al. Effect of 2 years of cortisol normalization on the impaired bone mass and turnover in adolescent and adult patients with Cushing's disease: a prospective study. Clin Endocrinol 58:302–308, 2003.
68. Faggiano A, Pivonello R, Spiezia S, et al. Cardiovascular risk factors and common carotid artery caliber and stiffness in patients with Cushing's disease during active disease and 1 year after disease remission. J Clin Endocrinol Metab 88:2527–2533, 2003.
69. Addison T. On the constitutional and local effects of disease of the supra-renal capsules. Med Classics 2:244–277, 1937.
70. Zelissen PMJ, Bast EJEG, Croughs RJM. Associated autoimmunity in Addison's disease. J Autoimmun 8:121–130, 1995.
71. Chin R Jr, Zekan JM. Adrenal insufficiency. Prob Crit Care 4:312–324, 1990.
72. Loriaux DL. Syndromes of adrenal insufficiency. In: Becker KL, ed. Principles and practice of endocrinology and metabolism. 3rd ed. Philadelphia: Lippincott Williams & Wilkins, 2001:739–743.
73. Kong M-F, Jeffcoate W. Eighty-six cases of Addison's disease. Clin Endocrinol 41:757–761, 1994.
74. Laureti S, Vecchi L, Santeusanio F, et al. Is the prevalence of Addison's disease underestimated? J Clin Endocrinol Metab 84:1762, 1999.
75. Betterle C, Greggio NA, Volpato M. Autoimmune polyglandular syndrome type 1. J Clin Endocrinol Metab 83:1049–1055, 1998.
76. Barker NW. The pathologic anatomy in twenty-eight cases of Addison's disease. Arch Pathol 8:432–450, 1929.
77. Ten S, New M, Maclaren N. Addison's disease 2001. J Clin Endocrinol Metab 86:2909–2922, 2001.
78. Baker JR, Jr. Autoimmune endocrine disease. JAMA 1997:278:1931–1937.
79. Dluhy RG. The growing spectrum of HIV-related endocrine abnormalities. J Clin Endocrinol Metab 70:563–565, 1990.
80. Brosnan CM, Gowing NFC. Lesson of the week: Addison's disease. BMJ 312:1085–1087, 1996.
81. Oelkers W. Current concepts: adrenal insufficiency. N Engl J Med 335:1206–1212, 1996.
82. Nerup J. Addison's disease—clinical studies. Acta Endocrinol 76:127–41, 1974.
83. Dorin RI, Qualls CR, Crapo LM. Diagnosis of adrenal insufficiency. Ann Intern Med 139:194–204, 2003.
84. Orth DN. Measurement of ACTH; CRH; and other hypothalamic and pituitary peptides. In: UpToDate Online Release 11.3 2004. Available at: http://www.uptodate.com. Accessed March 22, 2004.
85. Silva RC, Kater CE, Dib SA, et al. Autoantibodies against recombinant human steroidogenic enzymes 21-hydroxylase, side-chain cleavage and 17α-hydroxylase in Addison's disease and autoimmune polyendocrine syndrome type III. Eur J Endocrinol 142:187–194, 2000.
86. Falorni A, Nikoshkov A, Laureti S, et al. High diagnostic accuracy for idiopathic Addison's disease with a sensitive radiobinding assay for autoantibodies against recombinant human 21-hydroxylase. J Clin Endocrinol Metab 80:2752–2755, 1995.
87. Nieman LK, Orth DN. Treatment of adrenal insufficiency. In: UpToDate Online Release 11.3, 2003. Available at: http://www.uptodate.com. Accessed December 3, 2003.
88. De Bellis A, Bizzarro A, Rossi R, et al. Remission of subclinical adrenocortical failure in subjects with adrenal autoantibodies. J Clin Endocrinol Metab 76:1002–1007, 1993.
89. Esteban NV, Loughlin T, Yergey AL, et al. Daily cortisol production rate in man determined by stable isotope dilution/mass spectrometry. J Clin Endocrinol Metab 72:39–45, 1991.
90. Kraan GPB, Dullaart RPF, Pratt JJ, et al. The daily cortisol production reinvestigated in healthy men. J Clin Endocrinol Metab 83:1247–1252, 1998.
91. Symreng T, Karlberg BE, Kagedal B, et al. Physiological cortisol substitution of long-term steroid-treated patients undergoing major surgery. Br J Anaesth 53:949–954, 1981.
92. Scott RS, Donald RA, Espiner EA. Plasma ACTH and cortisol profiles in Addisonian patients receiving conventional substitution therapy. Clin Endocrinol 9:571–576, 1978.
93. Løvås K, Gebre-Medhin G, Trovik TS, et al. Replacement of dehydroepiandrosterone in adrenal failure: no benefit for subjective health status and sexuality in a 9-month, randomized, parallel group clinical trial. J Clin Endocrinol Metab 88:1112–1118, 2003.
94. Arlt W, Callies F, van Vlijmen JC, et al. Dehydroepiandrosterone replacement in women with adrenal insufficiency. N Engl J Med 341:1013–1020, 1999.
95. Ulick S. Cortisol as mineralocorticoid. J Clin Endocrinol Metab 81:1307–1308, 1996.
96. Ernst E. Harmless herbs? A review of the recent literature. Am J Med 104:170–178, 1998.
97. Anonymous. List of drug products that have been withdrawn or removed from the market for reasons of safety or effectiveness. Federal Register 64:10944–10947, 1999.
98. Galil K, Miller LA, Yakrus MA, et al. Abscesses due to mycobacterium abscessus linked to injection of unapproved alternative medication. Emerg Infect Dis 5:681–687, 1999.
99. Jusko WJ, Ludwig EA. Corticosteroids. In: Evans WE, Schentag JJ, Jusko WJ, eds. Applied pharmacokinetics: principles of therapeutic drug monitoring. 3rd ed. Vancouver, WA: Applied Therapeutics, 1992:27-1–27-34.
100. Derendorf H, Hochhaus G, Möllmann H, et al. Receptor-based pharmacokinetic-pharmacodynamic analysis of corticosteroids. J Clin Pharmacol 33:115–123, 1993.
101. Johnson M. Pharmacodynamics and pharmacokinetics of inhaled glucocorticoids. J Allergy Clin Immunol 97:169–176, 1996.
102. Giannotti B. Current treatment guidelines for topical corticosteroids. Drugs 36 (Suppl 5):9–14, 1988.
103. Cooper MS, Stewart PM. Current concepts: corticosteroid insufficiency in acutely ill patients. N Engl J Med 348:727–734, 2003.
104. Hamrahian AH, Oseni TS, Arafah BM. Measurements of serum free cortisol in critically ill patients. N Engl J Med 350:1629–1638, 2004.
105. Beishuizen A, Thijs LG. Relative adrenal failure in intensive care: an unidentifiable problem requiring treatment? Best Pract Res Clin Endocrinol Metab 15:513–531, 2001.
106. Annane D, Sébille V, Charpentier C, et al. Effect of treatment with low doses of hydrocortisone and fludrocortisone on mortality in patients with septic shock. JAMA 288:862–871, 2002.
107. Rossi SJ, Schroeder TJ, Hartharan S, et al. Prevention and management of the adverse effects associated with immunosuppressive therapy. Drug Saf 9:104–131, 1993.
108. Truhan AP, Ahmed AR. Corticosteroids: a review with emphasis on complications of prolonged systemic therapy. Ann Allergy 62:375–390, 1989.
109. Magiakou MA, Chrousos GP. Corticosteroid therapy, nonendocrine disease, and corticosteroid withdrawal. Curr Ther Endocrinol Metab 6:138–142, 1997.
110. Maxwell SRJ, Moots RJ, Kendall MJ. Corticosteroids: do they damage the cardiovascular system? Postgrad Med J 70:863–870, 1994.
111. Conn HO, Poynard T. Corticosteroids and peptic ulcer: meta-analysis of adverse effects during steroid therapy. J Intern Med 236:619–632, 1994.
112. Buchman AL. Side effects of corticosteroid therapy. J Clin Gastroenterol 33:289–294, 2001.
113. Piper JM, Ray WA, Daugherty JR, et al. Corticosteroid use and peptic ulcer disease: role of nonsteroidal anti-inflammatory drugs. Ann Intern Med 114:735–740, 1991.

114. Helfer EL, Rose LI. Corticosteroids and adrenal suppression. Drugs 38:838–845, 1989.

115. Melby JC. Systemic corticosteroid therapy: pharmacology and endocrinologic considerations. Ann Intern Med 81:505–512, 1974.

116. Livanou T, Ferriman D, James VHT. Recovery of hypothalamo-pituitary-adrenal function after corticosteroid therapy. Lancet 2: 856–859, 1967.

117. Mak V, Melchor R, Spiro SG. Easy bruising as a side-effect of inhaled corticosteroids. Eur Respir J 5:1068–1074, 1992.

118. Kanda F, Okuda S, Matsushita T, et al. Steroid myopathy: pathogenesis and effects of growth hormone and insulin-like growth factor-1 administration. Horm Res 56 (Suppl 1):24–28, 2001.

119. Hodge WG, Whitcher JP, Satariano W. Risk factors for age-related cataracts. Epidemiol Rev 17:336–346, 1995.

120. Leone FT, Fish JE, Szefler SJ, et al. Systemic review of the evidence regarding potential complications of inhaled corticosteroid use in asthma: collaboration of American College of Chest Physicians, American Academy of Allergy, Asthma, and Immunology, and American College of Allergy, Asthma, and Immunology. Chest 124:2329–2340, 2003.

121. Delcourt C, Cristol JP, Tessier F, et al. Risk factors for cortical, nuclear, and posterior subcapsular cataracts: the POLA study. Am J Epidemiol 151:497–504, 2000.

122. Vincent FM. The neuropsychiatric complications of corticosteroid therapy. Comprehensive Therapy 21:524–528, 1995.

123. BCDSP. Acute adverse reactions to prednisone in relation to dosage. Clin Pharmacol Ther 1972;13:694–698.

124. Picado C, Luengo M. Corticosteroid-induced bone loss. Drug Saf 1996;15:347–359.

125. Anonymous. Recommendations for the prevention and treatment of glucocorticoid-induced osteoporosis. Arthritis Rheum 39: 1791–1801, 1996.

126. Drug Interactions Facts. Available at: http://www.efactsweb.com. Accessed March 8, 2004.

127. Kyriazopoulou V, Parparousi O, Vagenakis AG. Rifampin-induced adrenal crisis in Addisonian patients receiving corticosteroid replacement therapy. J Clin Endocrinol Metab 59:1204–1206, 1984.

Thyroid Disorders

38

Betty J. Dong

The thyroid disorders discussed in this chapter include hyperthyroidism, hypothyroidism, and thyroid nodules. Thyroid hormones are responsible for the optimal growth, development, and function of all metabolic processes and body systems. Therefore, a deficiency or excess in thyroid hormone secretion can affect multiple organ systems and result in a wide variety of complaints and physical findings. It is also important to recognize that the clinical presentation of thyroid disorders, especially in older adults, can masquerade as many different illnesses (e.g., atrial fibrillation). It is essential to exclude an underlying thyroid disorder when considering the medical diagnosis. Thyroid disorders can also affect the treatment of concurrent illnesses (e.g., diabetes, depression, angina) and changes in thyroid function can alter the pharmacokinetics of drugs used in management of other illness.[1]

OVERVIEW OF THE THYROID

ANATOMY AND PHYSIOLOGY

The gland synthesizes, stores, and releases two major metabolically active hormones: triiodothyronine (T_3) and thyroxine (T_4). T_3 is more active than T_4 because the thyroid receptor protein within the cell nucleus has about a tenfold higher affinity for T_3 than for T_4. Approximately 35% to 40% of the secreted T_4 is peripherally monodeiodinated to active T_3, which provides 80% of the total daily production of T_3 and 40% of reverse T_3 (rT_3), which has little or no thyroid activity. Many acute conditions, chronic disorders, and drugs can reduce the peripheral conversion of T_4 to active T_3 and increase the conversion to inactive rT_3, which can cause diagnostic confusion if such laboratory findings are not properly recognized.[2]

The thyroid hormones circulate in the active, free (unbound) form and the protein-bound or inactive form. T_4 is 99.89% bound; only 0.02% is free. This high affinity for the plasma proteins [thyroxine-binding globulin (TBG), 80%; thyroxine-binding prealbumin (TBPA), 10%–15%; and albumin 4%–5%] accounts for the high serum concentration and the slow metabolic degradation ($t_{1/2} = 7$ days) of T_4. In hyperthyroidism, the half-life of T_4 is shortened to 3 to 4 days, and in hypothyroidism the half-life is prolonged to 9 to 10 days. Similar changes in half-life are described for T_3.[1] T_3 is three times more potent metabolically than T_4, but its biologic activity is similar because the lower affinity of T_3 for the plasma proteins results in a lower serum concentration and greater clearance ($t_{1/2} = 1.5$ days). About 0.2% of T_3 is free and active.

Hormone synthesis and release is achieved by an intricate negative feedback mechanism involving the gland, the hypothalamic-pituitary axis (Fig. 38.1), and autoregulation of iodide uptake. Low circulating levels of the thyroid hormone initiate the release of thyroid-stimulating hormone (TSH) or thyrotropin from the pituitary and secretion of thyrotropin-releasing factor (TRF) from the hypothalamus. Rising TSH levels increase iodide trapping by the gland, causing a subsequent increase in hormone synthesis and circulating hormone levels that shut off TRF and TSH secretion and prevent further hormone synthesis. As the hormone levels drop, the hypothalamic-pituitary centers release of TSH and TRF. Physiologic factors (i.e., dopamine, stress) can also influence the hypothalamic-pituitary axis and hormone synthesis.

The gland can also regulate its own uptake of iodide to protect against excessive hormone production if a large iodide load is ingested (i.e., radiographic iodine dye). This autoregulation, known as the Wolff–Chaikoff block, is not overcome by TSH stimulation and occurs when a critical intrathyroidal iodide concentration effect is established within the gland. The normal gland escapes from the block within 7 to 14 days, which prevents subsequent development of hypothyroidism and goiter. Escape results from a decrease in iodide transport or an iodide leak, both of which tend to decrease the intrathyroidal iodide concentration and remove the block to further hormone synthesis. In certain thyroid disorders (e.g., Hashimoto's thyroiditis), the gland cannot escape from the Wolff–Chaikoff block, causing hypothyroidism. Conversely, hyperthyroidism results if this critical block does not occur (as in multinodular goiter).

THYROID EVALUATION

The assessment of a patient with a suspected thyroid disorder should include the following symptoms of thyroid excess or deficiency:

Neck or thyroid symptoms (e.g., pain, tenderness, difficulty swallowing or breathing)

A history of familial thyroid abnormalities

A history of upper chest or neck irradiation during childhood

Examination of the thyroid for enlargement, consistency, and nodularity

Examination for thyroid hormone effects on target systems

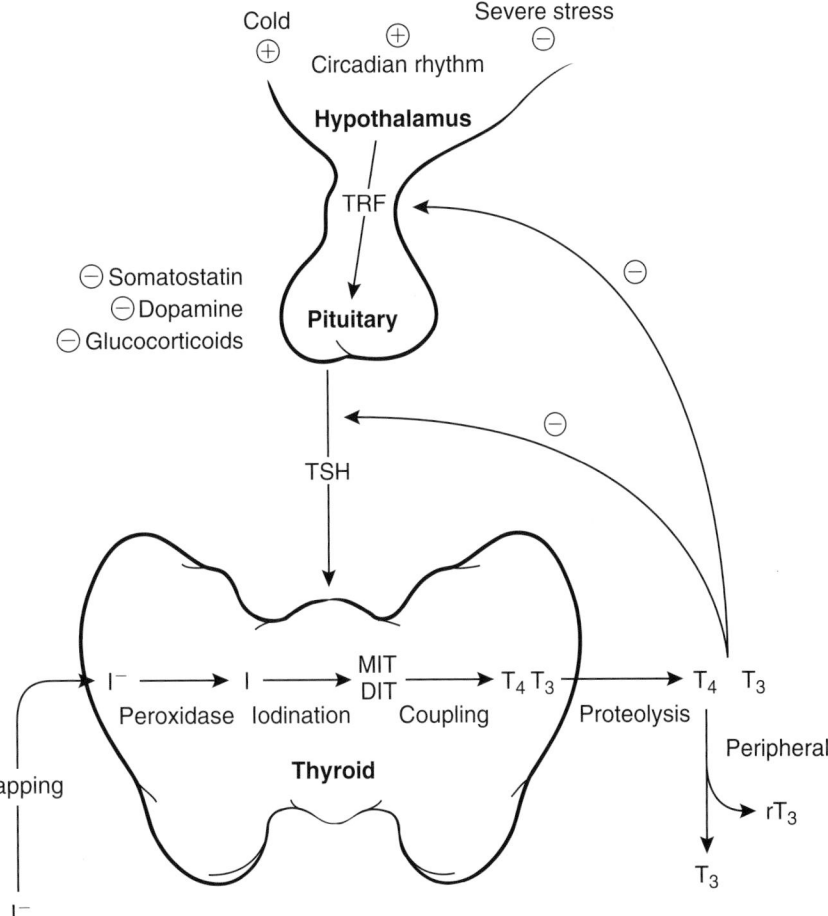

FIGURE 38.1 Hormone synthesis via negative feedback control on the hypothalamic–pituitary–thyroid axis. DIT, diiodotyrosine; MIT, monoiodotyrosine; rT_3, reverse triiodothyronine; T_3, triiodothyronine; T_4, thyroxine; TRF, thyrotropin-releasing factor; TSH, thyroid-stimulating factor. (−, inhibitory influence; +, stimulatory influence.)

Medication history for ingestion of thyroid, antithyroid
   drugs, or drugs that can cause or be altered by thyroid
   disease

Appropriate thyroid function tests

THYROID FUNCTION TESTS

Several laboratory tests are available to assess thyroid homeostasis and metabolic function.[2] These tests measure circulating T_4 and T_3 levels, iodine-trapping ability of the gland,
hypothalamic–pituitary function, autoimmunity, and various
nonspecific metabolic indices (Table 38.1). The normal
range depends on the laboratory and the assay used. The
most cost-effective screening test for thyroid disorders is a
TSH or thyrotropin level. Routine TSH screening for thyroid
illness is recommended, particularly in patients more than
50 years old.[3,4] A free thyroxine level (FT_4) or a free thyroxine index (FT_4I) can be obtained concurrently if the clinical
suspicion for thyroid disease is high. A total or free triiodothyronine level (TT_3 or FT_3) is helpful only in evaluating
hyperthyroidism and should not be obtained routinely. If the
screening TSH level is abnormal, subsequent determinations
of hormone levels are indicated. Thyroid antibodies confirm
the presence of an autoimmune thyroid disorder only if an
abnormal thyroid gland or clinical symptoms exist. A number of nonspecific indices, including the cholesterol, carotene, transaminase (e.g., serum glutamic-oxaloacetic transaminase [SGOT], serum glutamic-pyruvic transaminase
[SGPT]), creatine phosphokinase (CPK), and lactic dehydrogenase (LDH) levels, can be abnormal in thyroid dysfunction
because of impaired clearance in severe hypothyroidism or
increased elimination in hyperthyroidism. It should be appreciated that several drugs and clinical conditions can alter
laboratory values, interfere with proper interpretation of
these tests, and make evaluation of thyroid status difficult
(Table 38.2).[2,5,6] An algorithm for laboratory evaluation of
thyroid disorders is presented in Figure 38.2.

MEASUREMENTS OF CIRCULATING HORMONE LEVELS

Tests of circulating hormone levels can measure the free
(active) or total (free and protein-bound) concentrations of
T_4 and T_3 (Table 38.1).[2] Measurements of FT_4 concentrations are more accurate and should replace older measurements of the total thyroxine level (TT_4), which are affected
by changes in protein binding. FT_4 levels also can be estimated by calculation of FT_4I.

The total T_3 (free and bound T_3) is most useful in evaluating hyperthyroidism because it can be elevated when T_4
levels are normal (e.g., in T_3 toxicosis and before the development of elevated T_4 levels). The TT_3 is not reliable in
evaluating hypothyroidism or euthyroidism because it can
be normal or low. Therefore, a low TT_3 does not prove hypothyroidism because multiple factors (e.g., age and acute or
chronic disease) can cause a low TT_3 in the euthyroid patient
by inhibiting the peripheral conversion of T_4 to T_3. Interfer-

ence of the TT_3 by changes in protein binding can be corrected by calculation of the free T_3 index (FT_3I). Measurement of free T_3 (FT_3) is also helpful, but this test may not
always be available.

The FT_4I and FT_3I are indirect, calculated estimates of the
FT_4 and FT_3, as derived from TT_4 and TT_3 measurements,
respectively. The FT_4I and FT_3I correct for fluctuations in
TBG (Table 38.2), which do not accurately reflect the active
or free hormone levels and are unchanged in a euthyroid
state. An exception is in the euthyroid sick syndrome, where
the FT_4I or FT_3I can be falsely low. Two methods can be
used to calculate the index, and the method selected depends
on the laboratory performing the assays (Table 38.1).

THYROTROPIN OR THYROID-STIMULATING HORMONE

The sensitive TSH assay is the most accurate indicator of
euthyroidism and thyroid dysfunction (Table 38.1). Serum
TSH elevations often occur before overt clinical and laboratory manifestations of hypothyroidism are present. Therefore, the TSH can be elevated despite normal FT_4, TT_4, and
FT_4I, findings that indicate early subclinical hypothyroidism
or insufficient hormone replacement. Likewise, in subclinical hyperthyroidism or in over-replacement therapy, the TSH
is suppressed into the subnormal range, even though circulating hormone levels may be within the normal range. In overt
hyperthyroidism, the TSH is often undetectable. The TSH
also can be used to differentiate primary thyroid failure (elevated TSH) from secondary (central) pituitary deficiency
(absent or low normal TSH). Finally, TSH is invaluable in
excluding secondary thyroid failure in patients with the euthyroid sick syndrome. The sensitive TSH assays are not
affected by the high levels of human chorionic gonadotropins (HCG) found during pregnancy. However, factors that
affect dopamine, which physiologically controls TSH secretion, can alter the TSH level. Dopamine agonists (e.g., dopamine, levodopa, bromocriptine) and high-dose corticosteroids can suppress TSH secretion, and dopamine antagonists
(e.g., metoclopramide) can increase TSH secretion.[2,5] These
mild drug-induced alterations in TSH levels generally do
not interfere with the diagnosis of thyroid dysfunction in
patients with true thyroid disease.

THYROID ANTIBODIES

The presence of thyroid antibodies, antithyroglobulin
(ATgA) and thyroperoxidase (TPO), directed against the
thyroglobulin and the peroxidase component of the thyroid
gland usually indicates an underlying autoimmune process,
such as Graves disease or Hashimoto thyroiditis.[2] However,
because positive antibodies can occur in patients without
thyroid dysfunction or in patients with collagen vascular disorders, their presence is not diagnostic of thyroid illness in
the absence of clinical findings. The levels of ATgA and
TPO are consistently higher during the acute phases of autoimmune thyroid disease and decline during remission and
after therapy. TPO is the more sensitive of the two antibodies

TABLE 38.1	Thyroid Function Tests				
Test	**Normal Values**	**Measures**	**Hyperthyroidism**	**Hypothyroidism**	**Comments**
TT$_4$ (total thyroxine)	64–142 mmol/L (5–11 µg/dL)	Total T$_4$, both free and bound	↑	↓	Affected by changes in thyroxine-binding globulin (TBG)
FT$_4$ (free thyroxine)	9–24 pmol/L (0.7–1.9 ng/dL)	Direct measure of free T$_4$ by equilibrium dialysis or analog method	↑	↓	Levels reflect true thyroid status; not affected by changes in TBG.
FT$_4$I (free thyroxine index)	16–50 mmol/L (1.3–4.2) calculated index using product of RT$_3$U and TT$_4$	Indirect estimate of active free T$_4$ levels	↑	↓	Compensates for changes in TBG concentration; reflects true thyroid status except in euthyroid sick syndrome.
	107–118 mmol/L (6.5–12.5) calculated index by dividing TT$_4$ by T$_4$ uptake.		↑	↓	
RT$_3$U (resin T$_3$ uptake)	0.25–0.37 (25%–37%)	Indirect measure of degree of saturation of TBG sites by T$_4$	↑	↓	Affected by changes in TBG
T$_4$U (T$_4$ uptake)	0.6–1.2	Available binding sites on TBG, prealbumin, and albumin	↑	↓	Affected by changes in TBG, prealbumin, and albumin
TT$_3$ (total T$_3$)	1.1–2.0 nmol/L (70–132 ng/dL)	Total T$_3$, (free and bound)	↑	↓	Affected by changes in TBG; not useful in diagnosis of hypothyroidism.
FT$_3$I (free T$_3$ index)	0.28–0.75 nmol/L (18–49 ng/dL)	Product of RT$_3$U and TT$_3$; calculated estimate of active free T$_3$ levels	↑		See comments for FT$_4$I
RAIU (^{131}I radioactive-iodine uptake)	5%–15% at 5 hours 10%–35% at 24 hours	Iodine trapping ability of gland	↑	↓ or ↑ in subclinical hypothyroidism	Normal values vary depending on the degree of dietary iodide intake and on geographical locale; interfered by iodide intake (i.e., contrast dye)

(continues)

TABLE 38.1	Continued				
Test	**Normal Values**	**Measures**	**Hyperthyroidism**	**Hypothyroidism**	**Comments**
TSH (thyrotropin-stimulating hormone)	0.5–4.7 mIU/L (0.5–4.7 mIU/mL)	Pituitary TSH	↓	↑	Most sensitive indicator of adequate circulating hormone levels
Thyroid Antibodies ATgA (thyroglobulin antibody)	0%–8%	Autoimmune process	Often + (Graves disease)	Often + (Hashimoto thyroiditis)	TPO more sensitive than ATgA, elevated even with remission
TPO (thyroperoxidase antibody)	<100 IU/L (<100 IU/mL)	Autoimmune process	Often + (Graves disease)	Often + (Hashimoto thyroiditis)	
TRab (Thyroid-receptor antibodies)	Negative	IgG immunoglobulin in Graves disease	Often + (Graves disease)	Often negative	Indicates Graves disease, predictive for neonatal Graves disease during pregnancy
Thyroid scan	Isotopes scan with ^{123}I or ^{99}TcO$_4$	Detects hypofunctioning (cold) and hyperfunctioning (hot) nodules and estimates size of gland	Diffusely enlarged; can have hot areas	Cold areas might occur with Hashimoto disease	Not usually done unless discrete nodules are felt on physical examination

TABLE 38.2 | Summary of Laboratory Alterations by Drug/Disease States

Drugs/Disease	Mechanism	TT$_4$	RT$_3$U	FT$_4$/FT$_4$I	TT$_3$	^{131}I Uptake	TSH	Comments
Estrogens, oral contraceptives, pregnancy, heroin, methadone, clofibrate, acute and chronic active hepatitis, familial ↑TBG.	↑ serum TBG concentrations	↑	↓	No change	↑	No change	No change	FT$_4$/FT$_4$I corrects for TBG alterations, TSH indicates true thyroid status.
Glucocorticoids (stress doses)	↓ serum TBG concentrations, ↓TSH secretion, ↓T$_4$ to T$_3$ conversion	↓	↑	↓	↓	Slight ↓	→	Evaluate thyroid status after steroids are stopped.
Androgens, anabolic steroids, danazol, L asparaginase, nephrotic syndrome, cirrhosis, familial ↓TBG.	↓ serum TBG concentrations	↓	↑	No change	↓	No change	No change	FT$_4$/FT$_4$I corrects TBG alterations; TSH indicates true thyroid status.
Phenytoin in vitro, high dose heparin, furosemide, salicylates (level >15 mg/100 mL), phenylbutazone, diclofenac, halofenat, mitotane, chloralhydrate, 5-fluorouracil	Displacement of T$_4$ and T$_3$ from TBG	↓	↑ or little to no change	No change	↓	No change	No change	FT$_4$/FT$_4$I corrects for TBG changes; TSH indicates true thyroid status.
Serotonin reuptake inhibitors (e.g. sertraline)	↓ serum TBG concentrations; ? ↑T$_4$ clearance	↓/no change	↑ or ↓/no change	↓/no change	↓/no change	↑/no change	↑/no change	Sertraline reported to cause hypothyroidism
Iodide-containing compounds, contrast media, povidone-iodine, kelp, tincture of iodine, saturated solution potassium iodide (SSKI), Lugol solution, amiodarone (see below)	Dilution of total body iodide pools	No change if test not interfered by iodide (i.e., radioimmunoassay)	No change	No change	No change	→	No change	No change in thyroid status
Strong diuresis by furosemide, ethacrynic acid; iodine deficiency	Decrease total body iodide pools	No change	No change	No change	No change	Might be ↑	No change	No change in thyroid status

(continues)

TABLE 38.2	Continued						
Drugs/Disease	Mechanism	TT$_4$	RT$_3$U	FT$_4$/FT$_4$I	TT$_3$	^{131}I Uptake	TSH	Comments
Phenytoin carbamazepine, rifampin, phenobarbital	Hepatic enzyme inducer of T$_4$ metabolism	↓ or normal	↑ or no change	↓ or normal	No change	No change	No change in euthyroid patients not on T$_4$ replacement	No change in euthyroid patients not on T$_4$ replacement
Propranolol, old age, fasting, malnutrition, acute and chronic systemic illness (e.g., euthyroid sick syndrome)	Impair peripheral conversion of T$_4$ to T$_3$; ↑ rT$_3$	Normal or ↓	N/A	Normal or ↓	Usually low	No change	No change but in euthyroid sick, slight ↑ or ↓ in TSH might occur	Thyroid replacement not necessary
Dopamine, levodopa, high dose glucocorticoids, bromocriptine	Dopamine suppresses TSH secretion	No change	No change	No change	No change	No change	↓ TSH secretion	Not enough to interfere with diagnosis of hyperthyroidism
Amiodarone, ipodate, iopanoate	Impair pituitary and peripheral conversion of T$_4$ to T$_3$	↑	N/A	↑	↓	↓	Transient ↑	Thyroid abnormalities transient, should be normal within 3 months. Can cause thyroid dysfunction in predisposed patients.

See Table 38.1 for definitions.

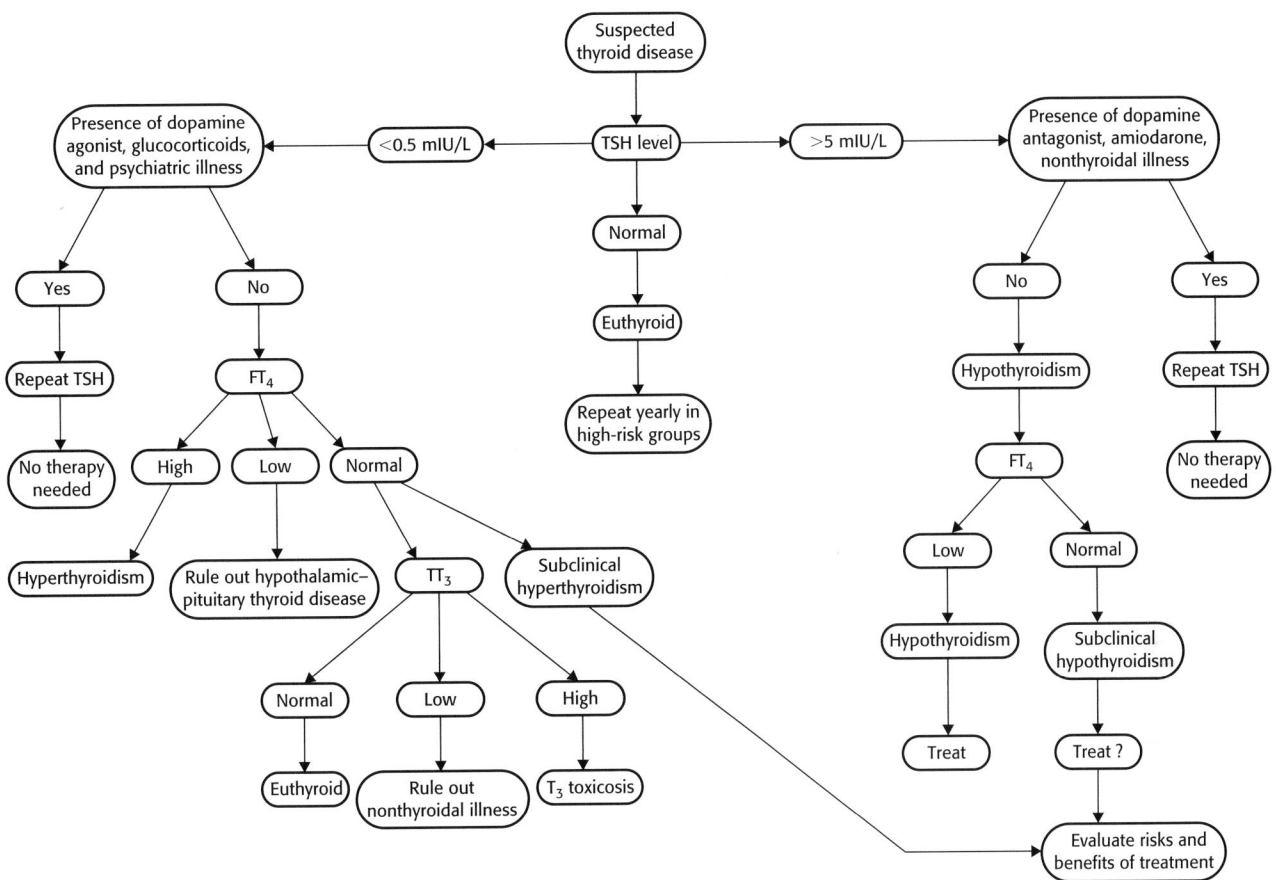

FIGURE 38.2 Algorithm for laboratory evaluation of thyroid disorders. FT$_4$, free thyroxine; TSH, thyroid-stimulating hormone; T$_3$, triiodothyronine; TT$_3$, total triiodothyronine.

because levels remain detectable after remission, whereas ATgA titers might revert to normal.

Thyroid receptor antibody (TRab) is an immunoglobulin G (IgG) capable of stimulating the thyroid gland and found in approximately 90% of patients with Graves disease. There is no need to run a TRab test on a patient with classic symptoms of Graves disease because the test is expensive (approximately $100) and offers no additional therapeutic or diagnostic information. The TRab will help confirm the diagnosis of Graves disease in clinically euthyroid patients with an atypical presentation (e.g., Graves ophthalmopathy).[2] The TRab should be monitored in all pregnant women with a history of Graves disease because a high maternal TRab titer offers predictive information about the risk of neonatal Graves disease. Finally, the presence or absence of TRab in patients with Graves disease may act as a prognostic indicator of the potential for disease relapse and remission.

RADIOACTIVE IODINE UPTAKE AND SCAN

The radioactive iodine uptake (RAIU) measures only the iodine-trapping ability of the gland without regard to the iodine's ultimate fate. After a tracer dose of radioactive iodine (RAI), the percentage of iodine uptake is measured at 5 and 24 hours. An elevated uptake (>35% at 24 hours)

typically occurs in hyperthyroidism, whereas a depressed uptake (<30% in 24 hours) is seen in hypothyroidism. However, an elevated uptake can also occur in early hypothyroidism, indicating an attempt by the failing gland to increase iodine uptake and subsequent hormone synthesis. Fluctuations in the total iodide pool, by dietary or therapeutic maneuvers, will falsely alter the true value of the RAIU (Table 38.2). A thyroid scan usually is obtained concurrently. An uptake and scan often is used to estimate a therapeutic dose of RAI therapy for hyperthyroidism. The scan provides an image of the gland, allowing visualization of hypofunctioning, noniodine-concentrating cold areas, or hyperfunctioning, iodine-concentrating hot areas in the gland. A scan is particularly helpful if discrete thyroid nodules or irregularities are palpable. However, most clinicians prefer to use a fine-needle aspiration rather than an uptake and scan to evaluate a thyroid nodule.

EUTHYROID SICK SYNDROME

Many acute and chronic nonthyroid disorders (e.g., starvation, acute depression and other psychiatric disorders, acute infection, chronic cardiac, pulmonary, renal, hepatic, and neoplastic disorders, and acquired immunodeficiency syndrome) are associated with impaired peripheral conversion of T_4 to T_3, causing abnormal and confusing thyroid function tests in euthyroid patients.[6]

This euthyroid sick syndrome, most common in hospitalized patients, requires appropriate recognition to avoid dangerous and unnecessary hormone replacement. Abnormalities in thyroid function tests vary, but they often include a low TT_4, TT_3, a low calculated FT_4 and FT_3 index, normal or elevated FT_4, and usually a normal or slightly elevated

TSH of less than 10 mIU per liter. The slight elevations in TSH concentrations tend to be transient and indicate a recovery phase. Less often, hyperthyroxinemia (e.g., psychiatric illness) occurs. An abnormal binding inhibitor in the sera of sick patients probably accounts for some of the abnormal alterations. Reversal of the abnormal thyroid function tests is a good prognostic indicator of recovery and decreased mortality. Thyroid hormone supplementation is dangerous, unwarranted, and might impair normal recovery of thyroid homeostasis.[7]

HYPERTHYROIDISM

DEFINITION

Hyperthyroidism or thyrotoxicosis is a syndrome caused by excessive production of both thyroid hormones and is characterized by increased metabolism of all body systems. Thyroid storm, a medical emergency, is an exaggerated form of thyrotoxicosis. A suppressed TSH level with normal thyroid hormone levels is defined as subclinical hyperthyroidism; symptoms may not always be present, particularly in elderly patients

TREATMENT GOALS: HYPERTHYROIDISM

- Reverse the signs and symptoms of hyperthyroidism, normalize thyroid hormone levels, minimize the deleterious effects of T_4 on organ systems, prevent thyroid storm, and improve overall functional capacity.
- Reverse hyperthyroid complaints.
- Reverse hyperthyroid physical findings.
- Normalize free T_4, T_3, and TSH levels.
- Reduce goiter size.
- Improve cardiac function and prevent systemic embolism.
- Preserve bone density and prevent osteoporosis.
- Improve emotional well-being and quality of life.
- Support placenta development and maintenance of pregnancy.
- Promote normal growth, and physical and mental development.

EPIDEMIOLOGY

OVERVIEW

Hyperthyroidism affects approximately 2% of women and 0.2% of men; the incidence of hyperthyroidism is reported to be 2.5 to 4.7 per 1,000 women.[8,9] Hyperthyroidism in children is rare, accounting for about 1% to 5% of cases.[10] It is unusual in the first 5 years of life; the peak incidence occurs between the ages of 10 and 12 years. The frequency of subclinical hyperthyroidism has ranged from 0.7% to 2% and is more common in women than men and in the elderly; the percentage who progress to overt hyperthyroidism is low.[11] The causes of hyperthyroidism and subclinical hyperthyroidism are presented in Table 38.3.

The most common cause of hyperthyroidism is Graves disease.[8,12] Graves disease can occur at any age, although

its peak onset is between ages 20 and 50 years. Like all other thyroid disorders, it is eight to ten times more common in women than in men; incidences of 80 per 100,000 women per year and 10 per 100,000 men have been reported.[12] There is a strong familial predisposition, but the mode of genetic transmission is unknown. The combination of pregnancy and Graves thyrotoxicosis is rare, affecting 0.2% to 1.4% of the pregnant population. Usually the thyrotoxicosis and treatment antedate the pregnancy because most hyperthyroid patients have reduced fertility. Neonatal thyrotoxicosis develops in 1% to 1.4% of these pregnant women.

The incidence of hyperthyroidism from toxic multinodular goiters (TMG) ranges from 9% to 16%; incidences of 5 to 16 per 100,000 have been reported.[8,13,14] This is the most common cause of new-onset hyperthyroidism in adults in the fifth or sixth decade of life. Single toxic adenomas

TABLE 38.3	Causes of Hyperthyroidism
Graves disease	Autoimmune (see Table 38.6)
Toxic nodules	Single and multinodular
Subacute thyroiditis	Inflammatory thyroiditis, including postpartum thyroiditis, viral thyroiditis (e.g., de Quervain, amiodarone
Drug-induced	Iodides (Jod-Basedow), amiodarone, lithium, cytokines
Neonatal thyrotoxicosis	Transplacental passage of TRab
Hashitoxicosis	Hyperthyroid phase of Hashimoto thyroiditis
T3 toxicosis	Preferential secretion of T3, often precedes T4 toxicosis
Tumors	Secretion of thyroid stimulating substances
Factitious	Self-administration of levothyroxine

TRab, thyroid receptor antibody; T_3, triiodothyronine; T_4, thyroxine.

are less common; an incidence of 1.6% was noted in the United States, and a higher incidence (9%) was noted in Europe.[14]

The incidence of hyperthyroidism from a subacute thyroiditis is variable. Postpartum thyroiditis (PPT) develops in 4% to 8% of women after delivery and in as many as 25% of women with insulin-dependent diabetes.[15,16] Cases of subacute thyroiditis (de Quervain's thyroiditis) tend to be seasonal and follow a viral infection.

The incidence of drug-induced thyroid dysfunction ranges from 6% for interferon-α, to 15% to 30% for lithium, and 2% to 24% for amiodarone.[17–24] Hyperthyroidism is less common than hypothyroidism. The incidence of amiodarone-induced hyperthyroidism is 10% in areas of endemic iodine deficiency but only 2% to 3% in iodine-sufficient areas such as the United States. Iodide-induced hyperthyroidism is known as "Jod-Basedow disease."

DRUG-INDUCED THYROTOXICOSIS

Iodine-induced thyrotoxicosis (Jod-Basedow) was first described in the 1800s in residents of iodine-deficient areas who became symptomatic after adequate iodine supplementation. Most cases occurred in patients with multinodular goiters and autonomous functioning nodules that were activated by the increased iodine supplements. Iodides do not cause the underlying thyroid disease; they produce thyrotoxicosis in abnormal thyroid glands that have lost the protective Wolff–Chaikoff block.[25] Hyperthyroidism has also been reported after injections of radiocontrast material or iodinated topical preparations.[16]

Lithium is rarely associated with the development of hyperthyroidism, probably through an immune-modulating ef-

fect.[16,21] Paradoxically, because lithium acts like iodides in blocking hormone release, lithium has been suggested for the treatment of hyperthyroidism if other options are not feasible.[26]

Amiodarone, which contains 37.2% iodine by weight, has been implicated in causing two types of hyperthyroidism that can occur abruptly at any time during the course of therapy.[19,20] Type I hyperthyroidism occurs in patients with predisposing risk factors (e.g., multinodular goiter with autonomous nodules, subclinical Graves disease) and is related to the high iodine content of amiodarone and loss of the protective Wolff–Chaikoff effect. Type II results from an inflammatory type of thyroiditis, causing leakage of large quantities of hormone into the circulation and subsequent hyperthyroidism. Management of amiodarone-induced hyperthyroidism is challenging since the optimal treatment selected would depend on the type of hyperthyroidism, a situation that is often difficult to identify. In addition, stopping the drug does not reverse symptoms promptly because of its long elimination half-life and sequestration in fat. Typically, the combination of thioamides, potassium perchlorate, and β-blockers are used to manage the hyperthyroidism. For type-II hyperthyroidism, glucocorticoids, β-blockers, and iodinated contrast agents are most useful. Similar to amiodarone, two types of hyperthyroidism have also been associated with interferon-α administration but hyperthyroid symptoms are usually transient, requiring only symptomatic control with β-blockers.[17,18]

Because hyperthyroxinemia is a normal laboratory finding in euthyroid patients receiving amiodarone, true thyrotoxicosis should be documented by elevations in serum FT_3 or TT_3 levels, suppression of the TSH level, and clinical symptoms. Worsening of cardiac symptoms requires investigation for amiodarone-induced hyperthyroidism. Typical laboratory findings in euthyroid patients on amiodarone include an elevated FT_4 or FT_4I, a subnormal T_3, and an initial transient elevated TSH level that returns to normal after the first 2 to 3 months of amiodarone therapy.

PATHOPHYSIOLOGY

Graves disease is an autoimmune disorder caused by an abnormal thyroid receptor IgG-stimulating immunoglobulin (e.g., TRab) that binds to the TSH receptor to cause uncontrolled thyroid hormone production.[8,12] Lymphocytic infiltration of the thyroid gland, cytokines including interleukin 1, 4, 8, 10, and interferon-γ, and ATgA and TPO antibodies provide further evidence for an autoimmune process. A defect in suppressor T lymphocytes may be responsible for the formation of the TRab found in the blood of patients with active disease. Cure and spontaneous remission are unlikely as long as the TRab is present; however, how long the TRab persists is unknown. In pregnancy, spontaneous remission and improvement of hyperthyroid symptoms can result from falls in the concentrations of TRab and thyroid antibody titers. Transplacental passage of TRab from the maternal circulation can produce fetal and neonatal hyperthyroidism, which resolves 1 to 2 months after delivery as the antibody levels decline.[27,28] Graves disease often occurs with other autoimmune processes, including Hashimoto thyroiditis, type I diabetes mellitus, Addison disease, vitiligo, and myasthenia gravis. Graves disease and Hashimoto thyroiditis have been postulated to be the same autoimmune process because Graves disease can undergo spontaneous remission to hypothyroidism. Precipitation of Graves disease has been reported after trauma, severe emotional stress, smoking, weight reduction involving diet restrictions, stimulants, thyroid hormone, and iodide administration (Jod-Basedow).[8,25]

Single or multiple nodules can produce hyperthyroidism because the nodules function independently of TSH control (autonomously).[14] Patients with autonomous nodules residing in an iodine-deficient area often experience toxemia when given an increased iodide substrate (e.g., iodinated contrast media, relocation to an iodine-sufficient area such as the United States).[14,25] Patients with a TMG often give a history of a large, firm, multinodular goiter and euthyroidism (normal thyroid status) before hyperthyroidism occurs. Similarly, a single adenoma can be quiescent for many years before becoming toxic. Multiple etiologic factors, including iodine deficiency, genetic abnormalities, and the immune system, have been implicated. Recent evidence suggests that the immune system may be involved, as in Graves disease, because TPO and TRab antibodies have been detected in patients with TMG.[14]

Hyperthyroidism caused by a subacute thyroiditis results from dumping or leakage of thyroid hormones into the circulation from an inflamed gland.[15,16] de Quervain's thyroiditis is a spontaneous, remitting, inflammatory thyroid condition that is believed to have a viral origin; positive antibody titers to Coxsackievirus, mumps, and other viruses have been identified. PPT is most likely to occur in women with positive thyroid antibodies; 30% to 50% of women with positive thyroid antibodies during pregnancy or at the time of delivery developed PPT. Thyrotoxicosis should be differentiated from Graves disease or other forms of hyperthyroidism. PPT may recur after subsequent pregnancies, and treatment does not prevent recurrences. Routine screening of women after pregnancy has been recommended. Amiodarone has also been associated with inflammatory thyroiditis.

T_3 thyrotoxicosis is characterized by normal levels of T_4 and elevated levels of T_3. T_3 toxicosis is seen in Graves disease, toxic goiters, and carcinomas, and is reported in children. Preferential T_3 secretion, producing toxicity, is more prevalent in iodine-deficient areas. Elevated T_3 levels often precede the onset of frank T_4 toxicosis after withdrawal of antithyroid medications in patients with Graves disease.

Subclinical hyperthyroidism is caused by the same disorders that cause overt hyperthyroidism.[11] A common cause of a suppressed TSH is partially treated Graves disease after RAI therapy. Nonthyroidal illness, medications (Table 38.2),

central hypothyroidism, and excessive l-thyroxine replacement therapy should be excluded as potential causes of subclinical hyperthyroidism. Treatment of subclinical hyperthyroidism is warranted.[11,29] Among patients more than 60 years of age with untreated subclinical hyperthyroidism, a threefold greater risk of developing atrial fibrillation occurred during a 10-year period.[30] Other concerns include cardiac ischemia, loss of bone density, and an increased risk of osteoporosis, especially problematic in postmenopausal women.[31,32]

CLINICAL PRESENTATION AND DIAGNOSIS

SIGNS AND SYMPTOMS

The clinical symptoms of hyperthyroidism (Table 38.4) in adults reflect increased adrenergic activity, primarily cardiovascular and neurologic. Not all manifestations are present in the same patient. Exogenous ingestion of sympathomimetics or agents with sympathomimetic activity intensify the hyperthyroid symptoms and should be avoided during active disease. Concurrent medical conditions (e.g., diabetes, cardiac conditions) can be exacerbated, and drug action (e.g., digoxin, warfarin, theophylline, insulin) can be altered by the thyrotoxicosis (Tables 38.2 and 38.5).[1]

Thyrotoxicosis-induced increases in heart rate (HR), stroke volume (SV), and cardiac output can cause new or worsening angina, atrial fibrillation, extrasystoles, or congestive heart failure (CHF; high output) that usually are resistant to conventional treatment until euthyroidism occurs. Clinically, a rapid bounding pulse, an elevated systolic blood pressure, a wide pulse pressure, cardiomegaly, and a systolic murmur are seen. Tachycardia, increased voltage, and a prolonged P-R interval are evident on an electrocardiogram (ECG). It is important to eliminate thyrotoxicosis as causing or exacerbating the cardiac disease, particularly in older adults, in whom cardiac findings can predominate and systemic arterial embolism is of concern.

Thyroid storm is a medical emergency characterized by accentuation of the hyperthyroid symptoms and the acute onset of high fever. If untreated, cardiovascular collapse and shock can occur. Gastrointestinal symptoms can be profound, producing diarrhea, vomiting, abdominal pain, and liver enlargement. Central nervous system involvement can cause agitation and psychosis, leading to apathy, stupor, and coma.[33,34]

Occasionally, a patient with severe toxemia may exhibit none of the classic hyperthyroid symptoms. This "apathetic" or masked hyperthyroidism can be a typical finding in older adults. Presenting symptoms of anorexia, fatigue, apathy, listlessness, dull eyes, extreme weakness, CHF, delayed speech and mentation, and low-grade fever are confusing in such patients and obscure the diagnosis. Likewise, premature atrial contractions, atrial fibrillation with embolism, or tremor might be the only clue to occult hyperthyroid-

TABLE 38.4	Signs and Symptoms of Hyperthyroidism and Hypothyroidism	
Body System	**Hyperthyroidism**	**Hypothyroidism**
General	Heat intolerance, weight loss, ↑ appetite, ↑sweating, weight gain due to ↑appetite.	Cold intolerance, weight gain despite ↓ appetite, hoarseness and lowering of the voice pitch, ↓ sweating, easy fatigability.
Head	Thinning of the hair; fine texture	Dry, brittle, and sparse hair; thinning of the lateral aspects of the eyebrows; puffy facies, large tongue.
Eyes	Prominence of the eyes, lid lag, lid retraction, can proceed to loss of visual acuity; Graves' ophthalmopathy	Edematous eyelids, ptosis
Neck	Soft diffusely enlarged goiter; or single or multiple nodules.	Goiter in primary hypothyroidism, none found in pituitary disorders
Cardiac	Palpitations, high output failure, angina, edema, ↑ pulse and systolic pressure, wide pulse pressure, presence of systolic murmurs.	Cardiac enlargement, poor heart sounds, pericardial pain, low output failure, dyspnea
Gastrointestinal	Diarrhea, loose bowels, or hyperdefecation	Constipation
Genitourinary	Amenorrhea or ↓ menstrual flow	Menorrhagia, dysmenorrhea
Extremities	Pretibial myxedema, Plummer's nails; hot, flushed, and moist skin; palmar erythema	Broad hands and feet, pretibial myxedema, cold and dry skin, brittle nails, yellowish skin tint.
Neuromuscular	Fatigue, weakness, tremor, rapid deep tendon reflexes	Muscle pain and weakness, paresthesias, delayed deep tendon reflexes
Emotional	Nervousness, irritability, emotional liability, insomnia, or shortened sleep cycles	Emotional instability, depression, lethargy, ↓ energy, ↑sleep requirements, mental sluggishness

ism in older adults. If the condition goes untreated, coma and death are certain. The presence of any new or worsening cardiac, neurologic, or failure-to-thrive symptoms in older adults warrant an evaluation for underlying thyroid disease. Occult thyrotoxicosis is confirmed easily by standard laboratory tests.

In children, the signs and symptoms are similar to those seen in the adult, with the notable exception of cardiovascular manifestation.[10] Excessive thirst, behavioral manifestations of restlessness, and inability to concentrate incur difficulties in school and family relationships and might be the initial presenting symptom.

Fetal hyperthyroidism usually appears during the second half of pregnancy and is characterized by tachycardia (HR >160/minute), craniosynostosis, frontal bossing, mental retardation, intrauterine growth retardation, premature delivery, and a mortality rate of approximately 16%.

The triad of hyperthyroidism, a diffusely enlarged and symmetric goiter, and infiltrative ophthalmopathy or dermopathy, characterizes Graves disease. A bruit, indicative of high blood flow, might be present in a severely toxic patient. Bruits usually are audible over the entire thyroid gland and disappear in euthyroidism. Not all of these clinical findings are present or necessary for the diagnosis.

The ocular findings are the most striking abnormalities of Graves disease.[35,36] Graves ophthalmopathy is not directly correlated with the thyroid status and can appear before, during, or even years after successful therapy of the hyperthyroidism. The ocular involvement can be unilateral or bilateral and might not reverse with achieving euthyroidism. Progression and worsening of the eye signs can occur abruptly after RAI therapy, particularly in patients who have mild symptoms before RAI therapy, and prophylaxis with systemic corticosteroids is indicated.[35,36] It is not known why the eyes and the orbital muscles are involved whereas other organ systems are spared. Mild eye symptoms are found in 50% of patients; the most severe forms occur in less than 5%. The ophthalmopathy is more severe and progressive in smokers, who have higher levels of TRab than nonsmokers. The ocular manifestations include the noninfiltrative and the characteristic infiltrative ophthalmopathy of Graves disease.

Drug	Hyperthyroidism	Hypothyroidism	Comments
TABLE 38.5	**Effect of Thyroid Status on Drug Action**		
Sympathomimetics (e.g., asthma and cold preparations)	↑ sensitivity to catecholamines; exacerbation of thyrotoxic symptoms, especially cardiac	Blunted response to sympathomimetics; insignificant	↑ hyperthyroid symptoms even if thyroid function tests normal
Digoxin and digitalis preparations	↑ volume of distribution and renal clearance of digoxin; might require ↑ doses to achieve therapeutic effect	↑ sensitivity to digoxin therapeutic and toxic effect; require ↓ digoxin to achieve therapeutic effect	Need to adjust doses as thyroid function changes to maintain efficacy and avoid toxicity
Insulin	↑ insulin metabolism/clearance; exacerbation of diabetes	Prolonged insulin effect; ↑ risk of hypoglycemia and ↓ insulin to control Type II diabetes	Need to adjust insulin doses in patients with type II diabetes as thyroid status changes
Warafin	↑ metabolism of clotting factors; ↓ half-life of clotting factors; require ↓ warfarin for anticoagulation	↓ metabolism of clotting factors; ↑ half-life of clotting factors; require ↑ warfarin for anticoagulation	Need to adjust doses as thyroid function changes to maintain efficacy and avoid toxicity
β-Blockers (propranolol, metoprolol, atenolol)	Increased metabolic clearance	Not significant	Might require higher doses for desired clinical response in hyperthyroidism.
Respiratory depressants (e.g., barbiturates, phenothiazines, narcotics)	Not significant	Increased sensitivity to the respiratory depressant effects of sedative hypnotic agents	Increased CO_2 retention, might precipitate myxedema coma use cautiously in hypothyroidism.
Theophylline	Not significant	↓ metabolic clearance	Might require less drug for clinical response, monitor for toxicity
L-thyroxine	↓ serum half-life to 3–4 days	↑ half life to 9–10 days	Changes in time to steady state levels and monitoring of thyroid function tests
Cortisol	↓ serum half-life to 50 minutes	↑ half life to 155 minutes	Might need ↑ steroids in management of hyperthyroidism

The noninfiltrative ocular abnormalities result from hyperactivity of the sympathetic system and can be found in any hyperthyroid condition. Increased sympathetic tone on Muller's superior palpebral muscle causes spasm and retraction of the upper lid, widening the palpebral fissure to give the characteristic stare or frightened expression. On physical examination, lid lag is present when the eyelid movement lags behind eye movement, and a narrow white rim of sclera becomes visible between the upper lid and the cornea. These ocular changes can cause symptoms of grittiness, dryness, tearing, itching, redness, and photophobia that improve with normalization of the hormone levels.

Exophthalmos or proptosis (protrusion of the cornea more than the normal 18–20 mm beyond the lateral margin of the orbit) is a characteristic feature of Graves ophthalmopathy that results from an increase in the orbital contents. Histologic examination reveal lymphocytic infiltration and deposition of mucopolysaccharides, fat, and water in all retrobulbar tissue, causing the globes to be firmer and harder than normal. Proptosis can produce a wide-eyed stare, leading to

increased tearing and irritation from the exposed conjunctiva. Soft tissue involvement can produce edema and swelling of the lids and periorbital tissue, causing chemosis, excessive tearing, photophobia, and conjunctivitis. Corneal scarring and ulceration result if the proptosis causes the lid to remain open, exposing and drying out the eye during sleep. Paralysis of extraocular muscles can limit eye movements, producing diplopia, loss of upward gaze, and loss of convergence. Blindness might result from venous congestion and hemorrhage of the retina and optic nerve.

The dermopathy of Graves disease, also known as ''pretibial myxedema,'' can occur with the infiltrative ophthalmopathy. Mucopolysaccharide infiltration of the skin causes the cutaneous thickening and hyperpigmentation (i.e., orange-peel skin) usually seen over the tibial aspects of the leg. Similar lesions can appear on the dorsa of the feet and hands. Pretibial myxedema usually is asymptomatic but can be painful or pruritic. Like the infiltrative ocular symptoms, pretibial myxedema can occur at any time in the course of the disease. If necessary, the clinical diagnosis can be con-

TABLE 38.6 | Characteristics of Graves Disease

Hyperthyroidism, goiter, and ophthalmopathy or dermopathy

Positive family history

Females > males patients

Elevated FT_4 or FT_4I, TT_4, TT_3

Suppressed /Undetectable TSH level

Positive ATgA, TPO, TRab

Unknown duration of disease

FT_4, free thyroxine level; FT_4I, free thyroxine index; TT_4, total thyroxine level; TT_3, triiodothyronine; TSH, thyroid-stimulating hormone; ATgA, antithyroglobulin antibody; TPO, thyroperoxidase antibody; TRab, thyroid receptor antibody; FT_3, free triiodothyronine.

firmed by tissue biopsy. Treatment with high-potency topical corticosteroids and plastic wrap often is effective.

DIAGNOSIS

Several organizations, including the American Thyroid Association (ATA), have established clinical guidelines for the diagnosis and management of hyperthyroidism.[3,4] The diagnosis of hyperthyroidism is confirmed by findings of abnormally high levels of FT_4 or TT_3 and an undetectable TSH. The presence of positive antibodies (i.e., ATgA and TPO), ophthalmopathy, or dermopathy confirm the diagnosis of Graves disease (Table 38.6). An elevated TT_3 and positive TRab can provide essential information in patients with atypical presentations. The RAIU is elevated but is not cost-effective or necessary for a diagnosis of Graves in a patient with positive antibodies and the classic presentation. On a scan, a diffusely enlarged, homogeneous hot gland is found.

The presence of palpable nodules in a normal or enlarged goiter requires exclusion of a TMG or toxic adenoma.[14] The diagnosis is confirmed by the presence of hyperthyroid indices, a suppressed TSH in a mildly symptomatic or asymptomatic person, and an RAIU and scan revealing hot nodules. In some cases, the rest of the thyroid may not be visible on the thyroid scan if normal thyroid tissue is suppressed by the hot nodule.

Conditions caused by subacute thyroiditis (e.g., PPT, amiodarone) can be confirmed by the presence of a low or undetectable RAIU, elevated thyroid hormone levels, and a suppressed or undetectable TSH level. de Quervain subacute thyroiditis must be suspected if there is the acute onset of gland tenderness or pain with swallowing, a recent history of flu-like symptoms, fever, malaise, and symptoms of hyperthyroidism or hypothyroidism.[16] Other laboratory abnormalities include an elevated erythrocyte sedimentation rate (ESR), negative thyroid antibodies, and leukocytosis.

THERAPEUTIC PLAN

The ATA, the American Association of Clinical Endocrinologists, and others have published clinical guidelines for

treatment of hyperthyroidism.[3,37] The major treatment modalities for the management of hyperthyroidism include thioamides, RAI, and surgery (Table 38.7).[38–42] In the United States, RAI therapy is the most commonly used treatment, except in younger patients, for whom thioamides are chosen. In contrast, thioamides are selected as the treatment of choice by European and Japanese endocrinologists. Surgery is often reserved as the last choice unless there are obstructive symptoms or concerns about malignancy. Each has its own advantages and limitations, so treatment must be individualized. The etiology of the hyperthyroidism, its severity, the patient's age, the size of the goiter, the presence of thyroid and medical complications, and social and economic issues are critical considerations for treatment selection. For example, all three treatment options are effective options for Graves disease but patients or physicians might prefer medications rather than RAI or surgery. Likewise, for management of a TMG, RAI or surgery is more effective than medications but certain factors (e.g., patient's concomitant medical conditions, patient or physician preference) may dictate that RAI rather than surgery be used. In some cases, therapy might be transient because the disease is self-limited (e.g., subacute thyroiditis, neonatal Graves disease, PPT, drug-induced hyperthyroidism). Treatment algorithms such as the one in Figure 38.3 enable healthcare providers to treat patients with hyperthyroidism effectively. Treatment adjuncts include iodides,[25] iodinated contrast media,[43] potassium perchlorate, adrenergic antagonists, corticosteroids, cholestyramine,[44] and rarely, lithium[26,38] (Table 38.7).

Patients with uncomplicated Graves disease, particularly children, may be treated medically with thioamides until remission occurs.[8–10] Theoretically, thioamides are preferred over RAI and surgery to treat the patient with uncomplicated Graves because they do not destroy the gland and they control the disease. Therefore, chronic thyroid replacement, which is likely with RAI or surgery, might not be necessary if thioamides are used. This advantage of thioamides might be irrelevant because the natural history of Graves disease appears to be eventual hypothyroidism even if no glandular destruction occurs. If RAI or surgery is selected, most older patients and all severely thyrotoxic patients should be pretreated with thioamides.[39–41] Pretreatment depletes the gland of stored hormones, reduces the hypermetabolic rate, and prevents leakage of hormone from the gland after RAI or during surgery, preventing thyroid storm. However, the final decision in the patient with uncomplicated Graves disease is often empiric, depending on available resources, the physician's experience, and the patient's personal preference. Treatment selection should be a joint patient and physician decision after a discussion of the benefits and risks of each method.

The optimal therapy of hyperthyroidism in patients with Graves ophthalmopathy is unresolved.[35,36] Endocrinologists at the University of California at San Francisco prefer thyroid ablation with RAI or surgery (less desirable) to remove the antigen source (i.e., gland) and believe that these meth-

TABLE 38.7 | **Management of Hyperthyroidism**

Method	Drug	Dose	Mechanism of Action	Toxicity	Comments
Thioamides	Propylthiouracil (PTU) 50-mg tablets; can be formulated for rectal administration	300–400 mg/day given q 6–8 hours initially, maintenance of 50–150 mg daily	Blocks organification of hormone synthesis, also inhibits peripheral conversion of T_4 to T_3; immunosuppressive	Skin rash, bitter taste, agranulocytosis, gastrointestinal symptoms, hepatocellular hepatitis	Remission rate of 20%–30%; onset of action approximately 2–4 weeks; used in pregnancy and during lactation
	Methimazole (Tapazole) 5- and 10-mg tablets; can be formulated for rectal administration	30–40 mg once daily initially, maintenance of 5–15 mg daily	Blocks organification of hormone synthesis; immunosuppressive	See PTU; secreted in breast milk; might be teratogenic (e.g., scalp defects); obstructive jaundice	DOC for once daily dosing; remission rate of 20%–30%; onset of action approximately 2–4 weeks; Appears to have little cross-sensitivity to PTU for maculopapular rash
Iodides	Lugol's solution 8 mg iodide/drop: Saturated solution of potassium iodide (SSKI) 50 mg/drop	6 mg iodide/day although larger doses are given; see surgery for iodide doses	Block hormone release; decreases gland vascularity and increases gland firmness to facilitate surgical removal	Hypersensitivity reactions—rash, rhinorrhea, parotid and submaxillary swelling; rarely anaphylactoid reactions. Contraindicated in pregnancy.	Provides symptomatic relief before onset of thioamides; use in thyroid storm and as a preoperative adjunct; DO NOT USE BEFORE RAI.
Adrenergic antagonists	Propranolol (Inderal) Metoprolol (Lopressor) Atenolol (Tenormin) Various tablet strengths; IV propranolol 1 mg/mL; Avoid β-blocker with ISA activity	Propranolol 20–40 mg po every 6 hours or equivalent β-blocker	Blocks the peripheral action of thyroid hormone, no effect on disease state. Blocks peripheral T_4 to T_3 conversion	Bradycardia, congestive heart failure, asthma, inhibits hyperglycemic response to hypoglycemia. Avoid in pregnancy	Provides rapid symptomatic relief while awaiting activity of thioamides, RAI, or surgery
	Diltiazem (Cardizem) 30, 60, 90, 120 mg tablets; sustained release tablets might not be as effective	60 mg po qid or 120 mg tid	Blocks the peripheral action of thyroid hormone, no effect on disease state	Hypotension, bradycardia, pedal edema	Alternative to patients unable to tolerate β-blockers (e.g., asthma, IDDM). Verapamil and dihydropyridine calcium channel blockers not as effective.
Radioactive iodine	¹³¹I	80–150 μCi/g thyroid tissue; usual dose of 8–10 mCi.	Destruction of the gland	Hypothyroidism, rarely radiation thyroiditis; fear of malignancy, leukemia, and genetic damage. Contraindicated in pregnancy.	Slow onset of action approximately 2–4 weeks, full effects seen within 3–6 months.

Surgery	Iodides, thioamides or β-blockers preoperatively to prevent storm and facilitate surgery	5–10 drops/day of iodides for 10–14 days before surgery; see β-blockers and thioamides dosing	Removal of the gland; total thyroidectomy might be surgery of choice to prevent recurrent hyperthyroidism.	Hypothyroidism, hypoparathyroidism complications of surgery and anesthesia	Incidence of hypothyroidism indirectly proportional to gland remnant left
Iodinated contrast media	Ipodate, iopanoic acid 500-mg tablets	500 mg–1 g po qd or 3 g q 3rd day po	Blocks T_4 to T_3 conversion; release of iodides. See iodides	Similar to iodides; nausea, vomiting, abdominal cramps, diarrhea, dizziness, headache.	Rapid onset of action; adjunct to thioamides, not for chronic use because effects not sustained
Ionic exchange resin	Cholestyramine 4 g oral powder packets	4 g po tid	Increases fecal excretion of T_4 by binding T_4 in the intestine	Gastrointestinal: bloating, flatulence, constipation; impairs absorption of concurrent medications	Adjunct to thioamides, useful when additional decline in hormones levels is desirable.
Monovalent anions	Potassium perchlorate 200-mg capsules	800–1,000 mg/day po in four divided doses for 2–6 weeks	Competitive inhibitor of iodide binding; discharges nonorganified iodide from the gland	Gastric irritation, nausea, vomiting, fever, rashes. Aplastic anemia, bone marrow suppression and nephrotic syndrome when used chronically	Useful short-term adjunct to thioamides for amiodarone induced hyperthyroidism
Lithium	Lithium carbonate, various dosage forms available	800–1,200 mg/day in 2–3 divided doses.	Acts similar to iodides to block hormone release	Nausea, vomiting, diarrhea, tremor, ataxia, dizziness, confusion, coma. Maintain normal serum levels. Avoid hyponatremia or sodium depletion.	Reserved for special situations when other agents contraindicated or ineffective.

q, every; T_3, triiodothyronine; T_4, thyroxine; DOC, drug of choice; RAI, radioactive iodine; IV, intravenously; ISA, intrinsic sympathomimetic activity; po, by mouth; qd, every day; qid, four times daily; tid, three times daily; IDDM, insulin-dependent diabetes mellitus.

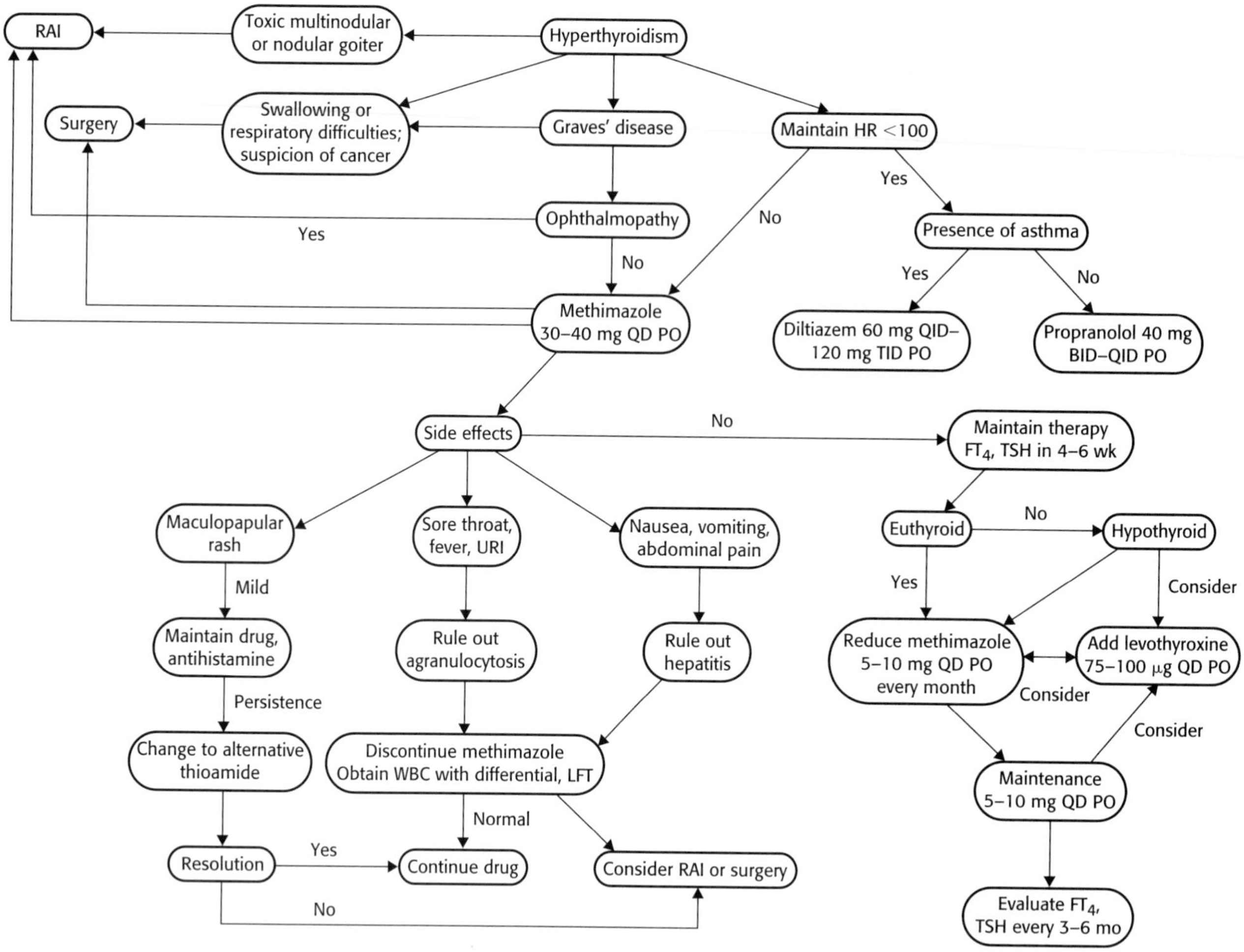

RAI ← Toxic multinodular or nodular goiter ← Hyperthyroidism

Surgery ← Swallowing or respiratory difficulties; suspicion of cancer ← Graves' disease

Hyperthyroidism → Maintain HR <100

Graves' disease → Ophthalmopathy → (Yes → RAI/Surgery)

Ophthalmopathy → No → Methimazole 30–40 mg QD PO

Maintain HR <100 → Yes → Presence of asthma; No → Methimazole 30–40 mg QD PO

Presence of asthma → Yes → Diltiazem 60 mg QID–120 mg TID PO; No → Propranolol 40 mg BID–QID PO

Methimazole 30–40 mg QD PO → Side effects

Side effects → No → Maintain therapy FT4, TSH in 4–6 wk

Side effects → Maculopapular rash; Sore throat, fever, URI; Nausea, vomiting, abdominal pain

Maculopapular rash → Mild → Maintain drug, antihistamine → Persistence → Change to alternative thioamide → Resolution

Sore throat, fever, URI → Rule out agranulocytosis → Discontinue methimazole Obtain WBC with differential, LFT

Nausea, vomiting, abdominal pain → Rule out hepatitis → Discontinue methimazole Obtain WBC with differential, LFT

Resolution → Yes → Continue drug; No → Consider RAI or surgery

Discontinue methimazole Obtain WBC with differential, LFT → Normal → Continue drug; → Consider RAI or surgery

Maintain therapy FT4, TSH in 4–6 wk → Euthyroid; Hypothyroid

Euthyroid → No → Hypothyroid

Euthyroid → Yes → Reduce methimazole 5–10 mg QD PO every month

Hypothyroid → Consider → Add levothyroxine 75–100 μg QD PO

Reduce methimazole 5–10 mg QD PO every month ↔ Consider ↔ Add levothyroxine 75–100 μg QD PO

Reduce methimazole → Maintenance 5–10 mg QD PO

Add levothyroxine → Consider → Maintenance 5–10 mg QD PO

Maintenance 5–10 mg QD PO → Evaluate FT4, TSH every 3–6 mo

FIGURE 38.3 Treatment algorithm for management of hyperthyroidism from Graves' disease or autonomous nodules (single or multinodular). FT4, free thyroxine; HR, heart rate; LFT, liver function test; RAI, radioactive iodine; TSH, thyroid-stimulating hormone; URI, upper respiratory tract infections.

ods are more effective than thioamides to prevent progressive ophthalmopathy. However, worsening ocular symptoms have been reported after all types of treatment, particularly after RAI in patients with preexisting eye symptoms. In the aforementioned patients, prophylactic systemic corticosteroids (e.g., prednisone 30–40 mg daily starting within a few days of RAI and continuing for approximately 2–3 weeks) is warranted to prevent further progression of the ophthalmopathy. Hypothyroidism can also aggravate preexisting eye complaints. Regardless of the method of treatment selected, hyperthyroidism control and hypothyroidism prevention are essential to prevent progression of the ophthalmopathy. Although thioamides can normalize thyroid hormone levels, single or toxic multinodular disease is best managed with definitive treatment, such as RAI or surgery, because spontaneous remission is unlikely.[14]

The usual treatment choices in children are thioamides and subtotal thyroidectomy, although all three methods (surgery, RAI, and thioamides) have been used.[10,45] The risks of surgery must be weighed against the benefits of speedy correction of the thyrotoxicosis and the lack of need for the rigid dosing schedules of the thioamides. RAI usually is not recommended because of fear of genetic damage, leukemia, and carcinogenesis, although these risks are unsubstantiated.[40] Thyroid carcinoma and dysfunction have been reported in children exposed to external head and neck irradiation, although similar results have not been shown with internal RAI.

Hyperthyroidism can be difficult to manage during pregnancy. Pregnancy is best postponed until the hyperthyroidism is controlled permanently with surgery or RAI to prevent disease flares and relapse during pregnancy and during and after delivery.[27,28] Spontaneous remission of the disease with improvement of symptoms can occur during pregnancy because of declines in TRab levels, and antithyroid medications often are not necessary. Untreated maternal thyrotoxicosis can result in abortion, perinatal death, and prematurity, so proper treatment is crucial. Thioamides can be used if precautions are taken. RAI and iodides are absolutely contraindicated, and surgery in the second trimester is an option.

Infants with neonatal Graves disease are extremely ill within hours of delivery. Supportive measures, including sedation, cooling, oxygen, fluid, and electrolyte replacement and short-term management of the hyperthyroidism by thioamides, iodides, or β-blockers, are required. Fortunately, the disease is self-limiting and symptoms disappear in 1 to 2 months as the level of TRab declines. Antithyroid drugs should be withdrawn at this time.

Subacute thyroiditis is self-limiting, and spontaneous recovery is common.[16] Treatment is symptomatic and consists of heat, rest, analgesics (e.g., nonsteroidal antiinflammatory drugs), and β-blockers, if necessary, to control the symptoms of hyperthyroidism. Thioamides are not effective because hormone leakage from the gland, rather than increased hormone synthesis, causes the elevated hormone levels. Corticosteroids are indicated for severe inflammation if analgesics are ineffective. In the hypothyroid phase, transient thyroid replacement might be necessary to suppress further TSH stimulation to the damaged gland and treat symptoms of hypothyroidism.

TREATMENT

PHARMACOTHERAPY

Thioamides. Thioamides can be used as long-term primary therapy for Graves hyperthyroidism, especially in adolescents and children, or given transiently to reduce thyroid hormone levels before definitive therapy with RAI or surgery.[8,9,38,39] Thioamides are the treatment of choice in patients with small goiters and mild disease and for whom a high remission rate is likely. The advantages of thioamides include the potential for remission without damage to the gland. Limitations include nonadherence, strict parental and physician supervision in children, low success rates, and the risks of adverse reaction.

The thioamides, propylthiouracil (PTU) and methimazole, prevent thyroid hormone synthesis by inhibiting the oxidation binding of iodide and its coupling to tyrosine residue. PTU (but not methimazole) also inhibits the peripheral deiodination of T_4 to T_3, so serum T_3 levels decline 20% to 30% more rapidly in severely thyrotoxic patients. TSH receptor antibody levels also are suppressed by thioamides via an unknown immunosuppressive mechanism of action.[38]

Thioamide selection is based largely on the prescriber's personal preference, although certain pharmacologic differences should dictate the choice. In most situations, methimazole is the preferred thioamide of choice rather than PTU for several reasons. Methimazole can be given as a single daily dose, which improves patient adherence. It is more potent than PTU and requires fewer tablets. It is also less expensive, better tolerated, and at low doses is less toxic than PTU.[39] Generally, PTU is preferred over methimazole in patients with thyroid storm or in those with severe hyperthyroidism because it blocks the peripheral conversion of T_4 to T_3 and, therefore, might have a faster onset of action. PTU, and not methimazole, has been considered the drug of choice in pregnancy because maternal use of methimazole

is associated with congenital skin defects (i.e., aplasia cutis). However, the association between methimazole and congenital skin defects is not sufficiently supported to preclude the use of this drug during pregnancy, and methimazole has been used without deleterious effects.[46–48] One study found that the risks of reversible aplasia cutis were similar in women receiving methimazole (2.7%) or PTU (3.0%) compared to 6% in hyperthyroid controls.[47] Furthermore, fetal umbilical cord thyroid hormone concentrations from mothers receiving either thioamide were similar.[49] Therefore, PTU or methimazole can be safely used in pregnancy. In lactating women, PTU is preferred over methimazole because insignificant amounts of PTU are excreted in the milk, whereas 7% to 16% of a methimazole dose is detected in breast milk.[39] Therefore, methimazole is the thioamide of choice except in patients unable to tolerate PTU and in the situations just identified, in which PTU might be preferable.

Methimazole is ten times as potent as PTU (100 mg PTU ≈ 10 mg methimazole), but they are equally effective if given in equipotent dosages. Both drugs are absorbed rapidly from the gastrointestinal tract, and peak plasma concentrations are reached within 30 minutes of ingestion. The serum half-lives of 4 to 6 hours for methimazole and 1 to 2 hours for PTU do not change as the thyroid status changes. However, the duration of action and frequency of dosing depend on the intrathyroidal half-life, not on the short plasma half-lives. The duration of action of methimazole is 24 to 36 hours, permitting once-daily administration. The intrathyroidal duration of PTU is much shorter, requiring initial dosing every 6 to 8 hours to be effective.

Initial therapy should begin with 30 to 40 mg per day orally of methimazole, given as a single daily dose or in three divided doses, if needed to limit gastrointestinal intolerance. Alternatively, 300 to 400 mg per day of PTU can be given in three to four divided doses. Dosage regimens for thioamides in children are similar to those used in adults. In neonates, PTU (5–10 mg/kg/day) or methimazole (0.5–1 mg/kg/day) is effective.[10] Initial single-dose regimens have been used successfully with PTU, but the best results can be obtained by multiple daily dosing until euthyroidism is achieved, then changing to a single-dose maintenance regimen. Patients experiencing severe toxemia or thyroid storm may need doses as high as 1,200 mg per day of PTU or its equivalent, given in divided doses. There are no intravenous preparations, although both drugs can be formulated for rectal administration.[50–52] Tapering of the thioamide dose should not begin until symptoms are reduced and T_4 levels are normal, usually 6 to 8 weeks (based on elimination of existing thyroid stores; $t_{1/2} \sim 7$ days). The initial dose can be reduced gradually, by one third each month, until a daily maintenance dosage of 5 to 15 mg of methimazole or 50 to 150 mg per day of PTU is reached. If symptoms do not resolve within the specified time, poor adherence, incomplete blockage of synthesis by insufficient dose, or an inadequate dosing interval should be considered as causes of failure. A change to methimazole is indicated if PTU was the initial drug because nonadherence is more likely to occur with PTU than with methimazole.

In pregnancy, the dangers of fetal goiter and hypothyroidism are reduced if initial doses of PTU are maintained at less than 300 mg per day (given in divided doses) and maintenance doses of 50 to 100 mg per day are used throughout pregnancy.[27,28] Equivalent doses of methimazole appear to be as safe as PTU with respect to fetal hypothyroidism and could be used if necessary, although methimazole might pose a rare teratogenic risk of aplasia cutis.[46–48] Clinically, the mother should be maintained in a comfortable, mildly hyperthyroid state (FT$_4$I or FT$_4$ in the upper ranges of normal) to prevent fetal thyroid suppression. The appearance of an enlarged maternal goiter during therapy is alarming because it implies the development of maternal and fetal hypothyroidism. The concomitant use of thyroid hormone is not helpful because the thyroid hormone does not cross the placenta and might make maternal management more difficult. Fortunately, the intellectual development of offspring exposed to antithyroid drugs in utero appears to be no different from that of unexposed siblings.[53,54]

A baseline FT$_4$ or FT$_4$I, TSH, and white blood cell (WBC) count with differential should be obtained before thioamides are started. A baseline WBC with differential can help ascertain the development of thioamide-induced agranulocytosis because hyperthyroidism can be associated with a relative reduction in the neutrophil count. Thyroid hormone levels should normalize within 6 to 8 weeks after the start of therapy and parallel the clinical response. The FT$_4$ or FT$_4$I and TSH should be monitored routinely at 4 to 8 weeks after the start of therapy and after any change in the dosing regimen. Once a stable thioamide maintenance dose is reached, thyroid function tests can be monitored routinely every 2 to 4 months.

The recommended duration of thioamide therapy for Graves disease is empiric, generally 12 to 18 months. Courses of 3 to 6 months have been proposed, but lower remission rates of 20% to 40% result.[39] Several studies suggest that the remission rate might improve with a longer duration of therapy.[39,55–57] An 18-month treatment period yielded higher remission rates (61.8%) than 6-month therapy (41.7%). A study in children noted a 25% increase in the remission rate when the duration was increased by 1 year.[58] Therefore, 12 months is the minimum treatment duration recommended to maximize remission potential. Longer treatment durations can be used if there are no adverse effects and the patient is willing to continue antithyroid therapy.

Disappointing remission rates of 15% to 80% after stopping thioamides have led to progressive disenchantment with the antithyroid drugs as definitive therapy for Graves disease. Permanent spontaneous remission is rare. It is unclear why some patients remain in remission while others relapse. No factors have been consistently predictive of successful long-term remission, and most studies have produced conflicting results. Factors associated with poor long-term remission rates include increased dietary intake of iodides, severe hyperthyroidism, a large goiter that does not regress with thioamide therapy, short duration of thioamide therapy, persistent high titers of TRab after stopping thioamides, recurrent hyperthyroidism, and presence of HLA antigen.[39,55–59]

An excellent indicator for remission is normalization of the goiter size during therapy. Patients with small goiters, mild and short duration of symptoms and illness, and disappearance of TRab during therapy have a better chance of remission.[39,55–59]

Factors associated with TRab titer reduction include therapy duration greater than 1 year, high blocking doses of thioamides, and concomitant administration of levothyroxine (l-thyroxine) with thioamides. High thioamide blocking doses (i.e., 600–800 mg PTU or 40–60 mg methimazole) given throughout therapy produced better remission rates (75.4%) than conventional therapy (41.6%) but produced greater toxicity, and therefore, cannot be recommended.[38,60]

The initial enthusiasm and optimism generated by a study showing that adding l-thyroxine to antithyroid therapy could reduce relapse rates by suppressing TSH receptor antibody levels have quieted. Hashizume et al.[61] first reported a startling recurrence rate of 1.7% in Japanese patients who received methimazole for 6 months, followed by combined l-thyroxine and methimazole for a year, and then l-thyroxine alone for 3 years, compared with a relapse rate of 34.7% in those not receiving l-thyroxine. Unfortunately, subsequent prospective studies, using similar designs, have been unable to demonstrate greater TSH receptor antibody suppression with combination thioamide/thyroxine therapy nor duplicate the favorable remission rates of Hashizume et al.[62–64] Therefore, the advantages of using a more complicated and expensive combination regimen are unsubstantiated. Some clinicians advocate the concomitant use of exogenous l-thyroxine during antithyroid therapy to prevent hypothyroidism and suppress goiter formation from excessive PTU or methimazole administration. Proper titration of the thioamide dosage should alleviate this problem, so concomitant l-thyroxine therapy is recommended only if proper titration is difficult.

Toxic reactions to PTU and methimazole occur in 1% to 5% of patients.[8,39] A pruritic maculopapular skin rash, without other systemic manifestations, is the most common adverse reaction. Therefore, all patients should be instructed to report symptoms of skin reactions. It is also important to distinguish a thioamide rash from a heat rash or hives caused by hyperthyroidism. In mild cases, the rash might disappear spontaneously despite continued therapy. Antihistamines can provide symptomatic relief of the pruritus. If the rash persists, the alternative thioamide can be substituted because little cross-sensitivity exists. However, if the rash is associated with systemic symptoms (i.e., fever, arthralgias) or if angioneurotic edema, hives, or other anaphylactoid reactions occur, substitution with another thioamide is not recommended because the risks of cross-sensitivity are high.

Hepatitis is more common than previously appreciated.[65–67] Hepatocellular and obstructive hepatitis have been reported with both agents; however, hepatocellular damage is more common with PTU, and obstructive jaundice occurs with methimazole, especially at doses greater than 40 mg per day. The incidence of PTU-induced hepatotoxicity is estimated to be less than 0.5%, but the true incidence is unknown. Approximately 30% of patients on PTU can have asymptomatic hepatic transaminase elevations.[65] Stopping PTU might not be necessary if the transaminases normalize within 3 months of a dose reduction. In contrast, PTU should be stopped immediately to ensure complete recovery in patients with clinical evidence of hepatitis. PTU-induced hepatitis typically is associated with nonspecific hepatocellular necrosis on liver biopsy. The prognosis appears worse in those less than 11 years or greater than 40 years of age, with duration of jaundice more than 7 days before onset of encephalopathy, and with significant elevations in serum bilirubin (>300 μmol/L, or 17.5 mg/dL) and prothrombin time (>50 seconds). Circulating autoantibodies and in vitro peripheral lymphocyte sensitization to PTU indicate a possible autoimmune cause. These idiosyncratic reactions typically occur early in therapy, although delayed reactions have been noted. It is reversible if detected early, although fatalities have been reported. Because of the severity of the reaction and potential for cross-sensitivity, substitution with the alternative thioamide is not recommended. Routine monitoring of liver function tests should be considered in patients with a history of liver disease and risk factors for hepatitis (e.g., alcoholism). All patients should be educated about the symptoms of hepatitis and instructed to avoid alcohol and to immediately report any symptoms of hepatitis to their health care providers.

Rarely, hypoprothrombinemia (with PTU), serologic abnormalities (lupus erythematosus, antinuclear antibody), lupus, and lupus-like syndromes have also been reported.[38,39] Recovery occurs after withdrawal of the drug or institution of steroids.

Agranulocytosis (<500 polymorphonuclear neutrophil leukocytes) is the most serious (but rare) adverse reaction to the thioamides. The incidence is between 0.5% and 6%.[39] The onset of fever greater than 101°F, malaise, gingivitis, and sore throat is so abrupt that routine WBC counts usually are not helpful. Although one study suggests that weekly monitoring of the WBC with differential during the first 3 months of therapy might identify early and asymptomatic agranulocytosis, routine monitoring is not indicated because it might hamper patient adherence and does not appear to be cost-effective.[68] All patients should be educated carefully about agranulocytosis and instructed to immediately report the onset of such symptoms to their healthcare provider. Patients greater than 40 years of age and those on high-dose methimazole (>40 mg/day) might be at greater risk of developing this toxic reaction, although it is not necessarily dose-related. Lower doses (<30 mg/day) of methimazole might be safer than any dose of PTU. Sex is not a predictive factor. This reaction is more likely to occur during the first 6 weeks of therapy, although it can occur at any time in the course of treatment. One study suggests that agranulocytosis might occur earlier with PTU therapy (i.e., 17.7 ± 9.7 days) than with methimazole therapy (36.9 ± 14.5 days).[68] Fortunately, complete resolution of symptoms and recovery of granulocytes are often seen within a few days to 3 weeks after the thioamides are stopped. Granulocyte colony-stimulating factor and corticosteroids might shorten the recovery period. If infection occurs, antibiotics, adrenal steroids, and possibly hospitalization are indicated. Rechallenge with the same drug or an alternative thioamide is not recommended because the risk of recurrent agranulocytosis outweighs the benefits of therapy. The degree of cross-sensitivity is not known.

Potassium Perchlorate. Potassium perchlorate is a monovalent anion that interferes with iodide binding and causes the discharge of nonorganified iodide from the gland. Because perchlorate is a competitive inhibitor of iodide, it is particularly useful for the short-term management of amiodarone-induced hyperthyroidism, but its antithyroid effect can be overcome by iodine administration. Short-term administration (e.g., 800 mg to 1 g/day for 2–6 weeks) is well tolerated, but irreversible aplastic anemia and nephrotic syndrome have limited the usefulness of the monovalent anions for chronic therapy of hyperthyroidism.

Iodides. Although the iodides have been known to provide symptomatic relief of thyrotoxicosis since the 1920s, their clinical use has been largely superseded by the thioamides and β-blockers. Iodides act by several mechanisms of action. They inhibit organification (Wolff–Chaikoff effect) and hormone release and decrease gland vascularity.[25,38] The rapid relief of thyrotoxic symptoms after 2 to 7 days of iodide administration suggests that inhibition of hormone release is the predominant mechanism of action, rather than a block in organification, which would not be apparent for several weeks. This rapid effect is advantageous for patients in thyroid storm and for those awaiting the onset of thioamide therapy. However, iodides should not be used before RAI therapy (or if RAI is considered as subsequent treatment) because iodides can block effective RAI retention by the gland for several weeks after use.

Iodides are routinely given 10 to 14 days before surgery to facilitate surgical removal of the hyperplastic gland by decreasing its vascularity and increasing its firmness. Preoperatively, the combination of β-blockers and iodides can also be used, although the established regimen of thioamides and iodides is preferable.

Stable iodine is available as Lugol's solution (5% iodine and 10% potassium iodide), containing 8 mg of iodide per drop, or as the more palatable saturated solution of potassium iodide (SSKI), containing 50 mg per drop (Table 38.7).

The major adverse effects of iodides are hypersensitivity reactions, including rash, drug fever, sialadenitis, conjunctivitis, rhinitis, and collagen vascular disorders. In patients with underlying thyroid disorders (e.g., multinodular goiter), iodides can produce hyperthyroidism from failure of the Wolff–Chaikoff block, or they can cause goiter and hypothyroidism (e.g., Hashimoto thyroiditis) in patients unable to escape from the Wolff–Chaikoff block.[25] Chronic iodide administration should be avoided throughout pregnancy because ingesting as little as 12 mg iodine has caused fetal goiter and asphyxiation. Vaginal povidone or topical iodine can produce high serum concentrations of iodine and should also be avoided.

Advantages of iodide therapy include simplicity, low cost, low toxicity, and no gland destruction. Limitations of treatment include escape, treatment relapse, allergic reactions, and interference with subsequent RAI therapy.

Adrenergic Antagonists. Because many of the signs and symptoms of thyrotoxicosis are mediated through the sympathetic nervous system, drugs that deplete or block the effects of thyroid hormones on tissue catecholamines can provide rapid symptomatic relief before thioamides, RAI, and surgery act. These agents do not affect the underlying disease process, so they should not be used as primary therapy.

Propranolol is the β-blocker most widely used and studied in the treatment of the hyperthyroidism and, therefore, the standard against which others are judged.[9,69] When propranolol is given orally in doses of 20 to 40 mg three to four times a day as necessary, symptomatic relief of palpitations, tachycardia, anxiety, sweating, tremor, and diarrhea occurs. However, weight loss remains unaffected. Patients with severe toxemia might need as much as 480 mg per day to achieve symptomatic relief and maintain the HR less than 100 beats per minute (bpm). Propranolol is also effective in controlling the neuromuscular manifestations of hyperthyroidism, especially periodic paralysis. It can be used as an adjunct to thioamides and RAI during therapy of neonatal thyrotoxicosis, pregnancy, or thyroid storm, and as a preoperative medication. Although β-blockers have been used successfully as sole agents preoperatively, they are not recommended in the patient with severe toxemia because inadequate control of severe thyrotoxicosis has resulted in storm. All the selective and nonselective β-blockers (e.g., nadolol, atenolol, metoprolol) appear to be equally effective in the symptomatic relief of hyperthyroidism. β-Blockers with intrinsic sympathomimetic activity (e.g., pindolol) are not recommended because they do not reduce the HR as much as β-blockers without intrinsic sympathomimetic activity. Chronic administration of β-blockers should be avoided during pregnancy, particularly in the last trimester, because of the risk of fetal respiratory depression, small placenta, intrauterine growth retardation, impaired responses to anoxic stress, and postnatal bradycardia and hypoglycemia. Propranolol is also excreted in breast milk and should be avoided during lactation. Such findings indicate that propranolol, like iodides, should be used only on a short-term basis during pregnancy.

The calcium-channel blockers, particularly diltiazem, might be a useful alternative when β-blockers are contraindicated (e.g., in patients with asthma, insulin-dependent diabetes). Oral diltiazem, 120 mg three times daily or 60 mg four times daily is well tolerated and appears to be as effective as propranolol in suppressing thyrotoxicosis symptoms.[70] However, verapamil has produced detrimental effects in thyrotoxicosis. The potential synergistic benefits and toxicity of the calcium blockers and β-blockers in the management of thyrotoxicosis are unknown.

Radioactive Iodine. RAI therapy is indicated in postadolescent patients, those with Graves ophthalmopathy or a history of thyroid surgery, those who are poor surgical candidates because of complicating nonthyroid illness, and those who fail or experience thioamide toxicity.[8,40] RAI is absolutely contraindicated in pregnancy because the RAI crosses the placenta and destroys the fetal thyroid gland, which begins functioning between the 12th and 14th weeks of life. RAI is the treatment of choice in older patients with cardiac disease and in those with TMGs. ^{131}I, which has a half-life of 8 days and delivers high-energy β-radiation to a maximal depth of 2 mm, is the isotope most commonly used. ^{125}I, which has less tissue penetration and a half-life of 60 days, has not resulted in a lower incidence of hypothyroidism, as was initially anticipated. Because ^{125}I emits γ rays that penetrate only a few microns, larger therapeutic doses are required, which increases considerably the total body radiation without reducing the incidence of hypothyroidism.

RAI dosage is calculated using a formula that incorporates an estimate of the gland size, the uptake of iodine at 24 hours, and the standard number of microcuries of iodine given per gram of thyroid tissue. At the University of California, patients receive approximately 80 to 150 μCi per gram of thyroid tissue. Despite this formula, the proper dosage (i.e., one that prevents recurrent hyperthyroidism and subsequent hypothyroidism) is difficult to calculate or predict.

$$^{131}I \text{ (mCi)} = [\text{Estimated gland weight (g)} \times 80 - 150 \text{ μCi/g}] \div 100\% \text{ 24-hour RAI}$$

Pretreatment with thioamides for approximately 1 month to deplete the gland of stored hormones or with β-blockers before and after RAI therapy is necessary to prevent exacerbations of thyrotoxicosis within 10 to 14 days after RAI. Older adults, patients with heart disease, and those with large intraglandular stores of hormones are at greatest risk.[40] Methimazole is the preferred thioamide to use prior to RAI therapy because PTU has been associated with poorer RAI retention and higher RAI failure rates than methimazole.[71–73] Therefore, to facilitate optimal ^{131}I uptake and retention, PTU should be stopped 1 week before, and methimazole 4 days before RAI therapy. Nevertheless, the RAI dose might have to be increased by 25% in patients pretreated with thioamides. β-Blockers and calcium-channel blockers can be used without compromising RAI therapy.

Iodides should not be used before RAI therapy because ^{131}I uptake and efficacy will be significantly impaired for several months. Lithium may be useful.[8,26]

Resolution of the hyperthyroidism is slow after RAI treatment. Improvement of symptoms might be apparent by 3 to 6 weeks after RAI; however, maximum effects do not occur until 3 to 4 months after an ablative dose. Because of this delayed onset, iodides, ipodate or other iodinated contrast media, thioamides, or β-blockers might be necessary for symptomatic control after RAI is given. If a second dose is required, a larger dose of RAI must be given to optimize gland uptake exposing the body to more radiation.

The lowest appropriate age limit for RAI therapy is controversial. After more than 25 years of extensive clinical experience, RAI is generally accepted as safe for most adult patients less than 35 years of age. Adolescents have also been safely treated with RAI, although its use is controversial.[10,40]

The major concerns about RAI therapy include carcinogenesis, leukemia, and genetic damage. So far, these hazards appear to be unfounded. Although a large retrospective cohort study found a small increase in cancer mortality, RAI did not result in a significant increase in total cancer mortality.[74] The radiation dose to the gonads in patients treated with ^{131}I for hyperthyroidism is generally less than 3 rads, which is not significantly different from gonadal irradiation received from commonly used diagnostic tests such as barium enemas and pyelograms. The major complication of RAI is hypothyroidism, which is most common the first year after therapy and increases at a constant rate of 2.5% per year thereafter, accounting for a 20-year incidence of 30% to 70%. Immediate side effects of ^{131}I therapy are minimal and might include mild thyroid pain and tenderness, temporary hair thinning, and (rarely) dysphagia. Exacerbation of Graves ophthalmopathy can occur after RAI therapy, and prophylactic systemic corticosteroids should be considered in patients with mild eye symptoms.[35,36] Generally, RAI therapy is effective, quick, easy, painless, and nontoxic.

Iodinated Contrast Media. An unlabeled use for iodinated contrast dye (e.g., ipodate, iopanoic acid, sodium tyropanoate, diatrizoate sodium) is the acute management of hyperthyroidism.[43] When ipodate is administered in a daily dose of 500 mg to 1 g orally or 3 g every third day to thyrotoxic patients, dramatic improvement in subjective and objective symptoms parallel the rapid fall in thyroid hormone levels. The changes in serum T_4, serum T_3, and rT_3 levels are consistent with inhibition of the peripheral deiodination of T_4 to T_3. Serum T_3 levels decline within 6 hours of ipodate administration, declining to 50% of baseline at 24 hours and 70% of baseline (nadir) at 48 hours. T_3 levels remain suppressed for 3 to 5 days after a single administration. Similarly, T_4 levels reach their nadir 3 days after administration and remain depressed for as long as 6 days after the last dose. When compared with PTU, ipodate produced earlier symptomatic and objective improvements and more rapid declines in T_3 hormone levels. Prolonged suppression

of T_3 and T_4 levels suggests that hormone secretion inhibition, caused by the released iodine, is an additional mechanism of action. Although similar inhibition of peripheral T_3 production is seen with most iodinated contrast media, ipodate (Oragrafin), which contains 61.4% iodine, is the most potent. Each gram of the iodinated contrast media contain between 600 and 650 mg of iodine.

Because the iodinated contrast dyes are relatively nontoxic agents, they are useful adjuncts to the thioamides in the management of severe thyrotoxicosis, thyroid storm, amiodarone-induced thyrotoxicosis,[75] or as an alternative in those allergic to thioamides. They may also be an effective preoperative preparation in lieu of iodides, but experience is limited.[76] However, chronic use of these agents is not indicated because the hormone level reductions seen within the first month of therapy are not sustained in most hyperthyroid patients.

NONPHARMACOLOGIC THERAPY
Surgery. Thyroidectomy is considered the treatment option of choice for patients in whom RAI or thioamides are contraindicated; in those with large goiters, causing cosmetic disfigurement, respiratory distress, or swallowing difficulties; in those with suspected malignancies; and in selected children and pregnant women.[8] Some argue that surgery may be underutilized since in one prospective randomized trial, surgery produced euthyroidism faster and resulted in a lower rate of relapse than with either RAI or thioamides.[41,42] Prior thyroid surgery should be considered a strong deterrent to further surgery because reoperation increases the hazard of vocal cord paralysis and hypoparathyroidism 10-fold and 30-fold, respectively. Other poor surgical candidates are patients with severe cardiac, respiratory, or debilitating diseases, and women in the third trimester of pregnancy (because surgery can precipitate spontaneous labor). Surgery can be performed safely in the second trimester after suitable preparation with thioamides or short-term use of β-blockers.

The ideal surgical endpoint is a 3- to 8-g remnant of thyroid tissue that produces neither a recurrence of the thyrotoxicosis nor hypothyroidism.[41] The risk of recurrent thyrotoxicosis is directly proportional to the amount of thyroid remnant left. Increasing the remnant gland size by 1 g decreases the risk of postoperative hypothyroidism by 10%; conversely, increasing the remnant size above 10 g increases the risk of recurrent disease without changing the risk of hypothyroidism. Although euthyroidism might not always be feasible, one series reported a 94% euthyroid success rate using a modified subtotal thyroidectomy. Subtotal thyroidectomy is the preferred operation for hyperthyroidism because it offers the best chance of euthyroidism. Others advocate a total thyroidectomy, despite the risk of hypothyroidism, to prevent recurrence of the hyperthyroidism. Surgery appears to be as safe as nonsurgical treatments for hyperthyroidism if it is performed by experienced surgeons on patients adequately prepared by the standard combination of thioamides, iodides, or β-blockers. In adequately prepared preoperative patients, operative mortality and risk of thyroid storm are low. Vocal cord paralysis and permanent hypoparathyroidism occur in less than 1% of patients after a subtotal thyroidectomy.

The major surgical complication is hypothyroidism, which occurs in the first 6 months to 3 years postoperatively, but it can develop insidiously as late as 10 years postoperatively. Incidences of 5% to 75% have been reported. The incidence of hypothyroidism is inversely proportional to the remnant of thyroid tissue left; remnants of 2 to 4 g result in an incidence of 70%.

The disadvantages of surgery include expense, need for hospitalization, risks of anesthesia, postoperative complications, and the patient's fear of surgery. These disadvantages may outweigh the advantages of rapid, definitive surgical intervention.

SPECIAL TREATMENT ISSUES

Subclinical Hyperthyroidism. Treatment of subclinical hyperthyroidism is controversial because the benefits of therapy are unproven.[11,29] Recommendations for therapy must be individualized and may be considered for those at the greatest risk for morbidity (e.g., adults >60 years of age, or those with cardiac disease, atrial fibrillation, or osteoporosis, especially postmenopausal women).[30-32] In patients without risk factors, observation and routine TSH monitoring may be the optimal plan because progression to overt hyperthyroidism is infrequent.

Exophthalmos and Ophthalmologic Complications. Because the pathogenesis and progression of ophthalmopathy are not well understood, treatment of ocular complaints often is symptomatic until euthyroidism occurs.[35]

Periorbital edema and chemosis (inflammation of the conjunctiva) respond to elevation of the head of the bed to promote diuresis. Protective glasses, methylcellulose and hydrocortisone drops, and avoidance of smoke and dust might alleviate photophobia and external irritation. In patients whose eyes do not completely close during sleep, taping the eyelids shut at night is essential to prevent corneal scarring and drying.

Systemic corticosteroids are indicated for progressive inflammatory exophthalmos and decreasing visual acuity. Prednisone (60–120 mg/day) administered in divided doses for 1 to 3 weeks often produces dramatic resolution of inflammatory eye symptoms. When symptoms resolve, the dosage can be tapered over 2 weeks and then gradually withdrawn. In addition to their antiinflammatory action, corticosteroids suppress TRab levels and decrease T_3 levels by impairing the peripheral conversion of T_4 to T_3. Immunosuppressive agents, such as cyclophosphamide and azathioprine, have not been as effective as steroids. External orbital radiation therapy, which achieves similar results, can be used in patients with contraindications to corticosteroids.

After euthyroidism is achieved and the eye symptoms are stable, lid or orbital surgery can provide cosmetic or visual corrections.

Atrial Fibrillation and Congestive Heart Failure. Hyperthyroidism or subclinical hyperthyroidism can cause new or worsening atrial fibrillation and CHF.[29-31] Therefore, routine thyroid function tests should be obtained in all patients presenting with these cardiac symptoms to exclude underlying thyroid disease. The atrial fibrillation and heart failure often are difficult to control until euthyroidism occurs.[77] A combination of medications, including β-blockers and calcium blockers, and larger doses of digoxin (Table 38.5) might be needed to slow the HR and correct the heart failure. Hyperthyroid patients tend to be clinically resistant to the digitalis glycosides, whereas hypothyroid patients are very sensitive. A larger loading and maintenance dose of digoxin is required in thyrotoxicosis because of hyperthyroidism-induced increases in the digoxin volume of distribution and clearance.[1]

Anticoagulation with warfarin is recommended in patients with hyperthyroidism-related atrial fibrillation, valvular disease, and heart failure because of the high incidence of systemic emboli. Smaller doses of warfarin (e.g., 2–3 mg) are needed for anticoagulation in hyperthyroidism (Table 38.5). An enhanced anticoagulant response occurs because the warfarin-induced decrease in clotting factor synthesis is combined with hyperthyroidism-induced increases in factor catabolism. The opposite occurs in hypothyroidism; the anticoagulant response decreases because of delayed catabolism of clotting factors. Therefore, thyrotoxic patients need less warfarin and myxedematous patients need more warfarin to achieve the same hypoprothrombinemic response.

The doses of digoxin and warfarin must be adjusted as euthyroidism occurs to prevent toxicity and maintain therapeutic efficacy. Spontaneous conversion to normal sinus rhythm after becoming euthyroid is less likely if the patient has underlying heart disease or if the duration of the atrial fibrillation persists more than 4 months after achieving euthyroidism.[77]

Thyroid Storm. The pathogenesis of storm is not well understood, but it appears to be an exaggerated form of thyrotoxicosis. Storm can be precipitated by childbirth, stress, infection, trauma, diabetic ketoacidosis, inadequate preparation before RAI or surgery, and nonadherence with antithyroid medication.[33,34]

Prompt recognition and immediate treatment can decrease the 100% mortality rate to 7% or better. Treatment is directed at five major areas:

1. Supporting vital functions with sedation, oxygen, fluids, and antipyretics, treating infection, correcting electrolyte abnormalities, and using corticosteroids (hydrocortisone 100–200 mg intravenously every 6 hours) for unsuspected hypoadrenalism. Peripheral conversion to T_3 is also reduced by corticosteroids.

2. Starting thioamides and iodides to block synthesis and release of hormones. Preferably, large doses of PTU (200–300 mg every 6 hours or 600–1,200 mg/day) or methimazole (30–40 mg every 6 hours) should be given.

Theoretically, iodides should be given 1 hour after thioamide administration so as not to interfere with the thioamide's effect and to prevent iodizing existing hormone stores, which will aggravate existing storm. Iodides (e.g., Lugol's solution 30–60 drops/day orally) and the combination of thioamides often control symptoms within 1 day. Lithium can be given in doses of 500–1,500 mg per day if iodides are contraindicated, but it offers no advantages over iodides. Cholestyramine has also been recommended.[44]

3. Blocking the metabolic effects by administering propranolol 20 to 80 mg orally every 6 hours or 0.5 to 2 mg intravenously every 4 hours or a comparable β-blocker, or diltiazem 60 to 120 mg orally three to four times a day.
4. Eliminating and correcting precipitating factors.
5. Removing circulating hormone by plasmapheresis, exchange transfusion, and dialysis when routine measures fail.

HYPOTHYROIDISM

DEFINITION

Hypothyroidism is a clinical syndrome caused by thyroid hormone deficiency and characterized by a slowing down of all body systems. An exaggeration of the signs and symptoms of severe and prolonged hypothyroidism, which can precede coma, is known as myxedema. Myxedema coma is the end stage of long-standing uncorrected hypothyroidism. Cretinism or congenital hypothyroidism is hypothyroidism that develops in utero or in the neonate that leads to developmental impairment. Subclinical hypothyroidism exists when TSH levels are elevated and thyroid hormone levels are normal, usually in a patient without symptoms of hypothyroidism.

Primary hypothyroidism, or failure of the thyroid gland to secrete sufficient thyroid hormones, is the most common type of hypothyroidism. Rarely, central or secondary causes of hypothyroidism result from pituitary or hypothalamic injury.

TREATMENT GOALS: HYPOTHYROIDISM

- Reverse hypothyroid complaints
- Reverse hypothyroid physical findings
- Normalize the FT_4 level
- Normalize the TSH level
- Reduce goiter size, if applicable
- Reduce diastolic blood pressure
- Reduce serum cholesterol levels
- Improve emotional well-being and quality of life
- Prevent the development of myxedema
- Support placenta development and maintenance of pregnancy
- In neonates and children, maintain normal growth and physical and mental development

EPIDEMIOLOGY

OVERVIEW

Hypothyroidism affects approximately 8 million Americans. An incidence of 1.4% in women with overt hypothyroidism, and less than 0.1% in men has been reported.[78] Women are five to seven times more likely to develop hypothyroidism than men. Patients with a family history of thyroid or autoimmune disorders (e.g., diabetes, rheumatoid arthritis), older adults, particularly women, and those with a history of medically treated thyroid disease (e.g., radioactive therapy, thyroidectomy) are at greater risk of overt hypothyroidism.

Goitrous forms include Hashimoto, thyroiditis, drug-induced thyroiditis, dyshormonogenesis, endemic thyroiditis, subacute thyroiditis, and multinodular goiters. Nongoitrous forms include cretinism (congenital hypothyroidism), idiopathic atrophy, or iatrogenic causes. Congenital hypothyroidism is reported in 1 in 4,000 births.

Hashimoto thyroiditis is the most common cause of goiter and hypothyroidism in the United States and is similar to Graves disease in prevalence. Like other thyroid disorders, it is more common in women than men and has a strong familial predisposition. Its occurrence peaks in middle age, although any age group is at risk.

Iatrogenic hypothyroidism, caused by RAI or surgery, is the next most common cause of hypothyroidism after Hashimoto thyroiditis. Virtually all patients receiving RAI and about 50% to 75% of patients undergoing total thyroidectomies develop hypothyroidism.[40,41] Therefore, all patients with a history of RAI or surgery should be routinely monitored for life for the development of hypothyroidism.

Postpartum thyroiditis, a type of subacute thyroiditis, can affect approximately 5% of women in the first year after delivery.[15,16] High-risk women include those with preexisting autoimmune disorders, including diabetes mellitus, autoimmune thyroiditis, collagen vascular disorders, and women with positive antibodies.

Pituitary causes [e.g., postpartum hemorrhage (Sheehan's syndrome), head injury, pituitary tumors, or idiopathic atrophy of the hypophysis] are uncommon. Concomitant disorders of the adrenals and gonads (Simmonds' disease or panhypopituitarism) may also occur. Hypothalamic hypothyroidism caused by inadequate secretion of TRF is rare.

DRUG-INDUCED HYPOTHYROIDISM

Iodides and iodide-containing compounds (i.e., povidone iodine, amiodarone, iodinated contrast media) can produce hypothyroidism and goiter in patients with underlying thyroid abnormalities.[5,19,78] Susceptible patients (e.g., those with cystic fibrosis, and untreated Hashimoto thyroiditis and those not receiving l-thyroxine with a history of RAI- or surgery-treated Graves disease) are inordinately sensitive to iodides and unable to normally escape from the Wolff–Chaikoff block to resume hormone synthesis. Older adults and patients on long-term amiodarone also appear to be at greater risk of amiodarone-induced hypothyroidism. Unfortunately, the goiter or hypothyroidism may not always be reversible after the iodides or amiodarone are stopped. l-Thyroxine can be given concurrently, if necessary, to treat the hypothyroidism and goiter.

The prevalence of amiodarone-induced hypothyroidism ranges from 1% to 9.8%.[19,20] Each 200-mg tablet of amiodarone contains 75 mg organic iodide, of which 6 to 12 mg free iodine is released. An iodine load is produced that is 100 times greater than the normal daily intake of 0.5 mg. Patients at risk for hypothyroidism include those with a family history of thyroid disease, a nontoxic multinodular goiter, or positive thyroid antibodies indicative of an autoimmune process (e.g., Hashimoto). No relationship is identified with the development of thyroid dysfunction and the cumulative dose or duration of therapy. Hypothyroidism usually develops within the first 2 years of therapy, or it may occur during the first year after therapy is stopped because of amiodarone's long half-life and accumulation in adipose tissue. Amiodarone-induced hypothyroidism may be difficult to recognize because symptoms of bradycardia and constipation can be attributed to either hypothyroidism or amiodarone. Suspected hypothyroidism is confirmed by an elevated TSH level greater than 10 mIU per liter and a reduction in FT_4 levels. Routine monitoring of thyroid function tests is recommended at baseline and every 6 months thereafter in patients receiving amiodarone.

Lithium-induced hypothyroidism and goiter have been reported in 5% to 50% of patients on chronic therapy.[5,22–24] Risk factors include a family history of thyroid illness, presence of thyroid antibodies, abnormal thyroid glands, and underlying thyroid illness, although a few cases have occurred in patients without any risk factors. The antithyroid effect of lithium is similar to that of the iodides and was first identified in patients receiving treatment for bipolar disorder. The onset of a nontender, diffuse goiter with or without hypothyroidism is variable and may appear after 5 months to 2 years of therapy. Regression of the goiter and reversal of hypothyroidism do not always occur after the lithium is stopped, but l-thyroxine can be added to permit continued lithium therapy.

The cytokines (e.g., interleukin-2 and interferon-α) have produced transient episodes of hypothyroidism.[17,18] Preexisting hypothyroidism can also worsen. Interleukin-2 has produced thyroid dysfunction in 10% to 41% of patients after two courses of therapy. Hypothyroidism can be persistent and require chronic replacement thyroid therapy. Positive thyroid antibodies have been reported in 20% of patients receiving interferon-α.

Thiocyanate is a well-known inhibitor of iodide trapping, particularly if high blood concentrations are present. Thiocyanate-induced hypothyroidism can result from long-term use of nitroprusside in patients with renal insufficiency. Plants such as rutabagas, cabbage, and turnips contain thiocarbamides that are metabolized in the body to thiocyanates. These dietary goitrogens do not produce a significant degree of hypothyroidism unless large amounts are ingested raw over a long period.

Goiters can result from the use of certain drugs with antithyroid activity (Table 38.8). The thioamides and the monovalent anions can produce goiter if excessive doses are used.

PATHOPHYSIOLOGY

Hashimoto thyroiditis, an autoimmune process resulting from defects in suppressor T lymphocytes, is characterized by diffuse enlargement and lymphocytic infiltration of the thyroid gland, an immunologic disturbance, and hypothyroidism.[78] ATgA and TPO antibodies usually are present. If the gland is able to maintain hormone synthesis in response to TSH stimulation, then euthyroidism is maintained. However, when the gland eventually fails to keep up with metabolic demands, goiter and hypothyroidism occur. Hashimoto disease often coexists with other autoimmune disorders, including Graves disease, pernicious anemia, rheumatoid arthritis, and other collagen vascular diseases. Some postulate that Graves and Hashimoto thyroiditis are actually the same

TABLE 38.8 | Drug-Induced Thyroid Disease

Drug	Mechanism	Drug-Induced Thyroid Effect	Comments
Nitroprusside	Metabolized to thiocyanate, an anion inhibitor	Goiter, hypothyroidism	Increased risk with renal failure and duration of use
Lithium	Inhibits hormone release	Goiter, hypothyroidism, hyperthyroidism	Usually in patients with untreated thyroid disease (e.g., Hashimoto's thyroiditis)
Iodides and iodine containing compounds (e.g., amiodarone, ipodate, iodinated contrast media)	Inability to escape from Wolff-Chaikoff block	Hypothyroidism, goiter	Usually in patients with untreated Hashimoto's thyroiditis or Graves' disease incompletely treated with RAI or surgery and not receiving thyroid replacement.
Iodides and iodine containing compounds (e.g., amiodarone, ipodate, iodinated contrast media)	Provides substrate to iodide-deficient autonomous thyroid tissue; loss of Wolff-Chaikoff block	Hyperthyroidism	Usually in patients with multinodular goiters and autonomous nodules (Jod-Basedow disease)
Amiodarone	Destruction thyroiditis with "dumping of hormones" into circulation. See also iodides	Hyperthyroidism	Associated with elevation of interleukin-6 levels.
Sertraline	Related to ↑ T$_4$ elimination	Hypothyroidism, TSH elevation	Prevalence unknown; unknown if occurs with other serotonin reuptake inhibitors
Sulfonylureas, sulfonamides, PAS, resorcinol, phenylbutazone	Inhibits organic binding and organification	Hypothyroidism, goiter	Rare cause of thyroid disease
Immunotherapy (e.g., interferon-α, interleukin-2)	Autoimmune process	Hypothyroidism, hyperthyroidism	Generally transient, resolves without treatment
Natural goitrogens cabbage, etc.	Contains thiocyanate and other goitrogens	Hypothyroidism, goiter	Rare, need large consumption of raw vegetables

RAI, radioactive iodine; T$_4$, thyroxine; TSH, thyroid-stimulating hormone; PAS, para-aminosalicylic acid.

disease because mild thyrotoxicosis can precede the onset of hypothyroidism. Findings of positive thyroid antibodies, similar histologic lymphocytic infiltration of the gland, and the presence of thyroid immunoglobulins that block rather than stimulate the TSH receptor strengthen the autoimmune association between Graves and Hashimoto thyroiditis. Likewise, hypothyroidism can be the result of long-standing Graves disease.

Congenital, nongoitrous hypothyroidism, produced by a deficiency of thyroid hormone in utero or in the neonate, may result from defective hormone synthesis, pituitary or hypothalamic dysfunction, or incomplete growth of the gland (agenesis).[78] Ectopic thyroid tissue, destruction of the gland by maternal autoantibodies, and destruction by RAI therapy are other possible causes of agenesis. Neonatal goitrous hypothyroidism has been reported after maternal ingestion of iodides and thioamide therapy.

"Endemic goiter" is a descriptive term for a goiter caused by an iodine deficiency during the growth years. The amount of dietary iodine deficiency determines the degree of nodularity and gland enlargement. Patients may be euthyroid or hypothyroid.

Dyshormonogenesis is a group of familial thyroid disorders resulting from abnormalities in the synthesis, delivery, or peripheral action of thyroid hormones. Impaired hormone synthesis can result from defects in iodine accumulation or iodide organification, from a dehalogenase deficiency, and from a coupling abnormality.

Approximately 200 cases of myxedema coma have been reported in elderly women with a history of long-standing hypothyroidism.[33] Myxedema coma can be precipitated by cold weather (hypothermia), stress (surgery), infection, trauma, acid-based disturbances, and unrecognized concomitant illness (i.e., diabetes and arteriosclerotic cardiovascular disease). Respiratory depressants of any kind (i.e., anesthetics, narcotics, phenothiazines, and sedative-hypnotics), which are metabolized slowly in the hypothyroid patient, can precipitate coma by aggravating preexisting hypothermia and carbon dioxide retention. Immediate and aggressive therapy is required to prevent a 15% to 20% mortality.[33]

Hypothyroidism from a subacute thyroiditis (e.g., PPT, de Quervain thyroiditis) occurs if long-standing inflammation of the gland prevents further hormone synthesis after the initial hormone stores are depleted.[15,78] Patients often undergo a mild thyrotoxic phase before transient hypothyroidism develops. Transient l-thyroxine therapy may be necessary, although permanent hypothyroidism can occur (e.g., PPT).

CLINICAL PRESENTATION AND DIAGNOSIS

SIGNS AND SYMPTOMS

Classic symptoms of hypothyroidism include weakness, fatigue, lethargy, cold intolerance, constipation, and weight gain (Table 38.4). Normochromic, normocytic anemia, or microcytic anemia caused by heavy menses in women may be present. In older adults, the diagnosis of hypothyroidism might be missed easily and is particularly difficult because symptoms may be absent, atypical, or wrongly attributed to normal aging. Hypothyroid symptoms from naturally occurring hypothyroidism (e.g., Hashimoto thyroiditis) can be insidious, remain unnoticed by the patient, and occur with amazing placidity over several months to years before the appearance of a terminal myxedematous state. In contrast, symptoms resulting from iatrogenic causes (e.g., RAI therapy or surgery) occur rapidly and rarely go unrecognized by the patient. It should be appreciated that hypothyroid patients are inordinately sensitive to medications such as digoxin and the respiratory and central nervous system effects of respiratory depressants, including anesthetics, narcotics, phenothiazines, and sedative-hypnotics (Table 38.5). Likewise, medical treatment of concurrent medical conditions (e.g., diabetes, hyperlipidemia, cardiac conditions) can be influenced by hypothyroidism (Table 38.5).[78]

Marked physical findings, usually present in myxedema, include a puffy and mask-like facies, edematous eyelids, thickened and doughy skin changes, especially over the pretibial aspects of the leg, hair loss from the lateral aspects of the eyebrows, a large tongue, cardiomegaly, and a yellowish tint to the skin. Myxedematous cachexia is characterized by intensifying hypothyroid signs and symptoms and often precedes the onset of myxedema coma. Significant clinical features of myxedema coma include hypothermia, hypoxia, carbon dioxide retention, hyponatremia, hypoglycemia, markedly delayed or absent deep tendon reflexes, altered sensorium ranging from stupor to coma, and shock. Paranoid psychosis has also been reported.[33,34]

The cardiovascular manifestations of hypothyroidism can mimic or exacerbate preexisting low-output CHF. Preexisting angina typically becomes quiescent; rarely, the severity and frequency of attacks can increase. Elevated cholesterol levels caused by impaired elimination might accelerate atherosclerotic changes, although this effect is speculative.[79] Clinical findings include cardiomegaly caused by loss of muscle tone and mucopolysaccharide deposition; dyspnea; edema; and pleural effusions caused by decreased cardiac output and stroke volume and reduced myocardial contractility. Characteristic ECG changes can resemble those of ischemia, and include slow rate and low voltage, flattened or inverted T waves, and, occasionally, increased P-R interval and widened QRS complex. Although glomerular filtration rate (GFR) and renal plasma flow are reduced by decreased cardiac output and blood volume, overt evidence of renal failure does not occur. In severe myxedema, changes in GFR and inappropriate antidiuretic hormone secretion delay water excretion, producing edema and hyponatremia.

A goiter should always be considered an abnormal finding. Goiters are produced by prolonged TSH stimulation, usually in response to low levels of circulating hormone. However, some patients with a goiter can be euthyroid because the thyroid gland might transiently increase hormone secretion in response to the elevated TSH level. A very large goiter (e.g., multinodular goiter), producing pressure symptoms, a choking sensation, pain and difficulty swallowing, or regurgitation of food and liquids from compression of the trachea or the esophagus, is an indication for surgical removal. Clinically, patients can be euthyroid but often develop hyperthyroidism or hypothyroidism in later years.[13,14]

Patients with Hashimoto thyroiditis can present with thyrotoxicosis in the early stages (Hashitoxicosis), euthyroidism and goiter, hypothyroidism and goiter, or hypothyroidism without goiter in the later stages of the disease. Euthyroidism occurs if the gland is able to compensate for the inherent block in hormone synthesis by increasing hormone synthesis in response to TSH stimulation. Asymptomatic thyroiditis, characterized by euthyroidism, absence of goiter, normal levels of circulating hormones, and positive antithyroid antibodies, may precede the clinical manifestations of overt goiter and hypothyroidism. Idiopathic atrophy of the thyroid and destruction of the gland represent the end stages of Hashimoto thyroiditis.

The clinical presentation of congenital hypothyroidism depends on the severity of the hypothyroidism, the age of onset, and the cause of the thyroid deficiency. Determining cord TSH levels at time of delivery is crucial because it permits early diagnosis of hypothyroidism. The clinical symptoms are so subtle that if the condition is not detected until the child is older, irreversible neurologic damage can occur. The earliest findings are a heavy expression, a piglike appearance of the eyes, hypothermia, prolonged jaundice, umbilical hernia, hoarseness, thick tongue, protuberant abdomen, constipation, and drooling. Delayed developmental characteristics, failure to thrive, poor appetite, and cretinoid facies might not be recognized until the infant is 3 to 6 months old and neurologic damage is irreversible.[80,81] Growth retardation, delayed physical development, and hypothyroid symptoms, similar to those seen in an adult, are of concern. Radiologic evidence of epiphyseal dysgenesis is pathognomonic of neonatal hypothyroidism.

DIAGNOSIS

Clinical guidelines for screening and diagnosing hypothyroidism have been established by the ATA and the American College of Physicians.[3,4] The ATA recommends measurement of the TSH level beginning at age 35 years and every 5 years thereafter, particularly in women. In adults, the diagnosis of hypothyroidism is confirmed by laboratory findings of a low FT_4I or FT_4 and an elevated TSH level (Table 38.1). Because T_3 levels can be normal in overt hypothyroidism, T_3 levels are not helpful or cost-effective and should not be obtained. In secondary hypothyroidism, FT_4 levels are low when the TSH level is low, and other features of pituitary or hypothalamic disease usually are apparent. The presence of positive antibodies indicates an underlying autoimmune process (e.g., Hashimoto thyroiditis). An RAIU is not necessary for diagnosis of autoimmune hypothyroidism; it is usually decreased, but an elevated uptake may be present in the early stages of hypothyroidism. Serum SGOT, LDH, CPK, carotene, cholesterol, and triglyceride levels may be elevated from impaired elimination.

THERAPEUTIC PLAN

The ATA and the American Association of Clinical Endocrinologists have published clinical guidelines for treatment of hypothyroidism.[3,4,11,37] Administering thyroid hormones provides adequate replacement therapy for hypothyroidism and prevents progression to myxedema coma. The average replacement dose often is quoted as 100 to 150 μg l-thyroxine daily, which parallels the normal thyroid production. However, such a simplistic approach is inappropriate and dangerous. Dosing requirements depend on several factors, including patient age and weight, severity and cause of the illness, presence or absence of cardiac disease, and hormone absorption. Any existing goiter usually regresses in size because TSH production is suppressed (Fig. 38.1). Hypothyroid patients on l-thyroxine can be treated effectively by the healthcare provider using a treatment algorithm (Fig. 38.4).

TREATMENT

PHARMACOTHERAPY

l-Thyroxine is the preparation of choice for hormone replacement, although other thyroid hormones preparations are available commercially (Table 38.9).[82] The initial dose of T_4 depends on the patient's age, the severity and duration of the hypothyroidism, and the presence or potential for un-

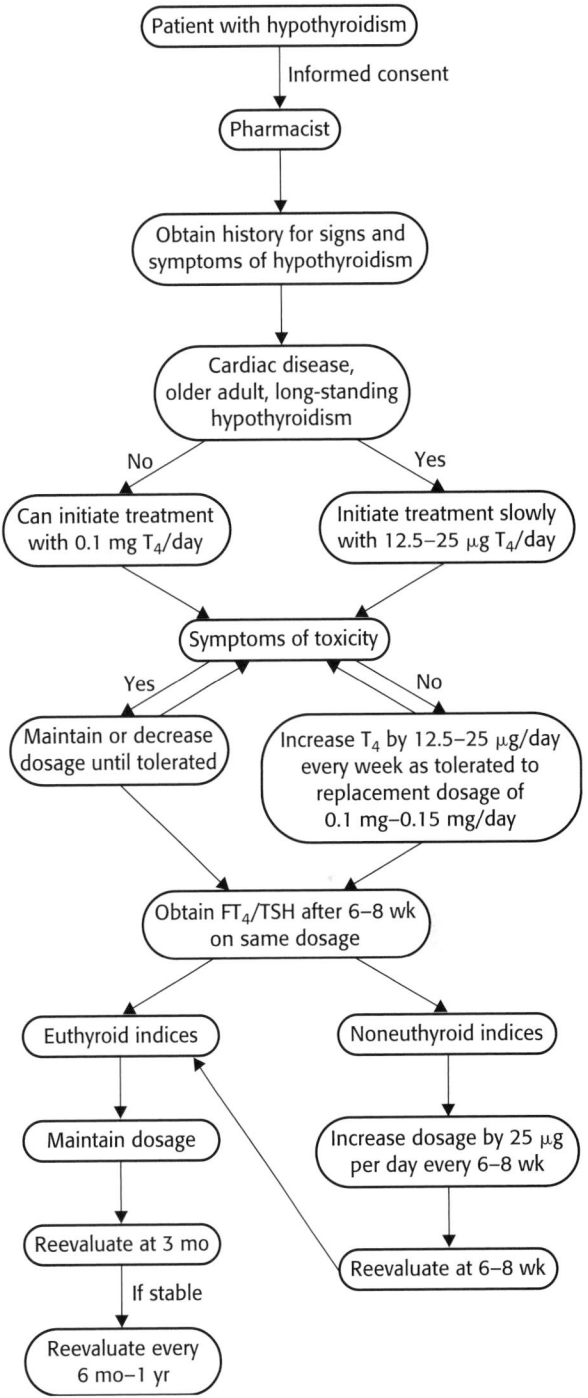

FIGURE 38.4 Treatment algorithm for management of hypothyroidism. FT_4, free thyroxine; T_4, thyroxine; TSH, thyroid-stimulating hormone.

derlying cardiac disease. In young, healthy patients with disease of short duration, l-thyroxine can be administered in nearly full replacement doses (e.g., 100–150 μg daily) without fear of precipitating cardiac toxicity. This dose can be adjusted as necessary, using the patient's symptoms and laboratory values obtained at steady state (i.e., after 6–8 weeks of therapy). However, in patients with long-standing and

TABLE 38.9	Thyroid Preparations in Treatment of Hypothyroidism				
Preparation[a]	**Content**	**Advantages**	**Disadvantages**	**Effect on Thyroid Tests**	**Comments**
Desiccated thyroid US Pharmacopeia 0.25, 0.5, 1, 1.5, 2, 3, 4, or 5 grains	Defatted, dried pig thyroid powder, containing 0.17%–0.23% iodine	Inexpensive	Poor standardization with variable hormonal content and T_4/T_3 ratios; deterioration with storage	Normal FT_4/FT_4I, TSH normal or ↑ TT_3	Obsolete product. Variable potency; problems inherent to all T_3 containing products; see T_3 comments.
Sodium l-thyroxine[a], (Levoxyl, Levothroid, Levo-T, Mylan Pharmaceuticals, Novothyrox, ThyroTab, Synthroid, Unithroid, Various) 0.0125, 0.025, 0.05, 0.075, 0.088, 0.1, 0.112, 0.125, 0.137, 0.15, 0.175, 0.2, 0.3 mg; Inj. 200, 500 μg	Synthetic, pure T_4	Stable, smooth action, relatively inexpensive; long $t_{1/2} = 7$ days); generics and branded FDA-approved products	Slow onset of action, cumulative effects; various drugs can impair absorption.	Normal thyroid function tests; TSH in normal range	Might be more potent than desiccated thyroid, should lower the T_4 dose by 0.5 grains to avoid toxicity when changing from >2 grains desiccated thyroid to l-thyroxine
Sodium l-thyronine, (Cytomel) 5, 25, 50 μg; Inj. 10 μg/mL (Triostat)	Synthetic, pure T_3	Uniform absorption, fast onset of action	Expensive, supraphysiologic T_3 levels can produce toxicity Requires bid daily dosing.	Low FT_4, normal or ↑ TT_3, normal TSH	Not DOC for hormone replacement, monitor T_3 and TSH levels
Liotrix 0.25, 0.5, 1, 2, 3 (Thyrolar)	Contains T_4 and T_3 in a ratio of 4 : 1 (mimics natural secretion of hormone)	Both short- and long-acting effects	Expensive	Normal thyroid function values	No real need for liotrix since T_4 is peripherally converted to T_3

[a] Approximate dosage equivalence: 1 grain desiccated thyroid = 0.1 mg l-thyroxine = 37.5 μg l-thyronine = liotrix-1 (See "Comments" column.)
T_4, thyroxine; T_3, triiodothyronine; FT_4, free thyroxine level; FT_4I, free thyroxine index; TSH, thyroid-stimulating hormone; TT_3, triiodothyronine level; injectable; FDA, Food and Drug Administration; bid, twice a day; DOC, drug of choice.

severe myxedema, in older adults, and in patients with cardiac disease (i.e., angina, CHF), who are likely to be extremely sensitive to the metabolic effects of thyroid hormone, minute doses of l-thyroxine must be instituted cautiously to avoid cardiovascular complications of heart failure, angina, tachycardia, and myocardial infarction. Subtherapeutic l-thyroxine doses can precipitate these complications, so careful monitoring is critical. Angina should be controlled before l-thyroxine therapy is attempted. If medically indicated, coronary bypass surgery can be performed safely in hypothyroid patients before l-thyroxine replacement. In the high-risk patient, initial doses should not exceed 25 μg T_4 daily. The patient should be instructed to report any cardiac symptoms immediately. If after 1 week the initial dose is well tolerated, the dose can be increased by similar increments every 1 to 2 weeks until therapeutic

levels are achieved. It is not necessary to monitor thyroid function tests at these subtherapeutic doses. Complete euthyroidism might never be achieved in high-risk patients without further compromising the cardiac status.

The daily maintenance dose of l-thyroxine for uncomplicated hypothyroidism is estimated to be 1.6 to 1.7 μg per kilogram, or about 0.7 to 0.8 μg per pound.[78,82] The average daily replacement dose is 100 to 125 μg daily in women and 125 to 150 μg in men. In older adults, lower doses of 50 to 100 μg daily (<1.6 μg/kg/day) might be sufficient to maintain euthyroidism. Lower replacement doses are usually sufficient in patients with hypothyroidism caused by RAI or surgery ablation than in those with spontaneous hypothyroidism.

It is generally accepted that approximately 75% of patients receiving adequate prepregnancy l-thyroxine replacement will require a 20% to 30% increase in their replacement dose during the first or second trimester to maintain a normal TSH level.[28] However, some have questioned whether levothyroxine requirements actually increase or are a consequence of the concomitant administration of iron and calcium containing products that decrease l-thyroxine absorption.[83]

Normal development of the fetal thyroid gland is independent of maternal thyroid hormones which do not cross the placenta. The greatest dangers to the fetus from inadequate maternal replacement therapy during the first trimester are poor placenta development and poor maintenance of the pregnancy. Although normal offspring have been reported in women who remained hypothyroid throughout pregnancy, congenital defects, abnormal fetal development, spontaneous abortions, stillbirths, and mental retardation[11,28] have been associated with maternal myxedema. If hormone replacement therapy is adequate and maternal euthyroidism (normal TSH and FT_4I, or FT_4 level) is achieved, a normal pregnancy is expected. TT_4 levels will be elevated because of pregnancy-induced TBG levels. After delivery, the prepregnancy dose of l-thyroxine can be reinstituted if necessary.

Malabsorption caused by short bowel syndrome, the concurrent administration of several drugs (Table 38.10) or soy protein supplements that impair thyroxine absorption can affect the daily l-thyroxine replacement dose.[84] Separating administration times of l-thyroxine and certain medications (e.g., calcium, iron, cholesterol resin binders, raloxifene) can minimize impairment of l-thyroxine absorption.[82,85,86] However, this strategy is not helpful with aluminum-containing antacids; if appropriate, these preparations should be avoided.[87] An increase in the daily l-thyroxine dose usually is necessary when enzyme inducers (e.g., phenytoin, carbamazepine), aluminum-containing products, and sertraline are given concurrently.[5,87,88]

Patients should notice improvement in typical hypothyroid symptoms after 3 to 4 weeks of daily medication adherence. Weight, skin, hair, and voice changes may not reverse for several months despite normalized thyroid function tests.

The TSH and FT_4 levels should be evaluated at steady state (e.g., after 2 to 3 months of daily dosing). Trough TSH levels, obtained before the next dose or at least 10 hours after the last dose, are recommended to minimize transient high peak FT_4 levels, suppressed TSH levels, and properly interpret laboratory results.[89] Once the dose has been established, therapy should be evaluated at yearly intervals to ensure that the current l-thyroxine dose is still appropriate. A dose reduction might be necessary in patients whose dose was determined before the availability of more potent products and the advent of the sensitive TSH assay, in adults as they age, or if there is significant weight loss. The FT_4 or FT_4I should be maintained within the normal range, and the TSH preferably between 1 and 2 mIU per liter. Suppression of TSH to undetectable levels (<0.05 mIU/L) should be avoided with replacement therapy to minimize over-replacement and subclinical signs of hyperthyroidism. Supraphysiologic doses may predispose patients to an increased risk of bone loss, osteoporosis, and cardiac arrhythmia.[29–32] However, TSH levels on a stable dose of l-thyroxine can be quite variable, and it is unknown if toxicity is produced and a dose adjustment is always necessary. Some clinicians arbitrarily accept TSH levels that vary from a suppressed TSH of 0.25 mIU per liter to a high of 5.0 mIU per liter. In addition, retrospective studies show no difference in morbidity and mortality between patients with normal and variable TSH levels.[29,90]

Currently, there are eight l-thyroxine preparations (Levothroid, Levoxyl, Levo-T, Mylan Pharmaceuticals, Novothyrox, Synthroid, ThyroTab, Unithroid) that have been approved by the Food and Drug Administration (FDA) as new drugs. Previous concerns about subpotent and unstable tablets have been corrected by the 2000 FDA requirement that all manufacturers marketing l-thyroxine must submit a New Drug Application demonstrating potency and stability.[91] Unithroid and the Mylan generic product are AB rated (interchangeable) while the others are BX rated. Bioequivalence between these FDA-approved reformulated products have yet to be demonstrated because there is controversy about the optimal method for determining levothyroxine bioequivalence and therapeutic interchangeability.[92] Data obtained prior to the FDA reformulation of levothyroxine found interchangeability and bioequivalence between a leading branded product and its competitor products using the current FDA criteria for bioequivalence of oral products.[93,94]

l-Thyroxine's potency, cost-effectiveness, lack of foreign protein antigenicity, and ease of dosing contribute to its popularity. Its long half-life of 7 days makes it amenable to once-a-day dosing, increasing patient compliance and allowing various convenient dosing schedules (e.g., daily except weekends). Once-weekly administration of l-thyroxine has been proposed for noncompliant patients but requires further study.[95] l-Thyroxine absorption is enhanced about 20% during fasting. The bioavailability of branded l-thyroxine preparations is 80%; the bioavailability of generic preparations is presumed to be similar. This similarity should be considered when changing from oral to intravenous or intramuscular dosing regimens. l-Thyroxine replacement may produce TT_4 levels in the hyperthyroid range in about 20% of patients; however, no dose adjustment is necessary if the TSH levels are normal and the patient is clinically euthyroid. T_3 levels often are within the normal range.[82]

T_3 is a chemically pure agent with predictable potency, excellent bioavailability, and a half-life of 1.5 days. T_3 may be used when short-term hormone replacement therapy is indicated (e.g., in patients who need repeat scans and RAIU after total thyroidectomy for thyroid cancer). The thyroid hormones must be eliminated completely before the scan. Because T_3 has a short half-life, it is rapidly eliminated after

TABLE 38.10	Medications and Conditions Affecting l-Thyroxine Replacement Doses		
Conditions	**Mechanism**	**Recommendation**	**Comments**
Resin binders (e.g., cholestyramine, colestipol)	Binds T_4 in gut, $\downarrow T_4$ absorption	Separate time of administration by 4–6 hours	$\uparrow$ dose of T_4 might be needed
Soy protein supplements	Binds T_4 in gut, $\downarrow T_4$ absorption	Take l-thyroxine on empty stomach	Inconsistent interaction
Aluminum containing preparations (e.g., sucralfate, aluminum containing antacids)	Binds T_4 in gut, $\downarrow T_4$ absorption	Separating time of administration by 4–6 hours might not be effective in avoiding this interaction	Avoid aluminum containing products or $\uparrow$ dose of T_4 might be needed
Iron sulfate	Binds T_4 in gut, $\downarrow T_4$ absorption	Separating time of administration by 4–6 hours might be effective in avoiding this interaction	Monitor and $\uparrow$ dose of T_4 if necessary
Calcium carbonate	Binds T_4 in gut, $\downarrow T_4$ absorption	Separate time of administration by 4–6 hours appears effective.	Interaction might not occur with all calcium preparations
Sertraline	Unknown mechanism, $\uparrow T_4$ elimination	Separating time of administration by 4–6 hours might not be effective in avoiding this interaction	$\uparrow$ dose of T_4 might be needed; similar effect with other serotonin reuptake inhibitors
Lovastatin	Binds T_4 in gut, $\downarrow T_4$ absorption	Change to another lipid lowering agent, monitor TFTs and $\uparrow$ dose if needed	Interaction not well documented and based on one case report
Raloxifene	Binds T_4 in gut, $\downarrow T_4$ absorption	Separate time of administration by 12 hours might be effective in avoiding this interaction	Interaction based on one case report
Enzyme Inducers (i.e., phenytoin, carbamazepine, rifampin, phenobarbital)	$\uparrow$ metabolism and clearance of thyroxine	$\uparrow$ dose of thyroxine to normalize TSH level; free T_4 level might remain low	Not significant in euthyroid individuals not on thyroxine therapy
Androgens	$\downarrow$ levels of TBG; higher free T_4 and lower TSH levels might occur	Might need to $\downarrow$ dose of T_4 by 25%–50% to normalize TSH	Not significant in euthyroid individuals not on thyroxine therapy
Pregnancy	$\uparrow$ levels of TBG and $\uparrow$ thyroxine demands	$\uparrow$ dose of T_4 by 20%–30% to achieve normal TSH level	Not significant in euthyroid individuals on birth control pills or on postmenopausal hormone replacement
Age	T_4 clearance $\downarrow$ with age	Lower doses (<1.6–1.7 µg/kg/day) might be effective in those >60 years old	Monitor TFT yearly; dose reduction with advancing age
Malabsorption (i.e., diarrhea, short bowel syndrome)	$\downarrow T_4$ absorption	$\uparrow$ dose of thyroxine, monitor TSH to adjust dosage.	High dose T_4 therapy might be necessary

T_4, thyroxine; TFT, thyroid function test; TSH, thyroid-stimulating hormone; TBG, thyroxine-binding globulin.

discontinuation, producing a short duration of tolerable hypothyroidism before the RAIU and scan. However, T_3 replacement is used infrequently these days since the availability of recombinant human thyrotropin reduces the need to withdraw thyroid replacement completely.[96]

Theoretically, T_3, rather than T_4, has been proposed as the drug of choice in patients with cardiovascular problems because its shorter half-life might permit any adverse effects on the heart to resolve more quickly (i.e., in 3–5 days) once T_3 is stopped (the half-life of T_4 is 7–10 days). However, because of the rapid absorption of T_3, supraphysiologic T_3 levels occur after ingestion, producing symptoms of mild toxicity in susceptible patients.[82] The greater cardiotoxic potential of T_3 outweighs its advantage of rapid elimination, so its use cannot be recommended. Because of its rapid onset of action (1–3 days), intravenous T_3 has also been recommended as the drug of choice for myxedema coma. However, its routine use in this condition is limited by concerns about its potentially greater cardiotoxicity. Also, mortality has occurred despite the higher T_3 levels achieved after T_3 administration.[33,34] T_3 is not recommended as routine thyroid replacement because of its high cost, the need for multiple daily dosing to ensure a uniform response, and greater difficulty in monitoring therapeutic and toxic responses. Approximately 25 to 37.5 μg of T_3 is equivalent to 0.1 mg of l-thyroxine.

T_3 administration does not change pretreatment T_4 levels, which, if not properly recognized, can cause therapeutic confusion and potential overreplacement despite adequate hormone replacement. T_3 administration is best monitored by TSH and TT_3 levels. Patients should not receive T_3 as routine hormone replacement therapy.

Nevertheless, the combination of T_3 and T_4 has been recommended after a small study found that the combination improved cognitive performance, mood, and physical well-being more than administration of T_4 alone.[97] However, recommendation of this dual approach is premature since three additional studies in patients with mostly primary thyroid failure, have failed to substantiate the benefits of a T_3 plus T_4 combination.[98–100] It is unclear if therapeutic benefits would be shown if a more physiologically sustained release preparation of T_3[101] was used or if predominately hypothyroid patients with no remaining thyroid tissue were studied (e.g., surgery or RAI-induced hypothyroidism). Further investigation is warranted.

Desiccated thyroid (USP) is obtained from animal thyroid glands (e.g., hog, cow, sheep). Because this preparation is standardized only by iodine content (0.17%–0.23% iodine), the hormone ratio of T_4 to T_3 may vary from 2:1 (hog) to 3:1 (cow or sheep). Therefore, variability in potency might result from changes in the ratio of the two hormones or from the quantity of organic iodine present. Patients taking dessicated thyroid suffer from problems inherent to all T_3-containing preparations. Improper or prolonged tablet storage, causing a loss of potency, can also contribute to an unpredictable response. Desiccated thyroid tablets appear to be stable for ≥5 years if they are kept dry. Inactive preparations, containing small amounts of T_4 and T_3 or iodinated casein, and tablets with excessive biological activity have been reported. Allergic reactions to the protein component might also occur. During therapy, the FT_4 levels (i.e., FT_4I or FT_4), TT_3, and TSH should remain within normal limits; however, thyroid function tests often are abnormal, especially if supraphysiologic levels of T_3 occur. For these reasons, desiccated thyroid is considered obsolete. However, desiccated thyroid remains on the market because this preparation is inexpensive and some patients prefer the "high" that results from the T_3 component. It is strongly recommended that all patients receiving desiccated thyroid be changed to l-thyroxine. Although 0.1 mg of l-thyroxine is

theoretically equivalent to 1 grain or 60 mg of desiccated thyroid, such equivalents might not be valid if dosage titrations were initially based on inactive desiccated thyroid preparations. In one study, 60 μg l-thyroxine was equivalent to 1 grain desiccated thyroid.[102] This disparity in equivalence is especially important when patients needing more than 2 grains daily of desiccated thyroid are changed to l-thyroxine. A theoretically equivalent dose of l-thyroxine might not be reasonable (e.g., 3 grains of desiccated thyroid equivalent to 300 μg of l-thyroxine) because of subpotent desiccated preparations, and dosage retitration is recommended.

Liotrix is a combination of synthetic T_4 and T_3 in a 4 to 1 ratio that mimics the natural secretion of hormones. It is available commercially as Thyrolar. Because this preparation approximates the normal thyroid production, it was once considered the agent of choice, before it was recognized that a significant amount of T_4 is converted peripherally to T_3. Liotrix is stable and chemically pure, is of predictable potency, and produces laboratory values similar to those seen after T_4 administration. In Thyrolar-1, 50 μg T_4 and 12.5 μg T_3 is equivalent to 1 grain thyroid. Because of its high cost, problems inherent to all T_3-containing preparations, and lack of therapeutic rationale, there is no advantage in using Liotrix.

SPECIAL TREATMENT ISSUES

Congenital Hypothyroidism. Normal growth and physical and mental development are determined by the age at which treatment is instituted, the initial dose of l-thyroxine, the serum thyroxine levels attained during therapy, and by how well euthyroidism is maintained.[80,81] The initial replacement dose of 10 to 17 μg/kg/day should raise the serum T_4 to more than 129 nmol per liter (10 μg/dL) within a week. The earlier treatment begins, the better the prognosis for normal mental and growth development. Mean IQ is higher in those who receive treatment before 3 months and achieve a serum T_4 level of more than 180 nmol per liter (14 μg/dL) in the first month than in those who do not. If treatment is delayed until 6 months to 1 year, mental development is impaired despite subsequent treatment. Despite early therapy, neurologic deficits also occur if replacement is inadequate to increase the serum TT_4 more than 103 mmol per liter (8 μg/dL) and to suppress the TSH into the normal range after 3 to 4 months of therapy. Dwarfism does not occur if therapy is delayed until age 5. Infants born athyreotic may have a poorer prognosis for normal mental development because of late detection compared with those born with an abnormal or ectopic thyroid gland.

The preparation of choice for hormone replacement is l-thyroxine. The appropriate T_4 replacement dose depends on the infant's age and the presence of risk factors (Table 38.11).[80,81] Full replacement doses can be started in the infant without cardiac disease or other complications. However, infants with long-standing and severe myxedema are extremely sensitive to minute doses of thyroid, necessitat-

TABLE 38.11	Dose of T₄ for Infants and Children
Age	**T₄ Dose (μg/kg/day)**
0–3 months	10–17
3–6 months	6–8
6–12 months	5–7
1–10 years	3–6
10–16 years	2–4

T₄, thyroxine.

ing initiation with very small doses of l-thyroxine to prevent toxicity (i.e., hyperactivity and irritability). In these infants, initial doses of T_4 should not exceed 25% to 33% of the normal recommended dose. If no toxicity occurs after 1 to 2 weeks, doses can be increased gradually by similar increments every 1 to 2 weeks until full replacement doses are achieved or until the dose is limited by toxicity.

Normal physical and mental development and reversal of hypothyroid signs and symptoms indicate the optimal replacement dose. Adequate replacement is achieved when the serum TT_4 level reaches 154 to 180 mmol per liter (12–14 μg/dL).[80,81] TSH normalization should not be used as the sole criterion because the hypothalamic-pituitary system is not responsive to the negative feedback effect of thyroid hormone, causing TSH to remain elevated for months despite proper or excessive hormone replacement. TSH should normalize within 3 to 4 months after the start of therapy; attempts to normalize TSH earlier may result in over-replacement, producing symptoms of over-metabolism, irritability, brain dysfunction, and premature craniosynostosis.

Subclinical Hypothyroidism. The prevalence of subclinical hypothyroidism ranges from 4% to 26%, and is higher in women more than 60 years of age.[11,103–105] It is debatable whether l-thyroxine therapy should be started in all patients with subclinical hypothyroidism since data supporting benefits of treatment are limited and not all patients will progress to overt hypothyroidism. The risk of developing overt hypothyroidism in untreated patients increases with the degree of TSH elevation, and is greatest (e.g., approximately 5%) in patients with a TSH more than 10 mIU per liter. Although many patients are older and asymptomatic, improvement in cardiac contractility, lipoprotein concentrations, and cognitive function have been reported.[11,103–105] The decision to start therapy should be based on several considerations, including the risks and benefits of treatment, the likelihood of overt hypothyroidism, the degree of TSH elevation, and history of thyroid disease. In patients receiving l-thyroxine therapy, the elevated TSH level could imply nonadherence or inadequate replacement, and the dose should be increased to normalize the TSH if nonadherence is not suspected. In patients with a history of partial thyroid ablation therapy (e.g., RAI, surgery), the likelihood of progression to overt

hypothyroidism is high, and replacement therapy is strongly encouraged. In patients with a negative history for thyroid illness, a normal gland, negative thyroid antibodies, TSH elevations less than 10 mIU per liter, and no lipid or cardiac abnormalities, l-thyroxine therapy can be withheld if close monitoring of the TSH level every 3 to 4 months is feasible. In patients with an abnormal gland, positive thyroid antibodies, lipid or end organ abnormalities, and TSH levels more than 10 mIU per liter, l-thyroxine replacement should be strongly considered if the potential benefits of improvement in cardiac contractility, lipoprotein concentrations, and cognitive function warrant the risks and expense of therapy.

Myxedema Coma. Treatment includes hormone replacement and supportive measures.[33,34] There are no comparative trials between l-thyroxine and T_3 in myxedema coma. However, T_4 generally is recommended because of greater clinical experience with its administration than T_3. Fatalities have also been reported after T_3 administration even though higher T_3 levels were achieved. Replacement therapy with large doses of l-thyroxine (400–600 μg intravenously) should be given to saturate the TBG. This dose can be reduced if there are cardiac risk factors. Maintenance doses of 50 to 100 μg intravenous T_4 daily should be started until the patient can take oral medications. Alternatively, T_3 10 to 20 μg can be given as an initial intravenous bolus, followed by 10 μg intravenously every 4 to 6 hours for up to 48 hours. Hydrocortisone 50 to 100 mg intravenously every 6 hours must be given to prevent adrenal crisis in case undetected hypopituitarism exists.

Supportive measures include assisted ventilation, glucose infusions for hypoglycemia, fluid restriction because of hyponatremia, and use of plasma expanders for shock and circulatory collapse. Heating blankets, which may further aggravate shock by vasodilatation, are not recommended. Finally, precipitating factors should be eliminated or corrected. If the proper treatment and support are provided, consciousness, restoration of normal vital functions, and normalization of TSH levels occur within 24 hours.

IMPROVING OUTCOMES

Patients must be aware that reversal of hypothyroid symptoms can be delayed for several weeks even if l-thyroxine adherence is excellent. Patients should be instructed about the proper timing of l-thyroxine in relation to meals and about drug interactions that can significantly impair l-thyroxine's efficacy. l-Thyroxine should be taken on an empty stomach to improve absorption.

PHARMACOECONOMICS

l-Thyroxine therapy is inexpensive, costing approximately $480 to $500 per year, depending on whether a brand name or generic preparation is prescribed. Approximately 8 to 12 million l-thyroxine prescriptions are filled annually. Yearly direct savings could amount to $356 to $534 million if a less costly brand or generic preparation is used instead of the top selling brand-name preparation. Costs for laboratory medical visits should also be included.

THYROID NODULES

EPIDEMIOLOGY

The discovery of asymptomatic single or multiple nodules in a normal or enlarged thyroid gland is common, affects women more than men, and occurs in about 5% to 7% of all adults more than 30 years old.[13,14] Its incidence may be as high as 50%, based on ultrasonography in patients without evidence of clinical thyroid disease. Benign nodules may be present in 10 to 20 million people in the United States.

PATHOPHYSIOLOGY

The pathogenesis is not well understood, but it may be related to iodide deficiency, irradiation, dietary goitrogens, and enzymatic defects. These nodules can be described as hypofunctioning ("cold") or autonomously functioning ("hot"). A significant increase in benign thyroid abnormalities (20%–33%) and thyroid cancers (6%–9%) has been observed in adults who received external irradiation to the thyroid, thymus, tonsils, adenoids, or upper head and neck region 20 to 25 years earlier.[13,14] Papillary, mixed papillary-follicular, and follicular malignancies and benign abnormalities, including focal hyperplasia, Hashimoto thyroiditis, adenomas, Graves disease, and colloid nodules have been reported. These malignant tumors are slow growing, and the prognosis is good if there are no metastases. Nonpalpable cancers have been found during surgery.

CLINICAL PRESENTATION AND DIAGNOSIS

Patients usually are asymptomatic and clinically euthyroid, although bothersome symptoms can occur. It is often difficult to determine clinically which nodule, if any, is cancerous. In general, 10% to 20% of cold nodules on thyroid scan are cancerous and hot nodules rarely are carcinogenic. The risk of malignancy is higher if a history of irradiation is present. Cold nodules in a multinodular goiter rarely are malignant; evidence of hypothyroidism or hyperthyroidism reduces but does not eliminate the risk of malignancy. A physician skilled in thyroid examinations should evaluate all patients with a history of childhood irradiation. A physical examination of the thyroid, baseline TSH, FT_4I or FT_4, and antibodies should be obtained even if the patient is clinically euthyroid and asymptomatic. If no abnormalities are found, routine yearly examinations are recommended. A fine-needle biopsy of the nodule, performed in the outpatient setting, can provide supporting information for or against surgery. Significant risk factors for malignancy are listed in Table 38.12.

TABLE 38.12	Risk Factors for Thyroid Cancer	
Evidence	**Lower Index of Suspicion**	**Higher Index of Suspicion**
History	Familial history of thyroid disease or endemic goiter	History of neck or head irradiation
Patient characteristics	Older women; multinodular goiter, soft nodule	Children, young adults, males; solitary firm dominant nodule >1 cm; vocal cord paralysis; enlarged lymph nodes; hoarseness
Laboratory characteristics	Negative thin-needle biopsy; positive thyroid antibodies; hot nodule on scan; cystic lesion on ultrasound	Positive thin-needle biopsy; ↑ thyroglobulin after thyroid surgery; ↑ serum calcitonin levels; cold nodule on scan; solid lesion on ultrasound.
L-thyroxine suppression therapy	Regression of nodule after 6–12 months of therapy	No regression, ↑ growth

THERAPEUTIC PLAN

A high index of suspicion for thyroid carcinoma requires surgical intervention. In euthyroid patients with a nodule that is likely to be benign, no history of thyroid irradiation, and a low index of suspicion for cancer, a trial of TSH suppression therapy is warranted to reduce growth of the existing nodule and may prevent growth of new nodules.[106,107] Higher doses of l-thyroxine (0.15–0.2 mg) may be required to achieve a suppressed TSH level of 0.1 to 0.5 mIU per liter, raising concerns about l-thyroxine toxicity.[29–32] There is also the potential for overt hyperthyroidism, especially if exogenous l-thyroxine is added to endogenous thyroxine overproduction (e.g., hot nodule). If significant regression of the nodule occurs after 6 to 12 months of therapy, treatment may be continued indefinitely. However, therapy usually does not shrink the gland to normal size. Any growth of the nodule during thyroid suppression therapy is alarming and requires rebiopsy or surgical removal because of the risk of malignancy. A clinically euthyroid patient with a suppressed TSH level should be the goal of therapy. However, the use of TSH suppression in preventing nodule growth and potential symptoms has produced mixed results, leading some to criticize such use.

KEY POINTS

- Hypothyroidism, hyperthyroidism, and nodular disease are common endocrine problems that affect 15% of women and 5% of men
- Practitioners should be alert to drugs that cause thyroid illness, interfere with proper laboratory interpretation, or interact with effective medical management
- Thyroid function tests are essential to detect, evaluate, and monitor thyroid disease in symptomatic patients and in older adults who have atypical symptoms
- TSH is the most sensitive test for monitoring thyroid function
- Many different treatment options are available for hyperthyroidism, hypothyroidism, and nodular disease
- l-Thyroxine is the preparation of choice for managing hypothyroidism
- Supraphysiologic T_4 doses can cause osteoporosis and cardiac arrhythmias
- Practitioners should integrate several patient and medication considerations in selecting the optimal treatment regimen for hyperthyroidism
- The preferred thioamide for managing hyperthyroidism is methimazole
- Rash, hepatotoxicity, and agranulocytosis can occur with thioamide therapy
- An understanding of the detection, evaluation, medical management, and education of patients with thyroid disease is essential

SUGGESTED READINGS

Cooper DS. Hyperthyroidism. Lancet 362:459–468, 2003.

Cooper DS. Antithyroid drugs for the treatment of hyperthyroidism caused by Graves' disease. Endocrinol Metab Clin N Am 27: 225–247, 1998.

Meier CA. Thyroid nodules: pathogenesis, diagnosis, and treatment. Baillière's Best Practice and Research. Clin Endocrinol Metab 14: 559–575, 2000.

Sarlis NJ, Gourgiotis L. Thyroid emergencies. Rev Endocr Metab Dis 4: 129–136, 2003.

Surks MI, Ortiz E, Daniels GH, et al. Subclinical thyroid disease. Scientific review and guidelines for diagnosis and management. JAMA 291:228–238, 2004.

REFERENCES

1. O'Connor P, Feely J. Clinical pharmacokinetics and endocrine disorders. Therapeutic implications. Clin Pharmacokinet 13:345–364, 1987.
2. Demers LM, Spencer CA. Laboratory Medicine Practice Guidelines. Laboratory support for the diagnosis and monitoring of thyroid disease. Thyroid 13:19–56, 2003.
3. Arbelle JE, Porath A. Practice guidelines for the detection and management of thyroid dysfunction. A comparative review of recommendations. Clin Endocrinol 51:11–18, 1999.
4. Ladenson PW, Singer PA, Ain KB, et al. American Thyroid Association guidelines for detection of thyroid dysfunction. Arch Intern Med 160:1573–1575, 2000.
5. Surks MI, Sievert R. Drugs and thyroid function. N Engl J Med 333:1688–1694, 1995.
6. Chopra IJ. Clinical review 86: euthyroid sick syndrome: is it a misnomer? J Clin Endocrinol Metab 82:329–334, 1997.
7. Stathatos N, Levetan C, Burman KD, et al. The controversy of the treatment of critically ill patients with thyroid hormone. Best Pract Res Clin Endocrinol Metab 15:465–478, 2001.
8. Cooper DS. Hyperthyroidism. Lancet 362:459–468, 2003.
9. Gittoes NJ, Franklyn JA. Hyperthyroidism. Current treatment guidelines. Drugs 55:543–553, 1998.
10. Zimmerman D, Lteif AN. Thyrotoxicosis in children. Med Clin North Am 27:109–126, 1998.
11. Surks MI, Ortiz E, Daniels GH, et al. Subclinical thyroid disease. Scientific review and guidelines for diagnosis and management. JAMA 291:228–238, 2004.
12. McIver B, Morris JC. The pathogenesis of Graves' disease. Med Clin North Am 27:73–89, 1998.
13. Meier CA. Thyroid nodules: pathogenesis, diagnosis, and treatment. Baillière's Best Practice and Research. Clin Endocrinol Metab 14:559–575, 2000.
14. Siegel RD, Lee SL. Toxic nodular goiter: toxic adenoma and toxic multinodular goiter. Med Clin North Am 27:151–168, 1998.
15. Stagnaro-Green A. Postpartum thyroiditis. Best Pract Res Clin Endocrinol Metab 18:303–316, 2004.
16. Ross DS. Syndromes of thyrotoxicosis with low radioactive iodine uptake. Med Clin North Am 27:169–185, 1998.
17. Koh LK, Greenspan FS, Yeo PP. Interferon-α induced thyroid dysfunction: three clinical presentations and a review of the literature. Thyroid 7:891–896, 1997.
18. Dalgard O, Bjoro K, Hellum K, et al. Thyroid dysfunction during treatment of chronic hepatitis C with interferon alpha: no association with either interferon dosage or efficacy of therapy. J Intern Med 251:400–406, 2002.
19. Harjai KJ, Licata AA. Effects of amiodarone on thyroid function. Ann Intern Med 126:63–73, 1997.
20. Martino E, Bartalena L, Bogazzi F, et al. The effects of amiodarone on the thyroid. Endocr Rev 22:240–254, 2001.
21. Barclay MI, Brownlie BE, Turner JG, et al. Lithium associated thyrotoxicosis: a report of 14 cases, with statistical analysis of incidence. Clin Endocrinol 40:759–764, 1994.

22. Bocchetta A, Mossa P, Velluzzi F, et al. Ten-year follow-up of thyroid function in lithium patients. J Clin Psychopharmacol 21: 594–598, 2001.

23. Kleiner J, Altshuler L, Hendrick V, et al. Lithium-induced subclinical hypothyroidism: review of the literature and guidelines for treatment. J Clin Psychiatry 60:249–255, 1999.

24. Dang AH, Hershman JM. Lithium-associated thyroiditis. Endocr Pract 8:232–236, 2002.

25. Roti E, Uberti ED. Iodine excess and hyperthyroidism. Thyroid 5: 493–500, 2001.

26. Bogazzi F, Bartalena L, Campomori A, et al. Treatment with lithium prevents serum thyroid hormone increase after thioamide withdrawal and radioiodine therapy in patients with Graves' disease. J Clin Endocrinol Metab 87:4490–4495, 2002.

27. Mestman JH. Hyperthyroidism in pregnancy. Best Pract Res Clin Endocrinol Metab 18:267–288, 2004.

28. Lazarus JH, Kokandi A. Thyroid disease in relation to pregnancy: a decade of change. Clin Endocrinol 53:265–278, 2000.

29. Toft AD. Clinical practice: subclinical hyperthyroidism. N Engl J Med 345:512–516, 2001.

30. Sawin CT, Geller A, Wolf PA, et al. Low serum thyrotropin concentrations as a risk factor for atrial fibrillation in older persons. N Engl J Med 331:1249–1952, 1994.

31. Biondi B, Palmieri EA, Lombardi G, et al. Effects of subclinical thyroid dysfunction on the heart. Ann Intern Med 137:904–914, 2002.

32. Greenspan SL, Greenspan FS. The effect of thyroid hormone on skeletal integrity. Ann Intern Med 130:750–758, 1999.

33. Sarlis NJ, Gourgiotis L. Thyroid emergencies. Rev Endocr Metab Dis 4:129–136, 2003.

34. Ringel MD. Management of hypothyroidism and hyperthyroidism in the intensive care unit. Crit Care Clin 17:59–74, 2001.

35. Bartalena L, Pinchera A, Marcocci C. Management of Graves' ophthalmopathy: reality and perspectives. Endocr Rev 21:168–199, 2000.

36. Bartalena L, Tanda ML, Piantanida E, et al. Relationship between management of hyperthyroidism and course of the ophthalmopathy. J Endocrinol Invest 3:288–294, 2004.

37. American Association of Clinical Endocrinologists. Medical guidelines for clinical practice for the evaluation and treatment of hyperthyroidism and hypothyroidism. Endocr Pract 8:458–469, 2002.

38. Streetman DD, Khanderia U. Diagnosis and treatment of Graves disease. Ann Pharmacother 37:1100–1109, 2003.

39. Cooper DS. Antithyroid drugs for the treatment of hyperthyroidism caused by Graves' disease. Endocrinol Metab Clin North Am 27: 225–247, 1998.

40. Kaplan MM, Meier DA, Dworkin HJ. Treatment of hyperthyroidism with radioactive iodine. Med Clin North Am 27:205–223, 1998.

41. Alsanea O, Clark OH. Treatment of Graves' disease: the advantage of surgery. Endocrinol Metab Clin North Am 29:321–337, 2000.

42. Torring O, Tallstedt L, Wallin G, et al. Graves' hyperthyroidism: treatment with antithyroid drugs, surgery, or radioiodine-a prospective, randomized study. J Clin Endocrinol Metab 81:2986–2893, 1996.

43. Fontanilla JC, Schneider AB, Sarne DH. The use of oral radiographic contrast agents in the management of hyperthyroidism. Thyroid 22:561–567, 2001.

44. Mercado M, Mendoza-Zubieta V, Bautista-Osorio R, et al. Treatment of hyperthyroidism with a combination of methimazole and cholestyramine. J Clin Endocrinol Metab 81:3191–3193, 1996.

45. Glaser NS, Styne DM. Predictors of early remission of hyperthyroidism in children. J Clin Endocrinol Metab 82:1719–1726, 1997.

46. Wing DA, Millar LK, Koonings PP, et al. A comparison of propylthiouracil versus methimazole in the treatment of hyperthyroidism in pregnancy. Am J Obstet Gynecol 170:90–95, 1994.

47. Momotani N, Ito K, Hamada N, et al. Maternal hyperthyroidism and congenital malformation in the offspring. Clin Endocrinol 20: 695–700, 1984.

48. Mandel SJ, Brent GA, Larsen PR. Review of antithyroid drug use during pregnancy and report of a case of aplasia cutis. Thyroid 4: 129–133, 1994.

49. Momotani N, Noh JY, Ishikawa N, et al. Effects of propylthiouracil and methimazole on fetal thyroid status in mothers with Graves' hyperthyroidism. J Clin Endocrinol Metab 82:3633–3636, 1997.

50. Jongjaroenprasert W, Akarawut W, Chantasart D, et al. Rectal administration of propylthiouracil in hyperthyroid patients: comparison of suspension enema and suppository form. Thyroid 12: 627–631, 2002.

51. Yeung SC, Go R, Balasubramanyam A. Rectal administration of iodide and propylthiouracil in the treatment of thyroid storm. Thyroid 5:403–405, 1995.

52. Nabil N, Miner DJ, Amatruda JM. Methimazole: an alternative route of administration. J Clin Endocrinol Metab 54:180–181, 1982.

53. Eisenstein Z, Weiss M, Katz Y, et al. Intellectual capacity of subjects exposed to methimazole or propylthiouracil in utero. Eur J Pediatr 151:558–559, 1992.

54. Messer PM, Hauffa BP, Olbricht T, et al. Antithyroid drug and Graves' disease in pregnancy: long term effects on somatic growth, intellectual development and thyroid function of the offspring. Acta Endocrinol 123:311–316, 1990.

55. Allannic H, Fauchet R, Orgiazzi J, et al. Antithyroid drugs and Graves' disease: a prospective randomized evaluation of the efficacy of treatment duration. J Clin Endocrinol Metab70:675–679, 1990.

56. Maugendre D, Gatel A, Campion L, et al. Antithyroid drugs and Graves' disease—prospective randomized assessment of long-term treatment. Clin Endocrinol 50:127–132, 1999.

57. Orgiazzi J, Madec AM. Reduction of the risk of relapse after withdrawal of medical therapy for Graves' disease. Thyroid 12: 849–853, 2002.

58. Lippe BM, Landaw EM, Kaplan SA. Hyperthyroidism in children treated with long term medical therapy: twenty-five percent remission every two years. J Clin Endocrinol Metab 64:1241–1245, 1987.

59. Vitti P, Rago T, Chiovato L, et al. Clinical features of patients with Graves' disease undergoing remission after antithyroid drug treatment. Thyroid 3:369–375, 1997.

60. Romaldini JH, Bromberg N, Werner RS, et al. Comparison of effects of high and low dosage regimens of antithyroid drugs in the management of Graves' hyperthyroidism. J Clin Endocrinol Metab 57:563–570, 1983.

61. Hashizume K, Ichikawa K, Sakurai A, et al. Administration of thyroxine in treated Graves' disease: effects on the level of antibodies to thyroid-stimulating hormone receptors and on the risk of recurrence of hyperthyroidism. N Engl J Med 324:947–953, 1991.

62. Rittmaster RS, Zwicker H, Abbott EC, et al. Effect of methimazole with or without exogenous l-thyroxine on serum concentrations of thyrotropin (TSH) receptor antibodies in patients with Graves' disease. J Clin Endocrinol Metab 81:3283–3288, 1996.

63. McIver B, Rae P, Beckett G, et al. Lack of effect of thyroxine in patients with Graves' hyperthyroidism who are treated with an antithyroid drug. N Engl J Med 334:220–224, 1996.

64. Hoermann R, Quadbeck B, Roggenbuck U, et al. Relapse of Graves' disease after successful outcome of antithyroid drug therapy: results of a prospective randomized study on the use of levothyroxine. Thyroid 12:1119–1128, 2002.

65. Liaw Y-F, Huang M-J, Fan K-D, et al. Hepatic injury during propylthiouracil therapy in patients with hyperthyroidism: a cohort study. Ann Intern Med 118:424–428, 1993.

66. Williams KV, Nayak S, Becker D, et al. Fifty years of experience with propylthiouracil-associated hepatotoxicity: what have we learned? J Clin Endocrinol Metab 82:1727–1733, 1997.

67. Woeber KA. Methimazole-induced hepatotoxicity. Endocr Pract 8: 222–224, 2002.

68. Tajiri J, Noguchi S, Murakami T, et al. Antithyroid drug-induced agranulocytosis: the usefulness of routine white blood cell count monitoring. Arch Intern Med 150:621–624, 1990.

69. Geffner DL, Hershman JM. Beta-adrenergic blockade for the treatment of hyperthyroidism. Am J Med 93:61–68, 1992.

70. Milner MR, Gelman KM, Phillips RA, et al. Double-blind crossover trial of diltiazem versus propranolol in the management of thyrotoxic symptoms. Pharmacotherapy 10:100–106, 1990.

71. Andrade VA, Gross JL, Maia AL. The effect of methimazole pretreatment on the efficacy of radioactive iodine therapy in Graves' hyperthyroidism: one-year follow-up of a prospective randomized study. J Clin Endocrinol Metab 86:3488–3493, 2001.

72. Imseis RE, Vanmiddlesworth L, Massie JD, et al. Pretreatment with propylthiouracil but not methimazole reduces the therapeutic efficacy of iodine-131 in hyperthyroidism. J Clin Endocrinol Metab 83:685–687, 1998.

73. Braga M, Walpert N, Burch HB, et al. The effect of methimazole on cure rates after radioiodine treatment for Graves' hyperthyroidism: a randomized clinical trial. Thyroid 12:135–139, 2002.

74. Ron E, Doody MM, Becker DV, et al. Cancer mortality following treatment for adult hyperthyroidism. JAMA 280:347–355, 1998.

75. Chopra IJ, Baber K. Use of oral cholecystographic agents in the treatment of amiodarone-induced hyperthyroidism. J Clin Endocrinol Metab 86:4707–4710, 2001.

76. Bogazzi F, Miccoli P, Berti P, et al. Preparation with iopanoic acid rapidly controls thyrotoxicosis in patients with amiodarone-induced thyrotoxicosis before thyroidectomy. Surgery 132:1114–1117, 2002.

77. Shimizu T, Koide S, Noh JY, et al. Hyperthyroidism and the management of atrial fibrillation. Thyroid 12:489–493, 2002.

78. Roberts CGP, Ladenson PW. Hypothyroidism. Lancet 363: 793–803, 2004.

79. Duntas LH. Thyroid disease and lipids. Thyroid 12:287–293, 2002.

80. LaFranchi S. Congential hypothyroidism: etiologies, diagnosis, and management. Thyroid 9:735–740, 1999.

81. Heyerdahl S, Oerbeck B. Congenital hypothyroidism: developmental outcome in relation to levothyroxine treatment variables. Thyroid 13:1029–1038, 2003.

82. Wiersinga WM. Thyroid hormone replacement therapy. Horm Res 56 (Suppl 1):74–81, 2001.

83. Chopra IJ, Baber K. Treatment of primary hypothyroidism during pregnancy: is there an increase in thyroxine dose requirement in pregnancy? Metabolism 52:122–128, 2003.

84. Bell DS, Ovalle F. Use of soy protein supplement and resultant need for increased dose of levothyroxine. Endocr Pract 7:193–194, 2001.

85. Siraj ES, Gupta MK, Reddy SS. Raloxifene causing malabsorption of levothyroxine. Arch Intern Med 163:1367–1370, 2003.

86. Singh N, Singh PN, Hershman JM. Effect of calcium carbonate on the absorption of levothyroxine. JAMA 283:2822–2825, 2000.

87. Liel Y, Sperber AD, Shany S. Nonspecific intestinal adsorption of levothyroxine by aluminum hydroxide. Am J Med 97:363–365, 1994.

88. McCowen KC, Garger JR, Spark R. Elevated serum thyrotropin in thyroxine-treated patients with hypothyroidism given sertraline [letter]. N Engl J Med 337:1010–1011, 1997.

89. Ain KB, Pucino F, Shiver TM, et al. Thyroid hormone levels affected by time of blood sampling in thyroxine-treated patients. Thyroid 3:81–85, 1993.

90. Leese GP, Jung RT, Guthrie C, et al. Morbidity in patients on l-thyroxine: a comparison of those with a normal TSH level to those with suppressed TSH. Clin Endocrinol 37:500–503, 1992.

91. Hennessey JV. Levothyroxine a new drug? Since when? How can that be? Thyroid 3:279–282, 2003.

92. Klein I, Danzi S. Evaluation of the therapeutic efficacy of different levothyroxine preparations in the treatment of human thyroid disease. Thyroid 12:1127–1132, 2003.

93. Escalante DA, Arem N, Arem R. Assessment of interchangeability of two brands of levothyroxine preparations with a third-generation TSH assay. Am J Med 98:374–378, 1995.

94. Dong BJ, Hauck WW, Gambertoglio JG, et al. Bioequivalence of generic and brand-name levothyroxine products in the treatment of hypothyroidism. JAMA 277:1205–1213, 1997.

95. Grebe SK, Cooke RR, Ford HC, et al. Treatment of hypothyroidism with once weekly thyroxine. J Clin Endocrinol Metab 82: 870–875, 1997.

96. Ladenson PW, Braverman LE, Mazzaferri EL, et al. Comparison of administration of recombinant human thyrotropin with withdrawal of thyroid hormone for radioactive iodine scanning in patients with thyroid carcinoma. N Engl J Med 337:888–896, 1997.

97. Bunevicius R, Kazanavicius G, Zalinkevicius R, et al. Effects of thyroxine as compared with thyroxine plus triiodotyronine in patients with hypothyroidism. N Engl J Med 340:424–429, 1999.

98. Clyde PW, Harari AE, Getka EJ, et al. Combined levothyroxine plus liothyronine compared with levothyroxine alone in primary hypothyroidism. JAMA 290:2952–2958, 2003.

99. Walsh JP, Shiels L, Lim BM, et al. Combined thyroxine/liothyronine treatment does not improve well-being, quality of life or cognitive function compared to thyroxine alone: a randomized controlled trial in patient with primary hypothyroidism. J Clin Endocrinol Metab 88:4543–4550, 2003.

100. Sawka AM, Gerstein HC, Marriott MJ, et al. Does a combination of T_4 and T_3 improve depressive symptoms better than T_4 alone in patients with hypothyroidism? Results of a double-blinded randomized controlled trial. J Clin Endocrinol Metab 88:4551–4555, 2003.

101. Hennemann G, Docter R, Visser TJ, et al. Thyroxine plus low-dose, slow-release triiodothyronine replacement in hypothyroidism: proof of principle. Thyroid 14:271–275, 2004.

102. Sawin CT, Hershman JM, Fernandez-Garcia R, et al. A comparison of thyroxine and desiccated thyroid in patients with primary hypothyroidism. Metabolism 27:1518–1525, 1978.

103. Chu JW, Crapo LM. The treatment of subclinical hypothyroidism is seldom necessary. J Clin Endocrinol Metab 86:4591–4599, 2001.

104. McDermott MT, Ridgway EC. Subclinical hypothyroidism is mild thyroid failure and should not be treated. J Clin Endocrinol Metab 86:4585–4590, 2001.

105. Col NF, Surks MI, Daniels GH. Subclinical thyroid disease. Clinical applications. JAMA 291:239–243, 2004.

106. Castro MR, Caraballo PJ, Morris JC. Effectiveness of thyroid hormone suppressive therapy in benign solitary thyroid nodules: a meta-analysis. J Clin Endocrinol Metab 87:4154–4159, 2002.

107. Wemeau JL, Caron P, Schvartz C, et al. Effects of thyroid-stimulating hormone suppression with levothyroxine in reducing the volume of solitary thyroid nodules and improving extranodular nonpalpable changes: a randomized, double-blind, placebo-controlled trial by the French Thyroid Research Group. J Clin Endocrinol Metab 87:4928–4934, 2002.

Parathyroid Disorders

39

Renu F. Singh and Betty J. Dong

TREATMENT GOALS: HYPERPARATHYROIDISM

- Reduce serum calcium levels.
- Reverse symptoms resulting from severe hypercalcemia.
- Correct dehydration.
- Increase urinary calcium excretion.
- Inhibit bone resorption.
- Treat underlying cause (when possible).

HYPERPARATHYROIDISM

DEFINITION

Primary hyperparathyroidism is an endocrine disorder characterized by excessive and incompletely regulated release of parathyroid hormone (PTH) from one or more parathyroid glands, resulting in hypercalcemia.

ETIOLOGY

The cause of primary hyperparathyroidism is unknown. It usually occurs sporadically. Primary hyperparathyroidism can be produced by three different pathologic lesions: (a) parathyroid adenoma, (b) hyperplasia, or (c) carcinoma(1)

1021

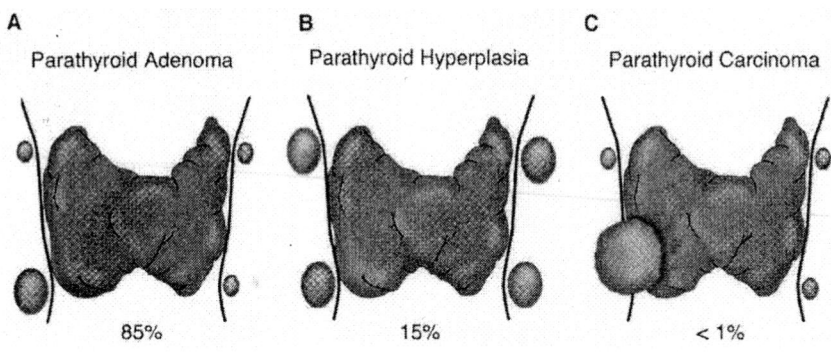

A Parathyroid Adenoma   85%

B Parathyroid Hyperplasia   15%

C Parathyroid Carcinoma   < 1%

FIGURE 39.1 Three pathologic causes of primary hyperparathyroidism include (A) adenoma; (B) hyperplasia; and (C) carcinoma. (From Sosa JA, Udelsman R. New directions in the treatment of patients with primary hyperparathyroidism. Curr Probl Surg 40:803–849, 2003,[1] with permission.)

(Fig. 39.1). A parathyroid adenoma is a benign encapsulated neoplasm that accounts for 80% to 90% of cases. Although this condition usually affects a single gland, 2% to 5% of patients with primary hyperparathyroidism have adenomas of two glands. Parathyroid hyperplasia is a proliferation of parenchymal cells and affects all of the parathyroid glands. Hyperplasia accounts for 10% of the cases of primary hyperparathyroidism. It is also associated with multiple endocrine neoplasia (MEN types 1 and 2) syndromes. The third lesion of the parathyroid is parathyroid carcinoma, which is a slow growing neoplasm, and accounts for 0.5% to 2% of cases.[1]

Of those patients diagnosed with primary hyperparathyroidism, 10% to 20% have an inherited hyperfunction of multiple parathyroid glands. These patients are usually diagnosed at an early age. Familial forms of primary hyperparathyroidism include MEN (types 1 and 2), neonatal severe primary hyperparathyroidism, hyperparathyroidism-jaw tumor syndrome, familial hypocalciuric hypercalcemia, and familial isolated hyperparathyroidism.[2]

Primary hyperparathyroidism should be distinguished from secondary and tertiary hyperparathyroidism because treatment is different. Secondary hyperparathyroidism oc-

curs from a physiologic parathyroid response to hypocalcemia. The most common cause of secondary hyperparathyroidism is chronic renal failure, which results in a low concentration of 1,25-dihydroxyvitamin D_3 from decreased renal production. Low levels of 1,25-dihydroxyvitamin D_3 reduces intestinal absorption of calcium, resulting in low serum calcium levels and increased serum phosphate levels (Fig. 39.2). Less common causes include malabsorptive and other metabolic disorders, where absorption of calcium and vitamin D are reduced. Tertiary hyperparathyroidism occurs from prolonged stimulation of the parathyroids, usually due to longstanding chronic renal failure leading to hypocalcemia. This causes the parathyroid glands to develop autonomous hyperfunction, with subsequent hypercalcemia, and loss of the parathyroid-calcium feedback inhibition loop.[1]

EPIDEMIOLOGY

Since routine screening for serum calcium became available in the 1970s in the United States, the incidence of new cases of hyperparathyroidism has increased. After diabetes mellitus and thyroid disease, primary hyperparathyroidism is the third most commonly diagnosed endocrine disorder. In the United States, primary hyperparathyroidism occurs in 25 per 100,000 people in the general population, resulting in 100,000 new cases per year. The peak incidence of hyperparathyroidism occurs between the 5th and 6th decades, although it can affect any age group. The majority of cases (60%–65%) occur in postmenopausal women, with the average age at diagnosis being 55 years.[3]

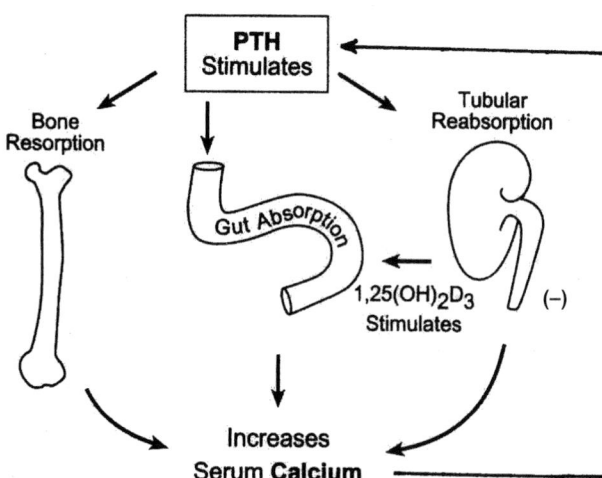

FIGURE 39.2 The parathyroid hormone stimulation and feedback loop. (From Sosa JA, Udelsman R. New directions in the treatment of patients with primary hyperparathyroidism. Curr Probl Surg 40:803–849, 2003,[1] with permission.)

PATHOPHYSIOLOGY

The parathyroid glands are four, pea-sized glands located posteriorly on the thyroid gland in the neck (Fig. 39.3). The glands secrete PTH, which is the principal regulator responsible for maintaining the extracellular calcium concentration within a narrow normal range. PTH is released from the parathyroid glands via a negative feedback system responsive to plasma calcium levels.[1] Normal plasma calcium is maintained by the action of PTH on bone, intestine, and

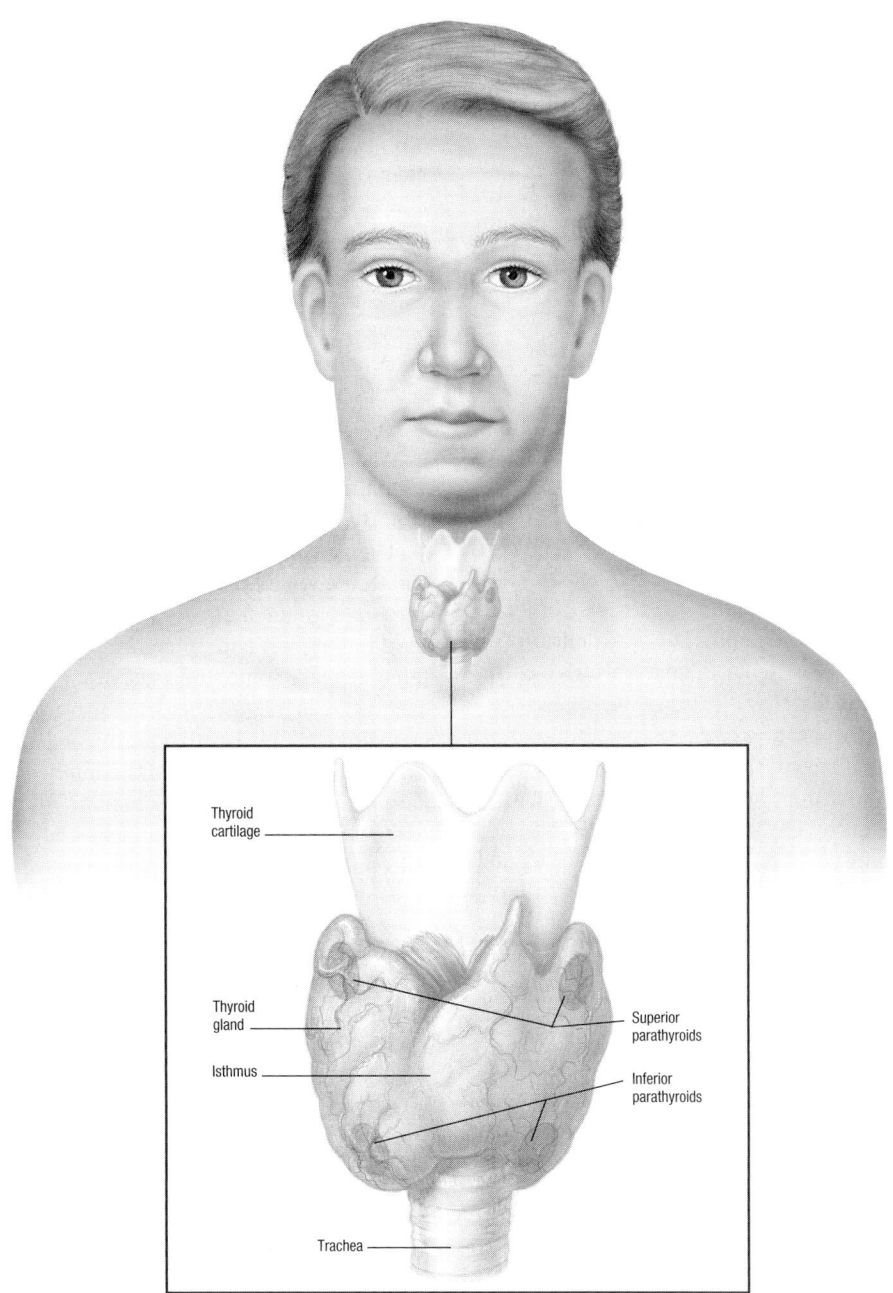

FIGURE 39.3 The thyroid and parathyroid glands. (From Anatomical Chart Co., with permission.)

kidney (Fig. 39.2). Low levels of serum calcium cause the parathyroid glands to release PTH, which stimulates bone resorption and increases the gastrointestinal absorption and renal tubular reabsorption of calcium, resulting in an overall increase in serum calcium levels. In addition, the kidney secretes 1,25-dihydroxyvitamin D_3, which also encourages intestinal absorption of calcium (Fig. 39.2). The hallmark of hyperparathyroidism is hypercalcemia, because the negative feedback cycle fails to suppress further PTH secretion.

Most of the total body calcium is in the form of hydroxyapatite in bone (99%), and only a small fraction of the calcium circulates in the bloodstream as the active (ionized) or inactive (bound) forms. Approximately 40% of the total serum calcium is bound, primarily to albumin, 15% is complexed with phosphate or other anions, and 45% is in the ionized active form. Therefore, reductions in serum albumin alter the concentration of protein-bound calcium and increase the free ionized fraction proportionally. The normal total serum calcium concentration is approximately 2.1 to 2.62 mmol per liter (8.5–10.5 mg/dL), depending on the assay. In patients with hypoalbuminemia, the serum calcium can be adjusted by adding 0.2 mmol per liter (0.8 mg/dL) for each 10 g per liter (1.0

g/dL) of albumin below a normal level of 40 g per liter (4.0 gm/dL) to the measured serum calcium:

$$\text{Serum Ca}_{\text{corrected}} \text{ (mg/dL)} = \text{Serum Ca}_{\text{observed}}$$
$$+ 0.8 (4 - \text{Serum albumin}_{\text{observed}}) \quad (39.1)$$

For example, for a patient with a serum albumin of 1.8 g per deciliter and an observed serum calcium level of 10, this equation would be: measured serum calcium [Serum Ca$_{\text{corrected}}$ (mg/dL) = 10 + 0.8(4 − 1.8) = 11.76]. This formula might not completely correct for albumin, and direct determination of ionized calcium levels may be useful.

In summary, PTH maintains normocalcemia by the following mechanisms:

- Releases calcium and phosphate from osteoclastic bone resorption.
- Increases calcium reabsorption from the renal tubule.
- Increases intestinal calcium absorption indirectly via vitamin D (1,25-dihydroxyvitamin D$_3$).
- Increases conversion of the metabolite 25-hydroxycholecalciferol to active vitamin D$_3$ (1,25-dihydroxycholecalciferol or 1,25-dihydroxyvitamin D$_3$ or calcitriol) by stimulating the activity of renal tubular 25-OH-1-α-hydroxylase.
- Increases renal bicarbonate excretion (bicarbonaturia), producing a metabolic acidosis that decreases the ability of circulating albumin to bind calcium, thus increasing free ionized calcium by physiochemical means.
- Increases renal phosphate excretion (phosphaturia) and prevents elevations in plasma phosphate levels from increased bone resorption.

Thus, a reciprocal relationship between calcium and phosphate exists. In hyperparathyroidism, serum calcium is elevated and hypophosphatemia occurs. Conversely, in hypoparathyroidism, hypocalcemia and hyperphosphatemia are seen.

CLINICAL PRESENTATION AND DIAGNOSIS

Most patients presenting with primary hyperparathyroidism in the United States today are asymptomatic. With the introduction of the automated serum screening chemistry panel in the early 1970s, elevations in serum calcium levels were routinely detected at physician office visits, and the biochemical diagnosis of primary hyperparathyroidism was made before symptoms appeared.

SIGNS AND SYMPTOMS

With only mildly elevated serum calcium (0.24 mmol/L, or 1 mg/dL above upper limits), most patients are asymptomatic or have nonspecific complaints of weakness and easy fatigability. High-risk older women might show confusion and dehydration. Before the routine use of serum calcium measurements, patients typically presented with symptoms resulting from severe hypercalcemia. These included the classic pentad of painful *bones,* kidney *stones,* abdominal

groans, psychic *moans,* and fatigue *overtones.*[1] Currently, less than 20% of patients with primary hyperparathyroidism have kidney stones, and less than 5% have evidence of osteitis fibrosa cystica. Serum calcium levels greater than 3 mmol per liter (12 mg/dL) commonly produce gastrointestinal symptoms (e.g., anorexia, nausea, and vomiting) and neurologic manifestations of proximal muscle weakness, delayed deep tendon reflexes, and altered mental status. Patients with hyperparathyroidism may be more prone to depression, obsession-compulsion, hostility, psychosis, and paranoid ideation.[4,5] Skeletal symptoms may include diffuse bone pain and arthralgias. Severe deforming bone disease, such as osteitis cystica, is rarely seen with primary hyperparathyroidism today but is still a problem with secondary hyperparathyroidism in patients with end-stage renal disease complicated by renal osteodystrophy. However, even patients with mild, asymptomatic disease have evidence of skeletal involvement with higher levels of bone resorption and formation markers.[6] Bone density studies reveal that hyperparathyroidism affects cortical bone (e.g., the distal one third radius site) and cancellous bone, such as the spine and femoral neck. Some studies have suggested that there may be an increase in fracture incidence in primary hyperparathyroidism, although this is still controversial and debated.[7]

The clinical spectrum and complications of primary hyperparathyroidism are presented in Table 39.1. The severity of the clinical manifestations, especially the degree of hypercalcemia, generally is proportional to the degree of hyperfunctioning tissue and the level of PTH elevation.

DIAGNOSIS AND CLINICAL FINDINGS

Because there are usually no abnormal physical findings on physical examination, in 80% to 90% of cases, the diagnosis of hyperparathyroidism is based on an elevated total serum calcium level (usually >2.62 mmol/L or 10.5 mg/dL) that is corrected for the patient's albumin concentration, and an elevated PTH level. The first-generation immunoradiometric assay for intact PTH levels (IRMA PTH-intact), one of the most sensitive PTH assays, should be used to confirm the diagnosis of hyperparathyroidism. The normal range of the IRMA PTH-intact assay is 10 to 65 pg per milliliter. However, normal levels may vary in different populations. African-Americans typically have higher normal PTH levels than whites. Normal PTH levels are also lower in younger adults and rise with age. A second-generation IRMA assay for PTH has been developed that measures the full-length PTH molecule and may provide increased diagnostic sensitivity for this disorder.[8]

Although there are many causes of hypercalcemia, few are associated with elevated PTH levels, making the differential diagnosis fairly clear. Nonhyperparathyroid causes of hypercalcemia should be eliminated (Table 39.2). However, hyperparathyroidism and malignancy account for over 90% of hypercalcemia cases.[9]

Drugs that can increase serum calcium concentrations include thiazide diuretics and lithium, which should be withdrawn, and the patient retested 3 months later.[8]

TABLE 39.1	Signs and Symptoms of Moderate to Severe Hypercalcemia^a and Hyperparathyroidism		
System	**Symptoms**	**Complications**	**Laboratory Tests**
General	Weakness, easy fatigability		
Gastrointestinal	Nausea, vomiting, anorexia, constipation, abdominal pain, weight loss	Peptic ulcer disease (10%–15%), chronic pancreatitis, cholelithiasis, fecal impaction, intestinal obstruction	↑ Amylase, ↑ gastrin
Genitourinary	Polyuria, nocturia, polydipsia, dehydration, uremia symptoms, renal colic pain	Nephrolithiasis, nephrocalcinosis (20%–30%), renal failure, pyelonephritis	Hematuria, inability to concentrate urine (low specific gravity), pyuria, ↓ Na, ↓ K, ↓ Mg
Skeletal	Vague aches and pains, arthralgias, localized swelling	Osteitis fibrosa cystica, chondrocalcinosis, pathologic fractures, bone cysts, calcium depositions leading to gout, pseudogout	Radiologic: subperiosteal bone resorption Dual energy absorptiometry: ↓ bone mineral density in regions of cortical bone
Neurologic	Emotional lability, slow mentation, poor memory, drowsiness, ataxia, coma	Depression, psychoses; headaches, myopathy (proximal), coma	Hyperactive deep tendon reflexes
Cardiovascular	Bradycardia	Hypertension (20%–60%), cardiac arrest, bundle branch block, heart block, enhanced digitalis sensitivity	Electrocardiographic intervals: ↓ Q-T, ↑ P-R, ↑ QRS
Metabolic	Dehydration	Hyperchloremic acidosis, insulin hypersecretion, decreased insulin sensitivity	↓ HCO_3, ↑ Cl
Others	Pruritus caused by ectopic calcifications in skin; ectopic calcifications in lungs, kidneys, cornea; red eyes	Anemia, band keratopathy, thrombosis, malignancies in gastrointestinal tract, breast, thyroid	

^{a} Moderate to severe hypercalcemia defined as serum calcium concentration ≥12 mg/dL.

Other abnormal laboratory findings in primary hyperparathyroidism include hypophosphatemia, hyperphosphaturia, hypercalciuria, low serum bicarbonate concentration, elevated serum chloride levels, elevations in serum alkaline phosphatase and osteocalcin (markers of bone formation), and urinary hydroxyproline and collagen cross-link residues (markers of bone resorption).

Once the diagnosis of primary hyperparathyroidism has been confirmed biochemically, a complete diagnostic evaluation of the target organs that are most likely to be affected by the disorder should be done, namely, the skeleton and the kidneys. Radiography (x-rays) rarely shows skeletal involvement, whereas bone densitometry is far more sensitive. Bone densitometry using dual energy x-ray absorptiometry should be used to measure bone density in the lumbar spine, hip, and forearm. A baseline renal assessment with renal ultrasound and/or abdominal x-ray can be useful to assess for kidney stones. A 24-hour urinary calcium measurement should also be obtained to measure the renal burden for handling calcium. Serum creatinine levels can be helpful in estimating creatinine clearance and renal function.

DISEASE COURSE

Most patients diagnosed with primary hyperparathyroidism today are asymptomatic. In general, patients who do not meet criteria for surgery do well without disease progression, suggesting a relatively benign disease course for most patients. The average serum calcium and PTH levels did not change in patients who were not treated with surgery when followed over a 10-year period.[10] However, 25% of the patients will have progression of the disease, which includes worsening hypercalcemia, hypercalciuria, and decreases in bone mass.[10] The main predictor for disease progression seems to be age; patients younger than 50 years of age are three times more likely to have worsening disease. Therefore, patients who do not undergo parathyroid surgery should be carefully monitored for disease progression.

A population-based study in the United States of patients with mild, asymptomatic primary hyperparathyroidism did not show an increase in overall mortality, although mortality was higher in patients in the highest quartile of serum calcium concentrations (i.e., 2.8–4 mmol/L; 11.2–16 mg/dL).[11] However, European studies suggest that primary

TABLE 39.2	Selected Causes of Hypercalcemia

Hyperparathyroidism

- Primary: parathyroid adenomas, hyperplasia, or carcinoma

- Secondary: chronic renal failure

- Tertiary: chronic renal failure

Granulomatous disease (sarcoidosis, tuberculosis, histoplasmosis, coccidiomycosis, leprosy)

Drugs

- Vitamin A or D toxicity or calcium intoxication

- Milk-alkali syndrome

- Lithium

- Thiazides and thiazidelike diuretics

- Estrogens, antiestrogens, testosterone in breast cancer

Malignancies

- Nonhematologic (breast, bronchus)

- Hematologic (myeloma, leukemia, lymphoma)

Endocrine (adrenal insufficiency, thyrotoxicosis, acromegaly, pheochromocytoma)

Immobilization

Bone disorders (Paget osteoporosis)

Familial hypocalciuric hypercalcemia

Parenteral nutrition

Aluminum excess

Acute and chronic renal disease

TABLE 39.3	Indications for Surgical Parathyroidectomy in Asymptomatic Primary Hyperparathyroidism

Patients <50 years of age

Serum calcium >1 mg/dL (0.25 mmol/L) above the upper limit of normal

Urinary calcium excretion >400 mg/day

Creatinine clearance reduced by >30%

Bone mineral density (lumbar, hip, or distal radius) >2.5 SD below peak bone mass (t-score −2.5)

When medical follow up is not possible or desirable

Source: Bilezikian JP, Potts JT Jr, Fuleihan GE, et al. Summary statement from a workshop on asymptomatic primary hyperparathyroidism: a perspective for the 21st century. J Clin Endocrinol Metab 87:5353–5361, 2002.

hyperparathyroidism may be associated with greater mortality, higher cardiovascular risks, dyslipidemia, and impaired glucose tolerance.[12,13] Also, it is unclear if there is an increased risk of fractures in primary hyperparathyroidism.[7] Some studies have found that parathyroid surgery in patients with primary hyperparathyroidism reduced hip and upper arm fractures in up to 50% of patients.[7] Although reduced bone mineral density may occur from primary hyperparathyroidism, an increased risk of fractures has not been a consistent finding in other long-term studies.[10,14] Further study is needed in this area to determine if patients with long-standing hyperparathyroidism are at increased risk of fractures.

PSYCHOSOCIAL ASPECTS

Depression occurs in 10% of patients undergoing parathyroidectomy for primary hyperparathyroidism.[5] Patients with hyperparathyroidism also report a higher incidence of other psychological symptoms, including obsession compulsion, psychosis, hostility, and paranoid ideation.[4] Many of these symptoms, especially depression, resolve within 1 month after parathyroid surgery.[4,5]

THERAPEUTIC PLAN

Parathyroid surgery is the only definitive treatment for primary hyperparathyroidism. A National Institutes of Health (NIH) consensus panel established and recently revised guidelines for the surgical and medical management of primary hyperparathyroidism.[9,15] All patients with symptomatic primary hyperparathyroidism, including target organ complications such as severe bone disease (osteitis fibrosa cystica), fractures, nephrolithiasis, nephrocalcinosis, or overt muscular dysfunction, are strongly advised to undergo parathyroidectomy. Certain asymptomatic patients should also receive surgical management (Table 39.3). In addition, patients with psychological symptoms, such as depression, should be considered for parathyroid surgery. Many psychological symptoms resolve or improve following parathyroidectomy. Patients who do not undergo parathyroidectomy for asymptomatic primary hyperparathyroidism should be followed closely, with serum calcium being checked twice a year, serum creatinine once a year, and bone mineral density scan (at three sites: forearm, hip, and lumbar spine) performed annually.[35]

In patients with secondary hyperparathyroidism, whenever possible, the underlying cause should be corrected. The goal of management is to reduce the synthesis and secretion of PTH by reducing serum phosphate levels and supplementing levels of calcium and vitamin D.[16] Parathyroidectomy is usually required in patients who develop tertiary hyperparathyroidism and severe metabolic bone disease.[3]

TREATMENT

SURGERY

The standard parathyroidectomy operation is bilateral exploration of the neck and all four parathyroid glands. In 15%

to 20% of patients with primary hyperparathyroidism, enlargement of more than one gland will be discovered. Recent advances in local anesthesia have allowed many surgeons to perform parathyroidectomy with local, rather than general, anesthesia. In addition, many minimally invasive procedures (MIPs) have become available. Technetium Tc 99m sestamibi scanning is one of the most accurate techniques (80%–90% sensitivity) for localizing abnormal parathyroid glands. Other methods of preoperative localization include ultrasound, computed tomography (CT), and magnetic resonance imaging (MRI). MIPs are reserved for sporadic primary hyperparathyroidism and only if a single adenoma is visualized preoperatively. The surgery is then performed under local anesthesia with identification and removal of the abnormal tissue. The other parathyroid glands are not explored or identified with a MIP. During surgery, a rapid intraoperative PTH (quick PTH) assay can provide serum PTH levels within 12 minutes. If the intraoperative serum PTH level decreases by 50%, the operation is completed. If the level does not decrease by 50%, the operation is extended, and a full neck exploration may be performed to assess for other overactive glands.

Most critical to the surgical treatment of primary hyperparathyroidism is an experienced and skilled surgeon. In competent hands, the evidence of postoperative complications (i.e., vocal cord paralysis, hypoparathyroidism, wound infection, hematoma) is minimal, and the cure rate for parathyroidectomy is greater than 95%.[1,17]

Postoperatively, serum calcium levels will normalize or fall below normal within 24 to 48 hours. Hypocalcemia is usually mild and transient. Serum calcium levels should be monitored daily until levels stabilize, around postoperative days 5 to 6. Serum calcium should be maintained above 2 mmol per liter (8 mg/dL). Hypocalcemic symptoms of tetany or pretetany should be treated intravenously with 10 to 20 mL of 10% calcium gluconate, infused slowly (not faster than 10 mL/minute) until symptoms are relieved. Modest degrees of postoperative hypocalcemia can be managed by ensuring an adequate calcium intake with dietary or elemental calcium in oral doses of 1 to 2 g per day in 3 to 4 divided doses. Postoperatively, most patients have a temporary hypocalcemia that normalizes quickly as the parathyroid glands begin to regain function. A small percentage of patients develop permanent hypoparathyroidism, necessitating treatment with vitamin D. Urinary calcium excretion and recurrent kidney stones are reduced by successful parathyroid surgery.[10] Neuromuscular symptoms, such as proximal muscle weakness, often are reversed by parathyroidectomy. Psychiatric symptoms, such as mental dullness, confusion, and loss of consciousness, may improve within days of parathyroidectomy. Symptoms of depression improve significantly within 1 month of surgery.[4,5] Significant improvements are also seen in bone mineral density in the lumbar spine and hip within 6 months of a parathyroidectomy, and in the femoral neck after 1 year.[10,18] Paradoxically, however, parathyroidectomy does not increase bone mineral density in radial bone, suggesting that bone loss in cortical bone may not be reversible in patients with primary hyperparathyroidism.[10] Parathyroid surgery does not produce any change in blood pressure or renal impairment.

Parathyroid transplantation might be indicated for the patient with secondary hyperparathyroidism (renal osteodystrophy), primary parathyroid hyperplasia, persistent or recurrent hyperparathyroidism, or radical head and neck surgery including thyroidectomy.

PHARMACOTHERAPY

There is no pharmacologic substitute for correction of the underlying disorder by surgery. However, some patients with asymptomatic primary hyperparathyroidism will not meet guideline criteria for surgery. Medical management of hypercalcemia is indicated in symptomatic patients before surgery, in patients who refuse or who are poor candidates for surgery, in those with life-threatening hypercalcemia, and in those with resistant or recurrent hyperparathyroidism despite previous neck surgery.

There are no medical therapies that effectively cure primary hyperparathyroidism. Pharmacotherapy is individualized based on the degree of hypercalcemia (mild, moderate, or severe) and severity of symptoms. Hypercalcemia is considered mild if the total serum calcium is less than 3 mmol per liter (12 mg/dL).[9] Asymptomatic patients with mild hypercalcemia generally do not benefit from normalization of their serum calcium levels, and hence, need not be acutely treated.[19] Asymptomatic patients with serum calcium levels between 3 and 3.4 mmol per liter (12–13.5 mg/dL) are considered to have moderate hypercalcemia and should receive surgery. However, patients who are poor surgical candidates or unwilling to undergo surgery may be treated with long-term hypocalcemic agents, including estrogens and progestins, selective estrogen-receptor blockers, bisphosphonates, or the newer calcimimetic agents. Serum calcium levels of 3.5 mmol per liter (14 mg/dL) or higher are considered severely hypercalcemic and potentially life-threatening. These patients, and symptomatic patients with calcium levels greater than 3 mmol per liter (12 mg/dL), should receive immediate and aggressive treatment. Immediate goals are to correct dehydration, increase renal calcium excretion, and reduce serum calcium levels. The acute management of severe hypercalcemia from any cause is reviewed in detail in Chapter 28. The safest and most effective treatment of severe hypercalcemia is rehydration with intravenous fluids, such as saline (Table 39.4). Hydration reduces the serum calcium level by dilution and diuresis. Patients with kidney failure require dialysis because diuresis is not possible. Once euvolemic, if necessary, a loop diuretic (e.g., furosemide) may be initiated to further lower the serum calcium. Thiazide diuretics should be avoided because they increase calcium

TABLE 39.4	Commonly Used Treatments of Hypercalcemia					
Method	**Mechanism of Action**	**Dosage**	**Onset of Calcium-lowering Effect**	**Maximal Effect**	**Adverse Effects**	**Comments**
Hydration with saline, replacement of depleted electrolytes	Increases calcium excretion	100–150 mL/hr IV saline	Hours	Decreases serum calcium by 1–2 mg/dL	Volume overload	Cautious administration in patients with congestive heart failure, renal failure; careful fluid and electrolyte monitoring is crucial
Hydration with saline and loop diuretic	Increases calcium excretion	Furosemide 10–20 mg IV q6–12h	Within 4 hrs	Decreases by 1–3 mg/dL	Volume depletion, serum calcium hypokalemia, hypomagnesemia	Avoid in dehydration; avoid thiazides, which decrease calcium excretion
Forced diuresis with saline	Increases calcium excretion	150–250 mL/hr IV saline plus furosemide 80–100 mg IV q1–2h	Hours	Decreases serum calcium by 2–4 mg/dL	Volume depletion hypokalemia, hypomagnesemia	Central venous pressure monitoring of fluid status and bladder catheterization needed; continuous electrolyte repletion crucial
Calcitonin (Miacalcin)	Inhibits bone resorption	4 IU/kg SQ or IM q12h; maximum of 8 IU/kg q6h	2–4 hrs	12–24 hr; decreases serum calcium by 1–2 mg/dL	Hypersensitivity reactions, nausea, abdominal cramps, flushing	Rapid rebound in hypercalcemia within 24–48 hr; combination with a bisphosphonate sustains calcium-lowering effect
Raloxifene (Evista)	Inhibits bone resorption	60 mg orally daily	4–8 wks	8 wks	Hot flashes, leg cramps	Effective in postmenopausal women with mild hyperparathyroidism
Pamidronate (Aredia)	Inhibits bone resorption	60–90 mg IV over 2–24 hrs	24–48 hrs	7–10 days	Fever, myalgias, hypophosphatemia	Do not repeat dose earlier than 7 days after initial dose; use with caution in renal dysfunction
Alendronate (Fosamax)	Inhibits bone resorption	10 mg orally daily	1 month	1–3 months	Esophageal irritation	Must take with a full glass of water on an empty stomach; avoid lying down for at least 30 min after administration
Zoledronic acid (Zometa)	Inhibits bone resorption	4 mg IV over 15 minutes	24–48 hrs	7–10 days	Fever, flulike symptoms, nausea, vomiting	Duration of infusion must not be less than 15 minutes (risk of renal function deterioration).
Cinacalcet (Sensipar)	Decreases PTH secretion	30 mg orally daily	24 hrs	1 wk	Nausea, vomiting	Approved for the treatment of secondary hyperparathyroidism in patients on dialysis; may cause increased seizure risk; take with food

IV, intravenously; SQ, subcutaneous; IM, intramuscularly; PTH, parathyroid hormone.

reabsorption. Although fluid rehydration and diuresis will reduce serum calcium levels, normocalcemia is rarely achieved in patients with severe hypercalcemia. Calcitonin, the most rapidly acting hypocalcemic agent, can acutely reduce renal calcium excretion by inhibiting bone resorption. Synthetic (salmon) and human calcitonin are available in the United States; however, most experience is with the more potent and longer-acting salmon calcitonin. Calcium levels decrease rapidly within 2 to 4 hours after administration of 4 IU per kilogram of calcitonin subcutaneously or intramuscularly every 12 hours. Doses can be increased to 8 IU per kilogram every 6 hours if the lower dosage is ineffective. The maximal calcium-lowering effect occurs within 12 to 24 hours of administration, but tolerance develops within 24 to 48 hours, limiting its usefulness.[20] Calcitonin is less potent than bisphosphonates and plicamycin, rarely lowering serum calcium more than 2 mg per deciliter. Normocalcemia is rarely achieved with calcitonin alone except in patients with mild hypercalcemia. The combination of a bisphosphonate and calcitonin produce a more rapid fall in serum calcium levels than a bisphosphonate alone. Therefore, this combination is especially useful in patients with severe hypercalcemia who require a rapid but sustained fall in serum calcium levels. Calcitonin is well tolerated. Flushing, mild nausea that is transient, and abdominal cramps are the most common side effects. Because of its potential for anaphylactoid reactions, the manufacturer recommends initial skin testing with 1 IU per 0.1 mL intracutaneously, especially in atopic patients or in those with a history of hypersensitivity to calcitonin. However, true allergic reactions are rare and treatment should not be withheld pending skin test results.

Chronic maintenance therapy to lower serum calcium levels may be considered in asymptomatic patients with only mild to moderately elevated serum calcium levels. However, there is little consensus among experts for which long-term pharmacologic agents should be used in primary hyperparathyroidism, if any, because long-term clinical outcomes (e.g., fracture risk or mortality) have not been shown. Most chronic therapies focus on maintaining normocalcemia in addition to reducing bone loss. Agents that have been used include estrogens and progestins, selective estrogen-receptor modulators, bisphosphonates, and the newer calcimimetic drugs. Table 39.5 summarizes the medication regimens used to treat hypercalcemia caused by primary hyperparathyroidism.

Numerous studies show that the chronic oral administration of estrogens and progestins with androgenic properties (e.g., norethindrone) reduce serum calcium levels minimally by 0.12 to 0.25 mmol per liter (0.5–1 mg/dL), reduce calciuria, and increase bone density in postmenopausal women with primary hyperparathyroidism.[21] Estrogens and progestins block PTH-mediated bone resorption without affecting circulating PTH levels. However, the discovery of the negative cardiovascular risks associated with estrogen therapy in postmenopausal women[22] has made it less favorable to use these agents in this population. A potential alternative is raloxifene (Evista), a selective estrogen-receptor modulator. Raloxifene binds to the estrogen receptor and acts as an estrogen agonist on bone and lipid metabolism and as an estrogen antagonist in the breast and uterus. It also appears to have similar effects as estrogen on calcium metabolism in postmenopausal women. In a short-term (8-week) study in 18 postmenopausal women with mild asymptomatic primary hyperparathyroidism, raloxifene reduced the serum calcium concentration by approximately 0.1 mmol per liter (0.4 mg/dL) from 2.7 mmol per liter (10.8 ± 0.2 mg/dL) to 2.6 mmol per liter (10.4 ± 0.2 mg/dL) and also reduced markers of bone turnover.[23] In three postmenopausal women with asymptomatic, mild hyperparathyroidism, a 12-month treatment of raloxifene reduced the total serum calcium and phosphate levels, and increased bone mineral density of the lumbar spine and femur neck by 3.4% and 2.5%, respectively.[24] Although levels of ionized calcium and intact PTH were lower at 6 months, both levels returned close to baseline values by 12 months. Overall, raloxifene seems to have a similar effect as estrogen therapy by modestly reducing serum calcium concentrations and increasing bone mineral density without sustained reductions in PTH level.

Because primary hyperparathyroidism is characterized by high bone turnover, bisphosphonates have also been used in the management of acute hypercalcemia. Bisphosphonates are stable pyrophosphate analogs that bind to hydroxyapatite in bone and act as potent inhibitors of PTH-mediated osteoclastic bone resorption. The calcium-lowering effect varies among bisphosphonates, and the effect is significantly weaker in patients with primary hyperparathyroidism than in patients with tumor-induced hypercalcemia. The first bisphosphonate to be used for this purpose was etidronate. Although effective for calcium lowering, etidronate impaired bone mineralization with chronic use, resulting in osteomalacia. Newer second-generation and third-generation bisphosphonates have improved efficacy, ease of use, and safety profiles so that etidronate is rarely used now for the treatment of hypercalcemia.

Pamidronate (Aredia), a second-generation bisphosphonate, is more potent than etidronate and is less likely to inhibit bone mineralization or osteoblast activity. It is the most widely used bisphosphonate for the treatment of hypercalcemia. Serum calcium levels start to fall within 24 to 48 hours after administration, but maximal effects may take up to 7 days. The higher the basal serum calcium level, the greater the reduction in serum calcium level after pamidronate treatment. Pamidronate is administered as a 60- or 90-mg intravenous infusion over 2 to 24 hours. Longer infusions are preferred in patients with preexisting renal dysfunction.[25] In the United States, pamidronate is available only intravenously. However, in countries where oral pamidronate is available, the intravenous route would still be preferred to minimize the gastrointestinal intolerance that occurs with oral administration. Repeat pamidronate doses should not be given before 7 days. Intravenous pamidronate may cause a mild, transient fever in 20% of patients, a small reduction in serum phosphate levels, and myalgias in 33% of patients. In postmenopausal hemodialysis patients with secondary hyperparathyroidism, pamidronate increased PTH levels after a single intravenous infusion, suggesting that pamidronate may worsen secondary hyperparathyroidism initially.[26] It is unclear whether these negative effects will continue with long-term use. Therefore, it seems prudent to avoid bisphosphonates in patients with secondary hyperparathyroidism due to renal failure.

Zoledronic acid (Zometa) is a third-generation parenteral bisphosphonate that is 100 to 800 times more potent than pamidronate in normalizing calcium levels. Normal calcium levels are also maintained longer with zoledronic acid.[9] Another advantage over pamidronate is its shorter infusion time. It is administered as a 4-mg intravenous infusion over 15 minutes. Zoledronic acid must not be infused faster than 15 minutes to avoid deterioration of renal function.[27] As with pamidronate, its calcium lowering effects are apparent after 24 to 48 hours, and a minimum of 7 days should elapse before repeating the dose to allow for maximal drug response.[27]

Second-generation oral bisphosphonates include alendronate, tiludronate, and risedronate. Currently, alendronate and risedronate are approved for the treatment of osteoporosis in the United States, although alendronate is approved in Europe for the treatment of mild hypercalcemia. Clinical trials of oral alendronate in small numbers of patients with primary hyperparathyroidism show significant increases (e.g., 4%–6%) in vertebral bone density.[28,29] However, its biochemical effects on serum calcium lowering are modest and not sustainable longer than 3 months.[28]

Cinacalcet (Sensipar), an oral calcimimetic drug, is the first medical therapy approved for the treatment of hypercalcemia from primary hyperparathyroidism and secondary hyperparathyroidism caused by chronic kidney disease requiring dialysis.[30] It acts by increasing the affinity of the calcium-sensing receptor (CaR) on the surface of the chief cell of the parathyroid gland to extracellular calcium. This leads to an increase in intracellular calcium, thereby decreasing the secretion of PTH. In turn, this results in lower serum calcium levels. When cinacalcet was given to patients with mild primary hyperparathyroidism (mean baseline serum calcium concentration 2.7 mmol/L or 10.6 mg/dL), serum calcium levels normalized after the second dose and remained normal throughout the study period.[31] In addition, serum PTH levels decreased by more than 50% within 2 to 4 hours after dosing.[31] Long-term clinical trials with cinacalcet have demonstrated normalization of the serum calcium levels for up to 3 years.[32] However, cinacalcet has not demonstrated any change in the bone mineral density as measured

by dual-energy x-ray absorptiometry. The most commonly reported side effects of cinacalcet are nausea and vomiting. Cinacalcet has also been shown to be effective in lowering PTH and serum calcium levels in patients with secondary hyperparathyroidism receiving hemodialysis.[33]

Plicamycin and gallium nitrate are rarely used today for management of hypercalcemia from primary hyperparathyroidism due to their toxicities and the availability of equally effective or superior but less toxic alternatives. Their use is limited to severe hypercalcemia unresponsive to the agents listed previously.

Plicamycin (mithramycin), an antitumor antibiotic that inhibits bone resorption, is the oldest and least expensive agent for producing a prolonged normocalcemic response. However, because of its high risk of toxicity and the availability of effective, more tolerable alternatives, plicamycin generally is reserved for patients who are intolerant or unresponsive to bisphosphonates. Serum calcium concentrations begin to fall 6 hours after a single 4-hour intravenous infusion of 25 μg per kilogram. Because maximum reductions in calcium levels might not occur for 2 to 4 days, it is advisable to wait at least 48 hours before administering additional doses to avoid hypocalcemia. However, repeated doses (i.e., 3 or 4) might be necessary. The duration of action is highly variable, ranging from 5 to 15 days. Nausea is a common side effect and can be minimized by slow intravenous infusion. Care should be used to prevent local extravasation of plicamycin. Plicamycin can also cause hepatotoxicity, with serum aminotransferase elevation seen in 20% of patients, nephrotoxicity (increased serum creatinine and blood urea nitrogen concentration, and proteinuria), and thrombocytopenia. These adverse effects are more likely after repeated administration. Plicamycin is contraindicated in patients with hepatic or renal dysfunction, bone marrow suppression, or coagulation disorders. However, lower doses of 12.5 μg/kg/day can be cautiously tried in patients with preexisting hepatic or renal dysfunction.

Gallium nitrate, a potent inhibitor of bone resorption, is approved for the treatment of hypercalcemia associated with malignancy. Gallium nitrate does not affect bone mineralization. In patients with malignancy-induced hypercalcemia, a continuous intravenous infusion of gallium nitrate 200 mg/m^2/day for 5 days was more effective than salmon calcitonin 8 IU per kilogram subcutaneously every 6 hours for 5 days in achieving a longer duration (6 vs. 1 day) of normocalcemia.[34] Although the usual dose of gallium nitrate is a 200-mg/m^2 24-hour infusion for 5 consecutive days, 100 mg/m^2 for 5 days may be warranted in patients with mild hypercalcemia. The onset of effect is 24 to 48 hours after the first dose, and the maximum response observed within 7 to 10 days. The major adverse effect associated with gallium nitrate is nephrotoxicity. It should be avoided in patients with a serum creatinine above 221 μmol per liter (2.5 mg/dL) or with the concomitant administration of nephrotoxic drugs such as aminoglycosides or amphotericin B. Patients should be well hydrated, and serum creatinine and blood urea nitrogen concentrations should be monitored. Other side effects include hypophosphatemia, hypocalcemia, and anemia (in high doses).

Although corticosteroids are usually not effective for treating hypercalcemia from primary hyperparathyroidism, they may be effective in managing malignancy-induced hypercalcemia.[20]

Dialysis should be considered for hypercalcemia complicated by renal failure. Peritoneal dialysis and hemodialysis with calcium-free dialysis fluid are equally effective in rapidly removing large quantities of calcium from the blood. Serum calcium levels might be reduced by 0.7 to 3 mmol per liter (3–12 mg/dL) over 24 to 48 hours. Because phosphate is also removed in dialysis, serum phosphate levels should be monitored after dialysis and supplemented if necessary. Vitamin D analogues may be indicated in patients with secondary hyperparathyroidism due to chronic renal failure. Paricalcitol has been approved for the prevention and the treatment of hyperparathyroidism associated with chronic renal failure (Table 39.5).

NONPHARMACOLOGIC THERAPY

In general, adults with hyperparathyroidism should adhere to the current standards for optimal calcium intake (1,000–1,500 mg/day in 3–4 divided doses).[35] In fact, there is concern that calcium restricted diets (<750 mg/day) may further stimulate PTH secretion. Many patients with primary hyperparathyroidism have low levels of 25-hydroxyvitamin D, and should receive adequate supplementation. Levels of 1, 25-dihydroxyvitamin D_3 below 20 ng per milliliter may also stimulate PTH secretion.[35] Doses of 400 to 600 IU/day of vitamin D are recommended, although serum calcium levels must be monitored frequently to prevent the development of hypercalcemia. Higher dosages of vitamin D or calcium should be avoided because hypercalcemia, hypercalciuria, and potentially, kidney stones can develop.[8] Prolonged bed rest and immobilization should also be avoided to prevent increased bone resorption, decreased bone formation, and subsequent hypercalciuria and hypercalcemia. Patients should also be advised to stay well hydrated to avoid worsening the hypercalcemia.

FUTURE THERAPIES

The newer calcimimetic drugs are the first medical agents that reduce PTH levels and serum calcium levels. It remains to be seen with future studies if such agents will reduce major health outcomes such as death, cardiovascular events, and bone disease.

IMPROVING OUTCOMES

PATIENT EDUCATION

Patients with asymptomatic, mild hyperparathyroidism who do not undergo parathyroidectomy should be advised to

follow-up with a clinician at least every 6 months. Patients with inconsistent or poor medical follow-up should be considered for parathyroid surgery. If long-term hypocalcemic agents are started, patients should be properly educated about each individual agent. With alendronate it is very important that patient be instructed to take the dose on an empty stomach (e.g., administer on arising in the morning) to maximize absorption. Also, the patient must take each dose with at least 6 to 8 oz of water, and avoid lying down for at least one-half hour after the dose to reduce the risk of esophageal erosions or ulcers.

METHODS TO IMPROVE ADHERENCE TO DRUG THERAPY

Treatment for acute hypercalcemia caused by primary hyperparathyroidism usually requires hospitalization. However, the availability of zoledronic acid, a bisphosphonate with an infusion time of 15 minutes, may allow a patient to be discharged earlier. Similarly, pamidronate may be administered over a minimum of 2 hours in patients with normal renal function.

DISEASE MANAGEMENT STRATEGIES TO IMPROVE PATIENT OUTCOMES

All patients who are surgical candidates should be strongly encouraged to undergo parathyroidectomy (Table 39.3). Patients with asymptomatic primary hyperparathyroidism who do not undergo parathyroid surgery must be monitored carefully. The parameters that should be followed and the frequency of monitoring have been previously discussed under "Therapeutic Plan."[35] The serum calcium levels should be measured twice yearly and the creatinine clearance estimated using the Cockcroft-Gault equation.[36] In addition, bone density of the lumbar spine, hip, and forearm should be obtained on a yearly basis. Studies have shown that up to 25% of asymptomatic patients develop indications for surgery during medical observation.[10]

Although consensus guidelines for primary hyperparathyroidism have been developed to identify potential candidates for parathyroid surgery, no similar recommendations have been made regarding specific long-term hypocalcemic treatments for nonsurgical patients. It is important to note that despite efficacy in reducing serum calcium levels and other biochemical markers, none of the pharmacologic agents used in primary hyperparathyroidism, including bisphosphonates and cinacalcet, have been shown to reduce the incidence of fractures, cardiovascular disease, or death. Further study is needed to determine if the long-term medical management of mild to moderate hypercalcemia due to primary hyperparathyroidism has an impact on these health indicators.

In selecting an appropriate approach to managing hypercalcemia secondary to hyperparathyroidism, a patient's

TABLE 39.5	Comparison of Vitamin D Preparations				
Preparation	**Abbreviation**	**Brand Name**	**Dosage**	**Characteristics**	**Activity**	**Comments**
Calciferol Ergocalciferol Capsules 50,000 IU Liquid 8,000 IU/mL Injection 500,000 IU/mL	Vitamin D_2	Calciferol, Drisdol	Initial: 50,000 IU/day Maintenance: 50,000–200,000 IU/day 1 mg = 40,000 IU 3 mg = 120,000 IU	Restores normocalcemia in 4–8 wk; maximal effects in 4–12 wk; long $t_{1/2}$; slow elimination; persists 6–18 wk after cessation	Biologically inactive; requires activation by hepatic 25-hydroxylation and renal 1-α-hydroxylase	Least expensive; bile salts needed for complete absorption in gut; short shelf-life
Dihydrotachysterol Tablets 0.125 mg, 0.2 mg, 0.4 mg Solution 0.2 mg/mL	DHT	Hytakerol	Initial: 0.75–2.5 mg/day Maintenance: 0.2–1.75 mg/day	Restores normocalcemia in 1–2 wk; maximal effect in 1–2 wk; persists 1–3 wk after cessation	Requires only hepatic 25-hydroxylation for activation; contains 1α-hydroxyl group so no kidney activation necessary	Three times more potent than vitamin D_2; main action is to increase intestinal calcium absorption; calcium supplementation recommended; more effective in chronic renal failure and hypoparathyroidism than vitamin D_2
Calcifediol (25-hydroxy-cholecalciferol) Capsules 20 μg 50 μg	25-(OH)-D_3	Calderol	Initial: 50 μg/day Maintenance: 50–100 μg/day	Restores normocalcemia in 2–4 wk; $t_{1/2}$ 16 days; persists 4–12 wks after cessation	Requires kidney for bioactivation	1.5 times as potent as vitamin D_2; preparation of choice in intestinal malabsorption and hepatobiliary disease; also effective in renal osteodystrophy; therapeutic blood level monitoring available
Calcitriol (1,25-dihydroxy-vitamin D_3) Capsules 0.25 μg, 0.5 μg Injection 1 μg/mL 2 μg/mL	1,25-(OH)$_2$-D_3	Rocaltrol, Calcijex	Initial: 0.25 μg/day Maintenance: 0.5–2 μg/day	Restores normocalcemia in 3–7 days; $t_{1/2}$ 5–8 hr; persists 3–5 days after cessation; dose may be increased by 0.5–1 μg/day q2–4 wks	Active	Expensive, and most potent preparation available; requires calcium supplementation in hypoparathyroidism; major advantage is rapid onset.
Paricalcitol Injection 2 μg/mL 5 μg/mL Capsules 1, 2, 4 μg	19-nor-1,25-(OH)$_2$-D_2	Zemplar	Initial: 0.04–0.1 μg/kg IV bolus 3 × /week (maximum 0.24 μg/kg) during hemodialysis	$t_{1/2}$ 15 hr; dosage may be increased q2–4wk	Active	Approved for prevention and treatment of secondary hyperparathyroidism associated with chronic renal failure; monitor serum calcium and phosphate levels monthly and parathyroid hormone levels q3mo
Doxercalciferol Capsules 2.5 μg Injection 2 μg/mL	1,25-(OH)$_2$-D_2	Hectorol	Initial: 10 μg 3 × /week at dialysis	$t_{1/2}$ 32–37 hr	Undergoes metabolic activation in vivo to active form (does not require kidneys for activation)	Approved for treatment of secondary hyperparathyroidism associated with chronic renal failure

IV, intravenously

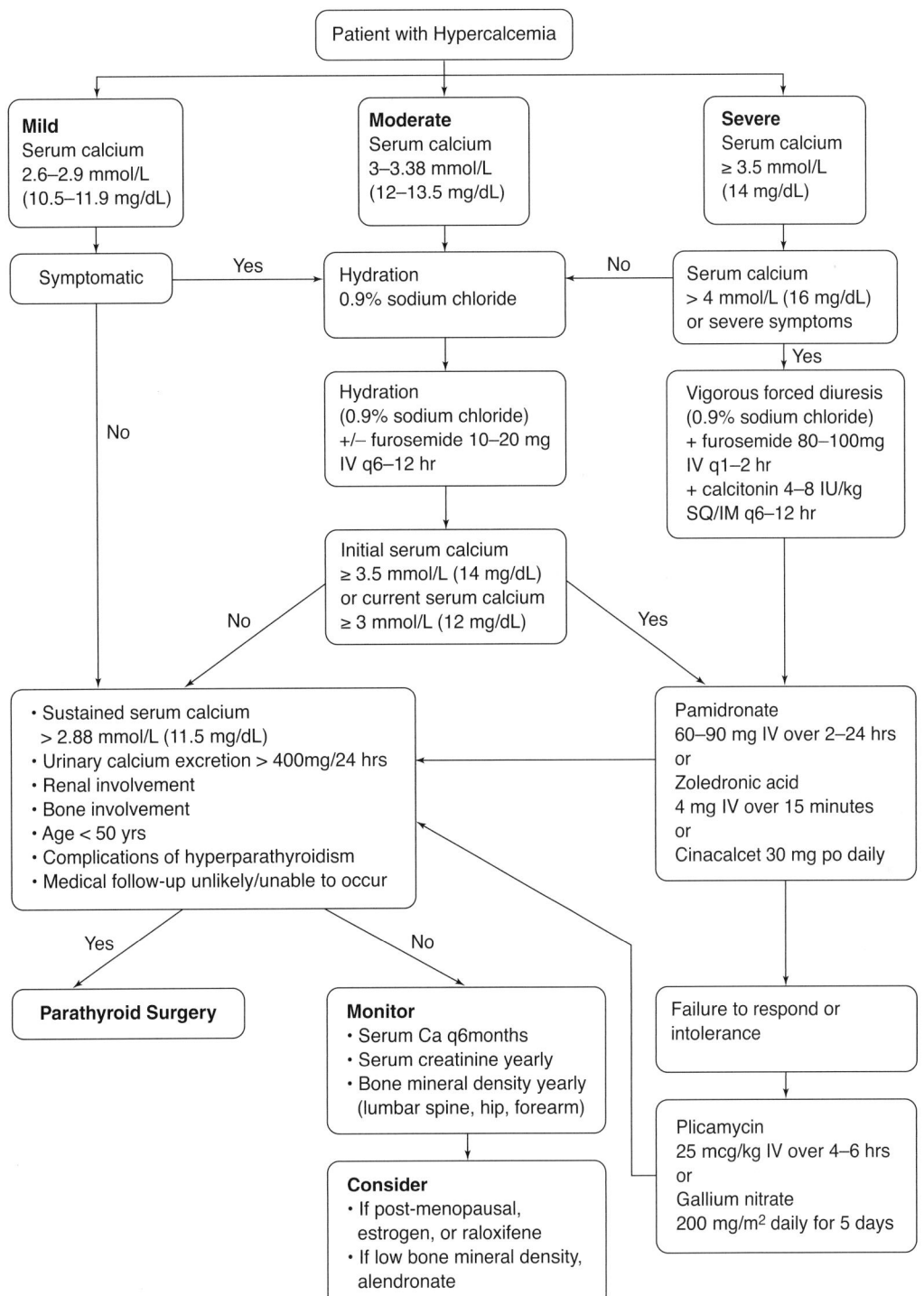

FIGURE 39.4 Algorithm for the management of hypercalcemia due to primary hyperparathyroidism.

serum calcium level and clinical status must be determined (Fig. 39.4). All patients with a serum calcium level of 3 mmol per liter (12 mg/dL) or higher should be hydrated immediately with intravenous saline. If the clinical symptoms and hypercalcemia are mild (serum calcium 2.6–2.9 mmol/L; 10.5–11.9 mg/dL), hydration alone often is suffi-

cient, without the addition of drug therapy. In moderate hypercalcemia (serum calcium 3–3.38 mmol/L; 12–13.5 mg/dL), hydration with saline should be followed by a saline diuresis, with or without the addition of furosemide, depending on the patient's fluid status. If subsequent serum calcium levels remain above 3 mmol per liter (12 mg/dL), pamidronate or zoledronic acid should be administered. If the serum calcium is greater than 3.5 mmol per liter (14 mg/dL) or if the patient is severely symptomatic, a rapidly acting agent, calcitonin, should be administered along with hydration. Concurrently, pamidronate or zoledronic acid should be initiated to provide a sustained effect. Alternatively, cinacalcet could be initiated to provide sustained reductions in serum calcium levels and PTH levels. Cinacalcet is preferred over bisphosphonates in patients with secondary hyperparathyroidism on hemodialysis because the latter has been noted to increase PTH levels initially. If the patient does not respond or cannot tolerate a bisphosphate, plicamycin, or gallium, nitrate can be considered if there are no contraindications (e.g., renal or hepatic dysfunction, thrombocytopenia, or coagulopathy). If the patient has marked hypercalcemia, but a less urgent reduction in serum calcium is appropriate (e.g., serum calcium >3.5 mmol/L, or 14 mg/dL, with mild to moderate symptoms), pamidronate or zoledronic acid might be started with saline (with or without furosemide) rather than calcitonin. Postmenopausal women should be considered for a selective estrogen-receptor modulator if there are no contraindications. In patients with asymptomatic primary hyperparathyroidism with low bone mineral density, alendronate may be a useful alternative to parathyroid surgery.

PHARMACOECONOMICS

Parathyroid surgery is the most cost-effective management of primary hyperparathyroidism for patients who meet surgery criteria (Table 39.3). Parathyroidectomy is also cost-effective in patients experiencing depressive symptoms with hyperparathyroidism because parathyroid surgery can eliminate or reduce the need for antidepressant medications in up to 54% of patients.[5]

For the management of hypercalcemia, saline hydration with or without a loop diuretic is an effective and inexpensive way to lower serum calcium. Calcitonin lowers serum calcium more rapidly, but it is more expensive. Therefore, it should be reserved for symptomatic patients or patients with markedly elevated serum calcium levels who require a rapid reduction. In addition, calcitonin's calcium-lowering effects are limited after 48 hours of therapy, thus, a bisphosphonate should be started simultaneously. A single 4-mg dose of zoledronic acid has a wholesale price of almost $1,000,[37] whereas a 60-mg dose of pamidronate is almost half the price of zoledronic acid.[37] However, because zoledronic acid may be infused over a 15-minute period versus a minimum 2-hour period for pamidronate, the additional monitoring time and required length of stay in the hospital or infusion center must also be considered in the cost decision.

TREATMENT GOALS: HYPOPARATHYROIDISM

- Increase serum calcium levels.
- Reverse hyperphosphatemia.
- Reverse signs and symptoms of hypocalcemia.
- Prevent complications resulting from hypocalcemia.
- Prevent vitamin D toxicity.

HYPOPARATHYROIDISM

DEFINITION

Hypoparathyroidism is an endocrine disorder characterized by decreased secretion or peripheral action of PTH, resulting in hypocalcemia and hyperphosphatemia.

ETIOLOGY/EPIDEMIOLOGY

The most common cause of hypoparathyroidism is damage to or removal of the parathyroid glands during surgical exci-

sion or exploration of the anterior neck. With an experienced surgeon, the risk of developing postoperative hypoparathyroidism is less than 5%.[1,17]

There are numerous other causes of hypoparathyroidism. Table 39.6 outlines other possible causes of hypocalcemia. Rare causes include idiopathic hypoparathyroidism, neonatal hypoparathyroidism, destruction of the parathyroid glands by radiation or metastatic disease, inactive PTH, and target organ resistance to PTH (pseudohypoparathyroidism). Nonparathyroid causes of hypocalcemia include functional hypoparathyroidism resulting from severe hypomagnese-

TABLE 39.6 | Selected Causes of Hypocalcemia

Hypoparathyroidism

  Postsurgical: thyroidectomy, parathyroidectomy, neck exploration

  Idiopathic

  Congenital (DiGeorge's Syndrome, velocardiofacial syndrome, autoimmune polyglandular syndrome type 1

  Neonatal (prematurity, asphyxia)

  Destruction of parathyroids (tumor, radiation)

  Pseudohypoparathyroidism (end-organ resistance to parathyroid hormone)

  Inactive parathyroid hormone

Magnesium deficiency (functional hypoparathyroidism)

Acute pancreatitis or malabsorption

Renal failure (secondary hypoparathyroidism)

Osteomalacia

Drugs: phenytoin, phenobarbital, cholestyramine; laxative abuse with phosphate enemas; aminoglycosidenephrotoxicity; foscarnet

Hyperphosphatemic states: rhabdomyolysis, chemotherapy (causing cell lysis), malignant hyperthermia

Vitamin D deficiency

mia. Because magnesium is needed for normal release of PTH and for the action of PTH peripherally, hypocalcemia might persist until the hypomagnesemia is corrected. Some causes of hypomagnesemia include starvation, prolonged intravenous feeding (parenteral nutrition), malabsorption, chronic alcoholism, diuretics, aminoglycosides, and *cis*-platinum therapy. Malabsorption and chronic pancreatitis can significantly reduce intestinal calcium and fat soluble vitamin absorption, especially of vitamin D.

The long-term use of anticonvulsants such as phenytoin, phenobarbital, and structurally related compounds increases the hepatic conversion of vitamin D_3 (cholecalciferol) and 25-hydroxycholecalciferol (25-OH-D_3) to biologically inactive metabolites, causing decreased concentrations of 25-OH-D_3, malabsorption of calcium, hypocalcemia, and osteomalacia. This risk is greater in patients on long-term combination anticonvulsant therapy, low dietary calcium intake, little sunlight exposure, diseases predisposing to vitamin D malabsorption, and in dark-skinned individuals because of their greater resistance to the irradiating effects of sunlight. Changes in serum calcium, alkaline phosphatase and phosphate levels, and the bony changes of osteomalacia should be monitored closely in these patients.

Another iatrogenic cause of hypocalcemia and osteomalacia is long-term administration of cholestyramine, which binds the bile acids necessary for vitamin D absorption from the intestine. Therapy with higher doses of vitamin D is necessary to overcome the inhibitory effects of cholestyramine on vitamin D absorption.

PATHOPHYSIOLOGY

Deficiency of PTH decreases bone resorption, causes hyperphosphatemia and hypophosphaturia, decreases intestinal absorption of calcium, decreases levels of active 1,25-$(OH)_2$-vitamin D, causes hypocalcemia and hypercalciuria, and causes metabolic alkalosis due to decreased bicarbonate excretion.

CLINICAL PRESENTATION AND DIAGNOSIS

SIGNS AND SYMPTOMS

The clinical manifestations of hypoparathyroidism are related to the severity and chronicity of hypocalcemia. Abrupt declines in serum calcium level (e.g., within the first 48 hours after parathyroidectomy) are much more likely to produce hypocalcemic symptoms than gradual reductions of calcium levels. Changes in acid-base status also affect the symptoms. Metabolic alkalosis worsens the hypocalcemia by increasing the plasma protein binding of calcium and decreasing the free ionized fraction. Conversely, metabolic acidosis improves the hypocalcemia by increasing the free, active, ionized calcium levels. The signs and symptoms of hypocalcemia and hypoparathyroidism are presented in Table 39.7.

DIAGNOSIS AND CLINICAL FINDINGS

Hypoparathyroidism should be suspected in the presence of hypocalcemia, hyperphosphatemia, low or undetectable levels of PTH, and a history of neck surgery. Serum phosphate concentrations may not always be elevated because of dietary restrictions, use of aluminum-containing phosphate binders, or increased mineral uptake by bone. Normal or elevated PTH levels with hypocalcemia excludes the diagnosis of true hypoparathyroidism and strongly suggests end-organ resistance to PTH (pseudohypoparathyroidism) or secretion of inactive PTH hormone. Serum magnesium levels should be checked to exclude the diagnosis of functional hypoparathyroidism. Other causes of hypocalcemia, including drugs, should be excluded (Table 39.6).

THERAPEUTIC PLAN

The primary treatments for hypoparathyroidism are high doses of calcium supplements, vitamin D or vitamin D analogues, and drugs that increase renal tubular reabsorption of calcium, such as thiazide diuretics. Renal production of 1,25-$(OH)_2$-vitamin D does not occur in any of the hypoparathyroid states because it is PTH-dependent (Fig. 39.5).[3] Hence, vitamin D supplementation with an active analogue is essential to ensure that vitamin D needs are met.

TABLE 39.7	Clinical Features of Hypocalcemia and Hypoparathyroidism		
System	**Signs and Symptoms**	**Complications**	**Comments**
Musculoskeletal	Circumoral and distal numbness and tingling, muscle twitching, hyperreflexia, positive Chvostek and Trousseau signs	Tetany: carpopedal spasms, laryngeal stridor, convulsions	Emergency treatment with intravenous calcium needed
Neurologic	Papilledema, increased cerebrospinal fluid pressure, basal ganglia calcifications, extrapyramidal symptoms, abnormal electroencephalogram	Epilepsy, parkinsonism; complication in 20% of patients with hypoparathyroidism	Improves with eucalcemia, increased sensitivity to dystonic reactions with phenothiazines
Psychiatric	Irritability, paranoia	Depression, psychosis, mental retardation in 20% of children	May improve with eucalcemia
Integument	Dry, scaly skin, coarse, friable dry hair, longitudinal nail ridges	Exfoliative dermatitis, atopic eczema, psoriasis, *candida* infection	May improve with eucalcemia
Ocular	Visual impairment and lens opacities	Lenticular cataracts most common sequelae of hypoparathyroidism	Eucalcemia halts progression of cataracts
Cardiac	Symptoms of heart failure, irregular rhythm, ↑ Q-T interval, T-wave peaks, and inversions	Cardiac dilation	Improves with eucalcemia
Others	Impaired dental development, intestinal malabsorption with steatorrhea		Improves with eucalcemia
Laboratory results	Increased creatine phosphokinase, lactate dehydrogenase, ↓ calcium, ↑ phosphate, urinary phosphate low, urinary calcium low to absent, parathyroid hormone low		

TREATMENT

PHARMACOTHERAPY

A daily intake of 1,000 to 2,000 mg elemental calcium in three or four divided doses usually is sufficient to maintain calcium homeostasis in patients with mild hypoparathyroidism. Symptomatic patients with serum calcium levels below 1.87 mmol per liter (7.5 mg/dL) often need concomitant therapy with vitamin D to maintain eucalcemia. Therapy directed at reducing serum phosphorus levels generally is not necessary because normalization of serum calcium levels reduces the renal threshold for phosphorus excretion and lowers serum phosphorus concentrations. However, if serum calcium levels remain low with high serum phosphorus concentrations after a few weeks of calcium supplementation, a phosphate binder should be added to bind and prevent absorption of dietary phosphorus, and a moderately restricted phosphorus diet should be initiated to allow increased calcium absorption.

If dietary intake is inadequate, effective calcium supplementation can be provided with various calcium-containing salts. Calcium gluconate, containing small amounts of calcium, is not very palatable because a large number of tablets must be administered to attain a therapeutic dose. Similarly, calcium chloride is most likely to cause gastric irritation. Calcium carbonate usually is preferred because it is well tolerated, fewer tablets are needed, and it is more effective than supplements containing small amounts of calcium (gluconate, lactate). Calcium must be in a soluble, ionized form in the intestine for absorption to occur. Ionization of calcium occurs in an acidic intestinal pH. Conversely, alkaline intestinal pH retards calcium absorption. Therefore, calcium carbonate is poorly absorbed in patients with achlorhydria, such as older adults, and should be administered with food in this

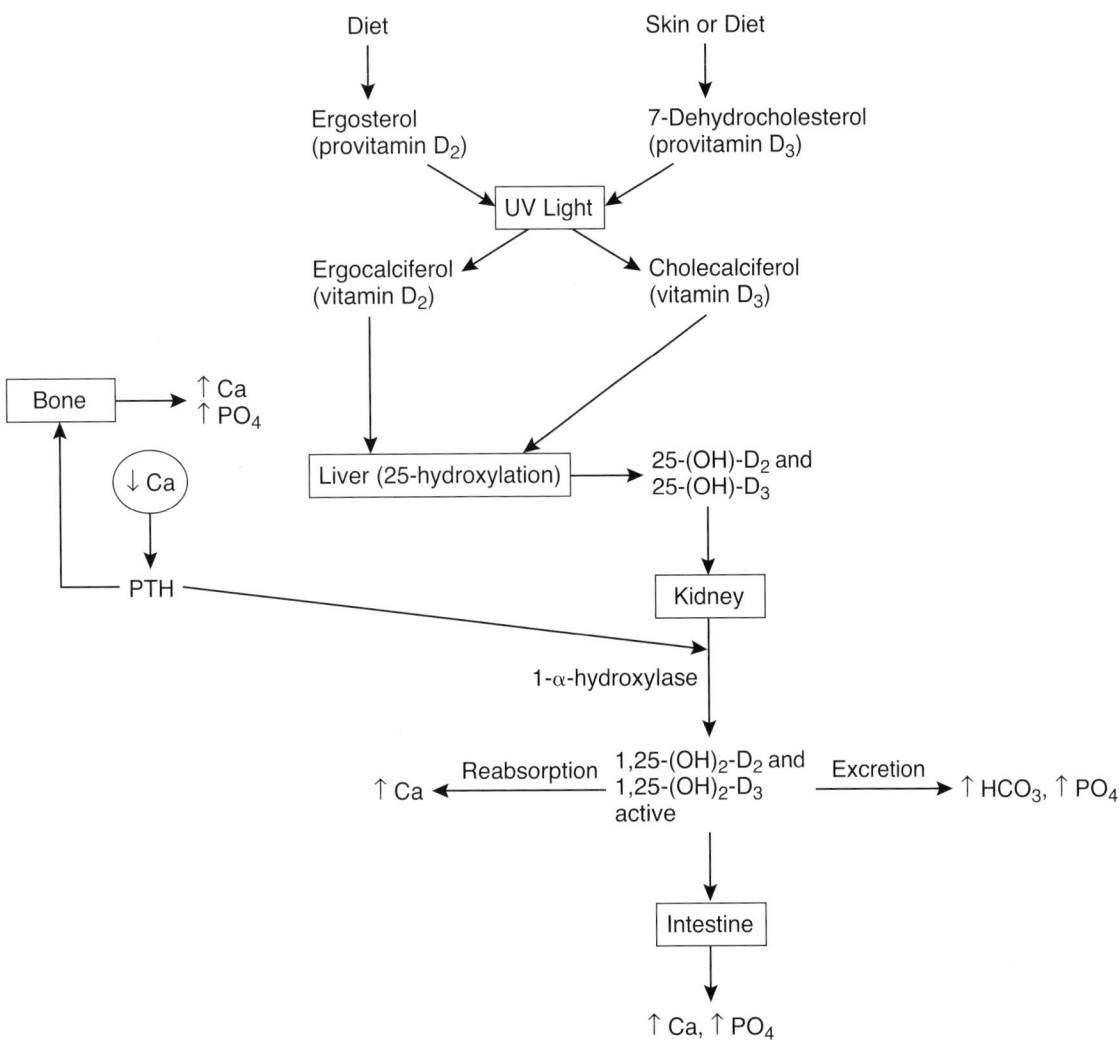

FIGURE 39.5 Relationship and metabolism of vitamin D to PTH and calcium.

population to facilitate absorption. Calcium absorption is also poor in patients with renal osteodystrophy, steatorrhea, or uremia.

The following salts provide 1 g calcium:

Calcium carbonate   2.5 g (40% calcium)
Tricalcium phosphate   2.6 g (39% calcium)
Calcium chloride   3.7 g (27% calcium)
Calcium acetate   4.0 g (25% calcium)
Calcium citrate   4.75 g (21% calcium)
Calcium lactate   7.7 g (13% calcium)
Calcium gluconate   11.0 g (9% calcium)

Constipation is a potential problem with all calcium supplements and may require management with regular bulk-forming agents and/or stool softeners.

Vitamin D should be started for hypocalcemic symptoms as soon as possible. The general term "vitamin D" refers to any form of vitamin D. Vitamin D metabolism is depicted in Figure 39.5. Vitamin D_3 (cholecalciferol) is produced in the skin after ultraviolet sunlight exposure. Provitamin D_2

(ergosterol) is absorbed from the distal ileum from dietary sources and undergoes metabolism by ultraviolet sunlight exposure to ergocalciferol (vitamin D_2). The active form of vitamin D is 1,25-dihydroxy-vitamin D, or 1,25-$(OH)_2$-D, which is activated in the kidney by the 1-α-hydroxylase enzyme after hepatic 25-hydroxylation; 1,25-$(OH)_2$-D_2 and 1,25-$(OH)_2$-D_3 are equally active. The selection of an appropriate vitamin D preparation depends on the cause of the hypocalcemia, onset of action, metabolism, duration of toxicity after discontinuation, and cost. The 1-hydroxylated forms of vitamin D are more potent and act more quickly because hepatic conversion to the active form is unnecessary. Serum calcium levels may increase from 1.5 mmol per liter (6 mg/dL) up to 2.2 mmol per liter (8.8 mg/dL) within a few days, rather than a few weeks for vitamin D_2 or vitamin D_3. In addition, serum calcium levels decrease more rapidly on discontinuation of 1-hydroxylated compounds, an advantage in the case of inadvertent overdose. However, the effects of vitamin D_2 or D_3 may take several weeks to months to disappear because they are stored in body fat and released slowly. Vitamin D products should not be interchanged without careful monitoring and consideration. In addition, considerable confusion occurs about dose equivalence because some preparations are dosed in international units, whereas others are dosed in weight (milligrams or micrograms); 1 mg vitamin D_2 (ergocalciferol) is equal to 40,000 IU.

Vitamin D_2 is commonly used in patients with long-standing hypoparathyroidism because it is the least expensive of all the preparations. Vitamin D_2 therapy can be initiated with 50,000 IU daily and then gradually increased to maintenance doses of 50,000 to 200,000 IU per day after steady-state serum calcium levels are achieved at each dose level. Maximal effects on serum calcium usually are achieved in 4 to 6 weeks, but can take up to 12 weeks. Because of its slow onset of effect, dosage titration must be gradual. Conversely, dihydrotachysterol (DHT) or calcitriol might be preferred in patients with newly diagnosed hypoparathyroidism due to its fast onset of action. Calcitriol increases serum calcium levels within 1 to 2 days after treatment begins, and dissipates equally quickly on discontinuation. Calcitriol may be dosed initially at 0.25 to 0.5 μg once or twice daily. Serum calcium levels may be measured every 1 to 2 days if rapid stabilization is needed, with dose adjustment every 2 to 3 days. Stabilization to a lower maintenance dosage is possible within 1 month. Calcitriol exerts its action more rapidly than vitamin D_2, DHT, or calcifediol (25-OH-D_3) because it bypasses renal and hepatic hydroxylation. DHT is a synthetic reduction product of tachysterol, a close isomer of vitamin D. DHT is hydroxylated in the liver to 25-hydroxy-DHT, the major circulating active form of the drug, and it does not undergo further hydroxylation by the kidney. The initial dose of DHT is 0.8 to 2.4 mg daily for several days, then a maintenance dosage of 0.2 to 1 mg daily. To shorten the time to maximal action, DHT is occasionally initiated with a loading dosage of four times the daily maintenance dose for 2 days, followed by two times the daily maintenance dose for 2 days. However, such an approach increases the risk of toxicity and must be monitored carefully. Patients with widely fluctuating serum calcium levels because of medication noncompliance may be better treated with a longer-acting vitamin D_2 or D_3 product.

Because PTH and hypophosphatemia stimulate activity of renal 1-α-hydroxylase enzyme, a suitable vitamin D preparation in patients with hypoparathyroidism (where there is absence of PTH and hyperphosphatemia) that already contains the 1-α-hydroxyl group (i.e., DHT or calcitriol) would be appropriate. DHT still must undergo 25-hydroxylation by the liver, and therefore, should be avoided in the setting of hepatic disease.

Conversely, patients with renal osteodystrophy or hypocalcemia secondary to chronic renal disease may have more predictable results with calcitriol or DHT. A new synthetic vitamin D analog, paricalcitol [19-nor-1-α-25-(OH)$_2$-D_2], contains the 1-α-hydroxyl group and 25-hydroxyl group and has been approved for treating hyperparathyroidism secondary to chronic renal failure. Paricalcitol may be less likely to result in hypercalcemic and hyperphosphatemic complications than calcitriol in patients on chronic hemodialysis while effectively reducing PTH serum levels. It is available as an intravenous injection only and can be administered on days of hemodialysis.

Antiseizure medications such as phenytoin and phenobarbital induce hepatic enzymes, resulting in decreased plasma concentrations of 25-hydroxylated ergocalciferol and cholecalciferol. If DHT or ergocalciferol is administered, higher doses may be needed. However, any change in antiseizure medication may also necessitate a change in the vitamin D dosage. Calcifediol [25-(OH)D_3], which does not require hepatic hydroxylation, and calcitriol may be more stable choices.

To avoid hypercalcemia, doses of all vitamin D preparations should be increased gradually and only after maximal effects are achieved. Serum calcium levels should be maintained between 2.12 and 2.25 mmol per liter (8.5–9 mg/dL), leaving a margin for fluctuations. Serum calcium and phosphorus levels should be checked weekly at initiation of vitamin D therapy, then monthly during dose adjustments and at least every 3 months thereafter. An abdominal radiograph or ultrasound should be considered before vitamin D therapy is started and should be repeated every few years to check for nephrocalcinosis or stone formation. Patients should be monitored carefully for early signs of vitamin D intoxication, which include lassitude, anorexia, thirst, constipation, and bone pain. Frequent adjustments in vitamin D doses might be necessary to prevent vitamin D intoxication. Higher doses of vitamin D are needed for patients on anticonvulsants, oral contraceptives, and glucocorticoids. Estrogens decrease serum calcium by preventing bone resorption. Glucocorticoids reduce intestinal absorption of calcium by antagonizing vitamin D, decrease bone resorption by antagonizing PTH, and reduce renal tubular absorption of calcium.

Toxicities of all vitamin D preparations include hypercalcemia, hypercalciuria, and nephrolithiasis, which can be prevented by close monthly monitoring of serum calcium, phosphorus, and alkaline phosphatase levels. Availability of 25-(OH)-D_3 and 1,25-(OH)$_2$-D_3 assays in specialized centers might help prevent toxicity from hypercalcemia.

Thiazide diuretics and sodium restriction have been shown to reduce urinary calcium excretion in patients with mild hypocalcemia, allowing calcium and vitamin D supplementation to be reduced. Serum calcium levels should be monitored carefully. This therapy might also protect against the development of kidney stones, a potential complication of the long-term management of hypoparathyroidism. Long-term studies are necessary to assess the role of this approach. Patients with hypoparathyroidism might be more sensitive to the calciuretic effects of loop diuretics such as furosemide, so they should be avoided.

Patients who suddenly develop hypocalcemia, such as after inadvertent parathyroidectomy during thyroid surgery, should be immediately treated with intravenous calcium.[3]

After the patient's airway is cleared, 1 mg/kg/hour of elemental calcium is administered intravenously until symptoms are relieved or until the serum calcium level increases above 1.87 mmol per liter (7.5 mg/dL). Serum calcium levels should be monitored every 6 hours. The plasma calcium level should increase by approximately 0.5 mg/dL/100-mg calcium load per 24 hours. A too vigorous treatment of the hypocalcemia can cause irreversible tissue calcification. Hypomagnesemia should be corrected, and oral calcium and vitamin D supplements should be started immediately. Drugs that exacerbate hypocalcemia (i.e., loop diuretics) should be avoided. Phenothiazines should be used cautiously because dystonic reactions can occur. Also, inadvertent hypercalcemia can precipitate cardiac arrhythmias in patients receiving digoxin, and such patients need ECG monitoring while receiving intravenous calcium therapy.

Transient hypocalcemia commonly occurs after neck exploration, with normocalcemia reestablished within 1 week. Such patients should be given oral calcium supplements and reassessed in a few weeks. Vitamin D therapy may not be necessary at that point.

NONPHARMACOLOGIC THERAPY

Parathyroid autografts or allografts have sometimes been transplanted into the forearm muscles or the sternomastoid muscles in patients in whom accidental removal or devascularization of the parathyroid glands has occurred during thyroid or parathyroid surgery. Half of these grafts fail, and there is a high incidence of late autograft-mediated recurrence of hyperparathyroidism.[3]

FUTURE THERAPIES

There has been some success in using synthetic human PTH for the long-term treatment of chronic hypoparathyroidism. In a 3-year comparison study with calcitriol and calcium, hypoparathyroid patients receiving twice daily subcutaneous PTH had serum calcium levels within or just below the normal range.[38] Bone mineral density showed no significant difference between the two groups over the study period. Overall, the PTH was very well tolerated with few side effects and may offer an effective alternative to calcitriol therapy.[38] Teriparatide [recombinant human parathyroid hormone (1-34)] is available for the treatment of osteoporosis.

IMPROVING OUTCOMES

Patients with long-standing hypoparathyroidism may start with the slow-acting vitamin D_2 (ergocalciferol). Patients with newly diagnosed hypoparathyroidism may need DHT or calcitriol for a more rapid response. Patients with autoimmune polyglandular syndrome type 1, a condition in which the efficacy of treatment may vary, are best treated with vitamin D analogues that have a short half-life, such as

calcitriol.[3] Close monitoring of serum calcium and phosphate levels is important in ensuring adequate vitamin D doses and preventing toxicity. The prognosis of hypoparathyroidism is excellent. Improvement of most symptoms can be expected with restoration of normal serum calcium levels. In surgery-associated hypoparathyroidism, vitamin D therapy usually is withdrawn after 6 to 8 weeks of treatment to assess if the patient can maintain a normocalcemic state. Such an approach minimizes the risk of vitamin D intoxication.

PATIENT EDUCATION

Oral calcium absorption is most efficient with single doses of 500 mg or less taken on an empty stomach. However, calcium carbonate has reduced bioavailability in achlorhydric patients, such as older adults. Such patients should be instructed to take this preparation with meals. Calcium carbonate may reduce absorption of various drugs, including levothyroxine, iron, tetracyclines, and fluoroquinolone antibiotics, and should not be administered simultaneously with these products. Dosing of oral calcium carbonate should be separated by at least 2 to 4 hours from administration of the previously mentioned agents. Calcium citrate does not reduce iron absorption. Fiber does not significantly reduce absorption of calcium, although combination with wheat bran may.[39] Certain preparations of calcium (bone meal and dolomite) can be contaminated by lead and other heavy metals, although most commercial calcium products are tested to ensure that significant heavy metal contamination is not present. Dietary calcium may be an alternative to supplements (250 mL skim or whole milk provides approximately 300 mg elemental calcium). However, patients intolerant to dairy products should use calcium supplements.

Constipation is common in patients receiving calcium supplements. Patients should be instructed to increase their fiber and fluid intake; if necessary, a stool softener or bulk-forming laxative may be added.

METHODS TO IMPROVE ADHERENCE TO DRUG THERAPY

Calcium carbonate has the highest amount of calcium per tablet. A tablet containing calcium carbonate 500 mg provides 40% elemental calcium, or 200 mg. Tablets containing the highest amounts of elemental calcium should be selected to reduce the number of calcium tablets needed per day. Calcium carbonate preparations generally are well tolerated and preferred over other calcium salts. Although preparations combining calcium with vitamin D are available commercially, the amount of vitamin D contained in such supplements generally is too low for treatment of hypoparathyroidism. Calcium doses need to be taken in divided doses (maximum 500 mg elemental calcium per dose) to ensure adequate gut absorption of calcium.

PHARMACOECONOMICS

A large number of inexpensive calcium products are available over-the-counter. Vitamin D preparations are more costly than calcium preparations. Calcitriol is slightly more expensive than DHT.[37] Ergocalciferol is available without a prescription in the United States, but its cost is comparable to calcifediol when administered in high dosages. The newer vitamin D analogue, doxercalciferol, is 30% more expensive than calcitriol, but has approval for use in secondary hyperparathyroidism due to chronic renal failure.

In addition to cost, vitamin D selection depends on its onset of action and metabolism, the duration of toxicity after discontinuation, and the cause of the hypocalcemia (Table 39.6).

KEY POINTS

HYPERPARATHYROIDISM

- Hyperparathyroidism results in hypercalcemia, hypercalciuria, and increased PTH
- The majority of patients with hyperparathyroidism are asymptomatic
- Parathyroid surgery is indicated for symptomatic hyperparathyroidism
- Intravenous hydration is the treatment of choice for hypercalcemia
- Calcitonin produces its calcium-lowering effect rapidly, but its effects are not sustained beyond 72 hours
- Parenteral bisphosphonates have a slower onset of action, but provide sustained lowering of serum calcium for at least 1 week
- Cinacalcet results in a rapid reductions in serum calcium and PTH levels for patients with primary and secondary hyperparathyroidism

HYPOPARATHYROIDISM

- Hypoparathyroidism is caused by decreased secretion of PTH, resulting in hypocalcemia and hyperphosphatemia
- The most common cause of hypoparathyroidism is surgical excision or exploration of the neck
- Treatment includes oral intake of calcium and vitamin D
- Vitamin D selection depends on the preparation's onset of action, metabolism, duration of toxicity after discontinuation, cost of treatment, and the cause of hypocalcemia

SUGGESTED READINGS

Bilezikian JP, Potts JT Jr, Fuleihan GE, et al. Summary statement from a workshop on asymptomatic primary hyperparathyroidism: a per-

spective for the 21st century. J Clin Endocrinol Metab 87: 5353–5361, 2002.
Bilezikian JP, Silverberg SJ. Asymptomatic primary hyperparathyroidism. N Engl J Med 350:1746–1751, 2004.
Marx SJ. Hyperparathyroidism and hypoparathyroid disorders. N Engl J Med 343:1863–1875, 2000.
NIH Conference 1991. Diagnosis and management of asymptomatic primary hyperparathyroidism: consensus development conference statement. Ann Intern Med 114:593–597. 1991.

REFERENCES

1. Sosa JA, Udelsman R. New directions in the treatment of patients with primary hyperparathyroidism. Curr Probl Surg 40:803–849, 2003.
2. Marx SJ, Simonds WF, Agarwal SK, et al. Hyperparathyroidism in hereditary syndromes: special expressions and special managements. J Bone Miner Res 17 (Suppl 2):N37–N43, 2002.
3. Marx SJ. Hyperparathyroidism and hypoparathyroid disorders. N Engl J Med 343:1863–1875, 2000.
4. Solomon BL, Schaaf M, Smallridge RC. Psychologic symptoms before and after parathyroid surgery. Am J Med 96:101–106, 1994.
5. Wilhelm SM. Major depression due to primary hyperparathyroidism: a frequent and correctable disorder. Am Surg 70:175–179, 2004.
6. Seibel MJ, Gartenberg F, Silverberg SJ, et al. Urinary hydroxypyridinium cross-links of collagen in primary hyperparathyroidism. J Clin Endocrinol Metab 74:481–486, 1992.
7. Vestergaard P, Mosekilde L. Parathyroid surgery is associated with a decreased risk of hip and upper arm fractures in primary hyperparathyroidism: a controlled cohort study. J Intern Med 255:108–114, 2004.
8. Bilezikian JP, Silverberg SJ. Asymptomatic primary hyperparathyroidism. New Engl J Med 350:1746–1751, 2004.
9. Potts JT Jr. Diseases of the parathyroid gland and other hyper- and hypocalcemic disorders. In: Braunwald E, Fauci AS, Kasper DL, Hauser SL, Lomgo DL, Jameson JL, eds. Harrison's principles of internal medicine. 15th ed. New York:McGraw-Hill, 2001:2205–2226.
10. Silverberg SJ, Shane E, Jacobs TP, et al. A 10-year prospective study of primary hyperparathyroidism with or without parathyroid surgery. N Engl J Med 341:1249–1255, 1999.
11. Wermers RA, Khosla S, Atkinson EJ, et al. Survival after the diagnosis of primary hyperparathyroidism: a population-based study. Am J Med 104:115–122, 1998.
12. Hedback G, Oden A. Increased risk of death from primary hyperparathyroidism-an update. Eur J Clin Invest 28:271–276, 1998.
13. Nilsson IL, Yin L, Lundgren E, et al. Clinical presentation of primary hyperparathyroidism in Europe—a nationwide cohort analysis on mortality from nonmalignant causes. J Bone Miner Res 17 (Suppl 2):N68–N74, 2002.
14. Larsson K, Ljunghall S, Krusemo UB, et al. The risk of hip fractures in patients with primary hyperparathyroidism: a population-based cohort study with a follow-up of 19 years. J Intern Med 234: 585–593, 1993.
15. Development Conference Panel. Diagnosis and management of asymptomatic primary hyperparathyroidism: Consensus Development Conference statement. Ann Intern Med 114:593–597, 1991.
16. Curhan G. Fooling the parathyroid gland - will there be health benefits? (editorial). N Engl J Med 350:1565–1567, 2004.
17. Allendorf J, Kim L, Chabot J, et al. The impact of sestamibi on the outcome of parathyroid surgery. J Clin Endocrinol Metab 88: 3015–3018, 2003.
18. Christiansen P, Steiniche T, Brixen K, et al. Primary hyperparathyroidism: effect of parathyroidectomy on regional bone mineral density in Danish patients: a three-year follow-up study. Bone 25: 589–595,1999.
19. Carroll MF, Schade DS. A practical approach to hypercalcemia. Am Fam Physician 67:1959–1966, 2003.
20. Kearns AE, Thompson GB. Medical and surgical management of hyperparathyroidism. Mayo Clin Proc 77:87–91, 2002.
21. Marcus R. The role of estrogens and related compounds in the management of primary hyperparathyroidism. J Bone Miner Res 17 (Supp 2):N146–N149, 2002.
22. Rossouw JE, Anderson GL, Prentice RL, et al. Risks and benefits of estrogen plus progestin in healthy postmenopausal women: Principal

results from the Women's Health Initiative. JAMA 288:321–333, 2002.

23. Rubin MR, Lee KH, McMahon DJ, et al. Raloxifene lowers serum calcium and markers of bone turnover in postmenopausal women with primary hyperparathyroidism. J Endocrinol Metab 88: 1174–1178, 2003.

24. Zanchetta JR, Bogado CE. Raloxifene reverses bone loss in postmenopausal women with mild asymptomatic primary hyperparathyroidism. J Bone Miner Res 16:189–190, 2001.

25. Aredia Package Insert. Rev. Aug 2004. Available at: http://www.pharma.us.novartis.com/product/pi/pdf/aredia.pdf Accessed February 5, 2005.

26. Lu K, Yeung L, Lin SH, et al. Acute effect of pamidronate on PTH secretion in postmenopausal hemodialysis patients with secondary hyperparathyroidism. Am J Kidney Dis 42:1221–1227, 2003.

27. Zometa Package Insert. Rev. Nov 2004. Available at: http://www.pharma.us.novartis.com/product/pi/pdf/Zometa.pdf Accessed February 5, 2005.

28. Parker CR, Blackwell PJ, Fairbairn KJ, et al. Alendronate in the treatment of primary hyperparathyroidism-related osteoporosis: a 2-year study. J Clin Endocrinol Metab 87:4482–4489, 2002.

29. Chow CC, Chan WB, Li JKY, et al. Oral alendronate increases bone mineral density in postmenopausal women with primary hyperparathyroidism. J Clin Endocrinol Metab 88:581–587, 2003.

30. Sensipar (cinacalcet) package insert. Amgen Inc, 2004.

31. Shoback DM, Bilezikian JP, Turner SA, et al. The calcimimetic cinacalcet normalizes serum calcium in subjects with primary hyperparathyroidism. J Clin Endocrinol Metab 88:5644–5649, 2003.

32. Peacock M, Scumpia S, Bolognese MA, et al. Long term control of primary hyperparathyroidism with cinacalcet HCL [abstract]. J Bone Miner Res 18 (Suppl 2):S17, 2003.

33. Block GA, Martin KJ, deFrancisco AL, et al. Cinacalcet hydrochloride for secondary hyperparathyroidism in patients receiving hemodialysis. N Engl J Med 350:1516–1525, 2004.

34. Warrell RP Jr, Israel R, Frisone M, et al. Gallium nitrate for acute treatment of cancer-related hypercalcemia: a randomized, double-blind comparison to calcitonin. Ann Intern Med 108:669–674, 1988.

35. Bilezikian JP, Potts JT Jr, Fuleihan GE, et al. Summary statement from a workshop on asymptomatic primary hyperparathyroidism: a perspective for the 21st century. J Clin Endocrinol Metab 87: 5353–5361, 2002.

36. Cockcroft DW, Gault MH. Prediction of creatinine clearance from serum creatinine. Nephron 16:31–41, 1976.

37. Drug Topics Red Book. Montvale, NJ: Medical Economics Company, 2004.

38. Winer KK, Ko CW, Reynolds JC, et al. Long-term treatment of hypoparathyroidism: a randomized controlled study comparing parathyroid hormone (1–34) versus calcitriol and calcium. J Clin Endocrin Metab 88:4214–4220, 2003.

39. National Institutes of Health Conference Statement. Optimal calcium intake. JAMA 272:1942–1948, 1994.

Diabetes

40

Stephen M. Setter, John R. White, Jr., and R. Keith Campbell

Diabetes mellitus was recognized as early as 1500 BC by Egyptian physicians, who described a disease associated with ''the passage of much urine.'' The word *diabetes* (the Greek word for siphon) was coined by Greek physician Aretaeus the Cappadocian around 2 AD. Aretaeus noticed that patients with diabetes had a disease that caused the siphoning of the structural components of the body into the urine. Although it was known for centuries that the urine of patients with diabetes was sweet, it was not until 1674 that a physician named Willis coined the term *diabetes mellitus* (from the Greek word for honey).

Diabetes mellitus is a complex syndrome that affects virtually every cell in the body and can lead to pathology in multiple organ systems. There is still much to be learned about diabetes mellitus, but recent pharmacologic and surgical advances have enhanced our understanding and treatment of this syndrome. The landmark Diabetes Control and Complications Trial (DCCT) showed conclusively that the level of glycemic control is closely correlated with the appearance and progression of retinopathy, nephropathy, and neuropathy in patients with type 1 diabetes.[1] The results of the 20-year United Kingdom Prospective Diabetes Study (UKPDS) confirmed the benefit of strict glycemic control in patients with type 2 diabetes.[2-5] Strict glycemic control is within reach of many patients with diabetes now that self-monitoring of blood glucose (SMBG) is commonly practiced and better education programs and new treatment protocols are available. The overall treatment goal for all patients with diabetes is to achieve glycemic control to prevent the long-term complications of diabetes. Individual management to achieve this goal varies between patients but generally involves SMBG, nutritional counseling, exercise, and training in self-management and problem solving.[6]

A thorough, positive, and empowering education program for the patient with diabetes that covers the disease, medication, monitoring, and hygiene is a major component of diabetes management. Studies have shown that poor diabetes control is often the result of medication error, misinterpretation of test results, and ignorance of the disease.[7] Patient education is extremely important. Healthcare providers must explain the importance of diet control, nutritional therapy, and the food exchange system. Patients need to develop a positive and proactive attitude, learn how to perform tests to monitor control, learn proper insulin injection technique, and keep records of factors that affect glycemic control. Healthcare providers need to answer patients' questions about the disease, blood testing, drug therapy, diet and nutrition products, and foot care and reinforce the information that other members of the team provide. The pharmacist is an invaluable asset to the diabetes healthcare team. Because patients with diabetes see pharmacists more often than any other health professional, the pharmacist is in a unique position to have a significant impact on their treatment and quality of life. Pharmacists must become competent in selecting, initiating, and individualizing drug therapy for the various types of diabetes. Thus, the pharmacist performs three significant functions: referral, monitoring, and education.

DEFINITION

Diabetes mellitus is a spectrum of conditions that includes hyperglycemia as a common finding. Diabetes was once thought of as a single disease, but it is clearly a heterogeneous group of disorders that are secondary to various genetic predispositions and precipitating factors. Not only does type 1 diabetes (formerly known as insulin-dependent diabetes [IDDM]) differ from type 2 diabetes (formerly known as non–insulin-dependent diabetes [NIDDM]), but there appears to be heterogenicity within each of the two types.[8] Recently the word *prediabetes* has been adopted by the American Diabetes Association to classify patients with impaired glucose tolerance or impaired fasting glucose.[9] Diabetes is a chronic disease characterized by disorders in carbohydrate, fat, and protein metabolism caused by an absolute or relative deficiency in the action of insulin and possible abnormally high amounts of glucagon and other counterregulatory hormones such as growth hormone, sympathomimetic amines, and corticosteroids. Insulin secretion in patients with type 1 diabetes is normally deficient to nonexistent, whereas those with type 2 disease may have normal, high, or low insulin secretion.

In addition to type 1 and type 2 diabetes, there are many other potential underlying causes for the development of diabetes. One particular type, known as latent autoimmune diabetes of the adult or informally known as type 1.5, is thought to be responsible for up to 12% of people diagnosed with type 2 diabetes.[10,11] This is a slowly progressive type 1 variant and is just one example of a type of diabetes that does not fit into the broad category of being type 1 or type 2.

Classifying the patient with diabetes into one of several categories in which hyperglycemia is a clinical finding is critical in developing a patient-specific treatment regimen. In the past many classification schemes were used, often resulting in confusion. In 1997 an expert panel revised the criteria for diagnosing and classifying diabetes mellitus. Table 40.1 summarizes the new etiologic classification system with the updated terminology, and the new diagnostic criteria for diabetes mellitus are outlined in Table 40.2. ''Prediabetes'' can be used to describe patients with a fasting plasma glucose level of 100 to 125 mg per dL (5.6 to 6.9 mmol/L) to be in a category known as impaired fasting glucose. When using the oral glucose tolerance test, values of 140 to 199 mg per dL (7.8 to 11.1 mmol/L) after a glucose load are referred to as impaired glucose tolerance.

Type 1 diabetes results from immune-mediated destruction of the β cells of the pancreas, resulting in eventual absolute insulin deficiency. Roughly 5% to 10% of people

TABLE 40.1	Diabetes Mellitus: Etiologic Classification

Type 1 diabetes (β-cell destruction, usually leading to absolute insulin deficiency)
  Immune-mediated
  Idiopathic

Type 2 diabetes (may range from predominantly insulin resistance with relative insulin deficiency to a predominantly secretory defect with insulin resistance)

Other specific types
  Genetic defects of β-cell function
    May involve chromosome 12, HNF–1α, 7, 20, HNF–4α, 13, 17, 2,
    mitochondrial DNA
    Others

  Genetic defects in insulin action
    Type A insulin resistance, leprechaunism, Rabson-Mendenhall syndrome, lipoatrophic diabetes, others

  Diseases of the exocrine pancreas
    Pancreatitis
    Trauma/pancreatectomy
    Neoplasia
    Cystic fibrosis
    Hemochromatosis
    Fibrocalculous pancreatopathy
    Others

  Endocrinopathies
    Acromegaly
    Cushing's syndrome
    Pheochromocytoma
    Others

  Drug- or chemical-induced
    Vacor
    Pentamidine
    Nicotinic acid
    Glucocorticoids
    Phenytoin thyroid hormone
    β-adrenergic agonist
    Thiazides
    Others

  Infections
    Congenital rubella
    Cytomegalovirus
    Others

  Uncommon forms of immune-mediated diabetes
    "Stiff-man" syndrome
    Anti-insulin receptor antibodies
    Others

  Other genetic syndromes sometimes associated with diabetes
    Down's syndrome
    Klinefelter's syndrome
    Turner's syndrome
    Others

Gestational diabetes mellitus

(From Expert Committee on the Diagnosis and Classification of Diabetes Mellitus. Report of the expert committee on the diagnosis and classification of diabetes mellitus. Diabetes Care 20:1183–1197, 1997; and Expert Committee on the Diagnosis and Classification of Diabetes Mellitus. Follow-up report on the diagnosis of diabetes mellitus. Diabetes Care 26:3160–3167, 2003.)

HNF, hepatocyte nuclear factor.

TABLE 40.2 | **Diabetes Mellitus: Diagnostic Criteria**

Symptoms of diabetes plus casual plasma glucose concentration >200 mg/dL (11.1 mmol/L). *Casual* is defined as any time of day without regard to time since last meal.

The classic symptoms of diabetes include polyuria, polydipsia, and unexplained weight loss.

Or

Fasting plasma glucose >126 mg/dL (7.0 mmol/L). *Fasting* is defined as no caloric intake for at least 8 hours.

Or

Two-hour plasma glucose >200 mg/dL during an oral glucose tolerance test. A 75-g glucose load or equivalent is recommended when performing this test.

(From Expert Committee on the Diagnosis and Classification of Diabetes Mellitus. Report of the expert committee on the diagnosis and classification of diabetes mellitus. Diabetes Care 20:1183–1197, 1997; and Expert Committee on the Diagnosis and Classification of Diabetes Mellitus. Follow-up report on the diagnosis of diabetes mellitus. Diabetes Care 26:3160–3167, 2003.)

with diabetes have type 1 disease.[12] Patients with type 1 disease are more likely to develop ketoacidosis than patients with type 2. Patients with type 2 usually have some degree of insulin resistance with variable insulin secretion. Insulin secretion is said to be relatively deficient because many patients may have normal to elevated levels of insulin; however, their blood sugar levels remain elevated because of tissue resistance to the action of the insulin. Many patients with type 2 diabetes can survive without insulin; however, up to 40% use insulin at some point during the disease course. Table 40.3 compares the two major clinical types of diabetes.

Because up to 80% of diabetic patients die of cardiovascular disease, in recent years a strong emphasis in treating diabetic patients has been placed on reducing cardiovascular risk factors. Diabetic patients should normalize blood pressure, blood lipids, and coagulation and inflammatory factors in addition to achieving tight management of blood glucose levels.

TREATMENT GOALS

- Because diabetes is an incurable disease (unless pancreatic transplants or islet cell transplants are performed), focus on controlling blood sugar levels in the normal or near-normal range and preventing the short- and long-term complications associated with this disease.
- Maintain normal growth and development in children.
- Promote SMBG at least three or four times a day in those with type 1 diabetes and a sufficient number of times daily or weekly to facilitate reaching glucose goals in patients with type 2 diabetes.
- Administer medical and nutritional therapy that balances food intake with physical activity and pharmacologic therapies.
- Prevent symptoms of hyperglycemia, such as polyuria, blurred vision, weight loss, recurrent infection, ketoacidosis, and hyperosmolar hyperglycemia, and prevent symptoms of hypoglycemia, including mood changes, mental confusion, and coma.
- Prevent long-term complications (microvascular and macrovascular disease) by keeping blood glucose levels as close to normal as possible.
- Maintain appropriate blood pressure and lipid values.
- Treat other physiologic derangements when present.
- Provide comprehensive and ongoing education and reevaluate the patient's understanding and ability to control his or her disease.
- Maintain a flexible and normal lifestyle.

EPIDEMIOLOGY

Diabetes mellitus is present in roughly 18.2 million U.S. citizens (6.3% of the population), but only 13 million with this disease are diagnosed.[13] Close to 675,000 people have type 1 diabetes, and the majority of those remaining have type 2 disease. Girls experience a peak incidence of type 1 diabetes between 10 and 12 years of age, whereas boys have a higher incidence between 12 and 14 years. Diabetes in people older than 20 accounts for 90% to 95% of all cases. Half of all new cases of diabetes occur in adults over the age of 55, and approximately 18% of the older population (60 and older) has diabetes.[13] Certain ethnic groups have a higher incidence of diabetes than Caucasians: African Americans have a 50% to 60% higher rate, Mexican Americans have a 110% to 120% higher rate, and the Pima Indians of Arizona have the highest rate

TABLE 40.3	Distinguishing Features of Two Major Types of Diabetes Mellitus	
	Type 1	**Type 2**
Age of onset	Usually but not always during childhood or puberty	Often over 35
Type of onset	Abrupt	Usually gradual
Prevalence	0.5%	Roughly 6%
Incidence	Less than 10%	90% or greater
Family history of diabetes	Rarely positive	Commonly positive
Primary cause	Pancreatic β-cell deficiency	Insulin resistance
Nutritional status at time of onset	Usually undernourished	Usually obese
Symptoms	Polydipsia, polyuria, polyphagia	May be none
Hepatomegaly	Common	Uncommon
Stability	Blood glucose fluctuates widely in response to small changes in insulin dosage, exercise, and infection.	Less marked blood glucose fluctuations
Cause	Unknown	Unknown
Proneness to ketosis	Common, especially if treatment is insufficient	Uncommon except in presence of unusual stress or sepsis
Insulin defect	Defect in secretion; secretion is impaired early in disease; secretion may be totally absent late in disease.	*Insulin deficiency:* Most patients show failure of insulin secretion to keep pace with inordinate demands engendered by obesity; may appear initially as failure to respond to glucose alone, suggesting impairment on the glucoreceptor of the pancreatic β-cell.
		Insulin resistance: Some patients have a defect in tissue responsiveness to insulin and evidence of hyperinsulinemia; in such patients, insulin resistance may be mediated by receptor or postreceptor defects.
Plasma insulin (endogenous)	Negligible to zero	Low, normal, or high
Vascular complications of diabetes and degenerative changes	Uncommon until diabetes has been present for at least 5 yr	Common
Usual causes of death	Degenerative complications (e.g., renal failure caused by diabetic nephropathy)	Accelerated atherosclerosis (e.g., myocardial infarction); to a lesser extent, microangiopathic changes in target tissues (e.g., renal failure)
Diet	Mandatory in all patients	If diet is used fully, antidiabetic drug therapy may not be needed.
Insulin	Necessary for all patients	Necessary for 20%–30% of patients
Oral agents	Rarely efficacious	Efficacious

known in the world, with about half of this population afflicted with diabetes.[12,14]

Patients who are diagnosed with diabetes include 2.8% of the U.S. population; the disease accounts for 5.8% of the total personal healthcare cost.[15] A new case of diabetes is diagnosed every 60 seconds, and 7% to 8% of hospital admissions are related to diabetes. The chance of developing diabetes doubles with every 20% increase above ideal body weight (IBW) and every decade of life. Diabetes is the leading cause of new cases of adult blindness; patients with diabetes are 25 times more prone to blindness than are nondiabetic patients. Patients with diabetes are 17 times more prone

to kidney disease, with diabetic nephropathy being the primary cause of end-stage renal disease in adults.[16] Patients with diabetes are two to four times more likely to develop heart disease and stroke than nondiabetic people and 25 times more prone to developing gangrene. Also, diabetes is the leading cause of nontraumatic lower limb amputations in the United States, and up to 50% of men with longstanding diabetes have erectile dysfunction.

The annual cost of diabetes in the United States is estimated at over $100 billion; most of these costs are related to hospitalization and the treatment of long-term complications.[17] As an example of the cost of diabetic complications, approximately one third of all cases of end-stage renal disease in the United States are the result of diabetes. The U.S. Renal Data System reported in 2003 that the cost of medical care for patients with end-stage renal disease was about $16.6 billion, with diabetes accounting for about $7.4 billion of this cost per year.[18]

PATHOPHYSIOLOGY

The etiology of diabetes is incompletely understood, and numerous factors are associated with its development; Table 40.4 summarizes some of these factors. Patients with type 1 diabetes have pancreatic β-cell dysfunction related to genetic defects or other external factors. The extrinsic factors affecting β-cell function include damage caused by viruses such as mumps or Coxsackie B4, by destructive cytotoxins and antibodies released by sensitized lymphocytes, or by autodigestion in the course of an inflammatory disorder involving the exocrine pancreas.

Genetic susceptibility to type 1 diabetes appears to be linked to two genes on chromosome 6. These genes control the production of human lymphocyte antigens (HLAs) DR3 and DR4, and people with either or both of these antigens have a greater chance of developing diabetes than does a person lacking the antigens.[19] Ninety-five percent of patients with type 1 diabetes have one or both of these antigens; however, 40% of patients without diabetes have one or both of these antigens. Conversely, patients who carry HLA-DQA1*0102 or HLA-DQB1*0602 are resistant to type 1 diabetes.[19]

The reaction of predisposed patients to environmental stimuli (β-cell cytotoxic virus or chemicals) is abnormal and leads to destructive autoimmune-mediated mechanisms, or these patients experience lack of regeneration after β cells are damaged. Intensive research is being done to test and identify the mechanisms involved. The majority of patients

who develop type 1 diabetes have circulating antibodies, islet cell antibodies, and insulin autoantibodies before overt type 1 disease develops.[20] The result is an absolute insulin deficiency.

On the other hand, many patients with type 2 diabetes have excess insulin secretion and are obese. In addition to hyperinsulinemia and obesity, many patients with type 2 disease have hypertension, dyslipidemia, and impaired fibrinolysis, a collection of conditions called syndrome X.[21] Patients with syndrome X are more likely to experience cardiovascular disease and develop long-term complications of diabetes. Hyperinsulinism and insulin resistance may be correlated with a decrease in insulin receptors, reduced insulin binding, or post–insulin-receptor signaling defects.

Insulin resistance is thought to be the primary underlying pathophysiologic defect in type 2 diabetes. Patients with type 2 diabetes and insulin resistance demonstrate the following two major metabolic defects: a decreased sensitivity of target tissues (primarily the liver and skeletal muscle) to the actions of insulin and a relative deficiency of endogenous insulin secretion.[22] Because the peripheral tissues (liver and muscle) are less able to respond to insulin, patients secrete higher levels of insulin in an attempt to compensate for the diminished activity of insulin, and plasma glucose levels rise. Impaired insulin secretion and increased glucagon contribute to continued hepatic glucose output, resulting in elevated fasting glucose levels.[23] Figure 40.1 illustrates the insulin resistance syndrome, which is also known as the metabolic syndrome or the dysmetabolic syndrome. Table 40.5 lists the criteria established by the National Cholesterol Education Program for the definition of the metabolic syndrome.

Blood glucose levels can be elevated by a variety of mechanisms. Some patients have elevated blood glucose levels because of excessive glucagon or abnormal and excessive hepatic glucose production. Others may have a defect in somatostatin or an excess of growth hormone, cortisol, epinephrine, or other hormones that influence blood glucose regulation. Numerous drugs have also been implicated in increasing blood glucose levels, including atypical antipsychotics, corticosteroids, diazoxide, phenytoin, glucagon, caffeine, cyclophosphamide, lithium, epinephrine and other

TABLE 40.4	Etiologic Factors Associated With Diabetes Mellitus

Obesity

Increasing age

Heredity

Emotional stress

Autoimmune β-cell damage

Endocrine diseases (e.g., Cushing disease)

Viral stress

Vasculitis in tissues highly perfused with capillaries (e.g., eye, kidney)

Insulin receptor or post-insulin receptor defects

Drugs (e.g., atypical antipsychotics, corticosteroids, thyroid, phenytoin, diazoxide, thiazide diuretics)

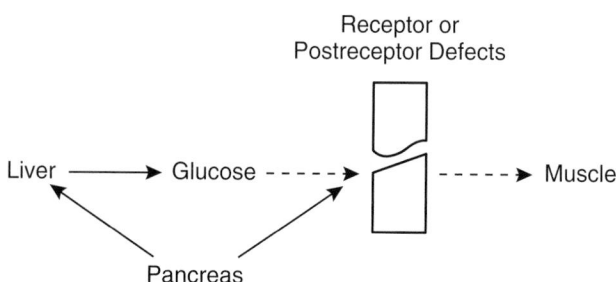

FIGURE 40.1 Characteristics of insulin resistance. Insulin resistance is defined by Polonsky et al as "a diminished ability of insulin to exert its biologic action across a broad range of concentrations."[23]

TABLE 40.5 | Metabolic Syndrome

Patient must have at least 3 of the following criteria:

- Fasting plasma glucose of 110 mg/dL or greater
- Serum triglycerides of 150 mg/dL or greater
- Serum high-density lipoprotein cholesterol of <40 mg/dL for men and <50 mg/dL for women
- Blood pressure 130/85 mm Hg or higher
- Waist girth of >102 cm or 40 inches (men) or >88 cm or 36 inches (women)

(From Expert Panel on Detection, Evaluation, and Treatment of High Blood Cholesterol in Adults. Executive summary of the third report of the National Cholesterol Education Program (NCEP) Expert Panel on Detection, Evaluation, and Treatment of High Blood Cholesterol in Adults (Adult Treatment Panel III). JAMA 285:2486–2497, 2001.)

catecholamines, estrogens, furosemide, thiazide diuretics, thyroid preparations, and sugar-containing medications. Other drugs may cause lower-than-normal blood glucose levels, including anabolic steroids, sulfonylureas, disopyramide, ethanol, monoamine oxidase inhibitors, propranolol, and large doses of salicylates.[24,25] Table 40.6 lists drugs associated with hyperglycemia or hypoglycemia and their clinical significance.

Numerous factors other than a relative or true lack of insulin may cause an increase in blood glucose. These include Cushing's disease, pheochromocytoma, aldosteronism, hyperthyroidism, pancreatitis, cirrhosis, pregnancy, emotional stress, and infections. Other factors can decrease blood glucose levels, such as an exogenous insulin excess, nonfasting reactive hypoglycemia, and fasting hypoglycemia.

Once hyperglycemia is established, elevated blood sugar values themselves can lead to glucotoxicity, which causes an increase in insulin resistance and reduces insulin secretion. When hyperglycemia is reduced by pharmacotherapeutic means, glucotoxicity is lessened and insulin secretion is reduced, with a concomitant reduction in insulin resistance. Nonpharmacologic methods can also improve glycemic control. Modest weight loss has been shown to reduce hepatic glucose production, improve insulin secretion, and increase peripheral insulin action, all of which tend to lessen insulin resistance.[26] These measures, when combined with proper nutrition and exercise, are particularly useful in controlling blood sugar levels in patients with type 2 diabetes.

There is still a great deal to learn about the specific cellular biochemical mechanisms involved in diabetes. The consequences of a lack of insulin or a lack of insulin effect are well known. The consequences of high blood glucose levels may be categorized into acute and chronic effects. The complex cellular effects of insulin provide numerous clues about the type of intervention that should be implemented to improve the prognosis of a patient with diabetes.

NORMAL INSULIN PRODUCTION AND EFFECTS

Insulin is a protein composed of 51 amino acids in two chains (A and B chains), connected by two disulfide bonds. Insulin is synthesized and stored in the β cells of the islets of Langerhans, which are located in the pancreas. The pancreas produces a parent protein called preproinsulin. Preproinsulin is cleaved to form a smaller protein, proinsulin. Proinsulin is cleaved to form equimolar amounts of C-peptide and insulin.[27] The normal human pancreas contains approximately 200 units of insulin, and a basal amount of insulin is secreted continuously at an hourly rate of approximately 0.5 to 1.0 units. Additional insulin is also released in response to blood glucose levels of 100 mg per dL or more. The average daily insulin secretory rate in the adult is 25 to 50 units. Insulin is cleared metabolically by the liver, peripheral tissues, and kidneys. Insulin follows first-order elimination kinetics, and the serum half-life is approximately 4 to 5 minutes.

The important metabolic sites that are sensitive to insulin include the liver, where glycogen is synthesized, stored, and broken down; skeletal muscle, where glucose oxidation produces energy; and adipose tissue, where glucose can be converted to fatty acids, glyceryl phosphate, and triglycerides. Insulin affects carbohydrate, protein, and lipid metabolism.

CARBOHYDRATE METABOLISM

In patients without diabetes, insulin acts in concert with glucagon, somatostatin, growth hormone, corticosteroids, epinephrine, and parasympathetic innervation to maintain blood glucose levels between 40 and 160 mg per dL (2.2 and 8.9 mmol/L) at all times. Three cell types, α cells, β cells, and δ cells, have been identified in the islets of Langerhans of the pancreas. The α cells produce glucagon, a hormone that acts to increase blood glucose levels. The β cells produce, store, and release insulin. The δ cells produce somatostatin, which inhibits both insulin and glucagon secretion and suppresses growth hormone. The suppression of glucagon by somatostatin decreases blood glucose levels, and its effect persists for roughly 60 to 120 minutes.

Euglycemia is maintained by the three previously identified hormones working in concert. Ingestion of a carbohydrate load results in a prompt increase in the amount of insulin release and a concomitant decrease in plasma glucagon. Glucagon is released in response to low blood glucose levels and protein ingestion. Glucagon release stimulates insulin secretion; insulin in turn inhibits glucagon release.

The presence of insulin favors the uptake and use of glucose by insulin-sensitive sites. In skeletal muscle, glucose uptake and subsequent energy production increase. In the liver, glucose uptake and the formation of glycogen increase in the presence of insulin.

A minimum blood glucose level of 40 mg per dL (2.2 mmol/L) is needed to provide adequate energy for the brain, which can use only glucose as energy and does not depend on the presence of insulin for its use. Glucose "spills" into the urine when blood glucose levels exceed the renal thresh-

TABLE 40.6 | Drugs That May Alter Blood Glucose Levels

Drug	Mechanism of Action	Clinical Significance
Drugs That May Increase Blood Glucose Levels		
Acetazolamide	Unknown, but may enhance insulin or sulfonylurea elimination	+
Alcohol (ethanol)	Glucose tolerance may worsen with chronic ingestion and may increase metabolism of tolbutamide. May result in chlorpropamide flush reaction or hypoglycemia.	+
Asparaginase	May inhibit insulin synthesis (diabetic ketoacidosis has been reported)	++
Atypical antipsychotics; in particular, clozapine, olanzapine, and risperidone	Unknown: possibly due to the development of insulin resistance; decreased insulin secretion due to direct β-cell inhibition via the 5-HT$_{1A}$ receptor	++/+++
β-Adrenergic antagonists	Inhibit insulin secretion; cardioselective agents less likely to produce this effect	++
Caffeine	High dosages may stimulate gluconeogenesis.	+
Calcium channel antagonists	Inhibit insulin secretion	+
Clonidine	May be related to release of growth hormone (transient and associated only with high dosages of clonidine)	+
Diazoxide	Inhibits insulin secretion; decreases use of insulin	+++
Diuretics	May be related to hypokalemia, leading to a decrease in insulin secretion. Thiazides show a greater increasing effect than loop diuretics, which show a greater effect than potassium-sparing diuretics.	++
Epinephrine-like agents (sympathomimetics, decongestants, anorexiants)	Increase glycogenolysis and gluconeogenesis	++
Glucagon	Increases glycogenolysis	+++
Glucocorticosteroids	Increase gluconeogenesis; depress insulin action	+++
Glycerol	Unknown, probably volume depletion (hyperglycemic hyperosmolar nonketotic coma has been reported)	++
Immunosuppressives (tacrolimus)	May induce insulin resistance	++
Interferon (α and β)	Unknown	+
Lithium salts	May decrease insulin secretion	+
Niacin	Unknown; may worsen insulin resistance	++
Nicotine	Vasoconstriction, leading to a decreased absorption of injected insulin	++
Oral contraceptives	Unknown; high-dose combination products can impair glucose tolerance (minimal effect with newer low-dose combination products)	++
Pentamidine	Toxic to pancreatic β cells	+++
Phenytoin	Inhibits insulin secretion	++
Protease inhibitors	Unknown; possibly pancreatic toxicity	+
Rifampin	Enhances tolbutamide metabolism	+
Sugar-containing syrups	Increase sugar load	++
Sympathomimetics	Increased glycogenolysis and gluconeogenesis	++
Thyroid hormones	Increase metabolic clearance of insulin and hypoglycemic agents	++
Drugs That May Cause Hypoglycemia		
Alcohol (ethanol)	Impairs gluconeogenesis and increases insulin secretion	+++
Anabolic steroids	Decrease glucose tolerance	+
Angiotensin-converting enzyme inhibitors	May improve insulin sensitivity, particularly in skeletal muscle	+

(continued)

TABLE 40.6	continued	
Drug	**Mechanism of Action**	**Clinical Significance**
β-Adrenergic antagonists	Inhibit glycogenolysis; attenuate signs and symptoms of hypoglycemia	++
Bishydroxy-coumarin	Inhibits hepatic clearance of tolbutamide and chlorpropamide	++
Chloramphenicol	May inhibit metabolism of sulfonylureas	++
Chloroquine	Unknown; hypoglycemia leading to death has been reported in overdose	++
Clofibrate	Unknown	+
Coumarins and dicumarol	Inhibit hepatic clearance of tolbutamide and chlorpropamide	++
Disopyramide	Unknown; appears to result from endogenous insulin secretion	++
Ethanol	Impairs gluconeogenesis and increases insulin secretion	+++
Gatifloxacin	May increase insulin release via blockade of ATP-sensitive K^+ channels	++
Growth hormone	Unknown	++
Monoamine oxidase inhibitors	May increase insulin release and decrease sympathetic response to hypoglycemia	+
Pentamidine	Cytolytic response in pancreas accompanied by insulin release	+++
Phenylbutazone	Reduces clearance of sulfonylureas	++
Salicylates	Increase insulin secretion and sensitivity; may alter pharmacokinetic disposition of sulfonylureas	++
Saquinavir	Unknown	+
Sulfonamides	Alter clearance of sulfonylureas	+
Triazole antifungals	Enhance the effect of sulfonylureas	+++

(From Skyler JS, Marks JB. Immune intervention in type 1 diabetes mellitus. Diabetes Rev 1:15–42, 1993.)
+, low probability of occurrence or low level of glucose alteration expected in most patients; ++, probability of occurrence in most patients is high, but degree of glucose alteration may or may not be clinically significant; +++, high probability of occurrence, clinically significant in many cases.

old of 180 mg per dL (9.9 mmol/L), resulting in energy and water loss.

PROTEIN METABOLISM

The presence of insulin favors the production of structural proteins from constituent amino acids. When glucose is present intracellularly in sufficient quantities for needed energy production, most structural proteins retain their integrity. In the absence of insulin, structural protein production is not favored, and intracellular glucose levels are insufficient to match energy demands. In an attempt to produce energy, skeletal muscle converts its structural proteins to constituent amino acids. The liberated amino acids are transported to the liver, where they are converted to glucose via gluconeogenesis. In patients with diabetes, glucose enters the blood but is not taken up by tissue because of a true or relative lack of insulin. Thus, hyperglycemia is escalated, and structural proteins are wasted.

FAT METABOLISM

The presence of insulin favors the production of triglycerides from free fatty acids. When insulin deficiency causes an energy deficit, free fatty acids are oxidized to β-hydroxybutyric acid, acetoacetic acid, and acetone. β-Hydroxybutyric acid can be used as an energy source, but in the absence of insulin, the production of the keto acids eventually is greater than their metabolism and excretion. If insulin is not given to the patient, metabolic ketoacidosis ensues. The keto acids cause the blood pH to decline, and diuresis secondary to the elimination of ketones and glucose causes dehydration. The body's neutralizing factors eventually are depleted, and the patient continues to deteriorate to the point of coma and possibly death. Figure 40.2 shows the clinical manifestations of the untreated patient with type 1 diabetes who completely lacks insulin.

Patients with type 2 diabetes may have an elevated, normal, or low level of circulating insulin, depending on the chronicity of their disease, and have a relative lack of effec-

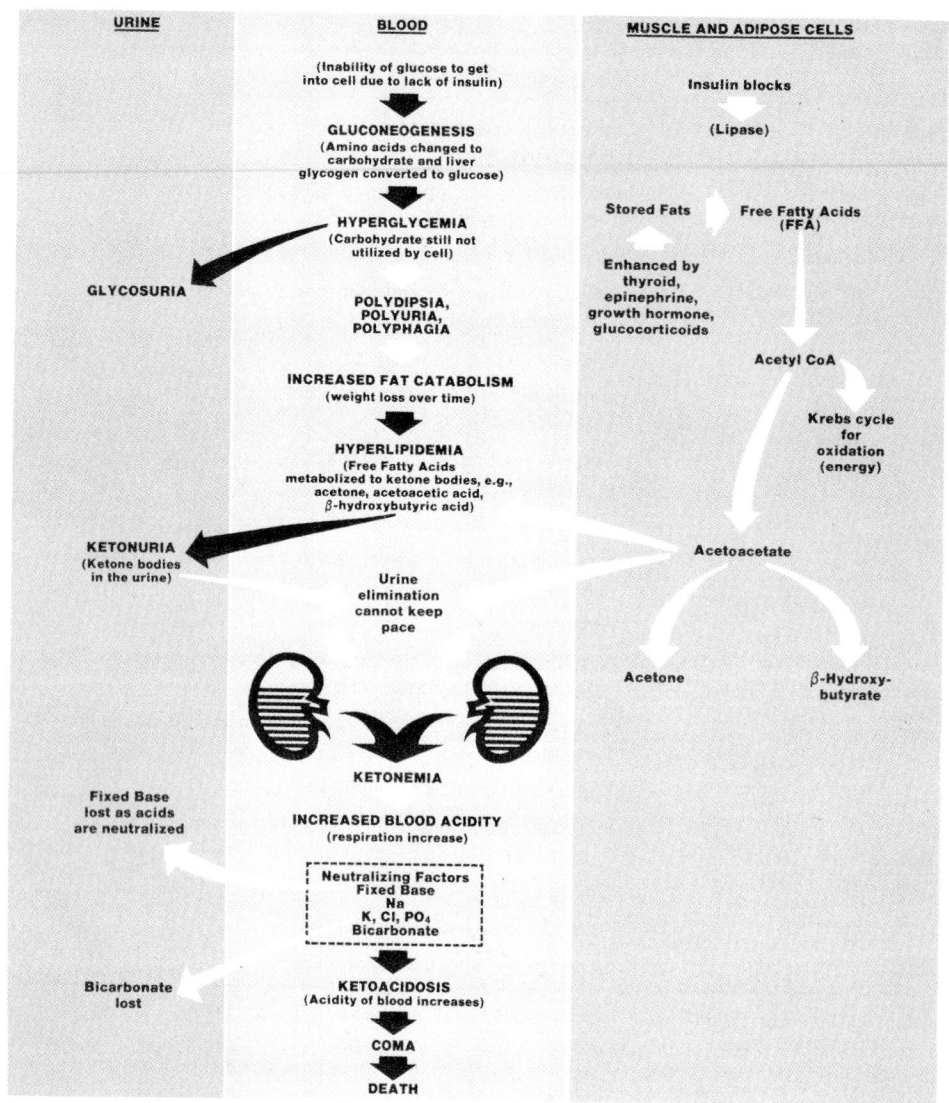

FIGURE 40.2 Clinical manifestations of a complete lack of insulin.

tive insulin. In patients with type 2 disease, insulin and glucose levels usually are adequate to prevent the development of ketoacidosis. However, glucose can accumulate in the blood and can reach extremely high levels [more than 400 mg/dL (22.2 mmol/L)], resulting in hyperosmolar hyperglycemic state (HHS), formerly known as nonketotic hyperosmolar syndrome or nonketotic hyperosmolar coma.

CLINICAL PRESENTATION AND DIAGNOSIS

SIGNS AND SYMPTOMS

Type 1 diabetes usually presents rapidly, typically with polydipsia, polyuria, polyphagia, weakness, weight loss, dry skin, and ketoacidosis (30% of all cases of diabetic ketoacidosis [DKA] occur in previously undiagnosed patients). On the other hand, type 2 diabetes typically is slow and insidious

in onset and often asymptomatic. Type 2 diabetes often is discovered when glucose is found in the urine or when elevated blood sugar is noticed during a routine examination. Patients with type 2 disease usually are over the age of 40 and often obese; however, with the recent rise in childhood and adolescent obesity, type 2 diabetes is becoming more common in younger patients. Careful examination of patients with type 2 diabetes often reveals glucosuria, proteinuria, postprandial hyperglycemia, microaneurysms, and possibly retinal exudates.

Other symptoms of hyperglycemia that are associated with diabetes include blurred vision, tingling or numbness of the extremities, slow-healing skin infections, itching, drowsiness, and irritability. Patients with these symptoms and patients who have a family history of diabetes should be screened for hyperglycemia. Table 40.7 lists testing recommendations in previously undiagnosed patients. Monilial infections of the vagina and anus, and a history of complica-

TABLE 40.7 | Screening Criteria for Diabetes

Testing should be considered in all patients age 45 yr and older. Repeat at 3-yr intervals.

Consider testing at younger age or test more often in patients who:

- Are obese (≥120% desirable body weight or body mass index ≥27 kg/m²)
- Have a first-degree relative with diabetes
- Are members of a high-risk ethnic group (e.g., African American, Hispanic, Native American)
- Have delivered a baby weighing >9 lb or have been diagnosed with gestational diabetes mellitus
- Are hypertensive (≥140/90 mm Hg)
- Have a high-density lipoprotein cholesterol level ≤35 mg/dL or a triglyceride level ≥250 mg/dL
- On previous testing had "prediabetes" (impaired glucose tolerance or impaired fasting glucose)
- Have polycystic ovary syndrome
- Have a history of vascular disease

(From Expert Committee on the Diagnosis and Classification of Diabetes Mellitus. Report of the expert committee on the diagnosis and classification of diabetes mellitus. Diabetes Care 20:1183–1197, 1997; and Expert Committee on the Diagnosis and Classification of Diabetes Mellitus. Follow-up report on the diagnosis of diabetes mellitus. Diabetes Care 26:3160–3167, 2003.)

tions during pregnancy are also warning signs to test for diabetes. Delivering a baby weighing more than 9 pounds is another risk factor for diabetes. The earlier diabetes is diagnosed, the more easily it can be controlled and the better the long-term prognosis.

DIAGNOSIS

Type 1 diabetes usually is easy to diagnose because patients present with all of the classic symptoms of diabetes and high amounts of glucose in the urine and blood. Type 2 diabetes is more of a challenge to diagnose because patients often do not present with the classic symptoms. Table 40.7 reviews the screening criteria for diabetes mellitus and Table 40.2 summarizes the diagnostic criteria developed by the Expert Committee on the Diagnosis and Classification of Diabetes Mellitus in 1997.[6] Basically, there are three ways in which diabetes can be diagnosed. Each method must be confirmed on another day by the same or a different method.

Fasting plasma glucose is the preferred method for testing for diabetes. It is fast, economical, and commonly used. Blood is drawn from the patient after an overnight fast. A normal level is 65 to 100 mg per dL (3.6 to 5.55 mmol/L), with minor variations between laboratories. The diagnosis of diabetes may be confirmed in patients with two or more fasting plasma glucose levels of 126 mg per dL (7 mmol/L) or higher.

A less common and more cumbersome test is the oral glucose tolerance test, which measures the patient's ability to handle a glucose load over a period of time. After an overnight fast, a morning fasting blood sugar is drawn and the patient ingests a 75-g glucose load. Then blood samples are drawn at half-hour intervals for 2 hours and then at 3 hours.[28] In normal subjects, the blood glucose returns to normal in less than 2 hours. In patients with diabetes, the glucose peak is higher and occurs much later than in those without diabetes; levels also decline at a slower rate. A normal result occurs when the 2-hour plasma glucose is less than 140 mg per dL (7.77 mmol/L) and the intervening values are below 200 mg per dL (11.1 mmol/L). Because of criteria that accept random or fasting glucose levels as diagnostic, this test is less commonly performed. Infections, stress, pregnancy, metabolic abnormalities, and certain drugs can impair glucose tolerance and produce abnormal results. These situations should be screened for when this test is used.

Diagnostic test results can be elevated by emotional stress, physical exertion, and stimulants such as tobacco, coffee, and tea. Therefore, caution should be exercised in using diagnostic tests for diabetes. A patient should not be diagnosed as having diabetes unless it is certain that the disease exists. Mislabeling a patient with this diagnosis leads to frustration, including problems with insurance coverage, driver's license limitations in some states, and possible employment limitations. Healthcare providers who are monitoring older adults should be alert to the fact that as a person ages, tolerance to glucose decreases. This results in some older adults being labeled as diabetic and being prescribed unnecessary medications.

MONITORING

SELF-MONITORING OF BLOOD GLUCOSE

The objective of diabetes treatment is to achieve normal or near-normal blood glucose levels through a program of education, diet, exercise, and medications. Achieving this objective requires active patient involvement. One of the easiest and most practical methods of monitoring glycemic control is SMBG. SMBG is acceptable to many patients and allows the patient to better understand the factors that affect blood glucose levels. It gives an accurate reflection of the blood glucose level after physical activity, before and after meals, and when the patient is taking medications or is ill. It also helps the patient to better understand diabetes and the objectives of therapy, assists in detecting and therefore avoiding hypoglycemia, helps the patient understand the symptoms of hypoglycemia and hyperglycemia, improves the relationship between the healthcare professional and the patient, and helps the patient to become a more active, informed participant in diabetes management.

The disadvantages of SMBG, which include the increased expense and the annoyance of obtaining a drop of blood, are greatly outweighed by the many advantages. Several devices are now available to help the patient obtain a drop of blood easily and almost painlessly.[29] Several methods of determining blood glucose levels are available, and selection of a specific product can be made on the basis of cost, ability to perform the test accurately, and flexibility of the system. The manual dexterity needed and the ease of reading the results are additional factors to consider. Some systems have extended memories so that record-keeping is easier, and newer products can download data to a computer, making trends much easier and more convenient for health professionals to analyze.

Because blood sugar maintenance is impossible without measurement and because it is convenient and less costly for the patient to self-monitor, SMBG is highly recommended for all patients with diabetes. Pregnant patients, patients who have difficulty bringing their diabetes under control, and patients with frequent hypoglycemia are all excellent candidates for SMBG. Also, blood glucose monitoring is a necessity for patients who are using continuous subcutaneous insulin infusion.

Most of the tests available for use by patients involve the glucose oxidase and peroxidase reaction to detect glucose. Some of the tests use a reflective photometer to read the strip and give a digital readout of the blood glucose values. Other methods have a color reaction on the strip, which is compared to a chart on the side of the bottle that the patient reads visually. Although the visually read strips are less expensive and are very portable, electronic blood glucose monitoring gives the patient a more accurate blood glucose determination. In general, the visually read strips are not recommended. Patients with type 1 diabetes generally should test their blood sugar levels three or four times daily.[30] The optimal monitoring frequency in patients with type 2 diabetes is not known, and testing frequency should be influenced by their dependence on oral or injectable therapy and their adherence to a diet and exercise program.

URINE TESTS

Patient-performed urine tests are available for evaluating glucose, ketones, and protein values. Glucosuria is observed in many conditions and is not a persistent finding in diabetes. It occurs when the renal threshold is exceeded [blood glucose level of 180 mg/dL (10 mmol/L) or higher], but this value is not consistent for all patients. In particular, older patients with diabetes may not spill any glucose into the urine despite greatly elevated blood sugar values. Older patients may have diabetes that may not be detected by urinalysis; therefore, urine testing in older adults would not reflect their level of glycemia accurately. Because of the problems inherent in urine glucose monitoring, this method is no longer recommended.

Available urine ketone tests include Acetest, Chemstrip K, and Ketostix. Urine ketone testing should be encouraged for the patient with diabetes during acute illness or stress, or when blood glucose levels are not well controlled. Patients with type 1 disease should test for urine ketones when blood sugar readings are greater than 240 mg per dL (13.3 mmol/

L) and should report moderate or higher ketone readings to their healthcare professional.

Finally, urine tests are available for measuring urine proteins. Constant routine monitoring of urine protein usually is not warranted. Urine protein tests are used primarily as a screening tool for the presence of diabetic nephropathy. Patients who test negative with standard dipstick methods may be further evaluated with an in-office microalbumin test (Micro-Bumintest) or by 24-hour urine collections. These methods are much more sensitive than the standard dipstick method. Patients who have had type 1 diabetes for 5 or more years should be screened annually for microalbuminuria, and patients with type 2 diabetes should be screened annually from the time of diagnosis.[31]

GLYCOSYLATED HEMOGLOBIN (A1C)

Hemoglobin glycosylation occurs when hemoglobin is exposed to ambient glucose concentrations in the blood. When higher concentrations of blood glucose are present, the percentage of glycosylated hemoglobin as measured by A1C increases because red blood cells are freely permeable to glucose. Because the average life span of the red blood cell is 120 days, the A1C reflects glycemic control for that time period and most precisely reflects the average blood sugar level for the previous 60 to 90 days. A1C is an important measure of long-term glycemic control and is directly correlated with the long-term complications of diabetes.

Typically, the patient without diabetes has an A1C in the range of 4% to 6%, and those with diabetes may have values as high as 20%. In general, each 1% rise in A1C value reflects an average serum blood sugar increase of 35 mg per dL (1.94 mmol/L). Therefore, an A1C value of 6% would correlate with an average blood sugar level of 135 mg per dL (7.5 mmol/L), and a person with a 9% value would have an average blood glucose value corresponding to approximately 240 mg per dL (13.3 mmol/L).

Studies show that when a patient with uncontrolled diabetes brings his or her blood glucose under strict control, there is a dramatic improvement in glycosylated hemoglobin. The DCCT confirmed that there is a strong correlation between glycosylated hemoglobin concentrations and the progression of microvascular disease in patients with type 1 diabetes. This test is particularly useful for patients who have poor compliance in record-keeping or who make an extra effort to achieve acceptable plasma glucose levels only at the time of the physician visit. The test can be performed at any time and is not affected by recent meals or physical activities. Glycohemoglobin testing should be performed in all patients with diabetes on a routine basis. The ideal frequency of testing has not been determined, although it is generally recommended that two to four tests be performed per year. The number of tests to do per year depends on the degree of glycemic control, the number of therapeutic changes made, and the physician's clinical judgment. The therapeutic goal recommended by the American Diabetes Association for glycosylated hemoglobin is less than 7%, with more strin-

TABLE 40.8	Glycemic Control Parameters	
Biochemical Index		**Goal**
Preprandial glucose (mg/dL)		90–130
Postprandial glucose <mg/dL)		<180
Hemoglobin A1C (%)		<7

(From Standards of medical care in diabetes. Diabetes Care 27 (Suppl 1):S15–S35, 2004.)

gent goals being appropriate for some individuals. Table 40.8 lists goals of therapy.

GLYCATED SERUM PROTEIN

Proteins in the bloodstream can become glycated, much like hemoglobin. The half-life of serum albumin ranges from 14 to 20 days and acts as a marker of glycemic control over a shorter time frame than the A1C.[30] The serum fructosamine assay, another method of measuring glycated albumin in the body, is highly correlated with A1C values. A serum fructosamine value gives information about the degree of glycemic control over the previous 2 to 3 weeks and may be invaluable in monitoring patients whose glycemic status must be verified over a shorter period of time. Patients who may benefit from this include pregnant patients, those undergoing major changes in therapy, and older adults.

HYPERGLYCEMIA

SHORT-TERM (ACUTE) EFFECTS

The short-term effects of hyperglycemia range from minor symptoms to life-threatening metabolic compromise. Short-term effects such as blurred vision, polydipsia, polyuria, an increased incidence of urinary tract infection, fatigue, or drowsiness may impair the quality of life of patients untreated or poorly treated for diabetes. Although these can lead to significant impairment (e.g., blurred vision), two life-threatening short-term complications necessitate prompt medical intervention: DKA and HHS.

Diabetic Ketoacidosis. The physiologic events that lead to DKA are described in Figure 40.2. DKA is a life-threatening condition that occurs secondary to an insulin deficit. DKA may occur in patients with diabetes who have an active infection, those who have discontinued insulin therapy, or those subjected to other forms of stress (e.g., acute myocardial infarction, stroke). DKA requires prompt and proper treatment and has a 5% to 10% mortality rate.[32]

Signs and symptoms of DKA include polydipsia, polyuria, fruity breath, dry mucous membranes, tachycardia, and hypotension. Consciousness may be mildly to severely impaired. Common laboratory findings include elevated serum glucose, creatinine, blood urea nitrogen, hyponatremia, ketonuria, and glucosuria.

Insulin is usually administered initially with an intravenous bolus dose between 0.1 and 0.2 units per kg, followed by a continuous infusion of 0.1 units/kg/hour. Normal saline (0.9% NaCl) is administered at a rate of 0.5 to 1 L per hour until blood pressure and pulse are stabilized, at which point normal saline is substituted. When blood glucose approaches normal, 5% dextrose in normal saline normal saline may be used. If potassium levels are elevated, supplemental potassium should not be administered. Once normokalemia has been achieved, 10 to 20 mEq per hour of potassium is needed for maintenance. Hypokalemic patients need additional potassium supplementation beyond the maintenance rate, based on serum potassium levels (typically 20 to 40 mEq/L fluid). Phosphate administration is controversial because it can promote hypokalemia and hypomagnesemia; however, it can be provided to patients with low phosphorus levels at a rate of 5 mmol per hour. Bicarbonate should be administered only to a patient whose arterial pH is less than 7.1 and in doses of up to 44 mEq per hour.[33]

Hyperosmolar Hyperglycemic State. HHS typically is characterized by blood glucose levels higher than 600 mg per dL (33.3 mmol/L) and has a mortality rate up to 30%. Older adults with type 2 diabetes are at increased risk of HHS and are much less likely to develop DKA. Certain diseases, such as infections or renal or cardiac disease, may precipitate HHS. Prompt recognition and treatment are needed to prevent death. After a major insult (e.g., acute myocardial infarction, infection), the body releases cortisol and epinephrine, which has the effect of worsening hyperglycemia. With increased glycemia, dehydration and hyperosmolarity develop and increased amounts of glucose are lost in the urine. Ketone bodies are not formed because of the presence of insulin. Dehydration and hyperosmolarity occur and can result in altered consciousness and lethargy, with coma being less commonly recognized (older terms for this syndrome included nonketotic hyperosmolar coma syndrome and nonketotic hyperosmolar syndrome).

Signs of dehydration in patients with HHS include tachycardia, dry skin, and orthostatic hypotension. The primary treatment consists of rehydration, insulin, electrolyte replacement, and treatment of the underlying cause. Because older patients with diabetes are more prone to develop HHS, health professionals must encourage regular serum glucose monitoring by older adults and advocate consistent recording and reporting of any upward trends in blood sugar levels.

LONG-TERM (CHRONIC) EFFECTS

Although the short-term metabolic effects of hyperglycemia are life-threatening and necessitate prompt attention, the long-term effects are insidious and often go unnoticed. Nonetheless, the prolonged effects are serious, often debilitating, and, if untreated, life-threatening over the long term. The chronic complications of diabetes include macrovascular disease (peripheral, cerebral, cardiovascular), microvascular disease (retinopathy and nephropathy), neuropathy (peripheral and autonomic), and foot problems. Although the molecular mechanisms leading to chronic complications have not been determined conclusively, several abnormal biochemical pathways have been suggested. Most salient in this list of deleterious pathways is the production of high concentrations of advanced glycosylation end products (AGE) and sorbitol. Additional pathways include the generation of reactive oxygen species (ROS), and the activation of diacylglycerol (DAG) and protein kinase C (PKC) isoforms. All pathways contribute to endothelial damage and destruction, thereby contributing to the development of microvascular complications.[34] Figure 40.3 shows how hyperglycemia and the activation of PKC-β may lead to microvascular complications of diabetes. This figure also shows where this pathway could be interrupted with a PKC-β inhibitor such ruboxistaurin, which is under development.[35]

There has been considerable debate about whether the lesions that develop within the diabetic patient's retina, kidneys, nerves, and vascular system result from a disorder in the structure and function of blood vessels or from prolonged hyperglycemia caused by inadequate metabolic control. Most of the data suggest that microvascular disease and neuropathy are linked to hyperglycemia.[1–5]

The causes of macrovascular disease associated with diabetes are less well understood. Ischemic heart disease accounts for approximately 40% of the mortality in this population, with cardiovascular disease and stroke accounting for an additional 25%.[36] Many patients with type 2 diabetes have hyperinsulinemia, are obese, and have hypertension along with high levels of triglycerides and low-density lipoprotein and low levels of high-density lipoprotein; all but hyperinsulinemia are known risk factors for cardiovascular disease. The role of hyperinsulinemia is not as clear, and definitive clinical trials assessing the role of hyperinsulinemia and exogenous insulin administration are needed to determine whether high insulin levels contribute to macrovascular disease.

Advanced Glycosylation End Products. Proteins throughout the body are non-enzymatically glycosylated at a rate proportional to the ambient glucose concentration. These glycosylated proteins are highly reactive, forming bonds with other glycosylated proteins, collagen, and other molecules, and eventually forming AGEs (Fig. 40.4). Once formed, AGEs are very stable and are incorporated into the basement membrane matrix of capillaries. This process causes the thickening of basement membranes and a reduction in the production of nitric oxide [formerly known as endothelium-derived relaxing factor (EDRF)], resulting in vasoconstriction.[37] The net result of this process is leakage across the basement membranes, which appears as hard exudates in the patient with diabetic retinopathy and as proteinuria in the patient with diabetic nephropathy. This process is thought to be one of the major pathways leading to the development of microvascular disease. To date there is no drug product available to alter the formation of AGEs; however, several products are under investigation.

Sorbitol and Aldose Reductase Inhibition. The sorbitol pathway may be another clinically important biochemical mechanism by which chronic complications develop in patients with diabetes.[38] Many cell lines, such as the Schwann cell in the nervous system, do not need insulin for glucose uptake. These cell types are subject to intracellular hyperglycemia during times of ambient hyperglycemia. Intracellular hyperglycemia causes an inordinately high fraction of glu-

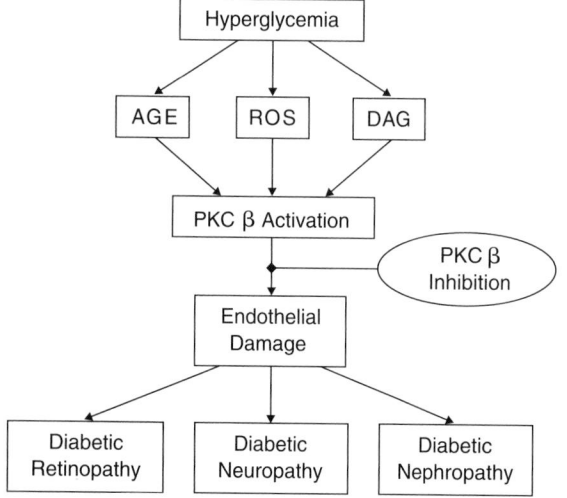

FIGURE 40.3 PKC-β activation and inhibition of diabetic microvascular complications. AGE, advanced glycosyllation end products; ROS, reactive oxygen species; DAG, diacylglyceral; PKC, protein kinase C.

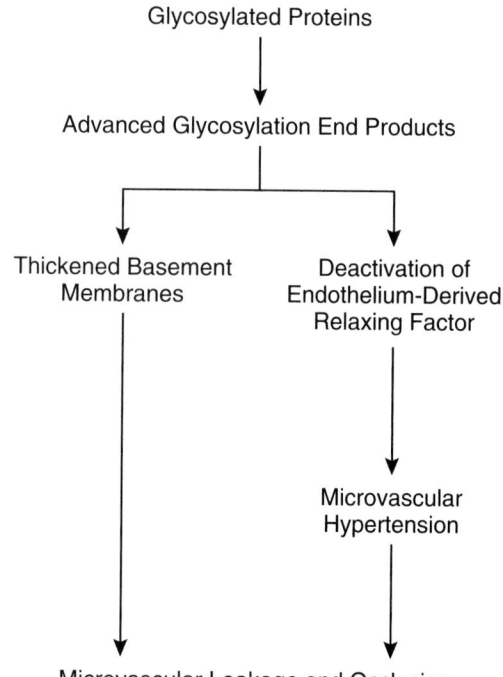

FIGURE 40.4 Advanced glycosylation end products and microvascular disease.

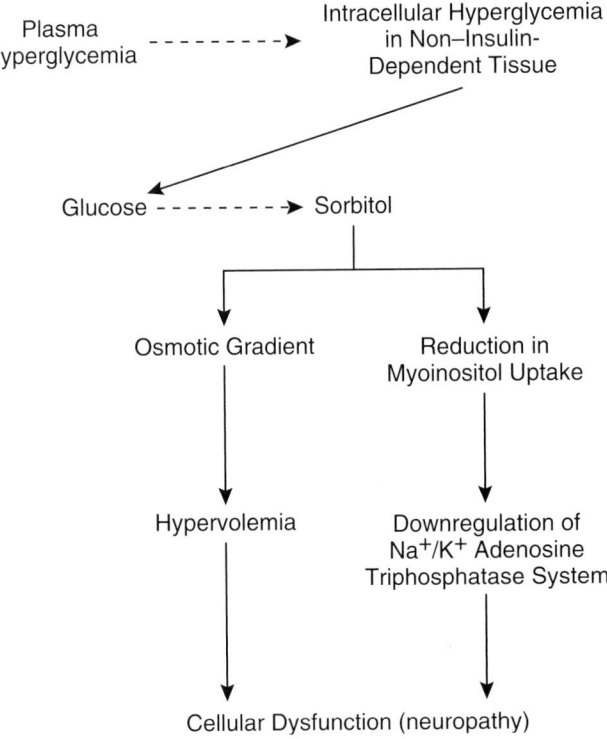

FIGURE 40.5 The sorbitol pathway.

cose to be shunted into the sorbitol pathway (Fig. 40.5), leading to the production of high concentrations of sorbitol via the enzyme aldose reductase. High concentrations of sorbitol cause a reduction in myoinositol uptake, which in turn results in the downregulation of the Na^+/K^+ adenosine triphosphatase system, leading to a reduction in energy production. Additionally, sorbitol creates an intracellular osmotic gradient, resulting in hypervolemia of the cell, further compromising cellular function. This pathway may play a substantial role in the development of diabetic neuropathy. Aldose reductase inhibitors currently in clinical studies include fidarestat and zenarestat.

DIABETES STUDIES

DIABETES CONTROL AND COMPLICATIONS TRIAL

The landmark DCCT conclusively determined that glycemic control affects the appearance and progression of chronic diabetic complications.[1] This study evaluated patients with type 1 disease. Patients were randomized to receive either conventional therapy (one or two insulin injections per day and avoidance of acute symptoms of hyperglycemia) or intensive therapy (three or more injections per day or subcutaneous insulin infusion pump therapy and strict glycemic control). The interim analysis showed an overwhelming support for intensive therapy, and the study was stopped 1 year earlier than initially planned. Results were reported in terms of relative risk reduction—what level of risk reduction for the

appearance or progression of a chronic complication is imparted by intensive therapy versus conventional therapy. The results are shown in Table 40.9. In addition to the significant chronic complications, the study also reported a threefold increase in hypoglycemic episodes and more weight gain in the patients who were treated with intensive insulin therapy.

Despite these potential drawbacks to intensive therapy, there is a renewed emphasis on strict but reasonable glycemic control to prevent the severe and debilitating chronic

TABLE 40.9	Results of Two Landmark Studies

Diabetes Control and Complications Trial

60% reduction in clinical neuropathy development

35% reduction in microalbuminuria development

56% reduction in albuminuria development

27% reduction in initial appearance of retinopathy

34%–76% reduction in clinically significant retinopathy

45% reduction in progression to severe retinopathy

34% reduction in low-density lipoprotein concentration

41% reduction in risk of macrovascular disease

300% increase in incidence of severe hypoglycemia

United Kingdom Prospective Diabetes Study

Intensive blood glucose control with sulfonylureas or insulin

    12% reduction of any diabetes-related endpoint

    25% reduction in microvascular complications

    29% reduction in photocoagulation

    21% reduction in progression to retinopathy

    34% reduction in progression to microalbinuria

    Mean 3.1-kg weight gain in intensive group over 10 yr

Intensive blood glucose control with metformin in overweight patients

    32% reduction in any diabetes-related endpoint

    42% reduction in risk of diabetes-related death

    36% reduction in mortality

    39% reduction of myocardial infarction

Effect of tight blood pressure control (≤150/85 mm Hg) in hypertensive patients

    24% reduction in any diabetes-related endpoint

    32% reduction in diabetes-related death

    44% reduction in fatal and nonfatal stroke

    37% reduction in microvascular disease

    34% reduction in deterioration of retinopathy

Effect of atenolol and captopril in risk reduction of microvascular and macrovascular complications

Both agents equally effective in maintaining blood glucose control

No differences in risk of macrovascular or microvascular disease between the two groups complications of diabetes. Strict glycemic control is particularly important before and during pregnancy and has been shown to reduce the incidence of perinatal complications and mortality in mothers with diabetes.

UNITED KINGDOM PROSPECTIVE DIABETES STUDY

The UKPDS was a 20-year study involving more than 4,000 patients with type 2 diabetes.[2–5] Four separate trials were conducted and involved the following four components: effects of intensive blood glucose control with sulfonylureas or insulin, effects of intensive blood glucose control with metformin in overweight patients, effect of tight blood pressure control in hypertensive diabetic patients, and the effects of atenolol and captopril on blood pressure control. In this study, intensive control was defined as achieving fasting plasma glucose levels of less than 6 mmol per L (108 mg/dL), and conventional treatment was treatment that resulted in a fasting plasma glucose level less than 15 mmol per L (270 mg/dL). Patients treated with conventional therapy were treated with diet and weight maintenance and with sulfonylureas, metformin, or insulin if severe or symptomatic hyperglycemia occurred. Blood sugar levels were controlled with chlorpropamide, glyburide, glipizide, or insulin in the intensively treated group. The following endpoints were evaluated: any diabetes-related endpoint (sudden death, death from hyperglycemia or hypoglycemia, fatal or nonfatal myocardial infarction); other cardiovascular events, amputation, or ophthalmic events; death related to diabetes including sudden death, stroke, peripheral vascular disease, renal disease, glycemic derangements, and death from myocardial infarction; or death from all causes. Single clinical endpoints examined included myocardial infarction, stroke, amputation, or death from peripheral vascular disease, and microvascular complications.

A1C values over a 10-year period were 7% in the intensive group and 7.9% in the conventional group, with all agents having similar efficacy in the intensively treated patients. Patients in the intensively treated group had a 12% lower risk of any diabetes-related endpoint and a 25% lower risk of microvascular complications than those in the conventionally treated group. No significant differences in the risk of diabetes-related deaths, all-cause mortality, myocardial infarction, stroke, amputation, or death from peripheral vascular disease were noted. As in the DCCT, significant reductions in the risk of progression of retinopathy and microalbuminuria were noted. See Table 40.9 for the results of the DCCT and UKPDS studies.[2–5]

THERAPEUTIC PLAN

The treatment objectives for diabetes are summarized in Table 40.10. In achieving the objectives, one must remember that diabetes is a heterogeneous condition, and that there is tremendous variation among patients. The treatment proto-

TABLE 40.10	Treatment Objectives for Diabetes Mellitus

Normalize glucose metabolism

Normalize glycosylated hemoglobin

Urine ketones negative

Fasting blood glucose 5–7.2 mmol/L (90–130 mg/dL)

1- to 2-hr postprandial glucose level <10 mmol/L (180 mg/dL)

Avoid symptoms of diabetes mellitus

Avoid hypoglycemia

Normalize nutrition and maintain reasonable weight

Achieve normal growth and development

Minimize or prevent complications

Accept diabetes with a realistic but positive attitude

Enjoy normal and flexible lifestyle

Promote emotional well-being; have patient take charge of condition

col must be individualized and can be developed only after the type of diabetes has been categorized. In general, glucose metabolism is normalized in patients who achieve excellent control. The DCCT verified that strict glycemic control is associated with a reduction in the occurrence and progression of chronic complications in patients with type 1 diabetes. The results of the UKPDS confirm that intensive control of blood sugar results in a decrease in long-term complications and mortality in patients with type 2 disease. Excellent blood sugar control in patients with either type 1 or type 2 diabetes significantly improves the patient's quality of life.

The formula to achieve these objectives combines a program of weight control or loss with an individualized exercise program and the use of medications. Diet, exercise, and medications are greatly enhanced by a program of education and weight control.

TREATMENT

Although therapies exist for treating the chronic complications of diabetes, prevention should always be the goal. As demonstrated by the DCCT and UKPDS, good glycemic control can have dramatic effects on the development and progression of complications and should be attempted unless otherwise contraindicated.

Diabetes affects virtually every organ of the body. Complications of diabetes often affect the eyes, nervous system, penile erectile function, kidneys, cardiovascular system, and extremities. Retinopathy can be treated successfully with laser photocoagulation. If retinal vitreous hemorrhage occurs, surgical vitrectomy can often restore vision. Diabetic cataracts may improve with strict glycemic control and may respond to treatment with aldose reductase inhibitors. Neuropathies may also respond to strict glycemic control, but

TABLE 40.11	Clinical Manifestations and Treatment of Neuropathies	
Disturbance	**Manifestation**	**Treatment**
Cardiovascular abnormalities	Orthostatic hypotension	Fludrocortisone
		Midodrine
Motor disturbance of gastrointestinal tract	Gastroparesis	Metoclopramide
		Erythromycin
	Constipation	Laxatives, stool softeners
	Diarrhea	Antidiarrheals
Genitourinary tract disturbances	Sexual dysfunction	Sildenafil
	Male: erectile dysfunction	Vardenafil
		Tadalafil
		Alprostadil (injection or penile suppository)
		Vacuum tumescent devices
		Testosterone
	Female: insufficient lubrication	Estrogen
		Vaginal lubricants
Peripheral neuropathy	Nerves of extremities	Amitriptyline
		Desipramine
		Imipramine
		Duloxetine
		Capsaicin cream
		Gabapentin
		Phenytoin
		Mexiletine

other therapeutic modalities often are necessary. Table 40.11 lists neuropathies and their treatment options.

Many men with diabetes experience partial or complete erectile dysfunction. Self-injection or intrapenile insertion of prostaglandins, vacuum tumescence devices, and surgical prosthetic implants are viable options for the man with impotence. A class of drugs called phosphodiesterase type 5 (PDE-5) inhibitors has recently revolutionized the treatment of erectile dysfunction.[39] These drugs selectively inhibit the PDE-5 enzyme, thereby enhancing the activity of nitric oxide, which increases blood flow to the penis, resulting in enhanced penile pressure and erection maintenance. Sildenafil, vardenafil, and tadalafil are three PDE-5 inhibitors currently available for the management of erectile dysfunction.

Patients with diabetes are more likely to develop nephropathy than those without diabetes; diabetic nephropathy is the most common cause of end-stage renal disease in the Western world.[18] Proteinuria is the first clinical manifestation, with progression to hypertension, azotemia, hypoalbuminemia, and edema. Dialysis or kidney transplantation may be necessary when the patient progresses to end-stage renal disease. Strict blood glucose control is necessary to reduce,

or possibly prevent, pathologic changes caused by hyperglycemia. Although many antihypertensive drugs have been evaluated for preventing and treating diabetic nephropathy, angiotensin-converting enzyme inhibitors (ACEIs) and angiotensin receptor blockers (ARBs) have a greater effect on reducing diabetic proteinuria and slowing creatinine clearance reduction than other types of antihypertensive medications.[40] Currently, many practitioners are treating patients who have diabetic proteinuria, with or without hypertension, with ACEIs or ARBs in an attempt to slow the progression of nephropathy.

Training the patient with diabetes to monitor foot care and vigorously treat any foot problems can reduce the incidence of infection and gangrene, which often necessitates amputation. Patients with diabetes are 15 to 40 times more likely to need lower limb amputation than those without the disease.[41] Ulceration of the foot with subsequent infection often is the initiating complaint. Peripheral vascular disease caused by atherosclerosis, deceased pain sensation caused by neuropathy, and poor immune function may all contribute to the development of foot lesions. Patients with diabetes should thus be instructed to monitor foot care daily, never go barefoot, strictly control their blood glucose levels, and avoid trauma to the feet by properly cutting their toenails and wearing shoes that fit properly. The hemorheologic agent pentoxifylline may improve impaired circulation, slow neuropathy development, improve healing, and correct blood flow defects common in patients with diabetes.[42] Cilostazol is an agent that can improve walking distance in those affected by intermittent claudication caused by underlying peripheral vascular disease.[43] Becaplermin gel, a topical agent that is a genetically engineered platelet-derived growth factor, may promote wound healing and decrease the time to complete ulcer closure in patients with neuropathic lower extremity ulcers.[44] Despite effective treatment modalities, prevention of foot ulcers is always preferred, because 20% of people with foot ulcers eventually require amputation.[45]

NONPHARMACOLOGIC THERAPY

Education. The patient with diabetes spends 365 days a year caring for the condition and monitoring the results of his or her efforts. Each patient with diabetes must understand the disease and be able to follow specific steps to treat the condition and evaluate whether the treatment protocol is achieving its objectives.

Patient education entails a health team approach that includes a physician, nurse, dietitian, pharmacist, and possibly a social worker, psychologist, and exercise physiologist. It is also important that the patient be educated continually and interact with other patients who also have diabetes. This can be achieved by active involvement in the Juvenile Diabetes Foundation or the local affiliate of the American Diabetes Association. The educational effort must be well organized and assess each individual patient's needs. It is also important that patients be evaluated periodically for their competence in performing blood tests, mixing and injecting insulin, rotating injection sites, using the diet exchange system, and following a prescribed physical activity program. Education should be broken down into at least three areas:

■ Initial management of the diabetes, which provides necessary information to bring the condition under control and gives the patient time to adjust to the condition. This level of education is based on the limitations of the patient and family to accept or assimilate all there is to know about diabetes at the time of diagnosis. During this time, the patient is taught the initial skills needed for basic self-care (insulin injection technique, recognition of signs and symptoms of hyperglycemia and hypoglycemia).

■ Home management of diabetes places emphasis on increasing knowledge and flexibility as some experience is gained in adapting to and living with diabetes. This level is essential for every patient but must be tailored to each person's needs and capacity. This type of educational experience is preferably offered in a non-hospital environment that is as close to home as possible.

■ Lifestyle improvement is the third area in which educational guidelines should be developed. This form of education deals with advanced learning and is viewed as enriching the patient's life with flexibility, insight, and

self-determination. This level also provides education on how to respond to special situations such as adjusting insulin dosages when traveling across time zones or using devices designed to assist visually impaired patients. Unfortunately, many patients with diabetes are left to discover this information by trial and error.

Physical Activity (Exercise). Exercise has many physical and psychological benefits and should be practiced in some form by most patients with diabetes. Although physicians nearly always recommend exercise as part of diabetes treatment, it is seldom prescribed or followed. Recently, more healthcare professionals have begun to understand how physical activity improves the control of diabetes. Programs are available specifically for patients with diabetes. Exercise improves insulin sensitivity or the body's ability to facilitate entry of glucose into the cell. This is particularly important in patients with type 2 diabetes. Exercise also lowers blood glucose levels by allowing glucose to penetrate the muscle cell and be metabolized without the assistance of insulin. Glucose can be used to varying degrees without insulin in all types of cells. Exercise also improves circulatory function, helps maintain normal body weight, and aids in breathing, digestion, and metabolism. An exercise log may help the patient maintain a regular daily schedule. Patients who monitor their own blood glucose become motivated to exercise because they easily see the beneficial effects of exercise on blood sugar control.

A physical activity program should be prescribed and followed by all patients with diabetes. Patients should be evaluated before the exercise prescription is determined. The patient's health, interests, preferences, and motivation to exercise should be taken into consideration in developing a specific method of exercising. If the patient's blood glucose level is greater than 300 mg per dL (16.7 mmol/L), exercise can result in an excessive rise in counterregulatory hormones that in the presence of inadequate insulin availability can decrease muscle glucose uptake and increase liver glucose production, causing more pronounced hyperglycemia. Therefore, patients with type 1 diabetes should know their blood glucose level before beginning exercise. If the blood glucose level is less than 300 mg per dL (16.7 mmol/L), injected insulin that has been absorbed subcutaneously can be absorbed more rapidly, resulting in excessive insulin, which, in combination with the exercise, can cause a serious drop in blood glucose. Patients over the age of 40 and those who have had diabetes for more than 25 years should have an exercise stress test, and an individualized graded exercise program should be prescribed. Patients with peripheral sensory neuropathy or vascular insufficiency should avoid exercise that may cause trauma to the feet. Patients with proliferative retinopathy should avoid strenuous exercise because it may induce hemorrhage and resultant blindness.

Exercise-induced hypoglycemia is another concern in patients who exercise. Consuming additional carbohydrate 30 minutes before exercise can help prevent hypoglycemia. Patients should also inject insulin at a non-exercise site (e.g., in the abdomen if the patient intends to run). The patient should log the exercise and monitor what effect it has on his or her blood glucose control. By doing this, the patient will be encouraged to engage in physical activity regularly. If hypoglycemia is a recurrent problem, a decrease in the insulin dose may be warranted. Patients should also be warned to wear an identification bracelet or necklace when exercising in case of an emergency. All patients should carry a quick source of carbohydrate with them when exercising in case hypoglycemia develops. General guidelines for all people with diabetes who exercise include the following: wear proper footwear and other protective clothing, avoid exercising in extreme temperatures, inspect feet daily and after each exercise session, and avoid exercise when glycemic control is erratic.[46]

Nutritional Therapy (Diet). Diet is one of the most challenging and difficult aspects of therapy to maintain consistently. For this reason, the American Diabetes Association in recent years has begun to focus on developing nutrition goals that can be achieved with a wide range of diets. Therefore, there is no one "diabetic diet" or "American Diabetes Association diet"; rather, nutritional and therapy goals are established for each patient, taking into consideration the patient's lifestyle, food preferences, cultural background, and other factors that may influence the foods consumed. Table 40.12 provides an overview of diabetes diet therapy and outlines the goals of medical nutrition therapy. The overall goal of nutrition therapy is to "assist people with diabetes in making changes in nutrition and exercise habits leading to improved metabolic control."[47]

Patients should be taught to read labels carefully because many sugarless and "diabetic" products actually contain a

---

TABLE 40.12   Diabetes Diet Therapy and Goals of Medical Nutritional Therapy

Maintain near-normal blood glucose levels by balancing food intake with insulin or oral glucose-lowering medications and activity levels.

Achieve optimal serum lipid levels.

Maintain reasonable weight for adults and growth and development rates in children and adolescents; meet increased metabolic needs during pregnancy and lactation or recovery from catabolic illnesses. ("Reasonable weight" is the weight a patient and healthcare provider acknowledge as achievable and maintainable; it need not be the same as the traditionally defined ideal body weight.)

Prevent and treat acute complications (e.g., hypoglycemia, short-term illness, exercise-related problems) and chronic complications (e.g., renal disease, neuropathy, hypertension, and cardiovascular disease).

Improve health by optimizing nutrition.

(From Evidence-based nutrition principles and recommendations for the treatment and prevention of diabetes and related complications (technical review). Diabetes Care 25:148–198, 2002.)

---

high number of calories and are not effective in helping those with diabetes achieve or maintain ideal body weight. Ingestion of animal (saturated) fats should be minimized because of the increased incidence of atherosclerotic disease in patients with diabetes. Some excellent studies have been done that show the importance of increasing fiber in the diet of patients with diabetes. However, each patient needs to see how he or she responds to the various types of fiber. Some fibers that have a high degree of pectin can cause constipation, while other fiber products, because of their bulk nature, can cause flatulence and diarrhea. Fiber may have a role in the prevention of colon cancer and can have a beneficial effect on lipid profile. Daily fiber intake of 20 to 35 g generally is recommended and should come from a variety of sources, such as whole grains, fruits, and vegetables.

To achieve the objectives of diet therapy, the patient must spend time with a dietitian to determine individual goals and outline a method to achieve those goals. Blood glucose monitoring, A1C, lipids, blood pressure, and renal function are all critical factors in assessing nutrition therapy. In general, protein should be restricted to 15% to 20% of total calories; in those with renal dysfunction, lower protein intakes may be advised. Protein should be derived from both animal and plant sources.

If 15% to 20% of total calories are derived from protein, then the remaining 80% to 85% will be derived from carbohydrates and fats. Specifically, carbohydrate and monounsaturated fat should provide 60% to 70% of total energy intake. In contrast to older dietary recommendations, there are no guidelines on how many calories should come from these latter sources. Simple sugars are no longer shunned, and complex carbohydrates are no longer the only type of carbohydrate recommended. It has been shown that fruits and milk have a lower glycemic index than most starches, and the glycemic response to bread, rice, and potatoes may be similar to that to sucrose. Adjustment of the type and proportion of carbohydrate intake is dictated by the goals for that individual patient and should take into account the patient's glucose and lipid profile. Nonnutritive sweeteners approved by the U.S. Food and Drug Administration (FDA) are safe for all patients with diabetes and include saccharin, aspartame, acesulfame potassium, and sucralose.

Of all the calories consumed, less than 10% should consist of saturated fats and up to 10% from polyunsaturated fats, and the consumption of trans unsaturated fatty acids should be minimized. The desired glucose, lipid, and body weight goals influence the amount of fat to consume. Patients with normal lipid levels and a reasonable weight should receive 30% or less of total calories from total fat and less than 10% of calories as saturated fat. If obesity and weight loss are concerns, a further reduction in fat intake is warranted.

Patients with diabetes need to learn the simple diabetic exchange system, which allows patients to eat a large variety of foods. Diet therapy with type 2 diabetes has a high degree of failure and often creates feelings of frustration, pessimism, and anger, which in turn result in poorly informed and inadequately motivated patients. Successful diet programs entail behavior modification. Patients should be encouraged to join groups such as Weight Watchers and to keep a diet log. For a period of 4 to 10 days, each time he or she eats, the patient should write down how much he or she eats and why (e.g., because of social pressure, loneliness, depression, or nervousness or because nourishment is truly needed). By using smaller plates, taking only one helping of food at a time, and being aware of why they eat, patients can change their dietary behavior.

One reason diet therapy may fail is that changes in the patient's diet are not accompanied by an appropriate change in the dose of insulin or other medication. The first steps in diet therapy should be to prescribe an exercise program, lower the medication dose, and put the patient on a diet containing fewer calories. Insulin overtreatment probably is one of the most common causes of inadequate diabetes control and weight gain. In one group of diabetic patients, 75% needed a reduction in insulin dose of at least 10%; 35% of the overtreated patients had large appetites, and 30% had hepatomegaly and headaches.[48] Patients taking too much insulin tend to eat up to that level of insulin and therefore gain weight. Also, many patients with type 2 diabetes already have excess serum insulin levels and may still feel hungry after eating a large meal, presumably because of their excess insulin levels.

Alcohol Use. If a patient's diabetes is well controlled, modest amounts of alcohol will not significantly alter blood glucose levels. In general, the same guidelines of alcohol use applicable to the general public apply to patients with diabetes. Two government agencies recommend that no more than two drinks per day for men and one drink a day for women are considered safe and reasonable.[49] Pregnant women and patients with a history of alcoholism or alcohol abuse should avoid alcohol. Likewise, if other medical conditions exist that could be exacerbated by alcohol (e.g., pancreatitis, neuropathy, hypertension), then abstention from alcohol would be prudent. Alcohol should always be ingested along with a meal, and patients taking insulin or secretagogues may be more susceptible to altered blood glucose levels when consuming alcohol. Two first-generation sulfonylureas, tolbutamide and chlorpropamide, have been reported to interact with alcohol, resulting in a disulfiram-like reaction. The second-generation agents (e.g., glyburide) do not appear to cause such a reaction.

Patients who consume alcoholic beverages must consider the caloric content of the beverage and should be encouraged to choose low-calorie drinks. The sugar content of wines and mixed drinks also must be considered.

Blood Pressure and Lipid Control. The presence of hypertension or dyslipidemia in patients with diabetes contributes to chronic complications such as nephropathy, retinopathy, cerebrovascular disease, and peripheral vascular and cardiovascular disease. In general, diabetes places patients at risk for atherosclerotic vascular disease, and this risk increases when hypertension or dyslipidemia is present. Obesity and smoking can further contribute to the development of vascular complications. Table 40.13 lists current guidelines for blood pressure and lipid control in patients with diabetes. The American Diabetes Association recommends that diabetic patients be prescribed a statin medication daily to reduce cardiovascular risks. In addition, an ACEI or ARB is recommended for most patients for a renoprotective effect.

Pancreas Transplantation. Whole organ kidney and pancreas transplantation is a surgical option for the treatment of select patients with uremia and type 1 diabetes. Pancreas transplantation typically occurs in three scenarios: simultaneous kidney and pancreas transplant, pancreas transplant after kidney transplantation, and solitary pancreas transplant alone. Approximately 85% to 90% of patients can achieve normal glycemic control with this procedure. Chapter 27 discusses pancreas transplantation. In addition, replacement of the damaged insulin-producing β cells with functioning islet cells (islet cell transplantation) is an emerging strategy for the treatment of type 1 diabetes.

PHARMACOTHERAPY

The therapeutic options available in the United States for managing diabetes mellitus have expanded greatly in the past few years. Currently, eight categories of FDA-approved medications for treating diabetes are available: insulin, sulfonylureas, biguanides, α-glucosidase inhibitors, thiazolidinediones, meglitinides/phenylalanines (short-acting secretagogues), amylin analogs, and incretin mimetics. All eight categories of medicines can treat patients with type 2 diabetes effectively, but insulin is the only medication essential for those with type 1 disease. In this chapter, the sulfonylureas and the short-acting "sulfonylurea-like" agents nateglinide and repaglinide will be referred to as secretagogues.

Because of the recent expansion in the number of antidiabetic drugs available, choosing the optimal medication or combinations for the management of hyperglycemia in pa-

TABLE 40.13	Treatment Goals for Blood Pressure and Lipids
Blood Pressure	
Adults	<130/80 mm Hg
Lipids	
Low-density lipoprotein	<100 mg/dL
Triglycerides	<150 mg/dL
High-density lipoprotein (men)	>40 mg/dL
High-density lipoprotein (women)	A goal of 10 mg/dL; higher may be appropriate

(From Standards of medical care in diabetes. Diabetes Care 27 (Suppl 1):S15–S35,2004.)

tients with diabetes is not easily reduced to a single treatment algorithm. Treating the patient with diabetes remains an art and entails constant reevaluation and assessment of the patient's response to proven therapies. Although some situations clearly warrant the use of one product over another, the choice of medications usually is not clear-cut, and cost considerations, the amount of glycemic lowering needed, compliance/adherence issues, and the patient's age, weight, and lipid profile all factor into the decision-making process.

Insulin. Insulin has been used since 1922 as monotherapy in patients with type 1 disease and since the late 1950s in combination or monotherapy in patients with type 2 diabetes. Typically, patients who have type 1 diabetes and need insulin initially tend to be younger than 30 years old, lean, markedly hyperglycemic, and prone to developing ketoacidosis.

Children with diabetes should begin giving their own injections around age 8 or 9, although parents should periodically administer insulin to stay in practice and should inject in areas that are difficult for the child to reach. All patients taking insulin therapy should be strongly encouraged to self-monitor their blood glucose levels. Insulin regimens should be tailored to each patient's individual needs, desired metabolic control, and age. Tighter glycemic control is best achieved with three or four insulin injections per day or with an insulin infusion pump, although not all patient populations are best served by regimens offering strict glycemic control (e.g., the very old, the very young).

Choice of Insulin. The time action profile, effects of mixing, species, strength, and cost of insulin all must be considered in choosing an insulin preparation. Factors to consider when choosing insulin are outlined in Table 40.14, and Table 40.15 summarizes the currently available insulin preparations.

Time Activity Profile. Insulins may be categorized in the following groups on the basis of their time activity profiles: rapid-acting, short-acting, intermediate-acting, and long-acting. Figure 40.6 shows the kinetic parameters of the four categories of insulin. Each patient may experience variations in clinical response to any particular class of insulin, and the characteristics of each insulin (time of onset, time to peak, duration of action) can vary from patient to patient.

TABLE 40.14 | Factors Considered in Comparing Insulins

Kinetic formulation and time activity profile

Species source (human, pork, beef)

Strength (U = 100, U = 500)

Methods of achieving long action (e.g., protein such as protamine)

Purity

Mixability

Cost

Manufacturer dependability and availability

Table 40.16 describes some of the factors that may alter the time activity profiles of insulin.

Rapid-acting insulins include the insulin analogs lispro, aspart, and glulisine. Human insulin analogs have a similar structure and function to human insulin but are developed with DNA recombinant technology. By altering the amino acid sequence in human insulin, manufacturers can create various alterations in the actions of insulin. For example, insulin lispro has the normal sequence of proline (Pro) and lysine (Lys) reversed at the 28th and 29th positions. The change in amino acid sequence results in rapid absorption from the subcutaneous tissues, resulting in a faster physiologic action than human regular insulin.[50] Rapid-acting insulins can be administered immediately before a meal and provides added flexibility, particularly for young patients and those with erratic meal schedules. Rapid-acting insulins may be safer and more predictable in regard to the development of hypoglycemia when compared to regular insulin.

The short-acting insulins include semilente, regular, and regular buffered insulins. Regular and buffered insulin formulations are clear and contain solubilized crystalline insulin. Regular insulin and the rapid-acting analogs are the only insulins that can be safely given intravenously, but regular is the only insulin used in this fashion because intravenous use of the rapid-acting analogues would be more expensive and would not provide any advantage over regular insulin. The only FDA-approved insulin for use in insulin pumps is the genetically engineered Velosulin BR (buffered regular human insulin of rDNA origin); however, human regular insulin has been safely used for many years, and insulin lispro and insulin aspart are commonly used with this mode of delivery with excellent results. Semilente is an amorphous precipitate of insulin and zinc in the form of a suspension, with a slightly delayed onset and peak and a greater duration of action than regular insulin.

Intermediate-acting insulins include neutral protamine Hagedorn (NPH) and lente insulins. NPH insulin preparations contain a suspension of zinc–insulin crystals and protamine, a protein derived from fish sperm. A few patients are or can become allergic to protamine. Lente insulin is composed of a 30:70 mixture of semilente and ultralente. The lente insulins are produced from various forms of the zinc–insulin complex and are particularly useful in patients sensitive to protamine. The available long-acting insulins include ultralente and the insulin analogue glargine. Insulin detemir is another long-acting insulin that recently gained FDA approval.

Currently, two strengths of insulin are available in the United States: U-100 and U-500. U-500 can be obtained only by prescription and must be special ordered from Eli Lilly. In Europe insulin is available only by prescription and in one strength, U-40. In the United States all of the insulin analogues are available with a prescription, while the non-analogue U-100 insulins can be purchased without a prescription.

TABLE 40.15	Insulin Preparations Available in the United States	
Product	**Manufacturer**	**Strength**
Rapid-acting		
Humalog (Insulin lispro)	Lilly	U–100
Novolog (Insulin aspart)	Novo-Nordisk	U–100
Apidra (Insulin glulisine)	Aventis	U–100
Short-acting		
Pork*		
Iletin II Regular	Lilly	U–100, U–500
Human		
Humulin Regular	Lilly	U–100
Novolin R	Novo-Nordisk	U–100
Velosulin Human R	Novo-Nordisk	U–100
Intermediate-acting		
Pork*		
Iletin II Lente	Lilly	U–100
Iletin II NPH	Lilly	U–100
Human		
Humulin L (Lente)	Lilly	U–100
Humulin N (NPH)	Lilly	U–100
Novolin L (Lente)	Lilly	U–100
Novolin N (NPH)	Lilly	U–100
Long-acting		
Human		
Humulin U (Ultralente)	Lilly	U–100
Lantus (Insulin glargine)	Aventis	U–100
Levemir (Detemir)	Novo-Nordisk	U–100
Fixed combinations (all are U–100 insulins)		
Human		NPH/Regular
Humulin 70/30	Lilly	70/30
Novolin 70/30	Novo-Nordisk	70/30
Humulin 50/50	Lilly	50/50
Novolog Mix 70/30	Novo-Nordisk	70/30 (aspart protamine/aspart)
Humalog Mix 75/25	Lilly	75/25 (lispro protamine/lispro)

*Pork insulin no longer available for human use beginning January 2006.

Species Source and Purity. Species source is becoming less of a concern as more and more patients are switched to or are started on human forms of insulin. The following sources of insulin are available: pork, biosynthetic human, semisynthetic human, and analogues of human insulin. Pork insulin is less antigenic than beef insulin, and therefore the manufacture of beef insulin and beef/pork mixtures has been discontinued.[51] Purified pork insulin has no clear advantages over human insulin, and its availability may cease in the near future.

Human insulin is the least antigenic of the available insulins and tends to be more soluble than animal insulins. This results in more rapid absorption and a shorter duration of action, so a patient being switched from one source of insulin to another should be monitored closely. Close monitoring is also needed for patients switching from a short-acting insulin to a rapid-acting insulin analogue such as lispro or aspart.

Biosynthetic insulin and semisynthetic insulin are therapeutically equivalent. Biosynthetic insulins include an insulin formed by recombinant DNA using *Escherichia coli* (Eli Lilly), insulin formed by biosynthetic recombinant DNA using baker's yeast (Novo-Nordisk), and semisynthetic insulin (Novo-Nordisk). Insulin is produced through recombinant processes by the insertion of the human gene for proin-

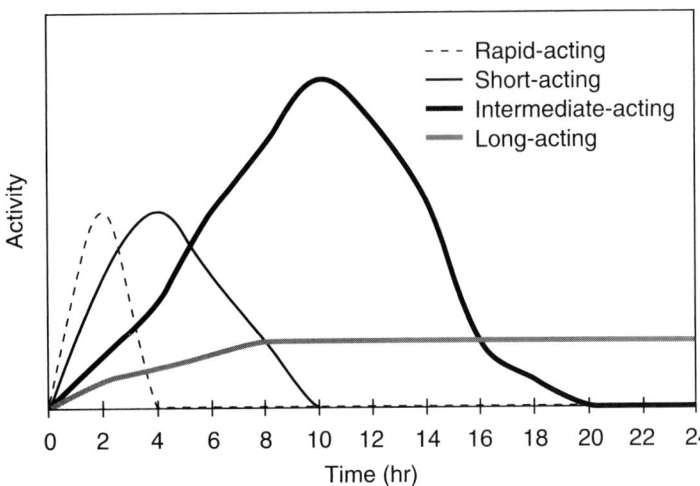

Insulin Type	Onset	Peak	Duration
Rapid-acting	0–0.25 hr	1–2 hr	2–4 hr
Short-acting	0.5–1 hr	2–4 hr	6–8 hr
Intermediate-acting	1–4 hr	6–10 hr	16–24 hr
Long-acting	4–6 hr	18 hr	24–36 hr

FIGURE 40.6 Time activity profiles for insulin.

sulin into the *E. coli* or baker's yeast genome. These genetically altered organisms are fermented in an appropriate medium that is conducive to the production of proinsulin (or a miniproinsulin). The proinsulin is harvested, enzymatically altered to form insulin, and purified. Human insulin is also produced via a semisynthetic method by the enzymatic transpeptidation of pork insulin at position 30 of the B chain with the substitution of threonine for alanine.

The recommendations for dosing insulin when changing from beef to human insulin or from conventional to purified insulin are summarized in Table 40.17. Human insulin is indicated for the patient types listed in Table 40.18. All patients with insulin allergy should be placed on human insulin.

Another factor that may affect insulin choice is purity. Most forms of insulin available today are highly purified and are unlikely to contain substances that affect the action of the insulin. All of the insulins listed in Table 40.15 are classified as highly purified because they have fewer than 10 parts per million of proinsulin. Highly purified insulins are less likely to produce lipoatrophy or cause insulin antibody formation.

Insulin Dosing. A number of dosing regimens are used in administering insulin to patients with type 1 diabetes (Fig. 40.7). Commonly used methods include the following:

1. Single daily injection of intermediate-acting insulin
2. Two daily injections of intermediate-acting insulin
3. Two daily injections of 70:30 (intermediate-acting:short-acting) premixed insulin
4. Two daily injections of split and mixed intermediate-acting and short-acting insulin
5. Three daily injections of short-acting (or rapid-acting) insulin in combination with a single injection of long-acting insulin (e.g., glargine)
6. Continuous subcutaneous insulin infusion (insulin infusion pump)
7. Sliding scale (multiple daily injections of short-acting or rapid-acting insulin)

The level of practitioner motivation, the ability of the patient to monitor glucose control and adjust doses, and the level of control desired affect the choice of regimen. The daily insulin need of the typical patient with type 1 diabetes is 0.5 to 1.0 units per kg. This total daily dosage may be given as one injection (method 1) or may be divided into several doses to more closely mimic physiologic insulin secretion. Premeal doses of insulin are adjusted; approximately

TABLE 40.16	Factors Affecting Serum Insulin Concentrations

Injection site (abdomen, arm, thigh)

Exercise (enhances absorption)

Depth of injection

Concentration of insulin

Increase in ambient temperature (increases absorption)

Massage of site (increases absorption)

Insulin antibodies (attract and hold insulin)

Variance in degrading enzymes at site (yields day-to-day variation)

Insulin interaction with receptors

TABLE 40.17	Recommendations for Dosing Insulin When Changing From Animal to Human Insulin or Conventional to Purified Insulin

Highly variable from patient to patient; patient should monitor blood glucose levels closely (decreases of 9%–20% reported).

Recommend 10% decrease of normal dosages.

Recommend 20% decrease if patient is receiving more than 50 units/day.

TABLE 40.18	Patients Who Should Use Human Insulin

Patients with severe insulin resistance (using >100–200 units/day)

Patients with insulin allergy (e.g., local cutaneous reactions, rashes)

Patients with lipoatrophy or lipohypertrophy

All patients with type 2 diabetes using insulin for a short period of time (e.g., during surgery, infections)

Any patient using insulin intermittently (e.g., patients with gestational diabetes, those on total parenteral nutrition)

All newly diagnosed patients with type 1 diabetes

Pregnant patients (antibodies are passed to the fetus)

1 to 2 units of insulin is given for each 50 mg per dL (2.78 mmol/L) of desired decrease in blood glucose levels.

Insulin can be delivered through different devices, the most common being the syringe. Insulin pumps, jet injectors, and insulin pens are additional methods of delivery. Inhaled insulin is under development and may become available in the near future. When syringes are used properly, the injections are not painful because of finer needles and the use of special coatings that allow easy insertion. Insulin pumps are small, computerized, externally worn devices that deliver a steady dose of insulin through a small plastic tube and a small needle that is inserted and taped into place in the abdominal region. A bolus dose of insulin can be given upon command before meals. Jet injectors force a pressurized stream of insulin through the skin, thereby avoiding puncturing of the skin. This mode of injecting may cause some skin bruising. Insulin pen devices are small and convenient and look much like old-fashioned cartridge pens. The insulin is stored in prefilled cartridges that can be replaced. Insulin pens can be adjusted easily to deliver a precise amount of insulin, and some devices are disposable. The insulin pen device is well suited for patients with limited coordination (e.g., older adults) and for people leading active lives.

Basal/Bolus Concept of Insulin Administration. To achieve maximal blood glucose control, insulin administration should closely mimic normal physiologic insulin release in a person without diabetes. As previously discussed, insulin is released at a constant rate throughout a 24-hour period, which is known as basal insulin secretion. When a meal is consumed, the pancreas releases additional insulin (bolus insulin) to cover the postprandial blood glucose excursion. Insulin regimens that mimic this pattern tend to result in optimal control. Obviously, the use of an insulin pump (method 6) mimics the normal pancreas most closely; however, injecting long-acting insulin (basal insulin) once or twice daily along with rapid-acting or regular insulin (bolus insulin) prior to each meal can produce superior blood glucose control as well (method 5) and is an example of maximally using the basal/bolus concept of insulin administration.

Method Comparison. Method 1, a single injection of intermediate-acting insulin in a patient with type 1 diabetes, is not sufficient to control blood glucose levels for a 24-hour period. This regimen usually results in hyperglycemia before the next dose and may cause hypoglycemia that coincides with peak levels about 8 hours after the dose. A dose that is high enough to cover the patient for 24 hours usually will also cause hypoglycemia at the peak. Ketoacidosis may be avoided, but erratic blood glucose swings are common. A1C levels attained with this regimen typically fall in the range of 11% to 13%, which is unacceptable blood glucose control.

Glycemic control with method 2 is slightly better than that with method 1. With method 2, two thirds of the total daily insulin requirement is injected before breakfast and one third is injected just before dinner. Intermediate-acting insulin is used. The chance of developing hypoglycemia is less with this method than with method 1, but the glycemic control attained is only slightly better than that of method 1.

Methods 3 and 4 provide average to above-average control with two injections per day. The only difference between the two methods is that with method 3, the patient can increase or decrease the individual doses but not alter the ratio of short-acting to intermediate-acting insulin. The patient usually takes two thirds of the total daily dose before breakfast and one third before dinner. The split and mixed regimen is initiated with a 70:30 mixture of intermediate-acting: short-acting insulin, but this ratio may be altered according to insulin needs. Blood sugar must be monitored before meals and at bedtime and the insulin dosage adjusted accordingly. Method 4 is preferred over method 3. A common variation of method 3 is to administer a mixed (intermediate-acting and short-acting) dose before breakfast, a dose of short-acting insulin before dinner, and a dose of intermediate-acting insulin at bedtime. Glycemic control expected with these methods may provide A1C values in the range of 7% to 9%.

Method 5 uses doses of short-acting or rapid-acting insulin before each meal in combination with one or two daily doses of a longer-acting insulin. Variations of this method include administering regular or a rapid-acting insulin analogue such as lispro, aspart, or glulisine before each meal, with a dose of intermediate-acting insulin or long-acting insulin (e.g., glargine) once daily. This regimen entails a great deal of patient motivation but provides excellent glycemic coverage and allows the patient a great deal of latitude with regard to meals.

Method 6, continuous subcutaneous insulin infusion, is an excellent method. Initially, it requires intensive patient training, but the increased flexibility and freedom are unparalleled by other dosage regimens. This method provides the patient with a continuous basal amount of insulin (0.5 to 1 units/hour) in combination with bolus doses to cover meals. Currently available pumps are about the size of a deck of cards and weigh only a few ounces. Insulin reaches the patient via a small plastic catheter and through a subcutaneous

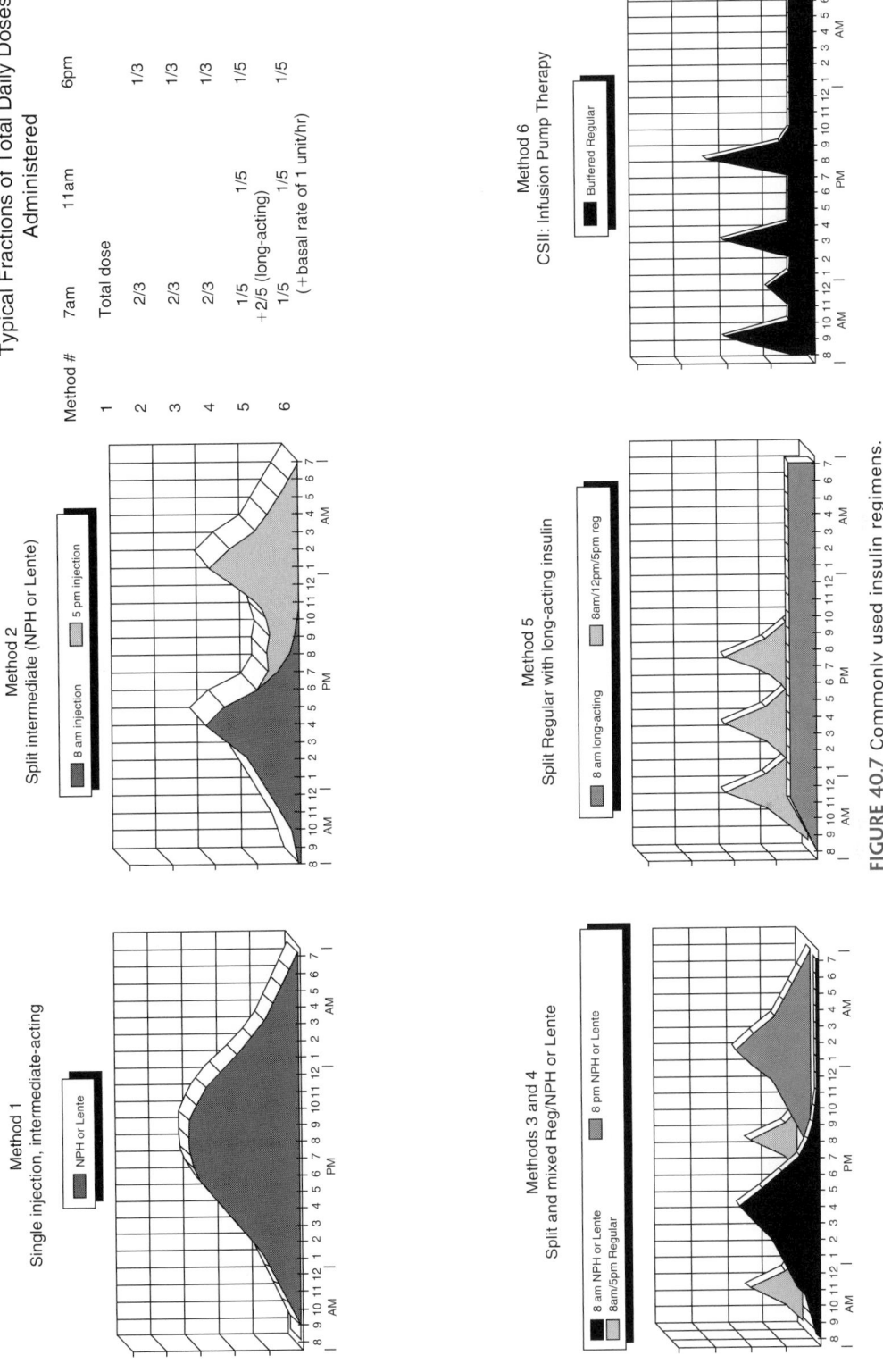

Typical Fractions of Total Daily Doses Administered

Method #	7am	11am	6pm
1	Total dose		
2	2/3		1/3
3	2/3		1/3
4	2/3		1/3
5	1/5 +2/5 (long-acting)	1/5	1/5
6	1/5	1/5 (+basal rate of 1 unit/hr)	1/5

Method 1
Single injection, intermediate-acting

NPH or Lente

Method 2
Split intermediate (NPH or Lente)

8 am injection   5 pm injection

Methods 3 and 4
Split and mixed Reg/NPH or Lente

8 am NPH or Lente   8 pm NPH or Lente
8am/5pm Regular

Method 5
Split Regular with long-acting insulin

8 am long-acting   8am/12pm/5pm reg

Method 6
CSII: Infusion Pump Therapy

Buffered Regular

FIGURE 40.7 Commonly used insulin regimens.

TABLE 40.19	Criteria for Prescribing Insulin Pumps

Selecting patients

Pregnant patients

Patients with early complications

Renal transplant recipients

Patients with difficult-to-control diabetes

Motivated patients with type 1 diabetes

Not suitable for children and patients with type 2 diabetes

All patients must be:

- Willing and highly motivated
- Capable of learning to use pump correctly
- Responsible for keeping records and following specific procedures
- Willing to perform and log blood tests daily
- Willing to be hospitalized for 2–4 days if necessary

Pump selection

Safety features (e.g., low-battery alarm)

Durability

Service level by manufacturer

Degree of training provided by manufacturer

Ease of use

Clinical features (e.g., programmable basal rates)

Cosmetic appeal

---

needle. Table 40.19 summarizes the criteria that are used for selecting patients for this method.[52] Factors to be considered when choosing a pump include safety and clinical features (e.g., low-battery alarm, programmable basal rates), durability, service level of manufacturer, ease of use, and cosmetic appeal. A1C values commonly achieved with methods 5 and 6 fall in the range of 5% to 7%.

Method 7, the sliding-scale method, is reserved for hospitalized patients who undergo frequent blood glucose monitoring. Patients who are acutely ill require more insulin than normal, and the scales used in these patients vary from institution to institution. The following is an example of a sliding scale that uses regular insulin for an adult: for a blood glucose level of less than 140 mg per dL, the subcutaneous insulin dosage would be 0 units; for 140 to 200 mg per dL, 2 units; for 201 to 300 mg per dL, 5 units; for 301 to 400 mg per dL, 10 Units; and for more than 400 mg per dL, 12 units. The scale is adjusted on the basis of the patient's response to various dosages of insulin. Disadvantages to using sliding-scale insulin regimens include the following: the insulin dose is based on a single glucose value without regard to patterns of response; it does not lead to stability of blood glucose levels; and it requires hyperglycemia to initiate therapy if given without basal insulin. Recently, the clinical utility of sliding-scale insulin regimens has come under scrutiny.

Interpretation of Blood Glucose Levels. Several problems may be encountered in SMBG. Proper patient technique and understanding of the particular method a patient uses should always be ascertained before the insulin dosage is adjusted. Patients using methods 3 through 6 should routinely check their blood glucose levels four times daily (before meals and at bedtime). Additionally, early morning (3 to 4 AM) and postprandial levels may be checked as needed. Patients who use method 1 should also be instructed to check their blood glucose levels; however, it is difficult to target particular out-of-range levels because only one dose is administered daily.

Generally, an increase in insulin dosage of 1 unit can be expected to decrease the blood glucose level by approximately 50 mg per dL (2.78 mmol/L). Some patients adjust their doses daily on the basis of the previous day's response. This approach may be reasonable for some, but it is probably more prudent to alter dosages only after a trend has been identified.

Two potential problems observed with the interpretation of morning fasting blood glucose levels include the dawn effect and the Somogyi phenomenon. The dawn effect results from a rise in blood glucose levels that increases insulin need starting at about 5 AM and continuing until about 9 AM. The early morning glucose rise can be caused by insufficient treatment, but in studies involving patients with continuous subcutaneous insulin infusion, the dawn phenomenon can still occur. Food ingestion is another factor that could influence the early morning rise. However, studies of fasting patients show that blood glucose levels can increase in the early morning. Although the phenomenon and its prevalence are not totally understood, it is a cause for concern for patients who are trying to achieve strict control. The most logical mechanism for the dawn phenomenon is an increased glucose production or decreased glucose utilization caused by the morning rise of cortisol levels, or other circadian influences.

In the Somogyi phenomenon, there is early morning hyperglycemia secondary to hypoglycemia. The patient with diabetes suffers an episode of hypoglycemia during sleep that results in the release of hormones that increase blood glucose levels such as cortisol, glucagon, and epinephrine. These hormones cause blood glucose levels to increase, and when the patient arises in the morning and tests his or her blood glucose, it is elevated. Because hypoglycemia is the precipitating cause of this phenomenon, the necessary step in treatment is to decrease the insulin dose.

The assessment of morning hyperglycemia must include an early morning (3 to 4 AM) blood glucose determination. If hypoglycemia is observed, then the bedtime or evening insulin dose should be decreased. If the level is within normal limits or high, then a slight increase in the evening insulin dose is warranted.

With the advent and availability of subcutaneous glucose sensors, achieving excellent glycemic control has become safer. Currently, MiniMed produces such a sensor that continuously monitors glucose levels in the interstitial fluid that under stable glucose levels corresponds to blood glucose levels.

Mixing and Storing Insulin. Insulin can be stored at room temperature for up to 1 month, and it should be injected at room temperature for patient comfort. Unused vials of insulin may be stored in the refrigerator, but they should not be exposed to extreme temperatures. Patients should be cautioned to store insulin properly when traveling in very hot or very cold climates.

Rapid-acting insulin and regular and NPH insulin are stable when mixed together in any ratio, and they are the mixture of choice when rapid or short- and intermediate-acting insulin is needed.[53] Patients should adhere to the following sequence when mixing NPH and rapid-acting/short-acting insulin:

1. Inject the appropriate quantity of air into the NPH insulin vial.
2. Inject the appropriate quantity of air into the rapid-acting insulin or regular insulin vial.
3. Withdraw the dose of rapid-acting or regular insulin.
4. Withdraw the dose of NPH insulin.

Insulin lispro or aspart can also be mixed in the same syringe with NPH insulin or insulin–zinc suspension insulins. As with regular insulin, the patient should always draw the rapid-acting insulin into the syringe first, then introduce the other insulin into the syringe. Regular and lente (also ultralente) insulin interact when mixed, the result being a blunting of the short-acting insulin. Patients should be instructed to either inject immediately after mixing or consistently inject after a measured period of time. The reaction between lente and regular insulin continues for 24 hours, so the response from an injection that is taken immediately after mixing may be significantly different from the response from an injection taken 24 hours after mixing. Velosulin regular insulins should not be mixed with lente insulins. The phosphate buffers precipitate the zinc from these formulations, resulting in an increased activity of short-acting insulin. Lente insulins may be mixed with each other in any ratio without affecting the time activity profile of the components, and mixtures of this nature remain stable for up to 18 months. Insulin glargine cannot be mixed with any type of insulin and should not be used in prefilled syringes.

Adverse Reactions to Insulin. The most common and serious reaction to insulin therapy is hypoglycemia. Previously, when less pure sources of insulin were used, lipoatrophy, insulin allergy, and insulin antibody formation were more common; they are now uncommon.

Hypoglycemia. All patients with diabetes should know the signs and symptoms of hypoglycemia, particularly patients on insulin therapy or oral secretagogue therapy. Factors that predispose the patient to hypoglycemia include insufficient food intake (skipping meals, vomiting, or diarrhea), poor timing of injections in relation to food intake, excessive exercise, inaccurate measurement of insulin, concomitant intake of hypoglycemic drugs, termination of diabetogenic conditions or drugs, and strict glycemic control. Symptoms of hypoglycemia include a parasympathetic response (nausea, hunger, or flatulence), diminished cerebral function known as neuroglycopenia (confusion, agitation, lethargy, or personality changes), sympathetic responses (tachycardia, sweating, or tremor), coma, and convulsions. Ataxia and blurred vision also are common. In older adults with decreased nerve function, patients with advanced neuropathy, patients who have had diabetes for 10 years or more, or patients receiving β-blockers, the symptoms of hypoglycemia sometimes are blunted or absent (usually sweating is preserved) and the condition may go undetected and untreated.

All manifestations of hypoglycemia are relieved rapidly by glucose administration. In unconscious patients, injections of glucagon or intravenous glucose or dextrose may be needed. Because of the potential danger of insulin reactions, the patient with diabetes should always carry packets of table sugar, candy, or glucose tablets for use at the onset of hypoglycemic symptoms. If a hypoglycemic person is mistakenly thought to be hyperglycemic and is given insulin, severe hypoglycemia and subsequent brain damage may result. Thus, when there is doubt as to whether a person with diabetes is hypoglycemic or hyperglycemic, sugar should be given initially until the condition can be evaluated accurately. Spouses or caregivers of patients with diabetes should be trained to administer glucagon in the event of hypoglycemia-induced unconsciousness. Glucagon (1 mg) should be administered subcutaneously or intramuscularly. Glucagon may cause nausea and vomiting; therefore, the unconscious patient should be positioned lying on his or her side or on his or her stomach to avoid aspiration.

Virtually every patient treated with insulin experiences hypoglycemia at some time. Ten percent of insulin-treated patients need assistance for at least one episode of severe hypoglycemia per year. Mortality secondary to hypoglycemia in insulin-treated patients may be as high as 3%.[54] Patients in the DCCT who were treated with intensive insulin therapy had an incidence of hypoglycemia three times higher than that of patients treated with conventional therapy.[1]

Lipohypertrophy. Lipohypertrophy is a problem encountered by patients who do not rotate injection sites. Fatty accumulations occur and usually resolve after the patient begins to rotate sites. Because this problem probably is not immunologic in nature, switching to a more highly purified product is not warranted.

Lipoatrophy. Atrophy of the fatty tissue (lipoatrophy) appears to be an immunologic process that may occur at the injection site or at a distant location. Female patients are affected more than male patients. The treatment of choice is to switch to human insulin. Human insulin should be injected directly into the atrophied area until the site has filled in.

After resolution, the patient should be instructed to continue to inject the area every 2 to 3 weeks to prevent recurrence.[55]

Oral Medications for Treating Type 2 Diabetes. Oral therapy is very efficacious in treating patients with type 2 diabetes, but most patients should first try a course of diet and exercise for 3 months before oral therapy is used. Certain situations dictate the use of intravenous therapy over oral agents in patients with type 2 diabetes (e.g., development of HHS) or temporary use of subcutaneous insulin (e.g., presence of severely elevated blood glucose levels), but the importance of diet and exercise cannot be overstated. Some patients with type 2 diabetes can manage their disease by losing weight and following a strict exercise program and diet. Even if oral medication is needed, patients who exercise regularly and are on a proper diet can manage their condition on less medicine than those not on a suitable diet or exercise program.

Secretagogues

Sulfonylureas. Sulfonylureas have been the mainstay of therapy for patients with type 2 diabetes since the late 1970s. This class of agents will continue to be widely used for treating diabetes, but as more is learned about the pathophysiology of insulin resistance and type 2 diabetes, agents with other mechanisms of action than the insulin secretagogues (e.g., incretin mimetics) will play an important role in diabetes treatment.

Sulfonylureas have shown both pancreatic and extrapancreatic effects but are useful only in patients with intact and functioning β cells.[56] Sulfonylureas increase insulin secretion directly and decrease glucagon release. They also may affect glucose levels by increasing insulin receptor binding affinity, increasing insulin effect by postreceptor action, and decreasing hepatic insulin extraction. The clinical effects of these extrapancreatic effects continue to be a subject of research and debate.

The following patient characteristics sometimes predict a positive clinical response to sulfonylureas: the patient is not diagnosed with diabetes until after age 40, the duration of diabetes is less than 5 years, the patient is near or above his or her ideal body weight, there has been no prior insulin treatment or the disease has been controlled with less than 40 units of insulin per day, and the fasting blood glucose level is less than 180 mg per dL (10 mmol/L).

The sulfonylureas available commercially are summarized in Table 40.20. Use typically results in a 1.5- to 2-unit drop in A1C. Chlorpropamide has the longest half-life of the first-generation agents and is associated in the highest incidence of adverse events; it is not recommended for newly diagnosed patients. The first-generation agents tend be less potent, so higher doses are needed. They also tend to displace drugs from protein-binding sites and are more likely to have drug interactions. Drug interactions with the first-generation agents include alcohol, anabolic steroids, β-blockers, dicoumarol, monoamine oxidase inhibitors, salicylates, and sulfonamides. Second-generation sulfonylureas are more po-

tent and tend to have fewer drug interactions because they bind nonionically and are present at much lower concentrations than the first-generation agents. Tolbutamide, tolazamide, and glipizide are metabolized to inactive or weakly active metabolites and are favored for use in patients with renal failure. The newest sulfonylurea, glimepiride, has similar effects as the other sulfonylureas and can be given once daily. Glimepiride is reported to have a lower incidence of hypoglycemia than other sulfonylureas, perhaps making it an attractive choice in older adults.[57]

The primary side effects of sulfonylureas include hypoglycemia and weight gain. The incidence of hypoglycemia is variable and depends on the agent and patient characteristics. One study reported a 20% chance of developing hypoglycemia for every 6 months of continuous sulfonylurea therapy.[56] Weight gain in the range of 1.8 to 2.8 kg has been observed in clinical studies. Conditions in which the sulfonylureas usually are contraindicated include acidosis, severe infections, major surgery, sulfa sensitivity, and pregnancy.

With proper patient selection, most patients respond adequately to sulfonylurea therapy.[58] Roughly 10% of all patients do not respond initially and are considered to be primary failures. Secondary failure that occurs with long-term use is most likely related to the natural progression of type 2 diabetes and β-cell dysfunction and has been reported to be in the range of 5% to 10% per year.[58]

In general, therapy should be started at a low dose that is gradually titrated until the desired effect is achieved. Low doses are given once daily before breakfast; higher doses are divided and given two or more times per day, depending on the half-life and formulation of the drug. Table 40.21 lists counseling points for each category of oral agents.

Meglitinides/Phenylalanines. The rapid-acting secretagogues repaglinide and nateglinide are unrelated to the sulfonylureas, although they have similar clinical effects: both cause an increase in insulin secretion from the pancreas and therefore require functioning β cells for their action.

Repaglinide is rapidly absorbed and eliminated (half-life less than 1 hour) and is most effective when given within 30 minutes before meals. Adverse events common with repaglinide therapy include weight gain and hypoglycemia, which is not surprising considering its mechanism of action. Modest weight gain has been reported (3.3%). Hypoglycemia appears to be more likely in sulfonylurea-naive patients with A1C values less than 8%, whereas those who have received sulfonylureas and have A1C values of 8% or more do not have an increased incidence in hypoglycemia. Antifungal agents such as ketoconazole and miconazole and the antibiotic erythromycin may inhibit the metabolism of repaglinide. Also, hepatic inducers of the CYP 3A4 isoenzyme (e.g., carbamazepine, barbiturates) can increase the metabolism of repaglinide.

Because repaglinide is metabolized by the liver and excreted via the feces, cautious use is advised in patients with hepatic impairment. In patients with renal compromise,

TABLE 40.20	Oral Diabetic Agents			
Generic Name	Brand Name	Mechanism of Action	Dosing	Side Effects
First-Generation Sulfonylureas				
Acetohexamide Chlorpropamide (not recommended)	Dymelor Diabinese	Stimulates release of insulin from pancreatic β cells	250 mg QD; titrate to a maximum of 1.5 g/day (divided) 250 mg QD; titrate to a maximum of 750 mg/day (divided) Initiate elderly patients at 100–125 mg QD	Hypoglycemia, weight gain, GI, blood dyscrasias, SIADH, disulfiram reaction Prolonged hypoglycemia, weight gain, GI, blood dyscrasias, disulfiram reaction, dilutional hyponatremia
Tolazamide	Tolinase		100–250 mg QD; titrate to a maximum of 500 mg BID	Hypoglycemia, weight gain, GI, blood dyscrasias, disulfiram reaction
Tolbutamide	Orinase		Adults over 65: 50–125 mg QD; titrate 1–2 g QD; titrate to a maximum of 3 g (divided)	Hypoglycemia, weight gain, GI, blood dyscrasias, disulfiram reaction, dilutional hyponatremia
Second-Generation Sulfonylureas				
Glimepiride	Amaryl (safe for elderly pts)	Stimulates release of insulin from pancreatic β cells *Glimepiride:* less weight gain, greater extrapancreatic effect, selective effects on K_{ATP} channels in the heart, less hypoglycemia	1–2 mg QD; titrate to a maximum of 8 mg/day	Weight gain, hypoglycemia, GI, blood dyscrasias, cholestatic jaundice
Glipizide	Glucotrol, Glucotrol XL (safe for elderly pts)	*Glipizide:* less hypoglycemia	5 mg QD; titrate to a maximum of 40 mg/day (divided) or 20 mg/day for Glucotrol XL	Weight gain, hypoglycemia, GI, blood dyscrasias, cholestatic jaundice, disulfiram reaction
Glyburide	Diabeta, Micronase Glynase (micronized),		2.5–5 mg QD; titrate to a maximum of 20 mg/day. Micronized: 1.5–3 mg QD; titrate to a maximum of 12 mg/day	Weight gain, hypoglycemia, GI, visual changes, blood dyscrasias, cholestatic jaundice, hepatitis, increased LFTs
Alpha-Glucosidase Inhibitors				
Acarbose Miglitol	Precose Glyset	Competitive and reversible inhibition of intestinal α-glucoside hydrolase and glucoside hydrolase and pancreatic α-amylase, resulting in delayed carbohydrate metabolism and absorption	*Acarbose* 25 mg TID with first bite of food of each main meal; titrate every 4–8 weeks to a maximum of 50–100 mg TID ≤ 60 kg: 50 mg TID; ≥60 kg: 100 mg TID *Miglitol* 25 mg TID with first bite of food of each main meal; titrate over 4–8 weeks up to 50 mg TID. If not at A_{1c} goal in 3 months, titrate up to 100 mg TID.	GI, increase in LFTs GI; use caution in patients with chronic intestinal disorders
Biguanide				
Metformin	Glucophage/Glucophage XR, Riomet 100 mg/mL	Decreases hepatic glucose production; increases peripheral insulin sensitivity	500 mg BID or 850 mg QD; titrate 500 mg weekly to a maximum of 2,500 mg/day or 850 mg every 2 weeks to a maximum of 2,550 mg/day	Weight loss, GI, megaloblastic anemia, lactic acidosis,^{a} dysgeusia (alterations in taste) Use caution in patients >80 years old. Monitor renal function.

(continues)

TABLE 40.20	Continued			
Generic Name	**Brand Name**	**Mechanism of Action**	**Dosing**	**Side Effects**
Thiazolidinediones				
Pioglitazone	Actos	Increases skeletal muscle cell sensitivity to insulin; decreases hepatic glucose production; decreases free fatty acids	*Pioglitazone* Monotherapy or use with metformin, sulfonylurea, or insulin. 15, 30, 45 mg QD (45-mg dose not approved for use with insulin)	Weight gain, edema, fluid retention, anemia Positive effect on lipid profile: increased HDL, decreased triglycerides, no change in LDL, decreased small dense LDL. Monitor LFTs Use caution in patients prone to or with heart failure.
Rosiglitazone	Avandia		*Rosiglitazone* Monotherapy or combination with metformin or sulfonylurea; 2 mg BID or 4 mg QD, if not at goal titrate to 4 mg BID or 8 mg QD after 3 months	Weight gain, fluid retention, edema, anemia May increase triglycerides, LDL, and HDL and decrease small dense LDL Use caution in patients prone to or with heart failure Monitor LFTs
Meglitinides/Phenylalanines "Glinides"				
Repaglinide (meglitinide)	Prandin	Increases insulin secretion by the pancreas "Sulfonylurea-like"	*Repaglinide* Monotherapy: 0.5 to 4 mg 30 minutes prior to each meal Combination therapy: with metformin, pioglitazone, rosiglitazone, or insulin	Hypoglycemia, weight gain
Nateglinide (phenylalanine)	Starlix		*Nateglinide* Monotherapy: 60–120 mg prior to each meal Combination therapy: with metformin or insulin	Hypoglycemia, weight gain; in phase 3 trials the incidence of hypoglycemia was 2.4% vs. 31% with repaglinide. Dose titration often unnecessary
Combination				
Glipizide + Metformin	Metaglip	See glipizide and metformin above.	2.5/250, 2.5/500, 5/500 Naive patients: 2.5/250 QD w/ meal. Fasting plasma glucose >280–320 mg/dL: 2.5/500 BID. One tab per day every 2 wks: Maximum 10/1,000 or 10/2,000 per day divided. Previously treated: 2.5/500 or 5/500 BID, Maximum 20/2,000	See glipizide and metformin above.
Glyburide + Metformin	Glucovance	See glipizide and metformin above.	Initial therapy: starting dose of 1.25/250 mg QD or BID with meals; can be increased to 10/2,000 mg. Previously treated patients: starting dose 2.5/500 mg or 5/500 mg BID with meals, can be increased to 20/2,000 mg.	See glyburide and metformin above.
Rosiglitazone + Metformin	Avandamet	See rosiglitazone and metformin above.	1/500, 2/500, 4/500 BID; maximum 8/2,000	See rosiglitazone and metformin above.

GI, gastrointestinal; SIADH, syndrome of inappropriate antidiuretic hormone; LFTs, liver function tests.

[a] No reports of lactic acidosis during more than 20,000 patient-years of exposure to metformin in clinical trials

(From Developed by WSU College of Pharmacy: Steve Setter, R. Keith Campbell, and John White.)

TABLE 40.21	Counseling Points for Oral Antidiabetic Agents

Sulfonylureas

Review signs and symptoms of hypoglycemia.

α-Glucosidase inhibitors

Take with first bite of each meal.

If a meal is missed, do not take dose.

May cause diarrhea, flatulence, abdominal pain, especially at initiation of therapy.

Report any persistent or severe signs or symptoms of gastrointestinal discomfort.

Biguanides

Take with food.

Mild gastrointestinal symptoms may be noted early in therapy.

Signs and symptoms of hypoglycemia should be reviewed if taking with secretagogues or insulin.

Report any unusual signs or symptoms to a healthcare professional (diarrhea, severe muscle pain or cramping, shallow and fast breathing, unusual tiredness and weakness, and unusual sleepiness may be signs of lactic acidosis).

Thiazolidinediones

Take with food.

Review signs and symptoms of hypoglycemia if taking with secretagogues or insulin.

Follow recommended schedule for liver function tests.

Report the following symptoms of hepatic dysfunction to a healthcare professional: nausea, vomiting, abdominal pain, fatigue, anorexia, or dark urine.

Meglitinides/Phenylalanines

Review signs and symptoms of hypoglycemia.

Take from 30 min to immediately before a meal.

If a meal is missed, do not take.

---

lower starting doses and longer intervals between dose increases also are recommended. Currently, repaglinide is approved for monotherapy use, or in combination with insulin, sulfonylureas, metformin, and thiazolidinediones. Its clinical effect is most pronounced in the first few weeks of therapy, with A1C reductions of 1.7% to 2.1% being reported.[59]

Nateglinide's peak concentration after oral administration is less than 1 hour, with hydroxylation and glucuronide conjugation responsible for the majority of its metabolism. Nateglinide should be administered within 30 minutes of a meal. As with repaglinide, if a meal is skipped, the dose of medication should be skipped as well. Similar to the sulfonylureas, if the rapid-acting secretagogues are combined with other antidiabetic agents, the risk of hypoglycemia may increase, and careful monitoring is advised. The incidence of hypoglycemia appears to be less with nateglinide (2.4%) than with repaglinide (up to 31%).

Biguanides. Metformin is a biguanide that lowers blood glucose by reducing hepatic glucose production and glycogen metabolism in the liver and enhancing insulin-mediated glucose uptake by skeletal muscle. Phenformin, a congener of metformin, was removed from the market because of a high incidence of lactic acidosis (64 cases per 100,000 patient-years). Approximately 5 to 9 patients per 100,000 patients treated with metformin develop lactic acidosis, mainly those with contraindications to its use.[60] Metformin has a much lower incidence of lactic acidosis, particularly when recommended prescribing guidelines are followed. Recently, it has been determined that most cases of metformin-associated lactic acidosis are related to underlying conditions and not due to metformin itself.[61]

Abdominal bloating, nausea, intestinal cramping, and diarrhea are common adverse effects of metformin, particularly when therapy is initiated. With continued use, many of these side effects dissipate. Side effects can be lessened by always taking the drug with food and starting with a low dose and slowly titrating to a maximum of 2,000 to 2,550 mg. In one dose-response trial, the greatest glycemic effect was observed at a dose of 2,000 mg per day; doses greater than that have less of an effect.[62] Metformin typically is started at 500 mg twice daily and then titrated every 1 to 2 weeks by 500 mg. If the patient is started on 850 mg, this can usually be given once daily and then titrated as needed. Metformin should always be taken with food.

Metformin is not metabolized and is secreted primarily by the renal tubules, so it is contraindicated in patients with renal dysfunction [serum creatinine greater than 1.5 mg/dL (132.6 μmol/L) in male patients or greater than 1.4 mg/dL (123.8 μmol/L) in female patients], laboratory evidence of hepatic dysfunction, acute or chronic lactic acidosis, or a history of alcoholism or binge drinking, or in patients who need pharmacologic management of congestive heart failure. Metformin should be withheld temporarily in patients experiencing conditions that may predispose them to acute renal failure or acidosis, such as cardiovascular collapse, acute myocardial infarction, or acute exacerbation of congestive heart failure, or undergoing a major surgical procedure. Lastly, metformin should be discontinued before intravenous iodinated contrast medium is administered and not restarted until 48 hours after the procedure, and upon documentation of normal renal function.

Monotherapy with metformin reduces fasting plasma glucose levels an average of 58 mg per dL (3.22 mmol/L) and A1C an average of 1.8%. Metformin is also associated with a reduction in triglyceride concentrations (16%), low-density lipoprotein cholesterol (8%), and total cholesterol (5%), and it is associated with a slight increase in high-density lipoprotein cholesterol (2%).[63] Many patients lose a small amount of weight when metformin is used, which is useful for the many overweight patients with type 2 diabetes.[51] Metformin can also be used in combination with insulin, secretagogues, thiazolidinediones, and α-glucosidase inhibitors for patients with type 2 diabetes. As with oral antidiabetic agents, the risk of hypoglycemia increases when it is used with insulin secretagogues or insulin. Metformin is also available in fixed-dose combinations with rosiglitazone, glyburide, and glipizide, and a liquid formulation.

α-Glucosidase Inhibitors. α-Glucosidase enzymes in the brush border of the small intestine, along with pancreatic α-amylase, are responsible for the hydrolysis of complex starches, oligosaccharides, trisaccharides, and disaccharides. Acarbose, an α-glucosidase and α-amylase inhibitor, works by reducing the rate of complex carbohydrate digestion and subsequent absorption of glucose, thereby lowering postprandial glucose excursion in patients with diabetes.[64] Acarbose is particularly effective for patients who experience postprandial hyperglycemia. Miglitol is another α-glucosidase inhibitor that works similarly to acarbose and likewise is effective in controlling postprandial hyperglycemia.

Dose-related side effects of the α-glucosidase inhibitors are mainly gastrointestinal and include flatulence, diarrhea, and abdominal pain. Slow titration of these agents may lessen the severity of side effects, and patients who continue to take the medicine may develop tolerance to the side effects. Although the α-glucosidase inhibitors by themselves are not considered hypoglycemic agents, when they are used in combination with insulin or a secretagogue, hypoglycemia can occur. Hypoglycemic episodes in patients taking α-glucosidase inhibitors must be treated with oral glucose tablets or gel because oral complex carbohydrates cannot be digested and absorbed.

Patients with inflammatory bowel disease, colonic ulceration, obstructive bowel disorders, or any gastrointestinal condition in which excess intestinal gas would be detrimental should not receive these agents. Patients with serum creatinine levels higher than 2 mg per dL (176.8 μmol/L) should not receive α-glucosidase inhibitors. The α-glucosidase inhibitors can interact with intestinal adsorbents such as charcoal, and supplemental pancreatic or intestinal enzyme replacements containing amylase, pancrelipase, or other related enzymes can decrease the effectiveness of α-glucosidase inhibitors.

Reductions in fasting plasma glucose of 5.4 to 20 mg per dL (0.3 to 1.11 mmol/L) and 38 to 50 mg per dL (2.11 to 2.78 mmol/L) have been reported with acarbose. Reductions in A1C of approximately 0.5% could be expected with the α-glucosidase class of medicines.

Thiazolidinediones. Pioglitazone and rosiglitazone are thiazolidinedione (TZD) agents, which are insulin sensitizers that lower blood glucose levels by enhancing the action of insulin and reducing insulin resistance. Their main action is on muscle tissue, where they increase glucose disposal; they act to a lesser degree in the liver, where they decrease hepatic glucose production.

Liver function testing is recommended prior to initiating therapy with a TZD, with periodic evaluations recommended

TABLE 40.22	**Thiazolidinediones (Pioglitazone and Rosiglitazone): Recommendations for Liver Enzyme Monitoring**

Check alanine aminotransferase (ALT) levels at the start of therapy. Do not initiate therapy ALT is >2.5 times the upper limit of normal.

If at any time levels are >3 times normal, recheck as soon as possible. If ALT levels remain >3 times the upper limit of normal or if the patient develops jaundice, discontinue therapy.

Monitor liver function tests every 2 months for the first 12 months, and periodically thereafter.

thereafter (Table 40.22). If signs or symptoms of liver impairment (e.g., nausea, jaundice) occur during therapy, the TZD should be discontinued and the origin of the problem identified. TZDs can lead to fluid retention and edema, thereby leading to or exacerbating heart disease. Patients at risk of heart disease should be closely monitored for signs and symptoms of heart disease such as weight gain or edema. The TZDs should not be used in patients with New York Heart Association class III or IV congestive heart failure. The TZDs are associated with a mild decrease in hemoglobin (approximately 3%) that is rarely associated with clinical effects; however, a slight decrease in hemoglobin in a patient with anemia could be problematic.

Pioglitazone is a substrate for and weak inducer of CYP 3A4. Theoretical drug interactions with other 3A4 substrates are possible. Rosiglitazone does not have drug interactions with any drugs metabolized by the major CYP isoenzyme.

TZDs are approved for combination use in patients on insulin or a sulfonylurea or metformin, and as triple therapy for those on metformin and a sulfonylurea. Reductions in A1C of approximately 0.5% are seen when TZDs are used as monotherapy, with drops of 1.4% and 1.8% reported when used in combination with insulin or sulfonylureas, respectively. Modest weight gain is reported when TZDs are used in combination with other oral agents or insulin.

Amylin Analogues. Amylin is a naturally occurring hormone that is secreted from the pancreatic β cells along with insulin when a meal is consumed.[65] This endogenous hormone assists with the regulation of blood glucose through the following mechanisms: (a) delays gastric emptying; (b) prevents rise in postprandial glucagon release; and (c) acts on the central nervous system to modulate appetite and satiety. Pramlintide, a synthetic analogue of amylin, is approved for the treatment of patients with type 1 and 2 diabetes. It is used as adjunctive treatment with insulin in patients with type 1 diabetes, and in type 2 patients who have not achieved glucose targets with insulin, sulfonylureas, and/or metformin.

Pramlintide is contraindicated in patients with gastroparesis or hypoglycemia unawareness. Insulin and pramlintide should never be mixed. Initial dosing in patients with type

1 diabetes is 15 μg, with 15-μg incremental titration to 30 to 60 μg as tolerated. In patients with type 2 diabetes therapy is initiated at 60 μg, with doses up to 120 μg as determined by glycemic response. Adverse reactions associated with pramlintide include nausea, vomiting, dyspepsia, anorexia, and headache.[66]

Incretin Mimetics. Incretin peptides such as glucose-dependent insulinotropic peptide-1 (GLP-1) are substances that are released from cells in the gastrointestinal tract in response to the ingestion of a meal.[67] Incretin mimetics reduce blood glucose levels by enhancing glucose-dependent insulin secretion, suppressing glucagon secretion, slowing gastric emptying, and reducing appetite through central nervous system mechanisms. Exenatide is a synthetic incretin mimetic that possess action similar to GLP-1. The net effect of exenatide is to reduce postprandial glucose excursion, improve A1C levels, and reduce appetite and weight, all beneficial effects for many patients with type 2 diabetes. Exenatide was recently approved for type 2 patients not achieving target A1C levels despite the use of insulin, sulfonylureas, or metformin. Exenatide is injected subcutaneously twice daily within 60 minutes of the morning and evening meals. Therapy is initiated with 5 μg; after a month, the dose can be titrated to 10 μg based on the patient's glycemic response. The most common adverse reactions are nausea and hypoglycemia, with diarrhea, headache, decreased appetite, and dizziness being less common.

Combination Therapy. Combination therapies are becoming much more common in the treatment of type 2 diabetes. A second agent may be given to a patient who is poorly controlled on a single agent, and sometimes a third drug is needed to achieve the clinical goal. In general, oral agents should not be substituted for one another, but rather a second or third drug should be added to the regimen. Clinical studies show that if antidiabetic drugs are simply substituted, no increase in therapeutic effect is seen and in many cases glycemic control is compromised. Insulin may be used in combination with sulfonylureas, rapid-acting secretagogues, α-glucosidase inhibitors, metformin, TZDs, repaglinide, nateglinide, as well as pramlintide in patients with type 1 or type 2 diabetes, and exenatide in patients with type 2 diabetes. Insulin needs may decrease when oral agents are added to the regimen, or the dose of oral agents may need to be decreased when insulin is added. It is becoming more common for fixed doses of combination oral products to be marketed, and such products may increase patient compliance, in addition to easing the transition to combination therapy when required.

Role of Aspirin. Aspirin has been shown to reduce the risk of myocardial infarction and other vascular adverse events (stroke, transient ischemic attack) through its inhibition of thromboxane A_2. Thromboxane A_2 is a potent platelet aggregator and vasoconstrictor. The use of enteric-coated aspirin (81 to 325 mg) is recommended in patients with diabetes who have evidence of large vessel disease (e.g., history of myocardial infarction, stroke, angina) and in those with a family history of coronary heart disease, cigarette smoking, hypertension, hyperlipidemia, obesity, or albuminuria. Contraindications to aspirin therapy include aspirin allergy, bleeding disorder, history of gastrointestinal bleeding, and active hepatic disease.

FUTURE THERAPIES

GLP-1 is rapidly metabolized by the enzyme dipeptidyl peptidase-IV (DPP-IV). Several oral DPP-IV inhibitors are under investigation. Molecules that are resistant to DPP-IV degradation, such as liraglutide and CJC-1131, are being studied. Many other drugs and insulin delivery methods are under investigation for the management of diabetes.

CONCLUSION

Diabetes mellitus is a complex, heterogeneous endocrine disorder that necessitates a health team effort to achieve treatment objectives. Through a combination of diet, exercise, medications, and most importantly education that results in the patient's taking charge of the condition, the outlook for the patient with diabetes is improving continually. Because of the rapid expansion of available therapeutic agents to treat this disease, the pharmacist's role in caring for patients with diabetes has expanded. Pharmacists can educate their patients about the proper use of medications, screen for drug interactions, explain monitoring devices, and make recommendations for ancillary products and services.

Healthcare providers must make a concerted effort to educate patients with diabetes about treatment and monitoring. Members of the team must communicate and reinforce the information they provide to the patient with diabetes. Providers should participate actively in diabetes associations, keep current on educational methods and programs relating to diabetes, and become active in the American Association of Diabetes Educators. Providers should familiarize themselves with all available diabetes care products. The opportunity for specialists in the care of diabetes is great, and those who participate will find that the rewards are even greater.

KEY POINTS

■ Diabetes is for the most part an incurable disease, so the overall goals of treatment include maintaining blood sugar levels in the normal or near-normal range and preventing the short- and long-term complications associated with this disease

■ Type 1 diabetes is seen primarily in children and adolescents, whereas type 2 diabetes most commonly affects those over age 45. However, with the increase in childhood and adolescent obesity, type 2 diabetes is becoming more common in younger individuals

- Measuring glycosylated hemoglobin (A1C) is the gold standard for monitoring patients with diabetes. All patients with diabetes should have this test performed one to four times yearly
- SMBG should be performed by most patients with diabetes. The results should be reviewed regularly with a healthcare professional
- Uncontrolled diabetes results in kidney, eye, and nerve disease that greatly compromises the quality of life of patients with diabetes, so normalization or near normalization of the blood glucose level is a primary treatment goal
- Educating the patient with diabetes is critical to the successful management of this chronic disease
- In addition to insulin, the therapeutic options to control diabetes include an array of agents that have various effects on the pancreas, muscle, and liver
- The successful treatment of diabetes requires a team approach that incorporates the expertise of physicians, nurses, pharmacists, and dietitians, among others

SUGGESTED READINGS

American Diabetes Association. Diagnosis and classification of diabetes mellitus. Diabetes Care 28 (Suppl 1):S37–S42, 2005.
American Diabetes Association. Technical reviews. Diabetes Care 28 (Suppl 1):S64–S66, 2005.
Hirsch IB. Insulin analogues. N Engl J Med 352:174–183, 2005.
Krentz AJ, Bailey CJ. Oral antidiabetic agents: current role in type 2 diabetes mellitus. Drugs 65:385–411, 2005.
Stoner GD. Hyperosmolar hyperglycemic state. Am Fam Phys 71:1723–1730, 2005.
Trachtenberg DE. Diabetic ketoacidosis. Am Fam Phys 71:1705–1714, 2005.

REFERENCES

1. Diabetes Control and Complications Trial Research Group. The effect of intensive treatment on the development and the progression of long-term complications in insulin-dependent diabetes mellitus. N Engl J Med 329:977–986, 1993.
2. UK Prospective Diabetes Study (UKPDS) Group. Intensive blood-glucose control with sulfonylureas or insulin compared with conventional treatment and risks of complications in patients with type 2 diabetes (UKPDS 33). Lancet 353:837–853, 1998.
3. UK Prospective Diabetes Study (UKPDS) Group. Effect of intensive blood glucose with metformin on complications in overweight patients with type 2 diabetes (UKPDS 34). Lancet 352:854–865, 1998.
4. UK Prospective Diabetes Study (UKPDS) Group. Tight blood pressure control and risk of macrovascular and microvascular complications in type 2 diabetes (UKPDS 38). Br Med J 317:703–713, 1998.
5. UK Prospective Diabetes Study (UKPDS) Group. Efficacy of atenolol and captopril in reducing risk of macrovascular and microvascular complications in type 2 diabetes (UKPDS 39). Br Med J 317:13–20, 1998.
6. American Diabetes Association. Standards of medical care for patients with diabetes mellitus. Diabetes Care 20 (Suppl 1):S5–S13, 1997.
7. Watkins JD, Robers DE, Williams TF, et al. Observation of medication errors made by diabetic patients at home. Diabetes 16:883, 1967.
8. Salans LB. Diabetes mellitus, a disease that is coming into focus. JAMA 247:590, 1982.
9. Expert Committee on the Diagnosis and Classification of Diabetes Mellitus. Follow-up report on the diagnosis of diabetes mellitus. Diabetes Care 26:3160–3167, 2003.
10. Hosszufalusi N, Vatay A, Rajczy K, et al. Similar genetic features and different islet cell autoantibody pattern of latent autoimmune diabetes in adults (LADA) compared with adult-onset type 1 diabetes with rapid progression. Diabetes Care 26:452–457, 2003.
11. Pozzilli P, Mario UD. Autoimmune diabetes not requiring insulin at diagnosis (latent autoimmune diabetes of the adult). Diabetes Care 24:1460–1467, 2001.
12. Diabetes 1996 vital statistics. Alexandria, VA: American Diabetes Association, 1996:1–102.
13. Centers for Disease Control and Prevention. National diabetes fact sheet; general information and national estimates on diabetes in the United States, 2003, revised ed. Atlanta: U.S. Department of Health and Human Services, Centers for Disease Control and Prevention, 2004.
14. Epidemiological correlates of NIDDM in Hispanics, whites, and blacks in the U.S. population. Diabetes Care 14 (Suppl 1):639–648, 1991.
15. Direct and indirect costs of diabetes in the United States in 1992. Alexandria, VA: American Diabetes Association, 1993.
16. Fioretto P, Steffes MW, Sutherland DER, et al. Reversal of lesions of diabetic nephropathy after pancreas transplantation. N Engl J Med 339:69–75, 1998.
17. Eastman RC, Javitt JC, Herman WH, et al. Model of complications of NIDDM. Diabetes Care 20:735–744, 1997.
18. United States Renal Data System. USRDS 2003 annual report. Bethesda, MD, 2003.
19. Atkinson MA, Maclaren NK. The pathogenesis of insulin-dependent diabetes mellitus. N Engl J Med 331:1428–1436, 1994.
20. Skyler JS, Marks JB. Immune intervention in type 1 diabetes mellitus. Diabetes Rev 1:15–42, 1993.
21. Reaven GM. Banting lecture 1988. Role of insulin resistance in human disease. Diabetes 37:1595–1607, 1988.
22. DeFronzo RA, Bonadonna RC, Ferrannini E. Pathogenesis of NIDDM. A balanced overview. Diabetes Care 15:318–368, 1992.
23. Polonsky KS, Sturis J, Bell GI. Non-insulin-dependent diabetes mellitus: a genetically programmed failure of the beta cell to compensate for insulin resistance. N Engl J Med 334:777–783, 1996.
24. White JR, Campbell RK. Drug/drug and drug/disease interactions and diabetes. Diabetes Educator 21:283–289, 1995.
25. Luna BL, Feinglos MN. Drug-induced hyperglycemia. JAMA 286:1945–1948, 2001.
26. Henry RR, Wallace P, Olefsky JM. Effects of weight loss on mechanisms of hyperglycemia in obese non-insulin-dependent diabetes mellitus. Diabetes 35:990–998, 1986.
27. Galloway JA, Potvin JH, Shuman CR, eds. Diabetes mellitus, 9th ed. Indianapolis: Lilly Research Laboratories, 1988.
28. The physician's guide to type II diabetes (NIDDM): diagnosis and treatment. Alexandria, VA: American Diabetes Association, 1992.
29. Buyer's guide to diabetes products, 1998. Alexandria, VA: American Diabetes Association, 1998.
30. Tests of glycemia in diabetes. Diabetes Care 20 (Suppl 1):S18–S20, 1997.
31. Diabetic nephropathy. Diabetes Care 20 (Suppl 1):S24–S27, 1997.
32. Lipsky M. Management of diabetic ketoacidosis. Am Fam Physician 49:1607–1612, 1994.
33. Fish LH. Diabetic ketoacidosis. Postgrad Med 93:75–96, 1995.
34. Brownlee M. Biochemistry and molecular cell biology of diabetic complications. Nature 414:813–820, 2001.
35. Setter SM, Campbell RK, Cahoon CJ. Biochemical pathways for microvascular complications of diabetes mellitus. Ann Pharmacother 37:1858–1866, 2003.
36. Stern MP. The effect of glycemic control on the incidence of macrovascular complications of type 2 diabetes. Arch Fam Med 7:155–162, 1998.
37. Brownlee M. Glycation products and the pathogenesis of diabetic complications. Diabetes Care 15:1838, 1992.

38. Frank R. The aldose reductase controversy. Diabetes 43:169–172, 1994.

39. Rosen RC. Overview of phosphodiesterase 5 inhibition in erectile dysfunction. Am J Cardiol 92 (Suppl);9M–18M, 2003.

40. Arauz-Pacheco C, Parrott MA, Raskin P. The treatment of hypertension in adult patients with diabetes (technical review). Diabetes Care 25:134–147, 2002.

41. Pecoraro RE, Reiber GE, Burgess EM. Pathways to diabetic limb amputation: basis for prevention. Diabetes Care 13:513–521, 1990.

42. Campbell RK. Clinical update on pentoxifylline therapy for diabetes-induced peripheral vascular disease. Ann Pharmacother 27:1099–1105, 1993.

43. Dawson DL, Cutler BS, Meisnner MH, et al. Cilostazol has beneficial effects in treatment of intermittent claudication. Circulation 98:678–686, 1998.

44. Steed DL and the Diabetic Ulcer Study Group. Clinical evaluation of recombinant human platelet-derived growth factor for the treatment of lower extremity diabetic ulcers. J Vasc Surg 21:71–81, 1995.

45. Bureau of Primary Health Care. LEAP Into Primary Care conference proceedings. Washington DC: Health Resources and Services Administration, 1995.

46. Clinical Practice Recommendations 2004. Physical activity/exercise and diabetes. Diabetes Care 27 (Suppl 1):S58–S62, 2004.

47. Evidence-based nutrition principles and recommendations for the treatment and prevention of diabetes and related complications (technical review). Diabetes Care 25:148–198, 2002.

48. Richter EA, Ruderman NB, Schneider SH. Diabetes and exercise. Am J Med 70:201, 1981.

49. US Department of Agriculture, US Department of Health and Human Services. Nutrition and your health: dietary guidelines for Americans, 4th ed. Hyattsville, MD: USDA Human Nutrition Information Service, 1995.

50. Campbell RK, Campbell LK, White JR. Insulin lispro: its role in the treatment of diabetes mellitus. Ann Pharmacother 30:1263–1271, 1996.

51. Galloway JA, Potvin JH, Shuman CR, eds. Diabetes mellitus, 9th ed. Indianapolis: Lilly Research Laboratories, 1988.

52. Continuous subcutaneous insulin infusion. American Diabetes Association. Diabetes Care 20 (Suppl 1):50, 1997.

53. Diabetes management therapies: a core curriculum for diabetes educators. In Franz MJ, ed. Pharmacologic Therapies. Chicago: American Association of Diabetes Educators, 2001.

54. White J, Campbell RK. The guide to mixing insulins. Hosp Pharm 26:1046–1050, 1991.

55. Valenta LJ, Elias AN. Insulin-induced lipodystrophy in diabetic patients resolved by treatment with human insulin. Ann Intern Med 102:790–791, 1985.

56. Gerich JE. Oral hypoglycemic agents. N Engl J Med 321:1232–1245, 1989.

57. Campbell RK. Glimepiride: role of a new sulfonylurea in the treatment of type 2 diabetes mellitus. Ann Pharmacol 32:1044–1052, 1998.

58. Porte D, Sherwin RS, Baron A, eds. Ellenberg & Rifkin's diabetes mellitus, 6th ed. McGraw-Hill, 2003.

59. Cheatham WW. Repaglinide: a new oral blood glucose lowering agent. Clin Diabetes 16:70–72, 1998.

60. Misbin RI, Green L, Stadel BV, et al. Lactic acidosis in patients with diabetes treated with metformin [letter]. N Engl J Med 338:265–266, 1997.

61. Stades AME, Heikens JT, Erkelens DW, et al. Metformin and lactic acidosis: cause or coincidence? A review of case reports. J Int Med 255:179–187, 2004.

62. Garber AJ, Duncan TG, Goodman AM, et al. Efficacy of metformin in type II diabetes: results of a double-blind, placebo-controlled, dose-response trial. Am J Med 102:491–497, 1997.

63. DeFronzo RA, Goodman AM, and the Multicenter Metformin Study Group. Efficacy of metformin in patients with NIDDM. N Engl J Med 333:541–549, 1995.

64. Santeusanio F, Compagnucci P. A risk-benefit appraisal of acarbose in the management of non-insulin-dependent diabetes mellitus. Drug Saf 11:432–444, 1994.

65. Samson M, Szarka LA, Camilleri M, et al. Pramlintide, an amylin analog, selectively delays gastric emptying: potential role of vagal inhibition. Am J Physiol Gastrointest Liver Physiol 278:946–951, 2000.

66. Ratner RE, Dickey R, Fineman M et al. Amylin replacement with pramlintide as an adjunct to insulin therapy improves long-term glycemic and weight control in type 1 diabetes mellitus: a 1-year, randomized controlled trial. Diabet Med 21;1204–1212, 2004.

67. Edwards CMB. GLP-1: target for a new class of antidiabetic agents? J Royal Soc Med 97:270–274, 2004.

Hyperlipidemia

41

Michael B. Doherty and Michael Bottorff

TREATMENT GOALS

- Reduce morbidity and mortality from coronary heart disease (CHD), and decrease mortality from all causes in patients with established CHD.
- Reduce new CHD events and CHD mortality in patients without established CHD.
- Decrease the risk of myocardial infarction (MI), unstable angina, stroke (in patients with established CHD), and transient ischemic attack (in patients with established CHD), and the need for coronary artery bypass grafts and angioplasty.

Cardiovascular diseases remain the number-one cause of death in the United States. According to the American Heart Association, approximately 38% of deaths in America are due to cardiovascular diseases (about 1 in every 2.6 deaths), and the total number of deaths due to cardiovascular disease continues to increase each year.[1] Over 70 million Americans have at least one form of cardiovascular disease (including hypertension, congenital heart diseases, and atherosclerosis). As a result, this country spends over $393 billion for cardiovascular disease treatment and disability. Risk factors that contribute to cardiovascular disease are common and numerous, and include gender, age, cigarette smoking, diabetes, hypertension, and dyslipidemia.[2] Many of these risk factors, including the dyslipidemias, are modifiable, and the drug therapy management of hyperlipidemia, in particular, has been associated with significant reductions in cardiovascular morbidity and mortality.[3] A variety of drugs, in addition to dietary measures, are available to modify the various lipid fractions. These drugs are often used as monotherapy, and increasingly are used in combination to achieve well-defined treatment goals and correspondingly significant reductions in cardiovascular morbidity and mortality.

DEFINITIONS

Dyslipidemias include either a low high density lipoprotein (HDL) cholesterol value or elevations in atherogenic lipo-
protein particles, including cholesterol, cholesterol esters, and triglycerides. The bulk of the epidemiologic evidence is for elevated total and low density lipoprotein (LDL) cholesterol (Fig. 41.1). The risk is highest with extreme elevations in cholesterol, but the relationship is continuous, and even cholesterol values previously considered "normal" have been associated with cardiovascular risk, even more so in patients with other known cardiovascular risk factors (Fig. 41.2).

The most widely adopted treatment guidelines for dyslipidemia are from the National Cholesterol Education Program Adult Treatment Panel III (NCEP ATP III).[2] Reducing LDL cholesterol is the primary focus of treatment, with secondary objectives that include lowering non-HDL cholesterol, by reducing triglycerides, increasing HDL cholesterol, or both.[4] Table 41.1 lists the NCEP ATP III normal and abnormal values for LDL cholesterol and triglycerides.

ETIOLOGY

Hyperlipidemia can be caused by primary causes (genetic predisposition) or secondary causes (diet, underlying disease, or medications). Primary hyperlipidemia is associated with high morbidity and mortality. A defect often occurs in lipid metabolism or transport in primary hyperlipidemia, resulting in reduced LDL receptor activity and accumulation of LDL cholesterol in the plasma, leading to atherogenesis.

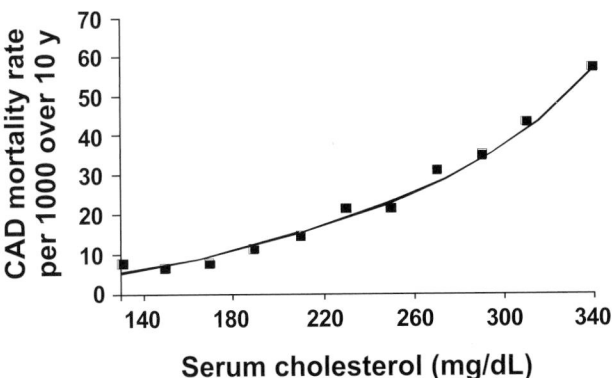

FIGURE 41.1 Total serum cholesterol levels and risk for coronary artery disease. Men screened for the Multiple Risk Factor Intervention Trial (n = 316,099). (From Neaton JD, Wentworth D. Serum cholesterol, blood pressure, cigarette smoking, and death from coronary heart disease. Overall findings and differences by age for 316,099 white men. Multiple Risk Factor Intervention Trial Research Group. Arch Intern Med 152:56–64, 1992.)

TABLE 41.1	ATP III Classification of LDL and Triglyceride Levels	
LDL-C (mg/dL)	Triglycerides (mg/dL)	Classification
<100	<150	Optimal/normal
100–129		Above optimal
130–159	150–199	Borderline high
160–189	200–499	High
≥190	≥500	Very high

Patients usually require medication in addition to diet and exercise education to achieve desired goals for LDL cholesterol.

Two types of genetic lipid receptor alterations can occur. A heterozygous receptor abnormality can occur when there is a mutant gene for the LDL receptor such that only half the LDL receptors are functional. Patients usually have cholesterol levels that are twice normal, causing an increased risk of premature heart disease, angina, or MI (generally by age 30 or 40). A homozygous receptor alteration occurs when two mutant genes for the LDL receptor are present, leaving patients with essentially no functional LDL receptors. Cholesterol levels can be as high as 1,000 mg per dL (25.9 mmol/L) and CHD may develop in the first or second decade of life.[5]

All patients should be evaluated for secondary causes of hyperlipidemia. Diseases such as diabetes mellitus, hypothyroidism, Cushing's syndrome, obstructive liver disease, nephrotic syndrome, and alcoholism are all common causes of high cholesterol.[6] Correction of the underlying disorder often results in improvement or normalization of the cholesterol profile. Therefore, in each case, correction of the underlying disorder should be attempted prior to initiating cholesterol therapy. Tables 41.2 and 41.3 list the conditions and drugs that are common causes of secondary hyperlipidemias.[6-8]

SPECIAL CONCERNS

Screening for hyperlipidemia is recommended for children older than 2 years whose parents or grandparents had documented CHD at or before the age 55 years or whose parents have serum cholesterol levels above 240 mg per dL (6.22 mmol/L). Obese children or those who smoke are judged to be at higher risk for CHD and should also be screened for hyperlipidemia. If a family history is not available, children can be screened for hyperlipidemia at the discretion of the healthcare provider. Medical treatment should be reserved for children over 10 years of age with LDL levels above 190 mg per dL (4.92 mmol/L) or LDL levels above 160 mg per dL (4.14 mmol/L) with multiple risk factors. The desired LDL level for children is less than 110 mg per dL (2.85 mmol/L). These values are lower than those for adults because during the first two decades of life, overall lipid levels are lower.

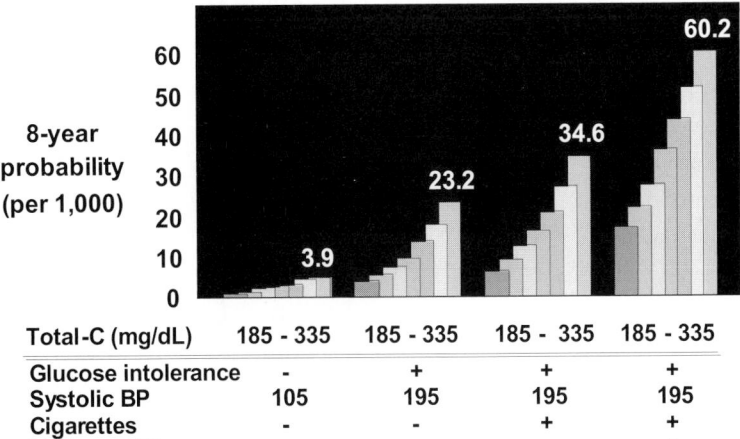

FIGURE 41.2 Cardiovascular disease risk according to cholesterol and risk factors (Framingham study). (From Kannel WB. High-density lipoproteins: epidemiologic profile and risks of coronary artery disease. Am J Cardiol. 52:9B–12B, 1983.)

Total-C (mg/dL)	185 - 335	185 - 335	185 - 335	185 - 335
Glucose intolerance	-	+	+	+
Systolic BP	105	195	195	195
Cigarettes	-	-	+	+
LVH on ECG	-	-	-	+

TABLE 41.2	Secondary Causes of Hyperlipidemia

Conditions Causing Hypertriglyceridemia	Conditions Causing Hypercholesterolemia
Acromegaly	Anorexia nervosa
Alcoholism	Cholestasis
Burns	Cushing's syndrome
Chronic renal failure	Growth hormone deficiency
Diabetes mellitus	Hypothyroidism
Glycogen storage disease	Myelomatosis (immunoglobulins A and G)
Hyperandrogenism in women	Nephrotic syndrome
Lipodystrophy	Obstructive liver disease
Pancreatitis	
Systemic lupus and polyclonal gammopathy	
Weight gain	

(From Stone N. Secondary causes of hyperlipidemia. Med Clin North Am 78:117–141, 1993; and Clark A, Holt J. Identifying and managing patients with hyperlipidemia. Am J Man Care 3:1211–1219, 1997.)

TABLE 41.3	Medications That Can Induce Hyperlipidemia

Medication	Total Cholesterol	LDL	HDL	TG	VLDL
Anabolic steroids	↑	↑	↓	—	—
Anticonvulsants	—	—	↑	—	—
Atypical antipsychotics	—	—	↓	↑	—
β-blockers (non-ISA)	—	—	↓	↑	↑
Corticosteroids	↑	↑	↑	↑	↑
Cyclosporine	↑	↑	—	—	—
Estrogen therapy	↓	↓	↑	↑	↑
Isotretinoin	↑	—	↓	↑	—
Phenothiazines	↑	—	↓	—	—
Progestins	↑	↑	↓	—	—
Protease inhibitors	↑	↑	—	↑	—
Retinoids	↑	↑	↓	↑	↑
Thiazide diuretics	↑	↑	—	↑	↑

LDL, low–density lipoprotein; HDL, high-density lipoprotein; VLDL, very low density lipoprotein; ISA, intrinsic sympathomimetic activity
Source: references 6, 7, and 8.

Treating hyperlipidemia in older patients can prolong life as well as improve the quality of life of these patients. In addition, it may reduce the need for expensive long-term care and help contain healthcare costs. Decisions about diagnostic or therapeutic interventions should not be based on the patient's chronologic age but rather on the patient's physiologic age, presence and severity of concomitant diseases, mental status, cognitive ability, and expectations for medical care.[9] Recently, clinical trials have helped clarify the role of lipid-lowering agents in the elderly. The Heart Protection Study (HPS) and the Prospective Study of Pravastatin in the Elderly at Risk (PROSPER), which evaluated simvastatin and pravastatin respectively, both demonstrated a reduction in CHD events in patients over 70 years of age. This reduction was seen in patients with both a history of vascular disease as well as those with risk factors for CHD.[10,11] A third trial, the Antihypertensive and Lipid-Lowering Treatment to Prevent Heart Attack Trial (ALLHAT), was designed to evaluate different antihypertensive classes in the elderly. ALLHAT also contained a lipid-lowering arm that was intended to compare pravastatin to usual care. ALLHAT did not show any differences in mortality or cardiovascular events, though this was most likely due to the small difference in lipid-lowering effects and the large number of "usual care" patients who were placed on lipid-lowering therapy due to the non-blinding of the study.[12]

Patients with diabetes have a very high risk for CHD. Much of this is the result of their high propensity for cardiovascular risk factors. The elevated risk is of such significance that the most recent NCEP ATP III guidelines classify diabetes as a cardiovascular risk equivalent.[2] The HPS demonstrated significant reductions in cardiovascular events in diabetic patients with and without a history of CHD. Independent of previous history of CHD, reduction in events was also seen in diabetic patients with LDL levels below 116 mg per dL (3 mmol/L) at baseline. Therefore, it is plausible to recommend lipid lowering with statins in diabetic patients regardless of their baseline LDL cholesterol.[10]

Hyperlipidemia is common after cardiac transplantation and affects about 70% of transplant recipients. Accelerated coronary artery disease remains a major cause of morbidity and mortality in patients who are alive more than 1 year after transplantation. Niacin is of benefit if the patient does not have impaired glucose tolerance. Resins interfere with cyclosporine absorption and raise triglyceride levels. Fibrates are well tolerated and reduce triglycerides. Statins have been shown to lower total cholesterol and LDL levels in transplant recipients, but they are not without risk. The incidence of rhabdomyolysis in heart transplant recipients treated with a statin and cyclosporine is about 1%. Pravastatin may be less likely to cause this adverse effect and should be considered first in this population.[13]

C-reactive protein (CRP) is an inflammatory biomarker that is often elevated in patients who experience acute coronary syndromes. Statins can lower CRP levels as well as lipid levels in patients with coronary artery disease. Reducing CRP levels to less than 2 mg per L with statin therapy has been shown to decrease a patient's risk for recurrent cardiovascular events. This benefit was seen regardless of the LDL level. CRP may be useful for determining whether to initiate or intensify lipid therapy, although the value of CRP as a monitoring tool in cholesterol management has not been fully established.[14]

PATHOPHYSIOLOGY

Cholesterol, a lipid, is an essential component of cell membranes and is a precursor in steroid hormone and bile acid metabolism. Cholesterol may be absorbed either from dietary sources or through endogenous manufacture; up to 60% of cholesterol in the body is through endogenous production, with the remainder coming from dietary sources. Thus, restrictions on dietary cholesterol will be only partially effective in reducing serum cholesterol values.[15]

Cholesterol, triglycerides, and other lipid particles are transported throughout the human body in the form of lipoproteins. These spherically shaped lipoproteins may be divided into five main categories: LDL, composed primarily of cholesterol; HDL, mostly containing cholesterol; very-low-density lipoproteins (VLDL), consisting mostly of triglycerides with some cholesterol esters; intermediate-density lipoproteins (IDLs), composed of triglycerides and cholesterol esters and also known as VLDL remnants; and dietary apolipoproteins obtained exogenously or assembled in the gut known as chylomicrons. Table 41.4 reviews these lipoproteins.

LDL typically accounts for 60% to 70% of circulating total cholesterol. Excess LDL, even more so in the presence of cardiovascular risk factors, is oxidized as it enters the vascular subendothelial space of primarily arterial walls. Oxidized LDL becomes cytotoxic and initiates the atherosclerosis process; thus, it plays a prominent role both as a predictor of cardiovascular disease and as a target for drug therapy. HDL cholesterol accounts for approximately 20% to 30% of total serum cholesterol. HDL is the so-called good cholesterol because it is involved in reverse cholesterol transport; that is, HDL accepts free cholesterol from peripheral tissues, including the vasculature, for transportation to the liver and kidney for metabolism and removal. VLDL is composed mainly of triglyceride and also contributes to approximately 10% to 15% of total serum cholesterol values. Triglycerides are constructed from free fatty acids and are used as an energy source. Using both dietary fat and excess carbohydrate, the liver produces and secretes VLDL as the primary source of circulating triglyceride.

There are two main pathways of cholesterol metabolism and transport, the endogenous and exogenous pathways (Fig. 41.3). The exogenous system involves the metabolism and transport of chylomicron particles and remnants. Cholesterol and triglycerides obtained from the diet are incorporated into triglyceride-rich chylomicrons in the intestinal endothelium;

they then enter the lymphatic system and are transported throughout the body. Once in the general circulation, chylomicrons can be hydrolyzed through an enzymatic process with lipoprotein lipase on the vascular endothelium, producing a chylomicron remnant and free fatty acids. The free fatty acids are absorbed into muscle and adipose tissue and used as a source of energy. The smaller chylomicron remnant contains less triglyceride and is therefore more concentrated in cholesterol. These cholesterol-rich chylomicron remnants contain apoproteins B-48 and E, which are recognized by hepatic LDL receptors for uptake into the liver for incorporation into bile salts. Bile salts are secreted into the intestine and help solubilize dietary fats to assist in their absorption.

Cholesterol and triglyceride produced in the body are transported by the endogenous pathway by VLDL, LDL, and HDL particles. The liver secretes triglycerides into the bloodstream as VLDL, which contains five times as much triglyceride as cholesterol. VLDL also contains the apolipoproteins B-100, E, and C-II. The B and E apolipoproteins interact with cell surface LDL receptors for uptake of VLDL and its remnants into various tissues. Apolipoprotein C-II serves as a cofactor for the enzyme lipoprotein lipase. Once VLDL is secreted from the liver into the bloodstream, the triglyceride component is hydrolyzed by vascular lipoprotein lipase into IDL and ultimately into LDL particles. By the time LDL particles are formed, they have had most of the triglyceride removed by lipoprotein lipase and are smaller and denser and contain primarily cholesterol. These LDL particles transport cholesterol to various body tissues, where they interact with LDL receptors for cellular uptake of cholesterol. The LDL particles are used for steroid synthesis or cell membrane construction. Excessive LDL may be deposited outside the cell and in the vascular endothelium, initiating the atherosclerotic process.

It is now recognized that there are different densities and types of LDL particles. In patients with metabolic syndrome and/or type 2 diabetes, there is a shift in LDL particle diameter toward a denser LDL particle that is more readily oxidized and more easily penetrates the vascular endothelium (Fig. 41.4). Small, dense LDL particles have been associated with a higher risk for cardiovascular disease.[17] Commercially available tests allow for the measurement of LDL particle number and density, but it is unclear whether drug therapy altering particle density would result in fewer cardiovascular events. Some LDL particles are surrounded by a plasminogen-like glycoprotein called apolipoprotein (a); these LDL particles are called Lp(a) and are strongly associated with cardiovascular disease.[18] Again, despite the associated risk, there is no clinical evidence that lowering Lp(a) reduces cardiovascular events.

HDL particles are rich in cholesterol and are involved in the process called reverse cholesterol transport. HDL acts as a repository for circulating free cholesterol in tissues and returns it to the liver and kidney for catabolism. Small HDL_3 particles are converted into larger HDL_2 particles by the

TABLE 41.4 | **Properties of Human Lipoproteins**

| Lipoprotein | Density (g/mL) | Electrophoretic Mobility | Origin | Composition | | | | | Major Lipo-proteins |
				Protein (%)	Phospho-lipid (%)	Cholesterol Ester (%)	Free Choles-terol (%)	TG (%)	
Chylomicron	<0.95	Origin	Gut	2	3	3	2	90	A-I, II, IV, III, B-48, E
VLDL	0.95–1.006	Pre-β	Liver gut	6	16	17	6	55	C-I, II, III, B-100, E
IDL	1.006–1.019	Pre-β, β	VLDL catabolism	18	22	32	8	20	B-100, E
LDL	1.019–1.063	β	IDL catabolism	20	22	44	8	6	B-100
Lp(a)	1.06–1.09	Pre-β	LDL	21	20	45	8	6	B-100 Apo-a
HDL	1.063–1.21	α	Liver, gut VLDL	44	26	20	5	5	A-I, II, C-I II, III

VLDL, very low density lipoprotein; IDL, intermediate-density lipoprotein; LDL, low-density lipoprotein; Lp(a), lipoprotein (a); HDL, high-density lipoprotein.
Source: reference 6.

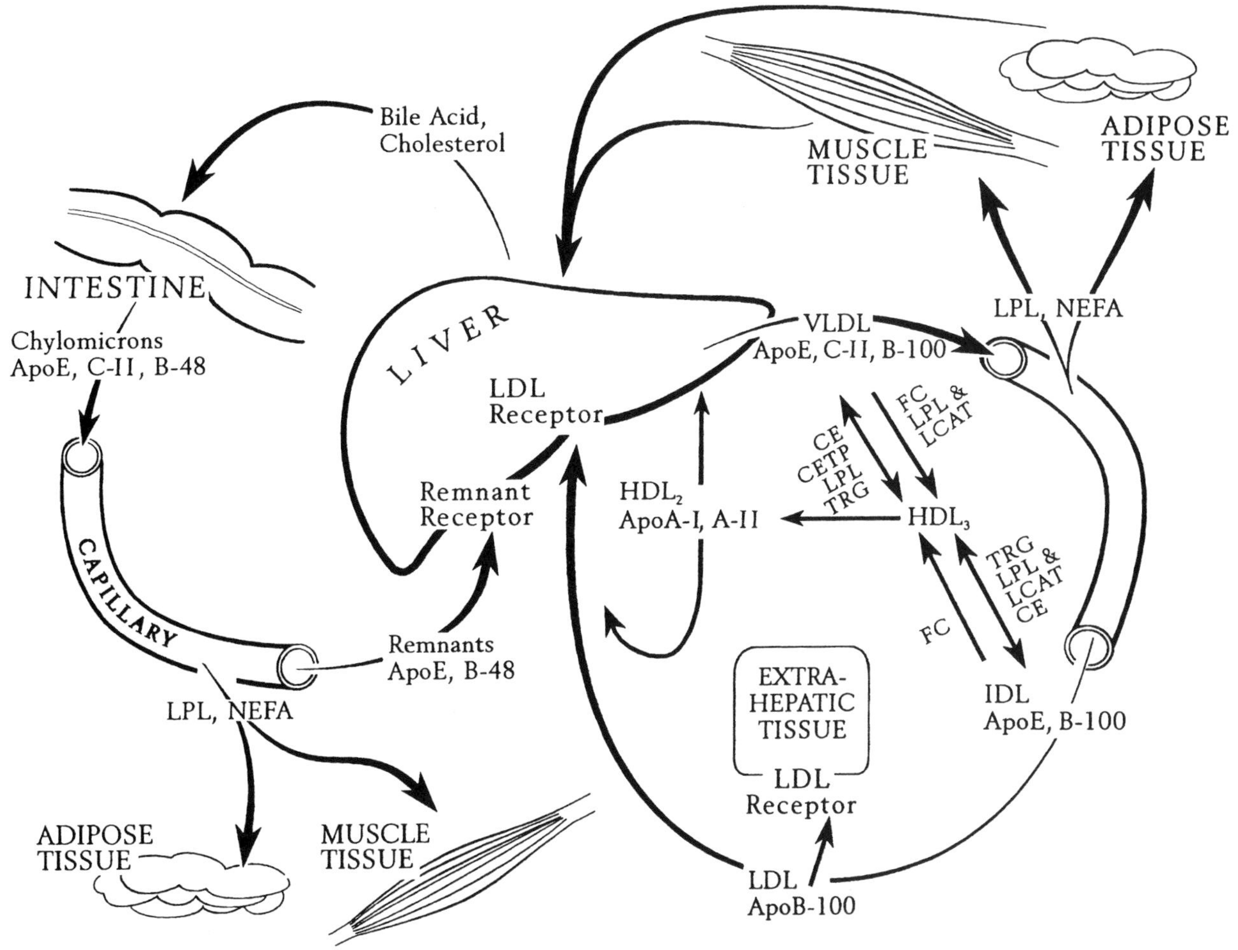

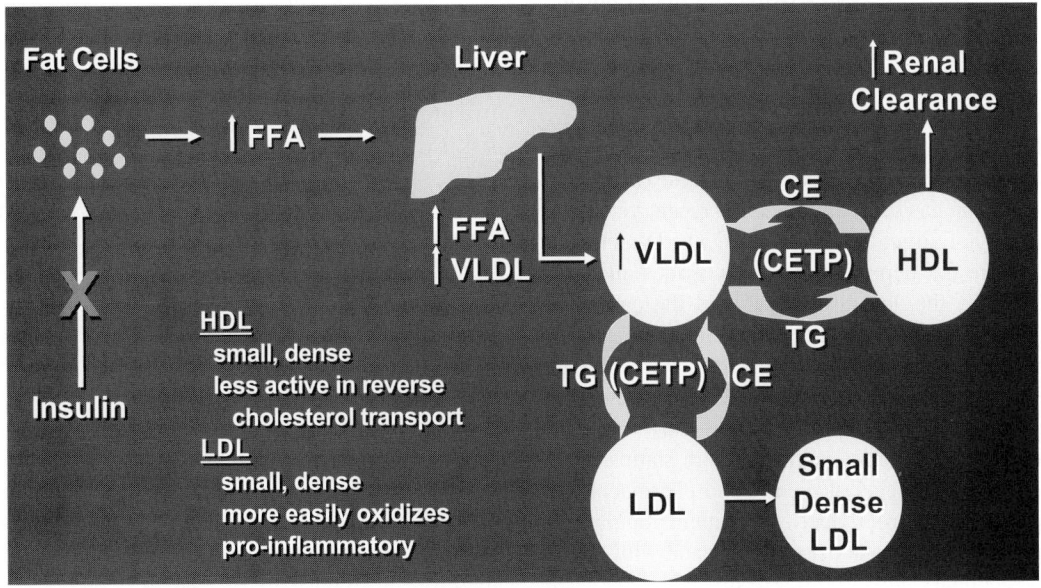

FIGURE 41.3 Diet therapy algorithm. LDL, low-density lipoprotein. (Adapted from Havel R, Rapaport E. Management of primary hyperlipidemia. N Engl J Med 332:1491–1498, 1995.)

FIGURE 41.4 Low-density lipoprotein (LDL) particle size in insulin resistance.

acquisition of triglycerides and cholesterol from peripheral cells. HDL particles contain apolipoproteins A-I, A-II, and C. Apolipoprotein A-I is most strongly associated with reduced cardiovascular risk.

Apolipoprotein A-I activates the transport of cholesterol from peripheral tissues to the liver by increasing the activity of the enzyme lecithin:cholesterol acyl transferase (LCAT) to convert HDL cholesterol to insoluble cholesterol esters. Cholesterol ester transfer protein (CTEP) activates the exchange of cholesterol esters from HDL particles for triglycerides in VLDL particles and remnants, enhancing their uptake and elimination by the liver.

CLINICAL PRESENTATION AND DIAGNOSIS

SIGNS AND SYMPTOMS

LDL cholesterol is the lipid component most closely associated with the risk of CHD. Increased serum cholesterol levels are also directly linked to the risk of CHD. Clinical trials have demonstrated that lowering serum cholesterol levels is associated with reduced morbidity and mortality. For every 1% reduction in total serum cholesterol, there is a 2% to 3% decrease in the risk of CHD.[2]

Hypertriglyceridemia has not been associated directly and independently with an increased risk of CHD, but it is generally indicative of an underlying lipid abnormality. A high triglyceride level usually results in a low HDL level, which is a known risk factor for CHD. A triglyceride level below 150 mg per dL (1.70 mmol/L) is considered normal according to NCEP ATP III; above 500 mg per dL (5.65 mmol/L) is defined as high. A triglyceride level above 500 mg per dL (5.65 mmol/L) poses an immediate risk for pancreatitis and thus warrants immediate treatment to lower triglycerides in some individuals.[2,6,7]

LDL cholesterol levels can be calculated from measured total cholesterol, HDL, and triglycerides by the Friedwald formula:

$$LDL = \text{Total Cholesterol} - \text{Triglycerides}/5 - \text{HDL} \quad (41.1)$$

This equation is not without limitations. Triglyceride levels above 400 mg per dL (4.52 mmol/L) result in a falsely low LDL value and the formula becomes invalid. The limitation of this equation has been minimized in recent years due to the availability of direct LDL measurements. Direct LDL measurements are not dependent on triglycerides and thus are not affected by the non-fasting status of the patient or restricted by the Friedwald equation. This allows for greater flexibility in screening patients, allowing an LDL level to be obtained for every patient, and prevents delays in initiating appropriate therapy due to incomplete lipid data.

A number of clinical trials, primarily with statins, have studied the combined effects of dietary and pharmacologic interventions for cholesterol reduction in patient populations with no existing CHD (primary prevention) and with established CHD (secondary prevention). The distinction between primary and secondary prevention has become less evident

because many patients considered as having risk for CHD actually have clinically undetectable atherosclerosis. As such, there is an ongoing emphasis on the risk of disease progression in patients with hypercholesterolemia, which has been promoted by the NCEP ATP III guidelines and newer clinical trials.

Some of the older studies (Lipid Research Clinic Coronary Primary Prevention Trial, Helsinki Heart Study, Coronary Drug Project Niacin Study, Oslo Study Diet and Antismoking Trial) conducted in the 1970s and early 1980s using interventions such as gemfibrozil, clofibrate, niacin, and cholestyramine were criticized for stating the benefit of cholesterol reduction on outcomes as a reduction in relative risk instead of absolute risk.[19–24] More recent trials using primarily 3-hydroxy-3-methylglutaryl co-enzyme A (HMG CoA) reductase inhibitors (statins) have been conducted on a broader range of patients, including women, older adults, and subjects with average cholesterol levels. This permitted interpretation of cholesterol reduction in these populations, which was found to be just as beneficial. These newer trials support the guidelines set forth by the NCEP ATP III and the ATP III modification.

Most experts agree that the apparent benefit of cholesterol reduction in study patients at risk for CHD warrants interventions in the general population for those at increased risk with or without evidence of preexisting CHD.[2] This position is strengthened by studies in patients with CHD or previous MI, where lipid-lowering interventions reduced the incidence of cardiac events and resulted in the regression of measurable coronary lesions.

DIAGNOSIS

Table 41.5 lists the NCEP ATP III classification for lipids and triglycerides. Treatment decisions are based on a patient's LDL level, risk factor status, presence of known CHD or CHD risk equivalents, and Framingham risk projection. The NCEP ATP III placed greater emphasis on multiple risk factors combined with the use of Framingham projections of 10-year absolute CHD risk (i.e., the percent probability of having a CHD event in 10 years) to identify patients with two or more risk factors for more intensive treatment.[2] Major risk factors are listed in Table 41.6, and the Framingham risk assessment for men and women is shown in Figure 41.5.

As a result of the many clinical trials published after the release of the NCEP ATP III guidelines in 2002, a modification to the guidelines was issued in 2004 that incorporated the results of these studies. This led to the development of new classifications for cardiovascular risk, as well as more aggressive management of hyperlipidemia.[25]

Patients are placed in one of four risk categories to determine the most appropriate intervention and goals of that intervention. Patients with known CHD and CHD risk equivalents have the highest risk for a future event. CHD risk equivalents (Table 41.7) carry a risk for major coronary events equal to that of established CHD, and these patients therefore are considered to be in a secondary prevention group. Patients with elevated cholesterol levels and multiple

TABLE 41.5	ATP III Classification of LDL, Total Cholesterol, HDL, and Triglycerides (mg/dL)
LDL Cholesterol	
<100	Optimal
100–129	Near optimal/above optimal
130–159	Borderline high
160–189	High
≥190	Very High
Total Cholesterol	
<200	Desirable
200–239	Borderline high
≥240	High
HDL Cholesterol	
<40	Low
≥60	High
Triglycerides	
<150	Normal
150–199	Borderline high
200–499	High
≥500	Very high

LDL, low-density lipoprotein; HDL, high-density lipoprotein.

risk factors (two or more) and a Framingham 10-year risk of 10% to 20% are at a moderately high risk. Patients with two or more risk factors and a Framingham 10-year risk below 10% are at a moderate risk. Finally, patients with zero or one risk factors but elevated cholesterol levels have a low

TABLE 41.6	Risk Factors for Coronary Heart Disease (CHD)
Positive Risk Factors	**Comments**
Age	Men ≥45 y; women ≥55 y
Family history of premature CHD	CHD in male first-degree relative <55 y; CHD in female-first degree relative <65y
Low HDL	<40 mg/dL
Hypertension	Blood pressure ≥140/90 mm Hg or on antihypertensive medication
Cigarette smoking	Current smoker
Negative Risk Factor	**Comments**
High HDL	≥60 mg/dL (if present, subtract a positive risk factor)

LDL, low-density lipoprotein; HDL, high-density lipoprotein.

risk. Patients with no known CHD are considered to be in the primary prevention group. In the modification to the guidelines, an additional group was identified that would benefit from more aggressive cholesterol lowering; very high risk. Very high-risk patients are those with established CHD and acute coronary syndromes or multiple risk factors, especially diabetes, smoking, and metabolic syndrome.

Positive risk factors are those that increase the risk of developing CHD. Factors such as age, sex, and family history cannot be modified. Hypertension and diabetes are risk factors that respond to medical intervention but remain positive risk factors for CHD even when controlled. Smoking is also a modifiable risk factor, but history of smoking is not counted as a positive risk factor, which is one reason why cessation is vital for patients who smoke.

Negative risk factors are those that, if present, reduce the risk of developing CHD. An HDL greater than or equal to 60 mg/dL is considered a negative risk. Therefore, when the HDL is elevated, one positive risk factor can be subtracted from the patient's total risk score.[2]

Intervention goals of dietary and drug therapy for patients with high LDL levels are listed in Table 41.8. Acute ischemic events such as an MI or surgical revascularization may reduce serum cholesterol levels below the true baseline. Levels should return to normal within 6 weeks. When making treatment decisions based on laboratory values, it is important to be working with a reliable laboratory. The laboratory should adhere to established standards for cholesterol management.[25]

The NCEP ATP III guidelines recommend screening all adults 20 years or older for elevated cholesterol levels by obtaining a fasting lipoprotein profile (total cholesterol, LDL, HDL, and triglyceride levels) every 5 years for primary prevention. In a non-fasting sample, only the total cholesterol and HDL values can be used unless a direct LDL was done. Therefore, the patient would need to undergo a follow-up fasting lipoprotein sample to allow for appropriate treatment based on LDL and to obtain an accurate triglyceride level. Figure 41.6 outlines screening guidelines for primary and secondary prevention. Monitoring and treatment decisions are based on total cholesterol, HDL, and LDL levels. Patients in the primary prevention category should be evaluated for secondary causes of hyperlipidemia. Information such as the patient's past medical history and current medication profile is important in making this determination. All patients should receive proper dietary and physical activity counseling, regardless of classification.

TREATMENT

Once a patient has been diagnosed with hyperlipidemia and classified according to the presence of risk factors, treatment options are the next area of consideration. No matter what the lipid disorder, therapeutic lifestyle change is a necessary part of any treatment plan. Secondary causes of hyperlipidemia such as hypothyroidism, diabetes, diet, and drugs

FIGURE 41.5 Framingham Risk Assessment of coronary heart disease risk in men **(A)** and women **(B)**. ATP III Framingham risk scoring. (From Executive Summary of The Third Report of The National Cholesterol Education Program (NCEP) Expert Panel on Detection, Evaluation, And Treatment of High Blood Cholesterol In Adults (Adult Treatment Panel III). JAMA 285:2486–2497, 2001.)

A.

Step 1: Age

Years	Points
20-34	-9
35-39	-4
40-44	0
45-49	3
50-54	6
55-59	8
60-64	10
65-69	11
70-74	12
75-79	13

Step 2: Total Cholesterol

TC (mg/dL)	Age 20-39	Age 40-49	Age 50-59	Age 60-69	Age 70-79
<160	0	0	0	0	0
160-199	4	3	2	1	0
200-239	7	5	3	1	0
240-279	9	6	4	2	1
280	11	8	5	3	1

Step 3: HDL-Cholesterol

HDL-C (mg/dL)	Points
60	-1
50-59	0
40-49	1
<40	2

Step 4: Systolic Blood Pressure

Systolic BP (mm Hg)	Points if Untreated	Points if Treated
<120	0	0
120-129	0	1
130-139	1	2
140-159	1	2
160	2	3

Step 5: Smoking Status

	Age 20-39	Age 40-49	Age 50-59	Age 60-69	Age 70-79
Nonsmoker	0	0	0	0	0
Smoker	8	5	3	1	1

Step 6: Adding Up the Points

Age	___
TC	___
HDL-C	___
Systolic BP	___
Smoking status	___
Point total	___

Step 7: CHD Risk

Point Total	10-Year Risk	Point Total	10-Year Risk
<0	<1%	11	8%
0	1%	12	10%
1	1%	13	12%
2	1%	14	16%
3	1%	15	20%
4	1%	16	25%
5	2%	17	30%
6	2%		
7	3%		
8	4%		
9	5%		
10	6%		

B.

Step 1: Age

Years	Points
20-34	-7
35-39	-3
40-44	0
45-49	3
50-54	6
55-59	8
60-64	10
65-69	12
70-74	14
75-79	16

Step 2: Total Cholesterol

TC (mg/dL)	Age 20-39	Age 40-49	Age 50-59	Age 60-69	Age 70-79
<160	0	0	0	0	0
160-199	4	3	2	1	1
200-239	8	6	4	2	1
240-279	11	8	5	3	2
280	13	10	7	4	2

Step 3: HDL-Cholesterol

HDL-C (mg/dL)	Points
60	-1
50-59	0
40-49	1
<40	2

Step 4: Systolic Blood Pressure

Systolic BP (mm Hg)	Points if Untreated	Points if Treated
<120	0	0
120-129	1	3
130-139	2	4
140-159	3	5
160	4	6

Step 5: Smoking Status

	Age 20-39	Age 40-49	Age 50-59	Age 60-69	Age 70-79
Nonsmoker	0	0	0	0	0
Smoker	9	7	4	2	1

Step 6: Adding Up the Points

Age	___
TC	___
HDL-C	___
Systolic BP	___
Smoking status	___
Point total	___

Step 7: CHD Risk

Point Total	10-Year Risk	Point Total	10-Year Risk
<9	<1%	20	11%
9	1%	21	14%
10	1%	22	17%
11	1%	23	22%
12	1%	24	27%
13	2%	25	30%
14	2%		
15	3%		
16	4%		
17	5%		
18	6%		
19	8%		

should be addressed, and the impact of treatment on the lipid profile should be measured before hyperlipidemia treatment is started.

NONPHARMACOLOGIC THERAPY

Therapeutic Lifestyle Changes. The NCEP ATP III recommends a comprehensive lifestyle modification to reduce CHD risk, which is called Therapeutic Lifestyle Changes (TLC). TLC encompasses behavior modification (including weight reduction, increased physical activity, and smoking cessation), reduced intake of saturated fats and cholesterol, and the use of plant stanols/sterols and viscous fiber.

Smoking cessation and hypertension management are interventions that have been proven to lower CHD risk and therefore should be addressed early in the patient's therapy. Cigarette smoking is associated with decreased levels of HDL cholesterol. Smoking cessation can increase HDL levels by 10% to 30% within several weeks of quitting. Controlling hypertension also decreases the risk of CHD. Aerobic exercise stimulates lipoprotein lipase activity, thereby de-

TABLE 41.7	Coronary Heart Disease (CHD) Risk Equivalents
Risk Equivalent	**Comments**
Other forms of athero-sclerotic disease	Peripheral arterial disease, abdominal aortic aneurysm, and symptomatic carotid artery disease
Diabetes	
Multiple risk factors that confer a 10-y risk for CHD >20%	

creasing the number of triglyceride particles and increasing levels of HDL cholesterol. Excess body weight is positively correlated with LDL cholesterol and negatively associated with HDL cholesterol. Weight loss stimulates lipoprotein lipase activity, decreasing triglyceride levels and increasing HDL levels. Another added benefit of weight reduction and increased physical activity is a decrease in blood pressure and the risk of developing diabetes mellitus.[26]

Diet is the cornerstone of treatment for hyperlipidemia. Efforts to reduce the dietary intake of total fat, saturated fat, and cholesterol and caloric intake beyond daily needs are the goals of diet therapy. Several dietary protocols have been developed, and most follow the recommendations of NCEP ATP III and the American Heart Association. These diets recommend reducing total fat intake to less than 30% of total daily calories and reducing saturated fat intake while increasing polyunsaturated and monounsaturated fats. Cholesterol consumption should be reduced and daily total caloric intake should be decreased to help patients reach and maintain an ideal body weight. Proteins and carbohydrates should be consumed in appropriate ratios for a balanced diet.

NCEP ATP III has developed a TLC diet (Table 41.9). Diet therapy alone can reduce cholesterol levels by 10% or more in compliant patients. A patient's response to diet therapy should be evaluated after 6 weeks. If LDL is not at goal, other options for lowering LDL such as viscous fiber and plant stanol/sterols can be added to the diet. TLC interventions should be given a 4- to 6-month trial to determine their effectiveness in lowering cholesterol levels (Fig. 41.7). Patients should receive dietary advice from trained professionals. Complying with dietary guidelines is difficult, so patients should receive encouragement and reinforcement at every visit to help them reach their goals. Involving family members in the process is helpful because they can offer additional support to the patient.[2,7]

Patients should be instructed on which foods to choose or avoid (Tables 41.10 and 41.11). Increased intake of fruits and vegetables should be encouraged. In general, highly processed foods and most snack products are high in calories and fat and should be avoided. Remind patients that a product that is low in fat or cholesterol is not necessarily low in calories. Oils, meats, dairy products, and condiments can also be a significant source of fat in the diet. Patients should read labels and check for the total calories, fat, and cholesterol content of a serving of the product. Converting fat content in grams to calories (9 kcal/g) reveals whether it represents more than 30% of calories.

Bran, fish oil, red wine, and other foods may lower serum cholesterol or reduce CHD risk. Confusion over health claims for these and other products led to the development of the U.S. Nutrition Labeling and Education Act of 1990. This act resulted in the U.S. Food and Drug Administration (FDA)'s final rule regarding seven accepted health claims, two of which address CHD risk reduction. First, fruits, vegetables, and grain products that contain fiber, particularly soluble fiber, are associated with a reduction in CHD risk. The

TABLE 41.8	NCEP ATP III Recommended Interventions Based on LDL Cholesterol Levels		
Risk Category	**LDL Cholesterol Goal**	**Initiate Therapeutic Lifestyle Changes**	**Consider Drug Therapy**
High risk: CHD or CHD risk equivalents (10-y risk, >20%)	<100 mg/dL (optional goal of <70 mg/dL for very high risk)	≥100 mg/dL	≥100 mg/dL (consider drug options if LDL-C <100 mg/dL)
Moderately high risk: 2 or more risk factors (10-y risk 10–20%)	<130 mg/dL (with an optional goal of <100 mg/dL	≥130 mg/dL	≥130 mg/dL (consider drug options if LDL-C 100–129 mg/dL)
Moderate risk: 2 or more risk factors (10-y risk <10%)	<130 mg/dL	≥130 mg/dL	>160 mg/dL
Low risk: 0 or 1 risk factors	<160 mg/dL	≥160 mg/dL	≥190 mg/dL (consider drug options if LDL-C 160–189 mg/dL)

LDL, low–density lipoprotein.
(From Third Report of the National Cholesterol Education Program [NCEP] expert panel on detection, evaluation and treatment of high blood cholesterol in adults [Adult Treatment Panel III] final report. Circulation 106:3143–3421, 2002; and Grundy SM, Cleeman JI, Merz CN, et al. Implications of recent clinical trials for the National Cholesterol Education Program Adult Treatment Panel III guidelines. Circulation 110:227–239, 2004.)

Primary Prevention

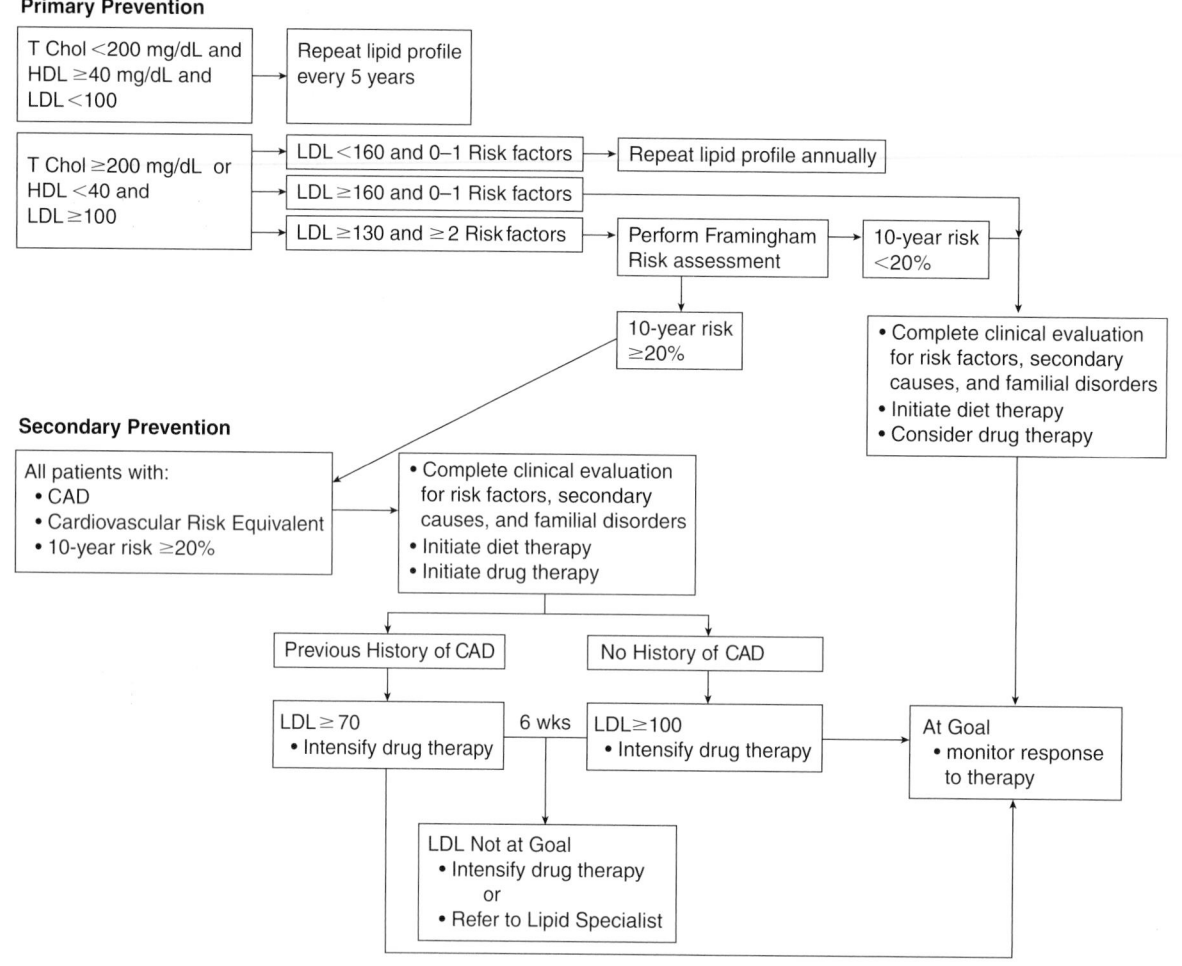

FIGURE 41.6 Screening algorithm. (Adapted from Havel R, Rapaport E. Management of primary hyperlipidemia. N Engl J Med 332:1491–1498, 1995.)

TABLE 41.9	Dietary Recommendations of NCEP ATP III for Treating Hyperlipidemia
Nutrient	**Recommended Intake**
Saturated fat[a]	<7%
Polyunsaturated fat[a]	<10%
Monounsaturated fat[a]	<20%
Total fat[a]	25–35%
Carbohydrate[a]	50–60%
Fiber	20–30 g/day
Protein[a]	~15%
Cholesterol	<200 mg/day
Total calories	To maintain optimal weight

[a]Percentage of total daily calories.
(From Third Report of the National Cholesterol Education Program [NCEP] expert panel on detection, evaluation and treatment of high blood cholesterol in adults [Adult Treatment Panel III] final report. Circulation 106:3143–3421, 2002.)

second claim states that diets low in saturated fats may reduce the risk of CHD. Conversely, antioxidant vitamins have not shown the ability to prevent CHD, as they were previously believed to. In fact, when antioxidant therapy is added to statin or niacin therapy, the protective benefits of these agents may be diminished.[27]

PHARMACOTHERAPY

Plant Stanols/Sterols. Plant stanols/sterols are found in butter substitutes such as Benecol and Take Control and can significantly lower LDL and triglyceride levels. Plant stanols/sterols displace cholesterol from micelles in the brush border of the small intestine, preventing its uptake and reducing the amount of cholesterol transported to the liver. As a result of diminished cholesterol delivery to the liver, there is an increased clearance of LDL from plasma. Plant stanols/sterols can reduce LDL by 10% to 15% and triglycerides by 5% but have little to no effect on HDL. Due to their intestinal action they can, however, block the absorption of fat-soluble vitamins. The NCEP ATP III guidelines recommend that plant stanols/sterols be incorporated into the diet to reduce plasma levels of LDL. Plant stanols/sterols should

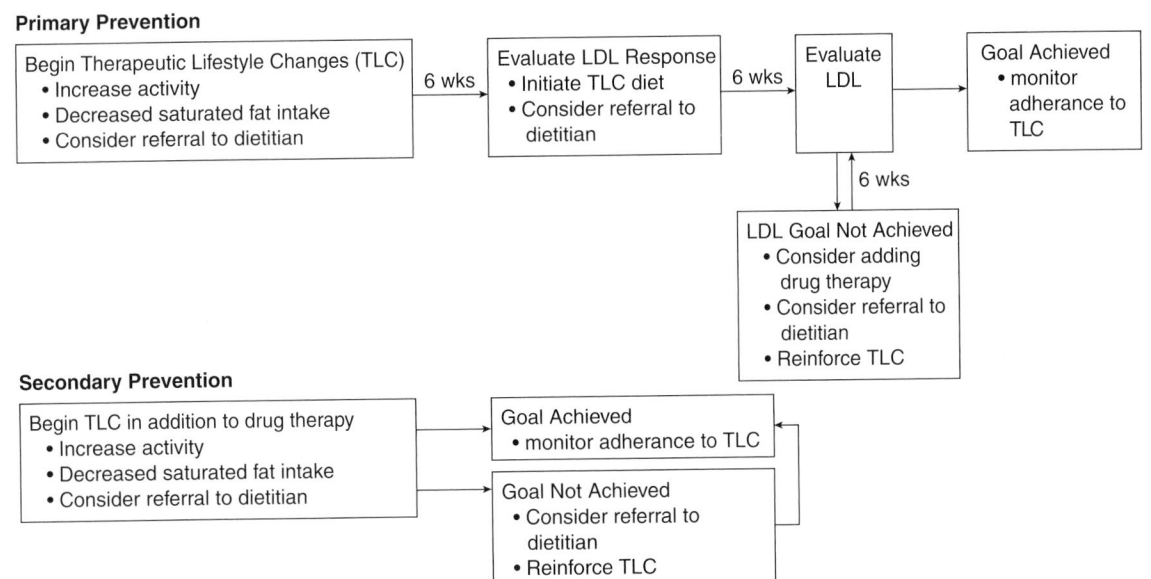

Primary Prevention

| Begin Therapeutic Lifestyle Changes (TLC) • Increase activity • Decreased saturated fat intake • Consider referral to dietitian | →6 wks→ | Evaluate LDL Response • Initiate TLC diet • Consider referral to dietitian | →6 wks→ | Evaluate LDL | → | Goal Achieved • monitor adherence to TLC |

↕ 6 wks

LDL Goal Not Achieved
• Consider adding drug therapy
• Consider referral to dietitian
• Reinforce TLC

Secondary Prevention

Begin TLC in addition to drug therapy
• Increase activity
• Decreased saturated fat intake
• Consider referral to dietitian

→ Goal Achieved
• monitor adherence to TLC

→ Goal Not Achieved
• Consider referral to dietitian
• Reinforce TLC

FIGURE 41.7 Therapeutic lifestyle modification algorithm. (Adapted from Havel R, Rapaport E. Management of primary hyperlipidemia. N Engl J Med 332:1491–1498, 1995.)

TABLE 41.10	Recommended Diet Modifications to Lower Blood Cholesterol	
Products	**Increase**	**Decrease**
Fruits and vegetables	Fresh, frozen, canned, or dried fruits and vegetables	Vegetables prepared in butter, creams, or other sauces
Meat, poultry, and fish	Fish, poultry without skin, lean cuts of beef, lamb, pork, or veal, shellfish	Fatty cuts of beef, lamb, pork, spare ribs, organ meats, regular cold cuts, sausage, hot dogs, bacon, sardines
Bread, cereals, and grains	Rice, pasta Whole-grain breads and cereals (oatmeal, whole wheat, rye, bran, multigrain) Homemade baked goods using unsaturated oils sparingly, angel food cake, low-fat crackers, low-fat cookies	Egg noodles Breads in which eggs are a major ingredient Commercial baked goods: pies, cakes, doughnuts, croissants, pastries, muffins, biscuits, high-fat crackers, high-fat cookies
Eggs	Egg whites (two egg whites equal one egg in recipes), cholesterol-free egg substitutes	Egg yolks
Dairy products	Skim or 1% fat milk (liquid, powdered, evaporated), buttermilk	Whole milk, regular, evaporated, condensed milk; cream, half-and-half, 2% milk, imitation milk products, most nondairy creamers, whipped toppings
	Nonfat or low-fat yogurt	Whole-milk yogurt
	Low-fat cottage cheese (1%–2%)	Whole-milk cottage cheese (4% fat)
	Low-fat cheeses, farmer or pot cheeses (all should be labeled no more than 2–6 g fat per ounce)	All natural cheeses (e.g., bleu, roquefort, camembert, cheddar, swiss), cream cheese, sour cream
	Sherbet, sorbet	Ice cream
Fats and oils	Baking cocoa	Chocolate
	Unsaturated vegetable oils; corn, olive, canola, safflower, sesame, soybean, sunflower oil; margarine or shortenings made from unsaturated oils, diet margarine	Butter, coconut oil, palm oil, lard, bacon fat
	Mayonnaise, salad dressings made with unsaturated oils, low-fat dressings	Dressings made with egg yolk
	Seeds and nuts	Coconut

The Expert Panel. Report of the National Cholesterol Education Program Expert Panel on Detection, Evaluation, and Treatment of High Blood Cholesterol in Adults. Arch Intern Med 148:36–69, 1988.

TABLE 41.11	Fatty Acid Composition of Vegetable Oils and Animal Fats

High in saturated fats

    Coconut oil

    Cocoa butter

    Palm kernel oil

    Palm oil

    Butterfat

    Beef tallow

High in monounsaturated fats, low in saturated fats

    Olive oil

    Peanut oil

    Canola (rapeseed) oil

High in polyunsaturated fats, low in saturated fats

    Soybean oil

    Corn oil

    Sunflower oil

    Safflower oil

American Medical Association Council on Scientific Affairs. Saturated fatty acids in vegetable oils, JAMA 263:693–695, 1990.

not be considered a primary therapy for hyperlipidemia but rather an integral component of therapeutic lifestyle changes to assist patients in achieving cholesterol goals.[2]

Bile Acid Resins. Bile acid resins exchange an anion, usually sodium, for bile acids in the intestinal tract. This interrupts the recycling of bile acid through enterohepatic circulation, causing hepatic cells to be stimulated to convert more cholesterol into bile acids. This process upregulates the LDL receptors and enhances LDL clearance from the plasma. Therefore, bile acids resins exert their primary effect on LDL cholesterol. Colestipol, cholestyramine, and colesevelam lower total cholesterol and LDL levels by 15% to 30%. HDL may be increased moderately by 3% to 5%. Triglycerides can be increased by 7% acutely, and 2% to 3% after prolonged therapy in patients with normal triglyceride levels. Clinicians should use resins with caution in patients with mild to moderate triglyceride elevations because the increase in triglycerides may be pronounced in these patients and may precipitate pancreatitis. Bile acid resins can decrease the risk of CHD, are safe, and have no long-term risks.[2,20,21]

Because resins are not absorbed from the gastrointestinal (GI) tract, they have no systemic effects. These agents are ideal for younger patients, including women considering pregnancy. The most common side effects involve the GI tract and include constipation, abdominal pain, belching, bloating, gas, heartburn, and nausea. These adverse effects do not occur as frequently with colesevelam. Constipation occurs in about 20% of patients and can be reduced with stool softeners and increased intake of soluble fiber. Psyllium can be used to increase dietary soluble fiber and has the added benefit of further reducing LDL levels. Resin doses should be titrated slowly to allow patients to develop tolerance to the GI complaints. Side effects may become more tolerable with prolonged therapy.

Resins are also known to interfere with the absorption of medications taken concurrently. Patients should take other medications at least 1 hour before or 4 hours after the resin. Interactions with digoxin, warfarin, thyroid hormones, thiazide diuretics, antibiotics, β-blockers, HMG CoA reductase inhibitors, iron salts, and phenobarbital have been documented.

Dosing is usually initiated at 4 g for cholestyramine, 5 g for colestipol, or six tablets of colesevelam, with maximum amounts of 24 g, 30 g, and seven tablets, respectively, generally given in two to four divided doses. A common regimen is to divide the total daily dosage by the number of meals the patient has each day. Resin powders should be given in at least 4 oz of a beverage or soup or sprinkled on a pulpy fruit. The dose should be sprinkled on top of the desired liquid to allow hydration before mixing. The drug should not be taken dry because of the risk of esophageal irritation or blockage. Colestipol beads are odorless and tasteless and may be preferable to some patients; 1-g tablets of colestipol are also available. Tablet formulations of these agents should be taken whole, not crushed.

The taste and side effects of resins make them difficult to tolerate as a lifelong regimen. This should be considered if the patient has a history of noncompliance. For this reason, bile acid resins typically are used as second- or third-line agents. The addition of low-dose resin therapy to other cholesterol-lowering agents can produce an additional 9% to 16% reduction in total cholesterol and LDL.

Ezetimibe. Ezetimibe acts at the brush border of the small intestines by binding to the receptor that is responsible for cholesterol uptake and therefore blocks intestinal cholesterol absorption. It does this without affecting the absorption of fat-soluble vitamins, bile acids, or triglycerides. When used alone it can reduce LDL by 18% and triglycerides by 6%, with minimal effect on HDL. When ezetimibe is combined with statin therapy, an additional LDL lowering of 10% to 20%, triglyceride lowering up to 10%, and a 1.5% rise in HDL can be seen.

Unlike bile acid resins, ezetimibe is systemically absorbed and has the potential for causing systemic side effects. While it has a long biological half-life (approximately 24 hours), limited systemic exposure occurs. Despite its absorption, the most common adverse effects are GI in nature, such as diarrhea and abdominal pain. It has also been associated with fatigue, back pain, and arthralgia. Ezetimibe has a very favorable side effect profile when used as monotherapy, but slight increases in the frequency of elevated liver function test results has been identified when used in combination with statins.[28] Ezetimibe also has a favorable drug interaction profile. It has not been associated with interactions with HMG CoA reductase inhibitors, fibric acid derivatives, digoxin, or warfarin. However, it cannot be taken concomitantly with bile acid resins because they will block its absorption.[29]

The customary dose of ezetimibe is 10 mg a day. It can be taken with or without food at a time that is most convenient for the patient. Doses of 20 mg a day have been evaluated and demonstrate an acceptable safety profile but are not routinely used because of limited additional clinical benefits. Ezetimibe is also commercially available in combination with simvastatin. This formulation is available in a number of simvastatin doses, all containing a fixed 10-mg dose of ezetimibe.

To date there have been no published primary or secondary prevention studies demonstrating ezetimibe's ability to prevent CHD when used alone or in combination with statins or other lipid-lowering agents. Therefore, ezetimibe should not be considered a first-line agent for treating hyperlipidemia. It could, however, be used as a first-line agent in a patient who cannot tolerate or has a contraindication to statin therapy.

Niacin. Niacin is a water-soluble B vitamin that exerts its lipid-lowering effect by inhibiting the production of VLDL particles in the liver. This results in a decrease in triglycerides and LDL. Niacin may also increase HDL levels by reducing its catabolism. Niacin lowers LDL by 5% to 25%, decreases triglycerides by 20% to 50%, and increases HDL by 15% to 35%.[2] These cholesterol-lowering effects are dose-related, and more than 1,500 mg per day of immediate-release niacin or 1,000 mg of extended-release niacin is usually required. Niacin is an ideal agent for patients who have elevated LDL and triglyceride levels and a normal or low HDL level. The Coronary Drug Project trial showed a decrease in the risk of recurrent MI in patients taking niacin. In the 15-year follow-up group, total mortality decreased by 11% in the niacin arm of the trial.[23]

Despite the favorable effects of niacin on the lipid profile, many patients cannot tolerate the medication's side effects. The most common symptoms with immediate-release niacin include flushing, tingling, itching, rash, and headaches, which are thought to be a result of prostaglandin-mediated vasodilation. These side effects are seen mainly at the beginning of therapy, with subsequent dosing changes, and when therapy is resumed after missed doses. Tolerance to these side effects quickly develops with continued dosing. Patients are instructed to take niacin with food to reduce GI side effects and with a low dose of aspirin (81 mg) 30 minutes before administration to reduce prostaglandin-mediated vasodilation. These side effects can also be minimized by slowly titrating to the recommended dose of 1,500 to 3,000 mg per day (Table 41.12).

Niacin can cause abdominal pain and discomfort. Some clinicians avoid niacin in patients with a history of peptic ulcer disease (PUD) because of concern that it may aggravate PUD or interfere with clinical presentation. Niacin is contraindicated in patients with chronic liver disease and active PUD. The over-the-counter sustained-release preparations that are available may decrease the prostaglandin-mediated side effects and GI discomfort, but they are generally less

TABLE 41.12	Schedule for Titrating Niacin	
Week	Immediate-Release Niacin	Extended-Release Niacin
1	125 mg BID	500 mg QHS
2	250 mg BID	500 mg QHS
3	500 mg BID	500 mg QHS
4	500 mg BID	500 mg QHS
5	1,000 mg BID	1,000 mg QHS
6	1,500 mg BID	1,000 mg QHS
8	—	1,500 mg QHS
12	—	2,000 mg QHS

BID, twice daily; QMS, at bed time

effective cholesterol-lowering agents and have been associated with an increase in the risk of hepatotoxicity.[30] The difference in toxicity may be the result of differences in the metabolism of the immediate-release and sustained-release formulations. A third formulation of niacin, extended-release niacin, offers many advantages over immediate- and sustained-release niacin, especially in terms of adverse effects. Although most of the adverse effects that patients experience with extended-release niacin are the same, it is associated with less flushing than the immediate-release preparation and less hepatotoxicity than the sustained-release one. These benefits are seen without sacrificing any lipid-lowering effects.[31]

Other adverse effects include elevations in liver function test results, uric acid levels, and blood glucose levels. For these reasons, niacin should be used with caution in patients with gout or diabetes. Elevation in liver enzymes can occur at any time, but it usually occurs if the niacin dose is increased too quickly. Patients should undergo baseline liver function tests when niacin is started and regular monitoring thereafter. NCEP ATP III guidelines recommend a maximum dose of immediate-release niacin of 3,000 mg per day, which is usually given in three divided doses, but niacin can be dosed up to 6,000 mg per day with appropriate monitoring.

Statins. The statins share a common mechanism of action: they bind to and inhibit the enzyme HMG-CoA reductase, the rate-limiting step in cholesterol biosynthesis (Fig. 41.8). The inhibition of HMG-CoA reductase activity results in a drop in intracellular cholesterol production, thus activating primarily hepatic LDL receptors and increasing the clearance of LDL from the bloodstream. There are currently six statins on the U.S. market, and they differ in their potency in lowering LDL cholesterol and triglycerides, their pharmacokinetic features, and potential for drug interactions. Lovastatin and simvastatin are administered as an inactive lactone, which after absorption is hydrolyzed into the active acid form. Atorvastatin, fluvastatin, pravastatin, and rosuvastatin are given as the active acid. A seventh statin, ceri-

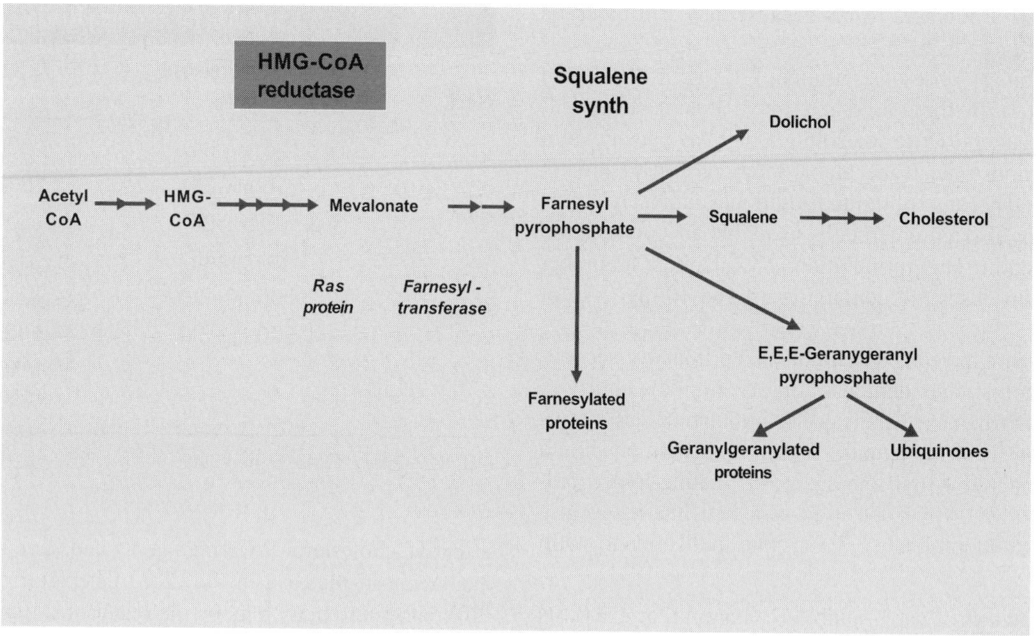

FIGURE 41.8 Cholesterol biosynthetic pathway.

vastatin, was on the U.S. market from 1998 until it was withdrawn in 2001 for excessive cases of muscle toxicity, including myopathy and fatal rhabdomyolysis, a rare but serious side effect also noted with other statins.[32]

Rosuvastatin, the most recently approved statin, is considered the most potent in lowering LDL cholesterol. Atorvastatin is the next most potent, followed by simvastatin. Lovastatin and pravastatin are similar in potency, and fluvastatin is considered the least potent of the statins. The relative effects of the available statins on LDL cholesterol, HDL cholesterol, and triglycerides are presented in Table 41.13. From the table, a few conclusions can be drawn:

1. Statins differ in their relative LDL-lowering potency. Doubling the dose of a statin on average provides additional LDL lowering of approximately 6%.
2. Statins lower serum triglyceride values in a manner similar to their LDL potency. The most significant triglyceride reductions are seen with the more potent statins on LDL (rosuvastatin and atorvastatin). The relationship between statin dose and triglyceride lowering is not as clear as the dose–response relationship with LDL.
3. Most statins are similar in their ability to raise HDL by 5% to 15%. Atorvastatin is a notable exception: at the upper end of its dosage range, atorvastatin loses its beneficial effect on raising HDL and has been reported to lower HDL in some patients. It is uncertain whether this effect blunts beneficial effects on other lipoprotein fractions, such as triglyceride and LDL lowering.

Statin selection is usually determined first by calculating the percentage of LDL reduction needed to reach the patient's LDL treatment goal. The choice of statin and the dose is often dictated by formulary considerations. Usually, more than one if not several statins could be selected to reach a given goal.

Statins may be grouped by how they are metabolized and eliminated, which corresponds to the potential for drug–drug interactions (Table 41.14). Simvastatin, lovastatin, and (to a lesser extent) atorvastatin are metabolized by the cytochrome P450 3A4 enzyme.[34] A number of drugs altering CYP3A4 activity are listed in Table 41.15. The interacting drug combinations blocking P450 metabolism increase the potential for both liver and muscle toxicity, producing increases in statin drug concentrations by as much as 20-fold. These combinations should be avoided or, if the interacting drug is to be used only temporarily (like a 7- to 10-day course of an antibiotic), the 3A4 statin should be temporarily discontinued and restarted upon completion of the antibiotic course. Numerous reports of statin myopathy in the literature can be traced to drug–drug interactions.[35] Drug interactions involving induction of CYP3A4 would be expected to reduce statin serum concentrations and effectiveness, requiring higher-than-expected doses to achieve the desired therapeutic response.

Fluvastatin is metabolized by the CYP2C9 pathway. Few drug interactions involving fluvastatin have been reported, but it may act as a CYP2C9 inhibitor and increase the International Normalized Ratio (INR) value in patients taking warfarin, another CYP2C9 metabolized drug.[36]

Pravastatin is more water-soluble, resulting in little P450 metabolism and fewer drug interactions. Increases in serum pravastatin concentrations have been noted with cyclosporine and gemfibrozil, possibly due to inhibition of biliary excretion. It is unclear whether these drug interactions are clinically important, however, because renal transplant pa-

TABLE 41.13	Efficacy of HMG-CoA Reductase Inhibitors			
Drug	**Dose (mg/day)**	**% Reduction LDL**	**% Increase HDL**	**% Reduction Triglycerides**
Atorvastatin	5	29	8	25
	10	36	7	13
	20	46	6	22
	40	50	3	30
	80	58	2	26
Fluvastatin	20	21	3	8
	40	26	3	12
	80	34	8.5	12.4
Lovastatin	20	24	7	10
	40	34	9	16
	80	40	10	19
Pravastatin	10	18	5	5
	20	25	16	13
	40	28	7	11
	80	37	3	19
Rosuvastatin	5	42	8	16
	10	47	9	19
	20	52	10	20
	40	57	10	23
Simvastatin	5	23	8	10
	10	28	6	9
	20	37	6	12
	40	40	12	19
	80	46	4	19

LDL, low-density lipoprotein; HDL, high-density lipoprotein.
(Adapted from McKenney JM, Hawkins D. Handbook on the management of lipid disorders. National Pharmacy Cholesterol Council, 2001.)

TABLE 41.14	Pharmacokinetic Properties of Statins					
Variable	**Atorvastatin**	**Fluvastatin**	**Lovastatin**	**Pravastatin**	**Rosuvastatin**	**Simvastatin**
Prodrug	No	No	Yes	No	No	Yes
Effect of food on absorption	No	No	Yes	No	No	No
Protein binding (%)	>98	98	>95	55–60	88	95
Active metabolites	Yes	No	Yes	No	No	Yes
Water solubility	No	No	No	Yes	Yes	No
Elimination	Hepatic	Hepatic	Hepatic	Renal/ Hepatic	Renal/ Hepatic	Hepatic
Plasma elimination half-life (h)	14	0.5–3	2–3	1.3–2.6	19	4
Major metabolic Isozyme	CYP3A4	CYP2C9	CYP3A4	None	CYP2C9/ CYP2C19	CYP3A4

(Adapted from Bottorff MB, Hansten P. Long-term safety of HMG-CoA reductase inhibition: role of metabolism. Arch Intern Med 160:2273–2280, 2000.)

TABLE 41.15	Representative Drugs Altering Statin Metabolism Through the CYP3A4 Pathway

Potent Inhibitors	Mild Inhibitors	Metabolic Inducers
Itraconazole (and other azole antifungal drugs)	Erythromycin (and other macrolides but not azithromycin)	Rifampin
Ritonavir (and other protease inhibitor HIV drugs)	Diltiazem/Verapamil	St. John's wort Carbamazepine
Cyclosporine	Grapefruit juice	Phenobarbital
Amiodarone		

tients receiving cyclosporine and pravastatin do not appear to be at an increased risk for myopathy.[13]

Rosuvastatin, the most recently FDA-approved statin, possesses the greatest degree of LDL lowering. It has water-solubility features similar to pravastatin, but rosuvastatin has a small degree of P450 metabolism by the CYP2C9 and CYP2C19 metabolic pathways. Although the extent of P450 metabolism is small, a recent change in the labeling recommends using lower doses in people of southeast Asian decent (e.g., Japanese, Chinese) due to higher-than-expected drug levels at any given dose. These populations are noted for having polymorphic CYP2C19 metabolism, resulting in impaired metabolism in up to 20% of the population. It is unclear at this time whether this is the mechanism of this observation. Rosuvastatin levels are also increased in patients with creatinine clearances below 30 mL per minute, resulting in a recommended starting dose of 5 mg, not to exceed 10 mg. There is also a drug interaction with cyclosporine, although not likely P450 in nature; it may involve biliary excretion

similar to pravastatin. Doses of rosuvastatin should be limited to 10 mg in patients taking cyclosporine as well.

Once the appropriate statin and dose are selected, the statin is usually given once a day in the evening, resulting in slightly more LDL reduction than the same daily dose given in the morning. The exception is with the statins having longer elimination half-lives, atorvastatin and rosuvastatin, which may be given at any time of day with similar response. The same daily statin dose given twice a day may produce slightly improved LDL lowering but introduces an additional dose per day and is rarely used. Some clinicians have tried alternate-day dosing in an attempt to reduce costs or side effects, but this is somewhat less effective and would usually require higher doses to reach the same level of LDL reduction; it may also be less convenient than taking the medication once a day.

There is a large clinical experience with the statins (Table 41.16).[10–12,37–45] The trials differ in the statin studied, the patient population evaluated, and the baseline CHD risk.

TABLE 41.16	Statin Outcome Trials

Trial	Intervention	Type	LDL-C Reduction (%)	HDL-C Increase (%)	CHD Risk Reduction (%)
AFCAPS/TexCAPS	Lovastatin	1°	25	6	37
WOSCOPS	Pravastatin	1°	26	5	31
ASCOT-LLA	Atorvastatin	1°	39	NA	36
CARE	Pravastatin	2°	32	5	24
LIPID	Pravastatin	2°	25	5	24
4S	Simvastatin	2°	35	8	34
AVERT	Atorvastatin	2°	47	7	36*
MIRACL	Atorvastatin	2°	40	5	16
HPS	Simvastatin	2°	32	3	24
A-Z Trial	Simvastatin 20 mg vs. 80 mg	2°	(18) relative	~13	~11
TNT	Atorvastatin 10 mg vs. 80 mg	2°	(24) relative	0	~22

NA = not available.
* Defined as reduction in total ischemic events.

Statins have been studied in five primary prevention trials (no known heart disease) and five secondary prevention trials (patients with established CHD). The PROSPER trial in an older population of patients included both patients with and without known heart disease. Most of the studies have been placebo-controlled, but three recent trials (PROVE-IT, A to Z, and TNT) have compared "lower-intensity" statin versus more aggressive statin therapy to lower LDL treatment goals than previously recommended by the NCEP. Taking these clinical trials in perspective, the following conclusions can be drawn:

1. Statin doses that reduce LDL cholesterol by 25% to 35% reduce future cardiovascular events by a similar percentage. The events reduced include fatal and non-fatal MI and fatal and non-fatal stroke, as well as a reduced need for revascularization procedures (angioplasty and bypass operations). This percentage event reduction is consistent irrespective of the statin used, the baseline LDL cholesterol value, and the baseline risk for CHD events.
2. High-risk patients treated to LDL levels below 70 mg per dL (1.81 mmol/L) have a better outcome than patients treated to LDL levels below 100 mg per dL (2.59 mmol/L), the previous treatment target for patients with established CHD or its equivalent.
3. Treatment benefits are clearly apparent after 1 to 2 years of therapy and persist throughout the 5-year duration for most of the trials.

Statins have become one of the most widely prescribed prescription drugs, in large part due to the numerous clinical trials documenting their efficacy. In addition, they are generally considered a safe and well-tolerated class of drugs. The most common side effects are GI and include nausea and abdominal pain. The two most important side effects requiring patient monitoring are liver and muscle related.

Statins are contraindicated in any patient with active hepatitis or unexplained elevations in liver function tests. Therefore, liver function tests should be done before starting statin therapy. Statins may subsequently produce persistent elevations in liver enzyme tests, resulting in drug discontinuation in up to 2% of patients. The likelihood of a measured liver function test abnormality increases with higher statin doses. If one or more of the transaminase values (AST, ALT) increases to greater than three times the upper limit of normal, statin therapy should either be reduced or discontinued. The vast majority of patients who have an elevated transaminase level are asymptomatic, so the test should be repeated to check for persistence. Many of the repeat values will return back to the normal range, not resulting in statin discontinuation. The term "transaminitis" was coined to reflect increases in transaminase values without apparent hepatotoxic consequences, because statins have only rarely been associated with liver toxicity.[46]

Patients more commonly report muscle symptoms associated with statin therapy. These have been defined by the American College of Cardiology, the American Heart Association, and the National Heart Blood and Lung Institute in a clinical advisory on statin safety published in the wake of the cerivastatin withdrawal.[47] These definitions are listed in Table 41.17. Myalgias occur fairly frequently in patients taking statins; the symptoms may be focal, such as leg cramps, or general and nonspecific, such as general weakness or easy fatigability. These symptoms may resolve with continued therapy or with dose reduction or temporary drug discontinuation. If the myalgias persist when the original statin is restarted at a reduced dose, then therapy with an alternate statin may be tried, and the addition of other forms of LDL-reduction therapy may be considered if higher doses of statin are not tolerated.

Creatine kinase (CK) determinations are useful in determining whether there is objective evidence of statin myositis in symptomatic patients. CK levels should be measured prior to initiating statin therapy to establish a baseline, because some patients may have unexplained mild elevations unrelated to statin therapy. Casual CK determinations in an asymptomatic patient are discouraged, given the unknown clinical significance of this finding. The absence of CK elevation in the presence of myalgias is usually interpreted as a benign finding. However, a recent study revealed histologic evidence of statin-related muscle toxicity in the absence of CK elevations, possibly indicating that CKs may not be sensitive enough to detect all types of statin-related myopathy.[48]

The exact mechanism of myositis/rhabdomyolysis is unknown and has been linked to a reduction in either tissue ubiquinone or ubiquinone precursors, including farnesyl and geranyl pyrophosphates.[49,50] There is insufficient evidence from placebo-controlled, randomized trials to promote the use of ubiquinone (Co-Q10) supplementation as a means to reverse or prevent muscle symptoms from statin therapy.

Since the withdrawal of cerivastatin, much has been published about the likelihood of the more serious side effect of statin therapy, myositis with or without rhabdomyolysis. Myositis/rhabdomyolysis may be more common in the presence of the following recognized risk factors that increase the potential occurrence:[47]

TABLE 41.17	Definition of Muscle Symptoms Associated With Statin Therapy
Myopathy	A general term referring to any disease of muscles
Myalgia	Muscle ache or weakness without creatinine kinase (CK) elevation
Myositis	Muscle symptoms with increased CK levels
Rhabdomyolysis	Muscle symptoms with marked CK elevations (typically greater than 10 times the upper limit of normal) and with creatinine elevation (usually with brown urine and urinary myoglobin)

Advanced age (particularly older women)
Small body frame
Multisystem disease (chronic renal insufficiency, especially diabetics)
Perioperative period
Hypothyroidism
Drug interactions

Evidence on the relative frequency of myositis/rhabdomyolysis may be derived from statin clinical trials, but these trials excluded patients possibly at risk (known drug interactions, comorbid clinical conditions) and some had run-in phases that excluded patients not tolerating the statin prior to study randomization, resulting in underestimates of risk. Other data evaluating statin safety come from the FDA's volunteer reporting system of adverse drug reactions. Reports of statin myositis/rhabdomyolysis are indexed to estimates of individual statin usage and standardized per million prescriptions. This type of analysis was useful in determining that cerivastatin was producing an unacceptable rate of rhabdomyolysis, resulting in its withdrawal.[32] An analysis of this database confirmed that rhabdomyolysis with statin use was most likely to be reported with gemfibrozil and cerivastatin, and that gemfibrozil was more likely than fenofibrate to cause rhabdomyolysis with other statins (Table 41.18).[51] The same FDA database was analyzed with a specific focus on rosuvastatin, the most recently approved statin.[52] Combined reports of proteinuria, rhabdomyolysis, nephropathy, and renal failure were low with all statins but occurred at a rate of approximately 30 per million prescriptions with rosuvastatin compared to 12 per million for simvastatin, 4 per million for atorvastatin, and 2 per million for pravastatin. Although the rate of these adverse reports with rosuvastatin was statistically higher than with other statins, the overall reporting rates for all statins are extremely small. In a similar analysis of 11 large managed care databases, the likelihood of hospitalization for rhabdomyolysis was most likely with gemfibrozil and cerivastatin (as expected), followed by cerivastatin alone; it was less likely with other statins used as monotherapy and least likely with pravastatin alone or in combination with any fibrate.[53]

The final source of statin-associated rhabdomyolysis comes from an analysis of case reports from the medical literature. In a recent review, the number of published cases as of 2001 totaled 74, of which only 15 were due to statin monotherapy. The majority were due to concomitant therapy known to increase the risk of statin myositis, including macrolide antibiotics, azole antifungals, cyclosporine, and fibrates, particularly gemfibrozil.[54]

In summary, we can make the following conclusions about the risk of serious muscle toxicity with the use of statins:

1. The overall rate appears to be low (<0.1%).
2. There do not appear to be substantial differences between currently available statins in terms of the risk of serious muscle toxicity.
3. The risk is increased in the presence of known interacting drugs, particularly inhibitors of CYP3A4 and statins metabolized by this enzyme (atorvastatin, lovastatin, and simvastatin).
4. Fibrates, in particular gemfibrozil, increase the risk of myositis/rhabdomyolysis.

Statins have rarely been associated with other adverse effects, including memory loss, ocular myasthenia, tendinopathy, and peripheral neuropathy. The overall incidence appears extremely small and poorly related to statin therapy.[55–58]

Mechanisms of Statin Benefit. Statins, in addition to their powerful ability to lower LDL cholesterol, have been associated with a variety of additional pharmacologic effects that may contribute to their overall clinical benefit. These include improvements in endothelial function, inhibition of prothrombotic forces, immunosuppression, atherosclerotic plaque stabilization, and an anti-inflammatory effect.[59,60] Of these, the anti-inflammatory effect, as assessed by lowering of plasma CRP levels, is the most studied. CRP values above 3 mg per liter are associated with a highest probability of a future cardiac event and are strongly correlated with cardiovascular risk determined by the Framingham risk model.[61,62] Statins, as a class effect, lower CRP, and the greatest reductions are observed in patients with the highest CRP levels at baseline, such as those with an acute coronary syndrome.[63] It is unclear whether the degree of CRP reduction is related to LDL cholesterol reduction, but statins have been shown to lower CRP as soon as 14 days after initiating therapy.[64] Thus, the anti-inflammatory effect of statin therapy may contribute to clinical benefit much earlier than other so-called pleiotropic effects such as plaque stabilization and slowing of atherosclerosis progression.

The role of CRP reduction in statin therapy is continuing to evolve. In the PROVE-IT trial, patients achieving CRP levels below 2 mg per liter had the lowest rates of future cardiac events, regardless of which statin was used and regardless of the LDL cholesterol level achieved.[65] Until further data are available, CRP testing is most helpful in assessing low levels of inflammation as a marker of future cardiovascular risk; CRP should not be used as a marker of statin response or as a guide to statin therapy adjustments.

TABLE 41.18	Statins and Rhabdomyolysis From FDA Database	
Medication	**No. Cases**	**Cases per Million Rx**
Fenofibrate		
With cerivastatin	14	140
With other statins	2	0.58
Gemfibrozil		
With cerivastatin	533	4,600
With other statins	57	8.6

Statin Combination Products. Lovastatin is available in a combination product with extended-release niacin under the trade name Advicor. This fixed-dose combination contains lovastatin doses of 10 to 40 mg and extended-release niacin (Niaspan) in doses of 500 to 2,000 mg. The maximum dose of 2,000 mg niacin and 40 mg lovastatin reduces LDL cholesterol by approximately 45%, reduces triglycerides by 40%, and increases HDL cholesterol by 40%.[66] These are the largest increases in HDL seen with any available therapy. Side effects seem to be mostly attributed to the niacin component of the combination, usually flushing and GI side effects.

Simvastatin is available in a fixed-dose combination with ezetimibe called Vytorin. The combination contains 10 mg ezetimibe combined with doses of simvastatin ranging from 10 to 80 mg. Across its dosage range, Vytorin reduces LDL cholesterol by 47% to 58%, increases HDL by 7% to 9%, and reduces triglycerides by 25% to 30%.[67] At comparable doses, Vytorin was more effective than atorvastatin at lowering LDL and raising HDL, with similar reductions in triglyceride levels. Ezetimibe may be used alone in patients who do not tolerate statin therapy, but its best use clinically is combined with statin therapy for patients who need but cannot tolerate higher statin doses or despite higher statin doses do not achieve their LDL cholesterol goals.

Other Benefits of Statin Therapy. In addition to the well-established reductions in cardiovascular morbidity and mortality (including stroke), statins are proposed through a variety of additional mechanisms to have other potential clinical uses. These include multiple sclerosis, colorectal cancer, osteoporosis and bone fractures, sepsis, and dementia.[68–71] Most of these data are observational, retrospective, or pilot data in small numbers of patients. It is premature at this time to recommend a statin for any of these indications or until a randomized, controlled clinical trial documents a benefit.

Fibric Acid Derivatives (Fibrates). Fibrates principally lower triglycerides by increasing the activity of lipoprotein lipase, the enzyme involved in hydrolysis of triglycerides from VLDL and IDL particles. This effect is mediated through stimulation of peroxisome proliferator-activated receptors (PPAR) of the α subtype.[72] Fibrates may also decrease the formation of VLDL and thereby have modest effects on lowering LDL cholesterol. Fibric acid derivatives generally provide a triglyceride reduction of 20% to 30%, decrease LDL by up to 20%, and increase HDL by 10% to 20%. Gemfibrozil, in a dose of 600 mg BID, was studied in the secondary prevention VA HIT trial in patients without elevated LDL levels and with reduced levels of HDL cholesterol.[73] Many of these patients had features of the metabolic syndrome. After a median follow-up of 5 years, a 6% increase in HDL and a 31% reduction in triglycerides was associated with a 22% risk reduction of nonfatal MI and death from coronary causes. Stroke and transient ischemic attacks were reduced by 29% and 59%, respectively, but total mortality was unaffected. Fenofibrate, the only other

fibrate available in the United States, has not yet been evaluated in a large-scale clinical outcome trial.

Gemfibrozil is available in generic form and is typically administered at the dose used in the VA HIT trial, 600 mg BID. Fenofibrate has undergone several dosage form alterations to improve bioavailability and reduce the effect of food. TriCor (fenofibrate) is available in 48-mg and 145-mg tablets and may be taken without regard to meals. Antara (fenofibrate) is available as 43-mg, 87-mg, and 130-mg capsules and should be taken with meals to improve absorption.

Fibrates are considered first-line therapy for patients with elevated triglycerides and may be used alone or in combination with statins in patients with mixed dyslipidemias. Fibrates are primarily eliminated by glucuronidation in the liver, with subsequent renal elimination of metabolites.[74] Fibrates are highly protein bound (>98%) and may interact with warfarin or other highly protein-bound drugs. Gemfibrozil appears more likely to interact with statins and increase the risk of myositis than fenofibrate, a clinical observation[51] that is now understood mechanistically. The hydroxy acid (active) form of atorvastatin, lovastatin, simvastatin, and rosuvastatin is metabolized by a non-P450 process termed glucuronidation. This metabolism is inhibited by gemfibrozil but not fenofibrate (Fig. 41.9).[75,76] There is considerable overlap in the glucuronidation isozymes involved in both statin and gemfibrozil metabolism, with no overlap involving fenofibrate. The increase in statin serum levels is approximately two- to three-fold (Fig. 41.10), which would be expected to increase the risk of myositis as observed in the FDA database. Since pravastatin is not glucuronidated, the observed increase in serum concentrations of pravastatin with gemfibrozil is speculative and may involve biliary excretion. There is no pharmacokinetic interaction between fenofibrate and statins, which may make this the preferred combination for safety reasons.[81,82]

Gemfibrozil and fenofibrate are generally well tolerated; the most common patient complaints are GI in nature. Fibrates uncommonly cause the same ''transaminitis'' seen with statins and rarely are associated with myositis; the effects on liver and muscle may be additive, and the risks of combination therapy with statins and fibrates must always be weighed against the benefits.

There are currently no outcome trials evaluating the combination of statin plus fibrate therapy, but the combination does appear to be particularly effective in shifting small, dense LDL particles toward larger, less atherogenic LDL particles while achieving aggressive LDL-lowering goals (Fig. 41.11).[83]

Fish Oils. Long-chain n-3 polyunsaturated fatty acids (PUFAs) are found in oily fish and fish oils and appear to protect against cardiovascular disease. There are several epidemiologic studies reporting that populations with at least weekly fish consumption have lower rates of cardiovascular disease.[84] There are two classes of PUFAs, the n-6 and the n-3, or ω-3 fatty acids. Both are considered essential fats, because they must come from dietary sources for incorporation into various body functions, including the production

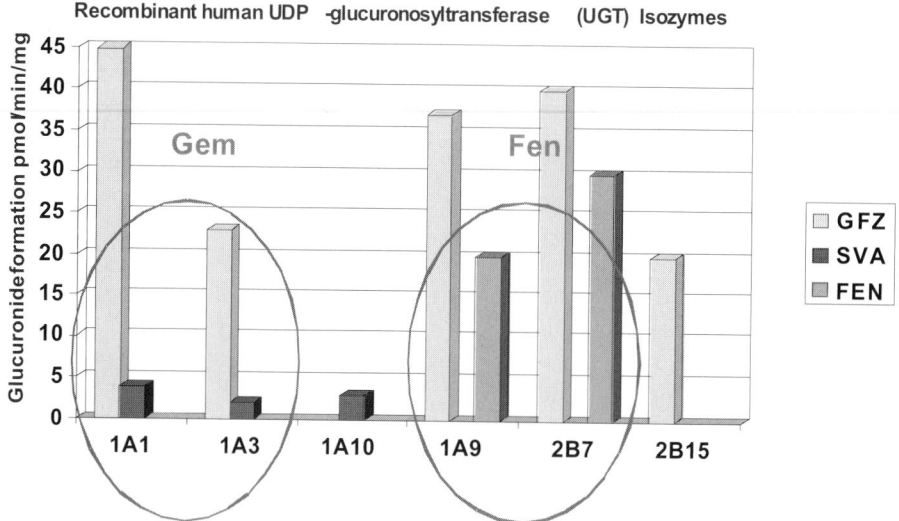

FIGURE 41.9 In vitro glucuronidation of simvastatin and gemfibrozil. (From Prueksaritanont T, Zhao JJ, Ma B, et al. Mechanistic studies on metabolic interactions between gemfibrozil and statins. J Pharmacol Exp Therapeut 301:1042–1051, 2002.)

of arachidonic acid and cellular membrane phospholipids.[85] The two major ω-3 fatty acids, eicosapentaenoic acid (EPA) and docosahexaenoic acid (DHA), are made in green plants, algae, and phytoplankton and are ingested directly from marine animals at the top of the food chain, mostly fatty fish such as salmon or herring. Plant α-linolenic acid may also be a source of ω-3 fatty acids. It can be found in certain vegetable oils (olive, canola, and flaxseed) and most nuts, including walnuts. The ω-3 fatty acids have been linked to a lower risk of cardiovascular disease through epidemiology studies, prospective dietary trials, and studies with ω-3 fatty

acid capsules. The benefits include a 25% to 30% reduction in triglyceride concentrations (requiring approximately 4 g/day of EPA/DHA), a decrease in platelet aggregation, and reductions in arrhythmias and sudden death (doses of approximately 1 g/day). The most common adverse effect of fish oil capsules is the fishy aftertaste, which may be reduced somewhat by storing the capsules in a refrigerator prior to consumption. Other side effects are GI, and there is some concern that excessive ingestion of fatty fishes may increase the exposure to toxins such as mercury. The supplements are essentially free of mercury.

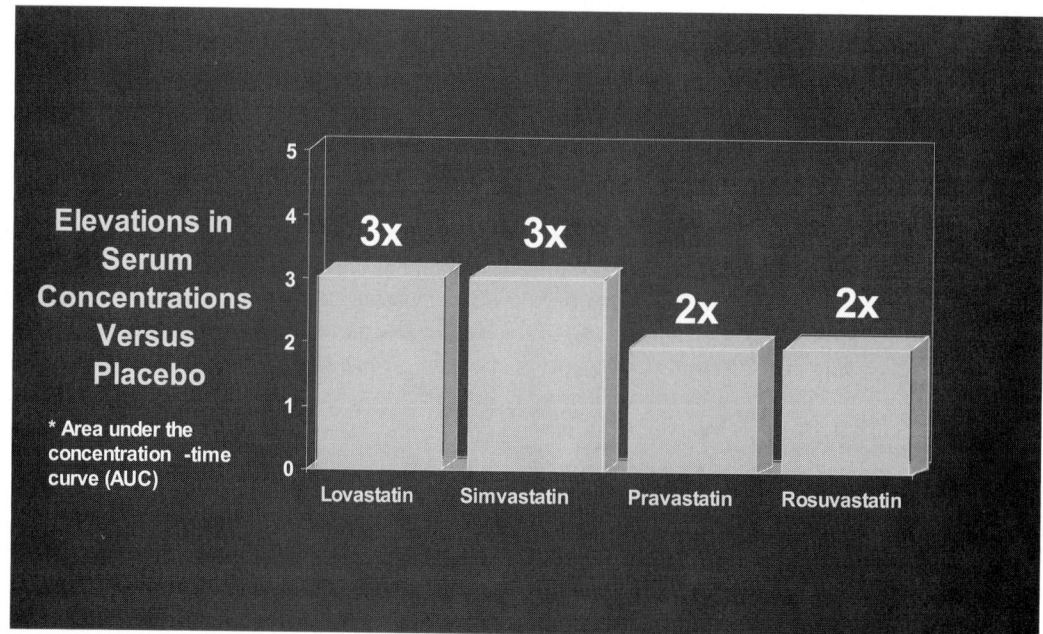

FIGURE 41.10 Effects of gemfibrozil on statin serum concentrations. From references 77, 78,79 and 80.

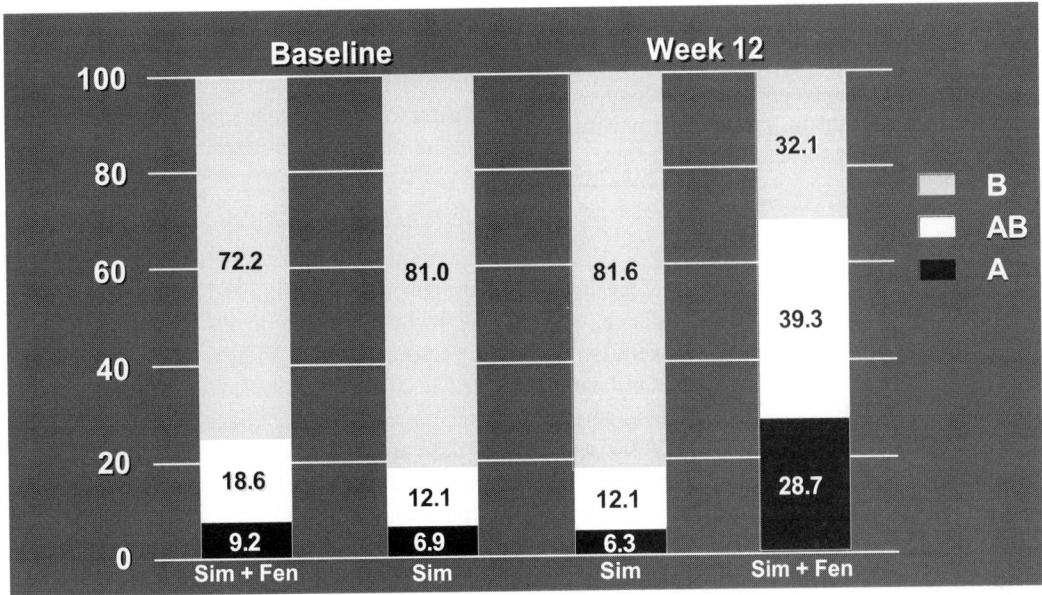

FIGURE 41.11 Statin plus fibrate combination and LDL particle size. **A.** LDL subclass A (predominance of larger, more buoyant particles ≥118 seconds). **B.** LDL subclass B (predominance of smaller, more dense particles <115 seconds). **AB.** LDL subclass AB (intermediate density between A and B for ≥115 and <118 seconds). (From Grundy SM, Vega GL, Yuan Z, et al. Effectiveness and tolerability of simvastatin plus fenofibrate for combined hyperlipidemia [the SAFARI trial]. Am J Cardiol 95:462–468, 2005.)

PHARMACOECONOMICS

Most of the statin trials have conducted post-hoc pharmacoeconomic studies, primarily based on concerns of the expense of statin therapy and the duration of therapy. In general, the higher the risk of the population treated, the greater the reduction in expensive procedures such as angioplasty and coronary artery bypass graft surgery and hospitalizations and treatment for stroke and acute coronary syndromes. Therefore, primary prevention trials will show a "higher cost" per patient for preventing events compared to secondary prevention trials. Table 41.19 shows the relative cost in various statin trials, events prevented, and costs per patient.[86] Treatment of dyslipidemias might be expected to become more cost-effective in the future. As more statins become available in generic form over the next few years, costs of therapy will continue to decline and procedure costs will undoubtedly continue to increase, providing a more favorable cost-effectiveness ratio. Secondly, the ability to detect and predict patients at the highest risk for future events will improve, allowing clinicians to target the highest-risk patients for therapy.

TABLE 41.19	Trials Examining Event Reduction and Pharmacoeconomics					
	Reductions per 1,000 Patients			**Cost Per Patient ($)**		
Study	**Deaths**	**Myocardial Infarction**	**Revascularization**	**Treatment**	**Offset**	**Net**
Primary Prevention						
WOSCOPS	5	19	8	3,700	100	3,600
AFCAPS	4	26	31	4,654	524	4,130
Secondary Prevention						
4S	32	47	59	4,650	3,900	780
CARE	11	18	47	5,550	1,660	3,890

(From Mark DB, Hlatky MA. Medical economics and the assessment of value in cardiovascular medicine: part II. Circulation 106:626–630, 2002.)

FUTURE THERAPIES

Several innovations in the management of dyslipidemias are on the horizon and are expected to improve our ability to manage patients with or at risk for cardiovascular disease.

MURAGLITAZAR

Type 2 diabetes is associated with a high risk of cardiovascular disease, in part due to a multitude of metabolic abnormalities that often include hypertension, insulin resistance, elevated triglycerides, low HDL cholesterol, and small, dense LDL particles. The thiazolidinediones (TZDs), rosiglitazone and pioglitazone, improve insulin sensitivity by being peroxisome proliferators-activated receptor gamma (PPARγ) agonists. The fibrates, gemfibrozil and fenofibrate, improve the dyslipidemia often seen in patients with either metabolic syndrome or type 2 diabetes through stimulation of the PPARα subtype. A number of drugs are in development that provide dual stimulation of varying degrees at both the PPARγ and PPARα receptors, thus improving insulin sensitivity, reducing triglycerides, raising HDL cholesterol, and shifting small dense LDL particles toward a less atherogenic profile.[87] Depending on the degree of receptor stimulation, muraglitazar would be expected to produce metabolic effects similar to combining a TZD with a fibrate.

PITAVASTATIN

Although six statins are currently on the U.S. market, a seventh is in development, pitavastatin, and may be available in the future. Compared to other statins, pitavastatin is considered potent and lowers LDL cholesterol from 34% to 47% over a dosage range of 1 to 4 mg.[88] Little has been published on the pharmacokinetic properties of pitavastatin, although it does appear to be somewhat lipid-soluble, and drug metabolism/interactions issues remain to be resolved.

RAISING HDL

Statins and fibrates are considered to have a mild ability to increase HDL; niacin is more potent but is poorly tolerated. A new group of agents—cholesterol ester transfer protein (CETP) inhibitors—are being investigated for their more pronounced effects in raising HDL cholesterol. The drug closest to potential market in the United States is torcetrapib. In a recent clinical trial, torcetrapib at a dose of 120 mg once a day increased HDL by 46%, with increases of 106% seen at a dose of 120 mg twice a day.[89] A 120-mg daily dose combined with atorvastatin 20 mg increased HDL by 61%. Torcetrapib alone reduced triglycerides by 18% to 26% and LDL cholesterol by 17%. Little is known about the metabolism of torcetrapib or its long-term safety.

OVER-THE-COUNTER STATINS

Simvastatin was recently granted over-the-counter (OTC) status in Great Britain, and both lovastatin and pravastatin are being evaluated for potential OTC status in the United States. While OTC approval would make clinically proven drugs available to a larger number of patients, there is considerable concern about safety, monitoring for response, and the need for more potent LDL lowering than OTC doses are likely to provide.[90]

PHARMACOGENETICS

In the future, pharmacogenetics will undoubtedly play a role in drug therapy selection and monitoring. Genetic variability may occur at multiple levels of cholesterol metabolism and drug response. The CYP2D6 polymorphism has been implicated in higher rates of adverse effects in people who are poor simvastatin metabolizers.[91] Polymorphisms in the paraoxonase enzyme carried on HDL particles may also determine the statin's ability to raise HDL; persons who were homozygous for the QQ allele had no HDL response to pravastatin.[92] As a final example, genetic variability in transporting enzymes involved in statin disposition may alter their efficacy and safety; different haplotypes in the alleles for organic anion-transporting polypeptides can result in two-fold higher statin concentrations.[93] Other potential sources for genetic variability are being determined, but due to the complexity of statin metabolism and statin response, it is unlikely that genetic testing will prove to be sole determinant of statin dose and response.

KEY POINTS

- Cardiovascular disease is one of the leading causes of morbidity and mortality in the United States
- One of the major risk factors for the development of CHD is hyperlipidemia
- Therapeutic lifestyle changes should be the foundation of all cholesterol-lowering interventions and should be incorporated into every treatment plan
- LDL cholesterol is the lipid component most closely associated with CHD risk and elevated serum cholesterol levels
- Low HDL levels are a risk factor for CHD
- Treatment decisions are based on a patient's LDL level, risk factor status, presence of CHD or cardiovascular risk equivalents, and cardiovascular risk assessment.
- Fruits, vegetables, and grain products that contain fiber, particularly soluble fiber, and a diet low in saturated fat and cholesterol are associated with a reduction in the risk of CHD
- The choice of which drug to begin should be based on the type of hyperlipidemia, past medical history, adverse effect profile of the drug, effectiveness of the drug, patient's adherence history, and cost
- Due to their LDL-lowering potency and abundance of clinical trials, statins are usually considered first-line therapy for the majority of patients with hyperlipidemia. Statins lower LDL cholesterol by up to 60%,

with 5% to 15% increases in HDL cholesterol and 15% to 30% reductions in triglycerides

- Intestinal cholesterol-lowering agents lower total cholesterol and LDL by 10% to 30% and increase HDL by 3% to 5%. Their effect on triglyceride levels varies according to the agent selected. These drugs are effective treatments for hypercholesterolemia but are usually not a first-line agent

- Fibrates are considered first-line therapy for patients with elevated triglyceride values. Fibrates are also used in combination therapy with statins in patients with persistently elevated triglyceride values. Certain statin/fibrate combinations increase the risk for myopathies

- Niacin decreases LDL by 10% to 25%, decreases triglycerides by 20% to 50%, and increases HDL by 15% to 35%, but it should be used with caution in patients with a history of chronic liver disease, PUD, gout, and diabetes. Niacin is effective in treating hypercholesterolemia and hypertriglyceridemia

ACKNOWLEDGMENT

The author acknowledges Camille W. Thornton and James M. Holt for their contributions to this chapter.

SUGGESTED READINGS

Cannon CP, Braunwald E, McCabe CH, et al. Comparison of intensive and moderate lipid lowering with statins after acute coronary syndromes. N Engl J Med 350:1495–1504, 2004.

Grundy SM, Cleeman JI, Merz CN, et al. Implications of recent clinical trials for the National Cholesterol Education Program Adult Treatment Panel III guidelines. Circulation 110:227–239, 2004.

Heart Protection Study Collaborative Group. MRC/BHF Heart Protection Study of cholesterol lowering with simvastatin in 20,536 high-risk individuals: a randomized placebo-controlled trial. Lancet 360:7–22, 2002.

Third Report of the National Cholesterol Education Program (NCEP) Expert Panel on Detection, Evaluation, and Treatment of High Blood Cholesterol in Adults (Adult Treatment Panel III) final report. Circulation 106:3143–3421, 2002.

REFERENCES

1. Heart Disease and Stroke Statistics, American Heart Association 2005; available at www.americanheart.org.
2. Third Report of the National Cholesterol Education Program (NCEP) expert panel on detection, evaluation and treatment of high blood cholesterol in adults (Adult Treatment Panel III) final report. Circulation 106:3143–3421, 2002.
3. Neaton JD, Wentworth D. Serum cholesterol, blood pressure, cigarette smoking, and death from coronary heart disease. Overall findings and differences by age for 316,099 white men. Multiple Risk Factor Intervention Trial Research Group. Arch Intern Med 152:56–64, 1992.
4. Kannel WB. High-density lipoproteins: epidemiologic profile and risks of coronary artery disease. Am J Cardiol 52:9B–12B, 1983.
5. Havel R, Rapaport E. Management of primary hyperlipidemia. N Engl J Med 332:1491–1498, 1995.
6. Stone N. Secondary causes of hyperlipidemia. Med Clin North Am 78:117–141, 1993.
7. Clark A, Holt J. Identifying and managing patients with hyperlipidemia. Am J Man Care 3:1211–1219, 1997.
8. Henkin Y, Como J, Oberman A. Secondary dyslipidemia: inadvertent effects of drugs in clinical practice. JAMA 267:961–968, 1992.
9. Welch G, Lascalzo J. Homocysteine and atherothrombosis. N Engl J Med 338:1042–1050, 1998.
10. Heart Protection Study Collaborative Group. MRC/BHF Heart Protection Study of cholesterol lowering with simvastatin in 20,536 high-risk individuals: a randomised placebo-controlled trial. Lancet 360:7–22, 2002.
11. Sheperd J, Blauw GJ, Murphy MB, et al. Pravastatin in elderly individuals at risk of vascular disease (PROSPER): a randomized controlled trial. Lancet 360:1623–1630, 2002.
12. The ALLHAT Officers and Coordinators for the ALLHAT Collaborative Research Group. Major outcomes in moderately hypercholesterolemic, hypertensive patients randomised to pravastatin vs. usual care. The Antihypertensive and Lipid-Lowering Treatment to Prevent Heart Attack Trial (ALLHAT-LLA). JAMA 288:2998–3007, 2002.
13. Kobashigawa JA, Katsnelson S, Laks H, et al. Effect of pravastatin on outcomes after cardiac transplantation. N Engl J Med 333:621–627, 1995.
14. Willerson JT, Ridker PM. Inflammation as a cardiovascular risk factor. Circulation 109 (Suppl):II2–10, 2004.
15. Denke MA. Cholesterol-reducing diets: a review of the evidence. Arch Intern Med 155:17–26, 1995.
16. Stone NJ, Blum CB. Pathophysiology of hyperlipoproteinemias. In: Management of lipids in clinical practice. National Lipid Association, 2005.
17. Coresh J, Kwiterovich PO. Small, dense low-density lipoprotein particles and coronary heart disease risk. A clear association with uncertain implications. JAMA 276:914–915, 1996.
18. Schaefer EJ, Lamon-Fava S, Jenner JL, et al. Lipoprotein (a) levels and risk of coronary heart disease in men. The Lipid Research Clinics Coronary Primary Prevention Trial. JAMA 271:999–1003, 1994.
19. Oliver M, Heady J, Morris J, et al. A cooperative trial in the primary prevention of ischemic heart disease using clofibrate. Br Heart J 40:1069–1118, 1978.
20. Lipid Research Clinics Program. The Lipid Research Clinics coronary primary prevention trial results. I. Reductions in incidence of coronary heart disease. JAMA 251:357–364, 1984.
21. Lipid Research Clinics Program. The Lipid Research Clinics coronary primary prevention trial results. II. The relationship of reduction in incidence of coronary heart disease to cholesterol lowering. JAMA 251:365–374, 19842000.
22. Frick M, Elo O, Haapa K, et al. Helsinki Heart Study; primary prevention trial with gemfibrozil in middle aged men with dyslipidemia. N Engl J Med 317:1237–1245, 1987.
23. Coronary Drug Project Research Group. Clofibrate and niacin in coronary heart disease. JAMA 231:360–381, 1975.
24. Hjermann I, Holme I, Velve Byrne K, et al. Effect of diet and smoking intervention on the incidence of coronary heart disease. Report from the Oslo Study Group of a randomized trial in healthy men. Lancet 11:1303–1310, 1981.
25. Grundy SM, Cleeman JI, Merz CN, et al. Implications of recent clinical trials for the National Cholesterol Education Program Adult Treatment Panel III guidelines. Circulation 110:227–239, 2004.
26. American Heart Association Nutrition Committee. Dietary guidelines for healthy American adults. Circulation 77:721A–724A, 1988.
27. Brown GB, Zhao XQ, Chait A, et al. Simvastatin and niacin, antioxidant vitamins, or the combination for the prevention of coronary disease. N Engl J Med 345:1583–1592, 2001.
28. Davidson M, McGarry T, Bettis R, et al. Ezetimibe coadministered with simvastatin in patients with primary hypercholesterolemia. J Am Coll Cardiol 40:135–138, 2002.
29. Kosoglou T, Statkevich P, Johnson-Levonas A, et al. Ezetimibe: a review of its metabolism, pharmacokinetics and drug interactions. Clin Pharmacokinet 44:467–494, 2005.
30. McKenney J, Proctor J, Harris S, et al. A comparison of the efficacy and toxic effects of sustained versus immediate-release niacin in hypercholesterolemic patients. JAMA 271:672, 1994.
31. Grundy S, Vegqa G, McGovern M, et al. Diabetes Multicenter Research Group. Efficacy, safety and tolerability of once-daily niacin for the treatment of dyslipidemia associated with type 2 diabetes: results of the Assessment of Diabetes Control and Evaluation of the Efficacy of Niaspan Trial. Arch Intern Med 162:1568–1576, 2002.

32. Staffa JA, Chang J, Green L. Cerivastatin and reports of fatal rhabdomyolysis. N Engl J Med 346:539–540, 2002.

33. McKenney JM, Hawkins D. Handbook on the management of lipid disorders. National Pharmacy Cholesterol Council, 2001.

34. Bottorff MB, Hansten P. Long-term safety of HMG-CoA reductase inhibition: role of metabolism. Arch Intern Med 160:2273–2280, 2000.

35. Worz CR, Bottorff MB. The role of cytochrome P450-mediated drug–drug interactions in determining safety of statins. Expert Opin Pharmacother 2:1119–1127, 2001.

36. Andrus MR. Oral anticoagulant drug interactions with statins: case report with fluvastatin and review of the literature. Pharmacotherapy 24:285–290, 2004.

37. Scandinavian Simvastatin Survival Study Group. Randomised trial of cholesterol lowering in 4444 patients with coronary heart disease: the Scandinavian Simvastatin Survival Study (4S). Lancet 344: 1383–1389, 1994.

38. Shepherd J, Cobbe M, Ford I, et al. Prevention of coronary heart disease with pravastatin in men with hypercholesterolemia. N Engl J Med 333:1301–1307, 1995.

39. Downs JR, Clearfield M, Weis S, et al. Primary prevention of acute coronary events with lovastatin in men and women with average cholesterol levels: results of AFCAPS/TexCAPS. JAMA 279: 1615–1622, 1998.

40. Sacks FM, Pfeffer MA, Moye LA, et al. The effect of pravastatin on coronary events after myocardial infarction in patients with average cholesterol levels. N Engl J Med 335:1001–1009, 1996.

41. The Long-Term Intervention With Pravastatin in Ischemic Disease (LIPID) study group. Prevention of cardiovascular events and death with pravastatin in patients with coronary heart disease and a broad range of initial cholesterol levels. N Engl J Med 339:1349–1357, 1998.

42. Sever PS, Dahlof B, Poulter NR, et al. Prevention of coronary and stroke events with atorvastatin in hypertensive patients who have average of lower-than-average cholesterol concentrations, in the Anglo-Scandinavian Cardiac Outcomes Trial Lipid Lowering Arm (ASCOT-LLA): a multicentre randomised controlled trial. Lancet 361:1149–1158, 2003.

43. Cannon CP, Braunwald E, McCabe CH, et al. Comparison of intensive and moderate lipid lowering with statins after acute coronary syndromes. N Engl J Med 350:1495–1504, 2004.

44. de Lemos JA, Blazing MA, Wiviott SD, et al. Early intensive vs. a delayed conservative simvastatin strategy in patients with acute coronary syndromes: Phase Z of the A to Z trial. JAMA 292: 1307–1316, 2004.

45. LaRosa JC, Grundy SM, Waters DD, et al. Intensive lipid lowering with atorvastatin in patients with stable coronary disease. N Engl J Med 352:1425–1435, 2005.

46. Dujovne C. Side effects of statins: hepatitis versus "transaminitis"—myositis versus "CPKitis." Am J Cardiol 89:1411–1413, 2002.

47. Pasternak RC, Smith SC, Bairey-Merz CN, et al. ACC/AHA/NHLBI clinical advisory on the use and safety of statins. Circulation 106: 1024–1028, 2002.

48. Phillips PS, Haas RH, Bannykh S, et al. Statin-associated myopathy with normal creatine kinase levels. Ann Intern Med 137:581–85, 2002.

49. Koumis T, Nathan JP, Rosenberg JM, et al. Strategies for the prevention and treatment of statin-induced myopathy: is there a role for ubiquinone supplementation? Am J Health Syst Pharm 61:515–519, 2004.

50. Flint OP, Masters BA, Gregg RE, et al. HMG CoA reductase inhibitor-induced myotoxicity: pravastatin and lovastatin inhibit the geranylation of low-molecular-weight proteins in neonatal rat muscle cell culture. Tox Appl Pharmacol 145:99–110, 1997.

51. Jones PH and Davidson MH. Reporting rate of rhabdomyolysis with fenofibrate + statin versus gemfibrozil + any statin. Am J Cardiol 95:120–122, 2005.

52. Alsheikh-Ali A, Ambrose MS, Kuvin JT, et al. The safety of rosuvastatin as used in common clinical practice: a post-marketing analysis. Circulation 2005;111:available online May 31, 2005.

53. Graham DJ, Staffa JA, Shatin D, et al. Incidence of hospitalized rhabdomyolysis in patients treated with lipid-lowering drugs. JAMA 292:2585–2590, 2004.

54. Omar MA, Wilson JP, Cox TS. Rhabdomyolysis and HMG-CoA reductase inhibitors. Ann Pharmacotherapy 35:1096–1107, 2001.

55. King DS, Wilburn AJ, Wofford MR, et al. Cognitive impairment associated with atorvastatin and simvastatin. Pharmacotherapy 23: 1663–1667, 2003.

56. Parmar B, Francis PJ, Ragge NK. Statins, fibrates and ocular myasthenia. Lancet 360:717, 2002.

57. Chazerain P, Hayem G, Hamza S, et al. Four cases of tendinopathy in patients on statin therapy. Joint Bone Spine 68:430–433, 2001.

58. Gaist D, Rodriguez LAG, Huerta C, et al. Are users of lipid-lowering drugs at increased risk of peripheral neuropathy? Eur J Clin Pharmacol 56:931–933, 2001.

59. Libby P, Aikawa M. Mechanisms of plaque stabilization with statins. Am J Cardiol 91:4B–8B, 2003.

60. Lefer DJ. Statins as potent anti-inflammatory drugs. Circulation 106: 2041–2042, 2002.

61. Ridker PM. Clinical application of C-reactive protein for cardiovascular disease detection and prevention. Circulation 107:363–369, 2003.

62. Albert MA, Glynn RJ, Ridker PM. Plasma concentration of C-reactive protein and the calculated Framingham coronary heart disease risk score. Circulation 108:161–165, 2003.

63. Kinlay S, Selwyn AP. Effects of statins on inflammation in patients with acute and chronic coronary syndromes. Am J Cardiol 91: 9B–13B, 2003.

64. Plenge JK, Hernandez TL, Weil KM, et al. Simvastatin lowers C-reactive protein within 14 days: an effect independent of low-density lipoprotein cholesterol reduction. Circulation 106: 1447–1452, 2002.

65. Ridker PM, Cannon CP, Morrow D, et al. C-reactive protein levels and outcomes after statin therapy. N Engl J Med 352:20–28, 2005.

66. Kashyap ML, McGovern ME, Berra K, et al. Long-term safety and efficacy of once-daily niacin/lovastatin formulation for patients with dyslipidemia. Am J Cardiol 89:672–678, 2002.

67. Ballantyne CM, Abate N, Yuan Z, et al. Dose-comparison of the combination of ezetimibe and simvastatin (Vytorin) versus atorvastatin in patients with hypercholesterolemia: the Vytorin versus Atorvastatin (VYVA) Study. Am Heart J 149:464–473, 2005.

68. Youssef S, Stuve O, Patarroyo JC, et al. The HMG Co-A reductase inhibitor atorvastatin promotes a Th2 bias and reverses paralysis in central nervous system autoimmune disease. Nature 420:78–84, 2002.

69. Poynter JN, Gruber SB, Higgins PDR, et al. Statins and the risk of colorectal cancer. N Engl J Med 352:2184–2192, 2005.

70. Yildirir A, Muderrisoglu H. Non-lipid effects of statins: emerging new indications. Curr Vasc Pharmacol 2:309–318, 2004.

71. Almog Y. Statins, inflammation and sepsis. Chest 124:740–743, 2003.

72. Tsimihodimos V, Miltiadous G, Daskalopoulou SS, et al. Fenofibrate: metabolic and pleiotropic effects. Curr Vasc Pharmacol 3: 87–98, 2005.

73. Rubins JB, Robins SJ, Collins D, et al. Gemfibrozil for the secondary prevention of coronary heart disease in men with low levels of high-density lipoprotein cholesterol. N Engl J Med 341:410–418, 1999.

74. Miller DB, Spence JD. Clinical pharmacokinetics of fibric acid derivatives (fibrates). Clin Pharmacokinet 34:155–162, 1998.

75. Prueksaritanont T, Zhao JJ, Ma B, et al. Mechanistic studies on metabolic interactions between gemfibrozil and statins. J Pharmacol Exp Therapeut 301:1042–1051, 2002.

76. Prueksaritanont T, Tang C, Qiu Y, et al. Effects of fibrates on metabolism of statins in human hepatocytes. Drug Metab Disp 30: 1280–1287, 2002.

77. Kyrklund C, Backman JT, Kivisto KT, et al. Plasma concentrations of active lovastatin acid are markedly increased by gemfibrozil but not by bezafibrate. Clin Pharmacol Ther 69:340–345, 2001.

78. Backman JT, Kyrklund C, Kivisto KT, et al. Plasma concentrations of active simvastatin acid are increased by gemfibrozil. Clin Pharmacol Ther 68:122–129, 2000.

79. Kyrklund C, Backman JT, Neuvonen M, et al. Gemfibrozil increases plasma pravastatin concentrations and reduces pravastatin renal clearance. Clin Pharmacol Ther 73:538–544, 2003.

80. Schneck DW, Birmingham BK, Zalikowski JA, et al. The effect of gemfibrozil on the pharmacokinetics of rosuvastatin. Clin Pharmacol Ther 75:455–463, 2004.

81. Martin PD, Dane AL, Schneck DW, et al. An open-label, randomized, three-way crossover trial of the effects of coadministration of rosuvastatin and fenofibrate on the pharmacokinetic properties of rosuvastatin and fenofibric acid in healthy male volunteers. Clin Therapeut 25:459–471, 2003.

82. Bergman AJ, Murphy G, Burke J, et al. Simvastatin does not have a clinically significant pharmacokinetic interaction with fenofibrate in humans. J Clin Pharmacol 44:1054–1062, 2004.

83. Grundy SM, Vega GL, Yuan Z, et al. Effectiveness and tolerability of simvastatin plus fenofibrate for combined hyperlipidemia (the SAFARI trial). Am J Cardiol 95:462–468, 2005.

84. Kris-Etherton PM, Harris WS, Appel LJ for the Nutrition Committee. Fish consumption, fish oil, omega-3 fatty acids and cardiovascular disease. Circulation 106:2747–2757, 2002.

85. Leaf A, Kang JX, Xiao YF, et al. Clinical prevention of sudden cardiac death by n-3 polyunsaturated fatty acids and mechanism of prevention of arrhythmias by n-3 fish oils. Circulation 107:2646–2652, 2003.

86. Mark DB, Hlatky MA. Medical economics and the assessment of value in cardiovascular medicine: Part II. Circulation 106:626–630, 2002.

87. Devasthale PV, Chen S, Jeon Y, et al. Design and synthesis of N-((4-methoxyphenoxy)carbonyl) –N-((4-(5-methyl-2-phenyl-4-oxazolyl)phenyl)methyl)glycine (Muraglitazar/BMS298585), a novel peroxisome proliferators-activated receptor α/γ dual agonist with efficacious glucose and lipid-lowering activities. J Med Chem 48:2248–2250, 2005.

88. Stein EA. Management of dyslipidemia in the high-risk patient. Am Heart J 144:S43–50, 2002.

89. Brousseau ME, Schaefer EJ, Wolfe ML, et al. Effects of an inhibitor of cholesteryl ester transfer protein on HDL cholesterol. N Engl J Med 350:1505–1515, 2004.

90. McKenney JM, Brown WV, Cohen JD, et al. The National Lipid Association surveys of consumers, physicians and pharmacists regarding an over-the-counter statin in the United States: is this a good idea? Am J Cardiol 94:16F–21F, 2004.

91. Mulder AB, van Lijf HJ, Bon MAM, et al. Associate of polymorphism in the cytochrome CYP2D6 and the efficacy and tolerability of simvastatin. Clin Pharmacol Ther 70:546–551, 2001.

92. Malin R, Laaksonen R, Knuuti J, et al. Paraoxonase genotype modifies the effect of pravastatin on high-density lipoprotein cholesterol. Pharmacogenetics 11:625–633, 2001.

93. Niemi M, Schaeffeler E, Lang T, et al. High plasma pravastatin concentrations are associated with single nucleotide polymorphisms and haplotypes of organic anion transporting polypeptide-C (OATP-C, SLC01B1). Pharmacogenetics 14:429–440, 2004.

CASE STUDIES

TOPIC: Topic: Diabetes Mellitus

THERAPEUTIC DIFFICULTY: Level 3
Stephen M. Setter and Jason L. Iltz

Chapter 40: Diabetes

■ Scenario

Patient and Setting: AJ, a 65-year-old African American male; ambulatory clinic

Chief Complaint: The patient has been experiencing a tingling sensation in his hands and some numbness in his feet.

■ History of Present Illness

The patient's abnormal sensations in his extremities began roughly 4 months ago and seem to be progressing.

Medical History: Diabetes diagnosed 12 years ago; hypertension (HTN) for 15 years; dyslipidemia; non-ST elevation myocardial infarction (MI) 3 years ago; depression × 3 years; history of angina prior to CABG

Surgical History: Four (quadruple) coronary artery bypass grafts (CABG) 3 years ago; renal cyst removed at age 45; appendectomy at age 12.

Family/Social History: Family History: Mother died at age 78 with CHF; father died of Alzheimer's disease at age 81
Social History: Divorced 7 years ago, lives alone. Cigarette smoker 2 packs/day for 45 years; 2–4 alcoholic drinks per day

Medications:
Hydrochlorothiazide (HCTZ), 50 mg BID
Propranolol, 40 mg BID
Nitroglycerin (NTG), 0.4 mg sublingual PRN for chest pain
Metformin, 500 mg bid
Niacin immediate release, 1 g TID (OTC, self-medicating)

Allergies: No known medication allergies

■ Physical Examination

GEN: Well-developed, well-nourished man in no apparent distress; alert and cooperative, somewhat flat affect

VS: BP 148/92, HR 54, RR 16, T 37°C, Wt 118 kg, Ht 183 cm
HEENT: WNL
COR: No heaves or thrills; regular rate and rhythm, 54/min S1 and S2 heard well without splits; no murmurs or rubs; neck veins nondistended

Pulses	R	L	
Carotid	2+	2+	no bruits (2+ = normal)
Femoral	2+	2+	no bruits
AT	1+	1+	no bruits
PT	1+	1+	no bruits

CHEST: No chest wall deformities; no vertebral tenderness; lungs resonant to percussion; vesicular breath sounds throughout, without crackles, rhonchi, wheezes, or rubs
ABD: Moderately protuberant, soft, nontender, no masses; liver and spleen not enlarged
GU: WNL
RECT: Deferred
EXT: 1+ edema bilateral LE, unable to discern 10 g monofilament on plantar surface of feet or on the distal half of the dorsal surface; capillary refill at 2 seconds
NEURO: Alert, cranial nerves II, III, VII, VIII, IX, X, XI, XII intact; deep tendon reflexes of biceps, knees, and ankles are normal; Romberg and Babinski negative; gait: walks easily without ataxia; no tremor or pronator drift noted

■ Results of Pertinent Laboratory Tests, Serum Concentrations, and Diagnostic Tests

Na 135 [135]	HCO$_3$ 26 [26]	Glu 10.82 mmol/L [195]
K 3.9 [3.9]	BUN 9.6 [27]	A1C 9.5% (<7.0%)
Cl 99 [99]	Cr 123 [1.4]	Hct 0.49 [49]
Plts 200 × 10^9	T Bili 8.55 [0.5]	Alb 40 [4.0]
[200 × 10^3]	TC 6.6 mmol/L [255 mg/dL]	Alk Phos 90 [90]
MCV 79 [79]	LDL 4.58 mmol/L [177 mg/dL]	Hgb 163 [16.3]
AST 65 [65]	HDL 0.80 mmol/L [31 mg/dL]	Uric Acid 452 [7.6]
ALT 40 [40]	TG 2.66 mmol/L [235 mg/dL]	
LDH 200 [200]	Ca 2.2 [8.8]	
Ggt 90 [90]	PO4 0.97 [3.0]	

Lkc differential: WNL
Urine dipstick (Uristix): 1+ protein
Ankle Brachial Index (ABI): L: 0.65, R: 0.75
Geriatric Depression Scale (GDS): 12 of 30

■ Problem List

Identify principal problems from the scenario in priority order (see Answers in back of book for correct list of problems).

■ SOAP Note

To be completed by the student (see Answers in back of book for correct SOAP Note).

■ QUESTIONS

(See Answers in back of book for correct responses.)

1. The probable cause of AJ's neuropathy is: (EO-1)
   a. Peripheral vasoconstriction secondary to smoking
   b. High-dose thiazide diuretic therapy
   c. Poorly controlled diabetes
   d. PAD

2. List signs and symptoms of hypoglycemia and hyperglycemia. (EO-2)

3. Which of the following Ankle Brachial Index (ABI) values is diagnostic for peripheral arterial disease? (EO-1)
   a. >1.3
   b. <1.3
   c. >0.9
   d. <0.9

4. Which laboratory parameters can be adversely affected by the use of niacin therapy? (EO-5, 9)

5. Describe the mechanisms of action of metformin. (EO-7)

6. Identify factors (medical conditions or drug therapies) that may predispose AJ to the development of hyperkalemia. (EO-4, 8, 10)

7. AJ is placed on atorvastatin 40 mg as a starting dose to assist in lowering his cholesterol. What are the appropriate counseling points to consider for this new therapy? (EO-10, 14)

8. Which of the following medications is FDA approved for the treatment of painful diabetic peripheral neuropathy? (EO-8, 11, 12)
   a. Duloxetine
   b. Gabapentin
   c. Amitriptyline
   d. Capsaicin

9. Which of the following medications can interact with ACEI therapy? (EO-9)
   a. Simvastatin
   b. Ibuprofen
   c. Glyburide
   d. Warfarin

10. AJ is forced to switch insurers. His current cholesterol treatment includes atorvastatin 40 mg daily. His new insurance company covers simvastatin only. Which of the following doses of simvastatin would be equivalent to atorvastatin 40 mg? (EO-17)
    a. 10 mg
    b. 20 mg
    c. 40 mg
    d. 80 mg

11. Which of the following ethic groups have the highest incidence of diabetes? (EO-3)
    a. Pima Indians
    b. African Americans
    c. Caucasians
    d. Pacific Islanders

12. AJ has uncontrolled hyperglycemia. Which of the following medication pairs can be associated with drug-induced hyperglycemia? (EO-10, 11)
    a. Niacin/thiazide diuretic
    b. ACEI/niacin
    c. ASA/ACEI
    d. HMG CoA Reductase Inhibitor/Beta Blocker

13. List absolute contraindications to metformin therapy. (EO-4, 6, 8)

14. Which of the following side effects is most often reported with the use of ACE inhibitors? (EO-10)
    a. Alopecia
    b. GI upset
    c. Nonproductive cough
    d. Headache

15. What psychosocial factors may affect AJ's adherence to both pharmacological and nonpharmacologic therapy? (EO-15)

16. Describe the health care provider's role relative to the proposed psychosocial factors identified. (EO-16)

17. Synthesize etiology, pathophysiology, epidemiology, therapeutic, and disease management concepts for diabetes utilizing a key points format. (EO-18)

CASE 16

TOPIC: Topic: Thyroid Disorder

THERAPEUTIC DIFFICULTY: Level 2
Trisha Ford and Matthew Machado

Chapter 38: Thyroid Disorders

■ Scenario

Patient and Setting: KZ, a 34-year-old female; primary care clinic

Chief Complaint: Complaints of fatigue, weight gain, menstrual irregularities, and cold intolerance

■ History of Present Illness

Patient was referred for evaluation of thyroid function tests. Her physical examination had been remarkable for a goiter, dry skin, and delayed relaxation of the deep tendon muscles.

Medical History: Hypertension (HTN) × 3 years; ventricular tachycardia (controlled with amiodarone for 1 year)

Surgical History: NA

Family/Social History: Father died of a stroke at 52; glass of red wine 2 to 3 nights a week

Medications:
Amiodarone, 200 mg PO QD
Lisinopril, 10 mg PO QD
TUMS, 1 tablet PO PRN

Allergies: No known medication allergies

■ Physical Examination

GEN: Well developed, well nourished
VS: BP 145/88, HR 65, RR 26, T 37.6°C, Wt 132 lb, Ht 5'8"
HEENT: WNL
COR: RRR
CHEST: WNL
ABD: WNL
GU: Deferred
RECT: Deferred
NEURO: Alert, 0 × 4

■ Results of Pertinent Laboratory Tests, Serum Drug Concentrations, and Diagnostic Tests

Na 136 (136)	Hct 0.35 (35)	AST 0.30 (18)	Glu 6.1 (110)
K 4.0 (4.0)	Hgb 80 (8.0)	ALT 0.5 (30)	Ca 2.2 (8.8)
Cl 100 (100)	Lkcs 8.2 × 10^9 (8.2 × 10^3)	LDH 1.7 (101)	PO_4 0.92 (2.8)
HCO3 26 (26)	Plts 200 × 10^9 (200 × 10^3)	Alk Phos 1.5 (90)	Mg (0.6) 1.2

BUN 2.6 (7.4)	MCV 80 (80)		Alb 40 (4.0)	Uric Acid 90 (1.5)
Cr 97 (1.1)	T Bili 58 (3.4)			

TSH: 54 (54)
Free T_4: 51 (3.9)
Total T_3: 1.3 (85)
Thyroid antibodies
Urinalysis: NA
Chest x-ray films: NA
ECG: NA

■ Problem List

Identify principal problems from the scenario in priority order (see Answers in back of book for correct list of problems).

■ SOAP Note

To be completed by the student (see Answers in back of book for correct SOAP Note).

■ QUESTIONS

(See Answers in back of book for correct responses.)

1. KZ is experiencing symptoms consistent with which of the following? (EO-1)
   a. Myxedema coma
   b. Menopause
   c. Hashimoto's
   d. Graves' disease

2. A potential cause for KZ's hypothyroidism is: (EO-3)
   a. Her cardiac history
   b. Amiodarone use
   c. Her age
   d. Family history

3. Which of the following is the most appropriate starting dose of oral levothyroxine for KZ? (EO-6)
   a. 25 μg
   b. 50 μg
   c. 75 μg
   d. 100 μg

4. When converting a patient from IV to PO levothyroxine, the recommended PO dose is _____ % of the IV dose? (EO-6)
   a. 25
   b. 50
   c. 75
   d. 100

5. Assuming KZ is to receive oral levothyroxine therapy, she should be counseled to do which of the following? (EO-14)
   a. Separate the levothyroxine dose from TUMS
   b. Discontinue the amiodarone

c. Take her levothyroxine with food

d. Separate the levothyroxine dose from lisinopril

6. KZ's primary care provider should follow up on her thyroid levels in: (EO-12)
   a. 1 week
   b. 2 weeks
   c. 4 weeks
   d. 6 weeks

7. KZ has had several follow-up visits to assess TSH levels and adjust her levothyroxine regimen—her current dose is levothyroxine 75 μg PO QD. On her most recent follow-up appointment KZ's TSH level was undetectable. Which of the following adjustments in her levothyroxine regimen is most appropriate? (EO-5)
   a. Increase the dose by 25 μg
   b. Keep the dose the same
   c. Decrease the dose by 25 μg
   d. Change levothryoxine to propylthiouracil

8. KZ has now developed hypothermia and does not recognize members of her family. She passed out at work and was picked up by EMTs who noted she was in respiratory distress. She is diagnosed with myxedema coma. What would be the most appropriate therapy for her myxedema coma at this time? (EO-12)
   a. Increase her oral levothyroxine dose
   b. IV levothyroxine
   c. IV steroids
   d. Liothryonine

9. List possible pharmacologic and nonpharmacologic treatment regimens that could be incorporated in KZ's treatment plan. (EO-11)

10. List signs and symptoms of hypothyroidism and identify those present in KZ. (EO-2)

11. Describe amiodarone's potential effect on thyroid function. (EO-7)

12. Summarize the pathophysiology of hypothyroidism and the therapeutic management of this condition using a key points format. (EO-18)

Acute Renal Disease

42

Myrna Y. Munar and Harleen Singh

DEFINITION

Acute renal failure (ARF) is generally defined as an abrupt and sustained decline in renal function that results in the inability of the kidneys to excrete nitrogenous waste, concentrate urine, regulate fluid and electrolyte balance, and maintain acid–base homeostasis.[1,2] However, more than 30 separate definitions of ARF are found in the literature due to lack of standardization and consensus, and the absence of a universal classification system for disease severity.[3,4] Nonconformity in the use of the terms acute tubular necrosis (ATN) versus ARF also exists. Although these terms are used interchangeably, ATN is a pathologic diagnosis resulting from ischemic or toxic injury to the kidneys, whereas ARF is a syndrome of multiple etiologies encompassing prerenal, intrinsic, and obstructive causes.[1,5] Severe renal failure requiring renal replacement therapy, including transplantation, is termed end-stage renal disease.

The Acute Dialysis Quality Initiative (ADQI) is under way to establish an evidence-based appraisal and a set of consensus recommendations to standardize and improve the quality of care delivered to patients with ARF requiring renal replacement therapy.[4] It is hoped that consensus criteria to define the presence and severity of ARF will be established.

The first signal in the detection of ARF is a change in serum creatinine (SCr), a surrogate marker of solute clearance by the kidneys. Although the rise in SCr lags behind the onset of renal injury, careful tracking of SCr allows early recognition, prompt management, and the greatest opportunity for reversal of or delay in disease progression. Many published studies base their definition of ARF on the SCr level. One broad definition is an increase in SCr for 2 weeks or less of 0.5 mg per deciliter (44.2 μmol/L) if the baseline is less than 2.5 mg per deciliter (221 μmol/L) or an increase in SCr by greater than 20% if the baseline value is greater than 2.5 mg per deciliter (221 μmol/L).[6] Other criteria for identifying patients with ARF are based on graded changes in SCr from baseline values (Table 42.1).[7,8] In critically ill patients, the Acute Physiology, Age, Chronic Health Evaluation (APACHE III) prognostic scoring system defines ARF as an SCr elevation greater than or equal to 0.5 mg/dL/day with urine output less than 410 mL per day and no preexisting chronic dialysis. Regardless of the criteria used to define ARF, smaller elevations in SCr may signal early signs of trouble.

The relationship between SCr and glomerular filtration rate (GFR) is curvilinear.[9] In patients with normal renal function, an increase in SCr from 1.0 to 2.0 mg per deciliter results in a fall in GFR from 100 to 40 mL/min/1.73 m². In contrast, in a patient with advanced renal failure, the same magnitude of increase in SCr from 6.0 to 8.0 mg per deciliter reflects a small reduction in GFR from 10 to 6 mL/min/1.73

TABLE 42.1	Serum Creatinine Values for Detection of Acute Renal Failure

Baseline	Change[a]
≤1.9	≥0.5
≥2.0 to ≤4.9	≥1.0
≥5.0	≥1.5

Data are given as mg/dL.

[a] Difference between maximum serum creatinine and baseline values.

(From Nash K, Hafeez A, Hou S. Hospital-acquired renal insufficiency. Am J Kidney Dis 39:930–936, 2002; and Hou SH, Bushinsky DA, Wish DB, et al. Hospital-acquired renal insufficiency: a prospective study. Am J Med 74:243–248, 1983.)

m^2. Therefore, the initial rise in SCr represents the greatest decline in renal function.

Clinicians should not use the SCr concentration as the sole means to assess kidney function.[10] Accumulation of nitrogenous waste, as indicated by an elevation in blood urea nitrogen (azotemia), and clinical evidence of declining renal function, such as decreased urine output and an inability to control volume, as well as derangements in electrolytes and acid–base balance, should also be taken into account. While SCr monitoring is routine in hospitalized patients, care must be taken when interpreting SCr values. The rate of SCr rise varies depending on the extent of renal injury, dietary intake, and the patient's muscle mass. SCr can be elevated without the presence of ARF in patients with a large muscle mass (such as body builders), after acute muscle injury, or during catabolic states.[2,5] Certain medications, such as trimethoprim and cimetidine, can cause false elevations in SCr by inhibiting its renal tubular secretion.

CLASSIFICATION

ARF is classified into three categories based on precipitating and etiologic factors: prerenal or hypoperfusion states, intrarenal or intrinsic renal parenchymal injury, and postrenal ARF or urinary obstructive disorders.[1] These standard classifications facilitate diagnosis and disease management. ARF can be further described according to the amount of urine produced per day as anuric ARF (<50 mL/day), oliguric ARF (50 to 400 mL/day), and nonoliguric (>400 mL/day). Although ARF is often thought of as a decrease in urine output, nonoliguric ARF accounts for up to 60% of cases of ARF.[11] Patients with nonoliguric ARF do not concentrate the urine that is produced and continue to retain urea, creatinine, and other waste products of metabolism.

ETIOLOGY

PRERENAL AZOTEMIA

Renal blood flow (RBF) is maintained at about 20% of cardiac output based on glomerular filtration needs.[12] Prerenal azotemia occurs when RBF decreases to a level adequate to sustain cells but inadequate to maintain normal GFR. Therefore, cellular injury does not occur and the GFR can be normalized rapidly once the pathologic state is corrected.[13] Reduced RBF may be secondary to any event that results in decreased renal perfusion or intense compensatory afferent arteriolar vasoconstriction.

Common causes of prerenal azotemia in the outpatient setting include conditions that result in a decline in effective blood volume, such as congestive heart failure, or a decline in intravascular volume, such as vomiting, diarrhea, poor fluid intake, fever, or the use of diuretics. Use of drugs that induce renal vasoconstriction, such as cyclosporine or tacrolimus, can also lead to prerenal azotemia. Elderly patients are susceptible to the development of prerenal azotemia because of decreased cardiac output due to myocardial dysfunction or pericardial disease, dehydration with insufficient fluid intake, and chronic use of drugs that alter intrarenal hemodynamics, such as nonsteroidal anti-inflammatory drugs (NSAIDs) and angiotensin-converting enzyme (ACE) inhibitors.[14] Heart failure, liver dysfunction, and sepsis are common causes of prerenal azotemia in hospitalized patients.[7,8] Anesthesia decreases effective blood volume, and when accompanied by a reduction in mean arterial pressure, can lead to a decrease in RBF, leading to prerenal azotemia in surgical patients.[1] Vascular diseases (e.g., renal artery emboli, atheroembolic renal disease) may reduce RBF and cause prerenal ARF. Thrombocytopenic purpura and hemolytic uremic syndrome may also lead to prerenal ARF, but more commonly they also cause significant glomerular injury. Various causes of prerenal azotemia are listed in Table 42.2.

Mild hypoperfusion, caused by volume depletion, leads to prerenal azotemia with a mild decrease in GFR. The kidneys attempt to increase intravascular volume by conserving salt and water through increased proximal and distal reabsorption as well as increased antidiuretic hormone (ADH) release. GFR is maintained initially, but only small amounts of concentrated urine are produced. Due to avid sodium reabsorption, urine sodium and the fractional excretion of sodium (FE_{Na}) are low (<1%). Urine is concentrated due to water conservation; thus, urine osmolality and the urine creatinine: plasma creatinine ratio are high. Because urea reabsorption is also increased, a disproportionate increase in blood urea nitrogen (BUN) relative to SCr occurs; therefore, the BUN: SCr ratio often is greater than 20:1. Other factors that may help to differentiate prerenal ARF from intrinsic or postrenal ARF are shown in Table 42.3.

Prerenal azotemia is rapidly reversible if the underlying cause is corrected.[1,5,15] Restoration of renal perfusion should reverse prerenal azotemia, but in some cases, prerenal ARF can lead to intrarenal, ischemic ATN. About 20% of cardiac output perfuses the kidneys, resulting in high oxygen delivery compared with total renal oxygen consumption. A high oxygen supply is required to support active ion and solute transport. The outer medulla of the kidney is the site of the

TABLE 42.2	Causes of Prerenal Acute Renal Failure

Decreased cardiac output
- Congestive heart failure
- Pericardial tamponade
- Pulmonary embolism
- Cardiomyopathy
- Myocardial infarction

Hypovolemia
- Major trauma
- Burns
- Hemorrhage (surgical, postpartum)
- Volume depletion (renal losses, skin, vomiting, diarrhea)
- Sequestration (hypoalbuminemia, pancreatitis, peritonitis)

Increased renal vascular resistance
- Renal vasoconstriction (norepinephrine, dopamine)
- Systemic vasodilation (sepsis, vasodilatory agents)
- Anesthesia
- Surgery

Systemic vasodilation
- Bacterial sepsis
- Antihypertensives
- Afterload reduction

Renovascular obstruction[a]
- Renal artery (atherosclerosis, thrombosis, embolism)
- Renal vein (thrombosis)

[a] In bilateral renal disease or single functioning kidney.
(From Conger JD, Brinner VA, Schrier RW. Acute renal failure: pathogenesis, diagnosis, and management. In: Schrier RW, ed. Renal and Electrolyte Disorders. 4th ed. Boston: Little Brown, 1992.)

lowest partial pressure of intrarenal oxygen (pO$_2$), existing on the brink of hypoxia. It is also the location of very active tubular segments, such as the thick ascending limb of the loop of Henle and the pars recta of the proximal tubule (Fig. 42.1; *see color insert*).[12] The outer medulla is at great risk for ischemia because of its low pO$_2$ and high metabolic activity, even in the setting of normal RBF.[12] The kidneys are vulnerable to changes in oxygen balance. A reduction in RBF, as in a prerenal state, compromises oxygen reserve and if prolonged can lead to the development of ischemic ATN. Clinically, this occurs when an insult such as hypotension and oliguria due to medications, sepsis, surgery, or bleeding occurs in the setting of a prerenal state. Rapid detection and correction of prerenal azotemia can prevent ischemic injury and the associated morbidity and mortality.

POSTRENAL ACUTE RENAL FAILURE

Obstruction of the collecting system generally must involve both kidneys (or a solitary kidney) to cause significant renal failure. Obstruction of the urinary tract may result from bladder outlet obstruction caused by prostate enlargement, tumor, or urethral stricture; urethral obstruction from tumor, stone, or fibrosis; or even crystal (uric acid, calcium oxalate) deposition in the tubules.[1] Several medications can lead to crystal-induced postrenal ARF, including acyclovir, sulfonamides, methotrexate, indinavir, and triamterene.[16] Obstruction should be considered in patients with acute anuria, particularly in those with a recent history of alternating polyuria and oliguria. Postrenal azotemia is simply an accumulation of nitrogenous wastes secondary to obstruction of urine flow. This disorder accounts for approximately 15% of cases of ARF.[17] Causes of postrenal azotemia are listed in Table 42.4. These causes should be ruled out initially because they are often easily corrected, preventing progression to intrinsic renal damage.

TABLE 42.3	Urinary Indices to Differentiate Causes of Acute Renal Failure		
	Prerenal	Acute Tubular Necrosis	Postrenal Obstruction
Protein	−	2–4+	−
WBC	−	2–4+	1+
RBC	−	2–4+	Variable
Casts	±	RTE, WBC	−
Osmolality (mOsm/kg)	>400	<350	<350
Specific gravity	>1.013	<1.013	−
U$_{Na}$ (mmol/L)	<20	>40	Variable
FE$_{Na}$ (%)	<1	>2	>1
BUN:SCr ratio	>20:1	<20:1	−
UCr:SCr ratio	>40	<20	<20
RFI	<1	>4	>1.5

WBC, white blood cell count; RBC, red blood cell count; U$_{Na}$, urine sodium concentration; FE$_{Na}$, fractional excretion of sodium; BUN, blood urea nitrogen; UCr, urine creatinine concentration; SCr, serum creatinine concentration; RFI, renal failure index; RTE, renal tubular epithelial.

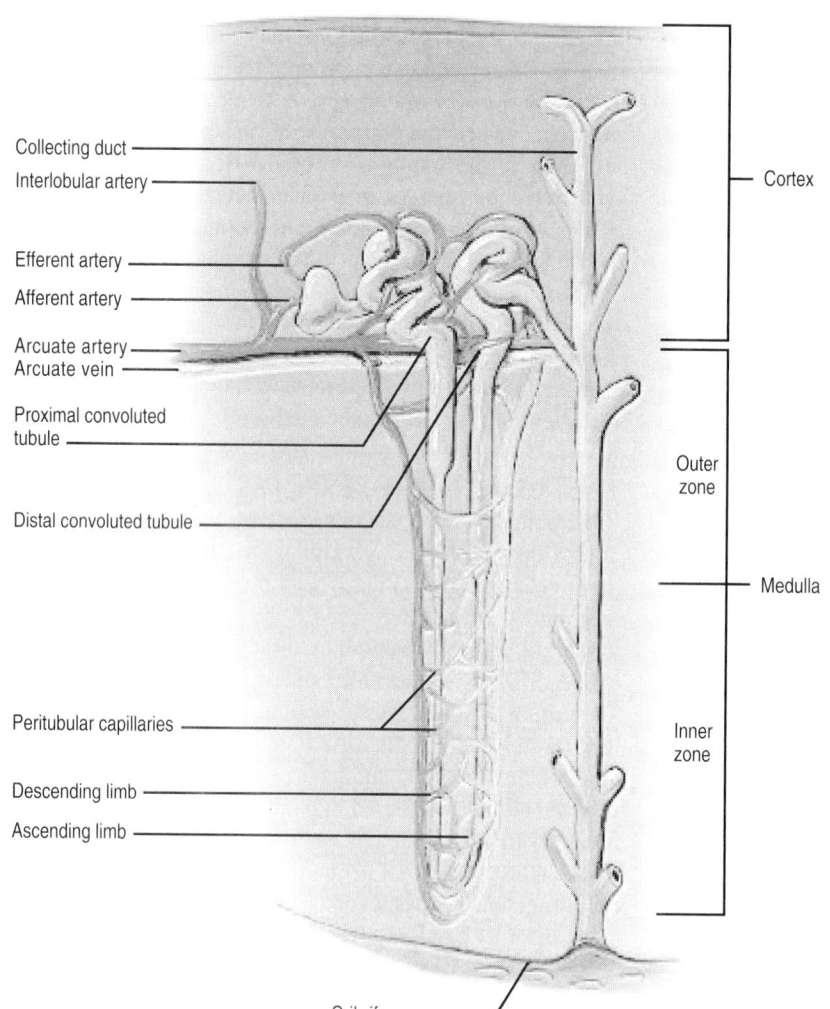

Collecting duct
Interlobular artery

Efferent artery
Afferent artery

Arcuate artery
Arcuate vein

Proximal convoluted
tubule

Distal convoluted tubule

Peritubular capillaries

Descending limb

Ascending limb

Cribriform area

Cortex

Outer
zone

Medulla

Inner
zone

FIGURE 42.1. The nephron (*see color insert*). (Reprinted with permission from Smith HW. The kidney: structure and functions in health and disease. New York: Oxford University Press, 1951.)

INTRINSIC ACUTE RENAL FAILURE

Intrinsic ARF is a decrease in renal function resulting from more severe or prolonged ischemic, toxic, or immunologic mechanisms (Table 42.5) and is associated with structural damage to glomeruli, tubules, vascular supply, or interstitial

TABLE 42.4	Causes of Postrenal Acute Renal Failure

Bilateral ureteral obstruction

Intraureteral (emboli, stones, crystals)

Extraureteral (tumor, retroperitoneal fibrosis)

Papillary necrosis (acute pyelonephritis)

Bladder obstruction

Mechanical (prostate hypertrophy, malignancy, infection)

Functional (anticholinergics, ganglionic blockers, neuropathy)

Urethral obstruction

tissue.[17] Such damage to the renal parenchyma often follows prerenal or postrenal azotemia, and if the degree of insult or the duration of hypoperfusion or obstruction is sufficient, it is not immediately reversible. Tubular dysfunction leads to impaired reabsorption of solutes and water; thus, an increase in urinary sodium concentration and fractional excretion of sodium and a defect in urinary concentrating ability with a decrease in urine osmolality are observed. Recovery from intrarenal disease commonly takes 10 to 14 days, but it may take 6 weeks to more than a year.[18] Ischemic or toxic ATN is a leading cause of ARF in hospitalized patients.[19] ATN is a histologic finding signifying necrotic damage to the renal tubules.

ACUTE RENAL FAILURE FROM THERAPEUTIC AGENTS

The kidneys are uniquely vulnerable to toxic injury because relative to their weight, they have the largest endothelial surface area and the highest blood flow of any organ. Con-

TABLE 42.5	Intrinsic Causes of Acute Renal Failure

Sequelae of prolonged prerenal azotemia

Nephrotoxic agents (drugs and radiocontrast)

Ischemic events

   Massive hemorrhage

   Pregnancy (preeclampsia, postpartum renal failure)

   Crush injury

   Septic shock

   Transfusion reaction

   Venous occlusion

   Arterial thrombosis

Glomerular

   Systemic lupus erythematosus

   Poststreptococcal glomerulonephritis

   Drug-induced vasculitis

   Malignant hypertension

Tubulointerstitial

   Acute tubular necrosis

   Acute interstitial nephritis

   Acute pyelonephritis

   Hyperuricemia

   Hypercalcemia

TABLE 42.6	Agents Associated with Nephrotoxicity

Acute Tubular Necrosis	Acute Tubulointerstitial Disease
Antibiotics:	Penicillins:
Aminoglycosides	Ampicillin, amoxicillin
Amphotericin B	Methicillin
Bacitracin and polymyxins	Nafcillin
Cephalosporins	Oxacillin
Sulfonamides	Penicillin
Metals:	Other antibiotics:
Bismuth	Cephalosporins
Mercurials	Erythromycin
Platinum	Rifampin
Radiocontrast media	Sulfonamides
Miscellaneous agents:	Metals:
Acetaminophen	Bismuth
Cisplatin	Gold
Cyclosporine	Miscellaneous agents:
Methotrexate	Captopril
Tacrolimus	Furosemide
Glomerulonephritis	Nonsteroidal anti-inflammatory drugs
Allopurinol	Phenytoin
Ampicillin	Thiazides
Captopril	Cimetidine
Cocaine	Allopurionol
Cyclophosphamide	5-aminosalicylates
Daunorubicin	
Gold	
Hydralazine	
Methicillin	
Penicillamine	
Penicillin	
Rifampin	
Thiazides	

centration of potential nephrotoxins occurs within the renal tubules through secretion and reabsorption, thus exposing the tubular lumen and peritubular cells to high concentrations of potential toxins. Renal medullary and papillary tissues are vulnerable to toxic damage because of a combination of low blood flow and extremely high solute concentration. Also, the kidneys are highly active metabolic organs capable of transforming innocuous substances, such as acetaminophen, into highly reactive metabolites.[20,21] The lesions associated with drug-induced nephropathy can be divided into six categories: prerenal failure, ATN, acute tubulointerstitial disease (ATID), crystal-induced ARF, glomerulonephritis, and thrombotic microangiopathy. The actual renal injury may result from a variety of insults. A list of drugs and chemicals associated with each of these lesions is provided in Table 42.6.

Blood from the renal arteries is delivered to the glomeruli via the afferent arterioles. The surface area and permeability of glomerular capillaries and glomerular hydrostatic pressure contribute to the formation of glomerular ultrafiltrate, which subsequently flows into the renal tubules. Maintenance of glomerular hydrostatic pressure is regulated by changes in glomerular afferent and efferent vasoconstriction or vasodilation. Medications can modify the vascular resistance of the afferent and efferent arterioles. ACE inhibitors and angiotensin II receptor antagonists block normal adaptive responses to renal hypoperfusion via predominant effer-

ent vasodilation. NSAIDs and potent vasoconstrictors such as cyclosporine and tacrolimus increase afferent vascular resistance. Use of these medications in the setting of decreased effective circulating volume (congestive heart failure, cirrhosis) or renovascular disease (renal artery stenosis) can lead to prerenal failure.

ATN is a nonspecific response to ischemia or direct toxic insult. ARF may be the result of tubular necrosis from cellular debris obstructing the proximal tubule. As intratubular pressure increases and glomerular filtration decreases, filtered wastes regain access to the circulation by leaking across transtubular membranes.[22–24] The type of cellular injury associated with ATN varies with the type of renal insult. In a study of 121 patients who developed ATN, hypotension (27%) and dehydration (27%) were the sole causes of ARF; more than one acute insult was identified in 62% of these patients.[25] In a study of 131 biopsies of drug-induced ARF, ATN occurred in 61.1% of cases.[26]

ATID, also known as acute interstitial nephritis, is characterized by interstitial edema and renal cellular infiltrates made up of monocytes, large and small lymphocytes, and plasma cells. Eosinophils may or may not be present. Tubular damage is evident by the presence of cellular infiltrates located along the tubular basement membrane or between tubular epithelial cells.[27] Drug-induced ATID appears to be a hypersensitivity reaction and often is associated with systemic signs of an allergic reaction such as fever, skin rash, eosinophilia, and arthralgia. Hypersensitivity is further suggested by the small number of patients developing the reaction, the lack of dose-related effect, extrarenal manifestations of hypersensitivity, and a sudden recurrence with reinstitution of therapy, accidental re-exposure to the drug, or exposure to a closely related medication.[28,29] Other less common causes of ATID include autoimmune diseases (e.g., lupus), infiltrative disease (e.g., sarcoidosis), and infectious agents (e.g., *Legionella pneumophila*).[1] Methicillin-induced ATID has long been the prototype of drug-induced ATID; however, this agent is infrequently used at present. While a large number of medications are associated with drug-induced ATID, the most common current causes include NSAIDs; penicillins and cephalosporins; rifampin; sulfonamides, including medications that include sulfa moieties (e.g., furosemide, bumetanide, and thiazide-type diuretics); cimetidine; allopurinol; ciprofloxacin and to a lesser degree other quinolone antibiotics; and 5-aminosalicylates (e.g., mesalamine).[30]

The onset of drug-induced ATID ranges from 1 to 5 days after second drug exposure to the same or a related drug to as long as several weeks after first drug exposure (e.g., NSAID). ARF caused by ATID is often reversible after the offending medication is discontinued or the underlying disease is treated. In cases of ATID in which infection can be excluded, corticosteroids may accelerate renal function recovery.

ARF caused by crystal deposition and intratubular obstruction occurs with certain commonly prescribed medications (acyclovir, sulfonamides, methotrexate, indinavir, and triamterene). Patients who require treatment with these medications may have risk factors that increase the likelihood of crystal deposition in the kidneys, such as volume depletion (chronic diarrhea, nausea, vomiting, febrile illness), third-spacing or sequestration of fluid (pancreatitis, ascites, pleural effusions), or decreased effective circulating volume (heart failure, sepsis). These factors result in renal hypoperfusion and sluggish tubular flow rates, leading to an increased risk of intratubular crystal deposition. Underlying renal impairment also increases the risk of crystal-induced ARF. Metabolic acid–base disturbances can exacerbate in-

trarenal crystal deposition by affecting urinary pH. Medications that are weak acids (sulfonamides, methotrexate, triamterene) can precipitate in an acidic urine, while indinavir precipitates in an alkaline urine.

Glomerulonephritis may be caused by several different mechanisms. In some cases, there is a direct dose-dependent effect on glomerular structures; in the majority, however, the glomerulus is involved through immunologic reactions. Drugs may act as haptens or antigens that either produce circulating antigen–antibody complexes or cause complex formation within the glomerulus. Damage to or alteration of the glomerular basement membrane produces proteinuria, a hallmark of this disease. The most common drug-induced lesion is membranous glomerulonephritis with proteinuria and nephrotic syndrome. Prompt treatment of glomerulonephritis using immunosuppressive agents or plasma exchange may reduce the risk of end-stage renal disease.[1]

Drug-induced thrombotic microangiopathy is a rare cause of severe ARF. Thrombotic microangiopathy involving the kidneys leading to renal impairment is referred to as hemolytic uremic syndrome (HUS), while predominant central nervous system involvement is referred to as thrombotic thrombocytopenic purpura (TTP). Patients who present with neurologic abnormalities as well as ARF are described by the comprehensive term HUS-TTP. Because of the similarities between HUS and TTP, the term ''thrombotic microangiopathy'' is also used to encompass these disorders.

Thrombotic microangiopathy is traditionally characterized by fever, microangiopathic hemolytic anemia (MAHA), thrombocytopenia, and variable signs of organ damage due to platelet thrombi in the microcirculation, such as encephalopathy or renal failure. A central feature in the pathogenesis of thrombotic microangiopathy is damage to endothelial cells in the microcirculation. Circulating antibodies and immunocomplexes can also contribute to endothelial injury. Toxic injury can lead to swelling and detachment of endothelial cells from the basement membrane. Exposure of the basement membrane to the circulation leads to platelet adhesion, aggregation, and activation, leading to platelet consumption, thrombocytopenia, and thrombi formation. Localized intravascular coagulation and fibrin deposition can occur at the site of vessel wall injury. Circulating red blood cells become trapped in the meshwork, causing red blood cells to fragment and leading to microangiopathic hemolytic anemia. Schistocytes, bur, or helmet cells are present on the peripheral blood smear. Variable signs of organ damage are evident, depending on the extent of thrombi and fibrin deposition and intravascular coagulation in the microvascular circulation.

Infections with Shiga-like toxin producing *Shigella dysenteriae* type 1 and verotoxin producing *Escherichia coli*, particularly the 0157:H7 serotype, are the most common cause of HUS, especially in children and in the elderly.[31] Toxins produced by these bacteria affect the gastrointestinal tract, resulting in bloody diarrhea. Atypical thrombotic microangiopathy is associated with other causes, including cancer, bone marrow and solid organ transplantation, pregnancy, and certain drugs.[32–36] Atypical thrombotic microangiopathy is not associated with a history of diarrheal prodrome.

Certain drugs have been associated with the development of thrombotic microangiopathy (Table 42.7). The main classes of drugs are antineoplastic agents and immunosuppressant medications used in bone marrow or organ transplantation. Thrombotic microangiopathy can also occur as a result of malignancy or transplantation. Among cancer chemotherapy treatments, most cases reported are associated with mitomycin C. Manifestations appear to be dose-related. Calcineurin inhibitors, such as cyclosporine, tacrolimus, and sirolimus, have been associated with post-transplantation thrombotic microangiopathy.[36–39] Platelet aggregation inhibitors, such as ticlopidine and clopidogrel, and other drugs, such as interferon-β and quinine, have also been associated with thrombotic microangiopathy.[40] Drug-associated atypical microangiopathy is generally managed by discontinuing the offending agent and plasma exchange to remove circulating antibodies and immunocomplexes. In the case of immunosuppression-induced thrombotic microangiopathy, it may be difficult to determine whether the situation is due to drug toxicity or transplant rejection. Careful dose reduction may be attempted if drug toxicity is highly suspected. Tacrolimus has been used successfully as an alternative medication in renal transplant patients who developed cyclosporine-induced thrombotic microangiopathy.[39,41,42]

The incidence of ARF in hospitalized patients attributed to medications is 16%.[7] The variety of drugs causing ARF has changed over the past two decades. New drugs that are nephrotoxic have been introduced, such as cyclosporine, tacrolimus, and other immunosuppressants, intravenous immune globulin, ACE inhibitors, angiotensin II receptor blockers, and newer versions of NSAIDs and antibiotics. Drug-induced nephrotoxicity has also been attributed to increased use of amphotericin B and pentamidine and higher doses of trimethoprim–sulfamethoxazole for AIDS-related infections. Aminoglycosides accounted for 82% of episodes of ARF in 1979, dropping to 29% in 1996.[7,8] This decline reflects careful use of regimens that avoid drug accumulation and the replacement of aminoglycosides with less nephrotoxic agents in the treatment of Gram-negative infections.

Aminoglycosides. Aminoglycosides are avidly concentrated within the renal cortex. After initial binding to tubular brush border membranes, they are vacuolized and taken up by the proximal tubular cells. Once within the cell, they are transported to lysosomes. Continued uptake results in lysosomal dysfunction and eventual degeneration, allowing lysosomal enzymes to act on other cell organelles. Drug uptake is saturable. Theoretically, the magnitude of drug toxicity can be manipulated by changing the frequency of drug administration. For a given total daily dose of any specific aminoglycoside, toxicity is greatest when the daily dose is divided into small multiple doses given two or three times a day, because maintaining a low serum concentration maximizes drug uptake. Tubular cell necrosis may result from continued exposure. On the other hand, the same daily dose given once daily saturates drug uptake, thus reducing the potential for toxicity.

The initial manifestations of nephrotoxicity include release of brush border and lysosomal enzymes, glycosuria, aminoaciduria, and tubular proteinuria. Defects in proximal tubular transport may be indicated by the presence of β_2-microglobulin. Hypokalemia, hypomagnesemia, and loss of concentrating ability may also be seen. Patients who develop aminoglycoside nephrotoxicity are most often nonoliguric. The occurrence of toxicity is most closely related to treatment duration and usually is seen after 7 to 10 days of therapy. Additional risk factors for the development of nephro-

TABLE 42.7	Drugs Associated with the Development of Thrombotic Microangiopathy

Antineoplastic Agents

Mitomycin

Tamoxifen

Bleomycin

Cisplatin

Deoxycoformycin

Lomustine (CCNU)

Daunorubicin

Cytarabine

Chlorozotocin

Zinostatin (neocarzinostatin)

Gemcitabine

Estramustine phosphate sodium

Other Drugs

Cyclosporine

Tacrolimus

Muromonab–CD-3 (OKT3)

Interferon

Ticlopidine

Clopidogrel

Simvastatin

Quinine

Oral contraceptives

Penicillin

Penicillamine

Rifampicin (Rifampin)

Metronidazole

Iodine

(Pisoni R, Ruggenti P, Remuzzi G. Drug-induced thrombotic microangiopathy. Incidence, prevention and management. Drug Saf 24:491–501, 2001.)

toxicity include age, dose, high trough serum concentrations, and low urine flow rates. Selecting patients correctly, based on culture and sensitivity data, withdrawing unnecessary therapy early, adjusting doses to ensure therapeutic levels, and maintaining good urine output during therapy help to minimize toxicity.[43–49]

Aminoglycoside dosing regimens have changed, with many medical centers adopting once-daily dosing of aminoglycosides in an attempt to simplify dosing, to take advantage of pharmacodynamic properties of concentration-dependent bactericidal activity and an extended post-antibiotic effect, and to reduce toxicities.

Several meta-analyses pooled data from studies comparing the incidence of nephrotoxicity between once-daily dosing and traditional twice- or three-times-a-day dosing regimens.[50–58] An advantage of meta-analysis is the ability to combine data from underpowered studies. Its limitations are that selection of data and the type of meta-analytic method used lead to inconsistent results. Reduced nephrotoxicity following once-daily aminoglycoside dosing was observed when a fixed-effects model was used for meta-analyses.[53,54] However, use of a random-effects model did not show a statistically significant difference in nephrotoxicity between once-daily and traditional dosing regimens.[51,52,55–58]

The results of prospective studies also show conflicting results. Once-daily versus twice-daily administration of aminoglycosides was evaluated in a prospective, randomized, double-blind study of 123 adults with suspected or proven Gram-negative sepsis.[59] Patients were treated with aminoglycosides for at least 72 hours. Nephrotoxicity developed in six patients in the twice-daily dosing group. No patients developed nephrotoxicity in the once-daily dosing group. In a similar study investigating the safety and efficacy of amikacin administered once daily versus twice daily in 136 adults with systemic infections, no difference was found in the incidence of nephrotoxicity.[60] A reduction in the incidence of nephrotoxicity was not consistently evident with once-daily dosing regimens. Nonetheless, once-daily dosing provides a cost-effective method for aminoglycoside administration by reducing costs of drug preparation and administration, and reducing or eliminating the need for drug concentration monitoring.[61,62]

Amphotericin B. Nephrotoxicity associated with amphotericin B administration is related to the dose and duration of therapy. Amphotericin B-induced nephrotoxicity was seen in up to 80% of patients treated with larger cumulative doses of 2 to 3 g. The incidence of nephrotoxicity in 494 hospitalized adults receiving conventional amphotericin B therapy (median cumulative dose 240 mg, interquartile range 113 to 500 mg) was 28% overall, with 12% of patients developing moderate to severe nephrotoxicity and 3% of patients with severe nephrotoxicity.[63] In the same epidemiologic study, it was determined that for each 10-mg increase in the mean daily amphotericin B dose, the adjusted rate of renal toxicity increased by a factor of 1.13. In a study of 643 inpatients,

the incidence rate of amphotericin B nephrotoxicity was similar at 27%.[64] Independent risk factors found in both studies included concomitant use of nephrotoxic medications such as amikacin or cyclosporine, mean daily dose greater than 35 mg, male sex, weight greater than 90 kg, a history of chronic renal disease, and acuity of illness.[63,64] Mortality was higher in patients who developed amphotericin B-associated ARF compared to patients who did not: 54% versus 16% (adjusted odds of death, 6.6).[65] The development of ARF can also increase length of stay (8.2 days) and the total cost of therapy ($29,823).[65]

The initial event triggering the development of nephrotoxicity is the interaction of amphotericin B with membrane sterols, disrupting cell membranes. Other cellular events that result in activation of second messenger systems, release of mediators, or activation of renal homeostatic mechanisms subsequently occur. The possibility of direct vasoconstriction of the renal vasculature has also been suggested. The occurrence of renal failure usually is associated with proximal tubular necrosis; however, glomerular function is also affected. Clinical manifestations of amphotericin B nephrotoxicity include azotemia, renal concentrating defects, distal renal tubular acidosis with potassium wasting, magnesium wasting resulting in hypomagnesemia, and modest proteinuria. If magnesium and potassium wasting occur concurrently, potassium replacement may not be successful unless magnesium deficiency is corrected first.

Because nephrotoxicity often limits a full course of therapy, many attempts to limit toxicity have been tried. To date, no regimen or manipulation in therapy has been found to attenuate the toxicity consistently. Encouraging results have been seen with daily sodium supplementation of 150 mEq. The effect of sodium supplementation on renal function was studied in 20 patients who received a 10-week course of amphotericin B.[66] Patients were randomized to receive pretreatment with 1 L of 0.9% saline or 5% dextrose in water intravenously over 1 hour in a double-blinded manner. A significant difference in renal function was observed between the two groups, with the 5% dextrose in water pretreatment group showing a significant increase in SCr levels, while SCr levels remained unchanged in the saline group. However, the saline group required significantly greater amounts of potassium supplementation to maintain normal serum potassium levels. Various methods of sodium supplementation have been tried, including 0.9% saline and antibiotics with a high sodium content, such as ticarcillin (5.2 mEq of sodium per gram of antibiotic) or piperacillin (1.9 mEq of sodium per gram of antibiotic). These antibiotics may be considered in patients who require concomitant antibiotics. Patients in whom sodium administration would exacerbate underlying disease (e.g., hypertension, congestive heart failure, edematous states) should not receive sodium supplementation. When sodium supplementation is used, special attention needs to be made to maintain potassium balance.

Alternate-day therapy may be used when toxicity is recognized, and discontinuation is recommended when the BUN exceeds 50 mg per dL.[43,67,68] In addition, new amphotericin products have been formulated to reduce nephrotoxicity. Liposomal amphotericin B has a lower potential for nephrotoxicity, although it is 20 to 50 times more expensive than conventional therapy.

Cyclosporine. Cyclosporine has a major role in the prevention of allograft rejection. However, its use has been associated with causing two different types of renal injury: acute nephrotoxicity and chronic nephrotoxicity. Acute nephrotoxicity is hemodynamically mediated and reversible with dose reduction or drug discontinuation. On the other hand, chronic nephrotoxicity is irreversible and characterized by progressive renal interstitial fibrosis. Acute nephrotoxicity can have four clinical presentations: asymptomatic increases in SCr without overt renal dysfunction, ARF, delayed graft function after renal transplantation, and recurrent or de novo HUS.[69] The most common presentation is a dose-dependent decline in GFR, with reversible increases in SCr and BUN concentrations. This toxicity can complicate treatment of renal transplant recipients because distinguishing between graft rejection and cyclosporine toxicity is difficult, even with the use of decision algorithms.[70,71] On the other hand, elevations in SCr in extrarenal allograft transplantation are likely due to cyclosporine. Enhanced toxicity may occur with the simultaneous use of acyclovir, ketoconazole, amphotericin B, aminoglycosides, and co-trimoxazole. Cyclosporine is extensively metabolized by the cytochrome P-450 enzyme system. Consequently, drugs that inhibit or induce this metabolic pathway can cause elevations or reductions in cyclosporine blood concentrations. Drugs that can increase cyclosporine blood levels include certain macrolide antibiotics such as clarithromycin and erythromycin; azole antifungal agents such as ketoconazole, fluconazole, and itraconazole; and calcium channel blockers such as verapamil, diltiazem, nicardipine, and amlodipine. Inducers of cyclosporine metabolism include rifampin, phenytoin, phenobarbital, carbamazepine, and isoniazid.

Functional nephrotoxicity can be reversed by dose reduction or drug withdrawal, although this leads to an increased risk of transplant rejection. Reduction in toxicity has also been attempted by prolonging the infusion time to up to 24 hours in patients receiving parenteral cyclosporine. Calcium channel blockers can attenuate the renal vasoconstrictive effects of cyclosporine by inducing afferent arteriolar vasodilation. Several studies have shown improvement in renal hemodynamics and/or renal function when calcium channel blockers were used in patients receiving cyclosporine.[72-74] Used in this manner, cyclosporine blood levels should be monitored because of the potential inhibitory effects of certain calcium channel blockers on drug metabolism.

Attempts have been made to monitor plasma levels of cyclosporine and to maintain trough concentrations of 100 to 250 ng per mL. In vitro data suggest that there is little immunosuppression in mixed lymphocyte cultures at concentrations below 100 ng per mL. On the other hand, many patients develop renal toxicity even though their cyclosporine trough concentrations are within the therapeutic range. Measurement of the area-under-the-drug concentration-time curve (AUC) is a better reflection of drug exposure than trough levels. An abbreviated AUC encompassing the first 4 hours of the dosing interval in the target range of 4,400 to 5,500 µg/hour/L was found to significantly reduce the risk of cyclosporine nephrotoxicity and acute rejection in the early posttransplantation period.[75] The search for a therapeutic window using pharmacokinetic monitoring continues to be an important function at transplantation centers.[76-78] Replacement of cyclosporine and other calcineurin inhibitors by nonnephrotoxic immunosuppressants such as sirolimus and mycophenolate mofetil are being investigated[79] (see Chapter 27).

Radiographic Contrast Media. The increased use of contrast media associated with intravenous pyelography, angiography, computed tomography, and other diagnostic and interventional radiographic procedures has led to greater recognition of this class of agents as an important cause of ARF. The diagnosis must be considered when one of these agents is used in a high-risk patient who subsequently develops any degree of renal failure. Mild nonoliguric renal failure may be transient, with SCr peaking in 3 to 5 days and returning to baseline within 10 to 14 days. Severe oliguric renal failure may occur within 24 hours of contrast administration, with a return to baseline within 3 weeks, residual renal impairment, or renal failure necessitating dialysis. High-risk patients include those with preexisting renal disease, especially in combination with diabetes mellitus.[80,81] Other confirmed risk factors include chronic renal failure, severe congestive heart failure, volume depletion, hypotension, and the amount and frequency of contrast media exposure.[82] Although a mathematical formula was developed to determine a contrast volume "limit" to minimize renal toxicity, contrast volume was found to be an independent risk factor only in azotemic, diabetic patients.[83,84] Suspected risk factors for contrast media-induced nephropathy include abnormal liver function tests, hypertension, generalized atherosclerosis, hyperuricemia, and proteinuria.[82] Multiple myeloma and diabetes without nephropathy are no longer considered to be risk factors for developing contrast-induced nephropathy.[80,85]

The overall risk of developing ARF from contrast media varies widely from less than 1% to over 70% depending on the type of contrast used, the diagnostic procedure itself, the presence or absence of risk factors, use and duration of hydration therapy, and concomitant medications. Contrast attenuates renal hemodynamics as well as renal tubular function, leading to a reduction in GFR.[86] The precise mechanism of nephrotoxicity is unknown, but may involve an interplay of several factors, including vasoactive substances such as endothelin and adenosine that modulate vasoconstriction and the production of oxygen free radicals that not only induce a renal vasoconstrictive effect but also cause a direct toxic effect on tubular cells. Intrarenal and medullary hypoxia results from increased metabolic demand and decreased RBF. These events can result in impaired renal perfusion, glomerular injury, tubular injury, and/or tubular obstruction.

Prevention is aimed at avoiding unnecessary procedures, providing vigorous hydration (particularly in high-risk patients), avoiding NSAIDs and other potential nephrotoxins, using low doses of contrast sufficient to ensure an interpretable study, and avoiding multiple procedures that involve the use of contrast. The use of hyperosmolar (1,500 mOsm/kg) or less hyperosmolar (750 mOsm/kg) nonionic contrast agents does not significantly influence the risk of nephrotoxicity in patients with normal renal function.[80,87–91] Clinical trials performed in patients with moderate renal insufficiency (SCr 1.4 to 2.4 mg/dL) have shown a lower incidence of renal dysfunction in patients receiving newer nonionic, low-osmolality agents than in those receiving ionic agents. Recently, a lower incidence of nephrotoxicity was reported when iso-osmolar, dimeric, nonionic (iodixanol) rather than low-osmolar, nonionic contrast was used in high-risk patients undergoing angiography.[92] However, because of greater expense, nonionic contrast agents should be restricted to high-risk patients, such as those with SCr >2 mg/dL, particularly if they are diabetic.[80,93]

Hydration with 0.45% sodium chloride (1 mL/kg/hr or 0.5 mL/kg/hr in patients with congestive heart failure) over 24 hours beginning 12 hours before the procedure and continued for 12 hours after the procedure resulted in a lower incidence of contrast-induced nephropathy than hydration with mannitol (25 g given intravenously 1 hour before contrast administration) or furosemide (80 mg intravenously).[94] While hydration has been shown to be beneficial, no conclusive evidence exists to support a protective role of mannitol or loop diuretics in preventing contrast-induced nephropathy. Indiscriminant use of these diuretics may induce volume depletion, which would enhance the nephrotoxicity of contrast media.

Oxygen free radicals are postulated to mediate contrast-induced nephropathy. Oxygen free radical formation is promoted in an acidic environment and inhibited at higher pH values. In animal models of ischemic renal failure, pretreatment with sodium bicarbonate was more protective than sodium chloride.[95] It is postulated that bicarbonate is a more efficacious anion for sodium than chloride in preventive hydration regimens. A prospective, single-center, controlled trial was conducted in 119 patients with stable renal function who were randomized to receive a 154 mEq per L infusion of either sodium chloride or sodium bicarbonate 1 hour before and for 6 hours after exposure to iopamidol (370 mg iodine/mL).[96] Contrast media-induced nephropathy occurred in only one patient (1.7%) receiving sodium bicarbonate versus eight patients (13.6%) receiving sodium chloride.

Other modalities used to prevent contrast-induced nephropathy include N-acetylcysteine and fenoldopam.[97,98] N-acetylcysteine is a thiol-containing antioxidant that acts primarily by scavenging oxygen free radicals. Several prospective, placebo-controlled studies have shown a statistically significant reduction in the incidence of nephrotoxicity with oral administration of N-acetylcysteine in patients with renal insufficiency undergoing angiographic procedures.[97,99–101] Data analysis of the above-mentioned studies showed that only a few patients would need to be treated with N-acetylcysteine to prevent one case of contrast-induced nephropathy.[102] In all of these studies, contrast-induced nephropathy was defined as an elevation in SCr levels from baseline values of 25% or more within 2 to 3 days of contrast administration. On the other hand, it has been suggested that N-acetylcysteine has a direct effect on decreasing SCr levels that may be independent of true alterations in GFR.[103]

Fenoldopam is a selective dopamine-1 receptor agonist that produces renal arterial, systemic, and peripheral vasodilation. It was approved by the U.S. Food and Drug Administration for the treatment of urgent and emergent hypertension. The renal vasodilatory effects increase RBF to the medulla of the kidney, which is thought to be beneficial in preventing contrast-induced nephropathy. However, the renal effects are short-lived. There has been shown to be an increase in renal plasma flow at 1 hour after the radiographic procedure in patients receiving fenoldopam; however, this difference was not maintained at 4 hours after the procedure.[98] The increase in renal plasma flow did not translate into a clinically significant effect on renal function. No difference in the incidence of nephrotoxicity occurred between patients receiving fenoldopam and patients receiving placebo. A single retrospective study showed a benefit of fenoldopam in preventing contrast-induced nephropathy, while prospective studies failed to show a benefit.[104–106] Results from the prospective, randomized multicenter Evaluation of Corlopam in Patients at Risk for Renal Failure—A Safety and Efficacy Trial (CONTRAST) showed a lack of effect of fenoldopam on the primary end point of contrast-induced nephropathy compared to placebo. No significant differences were observed in the secondary end points of 30-day mortality, dialysis, or rehospitalization. Based on these studies, fenoldopam should not be used to prevent nephrotoxicity in patients at risk for contrast-induced nephropathy.

Angiotensin-Converting Enzyme Inhibitors and Angiotensin II Receptor Antagonists. Acute reversible nonoliguric renal failure may occur after the initiation of ACE inhibitor therapy in patients with bilateral renal artery stenosis. An intact renin-angiotensin II system is required for the maintenance of GFR when renal perfusion pressure falls. Angiotensin II regulates GFR by two mechanisms. First, angiotensin II increases arterial pressure by producing vasoconstriction and sodium retention (via increased secretion of aldosterone and through a direct effect on the tubules), resulting in plasma volume expansion. Secondly, angiotensin II preferentially constricts the efferent arteriole, causing an increase in hydraulic pressure in the glomerular capillary, which acts to maintain glomerular filtration pressure. Maintenance of renal perfusion in patients with bilateral renal artery stenosis or renal artery stenosis in a solitary kidney, hypertension, congestive heart failure, and preexisting renal failure is highly dependent on angiotensin-mediated vasoconstriction. ACE inhibition leads to dilation of efferent arterioles, which causes an abrupt decline in renal function in those dependent on efferent tone to maintain GFR.[107,108] Patients with preexisting renal insufficiency and on ACE inhibitors experience an acute fall in GFR and a rise in SCr. Typically the rise in SCr begins within a few days after the initiation of therapy, and immediate discontinuation of therapy should improve renal function. ACE inhibitor-associated membranous glomerulopathy and interstitial nephritis has been reported. Patients who experienced proteinuria while taking captopril either were taking high doses of captopril or had preexisting renal disease.[109] Also, patients who developed acute interstitial nephritis while taking captopril were also taking furosemide.[110] Risk factors such as use of high doses of ACE inhibitors in renal disease, concomitant use of diuretics and NSAIDs, volume depletion, and sodium intake should be identified in patients being treated with ACE inhibitors who develop renal disease. Patients with diabetes and preexisting renal insufficiency are at a higher risk of developing an acute rise in SCr and hyperkalemia when treated with ACE inhibitors. Studies have reported an increase of 30% in SCr within the first 2 months in this patient population. However, the renal protective effects of both ACE inhibitors and angiotensin receptor blockers are associated with long-term preservation of renal function, and therefore discontinuation of ACE inhibitors may not be necessary in patients who have a less than 30% increase in SCr over baseline and potassium levels ≤5.6 mmol per L.[111–113]

Nonsteroidal Anti-Inflammatory Drugs. Local prostaglandin production promotes dilation of medullary blood vessels and maintains local blood flow. Although RBF is not dependent on the prostaglandins in normal patients, in hemodynamically stressed patients (e.g., patients with congestive heart failure, systemic hypotension, severe hemorrhage, pancreatitis, liver disease, volume depletion due to dehydration or diuretic use, third-space losses from burns, cardiogenic shock, old age), the compensatory prostaglandin vasodilation counteracts the neurohumoral vasoconstriction and preserves renal function.[114,115] Both traditional NSAIDs and selective COX-2 inhibitors inhibit renal prostaglandin synthesis and can cause renal ischemia and renal insufficiency by removing the vasodilatory effects of prostaglandins, allowing unopposed vasoconstriction.[115–117] Renal impairment is characterized by an increase in BUN, SCr, serum potassium, and weight, with a variable decrease in urinary output. These deleterious effects are reversible with the discontinuation of the offending agents.[118] Although selective COX-2 inhibitors spare the gastrointestinal tract compared to traditional NSAIDs, they have similar renal effects as nonselective NSAIDs. Therefore, these agents should be used carefully in patients with preexisting renal dysfunction, and patients should be monitored closely.[119–121] The association between NSAID-induced ARF with diuretic use may be related to the edematous state (and decreased effective blood volume) or stimulation of vasodilator prostaglandins. Cyclosporine increases urinary excretion of vasodilator prostaglandins, probably because of its renal vasoconstrictive effect, and increases the risk of NSAID-induced ARF.

Cisplatin. Cisplatin is highly concentrated in the proximal tubular cells. Intracellular transformation of the chloride ligands on the molecule into a highly reactive aquated compound is thought to occur because of the low intracellular chloride concentration. This transformed molecule is then able to alkylate purine and pyrimidine bases of DNA. ATN occurs because cellular degeneration results in a proximal tubular obstruction from cellular debris. The incidence and severity of renal toxicity is both dose- and duration-dependent. A rise in SCr and BUN levels may be preceded by proteinuria, tubular casts, enzymuria, and the presence of β_2-microglobulin in the urine. Cisplatin nephrotoxicity has been reduced with prehydration with saline. One such approach is administering 0.45% to 0.9% sodium chloride in 5% dextrose at a rate of 250 mL per hour beginning 2 hours before cisplatin is given. The cisplatin dose is administered in 250 mL of a 3% sodium chloride solution. Mannitol 12.5 g is given immediately before cisplatin and then infused at the rate of 10 g per hour for 3 hours. This technique provides enough chloride to prevent the aquation reaction within the cisplatin container and provides an osmotic diuresis to minimize exposure of proximal tubular cells.[43,122,123]

Sodium thiosulfate is a renal protective compound that has been reported to reduce cisplatin nephrotoxicity.[124] However, nausea and vomiting limit its use and may exacerbate the emetogenic effects of cisplatin. The ability of this agent to confer renal protection without diminishing cisplatin's antitumor activity depends on the route of cisplatin administration. When used in combination with intraperitoneal cisplatin, intravenous sodium thiosulfate confers renal protection without altering the local antitumor effects of cisplatin.[125] Intravenous sodium thiosulfate reacts covalently with and binds to the cisplatin that enters the systemic circulation from the peritoneal cavity. Intraperitoneal cisplatin remains active, but drug reaching the systemic circulation complexes with the sodium thiosulfate. The resulting complex lacks systemic or renal toxicity.

EPIDEMIOLOGY

The true incidence of ARF is difficult to quantitate because of lack of universal agreement on a definition. When identical criteria are used, the incidence of ARF in hospitalized patients was shown to increase over the past 20 years, with a reported frequency of 4.9% in 1983 and 7.2% in 2002.[7,8] The incidence is even higher among patients in the intensive care unit (ICU), with an overall incidence of 17.2% in the United States and 24.7% worldwide.[126,127] In the critically ill patient, ARF carries a dismal prognosis, with mortality as high as 66%.[128]

When hospital admissions for ARF are delineated as community-acquired or hospital-acquired, community-acquired ARF is 1.5 to 2 times more common than hospital-acquired ARF.[19,129] In the African American population, the incidence of community-acquired ARF is 3.5 times greater than that of hospital-acquired ARF.[130] Common causes of community-acquired ARF include intravascular volume depletion resulting in prerenal azotemia, infection, use of nephrotoxic medications, or urinary obstruction.[130] Most patients with community-acquired ARF have a treatable cause of renal failure and a more favorable prognosis. Hospital-acquired ARF is associated with higher mortality (Table 42.8).

Many factors are associated with the risk of developing ARF in both hospitalized and ICU patients, including older age, male gender, infection, sepsis, hypovolemia, hypotension, exposure to nephrotoxins, and preexisting chronic diseases. In ICU patients who develop ARF, disease severity as defined by higher mean APACHE scores, sepsis or septic shock, single-organ or multiple-organ failure, use of vasoactive medications, and mechanical ventilation were associated with poor prognosis. An increasing number of failing organs led to the higher mortality rate.[131,132] In one study,[19] the mortality rate attributed to ARF alone (excluding underlying disease as a cause of death) was 26.7%. In other studies, oliguric renal failure and the need for renal replacement therapy were found to be independent risk factors for mortality.[127,133]

The course of illness is highly variable, ranging from transient disease lasting less than 1 week and associated with full recovery of renal function to disease persisting for more than 6 weeks and necessitating dialysis and ICU management.[18] A few patients survive to hospital discharge free of dialysis.[134–136] Continuous hemofiltration and various modifications of continuous renal replacement therapy have become more popular over the past two decades. Despite these advances, survival in critically ill patients with ARF has not significantly improved, and optimal treatments and the preferred form of renal replacement therapy remain controversial.[8,18,137–139] Possible explanations for the lack of substantial improvement in survival may be that older patients, often with multiorgan failure and septicemia, are being hospitalized.[139] Also, more surgical procedures are being performed in older adults, thus contributing to the mortality statistics.

Patients with ARF often have other major medical problems necessitating aggressive drug therapy and often resulting in a high incidence of adverse drug reactions. In treating these patients, the clinician must be able to assess the degree of renal insufficiency, recognize pharmacologic agents that can worsen renal function, and adjust drug doses. Treating these patients entails an understanding of the underlying pathophysiology and consists of preventive measures, supportive care, and efforts to preserve renal function. This chapter examines the causes, clinical course, and treatment of ARF. Because there are many causes of ARF, only the major causes are discussed.

PATHOPHYSIOLOGY

NORMAL RENAL FUNCTION

A basic understanding of normal kidney function facilitates a clinical appreciation of ARF. The primary function of the kidney is to maintain the body's internal environment by regulating body fluid volume, electrolyte composition, and acid–base balance. The kidneys are also responsible for producing and secreting various hormones and enzymes. Erythropoietin is produced by the renal cortical cells and stimulates erythrocyte maturation in the bone marrow. Also, 1,25-dihydroxycholecalciferol (the active form of vitamin D) is formed in the proximal tubule cells and plays an important role in regulating body calcium and phosphate balance. Therefore, complications of renal disease reflect impairment of the normal physiologic functions of the kidney, primarily regulation of water and electrolyte balance, arterial blood pressure, erythrocyte production, and vitamin D activity, and excretion of metabolic waste products. A logical approach to understanding abnormal renal function is to divide the kidney into basic components of renal circulation, glomerular hemodynamics, and nephron function.

RENAL CIRCULATION

The renal arteries supply approximately one fifth of cardiac output to the kidneys. After reaching the kidney, the renal artery bifurcates into smaller arterial branches, eventually leading to afferent arterioles, which supply the glomeruli. As blood leaves the glomeruli, the capillaries coalesce into the efferent arteriole, which then bifurcates to form the peritubular capillary network. Thus, RBF passes through two extensive capillary networks, the glomerular bed and peritubular capillary bed. The peritubular capillary bed nourishes the tubular cells and brings substances to the tubules for secretion. The afferent arterioles supply blood to the glomerulus, and the efferent arterioles carry blood from the glomerulus (see Fig. 42.1).

GLOMERULAR HEMODYNAMICS

The glomerulus is located at the proximal end of the renal tubule and is the area where the afferent and efferent arterioles connect. The transcapillary hydrostatic pressure produced by glomerular surface area and vascular resistance across the arterioles is responsible for glomerular ultrafiltrate production. Afferent arteriolar tone is determined predominantly by the vasoconstrictor effects of angiotensin II and the vasodilator effects of prostaglandins. Efferent arteriolar tone is determined by local concentrations of angiotensin II.

Glomerular ultrafiltrate production is decreased by pathologic processes and medications that alter afferent or efferent arteriolar tone and reduce glomerular hydrostatic pressure (i.e., hypercalcemia, ACE inhibitors, and NSAIDs).

NEPHRON FUNCTION

Each nephron consists of a glomerular capillary network surrounded by Bowman's capsule, a proximal tubule, a loop of Henle, a distal tubule, and a collecting duct (see Fig. 42.1). There are about a million nephrons in each kidney. A plasma ultrafiltrate is formed in the glomerular capillary, with collection of the filtered fluid in Bowman's capsule. The filtrate then enters the proximal tubule, where approximately two thirds of the filtered sodium and water is reabsorbed. More than 90% of filtered bicarbonate and nearly all of filtered glucose and amino acids are also reabsorbed in the proximal tubule. The loop of Henle consists of the terminal portion of the proximal tubule, the thin descending and ascending limbs, and the thick ascending limb. The loop of Henle is responsible for urine dilution and is also the site of magnesium reabsorption. The distal tubule and collecting duct make the final adjustments in urine composition. Here, ADH regulates water reabsorption and aldosterone regulates sodium reabsorption and potassium excretion.

ABNORMAL RENAL FUNCTION

Although considerable experimental work using animal models has resulted in several theories, the pathogenesis of ARF remains unclear. Several mechanisms are thought to be involved in the development of renal dysfunction. Again, these theories can be categorized as circulatory, glomerular, or tubular events.

CIRCULATORY DISTURBANCES

Reduction of RBF, if severe enough, can lead to ischemia, which is the most common mechanism of ARF.[1,130,140] In response to reduced RBF, vasodilating prostaglandins (e.g., PGI_2 and PGE_2) reduce afferent arteriolar tone and increase blood flow to the kidney.[1] NSAIDs inhibit prostaglandin synthesis and limit the kidney's production of these vasodilatory substances. This is particularly detrimental in patients with congestive heart failure who have low effective arterial blood volume and in those with actual volume depletion.[141] Other clinical situations in which diminished RBF may lead to ischemic ARF include severe extracellular fluid volume depletion, systemic hypotension, severe hemorrhage, gastrointestinal losses, pancreatitis, liver disease, third-space losses from burns, cardiogenic shock, or surgical procedures in which repair of renal artery lesions entails aortic cross-clamping proximal to the renal arteries. Renal artery lesions or atheromatous disease may lead to structural changes and impair RBF. In these situations, GFR becomes dependent on angiotensin II for maintaining efferent arteriolar tone. The use of ACE inhibitors can decrease efferent arteriolar tone, thereby reducing glomerular capillary filtration pressure and ultimately GFR. When the ACE inhibitor is discontinued, the GFR usually increases rapidly.

α-Adrenergic receptor-mediated systemic vasoconstriction associated with norepinephrine or high-dose dopamine can also result in marked RBF reductions. Severe renal hypoperfusion also is associated with eclamptic complications of pregnancy.[142] Nephrotoxic agents, especially aminoglycosides, amphotericin B, and radiocontrast media, are commonly associated with the development of ARF. Finally, endotoxin-mediated renal vasoconstriction may occur in sepsis.[143]

In response to diminished RBF, the kidney attempts to maintain intravascular volume by conserving sodium and water through increased reabsorption in the proximal and distal tubules and by increasing ADH release. Despite these compensatory mechanisms, ischemia may occur if RBF diminishes to the extent that nutrient and oxygen supplies cannot meet metabolic demands of the renal tubular cells. During the ischemic insult, the lack of oxygen causes mitochondrial oxidative phosphorylation to stop, leading to depletion of adenosine triphosphate (ATP) stores.[144] Thus, cells with the greatest dependence on mitochondrial ATP production may be most susceptible to oxygen deprivation-induced ATP depletion.[145] In experimental models, renal epithelial cell ATP concentrations decrease shortly after ischemic insult. Exogenous administration of ATP results in accelerated recovery of ATP levels and a shortened duration of ARF.[146]

Severe ATP depletion may be expected to disable many energy-dependent processes, including active transport and the maintenance of intracellular homeostasis and cell structure.[140] Cellular volume regulation depends on Na-K adenosine triphosphatase (ATPase) pump activity, which is limited by decreased ATP during ischemia, such that accumulation of intracellular sodium and water leads to cell swelling and disruption of cell membranes.[147]

Calcium homeostasis is disrupted by low calcium ATPase concentrations. This may increase the intracellular calcium concentration, leading to further mitochondrial injury and exacerbating ATP depletion.[148] A high intracellular calcium concentration may activate phospholipases and proteases, which then alter membrane lipid composition, further contributing to cellular damage.[145]

During reperfusion, injury may worsen as oxygen free radicals are produced. This occurs when xanthine oxidase converts hypoxanthine to xanthine while donating an electron to generate superoxide radicals from the products of purine metabolism (e.g., adenosine monophosphate degradation).[145] Experimentally, oxygen free radicals increase membrane permeability via lipid peroxidation and may also cause oxidation of important sulfhydryl groups on proteins, including important renal transporter proteins.[149]

TUBULAR AND GLOMERULAR EVENTS

Besides intrarenal vasoconstriction, various other explanations for diminished renal function have been postulated.[2,140,150] These include back-leak of glomerular filtrate into peritubular fluid through damaged tubular epithelia,

TABLE 42.8	Summary of Epidemiology Studies of Acute Renal Failure

Patient Population	Location	Study Design	Study Period	Definition of ARF	Incidence n (%)
ICU	Belgium, university hospital	Retrospective, single center	16 months	Rise in SCr to ≥ 2 mg/dL	ARF = 30/185 patients with sepsis (16.2%) RRT = 21/30 patients (70%)
ICU	India, university hospital	Prospective, single center	12 months		Overall (8.6%) MICU (17.2%), burns (5.3%), pulmonary ICU (5.2%), stroke ICU (4.4%), SICU (3.1%), coronary ICU (1.3%)
ICU	US, urban, tertiary care, university hospital	Prospective, single center	10 months	Change in SCr of ≥0.5 mg/dL if baseline SCr ≤1.9 mg/dL; Change in SCr of ≥1.0 mg/dL if baseline SCr ≥2.0 to ≤4.9 mg/dL; Change in SCr of ≥1.5 mg/dL if baseline SCr ≥5.0 mg/dL	ARF = 254 patients/1,530 admissions (16.6%) ESRD = 57 patients/1,530 admissions (3.7%) No ARF = 1,219 patients/1,530 admissions (79.7%)
ICU	Germany, university hospital	Prospective, single center	69 months	Need for renal replacement therapy	n = 160 patients with ARF
ICU	Australia	Prospective, multicenter	3 months	Need for renal replacement therapy	n = 299 patients with severe ARF requiring acute renal replacement therapy
ICU	Finland, university hospital	Retrospective, single center	12 months	Need for renal replacement therapy	ARF = 62/3,447 admissions (1.8%)
Hospitalized African American patients	US, secondary & tertiary care hospital	Retrospective, single center	36 months	Rise in SCr ≥ 0.5 mg/dL from baseline Admission SCr ≥ 2.0 mg/dL when no history of renal disease was available	Community-acquired ARF = 79 patients (0.55%) Hospital-acquired ARF = 21 patients (0.15%)
ICU	16 countries	Prospective, multicenter	1 month	SCr ≥ 3.5 mg/dL and/or oliguria (daily urine output < 500 mL)	ARF = 348/1,411 patients (24.7%)
ICU	24 ICUs in Australia	Prospective, multicenter	3 months	Need for renal replacement therapy	Severe ARF = 116 (% not reported)
ICU	28 ICUs in France	Prospective, multicenter	12 months	SCr ≥ 3.5 mg/dL and/or oliguria (daily urine output < 500 mL)	ARF = 1,086/14, 116 admissions (7.7%)
ICU	ICU/hospital in Germany	Retrospective, single center	48 months	Need for renal replacement therapy	ARF = 154 patients (4.3% ICU; 0.6% hospitalized patients)
Hospitalized patients	US	Prospective, multicenter	54 months	Need for renal replacement therapy	ARF = 490 patients (5.4%)
ICU	20 ICUs in France	Prospective, multicenter	6 months	SCr ≥ 3.5 mg/dL, BUN ≥ 100 mg/dL or SCr and/or BUN increase ≥ 100% when baseline > 1.8 mg/dL and ≤ 3.4 mg/dL	ARF = 360 patients (7.0%)
Hospitalized patients	13 hospitals in Spain	Prospective, multicenter	9 months	SCr ≥ 2 mg/dL or mild to moderate CRF (SCr < 3 mg/dL) with sudden rise in SCr of 50% or more	ARF = 748 patients, % not reported

* Risk factors for ARF
** Risk factors for mortality

Mortality (%)	Risk Factors	Recovery	Reference	Citation
Overall 61/185 patients with sepsis (33%) 17 patients with ARF/61 non-survivors (28%) 17 patients requiring RRT/61 non-survivors (26%)	Older age, use of vasoactive medications, mechanical ventilation** Need for renal replacement therapy was independently associated with mortality		Hoste et al (2003)	Journal of the American Society of Nephrology 2003;14: 1022–1030
ARF=(62%)	Number of organ system failures, oliguria, septicemia**		Avasthi et al (2003)	Renal Failure 2003;25(1): 105–113
ARF = 86/254 (34%) ESRD = 8/57 (14%) No ARF = 109/1219 (9%)	Higher mean APACHE III scores, higher acute physiology scores, hypotension, tachycardia, tachypnea, higher WBC counts*		Clermont et al (2002)	Kidney International 2002;62:986–996
Daily HD = 22/80 (28%)* Alternate-day HD = 37/80 (46%) *(P=0.01)	Severity of underlying illness or coexisting condition, oliguria, sepsis**	Resolution of ARF in days: Daily HD=9±2* Alternate day HD=16±6 *(P=0.001)	Schiffl et al (2002)	New England Journal of Medicine 2002;346: 305–310
140/299 (46.8%)	Older age, higher mean APACHE II scores, higher acute physiology scores, higher baseline SCr, septic shock, mechanical ventilation, use of vasoactive drugs, higher bilirubin levels**	25/299 (8.3%) Required renal replacement therapy at the time of discharge. Survivors=159, therefore 134/159 (84.3%) did not require renal replacement therapy at the time of discharge	Silvester et al (2001)	Critical Care Medicine 2001;29:1910–1915
1172/3447 (34%)	History of hypotension, use of vasoactive drugs, oliguria**	Renal function recovered in 82% of survivors	Korkeila et al (2000)	Intensive Care Medicine 2000;26:1824–1831
Community-acquired ARF = 33% Hospital-acquired ARF = 59%	Oliguria, sepsis, ICU stay or mechanical ventilation, multiorgan failure**		Obialo et al (2000)	Archives of Internal Medicine 2000;160:1309–1313
Mortality 3 times higher in ARF patients than patients without ARF ICU 42.8%	Older age, presence of infection, CHF, respiratory failure, cardiovascular failure, lymphoma or leukemia, cirrhosis** Oliguric renal failure was an independent risk factor for mortality	48 patients (41.4%) survived to hospital discharge free of dialysis	de Mendonca et al (2000)	Intensive Care Medicine 2000;26:915.921
49.20%	Severity of illness, mechanical ventilation, inotrope/vasopressor support**		Cole et al (2000)	American Journal of Respiratory and Critical Care Medicine 2000;162:191–196
66%	Older age, presence of infection, male gender, multiorgan failure, mechanical ventilation**		Guerin et al (2000)	American Journal of Respiratory and Critical Care Medicine 2000;161:872–879
	ARF in ICU patients: higher APACHE II score* Mortality in ARF: single and multiorgan failure including cardiovascular, hepatic, respiratory, and neurologic failure, massive transfusions**		Schwilk et al (1997)	Intensive Care Medicine 1997;23:1204–1211
73%	Older age, multiorgan failure with sepsis, respiratory failure**		Hamel et al (1997)	Annals of Internal Medicine 1997;127:195–202
58%	Older age, male gender, previous hospitalization before ICU stay, sepsis*		Brivet et al (1996)	Critical Care Medicine 1996;24(2); 192–198
26.70%	Older age, male gender*		Liano et al (1996)	Kidney International 1996;50:811–818

tubular obstruction from cellular debris, and decreased glomerular capillary permeability. Urine flow and tubular capacity to reabsorb can be diminished by sloughing of the brush border membranes and cast formation within the tubular lumen. The sloughing of tubular membranes disrupts tubular integrity and allows back-leak of glomerular ultrafiltrate via disrupted tubular epithelium into the peritubular circulation. This increased permeability results in the return of urea, creatinine, and other waste products into the systemic circulation. Tubular obstruction also increases intratubular hydraulic pressure, which opposes glomerular filtration pressure, leading to an unfavorable glomerular filtration pressure gradient and reduced GFR.[150]

Another theory suggests that GFR declines because of an altered glomerular capillary ultrafiltration coefficient (K_f). Substantial reductions in the effective surface area for filtration cause a decrease in GFR. Experimental data indicate that the reduction in K_f may result from angiotensin II production.[17] Damage to the glomeruli can also result from immunologic reactions, and vascular occlusive diseases (e.g., HUS, renal artery thrombosis, or embolic diseases) are thought to cause glomerular damage by a mechanism similar to the mechanisms described earlier for ischemic events of the kidney.[17,150]

COMPLICATIONS

Complications of ARF are shown in Table 42.9. Before dialytic therapies were developed, the most common causes of death in patients with ARF were progressive uremia, hyperkalemia, and complications of volume overload. With the advent of dialysis, the most common causes of death are sepsis, cardiovascular and pulmonary dysfunction, and withdrawal of life-support measures.

CLINICAL PRESENTATION AND DIAGNOSIS

SIGNS AND SYMPTOMS
The clinical course of ARF often is divided into four sequential phases: initiation or injury, maintenance, diuresis, and

TABLE 42.9	Complications in Acute Renal Failure
Sodium and water imbalance	Carbohydrate intolerance
Acid–base imbalance	Hypertension
Potassium imbalance	Gastrointestinal disturbances
Anemia	Neuromuscular disturbances
Hemostatic defects	Renal osteodystrophy
Calcium and phosphate abnormalities	Dermatologic disorders
Hyperuricemia	Psychological disorders

recovery. Characteristic of the initiation phase is a significant change in hemodynamics and markedly decreased renal function. The maintenance phase of ARF usually lasts from several days to weeks and is commonly associated with oliguria. Treatment is focused on minimizing fluids and maintaining electrolyte balance until renal function returns. Impaired renal function may coexist with cellular repair processes. Surviving tubular cells regenerate new tubular cells necessary to restore functional capacity. This process probably is influenced by a variety of peptide growth factors.[151,152] Renal cells release growth factors, including epidermal growth factor and insulin-like growth factor, which may mediate repair of injured cells and recovery of renal function. Also, there appears to be some role for purine nucleotides in stimulating renal epithelial cell growth.[153]

Once kidney repair begins, it is typical to see a diuretic phase, which begins before measurable decreases in SCr and BUN. This diuresis is thought to result from the return of glomerular filtration function before complete correction of tubular reabsorption capacity. An osmotic diuretic effect may also result from accumulated uremic toxins and fluid during the oliguric phase. It is important to provide patients with adequate volume and electrolyte repletion during the diuretic phase of ARF.

DIAGNOSIS AND CLINICAL FINDINGS
Patient History and Physical Examination. Evaluation of the patient's history and physical examination often reveal the cause of ARF. For example, the findings of volume depletion or a recent history of exposure to a nephrotoxic medication or a radiocontrast agent could provide important diagnostic information necessary for prompt intervention. Additional diagnostic clues may include sudden anuria, suggesting postrenal ARF, or a rash in the case of allergic interstitial nephritis.

Urinalysis. Further important diagnostic information is obtained from a urinalysis and evaluation of various urine indices. A urinalysis usually is performed on a random sample of urine and consists of the following major components:

- Physical and chemical properties
- pH
- Concentrating ability
- Protein content
- Cells and casts
- Sodium excretion

Physical and Chemical Properties. The urine should be clear but usually has a faint yellow tinge from the presence of urochromes. Erythrocytes and white blood cells cause turbid urine. Agents that may cause urine to change color are shown in Table 42.10. Concentrated urine has a deepened color. Increasing amounts of bilirubin produce colors ranging from yellow-brown to deep olive green. Urine containing old blood, hemosiderin, or myoglobin is brown to black. Small amounts of red blood cells produce a characteristic

TABLE 42.10	Agents Causing Changes in Urine Color Not Related to Disease
Color	**Drug**
Darkening on standing	Cascara
	Chloroquine
	Levodopa
	Methocarbamol
	Methyldopa
	Metronidazole
	Nitrofurantoin
	Phenytoin
Red	Anthraquinone
	Daunorubicin
	Deferoxamine
	Doxorubicin
	Ibuprofen
	Prochlorperazine
	Phenolsulfonphthalein
Orange–brown	Rifampicin (Rifampin)
	Vitamin B
	Cascara
	Chloroquine
	Chlorzoxazone
	Furazolidone
	Ibuprofen
	Iron sorbitex
	Phenazopyridine
	Phenytoin
	Primaquine
	Quinine
	Senna
	Sulfamethoxazole
	Sulfasalazine
Blue-green	Amitriptyline
	Doan's Pills
	Indigo blue
	Methylene blue
	Resorcinol
	Triamterene
Deep yellow	Cascara
	Fluorescein
	Quinacrine
	Riboflavin

TABLE 42.11	Conditions Associated with Persistent Changes in Urine pH

Persistently Acid (pH < 7.0)

Metabolic acidosis

Respiratory acidosis

Pyrexia

Phenylketonuria

Alkaptonuria

Persistently Alkaline (pH >7.0)

Urinary tract infection with urea-splitting organisms

Metabolic alkalosis

Carbonic anhydrase inhibitors

Hyperaldosteronism

Cystinosis

smoky appearance. Patients with porphyria may void a normal-colored urine, but the sample may develop a deep purple or brownish color on standing. Food pigments, such as the pigment in beets, can color the urine red.[154,155]

pH. Urine pH varies between 4.5 and 8 in patients with healthy kidneys. The pooled daily urine specimen usually is acidic (pH 6). Decreased pulmonary ventilation during sleep causes respiratory acidosis and the development of a highly acidic urine. After meals, the urine becomes alkaline for a few hours. Thus, pH varies widely depending on the time of collection. Highly concentrated urine usually is strongly acidic and may be irritating. When urine stands it becomes alkaline as urea breaks down to ammonia. Therefore, a pH test should always be done on freshly voided urine. Urine that is persistently acid or alkaline may suggest the presence of systemic or urinary tract disease. Conditions associated with persistently acid or alkaline urine are listed in Table 42.11.[155] Some agents known to alter urine pH are listed in Table 42.12.[154]

TABLE 42.12	Agents Causing a Change in Urine pH	
Increased pH		**Decreased pH**
Acetohexamide		Ammonium chloride
Amiloride		Ascorbic acid
Amphotericin B		Corticotropin
Citrates (potassium or sodium)		Diazoxide
Epinephrine		Glucose
Niacinamide		Methenamine mandelate
Sodium bicarbonate		Metolazone
Triamterene		Niacin
		Sucrose

Concentrating Ability. Specific gravity is the most convenient way to measure the amount of dissolved solids in the urine (e.g., urea, sodium, and chloride) and provides an accurate assessment of renal concentrating ability. By definition, the specific gravity of urine is the ratio of urine weight to the weight of an equal volume of distilled water. In health, the specific gravity may range from 1.003 to 1.030. Concentrated and dilute urine have specific gravities greater than or less than 1.010, respectively. Specific gravity is a useful tool in differentiating between prerenal azotemia and ATN. Usually in prerenal azotemia, the kidney conserves sodium and water, leading to a specific gravity greater than 1.030. Conversely, during ATN, the kidney loses its ability to concentrate, leading to a lower urine specific gravity.

Osmolality measurement is more accurate and less influenced by large, dense molecules such as protein and radiographic contrast media. To test concentrating ability, the patient is either deprived of water for a number of hours or given vasopressin 10 units subcutaneously. Failure to concentrate urine to greater than 800 mOsm per kg or 1.020 specific gravity shows decreased concentrating ability. When renal function approaches 20% of normal, the specific gravity and osmolality become fixed and stabilize at 1.010 and 300 mOsm per kg, respectively. The term *isosthenuria* is used to describe urine that is consistently at 1.010 or 300 mOsm/kg.

Protein Content. Normally, nearly all filtered protein is reabsorbed or catabolized by the proximal tubular cells, and less than 150 mg of protein is excreted in the urine per day. Proteinuria is an important indicator of renal disease. Its evaluation entails a knowledge of factors that cause proteinuria without renal disease. Nonpathologic or functional proteinuria is transient and usually occurs in young adults. Proteinuria can occur with excessive exercise, exposure to cold, postural changes (such as standing from a recumbent position), and pregnancy. Proteinuria associated with renal disease results from numerous disorders (Table 42.13).[156] Proteinuria is a common characteristic of nearly every form of glomerular disease and contributes to several nephrotic syndrome complications.

Protein in the urine is measured by sulfosalicylic acid, heat and acetic acid, or dipstick methods. Because of its simplicity, the dipstick method often is used as a screening test for proteinuria. Various urine dipstick products are commercially available to detect and quantitate urine protein. In general, if protein losses exceed 3 g per day, a glomerular origin is suspected. Protein losses of less than 3 g per day are nondiagnostic, and the source is often unclear. The source of protein loss is also evaluated using electrophoresis, which differentiates prerenal, glomerular, or tubular origin.

Spot Protein/Creatinine Ratio. Protein is measured in a 24-hour collection of urine, with a normal value of <150 mg of protein per day. Overt proteinuria is defined as >500 mg of protein in a 24-hour urine collection. Patients excreting >3 g of protein per day are considered to have ne-

TABLE 42.13	Diseases Associated with Proteinuria

Infectious disease

  Poststreptococcal glomerulonephritis

  Infective endocarditis

  Syphilis

Neoplastic disease

  Lymphoma

  Leukemia

  Carcinoma (colon, lung, breast, stomach, kidney)

Multisystem and connective tissue diseases

  Systemic lupus erythematosus

  Polyarteritis

  Sarcoidosis

  Sjögren's syndrome

  Amyloidosis

  Diabetes mellitus

Miscellaneous conditions

  Allergic reactions (bee stings, serum sickness)

  Chronic allograft rejection

  Preeclampsia

(From Kaysen GA. Proteinuria and the nephrotic syndrome. In: Schrier RW, ed. Renal and Electrolyte Disorders. Boston: Little, Brown, 1992:681–726.)

phrotic-range proteinuria. An alternative to the cumbersome 24-hour urine collection is obtaining a random urine specimen or "spot urine" and calculating the spot protein to creatinine ratio as an estimate of daily urinary protein excretion.[157] The rationale is that a normal person excretes about 100 mg (0.1 g) of protein and 1,000 mg (1.0 g) of creatinine per day. The ratio correlates closely with daily protein excretion.[157–160] Therefore, the normal ratio is 100 mg protein to 1,000 mg creatinine, which equals 0.1 g protein per 1 g creatinine, or 0.1 g protein per day. Assuming that creatinine excretion remains constant (i.e., the denominator is 1 g creatinine), then a ratio of 2.0 equals a urinary protein excretion of 2 g per day, and a ratio of 3.0 equals a urinary protein excretion of 3 g per day. The numerator should be multiplied by a conversion factor (0.088 mmol/L = 1 mg/dL) when the urinary creatinine concentration is measured in mmol per L.

Conditions that alter creatinine excretion and cause deviations from a normal excretion of 1 g creatinine per day should be taken in to account when using this calculation. Theoretically, if creatinine excretion is low, as in the case of elderly patients with low muscle mass, then the spot protein/creatinine ratio will be a high value and the degree of proteinuria will be overestimated. Conversely, when creatinine excretion is high, then the ratio will be a low value and the degree of proteinuria will be underestimated. However, upon repeated measurements, the spot protein/creatinine ratio will be reproducible and can be used to monitor treatment-induced changes in proteinuria such as primary glomerular diseases, slowly progressive renal failure, and essential hypertension with albuminuria. Spot protein/creatinine ratios are used to monitor therapy in patients with diabetic nephropathy; however, one multicenter study of type I diabetic patients with overt proteinuria found lack of reproducibility in repeat measurements and wide variability at urinary protein excretion rates greater than 3.5 g per day.[161] Nonetheless, spot ratios have utility in clinic settings or circumstances where 24-hour urine collections are not feasible.[162]

Cells and Casts. Normal urine contains a small number of red blood cells, white blood cells, and hyaline casts. Casts are cylindrical elements with parallel sides that derive their shape and size from the tubular segment in which they were formed. Factors favoring cast formation are an acid pH, highly concentrated urine, proteinuria, and stasis within the tubules. The transparent hyaline casts are composed entirely of protein. Cellular casts represent red blood cells, white blood cells, or renal epithelial cells trapped within the protein matrix. Granular casts represent degraded cellular casts and usually indicate renal parenchymal damage.

Sodium Excretion. Renal tubular sodium reabsorption (i.e., the difference between the amount of sodium filtered and the amount excreted) is the predominant mechanism that regulates sodium excretion. Tubule reabsorption accounts for >99% of filtered sodium under normal conditions. For example, when the GFR is 2 mL per second (120 mL/min) and the plasma sodium concentration is 145 mmol per L, approximately 17 mmol of sodium is filtered per minute. Over the course of a day this is equivalent to about 25,000 mmol (or 575 g) of filtered sodium. However, only 100 to 250 mmol of sodium is excreted per day (<1%).

FE_{Na} is the fraction of filtered sodium excreted in urine, using creatinine as an estimate for GFR. Thus, FE_{Na} (%) is calculated as follows:

$$FE_{Na} = \frac{U_{Na} \times P_{Cr}}{U_{Cr} \times P_{Na}} x100 \qquad (42.1)$$

where U_{Na} is urine sodium concentration (mmol/L), Pcr is plasma creatinine concentration in milligrams per deciliter (μmol/L), Ucr is urine creatinine concentration in milligrams per deciliter (μmol/L), and P_{Na} is plasma sodium concentration (mmol/L).

FE_{Na} is a useful guide to distinguish whether an abrupt rise in BUN is the result of impaired renal perfusion (i.e., prerenal azotemia) or ATN. During ATN, tubular sodium transport is impaired and FE_{Na} values usually exceed 2%. FE_{Na} values less than 1% suggest prerenal azotemia. However, values between 1% and 2% may have little predictive value. FE_{Na} may be elevated in patients receiving diuretics. The renal failure index (RFI) has also been proposed to help differentiate prerenal ARF from ATN. The RFI is determined by dividing the urine sodium concentration by the urine/plasma creatinine ratio. RFI values less than 1 suggest prerenal failure and values >4 may indicate ATN.[163]

LABORATORY DATA

Determination of Glomerular Filtration Rate or Inulin Clearance. GFR is approximated by measuring the urinary excretion rate of a marker substance known to be filtered and excreted in equal amounts. Properties of the ideal marker substance are that it is neither absorbed nor secreted by the renal tubules and is filtered freely across glomerular membranes, not metabolized in renal tubules or produced by the kidneys, and not eliminated by nonrenal routes. These critical properties are satisfied ideally by inulin. To measure inulin clearance, a continuous intravenous infusion of inulin is given, then several samples of blood and urine are collected at specified times, and these samples are assayed for inulin concentrations. Because the filtered amount of inulin is equal to the amount of inulin excreted, the following equation applies:

$$GFR = \frac{U_{in}}{P_{in}} xV \qquad (42.2)$$

where GFR is glomerular filtration rate (mL/s), U_{in} is urine inulin concentration (μmol/L), P_{in} is plasma inulin concentration (μmol/L), measured at the midpoint of the collection period, and V is volume per unit time (i.e., the total urine volume collected divided by the total time of collection, in mL/second). Because GFR varies according to body size, values typically are expressed by standardizing them to body surface area. The average GFR in young men is approximately 2 mL/s/1.73 m^2 (120 mL/min/1.73 m^2). This value usually is 10% to 15% lower in women.

Inulin is mainly used for research purposes. Its clinical utility is limited by the intravenous route of administration, the need for collection of blood and urine samples, and the availability of an inulin assay within the clinical laboratory.

Creatinine Clearance. In clinical practice, creatinine clearance is the index of GFR most often used. Determination of creatinine clearance is convenient and inexpensive and can be easily calculated from a timed urine collection assayed for creatinine and a single SCr measurement. Measurement is most accurate if the urine collection interval is 24 hours and a blood sample is obtained at the midpoint of this timed collection. The calculation of creatinine clearance is similar to that of GFR, except that urine and SCr concentrations are substituted for inulin concentrations.

Creatinine production results from the nonenzymatic hydrolysis of muscle stores of creatine and creatine phosphate. Creatinine is produced at a fairly constant daily rate: approximately 1 mg creatinine is produced daily from about 20 g muscle.[164] Therefore, creatinine production depends on muscle mass and is influenced by age and gender. After age 20, creatinine production decreases by approximately 2 mg/kg/24 hours per decade of life in men and women.[165] Because creatinine is filtered by the glomerulus and is also secreted in the proximal tubule, its clearance approximates but is always greater than GFR.[166] If GFR is greater than 0.4 mL per second (25 mL/min), then creatinine clearance approximates GFR reasonably well. However, creatinine secretion is enhanced in patients with lower GFR, and especially in disease states affecting primarily the glomeruli (i.e., acute glomerulonephritis), leading to overestimation of GFR.

Often it is difficult to obtain accurate 24-hour urine collections. Therefore, creatinine clearance may be estimated using the following formula, derived by Cockroft and Gault[167]:

$$Ccr(men) = \frac{(140 - Age) \times Weight}{72 \times SCr} \quad (42.3)$$

where Ccr is creatinine clearance (mL/min), age is in years, weight is in kilograms, and SCr is the serum creatinine concentration (mg/dL). In women, Equation 42-3 is multiplied by 0.85. Factors other than a decreased GFR can alter the SCr level and must be considered in assessing renal function. Patients with decreased muscle mass as a result of old age or cachexia have a decreased creatinine production and therefore a low or normal SCr level, even though their renal function may be impaired.[168,169]

An equation developed by investigators of the Modified Diet and Renal Disease (MDRD) study incorporates serum albumin, ethnicity, and serum urea nitrogen concentration, in addition to sex, age, and SCr, to improve the accuracy of GFR estimates compared to other predictive equations.[9] The MDRD equation was developed from a randomly selected sample of 1,070 patients and validated in a separate group of 558 patients. The median absolute errors between actual and predicted GFR values (and the median percentage absolute errors) from the MDRD equation and the Cockroft-Gault equation were 3.8 mL/minute/1.73 m² (11.5%) and 6.8 mL/minute/1.73 m² (19.8%). The maximal R^2 value was 90.3% for the MDRD equation versus 84.2% for the Cockroft-Gault equation. Unexplained variance $(1 - R^2)$ decreased from 15.8% with the Cockroft-Gault equation to 9.7% with the MDRD method. The Cockroft-Gault equation overestimated GFR by 16%.

The MDRD equation offers several advantages over other equations, including the ability to predict GFR rather than creatinine clearance, use of a validated measure for measuring GFR (renal clearance of ^{125}I-iothalamate), use of the most widely accepted assay method for measuring SCr (kinetic alkaline picrate reaction), validation of the equation in a separate patient cohort, and prediction ability over a wide range of values. This method does not require collection of a timed urine sample or measurement of patient height and weight.

Creatine is the amino acid precursor of creatinine. Synthesis of creatine from glycine, arginine, and methionine occurs in the liver. Thus, patients with advanced liver disease have decreased creatine production and decreased body pools of creatine. This results in decreased creatinine production and SCr concentrations below expected values for any given level of renal function. In patients with liver disease, formulas that estimate renal function based on a SCr level should not be used because they will greatly overestimate renal function.[170] Creatine is also contained in meat. Cooking converts creatine to creatinine, which is absorbed and contributes to the total body creatinine pool. Patients who do not eat meat will have a lower intake of creatine and creatinine, which results in a smaller body pool of these substances. This accounts for a lower-than-usual SCr, even though these patients may have normal renal function.

Laboratory determination of SCr is based on the alkaline picrate method of Jaffe, modified for increased specificity and to accommodate automation.[165] Because this is a colorimetric test, other noncreatinine chromogens can result in overestimation of SCr. See Chapter 5 for further discussion. Some of these agents are listed in Table 42.14.[171] Large elevations in SCr levels without appreciable changes in the BUN should alert the clinician to possible laboratory interference. Some drugs (e.g., cimetidine) compete with creatinine for tubular secretion and thus result in elevated SCr concentrations.

Blood Urea Nitrogen. Urea nitrogen is derived from hepatic deamination of amino acids, causing liberation of ammonia, which combines with available carbon dioxide. Urea is eliminated primarily by the kidney through glomerular filtration and undergoes reabsorption in the proximal tubule. The extent of reabsorption depends on the urine flow rate, such that 40% of the filtered urea is reabsorbed with diuresis and 60% is reabsorbed with antidiuresis. Normal BUN concentrations are 3.6 to 5.4 mmol per L (10 to 15 mg/dL) but may increase to greater than 54 mmol per L (150 mg/dL) with severe renal failure. In general, BUN concentrations

TABLE 42.14	Agents That Cause a False Elevation in Serum Creatinine as Measured by the Jaffe Method
Acebutolol	Fluorescein
Acetoacetate	Fructose
Acetohexamide	Glucose
Acetone	Levodopa
Aminohippuric acid	Methyldopa
Ascorbic acid	Moxalactam
Cefamandole	Nitrofurantoin
Cefoperazone	Phenolsulfonphthalein
Cefoxitin	Pyruvate
Cephalothin	Sulfobromophthalein

(From Young DS. Effects of drugs on clinical laboratory tests. 3rd ed. Washington DC: American Association of Clinical Chemistry, 1990; and Siest G, Galteau MM. Drug Effects on laboratory test results. St. Louis: Year Book, 1988.)

TABLE 42.15	Factors Elevating Blood Urea Nitrogen without Renal Impairment
High-protein diet	Hypovolemia
Febrile illness with catabolism	Decreased cardiac output
Gastrointestinal bleeding	Steroids
Hyperthyroidism	Tetracyclines

greater than 36 mmol per L (100 mg/dL) are associated with a higher risk of complications during renal failure and the need for dialysis. BUN is less accurate than SCr levels or creatinine clearance in assessing renal function. The major limitations are related to a number of factors that can alter urea generation and urea clearance in the absence of changes in renal function. Urea generation depends on protein catabolism and therefore is altered by changes in dietary intake, liver disease, blood in the gastrointestinal tract, steroid-induced catabolism, and the antianabolic effect of most tetracyclines. Because the amount of urea reabsorbed is inversely proportional to the urine flow rate, low-flow states elevate BUN disproportionately to changes in SCr. Any factors that lower the absolute or effective blood volume (and hence RBF) increase BUN. Table 42.15 lists factors responsible for BUN elevation in the absence of renal impairment.[155,171] See Chapter 5 for further discussion.

Renal Imaging and Renal Biopsy. In patients who present with severe oliguria or anuria, a renal ultrasound is a useful examination to quickly rule out a urinary tract obstruction. The ultrasound may be followed by contrast studies to establish the precise location of an obstruction. Renal biopsy usually is not necessary in evaluating the patient with ARF. However, when prerenal and postrenal causes have been excluded by other measures (e.g., history, laboratory and imaging studies), histologic analysis may establish an intrarenal diagnosis and guide management.

THERAPEUTIC PLAN

PREVENTION

In the patient who suddenly develops oliguria with rising BUN and SCr concentrations, it is important to distinguish whether the underlying disease process is prerenal or postrenal, because rapid correction of these conditions can prevent progression to ischemic injury and development of ARF. Correction of volume deficits can lead to prompt restoration of renal perfusion. Therapeutic agents known to further reduce blood flow must be withdrawn and potential nephrotoxins, such as aminoglycosides, radiocontrast dye, NSAIDs, and ACE inhibitors, should be administered cautiously, if at all. Initial efforts should also be directed at ruling out urinary tract obstruction. Factors suggesting obstruction include a normal urinalysis, rapid changes in urine

output, and residual urine on postvoiding catheterization. If renal calculi are present, a radiograph of the abdomen will detect the 90% that are radiopaque. In the absence of obstruction, urinary indices provide the most reliable method of distinguishing prerenal azotemia from ATN.

Table 42.4 will help in distinguishing reversible prerenal failure from ATN, but its usefulness is limited after diuretics are administered or in patients with underlying chronic renal failure. It is important to differentiate between prerenal and intrinsic ARF on the basis of these clinical laboratory measurements. If prerenal azotemia is suspected, aggressive fluid resuscitation should result in an increased urine output. If urine flow does not increase, additional fluids should be given cautiously, if at all, because fluid overload is likely to ensue if ARF is already established. Also, a fluid challenge can be detrimental to the patient with intrinsic renal damage (ATN). Thus, the patient who presents with a high urinary sodium (in the absence of diuretic use) and FE_{Na} >2% probably has ATN and should not receive fluid resuscitation.

Preventing associated complications, such as infection and gastrointestinal bleeding, is very important. Careful maintenance of intravenous access, minimal use of indwelling urinary bladder catheters, and early recognition and treatment of wound and other infections are necessary. Monitoring for signs of blood loss (e.g., testing stools for occult blood, monitoring the hematocrit, and controlling gastric pH with H_2 antagonists or antacids) minimizes the morbidity associated with bleeding.

If potential nephrotoxic insults are likely to occur, specific preventive measures, such as hydration and volume repletion before and during nephrotoxin exposure, are recommended. For example, when using amphotericin B or aminoglycosides, ensuring that patients are well hydrated may eliminate or reduce the severity of renal damage. Other preventive measures to consider are therapeutic drug monitoring of aminoglycoside concentrations, fluid hydration before cisplatin therapy, and the use of allopurinol and urine alkalinization during high-dose chemotherapy to avoid uric acid nephropathy. Combination therapy with more than one nephrotoxic agent carries additional risk and should be avoided if possible. Substitution of less nephrotoxic agents should be considered in older adults and others at risk for renal dysfunction (Table 42.16). For example, in high-risk patients, it may be possible to avoid radiocontrast agents and use less invasive diagnostic techniques such as ultrasonography. Nephrotoxins should be avoided or discontinued, and doses of medications whose pharmacokinetics or pharmacodynamics are affected by renal dysfunction should be adjusted. Several common medications whose dose must be adjusted during renal insufficiency are listed in Table 42.17. Dose adjustments must be based on the degree of renal dysfunction and the characteristics of the medication. The goal is to maintain efficacious drug therapy while avoiding toxicity (see also Drug Dosing Issues later in this chapter).

TABLE 42.16	Preventing Acute Renal Failure

Identify patients at risk.

Older adults.

Patients with abnormal renal function or diabetes.

Volume-depleted patients

Avoid nephrotoxic agents.

Nonsteroidal anti-inflammatory drugs

Aminoglycosides

Amphotericin B

Angiotensin-converting enzyme inhibitors in volume depleted patients

Use prevention strategies.

Contrast media (extracellular fluid volume expansion)

Rhabdomyolysis (correct intravascular volume, urinary alkalinization, mannitol infusion)

Tumor lysis syndrome (allopurinol, diuresis, urinary alkalinization)

Surgical procedures (optimize volume status, avoid multiple insults and hypotension)

SUPPORTIVE CARE

ARF often persists for several days or weeks, necessitating prolonged supportive care. The minimum daily fluid needs include replacement of measurable losses (i.e., urine output, nasogastric suction, vomiting, chest tube drainage, and fistula output) and insensible losses through the skin and lungs (approximately 600 to 900 mL/day). The choice of fluid intake should be determined by the need for colloid or crystalloid, electrolytes, and calories.

FLUID MANAGEMENT

The normal kidney is critical to the maintenance of volume homeostasis, which permits constant circulatory and extracellular fluid volumes despite varying water and salt consumption and varying loss. The presence of pedal or sacral edema or pulmonary edema in the setting of ARF implies that water or salt intake has exceeded the injured kidney's ability to excrete the water and salt load. This situation can be anticipated in the oliguric or anuric patient but often complicates nonoliguric ARF as well. Most patients with ARF lose the ability to concentrate or dilute the urine and as a consequence excrete a constant volume of urine regardless of fluid intake. For example, a patient with ATN whose urine output is fixed at 500 mL per day but receives 1,000 mL per day of parenteral nutrition, along with various intravenous antibiotics, will gradually develop volume overload and edema unless the volume administered is adjusted. Volume status management is based on careful physical examination, and the patient must be examined daily to measure supine and standing blood pressure and pulse, skin turgor, and mucous membrane hydration; auscultate the lungs for evidence of pulmonary congestion; perform a general examination for sacral or pedal edema; review daily intake and output; and measure daily (serial) weight changes accurately. A bolus of normal saline (250 to 500 mL) may be used initially in most cases. The rate of fluid replacement is determined by the extent of hemodynamic compromise.

The prescription for fluid and sodium intake should be specified. In general, a patient who is euvolemic should be given an additional 300 to 500 mL per day of electrolyte-free water to replace insensible water losses. A sodium intake of less than 2 g per day should be prescribed. Patients with increased insensible fluid loss, such as those with burns or severe diarrhea, have much larger fluid needs. However, because insensible fluid losses cannot be measured accurately, the patient's volume status must be assessed accurately on a daily basis and the fluid prescription modified as necessary. The patient with clinical evidence of fluid overload should be restricted to a fluid intake less than the daily urine output. Patients with clinical evidence of volume depletion should be given additional volume to achieve a euvolemic state. Sustained hypovolemia may worsen renal injury or delay recovery from renal failure. Increased fluid needs should be anticipated during the polyuric recovery phase of ARF.

In the ICU, clinical assessment of volume status can be confounded by surgical wound loss, severe pneumonia, or edema caused by altered capillary permeability. Here, measurements of central venous pressure and capillary wedge pressure are important adjuncts to volume status monitoring. These patients often are receiving multiple parenteral medications that constitute a large obligatory volume load. Often these medications can be given slowly in a concentrated solution to minimize the volume administered. Likewise, the volume of parenteral nutrition should be adjusted to optimize calories and protein in a minimum volume. The clinician must keep in mind the solutions in which various medications are delivered.

ELECTROLYTE HOMEOSTASIS

Electrolyte abnormalities that occur in ARF include disorders of sodium, potassium, phosphate, magnesium, and calcium homeostasis. Hypernatremia and hyponatremia often are observed in patients with ARF. Because abnormal serum sodium concentrations are caused by disorders of water metabolism, sodium homeostasis is linked to volume management. Hyponatremia usually results from an excess of free water relative to solute, whereas hypernatremia results when free water intake is inadequate. It is important to keep track of the amount of free water delivered in intravenous solutions and to limit this free water whenever necessary. For example, administering 500 mL of 0.45% saline is equivalent to giving 250 mL of 0.9% (normal) saline and 250 mL of electrolyte-free water. Other sources of free water excess include parenteral and enteral feedings.

Hyperkalemia can be a serious consequence of ARF; potassium intake can exceed the injured kidney's reduced potassium excretory capacity. In addition, there can be shifts

TABLE 42.17	Selected Medications for Which Dose Adjustment is Needed in Renal Insufficiency

Antimicrobials

Aminoglycosides (amikacin, gentamicin, tobramycin)

Antifungal agents (fluconazole, flucytosine, itraconazole)

Antitubercular agents (ethambutol, pyrazinamide)

Antiviral agents (acyclovir, cidofovir, didanosine, famciclovir, foscarnet, ganciclovir, lamivudine, stavudine, zalcitabine, zidovudine)

Cephalosporins (cefamandole, cefazolin, cefmetazole, cefonicid, cefotaxime, cefotetan, cefoxitin, ceftazidime, ceftizoxime, cefuroxime, cephalothin)

Fluoroquinolones (ciprofloxacin, levofloxacin, ofloxacin)

Macrolides (clarithromycin, erythromycin)

Penicillins (ampicillin, methicillin, mezlocillin, penicillin, piperacillin, ticarcillin)

Tetracyclines (minocycline, tetracycline)

Others (aztreonam, chloramphenicol, imipenem, meropenem, trimethoprim–sulfamethoxazole, vancomycin)

Cardiovascular

Angiotensin-converting enzyme inhibitors (benazepril, captopril, enalapril, lisinopril, quinapril, ramipril)

Antiarrhythmic agents (bretylium, flecainide, procainamide, quinidine, sotalol)

β-blockers (acebutolol, atenolol, carteolol, nadolol, pindolol)

Others (digoxin, milrinone, nitroprusside)

Others

Analgesics (codeine, ketorolac, meperidine, morphine)

Barbiturates (phenobarbital, thiopental)

Gastrointestinal agents (cimetidine, famotidine, metoclopramide, ranitidine)

Hypoglycemic agents (acetohexamide, chlorpropamide, glyburide, insulin)

Neuromuscular blocking agents (neostigmine, pancuronium, pyridostigmine, tubocurarine, vecuronium)

Others (allopurinol, lithium carbonate, paroxetine, phenytoin)

---

between intracellular and extracellular compartments secondary to acid–base balance. Hyperkalemia usually is prevented by restricting daily potassium intake to less than 50 mEq. Certain food types, such as fruits, chocolates, and nuts, must be eliminated from the diet. Often, potassium is omitted from parenteral fluids, and it is important not to overlook nondietary exogenous sources of potassium; these include drugs such as potassium penicillin G and salt substitutes. Finally, drugs that impair renal potassium excretion, such as potassium-sparing diuretics, NSAIDs, and ACE inhibitors, should be avoided if possible.

If potassium restriction is inadequate to prevent hyperkalemia, sodium polystyrene sulfonate can be used to exchange sodium for potassium in the bowel and increase intestinal excretion of potassium. Although usually administered orally (15 to 30 gm in 20% sorbitol), in the presence of an ileus, potassium exchange resins are effective when given as an enema. Because these compounds exchange sodium for potassium, large sodium loads can worsen volume overload or cause hypernatremia. Repeated administration can lead to

diarrhea as a result of sorbitol intake, which may complicate acidosis by increasing intestinal bicarbonate loss. Persistent hyperkalemia despite potassium intake restriction and sodium polystyrene administration is an indication for dialysis. However, other endogenous causes of hyperkalemia (e.g., severe acidosis, insulinopenia, hemolysis, rhabdomyolysis, and ischemic tissue injury) should also be investigated.

Hypocalcemia may occur secondary to the hypomagnesemia associated with cisplatin, amphotericin B, or aminoglycoside administration. Hypomagnesemia also inhibits synthesis and release of parathyroid hormone, which may cause hypocalcemia. Decreased synthesis of 1,25-dihydroxyvitamin D by the injured kidney reduces intestinal calcium absorption and can contribute to hypocalcemia. In addition, hypocalcemia can result from frequently administered blood products preserved in citrate. Hypocalcemia is prevented and treated with generous calcium supplementation either orally (3 to 4 g/day in divided doses) or, for symptomatic hypocalcemia, as calcium acetate, calcium gluconate, or calcium chloride. Magnesium should be repleted (cautiously) orally or parenterally. Avoiding magnesium-containing antacids decreases the potential for hypermagnesemia.

Phosphorus accumulates during renal failure and may result in hyperphosphatemia. Although hyperphosphatemia is much more problematic in patients with chronic renal failure, high serum phosphorus levels can contribute to hypocalcemia. Restricting dietary phosphate and administering phosphate-binding antacids (e.g., calcium-containing antacids) usually maintains serum phosphate within the normal range.

TREATMENT

Three basic therapeutic interventions are currently used in ARF: pharmacologic, dialytic, and nutritional therapies. Despite considerable recent research, none of these has been found to improve mortality rates or hasten renal function recovery significantly. Thus, the initial care of a patient with ARF should focus on reversing the underlying cause, correcting fluid and electrolyte imbalances, and preventing further renal injury by providing supportive measures (Fig. 42.2).

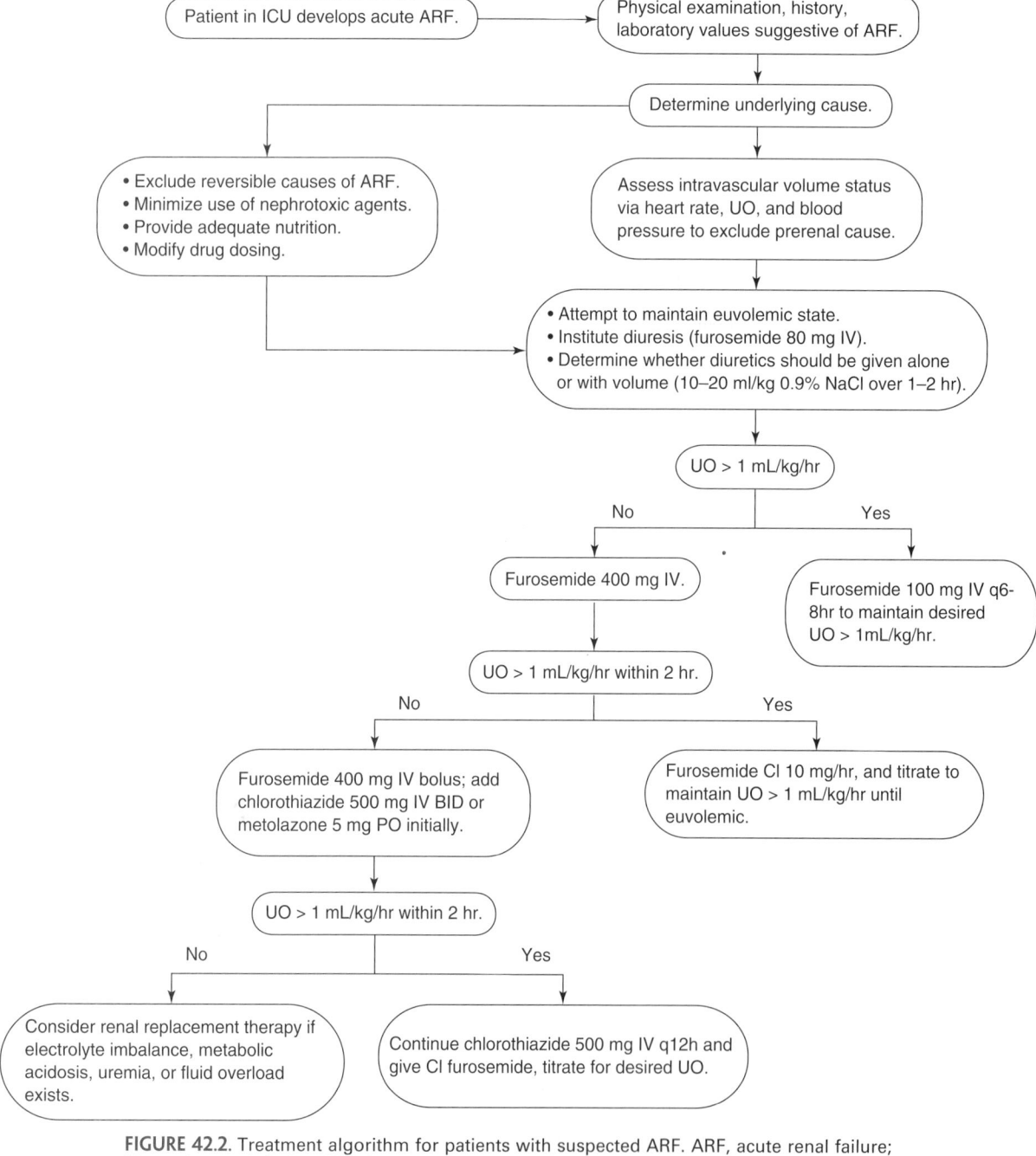

FIGURE 42.2. Treatment algorithm for patients with suspected ARF. ARF, acute renal failure; CI, continuous infusion; ICU, intensive care unit; UO, urine output.

PHARMACOTHERAPY

Therapeutic modalities for treating ARF are designed to increase RBF, increase urine output, maintain fluid and electrolyte balance, remove metabolic wastes, and slow or reverse kidney damage.

Diuretics. Although diuretic therapy (e.g., mannitol and furosemide) helps to protect the kidney from injury in experimental ischemia, most clinical trials have failed to show effectiveness of these agents in treating or preventing ischemic ARF. If administered early in the course of ARF, both furosemide and mannitol can convert oliguric ARF to a nonoliguric state. Because evidence suggests that nonoliguric ARF is associated with less morbidity and mortality, clinicians have often tried to convert oliguric ARF to nonoliguric ARF. However, no prospective controlled clinical trials confirm that pharmacologic conversion from oliguria to nonoliguria reduces mortality or time to recovery in established ARF. However, most clinicians would agree that nonoliguric patients are easier to manage than oliguric patients and have fewer complications, less need for dialysis, and shorter hospital stays than those with oliguric renal failure.[18] Maintaining a high urine output may prevent volume overload and allow increased nutritional support.

At present, loop diuretics or mannitol should be used to optimize fluid management in newly apparent intrinsic ARF. Diuretics should be avoided in the setting of contrast nephropathy and as routine prophylaxis of ARF because resultant hypovolemia could accelerate the progression from prerenal azotemia. Instead, urine flow rates and intravascular volume are greater after saline administration than after diuretic use.[94] It is also clear that high-dose diuretics are of no value when administered after intrinsic ARF is firmly established.[172,173]

Mannitol. Mannitol was the first pharmacologic substance used in ARF, and many nephrologists continue to use it to treat ARF. Proposed mechanisms of benefit include increased filtration pressure, improved urine flow rates, reduced tubular cell inflammation, and improved RBF caused by a decrease in renal vascular resistance.[18,172] Mannitol is also a free radical scavenger. Despite these theoretical benefits, there are several reports of mannitol-induced ARF, and consistent benefit in patients with ARF has not been found.

As soon as possible after a decrease in urine output is noted, a short course of mannitol might be tried. In adults, a wide range of mannitol doses sufficient to expand intravascular volume and increase renal perfusion pressure have been tried.[163] In general, 20% mannitol solution dosed at 0.5 g per kg can be infused over 30 to 60 minutes, then repeated in an hour if there is no response. If urine output follows, additional doses are titrated to maintain urine output. If diuresis does not occur and additional doses are given, intravascular volume overload and congestive heart failure may occur. Mannitol is recommended for prevention and early treatment of myoglobinuric ARF[174] and is used with adequate hydration to prevent cisplatin-associated nephrotoxicity.

Loop Diuretics. Loop diuretics usually are considered the diuretics of choice in patients with renal insufficiency.[175] The benefits of loop diuretics in early ARF are thought to result from decreased tubule obstruction, reduction of active transport processes and oxygen demand in the tubular cells, or renal vasodilation resulting in increased RBF.[150,176] All loop diuretics (i.e., furosemide, torsemide, ethacrynic acid, and bumetanide) affect the ascending limb of the loop of Henle to prevent sodium reabsorption. However, ethacrynic acid is not used in patients with renal failure because of accumulation and ototoxicity. Ethacrynic acid is reserved for patients allergic to sulfa medications. Diuretics have similar efficacy when given in equivalent doses. The equipotency ratio of intravenous bumetanide/torsemide/furosemide is 1: 20:40. In patients with renal failure, the ratio of equipotency of IV torsemide to furosemide is 1:1.[177] Bumetanide is an effective and potent loop diuretic and can be used in patients with ARF; however, its use in these patients has not been studied extensively. Torsemide and bumetanide have better oral bioavailability than furosemide. Compared to furosemide, torsemide's advantages include a high oral bioavailability (80% to 100%) and a long duration of activity (12 to 24 hours), allowing for less frequent dosing.

The use of furosemide has been evaluated in both animals and humans. Although the majority of experimental studies are not in models of well-established experimental ATN, the effects of loop diuretics in animal models are consistently positive. In various clinical trials, the use of furosemide in patients with oliguric ARF has been associated with a response rate of 40% to 100% for conversion to a nonoliguric state.[172,178] A meta-analysis of 19 studies found significantly greater survival in patients with early oliguric ATN who responded to diuretic therapy.[172] However, the use of a diuretic may simply predict better outcome on the basis of less severe injury rather than decreasing morbidity and mortality.[172] Studies clearly suggest that if any benefits are to be gained, therapy with diuretics or mannitol should begin during the first 24 hours after an insult.[175,176] Two reports have found possible deleterious effects when furosemide is used as prophylaxis to prevent contrast nephropathy.[94,179]

Although the use of loop diuretics remains controversial, they should be considered after an inadequate response to a fluid challenge. Recent trials have shown an increase in urine output with the use of loop diuretics in ARF patients. Increase in urinary output not only makes fluid management easier in critically ill patients, but can also be used as a prognostic tool to assess the severity of renal insult.[180] Because the window of opportunity may be narrow, an initial intravenous furosemide dose of 1.5 to 3 mg per kg (100 to 200 mg) should be infused over 15 to 30 minutes.[176,181] If urine output does not increase within an hour, the dose should be doubled and a thiazide added. If there is no response, therapy should be discontinued. Doses >500 mg are unlikely to be of benefit. If urine output increases, additional doses can be given to maintain urine flow. Patients who have a poor response to intermittent doses of a loop diuretic may benefit from a continuous furosemide infusion at a dose of 10 to 40 mg per hour, titrated according to the patient's urine output.[175,176] Continuous infusion of loop diuretics has been reported to be more effective than intermittent dosing. It is thought that maintaining effective amounts of diuretic within the luminal tubule will enhance the diuretic response.[175] Also, continuous infusion decreases the frequency of adverse reactions, such as myalgias and ototoxicity.[182,183] Before a continuous infusion of a loop diuretic is started, a loading dose should be given to decrease the time necessary to achieve therapeutic drug concentrations.

Diuretic Resistance. Patients with renal insufficiency often encounter a decreased response to loop diuretics often referred to as "diuretic resistance." Some common causes of diuretic resistance in ARF are excessive sodium intake, inadequate diuretic dose or inappropriate regimen, reduced bioavailability (from gastrointestinal edema), reduced RBF (drugs, intravascular depletion), increased sodium reabsorption, and nephrotic syndrome (in nephrotic syndrome, diuretics bind to proteins in the renal tubule, reducing diuretic effects).[184] Strategies to overcome diuretic resistance may include increasing the dose or the dosing frequency; continuous intravenous infusion of the diuretic; and concomitant administration of loop diuretics with diuretics that act at the distal convoluted tubule (thiazides) or the collecting duct (amiloride, triamterene, and spironolactone).[184,185] Combination of loop diuretics with a different site of action synergistically increases sodium excretion by blocking any compensatory increase in the distal sodium reabsorption. Metolazone and hydrochlorothiazide are frequently added to furosemide therapy.[186] In patients with severe renal impairment, careful selection of diuretics is important. Metolazone, unlike other thiazides, maintains the ability to produce effective diuresis at a GFR of less than 20 mL per minute.[187,188] Special consideration of disease states such as heart failure and cirrhosis (which increase sodium reabsorption) and careful use of drugs such as NSAIDs and ACE inhibitors (which can reduce RBF as a result of sodium and water retention) can help to maximize therapy and minimize diuretic resistance.

Vasoactive Agents

Dopamine. Dopamine is an endogenous catecholamine whose actions are mediated by stimulation of various dopaminergic and adrenergic receptors. The mechanisms by which dopamine modulates RBF depend on the rate of infusion. Dopaminergic effects occur at low doses of 0.5 to 1 μg/kg/minute. Activation of dopamine-1 and dopamine-2 receptors leads to intrarenal vasodilation and increased RBF. In addition, dopamine-1 receptor stimulation leads to diuresis via actions on the medullary ascending limb of the loop of Henle and brush border of the proximal tubule. Stimulation of β-1 adrenergic receptors occurs at doses of 1 to 3 μg/kg/minute, resulting in increased cardiac output and increased RBF. Because an increase in RBF with resultant diuresis occurs at lower infusion rates, these doses are referred to as "low-dose" or "renal-dose dopamine." Alpha-adrenergic effects (i.e., vasoconstriction) predominate at doses of 5 to 20 μg/kg/minute. Dopamine may also decrease renal oxygen demand by inhibiting Na-K ATPase and tubular sodium reabsorption. These effects not only contribute to natriuresis but are also thought to exert protective effects on the kidney by reducing renal ischemia. However, these protective effects have not been borne out in clinical trials.

The renal effects of low-dose dopamine were first shown more than four decades ago.[189] Many uncontrolled studies have shown the natriuretic and diuretic effects of dopamine, leading to the wide use of dopamine in the conversion from oliguric ARF to nonoliguric ARF.[190–193] In these situations, controlling volume, thereby reducing the complications of volume overload, facilitates patient management. Unfortunately, the increase in urine output has not been shown to translate into improved survival or delayed dialysis in patients with ARF.

Results of clinical studies assessing the use of renal-dose dopamine are controversial. Dopamine at a dose of 2 μg/kg/min was found to have no protective effect against radio-contrast nephrotoxicity in patients with underlying renal disease compared to those treated with saline.[194] Low-dose dopamine resulted in greater diuresis without a change in creatinine clearance, while low-dose dobutamine exhibited a greater improvement in estimated creatinine clearance without an increase in urine output.[195] It is widely assumed that dobutamine in combination with dopamine could improve cardiac index, cause arterial vasodilation, and maximize RBF and natriuresis in oliguric patients with left ventricular dysfunction. However, although urine output may be enhanced, it has not been established whether dopamine prevents ARF or improves outcome in this setting.[196]

Another trial[197,198] questioned the routine administration of dopamine. Patients in the anaritide ARF study received low-dose (<3 μg/kg/min), high-dose (>3 μg/kg/min), or no dopamine; there was no significant difference in the relative risk of mortality or the need for dialysis.[197,198] In a retrospective analysis, low-dose dopamine did not reduce the incidence of ARF, the need for dialysis, or 28-day mortality in septic shock patients with oliguria.[199] Similarly, no difference in mortality, need for renal replacement therapy, or peak serum creatinine levels were found in a prospective, randomized, double-blinded, placebo-controlled trial of low-dose dopamine in 324 ICU patients with systemic inflammatory response syndrome and oliguria.[200] A meta-analysis of 24 published studies found that dopamine did not prevent mortality, the onset of ARF, or the need for hemodialysis.[201] The impact of dopamine on clinical outcomes is not substantiated.

The routine use of dopamine for renal protection has fallen out of favor because of the lack of benefit on patient outcomes in clinical trials. Dopamine use is not without risks. Adverse effects include tachycardia and arrhythmias, which can occur even at low doses. Its β-adrenergic effects can increase oxygen demand, leading to tissue hypoxia and ischemia. Dopamine is also associated with poor gastric emptying and gastroduodenal motility, aggravating digestive intolerance to enteral feedings; an impairment of respiratory drive, hindering weaning from mechanical ventilation; and suppression of secretion and function of anterior pituitary hormones.[202] Extravasation can occur if dopamine is administered peripherally.

Calcium Channel Blockers. After ischemic ARF, calcium channel blockers may protect against ARF by inhibiting vasoconstrictive responses of the afferent arterioles and increasing GFR. In addition, calcium antagonists may prevent damage from elevated intracellular calcium after hypoxic injury. These agents have been examined extensively in experimental ARF models, yet few clinical studies confirm their beneficial effects. In 12 patients with ARF, Lumlertgul et al.[203] compared verapamil (100 μg/minute intrarenally for 3 hours) and furosemide (0.8 mg/kg/hour intravenously for 24 hours) with control subjects receiving only furosemide. The verapamil-treated group was found to have a more rapid recovery of GFR. Also, in the setting of renal transplantation, verapamil improves early graft function when administered to donors before kidney procurement. Diltiazem has been shown to prevent cyclosporine-induced nephrotoxicity, as evidenced by an improvement in serum creatinine on discharge, and a decrease in the onset and duration of dialysis.[204] Other studies have also found benefits of calcium channel blockers in renal transplant patients.[205,206]

Atrial Natriuretic Peptide. Atrial natriuretic peptide (ANP) is a hormone synthesized by the cardiac atria that increases GFR by dilating afferent arterioles while constricting efferent arterioles. The hormone also inhibits tubular reabsorption of sodium and chloride, redistributes renal medullary blood flow, and disrupts tubuloglomerular feedback. Anaritide is a 25-amino acid synthetic form of ANP. In a randomized, controlled trial, anaritide did not improve overall dialysis-free survival in critically ill patients with ATN.[197] Subgroup analysis revealed that anaritide exhibited different effects depending on baseline urine output. Anaritide improved dialysis-free survival in patients with oliguria while worsening dialysis-free survival in nonoliguric patients, possibly by causing drug-induced hypotension. The literature does not support the use of ANP as therapy for ARF.

DRUG DOSING ISSUES

In patients with renal failure, a number of factors can affect drug absorption: uremic gastroparesis, changes in gastric pH, gut wall edema, and alterations in first-pass metabolism. It is also important to appreciate some pharmacodynamic changes likely to occur in renal failure. For example, because the sensitivity of β-receptors decreases in renal failure, it may be necessary to increase the propranolol dose despite

an increased bioavailability. In renal failure, the volume of distribution may change because of changes in body composition and decreased plasma protein binding. Plasma protein binding reduction is clinically significant for agents highly bound to albumin. This may occur secondary to hypoalbuminemia, drug displacement from binding sites on albumin by accumulated organic acids, and diminished drug affinity by albumin. With reduced plasma protein binding, a higher therapeutic free (active) serum concentration occurs at a lower total serum concentration. Tissue binding may be reduced in renal failure. Altered tissue binding can affect drugs like digoxin, which has extensive tissue binding but little plasma protein binding. Decreased tissue binding will lower the volume of distribution. Therefore, a standard loading dose will produce a higher drug level and a greater pharmacologic effect. In addition, renal failure may increase or decrease nonrenal (hepatic) drug clearance and decrease renal drug metabolism and excretion. Finally, the degree to which a drug is removed via dialysis determines whether a supplemental dose is necessary.

Changes in renal function make it necessary to alter the dose or dosing interval for drugs excreted by the kidney. Renal insufficiency influences drug disposition through changes in drug bioavailability, reduced protein binding, altered apparent volume of distribution, and altered renal metabolism. Tailoring regimens to targeted drug concentrations and monitoring free or unbound concentrations may minimize risks of drug toxicity associated with renal failure.[207] For more extensive reviews, see Chapter 1 and the comprehensive tables published by Bennett[208] and Benet.[209,210]

Dosing guidelines have also been established for use in patients receiving intermittent hemodialysis or continuous renal replacement therapy.[211–213] However, many of these recommendations were determined in patients with chronic renal failure, and for drugs with significant nonrenal clearance (which may be preserved in ARF) it may be necessary to distinguish between acute and chronic renal failure. Drug clearance in conventional intermittent hemodialysis therapies is substantially different from that in continuous renal replacement therapy (hemofiltration). Dosing becomes even more complicated when newer renal replacement techniques are used that combine diffusive and convective drug loss. A more complete discussion of estimating clearance by dialysis appears in Chapter 44.

NUTRITIONAL SUPPORT

With renal failure, the kidney can no longer regenerate bicarbonate, and metabolic acidosis ensues. This acidosis accelerates proteolysis and branched-chain amino acid oxidation and can be corrected with sodium bicarbonate.[214] ARF in the setting of multiple organ failure is associated with lean body mass catabolism, malnutrition, and a high rate of mortality.[215] Attempting to enhance patient outcomes through nutritional support remains controversial. An early clinical study showed greater survival rates and enhanced recovery of renal function in patients receiving small doses of essential amino acids plus glucose than in patients receiving glucose alone.[216] Subsequent studies suggested that such supplementation might improve renal function and patient outcomes, but these results are not conclusive.

Unfortunately, the dietary restrictions needed to manage ARF may offset efforts to optimize nutritional support, and the possible benefits of avoiding short-term dialysis must be weighed against the potential increase in morbidity and mortality caused by impaired nutrition. The need for nutrition support varies according to the patient's nutritional status, degree of hypercatabolism, GFR, clinical condition, and plans for dialysis or ultrafiltration therapy. For example, very-low-protein diets (0.3 to 0.5 g essential amino acids/kg/day) have been advocated to prevent uremia and avoid dialysis in nonhypercatabolic patients with ARF and little or no protein depletion.[217] However, this essential amino acid regimen remains controversial, and this level of protein restriction is not recommended for more than 2 weeks. In the nonhypercatabolic patient with better residual renal function (i.e., GFR >10 mL/min), a mixture of essential and nonessential amino acids or protein may be provided at 0.6 to 0.8 g/kg/day. Amino acid or protein needs may be considerably higher in very ill or severely wasted hypercatabolic patients with ARF who are expected to need dialysis. Generally about 1.2 g amino acids/kg/day is prescribed for patients receiving intermittent hemodialysis, and protein needs may even be higher in patients receiving continuous renal replacement therapy. Parenteral nutrition often is necessary in patients with ARF, but the composition of the solution must be modified in accordance with the loss of renal function. In general, most clinicians agree that patients who are severely ill do better if they are given sufficient caloric intake (25 to 35 kcal/kg/day) to attenuate gluconeogenesis and minimize negative nitrogen balance. This can be provided with parenteral formulations. The biggest limitation of parenteral nutrition in patients with acute renal failure is fluid volume. Also, parenteral nutrition is more expensive than enteral nutrition. Although there are published studies evaluating enteral nutrition in patients with chronic renal failure on hemodialysis, these studies are lacking in ARF patients. Fiacccadori et al. conducted a study to determine the safety and efficacy of enteral nutrition in patients with ARF and concluded that enteral nutrition is a safe alternative method to provide nutrition in ARF.[218] However, patients on renal replacement therapy will require both enteral and parenteral nutrition to meet the recommended protein requirements. Again, the method of nutritional support in ARF should be determined by individual patient needs and monitored closely. Use of renal replacement therapy can substantially reduce the nutrient composition of nutrition regimens provided in ARF. In patients on continuous renal replacement, measurable amounts of vitamin C, copper, and chromium can be found in the ultrafiltrate. Therefore, supplementation with water-soluble vitamins and selected trace elements may be necessary in this patient population.[219] For further discussion of nutrition needs in ARF, see Chapter 29.

RENAL REPLACEMENT THERAPY

The early use of dialysis to treat ARF has been associated with increased survival. A small prospective study of casualties during the Vietnam War showed that patients whose BUN was maintained at less than 18 mmol per L (50 mg/dL) and whose SCr concentration was maintained at less than 442 (5 mg/dL) had a mortality rate of 37%, whereas those given dialysis for a BUN greater than 43 mmol per L (120 mg/dL) and SCr concentration greater than 884 μmol per L (10 mg/dL) had a mortality rate of 80%.[220] It is postulated that early dialysis provides a better biochemical environment for fighting infections and for wound healing. Intermittent hemodialysis, peritoneal dialysis, or continuous renal replacement therapy may be indicated in patients with neurologic signs and symptoms of uremia, severe hyperkalemia, volume overload, or severe acidosis.

For the past several decades, intermittent hemodialysis has been the conventional renal replacement therapy for severe ARF. Continuously administered (e.g., venovenous hemofiltration or hemodiafiltration) renal replacement therapies have emerged. The advantages of continuous renal replacement therapy over intermittent hemodialysis include more precise fluid and metabolic control, less hemodynamic instability, better removal of harmful cytokines, and the ability to deliver unlimited nutritional support. The drawbacks to continuous renal replacement therapy include the need for prolonged anticoagulation, and the procedure entails constant sophisticated surveillance. Continuous renal replacement therapy is reserved for critically ill patients with renal failure.

In ARF, the role of renal replacement therapy is to prevent complications of ARF and to provide temporary support until the renal insufficiency resolves. The decision to initiate dialysis and the frequency of dialysis should be based on the patient's clinical condition rather than a particular BUN or SCr. There is no consensus on the timing with dialysis intervention in ARF. Absolute indications for dialysis are pericarditis and uremic symptoms, because these can be resolved only by dialysis. Relative indications include volume overload, hyperkalemia, and acidosis. In these cases, dialysis should be instituted when other conservative approaches have failed or are impractical. Indications for dialytic intervention are summarized in Table 42.18.[221] In general, a reasonable goal is to maintain predialysis BUN at less than

TABLE 42.18	Indications for Renal Replacement Therapy "A E I O U"

Acid–base abnormalities (metabolic acidosis)

Electrolyte imbalance (hyperphosphatemia, hyperkalemia, hypermagnesemia)

Intoxications (lithium, methanol, theophylline)

Overload (fluid)

Uremia (maintenance of blood urea nitrogen <100 mg/dL)

29 mmol per L (80 mg/dL). Further details of the dialysis prescription are beyond the scope of this discussion and are covered in greater detail in Chapter 44.

FUTURE THERAPIES

Many experimental therapies have been explored for the treatment and prevention of acute renal injury. Different biomarkers have been studied in in vivo and in vitro models with both disappointing and promising results. These include various cytokines, growth factors, cell adhesion molecules, and several miscellaneous substances.

CYTOKINES

Anti-inflammatory cytokines have been shown to decrease acute renal insult in animal and human studies. Interleukin-10 (IL-10), a potent anti-inflammatory cytokine, may protect against renal ischemia and cisplatin-induced injury and may have a role in the treatment of acute renal failure in the future.[222]

GROWTH FACTORS

Renal regeneration to restore structural injury and renal function starts immediately after an acute renal insult. Several mitogenic growth factors, including epidermal growth factor, transforming growth factor-α, insulin-like growth factor, and hepatocyte growth factor, have been shown to promote regeneration of tubular cells.[152] When administered to animals subjected to ischemic renal injury, epidermal growth factor, insulin-like growth factor, and hepatocyte growth factor reduced the extent of kidney damage and accelerated recovery of renal function. On the basis of these animal data, various clinical trials evaluating the efficacy of insulin-like growth factor in ARF have been performed, with differing results.[223–225] Insulin-like growth factor may increase creatinine clearance in patients with less severe renal injury who do not need renal replacement therapy.[223]

INTRACELLULAR ADHESION MOLECULES

Intracellular adhesion molecule-1 (ICAM-1) mediates ischemic ARF by potentiating the adhesion of neutrophils to endothelial cells, resulting in tissue damage. Increased systemic levels of tumor necrosis factor and interleukin-1 may upregulate ICAM-1 after ischemia and reperfusion injury.[226] Administering a monoclonal antibody against ICAM-1 protects animals from ischemic ARF, even when it is given 2 hours after the ischemic event.[227] However, antibodies against ICAM-1 and leukocyte function associated antigen-1 (LFA-1) do not protect the rat kidney against toxic renal injury.[228]

IMPROVING OUTCOMES

Despite major advances in dialysis and intensive care, the mortality rate associated with ARF continues to be high, probably because the age of these patients continues to rise and coexisting illnesses are increasingly common. Therefore, clinicians should focus on preventing ARF. Identifying risk factors for developing ARF is the first step (see Table 42.16). Preventing postsurgical ARF begins with preoperative risk assessment and optimizing volume status. Avoiding intraoperative volume depletion, hypotension, and nephrotoxic agents is also an important preventive measure. Aggressive intravascular volume restoration reduces the incidence of ATN after trauma. Adequate hydration and high urinary flow rates protect against toxicity from chemotherapeutic agents.

In 1996, the French Study Group on ARF[137] identified the following seven variables that predicted ARF death in 20 French ICUs: advanced age, poor health before admission, hospitalization before ICU admission, development of ARF later in the ICU admission (as compared to early on), sepsis, oliguria, and elevated initial disease severity score. These same factors have been identified in almost every trial of this type and suggest that extra vigilance is needed when treating patients with these characteristics.[15,25]

BIOCOMPATIBLE MEMBRANES

The choice of dialysis membrane in ARF may affect morbidity and mortality. Cellulose-based membranes lead to activation of the alternative pathway of complement.[229] This can upregulate leukocyte adhesion molecules and aggravate tissue damage in ischemic kidneys. The inflammatory response can occur in the lungs as well as other organs. This can result in hemodynamic changes and hypersensitivity-like reactions during dialysis.

Cellulose-based membranes are classified as unsubstituted (cuprophane) membranes and substituted (cellulose acetate and cellulose diacetate) membranes. Unsubstituted cuprophane membranes are composed of chains of glucosan rings and free hydroxyl groups. Substituted cellulose membranes are obtained through chemical bonding of material (acetate) to the free hydroxyl groups. Cellulosynthetic membranes are produced by adding a synthetic material to liquefied cellulose. Synthetic membranes (e.g., polyacrylonitrile, polymethylmethacrylate, and polysulfone) activate complement to a lesser extent than cuprophane membranes.

Improved patient survival and more rapid recovery of renal function occurred when dialysis was performed using the biocompatible (polymethylmethacrylate) membranes compared to cuprophane.[230] Dialysis with biocompatible membranes has also been shown to result in better rates of survival and renal function recovery.[231,232] In a meta-analysis, synthetic membranes conferred a significant survival advantage over cellulose-based membranes.[233] Sensitivity analysis showed that specifically unsubstituted cellulose (cuprophane) membranes had a negative impact on survival.

INTERMITTENT HEMODIALYSIS VERSUS CONTINUOUS RENAL REPLACEMENT THERAPY

Intermittent hemodialysis is the most widely used renal replacement method for ARF. However, it has been suggested that decreased urine output, hypotensive episodes, and complement activation may perpetuate renal injury and delay renal function recovery in patients with ARF occurring during intermittent hemodialysis.[181] Removal of excess volume and urea may decrease urine output and increase the workload of the remaining functional nephrons (fractional reabsorption) and predispose the patient to worsening of tubular obstruction. In addition, hypotension further compromises RBF, which may cause further ischemic insults in the kidney. Furthermore, bioincompatible (cellulose) membranes used for conventional intermittent hemodialysis may activate the complement system and lead to mobilization of neutrophils, which infiltrate the kidney and prolong ATN.

Patients who are hemodynamically unstable, such as those with sepsis, are not suitable candidates for intermittent hemodialysis. Continuous renal replacement therapy is preferred in patients whose major complication is fluid overload, those who need ongoing administration of large volumes of fluids, or those whose blood pressure is unstable. However, continuous renal replacement therapy requires meticulous monitoring and is associated with complications related to access, anticoagulation, lack of portability, and higher costs.[221,234] The need for anticoagulation and the resultant hemorrhagic risk are significant disadvantages of either method of dialysis. More importantly, clinical trials have not demonstrated a survival advantage of continuous renal replacement therapy over intermittent hemodialysis in ICU ARF patients.[235,236] It is often pointed out that mortality from ARF remains high despite recent improvements in therapy. Dialysis techniques are discussed extensively in Chapter 44.

CONCLUSION

The normal kidney is a remarkable organ that maintains the internal environment of the body by regulating body fluid volume, electrolyte composition, acid–base balance, and hormone and enzyme production. Although it is highly vulnerable to a variety of toxins, the kidney has the unique ability to regenerate new tubular cells and often recover from iatrogenic misadventures. Many therapeutic approaches have been undertaken to prevent ischemic or nephrotoxic renal injury and, once ARF has developed, to enhance renal function recovery and reduce mortality. Unfortunately, data supporting the efficacy of many of these interventions are inadequate, probably because ARF has a wide spectrum of causes, often occurs along with other comorbid factors, and it occurs with varying severity and in a variety of clinical settings, and controlled studies are difficult to perform particularly when the mortality rate of a disorder approaches 50%. The goals of management are to remove underlying causes, prevent associated complications, provide symptomatic care, and normalize the internal environment through dietary restriction, drugs, and dialysis.

KEY POINTS

■ Prevention is the best treatment for ARF. To date, conventional therapy offers little benefit to patients with established ARF (i.e., mortality remains high and renal function recovery cannot be improved)
■ Early recognition and management of prerenal ARF is important in preventing progression to ATN
■ In nearly every epidemiologic study of ARF, patients with nonoliguric ARF have a significantly lower mortality rate than anuric or oliguric patients. However, conversion from anuria or oliguria to nonoliguria does not improve mortality. Attempts to increase urine output may avoid complications of a fluid overload state and may make patient management easier
■ Maintaining euvolemia is essential in treating established ARF
■ In ARF, appropriate dose adjustments are required for drugs that are renally cleared
■ Nephrotoxic drugs should be avoided; alternative agents should be used whenever possible (e.g., substitute a third-generation cephalosporin for an aminoglycoside)
■ When nephrotoxins must be administered, hydration can improve renal perfusion and reduce tubular workload
■ When necessary, renal replacement therapy is used to support the patient awaiting renal function recovery. When selecting dosing regimens, the clinician must account for drug removal during renal replacement therapy

SUGGESTED READINGS

Dishart MK, Kellum JA. An evaluation of pharmacological strategies for the prevention and treatment of acute renal failure. Drugs 59:79–91, 2000.
Esson ML, Schrier RW. Diagnosis and treatment of acute tubular necrosis. Ann Intern Med 137:744–752, 2002.
Rossert J. Drug-induced acute interstitial nephritis. Kidney Int 60: 804–817, 2001.

REFERENCES

1. Thadhani R, Pascual M, Bonventre JV. Acute renal failure. N Engl J Med 334:1448–1460, 1996.
2. Nissenson AR. Acute renal failure. Kidney Int 53:S7–S10, 1998.
3. Kellum JA, Levin N, Bouman C, et al. Developing a consensus classification system for acute renal failure. Curr Opin Crit Care 8:509–514, 2002.
4. Bellomo R, Kellum JA, Mehta R, et al. Acute Dialysis Quality Initiative II: the Vicenza conference. Curr Opin Crit Care 8:505–508, 2002.
5. Esson ML, Schrier RW. Diagnosis and treatment of acute tubular necrosis. Ann Intern Med 137:744–752, 2002.
6. Singri N, Ahya SN, Levin ML. Acute renal failure. J Am Med Wom Assoc 289:747–751, 2003.
7. Nash K, Hafeez A, Hou S. Hospital-acquired renal insufficiency. Am J Kidney Dis 39:930–936, 2002.
8. Hou SH, Bushinsky DA, Wish DB, et al. Hospital-acquired renal insufficiency: a prospective study. Am J Med 74:243–248, 1983.

9. Levey AS, Bosch JP, Lewis JB, et al. A more accurate method to estimate glomerular filtration rate from serum creatinine: a new prediction equation. Ann Intern Med 130:461–470, 1999.

10. Levey AS, Coresh J, Balk E, et al. National Kidney Foundation practice guidelines for chronic kidney disease: evaluation, classification, and stratification. Ann Intern Med 139:137–147, 2003.

11. Anderson RJ, Linas RL, Berns AS, et al. Nonoliguric acute renal failure. N Engl J Med 296:1134–1138, 1977.

12. Dishart MK, Kellum JA. An evaluation of pharmacological strategies for the prevention and treatment of acute renal failure. Drugs 59:79–91, 2000.

13. Conger JD, Schrier RW. Renal hemodynamics in acute renal failure. Annu Rev Physiol 42:603–614, 1980.

14. Pascual J, Liano F, Ortuno J. The elderly patient with acute renal failure. J Am Soc Nephrol 6:144–153, 1995.

15. Bullock ML, Umen AJ, Finkelstein M, et al. The assessment of risk factors in 462 patients with acute renal failure. Am J Kidney Dis 5:97–103, 1985.

16. Perazella MA. Crystal-induced acute renal failure. Am J Med 106:459–465, 1999.

17. Conger JD, Anderson RJ, Schrier RW, et al. Acute renal failure. In: Schrier RW, ed. Renal and electrolyte disorders. Boston: Little Brown, 1996:1069–1113.

18. Finn WF. Recovery from acute renal failure. In: Lazarus JM, Brenner BM, eds. Acute renal failure. 3rd ed. New York: Churchill Livingstone, 1993:553–596.

19. Liano F, Pascual J. Epidemiology of acute renal failure: a prospective, multicenter, community-based study. Kidney Int 50:811–818, 1996.

20. Matzke GR, Millikin SP. Influence of renal function and dialysis on drug disposition. In: Evans WE, Schentag JJ, Jusko WJ, eds. Applied pharmacokinetics: principles of therapeutic drug monitoring. 3rd ed. Vancouver: Applied Therapeutics, 1992: 8-1–8-49.

21. Duggin GG. Mechanisms in the development of analgesic nephropathy. Kidney Int 18:553–561, 1980.

22. Myers BD, Moran SM. Hemodynamically mediated acute renal failure. N Engl J Med 314:97–105, 1986.

23. Stein JH, Fried TA. Experimental models of nephrotoxic acute renal failure. Transplant Proc 17:72–80, 1985.

24. Solez K, Racusen LC, Olsen S. The pathology of drug nephrotoxicity. J Clin Pharmacol 23:484–490, 1983.

25. Rasmussen HH, Ibels LS. Acute renal failure. Multivariate analysis of causes and risk factors. Am J Med 73:211–218, 1982.

26. Fleury D, Vanhille P, Pallot IL, et al. Drug-induced acute renal failure: a preventable disease linked to drug misuse. Kidney Int 38:1238, 1990.

27. Antonovych TT. Drug-induced nephropathies. Pathol Annu 19(Pt 2):165–196, 1984.

28. Laberke HG. Drug-induced nephropathy, part II: tubulointerstitial lesions. In: Berry CL, ed. Current topics in pathology. New York: Springer-Verlag, 1980:1430–1496.

29. Revert L, Montoliu J. Acute interstitial nephritis. Semin Nephrol 8:82–88, 1988.

30. Rossert J. Drug-induced acute interstitial nephritis. Kidney Int 60:804–817, 2001.

31. Remuzzi G, Ruggenti P. The hemolytic-uremic syndrome. Kidney Int Suppl 53:S54–S57, 1998.

32. Moake JL, Byrnes JJ. Thrombotic microangiopathies associated with drugs and bone marrow transplantation. Hematol Oncol Clin North Am 10:485–497, 1996.

33. Majhail NS, Hix JK, Almahameed A. Carcinoma of the colon in a patient presenting with thrombotic thrombocytopenic purpura–hemolytic uremic syndrome. Mayo Clin Proc 77:873, 2002.

34. von Bubnoff N, Sandherr M, Schneller F, et al. Thrombotic thrombocytopenic purpura in metastatic carcinoma of the breast. Am J Clin Oncol 23:74–77, 2000.

35. Porta C, Danova M, Riccardi A, et al. Cancer chemotherapy-related thrombotic thrombocytopenic purpura; biological evidence of increased nitric oxide production. Mayo Clin Proc 74:570–574, 1999.

36. Young BA, Marsh CL, Alpers CE, et al. Cyclosporine-associated thrombotic microangiopathic/hemolytic uremic syndrome following kidney and kidney–pancreas transplantation. Am J Kidney Dis 28:561–571, 1996.

37. Robson M, Cote I, Abbs I, et al. Thrombotic microangiopathy with sirolimus-based immunosuppression: potentiation of calcineurin-inhibitor–induced endothelial damage? Am J Transplant 3:324–327, 2003.

38. Lin CC, King KL, Chao YW, et al. Tacrolimus-associated hemolytic uremic syndrome: a case analysis. J Nephrol 16:580–585, 2003.

39. Schmidt R, Venkat K, Dumler F. Hemolytic-uremic syndrome in a renal transplant recipient on FK 506 immunosuppression. Transplant Proc 7:382–384, 1991.

40. Pisoni R, Ruggenti P, Remuzzi G. Drug-induced thrombotic microangiopathy. Incidence, prevention and management. Drug Saf 24:491–501, 2001.

41. Abdalla AH, Al-Sulaiman MH, Al-Khader AA. FK-506 as an alternative in cyclosporine-induced hemolytic uremia syndrome. Transplantation 59:1737–1739, 1994.

42. Kaufman DB, Kaplan B, Kanwar YS, et al. The successful use of tacrolimus (FK506) in a pancreas/kidney transplant patient with recurrent cyclosporine-associated hemolytic uremic syndrome. Transplantation 59:1737–1739, 1995.

43. Bennett WM, Elzinga LW, Porter GA. Tubulointerstitial disease and toxic nephropathy. In Brenner BM, ed. The kidney. 5th ed. Philadelphia: WB Saunders, 1996:1430–1496.

44. Matzke GR, Lucarotti RL, Shapiro HS. Controlled comparison of gentamicin and tobramycin nephrotoxicity. Am J Nephrol 3:11–17, 1983.

45. Sawyers CL, Moore RD, Lerner SA, et al. A model for predicting nephrotoxicity in patients treated with aminoglycosides. J Infect Dis 153:1062–1068, 1986.

46. Williams PJ, Hull JH, Sarubbi FA, et al. Factors associated with nephrotoxicity and clinical outcome in patients receiving amikacin. J Clin Pharmacol 26:79–86, 1986.

47. Johnson MW, Mitch WE, Heller AH, et al. The impact of an educational program on gentamicin use in a teaching program. Am J Med 73:9–14, 1982.

48. Garrison MW, Rotschafer JC. Clinical assessment of a published model to predict aminoglycoside-induced nephrotoxicity. Ther Drug Monit 11:171–175, 1989.

49. Contreras AM, Gamba G, Cortes J, et al. Serial trough and peak amikacin levels in plasma as predictors of nephrotoxicity. Antimicrob Agents Chemother 33:973–976, 1989.

50. Galloe AM, Graudal N, Christensen HR, et al. Aminoglycosides: single or multiple daily dosing? A meta-analysis on efficacy and safety. Eur J Clin Pharmacol 48:39–43, 1995.

51. Barza M, Ioannidis JP, Cappelleri JC, et al. Single or multiple daily doses of aminoglycosides: a meta-analysis. Br Med J 312:338–345, 1996.

52. Munckhof WJ, Grayson ML, Turnidge JD. A meta-analysis of studies on the safety and efficacy of aminoglycosides given either once daily or as divided doses. J Antimicrob Chemother 37:645–663, 1996.

53. Ferriols-Lisart R, Alos-Alminana M. Effectiveness and safety of once-daily aminoglycosides: a meta-analysis. Am J Health Syst Pharm 53:1141–1150, 1996.

54. Freeman CD, Strayer AH. Mega-analysis or meta-analysis: an examination of meta-analysis with an emphasis on once-daily aminoglycoside comparative trials. Pharmacotherapy 16:1093–1102, 1996.

55. Hatala R, Dinh T, Cook DJ. Once-daily aminoglycoside dosing in immunocompetent adults: a meta-analysis. Ann Intern Med 124:717–725, 1996.

56. Hatala R, Dinh TT, Cook DJ. Single daily dosing of aminoglycosides in immunocompromised adults: a systematic review. Clin Infect Dis 24:810–815, 1997.

57. Ali MZ, Goetz MB. A meta-analysis of the relative efficacy and toxicity of single daily dosing versus multiple daily dosing of aminoglycosides. Clin Infect Dis 24:796–809, 1997.

58. Bailey TC, Little JR, Littenberg B, et al. A meta-analysis of extended-interval dosing versus multiple daily dosing of aminoglycosides. Clin Infect Dis 24:786–795, 1997.

59. Rybak MJ, Abate BJ, Kang SL, et al. Prospective evaluation of the effect of an aminoglycoside dosing regimen on rates of observed nephrotoxicity and ototoxicity. Antimicrob Agents Chemother 43:1549–1555, 1999.

60. Karachaliou I, Halkiadaki D. Prospective randomized study of once-daily versus twice-daily amikacin regimens in patients with systemic infections. Int J Clin Pharmacol Ther 36:561–554, 1998.

61. Hitt CM, Klepser ME, Nightingale CH, et al. Pharmacoeconomic impact of once-daily aminoglycoside administration. Pharmacotherapy 17:810–814, 1997.

62. McCormack JP. An emotional-based medicine approach to monitoring once-daily aminoglycosides. Pharmacotherapy 20:1524–1527, 2000.

63. Stephan H, Pestotnik SL, Lloyd JF, et al. The epidemiology of nephrotoxicity associated with conventional amphotericin B therapy. Am J Med 111:528–534, 2001.

64. Bates DW, Su L, Yu DT, et al. Correlates of acute renal failure in patients receiving parenteral amphotericin B. Kidney Int 60:1452–1459, 2001.

65. Bates DW, Su L, Yu DT, et al. Mortality and costs of acute renal failure associated with amphotericin B therapy. Clin Infect Dis 32:686–693, 2001.

66. Llanos A, Cieza J, Bernardo J, et al. Effect of salt supplementation on amphotericin B nephrotoxicity. Kidney Int 40:302–308, 1991.

67. Heidemann HT, Gerkens JF, Spickard WA, et al. Amphotericin B nephrotoxicity in humans decreased by salt repletion. Am J Med 75:476–481, 1983.

68. Sacks P, Fellner SK. Recurrent reversible acute renal failure from amphotericin. Arch Intern Med 147:593–595, 1987.

69. Burdmann EA, Yu L, Andoh TF, et al. Calcineurin inhibitors and sirolimus. In: De Broe ME, Porter GA, Bennett WM, et al, eds. Clinical Nephrotoxins. 2d ed. Dordrecht: Kluwer Academic Publishers, 2003:403–458.

70. Kahan BD. Clinical summation. An algorithm for the management of patients with cyclosporine-induced renal dysfunction. Transplant Proc 17:303–308, 1985.

71. Neild GH, Taube HE, Hartley RB, et al. Morphological differentiation between rejection and cyclosporin nephrotoxicity in renal allografts. J Clin Pathol 39:152–159, 1986.

72. van Riemsdijk IC, Mulder PG, de Fijter JW, et al. Addition of isradipine (Lomir) results in a better renal function after kidney transplantation: a double-blind, randomized, placebo-controlled, multicenter study. Transplantation 70:122–126, 2000.

73. Rodicio JL. Calcium antagonists and renal protection from cyclosporine nephrotoxicity: long-term trial in renal transplantation patients. J Cardiovasc Pharmacol 35:S7–S11, 2000.

74. Inigo P, Campistol JM, Lario S, et al. Effects of losartan and amlodipine on intrarenal hemodynamics and TGF-β(1) plasma levels in a crossover trial in renal transplant recipients. J Am Soc Nephrol 12:822–827, 2001.

75. Mahalati K, Belitsky P, West K, et al. Approaching the therapeutic window for cyclosporine in kidney transplantation: a prospective study. J Am Soc Nephrol 12:828–833, 2001.

76. Luke RG, Greifer I. Posttransplant risks of cyclosporine nephrotoxicity. Am J Kidney Dis 5:342–342, 1985.

77. Whiting PH, Simpson JG. The enhancement of cyclosporine A included nephrotoxicity by gentamicin. Biochem Pharmacol 32:2025–2028, 1983.

78. Burckart GJ, Canafax DM, Yee GC. Cyclosporine monitoring. Drug Intell Clin Pharm 20:649–652, 1986.

79. Pescovitz MD, Govani M. Sirolimus and mycophenolate mofetil for calcineurin-free immunosuppression in renal transplant recipients. Am J Kidney Dis 38:S16–S21, 2001.

80. Rudnick MR, Goldfarb S, Wexler L, et al. Nephrotoxicity of ionic and nonionic contrast media in 1196 patients: a randomized trial. The Iohexol cooperative study. Kidney Int 47:254–261, 1995.

81. Moore RD, Steinberg EP, Powe NR, et al. Nephrotoxicity of high-osmolality versus low-osmolality contrast media: randomized clinical trial. Radiology 182:649–655, 1992.

82. Erley CM, Porter GA. Radiocontrast agents. In: De Broe ME, Porter GA, Bennett WM, et al, eds. Clinical Nephrotoxins. 2d ed. Dordrecht: Kluwer Academic Publishers, 2003:483–494.

83. Cigarroa RG, Lange RA, Williams RH, et al. Dosing of contrast material to prevent contrast nephropathy in patients with renal disease. Am J Med 86:649–652, 1989.

84. Manske CL, Sprafka JM, Strony JT, et al. Contrast nephropathy in azotemic diabetic patients undergoing coronary angiography. Am J Med 89:615–620, 1990.

85. McCarthy CS, Becker JA. Multiple myeloma and contrast media. Radiology 183:519–521, 1992.

86. Heyman SN, Rosen S, Brezis M. Radiocontrast nephropathy: a paradigm for the synergism between toxic and hypoxic insults in the kidney. Exp Nephrol 2:153–157, 1994.

87. Schwab SJ, Hlatky MA, Pieper KS, et al. Contrast nephrotoxicity: a randomized controlled trial of nonionic and an ionic radiographic contrast agent. N Engl J Med 320:149–153, 1989.

88. Katholi RE, Taylor GJ, Woods WT, et al. Nephrotoxicity of nonionic low-osmolality versus ionic high-osmolality contrast media: a prospective double-blind randomized comparison in human beings. Radiology 186:183–187, 1993.

89. Barrett BJ, Parfrey PS, Vavasour HM, et al. Contrast nephropathy in patients with impaired renal function: high versus low osmolar media. Kidney Int 41:1274–1279, 1992.

90. Barrett BJ, Parfrey PS, McDonald JR, et al. Nonionic low-osmolality versus ionic high-osmolality contrast material for intravenous use in patients perceived to be at high risk: randomized trial. Radiology 183:105–110, 1992.

91. Barrett BJ, Carlisle EJ. Metaanalysis of the relative nephrotoxicity of high- and low-osmolality iodinated contrast media. Radiology 188:171–178, 1993.

92. Aspelin P, Aubry P, Fransson S, et al. Nephrotoxic effects in high-risk patients undergoing angiography. N Engl J Med 348:491–499, 2003.

93. Steinberg EP, Moore RD, Powe N, et al. Safety and cost effectiveness of high-osmolality compared to low-osmolality contrast material in patients undergoing cardiac angiography. N Engl J Med 326:425–430, 1992.

94. Solomon R, Werner C, Mann D, et al. Effects of saline, mannitol, and furosemide on acute decreases in renal function induced by radiocontrast dye. N Engl J Med 331:1416–1420, 1994.

95. Atkins JL. Effect of sodium bicarbonate preloading on ischemic renal failure. Nephron 44:70–74, 1986.

96. Merten GJ, Burgess WP, Gray LV, et al. Prevention of contrast-induced nephropathy with sodium bicarbonate: a randomized controlled trial. JAMA 291:2328–2334, 2004.

97. Tepel M, Van Der Giet M, Schwarzfeld C, et al. Prevention of radiographic contrast-induced reductions in renal function by acetylcysteine. N Engl J Med 343:180–184, 2000.

98. Tumlin JA, Wang A, Murray PT, et al. Fenoldopam mesylate blocks reductions in renal plasma flow after radiocontrast dye infusion: a pilot trial in the prevention of contrast nephropathy. Am Heart J 143:894–903, 2002.

99. Shyu KG, Cheng JJ, Kuan P. Acetylcysteine protects against acute renal damage in patients with abnormal renal function undergoing a coronary procedure. J Am Coll Cardiol 40:1383–1388, 2002.

100. Diaz-Sandoval LJ, Kosowsky BD, Losordo DW. Acetylcysteine to prevent angiography-related renal tissue injury (the APART trial). Am J Cardiol 89:356–358, 2002.

101. Kay J, Chow WH, Chan TM, et al. Acetylcysteine for prevention of acute deterioration of renal function following elective coronary angiography and intervention. JAMA 289:553–558, 2003.

102. Walker PD, Brokering KL, Theobald JC. Fenoldopam and N-acetylcysteine for the prevention of radiographic contrast material-induced nephropathy: a review. Pharmacotherapy 23:1617–1626, 2003.

103. Hoffman U, Fischereder M, Kruger B, et al. The value of N-acetylcysteine in the prevention of radiocontrast agent-induced nephropathy seems questionable. J Am Soc Nephrol 15:407–410, 2004.

104. Kini AS, Mitre CA, Kim M, et al. A protocol for prevention of radiographic contrast nephropathy during percutaneous coronary intervention: effect of selective dopamine receptor agonist fenoldopam. Catheter Cardiovasc Interv 55:169–173, 2002.

105. Allaqaband S, Tumuluri R, Malik AM, et al. Prospective randomized study of N-acetylcysteine, fenoldopam, and saline for prevention of radiocontrast-induced nephropathy. Catheter Cardiovasc Interv 57:279–283, 2002.

106. Stone GW, McCullough PA, Tumlin JA, et al., for the CONTRAST Investigators. Fenoldopam mesylate for the prevention of contrast-induced nephropathy. A randomized controlled trial. JAMA 290:2284–2291, 2003.

107. Packer M. Identification of risk factors predisposing to the development of functional renal insufficiency during treatment with converting-enzyme inhibitors. Cardiology 76:50–55, 1989.

108. Textor S, Gephardt G, Bravo EL, et al. Membranous glomerulopathy associated with captopril therapy. Am J Med 74:705–711, 1983.

109. Lewis E, the Captopril Collaborative Study Group. Proteinuria and abnormalities of the renal glomerulus in patients with hypertension. Clin Exp Pharmacol Physiol 7:105–115, 1982.

110. Cahan D, Ucci A. Acute renal failure, interstitial nephritis, and nephrotic syndrome associated with captopril. Kidney Int 25:160, 1984.

111. Ahmed A. Use of angiotensin-converting inhibitors in patients with heart failure and renal insufficiency: how concerned should we be by the rise in serum creatinine? J Am Geriatr Soc 50:1297–1300, 2002.

112. Bakris G, Weir M. Angiotensin-converting enzyme inhibitor-associated elevations in serum creatinine. Is this a cause for concern? Arch Intern Med 160:685–693, 2000.

113. Palmer B. Angiotensin-converting enzyme inhibitors and angiotensin receptor blockers: what to do if the serum creatinine and/or serum potassium concentration rises? Nephrol Dial Transplant 18:1973–1975, 2003.

114. Perneger T, Whelton P, Klag M. Risk of kidney failure associated with use of acetaminophen, aspirin, and nonsteroidal antiinflammatory drugs. N Engl J Med 331:1675–1679, 1994.

115. Whelton A. Nephrotoxicity of nonsteroidal anti-inflammatory drugs: physiological foundations and clinical implications. Am J Med 106:13S–24S, 1991.

116. Brater D. Effects of nonsteroidal anti-inflammatory drugs on renal function: focus on cyclooxygenase-2-selective inhibition. Am J Med 107:65S–71S, 1999.

117. Whelton A, Hamilton C. Nonsteroidal anti-inflammatory drugs: effects on kidney function. J Clin Pharmacol 31:588–598, 1991.

118. Blackshear J, Napier J, Davidman M, et al. Renal complications of nonsteroidal anti-inflammatory drugs: identification and monitoring of those at risk. Semin Arthritis Rheum 14:163–175, 1985.

119. Ahmad S, Kortepeter C, Brinker A, et al. Renal failure associated with the use of celecoxib and rofecoxib. Drug Saf 25:537–544, 2002.

120. Perazella M, Eras J. Are selective COX-2 inhibitors nephrotoxic? Am J Kidney Dis 35:937–940, 2000.

121. Wolf G, Porth H, Stahl R. Acute renal failure associated with rofecoxib [letter]. Ann Intern Med 133:394, 2000.

122. Litterst CL. Alterations in the toxicity of cis-dichlorodiamine-platinum-II and in tissue localization of platinum as a function of NaCl concentration in the vehicle of administration. Toxicol Appl Pharmacol 61:99–108, 1981.

123. Finley RS, Fortner CL, Grove WR. Cisplatin nephrotoxicity: a summary of preventative interventions. Drug Intell Clin Pharm 19:326–327, 1985.

124. Hirosawa A, Niitani H, Hayashibara K, et al. Effects of sodium thiosulfate in combination therapy of cis-dichlorodiammine platinum and vindesine. Cancer Chemother Pharmacol 23:255–258, 1989.

125. Howell S, Pfeifle C, Wung W, et al. Intraperitoneal cisplatin with systemic thiosulfate protection. Ann Intern Med 97:845–851, 1982.

126. Clermont G, Acker CG, Angus DC, et al. Renal failure in the ICU: comparison of the impact of acute renal failure and end-stage renal disease on ICU outcomes. Kidney Int 62:986–996, 2002.

127. de Medonca A, Vincent JL, Suter PM, et al. Acute renal failure in the ICU: risk factors and outcome evaluated by the SOFA score. Intens Care Med 26:915–921, 2000.

128. Guerin C, Girard R, Selli JM, et al. Initial versus delayed acute renal failure in the intensive care unit. Am J Respir Crit Care Med 161:872–879, 2000.

129. Feest TG, Round A, Hamad S. Incidence of severe acute renal failure in adults: results of a community-based study. Br Med J 306:481–483, 1993.

130. Obialo CI, Okonofua EC, Tayade AS, et al. Epidemiology of de novo acute renal failure in hospitalized African Americans. Arch Intern Med 160:1309–1313, 2000.

131. Lins RL, Elseviers M, Daelemans R, et al. Prognostic value of a new scoring system for hospital mortality in acute renal failure. Clin Nephrol 53:10–17, 2000.

132. Avasthi G, Sandhu JS, Mohindra K. Acute renal failure in medical and surgical intensive care units: a one-year prospective study. Ren Fail 25:105–113, 2003.

133. Hoste EAJ, Lameire NH, Vanholder RC, et al. Acute renal failure in patients with sepsis in a surgical ICU: predictive factors, incidence, comorbidity, and outcome. J Am Soc Nephrol 14:1022–1030, 2003.

134. Silvester W, Bellomo R, Cole L. Epidemiology, management, and outcome of severe acute renal failure of critical illness in Australia. Crit Care Med 29:1910–1915, 2001.

135. Korkeila M, Ruokonen E, Takala J. Costs of care, long-term prognosis and quality of life in patients requiring renal replacement therapy during intensive care. Intens Care Med 26:1824–1831, 2000.

136. Cole L, Bellomo R, Silvester W, et al. A prospective, multicenter study of the epidemiology, management, and outcome of severe acute renal failure in a ''closed'' ICU system. Am J Respir Crit Care Med 162:191–196, 2000.

137. Brivet FG, Kleinknecht DJ, Loirat P, et al. Acute renal failure in intensive care units: causes, outcome, and prognostic factors of hospital mortality: a prospective, multicenter study. Crit Care Med 24:192–198, 1996.

138. van Bommel EF, Leunissen KM, Weimar W. Continuous renal replacement therapy for the critically ill: an update. J Intens Care Med 9:265–280, 1994.

139. Elasy TA, Anderson RJ. Changing demography of acute renal failure. Semin Dial 9:438–443, 1996.

140. Brady HR, Brenner BM, Lieberthal W. Acute renal failure. In: Brenner BM, ed. The kidney. 5th ed. Philadelphia: WB Saunders, 1996:1200–1252.

141. Galler M, Folkert VW, Schlondorff D. Reversible acute renal insufficiency and hyperkalemia following indomethacin therapy. JAMA 246:154–155, 1981.

142. Grunfeld JP, Ganeval D, Bournerias F. Acute renal failure in pregnancy. Kidney Int 18:179–191, 1980.

143. Auguste LJ, Stone AM, Wise L. The effects of Escherichia coli bacteremia on in vitro perfused kidneys. Ann Surg 192:65–68, 1980.

144. Trifillis AL, Kahng MW, Trump BF. Metabolic studies of glycerol-induced acute renal failure in the rat. Exp Mol Pathol 35:1–13, 1981.

145. Weinberg JM. The cell biology of ischemic renal injury. Kidney Int 39:476–500, 1991.

146. Siegel N, Avison MJ, Reilly HF, et al. Enhanced recovery of renal ATP with postischemic infusion of ATP-$MgCl_2$ determined by ^{31}P. Am J Physiol 245:F530–F534, 1983.

147. Shanley PF, Brezis M, Spokes K, et al. Transport-dependent cell injury in the S3 segment of the proximal tubule. Kidney Int 29:1033–1037, 1986.

148. Brezis M, Shina A, Kidroni G, et al. Calcium and hypoxic injury in the renal medulla of the perfused rat kidney. Kidney Int 34:186–194, 1988.

149. Paller MS, Hoidal JR, Ferris TF. Oxygen free radicals in ischemic acute renal failure in the rat. J Clin Invest 74:1156–1164, 1984.

150. Conger JD, Brinner VA, Schrier RW. Acute renal failure: pathogenesis, diagnosis, and management. In: Schrier RW, ed. Renal and Electrolyte Disorders. 4th ed. Boston: Little Brown, 1992.

151. Humes HD, Cieslinski DA, Coimbra TM, et al. Epidermal growth factor enhances renal tubule cell regeneration and repair and accelerates the recovery of renal function in postischemic acute renal failure. J Clin Invest 84:1757–1761, 1989.

152. Schena FP. Role of growth factors in acute renal failure. Kidney Int Suppl 53:S11–S15, 1998.

153. Lake EW, Humes HD. Acute renal failure: directed therapy to enhance renal tubular regeneration. Semin Nephrol 14:83–97, 1989.

154. Young DS. Effects of drugs on clinical laboratory tests. 3rd ed. Washington DC: American Association of Clinical Chemistry, 1990.

155. Friedman RB, Young DS. Effects of disease on clinical laboratory tests. 2d ed. Washington DC: American Association of Clinical Chemistry, 1990.

156. Kaysen GA. Proteinuria and the nephrotic syndrome. In: Schrier RW, ed. Renal and Electrolyte Disorders. Boston: Little, Brown, 1992:681–726.

157. Ginsberg JM, Chang BS, Matarese RA, et al. Use of single voided urine samples to estimate quantitative proteinuria. N Engl J Med 309:1543–1546, 1983.

158. Schwab SJ, Christensen RL, Dougherty K, et al. Quantitation of proteinuria by the use of protein-to-creatinine ratios in single urine samples. Arch Intern Med 147:943–944, 1987.

159. Chahar OP, Bundella B, Chahar CK, et al. Quantitation of proteinuria by use of single random spot urine collection. J Indian Med Assoc 91:86–87, 1993.

160. Iyer RS, Shailaja SN, Bhaskaranand N, et al. Quantitation of proteinuria using protein-creatinine ratio in random urine samples. Indian Pediatr 28:463–467, 1991.

161. Rodby RA, Rohde RD, Sharon Z, et al. The urine protein to creatinine ratio as a predictor of 24-hour urine protein excretion in type 1 diabetic patients with nephropathy. The Collaborative Study Group. Am J Kidney Dis 26:904–909, 1995.

162. Chitalia VC, Kothari J, Wells EJ, et al. Cost–benefit analysis and prediction of 24-hour proteinuria from the spot urine protein-creatinine ratio. Clin Nephrol 55:436–447, 2001.

163. Mann HJ, Fuhs DW, Hemstrom CA. Acute renal failure. Drug Intell Clin Pharm 20:421–438, 1986.

164. Alleyne GA, Millward D, Scullard GH. Total body potassium, muscle electrolytes, and glycogen in malnourished children. J Pediatr 76:75–781, 1970.

165. Bjornsson TD. Use of serum creatinine concentrations to determine renal function. New York: ADIS Press, 1983.

166. Walser M, Drew HH, LaFrance ND. Creatinine measurements often yield false estimates of progression of chronic renal failure. Kidney Int 34:412–418, 1988.

167. Cockroft DW, Gault MH. Prediction of creatinine clearance from serum creatinine. Nephron 16:31–41, 1976.

168. Goldberg TH, Finklestein MS. Difficulties in estimating glomerular filtration rate in the elderly. Arch Intern Med 147:461–463, 1987.

169. Hatton J, Parr MD, Blouin RA. Estimation of creatinine clearance in patients with Cushing syndrome. Ann Pharmacother 23: 974–977, 1989.

170. Hull JH, Hak LJ, Koch CG. Influence of range of renal function and liver disease on predictability of creatinine clearance. Clin Pharmacol Ther 29:516–521, 1981.

171. Siest G, Galteau MM. Drug effects on laboratory test results. St. Louis: Year Book, 1988.

172. Levinsky NG, Bernard DB. Mannitol and loop diuretics in acute renal failure. In: Brenner BM, Lazarus JM, eds. Acute renal failure. New York: Churchill Livingstone, 1988:841–856.

173. Conger JD. Interventions in clinical acute renal failure: what are the data? Am J Kidney Dis 26:565–576, 1995.

174. Better OS, Stein JH. Early management of shock and prophylaxis of acute renal failure in traumatic rhabdomyolysis. N Engl J Med 322:825–829, 1990.

175. Brater DC. Diuretic therapy. N Engl J Med 339:387–395, 1998.

176. Majumdar S, Kjellstrand CM. Why do we use diuretics in acute renal failure? Semin Dial 9:454–459, 1996.

177. Risler T, Kramer B, Muller GA. The efficacy of diuretics in acute and chronic renal failure. Focus on torasemide. Drugs 41(Suppl 3): 69–79, 1991.

178. Shilliday IR, Quinn KJ, Allison ME. Loop diuretics in the management of acute renal failure: a prospective, double-blind, placebo-controlled, randomized study. Nephrol Dial Transplant 12: 2592–2596, 1997.

179. Weinstein JM, Heyman S, Brezis M. Potential deleterious effect of furosemide in radiocontrast nephropathy. Nephron 62:413–415, 1992.

180. Schetz M. Should we use diuretics in acute renal failure? Best Pract Res Clin Anaesthesiol 18:75–89, 2004.

181. Klahr S, Miller SB. Acute oliguria. N Engl J Med 338:671–675, 1998.

182. Yellton S, Gaylor M, Murray K. The role of continuous infusion loop diuretics. Ann Pharmacother 29:75–89, 1995.

183. Rudy DW, Voelker JR, Greene PK, et al. Loop diuretics for chronic renal insufficiency: a continuous infusion is more efficacious than bolus therapy. Ann Intern Med 115:360–366, 1991.

184. Ellison DH. The physiologic basis of diuretic synergism: its role in treating diuretic resistance. Ann Intern Med 114:886–894, 1991.

185. Ellison DH. Diuretic drugs and the treatment of edema: from clinic to bench and back again. Am J Kidney Dis 23:623–643, 1994.

186. Fliser D, Schroter M, Neubeck M, et al. Coadministration of thiazides increases the efficacy of loop diuretics even in patients with advanced renal failure. Kidney Int 46:482–488, 1994.

187. Witte MK, Stork JE, Blumer JL. Diuretic therapeutics in the pediatric patient. Am J Cardiol 57:44A–53A, 1986.

188. Wells TG. The pharmacology and therapeutics of diuretics in the pediatric patient. Pediatr Clin North Am 37:463–504, 1990.

189. Goldberg LI, McDonald RH, Zimmerman AM. Sodium diuresis produced by dopamine in patients with congestive heart failure. N Engl J Med 269:1060–1064, 1963.

190. Henderson IS, Beattie TJ, Kennedy AC. Dopamine hydrochloride in oliguric states. Lancet 2:827–829, 1980.

191. Parker S, Carlon GC, Isaacs M, et al. Dopamine administration in oliguria and oliguric renal failure. Crit Care Med 9:630–632, 1981.

192. Lindner A. Synergism of dopamine and furosemide in diuretic resistant oliguric acute renal failure. Nephron 33:121–126, 1983.

193. Graziani G, Cantaluppi, A, Casati, S, et al. Dopamine and frusemide in oliguric acute renal failure. Nephron 37:39–42, 1984.

194. Weisberg LS, Kurnik PB, Kurnik BR. Dopamine and renal blood flow in radiocontrast-induced nephropathy in humans. Ren Fail 15: 61–68, 1993.

195. Duke GJ, Briedis JH, Weaver RA. Renal support in critically ill patients: low-dose dopamine or low-dose dobutamine? Crit Care Med 22:1919–1925, 1994.

196. Denton MD, Chertow GM, Brady HR. ''Renal-dose'' dopamine for the treatment of acute renal failure: scientific rationale, experimental studies and clinical trials. Kidney Int 50:4–14, 1996.

197. Allgren RL, Marbury TC, Rahman SN, et al. Anaritide in acute tubular necrosis. Auriculin Anaritide Acute Renal Failure Study Group. N Engl J Med 336:828–834, 1997.

198. Chertow GM, Sayegh MH, Allgren RL, et al. Is the administration of dopamine associated with adverse or favorable outcomes in acute renal failure? Auriculin Anaritide Acute Renal Failure Study Group. Am J Med 101:49–53, 1996.

199. Marik PE, Iglesias J. Low-dose dopamine does not prevent acute renal failure in patients with septic shock and oliguria. NORA-SEPT II Study Investigators. Am J Med 107:387–390, 1999.

200. Bellomo R, Chapman M, Finfer S, et al. Low-dose dopamine in patients with early renal dysfunction: a placebo-controlled randomised trial. Australian and New Zealand Intensive Care Society (AN-ZICS) Clinical Trials Group. Lancet 356:2139–2143, 2000.

201. Kellum JA, M Decker J. Use of dopamine in acute renal failure: a meta-analysis. Crit Care Med 29:1526–1531, 2001.

202. Debaveye YA, Van den Berghe GH. Is there still a place for dopamine in the modern intensive care unit? Anesth Analg 98:461–468, 2004.

203. Lumlertgul D, Hutdagoon P, Sirivanichai C, et al. Beneficial effect of intrarenal verapamil in human acute renal failure. Ren Fail 11: 201–208, 1989.

204. Tenschert W, Harfmann P, Meyer-Moldenhauer WH, et al. Kidney protective effect of diltiazem after renal transplantation with long cold ischemia time and triple-drug immunosuppression. Transplant Proc 23:1334–1335, 1991.

205. Donnelly PK, Feehally J, Jurewicz A, et al. Renal transplantation: nifedipine for the nonstarters? A prospective randomised study. Transplant Proc 25:600–601, 1993.

206. Barenbrock M, Colmorgen U, Firschka E, et al. A multicenter, randomized, double-blind, placebo-controlled, two-year trial to study the effect of nitrendipine on chronic renal transplant function. Clin Nephrol 43:388–391, 1995.

207. Toto RD. Approach to the patient with acute renal failure. In: Greenberg A, ed. Primer on Kidney Diseases. San Diego: Academic Press, 1998:253.

208. Bennett WM, Aronoff GR, Berns JS, et al. Drug prescribing in renal failure. 4th ed. Philadelphia: American College of Physicians, 1999.

209. Benet LZ, Williams RL. Design and optimization of dosage regimens: pharmacokinetic data. In: Gilman AG, Rall TW, Nies AS, et al, eds. The pharmacologic basis of therapeutics. 8th ed. New York: Pergamon, 1990:1650–1735.

210. Benet LZ, Massoud N. Pharmacokinetics. In: Benet LZ, Massoud N, Gambertoglio JG, eds. Pharmacokinetic basis for drug treatment. New York: Raven, 1984:1–28.

211. Bickley SK. Drug dosing during continuous arteriovenous hemofiltration. Clin Pharm 7:198–206, 1988.

212. Bressolle F, Kinowski JM, de la Coussaye JE, et al. Clinical pharmacokinetics during continuous haemofiltration. Clin Pharmacokinet 26:457–471, 1994.

213. Reetze-Bonorden P, Bohler J, Keller E. Drug dosage in patients during continuous renal replacement therapy. Pharmacokinetic and therapeutic considerations. Clin Pharmacokinet 24:362–379, 1993.

214. Hara Y, May RC, Kelly RA, et al. Acidosis, not azotemia, stimulates branched-chain, amino acid catabolism in uremic rats. Kidney Int 32:808–814, 1987.

215. Hak LJ. Nutrition in renal failure. In: Torosian MH, ed. Nutrition for the hospitalized patient: basic science and principles of practice. New York: Marcel Dekker, 1995:499–503.

216. Abel RM, Beck CH, Jr, Abbott WM, et al. Improved survival from acute renal failure after treatment with intravenous essential L-amino acids and glucose. Results of a prospective, double-blind study. N Engl J Med 288:695–699, 1973.

217. Kopple JD. The nutrition management of the patient with acute renal failure. JPEN 20:3–12, 1996.

218. Fiaccadori E, Maggiore U, Giacosa R, et al. Enteral nutrition in patients with acute renal failure. Kidney Int 65:999–1008, 2004.

219. Story D, Ronco C, Bellomo R. Trace element and vitamin concentrations and losses in critically ill patients with continuous venovenous hemofiltration. Crit Care Med 27:220–223, 1999.

220. London RE, Burton JR. Posttraumatic renal failure in military personnel in southeast Asia. Am J Med 53:137–142, 1972.

221. Mehta RL. Continuous renal replacement therapies in the acute renal failure setting: current concepts. Adv Ren Replace Ther 4(Suppl 1):81–92, 1997.

222. Deng J, Kohda Y, Chiao H, et al. Interleukin-10 inhibits ischemic and cisplatin-induced acute renal injury. Kidney Int 60:2118–2128, 2001.

223. Franklin SC, Moulton M, Sicard GA, et al. Insulin-like growth factor I preserves renal function postoperatively. Am J Physiol 272: F257–259, 1997.

224. Kopple JD, Hirschberg R, Guler HP, et al. Lack of effect of recombinant human insulin-like growth factor-1 (IGF-1) in patients with acute renal failure (ARF) [abstract]. J Am Soc Nephrol 7:1375, 1996.

225. Hirschberg R, Kopple J, Lipsett P, et al. Multicenter clinical trial of recombinant human insulin-like growth factor I in patients with acute renal failure. Kidney Int 55:2423–2432, 1999.

226. Kelly KJ, Williams WW, Jr, Colvin RB, et al. Intercellular adhesion molecule-1-deficient mice are protected against ischemic renal injury. J Clin Invest 97:1056–1063, 1996.

227. Kelly KJ, Williams, WWJ, Colvin RB, et al. Antibody to intercellular molecule-1 protects the kidney against renal injury. Proc Natl Acad Sci USA 91:812–816, 1994.

228. Ghielli M, Verstrepen WA, De Greef KE, et al. Antibodies to both ICAM-1 and LFA-1 do not protect the kidney against toxic (HgCl2) injury [erratum appears in Kidney Int 58:2257, 2000]. Kidney Int 58:1121–1134, 2000.

229. Hakim RM, Fearon DT, Lazarus JM. Biocompatibility of dialysis membranes: effects of chronic complement activation. Kidney Int 26:194–200, 1984.

230. Hakim RM, Wingard RL, Parker RA. Effect of the dialysis membrane in the treatment of patients with acute renal failure. N Engl J Med 331:1338–1342, 1994.

231. Schiffl H, Lang SM, Konig A, et al. Biocompatible membranes in acute renal failure: prospective case-controlled study. Lancet 344: 570–572, 1994.

232. Himmelfarb J, Tolkoff Rubin N, Chandran P, et al. A multicenter comparison of dialysis membranes in the treatment of acute renal failure requiring dialysis. J Am Soc Nephrol 9:257–266, 1998.

233. Subramanian S, Venkataraman R, Kellum JA. Influence of dialysis membranes on outcomes in acute renal failure: a meta-analysis. Kidney Int 62:1819–1823, 2002.

234. Manns B, Doig CJ, Lee H, et al. Cost of acute renal failure requiring dialysis in the intensive care unit: clinical and resource implications of renal recovery. Crit Care Med 31:449–455, 2003.

235. Mehta RL, McDonald B, Gabbai FB, et al. A randomized clinical trial of continuous versus intermittent dialysis for acute renal failure. Kidney Int 60:1154–1163, 2001.

236. Silvester W. Outcome studies of continuous renal replacement therapy in the intensive care unit. Kidney Int Suppl 66:S138–141, 1998.

Chronic Kidney Disease

43

Sarah R. Tomasello

TREATMENT GOALS: CHRONIC KIDNEY DISEASE

Research has shown that kidney disease can be delayed and slowed by early identification and intervention. With the increasing prevalence of patients with kidney disease, as well as patients with diabetes and hypertension, more patients at risk will be seen in primary care settings.[1] The appropriate treatment of patients at risk and patients with already documented kidney disease should be provided through a multidisciplinary approach.

- Identify patients at risk for kidney disease; screen patients with hypertension or diabetes
- Slow the progression of nephropathy by
  - Initiating an angiotensin-converting enzyme inhibitor (ACE-I) or an angiotensin receptor antagonist (ARB) if appropriate
  - Controlling hypertension and hyperlipidemia
  - Treating dyslipidemia
- Initiate therapies to decrease morbidity and mortality
- Promote smoking cessation
- Treat sequelae of chronic kidney disease, including
  - Secondary hyperparathyroidism
  - Anemia
  - Fluid and electrolyte disturbances
- Treat comorbid disease states
- Promote lifestyle modifications, including
  - Low-salt diet
  - Healthful eating
  - Possible protein or fluid restriction
  - Avoidance of excessive alcohol intake
- Avoid nephrotoxic drugs
- Ensure that dosing of all medications is appropriate for the level of kidney function
- Educate patients and providers about chronic kidney disease and promote early intervention

DEFINITION

The term *chronic kidney disease (CKD)* is a relatively new way to refer to a very old problem. Many terms have been used in the past, including *chronic renal insufficiency or failure*, *end-stage renal disease*, and *nephropathy*. The terms *renal*, *nephro-*, and *kidney* were used interchangeably. The name *chronic kidney disease* was proposed by the National Kidney Foundation–Kidney Disease Quality Outcome Initiative (K/DOQI) as a way of simplifying and codifying the language used to communicate about the disease.[2]

CKD is defined as either of the following conditions for a minimum of 3 months: glomerular filtration rate (GFR) less than 60 mL/min/1.73 m², or old damage to the kidney(s) with or without a decrease in GFR. This damage may be evidenced by abnormalities in the composition of blood or urine, or by changes seen in imaging studies[3] (Table 43.1). The K/DOQI[2] Working Group further categorizes the extent of kidney disease according to the presence of kidney damage and the GFR. Stage 1 CKD is defined as the presence of kidney damage even though GFR may be normal or even increased (≥90 mL/min/1.73 m²). Stage 2 CKD is evidenced by a GFR between 60 and 89 mL/min/1.73 m². Patients with stage 3 CKD may or may not have kidney damage, while their GFR is reduced to between 30 and 59 mL/min/1.73 m². CKD patients with stage 4 disease also may not have intrinsic kidney damage, but their GFR is severely reduced to between 15 and 29 mL/min/1.73 m². The last stage, stage 5, is also known as end-stage kidney disease (ESKD). This condition, formerly known as end-stage renal disease (ESRD), is defined as a GFR less than 15 mL/min/1.73 m² *or* the need for renal replacement therapy (RRT) for survival.

Most forms of kidney disease will cause irreversible, progressive deterioration of kidney function if not identified and treated properly. Depending on the cause, the disease may progress to complete loss of function over months to

TABLE 43.1	Classification of Chronic Kidney Disease	
Classification	**Damage**	**GFR (mL/min)**
Increased risk of kidney disease	Risk factors for CKD (diabetes, HTN, family history of CKD)	≥90
Stage I	Kidney damage with normal GFR	≥90
Stage II	Kidney damage with mild decrease in GFR	60–89
Stage III	Moderate decrease in GFR	30–59
Stage IV	Severe decrease in GFR	15–29
Stage V	Kidney failure	<15

CKD, chronic kidney disease; GFR, glomerular filtration rate; HTN, hypertension.
(From National Kidney Foundation. K/DOQI clinical practice guidelines for chronic kidney disease: evaluation, classification, and stratification. Am J Kidney Dis 39 (2 Suppl 1):S1–S266, 2002, with permission.)

years. As the extent of deterioration increases, the kidney is unable to perform normal homeostatic functions. This leads to fluid and electrolyte abnormalities, acid-base disturbances, hormonal dysregulation, and other systemic disturbances. When the GFR falls to below 15 mL/min/1.73 m², patients generally require some form of RRT for survival. Options for RRT include hemodialysis, peritoneal dialysis, and kidney transplantation (see Chapter 44). Although patients may be maintained on dialysis or may receive a kidney transplant, they have increased risks of morbidity and mortality. For example, in patients on dialysis, a 9% annual mortality rate from cardiovascular disease has been documented.[4]

EPIDEMIOLOGY

In 2002, it was estimated that approximately 20 million people had chronic kidney disease[5,6] (Table 43.2). With the rate of rise of diabetes and hypertension in the population, it is easy to imagine the corresponding rise in the incidence of CKD. Early stages of CKD are often asymptomatic, making prevalence and incidence difficult to determine. Calculating the prevalence of stage 5 CKD is much easier in that these data are tracked through the US Renal Data System (USRDS). It is a government-funded network that collects and reports data on patients with ESKD who are receiving benefits through Medicare. According to the Annual Data Report (ADR) for 2003, the prevalence of ESKD will likely double from 2000 to 2010.[7] This implies that more than 650,000 people will require RRT or transplantation by this time.

Diabetes and hypertension are the two most common causes of ESKD. Patients with hypertension but without diabetes are two to three times more likely to develop CKD than are patients without either disease. Furthermore, patients with diabetes have a 14% to 35% greater risk of developing CKD than do hypertensive patients, indicating that a higher risk for CKD is associated with diabetes than with hypertension. In 2004, the three main causes of ESKD were diabetes (45%), hypertension (30%), and glomerulonephritis (20%). The overall prevalence rate of ESKD is 1,435 per million population. In African-Americans, it is three times this, at 4,467. Rates of ESKD may be leveling off, except for the rate among the elderly. In fact, the rate for glomerulonephritis (GN) has actually declined. As in the past, the prevalence of ESKD is higher within African-American, Asian American, and Native American populations than in whites. The rate for African-Americans appears to be slowing whereas the rates for Asians and Hispanics are rising.[6, 8]

CKD carries a poor prognosis. If it is treated in the early stages, progression to ESKD may be delayed, and some complications of the disease may be avoided. For these goals to be achieved, it is imperative that patients at risk for CKD or those in the early stages of the disease, be identified. This task is made even more difficult by the fact that many patients do not even realize that they have CKD. One study found that less than one half of patients with stages 1 to 4 CKD were aware that they had kidney dysfunction. Patients who were unaware were more likely to be older, diabetic, hypertensive, and of a non-Hispanic black race. They were also more likely to have a higher urinary albumin-to-creatinine ratio (UACR) and a higher hemoglobin A1C level.[9] Timely identification and treatment are paramount. Without treatment, progressive, irreversible damage is likely and will result in ESKD.

Chronic renal disease is costly. In the United States, medical care provided to patients with ESKD incurred more than $11 billion in direct expenditures in 1997. In the year 2002, Medicare alone spent $17 billion on the ESKD program. This represents 6.7% of the total Medicare budget. In addition to Medicare, some coverage comes from employer group health plans (EGHPs). These plans contributed an additional $260 million to the medical care of patients with ESKD in 2002.[6] It is important to consider that these cost estimates are provided only for those patients in stage 5 CKD. When costs for the management of chronic kidney disease stages 1 to 4 and acute renal failure are considered in conjunction with ESKD, it can be seen that a sizable quantity of health care resources are spent on the treatment of patients with kidney disease.

TABLE 43.2	Prevalence of Chronic Kidney Disease	
Stage CKD	Number of People	Percentage of Population
1	5,900,000	3.3
2	5,300,000	3.0
3	7,600,000	4.3
4	400,000	0.2
5	300,000	0.2
All stages	19.2 million	11

CKD, chronic kidney disease.
(Adapted from Coresh J, Astor BC, Greene T, et al. Prevalence of chronic kidney disease and decreased kidney function in the adult US population: Third National Health and Nutrition Examination Survey. Am J Kidney Dis 41:1–12, 2003.)

ETIOLOGY

Chronic kidney disease may result from a primary intrinsic kidney disease, from anatomic or obstructive abnormalities, as a secondary complication of another systemic disease, or from acute kidney failure that never fully resolves. As was mentioned previously, the major diseases that lead to chronic kidney failure and new cases of ESKD are diabetes,

TABLE 43.3	Causes of Chronic Kidney Disease
Disease or Cause	**Description/Type**
Diabetes	Type 1 and type 2
Congenital anomalies	Polycystic kidney disease
Vasculitis or secondary glomerular nephritis	Lupus erythematosus, scleroderma, hemolytic-uremic syndrome
Glomerulonephritis	Acute or chronic, IgA nephropathy
Neoplasms or tumors	Wilms tumor, multiple myeloma
Drug induced	Analgesic abuse, radiocontrast media

IgA, immunoglobulin A.
(Adapted from Brenner B. The kidney. 5th ed. Philadelphia: WB Saunders, 1996.)

hypertension, and glomerulonephritis. Less common causes of ESKD are detailed in Table 43.3. Notably, diabetes mellitus (DM) now accounts for nearly 45% of new ESKD cases.[6] Approximately 20% to 40% of patients with diabetes develop kidney disease.[10] Although patients with type 1 diabetes have a much higher risk of developing CKD, type 2 diabetes is far more prevalent; therefore, many more patients with type 2 diabetes have ESKD. Patients who have received kidney transplants account for an expanding fraction of the CKD population. Although kidney transplant may cure ESKD, the transplanted kidney may eventually fail for a number of reasons, including recurrent damage from the original systemic disorder, acute or chronic rejection, and drug-related nephrotoxicity associated with the use of certain immunosuppressants (e.g., cyclosporine, tacrolimus). Kidney transplant recipients are a very complex subset of patients; however, many of the issues managed in CKD remain pertinent to this population.

PATHOPHYSIOLOGY

Several aspects of the anatomy and physiology of the kidney are reviewed in Chapter 42. The reader is referred to this material as background for the following discussion on the pathogenesis and pathophysiology of chronic kidney disease.

GLOMERULAR HYPERFILTRATION AND INTRAGLOMERULAR HYPERTENSION

The nephron, the functional unit of the kidney, comprises the glomerulus and the tubules. Approximately 1 million nephrons are located in each kidney. When the number of functioning nephrons is reduced because of insult or disease, the remaining nephrons compensate by enlarging (hypertrophy) and by increasing their individual GFRs. Through escalation of glomerular blood flow and intraglomerular capillary pressure, a state of increased glomerular perfusion can

be attained. This occurs with simultaneously induction of a degree of intraglomerular hypertension.[11] Referred to as *renal reserve capacity*, these glomerular adaptations accomplish the short-term goal of improving or restoring total GFR. Unfortunately, sustained elevations of blood flow and pressure within the glomeruli cause damage to remaining nephrons, ultimately leading to their demise.[12] Glomerular injury is also believed to result from increased capillary permeability (reduced permselectivity), which allows proteins and other macromolecules to leak through capillaries into the renal tubules. Microalbuminuria is one of the earliest clinical manifestations of glomerular damage. This process in turn may promote the secretion of proinflammatory mediators and induce renal mesangial cells to deposit an extracellular glycoprotein matrix,[13] leading to a type of renal fibrosis and scarring called *sclerosis*. Sclerosis may involve the entire nephron (nephrosclerosis), extending from the glomerulus (glomerulosclerosis) to the tubules and interstitium.

PROGRESSIVE NATURE

Many diseases or insults may cause the initial damage that begins the progressive decline of renal function. Hyperglycemia, systemic hypertension, dyslipidemia, and excessive dietary protein are some examples. Aggressive treatment or elimination of the primary disease may potentially retard or interrupt the progression of renal disease. Toward this end, *early* intervention appears to be crucial in maximizing the success of preventive efforts. Intensive control of blood glucose has been shown to reduce or slow the onset of diabetic nephropathy in patients with insulin-dependent diabetes[14] and in those with type 2 diabetes.[15–17] Numerous studies have shown that controlling blood pressure decreases proteinuria and delays the progression of nephropathy in diabetic and nondiabetic patients.[18–20]

PROTEINURIA

Because protein (mostly albumin) is a relatively large molecule, it generally is not filtered in the glomerulus but is returned to systemic circulation via the efferent arteriole. The presence of small amounts of protein in the urine (microalbuminuria) or larger amounts (proteinuria) is due to damage within the glomerulus. Although this may be the result of a self-limiting situation (e.g., acute muscle breakdown), it occurs more often as a result of injury caused by a disease process such as diabetes or hypertension. Both of these disease states may lead to intraglomerular hypertension and altered glomerular permeability. Filtering of protein in the glomerulus causes direct damage, and protein deposition evokes an inflammatory response that may cause more damage in the glomerulus or the tubules. The association of proteinuria with direct kidney damage is so strong that clinicians often use the degree of albuminuria as a measure of nephropathy. Furthermore, testing for the presence of microalbuminuria is suggested as a screening tool for nephropathy in those persons at risk for kidney disease.[2] Recently, proteinuria has been identified as a risk factor for cardiovascular disease (CVD).[21] Although the exact mechanism of damage is unknown, numerous factors have been implicated. These factors include insulin resistance, inflammation, and endothelial dysfunction, as well as alterations in the coagulation cascade. As is discussed later, diseases such as diabetes and hypertension cause proteinuria. Additionally, cigarette smoking has been shown to increase urinary albumin excretion (UAE) and is directly correlated with progression of nephropathy.[22]

DIABETES-ASSOCIATED CHRONIC KIDNEY DISEASE (DIABETIC NEPHROPATHY)

In the Western hemisphere, DM is the single most important disease leading to ESKD. The incidence of diabetic nephropathy peaks after 10 to 15 years of diabetes; however, functional renal abnormalities are often present within 2 years of the onset of type 1 DM. Because the diagnosis of type 2 DM is often delayed by actual onset, renal changes are usually present at diagnosis in this population. Aside from hyperglycemia, comorbidities such as hypertension and hyperlipidemia are common in patients with diabetes and are believed to contribute to progression of nephropathy in most cases. As was alluded to earlier, in a large proportion of patients with diabetes, disease progresses to ESKD. This fraction is disproportionately high in certain racial groups such as Pima Indians, Native Americans, Hispanics, and Asian/Pacific Islanders. Therefore, racial or hereditary factors are believed to influence the likelihood that end-stage diabetic nephropathy will occur.

The pathophysiology of diabetic nephropathy is complex and involves the formation of advanced glycation end products (AGEs). Hyperglycemia leads to a nonenzymatic reaction between sugar and protein.[23–26] These complexes accumulate because of decreased renal function. AGEs cause expansion of the mesangium, damage to the glomerular basement membrane, cytokine release, and gene expression. Other alterations, such as changes in endothelium-dependent vasodilation, may play a role in the development of diabetic nephropathy. The result of these changes is glomerulosclerosis.[27] In the initial stages of diabetic nephropathy, a period of hyperfiltration (improved functioning) may occur. With loss of some nephrons, the remaining "healthy" nephrons hypertrophy and hyperfilter to compensate for the loss. Eventually, however, these nephrons become overwhelmed and also stop functioning. Therefore, after an initial phase of apparent improvement, kidney function begins to decline. Diabetic nephropathy may progress slowly. However, in the presence of hypertension, increased urinary albumin excretion, hyperglycemia, and/or dyslipidemia, it may progress at an extraordinary rate—as high as 2 to 20 mL/min/year.[28–30] Additionally, cigarette smoking has been shown to increase

the rate of progression of CKD in patients with diabetes who have an increased urinary albumin excretion.[22] If patients are treated early, progression of diabetic nephropathy may be slowed or even arrested. If, however, the GFR drops to below approximately 40 mL per minute, progressive and irreversible decline is likely. No therapy has been found so far that can cause regression of diabetic nephropathy—only slow progression or delay the onset. This fact highlights the need for screening of patients at risk for kidney disease, so that preventive measures can be started early.

HYPERTENSION

Moderate to severe hypertension is strongly correlated with the risk of developing ESKD, consistent with observations that systemic hypertension may both cause and result from renal disease. Assuming that an elevated systemic blood pressure is transmitted to the glomerulus, systemic hypertension may be anticipated to exacerbate CKD progression by contributing to intraglomerular hypertension and hyperfiltration. Bakris et al[31] reviewed nine clinical trials undertaken to evaluate the progression of nephropathy and found a linear relationship between an increase in blood pressure and the rate of decline in kidney function. Arteriosclerosis, another hypertensive complication, may also contribute to nephron loss through ischemic mechanisms. Antihypertensive therapies have been postulated to protect against glomerulopathy by several mechanisms, including reduction in blood pressure or blood flow reaching the glomerulus, attenuation of intraglomerular hypertension via reductions in afferent or efferent arteriolar tone, alteration of nonhemodynamic factors such as membrane permselectivity, inflammation, and oxidative stress, or possibly some combination of these mechanisms.[11]

Hypertension is present in most patients with CKD. If it is not the preexisting cause of renal failure, hypertension invariably develops along the course of renal disease and may accelerate its progression.[11,32,33] The kidney plays a major role in the control of blood pressure by regulating sodium retention, extracellular fluid volume, and the renin-angiotensin system. Expanded extracellular fluid (ECF) volume is presumed to be a major factor contributing to hypertension in most patients with CKD, followed by elevated renin-angiotensin activity. Imbalances between endogenous vasoconstrictive (e.g., endothelin) and vasodilatory substances (e.g., nitric oxide) have also been recognized as a probable factor underlying hypertension in CKD.[34,35] Increased pulse pressure and isolated systolic hypertension are also more common in the CKD population, consistent with the concept of expanded ECF volume and reduced vascular compliance.

Hypertension significantly increases the risk for cardiac disease and stroke in the general population. This holds true for the ESKD population as well, in whom cardiovascular mortality is 10 to 20 times higher.[36] It seems reasonable to suspect that cardiovascular risk actually begins to increase *before* a patient enters ESKD, in parallel with or as a consequence of chronic renal disease. Risk factors common to the progression of both cardiovascular and renal disease are present in most of those with CKD and often include hypertension, hyperlipidemia, diabetes, and altered neurohumors (e.g., renin-angiotensin, endothelin, nitric oxide).[37] Elevated homocysteine levels and possibly oxidative stress are implicated as promoting cardiovascular disease in several populations and are suspected to rise progressively during the course of CKD as well.[38,39]

Hypertension is an important risk factor for the progression of renal disease. As was discussed in earlier sections, renal damage is thought to result from exaggerated intraglomerular hypertension and hyperfiltration, perhaps in conjunction with ischemic damage caused by arteriosclerotic changes in renal vasculature. As renal disease advances, good control of hypertension can be challenging to achieve, but this control is very important in minimizing or slowing end-organ damage.

Differences in Antihypertensive Agents. In theory, correction of hypertension by any agent *should* help reduce the risk of nephropathy. However, all antihypertensives do not appear to provide equal protection against the progression of kidney disease. Different antihypertensives alter glomerular hemodynamics to differing extents, depending on the interplay of their effects on systemic hemodynamics and afferent versus efferent arteriolar tone. Accumulating data suggest that for any given level of systemic blood pressure reduction, ACE-Is, ARBs and nondihydropyridine calcium channel blockers (diltiazem and verapamil) produce superior antiproteinuric and renoprotective effects, especially in patients with diabetes[40-42] and those with established proteinuria.[43,44] Beyond effective blood pressure control, the advantage of ACE-Is is believed to result from preferential dilation of the efferent renal artery, which should lower intraglomerular hypertension more consistently than can be achieved by other agents that dilate the afferent arteriole. The use of antihypertensives in CKD is discussed in greater detail later in this chapter.

CARDIOVASCULAR DISEASE

As has already been mentioned, patients with CKD tend to have many risk factors for CVD, including hypertension, dyslipidemia, and proteinuria. Additional predisposing factors include anemia, malnutrition, diabetes, and hyperparathyroidism. Types of heart disease include left ventricular hypertrophy, ischemic heart disease, and heart failure. In a study[45] of patients with an average creatinine clearance of 36 mL per minute, 46% were found to have CVD, 33% had ischemic heart disease or suffered an acute myocardial infarction, and 10% had heart failure. Another study[46] in patients with an average creatinine clearance of 30 mL per minute found that approximately 39% had CVD.

Left ventricular hypertrophy (LVH) may begin early in the course of kidney disease[47-49] and is correlated with a decline in hemoglobin levels or an increase in systolic blood pressure.[48] One study found that for every 1 mg per dL decrease in hemoglobin, a 6% increase in the risk of LVH occurred.[50] Other risk factors for LVH include age, hypertension, volume overload, and CKD.[51,52] Levin et al. found that 38.9% of the predialysis population had LVH.[50] Foley et al. found that 74% of patients had LVH at the initiation of dialysis.[53] These numbers are a matter of concern in that LVH is an independent predictor of CVD[54] and leads to diastolic dysfunction, which may increase complications during hemodialysis.[55] In fact, 50% of deaths in patients on dialysis are due to CVD, and 80% of patients newly on dialysis develop heart failure within the first year.[52] Hospitalization rates for cardiac disease are two to seven times higher in patients with CKD than in the rest of the population.[8] Patients with chronic kidney disease are nearly twice as likely to have a fatal cardiac event than are those without CKD,[56] and in general, they have poorer outcomes and prognoses after an acute event[57-61] (Table 43.4)

Dysregulation of calcium and phosphorus may be yet another risk factor for the development of CVD.[62,63] An increase in serum phosphorous levels has been shown to stimulate vascular calcification.[64] At the initiation of dialysis, one study found that 47% of patients had severe coronary or aortic calcification.[62] In patients with stage 5 CKD, studies have found a linear relationship between serum phosphorous levels and mortality. Each 1 g per dL increase in phosphorus correlated with an increase in mortality of 6% to 8%.[65,66] Additionally, Ganesh et al. showed a 41% increase in relative risk of death from coronary artery disease (CAD) and a 20% increase in sudden death among patients with a serum phosphorous level greater than 6.5 mg per dL.[67] In addition to serum phosphorus, serum calcium and the calcium X phosphorous product may play a role in vascular calcification. It

TABLE 43.4	In-Hospital Mortality Following Acute Myocardial Infarction	
Stage of CKD	**In-Hospital Mortality Rate**	**1-Year Mortality Rate (elderly)**
Normal kidney function	2%	24%
Mild CKD	6%	46%
Moderate CKD	14%	66%
Severe CKD	21%	*
ESRD on dialysis	30%	*

CKD, chronic kidney disease; ESRD, end-stage renal disease.
(Adapted from Wright R, Reeder G, Herzog C, et al. Association of creatinine and creatinine clearance in acute myocardial infarction with subsequent mortality. J Am Coll Cardiol 42:1535–1543, 2003.)

is suggested that the calcium phosphorous product be maintained below 55 mg^2 per dL^2 to minimize the physiochemical interaction and reduce precipitation.[68]

HYPERLIPIDEMIA

Dyslipidemia is more prevalent in patients with CKD than in the general population (30% vs. 20%).[4] In patients with nephrotic range proteinuria (>3 g/24 hours), the incidence may be as high as 70% to 100%[69] because of increased hepatic lipoprotein synthesis.[70] In these patients, the degree of proteinuria is directly proportionate to the increase in total cholesterol. Dyslipidemia may lead to the progression of CKD caused by oxidation and deposition of lipoproteins in the glomerulus and the mesangial cells. Oxidized low-density lipoprotein (LDL) may cause synthesis of inflammatory cytokines, vasoactive substances, and macrophage chemotactic factors. These changes eventually lead to glomerular scarring. Common abnormalities seen in patients with CKD include increased LDL, decreased HDL, and elevated triglycerides. These changes have been directly correlated with the development[71] and progression[72,73] of nephropathy. In one study, the relative risk of nephropathy was 2.6 when the serum LDL level was greater than 160 mg per dL, and 3 when the triglyceride level was greater than 200 mg per dL.[71]

Dyslipidemia may be detected early in chronic kidney disease—in stages 3 or 4.[74] Alterations in lipid profile commonly include an increase in very low-density lipoprotein, intermediate lipoprotein, triglycerides, and small, dense low-density lipoprotein, with a decrease in high-density lipoprotein.[75] These alterations have been associated with an increased risk for CAD and atherosclerosis. Other metabolic abnormalities may contribute to the increased risk of CAD. These factors include diabetes mellitus, hypertension, hyperhomocystinemia, elevated lipoprotein (a), and derangements in calcium and phosphate levels.[4,62,76–78] The increased incidence of events makes CKD a risk factor for CVD. In addition to being at greater risk for CVD, patients with CKD seem to have a higher mortality rate after an acute coronary event.[61]

DRUG EXACERBATION OF CHRONIC KIDNEY DISEASE AND OTHER REVERSIBLE FACTORS

Residual kidney function, as measured by GFR, is usually assumed to decline at a constant rate within a given person, although the rate of loss varies considerably between individuals. Patient features that have been identified to predict more rapid progression of renal disease include race (African-American), hypertension, low serum high-density lipoprotein (HDL) cholesterol, overt proteinuria, and diabetic microalbuminuria.[72] Exceptions to this generalization are noted, particularly when treatment to forestall GFR decline has been successful. As an example, if a patient exhibits a

TABLE 43.5	Drugs or Abnormalities That Cause Renal Dysfunction
Reduction in Renal Blood Flow	**Direct Nephrotoxin**
Diuretics	Antimicrobials: amphotericin, indinavir, tenofovir, aminoglycosides
ACE-Is/ARBs	Radiocontrast dyes (high-osmolar, high-volume)
NSAIDs	Anticancer agents: cisplatin, ifosfamide, high-dose methotrexate
Antihypertensives	Immunosuppressants: cyclosporine, tacrolimus
Volume loss, dehydration	
Urinary obstruction	

ACE-Is, angiotensin-converting enzyme inhibitors; ARBs, angiotensin receptor blockers; NSAIDs, nonsteroidal anti-inflammatory drugs.

stable decline in GFR of 4 mL per minute per year, one would predict that in the absence of successful intervention, the GFR would drop over the next 7 to 8 years from a present value of 40 mL per minute to 10 mL per minute. After this point, dialysis would become necessary within 1 year. However, if institution of ACE-I therapy were to slow the rate of decline by 50% (i.e., 2 mL/min/year), the need for dialysis could be delayed for 15, rather than 8, years.

Abrupt worsening or acceleration of GFR decline may be a signal that new factors have begun to hasten kidney deterioration. This is a situation of an acute insult superimposed on chronic kidney disease. Because the responsible factors are often reversible or correctable, potential causes should be sought and eliminated when renal function acutely worsens over a previously established rate of decline. Examples of acute drug and nondrug causes of exacerbation of renal dysfunction are described in Table 43.5. Several of these are included among the causes of acute renal failure (ARF), as described in Chapter 42. In the setting of decreased kidney reserve, drugs capable of inducing tubular necrosis, reducing kidney perfusion, or decreasing volume status should be used with particular caution. Because the kidneys are very sensitive to changes in perfusion or volume status, drugs that may alter these parameters should be used with caution. Agents such as ACE-Is, diuretics, and some other antihypertensives may be viewed as either nephroprotective or nephrotoxic, depending on the dose and clinical context of their use.

HISTOLOGIC FEATURES

Hallmark lesions of type 1 diabetic nephropathy include glomerular basement membrane thickening, glomerular hypertrophy, mesangial matrix expansion, and hyalinization or sclerosis of glomerular capillaries. Histologic findings in type 2 DM often include these lesions, as well as a mixture of others. Hypertensive kidney disease is typified by arteriolar thickening and vascular luminal narrowing, which promote ischemic damage in glomeruli and tubules. Deposition of hyaline, a proteinaceous material, is often observed throughout the nephron and leads to nephrosclerosis. In some forms of glomerulonephritis and immune-mediated renal disease, glomerular deposition of immune complexes or antibodies occurs in patterns that can be characterized only by special staining or electron microscopy techniques. A variety of histologic findings are associated with other types of intrinsic renal disease; a full discussion of these is beyond the scope of this chapter.

METABOLIC AND SYSTEMIC CONSEQUENCES OF CHRONIC KIDNEY DISEASE

The extent to which renal dysfunction reduces urinary solute excretion has been found to vary for different substances. For example, rises in urea and creatinine are observed early in CKD and inversely correlate with GFR, whereas the renal excretion of potassium, urate (uric acid), phosphorus, and hydrogen ion is generally preserved until GFR falls to below 25% of normal. Excretion of these solutes may be enhanced by increased tubular secretion or reduced reabsorption until GFR is 25 to 30 mL per minute or less, at which point accumulation becomes unavoidable and plasma levels of these solutes begin to rise. Finally, the renal handling of other solutes (e.g., Na^+, Cl^-) may be well preserved late into CKD but differs substantially among the various types of renal disease.

Azotemia refers to the systemic accumulation of nitrogenous wastes, such as blood urea nitrogen (BUN) and creatinine. Uremia is a clinical syndrome that encompasses not only a symptomatic degree of azotemia, but also a constellation of signs and symptoms due to the effects of ESKD on other organ systems. Although the concentration of urea may be loosely correlated with the degree of renal impairment and the overall severity of symptoms, no specific uremic toxins have been identified as being responsible for all the complications of the uremic syndrome. In addition to urea, other substances have been found to accumulate in uremia, including ammonia, guanidine, guanidinosuccinic acid, methyl guanidine, phenols, myoinositol, and others.[11]

Of the numerous complications of CKD listed in Table 43.6, the pathophysiology of only the most common and clinically relevant features is discussed here. The therapeutic management of each of these complications is discussed in the next section of this chapter.

VOLUME, SODIUM, AND WATER BALANCE
Because daily sodium intake usually exceeds requirements, the kidneys are able to maintain sodium balance by simply

TABLE 43.6	Uremic Complications of Chronic Kidney Disease

Fluid—electrolyte

　Volume control: hypervolemia, impaired sodium–water regulation

　Electrolytes: hyperkalemia, hypermagnesemia, hyperphosphatemia, hypocalcemia, hypercalcemia

Metabolic—nutritional

　Acid-base status: chronic metabolic acidosis, elevated anion gap acidosis

　Protein: azotemia, hypoalbuminemia, protein malnutrition

　Carbohydrate: prolonged insulin action, peripheral insulin resistance, glucose intolerance

　Lipid: dyslipidemia, hyperlipidemia

Endocrine

　Hyperparathyroidism; deficiency in erythropoietin, calcitriol, and gonadal hormones

Hematologic

　Anemia, thrombocytopenia, impaired hemostasis, uremic bleeding

Cardiovascular

　Hypertension, left ventricular hypertrophy, congestive heart failure, pericarditis, arrhythmias

Musculoskeletal

　Osteodystrophy, hyperuricemia, amyloidosis, extraskeletal calcification

Gastrointestinal

　Dyspepsia, peptic ulcer disease, anorexia, nausea and vomiting, uremic fetor, constipation

Neurologic

　Peripheral neuropathy, altered mentation, uremic seizures, restless legs syndrome, poor sleep

Dermatologic

　Pruritus, discoloration, dryness/scaliness of skin

Infectious

Impaired immune response, increased susceptibility to infection

Psychosocial

　Loss of autonomy, depression, loss of employment, financial hardships

(Adapted from American Diabetes Association. Standards of medical care for patients with diabetes mellitus [erratum appears in Diabetes Care 26:972, 2003]. Diabetes Care 26 (Suppl 1):S33–S50, 2003.)

reducing urinary Na^+ reabsorption (i.e., increasing the fractional excretion of sodium, or FE_{Na}). Conversely, if sodium intake is below output, the kidney is usually able to increase its conservation of sodium, except in certain salt-wasting nephropathies. At creatinine clearances below 25 mL per minute, however, renal adaptation to wide fluctuations in sodium or water intake is sluggish and incomplete. The kidney becomes unable to concentrate or dilute urine efficiently, and urinary excretion of water and salt tends to become fixed at nearly iso-osmotic concentrations, in volumes of about 2 L per day. Because iso-osmotic fluid reabsorption is preserved until late in CKD, serum sodium concentrations are maintained within normal limits. In contrast, regulation of volume status becomes significantly impaired. As ESKD is neared, daily urine volumes decrease further in most patients. When salt and water intakes are below output, volume depletion may rapidly develop. Intake often exceeds output, leading to volume retention, which exacerbates hypertension. As volume overload worsens, weight gain, edema, and finally, pulmonary congestion or other cardiovascular complications may develop.

ELECTROLYTE BALANCE: POTASSIUM AND MAGNESIUM

Potassium is carefully regulated in the body. Only a small amount—approximately 2%—is extracellular. Potassium is moved into and out of cells via sodium, potassium adenosine triphosphatase (Na^+,K^+-ATPase) pumps. Various factors may upregulate or downregulate the number of pumps on the cell membrane, causing a shift in potassium to other mechanisms. Insulin and β_2-agonists increase the movement of potassium intracellularly, and hyperparathyroidism and hypertonicity may cause potassium to shift to the extracellular compartment. Roughly 90% to 95% of daily intake is excreted in the urine via tubular secretion; 5% to 10% is eliminated in the feces.[79] As the degree of kidney failure progresses, an adaptive increase in colonic elimination of potassium occurs; in patients with ESKD, this increase may be up to twofold to threefold greater than that in subjects with normal kidney function.[80,81] This increased gastrointestinal secretion and an increase in distal tubular secretion prevent hyperkalemia until kidney function declines to 10 to 15 mL per minute. Factors that increase the risk of hyperkalemia include an increase in potassium intake and use of drugs that impair potassium excretion (ACE-Is, potassium-sparing diuretics), or drugs or conditions that shift potassium to the extracellular fluid from the intracellular fluid (β-blockers, metabolic acidosis).

The primary route of magnesium excretion is renal. Mild, asymptomatic elevations in serum magnesium may occur in patients with advanced CKD. Provided that dietary intake is not unusually excessive, life-threatening hypermagnesemia is uncommon. However, pharmaceutical sources of magnesium such as antacids and magnesium-based cathartics can markedly elevate serum magnesium levels when used on a long-term basis or in large quantities. Because many of these products are available over-the-counter, thorough medication histories and patient education sessions are paramount.

ACID-BASE REGULATION

A normal adult who consumes a mixed diet generates approximately 1 mEq per kg of metabolic acid daily. This hydrogen ion is rapidly buffered by circulating bicarbonate and is excreted by the lungs as respiratory acid (CO_2). Bicar-

bonate lost during this process is regenerated by the kidney through the excretion of acid (H^+), which must be buffered by ammonia (forming NH_4^+) or other urinary buffers. In kidney disease, renal ammonia formation (ammoniagenesis) is generally impaired as a consequence of reduced nephron mass. Because urinary acid secretion and renal regeneration of bicarbonate are coupled with the availability of ammonia, these associated processes become impaired in CKD. Bicarbonate is also filtered into the urine and must be reclaimed by reabsorption; however, this tends to remain intact until CKD is far advanced. The metabolic acidosis of CKD typically begins as a normal anion gap acidosis, characterized by low serum bicarbonate and mild hyperchloremia. As GFR falls to below 10 mL per minute, various organic acids accumulate, and the picture evolves toward that of an "elevated anion gap" acidosis, with bicarbonate levels near 12 to 15 mEq per L. The metabolic acidosis appears to be clinically tolerated, but it is thought to promote bone resorption and to contribute to a chronic catabolic state through stimulation of branched-chain amino acid breakdown.[11] In addition, patients with renal disease may not withstand acute acid-base challenges well (such as sepsis or ketoacidosis) because their overall buffer reserve is diminished.

ANEMIA OF CHRONIC KIDNEY DISEASE

Erythropoietin (EPO) is a hormone that is produced and secreted by the granular cells of the kidney in response to hypoxia or ischemia. When secreted, EPO travels to the bone marrow and causes the proliferation and differentiation of committed erythroid progenitor cells. Additionally, EPO prevents apoptosis of these cells, allowing them to mature.[82,83] The primary cause of anemia in CKD is the diminished production of EPO by the failing kidneys. Other causes include frequent phlebotomy, malnutrition, iron or vitamin deficiencies, and, for those patients on hemodialysis, blood loss in the dialytic circuit. Another contributing factor to anemia is the shortened life cycle of red blood cells in uremia. Ly et al[84] demonstrated that the life span of red blood cells in patients on hemodialysis is only approximately 60% that in healthy controls.

The National Kidney Foundation K/DOQI guidelines[85] define anemia as a hemoglobin level less than 12 g per dL in men and postmenopausal women, and less than 11 g per dL in premenopausal women and prepubertal patients. Although anemia may be present as early as stage 1 kidney disease,[48,86,87] it may not become clinically evident until patients reach stage 3 or 4.[88–90] In one study, 26.7% of patients with stage 1 CKD were anemic and 75% with stage 5 were anemic.[91] Another study[48] found an even higher incidence, at approximately 87%, in patients with a creatinine clearance below 25 mL per minute. The detrimental effects of anemia are well documented (Table 43.7). Research has demonstrated that anemia is a risk factor for stroke,[92] left ventricular hypertrophy and dysfunction,[50] and cardiovascular disease.[93] Subjectively, anemia causes fatigue and decreased energy, decreased exercise tolerance, and an overall decreased health-

TABLE 43.7	Detrimental Effects of Anemia in Patients With CKD

Decreased	Increased
Exercise capacity	Depression
Skeletal muscle oxidative capacity	Sleep/awake pattern
Coagulation	Cardiac output
Immune response	LVH
Cognitive function	Cardiac failure
Sexual function	Myopathy
Appetite/nutrition	Morbidity
QOL	Mortality
Growth in children	Angina

CKD, chronic kidney disease; QOL, quality of life; LVH, left ventricular hypertrophy.

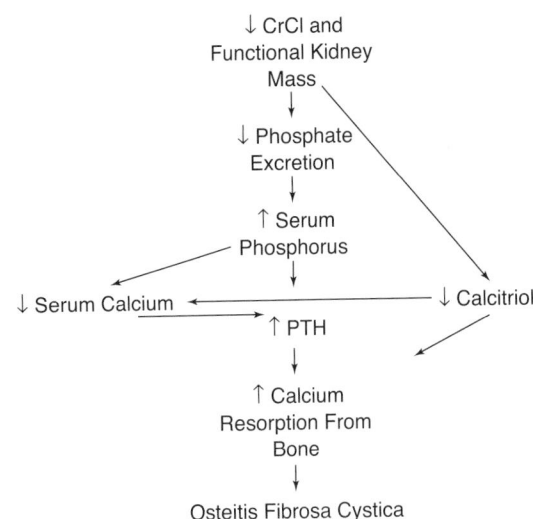

FIGURE 43.1 Mechanism of secondary hyperparathyroidism.

related quality of life.[94] The combination of CKD plus anemia increases the risk of stroke[95] and for every 1 g per dL decrease in hemoglobin, the relative risk of death increases by 1.14.[96] It must be noted that anemia of CKD is associated with an increase in morbidity and mortality,[97–99] and the combination of CKD and anemia places patients at higher risk for all-cause mortality than is predicted by assessment of each factor independently.[100] In May of 1995, it was estimated that 15.9% of Medicare patients who were beginning dialysis had a hemoglobin level greater than or equal to 11 g per dL. This figure rose to 29% in June of 2003.[101] Although this is a positive trend, there is much room for improvement in the treatment of patients with anemia of CKD.

CALCIUM, PHOSPHORUS, AND BONE HOMEOSTASIS

Abnormalities of bone metabolism and bone disease of CKD are complex. The process is described here and may be seen in Figure 43.1. As GFR decreases, excretion of solutes is impaired. Phosphorus may begin to accumulate in the early stages of CKD—stages 3 and 4. Hyperphosphatemia causes a decrease in serum calcium brought about through a physiochemical interaction and complexation. Reduction in serum calcium triggers the parathyroid gland to synthesize and secrete more parathyroid hormone (PTH). PTH in turn causes an increase in osteoclast activity in the bone, breaking down bone to release calcium and restore serum levels. These abnormalities are compounded by a relative deficiency of vitamin D. The failing kidneys are not able to convert vitamin D to the active form—1,25-dihydroxycholecalciferol (vitamin D_3). Under normal conditions, active vitamin D facilitates the absorption of calcium in the gastrointestinal tract (raising serum calcium levels) and also acts as a negative feedback loop to downregulate the production of PTH. In normal kidney function, elevated PTH levels cause increased secretion of phosphate in the tubule and hence, increased excretion of phosphate. The failing kidneys, however, are unable to

increase excretion, and hyperphosphatemia continues. The end results of this dysfunction often include hyperphosphatemia, hypocalcemia or hypercalcemia, hyperparathyroidism, and the bone disease called *osteitis fibrosa cystica*. This is one of the types of bone disease that are collectively known as *renal osteodystrophy*.

Other types of renal osteodystrophy include osteomalacia and adynamic bone disease. Osteomalacia, which is sometimes referred to as "softening" of the bone, is the result of demineralization. One cause of this abnormality is aluminum toxicity. Adynamic bone disease is referred to as a "low-turnover" subtype of renal osteodystrophy. This condition is associated with low PTH levels, which usually result from overzealous suppressive treatment. Osteoporosis, osteosclerosis, and mixed forms of bone disease can also plague patients with ESKD. These disturbances in bone and calcium phosphate metabolism progress insidiously, but they eventually lead to increased fracture rates (especially hip), bone pain, muscle weakness, musculoskeletal discomfort, and pathologic calcification of soft tissue, organs, nerves, and blood vessels.

A great deal of research is being done to elucidate the exact mechanism and to identify treatments to prevent vascular calcification. It is thought that this process is contributing to the increased risk of CVD and death in patients with CKD.[102,103] It is thought that the chemical interaction between phosphorus and calcium leads to precipitation and calcification. Multiplying the serum calcium (corrected for hypoalbuminemia) with the serum phosphorous levels yields what has been termed the "calcium X phosphorus product." Presumably, the higher the product, the more likely it is that calcium and phosphorus will come into contact in the blood. This would then lead to complexation and precipitation. The exact number at which this process occurs is still unknown. In previous studies, it was believed to be 70 mg^2 per dL^2. The K/DOQI guidelines now recommend that the product be maintained at below 55 mg^2 per dL^2.

The treatment of patients with disorders of bone metabolism is discussed in a later section. It should be noted, however, that among patients with ESKD, it has been shown that those with serum phosphorous levels greater than 6.5 mg per dL had a 56% higher risk of death than did patients with lower phosphorous levels. Additionally, for every 10 mg^2 per dL^2 increase in calcium X phosphorous product, an 11% increase in the incidence of sudden death was observed.[67] High serum levels of PTH were also correlated with an increased risk of death. A study of younger patients on hemodialysis found a correlation between elevated levels of calcium and phosphorus and the presence of coronary calcification.[104] The use of calcium-containing phosphate binders is thought to contribute to the process of calcification.[105,106] A recent study[102] found that despite the use of phosphate binders, 70% of patients on hemodialysis continued to be hyperphosphatemic. A separate study showed that compliance with phosphate binders is abysmal, with only 11 of 188 patients being compliant with their drug regimens.[107] Other studies of patients with stage 5 CKD have found that nearly 60% had cardiac calcification.[108,109] Although these complications are well recognized in patients with long-term ESKD, the belief is growing that these complications begin at earlier stages in chronic renal disease and should be amenable to intervention before the point of ESKD.[55] It is obvious that early intervention is necessary to prevent calcification; no medical treatment is available for use after it has developed. This underscores the importance of early identification and treatment of patients with CKD.

It must be noted that renal degradation of PTH is impaired in advanced renal disease, as is clearance of inactive PTH metabolites. In these patients, measurement of the active N-terminus moiety, called *intact parathyroid hormone (iPTH)*, provides a more accurate reflection of parathyroid status than is provided by nonspecific assays.

UREMIC BLEEDING

It has long been known that uremia can lead to an increased propensity for bleeding.[110] Purpura, epistaxis, and bleeding from venous and arterial access sites have been reported.[111] More serious, life-threatening bleeding includes hemorrhaging from gastrointestinal and genitourinary sites, as well as subdural hematomas.[110] The incidence and severity of bleeding have decreased over time as improvements have occurred in dialytic therapy and in the synthesis of recombinant erythropoietin, and as management of anemia has improved. The exact cause of uremic bleeding is still unknown but appears to be multifactorial. Some possible causes are listed in Table 43.8. Decreased platelet numbers and platelet adhesion and aggregation all play a key role in bleeding diathesis.[111] Degree of platelet dysfunction and risk of bleeding are best measured by a skin bleeding time test. Bleeding risk is not correlated with coagulation tests, the findings of which are generally within normal limits.

Because uremia is the accumulation of substances in the blood, much research has focused on identifying the compounds that are responsible for platelet abnormalities. One

TABLE 43.8	Potential Causes of Uremic Bleeding

Defects in platelet function and cellular metabolism

Defects of vascular endothelial/smooth muscle cell metabolism

Defects of platelet-vessel wall interactions

Anemia of chronic kidney disease

(From Weigert AL, Schafer AI. Uremic bleeding: pathogenesis and therapy. Am J Med Sci 316:94–104, 1998.)

such compound is guanidinosuccinic acid, a byproduct of ammonia detoxification.[112] Accumulation causes an increase in nitric oxide, which has been shown to decrease platelet function by interfering with the interaction of fibrinogen and the platelet GP IIb/IIIa receptor.[113]

ENDOCRINE AND HORMONAL ABNORMALITIES

Abnormalities in female and male gonadal hormones are common in ESKD and result in high incidences of infertility and sexual dysfunction.[114] Hyperprolactinemia is common, and gonadotropin, follicle-stimulating hormone (FSH), and luteinizing hormone (LH) levels may be low in both men and women. Women may cease to ovulate or menstruate, or they may do so irregularly. Although pregnancy is still possible, these are considered high-risk cases and only 40% result in successful deliveries. Decreased libido and erectile dysfunction are common among men with ESKD, which may be related not only to reduced testosterone levels but also to concurrent malaise, anemia, and vascular and neurologic abnormalities.

The regulation and function of other hormonal systems that are affected by ESKD have been discussed separately, including parathyroid hormone, calcitriol, erythropoietin, and insulin disposition and action. Many patients with ESKD exhibit a form of secondary hypothyroidism called *sick euthyroid syndrome*, which is characterized by low T3 and total T4 levels, but normal free T4 index and thyroid-stimulating hormone (TSH) levels.[115] Evaluation of thyroid abnormalities in ESKD is complicated by alterations in hormone protein binding and the frequent presence of concurrent diseases with overlapping symptoms.

GASTROINTESTINAL DISEASE

Patients with advanced renal failure commonly have gastrointestinal complications such as anorexia, nausea, and vomiting. These symptoms become pronounced as ESKD advances, to a degree that often prompts initiation of dialysis. Patients may complain of a metallic or salty taste, and their breath may smell of ammonia, referred to as *uremic fetor*. Uremic patients have high concentrations of urea in their saliva, which undergoes conversion to ammonia in the presence of bacterial ureases. As a consequence of the irritating effects of ammonia and probably other factors, mucosal and submucosal ulcerations often develop along the alimentary tract; these may take the form of stomatitis, parotitis, esophagitis, erosive gastritis, or colitis. Coupled with defects in hemostasis, blood loss from gastrointestinal sites is thought to contribute significantly to anemia in advanced CKD. In diabetic patients with uremia, it is not uncommon for gastroparesis to be superimposed on the aforementioned abnormalities, compounding nausea, vomiting, and gastroesophageal reflux. Constipation is a nearly universal complaint in ESKD, which partly stems from the use of constipating medications, along with fluid and dietary restrictions.

PRURITUS AND DERMATOLOGIC ABNORMALITIES

Generalized pruritus is common in CKD and may be one of the most recalcitrant and frustrating symptoms that patients experience. One study found that 66% of patients on hemodialysis currently had pruritus or had experienced it in the past.[116] Additionally, this study found that pruritus had adverse effects on patient quality of life. The cause of pruritus is still not well understood, and a large number of factors have been implicated (Table 43.9). Some of these include dry skin, accumulation of uremic wastes, elevations in serum calcium X phosphate product (leading to integumentary calcification), increased levels of histamine and serotonin, alterations in opioid receptors, and alterations in the immune system.[117–119] For patients on hemodialysis, the use of membranes that are less biocompatible has been thought to contribute to the disorder.

Although pruritus is the most prevalent dermatologic disorder in uremia, other changes may be seen as a consequence of CKD or as a consequence of medical procedures. A sallow yellowish or bronze pigmentation of the skin is common, as is pallor in extremely anemic patients. Bruises and hematomas reflect the heightened bleeding tendency and become even more evident as patients begin to undergo frequent venipunctures and invasive procedures.

MUSCULOSKELETAL AND NEUROLOGIC ISSUES

Uric acid is the end product of purine metabolism. It circulates primarily as urate, is filtered at the glomerulus, and is almost completely reabsorbed in the proximal tubules. Renal excretion of uric acid is impaired when the GFR falls to below 25 to 30 mL per minute, resulting in elevated serum uric acid levels. Potential complications from hyperuricemia include gouty attacks, uric acid kidney stones, and urate nephropathy.[11] More than 60% of uremic patients exhibit some evidence of peripheral neuropathy when GFR falls to below 5 mL per minute.[120] Early symptoms may include tingling or numbness, paresthesias, painful cramps, and restless leg syndrome (an intense, irresistible urge to move the legs). In severe cases, reduced or absent tendon reflexes, proximal muscle wasting, weakness, and ataxia may develop. Uremic polyneuropathy is presumed to involve axonal degeneration of motor and sensory nerve fibers, but it generally improves or stabilizes with institution of renal replacement therapies. Diabetic neuropathy is commonly superimposed on uremic polyneuropathy.

CLINICAL PRESENTATION AND DIAGNOSIS

SIGNS AND SYMPTOMS

Most patients experience few symptoms of CKD until less than 25% of normal renal function remains. CKD can therefore progress insidiously over months to years, evident only through abnormal biochemical parameters, such as gradually rising levels of BUN and serum creatinine values. Nonspecific complaints such as malaise, fatigue, and nocturia may be noted. Urine output may or may not be diminished. Hypertension may develop and, if discovered, presents a critical opportunity for investigation of renal implications. Unless patients are recognized to be at risk of and are monitored for kidney disease, they usually do not seek medical attention until the onset of uremic symptoms. At this point, interventions to forestall progression to ESKD are largely unfruitful.

DIAGNOSIS

Recently, the National Kidney Foundation (NKF) initiated the Kidney Early Evaluation Program (KEEP).[121] This is a community-based program created to screen people at risk for kidney disease. The program is executed by local agencies affiliated with the NKF. Of note, approximately one half of those screened have displayed evidence of kidney disease. Programs such as this that are detecting kidney disease in the early stages may have a great impact on outcomes because they refer patients for appropriate follow-up and management.

When a patient is newly discovered to have renal dysfunction, an effort should be made to discern whether this is the result of a long-standing chronic process, an acute reversible form of renal failure, or a combination of both. Several other systemic diseases can manifest initially with renal dysfunction. Diagnostic tests to rule out other causes such as autoimmune, malignant, and thrombotic disorders may be necessary. An extensive history should be conducted to gather informa-

TABLE 43.9	Possible Causes of Uremic Pruritus
Dry skin	Increased levels of histamine
Accumulation of uremic wastes	Increased levels of serotonin
Precipitation of calcium in the skin	Alterations in κ receptors
Hyperparathyroidism	Alterations in the immune system
Hypervitaminosis A	

(Adapted from Kuypers D, Claes K, Evenpoel P, et al. A prospective proof of concept study of the efficacy of tacrolimus ointment on uraemic pruritus (UP) in patients on dialysis therapy. Nephrol Dial Transplant 19:1895–1901, 2004; Momose A, Kudo S, Sato H, et al. Calcium ions are abnormally distributed in the skin of hemodialysis patients with uraemic pruritus. Nephrol Dial Transplant 19:2061–2066, 2004; Murphy M, Reaich D, Pai P, et al. A randomized, placebo-controlled, double-blind trial of ondansetron in renal itch. Br J Dermatol 148:314–317. 2003.)

tion on exposure to nephrotoxins (especially drugs), previously unrecognized urinary tract symptoms, or risk factors for renal disease. A renal biopsy can provide information that is helpful in confirming the cause of renal disease, its extent, and the overall prognosis, especially when causes other than diabetes or hypertension are suspected. In general, biopsies are performed only if a treatable form of systemic disease is suspected and the information gained will alter or guide therapeutic decisions. Renal ultrasound (sonography) can assist the clinician in assessing kidney size and in ruling out obstructive processes often associated with hydronephrosis. Small kidney size generally implies a long-standing, irreversible, or advanced form of the disease. Renal arteriography may be considered for use in ruling out the presence of renal artery stenosis or other vascular or perfusion abnormalities. Although serum creatinine values may provide a rough estimate of remaining GFR, measured urinary creatinine clearance studies more accurately assess residual renal function. Although urinalysis is usually less informative in differentiating chronic renal disease subtypes as compared with its usefulness in ARF, quantifying the amount of proteinuria is important as a prognostic feature, or in establishing a baseline for antiproteinuric interventions. Metabolic and hematologic panels aid the clinician in assessing the degree of multiorgan involvement that has occurred as part of the uremic syndrome.

Initial assessment should involve determination of the severity of disease, comorbid conditions, complications related to loss of kidney function, risk or progression of the disease, and risk for CVD.[2] Identification of factors that may aggravate progression of renal disease is crucial. Correction of reversible factors may help partially restore renal function toward baseline and preserve remaining function. Destabilizing variables might include the initiators of ARF superimposed on CRF, as well as uncontrolled hypertension or excessive protein intake. Depending on how advanced renal failure is, efforts to reduce proteinuria, correct dyslipidemia, and optimize glycemic control (in patients with diabetes) may prove very helpful with respect to retarding progression to ESKD.

NEPHROTIC SYNDROME

Nephrotic syndrome is the metabolic and clinical consequence of continued heavy proteinuria, usually greater than 3.5 grams of protein per day. In addition to proteinuria, this syndrome is characterized by hypoalbuminemia, edema, hyperlipidemia, and hypercoagulability. A variety of glomerulonephropathies have been associated with nephrotic syndrome, including those caused by systemic, metabolic, and endocrine diseases; allergens; microorganisms; drugs; and toxins.[11]

Increased glomerular permeability to plasma protein leads to each of the clinical and metabolic derangements associated with nephrotic syndrome.[81] Hypoalbuminemia is the direct result of albumin loss in the urine, which accounts for 60% to 90% of urinary protein. Loss of larger-molecular-weight proteins, including immunoglobulins, is associated with abnormalities in immune response and increased sus-

ceptibility to serious infection. Enhanced hepatic synthesis of lipoproteins is thought to result from hypoalbuminemia and a reduction in colloid oncotic pressure, inducing a hyperlipidemic state that is suspected to increase risk of ischemic heart disease.[82] Edema is due to sodium retention by the kidney and reduction in intravascular colloid oncotic pressure. Edema seen with nephrotic syndrome is marked by a distribution pattern that includes the face and periorbital region, particularly in the morning. Edema of the lower extremities can be seen as the day progresses. Numerous defects in clotting factors, the fibrinolytic system, and platelet function are responsible for the hypercoagulable state.

PSYCHOSOCIAL ASPECTS

Numerous studies have shown that the development of ESKD is often accompanied by significant losses in quality of life, functional status, and autonomy.[122] In turn, at least one study in this population has found that impairments in mental status, performance status, and quality of life are independently correlated with risk of mortality.[123] Many challenges to maintaining quality of life are rooted in medical causes, but they are compounded by constraints within the health care delivery system, the type of RRT administered, financial difficulties, and societal misunderstanding of renal disease. Several barriers, both practical and artificial, exist against employing patients with ESKD. Although these are not insurmountable, less than 10% of patients with ESKD who are younger than 60 years of age are able to maintain gainful employment.[123]

THERAPEUTIC PLAN

SLOWING THE PROGRESSION OF CHRONIC KIDNEY DISEASE

The interrelationship that chronic kidney disease shares with diabetes, hypertension, and hyperlipidemia is becoming increasingly recognized. Through recently developed clinical practice guidelines, the groundwork for an integrated approach to management of these disease states has been laid. These guidelines represent a collaborative effort and consensus between the National Heart, Lung and Blood Institute [through Joint National Committee (JNC)-VII],[124] the National Cholesterol Education Program (through Adult Treatment Panel III),[125] the NKF, and the American Diabetes Association (ADA). The K/DOQI has formed committees that are charged with researching various issues of CKD and providing practice guidelines. Such guidelines on a variety of issues involved in treating patients with CKD have been published (Table 43.10).

Strategies for slowing kidney disease progression are often divided into measures for patients with diabetes versus those for nondiabetic individuals. In practice, however, these groupings differ primarily in the threshold for their implementation and in the amount of clinical evidence that sup-

TABLE 43.10	Guidelines for the Management of Chronic Kidney Disease and Associated Complications

The National Kidney Foundation, Disease Outcomes Quality Initiative (NKF-K/DOQI)

1. K/DOQI Clinical Practice Guidelines for Chronic Kidney Disease: Evaluation, Classification, and Stratification. [Am J Kidney Dis 39 (Suppl 2):S1–S266, 2002]

2. K/DOQI Clinical Practice Guidelines for the Management of Dyslipidemias in Patients with Kidney Disease. [Am J Kidney Dis 41 (4 Suppl 3):S1–S91, 2003]

3. Clinical Practice Guidelines for the Management of Anemia of Kidney Disease. [Am J Kidney Dis 37 (1 Suppl 1):S182–S238, 2001]

4. Clinical Practice Guidelines for the Nutrition in Patients with Chronic Kidney Disease. [Am J Kidney Dis 36 (6 Suppl 2):S1–S140, 2000]

5. NKF-K/DOQI Clinical Practice Guidelines for Peritoneal Dialysis Adequacy. [Am J Kidney Dis 37 (1 Suppl 1):S65–S136, 2001]

6. NKF-K/DOQI Clinical Practice Guidelines for Hemodialysis Adequacy. [Am J Kidney Dis 37 (1 Suppl 1):S1–S64, 2001]

7. NKF-K/DOQI Clinical Practice Guidelines for Vascular Access. Update 2000. [Am J Kidney Dis 37 (1 Suppl 1):S137–S181, 2001]

8. Clinical Practice Guidelines on Hypertension and Antihypertensive Agents in Chronic Kidney Disease. [Am J Kidney Dis 43 (5 Suppl 1):S1–S290, 2004]

9. Bone Metabolism and Disease in Chronic Kidney Disease. [Am J Kidney Dis 42 (4 Suppl 3):S1–S201, 2003]

TABLE 43.11	Potential Alternatives to Nephrotoxic Therapies
Nephrotoxin	**Possible Alternative or Kidney-Sparing Approach***
Aminoglycoside	Fluoroquinolones, aztreonam, imipenem, meropenem, ceftazidime, cefepime
	Once-daily "pulse" dosing strategies
Cyclosporine, tacrolimus	Sirolimus
Amphotericin B	Liposomal or lipid complex formulations
	Itraconazole, fluconazole, voriconazole
	Caspofungin, micafungin
Cisplatin	Carboplatin
	Nephroprotection with amifostine
Radiocontrast media	Low-osmolality or nonionic contrast agents, low volume
	Nephroprotection protocols (hydration, bicarbonate, N-acetylcysteine, theophylline)

* Appropriateness of these alternatives depends on the specific patient, indication, and situation.

ports their beneficial role. Obviously, measures that target glycemic control pertain to the diabetic population. It is important residual kidney function be preserved at all stages of CKD. In addition to treating patients with risk factors and comorbid diseases, minimizing exposure to nephrotoxins is recommended. Table 43.11 offers some suggestions.

MONITORING PROGRESSION OF CHRONIC KIDNEY DISEASE

When a patient is identified to have renal disease, regular periodic assessments should be performed to determine the rate of GFR decline and to confirm the efficacy of interventions intended to slow renal demise. Regular monitoring also facilitates the detection of sudden deteriorations in GFR due to reversible factors. Early detection and management of complications that begin to develop before ESKD (e.g., anemia, bone disease, malnutrition, hypertension, heart disease) may help minimize morbidity and mortality. Maintaining an accurate gauge of renal status should help prompt the adjustment of dose or regimen for renally eliminated drugs, preventing toxicity or dangerous drug accumulation.

In the past, the reciprocal of SCr (1/SCr) has been used to quantify the degree of renal dysfunction. The accuracy of this approach has been debated because the relationship between SCr and GFR is subject to several nonrenal influences (lean body mass, liver disease, etc.). Additionally, other variables, such as age, race, and sex, have been determined to affect the estimation of GFR. As GFR declines, even measured creatinine clearance values tend to overestimate GFR because of the increasing contribution of tubular secretion to overall creatinine excretion. Although no surrogate marker of renal function is fail proof, GFR estimation and assessment of metabolic status are advocated at 3-month intervals, if not more often. Serial measures of proteinuria appear to be less precise than GFR in monitoring progression of renal disease but are valuable in establishing the presence and gross extent of nephropathy and in assessing antiproteinuric interventions.

TREATMENT

TREATMENT OF DIABETIC NEPHROPATHY

Diabetic nephropathy is caused mainly by the presence of hyperglycemia, as has been previously discussed. In this situation, the best way to prevent or slow renal damage is to prevent hyperglycemia.[14,23] Several trials[14–17] have shown that minimizing hyperglycemia can delay the onset and slow the progression of the microvascular and macrovascular complications of diabetes. The Diabetes Control and Complications Trial Research Group (DCCT trial) demonstrated that patients with type 1 diabetes who maintain hemoglobin A1C levels at approximately 7% (vs. 9%) delayed the onset and progression of retinopathy, nephropathy, and neuropathy.[14] Group et al.[126] conducted a similar trial with patients with type 2 diabetes and showed similar results. It is interesting to note that in this study the difference in hemoglobin A1C was very small—7% vs. 7.9%. This small difference resulted in a decrease of 35% in the relative risk of microvascular disease.[15] Given the results of these studies, the American Diabetes Association recommends that hemoglobin A1C be maintained at less than 7%.[10] In vitro as well as in vivo studies have shown that ACE-Is prevent the formation of AGEs, regardless of glycemic control.[26,127,128] The mechanism of inhibition is still unclear but may be secondary to chelation or a decrease in reactive oxygen species.[128] Other studies using angiotensin receptor antagonists have shown similar benefits.[127] Additionally, research in animal models has identified several other agents that are effective against AGEs but have yet to be used in trials with humans.[24]

Some research and debate have focused on the use of ACE-Is and ARBs. Given the properties of ACE-Is and ARBs, they are considered first-line agents in the treatment of patients with diabetic nephropathy, regardless of whether or not the patient is hypertensive. The renoprotective effects have been proved beyond their effects on blood pressure.[40,129,130] The ADA recommends that all patients with type 1 diabetes with microalbuminuria should take an ACE-I.[10] The ADA recommends the use of ARBs as first-line agents in the treatment of nephropathy in patients with type 2 diabetes. In a review of the current literature[131] on the use of ACE-Is and ARBs,[132] ACE-Is were noted to show a reduction in all-cause mortality, but ARBs did not. This discrepancy may be attributed to the small number of trials using ARBs that focused on mortality as an outcome.

Both classes of drugs—ACE-Is and ARBs—appear to be efficacious in slowing the progression of albuminuria and ne-

phropathy. ACE-Is may be favorable in that many are available generically, thus lowering the cost to the patient; ARBs appear to result in a lower incidence of cough and may be an alternative for those patients who cannot tolerate an ACE-I. Second-line therapy for the treatment of patients with diabetic nephropathy and proteinuria is the use of nondihydropyridine calcium channel blockers (NDCCBs). Diltiazem and verapamil have been shown to attenuate permeability changes in the glomerulus and to have an effect on rates of decline in GFR similar to that associated with treatment with an ACE-I.[133] It should be noted that evidence suggests that some dihydropyridine calcium channel blockers increase the risk of myocardial infarction and other cardiovascular events.[134-136] Because these agents have not been shown to significantly decrease proteinuria, they should not be used in the management of diabetic nephropathy.

Patients with diabetic nephropathy often have additional risk factors such as dyslipidemia and hypertension. These diseases should be addressed as well. Because CVD is the primary cause of mortality in patients with CKD, it should be noted that treating patients with hyperglycemia in conjunction with other risk factors significantly decreased the incidences of nephropathy and CVD.[137] Multifactorial interventional studies designed to control diet, exercise, smoking cessation, hyperglycemia, and dyslipidemia, and to administer ACE-Is, vitamins, and low-dose aspirin have shown a decrease in the progression of microvascular and macrovascular disease.[137,138] The treatment of patients with hypertension and hyperlipidemia is discussed in other sections.

TREATMENT OF HYPERTENSION WITH ANTIHYPERTENSIVE AGENTS

The K/DOQI Clinical Practice Guidelines on Hypertension and Antihypertensive Agents in Chronic Kidney Disease were published in May of 2004.[139] These guidelines were developed for use in patients with CKD at stages 1 to 4. Stage 5 CKD will be addressed separately, in forthcoming guidelines, because patients with ESKD may have different needs.

TREATMENT GOALS: HYPERTENSION

- Decrease blood pressure to less than 130/80 mm Hg.
- Reduce proteinuria.
- Slow progression of kidney disease.
- Reduce CVD risk.

It has been proven that treatment with ACEI-ARBs slows the progression of CKD even in the absence of hypertension. Patients who have a spot urine total protein-to-creatinine ratio greater than 200 mg per g, or microalbuminuria, should be treated with moderate to high doses of an ACE-I or ARB,

regardless of whether or not they are diabetic or hypertensive. Additionally, patients with diabetes should receive an ACE-I or an ARB, unless a specific contraindication exists (Table 43.12). Patients who do not have proteinuria or diabetes, similar to those discussed by JNC VII,[124] should be

TABLE 43.12	Cautions and Contraindications With ACE-Is and ARBs

Contraindication	Caution
Pregnancy	History of cough
History of allergy (both) or angioedema (ACE-I)	Concomitant drugs causing hyperkalemia
Bilateral renal artery stenosis	Angioedema with ACE-I (ARB)

ACE-Is, angiotensin-converting enzyme inhibitors; ARBs, angiotensin receptor blockers.
(Adapted from American Diabetes Association. Standards of medical care for patients with diabetes mellitus [erratum appears in Diabetes Care 26:972, 2003]. Diabetes Care 26 (Suppl 1):S33–S50, 2003.)

treated first with a diuretic. Specifically, JNC VII recommends the use of thiazide diuretics as first-line therapy because substantial data have revealed a resultant decrease in morbidity and mortality in hypertensive patients. Thiazides may be less effective in patients with CKD stage 4 (GFR <30 mL/min), who may require a loop diuretic. A combination of a thiazide and a loop diuretic may be necessary for patients with significant edema or hyporesponsiveness to a single agent. Calcium channel blockers are the preferred agents in transplant patients with CKD, followed by β-blockers and ACE-Is. Both K/DOQI and JNC VII guidelines emphasize that most patients with CKD and hypertension will require therapy with two or more antihypertensive agents to achieve target blood pressure less than 130/80 mm Hg. For patients with more severe hypertension [systolic blood pressure (SBP) >150 mm Hg], two agents should be used at initiation. Potassium-sparing diuretics should be used

with caution in CKD stages 4 and 5, as well as in patients who are receiving other agents that can cause hyperkalemia. In addition to use of pharmacologic agents, guidelines recommend initiation of lifestyle modifications. These include weight loss if obese, smoking cessation, moderation of alcohol intake, exercise, and adherence to the DASH diet (Dietary Approaches to Stop Hypertension).[140]

Monitoring of Antihypertensive Therapies. Appropriate monitoring consists of calculation of GFR, measurement of blood pressure, and assessment of serum electrolyte levels (especially potassium). Generally, assessment should be conducted every 12 weeks. More frequent evaluation (every 4 weeks) may be necessary if serum creatinine is rising, if hypertension is uncontrolled, or if serum potassium levels are out of the target range.

Differences in Antihypertensive Therapies. With few exceptions, the K/DOQI guidelines reiterate the recommendations of the JNC VII guidelines. The use of ACE-Is, ARBs, and calcium channel blockers is reviewed in the section on diabetic nephropathy. Diuretics are discussed in the section on fluid management. Other agents that may be used as adjunct therapy are briefly described here. A more thorough review of JNC VII and antihypertensive agents can be found in Chapter 20.

As has previously been discussed, ACE-Is or ARBs are recommended in the presence of diabetes, proteinuria, or established nephropathy (Table 43.13). NDCCBs are second-line agents for the treatment of proteinuria. Other agents may be added as adjunct therapy to control blood pressure. The choice of agents should be guided by compelling indications or comorbid diseases (see Chapter 20). In clinical practice, the use of adjunctive agents is generally the same for hypertensive patients without CKD. Care should be taken to regularly monitor patients with CKD for adverse events,

TABLE 43.13	K/DOQI Recommendations for Antihypertensive Therapy	

Type of Kidney Disease	Preferred Agents	Other Agents
Diabetic nephropathy or spot urine total protein-to-creatinine ratio ≥200 mg/g	ACE-I or ARB	Diuretic, then β-blocker or CCB
Nondiabetic CKD with spot urine total protein-to-creatinine ratio <200 mg/g	Diuretic	ACE-I, ARB, β-blocker, or CCB
CKD in the transplant recipient	None preferred	CCB, diuretic, β-blocker, ACE-I, or ARB

ACE-I, angiotensin-converting enzyme inhibitor; ARB, angiotensin receptor blocker; CCB, calcium channel blocker; CKD, chronic kidney disease; K/DOQI, Kidney Disease Outcomes Quality Initiative
(From Kidney Disease Outcomes Quality Initiative K/DOQI clinical practice guidelines on hypertension and antihypertensive agents in chronic kidney disease. Am J Kidney Dis 43 (5 Suppl 1):S1–S290, 2004, with permission.)

worsening of kidney function, or other effects such as hyperkalemia. It is prudent to begin therapy of antihypertensive patients with small doses and titrate to effect. This helps to prevent abrupt changes in hemodynamics within the kidney and therefore reduces the risk of exacerbating kidney dysfunction.

β-Adrenergic blocking agents lower blood pressure primarily by reducing cardiac output. They also inhibit renin release and thus may be especially useful in the setting of renovascular hypertension or renal failure, or in combination with renin-activating agents (such as diuretics). Although β-blockers reduce renal blood flow, renal autoregulatory mechanisms generally prevent clinically significant reductions in GFR from occurring. The nonselective β-blockers are believed to promote hyperkalemia by inhibiting β_2-mediated K^+ translocation across cell membranes. In practice, β-blocker–associated elevations in serum K^+ are usually observed only when other risk factors for hyperkalemia are also present. Selective β_1-antagonists are preferred. Labetalol and carvedilol combine α-blockade with nonselective β-blocking effects, do not directly produce significant alterations in GFR, and are thought to be tolerated comparably by CKD and non-CKD populations.

Other Adrenergic Blocking Agents. The centrally acting α_2-adrenergic agonists (methyldopa, clonidine, guanabenz, and guanfacine) are useful in reducing blood pressure in patients with chronic renal failure. Because methyldopa and its active metabolite accumulate with decreased renal function, dosing adjustments and cautious titration are necessary. At creatinine clearances below 50 mL per minute, reduction in clonidine dosage should also be considered, along with extended observation for symptoms of prolonged accumulation (excessive hypotension, bradycardia, somnolence, etc.). Guanabenz and guanfacine tend to produce sedation and xerostomia (dry mouth), making adherence to fluid restrictions difficult for some patients. The α_1-adrenergic antagonists (prazosin, terazosin, doxazosin) reduce blood pressure by producing arterial and venous vasodilation. Because of an association with increased mortality,[141] these agents are generally not used unless there is a compelling indication (e.g., benign prostatic hypertrophy).

Other Antihypertensives. The direct-acting vasodilators, hydralazine and minoxidil, decrease peripheral vascular resistance. Blood pressure reduction is usually accompanied by compensatory activation of the sympathetic nervous system and renin release, leading to reflex tachycardia, increased cardiac output, and fluid retention. Because of these secondary effects, hydralazine and minoxidil are commonly used in combination with agents that counteract fluid retention (e.g., diuretics) and tachycardia (e.g., β-blockers, which also blunt renin release).

TREATMENT OF PROTEINURIA

Given the detrimental effects of proteinuria, much research has been undertaken to evaluate the benefits of lowering total daily protein excretion in the urine and the use of different agents and therapies to achieve this goal. As was previously mentioned, protein is the specific target for renoprotective treatment.[142] Several strategies have been tried to decrease proteinuria and therefore decrease the rate of decline to ESKD, as well as to reduce morbidity and mortality. Table 43.14 lists some of the therapies that have been tried

TABLE 43.14	K/DOQI Antiproteinuric Therapies: Stratified Level of Recommendation		
Level 1*	**Level 2**	**Level 3**
Control BP	Restrict Na intake	Decrease homocysteine level
Provide ACE-I therapy	Control fluid intake	Give antioxidant therapy
Administer ARB treatment	Provide NDH-CCB therapy	Use sodium bicarbonate for metabolic acidosis
Provide combination ACE-I and ARB	Control lipids	Give NSAIDs for nephrotic syndrome
Avoid DHCCB	Administer an aldosterone antagonist	Other (avoid iron overload, intake of caffeine, etc.)
Provide β-blocker therapy	Assist with smoking cessation	
Control protein intake	Avoid estrogen/progestin	
	Assume supine/recumbent position	
	Reduce obesity	

ACE-I, angiotensin-converting enzyme inhibitor; ARB, angiotensin receptor blocker; BP, blood pressure; DHCCB, dihydropyridine calcium channel blocker; Na, sodium; NDH-CCB, nondihydropyridine calcium channel blocker; NSAIDs, nonsteroidal anti-inflammatory drugs.

* Level 1, strongest evidence, good evidence, little evidence or opinion.

(Adapted from Wilmer W, Rovin B, Hebert C, et al. Management of glomerular proteinuria: a commentary. J Am Soc Nephrol 14:3217–3232, 2003.)

and the level of evidence available to support their use. It has been shown that ACE-Is and ARBs reduce proteinuria beyond their blood pressure–lowering effects.[15,16,30,40,130] A meta-analysis[143] showed a benefit in patients with diabetes (decrease progression of CKD) and in those who do not have diabetes (decrease incidence of ESKD, decrease mortality). Although there are fewer studies on these, ARBs have been shown to be renoprotective and antiproteinuric.[144,145] A number of studies using ACE-Is and ARBs have been conducted with the primary end points of decreasing proteinuria, slowing kidney disease progression, and decreasing morbidity and mortality. Strippoli et al[131] reviewed 43 controlled trials that used ACE-Is, ARBs, or both, for the treatment of patients with diabetic nephropathy. ACE-Is and ARBs have consistently shown benefit in slowing the progression of nephropathy and in decreasing microalbuminuria. In addition, ACE-Is reduced the risk for all-cause mortality by 20%. Several studies have evaluated the effects of using an ACE-I and an ARB in combination. These studies have shown that ACE-Is plus ARBs have a synergistic effect on proteinuria.[146–155] The ACE-Is and the ARBs have the greatest body of supporting evidence regarding decreasing proteinuria secondary to diabetic nephropathy; however, in nondiabetic patients, both ACE-Is and NDCCBs are the preferred agents for use in reducing proteinuria.[124] For maximal effect, ACE-Is should be titrated to higher doses.[18] ACE-Is may cause a small increase in serum creatinine levels, which results from an initial decrease in intraglomerular pressure caused by efferent arteriolar dilation. Generally, this increase in serum creatinine is transient and levels return to baseline within several weeks. If, however, a sharp rise is noted or persists, the drug should be withdrawn.

Protein Intake and Therapeutic Implications. A high-protein diet has been found to increase renal blood flow and GFR by several potential mechanisms. One could therefore theorize that excessive protein intake would heighten glomerular hyperfiltration and hence, long-term risk of renal disease. Conversely, protein restriction might help limit hyperfiltration and kidney disease in certain individuals. Over the past decade, the effect of dietary protein restriction on the progression of renal disease has been the subject of several clinical investigations, which have yielded conflicting findings.

Early animal and pilot clinical studies in humans with moderate to severe diabetic nephropathy had demonstrated that moderate to strict protein restriction could significantly reduce the rate and number of patients progressing toward ESKD.[156,157] However, two larger trials subsequently failed to show a similar benefit from moderate to marked degrees of protein restriction, over a 3-year study period.[158,159] These landmark studies, one of which is known as the Modification of Diet in Renal Disease (MDRD) study,[158] were conducted in populations with largely nondiabetic forms of advanced renal disease. Because of the divergent findings between trials, considerable controversy exists over the value of dietary protein restriction in slowing CKD progression. Disagreement between the MDRD and earlier findings has been partially attributed to differences in the study populations and study designs, including the use of additional interventions in later trials, which helped lower the rate of disease progression in control groups (e.g., aggressive blood pressure control, the use of ACE-Is, levels of protein intake within "control" groups that were well below usual dietary practice in the United States and Europe).

Reanalysis of the original MDRD findings now favors the argument that protein restriction was indeed beneficial in retarding CKD progression, particularly in persons with moderate disease (GFR 25–55 mL/min) or a rapidly declining GFR at enrollment.[160] Similar to the pattern of response described earlier with interventions that reduce hyperfiltration, small reductions in GFR were noted after the initiation of protein restriction; these were later followed by slower rates of GFR decline when compared with controls. Unfortunately, the primary 3-year end point may have proved too early to demonstrate differences in absolute outcome between groups caused by initial losses in GFR experienced by treatment groups. With extended follow-up, the renal-sparing benefits of protein restriction might have become fully apparent, as the reduced rate of GFR decline in restricted groups began to compensate for early drops in GFR. Two meta-analyses examining the effects of dietary protein restriction on CKD progression also support the notion that dietary protein restriction is beneficial for some patients, especially those with diabetes and nondiabetic patients with moderate to severe disease.[161,162] In contrast, others maintain that the benefit is modest, relative to other interventions such as control of hypertension.[161] Given that numerous studies have demonstrated that hypoalbuminemia is correlated with an increase in morbidity and mortality in patients on dialysis,[163,164,165–167] imposition of a protein restriction must be executed cautiously. The only treatment for hypoalbuminemia is proper nutrition, which is extremely difficult to provide in patients with CKD, who may be subject to dietary restrictions such as sodium, potassium, phosphate, fat, and cholesterol. In practice, most nephrologists advise patients with CKD to avoid *excessive* protein intake but do not impose a protein restriction. In fact, as patients progress to ESKD, their protein requirements increase because of increased catabolism and loss during dialysis. It is recommended that these patients consume between 1.2 and 1.3 g/kg/day of protein.[168]

TREATMENT OF DYSLIPIDEMIA

The benefits of treating dyslipidemia in patients with CKD have been demonstrated through many studies. Specifically, studies suggest that hydroxymethylglutaryl coenzyme A reductase inhibitors (HMG-CoA, statins) are particularly beneficial. Statins may decrease proliferation of mesangial[169–171] and proximal tubular cells, reducing glomerulosclerosis.[172]

They may also decrease the inflammatory response stimulated by endothelin-1.[173] They have been shown to have an antiproteinuric effect,[169,174] as well as the ability to slow progression of renal dysfunction.[46,175,176] Studies have shown decreases in carotid intimal thickening (a marker of total body atherosclerosis).[177] Statins have also been shown to decrease plasma homocysteine levels; fibrates may have the opposite effect. In a meta-analysis of 13 trials with a total of 362 patients, Fried et al found a small beneficial effect on kidney function with improvement of the lipid profile.[178] Post hoc analysis of several other trials showed that treatment of patients with hyperlipidemia with statins improved kidney function.[46,179]

In a trial of atorvastatin versus placebo, atorvastatin reduced proteinuria from 2.2 to 1.2 g per day (vs. 2.0 to 1.8 in placebo). Creatinine clearance declined less in the treatment arm than in the placebo group—1.2 mL per minute versus 5.8 mL per minute.[180] Studies involving other statins have shown a decrease in urinary albumin excretion[173,181] and an increased GFR.[182] Most important is the fact that treatment of dyslipidemia in CKD patients with ischemic heart disease has been shown to decrease mortality.[183,184] This is significant in that CVD is a major cause of mortality in patients with CKD. In a study of patients with predominantly mild to moderate CKD, it was found that although 85% of the patient population had dyslipidemia (high LDL, low HDL, and/or high triglyceride levels), only about 15% were being treated for these abnormalities.[185]

Guidelines. In April of 2003, the K/DOQI published guidelines for the management of dyslipidemia in patients with kidney disease.[186] The definition of dyslipidemia was taken directly from the Adult Treatment Panel III Guidelines of the National Cholesterol Education Program (ATP/NCEP[125]) (Table 43.15). The K/DOQI guidelines highlight the many risk factors for CVD in addition to dyslipidemia, such as hypertension, tobacco use, obesity, and diabetes. It is recommended that treatment for patients with these other risk factors be initiated. Additionally, these risk factors should be evaluated every year.

Evaluation. The K/DOQI guidelines were created for patients at all stages of CKD (1–5), as well as for all renal transplant recipients regardless of lipid levels. They follow the ATP III guidelines, with only a few modifications (Table 43.16). One important difference is that K/DOQI considers CKD as a risk factor for CHD. Also, it is noted that practitioners should closely monitor patients and watch for complications of therapy. According to the guidelines, total cholesterol should be less than 200 mg per dL, LDL less than 100 mg per dL, triglycerides less than 150 mg per dL, and HDL more than 40 mg per dL. To assess patients, a fasting lipid profile should be obtained at the presentation of CKD, when there is a change of status, and yearly thereafter. Thera-

TABLE 43.15 Definition of Dyslipidemia

Dyslipidemia	Level (mg/dL)
Total cholesterol	
Desirable	<200
Borderline high	200–239
High	≥240
Low-density lipoprotein (LDL) cholesterol	
Optimal	<100
Near optimal	100–129
Borderline	130–159
High	160–189
Very high	≥190
Triglycerides	
Normal	<150
Borderline high	150–199
High	200–499
Very high	≥500
High-density lipoprotein (HDL) cholesterol	
Low	<40

(From Kidney Disease Outcomes Quality Initiative G. K/DOQI clinical practice guidelines for management of dyslipidemias in patients with kidney disease. Am J Kidney Dis 41 (4 Suppl 3):I–IV, Year, with permission.)

TABLE 43.16 Dyslipidemia Guideline Differences Between K/DOQI and ATP III K/DOQI's Recommendations

CKD is a CHD risk equivalent	Consider complications of lipid-lowering agents that may occur because of reduced renal function
Evaluation of dyslipidemia should occur at presentation of CKD, then annually	Consider that there may be other indications for lipid-lowering agents besides preventing ACVD
Initiate drug therapy if LDL is between 100 and 129 mg/dL after 3 months of TLC	Consider the treatment of proteinuria to improve the lipid profile
Initial drug therapy should be a statin	Fibrates may be used in CKD stage 5
Guidelines needed for patients >18 years old	

ACVD, atherosclerotic cardiovascular disease; ATP III, adenosine triphosphate III; CHD, coronary heart disease; CKD, chronic kidney disease; K/DOQI, Kidney Disease Outcomes Quality Initiative; TLC, therapeutic lifestyle changes.
(Adapted from Seliger S, Weiss N, Gillen D, et al. HMG-CoA reductase inhibitors are associated with reduced mortality in ESRD patients. Kidney Int 61:297–304, 2002.)

TABLE 43.17	Treatment Guidelines for Dyslipidemias of CKD			
Dyslipidemia	**Goal**	**Initiate**	**Increase**	**Alternative**
TG ≥500 mg/dL	<500	TLC	Fibrate or niacin	Fibrate or niacin
LDL 100–129	<100	TLC	Low-dose statin	Bile acid seq or niacin
LDL ≥130	<100	TLC + low-dose statin	Max-dose statin	Bile acid seq or niacin
TG ≥200 and non-HDL ≥130	Non-HDL <130	TLC + low-dose statin	Max-dose statin	Fibrate or niacin

CKD, chronic kidney disease; HDL, high-density lipoprotein; LDL, low-density lipoprotein; seq, sequestrants; TG, triglycerides; TLC, therapeutic lifestyle changes.
(From Seliger S, Weiss N, Gillen D, et al. HMG-CoA reductase inhibitors are associated with reduced mortality in ESRD patients. Kidney Int 61:297–304, 2002, with permission.)

peutic lifestyle modifications should be recommended for all dyslipidemic patients. These include healthful eating, increased physical activity, smoking cessation, and moderation of alcohol intake. Additionally, other modifiable risk factors should be addressed such as hypothyroidism, excessive alcohol intake, and uncontrolled diabetes. Table 43.17 highlights recommendations for treatment based on the type of dyslipidemia. When drug therapy is recommended, the statins are considered first-line agents because of their beneficial effects on renal function. Fibrates can be used in stage 5 if patients have triglycerides greater than 500 mg per dL, or in stages 1 to 4 if the non-HDL level is still greater than 130 mg per dL and patients do not tolerate a statin. Gemfibrozil is the fibrate of choice, as other fibrates may cause a reversible increase in serum creatinine.[187,188] Gemfibrozil decreases triglycerides and increases HDL but has minimal effects on LDL,[189] making it a particularly effective treatment for patients with hypertriglyceridemia. Because of the increased risk of rhabdomyolysis, fibrates and statins should not be used in combination.

Considerations in Patients With CKD. Some issues require special consideration when treating members of the CKD population. The phosphate binder sevelamer has been shown to lower serum LDL concentrations. Although it is not indicated for the treatment of patients with dyslipidemia, this characteristic may make the drug more desirable when a choice must be made among the available phosphate binders. Because of accumulation of drugs or their metabolites that causes kidney dysfunction, interactions that increase drug levels are particularly important. The serum concentration of most statins may be increased by agents that inhibit the cytochrome P-450 3A4 isozyme. Such drugs include azole antifungal agents, macrolide antibiotics, fibrates, calcium channel blockers, niacin, and grapefruit juice. Cyclosporine and tacrolimus, which are commonly prescribed to renal transplant recipients, do elevate statin levels. Pravastatin and fluvastatin are the least affected and may be the drugs of choice in this population. Bile acid sequestrants (BSAs) are second-line agents that must be used with caution in renal

transplant recipients. If given at the same time, these agents may bind immunosuppressive agents, placing the patient at risk for organ rejection. Care must be taken to stagger the administration of the BSA to ensure proper absorption of cyclosporine (and other immunosuppressants).

Dyslipidemia remains a serious risk factor for the development of CVD, and CVD remains a major cause of mortality for patients with CKD. The number of patients with CKD who have untreated dyslipidemia is distressing. This fact highlights the need for patient as well as provider education to improve awareness. Additionally, other risk factors for CVD, such as smoking, hypertension, obesity, and uncontrolled diabetes, should be addressed.

TREATMENT OF METABOLIC AND SYSTEMIC CONSEQUENCES OF CHRONIC KIDNEY DISEASE

DIURETICS AND VOLUME MANAGEMENT

Until patients become dialysis dependent, diuretic therapy is a mainstay of fluid and volume management. When used as single agents, thiazides lose much of their diuretic efficacy after GFR falls to below 20 to 30 mL per minute; however, their vasodilatory actions can still modestly contribute to blood pressure reduction. At this point, loop diuretics such as furosemide, bumetanide, and torsemide become drugs of choice in maintaining volume balance. These agents enter the urine through tubular secretion, producing dose-dependent diuretic responses that require a "threshold" urinary concentration to be present. In patients with CKD, drug entry into urine and at the site of action is impaired. Administration of doses two to ten times higher than those given to patients with normal renal function may be required to produce a comparable diuretic response.

Clinical resistance to loop diuretics may occur as the result of impaired drug entry into the urine (due to diminished tubular secretion or renal perfusion), rebound sodium retention at distal tubular sites, altered protein binding, concurrent use of nonsteroidal anti-inflammatory drugs (NSAIDs), or other factors.[12,93,94] One of the first steps required in overcoming diuretic resistance has traditionally been to escalate the dose until an effective diuresis is achieved, thereby establishing a "threshold" diuretic dose. In this circumstance, administration of a single larger dose of loop diuretic will more reliably elicit a diuresis than the same total amount divided into smaller intermittent doses that are below the threshold. The use of longer-acting agents (e.g., torsemide) or repeated doses of shorter-acting agents (furosemide, bumetanide) may further improve diuretic responsiveness by maintaining urinary drug levels and by reducing compensatory postdiuresis sodium retention. Repeat doses that are administered later in the day should be no smaller than the threshold effective dose. Although no loop diuretic is clearly superior, some differences exist between agents. The bioavailability of torsemide and bumetanide is nearly complete, whereas that of oral furosemide averages only 50% (range, 20% to 80%). Conversion from parenteral to oral furosemide dosing should account for this difference and generally requires a doubling of dose. In addition, severe gastrointestinal edema may reduce the bioavailability and efficacy of these agents, necessitating initial intravenous therapy, especially in the case of furosemide. In severe renal impairment, nonrenal clearance is more significant for bumetanide than for furosemide, and the usual milligram equivalency ratio of bumetanide to furosemide is reduced from 1:40 mg to 1:20 mg. Furosemide is highly protein bound and as such becomes bound to urinary albumin, reducing active urinary levels. In patients with high urine protein content (e.g., nephrotic syndrome), dose escalation becomes necessary, to overcome protein binding in the tubular fluid and to achieve desired diuretic responses. Although ototoxicity is possible with any of these agents, a slightly greater incidence is associated with furosemide, partly because of the higher doses and systemic accumulation noted in CKD. The risk of ototoxicity is generally greatest with high-dose intravenous bolus/infusion regimens, and when additional ototoxins are used concurrently, such as with aminoglycosides or cisplatin. Because of its even greater ototoxic potential, ethacrynic acid is generally reserved for patients with an established hypersensitivity to sulfa-based thiazides or other loop diuretics.

The addition of metolazone (or another thiazide) to a loop diuretic can greatly enhance diuretic response, presumably by blunting distal tubular sodium reabsorption. Many clinicians prefer to institute combination therapy before escalating to extremely high doses of loop diuretic. These synergistic combinations occasionally result in an exaggerated diuretic response associated with large urinary sodium, potassium, and magnesium losses. Volume status, blood pressure, and electrolytes should therefore be closely monitored in robust responders. If thiazides and loop diuretics are used in combination, their administration should be timed to ensure that both drugs are simultaneously present in the tubule. When both agents are being given by the same route (oral or intravenous), simultaneous administration is appropriate. However, an oral agent (usually the thiazide or metolazone) should be given at least 30 to 60 minutes before an intravenous loop diuretic, to allow adequate time for its absorption. Finally, if a patient fails to respond to escalation of a loop diuretic and to combination therapy, inpatient therapy with escalating IV bolus or continuous infusion loop diuretic may become necessary. Following administration of an effective loading bolus, continuous infusions of loop diuretic are thought to maintain urine drug concentrations and diuretic response more effectively than intermittent boluses.

Bed rest is beneficial in mobilizing interstitial fluid to the intravascular compartment. By expanding central blood volume, renal perfusion improves and enhances delivery of sodium and diuretic to the tubule. For this reason, diuretics are best given immediately after one arises from daily sleep (or even before bedtime, if patients are able to withstand arising to urinate). Patients with edema or diminishing diuretic responsiveness should be placed on a salt-restricted diet to assist in reducing positive sodium balance or rebound sodium retention (2 g/day of sodium). On a practical basis, this means no added salt to the home-cooked diet, as well as restricted intake of processed foods, especially meals from fast food restaurants. Significant reductions in dietary sodium intake are best instituted gradually in CKD, because renal adaptation to abrupt changes in volume status is inefficient. As urinary volume diminishes, restriction of daily fluid intake becomes necessary to prevent volume overload. Fluid intake is generally allowed, to match the daily urine output plus insensible losses (which average 500 mL/day under usual conditions).

HYPERKALEMIA

Patients with moderate or severe CKD may chronically have higher than normal potassium levels (4.5–5.5 mEq/L). Because of chronically elevated levels, many of these patients are able to tolerate high serum potassium levels without symptoms. Acute management of hyperkalemia should always be based on the clinical situation, not only on the serum level. If present, symptoms may include muscle weakness, paresthesias, and confusion. The hallmark signs of hyperkalemia are electrocardiographic (ECG) changes, specifically peaked T waves and a widened QRS complex. These changes are typically seen with serum potassium levels greater than 7 mEq per L. The presence of ECG changes signifies a medical emergency. The treatment of patients with acute hyperkalemia is reviewed in Chapter 28.

Chronic hyperkalemia is managed through dietary potassium restriction to approximately 1 mEq/kg/day and by curtailing the use of medications that can interfere with potassium excretion (e.g., ACE-Is, ARBs, potassium-sparing diuretics, β-blockers, trimethoprim). The addition of a potassium-binding resin such as sodium polystyrene sulfonate (Kayexalate, SPS Suspension) may become necessary when semiurgent lowering is needed or control cannot be maintained by dietary measures and the elimination of offending medications. This product acts to bind potassium in the gastrointestinal tract in exchange for sodium. For this reason, SPS must be used judiciously in patients with congestive heart failure because of the high sodium load. When given orally, SPS Suspension is typically administered as a commercially available suspension in sorbitol, which serves not only as a vehicle but also as a cathartic to hasten resin removal. Rarely, the sorbitol has been associated with bowel necrosis. To avoid sorbitol, an enema may be compounded from a powdered preparation. Maintenance doses usually range from 15 to 60 g per day (dosed by SPS content) in divided doses after meals or at bedtime. For both methods of administration, the onset of action is delayed until a bowel movement occurs.[79] Constipation itself may interfere with gut potassium secretion and should therefore be prevented, with care taken to avoid bulk laxatives that contain significant amounts of potassium. For patients with ESKD who are receiving hemodialysis, an additional management option is to modify the hemodialysis bath to promote greater potassium removal.

ACID–BASE MANAGEMENT AND SYSTEMIC ALKALINIZERS

Metabolic acidosis can be corrected by the administration of sodium bicarbonate or sodium citrate. The required amount of buffer varies among individual patients and according to whether additional forms of renal tubular acidosis (RTA) are present, but it is generally titrated to achieve serum bicarbonate levels near 20 mEq per L (mmol/L). Bicarbonate doses typically range from 20 to 40 mEq per day (0.5 to 2.0 mEq/kg/day); however, much higher doses may be needed when proximal (type 2) RTA is present.[11] Sodium bicarbonate is available in oral tablet and powder forms; each 325-mg tablet provides 4 mEq of bicarbonate. After oral administration, the bicarbonate reacts with gastric hydrochloric acid, generating carbon dioxide, which must be eliminated through belching. For patients in whom the elimination of stomach gas is difficult or painful, the use of Shohl's solution (a combination of sodium citrate and citric acid) provides an alternative buffer source. The sodium citrate in this formulation combines with hydrochloric acid to form citric acid, which is then absorbed and metabolized to carbon dioxide and water, without the generation of stomach gas. Per milliliter, Shohl's solution contains 1 mEq of sodium and 1 mEq of basic buffer. The use of potassium citrate solutions in patients with CKD should be avoided because of their potential to precipitate hyperkalemia. Citrate may also enhance the absorption of aluminum salts. Thus, citrates (e.g., sodium citrate, calcium citrate) and aluminum-based products (e.g., sucralfate, aluminum hydroxide) should be administered 2 to 3 hours apart to reduce the risk of chronic aluminum intoxication. In patients on hemodialysis, the inclusion of bicarbonate in the dialysis bath provides an additional source of alkaline buffer.

ANEMIA

Before the introduction of recombinant human erythropoietin (epoetin alfa [EPO]) in the late 1980s, anabolic steroids and red cell transfusions were the primary modalities by which anemia was treated in the CRD population. Anabolic steroids were only marginally effective, RBC transfusions were (and are still) costly, and each of these approaches was associated with significant safety concerns. The synthesis of epoetin revolutionized anemia management in the ESRD population, but despite more than a decade of clinical use, opinions are still evolving regarding the most appropriate manner of EPO use, optimal therapeutic hemoglobin (or hematocrit) goals, and their associated risk-benefit ratios. Today, three erythropoietic products are available in the United States. Epoetin alfa, a recombinant molecule with the same structure as endogenous erythropoietin, is manufactured under two name brands (Procrit, Epogen).[190,191] In 2001, a new molecule was synthesized with the same basic structure as erythropoietin but with two additional carbohydrate chains containing sailic acid residues (darbepoetin alfa, Aranesp). This modification gives darbepoetin [also known as a novel erythropoiesis-stimulating protein (NESP)], an increased half-life compared with epoetin alfa. This characteristic allows it to be dosed less frequently than epoetin was traditionally dosed.[192] All three products have the same mechanism of action—stimulation of the production and differentiation of erythrocytes. Procrit and Epogen are the same molecule but with different FDA-approved indications. Only Epogen and Aranesp are approved for the treatment of patients with anemia of chronic kidney disease.

The benefits of treating anemia are tremendous. Studies have demonstrated enhanced energy, exercise capacity, quality of life, and sense of well-being; improvement in the ability to perform activities of daily living and carry on relationships with others; and a decrease in fatigue, frustration, and depressive symptoms.[193–195] Treatment with EPO predialysis improved health-related quality of life, including the areas of physical functioning, activities of daily living, social activity, and cognitive function.[94] Increasing the level of hemoglobin may delay the progression of renal disease[196–200] and decrease the risk of hospitalization. Additionally, it has been shown that exercise capacity, cognitive function, cardiac function, and quality of life are improved when hematocrit is corrected to more than 30%.[201–204] Correcting the anemia associated with CKD not only may cause regression of left ventricular hypertrophy[49,205,206] but also may improve clinical symptoms of heart failure.[207] Correction of anemia has been shown to decrease morbidity and mortality.[197,208] In one study,[97] a linear relationship was noted between the relative risk of death and each gram per deciliter improvement in hemoglobin. In a cost analysis, patients who received erythropoietic therapy had lower treatment costs than did controls.[197] Given the positive outcomes associated with treating anemia, it is distressing that in an observational study of Medicare patients who were begin-

TABLE 43.18	Initial Evaluation of Anemia of CKD

Hemoglobin [hematocrit (HCT)]

Red blood cell (RBC) indices

Reticulocyte count

Iron parameters

    Transferrin saturation percentage (TSAT)

    Ferritin

Test for occult blood in stool

(It is not cost effective to draw EPO levels as they will seldom be elevated. If elevated, they are not high enough to compensate for the degree of anemia.)

(Adapted from Foundation NK. K/DOQI clinical practice guidelines for anemia of chronic kidney disease. Am J Kidney Dis 37 (Suppl 1):S182–S238, 2000.)

ning dialysis, 60% of patients had hematocrit lower than 30%, and only 15.6% had claims for epoetin.[209]

Evaluation. Patients with CKD should be evaluated for anemia when their hemoglobin levels fall below the target range. A thorough workup should be conducted to rule out other causes of anemia (Table 43.18). The K/DOQI guidelines suggest using hemoglobin as a more accurate measure of anemia than hematocrit. Reasons for this include (1) that hematocrit is susceptible to change depending on the handling of the blood sample, (2) that factors such as hyperglycemia can affect hematocrit levels, and (3) that greater assay variability occurs in the measurement of hematocrit.[210]

Goal. The goal of therapy is to decrease the incidence of left ventricular hypertrophy, expand exercise capacity, enhance quality of life, improve cognitive function, and decrease morbidity and mortality. K/DOQI recommends that hemoglobin be maintained at between 11 and 12 g per dL (hematocrit 33%–36%).[210] This recommendation was based on the results of several studies showing decreased risks of hospitalization,[201] morbidity,[211,212] and mortality.[201,204] Some debate has arisen as to whether this is the optimal target for

patients with CKD. Some studies have shown a benefit when hemoglobin was raised closer to normal values[213,214]; another study showed higher mortality rates at these levels.[215] Until more evidence becomes available K/DOQI recommends the goal of 11 to 12 mg per dL.

Dosing. Both epoetin alfa and darbepoetin alfa can be given intravenously (IV) or subcutaneously (SQ). Dosing epoetin alfa subcutaneously has been shown to decrease the total dose and prolong the dosing interval.[216] For this reason, SQ dosing is preferred, although in patients on hemodialysis, epoetin is generally given intravenously during the treatment session in consideration of patient comfort. For epoetin alfa, the dose varies with route of administration; the dose is the same with darbepoetin alfa (Table 43.19).

Titration. With each product, doses should be titrated so the hemoglobin goal of 11 to 12 g per dL is achieved. Generally, this is done in increments of approximately 25%. Increases should not be made more frequently than every 4 weeks to allow the body time to respond. Dose decreases may be made every 2 weeks as necessary.

Conversion. Because both products appear efficacious in treating patients with anemia of CKD, the choice of agents may depend on cost considerations and compliance issues. Patients with CKD stages 1 to 4 may benefit from a longer dosing interval, allowing less frequent clinic visits; patients on hemodialysis may not accept an SQ injection. In patients who need to be switched from one product to the other, conversion of 200 IU of epoetin to 1 μg of darbepoetin has been proposed.[192]

Adverse Effects. Reported adverse effects of EPO include hypertension,[217,218] seizures,[219,220] and vascular access clotting.[215] Seizures appear to be related to hypertension, and increased vascular access clotting has been reported only occasionally.[215] Hypertension is a more widespread adverse event. It is estimated that hypertension occurs in approximately one quarter to one third of patients who receive EPO therapy.[221–224] The mechanisms by which EPO causes hypertension are not fully understood. One hypothesis is that

TABLE 43.19	Dosing of Epoetin and Darbepoetin in CKD	
Drug	CKD Stages 1–4, CKD Stage 5 Not on Dialysis or on Peritoneal Dialysis	CKD Stage 5 on Hemodialysis
Epoetin alfa	80–120 units/kg/wk divided in 2 to 3 doses[210] or total dose given weekly[270]	50–150 units/kg given three times a week[210]
Darbepoetin alfa	0.45 μg/kg/wk[271] or 0.75 μg/kg given every other week[272]	0.45 μg/kg/wk[271] or 0.75 μg/kg given every other week[272]

(Adapted from Epogen Package insert. 2004; Aranesp (darbepoetin alfa) package insert. Thousand Oaks, Calif: Amgen Inc, 2004.)

anemia causes vasodilation as the result of hypoxia. When anemia is corrected with EPO, the vasodilatory response is no longer required and vasoconstriction ensues.[225] This hypothesis is supported by the finding that higher concentrations of erythropoietin are directly related to a decrease in renal blood flow.[226] The mechanism by which EPO vasoconstricts is also unclear; however, vasoconstriction may be due to the release of endothelin from cells and/or an increase in calcium in the vasculature.[227–229] Another study found that EPO impairs endothelial function via a cyclooxygenase pathway.[230] Another possibility is that the rise in hematocrit raises blood viscosity,[231] although some studies refute this hypothesis.[232] In trying to determine the cause of hypertension, some studies have found an association between the incidence of hypertension and the rate of rise of hemoglobin[219,233]; other studies have found no association.[234,235]

Hyporesponsiveness. A number of factors may decrease the body's ability to respond to erythropoietic agents (Table 43.20). The most common of these is iron deficiency. Iron deficiency may be caused by the increased iron usage that results from administration of erythropoietic agents. Other causes include poor oral intake and blood loss from the gastrointestinal tract or the dialyzer circuit. Other common causes of hyporesponsiveness include infection/inflammation, elevated aluminum levels, hyperparathyroidism, and folate or vitamin B_{12} deficiency.[236] Additionally, some studies suggest that therapy with ACE-Is may decrease serum EPO levels and decrease its effect.[237,238] These studies are reinforced by the fact that ACE-Is are sometimes used to treat erythrocytosis in post–renal transplant patients. A look at the studies of ACE-Is reveals that angiotensin II increases production of erythropoietin,[239] most likely because of vasoconstriction of the afferent arteriole and the subsequent decrease in perfusion pressure. Patients treated with an ACE-I were found to require significantly more epoetin alfa than those not on an ACE-I.[240,241] However, given the docu-

mented benefits of ACE-I therapy on both renal and cardiac function, these agents should not be discontinued unless the risks outweigh the benefits.

Hyporesponsiveness to EPO therapy requires a thorough evaluation of all factors that can blunt the response. Any modifiable causes should be treated appropriately. In patients on hemodialysis, some strategies that have been used to treat hyporesponsiveness include L-carnitine and ascorbic acid supplementation. A wealth of data reveals that the benefits associated with use of L-carnitine for this condition are not very clear. At this time, K/DOQI recommends it only as a last-line agent to be used under very specific circumstances. For patients with functional iron deficiency (see iron therapy), another option is a trial of intravenous ascorbic acid. It is thought that ascorbic acid acts as an electron donor to convert Fe^{2+} into the more usable Fe^{3+}. Evidence of this is seen in decreased ferritin levels and a corresponding increase in transferring saturation. Additionally, hemoglobin levels have trended upward.[242–246] Doses of IV ascorbic acid have ranged from 200 to 500 mg given thrice weekly after hemodialysis for 2 to 6 months.

Iron Therapy. Iron is necessary for the formation of hemoglobin and erythropoiesis. Iron deficiency may develop owing to frequent phlebotomy, gastrointestinal bleeding, blood remaining in the hemodialysis circuit, or decreased absorption from the gastrointestinal tract. K/DOQI recommends that iron parameters be evaluated before erythropoietic agents are initiated. In fact, erythropoietic agents may induce iron deficiency secondary to the increased usage of iron in the formation of hemoglobin and red blood cells.

Evaluation. Iron studies include serum iron level, total iron-binding capacity (TIBC), percent transferrin saturation (TSAT), and ferritin level. Clinically, the two parameters that are most useful are the TSAT and ferritin. The TSAT indicates the percentage of transferrin that is bound by iron. This iron is readily available for use in erythropoiesis. The TSAT should be maintained at between 20% and 50% (K/DOQI). Ferritin is the stored form of iron, primarily in the liver, spleen, bone marrow, and reticuloendothelial cells. In patients with CKD, the ferritin level should be between 100 and 800 ng per mL. Caution should be used in interpreting the serum ferritin levels, as ferritin is an acute-phase reactant. In situations such as stress, inflammation, or infection, ferritin is released into the serum, causing increased levels (hyperferritinemia). In such instances, the laboratory assay may suggest that the patient is iron overloaded, although the patient's TSAT may be within normal limits or even low (Table 43.21).

Dosing. For patients with CKD who are not on hemodialysis, oral iron may be sufficient.[247] It can be given as 200 mg of elemental iron per day in two to three divided doses. Iron has poor oral bioavailability. Care should be taken to avoid concomitant administration of medication, such as phos-

TABLE 43.20	Causes of Hyporesponsiveness to Erythropoietin[222]

Iron deficiency

Infection/inflammation

Chronic blood loss

Osteitis fibrosa

Aluminum toxicity

Hemoglobinopathies

Folate or B_{12} deficiency

Multiple myeloma

Malnutrition

Hemolysis

Angiotensin-converting enzyme inhibitor

TABLE 43.21	Interpretation of Iron Parameters		
Ferritin	**TSAT**	**Evaluation**	**Recommendation**
<100 ng/mL	<20%	Iron deficiency	Load with iron
100–600 ng/mL	20%–50%	Iron replete	Give maintenance iron
>800 ng/mL	>50%	Iron overload	Hold iron for 3 months
>800 ng/mL	<20%	Functional iron deficiency	May try ascorbic acid or careful administration of iron

TSAT, transferrin saturation.

phate binders, that may further impair absorption. Intravenous iron products have been shown to be safe and effective in predialysis patients,[248] although additional clinic visits or home care may be required for administration. Stage 5 patients on hemodialysis may require intravenous iron therapy because of additional blood loss in the dialysis circuit. For patients on hemodialysis or for other patients who need more aggressive dosing, intravenous iron may be preferred. When repletion is necessary, the products are dosed until 1 g has been given (see below). Optimally, after repletion, maintenance iron is started.

The first intravenous iron preparation available in the United States was iron dextran. The most favorable characteristic of iron dextran is that it can be administered as a single infusion of 1 g over 6 hours. The unfavorable aspect is that it has been associated with anaphylactic reactions. These reactions are most likely due to the large dextran moiety. Because of the increased risk of anaphylaxis, a test dose of 25 mg must be administered before the infusion can be started. Two newer agents are now available—sodium ferric gluconate (Ferrlecit)[249] and iron sucrose (Venofer).[250] These preparations were originally approved to be dosed in increments of 125 or 100 mg, respectively, to be given three times a week during hemodialysis, for a total dose of 1 g for repletion. Since they were approved by the US Food and Drug Administration (FDA), studies have supported the use of these agents in larger doses[251,252] for accelerated repletion. As has been noted, when replete, maintenance iron

should be instituted to ensure optimal iron availability for erythropoiesis.

Monitoring. In stage 5 CKD, serum TSAT and ferritin levels should generally be obtained once every 3 months. Levels may be drawn sooner if a loading dose (repletion) is given, or if clinically indicated. After a repletion regimen of 1 g of iron, it is important for the clinician to wait approximately 2 weeks before obtaining levels. Checking levels sooner may give erroneous results because the body requires time to process the iron and store it as ferritin. Iron studies may be obtained at any time during the maintenance phase.

BONE METABOLISM AND DISEASE

In October of 2003, the first guidelines for the treatment of bone metabolism and disease were published by the K/DOQI.[253] These guidelines provide recommendations for the evaluation, treatment, and monitoring of bone metabolism to prevent secondary hyperparathyroidism and renal osteodystrophy.

Goals. The recommendations focus on normalizing biochemical markers such as calcium, phosphorus, alkaline phosphatase, and parathyroid hormone. The ultimate goal is to prevent bone disease and metastatic calcification.

Evaluation. The evaluation of patients with these disorders should begin when the GFR falls to below 60 mL per minute. It should include measurement of serum calcium, phospho-

TABLE 43.22	Evaluation of Calcium, Phosphate, and PTH	
Stage of Kidney Disease	**Measurement of PTH**	**Measurement of Calcium and Phosphorus**
3	Every 12 months	Every 12 months
4	Every 3 months	Every 3 months
5	Every 3 months	Every month
Kidney transplant	Monthly for 3 months, then every 3 months	Every 2 weeks for 3 months, then every month

PTH, parathyroid hormone.
(From National Kidney Foundation. K/DOQI clinical practice guidelines for bone metabolism and disease in chronic kidney disease. Am J Kidney Dis 42 (4 Suppl 3):S1–S201, 2003, with permission.)

rus, and intact PTH. The reader should refer to Table 43.22 for information regarding the timing of subsequent monitoring.

Treatment. Early conservative management consists of restriction of dietary phosphorus through reduced intake of foods high in phosphorus, such as meat, milk, legumes, beer, and colas. Although dietary protein sources tend to be rich in phosphate, institution of a low-protein diet should be instituted only with proper nutrition counseling. Restricting protein may lead to malnutrition and hypoalbuminemia, which has been correlated with morbidity and mortality in patients with ESKD.

As renal failure progresses and GFR falls to below 30 mL per minute, dietary restriction alone becomes inadequate to prevent hyperphosphatemia. The use of phosphate-binding agents that decrease absorption of dietary phosphorus and promote removal of phosphate through the gut generally becomes necessary, as does acceptance of the goals of slightly higher serum phosphorus (Table 43.23). The divalent and trivalent cations Mg^{2+}, Ca^{2+}, and Al^{3+} can all work effectively as phosphate binders when given during or immediately preceding mealtime (Table 43.24).

Because systemic absorption of each of these cations occurs to some extent, calcium salts have emerged as preferred agents and often serve a dual purpose as a calcium supplement. Before the 1990s, aluminum salts were a mainstay of phosphate-binding regimens; however, accumulation syndromes, associated with encephalopathy, osteomalacia, myopathy, and microcytic anemia, were common. Short courses are used when the calcium X phosphorus product precludes the use of calcium binders and when sevelamer is not effective enough. It should be noted that the coadministration of citrate increases absorption, so use of products that contain citrate should be avoided in patients with CKD.[254] Aluminum-based binders are now reserved for short-term use in severely hyperphosphatemic patients or in hypercalcemic patients, in whom the initiation or escalation of calcium salts could present the danger of raising the calcium phosphate product to beyond 55 mg^2 per dL^2. Of the presently available

calcium salts, calcium carbonate and calcium acetate are the most commonly used as phosphate binders in patients with CKD. Because the efficiency of phosphate binding depends on solubilization of the calcium salt, the use of products not meeting US Pharmacopeia (USP) dissolution standards (such as those marketed as dietary supplements) may compromise therapeutic efficacy. The selection of dietary phosphorus–binding agents is discussed more fully in Chapter 28. Patients should be counseled about the importance of taking these agents immediately before or with meals and snacks, and about separating their administration from that of other drugs for which absorption could be impaired by simultaneous ingestion. Some patients learn to successfully ''titrate'' their phosphate binder dose according to dietary variations in phosphate intake, but others require more stringent dosing instructions. The initiation of dialytic therapies affords the additional removal of about 500 mg (16 mmol) phosphate per hemodialysis session, and helps compensate for the liberalization of protein intake usually implemented after dialysis is begun.

Calcium-based products are relatively inexpensive and are often used as initial therapy for patients with hyperphosphatemia. They have been used extensively in the past to treat hyperphosphatemia. Recently, the use of calcium-based products is limited by the concern for metastatic calcification. K/DOQI recommends limiting calcium intake to less than 2,000 mg per day. Of this amount, 1,500 mg may come from phosphate binders and 500 mg from the patient's diet. Additionally, calcium-based products should be discontinued if the serum calcium increases to above 10.2 mg per dL, or if the calcium X phosphorous product is greater than 55 mg^2 per dL^2. Alternatives to calcium-, magnesium-, and aluminum-based products include sevelamer (Renagel)[255] and lanthanum (Fosrenol).[256]

Sevelamer and lanthanum are two relatively new agents that do not contain calcium, aluminum, or magnesium. Both agents appear to be nontoxic and are not well absorbed. Both agents may cause gastrointestinal side effects, although no trial has been conducted to directly compare the two agents.

TABLE 43.23	Goals for Biochemical Markers of Bone Disease in CKD		
Stage of Kidney Disease	Serum Phosphorus (mg/dL)	Serum Calcium* (mg/dL)	Serum Intact PTH (pg/mL)
3	2.7–4.6	normal range for the laboratory used	35–70
4	2.7–4.6	normal range for the laboratory used	70–110
5	3.5–5.5	8.4–9.5	150–300

CKD, chronic kidney disease; PTH, parathyroid hormone.
*corrected for hypoalbuminemia
(From Ganesh S, Stack A, Levin N, et al. Association of elevated serum PO4, CaXPO4 product, and parathyroid hormone with cardiac mortality risk in chronic hemodialysis patients. J Am Soc Nephrol 12:2131–2138, 2001, with permission.)

TABLE 43.24	Phosphate Binding Agents		
Agent, Trade Name, and Dosage Form	**Elemental Mineral Content/Unit**		**Usual Dosing and Instructions**
Calcium-based products	**Ca content**		
Calcium carbonate (40% Ca)			Initial, then titrate: Elemental Ca^{2+} 500 mg–1 g with each meal plus 200–500 mg with high-PO_4 snacks
Tums 500 mg, 750 mg, 1,000 mg	200 mg, 300 mg, 400 mg		Chewing encouraged if chewable product (and dentition intact)
Oscal-500	500 mg		
$CaCO_3$ (various) 1,250 mg	500 mg		
Caltrate-600	600 mg		
$CaCO_3$ 1,250 mg/5 mL	500 mg/5 mL		Sorbitol content may cause diarrhea
CalCarb HD 6.5-g packets	2,400 mg/packet		Can be mixed into food
Calcium acetate (25% Ca)			
Phoslo 667 mg	167 mg		Initial: 2 tablets TID with meals. Large tablet—chew if possible
Calcium citrate (21% Ca) Citracal 950 mg	200 mg; 500 mg		Not commonly used
			Separate from Al^{3+}-containing products by at least 2 hr
Aluminum-based products	*All products*		
Aluminum hydroxide	Dosed by $Al(OH)_3$ content as labeled		Initial, then titrate: 300–900 mg $Al(OH)_3$ with meals and 300–400 mg with high-PO_4 snacks
Amphojel 600-mg Tablets			
Amphojel 320 mg/5 mL Liquid			Separate from citrate-containing products (Shohl's, Ca citrate)
AlternaGEL 600 mg/5 mL Liquid			
Alu-Cap 400 mg			Reserved for temporary use in patients with serum PO_4 >6.5, serum Ca^{2+} >10.2, or (Ca^{2+} × PO_4) product >55
Alu-Tab 500 mg			
Dialume 500 mg capsules			Tend to be constipating
Aluminum carbonate gel, basic	500 mg $Al(OH)_3$ equivalent		Caution: May interfere with absorption of other medicines
Basaljel 608 mg tablets, capsules			
Basaljel Liquid	400 mg $Al(OH)_3$/5 mL equivalent		
Sucralfate, Carafate 1-g tablet			Not indicated as phosphate binder, but may decrease serum PO_4^{2+} in use as antiulcer agent
Carafate 1 g/10 mL suspension			
Aluminum and calcium free			Significant Al^{3+} absorption possible with long-term use
Sevelamer, Renagel 400 and 800 mg tablets			Dose based on PO_4 levels. May cause bloating and diarrhea. Use cautiously in conditions of impaired gastric motility. Caution: May interfere with absorption of other medicines
Lanthanum, Fosrenol 250, 500, 750 and 1000 mg tablets			Chewable tablets. Dose based on PO_4 levels

Sevelamer may cause decreased absorption of other drugs. Although this interaction has not been tested for all drugs, care should be taken to separate the administration of sevelamer from that of other agents. Lanthanum does not appear to share this property. It is interesting to note that sevelamer has been shown to have lipid-lowering effects. Although it has not been shown to be cost-effective when compared with the combination of calcium carbonate and atorvastatin, the fact that it has a favorable effect on lipid levels is certainly a benefit. Again, no clinical trials have directly compared sevelamer with lanthanum. Some studies have shown that sevelamer is not very effective as monotherapy for hyperphosphatemia,[257,258] although lanthanum is effective in this capacity.[259–261]

Options besides calcium-containing binders are very important in the treatment of patients with hyperphosphatemia. Excessive calcium intake has been directly correlated with the development of vascular calcification. In a long-term study of sevelamer versus calcium carbonate, nearly one third of patients who received calcium displayed evidence of aortic and coronary artery calcification; however, no one in the sevelamer group did.[262] Although hyperphosphatemia is an independent risk factor for death in patients on hemodialysis,[67,263] it may be that treatments for the abnormality are actually increasing the risk of death. Despite evidence that shows the deleterious effect of secondary hyperparathyroidism, many patients remain uncontrolled. A recent study[62] found that despite the use of phosphate binders, 70% of patients on hemodialysis continued to be hyperphosphatemic. A separate study showed that compliance with phosphate binders is abysmal, with only 11 of 188 patients being compliant with their phosphate binders.[107] It is clear that additional safe and well-tolerated therapies are needed to treat patients with hyperphosphatemia and secondary hyperparathyroidism. Such therapies must be accompanied by patient and provider education to ensure compliance and better outcomes.

Vitamin D deficiency may be present early in CKD. If PTH levels are elevated at initial presentation, 25-hydroxyvitamin D (vitamin D_2) levels should be obtained. K/DOQI recommends that therapy with ergocalciferol (vitamin D_2) should be initiated if levels are below 30 ng per mL (Table 43.25). Calcitriol (1,25-dihydroxyvitamin D_3) offers some advantages over other forms of vitamin D, such as ergocalciferol (vitamin D_2) and cholecalciferol (vitamin D_3). Not only is calcitriol the most potent and specific congener that becomes deficient in renal disease, but it directly suppresses PTH suppression and has a shorter onset and duration of action than the others. The potential for vitamin D intoxication is a major hazard associated with pharmacologic doses of vitamins D_2 and D_3; it can induce sustained hypercalcemia and hyperphosphatemia that may require weeks to resolve. Hyperparathyroidism should be treated when the PTH level is above the target range for the level of kidney dysfunction (Table 43.23). Therapy with vitamin D_3 sterols should be initiated only when serum calcium and phosphorus

TABLE 43.26 Vitamin D_3 Analogues and Initial Doses*

Drug	Oral Dose	Intravenous Dose
Calcitriol	0.5–1.5 μg	0.5–1.5 μg
Doxercalciferol	5 μg	2 μg
Paricalcitol	†	2.5–5.0 μg

* Dose per each hemodialysis session.
† Formulation in trials, not commercially available at this time.

levels are within target range. In fact, it is important to note that vitamin D therapy should be discontinued if these levels are increased, if the calcium-phosphorous product is greater than 55 mg^2 per dL^2, or if the PTH level falls to below the lower limit of normal. It is imperative that vitamin D analogs be stopped if the PTH level is below goal; oversuppression may lead to adynamic bone disease.

Three vitamin D_3 analogs are available in the United States (Table 43.26). The first agent to be synthesized was calcitriol. Compared with the two newer agents, calcitriol has an increased incidence of hypercalcemia. This effect is due to the drug's affinity for intestinal and parathyroid vitamin D receptors. In contrast, paricalcitol and doxercalciferol are newer agents that are more selective for parathyroid receptors and may be less likely to cause hypercalcemia. It should also be noted that giving any of these agents as daily oral therapy may cause more hypercalcemia than is caused by intermittent intravenous therapy. Given these differences, calcitriol may be the agent of choice in patients with serum calcium levels below or on the low end of the normal range. A new strategy in controlling secondary hyperparathyroidism is the use of the calcimimetic agent, cinacalcet (Sensipar[264]). Cinacalcet acts by increasing the sensitivity of the calcium-sensing receptor on the parathyroid gland. This stimulation enhances the perception of serum calcium, causing a decrease in PTH synthesis and release. Cinacalcet has been shown to be beneficial in decreasing PTH levels and maintaining calcium and phosphorous levels with or without concomitant treatment with vitamin analogs.[265]

In situations where other treatments have failed, parathyroidectomy is a last-line option. This is indicated when PTH levels are consistently greater than 800 pg per mL, and levels of calcium and phosphorus are above the target range. Parathyroidectomy is neither completely safe nor effective. Occasionally, surgical complications may occur, and if a portion of the gland remains intact after surgery, hyperparathyroidism will recur. The last concern is that removal of the parathyroid gland may cause precipitous, persistent decreases in serum calcium and phosphorus. This syndrome is sometimes known as *hungry bone syndrome*, because the bone resorbs as much calcium and phosphorus as possible. Frequent monitoring and supplementation are essential.

BLEEDING AND HEMOSTATIC DEFECTS

In the absence of clinical bleeding or in situations of increased risk for bleeding (e.g., invasive or surgical proce-

TABLE 43.25 Dosing of Ergocalciferol

Vitamin D_2 Level (ng/mL)	Ergocalciferol Dose (IU)
<5	50,000 weekly × 12 doses, then monthly × 3 doses
5–15	50,000 weekly × 4 doses, then monthly × 5 doses
16–30	50,000 monthly × 6 doses

dures), no specific therapy is required. In general, bleeding diathesis may be reduced by adequate treatment of patients in the uremic state through hemodialysis or peritoneal dialysis, and by avoidance of unnecessary agents with antiplatelet effects. Through EPO therapy (or transfusion), correction of hematocrit to levels to above 30% may help enhance platelet–endothelium interactions. Although the benefit has largely been attributed to improved intravascular dispersion of platelets by red blood cell (RBC) mass, EPO has been proposed to increase the expression of platelet membrane GPIIb-IIIa receptors.[113]

Acute treatment for severe bleeding necessitates RBC transfusion and, in life-threatening circumstances, administration of cryoprecipitate. The role of platelet transfusion is more controversial, given that repeated platelet transfusions are likely to promote the development of antiplatelet antibodies. Moreover, platelets transfused into uremic environment are thought to become deficient in function, in the manner described in earlier sections for native platelets. Relatively rapid improvements in bleeding time can be produced in most uremic patients through the administration of desmopressin (DDAVP) 0.3 μg per kg by IV infusion. Desmopressin is thought to increase the release of von Willebrand factor (vWF), a glycoprotein that complexes with factor VIII from endothelial storage sites. Desmopressin has proved clinically useful and well tolerated in the prophylaxis and acute management of uremic bleeding episodes. Unfortunately, its effects are short-lived (4 to 24 hours), and repeated short-term administration of desmopressin eventually leads to tachyphylaxis, presumably due to depletion of vWF stores. Conjugated estrogens may be useful in reducing bleeding time, particularly when a more prolonged effect is desired. The mechanisms by which estrogens serve to shorten bleeding time are not completely understood but are believed to involve reductions in nitric oxide or precursor synthesis, possibly through estrogen-receptor–mediated control of nuclear transcription pathways. The hemostatic benefit of estrogens is dose dependent; however, the optimal dose of conjugated estrogens for control of uremic bleeding is unclear, in that reportedly effective doses have ranged widely (10 to 60 mg/day; 0.1 to 0.6 mg/kg/day).[266] With repeated dosing, hemostatic effects generally begin within 24 hours, peak at 5 to 7 days, and may persist for longer than 1 week after discontinuation. Because high doses are usually needed, estrogen-related adverse effects may limit their long-term usefulness in uremic bleeding.

GASTROINTESTINAL COMPLICATIONS

Antacids were once used heavily in patients with CKD for relief of dyspepsia or gastrointestinal irritation. In the setting of renal insufficiency, many of these agents present potential problems. Bicarbonate-based products may cause the inadvertent administration of large sodium loads, but they may be useful in controlling metabolic acidosis. When magnesium-containing antacids or cathartics are given on a long-term basis to patients with renal failure, accumulation of magne-

sium becomes a concern, as creatinine clearance falls to below 30 mL per minute. Serum magnesium levels may rise to above 6 mEq per L (3 mmol/L), leading to central nervous system depression, lethargy, somnolence, and loss of deep tendon reflexes. Dialysis removes magnesium effectively and may be indicated in cases of severe toxicity. As was discussed in earlier sections, long-term use of aluminum-based antacids or phosphate binders may lead to aluminum intoxication syndromes.

H_2-receptor antagonists have largely replaced long-term antacid use for dyspepsia in those with CKD and other populations. Most of these agents are eliminated renally, hence dosage reduction has traditionally been recommended at creatinine clearance less than 30 to 50 mL per minute; however, their elimination by active tubular secretion helps preserve renal drug clearance at reduced GFRs. Most accumulation-related adverse experiences have been reported in association with cimetidine and ranitidine; they consisted primarily of encephalopathy and mental status alterations. When one is evaluating H_2-antagonist dose, it is appropriate to remember that these agents have a wide dosing range depending on their therapeutic purpose; therefore, renal dose reductions may not be called for in situations where aggressive acid suppression is needed. Proton pump inhibitors do not undergo significant pharmacokinetic alterations in CKD. Their use could be anticipated to reduce the efficacy of calcium carbonate–based phosphate binders, which are dependent on gastric acidity for solubilization; however, available data do not consistently support a significant degree of interference.

Constipation is a common complaint in advanced CKD and is likely to be exacerbated by diet and fluid restrictions, Al^{3+}- or Ca^{2+}-based phosphate-binding agents, iron supplements, calcium channel blockers, and other medications. Bulk-forming laxatives are not first-line agents, as they are in the general population, because concomitant fluid restrictions reduce their efficacy and safety; some products also contain significant amounts of potassium. The use of cathartics that are magnesium or phosphate based (e.g., Phospho-Soda) should be minimized because of their potential for systemic accumulation. Long-term use of stimulant laxatives is permitted to a greater extent in patients with CKD than in the general population. Lactulose and the osmotic cathartic sorbitol are also prescribed, but they may generate patient disfavor because of the flatulence and bloating that often accompany their use.

UREMIC PRURITUS

The uremic milieu and the use of dialyzer membranes that are less biocompatible have been implicated in the pathogenesis of uremic pruritus (UP). This appears to be true, and with the improvements in hemodialysis adequacy and more compatible dialyzer membranes, a decrease in the incidence of pruritus has been reported.[267] Still, UP is a significant issue, especially in the dialysis population. A variety of topical and systemic therapies have been reported as beneficial

TABLE 43.27	**Management of Uremic Pruritus: Empiric and Anecdotal Approaches**

Rule out drug, diet, and environmentally induced causes

Administer topical therapies

Emollients and moisturizers: lanolin-based products, hypoallergenic lotion, superfatted soaps, oatmeal baths

Counterirritants: camphorated or mentholated lotions, capsaicin

Use topical antihistamines, topical anesthetics* (caution if widespread application)

Recommend phototherapy (ultraviolet B exposure; not commonly used)*

Give systemic therapies

Antihistamines (H$_1$ and H$_2$), serotonin-blocking antihistamines (cyproheptadine)

Administer opiate antagonists

Naltrexone

Perform toxin adsorption/removal*

Oral cholestyramine, activated charcoal

Optimize intensity of dialysis

Optimize control of hyperparathyroidism

Serum phosphate and calcium levels

Use erythropoietin therapy

---

* Anecdotal approaches.
(Adapted from Zucker I, Yosipovitch G, David M, et al. Prevalence and characterization of uremic pruritis in patients undergoing hemodialysis: uremic pruritis is still a major problem for patients with end-stage renal disease. J Am Acad Dermatol 49:842–846, 2003.)

in reducing or relieving uremic pruritus (Table 43.27). Unfortunately, none of these has proved uniformly effective, often necessitating a trial-and-error approach.

Topical therapies that moisten dry, scaly skin or produce a counterirritant effect are generally safe and are an appropriate initial measure that may provide partial relief. Ensuring optimal control of serum phosphate and calcium levels, along with minimizing secondary hyperparathyroidism, may help reduce the overall tendency toward severe itching episodes but usually does not lead to immediate symptomatic improvement. Although an increase in serotonin has been implicated in the pathogenesis of UP, the 5-HT$_3$ antagonist ondansetron did not prove effective in a randomized, placebo-controlled trial.[119] The same situation appears true for the opioid antagonist, naltrexone. Although the use of large quantities of antihistamine and antiserotonergic agents (systemically or topically) is common, patients should be monitored for intoxication syndromes and the inability to adhere to fluid restrictions because of the xerostomia that these drugs tend to produce. Cyclosporine, an immunosuppressant, has been reported, anecdotally, to provide relief from UP. A similar agent, tacrolimus, also proved effective when used topically in a small study.[117] These findings have not been confirmed in larger, controlled trials.

For all the theories that have been proposed to explain UP, nearly as many treatments have been tried. Unfortunately, these treatments have shown conflicting results, and the disorder remains a significant problem, especially in the dialysis population. At this time, it appears that beneficial treatments include improving dialysis adequacy; controlling calcium, phosphorous, and parathyroid hormone levels; avoiding hypervitaminosis; and moisturizing the skin. Agents such as antihistamines, antiserotonergics, opioid antagonists and calcineurin inhibitors have shown conflicting results and may cause unwanted adverse effects.

MUSCULOSKELETAL COMPLAINTS

Control of acute gouty attacks is often achieved through cautious use of traditional agents such as NSAIDs (e.g., indomethacin) and colchicine. Upon initiation of an NSAID, patients should be monitored closely for bleeding, worsened renal function, and loss of diuretic efficacy. When used on a long-term basis in the setting of renal impairment, colchicine accumulation can induce a peripheral neuropathy that may be mistakenly attributed to other factors. For long-term prevention of gouty attacks, uricosurics lose much of their efficacy in advanced CKD. Allopurinol, which decreases uric acid production, is the preferred prophylactic agent because it possesses an active metabolite (oxypurinol) that is renally eliminated; doses are usually reduced to 100 to 200 mg daily in advanced CKD.

DIETARY SUPPLEMENTS

Proper nutrition is essential for the health and well-being of patients. Educating patients about healthful eating, dietary and fluid restrictions, and the appropriate use of nutritional supplements, vitamins, and phosphate binders is essential in assuring compliance. Dietitians are integral members of most specialized care teams and can complement the pharmacist's efforts. As previously mentioned, dietary restrictions may include fluids, sodium, potassium, phosphorus, fats, and cholesterol.

Supplementation with moderate quantities of B-complex vitamins, folic acid, and other water-soluble vitamins is usually recommended in predialysis and dialysis patients because dietary intake of these nutrients is generally inadequate on restricted diets, and removal is enhanced by dialysis. Serum levels of vitamins A and E have been noted to be elevated in uremic patients. Although the clinical significance of this is not clear, routine supplementation of vitamins A, E, and K is not generally advised in advanced CKD. Recently, high-dose tocopherol (vitamin E) has been advocated for numerous maladies (e.g., restless leg syndrome, antioxidant protection); however, the long-term safety of pharmacologic doses of tocopherol has not yet been rigorously assessed in the ESKD setting. Variable derangements of trace mineral balance have been observed in uremic and dialysis patients and may be influenced by the trace mineral content of dialysate water sources. Supplementation of trace minerals has not been routine in CKD; if undertaken, the potential for prolonged accumulation and associated toxicities should be considered.

PHARMACOKINETIC CONSIDERATIONS AND DRUG DOSING

The presence of renal failure may alter all of the pharmacokinetic parameters of drugs, that is, absorption, distribution, metabolism, and excretion. Quantifying and predicting alterations is difficult because of high interpatient variability and a lack of data. Excretion is the easiest parameter to quantify, and most research has been performed in this area. For renally eliminated agents, a major clinical concern is the potential for drug accumulation and heightened risk of related systemic toxicities, especially when normal doses are used. In addition, some drugs damage the kidney, hence their use may further compromise renal function. Because several nephrotoxins also happen to be eliminated renally, both of these aspects may dictate the need for cautious use in the setting of CKD. A complete discussion of CKD-associated pharmacokinetic and pharmacodynamic alterations is beyond the scope of this chapter, but fundamental principles and classic examples are briefly summarized. Issues specific to drug removal and dosing requirements in hemodialysis and peritoneal dialysis recipients are discussed in Chapter 44.

PHARMACOKINETIC CHANGES

Absorption. Chronic kidney disease may alter the absorption of several agents. Drug absorption may be reduced in the presence of severe gastrointestinal edema, as could occur in nephrotic syndrome or fluid overload (digoxin, verapamil). However, a more clinically significant cause of impaired drug absorption may result from concurrent administration of alkaline therapy or phosphorus-binding agents (fluoroquinolones, iron, itraconazole). Gastroparesis is common among diabetic patients with CKD and may retard or reduce drug absorption. Most of the changes in absorption are believed to be of minor clinical significance, but judicious use and careful monitoring are warranted.

Distribution. In CKD, the distribution of drugs may be altered because of alterations in plasma protein binding or changes in the volume of distribution secondary to changes in volume status. Hypoalbuminemia due to malnutrition or nephrotic syndrome may cause an increased free fraction of drug. Additionally, uremia may alter the binding capacity of albumin secondary to the accumulation of endogenous substances that compete for binding sites. Drug-binding alterations have been characterized most consistently in long-standing uremia, whereas changes in stages 1 to 4 CKD or acute renal failure has proved less predictable. In situations of hypoalbuminemia or uremia, an increased free fraction of drug may lead to an increased effect; however, an increased

fraction is available for elimination as well. This confounds the assessment of changes made on the basis of alterations in protein binding or the measurement of serum total serum levels. Phenytoin is one such example. Although several formulas have been derived to correct levels, obtaining a free fraction phenytoin level is the most accurate measure. Digoxin is another agent that may need changes in dosing because of alterations in distribution.

Metabolism. Alterations in metabolism secondary to CKD may be due to changes in the metabolic function of the kidney or changes in the excretory function of the kidney. The latter refers to the accumulation of the parent drug or the metabolite caused by decreased renal elimination. The net effects of accumulation vary according to the characteristics of both parent and metabolite compounds. For example, drugs such as meperidine or procainamide have metabolites that accumulate in patients with renal dysfunction. Normeperidine is inactive but has been associated with adverse events; N-acetyl procainamide is active and contributes to the therapeutic efficacy of procainamide.

Although the kidney is not generally thought of in connection with metabolism, it is increasingly becoming recognized as a site of both metabolism and detoxification. It has long been recognized that the kidney plays a significant role in the breakdown of insulin. Theoretically, as CKD progresses, a decreased dose of exogenous insulin or oral hypoglycemic agents may become necessary. Clinically, the prolonged half-life of insulin is generally offset by insulin resistance in these patients. Care should be taken to monitor patients as CKD progresses, in case dose adjustment is needed. In addition to breaking down insulin, the kidney possesses a small percentage of the cytochrome P-450 enzymes. Much research is being conducted to explore the clinical significance of this system and the ramifications of it in CKD.

Excretion. The processes of glomerular filtration, tubular secretion, and renal metabolism may contribute by differing extents to the renal elimination of a drug. Apart from issues discussed previously, the presence of renal disease has the greatest implications for drug dosing when a significant fraction (>30%) of parent drug or active metabolite elimination is renal and compensatory elimination pathways are impaired or absent. The most commonly used gauge for approximating renal drug elimination capacity is the measured or estimated creatinine clearance. Despite the fact that creatinine clearance is an imperfect surrogate marker of renal drug clearance, in most medical centers, it remains the most practical approach through which dosing adjustments are guided. Most drug dosing guidelines are based on (1) specific ranges of creatinine clearance, (2) individualized approximations of drug clearance based on pharmacokinetic formulas that correlate creatinine clearance with drug clearance, or (3) pharmacokinetic individualization based on measured in vivo drug concentrations. Maintenance dosing adjustments may be accomplished through alteration of dose, reduction in frequency, or a combination of both, depending on the significance of peak-to-trough serum level fluctuations and other factors, such as convenience and available dosage increments.

PHARMACODYNAMICS

Drug response has been noted to be both increased (morphine, codeine, alprazolam) and decreased (digoxin, propranolol) in uremic patients. Although many of these apparent alterations in drug response may be accounted for by close examination of changes in disposition, it appears that sensitivity to the action of some drugs is affected by the uremic state. These pharmacodynamic alterations are difficult to predict but may account for some of the idiosyncratic reactions reported in patients with CKD.

As has been discussed, many alterations in pharmacokinetic parameters and drug disposition occur in the body. Most of these changes have not been adequately quantified and are subject to high interpatient variability. This fact makes it imperative that patients be closely monitored for subjective and objective signs of efficacy and toxicity. Additionally, with many therapeutic agents, it is prudent to start with a low dose and titrate upward to desired effect. (This does not hold true for agents such as antimicrobials, with which a minimum concentration must be achieved at initiation.)

PRACTICAL CLINICAL APPROACH

Several equations have been developed to quantify kidney function. Most of the published literature on dosing guidelines in kidney dysfunction describes use of the Cockcroft-Gault[268] method of estimating creatinine clearance. Recently, the MDRD equation[269] was derived to estimate glomerular filtration rate. This equation is now frequently used in clinical practice. Some differences may exist when the estimated creatinine clearance is compared with the estimated glomerular filtration rate. Although the difference is generally small, clinical judgment should be applied when one is using the MDRD-derived GFR to determine a drug dose that was based on creatinine clearance.

Dosage recommendations are sometimes based on estimated creatinine clearance values that have been normalized to weight or body surface area, and calculations are adjusted accordingly. Values for creatinine clearance (and therefore drug clearance) that have been calculated from serum creatinine carry an inherent margin of error averaging 10% to 25%. Doses should be determined on the basis of calculations, as well as through clinical judgment. For each drug, the risks of underestimation versus overestimation of dosage requirements should be weighed. This is especially important when calculated drug clearance values fall near cutoff values for dose adjustment, or when renal function appears to be changing. Finally, it is not uncommon to find conflicting recommendations for dosage adjustment from different resources. Clinical judgment and scrutiny of the conditions and patient characteristics from which dosage guidelines were

derived may help in selection of the most appropriate strategy. If therapeutic drug level monitoring is not feasible, monitoring parameters for both therapeutic failure and accumulation-related toxicities should be identified and closely followed.

With few important exceptions, most drugs in clinical use do not routinely require dosage adjustment until creatinine clearance values fall below 50 to 60 mL per minute. However, several renally eliminated agents of narrow therapeutic index merit dosage individualization at even milder degrees of renal impairment. These include but are not limited to aminoglycosides, digoxin, metformin, procainamide, foscarnet, ganciclovir, cidofovir, flucytosine, carboplatin, lepirudin, and vancomycin. References should be routinely consulted to ascertain the need for dosage adjustment (Table 43.28), especially at creatinine clearance values below 60 mL per minute. Knowing the fraction of drug or active metabolite that is renally eliminated under normal circumstances can help the clinician to more efficiently identify drugs that require renal dosage adjustment. Drug interactions and impairment of alternate elimination pathways may increase the significance of renal impairment.

AMINOGLYCOSIDE DOSING

The aminoglycoside antibiotics (AGs) are useful in patients with conditions ranging from CKD to gram-negative infec-

TABLE 43.28	Useful Resources in Determination of Renal Dosing Requirements

Compendia

Manufacturer's product literature

American Hospital Formulary System (AHFS) Drug Information

Drug Facts and Comparisons

Micromedex

Clinical Pharmacology

Martindale's *The Extra Pharmacopoeia*

Pocket Guides

Bennett WM, et al, eds. *Drug Prescribing in Renal Failure.* 4th ed. American College of Physicians, 1999

Gilbert DN, Moellering RC, Sande MA, eds. *The Sanford Guide to Antimicrobial Therapy.* Vienna, Va: Antimicrobial Therapy, Inc.

Review Articles

Talbert RL. Drug dosing in renal insufficiency. J Clin Pharmacol 34:99–110, 1994.

St Peter WL, Redic-Kill KA, Halstenson CE. Clinical pharmacokinetics of antibiotics in patients with impaired renal function. Clin Pharmacokinet 22:169–210, 1992.

tions, as well as for use as synergistic therapy to treat gram-positive infections. Unfortunately, aminoglycosides may be nephrotoxic, causing direct damage to the proximal tubule epithelial cells. This damage is associated with constant tubular exposure and total cumulative doses. Fortunately, these drugs exhibit concentration-dependent microbe killing, enhanced tissue penetration, and a long postantibiotic effect. These characteristics imply that AGs can be dosed to achieve high peak concentrations and low trough concentrations without sacrificing efficacy. The dosing strategy in patients with CKD is the same as that used in patients with normal kidney function, with the exception that as kidney function declines, the dosing interval must be lengthened accordingly. Oftentimes, these drugs are dosed "randomly" according to desired peak and trough levels. After drug levels are measured, an appropriate dose and dosing interval can be calculated for the individual patient. This regimen should achieve desired peak levels while minimizing trough levels and therefore minimizing tubular exposure to the drug.

FUTURE THERAPIES

Many agents are under investigation for use in delaying or decreasing the progression of kidney disease. Some of these include receptor antagonists of endothelin and antagonists of the advanced glycation end products. Ongoing and future studies of other presently available therapies should help clarify the optimal strategies for retarding the progression of CKD and its related comorbidities. Such agents include those under investigation for use with antilipemic agents and calcimimetics. At this time, it appears that current therapies can be used to delay progression in most patients with CKD (patients with diabetes and hypertension). One challenge that remains is educating the public to increase awareness.

IMPROVING OUTCOMES

PATIENT EDUCATION

Patients with advanced renal disease are expected to understand and follow complex dietary, medication, and physical care regimens. Data indicate that intense educational effort in ESKD is associated with increased patient autonomy, improved quality of life, increased compliance with therapies, and clinician ability to delay initiation of dialysis.[122] The need for renal replacement therapy (RRT) can often be predicted more than 1 year in advance, providing ample opportunity for early education of patients who face ESKD (and their caregivers). Patient referral to a renal care specialty team may help ensure that the patient gains an adequate understanding of kidney disease and participates in decisions regarding options for renal replacement modality. Educational programs generally emphasize patient comprehension of: the most common complications of kidney disease (anemia, bone disease, hypertension), measures to slow progres-

sion of renal disease (if still feasible), dietary management (protein, phosphorus, potassium, sodium, and fluid restrictions), medication management (reason for use, manner of use, and precautions), choice of RRT modality and physical preparation for this (e.g., catheter or fistula placement, transplantation referral), options for medical care and prescription coverage, and possibilities for vocational support. Individuals with renal disease could be considered fortunate, in that the renal community offers numerous organizations from which one can draw educational information, psychosocial support, and financial guidance. A partial list of organizations and programs that offer patient-focused resources for those suffering from renal disease is provided in Table 43.29. Numerous resources oriented toward renal health professionals exist, some of which are also accessible through these sites.

Health care providers can address several facets of medication use to foster patient acceptance, compliance, and safety. For those who are receiving nephroprotective medications as part of an effort to forestall ESKD, continued reinforcement and encouragement regarding the rationale for therapy may be necessary. Patients should understand that the safety and elimination of medication might change as their renal disease progresses, necessitating dosage adjustments or a change to alternative medications; anyone prescribing or dispensing medication to patients with CKD should be made aware of their *present* renal status. Patients should be encouraged to seek advice before using over-the-counter products because even over-the-counter products may worsen renal function (e.g., NSAIDs), prove dangerous (e.g., certain antacids, laxatives, NSAIDs), or require dosing precautions (e.g., H_2-antagonists used in excessive quantity).

TABLE 43.29	Patient-Focused Organizations and Resources
American Association of Kidney Patients	www.aakp.org
The Life Options Rehabilitation Council	www.lifeoptions.org
National Kidney Foundation	www.kidney.org
The Renal Association	www.renal.org
Kidney Dialysis Foundation	www.kdf.org
American Diabetes Association	www.diabetes.org
National Kidney and Urologic Diseases Information Clearinghouse/NIDDK	www.niddk.nih.gov
IgA Nephropathy Foundation American Kidney Fund	www.igan.org
Web-based link site and search engines	
Kidney Information Clearing House	www.renalnet.org.
The Nephron Information Center	www.nephron.com

The use of herbal products and dietary supplements without professional guidance should be discouraged.

METHODS FOR IMPROVING PATIENT ADHERENCE TO DRUG THERAPY

Patients with CKD are often prescribed numerous medications, often from different providers and specialists. This creates a situation wherein each prescriber is unaware of the patient's entire medication regimen. Given that the likelihood of drug interactions and drug-related misadventures increases with regimen complexity, a role for regular review of medication profiles becomes evident. Patients should be encouraged to communicate and verify information about their *actual* medication regimen (including the use of non-prescription products) on a regular basis because dosing changes are often communicated verbally from prescriber to patient, and medical records or dispensing profiles may not reflect actual practice.

Examples of instructions specific to medications commonly used in the CKD population are included in Table 43.30. Cognitive deficits and patient misunderstanding of the medication regimen are common barriers to compliance.

TABLE 43.30	Medication Counseling in Chronic Renal Disease: Some General Points

General Information

Ensure that all prescribers are aware of your kidney disease. Continue to inquire about special dosing for kidney disease (with new prescriptions and as kidney function changes). Seek advice before self-medication with over-the-counter agents, especially laxatives, antacids, nonsteroidal anti-inflammatory drugs, and herbal products. Vaccination yearly against influenza and every 5 years against pneumococcus is recommended. Ingestion of medications with soft, juicy foods may facilitate adherence to fluid restrictions.

Specific Medications

Calcium products that are being used as phosphate binders should be taken with or immediately after a meal; $CaCO_3$-based binders are best taken immediately before the meal. Calcium products that are being used for calcium supplementation should be taken at least 2 hours apart from meals. Phosphate binders may interfere with the absorption of other medications; inquire specifically.

Patients on Hemodialysis

Check to see whether medication should be specifically taken before or after dialysis (because some drugs are removed by dialysis); avoid changes in this "routine" unless approved by physician. Long-acting antihypertensives: Ask physician if you should take before dialysis on hemodialysis days. Hepatitis B vaccination series and boosters are recommended (often performed at hemodialysis center). If epoetin is administered subcutaneously, patients may require instructions on self-administration and appropriate storage.

Reviewing the rationale for use of a medication and discussing the results of examinations, laboratory tests, and diagnostic tests may help reinforce to the patient the value of compliance with diet, medication, and other treatments. Some patients are motivated by tradeoffs between dietary restriction and medication regimen complexity. For example, learning to estimate intake of dietary phosphorus and accordingly titrating the phosphate binder dose may afford flexibility and autonomy to patients who are capable of managing such alternatives. Patients are generally more willing to comply with dietary and medication treatment plans if they understand the usefulness and the consequences of noncompliance. Because of time constraints, physicians may not be able to provide this counseling to patients. Pharmacist intervention may play a vital role in this aspect of patient care.

KEY POINTS

- Chronic kidney disease is a significant and growing source of morbidity, mortality, and health care expenditure in the United States and worldwide
- The major causes of ESKD are diabetes mellitus and hypertension
- Much has been learned about the pathophysiology of CKD in the past decade; guidelines have been developed to treat many causes as well as complications of CKD
- Advanced CKD and uremia affect several organ systems, leading to secondary metabolic, hematologic, cardiovascular, skeletal, neuromuscular, gastrointestinal, endocrine, and other complications
- A critical area for improvement is the earlier recognition of kidney disease and screening of those at risk for CKD, followed by aggressive intervention to forestall progression to ESKD. This requires greater provider and patient awareness
- Pharmacologic therapies are a mainstay in managing the complications of uremia, but they should be coupled with dietary and lifestyle modifications for optimal results
- Medication regimen complexity and altered drug disposition in the CKD population provide a significant opportunity for pharmacists to improve patient outcomes, both on an individual level and at a population level

ACKNOWLEDGMENTS

The author acknowledges the contributions of Amy Galpin Krauss and Lawrence J. Hak, who authored the corresponding chapter in the seventh edition. Portions of that chapter have been used in this edition.

SUGGESTED READINGS

Kidney Disease Outcomes Quality Initiative. K/DOQI clinical practice guidelines on hypertension and antihypertensive agents in chronic kidney disease. Am J Kidney Dis 43 (5 Suppl 1):S1–S290, 2004.

Kidney Disease Outcomes Quality Initiative G. K/DOQI clinical practice guidelines for management of dyslipidemias in patients with kidney disease. Am J Kidney Dis 41 (4 Suppl 3):I–IV, 2003.

National Kidney Foundation. K/DOQI clinical practice guidelines for anemia of chronic kidney disease. Am J Kidney Dis 37 (Suppl 1): S182–S238, 2000.

National Kidney Foundation. K/DOQI clinical practice guidelines for bone metabolism and disease in chronic kidney disease [see comment]. Am J Kidney Dis 42 (4 Suppl 3):S1–S201, 2003.

National Kidney Foundation. K/DOQI clinical practice guidelines for chronic kidney disease: evaluation, classification, and stratification. Am J Kidney Dis 39 (2 Suppl 1):S1–S266, 2002.

Zillich ASJ, Saseen JJ, DeHart R, et al. Caring for patients with chronic kidney disease: a joint opinion of the ambulatory care and the nephrology practice networks of the American College of Clinical Pharmacy. Pharmacotherapy 25:123–143, 2005.

REFERENCES

1. Zillich ASJ, Saseen JJ, DeHart R, et al. Caring for patients with chronic kidney disease: a joint opinion of the ambulatory care and the nephrology practice networks of the American College of Clinical Pharmacy. Pharmacotherapy 25:123–143, 2005.

2. National Kidney Foundation. K/DOQI clinical practice guidelines for chronic kidney disease: evaluation, classification, and stratification. Am J Kidney Dis 39 (2 Suppl 1):S1–S266, 2002.

3. National Kidney F. K/DOQI clinical practice guidelines for chronic kidney disease: evaluation, classification, and stratification. Am J Kidney Dis 39 (2 Suppl 1):S1–266, 2002.

4. Gupta R, Birnbaum Y, Uretsky BF. The renal patient with coronary artery disease: current concepts and dilemmas. J Am Coll Cardiol 44:1343–1353, 2004.

5. Coresh J, Astor BC, Greene T, et al. Prevalence of chronic kidney disease and decreased kidney function in the adult US population: Third National Health and Nutrition Examination Survey. Am J Kidney Dis 41:1–12, 2003.

6. US Renal Data System. Excerpts from the USRDS 2002 annual report: atlas of end-stage renal disease in the United States. Am J Kidney Dis 41 (Suppl 2):S1–S256, 2003.

7. System USRD. Excerpts from the USRDS 2002 Annual Report: atlas of end-stage renal disease in the United States. Am J Kidney Dis 41 (Suppl 2):S1–S256, 2003.

8. System USRD. USRDS 2004 Annual Data Report: atlas of end-stage renal disease in the United States. Bethesda, MD: National Institutes of Health, National Institute of Diabetes and Digestive and Kidney Diseases, 2004.

9. Nickolas T, Frisch G, Opotowsky A, et al. Awareness of kidney disease in the US population: Findings from the National Health and Nutrition Examination Survey (NHANES) 1999 to 2000. Am J Kidney Dis 44:185–197, 2004.

10. American Diabetes Association. Standards of medical care for patients with diabetes mellitus [erratum appears in Diabetes Care 26: 972, 2003]. Diabetes Care 26 (Suppl 1):S33–S50, 2003.

11. Brenner B. The kidney. 5th ed. Philadelphia: WB Saunders, 1996.

12. Remuzzi G, Ruggenenti P, Benigni A. Understanding the nature of renal disease progression. Kidney Int 51:2–15, 1997.

13. Peten E, Striker L. Progression of glomerular disease. J Intern Med 236:241–249, 1994.

14. Diabetes Control and Complications Trial Research Group. The effect of intensive treatment of diabetes on the development and progression of long-term complications in insulin-dependent diabetes mellitus. N Engl J Med 329:978–986, 1993.

15. UK Prospective Diabetes Study (UKPDS) Group. Intensive blood-glucose control with sulfonylureas or insulin compared with conventional treatment and risk of complications in type 2 diabetes (UKPDS 33). Lancet 352:837–853, 1998.

16. UK Prospective Diabetes Study (UKPDS) Group. Effect of intensive blood-glucose control with metformin on complications in overweight patients with type 2 diabetes (UKPDS 34). Lancet 352: 854–865, 1998.

17. Ohkubo Y, Kishikawa H, Araki E, et al. Intensive insulin therapy prevents the progression of diabetic microvascular complications in Japanese patients with non-insulin dependent diabetes mellitus: a randomized prospective 6 year study. Diabetes Res Clin Pract 28: 103–117, 2003.

18. Jafar T, Stark P, Schmid C, et al. Proteinuria as a modifiable risk factor for the progression of non-diabetic renal disease. Kidney Int 60:2001.

19. Boero R, Rollino C, Massara C, et al. The verapamil versus amlodipine in nondiabetic nephropathies treated with trandolapril (VVANNTT) study. Am J Kidney Dis 42:67–75, 2003.

20. Wright JT Jr, Bakris G, Greene T, et al. Effect of blood pressure lowering and antihypertensive drug class on progression of hypertensive kidney disease: results from the AASK trial [see comment]. JAMA 288:2421–2431, 2002.

21. Lydakis C, Lip GY. Microalbuminuria and cardiovascular risk. QJM 91:381–391, 1998.

22. Chuahirun T, Khanna A, Kimball K, et al. Cigarette smoking and increased urine albumin excretion are interrelated predictors of nephropathy progression in type 2 diabetes. Am J Kidney Dis 41: 13–21, 2003.

23. Sugiyama S, Miyata T, Horie K, et al. Advanced glycation end-products in diabetic nephropathy. Nephrol Dial Transplant 11: 91–94, 1996.

24. Williams ME. New therapies for advanced glycation end product nephrotoxicity: current challenges. Am J Kidney Dis 41 (3 Suppl 1):S42–S47, 2003.

25. Sakurai S, Yonekura H, Yamamoto Y, et al. The AGE-RAGE system and diabetic nephropathy. J Am Soc Nephrol 14 (8 Suppl 3): S259–S263, 2003.

26. Forbes J, Cooper M, Thallus V, et al. Reduction of the accumulation of advanced glycation end products by ACE inhibition in experimental diabetic nephropathy. Diabetes 51:3274–3282, 2002.

27. Heidland A, Sebekova K, Schnizel R. Advanced glycation end-products and the progressive course of renal disease. Am J Kidney Dis 38:S100–S106, 2001.

28. Mogensen C. Long-term antihypertensive treatment inhibiting progression of diabetic nephropathy. BMJ 285:685–688, 1982.

29. Parving H, Andersen A, Smidt U, et al. Early aggressive antihypertensive treatment reduces rate of decline in kidney function in diabetic nephropathy. Lancet 1:1175–1179, 1983.

30. Viberti G, Wheeldon N. Microalbuminuria reduction with valsartan in patients with type 2 diabetes mellitus. Circulation 106:672–678, 2002.

31. Bakris GL, Weir MR, Secic M, et al. Differential effects of calcium antagonist subclasses on markers of nephropathy progression. Kidney Int 65:1991–2002, 2004.

32. Peterson J, Adler S, Burkart J, et al. Blood pressure control, proteinuria, and the progression of renal disease. The Modification of Diet in Renal Disease Study. Ann Intern Med 123:754–762, 1995.

33. Whelton P, Perneger T, He J, et al. The role of blood pressure as a risk factor for renal disease: a review of the epidemiologic evidence. J Hum Hypertens 10:683–689, 1996.

34. Kone B. Nitric oxide in renal health and disease. Am J Kidney Dis 30:311–333, 1997.

35. Kohan D. Endothelins in the normal and diseased kidney. Am J Kidney Dis 29:2–26, 1997.

36. Meyer K, Levey A. Controlling the epidemic of cardiovascular disease in chronic renal disease: report from the National Kidney Foundation Task Force on Cardiovascular Disease. J Am Soc Nephrol 9:S31–S42, 1998.

37. Coresh J, Longenecker J, Miller E, et al. Epidemiology of cardiovascular risk factors in chronic renal disease. J Am Soc Nephrol 9: S24–S42, 1998.

38. Ninomiya T, Kiyohara Y, Kubo M, et al. Hyperhomocysteinemia and the development of chronic kidney disease in a general population: the Hisayama study. Am J Kidney Dis 44:437–445, 2004.

39. Busch M, Franke S, Muller A, et al. Potential cardiovascular risk factors in chronic kidney disease: AGEs, total homocysteine and metabolites, and the C-reactive protein. Kidney Int 66:338–347, 2004.

40. Lewis E, Hunsicker L, Bain R, et al. The effect of angiotensin-converting-enzyme inhibition on diabetic nephropathy. N Engl J Med 329:1456–1462, 1993.

41. Kasiske B, Kalil R, Ma J, et al. Effect of antihypertensive therapy on the kidney patients with diabetes: a meta-regression analysis. Ann Intern Med 118:129–138, 1993.

42. Mogensen C, Keane W, Bennett W, et al. Prevention of diabetic nephropathy with special reference to microalbuminuria. Lancet 346:1080–1084, 1995.

43. The GISEN Group. Randomized placebo-controlled trial of the effect of ramipril on decline in glomerular filtration rate and risk of terminal renal failure in proteinuric, non-diabetic nephropathy. Lancet 349:1857–1863, 1997.

44. Machio G, Alberti D, Janin G, et al. Effect of the angiotensin-converting enzyme inhibitor benazepril on the progression of chronic renal insufficiency. N Engl J Med 330:877–884, 1996.

45. Levin A, Djurdjev O, Barrett B, et al. Cardiovascular disease in patients with chronic kidney disease: getting to the heart of the matter. Am J Kidney Dis 38:1398–1407, 2001.

46. Tonelli M, Moye L, Sacks F, et al. Effect of pravastatin on loss of renal function in people with moderate chronic renal insufficiency and cardiovascular disease. J Am Soc Nephrol 14:1605–1613, 2003.

47. Levin A, Singer J, Thompson CR, et al. Prevalent left ventricular hypertrophy in the pre-dialysis population: identifying opportunites for intervention. Am J Kidney Dis 27:347–354, 1996.

48. Levin A, Thompson CR, Ethier J, et al. Left ventricular mass index increase in early renal disease: impact of decline in hemoglobin. Am J Kidney Dis 34:125–134, 1999.

49. Portoles J, Torralbo A, Martin P, et al. Cardiovascular effects of recombinant human erythropoietin in predialysis patients. Am J Kidney Dis 29:541–548, 1997.

50. Levin A, Singer J, Thompson C, et al. Prevalent left ventricular hypertrophy in the pre-dialysis population: identifying opportunites for intervention. Am J Kidney Dis 27:347–354, 1996.

51. Levin A. Anemia and left ventricular hypertrophy in chronic kidney disease populations: a review of the current state of knowledge. Kidney Int Suppl 61 (Suppl 80):S35–S38, 2002.

52. Al-Ahmad A, Rand W, Manjunath G, et al. Reduced kidney function and anemia as risk factors for mortality in patients with left ventricular dysfunction. J Am Coll Cardiol 38:955–962, 2001.

53. Foley R, Parfrey P, Harnett J, et al. Clinical and echocardiographic disease in patients starting end-stage renal disease therapy. Kidney Int 47:186–192, 1995.

54. Parfrey P, Foley R, Harnett J, et al. Outcome and risk factors for left ventricular disorders in chronic uraemia. Nephrol Dial Transplant 11:1277–1285, 1996.

55. Bahlmann J, Schoter KH, Scigalla P, et al. Morbidity and mortality in hemodialysis patients with and without erythropoietin treatment: a controlled study. Contrib Nephrol 88:90–106, 1991.

56. Weiner DE, Tighiouart H, Stark PC, et al. Kidney disease as a risk factor for recurrent cardiovascular disease and mortality. Am J Kidney Dis 44:198–206, 2004.

57. Foley R, Levey A, Sarnak M. Clinical epidemiology of cardiovascular disease in chronic renal failure. Am J Kidney Dis 32 (Suppl 3):S112–S119, 1998.

58. Chertow G, Normand S, Silva L, et al. Survival after acute myocardial infarction in patients with end-stage renal disease: results from the cooperative cardiovascular project. Am J Kidney Dis 35:1217–1220, 2000.

59. Mann J, Gerstein H, Pogue J, et al. Renal insufficiency as a predictor of cardiovascular outcomes and the impact of ramipril: the HOPE randomized trial. Ann Intern Med 134:629–636, 2001.

60. Hemmelgarn B, Ghali W, Quan H, et al. Poor long-term survival after coronary angiography in patients with renal insufficiency. Am J Kidney Dis 37:64–72, 2001.

61. Wright R, Reeder G, Herzog C, et al. Acute myocardial infarction and renal dysfunction: a high risk combination. Ann Intern Med 137:563–570, 2002.

62. Block G, Port FK. Calcium phosphate metabolism and cardiovascular disease in patients with chronic kidney disease. Semin Dial 16:140–147, 2003.

63. Goodman W, London G, the Vascular Calcification Work Group. Vascular calcification in chronic kidney disease. Am J Kidney Dis 43:572–579, 2004.

64. Giachelli C, Jono S, Shioi A, et al. Vascular calcification and inorganic phosphate. Am J Kidney Dis 38:S34–S37, 2001.

65. Klassen P, Lowrie E, Reddan D, et al. Association between pulse pressure and mortality in patients undergoing maintenance hemodialysis. JAMA 287:1548–1555, 2002.

66. Block GA, Hulbert-Shearon TE, Levin N, et al. Association of serum phosphorous and calcium X phosphate product with mortality risk in chronic hemodialysis patients: a national study. Am J Kidney Dis 31:607–617, 1998.

67. Ganesh S, Stack A, Levin N, et al. Association of elevated serum PO4, CaXPO4 product, and parathyroid hormone with cardiac mortality risk in chronic hemodialysis patients. J Am Soc Nephrol 12:2131–2138, 2001.

68. National Kidney Foundation. K/DOQI clinical practice guidelines for bone metabolism and disease in chronic kidney disease. Am J Kidney Dis 42 (4 Suppl 3):S1–S201, 2003.

69. Appel G, Appel A. Angiotensin II receptor antagonists: role in hypertension, cardiovascular disease, and renoprotection. Prog Cardiovasc Dis 47:105–115, 2004.

70. Wheeler D, Bernard D. Lipid abnormalities in the nephrotic syndrome: causes, consequences, and treatment. Am J Kidney Dis 23:331–346, 1994.

71. Orchard T, Forrest K, Kuller L, et al, Pittsburgh Epidemiology of Diabetes Complications Study Group. Lipid and blood pressure treatment goals for type 1 diabetes: 10-year incidence data from the Pittsburgh Epidemiology of Diabetes Complications Study. Diabetes Care 24:1053–1059, 2001.

72. Hunsicker L, Adler S, Caggiula A, et al. Predictors of the progression of renal disease in the modification of diet in renal disease study. Kidney Int 51:1908–1919, 1997.

73. Yang W, Song N, Ying S, et al. Serum lipid concentrations correlate with the progression of chronic renal failure. Clin Lab Sci 12:104–108, 1999.

74. Attman P, Alaupovic P. Lipid and apolipoprotein profiles of uremic dyslipoproteinemia: relation to renal function and dialysis. Nephron 57:401–410, 1991.

75. Wanner C, Quaschning T. Dyslipidemia and renal disease: pathogenesis and clinical consequences. Curr Opin Nephrol Hypertens 10:195–201, 2001.

76. O'Neal D, Lee P, Murphy B, et al. Low-density lipoprotein particle size distribution in end-stage renal disease treated with hemodialysis or peritoneal dialysis. Am J Kidney Dis 27:84–91, 1996.

77. Moustapha A, Naso A, Nahlwi M, et al. Prospective study of hypercholesterolemia as an adverse cardiovascular risk factor in end-stage renal disease. Circulation 97:138–141, 1998.

78. Stenvinkel P, Heimburger O, Paultre F, et al. Strong association between malnutrition, inflammation, and atherosclerosis in chronic renal failure. Kidney Int 55:1899–1911, 1999.

79. Ahmed J, Weisberg L. Hyperkalemia in dialysis patients. Semin Dial 14:348–356, 2001.

80. Sandle G, Gaiger E, Tapster S, et al. Evidence for large intestinal control of potassium homeostasis in uraemic patients undergoing long-term dialysis. Clin Sci 73:247–252, 1987.

81. Martin R, Panese S, Virginillo M, et al. Increased secretion of potassium in the rectum of man with chronic renal failure. Am J Kidney Dis 8:105–110, 1986.

82. Gregoli PA, Bondurant MC. Function of caspases in regulating apoptosis caused by erythropoietin deprivation in erythroid progenitors. J Cell Physiol 178:133–143, 1999.

83. Sui X, Krantz SB, Zhao ZJ. Stem cell factor and erythropoietin inhibit apoptosis of human erythroid progenitor cells through different signalling pathways. Br J Haematol 110:63–70, 2000.

84. Ly J, Marticorena R, Donnelly S. Red blood survival in chronic renal failure. Am J Kidney Dis 44:715–719, 2004.

85. Anonymous IV. NKF-K/DOQI clinical practice guidelines for anemia of chronic kidney disease: update 2000 [erratum appears in

Am J Kidney Dis 38:442, 2001]. Am J Kidney Dis 37 (1 Suppl 1): S182–S238, 2001.

86. Astor BC, Muntner P, Levin A, et al. Association of kidney function with anemia: the Third National Health and Nutrition Examination Survey (1988–1994). Arch Intern Med 162:1401–1408, 2002.
87. Hsu C, McCulloch C, Curhan G. Epidemiology of anemia associated with chronic renal insufficiency among adults in the United States: results from the Third National Health and Nutrition Examination Survey. J Am Soc Nephrol 13:504–510, 2002.
88. Owen WF Jr. Patterns of care for patients with chronic kidney disease in the United States: Dying for improvement. J Am Soc Nephrol 14:S76–S80, 2003.
89. Radtke HW, Claussner A, Erbes PM, et al. Serum erythropoietin concentration in chronic renal failure: relationship to degree of anemia and excretory function. Blood 54:877–884, 1979.
90. Jungers PY, Robino C, Choukroun G, et al. Incidence of anaemia and use of epoetin therapy in pre-dialysis patients: a prospective study in 403 patients. Nephrol Dial Transplant 17:1621–1627, 2002.
91. McClellan W, Aronoff SL, Bolton WK, et al. The prevalence of anemia in patients with chronic kidney disease. Curr Med Res Opin 20:1501–1510, 2004.
92. Abramson JL, Jurkovitz CT, Vaccarino V, et al. Chronic kidney disease, anemia, and incident stroke in a middle-aged, community-based population: the ARIC study. Kidney Int 64:610–615, 2003.
93. Foley RN, Parfrey PS, Sarnak MJ. Clinical epidemiology of cardiovascular disease in chronic renal failure. Am J Kidney Dis 32 (Suppl 3):S112–S119, 1998.
94. Revicki DA, Brown RE, Feeny DH, et al. Health-related quality of life associated with recombinant human erythropoietin therapy for predialysis chronic renal disease patients. Am J Kidney Dis 25: 548–554, 1995.
95. Abramson J, Jurkovitz C, Vaccarino V, et al. Chronic kidney disease, anemia, and incident stroke in a middle-aged, community-based population: the ARIC study. Kidney Int 64:610–615, 2003.
96. Foley R, Parfrey P, Harnett J, et al. The impact of anemia on cardiomyopathy, morbidity and mortality in end-stage renal disease. Am J Kidney Dis 28:53–61, 1996.
97. Foley RN, Parfrey PS, Harnett JD, et al. The impact of anemia on cardiomyopathy, morbidity and mortality in end-stage renal disease. Am J Kidney Dis 28:53–61, 1996.
98. Xia H, Ebben J, Ma JZ, et al. Hematocrit levels and hospitalization risks in hemodialysis patients. J Am Soc Nephrol 10:1309–1316, 1999.
99. Ma JZ, Ebben J, Xia H, et al. Hematocrit level and associated mortality in hemodialysis patients. J Am Soc Nephrol 10:610–619, 1999.
100. Al-Ahmad A, Rand WM, Manjunath G, et al. Reduced kidney function and anemia as risk factors for mortality in patients with left ventricular dysfunction. J Am Coll Cardiol 38:955–962, 2001.
101. System USRD. USRDS 2004 annual data report: atlas of end-stage renal disease in the United States. Bethesda, Md: National Institutes of Health, National Institute of Diabetes and Digestive and Kidney Diseases, 2004.
102. Block GA, Port FK. Re-evaluation of risks associated with hyperphosphatemia and hyperparathyroidism in dialysis patients: recommendations for a change in management. Am J Kidney Dis 35: 1226–1237, 2000.
103. Raggi P, Boulay A, Chasan-Taber S, Amin N, Dillon M, Burke SK, Chertow GM. Cardiac calcification in adult hemodialysis patients. A link between end-stage renal disease and cardiovascular disease? J Am Coll Cardiol. 39:695-701, 2002
104. Goodman W, Goldin J, Kuizon B, et al. Coronary-artery calcification in young adults with end-stage renal disease who are undergoing dialysis. N Engl J Med 342:1478–1483, 2000.
105. Zacharias J, Fontaine B, Fine A. Calcium use increases risk of calciphylaxis: a case-control study. Perit Dial Int 19:248–252, 1999.
106. Mazhar A, Johnson R, Gillen D, et al. Risk factors and mortality associated with calciphylaxis in end-stage renal disease. Kidney Int 60:324–332, 2001.
107. Tomasello S, Dhupar S, Sherman R. Phosphate binders, K/DOQI guidelines, and compliance: the unfortunate reality. Dial Transplant 33:236–240, 2004.

108. Braun J, Olendorf M, Moshage W, et al. Electron beam computed tomography in the evaluation of cardiac calcification in chronic dialysis patients. Am J Kidney Dis 27:394–401, 1996.
109. Ribeiro S, Ramos A, Brandero A, et al. Cardiac valve calcification in hemodialysis patients: role of calcium-phosphate metabolism. Nephrol Dial Transplant 13:2037–2040, 1998.
110. Lewis J, Zucker M, Ferguson J. Bleeding tendency in uremia. Blood 11:1073, 1956.
111. Remuzzi G. Bleeding in renal failure. Lancet 1:1205–1208, 1988.
112. Cohen B, Stein I, Bonas J. Guanidinosuccic aciduria in uremia. Am J Med 45:63, 1968.
113. Gawaz MP, Dobos G, Spath M, et al. Impaired function of platelet membrane glycoprotein IIb-IIIa in end-stage renal disease. J Am Soc Nephrol 5:36–46, 1994.
114. Hou S. What are the clinically important consequences of ESRD-associated endocrine dysfunction? Semin Dial 10:11–13, 1997.
115. Amorosa L. Thyroid function in end-stage renal disease. Semin Dial 10:13–16, 1997.
116. Zucker I, Yosipovitch G, David M, et al. Prevalence and characterization of uremic pruritus in patients undergoing hemodialysis: uremic pruritus is still a major problem for patients with end-stage renal disease. J Am Acad Dermatol 49:842–846, 2003.
117. Kuypers D, Claes K, Evenpoel P, et al. A prospective proof of concept study of the efficacy of tacrolimus ointment on uraemic pruritus (UP) in patients on dialysis therapy. Nephrol Dial Transplant 19:1895–1901, 2004.
118. Momose A, Kudo S, Sato H, et al. Calcium ions are abnormally distributed in the skin of hemodialysis patients with uraemic pruritus. Nephrol Dial Transplant 19:2061–2066, 2004.
119. Murphy M, Reaich D, Pai P, et al. A randomized, placebo-controlled, double-blind trial of ondansetron in renal itch. Br J Dermatol 148:314–317, 2003.
120. Young G, Bolton C. Peripheral nervous system complications in hemodialysis patients. Semin Dialysis 10:46–51, 1997.
121. National Kidney Foundation. Kidney early evaluation program. Am J Kidney Dis 42 (Suppl 4):S1–S60, 2003.
122. Latham C. Is there data to support the concept that educated, empowered patients have better outcomes? J Am Soc Nephrol 9: S141–S144, 1998.
123. DeOreo P. Hemodialysis patient-assessed functional health status predicts continued survival, hospitalization, and dialysis-attendance compliance. Am J Kidney Dis 30:204–212, 1997.
124. Chobanian A, Bakris G, Black H, et al. The seventh report of the Joint National Committee on prevention, detection, evaluation, and treatment of high blood pressure. JAMA 289:2534–2573, 2003.
125. National Cholesterol Education Program Expert Panel on Detection, Evaluation, and Treatment of High Blood Cholesterol in Adults. Third report of the National Cholesterol Education Program (NCEP) Expert Panel on Detection, Evaluation, and Treatment of High Blood Cholesterol in Adults (Adult Treatment Panel III) final report [see comment]. Circulation 106:3143–3421, 2002.
126. Group TAiiDNT. Should all patients with type 1 diabetes mellitus and microalbuminuria receive angiotensin-converting enzyme inhibitors? Ann Intern Med 134:370–379, 2001.
127. Miyata T, van Ypersele de Strihou C, Ueda Y, et al. Angiotensin II receptor antagonists and angiotensin-converting enzyme inhibitors lower in vitro the formation of advanced glycation end products: biochemical mechanisms. J Am Soc Nephrol 13:2478–2487, 2002.
128. Brownlee M. Biochemistry and molecular biology of diabetic complications. Nature 414:813–820, 2001.
129. Ravid M, Savin H, Jutrin I, et al. Long-term stabilizing effect of angiotensin-converting enzyme inhibition on plasma creatinine and on proteinuria in normotensive type II diabetic patients. Ann Intern Med 118:577–581, 1993.
130. Parving H, Lehnert H, Brochner-Mortensen J, et al. The effect of irbesartan on the development of diabetic nephropathy in patients with type 2 diabetes. N Engl J Med 345:870–878, 2001.
131. Strippoli GF, Craig M, Deeks JJ, et al. Effects of angiotensin converting enzyme inhibitors and angiotensin II receptor antagonists on mortality and renal outcomes in diabetic nephropathy: systematic review. BMJ 329:828, 2004.
132. Molitch M, DeFronzo R, Franz M, et al. Nephropathy in diabetes. Diabetes Care 27 (Suppl 1):S79–S83, 2004.

133. Smith AC, Toto R, Bakris GL. Differential effects of calcium channel blockers on size selectivity of proteinuria in diabetic glomerulopathy. Kidney Int 54:889–896, 1998.

134. Psaty M, Heckbert T, Koepsell T, et al. The risk of myocardial infarction associated with antihypertensive drug therapies. J Am Med Assoc 274:620–625, 1995.

135. Pahor M, Psaty M. Health outcomes associated with calcium antagonists compared with other first line antihypertensive therapies: a meta-analysis of randomised control trials. Lancet 356:1949–1954, 2000.

136. Opie L, Messerli F. Nifedipine and mortality: grave defects in the dossier. Circulation 92:1068–1073, 1995.

137. Gaede P, Vedel P, Larsen N, et al. Multifactorial intervention and cardiovascular disease in patients with type 2 diabetes. N Engl J Med 348:383–393, 2003.

138. Gaede P, Vedel P, Parving H, et al. Intensified multifactorial intervention in patients with type 2 diabetes mellitus and microalbuminuria: the Steno type 2 randomised study. Lancet 353:617–622, 1999.

139. Kidney Disease Outcomes Quality I. K/DOQI clinical practice guidelines on hypertension and antihypertensive agents in chronic kidney disease. Am J Kidney Dis 43 (5 Suppl 1):S1–S290, 2004.

140. Harsha D, Lin P, Obarzanek E, et al. Dietary approaches to stop hypertension: a summary of study results. J Am Diet Assoc 99 (Suppl 8):S35–S39, 1999.

141. Barzilay JI, Davis BR, Bettencourt J, et al. Cardiovascular outcomes using doxazosin vs. chlorthalidone for the treatment of hypertension in older adults with and without glucose disorders: a report from the ALLHAT study. J Clin Hypertens (Greenwich) 6: 116–125, 2004.

142. Ruggenenti P, Perna A, Remuzzi G, GISEN Group Investigators. Retarding progression of chronic renal disease: the neglected issue of residual proteinuria. Kidney Int 63:2254–2261, 2003.

143. Pedrini M, Levey A, Lau J, et al. The effect of dietary protein restriction on the progression of diabetic and nondiabetic renal diseases. Ann Intern Med 124:627–632, 1996.

144. Lewis E, Hunsicker L, Clarke W, et al. Renoprotective effect of the angiotensin-receptor antagonist irbesartan in patients with nephropathy due to type II diabetes. N Engl J Med 345:851–860, 2001.

145. Brenner B, Cooper M, de Zeeuw D, et al. Effects of losartan on renal and cardiovascular outcomes in patients with type 2 diabetes and nephropathy. N Engl J Med 345:861–869, 2001.

146. Laverman G, Navis G, Henning R, et al. Dual renin-angiotensin system blockade at optimal doses for proteinuria. Kidney Int 62: 1020–1025, 2002.

147. Hebert L, Falkenhain M, Nahman N, et al. Combination ACE inhibitor and angiotensin II receptor antagonist in diabetic nephropathy. Am J Nephrol 19:1–6, 1999.

148. Mogensen C, Neldam S, Takkanen I, et al. Randomised controlled trial of dual blockade of renin-angiotensin system in patients with hypertension, microalbuminuria, and non-insulin dependent diabetes: the candesartan and lisinopril microalbuminuria (CALM) study. BMJ 321:1440–1444, 2000.

149. Jacobsen P, Anderson S, Rossing K, et al. Dual blockade of the renin-angiotensin system versus maximal recommended dose of ACE inhibition in diabetic nephropathy. Kidney Int 63:1874–1880, 2003.

150. Jacobsen P, Rossing K, Parving HH. Single versus dual blockade of the renin-angiotensin system (angiotensin-converting enzyme inhibitors and/or angiotensin II receptor blockers) in diabetic nephropathy. Curr Opin Nephrol Hypertens 13:319–324, 2004.

151. Cetinkaya R, Odabas AR, Selcuk Y. Anti-proteinuric effects of combination therapy with enalapril and losartan in patients with nephropathy due to type 2 diabetes. Int J Clin Pract 58:432–435, 2004.

152. Panos J, Michelis MF, DeVita MV, et al. Combined converting enzyme inhibition and angiotensin receptor blockade reduce proteinuria greater than converting enzyme inhibition alone: insights into mechanism. Clin Nephrol 60:13–21, 2003.

153. Segura J, Christiansen H, Campo C, et al. How to titrate ACE inhibitors and angiotensin receptor blockers in renal patients: according to blood pressure or proteinuria? Curr Hypertens Rep 5: 426–429, 2003.

154. Nakao N, Yoshimura A, Morita H, et al. Combination treatment of angiotensin-II receptor blocker and angiotensin-converting-enzyme inhibitor in non-diabetic renal disease (COOPERATE): a randomised controlled trial. Lancet 361:117–124, 2003.

155. Kincaid-Smith P, Fairley KF, Packham D. Dual blockade of the renin-angiotensin system compared with a 50% increase in the dose of angiotensin-converting enzyme inhibitor: effects on proteinuria and blood pressure. Nephrol Dial Transplant 19:2272–2274, 2004.

156. Zeller K. Low-protein diets in renal disease. Diabetes Care 14: 856–866, 1991.

157. Zeller K. Effect of restricting dietary protein on the progression of renal failure in patients with insulin-dependent diabetes mellitus. N Engl J Med 324:78–84, 1991.

158. Klahr S, Levey AS, Beck GJ, et al. The effects of dietary protein restriction and blood-pressure control on the progression of chronic renal disease. Modification of Diet in Renal Disease Study Group [see comment]. N Engl J Med 330:877–884, 1994.

159. Locatelli F, Alberti D, Graziani G, et al. Prospective, randomized multicentre trial of effect of protein restriction on progression of chronic renal insufficiency. Lancet 337:1299–1304, 1991.

160. Levey AS, Adler S, Caggiula AW, et al. Effects of dietary protein restriction on the progression of advanced renal disease in the Modification of Diet in Renal Disease Study. Am J Kidney Dis 27: 652–663, 1996.

161. Kasiske B, Lakatua J, Ma J, et al. A meta-analysis of the effects of dietary protein restriction on the rate of decline in renal function. Am J Kidney Dis 31:954–961, 1998.

162. Levey A, Greene T, Beck G, et al. Dietary protein restriction and the progression of chronic renal disease: what have all of the MDRD study shown? J Am Soc Nephrol 10:2426–2439, 1999.

163. US Renal Data System. Comorbid conditions and correlations with mortality risk among 3399 incident hemodialysis patients. Am J Kidney Dis 20:32–38, 1992.

164. Port F. Morbidity and mortality in dialysis patients. Kidney Int 46: 1728–1737, 1994.

165. Barrett B, Parfey P, Morgan J. Prediction of early death in end-stage renal disease patients starting dialysis. Am J Kidney Dis 214–222, 1997.

166. Churchill D, Taylor D, Cook R. Canadian hemodialysis morbidity study. Am J Kidney Dis 19:214–234, 1992.

167. Ikizer T, Hakim R. Nutrition in end-stage renal disease. Kidney Int 50:343–357, 1996.

168. Kopple JD. National Kidney Foundation K/DOQI clinical practice guidelines for nutrition in chronic renal failure. Am J Kidney Dis 37 (1 Suppl 2):S66–S70, 2001.

169. Tonolo G, Melis M, Formato M, et al. Additive effects of simvastatin beyond its effects on LDL cholesterol in hypertensive type 2 diabetic patients. Eur J Clin Invest 30:980–987, 2000.

170. Harris K, Purkenson M, Yates J, et al. Lovastatin ameliorates the development of glomerulosclerosis and uremia in experimental nephrotic syndrome. Am J Kidney Dis 15:16–23, 1990.

171. Grandaliano G, Biswas P, Choudhury G, et al. Simvastatin inhibits PDGF-induced DNA synthesis in human glomerular mesangial cells. Kidney Int 44:503–508, 1993.

172. Massy Z, Guijarro C, O'Donnell M, et al. Lipids, 3-hydroxy-3-methylglutaryl coenzyme A reductase inhibitors, and progression of renal failure. Adv Nephrol Necker Hosp 27:39–57, 1997.

173. Lee T, Su F, Tsai C. Effect of pravastatin on proteinuria in patients with well hypertension. Hypertension 40:67–73, 2002.

174. Albert M, Danielson E, Rifai N, et al. Effect of statin therapy on C-reactive protein levels: the pravastatin inflammation/CRP evaluation (PRINCE): a randomized cohort study. JAMA 286:64–70, 2001.

175. Imai Y, Suzuki H, Saito T, et al. The effect of pravastatin on renal function and lipid metabolism in patients with renal dysfunction with hypertension and hyperlipidemia. Pravastatin and Renal Function Research Group. Clin Exp Hypertens 21:1345–1355, 1999.

176. Youssef F, Seifalian A, Jagroop A, et al. The early effect of lipid-lowering treatment on carotid and femoral intima media thickness (IMT). Eur J Vasc Endovasc Surg 23:358–364, 2002.

177. Fathi R, Isbel N, Short L, et al. The effect of long-term aggressive lipid lowering on ischemic and atherosclerotic burden in patients with chronic kidney disease. Am J Kidney Dis 43:45–52, 2004.

178. Fried L, Orchard T, Kasiske B. Effect of lipid reduction on the progression of renal disease: a meta analysis. Kidney Int 59:260–269, 2001.

179. Athyros V, Papageorgiou A, Elisaf M, et al, Greace Study Collaborative Group. Statins and renal function in patients with diabetes mellitus. Curr Med Res Opin 19:615–617, 2003.

180. Bianchi S, Bigazzi R, Caiazza A, et al. A controlled, prospective study of the effects of atorvastatin on proteinuria and progression of kidney disease. Am J Kidney Dis 41:565–570, 2003.

181. Tonolo G, Ciccarese M, Brizzi P, et al. Reduction of albumin excretion rate in normotensive microalbuminuric type 2 patients during long-term simvastatin treatment. Diabetes Care 20:1891–1895, 1997.

182. Athyros V, Mikhailidis D, Papageorgiou A, et al. The effect of statins versus untreated dyslipidaemia on renal function in patients with coronary heart disease. A subgroup analysis of the Greek atorvastatin and coronary heart disease evaluation (GREACE) study [see comment]. J Clin Pathol 57:728–734, 2004.

183. Foundation MRCBH. Heart protection study of cholesterol lowering with simvastatin in 20,536 high risk individuals: a randomized placebo controlled trial. Lancet 360:7–22, 2002.

184. Seliger S, Weiss N, Gillen D, et al. HMG-CoA reductase inhibitors are associated with reduced mortality in ESRD patients. Kidney Int 61:297–304, 2002.

185. Ozsoy R, Kastelein J, Arisz L, et al. Atorvastatin and the dislipidemia of early renal failure. Atherosclerosis 166:187–194, 2003.

186. Kidney Disease Outcomes Quality Initiative G. K/DOQI clinical practice guidelines for management of dyslipidemias in patients with kidney disease. Am J Kidney Dis 41 (4 Suppl 3):I–IV, 2003.

187. Lipscombe J, Lewis G, Cattran D, et al. Deterioration in renal function associated with fibrate therapy. Clin Nephrol 55:39–44, 2001.

188. Broeders N, Knoop C, Antoine M, et al. Fibrate-induced increase in blood urea and creatinine: is gemfibrozil the only innocuous agent? Nephrol Dial Transplant 15:1993–1999, 2000.

189. Bloomfield R, Robins S, Wittes J, et al. Gemfibrozil for the secondary prevention of coronary heart disease in men with low levels of high-density lipoprotein cholesterol. N Engl J Med 341:410–418, 1999.

190. Procrit (epoetin alfa) package insert. Thousand Oaks, Calif: Amgen Inc, 2004.

191. Epogen (epoetin alfa) for Injection package insert. Thousand Oaks, Calif: Amgen Inc, 2004.

192. The NESP Usage Guidelines Group. Practical guidelines for the use of NESP in treating renal anaemia. Nephrol Dial Transplant 16 (Suppl 3):22–28, 2001.

193. Provenzano R, Garcia-Mayol L, Suchinda P, et al. Once-weekly epoetin alfa for treating the anemia chronic kidney disease. Clin Nephrol 61:392–405, 2004.

194. Lim VS, DeGowin RL, Zavala D, et al. Recombinant human erythropoietin treatment in pre-dialysis patients. Ann Intern Med 110:108–114, 1989.

195. Marrades R, Campistol J. Effects of erythropoietin on muscle O2 transport during exercise in patients with chronic renal failure. J Clin Invest 97:2092–2100, 1997.

196. Jungers P, Choukroun G, Oualim Z, et al. Beneficial influence of recombinant human erythropoietin therapy on the rate of progression of chronic renal failure in predialysis patients. Nephrol Dial Transplant 16:307–312, 2001.

197. Collins AJ. Anaemia management prior to dialysis: cardiovascular and cost-benefit observations. Nephrol Dial Transplant 18 (Suppl 2):ii2–ii6, 2003.

198. Kuriyama S, Tomonari H, Yoshida H, et al. Reversal of anemia by erythropoietin therapy retards the progression of chronic renal failure, especially in nondiabetic patients. Nephron 77:176–185, 1997.

199. Silverberg D, Wexler D, Blum M, et al. The correction of anemia in severe resistant heart failure with erythropoietin and intravenous iron prevents the progression of both the heart and the renal failure and markedly reduces hospitalization. Clin Nephrol 58 (Suppl 1):S37–S45, 2002.

200. Kleinman KS, Schweitzer SU, Perdue ST, et al. The use of recombinant human erythropoietin in the correction of anemia in predialysis patients and its effect on renal function: a double-blind, placebo-controlled trial. Am J Kidney Dis 14:486–495, 1989.

201. Xia H, Ebben J, Ma J, et al. Hematocrit levels and hospitalization risks in hemodialysis patients. J Am Soc Nephrol 10:1309–1316, 1999.

202. Ma J, Ebben J, Xia H, et al. Hematocrit level and associated mortality in hemodialysis patients. J Am Soc Nephrol 10:610–619, 1999.

203. Collins A, Li S, Ebben J, et al. Hematocrit levels and associated mortality in hemodialysis patients. Am J Kidney Dis 36:282–293, 2000.

204. Ma J, Ebben J, Xia H, et al. Hematocrit levels and hospitalization risks in hemodialysis patients. J Am Soc Nephrol 10:610–619, 1999.

205. Hayashi T, Suzuki A, Shoji T, et al. Cardiovascular effect of normalizing the hematocrit level during erythropoietin therapy in predialysis patients with chronic renal failure. Am J Kidney Dis 35:250–256, 2000.

206. Kuriyama S, Tomonari H, Yoshida H, et al. Reversal of anemia by erythropoietin therapy retards the progression of chronic renal failure, especially in nondiabetic patients. Nephron 77:176–185, 1997.

207. Silverberg DS, Wexler D, Blum M, et al. The correction of anemia in severe resistant heart failure with erythropoietin and intravenous iron prevents the progression of both the heart and the renal failure and markedly reduces hospitalization. Clin Nephrol 58 (Suppl 1):S37–S45, 2002.

208. Fink J, Blahut S, Reddy M, et al. Use of erythropoietin before the initiation of dialysis and its impact on mortality. Am J Kidney Dis 37:348–355, 2001.

209. Xue J, St. Peter W, Ebben J, et al. Anemia treatment in the pre-ESRD period and associated mortality in elderly patients. Am J Kidney Dis 40:1153–1161, 2002.

210. Anonymous. IV. NKF-K/DOQI clinical practice guidelines for anemia of chronic kidney disease: update 2000 [erratum appears in Am J Kidney Dis 38:442, 2001]. Am J Kidney Dis 37 (1 Suppl 1):S182–S238, 2001.

211. Locatelli F, Conte F, Marcelli D. The impact of haematocrit levels and erythropoietin treatment on overall and cardiovascular morbidity and mortality—the experience of the Lombardy Dialysis Registry. Nephrol Dial Transplant 13:1642–1644, 1998.

212. Portoles J, Torralbo A, Martin P, et al. Cardiovascular effects of recombinant human erythropoietin in predialysis patients. Am J Kidney Dis 29:541–548, 1997.

213. Hayashi T, Suzuki A, Shoji T, et al. Cardiovascular effect of normalizing the hematocrit level during erythropoietin therapy in predialysis patients with chronic renal failure. Am J Kidney Dis 35:250–256, 2000.

214. Moreno F, Sanz-Guajardo D, Lopez-Gomez J, et al. Increasing the hematocrit has a beneficial effect on quality of life and is safe in selected hemodialysis patients. J Am Soc Nephrol 11:335–342, 2000.

215. Besarb A, Kline B, Browne J, et al. The effects of normal as compared with low hematocrit values in patients with cardiac disease who are receiving hemodialysis and epoetin. N Engl J Med 39:584–590, 1998.

216. McClellan WM, Frankenfield DL, Wish JB, et al. Subcutaneous erythropoietin results in lower dose and equivalent hematocrit levels among adult hemodialysis patients: results from the 1998 End-Stage Renal Disease Core Indicators Project. Am J Kidney Dis 37:E36, 2001.

217. Canadian Erythropoietin Study Group. Effect of recombinant human erythropoietin therapy on blood pressure in hemodialysis patients. Am J Nephrol 11:23–26, 1991.

218. Abraham P, Macres M. Blood pressure in hemodialysis patients during amelioration of anemia with erythropoietin. J Am Soc Nephrol 2:927–936, 1991.

219. Eschbach J, Egrie J, Downing M, et al. Correction of the anaemia of end-stage renal disease with recombinant human erythropoietin. N Engl J Med 316:73–78, 1987.

220. Eschbach JW, Egrie JC, Downing M, et al. Correction of the anaemia of end-stage renal disease with recombinant human erythropoietin. N Engl J Med 316:73–78, 1987.

221. Raine A. Effects of erythropoietin on blood pressure. Am J Kidney Dis 18 (4 Suppl 1):76–83, 1991.

222. Foundation NK. K/DOQI clinical practice guidelines for anemia of chronic kidney disease. Am J Kidney Dis 37 (Suppl 1):S182–S238, 2000.

223. Borne P van de, Tielemans C, Vanherweghem J, et al. Effect of recombinant human erythropoietin therapy on ambulatory blood pressure and heart rate in chronic haemodialysis patients. Nephrol Dial Transplant 7:34–49, 1992.

224. Teehan B, Krantz S, Stone W, et al. Double-blind, placebo-controlled study of the therapeutic use of recombinant human erythropoietin for anemia associated with chronic renal failure in predialysis patients. Am J Kidney Dis 18:50–59, 1991.

225. Schwartz A, Terzian L, Kahn B. Erythropoietin for the anemia of chronic renal failure. Am Fam Physician 37:211–215, 1998.

226. Schmieder R, Hilgers K. Endogenous erythropoietin correlates with blood pressure in essential hypertension. Am J Kidney Dis 29: 376–382, 1997.

227. Carlini R, Rothstein M. Intravenous erythropoietin (rHuEPO) administration increases plasma endothelin and blood pressure in hemodialysis patients. Am J Hypertens 6:103–107, 1993.

228. Carlini RG, Dusso AS, Obialo C, et al. Recombinant human erythropoietin (rHuEPO) increases endothelin-1 release by endothelial cells. Kidney Int 43:1010–1014, 1993.

229. Neusser MT, Zidek W. Erythropoietin increases cytosolic free calcium concentration in vascular smooth muscle cells. Cardiovasc Res 27:1233–1236, 1993.

230. Wada Y, Matsuoka H, Tamai O, et al. Erythropoietin impairs endothelium-dependent vasorelaxation through cyclooxygenase-dependent mechanisms in humans. Am J Hypertens 12:980–987, 1999.

231. Lechre D, Schmidt R, Zoellner K, et al. Rheology in whole blood and in red blood cells under recombinant human erythropoietin therapy. Contrib Nephrol 76:299–305, 1989.

232. Johnson W, McCarthy J, Yanagihara T, et al. Effects of recombinant human erythropoietin on cerebral and cutaneous blood flow and on blood coagulability. Kidney 38:919–924, 1990.

233. Raine A, Roger S. Effects of erythropoietin on blood pressure. Am J Kidney Dis 18 (4 Suppl 1):76–83, 1991.

234. Conlon P, Kovalik E, Schumm D, et al. Normalization of hematocrit in hemodialysis patients with cardiac disease does not increase blood pressure. Ren Fail 22:435–444, 2000.

235. Akizawa T, Koshikawa S, Takaku F, et al. Clinical effect of recombinant human erythropoietin on anemia associated with chronic renal failure: a multi-institutional study in Japan. Int J Artif Organs 11:343–350, 1988.

236. Drueke T. Modulating factors in the hematopoietic response to erythropoietin. Am J Kidney Dis 18 (4 Suppl 1):87–92, 1991.

237. Jensen J, Eiskjaer H, Masden B, et al. Effect of captopril on the renal veno-arterial gradient of erythropoietin and oxygen in unilateral renal artery disease. Scand J Clin Lab Invest 53:859–865, 1993.

238. MacDougall I. The role of ACE inhibitors and angiotensin II receptor blockers in the response to erythropoietin. Nephrol Dial Transplant 14:1836–1841, 1999.

239. Freudenthaler SM, Korner T, Gleiter CH. Angiotensin II increases erythropoietin production in healthy human volunteers. Eur J Clin Invest 29:816–823, 1999.

240. Dhondt AV, Ringoir S. Angiotensin-converting enzyme inhibitors and higher erythropoietin requirement in chronic haemodialysis patients. Nephrol Dial Transplant 10:2107–2109, 1995.

241. Matsumura M, Nomura H, Koni I, et al. Angiotensin-converting enzyme inhibitors are associated with the need for increased recombinant human erythropoietin maintenance doses in hemodialysis patients. Nephron 77:164–168, 1997.

242. Tarng D, Wei Y, Huang T, et al. Intravenous ascorbic acid as an adjuvant therapy for recombinant erythropoietin in hemodialysis patients with hyperferritinemia. Kidney Int 55:2477–2486, 1999.

243. Tarng D, Huang T. A parellel, comparative study of intravenous iron versus intravenous ascorbic acid for erythropoietin-hyporesponsive anaemia in hemodialysis patients with iron overload. Nephrol Dial Transplant 13:2867–2872, 1998.

244. Sezer S, Ozdemir F, Yakupoglu U, et al. Intravenous ascorbic acid administration for erythropoietin-hyporesponsive anemia in iron loaded hemodialysis patients. Artif Organs 26:366–370, 2002.

245. Gastaldello K, Vereerstraeten A, Nzame-Nze T, et al. Resistance to erythropoietin iron-overloaded haemodialysis patients can be overcome by ascorbic acid administration. Nephrol Dial Transplant 10 (Suppl 6):44–47, 1995.

246. Keven K, Kutlay S, Nergizoglu G, et al. Crossover study of the effects of vitamin C on EPO response in hemodialysis patients. Am J Kidney Dis 41:1233–1239, 2003.

247. Trivedi H, Brooks B. Erythropoietin therapy in pre-dialysis patients with chronic renal failure: lack of need for parenteral iron. Am J Nephrol 23:78–85, 2003.

248. Silverberg DS, Iaina A, Peer G, et al. Intravenous iron supplementation for the treatment of the anemia of moderate to severe chronic renal failure patients not receiving dialysis. Am J Kidney Dis 27: 234–238, 1996.

249. Ferrlecit (sodium ferric gluconate) package insert. Corona, Calif: Watson Pharma, 2004.

250. Venofer (iron sucrose) package insert. Shirley, NY: American Regent, 2004.

251. Folkert VW, Michael B, Agarwal R, et al. Chronic use of sodium ferric gluconate complex in hemodialysis patients: safety of higher-dose (> or = 250 mg) administration. Am J Kidney Dis 41: 651–657, 2003.

252. Blaustein DA, Schwenk MH, Chattopadhyay J, et al. The safety and efficacy of an accelerated iron sucrose dosing regimen in patients with chronic kidney disease. Kidney Int Suppl 87:S72–S77, 2003.

253. National Kidney Foundation. K/DOQI clinical practice guidelines for bone metabolism and disease in chronic kidney disease [see comment]. Am J Kidney Dis 42 (4 Suppl 3):S1–S201, 2003.

254. Walker JA, Sherman RA, Cody RP. The effect of oral bases on enteral aluminum absorption. Arch Intern Med 150:2037–2039, 1990.

255. Renagel Package Insert. Cambridge, Mass: Genzyme Corporation, 2005.

256. Fosrenol Package Insert. Wayne, Pa: Shire US Inc, 2005.

257. Hergesell O, Ritz E. Phosphate binders in uremia: pharmacodynamics, pharmacoeconomics, pharmacoethics. Nephrol Dial Transplant 17:14–17, 2002.

258. Chertow G, Dillon M, Burke S, et al. A randomized trial of sevelamer hydrochloride (RenaGel) with and without supplemental calcium. Clin Nephrol 51:18–26, 1999.

259. D'Haese P, Spasovski G, Sikole A, et al. A multicenter study on the effects of lanthanum carbonate (Fosrenol™) and calcium carbonate on renal bone disease in dialysis patients. Kidney Int 63 (Suppl 85):S73–S78, 2003.

260. Joy M, Finn W. Randomized, double-blind, placebo-controlled, dose-titration, phase III study assessing the efficacy and tolerability of lanthanum carbonate: a new phosphate binder for the treatment of hyperphosphatemia. Am J Kidney Dis 42:96–107, 2002.

261. Finn WF, Joy MS, Hladik G, et al. Efficacy and safety of lanthanum carbonate for reduction of serum phosphorous in patients with chronic renal failure receiving hemodialysis. Clin Nephrol 62: 193–201, 2004.

262. Braun J, Asmus H, Holzer H, et al. Long-term comparison of a calcium-free phosphate binder and calcium carbonate—phosphorous metabolism and cardiovascular calcification. Clin Nephrol 62: 104–115, 2004.

263. Block G, Hulbert-Shearon T, Levin N, et al. Association of serum phosphorous and calcium X phosphorous product with mortality risk in end-stage renal disease. Am J Kidney Dis 31:607–617, 1998.

264. Sensipar (cinacalcet) package insert. Thousand Oaks, Calif: Amgen Inc, 2004.

265. Block GA, Martin KJ, de Francisco AL, et al. Cinacalcet for secondary hyperparathyroidism in patients receiving hemodialysis [see comment]. N Engl J Med 350:1516–1525, 2004.

266. Heunisch C, Resnick DJ, Vitello JM, et al. Conjugated estrogens for the management of gastrointestinal bleeding secondary to uremia of acute renal failure. Pharmacotherapy 18:210–217, 1998.

267. Mettang T, Pauli-Magnus C, Alscher DM. Uraemic pruritus—new perspectives and insights from recent trials. Nephrol Dial Transplant 17:1558–1563, 2002.

268. Cockcroft DW, Gault MH. Prediction of creatinine clearance from serum creatinine. Nephron 16:31–41, 1976.

269. Levey AS, Bosch JP, Lewis JB, et al. A more accurate method to estimate glomerular filtration rate from serum creatinine: a new prediction equation. Modification of Diet in Renal Disease Study Group [see comment]. Ann Intern Med 130:461–470, 1999.

270. Provenzano R, Garcia-Mayol L, Suchinda P, et al. Once-weekly epoetin alfa for treating the anemia chronic kidney disease. Clin Nephrol 61:392–405, 2004.

271. Locatelli F, Olivares J, Walker R, et al, European/Australian Nesp Study Group. Novel erythropoiesis stimulating protein for treatment of anemia in chronic renal insufficiency. Kidney Int 60: 741–747, 2001.

272. Suranyi MG, Lindberg JS, Navarro J, et al. Treatment of anemia with darbepoetin alfa administered de novo once every other week in chronic kidney disease. Am J Nephrol 23:106–111, 2003.

Dialysis Options and Pharmacotherapy for End-Stage Renal Disease

44

Joanna Q. Hudson and Harold J. Manley

TREATMENT GOALS

- Provide patient education about dialysis options and management of secondary complications prior to development of end-stage renal disease (ESRD).
- Increase the percentage of arteriovenous fistulas constructed as the permanent access site for patients to receive hemodialysis.
- Provide adequate dialysis as defined by the NKF-K/DOQI clinical practice guidelines for hemodialysis and peritoneal dialysis while minimizing complications.
- Regularly evaluate the patient's candidacy for kidney transplantation.
- Treat coexisting medical conditions such as diabetes mellitus, hypertension, and cardiovascular disease.
- Treat secondary complications of ESRD, including hypertension, anemia, metabolic acidosis, malnutrition, electrolyte abnormalities, hyperparathyroidism, and renal osteodystrophy.

- Improve the patient's quality of life through rehabilitation and maximizing his or her ability to function independently and engage in productive activities.
- Decrease hospitalization rates and overall morbidity and mortality.
- Optimize patient compliance with the complicated pharmacotherapeutic regimens.

DEFINITIONS

End-stage renal disease (ESRD) is the final stage of chronic kidney disease (CKD), known as stage 5 CKD, and is defined by a glomerular filtration rate (GFR) of less than 15 mL per minute per 1.73 m^2 and the need for renal replacement therapy, either dialysis or transplantation, to sustain life.[1] While the goal for patients with earlier stages of CKD is to delay progression of kidney disease to this final stage, many patients ultimately develop ESRD and must rely on chronic dialysis to maintain fluid and solute control. Renal replacement therapies for patients with ESRD include chronic hemodialysis, peritoneal dialysis, and kidney transplantation. During hemodialysis, anticoagulated blood is pumped through an extracorporeal system that includes a hemodialyzer as the semipermeable membrane for solute transport. A salt solution, known as the dialysate, is pumped on the opposite side of this semipermeable membrane to promote diffusion of solutes able to traverse the membrane. With peritoneal dialysis, this semipermeable membrane is the patient's own peritoneal cavity. These dialysis modalities are described in detail in this chapter. A brief discussion of renal replacement therapies available for the population with acute kidney disease is also included. Kidney transplantation is discussed in Chapter 27.

Throughout this chapter, guidelines developed by the National Kidney Foundation (NKF) known collectively as the NKF Kidney Disease Outcome Quality Initiative (NKF-K/DOQI) guidelines, will be referenced, with particular emphasis on aspects of the guidelines specific to hemodialysis and peritoneal dialysis.[2,3]

ETIOLOGY

ESRD can be caused by an acute irreversible insult to the kidney, a primary kidney disease, or a systemic illness. Diabetes mellitus continues to be the leading cause of ESRD in the United States, with an incidence rate that has almost doubled between the years 1990 and 2001.[4,5] During this same period, the incidence of ESRD caused by hypertension, the second leading cause of ESRD in the United States, increased by almost 50%. Glomerulonephritis, cystic kidney disease, and HIV-related nephropathy are among the other etiologies. Although the number of new cases of ESRD attributed to these other etiologies (i.e., incidence) is less than from diabetes and hypertension, the total number of ESRD patients with these conditions as the primary cause of their kidney disease (i.e., prevalence) has increased in the past

TABLE 44.1 Causes of End-Stage Renal Disease[a]

Cause of ESRD	Incidence %
Diabetes[b]	44
Hypertension[b]	27
Glomerulonephritis	8
Cystic kidney disease	2
Other urologic	2
Other cause	12
Unknown	4

[a] Based on data from 100,359 incident patients.
[b] Primary causes in the United States.
(Data from USRDS: the United States Renal Data System. Am J Kidney Dis 42 (Suppl 5):1–230, 2003.)

decade. This is due, in part, to the decrease in mortality among ESRD patients. Other causes of ESRD are listed in Table 44.1.[5] Etiologies of CKD and ultimately ESRD are also presented in Chapter 43.

Once patients have progressed to ESRD, concomitant disease states and conditions (e.g., diabetes, hypertension, cardiovascular disease) must be considered when choosing the dialysis modality and the aggressiveness of dialysis therapy. For example, the recommended "dialysis dose" (Kt/V) may be higher for patients with diabetes. Conversely, the effect of dialysis therapy on these disease states must also be taken into account, such as the effect of the dialysis procedure on blood pressure when evaluating the efficacy of antihypertensive medications.

EPIDEMIOLOGY

Based on data from the most recent United States Renal Data System (USRDS), a national database of all Medicare-treated patients with ESRD, a total of 96,295 new patients initiated ESRD treatment in 2001, and as of the end of the year, a total of 406,081 patients were being treated for ESRD: 292,215 undergoing dialysis treatment and 113,866 with kidney transplants.[5] African-Americans have a four-fold higher incidence rate compared to whites, a trend also observed in Native Americans (three-fold higher) and Hispanics (two-fold). The greatest increase in ESRD by age is in the population 65 and older.[5]

It is projected that by 2030, there could be an increase of 460,000 new ESRD cases per year with prevalence estimates of approximately 2.24 million, the majority of cases being attributed to diabetes.[5] With the increasing incidence of ESRD and health care expenditures necessary to manage the ESRD population, improving the outcomes and quality of care of patients with ESRD is a national priority. Initiatives such as "Healthy People 2010" have identified CKD as one of the areas of emphasis in an effort to decrease the number of patients reaching ESRD.[6]

Despite the overall improvement in survival rates of ESRD patients, morbidity and mortality in the U.S. ESRD population remain high, with an annual mortality rate of 20% to 25%.[5] Cardiovascular disease and sepsis are the leading causes of death in this patient population.[5] Overall life expectancy of ESRD patients is only one-third to one-sixth that of the general U.S. population. African-American ESRD patients have a higher survival rate compared to other demographic groups. While still less than the general population, kidney transplant recipients have expected lifetimes that are two to three times higher than for patients on dialysis.

There is considerable variability internationally and throughout the United States in terms of outcomes of dialysis patients and dialysis practices. To better characterize and understand such differences, collaborative efforts such as the Dialysis Outcomes and Practice Patterns Study (DOPPS) have been initiated. DOPPS is an ongoing observational study of hemodialysis patients in 12 countries, seeking to identify dialysis practices that contribute to improved mortality rates, hospitalization rates, health-related quality of life, and vascular access outcomes.[7] The hypothesis is that differences in practice patterns among various regions and nations may have direct correlations with the differences in patient outcomes. Thus far, data have been collected on more than 80,000 hemodialysis patients, and results from several analyses using these data have been published.[7-11] Findings from such an evaluation may provide better insight into specific areas for national and regional changes in the current treatment approaches for ESRD.

PATHOPHYSIOLOGY

The precise mechanism of kidney damage ultimately leading to ESRD depends on the etiology (Chapter 43). The time course of progression from the earlier stages of CKD to irreversible kidney failure or ESRD is generally months to years, depending on the underlying cause and effectiveness of interventions to delay such progression. Once kidney function has decreased to approximately less than 25% of normal (i.e., stage 4 CKD), progression to ESRD is inevitable, although the goal is to prolong the period until patients require renal replacement therapy.[12] Uremia is the clinical syndrome that develops in patients with severe kidney disease, and management of the associated symptoms often requires dialysis therapy.

The kidneys are involved not only in fluid and electrolyte homeostasis but also in the production and metabolism of many peptide hormones, including insulin, erythropoietin,

parathyroid hormone (PTH), and 1,25-dihydroxyvitamin D_3 (calcitriol). As such, ESRD leads to some predictable secondary complications that occur in the majority of patients, regardless of the etiology of kidney disease. These complications include hypertension, electrolyte abnormalities, metabolic acidosis, anemia, secondary hyperparathyroidism, renal osteodystrophy, malnutrition, and cardiovascular complications. In addition to providing adequate dialysis, appropriate management includes aggressive treatment of these secondary complications, often requiring implementation of complex pharmacotherapy regimens. USRDS data have shown that patients requiring hemodialysis use a median of 8 different medications and that more than 34% of patients are prescribed 10 or more medications.[13] It is clear that there is a role for pharmacists in the care of this growing population.

CLINICAL PRESENTATION

SIGNS AND SYMPTOMS

A reduction in GFR to the extent associated with ESRD (GFR <15 mL/min/1.73 m²) leads to azotemia and uremia (accumulation of nitrogenous waste products and of uremic toxins). Symptoms of ESRD include those associated with uremia as well as manifestations of the secondary complications that develop. Uremic symptoms include nausea, vomiting, anorexia, bleeding, neuropathy, malaise, pruritus, mental lassitude, and inability to concentrate. The constellation of signs and symptoms associated with uremia has been attributed in part to the accumulation of compounds that are collectively labeled as uremic toxins. Uremic solutes can be classified as small (300 to 500 Daltons) and water-soluble compounds, larger "middle" molecules (1,500 to 5,000 Daltons), or protein-bound solutes. Most potential uremic toxins are products of protein metabolism. Among the list of potential uremic toxins are urea, polyamines, guanidines, parathyroid hormone, myoinositol, and β_2-microglobulins. A cause-and-effect relationship between these specific compounds and the clinical manifestations of uremia has not been clearly established. Nonetheless, throughout the history of renal replacement therapy, the dialysis prescription has been based on the removal of these "uremic toxins."

Essentially every organ system is affected by kidney failure due to alterations in the excretory functions of the kidney as well as metabolic functions. Fluid accumulation contributes to development or worsening of hypertension and complications such as pericarditis. Electrolyte abnormalities, including hyperkalemia and metabolic acidosis, are more common with severe kidney disease. Cardiac manifestations including left ventricular hypertrophy (LVH) and atherosclerosis are of concern, given the high mortality associated with cardiovascular disease in ESRD patients. Anemia occurs in most patients with ESRD due to erythropoietin deficiency and leads to symptoms of fatigue and dyspnea; it is also associated with decreased quality of life and development of LVH.[14,15] Altered calcium and phosphorus homeostasis and decreased production of active vitamin D (1,25-dihydroxyvitamin D_3, known as calcitriol) contribute to development of secondary hyperparathyroidism, renal osteodystrophy, and metastatic calcifications. Gastrointestinal symptoms are common in advanced kidney disease and include nausea, vomiting, anorexia, diarrhea, and gastric and colonic ulcerations. Restless leg syndrome and other patterns of sensory and motor dysfunction are among the neuromuscular disturbances of ESRD. Other manifestations include blunted immune response, glucose intolerance secondary to peripheral resistance to insulin, pruritus, and sexual dysfunction. A complete review of systems in patients with kidney disease is necessary to identify all clinical manifestations of the disease, including the common secondary complications.

DIAGNOSIS AND CLINICAL FINDINGS

ESRD is diagnosed when the GFR is less than 15 mL per minute per 1.73 m^2 and therapeutic interventions to control fluid and electrolyte abnormalities and other manifestations of uremic syndrome become ineffective when used alone. It is at this point that renal replacement therapy with dialysis or transplantation becomes necessary. Some patients remain relatively asymptomatic, and the extent of their disease can be realized only by evaluation of objective data.

Quantification of kidney function provides an objective assessment; however, the limitations of the methods used to estimate kidney function must be considered. While the serum creatinine level is commonly used as a marker of underlying kidney dysfunction, use of serum creatinine alone to quantify the extent of kidney function is not recommended. The serum creatinine is affected by factors such as muscle mass, ingestion of creatine from dietary sources, and diurnal variation. Assessment of kidney function using equations to estimate GFR [i.e., Cockcroft-Gault and Modification of Diet in Renal Disease (MDRD) equations], which take into account the serum creatinine level and variables including age, gender, race, and body size, is recommended.[1,16] These prediction equations are preferred over more labor-intensive methods to measure creatinine clearance (i.e., urine collection methods) due to the problems with appropriate collection of urine and failure of this method to provide a more accurate assessment when compared to prediction equations. These collection methods, however, are recommended in select populations such as those with unique dietary intake (vegetarians, creatine supplementation) or decreased muscle mass (e.g., malnourished patients) and are often used to determine the point at which to initiate dialysis based on GFR (see section "Indications for Dialysis" later in the chapter).[1]

Urinalysis is a useful test to identify markers of kidney damage and should be done early in the course of CKD so that appropriate strategies for delaying progression can be implemented (Chapter 43). By the time patients progress to ESRD, identification of these markers may help to determine the etiology of the disease, but delaying progression is no longer a primary goal of therapy. Proteinuria, specifically albuminuria and an elevated protein to creatinine ratio, is a sensitive marker of kidney disease from the early to advanced stages. Other markers include the presence of red blood cells, white blood cells, or casts in the urine sediment. Abnormalities identified with imaging studies are suggestive of urologic or intrinsic kidney disease (e.g., structural abnormalities). Imaging studies are generally done in patients at risk of developing CKD due to urinary tract stones, infections, obstruction, or polycystic kidney disease. Kidney size is also indicative of the stage and type of CKD: large kidneys are commonly observed in patients with polycystic kidney disease and small kidneys are associated with the progressive decline in kidney function due to other causes.

Laboratory abnormalities observed in patients with ESRD are generally consistent with decreased elimination [e.g., increased serum creatinine, blood urea nitrogen (BUN)] and development of secondary complications (Table 44.2). Hyperkalemia is the most worrisome electrolyte abnormality and is a clear indication for dialysis when other medical interventions to control potassium are ineffective. Secondary complications become more severe at stage 5 CKD (or ESRD), as observed with worsening laboratory values (Table 44.2) indicative of complications such as anemia, secondary hyperparathyroidism, and metabolic acidosis. Ideally, interventions to manage these secondary complications are implemented before patients develop ESRD; unfortunately, early initiation of therapy is not common. Referral to a nephrologist is clearly recommended at stage 4 CKD (GFR <30 mL/min/1.73 m^2) but is often advisable earlier, during stage 3 (GFR <60 mL/min/1.73 m^2), to implement measures to delay progression, address secondary complications, and prolong the time before dialysis is necessary.

Regardless of the etiology of kidney disease, once progression to ESRD has occurred, recovery of kidney function is no longer possible and renal replacement therapy with transplantation (Chapter 27) or dialysis is required. A complete evaluation is necessary to determine the point at which dialysis should be initiated based on the specific indications for dialysis (refer to the section, "Indications for Dialysis" later in this chapter).

PSYCHOSOCIAL ASPECTS

Initial responses to the diagnosis of ESRD may include shock, grief, and denial, among others. Such responses will likely be more dramatic in individuals who initially present with ESRD as opposed to those who were identified early and have had appropriate education and counseling throughout the course of their disease. It is also very difficult for patients to accept that dialysis is not curative, but rather a life-long maintenance therapy, unless kidney transplantation is a possibility.

Among the major stresses of dialysis are the procedure itself, the overall medical treatment, which includes medica-

TABLE 44.2	Secondary Complications and Associated Laboratory Abnormalities in Patients With End-Stage Renal Disease
Secondary Complication	**Associated Laboratory Abnormalities**
Electrolyte disturbances	↑ Potassium, SCr, BUN, phosphorus, calcium,[a] magnesium, ↑ or ↓ sodium
Metabolic acidosis	↓ Bicarbonate, pH
Anemia	↓ Hgb/Hct, iron indices (TSat, Ferritin, serum iron), erythropoietin concentration[b]
Secondary hyperparathyroidism & metabolic abnormalities	↑ PTH, phosphorus, calcium[a] ↓ Active vitamin D (calcitriol)
Cardiovascular	
LVH, heart failure	↑ BNP
Dyslipidemia	↑ Total cholesterol, LDL, triglycerides
Malnutrition	↓ Albumin, ↓ cholesterol, ↓ carnitine[b]
Other	↑ CRP, myoglobin, cardiac troponin T, insulin

SCr, serum creatinine; BUN, blood urea nitrogen; Hgb, hemoglobin; Hct, hematocrit; TSat, transferrin saturation; PTH, parathyroid hormone; LVH, left ventricular hypertrophy; BNP, brain natriuretic peptide; LDL, low-density lipoprotein; CRP, C-reactive protein

[a] May be decreased, particularly in earlier stages of chronic kidney disease.
[b] Not routinely measured in patients with chronic kidney disease.

tions and diet, time constraints associated with time on hemodialysis or performing peritoneal dialysis exchanges, loss of employment, hospitalizations, changes in sexual function, and fear of death. As a result of these physical and psychological stresses, the psychosocial disorders seen include delirium, depression, anxiety, social withdrawal, suicide, uncooperative behavior, sexual dysfunction, and psychosis.[17,18] Nonadherence to treatment is also common. Alcohol use may be more frequent than reported at initiation of dialysis, particularly in men, and such use may be influenced by other comorbid conditions that are now more prevalent in the ESRD population (e.g., HIV infection).[19]

Depression and anxiety are common in patients with ESRD, but they are often not diagnosed or are considered less important than other pending medical problems associated with kidney failure.[17,20] Patient education and counseling by professionals knowledgeable about kidney disease and the associated psychological disorders early in the course of kidney disease may prevent depression and other psychosocial disorders from developing as patients progress to ESRD and require dialysis. Often the nephrologist becomes the primary care provider for the patient receiving chronic dialysis; however, referral of these patients to specialists for evaluation and appropriate treatment of psychosocial disorders is warranted.

The patient's quality of life is also an important consideration and should be assessed periodically. Health-related quality of life (HRQOL) refers to the measure of a patient's functioning, well-being, and general health perception in each of three domains: physical, psychological, and social.[21] Two quality-of-life instruments used for assessment are the Medical Outcomes Study 36-Item Short-Form Health Survey (SF-36) and the Kidney Disease QOL questionnaire.[22,23]

Interestingly, differences in quality of life have been reported based on ethnicity.[24,25] For example, results from DOPPS for 6,151 hemodialysis patients showed higher HRQOL scores in African-Americans.[25] Measures such as physical rehabilitation (e.g., exercise programs) may improve HRQOL and the negative outcomes associated with poor quality of life (e.g., hospitalization, morbidity, poor quality of self-care).[25–27]

THERAPEUTIC PLAN

The goals of ESRD care are to provide adequate renal replacement therapy for fluid and solute control, to manage secondary complications, and to decrease morbidity and mortality. To achieve these goals, a therapeutic plan that includes early planning for dialysis is essential. Once patients progress to stage 4 CKD (GFR <30 mL/min/1.73 m^2), referral to a nephrologist is recommended to begin preparation for renal replacement therapy. Ideally, prior to this point, secondary complications such as fluid and electrolyte abnormalities, anemia, secondary hyperparathyroidism and the associated metabolic disturbances, metabolic acidosis, and other complications of kidney disease have been evaluated and appropriate interventions implemented by either the patient's primary care provider or a nephrologist. Unfortunately, in many cases early intervention has not occurred prior to progression to stage 5 CKD (or ESRD), and preparation for dialysis becomes more urgent rather than anticipatory.[28]

Preparation for dialysis includes patient and family education regarding dialysis modalities (i.e., peritoneal dialysis and hemodialysis) to allow the patient to make an informed decision about the appropriate modality. This includes providing information about the risks and benefits as well as advantages and disadvantages of hemodialysis and peritoneal dialysis. Transplantation should also be discussed (Chapter 27). Some patients may be a candidate for only one particular dialysis modality (see section, ''Choice of Dialytic Modality'' later in this chapter). Often the social worker, as part of the multidisciplinary team, provides patient education about dialysis options and logistics of coordinating initiation of dialysis (e.g., transportation, financial and social resources); however, all team members should play an active role in this process.

Adequate preparation for dialysis requires an evaluation for vascular access placement, depending on the type of dialysis selected. An arteriovenous (AV) fistula is preferred as opposed to an AV graft in patients scheduled to begin hemodialysis due to the longer lifespan of AV fistulas and decreased likelihood of infection.[29] Early planning is essential, since an AV fistula requires several months to mature. Measures should be taken to preserve the potential site for hemodialysis access (e.g., nondominant arm) prior to access placement in patients to begin this dialysis modality by avoiding venipuncture and blood pressure measurements using that extremity. Unfortunately, many patients are not diagnosed or are not referred to a nephrologist early enough to implement these strategies. In these situations dialysis may be needed immediately or in a very short time period, requiring placement of a temporary access site as opposed to the preferred method of placing an AV fistula or graft. This increases the risk of access complications (see section, ''Vascular Access Complications'' later in this chapter). Placement of an AV fistula is more likely in patients referred early to a nephrologist.[28] The catheter used for peritoneal dialysis may be placed within a relatively short window of time prior to the start of dialysis; however, early planning is still warranted. Once the patient has been educated about the selected dialysis modality and a viable access site has been placed, the time point at which dialysis is initiated will depend on kidney function and the extent of uremic symptoms (see section, ''Indications for Dialysis'' later in this chapter).

With the growing number of patients with CKD at risk for developing ESRD and the extent of problems that develop in this population, a multidisciplinary approach to patient care is essential. The federal government mandates that this multidisciplinary group include nephrologists, nurses, dietitians, and social workers, but certainly there is a need for intervention by other health care professionals, including pharmacists, case managers, and other allied health practitioners. The potential for drug-related problems is high in this patient population because of the large number of medications (range of 8 to 12 medications per day) often prescribed to manage the primary disease and the associated secondary complications.[13,30,31] The therapeutic plan for patients with ESRD should include a complete evaluation of medications, both prescription and nonprescription. Pharmacists can play

a role by educating patients with severe kidney dysfunction about medications to avoid (e.g., nonsteroidal anti-inflammatory agents, metformin) and by providing information about the medications commonly prescribed to manage secondary complications (e.g., phosphate binders, antihypertensive agents). This education needs to be continually reinforced once the patient begins dialysis.

TREATMENT

Renal replacement therapy, predominantly dialysis, is the primary treatment option for ESRD to manage fluid and electrolyte abnormalities and control uremic symptoms. While dialysis cannot mimic all aspects of kidney function, such as endocrine function, it can maintain reasonable fluid and electrolyte homeostasis if the dialysis prescription is appropriately adjusted. Other therapies are used in conjunction with dialysis to manage secondary complications of ESRD that occur as a result of the altered metabolic and endocrine functions of the kidney. Such therapies include dietary and pharmacologic interventions for anemia, secondary hyperparathyroidism, altered calcium and phosphorus homeostasis, cardiovascular disorders, and clinical manifestations that occur in the presence of uremia, such as bleeding and gastrointestinal disorders.

PHARMACOTHERAPY

Specific drug therapy for patients with ESRD includes agents used to treat secondary complications. These therapies have been previously discussed (see Chapter 43), but treatment considerations specific to the ESRD population are addressed later in this chapter (see section, ''Pharmacotherapeutic Considerations for Patients on Dialysis'').

NONPHARMACOLOGIC THERAPY

In conjunction with hemodialysis and peritoneal dialysis, dietary intervention is a necessary nonpharmacologic therapy to manage the complications of ESRD. For this reason, a dietitian is an integral part of the health care team, as mandated by the federal government. Specific dietary recommendations are tailored to help control diabetes, hypertension, hyperlipidemia, calcium and phosphorus homeostasis, and malnutrition and to minimize the accumulation of fluid and certain electrolytes (e.g., potassium) in the dialysis population. Frequent reassessment by a dietitian knowledgeable about ESRD and continued patient education are necessary to ensure that patients comply with recommended dietary interventions.

Exercise programs for ESRD patients have also been advocated as a routine nonpharmacologic strategy based, in part, on evidence of the association of a sedentary lifestyle with risk of mortality in this population.[32] Improvements in physical fitness and well-being have been observed with formally structured exercise programs, including use of stationary bikes during dialysis and outpatient exercise training.[27] Other exercises include those specific for patients with newly placed vascular access sites for hemodialysis, such as squeezing a ball three or four times a day, which increases blood flow through the site and promotes its maturation to allow for use during dialysis.

DIALYSIS

PRINCIPLES

Hemodialysis and peritoneal dialysis are renal replacement therapies that have become the mainstay of chronic management for patients with ESRD. Since the development of dialysis therapy in the 1960s and its more widespread use in the United States in the early 1970s, dialysis has evolved substantially as an essential treatment for patients with both acute and chronic kidney disease. Dialysis is a process designed to mimic the kidney's functions of fluid and solute removal. Technological advances in these modalities have resulted in increased clearance of uremic toxins and other endogenous substances.

The three basic components of a dialysis system are a blood compartment, a dialysate compartment, and a semipermeable membrane (or dialyzer) that separates the blood and dialysate compartments. The transport mechanisms responsible for fluid and solute transfer across the membrane are diffusion and convection. Diffusion involves the passive movement of a solute down its concentration gradient (i.e., from the area of higher to lower concentration). Therefore, a substance will move from the blood to the dialysate or from the dialysate to the blood, depending on the concentration of the particular substance in each compartment. Variations in process-specific factors such as blood and dialysate flow rates, membrane characteristics, and duration of dialysis sub-

stantially alter solute and drug clearances during dialysis. Drug characteristics affecting clearance include molecular size, steric hindrance, protein binding, and volume of distribution.[33]

During hemodialysis, anticoagulated blood and a physiologic salt solution (i.e., dialysate) are perfused on opposite sides of a semipermeable membrane.[34] With peritoneal dialysis, the semipermeable membrane is the patient's own peritoneal cavity. Anticoagulation is not required since peritoneal dialysis is not an extracorporeal process; however, heparin may be added to the dialysate to prevent fibrin formation. With both hemodialysis and peritoneal dialysis, waste products of protein metabolism and other toxins move from the blood compartment into the dialysate by passive diffusion along concentration gradients. Conversely, if a substance is present in the dialysate in a higher concentration than in the blood (e.g., bicarbonate), this solute will diffuse from the dialysate into the systemic circulation. Substances too large to traverse the pores of the membrane (e.g., protein, protein-bound solutes) are not removed during this process.

Ultrafiltration is the process by which water and nonprotein plasma move down the hydrostatic pressure gradient from the blood into the dialysate. This is the primary mode for removal of excess body fluids. As plasma water moves across the membrane, solutes dissolved in this solvent are also transported, a process known as convection. Ultrafiltration (expressed in mL/hour/mm/Hg) during hemodialysis can be maximized by increasing the hydrostatic pressure gradient (mm Hg) across the dialysis membrane. The amount of fluid removed with each mm Hg increase in transmembrane pressure is specified by the ultrafiltration coefficient (Kuf) reported for each dialysis filter (Table 44.3): the higher the Kuf, the greater the ultrafiltration rate. If a patient needs

TABLE 44.3	**Characteristics of Selected Dialyzers**				
Manufacturer and Model	**Membrane**	**Surface Area (m²)**	**Ultrafiltration Coefficient [Kuf] (mL/hour/mm Hg)**	**Clearance (Qb = 200 mL/min)[a]**	
				Urea	**Vitamin B₁₂**
Baxter					
CT 110 G	CTA	1.1	22	185	109
CT 190G	CTA	1.9	36	192	137
Fresenius					
F 40	PS	0.7	20	165	75
F 60	PS	1.25	40	185	115
Toray					
BK-3–2.0A	PMMA	2.0	11	190	100
BK-2.1U	PMMA	2.1	19	194	125

CTA, cellulose triacetate; PS, polysulfone; PMMA, polymethylmethacrylate.
[a]At a blood flow (Qb) of 200 mL/min.

a larger amount of fluid removal during each dialysis session, one option is to select a dialyzer with a larger ultrafiltration coefficient.

With hemodialysis, the membrane that separates the blood from the dialysate compartment can be selected to attain the optimal diffusion and ultrafiltration goals. In contrast, with peritoneal dialysis, the dynamics of fluid and solute transport depend on the patient's own peritoneal membrane, a condition that cannot be altered. Ultrafiltration during peritoneal dialysis can be enhanced by changing the dextrose concentration in the dialysate. An increase in dextrose concentration increases the osmolality of the peritoneal compartment, resulting in an increase in fluid removal. Solute transported during peritoneal dialysis is affected by the thickness of the peritoneal membrane, the effective surface area of the membrane that is exposed to the dialysate, the peritoneal capillary blood flow, the dialysate flow rate, the volume of instilled dialysate, and the temperature of the dialysate.[35] The specifics of hemodialysis and peritoneal dialysis are explained in more detail later in this chapter.

Extracorporeal procedures have also been designed for patients with acute kidney failure who are hemodynamically unstable and not able to withstand the large fluctuations in fluid that occur with intermittent hemodialysis procedures. These procedures are known as continuous renal replacement therapies (CRRT) and are less aggressive modalities performed over a prolonged time period (e.g., 12 to 24 hours) when compared to intermittent dialysis procedures, which are generally performed over a 3- to 5-hour period. Blood flow and dialysate flow rates (when applicable) are lower with CRRT than with intermittent hemodialysis procedures. The lower blood and dialysate flow rates and the prolonged duration allow for more gradual removal of fluid and solutes. The terminology used to characterize the available types of CRRT indicates the vascular access site and driving force for the extracorporeal circuit (arterial or venous) and the specific procedure of CRRT: hemofiltration, hemodialysis, or hemodiafiltration (Table 44.4). CRRT procedures vary in the degrees of diffusion and ultrafiltration that occur during the process. The slow continuous ultrafiltration (SCUF) and

hemofiltration procedures do not incorporate a dialysate component on the opposite side of the membrane, but rather rely solely on ultrafiltration for fluid removal. The SCUF procedure is used for fluid control in the management of refractory edema in patients with or without acute kidney failure. Hemofiltration procedures use higher ultrafiltration rates to also achieve solute removal when compared to SCUF and generally require administration of replacement fluids. The hemodialysis and hemodiafiltration procedures incorporate a dialysate component; therefore, diffusion and ultrafiltration are the transport mechanism for these procedures, with the extent of ultrafiltration generally higher with hemodiafiltration. These procedures are most often performed in the intensive care unit setting.

INDICATIONS FOR DIALYSIS

The absolute and relative indications for dialysis are listed in Table 44.5. The timing of initiation of dialysis depends on the severity of uremic symptoms and laboratory abnormalities and differs for patients with acute versus chronic kidney disease. Dialysis (or CRRT) is required for patients with acute kidney failure in whom recovery of kidney function will be delayed or perhaps is not a realistic outcome. For the latter group, preparation for chronic dialysis is necessary. Indications for emergent dialysis in the acute kidney disease population include fluid overload, hyperkalemia, metabolic acidosis, pericarditis, and severe uremic symptoms that cannot be managed with other recommended therapies (e.g., diuretics, bicarbonate administration). Dialysis (or CRRT) is often initiated in the acute setting when the BUN exceeds 70 to 100 mg per dL (25 to 35 mmol/L) or the GFR is less than 15 to 20 mL per minute per 1.73 m². Factors that

TABLE 44.4	Continuous Renal Replacement Therapies (CRRT)
Procedure Abbreviation	**Procedure Name**
SCUF	Slow continuous ultrafiltration
CAVH	Continuous arteriovenous hemofiltration
CVVH	Continuous venovenous hemofiltration
CAVHD	Continuous arteriovenous hemodialysis
CVVHD	Continuous venovenous hemodialysis
CAVHDF	Continuous arteriovenous hemodiafiltration
CVVHDF	Continuous venovenous hemodiafiltration

TABLE 44.5	Indications for Dialysis[a]

- Severe uremic symptoms [persistent nausea and vomiting, anorexia, altered mental status, confusion, asterixis, myoclonus (indicative of encephalopathy and/or neuropathy), bleeding diathesis]
- Pericarditis
- Fluid overload or pulmonary edema refractory to diuretics
- Hypertension poorly responsive to antihypertensive medications
- Metabolic acidosis
- Hyperkalemia
- Blood urea nitrogen >100 mg/dL (35 mmol/L)
- Plasma creatinine >12 mg/dL (>1,060 μmol/L)
- Weekly Kt/V[b] <2.0[3]
- Persistent protein–energy malnutrition attributed to low nutrient intake

[a] Earlier initiation of dialysis may be advocated in patients with diabetes.
[b] For patients with chronic kidney disease [see the section on Adequacy of Dialysis for explanation of Kt/V]. A weekly Kt/V of 2.0 approximates a creatinine clearance of 9 to 14 mL/min/1.73 m².

influence the urea concentration (e.g., nutritional status, gastrointestinal bleeding, corticosteroids) and the assessment of kidney function (e.g., serum creatinine) must also be considered. For example, a patient with a low BUN may be severely undernourished, making assessment of the patient's uremic status by BUN levels alone unreliable. Use of the serum creatinine alone is also not a reliable indicator of kidney function. The overall clinical presentation of the patient must be evaluated in the context of objective findings when deciding whether to initiate dialysis. For example, a patient with a BUN of more than 70 mg per dL (>25 mmol/L) without uremic symptoms may not require dialysis. In contrast, a patient with a BUN less than 70 mg per dL (<25 mmol/L) may have uremic symptoms that warrant dialysis. These scenarios underscore the importance of considering objective and subjective findings when deciding whether to initiate dialysis.

The timing of initiation of dialysis in patients with CKD depends on the severity of symptoms and indications (Table 44.5), as discussed for patients with acute kidney disease; however, documentation of creatinine clearance below a specific level (<10 mL/min/1.73 m² in nondiabetics and less than 15 mL/min/1.73 m² in diabetics) is necessary for Medicare reimbursement, a factor that plays a significant role in dialysis initiation in the United States and is not without problems.[2,3,36] Guidelines suggest that dialysis should be started in nondiabetic patients with one or more uremic symptoms when their creatinine clearance is 9 mL/min/1.73 m², and perhaps even earlier (creatinine clearance 9 to 14 mL/min/1.73 m²) in patients with diabetes.[3] The average of the creatinine clearance and urea clearance is often used to assess filtration or GFR. This is based on the fact that creatinine is not only filtered but also secreted, potentially leading to an overestimation of GFR in patients with severe kidney disease. Since urea is filtered and reabsorbed, the average of creatinine and urea clearance provides a more accurate estimate of GFR. The NKF-K/DOQI guidelines recommend that chronic dialysis be initiated when the weekly renal Kt/V falls below 2.0 (see section, "Adequacy of Dialysis" later in this chapter).[3,37] A weekly Kt/V of 2.0 approximates a urea clearance of 7 mL per minute and a creatinine clearance that varies between 9 and 14 mL/min/1.73 m². This equates to a GFR of 10.5 mL/min/1.73 m² when calculated by the mean of the urea and creatinine clearances.

Evaluation of nutritional status is also important in the decision of when to start dialysis. The NKF-K/DOQI guidelines suggest that initiation of chronic dialysis or transplantation be considered if a patient has persistent protein–energy malnutrition despite attempts to optimize protein and energy intake, and low nutrient intake is the only identifiable cause of the malnutrition.[2,3] Therefore, evaluation of nutritional markers, including albumin, prealbumin, body mass index, and protein intake, should be performed in patients at risk for malnutrition. Other conditions that may support the initiation of dialysis when present in conjunction with more absolute indications include persistent pruritus, restless leg syndrome, and severe anemia unresponsive to erythropoietic

therapy. Patients with drug intoxication may also require emergent dialysis therapy if the characteristics of the specific agent make it likely to be removed by the dialysis procedure.

The goal of dialysis is to enhance quality of life and ideally to prolong survival. Late initiation of dialysis in patients with ESRD is associated with high rates of mortality and hospitalization; therefore, early referral to a nephrologist for timely initiation of dialysis is advocated.[38,39] Patients with stage 4 CKD (GFR <30 mL/min/1.73 m²) should be referred to a nephrologist for preparation for dialysis therapy. This includes patient education about renal replacement therapy (including dialysis modalities and transplantation) and early planning of dialysis access (e.g., AV fistula). The topic of timing of dialysis initiation continues to be of interest as more efforts are made to identify patients with CKD early and begin appropriate interventions. The IDEAL (Initiating Dialysis Early and Late) study will evaluate whether the timing of dialysis initiation has an effect on survival in ESRD patients and the effect of early (GFR 10 to 14 mL/min/1.73 m²) versus late (GFR 5 to 7 mL/min/1.73 m²) dialysis on nutritional and cardiac morbidity, quality of life, and economic cost.[40]

In some situations the decision of whether to start dialysis at all or whether to discontinue dialysis must be made. Patient conditions that force such ethical decisions include dementia, severe mental illness, malignancies, severe multiorgan disease, and advanced age.[41,42] The effect of dialysis initiation on the patient's quality of life, considered in the context of the expected outcomes from other comorbid conditions, certainly factors into the decision. Given the frequency of these situations, the ethical dilemmas involved in such decisions, and the annual mortality attributed to discontinuation of dialysis (approximately 20%), the Renal Physicians Association and the American Society of Nephrology (RPA/ASN) developed guidelines for appropriate initiation and withdrawal of dialysis in patients with acute and chronic kidney disease.[43] These guidelines are based on the principles of "shared-decision making" involving the nephrologist and patient and/or family. While guidelines cannot solve all such dilemmas facing the nephrologist, they at least outline specific questions and factors to consider when deciding whether to start dialysis or discontinue this treatment.

CHOICE OF DIALYTIC MODALITY

Acute Dialysis. The choice of dialysis modality in acute situations is often limited to intermittent hemodialysis or CRRT for patients who are hemodynamically unstable. While peritoneal dialysis is an option in this setting, it is not often used due to the logistics of placing a peritoneal catheter, contraindications to acute peritoneal dialysis (e.g., recent abdominal surgery), and the risk of peritonitis. The dialysis prescription in the acute setting depends on the patient's comorbid conditions and hemodynamic status and may be altered frequently as the patient's clinical status changes.

Chronic Dialysis. Before the patient is given a choice of hemodialysis or peritoneal dialysis, it must be decided whether that patient is indeed a candidate for either modality. Contraindications (absolute or relative) to peritoneal dialysis are more specifically defined than for hemodialysis. According to the NKF-K/DOQI Guidelines for Peritoneal Dialysis Adequacy, absolute contraindications to peritoneal dialysis include documented loss of peritoneal function or extensive abdominal adhesions that limit dialysate flow (e.g., fibrosis of the peritoneal membrane), physical or mental handicaps that logistically prevent manipulation of the equipment for peritoneal dialysis (in the absence of a support person who can do the procedures), and mechanical defects that prevent effective peritoneal dialysis or increase the risk of infection (e.g., surgically irreparable hernia, omphalocele, gastroschisis, diaphragmatic hernia, and bladder exstrophy).[3] Relative contraindications for peritoneal dialysis include recent abdominal surgery, peritoneal leaks, body size limitations, intolerance to the peritoneal dialysis volumes necessary to achieve an adequate peritoneal dialysis dose, inflammatory or ischemic bowel disease, abdominal wall or skin infection, morbid obesity (in short individuals), severe malnutrition, and frequent episodes of diverticulitis.[3] Patient-specific factors must be considered in the context of these guidelines when deciding whether peritoneal dialysis is a viable dialysis option. If peritoneal dialysis is contraindicated, then plans must be made to begin hemodialysis for chronic management of ESRD. Problems with acquiring and maintaining a viable vascular access site and access infections are primary reasons a patient may not be able to start or to continue chronic hemodialysis.

Patients in whom peritoneal dialysis may be preferable include those with particular disease states or conditions where the aggressive fluid and electrolyte shifts that occur with intermittent hemodialysis may be intolerable. With peritoneal dialysis, the rate of ultrafiltration is slower, which reduces the risk of hypotension and rapid fluctuations in fluids and electrolytes, a potential advantage for patients with heart failure, coronary artery disease, or variable blood pressure (i.e., uncontrolled hypertension, frequent hypotensive episodes). Patients with diabetes are not prohibited from selecting peritoneal dialysis as a modality despite the increased glucose load. Prudent monitoring of blood glucose, with appropriate adjustments in insulin administration (systemic and intraperitoneal), is necessary, which underscores the importance of patient education to improve compliance with more complex regimens. Peritoneal dialysis is the primary dialysis modality used in children requiring renal replacement therapy. Advantages and disadvantages of peritoneal dialysis compared to hemodialysis are listed in Table 44.6.

For patients without contraindications to either dialysis modality or without compelling disease states or conditions that make one modality more favorable, the decision of hemodialysis versus peritoneal dialysis is made by the patient. Ideally, patients with ESRD have been identified and re-

TABLE 44.6	Potential Advantages and Disadvantages of Peritoneal Dialysis Compared to Intermittent Hemodialysis
Advantages	**Disadvantages**
Steady-state biochemical parameters	Excessive glucose load (weight gain, hyperglycemia)
Hemodynamic stability (slow and sustained ultrafiltration)	Continued need for sterile environment for exchanges
Improved clearance of larger molecules (e.g., β_2-microglobulin)	Requires patient motivation for compliance
Preservation of residual kidney function	Higher protein and amino acid losses
Systemic heparin not required	Peritonitis risk
Anemia of chronic kidney disease not as severe (less blood loss)	Risk of catheter complications
No machine dependence (unless on cycler)	Mechanical problems (e.g., leaks)
Self-care allows for more flexibility in schedule (e.g., travel, work)	Increased intraabdominal pressure
Ability to administer antibiotics and insulin in the peritoneal cavity (intraperitoneal administration)	Dependent on characteristics of the patient's peritoneal cavity (e.g., high transporter, low transporter) and associated complications (e.g., loss of ultrafiltration from fibrosis)
Vascular access not required	Requires maintenance of peritoneal dialysis supplies (home storage, adequate supply when traveling)
Fewer dietary restrictions	Body image problems with peritoneal dialysis catheter

ferred to a nephrologist early (stage 4 CKD) to allow time to educate the patient and family members about each modality so they can make an informed decision. Health care providers with specialized training in nephrology (e.g., social workers, nurses) are the most appropriate personnel to provide this education.

Options for dialysis include peritoneal dialysis, in-center hemodialysis, and home hemodialysis. Home hemodialysis is done by the patient and a designated family member or other support person in the home environment. While less common than in-center hemodialysis, home hemodialysis allows more flexibility in the dialysis schedule and permits more frequent hemodialysis. It may be beneficial for the patient to visit a hemodialysis center and talk with other patients who are undergoing hemodialysis. Videotapes and reading materials are also available from the NKF to inform patients and family members about their disease and the various treatment options.[44] Personal, economic, and psychosocial factors influence the patient's choice of modality. Patients with a more active lifestyle may opt for peritoneal dialysis (or home hemodialysis) to provide more flexibility in their schedule. Patients who prefer home hemodialysis but have no assistant may also select peritoneal dialysis. Other patients may decide that they do not want the responsibility of performing their own dialysis and prefer to come to a dialysis clinic three times per week for hemodialysis. Patient compliance is certainly important with both hemodialysis and peritoneal dialysis; however, peritoneal dialysis is more labor-intensive on the part of the patient, and compliance with daily exchanges and aseptic technique is critical. As such, technique failure is much more common with peritoneal dialysis than hemodialysis. Noncompliance leads to inadequate dialysis and frequent episodes of peritonitis, which are common reasons patients may have to switch from peritoneal dialysis to hemodialysis. When deciding whether a patient can perform peritoneal dialysis, an assessment as to whether a patient's home environment is suitable for peritoneal dialysis is also necessary.

Despite the potential advantages of peritoneal dialysis, hemodialysis remains the predominant dialysis modality in the United States. With the growing number of patients expected to develop ESRD, there is a need to educate patients earlier about dialysis modalities and encourage selection of peritoneal dialysis if the patient is a candidate to prevent overburdening hemodialysis centers.[45]

One potential advantage of interest with peritoneal dialysis is preservation of the patient's residual kidney function. Maintenance of some degree of kidney function, even as low as a GFR of less than 10 to 15 mL per minute with ESRD, has significant clinical importance, including a substantial contribution to the removal of small solutes and middle molecules.[46] Patients on peritoneal dialysis tend to preserve their residual kidney function for a longer period than those on hemodialysis.[46–48] This may be because of better removal of toxins involved in residual nephron damage,

preservation or enhancement of growth factors that are beneficial to the maintenance of GFR and renal blood flow, less ischemic injury to the kidneys because of a more stable hemodynamic status, and lack of membrane-induced inflammatory changes (e.g., production of tumor necrosis factor and interleukin-1), which may cause vascular or immunologic renal injury.[46–48] In addition, the increased removal of sodium, potassium, phosphate, and hydrogen ions with peritoneal dialysis allows for less restrictive fluid and dietary intake.

There has been much debate over whether hemodialysis or peritoneal dialysis is associated with better survival; this debate continues, given the problems with making uniform comparisons between the two modalities.[49–52] This question has been particularly raised in the diabetic ESRD population, since this group is known to have a worse prognosis than nondiabetic patients on dialysis.[53] Diabetic patients often start dialysis with advanced comorbid conditions (e.g., coronary artery disease) that progress during dialysis therapy. Survival differences have been shown to vary based on other factors, including age, cause of ESRD (specifically, diabetic vs. nondiabetic etiologies), and other comorbidities.[52] When controlling for these factors, hemodialysis was associated with an increased risk of death in nondiabetic patients and younger diabetic patients (age 18 to 44 years) who did not have other comorbidities. In contrast, an increased risk of mortality with peritoneal dialysis was observed for diabetic patients more than 45 years of age.[52] Similar evaluations done in patients with HIV-associated nephropathy did not find any difference in mortality in patients managed with hemodialysis versus peritoneal dialysis, and supported the choice of dialysis modality in these patients.[49] In contrast, higher mortality was observed for patients with coronary artery disease and patients with heart failure who were started on peritoneal dialysis when compared to patients with these comorbid conditions started on hemodialysis.[50,54,55] Differences in patient populations and study design make it difficult to make definitive conclusions regarding the choice of dialysis modality based on survival data. Additional studies are needed to better characterize the factors associated with mortality in the dialysis population. Efforts are being made through the recommendation of the NKF-K/DOQI Guidelines on Peritoneal Dialysis Adequacy to collect information on outcomes that can be used to make more evidence-based conclusions related to survival.[3]

HEMODIALYSIS

HEMODIALYSIS SYSTEM

Hemodialysis is an extracorporeal process used to correct fluid and electrolyte abnormalities and remove uremic toxins. It does not correct endocrine abnormalities of kidney disease (e.g., erythropoietin and vitamin D production), but adequate dialysis can facilitate management of the secondary complications associated with such endocrine abnormalities. The

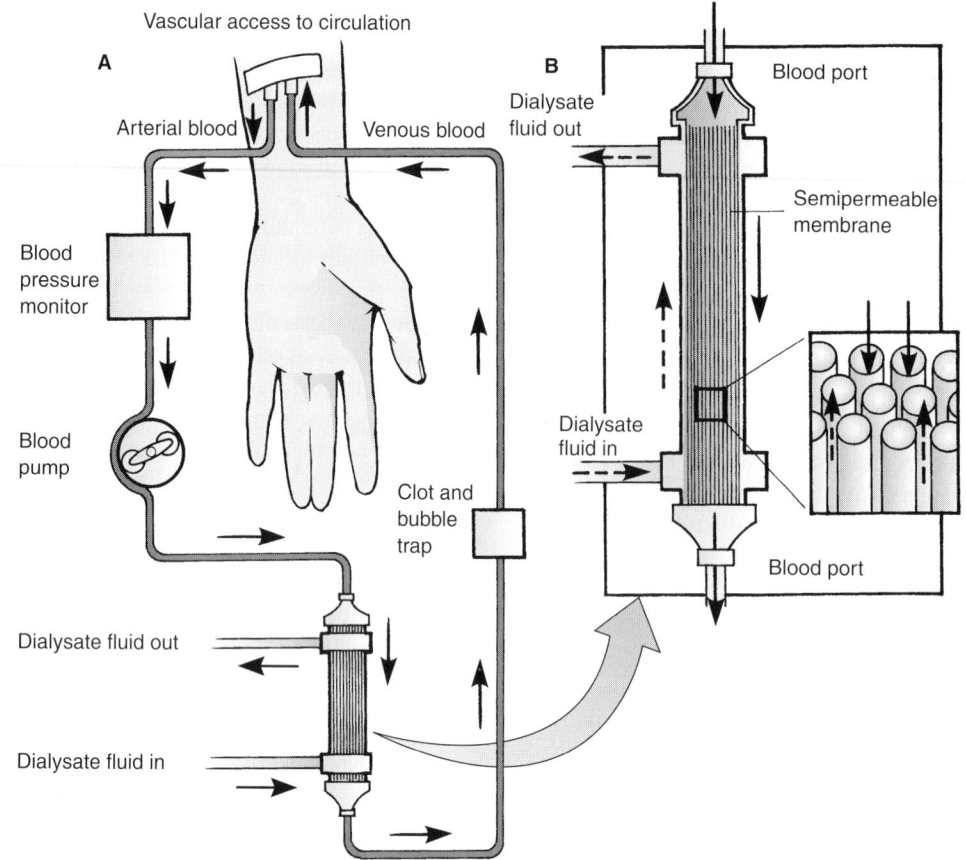

FIGURE 44.1. Hemodialysis schematic (see color insert). An external pump provides the driving force for blood flow from the patient's arterial access site **(A)** through the dialyzer **(B)**, where diffusion and ultrafiltration occur. Filtered blood is pumped back to the patient through the venous access. Dialysate flow moves in the opposite direction across the semipermeable membrane (dialyzer). (From Smeltzer SC, Bare BG. Textbook of medical-surgical nursing, 9th ed. Philadelphia: Lippincott Williams & Wilkins, 2000.)

general principles of diffusion and ultrafiltration used with both hemodialysis and peritoneal dialysis have previously been discussed (see earlier section, ''Dialysis Principles'').

To apply these principles with a hemodialysis system, two major components are involved: a blood circuit and a dialysate circuit (Fig. 44.1; *see color insert*). A dialysis machine is used to pump blood and warmed dialysate (approximately 37°C) on opposite sides of a semipermeable membrane or dialyzer. Diffusion occurs due to differences in solute concentration in the blood and dialysate. For example, a standard potassium concentration in the dialysate of 3 mEq per liter (3 mmol/L) is less than the blood concentration of most patients at the start of dialysis (e.g., >4 to 4.5 mEq/L; 4 to 4.5 mmol/L). The concentration gradient created promotes transport of potassium from the area of higher concentration (the blood) to the area of lower concentration (the dialysate). The concentration gradient is maintained throughout the dialysis procedure as fresh dialysate continuously circulates through the dialyzer. Diffusion is maximized by maintaining high blood and dialysate flow rates (blood flow 200 to 500 mL/min; dialysate flow 500 to 800

mL/min) and pumping the two solutions in opposite directions. The higher the concentration gradient for a given solute, the greater the diffusion; therefore, concentrations of certain substances in the dialysate can be altered based on the need for more or less removal (e.g., potassium, calcium).

The dialysate solution consists of purified water with electrolytes and other physiologic substances (Table 44.7).

TABLE 44.7	Composition of Hemodialysate Solution
Solute	**Concentration Range**
Sodium	135–145 mEq/L
Potassium	0–4 mEq/L
Chloride	100–124 mEq/L
Calcium	2.5–3.5 mEq/L
Magnesium	0.5–1.5 mEq/L
Bicarbonate	30–38 mEq/L
Dextrose	0–200 mg/dL

Bicarbonate or acetate is added to the dialysate in concentrations to promote diffusion from dialysate to blood, thus correcting metabolic acidosis. The dialysate is prepared from a commercially available concentrated liquid or dried salts and treated water. The most common method of water purification for the dialysate solution is reverse osmosis, where water is pressured across a membrane to remove impurities. Deionizers may also be incorporated to remove inorganic charged ions and nonionic contaminants.

Ultrafiltration (and thus convective clearance) can be added by generating a transmembrane pressure within the dialyzer, measured in mm Hg. The extent of ultrafiltration achieved at a given transmembrane pressure depends on the characteristics of the dialyzer, specifically the ultrafiltration coefficient or Kuf (Table 44.3). The Kuf is the volume of fluid (in mL) per hour that will be transferred across the dialyzer per mm Hg of transmembrane pressure (mL/hour/mm Hg). The greater the Kuf, the greater the ultrafiltration rate. For example, for every 1 mm Hg of transmembrane pressure, fluid removal for the Fresenius F60 will be 40 mL per hour (Table 44.3).

The hemodialysis system also includes a number of safety devices, pump controllers, pressure and flow monitors, air leak detectors, patient blood pressure monitors, systems to change the composition of the dialysate, and systems to monitor blood chemistry. The tubing segment that carries blood from the patient to the dialyzer is generally referred to as the "arterial side," while the segment that carries blood from the dialyzer to the patient is referred to as the "venous side." Medications can be administered via access ports on the tubing (generally on the "venous side"), providing a convenient means for giving intravenous medications during hemodialysis. Generally, anticoagulation is achieved by infusing heparin continuously or intermittently into tubing on the arterial side of the dialyzer. A 1-L bag of normal saline is also connected to the tubing of the dialysis system to allow for immediate infusion of replacement fluid by opening an access port. This measure is required when too much fluid has been removed during the dialysis procedure, as indicated by hypotensive episodes and/or excessive cramping.

VASCULAR ACCESS

A permanent access site is preferred for long-term hemodialysis therapy using one of two available types of access: an AV fistula or AV graft. The NKF-K/DOQI Guidelines on Vascular Access recommend placement of an AV fistula due to the excellent patency and lower risk of complications compared to the AV graft.[56] Despite such recommendations, graft use was found to be more prevalent that fistulas in dialysis centers evaluated in DOPPS and was associated with a higher relative risk of failure.[56]

Creation of a fistula involves anastomosis of a vein and an artery, whereas creation of an AV graft involves grafting a synthetic material [polytetrafluoroethylene (PTFE)] under the skin to make the connection between the artery and vein

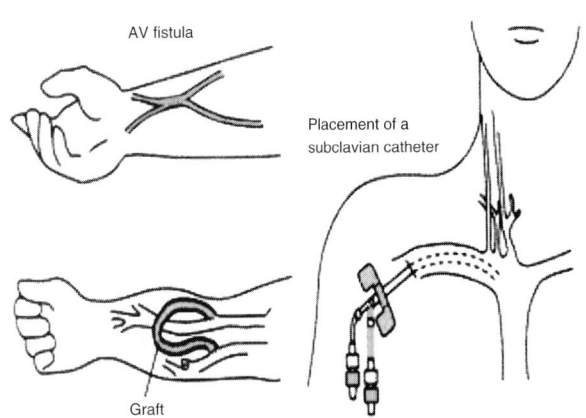

FIGURE 44.2. Vascular access for hemodialysis. Permanent access sites are preferred for chronic hemodialysis therapy. Creation of the site requires attachment of an artery and vein either surgically (AV fistula) or using a synthetic material, typically made of polytetrafluoroethylene, grafted under the skin (AV graft). The AV graft shown in this figure is a loop graft. A straight graft (not shown) is another type of AV graft. Temporary access sites, if needed, require catheter insertion into the internal jugular, subclavian (shown here), or femoral vein. (From http://www.ghsrenal.com/ghsfiles/2hemo dialysiswebsite_files/image006.gif)

and provide a site for blood access (Fig. 44.2). The preferred anatomic connections are the radial artery and cephalic vein or the brachial artery and cephalic vein. It is best to begin with more distal locations (radial artery and cephalic vein) so that the proximal site is preserved for future placement of a permanent access if the distal sites fail. The basic premise of creating a permanent access is that the venous segment will be exposed to the higher arterial pressures and over time will dilate and develop a thickened wall to withstand the needle sticks required for frequent hemodialysis. While AV fistulas are preferred, the problem lies in establishing a viable site in a patient population with a high prevalence of diabetes and vascular disease.

Adequate planning is necessary for permanent access placement to allow scheduling of the procedure and sufficient time for maturation of the site. An AV fistula requires a longer time to mature than an AV graft (2 months vs. 2 weeks), and is often one reason that AV grafts are inappropriately selected as the type of access despite evidence in support of the AV fistula. Unfortunately, patients are often not diagnosed with CKD early enough to plan or are lost to follow-up and present in the hospital with conditions that warrant immediate dialysis. In these situations a temporary access using a catheter, typically inserted into the internal jugular, subclavian, or femoral vein, is used. This type of access is also necessary for patients who no longer have viable sites for placement of a permanent access. Problems with temporary access for hemodialysis include infection (most common), venous stenosis, thrombosis, and short duration of use. If a temporary access must be used, a tunneled cuffed venous catheter is recommended. Vascular access complications are discussed in more detail in the section on Complications of Hemodialysis.

DIALYSIS PRESCRIPTION

Patients with ESRD receiving in-center intermittent hemodialysis are typically dialyzed three times per week for 3 to 5 hours. The dialysis prescription must be specified by the nephrologist and regularly reassessed to ensure the patient receives adequate dialysis. The components of the dialysis prescription are as follows: blood and dialysate flow rates (blood flow 200 to 500 mL/min; dialysate flow 500 to 800 mL/min), dialyzer, dialysate solution (e.g., variations in potassium or calcium concentrations), time of dialysis (generally 3 to 5 hours), the anticoagulation regimen if required, and the patient's dry weight. Adjustments in these components are made to achieve the target Kt/V (refer to the section "Adequacy of Hemodialysis" later in this chapter and avoid volume overload and volume depletion (i.e., keep the patient hemodynamically stable).

The patient's dry weight is defined as the weight at which the patient is hemodynamically stable and serves as the target weight to achieve by the end of each hemodialysis session. Through trial and error, a postdialysis target weight is determined for every patient on hemodialysis, such that 0 to 5 kg typically is removed during each dialysis session. Patients are weighed before each hemodialysis session to determine the amount of fluid removal required to achieve this target weight. For example, a patient weighing 83 kg prior to hemodialysis whose target dry weight is 80 kg will require 3 kg (6.6 lb) of fluid removal during the hemodialysis session. This equates to approximately 3 L of fluid (1 L is approximately 1 kg or 2.2 lb). The target volume to be removed (in this case 3 L) and the time of dialysis are programmed into the dialysis machine, which is designed to provide precise volumetric fluid removal. Using this information, a transmembrane pressure is then calculated based on the desired ultrafiltration rate. The patient's dry weight must be reevaluated regularly and altered as the patient gains or loses nonfluid weight to avoid removing excessive or inadequate fluid during hemodialysis.

The dialyzer contains four ports: two for inflow and outflow of blood and two for inflow and outflow of dialysate in countercurrent directions (Fig. 44.1). The semipermeable membrane consists in most cases of hollow fibers made of one of four materials: cellulose, substituted cellulose, cellulosynthetic (hemophane), or synthetics. Flat-plat dialyzers are also available but not as commonly used as the hollow fiber dialyzers. The cellulose-based dialyzers differ from the synthetics in that they generally have smaller pore size (thereby restricting removal of larger-molecular-weight substances and drugs) and are more likely to cause dialyzer reactions (see section, "Complications of Hemodialysis" later in this chapter). For these reasons, synthetic "biocompatible" dialyzers have become more commonly used and have replaced the cellulose-based membranes. Synthetic

membranes include polyacrylonitrile, polysulfone, polycarbonate, polyamide, and polymethylmethacrylate. Dialyzers are also characterized by their permeability to solutes and water, as indicated by the terminology "high efficiency" and "high flux." A high-efficiency dialyzer generally has a relatively large surface area and can remove low-molecular-weight substances very well (e.g., urea, with a molecular weight of about 60 daltons), but not necessarily high-molecular-weight solutes (e.g., β_2-microglobulin, with a molecular weight of 11,800 daltons). High-flux dialyzers have larger pores capable of removing higher-molecular-weight substances and Kuf values more than 10 mL/hour/mm/Hg. These high-flux membranes are being more commonly used in clinical practice. It is important to consider the effect of membrane selection not only on uremic toxins (a desired effect) but also on drug removal. Table 44.3 shows only a few of the available dialyzers. Generally, a given dialysis center or hospital purchases only two or three different dialyzers. Selection for a particular patient is based on the extent of fluid and solute removal desired. Each dialyzer comes with a specification sheet that includes the information listed in Table 44.3 and additional information on clearance of low- and high-molecular-weight solutes at typical blood and dialysate flow rates used in clinical practice. Urea clearance of a given dialyzer is important to consider, since the urea removal by dialysis is the measure of dialysis adequacy.

The duration of intermittent dialysis procedures generally is 3 to 5 hours. Time of dialysis is one of the most important determinants of solute clearance, yet there are logistical limitations to how long a patient can be dialyzed. For example, most dialysis centers have two or three shifts of patients scheduled to dialyze per day. With the availability of high-efficiency and high-flux dialyzers in conjunction with other technological advances, the duration of dialysis required to provide adequate dialysis has decreased (e.g., from a duration of up to 12 hours to 3 to 5 hours per session). Changes in time of dialysis within the realistic range of 3 to 5 hours are made as necessary to maintain the target Kt/V (see section, "Adequacy of Hemodialysis" later in this chapter).

Diffusion and ultrafiltration usually occur simultaneously during standard hemodialysis procedures; however, for select patients these two processes may be performed in sequence. This form of sequential hemodialysis therapy is particularly beneficial for patients who have extensive fluid gains between dialysis periods, as well as for patients with poor cardiac function who are unable to tolerate simultaneous, extensive ultrafiltration. The primary problem of long-term sequential dialysis treatment is that the reduced diffusion time may not allow adequate removal of uremic waste products.

Dialysis for acute kidney failure is used to prevent morbidity associated with complications of the disease and ideally is required only temporarily until kidney function improves. The dialysis prescription is considerably different than that for a patient with ESRD. Daily or as-needed dialysis may be required to manage fluid and electrolyte status as opposed to the intermittent three-times-per-week schedule for an ESRD patient. The CRRT modalities may be prescribed to provide a renal replacement therapy more suitable for a hemodynamically unstable patient. The dialysis prescription in the acute care setting is more individualized and subject to frequent changes, a much different scenario than in the chronic dialysis setting.

ADEQUACY OF HEMODIALYSIS

Dialysis Dose. In the early years of hemodialysis, the dialysis prescription was not individualized. In the late 1980s and early 1990s, it became evident that inadequate dialysis was associated with an increase in the frequency of adverse clinical outcomes and high mortality rates.[57,58] In response to the widespread concern about underdialysis, a number of investigators attempted to quantitatively define adequate dialysis using a surrogate marker. The ideal marker of uremia has the following characteristics: it accumulates in kidney failure, it is removed by dialysis, its production and elimination are representative of other potential toxins not typically measured in clinical practice, it demonstrates a concentration-dependent clinical outcome, and it is easily measured in blood, urine, and dialysate.[59] Urea, or BUN, serves as such a marker and is the only solute for which the concentration has been correlated with outcomes.[60–62]

In 1974 a multicenter study was initiated by the National Institutes of Health to evaluate quantitative methods for prescribing hemodialysis therapy: the National Cooperative Dialysis Study (NCDS).[62] In this study of 151 patients, four treatment groups were studied according to two parameters: dialysis treatment time (2.5 to 3.5 hours vs. 4.5 to 5.0 hours) and time-averaged BUN concentration (TAC) or the area under the BUN curve divided by time (TAC 20 to 50 mg/dL vs. 50 to 100 mg/dL). BUN concentration was considered a surrogate marker for small molecules. Patients in the low-dialysis-dose group (TAC 50 to 100 mg/dL) had more withdrawals from dialysis and more hospitalizations compared to the high-dialysis dose group (TAC 20 to 50 mg/dL). A post hoc analysis of the NCDS findings also indicated that reducing the dialysis time increased the hospitalization rate by 181%, especially for patients who had received the low dose of dialysis.[63] The results of the NCDS revealed that four factors were independently associated with greater morbidity: BUN concentration (a higher TAC urea), protein catabolic rate (PCR; a lower PCR rate or dietary protein intake), the presence of comorbid conditions, and shorter dialysis time.

From the NCDS, a study method to quantify dialysis was developed and the term Kt/V was introduced.[62] The Kt/V is now accepted as the measure of dialysis adequacy. Kt/V is a dimensionless parameter that takes into account dialyzer urea clearance (K), the duration of the dialysis procedure (t), and the patient's urea volume of distribution (V). This yields the prescribed fractional clearance of urea from total

body water. The NKF-K/DOQI Guidelines on Hemodialysis Adequacy recommend formal urea kinetic modeling to determine the delivered dialysis dose (Kt/V), based on either two or three BUN samples, as the best method for routine measurement of the dose of hemodialysis.[2] The complexity of these methods warrants use of computational software. One simpler method that is acceptable incorporates the predialysis and postdialysis BUN concentrations along with the change in the patient's weight:

$$Kt/V = -\ln(R - 0.008t) \qquad (44.1)$$
$$+ (4 - 3.5R)x\,\frac{UF}{Weight_{post}}$$

where R is the ratio of postdialysis BUN to predialysis BUN, t is the duration of dialysis in hours, and UF is the predialysis weight minus the postdialysis weight.[64] This equation takes into consideration the efficiency of the treatment as a function of the treatment time and the convective removal of urea in the ultrafiltrate (UF/Weight).

As an alternative to the Kt/V, the fractional urea clearance during a single dialysis session may be approximated by calculating the urea reduction ratio (URR)[65]:

$$URR = \frac{BUN_{predialysis} - BUN_{postdialysis}}{BUN_{predialysis}} \times 100$$
$$(44.2)$$

Therefore, URR is the percentage reduction in blood urea concentration during the course of one dialysis session. It offers the advantage of determining dialysis dosage independent of patient size, dialysis time, blood and dialysis flow rates, and dialyzer urea clearance. The URR, however, does not account for the contribution of ultrafiltration to the final delivered dose of dialysis.

In the NCDS, a Kt/V of less than 0.8 was associated with high morbidity, while values between 1.0 and 1.2 had a lower rate of morbidity.[62,64] Based on these data, the NKF-K/DOQI guidelines recommend a minimum acceptable delivered Kt/V of at least 1.2 for both adult and pediatric hemodialysis patients.[2] This corresponds to an average URR of 65%. Ideally, the delivered dose should be consistent with the prescribed dialysis dose; however, the delivered dose of dialysis, when accurately measured, is generally lower than the prescribed dose. Therefore, to achieve the recommended dose of dialysis, the prescribed Kt/V and URR should be 1.3 and 70% URR, respectively. Diabetic patients may respond better to even higher doses.[66]

For a patient starting hemodialysis, the initial prescribed dialysis dose is determined using information on the available dialyzer (the urea clearance for that dialyzer, or K), the volume of distribution of urea (determined using estimating equations or a nomogram approach specific for males or females),[64] and the target Kt/V of 1.3. With this information, the time of dialysis is calculated. Calculation of the delivered dialysis dose should be done at least monthly in hemodialysis patients and requires measurement of a predialysis and postdialysis BUN. The evaluation of dialysis adequacy must include BUN, PCR, and Kt/V (or URR). The goal of adequate dialysis is not only high urea removal but also adequate dietary protein (i.e., ≥1.2 g/kg/day) and caloric intake (i.e., ≥35 kcal/kg/day). The patient's residual kidney function must be considered in such an assessment to allow a more valid estimation of clearance values.

Data from two large prospective trials have recently been published that include an evaluation of dialysis dose: the NIH-sponsored hemodialysis (HEMO) study and DOPPS.[67,68] Interestingly, data from the HEMO study, which evaluated outcomes of high and low dialysis dose, found a survival benefit associated with a higher dialysis dose (URR >75%) in women but not in men.[68] This trend has been supported by data from DOPPS, designed to evaluate international practice patterns in dialysis patients and their effect on outcomes.[67,69] These findings warrant additional investigation into gender-related differences. DOPPS also showed that a shorter time of dialysis (<3.5 hours) was associated with a significantly higher mortality risk compared to longer times of dialysis.[67,69] The effect of longer dialysis times (>4.5 hours) could not be evaluated in this study due to inadequate numbers of patients. DOPPS also supported achievement of a Kt/V more than 1.2 due to an increased relative risk of mortality at values below this target.[67,69] Other factors associated with an increased relative risk of mortality included poor anemia management, hyperphosphatemia, low albumin, and use of catheters for vascular access.[69]

Causes of Inadequate Dialysis. Numerous factors may lead to the delivery of a dialysis dose less than prescribed. Among these are use of an estimated volume of distribution of urea less than the patient's actual volume to determine the initial dialysis prescription, an actual blood flow rate less than prescribed, time of dialysis less than prescribed, lower clearance of urea by the dialyzer than indicated by the manufacturer, access recirculation, and error in blood sampling (e.g., obtaining the postdialysis BUN sample >5 minutes after the end of dialysis; rebound phenomenon). Adjustment of conditions during dialysis due to complications or other factors can contribute to the decrease in the delivered dialysis dose. For example, a patient who experiences hypotension during dialysis may require a reduction in the blood flow rate. Other complications and confounders in a given dialysis center may lead to a shorter time of dialysis than prescribed (e.g., patient refusing to complete full dialysis time). Recirculation of urea may occur during hemodialysis if blood returned to the patient is then pumped immediately back into the arterial side and delivered to the dialyzer. This makes for an inefficient dialysis and causes a reduction in the delivered dialysis dose. To minimize the risk of recirculation, the arterial and venous needles must not be placed in close proximity to one another.

The method used for drawing the BUN samples is critical to minimize inaccuracies in calculating the dialysis dose. Dilution of the predialysis sample may occur if it is drawn

from a needle that has been flushed with saline or heparin. When obtaining the postdialysis sample, the blood pump should be slowed to approximately 50 to 100 mL per minute for at least 10 to 20 minutes.[70] After this period, the pump can be stopped and the sample collected. A rebound (or increase) in urea concentration following dialysis is generally observed as urea redistributes into the blood (i.e., as equilibrium between blood and tissue compartments is reestablished). A delay in obtaining the postdialysis sample may lead to underestimation of the delivered dialysis dose due to the expected increase in urea concentration following dialysis (the rebound phenomenon).

If blood sampling is done correctly and it is determined that a patient is underdialyzed, strategies to increase the delivered dialysis dose include increasing the time of dialysis, changing the dialyzer to one with a greater reported urea clearance (greater K), and increasing the blood or dialysate flow rates to achieve the prescribed Kt/V (or URR), considering the limitations in the extent of improvement in urea clearance that each of these changes may achieve.

COMPLICATIONS OF HEMODIALYSIS

Vascular Access Complications. Vascular access complications have been referred to as the Achilles' heel of dialysis and often prevent continuation of hemodialysis.[29,56] Efforts to increase AV fistula placement over AV grafts and temporary catheters are being made, since AV fistulas have greater survival rates and are associated with fewer complications.[29] Among the most common complications with vascular access are stenosis, thrombosis, and infection.

Significant stenosis, or low arterial blood flow, occurs when there is at least a 50% reduction in vessel diameter along with a hemodynamic, functional, or clinical abnormality, such as elevated static or dynamic pressures, decreased blood flow, elevated access recirculation, a swollen extremity, or unexplained reduction in Kt/V.[29] Venous stenosis also increases the risk of thrombosis (>90% of thrombosed grafts are associated with stenosis). Treatment options include percutaneous transluminal angioplasty and surgical revision. Treatment of significant stenoses reduces the rate of thrombosis and graft loss and prolongs the average life of the access site. Thrombosis of an AV graft should be corrected with surgical thrombectomy or with thrombolysis (e.g., alteplase, reteplase) or mechanical thrombolysis.[29] Data on treatment of thrombosis in an AV fistula are limited, and generally the decision is based on expertise at a given institution or center. Thrombolytic agents, including alteplase and reteplase, have been successfully used to restore flow in occluded dialysis catheters.[71,72] Use of warfarin has been considered for some hemodialysis patients in an effort to prevent thrombosis; however, the risk of bleeding outweighed the potential benefit of maintaining graft patency.[73–75] In DOPPS, warfarin-treated patients had an increased relative risk of graft failure.[75] Agents associated with improved graft patency in this analysis were calcium channel blockers and aspirin, while angiotensin-converting enzyme (ACE) inhibitors were associated with better fistula patency.

Infection. Infection accounts for approximately 20% of access complications and is the second leading cause of mortality in the hemodialysis population.[76,77] *Staphylococcus aureus* and *S. epidermidis* are the pathogens most often responsible for infection at the vascular access site, with or without associated bacteremia.[76,77] *Streptococcus* species, gram-negative organisms, and *Enterococcus* species are among the other potential organisms. Vascular access-related bacteremia can be life-threatening and has a high mortality rate.[77] The infection rate is highest in catheters, followed by AV grafts then AV fistulas, another reason why AV fistulas are preferred.

Treatment requires empiric antibiotic therapy (i.e., gram-negative and staphylococcal and streptococcal coverage) based on common pathogens, followed by more specific therapy based on the culture and sensitivity data. Localized infections can be treated with antibiotic therapy alone. Surgical revision of the access site may also be required with more extensive infection. Catheters have low salvage rates when antibiotics are used alone. The duration of therapy is based on the organism and severity (e.g., presence of bacteremia), with required treatment durations ranging from 2 to 6 weeks. Complications of infected access sites include endocarditis, osteomyelitis, septic arthritis, septic pulmonary emboli, and sepsis syndrome.

Approximately 20% to 25% of hemodialysis patients have a catheter as their vascular access for dialysis therapy, placing these patients at greater risk for infection and bacteremia. Not only are catheters more likely to become infected compared with fistulas and grafts, but they are also associated with an increased risk of hospitalization and death.[78] In many patients systemic antibiotics alone do not eradicate the infection. Catheter removal is often necessary, with replacement of the catheter occurring at a later time or immediately if the infected catheter is exchanged with a new catheter over a guidewire.

Antibiotic lock solutions have more recently been investigated as a strategy to treat catheter-related infections. Various regimens have been evaluated in patients with central vein catheters used for parenteral nutrition and chemotherapy, and now more recently in the hemodialysis population.[79,80] An antibiotic lock solution typically contains a concentrated amount of antibiotic along with heparin and is instilled into the infected catheter or port and left to dwell between dialysis sessions. Various strategies have been adopted for prevention and treatment of infected catheters.[79,80] Stability of the antibiotic solution must be considered, given the duration of the dwell time in the catheter. Antibiotics (and concentrations) generally selected for this purpose include vancomycin (1 to 5 mg/mL), gentamicin (0.4 to 1 mg/mL), cefazolin (5 mg/mL), and ceftazidime (2 to 5 mg/mL), although other agents and concentrations have been used.[79–81] Gentamicin concentrations more than 10 mg/

mL should not be mixed with heparin, since precipitation occurs at this concentration.[81] These antibiotic lock solutions can be given with or without systemic antibiotic therapy, depending on whether used for prophylaxis or treatment. Systemic antibiotic therapy is necessary for patients with bacteremia.

Prudent use of vancomycin must also be considered in this population, since vancomycin-resistant enterococci (VRE) and vancomycin-resistant *S. aureus* (VRSA) have been identified in hemodialysis patients.[82–84] The first case of VRSA in the United States was reported in a hemodialysis patient.[82] The percentage of centers reporting one or more patients infected or colonized with VRE increased from 12% in 1995 to 31% in 2001.[85] The nasal carriage of *S. aureus* has been identified as a risk factor for the development of infections (e.g., bacteremia) in patients on hemodialysis. A recent meta-analysis found that administration of mupirocin was effective for reducing the incidence of *S. aureus* infections in hemodialysis patients (78% reduction).[86]

Hypotension. Intradialytic (during dialysis) hypotension is a common complication of hemodialysis, occurring in approximately 10% to 30% of hemodialysis treatments, and leads to several complications, including nausea, vomiting, cramping, angina, neurologic manifestations, and extreme fatigue and weakness.[87,88] It also leads frequently to premature termination of dialysis, significant patient morbidity, increased nursing time, as well as increased health care costs. Conditions that increase the risk of frequent hypotensive episodes during hemodialysis include diabetes, autonomic insufficiency, heart disease (including LVH), and advanced age.[87,88] Aggressive ultrafiltration during a given hemodialysis session is also a risk factor for intradialytic hypotension, as the combination of high ultrafiltration and a decrease in extracellular osmolality due to solute removal leads to a decrease in intravascular volume. Other potential causes of the acute drop in blood pressure include enhanced nitric oxide production and a surge in serotonin levels.[89,90]

Various nonpharmacologic and pharmacologic strategies have been used to manage hypotensive episodes. Acute management includes placing patient in the Trendelenburg position, decreasing the ultrafiltration rate, and administering normal saline, hypertonic saline, and mannitol. Medications that have been investigated to prevent hypotension in patients with frequent episodes include vasopressin, caffeine, carnitine, ephedrine sulfate, fludrocortisone, sertraline, and midodrine.[88] These strategies have been used with various degrees of success, and no universal recommendations can be made for all patients on hemodialysis who experience hypotension. It may be prudent to avoid giving antihypertensive agents prior to initiation of hemodialysis in patients who experience frequent hypotensive episodes during the procedure.

Cardiovascular Complications. Cardiovascular disease is the most common cause of mortality among the dialysis population, accounting for 50% of deaths.[5] Myocardial infarction, coronary artery disease, moderate to severe heart failure, vascular stroke, and peripheral vascular disease are present in one third or more of hemodialysis patients.[14,91,92] The hemodialysis procedure is associated with both acute (e.g., hypotension, sudden death) and chronic (e.g., LVH, heart failure, coronary artery disease) cardiovascular complications. Most patients on hemodialysis have LVH, which is the most important pathogenic factor in the development of diastolic dysfunction.[92,93] Because LVH often is associated with left atrial dilation, patients are at risk for the development of atrial fibrillation. Patients on hemodialysis are often in a state of volume overload, predisposing the patient to pulmonary congestion and edema. During rapid intradialytic fluid removal, the left ventricular pressure is reduced rapidly, and this may result in intradialytic hypotension. In patients with significant vascular disease (e.g., coronary, carotid, or peripheral artery disease), prolonged hypotension may lead to ischemic symptoms and possibly myocardial infarction and stroke. Large and rapid changes in intravascular volume should be avoided during dialysis. Ideally, hypertension and anemia should be treated aggressively before dialysis to reduce the degree of LVH and associated complications.[94]

Cardiac arrhythmias (atrial and ventricular) are a cause of sudden death during hemodialysis. Coronary artery disease and LVH increase the patient's risk of arrhythmias and sudden death during dialysis. The hemodialysis process itself causes fluctuations in electrolytes and fluid volume that increase the likelihood of cardiac arrhythmias in patients predisposed to cardiac abnormalities. Hypotension and chronic intermittent ischemia are implicated in the arrhythmias observed during hemodialysis.[95] Patients receiving digitalis are at an even greater risk.

If an arrhythmia occurs during hemodialysis, the procedure should be immediately stopped and blood returned to the patient if possible. Interventions consistent with emergency management of arrhythmias should be implemented (e.g., antiarrhythmic agents, cardioversion).[95]

Dialyzer Reactions. There are two types of dialyzer reactions, type A and type B. Type A is an anaphylactoid or allergic reaction to some component of the hemodialysis circuit; it develops within the first 20 minutes of a dialysis session and is thought to be IgE-mediated.[96] Signs and symptoms are similar to those of a drug-induced anaphylactic reaction and may result from sensitization to a component of the extracorporeal circuit. Patients receiving ACE inhibitors are at an increased risk of developing type A dialyzer reactions when dialyzed using the polyacrylonitrile membrane (AN69). This negatively charged membrane may promote bradykinin release. Reduced degradation of bradykinin in the presence of ACE inhibition leads to anaphylactoid reactions. Although the potential for this interaction between ACE inhibitors and the AN69 membrane has been documented for some time, the combination is still used and anaphylactoid reactions continue to be reported in clinical practice.[97] Treatment involves immediate discontinuation of

dialysis and the institution of standard therapy for anaphylactic reactions, such as epinephrine, antihistamines, corticosteroids, and, if necessary, ventilatory support.

Type B reactions occur within 20 to 60 minutes of initiating dialysis and involve primarily chest and back pain. Usually, symptoms subside with continued dialysis. However, in severe cases, dyspnea may develop, necessitating discontinuation of dialysis. Type B reactions may be caused by intradialytic complement activation and are associated more with cellulose-based dialyzers as opposed to synthetic high-flux dialyzers.[96]

The effect of dialyzer reuse of patient outcomes has also been questioned, since it remains a common practice in the United States.[98,99] Reuse of dialyzers refers to repeated use of a dialyzer for the same patient. This involves a process of rinsing, use of a cleansing agent (e.g., bleach, hydrogen peroxide), performance testing to assess the number of reuses, disinfection, and proper storage between hemodialysis sessions. A sterilization process using either chemical (e.g., Renalin, formaldehyde) or heat sterilization is used to disinfect the dialyzer. With repeated dialyzer use, the effective clearance (K) is reduced. It is currently recommended that dialyzers be discarded once the total cell volume of the dialyzer drops below 80% of the initial value.[2] With reuse, there is also a small potential risk of death from sepsis caused by inadequate sterilization of the dialyzer. The use of high-flux synthetic membrane dialyzers has been associated with a lower mortality risk, particularly when exposed to bleach.[98] Dialyzer reuse may be performed safely under the established sterilization guidelines of the Association for the Advancement of Medical Instrumentation.[2]

Muscle Cramps. The pathogenesis of muscle cramping during hemodialysis is not well understood; however, a common cause is aggressive ultrafiltration during hemodialysis, leading to plasma volume contraction. This complication develops frequently in patients who experience a drop in weight during dialysis below their targeted dry weight or who have an acute lowering in the plasma sodium concentration.[100] Other associated factors include hypotension, hyponatremia, hypovolemia, and carnitine deficiency.[100]

Dialysis-associated muscle cramps may be acutely relieved by boluses of normal saline, hypertonic saline, or osmotic agents (dextrose solutions, mannitol). Sodium profiling (varying the sodium concentration during dialysis) and varying the degree of ultrafiltration have also been effective.[101] Other treatment strategies include administration of vitamin E (400 IU) and quinine (200 to 300 mg at bedtime).[100] The adverse effect profile of quinine must be weighed against the potential benefit in treating muscle cramps. The combination of vitamin E and vitamin C has also shown benefits in reducing the incidence of hemodialysis-associated muscle cramps when used short term (8 weeks of therapy).[102] The association of carnitine deficiency with development of muscle cramps has prompted investigation of the effects of carnitine supplementation.[103,104] Administration of low-dose l-carnitine (500 mg/day) to hemodialysis patients is effective in improving muscular symptoms.[104] Chronic leg cramps are also frequently reported in the ESRD population.[100]

Dialysis Dysequilibrium Syndrome. Dialysis disequilibrium syndrome is one of a number of central nervous system abnormalities seen in patients with ESRD. It occurs predominantly in patients who are undergoing rapid dialysis or patients who have recently started hemodialysis. Although the exact mechanism is unclear, the signs and symptoms of dialysis disequilibrium syndrome are caused by the increased intracranial pressure that results from dialysis-induced cerebral edema. Changes in the intracellular pH have also been proposed as a potential mechanism.[100] Younger patients, especially children, and those with a previous neurologic disorder (e.g., head trauma, stroke, malignant hypertension) appear to be at a higher risk for this syndrome. The minor disequilibrium symptoms include headache, restlessness, blurred vision, dizziness, nausea, vomiting, and muscular twitching. Major signs and symptoms include disorientation, hypertension, tremors, and seizures.

Limiting the targeted reduction in urea concentration to approximately 30% for patients who require acute dialysis or who are new to dialysis may be warranted to prevent this syndrome. Other preventive strategies include use of a dialysate sodium concentration of at least 140 mEq per liter and a glucose of at least 200 mg per dL.[100] Treatment is supportive and based on the severity of symptoms (e.g., administration of hypertonic saline in mild cases; seizure control in severe cases).

β$_2$-Microglobulin Amyloidosis. Patients who receive long-term hemodialysis (typically for 10 or more years) commonly suffer from a syndrome of pain and osteoarthropathy called dialysis-related amyloidosis, caused primarily by the deposition of β$_2$-microglobulin-containing amyloid in joints and soft tissue.[105] Patients on hemodialysis have serum β$_2$-microglobulin concentrations that may reach 60 times the normal values of 1 to 3 mg per liter.[106] Dialysis-related amyloidosis may cause carpal tunnel syndrome, destructive arthropathy of the medium-sized joints (e.g., knees, wrists, shoulders, pelvis, vertebral column), and periarticular cystic bone lesions.[105] Amyloidosis was also identified as an independent risk factor for mortality in a small sample of hemodialysis patients.[107] The risk of carpal tunnel syndrome is related to the duration of dialysis. The incidence in patients receiving hemodialysis for less than 8 years was relatively low, but it increased to 30% to 50% after 15 years and approached 100% after 20 years of hemodialysis with biocompatible dialyzers.[106,108] Advanced glycosylation end products (AGEs), which accumulate in patients with ESRD, have recently been implicated in the pathogenesis of β$_2$-microglobulin amyloidosis.[109] Although carpal tunnel syndrome can be treated surgically, there is no established treatment for amyloidosis. Dialysis-related amyloidosis is less common in patients who are dialyzed with biocompatible

synthetic membranes (e.g., polyacrylonitrile); therefore, attempts should be made to maximize removal of β$_2$-microglobulin using high-flux biocompatible membranes (e.g., polysulfone, polyacrylonitrile, cellulose triacetate, and polymethylmethacrylate).[108]

Pruritus. Pruritus (itching) is a common problem in patients with ESRD and may often be worse during the dialysis procedure. Uremic pruritus has been attributed to numerous factors, including inadequate dialysis, skin dryness, secondary hyperparathyroidism, increased vitamin A and histamine plasma concentrations, and increased sensitivity to histamine.[110,111] Itching that worsens during hemodialysis may be due to hypersensitivity to the dialyzer or blood circuit.

Therapy for pruritus is largely empirical. The most practical treatment is adequate dialysis, despite the fact that a correlation between pruritus and adequate dialysis (Kt/V) has not been shown.[111] Control of serum phosphorus and calcium (consistent with guidelines for management of secondary hyperparathyroidism) may also be of benefit. Antihistamine treatment does not consistently improve symptoms, but a trial may be warranted, as some patients do experience relief with this therapy. Other therapies include activated charcoal and cholestyramine; however, drug interactions and extra fluid required for the administration of these agents may preclude use. Some patients gain relief from topical administration of emollients, although dry skin does not appear to be a predominant factor in pruritus. Nonpharmacologic therapies that have been tried with some benefit include acupuncture and ultraviolet B therapy.[110]

Other Complications. Following the hemodialysis procedure, patients often report postdialytic symptoms, including weakness and fatigue. These symptoms are likely caused in part by intradialytic cytokine and complement activation and may be reduced by the use of biocompatible polymer membranes (e.g., polysulfone, polyacrylonitrile, polymethylmethacrylate) as opposed to cellulosic membranes.

Bleeding following the dialysis procedure is another potential complication of hemodialysis. It may be due in part to the method of anticoagulation used during the procedure. Aluminum accumulation was at one time a concern; however, improved techniques for processing of the water used for the dialysate solution and less frequent use of aluminum-containing phosphate binders have decreased the incidence of aluminum toxicity in dialysis patients.

PERITONEAL DIALYSIS

Peritoneal dialysis has undergone several modifications over the past 30 years. The introduction of continuous ambulatory peritoneal dialysis (CAPD) led to an increase in the proportion of patients receiving peritoneal dialysis; however, adverse events such as peritonitis were common and a predominant reason for patients to switch to hemodialysis. During the 1990s an automated process of peritoneal dialysis using cyclers was introduced in an attempt to enhance patient acceptance and improve the delivered dose of dialysis.[112] Currently in the United States, the number of patients prescribed automated peritoneal dialysis surpasses those prescribed traditional CAPD.[4] Regardless of the specific modality of peritoneal dialysis, the principles of fluid and solute removal (including drugs) with peritoneal dialysis are similar.

PERITONEAL MEMBRANE

The peritoneal cavity contains a single-layer membrane that lines the abdomen and the visceral organs. The side of the peritoneal cavity that covers the abdominal wall is called the parietal surface, and the visceral surface covers the visceral organs. The peritoneal surface area of adults approximates the body surface area and ranges from 1 to 2 m^2. The adult peritoneal cavity contains approximately 100 mL of lipid-rich fluid that acts as a lubricating agent. The peritoneal space can accommodate several liters of fluid, as noted in conditions of ascites or by instillation of dialysate solution.[113,114]

The peritoneal membrane has pores that are large enough to allow the passage of middle- to high-molecular-weight compounds. Therefore, peritoneal dialysis clears larger substances more effectively than conventional cellulosic hemodialysis membranes. The routes of absorption from the peritoneal cavity differ for small solutes and macromolecules (molecular weights >20,000 Daltons), such as albumin and dextrans. Whereas small solutes diffuse down their concentration gradient into the systemic circulation, macromolecules are absorbed primarily via the subdiaphragmatic lymphatic system.[115] With chronic peritoneal dialysis, the character of the mesothelial layer may change, mostly because of the hyperosmolarity of the dialysate solutions.[113] These alterations may lead to peritoneal fibrosis (thickening), decreased permeability, and diminished ultrafiltration.[114,116] Just as with hemodialysis, regular evaluation of the delivered dose of dialysis (i.e., the adequacy of dialysis) is required to determine whether such changes in the peritoneal membrane have occurred.

MECHANICS OF PERITONEAL DIALYSIS

Like hemodialysis, peritoneal dialysis has three basic components: a blood compartment (systemic circulation), a dialysate compartment (peritoneal cavity), and a semipermeable membrane that separates the blood and dialysate compartments (peritoneal membrane). In peritoneal dialysis, the dialysis solution is instilled into the peritoneal cavity via an indwelling catheter. In the presence of dialysate, solute transfer occurs via diffusion and convection bidirectionally across the peritoneal membrane to and from the blood compartment.[113] Because the dialysis fluid contains an osmotic agent (i.e., glucose or polyglucose), fluid is pulled from the intravascular space into the peritoneal cavity by ultrafiltration. This osmotic effect is lost as the dialysate glucose is ab-

sorbed, especially if the time during which dialysate resides in the peritoneal cavity (the dwell time) is prolonged.

PERITONEAL ACCESS DEVICES AND PLACEMENT TECHNIQUES

Permanent access to the peritoneal cavity for peritoneal dialysis may be accomplished by several techniques. The first catheter developed for long-term peritoneal dialysis was described by Tenckhoff in 1968. Several catheters for long-term peritoneal dialysis have been introduced in the past few years.[117] The multiple types of indwelling catheters and administration sets are designed to prevent contamination and to reduce infectious complications. Chronic (permanent) indwelling catheters are made of silicone rubber, polyurethane, and other soft materials. The Tenckhoff catheter, which is the most commonly used peritoneal catheter, has two sections, intraperitoneal and extraperitoneal. The intraperitoneal portion is placed via a surgical procedure in the left or right lower peritoneum, preferably in one of the pelvic gutters just above the hips.[113] The extraperitoneal end is passed through subcutaneous layers and placed approximately halfway between the umbilicus and the pubis in the caudal direction. The indwelling catheter is then immobilized to allow healing, prevent leaks, and act as a barrier against migration of skin microorganisms. For this purpose, one or preferably two Dacron cuffs are placed above or below the abdominal muscle layers, and the patient is allowed to heal before peritoneal dialysis is begun (Fig. 44.3; see color insert).[118] During this healing period, the patient undergoes training for self-administration of dialysis and care of the catheter using sterile technique. The waiting period between catheter placement and dialysis initiation varies among patients. The healing period is usually 4 to 6 weeks for patients with potentially impaired wound healing, such as diabetic patients and those receiving high-dose steroids. A young and otherwise healthy patient can often start dialysis 2 weeks after catheter placement. Patients who are about to undergo continuous cycling peritoneal dialysis may start even sooner, because they can initially use smaller volumes of dialysate with no daytime dwell period.

DIALYSATE SOLUTIONS

The peritoneal dialysis solution is a hypertonic osmolar solution that either contains dextrose (1.5%, 2.5%, or 4.25%) or polyglucose (icodextrin 7.5%), which is necessary to create a diffusive gradient between the peritoneal and blood compartments and to augment ultrafiltration.[119] The dialysate also contains electrolytes such as sodium, potassium, chloride, magnesium, and calcium.[120] Although other osmotic agents have been used experimentally, including glycerol and amino acids, none are available commercially in the United States.[119] A variety of additives, including potassium, calcium, and lactate, may be added to the dialysate to control the balance of electrolytes and to correct the metabolic acidosis associated with ESRD.[120]

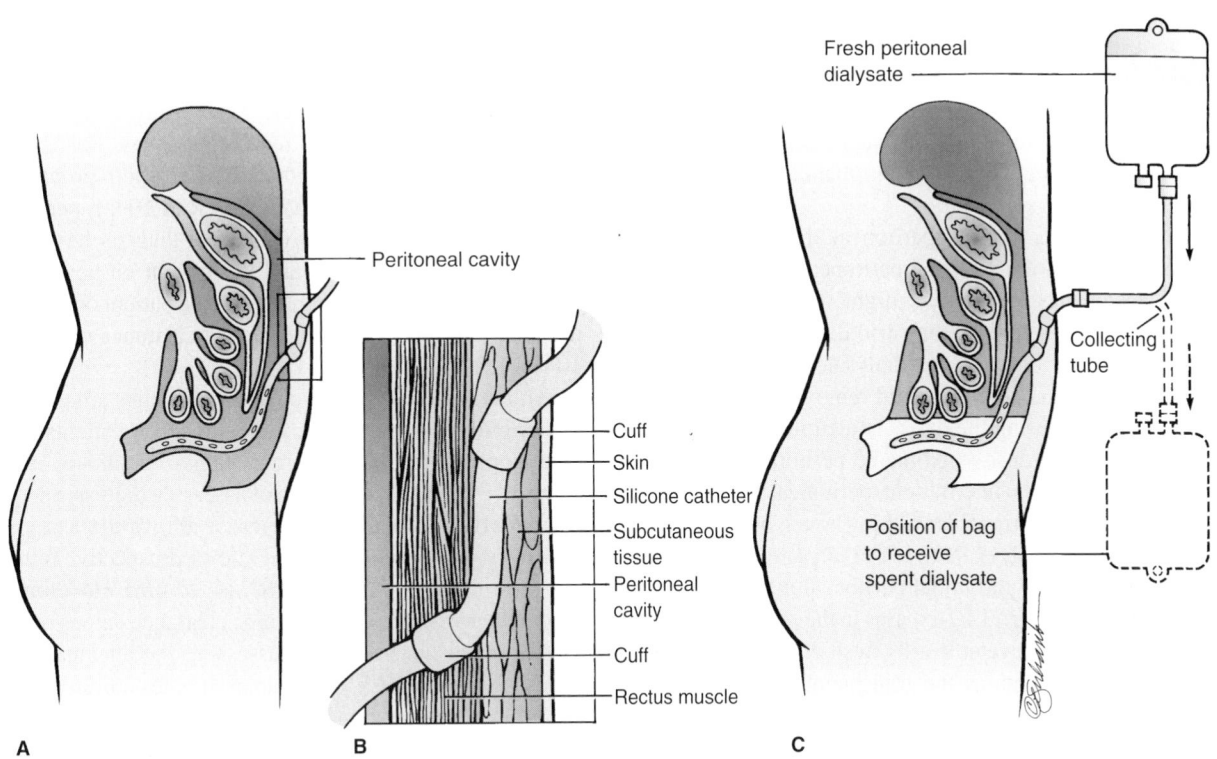

FIGURE 44.3. Peritoneal dialysis schematic and catheter placement (see color insert). (From Smeltzer SC, Bare BG. Textbook of medical-surgical nursing, 9th ed. Philadelphia: Lippincott Williams & Wilkins, 2000.)

CONTINUOUS AMBULATORY PERITONEAL DIALYSIS

In CAPD, as the name implies, patients are dialyzed continuously, 24 hours a day, 7 days a week. A typical CAPD regimen involves four daily exchanges: three with a dialysate dwell time of about 4 to 6 hours and one with an overnight dwell time of about 10 to 12 hours.[112,113] Given its demanding and time-consuming nature, the patient must be reliable and highly motivated. Omission of only a few exchanges per week reduces the urea clearance (the marker of dialysis adequacy), with the potential of increasing morbidity and mortality. Commercial CAPD solutions are available in volumes of 1 to 3 L in flexible polyvinyl chloride plastic bags similar to those of large-volume parenterals. The bags have a port for connecting an administration set and a port for administering excipients (e.g., insulin, antibiotics).

The fresh dialysate bag is connected to the permanent indwelling catheter via an administration set. A volume of dialysate (commonly 2 L) is warmed to body temperature and infused by gravity into the peritoneal cavity over 10 to 20 minutes (Fig. 44.3). The dialysate is warmed to prevent pain and cramping during the initial minutes of an exchange. Depending on the catheter and administration set, the empty bag is either removed and tucked inside the patient's clothing or carried inside a separate belt underneath the clothing while still connected to the catheter.[113,114] After the prescribed

dwell time, the same bag is connected to the administration set and placed at a level lower than the peritoneal cavity to allow drainage by gravity, which also takes 10 to 20 minutes. When the drainage has ceased, the tubing is again clamped, and using sterile technique (mask and gloves), the patient disconnects the bag of drained fluid. Then a fresh bag of sterile dialysate fluid is connected to the tubing and allowed to infuse into the peritoneal cavity. Fresh, unused dialysate is clear and colorless; spent or used dialysate is clear and straw-colored. During bouts of peritonitis (see section, ''Peritonitis'' later in this chapter), the spent dialysate becomes cloudy; this is considered a diagnostic sign of infection.

AUTOMATED PERITONEAL DIALYSIS

In 2002, there were about 24,903 peritoneal dialysis patients in the United States.[4] Of these, 10,937 (43.9%) were treated with CAPD and 13,966 (56.1%) were treated with some type of automated peritoneal dialysis. The four main forms of automated peritoneal dialysis are continuous cycling peritoneal dialysis, daily ambulatory peritoneal dialysis, nightly intermittent peritoneal dialysis, and nightly tidal peritoneal dialysis.[112] These procedures involve the use of a dialysate cycling machine, which automatically instills and drains the peritoneal dialysate solutions. The patient attaches the dialysis catheter to tubing attached to a cycle machine that performs the majority of exchanges automatically at night. The purpose of automated peritoneal dialysis is to promote maximum clearance and ultrafiltration. Automated peritoneal dialysis allows for multiple exchanges to occur without the need to disconnect and reconnect, and is convenient for patients due to the nighttime dialysis exchanges. Other advantages are improved patient compliance and decreased peritonitis rates.[121]

With continuous cycling peritoneal dialysis, the most common variation of automated peritoneal dialysis, four or five 2-L exchanges are done at night while the patient is sleeping over an 8- to 10-hour period. In the daytime, the patient may carry 0 to 2 L of dialysate in the peritoneal cavity. When greater solute or fluid removal is necessary, a second exchange during the day is sometimes added; this is often termed "high-dose" automated peritoneal dialysis.

Patients on nightly intermittent peritoneal dialysis perform no exchanges during their waking hours, but while they sleep, six to eight 2.5-L exchanges of dialysate are delivered by the cycler. With nightly tidal peritoneal dialysis, a minimal dwell volume (often 1 L) remains in the peritoneal cavity during the night. The cycler instills fresh dialysate at regular intervals, which maintains the transmembrane solute gradient to enhance solute removal and prevents formation of a stagnant fluid layer at the peritoneal membrane.[122] This therapy is prescribed for patients who have difficulty completely draining the dialysate fluid from the peritoneal cavity because of pain, since the number of drain procedures is reduced with nightly tidal peritoneal dialysis. One of the drawbacks is the need for larger amounts of dialysate in a 24-hour period, and therefore this therapy is used infrequently.

ADEQUACY OF PERITONEAL DIALYSIS

During the early years of this therapy, patients on CAPD routinely received a standard daily therapy consisting of four 2-L exchanges. For the purpose of quantifying the dialysis dosage, creatinine rather than urea was proposed as a marker.[123] On the basis of clinical experience, a normalized weekly creatinine clearance of about 60 L per 1.73 m^2 of body surface area has been suggested as minimally adequate.[3,124] The weekly Kt/V for the standard CAPD regimen of four daily 2-L exchanges is approximately 1.7 (1.5 to 1.8) per week, compared to a weekly Kt/V of 3.0 to 3.6 for hemodialysis (based on thrice-weekly hemodialysis and a per-treatment Kt/V of approximately 1.2).[3,124] The low CAPD Kt/V is similar to that of the low-dose hemodialysis regimen used in the NCDS (i.e., high-failure) groups; however, the mortality rates in the peritoneal dialysis population are equal to or lower than those of the hemodialysis population.[125] There are two possible explanations for this incongruity. First, because of the continuous nature of peritoneal dialysis, the concentrations of blood urea (or other uremic toxins) during CAPD are at a fairly constant steady state, whereas a sawtooth profile is observed with hemodialysis (i.e., peak predialysis concentrations followed by trough

postdialysis concentrations).[126] The second possible reason for the discrepant minimum dialysis dosage needs is that residual kidney function is better preserved during peritoneal dialysis than during hemodialysis.[46–48] To illustrate, in calculating Kt/V for urea, the clearance of urea (or K) should include both dialyzer and renal clearances. For example, peritoneal dialysis and hemodialysis may both provide a dialysis dose that is equivalent to a GFR of 10 mL per minute. However, if the patient on peritoneal dialysis has a native GFR of 5 mL per minute and the patient on hemodialysis has lost all residual kidney function, the patient on peritoneal dialysis will have a higher total urea clearance of 15 versus 10 mL per minute.

Although both urea and creatinine kinetics are associated with clinical outcome in peritoneal dialysis patients, creatinine appears to be a more sensitive predictor of outcome.[126,127] The Kt/V method of assessing dialysis adequacy offers two additional advantages: it allows the assessment of dietary protein intake, and it allows prospective prescription of a dialysis dose.[3,124] The use of urea modeling (Kt/V) together with weekly creatinine clearance values provides a comprehensive method of assessing the adequacy of dialysis. A weekly Kt/V of 2.0 approximates a urea clearance of 7 mL per minute and a creatinine clearance that varies between 9 and 14 mL/min/1.73 m^2. Urea clearance should be normalized to total body water (V) and creatinine clearance should be expressed per 1.73 m^2 of body surface area. The GFR, which is estimated by the arithmetic mean of the urea and creatinine clearances, will be approximately 10.5 mL/min/1.73 m^2 when the weekly Kt/V urea is about 2.0. The NKF-K/DOQI Guidelines for Peritoneal Dialysis Adequacy recommend that for CAPD patients, the delivered peritoneal dialysis dose should be a total Kt/V urea of at least 2.0 per week and a total creatinine clearance of at least 60 L/week/1.73 m^2 for high and high-average transporters and 50 L/week/1.73 m^2 in low and low-average transporters.[3,124] Total Kt/V urea and total creatinine clearance assessments include the contribution of peritoneal dialysis and residual kidney function. For patients receiving nightly intermittent peritoneal dialysis, the weekly delivered peritoneal dialysis dose should be a total Kt/V urea of at least 2.2 and a weekly total creatinine clearance of at least 66 L/week/1.73 m^2. For continuous cycling peritoneal dialysis patients, the weekly delivered peritoneal dialysis dose should be a total Kt/V urea of at least 2.1 and a weekly total creatinine clearance of at least 66 L/week/1.73 m^2.[3,124]

Peritoneal dialysis adequacy, as assessed by total Kt/V urea and total creatinine clearance, should be determined at least twice during the first 6 months of initiating peritoneal dialysis. Afterwards, adequacy tests should be performed at every 4 months, unless the prescription has been changed or there has been a significant change in the patient's clinical status (e.g., peritonitis episode within the past few months). Patients should be monitored monthly for protein–calorie malnutrition; the monitoring should include body weight (measured with an empty peritoneum) and serum concentrations of albumin and transferrin. In addition, dietary intake should be monitored at least every 6 months.[3,124]

COMPLICATIONS OF PERITONEAL DIALYSIS

The most common complication in peritoneal dialysis patients is infection, either peritonitis (infection of the peritoneal membrane) or exit-site and tunnel infections of the peritoneal dialysis catheter. Since 1983 the International Society of Peritoneal Dialysis (ISPD) has published evidence-based guidelines for treatment and prevention of peritoneal dialysis-associated infections.[121,128] The most recent guidelines are organized into five sections: prevention of peritoneal dialysis-related infections, prevention of exit-site and tunnel infections, initial management of peritonitis, subsequent management of peritonitis (organism-specific), and future research.[121] For purposes of this chapter, only the first four sections are presented. These guidelines serve as a basis for treatment of infection in the peritoneal dialysis population, but each dialysis clinic should examine its own patterns of infection, causative organisms, and antibiotic sensitivities and adapt its prevention and treatment protocols as necessary.

Peritonitis. Peritonitis is the most prevalent infectious complication of peritoneal dialysis, occurring at a rate of one to two episodes per patient-year.[114,121] Breakdown in aseptic technique during dialysis exchanges is one of the major risk factors for the development of peritonitis. The peritonitis-causing organism may enter directly through the catheter lumen or migrate along the catheter through a tunnel. The development of catheter biofilms or exit-site infections may also contribute to peritonitis. Rarely, peritonitis is caused by intestinal or genitourinary sources or from hematogenous seeding. Peritonitis may necessitate discontinuation of peritoneal dialysis and a switch to hemodialysis for a particular patient and can be the cause of significant morbidity and mortality in the peritoneal dialysis population.[121]

Patients on peritoneal dialysis have many immune deficiencies. In addition, the presence of a low-pH, hyperosmolar dialysate solution inhibits phagocytosis, chemotaxis, bactericidal killing, free oxygen radical generation, and leukotriene synthesis of peripheral neutrophils and peritoneal macrophages.[129,130] This diminished intraperitoneal immune capacity may contribute to the development of peritonitis. Bacterial colonization of the nares with *S. aureus* is a risk factor for both exit-site infection and peritonitis.[121] Recurrent peritonitis occurs in up to one third of the patients and is a major cause of technique failure (i.e., discontinuation of this dialysis modality).[114]

Peritonitis associated with peritoneal dialysis is typically less serious than that caused by gastrointestinal perforation. Most cases of peritonitis are of bacterial origin, although other forms, such as chemical, viral, mycobacterial, and fungal, have occurred. The most frequent pathogens are *S. aureus* and *S. epidermidis*, accounting for nearly 60% of peritonitis episodes.[131] Gram-negative organisms, mostly Enterobacteriaceae, *Pseudomonas* species, and *Acinetobacter* species, cause up to 35% of cases. Polymicrobial peritonitis accounts for 5% of cases and may be indicative of intraabdominal viscus perforation. Sterile peritonitis may be caused by a transient allergic reaction to some component of the peritoneal dialysis catheter or poor laboratory culture techniques.[121,131]

Initial Assessment. Cloudy effluent and abdominal pain often result from peritoneal dialysis-associated peritonitis, but not all patients will present with these symptoms. If a patient presents with either symptom, peritonitis should be considered. Other noninfectious causes of abdominal pain (e.g., pancreatitis) and cloudy effluent (e.g., chemical peritonitis, hemoperitoneum) should be ruled out.[121] The effluent may be clear or may remain cloudy after microbiologic cure.[131] When peritonitis is suspected, a Gram stain of the dialysate should be obtained. Culture of the spent dialysate must also be obtained, but therapy should not await the results. Diagnosis of peritonitis is confirmed when more than 50% of white cells in the effluent sample are polymorphonuclear cells and there is a positive dialysate culture.[131] The majority of cultures will become positive after the first 24 hours, and in more than 75% of cases diagnosis can be established in less than 3 days.[121]

Empiric Therapy. Because peritoneal dialysis-associated peritonitis is less severe than other forms of peritonitis, it usually is treated on an outpatient basis. However, the following circumstances may necessitate hospitalization: inability or unwillingness to self-administer antibiotics, noncompliance with therapy or follow-up, and presence of significant systemic symptoms, such as fever, vomiting, abdominal pain, or hypotension.[116] Once peritonitis has been diagnosed, two or three rapid dialysis exchanges of 20 minutes each may provide symptomatic benefit. Also, the addition of heparin (1,000 U/L) to the fresh dialysate may reduce the number of subsequent peritoneal adhesions and reduce postinfectious complications.[131] If the organism is sensitive to a first-generation cephalosporin and the patient is relatively asymptomatic, then oral antibiotic therapy may be possible if for some reason intraperitoneal or intravenous antibiotic therapy is not feasible. Oral therapy is not suitable for more severe cases of peritonitis.[121]

Before the causative organism is determined, empiric broad-spectrum antibiotic therapy must be initiated against common gram-positive or gram-negative bacteria, which cause approximately 90% of all CAPD peritonitis cases.[121] Typically, a first-generation cephalosporin (e.g., cefazolin) in combination with an antibiotic for broad gram-negative coverage (e.g., aminoglycoside, ceftazidime, cefepime, or a carbapenem) will be suitable. However, the selection of empiric antibiotics must be made in light of both the patient's and the dialysis clinic's history of causative microorganisms and antibiotic sensitivities. For example, a program should use vancomycin for gram-positive coverage if it has a high rate of methicillin-resistant organisms. Gram-negative coverage can also be provided with a fluoroquinolones if local sensitivities support such use.

Extended courses of aminoglycoside therapy may increase the risk for both vestibular toxicity and ototoxicity, but short-term aminoglycoside therapy appears to be safe and inexpensive while providing good gram-negative coverage. There does not appear to be convincing evidence that short courses of aminoglycosides harm residual kidney function. The ISPD guidelines suggest that repeated or prolonged courses of aminoglycoside therapy may not be advisable if an alternative approach is possible.

Intraperitoneal antibiotic administration is favored over the intravenous route. Current antibiotic dosing recommendations for CAPD and automated peritoneal dialysis patients are provided in Tables 44.8, 44.9, and 44.10.[121] Antibiotic regimens are different for CAPD and automated peritoneal dialysis patients, as the transfer of solutes across the peritoneal membrane differs in these two groups of patients. These types of peritoneal dialysis involve very different exchange characteristics with varying dialysate volumes and dwell durations. Subsequently, the disposition of drugs differs considerably between CAPD and automated peritoneal dialysis.

Gram-Positive Organisms on Culture. If a gram-positive organism is identified on culture, the choice of therapy should be guided by the sensitivity pattern of the organism.[121] Coagulase-negative staphylococci, especially *S.*

TABLE 44.8	Oral Antibiotics Used in Peritoneal Dialysis-Associated Exit-Site and Tunnel Infections
Drug	**Typical Dose**
Amoxicillin	250–500 mg BID
Cephalexin	500 mg BID
Ciprofloxacin	250–500 mg BID
Clarithromycin	250–500 mg BID
Dicloxacillin	250–500 mg BID
Fluconazole	200 mg QD
Flucytosine	2 g load, then 1 g QD
Isoniazid	300 mg QD
Linezolid	600 mg BID
Metronidazole	400 mg BID for <50 kg; 400–500 TID for >50 kg
Ofloxacin	400 mg 1st day, then 200 mg QD
Pyrazinamide	35 mg/kg QD (given as BID or once daily)
Rifampin	450 mg QD for <50 kg, 600 mg QD for >50 kg
Trimethoprim/ sulfamethoxazole	80/400 mg QD

(Adapted from Piraino P, Bailie GR, Bernardini J, et al. Peritoneal dialysis-related infections recommendations: 2005 update. Perit Dial Int 25:107–131, 2005.)

epidermidis, are the most common organisms and are associated with mild abdominal pain. The peritonitis is usually caused by touch contamination of the peritoneal dialysis catheter. It generally responds well to antibiotic therapy and is seldom related to a catheter infection. Streptococcal and enterococcal peritonitis generally cause severe pain. Treatment with ampicillin 125 mg per liter in each exchange is the preferred antibiotic in this scenario. An aminoglycoside (given once daily intraperitoneally as 20 mg/L) may be added for synergy for enterococcal peritonitis. If VRE are ampicillin-susceptible, ampicillin remains the drug of choice for enterococcal peritonitis. Linezolid or quinupristin/dalfopristin should be used to treat VRE peritonitis. Quinupristin/dalfopristin is not active against *E. faecalis* isolates. Bone marrow suppression usually occurs after 10 to 14 days of therapy of linezolid, and more prolonged therapy can also result in neurotoxicity. Peritonitis caused by *S. aureus* is often severe and a result of a catheter infection, although it may be due to touch contamination. *S. aureus* infections usually can be managed with continuation of the first-generation cephalosporin and the addition of oral rifampin 600 mg per day. If MRSA is identified, vancomycin therapy must be used. If vancomycin-resistant *S. aureus* is identified, linezolid, daptomycin, or quinupristin/dalfopristin must be used. The usual duration of therapy is 3 weeks for *S. aureus* infections and 2 weeks for all other gram-positive species.

Gram-Negative Organisms on Culture. The choice of therapy for Gram-negative organisms should be guided by the sensitivity pattern of the organism. Single-organism gram-negative peritonitis may be due to touch contamination, exit-site infection, or possibly a bowel source, such as constipation, colitis, or transmural migration.[121] If a single gram-negative organism, such as *Escherichia coli*, *Klebsiella*, or *Proteus*, is isolated, the antibiotic can be chosen based on sensitivities, safety, and convenience. Often, ceftazidime or cefepime is indicated based on in vitro sensitivity testing. *Pseudomonas aeruginosa* peritonitis is generally severe and often associated with infection of the catheter. If catheter infection is present or has preceded peritonitis, catheter removal is necessary. Antibiotics must be continued while the patient receives hemodialysis for 2 weeks. In the presence of *Pseudomonas* or *Stenotrophomonas* species, dual therapy is required (e.g., ceftazidime plus an aminoglycoside, ciprofloxacin, or aztreonam). If an extended-spectrum penicillin is to be used with an aminoglycoside, it is best to administer the penicillin intravenously to avoid intraperitoneal inactivation of the aminoglycoside. Peritonitis caused by *Pseudomonas* or *Stenotrophomonas* often necessitates removal of the peritoneal catheter and 2 weeks of antibiotic therapy.

Polymicrobial Peritonitis. In the presence of a polymicrobial infection, surgical abdominal exploration should be considered.[121] In cases of multiple enteric organisms, where the intestines are thought to be the source, the therapy of choice is metronidazole in combination with ampicillin and ceftazidime or an aminoglycoside in the recommended doses. Poly-

TABLE 44.9	Intraperitoneal Antibiotic Dosing Recommendations for Continuous Ambulatory Peritoneal Dialysis Patients

For patients with residual kidney function (defined as a urine output of >100 mL/day), the dose of drugs dependent on renal elimination should be empirically increased by 25%.

	Intermittent (per exchange, once daily)	Continuous (mg/L, all exchanges)
Aminoglycosides		
Amikacin	2 mg/kg	LD 25, MD 12
Gentamicin	0.6 mg/kg	LD 8, MD 4
Tobramycin	0.6 mg/kg	LD 8, MD 4
Cephalosporins		
Cefazolin	15 mg/kg	LD 500, MD 125
Cefepime	1 g	LD 500, MD 125
Cephradine	15 mg/kg	LD 500, MD 125
Ceftazidime	1,000–1,500 mg	LD 500, MD 125
Ceftizoxime	1,000 mg	LD 250, MD 125
Penicillins		
Ampicillin	ND	MD 125
Oxacillin	ND	MD 125
Nafcillin	ND	MD 125
Amoxicillin	ND	LD 250–500, MD 50
Penicillin G	ND	LD 50,000 units, MD 25,000 units
Quinolones		
Ciprofloxacin	ND	LD 50, MD 25
Others		
Vancomycin	15–30 mg/kg q5–7d	LD 1,000, MD 25
Aztreonam	ND	LD 1,000, MD 250
Antifungals		
Amphotericin	NA	1.5
Combinations		
Ampicillin/sulbactam	2 g q12h	LD 1,000, MD 100
Imipenem/cilistatin	1 g BID	LD 500, MD 200
Quinupristin/dalfopristin	25 mg/L in alternate bags[a]	

LD, loading dose in mg; MD, maintenance dose in mg; NA, not applicable; ND, no data.
[a] Stable in dialysate at concentrations from 150 to 600 mg/L.
(Adapted from Piraino P, Bailie GR, Bernardini J, et al. Peritoneal dialysis-related infections recommendations: 2005 update. Perit Dial Int 25:107–131, 2005.)

microbial peritonitis due to multiple gram-positive organisms is most likely due to contamination or catheter infection; the patient's technique should be reviewed and the exit site carefully examined. Polymicrobial peritonitis due to contamination generally resolves with antibiotics without catheter removal, unless the catheter is the source of the infection.

Fungal Organisms on Culture. Fungal peritonitis is a serious infection leading to death in approximately 25% or more of episodes.[121] Initial therapy should include prompt catheter removal and antifungal therapy with the combination of amphotericin B and flucytosine until the culture results with susceptibilities are available. Caspofungin, fluconazole, or voriconazole may replace amphotericin B, based on the species identification and minimum inhibitory concentration (MIC) values. Intraperitoneal use of amphotericin causes chemical peritonitis and pain, while intravenous use leads to poor peritoneal administration. Voriconazole is an alterna-

TABLE 44.10	Intraperitoneal Dosing of Antibiotics for Automated Peritoneal Dialysis Patients
Drug	**Intraperitoneal (IP) Dose**
Vancomycin	Loading dose 30 mg/kg IP in long dwell, repeat dosing 15 mg/kg IP in long dwell every 3–5 days, following levels
Cefazolin	20 mg/kg IP every day, in long day dwell
Tobramycin	Loading dose 1.5 mg/kg IP in long dwell, then 0.5 mg/kg IP each day in long day dwell.
Fluconazole	200 mg IP in one exchange per day every 24–48 h
Cefepime	1 g IP in one exchange per day

(Adapted from Piraino P, Bailie GR, Bernardini J, et al. Peritoneal dialysis-related infections recommendations: 2005 update. Perit Dial Int 25:107–131, 2005.)

tive for amphotericin B when filamentous fungi has been cultured; it can be used alone for candidal peritonitis (with catheter removal).

Exit-Site and Tunnel Infections. Exit-site and tunnel infections occur at a rate of about one episode every 1 to 2.5 patient-years.[132] Exit-site and tunnel infections are most commonly caused by S. aureus and P. aeruginosa but may be caused by a variety of microorganisms.

An exit-site infection is defined by the presence of purulent drainage, with or without erythema of the skin, at the catheter–epidermal interface. Other symptoms include heat, drainage, odor, tenderness, and pain. A tunnel infection may present with erythema, edema, or tenderness over the subcutaneous pathway, but is often clinically occult and usually occurs in the presence of an exit-site infection. A tunnel infection rarely occurs alone and often precedes the development of peritonitis. It may be difficult to differentiate between exit-site and tunnel infections.[121]

Treatment of exit-site infections has included systemic and intraperitoneal antibiotics, topical antibiotics and disinfectants, débridement of the infected subcutaneous cuff, and catheter removal.[113,121] If empiric antibiotic therapy is initiated, it should include coverage for S. aureus and possibly P. aeruginosa if the patient has had a P. aeruginosa infection in the past.[121] If empiric antibiotics are not given, results from a Gram stain of exit-site drainage can guide initial therapy. Oral antibiotic therapy has been shown to be as effective as intraperitoneal antibiotics. Antibiotic therapy must be continued for at least 2 weeks, until the exit site appears entirely normal. If antibiotic therapy fails to resolve the infection or if peritonitis develops, the catheter may need to be replaced.[121]

Prevention of Peritoneal Dialysis-Related Infections. Every effort should be made to reduce peritoneal dialysis-related infections, as they may lead to dialysis tech-

nique failure, hospitalization, and, in some cases, death.[121] Dialysis clinics should monitor all peritoneal dialysis-related infections as part of a continuous quality improvement program. Infection rates for the dialysis clinic as well as for individual organisms should also be determined and compared to published reports. The ISPD guidelines recommend that the peritonitis rate should be no more than one episode every 18 months (0.67 per year at risk).[121]

Because peritoneal dialysis entails frequent manipulation of the dialysis catheter through repeated connections and disconnections of the administration set, the patient and/or caregiver must be trained to use aseptic technique. Recent advances in the disconnect systems using the flush-before-fill technique (e.g., Y-connector set) have limited the manipulations needed during exchanges, thus reducing the incidence of peritonitis and exit-site and tunnel infections caused by touch contamination, mainly by reducing S. epidermidis, polymicrobial, and other gram-positive infections.[132,133] Unfortunately, the rates of S. aureus and gram-negative infections have not changed.[133,134]

Methods to reduce a center's infection rate may include root cause analyses for each episode and possibly retraining patients to perform aseptic technique during peritoneal dialysis exchanges. At the time of peritoneal dialysis catheter placement, patients should be free of constipation and prophylactic antibiotics (vancomycin 1 g or cefazolin 1 g intravenously) should be administered in an effort to reduce the risk of infection.[121] Prophylactic vancomycin is superior to cefazolin in prevention of peritonitis, but each center must weigh the risk of developing vancomycin-resistant organisms and use vancomycin judiciously. Prophylactic antibiotics before abdominal procedures (ampicillin 1 g plus a single dose of an aminoglycoside, with or without metronidazole) or dental procedures (amoxicillin 2 g) may also be administered. Finally, appropriate peritoneal dialysis catheter care is essential in prevention of peritoneal dialysis-associated infections. Appropriate peritoneal dialysis catheter care includes antibacterial soap and water or an antiseptic (povidone–iodine or chlorhexidine) to clean the exit site (hydrogen peroxide is drying and should be avoided); immobilization of the catheter to prevent pulling and trauma; and daily application of topical antibiotics (e.g., mupirocin cream or ointment, gentamicin ointment, or ciprofloxacin otic solution) to the skin around the exit site to reduce S. aureus and P. aeruginosa (gentamicin and ciprofloxacin only). Mupirocin ointment should be avoided in patients with polyurethane peritoneal dialysis catheters, as structural damage to the catheter may occur.[121]

The nasal carriage of S. aureus is an established predisposing factor for peritonitis and tunnel and exit-site infections.[121] Up to 60% of patients on dialysis are nasal carriers of this organism, compared to 10% to 30% of the general population; the rate is even higher among diabetic patients.[134] Eradicating nasal S. aureus with intranasal mupirocin 2% ointment, administered twice daily for 5 days of every month, can reduce the incidence of peritonitis and exit-site infection by *S. aureus*;[135] however, the incidence of infections with other gram-positive and gram-negative bacteria may simultaneously increase. Rifampin 300 mg twice daily for 5 consecutive days every 12 weeks can prevent peritonitis and exit-site infections without a significant effect on nasal carriage of *S. aureus*.[136] Thus, patients with recurrent CAPD infections may benefit from one of these intermittent treatment regimens.

Cardiovascular Complications. Many of the cardiovascular complications of ESRD that are associated with hemodialysis are less prevalent in peritoneal dialysis patients.[137] The continuous nature of CAPD prevents the large, rapid volume shifts of hemodialysis, thus minimizing the risk of rapid reduction in left ventricular pressure and hypotension. However, aggressive fluid removal with the use of hypertonic (4.25% hydrous dextrose) solutions occasionally results in hypotension, usually orthostatic hypotension.[138] Compared with patients not on dialysis, patients on CAPD have lower left ventricular end-diastolic and end-systolic volumes, a lower stroke index and cardiac index, and a faster myocardial contraction speed.[137]

Recently a national cohort of 107,922 patients starting dialysis therapy between May 1995 and July 1997 were classified on the basis of coronary artery disease (CAD) presence and followed until death or the end of 2 years.[50] Among patients with diabetes, patients with CAD treated with peritoneal dialysis had a 23% higher relative risk of death compared with similar hemodialysis patients, whereas patients without CAD receiving peritoneal dialysis had a 17% higher relative risk of death compared with hemodialysis. Among patients without diabetes, patients with CAD treated with peritoneal dialysis had a 20% higher relative risk of death compared with hemodialysis patients, whereas patients without CAD had similar survival on peritoneal dialysis or hemodialysis. It was concluded that the mortality risk for new ESRD patients with CAD differed by treatment modality. For both the diabetic and nondiabetic patients, those with CAD treated with peritoneal dialysis had significantly poorer survival compared with patients receiving hemodialysis.

Evaluation of the same data set also revealed that mortality risks were significantly higher for patients with congestive heart failure (CHF) treated with peritoneal dialysis than for those treated with hemodialysis.[54] Among patients without CHF, the adjusted mortality risk was higher only for diabetic patients treated with peritoneal dialysis compared with hemodialysis; nondiabetics had similar survival on peritoneal dialysis or hemodialysis. The authors concluded that new ESRD patients with a clinical history of CHF experienced poorer survival when treated with peritoneal dialysis compared with hemodialysis. These more recent data suggest that peritoneal dialysis may not be the optimal choice for new ESRD patients with CHF, perhaps through impaired volume regulation and worsening cardiomyopathy.

In a report from the Netherlands Cooperative Study on the Adequacy of Dialysis, a multicenter, prospective, obser-vational, cohort study in which new patients with ESRD were monitored until transplantation or death, a decrease in mortality rate was observed for the period of 24 to 48 months in the hemodialysis patients, while an increase in mortality was observed during that same time for patients on peritoneal dialysis. This favorable effect of hemodialysis was particularly notable for patients more than 60 years of age and occurred in patients with and without cardiovascular risk factors.[55]

Additional studies are needed to better characterize the factors associated with mortality in the dialysis population; however, these studies provide some evidence that hemodialysis should be considered for ESRD patients with certain comorbid conditions.

Increased Intraabdominal Pressure. The infusion of peritoneal dialysate increases the intraabdominal pressure up to five times without a significant increase in pressure inside the stomach or at the lower esophageal sphincter.[120,139] This increased intraabdominal pressure can increase the stress on structures of the abdomen and lead to a number of complications, including a sensation of bloating and symptoms of esophageal reflux.[116,120] The dialysate-induced increase in intraabdominal pressure can push against the diaphragm in a manner similar to that observed during pregnancy or obesity. The resulting upward displacement of the diaphragm decreases the functional residual capacity of the lungs. If severe enough, it may lead to small airway collapse, ventilation/perfusion mismatch, and arterial hypoxemia. Paradoxically, a less severe displacement may actually improve the efficiency of diaphragmatic contraction and improve ventilation.[139] A serious complication of peritoneal dialysis is the leakage of dialysate across the diaphragm, resulting in hydrothorax (i.e., fluid in the pleural cavity).[120] Although mild hydrothorax may be asymptomatic, life-threatening respiratory compromise may occur in severe cases.[139] The most common clinical manifestations include dyspnea, chest pain, hypotension, and, in rare instances, atrial fibrillation.[140]

The goal of treatment is to resolve the pleural effusion and prevent its recurrence. CAPD should be discontinued temporarily until the effusion regresses spontaneously.[139] For severe dyspnea or cardiovascular instability, a chest tube may be placed to allow drainage of fluid.[140] If hydrothorax recurs, surgical repair may be necessary. Alternatively, the pleural space can be closed off with talcum powder, iodized talc, triamcinolone acetonide, fibrin adhesive, or autologous blood instillation.

The increased intraabdominal pressure places excess stress on the lumbar vertebrae. In the presence of poor abdominal muscle tone, the spinal stress increases, leading to back pain or sciatica. Treatment involves the use of smaller dialysate volumes, although this may compromise dialysis adequacy. The optimal solution may be to start the patient on nightly intermittent peritoneal dialysis.[139]

Hernias. Up to one quarter of patients on CAPD develop a hernia, most commonly at the site of the incision for catheter insertion, the inguinal canal, or the umbilicus.[120,139] If the hernia is left untreated, bowel incarceration and strangulation may ensue, necessitating emergency surgery. Hernia treatment usually involves surgical correction.[120,141]

Loss of Ultrafiltration. Although rare, a loss of ultrafiltration is troublesome because it may necessitate discontinuation of peritoneal dialysis. There are two types of ultrafiltration failure. Most cases are type I failure, in which the permeability of the peritoneal membrane to glucose is increased, resulting in rapid absorption of intraperitoneal glucose and loss of transmembrane osmotic gradient. Although the ability to remove fluid is lost, the clearance of other solutes, such as creatinine or urea, is maintained or even increased because their removal depends on diffusion. Type I ultrafiltration failure usually occurs in patients who are on long-term CAPD but can also occur during bouts of peritonitis, when peritoneal permeability and intraperitoneal glucose absorption increase. Treating type I ultrafiltration failure involves the use of hypertonic dialysate (4.25%) and more frequent dialysis exchanges.[120,130]

Type II ultrafiltration failure is caused by a reduction in effective peritoneal surface area that results from extensive scar tissue formation (fibrosis) and peritoneal adhesions. Permeability to glucose remains normal or is decreased. Type II failure most commonly results from severe and prolonged peritonitis, usually caused by *S. aureus* or a fungus, and often necessitates discontinuation of CAPD.[130]

FUTURE THERAPIES

Patients with ESRD typically receive in-center intermittent hemodialysis three times per week for 3 to 5 hours, or some variant of peritoneal dialysis. There is a small subset of hemodialysis patients, approximately 250 to 300 nationwide, who dialyze at home daily.[4] While there are many variants of daily dialysis, this treatment may become more widespread because it has been shown that increased frequency and longer duration of treatment results in improved patient outcomes.[142–146] A multicenter trial sponsored by the National Institutes of Health, which began in July 2005, will investigate the long-term outcomes and cost-effectiveness of this therapy.

Advances in peritoneal dialysis involve using continuous-flow peritoneal dialysate.[147] This technique maintains a fixed intraperitoneal volume and rapid, continuous movement of dialysate into and out of the peritoneal cavity. This peritoneal dialysis prescription requires two peritoneal dialysis catheters, an inlet and an outlet catheter, and a means of generating a large volume of sterile dialysate. Dialysate is generated via conventional hemodialysis equipment or sorbent technology. Clearance of small solutes is three to eight times greater than with automated peritoneal dialysis and approximates that with daily hemodialysis.[147,148] Potential applications include daily home dialysis, treatment of

acute renal failure in the intensive care unit, and ultrafiltration of ascites.[147]

PHARMACOTHERAPEUTIC CONSIDERATIONS FOR PATIENTS ON DIALYSIS

Management of secondary complications of CKD is discussed in Chapter 43. A key consideration for all such complications is early intervention, prior to the development of the final stage or ESRD. While in many cases the principles of managing these complications are the same regardless of the stage of CKD, there are some unique considerations for patients requiring dialysis, either hemodialysis or peritoneal dialysis. This section will highlight some of the special considerations for common secondary complications in patients with ESRD.

ANEMIA

Most patients with ESRD will require erythropoietic therapy (i.e., epoetin alfa or darbepoetin alfa) to correct the relative deficiency in endogenous erythropoietin. In many cases patients have not received erythropoietic or iron supplementation prior to the start of dialysis and have hemoglobin and hematocrit values below target values—hemoglobin less than 11 to 12 g per dL (110 to 120 g/L), hematocrit less than 33% to 36%.[149] Conditions associated with poor anemia management are also prevalent in the ESRD population, including LVH, with a reported prevalence of 74% by the time patients start dialysis.[150] Fortunately, anemia is well recognized as a complication in the ESRD population, and most dialysis centers have anemia management protocols in place to achieve the target hemoglobin, hematocrit, and iron indices recommended by the NKF-K/DOQI Clinical Practice Guidelines for Anemia.[151] Dialysis centers are reimbursed for medications administered in conjunction with dialysis treatments (depending on reported outcome measures), which avoids some, but certainly not all, of the challenges with reimbursement that exist when implementing erythropoietic therapy for patients with CKD not on dialysis. Patients on hemodialysis receive erythropoietic therapy either intravenously, typically three times per week, or subcutaneously, generally one to three times per week. The NKF-K/DOQI guidelines recommend subcutaneous administration, but many dialysis centers continue to administer these agents by the intravenous route. The subcutaneous route of administration is common in patients receiving peritoneal dialysis since they do not have regular intravenous access.

With regard to iron status, patients with ESRD generally are in environments where more consistent monitoring of iron status is done (e.g., monthly or quarterly). Patients with iron indices below the target values, transferrin saturation (TSat) less than 20% to 50%, serum ferritin less than 100 to 800 ng per mL (<224.7 to 1,797 pmol/L), will typically receive a 1-g course of intravenous iron therapy (in divided doses). Iron dextran (INFeD, Dexferrum) has been replaced in many centers with newer agents [sodium ferric gluconate (Ferrlecit), iron sucrose (Venofer)] that have a better safety profile and less risk of anaphylactic reactions.[152,153] Maintenance iron (weekly or monthly) in doses ranging from 25 to 200 mg, depending on the formulation used, is also a common method of supplementation to avoid iron deficiency.[154] Oral iron supplementation of at least 200 mg of elemental iron per day remains a common regimen in patients receiving peritoneal dialysis since regular intravenous access is not available; however, intravenous iron may be required in patients below the recommended target iron indices despite oral therapy.

Reasons for lack of response to erythropoietic therapy or resistance to therapy in addition to iron deficiency include active inflammation, severe hyperparathyroidism, and aluminum overload (although now less common). A factor that contributes even more to development of anemia in the hemodialysis population is the blood loss with regular hemodialysis therapy. This may account for some of the differences in the requirement for erythropoietic therapy in the hemodialysis population when compared to patients on peritoneal dialysis. Specifically, lower doses and less frequent administration of erythropoietic therapy are required in the peritoneal dialysis population.[155,156] Providing adequate dialysis may also improve anemia management, as demonstrated in the hemodialysis population. Reduced doses of erythropoietic agents were required in iron-replete hemodialysis patients receiving adequate dialysis as measured by Kt/V.[156] Improved response to erythropoietic therapy with carnitine administration has also been shown, although inconsistently.[157,158] The NKF-K/DOQI nutrition guidelines support a trial of L-carnitine (approximately 1 g intravenously or orally following dialysis) for patients not responding to relatively large doses of erythropoietic therapy.[37]

HYPERTENSION

Hypertension is a major modifiable cardiovascular risk factor in patients with ESRD but is still found in up to 80% of hemodialysis and 50% of peritoneal dialysis patients.[92,159] Inadequate blood pressure control accelerates atherosclerosis and contributes to cardiovascular mortality, the leading cause of death in patients with ESRD.[5] In fact, the mortality rate from cardiovascular disease is 10 to 20 times higher in the ESRD population than in the general population.[91,92] The mechanism of hypertension in the ESRD population is due not only to extracellular volume expansion, but also to other contributing factors, including increased sympathetic activity, elevated levels of endothelin-1, erythropoietin use, hyperparathyroidism, and structural changes in the arteries (e.g., metastatic calcification).[92,159] Blood pressure patterns in ESRD patients also lack the diurnal variation seen in the general population. The timing of blood pressure monitoring relative to hemodialysis is also a consideration, since variations occur during the hemodialysis procedure with ultrafiltration; hence, the predialysis and postdialysis blood pressure measurements may be substantially different. Increased risk of mortality in the ESRD population has been associated with both a high and low predialysis and postdialysis systolic blood pressure reading, referred to as a bimodal or "U-shaped" relationship.[160]

Recently, NKF/KDOQ1 guidelines were made available on the target blood pressure in dialysis patients.[161] Predialysis and postdialysis blood pressure goals should be <140/90 mm Hg and <130/80 mm Hg, respectively.[161] Blood pressure control requires management of fluid status (i.e., dry weight), antihypertensive medications, and a multidisciplinary approach. Patients should be educated by a dietitian on a low-sodium diet (2–3 g/day) and avoid medications that increase thirst. Removal of excess fluid from patients may require increased ultrafiltration or longer or more frequent dialysis treatments per week. Initial medication therapy should include ACE inhibitors or angiotensin II receptor blockers, as these agents also cause greater regression of LVH, reduce sympathetic nerve activity, reduce pulse wave velocity, may improve endothelial function, and may reduce oxidative stress.[161] However, dialysis patients oftentimes require several medications to control their blood pressure. Additional antihypertensive medications should be selected based on the individual dialysis patient's "compelling indications" (e.g., beta-blocker use in patients with heart failure, angina, or postmyocardial infarction) and dialyzability characteristics.[161] Patients should be counseled to take their antihypertensive medications at night, because it may reduce the nocturnal surge of blood pressure and minimize intradialytic hypotension.[161] Reasons for poorly controlled blood pressure in dialysis patients include physician satisfaction with the predialysis blood pressure level, patient noncompliance with restrictions on fluid and sodium intake, inadequate ultrafiltration during dialysis, inadequate dialysis, inappropriate antihypertensive therapy or noncompliance with therapy, and underlying secondary forms of hypertension.[159,162]

Hypertension in patients on dialysis can be treated by dialytic removal of sodium and water in conjunction with reduction in salt and fluid intake to maintain extracellular fluid volume (e.g., maintain the patient's dry weight). Antihypertensive therapy should be added as needed to improve blood pressure control. Fluid volume may be better controlled early in the course of peritoneal dialysis compared with hemodialysis, related in part to the patient's residual kidney function.[47] Furthermore, because of the slow correction and more stable control of sodium and water balance with peritoneal dialysis, management of hypertension may be easier; in fact, a significant number of patients on peritoneal dialysis may not need antihypertensive agents. It is reasonable also to follow recommendations from the seventh report of the Joint National Committee on the Prevention and Treatment of Hypertension (JNC-7) specific to lifestyle modifications (e.g., reduced saturated fat and cholesterol intake, smoking cessation).[163] Counseling by a dietitian is a routine component in caring for the patient with ESRD, given the extensive fluid and dietary restrictions necessary not only for blood pressure control but also for other secondary complications of ESRD (e.g., hyperphosphatemia).

The selection of antihypertensive therapy should take into consideration other comorbid conditions such as diabetes mellitus, coronary heart disease, myocardial infarction, and depression and the side effect profile. Lower starting doses are necessary in older adults and for agents predominantly eliminated by the kidney. Agents that are removed by dialysis may be given after the dialysis procedure for hemodialysis patients. In general, blood pressure can be reduced effectively by all classes of antihypertensive agents other than diuretics (e.g., ACE inhibitors, angiotensin receptor antagonists, long-acting calcium channel blockers, β-blockers). High doses of individual medications and combination therapy may be required. Agents including sympathetic nervous system active agents (prazosin, clonidine) or vasodilators (minoxidil, hydralazine) may be added for patients unresponsive to more standard therapies (e.g., ACE inhibitors, angiotensin receptor antagonists, calcium channel blockers, β-blockers). Side effects of these agents such as postural hypotension (e.g., prazosin) and reflex tachycardia (e.g., minoxidil) must be considered when individualizing therapy.

HYPERLIPIDEMIA AND ATHEROSCLEROSIS

The increased incidence of atherosclerotic cardiovascular disease in patients with CKD compared to the general population supports the recommendation that CKD patients be considered in the highest risk category when evaluated for specific interventions.[164] Management of dyslipidemia in patients with CKD is based on the report from the National Cholesterol Education Program (NCEP III) and the NKF-K/DOQI guidelines for dyslipidemia in patients with CKD.[164,165] Although diet therapy is a reasonable first-step approach, it may not be successful in many patients with ESRD because of noncompliance. A dietitian well versed in management of kidney disease should be consulted.

Since cardiovascular diseases such as myocardial infarction, cardiac failure, and stroke account for the majority of deaths in the ESRD population, hypercholesterolemia should be treated aggressively. Goals for patients with stage 5 CKD based on lipid abnormality and the suggested therapies are listed in Table 44.11. Statins are indicated to lower LDL to acceptable levels in CKD patients based on efficacy and additional benefits observed in the general population, including the reduction in cardiovascular events and all-cause mortality.[92,164] Drug therapy for hypertriglyceridemia includes a fibrate or niacin. In general, fibrates are better tolerated than nicotinic acid. Caveats of using these agents (e.g., dose titration and monitoring for adverse effects) may be found in Chapter 41. Sevelamer (Renagel), used as a phosphate-binding agent in patients with ESRD, also has been shown to significantly decrease LDL cholesterol.[166]

Cardiovascular Considerations. In addition to traditional cardiac risk factors (e.g., hypertension, diabetes), patients with ESRD have other factors that increase the risk of cardiovascular events. Among these are hyperhomocystinemia, elevated levels of C-reactive protein, increased oxidant stress, and hemodynamic overload.[92] Homocysteine levels are elevated in both hemodialysis and peritoneal dialysis patients, with estimates of elevated levels in more than 90% of patients.[167] Pharmacologic doses of folic acid (i.e., 5 to 15 mg/day) reduce homocysteine levels in patients on dialysis, although this finding is not consistent and no studies clearly demonstrate that lowering homocysteine levels leads to improved cardiovascular outcomes.[167–169] Further research should focus on identifying better methods to treat hyperhomocystinemia and evaluate the effects of treatment on patient outcomes and survival before routine interventions to lower homocysteine in this population can be recommended.

Other factors predisposing to chronic cardiovascular complications in ESRD patients include predialytic hypertension, chronic anemia, hyperparathyroidism, disorders of calcium, phosphorus, and vitamin D, volume overload, and high-output cardiac failure. Myocardial calcification and fibrosis contribute to the development of heart failure (especially diastolic dysfunction). In addition to considerations in

TABLE 44.11	Management of Dyslipidemias in ESRD Patients			
Dyslipidemia	Goal	Initial Therapy	Modification in Therapy	Alternative
TG ≥500 mg/dL (≥5.65 mmol/L)	TG <500 mg/dL (<5.65 mmol/L)	TLC	TLC + fibrate or niacin	Fibrate or niacin
LDL 100–129 mg/dL (2.59–3.34 mmol/L)	LDL <100 mg/dL (<2.59 mmol/L)	TLC	TLC + low-dose statin	Bile acid sequestrant or niacin
LDL ≥130 mg/dL (≥3.37 mmol/L)	LDL <100 mg/dL (<2.59 mmol/L)	TLC + low-dose statin	TLC + max-dose statin	Bile acid sequestrant or niacin
TG ≥200 mg/dL (2.26 mmol/L) and non-HDL ≥130 mg/dL (≥3.37 mmol/L)	Non-HDL <130 mg/dL (<3.37 mmol/L)	TLC + low-dose statin	TLC + max-dose statin	Fibrate or niacin

TLC, therapeutic lifestyle changes.

(From K/DOQI clinical practice guidelines for management of dyslipidemias in patients with kidney disease. Am J Kidney Dis 41 (Suppl 3):I–IV, S1–91, 2003.)

the general population to reduce cardiovascular complications (e.g., treatment of hypertension, hyperlipidemia, smoking cessation), these other unique factors need to be addressed in patients with ESRD.

METABOLIC ACIDOSIS

Metabolic acidosis is common in patients with ESRD and is the result of reduced acid secretion in conjunction with decreased bicarbonate production. Bicarbonate levels in ESRD patients are determined by factors such as the rate of endogenous acid production, characteristics of the dialysis prescription, organic anion loss during dialysis, and loss or gain from the gastrointestinal tract.[170,171] Uncorrected chronic metabolic acidosis has significant negative clinical effects on bone turnover through direct actions of bone, stimulation of PTH secretion, and suppression of vitamin D synthesis. Hyperkalemia is also a result of metabolic acidosis. Acidosis also stimulates protein catabolism and amino acid oxidation and may worsen uremia.[171]

Several technical problems with measuring bicarbonate must be considered when interpreting laboratory data. Underfilling of sample tubes and transport of samples to facilities off site that result in long delays in the measurement (a common practice with dialysis centers) can result in falsely low values for bicarbonate (as total CO_2) reported by the laboratory.[171] This is thought to be due to the increased probability of air coming in contact with blood during these situations. For more accurate values, blood should not be allowed to have contact with air, delays in processing of the sample should be avoided, and the same laboratory and methods of analysis should be used for serial measurements.[37,171]

The goals of therapy of metabolic acidosis in patients with ESRD are to normalize the pH of the blood (pH of approximately 7.35 to 7.45) and to maintain the serum bicarbonate within the normal range (22 to 28 mEq/L; 22 to 28 mmol/L). In patients on hemodialysis, the goal of therapy is to maintain a predialysis or stabilized bicarbonate concentration of at least 22 mEq per L (22 mol/L).[37] Acid–base homeostasis in patients on dialysis is accomplished by bicarbonate transfer (as bicarbonate or lactate) across the dialysis membrane (i.e., from an area of higher concentration in the dialysate to the area of lower concentration in the blood). Dialysate bicarbonate concentrations of more than 38 mEq per L are used to safely increase predialysis serum bicarbonate concentrations. Oral administration of sodium bicarbonate (approximately 2 to 4 g/day or 25 to 50 mEq/day) may also be used, although this practice in more common in CKD patients not requiring dialysis.[37]

SECONDARY HYPERPARATHYROIDISM AND RENAL OSTEODYSTROPHY

Secondary hyperparathyroidism and associated metabolic abnormalities are common early in the course of CKD and worsen as kidney function declines. Specifically, phosphorus excretion by the kidney further declines, leading to more severe hyperphosphatemia in ESRD patients. Conversion of vitamin D to its active form (1,25-dihydroxyvitamin D_3 or calcitriol) by the kidney is further impaired. Calcium irregu-

larities may shift from hypocalcemia in the earlier stages of CKD to hypercalcemia as kidney disease progresses, due in large part to the use of calcium-containing phosphate binders. Negative outcomes, including metastatic calcification of joints, vessels, and soft tissue and increased mortality, have been associated with hyperphosphatemia and an elevated calcium and phosphorus product.[172,173]

In the ESRD population, bone disease is a long-term manifestation of secondary hyperparathyroidism. Fractures frequently occur and are associated with an increased risk of mortality.[174] Bone disease in dialysis patients most often manifests as osteitis fibrosa cystica, a high-turnover bone disease. Osteomalacia and adynamic lesions (caused by low bone turnover) have also been characterized. The incidence of adynamic lesions has increased over the past 10 years, predominantly because of aggressive management of osteitis fibrosa cystica with vitamin D therapy. Renal osteodystrophy often progresses insidiously for several years before patients become symptomatic. When bone pain and skeletal fractures occur, the disease is not easily amenable to treatment.

As is the case for many secondary complications of CKD, secondary hyperparathyroidism is poorly managed prior to the development of ESRD, increasing the risk of bone disease and other negative outcomes associated with this disorder.[149,175] Efforts should be made to intervene well before patients progress to ESRD, using recommendations from the NKF-K/DOQI Guidelines on Bone Metabolism and Disease as a basis for management.[175] Goals of management of secondary hyperparathyroidism and the associated metabolic abnormalities are to control serum phosphorus and PTH concentrations and normalize the serum calcium concentration. These general goals apply to all states of CKD; however, specific targets for calcium, phosphorus, and PTH differ in patients with ESRD.[175] Goals specific to stage 5 CKD or ESRD (and the comparison with earlier stages of CKD) are a calcium level of 8.4 to 9.5 mg per dL (2.1 to 2.38 mmol/L) (narrower range), a phosphorus level of 3.5 to 5.5 mg per dL (1.13 to 1.78 mmol/L) (slightly higher range), an intact PTH level of 150 to 300 pg per dL (higher target to maintain normal bone turnover), and a Ca × P of 55 mg^2 per dL^2 (same target goal).

When evaluating PTH levels, it is important to know the assay used. Some assays (e.g., immunoradiometric assay for intact PTH) measure not only the intact molecule, but also fragments with variable activity. A new assay called the whole PTH or Bio-Intact PTH that detects the full-length PTH molecule is now being used by some dialysis centers. The target Bio-Intact PTH is approximately half the recommended intact PTH (i.e., the target intact PTH value of 150 to 300 pg/mL corresponds with a Bio-Intact PTH of 75 to 150 pg/mL).[176]

As for all stages of CKD, dietary intervention is critical. The NKF-K/DOQI guidelines recommend phosphorus restriction to 800 to 1,000 mg per day.[175] The challenge with dietary restriction of phosphorus is limiting phosphorus while providing enough protein to prevent malnutrition in patients on dialysis who have higher protein needs (see section, "Nutrition" later in this chapter). Removal of phosphorus does occur with hemodialysis and peritoneal dialysis (approximately 2 to 3 g per week, depending on the dialysis prescription); however, dialysis alone does not adequately control hyperphosphatemia. Dietary restriction and phosphate binders are also required.

In an effort to maintain the recommended calcium target, the NKF-K/DOQI guidelines recommend that the total dose of elemental calcium provided by calcium-containing binders not exceed 1,500 mg per day and the total daily intake from both binders and dietary sources not exceed 2,000 mg.[175] Sevelamer (Renagel) is a nonelemental phosphate binder that is frequently used in patients with ESRD and is not associated with cardiovascular calcifications.[177] It also has a cardiovascular benefit through its observed decrease in LDL cholesterol.[166] A more detailed discussion of the available phosphate-binding agents is found in Chapter 43. The dialysate calcium concentration recommended to further reduce the calcium load is 2.5 mEq per L (1.25 mmol/L).[175]

Vitamin D supplementation is often necessary in patients with ESRD to achieve the target level for intact PTH. The vitamin D analogues paricalcitol (Zemplar), also referred to as 19-nor-1,25-dihydroxyvitamin D_2, and doxercalciferol (Hectorol), or 1-α-hydroxyvitamin D_2, are commonly part of the protocol for management of secondary hyperparathyroidism in chronic dialysis centers. These agents are vitamin D_2 compounds and vary in their affinity for the vitamin D receptor compared to calcitriol. They were developed to retain the suppressive effect on PTH release while decreasing the potential for hypercalcemia relative to calcitriol. Recommended doses for patients with ESRD are listed in Table 44.12.

Cinacalcet (Sensipar) is a calcimimetic agent (currently the only agent in its class) that works by increasing sensitivity of the calcium-sensing receptor of the parathyroid gland to extracellular calcium, resulting in decreased secretion of PTH.[178] Currently this agent is approved for treatment of secondary hyperparathyroidism only in patients with ESRD. Cinacalcet does have the potential to cause hypocalcemia and should not be started if the calcium level is less than 8.4 mg per dL (<2.1 mmol/L). The recommended starting dose in patients with ESRD is 30 mg once daily, with dose titrations made in approximately 30-mg increments every 2 to 4 weeks up to 180 mg per day or until the target PTH (150 to 300 pg/mL) is achieved. Doses up to 300 mg per day have been safely administered. The potential for drug interactions should be evaluated in all patients, since cinacalcet is metabolized by cytochrome P450 enzymes CYP3A4, CYP2D6, and CYP1A1, and is a strong inhibitor of CYP2D6. This agent may be used alone or in combination with vitamin D and phosphate binders. The challenge clinically is to determine how to best use this agent in conjunction with existing therapies and in the context of the current NKF-K/DOQI guidelines, which were developed prior to approval of cinacalcet and do not include this agent in the recommended treatment algorithms.[175]

The NKF-K/DOQI guidelines for bone metabolism and disease recommend surgery in cases of persistently elevated intact PTH levels (>800 pg/mL) associated with hypercalcemia and/or hyperphosphatemia that are refractory to medical therapy.[175] Subtotal parathyroidectomy or total parathyroidectomy, with transplantation of some parathyroid tissue to an accessible site (e.g., the forearm), is the most common surgical procedure. Postoperative hypocalcemia, hypophosphatemia, and hypomagnesemia may be severe and necessitate treatment with supplemental calcium and calcitriol for weeks or months. After surgery, continual efforts to prevent hyperphosphatemia and the recurrence of secondary hyperparathyroidism may be necessary.

TABLE 44.12	Dosing Recommendations for Vitamin D in Patients with ESRD		
PTH (pg/mL)	IV & PO Calcitriol (dose per hemodialysis)[a]	IV Paricalcitol (dose per hemodialysis)	PO & IV Doxercalciferol (dose per hemodialysis)[a]
300–600[b]	0.5–1.5 μg PO or IV	2.5–5.0 μg	5 μg PO / 2 μg IV
600–1,000[b]	1–4 μg PO / 1–3 μg IV	6.0–10 μg	5–10 μg PO / 2–4 μg IV
>1,000[c]	3–7 μg PO / 3–5 μg IV	10–15 μg	10–20 μg PO / 4–8 μg IV

PTH, parathyroid hormone; PO, orally; IV, intravenously.

[a] Oral doses of calcitriol (0.5–1.0 μg) or doxercalciferol (2.5–5.0 μg) may be used in peritoneal dialysis patients two or three times weekly. Alternative is daily calcitriol at 0.25 μg QD; [b] if serum calcium is <9.5 mg/dL, phosphorus is <5.5 mg/dL, and Ca × P is <55 mg²/dL²; [c] if serum calcium is <10 mg/dL, phosphorus is <5.5 mg/dL, and Ca × P is <55 mg²/dL².

(From Eknoyan G, Levin A, Levin NW. Bone metabolism and disease in chronic kidney disease. Am J Kidney Dis 42 (Suppl 3):1–201, 2003.)

NUTRITION

Protein–energy malnutrition is a common finding among patients with ESRD and is not often appropriately recognized or addressed in the earlier stages of CKD. Protein–energy intake is often insufficient due to the dietary restrictions implemented in the earlier stages of CKD (e.g., protein restriction to delay progression) and the changes that occur in the presence of uremia, such as anorexia and taste alterations. Certain conditions, such as acidosis and inflammatory conditions, worsen as CKD progresses to ESRD and create a catabolic environment. In addition, dialysis not only removes uremic toxins (the desired effect) but also promotes loss of nutrients, including amino acids, proteins (particularly with peritoneal dialysis) and vitamins. Supplementation of water-soluble vitamins (vitamins B and C and folic acid) to account for losses during dialysis is routine in both hemodialysis and peritoneal dialysis patients. In the pediatric population, additional factors that contribute to impaired growth include calcitriol deficiency and tissue resistance to the actions of growth hormone and insulin-like growth factor.[37] Protein–energy malnutrition may be indicated by reduced energy stores (subcutaneous fat stores), reduced muscle mass, decreased BUN (marker of dietary protein intake), low serum concentrations of albumin, transferrin, and other visceral proteins, abnormalities in the plasma and intracellular amino acids profiles, and low cholesterol (marker of dietary intake).

While there are many negative outcomes of malnutrition, hypoalbuminemia and protein–energy malnutrition are both independently predictive of mortality in dialysis patients.[37,179,180] The risk of death increases exponentially with decreasing serum albumin values. With a reference value of 4 g per dL (40 g/L), a serum albumin value of 3.5 to 4.0 g per dL (35 to 40 g/L), which is still within the normal reference range for most laboratories, is associated with a two-fold increase in the mortality rate.[65] The mortality risk increases nearly 7-fold when the albumin concentration is 3.0 to 3.5 g per dL (30 to 35 g/L) and 15-fold when it is 2.5 to 3.0 g per dL (25 to 30 g/L).

Prevention of protein–energy malnutrition includes regular dietary counseling and ensuring adequate protein and calorie intake. Optimizing the dialysis dose and avoiding metabolic acidosis and catabolic diseases such as infections may also minimize the likelihood of protein–energy malnutrition. The NKF-K/DOQI nutrition guidelines recommend a daily dietary protein intake of 1.2 g per kg body weight for hemodialysis patients.[37] This higher protein requirement compared to the general population is due to a higher protein catabolism as a result of metabolic acidosis, infections, the blood–dialyzer interaction (especially with bioincompatible membranes), and losses of protein and amino acid in the dialysate.

The recommended daily intake for patients on chronic peritoneal dialysis is higher, at 1.2 to 1.3 g per kg body weight, due to the increased protein loss that occurs with this modality.[37] Daily protein and amino acid losses with peritoneal dialysis range from 5 to 15 g and 3 g, respectively, and may be increased with peritonitis.[37] The recommended total daily energy intake in both hemodialysis and peritoneal dialysis patients is of 35 kcal per kg body weight. For peritoneal dialysis patients, this includes intake from both the diet and that obtained from the glucose absorbed from peritoneal dialysate solution. Unfortunately, most patients have nutritional intakes below the recommended level; thus, the prevalence of protein–energy malnutrition is high in this population.

Nutritional intervention for the management of protein–energy malnutrition in nondialysis patients may also be generally applied to hemodialysis and peritoneal dialysis patients. Total parenteral nutrition support for hemodialysis or peritoneal dialysis patients, however, is associated with many complications, ranging from the lack of vascular access, fluid overload, and electrolyte abnormalities, to economic and logistical consequences. Therefore, prior to implementation of parenteral nutrition, counseling to increase dietary protein and energy intake, nutritional supplements, and tube feeding should be considered. Intradialytic parenteral nutrition may be considered in hemodialysis patients who have evidence of protein–energy malnutrition and who have inadequate dietary intake; who cannot administer or tolerate adequate oral nutrition, including food supplements or tube feeding; and who are expected to have their nutritional needs met with the combination of intradialytic parenteral nutrition and oral or enteral intake.[37] An advantage of intradialytic parenteral nutrition is that administration during hemodialysis reduces the risk of fluid overload, since ultrafiltration may be adjusted to compensate for the extra fluid administered. Unfortunately, this nutritional support method is limited to 3 days per week and may not meet the patient's nutritional needs.

Administration of amino acids to patients on peritoneal dialysis, referred to as intraperitoneal amino acid administration, is also considered a form of nutritional support. Amino acids are added to a peritoneal dialysis exchange to allow for uptake during the exchange; the extent of uptake depends on the concentration and dwell time. For example, a peritoneal dialysis exchange volume of 2 L containing 1.1% amino acids that is allowed to dwell for 5 to 6 hours will provide approximately 17 to 18 g of amino acids.[37] Patients with evidence of protein–energy malnutrition and an inadequate daily protein intake; patients who cannot administer or tolerate adequate oral protein nutrition, including food supplements, or enteral tube feeding; and patients in whom the combination of oral or enteral intake with intraperitoneal amino acid administration will meet the individual's nutritional goals may benefit from intraperitoneal amino acid administration. This form of nutritional support may reduce glucose and lipid levels in patients who have difficulty with control of hyperglycemia, hypercholesterolemia, or hypertriglyceridemia that is related to the extensive carbohydrate absorption from peritoneal dialysate solution. Data on outcomes with intraperitoneal amino acid administration are limited.

For children on hemodialysis or peritoneal dialysis, the energy requirements should be at the Recommended Dietary Allowance (RDA) for their chronologic age, with subsequent changes made based on response. The protein requirement should also be based on the RDA for age, but an additional 0.4 g/kg/day should be added for hemodialysis patients. The additional amount to add for peritoneal dialysis patients should be based on estimated protein losses with the prescribed peritoneal dialysis regimen.[37] Recombinant human growth hormone may be considered for pediatric dialysis patients whose growth does not meet expectations based on age and other parameters.

DRUG DOSING CONSIDERATIONS FOR PATIENTS ON DIALYSIS

Patients who receive chronic dialysis therapy are commonly prescribed medications that depend substantially on the kidney for elimination (i.e., the fraction excreted unchanged by the kidney, or Fe, exceeds 60%) and therefore require dose adjustment.[181] Furthermore, the effects of hemodialysis and peritoneal dialysis on drug disposition must be considered. Drug characteristics that make a given drug more likely to be removed by dialysis (hemodialysis or peritoneal dialysis) include a low molecular weight, low protein binding, a small volume of distribution, a rapid rate of equilibration between tissue-binding sites and blood, and a limited amount of non-renal metabolism and excretion.[33] With hemodialysis, multiple dialyzers are available that differ in composition and hence the degree to which a given drug is removed during the dialysis procedure. The specific dialysis conditions may also vary substantially (e.g., the extent of diffusion or ultrafiltration prescribed).

Variations in dialysis conditions make references with yes-or-no information in terms of the dialyzability of a given drug incomplete. Rather, references that provide quantitative estimates of the effect of hemodialysis or peritoneal dialysis on the elimination half-life or total body clearance of a drug should be used when available. This clearance information, together with the estimated patient-specific pharmacokinetic parameters, can be used to design a dosing regimen for a given patient using the concept that total clearance of a drug is the sum of the patient's clearance (i.e., from residual kidney function and hepatic clearance) and clearance by dialysis. The additional effect of dialysis clearance usually is not considered important unless the procedure increases overall plasma clearance by at least 30% or the fractional drug removal by dialysis is >0.30.[182] Accurate information on the dialysis kinetics of many drugs is not readily available, and reasonable estimates need to be made based on the dialysis conditions and drug characteristics. Consideration of drug transport across the peritoneal membrane must also be considered with intraperitoneal administration of drug (e.g., antibiotics for treatment of peritonitis), as drug absorption may be significant for certain agents, affecting drug

selection and the dosing regimen (see section, ''Peritoneal Dialysis'' earlier in the chapter).

IMPROVING OUTCOMES

PATIENT EDUCATION

Patient education about kidney disease and the associated secondary complications should begin early (stages 3 and 4 CKD). Early intervention is necessary to provide patients and their family and support network with the information necessary to make informed decisions about dialysis modalities (hemodialysis vs. peritoneal dialysis) and to improve patient compliance with pharmacologic and nonpharmacologic therapies. Patients with ESRD are instructed on stringent dietary and fluid restrictions, have a large medication burden, and are asked to make changes in their lifestyle to accommodate dialysis. Given the extent of the lifestyle changes often necessary, it is not surprising that many patients are noncompliant not only with diet and medications but also with dialysis treatments. It is not uncommon for patients to cut short the dialysis time (with hemodialysis) or decrease the number of exchanges (with peritoneal dialysis). This noncompliance manifests as inadequate dialysis (low Kt/V) and poor patient outcomes (mortality).[9]

It has been estimated that approximately 50% of hemodialysis patients do not adhere to at least part of their dialysis regimen.[183] DOPPS found that nonadherence with hemodialysis was associated with increased mortality risk and increased hospital admissions.[9] Educational initiatives improve the quality of life of dialysis patients (including both the psychosocial and functional domains). Other specific improvements include decreased use of medical services, maintenance of employment, consumer satisfaction with care, and cost benefits.[184] The potential improvement in patient outcomes may be more likely when educational initiatives are implemented early and consistently enforced, although there may be other patient-specific factors that affect the outcome of these initiatives. For example, in one evaluation, dialysis patients with a low level of perceived control had poor adherence and did worse following educational sessions; however, patients with a higher level of perceived control had improved adherence.[183] The best method may be one that uses a combination of patient education and cognitive behavioral strategies while allowing patients to feel more in control of their health and decisions.

To assist in patient education, organizations such as the National Kidney Foundation have developed educational materials and an interactive patient education program that addresses many of the fears and concerns patients may have about kidney disease and dialysis. It encourages patients and family to be actively involved in decision making and their overall care. Specific topics include kidney disease, hemodialysis, peritoneal dialysis, transplantation, nutrition, and lifestyle issues. Health care providers involved in the care of patients with CKD (and ESRD) are encouraged to learn more about these and similar programs that they may recommend for their patients.[30,44]

METHODS TO IMPROVE ADHERENCE TO DRUG THERAPY

Patients on dialysis require many medications (range of 8 to 12) to manage comorbid conditions and secondary complications of ESRD, including the medications received during dialysis (e.g., erythropoietic therapy, vitamin D).[30] It is not surprising that noncompliance with drug therapy is a problem and medication-related problems are common in the ESRD population.[31,185] The most prevalent medication-related problems identified in this setting include errors in dosing, adverse drug reactions, and indications for which appropriate medications are not prescribed (e.g., cardiovascular disorders).[31] Other factors contributing to nonadherence with medication regimens include frequent dosing, patient's perception of treatment benefits, poor patient–physician communication, lack of motivation, poor socioeconomic background, lack of family and social support, and younger age.[185]

Regular involvement of a clinical pharmacist has been shown to be a cost-effective means to address such problems.[31,186,187] While intervention by clinical pharmacists with knowledge of the unique problems in patients with ESRD is logical, pharmacists have not been formally identified as part of the dialysis health care team (e.g., nephrologists, nurses, dietitians, social workers) as indicated by the federal government (the payer of a large portion of dialysis care). In environments where clinical pharmacy services are not readily available, other practitioners involved in this setting (e.g., nephrologists, nurses) must make every effort to regularly review medication profiles and provide consistent patient counseling. Strategies that may serve to improve compliance include simplification of medication regimens (when possible), establishing a partnership with the patient, and increasing awareness through education and feedback.

DISEASE MANAGEMENT STRATEGIES TO IMPROVE PATIENT OUTCOMES

While dialysis therapies have turned ESRD from a fatal disease into one for which there are now therapeutic options, survival of the ESRD population remains much lower than that of the general population.[5,150] Efforts to improve the delivery of adequate dialysis (as measured by Kt/V) are being made, since lower Kt/V values are associated with increased mortality.[57] The nephrology community is acutely aware of the increase in the number of patients with CKD (and ultimately ESRD). Because nephrology practitioners already are heavily burdened with the care of patients with ESRD, it is clear that nephrologists alone cannot manage the expected increased number of patients. Efforts are being made to increase awareness among other practitioners who regularly see patients at risk for developing ESRD (e.g., primary care physicians). Interventions should focus on improving measures associated with higher mortality at the start of dialysis (e.g., improve hemoglobin and albumin). Any intervention to reduce cardiovascular risk is advocated, since cardiovascular disease is the leading cause of mortality in the ESRD population. Application of the NKF-K/DOQI guidelines and continued research to determine whether the targeted outcomes improve mortality in ESRD patients are needed. A multidisciplinary approach to management of dialysis patients has led to improved outcomes, and there is some evidence that such a management strategy has a positive effect on survival in dialysis patients.[188]

Through more widespread educational efforts, earlier referral of patients with CKD to health care providers with specialized training in nephrology, and better management of complications of ESRD such as anemia and secondary hyperparathyroidism by a multidisciplinary team of providers, improvements in the management of ESRD may be realized.

PHARMACOECONOMICS

CKD ultimately progressing to ESRD is a public health problem in the United States, with incidence and prevalence expected to rise.[5] The cost of treating patients with ESRD is substantial, with most of this cost paid by the federal government. Based on data reported from 2001, the cost of ESRD care was $22.8 billion, with approximately 68% of this cost carried by Medicare.[5] Payment for ESRD care accounted for 6.3% of all Medicare expenditures in 2001, which was an increase of 1.5% in a decade. A consistent increase in the percentage of the Medicare budget dedicated to ESRD care has been observed over the past decade. Non-Medicare expenditures in 2001 were $7.4 billion, an increase of $5.2 billion in 10 years.[5] Factors such as the higher prevalence of ESRD, reimbursement structure, and the prevalence of diabetes as a cause of ESRD (with higher associated costs) contributed to this increase. In 2000, outpatient pharmacy-related costs accounted for approximately $66.3 million of the ESRD Medicare budget.[189] The cost of intravenous iron and vitamin D has increased, due primarily to increased use of the newer intravenous iron products iron sucrose (Venofer) and sodium ferric gluconate (Ferrlecit) and the intravenous vitamin D analogue paricalcitol (Zemplar). Changes in the reimbursement structure will need to be made if the number of patients with ESRD increases as predicted.[1,6]

KEY POINTS

- ESRD may result from primary injury to the nephron, systemic diseases (e.g., diabetes, hypertension), or exposure to toxic substances
- Patients with ESRD require renal replacement therapy with hemodialysis, peritoneal dialysis, or kidney transplantation
- The incidence and prevalence of ESRD (stage 5 CKD) is expected to increase, with estimated prevalence rates of approximately 2.2 million by 2030, the majority of cases being attributed to diabetes

- The availability of dialysis has led to a substantial reduction in morbidity and mortality for patients with ESRD; however, hemodialysis and peritoneal dialysis are associated with a number of medical and mechanical complications that can affect morbidity and mortality
- The choice of dialysis modality depends on comorbid conditions and patient preference
- The annual mortality rate in patients with ESRD remains relatively high (20% to 25%); death is primarily due to cardiovascular disease. The overall life expectancy of ESRD patients is only one-third to one-sixth that of the general U.S. population
- General goals of therapy for secondary complications of CKD (e.g., anemia, secondary hyperparathyroidism) apply to patients with ESRD (or stage 5 CKD); however, there are some factors unique to this population that should be considered when designing a treatment regimen
- NKF-K/DOQI guidelines are available specific to dialysis adequacy (for both hemodialysis and peritoneal dialysis) and vascular access, and for management of secondary complications of chronic kidney disease, including anemia, bone disease, nutrition, dyslipidemias, cardiovascular disease, and hypertension. These guidelines provide a basis for care of patients with ESRD
- A multidisciplinary approach to patient care is necessary to address the complex dietary, lifestyle, medication, and dialysis-related treatments in patients with ESRD
- The effects of hemodialysis and peritoneal dialysis on the pharmacokinetics of certain medications should be considered when designing a drug dosing regimen for individual patients
- With the increasing incidence of ESRD and health care expenditures necessary to manage the ESRD population, improving the outcomes and quality of care of patients with ESRD is a national priority

SUGGESTED READINGS

Eknoyan G, Levin A, Levin NW. Bone metabolism and disease in chronic kidney disease. Am J Kidney Dis 42 (Suppl 3):1–201, 2003.

Levey AS, et al. Controlling the epidemic of cardiovascular disease in chronic renal disease: what do we know? What do we need to learn? Where do we go from here? National Kidney Foundation Task Force on Cardiovascular Disease. Am J Kidney Dis 32:853, 1998.

NKF-DOQI clinical practice guidelines for anemia of chronic kidney disease, update 2000 [erratum in Am J Kidney Dis 38:442, 2001]. Am J Kidney Dis 37 (Suppl 1):S182, 2001.

NKF-DOQI clinical practice guidelines for hemodialysis adequacy. Am J Kidney Dis 30 (Suppl 2):S15–66, 1997.

NKF-DOQI clinical practice guidelines on managing dyslipidemias in chronic kidney disease. Am J Kidney Dis 41 (Suppl 3):S1–77, 2003.

NKF-DOQI clinical practice guidelines for nutrition in chronic renal failure. Am J Kidney Dis 35 (Suppl 2):S1–140, 2000.

NKF-DOQI clinical practice guidelines for peritoneal dialysis adequacy. Am J Kidney Dis 30 (Suppl 2):S67–136, 1997.

NKF-DOQI clinical practice guidelines for vascular access. Am J Kidney Dis 30 (Suppl 3):S150–191, 1997.

REFERENCES

1. NKF-K/DOQI clinical practice guidelines for chronic kidney disease: evaluation, classification, and stratification. Am J Kidney Dis 39 (Suppl 1):S1–266, 2002.
2. NKF-K/DOQI clinical practice guidelines for hemodialysis adequacy, update 2000. Am J Kidney Dis 37 (Suppl 1):S7–S64, 2001.
3. NKF-K/DOQI clinical practice guidelines for peritoneal dialysis adequacy, update 2000. Am J Kidney Dis 37 (Suppl 1):S65–S136, 2001.
4. U.S. Renal Data System, USRDS 2004 Annual Data Report. Atlas of end-stage renal disease in the United States, National Institutes of Health, National Institute of Diabetes and Digestive and Kidney Diseases. Bethesda, MD, 2004.
5. USRDS: the United States Renal Data System. Am J Kidney Dis 42 (Suppl 5):1–230, 2003.
6. U.S. Department of Health and Human Services. Healthy people 2010. 2nd ed. With Understanding and Improving Health and Objectives for Improving Health. Washington, DC: U.S. Government Printing Office, November 2000.
7. Goodkin D, Young E. An update on the Dialysis Outcomes and Practice Patterns Study (DOPPS). Contemp Dialysis Nephrol (October):36–41, 2001.
8. Goodkin DA, Bragg-Gresham JL, Koenig KG, et al. Association of comorbid conditions and mortality in hemodialysis patients in Europe, Japan, and the United States: the Dialysis Outcomes and Practice Patterns Study (DOPPS). J Am Soc Nephrol 14:3270–3277, 2003.
9. Saran R, Bragg-Gresham JL, Rayner HC, et al. Nonadherence in hemodialysis: associations with mortality, hospitalization, and practice patterns in the DOPPS. Kidney Int 64:254–262, 2003.
10. Rayner HC, Pisoni RL, Bommer J, et al. Mortality and hospitalization in haemodialysis patients in five European countries: results from the Dialysis Outcomes and Practice Patterns Study (DOPPS). Nephrol Dial Transplant 19:108–120, 2004.
11. Pisoni RL, Bragg-Gresham JL, Young EW, et al. Anemia management and outcomes from 12 countries in the Dialysis Outcomes and Practice Patterns Study (DOPPS). Am J Kidney Dis 44:94–111, 2004.
12. Mackenzie HS, Brenner BM. Current strategies for retarding progression of renal disease. Am J Kidney Dis 31:161–170, 1998.
13. U.S. Renal Data System. Medication use among dialysis patients in the dialysis morbidity and mortality study. USRDS 1998 Annual Data Report, National Institutes of Health, National Institute Diabetes and Digestive and Kidney Diseases. Bethesda, MD, 1998.
14. Levin A, Thompson CR, Ethier J, et al. Left ventricular mass index increase in early renal disease: impact of decline in hemoglobin. Am J Kidney Dis 34:125–134, 1999.
15. Foley RN, Parfrey PS, Morgan J, et al. Effect of hemoglobin levels in hemodialysis patients with asymptomatic cardiomyopathy. Kidney Int 58:1325–1335, 2000.
16. Levey AS, Bosch JP, Lewis JB, et al. A more accurate method to estimate glomerular filtration rate from serum creatinine: a new prediction equation. Modification of Diet in Renal Disease Study Group. Ann Intern Med 130:461–470, 1999.
17. Kimmel PL. Depression in patients with chronic renal disease: what we know and what we need to know. J Psychosom Res 53:951–956, 2002.
18. Levy NB. Psychiatric considerations in the primary medical care of the patient with renal failure. Adv Ren Replace Ther 7:231–238, 2000.
19. Hegde A, Veis JH, Seidman A, et al. High prevalence of alcoholism in dialysis patients. Am J Kidney Dis 35:1039–1043, 2000.
20. Wang PL, Watnick SG. Depression: a common but underrecognized condition associated with end-stage renal disease. Semin Dial 17:237–241, 2004.
21. Valderrabano, F Jofre R, Lopez-Gomez JM. Quality of life in end-stage renal disease patients. Am J Kidney Dis 38:443–464, 2001.
22. Hays RD, Kallich JD, Mapes DL, et al. Development of the kidney disease quality of life (KDQOL) instrument. Qual Life Res 3:329–338, 1994.

23. Walters BA, Hays RD, Spritzer KL, et al. Health-related quality of life, depressive symptoms, anemia, and malnutrition at hemodialysis initiation. Am J Kidney Dis 40:1185–1194, 2002.

24. Unruh M, Miskulin D, Yan G, et al. Racial differences in health-related quality of life among hemodialysis patients. Kidney Int 65: 1482–1491, 2004.

25. Lopes AA, Bragg-Gresham JL, Satayathum S, et al. Health-related quality of life and associated outcomes among hemodialysis patients of different ethnicities in the United States: the Dialysis Outcomes and Practice Patterns Study (DOPPS). Am J Kidney Dis 41: 605–615, 2003.

26. Mapes DL, Lopes AA, Satayathum S, et al. Health-related quality of life as a predictor of mortality and hospitalization: the Dialysis Outcomes and Practice Patterns Study (DOPPS). Kidney Int 64: 339–349, 2003.

27. Kouidi E, Grekas D, Deligiannis A, et al. Outcomes of long-term exercise training in dialysis patients: comparison of two training programs. Clin Nephrol 61 (Suppl 1):S31–38, 2004.

28. Allon M, Robbin ML. Increasing arteriovenous fistulas in hemodialysis patients: problems and solutions. Kidney Int 62:1109–1124, 2002.

29. NKF-K/DOQI clinical practice guidelines for vascular access, update 2000. Am J Kidney Dis 37 (Suppl 1):S137–141, 2001.

30. Manley HJ, Garvin CG, Drayer DK, et al. Medication prescribing patterns in ambulatory haemodialysis patients: comparisons of USRDS to a large not-for-profit dialysis provider. Nephrol Dial Transplant 19:1842–1848, 2004.

31. Manley HJ, Drayer DK, Muther RS. Medication-related problem type and appearance rate in ambulatory hemodialysis patients. BMC Nephrol 4:10, 2003.

32. O'Hare AM, Tawney K, Bacchetti P, et al. Decreased survival among sedentary patients undergoing dialysis: results from the Dialysis Morbidity and Mortality Study wave 2. Am J Kidney Dis 41:447–454, 2003.

33. Cheung A. Hemodialysis and hemofiltration. In: Greenberg A, ed. Primer on Kidney Diseases, 3rd ed. San Diego: Academic Press, 2001:396–404.

34. Ahmad S. Manual of Clinical Dialysis. London: Science Press Ltd, 1999.

35. Zawada E. Initiation of dialysis. In: Daugirdas J, ed. Handbook of dialysis. Philadelphia: Lippincott Williams & Wilkins, 2001.

36. NKF-DOQI clinical practice guidelines for hemodialysis adequacy. National Kidney Foundation. Am J Kidney Dis 30 (Suppl 2): S15–66, 1997.

37. Kopple JD. NKF-K/DOQI clinical practice guidelines for nutrition in chronic renal failure. Am J Kidney Dis 37 (Suppl 2):S66–70, 2001.

38. Caskey FJ, Wordsworth S, Ben T, et al. Early referral and planned initiation of dialysis: what impact on quality of life? Nephrol Dial Transplant 18:1330–1338, 2003.

39. Kazmi WH, Obrador GT, Khan SS, et al. Late nephrology referral and mortality among patients with end-stage renal disease: a propensity score analysis. Nephrol Dial Transplant 19:1808–1814, 2004.

40. Cooper BA, Branley P, Bulfone L, et al. The Initiating Dialysis Early and Late (IDEAL) study: study rationale and design. Perit Dial Int 24:176–181, 2004.

41. Rombola G. Dialysis for everybody? At any cost? J Nephrol 15 (Suppl 6):S33–42, 2002.

42. Stack AG, Messana JM. Renal replacement therapy in the elderly: medical, ethical, and psychosocial considerations. Adv Ren Replace Ther 7:52–62, 2000.

43. Moss AH. Shared decision-making in dialysis: the new RPA/ASN guideline on appropriate initiation and withdrawal of treatment. Am J Kidney Dis 37:1081–1091, 2001.

44. NKF, People Like Us, Live Educational Program at http:// www.kidney.org/patients/live.cfm. Accessed Dec. 11, 2004.

45. Thodis E, Passadakis P, Vargemezis V, et al. Peritoneal dialysis: better than, equal to, or worse than hemodialysis? Data worth knowing before choosing a dialysis modality. Perit Dial Int 21: 25–35, 2001.

46. Chandna SM, Farrington K. Residual renal function: considerations on its importance and preservation in dialysis patients. Semin Dial 17:196–201, 2004.

47. Alloatti S, Manes M, Paternoster G, et al. Peritoneal dialysis compared with hemodialysis in the treatment of end-stage renal disease. J Nephrol 13:331–342, 2000.

48. Rottembourg J. Residual renal function and recovery of renal function in patients treated by CAPD. Kidney Int (Suppl) 40:S106–110, 1993.

49. Ahuja TS, Collinge N, Grady J, et al. Is dialysis modality a factor in survival of patients with ESRD and HIV-associated nephropathy? Am J Kidney Dis 41:1060–1064, 2003.

50. Ganesh SK, Hulbert-Shearon T, Port FK, et al. Mortality differences by dialysis modality among incident ESRD patients with and without coronary artery disease. J Am Soc Nephrol 14:415–424, 2003.

51. Vonesh EF, Moran J. Mortality in end-stage renal disease: a reassessment of differences between patients treated with hemodialysis and peritoneal dialysis. J Am Soc Nephrol 10:354–365, 1999.

52. Vonesh EF, Snyer JJ, Foley RN, et al. The differential impact of risk factors on mortality in hemodialysis and peritoneal dialysis. Kidney Int 66:2389–2401, 2004.

53. USRDS 2000 Annual Data Report. Am J Kidney Dis 36 (Suppl 2): S1–S239, 2000.

54. Stack AG, Molony DA, Rahman NS, et al. Impact of dialysis modality on survival of new ESRD patients with congestive heart failure in the United States. Kidney Int 64:1071–1079, 2003.

55. Termorshuizen F, Korevaar JC, Dekker FW, et al. Hemodialysis and peritoneal dialysis: comparison of adjusted mortality rates according to the duration of dialysis: analysis of The Netherlands Cooperative Study on the Adequacy of Dialysis 2. J Am Soc Nephrol 14:2851–2860, 2003.

56. Young EW, Dyskstra DM, Goodkin DA, et al. Hemodialysis vascular access preferences and outcomes in the Dialysis Outcomes and Practice Patterns Study (DOPPS). Kidney Int 61:2266–2271, 2002.

57. Bloembergen WE, Stannard DC, Port FK, et al. Relationship of dose of hemodialysis and cause-specific mortality. Kidney Int 50: 557–565, 1996.

58. Held PJ, Port FK, Wolfe RA, et al. The dose of hemodialysis and patient mortality. Kidney Int 50:550–556, 1996.

59. Ringoir S. An update on uremic toxins. Kidney Int (Suppl) 62: S2–4, 1997.

60. Lowrie EG, Laird NM, Parker TF, et al. Effect of the hemodialysis prescription of patient morbidity: report from the National Cooperative Dialysis Study. N Engl J Med 305:1176–1181, 1981.

61. Laird NM, Berkey CS, Lowrie EG. Modeling success or failure of dialysis therapy: the National Cooperative Dialysis Study. Kidney Int (Suppl) 13:S101–106, 1983.

62. Gotch FA, Sargent JA. A mechanistic analysis of the National Cooperative Dialysis Study (NCDS). Kidney Int 28:526–534, 1985.

63. Harter HR. Review of significant findings from the National Cooperative Dialysis Study and recommendations. Kidney Int (Suppl) 13:S107–112, 1983.

64. Daugirdas JT, Depner TA. A nomogram approach to hemodialysis urea modeling. Am J Kidney Dis 23:33–40, 1994.

65. Lowrie EG, Lew NL. Death risk in hemodialysis patients: the predictive value of commonly measured variables and an evaluation of death rate differences between facilities. Am J Kidney Dis 15: 458–82, 1990.

66. Collins AJ, Ma JZ, Umen A, et al. Urea index and other predictors of hemodialysis patient survival. Am J Kidney Dis 23:272–282, 1994.

67. Saran R, Canaud BJ, Depner TA, et al. Dose of dialysis: key lessons from major observational studies and clinical trials. Am J Kidney Dis 44 (Suppl 3):47–53, 2004.

68. Port FK, Wolfe RA, Hulbert-Shearon TE, et al. High dialysis dose is associated with lower mortality among women but not among men. Am J Kidney Dis 43:1014–1023, 2004.

69. Port FK, Pisoni RL, Bragg-Gresham JL, et al. DOPPS estimates of patient life years attributable to modifiable hemodialysis practices in the United States. Blood Purif 22:175–180, 2004.

70. Daugirdas JT, Kjellstrand CM. Chronic hemodialysis prescription: A urea kinetic approach. In: Daugirdas J, ed. Handbook of dialysis. Philadelphia: Lippincott Williams & Wilkins, 2001:121–147.

71. Zacharias JM, Weatherstone CP, Spewark CR, et al. Alteplase versus urokinase for occluded hemodialysis catheters. Ann Pharmacother 37:27–33, 2003.

72. Falk A, Samson W, Uribarri J, et al. Efficacy of reteplase in poorly functioning hemodialysis catheters. Clin Nephrol 61:47–53, 2004.

73. Crowther MA, Clase CM, Margetts PJ, et al. Low-intensity warfarin is ineffective for the prevention of PTFE graft failure in patients on hemodialysis: a randomized controlled trial. J Am Soc Nephrol 13:2331–2337, 2002.

74. O'Shea SI, Lawson JH, Reddan D, et al. Hypercoagulable states and antithrombotic strategies in recurrent vascular access site thrombosis. J Vasc Surg 38:541–548, 2003.

75. Saran R, Dykstra DM, Wolfe RA, et al. Association between vascular access failure and the use of specific drugs: the Dialysis Outcomes and Practice Patterns Study (DOPPS). Am J Kidney Dis 40:1255–1263, 2002.

76. Butterly DW, Schwab SJ. Dialysis access infections. Curr Opin Nephrol Hypertens 9:631–635, 2000.

77. Marr KA, Kong L, Fowler VG, et al. Incidence and outcome of *Staphylococcus aureus* bacteremia in hemodialysis patients. Kidney Int 54:1684–1689, 1998.

78. Pastan S, Soucie JM, McClellan WM. Vascular access and increased risk of death among hemodialysis patients. Kidney Int 62:620–626, 2002.

79. Poole CV, Carlton D, Bimbo L, et al. Treatment of catheter-related bacteraemia with an antibiotic lock protocol: effect of bacterial pathogen. Nephrol Dial Transplant 19:1237–1244, 2004.

80. Allon M. Dialysis catheter-related bacteremia: treatment and prophylaxis. Am J Kidney Dis 44:779–791, 2004.

81. Krishnasami Z, Carlton D, Bimbo L, et al. Management of hemodialysis catheter-related bacteremia with an adjunctive antibiotic lock solution. Kidney Int 61:1136–1142, 2002.

82. *Staphylococcus aureus* resistant to vancomycin, United States, 2002. MMWR 51:565–567, 2002.

83. Atta MG, Eustace JA, Song X, et al. Outpatient vancomycin use and vancomycin-resistant enterococcal colonization in maintenance dialysis patients. Kidney Int 59:718–724, 2001.

84. Barbosa D, Lima L, Silbert S, et al. Evaluation of the prevalence and risk factors for colonization by vancomycin-resistant *Enterococcus* among patients on dialysis. Am J Kidney Dis 44:337–343, 2004.

85. Tokars JI, Finelli L, Alter MJ, et al. National surveillance of dialysis-associated diseases in the United States, 2001. Semin Dial 17:310–319, 2004.

86. Tacconelli E, Carmeli Y, Aizer A, et al. Mupirocin prophylaxis to prevent *Staphylococcus aureus* infection in patients undergoing dialysis: a meta-analysis. Clin Infect Dis 37:1629–1638, 2003.

87. Daugirdas JT. Pathophysiology of dialysis hypotension: an update. Am J Kidney Dis 38 (Suppl 4):S11–17, 2001.

88. Perazella MA. Pharmacologic options available to treat symptomatic intradialytic hypotension. Am J Kidney Dis 38 (Suppl 4):S26–36, 2001.

89. Sarkar SR, Kaitwatcharachai C, Levin NW. Nitric oxide and hemodialysis. Semin Dial 7:224–228, 2004.

90. Dheenan S, Venkatesan J, Grubb BP, et al. Effect of sertraline hydrochloride on dialysis hypotension. Am J Kidney Dis 31:624–630, 1998.

91. Foley RN, Parfrey PS, Sarnak MJ. Epidemiology of cardiovascular disease in chronic renal disease. J Am Soc Nephrol 9 (Suppl):S16–23, 1998.

92. Levey AS, Beto JA, Coronado BE, et al. Controlling the epidemic of cardiovascular disease in chronic renal disease: what do we know? What do we need to learn? Where do we go from here? National Kidney Foundation Task Force on Cardiovascular Disease. Am J Kidney Dis 32:853–906, 1998.

93. Zoccali C, Benedetto FA, Tripepi G, et al. Cardiac consequences of hypertension in hemodialysis patients. Semin Dial 17:299–303, 2004.

94. Levin A, Singer J, Thompson CR, et al. Prevalent left ventricular hypertrophy in the predialysis population: identifying opportunities for intervention. Am J Kidney Dis 27:347–354, 1996.

95. McCullough PA, Sandberg KR. Chronic kidney disease and sudden death: strategies for prevention. Blood Purif 22:136–142, 2004.

96. Salem M, Ivanovich PT, Ing TS, et al. Adverse effects of dialyzers manifesting during the dialysis session. Nephrol Dial Transplant 9 (Suppl 2):127–137, 1994.

97. Kammerl MC, Schaefer RM, Schweda F, et al. Extracorporal therapy with AN69 membranes in combination with ACE inhibition causing severe anaphylactoid reactions: still a current problem? Clin Nephrol 53:486–488, 2000.

98. Port FK, Wolfe RA, Hulbert-Shearon TE, et al. Mortality risk by hemodialyzer reuse practice and dialyzer membrane characteristics: results from the USRDS dialysis morbidity and mortality study. Am J Kidney Dis 37:276–286, 2001.

99. Agodoa LY, Wolfe RA, Port FK. Reuse of dialyzers and clinical outcomes: fact or fiction. Am J Kidney Dis 32 (Suppl 4):S88–92, 1998.

100. Bregman H, Ing TS. Complications during hemodialysis. In: Daugirdas J, ed. Handbook of dialysis. Philadelphia: Lippincott Williams & Wilkins, 2001:148–168.

101. Al-Hilali N, Al-Humoud HM, Ninan VT, et al. Profiled hemodialysis reduces intradialytic symptoms. Transplant Proc 36:1827–1828, 2004.

102. Khajehdehi P, Majerlou M, Behzadi S, et al. A randomized, double-blind, placebo-controlled trial of supplementary vitamins E, C and their combination for treatment of haemodialysis cramps. Nephrol Dial Transplant 16:1448–1451, 2001.

103. Bellinghieri G, Santoro D, Calvani M, et al. Carnitine and hemodialysis. Am J Kidney Dis 41 (Suppl 1):S116–122, 2003.

104. Sakurauchi Y, Matsumoto Y, Shinzato T, et al. Effects of L-carnitine supplementation on muscular symptoms in hemodialyzed patients. Am J Kidney Dis 32:258–264, 1998.

105. Drueke TB, Beta2-microglobulin and amyloidosis. Nephrol Dial Transplant 15 (Suppl 1):17–24, 2000.

106. Kay J. Musculoskeletal and rheumatic diseases. In: Daugirdas J, ed. Handbook of dialysis. Philadelphia: Lippincott Williams & Wilkins, 2001: 637–651.

107. Sengul S, Arat A, Ozdemir FN. Renal amyloidosis is associated with increased mortality in hemodialysis patients. Artif Organs 28:846–852, 2004.

108. Koda Y, Suzuki M, Hirasawa Y. Efficacy of choice of dialysis membrane. Nephrol Dial Transplant 16 (Suppl 4):23–26, 2001.

109. Zoccali C, Mallamaci F, Tripepi G. AGEs and carbonyl stress: potential pathogenetic factors of long-term uraemic complications. Nephrol Dial Transplant 15 (Suppl 2):7–11, 2000.

110. Robertson KE, Mueller BA. Uremic pruritus. Am J Health Syst Pharm 53:2159–2170, 1996.

111. Zucker I, Yosipovitch G, David M, et al. Prevalence and characterization of uremic pruritus in patients undergoing hemodialysis: uremic pruritus is still a major problem for patients with end-stage renal disease. J Am Acad Dermatol 49:842–846, 2003.

112. Brophy DF, Mueller BA. Automated peritoneal dialysis: new implications for pharmacists. Ann Pharmacother 31:756–764, 1997.

113. Bailie GR, Eisele G. Continuous ambulatory peritoneal dialysis: a review of its mechanics, advantages, complications, and areas of controversy. Ann Pharmacother 26:1409–1420, 1992.

114. Gokal R. Peritoneal dialysis. In: Greenberg A, ed. Primer on Kidney Diseases, 3rd ed. San Diego: Academic Press, 2001:405–413.

115. Mactier R. Peritoneal cavity lymphatics. In: Nolph KD, ed. Peritoneal Dialysis, 3rd ed. Boston: Kluwer, 1989:28–47.

116. Niezgoda JA, Wolfson AB. Continuous ambulatory peritoneal dialysis. Emerg Med Clin North Am 12:759–769, 1994.

117. Ash SR. Chronic peritoneal dialysis catheters: overview of design, placement, and removal procedures. Semin Dial 16:323–334, 2003.

118. La Greca FM, Ronco C. Proceedings of the 6th International Course on peritoneal dialysis. Perit Dial Int 17 (Suppl 2):S47–S83, 1997.

119. Crawford-Bonadio TL, Diaz-Buxo JA. Comparison of peritoneal dialysis solutions. Nephrol Nurs J 31:499–509, 1004.

120. Teitelbaum I, Burkart J. Peritoneal dialysis. Am J Kidney Dis 42:1082–1096, 2003.

121. Piraino P, Bailie GR, Bernardini J, et al. Peritoneal dialysis-related infections recommendations: 2005 update. Perit Dial Int 25:107–131, 2005.

122. Flanigan MJ. Nightly tidal peritoneal dialysis prescription and power. Contrib Nephrol 129:115–122, 1999.

123. Gotch FA. Adequacy of peritoneal dialysis. Am J Kidney Dis 21:96–98, 1993.

124. NKF-DOQI clinical practice guidelines for peritoneal dialysis adequacy. National Kidney Foundation. Am J Kidney Dis 30 (Suppl 2):S67–136, 1997.

125. Coles GA, Williams JD. What is the place of peritoneal dialysis in the integrated treatment of renal failure? Kidney Int 54:2234–2240, 1998.

126. Keshaviah P. Urea kinetic and middle molecule approaches to assessing the adequacy of hemodialysis and CAPD. Kidney Int (Suppl) 40:S28–38, 1993.

127. Brandes JC, Piering WF, Beres JA, et al. Clinical outcome of continuous ambulatory peritoneal dialysis predicted by urea and creatinine kinetics. J Am Soc Nephrol 2:1430–1435, 1992.

128. Keane WF, Bailie GR, Boeschoten E, et al. Adult peritoneal dialysis-related peritonitis treatment recommendations: 2000 update. Perit Dial Int 20:396–411, 2000.

129. Parker TF 3rd. Role of dialysis dose on morbidity and mortality in maintenance hemodialysis patients. Am J Kidney Dis 24:981–989, 1994.

130. Chaimovitz C. Peritoneal dialysis. Kidney Int 45:1226–1240, 1994.

131. Vas SI. Treatment of peritonitis. Perit Dial Int 14 (Suppl 3):S49–55, 1994.

132. Twardowski Z. Peritoneal catheter exit-site and tunnel infections. In: Nissenson AR, Fine RD, eds. Dialysis therapy. 2nd ed. Philadelphia: Hanley & Belfus, 1993:165–168.

133. Holley JL, Bernardini J, Piraino B. Infecting organisms in continuous ambulatory peritoneal dialysis patients on the Y-set. Am J Kidney Dis 23:569–573, 1994.

134. Morbidity and mortality of renal dialysis: an NIH consensus conference statement. Consensus Development Conference Panel. Ann Intern Med 121:62–70, 1994.

135. Nasal mupirocin prevents *Staphylococcus aureus* exit-site infection during peritoneal dialysis. Mupirocin Study Group. J Am Soc Nephrol 7:2403–2408, 1996.

136. Zimmerman SW, Ahrens E, Johnson CA, et al. Randomized controlled trial of prophylactic rifampin for peritoneal dialysis-related infections. Am J Kidney Dis 18:225–231, 1991.

137. Wizemann V, Timio M, Alpert MA, et al. Options in dialysis therapy: significance of cardiovascular findings. Kidney Int (Suppl) 40:S85–91, 1993.

138. Maiorca R, Cancarini GC, Brunori G, et al. Morbidity and mortality of CAPD and hemodialysis. Kidney Int (Suppl) 40:S4–15, 1993.

139. Bargman JM. Complications of peritoneal dialysis related to increased intraabdominal pressure. Kidney Int (Suppl) 40:S75–80, 1993.

140. Spinowitz B, Charytan C, Gupta B. Hydrothorax and peritoneal dialysis. In: Nissenson AR, Fine RN, eds. Dialysis therapy. 2nd ed. Philadelphia: Hanley & Belfus, 1993:189–191.

141. Spinowitz B, Charytan C. Abdominal hernias in CAPD. In: Nissenson AR, Fine RN, eds. Dialysis therapy. 2nd ed. Philadelphia: Hanley & Belfus, 1993:187–188.

142. Pierratos A, Ouwendyk M, Francoeur R, et al. Nocturnal hemodialysis: three-year experience. J Am Soc Nephrol 9:859–868, 1998.

143. Lockridge RS Jr, Spencer M, Craft V, et al. Nocturnal home hemodialysis in North America. Adv Ren Replace Ther 8:250–256, 2001.

144. Lacson E Jr, Diaz-Buxo JA. Daily and nocturnal hemodialysis: how do they stack up? Am J Kidney Dis 38:225–239, 2001.

145. Mohr PE, Neumann PJ, Franco SJ, et al. The case for daily dialysis: its impact on costs and quality of life. Am J Kidney Dis 37:777–789, 2001.

146. Hanly PJ, Pierratos A. Improvement of sleep apnea in patients with chronic renal failure who undergo nocturnal hemodialysis. N Engl J Med 344:102–107, 2001.

147. Diaz-Buxo JA. Continuous-flow peritoneal dialysis: update. Adv Perit Dial 20:18–22, 2004.

148. Amerling R, Dell'Aquila R, Bonello M, et al. Continuous flow peritoneal dialysis: principles and applications. Semin Dial 16:335–340, 2003.

149. St Peter WL, Schoolwerth AC, McGowan T, et al. Chronic kidney disease: issues and establishing programs and clinics for improved patient outcomes. Am J Kidney Dis 41:903–924, 2003.

150. Foley RN, Parfrey PS, Harnett JD, et al. Clinical and echocardiographic disease in patients starting end-stage renal disease therapy. Kidney Int 47:186–192, 1995.

151. NKF-K/DOQI clinical practice guidelines for anemia of chronic kidney disease, update 2000. Am J Kidney Dis 37 (Suppl 1):S182–238, 2001.

152. Aronoff GR, Bennett WM, Blumenthal S, et al. Iron sucrose in hemodialysis patients: safety of replacement and maintenance regimens. Kidney Int 66:1193–1198, 2004.

153. Michael B, Coyne DW, Folkert VW, et al. Sodium ferric gluconate complex in haemodialysis patients: a prospective evaluation of long-term safety. Nephrol Dial Transplant 19:1576–1580, 2004.

154. Besarab A, Amin N, Ahsan M, et al. Optimization of epoetin therapy with intravenous iron therapy in hemodialysis patients. J Am Soc Nephrol 11:530–538, 2000.

155. Coronel F, Herrero JA, Montenegro J, et al. Erythropoietin requirements: a comparative multicenter study between peritoneal dialysis and hemodialysis. J Nephrol 16:697–702, 2003.

156. Movilli E, Cancarini GC, Zani R, et al. Adequacy of dialysis reduces the doses of recombinant erythropoietin independently from the use of biocompatible membranes in haemodialysis patients. Nephrol Dial Transplant 16:111–114, 2001.

157. Golper TA, Goral S, Becker BN, et al. L-carnitine treatment of anemia. Am J Kidney Dis 41 (Suppl 4):S27–34, 2003.

158. Kletzmayr J, Mayer G, Legenstein E, et al. Anemia and carnitine supplementation in hemodialyzed patients. Kidney Int (Suppl) 69:S93–106, 1999.

159. Mailloux LU, Haley We. Hypertension in the ESRD patient: pathophysiology, therapy, outcomes, and future directions. Am J Kidney Dis 32:705–719, 1998.

160. Zager PG, Nikolic J, Brown RH, et al. U-curve association of blood pressure and mortality in hemodialysis patients. Medical Directors of Dialysis Clinic, Inc. Kidney Int 54:561–569, 1998.

161. National Kidney Foundation. N/DOQI clinical practice guidelines for cardiovascular disease in dialysis patients. Am J Kidney Dis 45:S1–S154, 2005.

162. Horl MP, Horl WH. Hemodialysis-associated hypertension: pathophysiology and therapy. Am J Kidney Dis 39:227–244, 2002.

163. Chobanian AV, Bakris GL, Black HR, et al. Seventh report of the Joint National Committee on Prevention, Detection, Evaluation, and Treatment of High Blood Pressure. Hypertension 42:1206–1252, 2003.

164. K/DOQI clinical practice guidelines for management of dyslipidemias in patients with kidney disease. Am J Kidney Dis 41 (Suppl 3):I-IV, S1–91, 2003.

165. Executive Summary of the Third Report of The National Cholesterol Education Program (NCEP) Expert Panel on Detection, Evaluation, and Treatment of High Blood Cholesterol In Adults (Adult Treatment Panel III). JAMA 285:2486–2497, 2001.

166. Wilkes BM, Reiner D, Kern M, et al. Simultaneous lowering of serum phosphate and LDL-cholesterol by sevelamer hydrochloride (RenaGel) in dialysis patients. Clin Nephrol 50:381–386, 1998.

167. Shemin D, Bostom AG, Selhub J. Treatment of hyperhomocysteinemia in end-stage renal disease. Am J Kidney Dis 38 (Suppl 1):S91–94, 2001.

168. Gonin JM, Nguyen H, Gonin R, et al. Controlled trials of very high dose folic acid, vitamins B12 and B6, intravenous folinic acid and serine for treatment of hyperhomocysteinemia in ESRD. J Nephrol 16:522–534, 2003.

169. Wrone EM, Hornberger JM, Zehnder JL, et al. Randomized trial of folic acid for prevention of cardiovascular events in end-stage renal disease. J Am Soc Nephrol 15:420–426, 2004.

170. Gennari FJ. Acid–base balance in dialysis patients. Semin Dial 13:235–239, 2000.

171. Mehrotra R, Kopple JD, Wolfson M. Metabolic acidosis in maintenance dialysis patients: clinical considerations. Kidney Int (Suppl) 88:S13–25, 2003.

172. Block GA, Klassen PS, Lazarus JM, et al. Mineral metabolism, mortality, and morbidity in maintenance hemodialysis. J Am Soc Nephrol 15:2208–2218, 2004.

173. Goodman WG, London G, Amann K, et al. Vascular calcification in chronic kidney disease. Am J Kidney Dis 43:572–579, 2004.

174. Mittalhenkle A, Gillen DL, Stehman-Breen CO. Increased risk of mortality associated with hip fracture in the dialysis population. Am J Kidney Dis 44:672–679, 2004.

175. Eknoyan G, Levin A, Levin NW. Bone metabolism and disease in chronic kidney disease. Am J Kidney Dis 42 (Suppl 3):1–201, 2003.

176. Goodman WG. New assays for parathyroid hormone (PTH) and the relevance of PTH fragments in renal failure. Kidney Int (Suppl) 87:S120–124, 2003.

177. Braun J, Asmus HG, Holzer H, et al. Long-term comparison of a calcium-free phosphate binder and calcium carbonate–phosphorus metabolism and cardiovascular calcification. Clin Nephrol 62: 104–115, 2004.

178. Block GA, Martin KJ, de Francisco AL, et al. Cinacalcet for secondary hyperparathyroidism in patients receiving hemodialysis. N Engl J Med 350:1516–1525, 2004.

179. Owen WF Jr, Lew NL, Liu Y, et al. The urea reduction ratio and serum albumin concentration as predictors of mortality in patients undergoing hemodialysis. N Engl J Med 329:1001–1006, 1993.

180. Cooper BA, Penne EL, Bartlett LH, et al. Protein malnutrition and hypoalbuminemia as predictors of vascular events and mortality in ESRD. Am J Kidney Dis 43:61–66, 2004.

181. Arnoff GR, Brier ME, Golper TA, et al. Drug prescribing in renal failure. Dosing guidelines for adults. 4th ed. Philadelphia: American College of Physicians, 1999.

182. Joy MS, Matzke GR, Armstrong DK, et al. A primer on continuous renal replacement therapy for critically ill patients. Ann Pharmacother 32:362–375, 1998.

183. White RB. Adherence to the dialysis prescription: partnering with patients for improved outcomes. Nephrol Nurs J 31:432–435, 2004.

184. Latham CE. Is there data to support the concept that educated, empowered patients have better outcomes? J Am Soc Nephrol 9 (Suppl):S141–144, 1998.

185. Loghman-Adham M. Medication noncompliance in patients with chronic disease: issues in dialysis and renal transplantation. Am J Manag Care 9:155–171, 2003.

186. Grabe DW, Low CL, Bailie GR, et al. Evaluation of drug-related problems in an outpatient hemodialysis unit and the impact of a clinical pharmacist. Clin Nephrol 47:117–121, 1997.

187. Manley HJ, Carroll CA. The clinical and economic impact of pharmaceutical care in end-stage renal disease patients. Semin Dial 15: 45–49, 2002.

188. Ravani P, Marinangeli G, Tancredi M, et al. Multidisciplinary chronic kidney disease management improves survival on dialysis. J Nephrol 16:870–877, 2003.

189. U.S. Renal Data System. USRDS 2002 Annual Data Report: Atlas of End-Stage Renal Disease in the United States. National Institutes of Health, National Institute of Diabetes and Digestive and Kidney Diseases, Bethesda, MD, 2002.

CASE 17

TOPIC: Chronic Kidney Disease

THERAPEUTIC DIFFICULTY: Level 2
Susan Krikorian

Chapter 43: Chronic Kidney Disease

■ Scenario

Patient and Setting: HG, a 55-year-old white female seen at her regularly scheduled PCP office visit

Chief Complaint: Increasing fatigue and joint pain for several weeks, 2 lb weight gain and slight swelling of her ankles within the last week.

■ History of Present Illness

Patient attributed several weeks of increasing joint pain and fatigue to arthritis and started taking 2 tablets acetaminophen (APAP) 650 mg q 6 hours PRN with no relief; HgA1c 12% (1 week ago).

Medical History: Type 1 DM since childhood; HTN for 20 years; diabetic nephropathy (microalbuminuria detected 2 years ago); chronic kidney disease (baseline SCr 1.6, 6 months ago); medication nonadherence; seasonal allergies

Surgical History: TAH (10 years ago)

Family/Social History: Father age 83 with HTN and CAD; mother age 83 with HTN. Married with two children; occasional alcohol use; smoked 1 pack/day × 20 years; quit tobacco 1 year ago

Medications:
Regular/NPH 70/30(Humulin) insulin, 30 U sc AM, 20 U sc PM
HCTZ, 50 mg PO QD
Lisinopril, 20 mg PO QD
Calcium carbonate, 1,500 mg PO TID w/meals
Calcitriol, 0.25 µg PO QD
APAP, 650 mg ii tabs q6h PRN for joint pain

Allergies: Amoxicillin (rash); radiocontrast dye (pruritis)

■ Physical Examination

GEN: Looks older than her stated age and appears in moderate discomfort

VS: BP 154/90, HR 85, RR 18, T 37.8°C, Wt 59 kg, Ht 162 cm
HEENT: PERRLA, EOMI
COR: RRR, nl S1, S2 no rubs or gallops
CHEST: CTA
ABD: Soft, NT/ND, (−) HSM
GU: Deferred
RECT: Deferred
EXT: Trace ankle edema bilaterally, good distal pulses, restricted ROM in joints; pain assessment 7/10
NEURO: A and O × 3

■ Results of Pertinent Laboratory Tests, Serum Drug Concentrations, and Diagnostic Tests

Na 140 (140)
K 5.2 (5.2)
Cl 100 (100)
HCO_3 20 (20)
BUN 10 (28)
SCr 167 (1.9)
Ferritin: Pending
Serum Iron: Pending
TSAT: Pending
ANA: negative
Urinalysis: + protein, hyaline casts
Urine output: 10mL/hour
Guaiac stool: negative
Chest x-ray: unremarkable
ECG: normal tracings
Estimated GFR = 29 mL/min/ 1.73 m² (using MDRD formula)

Hct 0.28 (28)
Hgb 90 (9.0)
Lkcs 7.5×10^9 (7.5×10^3)
Plts 210×10^3 (210×210^3)

■ Problem List

Identify principal problems from the scenario in priority order (see Answers in back of book for correct list of problems).

■ SOAP Note

To be completed by the student (see Answers in back of book for correct SOAP Note).

■ QUESTIONS

(See Answers in back of book for correct responses.)

1. List the possible causes of CKD in this patient. (EO-1)

2. Based on this patient's estimated GFR, she is classified into which of the following stages of CKD? (EO-2, 3, 5)
   a. Stage 2
   b. Stage 3
   c. Stage 4
   d. Stage 5 or end-stage kidney disease (ESKD)

3. Describe why monotherapy with HCTZ is not recommended for this patient. (EO-7, 8, 9, 11, 13)

4. Explain how CKD leads to abnormalities in calcium, phosphorus, active vitamin D, and iPTH and identify the therapeutic options to address these abnormalities. (EO-12)

5. Describe the role of sevelamer or lanthanum in the management of hyperphosphatemia. (EO-10, 12)

6. The patient exhibits persistent pain and disability associated with renal osteodystrophy not controlled with APAP. Provide your recommendation for short-term use of an opiate. Why is the opiate meperidine avoided in this setting? (EO-6, 10, 13)

7. Based on this patient's estimated GFR (and stage of CKD) the target range for intact PTH (iPTH) is which of the following? (EO-7, 13)
   a. 35–70 pg/mL
   b. 70–110 pg/mL
   c. 150–300 pg/mL
   d. 400–700 pg/mL

8. In this case, describe the role of ACE inhibitors in the prevention of diabetic nephropathy. (EO-5, 8, 12, 13)

9. Which of the following is the target Hgb in a patient with anemia of CKD treated with erythropoietic therapy? (EO-5, 8)
   a. 9–10 g/dL
   b. 11–12 g/dL
   c. 13–14 g/dL
   d. 15–16 g/dL

10. List the parameters that should be monitored to determine response to erythropoietic and iron therapy in this patient. (EO-5, 8, 12)

11. What are the options for erythropoietic therapy in this patient and the appropriate starting doses? (EO-5, 12)

12. Describe the recommended strategy for making dosing adjustments to erythropoietic therapy. (EO-5, 12)

13. List psychosocial factors that may influence this patient's deterioration of kidney function. (EO-5, 13, 15)

14. Describe the health care provider's role in promoting medication adherence in this case. (EO-14, 15, 16)

15. Summarize etiology, pathophysiology, epidemiology, therapeutic, and disease management concepts for CKD utilizing a key points format. (EO-18)

CASE 18

TOPIC: Dialytic and Pharmacotherapy for End-Stage Kidney Disease

THERAPEUTIC DIFFICULTY: Level 3
Joanna Q. Hudson and Harold J. Manley

Chapter 44: Dialytic and Pharmacotherapy for End-Stage Kidney Disease

■ Scenario

Patient and Setting: BC, a 62-year-old black male; outpatient peritoneal dialysis clinic

Chief Complaint: Painful continuous ambulatory peritoneal dialysis (CAPD) exchanges, "hazy" dialysate fluid, fatigued, feverish, decreased appetite; "I cannot do all my exchanges—I feel too bad."

■ History of Present Illness

Four-day history of painful sensation during exchanges, cloudy effluent drained from peritoneal cavity; fatigued, feverish × 2 days, swollen ankles; brought effluent and 24-hour urine collection for assessment of dialysis adequacy and residual kidney function; dextrose content of dialysate fluid increased from 1.5% to 2.5% for daytime exchanges and from 2.5% to 4.25% for the nighttime exchange 2 weeks ago per verbal instructions by nephrologist; has become less motivated to do exchanges in last 6 months per spouse

Medical History: End-stage kidney disease secondary to type 2 diabetes; CAPD × 5 years; peritonitis—approximately 1 episode per year; type 2 diabetes mellitus × 14 years, hypertension × 4 years.

Surgical History: Amputation of R middle digit 2 years ago

Family/Social History: Family History: Father, myocardial infarction (MI), age 53
Social History: Nonsmoker, denies alcohol use

Medications:
Enalapril, 10 mg PO QD
Epoetin alfa, 4,000 Units SC BIW (Monday, Thursday)
Ferrous sulfate, 325 mg PO TID
Nephrocaps, 1 PO QD
NPH insulin, 8 Units SC QAM
Metoclopramide, 5 mg PO AC and HS
Dextrose solution 2.25%, 2 L IP (8 AM, 1 PM, 6 PM)
Dextrose solution 4.25%, 2 L IP 11 PM
Calcium carbonate, 1,500 mg PO with meals
Calcitriol, 0.25 μg PO QD
Enteric-coated aspirin, 81 mg PO QD

Allergies: No known medication allergies

■ Physical Examination

GEN: Well-developed male in no acute distress
VS: BP 138/88, HR 75, RR 14, T 38°C, Wt 84 kg, Normal weight: 80 kg, Ht 172 cm
HEENT: WNL
COR: WNL
CHEST: Few rales in lower third of lung fields
ABD: Abdominal tenderness and guarding
GU: WNL
RECT: WNL
EXT: 1+ edema in ankles
NEURO: WNL

■ Results of Pertinent Laboratory Tests, Serum Drug Concentrations, and Diagnostic Tests

Na 142 (142)	BUN 35 (98)	Hgb 114 (11.4)	Ca 2.45 (9.8)
K 5.2 (5.2)	CR 601 (6.8)	Hct 0.34 (34.2)	PO$_4$ 1.73 (6.9)
Cl 104 (104)	Glu 10.6 (190)	Plts 230 × 10^9 (230 × 10^3)	Mg 0.91 (2.2)
HCO$_3$ 22 (22)	HgA$_{1C}$ 0.062 (6.2)	Lkcs 9.7 × 10^9 (9.7 × 10^3)	Alb 36 (3.6)

Intact PTH 450 (450)
Total Cholesterol 6.2 (240)
LDL Cholesterol 4.8 (184)
HDL Cholesterol 0.72 (28)
Triglycerides 1.6 (140)
Dialysate effluent: WBC 200/mm³, neutrophils 110 /mm³, (Gram stain and culture pending)
Measured Kt/V = 1.1
Weekly creatinine clearance = 45 L/1.73 m²
Urine volume in 24 hours = 300 mL

■ Problem List

Identify principal problems from the scenario in priority order (see Answers in back of book for correct list of problems).

■ SOAP Note

To be completed by the student (see Answers in back of book for correct SOAP Note).

■ QUESTIONS

(See Answers in back of book for correct responses.)

1. Identify subjective and objective findings in BC consistent with peritonitis. (EO-2, 5)

2. The best antibiotic selection for empiric treatment of peritonitis in BC is: (EO-12)
   a. Cefazolin alone
   b. Gentamicin alone
   c. Cefazolin + gentamicin
   d. Vancomycin + gentamicin

3. Which of the following is the most likely pathogen of peritonitis in BC? (EO-1)
   a. *E. coli*
   b. *P. aeruginosa*
   c. *S. epidermidis*
   d. Candidiasis

4. Compared to intravenous (IV) administration, intraperitoneal (IP) administration of antibiotics for treatment of CAPD peritonitis: (EO-7, 8)
   a. Requires a longer time for resolution of infection
   b. Is the preferred method of administration
   c. Results in greater systemic drug concentrations
   d. Places patients at increased risk of systemic toxicity

5. Which of the following would be the appropriate antibiotic selection if BC's culture reveals *Pseudomonas*? (EO-12)
   a. Gentamicin alone
   b. Vancomycin alone
   c. Ceftazidime + gentamicin
   d. Fluconazole + gentamicin

6. Discuss possible options for prevention of CAPD infections in BC. (EO-7, 12)

7. Identify laboratory findings in BC that are suggestive of inadequate dialysis. (EO-11)

8. Based on the NKF-K/DOQI guidelines for management of dyslipidemia in kidney disease, BC's target LDL level is: (EO-8)
   a. <100 mg/dL
   b. <130 mg/dL

c. <160 mg/dL
d. <190 mg/dL

9. Which of the following is least likely to influence the potential for drug removal during CAPD? (EO-6)
   a. Protein binding
   b. Volume of distribution
   c. Bioavailability
   d. Molecular weight

10. If BC is switched to hemodialysis as his long-term renal replacement therapy, which of the following types of vascular access would be preferred? (EO-8, 12)
    a. AV graft
    b. AV fistula
    c. Catheter inserted in subclavian vein
    d. Catheter inserted in femoral vein

11. Evaluate BC's current regimen for management of the anemia of chronic kidney disease. (EO-11)

12. What pharmacoeconomic factors should be considered in BC's situation? (EO-17)

13. Identify psychosocial factors that may influence BC's adherence with his CAPD exchanges. (EO-15)

14. Summarize therapeutic, pathophysiologic, and disease management concepts for peritonitis using a key points format. (EO-18)

Peptic Ulcer Disease and Gastroesophageal Reflux Disease

45

Kristina L. Butler

TREATMENT GOALS: PEPTIC ULCER DISEASE AND GASTRO-ESOPHAGEAL REFLUX DISEASE

- Relieve pain, enhance ulcer healing, prevent ulcer recurrence, prevent primary complications such as gastrointestinal (GI) bleeding or perforation, and prevent secondary complications such as cough, asthma exacerbation, stricture, and adenocarcinoma.
- Apply pharmacotherapy to neutralize stomach acid (antacids), protect the stomach mucosa (sucralfate, misoprostol), and/or prevent gastric acid secretion [histamine H_2 receptor antagonists (H_2RAs), proton pump inhibitors (PPIs)]. Prokinetic agents (metoclopramide) may be considered for some patients with gastroesophageal reflux disease (GERD).
- Detect and eradicate *Helicobacter pylori* infection when present with peptic ulcer disease (PUD), using appropriate diagnostic tests and treatment regimens.
- Avoid use of ulcerogenic drugs, namely, nonsteroidal anti-inflammatory drugs (NSAIDs) and aspirin.
- Encourage nonpharmacologic measures that can decrease gastric acid secretion and increase lower esophageal sphincter (LES) pressure, such as smoking cessation and limiting intake of certain foods/beverages.

DEFINITION

Peptic ulcer disease broadly refers to a group of disorders characterized by the presence of ulcers in any portion of the GI tract exposed to acid in sufficient duration and concentration. Although these ulcerations most commonly occur in the small intestine [duodenal ulcer (DU)] or stomach [gastric ulcer (GU)], PUD also includes Barrett ulcer of the esophagus (Barrett's esophagus or Barrett's metaplasia), some types of Meckel's diverticulum, and other upper GI ulcers.[1] Any symptomatic clinical condition or histologic presentation of damage to the esophageal mucosa by retrograde flow of gastric contents into the esophagus is described as

GERD.[2] For the purposes of this chapter, unless otherwise specified, PUD refers to DU and GU, and GERD addresses upper GI disease.

During the first part of the 20th century, psychological stress and dietary factors were thought to be key factors in the pathogenesis of PUD, leading to the use of hospitalization, bed rest, and bland diets as therapy. Investigators and clinicians later recognized the pathogenic role of gastric acid and the imbalance between aggressive and protective factors in the GI tract (Table 45.1). With a focus on gastric acid as the primary cause of GI ulcers, PUD treatment included the use of antacids, then histamine H_2RAs, and eventually PPIs. Although these acid suppressive therapies were shown to be

TABLE 45.1	Factors That Contribute to Peptic Ulcer Disease

Aggressive Factors

Hydrochloric acid, pepsin

Helicobacter pylori

Nonsteroidal anti-inflammatory drugs, aspirin

Gastric mucosal ischemia

Protective Factors

Preepithelial mechanisms

   Mucus secretion

   Bicarbonate secretion

   Phospholipids (hydrophobic layer at luminal surface)

   Fibrin-mucus cap

Epithelial mechanisms

   Intracellular tight junctions and apical cell membranes

   Basolateral membrane ion pumps

   Rapid restitution (healthy cells migrate to close minor mucosal defects)

   Epithelial cell regeneration and proliferation

   Angiogenesis (formation of vessels within the injured microvascular bed)

Postepithelial mechanisms

   Mucosal blood flow

Normal pyloric function (motility)

(From Spechler SJ. Peptic ulcer and its complications. In: Feldman M, Friedman LS, Sleisenger MH, eds. Sleisenger and Fordtran's gastrointestinal and liver disease: pathophysiology/diagnosis/management. 7th ed. Philadelphia: WB Saunders, 2002:747–772.)

effective in healing acute peptic ulcer (PU), most patients experienced recurrences. During the 1980s, investigators discovered that most PUs were associated with gastric infections with *H. pylori* bacteria or with the use of NSAIDs. Elimination of these factors not only improves ulcer healing, but also prevents recurrence. Unlike for PUD, several factors usually contribute to GERD, but the best therapy for most patients is a combination of lifestyle changes and acid suppressive therapy.

EPIDEMIOLOGY

Approximately 500,000 new cases and 4 million recurrences of PU are reported each year, contributing to the approximately 10% of Americans who will develop PUD during their lifetime.[3,4] Men are affected to a slightly greater extent than women with lifetime prevalence rates of 12% compared with 9%, respectively, although this difference appears to be decreasing in the United States.[5] In Western developed countries, DU is about 1.5 times more common than GU.[6] Before the 19th century, PUD appears to have been a rare disorder, with the first cases of perforated PUs described in

the early 1800s. Incidence increased through the first half of the 20th century until the late 1960s, when the overall incidence of PUD began to decline.[7] This decreasing incidence has been associated with the declining prevalence of *H. pylori*, particularly in developed countries.[8] Although ulcer-related hospitalizations, surgeries, and deaths in the United States have also declined since the 1960s, the decrease in hospitalizations and surgeries may be the result of improvements in diagnosis and treatment for PUD, as well as changes in hospitalization criteria and the shift to ambulatory care. Despite the decrease in uncomplicated PUD, the rate of hospitalization for ulcer *complications* has not changed substantially and appears to be increasing when associated with GU. This rise in hospitalization is most evident in the elderly, and is thought to be largely due to high rates of NSAID use in this population.

Although GERD is one of the most prevalent GI diseases affecting both adults and children, incidence and prevalence rates are generally only estimates because not all patients seek medical treatment, erosive and nonerosive disease cannot be differentiated by clinical history alone, and there is currently no gold standard for the recognition or exclusion of GERD. In general, men and women are equally affected by GERD; population-based studies show that up to 15% of persons report having the hallmark symptom of epigastric burning sensation, more commonly referred to as "heartburn," at least once a week, and about 7% have it daily. The prevalence appears to be highest in Caucasians, North Americans, and Europeans, and adults over the age of 40.[9] Heartburn is commonly reported during pregnancy, with approximately 48% to 79% of women reporting daily symptoms.[2] Although men and nonpregnant women are equally effected by GERD, men are two to three times as likely to develop esophagitis and are ten times as likely to develop Barrett's metaplasia.[10] Fortunately, less than 15% of all patients with GERD suffer from severe esophagitis; however, some patients with esophageal damage may not experience significant symptoms or may present with atypical symptoms.[11]

ETIOLOGY

PEPTIC ULCER DISEASE

PUD occurs when aggravating factors, most commonly *H. pylori* or NSAIDs (Table 45.2), combine with the caustic effects of gastric acid and pepsin, which disrupts the normal defense mechanisms of the GI mucosa.[12] The relative effect of these causative factors varies considerably among different populations, and even within populations on the basis of age and other factors. The most common forms of PUD vary according to cause and clinical presentation (Table 45.3).

Helicobacter pylori. Since the identification of *H. pylori* from mucosal biopsies of patients with chronic gastritis, it has been shown that this infection is causally linked with many GI diseases, including up to 75% of PUs.[13–15] Trans-

TABLE 45.2 | Potential Causes of Peptic Ulcer Disease

Helicobacter pylori

Nonsteroidal anti-inflammatory drugs (NSAIDs), aspirin

Stress-related erosive syndrome (SRES; "stress ulcers")

Hypersecretory conditions (e.g., Zollinger-Ellison's syndrome)

Other ulcerogenic medications (e.g., alcohol, bisphosphonates, corticosteroids, erythromycin, iron salts, potassium chloride, zidovudine)

Cigarette smoking

Viral infections (e.g., cytomegalovirus, herpes simplex)

Other bacterial infections (e.g., tuberculosis)

Radiation

Chemotherapy

Illicit drug use (e.g., crack cocaine)

Vascular insufficiency

Genetic predisposition

Idiopathic causes

(From Spechler SJ. Peptic ulcer and its complications. In: Feldman M, Friedman LS, Sleisenger MH, eds. Sleisenger and Fordtran's gastrointestinal and liver disease: pathophysiology/diagnosis/management. 7th ed. Philadelphia: WB Saunders, 2002:747–772.)

mission appears to be human to human, most likely through the fecal–oral route. In developed countries, however, infection with *H. pylori* is uncommon before age 10 and increases to 10% in 18- to 30-year-olds, compared with 50% in those older than 60. Factors that influence the rate of *H. pylori* infection include birth in a developing country, low socioeconomic status, crowded living conditions, large families, unsanitary living conditions, unclean food or water, presence of infants in the home, and exposure to gastric contents of infected persons.[16] Although only 15% of persons infected with *H. pylori* develop clinical manifestations of PU, the causal relationship is supported by evidence that most non-NSAID ulcers are infected with *H. pylori*, and eradication of the bacteria significantly decreases ulcer recurrence.[13,17] Both host-specific factors and bacterial strain variability are likely to be involved in the pathogenesis of PUD.[18,19]

Nonsteroidal Anti-Inflammatory Drugs. The role of long-term NSAID (including aspirin) use in various GI tract injuries has been well documented.[20–22] NSAID-induced GI toxicity is of concern because of the frequent and often long-term use of this class of drugs, both as prescription and as over-the-counter (OTC) medications. Although superficial gastric lesions such as petechiae and erosions are common with NSAID use, especially early in the course of therapy, these lesions usually heal within a few days and decrease with long-term NSAID use. In contrast, GUs are generally of greater clinical importance because of their potential to bleed or perforate; DUs occur less often with NSAID use and may be the result of a different mechanism. NSAIDs may also exacerbate inflammatory bowel disease or cause

colonic ulcers.[20,21] During the first 3 months of NSAID use, endoscopically documented DUs and GUs occur in 4% to 15% and 10% to 40% of patients, respectively.[20] However, only 2% to 4% of long-term NSAID users will develop uncomplicated ulcers that lead to symptoms, and only 0.5% will have a serious complication.[20,23–25]

Patients with a history of PUD, upper GI bleeding, or NSAID-related complications, or those taking concurrent ulcerogenic medications (e.g., corticosteroids) or agents that increase bleeding risk (e.g., warfarin, clopidogrel), are at greatest risk for serious GI complications.[20,22] Although it appears that these may not be independent risk factors, patient age, smoking status, chronic excessive alcohol use, presence of cardiovascular disease, or other chronic medical conditions that lead to poor general health also increase the risk of GI complications with NSAIDs. Use of antacids or H$_2$RAs by asymptomatic patients may actually increase the risk for serious complications because, although they may not completely prevent GI bleeding, these agents may mask symptoms associated with GI complications.[22]

Hypersecretory Conditions. Rarely, PUD results from hypersecretory conditions in which the stomach secretes large quantities of gastric acid and overwhelms the body's normal defense mechanisms. Zollinger-Ellison's syndrome (ZES), which is associated with recurrent ulcerations caused by a gastrinoma (gastrin-producing tumor), accounts for less than 0.1% of patients with DU.[26] Men and women are equally at risk. The mean age of diagnosis is 50 years, although much older or younger patients may present. Systemic mastocytosis is a rare disorder characterized by mast cell infiltration of a number of organs; approximately 40% of persons with systemic mastocytosis develop DUs. Such disorders should be considered in any patient with recurrent PUs in the absence of *H. pylori* or NSAID use, particularly if there is associated diarrhea, and if the ulcer is severe or complicated or involves the postbulbar duodenum.

Stress-Related Erosive Syndrome. Physiologic stress from shock, sepsis, serious burn injury, head injury with increased intracranial pressure, severe trauma, quadriplegia due to acute cervical spine injury, acute renal failure, cirrhosis, multiorgan failure, respiratory failure/ventilator dependency, or coagulopathy can cause stress-related erosive syndrome (SRES); the latter two are strong independent risk factors for hemorrhage.[1,27–31] A small number of ulcers may develop as quickly as 48 to 72 hours after the onset of injury or severe stress; larger amounts of blood loss usually occur 3 or more days after the initial injury or stress event. Although studies using endoscopic examination of severely ill patients have found gastroduodenal mucosal lesions in more than 75% of cases, when untreated, only a very small proportion of patients develop clinically important consequences; perhaps this is a result of advances in the medical management of critically ill patients.[32] In contrast to *H. pylori* or NSAID-induced ulcers, the mucosa surrounding these lesions is not involved in an inflammatory process, and associated bleeding is usually superficial but progressive. When accompa-

TABLE 45.3	Causes, Characteristics, and Clinical Features of Peptic Ulcer Disease, and Gastroesophageal Reflux Disease			
Feature	DU	GU	SRES	GERD
Most common cause	*H. pylori* (NSAID less common)	NSAIDs (*H. pylori* less common)	Physiologic stress	↑ LES relaxation frequency or ↓ LES pressure
Dependence on intragastric pH	More dependent	Less dependent	Less dependent	Less dependent
Deep ulcers	No	Yes	No	No
Severe GI bleeding	No	Yes	Yes	No
Pain	Consistently	Consistently	Rarely (usually asymptomatic)	Frequently
Location of most common pain	Consistently epigastric	Frequently epigastric (often more diffuse)	N/A	Frequently substernal, may radiate to neck
Severe	Frequently	Frequently	N/A	Infrequently
Description	Gnawing, burning, aching	Gnawing, burning	N/A	Warm or burning
Episodes	Clustered	Intermittent	N/A	Intermittent
Worse at night	67%	33%	N/A	Frequently
Impact of food	Relieved	Worsened/no change	N/A	Worsened by certain foods
Relieved by antacids	Consistently	Frequently	N/A	Frequently
Nausea	Infrequently	Frequently	N/A	Rarely
Vomiting	Infrequently	Frequently	N/A	Rarely
Anorexia	Rarely	50%	N/A	Rarely
Weight changes	Increases are more common	50%	N/A	Rarely
Bloating	Frequently	Frequently	N/A	Frequently
Belching	Frequently	Frequently	N/A	Frequently
Heartburn	Frequently	Rarely	N/A	Consistently

DU, duodenal ulcer; GU, gastric ulcer; SRES, stress-related erosive syndrome; GERD, gastroesophageal reflux disease; NSAID, nonsteroidal anti-inflammatory drug; LES, lower esophageal sphincter; GI, gastrointestinal.

nied by acute upper GI bleeding, SRES is associated with significant morbidity and mortality.

Other Factors. Although epidemiologic evidence links cigarette smoking to PUD and its complications, it remains unclear whether smoking is an independent risk factor.[1,12,33,34] Cigarette smoking appears to increase the risk of PUD with *H. pylori* infection, but not after eradication. Similarly, cigarette smoking has been reported to increase the risk of NSAID-induced GI complications.[22] Smoking impairs ulcer healing and promotes recurrence in a dose-dependent manner, requiring longer treatment periods and/or higher doses of antisecretory agents.[35] Smoking also appears to increase the risk of complications and the need for surgery.

No published studies have established a convincing link between diet or alcohol and PUD. Although the ingestion of certain foods such as coffee, tea, cola beverages, alcoholic beverages, milk, and spicy cuisine may increase gastric acid secretions and cause dyspepsia, the evidence that such foods or beverages cause PU is virtually nonexistent.[1,34] Therefore, although it was once traditional to prescribe a bland diet for patients with PU, beverage restriction and bland diets have not been shown to confer any benefit in preventing or treating PUD.

The role of psychological factors in PUD is controversial. Clinical observations have long supported the belief that emotional stress might cause or exacerbate PU; however, controlled studies have failed to document a causal effect. Although major psychological stress has been reported to increase basal acid secretion and may predispose the GI mucosa to injury, psychological stress alone does not appear to be sufficient to cause PUD in most persons, because eradication of *H. pylori* and elimination of NSAIDs generally prevents ulcer recurrence, regardless of emotional factors.

A number of genetic factors have been proposed to explain familial aggregation of PUD; however, the genes responsible for this apparent ulcer predisposition are not known. Data suggest that *H. pylori* infection is the more likely explanation for familial clustering of PUD.[36] Some proposed genetic markers for PUD might actually represent a genetic susceptibility to *H. pylori* infection rather than a specific susceptibility to PU.

Several chronic illnesses have been associated with PUD; however, considerable overlap may be noted with other causes, such as NSAID and corticosteroid use in arthritis, or smoking and corticosteroid use in chronic pulmonary disease.[1] DU and GU are increased in patients with cirrhosis, but a causal relationship has not been confirmed, and drinkers without cirrhosis do not have increased risk of PUD. Chronic renal failure has also been proposed as a risk factor for PUD, but studies on this issue are conflicting. Similarly, Addison's disease, Cushing's disease, hyperparathyroidism, atrophic gastritis, pernicious anemia, and coronary artery disease have been suggested as being associated with PUD, but supporting evidence is lacking.

GASTROESOPHAGEAL REFLUX DISEASE

Unlike with PUD, the roles of *H. pylori* and NSAIDs in GERD are controversial. NSAID use has been associated with peptic strictures,[37] and observational data showed a small but statistically significant increase in reflux esophagitis in veterans using NSAIDs.[38] With regard to *H. pylori*, epidemiologic data suggest a protective role for *H. pylori* infection in that patients with GERD and *H. pylori* are less likely to develop esophagitis or Barrett's metaplasia than are GERD patients without the infection. Additionally, the incidences of GERD and esophagitis increase after antibiotic eradication of *H. pylori*, and the presence of *H. pylori* may improve the efficacy of antisecretory therapy in healing esophagitis and maintaining remission.[2] Whether or not *H. pylori* infection should be treated in patients with GERD remains unresolved because of the conflicting risks of treatment with GERD and the benefits of treatment associated with PUD. Another difference between GERD and PUD is the role of dietary factors and alcohol. Many foods and beverages can contribute to or decrease GERD through mechanisms discussed in the next section, as can various medications, some hormones, and other physiologic factors (Table 45.4).[2,39]

Most conditions that predispose patients to the development of GERD are associated with abnormalities of the antireflux barrier or esophageal acid clearance. Pregnancy is the most common condition that predisposes patients to GERD; as the uterus enlarges, an increase in the abdominal pressure occurs, which promotes reflux of the gastric contents retrograde up the esophagus. Additionally, increases in progesterone levels are associated with decreases in resting LES pressure and slow gastric emptying. Patients with mixed connective tissue disorders (e.g., scleroderma) commonly have impaired esophageal function, characterized by diminished peristalsis in the smooth muscle segment of the esophagus and decreased or absent LES pressure. Changes in gastric emptying associated with diabetic gastroparesis, intestinal pseudo-obstruction, and collagen vascular disorders may also increase the risk of GERD. Patients with hypersecretory conditions, such as ZES, are also at risk for GERD because of associated abnormalities in the quality and quantity of the refluxate (in contrast to abnormalities of the antireflux barrier or esophageal acid clearance).[2]

PATHOPHYSIOLOGY

PUD occurs when various processes affect the regulation of gastric acid and pepsin, or when the epithelial defense and healing mechanisms are altered (Fig. 45.1; *see color insert*). Abnormal gastric motility can also contribute to PUD and is the key factor in GERD.

GENERAL PHYSIOLOGY AND PATHOPHYSIOLOGY

Regulation of Gastric Acid Secretion. As proposed by Schwarz in 1910 with his famous dictum, "no acid, no ulcer," gastric acid is a requirement for PUD. Acid secretion is a complex, integrated process that can be modified at several points. Basal acid production occurs in a circadian pattern, with highest levels occurring during the night (average diurnal pH as low as 1.4), and lowest levels during morning hours.[40] Basal acid output usually ranges from 0 to 5 mEq per hour, but can rise to 20 mEq per hour or higher with maximal acid output or in response to a meal. The stimulation and inhibition of gastric acid secretion by parietal cells are mediated by three pathways: neurocrine, paracrine, and endocrine (Fig 45.2).[41]

Parietal cells, located in the walls of the oxyntic mucosa, secrete hydrochloric (HCl) acid when the hydrogen-potassium ion adenosine triphosphatase (H^+/K^+-ATPase) proton pump is activated. During rest, this enzyme is located within the cytoplasm of the parietal cell, but it translocates to the canalicular membrane upon activation. Active proton pumps then exchange one potassium ion (K^+) for one hydrogen ion (H^+) from the cytoplasm. The stomach contains approximately 1 billion parietal cells that can secrete H^+ ions into the gastric lumen against a 3 million:1 concentration gradient, producing acid concentrations as high as 160 mEq per L.[40] The parietal cell has several receptors for stimulation of H^+ ion production, including histamine (H_2), gastrin, and acetylcholine (the muscarinic, M_3 receptor).

The principal neurocrine transmitter, acetylcholine, is released from postganglionic vagal neurons in the stomach. The endocrine pathway involves the secretion of gastrin from antral gastrin cells (G-cells) in the pyloric mucosa. Gastrin has many physiologic actions, such as stimulation of pepsinogen secretion, hepatic bile flow, and secretions of the pancreas, including insulin. Gastrin also stimulates gas-

| TABLE 45.4 | Factors That Affect Lower Esophageal Sphincter (LES) Pressure and Contractility |

	Aggravating/Protecting Factor			
Mechanism	Foods and Beverages	Medications	Hormones and Physiologic Factors	Other
Increased GERD				
Decreased resting LES pressure	Caffeinated beverages Citrus juices Chocolate Ethanol Fatty foods/meal Garlic Mint Onion Sugar Tomato and tomato juices	Anticholinergics α-blockers β-agonists Barbiturates Benzodiazepines Caffeine Calcium channel blockers Dopamine Estrogen Isoproterenol Opioids Nicotine Nitrates Phentolamine Progesterone Theophylline	Cholecystokinin Estrogen Gastric acidification Gastric inhibitory polypeptide Glucagon Progesterone Prostaglandins (E_1, E_2, A_2) Secretin Serotonin Vasoactive intestinal peptide (VIP)	Pregnancy
Increased transient LES relaxation frequency	Fatty foods/meals	Sumatriptan	Cholecystokinin l-Arginine	
Direct mucosal irritant	Alcohol Caffeine-containing beverages/foods Carbonated beverages Citrus products Spicy foods Tomato-based products	Aspirin NSAIDs Tetracycline Quinidine Potassium chloride tablets Iron salts		Reclining after meals
Increased intra-abdominal pressure	Carbonated beverages Chewing gum after meals Consuming fluids with meals Eating rapidly Large meal size Smoking after meals			Bending over Constipation Exercise Lifting Obesity Overeating Pregnancy Restrictive abdominal clothing Straining (bowel movements)
Decreased GERD				
Increased resting LES pressure	High-protein foods/meals	α-agonists β-blockers Cholinergic agents Dopamine antagonists Gastrinlike agents Parasympathomimetic agents Prokinetic agents Sympathomimetic agents	Gastric alkalinization Gastrin Motilin Prostaglandin $F_{2\alpha}$ Substance P	
Decreased transient LES relaxation frequency		Atropine Baclofen Morphine	L-nitroarginine methyl ester (L-NAME) Serotonin	
Direct mucosal buffer	Chewing gum or sucking on a lozenge after meals Nonfat or low-fat milk			
Decreased intra-abdominal pressure	Smaller meal size			Elevate head of bed 4–6 inches Wear loose clothing around abdomen Lose weight if overweight

GERD, gastroesophageal reflux disease; NSAIDs, nonsteroidal anti-inflammatory drugs.

(From Kahrilas PJ, Pandolfin JE. Gastroesophageal reflux disease and its complications, including Barrett's metaplasia. In: Felman M, Friedman LS, Sleisenger MH, eds. Sleisenger and Fordtran's gastrointestinal and liver disease: pathophysiology/diagnosis/management. 7th ed. Philadelphia: WB Saunders, 2002:599–622; Kim SL, Hunter JG, Wo JM, et al. NSAIDs, aspirin, and esophageal strictures: are over-the-counter medications harmful to the esophagus? J Clin Gastroenterol 29:32–34, 1999; with permission.)

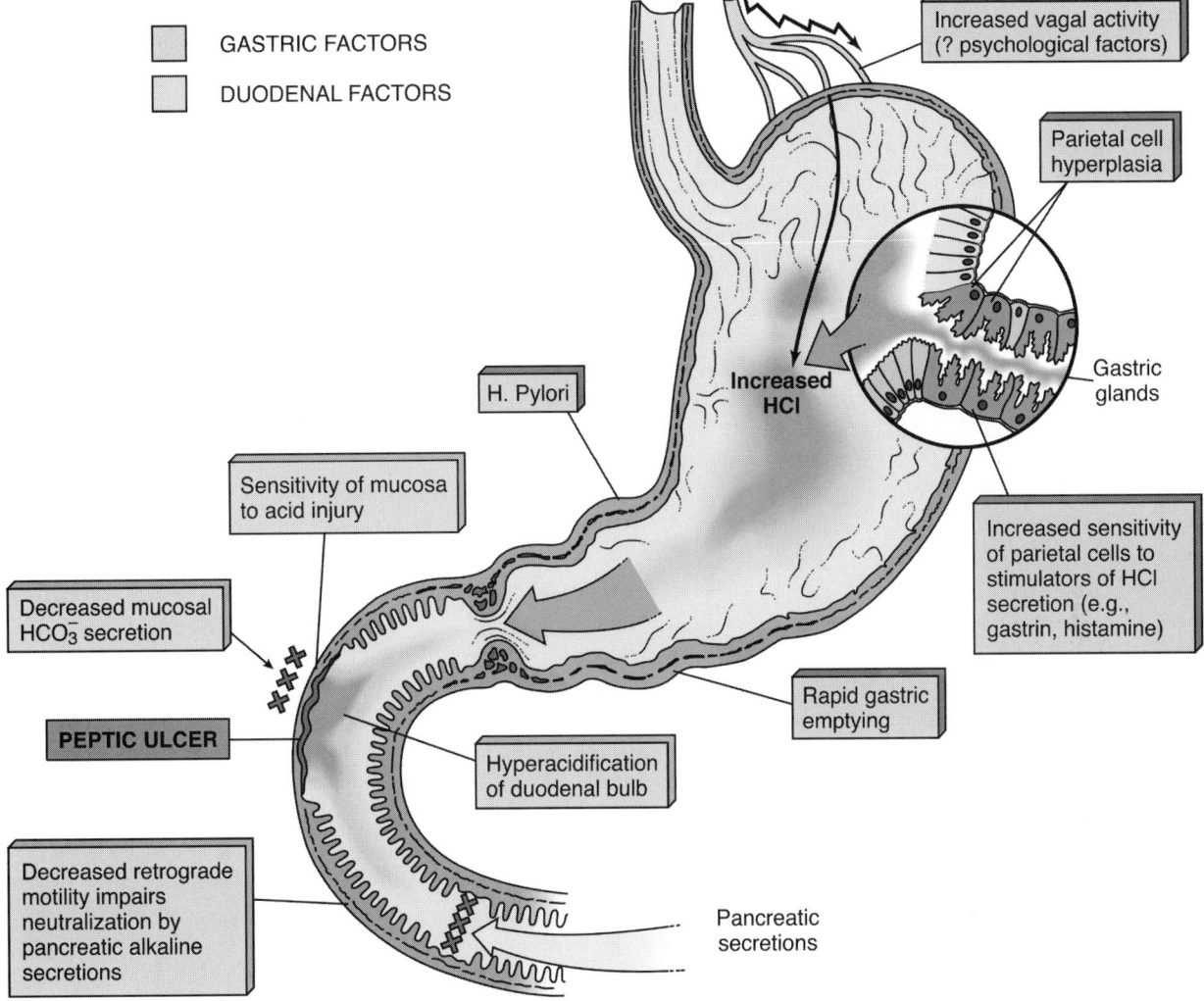

GASTRIC FACTORS

DUODENAL FACTORS

Increased vagal activity
(? psychological factors)

Parietal cell
hyperplasia

Increased
HCl

Gastric
glands

H. Pylori

Sensitivity of mucosa
to acid injury

Increased sensitivity
of parietal cells to
stimulators of HCl
secretion (e.g.,
gastrin, histamine)

Decreased mucosal
HCO₃⁻ secretion

PEPTIC ULCER

Rapid gastric
emptying

Hyperacidification
of duodenal bulb

Decreased retrograde
motility impairs
neutralization by
pancreatic alkaline
secretions

Pancreatic
secretions

FIGURE 45.1 Gastric and duodenal factors in the pathogenesis of duodenal peptic ulcers (*see color insert*). (Reprinted from Rubin E, Farber JL. Pathology. 3rd ed. Philadelphia: Lippincott Williams & Wilkins, 1999, with permission.)

tric and intestinal motility, and increases LES pressure, which promotes closure of the sphincter. The role of gastrin in gastric acid secretion is twofold: gastrin directly stimulates HCl acid secretion through action at the gastrin receptors on the parietal cell, but more importantly, gastrin is a potent activator of the enterochromaffin-like (ECL) cell, which releases histamine. Histamine, the primary paracrine transmitter and apparent dominant pathway, which in turn activates the H_2 receptors on the parietal cell. Adenylate cyclase is then activated, which produces increased levels of adenosine 3′,5′-cyclic monophosphate (cAMP) from ATP and the subsequent generation of H^+ ions. The proton pump then becomes mobilized and activated, as described earlier.[41]

The discovery that different factors and their corresponding receptors lead to the activation of different signaling pathways explains the potentiation of acid secretion that occurs when acetylcholine, histamine, and gastrin are combined. Additionally, this explains why blocking of one recep-

tor type (H_2) decreases acid secretion, regardless of which factor was involved in the stimulation. However, it also explains why blocking only one pathway may not be as effective as blocking the final common step of acid secretion.

Autoregulatory mechanisms prevent postprandial acid hypersecretion. With the ingestion of a meal, gastrin release stimulates gastric acid secretion (as detailed earlier), decreasing intraluminal pH, which then stimulates the release of somatostatin from antral D-cells. Somatostatin then acts via a paracrine pathway to inhibit the G-cells from releasing more gastrin, and may directly inhibit acid secretion from parietal cells and suppress histamine release from ECL cells (Fig. 45.2).[41] Other neurotransmitters, such as vasoactive intestinal peptide (VIP), galanin, serotonin, and pituitary adenylate cyclase–activating peptide, may also be important in the direct and indirect regulation of gastric acid secretion.

Approximately 30% to 50% of patients with DU are hypersecretors of gastric acid, particularly those with *H. pylori*

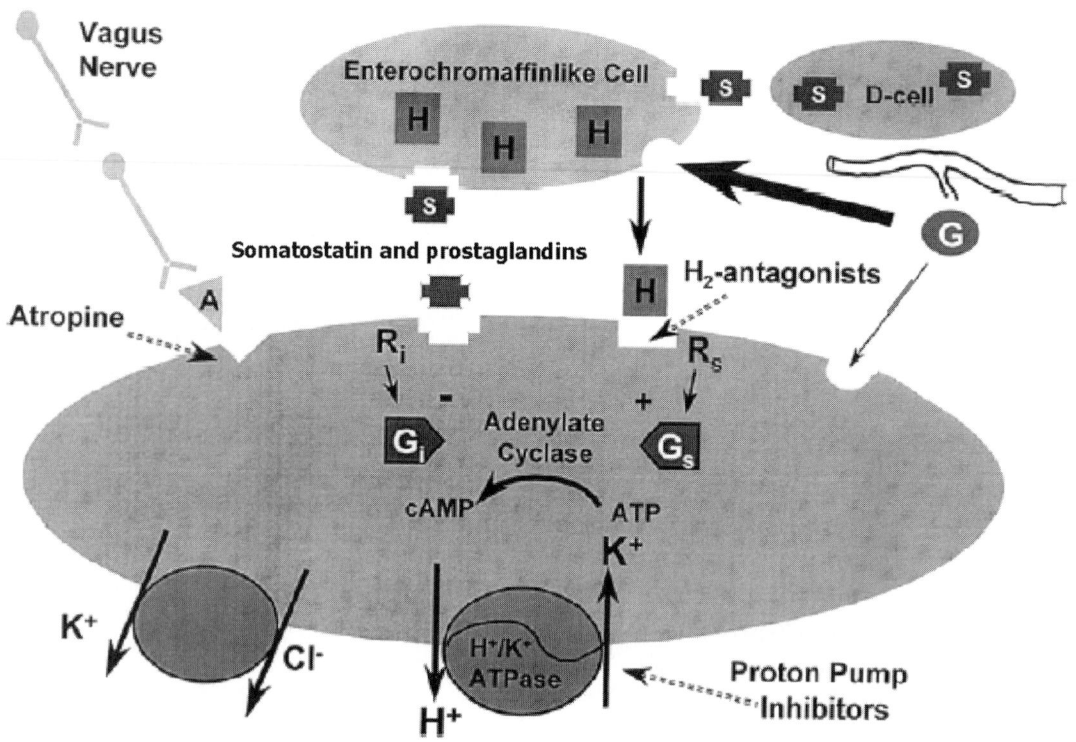

FIGURE 45.2 Schematic representation of the factors that influence gastric acid secretion by the parietal cell, depicting neurocrine [acetylcholine and other neurotransmitters (A) from vagal efferent neurons], paracrine [histamine (H) from gastric enterochromaffinlike (ECL) cells and somatostatin (S) from D-cells], and endocrine [circulating gastrin (G)] factors. *Dashed arrows* indicate potential sites of pharmacologic inhibition of acid secretion, via receptor antagonism or inhibition of H^+,K^+-adenosine triphosphatase (ATPase). (Reprinted from Wolfe MM, Sachs G. Acid suppression: optimizing therapy for gastroduodenal ulcer healing, gastroesophageal reflux disease, and stress-related erosive syndrome. Gastroenterology 118:S10, 2000, with permission.)

infection.[42] Factors such as increased parietal cell mass, increased basal secretory drive, and increased postprandial secretory drive account for this acid hypersecretion, which may be affected by enhanced sensitivity of the parietal cell to secretagogues or vagal stimulation, as well as impaired acid inhibitory mechanisms. Gastrinomas, such as those in ZES, cause high gastrin levels and basal acid hypersecretion. Fasting and meal-stimulated gastrin levels are also elevated in patients with DU and *H. pylori* infection. In contrast to what is seen with DU and *H. pylori*–associated PUD, patients with GU often have normal or reduced rates of acid secretion, which reflect a low–normal parietal cell mass.

Pepsin. Not only do acid and pepsin work together to facilitate peptic digestion of dietary protein in the stomach, but pepsin also contributes to ulcer formation by disrupting the mucus–bicarbonate barrier. Stimulated by similar pathways as those involved in gastric acid secretion, gastric mucosal cells secrete two types of proteolytic proenzymes: pepsinogen I (PI) and pepsinogen II (PII); PI secretion is directly proportional to the rate of gastric acid secretion. Pepsin is activated by acidic pH (optimal pH 1.8 to 3.5), inactivated reversibly at pH 5, and denatured at pH 7 to 8.[1,42] Hypergas-

trinemia and *H. pylori* infection in DU are associated with increased serum PI concentrations, while serum levels of PII are elevated in GU.

Alteration of Mucosal Defense and Healing. Although the gastric mucosa is continuously exposed to acid, pepsin, and other noxious agents, ulceration is a relatively abnormal event. The mechanisms that are employed to resist acid-peptic assault can be divided into three major components: preepithelial, epithelial, and postepithelial defense mechanisms (Table 45.1).[1] Gastric epithelial cells and duodenal Brunner's glands secrete mucus and bicarbonate, and additional bicarbonate from the blood enters the unstirred water layer through paracellular diffusion. The phospholipids contained in the mucus and the unstirred bicarbonate-rich water near the mucosal surface may protect the mucosa by forming hydrophobic layers that repel and neutralize acid. Within the mucous layer, glycoproteins also form a physical barrier to the diffusion of pepsin. As a result of these preepithelial defense mechanisms, the epithelial surface's pH can normally be maintained in the neutral range, even when pH in the lumen falls to below 2. Patients with DU, however, have decreased production of bicarbonate by the duodenum.

Intracellular tight junctions, apical cell membranes, and basolateral membrane ion pumps further help prevent hydrogen ions from crossing the gastric mucosa. If damaged, mucus, fibrin, and cellular debris are released from the mucosa to form a protective cap that clings to the injured epithelium and impedes further contact with acid. At the same time, healthy cells migrate to close minor mucosal defects, new cells are formed because of rapid regeneration and proliferation, and vessels are formed within the injured microvascular bed to repair the mucosa. If hydrogen ions do cross the gastric mucosa, gastric mucosal blood flow removes them rapidly. Endogenous prostaglandins (PGs) are primarily responsible for preserving this mucosal integrity and repair by stimulating mucus and bicarbonate secretion, maintaining gastric mucosal blood flow, and activating mucosal proliferation to prevent deep mucosal injury.

Abnormal Gastric Motility. The rate at which stomach contents move to the duodenum is defined as gastric motility. In contrast, duodenal motility affects the clearance of gastric, biliary, and pancreatic sections from the duodenum.[1] Abnormal motility patterns allow the contents of the duodenum, including bile salts and pancreatic enzymes, to reflux into the stomach, which contributes to GU. For some patients with DU, a relative increase may be noted in the acidity of the proximal duodenum, caused by accelerated gastric emptying. Conversely, delayed gastric emptying increases the stomach's exposure to acid, pepsin, and refluxed duodenal content. For some patients, these motility abnormalities may increase the severity of gastric injury induced by *H. pylori* or NSAIDs. Alterations in gastric motility may also affect gastric acid secretion, in that the location of food and other gastric contents within the GI tract is another factor that both positively and negatively regulates acid and digestive enzyme secretion.

A competent esophagogastric junction for prevention of gastroesophageal reflux requires numerous anatomic and physiologic mechanisms, including intrinsic LES pressure, extrinsic compression of the LES by the crural diaphragm, intra-abdominal location of the LES, integrity of the phrenoesophageal ligament, and maintenance of the acute angle of His between the distal esophagus and proximal stomach with its flap valve function.[2] It is thought that the prominent mechanism may vary, depending on the situation. For example, the intra-abdominal segment of the LES may be the most important factor to prevent reflux during swallowing, but basal LES pressure may play a larger role if the patient is reclined. Because these mechanisms are additive in their protective effects, if several components are compromised, the risk of damage caused by increasingly abnormal esophageal acid exposure is heightened.

ETIOLOGY-SPECIFIC PATHOPHYSIOLOGY

Helicobacter pylori. *H. pylori* is a spiral-shaped, flagellated, pH-sensitive, urease-producing, microaerophilic, gram-negative organism that uses its shape and flagella to burrow through the mucosal layer to the neutral-pH environment of the gastric epithelial cell surface.[1,13,43] *H. pylori* can be found on any surface of the gastric mucosa but favors the metaplastic gastric epithelium in the duodenal bulb. High duodenal acid levels promote gastric metaplasia, which then provides a favorable environment for *H. pylori* colonization. Colonization leads to inflammation of the mucosa, promoting more gastric metaplasia, which then results in more extensive *H. pylori* colonization. The result of this vicious circle is that the mucosa becomes highly susceptible to ulceration. *H. pylori* strains differ in the severity of inflammation produced, and those strains that cause the most severe inflammation are the most likely to cause symptomatic disease.[6] Although strains vary in virulence, all strains may cause inflammation, PU, or gastric cancer.

Acute *H. pylori* infection is accompanied by transient hypochlorhydria, which allows bacteria to survive in the acidic environment of the stomach. One theory of how *H. pylori* induces hypochlorhydria is that the bacteria produce large quantities of urease, which hydrolyzes urea contained in gastric secretions, converting it to ammonia and bicarbonate; this creates a neutral microenvironment and protects the organism from the lethal effects of the acid.[13] The bacteria may also produce acid-inhibitory proteins. Once a stable microenvironment is created, *H. pylori* attaches to the gastric epithelium with adherence pedestals, preventing it from being shed through the normal mucosal defense and healing processes, and periodic emptying of gastric contents.

Before the discovery of *H. pylori*, when PUD was considered a disorder of gastric acid homeostasis, many studies focused on identifying abnormalities in acid secretion. It is now thought that many of the abnormalities most commonly seen with DU (e.g., increased basal acid secretion, elevated fasting and meal-stimulated gastrin levels) may not be the primary problem, but rather, may be a reversible consequence of *H. pylori* infection.[44] Although more than 80% of patients with DU and more than 60% of patients with GU are infected with *H. pylori*,[45] bacterial, environmental, and host factors are likely important in determining infection outcome.[6] The exact role of the infection in many of the physiologic abnormalities identified in PUD remains unclear. Direct mucosal damage is thought to be one of the mechanisms by which *H. pylori* contributes to PUD. Bacterial enzymes, such as lipases and proteases, degrade the gastric mucosa, and urease produces ammonia, which may be toxic to gastric epithelial cells. Bacterial adherence, as described earlier, enhances the uptake of toxins by the epithelial cells, and the protein toxin Vac A, which is present in about 50% of *H. pylori* strains, causes cellular vacuole formation. The second proposed mechanism by which *H. pylori* leads to PUD is via an altered immune/inflammatory response, in which bacteria damage the epithelial cells directly by cell-mediated immune mechanisms and indirectly by the activation of neutrophils or macrophages that attempt to phagocytose the bacteria or bacterial products.[46]

Hypergastrinemia that leads to increased gastric acid production is the third way that *H. pylori* is proposed to induce PUD.[47] This appears to be mediated by the following pathways: cytokines, such as tumor necrosis factor (TNF-α); products of *H. pylori*, including ammonia; and decreased expression of protective factors such as somatostatin, which may also result from the cytokines.[47] Unlike with PUD, in patients with gastric cancer, *H. pylori* infection appears to promote gastric atrophy, which leads to decreased acid output.

Nonsteroidal Anti-Inflammatory Drugs. The exact mechanism by which NSAID therapy contributes to PUD is not known, but the two major ulcerogenic components are (1) the direct or topical effects of acid on the gastric mucosa, and (2) the systemic inhibition of the synthesis of protective endogenous PGs, of which the latter is most significant.[20] The conversion of arachidonic acid to PGs is mediated by the enzyme cyclooxygenase (COX), which is inhibited by NSAIDs (Fig. 45.3). The two following subtypes of the COX enzyme exist in humans: COX-1, which is found in many body tissues such as the stomach and intestines, kidneys, and platelets; and COX-2, which under normal physiologic conditions is not detectable but is induced during acute and chronic inflammation.[20,21] COX-1 produces protective PGs important for the regulation of physiologic processes such as GI cytoprotection, renal function, and vascular homeostasis. Inflammatory stimuli such as cytokines upregulate COX-2, which produces PGs involved in the processes of inflammation and pain. All NSAIDs inhibit both COX-1 and COX-2 to varying degrees.

A number of other mechanisms might also contribute to the development of NSAID-related mucosal injury. TNF-α may signal the adherence of neutrophils within the gastric microcirculation, which can damage the vascular endothelium and cause a reduction in mucosal blood flow, or it might liberate oxygen-derived free radicals and proteases.[21]

Inflammatory leukotrienes may also stimulate neutrophil adherence and contribute to mucosal injury.

In gastric acid, weakly acidic NSAIDs (e.g., aspirin) exist in their un-ionized form, which allows them to easily enter the gastric cells. Within the cell's neutral pH environment, H^+ ions dissociate, resulting in a negatively charged NSAID molecule that cannot pass back across the cell membrane. Through this mechanism, NSAIDs may rapidly become concentrated in the mucosa and cause superficial injury (e.g., petechiae, erosions) within minutes of ingestion. NSAID metabolites, which are excreted in bile, can also cause topical injury to the GI mucosa.[1] Although superficial NSAID-related GI injury may be decreased with the use of prodrugs, salicylate derivatives, enteric-coated preparations, or non-oral routes of administration, these preparations do not significantly reduce the risk of PUD, which reinforces that the main cause of NSAID-related ulceration is the systemic inhibition of PGs.

Not only can NSAIDs cause new ulcers, they can also inhibit the healing of preexisting lesions by interfering with cellular restitution. Through their inhibition of platelet aggregation, NSAIDs may also increase the risk that PUs will bleed. The pathogenesis of NSAID-related ulcers of the duodenum and colon is not as well understood as that in the stomach, but it appears that enteric bacteria and enterohepatic NSAID recirculation contribute more significantly than does PG inhibition to the formation of ulcers at these sites.[21]

Zollinger-Ellison's Syndrome and Other Hypersecretory Conditions. Rarely, PUD results from hypersecretory conditions in which the extensive amount of gastric acid produced overwhelms the normal epithelial defense mechanisms, leading to ulcer formation.[1,26] Additionally, the large amounts of gastric acid that pass into the duodenum can damage the intestinal mucosa and denature pancreatic digestive enzymes, causing malabsorption and diarrhea. In contrast to chronic PUD, in which gastrin levels are not elevated,

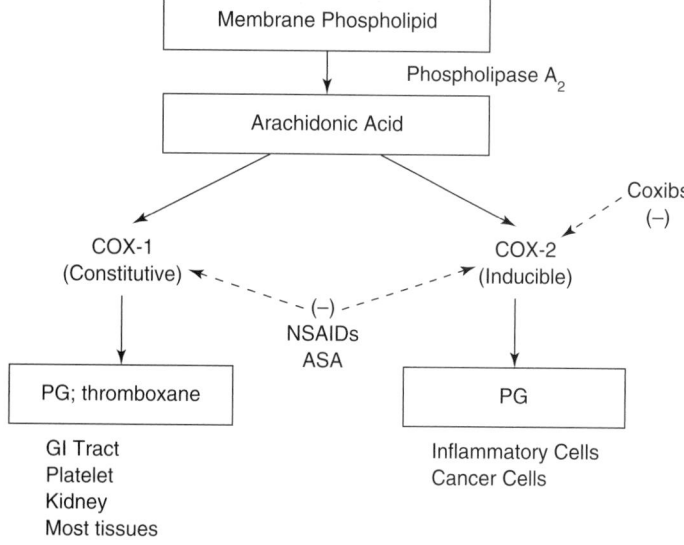

FIGURE 45.3 Mechanism of action of traditional nonsteroidal anti-inflammatory drugs (NSAIDs) and cyclooxygenase-2 selective inhibitors (coxibs). Cyclooxygenase-1 (COX-1) is constitutively expressed and produces protective prostaglandins (PGs) in the gastrointestinal (GI) tract, platelets, kidneys, and most tissues; its expression may also be regulated. Cyclooxygenase-2 (COX-2) is induced at sites of inflammation and produces PGs for inflammation and pain in inflammatory cells, and in the kidneys, female reproductive system, brain, and cancer cells. *Dashed arrows* indicate potential sites of pharmacologic inhibition in the arachidonic acid pathway, via inhibition of COX-1 or COX-2.

patients with ZES have a gastrin-producing pancreatic adenoma (gastrinoma) that causes recurrent ulcerations, most commonly DUs located in the region of the pancreas. Gastrin not only has potent effects on gastric acid secretion, but it is also able to stimulate growth of the gastric mucosa. ECL and parietal cell hyperplasia often occurs in patients with ZES.

A rare primary form of antral G-cell hyperfunction not associated with *H. pylori* may manifest as gastric acid hypersecretion, elevated fasting serum gastrin levels, and marked postprandial hypergastrinemia. The mast cells, which are numerous in systemic mastocytosis, release histamine. The elevated serum levels of histamine appear to cause profound gastric acid hypersecretion, which has been observed in some patients. Similar to mast cells, basophils contain histamine; occasionally, myeloproliferative disorders associated with basophilia (e.g., polycythemia vera, basophilic chronic myelogenous leukemia) have been accompanied by gastric acid hypersecretion and PUD.[1,26]

Stress-Related Erosive Syndrome. The main pathology of SRES is impaired mucosal resistance to peptic injury. Reduced gastric blood flow causes mucosal ischemia, which can lead to local acidosis, free radical formation, diminished acid-buffering capacity, decreased mucosal secretion of mucus and bicarbonate, and impaired rapid restitution. These effects allow acid in the lumen to reenter the mucosa (so-called acid ''back-diffusion'') and cause further injury. Unlike other ulcer types described previously, little inflammation of the surrounding mucosa has been noted with SRES ulcers. Gastric acid appears necessary for the formation of lesions, but acid hypersecretion is not usually present.[48] Cushing's ulcers (those that occur with acute head injuries) differ from other SRES ulcers in this regard because they are associated with hypergastrinemia and hypersecretion of gastric acid. Although most of these ulcers are asymptomatic gastric erosions, deep GUs and DUs that can become complicated by life-threatening hemorrhage and perforation are possible.

Gastroesophageal Reflux Disease. Esophageal damage is primarily related to the reflux of noxious gastric contents such as gastric acid, pepsin, bile acids, and pancreatic enzymes. Unlike some types of PUD, GERD is not usually associated with hypersecretion of acid; instead, the problem is that the acid produced remains in contact with the esophageal mucosa for extended periods. In most cases, GERD is due to defective LES pressure, which may be related to spontaneous transient LES relaxations, transient increases in intra-abdominal pressure, or an atonic LES. Problems with other normal mucosal defense mechanisms and gastric emptying, as described earlier, may also contribute to the development of GERD, although to a much lesser degree.[2]

It is thought that transient LES relaxations are the most frequent mechanism that causes reflux in the majority of patients.[2] These episodes persist for longer periods (>10 seconds) than do swallowing-induced LES relaxations, occur independently of swallowing, and are not accompanied by peristalsis, but they are associated with normal diaphragmatic inhibition. A decrease in resting LES tone or pressure is another significant mechanism for reflux, although few patients with GERD have a resting LES pressure of less than 10 mm Hg (normal is 10 to 30 mm Hg, relative to intragastric pressure).[2] In addition to the numerous physiologic, pharmacologic, and dietary agents that affect resting LES pressure and transient LES relaxation frequency (Table 45.4), distention of the proximal stomach and increased intra-abdominal pressure are key stimuli for reflux.

''Esophageal acid clearance time'' refers to the duration of time that the esophageal mucosa remains acidified (pH <4) after an episode of gastric acid reflux. Prolonged acid exposure has been shown to correlate with the severity of esophagitis and the presence of Barrett's metaplasia. Acid clearance involves peristalsis and neutralization with swallowed saliva. Impaired esophageal emptying in GERD is evident in the observation that symptoms improve with change to an upright posture, which demonstrates the role of gravity in augmenting fluid emptying. Peristaltic dysfunction and re-reflux associated with hiatal hernias have been identified as two mechanisms of impaired esophageal emptying. As esophagitis increases in severity, so does the incidence of peristaltic dysfunction, but unfortunately, healing of the esophagitis through acid inhibition or by antireflux surgery has not been shown to reverse peristaltic dysfunction. It is thought that acute dysfunction may be partially reversible, but that chronic disease associated with strictures or extensive fibrosis is not.[2] Patients with nonreducing hiatal hernias also have impaired esophageal emptying, with evidence of retrograde flow of fluid from the hernia.

Saliva contains bicarbonate, as well as growth factors that may enhance mucosal repair. Periods of diminished salivation, such as those occuring during sleep, reduce acid neutralization and are associated with more frequent reflux events. Use of substances that increase salivation, such as oral lozenges, chewing gum, or bethanechol chloride, accelerates acid clearance; however, hyposalivation prolongs acid clearance.[2] Cigarette smokers have prolonged esophageal acid clearance times (50% longer than nonsmokers) that are attributed to hyposalivation.

Mucosal defense and healing processes of the esophagus are somewhat similar to those of the stomach and small intestine; however, preepithelial mechanisms play a minimal role in the esophagus. Therefore, the burden of defense shifts to the integrity of the squamous epithelium, which (1) provides a structural barrier to prevent acid diffusion, and (2) exhibits metabolic specialization, neutralizing hydrogen ions within the intercellular space and cytoplasm. The 25 to 30 cell layers are divided into a proliferating basal cell layer, a midzone layer of metabolically active cells, and a layer of dead squamous cells (5 to 10 cells thick). The epithelium also contains sparse bicarbonate-secreting submucosal glands. Increased vascular perfusion is the main postepithelial defense, in that it provides nutrients and bicarbonate and removes hydrogen ions.[2]

CLINICAL PRESENTATION AND DIAGNOSIS

SIGNS AND SYMPTOMS

Duodenal and Gastric Ulcer. The clinical findings of PUD are somewhat nonspecific and variable, with slight distinctions that make differentiation and diagnosis according to symptoms alone difficult. Patients can be asymptomatic or may experience anorexia, nausea, vomiting, belching, bloating, and heartburn; epigastric pain is the hallmark and most frequent symptom of DU and GU (Table 45.3); however, the mechanism by which PU causes pain is not clear.[1] Patients with endoscopically documented PUs are often asymptomatic; in contrast, pain syndromes indistinguishable from those of classic PUD occur frequently in patients who have no demonstrable ulcer [nonulcer dyspepsia (NUD)] and patients who have healed PU but who still experience ulcer-type pain.

Patients with DU commonly complain of epigastric pain or tenderness between the xiphoid and umbilicus that is burning, gnawing, and aching, often relieved with food intake, and worse when the stomach is empty, such as between meals and at night, although pain upon awakening in the morning is unusual. Some patients describe episodes of pain that occur in clusters lasting from several days to weeks, followed by longer pain-free intervals. Anorexia and weight loss occur infrequently in uncomplicated DU, and in fact patients often describe hyperphagia and weight gain, perhaps because eating typically relieves the pain.

Patients with GU typically complain of diffuse burning or gnawing pain over the midepigastrium, which tends to occur sooner after meals than does DU pain, with less reliable relief provided by antacids. Eating may provide little relief or may even precipitate pain in some patients with GU. Only one-third of patients with GU describe pain that awakens them from sleep, but anorexia and weight loss may occur in up to 50% of patients. These symptoms may be related to the delayed gastric emptying that can accompany GU, even in the absence of mechanical gastric outlet obstruction. Because benign and malignant GUs may manifest with similar degrees of pain, anorexia, and weight loss, it is not possible for the clinician to distinguish between them on the basis of history alone.

Patients with DU or GU may occasionally describe pain that radiates to other areas, such as the back or lower abdomen, and some patients may perceive abdominal pressure or a hunger sensation. Changes in the character of a patient's pain may be a sign of complications, such as penetration, perforation, gastric outlet obstruction, or hemorrhage. Some patients may have a "silent ulcer" and do not experience symptoms with active disease, especially with recurrences. Many NSAID-induced ulcers and ulcers in older adults bleed with no previous symptoms. In addition to their role in promoting PU, it has been proposed that NSAIDs may mask the pain of PUD. Therefore, the presence or absence of pain is not reliable in diagnosing or assessing the effectiveness of treatment in patients with PUD. Because numerous other GI disorders may cause pain similar to PU, if a patient's symptoms suggest PUD, objective tests are necessary to confirm the diagnosis.

Zollinger-Ellison's Syndrome. Most patients with ZES present with epigastric discomfort, a complication of PU (e.g., bleeding), or chronic diarrhea; however, the clinical manifestation of ZES can be elusive, and, as a result, ZES is frequently misdiagnosed. For patients with one or more of the following features, in whom an alternate diagnosis cannot be easily established, ZES should be considered: postbulbar DU; multiple DUs or jejunal ulcers; PUD in association with chronic watery diarrhea; PUD refractory to medical therapy; history of PUD and nephrolithiasis; recurrent PUD in the absence of *H. pylori* or NSAID use; or family history of PUD and hypercalcemia. Erosive esophagitis also may occur and can be difficult to manage in ZES.

Stress-Related Erosive Syndrome. Unlike chronic PU, SRES lesions are characteristically asymptomatic. Blood loss, represented by gross examination of gastric contents or positive guaiac findings of nasogastric aspirate, is usually the first sign of ulceration. Not all patients with minor blood loss progress to clinically important bleeding, but when hemorrhage occurs, the associated mortality ranges from 50% to 80%.[1,27,31]

Gastroesophageal Reflux Disease. Patients with GERD may present with typical, atypical, or complicated symptoms. The most common typical symptoms of GERD are heartburn and regurgitation. Heartburn (pyrosis) is characterized by a discomfort or burning sensation behind the sternum that starts above the epigastrium and may radiate toward the neck. Heartburn is an intermittent symptom, most commonly experienced within 60 minutes of eating, during exercise, while bending over, or when lying recumbent. Regurgitation is defined as the effortless return of esophageal or gastric contents into the pharynx without nausea or retching; it is often associated with the presence of sour or burning fluid in the throat or mouth that may also contain undigested food particles. Bending, belching, or moving in a way that increases intra-abdominal pressure can provoke regurgitation.[2] Less common typical symptoms of GERD include water brash and globus sensation. Water brash (hypersalivation) results from a vagal reflex that is triggered by esophageal acidification. Globus sensation is the perception of a lump or fullness in the throat that is felt irrespective of swallowing.

Atypical symptoms include chronic hoarseness, pharyngitis, cough, nonallergic asthma, and chest pain. Otolaryngologic manifestations of GERD are caused by refluxed acid that reaches the proximal esophagus and subsequent regurgitation into the hypopharynx, which contributes to laryngeal mucosal breakdown and a spectrum of diseases such as chronic hoarseness, posterior laryngeal erythema and edema, and contact ulceration of the vocal folds.[2] Patients with asthma or cough that is not responding to standard medical therapies should be evaluated for GERD as a possible cause for their symptoms. Pulmonary symptoms, including cough, are thought to be a vagally mediated bronchospasm in response to stimulation of the esophageal mucosa by refluxed acid. A less common cause of pulmonary symptoms is aspiration of refluxate into the lungs, causing chemical irritation, which may present as pneumonia or pulmonary fibrosis.[49] Patients who present with chest pain must undergo further workup to distinguish GERD-associated chest pain from pain of cardiac origin. Once cardiac ischemia has been ruled out, the cause of chest pain in these persons can be difficult to establish, and GERD is often implicated. The mechanism by which GERD induces chest pain is unclear, but evidence suggests that esophageal afferent nerves discriminate poorly among stimuli, such that distention and reflux may be perceived as chest pain or heartburn.

Complicated symptoms, such as continual pain, dysphagia (difficulty swallowing), or odynophagia (painful swallowing), may indicate complicated disease and usually occur in patients with more severe esophagitis.[50] Dysphagia in patients with GERD may be caused by esophageal stricture or malignancy but can also occur with esophageal diverticulum, esophageal spasm, obstruction, infection, peristaltic dysfunction, or simple mucosal inflammation. Odynophagia is not common in GERD and should prompt a search for other causes; when it does occur in GERD, it is likely related to an esophageal ulcer or deep erosion.[2]

Although the symptoms of GERD are often relieved by drinking water or using antacids, for some persons, symptoms can occur frequently and have a negative impact on normal activities and perceived quality of life. Only a loose correlation has been found between frequency of GERD symptoms and degree of esophageal acid exposure and presence and extent of mucosal injury; some patients with severe esophagitis or Barrett's metaplasia deny having any symptoms of GERD.

DIAGNOSIS AND CLINICAL FINDINGS

Radiology and Endoscopy for Peptic Ulcer Disease. The definitive diagnosis of PUD depends on radiologic or endoscopic visualization of the ulcer (esophagogastroduodenoscopy, or upper GI endoscopy). Use of these studies can help the clinician to distinguish GU from DU, and to differentiate PUD from other acid-related GI disorders. Historically, single-contrast barium examination of the upper GI tract was the standard test for diagnosing PUD, but its use is much less common since the introduction of flexible endoscopy. Endoscopy is considered the "gold standard," and in comparative tests, it has been found to be more sensitive for identifying PUs and other mucosal lesions (95%) than is single-contrast (60% to 80%) or double-contrast (80% to

90%) radiography.[51,52] Endoscopy also allows direct inspection, visualization of superficial erosions and sites of active bleeding, and biopsy of suspicious lesions and tissue for cultures and histology from the esophagus, stomach, and duodenum.[1] As a result, endoscopy has become the recommended first-line test for confirming the presence of PU in patients with dyspeptic symptoms, although many providers initially test patients who present with dyspepsia for *H. pylori* (see later) and empirically manage the ulcer by using therapy to eradicate the infection, if present.[6,53] Endoscopic examination is also the most reliable method for detecting acute SRES. Some argue that the lower cost, good safety, and greater availability of contrast imaging make it the initial diagnostic procedure of choice in patients with assumed uncomplicated PUs. However, if complications are suspected or if a definitive diagnosis is desired, endoscopy is the preferred procedure. For patients who have GU or suspicious (e.g., cancerous) lesions identified on radiography, subsequent endoscopy for confirmation and biopsy is required; therefore, the use of endoscopy as first-line testing might actually save time, decrease the number of procedures required, and decrease the overall cost of diagnosis. Some patients with complicated PUD, however, also require barium contrast studies, which occasionally offer important information about gastroduodenal anatomy that endoscopy cannot fully provide. Endoscopic ultrasound can also be used to examine ulcer depth and fibrosis.[54] Follow-up with radiography or endoscopy after treatment to document healing should not be performed routinely; if endoscopic, histologic, or cytologic tests suggest malignancy, then follow-up endoscopy is recommended.[55]

Laboratory Tests for Peptic Ulcer Disease. Routine laboratory tests do not contribute to the diagnosis of uncomplicated PUD. Hemoglobin, hematocrit, and fecal occult blood tests can be helpful in detecting bleeding. If patients do not respond to therapy, or if hypersecretory conditions are suspected, acid secretory studies and fasting serum gastrin concentrations are recommended, but they should not be included as part of the routine workup of uncomplicated disease.

Testing for *Helicobacter pylori*. The tests used to diagnosis *H. pylori* can be categorized as invasive or noninvasive (Table 45.5).[6,13,56–61] The appropriate test should be selected according to the clinical situation of each patient.

Invasive Screening Methods. Most invasive tests use tissue obtained by endoscopic biopsy; moderately less invasive methods (e.g., small bowel biopsy tube or capsule, biopsy forceps via a modified nasogastric tube) are available but are not as commonly used. Until relatively recently, the preferred diagnostic method was histologic examination of the mucosal biopsy specimen for the presence of *H. pylori* or gastritis. For the best diagnostic outcome, this method required numerous samples (at least three), proper mounting and preparation of the samples, and use of an appropriate

TABLE 45.5	Diagnostic Tests for *Helicobacter pylori*
Test	**Comments**
Serology	• Noninvasive; detects antibodies to *H. pylori* in blood • Inexpensive; rapid; represents the entire mucosa (no sampling errors) • Does not differentiate active and past infection; possible cross-reactivity with similar bacteria, so specificity is generally lower than urea breath test (UBT) or endoscopic tests
Urea breath test	• Noninvasive ingestion of labeled carbon 13 or 14 • Less expensive than endoscopy; represents the entire mucosa (no sampling errors); may be used to monitor response to therapy • Results often take 2 days to return; potential for false-negative after antibiotic, bismuth, or proton pump inhibitor (PPI) use
Stool antigen test	• Noninvasive; detects *H. pylori* antigen in stool • Inexpensive; rapid • Posttreatment testing may have variable accuracy; potential for false-negative after antibiotic, bismuth, or PPI use
Rapid urease	• Invasive; endoscopic biopsies of multiple sites tested with the use of urea-rich medium with pH-sensitive dye • Test of choice when endoscopy is used; easily performed; rapid results; high sensitivity and specificity • Expensive; patient discomfort; potential for false-negative after antibiotic, bismuth, or PPI use; patchy distribution of *H. pylori* can cause false-negative results
Histology	• Invasive; endoscopic biopsies of multiple sites with proper mounting and preparation of the samples; special stains (e.g., Genta or El-Zimaity "triple" stains) needed • "Gold standard"; high sensitivity and specificity • Expensive; patient discomfort; patchy distribution of *H. pylori* can cause false-negative results
Culture	• Invasive; endoscopic biopsies of multiple sites; bacteria cultured • Tests antibiotic sensitivity/resistance; high specificity • Expensive; patient discomfort; results often take a week or longer to return; patchy distribution of *H. pylori* can cause false-negative results

stain (e.g., Genta or El-Zimaity "triple" stains); when these criteria were met, histologic examination could detect chronic or chronic active inflammation and the presence of *H. pylori,* even with a low density of bacteria, a small specimen, or other sample quality issues.[13,56] Another endoscopic method of diagnosing *H. pylori* involves the detection of urease activity in the tissue specimen. Rapid urease tests check for the presence of *H. pylori* by placing mucosal biopsy specimens on a urea-rich medium with pH-sensitive dye; if *H. pylori* is present, urease from the bacteria produces bicarbonate and ammonia, the latter of which causes a change in the color of the indicator. Recent use of antibiotics, bismuth, or PPIs may cause a false-negative rapid urease test. Endoscopic biopsies may also isolate the organism for antibiotic sensitivity testing; however, currently, this test is not widely available, and laboratory personnel with experience are required to successfully culture *H. pylori*. Cultures may become necessary in the future in the selection of appropriate options for those who do not respond to therapy, especially if the frequency of resistance to antibiotics increases. If endoscopy is clinically indicated to diagnose PU, mucosal biopsy specimens should be obtained at that time for a rapid urease test and histology, if necessary. Rapid urease tests are the easiest and least expensive of the biopsy tests and should be performed first; extra biopsies from normal-appearing mucosa should be taken and can be held for examination of histology if the rapid urease test is negative. If endoscopy is not indicated for other clinical reasons, it should not be performed exclusively to diagnose *H. pylori* infection, due to the high sensitivity and the availability of noninvasive testing.

Noninvasive Screening Methods. Chronic infection with *H. pylori* leads to an immunoglobulin G (IgG) antibody response that can be reliably, quantitatively, rapidly, and inexpensively measured through noninvasive serologic tests. These are sometimes considered "passive" tests because they determine whether a patient has ever been infected with the bacterium; however, these are the initial screening tests of choice in patients with new-onset dyspepsia who have no symptoms of complications. Office-based serologic tests are available, but these are less sensitive than laboratory serologic tests.[60] Although IgG antibodies for *H. pylori* can be detected in urine, saliva, and gingival transudate, no reliable tests are currently available in the United States.[13,60] Testing for other immunoglobulin (e.g., IgA, IgM) antibodies is also not recommended because it is unreliable. Although serologic tests are very useful in the initial diagnosis of *H. pylori,* they are not helpful in confirming bacterial eradication following therapy because it can take 6 to 24 months for serologic tests to become negative after antibiotic therapy has completed.[57,62] If there is concern that a positive serologic test is a reflection of a previous infection and does not accurately represent current status, other noninvasive ''active'' tests can be used to document active infection.

Similar to the rapid urease test, urea breath tests (UBTs) use the urease enzyme of *H. pylori* to diagnose active infection. Urea labeled with [13]C (nonradioactive isotope) or [14]C (radioactive isotope) is ingested; in patients infected with the bacterium, labeled bicarbonate will be produced and excreted by the lungs as labeled carbon dioxide. Although this test has been found to be highly accurate, if there are small numbers of bacteria, the amount of labeled bicarbonate produced may be insufficient to be detected, causing a false-negative result. Recent use of antibiotics or bismuth (within the previous 4 weeks) or PPIs (within the previous 1 to 2 weeks) can also lead to false-negative findings.[13,56–58,63] Urea blood tests are available for patients who cannot breathe into a container for the UBT.[64] Another noninvasive diagnostic test is a stool antigen test (HpSA test), which has been shown to have accuracy in the initial diagnosis of *H. pylori* similar to that of the UBT.[65] Individual studies have suggested that there may be some variation in reliability among the actual HpSA tests, depending on the reagent used.[13] Similar to several of the other tests, HpSA is susceptible to inaccuracy with low bacterial load; during concomitant administration of PPIs, bismuth, or antibiotics; and in patients with GI bleeding.[6,66]

Approach to Screening. Tests for the detection of *H. pylori* should be performed only if the decision has been made to treat patients with positive results.[61] Patients with newly diagnosed GU or DU should be tested for the infection, as should patients with complicated PUD or a history of PUD who are currently receiving maintenance therapy with antisecretory agents. The role of testing for *H. pylori* in patients taking NSAIDs is controversial; however, screening to prevent gastric cancer may be cost-effective in patients with risk factors or a strong family history.[61] Currently, asymptomatic persons should be screened for *H. pylori* only if they have first-degree relatives with gastric cancer or PUD; then, positive tests (e.g., UBT, HpSA) should be confirmed before therapy is initiated. Posttreatment assessment to confirm eradication is not recommended or required in most cases, except for patients with complications. If confirmation of successful treatment is desired, UBT can be used, but it must be delayed at least 4 weeks after completion of therapy so that misinterpretation of bacterial suppression as eradication can be avoided. Data are conflicting regarding the accuracy of HpSA for posttreatment testing, particularly when it is used sooner than 4 weeks after therapy.[67,68] As such, waiting 6 to 12 weeks is recommended before retesting with HpSA to reliably confirm eradication.[6]

Zollinger-Ellison's Syndrome. Unlike chronic PUD, where gastrin levels are not elevated, patients with ZES have a gastrinoma (gastrin-secreting tumor). Therefore, evaluating the gastrin level is necessary for the diagnosis of ZES. Not only is gastrin analysis useful for diagnosing ZES, it can also be used to monitor the efficacy of antisecretory medications (discussed later in this chapter). Patients with ZES have extremely elevated fasting blood levels of gastrin (typically above 1,000 pg per mL) and increased basal acid output (over 10 mEq per hour, with an average of 40 mEq per hour); however, many patients with gastrinoma may have less elevated fasting gastrin levels.[26] Patients with elevated fasting gastrin levels, but levels below 1,000 pg per mL, should be evaluated for other conditions that can cause gastrin levels to be in this range. Antisecretory medications such as PPIs can cause false-positive gastrin results; therefore, they should be discontinued for at least 1 week before the fasting gastrin level is measured. Hyperlipidemia may also cause false reports of elevated serum gastrin levels by interfering with the gastrin assay. Many medical conditions have been associated with increased fasting gastrin levels, including vagotomy without gastric resection, small bowel resection (transiently), renal failure (due to reduced gastrin clearance), and primary hyperparathyroidism. When the fasting serum gastrin level is only modestly elevated and the diagnosis of ZES is questionable, a secretin provocative test can be used to confirm the diagnosis.[26]

Gastroesophageal Reflux Disease. The diagnosis of GERD is based largely on clinical history, including associated risk factors and symptoms. Esophageal studies are sometimes required, however, to detect (a) mucosal injury and esophagitis, (b) presence of reflux, or (c) peristaltic dysfunction or decreased LES pressure. Selection of the appropriate test depends on which of these problems needs to be defined. Patients with typical symptoms of reflux do not usually require invasive evaluation; they may benefit from empiric lifestyle modifications and pharmacotherapy. As described earlier, patients with certain atypical symptoms should first be evaluated for cardiac or respiratory causes of their symptoms.[2] Once these causes have been excluded, esophageal studies are needed to diagnose GERD. Other patients who should undergo diagnostic evaluation for determination of the presence of mucosal injury include those who have failed empiric therapy, and those with recurrent or complicated disease.[69]

Diagnostic options for determining whether mucosal injury has occurred include air-contrast barium esophagogram and upper GI endoscopy. Endoscopy is the most commonly used method to assess the severity of esophageal damage. As with PUD, endoscopy allows direct visualization and biopsy of the mucosa, the latter of which is used for histology, which can be an important tool in the diagnosis of mild GERD when the mucosa may appear relatively normal. Endoscopic biopsies are also important in distinguishing between esophagitis and Barrett's metaplasia. Barium esophagograms are most useful for detecting esophageal strictures or obstructions in patients who present with dysphagia; they may detect hiatal hernia and esophageal motor dysfunction, although endoscopy is used to detect these as well.[50,70]

Unfortunately, normal biopsy findings do not rule out GERD, and the detection of mucosal injury does not necessarily mean that reflux is the cause of the patient's symptoms. To establish a causal relation between patient symptoms and abnormal esophageal acid exposure, especially in the absence of mucosal injury, provocative tests such as an acid perfusion test (Bernstein test), the standard acid reflux test, scintigraphic determination of reflux, or maneuvers to induce reflux during barium esophagograms can be used.[69] Although these tests may establish that symptoms are related to GERD, they do not differentiate between degrees of reflux or esophagitis, and they have relatively poor sensitivity and specificity; therefore, they are not routinely used in the diagnosis of GERD. If the goal is to establish the presence of acid above the LES as the cause of symptoms or esophageal damage, the preferred test is a 24-hour ambulatory esophageal pH study, which documents the amount of time the esophageal pH is low. Although this test is typically performed over 24 hours, shorter monitoring periods have been studied and may be adequate in some patients.[71] Ambulatory pH monitoring is useful in patients who have not responded or who have had an incomplete response to empiric therapy, have symptoms without evidence of mucosal injury, or have atypical symptoms.[69,70] In these patients, this test may be the only way to prove that their symptoms are caused by GERD. Because ambulatory pH testing also defines the pattern of reflux, it can provide prognostic information as well. For example, supine or combined supine-upright GERD is associated with more severe resistant esophagitis than is reflux that occurs only while patients are upright.[72] The use of ambulatory pH testing for the evaluation of "bile" or "alkaline" reflux is being investigated, although the clinical importance of this type of reflux is controversial.[69,73]

Although it is not useful for the routine diagnosis of GERD, esophageal manometry can be used to evaluate peristalsis and assess the function of the LES; therefore, it should be used in antireflux surgery candidates to determine which procedure is most appropriate. Manometry has also shown correlation between more severe disease and a high percentage of abnormal contractions, the presence of a hypotensive LES, or both; these findings have been associated with poor response to therapy.

COMPLICATIONS

Peptic Ulcer Disease. Approximately 25% of patients with PU will have a major complication such as hemorrhage, perforation, penetration, or obstruction.[6] Gastric cancer is also associated with GU. When ulcers are deep enough to affect the arterial vessels, hemorrhage can occur. It is the most common complication of PU, affecting approximately 15% of patients with PUD, and it has a mortality rate of about 10%.[6] Patients with bleeding PUs may present with

melena, hematemesis, or both. Less commonly, patients may have rapid bleeding that manifests as hematochezia.[74] Approximately 7% of PUs will perforate into the peritoneal cavity.[6] This complication and its associated peritonitis are life-threatening events, particularly since they are most common in the elderly. NSAID use, smoking, and use of crack cocaine are all strong independent risk factors for perforation. Up to 10% of patients experience perforation accompanied by hemorrhage. Penetration occurs when the ulcer bores through the wall of the stomach or duodenum but instead of perforating into the peritoneal cavity, it burrows into an adjacent organ; this is seen in DUs that penetrate into the pancreas, or in GUs that involve the left lobe of the liver. Fistulas caused by penetrating PUs are rare. PUs can also cause gastric outlet obstruction as a result of the swelling and edema that occur with active disease or as a consequence of the scarring that is associated with ulcer healing, although this is an uncommon complication.

Strong evidence from epidemiologic studies indicates that asymptomatic *H. pylori* infection is associated with chronic atrophic gastritis, gastric mucosa–associated lymphoid tissue (MALT) lymphoma, and gastric adenocarcinoma in some persons.[13,14,75,76] Additionally, serologic data have shown an association between the bacterium and gastric cancer.[13,75] In 1994, the World Health Organization concluded that *H. pylori* infection is a group I carcinogen in humans.[14,75] Normal gastric tissue does not include lymphoid tissue, but after *H. pylori* infection, some patients can develop MALT, with lymphoid hyperplasia and clonal expansion of B-cells, which are thought to then give rise to lymphoma. Gastric carcinoid tumors arise from GI neuroendocrine cells, mainly ECL cells. Pernicious anemia and chronic atrophic gastritis are risk factors for the development of ECL cell tumors, likely because of the secondary hypergastrinemia that occurs in these patients with low acid output, which causes ECL cell hyperplasia. The development of atrophic gastritis and gastric carcinoma typically occurs over 20 to 40 years, but in affected persons, careful evaluation and close follow-up are recommended.

Zollinger-Ellison's Syndrome. Gastrinomas, such as those associated with ZES, are malignant in 30% to 50% of patients, with regional lymph nodes, liver, spleen, and bone being the most common sites of metastasis.[26] ECL cell carcinoids can also be seen occasionally in ZES. Patients with ZES and pernicious anemia are more likely to develop gastric carcinoid tumors than are people without either condition. Extensive biopsy sampling of both the greater and the lesser curve of the stomach may help detect ECL cell hyperplasia or early carcinoid tumor formation in ZES.

Stress-Related Erosive Syndrome. Hemorrhage is the most common complication of SRES. Although the bleeding tends to occur from superficial mucosal capillaries, rather than from deeper arterial vessels, it is often progressive and severe enough to require blood transfusions. SRES hemorrhage may be associated with significant morbidity and mortality.

Gastroesophageal Reflux Disease. Although GERD may lead to esophageal bleeding, such blood loss is usually chronic and rather minor, although it can lead to anemia. The severe complications associated with GERD consist of esophagitis, esophageal stricture, and Barrett's metaplasia, with the associated risk of esophageal adenocarcinoma.[2] Strictures are most common in the distal esophagus and are generally 1 to 2 cm long. As mentioned previously, observational studies suggest that the use of aspirin or NSAIDs may increase the risk of esophageal stricture.[37] In some patients with GERD, columnar-type epithelium replaces the squamous epithelial lining of the esophagus during the reparative process. This condition is referred to as Barrett's esophagus or Barrett's metaplasia, and it is more likely to occur in patients affected by GERD for years.

THERAPEUTIC PLAN

The goals of treatment for PUD are to relieve pain, enhance ulcer healing, prevent ulcer recurrence, and decrease the risk of complications, such as those discussed earlier. The cause of the ulcer (*H. pylori*, NSAID, or other), whether it is a new or recurrent ulcer, and the presence or absence of complications must be taken into account in the treatment of patients with PUD. With GERD, the goals of treatment are to decrease or eliminate symptoms; reduce the frequency, duration, and recurrence of reflux; promote the healing of injured mucosa; and reduce the risk of complications. For both PUD and GERD, therapy is usually directed at eliminating or reducing the aggravating factors and enhancing the natural defense mechanisms.

Drug therapies for PUD and GERD are primarily oriented toward neutralizing (antacids) or reducing the amount of acid secreted (H2RAs, PPIs), or protecting the gastric mucosa from the effects of acid (sucralfate, PGs). In patients with documented *H. pylori* infection and active ulcer or history of ulcer-related complications, the goal of therapy is to eradicate the bacterium and heal the ulcer. Prokinetic agents have also been evaluated in the treatment of GERD, although the side effects of available agents limit their usefulness.

TREATMENT

NONPHARMACOLOGIC THERAPY
Although excellent drug therapy is available for PUD and GERD, other measures involving lifestyle modifications and avoidance of ulcerogenic drugs are important for optimizing therapy. Patients should be advised to stop smoking and avoid alcohol intake because both can impair ulcer healing. NSAIDs, including aspirin, should be avoided when possible

in patients with or at high risk for PUD; acetaminophen, opioids, nonacetylated salicylates (e.g., salsalate), and newer "GI-safe" NSAIDs are alternative analgesics. Foods and beverages that aggravate symptoms of ulcers or reflux should be avoided, as should behaviors and medications that are known to increase symptoms, particularly with GERD (Table 45.4); nonpharmacologic therapy is key with this condition.[1,2,69] Psychological stress management may also reduce symptoms.

Surgical procedures for the management of PUD and GERD are becoming very uncommon with the availability of highly effective pharmacologic therapies and the recognition that ulcer recurrence is uncommon if *H. pylori* infection and NSAID use are eliminated. Some patients, however, may require surgical management of their disease, especially those with GERD who have pharmacotherapy-nonresponsive esophagitis, stricture, bleeding, or pulmonary complications. Complications associated with surgery have decreased as laparoscopic procedures have become available; however, the role of surgery in the long-term management of GERD remains controversial.[77]

Immunizations for *H. pylori* are being investigated. To protect against bacterial infection, the mucosal surface generates an adaptive immune response in which IgA is produced. Because vaccines that are administered parenterally usually result in the production of IgM and IgG, research has focused on oral vaccines for *H. pylori*. More information regarding *H. pylori* vaccines can be found elsewhere.[78]

PHARMACOTHERAPY
Numerous agents are used in the management and prevention of PUD, the eradication of *H. pylori*, and the treatment of patients with GERD (if symptoms persist despite nonpharmacologic approaches). Patients with risk factors for ulcer recurrence (despite elimination of known risk factors, such as NSAID use and *H. pylori*) or history of ulcer complications, or those who fail *H. pylori* eradication therapies may require maintenance antisecretory therapy after the ulcer has initially healed; in some cases, treatment may be needed indefinitely.

Antiulcer Agents.
Proton Pump Inhibitors. The PPIs decrease basal and stimulated gastric acid secretion through inhibition of the final step of acid secretion by the parietal cell—the H^+/K^+-ATPase proton pump.[1,41,79,80] These agents (esomeprazole, lansoprazole, omeprazole, pantoprazole, and rabeprazole) are the most effective and most widely used antisecretory agents, particularly with the availability of omeprazole as an OTC medication. All medications in this class are weak bases that must be activated by acid to inhibit the proton pump. Ironically, these prodrugs are acid-labile compounds that can be degraded by stomach acid during oral administration and therefore are available as enteric-coated, delayed-release formulations. Once the drug reaches the higher pH of the duodenum, the enteric coating dissolves and the un-

protonated prodrug readily penetrates the cell membranes, specifically that of the parietal cell. As it transverses the parietal cell and is exposed to intracellular acid, the prodrug becomes protonated and is no longer able to freely cross the cell membranes; thus, the activated PPI becomes trapped in the parietal cell. Once formed, the active sulfonamide moiety covalently binds to H^+/K^+-ATPase and inhibits acid secretion.

Although PPIs have a relatively short (less than 2 hours) plasma half-life, their associated acid inhibition is long (more than 24 hours) because of noncompetitive and irreversible inhibition of the proton pump. It may, however, take several days to reach steady state; thus PPIs are not generally recommended for immediate symptom relief. Additionally, for PPIs to be most effective, they should be taken consistently; some patients may benefit from receiving twice-daily doses for the first 2 or 3 days of therapy.[41] After a PPI has been discontinued, acid secretion does not return to preinhibition levels for a few days. Rebound acid hypersecretion may occur after cessation of PPI therapy, likely caused by heightened gastrin secretion during acid suppression, which increases the number of ECL cells responsible for histamine release.[80] Further research is needed to determine the frequency, duration, and clinical importance of rebound hypersecretion after PPI therapy is stopped. Food may delay the absorption of some agents, but because PPIs require accumulation and acid activation, and because they inhibit only proton pumps that are actively secreting acid, they are most effective when taken on an empty stomach, shortly before meals (e.g., before breakfast). Although liver failure can delay PPI clearance, dose adjustments are generally not necessary because of the wide safety margins of these agents. Dose adjustments in patients with renal insufficiency are not required because the renally excreted metabolites are inactive.

The PPIs are metabolized in the liver by the cytochrome P-450 (CYP) enzyme system (mainly CYP2C19), but clinically significant drug–drug interactions related to this pathway are uncommon. Omeprazole and esomeprazole can increase levels of warfarin, phenytoin, and diazepam.[1,80] PPIs cause an increase in gastric pH that can affect the absorption of many medications, mainly those with pH-dependent dosage forms. With the exception of ketoconazole or digoxin, however, this antisecretory action has little clinical significance. PPIs do not appear to affect the absorption of most dietary minerals,[81,82] and although antisecretory therapy has been shown to decrease the absorption of protein-bound, but not unbound, cobalamin (vitamin B_{12}), most available studies have found that serum cobalamin levels are not significantly affected by long-term antisecretory therapy.[1] All PPIs are very safe and well tolerated; the most frequently reported side effects are headache and diarrhea, which occur at rates similar to those with H₂RAs.[1,41,80] Serious side effects with PPI therapy are rare.

With standard doses of PPIs, healing rates for DU of 80% to 100% can be achieved with 4 to 8 weeks of therapy (Table 45.6). Healing rates for GU with the same doses and duration of therapy appear to be somewhat lower (70% to 85%). The PPIs also are very effective in treating GERD and are used extensively in the long-term treatment of hypersecretory conditions such as ZES. No single PPI has been shown to be clearly superior to the others in healing efficacy.[1,80,83] PPIs appear to heal PUs more rapidly and frequently than do H₂RAs, and in contrast to H₂RAs, tolerance does not develop during PPI therapy.[80] However, for PUs that are not related to NSAID use (discussed later), it is unclear whether the slightly faster healing rate with PPIs justifies their higher cost compared with those of other available agents, although the availability of OTC omeprazole has significantly reduced the intensity of this debate. In most cases, short-term therapy is sufficient because eradication of *H. pylori* or elimination of NSAIDs significantly decreases ulcer recurrence. Long-term PPI therapy may be necessary, however, for patients with PUs associated with hypersecretory conditions, those who cannot discontinue NSAIDs, and persons with complicated PUD. Although many consequences of prolonged hypochlorhydria are proposed to have some theoretical merit (e.g., hypergastrinemia, hastened gastric atrophy in patients with *H. pylori* infection, GI bacterial overgrowth and risk for enteric infections), studies have not established an association between long-term PPI use and increased risk for gastric cancer or other serious safety concerns.[1,41]

Histamine H₂ Receptor Antagonists. The development and use of H₂RAs significantly enhanced the management of PUD when cimetidine was introduced in 1977. These agents (cimetidine, famotidine, nizatidine, and ranitidine) competitively and reversibly bind the H₂ receptors on the parietal cell, decreasing histamine-stimulated, basal, and postprandial gastric acid secretion.[1,41] All these agents are available on an OTC basis without prescription, and they are equally effective in the eradication of *H. pylori* (discussed later), as well as in the acute treatment of DU and GU; the maintenance treatment of ulcers, hypersecretory conditions, and erosive and nonerosive GERD; and the prevention of upper GI bleeding caused by SRES (Table 45.6). H₂RAs may be given in divided or single daily doses for acute and maintenance therapy of patients with DU and GU, with similar efficacy rates. Evening administration is especially effective in suppressing nocturnal basal acid output, which has been shown to correlate with increased PU healing. Treatment of GERD with H₂RAs usually requires higher doses that are divided throughout the day. The H₂RAs differ slightly with regard to their potential for drug interactions, adverse effects, and pharmacokinetic properties, the latter of which are mostly clinically insignificant.[41] The H₂RAs are well absorbed when dosed orally and may be taken with or without food; however, concomitant dosing of antacids or sucralfate can decrease H₂RA absorption by 10% to 20%. Cigarette smokers may require higher doses or longer durations of treatment. Decreased doses may be required in patients with moderate to severe renal insufficiency, but dosage adjust-

TABLE 45.6	Pharmacotherapeutic Agents Used to Eradicate *Helicobacter pylori* Infection, Heal Ulcers, Maintain Ulcer Healing, or Treat Gastroesophageal Reflux Disease

Drug	Eradication of *H. pylori* Infection	Ulcer Healing[a]	Maintenance of Ulcer Healing	Prevention of NSAID-induced Ulcers	Treatment/ Maintenance of Erosive GERD	Treatment of Nonerosive GERD
Proton Pump Inhibitors (PPIs)[b]						
Esomeprazole	40 mg once daily		20–40 mg once daily		20 mg once or twice daily	
Lansoprazole	30 mg twice daily		30 mg once daily		30 mg once or twice daily	
Omeprazole	40 mg once daily or 20 mg twice daily		20 mg once daily		20 mg once or twice daily	
Pantoprazole	40 mg twice daily		40 mg once daily		40 mg once or twice daily	
Rabeprazole	20 mg twice daily		20 mg once daily		20 mg once or twice daily	
H₂ Receptor Antagonists (H₂RAs)[c,d]						
Cimetidine	400 mg twice daily or 800 mg once daily at bedtime	800 mg once daily	400 mg once daily	N/A	400 mg every 6 hours	400 mg twice daily
Famotidine	20 mg twice daily or 40 mg once daily at bedtime	40 mg once daily	20 mg once daily	N/A	40 mg every 12 hours	20 mg twice daily
Nizatidine	150 mg twice daily or 300 mg once daily at bedtime					
Ranitidine		300 mg once daily	150 mg once daily	N/A	150 mg every 6 hours	150 mg twice daily
Other Agents						
Ranitidine bismuth citrate[e–g]	400 mg twice daily		N/A		N/A	N/A
Bismuth subsalicylate (BSS)[e,g]	525 mg four times daily		N/A		N/A	N/A
Sucralfate (S)[h]	1 g four times daily or 2 g twice daily	1 g four times daily or 2 g twice daily	1 g twice daily (DU); 1 g four times daily or 2 g twice daily (GU)	N/A	N/A	N/A
Misoprostol	N/A	N/A	N/A	(at least) 200 µg three times daily	N/A	N/A
Antacids	Adjunctive therapy for symptomatic relief only					
Antibiotics						
Amoxicillin (A)[i]	500 mg four times daily or 1,000 mg twice or three times daily[i]	N/A (unless associated with documented *H. pylori* infection)				
Clarithromycin (C)[k]	500 mg twice or three times daily[i]	N/A (unless associated with documented *H. pylori* infection)				
Metronidazole (M)	250 mg four times daily or 500 mg twice daily	N/A (unless associated with documented *H. pylori* infection)				

| | **TABLE 45.6** | continued | | | | | |

Drug	Eradication of *H. pylori* Infection	Ulcer Healing[a]	Maintenance of Ulcer Healing	Prevention of NSAID-induced Ulcers	Treatment/ Maintenance of Erosive GERD	Treatment of Nonerosive GERD
Tetracycline (T)[l]	500 mg twice or four times daily	N/A (unless associated with documented *H. pylori* infection)				

NSAID, nonsteroidal anti-inflammatory drug; GERD, gastroesophageal reflux disease; DU, duodenal ulcer; GU, gastric ulcer.

[a] In general, DUs should be treated for 4 weeks and GUs for 8 weeks; larger ulcers may require prolonged therapy with a PPI.
[b] Once-daily dosing should be administered before breakfast; if second dose is necessary, should be given before evening meal.
[c] Once-daily dosing should be administered between the evening meal and bedtime; if second dose is necessary, should be administered between breakfast and lunch; additional doses should be spaced evenly throughout the day.
[d] Dosing adjustments required for moderate to severe renal insufficiency.
[e] Not interchangeable.
[f] Not available in the United States.
[g] Also has some antimicrobial activity.
[h] Should be separated from meals and potentially interacting medications by 2 hours.
[i] Not ampicillin.
[j] Higher doses used with two-drug regimens.
[k] Not azithromycin.
[l] Not doxycycline.

ments are rarely required in patients with impaired hepatic function, unless it is accompanied by renal failure.

The H_2RAs are very safe and well tolerated, with less than 4% of patients reporting adverse effects; serious side effects are extremely uncommon.[84] Most reported adverse events occur with cimetidine, probably because it was the first H_2RA to be used, and it has the largest quantity of postmarketing data; however, no single agent has a clear-cut safety advantage over the others. Side effects with H_2RAs may be related to their potential inhibition of H_2 receptors in organs other than the stomach. For example, H_2 receptors in the heart mediate inotropic and chronotropic effects, and, very rarely, H_2RAs have been associated with hypotension, bradyarrhythmias and tachyarrhythmias, atrioventricular conduction abnormalities, and cardiac arrest. These highly uncommon reactions occurred primarily in patients who were seriously ill. Some had received the H_2RAs by rapid intravenous (IV) bolus injection; therefore, if H_2RAs are administered through the IV route, rapid boluses should be avoided. Central nervous system (CNS) symptoms, such as sedation, dizziness, and headache, are the most common side effects reported by ambulatory patients taking H_2RAs.[84,85] The more serious CNS problems associated with H_2RAs (e.g., depression, memory problems, confusion, psychosis, and hallucinations) most often affect hospitalized elderly patients. Myelosuppression is a rare, idiosyncratic reaction that affects less than 1% of patients who take H_2RAs; however, it may be advisable to avoid the use of H_2RAs in patients with other risk factors for bone marrow suppression.[1] Cimetidine has weak antiandrogenic activity and has been reported to cause gynecomastia and impotence; however, this has not been observed with the other H_2RAs and appears to be related to the dose and duration of cimeti-

dine therapy—it occurs in almost half of patients treated on a long-term basis with high doses.[84] Routine monitoring of liver enzymes with H_2RA use is not necessary, even though transient, mild, asymptomatic elevations of hepatic aminotransferases may occur, because many of these laboratory abnormalities will resolve spontaneously, even with continued H_2RA use. Rarely, hepatitis has been reported, but it resolved with discontinuation of the drug in all cases. H_2RAs compete with creatinine for renal tubular secretion, but the associated small increases in serum creatinine do not reflect a change in glomerular filtration rate and are generally clinically insignificant.[1] Drug interactions mediated by the CYP system have been reported with theophylline, phenytoin, lidocaine, quinidine, and warfarin, when taken with cimetidine and ranitidine, although less frequently with the latter.[86] Famotidine and nizatidine do not appear to have any significant drug–drug interactions. The clinical significance of the interaction of H_2RAs with ethanol remains uncertain.

Patients have been observed to develop tolerance to the antisecretory effects of H_2RAs rather frequently and quickly; this cannot be overcome by dose increases. Because H_2RAs competitively inhibit the histamine H_2 receptor, it is proposed that their effect could be lessened with increased release of histamine from upregulated ECL cell activity that accompanies antisecretory-induced hypergastrinemia. Upregulated ECL cell activity may also contribute to rebound hypersecretion of gastric acid after discontinuation of H_2RA therapy, which, although somewhat controversial, may cause a short-lived (<9 days) increase in nocturnal gastric acid output.[1]

Sucralfate. Sucralfate is a complex aluminum salt of sulfated sucrose that, when exposed to gastric acid, forms sulfate anions that can bind electrostatically to positively charged proteins in damaged tissue, creating a viscous layer that adheres to ulcer craters and creates a protective barrier to prevent further acid-peptic attack.[1] Other proposed beneficial actions of sucralfate include the enhancement of mucosal PG levels, the stimulation of mucus and bicarbonate secretion, the binding of bile salts and epidermal growth factors, and the promotion of angiogenesis. Although the ionized sucralfate molecule also releases aluminum hydroxide, it has little acid-neutralizing capacity. Sucralfate has been shown to have similar efficacy as H_2RAs in the healing of DU and GU, although it has not been approved by the US Food and Drug Administration (FDA) for the latter.[87] Significantly less published literature is available for sucralfate than can be found on the antisecretory agents. Sucralfate is only minimally absorbed (3% to 5%) and has few side effects, of which constipation and other GI complaints are the most common. Prolonged sucralfate use or combination with aluminum-containing antacids may increase the risk for hypophosphatemia and the potential for aluminum toxicity, particularly in patients with renal insufficiency. Rarely, gastric bezoar formation has been reported.[1] A significant limitation to the use of sucralfate is its complicated dosing regimen, which involves four tablets a day, separated from meals and potentially interacting medications (e.g., phenytoin, warfarin, digoxin, theophylline, quinidine, fluoroquinolones, macrolide antibiotics) by at least 2 hours.[86]

Misoprostol. As discussed in the Pathophysiology section, PGs have several beneficial effects for patients with PUD. Misoprostol is a PGE_1 analog with antisecretory effects at low doses (50 to 200 μg) and cytoprotective effects at higher doses (above 200 μg). Misoprostol is not indicated for the treatment of PUD in the United States, but it has been shown to have efficacy comparable with that of H_2RAs or sucralfate in healing DU and GU, and to PPIs for the treatment of active NSAID-induced ulcer.[1] Problems with PG side effects (e.g., abdominal cramping, frequent diarrhea, abortifacient actions) and the availability of safe and effective antisecretory agents have significantly decreased the role of PGs in the treatment of patients with PUD. Misoprostol is mainly used for the prevention of NSAID-induced GU in patients at high risk for complications; it should be dosed with or after meals to decrease GI side effects. Misoprostol is contraindicated in pregnant women, and when it is used in women of childbearing years, adequate contraceptive measures should be employed and a negative serum pregnancy test should be documented within 2 weeks of initiation of therapy.

Bismuth Compounds. Bismuth compounds such as bismuth subsalicylate (BSS) (e.g., Pepto-Bismol) and colloidal bismuth subcitrate are commonly used to treat patients with a variety of GI symptoms, including nausea, heartburn, dyspepsia, and diarrhea. Bismuth compounds have shown some efficacy in healing PUs, possibly by forming complexes with mucus to ''coat'' ulcer craters and protect the ulcer from damaging acid and pepsin. These agents may increase mucosal PG synthesis and bicarbonate secretion, and they have documented antimicrobial actions against *H. pylori* (discussed later in the chapter).[1] The risk of bismuth neurotoxicity increases with high doses and extended duration of therapy, especially in patients with renal insufficiency. The most common side effect of the bismuth compounds is blackened stools.[13] BSS should be used cautiously in patients with bleeding disorders, those on high-dose salicylate therapy, and persons with salicylate sensitivity. Monotherapy with bismuth-containing preparations in the treatment of patients with PUD is rare, but they may be used in combination with antibiotics and other antiulcer agents for the treatment of patients with PUD associated with *H. pylori* infection.

Antacids. Antacids provide symptomatic relief and hasten ulcer healing by binding bile salts and neutralizing gastric acid, which leads to the inactivation of pepsin when gastric pH is greater than 4. Aluminum-containing agents may also help cure PUs by suppressing *H. pylori* and enhancing mucosal defenses. Antacids may also increase mucosal PG levels, stimulate mucus and bicarbonate secretion, and enhance angiogenesis. Because antacids are not as convenient, palatable, well tolerated, or effective as antisecretory agents, they have taken a secondary role in the management and treatment of PUD and GERD. Nonetheless, antacids are easily accessed (available OTC) and provide symptomatic relief for a wide variety of dyspeptic symptoms.

Common antacid preparations include sodium bicarbonate, calcium carbonate, and salts of aluminum and magnesium; magnesium salts have the longest neutralizing effect of the class. Although calcium stimulates gastrin release, the clinical importance of acid rebound with calcium-containing antacids is controversial. Frequent administration of antacid is necessary to buffer the constant secretion of acid produced by the stomach. The stomach in a fasting state empties its contents into the duodenum as often as every 15 to 30 minutes, limiting the amount of antacid in the stomach. A regimen that requires the taking of antacids 1 hour after a meal and at bedtime maximizes the buffering ability of the antacid because food acts as a buffer for about an hour and prolongs the antacid-neutralizing effect for an additional 2 hours.

Antacid adverse effects are primarily GI in nature and dose dependent, and they often contribute to noncompliance. High calcium intake in patients with systemic alkalosis may be associated with the milk-alkali syndrome, producing hypercalcemia, hyperphosphatemia, increased blood urea nitrogen and creatinine, alkalosis, renal insufficiency, and renal calcinosis. The alkalosis may be produced by prolonged vomiting or may be caused by sodium bicarbonate, which produces gas resulting from carbon dioxide formation in the stomach. Magnesium-containing antacids can cause significant diarrhea; aluminum salts cause constipation. In magnesium-aluminum combination products, diarrhea usually predominates and may require alternation with doses of aluminum-containing antacids. Aluminum salts bind to dietary phosphorus in the intestinal tract and may cause hypophosphatemia in patients with low dietary phosphate intake; long-term complications may include osteopenia and osteoporosis. The combination of aluminum-containing antacids with sucralfate may increase the risk for hypophosphatemia and the potential for aluminum toxicity. All antacids must be used cautiously, if at all, in patients with renal insufficiency, because of the risks of hypermagnesemia, hypercalcemia, hyperaluminumemia, and alkalosis.[88] Antacids may cause drug interactions, usually by interfering with absorption or chelation of the drug. Clinically significant drug–drug interactions occur when antacids are administered concomitantly with warfarin, digoxin, ketoconazole, tetracycline, ferrous sulfate, quinidine, isoniazid, and fluoroquinolones; most of these can be avoided by separating the antacid from the other drug by 2 hours.

Anticholinergics. Although anticholinergic medications inhibit basal and meal-stimulated gastric acid secretion, they do so at a substantially lower rate than do other antisecretory agents.[41] The significant adverse effects of the nonselective anticholinergic agents (e.g., atropine) limit their use in PUD. Although adverse effects are less common with the selective M_1 antagonists (pirenzepine and telenzepine), these agents have limited efficacy and essentially no role in the treatment of patients with PUD, nor are they available in the United States.[1]

Treatment of *Helicobacter pylori*. The basic premise of therapy for *H. pylori* is that if infection is diagnosed in patients with active ulcer or a history of complications, it should be treated, because eradication (absence of the organism at least 4 weeks after completion of antibiotic therapy) decreases ulcer recurrence to less than 10% in 1 year and facilitates ulcer healing.[13,89] Data are conflicting with regard to *H. pylori* eradication in patients with dyspepsia or NUD. Empiric eradication therapy without *H. pylori* testing is strongly discouraged because the prevalence of the bacterium is low in Western developed countries, especially in young patients with symptoms of dyspepsia. Additionally, the medications are not without side effects, and widespread antibiotic use may increase the risk of antibiotic resistance.[89]

Although *H. pylori* infection is easily suppressed, sustained cure rates of better than 80% to 90% require the use of regimens that combine two or three antimicrobial agents (including bismuth compounds) with antisecretory agents.[61,90–94] Antisecretory agents not only speed relief of symptoms and ulcer healing, they also increase the efficacy of bacterial eradication with antibiotics (possibly by increasing antibiotic concentrations, enhancing activity or stability in the gastric mucosa); however, antisecretory agents do not offer a cure for *H. pylori* when used alone (e.g., as monotherapy without an antibiotic).[95] Although three- and four-drug regimens may be more complex and may cause more side effects (namely, those containing bismuth compounds), their efficacy is much higher than that of two-drug regimens,

which are not currently recommended as first-line treatment.[13,96] Regimens that contain a single antibiotic are less effective than regimens with two or more antibiotics, and concern regarding antibiotic resistance limits the use of these regimens as first-line therapies.[96] Primary resistance of *H. pylori* to metronidazole monotherapy is fairly common in the United States, and clarithromycin resistance is increasingly reported, so local resistance patterns may need to be considered, as should an individual patient's past antibiotic use, particularly if the initial eradication therapy has failed.[96] Most studies have shown better efficacy rates with treatment regimens of 10 to 14 days compared with regimens of 7 days or less.[97] Despite the extensive number of studies that have been conducted on different *H. pylori* eradication regimens, it must be recognized that these studies are difficult to directly compare, and that study results can vary substantially depending on the method used to analyze the results, the regimen used for eradication of bacteria, the geographic diversity of the patients studied, and even small differences in the combinations, doses, or durations of the agents used. Only regimens with consistent data should be used in clinical practice.[13] Agents with significant adverse effects or complicated dosing regimens that could decrease compliance should be reserved for second- or third-line therapies, if possible. Regardless of the regimen selected, patients should be counseled to complete the full course of therapy to maximize efficacy. Eradication regimens should be based on efficacy, tolerability, the likelihood of compliance/adherence, potential drug interactions (or lack thereof), drug allergies, and antibiotic resistance and cost, and such regimens should be individualized for each patient (Tables 45.6 and 45.7).

Antibiotics Used in the Eradication of *Helicobacter pylori*. Although *H. pylori* has very good in vitro sensitivity to most antibiotics, including amoxicillin, metronidazole (or tinidazole, a nitroimidazole not available in the United States that has comparable efficacy), tetracycline, macrolide antibiotics, and fluoroquinolones, in vivo sensitivity of these agents is suboptimal. Clarithromycin is the most effective single antibiotic in vivo, but it has an eradication rate of only 40% to 70%. The difference seen between high in vitro and low in vivo efficacy may be partially due to the degradation of the antimicrobial agent in gastric acid, or it may be caused by insufficient penetration into the gastric mucosa.[13,96] Tetracycline is active at low pH and the activity of metronidazole is not dependent on pH. Even with antisecretory cotherapy, which increases antibiotic efficacy and promotes ulcer healing (as discussed earlier), amoxicillin and clarithromycin are the only antibiotics approved for use in two-drug regimens, and these regimens are not considered first-line therapy.

In addition to their topical GI protective effects, bismuth compounds act as topical antimicrobials that disrupt the integrity of the *H. pylori* cell wall; in so doing, they demonstrate antibacterial activity when sufficient mucosal concentrations are reached (lasting about 2 hours after dosing).[13]

TABLE 45.7	Regimens for Eradicating *Helicobacter pylori*				
Regimen	**Duration**	**Efficacy**	**Compliance[a]**	**Adverse Effects**	

1 Antibiotic[b] + 1 Adjunctive Agent

Regimen	Duration	Efficacy	Compliance	Adverse Effects
A + PPI	14 days[c]	<70%–80%	Likely	Low-medium
C + PPI	14 days[c]	>70%–90%	Likely	Low-medium
C + RBC[d]	14 days[d]	>70%–90%	Likely	Low-medium
2 Antibiotics + 1 Adjunctive Agent				
C + A + PPI	10–14 days[c]	>80%–>90%	Likely	Low-medium
C + M + PPI	10–14 days[c]	>80%–>90%	Likely	Medium
C + T + PPI	14 days[c]	>80%–90%	Likely	Medium
A + M + PPI	14 days[c]	>80%–90%	Likely	Medium
A + T + PPI	14 days[c]	>80%–90%	Likely	Medium
M + T + PPI	14 days[c]	>80%–90%	Likely	Medium
C + M + H₂RA or RBC[e]	14 days[d]	>80%–90%	Unlikely	Medium
C + A + H₂RA or RBC[e]	14 days[d]	>80%–90%	Unlikely	Medium
C + T + H₂RA or RBC[e]	14 days[d]	>80%–90%	Unlikely	Medium
T + M + S	14 days[d]	>80%–90%	Unlikely	Medium
M + T + BSS	14 days	>80%–90%	Unlikely	Medium-high
M + A + BSS	14 days	>80%–90%	Unlikely	Medium-high
C + T + BSS	14 days	>80%–90%	Unlikely	Medium-high
C + A + BSS	14 days	>80%–90%	Unlikely	Medium-high
2 Antibiotics + 2 Adjunctive Agents				
M + T + PPI + BSS	7–10 days[c]	>80%–>90%	Unlikely	Medium-high
M + C + PPI + BSS	7–10 days[c]	>80%–>90%	Unlikely	Medium-high
M + T + H₂RA + BSS	14 days[d]	>80%–>90%	Unlikely	Medium-high
M + A + H₂RA + BSS	14 days[d]	>70%–90%	Unlikely	Medium-high

A, amoxicillin; PPI, proton pump inhibitor; C, clarithromycin; RBC, ranitidine bismuth citrate; M, metronidazole; T, tetracycline; H₂RA, H₂ receptor antagonist; BSS, bismuth subsalicylate.
[a] Based on pill burden, frequency of administration, and significant adverse effects.
[b] Higher antibiotic doses used with two-drug regimens.
[c] Duration of conventional antiulcer dosage of PPI may be extended to 28 days when patients with active PU are treated.
[d] Duration of adjunctive agent should/may extend an additional 2 weeks after antibiotics are completed.
[e] Not available in the United States.
From references 13 and 90–100.

Despite this antimicrobial effect, when used in *H. pylori* regimens, bismuth is more commonly categorized as an adjunctive agent (Table 45.7). Although BSS is available in the United States, the bismuth product available in other parts of the world is bismuth subcitrate, which has been more extensively tested for *H. pylori* than has BSS. Bismuth subcitrate is also available as a component of ranitidine bismuth citrate (discussed later); however, this product is no longer available in the United States. Although the two forms of bismuth have not been studied for equivalency, BSS has proven efficacy in several *H. pylori* regimens.

H. pylori resistance to amoxicillin and tetracycline is rare in Western countries.[13] Primary resistance is most common with metronidazole (10% to 50%), and regimens that include

this agent are generally associated with lower cure rates.[13,98] Metronidazole resistance may be overcome by increasing the dose (e.g., to 500 mg three times daily).[99] In the United States, less than 15% of *H. pylori* infections are resistant to clarithromycin, although acquired resistance may occur in as many as 66% of treatment failures, but unlike for metronidazole, there is no evidence that increasing the dose will overcome resistance.[13]

Few data are available by which the tolerability of the many eradication regimens can be compared. In general, regimens with four drugs, mainly those containing bismuth, have the highest rates of adverse effects, and PPI-based three-drug regimens are very well tolerated. Metronidazole has the potential for a disulfiram (Antabuse)-like effect with ingestion of ethanol-containing beverages or products. The most common adverse effects with *H. pylori* eradication regimens are taste perversion (clarithromycin and metronidazole), diarrhea, nausea/vomiting, and abdominal pain. Tetracycline is contraindicated in children younger than 8 years of age because of the risk of tooth discoloration.[13]

Adjunctive Agents Used in the Eradication of *Helicobacter pylori*. H_2RAs have been used to promote the healing of PUs for many years. In vitro, PPIs inhibit the growth of *H. pylori* at pH less than 7, which is most important when one is considering the effect that PPIs have on the accuracy of various diagnostic tests for *H. pylori*. In the treatment of *H. pylori*, H_2RAs and PPIs are not effective as monotherapy, but they are useful for increasing gastric pH, which may enhance the local immune response and make acid-sensitive drugs (clarithromycin and amoxicillin) more effective. Intragastric concentrations of antibacterial agents may increase because of the lower volumes of gastric juice seen with antisecretory drugs. In general, regimens with PPIs have been shown to be as, or slightly more, effective than those with H_2RAs. Ranitidine bismuth citrate is a novel compound with characteristics of both an H_2RA and bismuth, and the combination of ranitidine bismuth citrate with other antibiotics has been shown to be as good as, and possibly superior to, the same antibiotics combined with a PPI.[92,100] Ranitidine bismuth citrate is no longer available in the United States, however. The manufacturer voluntarily removed it from the market in 1999 based on a lack of market interest in the product.

Therapeutic Regimens Used in the Eradication of *Helicobacter pylori*. Regimens to treat *H. pylori* may be classified by the number of antibiotics and adjunctive agents employed (Tables 45.6 and 45.7). Although two-drug regimens one antibiotic and one adjunctive agent) were the first therapies approved for *H. pylori* management, these regimens are no longer recommended because low cure rates and a high frequency of clarithromycin resistance among the treatment failures. Regimens with three drugs (two antibiotics plus one adjunctive agent) are now the most widely used because they provide high cure rates. The most popular triple therapies combine a PPI with any two of amoxicillin, metronidazole, and clarithromycin; tetracycline may also be used in place of amoxicillin or metronidazole.[13] If a three-drug regimen is ineffective because of clarithromycin or metronidazole resistance, high-dose, four-drug therapy may be highly effective. Although it is intuitive that metronidazole-containing regimens would be effective against strains resistant to clarithromycin, they have also been shown to be effective against metronidazole-resistant strains.[99] Guidelines for treating pediatric patients with *H. pylori* may be found elsewhere.[101]

Treatment and Prevention of NSAID-Induced Ulcers

Treatment of NSAID-Induced Ulcers. When PU is associated with the use of NSAIDs, the NSAID should be discontinued if possible, because with standard regimens of PPI, H_2RA, or sucralfate (Table 45.6), most uncomplicated NSAID-induced ulcers will heal and will not recur if the offending agent has been stopped.[1,20,21,89] For patients with severe inflammatory conditions, however, it may not be feasible to stop NSAID therapy. Numerous studies have shown that NSAID-induced PUs can heal with antisecretory therapy, even if NSAID treatment continues, but that healing occurs at a slower rate.[1,20,21] PPIs have been shown to be superior to H_2RAs for healing and as maintenance therapy for PUs in patients who continue to use NSAIDs.[1,102,103]

Prevention of NSAID-Induced Ulcers. Although the most effective way to prevent NSAID-induced ulcers is to avoid the use of NSAIDs, in high-risk patients who need to continue NSAID therapy, several options are available to decrease the risk of clinically important PU complications. It is important that the clinician (1) identify patients who are at high risk for serious complications with NSAID therapy, and (2) recognize that dyspepsia does not correlate with the development of clinically significant NSAID-related mucosal damage.

Although conventional doses of H_2RAs are effective for preventing DU, they may not be as effective with GU in patients who remain on long-term NSAID therapy.[1,20,21] Evidence suggests that high-dose H_2RAs may be more effective than standard doses in preventing both DU and GU; however, the use of H_2RAs in the prevention of NSAID-induced PU is generally not recommended.[41] PPIs have been shown to decrease the incidence of both DU and GU associated with continued NSAID use.[20,41,89] This demonstrated efficacy, combined with their ease of administration, infrequent adverse effects, and excellent safety profile, makes PPIs a popular choice for prevention of NSAID-induced ulcers in high-risk patients. However, large-scale studies are still needed to demonstrate that PPIs protect against PU complications.

Use of misoprostol has been shown to prevent both DU and GU and their complications in patients who take NSAIDs.[1,20,41,89] The PGE_1 analogue's benefit is likely related to its ability to replenish the mucosal PGs that have been decreased by the NSAID. Unfortunately, the adverse effects of the medication (discussed previously) limit its use, despite its efficacy. Lower doses may provide adequate protection with better tolerability, but as with the adverse effects of misoprostol, the ability to prevent GU is dose related.[104] Although misoprostol has been shown to decrease the incidence of serious PUD complications, it did not prevent 60% of adverse events in one study.[105]

Anti-inflammatory agents that have enhanced selectivity for COX-2 ("COX-2 inhibitors" or "coxibs") decrease, but do not eliminate, the GI-related toxicity associated with NSAIDs. Although most NSAID toxicities, including GI effects and renal dysfunction, have been associated with the inhibition of COX-1, agents with higher selectivity for COX-2 may adversely affect renal function and blood pressure and may increase risk for cardiovascular adverse events; thus, they should be used only in appropriate patients.[106,107]

For high-risk patients who require analgesic or anti-inflammatory therapy, non-NSAID analgesics such as acetaminophen should be considered whenever possible. If an NSAID is required, the drug should be used at the lowest effective dose, and if a nonselective NSAID is used, those with potentially lower risk of ulcerogenesis such as etodolac or the nonacetylated salicylates may be preferred. Cotherapy with misoprostol or a PPI is recommended with NSAID therapy in high-risk patients. Alternatively, new NSAIDs that have less GI toxicity (e.g., COX-2 inhibitors) may provide effective analgesia with reduced risk of PUD; however, their overall safety remains controversial, particularly in light of recent findings with increased cardiovascular events.

Treatment of Refractory Ulcers. Although most PUs heal within 4 to 8 weeks of initiation of antisecretory therapy, a small but significant number of patients have persistent (or "refractory") ulcers, despite prolonged conventional treatment (e.g., 12 weeks with therapeutic doses of antisecretory agents) or several courses of H. pylori treatment. Unfortunately, a standardized definition for a refractory PU is lacking, which complicates the interpretation of clinical treatment trials in that different investigators use different diagnostic criteria. The location of the ulcer, the type of antiulcer therapy used, the duration of therapy, whether H. pylori infection was successfully eradicated, and whether NSAID therapy is being continued should all be taken into consideration before an ulcer is declared to be refractory, although the specific circumstances in which an ulcer would be considered refractory remain unclear. Poor adherence/compliance, cigarette smoking, large ulcers, use of NSAIDs, resistant H. pylori infections, and hypersecretory conditions may contribute to refractory PUD; nonulcerative causes of dyspepsia, including malignancy, should also be considered and excluded as appropriate. Most refractory ulcers will be healed with higher PPI doses, even if they did not respond to standard doses of PPIs or to conventional or high-dose H$_2$RAs.[1,41] Combination therapy has not been proven to be more effective than monotherapy.

Treatment of Zollinger-Ellison's Syndrome. PPIs are the first-line therapy used to control gastric acid secretion in patients with a confirmed diagnosis of ZES; they decrease the risks of PU complications and other acid-peptic disease (e.g., esophagitis). H$_2$RAs may be considered for second-line therapy.[26] Antisecretory agents should be dose-adjusted so that a basal acid output of less than 10 mEq per hour (below 5 mEq per hour in patients with previous acid-reducing gastric surgery) is maintained. If basal acid output before the next scheduled dose is zero, doses can be carefully reduced, if this is desired. High doses of PPIs or H$_2$RAs are usually needed in ZES to control acid secretion (generally two to four times standard ulcer-healing doses, but possibly even higher); divided dosing is usually needed to maintain 24-hour acid suppression. Once acid secretion is well controlled, doses may be safely tapered to approximately half the starting dose in some patients. Even patients with ZES who have undergone successful gastrinoma resection usually continue to require long-term control of gastric acid secretion with antisecretory drugs, because of the increased parietal cell mass that occurs with long-term hypergastrinemia. Octreotide, a long-acting somatostatin analog, inhibits gastric acid and gastrin production, as well as release of secondary peptides by the gastrinoma.[26,108] Octreotide is rather expensive, requires administration by IV or subcutaneous injection, and is only modestly effective as monotherapy; therefore, its role in ZES therapy is currently somewhat limited.

Once adequate control of gastric acid secretion has been achieved, imaging studies [e.g., endoscopic ultrasound, magnetic resonance imaging, spiral/helical computed tomography, and somatostatin receptor scintigraphy (OctreoScan)] should be performed to locate the tumor and stage the disease; biopsies may also be used to confirm metastases. If a metastatic lesion is found, management then focuses on palliative antitumor therapy provided through a combination of chemotherapy, hormonal therapy with a somatostatin analog, and surgical debulking. It is important that uninterrupted gastric acid suppression be continued, even during hospitalization for resection surgery or chemotherapy; the availability of IV pantoprazole has been useful for this and other conditions in which antisecretory agents are needed for patients who cannot take oral medications.

Prophylaxis of Stress-Related Erosive Syndrome. Because it is not currently practical to measure the gut perfusion and protective function of all critically ill patients, a prophylactic approach is used to decrease the risk of severe complications associated with SRES. It remains controversial whether all intensive care unit (ICU) patients require SRES prophylaxis; however, patients with sepsis, shock, trauma, respiratory failure, coagulopathy, quadriplegia, extensive burns, head trauma, or recent neurosurgery have an increased risk for serious GI bleeding events and are often targeted for prophylaxis. Patients who have a history of PUD, cirrhosis, or acute renal failure should also be candidates for prophylaxis.[30,31,41] The literature on the topic of prophylactic therapy for SRES is confusing and often contradictory because there are many discrepancies in the criteria used to determine the presence of bleeding, as well as major differences in the patient populations studied. Generally, the literature suggests that acid-suppressive agents, including antacids (titrated to an intragastric pH greater than 4), sucralfate (usually given by nasogastric or nasoduodenal tube), and IV H$_2$RAs, significantly decrease the risk of GI bleeding in critically ill patients compared with placebo.[1,30,31] Small recent trials that have studied PPIs (IV, oral capsules opened and administered by nasogastric or gastrostomy tube, or suspension provided by nasogastric tube) and active comparators suggest that PPIs are superior to traditional agents in preventing GI bleeding in patients at risk for SRES.[30,31,41] Some data show that critically ill patients treated with sucralfate may have a lower overall mortality rate compared with those treated with antacids or H$_2$RAs, perhaps related to the lower rate of nosocomial pneumonia associated with sucralfate than with antisecretory agents. Patients with higher gastric pH resulting from antacids and antisecretory agents may have increased growth of gram-negative bacteria in the stomach, and if severely ill patients aspirate these bacteria into the airway, they may develop pneumonia; sucralfate, however, does not raise intragastric pH significantly. Studies on this issue are not definitive, however, and there is still much dispute regarding the contribution of SRES prophylaxis to nosocomial pneumonia in critically ill patients.[1] Discontinuing SRES prophylaxis is often possible when patients show improvement in their overall medical condition (e.g., starting oral intake, extubation, or discharge from ICU).

Treatment of Gastroesophageal Reflux Disease
Treatment of Erosive Gastroesophageal Reflux Disease. Although many patients regularly report symptoms of GERD, few seek medical care for their condition; most instead treat themselves or ignore their symptoms.[2,70] Along with lifestyle modifications (discussed previously), nonprescription therapy for GERD often includes antacids and on-demand use of OTC H_2RAs. Patients with severe symptoms of GERD or erosive esophagitis should be treated with scheduled doses of antisecretory agents (Table 45.6). These agents raise intragastric pH to greater than 4 during the periods of the day in which reflux is most likely to occur. Studies have found that patients with greater esophageal acid exposure require longer periods of acid suppression for healing.[2] Results of clinical trials evaluating the effectiveness of acid suppression are variable, partly because the efficacy of GERD therapy varies according to disease severity, and in these trials, disease severity and the definition of esophagitis were not consistent. Comparison of the therapeutic effect of antisecretory agents with placebo response provides an indirect measure of disease severity in the population studied. For healing esophagitis, the H_2RAs provide only 10% to 24% relative benefit compared with placebo, regardless of esophagitis severity or the dose of H_2RA used. In contrast, PPIs show increasing therapeutic gain with increasing disease severity, and their efficacy is dose and potency dependent.[2,41,70,109] Twice-daily regimens may be required in patients who have insufficient response to once-daily PPIs.

In spite of the recognition that delayed gastric emptying is often a component of GERD, the prokinetic agents (metoclopramide and cisapride) have limited usefulness in GERD because they demonstrate no advantage over antisecretory agents and are associated with significant adverse effects (significant CNS adverse effects with metoclopramide and serious cardiac arrhythmias with cisapride).[2] Although perhaps more effective than metoclopramide, cisapride is available in the United States only through an investigational limited access program from the manufacturer. This restriction is the result of its cardiotoxic effects, which are increased when it is used in combination with other drugs metabolized by the CYP system. Currently, there is an interest in developing other agents, similar to cisapride, in the hopes of finding a safe and effective prokinetic agent

for GERD. Even though several pharmacologic agents have been reported to inhibit LES relaxation (Table 45.4), none is considered clinically useful in this capacity. Several agents that have shown an ability to decrease transient LES relaxations are being studied, including loxiglumide [(a cholecystokinin A antagonist)], n-monomethyl-l-arginine [a nitric oxide (NO) synthase inhibitor], an l-Baclofen [a γ-aminobutyric acid B (GABA$_B$) receptor agonist]; l-Baclofen is already approved for the treatment of spastic disorders and chronic hiccups, and it will likely be the first agent clinically tested to target transient LES relaxation.[2]

Maintenance Therapy of Erosive Gastroesophageal Reflux Disease. Although almost all severe esophagitis can be healed with PPIs, recurrence occurs within 6 months of therapy discontinuation in approximately 80% of patients and is related to the initial severity of esophagitis. Because of this high rate of relapse, maintenance therapy with PPIs is usually indicated; evidence suggests that H_2RAs are significantly less effective as maintenance therapy.[2,41,70] Few data support the use of step-down therapy for maintenance treatment in esophagitis, which initially requires a PPI; despite the need for a periodic increase or decrease in a patient's PPI dose, the median doses required to maintain remission are generally at or near the doses required for healing the esophagitis.[2]

Treatment of Nonerosive Gastroesophageal Reflux Disease. Compared with the number of trials that have studied erosive GERD, relatively few studies have assessed therapy for nonerosive GERD. Symptom response is the primary outcome in this population, because endoscopic healing is not an applicable end point. Similar to the results seen in erosive GERD, PPIs have consistently been shown to provide better symptom relief in nonerosive GERD than H_2RAs or cisapride, although elimination of heartburn appears to be more difficult to achieve than the cure of esophagitis, disproving the theory that nonerosive disease is more responsive to treatment than erosive disease.[2] However, data on endoscopy-negative GERD and less severe esophagitis do support a less aggressive therapeutic approach to maintain remission, and suggest that intermittent or on-demand therapy may be adequate for symptom control in this population.[2,41,70]

Treatment of Complications. For patients with ulcer hemorrhage, therapeutic endoscopy (injection with epinephrine alone or with saline or alcohol, or electrocoagulation) is highly effective for achieving hemostasis (90% of cases) and is the standard of care.[110] Bleeding related to esophageal varices may be treated with endoscopic injection of the varix with a sclerosing agent or banding of the varix.[111] The use of antisecretory agents in the treatment of bleeding PUs makes sense because of their theoretical ability to decrease peptic damage to injured blood vessels, prevent peptic digestion of blood clots, and improve platelet function, which is impaired by acid. However, numerous studies with H$_2$RAs in this setting have showed no significant benefit in controlling hemorrhage, and results with PPIs have been mixed. The availability of IV PPIs will likely increase the use of this therapy as an adjunct to endoscopic treatment for bleeding PUs, because more positive studies have been seen with this form of administration.[1,111] The traditional therapy for perforated PU is surgery to close the perforation and irrigate the peritoneal cavity, and administration of IV broad-spectrum antibiotics.[1] Penetrating PUs are currently not treated any differently than nonpenetrating PUs, largely because clinicians rarely have confirmation that they are dealing with a penetrating ulcer; diagnosing this complication generally requires surgery or imaging procedures such as computed tomography.

IMPROVING OUTCOMES

PATIENT EDUCATION

Patients with PUD or GERD should be educated regarding their disease, including cause, diagnosis, treatment, alarm symptoms, and follow-up if needed. Patients should be counseled to decrease or eliminate factors that may cause or exacerbate PUD, GERD, or their symptoms, such as NSAIDs, psychological stress, smoking, and certain foods and beverages. Patient compliance should be assessed, and the simplest, most effective regimen should be used whenever possible. Completion of therapy as prescribed (even if the patient is feeling better) should be emphasized to all patients, especially those receiving antibiotics as part of an *H. pylori* treatment regimen. As with any medication selection, consideration of patients' drug allergies and potential drug–drug, drug–food, or drug–disease interactions must be applied when therapies for PUD and GERD are chosen, particularly with *H. pylori* eradication regimens. Similarly, patients who use oral contraceptives should be made aware of the potential of antibiotics to decrease the efficacy of birth control pills, and they should be advised appropriately. Patients who are prescribed metronidazole should be counseled to avoid consuming ethanol beverages or products that contain ethanol during, and for at least 3 days after completion of metronidazole treatment. Adverse effects (potential and common) should be considered in medication selection; patients should be counseled regarding these, especially if compliance could be negatively affected. Specifically, if bismuth-containing compounds are used in *H. pylori* eradication regimens, patients should be made aware of an expected change in stool color. If a patient is not responsive to *H. pylori* eradication therapy, noncompliance and the possibility of antibiotic resistance should be assessed.

METHODS TO IMPROVE ADHERENCE TO DRUG THERAPY

The importance of therapy to improve PUD or GERD symptoms and healing and to avoid complications should be emphasized to patients to enhance compliance. In conditions

that require more complex therapies, such as *H. pylori* eradication regimens, the short-term nature of the therapy should be highlighted to encourage patient adherence. Compliance tends to decrease with multiple medications, increased frequency of administration, increased duration of treatment, and intolerable adverse effects.[112] As discussed earlier, patients should be made aware of potential adverse effects and drug interactions of their medications, as well as the risks of incomplete courses of therapy, including suboptimal disease treatment, incomplete ulcer healing, and the risk of antibiotic resistance. Regimens should be well tolerated and simple, while retaining excellent efficacy to improve adherence. Reminder tools (pill boxes, calendars, timers) may be used if patients need additional assistance in being compliant with their medication regimen.

PHARMACOECONOMICS

Annual health care costs of PUD and GERD in the United States have been estimated at over $15 billion (in 1998 dollars).[113] The GI disease with the highest direct and indirect costs is GERD (including Barrett's esophagus) at over $10 billion, while the annual health care (direct and indirect) costs of PUD have been estimated at $5 to $6 billion.[4,113] For GERD (with and without Barrett's esophagus), 62% of the total direct costs are from the cost of pharmaceuticals. In comparison, drug therapy is only 20% of the total direct costs of PUD.[113] The bulk of the direct costs for PUD come from hospitalizations and physician office visits.[4,113] Pharmacoeconomic modeling suggests that eradication of *H. pylori* is superior to conventional treatment with H$_2$RAs, mainly because eradication decreases the need for continued treatment and PUD recurrence. Comparisons between and among the H$_2$RAs and PPIs is difficult; differences in health care models (e.g., United States vs. Canada vs. European countries) and even differences in formulary coverage can greatly affect the costs of these agents, which can influence which single agent is most cost-effective for an individual patient. In general, it has been suggested that a more costly agent with better efficacy may lead to greater cost savings over the long term because of the lower rates of recurrence and complications associated with more effective agents. With the availability of OTC omeprazole, the difference in acquisition cost between PPIs and H$_2$RAs is less significant, making the choice between PPIs and H$_2$RA less of an issue. Because no one PPI has been shown to have superior clinical efficacy over another, selection of the agent with the lowest acquisition cost is preferred.

CONCLUSION

Eradication of *H. pylori* and discontinuation of NSAID use are important factors in the treatment of PUD, as these interventions are associated with ulcer healing and decreased recurrence. When antiulcer agents are needed for treatment, prevention, or maintenance of PUD (including ZES and SRES) and GERD, PPIs are considered first-line agents because of their efficacy, safety, tolerability, and, because of the availability of OTC omeprazole, cost-effectiveness. H$_2$RAs are also effective and safe therapies for many ulcerative conditions. Sucralfate, misoprostol, and antacids are less commonly used because of their complex dosing regimens, greater adverse effects, and lower efficacy.

KEY POINTS

- PUD is a group of disorders characterized by the presence of ulcers in any portion of the GI tract that has undergone acid exposure of sufficient duration and concentration. GERD is any symptomatic clinical condition or histologic presentation caused by damage to the esophageal mucosa resulting from retrograde flow of gastric contents into the esophagus

- *H. pylori* infection and NSAID use are the most common causes of PUD. It is suggested that *H. pylori* infection contributes to gastric mucosal injury through direct mechanisms, alterations in the immune/inflammatory response, and hypergastrinemia that leads to increased acid secretion. The ulcerogenic effects of NSAIDs are thought to be related to direct/topical irritation of the gastric epithelium and systemic inhibition of PG synthesis, which serve to weaken endogenous GI mucosal defenses

- The goals of treatment for PUD are to relieve pain, promote ulcer healing, prevent ulcer recurrence, prevent primary complications such as GI bleeding or perforation, and prevent secondary complications such as cough, asthma exacerbation, stricture, and adenocarcinoma

- Antiulcer and antibiotic therapy can effectively treat patients and reduce the recurrence of PUD when *H. pylori* infection is present. NSAID-induced ulcers can be treated by removal of the ulcerogenic drug (if possible) or the use of agents that prevent gastric acid secretion (H$_2$RAs, PPIs) or protect the stomach mucosa (sucralfate, misoprostol) when NSAIDs are used in high-risk patients. GERD is most commonly pharmacologically treated with antacids and antisecretory agents. Prokinetic agents may be considered in some cases of GERD

- Nonpharmacologic modifications such as smoking cessation, reduction of psychological stress, and avoidance of food/beverages that exacerbate symptoms may be beneficial with active or chronic PUD or GERD

SUGGESTED READINGS

DeVault KR, Castell DO. Updated guidelines for the diagnosis and treatment of gastroesophageal reflux disease. Am J Gastroenterol 100:190–200, 2005.

Peterson WL, Fendrick AM, Cave DR, et al. *Helicobacter pylori*–related disease: guidelines for testing and treatment. Arch Intern Med 160:1285–1291, 2000.

Shiotani A, Graham DY. Pathogenesis and therapy of gastric and duodenal ulcer disease. Med Clin North Am 86:1447–1466, 2002.

Wolfe MM, Sachs G. Acid suppression: optimizing therapy for gastroduodenal ulcer healing, gastroesophageal reflux disease, and stress-related erosive syndrome. Gastroenterology 118:S9–S31, 2000.

REFERENCES

1. Spechler SJ. Peptic ulcer and its complications. In: Feldman M, Friedman LS, Sleisenger MH, eds. Sleisenger and Fordtran's gastrointestinal and liver disease: pathophysiology/diagnosis/management. 7th ed. Philadelphia: WB Saunders, 2002:747–772.
2. Kahrilas PJ, Pandolfin JE. Gastroesophageal reflux disease and its complications, including Barrett's metaplasia. In: Felman M, Friedman LS, Sleisenger MH Eds. Sleisenger and Fordtran's gastrointestinal and liver disease: pathophysiology/diagnosis/management. 7th ed. Philadelphia: WB Saunders, 2002:599–622.
3. Munnangi S, Sonnenberg A. Time trends of physician visits and treatment patterns of peptic ulcer disease in the United States. Arch Intern Med 157:1489–1494, 1997.
4. Sonnenberg A, Everhart JE. Health impact of peptic ulcer in the United States. Am J Gastroenterol 92:614–620, 1997.
5. Isenberg JI, Soll AH. Epidemiology, clinical manifestations, and diagnosis of peptic ulcer. In: Bennett JC, Plum F, eds. Cecil textbook of medicine. 20th ed. Philadelphia: WB Saunders, 1996:664–666.
6. Shiotani A, Graham DY. Pathogenesis and therapy of gastric and duodenal ulcer disease. Med Clin North Am 86:1447–1466, 2002.
7. Sonnenberg A. Temporal trends and geographical variations of peptic ulcer disease. Aliment Pharmacol Ther 9(Suppl 2):3–12, 1995.
8. Parsonnet J. The incidence of *Helicobacter pylori* infection. Aliment Pharmacol Ther 9(Suppl 2):45–51, 1995.
9. Sonnenberg A, El-Serag HB. Clinical epidemiology and natural history of gastroesophageal reflux disease. Yale J Biol Med 72:81–92, 1999.
10. Wienbeck M, Barnert J. Epidemiology of reflux disease and reflux esophagitis. Scan J Gastroenterol Suppl 156:7–13, 1989.
11. Kitchin LI, Castell DO. Rationale and efficacy of conservative therapy for gastroesophageal reflux disease. Arch Intern Med 151:448–454, 1991.
12. Kurata JH, Nogawa AN: Meta-analysis of risk factors for peptic ulcers: nonsteroidal anti-inflammatory drugs, *Helicobacter pylori,* and smoking. J Clin Gastroenterol 24:2–17, 1997.
13. Peterson WL, Graham DY. *Helicobacter pylori.* In: Feldman M, Friedman LS, Sleisenger MH, eds. Sleisenger and Fordtran's gastrointestinal and liver disease: pathophysiology/diagnosis/management. 7th ed. Philadelphia: WB Saunders, 2002:732–743.
14. Kuipers EJ. *Helicobacter pylori* and the risk and management of associated diseases: gastritis, ulcer disease, atrophic gastritis and gastric cancer. Aliment Pharmacol Ther 11(Suppl 1):71–88, 1997.
15. Laine I, Hopkins RJ, Girardi LS. Has the impact of *Helicobacter pylori* therapy on ulcer recurrence in the United States been overstated? A meta-analysis of rigorously designed trials. Am J Gastroenterol 93:1409–1415, 1998.
16. Pounder RE, Ng D. The prevalence of *Helicobacter pylori* infection in different countries. Aliment Pharmacol Ther 9(Suppl 2):33–39, 1995.
17. Graham DY, Lew GM, Klein PD, et al. Effect of treatment of *Helicobacter pylori* infection on the long-term recurrence of gastric or duodenal ulcer: a randomized controlled study. Ann Intern Med 116:705–708, 1992.
18. Go MF. What are the host factors that place an individual at risk for *Helicobacter pylori*–associated disease? Gastroenterology 113(Suppl):S15–S20, 1997.
19. Mobley HLT. *Helicobacter pylori* factors associated with disease development. Gastroenterology 113(Suppl):S21–S28, 1997.
20. Cryer B. Nonsteroidal anti-inflammatory drug injury. In: Feldman M, Friedman LS, Sleisenger MH, eds. Sleisenger and Fordtran's gastrointestinal and liver disease: pathophysiology/diagnosis/management. 7th ed. Philadelphia: WB Saunders, 2002:408–426.

21. Wallace JL. Nonsteroidal anti-inflammatory drugs and gastroenteropathy; the second hundred years. Gastroenterology 113(Suppl): S67–S77, 1997.

22. Singh G, Rosen DR, Morfield D, et al. Gastrointestinal tract complications of nonsteroidal anti-inflammatory drug treatment in rheumatoid arthritis. Arch Intern Med 156:1530–1536, 1996.

23. Gabriel SE, Jaakkimainen L, Bombardier C. Risk for serious gastrointestinal complications related to use of nonsteroidal anti-inflammatory drugs: a meta-analysis. Ann Intern Med 115:787–796, 1991.

24. Singh G, Triadafilopoulos G. Epidemiology of NSAID-induced gastrointestinal complications. J Rheumatol 26:18–24, 1999.

25. Peura DA, Lanza FL, Gostout CJ. The American College of Gastroenterology Bleeding Registry: preliminary findings. Am J Gastroenterol 11:282–291, 1997.

26. Pisegna JR. Zollinger-Ellison syndrome and other hypersecretory states. In: Feldman M, Friedman LS, Sleisenger MH, eds. Sleisenger and Fordtran's gastrointestinal and liver disease: pathophysiology/diagnosis/management. 7th ed. Philadelphia: WB Saunders, 2002:782–796.

27. Cook DJ, Fuller HD, Guyatt GH, et al. Risk factors for gastrointestinal bleeding in critically ill patients. Canadian Critical Care Trials Group. N Engl J Med 330:377–381, 1994.

28. Goldin GF, Peura DA. Stress-related mucosal damage. What to do or not to do. Gastrointest Endosc Clin North Am 6:505–526, 1996.

29. Fisher RL, Pipkin GA, Wood JR. Stress-related mucosal disease: pathophysiology, prevention, and treatment. Crit Care Clin 11: 323–345, 1995.

30. Tryba M, Cook D. Current guidelines on stress ulcer prophylaxis. Drugs 54:581–596, 1997.

31. Spirt MJ. Acid suppression in critically ill patients: what does the evidence support? Pharmacotherapy 23:S87–S93, 2003.

32. Beejay U, Wolfe MM. Acute gastrointestinal bleeding in the intensive care unit. Gastroenterol Clin North Am 29:309–336, 2000.

33. Svanes C, Soreide JA, Skarstein A, et al. Smoking and ulcer perforation. Gut 2:177–180, 1997.

34. Aldoori WH, Giovannucci EL, Stampfer MJ, et al. A prospective study of alcohol, smoking, caffeine, and the risk of duodenal ulcer in men. Epidemiology 4:420, 1997.

35. Sonnenberg A, Muller-Lissner A, Vogel E, et al. Predictors of duodenal ulcer healing and relapse. Gastroenterology 81:1061–1067, 1981.

36. Parente F, Maconi G, Sngaletti O, et al. Behaviour of acid secretion, gastrin release, serum pepsinogen I, and gastric emptying of liquids over six months from eradication of Helicobacter pylori in duodenal ulcer patients: a controlled study. Gut 37:210–215, 1995.

37. Kim SL, Hunter JG, Wo JM, et al. NSAIDs, aspirin, and esophageal strictures: are over-the-counter medications harmful to the esophagus? J Clin Gastroenterol 29:32–34, 1999.

38. El-Serag HB, Sonnenberg A. Associations between different forms of gastro-oesophageal reflux disease. Gut 41:594–599, 1997.

39. Weinberg DS, Kadish SL. The diagnosis and management of gastroesophageal reflux disease. Med Clin North Am 80:411–429, 1996.

40. Sachs G. Physiology of the parietal cell and therapeutic implications. Pharmacotherapy 23(Suppl):S68–S73, 2003.

41. Wolfe MM, Sachs G. Acid suppression: optimizing therapy for gastroduodenal ulcer healing, gastroesophageal reflux disease, and stress-related erosive syndrome. Gastroenterology 118:S9–S31, 2000.

42. Feldman M. Gastric secretion. In: Feldman M, Friedman LS, Sleisenger MH, eds. Sleisenger and Fordtran's gastrointestinal and liver disease: pathophysiology/diagnosis/management. 7th ed. Philadelphia: WB Saunders, 2002:715–731.

43. Peura DA. Ulcerogenesis: integrating the roles of Helicobacter pylori and acid secretion in duodenal ulcer. Am J Gastroenterol 92(Suppl):S8–S16, 1997.

44. El-Omar EM, Penman ID, Ardill JE, et al. Helicobacter pylori infection and abnormalities of acid secretion in patients with duodenal ulcer disease. Gastroenterology 109:681–691, 1995.

45. Marshall BJ. Helicobacter pylori. Am J Gastroenterol 89(Suppl): S116–S128, 1994.

46. Ernst PB, Crowe SE, Reyes VE. How does Helicobacter pylori cause mucosal damage? The inflammatory response. Gastroenterology 113(Suppl):S35–S42, 1997.

47. Calam J, Gibbons A, Healey ZV, et al. How does Helicobacter pylori cause mucosal damage? Its effect on acid and gastrin physiology. Gastroenterology 113(Suppl):S43–S49, 1997.

48. Fisher RL, Pipkin GA, Wood JR. Stress-related mucosal disease: pathophysiology, prevention, and treatment. Crit Care Clin 11: 323–345, 1995.

49. Simpson WG. Gastroesophageal reflux disease and asthma. Diagnosis and management. Arch Intern Med 155:798–803, 1995.

50. Larsen RR. Gastroesophageal reflux disease: gaining control over heartburn. Postgrad Med 101:181–187, 1997.

51. Levine MS. Role of the double-contrast upper gastrointestinal series in the 1990s. Gastroenterol Clin North Am 24:289–308, 1995.

52. Glick SN. Duodenal ulcer. Radiol Clin North Am 32:1259–1274, 1994.

53. Committee on Endoscopic Utilization, American Society for Gastrointestinal Endoscopy (ASGE). Appropriate use of gastrointestinal endoscopy. Oak Brook, Ill: ASGE, August 1992.

54. Yamao K, Nakazawa S, Yoshino J, et al. Evaluating gastric ulcer healing by endoscopic ultrasonography. Endoscopy 26:798–799, 1994.

55. Kochman ML, Elta GH. Gastric ulcers—when is enough enough? Gastroenterology 105:1582–1584, 1993.

56. Cohen H, Laine L. Endoscopic methods for the diagnosis of Helicobacter pylori. Aliment Pharmacol Ther 11(Suppl):S3–S9, 1997.

57. Atherton JC. Non-endoscopic tests in the diagnosis of Helicobacter pylori. Aliment Pharmacol Ther 11(Suppl):S11–S20, 1997.

58. Megraud F. How should Helicobacter pylori infection be diagnosed? Gastroenterology 113(Suppl):S93–S98, 1997.

59. Cutler AF, Havstad S, Ma CK, et al. Accuracy of invasive and non-invasive tests to diagnose Helicobacter pylori infection. Gastroenterology 109:136–141, 1995.

60. Vakil N, Vaira D. Non-invasive tests for the diagnosis of H. pylori infection. Rev Gastroenterol Disord 4:1–6, 2004.

61. Peterson WL, Fendrick AM, Cave DR, et al. Helicobacter pylori–related disease. Guidelines for testing and treatment. Arch Intern Med 160:1285–1291, 2000.

62. Feldman M, Cryer B, Lee E, et al. Role of seroconversion in confirming cure of Helicobacter pylori infection. JAMA 280:363–365, 1998.

63. Laine L, Estrada R, Trujillo M, et al. Effect of proton-pump inhibitor therapy on diagnostic testing for Helicobacter pylori. Ann Intern Med 129:547–550, 1998.

64. Cutler AF, Toskes P. Comparison of [13C]urea blood test to [13C]urea breath test for the diagnosis of Helicobacter pylori. Am J Gastroenterol 94:959–961, 1999.

65. Vaira D, Malfertheiner P, Megraud F, et al. Diagnosis of Helicobacter pylori infection with a new non-invasive antigen-based assay. Lancet 354:30–33, 1999.

66. Manes G, Balzano A, Iaquinto G, et al. Accuracy of the stool antigen test in the diagnosis of Helicobacter pylori infection before treatment and in patients on omeprazole therapy. Aliment Pharmacol Ther 15:73–79, 2001.

67. Vaira D, Vakil N, Menegatti M, et al. The stool antigen test for detection of Helicobacter pylori after eradication therapy. Ann Intern Med 136:280–287, 2002.

68. Gisbert JP, Pajares JM. Stool antigen test for the diagnosis of Helicobacter pylori infection: a systematic review. Helicobacter 9: 347–368, 2004.

69. DeVault KR, Castell DO, for the Practice Parameters Committee of the American College of Gastroenterology. Guidelines for the diagnosis and treatment of gastroesophageal reflux disease. Arch Intern Med 155:2165–2173, 1995.

70. Fennerty MB, Castell D, Fendrick AM, et al. The diagnosis and treatment of gastroesophageal reflux disease in a managed care environment: suggested disease management guidelines. Arch Intern Med 156:477–484, 1996.

71. Dobhan R, Castell DO. Prolonged intraesophageal pH monitoring compared with 16-hour overnight recording. Dig Dis Sci 37: 857–864, 1992.

72. Orr WC, Allen ML, Robinson M. The pattern of nocturnal and diurnal esophageal acid exposure in the pathogenesis of erosive mucosal damage. Am J Gastroenterol 89:509–512, 1994.

73. Waring JP, LeGrand J, Chinichian A, et al. Duodenogastric reflux in patients with Barrett's esophagus. Dig Dis Sci 35:759–762, 1990.

74. Wara P, Stodkilde H. Bleeding pattern before admission as guideline for emergency endoscopy. Scand J Gastroenterol 20:72–78, 1985.

75. Asaka M, Takeda H, Sugiyama T, et al. What role does *Helicobacter pylori* play in gastric cancer? Gastroenterology 113(Suppl): S56–S60, 1997.

76. Thiede C, Morgner A, Alpen B, et al. What role does *Helicobacter pylori* eradication play in gastric MALT and gastric MALT lymphoma? Gastroenterology 113(Suppl):S61–S64, 1997.

77. Castell DO. Long-term management of GERD: the pill, the knife or the endoscope? Gastrointest Endosc 40:252–253, 1994.

78. Czinn SJ. What is the role for vaccination in *Helicobacter pylori*? Gastroenterology 113(Suppl):S149–S153, 1997.

79. Berardi RR, Welage LS. Proton pump inhibitors in acid-related disease. Am J Health Syst Pharm 55:2289–2298, 1998.

80. Welage LS. Pharmacologic properties of proton pump inhibitors. Pharmacotherapy 23:S74–S80, 2003.

81. Serfaty-Lacrosniere C, Wood RJ, Voytko D, et al. Hypochlorhydria from short-term omeprazole treatment does not inhibit intestinal absorption of calcium, phosphorus, magnesium, or zinc from food in humans. J Am Coll Nutr 14:364–368, 1995.

82. Koop H, Bachem MG. Serum iron, ferritin, and vitamin B12 during prolonged omeprazole therapy. J Clin Gastroenterol 14: 288–292, 1992.

83. Vakil N, Fennerty MB. Direct comparative trials of the efficacy of proton pump inhibitors in the management of gastro-oesophageal reflux disease and peptic ulcer disease. Aliment Pharmacol Ther 18:559–568, 2003.

84. Sax MJ. Clinically important adverse effects and drug interactions with H2-receptor antagonists: an update. Pharmacotherapy 7: S110–S115, 1987.

85. Lipsy RJ, Fennerty B, Fagan TC. Clinical review of histamine 2 receptor antagonists. Arch Intern Med 150:745–751, 1990.

86. Welage LS, Berardi RR. Drug interactions with antiulcer agents: considerations in the treatment of peptic ulcer disease. J Pharm Pract 7:177–195, 1994.

87. McCarthy DM. Sucralfate. N Engl J Med 325:1017–1025, 1991.

88. Thomson MICROMEDEX.

89. Soll AH. Medical treatment of peptic ulcer disease: practice guidelines. JAMA 275:622–629, 1996.

90. Howden CW, Hunt RH. Guidelines for the management of *Helicobacter pylori* infection. Ad Hoc Committee on the Practice Parameters of the American College of Gastroenterology. Am J Gastroenterol 93:2330–2338, 1998.

91. Laheij RJF, VanRossum LGM, Jansen JBMJ, et al. Evaluation of treatment regimens to cure *Helicobacter pylori* infection: a meta-analysis. Aliment Pharmacol Ther 13:857–864, 1999.

92. Gisbert JP, Gonzalez L, Calvet X, et al. Helicobacter pylori eradication: proton pump inhibitor vs. ranitidine bismuth citrate plus two antibiotics for 1 week: a meta-analysis of efficacy. Aliment Pharmacol Ther 14:1141–1150, 2000.

93. Gisbert JP, Gonzalez L, Calvet X, et al. Proton pump inhibitor, clarithromycin and either amoxycillin or nitroimidazole: a meta-analysis of eradication of *Helicobacter pylori*. Aliment Pharmacol Ther 14:1319–1328, 2000.

94. Graham DY. Therapy of *Helicobacter pylori*: current status and issues. Gastroenterology 118:S2–S8, 2000.

95. Peterson WL. The role of antisecretory drugs in the treatment of *Helicobacter pylori* infection. Aliment Pharmacol Ther 11(Suppl 1):S21–S25, 1997.

96. Salcedo JA, Al-Kawas F. Treatment of *Helicobacter pylori* infection. Arch Intern Med 158:842–851, 1998.

97. Calvet X, Garcia N, Lopez T, et al. A meta-analysis of short versus long therapy with a proton pump inhibitor, clarithromycin, and either metronidazole or amoxycillin for treating *Helicobacter pylori* infection. Aliment Pharmacol Ther 14:603–609, 2000.

98. Dore MP, Leandro G, Realdi G, et al. Effect of pretreatment antibiotic resistance to metronidazole and clarithromycin on outcome of *Helicobacter pylori* therapy: a meta-analytical approach. Dig Dis Sci 45:68–70, 2000.

99. Graham DY, Osato MS, Hoffman J, et al. Metronidazole-containing quadruple therapy for infection with metronidazole-resistant *Helicobacter pylori*: a prospective study. Aliment Pharmacol Ther 14:745–750, 2000.

100. Van Oijen AH, Verbeek AL, Jansen JB, et al. Treatment of *Helicobacter pylori* infection with ranitidine bismuth citrate- or proton pump inhibitor–based triple therapies. Aliment Pharmacol Ther 14: 991–999, 2000.

101. Robinson DH, Abdel-Rahman SM, Nahata MC, et al. Guidelines for the treatment of *Helicobacter pylori* in the pediatric patient. Ann Pharmacother 31:1247–1249, 1997.

102. Yeomans ND, Tulassay Z, Juhasz L, et al. A comparison of omeprazole with ranitidine for ulcers associated with nonsteroidal anti-inflammatory drugs. Acid Suppression Trial: Ranitidine Versus Omeprazole for NSAID-Associated Ulcer Treatment (ASTRONAUT) study group. N Engl J Med 338:719–726, 1998.

103. Agrawal NM, Campbell DR, Safdi MA, et al. Superiority of lansoprazole versus ranitidine in healing nonsteroidal anti-inflammatory drug-associated gastric ulcers: results of a double-blind, randomized, multicenter study. NSAID-associated gastric ulcer study group. Arch Intern Med 160:1455–1461, 2000.

104. Raskin JB, White RH, Jackson JE, et al. Misoprostol dosage in the prevention of nonsteroidal anti-inflammatory drug-induced gastric and duodenal ulcers: a comparison of three regimens. Ann Intern Med 123:344–350, 1995.

105. Silverstein FE, Graham DY, Senior FR, et al. Misoprostol reduces serious gastrointestinal complications in patients with rheumatoid arthritis receiving nonsteroidal anti-inflammatory drugs. Ann Intern Med 123:241–249, 1995.

106. Sowers JR, White WB, Pitt B, et al. The effects of cyclooxygenase-2 inhibitors and nonsteroidal anti-inflammatory therapy on 24-hour blood pressure in patients with hypertension, osteoarthritis, and type 2 diabetes mellitus. Arch Intern Med 165:161–168, 2005.

107. Bombardier C, Laine L, Reicin A, et al. Comparison of upper gastrointestinal toxicity of rofecoxib and naproxen in patients with rheumatoid arthritis. VIGOR Study Group. N Engl J Med 343: 1520–1528, 2000.

108. Mozell EJ, Cramer AJ, O'Dorsio TM, et al. Long term efficacy of octreotide in the treatment of Zollinger-Ellison syndrome. Arch Surg 127:1019–1026, 1992.

109. Kahrilas PJ. Gastroesophageal reflux disease. JAMA 276:983–988, 1996.

110. Chung SC, Leung JW, Sung JY, et al. Injection or heat probe for bleeding ulcer. Gastroenterology 100:33–37, 1991.

111. Pisegna JR. Treating patients with acute gastrointestinal bleeding or rebleeding. Pharmacotherapy 23:S81–S86, 2003.

112. Malfertheiner P. Compliance, adverse events and antibiotic resistance in *Helicobacter pylori* treatment. Scand J Gastroenterol 28(Suppl 196):S34–S37, 1993.

113. Sandler RS, Everhart JE, Donowitz M, et al. The burden of selected digestive diseases in the United States. Gastroenterology 122:1500–1511, 2002.

Inflammatory Bowel Disease

Rosemary R. Berardi

TREATMENT GOALS

- Maintain or improve quality of life.
- Terminate the acute attack and induce clinical remission.
- Maintain remission during quiescent symptom-free periods.
- Control symptoms during chronic symptomatic periods.
- Prevent or control complications.
- Avoid surgery, if possible.
- Use the most cost-effective drug treatment.

DEFINITION

Inflammatory bowel disease (IBD) describes two major chronic, nonspecific inflammatory disorders of the gastrointestinal (GI) tract, ulcerative colitis (UC), and Crohn's disease (CD), the causes of which remain unknown.[1] UC is usually limited to the colon and rectum (Fig. 46.1). It may affect the rectum alone (proctitis), only the descending and sigmoid colon and rectum (proctosigmoiditis), or the entire colon (pancolitis, universal). In contrast, CD may affect any part of the GI tract (Fig. 46.1) from mouth to anus; it may involve only the terminal ileum (ileitis), regions of the small intestine (regional enteritis), only the colon (colitis), or both the small bowel and the colon (ileocolonic). When only the colon is affected, CD can be difficult to distinguish from UC. The anatomic location is important as the response to drug therapy may vary according to the site of involvement.

Both UC and CD are characterized by recurrent acute inflammatory episodes and periods of remission.

CAUSES AND RISK FACTORS

The cause of IBD remains unknown. However, there is sufficient evidence to support the theory that proinflammatory antigenic triggers within the intestinal lumen activate the immune response and are influenced by genetic and environmental factors.[1]

PROINFLAMMATORY ANTIGENIC TRIGGERS

The specific proinflammatory antigenic trigger in IBD remains elusive, but microbial, dietary, and autoimmune factors have been implicated. Various microbial pathogens, including *Mycobacterium paratuberculosis,* have been

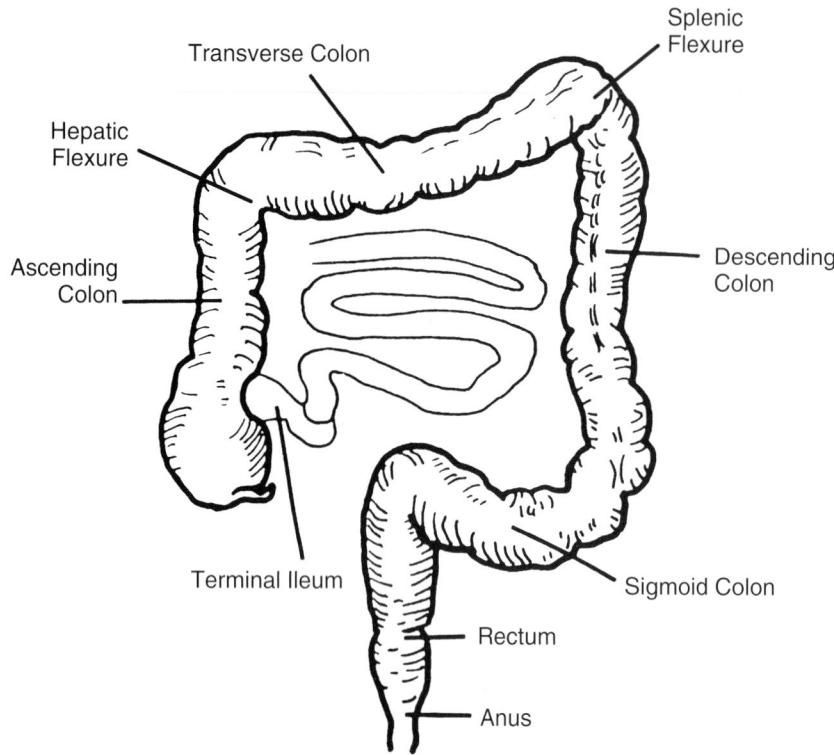

FIGURE 46.1 Anatomic location of various segments of the bowel.

proposed as antigenic triggers in IBD.[2] It has also been hypothesized that normal nonpathogenic colonic flora can stimulate an abnormal immune response. There is no conclusive evidence, however, to support any one specific pathogen or nonpathogenic microbe as having a causative role in UC or CD.[1] Milk, refined sugars, and chemical food additives have been suggested as antigenic triggers. However, there is little evidence to indicate that any food plays an important role as a cause of IBD.[1] In the past, a lactase deficiency in patients with IBD may have been construed as a milk allergy. The autoimmune hypothesis suggests that the patient mounts an appropriate immune response to a microbial or dietary antigen, but because of similarities between the luminal antigen and the epithelial cell proteins, the patient's immune system attacks and destroys the intestinal epithelial cells.[1] Whether antibodies play a causative role in IBD or serve as markers of immune activation remains unclear.

GENETIC INFLUENCES

It has become increasingly clear that there is a genetic basis for IBD. The most important risk factor is a positive family history; 15% of patients have first-degree relatives who also have IBD.[1] However, the incidence of CD among first-degree relatives is higher than that of UC. Studies with monozygotic twins also support the presence of a genetic influence. Although a pattern of inheritance has not been confirmed, positive associations of UC and CD have been established with human leukocyte antigen (HLA) class II genes.[1,3] Genome-wide scanning and gene analysis indicate

that four areas of linkage have been replicated on chromosomes 16, 12, 6, and 14.[3] Specific genetic markers have also been implicated as predictors of disease severity. Continued investigation in medical genetics should provide important insight into the susceptibility, pathogenesis, severity, and treatment of IBD.

ENVIRONMENTAL FACTORS

A number of environmental factors have been proposed as contributing to the development of IBD. These include cigarette smoking, the use of medications such as nonsteroidal anti-inflammatory drugs (NSAIDs), and psychological factors. Cigarette smoking is an established risk factor for CD.[1,4] Patients who smoke have a more severe disease course, require more immunosuppressive drug therapy, and have a more rapid recurrence after surgery than do nonsmokers. Exsmokers are also at increased risk, but the risk is less than that for current smokers. In contrast to CD, smoking reduces the risk of UC.[1,4] However, former smokers are at increased risk when compared with those who have never smoked. How smoking protects patients with UC is unknown, but it probably involves nicotine. NSAIDs can cause a variety of effects in patients with IBD, ranging from asymptomatic mucosal inflammation to strictures, obstruction, perforation, and hemorrhage.[5] NSAIDs have also been linked to colitis in patients without previous IBD and may activate quiescent disease.[5,6] It is unclear whether selective cyclooxygenase-2 (COX-2) inhibitors have a similar effect in IBD.[6] Emotional and psychological factors have been implicated in the origin of IBD, but there is no evidence that stress is causative and that psychotherapy is effective.[7]

EPIDEMIOLOGY

The epidemiology of UC is similar to that of CD in many ways (Table 46.1).[1] Both diseases are more common in Western populations and in urban rather than rural areas. The incidence of UC in the United States (US) has leveled off, but that of CD is still increasing. This increase, however, may reflect improved disease awareness, diagnosis, and reporting. A higher rate of IBD has been reported among the Jewish population born in the US and Europe than in Israeli-born Jewish people. In the United States, UC and CD are more prevalent in whites, but the gap between African-Americans and whites is narrowing. UC and CD have been reported in different members of the same family. IBD can occur at any age, but the peak age of onset is the teens or early twenties; a second, more controversial peak may occur later in life. UC is more common than CD in children younger than 10 years of age.

PATHOPHYSIOLOGY

The pathophysiologic changes that occur in IBD, including mucosal inflammation and tissue damage, are primarily confined to specific anatomic locations within the GI tract

(Table 46.2) and are related to mediators released in the inflammatory process. Similarities between UC and CD suggest that, although they both have histologic characteristics of an acute inflammation, they may be heterogeneous disorders with different antigenic triggers.[1,8] Abnormal immunologic findings appear with the active inflammatory process and subside with quiescence. Although UC and CD involve the bowel, both diseases are associated with extraintestinal manifestations and complications.

ALTERED MUCOSAL IMMUNE RESPONSES
Alterations in the mucosal immune system are central to the pathophysiology of IBD. However, no consistent immunologic abnormality has been established as the primary defect in UC or CD. Because the inflammatory process is a component of wound healing, the inflamed mucosa activates the typical inflammation-associated genes and genes associated with wound healing.[1] Proinflammatory antigenic triggers in the intestinal lumen activate macrophages and T-helper 1 (Th1) lymphocytes to release numerous endogenous proinflammatory mediators (e.g., cytokines, arachidonic acid metabolites, growth factors) of inflammation.[1,8] Cytokines, neuropeptides, and leukotrienes (Fig. 46.2) frequently correlate with disease activity and provide a rationale for drug therapy. Many mediators of tissue damage also serve to amplify the immune response and promote further inflammation. Increased production of potent proinflammatory cytokines, including interleukin-1 (IL-1), interleukin-12 (IL-12), tumor necrosis factor (TNF), platelet-activating factor (PAF), and interferon-γ (IFN-γ), stimulates epithelial, endothelial, and

TABLE 46.1	Epidemiology of Ulcerative Colitis and Crohn's Disease	
Factor	Ulcerative Colitis	Crohn's Disease
Incidence (per 100,000)	2–10	1–6
Prevalence (per 100,000)	35–100	10–100
Urban-rural	More common in urban than rural areas	More common in urban than rural areas
Ethnicity	More common in Jewish than non-Jewish people	More common in Jewish than non-Jewish people
Race	More common in whites than African-Americans, Asians, Hispanics, or Native Americans	More common in whites than African-Americans, Asians, Hispanics, or Native Americans
Gender	Slightly more common in men than in women	Slightly more common in women than in men
Age of onset, years	15–25, 55–65	15–25, 55–65
Cigarette smoking	Less common in smokers than in nonsmokers	More common in smokers than in nonsmokers
Socioeconomic status	More common in higher socioeconomic status	More common in higher socioeconomic status

(From Stenson WF, Korzenik J. Inflammatory bowel disease. In: Yamada T, Alpers DH, Kaplowitz N, et al, eds. Textbook of gastroenterology. 4th ed. Philadelphia: Lippincott Williams & Williams, 2003:1699–1759.)

| TABLE 46.2 | Anatomic, Pathologic, and Clinical Features of Ulcerative Colitis and Crohn's Disease | | |

Feature	Ulcerative Colitis	Crohn's Disease
Anatomic		
Small bowel only	+	+++
Small bowel and colon	+	++++
Colon only	++	++
Anorectal area only	++++	+
Diffuse, continuous involvement	++++	++
Cobblestoning	+	++++
Pathologic		
Transmural	+	++++
Fissures and fistulas	++	+++
Crypt abscesses	++++	++
Strictures	+	+++
Shortening of the colon	+++	+
Pseudopolyps	+++	+
Clinical		
Rectal bleeding	++++	++
Diarrhea	++++	++++
Abdominal pain	++	++++
Malaise, fever	++	++++
Weight loss	+++	++++
Extraintestinal manifestations	++	++
Perianal disease	++	+++
Intestinal obstruction	+	+++
Toxic megacolon	+++	++
Risk of malignancy	+++	++

Frequencies represent estimates and are categorized in the following ways: ++++, consistent; +++, frequent; ++, infrequent; and +, rare. None of the features is always present or always absent.

mesenchymal cells and activates immune cells. The chemotactic cytokines, interleukin-8 (IL-8), macrophage chemotactic and activating factor (MCAF), and other chemotactic substances such as leukotriene B_4 (LTB_4), serve to increase macrophage and neutrophil migration from the circulation into the inflamed mucosa. This process may be related to ischemic injury involving the release of superoxide and other reactive oxygen species. Anti-inflammatory mediators include interleukin-4 (IL-4) and interleukin-10 (IL-10).

DISEASE LOCATION AND MUCOSAL INFLAMMATION

UC affects primarily the mucosa and the submucosa of the rectum and the left colon, with the rectum involved histologically in more than 90% of cases.[1] Distal UC may be described as proctitis or proctosigmoiditis, depending on the location of

mucosal inflammation. Lesions usually develop in the rectum and spread proximally; however, initial disease may involve the entire colon (Fig. 46.1). In 5% to 10% of patients, the entire colon is affected, and disease may involve a minimal portion of the terminal ileum (backwash ileitis). In severe forms of UC, deeper layers of the colon may be involved. The inflammatory process in UC is continuous, with no intervening areas of normal mucosa. Chronic recurrent mucosal inflammation with concomitant tissue repair may lead to characteristic findings such as the formation of crypt abscesses, pseudopolyps, shortening of the colon (foreshortening), and a "lead-pipe" appearance (Table 46.2). Dysplasia may represent a premalignant change and a risk of carcinoma.

The distal ileum and the right colon (Table 46.2) are the most common sites of involvement in CD.[1] Although the terminal ileum (TI) is usually involved, other areas of the

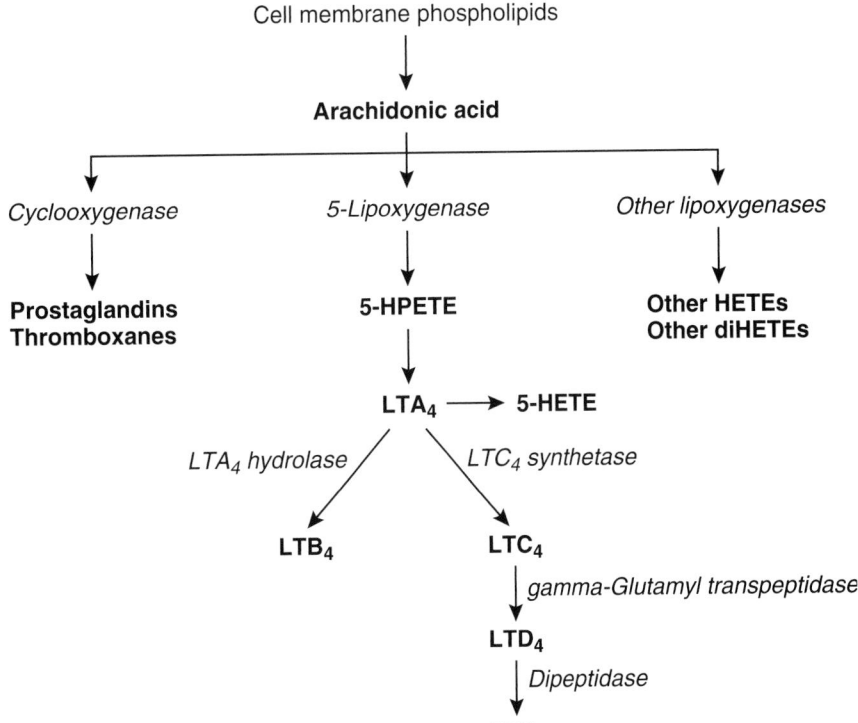

FIGURE 46.2 Arachidonic acid metabolism and leukotriene formation. LTA_4–LTE_4, leukotrienes A_4 to E_4; 5-HETE, 5-hydroxyeicosatetraenoic acid; 5-HPETE, 5-hydroxyperoxyeicosatetraenoic acid; HETE, hydroxyeicosatetraenoic acid; diHETE, dihydroxyeicosatetraenoic acid.

small bowel may be affected. The small bowel and colon are involved in 40% to 55% of patients, with about 30% to 40% having small bowel disease only, and 15% to 25% having only colonic involvement. In most patients with CD of the colon, the rectum is spared. Sections of bowel that appear normal by radiography or colonoscopy may have histologic features of CD. In contrast to UC, CD is characterized by chronic inflammation that extends through all layers of the bowel wall, as well as the mesentery and regional lymph nodes.[2] The transmural process can lead to the formation of fissures and fistulas, along with a thickened, edematous bowel, which can result in obstruction (Table 46.2). The disease often involves segments of the bowel separated by normal-appearing bowel, called ''skip lesions.'' In advanced cases, the mucosa has a nodular or ''cobblestoned'' appearance. Although certain anatomic and pathologic features enable CD of the colon to be distinguished from UC, this distinction is not possible in about 20% of cases.

EXTRAINTESTINAL MANIFESTATIONS

Many extraintestinal manifestations (Table 46.3) are associated with IBD and may precede or accompany the underlying intestinal disorder.[1,9,10] These manifestations may be related to the clinical activity of the inflammatory process, its anatomic location, or the disordered physiology of the small intestine. Arthritic, skin, and eye manifestations occur more often in patients with UC and Crohn colitis than in patients with CD of the small intestine. The arthritis is usually asymmetric and affects the joints of the knees, hips, ankles, wrists, and elbows. In most patients, it tends to parallel the activity and severity of the bowel disease, often subsiding with therapy, colectomy, or spontaneous remission.[1] In contrast, ankylosing spondylitis may appear years before bowel symptoms and runs a course independent of the intestinal disease. Osteoporosis occurs in both UC and CD and may be attributed to numerous factors, including malnutrition, malabsorption, smoking, and the continuous use of corticosteroids.[1] Thromboembolic events (e.g., deep vein thrombosis, pulmonary emboli) result from abnormalities of clotting factors during active episodes and may complicate the course of UC and CD.[1] Minor abnormalities in hepatic transaminases commonly occur in patients with IBD, but clinically significant liver disease is uncommon. Cirrhosis, chronic hepatitis, and sclerosing cholangitis, although infrequent, tend to occur more often in UC. Cholelithiasis may occur in CD with ileal involvement or resection and results from diminished bile salt reabsorption. Nephrolithiasis also occurs in ileal CD and results from increased oxalate absorption secondary to malabsorption of fatty acids. Renal amyloid may cause nephrotic syndrome and renal failure in CD.

GASTROINTESTINAL COMPLICATIONS

GI complications associated with IBD include local intestinal complications, toxic megacolon, and colorectal cancer. The incidence of each complication varies with disease type (UC or CD), location, and severity (Table 46.2).

Local Intestinal Complications. Local complications arise from the intestinal component of IBD and include pseudopolyps, perianal fissures, abscesses, fistulas, strictures, ob-

TABLE 46.3	Extraintestinal Manifestations of Inflammatory Bowel Disease	
Manifestation	**Incidence (%)**	**Related to Intestinal Disease Activity**
Arthritis/arthralgias	25–30	Yes
Aphthous mouth ulcers	5–10	Yes
Episcleritis or uveitis (iritis)	5–10	Yes
Erythema nodosum	1–5	Yes
Pyoderma gangrenosum	1–5	Usually
Sacroiliitis	10–15	No
Ankylosing spondylitis	1–2	No
Osteoporosis	50	No
Thromboembolic events	1–2	No
Abnormal liver transaminases	30–50	No
Liver disease	1–3	No
Sclerosing cholangitis	1–4	No
Cholelithiasis[a]	20–30	No
Nephrolithiasis[a]	25–35	No
Renal disease[a]	1–3	No

In general, the extraintestinal manifestations in ulcerative colitis and Crohn's colitis are similar in type and prevalence.

[a]This manifestation is seen primarily in Crohn's disease of the small intestine.

(From Stenson WF, Korzenik J. Inflammatory bowel disease. In: Yamada T, Alpers DH, Kaplowitz N, et al, eds. Textbook of gastroenterology. 4th ed. Philadelphia: Lippincott Williams & Williams, 2003:1699–1759; Orchard T. Extraintestinal complications of inflammatory bowel disease. Curr Gastroenterol Rep 5:512–517, 2003; van Bodegraven AA, Pena AS. Treatment of extraintestinal manifestations in inflammatory bowel disease. Curr Treat Opt Gastroenterol 6:201–212, 2003.)

struction, colonic perforation, and massive hemorrhage.[1] The incidences of abscess and fistula formation are higher in CD than in UC; these complications may occur as the initial presentation of the disease. Perianal fistulas are common, but fistulas can also arise from one section of the GI tract and can connect to another (e.g., enteroenteric, enterocolonic) or to other organs (e.g., enterocutaneous, enterovaginal). Small bowel obstruction is a common complication of CD that results from inflammation and edema of the involved intestine or narrowing of the bowel secondary to scar formation. Colonic perforation is uncommon in CD but may complicate toxic megacolon in UC. The risk of perforation and peritonitis is greatest during an initial severe attack and is associated with a high rate of mortality.

Toxic Megacolon. Toxic megacolon may occur in CD of the colon but is more likely to complicate severe attacks of UC.[1,11] This serious complication is preceded by a rapidly deteriorating clinical course and is associated with a high mortality. It is characterized by acute dilation of the transverse colon to a diameter greater than 6 cm with accompanying systemic toxicity.[1] The pathogenesis of the acute dilation is related to the deep inflammatory process, which involves all layers of the colon and results in the inability of the colon to contract. Toxic megacolon may be triggered by drugs that impair colonic motility (e.g., anticholinergics, narcotic analgesics, antidiarrheals) or by severe electrolyte abnormalities such as hypokalemia.[1,11] Toxic megacolon may occur with the initiation of drug therapy, or it may result from an increase in the doses of these agents.

Colorectal Cancer. The risk of colorectal cancer is greater in patients with IBD than in the general population, with a higher incidence observed in UC than in CD.[1] The risk of developing cancer in UC increases when the duration of the disease is longer than 8 to 10 years, and when the disease involves the entire colon.[1] Patients with long-standing UC are at risk of developing cancer even if they have only mild symptoms, or if the disease has been quiescent. Because colorectal cancer is virulent, surveillance conducted by colonoscopy with biopsy is recommended every 1 to 2 years in most patients with extensive colitis of 8 to 10 years' duration.[1] A prophylactic total colectomy cures UC and prevents colorectal cancer.

CLINICAL PRESENTATION AND DIAGNOSIS

SIGNS AND SYMPTOMS

Ulcerative Colitis. The predominant symptoms in UC are bloody diarrhea and abdominal pain.[1] The clinical features,

TABLE 46.4	Clinical Features of Ulcerative Colitis Based on Disease Severity		
	Mild	**Moderate**	**Severe**
Frequency	55%–60%	20%–25%	15%–20%
Location	Rectum and distal colon	Rectum and 1/3 to 1/2 of colon	Rectum and entire colon
Diarrhea	<4 stools/day	4–6 stools/day	>6 stools/day
Abdominal pain	Uncommon	Common	Severe
Rectal bleeding	Intermittent	Common	Severe
Weight loss	Uncommon	<10 lb	>10 lb
Fever	Uncommon	Intermittent	Persistent
Bowel sounds	Normal	Normal	Absent
Tachycardia	Uncommon	Frequently	Common
Anemia	Uncommon	Hct >30%	Hct <30%
Leukocytosis	Uncommon	Common	Common
Albumin	Normal	Normal	Reduced
Extraintestinal manifestations	Uncommon	Common	Severe
Risk of malignancy	Not increased	Increased after 8–10 yr	Increased after 8–10 yr
Mortality (acute attack)	<0.5%	2%	10%–25%

Hct, hematocrit.

however, vary with disease severity (Table 46.4). Because most patients with mild UC have disease confined to the rectum, bleeding and abdominal pain are uncommon. Patients with moderate disease often present with diarrhea and varying degrees of rectal bleeding. Abdominal pain and cramping is prominent but is often relieved by defecation. Severe UC is a serious and potentially life-threatening disease characterized by a sudden onset of profuse diarrhea, bleeding, and severe abdominal pain. The patient is usually febrile, dehydrated, and profoundly weak. Blood loss can result in rapid pulse, low blood pressure, and anemia.

Crohn's Disease. The predominant symptoms of CD are abdominal pain, diarrhea, and weight loss.[1] The clinical features of CD vary but usually reflect the anatomic location of the disease (Table 46.5). Acute symptoms may be mild, moderate, or severe, depending on the extent of involvement. Abdominal pain tends to be steady and localized to the right lower quadrant. A colicky or cramping pain, usually associated with bowel movements, may be superimposed upon the steady pain. When CD is confined to the small bowel, diarrhea often occurs without bleeding. With colonic disease, diarrhea is often accompanied by rectal bleeding, urgency, and tenesmus. Most patients have recurrent episodes of diarrhea, abdominal pain, and fever that last from a few days to several months. Weight loss and nutritional deficiencies occur, to varying degrees, in most patients because of food avoidance, malabsorption, and malnutrition. Prolonged periods of poor nutrition and disease can result in dehydration, acid-base and electrolyte disturbances, protein-calorie malnutrition, and deficiencies of vitamins D, K, B_{12}, and folic

TABLE 46.5	Clinical Features of Crohn's Disease Based on Disease Location		
	Small Bowel	**Ileocolitis**	**Colitis**
Diarrhea	>90%	>90%	>90%
Abdominal pain	Common	Common	Very common
Malnutrition	Common	Common	Less common
Fistula	10%–20%	30%–50%	10%–30%
Obstruction	30%–40%	40%–50%	10%–20%
Perianal disease	Uncommon	Common	Very common

acid. Perianal fissures, fistulas, and abscesses may accompany the initial attack. A low-grade fever occurs in more than 50% of patients in the absence of complications. Anemia is associated with chronic blood loss. Fatigue and malaise may negatively influence work performance.

DIAGNOSIS AND CLINICAL FINDINGS

The diagnosis of IBD relies on the clinical picture, the endoscopic appearance of the intestinal mucosa, and histologic assessment.[1] A diagnosis of IBD should be considered in all patients who present with persistent abdominal pain and diarrhea or bloody diarrhea. Clinical findings vary with the location and severity of the disease (Tables 46.4 and 46.5). Rebound tenderness is often present over the abdominal area of disease activity. Occasionally, fever, weight loss, extraintestinal manifestations, and intestinal complications overshadow the intestinal symptoms. Laboratory tests are usually nonspecific and do not establish the diagnosis. Leukocytosis and an elevated erythrocyte sedimentation rate may reflect the inflammatory process. Electrolyte abnormalities, particularly hypokalemia, occur when there is severe diarrhea. Hypoalbuminemia may reflect the patient's poor nutritional status and overall clinical condition. The blood count may reveal anemia from blood loss, nutritional deficiencies, or chronic disease. Colonoscopy or sigmoidoscopy with biopsy confirms the diagnosis of IBD, differentiates UC from CD, and establishes the extent and severity of disease (Table 46.2). Barium contrast studies are used in CD when involvement of the small bowel or fistula is suspected. A plain film radiograph of the abdomen may be indicated in patients in whom a barium enema and endoscopy are contraindicated. Computed axial tomography and ultrasonography are useful in diagnosing abscess, fluid collection, and intestinal obstruction.

CLINICAL COURSE AND PROGNOSIS

Most patients with IBD follow a chronic course of intermittent acute attacks of active disease (exacerbations) with periods of quiescence (remission). A small number of patients suffer from a continuous course of persistent symptoms and no remission.

Ulcerative Colitis. The initial attack of UC is often abrupt, with symptoms ranging from nonbloody diarrhea to fulminant diarrhea and colonic hemorrhage. Arthritis and arthralgias occur in about 10% of patients at initial presentation.[1] Most patients have highly variable intermittent attacks with varying intervals of asymptomatic remission. Patients with mild initial disease or proctitis follow a benign course but are at risk for extension of their disease and progression to pancolitis.[1] Morbidity is greatest when the onset of symptoms is severe, colonic involvement is extensive, or toxic megacolon develops. Patients with severe initial disease, pancolitis, or toxic megacolon have a 40% chance of requiring a colectomy.[1] The life expectancy for most patients with UC is similar to that of the general population.[1] Disease-related complications and colorectal cancer may complicate the clinical course and alter the prognosis.

Crohn's Disease. CD, like UC, follows a clinical course of acute exacerbations and remissions. About 60% of patients require surgery within 10 years of the initial diagnosis; of these, about half eventually require another operation.[1] Patients with a young age of onset are more likely to have a complicated course and to require surgery. Psychosocial factors may influence the clinical course, as acute flares of activity often occur in association with stressful events. The prognosis for CD is not as favorable as that for UC because of the variable nature of the disease, the less than optimal response to drug therapy, the need for surgery, and the high rate of postoperative disease recurrence. Life expectancy is near normal, but mortality is increased in younger patients. Morbidity is increased when peritonitis or sepsis develops.

Pregnancy, Lactation, Fertility. In most patients with IBD, pregnancy does not significantly alter the course of disease, nor does the disease adversely affect the outcome of pregnancy or fertility.[1] Although none of the medications used to treat patients with IBD affect female fertility, sulfasalazine (SASP) causes reversible infertility in men.[12] Of concern are the potential undesirable effects on the fetus when women with IBD take medications throughout their pregnancy. Although the aminosalicylates and corticosteroids (prednisone, methylprednisolone, and hydrocortisone) are not associated with an increased risk of fetal complications,[12,13] it is advisable to minimize exposure to these drugs if at all possible. Women who are pregnant and taking SASP should receive folic acid supplementation of 1 mg twice daily.[1] Less is known about the safety of balsalazide and budesonide during pregnancy. Metronidazole appears to be safe for use in the second and third trimesters.[1,12] Azathioprine (ASA), 6-mercaptopurine (6-MP), cyclosporine, and methotrexate (MTX) should be avoided in pregnancy because of the risk of fetal growth retardation, prematurity, or congenital malformation.[12,14] One report indicates that there was no teratogenicity or toxicity when infliximab was used during pregnancy.[15] Breast-feeding is not recommended in mothers treated with these medications.

Children and Adolescents. When IBD begins in childhood, the clinical course is similar to that observed when onset occurs later in life. However, growth retardation is more common in children with CD than those with UC. Because malnutrition contributes to growth failure, nutritional supplementation must be aggressively pursued. Medications used in the treatment of children with IBD are similar to those used in adult patients.[16,17] However, prolonged use of high-dose corticosteroids may suppress growth and cause other steroid-related side effects. Although metronidazole and the immunomodulators have been used in children, they should be avoided because of potentially serious complications.

PSYCHOSOCIAL ASPECTS

UC and CD are chronic relapsing diseases that may profoundly affect the physical, emotional, social, educational, and professional activities of the patient.[7] Many patients with IBD express concerns related to symptoms, body image, surgery, and cancer. Stressful life events may exacerbate their symptoms. Patients with CD have a more impaired quality of life than do those with UC because of the uncertain nature of the disease, fear of numerous hospitalizations and surgeries, fear of work loss and possible unemployment, medication side effects, and fatigue.[7,18] Anxiety and depression also contribute to a diminished quality of life.[7,19] Disease activity and severity are directly related to an impaired sense of well-being, but sustained remission translates into an improved quality of life.[19] Health-related quality of life (HRQOL) questionnaires have been developed to assess the perception of psychosocial well-being in the patient with IBD.[20]

THERAPEUTIC PLAN

UC and CD are chronic conditions that are not curable with currently available drug therapy. The approach selected for the treatment of patients with UC or CD is based on an assessment of disease activity (active or quiescent), location (e.g., rectum, colon, small bowel), and severity (mild, moderate, severe). Disease severity is determined by evaluating the signs and symptoms related to mucosal inflammation, extraintestinal manifestations, and obstructive or fistulizing processes, and by assessing the global impact of disease on the patient's quality of life. Disease activity indices, often used to assess CD activity and response to treatment in research studies, are not recommended for clinical monitoring.[1] Medical therapy is empirically assessed by evaluating the patient's response to the most troublesome problems (e.g., diarrhea, abdominal pain). Recommendations for the treatment of UC and CD are presented in Figures 46.3 and 46.4, respectively.

GENERAL APPROACH

Patients with IBD should receive adequate rest during an active flare of the disease. Patients with CD who smoke

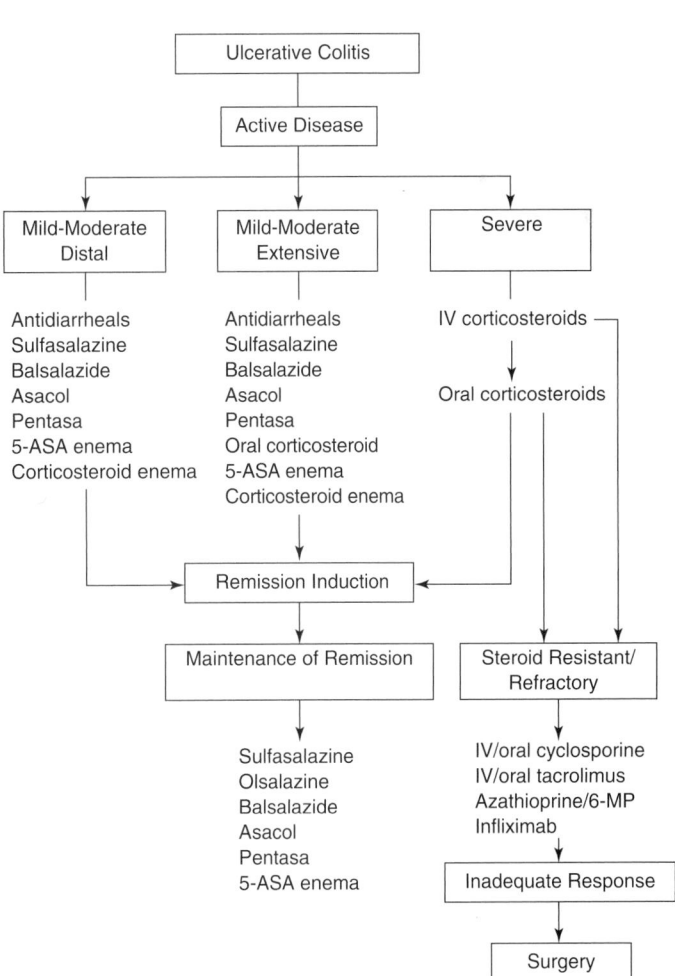

FIGURE 46.3 Algorithm for managing ulcerative colitis. 5-ASA, 5-aminosalicylic acid; 6-MP, 6-mercaptopurine; IV, intravenous.

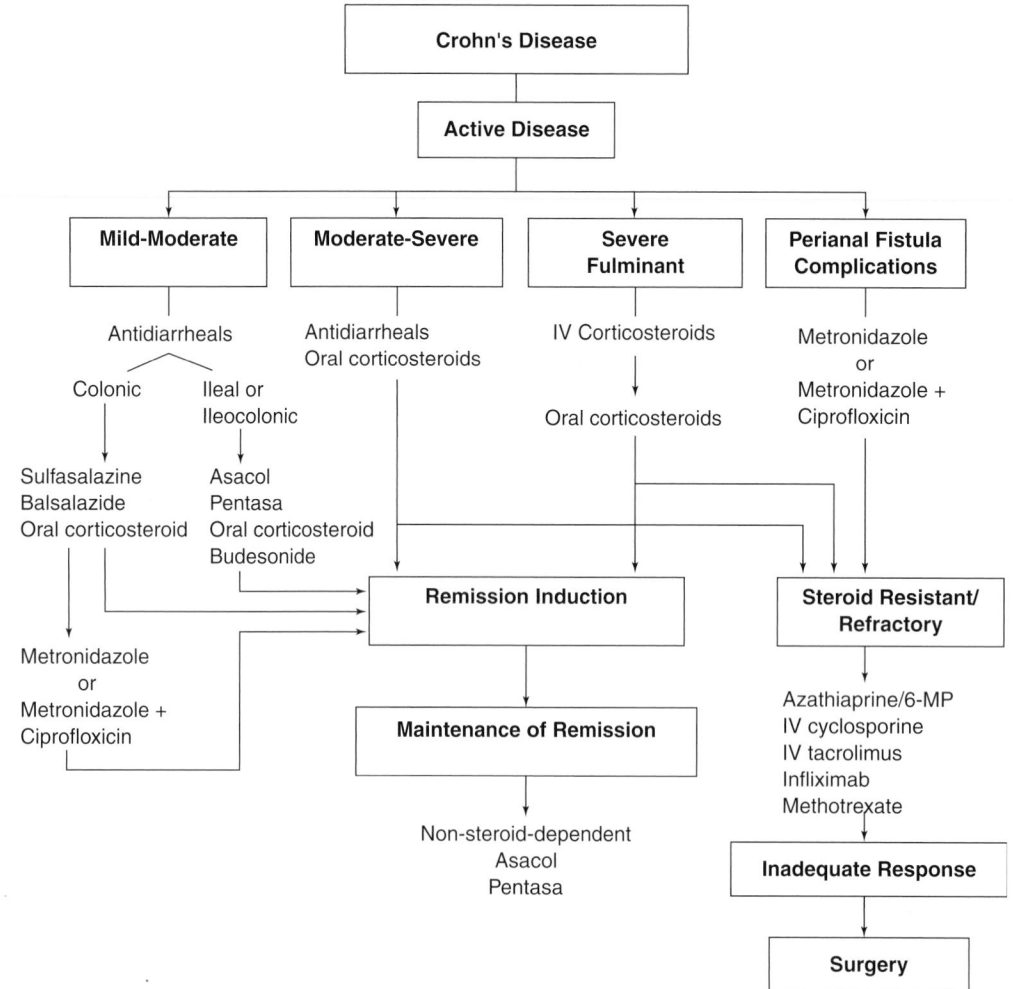

FIGURE 46.4 Algorithm for managing Crohn's disease. 6-MP, 6-mercaptopurine; IV, intravenous.

should be encouraged to stop, as smoking may reduce the response to drug treatment. Symptomatic treatment with an antidiarrheal, antispasmodic, or analgesic should be initiated in patients with mild to moderate disease. Psychosocial support should be incorporated into the daily care plan.

ULCERATIVE COLITIS

Severe Active Disease. The mainstay of therapy for severe active UC consists of bowel rest, aggressive intravenous fluid and electrolyte replacement, and intravenous corticosteroids (Table 46.6).[1,21,22] Patients with significant anemia should receive a blood transfusion. In the presence of a fever and leukocytosis, bacterial cultures should be obtained and the patient started on an intravenous broad-spectrum antibiotic directed at enteric gram-negative enterococci, and anaerobic pathogens. If the patient improves during the next 7 to 10 days, the intravenous steroid should be switched to an oral regimen and the dose tapered gradually. Failure to improve during this time is an indication for surgery (colectomy) or a trial of intravenous cyclosporine 2 to 4 mg/kg/day (Table

46.6). If a beneficial response to intravenous cyclosporine occurs (average time to response is 7 days), the patient should be switched to oral cyclosporine at a dose of 4 to 8 mg/kg/day for about 3 months. Patients with severe UC which is unresponsive to conventional treatments may benefit from a trial of infliximab.

Mild to Moderate Active Extensive Disease. The oral aminosalicylates are the drugs of choice for mild to moderate extensive active UC (Tables 46.6 and 46.7).[1,23,24] Treatment is usually initiated with SASP, because it is the least expensive and most data indicate equivalent efficacy among the available aminosalicylates.[23] Although most patients do respond to oral doses of 3 to 4 g per day of SASP, dose-related side effects usually offset a dose-response effect.[23,24] Side effects can be minimized by initiating treatment at a lower dose and gradually increasing the dose by 500 mg every 2 to 3 days (Table 46.6), administering SASP with meals, or using the enteric-coated tablet. Balsalazide or 5-acetylsalicylic acid (5-ASA) preparations (Asacol or Pentasa) should

TABLE 46.6	Drug Regimens Used to Treat Inflammatory Bowel Disease		
	Route of Administration	**Active Disease**	**Maintenance of Remission**
Aminosalicylates			
Sulfasalazine	Oral	3–4 g/day	2–4 g/day
Olsalazine	Oral	2–3 g/day	1 g/day
Balsalazide	Oral	2–6.75 g/day	2–6.75 g/day
Asacol	Oral	2.4–4.8 g/day	0.8–4.8 g/day
Salofalk/Claversal	Oral	1.5–3 g/day	0.75–1.5 g/day
Pentasa	Oral	2–4 g/day	1.5–4 g/day
Mesalamine enema	Rectal	1–4 g/bedtime	1–2 g/bedtime
Mesalamine suppository	Rectal	1–1.5 g/day	0.5–1 g/bedtime
Corticosteroids			
Methylprednisolone	IV	48–60 mg/day	Not indicated
Prednisolone	IV	60–80 mg/day	Not indicated
Hydrocortisone	IV	300 mg/day	Not indicated
Prednisone	Oral	20–60 mg/day	Not indicated
Budesonide	Oral	9 mg/day	Not indicated
Hydrocortisone enema	Rectal	100–200 mg/day	Not indicated
Immunosuppressants			
Azathioprine	Oral	2–3 mg/kg/day	2–3 mg/kg/day
6-Mercaptopurine	Oral	1–1.5 mg/kg/day	1–1.5 mg/kg/day
Cyclosporine	IV	2–4 mg/kg/day	Not indicated
	Oral	4–8 mg/kg/day	Not indicated
Tacrolimus	IV	0.01 mg/kg/day	Not indicated
	Oral	0.1–0.2 mg/kg/day	Not indicated
Methotrexate	IM	25 mg/wk	25 mg/wk
	Oral	15–25 mg/wk	15–25 mg/wk
Infliximab	IV	5 mg/kg	5–10 mg/kg
Antibiotics			
Metronidazole	Oral	10–20 mg/kg/day	Not indicated
Ciprofloxacin	Oral	1–1.5 g/day	Not indicated

be used in patients who are intolerant of SASP; the cost of the drug usually determines which agent is selected.[23,24] Symptomatic improvement with the oral aminosalicylates usually takes 3 to 4 weeks. If an immediate response is required, or if the response to an aminosalicylate is inadequate, the treatment of choice is an oral corticosteroid (prednisone) instituted at a dosage of 40 mg per day. When clinical improvement occurs (after several days to several weeks), the prednisone dose should be gradually tapered (5 to 10 mg every 1 to 2 weeks) until 20 mg per day is achieved. In some patients, it may be necessary to taper the dose to below 20 mg per day more slowly, or to use alternate-day dosing as part of the taper.[1,23] Maintenance therapy with an oral aminosalicylate should be initiated 3 to 4 weeks before prednisone is discontinued.

Mild to Moderate Active Distal Disease. The treatments of choice for mild to moderate active distal UC (proctitis, proctosigmoiditis, left-sided colitis) are oral aminosalicylates, rectally administered 5-ASA, and corticosteroid enemas; they are all effective (Table 46.6).[1,23,25] The selection of a specific treatment depends on the extent of disease, the patient's preference for an oral or topical dosage form, and the cost of drug therapy. The monthly cost of 5-ASA enemas, as well as patient acceptance and compliance, should be considered when less costly and more convenient treatment alternatives are available. Although the response to an oral aminosalicylate is slower than the response to a corticosteroid or a 5-ASA enema, the oral dosage form may be more effective in patients with disease that extends to the splenic flexure. If an oral aminosalicylate is selected, the

TABLE 46.7	Comparison of Aminosalicylate Preparations		
Product	**Trade Name**	**Formulation**	**Delivery**
Sulfasalazine	Azulfidine, various	5-ASA linked to sulfapyridine carrier by azo-bond	Colon
Balsalazide	Colazal	5-ASA linked to aminobenzoyl-alanine carrier by azo-bond	Colon
Olsalazine	Dipentum	Two 5-ASAs linked by azo-bond	Colon
Mesalamine	Asacol	5-ASA coated with Eudragit-S; delayed release (pH >7)	Distal ileum-colon
Mesalamine	Pentasa	5-ASA encapsulated in ethylcellulose microgranules; sustained release	Duodenum-colon
Mesalamine	Salofalk, Claversal	5-ASA coated with Eudragit-L; delayed release (pH >6)	Mid-ileum
Mesalamine	Rowasa	Enema; 60-mL suspension	Left colon-rectum
Mesalamine	Rowasa, Canasa	Suppository	Rectum

(From Sandborn WJ, Hanauer SB. Systematic review: the pharmacokinetic profiles of oral mesalazine formulations and mesalazine pro-drugs used in the management of ulcerative colitis. Aliment Pharmacol Ther 17:29–42, 2003; Wadworth AN, Fitton A. Olsalazine: a review of its pharmacodynamic and pharmacokinetic properties, and therapeutic potential in inflammatory bowel disease. Drugs 41:647–664, 1991; Ragunath K, Williams JG. Review article: balsalazide therapy in ulcerative colitis. Aliment Pharmacol Ther 15:1549–1554, 2001; Clemett D, Markham A. Prolonged-release mesalamine: a review of its therapeutic potential in ulcerative colitis and Crohn's disease. Drugs 59:926–956, 2000.)

newer and more costly dosage forms (Asacol, Pentasa, balsalazide) should be reserved for those who are intolerant of SASP. 5-ASA rectal suppositories and corticosteroid foams (10% hydrocortisone) should be reserved for patients with proctitis. In patients unresponsive to a single agent, a combination of two 5-ASA dosage forms (oral and rectal) may be used, but combined therapy does not offer a clear advantage over single treatment for most patients.[25] Oral SASP may also be combined with a topical corticosteroid. Maintenance therapy should be considered once remission has been achieved. Patients who do not respond after 4 to 8 weeks of treatment with an oral aminosalicylate, topical corticosteroid, or 5-ASA enema, or a combination of oral and rectal dosage forms, should be given oral corticosteroids.

Maintenance of Remission. Most patients with UC are potential candidates for maintenance therapy because 70% of patients given no such treatment can expect to relapse over a 12-month period.[26] Patients with a single, mild active episode are usually placed on maintenance therapy for 1 year and are then reevaluated.[1] Lifetime maintenance therapy is recommended for patients who have multiple recurrences or difficulty controlling their disease. The oral aminosalicylates are all effective, and their efficacy is a function of the daily dose (Table 46.6). Frequent relapses may require higher maintenance doses. 5-ASA enemas may be used to maintain remission in patients with distal (left-sided) disease, and suppositories are effective for proctitis. Oral and rectal corticosteroids are ineffective in maintaining remission and should

not be used. Patients with severe or frequent recurrences and those who require cyclosporine for an acute attack require maintenance therapy with AZA/6-MP (Table 46.6). AZA/6-MP should be started once the acute disease is brought under control with intravenous cyclosporine; it takes 3 to 6 months to obtain the optimal effect.

Steroid-Dependent and Refractory Disease. A small number of patients with UC are unable to discontinue corticosteroids (steroid-dependent) or do not respond to corticosteroids (refractory).[1] If the patient is taking more than 15 mg per day of prednisone for 6 months or longer, treatment with an immunosuppressant or surgery should be considered.[1,26] The use of bridge therapy with cyclosporine or tacrolimus and the addition of AZA or 6-MP may permit withdrawal of the corticosteroid in those wishing to avoid a colectomy. The immunosuppressant should be discontinued if the corticosteroid cannot be tapered after 6 months. In those patients who do respond, an attempt to taper the immunosuppressant should be considered after several years because of the risk of malignancy associated with long-term use. Some clinicians, however, will continue the immunosuppressant indefinitely because recurrence occurs within a few months following withdrawal.

CROHN'S DISEASE

Severe Fulminant Disease. The usual approach to treating patients with severe fulminant CD is similar to that for severe UC once an abscess or intestinal obstruction has been excluded. Intravenous corticosteroids are usually given intermittently in dosages similar to those used in UC (Table 46.6).[1,27–29] Patients who fail to improve within 10 days may respond to intravenous cyclosporine or tacrolimus, but evidence is insufficient to support their routine use.[27] Patients who respond to intravenous steroids should be switched to an oral corticosteroid until symptomatic relief is obtained, then gradually tapered. In patients whose symptoms worsen when corticosteroids are withdrawn, consideration should be given to the addition of AZA or 6-MP in preparation for an attempt to withdraw or reduce the corticosteroid dose. Nutritional support (total parenteral nutrition or elemental tube feedings) is indicated for patients who are unable to maintain adequate oral nutrition for longer than 5 to 7 days. Failure to respond to drug therapy is an indication for surgery.

Moderate to Severe Active Disease. Therapy for patients with moderate to severe active CD should be initiated with oral prednisone 40 to 60 mg per day until symptoms resolve (usually 1 to 4 weeks).[1,27–29] When a clinical response is achieved, the corticosteroid dose should be gradually tapered. In patients who are unable to discontinue oral corticosteroids, AZA or 6-MP should be added to the regimen in an attempt to lower the steroid dose. Infliximab (Table 46.6) is a logical choice for patients who fail treatment with corticosteroids and immunomodulators. A beneficial response may last for up to 12 weeks, if it is combined with AZA or 6-MP.

Mild to Moderate Active Disease. Drugs used to treat patients with mild to moderate active CD include aminosalicylates, conventional corticosteroids (prednisone), budesonide, and antibiotics.[1,27,30,31] The traditional approach is to start with an oral aminosalicylate.[1,27] Because Pentasa and Asacol release 5-ASA in the small bowel (Table 46.7), they are preferred to the azo-bond prodrugs for patients with ileitis or ileocolitis. Although sulfasalazine is effective for mild to moderate active CD of the colon, intolerance to dose-related side effects may limit its use. Balsalazide avoids many of these side effects and is an acceptable option. Metronidazole or ciprofoxacin (500 mg twice daily) is usually used as the next step for those who fail to respond to an aminosalicylate (Table 46.6). However, controlled trials do not consistently demonstrate efficacy other than in patients with colonic disease.[30,31]

Oral corticosteroids are typically used as first-line agents for patients with ileal, colonic, or ileocolonic disease with higher levels of disease activity, or for those who have failed aminosalicylate and antibiotic therapy.[1] When a patient has failed aminosalicylate therapy, the corticosteroid should be added to the regimen. Dosage regimens for the aminosalicylates and the oral corticosteroids are the same as those used to treat patients with UC (Table 46.6). Oral budesonide is an option for patients who experience significant corticosteroid-related side effects, or when long-term corticosteroid treatment is anticipated. Although budesonide has fewer side effects, it is more costly than prednisone. The response to initial therapy should be evaluated after several weeks and the treatment continued until remission or failure to improve is noted. The clinical response may take as long as 3 to 4 weeks when an aminosalicylate or an antibiotic is used.[1] If remission is achieved, maintenance therapy should be initiated.

An alternative evidenced-based approach to treating patients with mild to moderate CD suggests that sulfasalazine or balsalazide should be considered as first-line treatment for patients with disease restricted to the left side of the colon, and that budesonide should be used as first-line therapy for patients with diseases involving the ileum or ascending colon.[31] With this approach, conventional oral steroids are reserved for patients with high disease activity, those with left-sided colonic disease who are allergic or intolerant to sulfasalazine, and those who do not respond to budesonide treatment.

Maintenance of Remission. Maintenance therapy with Pentasa or Asacol is recommended for patients brought into remission by corticosteroids, with the knowledge that even with higher treatment doses, their benefit may be limited.[1,27,31,32] Although there is no role for higher doses of corticosteroids, steroid-dependent patients are often maintained in clinical remission with lower daily doses. Maintenance therapy with AZA or 6-MP is recommended for patients brought into remission on these drugs, but the risk of malignancy must be weighed against the benefits. Infliximab and MTX may be suitable options. Because of efficacy and safety issues, another strategy is to suspend therapy in patients with mild to moderate CD once remission has been achieved, then restart treatment when active disease returns.[31] The 5-ASA preparations are effective in preventing postsurgical relapse and recurrence in patients with CD.[33]

Steroid-Dependent and Refractory Disease. Approximately 50% of patients with CD who are treated with corticosteroids will become steroid dependent or resistant after the short-term course.[27] AZA or 6-MP is preferred initially, as these agents are usually effective in permitting a reduction in the corticosteroid dose.[1,34] Failure to respond to AZA or 6-MP will require an alternative drug such as MTX or infliximab. High intravenous doses of cyclosporine (8 mg/kg/day) may be used on a short-term basis in patients who are unresponsive to AZA, 6-MP, MTX, or infliximab; when surgery is to be deferred; or when bridge therapy is necessary to cover a patient until AZA or 6-MP takes effect.[34]

Perianal and Fistulizing Disease. Fistulas that develop in patients with CD are of two types: external (perianal) and internal (those that connect two internal organs).[35] Most patients with a perianal fistula present with an abscess, which either drains spontaneously or must be drained surgically.[1,35,36] Corticosteroids should be avoided in patients with internal or external fistula as they may interfere with fistula healing.[35] Antibiotics are usually effective and they improve quality of life. Although most patients with perianal or internal fistula respond to metronidazole alone or in combination with ciprofloxacin (Table 46.6), symptoms usually recur upon discontinuation of the antibiotic.[35] Therefore, AZA or 6-MP is usually added to the antibiotic regimen if the fistula persists. AZA or 6-MP is frequently used before initiation of infliximab therapy because these agents are usually effective in healing and maintaining closure of the fistula, and they are less costly.[35,36] Patients who are unresponsive to antibiotics and AZA/6-MP or those with fulminant disease should be given infliximab to achieve fistula closure (Table 46.6). Those patients with more complex disease may require maintenance treatment every 8 weeks or higher doses (10 mg/kg). Refractory fistulas may respond to MTX, cyclosporine, or tacrolimus followed by AZA or 6-MP.[35,36]

TREATMENT

PHARMACOTHERAPY

Antidiarrheals, Antispasmodics, Analgesics. Antidiarrheals, antispasmodics, and analgesics provide symptomatic relief without affecting IBD activity.[1] Antidiarrheals, such as diphenoxylate and loperamide, are useful in patients with mild chronic IBD, but they should be used cautiously in severe IBD because they may precipitate toxic megacolon. In addition, they may be ineffective in severe disease because diarrhea results from loss of colonic absorptive capacity due to widespread destruction of the colonic mucosa. Cholestyramine is the drug of choice for patients with CD who have bile salt diarrhea resulting from resection of the terminal ileal. It is also used in CD to prevent the formation of oxalate kidney stones and steatorrhea. Octreotide may be used to enhance fluid and electrolyte absorption in refractory diarrhea, but its usefulness is limited. Antispasmodics such as tincture of belladonna or opium, dicyclomine, or propantheline may be effective in reducing cramps and rectal urgency, but these agents should be avoided in patients with intestinal obstruction or severe disease. Analgesics should not become the mainstay of long-term pain control. If narcotics are used to relieve severe pain, they should be scheduled around the clock.

Aminosalicylates. A number of oral aminosalicylate formulations have been designed to prevent orally administered 5-ASA from being absorbed and to permit its release in the ileum or colon for topical treatment (Table 46.7). Preparations used to treat patients with IBD include azo-bond prodrugs (SASP, balsalazide, olsalazine), a delayed-release 5-ASA (Asacol), and a sustained-release 5-ASA (Pentasa) dosage form (Table 46.8).

Azo-bond Prodrugs. The prodrugs (SASP, olsalazine, balsalazide) contain an azo-bond that is cleaved by colonic bacterial azo-reductase enzymes to release 5-ASA. Diarrhea or concomitant antibiotics may reduce the breakdown of the prodrug in the colon, and bacterial overgrowth (if present) may permit metabolism in the small bowel.[37]

SASP, the prototype aminosalicylate, is minimally absorbed in the proximal small bowel (Fig. 46.5), with 5% of the parent drug excreted in the urine and 1% in the feces.[37] The remainder of the parent drug passes unchanged into the colon, where 5-ASA and sulfapyridine are released. One gram of SASP releases 400 mg of 5-ASA. Most of the liberated 5-ASA remains in the colon and is excreted in the feces.

	Ulcerative Colitis		**Crohn's Disease**		
Drug	**Active**	**MTN**	**Active**	**MTN**	**Fistula**
Sulfasalazine	++	++	+	−	−
Olsalazine	++	++	+	−	−
Balsalazide	++	++	+	−	−
Asacol	++	++	+	+	−
Pentasa	++	++	+	+	−
Corticosteroids	++	−	++	−	−
Metronidazole	−	−	+	−	−
Ciprofloxacin	−	−	+	−	+
Azathioprine/6-MP[a]	+	+	+	+	+
Cyclosporine[a]	+	−	+	−	+
Methotrexate[a]	−	−	+	+	−
Infliximab[a]	+	+	+	+	+

TABLE 46.8 Efficacy of Drugs Used to Treat Ulcerative Colitis and Crohn's Disease

Active, active disease; MTN, maintenance of remission; ++, effective; +, likely to be effective; −, documented efficacy lacking.
[a]Severe, resistant, or refractory disease.

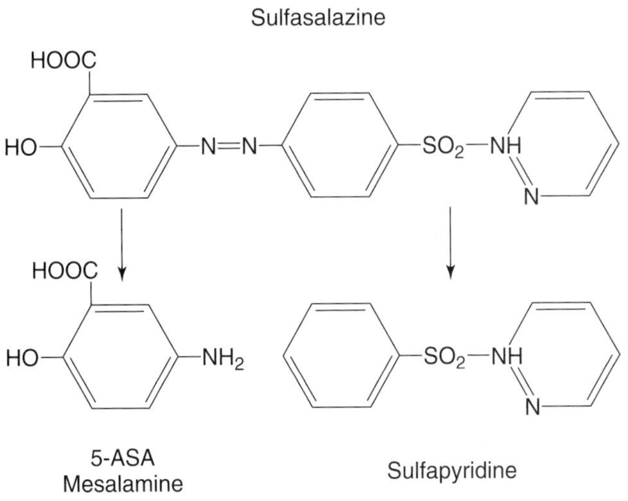

FIGURE 46.5 Structures of sulfasalazine, 5-aminosalicylic acid (5-ASA), and sulfapyridine.

Sulfapyridine is absorbed, metabolized, in part by acetylation in the liver, and excreted in the urine. The exact mechanism by which SASP acts in IBD is uncertain, but 5-ASA, the primary active moiety, interferes with arachidonic acid metabolism and may act as a free radical scavenger.[1]

SASP is associated with dose-dependent and dose-independent side effects (Table 46.9). The dose-related effects occur in about 50% of patients and are related to the SASP dose, serum sulfapyridine concentrations, and acetylator status.[1,38] Side effects usually develop within the first few weeks of treatment and increase with doses of 4 g or more per day, but they resolve when the drug is discontinued. Dose-related side effects can be minimized by gradually increasing the daily dose (begin at 500 mg twice daily and increase to 1 g four times daily over a week) or by using lower daily doses. Dyspepsia can be avoided by taking the drug with meals or by using the enteric-coated dosage form. SASP alters sperm morphology and motility and sperm counts, leading to male infertility, but this is reversible within 3 months of discontinuation of the drug.[1] Dose-independent side effects include hypersensitivity reactions typical of the sulfonamides, and they are not related to the SASP dose, serum sulfapyridine concentrations, or acetylator status.[1,38] A hypersensitivity reaction to 5-ASA occurs in about 10% to 20% of patients. Patients allergic to aspirin should not take 5-ASA. Nephrotoxicity may occur with any 5-ASA preparation and is increased with high daily doses, concomitant 5-ASA–liberating medications, and preexisting renal disease.[1] SASP inhibits folic acid absorption and metabolism; therefore, folic acid supplementation of 1 to 2 mg per day is recommended, especially for patients on other medications that interfere with folic acid and those with inadequate nutrition.[1] Interactions between SASP and highly protein-bound drugs (e.g., warfarin) may lead to displacement of these drugs from their protein binding sites. The

importance of drug interactions with digoxin or iron is not known.

The efficacy of SASP as a single agent to treat patients with mild to moderate active UC and to maintain remission is well established, but its effectiveness varies inversely with the total daily dose.[1,23,25,26] Patients who respond to SASP usually do so in 3 to 4 weeks. In most patients, the optimal treatment dose is 4 g per day, and the maintenance dose is 2 g per day given in divided daily doses.[1] SASP is modestly effective in treating mild to moderate active CD, but patients with ileal disease respond less favorably than those with colonic involvement.[1,30,31] The release of 5-ASA in the colon (and not in the ileum) accounts for the difference in efficacy. Although it is often used, evidence is insufficient to support the efficacy of SASP in maintaining remission in nonsurgical or postoperative patients with CD.[1,27,32,33]

Olsalazine, on a molar basis, delivers twice as much 5-ASA to the colon as SASP (Table 46.7). Its efficacy in treating patients with active UC and in maintaining remission is similar to that of SASP when equivalent 5-ASA doses are used.[39] However, the higher treatment dosages (Table 46.6) are seldom used because they are associated with dose-related secretory diarrhea.[23,24,39] Olsalazine is used for maintenance of remission in UC when patients are intolerant of SASP.

Balsalazide (Table 46.7) has a similar efficacy to SASP when used to induce and maintain remission in UC.[24,40] When compared with Asacol 2.4 g per day, balsalazide 6.75 g per day tends to achieve a quicker response and a higher rate of complete remission, but differences between the two treatments are not clinically important.[24,40,41] The efficacy of balsalazide in treating patients with CD is similar to that of SASP. The major advantages of balsalazide over SASP are its improved safety profile and patient tolerability (Table 46.9).[40] The type and frequency of side effects, however, are similar to those associated with 5-ASA. Balsalazide should be considered in patients taking SASP who experience troublesome side effects.

Delayed-Release Dosage Forms. Asacol is a delayed-release oral dosage form that delivers 5-ASA to the distal ileum and proximal colon when the intestinal pH is sufficient (pH >7) to dissolve the enteric coating (Table 46.7).[24] Because intestinal pH and motility vary in IBD, Asacol may not provide reliable site-specific release of 5-ASA.[37] Intact and partially intact tablets have been reported in the stool.[36] The most commonly reported side effects associated with 5-ASA are presented in Table 46.9. Interstitial nephritis has been reported and is believed to be related to increased systemic absorption of 5-ASA from the delayed-release and sustained-release dosage forms.[24,42] However, the frequency of renal insufficiency is low in large safety databases for Asacol and Pentasa.[24] Treatment of patients with UC and CD is usually initiated at 2.4 g per day in three divided doses; this may be increased to 4.8 g per day, if necessary (Table 46.6). Asacol is as effective as SASP in inducing and

TABLE 46.9	Side Effects of Medications Used to Treat Inflammatory Bowel Disease

Sulfasalazine	Corticosteroids	Azathioprine/6-P	Cyclosporine	Balsalazide
Dose-dependent	**Major**	Nausea	Tremor	Headache
Nausea	Infection	Diarrhea	Paresthesias	Abdominal pain
Vomiting	Hypertension	Fever	Headache	Dyspepsia
Dyspepsia	Psychosis	Skin rash	Nausea	Nausea
Diarrhea	Hypokalemia	Infection	Anorexia	Diarrhea
Anorexia	Hyperglycemia	Arthralgias	Hypertrichosis	Dizziness
Headache	Osteoporosis	Pancreatitis	Gingival hyperplasia	
Malaise	Cataracts	Hepatitis	Nephrotoxicity	
Male infertility	Glaucoma	Bone marrow suppression	Hypertension	
Dose-independent	**Minor**			
Fever	Moon face			
Skin rash	Acne			
Hemolytic anemia	Hirsutism			
Agranulocytosis	Insomnia			
Pulmonary complications	Skin striae			
Hepatitis	Weight gain			
Pancreatitis	Easy bruising			
Neurological toxicity	Buffalo hump			
Aplastic anemia	Swollen ankles			

Budesonide	Infliximab	Mesalamine (5-ASA)	Metronidazole	Methotrexate
Moon face	Upper respiratory and other infections	Fever	Dyspepsia	Nausea
Acne		Skin rash	Metallic taste	Vomiting
Easy bruising	Tuberculosis	Nausea	Skin rash	Diarrhea
Nausea	Acute infusion reaction	Diarrhea	Dark urine	Stomatitis
Hirsutism		Pancreatitis	Glossitis	Headache
Headache	Delayed hypersensitivity reaction	Hepatitis	Disulfiram-like reaction	Fever
Buffalo hump		Nephrotoxicity	Perhipheral neuropathy	Alopecia
	Lupus-like reaction	Headache	Neutropenia	Pulmonary fibrosis
		Alopecia	Pancreatitis	Bone marrow suppression
				Hepatic fibrosis/cirrhosis

maintaining remission in mild to moderate active UC.[24,26,43] Asacol is modestly effective in treating patients with mild to moderate active CD, but not all clinical trials show a clear benefit when compared with placebo.[27,30,31] The efficacy of Asacol in maintaining remission in CD is equivocal, although benefit has been observed in postsurgical patients and those with ileal involvement.[32,44]

Sustained-Release Dosage Forms. Pentasa microgranules release 5-ASA slowly and continuously throughout the small bowel and colon in a time-dependent rather than a pH-dependent manner (Table 46.7). About 20% to 50% of the 5-ASA is released in the small bowel; the remainder is released in the colon.[45] Small beads may be left in the stool after the

5-ASA has been released. The efficacy of Pentasa in treating patients with mild to moderate active UC and in maintaining remission is established (Table 46.6) and is similar to that of SASP.[24,26,43,46] The efficacy of Pentasa in CD is similar to that of Asacol, with only modest benefits achieved in mild to moderate active disease and equivocal results observed in maintaining remission.[27,31,32,46] Pentasa may benefit patients with ileal disease because its release of 5-ASA in the small bowel increases the local concentration and distribution of 5-ASA in the ileum.

Topical Aminosalicylates. Topical (rectal) administration of 5-ASA exerts a local anti-inflammatory effect and is associated with fewer side effects than are caused by oral SASP or 5-ASA, because less than 15% of the rectally administered 5-ASA dose is systemically absorbed.[23] Anal irritation or a hypersensitivity reaction to 5-ASA or the sulfite contained in the topical suspension may occur. 5-ASA enemas are the treatment of choice for patients with mild to moderate active distal (left-sided) UC because they are as effective as oral SASP and more effective than rectal corticosteroids.[23,25] Most patients who are intolerant of SASP will tolerate the 5-ASA enema or suppository. Patients who are unresponsive to oral SASP and oral or rectal corticosteroids may respond to rectal 5-ASA alone or in combination with oral therapy.[23] The enema should be administered at bedtime and retained for 8 hours. Improvement occurs within a week, but the usual course of therapy extends over 3 to 6 weeks, depending on symptoms and endoscopic findings. Rectal suppositories are indicated for proctitis and should be retained for 1 to 3 hours or longer for maximum benefit. Lower daily doses of the enema and the suppository (Table 46.6), as well as alternate-day dosing, are effective in maintaining remission.[26] Maintenance of remission may also be achieved by combining oral 5-ASA and intermittent 5-ASA enemas. Although widely used, topical 5-ASA preparations have not been evaluated in patients with left-sided colonic CD.

Corticosteroids. The efficacy of systemic and topical conventional corticosteroids in treating patients with active UC and CD has been well established (Table 46.8), but their clinical benefits are offset by serious and predictable side effects (Table 46.9).[1,47-50] Newer corticosteroids such as budesonide preserve the benefits of steroids while minimizing long-term risks. The exact mechanism by which corticosteroids act to suppress intestinal inflammation is unknown, but theories include interaction with the immune system, inhibition of prostaglandins and proinflammatory cytokines, and stabilization of lysosomal membranes.[48] The dosage regimen and route of administration (intravenous, oral, topical) vary with disease severity and activity (Table 46.6).

Intravenous Corticosteroids. The continuous or intermittent intravenous infusion of a corticosteroid induces remission within 7 to 10 days in most patients with severe active UC or CD.[1,48] However, results are not always so dramatic and remission is more difficult to achieve in patients with CD. Although few studies have assessed the relative value and specific dose of the available parenteral agents, methylprednisolone (in divided daily doses) is often preferred (Table 46.6). Higher intravenous doses or pulsed intravenous administration appears to be no more effective than standard continuous or intermittent intravenous regimens.

Oral Corticosteroids. Oral corticosteroids (Table 46.6) are the mainstay of treatment for patients with IBD, especially those with CD.[47-49] A favorable response to treatment with an oral corticosteroid (prednisone 40 to 60 mg per day, or equivalent) is defined as clinical improvement within 30 days.[47] CD patients with ileal or ileocolonic disease respond more favorably to oral corticosteroids than do patients with colonic involvement. Although most patients with CD respond initially, a small number are steroid resistant.[47] A larger number of patients become steroid dependent as they experience recurrent symptoms while the corticosteroid dose is being tapered, or shortly after withdrawal.[48,49] Some clinicians maintain patients with CD on a minimum steroid dose for 1 to 2 months before beginning the steroid taper. Continuing the corticosteroid after remission induction, however, does not alter the frequency of recurrence or relapse after surgery because corticosteroids are not effective in maintenance of remission.[1,48,49] AZA and 6-MP have corticosteroid-sparing effects that can facilitate the withdrawal of corticosteroids.

The use of corticosteroids in patients with IBD is associated with an increased incidence of a variety of side effects (Table 46.9).[48-50] Older patients with CD who are given corticosteroids are at increased risk of developing hypertension, hypokalemia, and altered mentation. Patients with fistula, abscess, or malnutrition are at increased risk for infection and fluid and electrolyte disturbances. Osteoporosis is present in about 30% to 60% of patients with CD, and it occurs at a somewhat lower rate in patients with UC.[48,49] Although the inflammatory process itself can lead to reduced bone mineral density, the risk is compounded by the use of corticosteroids.[51] Therefore, patients with IBD, especially those who are given corticosteroids, should receive treatment to increase bone mineral density and reduce fracture risk. For most patients with IBD, a single morning dose is as effective as a divided daily dose, but some patients with CD respond best when the total daily dose is divided (the largest portion of the dose should be taken in the morning). Because a reduction in side effects often parallels a decrease in therapeutic effect, alternate-day therapy may not be effective in some patients. In addition, it does not minimize some of the long-term side effects (cataracts, osteoporosis).[48] However, growth-stunted children who require maintenance corticosteroids may benefit from this regimen.

Topical Corticosteroids. Topical (rectal) corticosteroids are effective in mild to moderate distal (left-sided) UC (Table 46.6).[23,25] Although enemas may spread to the middle of the descending colon (Fig. 46.1), their use should be limited to left-sided colitis or proctosigmoiditis.[1] Rectal foams are convenient in patients who are unable to retain an enema because of local inflammation, tenesmus, or diarrhea. Because foams do not spread beyond the sigmoid colon, they should be used only when disease is confined to the sigmoid or rectum. Retention enemas should be administered at bedtime to permit overnight contact with the inflamed mucosa. An additional dose may be given in the morning after the first bowel movement. Once remission occurs, usually within 2 to 3 weeks, an alternate-night schedule may be used for an additional 2 weeks. Topical administration results in absorption of up to 50% of the corticosteroid, but the degree of adrenal suppression and extent of side effects are less than those seen with the equivalent oral dose of the same drug. Whether acute intestinal inflammation alters drug absorption is unclear.

Budesonide. Budesonide is a corticosteroid with a high affinity for glucocorticoid receptors.[48] The oral enteric-coated controlled-release dosage form slowly releases the drug into the distal ileum and ascending colon, where it acts topically and undergoes a high first-pass metabolism, which is responsible for a reduction in its systemic corticosteroid side effects. Intestinal and hepatic metabolism by cytochrome P 450 (CYP) 3A4 convert budesonide to inactive metabolites and results in a systemic bioavailability of about 10%.[48] Budesonide (9 mg once daily in the morning) is indicated for the treatment of patients with mild to moderate active CD of the terminal ileum, cecum, and ascending colon (Table 46.6).[52] In comparative studies, budesonide outperformed 5-ASA (Pentasa) in induction of remission, but it is slightly less effective than conventional corticosteroids.[48,52,53] Corticosteroid-dependent patients are more likely to remain in remission on budesonide than are those receiving 5-ASA.[52,54] However, lower doses (6 mg per day and 3 mg per day) are ineffective in maintaining long-term remission in non–corticosteroid-dependent patients.[48,52] Budesonide is not indicated for isolated colonic CD. Although the side-effect profile of budesonide is significantly better than those of conventional corticosteroids, many minor signs and symptoms (Table 46.9) and a loss of bone mineral density do occur.[48,52,55] Concomitant treatment with drugs that inhibit CYP450 3A4 (e.g., ketoconazole, itraconazole, cyclosporine, erythromycin) or with grapefruit juice may inhibit the biotransformation of budesonide and increase systemic exposure to the parent drug.

Immunomodulators

Azathioprine and 6-Mercaptopurine. AZA and its metabolite, 6-MP, are established medications for the treatment of active, steroid-refractory or steroid-dependent IBD, and fistulizing CD (Table 46.8).[56–58] AZA is a prodrug that is converted in the liver to 6-MP. 6-MP is subsequently metabolized in the liver and gut by one of three enzymes: thiopurine S-methyltransferase (TPMT), which catalyzes 6-MP to the inactive metabolite, 6-methyl-MP (6-MMP); xanthine oxidase, which converts 6-MP to thiourate; and hypoxanthine-guanine-phosphoribosyltransferase, which metabolizes 6-MP to 6-thioguanine (6-TG) nucleotides.[57] AZA and 6-MP have similar therapeutic and toxic effects. The therapeutic efficacy and hematologic toxicity of 6-MP are related to serum concentrations of 6-TG.[38,57] TPMT exhibits genetic polymorphism; low levels are associated with high levels of 6-TG and, as a consequence, increased therapeutic efficacy and bone marrow suppression.[38,57] Conversely, high TPMT levels are associated with lack of response and fewer side effects. The specific mechanism by which 6-MP acts in IBD is uncertain, but is most likely related to its ability to competitively inhibit nucleotide biosynthesis.

AZA and 6-MP are effective when used in conjunction with corticosteroids to reduce the steroid dose and as single agents to maintain remission once the corticosteroid has been withdrawn (Table 46.8).[57,58] The typical starting dose of 6-MP (0.25 to 0.5 mg/kg/day) is one-half that of AZA (0.5 to 1.0 mg/kg/day).[57] These lower daily doses are then increased within 2 weeks to the full therapeutic dose (Table 46.6). Because allopurinol blocks the metabolism of 6-MP via the inhibition of xanthine oxidase, a 50% reduction in the AZA/6-MP daily dose is recommended.[57] A beneficial response to AZA/6-MP requires 3 to 4 months.[57,58] However, intravenous administration of AZA may reduce the response time to a few weeks.[59] The patient is considered to be in remission when disease activity does not flare upon withdrawal of corticosteroids. If effective and tolerated, AZA/6-MP can be used to maintain remission for up to 5 years.[57] Unfortunately, relapse often occurs upon withdrawal, and there is concern about the long-term safety of these agents.[57]

The short- and long-term toxicities of AZA/6-MP often limit their use (Table 46.9).[57,58] About 5% to 10% of patients discontinue treatment on their own within the first month because of side effects.[57] These side effects may be dose dependent (e.g., bone marrow suppression) or dose independent (e.g., pancreatitis, hepatitis). The potential for bone marrow suppression requires that blood counts be monitored regularly, especially when therapy is initiated (Table 46.10). In the future, 6-MP metabolite concentrations and TPMT genotyping may enable clinicians to optimize AZA/6-MP therapy in patients with IBD.[60] Long-term treatment is associated with immunosuppression and serious opportunistic infection. A theoretical risk of developing cancer, particularly non-Hodgkin lymphoma, exists after long-term treatment with AZA/6-MP, but this risk has not been confirmed in patients with IBD.[61,62]

Cyclosporine and Tacrolimus. Cyclosporine and tacrolimus are used as rescue therapy in patients with severe active IBD that is resistant or refractory to corticosteroid therapy and in patients with CD who have fistulizing disease (Table 46.8).[63–69] Both drugs act as potent inhibitors of cell-mediated immunity by blocking the production of IL-2 and other proinflammatory cytokines. In patients with UC who are trying to avoid a colectomy, cyclosporine and tacrolimus have a rapid onset of action, thereby serving as a ''bridge'' until AZA or 6-MP takes effect. In CD, cyclosporine and tacrolimus are used as a last resort for patients who are resistant to infliximab and have limited surgical options.

Patients with severe UC should be started on a continuous infusion of cyclosporine at a dose of 4 mg/kg/day and adjusted to whole blood concentrations of 250 to 400 ng per mL (Table 46.6).[63,65] A lower 2 mg per kg dose appears to be as effective as 4 mg per kg and reduces the risk of toxicity.[66] If no response occurs after 7 days, treatment should be stopped. If the patient responds, treatment should be continued for 1 to 2 weeks. The patient should then be switched to oral cyclosporine for 3 months, targeting trough concen-

TABLE 46.10	Recommended Laboratory Tests for Monitoring the Side Effects of Drugs Used to Treat Inflammatory Bowel Disease
Drug	**Recommendations**
5-Acetylsalicylic acid dosage forms	Complete blood count, serum creatinine, liver transaminases before initiation of therapy. Monitor serum creatinine at 6 and 12 months; repeat yearly thereafter.
Azo-bond prodrugs	Complete blood count, serum creatinine, liver transaminases before initiation of therapy.
Azathioprine and 6-mercaptopurine	Complete blood count, serum creatinine, liver transaminases before initiation of therapy. Monitor complete blood count at 2 and 4 weeks; repeat every 3 months thereafter.
Corticosteroids	DEXA scan before initiation of therapy; repeat based on corticosteroid use and T-score.
Cyclosporine	Complete blood count, serum creatinine, serum electrolytes (including magnesium), serum albumin, serum cholesterol, liver transaminases, erythrocyte sedimentation rate, pregnancy test, and blood pressure before initiation of intravenous therapy. Monitor blood pressure every 4 hours; monitor cyclosporine level, serum creatinine, potassium, magnesium, and cholesterol every other day if within normal range, or daily if abnormal. For outpatients, monitor complete blood count, serum chemistry (see intravenous use), erythrocyte sedimentation rate, and cyclosporine trough level weekly for first month, then every 2–4 weeks.
Methotrexate	Complete blood count and liver transaminases every 3 months; repeat liver transaminases monthly if elevated. If elevated for 3 consecutive months, or if greater than 3 times the upper limit of normal, discontinue drug or recommend liver biopsy. Recommend liver biopsy after 1.5 g of methotrexate or 2 years of treatment.

DEXA, dual-energy x-ray absorptiometry.

trations of 100 to 200 ng per mL (Table 46.6).[63,65] During this time, treatment with AZA or 6-MP should be initiated so that cyclosporine can be discontinued. The role of cyclosporine in CD is limited, as lower oral doses (5 mg/kg/day) are ineffective and higher doses (7.5 mg/kg/day), although effective, are unacceptable for long-term use.[1] Compared with cyclosporine, data regarding the use of tacrolimus in IBD is limited. However, initial studies suggest that tacrolimus is effective in steroid-resistant or refractory disease and may have a beneficial effect over the long term.[67–69] Target whole blood trough concentration is 5 to 10 ng per mL.

The use of cyclosporine or tacrolimus must be weighed against the risk of irreversible nephropathy (particularly with higher doses) and other serious side effects (Table 46.9). In most cases, side effects with cyclosporine and tacrolimus are similar, dose dependent, and reversible. Severe immunosuppressant-related infections may complicate treatment, especially if the patient is receiving concomitant corticosteroids. Patients who are receiving cyclosporine (or tacrolimus) should be monitored closely for side effects (Table 46.10) and for drug interactions with medications that interact with hepatic CYP P450 isoenzymes. Detailed guidelines

for using and monitoring cyclosporine therapy in severe IBD have been published.[65]

Methotrexate. MTX, a folic acid antagonist, is usually reserved for patients with CD who fail to respond to or are intolerant of AZA/6-MP.[70,71] Among its numerous immunosuppressant effects, MTX interferes with leukotriene B_4 and IL-1 activity. When given weekly as an oral or intramuscular injection (Table 46.6), it tends to act more rapidly (2 to 8 weeks) than AZA/6-MP. MTX alleviates symptoms and reduces the requirements for corticosteroids in patients with resistant or refractory active CD and appears to be effective as maintenance therapy (Table 46.8).[70,71] However, symptomatic relapses occur when the drug is withdrawn. Of major concern are the major side effects (Table 46.9), especially hepatic injury and bone marrow suppression, which require careful monitoring (Table 46.10) and limit its use.

Infliximab. Infliximab, a chimeric monoclonal antibody to TNFα (anti-TNFα) is an option for patients with active UC and CD or fistulizing CD that is unresponsive to other treatments or resistant to steroids (Table 46.8).[1,72–74] Its mechanism of action confirms the central role of TNFα in the inflammatory process. An intravenous infusion of 5 mg per kg given at 0, 2, and 6 weeks is the preferred induction strategy for patients with moderate to severe active disease or fistula.[72,73] Patients who receive a three-dose induction are less likely to form human antichimeric antibodies (HACAs) or to develop an infusion or delayed hypersensitivity reaction.[72] Coadministration of AZA/6-MP or MTX may have a synergistic effect on clinical response, reduce HACA and antinuclear antibody (ANA) formation, and reduce the risk for an acute infusion or delayed hypersensitivity reaction.[72] Pretreatment with diphenhydramine (25 to 50 mg orally or intravenously) and, in selected cases, acetaminophen or corticosteroids, is recommended for patients with a history of infusion reactions and those at risk for a delayed hypersensitivity reaction.[72]

Maintenance therapy (Table 46.6), if required, is given every 8 weeks and appears to be effective for most patients.[72,74] The maintenance dose and interval should be individualized because some patients may benefit from a 10 mg per kg dose, but others may require shorter (4 to 6 weeks) or longer (12 weeks) treatment intervals.[72,74] The beneficial response declines with repeated dosing, and the incidence of side effects increases with repeated infusions (Table 46.9). An infusion of infliximab is very expensive, and its high cost may limit its use as maintenance therapy. Because reactivation of latent tuberculosis has been reported following administration of infliximab, patients should be given a purified protein derivative skin test before treatment is begun.[72,76] If findings are positive, the patient should undergo a chest x-ray. Detailed guidelines for infliximab treatment in CD have been published.[72]

Antibiotics. Metronidazole, when used as a single agent, is effective for remission induction in mild to moderate active colonic CD (Table 46.8), but it is less effective in patients with ileal disease.[27,28,31] The mode by which metronidazole acts in CD is unclear but is probably related to its immunosuppressive and antimicrobial properties. Effective doses range from 10 to 20 mg/kg/day (Table 46.6) and are usually given in two or three divided doses. Higher doses may be required in patients with CD who have a perianal fistula.[28,35] Metronidazole may reduce postoperative recurrence, but treatment is associated with a number of side effects (Table 46.9).[28] Peripheral neuropathy occurs in up to 50% of patients and is dose dependent. Ciprofloxacin (Table 46.6) may be used as an alternative to metronidazole because of its better tolerability, or it may be combined with metronidazole.[27,28,77] However, the addition of metronidazole and ciprofloxacin to budesonide does not appear to provide any added benefit.[78]

NONPHARMACOLOGIC THERAPY

Nutrition. Replacement of vitamins, minerals, and other nutrients is indicated whenever clinical or laboratory evidence of deficiency is found.[1,79,80] Iron, folic acid, and B_{12} deficiencies should be identified and treated appropriately.

Fat malabsorption in CD may contribute to malabsorption of vitamins A, D, and K; replacement of these vitamins may be necessary. Patients with CD involving the small bowel may present with deficiencies of calcium, magnesium, B vitamins, and vitamin C. Lactose-intolerant patients should avoid dairy products or use lactase-containing preparations. The use of enteral or parenteral nutrition as adjunct therapy in IBD to restore a balanced nutritional state is well established. Parenteral nutrition should be used to improve the nutritional status of patients with IBD who cannot be fed enterally, and in patients in whom bowel rest may be of value.

Surgery. Surgery is indicated in UC after drug therapy proves ineffective, when actual or impending complications (e.g., toxic megacolon, colonic perforation, hemorrhage, anal complications) occur, and when reducing the risk of colorectal cancer is the goal.[1,81] In contrast to CD, a colectomy in UC is a curative procedure. Although a prophylactic colectomy has been recommended for children and adults with pancolitis, the most reasonable approach is periodic colonoscopy and histologic examination of biopsy specimens for precancerous changes. Surgery in CD is influenced by the site of involvement, postoperative recurrences, and related intestinal complications (e.g., obstruction, strictures, fistulas, abscess formation, perforation, hemorrhage).[1,82] Approximately 60% of patients with CD require surgery within 10 years of initial symptoms.[1] Increasing losses of the small bowel through resection and disease may limit its absorptive surface, resulting in malabsorption and malnutrition.

ALTERNATIVE THERAPIES

Patients with IBD commonly use complementary and alternative medicines (CAM) because of the side effects associated with conventional drug treatment, the chronicity of the disease, and, for many, an impaired quality of life.[83,84] Patients generally combine CAM with conventional medicine and herbal medicines with special diets (e.g., gluten free) or dietary manipulations, as well as other alternative approaches (e.g., homeopathy, naturopathy, Tai chi, chiropractic treatment, massage, meditation).[83] Common therapies include acidophilus, flaxseed, garlic, aloe vera, salmon oil, cat's claw, primrose oil, fenugreek, and slippery elm.[83,84] Some herbal medicines (e.g., slippery elm, fenugreek) contain biologically active antioxidants, which may produce a therapeutic effect in patients with IBD.[84]

FUTURE THERAPIES

An explosion in knowledge related to our understanding of the immune and inflammatory mechanisms in IBD has led to the development of new agents (most of them directed at

TABLE 46.11	Potential New Biological Agents for the Treatment of Patients with Inflammatory Bowel Disease
Agent	**Molecular Derivation/Proposed Mechanism of Action**
Adalimumab	Recombinant human IgG antitumor necrosis factor monoclonal antibody; upregulates T-lymphocyte apoptosis.
Alicaforsen	Antisense oligonucleotide to ICAM-1 mRNA; downregulates T-lymphocyte trafficking.
Interleukin-10	Plant-derived interleukin-10; downregulates T-lymphocyte proliferation.
Natalizumab	Humanized mouse antihuman α4 integrin monoclonal antibody; downregulates T-lymphocyte trafficking.
Onercept	Human recombinant p55 tumor necrosis factor–binding protein; upregulates T-lymphocyte apoptosis.

From Rutgeerts P, Van Deventer S, Schreiber S. Review article: the expanding role of biological agents in the treatment of inflammatory bowel disease—focus on selective adhesion molecule inhibition. Aliment Pharmacol Ther 17:1435–1450, 2003; Caprilli R, Viscido A, Guagnozzi D. Review article; biological agents in the treatment of Crohn's disease. Aliment Pharmacol Ther 16:1579–1590, 2002; Sandborn WJ, Yednock TA. Novel approaches to treating inflammatory bowel disease: targeting alpha-4 integrin. Am J Gastroenterol 98:2372–2382, 2003; Ghosh S, Goldin E, Gordon F, et al. Natalizumab for active Crohn's disease. N Engl J Med 348;24–32, 2003.)

CD) that selectively target key pathogenic processes.[85–92] Numerous biological agents are under investigation; some of the most promising are listed in Table 46.11. Natalizumab appears to be effective and well tolerated in active CD and may be of some benefit in active UC.[85–88] In addition to biologicals, other therapies, including probiotics, thalidomide, essential fatty acids, heparin, and nicotine, are being evaluated for use in UC.[91] Investigation into the genetic causes of IBD may eventually permit dosing based on genotype and pharmacogenetic parameters and may reveal novel mechanisms for optimizing therapy.[60,89]

IMPROVING OUTCOMES

PATIENT EDUCATION

Patient education, the cornerstone of successful treatment in IBD, should focus on the disease, drug therapy, and CAM. The patient should be advised of the important side effects associated with specific drugs and should be informed about when to contact the health care practitioner. Alternatively, the patient must understand the importance of adherence to drug therapy, especially during asymptomatic periods of remission. Patients with IBD should avoid the use of NSAIDs and should stop smoking. Patients with CD who smoke must understand the detrimental effects smoking has on the disease and on the effects of drug treatment.[4,93] Patients should be counseled to maintain adequate nutrition and to limit *only* those foods that consistently produce symptoms.

METHODS TO IMPROVE ADHERENCE TO DRUG THERAPY

Medication nonadherence in IBD is about 20% for short-term and 50% for long-term treatment and is a key determi-

nant of treatment failure.[94,95] Although data are limited in patients with IBD, demographic, clinical, and psychosocial factors, as well as the patient–physician relationship, are important predictors of medication nonadherence.[94,95] Patients are more likely to adhere to treatment if they have confidence in their health care practitioner and believe that the treatment is necessary. Depression and anxiety are common in patients with IBD and may go unrecognized. Recognition and appropriate treatment not only improves psychological well-being, but may improve compliance as well. Medication adherence is improved by monitoring the patient closely for drug efficacy, side effects, and nonadherence. Specific methods to improve medication adherence in patients with IBD include selecting medications with similar efficacy but less problematic side effects (e.g., 5-ASA in place of SASP, or budesonide in place of prednisone); when possible, using drug regimens that require less frequent dosing (e.g., SASP twice daily instead of four times daily for maintenance); selecting dosage forms that are more likely to enhance adherence (e.g., oral 5-ASA instead of a 5-ASA rectal enema); and, in cases where drug costs are a factor, identifying less expensive medications with similar efficacy (e.g., SASP instead of 5-ASA, or prednisone instead of budesonide) or assisting with a patient drug program. Closer attention to these issues may reduce medication nonadherence and improve health outcomes.

DISEASE MANAGEMENT STRATEGIES AND IMPROVING PATIENT OUTCOMES

Health care practitioners should work with the patient with IBD to develop a psychosocial plan that includes patient education, coping strategies, stress reduction techniques, social/family support, self-help groups, and psychological referral when appropriate. Adherence to drug therapy, smoking cessation, and, in some cases, surgery should improve the overall health status of the patient. Quality-of-life-parameters, including social activities, work or occupation, hobby or recreation, ability to sleep, sexual relationships, and indoor or outdoor activities, should also be evaluated so that improvement in patient outcomes is ensured. A number of clinical trials in CD have assessed HRQOL and have shown improvement in patients receiving newer and often more expensive medications, including 5-ASA preparations (Asacol, Pentasa), budesonide, cyclosporine, infliximab, and MTX.[18,96] Clinicians should be cognizant of the many strategies that influence quality of life and improve patient outcomes; they should incorporate these techniques into treatment plans for patients with IBD.

PHARMACOECONOMICS

Impaired quality of life, work loss, surgery, and hospitalization rank among the most important factors that contribute to the cost and burden of care for patients with IBD.[18,19, 97,98] Newer and more efficacious medications that have been shown to improve quality of life and patient outcomes are very expensive. However, these more costly medications may, in fact, be cost saving if they decrease health care costs (e.g., physician visits, hospitalizations, surgery). It is hoped that pharmacoeconomic evaluation of these expensive drugs will eventually be undertaken and that it will confirm their cost benefit in the treatment of patients with IBD.

KEY POINTS

- The goal of medical therapy in IBD is to improve quality of life. This is best accomplished by inducing and maintaining remission, controlling symptoms, and preventing or controlling complications
- Drug selection, dose, and route of administration are determined by the location, extent, and severity of intestinal involvement
- Maintenance of adequate nutrition is an important goal in patients with IBD, especially when there is extensive intestinal involvement or bowel resection
- Psychosocial factors are an important component of treatment in IBD and should constitute a part of the daily care plan
- Antidiarrheals should be used with caution in severe IBD because they may precipitate toxic megacolon
- SASP may cause dose-dependent and dose-independent side effects, including infertility in men
- The 5-ASA oral formulations are more effective than SASP in the treatment of patients with CD with ileal involvement, but they are similar to SASP when colonic CD and UC are treated
- Patients with severe IBD should be treated with intravenous corticosteroids. Failure to improve after 7 to 10

days signals the need for surgery or intravenous immunosuppressive therapy
- Metronidazole or ciprofloxacin is most beneficial for treating patients with mild to moderate active colonic or fistulizing CD
- ASA/6-MP should be used to treat patients with steroid-dependent or refractory UC and CD, and those with fistulizing CD
- Cyclosporine should be used only as "rescue" therapy, or as a "bridge" to other agents (e.g., AZA and 6-MP, which take longer to act)
- Parenteral nutrition may be used only to improve the nutritional status of severely ill patients with IBD who cannot be fed enterally and patients for whom bowel rest may be of value
- A colectomy is curative in UC and may rid the patient of systemic complications
- Surgery in CD is not curative and is influenced by response to drug therapy and impending complications
- Patient education and improvement in health-related quality-of-life parameters contribute to improvement in outcomes for patients with IBD

SUGGESTED READINGS

Egan LJ, Sandborn WJ. Advances in the treatment of Crohn's disease. Gastroenterology 126:1574–1581, 2004.
Nielsen OH, Vainer B, Rask-Madsen J. Review article: the treatment of inflammatory bowel disease with 6-mercaptopurine or azathioprine. Aliment Pharmacol Ther 15:1699–1708, 2001.
Yang YX, Lichenstein GR. Corticosteroids in Crohn's disease. Am J Gastroenterol 97:803–823, 2002.

REFERENCES

1. Stenson WF, Korzenik J. Inflammatory bowel disease. In: Yamada T, Alpers DH, Kaplowitz N, et al, eds. Textbook of gastroenterology. 4th ed. Philadelphia: Lippincott Williams & Williams, 2003: 1699–1759.
2. Chamberlin W, Graham DY, Hulten K, et al. Review article: *Mycobacterium avium subsp. paratuberculosis* as one cause of Crohn's disease. Aliment Pharmacol Ther 15:337–346, 2001.
3. Ahmad T, Tamboli CP, Jewell D, et al. Clinical relevance of advances in genetics and pharmacogenetics of IBD. Gastroenterology 126:1533–1549, 2004.
4. Odes HS, Fich A, Reif S, et al. Effects of current cigarette smoking on clinical course of Crohn's disease and ulcerative colitis. Dig Dis Sci 46:1717–1721, 2001.
5. Felder JB, Korelitz BI, Rajapskes R, et al. Effects of nonsteroidal anti-inflammatory drugs on inflammatory bowel disease: a case-control study. Am J Gastroenterol 95:1949–1954, 2000.
6. Gleeson MH, Davis AJM. Non-steroidal anti-inflammatory drugs, aspirin and newly diagnosed colitis: a case-control study. Aliment Pharmacol Ther 17:817–825, 2003.
7. Talal AH, Drossman DA. Psychosocial factors in inflammatory bowel disease. Gastroenterol Clin North Am 24:699–716, 1995.
8. Abreu MT. The pathogenesis of inflammatory bowel disease: translational implications for clinicians. Curr Gastroenterol Rep 4: 481–489, 2002.
9. Orchard T. Extraintestinal complications of inflammatory bowel disease. Curr Gastroenterol Rep 5:512–517, 2003.
10. van Bodegraven AA, Pena AS. Treatment of extraintestinal manifestations in inflammatory bowel disease. Curr Treat Opt Gastroenterol 6:201–212, 2003.

11. Gan SI, Beck PL. A new look at toxic megacolon: an update and review of incidence, etiology, pathogenesis, and management. Am J Gastroenterol 98:2363–2371, 2003.
12. Tilson RS, Friedman S. Inflammatory bowel disease during pregnancy. Curr Treat Opt Gastroenterol 6:227–236, 2003.
13. Norgard B, Czeizel AE, Rockenbauer M, et al. Population-based case control study of the safety of sulfasalazine use during pregnancy. Aliment Pharmacol Ther 15;483–486, 2001.
14. Norgard B, Pedersen L, Fonager K, et al. Azathioprine, mercaptopurine and birth outcomes: a population-based cohort study. Aliment Pharmacol Ther 17:827–834, 2003.
15. Katz A, Lichenstein G, Keenan G, et al. Outcome of pregnancy in women receiving Remicaide (infliximab) for treatment of Crohn's disease or rheumatoid arthritis. Gastroenterology 120:A69, 2001.
16. Winter HS, Ng S. Consensus conference on the evaluation of drugs to treat children with inflammatory bowel disease. Inflamm Bowel Dis 4:101–131, 1998.
17. Kim SC, Ferry GD. Inflammatory bowel disease in pediatric and adolescent patients: therapeutic and psychosocial considerations. Gastroenterology 126:1550–1560, 2004.
18. Cohen RD. The quality of life in patients with Crohn's disease. Aliment Pharmacol Ther 16:1603–1609, 2002
19. Lichenstein GR, Yan S, Bala M, et al. Remission in patients with Crohn's disease is associated with improvement in employment and quality of life and a decrease in hospitalizations and surgeries. Am J Gastroenterol 99:97–101, 2004.
20. Kanwal F, Gralnek IM. Measuring health-related quality of life in gastroenterology and hepatology. Evidence-Based Gastroenterol 4:65–81, 2003.
21. Rizzelo F, Gionchetti P, Venturi A, et al. Review article: medical treatment of severe ulcerative colitis. Aliment Pharmacol Ther 17 (Suppl 2):7–10, 2003.
22. Hanauer SB. Medical therapy for ulcerative colitis 2004. Gastroenterology 126:1582–1592, 2004.
23. Gionchetti P, Amadini C, Rizzelo F, et al. Review article: treatment of mild to moderate ulcerative colitis and pouchitis. Aliment Pharmacol Ther 16 (Suppl 4):13–19, 2002.
24. Sandborn WJ. Rational section of oral 5-aminosalicylate formulations and prodrugs for the treatment of ulcerative colitis. Am J Gastroenterol 97:2939–2941, 2002.
25. Vecchi M, Saibeni S, Devani M, et al. Review article: diagnosis, monitoring and treatment of distal colitis. Aliment Pharmacol Ther 17 (Suppl 2):2–6, 2003.
26. Kamm MA. Review article: maintenance of remission in ulcerative colitis. Aliment Pharmacol Ther 16 (Suppl 4):21–24, 2002.
27. Egan LJ, Sandborn WJ. Advances in the treatment of Crohn's disease. Gastroenterology 126:1574–1581, 2004.
28. Parkes M, Jewell DP. Review article: the management of severe Crohn's disease. Aliment Pharmcol Ther 15:563–571, 2001.
29. Scribano M, Prantera C. Review article: medical treatment of moderate to severe Crohn's disease. Aliment Pharmacol Ther 17 (Suppl 2):23–30, 2003.
30. Lofberg R. Review article: medical treatment of mild to moderately active Crohn's disease. Aliment Pharmacol Ther 17 (Suppl 2):18–22, 2003.
31. Sandborn WJ, Feagan BG. Review article: mild to moderate Crohn's disease—defining the basis for a new treatment algorithm. Aliment Pharmacol Ther 18:263–277, 2003.
32. Baincone L, Tosti C, Fina D, et al. Review article: maintenance treatment of Crohn's disease. Aliment Pharmacol Ther 17 (Suppl 2):31–37, 2003.
33. Cottone M, Orlando A, Viscido A, et al. Review article: prevention of postsurgical relapse and recurrence in Crohn's disease. Aliment Pharmacol Ther 17 (Suppl 2):38–42, 2003.
34. Rizzello F, Gionchetti P, Venturi C, et al. Review article: the management of refractory Crohn's disease. Aliment Pharmacol Ther 16 (Suppl 4):40–47, 2002.
35. Present DH. Crohn's fistula: current concepts in management. Gastroenterology 124:1629–1635, 2003.
36. Dubinsky MC, Fleshner PP. Treatment of Crohn's disease of inflammatory, stenotic, and fistulizing phenotypes. Curr Treat Opt Gastroenterol 6:183–200, 2003.
37. Sandborn WJ, Hanauer SB. Systematic review: the pharmacokinetic profiles of oral mesalazine formulations and mesalazine pro-drugs

used in the management of ulcerative colitis. Aliment Pharmacol Ther 17:29–42, 2003.
38. Cunliffe RN, Scott BB. Review article: monitoring for drug side-effects in inflammatory bowel disease. Aliment Pharmacol Ther 16:647–662, 2002.
39. Wadworth AN, Fitton A. Olsalazine: a review of its pharmacodynamic and pharmacokinetic properties, and therapeutic potential in inflammatory bowel disease. Drugs 41:647–664, 1991.
40. Ragunath K, Williams JG. Review article: balsalazide therapy in ulcerative colitis. Aliment Pharmacol Ther 15:1549–1554, 2001.
41. Pruitt R, Hanson J, Safdi M, et al. Balsalazide is superior to mesalamine in the time to improvement of signs and symptoms of acute mild to moderate ulcerative colitis. Am J Gastroenterol 97:3078–3086, 2002.
42. Corrigan G, Stevens P. Review article: interstitial nephritis associated with the use of mesalazine in inflammatory bowel disease. Aliment Pharmacol Ther 14:1–6, 2000.
43. Sutherland L, Roth D, Beck P, et al. Oral 5-aminosalicylic acid for inducing remission in ulcerative colitis. Cochrane Database of Syst Rev 2:CD00544, 2000.
44. Camma C, Giunta M, Rosselli M, et al. Mesalamine in the maintenance treatment of Crohn's disease: a meta-analysis adjusted for confounding variables. Gastroenterology 113:1465–1473, 1997.
45. Layer PH, Goebell H, Keller J, et al. Delivery and fate of oral mesalamine microgranules within the human small intestine. Gastroenterology 108:1427–1433, 1995.
46. Clemett D, Markham A. Prolonged-release mesalamine: a review of its therapeutic potential in ulcerative colitis and Crohn's disease. Drugs 59:926–956, 2000.
47. Faubion WA Jr, Loftus EV Jr, Harmsen WE, et al. The natural history of corticosteroid therapy for inflammatory bowel disease: a population-based study. Gastroenterology 121:255–260, 2001.
48. Yang YX, Lichenstein GR. Corticosteroids in Crohn's disease. Am J Gastroenterol 97:803–823, 2002.
49. Rutgerts PJ. Review article: the limitations of corticosteroid therapy in Crohn's disease. Aliment Pharmacol Ther 15:1515–1525, 2001.
50. Buchman AL. Side effects of corticosteroid therapy. J Clin Gastroenterol 33:289–294, 2001.
51. Berstein CN, Leslie WD, Leboff MS. AGA technical review on osteoporosis in gastrointestinal disease. Gastroenterology 124:785–794, 2003.
52. Kane SV, Schoenfeld P, Sandborn WJ, et al. Systematic review: the effectiveness of budesonide therapy for Crohn's disease. Aliment Pharmacol Ther 16:1509–1517, 2002.
53. Thomsen O, Cortot A, Jewell D, et al. A comparison of budesonide and mesalamine for active Crohn's disease. N Engl J Med 339:370–374, 1998.
54. Cortot A, Colombel JF, Rutgeerts P, et al. Switch from systemic steroids to budesonide in steroid-dependent patients with inactive Crohn's disease. Gut 48:186–190, 2001.
55. Cino M, Greenberg GR. Bone mineral density in Crohn's disease: a longitudinal study of budesonide, prednisone, and nonsteroid therapy. Am J Gastroenterol 97:915–921, 2002.
56. Fraser AG, Orchard TR, Jewell DP. The efficacy of azathioprine for the treatment of inflammatory bowel disease: a 30 year review. Gut 50:485–489, 2002.
57. Nielsen OH, Vainer B, Rask-Madsen J. Review article: the treatment of inflammatory bowel disease with 6-mercaptopurine or azathioprine. Aliment Pharmacol Ther 15:1699–1708, 2001.
58. Sandborn W, Sutherland L, Pearson D, et al. Azathioprine or 6-mercaptopurine for inducing remission of Crohn's disease. Cochrane Database Syst Rev 2:CD000545, 2000.
59. Sandborn WJ, Zins BJ, Tremaine WJ, et al. An intravenous loading dose of azathioprine decreases the time to response in patients with Crohn's disease. Gastroenterology 109:1808–1817, 1995.
60. Dubinsky MC, Lamothe S, Yang HY, et al. Pharmacogenomics and metabolite measurement for 6-mercaptopurine therapy in inflammatory bowel disease. Gastroenterology 118:705–713, 2000.
61. Fraser AG, Orchard TR, Robinson EM, et al. Long-term risk of malignancy after treatment of inflammatory bowel disease with azathioprine. Aliment Pharmacol Ther 16;1225–1232, 2002.
62. Bebb JR, Logan PH. Review article: does the use of immunosuppressive therapy in inflammatory bowel disease increase the risk of developing lymphoma? Aliment Pharmacol Ther 15:1843–1849, 2001.

63. Hawthorne AB. Cyclosporin and refractory colitis. Eur J Gastroenterol Hepatol 15:239–244, 2003.

64. Cohen RD, Stein R, Hanauer SB. Intravenous cyclosporin in ulcerative colitis: a five-year experience. Am J Gastroenterol 94:1587–1592, 1999.

65. Kornbluth A, Present DH, Lichtiger S, et al. Cyclosporin for severe ulcerative colitis: a user's guide. Am J Gastroenterol 92:1424–1428, 1997.

66. Van Assche G, DHaens G, Vermeire NM, et al. Randomized, double-blind comparison of 4 mg/kg versus 2 mg/kg intravenous cyclosporine in severe ulcerative colitis. Gastroenterology 125:1025–1031, 2003.

67. Ierardi E, Principi M, Francavilla R, et al. Oral tacrolimus long-term therapy in patients with Crohn's disease and steroid resistance. Aliment Pharmacol Ther 15:371–377, 2001.

68. Baumgart DC, Wiedenmann B, Dignass AU. Rescue therapy with tacrolimus is effective in patients with severe and refractory inflammatory bowel disease. Aliment Pharmacol Ther 17:1273–1281, 2003.

69. Sandborn WJ, Present DH, Isaacs KL, et al. Tacrolimus for the treatment of inpatients with Crohn's disease; a randomized, placebo-controlled trial. Gastroenterology 125:380–388, 2003.

70. Feagan BG, Rochon J, Fedorak RN, et al. Methotrexate for the treatment of Crohn's disease. N Engl J Med 332:292–297, 1995.

71. Feagan BG, Febork RN, Irvine EJ, et al. A comparison of methotrexate with placebo for the maintenance of remission in Crohn's disease. North American Crohn's Study Group Investigators. N Engl J Med 342:1627–1632, 2000.

72. Sandborn WJ, Hanauer SB. Infliximab in the treatment of Crohn's disease: a user's guide. Am J Gastroenterol 97:2962–2972, 2002.

73. Present DH, Rutgeerts P, Targan S, et al. Infliximab for the treatment of fistulas in patients with Crohn's disease. N Engl J Med 340:1398–1405, 2003.

74. Hanauer SG, Feagan BG, Lichtenstein GE, et al. Maintenance infliximab for Crohn's disease; the ACCENT I randomized trial. Lancet 359:1541–1549, 2002.

75. Farrell RJ, Alsahi M, Jeen TY, et al. Intravenous hydrocortisone premedication reduces antibodies to infliximab in Crohn's disease: a randomized controlled trial. Gastroenterology 124:917–924, 2003.

76. Keane J, Gershon S, Wise RP, et al. Tuberculosis is associated with infliximab, a tumor necrosis factor alpha-neutralizing agent. N Engl J Med 345:1098–1104, 2001.

77. Arnold GL, Beaves MR, Pryjdun VO, et al. Preliminary study of ciprofloxacin in active Crohn's disease. Inflamm Bowel Dis 8:10–15, 2002.

78. Steinhart AH, Feagan BG, Wong CJ, et al. Combined budesonide and antibiotic therapy for active Crohn's disease: a randomized controlled trial. Gastroenterology 123:33–40, 2002.

79. Goh J, O'Morain A. Review article: nutrition and adult inflammatory bowel disease. Aliment Pharmacol Ther 17:307–320, 2003.

80. Forbes A. Review article: Crohn's disease—the role of nutritional therapy. Aliment Pharmacol Ther 16 (Suppl 4):48–52, 2002.

81. Nicholls RJ. Review article: ulcerative colitis—surgical indications and treatment. Aliment Pharmacol Ther 16 (Suppl 4):25–28, 2002.

82. Poggioli G, Pierangeli F, Laureti S, et al. Review article: indication and type of surgery in Crohn's disease. Aliment Pharmacol Ther 16 (Suppl 4):59–64, 2002.

83. Hilsden RJ, Verhoef MJ, Best A, et al. Complementary and alternative medicine use in Canadian patients with inflammatory bowel disease; results from a national survey. Am J Gastroenterol 98:1563–1568, 2003.

84. Langmead L, Dawson C, Hawkins C, et al. Antioxidant effects of herbal therapies used by patients with inflammatory bowel disease: an in vitro study. Aliment Pharmacol Ther 16:197–205, 2002.

85. Rutgeerts P, Van Deventer S, Schreiber S. Review article: the expanding role of biological agents in the treatment of inflammatory bowel disease—focus on selective adhesion molecule inhibition. Aliment Pharmacol Ther 17:1435–1450, 2003.

86. Caprilli R, Viscido A, Guagnozzi D. Review article; biological agents in the treatment of Crohn's disease. Aliment Pharmacol Ther 16:1579–1590, 2002.

87. Sandborn WJ, Yednock TA. Novel approaches to treating inflammatory bowel disease: targeting alpha-4 integrin. Am J Gastroenterol 98:2372–2382, 2003.

88. Ghosh S, Goldin E, Gordon F, et al. Natalizumab for active Crohn's disease. N Engl J Med 348;24–32, 2003.

89. Dubinsky MC, Feldman EJ, Abreu MT, et al. Thioguanine: a potential alternative for IBD patients allergic to 6-mercaptopurine or azathioprine. Am J Gastroenterol 98:1058–1063, 2003.

90. Ford AC, Towler RJ, Moayyedi P, et al. Mycophenolate mofetil in refractory inflammatory bowel disease. Aliment Pharmacol Ther 17:1365–1369, 2003.

91. Cohen RD. Evolving medical therapies for ulcerative colitis. Curr Gastroenterol Rep 4:497–505, 2002.

92. Seegers D, Bouma G, Pena S. Review article: a critical approach to new forms of treatment of Crohn's disease and ulcerative colitis. Aliment Pharmacol Ther 16 (Suppl 4):53–58, 2002.

93. Cosnes J, Beaugerie L, Carbonnel F, et al. Smoking cessation and the course of Crohn's disease: an interventional study. Gastroenterology 120;1093–1099, 2001.

94. Sewitch MJ, Abrahamowicz M, Barkun A, et al. Patient nonadherence to medication in inflammatory bowel disease. Am J Gastroenterol 98:1535–1544, 2003.

95. Shale MJ, Riley SA. Studies of compliance with delayed-release mesalazine therapy in patients with inflammatory bowel disease. Aliment Pharmacol Ther 18:191–199, 2003.

96. Van Balkom BPJ, Schoon EJ, Stockbraugger RW, et al. Effects of anti-tumour necrosis factor-α therapy on the quality of life in Crohn's disease. Aliment Pharmacol Ther 16:1101–1107, 2002.

97. Longobardi T, Jacobs P, Wu L, et al. Work losses related to inflammatory bowel disease in Canada: results from a national population health survey. Am J Gastroenterol 98:844–849, 2003.

98. Bloomquest P, Feltelius N, Lofberg R, et al. A 10-year survey of inflammatory bowel diseases—drug therapy, costs and adverse reactions. Aliment Pharmacol Ther 15:475–481, 2001.

Nausea and Vomiting

Bruce D. Clayton and Bernadette K. Brown

TREATMENT GOALS: NAUSEA AND VOMITING

- Review the cost-effectiveness of medications used regularly in a particular practice setting.
- Analyze the usage patterns, efficacy, and pharmacoeconomics of medications used.
- Develop treatment protocols for the practice setting based on outcomes and cost-effectiveness.
- Treat the cause of nausea and vomiting, if this can be identified.
- Assess the contribution of concurrent diseases to the occurrence of nausea and vomiting.
- Assess for fluid and electrolyte loss.
- Individualize appropriate symptomatic drug treatment after considering contraindications and adverse drug effects.
- For patients undergoing clinical events in which nausea and vomiting are likely to occur (i.e., chemotherapy, surgery, radiation, motion sickness), maintain adequate hydration; recommend that the patient eat small, light meals, avoiding sweet, greasy, or spicy foods; premedicate with an antiemetic regimen specific for the patient and the chemotherapy to be administered; ensure that the patient has adequate knowledge of nonpharmacologic preventive measures; and educate the patient about the risks and benefits of the medications that will be used.

DEFINITION

Nausea is the subjectively unpleasant sensation of the awareness of the urge to vomit. It is often preceded or accompanied by a variety of autonomic signs such as pallor, sweating, tachycardia, salivation, and increased respiratory rate.

Vomiting or emesis is the reflex expulsion of the stomach contents via the esophagus and mouth, and it is usually associated with nausea and retching. Nausea and retching can occur without expulsion, and occasionally expulsion occurs without prior nausea and retching. This is known as projectile vomiting.

Retching is the involuntary but unsuccessful effort to vomit. It involves mainly the respiratory muscles of the abdomen, diaphragm, and chest and often is accompanied by bradycardia.

Nausea, vomiting, and retching are three separate clinical conditions. Each should be assessed independently.

PATHOPHYSIOLOGY

The vomiting reflex is found in many species and probably evolved as a protective mechanism to limit the effects of ingested toxic materials.[1] In humans, the tendency to experience nausea and vomiting varies greatly. Causes of nausea and vomiting are listed in Table 47.1.

The principal anatomic elements involved in vomiting are shown diagrammatically in Figure 47.1. Coordination of the vomiting reflex occurs in the vomiting center (VC), located in the lateral reticular formation of the medulla. Afferent fibers from sensory receptors in the pharynx, stomach, intestines, and other viscera connect directly with the VC through the vagus and splanchnic nerves, and produce vomiting when stimulated. The center also responds to stimuli originating in other tissues, such as the cerebral cortex, vestibular apparatus of the inner ear, and blood. These so-called central stimuli are believed to travel first to the chemoreceptor

TABLE 47.1	Causes of Vomiting

1. Ingestion of certain substances present in food and the environment
2. Ingestion of certain drugs, particularly opiates, general anesthetics, and antineoplastic drugs
3. Motion or other effects on the vestibular apparatus
4. Infection—part of the prodrome of many infections
5. Respiratory problems such as violent coughing
6. Cardiovascular disease such as myocardial infarction
7. Disorders of the gastrointestinal tract:
   a. Gastrointestinal tract obstruction
   b. Mucosal lesions such as ulcers, inflammation, and atrophy
   c. Liver disease
   d. Pancreatic and small intestinal diseases
   e. Diseases of the components of the gut wall (collagen, smooth muscle, nerve)
   f. Peritonitis
8. Renal diseases such as renal failure, pyelonephritis, uremia, and uremic colic
9. Metabolic and endocrine disorders such as diabetic ketoacidosis, hyperparathyroidism, adrenal insufficiency, and pregnancy
10. Gynecologic disorders such as pelvic inflammation and complications of pregnancy
11. Normal pregnancy
12. Neurologic disorders such as increased cranial pressure, hemorrhage, epilepsy, meningitis, migraine, vertigo and Meniere's syndrome, and brain metastases
13. Psychiatric disorders including bulimia, rumination, and anorexia nervosa
14. Drug withdrawal syndromes
15. Radiation therapy

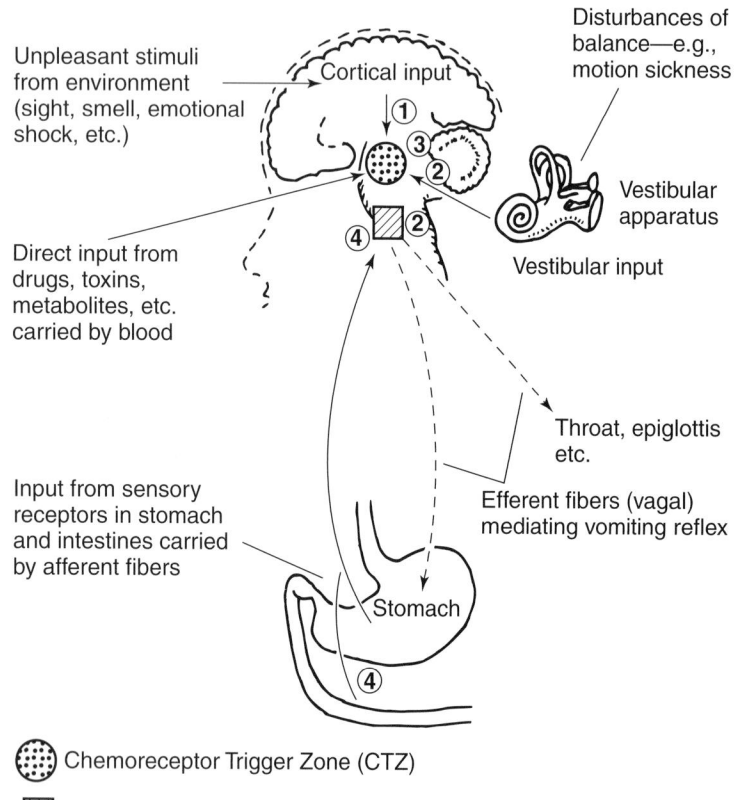

Chemoreceptor Trigger Zone (CTZ)

Vomiting Center

FIGURE 47.1 Anatomic structures involved in the vomiting reflex. Sites of action of common antiemetic drugs are labeled as follows: site of action of sedative (1), site of action of antihistamines and anticholinergics (2), site of action of dopamine antagonists (3), and proposed sites of action of serotonin antagonists and neurokinin-1 antagonists (4). The vomiting reflex is mediated through the vomiting center. This center receives impulses from afferent fibers from the stomach and intestines and from fibers in the chemoreceptor trigger zone. It sends out impulses via afferent fibers to the muscles of the throat, epiglottis, and stomach, as shown in Figure 47.2.

trigger zone (CTZ), which then activates the VC to induce vomiting. The CTZ is located in the medullary region known as the area postrema, located on the caudal margin of the fourth ventricle. An important function of the CTZ is to sample blood and spinal fluid for potentially toxic substances and, when detected, to initiate the vomiting reflex. It is, therefore, appropriate that the CTZ is located in the area postrema, a region of the brain that is not protected by the blood-brain barrier. The CTZ cannot initiate emesis independently but only by stimulating the VC.[2] The VC and the CTZ are bilateral and are much smaller than shown in Figure 47.1.

The higher centers of the brain can be a source of stimulus or inhibition of the VC (Fig. 47.1). Vomiting can occur as a conditioned response (e.g., the pretreatment nausea that occurs in some patients about to receive a course of anticancer chemotherapy) or as a reaction to unpleasant sights and smells. The cerebrum can greatly modify the vomiting response to stimuli from other sources such as visceral or vestibular nerve pathways, enhancing or repressing vomiting. The large placebo response seen in many trials of antiemetics can be explained in these terms, as can repression of motion sickness by the patient's concentration on some mental activity. Psychological factors can thus play an important role in nausea and vomiting, although they are usually outweighed by physical factors.

Anatomically, the VC is well placed to coordinate the various efferent functions associated with vomiting (Fig. 47.1). When the VC is stimulated, efferent impulses are sent to the salivary, vasomotor, and respiratory centers and to cranial nerves VIII and X. The vomiting reflex begins with a sudden deep inspiration that increases abdominal pressure (Fig. 47.2), which is further increased by contraction of the abdominal muscles. The soft palate rises and the epiglottis closes, preventing the aspiration of vomitus into the lungs. The pyloric sphincter contracts and the cardiac sphincter and esophagus relax, allowing stomach contents to be expelled. The flow of saliva increases to aid the expulsion.[3]

Drugs that exert an emetic effect by acting on the CTZ include apomorphine, digitalis glycosides, morphine, the ergot alkaloids, anesthetics, and many antineoplastic agents. There are considerable interspecies differences in the sensitivity of the CTZ to emetic drugs and great variation in the extent to which emesis is stimulated by other routes, such as stimulation of the sensory receptors of the viscera. Apomorphine is the only drug that produces vomiting solely by direct action on the CTZ in all species. The complexity of the pharmacology of emetic drugs is illustrated by morphine, which can act on the CTZ directly or indirectly via the vestibular afferent system. It can also antagonize the emetic action of other drugs by direct depression of the VC.

The neurochemical control of vomiting is not completely understood; however, five neurotransmitter systems appear to play significant roles in mediating the emetic response: (a) dopaminergic, (b) histaminic, (c) cholinergic, (d) 5-hydroxytryptamine$_3$ (5-HT$_3$), and (e) substance P. Dopamine receptors are found in the CTZ and the gastrointestinal (GI) tract. Dopamine agonists (apomorphine and levodopa) produce emesis by acting on the CTZ and peripheral dopamine receptors that stimulate the CTZ, whereas dopamine antagonists (the phenothiazines, butyrophenones, and metoclopramide) block emesis. Histamine (H$_1$ and H$_2$) receptors also are found in the CTZ, but histamine receptor blockade results in antiemetic activity limited to vestibular causes. The neurotransmitters involved in motion sickness are better understood. The sensory disorientation that occurs

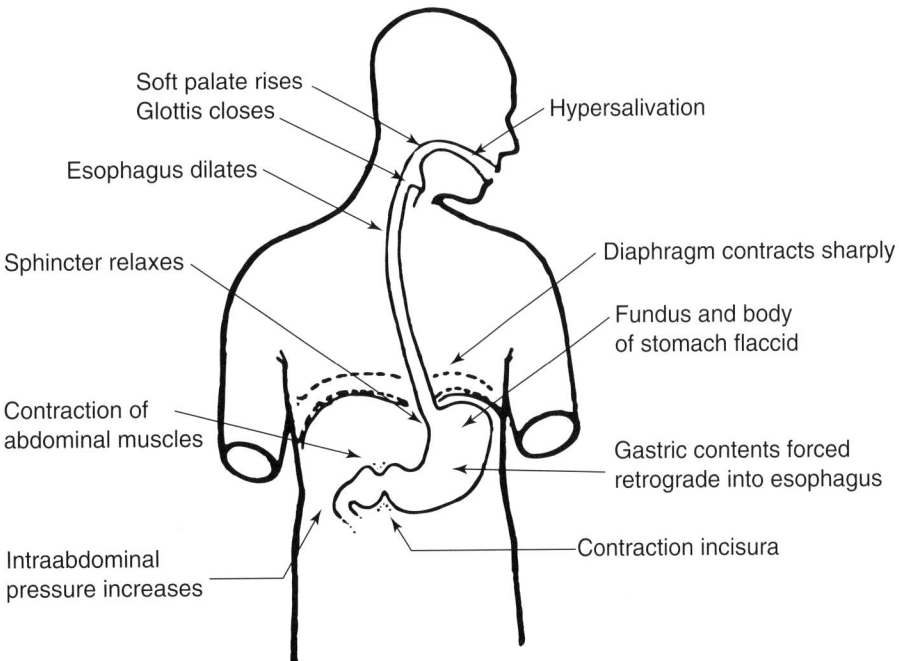

FIGURE 47.2 The mechanism of the complex act of vomiting. (From Whelan G. Targeting therapy: the patient with nausea, retching and vomiting. Curr Ther 26:26, 1985.)

in motion sickness results in an imbalance in cholinergic and adrenergic activity in the region of the medulla near the VC and CTZ. The result is excess acetylcholine that affects the VC directly or, more likely, via an effect on the CTZ.[1] Studies indicate that serotonergic receptors (subtypes 5-HT$_3$ and 5-HT$_4$) appear to be principal mediators in the emetic reflex. High concentrations of the 5-HT$_3$ receptors have been identified in the area postrema-nucleus tractus solitarii region of the medulla.[4] About 90% of the 5-HT$_3$ in the adult human body is located in the enterochromaffin cells of the GI tract, and the remainder is present in the central nervous system and the platelets. It is thought that chemotherapeutic agents (e.g., cisplatin) produce nausea and vomiting by releasing serotonin from the enterochromaffin cells and that the released serotonin then activates 5-HT$_3$ receptors located on afferent vagal nerve terminals to initiate the vomiting reflex.[5] The serotonin antagonists act as antiemetics by selectively inhibiting 5-HT$_3$ receptors.

Another mediator thought to play a role in the emetic reflex is substance P. Substance P is a neuropeptide that belongs to the tachykinin family. It is found in high concentrations in the nucleus tractus solitarius and area postrema of the central nervous system, and it coexists with serotonin in the enterochromaffin cells and vagal afferent nerves of the GI tract.[6] The actions of substance P are mediated through the neurokinin-1 (NK$_1$) receptor.[7] Aprepitant is a potent, selective NK$_1$ antagonist that blocks the effects of substance P in the CNS.[8] It has no affinity for serotonin, dopamine, or corticosteroid receptors.[9]

Other receptors may initiate emesis for drugs such as the digitalis glycosides, copper sulfate, and the opiates. Other neurotransmitters and peptides, including enkephalin, arginine vasopressin, substance P, peptide YY, and catecholamines, stimulate the CTZ and may play a role in triggering emesis.[3] Emesis is thus mediated through a variety of receptor types, and it is probable that more pathways will be discovered leading to more effective and more disease-specific antiemetic therapy.

CLINICAL PRESENTATION AND DIAGNOSIS

SIGNS AND SYMPTOMS
The signs and symptoms of vomiting-induced metabolic disturbances include the following:

- Dehydration, suggested by oliguria, weight loss, mental confusion, and reduced skin turgor
- Sodium depletion, suggested by thirst and hypotension
- Potassium depletion, suggested by muscle weakness or cardiac rhythm disturbances
- Alkalosis, which can result from loss of hydrogen ions in the vomitus, and the concentration of extracellular fluid secondary to fluid loss

Sodium, potassium, and chloride depletion result mainly from loss in the vomitus but also from other metabolic disturbances.

DIAGNOSIS
An accurate diagnosis is essential before treatment for nausea and vomiting begins because symptomatic therapy may be contraindicated (e.g., in GI obstruction, acute appendicitis, or cerebral edema), or assessment of the underlying disease could be complicated by the sedative properties of most antiemetic therapy. The causes of vomiting should be kept in mind (Table 47.1) in developing the treatment plan.

The appearance, frequency, and timing of nausea and vomiting, together with associated specific and nonspecific symptoms such as jaundice, dehydration, diarrhea, weight loss, pain, and fever are important in making a diagnosis. Blood in the vomitus, an important sign, can be fresh and bright red (as from an esophageal tear) or altered, having the appearance of coffee grounds (indicating a GI bleed). Bile in the vomitus gives it a green or yellow color and suggests that the pyloric sphincter is open, allowing reflux of duodenal contents into the stomach.

The cause of vomiting usually is obvious (e.g., pregnancy, motion, or the use of certain drugs), but in some cases diagnosis can be difficult, especially if psychogenic factors are involved. With unexplained vomiting, the first step in assessment is eliminating the possibility of upper GI tract lesions or systemic conditions such as meningitis or uremia. The need to treat the sequelae of prolonged vomiting, such as fluid and electrolyte depletion, should also be assessed.

Chronic vomiting, with or without weight loss, can be psychogenic. This is suggested when the vomiting has been occurring for some time (especially if the patient has delayed seeking help), there is a family history of vomiting, the patient is able to suppress vomiting, or vomiting rarely occurs in a public place.

THERAPEUTIC PLAN

The patient experiencing nausea or vomiting is in acute need of pharmaceutical care. The health care provider's primary goals are to recognize patients and circumstances that have a higher incidence of nausea and vomiting and prevent or minimize the frequency of nausea and vomiting. The health care provider must use the accumulated knowledge about the causes and impact of nausea and vomiting to design an individualized pharmaceutical care plan that addresses drug efficacy, disease remission, and patient well-being to effectively treat this disorder with minimal patient morbidity. In preparation for individualized patient therapy, health care providers should do the following:

- Treat the cause if it can be identified.
- Assess for fluid and electrolyte loss. In most cases this entails giving adequate fluids orally, particularly those

containing glucose. If fluid loss leads to metabolic disturbances, the patient should be hospitalized and given appropriate intravenous fluids.

- Give appropriate symptomatic drug treatment after considering contraindications and potential for adverse drug reactions. The choice of drug and dose must be individualized.
- For unexplained vomiting, continue with diagnostic examinations.[10]

TREATMENT

PHARMACOTHERAPY

Antiemetic Drugs. Considerable effort has been spent in developing antinausea drugs. In the past, most research focused on treating motion sickness and nausea of pregnancy (hyperemesis gravidarum), but more recently it has focused on treating nausea and vomiting associated with surgery and cancer chemotherapy. Nausea and vomiting are common complications of chemotherapeutic regimens, often so severe as to cause the patient not to return for further treatment.

When selecting drugs to treat nausea and vomiting, it is important to remember that therapy must be individualized. These disorders can be caused by a variety of stimuli, and correlations between serum levels and efficacy have not been established for most antiemetics. For these reasons, treatment regimens should be regarded only as guidelines.

Dopamine Antagonists. The dopamine D_2 receptor antagonists include the phenothiazines, butyrophenones, and substituted benzamides (e.g., metoclopramide). The antiemetic action of the compounds is thought to result, at least in part, from inhibition of dopamine receptors in the CTZ. Unfortunately, the antiemetics that act as dopamine antagonists may also produce symptoms of dystonia, parkinsonism, akathisia, and tardive dyskinesia because the extrapyramidal nigrostriatal system is highly innervated by dopaminergic fibers.[11]

Phenothiazines. The phenothiazines have been the most widely used antiemetics since the 1950s. Two key modifications of the phenothiazine heterocyclic structure improve antiemetic activity. Halogenation (prochlorperazine, perphenazine) or thiethylation (thiethylperazine) of position 2 (R1), in combination with the attachment of a piperazine side chain at the 10 position (R2), enhances antiemetic (and extrapyramidal) activity. The phenothiazines also have varying amounts of anticholinergic and antihistaminic activity that may inhibit the vestibular pathway and the VC of the brain.[12]

Adverse effects of the phenothiazines include orthostatic hypotension and excessive sedation, which may limit use in ambulatory patients. Extrapyramidal effects occur most often with perphenazine, but are readily controlled with diphenhydramine or benztropine. The phenothiazines can be given orally, parenterally, and rectally. The latter routes are useful when vomiting precludes oral administration.

Phenothiazines are used primarily to treat mild to moderate nausea and vomiting associated with anesthesia and surgery, radiation therapy, and cancer chemotherapy. Prochlorperazine has been the phenothiazine most widely used and studied as an antiemetic. Onset of action is 10 to 20 minutes for intramuscular administration, 30 to 40 minutes for oral tablet administration, and 60 minutes for rectal suppository administration. The duration of action is 3 to 4 hours regardless of the route. Prochlorperazine has routinely been administered in a dose of 10 mg every 4 to 6 hours, orally or intramuscularly, or 25 mg every 6 hours rectally to provide optimal antiemetic efficacy. At these doses, comparative studies of cancer chemotherapy indicate that it is more effective than placebo, equivalent in potency to low-dose metoclopramide (0.1 to 0.3 mg/kg/dose) and droperidol, and less effective than tetrahydrocannabinol (THC), high-dose metoclopramide (1 to 3 mg/kg/dose), and nabilone.[7] Studies have demonstrated significantly greater antiemetic activity when doses of 30 to 40 mg of prochlorperazine were administered by slow intravenous infusion. There was no substantial increase in adverse effects if diphenhydramine was administered prophylactically to prevent extrapyramidal reactions.[12–14]

Butyrophenones. The butyrophenones, like the phenothiazines, are dopamine D_2 receptor antagonists and are effective antiemetic agents with similar uses and side effects. The main side effect is sedation, although extrapyramidal side effects do occur. The butyrophenones are less likely to produce hypotension than the phenothiazines. Droperidol is an effective antiemetic for use in cytotoxic therapy and in combination with fentanyl for postoperative nausea and vomiting (PONV), but it is for parenteral administration only. The onset of pharmacologic action of droperidol occurs within 3 to 10 minutes, but peak pharmacologic effects may not be apparent until 30 minutes after injection. Duration of antiemetic action is 2 to 4 hours, but sedating and tranquilizing effects may persist for up to 12 hours after a single dose. In 2001, the US Food and Drug Administration (FDA) added a black box warning to the prescribing information for droperidol.[15] This warning was issued due to reports of serious and sometimes fatal cardiac arrhythmias associated with droperidol use. Prolongation of the QT interval and torsades de pointes occurred at doses less than 2.5 mg, the manufacturer's minimum recommended dosage. The FDA warning recommends that a 12-lead electrocardiograph (ECG) be obtained before administration of the drug to determine if a prolonged QT interval is present. If present, droperidol should not be administered. If a prolonged QT interval is not present and droperidol is used, the patient should be monitored with an ECG continuously for 2 to 3 hours after completing treatment. Despite the efficacy of droperidol for PONV, its use has been severely restricted since the black box warning was added.

Haloperidol is used occasionally as an antiemetic. It is usually given in doses of 1 to 3 mg orally or intramuscularly every 3 hours. Oral bioavailability is 60%. Peak plasma concentrations occur within 2 to 6 hours. Haloperidol appears to undergo first-pass metabolism and enterohepatic recirculation. After intramuscular administration, peak plasma concentrations occur within 10 to 20 minutes, with peak pharmacologic action within 30 to 45 minutes.

Metoclopramide. Metoclopramide has dual action as an antagonist of dopamine D_2 and 5-HT_3 receptors, protecting against the emetic effects of dopamine and serotonin agonists. The action of metoclopramide is more selective than that of the phenothiazines in that it shows neuroleptic activity only at very high doses. Via a peripheral action, possibly as a partial agonist of enteric postsynaptic neurons,[16] metoclopramide also increases the motility of the stomach and small intestine and relaxes the pyloric sphincter, increasing the activity of the upper regions on the GI tract. The antidopaminergic and antiserotonergic effects of metoclopramide on the gut compliment the central antiemetic effect and are particularly useful in treating nausea and vomiting associated with GI cancer, gastritis, peptic ulcer, radiation sickness, and migraine headaches. Metoclopramide is contraindicated in patients with intestinal obstruction who are at high risk for colonic rupture. It appears to be of little value in treating motion sickness, although it has been widely used for this purpose in Europe.

Early clinical trials of metoclopramide at doses of 0.1 to 0.3 mg/kg showed only minimal antiemetic effect for a variety of antineoplastic agents, but high-dose (1 to 3 mg/kg) metoclopramide therapy was much more effective as an antiemetic.[17] There are no major differences in the pharmacokinetics of conventional- and high-dose metoclopramide.[18] Oral doses are rapidly absorbed, but variable first-pass metabolism provides an oral bioavailability of 32% to 100%.[19] Peak levels occur in about 1 hour. High lipophilicity results in a large volume of distribution (2.8 to 4.5 L/kg). Approximately 85% of an orally administered dose appears in the urine within 72 hours. Of the 85% eliminated in the urine, about half is present as free or conjugated metoclopramide. The terminal half-life is 4.5 to 8.8 hours. One study to date indicates that there is substantial pharmacokinetic variability between patients with various cancers. The authors attribute this variability primarily to differences in body weight and serum alkaline phosphatase levels.[20] Although an early study indicated that serum levels greater than 800 ng/mL were necessary to achieve maximum protection against cisplatin-induced emesis, more recent trials have failed to show that serum metoclopramide concentrations predict antiemetic response or adverse effects.

Several studies have investigated routes of administration for optimal antiemetic therapy, ease and expense of administration, and frequency of adverse effects. Although optimal doses and time schedules have not been delineated completely, the studies indicate that oral, continuous intravenous, and intermittent intravenous administration provide comparable antiemetic activity against a variety of chemotherapeutic agents. Oral therapy tends to be associated with a greater

frequency of loose stools than intravenous administration, and scheduled dosing may be difficult if vomiting occurs. Rectal administration shows significant variation in the bioavailability of extemporaneously compounded suppositories (30% to 86%) but can be successful in reducing the frequency of emesis as described in a case report of one patient.[21] Other points such as legal aspects of compounding, formulation stability, and cost must also be considered.[22]

Adverse effects associated with metoclopramide therapy include diarrhea, sedation, dizziness, and extrapyramidal symptoms. Diarrhea occurs in about 50% of patients receiving high-dose metoclopramide and cisplatin, but this may be related to cisplatin therapy. Mild sedation is observed in most patients who receive higher doses. The extrapyramidal symptoms include akathisia, restlessness, and dystonic reactions (including torticollis, oculogyric crisis, and Parkinson-like symptoms). The overall frequency is 3% to 5%, but as many as 30% of men under the age of 30 years may suffer from extrapyramidal effects. Extrapyramidal symptoms subside within 5 minutes of intravenous diphenhydramine administration. When high-dose metoclopramide is used as an antiemetic, many cancer chemotherapy protocols now include routine doses of diphenhydramine to minimize extrapyramidal symptoms (see Chemotherapy-Induced Nausea and Vomiting).

Serotonin Receptor Antagonists. The serotonin (5-HT_3) receptor antagonists have made a major impact in the treatment of emesis associated with cancer chemotherapy, radiation therapy, and PONV. Four serotonin (5-HT_3) receptor antagonists (ondansetron, granisetron, dolasetron, and palonosetron) are now available. Table 47.2 compares the pharmacokinetic properties of these agents. Serum concentrations do not correlate with antiemetic efficacy, and there does not appear to be accumulation after multiple dosing. Ondansetron is extensively metabolized with only 5% recovered in the urine as unchanged drug. The primary metabolic pathway is hydroxylation of the indole ring followed by glucuronide or sulfate conjugation.[23] Granisetron is metabolized by *N*-demethylation and aromatic ring oxidation followed by conjugation. Animal studies suggest that some of the metabolites may also have 5-HT_3 receptor antagonist activity. In normal volunteers, approximately 12% is eliminated unchanged in the urine in 48 hours. The remainder is excreted as metabolites, 49% in the urine and 34% in the feces. Dolasetron is rapidly (half-life less than 10 minutes) reduced to hydrodolasetron, the primary active agent, by carbonyl reductase. Hydrodolasetron is further metabolized by oxidation of the indole ring; *N*-oxidation also occurs before it is excreted as glucuronide, sulfate conjugates, and *N*-oxide.[24,25] Two-thirds of the administered dose is eliminated in the urine and one-third in the feces. Palonosetron is approximately 50% metabolized to form two primary metabolites: N-oxide-palonosetron and 6-S-hydroxy-palonosetron, each of which is essentially inactive as a serotonin

TABLE 47.2	Pharmacokinetics of Serotonin Antagonists

Variable	Ondansetron PO[a]	Ondansetron IV[b]	Granisetron PO[c]	Granisetron IV[d]	Dolasetron PO (Hydrodolasetron)	Dolasetron IV (Hydrodolasetron)	Palonosetron IV
Bioavailability	56%		NA		75%		
Half-life (hr)							
Cancer patients		4.0		9	7.9[e]	7.5[h]	40[l,n]
Volunteers 40[g,h]							
20–40 yrs	3.3	3.5	6.2[k]	4.9	8.1[f]	7.3[l]	
60–75 yrs[g]	4.5	4.7		7.7	7.2[g]	6.9[i]	
>75 yrs[g]	5.5	5.5					
Liver impairment[n]							
Moderate		9.2	NA	NA	NA	NA	NA
Severe		20.6	NA	NA	11	11.7	NA
Protein binding	70%–76%		65%		69%–77%		62%
Volume of distribution (L/kg)			3.97		5.8		8.3

[a]Single 8-mg oral dose.
[b]Single 0.15 mg/kg IV dose.
[c]single 1-mg oral dose.
[d]Single 40-μg/kg IV dose.
[e]25–200-mg oral dose.
[f]Single 1.8-mg/kg IV dose.
[g]No dose adjustment is required in the elderly.
[h]Population not identified other than healthy volunteers.
[i]No age differentiation with 39 normal volunteers.
[j]200-mg oral dose. [k]Single 100-mg IV dose.
[l]2.4-mg/kg oral dose.
[m]Single 2.4-mg/kg IV dose.
[n]No dose adjustment required.
PO, by mouth; IV, intravenous.
(From product information for Zofran. Research Triangle Park, NC: GlaxoWellcome, December 1996; product information for Anzemet. Kansas City, MO: Hoechst Marion Roussel, October, 1997; product information for Aloxi. Bloomington, MN: MGI Pharma, Inc., July, 2003; product information for Kytril. Nutley, NJ: Roche Laboratories, Inc., December, 2000.)

antagonist. Over 80% of the palonosetron and metabolites are excreted in the urine.[26]

Ondansetron, granisetron, dolasetron, and palonosetron are metabolized by the cytochrome P-450 2D6 isoenzyme of the hepatic cytochrome P-450 enzyme system[27]; inducers or inhibitors of these enzymes may change the clearance and the half-life of these serotonin antagonists. Blood levels of hydrodolasetron increased 24% when dolasetron was coadministered with cimetidine for 7 days and decreased 28% with coadministration of rifampin for 7 days.[24] At this time, no dosage adjustments are recommended, only close monitoring for adverse effects. Ondansetron, granisetron, dolasetron, and palonosetron do not induce or inhibit the cytochrome P-450 enzyme system.[23,24,26,28] A particular advantage of this group of antiemetics is minimal dopaminergic blockade, demonstrated by few reports of extrapyramidal adverse effects.[23,24,29,30]

Tables 47.3 and 47.4 compare the frequency of adverse effects of the serotonin antagonists. Note that the clinical studies cited for frequency of adverse effects of granisetron used a dose of 40 μg per kilogram. Because no statistical difference in antiemetic efficacy has been demonstrated between 10 and 40 μg per kilogram, the recommended dose in the United States is now 10 μg per kilogram.[28]

Case reports indicate that the serotonin antagonists may induce ECG interval changes (PR, QTc, JT prolongation, and QRS widening). These changes are dose related; some patients have interval prolongations for 24 hours or more. There have been rare reports of interval prolongation leading to heart block and cardiac arrhythmias. Serotonin antagonists should be administered with caution in patients who have or may develop prolonged conduction intervals. This side effect is more common in patients with hypokalemia or hypomagnesemia and those taking diuretics, antiarrhythmic drugs, or other drugs that lead to QT prolongation and in patients on a cumulative high-dose anthracycline therapy.[24,26] Concern has been expressed that with the restrictions placed on the use of droperidol (see "Butyrophenones") due to arrhythmias, there may be an increased incidence of arrhythmias secondary to the serotonin antagonists since the use of droperidol for PONV is being replaced by the serotonin antagonists.[31–33]

TABLE 47.3	Frequency of Adverse Effects Reported in Clinical Trials after Oral Administration[a]		
	Ondansetron 8 mg bid	Granisetron 2 mg qd	Dolasetron[b] 100 mg qd
CINV[c]			
Headache	24%	20%	22.9%
Fatigue	13%	NA	5.7%
Constipation	9%	14%	NA
Diarrhea	6%	9%	5.3%
Dizziness	5%	NA	3.1%
Asthenia	NA	18%	NA
Dyspepsia	NA	6%	2.2%
PONV			
Headache	9%	NA[d]	7%
Fever	8%		3.5%
Dizziness	7%		4.4%

[a]Adverse effects listed are those that had a reported incidence higher than the incidence reported with placebo.

[b]Dolasetron not compared against placebo in CINV studies.

[c]Ondansetron and cyclophosphamide regimen, granisetron and cyclophosphamide or cisplatin regimen, dolasetron and cyclophosphamide or doxorubicin regimen.

[d]Granisetron not tested in PONV.

bid, twice a day; qd, every day; CINV, chemotherapy-induced nausea and vomiting; PONV, postoperative nausea and vomiting. (From product information for Zofran. Research Triangle Park, NC: GlaxoWellcome, December, 1996; product information for Anzemet. Kansas City, MO: Hoechst Marion Roussel, October, 1997; product information for Kytril. Nutley, NJ: Roche Laboratories, Inc. December, 2000.)

Cisplatin, a potent serotonin agonist, is well recognized for its almost 100% emetic potential when administered to patients without emesis prophylaxis. Therefore, it is the primary agent against which the efficacy of antiemetics is measured. The serotonin antagonists have been shown to actively control nausea and vomiting associated with cisplatin and several other emetogenic chemotherapeutic agents in animals and humans. Comparative studies between ondansetron and metoclopramide conclude that ondansetron is more effective than metoclopramide in the control of high-dose cisplatin-induced nausea and vomiting.[29,34–37] Several single-center and multicenter, double-blind, randomized studies comparing the efficacy and safety of ondansetron, granisetron, and dolasetron in controlling cisplatin-induced acute emesis conclude that there are no significant differences between any of the treatment groups with respect to emetic control, nausea, or adverse reactions. These studies also bear out the impact of the dose of highly emetogenic agents (cisplatin) and moderately emetogenic agents (cyclophosphamide, doxorubicin) in comparing studies with different rates of control of emesis and nausea. For higher-dose cisplatin, 35% to 50% of patients receiving serotonin antagonists have

no episodes of emesis, and 50% to 70% have two or fewer episodes of emesis. Emesis is controlled in 50% to 70% of patients receiving moderately emetogenic chemotherapy. Headache is the most frequently reported drug-related adverse effect, occurring in 9% to 24% of all patients.[38–47] More recently, the serotonin antagonists have been shown to be more effective against chemotherapy-induced nausea and vomiting (CINV) when combined with dexamethasone (see "Corticosteroids") than when administered as monotherapy.

The serotonin antagonists have become a common choice for preventing and treating PONV. Ondansetron, granisetron, and dolasetron are approved by the FDA for PONV. Palonosetron is currently approved only for acute and delayed chemotherapy-induced nausea and vomiting. When used properly, these drugs have very few adverse effects. The expense of the serotonin antagonists limits their cost-effectiveness for preventing and treating PONV, but their therapeutic efficacy must be considered in evaluating potential drug therapy (see "Postoperative Nausea and Vomiting").

Neurokinin-1 Receptor Antagonists. Aprepitant is the first oral NK$_1$ receptor antagonist available in the United States. Aprepitant blocks the effects of Substance P by competitively blocking NK$_1$ receptors in the brain.[8] It is indicated for the prevention of acute and delayed chemotherapy-induced nausea and vomiting caused by highly emetogenic antineoplastic agents. It is used in combination with a corticosteroid and a 5-HT$_3$ receptor antagonist. The recommended dose interval for aprepitant is 125 mg orally on day 1, followed by 80 mg on days 2 and 3 of the chemotherapy cycle 1 hour prior to chemotherapy.[48] Aprepitant exhibits nonlinear kinetics, thus requiring lower doses on days 2 and 3. The oral dosage form has about 65% bioavailability, with a C$_{max}$ at approximately 4 hours on each day of administration.[9] Food does not affect the bioavailability. Aprepitant is highly protein bound (>95%) and extensively metabolized by the liver. Aprepitant is metabolized primarily by cytochrome P-450 3A4 (CYP3A4) and to a lesser extent by CYP1A2 and CYP2C19. Aprepitant is eliminated primarily by metabolism; aprepitant is not renally excreted. The elimination half-life ranges from 9 to13 hours.[9]

Aprepitant is an inhibitor and an inducer of CYP3A4. Caution should be used if administering aprepitant with other substrates or inhibitors of CYP3A4 (e.g., docetaxel, paclitaxel, etoposide, irinotecan, ifosfamide, imatinib, vinorelbine, vinblastine, vincristine, ketoconazole, itraconazole, rifampin, carbamazepine, phenytoin, clarithromycin, ritonavir, and midazolam). Oral doses of dexamethasone and methylprednisolone should be reduced by approximately 50% when prescribed concurrently with aprepitant. Intravenous methylprednisolone doses should be reduced by 25%.[49] Female patients receiving aprepitant who take oral contraceptives should be advised to use an alternate or additional method of birth control.[9] Patients receiving warfarin therapy

TABLE 47.4	Frequency of Adverse Effects Reported in Clinical Trials after Intravenous Administration[a]			
	Ondansetron	**Granisetron**	**Dolasetron**	**Palonosetron**
CIE[b,c]				
Headache	25%	14%	24.3%	9%
Diarrhea	8%	4%	12.4%	1%
Fever	7%	NA	4.3%	NA
Fatigue	NA	NA	3.6%	<1%
Constipation	2%	NA	6%	5%
PONV[d]				
Headache	17%	8.6%	9.4%	NA[e]
Dizziness	12%	4.1%	5.5%	
Drowsiness	8%	NA	2.4%	

[a]Adverse effects listed are those that had a reported incidence higher than the incidence reported with placebo [b]Chemotherapy received was predominately cisplatin [c]Doses (single dose): ondansetron (32 mg), granisetron (40 μg/kg), dolasetron (1.8 mg/kg), palonosetron (0.25 mg). [d]Doses (single dose): ondansetron (4 mg), granisetron (1 mg), dolasetron (12.5 mg). [e]Palonosetron not tested in PONV. CINV, chemotherapy-induced nausea and vomiting; PONV, postoperative nausea and vomiting. (From product information for Zofran. Research Triangle Park, NC: GlaxoWellcome, December, 1996; product information for Anzemet. Kansas City, MO: Hoechst Marion Roussel, October, 1997; product information for Aloxi. Bloomington, MN: MGI Pharma, Inc., July, 2003; product information for Kytril. Nutley, NJ: Roche Laboratories, Inc., December, 2000.)

should be instructed to have an International Normalized Ratio (INR) checked approximately 7 to 10 days after aprepitant therapy, since coadministration with aprepitant may result in increased metabolism of warfarin and a reduced INR.[9]

Clinically, aprepitant has been studied in combination with other antiemetics to prevent emesis from highly emetogenic chemotherapy. When given to prevent acute and delayed CINV in patients receiving high-dose cisplatin chemotherapy, studies have shown that aprepitant added to standard therapy (dexamethasone plus a 5-HT$_3$ antagonist) provides superior results than the standard therapy alone.[7,50–53] Two studies have shown that this effect was sustained over multiple cycles of chemotherapy.[52,53] Aprepitant appears to be well tolerated, with GI side effects (anorexia, diarrhea, constipation, abdominal pain), headache, dizziness, hiccups, and asthenia reported.[54] Of note, aprepitant appears to be most effective in reducing delayed CINV.[7,51,54] Though aprepitant's place in the prevention of CINV in patients receiving other types of less emetogenic chemotherapy is yet to be determined, it is expected that it will quickly find a role in prevention of CINV in patients receiving highly emetogenic chemotherapy.

Anticholinergic Drugs. Anticholinergic drugs include muscarinic antagonists such as scopolamine and H$_1$ receptor antagonist antihistamines. Scopolamine and other anticholinergic agents have long been used to prevent and treat PONV because they decrease the volume of gastric secretions and reduce GI motility. Anticholinergic drugs are also used to treat motion sickness and, in the case of the antihistamines,

for treating nausea and vomiting associated with pregnancy. The antiemetic effects of the antihistamines result primarily from their anticholinergic activity, not the blocking of histamine receptors.[55]

The most commonly used anticholinergic antiemetic drugs include scopolamine (hyoscine) and the antihistamines promethazine, diphenhydramine, cyclizine, and meclizine. The choice of drug depends on the period for which antinausea protection is needed and the side effects. Clinical studies indicate that oral scopolamine (0.2 to 0.6 mg) is the drug of choice for brief periods of motion and an antihistamine is the drug of choice for longer periods.[1] Of the antihistamines, promethazine (25 mg) is the drug of choice.[55] Although higher doses have a longer duration of action, sedation usually is a problem. Cyclizine (50 mg) has fewer side effects than promethazine, but it has a shorter duration of action and is less effective for severe conditions. Meclizine (50 mg) is similar to cyclizine, and both drugs are used when nausea is mild and protection is needed for short periods. Diphenhydramine has a long duration, but excessive sedation usually is a problem. For very severe conditions, sympathomimetic drugs such as ephedrine are used in combination with scopolamine or antihistamines.

The transdermal (patch) delivery system for administering scopolamine has produced good results.[56] The 2-mm thick patch with a surface area of 2.5 cm^2 contains 1.5 mg of scopolamine. Part of the dose is contained in the hypoallergenic contact adhesive and is released immediately to saturate skin-binding sites and initiate absorption. The remainder of the dose is contained in a reservoir separated from the contact surface by a membrane that releases the drug at a constant rate of about 5 μg per hour for a period of approximately 66 hours. The patch is backed by a water-resistant layer. The manufacturers recommend that the patch be applied to the postauricular skin (a highly permeable skin site of the body) 4 to 6 hours before the user expects to be in motion.

About 67% of people using transdermal scopolamine complain of dryness of the mouth, although this is not a contraindication. Drowsiness occurs in about 17% of patients, and blurred vision is experienced by about 12% of users and probably results in some cases from transfer of drug to the eyes by the fingers. Potential users should be advised to try the patch before using them in a travel situation and to wash their hands after applying the patch. The patch should not be used in children and adolescents, during pregnancy, in patients with glaucoma or a family history of glaucoma, and in those with psychosis.

A gel form of scopolamine for topical use has been compounded by many pharmacists and used at a time when production problems caused the patch to be temporarily withdrawn from the market. This dosage form has similar effects as the marketed patch.[57]

Corticosteroids. A variety of studies have shown that dexamethasone and, to a lesser extent, prednisolone and methylprednisolone can be effective antiemetics as single agents or in combination with other antiemetics. The antiemetic mechanism of action is unknown, but it has been suggested that the drugs act by inhibiting prostaglandin synthesis in the hypothalamus. Other actions of the corticosteroids (i.e., mood elevation, increased appetite, and a sense of well-being) may be responsible for patient acceptance and positive outcomes.[58]

When administered as an antiemetic for chemotherapy-induced vomiting, the antiemetic effects of dexamethasone are comparable to those of high-dose metoclopramide (1 to 3 mg/kg) in controlling nausea and vomiting associated with low-dose cisplatin (less than 60 mg/m^2) therapy and standard doses of chemotherapeutic agents with moderately emetogenic activity. However, metoclopramide appears to be more effective than dexamethasone against high-dose cisplatin (120 mg/m^2) and other highly emetogenic cancer chemotherapy agents. Dexamethasone also appears to be more effective against emesis induced by moderately emetogenic agents than standard doses of oral prochlorperazine (10 mg).[58] The overall antiemetic activity can be improved when dexamethasone is added to metoclopramide and prochlorperazine therapy.[59] A randomized, double-blind, parallel-group study comparing ondansetron plus dexamethasone with metoclopramide plus dexamethasone demonstrated that ondansetron plus dexamethasone is highly effective and is superior to metoclopramide plus dexamethasone in preventing carboplatin-induced emesis.[60] Recent studies have demonstrated significantly less nausea and vomiting with the combination of dexamethasone plus a serotonin antagonist for both moderately emetogenic chemotherapy[61–63] and highly emetogenic chemotherapy.[64,65] The dexamethasone dose used in these studies ranged from 8 to 20 mg. Oral dolasetron and dexamethasone have been shown to be as effective in preventing emesis as intravenously administered antiemetics.[64]

When used in PONV, a quantitative systematic review of 17 trials with 1,946 patients demonstrated that a single prophylactic dose of dexamethasone is more effective than placebo and without clinically significant toxicity. Dexamethasone appears to be more effective in late emesis (i.e., up to 24 hours) than in emesis occurring within 6 hours postoperatively. The combination of dexamethasone with a serotonin antagonist is also more effective in lowering the absolute risk of PONV.[66]

The advantage of the steroids, apart from their efficacy, is their relative lack of side effects with short-term use. Lethargy, weakness, euphoria, a sense of well-being, insomnia, increased appetite, and generalized swelling are the more common side effects of corticosteroids. Other rare effects reported include headache, metallic taste, abdominal discomfort, itchy throat, and a swollen feeling in the mouth. Adverse effects associated with the long-term use of corticosteroids are not applicable in this setting. Dexamethasone is also reported to significantly decrease the incidence of diarrhea and sedation associated with metoclopramide therapy.[59] Further trials are needed to establish the optimal dosing regimens for use with the various antineoplastic agents and the advantages of combining corticosteroids with other antiemetics.

Cannabinoids. In light of numerous reports that smoking marijuana reduces nausea, the antiemetic properties of the active ingredients delta-8- and 9-THC (dronabinol) and synthetic analogs such as nabilone and levonantradol have been studied extensively. Proposed mechanisms of action are that the cannabinoids act in the cerebral cortex to inhibit pathways to the VC, exert an anticholinergic effect on cholinergic terminals in Auerbach plexus, and possibly mediate the prostaglandin cyclic nucleotide system.[67] Other studies indicate that there is no dopaminergic antagonist activity.[68]

Pharmacokinetic studies of THC show that absorption from the GI tract is slow and erratic, with bioavailability less than 10%, although this may depend on the formulation. THC is highly protein bound (97%). Peak plasma concentrations are attained in about 1 hour after oral administration with serum levels in the 5 to 10 ng/mL range producing antiemetic activity. Higher serum levels are associated with greater antiemetic effect but with substantially more adverse effects. The terminal half-life of THC is 20 to 30 hours, but other active metabolites take 1 to 2 days for elimination. Patients report a correlation with the peak serum concentrations and a euphoric high. The high following oral administration usually begins 30 to 60 minutes after ingestion, peaks in 1 to 3 hours, and lasts for 4 to 6 hours. Smoking THC cigarettes raises bioavailability (to about 20%), with onset of action in 6 to 12 minutes. Peak levels are attained in 30 to 120 minutes with a duration lasting 3 to 4 hours. Normal behavior is observed 24 hours after administration.[67,68]

THC has been shown to be more effective than placebo and as effective as prochlorperazine in patients receiving moderately emetogenic chemotherapy. It is less effective than metoclopramide and associated with more side effects when used to prevent emesis secondary to cisplatin therapy. Most common adverse effects associated with THC therapy include dry mouth, sedation, orthostatic hypotension, dizziness, and confusion. Dysphoric effects such as depressed mood, dreaming or fantasizing, perception distortion, and elated mood are more common with doses greater than 5 mg/m^2. Younger patients appear to tolerate these side effects better than older patients or patients who have not previously used marijuana.[69] Voth and Schwartz[70] evaluated research published between 1975 and 1996 on the medical uses, complications, and legal precedents for the use of THC and crude marijuana. They concluded that pure THC is beneficial in treating nausea associated with cancer chemotherapy, but with the availability of other effective antiemetic agents and pure THC (dronabinol) as a prescription, crude marijuana need not be made available for medicinal purposes. Tramer et al[71] completed a meta analysis of 30 randomized controlled trials published between 1975 and 1997 that included 1,366 patients. Sixteen of the studies tested oral nabilone, 13 tested oral dronabinol, and 1 tested intramuscular levonantradol. Analysis indicated that cannabinoids were more effective antiemetics than the comparators (e.g., prochlorperazine, metoclopramide, placebo) for moderately emetogenic chemotherapy, but there were also substantial side effects. Beneficial side effects included sedation (30%), a sensation of a ''high'' (20%), and euphoria (15%). Severe adverse effects that can be directly attributed to the cannabinoids included dysphoria or depression (13%), hallucinations (6%), and paranoia (9%). Approximately 9% of patients treated with cannabinoids discontinued treatment who would not have stopped treatment had they taken a placebo or another antiemetic.

Nabilone is rapidly and well absorbed orally (96%) with an elimination half-life of about 2 hours. Studies indicate that nabilone is more effective than placebo and prochlorperazine against moderately emetogenic chemotherapeutic agents. However, it is not as effective as metoclopramide with vomiting associated with cisplatin therapy. Nabilone has been reported to have fewer euphoric effects than THC.[72]

Because of the mind-altering effects of the cannabinoids and the potential for abuse, these agents have been used as antiemetics only in patients receiving chemotherapy. The cannabinoids have more utility in younger patients who are refractory to other antiemetic regimens and in whom combination therapy may be more effective.

Benzodiazepines. The benzodiazepines, diazepam, lorazepam, and midazolam, are effective in reducing not only the frequency of nausea and vomiting but also the anxiety

often associated with chemotherapy[73,74] and surgery.[75] This action probably results from a combination of effects, including sedation, reduction in anxiety, possible depression of the VC, and an amnesic effect. Of these, the amnesic effect appears to be the most important in treating patients with cancer, and in this respect, lorazepam and midazolam are superior to diazepam. The sedative and amnesic effects are dose-related with higher doses (4 mg or above) of lorazepam inducing amnesic effects that persist for a longer period and occur in a larger percentage of patients. Amnesia does not correlate well with sedation. Sedation may remain high while the amnesic effects decline.

After intravenous administration of lorazepam or midazolam, the onset of sedative, anxiolytic, and amnesic action usually occurs within 1 to 5 minutes. The duration of action after intravenous administration of midazolam usually is less than 2 hours; however, dose-dependent actions may persist for up to 6 hours in some patients. After intramuscular administration, the onset of action of lorazepam is 15 to 30 minutes and the duration of action is 12 to 24 hours. After intramuscular administration of midazolam, onset of action occurs within 5 to 15 minutes but may not be maximal for 20 to 60 minutes; the duration of action is about 2 hours, although the range is 1 to 6 hours. The onset of action of orally administered lorazepam is about 30 minutes with peak activity occurring within 2 hours. Duration of action is 4 to 6 hours. The elimination half-life of lorazepam is 10 to 20 hours with no active metabolites, whereas that of midazolam is 1 to 12 hours with active metabolites.

Clinically, midazolam and lorazepam are most useful in combination with other antiemetics such as the serotonin antagonists, metoclopramide, and dexamethasone. The anxiolytic and amnesic effects results in increased patient satisfaction and decreased anxiety.[76] The greatest benefit from benzodiazepine therapy is derived by patients who have not received prior chemotherapy and who have not developed negative conditioning by episodes of nausea and vomiting (see ''Anticipatory Nausea and Vomiting''). Side effects associated with benzodiazepine therapy are drowsiness and dizziness. Patients should not be left unattended in the sedated, amnesic state because vomiting may still occur and could lead to aspiration. Because of its short half-life and short duration of action, midazolam may be the more appropriate adjunctive antiemetic for outpatient use.

TREATMENT OF SELECTED CAUSES OF NAUSEA AND VOMITING

Chemotherapy-Induced Nausea and Vomiting. CINV is the most unpleasant adverse effect associated with the use of antineoplastic agents. Many patients regard it as the most stressful aspect of their disease, more so even than the prospect of dying. Because the object of therapy in many cases is to prolong life, the effect of CINV on the quality of life must be considered. Also, many patients whose prognosis is good, find it difficult to adhere with chemotherapy regimens and may request that they be discontinued because of CINV. Before contemporary treatment regimens for CINV were tested, one multicenter survey found that as many as 10% of patients refused to continue with chemotherapy because of nausea and vomiting.[77]

Three types of emesis have been identified in patients receiving chemotherapy:

- Anticipatory nausea and vomiting
- Acute CINV
- Delayed emesis

Patients may also have emesis for reasons other than chemotherapy, perhaps induced by medications such as analgesics, or tumor-related complications such as intestinal obstruction. Addressing these matters usually is more important than selecting antiemetic therapy.[78] Apart from distressing the patient, severe vomiting complicates the patient's medical condition, causing dehydration, metabolic alkalosis, electrolyte deficiencies, nutritional impairment including cachexia, and physical injury, including esophageal tears and bone fractures.

Anticipatory Nausea and Vomiting. The patient's fear of CINV may lead to anticipatory nausea or vomiting (ANV). Anticipatory nausea alone has been reported in up to 78% of patients[79] and anticipatory vomiting in up to 38%.[80] Patients who develop ANV are more likely to have increased pretreatment anxiety, greater posttreatment dizziness and vomiting, and a delayed onset of postchemotherapy nausea and vomiting.[79] Patients who experience ANV are more likely to be younger and to have received twice as many courses of chemotherapy with more drugs for about three times longer than patients who do not experience ANV.[80,81] ANV correlates with the emetic potential of chemotherapy regimens and with the severity of nausea and vomiting after chemotherapy. Although considerable interpatient variability is observed, the onset of ANV usually starts 2 to 4 hours before treatment and is most severe at the time of drug administration.[82] It is believed that ANV is a conditioned response triggered by the sight or smell of the clinic or hospital or by the knowledge that treatment is imminent. ANV tends to become more severe as treatments progress unless behavior therapy modifies the conditioned response.[83] Such treatments include progressive muscle relaxation, mind diversion, hypnosis, self-hypnosis, and systematic desensitization. People with a negative attitude toward therapy, such as the belief that it will be of no benefit, are more likely to develop ANV than those with a positive attitude. A positive relationship between the patient and health care professionals is important in the success of behavioral treatment of CINV. The patient must be able to communicate freely with the staff about real and imagined fears about therapy and thereby develop positive attitudes toward their treatment. In this age of managed care, health maintenance organizations, and rotating medical staff in teaching hospitals and clinics, the patient may not always see the same health care provider.[83]

Complications associated with ANV underscore the need to accompany the initial course of emesis-producing chemotherapy with the most effective antiemetic regimen and continue vigorous therapy with each subsequent cycle of chemotherapy.[62,78] Adding lorazepam to antiemetic regimens induces an amnesic effect about chemotherapy and emesis in some patients[84] and has received subjective support from patients.[85] If delayed emesis is associated with any of the agents in the chemotherapeutic regimen, effective antiemetic therapy should be continued long enough to reduce the frequency of nausea and emesis, thus minimizing the risk of preconditioning the patient against further chemotherapy and ANV.

Acute Chemotherapy-Induced Nausea and Vomiting. The choice of antiemetic therapy for patients receiving antineoplastic therapy should take into account both patient and drug factors.

Patient Factors. The incidence and severity of CINV generally are greater among people of advanced age, those in poor general health (especially if cachetic), and those with metabolic disturbances, (i.e., dehydration, uremia, GI tract obstruction, or infection). Patient age can also influence the response to antiemetic drugs. For example, patients under age 30 are more sensitive to the extrapyramidal effects of dopaminergic blockade from phenothiazines or high-dose metoclopramide than older patients. However, younger patients tolerate cannabinoids better than older people. Patients who have a history of chronic heavy alcohol usage (more than five mixed drinks per day) tolerate chemotherapy with fewer bouts of emesis than those without this history.[78] Patients who are prone to motion sickness seem to be more sensitive to the emetic effects of cytotoxic agents. Because these two types of emesis are mediated by different mechanisms, this correlation probably reflects a psychogenic component. Finally, the patient's mental outlook and attitude toward therapy can influence the frequency and severity of emetic reactions considerably.

Drug Factors. The emetogenic potential of antineoplastic drugs varies greatly, ranging from more than 90% in the case of cisplatin to 10% or less with chlorambucil. Table 47.5 classifies chemotherapeutic agents in terms of emetogenicity, although emetogenicity is also influenced by the dose, duration, and frequency of courses. The effects of combinations of chemotherapeutic agents on vomiting are poorly understood.

The extensive literature on testing antiemetics for use with antineoplastic agents often is difficult to interpret. Comparisons between trials are difficult because of differences in protocol, cytotoxic drugs, and patient characteristics.[73,86] Most prospective clinical trials that test efficacy of antiemetics use patients who have not had prior exposure to chemotherapy (chemotherapy-naive patients). Success rates of antiemetic regimens are substantially more variable after multiple courses of chemotherapy. Some studies rely en-

TABLE 47.5	Relative Emetic Activity of Chemotherapeutic Agents

1. Very high emetic incidence (>90%)
   Carmustine >250 mg/m²
   Cisplatin >50 mg/m²
   Cyclophosphamide >1,500 mg/m²
   Dacarbazine >500 mg
   Dactinomycin
   Lomustine >60 mg
   Mechlorethamine
   Streptozocin
2. High emetic incidence (60%–90%)
   Carboplatin
   Carmustine <250 mg/m²
   Cisplatin <50 mg/m²
   Cyclophosphamide >750 mg/m² <1,500 mg/m²
   Cytarabine >1 g/m²
   Dacarbazine <500 mg
   Doxorubicin >60 mg/m²
   Ifosfamide >1.5 g
   Lomustine <60 mg
   Methotrexate >1,000 mg/m²
   Procarbazine (oral)
3. Moderate emetic incidence (30%–60%)
   Cyclophosphamide <750 mg/m²
   Cyclophosphamide (oral)
   Doxorubicin 20–60 mg/m²
   Epirubicin <90 mg/m²
   Hexamethylmelamine (oral)
   Idarubicin

Ifosfamide
Irinotecan
Methotrexate 250–1,000 mg/m²
Mitoxantrone <15 mg/m²
4. Low emetic incidence (10%–30%)
   Capecitabine
   Docetaxel
   Etoposide
   5-Fluorouracil <1,000 mg/m²
   Gemcitabine
   Methotrexate >50 mg/m² <250 mg/m²
   Mitomycin
   Paclitaxel
   Topotecan
5. Very low emetic incidence (<10%)
   Bleomycin
   Busulfan
   Chlorambucil (oral)
   2-Chlorodeoxyadenosine
   Fludarabine
   Hydroxyurea
   Methotrexate <50 mg/m²
   L-phenylalanine mustard (oral)
   Thioguanine (oral)
   Vinblastine
   Vincristine
   Vinorelbine

(Data from Hesketh P, Kris M, Grunberg S, et al. Proposal for classifying the acute emetogenicity of cancer chemotherapy. J Clin Oncol 15:103–109, 1997; Hesketh PJ. Defining the emetogenicity of cancer chemotherapy regimens: relevance to clinical practice. The Oncologist 4:191–196, 1999; Farley P, Dempsey C, Shillington A, et al. Patients' self-reported functional status after granisetron or ondansetron therapy to prevent chemotherapy-induced nausea and vomiting at six cancer centers. Am J Health Syst Pharm 54:2478–2482, 1997.)

tirely on objective data alone (i.e., the frequency of vomiting and the volume of vomitus) without investigating patient attitudes, performance capabilities, or quality of life issues. A patient who vomits only occasionally but experiences nausea continually may have a poorer quality of life than someone who vomits more frequently but has little intervening nausea. Hesketh et al[87,88] have proposed a classification of emetogenicity of chemotherapeutic agents that may serve as a framework to allow more accurate comparisons of the antiemetic effects of medicines with subsequent development of treatment guidelines.

It is clear that major progress has occurred in treating CINV,[89] and the following general recommendations can be made:

■ Antiemetics are most effective when administered prophylactically against nausea and vomiting. Most nausea and vomiting starts 1 to 4 hours after chemotherapy is initiated; therefore, in general, antiemetics should be administered 30 to 60 minutes before chemotherapy is administered. Doses, efficacies, and severity of adverse effects of primary antiemetic drugs are given in Table 47.6. Therapy must be individualized, and the doses and treatment schedules given are meant as guidelines only. All antiemetics except antimuscarinics (anticholinergics and antihistamines) have been found useful in treating CINV.

■ All patients being treated with moderate to very high emetogenic chemotherapeutic agents (Table 47.5) should receive prophylactic antiemetic therapy before antineoplastic therapy is initiated. Combinations of ondansetron, granisetron, dolasetron, or palonosetron plus dexamethasone, plus lorazepam, plus prochlorperazine are the drugs of choice in treating cisplatin-induced emesis.[90] An alter-

| TABLE 47.6 | Efficacy, Dose, and Toxicity of Antiemetics Used in the Treatment of Chemotherapy-Induced Nausea and Vomiting (CINV) |

	Antiemetic	Dosage Range	Adverse Drug Activity[a] (doses must be individualized)[b] Effects[c]
Phenothiazines			
Prochlorperazine	+ +	5–10 mg q2–4h PO; 5–10 mg q 3–6 h IM./IV[d]; 25 mg pr q6h	+/+ +
Chlorpromazine	+ +	25–50 mg q3–6h PO 25 mg q4–6h PO/IM/IV[d]/pr	+/+ +
Butyrophenones			
Droperidol	+ +	1–3 mg q4–6h IV or 5 mg IV 30 min prior to chemotherapy then continuous infusion of 1–1.5 mg/hr for 9–12 hr	+/+ +
Haloperidol	+ +	1–3 mg q4–6h PO/IM/IV[d]	+/+ +
Metoclopramide (high dose) doses after chemotherapy	+ + +	1–3 mg/kg IVPB over 15 min 0.5 hr before and q2h × 3–4 doses	+ +
Corticosteroids			
Dexamethasone	+ + +	4–25 mg PO/IV before chemotherapy and q4–6h × 1–2 days	0/+
Methylprednisolone	+ + +	125–500 mg PO/IV 2 hr before chemotherapy and 2 hr after or as infusion	0/+
Benzodiazepines			
Lorazepam	+ +/+ + +	1–4 mg q4–6h PO/IV; can commence when patient arrives for chemotherapy	+/+ +
Cannabinoids			
Δ-9-THC (Dronabinol)	+ +[e]	5–15 mg/m² q4h PO; commence night before chemotherapy	+ +/+ + +
Serotonin Antagonists			
Granisetron	+ + +	1 mg PO within 60 min before starting chemotherapy Repeat once at 12 hr	+ +
		10 µg/kg IVPB over 5 min within 30 min before starting chemotherapy	
Ondansetron	+ + +	8 mg PO q4h × 3 doses beginning 30 min before start of emetogenic chemotherapy. Follow chemotherapy with 8 mg q8h for 1–2 days. 32 mg IVPB as a single dose, or 0.15 mg/kg IVPB q4h × 3 doses. Infuse dose over 15 min beginning 30 min before start of emetogenic chemotherapy.	+ +
Dolasetron	+ + +	100 mg PO within 60 minutes before chemotherapy 1.8 mg/kg or 100 mg IVPB over up to 15 min within 30 min before starting chemotherapy[f]	+ +
Palonosetron	+ + +	0.25 mg IV over 30 seconds, 30 minutes before the start of chemotherapy	+ +
Neurokinin-1 Antagonist			
Aprepitant	+ + +[g]	125 mg PO 1 hr before chemotherapy on day 1; 80 mg PO once daily in the morning on days 2 and 3	+/+ +

[a]Antiemetic activity against cisplatin: 0, little or none, to + + +, high. [b]Doses are examples only and represent the ranges given in the references cited in the text. Best results are usually obtained with a combination of antiemetics. Frequently dosing is begun before chemotherapy. [c]0, little or none, to + + +, high incidence. [d]Can be administered by slow (15–20 min) IV administration. [e]May have marked efficacy in young patients. [f]May also be given undiluted IV as 100mg/30 sec. [g]When aprepitant is used in combination with a corticosteroid and serotonin antagonist.

qh, each hour; PO, by mouth; IM, intramuscularly; IV, intravenously; pr, per rectum; IVPB, intravenous piggyback.

native for the patient who cannot tolerate serotonin receptor antagonists is high-dose metoclopramide, dexamethasone, and diphenhydramine.[78,91–94] Based on current clinical evidence, aprepitant, the NK_1 antagonist, should also be added to these regimens. Antiemetic therapy should be continued for 2 to 4 days to prevent or minimize delayed vomiting (see "Delayed Emesis").

■ Emesis induced by moderately emetogenic agents such as methotrexate and 5-fluorouracil can be treated prophylactically with prochlorperazine and dexamethasone, and therapy should be continued for 24 hours.[95]

■ Since antiemetics have adverse effects and do place the patient at some risk, pretreatment is not recommended when low-risk emetogenic agents are administered. Prochlorperazine can be used as needed in these patients.

■ Second-line treatment of any emesis may include phenothiazines, butyrophenones, benzodiazepines, and cannabinoids. Nonpharmacologic measures can be used at any time as adjunct treatments.

The rationale for using combinations of antiemetic agents is based on the assumption that cytotoxic agents produce emesis by multiple mechanisms. Antiemetics also act by multiple mechanisms, and a combination could have a synergistic action. Side effects also are a factor in the choice of an antiemetic. Combinations of drugs acting by different mechanisms are less likely to produce adverse reactions than the highest dosage of a single drug. In some cases a second antiemetic agent may reduce the side effects of the first drug (e.g., dexamethasone, diphenhydramine, or lorazepam is added to high-dose metoclopramide).

The availability of the 5-HT_3 antagonists has made a significant impact in reducing the frequency of nausea and vomiting episodes in patients receiving moderately and highly emetogenic chemotherapy. Unfortunately, the cost of the wide use of serotonin receptor antagonists for most cases of CINV, regardless of emetogenicity, has become prohibitive. These high costs have necessitated the development of guidelines for using the antiemetic agents.[96–98] Multidisciplinary teams of physicians, nurses, and pharmacists have developed highly successful guidelines[99,100] for use of antiemetics based on the emetic potential of the chemotherapy, lower effective ondansetron doses,[98,99] higher effective doses of non–5-HT_3 antagonist antiemetics,[101] use of oral rather than parenteral dosage forms,[64,102] and avoidance of treatment of delayed-onset nausea and vomiting with 5-HT_3 antagonists.[90,103]

There has been a general perception among health care providers that the 5-HT_3 receptor antagonists improve the patient's quality of life because the frequency of nausea and vomiting is reduced by these agents. Assessment tools can be used to measure the impact of chemotherapy and antiemetics on patients' quality of life.[104,105] Comparison with preserotonin antagonist studies is difficult because of differing patient populations, use of much more aggressive chemotherapy, newer antineoplastic agents, and the avail-

ability of the new antiemetics. The serotonin antagonists have also brought the concept of delayed emesis much more clearly into focus as a separate entity (see "Delayed Emesis"), and preventing delayed emesis is much less successful than preventing acute emesis. de Boer-Dennert et al[106] repeated a study published in 1983 that cited nausea and vomiting as the two most distressing side effects associated with chemotherapy. The new study, following the use of serotonin antagonists, reported that nausea, hair loss, and vomiting were the three most distressing side effects of chemotherapy, even though the incidence and severity of acute nausea and vomiting were reduced significantly.

The Functional Living Index–Emesis (FLIE) provides an assessment of the impact of CINV on a patient's daily functioning.[105] A multicenter study was conducted to measure the impact of serotonin antagonists on quality of life and to determine whether there was a difference in scores between those treated with ondansetron or granisetron. The study demonstrated significantly lower FLIE scores in patients who had nausea and vomiting after chemotherapy but no difference in scores of patients receiving granisetron or ondansetron.[107] In a study that evaluated the use of aprepitant and the FLIE questionnaire, it demonstrated that patients who received aprepitant reported minimal or no effect of CINV on daily functioning (74.7%) when compared to patients receiving standard therapy (63.5%).[50]

The European Organization for Research and Treatment of Cancer (EORTC) Core Quality of Life Questionnaire (QLQ-C30) is another quality of life assessment tool consisting of 30 questions that measure five functional domains, a global quality of life domain, three symptom domains, five additional symptoms, and an item on financial status.[108] It has been shown that patients who received moderately or highly emetogenic chemotherapy who developed CINV had significantly lower physical, role, and social function scores and lower global quality of life scores than did those who were emesis-free.[109] It has been suggested that pretreatment quality scores could predict which patients are at greater risk for CINV, so that additional measures may be taken to minimize the severity of CINV.

Delayed Emesis. Delayed emesis is a distinct syndrome that occurs 24 or more hours after chemotherapy is administered. It has been reported in as many as 93% of patients receiving high-dose cisplatin. It is particularly severe in patients receiving doses greater than 100 mg per square meters. Symptoms may occur 24 to 120 hours after cisplatin administration but are most severe at 48 to 72 hours. Patients who have incomplete control of acute emesis often experience delayed emesis. Delayed nausea and vomiting usually are less severe than those that may occur acutely but can still be important in developing ANV and reducing activity, nutritional state, and hydration. The causes of delayed nausea and vomiting are not known, but different mechanisms appear to play a role in acute and delayed emesis.[110] Symptoms may be caused directly by the action of chemotherapeutic agents or their metabolites on the nervous system or GI tract.[111] In addition to delayed emesis caused by chemotherapy or its metabolites, episodes of delayed vomiting often are associated with provocative events such as brushing teeth, using mouthwash, manipulating dentures, seeing food, and, in the morning, standing up after getting out of bed. A combination of prochlorperazine (10 mg), lorazepam (0.5 mg), and diphenhydramine (50 mg) all given orally 1 hour before breakfast, lunch, and dinner has been reported to be successful in controlling delayed emesis secondary to cisplatin therapy.[112] The combination of oral dexamethasone and metoclopramide has been shown to decrease the frequency of delayed vomiting.[113] The Italian Group for Antiemetic Research found similar protection in treating cisplatin-induced delayed emesis when ondansetron plus dexamethasone or high-dose metoclopramide plus dexamethasone was used. Their study also reinforced the observation that patients who had complete control of acute emesis had a much lower incidence of delayed-onset emesis.[114] The 5-HT$_3$ receptor antagonists have been no more effective than placebo in controlling delayed emesis secondary to cisplatin therapy when given alone.[115–117] Recent studies indicate that adding aprepitant, the NK$_1$ antagonist, significantly reduces the incidence of delayed emesis. The addition of aprepitant has been reported to control delayed emesis in 67% of patients compared to 47% control in patients receiving standard (serotonin antagonist plus dexamethasone) antiemetic therapy.[50] In another study, there was 63% control in the aprepitant plus standard therapy (granisetron and dexamethasone) compared with control in 29% of patients who received only standard therapy.[51]

It has been noted that if complete 24-hour control after cisplatin administration is not achieved, emesis usually begins at 17 to 22 hours. This raises the question of whether this is the start of delayed emesis, even though, by definition, 24 hours had not passed.[64,118] Gralla et al[118] devised a study that demonstrated that ondansetron plus dexamethasone started 16 hours after cisplatin administration was more successful (62% vs. 52%) than metoclopramide plus dexamethasone[113] in controlling delayed vomiting.

Postoperative Nausea and Vomiting. PONV is a complication of many surgical procedures. Over the past few years, this disorder has received greater attention because of the increase in outpatient surgical procedures. PONV can lengthen the patient's recovery time and significantly delay release from an ambulatory surgical center, even to the point of necessitating hospital admission.[119] Serious complications of PONV are uncommon, but the patient can become dehydrated or experience electrolyte abnormalities that can delay wound healing or lead to other complications. The overall incidence for all surgeries and all types of patients is 25% to 30%.[120] However, PONV occurs in as many as 70% of high-risk patients. Risk factors for PONV in adults include female sex, nonsmoking status, previous history of PONV or motion sickness, use of volatile anesthetics within the previous 2 hours, use of nitrous oxide, use of intraoperative or postoperative opioids, duration of surgery, and the type of surgery. Surgeries in which there is a higher risk of PONV include: laparoscopy, ear-nose-throat, neurosurgery, breast, strabismus, laparotomy, plastic surgery, dental surgery, and orthopaedic shoulder procedures.[75] Use of regional anesthesia, propofol for induction and maintenance of anesthesia, intraoperative supplemental oxygen, and hydration; avoidance of nitrous oxide and volatile anesthetics; and minimal use of neostigmine and opioids can significantly reduce the incidence of PONV.[75]

Patients who are considered to be at moderate to high risk for PONV should be considered for prophylactic antiemetic therapy. In addition to minimizing risk factors listed above, a "multimodal treatment approach" is recommended because of the variety of receptor types associated with PONV. Therapy may include hydration, supplemental oxygen, a benzodiazepine for anxiolysis, a combination of antiemetics (e.g., droperidol, dexamethasone, serotonin antagonist [Table 47.7]), total IV anesthesia (e.g., propofol and remifentanil) and analgesia with a nonsteroidal anti-inflammatory drug (NSAID) (e.g., ketorolac) rather than an opioid.[75] Nonpharmacologic techniques prior to surgery using acupuncture, transcutaneous electrical nerve stimulation, and acupoint stimulation have also been shown to reduce PONV.[75]

Patients who did not receive prophylaxis or in whom it was not effective must be evaluated to identify factors that induce emesis. Blood draining down the throat, patient-controlled opiate analgesia, or GI obstruction are potential causes of PONV. If no inciting factors are identified, rescue antiemetics may be indicated (Table 47.8).

TABLE 47.7	Antiemetics Used to Treat Postoperative Nausea and Vomiting*a*	
Drug	**Dose**	**Timing of Administration**
Dolasetron	12.5 mg IV	At end of surgery
Granisetron	0.35–1 mg IV	At end of surgery
Ondansetron	4–8 mg IV	At end of surgery
Dexamethasone	5–10 mg IV	Before induction
Droperidol	0.625–1.25 mg IV	At end of surgery
Dimenhydrinate	1–2 mg/kg IV	
Prochlorperazine	5–10 mg IV	At end of surgery
Promethazine	12.5–25 mg IV	At end of surgery
Scopolamine	Transdermal patch	Evening prior to surgery or 4 hr before end of anesthesia

*a*Use smallest dose.

IV, intravenously.

(From Gan TJ, Meyer T, Apfel CC, et al. Consensus guidelines for managing postoperative nausea and vomiting. Anesth Analg 97:62–71, 2003, with permission.)

TABLE 47.8	Rescue Treatment of Postoperative Nausea and Vomiting (PONV) When Initial Therapy Fails
Initial Therapy	**Follow-up Treatment**
No prophylaxis or dexamethasone	Administer small-dose 5-HT$_3$ antagonist[a]
5-HT$_3$ antagonist[a] plus second agent[b]	Use drug from different class
Triple therapy with 5-HT$_3$ antagonist[a] plus two other agents when PONV occurs <6 hr after surgery	Do not repeat initial therapy; Use drug from a different class or propofol 20 mg as needed in postanesthesia care unit
Triple therapy with 5-HT$_3$ antagonist[a] plus two other agents when PONV occurs >6 hr after surgery	Repeat 5-HT$_3$ antagonist[a] and droperidol (not dexamethasone or transdermal scopolamine)
	Use drug from different class

[a]Small-dose 5-HT antagonist dosing: ondansetron 1.0 mg, dolasetron 12.5 mg, granisetron 0.1 mg. [b]Alternative therapies for rescue: droperidol 0.625 mg IV, dexamethasone 2–4 mg IV, and promethazine 12.5 mg IV.
(From Gan TJ, Meyer T, Apfel CC, et al. Consensus guidelines for managing postoperative nausea and vomiting. Anesth Anal 97:62–71, 2003, with permission.)

Many other therapies for PONV have been reported. Metoclopramide has been used extensively for PONV for many years. A quantitative systematic review of randomized, placebo-controlled studies, however, could not document clinically relevant antiemetic effect from metoclopramide in the dose range recommended (e.g., 5 to 30 mg) for the prevention of PONV. There was also no evidence of an increased risk of adverse reactions with metoclopramide when compared with placebo.[121] The use of ginger as an antiemetic in day surgery has been evaluated, but a systematic review of randomized clinical trials[122] cited a lack of literature supporting the use of ginger in PONV.[122,123] Cannabinoids have also not been shown to control emesis associated with PONV.[124]

Motion Sickness. Motion sickness is not a true sickness but rather a normal response to an abnormal situation. Any healthy person can experience this response given the right type and degree of stimulation. The susceptibility to motion sickness varies greatly, with approximately one-third of people being very sensitive, one-third reacting only to rough conditions, and one-third reacting only to extreme conditions. Although there is no question about the physical basis of motion sickness, it is also very clear that psychological factors play an important part in suppressing and enhancing the tendency to be sick.

The stimuli that produce motion sickness arise in the labyrinth of the inner ear. They are carried by afferent fibers that synapse in the vestibular region of the medulla where they are thought to stimulate the release of an excessive amount of acetylcholine that acts on the CTZ, which then stimulates the VC.[1,125] A proposed theory suggests that motion sickness arises when there is conflict between the sensory information being transmitted by the eyes, vestibular system, and nonvestibular proprioceptors, particularly as it relates to previous experience. As a result of this conflict, an imbalance of cholinergic and sympathetic transmitters occurs in the medulla, which can be corrected by giving anticholinergic drugs or sympathomimetics. The vestibular system plays the central

role. True immunity to motion sickness is possible only in a person who lacks a normally functioning peripheral vestibular system.

Nausea is the most common symptom of motion sickness, but most patients experience several other symptoms including pallor, yawning, restlessness, and cold sweats. Vomiting does not inevitably result from nausea because elimination of the offending stimulus can prevent it. The importance of conflicting sensory stimuli as a cause of motion sickness is illustrated in a practical way by the relief obtained when the person can establish a satisfactory stable visual reference. For example, looking out of a car window (particularly from the front seat) can give marked relief, whereas reading in a car (particularly in the rear seat) can provoke motion sickness.

Despite the very extensive literature on anti–motion sickness drug testing, there is a distinct lack of basic clinical pharmacology such as dose-response relationships and pharmacokinetic parameters. In accordance with the sensory conflict theory of motion sickness, drugs used to treat motion sickness would need to block acetylcholine or enhance norepinephrine activity in the central nervous system. Drugs that have proved effective include sympathomimetics and anticholinergics (Table 47.9). The choice of drug or drug combination depends on the expected duration and severity of the reaction. For severe conditions, as might be experienced by an astronaut adapting to weightlessness, combinations of scopolamine and dexamphetamine or amphetamine have shown the greatest efficacy.[126] Such combinations have the advantage that the stimulatory effects of the amphetamine offset the drowsiness caused by the scopolamine. Unfortunately, the tendency for amphetamines to be abused limits their usefulness in this disorder. Combinations of ephedrine and promethazine also are very effective and have been ranked just below the amphetamine-scopolamine combination.[55] Doses are given in Table 47.9.

Of the single drugs, oral scopolamine (0.2 to 0.6 mg) is the most effective for short periods of exposure (less than

TABLE 47.9	Doses and Duration of Action of Anti–Motion Sickness Drugs		
Severity of Sickness	**Drug**	**Oral Dose**[a]	**Duration of Action (hr)**
Severe	Scopolamine and dexamphetamine	0.2–0.6 mg scopolamine and 5–10 mg dexamphetamine[b]	6
Severe	Promethazine and ephedrine	25 mg promethazine and 25 mg TID ephedrine	12
Severe	Scopolamine	0.2–0.6 mg q6h[c]	4
Severe	Promethazine	25 mg tid	12
Moderate	Dimenhydrinate	50 mg 2–3 × daily	6
Mild	Cyclizine	50 mg 2–3 × daily	4
Mild	Meclizine	50 mg 2–3 × daily	6

[a]Anti–motion sickness drugs are most effective if therapy is initiated before exposure to motion. Usually therapy should be initiated about 30 min before departure and repeated if necessary.
[b]Used only under special circumstances (e.g., by service personnel). [c]Not more than four doses should be taken in 24 hr.
qh, each hour; tid, three times daily.

6 hours). Unfortunately, the commercially prepared oral dosage form is not available in the United States. For longer periods or for moderate to mild conditions, the antihistamines are the drugs of choice. Of these, promethazine (25 mg) and dimenhydrinate (50 to 100 mg) appears to be the most effective.[55] Transdermal scopolamine has been used successfully to treat motion sickness of several days' duration. It can be applied before entering situations in which motion sickness is likely to occur. All anti–motion sickness drugs are more effective if used prophylactically rather than after sickness has developed.

For patients with severe motion sickness, the oral route may be unavailable and therapy can be given by the intramuscular route. Scopolamine (0.2 mg) or promethazine (50 mg) (adult doses) may be given. Promethazine probably is the preferred injectable medication for acute motion sickness, and transdermal scopolamine could be used if a rapid onset is not necessary.

In therapeutic doses, all drugs used to treat motion sickness cause side effects. Anticholinergic drugs produce dry mouth, sedation, and blurred vision. The sympathomimetics produce tachycardia. In the case of scopolamine, the total dose should not exceed 1 mg in 24 hours because of effects on the central nervous system.

Nonpharmacologic therapy has also proven very successful in preventing and treating motion sickness. Behavioral modification can be effective for people whose employment involves frequent exposure to motion (e.g., pilots, sailors). Powdered ginger root was used in a double-blind, placebo-controlled study in passengers on an ocean cruise and found to significantly reduce the tendency to vomit and have cold sweats.[127] Acupuncture and acupressure have also been studied extensively. In acupressure techniques, a wristband with a pressure button located over the Neiguan (P6) Acupoint is worn by the patient. This technique has been effective in preventing motion sickness and treating PONV.[128]

Psychogenic Vomiting. Psychogenic vomiting can be self-induced or it can occur involuntarily in response to situations that the person considers threatening or distasteful (e.g., eating food whose origin is considered repulsive).

When a person presents with chronic or recurrent vomiting, a diagnosis of psychogenic vomiting is made after all other possible causes are eliminated (Table 47.1). The person with psychogenic vomiting usually does not lose weight and can control vomiting in certain situations (e.g., in public). It may not be possible to identify the causes of psychogenic vomiting and resolve the problem. A short course of an antiemetic drug such as metoclopramide or antianxiety drugs may be prescribed, along with counseling to treat psychogenic vomiting.

CONCLUSION

Nausea and vomiting ranges from a minor inconvenience of a transient GI infection to a severe and limiting adverse reaction to drug therapy. The consequences of vomiting can be severe. The cause of the nausea and vomiting should be determined before treatment is begun, and specific therapy should be chosen for each cause. Drug regimens specifically designed for the patient and the cause of nausea and vomiting, based on valid clinical studies, have a high success rate in treating this disorder. However, care should be taken to minimize any side effects from the antiemetic drugs.

KEY POINTS

NAUSEA AND VOMITING

- An accurate diagnosis is essential before treatment of nausea and vomiting begins
- Treat the cause if it can be identified

■ Assess for fluid and electrolyte loss

CHEMOTHERAPY-INDUCED NAUSEA AND VOMITING

■ There are three types of CINV: ANV, acute CINV, and delayed emesis
■ The emetogenic potential of antineoplastic drugs varies significantly (Table 47.5)
■ Antiemetics are most effective when administered 30 to 60 minutes before chemotherapy is administered
■ All patients being treated with moderate to very high emetogenic chemotherapeutic agents should receive prophylactic antiemetic therapy. Combinations of a serotonin antagonist plus dexamethasone, plus aprepitant, plus lorazepam, plus prochlorperazine are the drugs of choice
■ Emesis induced by moderately emetogenic agents may be treated prophylactically with dexamethasone and prochlorperazine
■ Prochlorperazine or dexamethasone alone is recommended if needed if the chemotherapy is of low emetic potential

POSTOPERATIVE NAUSEA AND VOMITING

■ The causes of PONV are multifactorial
■ A review of the patient's previous history can help determine who would benefit from prophylactic antiemetic therapy
■ Maintaining good hydration and adequate blood pressure and avoiding excess movement of the patient limit the incidence of PONV
■ No one medication or combination has been found to be the therapy of choice for PONV. Scopolamine, phenothiazines, droperidol, and the serotonin antagonists often are used to prevent PONV
■ The serotonin antagonists have good success rates and the fewest side effects, but are the most expensive

MOTION SICKNESS

■ Antiemetics are most effective when administered 30 to 60 minutes before activities that may induce motion sickness
■ Anticholinergic drugs have been studied the most extensively and are most frequently recommended (e.g., scopolamine, promethazine, dimenhydrinate)
■ Patients who experience motion sickness routinely because of their occupation might best be treated with behavioral therapy rather than drugs

SUGGESTED READINGS

American Society of Health-System Pharmacists, ASHP therapeutic guidelines on the pharmacologic management of nausea and vomiting in adult and pediatric patients receiving chemotherapy or radiation therapy or undergoing surgery. Am J Health Syst Pharm 56: 729–764, 1999.

Gan TJ, Meyer T, Apfel CC, et al. Consensus guidelines for managing postoperative nausea and vomiting. Anesth Analg 97:62–71, 2003.

Hesketh PJ. Defining the emetogenicity of cancer chemotherapy regimens: relevance to clinical practice. The Oncologist 4:191–196, 1999.

Kovac AL. Benefits and risks of newer treatments for chemotherapy-induced and postoperative nausea and vomiting. Drug Safety 26: 227–259, 2003.

REFERENCES

1. Barnes JH. The physiology and pharmacology of emesis. Mol Aspects Med 7:397–508, 1984.
2. Grunberg SM. Control of chemotherapy-induced emesis. N Engl J Med 329:1790–1796, 1993.
3. Mitchelson F. Pharmacological agents affecting emesis. Drugs 43: 295–315, 1992.
4. Cubeddu LX, Hoffmann IS, Fuenmayor NT, et al. Efficacy of ondansetron (GR38032F) and the role of serotonin in cisplatin-induced nausea and vomiting. N Engl J Med 322:810–816, 1990.
5. Bermudez J, Boyle EA, Miner WD, et al. The antiemetic potential of the 5-hydroxytryptamine$_3$ receptor antagonist BRL 43694. Br J Cancer 58:644–650, 1988.
6. Veyrat-Follet C, Farinotti R, Palmer JL. Physiology of chemotherapy-induced emesis and antiemetic therapy. Drugs 53:206–234, 1997.
7. Hesketh PJ, Grunberg SM, Gralla RJ, et al. The oral neurokinin-1 antagonist aprepitant for the prevention of chemotherapy-induced nausea and vomiting: a multinational, randomized, double-blind, placebo-controlled trial in patients receiving high dose cisplatin-the aprepitant protocol 052 study group. J Clin Oncol 22:5512–5519, 2003.
8. Dando TM, Perry CM. Aprepitant: a review of its use in the prevention of chemotherapy-induced nausea and vomiting. Drugs 64: 777–794, 2004.
9. Merck & Co. Inc. EMEND® (aprepitant) capsules: prescribing information. USA [online]. Available at: http://www.merck.com. Accessed May 24, 2004.
10. Malagelada JR, Camilleri M. Unexplained vomiting: a diagnostic challenge. Ann Intern Med 101:211–218, 1984.
11. Wampler G. Pharmacology and clinical effectiveness of phenothiazines and related drugs for managing chemotherapy-induced emesis. Drugs 25(Suppl 1):35–51, 1983.
12. Carr B, Doroshow J, Blayney D, et al. Toxicity and dose-response studies of prochlorperazine for cisplatin-induced emesis [abstract]. Proc Am Soc Clin Oncol 5:252, 1986.
13. Olver IN, Bishop JF, Hollcoat BL, et al. A phase-I dose finding study for intravenous prochlorperazine as an antiemetic for chemotherapy induced emesis [abstract]. Proc Am Soc Clin Oncol 7:287, 1988.
14. Carr BI, Somlo G, McDevitt J, et al. Pharmacokinetic profiles of high- and low-dose prochlorperazine [abstract]. Proc Am Soc Clin Oncol 7:294, 1988.
15. Food and Drug Administration. Box warning of droperidol. Available at: http://www.fda.gov/medwatch/SAFETY.2001/inapsine.htm. Accessed May 25, 2004.
16. Fozard JR. Neuronal 5-HT receptors in the periphery. Neuropharmacology 23:1473–1486, 1984.
17. Gralla RJ. Metoclopramide: a review of antiemetic trials. Drugs 25: 63–73, 1983.
18. McGovern EM, Grevel J, Bryson SM. Pharmacokinetics of high-dose metoclopramide in cancer patients. Clin Pharmacokinet 11: 415–424, 1986.
19. Bateman DN. Clinical pharmacokinetics of metoclopramide. Clin Pharmacokinet 8:523–529, 1983.
20. Grevel J, Whiting B, Kelman AW, et al. Population analysis of the pharmacokinetic variability of high-dose metoclopramide in cancer patients. Clin Pharmacokinet 14:52–63, 1983.
21. Parrish RH, Bonzo SM. Use of metoclopramide suppositories. Clin Pharm 2:395–396, 1983.
22. Tami JA, Waite WW. Metoclopramide suppository considerations. Drug Intell Clin Pharm 22:268–269, 1988.

23. Product information for Zofran. Research Triangle Park, NC: GlaxoWellcome, December 1996.
24. Product information for Anzemet. Kansas City, MO: Hoechst Marion Roussel, October, 1997.
25. Balfour JA, Goa KL. Dolasetron. Drugs 54:273–298, 1997.
26. Product information for Aloxi. Bloomington, MN: MGI Pharma, Inc., July, 2003.
27. Sanwald P, David M, Jow J. Characterization of the cytochrome P-450 enzymes involved in the in vitro metabolism of dolasetron. Drug Metab Dispos 24:602–609, 1996.
28. Product information for Kytril. Nutley, NJ: Roche Laboratories, Inc., December, 2000.
29. Marty M, Pouillart P, Scholl S. Comparison of the 5-hydroxytryptamine$_3$ (serotonin) antagonist ondansetron (GR38032F) with high-dose metoclopramide in the control of cisplatin-induced emesis. N Engl J Med 322:816–821, 1990.
30. Mathews H. Extrapyramidal reaction caused by ondansetron. Ann Pharmacother 30:196, 1996.
31. Kantor GS. Arrhythmia risk of antiemetic agents. Anesthesiology 97:286, 2002.
32. White PF. Droperidol: A cost-effective antiemetic for over thirty years. Anesth Analg 95:780–790, 2002.
33. Miller DR. Arrhythmogenic potential of antiemetics: perspective on risk-benefits. Can J Anesth 50:215–220, 2003.
34. De Mulder PHM, Selynaeve C, Vermorken JB, et al. Ondansetron compared with high-dose metoclopramide in prophylaxis of acute and delayed cisplatin-induced nausea and vomiting. Ann Intern Med 113:834–840, 1990.
35. Hesketh PJ. Comparative trials of ondansetron vs. metoclopramide in the prevention of acute cisplatin-induced emesis. Semin Oncol 19(Suppl 10):33–40, 1992.
36. Sledge G Jr, Einhorn L, Nagy C. Phase III double-blind comparison of intravenous ondansetron and metoclopramide as antiemetic therapy for patients receiving multiple-day cisplatin-based chemotherapy. Cancer 70:2524–2528, 1992.
37. Tsavaris N, Charalambidis G, Ganas N, et al. Ondansetron versus metoclopramide as antiemetic treatment during cisplatin-based chemotherapy. Acta Oncol 34:243–246, 1995.
38. Ruff P, Paska W, Goedhals L, et al. Ondansetron compared with granisetron in the prophylaxis of cisplatin-induced acute emesis: a multicenter double-blind, randomized, parallel-group study. Oncology 51:113–118, 1994.
39. Jantunen I, Muhonen T, Kataja V, et al. 5-HT3 receptor antagonists in the prophylaxis of acute vomiting induced by moderately emetogenic chemotherapy: a randomized study. Eur J Cancer 29A:1669–1672, 1993.
40. Noble A, Bremer K, Goedhals L, et al. A double-blind, randomized, crossover comparison of granisetron and ondansetron in 5-day fractionated chemotherapy: assessment of efficacy, safety and patient preference. Eur J Cancer 30A:1083–1088, 1994.
41. Gebbia V, Cannata G, Testa A, et al. Ondansetron versus granisetron in the prevention of chemotherapy induced nausea and vomiting: results of a prospective, randomized trial. Cancer 74:1945–1952, 1994.
42. Navari R, Gandara D, Hesketh S, et al. Comparative clinical trial of granisetron and ondansetron in the prophylaxis of cisplatin-induced emesis. J Clin Oncol 13:1242–1248, 1995.
43. Park J, Rha S, Yoo N, et al. A comparative study of intravenous granisetron versus intravenous and oral ondansetron in the prevention of nausea and vomiting associated with moderately emetogenic chemotherapy. Am J Clin Oncol 20:569–572, 1997.
44. Hesketh P, Navari R, Grote T, et al. Double-blind, randomized comparison of the antiemetic efficacy of intravenous dolasetron mesylate and intravenous ondansetron in the prevention of acute cisplatin-induced emesis in patients with cancer. J Clin Oncol 14:2242–2249, 1996.
45. Fauser AA, Duclos B, Chemaissani A, et al. Therapeutic equivalence of single oral doses of dolasetron mesylate and multiple doses of ondansetron for the prevention of emesis after moderately emetogenic chemotherapy. Eur J Cancer 32A:1523–1529, 1996.
46. Pater J, Lofters W, Zee B, et al. The role of the 5-HT3 antagonists ondansetron and dolasetron in the control of delayed onset nausea

and vomiting in patients receiving moderately emetogenic chemotherapy. Ann Oncol 8:181–185, 1997.
47. Audhuy B, Cappelaere P, Martin M, et al. A double-blind, randomized comparison of the anti-emetic efficacy of two intravenous doses of dolasetron mesylate and granisetron in patients receiving high dose cisplatin chemotherapy. Eur J Cancer 32A:807–813, 1996.
48. Chawla SP, Grunberg SM, Gralla RJ, et al. Establishing the dose of the oral NK1 antagonist aprepitant for the prevention of chemotherapy-induced nausea and vomiting. Cancer 97:2290–2300, 2003.
49. McCrea JB, Majundar AK, Goldberg MR, et al. Effects of the neurokinin1 receptor antagonist aprepitant on the pharmacokinetics of dexamethasone and methylprednisolone. Clin Pharmacol Ther 74:17–24, 2003.
50. Poli-Bigelli S, Rodrigues-Pereira J, Carides AD, et al. Addition of the neurokinin 1 receptor antagonist aprepitant to standard antiemetic therapy improves control of chemotherapy-induced nausea and vomiting. Cancer 97:3090–3098, 2003.
51. Campos D, Rodrigues-Pereira J, Reinhardt RR, et al. Prevention of cisplatin-induced emesis by the oral neurokinin-1 antagonist, MK-869, in combination with granisetron and dexamethasone or with dexamethasone alone. J Clin Oncol 19:1759–1767, 2001.
52. Olver IN. Aprepitant in antiemetic combinations to prevent chemotherapy-induced nausea and vomiting. Int J Clin Pract 58:201–206, 2004.
53. de Wit R, Herrstedt J, Rapoport B, et al. Addition of the oral NK1 antagonist aprepitant to standard antiemetics provides protection against nausea and vomiting during multiple cycles of cisplatin-induced chemotherapy. J Clin Oncol 21:5505–5511, 2003.
54. Van Belle S, Lichinitser MR, Navari RM, et al. Prevention of cisplatin-induced acute and delayed emesis by the selective neurokinin-1 antagonists L-758,298 and MK-869. Cancer 94:3032–3055, 2002.
55. Wood CD. Antimotion sickness and antiemetic drugs. Drugs 17:471–479, 1985.
56. Clissold SP, Heel RC. Transdermal hyoscine (scopolamine): a preliminary review of its pharmacodynamic properties and therapeutic efficacy. Drugs 29:189–207, 1985.
57. Allen LV. Scopolamine topical gel for travelers. US Pharmacist March:22–23, 1995.
58. Cersosimo RJ, Karp DD. Adrenal corticosteroids as antiemetics during cancer chemotherapy. Pharmacotherapy 6:118–127, 1986.
59. Kris MG, Gralla RJ, Tyson LB, et al. Improved control of cisplatin-induced emesis with high-dose metoclopramide and with combinations of metoclopramide, dexamethasone and diphenhydramine. Cancer 55:527–534, 1985.
60. du Bois A, McKenna C, Andersson H, et al. A randomised, double-blind, parallel-group study to compare the efficacy and safety of ondansetron (GR38032F) plus dexamethasone with metoclopramide plus dexamethasone in the prophylaxis of nausea and emesis induced by carboplatin chemotherapy. Oncology 54:7–14, 1997.
61. Italian Group for Antiemetic Research. Dexamethasone, granisetron, or both for the prevention of nausea and vomiting during chemotherapy for cancer. N Engl J Med 332:1–5, 1995.
62. Italian Group for Antiemetic Research. Persistence of efficacy of three antiemetic regimens and prognostic factors in patients undergoing moderately emetogenic chemotherapy. J Clin Oncol 13:2417–2426, 1995.
63. Kirchner V, Aapro M, Terrey J-P, et al. A double-blind crossover study comparing prophylactic intravenous granisetron alone or in combination with dexamethasone as antiemetic treatment in controlling nausea and vomiting associated with chemotherapy. Eur J Cancer 33:1605–1610, 1997.
64. Kris M, Pendergrass K, Navari R, et al. Prevention of acute emesis in cancer patients following high-dose cisplatin with the combination of oral dolasetron and dexamethasone. J Clin Oncol 15:2135–2138, 1997.
65. Pectasides D, Mylonakis A, Varthalitis J, et al. Comparison of two different doses of ondansetron plus dexamethasone in the prophylaxis of cisplatin-induced emesis. Oncology 54:1–6, 1997.
66. Henzi I, Walder B, Tramer MR. Dexamethasone for the prevention of postoperative nausea and vomiting: a quantitative systematic review. Anesth Analg 90:186–194, 2000.

67. Vincent BJ, McQuiston DJ, Einhorn LH, et al. Review of cannabinoids and their antiemetic effectiveness. Drugs 25(Suppl 1):52–62, 1983.
68. Anderson PO, McGuire GG. Delta-9-tetrahydrocannabinol as an antiemetic. Am J Hosp Pharm 38:639–646, 1981.
69. Devine ML, Dow GJ, Greenberg BR, et al. Adverse reactions to delta-9-tetrahydrocannabinol given as an antiemetic in a multicenter study. Clin Pharm 6:319–322, 1987.
70. Voth E, Schwartz R. Medicinal applications of delta-9-tetrahydrocannabinol and marijuana. Ann Intern Med 126:791–798, 1997.
71. Tramer MR, Carroll D, Campbell FA, et al. Cannabinoids for control of chemotherapy induced nausea and vomiting: quantitative systematic review. Br Med J 323:16–21, 2001.
72. Ward A, Holmes B. Nabilone: a preliminary review of its pharmacological properties and therapeutic use. Drugs 30:127–144, 1985.
73. Kearsley JH, Tattersall MH. Recent advances in the prevention and reduction of cytotoxic-induced emesis. Med J Aust 143:341–346, 1985.
74. Bishop JF, Oliver IN, Wolf MM, et al. Lorazepam: a randomized double-blind crossover study of a new antiemetic in patients receiving cytotoxic chemotherapy and prochlorperazine. J Clin Oncol 2:691–695, 1984.
75. Gan TJ, Meyer T, Apfel CC, et al. Consensus guidelines for managing postoperative nausea and vomiting. Anesth Analg 97:62–71, 2003.
76. Kris MG, Gralla RJ, Clark RA, et al. Consecutive dose-finding trials adding lorazepam to the combination of metoclopramide plus dexamethasone: improved subjective effectiveness over the combination of diphenhydramine plus metoclopramide plus dexamethasone. Cancer Treat Rep 69:1257–1262, 1985.
77. Penta JS, Poster DS, Bruna S, et al. Cancer chemotherapy induced nausea and vomiting in adult and pediatric patients. Am Soc Clin Oncol 4:396, 1981.
78. Gralla RJ, Tyson LB, Kris MG, et al. The management of chemotherapy-induced nausea and vomiting. Med Clin North Am 70:289–301, 1987.
79. Chin S, Kucuk O, Peterson R, et al. Variables contributing to anticipatory nausea and vomiting in cancer chemotherapy. Am J Clin Oncol 15:262–267, 1992.
80. Moher D, Arthur AZ, Pater JL. Anticipatory nausea and/or vomiting. Cancer Treat Rev 11:257–264, 1984.
81. Alba E, Roma B, de Andres L, et al. Anticipatory nausea and vomiting: prevalence and predictors in chemotherapy patients. Oncology 46:26–30, 1989.
82. Dolgin MJ, Katz ER, McGinty K, et al. Anticipatory nausea and vomiting in pediatric cancer patients. Pediatrics 75:547–552, 1985.
83. Stoudemire A, Cotanch P, Laszlo J. Recent advances in the pharmacologic and behavioral management of chemotherapy-induced emesis. Arch Intern Med 144:1029–1033, 1984.
84. Laszlo J, Clark RA, Hanson DC, et al. Lorazepam in cancer patients treated with cisplatin: a drug having antiemetic, amnesic and anxiolytic effects. J Clin Oncol 3:864–869, 1985.
85. Kris MG, Gralla RJ, Clark RA, et al. Consecutive dose-finding trials adding lorazepam to the combination of metoclopramide plus dexamethasone: improved subjective effectiveness over the combination of diphenhydramine plus metoclopramide plus dexamethasone. Cancer Treat Rep 69:1257–1262, 1985.
86. Pater JL, Willian AR. Methodologic issues in trials of antiemetics. J Clin Oncol 2:484–497, 1984.
87. Hesketh P, Kris M, Grunberg S, et al. Proposal for classifying the acute emetogenicity of cancer chemotherapy. J Clin Oncol 15:103–109, 1997.
88. Hesketh PJ. Defining the emetogenicity of cancer chemotherapy regimens: relevance to clinical practice. The Oncologist 4:191–196, 1999.
89. O'Brien MER, Cullen MH. Are we making progress in the management of cytotoxic drug-induced nausea and vomiting? J Clin Pharmacol Ther 13:19–31, 1988.
90. Berard C, Mahoney C. Cost-reducing treatment algorithms for antineoplastic drug-induced nausea and vomiting. Am J Health Syst Pharm 52:1879–1885, 1995.
91. Smith DB, Newlands ES, Spruyt OW, et al. Ondansetron (GR380032F) plus dexamethasone: effective antiemetic prophylaxis for patients receiving cytotoxic chemotherapy. Br J Cancer 61:323–324, 1990.
92. Cunningham D, Turner A, Hawthorn J, et al. Ondansetron with and without dexamethasone to treat chemotherapy-induced emesis. Lancet 1:1323, 1989.
93. Italian Group for Antiemetic Research. Ondansetron + dexamethasone vs metoclopramide + dexamethasone + diphenhydramine in prevention of cisplatin-induced emesis. Lancet 340:96–99, 1992.
94. Chevallier B. The control of acute cisplatin-induced emesis: a comparative study of granisetron and a combination regimen of high-dose metoclopramide and dexamethasone. Br J Cancer 68:176–180, 1993.
95. Craig JB, Powell BL. Review: the management of nausea and vomiting in clinical oncology. Am J Med Sci 293:34–44, 1987.
96. Browman GP, Levine MN, Mohide EA, et al. The practice guidelines development cycle: a conceptual tool for practice guidelines development and implementation. J Clin Oncol 13:502–512, 1995.
97. Mahoney CD, Berard CM, Simas EA, et al. Implementing a chemotherapy practice standard in an integrated health care system. Hosp Pharm 33:954–960, 1998.
98. Osoba D, Warr DG, Fitch MI, et al. Guidelines for the optimal management of chemotherapy-induced nausea and vomiting: a consensus. Can J Oncol 5:381–399, 1995.
99. American Society of Health-System Pharmacists, ASHP therapeutic guidelines on the pharmacologic management of nausea and vomiting in adult and pediatric patients receiving chemotherapy or radiation therapy or undergoing surgery. Am J Health-Syst Pharm 56:729–764, 1999.
100. National comprehensive cancer network antiemesis practice guidelines, Vol. 2. NCCN proceedings. Oncology 11:57–89, 1997.
101. Trovato J, Stull D, Finley R. Outcomes of antiemetic therapy after the administration of high-dose antineoplastic agents. Am J Health Syst Pharm 55:1269–1274, 1998.
102. Perez E, Hesketh P, Sandbach J, et al. Comparison of single-dose oral granisetron versus intravenous ondansetron in the prevention of nausea and vomiting induced by moderately emetogenic chemotherapy: a multicenter, double-blind, randomized parallel study. J Clin Oncol 16:754–760, 1998.
103. Nolte M, Berkery R, Pizzo B. Assuring the optimal use of serotonin antagonist antiemetics: the process for development and implementation of institutional antiemetic guidelines at Memorial Sloan-Kettering cancer center. J Clin Oncol 16:771–778, 1998.
104. Schipper H, Clinch J, McMurray A, et al. Measuring the quality of life of cancer patients. The functional living index, cancer: development and validation. J Clin Oncol 2:472–483, 1984.
105. Lindley CM, Hirsch JD, O'Neill CV, et al. Quality of life consequences of chemotherapy-induced emesis. Qual Life Res 1:331–340, 1992.
106. de Boer-Dennert M, de Wit R, Schmitz P, et al. Patient perceptions of the side effects of chemotherapy: the influence of 5HT3 antagonists. Br J Cancer 76:1055–1061, 1997.
107. Farley P, Dempsey C, Shillington A, et al. Patients' self-reported functional status after granisetron or ondansetron therapy to prevent chemotherapy-induced nausea and vomiting at six cancer centers. Am J Health Syst Pharm 54:2478–2482, 1997.
108. Osoba D, Zee B, Pater J, et al. Psychometric properties and responsiveness of the EORTC Quality of Life Questionnaire (QLQ-C30) in patients with breast, ovarian and lung cancer. Qual Life Res 3:353–364, 1994.
109. Osoba D, Zee B, Warr D, et al. Quality of life studies in chemotherapy-induced emesis. Oncology 53(Suppl 1):92–95, 1996.
110. Morrow G, Hickok J, Burish T, et al. Frequency and clinical implications of delayed nausea and delayed emesis. Am J Clin Oncol 19:199–203, 1996.
111. Kris MG, Gralla RJ, Clark RA, et al. Incidence, course, and severity of delayed nausea and vomiting following the administration of high dose cisplatin. J Clin Oncol 3:1379–1384, 1985.
112. Sridhar KS, Donnelly E. Combination antiemetics for cisplatin chemotherapy. Cancer 61:1508–1517, 1988.
113. Kris MG, Gralla RJ, Tyson LB, et al. Controlling delayed vomiting: double blind, randomized trial comparing placebo, dexamethasone alone and metoclopramide plus dexamethasone in patients receiving cisplatin. J Clin Oncol 7:108–114, 1989.

114. Italian Group for Antiemetic Research. Ondansetron versus metoclopramide, both combined with dexamethasone, in the prevention of cisplatin-induced delayed emesis. J Clin Oncol 15:124–130, 1997.

115. Kris MG, Tyson LB, Clark RA, et al. Oral Ondansetron for the control of delayed emesis after cisplatin. Cancer 70(Suppl): 1012–1016, 1992.

116. Pater J, Lofters W, Zee B, et al. The role of the 5-HT3 antagonists ondansetron and dolasetron in the control of delayed onset nausea and vomiting in patients receiving moderately emetogenic chemotherapy. Ann Oncol 8:181–185, 1997.

117. Hesketh P. Management of cisplatin-induced delayed emesis. Oncology 53(Suppl 1):73–77, 1996.

118. Gralla R, Rittenberg C, Peralta M, et al. Cisplatin and emesis: aspects of treatment and a new trial for delayed emesis using oral dexamethasone plus ondansetron beginning at 16 hours after cisplatin. Oncology 53(Suppl 1):86–91, 1996.

119. Gold BS, Kitz DS, Lecky JH, et al. Unanticipated admission to the hospital following ambulatory surgery. JAMA 262:3008–3010, 1989.

120. Watcha MF, White PGF. Postoperative nausea and vomiting: its etiology, treatment and prevention. Anesthesiology 77:162–184, 1992.

121. Philips S, Ruggier R, Hutchinson SE. *Zingiber officinale* (ginger): an antiemetic for day case surgery. Anaesthesia 48:111–120, 1993.

122. Ernst E, Pittler MH. Efficacy of ginger for nausea and vomiting: a systematic review of randomized clinical trials. Br J Anaesth 84: 367–371, 2000.

123. Henzi I, Walder B, Tramer MR. Metoclopramide in the prevention of postoperative nausea and vomiting: a quantitative systematic review of randomized, placebo-controlled studies. Br J Anaesth 83: 761–771, 1999.

124. Lewis, IH, Campbell DN, Barrowcliffe MP. Effect of nabilone on nausea and vomiting after total abdominal hysterectomy. Br J Anaesth 73:244–264, 1994.

125. Reason JT, Brand JJ. Motion sickness. New York: Academic Press, 1975.

126. Wood CD, Manno JE, Wood MJ, et al. Mechanisms of antimotion sickness drugs. Aviat Space Environ Med 58(Suppl):A262–265, 1987.

127. Grontved A, Brask T, Kambskard J, et al. Ginger root against seasickness: a controlled trial on the open sea. Acta Otolaryngol 105: 45–49, 1988.

128. Stein DJ, Birnback DJ, Danzer BI, et al. Acupressure versus intravenous metoclopramide to prevent nausea and vomiting during spinal anesthesia for cesarean section. Anesth Analg 84:821–825, 1997.

Constipation and Diarrhea

48

Valerie W. Hogue and Yolanda B. McKoy-Beach

Constipation and diarrhea are common disorders of the gastrointestinal system that most people experience at some time in their lives. Generally, these symptoms are self-limiting and may not necessitate intervention. However, patients may consider intervention necessary because of their beliefs and attitudes toward normal bowel function. Constipation and diarrhea can affect the ability to carry out work or school responsibilities, and loss of productivity usually necessitates prompt and effective intervention.

Symptoms of diarrhea and constipation may result from various disease states, medications, dietary changes, food or water contamination, and even psychological distress. Many over-the-counter (OTC) products are available in the United States for resolving the symptoms. The pharmacist's consultation is important for proper use of these products during self-treatment. The pharmacist must ascertain the possible cause of these symptoms to prevent masking a serious medical problem and to deter laxative and antidiarrheal abuse.

CONSTIPATION AND DIARRHEA

DEFINITION

The definitions of diarrhea and constipation have been debated for several years, primarily because of variations in the definition of normal bowel habits. Most clinicians agree that no single definition describes either medical problem effectively.

Clinicians generally incorporate two primary aspects in the definition of constipation: difficulty passing stools and infrequent stools. However, patients may describe constipation as less frequent defecation than is normally observed, lower stool volume, difficulty passing stool, hard or firm stool, straining upon defecation, a sensation of incomplete evacuation of bowel, or the lack of an urge to stool. A study of young adults not seeking health care were surveyed about their definition of constipation. They emphasized function (straining) and consistency (hard stools) rather than the number of stools in their definition.[1] Therefore, determining the patient's definition is essential.

Diarrhea has been described more consistently than constipation. Generally, it is defined as three or more loose or unformed bowel movements per day, accompanied by symptoms of fever, abdominal cramps, or vomiting. It has been further described as a condition of abnormal increases in stool weight and liquidity. An increase in stool water excretion above 150 mL every 24 hours is an objective parameter for acute diarrhea.[2]

TREATMENT GOALS: CONSTIPATION AND DIARRHEA

- For diarrhea, alleviate the loose stools and accompanying symptoms.
- For constipation, relieve the difficulty in passing stools and the irregularity of bowel movements.
- Prevent complications associated with diarrhea, including dehydration and electrolyte losses.
- Prevent complications associated with constipation, including hemorrhoids and anal fissures.
- Restore normal bowel habits by increasing or decreasing frequency of defecation based on presenting problem.
- Restore normal bowel consistency.

EPIDEMIOLOGY

CONSTIPATION
Constipation may result from underlying systemic disorders or general lifestyle factors (Table 48.1). Diseases producing constipation may be localized to the gastrointestinal tract or anorectum (Table 48.2). Drugs, including the chronic use of laxatives, may induce constipation (Table 48.3). In addition, psychological factors may cause changes in bowel habits, leading to constipation.[3]

DIARRHEA
Diarrhea may be caused primarily by inhibition of ion absorption, stimulation of ion secretion, retention of fluid in the intestinal lumen, and disorders of intestinal motility. Retention of fluid in the bowel lumen may be precipitated by carbohydrate malabsorption, disaccharidase deficiencies, lactulose therapy, poorly absorbable salts (magnesium sulfate, sodium phosphate, sodium citrate, antacids), and ingestion of mannitol or sorbitol. Secretagogues from tumors such as vasoactive intestinal polypeptide (VIP), serotonin, and calcitonin may be mediators of secretory diarrhea. Certain medications may act as mediators also (Table 48.4). Disorders of motility may lead to symptoms of diarrhea in irritable bowel syndrome (IBS), diabetic neuropathy, or thyrotoxicosis. Bacterial and viral infections often cause diar-

rhea [e.g., travelers' diarrhea (TD)]. Food intolerance associated with disaccharidase (lactose) deficiency also may result in diarrhea.[4]

EPIDEMIOLOGY

CONSTIPATION
Although constipation is a common disorder, its prevalence is difficult to define because it lacks a standard definition. However, several studies have assessed its prevalence based on patients' self-report. The incidence of self-reported constipation, diarrhea, and defecation frequency in the United States was estimated from the results of a national, population-based survey.[5] Respondents ranged in age from 25 to 74 years. The majority of the respondents reported daily defecation (73.3% of European Americans, 63.7% of African-Americans). The frequency of defecation differed significantly with regard to race and sex but not age. Regardless of sex or race, self-reported constipation was positively correlated with age. This difference may reflect a difference in the perception of constipation by older adults because the frequency of defecation did not change as age progressed.

In a study of 15,014 men and women aged 12 to 74 years, the overall incidence of self-reported constipation was 12.8% in the United States population.[6] It was ob-

TABLE 48.1	General, Systemic, and Psychological Causes of Constipation

Lifestyle Factors
   Inadequate fluid intake
   Decreased food intake
   Ignored defecation urge
   Immobility
External Factors
   Medications
Endocrine and Metabolic
   Hypothyroidism
   Hypercalcemia
   Porphyria
Neurologic
   Parkinson's disease
   Multiple sclerosis
   Spinal lesions
   Damage to sacral parasympathetic nerves
   Autonomic neuropathy
   Autonomic failure
Psychological
   Depression
   Eating disorders (e.g., anorexia nervosa)
   Misconceptions about "inner cleanliness"
   Denied bowel activity

(From Lennard-Jones JE. Constipation. In: Feldman M, Friedman LS, Sleisenger MH. Gastrointestinal and liver disease: pathophysiology/diagnosis/management. 7th ed. Philadelphia: WB Saunders, 2002: 185, with permission.)

TABLE 48.2	Gastrointestinal Causes of Constipation and Related Symptoms

Gastrointestinal tract
   Obstruction
   Aganglionosis (Hirschsprung's disease, Chagas' disease)
   Myopathy
   Neuropathy
   Systemic sclerosis
   Megarectum or megacolon
Anorectum
   Anal atresia or malformation
   Hereditary internal anal sphincter myopathy
   Anal stenosis
   Weak pelvic floor
   Large rectocele
   Internal intussusception
   Anterior mucosal prolapse
   Prolapse
   Solitary rectal ulcer

(From Lennard-Jones JE. Constipation. In: Feldman M, Friedman LS. Gastrointestinal and liver disease: pathophysiology/diagnosis/management. 7th ed. Philadelphia: WB Saunders, 2002:185, with permission.)

served most often in African-Americans (17.3%), women (18.2%), and people over 60 years of age (23%). Another study of 10,018 adults reported an overall prevalence of 14.7% .[7]

DIARRHEA

It has been estimated that the incidence of diarrhea in the United States and other industrialized nations is, on average, one episode per person annually.[8] It is of special concern in older adults because the majority of deaths associated with diarrheal illnesses in the United States occur in this population. In addition, adults who care for infants in day care facilities, international travelers, immunocompromised patients, and those exposed to contaminated food and water are at greater risk.[9]

PATHOPHYSIOLOGY

An understanding of the normal physiologic flow rate of fluid and electrolytes and the process of defecation is the

TABLE 48.3	Medication-induced Constipation

Antacids (e.g., calcium and aluminum-containing)
Anticholinergics
Barium sulfate
Bismuth
Calcium channel blockers (e.g., verapamil, diltiazem)
Central α-adrenergic agonists (e.g., clonidine, guanabenz, guanfacine)
Clozapine
Diuretics
Ganglionic-blocking agents
Iron
Laxatives (overuse)
Monoamine oxidase inhibitors
Opiates
Phenothiazines
Resins (e.g., cholestyramine, colestipol, polystyrene sulfonate)
Sucralfate
Tricyclic antidepressants
Vincristine

(From Tedesco FJ, DiPiro JT. Laxative use in constipation. Am J Gastroenterol 80:303–309, 1985, with permission.)

TABLE 48.4	Medication-induced Diarrhea

Acarbose

Antacids (magnesium-containing)

Antibiotics

Antineoplastic agents

Auranofin

β-Blockers

Colchicine

Didanosine

Guanethidine

H_2 Antagonists

Laxatives

Metformin

Metoclopramide

Misoprostol

Protease Inhibitors

Proton Pump Inhibitors

Quinidine

Reserpine

Tacrine

Tacrolimus

(From Hogue VW. The management of constipation and diarrhea. Drug Store News for the Pharmacist 6:56–64, 1996, with permission; Copyright Drug Store News for the Pharmacist, March 1996.)

basis for discussing the development of constipation and diarrhea. Three major aspects of bowel function exist: colonic absorption, colonic motility, and defecation reflexes.

The daily volume of fluid traversing the duodenum is 9 L for people consuming three meals daily. Approximately 8 L of fluid per day are absorbed by the small bowel. However, the colon absorbs 0.9 to 1.4 L per day, which is 90% of the fluid presented initially. The absorptive capacity of the colon exceeds that of the small intestine, which absorbs only 75% of the fluid presented initially. Daily fecal output is less than 200 mL, which contains approximately 5 mEq sodium and 8 mEq potassium.

Colonic motility involves three patterns of muscle contractions controlled by the autonomic nervous system: (a) nonpropulsive segmental contractions, which churn the contents of the lumen; (b) short-segment propulsive contractions, which move contents forward and backward, promoting absorption; and (c) long-segment propulsive contractions, which move contents forward over long distances. The urge to defecate occurs when gastric filling and increased physical activity trigger the gastroenteric reflex to produce massive peristalsis. The feces move from the sigmoid colon to the rectum, producing an urge to defecate. This occurs most often after breakfast.[10]

Defecation is initiated by the distension of the rectum by feces. Normally, the rectum can differentiate distension produced by fluids, flatus, and feces by defecation reflexes. Evacuation occurs after the internal and external anal sphincters relax in conjunction with the contraction of the rectosigmoid segment and increased intraabdominal pressure. Voluntary relaxation of the external anal sphincter allows evacuation of the bowel. Conversely, voluntary contraction of the sphincter inhibits defecation.[10]

CONSTIPATION

An intact nervous system is vital for normal defecation. Many patients develop constipation secondary to colonic motility disorders caused by congenital or acquired abnormalities of the nervous system. Outlet obstruction, a mechanism of constipation, may be secondary to a hyperactive rectosigmoid junction, increased storage capacity of the rectum, rectal spasticity, and hypertonicity of the anal canal.[3]

DIARRHEA

Four physiologic mechanisms may contribute to the development of diarrhea: (a) increased osmolality, (b) intestinal ion secretion, (c) impaired absorption, and (d) inflammatory and ulcerative processes. An understanding of the mechanisms of fluid loss aids in comprehending the mechanism of action of antidiarrheals.[4]

Increased Osmolality (Osmotic Diarrhea). In general, osmotic diarrhea is caused by the retention of fluid by nonabsorbable solutes in the bowel lumen. Peristalsis is stimulated by the increased fluid volume in the lumen, resulting in increased transit of the fecal matter by the colon. Because the colon is very efficient in the reabsorption of sodium chloride and water, increased transit through the colon promotes diarrhea.

Osmotic diarrhea also is evident when enzymes, such as lactase, are deficient. Lactase deficiency is common among certain racial groups, such as those of African and Asian descent. Lactase is responsible for the degradation of lactose to glucose and galactose, which are absorbed by the mucosa. In the absence of this enzyme, lactose retains fluid, thereby increasing the volume of water in the stool.

Intestinal Ion Secretion (Secretory Diarrhea). Two factors contribute to secretory diarrhea: (a) inhibition of ion absorption and (b) intestinal ion secretion. As a result, the stool contains an excess of monovalent ions and water. Enterotoxins produced by certain bacteria stimulate intestinal fluid secretion. Laxatives, such as senna and dioctyl sodium sulfosuccinate, may also cause this type of diarrhea. Certain hormones, such as serotonin, calcitonin, prostaglandin E_1, and VIP, have been implicated as mediators of secretory diarrhea.[2]

Altered Intestinal Motility. Changes in intestinal motility may affect fluid and electrolyte absorption within the gut lumen. Increased activity may reduce the surface area and limit the contact time for nutrient absorption.

Inflammatory and Ulcerative Processes. Inflammation and ulceration of the intestinal mucosa often result in the release of mucus, serum proteins, and blood into the lumen. The absorption of water and electrolytes is impaired. This malabsorption is the presumed cause of diarrhea in patients with ulcerative colitis.

Consequences of Diarrhea. Although diarrhea may be uncomplicated and self-limiting, persistent diarrhea may cause serious consequences. Sodium and water deficits secondary to fluid loss are common in persistent diarrhea. Potassium losses of approximately 6 to 7 mEq per kilogram may be observed in untreated patients, and places the patient at risk of developing paralytic ileus and cardiac arrhythmias if potassium is not replaced appropriately. Fecal loss of bicarbonate and impaired renal excretion of acids may cause metabolic acidosis.

CLINICAL PRESENTATION AND DIAGNOSIS

CONSTIPATION

The clinician must obtain a complete history to diagnose constipation. During the interview, the patient's definition of normal bowel function must be ascertained to determine the impact of the change in bowel habit. The onset and duration of constipation, a description of the stool, and the presence of symptoms are necessary information. Medication use should be determined, especially that of OTC laxatives. The physical examination should include an abdominal examination, a digital examination of the rectum, and a proctosigmoidoscopy. A barium enema should be initiated in chronically constipated patients and patients with a recent history of constipation to determine if an obstruction is present.

DIARRHEA

A careful history and physical examination are essential for the diagnosis of diarrhea. Ascertaining the duration of diarrhea, the description of the stool (consistency, color, odor, presence or absence of melanic stool), the frequency of bowel movements, associated symptoms, and any underlying disorders is essential to obtaining a thorough history. Distinguishing between large-stool and small-stool diarrhea helps determine whether the underlying disorder originates from the small bowel, proximal colon, the left colon, or rectum.

Several signs and symptoms of diarrhea suggest underlying disease states. Generally, the passage of blood may indicate inflammatory, infectious, or neoplastic disease. Pus or exudate in the stool may indicate inflammation or infection.

Infection caused by *Shigella* has a characteristic blood-tinged mucus without an odor. *Salmonella* sp. infections and *Escherichia coli* infections in infants usually are characterized by green, soupy stools. Passage of nonbloody mucus often suggests IBS, particularly when it is associated with intermittent diarrhea and constipation. Fecal incontinence and nocturnal diarrhea are associated with rectal sphincter dysfunction secondary to neurologic problems. Less specific signs of diarrhea associated with a patient's desire to lose weight may suggest laxative abuse.

PSYCHOSOCIAL ASPECTS

The decision to self-medicate for constipation or diarrhea depends largely on the patient's perception of abnormal bowel habits. In a survey of public perceptions of digestive health and disease, researchers found that 62% of American respondents believed that a bowel movement each day is necessary for good digestive health.[11] This idea may have been influenced by the notion of autointoxication, which stated that noxious substances in the colon increase cellular degeneration and promote aging.[10] Although this notion is obsolete, the belief appears to be common among older adults, whose concern for regularity of bowel movements is shown by their frequent use of laxatives.

Normal bowel habits may range between 3 and 21 stools per week.[12] This demonstrates a wide variation of bowel habits among healthy people and may suggest an equivalent variation in laxative use.

THERAPEUTIC PLAN

Constipation and acute, nonspecific diarrhea often are self-limiting and self-managed. The American Gastroenterological Association has developed guidelines for the management of constipation.[13] Specific disorders such as acute infectious diarrhea (including TD) and IBS have recommendations for their management that are described later in this chapter.

TREATMENT OF CONSTIPATION

PHARMACOTHERAPY

The classification of laxatives is controversial. They have been categorized primarily by their mechanism of action, although the exact mechanisms are unclear. Most laxatives alter intestinal fluid and electrolyte transport mechanisms, thereby causing defecation.[14] The therapeutic options are many. Agents available for use are varied and include bulk-forming agents, hyperosmotic agents, stool softeners, lubricants, saline, and stimulant laxatives (Table 48.5). Several dosage forms are available for laxatives. Some agents, such

TABLE 48.5	Laxatives for the Management of Constipation

Laxative Category	Dosage Per Day		Dosage Form	Onset of Action	Patient Information
	Adult	Pediatric			
Bulk-forming					
Bran	>12 yr: up to 14 g	6–11 yr: up to 7 g 2–5 yr: up to 3.5 g	O	12–72 hr	Should be administered with 240 mL liquid/dose; additional fluid intake encouraged; recommended in pregnancy.
Karaya	>12 yr: up to 14 g		O		
Malt soup extract	>12 yr: up to 64 g	6–11 yr: up to 32 g 2–5 yr: up to 16 g	O		
Methylcellulose and sodium carboxymethyl-cellulose	>12 yr: up to 6 g	6–11 yr: up to 3 g	O		
Psyllium hydrophilic mucilloid	>12 yr: up to 30 g	6–11 yr: up to 15 g	O		
Stimulants					
Bisacodyl[a]	>12 yr: 5–15 mg >12 yr: 10 mg	>3 yr: 0.3 mg/kg 2–11 yr: 5–10 mg <2 yr: 5 mg	O RS	6–12 hr 15 min–2 hr	May cause a pink or red discoloration of the urine. May cause skin rash; discontinue medication and contact pharmacist or physician. Tablets should not be chewed.
Dehydrocholic acid	>12 yr: 750–1,500 mg		O		
Sennosides[a]	>12 yr: 12–75 mg >12 yr: 30–60 mg	6–11 yr: 6–33 mg 2–6 yr: 3–12.5 mg	O RS		
Saline agents					
Magnesium citrate	>12 hr: 11–25 g	6–11 yr: 5.5–12.5 g 2–5 yr: 2.7–6.25 g	O	30 min–6 hr	
Magnesium hydroxide	>12 yr: 2.4–4.8 g	6–11 yr: 1.2–2.4 g 2–5 yr: 0.4–1.2 g	O		
Magnesium sulfate	>12 yr: 10–30 g	6–11 yr: 5–10 g 2–5 yr: 2.5–5 g	O		
Sodium phosphate, monobasic	>12 yr: 9.1–20.2 g >12 yr: 18.24–20.16 g	10–11 yr: 4.5–10.1 g 5–9 yr: 2.2–5.05 g 2–11 yr: 9.12–10.08 g	O RE	2–15 min	
Sodium phosphate dibasic	>12 yr: 3.42–7.5 g >12 yr: 6.84–7.56 g	10–11 yr: 1.71–3.78 g 5–9 yr: 0.86–1.89 g 2–11 yr: 3.42–2.78 g	O RE	2–15 min	

(continued)

TABLE 48.5	continued					
	Dosage Per Day		**Dosage Form**	**Onset of Action**	**Patient Information**	
Laxative Category	**Adult**	**Pediatric**				
Hyperosmotic agents						
Glycerin	>12 yr: 3 g	>6 yr: 2–3 g	RS	15–30 min	May cause rectal burning or irritation.	
		5–15 mL	RE			
		<6 yr: 1–1.7 g	RS			
		2–5 mL	RE			
Lactulose	>12 yr: 10–20 g, then up to 40 g	<12 yr: 5 g[b]	O, RE		May be mixed in fruit juice to increase palatability. May cause belching, flatulence, or abdominal cramps. Pediatric dose should be given after breakfast.	
Polyethylene glycol 3350	17 g	No recommendation	O		Take with 240 mL water, soda, coffee, or tea on full or empty stomach. Expect bowel movement in 2 to 4 days.	
Lubricants						
Mineral oil	>12 yr: 15–45 mL	6–11 yr: 5–15 mL	O	6–8 hr	Should not be administered to children <6 yr, pregnant women, or debilitated patients. Bedtime doses should be avoided. May cause pruritus ani, especially when administered rectally.	
	>12 yr: 120 mL	6–11 yr: 30–60 mL	RE			
Surfactants						
Dioctyl sulfosuccinate (calcium, potassium, sodium)	No official recommendation		O, RE		Oral solutions may be diluted with 120 mL milk, fruit juice, or infant formula; solutions may cause throat irritation.	
Tegaserod	12 mg	No recommendation	O		Take before meals	
					Divide dose twice daily	
					Watch for symptoms of diarrhea	

[a] The U.S. Food and Drug Administration (FDA) has proposed the reclassification of these agents from category I (generally recognized as safe and effective and not misbranded) to category III (further testing is needed).

[b] Use currently is not included in the FDA-approved labeling.

O, oral; RE, rectal enema; RS, rectal suppository.

(From Anonymous. Safety of stool softeners. Med Lett 19:45–46, 1977, with permission.)

as psyllium and senna, are uniquely formulated in wafers and tea bags, respectively.

In general, there are no differences in efficacy between laxatives, but there are differences in their uses. One study suggests that the stool-softening and laxative effect of psyllium (a bulk-forming agent) compared with that of docusate sodium (a stool softener) was significantly better in patients with chronic idiopathic constipation.[15] More study is needed to verify if there is a significant clinical difference between these and other laxatives.

Bulk-forming Laxatives. Bulk-forming agents include nonabsorbable polysaccharide and cellulose derivatives. These agents swell in water, forming an emollient gel that increases bulk in the intestines. Peristalsis is stimulated by the increased fecal mass that decreases the transit time. It is proposed that microflora metabolize polysaccharides to osmotically active metabolites. The metabolites may alter intestinal motility and electrolyte transport.

Bulk-forming agents generally produce a laxative effect within 12 to 24 hours, but they may take 2 to 3 days to exert their full effect. They are generally safe with minimal side effects associated with their use. Flatulence may occur if doses are increased rapidly. Intestinal and esophageal obstruction may occur if insufficient liquid is administered with the dose. Therefore, the Food and Drug Administration (FDA) has tentatively ruled that psyllium in a granular dosage form poses an unacceptable risk for the development of esophageal obstruction, and has proposed to reclassify it as not generally recognized as safe and effective.[16] Granular dosage forms include, but is not limited to: (a) any granules that are swallowed dry prior to drinking liquid; (b) any granules that are dispersed, suspended, or partially dissolved in liquid prior to swallowing; (c) any granules that are chewed, partially chewed, or unchewed, and then followed with liquid; and (d) any granules that are sprinkled over food. Patients using the nongranular powder form should be cautioned to take each dose with at least one 240-mL glass of liquid.

Bulk-forming laxatives should not be recommended for patients with intestinal stenosis, ulceration, or adhesions. Rare reports of allergic reactions to karaya have been noted, characterized by urticaria, rhinitis, dermatitis, and bronchospasm.[14]

Hyperosmotic Agents. Glycerin, lactulose, and polyethylene glycol are hyperosmotic laxatives. They increase osmotic pressure within the intestinal lumen, which results in luminal retention of water, softening the stool. Lactulose is an unabsorbed disaccharide metabolized by colonic bacteria primarily to lactic, formic, and acetic acids. It has been proposed that these organic acids may contribute to the osmotic effect.[14] Polyethylene glycol (PEG) 3350 laxative is a synthetic polyglycol, which is absorbed in only trace amounts,

and is not metabolized to hydrogen or methane by colonic bacteria.[17]

Glycerin is available only for rectal administration (suppository or enema) for treating acute constipation. Its laxative effect occurs within 15 to 30 minutes. Lactulose may take effect in 24 to 48 hours. It should be reserved for acute constipation because it is as effective as other less costly medications. Polyethylene glycol laxative is available as a powder for solution that should be dissolved in 8 ounces of water, soda, coffee, or tea, then ingested. Its laxative effect occurs in 48 to 96 hours and should be used for 2 weeks or less.[18]

Side effects of glycerin include rectal irritation and burning and hyperemia of the rectal mucosa may occur. Lactulose is associated with flatulence, abdominal cramps, and diarrhea. Caution should be exercised when this agent is administered because it may also cause significant electrolyte imbalances and dehydration.[19] Whereas nausea, abdominal bloating, cramping, and flatulence may occur with PEG, there may be fewer symptoms than with lactulose because it does not cause fermentation in the gastrointestinal tract.[20] Studies directly comparing the side effect profile of lactulose versus PEG are needed. Its use is contraindicated in patients with known or suspected bowel obstruction.

Stool Softeners. Stool softeners are also called emollient laxatives. They include calcium, potassium, and sodium salts of dioctyl sulfosuccinate. Stool softeners are anionic surfactants that lower the fecal surface tension allowing water and lipid penetration. It has been proposed that these agents stimulate water and electrolyte secretion into the colon.[14]

Softening of the feces generally occurs after 1 to 3 days. Some products (e.g., docusate sodium with casanthrol) combine a stool softener with a laxative. Adverse effects are rare with docusate preparations. Mild gastrointestinal cramping may occasionally develop. Throat irritation has occurred following use of the docusate sodium solution.[21]

Lubricants. The primary lubricant laxative is mineral oil. Its mechanism of action involves lubrication of the feces and hindrance of water reabsorption in the colon. Mineral oil is indigestible and its absorption is limited considerably in the nonemulsified formulation. Greater absorption from the emulsion formulation has been reported, but the clinical significance is unsubstantiated.

The onset of action of orally administered mineral oil is 6 to 8 hours. Although adverse effects occur rarely with mineral oil, potentially significant effects may occur. Chronic use of mineral oil has been reported to cause impaired absorption of fat soluble vitamins (A, D, E, and K). Aspiration of the product may cause a lipoid pneumonia, so its oral use should be avoided in young children (<6 years), older adults, and debilitated patients. Administration at bedtime should be avoided to prevent aspiration. Foreign-body reactions in the lymphoid tissue of the intestinal tract have resulted from its limited amount of absorption. Seepage of the product from the rectum following high-dose oral or rectal administration may cause pruritus ani, increased infection, and decreased healing of anorectal lesions.[14,19]

Saline Laxatives. Magnesium, sulfate, phosphate, and citrate salts are used when rapid bowel evacuation is needed. The mechanism of action of these poorly absorbed ions is unclear, but it is believed that they produce an osmotic effect that increases intraluminal volume and stimulates peristalsis. Magnesium may cause cholecystokinin release from the duodenal mucosa, promoting increased fluid secretion and motility of the small intestine and colon.[22]

The laxative effect of the orally administered magnesium and sodium phosphate salts occurs within 0.5 to 6 hours. Phosphate-containing rectal enemas evacuate the bowel within 2 to 15 minutes.

Saline laxatives are safe for short-term management of constipation. They are useful in preparing for endoscopic examinations, eliminating parasites and toxic anthelmintics before or after therapy, removing poisons, and treating fecal impaction. They may cause significant fluid and electrolyte imbalances when used for prolonged periods or in certain patients. Dehydration may result from repeated administration without appropriate fluid replacement. The risk of hypermagnesemia in patients with renal dysfunction should be considered when magnesium salts are initiated because 10% to 20% of the dose may be absorbed systemically. Caution should be exercised when administering the sodium phosphate salts to patients with congestive heart failure when sodium restriction is necessary. These agents are not recommended for children under 2 years of age because of the potential for hypocalcemia in this population.

Stimulant Laxatives. Anthraquinone (sennosides) and diphenylmethane (bisacodyl) derivatives, castor oil, and dehydrocholic acid are stimulant laxatives. They are called stimulants because they stimulate peristalsis via mucosal irritation or intramural nerve plexus activity, which results in increased motility. Although this has been long regarded as the mechanism of action for these agents, their activity actually may be related to their effect on the colonic mucosal cells. It is proposed that stimulant laxatives modify the permeability of these cells, resulting in intraluminal fluid and electrolyte secretion.

Defecation occurs 6 to 12 hours after oral administration of these agents. Therefore, a single bedtime dose promotes a morning bowel movement. Unlike the other stimulant laxatives, dehydrocholic acid is administered at least three times daily. Rectal administration of bisacodyl and senna produces catharsis within 15 minutes to 2 hours.

Adverse effects of these medications include abdominal cramps, nausea, electrolyte disturbances (e.g., hypokalemia,

hypocalcemia, metabolic acidosis, or alkalosis), and rectal burning and irritation with suppository use. Anthraquinone derivatives have been noted to cause melanosis coli (discoloring of colonic mucosa), which is harmless and reversible. Hypersensitivity reactions may occur (rarely) with phenolphthalein and dehydrocholic acid, causing dermatologic manifestations (e.g., skin eruptions, rash, pigmentation, pruritus). These agents may also cause a pink or red discoloration of the urine.

Chronic use of stimulant laxatives should be discouraged and use beyond 1 week should be avoided. These agents may produce a "cathartic colon" if used for several years (15–40 years). The colon develops abnormal motor function, and the condition resembles ulcerative colitis on roentgenogram. Usually, discontinuation of laxative use restores normal bowel function. Several stimulant laxatives have been removed from the market by the FDA because they were classified as "not generally recognized as safe and effective" in animal carcinogenicity studies. Although only insignificant amounts distribute into the milk of nursing mothers, stimulant laxatives should be avoided during lactation.[23]

Other Agents. Tegaserod maleate is a 5-hydroxytryptamine or serotonin subtype-4 (5-HT$_4$), partial receptor agonist. It binds to 5-HT$_4$ receptors, present largely in the gastrointestinal tract, stimulating intestinal peristalsis and secretion. It is indicated for patients less than 65 years of age with chronic constipation and IBS with constipation (see "Irritable Bowel Syndrome").

The recommended oral dose of tegaserod in patients with chronic idiopathic constipation is 6 mg twice daily (bid) before meals for up to 12 weeks of therapy. Common side effects of tegaserod include diarrhea, which may be severe in some patients, abdominal pain, and headaches.[24]

Inhibition of cytochrome P450 isoenzymes 1A2 and 2D6 may occur with tegaserod. However, there are no clinically significant drug interactions reported with its concomitant use. Although not clinically significant, tegaserod may reduce digoxin levels by 15%. Therefore, monitoring is important in patients who begin tegaserod and are dosed at the lower limit of normal with digoxin.[25]

Tegaserod is contraindicated in patients with severe renal impairment, moderate to severe hepatic impairment, a history of bowel obstruction, symptomatic gallbladder disease, suspected sphincter of Oddi dysfunction, or abdominal adhesions. It should be discontinued if severe diarrhea, hypotension, syncope, or sudden worsening of abdominal pain occurs. Tegaserod should also be discontinued immediately in persons who develop rectal bleeding, bloody diarrhea, or new or worsening abdominal pain, which may suggest ischemic colitis.[25,26]

The efficacy, safety, and tolerability of tegaserod has been demonstrated in a multicenter, double-blind, placebo-controlled study. Patients were randomized to receive treatment with tegaserod 2 mg bid, 6 mg bid, or placebo. A total of 1,348 patients were enrolled in the study. Patients were considered to have responded to treatment if the number of bowel movements increased from baseline. The study demonstrated that the response rate was significantly higher in the tegaserod-treated patients than placebo. The response rates were 41.4% in the 2 mg bid group, 43.2% in the 6 mg bid group, and 25.1% in the placebo group.[24]

Data suggest a role for other agents in treating constipation. Naloxone and cisapride have been used to treat chronic idiopathic constipation. It has been postulated that endogenous opiates regulate colonic propulsive activity.[27] Consequently, the role of opiate receptor antagonists in treating constipation has been investigated. Naloxone (an opiate receptor antagonist) has reversed chronic idiopathic constipation at intravenous and oral doses of 20 to 30 mg per day.[28] In addition, naloxone causes acceleration of colonic transit, although it has not been shown to affect the number of bowel movements per 48 hours.[29] Further studies are needed to define the role of this agent in treating chronic constipation.

Cisapride is a piperidinyl benzamide that is chemically related to metoclopramide. It is a prokinetic agent that enhances gastrointestinal motility throughout the entire length of the gastrointestinal tract. The mechanisms by which cisapride facilitates gastrointestinal motility have not been elucidated. However, a proposed mechanism involves its enhancement of acetylcholine release in the myenteric plexus of the gut.[30] Cisapride has no antidopaminergic effects.

In 2000, the FDA required the manufacturer of cisapride to discontinue active marketing of the drug due to reports of cardiac arrhythmias, some resulting in death.[31] It is available through the manufacturer under a limited-access program for patients in the treatment of severe chronic constipation, gastroesophageal reflux disease, gastroparesis, and pseudo-obstruction.[32]

Cisapride, in oral doses of 5 to 20 mg, is absorbed rapidly and almost completely from the gastrointestinal tract. The oral bioavailability is approximately 40% to 50% and is enhanced by food. Its tissue distribution in humans is not known, however, it is metabolized extensively to metabolites with minimal pharmacologic activity. Its elimination half-life after oral administration is approximately 7 to 10 hours. Some evidence suggests that the half-life of cisapride may increase in older adults and those with hepatic impairment.[30]

Cisapride at a dose of 20 mg bid daily was investigated in patients with chronic idiopathic constipation or chronic laxative use. Cisapride increased stool frequency by 50% and reduced mean laxative intake by half.[33] In another study, cisapride was used to treat constipation at doses of 5 and 10 mg three times daily for 12 weeks. Stool frequency was increased by approximately 70% with both doses, compared to 43% with placebo.[34]

Common side effects include abdominal cramping, borborygmi (intestinal rumbling), and diarrhea. Central nervous system (CNS) side effects, such as somnolence and fatigue, have been reported less often.

Concomitant administration of cisapride with other drugs may result in significant drug interactions. Cimetidine coadministration may cause a 45% increase in the bioavailability of cisapride.[30] Cisapride may enhance acenocoumarol absorption; therefore, monitoring coagulation times is advisable with anticoagulants.[30] Cisapride can accelerate gastric emptying, therefore patients should be monitored during concomitant use of agents with narrow therapeutic index (e.g., digoxin and phenytoin).

NONPHARMACOLOGIC THERAPY

Some of the primary causes of constipation may necessitate nonpharmacologic intervention for symptom relief. Deficient fluid and fiber intake have been suggested as causative factors. However, two large-scale studies have not demonstrated an association between fiber consumption and self-reported constipation.[5,6] Fiber may be useful in preventing constipation. Fiber increases stool bulk, based on the ability of the polysaccharides to absorb and retain water and the extent of bacterial fermentation of these polysaccharides in the gut. A dietary bulk-forming agent such as bran may be useful in preventing constipation because it is only partially fermented by bacteria, resulting in increased stool bulk, accelerated transit time, and promotion of normal defecation.

Fiber intake may also have other health benefits. The FDA has ruled that labels on certain foods (i.e., breakfast cereals) containing soluble fiber from psyllium seed husk (PSH) may claim that, as part of a diet low in saturated fat and cholesterol, they can reduce the risk of coronary heart disease.[35] The ruling is based on evidence that consumption of approximately 7 g per day soluble fiber from PSH showed significant lowering of total and low-density lipoprotein cholesterol.

Increased fiber intake should be recommended cautiously. Rapid increases in dietary roughage may cause abdominal bloating and flatulence. Adequate fluid intake is also necessary to prevent fecal impaction. Generally, 240 to 360 mL fluid with each tablespoon of bran is sufficient.

Immobility and inactivity, common among debilitated patients and older adults, are risk factors for the development of constipation.[36] Regular exercise such as walking or jogging may improve constipation associated with a sedentary lifestyle. Pharmacologic intervention (e.g., laxatives) may be necessary if lifestyle modifications are unsuccessful.

TREATMENT OF ACUTE, NONSPECIFIC DIARRHEA

For most people, diarrhea is a transient, self-limiting complaint. This form of diarrhea is often called acute, nonspe-

TABLE 48.6	Recommended Over-the-Counter Antidiarrheals	
Medication	**Dosage**	**Maximum Dosage per Day**
Bismuth Subsalicylate	>12 yr: 30 mL every 30 min to 1 hr as needed.	Up to 8 doses for all ages
	9–12 yr: 15 mL every 30 min to 1 hr as needed	
	6–9 yr: 10 mL every 30 min to 1 hr as needed	
	3–6 yr: 5 mL every 30 min to 1 hr as needed	
Kaolin	>12 yr: 26.2 g after each stool	262 g
	<12 yr: consult physician	
Loperamide[a]	>12 yr: 4 mg at onset, then 2 mg after each loose stool	8 mg;[b] 16 mg
	9–11 yr: 2 mg at onset, then 1 mg after each loose stool	6 mg
	6–8 yr: 1 mg at onset, then 1 mg after each loose stool	4 mg
	<6 yr:[c] 1 mg at onset, then 1 mg after each loose stool	3 mg

[a] Therapy should not exceed 2 days.
[b] Travelers diarrhea. [c] Use only under medical supervision.
(From Antidiarrheal Drug Products for Over-the-Counter Human Use; Final Monograph. FDA Federal Register, April 17, 2003; 68; 74: 18869–18882; Drug Information Handbook 2002–2003, with permission.)

cific diarrhea that is not caused by underlying diseases or etiologic agents. However, the symptoms may often interfere with activities and contribute to loss of productivity. The management of acute, nonspecific diarrhea consists of adequate oral rehydration and symptom relief. Several nonprescription agents are effective in managing the associated symptoms of diarrhea (Table 48.6).

PHARMACOTHERAPY

Various medications, prescription and OTC, are available for the symptomatic relief of diarrhea. The FDA reevaluated the safety and efficacy of OTC products for diarrhea. The Advisory Review Panel on OTC Laxative, Antidiarrheal, Emetic, and Antiemetic Drug Products reviewed several products for their safety and efficacy. The FDA evaluated the panel's recommendations and published final rulings.[37] The FDA ruled that placebo-control studies were needed to establish the effectiveness of attapulgite, polycarbophil, and calcium polycarbophil. Currently, the only OTC products considered safe and effective treatments of diarrhea are kaolin (without pectin), loperamide, and bismuth subsalicylate (see Travelers' Diarrhea).

Kaolin is a naturally occurring hydrated aluminum silicate with adsorbent properties. It is effective in treating acute nonspecific diarrhea based on its ability to improve stool consistency within 24 to 48 hours. Kaolin is no longer approved for OTC use in combination with pectin for treating diarrhea. Studies have not demonstrated that the fixed combination (kaolin and pectin) is more effective than kaolin alone. Kaolin has minimal side effects. Recommended doses for adults and children older than 12 years are listed in Table 48.6.

Loperamide is a synthetic congener of meperidine, which decreases gastrointestinal motility by its effect on the circular and longitudinal muscles of the intestines. CNS penetration of the drug is low. It does not elicit the CNS side effects associated with opiate use and lacks potential for abuse.

Loperamide relieves symptoms of acute nonspecific diarrhea, and it is effective in treating nondysenteric TD.[38–40] It has been compared with attapulgite in acute diarrhea.[39] The dose of loperamide used was 4 mg initially, then 2 mg after every unformed stool, not exceeding 8 mg in 24 hours. Attapulgite was administered initially as 3 g, followed by up to 6 g after each unformed stool, to a maximum dose of 9 g in 24 hours. The mean number of unformed stools was significantly lower in the loperamide group in the first and second 12-hour intervals. However, no significant difference was observed in duration of relief from diarrhea after the initial dose.

Although generally well tolerated, loperamide can cause abdominal pain, constipation, drowsiness, fatigue, dry mouth, nausea, and vomiting. Doses for adults should not exceed 8 mg per day for OTC use; however, maximum daily doses of 16 mg are permitted under medical supervision. Children under 6 years of age should not receive loperamide unless medically supervised. The medication should be discontinued after 48 hours if clinical improvement is not evident.

Opiates (opium powder, tincture, and paregoric) have been used extensively to treat acute, nonspecific diarrhea. Opiates contain morphine, which promotes increased smooth muscle tone of the gastrointestinal tract, inhibits gastrointestinal motility and propulsion, and reduces digestive secretions. Paregoric is commonly used at doses of 5 to 10 mL one to four times daily for adults and 0.25 to 0.5 mL per kilogram one to four times daily for children.[41] Opium tincture contains 25% more morphine than paregoric; therefore, the dose is 0.3 to 1 mL four times daily with a maximum daily dosage of 6 mL.

Other derivatives of morphine, such as codeine and the meperidine congener diphenoxylate, can be used for diarrhea. At doses of 15 to 30 mg orally every 6 hours, codeine reduces the frequency of loose stools. However, its use has been limited in favor of the various nonnarcotic alternatives for diarrhea currently available. Diphenoxylate, which has activity similar to that of morphine on intestinal smooth muscle, is used in combination with atropine sulfate at doses of 2.5 to 5 mg orally four times daily. Unlike loperamide, diphenoxylate can produce euphoria and suppress opiate withdrawal symptoms at high doses. Consequently, abuse potential exists with diphenoxylate alone. Atropine sulfate has been added to discourage abuse.

NONPHARMACOLOGIC THERAPY

Fluid losses in acute, nonspecific diarrhea in adults generally are not severe and necessitate only simple replacement of fluid and electrolytes lost in the stool. However, special consideration should be given to older and immunocompromised patients. Patients should be advised to ingest 2 to 3 L clear liquids (e.g., flat ginger ale and decaffeinated cola, tea, broth, or gelatin) within the first 24 hours. For 24 hours, the diet should consist of bland foods including rice, soup, bread, salted crackers, cooked cereals, baked potatoes, eggs, and applesauce. A regular diet may be resumed after 2 to 3 days.

Untreated diarrhea in the pediatric population is a major cause of morbidity and mortality, especially in developing countries. Infants and young children are more susceptible to the acute losses of fluid caused by diarrhea because the intestinal surface area of infants and children is greater in relation to their body size. Consequently, oral rehydration solutions (ORSs) are recommended for acute diarrhea. Infants and children with a 5% to 7.5% weight loss should receive an ORS at a dosage of 40 to 50 mL per kilogram administered in the first 4 to 6 hours. Oral maintenance can be administered at a rate of 150 mL/kg/day after rehydration is achieved.[42] The World Health Organization (WHO) provides the standard ORS, which contains glucose (20 g/L), sodium (90 mEq/L), potassium (20 mEq/L), chloride (80 mEq/L), and citrate (10 mEq/L) as a base. It is prepared by mixing one packet with 1 L boiled or treated water. The solution should be discarded within 12 hours if kept at room temperature and within 24 hours if refrigerated. Packets are available in stores or pharmacies in all developing countries. Other ORSs are available commercially in the United States as ready-to-use preparations.

TREATMENT OF INFECTIOUS DIARRHEA

The role of antiperistaltic agents in infectious diarrhea has been questioned. The body normally defends itself from invading bacteria by eliminating these organisms during diarrhea. Antiperistaltic agents, such as diphenoxylate and loperamide, inhibit this process by increasing gastrointestinal transit time. Therefore, these agents are not recommended for treating diarrhea induced by invasive organisms such as enterotoxigenic *E. coli* (ETEC), *Salmonella,* or *Shigella.*[43,44] They should also be avoided in patients with fecal leukocytes, fever, or blood in the stools. The risk of toxic megacolon exists when these agents are given to patients with pseudomembranous colitis or ulcerative colitis.[44]

Although infectious diarrhea can be treated with antimicrobial therapy, the use of these agents is controversial. However, antimicrobial therapy is indicated when diarrhea persists for more than 48 hours, when the patient passes six or more loose stools in 24 hours, or when diarrhea is associated with fever, blood, or pus in the stools. Table 48.7 describes the common organisms and their therapy.

TREATMENT OF DIARRHEA IN IMMUNOCOMPROMISED PATIENTS

Diarrhea in immunocompromised patients (e.g., acquired immunodeficiency syndrome [AIDS], organ transplant, or chemotherapy) poses a challenge. Chronic diarrhea is identified in 30% to 70% individuals with human immunodeficiency virus (HIV)/AIDS.[45] The incidence and severity of the diarrhea increases in those persons with advanced HIV infection. Forty-nine percent of individuals with CD4 counts below 50 cells/mm^3 develop diarrhea within 1 year and 96% by 3 years.[46] It is commonly due to opportunistic infections, and the most common opportunistic pathogens identified are microsporidia, cytomegalovirus (CMV), cryptosporidia, mycobacterium avium complex (MAC). Less common pathogens are *Isospora* sp., *Cyclospora* sp., and enteric organisms (e.g., *Salmonella* sp., *Shigella* sp., and group A rotavirus). However, in 15% to 46% of HIV-infected persons no organism is identified.[45]

Generally, these patients experience symptoms that are refractory to conventional therapy. Some patients may respond to opium tincture when loperamide is not successful.[9] Somatostatin, a cyclic peptide hormone, is useful in treating diarrhea in these patients because it promotes intestinal absorption of water and electrolytes, prolonging the gastrointestinal transit time, and decreasing endogenous fluid secretion in the jejunum.[5] It should be recommended only after other therapies have failed because it is given subcutaneously and is expensive. Octreotide, a synthetic analog of somatostatin, was found to be effective in a small prospective, open label study. Fifty-one HIV-positive individuals with uncontrolled diarrhea received octreotide 50 μg every 8 hours for 48 hours. A decrease in daily stool volume was experienced by 41.2% of the patients.[47] However, further

TABLE 48.7	Antimicrobial Therapy for Common Causes of Infectious Diarrhea	
Organism	**Suggested Antimicrobial Therapy**	**Duration**
Salmonella		
Uncomplicated	None	
Hyperpyrexia and systemic toxicity	TMP/SMX 160/800 mg PO bid	5–7 days
	Fluoroquinolones[a]	
Shigella	TMP/SMX 160/800 mg PO bid (if acquired in the United States)	3 days
	Fluoroquinolones[a] (if acquired internationally)	3–5 days
Enteropathogenic E. coli	Fluoroquinolones[a]	3–5 days
Enterotoxigenic E. coli	Fluoroquinolones[a]	1–5 days
Enteroinvasive E. coli	TMP/SMX 160/800 mg bid (if acquired in the United States)	3 days
	Fluoroquinolones[a] (if acquired internationally)	3–5 days
Enterohemorrhagic E. coli	Antimicrobials usually withheld except in particularly severe cases	
Campylobacter spp.	Erythromycin stearate 500 mg PO bid	5 days
	Fluoroquinolones,[a] if susceptible	
	Azithromycin (for quinolone-resistant cases)	
Yersinia spp.	Fluoroquinolones[a]	3–5 days
	Ceftriaxone 1 g IV qd (severe cases)	5 days
Noncholera Vibrio	Fluoroquinolones[a]	3–5 days
Clostridium difficile	Vancomycin 125–500 mg PO qid	10 days
Giardia lamblia	Metronidazole 250 mg PO qid	7 days
	Quinacrine 100 mg PO tid (where available)	7 days
	Tinidazole 2 g single dose (where available)	
Cryptosporidium		
Uncomplicated	None	
Severe	Paromomycin 500 mg PO tid	7 days
Isospora	TMP/SMX 160/800 mg PO bid	7 days
Cyclospora	TMP/SMX 160/800 mg PO bid	7 days

[a] Oral fluoroquinolones include norfloxacin 400 mg, ciprofloxacin 500 mg, and ofloxacin 300 mg at bid dosing.
bid, twice a day; IV, intravenous; PO, by mouth; qd, every day; qid, four times daily
TMP/SMX, trimethoprim-sulfamethoxazole.
(From DuPont HL. Guidelines on acute infectious diarrhea in adults. Am J Gastroenterol 92:1962–1975, 1997, with permission.)

studies are needed to define the role of octreotide in AIDS-related diarrhea.

When the cause of diarrhea is a microorganism, it is often difficult to identify a pathogen or control symptoms even when a pathogen is known. In addition, AIDS patients often have a poor prognosis. Empiric treatment with antimicrobial therapy is indicated. Specific antimicrobial therapy for infectious diarrhea in immunocompromised patients is described in Table 48.8.

Prevention of exposure to some of these opportunistic pathogens (e.g., enteric organisms) should be recommended to patients. Exposure to animals less than 6 months

TABLE 48.8	Indications for Specific Antimicrobial Therapy in Infectious Diarrhea in Immunocompromised[a] Patients
Indication for Antimicrobial Therapy	**Suggested Antimicrobial Therapy**
Shigellosis	[c]Floroquinolone IV or PO for 3–7 days or TMP-SMX 160/800 mg PO BID for 3–7 days (If acquired in the US). If acquired during international travel, treat as febrile dysentery; check for susceptibility of drug used.
Intestinal salmonellosis	Quinolone[b] NF 400 mg, CF 500–750 mg, OF 300–400 mg PO BID for 14 days; repeat stool cultures 1 wk after treatment.
Cryptosporidium diarrhea	Paromomycin 500 mg PO qid with food for 14–28 days, then 500 mg bid indefinitely; with treatment failures, may try azithromycin 2.4 g PO day 1, then 1.2 g/day for 27 days, then 600 mg/day for maintenance treatment given indefinitely.
Isospora diarrhea	320 mg TMP/1600 mg SMX PO bid for 2–4 wk, then 160–320 mg TMP/800–1,600 mg SMX PO qd.
Cyclospora diarrhea	TMP/SMX 160/800 mg PO qid for 10 days, then 160/800 mg three times a week indefinitely.
Microsporidiosis	Albendazole 400 mg PO BID ≥4 wk or until CD4 >200 cells/mm^3
Cytomegalovirus diarrhea	Ganciclovir 5 mg/kg IV q12hr or q8hr 21–28 days and foscarnet 60 mg/kg IV q8hr or 90 mg/kg IV q12hr for 21–28 days.
Mycobacterium avium-intracellulare complex	Clarithromycin 500 mg PO BID or [c]Azithromycin 500–600 mg po qd, ethambutol PO 15 mg/kg/day, plus one of the following: CF 500–750 mg PO BID, clofazimine PO 100 mg/day, rifampin 600 mg PO qd, or rifabutin 300 mg/day PO indefinitely

[a] Patients with AIDS, after organ transplantation, and during cancer chemotherapy.

[b] Fluoroquinolones include norfloxacin (NF), ciprofloxacin (CF), and ofloxacin (OF).

AIDS, acquired immunodeficiency syndrome; bid, twice a day; CF, ciprofloxacin; IV, intravenous; NF, norfloxacin; OF, ofloxacin; PO, by mouth; q, each, every; qid, four times daily; TMP/SMX, trimethoprim-sulfamethoxazole.

[c] Source: 2004 Treating Opportunistic Infections Among HIV Infected Adults and Adolescents. The National Institutes of Health and the HIV Medicine Association/Infectious Disease Society of America December 16, 2004: 1–35.

(From DuPont HL. Guidelines on acute infectious diarrhea in adults. The Practice Parameters Committee of the American College of Gastroenterology. Am J Gastroenterol 92:1962–1975, 1997, with permission.)

of age, especially those with diarrhea, should be avoided by HIV-infected individuals because of the risk of cryptosporidium. Undercooked and raw meats and raw eggs should not be consumed due to the risk of Salmonella infection.[48]

Drug-induced diarrhea can occur in HIV/AIDS patients. Highly Active Antiretroviral Therapy (HAART), which often includes the use of protease inhibitors, improves immune function, and reduces gastrointestinal opportunistic infections. Although these agents can cause diarrhea, their exact mechanism is unknown. The incidence of protease inhibitor-associated diarrhea ranges from 0% to 56%. The occurrence of diarrhea is greater the first few weeks of therapy with many patients becoming tolerant as therapy continues. Protease inhibitor-associated diarrhea can be managed with diet, OTC preparations, and prescription medications (Table 48.9).[46]

ALTERNATIVE THERAPIES

Several OTC products are marketed as herbal remedies for constipation, diarrhea, and other common ailments of the gastrointestinal tract. Although products for constipation contain roots and bark of various plants and trees, their main ingredients often include aloe, psyllium seed, senna, or cascara sagrada. Some products also contain prune concentrate. Prunes are high in fiber and well regarded as a dietary inter-

TABLE 48.9	Management of Protease Inhibitor-Associated Diarrhea

Oat Bran 1,500 mg bid increases intestinal transit time bloating and flatulence decrease colonic pH

Psyllium 1 tablespoon daily holds water in the stool bloating and flatulence or two bars daily causing distention

Loperamide 4 mg daily initially, then slows intestinal motility abdominal pain, discomfort

  2 mg after each

  loose stool

  max 16 mg/d

Calcium Carbonate 500 mg bid Constipation Gastrointestinal. irritation nausea, vomiting, constipation

Provir (SP–303) 500 mg qid Unknown No side effects known

+ Diphenoxylate/5 mg qid Inhibit gastrointestinal motility nausea, vomiting, abdominal Atropine pain

Pancreatic enzymes 1–2 tabs reduces amount of fat in the nausea, abdominal cramps with meals stool

bid, twice daily; qid, four times daily.
(From Fish DN, Sherman DS, Managemet of protease inhibitor-associated diarrhea. Clin Infect Dis 30:908–914, 2000, with permission.)

vention for constipation. Rhubarb root often is included in many herbal products for constipation because of its natural laxative effect.[49,50]

Many herbal remedies for diarrhea include substances known as tannins. They have astringent properties, thereby reducing intestinal inflammation and restricting secretions. Edible berry plants (i.e., blackberry, blueberry, and raspberry) are commonly used. Dried blueberries are recommended over fresh berries because the latter are high in fiber and may produce a laxative effect. Table 48.10 describes herbs commonly used for constipation and diarrhea and their therapeutic ingredients.[49,50]

Disorders leading to chronic constipation may be aided by other alternative therapies for relief of symptoms. Patients who experience pelvic floor dyssynergia (an inability to relax the pelvic floor muscles during defecation) may benefit from biofeedback training. Patients with diarrhea or abdominal pain associated with IBS may also respond to biofeedback, in addition to hypnosis, cognitive and behavioral treatment, relaxation and stress management, or psychotherapy.[50]

IMPROVING OUTCOMES

PATIENT EDUCATION AND IMPROVING ADHERENCE TO DRUG THERAPY

To provide patient medication counseling for constipation, the pharmacist must determine the patient's perception of nor-mal bowel habits. Only then can the pharmacist determine whether nonpharmacologic or pharmacologic treatment is appropriate. A discussion of bowel habits should emphasize that although constipation often is self-limiting, it may be a symptom of a more serious disease. Consequently, counseling should include questions about the onset and duration of constipation and a history of medical illnesses. The patient's medication profile should be reviewed for possible drug-induced constipation and for a history of the patient's laxative use. Diet and lifestyle activities are ascertained because the lack of exercise and fiber is associated with the development of constipation. Finally, educating patients (especially children) to respond to the urge to defecate is essential.

Several patient education materials are available in print and online for constipation and diarrhea. The National Digestive Diseases Information Clearinghouse has several publications for order via facsimile or electronic mail. Flow-charts for self-diagnosis and care of problems such as diarrhea and constipation are available online from the American Academy of Family Physicians. In addition, the International Foundation for Functional Gastrointestinal Disorders provides support and educational information for people affected by gastrointestinal disorders such as constipation, diarrhea, and IBS.

DISEASE MANAGEMENT STRATEGIES TO IMPROVE PATIENT OUTCOMES

When recommending an appropriate product, the health care provider should consider the following:

- Laxative use should not exceed 1 week of self-medication.
- Laxatives are inappropriate in the presence of abdominal pain or cramping, nausea, vomiting, or bloating.
- Daily administration of bulk-forming agents should be the first choice in uncomplicated chronic constipation.
- The following should be used for 1 week or less: a low-dose saline laxative, stimulant laxative at bedtime, or glycerin suppository.
- Institutionalized or bedridden patients may need laxatives in addition to daily bulk-forming agents to prevent fecal impaction (e.g., weekly intermittent doses of stimulant laxatives, lactulose 30 mL/day, or milk of magnesia).
- Mineral oil should be avoided in older adults, young children (<6 years), and debilitated patients because of the risk of aspiration.
- Patients with a history of myocardial infarction, anal fissures, hernias, or colorectal surgery are candidates for prophylactic laxative therapy to prevent straining. Acceptable agents include docusate, milk of magnesia, glycerin suppository, and bulk-forming products.
- Pregnant patients should use only bulk-forming agents and stool softeners if a laxative is needed.
- Patient education for acute diarrhea should include information about the prevention of subsequent episodes (especially for pediatric diarrhea and TD). Pharmacists should inform the parents of children to do the following:
- Keep ORSs in the home at all times.

TABLE 48.10	Common Herbal Remedies for Constipation and Diarrhea				
Herb	**Active Therapeutic Ingredient**	**Effect**	**Dosage**	**Comments**	
Constipation					
Buckthorn bark	Anthraquinone derivatives: glucofrangulin A and B, frangulin A and B	Stimulant (gentle)	1 g	Bark must be aged 1 yr before use.	
Plantago seed (psyllium seed)	*Plantago psyllium L* or *Plantago indica L*	Bulk-producing (gentle)	7.5 g (2 rounded teaspoons)	Stir husks into glass of water, juice, or milk; drink before mixture thickens. Patients should drink plenty of fluids. May have positive effects on cholesterol.	
Senna	Dianthrone glycosides: sennosides A, A₁, B, C, D, G	Stimulant	0.5–2 g to prepare a bitter tea	A more palatable beverage can be prepared by soaking leaflets in cold water for 10–12 hr.	
Rhubarb	Dried rhizome and root of *Rheum officinale*	Stimulant (potent)	None described	Differs from common garden rhubarb. Causes intestinal griping or colic and is rarely used.	
Diarrhea					
Blackberry leaves	Tannin (8%–14%)	Astringent	Boiling water over 1–2 teaspoons of leaves	Drink up to 6 times/day.	
Blueberry leaves	Tannin (up to 6.7%)	Astringent	Same		
Raspberry leaves	Tannin	Astringent	Same		
Dried blueberries	Tannin	Astringent	Chew and swallow 3 tablespoons		
	Pectin	Adsorbent			

From Tyler VE. Herbs of choice: the therapeutic use of phytomedicinals. New York: Haworth Herbal Press, 2000:62–65, with permission.)

■ Use of newer dosage forms (e.g., freezer pops) and more palatable flavors to enhance compliance.
■ Pack a diarrhea prevention kit when traveling that includes oral rehydration packets, water purification tablets, antidiarrheal medications, and a thermometer.
■ Monitor children for signs and symptoms of diarrhea upon the initiation of any antibiotic medication.
■ Recognize the importance of early intervention of acute diarrhea to prevent complications of dehydration and electrolyte losses.

PHARMACOECONOMICS

The financial impact of constipation and diarrhea in the United States is significant. Currently, an estimated $2 billion is spent on antacids and digestive aids, primarily antidiarrheals and laxatives.[51] One factor contributing to the increased usage is the rise in patient self-treatment with OTC products. A survey of consumer OTC usage trends revealed that of 1,356 household respondents, 26% used products for constipation and 28% used products for diarrhea over a 6-month period.[52] People over the age of 60 years and women used nonprescription laxatives more often. No correlation was observed in these two populations with the use of antidiarrheals.

In a study of 1,059 rural older adults taking OTC medications, 9.7% of those interviewed used laxatives. Results indicated that the use of laxatives was significantly associated with a higher number of physician visits, hospitalizations, emergency room visits, and number of prescriptions 6 months before the interview. The use of home health services was also significantly associated with laxative use.[53]

RELATED DISORDERS

Two disorders related to uncomplicated constipation and diarrhea warrant special discussion: TD and IBS. Although treating these disorders often incorporates several of the therapeutic interventions mentioned previously, they are unique and specific disorders.

TRAVELER'S DIARRHEA

DEFINITION AND EPIDEMIOLOGY

Each year 10% of the American population travels to other countries. Specifically, more than 8 million travel to developing countries.[54] Often their excursions are interrupted by TD, an infectious disease of the gastrointestinal tract in people traveling outside their home country that result in a twofold or greater increase in the frequency of unformed bowel movements with associated symptoms. The risk of TD depends on the traveler's destination. Approximately 20% to 50% of travelers develop TD.[42] The disease affects primarily people traveling from industrialized nations to developing countries. People traveling from the United States, Canada, or northern Europe would be at risk of developing TD when traveling to Latin America, Africa, the Middle East, or Asia. The incidence is slightly greater in young adults than in older adults.

CLINICAL PRESENTATION AND DIAGNOSIS

The abrupt onset of diarrhea generally is self-limiting, with a median duration of 3 to 5 days. Although persistent diarrhea is uncommon in TD, 10% of the cases may continue for more than 1 week. Travelers should be aware that TD may occur more than once during a trip, so appropriate precautions should be taken throughout the travel period. TD develops from food or water that is contaminated with fecal material containing bacteria, viruses, parasites, or combinations of microbes. The most common offending organism is enterotoxigenic *E. coli,* which accounts for more than 40% of cases. *Salmonella* and *Shigella* species and *Campylobacter jejuni* also cause TD. Other potential bacterial pathogens include *Aeromonas hydrophila, Yersinia enterocolitica, Plesiomonas shigelloides, Vibrio parahaemolyticus,* and other *Vibrio* species. Viruses such as rotavirus and Norwalk virus often contaminate water, but they are not common causes of TD in adults. Parasitic enteric pathogens including *Giardia lamblia, Entamoeba histolytica,* and *Cryptosporidium* cause fewer cases of TD.

PREVENTION

PHARMACOTHERAPY

Although there is a consensus in the health community about food and water precautions for TD prevention, chemoprophylaxis for TD prevention is controversial. Several studies have provided data that demonstrate efficacy for antimicrobial and nonantimicrobial agents in decreasing the incidence of diarrhea. The nonantimicrobial agent bismuth subsalicylate has been approved to relieve symptoms of TD.[37] It has been shown to prevent diarrhea in up to 65% of subjects receiving two tablets (524 mg) four times daily for 21 days beginning on the first day of travel. Lower protection rates (40%) were observed in subjects receiving one tablet (262 mg) four times daily.[55] In a previous trial of the liquid preparation, 60 mL four times daily for 3 weeks resulted in a 62% reduction in illness.[56] Bismuth subsalicylate has side effects, including darkening of the tongue and stool and mild tinnitus. Patients taking aspirin concurrently for arthritis may be at increased risk for developing tinnitus secondary to the salicylate component in bismuth subsalicylate. This agent is contraindicated in patients with renal insufficiency, gout, or allergies to aspirin. Caution should be exercised when administering this medication to adolescents and children with chicken pox or flu because of the risk of Reye's syndrome. This agent is not indicated for children less than 3 years old. Patients with AIDS may be at greater risk of developing encephalopathy from consuming excessive dosages of bismuth subsalicylate.[57] Concurrent use of anticoagulants, probenecid, or methotrexate is contraindicated with this agent. Bismuth subsalicylate appears to be effective for TD prophylaxis and is recommended by the Centers for Disease Control for use not longer than 3 weeks.

Several antibiotics have been investigated for TD chemoprophylaxis. One of the earliest antimicrobials studied was doxycycline. Doses of 100 mg per day for 21 days are effective in areas where ETEC were sensitive to the drug.[58,59] However, the protection rate decreased in geographic areas with resistant strains.[58] In addition, side effects including photosensitivity and diarrhea and contraindications in pregnancy and lactation and in children (<8 years of age) increase its risk to benefit ratio for prophylactic use.

Trimethoprim-sulfamethoxazole (TMP/SMX) in regimens of 160/800 mg bid for 21 days and daily for 14 days has demonstrated efficacy in preventing TD.[60,61] TMP alone at dosages of 200 mg daily for 14 days is effective for diarrhea prevention.[61] Although better compared with placebo, the protection rate of TMP alone was less than that of the combination (95% vs. 52%). Side effects noted in the studies were primarily dermatologic, including rashes and skin eruptions. Because TMP/SMX can cause serious skin eruptions such as Stevens-Johnson syndrome, the risk of taking these agents for TD prophylaxis is of concern.

Quinolone carboxylic acid derivatives are useful for TD chemoprophylaxis. Norfloxacin, ciprofloxacin, and levofloxacin have been studied widely. Norfloxacin 400 mg orally once daily for 14 days is effective.[62] Fewer patients developed diarrhea on norfloxacin than on placebo (7% vs. 61%). Norfloxacin provided an 88% protection rate. Resistance was not evident among aerobic Gram-negative bacilli. Adverse reactions were limited to one case of a generalized rash 11 days after therapy with norfloxacin, which resolved on discontinuation. In another study, ciprofloxacin 500 mg daily was compared with placebo in people traveling to Tunisia.[63] Ciprofloxacin provided a 94% protection rate and was well tolerated. One case of serious sunburn was observed that may have been drug related. Ciprofloxacin did not appear to affect aerobic bacterial flora 5 weeks after travel.

Azithromycin, a macrolide antibiotic, has been shown to be a safe and effective alternative for the treatment of TD in pregnant women, children, and those who do not respond to fluoroquinolones. Azithromycin has good activity against the common bacterial enteric pathogens and it achieves high intracellular concentrations.[64] The azithromycin dose is 1,000 mg once or 500 mg once daily for 3 days.[65]

A randomized, double-blind trial compared the effectiveness of azithromycin 1,000 mg single dose to levofloxacin 500 mg single dose for the treatment of TD. Out of 217 patients, 9.5% in the azithromycin group and 7.5% in the levofloxacin group, failed treatment following 4 days of treatment. It was concluded that both antimicrobials were safe and effective for the treatment of TD.[66]

Rifaximin is a rifamycin derivative that inhibits bacterial ribonucleic acid (RNA) synthesis. It has been found to have activity against Gram-positive and Gram-negative organisms. The drug is approved for TD in persons at least 12 years of age when TD is caused by noninvasive strains of *E. coli*. It is recommended that rifaximin not be used when *Campylobacter jejuni*, *Shigella*, or *Salmonella* are the suspected causative pathogens.[65,67] The oral bioavailability of rifaximin is low, with less than 0.4% of the oral rifaximin being absorbed. It is contraindicated in persons allergic to rifamycins. Like rifamycins, it is a mild inducer of cytochrome P450 (CYP) enzyme system 3A4; however, there are no clinically significant drug interactions associated with its concomitant use. Rifaximin is dosed 200 mg three times a day for the treatment of TD.[67]

A randomized, double-blind clinical trial of 187 patients was conducted to demonstrate rifaximin safety and effectiveness of rifaximin at 400 mg bid compared to ciprofloxacin 500 mg bid in TD. Ninety-three subjects received rifaximin and 94 received ciprofloxacin. Both drugs demonstrated effectiveness in the treatment of TD. The duration of diarrhea was approximately 1 day for both agents.[68]

Although prophylactic management of TD with antimicrobial agents has demonstrated benefits, the uncertainty of the risk of widespread use must be evaluated. These agents have the potential for side effects such as skin rashes, photosensitivity reactions, blood disorders, Stevens-Johnson syndrome, and staining of the teeth in children. In addition, infections secondary to antimicrobial therapy (e.g., *Candida* vaginitis, antibiotic-associated colitis, and *Salmonella* enteritis) are a risk. Therefore, prophylactic antimicrobial agents are not recommended for travelers. Alternatively, instructing travelers about proper food and water precautions and early treatment of TD provide better outcomes without the risks associated with widespread prophylaxis.

NONPHARMACOLOGIC THERAPY

Instructing travelers about safe food and water precautions is the mainstay of TD prevention. Travelers should be advised to avoid drinking or brushing their teeth with tap water. Ice cubes should be avoided because they may have been made with contaminated water. Boiled water (as in hot tea or coffee), carbonated beverages, beer, and wine generally are safe to consume. Two reliable methods of purification are vigorous boiling of water and chemical disinfection with iodine. Chemical disinfection can be accomplished by using tincture of iodine or tetraglycine hydroperiodide tablets. These tablets are available in pharmacies. However, disinfection with iodine often leaves an unpleasant taste. Foods that should be avoided are undercooked or raw foods, salads, and unpasteurized milk and milk products. Foods safe for consumption include bread or crackers, peeled fruit or vegetables, and well-cooked foods.[42]

TREATMENT

Approaches to treating TD include many of the remedies for treating acute nonspecific diarrhea: fluid replacement and symptomatic relief with adsorbents, antimotility agents, and short-term antimicrobial therapy. The self-limiting nature of TD generally allows successful management with nonspecific agents. However, antimicrobial agents may be useful in persistent diarrhea.

Bismuth subsalicylate is effective for relieving symptoms of mild to moderate TD. Doses of 30 mL every 30 minutes for 8 doses generally are effective in relieving abdominal pain and cramping and reducing unformed stools.[69,70] Bismuth subsalicylate has not been shown to improve the nausea and vomiting of TD.

Loperamide, an antimotility agent, is approved for the symptomatic relief of TD at doses up to 8 mg per day. Loperamide was compared with bismuth subsalicylate for treating TD.[70] Doses of loperamide were administered at 4 mg initially, then 2 mg after each unformed stool, and bismuth subsalicylate was administered at recommended doses. Loperamide demonstrated significantly more relief (disappearance) of diarrhea and abdominal pain and a greater decrease in severity of symptoms than bismuth subsalicylate. There was no significant difference in the duration of diarrhea. Loperamide-treated patients with shigellosis did not experience prolongation of diarrhea.[70] This is consistent with the results of a study involving 43 patients; two patients infected with *Shigella* sp. were treated with loperamide without prolongation of diarrhea.[71]

Although using antimicrobial agents to treat TD is controversial, they may be appropriate in patients who develop persistent diarrhea. Travelers with diarrhea unresponsive to conventional therapy, three or more loose stools in an 8-hour period, and associated symptoms of nausea, vomiting, abdominal cramps, fever, or blood in the stools may benefit from a short course of therapy. Selection of an appropriate agent may depend on the traveler's symptoms, the location of travel, the climate, and the type of chemoprophylaxis received before treatment. The recommended duration of treatment is 3 days.[42]

TMP/SMX (160 mg/800 mg bid) or TMP (200 mg bid) alone for 3 to 5 days is effective in reducing the number of unformed stools and decreasing symptoms, including abdominal cramps, pain, and nausea.[72] The efficacy of ciprofloxacin (500 mg bid) and TMP/SMX (160 mg/800 mg bid), each for 5 days, was compared with that of placebo.[73] Both agents were equally effective. Ciprofloxacin may offer an alternative for patients with hypersensitivity to TMP/SMX. As resistance to TMP/SMX increases, fluoroquinolones may have greater benefit.

In general, fluoroquinolones are the drugs of choice for adults traveling to high-risk areas (e.g., Latin America, Africa, the Middle East, and Asia).[42] Data suggest the use of combination therapy with antimotility agents (loperamide) and antibiotics (TMP/SMX) initially in patients with moderate to severe diarrhea.[74] However, further study on the efficacy and safety is warranted.

FUTURE THERAPIES

Future developments in TD prophylaxis and treatment may include the use of poorly absorbed antimicrobial agents such as bicozamycin and oral aztreonam.[75,76] These agents should be safe in pregnant women and children. Zaldaride maleate, an intestinal calmodulin inhibitor, is another agent under investigation for TD because of its antisecretory properties.[77] However, more data about the safety and efficacy of these agents are needed.

IRRITABLE BOWEL SYNDROME

DEFINITION

IBS is one of the most common disorders of the gastrointestinal tract among young to middle-aged adults. It is defined as a combination of chronic or recurrent gastrointestinal symptoms not explained by structural or biochemical abnormalities, attributed to the intestines, and associated with

symptoms of pain and disturbed defecation or symptoms of bloating and distension.[78]

EPIDEMIOLOGY AND PATHOPHYSIOLOGY

The impact of IBS on health care is significant. It is estimated that IBS accounts for 2.4 to 3.5 million physician visits and more than 2.2 million prescriptions annually in the United States.[79–81] In a recent study, health care costs attributed to IBS in 1 year were $742, compared with $429 for patients without IBS.[82] Loss of work days was three times greater in people with IBS than in those without bowel symptoms.[83]

Although this syndrome comprises 41% of all functional gastrointestinal disorders, little is known about the pathogenesis of IBS. It is believed that IBS results from disordered intestinal motility and increased visceral sensitivity with psychological stress contributing to its recurrence and exacerbation.[78,84]

CLINICAL PRESENTATION AND DIAGNOSIS

Clinical manifestations of IBS may vary. The diagnosis is made by identifying symptom-based criteria, known as the Rome II criteria (Table 48.11), and excluding symptoms of diseases that may mimic IBS. A physical examination and a medical history are warranted to exclude other diagnoses.

TABLE 48.11	Rome II Diagnostic Criteria for Irritable Bowel Syndrome

At least 3 mos of noncontinuous, abdominal pain or discomfort in the preceding 12 months that is accompanied by two of three characteristics:

Relieved with defecation or

Associated with change in frequency of stool or

Associated with a change in consistency of stool

Symptoms that collective suggest a diagnosis of IBS

Altered stool frequency (for research purposes *altered* may be defined as more than three bowel movements each day or fewer than three bowel movements each week)

Altered stool form (lumpy/hard or loose/watery stool)

Altered stool passage (straining, urgency, or feeling of incomplete evacuation)

Passage of mucus

Bloating or feeling of abdominal distension

IBS, irritable bowel syndrome.
(From the American Gastroenterological Association Patient Care Committee. Irritable bowel syndrome: a technical review for practice guideline development. Gastroenterology 123:2108–2131, 2002.)

Additional diagnostic tests can be initiated to determine if "alarm signs" or "red flags" are present, such as family history of IBS, colon or rectal cancer, weight loss, fever, anemia, blood in stool, and abnormal physical and blood work. A diagnosis can be made based on the patient's symptomatic subgroup (Table 48.11).

THERAPEUTIC PLAN

Treatment should be initiated to alleviate the predominant symptom (i.e., constipation, diarrhea, or pain, gas, or bloating). Therapy generally should be reassessed after 3 to 6 weeks (Table 48.12).

TREATMENT

PHARMACOTHERAPY

Several pharmacologic agents have been investigated for treating IBS symptoms. Bulk-forming laxatives generally are recommended for patients with constipation. Cisapride, on a limited-access basis, has been used in these patients; however, its widespread use has been minimal due to serious side effects.[31,85] Newer agents for the management of IBS symptoms have gained interest because they provide options for treating either symptom.

In treating diarrhea, data suggest that the opiate agonist loperamide is safe and effective. Studies demonstrate that patients with IBS taking loperamide experience improvement in diarrhea associated with decreases in stool frequency, passage of unformed stools, and incidence of urgency.[86,87] In patients with IBS and constipation, loperamide may worsen the symptoms.[87] An appropriate dose for loperamide in IBS has not been determined. However, doses ranging from 2 mg bid to 4 mg four times daily have been used for relief of symptoms. Cholestyramine, a bile acid sequestrant, may be beneficial in patients with IBS and diarrhea, and a history of cholecystectomy or idiopathic bile acid malabsorption.[78]

Antispasmodics (anticholinergic agents) are commonly used in the United States for treating symptoms of abdominal pain associated with IBS. These agents suppress the postprandial contractile response of the gastrointestinal tract, thereby reducing its tone and motility. Examples of these agents are belladonna alkaloids, dicyclomine hydrochloride, and hyoscyamine sulfate. Before therapy with these agents is initiated, patients should be informed of their anticholinergic side effects. Antispasmodic medications may be contraindicated in patients with a history of cardiac arrhythmia, glaucoma, and urinary retention.

Serotonin-receptor modulators have been used based on the role of serotonin in normal gastrointestinal function. Two new agents, alosetron and tegaserod, are available for use in IBS (Table 48.12). These agents work as an antagonist to serotonin-3 (5-HT_3) and a partial agonist to serotonin-4 (5-HT_4) receptors, respectively. Antagonism of 5-HT_3 receptors reduce colonic transit, reduce visceral pain, and decrease small intestinal secretion. An agonist of the 5-HT_4 receptors can cause peristaltic reflex in the gastrointestinal tract.[88]

Alosetron was reapproved by the FDA in June 2002 after being withdrawn in 2000 because 1 in 700 patients who took alosetron experienced ischemic colitis, and some patients died.[89] It is indicated for women who have severe diarrhea-predominate IBS for at least 6 months, and who have not responded to conventional therapy. Alosetron is available under restricted conditions for use via the Prescribing Program for Lotronex. Enrollment and prescribing information

TABLE 48.12	Initial Treatment of Irritable Bowel Syndrome		
	Symptomatic Subgroup		
	Constipation	**Diarrhea**	**Pain, Gas, or Bloating**
Review diet history	Yes	Yes	Yes
Additional tests	No	Lactose-H_2 breath test	Plain abdominal radiograph
Therapeutic trial	Increase roughage	Loperamide	Antispasmodic (e.g., dicyclomine, hyoscyamine, glycopyrrolate)
	Osmotic	Alosetron[b]	
	Laxative (e.g., milk of magnesia, sorbitol, polyethylene glycol)		Antidepressants[c]
	Tegaserod[a]		

[a] Tegaserod is effective in women with constipation-predominate IBS. The FDA-approved dose is 6 mg bid for up to 12 weeks.

[b] Alosetron is recommended in women with diarrhea-predominate IBS. The FDA approved dose is 1mg qd for 4 wks.

[c] Low dose tricyclic antidepressants (e.g., amitriptyline, desipramine, doxepin, nortriptyline) are recommended when there is recurrent pain.

bid, twice a day; FDA, Food and Drug Administration; IBS, irritable bowel syndrome; qd, every day.

(From American Gastroenterological Association Patient Care Committee. Irritable bowel syndrome: a technical review for practice guideline development. Gastroenterology 123:2108–2131, 2002.)

is available at http://www.lotronex.com. This agent should be initiated at 1 mg once a day for 4 weeks. If alosetron is not effective after 4 weeks at 1mg once a day, then the dose may be increased to 1 mg bid. Constipation, nausea, anorexia, dizziness, headache, flatulence, and abdominal pain are the most frequently reported side effects. Its use is contraindicated in persons with a history of intestinal obstruction, active diverticulitis, or a history of diverticulitis and Crohn disease.[88]

Alosetron has been evaluated for the treatment of diarrhea-predominate IBS in women. Six hundred and forty-seven women were randomized to received alosetron (1 mg) or placebo for 3 months. A greater number of patients in the alosetron treatment group reported relief of pain, discomfort, and stool frequency. These patients also had improvement in stool consistency and a decrease in urgency.[90]

Tegaserod was approved by the FDA for treatment in women with constipation-predominate IBS for up to 12 weeks when fiber, laxatives, and antispasmodic agents have failed. Two randomized, double-blinded, placebo-control trials have been conducted to determine its safety and effectiveness. In both studies, patients were enrolled if they had IBS according to Rome II criteria and had constipation-predominate IBS of at least 3 months. Both studies found significant improvement in bloating, abdominal pain, discomfort, and constipation with the administration of tegaserod (6 mg bid) versus placebo. The recommended dose is 6 mg bid for 4 to 6 weeks; however, treatment may continue for an additional 4 to 6 weeks if symptoms persist. The most common side effects reported are diarrhea, headache, nausea, vomiting, and dizziness.[91,92]

Psychotropic medications, such as tricyclic antidepressants, are indicated for patients who experience severe or refractory symptoms with associated depression or panic attacks. These patients have generally failed psychological treatment methods (e.g., cognitive and behavioral treatment, hypnosis, relaxation and stress management, or psychotherapy).

Doses used for IBS are often lower than those used for depression. Although selective serotonin reuptake inhibitors have been used clinically because of their favorable side effect profile, no published controlled studies are available for review. Anxiolytics have been used but generally are not recommended because of their potential for physical dependence and drug interactions.[78]

NONPHARMACOLOGIC THERAPY

Treating IBS incorporates lifestyle modifications and pharmacologic management based on the patient's predominant symptoms. Although its use is controversial, it is recommended that patients with IBS and constipation increase their dietary fiber intake to 25 g per day. Patients with symptoms of diarrhea should avoid foods that may aggravate diarrhea such as dairy products, caffeine, alcoholic beverages, sorbitol-containing foods, and fatty foods. If symptoms of bloating and gas persist, avoiding gas-producing foods (e.g.,

beans, cabbage, and certain fruits) may be helpful. Certain medications may aggravate gastrointestinal symptoms and should be avoided (e.g., stimulant laxatives and antacids).[89]

KEY POINTS

- Constipation and diarrhea are common disorders of the gastrointestinal tract that are more often self-reported by older adults
- It is essential to counsel patients on the self-management of constipation and diarrhea
- The primary goals in the management of constipation and diarrhea should be to relieve symptoms, prevent complications, and restore normal bowel habits. These disorders often are self-limiting, therefore intervention may be of short duration
- Definitions of constipation vary but most often incorporate straining, hard or firm stool, less frequent defecation, and a feeling of incomplete evacuation
- Diarrhea generally is defined as three or more loose or unformed bowel movements per day with symptoms of fever, abdominal cramps, or vomiting
- Agents available for treating constipation include bulk-forming agents, hyperosmotic agents, stool softeners, lubricants, saline, stimulant laxatives, and tegaserod
- Laxatives should not be used for more than 1 week without medical supervision, nor should they be used in the presence of abdominal pain or cramping, nausea, or vomiting
- Patients should be instructed to increase fluid intake and participate in regular exercise to prevent constipation
- Infants and young children are more susceptible to acute losses of fluid from diarrhea and may need ORSs
- Kaolin is an agent with adsorbent properties used to treat acute nonspecific diarrhea
- Loperamide should be discontinued after 48 hours if clinical improvement of diarrhea is not observed
- People from industrialized nations traveling to developing countries often experience TD
- Safe food and water precautions are the mainstay of TD prevention. Prophylactic antimicrobial agents are not recommended for travelers
- TD can be managed successfully with bismuth subsalicylate and loperamide. Persistent TD may necessitate 3 days of antimicrobial therapy
- The diagnosis of IBS can be made using the Rome II criteria. Treatment is based on predominant symptoms
- Constipation-predominant IBS can be safely managed with bulk-forming agents or tegaserod. Diarrhea-predominant IBS is managed primarily with loperamide; however, alosetron is recommended in those patients who do not respond to conventional treatment. Abdomi-

nal pain is relieved by antispasmodics. Psychotropic medications are reserved for patients who are refractory to other medications and have certain psychiatric disorders

SUGGESTED READINGS

Centers for Disease Control and Prevention. Health Information for International Travel 2003–2004. Atlanta: US Department of Health and Human Services, Public Health Service, 2003.

Lembo A, Camilleri M. Chronic constipation. N Engl J Med 349: 1360–1368, 2003.

Mertz HR. Irritable bowel syndrome. N Engl J Med 349:2136–2146, 2003.

Oldfield E. Evaluation of chronic diarrhea in patients with human immunodeficiency virus infection. Rev Gastroenterol Disord 2:176–187, 2002.

REFERENCES

1. Sandler RS, Drossman DA. Bowel habits in young adults not seeking health care. Dig Dis Sci 32:841–845, 1987.
2. Binder HJ. Pathophysiology of acute diarrhea. Am J Med 88 (Suppl 6A):2S–4S, 1990.
3. Lennard-Jones JE. Constipation. In: Feldman M, Friedman LS, Sleisenger MH. Gastrointestinal and liver disease: pathophysiology, diagnosis, and management. 7th ed. Philadelphia: WB Saunders, 2002:181–210.
4. Schiller LR, Sellin JH. Diarrhea. In: Feldman M, Friedman LS, Sleisenger MH. Gastrointestinal and liver disease: pathophysiology, diagnosis, and management. 7th ed. Philadelphia: WB Saunders, 2002:131–153.
5. Everhart JE, Liang V, Johannes RS, et al. A longitudinal survey of self-reported bowel habits in the United States. Dig Dis Sci 34: 1153–1162, 1989.
6. Sandler RS, Jordan MC, Shelton BJ. Demographic and dietary determinants of constipation in the US population. Am J Public Health 80:185–189, 1990.
7. Stewart WF, Leberman JN, Sandler, et al. Epidemiology of Constipation (EPOC) Study in the United States: Relation of clinical subtypes to sociodemographic features. Am J Gastroenterol 94: 3530–3540, 1999.
8. Garthwright W, Archer D, Kvenberg J. Estimates of incidence and cost of intestinal infectious diseases in the United States. Public Health Rep 103:107–115, 1988.
9. DuPont HL. Guidelines on acute infectious diarrhea in adults. The Practice Parameters Committee of the American College of Gastroenterology. Am J Gastroenterol 92:1962–1975, 1997.
10. Koch TR. Constipation. In: Haubrich WS, Schaffner F, Berk JE. Bockus gastroenterology. 5th ed. Philadelphia: WB Saunders, 1995: 103–104.
11. Ruben BD. Public perceptions of digestive health and disease. Pract Gastroenterol 10:35–40, 1986.
12. Cohnell AM, Hilton C, Irvin G, et al. Variation of bowel habit in two population samples. BMJ 2:1095–1102, 1965.
13. American Gastroenterological Association medical position statement: Guidelines on constipation. Gastroenterology 119:1761–1778, 2000.
14. Jafri S, Pasricha PJ. Agents used for diarrhea, constipation, and inflammatory bowel disease; agents used for biliary and pancreatic disease. In: Hardman JG, Limbird LE, Gilman AG. Goodman & Gilman's the pharmacological basis of therapeutics. 10th ed. New York: McGraw-Hill, 2002:1037–1047.
15. McRorie JW, Daggy BP, Morel JG, et al. A clinical study comparing stool softening and laxative efficacy of psyllium vs. docusate sodium. Gastroenterology 112 (Suppl):A787, 1997.
16. Anonymous. Laxative drug products for over the counter human use: proposed amendment to the tentative final monograph federal register. Proposed Rule. August 5, 2003; Vol. 68, No. 150.
17. Lembo A, Camilleri M. Chronic constipation. N Engl J Med 349: 1360–1368, 2003.
18. Polyethylene glycol 3350, NF powder for solution; prescribing information. Available at http://www.drugs.com/PDR/MiraLax_Powder_for_Oral_Solution.html.
19. Tedesco FJ, Dipiro JT. Laxative use in constipation. Am J Gastroenterol 80:303–309, 1985.
20. DiPalma JA, DeRidder PH, Orlando RC, et al. A randomized, placebo-controlled multicenter study of the safety and efficacy of a new polyethylene glycol laxative. Am J Gastroenterol 95:446–450, 2000.
21. Anonymous. Safety of stool softeners. Med Lett 19:45–46, 1977.
22. Donowitz M. Current concepts of laxative action: mechanisms by which laxatives increase stool water. Clin Gastroenterol 1:777–784, 1979.
23. Anonymous. Laxatives. Replacing danthron. Drug Ther Bull 26: 53–56, 1988.
24. Johanson, JF, Wald A, Tougas G. Effect of tegaserod in chronic constipation: a randomized double-blind, controlled trial. Clin Gastroenterol Hepatol 2:796–805, 2004.
25. Rivkin A. Tegaserod maleate in the treatment of irritable syndrome: A clinical review. Clin Ther 25:1952–1971, 2003.
26. Brinker AD, Mackney CA, Prizont R. Tegaserod and ischemic colitis. N Engl J Med 351:1361–1364, 2004.
27. Hedner T, Cassieto J. Opioids and opioid receptors in peripheral tissues. Scand J Gastroenterol 130 (Suppl):36–40, 1987.
28. Kreek MJ, Schaefer RA, Hahn EF, et al. Naloxone, a specific opioid antagonist, reverses chronic idiopathic constipation. Lancet 1: 261–262, 1983.
29. Kaufman PN, Krevsky B, Malmud LS, et al. Role of opiate receptors in the regulation of colonic transit. Gastroenterology 94: 1351–1356, 1988.
30. Baron JA, Jessen LM, Colaizzi JL, et al. Cisapride: a gastrointestinal prokinetic drug. Ann Pharmacother 28:488–500, 1994.
31. Anonymous. FDA updates warnings for cisapride. FDA Talk Paper T00-6; January 24, 2000.
32. Anonymous. Limited-access protocol for the use of cisapride in the treatment of gastroesophageal reflux disease and other gastrointestinal motility disorders. Protocol No. CIS-USA-154. Janssen Pharmaceutica.
33. Muller-Lissner SA. Treatment of chronic constipation with cisapride and placebo. Gut 28:1033–1038, 1987.
34. Verheyen K, Vervaeke M, Demyttenaere P, et al. Double-blind comparison of two cisapride dosage regimens with placebo in the treatment of functional constipation. Curr Ther Res 41:978–985, 1987.
35. Anonymous. Psyllium health claims: final rule. Federal Register 1998 Feb 18:63 FR 8103.
36. Kinnunen O. Study of constipation in a geriatric hospital, day hospital, old people's home and at home. Aging 3:161–170, 1991.
37. Anonymous. Antidiarrheal drug products for over-the counter human use: final monograph. Federal Register 2003 68:18869–18882.
38. DuPont HL, Sanchez JF, Ericsson CD, et al. Comparative efficacy of loperamide hydrochloride and bismuth subsalicylate in the management of acute diarrhea. Am J Med 88 (Suppl 6A):15S–19S, 1990.
39. Dupont HL, Ericsson CD, DuPont MW, et al. A randomized open-label comparison of non-prescription loperamide and attapulgite in the symptomatic treatment of acute diarrhea. Am J Med 88 (Suppl 6A):20S–23S, 1990.
40. Johnson PC, Ericsson CD, DuPont HL, et al. Comparison of loperamide with bismuth subsalicylate for the treatment of acute traveler's diarrhea. JAMA 225:757–760, 1986.
41. Anonymous. Opium preparations. American Hospital Formulary Service Drug Information 2004. Bethesda, MD: American Society of Health-Systems Pharmacists, 2004:2768, Section 56.10.
42. Centers for Disease Control and Prevention. Health Information for International Travel 2003–2004. Atlanta: US Department of Health and Human Services, Public Health Service, 2003.
43. DuPont HL, Hornick RB. Adverse effect of lomotil therapy in shigellosis. JAMA 226:1525–1528, 1973.
44. Brown JW. Toxic megacolon association with loperamide therapy. JAMA 241:501–502, 1979.
45. Oldfield, E. Evaluation of chronic diarrhea in patients with human immunodeficiency virus infection. Rev Gastroenterol Disord 2: 176–187, 2002.

46. Fish DN, Sherman DS. Management of protease inhibitor-associate diarrhea. Clin Infect Dis 30:908–914, 2000.

47. Cello JP, Grendell JH, Basuk P, et al. Effect of octreotide on refractory AIDS-associated diarrhea. Ann Intern Med 115:705–710, 1991.

48. 2001 Guidelines for the prevention of opportunistic infections in person infected with HIV. United Public Health Services-Infectious Disease Society of America November 28, 2001:1–64.

49. Tyler VE. Herbs of choice: the therapeutic use of phytomedicinals. New York: Haworth Herbal Press, 1999:62–65.

50. Tyler VE. The honest herbal: a sensible guide to the use of herbs and related remedies. 3rd ed. 1993:336–351.

51. Gannon K. The next five years: the hot and not so hot OTC drugs. Drug Top (May 7):28–32, 1990.

52. Gannon K. Who's buying what in OTCs. Drug Top (Jan. 8):32–48, 1990.

53. Stoehr GP, Ganguli M, Seaberg EC, et al. Over-the-counter medication use in an older rural community: the Movies Project. J Am Geriatr Soc 45:158–165, 1997.

54. Salata RA, Olds GR. Infectious diseases in travelers and immigrants. In: Warren KS, Mahmoud AF. Tropical and geographic medicine. 2nd ed. New York: McGraw-Hill, 1990:228.

55. DuPont HL, Ericsson CD, Johnson PC. Prevention of travelers' diarrhea by the tablet formulation of bismuth subsalicylate. JAMA 257:1347–1350, 1987.

56. DuPont HL, Sullivan P, Evans DG, et al. Prevention of travelers' diarrhea (emporiatric enteritis): prophylactic administration of bismuth subsalicylate. JAMA 243:237–241, 1980.

57. Mendelowitz PC, Hoffman RS, Weber S. Bismuth absorption and myoclonic encephalopathy during bismuth subsalicylate therapy. Ann Intern Med 112:140–141, 1990.

58. Sack DA, Kaminsky DC, Sack RB, et al. Prophylactic doxycycline for travelers' diarrhea: results of a prospective double-blind study of Peace Corps volunteers in Kenya. N Engl J Med 298:758–763, 1978.

59. Sack RB, Frochlich JL, Zulich AW, et al. Prophylactic doxycycline for travelers' diarrheas: results of a prospective double-blind study of Peace Corps volunteers in Morocco. Gastroenterology 76:1368–1373, 1979.

60. DuPont HL, Evans DG, Rios N, et al. Prevention of traveler's diarrhea with trimethoprim-sulfamethoxazole alone. Gastroenterology 84:75–80, 1983.

61. DuPont HL, Galindo E, Evans DG, et al. Prevention of traveler's diarrhea with trimethoprim-sulfamethoxazole and trimethoprim alone. Gastroenterology 84:75–80, 1983.

62. Johnson PC, Ericsson CD, Morgan DR, et al. Lack of emergency of resistant fecal flora during successful prophylaxis of travelers' diarrhea with norfloxacin. Antimicrob Agents Chemother 30:671–674, 1986.

63. Rademaker CM, Hoepelam IM, Wolfhagen MJ. Results of a double-blind placebo-controlled study using ciprofloxacin for prevention of traveler's diarrhea. Eur J Clin Microbiol Infect Dis 8:690–694, 1989.

64. Gordillo ME, Sing KV, Murray BE. In vitro activity of azithromycin against bacterial enteric pathogens. Antimicrob Agents Chemother 37:1203–1205, 1993.

65. Anonymous. Rifaximin for traveler's diarrhea. Med Lett 74–75, 2004.

66. Adachi JA, Ericsson CD, Jiang ZD. Azithromycin found to be comparable to levofloxacin for the treatment of us travelers with acute diarrhea acquired in Mexico. Clin Infect Dis 37:1165–1171, 2003

67. Gillis JC, Brogden RN. Rifaximin. A review of its antibacterial activity, pharmacokinetic properties and therapeutic potential in conditions mediated by gastrointestinal bacteria. Drugs 49:467–484, 1995.

68. DuPont HL, Jiang ZD, Ericsson CD, et al. Rifaximin versus ciprofloxacin for the treatment of traveler's diarrhea: a randomized, double-blind clinical trial. Clin Infect Dis 33:1807–1815, 2001.

69. DuPont HL, Sullivan P, Pickering LK, et al. Symptomatic treatment of diarrhea with bismuth subsalicylate among students attending a Mexican university. Gastroenterology 73:715–718, 1997.

70. Johnson PC, Ericsson CD, DuPont HL. Comparison of loperamide with bismuth subsalicylate for the treatment of acute traveler's diarrhea. JAMA 255:757–760, 1986.

71. Van Loon FP, Bennish ML, Butler C. Double-blind trial of loperamide for treating acute watery diarrhea in expatriates in Bangladesh. Gut 30:492–495, 1989.

72. DuPont HL, Reves RR, Galindo E, et al. Treatment of traveler's diarrhea with trimethoprim/sulfamethoxazole and with trimethoprim alone. N Engl J Med 307:841–844, 1982.

73. Ericsson CD, Johnson PC, DuPont HL, et al. Ciprofloxacin or trimethoprim-sulfamethoxazole as initial therapy for traveler's diarrhea. Ann Intern Med 106:216–220, 1987.

74. Ericsson CD, DuPont HL, Mathewson JJ, et al. Treatment of travelers' diarrhea with sulfamethoxazole and trimethoprim and loperamide. JAMA 263:257–261, 1990.

75. Ericksson CD, DuPont HL, Sullivan P, et al. Bicozamycin, a poorly absorbable antibiotic, effectively treats traveler's diarrhea. Ann Intern Med 98:20–25, 1983.

76. DuPont HL, Ericsson CD, Mathewson JJ, et al. Oral aztreonam, a poorly absorbed yet effective therapy for bacterial diarrhea in U.S. travelers to Mexico. JAMA 267:1932–1935, 1992.

77. DuPont HL, Ericsson CD, Mathewson JJ, et al. Zaldaride maleate: an intestinal calmodulin inhibitor in the therapy of traveler's diarrhea. Gastroenterology 104:709–715, 1993.

78. American Gastroenterological Association Patient Care Committee. Irritable bowel syndrome: a technical review for practice guideline development. Gastroenterology 123:2108–2131, 2002.

79. Everhart JE, Renault PF. Irritable bowel syndrome in office-based practice in the United States. Gastroenterology 100:998–1005, 1991.

80. Sandler RS. Epidemiology of irritable bowel syndrome in the United States. Gastroenterology 99:409–415, 1990.

81. Greco AM. Diagnosis and management of irritable bowel syndrome. US Pharmacist 28:85–92, 2003.

82. Talley NJ, Gabriel SE, Harmsen WS, et al. Medical costs in community subjects with irritable bowel syndrome. Gastroenterology 109:1736–1741, 1995.

83. Drossman DA, Li Z, Andruzzi E, et al. U.S. household survey of functional gastrointestinal disorders: prevalence, sociodemography and health impact. Dig Dis Sci 38:1569–1580, 1993.

84. McGill B. Functional diarrhea. Evaluation and management. Pract Gastroenterol 4:16–20, 1980.

85. Van Outryve M, Milon R, Toussaint J, et al. "Prokinetic" treatment of constipation-predominant irritable bowel syndrome. A placebo-controlled study of cisapride. Clin Gastroenterol 13:49–57, 1991

86. Cann PA, Read NW, Holdsworth CD, et al. Role of loperamide and placebo in the management of irritable bowel syndrome. Dig Dis Sci 29:239–247, 1984.

87. Hovdenak N. Loperamide treatment of the irritable bowel syndrome. Scand J Gastroenterol 130 (Suppl):81–84, 1987.

88. Lembo A, Weber HC, Farraye FA, et al. Alosetron in irritable bowel syndrome: Strategies for its use in a common gastrointestinal disorder. Drugs 63:1895–1905, 2003.

89. Mertz HR, Irritable bowel syndrome. N Engl J Med 349:2136–2146, 2003.

90. Camilleri M, Northcutt AR, Kong S, et al. Efficacy and safety of alosetron in women with irritable bowel syndrome: a randomised, placebo-controlled trial. Lancet 355:1035–1040, 2000.

91. Muller-Lissner SA, Fumagalli KD, Bardhan KD, et al. Tegaserod a 5-HT4 receptor partial agonist, relieves symptoms in irritable bowel syndrome patients with abdominal pain, bloating and constipation. Aliment Pharmacol Ther 15:1655–1666, 2001.

92. Novick, J, Miner P, Krause R, et al. A randomized, double-blind, placebo-controlled trial of tegaserod in female patients suffering from irritable bowel syndrome with constipation. Aliment Pharmacol Ther 16:1877–1888, 2002.

CASE 19

TOPIC: Peptic Ulcer Disease

THERAPEUTIC DIFFICULTY: Level 1
Kristina Butler

Chapter 45: Peptic Ulcer Disease

■ Scenario

Patient and Setting: EC, a 23-year-old Caucasian female; primary care physician's office

Chief Complaint: Epigastric pain described as intense burning or gnawing sensation that is worse at night and between meals; better with food; started 3 weeks ago during midterms; occasional mild cramping sensation

■ History of Present Illness

Pain increasingly persistent over the last few weeks; has been using OTC antacids without maximal relief; denies "heartburn" symptoms, changes in bowel movements

Medical History: Asthma (exercise-induced), allergic rhinitis, menstrual migraine (last migraine 2 months ago)

Surgical History: Tonsillectomy and adenoidectomy

Family/Social History: Family History: Mother alive w/ hypertension (HTN); father alive s/p aortic valve replacement d/t aortic stenosis from congenital bicuspid aortic valve
Social History: nonsmoker, 3–4 glasses of wine a week; 1–2 diet colas a day; nursing student

Medications:
Levonorgestrel/EE, 0.15 mg/0.03 mg PO daily × 84 days (then 7 days of placebo)
Albuterol, 90 µg MDI, 1–2 puffs 30 minutes prior to exercise
Loratadine (OTC), 10 mg daily
Sumatriptan, 50 mg 1/2–1 tablet PO at onset of migraine, may repeat after 2 hours
Ibuprofen (OTC), 200mg 1–2 tablets PO q6h PRN pain (rare use)

Allergies: Penicillin

■ Physical Examination

GEN: Well-developed, well-groomed, alert young woman in mild discomfort
VS: BP 118/72, HR 82, RR 14, T 37.2°C (99°F), Wt 59 kg, Ht 162.5 cm (5'4")
HEENT: Sinuses mildly tender, nose moderately congested, fair amount of clear discharge bilaterally, turbinates pale pink and mildly swollen
COR: WNL
CHEST: Clear to percussion and auscultation
ABD: Normal sounds, soft, mild epigastric tenderness, no hepatosplenomegaly, no masses
GU: Deferred
RECT: Heme negative, no masses or tenderness
EXT: WNL
NERUO: Alert, oriented × 4

■ Results of Pertinent Laboratory Tests, Serum Drug Concentrations, and Diagnostic Tests

Hct 0.41 (41)
Hbg 134 g/L (13.4)
Lkcs 300 × 10³/mm³ (300 × 10⁹/L)
MCV 88 (88)
Serology: positive for *Helicobacter pylori*

■ Problem List

Identify principal problems from the scenario in priority order (see Answers in back of book for correct list of problems).

■ SOAP Note

To be completed by the student (see Answers in back of book for correct SOAP Note).

■ QUESTIONS

(See Answers in back of book for correct responses.)

1. The probable cause of EC's peptic ulcer is: (EO-1)
   a. NSAID use
   b. Psychological stress
   c. *H. pylori*
   d. Alcohol consumption

2. List signs and symptoms of PUD in EC. (EO-2)

3. Which of the following tests for the detection of *H. pylori* does NOT require endoscopy? (EO-5)

a. Serology (antibody detection)
b. Histology (microbiologic examination)
c. Bacteria culture
d. Rapid urease

4. Describe the mechanism of action of the pharmacologic and nonpharmacologic interventions in this case. (EO-7)

5. List factors to consider when selecting the optimal treatment regimen for EC? (EO-8)

6. Identify potential or actual drug interactions with EC's treatment regimen for peptic ulcer. (EO-4, 8, 9)

7. Which of the following would be LEAST likely to interact with EC's pharmacologic treatment regimen? (EO-9)
a. Paroxetine
b. Dihydroergotamine
c. Warfarin
d. Diazepam

8. Which of the following would be a common adverse effect of EC's treatment regimen? (EO-10, 14)
a. Hepatic failure
b. Leukopenia
c. GI side effects
d. Seizures

9. If EC's ulcer persisted or redeveloped, which of the following would be recommended as an option for follow-up? (EO-12)
a. Serology test to confirm failure to eradicate *H. pylori* infection
b. Second course of original treatment regimen, but for extended duration
c. Empiric treatment with PPI and H2RA
d. Endoscopy and bacteria culture to determine antibiotic sensitivity

10. With regard to EC's treatment regimen, EC should be counseled about which of the following points? (EO-4, 8, 9, 10, 14)
a. Regimen can be stopped as soon as symptoms improve.
b. When taking oral contraceptives, barrier contraceptive method(s) should be used during course of antibiotics and for 1 week after.
c. Long-term use of PPIs should be avoided due to increased risk of gastric cancer.
d. All NSAID agents should be avoided.

11. Describe the psychosocial factors that may affect EC's adherence to both pharmacologic and nonpharmacologic therapy. (EO-15)

12. Describe the health care provider's role relative to the proposed psychosocial factors identified. (EO-16)

13. Which of the following pharmacoeconomic considerations is the LEAST likely to be a factor for an uncomplicated peptic ulcer such as EC's? (EO-17)
a. Cost of pharmacotherapy (direct medical)
b. Travel, lost wages for frequent office visits (direct nonmedical)
c. Decreased productivity (indirect personal)
d. Pain and discomfort (intangible personal)

14. Summarize therapeutic, pathophysiologic, and disease management concepts for peptic ulcer disease utilizing a key points format. (EO-18)

CASE 20

TOPIC: Ulcerative Colitis

THERAPEUTIC DIFFICULTY: Level 3
Beth Welch

Chapter 46: Inflammatory Bowel Disease

■ Scenario

Patient and Setting: TA, a 20-year-old black female; ambulatory care facility

Chief Complaint: Abdominal pain, blood and mucous in stools

■ History of Present Illness

Blood and mucous in stools over several months; over past few days increasing abdominal pain relieved with defecation; increasing stool frequency now at 6 stools per day; denies travel, hospitalizations, or recent antibiotics.

Medical History: DVT 2 months ago; asthma for 12 years (step 2: mild persistent by National Heart, Lung, and Blood Institute; FEV1 82%, PEF 25%); history of Chlamydia 1 year ago

Surgical History: None

Family/Social History: Family History: Mother and father alive and well without history of inflammatory bowel disease (IBD)
Social History: College student; quit smoking 2 months ago; alcohol 1–2 drinks on weekends; sexually active with multiple partners

Medications:

Flunisolide MDI, 2 puffs (500 μg) BID

Albuterol MDI, 1–2 puffs q4–6h PRN and prior to exercise

Warfarin, 5 mg QD

Loestrin, 1/20 QD

Allergies: No known drug allergies

■ Physical Examination

GEN: Overweight, tired-appearing female in NAD

VS: BP 110/68, HR 85, RR 20, T 37.2°C, Wt 75 kg (2 months earlier 79 kg), Ht 160 cm

HEENT: PERRLA, EOMI, negative for iritis, conjunctivitis, or uveitis

COR: RRR, normal s1 and s2

CHEST: CTA, no rales, wheezes, or rhonchi

ABD: + BS, NTND, No masses, no hepatosplenomegaly

GU: WNL, no lesions

RECT: Tender, no hemorrhoids, masses, fissures, or lesions, Guaiac +

EXT: No edema, peripheral pulses intact

NEURO: A and O × 4

■ Results of pertinent Laboratory Tests, Serum Drug Concentrations, and Diagnostic Tests

Na 137 (137)	Hct 0.311 (31.1)	AST 0.53 (32)	Glu 5.0 (90)
K 3.3 (3.3)	Hgb 100 (10.0)	ALT 0.47 (28)	
Cl 97 (97)	Lkcs 8.2 × 10⁹	LDH 1.8 (110)	
	(8.2 × 10³)		
HCO3 26 (26)	Plts 455 × 10⁹	Alk Phos 1.7 (100)	
	(455 × 10³)		
BUN 3.9 (11)	MCV 78 (78)	Alb 30 (3.0)	
CR 97 (1.1)	MCH 24 (24)	T Bili 13.7 (0.8)	
PT 12.7			
INR 2.7			
ANA +			
ESR 70			

Stool: RBC, WBC, culture negative

Sigmoidoscopy: granular, edematous, and friable mucosa with continuous ulcerations extending from anus to 20 cm proximally; barium enema shows confluent disease extending from rectum to transverse colon.

■ Problem List

Identify principal problems from the scenario in priority order (see Answers in back of book for correct list of problems).

■ SOAP Note

To be completed by the student (see Answers in back of book for correct SOAP Note).

■ QUESTIONS

(See Answers in back of book for correct responses.)

1. What epidemiologic factor does TA possess that is consistent with a higher incidence of ulcerative colitis? (EO-3)
   a. Black race
   b. Age of onset
   c. Female gender
   d. Family history

2. List anatomic, pathologic, and clinical findings that point to the diagnosis of ulcerative colitis versus Crohn's Disease. (EO-1, 2, 5)

3. Describe the role of smoking in ulcerative colitis and Crohn's disease. How could TA's past smoking have interacted with her disease presentation? (EO-1, 3)

4. Based on TA's clinical and anatomic features, how would her ulcerative colitis best be classified? (EO-2, 5)
   a. Mild continuous disease affecting the rectum and distal colon
   b. Moderate continuous disease affecting the rectum and proximal colon
   c. Moderate continuous disease affecting the rectum and distal colon
   d. Severe continuous disease affecting the rectum and distal colon

5. Which of the following is a common gastrointestinal complication of ulcerative colitis? (EO-1)
   a. Toxic megacolon
   b. Fistula
   c. Stricture
   d. Fissure

6. List the therapeutic endpoints of treatment for TA. (EO-16, 18)

7. Based on location and severity of TA's disease, which of the following pharmacologic treatments would be most appropriate to use first-line? (EO-7, 8, 12)
   a. Mesalamine suppository
   b. Oral corticosteroids
   c. IV steroids
   d. Sulfasalazine

8. Describe the mechanism of action of the pharmacologic interventions for ulcerative colitis used in this case. (EO-7)

9. Which of the following reasons support the use of sulfasalazine over mesalamine in TA? (OE-7, 8, 17)
   a. Improved efficacy of sulfasalazine over mesalamine
   b. Decreased cost of sulfasalazine
   c. Potential for allergy with mesalamine
   d. Location of disease

10. Which of the following is a dose-independent side effect of sulfasalazine? (EO-10)
    a. Nausea
    b. Headache
    c. Malaise
    d. Fever

11. Sulfasalazine may _____ the therapeutic effects of warfarin by _____. (EO-9)
    a. Decrease; enzyme induction
    b. Increase; protein displacement
    c. Increase; enzyme inhibition
    d. Decrease; protein displacement

12. List the side effects and laboratory monitoring parameters for agents used in the treatment of ulcerative colitis. (EO-10)

13. Antidiarrheals are useful in the treatment of IBD because they do which of the following? (EO-8, 12)
    a. Maintain remission of chronic IBD
    b. Provide symptomatic relief in mild chronic IBD
    c. Improve the absorptive capacity of the colon in severe disease
    d. Reduce disease flares when used chronically

14. Explain the role of surgical interventions used in the treatment of IBD. (EO-8, 12)

15. Describe the psychosocial aspects of IBD and interventions the health care practitioner can make to improve patient outcomes. (EO-15, 16)

16. Describe options available for patients with refractory ulcerative colitis. (EO-8, 12)

17. Summarize therapeutic, pathophysiologic, and disease management concepts for inflammatory bowel disease utilizing a key points format. (EO-18)

Hepatitis: Viral and Drug-Induced 49

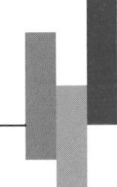

Mary F. Hebert

DEFINITION

Hepatitis is inflammation of the liver that can be caused by viruses (e.g., hepatitis A, hepatitis B, or hepatitis C), medications (e.g., methyldopa or isoniazid), or immunologic abnormalities (e.g., autoimmune hepatitis). Hepatitis can occur as acute or chronic disease. Chronic disease generally is defined as that persisting for 6 months or longer.

VIRAL HEPATITIS

There is a great deal of overlap between the symptoms and incubation periods for the various hepatitis viruses, therefore symptoms and time course alone cannot be used for differentiating between the virus types. Viral serologies are needed to distinguish between infections caused by each of the viruses. There are many hepatitis viruses, including all the letters of the alphabet from A to G. Although each of the viruses from A to G is mentioned briefly (Table 49.1), this chapter focuses on hepatitis A, B, and C viruses.

DRUG-INDUCED HEPATITIS

Drug-induced liver injury is highly variable in the type of reactions seen and individual patient susceptibility. Drug-induced liver injury is most often asymptomatic until extensive damage is done. For some agents, elevations in serum aminotransferases can be transient despite continuation of therapy. For others, continuation of the offending agent can result in extensive hepatocellular necrosis and death. Although other types of drug-induced liver injury occur (Table 49.2), this chapter addresses only drug-induced hepatitis. (For further discussion on other types of drug-induced liver injury, such as hepatocellular necrosis and cholestasis, see Chapter 2.)

TREATMENT GOALS: VIRAL HEPATITIS

Viral hepatitis can be prevented by avoiding exposure to the infectious agent (e.g., avoiding contaminated food and water, practicing good personal hygiene, avoiding reuse of intravenous needles, practicing safe sex, avoiding recapping needles after phlebotomy, and using sterile technique with acupuncture and tattooing).

- Prevent hepatitis viral infection by following postexposure prophylaxis regimens.
- If preventive measures fail, clear the virus as measured by polymerase chain reaction.
- Improve or normalize serum aminotransferases.
- Improve or normalize histologic changes associated with hepatitis.
- Prevent progression of hepatic disease.
- Maintain compliance with therapy.
- Minimize and manage adverse effects associated with therapy.
- Manage the complications of end-stage liver disease.

TABLE 49.1	Hepatitis Viruses			
Virus	**Other Names**	**Family**	**Type**	**Usual Route of Transmission**
Hepatitis A	Infectious hepatitis	Picornavirus	RNA	Oral-fecal
Hepatitis B	Serum hepatitis	Hepadnaviridae	DNA	Blood or sexual
Hepatitis C	Non-A, non-B	Flaviviridae	RNA	Blood
Hepatitis D	Delta hepatitis	Delta viridae	RNA	Blood or sexual
Hepatitis E		Caliciviridae	RNA	Fecal-oral
Hepatitis F	Toga virus			Fecal-oral
Hepatitis G		Flaviviridae	RNA	Blood or sexual

TREATMENT GOALS: DRUG-INDUCED HEPATITIS

Avoid, if possible, giving agents known to cause hepatitis to patients with liver disease (risks and benefits should be weighed before therapy is started).

- Detect drug-induced hepatitis early and discontinue the offending agent.
- Avoid significant liver damage.
- Treat drug-induced liver disease as clinically appropriate.

EPIDEMIOLOGY

VIRAL HEPATITIS

Hepatitis A. In epidemic years, 35,000 cases of hepatitis A have been reported.[1] It takes approximately 2 to 7 weeks (average 4 weeks) from the time of infection to the development of hepatitis symptoms such as anorexia, nausea, diarrhea, fever, fatigue, jaundice, malaise, and right upper quadrant pain.[2-4] The contagious period for hepatitis A appears to start 2 weeks before and continues through 1 week after the onset of symptoms.[5-7] Because high concentrations of hepatitis A are found in the stool of infected people, the usual mode of transmission is by direct fecal-oral contact or fecal contamination of food or water. There is no carrier state for hepatitis A. Therefore, transmission of hepatitis A through a blood transfusion is uncommon.[8-13]

TABLE 49.2	Types of Drug-Induced Liver Injury
Type	**Example**
Hepatocellular necrosis	Acetaminophen overdose
Hepatitis (acute or chronic)	Isoniazid
Cholestasis	Estrogen
Fatty liver	Corticosteroids
Fibrosis	Methotrexate
Vascular lesions	Azathioprine
Tumors	Anabolic steroids
Granulomatous	Diltiazem

Hepatitis B. It is estimated that 1.25 million people in the United States are chronically infected with hepatitis B virus.[14] Approximately 78,000 people per year become acutely infected with the hepatitis B virus in the United States. Of those infected, 70% become symptomatic; 26% are hospitalized; 90% of infants infected at birth, 30% of children infected at age 1 to 5 years, and 6% of those infected over 5 years of age develop chronic infections; and 1% from acute disease and 15% to 25% from chronic disease die each year.[14] Patients with cirrhosis are at a much greater risk for developing liver cancer (12 to 300 times normal risk).

Hepatitis B can be transmitted by blood or sexual exposure.[15,16] Hepatitis B transmission through infected blood exposures can occur when contaminated fluid splashes into an eye or when sterile techniques are not used with intravenous needles, tattooing, body piercing, or acupuncture.[17-21] The virus remains in the blood approximately 6 weeks with an acute infection. In addition, a carrier state exists for hepatitis B.[22] A carrier is a person who is persistently (more than 6 months) hepatitis B surface antigen (HBsAg) positive. Patients who test positive for HBsAg are potentially infectious, but those testing positive for hepatitis B e antigen (HBeAg) have the highest degree of infectivity.[23] The incubation period from the time of infection to the onset of symptoms is 4 months on average but ranges from 1.5 to 5 months.[23]

Hepatitis C. Almost 4 million people in the United States are thought to be infected with the hepatitis C virus (HCV).[24] An estimated 25,000 hepatitis C infections occur in the United States each year; 75% to 85% of these infections go on to become chronic infections.[25,26] When HCV replicates, it produces a large number of genetically slightly different viruses, called quasispecies. It is thought that this is the reason for the high rate of infections becoming chronic. Approximately 1% to 5% of patients with chronic hepatitis C develop hepatocellular carcinoma after 20 years of infection. Once cirrhotic, 1% to 4% of the patients per year develop hepatocellular carcinoma.[24] Hepatitis C is the leading indication for liver transplantation in the United States.[26] Hepatitis C appears to be transmitted primarily through infected blood exposures such as blood transfusions or needlesticks.[27–29] Currently, transfusion-related cases of hepatitis C occur in less than one per million transfused units of blood.[26] Although less efficient, perinatal (mother to infant) and sexual transmission also occur.[30,31] In 2001, when evaluating all the hepatitis C cases reported in the United States which included risk factor information, 6.6% of the cases were attributed to sexual exposure.[32] Although sexual exposure is believed to be a risk factor for transmission of hepatitis C, the exact risk is unclear due to conflicting data.

DRUG-INDUCED HEPATITIS

Drug-induced liver disease is rare, although as many as 1,000 agents have been associated with the various types of hepatic disease. Some agents or their metabolites have been found to be directly hepatotoxic, whereas others appear to produce an allergic reaction that results in hepatic injury. Between 1 in 600 and 1 in 3,500 hospital admissions and 2% to 3% of all admissions for drug-induced adverse reactions are related to drug-induced hepatic injury. In addition, approximately 5% of hospital admissions for jaundice, 20% to 50% of nonviral chronic hepatitis, and 15% to 30% of fulminant hepatic failure cases appear to be drug induced.[33,34] Many factors affect drug-induced hepatotoxicity. Some of the factors associated with an increased susceptibility to drug-induced liver injury are listed in Table 49.3.

PATHOPHYSIOLOGY

VIRAL HEPATITIS

Hepatitis A. Hepatitis A infections are asymptomatic in approximately one third of the patients. Another third develop mild nonspecific symptoms, and the last third develop more severe symptoms including jaundice. Adults are more likely to be symptomatic than children. In the hepatitis A cases reported in the United States in 2001, 71% were jaundiced, 22% required hospitalization, and 0.4% died.[32] A month after infection, patients typically experience the acute onset of symptoms that last about 4 weeks. Patients with more severe symptoms have an increase in their serum aspartate aminotransferase (AST), alanine aminotransferase (ALT), and bilirubin, which resolve over 4 to 6 months. About 15% of infections with hepatitis A result in prolonged or relapsing symptoms over 6 to 9 months.[1]

Hepatitis B and C. Hepatitis B infections are asymptomatic in approximately one third of patients. Acute hepatitis

occurs in the others with progression to fulminant hepatitis in less than 1%. Acute hepatitis B infection results in 26% of patients requiring hospitalization, and 1% die.[32] Of the adults infected, chronic hepatitis B infection develops in 6%. Some of those chronically infected have no symptoms, and others go on to develop cirrhosis or hepatocellular carcinoma. About 15% to 40% of those chronically infected with hepatitis B go on to develop cirrhosis. Eighty percent of patients with hepatitis C acute infection are asymptomatic. Unfortunately, 75% to 85% of the infections become chronic, and approximately 20% of patients develop chronic liver disease. Less than 3% of patients each year die from chronic HCV-related liver disease.[26] The 5-year survival of patients with chronic hepatitis C and compensated cirrhosis is 91%. In contrast, those with decompensated cirrhosis (concomitant liver failure, ascites, coagulopathy, and/or encephalopathy) have a 5-year survival of 50%.[24]

Acute hepatitis B is typically associated with high elevations in AST and ALT (more than a 100-fold increase over normal) and bilirubin (20-fold increase over normal). Serum AST, ALT, and bilirubin increase in acute hepatitis C infection, but the increases tend not to be as high as in hepatitis B. Jaundice is a common (64%) finding in acute hepatitis but is rare with chronic hepatitis unless the liver disease becomes severe. However, chronic hepatitis is associated with mild elevations in AST and ALT (up to 20 times normal), and generally normal alkaline phosphatase and γ-glutamyltransferase. Platelet and white blood cell counts remain normal until the liver disease becomes severe and splenomegaly develops. Liver biopsies, although not always performed, can be helpful in determining the severity of disease, establishing the cause, and predicting the outcome of therapy, particularly with hepatitis C. Chronic hepatitis is associated with an inflammatory infiltrate with mononuclear cells in the liver. There may also be hepatocyte necrosis.

DRUG-INDUCED HEPATITIS

Several different types of hepatitis have been reported as adverse drug reactions (Table 49.3). Nonspecific hepatitis is characterized by focal hepatocellular necrosis with a mononuclear infiltrate and variable amounts of portal inflammation. Viral-like hepatitis is characterized by an inflammatory infiltrate, variable amounts of hepatocyte necrosis, bile stasis, and lobular disarray. Severe cases can exhibit bridging submassive or massive necrosis. Granulomatous hepatitis is characterized by aggregates of epithelioid histiocytes with variable types and amounts of inflammatory cells. Autoimmune-like hepatitis is characterized by a hepatitis picture with positive antinuclear antibodies. Inflammation may be severe, and an elevated number of plasma cells may be seen in the liver biopsy. Cholestatic hepatitis is characterized by prominent cholestasis, variable amounts of hepatocellular necrosis, and portal and lobular mononuclear, neutrophilic, or eosinophilic inflammation. Some medications have been reported to cause more than one type of liver injury.

TABLE 49.3 | **Drug-Induced Hepatitis**

Agent	Type of Hepatitis Reaction	Time to Onset (frequency of hepatitis or jaundice)	Host Factors That Increase Susceptibility to Liver Damage	Expected Outcome	Comments
ACE inhibitors	Cholestatic hepatitis	1 wk to 20 mo (<1%)		Slow recovery after discontinuation, submassive necrosis and fulminant liver failure have occurred with continued therapy	
Allopurinol	Viral-like or granulomatous hepatitis	<5 wk	Diuretic use	Rarely fatal	
Amiodarone	Alcoholic-like, cholestatic, and granulomatous hepatitis	1 mo to several years (1%)	Renal disease	Insidious onset, hepatotoxicity may persist for several months after discontinuation, death from liver failure has been reported	
Aspirin	Nonspecific or viral-like hepatitis	Several days to wk (0.1%–0.5%)	Chronic rheumatic disease Children with acute rheumatic fever Low albumin Defect in mitochondrial β-oxidation	Reversible with stopping drug	Dose-dependent reaction, most common with concentrations >25 mg/dL (3–5 g/day for adults), can occur with concentrations <10 mg/dL in 2% of the reactions
Carbamazepine	Granulomatous or cholestatic hepatitis	(5%–10%)[a]		Mild asymptomatic increases in liver functions tests are common, more severe cases can take months to resolve	
Dantrolene	Viral-like acute or chronic hepatitis	>1 mo (1%–2%)	Age >30 years	22%–28% fatal	Monitor liver function tests in all patients on dantrolene
Diclofenac	Nonspecific acute or autoimmunelike chronic hepatitis	1 wk to 14 mo (<1%)		Most resolve with stopping the drug, fatalities from massive necrosis have occurred	Monitor liver function tests every 3–6 mo, discontinue if >3-fold increase
Disulfiram	Acute viral-like hepatitis	<2 mo (<1%)	Women	Fulminant hepatic failure has occurred	
Erythromycin estolate	Cholestatic hepatitis	1–4 wk (0.1%–0.5%)		Usually rapid and complete resolution after discontinuation, fulminant hepatic failure has been reported	Less common with other erythromycin salts
Etretinate	Chronic hepatitis	1 mo (1.5%)		Commonly causes transient increases in liver function tests, more serious reactions have occurred	

Drug	Histologic pattern	Onset (incidence)	Risk factors	Clinical course	Comments
Halothane	Viral-like acute hepatitis	Several days to 3 wk after exposure, shortened to a few days after repeat exposure (<0.001%)	Repeat exposures, Female, Obesity, Older adults	Usually mild, subclinical increase in liver function tests, acute hepatitis is rare, but fatal in 80% of cases	If repeat anesthetic exposure is necessary, avoid halothane
Isoniazid	Viral-like hepatitis	Most cases <2 mo, can be delayed as long as 1 year (<1%)	Age >50 years, Women	Reactions range from mild acute reactions to liver failure and death, case fatality rate approximately 10%	
MAO inhibitors	Acute viral-like hepatitis	(<1%)		Frequently fatal	
Methyldopa	Acute and chronic viral-like, cholestatic, and/or autoimmunelike hepatitis	<3 mo (0.1%–0.5%)		Usually transient, asymptomatic increases in liver function tests, recovery can take months, fatal massive necrosis is not uncommon	Rechallenge has been fatal in some cases
Niacin	Hepatitis	<3 mo, sometimes within days (50%)[a]		Fulminant failure has been reported in some patients	
Nitrofurantoin	Autoimmune-like or granulomatous hepatitis	Usually <1 mo, delayed cases have been reported (<1%)	Women (although this may reflect usage pattern)	Usually complete recovery following discontinuation, fatalities have been reported particularly if continued despite evidence of liver injury	
Oxacillin	Nonspecific focal hepatitis	>1 wk		Resolution within several weeks following discontinuation	Associated with high dose intravenous therapy
Phenytoin	Viral-like acute or chronic and granulomatous hepatitis	Usually 4–6 wk, may occur as early as 1–2 wk (0.5%–1%)		Usually resolves with stopping drug, advanced cases may be slow to resolve or progress and be fatal over weeks to months	Often associated with fever, malaise, rash, and eosinophilia
Procainamide	Granulomatous hepatitis			Usually resolves with discontinuation of agent	
Quinidine	Granulomatous, or hepatocellular-cholestatic hepatitis	1–2 wk		Usually reversible with discontinuation	
Rifampin	Viral-like acute hepatitis	(<1%)	Concomitant administration of isoniazid, Slow acetylators		
Sulfonamides	Nonspecific, autoimmunelike or granulomatous chronic hepatitis	Usually <2 wk, may be delayed (0.5%–1%)	HIV infection	Usually complete recovery within weeks to a few months after discontinuation, a few deaths have been reported	
Tetracycline	Viral-like hepatitis			Reaction is often progressive	
Trazodone	Chronic hepatitis			Reversible with discontinuation	

[a] Hepatitis incidence not found; percentage reported for patients with elevated liver function values.
ACE, angiotensin-converting enzyme; MAO, monoamine oxidase; HIV, human immunodeficiency virus.

CLINICAL PRESENTATION AND DIAGNOSIS

SIGNS AND SYMPTOMS

Viral Hepatitis

Hepatitis A. Hepatitis A is associated with the abrupt onset of symptoms, including fever in about 50% of patients, nausea, anorexia, diarrhea, fatigue, malaise, abdominal discomfort, dark urine, and jaundice. The severity of illness appears to be age dependent. In most cases, children have no symptoms, whereas adults usually experience symptoms and have jaundice. Hepatitis A viral infection generally is considered the most benign of the three viruses presented here. The fatality rate for hepatitis A infection is less than 1%.[23]

Hepatitis B and C

Acute Hepatitis. After the incubation period, patients who become symptomatic characteristically develop nonspecific, flu-like symptoms such as malaise, fatigue, weakness, anorexia, nausea, vomiting, and right upper quadrant abdominal pain (over the liver). These symptoms start about a week before jaundice develops. The onset of clinical symptoms is insidious and usually continues for a few weeks after the development of dark urine, jaundice, and serum bilirubin values of 2.5 mg per deciliter or more. The appearance of jaundice or dark urine often prompts a visit to the doctor. Before that, patients often feel as if they have had a very bad flu. A small percentage of patients develop fulminant viral hepatitis with symptoms of liver failure and encephalopathy. The fatality rate from fulminant viral liver failure is approximately 1% to 1.5% of those infected.[23]

Chronic Hepatitis. For many patients, chronic hepatitis is asymptomatic. Other patients experience mild intermittent symptoms. Sometimes the diagnosis of chronic hepatitis is not made until the patient develops cirrhosis.[60,61] The most common symptoms of chronic hepatitis are fatigue, weakness, and malaise. In a small subset of these patients, the fatigue is so severe that it impairs their ability to perform daily activities. Although less common, some patients experience tenderness in the right upper quadrant of the abdomen, nausea, anorexia, and muscle or joint pain. Once cirrhosis develops, the fatigue, anorexia, weight loss, and weakness become more severe. In addition, patients may develop ascites, jaundice, muscle wasting, hepatic encephalopathy, and esophageal varices (see Chapter 50 for further discussion). A small group of patients can develop extrahepatic symptoms of chronic viral hepatitis such as arthritis and urticaria. Death from chronic liver disease from hepatitis B occurs in 15% to 25% of chronically infected persons.[14]

Drug-Induced Hepatitis.

The signs and symptoms of drug-induced hepatitis are highly variable and can present as acute or chronic disease. Some patients may have only asymptomatic transient elevations in their serum aminotransferases, while others progress to fulminant hepatic failure. Patients may develop fever, rash, arthralgias, nausea,

jaundice, abdominal complaints, lymphadenopathy, hepatomegaly, and eosinophilia. All patients have elevations in at least some liver tests (AST, ALT, alkaline phosphatase, and bilirubin). The magnitude of the elevations and the enzymes involved depend on the offending agent and the severity and stage of the liver damage. Patients with very severe liver injury can develop encephalopathy and symptoms of portal hypertension such as ascites and esophageal varices (see Chapter 50 for further discussion). The case fatality rate for drug-induced hepatic injury is approximately 5% overall. Unfortunately, the fatality rate for some agents is much higher.

DIAGNOSIS

Viral Hepatitis

Hepatitis A. The diagnosis of acute hepatitis A cannot be made on clinical symptoms alone. Diagnosis is based on measurement of immunoglobulin M (IgM) antibodies to hepatitis A in the serum. Later, IgG antibodies to hepatitis A appear in the serum and protect against reinfection.

Hepatitis B. Several markers can be measured for diagnosis of hepatitis B. HBsAg can be measured in the serum 30 to 60 days after exposure to the hepatitis B virus. Antibodies against HBsAg develop in response to an infection with hepatitis B and provide long-term immunity. IgM antibodies against the hepatitis B core antigen also develop in response to an acute hepatitis B infection and persist for about 6 months. The IgM antibodies against the core antigen can be used as a marker for acute hepatitis B infection. HBeAg is a marker of rapid viral replication. The development of antibodies to HBeAg correlates with loss of replicating virus and decreased infectivity of the virus.

Hepatitis C. HCV infections can be diagnosed by detection of antibodies against the HCV, or HCV RNA in the patient's serum. Antibodies against hepatitis C can be measured 4 to 8 weeks after infection but depends on the assay.[27] Antibodies to HCV can be detected in 97% of persons by 6 months after exposure. HCV RNA can be measured within 1 week of infection.[25] About 15% of patients that test positive for antibodies against hepatitis C will test negative for HCV RNA. These patients have resolved infection.

Drug-Induced Hepatitis. The diagnosis of drug-induced liver injury requires exclusion of other causes because the symptoms of drug-induced hepatitis can be quite similar to those of hepatitis from other origins. Ultimately, the diagnosis depends on the history of exposure, time course, consistent clinical and laboratory findings, exclusion of other causes, and resolution of the injury after discontinuation of the offending agent. Although rechallenge with the suspected etiologic agent can confirm drug-induced injury, this usually is not done and should not be recommended because of the risk of further injury and the availability of alternative agents in most cases.

Often the pharmacist is asked to evaluate if the patient's medications could be contributing to liver disease. Although this is difficult to determine with any level of certainty, the first step in the evaluation is to determine for each medication (prescription and over-the-counter) the scope of liver injury that has been reported in the literature. A comparison between the time course, frequency, and type of injury the patient is exhibiting and those that have been reported in the literature is helpful in determining the likelihood that a particular reaction is drug induced.

PSYCHOSOCIAL ASPECTS

Three main psychosocial issues should be addressed in patients with chronic hepatitis B or C. The first is related to the disease process itself. Many patients become depressed following their diagnosis. Because hepatitis B and C are potentially life-threatening diseases with limited cure rates, even if patients are given information about the options, they often walk away with the perception that they are terminally ill and about to die. Patients may need to be told more than once that chronic hepatitis is a slowly progressive disease, that most patients live for many years after diagnosis, that treatments are available that provide clinical improvement or cure in some patients, that lifestyle changes such as discontinuation of ethanol consumption and illegal drug use may be helpful in prolonging life, and that for patients who do not respond to therapy, liver transplantation may be an option.

The second psychosocial issue is related to compliance with drug therapy. Although most patients are compliant with their treatment regimens, for some the adverse effects are prohibitive. It is helpful to educate patients about the severity and types of expected adverse effects before starting treatment. Patients should be encouraged to continue therapy as clinically appropriate and taught which symptoms are expected to decline with continued treatment. Finally, because patients with chronic viral hepatitis (particularly B) can transmit the virus to their partners through sexual contact, education about safe sex practices is important. Changes in sexual practices for people with chronic hepatitis C in monogamous relationships are controversial because the sexual transmission rate is believed to be low.

TREATMENT

PHARMACOTHERAPY
Viral Hepatitis
Hepatitis A: Preexposure Prophylaxis. The Centers for Disease Control currently recommend hepatitis A vaccination of persons over 2 years of age, traveling to areas with increased rates of hepatitis A. This includes areas of the world endemic with hepatitis A, particularly rural areas of developing countries with poor sanitation. Other populations where vaccination is recommended include ''men who have sex with men, injecting and noninjecting drug users, persons with clotting-factor disorders (e.g., hemophilia), persons with chronic liver disease, and children living in areas with increased rates of hepatitis A during the baseline period from 1987–1997.''[1] The two available inactivated hepatitis A vaccines should be administered into the deltoid muscle. The vaccine takes about 4 weeks to induce a protective immune response and lasts at least 20 years. The most common side effects of the hepatitis A vaccine are soreness at the injection site, headache, fatigue, and anorexia, which usually are mild and resolve within 2 days. Although rare, anaphylactic reactions have been reported. Children younger than 2 years of age making multiple visits or planning to live in hepatitis A endemic areas for long periods of time and those 2 years of age and older needing only short-term protection, should receive IM immune globulin. A single 0.02-mL per kilogram dose generally is adequate for short trips (less than 3 months), but 0.06 mL per kilogram every 5 months is necessary for longer visits.[62] Guidelines for travel prophylaxis are summarized in Table 49.4. IM injection of immune globulin can result in pain, swelling, and muscle stiffness at the injection site. Less commonly, urticaria, angioedema, headache, malaise, fever, and nephrotic syndrome have been reported.

TABLE 49.4	Hepatitis Travel Prophylaxis			
Hepatitis Type	**When to Give Prophylaxis**	**Comments**	**Age**	**Recommendation**
Hepatitis A	Travelers to hepatitis A endemic areas	Visit >3 mo or repeat visits	≥2 yr	Hepatitis A vaccine
		Visit <3 mo	All	Immune globulin 0.02 mL/kg IM single dose
		Visit >3 mo or repeat visits	<2 yr (or ≥2 yr and not vaccinated)	Immune globulin 0.06 mL/kg IM every 5 mo
Hepatitis B	Travelers to hepatitis B endemic areas	Visit >6 mo or short visits with high-risk of blood or sexual exposure to hepatitis B	All	Hepatitis B vaccine

IM, intramuscular.

Severe reactions including anaphylactic shock have been reported rarely. Patients who need repeat doses of immune globulin in a developing country should make sure that the product they receive meets licensing requirements for the United States. Immune globulin products produced in developing countries may not meet US standards for purity.

Hepatitis A: Postexposure Prophylaxis. The need for immune globulin postexposure prophylaxis for hepatitis A virus depends on the nature of the exposure. Immune globulin prophylaxis for hepatitis A is recommended for patients with household or sexual contact, or by sharing illegal drugs with people infected with hepatitis A, employees or attendees of a day care center if other children or employees are diagnosed as having a hepatitis A infection, those in close contact with people infected with hepatitis A in prisons or other group facilities, coworkers of a food handler infected with hepatitis A, and patrons of a restaurant in which a food handler infected with hepatitis A (with poor hygienic practices or diarrhea) has been preparing food, without wearing gloves, that will not be cooked before eaten. In addition, patients must be identified and treated within 2 weeks of exposure.[23] Immune globulin (0.02 mL/kg IM) has been found to be 80% to 90% effective in preventing hepatitis A infections after exposure if it is given early in the incubation period.[63,64] Giving immune globulin more than 2 weeks after exposure is not recommended.

Hepatitis B: Preexposure Prophylaxis. Hepatitis B vaccine is routinely given to infants and children in the United States. Immunization of previously unvaccinated adolescents at age 11 to 12 years is also recommended. Patients who have not received the hepatitis B vaccine series and plan to live in an area with high levels of endemic hepatitis B virus for longer than 6 months, or short-term travelers with a high likelihood of exposure to hepatitis B through blood or sexual contact with natives of a hepatitis B endemic area, should receive the hepatitis B vaccine series. Guidelines for travel prophylaxis are summarized in Table 49.4. In addition, people at high risk for exposure to hepatitis B (e.g., infants born to infected mothers, infants/children of immigrants from areas with high rates of hepatitis B virus infection, persons engaging in illegal drug use, sexually active persons with multiple partners or a diagnosis of a sexually transmitted disease, homosexual men, sexual and household contacts of infected patients, health care and public safety workers, persons receiving clotting factor concentrates, persons in drug treatment programs or long-term correctional facilities and patients on hemodialysis) should also receive the hepatitis B vaccine series.

Hepatitis B: Postexposure Prophylaxis. Hepatitis B immune globulin (HBIG) is produced from plasma that contains high titers of antibody against HBsAg. It is used to provide passive immunity against hepatitis B infection. The Immunization Practices Advisory Committee (ACIP) recommends HBIG for unvaccinated patients or those with an inadequate response to the hepatitis B vaccine who are exposed to HBsAg-positive individuals through a needlestick or human bite, direct mucous membrane contact (oral or ophthalmic), birth (neonates), sexual or intimate contact, and household exposure for infants younger than 12 months old. Prophylaxis of other household contacts is not routinely necessary unless there is an identifiable exposure to blood such as sharing razors or toothbrushes.[23] HBIG is 75% effective in preventing transmission of acute hepatitis B infection through sexual contact.[65] Because HBIG provides only short-term protection against hepatitis B, the hepatitis B vaccine series or booster doses should also be given to these patients as appropriate. HBIG (0.06 mL/kg for adults and children) should be administered by IM injection, preferably into the deltoid muscle or the anterolateral aspect of the thigh as soon after exposure to the hepatitis B virus as possible. The value of HBIG when given more than 7 days after the exposure is unclear. Newborns of hepatitis B surface antigen positive mothers should receive HBIG 0.5 mL IM within 12 hours of birth. The most common adverse reactions of HBIG are local pain, swelling, and erythema at the injection site. Allergic reactions, body and joint pain, muscle cramps, malaise, and fever have also been reported.

The hepatitis B vaccine is a recombinant product in which common baker's yeast is used to produce a noninfectious subunit of HBsAg. The series of three IM injections (second and third doses are given 1 and 6 months, respectively, after the first dose) produces an adequate antibody response in 90% of adults and 95% of children. An alternate two-dose regimen (second dose follows the first dose by 4 to 6 months) for hepatitis B vaccine (Recombivax HB) has been approved for adolescents (11 to 15 years of age). This regimen requires a higher dose than the three-dose regimen. Clinical trials have demonstrated that the hepatitis B vaccine is 80% to 95% effective in preventing hepatitis B infection in high-risk groups.[66,67] Infants with perinatal exposures should receive the hepatitis B vaccine in combination with HBIG, which has been shown to be 85% to 95% effective in preventing the hepatitis B carrier state.[67–70] The deltoid muscle is the recommended location for injection for adults and children because injections into the buttocks produce a lower response rate.[71] The anterolateral thigh muscle should be used for infants and neonates. Table 49.5 describes the available hepatitis B vaccine products and dosing information. Larger doses (two to four times the normal dosage) or one additional dose (total four doses) are needed to produce an adequate immune response in many immunocompromised patients or those on hemodialysis.[72,73] Some immunocompromised patients do not respond to the vaccine even when higher doses are given. Local reactions, such as soreness, pain, ecchymosis, and swelling are the most common side effects of the hepatitis B vaccine. Mild systemic symptoms such as fever, malaise, headache, and fatigue have also been reported. Allergic reactions such as rash, anaphylaxis, and serum sickness, although uncommon, have been reported. The hepatitis B vaccine is contraindicated in patients allergic

TABLE 49.5	Hepatitis B Vaccine		
Trade Name	**Patients**	**Product Concentration**	**Dose**
Recombivax HB	0–19 yr 2-dose regimen only approved for 11–15 yr	5µg/0.5ml 10 µg/mL	5 µg 10 µg
	≥20 yr Dialysis or immunocompromised	10 µg/mL 40 µg/mL	10 µg 40 µg

Engerix-B	≤10 yr
	11–19 yr
	≥20 yr
	Dialysis or
	   immunocompromised
		10 µg/0.5 mL
		10 µg/0.5 mL or 20 µg/mL
		20 µg/mL
		20 µg/mL
			10 µg
			10–20 µg
			20 µg
			40 µg (divided
			   between two sites)

All regimens are three-dose regimens except the two-dose alternative regimen for 11–15 year olds.

to yeast or any of the other ingredients contained in the vaccine.

Chronic Hepatitis B. Interferon was the first approved agent used to treat chronic hepatitis B. Several types of interferons are commercially available (interferon α-2a and α-2b, interferon α-n3, interferon alfacon-1, interferon β-1a and β-1b, and interferon γ-1b). Interferon has antiviral and immune stimulatory properties that may be beneficial in treating viral hepatitis. Interferon α-2b [5 million international units (IU) subcutaneously daily or 10 million IU three times weekly for 16 weeks for HBeAg-positive patients and 12 months for HBeAg-negative patients] has been used to treat chronic hepatitis B infection with some success. Virologic response (loss of HBeAg and hepatitis B DNA) occurred in 33% to 37% of the patients and 7% to 12% of controls. In addition, 43% to 44% had a biochemical response (normalization of serum ALT), as compared to 19% of controls. Sustained virologic response after discontinuation of therapy was 34% to 37%.[74,75] Interferon treatment often is associated with flu-like symptoms (fever, fatigue, headache, and myalgia). Dosing the interferon at bedtime can improve the tolerability of this drug. Acetaminophen should be used for fever and headache management. However, patients with liver disease should limit the amount of acetaminophen to 2 g per day for adults. Gastrointestinal symptoms (nausea, diarrhea, and anorexia), arthralgias, weakness, alopecia, and rigors also are common. Anemia, leukopenia, and thrombocytopenia are significant problems that can be dose limiting. Although less common, depression can be a very serious problem in these patients. Suicides have been reported as a result of depression associated with interferon therapy. Interferon can also induce various autoimmune diseases. Some patients also have photosensitivity reactions while on interferon and should be counseled on the use of sunscreen and protective clothing. Interferon therapy should be reduced or discontinued if the patient develops anemia, leukopenia, thrombocytopenia, depression, or autoimmune disease. Interferon can be quite difficult to tolerate:

10% to 40% of patients need dose reduction and 5% to 10% need discontinuation of therapy.[24] The pharmacokinetic disposition of interferon α-2a or -α-2b can be modified by attaching a monomethoxy-polyethylene glycolpolymer to the interferon molecule. The resulting compound, often referred to as peginterferon α-2a or -α-2b, respectively, exhibits a significantly longer elimination half-life, which allows for once a week dosing, compared to the daily or three times weekly administration with "conventional" interferons. Peginterferon α–2a is FDA approved for the treatment of chronic hepatitis B. Peginterferon α–2a for the treatment of hepatitis B e antigen (HBeAg)-positive chronic hepatitis B patients was reported to result in clearance of HBeAg in 37% and 35% of the patients at a dose of 90 µg and 180 µg weekly, respectively.[76] Determination of peginterferon's role in therapy will require further investigation.

Another class of agents has recently come on the scene for treating hepatitis B. Lamivudine [(−)2′,3′-dideoxy,3′-thiacytidine (3TC)], is an irreversible inhibitor of reverse transcriptase that blocks hepatitis B viral replication. Chronic hepatitis B treatment in HBeAg-positive patients with lamivudine 100 mg orally daily for 52 weeks results in loss of HBeAg in 17% to 32% (vs. 6% to 11% in controls), HBeAg seroconversion in 16% to 18% (vs. 4% to 6% in controls), normalization of ALT in 41% to 72% (vs. 7% to 24% in controls), and histologic improvement in 49% to 56% (vs. 23% to 25% in controls).[77–79] One of the greatest concerns with lamivudine is the high incidence of hepatitis B viral mutation and drug resistance. The most common adverse effects are headache, malaise, fatigue, nausea, vomiting, diarrhea, neuropathy, cough, congestion, and musculoskeletal pain. Less common but serious adverse events include neutropenia, anemia, thrombocytopenia, pancreatitis, and increased liver function tests. One study found that 100-mg lamivudine daily had comparable adverse reaction rates to placebo.[78] Dose adjustments must be made for patients with renal insufficiency.

Adefovir is an acyclic nucleotide analogue with antiviral activity against hepatitis B. In the treatment of chronic hepatitis B, HBeAg-positive patients, adefovir 10 mg daily for 48 weeks has resulted in loss of HBV DNA in 21% (vs. 0% in controls), loss of HBeAg in 24% (vs. 11% in controls), HBeAg seroconversion in 12% (vs. 6% in controls), normalization of ALT in 48% (vs. 16% in controls), and histologic improvement in 53% (vs. 25% in controls).[80] In the treatment of chronic hepatitis B HBeAg-negative patients, adefovir 10 mg daily for 48 weeks resulted in histologic improvement in 64% of patients (vs. 33% of controls) and loss of HBV DNA in 51% of patients (vs. 0% of controls).[81] Viral resistance appears to be much less common with adefovir than with lamivudine.[80] The most common adverse effects associated with adefovir include: nausea, diarrhea, vomiting, dyspepsia, headache, and weakness. Pruritus and rash have also been reported. Nephrotoxicity has been reported with adefovir. Patients receiving high doses and those with renal dysfunction appear to be at greater risk. Dose adjustment is necessary in patients with renal insufficiency. Exacerbation of hepatitis has been reported following discontinuation of adefovir.

Entecavir (Baraclude) is a guanosine nucleoside analog with selective activity against hepatitis B virus. Entecavir has been FDA approved for the treatment of nucleoside naïve (0.5 mg orally once a day) or lamivudine-resistant patients (1 mg orally once a day) with chronic hepatitis B. Entecavir is eliminated by the kidneys and requires dose adjustment in the setting of renal dysfunction.

Hepatitis C. Treatment of chronic hepatitis C is recommended for those at risk for developing cirrhosis.[82] Response to treatment of chronic hepatitis C is affected by many factors. Factors associated with poor response to treatment with peginterferon plus ribavirin include: genotype 1, age older than 40 years, body weight more than 75 kg, pretreatment viral load greater than 2 million copies per milliliter, pretreatment ALT more than three-fold higher than normal, cirrhosis, and lack of early virologic response (no detectable HCV RNA or 2 $\log_{10}$ drop in HCV RNA) at 12 weeks of treatment.[83] Optimizing medication selection, dose, and duration of treatment requires knowledge of the hepatitis C genotype. For those patients that are treatment naïve (have not previously been treated) for hepatitis C and have chronic hepatitis C genotype 1, peginterferon (α–2a or α–2b) plus ribavirin 1,000 to 1,200 mg per day has been reported to result in sustained viral response (SVR) of 42% to 46%, which is superior to conventional interferon plus ribavirin treatment. A sustained virologic response is defined as no detectable HCV RNA in the serum for at least 6 months after discontinuing treatment. In addition, 48 weeks of therapy was found to result in a higher percentage of patients achieving SVR than 24 weeks of treatment for those patients with HCV genotype 1.[82]

In contrast, those patients with chronic hepatitis C genotypes 2 or 3 are more likely to be successfully treated than those with genotype 1. For patients with genotypes 2 or 3, interferon (conventional or pegylated) plus a lower dose of ribavirin (800 mg per day) results in sustained viral response

in approximately 80% of patients. In addition, a shorter duration of treatment will result in similar response rates in patients with genotypes 2 or 3. Twenty-four weeks of treatment with peginterferon plus ribavirin produce SVR in 73% of patients and 48 weeks of treatment produce SVR in 78% of the patients.[82]

Early virologic response to HCV treatment, defined as a 2 $\log_{10}$ or greater drop in viral load from baseline by 12 weeks of treatment is predictive of sustained viral response. Those patients who do not have early virologic response to HCV treatment are highly unlikely to respond to continued treatment even after 1 year. Treatment need not be extended beyond 12 weeks in patients that do not have an early virologic response.[82]

Retreatment of patients with chronic hepatitis C is particularly challenging. A decision as to whether to proceed with retreatment must take into account multiple factors including: factors predicting the likelihood of response, what initial treatment they received, whether they had response to initial treatment, how well they tolerated the initial treatment, and whether or not they adhered to the initial treatment. Overall, only 15% to 20% of patients having no response to conventional interferon plus ribavirin will have sustained viral response with peginterferon plus ribavirin.[82] Those with genotype 2 or 3 are more likely to respond than genotype 1. Further studies are needed to evaluate optimal treatment strategies for those who relapsed following discontinuation of treatment and for those who had no response to initial treatment.

One disturbing side effect of ribavirin is hemolytic anemia, which is commonly observed within the first 2 to 4 weeks of therapy. The anemia can be associated with a significant number of cardiac and pulmonary events. Central nervous system side effects such as insomnia, depression, and irritability also are common. Allergic reactions such as rash and pruritus may also occur. Ribavirin is highly teratogenic and embryotoxic, and therefore should not be used in women who are pregnant or in men whose female partners are pregnant. Effective contraception should also be used in women of child bearing potential, and male patients and their female partners during treatment with ribavirin and for 6 months after stopping therapy. Ribavirin is eliminated by the kidneys and not removed by dialysis. Dose reduction or discontinuation should be instituted for patients who develop anemia, leukopenia, thrombocytopenia, or depression. Ten percent to 14% of patients receiving pegylated interferon and ribavirin in registration trials required discontinuation of treatment due to side effects.[82] Major side effects of combination treatment include flulike symptoms (headache, fever, fatigue, myalgia, nausea), hematologic side effects (anemia, leukopenia, thrombocytopenia), and depression. Since depression is a common problem in patients in hepatitis C and a significant side effect associated with hepatitis C treatment, patients should be assessed prior to treatment and at regular intervals during treatment. The serotonin reuptake inhibitors may be of benefit in this setting.

Drug-induced Hepatitis. The most important step that can be taken in a suspected clinically significant drug-induced liver injury is discontinuation of the offending agent. Management of the liver injury should be supportive (see Chapter 50 for management of severe liver disease).

NONPHARMACOLOGIC THERAPY

The development of end-stage liver disease and cirrhosis can be hastened in some patients by ethanol consumption.[24] In addition, many liver transplantation programs and insurance carriers require very long periods of ethanol abstinence before transplantation regardless of the cause of liver disease. Therefore, it is very important for patients to be counseled on the need to discontinue all alcohol consumption.

ALTERNATIVE THERAPIES

Interest in herbal remedies for treating liver disease and other medical problems appears to be growing. Several herbal remedies have been reported to cause liver dysfunction, such as germander (*Teucrium chamaedrys*), chaparral (*Larrea divaricata*), skullcap (*Scutellaria lateriflora*), chaso (green tea, cassiae torae semen, leaves of lotus, *fructus lycii, F. crataegi*, and chrysanthemum flowers), onshido (extract of *Gynostemma pentaphyllum makino*, green tea, aloe, *F. crataegi* fructus, and raphani semen) and valerian (*Valeriana officinalis*).[84–88] Milk thistle (*Silybum marianum*), however, has been used to treat liver disease.[89] Several clinical studies have reported positive results with silymarin (derived from the milk thistle plant), suggesting that it decreases complications and hastens recovery from hepatitis. Most clinical studies have been with small numbers of patients, a wide range of causes and severity of illness studied within each study, and in most cases the lack of control or evaluation of ethanol consumption.[89] Herbal remedies with claims of beneficial effects for the liver include ji gu cao pill (*Fructus abri* 40%, *Agkistrodan* 15%, *Margarita* 3%, *Calculus Bovis* 10%, *Radix Angelicae Sinensis* 10%, *Fructus Lycii Chinensis* 7%, and *Radix Salviae Miltiorrhizae* 15%), li gan pian liver strengthening tablets (*Herba Jinqiancao* 70% and *Fellis Bovis* 30%), yin chen hao tang (*Herba Artemisiae Scopariae* 43%, *Fructus Gardeniae* 28.5%, *Radix Rhizoma Rhei* 28.5%), ta chai hu tang (*Bupleurum falcatum*), and jujube (*Zizyphus jujuba*). Many studies have been conducted evaluating the effects of medicinal herbs for the treatment of HCV infections.[90] Some agents appear to show promise in the treatment of hepatitis C, but due to limitations in study design, it is unclear what, if any, role the medicinal herbs will have in the treatment of hepatitis C. Controlled clinical trials are needed to determine their efficacy and safety.

FUTURE THERAPIES

Several new antiviral agents appear to have efficacy against the hepatitis B virus. One of the promising new agents for treating chronic hepatitis B and possibly preventing hepatitis B recurrence after liver transplantation is famciclovir, a prodrug of penciclovir. Famciclovir has been shown to dramatically reduce hepatitis B viral DNA levels.[91] Other therapies, such as emtricitabine, telbivudine, elvucitabine, valtorcitabine, and thymosin, are being studied for treatment of hepatitis B. Another area of continued research is in combination treatments. Additional controlled trials are necessary to determine the place in therapy for the new agents.

IMPROVING OUTCOMES

Patient education for hepatitis should address several points. First, the ways to avoid exposure to and transmission of hepatitis should be addressed for travelers and patients with hepatitis. Avoiding food or beverages that may be contaminated with hepatitis A is important. In particular, water (or ice), uncooked shellfish, and uncooked fruits or vegetables that patients did not peel themselves may be contaminated with the hepatitis A virus and result in transmission. Second, educating patients about prescribed medication regimens, expected side effects, and side effect management is essential. For some medications, such as interferon, detailed education on administration technique and product handling is necessary. In addition to safe sex counseling, patients receiving ribavirin, a known teratogen, need to be informed about the risk to the fetus in the event of pregnancy. Because of the long half-life of ribavirin, the risk of teratogenicity extends 6 months after discontinuation of treatment. Compliance is another important area for patient education, particularly for patients receiving the three-dose hepatitis B vaccine series, which extends over 6 months, and for those receiving antiviral therapy because efficacy is diminished with nonadherence.

PHARMACOECONOMICS

Hepatitis A vaccination has been shown to be cost-effective in the following populations (cost/year of life saved): patients with chronic hepatitis C in highly endemic regions (cost savings), men who have sex with men (cost savings), children in endemic regions ($12,780), adolescents ($13,933), food service workers ($14,206), patients with chronic hepatitis C in moderate endemic regions ($39,922 at age 50 years) and universal vaccination of children ($40,923).[84] General screening prior to vaccination for hepatitis A antibodies is not cost-effective.[92] Hepatitis A vaccine is the most cost-effective prevention strategy for travelers that visit endemic regions for three or more times in 10 years or for more than 6 months. In contrast to those visiting endemic regions less than three times in 10 years or for less than 6 months, immune globulin is more cost-effective.[93]

The pharmacoeconomics of hepatitis B affects how we monitor before and after vaccination. Routine testing of patients for antibodies to hepatitis B core antigen or antibodies to HBsAg before vaccination is a cost-effectiveness issue that must be resolved at each center. It may be reasonable to screen high-risk patients before vaccination but not low-risk patients. This decision depends on the cost of the vaccine, the cost of testing, and the expected prevalence of immunity. Postvaccination testing for immune response to the hepatitis B vaccine is not recommended for healthy people because of the very high expected response rate (90%). However, people who would be expected to have a suboptimal response (e.g., immunocompromised patients and those on hemodialysis) would be advised to have postvaccination testing for antibody response to the vaccine 1 to 6 months after completion of the series. Revaccination of those who did not have an adequate response to the initial series with one additional dose results in 15% to 25% of the patients having an adequate antibody response. Repeating the entire series (three additional doses) results in 30% to 50% having an adequate antibody response.[94]

The cost-effectiveness of a universal hepatitis B vaccination program is dependent on a number of assumptions made in the analysis. One very important factor in assessing cost-effectiveness is the hepatitis B carrier rate in the country of interest. The United States is considered to be a country with low hepatitis B chronic infection (0.5% to 2%). For countries with low levels of chronic hepatitis B, studies have reported a wide range of costs ($639 to $23,179) per discounted life-year gained. Overall, universal hepatitis B vaccination programs have been found to be cost-effective.[95] General screening for hepatitis B antibodies prior to vaccination is not cost-effective.[93] The two-dose hepatitis B vaccination regimen for adolescents has been found to improve compliance leading to higher protection rates. The two-dose vaccination regimen has been found to be cost-effective in the private sector and in public schools with the average cost per year of life gained reported to be $964 and $1,246 respectively.[96]

The cost-effectiveness of interferon treatment for patients with chronic HBeAg positive has been studied. A meta analysis evaluating the cost-effectiveness of interferon α-2b found that it prolonged life at a reasonable marginal cost per year of life saved in patients with chronic hepatitis B (HBeAg positive).[97] Wong[98] reported that interferon treatment was expected to prolong life expectancy by 4.8 years and decrease lifetime costs by $6,300. Brooks et al [99] reported that using a 1-year decision-tree model that lamivudine was more cost-effective than interferon for treatment of chronic hepatitis B. Crowley et al[100] reported that having both interferon and lamivudine available for treatment of chronic HBeAg-positive patients as compared to interferon alone or no treatment is cost-effective. Although interferon and lamivudine have similar efficacy rates, lamivudine treatment for chronic HBeAg-positive patients is expected to increase the number of patients that can be treated because it has far fewer side effects than interferon. Because of this advantage, the availability of lamivudine is expected to reduce overall chronic hepatitis B disease progression and increase life expectancy over the long-term. Pharmacoeco-

nomic studies of peginterferon and adefovir for the treatment of chronic hepatitis B and evaluation of patients with chronic hepatitis B who are e antigen negative need to be performed.

Advances in treatment of hepatitis C have significantly improved efficacy in this debilitating infection. Along with the advancement in treatment efficacy has come substantial increases in the drug costs. The pharmacoeconomic analysis or hepatitis C treatment is highly dependent on the assumptions made by the investigators. For example, assumptions made regarding the natural history of disease progression such as the percentage of patients with chronic disease that will go on to develop cirrhosis, the severity of disease at the initiation of treatment ranging from mild disease to cirrhosis, genotype 1 versus 2 and 3, sex, and the percent of patients expected to respond to treatment have ranged widely and have significant impact on the incremental cost-effectiveness ratio, survivorship, and quality-adjusted life years (QALY) gained. The QALY is a method used to quantitate improvement in quality of life in which the change in life expectancy is adjusted for quality of life. The cost-effectiveness ratio is the amount of money it takes to gain 1 year of quality-adjusted life.

The pharmacoeconomics of the various treatment strategies for chronic hepatitis C have been reported. Wong et al[101] reported that the combination of interferon α-2b plus ribavirin is more cost-effective than interferon monotherapy with reported cost of QALY gained was found to be $4,400 and $5,400, respectively. For treatment of chronic hepatitis C genotype 1, the combination of peginterferon with ribavirin has been shown to be more effective than conventional interferon plus ribavirin. Sullivan et al[102] found that in the treatment of chronic hepatitis C genotype 1 patients, the incremental cost-effectiveness ratio with peginterferon α-2A plus ribavirin as compared with interferon alfa-2B plus ribavirin was $2,600 per QALY gained. Salomon et al[103] reported that the incremental cost-effectiveness of peginterferon plus ribavirin versus peginterferon monotherapy for men ranged from $26,000 to $64,000 per QALY gained for genotype 1 and from $10,000 to $28,000 per QALY for other genotypes based on an assumed 30-year incidence of progression to cirrhosis from 13% to 46%. Similarly for women, the incremental cost-effectiveness ranged from $32,000 to $90,000 for genotype 1 and $12,000 to $42,000 for other genotypes assuming 1% to 29% of women will progress to cirrhosis over 30 years. The dramatic difference in results between Sullivan et al[102] and Salomon et al[103] reflect the different comparator groups, the assumptions regarding severity of illness at initiation of treatment, differences in assumed treatment response rates, whether or not the investigators accounted for early discontinuation of treatment based on lack of virologic response or adverse events, and assumed percent of patients that will progress to cirrhosis. Wong et al[104] reported that testing for early virologic response at 12 weeks as compared to continued treatment with peginterferon plus ribavirin for 48 weeks results in savings of $15,116 to $16,268. For genotype 1, chronic hepatitis C-infected patients, early virologic testing at 12 weeks with discontinuation of treatment for nonresponders is cost effective. For genotype 2 and 3 chronic hepatitis C-infected patients, early virologic testing at 12 weeks with discontinuation of treatment for nonresponders results in similar costs to continuation of treatment for the full 24 weeks without testing.

KEY POINTS

Viral hepatitis can be prevented through precautions such as avoiding contaminated food and water, practicing good personal hygiene, not reusing intravenous needles, practicing safe sex, avoiding recapping needles after blood drawing, and using sterile technique and supplies with acupuncture, tattooing, or body piercing.

■ When traveling to hepatitis A and B endemic areas of the world, follow prophylaxis regimens to avoid hepatitis transmission

■ Treating chronic hepatitis B and C can promote clearance of the virus, improve liver function tests, improve liver histology, and prolong life

■ Maintaining compliance with therapy is essential for therapeutic efficacy, particularly for completion of the hepatitis B vaccine series and antiviral therapy

■ Many patients have difficulty tolerating interferon therapy. Evening dosing and judicious use of acetaminophen (less than 2 g/day) for fevers and headaches may improve tolerability

■ The teratogenicity during and 6 months after ribavirin therapy must be discussed with patients

■ The risks and benefits should be weighed before agents with hepatotoxic potential are initiated in patients with preexisting liver disease

■ Early detection and discontinuation of agents causing hepatitis may minimize liver injury

■ When a patient presents with possible drug-induced hepatitis, assessing all agents the patient has been taking for hepatotoxic potential (focusing on duration of exposure, type of injury, and clinical and laboratory findings) is helpful in determining the most likely culprit. However, exclusion of other causes and resolution of symptoms after discontinuation of the offending agent ultimately are necessary to confirm the cause

■ Treatment of end-stage liver disease caused by hepatitis should be supportive

SUGGESTED READINGS

Craig AS, Schaffner W. Prevention of hepatitis A with the hepatitis A vaccine. N Engl J Med 350:476–481, 2004.

Dufour DR, Lott JA, Nolte FS, et al. Diagnosis and monitoring of hepatic injury II. Recommendations for use of laboratory tests in screening and monitoring. Clin Chem 46:2050–2068, 2000.

Lee WM. Drug-induced hepatotoxicity. N Engl J Med 349:474–485, 2003.

Lok AS, McMahon BJ. Chronic hepatitis B: update of recommendations. Hepatology 39:1–5, 2004.

Strader DB, Wright T, Thomas DL, Seeff LB. Diagnosis, management, and treatment of hepatitis C. Hepatology 39:1147–1171, 2004.

REFERENCES

1. CDC hepatitis A fact sheet. Available at: http://www.cdc.gov/ ncidod/diseases/ hepatitis/a/fact.htm. Accessed January 15, 2004.
2. Havens WP Jr. Period of infectivity of patients with experimentally induced infectious hepatitis. J Exp Med 83:2521, 1946.
3. Giles JP, Liebharber H, Krugman S, et al. Early viremia and viruria in infectious hepatitis. Virology 24:107–108, 1964.
4. Havens WP Jr, Ward R, Drill LA, et al. Experimental production of hepatitis by feeding icterogenic materials. Proc Soc Exp Biol Med 57:206, 1944.
5. Dienstag JL, Feinstone SM, Kapikian AZ, et al. Fecal shedding of hepatitis-A antigen. Lancet 1:765–767, 1975.
6. Rakela J, Mosley JW. Fecal excretion of hepatitis A virus. J Infect Dis 135:933–938, 1977.
7. Hollinger FB, Bradley DW, Maynard JE, et al. Detection of hepatitis A viral antigen by radioimmunoassay. J Immunol 115: 1464–1466, 1975.
8. Krugman S, Giles JP, Hammond J. Infectious hepatitis: evidence for two distinctive clinical epidemiological and immunological types of infection. JAMA 200:365–373, 1967.
9. Barbara JA, Howell DR, Briggs M, et al. Post-transfusion hepatitis A. Lancet 1:738, 1982.
10. Hollinger FB, Khan NC, Oefinger PE, et al. Posttransfusion hepatitis type A. JAMA 250:2313–2317, 1983.
11. Corey L, Holmes KK. Sexual transmission of hepatitis A in homosexual men: incidence and mechanism. N Engl J Med 302: 435–438, 1980.
12. Neefe JR, Stokes J Jr. An epidemic of infectious hepatitis apparently due to a waterborne agent. JAMA 128:1063, 1945.
13. Denes AE, Smith JC, Hindman SH, et al. Foodborne hepatitis A infection: a report of two urban restaurant-associated outbreaks. Am J Epidemiol 105:156, 1977.
14. CDC hepatitis B fact sheet. Available at: http://www.cdc.gov/ ncidod/diseases/ hepatitis/b/fact.htm. Accessed January 15, 2004.
15. Beeson PB. Jaundice occurring one to four months after transfusion of blood or plasma: report of 7 cases. JAMA 121:1332, 1943.
16. Alter MJ, Margolis HS. The emergence of hepatitis B as a sexually transmitted disease. Med Clin North Am 74:1529–1541, 1990.
17. Kew MC. Possible transmission of serum (Australia-antigen-positive) hepatitis via the conjunctiva. Infect Immun 7:823–824, 1973.
18. Seeff LB, Zimmerman HJ, Wright EC, et al. Hepatic disease in asymptomatic parenteral narcotic drug abusers: a Veterans Administration collaborative study. Am J Med Sci 270:41–47, 1975.
19. Roberts RH, Stul H. Homologous serum jaundice transmitted by a tattooing needle. Can Med Assoc J 62:75–78, 1950.
20. Johnson CJ, Anderson H, Spearman J, et al. Ear piercing and hepatitis: nonsterile instruments for ear piercing and the subsequent onset of viral hepatitis. JAMA 227:1165, 1974.
21. Carron H, Epstein BH, Grand B. Complication of acupuncture. JAMA 228:1552–1554, 1974.
22. Tiku ML, Bentner KR, Ramirez RI, et al. Distribution and characteristics of hepatitis B surface antigen in body fluids of institutionalized children and adults. J Infect Dis 134:342–347, 1976.
23. Protection against viral hepatitis recommendations of the immunization practices advisory committee (ACIP). MMWR Morb Mortal Wkly Rep 39:1, 1990.
24. National Institutes of Health. Consensus development statement. Management of hepatitis C, 1997. http://consensus.nih.gov/1997/ 1997HepatitisC105html.htm. Accessed Oct. 22, 2005.
25. Kato N, Yokosuka O, Hosoda K, et al. Detection of hepatitis C virus RNA in acute non-A, non-B hepatitis as an early digestive tool. Biochem Biophys Res Commun 192:800–807, 1993.
26. CDC hepatitis C fact sheet. Available at: http://www.cdc.gov/ ncidod/diseases/ hepatitis/c/fact.htm. Accessed January 15, 2004.
27. Alter HJ, Purcell RH, Shih JW, et al. Detection of antibody to hepatitis C virus in prospectively followed transfusion recipients with acute and chronic non-A, non-B hepatitis. N Engl J Med 321: 1494–1500, 1989.
28. Seeff LB. Hepatitis C from a needlestick injury. Ann Intern Med 115:411, 1991.

29. Ko YC, Ho MS, Chiang TA, et al. Tattooing as a risk of hepatitis C infection. J Med Virol 38:288–291, 1992.
30. Everhart JE, Di Bisceglie AM, Murray LM, et al. Risk for non-A, non-B (type C) hepatitis through sexual or household contact with chronic carriers. Ann Intern Med 112:544–545, 1990.
31. Thaler MM, Park CK, Landers DV, et al. Vertical transmission of hepatitis C virus. Lancet 338:17–18, 1991.
32. Center for disease control and prevention. Hepatitis surveillance report no. 58. Atlanta, GA: US Department of Health and Human Services, Center for Disease Control and Prevention, 2003.
33. Lewis JH, Zimmerman HJ. Drug-induced liver disease. Med Clin North Am 73:775–792, 1989.
34. Bass NM, Ockner RK. Drug-induced liver disease. In: Zakim D, Boyer TD. Hepatology: A textbook of liver disease. 3rd ed. Philadelphia: WB Saunders, 1996:962.
35. Lee WM. Drug-induced hepatotoxicity. N Engl J Med 333: 1118–1127, 1995.
36. Hagley MT, Hulisz DT, Burns CM. Hepatotoxicity associated with angiotensin-converting enzyme inhibitors. Ann Pharmacother 27: 228–231, 1993.
37. Swank LA, Chejfec G, Nemchausky BA. Allopurinol-induced granulomatous hepatitis with cholangitis and a sarcoid-like reaction. Arch Intern Med 138:997–998, 1978.
38. Kalantzis N, Gabriel P, Mouzas J, et al. Acute amiodarone hepatitis. Hepatogastroenterology 38:71–74, 1991.
39. Wolfe JD, Metzger AL, Holdstein RC. Aspirin hepatitis. Ann Intern Med 80:74–76, 1974.
40. Horowitz S, Patwardhan R, Marcus E. Hepatotoxic reactions associated with carbamazepine therapy. Epilepsia 29:149–154, 1988.
41. Utili R, Boitnott JK, Zimmerman HJ. Dantrolene-associated hepatic injury. Gastroenterology 72:610–616, 1977.
42. Iveson TJ, Ryley NG, Kelly PM, et al. Diclofenac-associated hepatitis. J Hepatol 10:85–89, 1990.
43. Schade RR, Gray JA, Dekker A, et al. Fulminant hepatitis associated with disulfiram. Report of a case. Arch Intern Med 143: 1271–1273, 1983.
44. Carson JL, Strom BL, Duff A, et al. Acute liver disease associated with erythromycins, sulfonamides and tetracyclines. Ann Intern Med 119:576–583, 1993.
45. Sanchez MR, Ross B, Rotterdam H, et al. Retinoids hepatitis. J Am Acad Dermatol 28:853–858, 1993.
46. Neuberger JM. Halothane and hepatitis: a model of immune mediated drug hepatotoxicity. Clin Sci 72:263, 1987.
47. Black M, Mitchell JR, Zimmerman HJ, et al. Isoniazid-associated hepatitis in 144 patients. Gastroenterology 69:289–302, 1975.
48. DaPrada M, Kettler R, Keller HH, et al. Preclinical profiles of the novel reversible MAO-A inhibitors, moclobemide and brofaromine, in comparison with irreversible MAO inhibitors. J Neural Transm 28:5, 1989.
49. Rodman JS, Deutsch DJ, Gutman SI. Methyldopa hepatitis. A report of six cases and review of the literature. Am J Med 60: 941–948, 1976.
50. Mullin GE, Greenson JK, Mitchell MC. Fulminant hepatic failure after ingestion of sustained release nicotinic acid. Ann Intern Med 111:253–255, 1989.
51. Sharp JR, Ishak KG, Zimmerman HJ. Chronic active hepatitis and severe hepatic necrosis associated with nitrofurantoin. Ann Intern Med 92:14–19, 1980.
52. Onorato IM, Axelrod JL. Hepatitis from intravenous high-dose oxacillin therapy: findings in an adult population. Ann Intern Med 89: 497–500, 1978.
53. Roy AK, Mahoney HC, Levine RA. Phenytoin-induced chronic hepatitis. Dig Dis Sci 38:740–743, 1993.
54. Rotmensch HH, Yust I, Siegman-Igra Y, et al. Granulomatous hepatitis: a hypersensitivity response to procainamide. Ann Intern Med 89:646–647, 1978.
55. Knobler H, Levij IS, Gavish D, et al. Quinidine-induced hepatitis: a common and reversible hypersensitivity reaction. Arch Intern Med 146:526–528, 1986.
56. Scheuer PJ, Summerfield JA, Lal S, et al. Rifampicin hepatitis. Clinical and histological study. Lancet 1:421–425, 1974.
57. Ivarson I, Lundlin P. Multiple attacks of jaundice associated with repeated sulfonamide treatment. Acta Med Scand 206:219, 1979.
58. Peters RL, Edmondson HA, Mikkelsen WP, et al. Tetracycline-induced fatty liver in nonpregnant patients: a report of six cases. Am J Surg 113:622–632, 1967.
59. Beck PL, Bridges RJ, Demetrick DJ, et al. Chronic active hepatitis associated with trazodone therapy. Ann Intern Med 118:791–792, 1993.
60. Redeker AG. Viral hepatitis: clinical aspects. Am J Med Sci 270: 9–16, 1975.
61. Merican I, Sherlock S, McIntyre N, et al. Clinical, biochemical and histological features in 102 patients with chronic hepatitis C virus infection. Q J Med 86:119–125, 1993.
62. Centers for Disease Control, Department of Health and Human Services. Vaccine recommendations for travelers health-care provider information, 1996. http://www2.ncid.cdc.gov/travel/yb/utils/ybGet.asp?section = intro&obi = cert-requirements1.htm& cssNav = browseoyb. Accessed Oct. 21, 2005.
63. Drake ME, Ming C. Gamma globulin in epidemic hepatitis: comparative value of two dosage levels approximately near the minimal effective level. JAMA 155:1302, 1954.
64. Mosley JW, Reisler DM, Brachott D, et al. Comparison of two lots of immune serum globulin for prophylaxis of infectious hepatitis. Am J Epidemiol 87:539–550, 1968.
65. Redeker AG, Mosley JW, Gocke DJ, et al. Hepatitis B immune globulin as a prophylactic measure for spouses exposed to acute type B hepatitis. N Engl J Med 293:1055–1059, 1975.
66. Szmuness W, Stevens CE, Harley EJ, et al. Hepatitis B vaccine: demonstration of efficacy in a controlled clinical trial in a high-risk population in the United States. N Engl J Med 303:833–841, 1980.
67. Stevens CE, Taylor PE, Tong MJ, et al. Yeast-recombinant hepatitis B vaccine: efficacy with hepatitis B immune globulin in prevention of perinatal hepatitis B virus transmission. JAMA 257: 2612–2616, 1987.
68. Beasley RP, Hwang LY, Lee GC, et al. Prevention of perinatally transmitted hepatitis B virus infections with hepatitis B immune globulin and hepatitis B vaccine. Lancet 2:1099–1102, 1983.
69. Wong VC, Ip HM, Reesink HW, et al. Prevention of the HB$_s$Ag carrier state in newborn infants of mothers who are chronic carriers of HB$_s$Ag and HB$_e$Ag by administration of hepatitis-B vaccine and hepatitis-B immunoglobulin: double-blind randomised placebo-controlled study. Lancet 1:921–926, 1984.
70. Stevens CE, Toy PT, Tong MJ, et al. Perinatal hepatitis B virus transmission in the United States: prevention by passive-active immunization. JAMA 253:1740–1745, 1985.
71. CDC. Suboptimal response to hepatitis B vaccine given by injection into the buttock. MMWR 34:105, 1985.
72. Stevens CE, Alter HJ, Taylor PE, et al. Hepatitis B vaccine in patients receiving hemodialysis. Immunogenicity and efficacy. N Engl J Med 311:496–501, 1984.
73. Collier AC, Croey L, Murphy VL, et al. Antibody to human immunodeficiency virus and suboptimal response to hepatitis B vaccination. Ann Intern Med 109:101–105, 1988.
74. Perrillo RP, Schiff ER, Davis GL, et al. A randomized, controlled trial of interferon alfa-2B alone and after prednisone withdrawal for treatment of chronic hepatitis B. N Engl J Med 323:295–301, 1990.
75. Wong DK, Cheung AM, O'Rourke K et al. Effect of alpha-interferon treatment in patients with hepatitis B e antigen-positive chronic hepatitis B. Ann Intern Med 119:312–323, 1993.
76. Cooksley WGE, Piratvisuth T, Lee SD et al. Peginterferon α–2a (40 kDa): an advance in the treatment of hepatitis B e antigen-positive chronic hepatitis B. J Viral Hep 10:298–305, 2003.
77. Dienstag JL, Schiff ER, Wright TL, et al. Lamivudine as initial treatment for chronic hepatitis B in the United States. N Engl J Med 341:1256–1263, 1999.
78. Lai CL, Chien RN, Leung NW, et al. A one-year trial of lamivudine for chronic hepatitis B. N Engl J Med 339:61–68, 1998.
79. Schalm SW, Heathcoate J, Cianciara J, et al. Lamivudine and alpha interferon combination treatment of patients with chronic hepatitis B infection: a randomized trial. Gut 46:562–568, 2000.
80. Marcellin P, Chang T-T, Lim SG, et al. Adefovir dipivoxil for the treatment of hepatitis B e antigen-positive chronic hepatitis B. N Engl J Med 348:808–816, 2003.
81. Hadziyannis SJ, Tassopoulos NC, Heathcote EJ, et al. Adefovir dipivoxil for the treatment of hepatitis B e antigen-negative chronic hepatitis B. N Engl J Med 348:800–807, 2003.

82. NIH consensus statement on management of hepatitis C: 2002. NIH Consensus and State-of-the-Science-Statements, volume 19, number 3, June 10–12, 2002.

83. Fried NW, Shiffman ML, Reddy KR, et al. Peginterferon alfa-2a plus ribavirin for chronic hepatitis C virus infection. N Engl J Med 347:975–982, 2002.

84. Adachi M, Saito H, Kobayashi H, et al. Hepatic injury in 12 patients taking herbal weight loss AIDS Chaso or onshido. Ann Intern Med 139:488–492, 2003.

85. Dunbabin DW, Tallis GA, Popplewell PY, et al. Lead poisoning from Indian herbal medicine (Ayurveda). Med J Aust 157:835–836, 1992.

86. Pauwels A, Thierman-Duffaud D, Azanowsky JM, et al. Acute hepatitis caused by wild germander: hepatotoxicity of herbal remedies. Two cases. Gastroenterol Clin Biol 16:92–95, 1992.

87. Gordon DW, Rosenthal G, Hart J, et al. Chaparral ingestion: the broadening spectrum of liver injury caused by herbal medications. JAMA 273:489–490, 1995.

88. MacGregor FB, Abernethy VE, Dahabra S, et al. Hepatotoxicity of herbal remedies. Br Med J 299:1156–1157, 1989.

89. Flora K, Hahn M, Rosen H, et al. Milk thistle (*Silybum marianum*) for the therapy of liver disease. Am J Gastroenterol 93:139–143, 1998.

90. Liu J, Manheimer E, Tsutani K, et al. Medicinal herbs for hepatitis C virus infection: a Cochrane hepatobiliary systemic review of randomized trials. Am J Gastroenterol 98:538–544, 2003.

91. Main J, Brown JL, Howells C, et al. A double blind, placebo-controlled study to assess the effect of famciclovir on virus replication in patients with chronic hepatitis B virus infection. J Viral Hepat 3:211–215, 1996.

92. Rosenthal P. Cost-effectiveness of hepatitis A vaccination in children, adolescents, and adults. Hepatology 37:44–51, 2003.

93. Jacobs RJ, Saab S, Meyerhoff AS, et al. An economic assessment of pre-vaccination screening for hepatitis A and B. Public Health Rep 118:550–558, 2003.

94. Hadler SC, Francis DP, Maynard JE, et al. Long term immunogenicity and efficacy of hepatitis B vaccine in homosexual men. N Engl J Med 315:209–214, 1986.

95. Beutels P, Economic evaluations of hepatitis B immunization: a global review of recent studies (1994–2000). Health Econ 10:751–774, 2001.

96. Levaux HP, Schonfeld WH, Pellissier JM, et al. Economic evaluation of a 2-dose hepatitis B vaccination regimen for adolescents. Pediatrics 108:317–325, 2001.

97. Wong JB, Koff RS, Tine F, et al. Cost-effectiveness of interferon-α2B treatment for hepatitis B e antigen-positive chronic hepatitis B. Ann Intern Med 122:664–675, 1995.

98. Wong JB. Interferon treatment for chronic hepatitis B or C infection: costs and effectiveness. Acta Gastroenterol Belg 61:238–242, 1998.

99. Brooks EA, Lacey LF, Payne SL, et al. Economic evaluation of lamivudine compared with interferon-alpha in the treatment of chronic hepatitis B in the United States. Am J Manag Care 7:677–682, 2001.

100. Crowley S, Tognarini D, Desmond P, et al. Introduction of lamivudine for treatment of chronic hepatitis B: expected clinical and economic outcomes based on 4-year clinical trial data. J Gastroenterol Hepatol 17:153–164, 2002.

101. Wong JB, Poynard T, Ling MH, et al. Cost-effectiveness of 24 or 48 weeks of interferon alpha-2b alone or with ribavirin as initial treatment of chronic hepatitis C. International Hepatitis Intervention Group. Am J Gastroenterol 95:1524–1530, 2000.

102. Sullivan SD, Jensen DM, Bernstein DE, et al. Cost-effectiveness of combination peginterferon alfa-2a and ribavirin compared with interferon alfa-2b and ribavirin in patients with chronic hepatitis C. Am J Gastroenterol 99:1490–1496,2004.

103. Salomon JA, Weinstein MC, Hammitt JK, et al. Cost-effectiveness of treatment for chronic hepatitis C infection in an evolving patient population. JAMA 290:228–237, 2003.

104. Wong JB, Davis GL, McHutchison JG, et al., and the International Hepatitis Interventional Therapy Group. Economic and clinical effects of evaluating rapid viral response to peginterferon alfa-2b plus ribavirin for the initial treatment of chronic hepatitis C. Am J Gastroenterol 98:2354–2362, 2003.

Cirrhosis

J. Richard Brown

DEFINITION

Cirrhosis is defined as irreversible chronic injury of the liver characterized by diffuse fibrosis and the formation of regenerative nodules. Areas of necrosis and regeneration of hepatic parenchyma impart the classic glandular or nodular appearance of the liver. Necrosis of hepatocytes leads to deposition of connective tissue, which distorts the vasculature and alters the flow of blood through the liver, resulting in portal hypertension. These pathologic changes are the end result for many types of chronic liver injury.

TREATMENT GOALS

- Currently, there is no specific pharmacotherapy that will cure cirrhosis.
- Management is limited to the prevention or treatment of complications.
- The primary goal of therapy is to prevent symptoms and maintain a reasonable quality of life.
- Specific complications of the disease are treated to reduce morbidity and the need for frequent hospitalizations.
- Once the diagnosis of cirrhosis is established, it is of utmost importance therapeutically that patients discontinue consumption of all alcohol.

EPIDEMIOLOGY

Although cirrhosis is frequently encountered in medicine, it is difficult to cite an accurate incidence because patients often have no symptoms until the later stages of disease. Postmortem data from various hospitals show an incidence of 3% to 15%. In 1989, cirrhosis was the ninth leading cause of death in the United States.[1] Worldwide, the annual death rate from cirrhosis of all causes is as high as 15 to 40 per 100,000 people.[2] However, death and hospitalization rates of patients with chronic liver disease and cirrhosis are on the decline in the United States. In 1989, chronic liver disease was the underlying cause of death for 26,720 people and a contributing cause of death for an additional 14,101 people. From 1980 through 1989 the age-adjusted death rate for chronic liver disease decreased 23%, from 13.5 to 10.4 per 100,000 people. Chronic liver disease appeared as the first diagnosis in an estimated 72,232 hospitalizations in 1989 and as a secondary diagnosis in an additional 218,156 hospitalizations. From 1980 through 1989 the hospitalization rate attributed to chronic liver disease and cirrhosis declined 44%, from 50.6 to 28.2 per 100,000 people.[3] Centers for Disease Control and Prevention data from 2001 reported 27,035 deaths, or 9.5 per 100,000. In 2000, 360,000 discharges from chronic liver disease and cirrhosis were recorded. In 2002, chronic liver disease and cirrhosis was the 12th leading cause of death in the United States, accounting for 1.2% of all deaths recorded.[4]

Table 50.1 lists the relative frequencies of the various types of cirrhosis encountered in the clinical setting. The largest percentage is alcohol-related cirrhosis, which occurs principally in patients between 40 and 60 years of age and is more common in men. (The management of alcoholism is discussed in greater detail in Chapter 58.) In the United

TABLE 50.1	Cirrhosis: Incidence and Causes	
Type	Frequency (%)	Causes
Alcohol-associated	60–70	Alcohol abuse and protein deficiency inducing fatty changes, inflammation, and scarring of liver
Biliary (primary and secondary)	10–15	Obstruction of bile flow (e.g., immune complexes, stones, and carcinoma); often secondary to long-standing bacterial infection
Postnecrotic	10–15	Scarring following massive hepatic necrosis, such as that seen in chronic viral hepatitis, after exposure to hepatotoxic drugs, or in immune-mediated hepatitis
Cryptogenic	10–15	Unknown
Metabolic	5–10	Excessive iron (hemochromatosis) or excessive copper (Wilson's disease) deposition, α_1-antitrypsin deficiency, other inborn errors of metabolism

States, 50% to 90% of these patients have a history of chronic alcoholism. The quantity of ethanol needed to cause cirrhosis is 80 g per day for 5 years. With approximately 11 to 12 g in the average drink, six or seven drinks per day over this period could be considered a factor in the development of cirrhosis. In developing countries, children often acquire hepatitis B by maternal transmission.[1,2,5]

PATHOPHYSIOLOGY

Several major types of cirrhosis have been described (Table 50.1), but cirrhosis associated with chronic hepatitis C infection is currently the most commonly encountered form in the United States, followed by alcohol-related cirrhosis.[5,6] (Viral hepatitis is discussed further in Chapter 49.) Alcoholic liver disease usually begins with severe fatty changes in the liver (steatosis). In the early stages this fatty infiltration is not associated with fibrosis and scarring. Later stages are marked by a prominent inflammation, an increase in fibrous tissue, and a progressive shrinkage, nodularity, and hardening of the liver.

In experimental animal models, dietary derangements can induce significant fatty changes in the liver, with subsequent development of cirrhosis. Therefore, it is often claimed that dietary indiscretion in alcoholics may be an important underlying associated cause of cirrhosis. This concept is supported by the observation that when a chronic alcoholic is hospitalized and placed on an appropriate diet, excess fat can be mobilized and the liver structure and function may return to normal. This reversibility is less clear if fibrosis is present. Other evidence implicates alcohol as a direct hepatotoxin. One group of investigators showed development of cirrhosis in baboons that were maintained on a balanced diet but given large daily doses of alcohol.[7]

Biliary cirrhosis is caused by chronic obstruction of bile flow (cholestasis). Primary biliary cirrhosis (PBC) follows long-standing cholestasis that is generally of unknown origin, but it may have an underlying immunologic basis with elevated immunoglobulin M (IgM), autoantibodies, and circulating complement-fixing immune complexes. The presence of antimitochondrial antibodies is the serologic hallmark for PBC. Secondary biliary cirrhosis may be caused by bile stones or a tumor obstructing bile flow, leading to an inflammatory reaction and scarring.

Other causes of cirrhosis are related to chronic viral hepatitis (e.g., chronic hepatitis B), autoimmune hepatitis, and various metabolic disorders (Table 50.1). In 10% to 15% of cirrhotic patients, the cause is never determined. This is referred to as cryptogenic cirrhosis.

The liver has a unique blood supply. The hepatic artery, which supplies oxygen-rich blood, provides approximately 20% of the blood supply to the liver. The remaining 80% of the blood supply comes from the portal vein. The portal vein, formed from the confluence of the splenic and mesenteric veins, provides nutrient-rich blood that comes from the gastrointestinal (GI) tract. A second set of microvasculature (or sinusoids) runs throughout the liver and then rejoins to empty into the hepatic veins and eventually the inferior vena cava. The main function of the portal venous system is to act as a pathway for detoxification and metabolism by the liver of substances absorbed from the GI tract. The anatomy of the portal system allows for first-pass (presystemic) metabolism of orally administered drugs such as propranolol, verapamil, and morphine.

With the development of cirrhosis, fibrosis, and the formation of regenerative nodules, the normal flow of blood through the liver parenchyma is impeded, resulting in a dramatic rise in the portal venous pressure and that of its tributaries. This is referred to as portal hypertension. Blood may also be shunted around the liver via collateral veins in the distal esophagus and gastric fundus. The increase in blood flow through these normally low-pressure tributaries results in engorgement of the submucosal veins, commonly referred to as esophageal and gastric varices.

CLINICAL PRESENTATION AND DIAGNOSIS

DIAGNOSIS

The diagnosis of cirrhosis is usually made based upon clinical, laboratory, and radiologic data. Cirrhosis can be confirmed and staged based on histologic evidence from liver biopsy.

SIGNS AND SYMPTOMS

Cirrhosis is insidious in its development and is often asymptomatic until the late stages of disease. Up to 50% of all cases are discovered only at postmortem examination. Many patients seek medical help, complaining of vague, nonspecific symptoms such as weight loss, loss of appetite, nausea, vomiting, and ill-defined digestive disturbances. Others enter the hospital acutely ill with the full syndrome of acute hepatitis (a precursor to cirrhosis). These patients have jaundice (bilirubin levels range from 2 mg per deciliter to more than 40 mg per deciliter), mildly elevated serum alanine and aspartate aminotransferase (ALT and AST) and alkaline phosphatase levels, a low serum albumin level, evidence of impaired coagulation (prolonged prothrombin time and elevated INR), and right upper quadrant pain. In the later stages of cirrhosis, patients may have the complications of cirrhosis: ascites, variceal bleeding, and hepatic encephalopathy. The clinical manifestations include visible collateral venous engorgement on the abdominal wall (caput medusa), testicular atrophy, parotid gland enlargement, nail clubbing, skin hyperpigmentation, amenorrhea, jaundice, edema, palmar erythema, fetor hepaticus, loss of body hair, spider angiomas, gynecomastia, ascites, splenomegaly, and muscle wasting. Patients can also experience intense pruritus due to hyperbilirubinemia. Hepatocellular carcinoma develops in as many as 10% of subjects with long-standing cirrhosis.

Ascites. Ascites, characterized by the accumulation of protein-rich fluid in the peritoneal cavity, is one of the most striking features of cirrhosis. Complaints associated with ascites include a rapidly developing inability to fit into one's clothes, weight gain, abdominal and low-back pain, gastroesophageal reflux, and shortness of breath secondary to impaired diaphragm movement or the development of pleural effusions. The amount of fluid in the abdomen can vary from a few liters to 20 liters or more, leading to a large protuberant abdomen and an umbilical hernia. Ascitic fluid is a good medium for bacterial growth. Infection of the peritoneal cavity can occur spontaneously (spontaneous bacterial peritonitis). An unexplained high fever or elevated white blood cell count is an indication for obtaining a sample of the ascitic fluid for bacterial culture or initiating empiric antibiotic therapy.

Several mechanisms have been postulated to explain the formation of ascites (Fig. 50.1), none of which is fully accepted as the definitive answer.[8,9] Most agree that disruption of hepatic architecture and blood flow caused by inflammation, cell necrosis, fibrosis, or obstruction leads to hemodynamic alterations, causing an elevated lymphatic pressure within the hepatic sinusoids, which eventually causes excessive transudation (weeping) of protein-rich fluid from the surface of the liver into the peritoneal cavity. According to the underfill theory, both the lymphatic leakage and high prehepatic venous pressure (portal hypertension) cause a net flow of volume from the vascular space to the peritoneal cavity via hydrostatic forces. The high protein content of the ascitic fluid may also help to draw fluid out of the vasculature. As a result, effective vascular volume throughout the body decreases, causing secondary sodium and water retention by the kidney. The renin angiotensin system is a major mediator of the sodium and water retention, ultimately causing release of aldosterone from the adrenal gland. Antidiuretic hormone (ADH) release may also increase. Serum levels of aldosterone and ADH remain elevated because of impaired metabolism secondary to liver failure. These processes are accentuated by a reduced oncotic pressure within the intravascular space due to hypoalbuminemia. A major

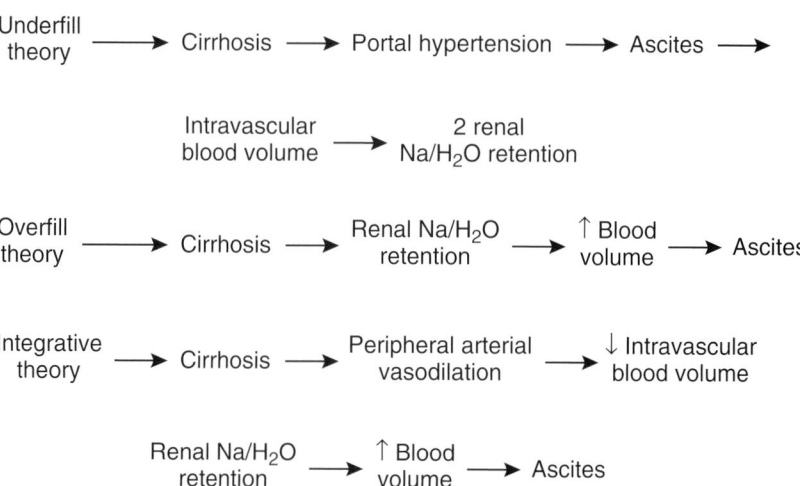

FIGURE 50.1 Mechanisms of ascites development.

inconsistency with the underfill theory is that some patients have an increased, not decreased, total intravascular volume, and not all patients have demonstrable hyperaldosteronism.

According to the overfill theory, the primary defect in ascites formation is excessive renal reabsorption of sodium and water. As plasma volume expands, ascites results from overflow of fluid out of the splanchnic circulation and increased pressure in the portal system. This implies that an unknown primary renal stimulus initiates the volume expansion. Increased sympathetic activity and a variety of hormonal substances have been proposed as factors affecting renal function in cirrhotic patients.[10]

Schrier et al[8] proposed an integration of these two theories, citing a possible systemic intravascular vasodilation that causes a relative decrease in effective plasma volume or pressure, followed by excessive renal retention of sodium and water. Central blood volume has a primary influence on renal circulation. In cirrhotic patients, there is reduced circulating volume even in patients who have not yet developed ascites. This volume reduction results from vasodilation of the peripheral vascular system. Sensing a shift from the central circulation, the kidneys and arterial baroreceptors activate vasoconstrictive systems to enhance sodium reabsorption. The renin-angiotensin-aldosterone system and the release of vasopressin act to increase central vascular filling.[9] It is believed that both intrahepatic hypertension and a primary renal defect are responsible for the early stages of ascites.[7]

Hypoalbuminemia, secondary to decreased hepatic synthesis and lymphatic leakage into the peritoneum, may further contribute to accumulation of ascites. A low serum albumin concentration reduces serum oncotic pressure, which favors the flow of fluid from the vasculature into the extravascular space. Not all patients with cirrhosis have hypoalbuminemia, but those who do may have both ascites and extensive peripheral edema with a relative systemic hypovolemia. Ascites from portal hypertension can be distinguished from other causes (hepatoma, pancreatic ascites, biliary ascites) by evaluation of a serum albumin ascites gradient. This gradient is calculated by subtracting the ascitic fluid albumin value from the serum albumin value. If the value of the gradient exceeds 1.1 g per dL, the patient has portal hypertension with 97% certainty.[10] Patients often have hyponatremia from retention of free water, induced by elevated ADH levels. Hypokalemia may develop secondary to hyperaldosteronism or excessive vomiting.

Gastrointestinal Bleeding. GI hemorrhage occurs in about one fourth to one third of patients. About one third of these patients die of the initial hemorrhage. Even nonfatal GI hemorrhages can be massive. The major cause of GI bleeding associated with cirrhosis is shunting of blood away from the high-pressure portal system to low-pressure collaterals in the esophagus or gastric fundus (esophageal or gastric varices respectively), rectum (hemorrhoids), and other parts of the GI tract. The increased blood flow causes these

veins to become enlarged and tortuous, which means they can easily rupture. The risk of bleeding can be compounded by a coagulopathy from a deficiency of vitamin K–dependent clotting factors (II, VII, IX, X). Esophageal varices account for about 50% to 60% of the cases of GI bleeding in patients with cirrhosis, while peptic ulcer disease accounts for another 25%. The presence of varices in the cirrhotic patient accounts for a 20% higher 2-year mortality rate and a 30% higher 5-year mortality rate.

Hepatic Encephalopathy. Hepatic encephalopathy is a spectrum of neuropsychiatric abnormalities seen in patients with liver failure. Other neurologic or metabolic causes of encephalopathy must be excluded first.

Reversal of the day–night sleep cycle (insomnia or hypersomnia) usually precedes other symptoms. Other manifestations range from forgetfulness, mental confusion, personality changes, hyperreflexia, asterixis (characteristic flapping of the fingers when the hands are dorsiflexed) to somnolence, confusion, and coma. Hepatic encephalopathy can be divided into five stages—stage 0, no abnormality; stage 1, mild impairment (insomnia or hypersomnia, reversal of sleep pattern); stage 2, moderate impairment (slow responsiveness, lethargy); stage 3, severe impairment (somnolence, confusion, semistupor); and stage 4, coma (stupor, unconsciousness).

As the disease progresses, a characteristic sweet, pungent odor (fetor hepaticus) may be present on the patient's breath. The cause of the odor is unclear but may be related to exhalation of mercaptans.

The diagnosis of hepatic encephalopathy may be complicated by other neurologic disorders, including alcohol withdrawal-induced tremors, Wernicke's disease (mental disturbances, ataxia, and nystagmus from acute thiamine deficiency), Korsakoff's syndrome (psychosis and confabulation from chronic thiamine deficiency), and cerebellar damage from chronic alcohol ingestion. The presence of asterixis is a major differentiating factor.

The pathogenesis of hepatic encephalopathy is not well understood, but it may be related in part to increased arterial and central nervous system (CNS) ammonia levels. No direct cause-and-effect relationship has been shown between encephalopathy and blood ammonia concentration. Elevation of blood ammonia is seen in 60% to 80% of encephalopathic patients. When factors that influence ammonia production are decreased, the patient's sensorium often clears. Ingestion of a protein-rich (more than 70 g per day) diet or bleeding into the GI tract (e.g., esophageal bleeding) introduces a source of protein into the intestinal tract. Ammonia is produced in the lower GI tract when these proteins and urea are metabolized by bacterial enzymatic action. The ammonia is then absorbed into the bloodstream. Normally, the liver converts the ammonia into glutamine and urea for excretion by the kidney, but when the liver is failing or the blood is being shunted away from it, as in advanced cirrhosis, serum ammonia levels increase and encephalopathy ensues. Hypo-kalemia can also contribute to renal ammonia production.

Hypokalemia should be promptly corrected. It is theo-rized that the cerebrotoxicity of ammonia results from inhibi-tion of oxidative metabolism by the citric acid cycle in the brain. Alpha-ketoglutarate combines with ammonia to pro-duce high CNS levels of glutamine (a byproduct of ammonia metabolism) while robbing the citric acid cycle of the α-ketoglutarate needed for production of high-energy adeno-sine triphosphate (ATP), impairing brain energy metabo-lism. Cerebrospinal fluid (CSF) glutamine levels are occa-sionally measured to confirm hepatic encephalopathy.

An alternative explanation for the pathogenesis of hepatic encephalopathy concerns derangements in plasma and brain amino acid patterns.[11–15] Characteristically, there is a rela-tive elevation in methionine and aromatic amino acid (AAA) levels (e.g., phenylalanine, tyrosine, and tryptophan) and a corresponding relative deficiency in branched-chain amino acids (BCAA; e.g., valine, leucine, and isoleucine). These derangements lead to an imbalance of brain neurotransmit-ters, causing elevated levels of serotonin, octopamine, and phenylethanolamine and a decrease in dopamine and possi-bly norepinephrine. Serotonin is an end product of trypto-phan metabolism, whereas phenylethanolamine and octo-pamine are byproducts of phenylalanine and tyrosine metabolism.

Although the exact reason for these derangements in plasma and brain amino acids is unknown, a number of ob-servations have been made.[9–11] The normal ratio of BCAAs to AAAs is 4:1 to 6:1. In both sepsis and liver failure, cata-bolic states lead to a negative nitrogen balance and preferen-tial use of BCAAs as a source of energy. As ammonia levels rise, glucagon secretion is stimulated, which in turn stimu-lates hepatic gluconeogenesis to convert amino acids into glucose for energy. In response to gluconeogenesis, insulin is secreted, which leads to increased uptake and metabolism of BCAAs by skeletal muscle. As liver failure progresses, the liver can no longer store or release glucose in adequate amounts, so greater quantities of BCAAs must be metabo-lized by skeletal muscle for energy.

Simultaneously, the plasma clearance of AAAs and me-thionine, which depends on hepatic metabolism, is dimin-ished. The net result is an alteration of the BCAA:AAA ratio. In acute liver failure the AAAs rise dramatically while BCAAs remain normal. In chronic hepatic disease the AAAs remain abnormally high while BCAA concentrations drop to low levels, further lowering the BCAA:AAA ratio. Although controversial, BCAA supplementation is used in an effort to restore the BCAA:AAA ratio. If patients are protein intol-erant, this approach may offer some merit.[16]

In addition to alterations in amino acid metabolism, there appears to be a derangement of the blood–brain barrier dur-ing chronic liver disease. In people with hepatic encephalop-athy, there is a selective increase in transport of AAAs across the blood–brain barrier, possibly via an exchange of CSF glutamine (from ammonia metabolism) for AAAs in the

plasma. The arterial concentration of ammonia and other amines may be accentuated by excessive dietary protein con-sumption, GI hemorrhage (source of protein), overdiuresis leading to dehydration, or other conditions that lead to severe electrolyte imbalance and metabolic alkalosis.

An entirely different avenue of research suggests that the γ-aminobutyric acid (GABA) benzodiazepine receptor com-plex is involved in the pathogenesis of hepatic encephalopa-thy.[17] GABA is the primary inhibitory neurotransmitter in the CNS. According to this theory, an increase in CNS GA-BAergic neurotransmission may partially account for the be-havioral and electrophysiologic manifestations of encepha-lopathy. This hypothesis is based on the observation that an accentuation of CNS inhibitory neurotransmitter tone can cause ataxia, sedation, and coma. Although GABA levels do not seem to be elevated in patients with encephalopathy, it is speculated that other endogenous or exogenous GABA-like ligands may be involved. Not surprisingly, these patients also demonstrate unusual sensitivity to benzodiazepine-like drugs that elicit GABAergic-like activity.

Other Associated Disorders. Anemia and other hemato-logic disorders commonly accompany cirrhosis. Chronic al-cohol abusers tend to malabsorb folic acid and iron. In addi-tion, their diets may be deficient in both iron and folate. Iron deficiency may be aggravated by a blocking of iron uptake into the bone marrow induced by chronic alcoholism and by slow GI bleeding caused by gastritis. Thrombocytopenia and leukopenia may occur because of folic acid deficiency and alcohol-related bone marrow suppression. Hypersplenism, secondary to portal hypertension, may also contribute.

Endocrine disorders are seen in advanced cirrhosis be-cause of the liver's inability to metabolize the steroid hor-mones of the adrenals and gonads. In men, increased circu-lating estrogen levels cause gynecomastia, testicular atrophy, loss of male-pattern body hair, impotence, spider angiomas, and palmar erythema.

The concurrent impairment of renal function with hepatic failure is called hepatorenal syndrome (HRS). HRS develops in about 4% of patients with decompensated cirrhosis and is associated with a poor prognosis; more than 95% of these patients die within a few weeks after the onset of azotemia. HRS is characterized by increased renal vascular resistance and decreased systemic vascular resistance. The complex hemodynamic changes occur in response to vasoactive agents that produce different effects on the systemic and renal circulation. The vasoactive agents and systems in-volved in HRS are the renin-angiotensin-aldosterone system, the sympathetic nervous system, ADH, and the renal prosta-glandin and kinin systems.

HRS may occur acutely or progressively. The acute onset generally occurs in patients with end-stage cirrhosis or with other complications such as encephalopathy, bacterial infec-tions, and bleeding. Clinical symptoms include oliguria that develops within a few days, along with a rapid increase in plasma urea and creatinine levels, tense ascites, dilutional hyponatremia, hypotension, and jaundice. A slower progressive type involving other chronic types of renal conditions associated with liver disease exhibits a gradual decrease in glomerular filtration rate that may last for several weeks or months. These patients may also demonstrate ascites that is poorly responsive to diuretics.[18]

PSYCHOSOCIAL ASPECTS

It is generally accepted that more than 90% of Americans drink alcohol at some time. The social drug clearly is the most widely abused substance in our society. Problems associated with the chronic use of alcohol are impressive in their pathologic magnitude and the costs incurred by society. For the alcoholic patient with cirrhosis, psychological therapy with consideration for structured rehabilitation should be a component of the overall care plan.

THERAPEUTIC PLAN

Management of cirrhosis is largely symptomatic (Table 50.2). Patients with complications of cirrhosis such as ascites, hepatic encephalopathy, and esophageal varices should receive appropriate treatment. Treatment of chronic hepatitis B or C may slow the progression of disease. Liver transplantation should be considered for patients with end-stage liver disease. Patients and their caregivers should be referred to a transplant center to determine whether liver transplantation will be a viable option (see Chapter 27).

All patients with liver disease should refrain from further alcohol consumption. Other potentially hepatotoxic drugs should also be discontinued. Acetaminophen-induced hepatotoxicity may be more common in alcoholic patients due to compromised nutritional intake and diminished hepatic reserves. Acetaminophen can be safely used, if the dose is limited to less than 2 g per day. The use of aspirin or nonsteroidal anti-inflammatory drugs may worsen gastritis or precipitate GI bleeding or renal dysfunction. Other analgesics, such as narcotics, may lead to profound CNS and respiratory depression if liver function is severely compromised or the patient is obtunded. If the patient experiences nausea, antiemetics may be used with caution. Phenothiazine-type antiemetics (e.g., prochlorperazine, promethazine) have been associated with cholestasis and can also cause altered sensorium. Benzodiazepines, sedatives, hypnotics, and other drugs that can alter sensorium should be avoided, as they may worsen or precipitate hepatic encephalopathy.

TREATMENT

PHARMACOTHERAPY

Vitamin Supplementation. Specific vitamin supplementation is essential in most cirrhotic patients, especially those with a recent history of alcohol abuse. Replacement of thiamine at 50 to 100 mg per day along with a balanced diet may improve mentation, decrease symptoms of nutritional polyneuropathy, and improve gait disorders.

Continuation of thiamine therapy beyond 1 or 2 weeks is of questionable value because it is a water-soluble vitamin whose stores are rapidly replaced. Up to 1 g per day is occasionally needed if the patient displays severe nystagmus, Wernicke's encephalopathy, or oculogyric crisis. Iron replacement and folic acid supplements may be needed if the patient is anemic or folate-deficient. Iron deficiency can be determined by a blood smear and measurement of serum iron, total iron-binding capacity, and ferritin concentrations (see Chapter 31).

Vitamin K 10 mg subcutaneously daily for 3 days is given if the prothrombin time/INR is elevated. Lack of response to vitamin K implies an impaired synthetic capacity that accompanies vitamin K deficiency from advanced liver disease. If the prothrombin time/INR is not reversed after three to five doses of vitamin K, further doses should be avoided because there may be a paradoxical lengthening of the prothrombin time from excessive vitamin K. This paradoxical effect is thought to be a result of consumptive processes induced by overstimulation of the production of clotting factors, leading to an eventual depletion of the body stores. Vitamin K_1, or phytonadione (AquaMephyton), gives a more rapid response when given parenterally than either vitamin K_3 (menadione) or vitamin K_4 (menadiol). Neither menadione nor menadiol is available in the United States. If giving phytonadione parenterally, the subcutaneous route is preferred, but it may also be given by very slow intravenous infusion in 50 mL of 5% dextrose in water over 15 to 20 minutes. Intramuscular injections are contraindicated if the patient has a prolonged prothrombin time/INR or is thrombocytopenic because of the possibility of hematoma and other bleeding complications. Because phytonadione is a colloidal suspension, there is a small risk of development of fever, chills, and even anaphylactic reactions with rapid intravenous injection. If the patient is malabsorbing fats or is cholestatic, the absorption of fat-soluble vitamins (A, D, E, and K) from the GI tract may be compromised. Subcutaneous phytonadione would be the preferred route in this setting. Patients should be assessed for signs and symptoms of vitamin deficiency and should receive vitamin supplementation if found deficient (see Chapter 29).

Ascites. Ascites reversal, especially with drug therapy, is a time-consuming process that entails weeks or months of conservative management including bed rest to decrease plasma renin release, sodium restriction (500 mg to 2 g per day), and, in some cases, fluid restriction. Approximately 5% of patients have a spontaneous diuresis with bed rest alone, while another 10% to 25% respond to salt restriction.[9] Fluid restriction is warranted only in cases of hyponatremia (serum sodium below 120 mmol/L) because excessive fluid restriction may lead to decreased renal blood flow and prere-

TABLE 50.2	**Drugs Used in Cirrhotic Patients**		
Drug	**Reason**	**Dose**	**Monitoring Parameters**
Thiamine	Reverse or prevent mental confusion secondary to thiamine deficiency (Wernicke's syndrome) and decrease peripheral neuropathies	100–200 mg/day, occasionally higher	Mental status Decrease in nystagmus, peripheral neuropathies; >10 days of therapy is unwarranted
Vitamin K (phytonadione)	Prevent bleeding secondary to decreased production of factors II, VII, IX, and X (vitamin K–dependent factors)	10 mg/day, not to exceed 3 doses	Hypersensitivity (fever, chills, anaphylaxis, flushing, sweating) Prothrombin time/INR
Spironolactone	Diuresis in ascites; specific for antagonism of preexisting hyperaldosteronism	100–400 mg/day, occasionally higher; may be given as a single daily dose	Weight (avoid more than 1-kg weight loss per day) Mental status Serum K^+ Urine Na^+ and K^+ (Na^+ should not exceed K^+ at therapeutic doses) Abdominal girth Blood urea nitrogen (increased in dehydration) Gynecomastia (prolonged use) Blood pressure
Loop diuretics furosemide	Diuresis in ascites used in combination with spironolactone	Start at 40 mg, titrate to 1-kg weight loss per day; occasionally very high doses (200–600 mg/day) needed	Same as spironolactone except urine electrolytes are of no value Possible hearing loss with rapid IV bolus
Vasopressin	Vasoconstrictor for esophageal bleeding	0.2–0.4 units/min IV infusion	Rate of GI bleeding Signs of ischemia (chest pain, elevated blood pressure, bradycardia) GI cramping Serum Na^+
Sodium tetradecyl sulfate, ethanolamine oleate, or sodium morrhuate	Sclerosing agents for esophageal variceal bleeding	0.5–2 mL of 1–1.5% tetradecyl, 5% ethanolamine, or 5% sodium morrhuate solution in each varix about 2 cm apart	Signs of GI bleeding Chest pain, fever, local ulceration
Propranolol	Prevent GI bleeding	20–320 mg/day titrated to 55–60 bpm resting pulse rate if tolerated	Signs of GI bleeding Mental changes Vital signs: pulse, blood pressure Signs of congestive heart failure, bradycardia Signs of bronchospasm Renal function
Lactulose	Hepatic encephalopathy; converted to acids to lower bowel pH and prevent absorption of NH_3	20–30 g QID or 300 mL lactulose QS to 700–1,000 mL as rectal enema titrated to 3–4 soft stools per day	Mental status, liver flap (asterixis), diarrhea
Neomycin	Hepatic encephalopathy; sterilizes gut to prevent bacterial breakdown of protein and thus decreases serum NH_3 levels	2–6 g/day, orally or rectally	Mental status, liver flap (asterixis) Diarrhea, bacterial overgrowth Renal function Signs of ototoxicity

(continued)

TABLE 50.2	continued		
Drug	**Reason**	**Dose**	**Monitoring Parameters**
Rifaximin[b]	Hepatic encephalopathy; decreases urease producing, bacteria	400 mg orally three times daily	Mental status, liver flap (asterixis)
Hepatamine, Hepatic-Aid, and Nutihep[a]	Hepatic encephalopathy; replace branched-chain amino acids	Titrate to caloric and nitrogen needs	Mental status Serum ammonia, cerebrospinal fluid glutamine Serum amino acid levels (branched-chain: aromatic amino acid ratio) Electrolyte balance
Dopamine[a]	Hepatorenal syndrome	1–4 µg/kg/min	Mental status, liver flap (asterixis) Urine output Blood pressure
Colchicine[a,b]	Anti-inflammatory and antifibrotic effects	0.6 mg PO BID or 1 mg PO QD 5 days/wk	Nausea, abdominal pain, diarrhea
Cefotaxime, norfloxacin[a], ciprofloxacin, trimethoprim/ sulfamethoxazole	Treatment or prevention of spontaneous bacterial peritonitis	Norfloxacin 400 mg daily or 400 mg BID (ciprofloxacin 750 mg weekly, TMP/SMX 1 DS QD, M through F)	Reduction in incidence of SBP
Flumazenil[a,b]	Acute reversal of hepatic encephalopathy	0.2–0.4 mg titrated to response	Reversal of mental obtundation
Octreotide	Treat GI bleeding	50-µg bolus, 50–200-µg/hr infusion for 5 days	Diarrhea Improvement in GI bleeding
Midodrine	Hepatorenal syndrome (investigational use)	Dosed orally to maintain increase of 15 mm Hg in mean arterial pressure	Blood pressure Glomerular filtration rate Renal sodium excretion

[a]Not recommended for all patients. [b]Investigational use only; efficacy unclear.

nal azotemia. Hospitalization usually is recommended for refractory patients for the following reasons: intensive education on medications and diet; close monitoring of serum and urine electrolytes, urea nitrogen, and creatinine; and investigation of the cause of the liver disease.

Diuretics are the cornerstone of drug therapy for the treatment of ascites. Diuresis must be slow and controlled to minimize complications. If urinary losses exceed the volume of fluid reabsorbed from ascites or peripheral edema, volume depletion with hypotension and renal insufficiency can develop. In patients treated with sodium restriction alone, no more than 300 mL of ascites can be reabsorbed per day. Even with the use of a diuretic, the maximum rate of reabsorption is 1,440 mL per 24 hours.[19,20] Diuresis should be limited to 0.2 to 0.3 kg weight loss per day in those without edema and 0.5 to 1 kg per day in patients with edema. Others allow a slightly more liberal diuresis of 0.75- to 2-kg weight loss per day.[20] These recommendations assume that each liter of volume lost is equivalent to a 1-kg weight loss. In patients with concurrent peripheral edema, a greater diuresis may be acceptable for the first 1 to 2 days because peripheral edema equilibrates more readily with the vasculature than does ascitic fluid. Other monitoring parameters include urine output, changes in abdominal girth, postural blood pressures, blood urea nitrogen, serum creatinine, increase in the urine-

potassium:sodium ratio from pretreatment baseline, and mental status changes.

Although slow diuresis with any diuretic may be acceptable for treating ascites, typically the first diuretic given is spironolactone with or without furosemide. Spironolactone is a gentle, slow-acting diuretic that antagonizes the effects of the hyperaldosteronism that exists in many of these patients. In contrast to the small doses of spironolactone that are used as an adjunct in hypertension and congestive heart failure, the initial dose for the treatment of ascites is usually 50 to 100 mg per day. A 3- to 5-day lag period exists for the onset and maximum response from spironolactone, so frequent dose adjustments prior to this time period should be avoided. Doses are titrated upward in 50- to 100-mg increments every 3 to 5 days, with 400 mg per day being required in approximately 75% of patients. The delayed onset and long duration of spironolactone result from the long half-life (approximately 17 to 20 hours) of its active metabolite, canrenone. For patient convenience and to improve compliance, once-daily dosing is recommended. Multiple daily doses are not necessary unless the patient cannot swallow the necessary number of tablets at one time without gastric distress.

Other concomitant diuretics such as furosemide offer an additional mechanism of diuresis. Runyon et al advocated the use of furosemide initially or early in treatment in a ratio of 40 mg to every 100 mg of spironolactone, given once daily in the morning to avoid nocturnal diuresis.[21] An added advantage of this combined approach is to maintain potassium balance in the face of diuresis.

Triamterene (Dyrenium) and amiloride (Midamor) are potassium-sparing diuretics that have a slightly more rapid onset of action, but they are not specific inhibitors of aldosterone. The relative efficacy of these potassium-sparing diuretics compared to spironolactone has not been evaluated extensively. They may be useful in patients who develop gynecomastia with spironolactone. The new and more selective aldosterone antagonist eplerenone (Inspra) is associated with less gynecomastia, but it has not been adequately studied in this patient population.

Besides the general monitoring parameters cited for diuretic therapy, serum and urine electrolyte levels, especially potassium, must be monitored. If hyperaldosteronism is present, it is not uncommon to see very little or no urinary sodium excretion and large urinary potassium losses. One measure of having achieved the desired spironolactone dose is a reversal of the urine electrolyte pattern to normal (i.e., sodium loss greater than potassium loss). Patients with urine sodium:potassium ratios greater than 1 tend to respond to lower doses of spironolactone (100 to 150 mg per day); those with ratios less than 1 often need larger doses, averaging 400 mg per day.[9]

Hyperaldosteronism, if present, may also cause a reduction in the serum potassium concentration. Although the use of spironolactone with potassium supplements is usually contraindicated in treatment of other diseases because of a high risk of inducing hyperkalemia, this combination may be necessary early in the treatment of ascites, especially if the patient has additional GI losses of potassium secondary to vomiting or diarrhea. Serum potassium must be monitored daily to avoid hypokalemia or hyperkalemia. Because these patients often are placed on a low-sodium diet, the use of salt substitutes that contain potassium use should be discouraged to further limit the complexity of potassium supplementation in this setting. Long-term use of spironolactone increases the risk of gynecomastia, a problem that is common in cirrhosis independent of diuretic use. Patients should be informed of this side effect of spironolactone.

High doses of spironolactone alone may not produce the desired diuresis in some patients or may cause hyperkalemia. In this situation, the addition of more potent diuretics such as thiazides or loop diuretics may be warranted. Some patients are especially refractory, often requiring several hundred milligrams per day of furosemide to obtain the desired weight loss of 0.5 to 1 kg per day. One drawback to the use of thiazides and loop diuretics is that they cause a significant natriuresis, which interferes with the ability to interpret urine electrolytes. Intravenous furosemide should be avoided if possible because it can decrease glomerular filtration rates and adds additional unnecessary cost.[22] Use of nonsteroidal anti-inflammatory drugs and COX-2 inhibitors should be avoided because they may blunt the effects of diuretics and decrease renal blood flow.

Paracentesis (aspiration of peritoneal fluid with a needle), except for the removal of small volumes (250 to 1,500 mL) to decrease pain and respiratory distress from abdominal distention, has traditionally been discouraged because of the risk of abdominal perforation and infection. If a large volume is removed, 15% to 100% (mean 58%) of the fluid may reaccumulate over the next 24 to 48 hours, leading to transient hypovolemia and the possibility of shock, encephalopathy, or acute renal failure.[19]

More recently, the combination of a therapeutic paracentesis with or without intravenous albumin infusion (to maintain volume in the vascular space) has become an accepted mode of therapy.[23–26] A typical regimen is the removal of 4 to 6 L per day via paracentesis, with replacement of 40 to 50 g albumin after each paracentesis (approximately 10 to 12.5 g of albumin per liter of ascites fluid removed). Paracentesis with albumin replacement is superior to diuretic therapy; it decreases ascites faster and shortens the hospital stay without significant worsening of hepatic, renal, or cardiovascular function. Single large-volume (about 5 L) paracentesis without albumin replacement also appears to be safe in patients with painful, tense ascites,[27] but repeated large-volume paracentesis without albumin replacement may result in hyponatremia or renal impairment in some patients.[24] Another possible concern is an increased risk of spontaneous bacterial peritonitis secondary to reduced ascitic fluid opsonic activity.[21] Arguments about the high cost of albumin are counterbalanced by the decreased length of hospital stay. The use of dextran as a volume expander after paracentesis has been evaluated as an alternative to albumin.[23] It has been shown to help prevent the asymptomatic abnormalities in laboratory values at a lower cost,[22] although its use remains controversial.[28,29] Albumin has also been used without paracentesis in an attempt to increase intravascular volume and induce diuresis. The drawbacks to this treatment are a short duration of response, the risk of inducing variceal hemorrhage, and high cost. Generally, treatment with albumin without paracentesis is to be avoided unless all other therapies have failed. In Europe, ascites recirculation (removal, concentration, and reinfusion of peritoneal fluid) has been found to be safe and effective.[30] The possibility of reaccumulation of ascites after paracentesis necessitates continuation of a low-sodium diet and diuretics.

The peritoneovenous (LeVeen or Denver) shunt, in use extensively for the past 20 to 25 years, was devised for use in diuretic-refractory ascites.[31,32] This type of shunt consists of a surgically implanted one-way valve in the abdominal wall, an intra-abdominal cannula, and an outflow tube tunneled subcutaneously from the valve to a vein that empties directly into the inferior vena cava. As the diaphragm descends, the pressure in the intrathoracic veins drops and intraperitoneal pressure rises. This pressure differential pushes ascitic fluid via the shunt into the venous system. The results may be dramatic, with urine output as high as 15 L occurring during the first 24 hours. Supplemental diuresis with furosemide may be needed to prevent vascular overload. However, use of this procedure is limited by such complications as fever, shunt occlusion, hypokalemia, infection, shunt leak, disseminated intravascular coagulopathy, and less often variceal hemorrhage, bowel obstruction, pulmonary edema, and pneumothorax.[31] A Veterans Administration Cooperative study involving 3,860 patients showed a lack of improvement in survival and significant morbidity rates in patients treated with a peritoneovenous shunt compared with those treated with diuretic therapy.[32] However, shunting alleviated disabling ascites more rapidly than medical management did.

A more widely accepted shunting approach is the transjugular intrahepatic portosystemic shunt (TIPS). A transjugular approach is used to place a stent within the liver that creates a low-resistance conduit between a branch of the portal vein and the hepatic vein. Blood will flow directly through the TIPS and decompress the portal venous system. Adverse effects of the TIPS include worsened hepatic encephalopathy, hepatic ischemia, and bleeding. The value of the TIPS in refractory ascites has been evaluated. In this study, the TIPS in combination with medical treatment was proven superior to medical management alone; however, the TIPS did not improve either survival or the quality of life.[33] These relatively aggressive shunting options are generally reserved for patients with ascites refractory to medical intervention.

Spontaneous Bacterial Peritonitis. Spontaneous bacterial peritonitis (SBP) is infection of the ascitic fluid in the absence of an intra-abdominal source (e.g., bowel perforation or abscess). SBP occurs in approximately 30% to 40% of cirrhotic patients.[34] Although some patients are asymptomatic, commonly observed signs and symptoms include fever, chills, vomiting, abdominal pain or tenderness, decreased bowel sounds, worsened renal function, and encephalopathy. The diagnosis of SBP is made by evaluating a small sample of the ascitic fluid. A polymorphonuclear cell count greater than 250 cells per cubic millimeter of ascitic fluid or a positive bacterial culture is diagnostic for SBP.[35,36]

SBP is thought to be the consequence of alterations in the immune defense of patients with advanced liver disease. It is believed that the gut is the main source of infecting bacteria in SBP; however, hematogenous spread from the urinary or respiratory tract or skin can occur. Bacterial translocation (passage of bacteria from the lumen of the GI tract to extraintestinal sites such as the peritoneum) is an important step in the pathogenesis of SBP. Bacterial overgrowth and bowel wall edema from portal hypertension contribute to the translocation of bacteria. Mesenteric lymph nodes and the hepatic reticuloendothelial filtering system would normally kill translocated bacteria, but in cirrhotic patients, some bacteria can escape this and reach the ascitic fluid. Defects in the local immune response such as decreased opsonization and phagocytosis by macrophages further contribute to infection of the ascitic fluid.[35]

Predisposing factors for SBP include a previous episode of SBP, the severity of underlying liver disease, GI hemorrhage, and an ascitic fluid total protein concentration of 1 g per dL or less.

Enteric gram-negative bacilli such as *Escherichia coli* and *Klebsiella pneumoniae*, and *Streptococcus pneumoniae* are the most common organisms seen with SBP. Anaerobic bacteria, *Pseudomonas* sp, *Staphylococcus* sp, and fungi are not common pathogens in SBP. Infection in SBP is usually monobacterial. If multiple species of bacteria or anaerobic bacteria are cultured, secondary bacterial peritonitis (e.g., bowel perforation) should be considered.

Empiric therapy has traditionally been ampicillin or a first-generation cephalosporin in combination with an aminoglycoside. More recently, the use of less toxic alternative agents such as ampicillin/sulbactam, ticarcillin/clavulanate, piperacillin/tazobactam, second- and third-generation cephalosporins, and quinolones have also resulted in favorable outcomes. Caution is advised with the use of cefotetan and other cephalosporins with a methylthiotetrazole (MTT) side chain, which can interfere with vitamin K and cause a hypoprothrombinemic state. Cefotaxime 2 g every 8 hours is generally accepted as the current drug of choice for SBP.[37,38] The antibiotic regimen should be tailored based upon culture and sensitivity results. Duration of therapy is approximately 5 days because of the relatively low inoculum of organisms in the ascitic fluid.[39] Administration of intravenous albumin in patients with SBP has been shown to reduce the mortality rate and decrease the incidence of renal dysfunction.

SBP is associated with significant morbidity and mortality. Recurrence of SBP is common following treatment. Long-term prophylaxis with antibiotics to prevent recurrent SBP has been evaluated in several clinical trials. Norfloxacin 400 mg once daily has been used successfully in high-risk patients. This fluoroquinolone results in a selective intestinal decontamination that decreases gram-negative bacilli but preserves the remaining normal flora. Norfloxacin has been shown to markedly reduce the incidence of SBP in patients with previous episodes of SBP.[40] Twice-daily dosing for the first 7 days of a prophylaxis regimen may be needed in patients experiencing a GI hemorrhage.[41] Other regimens such as trimethoprim/sulfamethoxazole 1 double-strength tablet daily given 5 days per week or ciprofloxacin 750 mg once a week have been shown to be effective in preventing SBP.[42,43] When a fluoroquinolone is chosen, it is important that concomitant administration with medications containing divalent and trivalent cations be avoided to minimize the drug–drug interaction.

Gastrointestinal Bleeding. Bleeding from esophageal or gastric varices is one of the most feared complications of portal hypertension. Variceal hemorrhage is a grave sign and may be difficult to stop. Mortality from a single bleeding episode is approximately 17% to 57%.[44]

Varices are portosystemic collateral veins that are dilated due to portal hypertension. Varices are present in up to 60% of patients with cirrhosis, but bleeding occurs in only about one third of patients. Factors associated with increased risk of a variceal hemorrhage include continued alcohol consumption, poor liver function, and large varices seen on endoscopy.

In the setting of an acute bleed, multiple blood transfusions and intravenous fluids may be necessary to maintain circulatory volume. Balloon tamponade, pharmacologic therapy, and endoscopic intervention are methods to stop bleeding.

Application of direct pressure with a balloon tube (Linton, Minnesota, or Sengstaken Blakemore tube) that can be inflated in the esophagus and/or stomach can slow bleeding. As the balloon is inflated, the varix is compressed between the balloon and the esophageal wall, slowing or even stopping bleeding. While bleeding is stopped in 40% to 80% of patients, it is only a temporary measure. This procedure is complicated by vomiting, a high risk of aspiration, ischemia of the esophageal mucosa, perforation, and recurrence of bleeding as soon as the balloon is deflated.

Endoscopic therapies include sclerotherapy and variceal ligation. Injection of sclerosing agents into esophageal varices has revolutionized the care of patients with bleeding varices.[45–50] This approach is considered by many to be the therapy of choice. The most commonly used sclerosing agents in the United States are sodium tetradecyl sulfate (Sotradecol), ethanolamine oleate (Ethamolin), and sodium morrhuate (Scleromate). Injection of these agents into a bleeding varix leads to an intense inflammatory response, thrombus formation, and cessation of bleeding within 2 to 5 minutes. A more permanent fibrotic obliteration of the vessel develops over several days.

Sclerotherapy controls acute variceal bleeding in 90% to 95% of patients.[45] A single treatment controls bleeding in 90% of patients; the remainder may require multiple treatments over several weeks.

Success rates are lower in actively bleeding patients than in those in whom bleeding was controlled initially by more conservative methods. Failure of therapy is defined as continuation of bleeding after two injections of a sclerosing agent during a single admission.[51] Compared with portacaval and splenorenal shunt procedures, sclerotherapy is almost equally effective in stopping bleeding, there is no difference in survival, and there is much lower morbidity.[47,48] Prophylactic sclerotherapy in patients with endoscopic evidence of varices but no history of past or current bleeding is of no clinical benefit.[49,50]

A 0.5% to 3% solution of tetradecyl sulfate or a premixed solution of ethanolamine 5% or morrhuate 5% for injection is used. After the endoscope is passed, approximately 0.5 to 2 mL of the sclerosing solution is injected into each varix at points about 2 to 4 cm apart. If bleeding recurs, therapy can be repeated. Although it appears that sclerotherapy is effective in stopping acute bleeding and preventing rebleeding, more than 50% of patients will rebleed, and the long-term mortality is not lower than with conventional therapy. Side effects associated with sclerotherapy include pericardi-

tis, chest pain, dysphagia, pyrexia, cardiac tamponade, formation of esophagobronchial or tracheoesophageal fistulas, and local ulcerations.

Following sclerotherapy, prophylaxis with antacids, histamine-2 (H2) antagonists, proton pump inhibitors, or sucralfate may be initiated. Dosing of these drugs is the same as that recommended for treating peptic ulcer disease or reflux esophagitis (see Chapter 45). Careful monitoring of mental status in those who are treated with cimetidine is warranted because cirrhosis may predispose patients to the mental confusion associated with this agent.[52] With the available acid-suppressing alternatives, one could make an argument for avoiding cimetidine altogether in this setting. The pharmacokinetics of ranitidine may also be altered in cirrhosis, resulting in its accumulation.[53] Sucralfate suspension has been used to prevent ulcers at the sclerosis site. Investigators using endoscopy have shown that the drug complex seems to coat the varices, decreasing ulcer formation.[54] The aluminum component of sucralfate may complex with coadministered norfloxacin or ciprofloxacin, resulting in poor absorption. The importance of divalent and trivalent cations complexing with quinolones could be questioned in SBP prophylaxis because of local intestinal rather than systemic action. However, because the complex does not enter bacteria as well,[55] it is prudent to space the administration of these agents even with SBP prophylaxis.

A newer endoscopic technique for control of variceal bleeds is endoscopic variceal banding therapy or ligation. The success rate of this procedure may be as high as 90%.[56] The procedure involves the endoscopic placement of a small rubber band over a distal varix. A large varix is drawn by suction aspiration into the end portion of the sleeve, and the rubber band is released over the base of the varix. A specially modified endoscope that carries a triggering device and rubber band on a small sleeve over the objective end of the scope is required. Endoscopic variceal banding therapy has a control rate of 86% for acute bleeding. It has also been associated with a lower complication rate, although the risk of rebleeding may be slightly higher than with sclerotherapy.[57,58]

Historically, the hormone vasopressin (ADH) was used to treat bleeding varices before the advent of sclerotherapy and octreotide. Vasopressin decreases portal blood flow and pressure by constricting portal and other splanchnic arterioles. This slows or stops bleeding long enough to allow thrombus formation at the site of bleeding in 60% to 80% of patients. The use of this drug is declining and it remains controversial because the benefits in terms of morbidity and mortality have never been proven.[59] Sclerotherapy has been shown consistently to be more effective than vasopressin, but vasopressin may be given first to slow bleeding and facilitate endoscopic visualization of the bleeding varix.

The major limitation to vasopressin therapy is its side effects. The intense vasoconstriction decreases cardiac output and may cause coronary ischemia. This is especially problematic in patients with coronary artery disease or hypertension; however, ischemic changes have also been reported in patients with no prior evidence of ischemic disease. Bradycardia caused by stimulation of the vagus nerve is the most widely observed side effect of vasopressin. It may also produce skin blanching, GI cramping, and even bowel necrosis. Women may experience uterine pain similar to menstrual cramps. Finally, vasopressin may lead to excess water retention and a dilutional hyponatremia.[59]

A continuous intravenous infusion starting at 0.2 to 0.4 units per minute and direct intra-arterial infusion via a catheter into the superior mesenteric artery at 0.05 to 0.4 units per minute have been tried. The maximum recommended intravenous infusion rate is 0.9 units per minute. Infusions may be continued for up to 72 hours, with a slow tapering of the dose over time. The results have been varied, with some authors claiming up to 50% to 70% effectiveness.[59] Others claim poor response and a high incidence of complications, including bleeding from the site of catheter insertion and septicemia.[60]

A combination of vasopressin infusion and intravenous nitroglycerin (10 to 50 μg per minute titrated according to blood pressure to a maximum of 400 μg per minute)[61] or sublingual nitroglycerin (0.6 mg every 30 minutes for 6 hours)[62] may cause an additional decrease in portal pressure. In the study using intravenous nitroglycerin, there was less bleeding with combination therapy; in the trial with sublingual nitroglycerin, the rate of bleeding cessation was equal to that with vasopressin alone. In both studies, combination therapy led to a marked reduction in cardiac complications.

Somatostatin and its analogue, octreotide, have also been evaluated in controlling variceal bleeding. Somatostatin reduces portal pressure and blood flow after a bolus dose followed by continuous intravenous administration. It offers efficacy equal to that of vasopressin, with considerably fewer side effects.[63] Its use is limited only by its higher acquisition cost.[47,64] Somatostatin dosing consists of a 250-μg bolus followed by an infusion of 250 μg per hour. The equally effective somatostatin analogue, octreotide, is dosed with a 50-μg bolus and continued as an infusion at a rate of 50 μg per hour for 5 days. Octreotide is considered the agent of choice in the management of acute variceal bleeding used alone and with endoscopic sclerotherapy or banding.[65,66]

Bleeding from other GI sites, especially bleeding caused by gastritis and peptic ulcer, usually is treated with nasogastric suction, H_2 receptor antagonists, or proton pump inhibitors or hourly antacids.[67] Occasionally, 20 units of vasopressin, 1 to 2 (4 to 8 mg) ampules of norepinephrine, or ice is used in a gastric lavage to cause localized vasoconstriction in an attempt to slow bleeding. No evidence documents these latter maneuvers to be any more effective than tap water lavage or acid suppression alone; therefore, their use is generally discouraged.

It has been suggested that because propranolol, nadolol, and possibly other nonselective β-adrenergic blockers decrease portal venous pressure, they may prevent GI bleeding associated with portal hypertension.[68–73] Primary prophy-

laxis is defined as treatment of patients with known varices but without a history of active bleeding. Secondary prophylaxis involves administering the drug after resolution of an acute bleeding episode to prevent subsequent bleeding. Although data are limited, overall analysis of the benefit of primary therapy is positive.[68–70] For example, in the European Cooperative study group, after a median dose of 160 mg per day (range 40 to 320 mg), 74% of patients in the propranolol group were free of bleeding after 2 years, compared with 39% in the placebo group. Two-year survival was 72% in the treated patients and 37% in the untreated subjects.[70] Propranolol also appears to be a cost-effective approach, with savings between $450 and $14,600 over 5 years in 1997 dollars.[71]

The results for secondary prophylaxis are also encouraging but somewhat more complex. Lebrec et al[72] showed that oral propranolol in doses that reduced the heart rate by 25% to a resting rate of 50 to 60 beats per minute led to a significantly lower frequency of rebleeding than did placebo, during a 2-year study in chronic alcoholic patients with a history of esophageal bleeding. Only 21% of patients in the propranolol group had recurrence of bleeding, compared to 68% in the placebo group. Cumulative survival was 90% in the propranolol group and 57% in the placebo group. None of the patients showed deterioration of hepatic or renal function while taking propranolol. Because propranolol may decrease cardiac output and liver blood flow, patients should be monitored closely.

A similar study by Burroughs et al[73] failed to confirm the findings of Lebrec. However, the patients in Burroughs et al's study had more severe liver disease and some had cirrhosis from causes other than chronic alcoholism. Selective β-blockade with atenolol or metoprolol appears to be less effective than sclerotherapy in arresting acute variceal bleeding.[68,69]

A follow-up study by Poynard et al[74] confirmed the benefits of propranolol, with 71% of subjects free of bleeding at 1 year and 57% at 2 years. In this study, five factors were identified that increased the risk of rebleeding: hepatocellular carcinoma, continued alcohol abuse, lack of suppression of pulse rate by propranolol, a history of rebleeding, and noncompliance with drug therapy. Of particular concern, 12 of 14 (86%) patients who discontinued β-blocker therapy abruptly had an episode of rebleeding. The time of greatest risk for rebleeding is within the first 3 to 4 days after stopping therapy, but it may occur up to 150 days later.[68,69,74–76] It is not possible to be certain that drug discontinuation is responsible for rebleeding in the delayed rebleeding cases.

A randomized controlled study by Teres et al[77] in Barcelona compared sclerotherapy with propranolol in the prevention of rebleeding for varices. Although the incidence of rebleeding was less with sclerotherapy (26 of 58 subjects) than with propranolol (37 of 58 subjects) titrated to reduce the resting heart rate by 25%, complications were significantly more common and of greater severity with sclerotherapy. The authors could not recommend either approach on the basis of the study findings.

Another published trial compared isosorbide-5-mononitrate with propranolol in long-term follow-up (128 patients followed up over 7 years). Isosorbide-5-mononitrate was as effective as propranolol in reducing mortality.[78] Additional perspective on this approach was offered in an accompanying editorial.[79] However, at least one trial comparing isosorbide mononitrate to nadolol showed a greater risk of bleeding with the nitrate.[80] Currently, β-blockade alone seems more established and safer than nitrates when used alone or when combined with β-blockade. Because patients with cirrhosis often have a low blood pressure, β-blockers should always be used with extreme caution.

Surgical treatment may be needed for patients who have repeated GI bleeding (especially esophageal varices) or those who have bleeding that cannot be stopped by the more conservative measures already described.[45] A portacaval shunt involves anastomosis of the portal vein directly to the inferior vena cava, thus bypassing the cirrhotic liver. This surgical procedure decreases portal hypertension. Unfortunately, these patients often have a poor prognosis because the blood that normally flows to the liver for detoxification and metabolism is now shunted away from the liver. If they survive the initial surgery, patients may die of sepsis or develop hepatic failure and encephalopathy. The Warren (distal splenorenal) shunt decompresses the varices by shunting splenic blood flow to the renal vein and does not alter hepatic perfusion as much. The TIPS procedure also effectively decompresses the portal system and is an option in the treatment of and prevention of variceal bleeding.

Hepatic Encephalopathy. Clinical manifestations of hepatic encephalopathy should be recognized and addressed promptly, because most are reversible with appropriate therapy.[81] If the patient exhibits signs of hepatic encephalopathy (e.g., confusion, drowsiness, asterixis), lactulose is indicated, as well as dietary protein restriction to approximately 0.8 to 1 g per kilogram per day. Use of CNS depressants (e.g., benzodiazepines, narcotics) should be minimized or avoided; this is especially true of benzodiazepines. Except for cautious use of spironolactone or furosemide, diuretics usually should be withheld at this stage because hypovolemia, hypokalemia, and metabolic alkalosis may aggravate encephalopathy.

Lactulose is a synthetic disaccharide of galactose and fructose that is neither absorbed nor hydrolyzed in the small bowel. It is degraded by colonic bacteria to lactic, acetic, and formic acid, thus lowering the pH of the colonic contents. The effect of lactulose was originally attributed to replacement of proteolytic bacteria such as *E. coli*, *Proteus*, and *Bacteroides* with organisms such as *Lactobacillus* that thrive in a more acidic medium and lack urease and other enzymes that are used in the production of ammonia. However, most investigators have not found a marked change in the colonic flora and have attributed the effects of lactulose solely to the change in pH of the colonic contents. As the colon becomes more acidic, this favors the conversion from

ammonia to ammonium. Ammonium is a charged particle and is not absorbed. There may also be back-diffusion of ammonia from the blood to the intestinal lumen under acidic pH conditions. Regardless of which mechanisms are in effect, lactulose therapy results in a decrease in arterial ammonia levels.[82]

Each 15 mL of lactulose oral liquid contains 10 g lactulose; it is usually given in a dose of 30 to 40 mL three or four times daily (approximately 45 to 90 g per day). Retention enemas of 300 mL of lactulose syrup diluted with 700 mL of tap water can also be used.[83] The onset of effect by either route is 12 to 48 hours, with an endpoint of two or three loose stools daily and an improvement in mental capacity. The success rate with lactulose has been reported to be around 85%. Patient tolerance can be improved by diluting the drug in water, fruit juice, or carbonated beverages. Patients may require prolonged therapy to prevent recurrence of symptoms.

The most common complaints of patients treated with lactulose are nausea (because of the sweet taste of the drug), gaseous distention, bloating, belching, or diarrhea caused by osmotic effects in the bowel. Diarrhea may account for part of the therapeutic effects of lactulose by flushing out toxins,[84] but compared with sorbitol, lactulose is more effective in treating the encephalopathy, indicating that other mechanisms are working such as decreasing ammonia levels. Excessive diarrhea may lead to dehydration and electrolyte abnormalities such as hypernatremia. Patients should be closely monitored during lactulose therapy to avoid these fluid and electrolyte abnormalities.

Neomycin, an alternative to lactulose, is an aminoglycoside antibiotic that kills the urease-producing bacteria in the colon, thus reducing the production of intestinal ammonia. Neomycin is given at a dose of 1 to 2 g four times a day. When the patient improves, the dose may be lowered to 2 to 4 g per day. For patients who cannot take medications orally, a retention enema of 2 to 4 g in 200 mL of saline thickened with methylcellulose may be used twice a day.

One well-controlled study failed to show a clear superiority of neomycin (83% effective) or lactulose (90% effective) in treating acute encephalopathy. For long-term use, lactulose has the potential advantage of less toxicity, but it is considerably more expensive.[85] The possibility that sterilization of the gut by neomycin might decrease the effectiveness of lactulose appears to be of minimal consequence;[86] in fact, the two drugs are more effective when used together.[87]

Even though neomycin is not well absorbed from the GI tract, approximately 1% to 3% of a dose is absorbed.[79] Neomycin can cause nephrotoxicity and ototoxicity in patients on chronic therapy.[88,89] Most of these patients had been taking neomycin for at least 8 months and had coexisting renal dysfunction. An auditory test should be performed at baseline and annually to assess for hearing impairment.

Other oral antibiotics that have been evaluated with some success include metronidazole, vancomycin, and rifaximin, a derivative of rifamycin.[81]

There are multiple approaches to the management of hepatic encephalopathy. Avoiding the use of drugs that can alter sensorium is of paramount importance. Lactulose is typically the drug of choice. Neomycin or rifaximin are alternatives for patients who are intolerant to lactulose or in whom the effects of lactulose are waning. Dietary interventions such as protein restriction and avoiding large protein loads are also useful.

Therapeutic Value of γ-Aminobutyric Acid Antagonists.
Some investigators believe that endogenous or exogenous GABAergic-like compounds that stimulate the GABA–benzodiazepine receptor complex in the brain may be responsible for symptoms of encephalopathy.[17,90] Preliminary data suggest that the benzodiazepine antagonist flumazenil may be valuable in both short-term and long-term management of hepatic encephalopathy.

In 14 subjects, 71% showed short-term improvement in symptoms after intravenous administration of flumazenil.[91] Arousal was greatest in patients with deeper coma (stage III or IV encephalopathy). Although response was rapid, the duration of effect was only 1 to 2 hours. The usual dose was 0.2 to 0.4 mg, with some subjects receiving up to 10 doses.

A single case report describes the long-term use of oral therapy.[92] A patient given 25 mg twice daily experienced complete reversal of symptoms for 14 months. Previously, this patient had experienced 12 episodes of coma over a 2-year period. Discontinuation of the drug led to a recurrence of symptoms within 48 hours.

A randomized double-blind placebo-controlled crossover trial from Canada showed a significant clinical improvement in 5 of 11 (45%) patients with hepatic coma receiving flumazenil in the initial treatment phase and 1 of 2 (50%) in the crossover phase of the study. The authors concluded that the agent is efficacious and safe for reversing neurologic symptoms in cirrhotic patients with hepatic coma.[93] This trial has been criticized.[94] A recent analysis of this approach has also shown efficacy, but it is short-lived and not associated with mortality reduction. Thus, the use of a benzodiazepine receptor antagonist in these patients remains investigational and controversial[95] and is not the standard of care.

Therapeutic Value of Corticosteroids. Cirrhotic patients with biopsy-proven alcoholic hepatitis may benefit from the anti-inflammatory effects of corticosteroid therapy. The beneficial effect may be related to the corticosteroid's inhibition of cytokine production.

The efficacy of steroids in treating liver disease remains controversial. Clinical trials have shown conflicting results with regard to mortality. A meta-analysis of the randomized trials was completed to determine the efficacy of steroids on short-term mortality in patients with alcoholic hepatitis. The combined data indicated that steroids provide a protective efficacy of 27% in patients with hepatic encephalopathy. This figure increased in patients without active GI bleeding. Among subjects without hepatic encephalopathy, steroids had no protective efficacy. These data suggest that only patients with severe disease would benefit from steroid therapy. Patients with severe disease are defined as those with hepatic encephalopathy or a discriminant function higher than 32 [discriminant function = 4.6 (Patient's prothrombin time − control prothrombin time) + bilirubin]. Patients with severe disease who have active GI bleeding or need treatment for active infection should be excluded from steroid therapy.[96]

Prednisolone is the most studied and appears to be the preferred corticosteroid. The typical dosing regimen is 40 mg per day for 4 weeks and is then tapered over 2 to 4 weeks.[97] Overall, the available data on this subject are less than consistent in their conclusions and outcomes. The American College of Gastroenterology consensus position on steroid use in hepatitis related to alcohol was recently published.[98]

Hepatorenal Syndrome

Therapeutic Value of Vasoactive Agents. HRS is the development of renal failure in patients with cirrhosis. Dopamine and norepinephrine are important neurotransmitters in the CNS, the periphery, and the kidneys. Some of the neurologic manifestations of hepatic failure, and HRS, may be caused by accumulation of other γ-hydroxylated phenylethylamines such as octopamine and serotonin. These compounds may replace normal transmitters and act as false neurotransmitters in sympathetic nerve terminals. Precursors of false neurotransmitters, such as phenylalanine and tyrosine (Fig. 50.2), are produced from protein in the gut by bacterial amino acid decarboxylases. Normally, these precursors are metabolized rapidly in the liver by monoamine oxidase, allowing norepinephrine that is formed elsewhere in the body to predominate. When hepatic function is impaired or when blood is shunted away from the liver, these false neurotransmitters may replace normal transmitters. Systemically, this may lead to lowered peripheral vascular resistance and shunting of blood away from the kidney. Similarly, asterixis and other signs of hepatic encephalopathy might result from displacement of transmitters such as dopamine and norepinephrine in the basal ganglia and other areas in the brain.

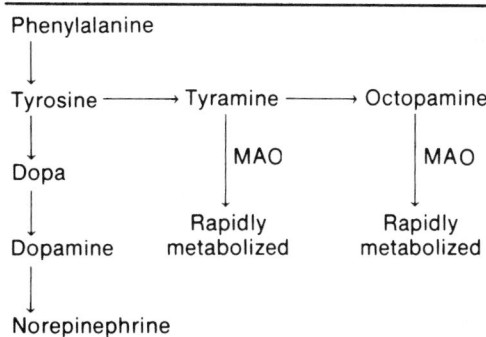

FIGURE 50.2 Synthetic pathway of neurotransmitters. Monoamine oxidase (MAO) action occurs mainly in the liver and is depressed in hepatic disease and shunting.

If the displacement of normal central and peripheral transmitters by less active amines can account for hepatic coma and its cardiovascular complications, then the restoration of normal transmitter stores might restore normal function. For hospitalized patients, this is accomplished with low-dose infusions of dopamine at 1.3 to 5 μg per kilogram per minute.[99] This may increase renal blood flow and help to reverse HRS. Failure to improve urine output or increase blood pressure within the first 24 hours of dopamine treatment is a poor prognostic sign. Because dopamine does not cross the blood–brain barrier, encephalopathy will not improve. However, as shown in Figure 50.2, dopamine is also a precursor to norepinephrine, which may help to restore natural neurotransmitter balance.

Use of the alpha agonist midodrine in combination with octreotide has also shown efficacy in reducing mortality in HRS.[100] Although not universally effective, this combination is becoming established as a trial modality to offer patients with this often fatal complication. There is no structural abnormality of the kidneys in HRS; rather, it is most likely due to humoral imbalances from liver failure. HRS is associated with a mortality rate that approaches 100%. While many therapeutic methods have been tried to improve renal function, most have either a minor or a temporary effect, with the exception of liver transplantation.

Pharmacotherapy of Primary Biliary Cirrhosis. Colchicine, a drug with both anti-inflammatory and antifibrotic properties, has been evaluated as a potential disease-modifying agent. In one study, 57 patients with biopsy-proven PBC were treated with 0.6 mg colchicine twice daily or placebo.[101] The colchicine-treated patients had a significant improvement in biochemical parameters (serum bilirubin and aminotransferase levels) but no difference in histologic progression when compared to placebo. A second group of investigators conducted a randomized, double-blind, placebo-controlled trial of colchicine, 1 mg per day, 5 days per week, in 100 patients with cirrhosis caused by alcohol abuse or a history of hepatitis.[102] Median survival was 3.5 years in the placebo group and 11 years in the colchicine-treated patients, while deaths from liver failure were 24% in the placebo group and 15% in the treatment group. Side effects in both trials were mild, consisting primarily of nausea, abdominal pain, and diarrhea. Although these results are encouraging, flaws in the study design and the small number of subjects treated prevent widespread endorsement of colchicine therapy at this time.

Numerous other drugs have been tried in treating PBC, including penicillamine, chlorambucil, azathioprine, cyclosporine, corticosteroids, and methotrexate.[103] Each of these therapies is based on the hope that anti-inflammatory or immunomodulating effects may alter the disease process. Cyclosporine showed modest improvement in symptoms, enzyme levels, and histologic findings in a controlled trial of PBC. However, toxicity with this drug is a limiting factor in therapy. Sequestration of copper by penicillamine may have a therapeutic effect, but most of the trials with these drugs have been limited by a small sample size without adequate controls, and the improvement obtained has been only marginal. At this time, none of these drugs can be recommended.

A controlled, multicenter trial with ursodeoxycholic acid also showed improvement in symptoms, enzyme levels, and histologic findings in some patients, but there was little effect in patients with advanced disease.[104] Ursodiol may be effective in slowing the progression of PBC and may decrease the need for transplantation.[105] Ursodiol (ursodeoxycholic acid) is a naturally occurring bile acid with choleretic properties. The dose of ursodiol in the treatment of PBC is 13 to 15 mg per kilogram per day given in four divided doses.

NONPHARMACOLOGIC THERAPY

It is imperative to provide adequate nutritional support in patients with liver disease. Positive nitrogen balance must be established without exacerbating hepatic encephalopathy. Diets high in BCAAs and low in AAAs and methionine may help to restore normal amino acid balance and reduce encephalopathy.[13–15,106] HepatAmine is an 8% amino acid solution that contains more BCAAs than standard parenteral amino acid solutions. The ratio of BCAAs to AAAs in HepatAmine is 37:1, compared to 5:1 with crystalline amino acid solutions. The indications for use and the efficacy of this special amino acid formulation are debated. The expense and questionable efficacy have limited its use to select patients with life-threatening encephalopathy refractory to conventional therapy. An amino acid screen can be used to assess the BCAA:AAA ratio in patients. The cost of an amino acid screen is approximately equal to 1 day's therapy with HepatAmine.

For the awake patient without central venous access, therapy with enteral nutrition is preferred. One such dietary supplement is Nutrihep, a calorically dense product with a high calorie to nitrogen ratio that helps maintain protein utilization for lean muscle mass in liver disease. This product provides a 50:50 ratio of aromatic and branch amino acids. Use of oral BCAAs has been limited because of its questionable efficacy, its expense, and its disagreeable taste. The American Society of Parenteral and Enteral Nutrition (ASPEN) has published guidelines for nutritional supplementation in patients with liver disease.[107] Growth hormone resistance has also been associated with the protein catabolic state seen in cirrhosis. From the limited data available, it appears that treatment with growth hormone can improve nitrogen utilization.[108] In addition, because *Helicobacter pylori* has strong urease activity, there is evidence that supports treatment. If present, *H. pylori* eradication can reduce hyperammonemia.[109]

ALTERNATIVE THERAPY

The use of herbal supplements and other alternative remedies have become popular in patients with liver disease. The naturally occurring whole extract of the milk thistle (*Silybum marianum*) is known as silymarin. This flavonoid complex has been shown to have a liver-protective effect in experimental models of hepatotoxicity from acetaminophen, ethanol, carbon tetrachloride, and phenylhydrazine. Use of silymarin has been popularized by the lay press and internet sources, with some scientific validation of efficacy. Silymarin has been found to prevent lipid peroxidation, changes in the phospholipid composition of membranes, and hepatic glutathione depletion. It also appears to normalize hepatic function markers in patients with alcoholic liver disease. This positive effect may be attributed to an isomer of the silymarin complex, silibinin, on inhibiting leukotriene formation by Kupffer cells.[110] There is the potential for silymarin to inhibit the activity of cytochrome P-450 3A4 (CYP3A4) and P-glycoprotein. Studies have confirmed this inhibitory effect, but the clinical significance has yet to be conclusively shown.[111,112] Caution is thus advised when it is used with any drugs that are substrates for CYP3A4 or P-glycoprotein.

Zinc deficiency is observed in patients with chronic liver disease, and zinc sulfate is often given to reverse this deficiency. Zinc may also improve dysgeusia and thus improve appetite. Zinc supplementation has also been suggested to improve cirrhosis-related hepatic encephalopathy, but outcomes data are inconclusive.[113]

IMPROVING OUTCOMES

The outcome for patients with cirrhosis depends on the stage of disease and the presence of complications. Once the diagnosis of liver disease has been established, consumption of alcohol should stop. If the patient continues to drink alcohol, the prognosis is poor. Adherence to a low-sodium, protein-restricted diet is important in minimizing the formation of ascites and maintaining adequate nitrogen balance. Compliance with the prescribed medical regimen is critical in the management of the complications arising from cirrhosis. A multidisciplinary approach can improve the outcome of this complex disease. It is also important to develop a rapport with family members and other caregivers to ensure their support of the treatment plan and lessen the risk of noncompliance and recidivism.

PROGNOSIS

In a series of 1,155 patients with cirrhosis from a variety of causes, the over-5-year survival was about 40%.[114] The causes of death were liver failure in 49%, hepatocellular carcinoma in 22%, bleeding in 14%, HRS in 8%, and other causes. Patients who entered the study with compensated cirrhosis (absent or mild symptoms) became symptomatic at a rate of 10% per year. Survival was higher in this group of patients (54% at 6 years). Patients who entered the study

with symptoms already present (ascites, history of bleeding, or encephalopathy) had a survival of only 21% at 6 years and a much higher incidence of hepatocellular carcinoma. The severity of disease can be classified according to various systems. The Child-Pugh score and the Model for Endstage Liver Disease (MELD) score can be used to assess surgical risk and short- and long-term mortality in patients with cirrhosis.[115–118] Given the irreversible nature of cirrhosis and the high morbidity and mortality, liver transplantation may be an option for select patients with end-stage liver disease.

PHARMACOECONOMICS

The management of cirrhosis can have a major economic impact, primarily because of the chronicity and progressive nature of the disease. Patients who do not abstain from alcohol and do not adhere to their diet and drug therapy can be expected to have multiple hospital admissions as the disease progresses. Management of patients with end-stage liver disease is expensive. The preventive approaches discussed in this chapter, such as SBP prophylaxis, diuretics, treatment of hepatic encephalopathy, vitamin supplementation, and dietary modification, are cost-effective and must be implemented early in the care plan.

KEY POINTS

- In the United States, cirrhosis is the 12th most common cause of death in people over age 40
- Despite extensive investigation, no effective drug therapy has been found to reverse cirrhosis
- Discontinuation of alcohol intake in patients with proven cirrhosis is of the utmost importance. Use of naltrexone in an effort to decrease craving may prove valuable in this setting[119]
- Although therapy for cirrhosis focuses mainly on symptom management, other forms of chronic liver disease, such as viral hepatitis and autoimmune hepatitis, can be successfully treated
- Portal hypertension, a complication of cirrhosis, can manifest as ascites, hepatic encephalopathy, esophageal varices, and hepatorenal syndrome
- Although the fibrosis from advanced cirrhosis is irreversible, it is estimated that 70% or more of liver tissue must be destroyed before the body is unable to eliminate drugs and toxins via the liver.[120] Unfortunately, it is difficult to tell which patients have reached this stage of involvement. Practitioners should always be aware of the potential inability of patients with advanced liver disease to metabolize various drugs normally cleared by the liver, and should adjust doses accordingly
- Limited pharmacokinetic dosing research and guidance are available for the aging liver and the diseased

liver.[121,122] Dose reductions continue to be made empirically because data quantifying the degree of adjustment necessary in liver disease generally are unavailable

SUGGESTED READINGS

Carithers RL Jr. Liver transplantation. Liver Transplant 6:122–135, 2000.

Gerber T, Schomerus H. Hepatic encephalopathy in liver cirrhosis: pathogenesis, diagnosis and management. Drugs 60:1353–1370, 2000.

Gines P, Arroyo V. Hepatorenal syndrome. J Am Soc Nephrol 10: 1833–1839, 1999.

Mowat C, Stanley AJ. Spontaneous bacterial peritonitis: diagnosis, treatment and prevention. Aliment Pharmacol Ther 15:1851–1859, 2001.

Runyon BA. AASLD Practice guideline: management of adult patients with ascites due to cirrhosis. Hepatology 39:1–16, 2004.

Sharara AI, Rockey DC. Gastroesophageal variceal hemorrhage. N Engl J Med 345:669–681, 2001.

REFERENCES

1. Trends in mortality from cirrhosis and alcoholism: United States. MMWR 35:703–705, 1983.
2. World Health Statistics Annual. Geneva: World Health Organization, 1985.
3. Deaths and hospitalizations from chronic liver disease: United States. MMWR 41:969–973, 1993.
4. http://www.CDC.gov/nchs/fastats/liverdis.htm. Accessed Sept. 24, 2004.
5. Cotran R, Kumar V, Robbins S. Pathological Basis of Disease. 4th ed. Philadelphia: WB Saunders, 1989:941–957.
6. Sloan K, Straits-Troster K, Dominitz JA, et al. Hepatitis C tested prevalence and comorbidities among veterans in the US Northwest. J Clin Gastroenterol 38:279–284, 2004.
7. Rubin E, Lieber C. Fatty liver, alcoholic hepatitis, and cirrhosis produced by alcohol in primates. N Engl J Med 290:128, 1974.
8. Schrier R, Arroyo V, Bernardi M, et al. Peripheral arterial vasodilation hypothesis: a proposal for the initiation of renal sodium and water retention in cirrhosis. Hepatology 8:1151–1157, 1988.
9. Rocco V, Ware A. Cirrhotic ascites: pathophysiology, diagnosis, and management. Ann Intern Med 105:573–585, 1986.
10. Porayko M, Wiesner R. Management of ascites in patients with cirrhosis. Postgrad Med 92:156, 1992.
11. Wood LJ, Massie D, McLean AJ, et al. Renal sodium retention in cirrhosis: tubular site and relation to hepatic dysfunction. Hepatology 8:831, 1988.
12. Runyon B, Montano A, Akriviadis E, et al. The serum ascites albumin gradient in the differential diagnosis of ascites is superior to the exudate transudate concept. Ann Intern Med 117:215, 1992.
13. Fraser C, Arieff A. Hepatic encephalopathy. N Engl J Med 313: 869–873, 1985.
14. Bode J, Shafer K. Pathophysiology of chronic hepatic encephalopathy. Hepatogastroenterology 32:259–265, 1985.
15. Sax H, Talamini M, Fischer J. Clinical use of branched-chain amino acids in liver disease, sepsis, trauma and burns. Arch Surg 121:358–366, 1986.
16. Horst D, Grace N, Conn HO, et al. Comparison of dietary protein with an oral branched chain-enriched amino acid supplement in chronic portal-systemic encephalopathy: a randomized controlled trial. Hepatology 4:279–287, 1984.
17. Basile A, Gammal S. Evidence for the involvement of benzodiazepine receptor complex in hepatic encephalopathy; implications for treatment with benzodiazepine receptor antagonists. Clin Neuropharmacol 11:401–422, 1988.
18. Badalamenti S, Graziani G, Salerno F, et al. Hepatorenal syndrome: new perspectives in pathogenesis and treatment. Arch Intern Med 153:1957–1967, 1993.
19. Shear L, Ching S, Gabuzda G. Compartmentalization of ascites and edema in patients with hepatic cirrhosis. N Engl J Med 282: 1391–1396, 1970.
20. Pockros P, Reynolds T. Rapid diuresis in patients with ascites from chronic liver disease: the importance of peripheral edema. Gastroenterology 90:1827–1833, 1986.
21. Runyon B. Care of patients with ascites. N Engl J Med 330: 337–342, 1994.
22. Daskalopoulos G, Laffi G, Morgan T, et al. Immediate effects of furosemide on renal hemodynamics in chronic liver disease with ascites. Gastroenterology 92:1859, 1987.
23. Gines P, Arroyo V, Quintero E, et al. Comparison of paracentesis and diuretics in the treatment of cirrhotics with tense ascites; results of a randomized study. Gastroenterology 93:234–241, 1987.
24. Gines P, Tito L, Arroyo V, et al. Randomized comparative study of therapeutic paracentesis with and without intravenous albumin in cirrhosis. Gastroenterology 94:1493–1502, 1988.
25. Panos MZ, Moore K, Vlavianos P, et al. Single, total paracentesis for tense ascites: sequential hemodynamic changes and right atrial size. Hepatology 11:662, 1990.
26. Tito LI, Gines P, Arroyo V, et al. Total paracentesis associated with intravenous albumin in the management of patients with cirrhosis and ascites. Gastroenterology 98:146, 1990.
27. Pinto P, Amerian J, Reynolds T. Large-volume paracentesis in nonedematous patients with tense ascites: its effect on intravascular volume. Hepatology 8:207–210, 1988.
28. Runyon B, Antillon M, Montano A. Effect of diuresis versus therapeutic paracentesis on ascitic fluid opsonic activity and serum complement. Gastroenterology 97:158–162, 1989.
29. Vermelulen LC, Ratko TA, Erstad BL, et al for the UHC Consensus Exercise on the Use of Albumin, Nonprotein Colloid and Crystalloid Solutions. A paradigm for consensus: the University Hospital Consortium guidelines for the use of albumin, nonprotein colloid and crystalloid solutions. Arch Intern Med 155:373–379, 1995.
30. Smart H, Triger D. A randomised prospective trial comparing daily paracentesis and intravenous albumin with recirculation in diuretic refractory ascites. J Hepatol 10:191–197, 1990.
31. Epstein M. Peritoneovenous shunt in the management of ascites and the hepatorenal syndrome. Gastroenterology 82:790–799, 1980.
32. Stanley M, Ochi S, Lee K, et al. Peritoneovenous shunting as compared with medical treatment in patients with alcoholic cirrhosis and massive ascites. N Engl J Med 321:1632–1638, 1989.
33. Sanyal A, Genning C, et al. The North American Study for the Treatment of Refractory Ascites. Gastroenterology 124:634–641, 2003.
34. Gines P, Arrovo V, Rodes J. Pharmacotherapy of ascites associated with cirrhosis. Drugs 43:325, 1992.
35. Conn H, Fessell JM. Spontaneous bacterial peritonitis in cirrhosis: variations on a theme. Medicine 50:161, 1991.
36. Friedman SL. Cirrhosis of the liver and its major sequelae. In: Cecil Textbook of Medicine. 20th ed. Philadelphia: WB Saunders, 1996:795.
37. Ariza J, Xiol X, Esteve M, et al. Aztreonam versus cefotaxime in the treatment of gram-negative spontaneous bacterial peritonitis in cirrhotic patients. Hepatology 14:91–98, 1991.
38. Felisart J, Rimola A, Arroyo V, et al. Cefotaxime is more effective than is ampicillin-tobramycin in cirrhotics with severe infections. Hepatology 5:457–462, 1985.
39. Fong TL, Akriviadis EA, Runyon BA, et al. Polymorphonuclear cell count response and duration of antibiotic therapy in spontaneous bacterial peritonitis. Hepatology 9:423–426, 1989.
40. Gines P, Rimola A, Planas R, et al. Norfloxacin prevents spontaneous bacterial peritonitis recurrence in cirrhosis: results of a double-blind, placebo-controlled trial. Hepatology 12:716–724, 1990.
41. Soriano G, Guarner C, Tomas A, et al. Norfloxacin prevents bacterial infection in cirrhotics with gastrointestinal hemorrhage. Gastroenterology 103:477, 1991.
42. Singh N, Gayowski T, Yu VL, et al. Trimethoprim-sulfamethoxazole for the prevention of spontaneous bacterial peritonitis in cirrhosis: a randomized trial. Ann Intern Med 122:595–598, 1995.
43. Rolachon A, Cordier L, Bacq Y, et al. Ciprofloxacin and long-term prevention of spontaneous bacterial peritonitis: results of a prospective controlled trial. Hepatology 22:1171–1174, 1995.

44. Zaman A. Current management of esophageal varies. Curr Treat Options Gastroenterol 6:499–507, 2003.

45. Terblanche J, Burroughs A, Hobbs K. Controversies in the management of bleeding esophageal varices. N Engl J Med (part 1) 320: 1393–1397, 1989; (part 2) 320:1469–1475, 1989.

46. Cello J, Crass R, Grendell J, et al. Management of the patient with hemorrhaging esophageal varices. JAMA 256:1480–1484, 1986.

47. Rice T. Treatment of esophageal varices. Clin Pharm 8:122–131, 1989.

48. Henderson J, Kutner M, Millikan W, et al. Endoscopic variceal sclerosis compared with distal splenorenal shunt to prevent recurrent variceal bleeding in cirrhosis. Ann Intern Med 112:262–269, 1990.

49. Santangelo W, Dueno M, Estes B, et al. Prophylactic sclerotherapy of large esophageal varices. N Engl J Med 318:214–216, 1988.

50. Sauerbruch T, Wotzka R, Kopcke W, et al. Prophylactic sclerotherapy before the first episode of variceal hemorrhage in patients with cirrhosis. N Engl J Med 319:8–15, 1988.

51. Goff J. Gastroesophageal varices: pathogenesis and therapy of acute bleeding. Gastroenterol Clin North Am 22:779, 1993.

52. Ziemniak J, Bernhard H, Schentag J. Hepatic encephalopathy and altered cimetidine kinetics. Clin Pharmacol Ther 34:375, 1983.

53. Gonzalez-Martin G, Paulos C, Veloso B, et al. Ranitidine disposition in severe hepatic cirrhosis. Int J Clin Pharmacol Toxicol 25: 139–142, 1987.

54. Roark G. Treatment of postsclerotherapy esophageal ulcers with sucralfate. Gastrointest Endosc 30:9–10, 1984.

55. Lecomte S, Baron MH, Chenon MT, et al. Effect of magnesium complexation by fluoroquinolones on their antibacterial properties. Antimicrob Agents Chemother 38:2810–2816, 1994.

56. Stiegmann GV, Goff JS, Sun JH, et al. Endoscopic ligation of esophageal varices. Am J Surg 159:21–26, 1990.

57. Van Stiegmann G, Cambre T, Sun JH. A new endoscopic elastic band ligating device. Gastrointest Endosc 32:230–233, 1986.

58. Stiegmann GV, Goff JS, Michaletz-Onody PA, et al. Endoscopic sclerotherapy as compared with endoscopic ligation for bleeding esophageal varices. N Engl J Med 326:1527–1532, 1992.

59. Stump D, Hardin T. The use of vasopressin in the treatment of upper gastrointestinal haemorrhage. Drugs 39:38–53, 1990.

60. Fogel M, Knaver C, Andres L, et al. Continuous intravenous vasopressin in active upper gastrointestinal bleeding: a placebo controlled trial. Ann Intern Med 96:565–569, 1982.

61. Gimson A, Westaby D, Hegarty J, et al. A randomized trial of vasopressin plus nitroglycerin in the control of acute variceal hemorrhage. Hepatology 6:410–413, 1986.

62. Tsai Y, Lay C, Lai K, et al. Controlled trial of vasopressin plus nitroglycerin versus vasopressin alone in bleeding esophageal varices. Hepatology 6:406–409, 1982.

63. Imperiale T, Teran J, McCullough A. A meta-analysis of somatostatin versus vasopressin in the management of acute esophageal variceal hemorrhage. Gastroenterology 109:1289–1294, 1995.

64. Lamberts SWJ, Von der Lely A, Herder WW, et al. Octreotide. N Engl J Med 334:246–254, 1996.

65. Bhasin DK, Siyad I. Variceal bleeding and portal hypertension: new lights on old horizon. Endoscopy 36:120–129, 2004.

66. de Franchis R. Somatostatin, somatostatin analogues and other vasoactive drugs in the treatment of bleeding oespophageal varices. Dig Liver Dis 36(Suppl 1):S93–100, 2004.

67. Laine L, Peterson W. Bleeding peptic ulcer. N Engl J Med 331: 717–727, 1994.

68. Lewis J, Davis J, Allsopp D, et al. Beta-blockers in portal hypertension: an overview. Drugs 37:62–69, 1989.

69. Hayes P, Davis J, Lewis J, et al. Meta-analysis of value of propranolol in prevention of variceal hemorrhage. Lancet 336:153–156, 1990.

70. Pascal J, Cales P. Propranolol in the prevention of first upper gastrointestinal tract hemorrhage in patients with cirrhosis of the liver and esophageal varices. N Engl J Med 317:856–861, 1987.

71. Teran JC, Imperiale TF, Mullen KD, et al. Primary prophylaxis of variceal bleeding in cirrhosis: a cost effectiveness analysis. Gastroenterology 112:473–482, 1997.

72. Lebrec O, Poynard T, Bernuau J, et al. A randomized controlled study of propranolol for prevention of recurrent gastrointestinal bleeding in patients with cirrhosis. Hepatology 4:355–384, 1984.

73. Burroughs A, Jenkins W, Sherlock S, et al. Controlled trial of propranolol for the prevention of recurrent gastrointestinal bleeding in patients with cirrhosis. N Engl J Med 309:1539–1542, 1983.

74. Poynard T, Lebrec D, Hillon P, et al. Propranolol for prevention of recurrent gastrointestinal bleeding in patients with cirrhosis: a prospective study of factors associated with rebleeding. Hepatology 7: 447–451, 1987.

75. Lebrec D, Bemuau J, Rueff B, et al. Gastrointestinal bleeding after abrupt cessation of propranolol administration in cirrhosis. N Engl J Med 307:560, 1982.

76. Alabaster S, Gogel H, McCarthy D. Propranolol withdrawal and variceal hemorrhage. JAMA 250:3047, 1983.

77. Teres J, Bosch J, Bordas J, et al. Propranolol versus sclerotherapy in preventing variceal rebleeding: a randomized controlled trial. Gastroenterology 105:1508–1514, 1993.

78. Angelico A, Carli L, Piat C, et al. Effects of isosorbide-5-mononitrate compared with propranolol on first bleeding and long-term survival in cirrhosis. Gastroenterology 113:1632–1639, 1997.

79. Groszmann RJ. Beta adrenergic blockers and nitro vasodilators for the treatment of portal hypertension: the good, the bad, the ugly [editorial]. Gastroenterology 113:1794–1797, 1997.

80. Borroni G, Salerno F, Cassaniga M, et al. Nadolol is superior to isosorbide mononitrate for the prevention of the first variceal bleeding in cirrhotic patients with ascites. J Hepatol 37:315–321, 2002.

81. Riordan SM, Williams R. Treatment of hepatic encephalopathy. N Engl J Med 337:473–479, 1997.

82. Avery GS, Davies EF, Brogden RN. Lactulose: a review. Drugs 4: 7–48, 1972.

83. Kersh ES, Rifkin H. Lactulose enemas. Ann Intern Med 78:81–84, 1973.

84. Rodgers JB Jr, Kiley JE, Balint JA. Comparison of results of long-term treatment of chronic hepatic encephalopathy with lactulose and sorbitol. Am J Gastroenterol 60:459–465, 1973.

85. Conn HO, Leevy CM, Vlahcevic J, et al. Comparison of lactulose and neomycin in the treatment of chronic portal systemic encephalopathy. Gastroenterology 72:573, 1977.

86. Conn HO. Interactions of lactulose and neomycin. Drugs 4:4–6, 1972.

87. Weber F, Fresard K, Lally B. Effects of lactulose and neomycin on urea metabolism in cirrhotic subjects. Gastroenterology 82: 213–217, 1982.

88. Breen K, Bryant R, Levinson J, et al. Neomycin absorption in man. Ann Intern Med 76:211–218, 1972.

89. Berk D, Chalmer T. Deafness complicating antibiotic therapy of hepatic encephalopathy. Ann Intern Med 73:393–396, 1970.

90. Basile AS, Hughes RD, Harrison PM, et al. Elevated brain concentrations of 1,4–benzodiazepines in fulminant hepatic failure. N Engl J Med 325:473–478, 1991.

91. Bansky G, Meier P, Riederer E, et al. Effects of the benzodiazepine receptor antagonist flumazenil in hepatic encephalopathy in humans. Gastroenterology 97:744–750, 1989.

92. Ferenci P, Grimm G, Meryn S, et al. Successful long-term treatment of portal-systemic encephalopathy by benzodiazepine antagonist flumazenil. Gastroenterology 96:240–243, 1989.

93. Pomier LG, Giguere JF, Lavoie J, et al. Flumazenil in cirrhotic patients in hepatic coma. Hepatology 19:32–37, 1994.

94. Sterling R, Shiffman M, Schubert M. Flumazenil for hepatic coma: the elusive wake-up call? Gastroenterology 107:1204–1205, 1994.

95. Goulenok C, Bernard B, Cadranel J, et al. Flumazenil vs. placebo in hepatic encephalopathy in patients with cirrhosis: a meta-analysis. Alimentary Pharmacol Ther 16:361–372, 2002.

96. Imperiale T, McCullough A. Do corticosteroids reduce mortality from alcoholic hepatitis? Ann Intern Med 113:299–307, 1990.

97. Ramond M, Poynard T, Rueff B, et al. A randomized trial of prednisolone in patients with severe alcoholic hepatitis. N Engl J Med 326:507–512, 1992.

98. McCullough AJ, O'Connor JF, et al. Alcoholic liver disease: proposed recommendations for the American College of Gastroenterology. Am J Gastroenterol 93:2022–36, 1998.

99. Chan TYK. Beneficial effects of low-dose dopamine in cirrhosis and renal insufficiency. Ann Pharmacother 29:433, 1995.

100. Angeli P, Volpin R, Gerunda G, et al. Reversal of type 1 hepatorenal syndrome with the administration of midodrine and octreotide. Hepatology 29:1690–1697, 1999.

101. Bodenheimer H, Schaffner F, Pezzullo J. Evaluation of colchicine therapy in primary biliary cirrhosis. Gastroenterology 95:124–129, 1988.

102. Kershenobich D, Vargas F, Barcia-Tsao G, et al. Colchicine in the treatment of cirrhosis of the liver. N Engl J Med 318:1709–1713, 1988.

103. Stavinoha M, Soloway R. Current therapy of chronic liver disease. Drugs 39:814–840, 1990.

104. Fennerty MB. Primary sclerosing cholangitis and primary biliary cirrhosis. Postgrad Med 94:81, 1993.

105. Poupon R, Poupon R, Balkau B, et al. Ursodiol for the long-term treatment of primary biliary cirrhosis. N Engl J Med 333:1342–1347, 1994.

106. Horst D, Grace N, Conn H, et al. Comparison of dietary protein with an oral, branched chain–enriched amino acid supplement in chronic portal-systemic encephalopathy: a randomized controlled trial. Hepatology 4:279–287, 1984.

107. Guidelines for the use of parenteral and enteral nutrition in adult and pediatric patients. JPEN J Parenter Enteral Nutr 26(Suppl 1):65–67SA, 2002.

108. Donaghy A, Ross R, Wicks C, et al. Growth hormone therapy in patients with cirrhosis: a pilot study of efficacy and safety. Gastroenterology 113:1617–1622, 1997.

109. Miyaji H, Ito S, Azuma T. Effects of *Helicobacter pylori* eradication therapy on hyperammonaemia in patients with liver cirrhosis. Gut 40:726–730, 1997.

110. Dehmlow C, Erhard J, De Groot H. Inhibition of Kupffer cell function as an explanation for hepatoprotective properties of silibinin. Hepatology 23:749–754, 1996.

111. Zhou S, Lim L, Chowbay B. Herbal modulation of P-glycoprotein. Drug Metab Rev 36:57–104, 2004.

112. DiCenzo R, Selton M, Jordan K, et al. Coadministration of milk thistle and indinavir in healthy subjects. Pharmacotherapy 23:866–870, 2003.

113. Riggio O, Ariosto F, Merli M, et al. Short-term oral zinc supplementation does not improve chronic hepatic encephalopathy. Dig Des Sci 36:1204–1208, 1991.

114. D'Amico G, Morabito A, Pagliaro L, et al. Survival and prognostic indicators in compensated and decompensated cirrhosis. Dig Dis Sci 31:468–475, 1986.

115. Pugh RN, Murray-Lyon IM, Dawson JL, et al. Transection of the oesophagus for bleeding esophageal varicies. Br J Surg 60:646–649, 1973.

116. Infante-Rivard C, Esnaola S, et al. Clinical and statistical validity of conventional prognostic factors in predicting short-term survival among cirrhotics. Hepatology 7:660–664, 1987.

117. Albers I, Volpin R, et al. Superiority of the Child-Pugh classification to quantitative liver function tests for assessing prognosis of liver cirrhosis. Scand J Gastroenterol 24:269–276, 1989.

118. Kamath PS, Wiesner RH, et al. A model to predict survival in patients with end-stage liver disease. Hepatology 33:464–470, 2001.

119. Approval of Naltrexone for Use in Chronic Alcoholism. Washington, DC: Food and Drug Administration, January 1995.

120. Bass N, Williams R. Guide to drug dosage in hepatic disease. Clin Pharmacokinet 15:396–420, 1988.

121. LeCouteur DG, Mclean AJ. The aging liver: drug clearance and an oxygen diffusion barrier hypothesis. Clin Pharmacokinet 34:359–373, 1998.

122. Morgan DJ, McLean AJ. Clinical pharmacokinetic and pharmacodynamic considerations in patients with liver disease. Clin Pharmacokinet 29:370–391, 1995.

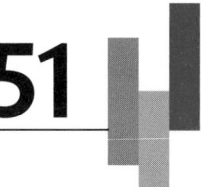

Pancreatitis

Jennifer W. Beall and Paula A. Thompson

Pancreatic inflammatory disease may be classified as either acute or chronic based on the reversibility of the functional and structural changes that arise within the gland. Although these are usually treated as discrete clinical entities, they may actually be part of a continuum of pancreatic disease.[1,2] Following an acute attack of pancreatitis, the pancreas will usually recover normal exocrine and endocrine function and morphology once the underlying cause of acute inflammation is eliminated. While most attacks have a mild, self-limited course, severe disease complicated by multiple organ system failure and life-threatening infection may develop. Although pancreatic necrosis can result in transient or, occasionally, permanent impairment of gland function and structure, acute pancreatitis rarely progresses to chronic disease.[3,4]

In contrast, the persistent inflammation from chronic pancreatitis is associated with a permanent and often progressive loss of pancreatic exocrine and endocrine function, and irreversible structural damage. Recurrent exacerbations of pancreatitis, which frequently complicate chronic disease, are virtually impossible to distinguish clinically from discrete attacks of acute pancreatitis.[4,5]

Reliable incidence and prevalence data are difficult to obtain. The incidence of both acute and chronic forms varies considerably among geographic areas as a consequence of differences in regional environmental and genetic factors.[5,6]

Both acute and chronic pancreatitis will be discussed after a brief review of pancreatic anatomy and physiology. An understanding of normal structure and function is necessary background for this discussion.

ANATOMY

The adult pancreas is a flattened and elongated gland, usually ranging from 12 to 20 cm in length and weighing 70 to 110 g. It is lobular, like the salivary glands, and its lack of a fibrous capsule makes it soft in texture. The pancreas lies retroperitoneally, the head nestled within the curve of the duodenum as it exits the stomach and the tail extending obliquely to the left (Fig. 51.1).[7,8]

Blood is supplied to the pancreas by the celiac and superior mesenteric arteries, and the blood ultimately drains into the hepatic portal vein. The lymphatic vessels draining the

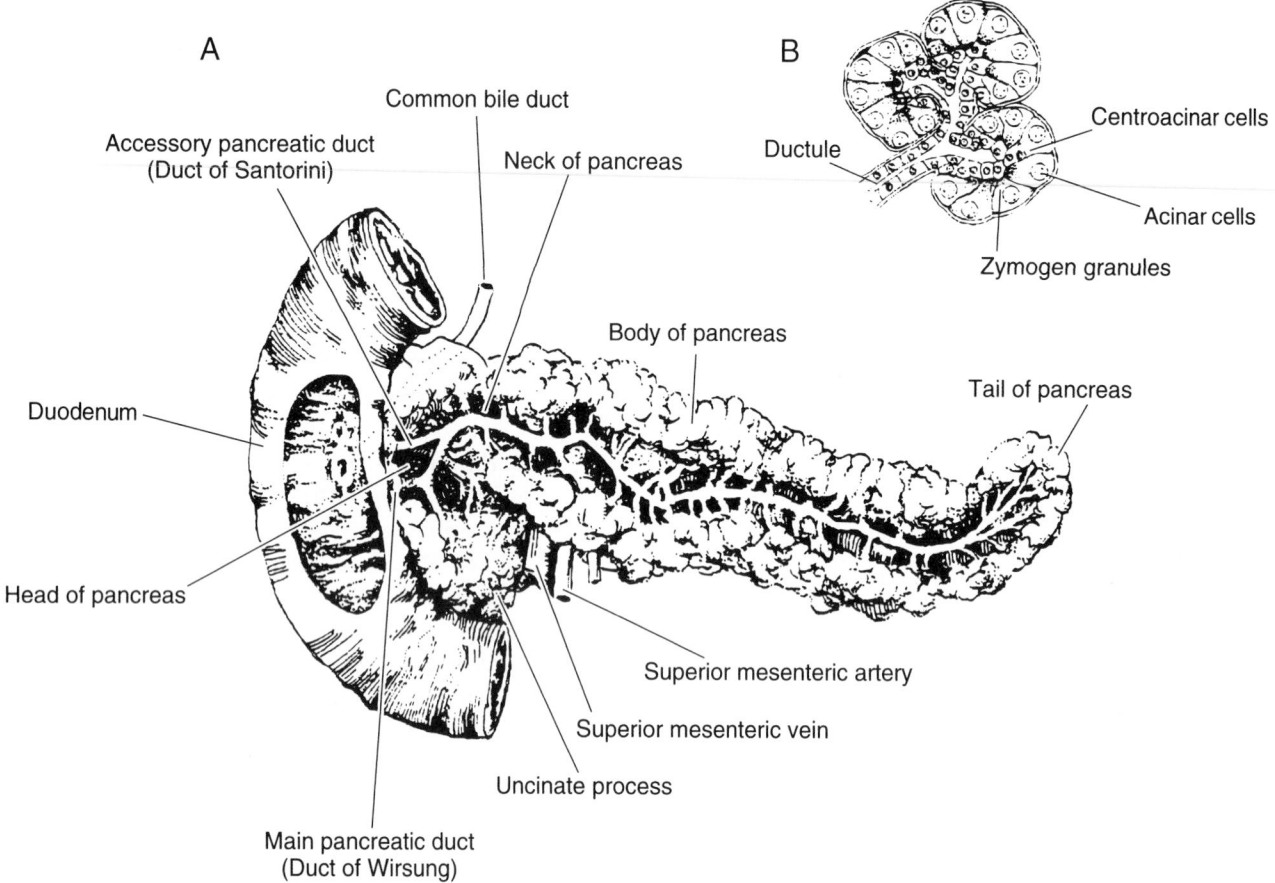

A

Accessory pancreatic duct
(Duct of Santorini)

Common bile duct

Neck of pancreas

Duodenum

Body of pancreas

Tail of pancreas

Head of pancreas

Superior mesenteric artery

Superior mesenteric vein

Uncinate process

Main pancreatic duct
(Duct of Wirsung)

B

Ductule

Centroacinar cells

Acinar cells

Zymogen granules

FIGURE 51.1 Structure of the pancreas. **A.** Dissected to show ductal system. **B.** Enlargement of a representative acinus.

pancreas terminate primarily in the pancreatosplenic and pancreatoduodenal lymph nodes. Sympathetic innervation is predominately through splanchnic neurons synapsing in the celiac plexus, and parasympathetic innervation is derived from the vagus nerve.[7,8]

The pancreas contains exocrine (about 80%) and endocrine (about 2%) tissue. The remaining 18% of the gland is ductular. The secretory unit of the exocrine pancreas is the acinus (Latin for "berries in a cluster"). Each acinus consists of 20 to 50 pyramid-shaped cells surrounding a central lumen. The acini are connected to the main pancreatic duct through a network of interconnecting ductules. The islets of Langerhans (pancreatic islets) make up the endocrine pancreas and are composed of four major cell types, each apparently secreting a single hormone. Approximately 50% to 80% of the islet cell mass is comprised of β cells, which secrete insulin. Glucagon, somatostatin, and pancreatic polypeptide are secreted by α cells, δ cells, and PP cells, respectively. Insulin and glucagon are critical in the regulation of carbohydrate metabolism (see Chapter 40). In addition to the systemic effects exerted by each of these hormones, they also play a role in the regulation of pancreatic exocrine secretion. Insulin may potentiate the actions of stimulatory factors, while glucagon, somatostatin, and pancreatic polypeptide exert inhibitory effects.[7]

PHYSIOLOGY

OVERVIEW OF EXOCRINE FUNCTION

Pancreatic exocrine function is complex and incompletely understood. During the course of a day, the pancreas can secrete 1 to 2.5 liters of isosmotic alkaline fluid containing over 20 enzymes and proenzymes (zymogens). This fluid, commonly termed "pancreatic juice," is produced by acinar and ductular cells. The acinar cells synthesize and secrete the digestive enzymes. Proximal ductular cells, termed centroacinar cells, extend into the lumen of the acinus and are primarily responsible for secretion of water and electrolytes. The intralobular ductules draining the acini coalesce with interlobular ductules, ultimately emptying into the main pancreatic duct. The main pancreatic duct and the common bile duct enter the duodenum at the ampulla of Vater (hepatopancreatic ampulla). The sphincter of Oddi (sphincter of the hepatopancreatic ampulla) regulates flow from both ducts.[9–11]

SECRETION OF WATER AND ELECTROLYTES

The principal cations of pancreatic juice are sodium and potassium, which are secreted at fixed concentrations similar to their plasma concentrations. The principal anions are bi-

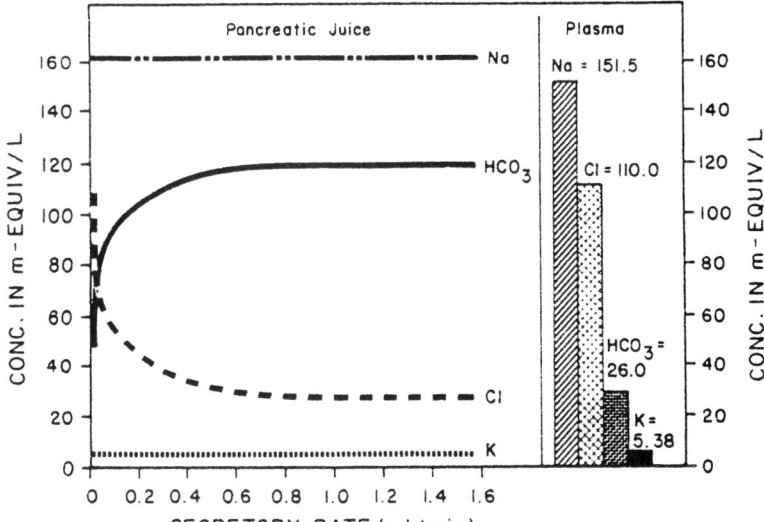

FIGURE 51.2 Relationship between ion concentration in pancreatic juice and secretory flow rate. (Reprinted with permission from Pandol S, Pancreatic physiology. In: Sleisenger MH, Fordtran JS. Gastrointestinal Disease: Pathophysiology, Diagnosis, Management. 5th ed. Philadelphia: WB Saunders, 1993:1586.)

carbonate and chloride, which vary reciprocally in concentration, maintaining the sum of the two fairly constant at approximately 150 mEq per liter (Fig. 51.2). Bicarbonate is secreted by the centroacinar cells, whereas secretions from the acinar cells are rich in chloride. The relative concentration of each reaching the duodenum depends on the amount secreted and the exchange of bicarbonate for chloride in the ductules. The concentration of bicarbonate, physiologically the most important of the electrolytes, increases with increasing flow rates. Flow rates range from a basal level of 0.2 to 0.3 mL per minute to 4 mL per minute during stimulation. At maximal rates of secretion, bicarbonate concentration approaches 120 mEq per liter, and the pH of the resulting pancreatic juice is approximately 8.3. This alkalinity buffers the acidic chyme delivered to the duodenum from the stomach and maintains a pH that is optimal for the functioning of pancreatic enzymes. Other ions present in pancreatic juice include calcium and trace amounts of magnesium, zinc, phosphate, and sulfate. Water enters the ductules passively down the concentration gradient established by the active transport of solute, maintaining iso-osmolality.[9–11]

ENZYMES

Protein represents up to 10% of pancreatic juice, and over 90% of this protein consists of digestive enzymes and proenzymes.[9–11] These enzymes are synthesized in the rough endoplasmic reticulum of the acinar cells and are stored in secretory vesicles (zymogen granules) prior to their release by exocytosis. There are four major categories of enzymes, corresponding to the four classes of organic compounds found in food: proteins, carbohydrates, lipids, and nucleic acids (Table 51.1). The proteases and phospholipases are secreted as inactive zymogens that become active in the intestinal lumen through the action of enterokinase produced by the duodenal mucosa. Enterokinase cleaves a small frag-

ment of trypsinogen to form active trypsin, which can then activate other zymogens, including additional trypsinogen molecules.

The pancreas is protected from autolysis not only by secretion of proteolytic enzymes in zymogen form, but also by the presence of trypsin inhibitor, which binds to trypsin in a 1:1 ratio, rendering it inactive. This protein is present

TABLE 51.1	Major Digestive Enzymes Secreted by the Pancreas

Proteolytic

Trypsinogen$^{\text{Enterokinase, Trypsin}}$ trypsin

Chymotrypsinogen^{Trypsin} chymotrypsin

Proelastase^{Trypsin} elastase

Procarboxypeptidase A^{Trypsin} carboxypeptidase A

Procarboxypeptidase B ^{Trypsin} carboxypeptidase B

Amylolytic

α-Amylase

Lipolytic

Lipase

Procolipase^{Trypsin} colipase [cofactor essential for optimal lipase activity]

Prophospholipase A$_2$^{Trypsin} phospholipase A$_2$

Carboxylesterase lipase

Nucleolytic

Deoxyribonuclease (DNAse)

Ribonuclease (RNAse)

(Adapted from Pandol SJ. Pancreatic physiology and secretory testing. In: Feldman M, Sleisenger MH, Scharschmidt BF. Gastrointestinal and Liver Disease: Pathophysiology, Diagnosis, Management. 6th ed. Philadelphia: WB Saunders, 1998:871.)

in sufficient quantity to protect against small amounts of trypsin, which may become active in the ductules, but its activity is insignificant in the duodenal lumen.[9,10,12]

REGULATION OF EXOCRINE FUNCTION

A discussion of all the putative regulatory factors of pancreatic exocrine function, both neural and hormonal, is beyond the scope of this text. The roles of secretin, cholecystokinin (CCK), and cholinergic neurons in pancreatic secretions have been well established and will be reviewed briefly.

Secretin, a peptide hormone released from the mucosa of the duodenum and jejunum, stimulates bicarbonate and water secretion, primarily in response to the presence of acid in the small intestine. The pH threshold for secretin release is 4.5. The presence of bile salts and some fatty acids within the intestinal lumen can also trigger secretin release. In addition to its effect on bicarbonate, secretin may cause a weak stimulation of pancreatic enzyme release.[9-11]

CCK, also a peptide hormone secreted by the mucosa of the small bowel, causes the release of an enzyme-rich juice from the pancreas. Production of CCK occurs when amino acids or fatty acids enter the duodenum. Intravenous administration of CCK also stimulates enzyme release, while pancreatic response is substantially reduced by the administration of CCK antagonists. The combined release of secretin and CCK potentiates the pancreatic response, increasing bicarbonate and volume secretion.[9-11]

Inhibitory mechanisms are less well understood than stimulatory ones. Intravenous infusions of amino acids or glucose inhibit pancreatic function, probably due at least in part to the release of glucagon and somatostatin from islet cells. Pancreatic polypeptide may also decrease exocrine function by modulating cholinergic pathways, although the physiologic significance of this has not been delineated. The presence of lipids in the colon inhibits CCK-stimulated pancreatic output, possibly acting through a mediator called peptide YY.[9-11,13] A negative feedback loop has also been hypothesized whereby trypsin in the intestinal lumen inactivates a CCK-releasing peptide, decreasing CCK release and pancreatic enzyme secretion.[9,10,12,14] Increasing our understanding of these inhibitory mechanisms may help to guide the development of effective therapeutic modalities for pancreatitis.

Phases of Pancreatic Secretion. Pancreatic function can best be described in terms of interdigestive (fasting) and digestive (postprandial) periods. Digestive secretion can be further subdivided into cephalic, gastric, and intestinal phases. The pancreas is not quiescent between meals, but rather displays a basal secretion that is cyclical. Although overall secretion is low, there are fluctuations that parallel changes in gastrointestinal motility.[9-11]

Vagal nerves mediate the cephalic phase, in which pancreatic secretion can be stimulated by the sight, smell, or taste of food. In sham feeding experiments (patients chew food without swallowing it), pancreatic enzyme secretion increased to approximately 50% of the maximal secretion elicited by intravenous CCK. Gastric acid production is also stimulated during this phase, triggering secretin release, which increases bicarbonate and enzyme secretion. The gastric phase begins when food enters the stomach. Gastric distention causes increased pancreatic secretion, mediated through a gastropancreatic vagovagal reflex. The most important phase is triggered when chyme enters the small intestine. This intestinal phase is regulated by the hormones secretin and CCK and by enteropancreatic vagovagal reflexes triggered by volume or hyperosmolality in the gut. During all phases of pancreatic secretion, it is the interplay of neural and hormonal factors that result in the coordinated response of the pancreas to feeding.[9-12]

This brief overview of normal anatomy and physiology should serve to clarify the subsequent discussions of acute and chronic pancreatitis.

ACUTE PANCREATITIS

DEFINITION

Acute pancreatitis is an acute inflammatory process of the pancreas with variable involvement of other regional tissues or remote organ systems.[15] The inflammation may remain localized in the pancreas or may involve tissues elsewhere.[16] Approximately 80% of patients have interstitial pancreatitis, which is characterized by interstitial edema resulting from inflammatory cells, yet there is no destruction to the architecture of the gland.[17-20] The remaining patients develop necrotizing pancreatitis, with diffuse or focal areas of nonviable pancreatic parenchyma and large areas of peripancreatic fat necrosis.[16,18] Thrombus is also common in acute necrotizing pancreatitis.

Acute pancreatitis can also be classified clinically as mild or severe.[16] Although interstitial pancreatitis may be associated with serious systemic toxicity, its clinical course is usually mild, with minimal organ dysfunction and a resultant mortality of less than 2%. In contrast, the mortality of severe acute pancreatitis, involving organ failure or local complications such as abscess or pseudocyst, is 10% to 30%.[17,18] Severe pancreatitis is most often the clinical expression of pancreatic necrosis.

ETIOLOGY

Acute pancreatitis is associated with many other disease processes and events (Table 51.2). Biliary tract stone disease and ethanol abuse account for 60% to 80% of acute bouts of pancreatitis, with the incidence of each depending on the patient population being evaluated.[6,17] Women tend to have pancreatitis as a result of biliary tract stone disease, whereas ethanol abuse is more often associated with pancreatitis in men.[6,17] A number of miscellaneous causes account for 10% to 15% of pancreatitis attacks, with another 10% to 15% of cases classified as idiopathic.[17,21] However, recent studies suggest that up to two thirds of idiopathic cases may be caused by biliary microlithiasis.[6]

EPIDEMIOLOGY

The incidence of acute pancreatitis varies widely and depends on the incidence of precipitating factors in a population.[6] The incidence of acute pancreatitis in the United States is thought to range from 54 to 238 episodes per 1 million people per year.[22] Disease incidence has been extensively studied in the United Kingdom and appears to have increased 10-fold from the 1960s to the 1980s.[21] This may reflect an increase in alcohol abuse and diagnostic advances.

Cholelithiasis increases a patient's relative risk of developing acute pancreatitis; however, the condition develops in only a few patients with this condition.[23] Biliary pancreatitis may be associated with recurrent episodes of acute disease, but chronic pancreatitis is rare. In contrast, many patients with alcoholic pancreatitis have consumed large amounts of alcohol for many years before the initial onset of symptoms. Pancreatitis in an alcoholic patient was previously thought to be an acute exacerbation of chronic pancreatitis. However, despite continued abuse of alcohol, not all will progress from acute to chronic disease.[6,15,21] Because clinical pancreatitis develops in only 5% of alcoholics, unidentified factors must affect susceptibility to pancreatic injury.[21]

Gallstones are the most common obstructive cause of acute pancreatitis, but inflammation may also result from other lesions that interfere with the flow of pancreatic juice through the ductal system. Thus, pancreatitis may result from ductal strictures, sphincter of Oddi dysfunction, or tumors of the pancreas, ampulla, or duodenum.[3,21] Blunt trauma to the abdomen may also cause pancreatitis by disrupting the pancreatic ductal system. Similarly, pancreatitis can occur as a postoperative complication of procedures that involve manipulation of the pancreas or during endoscopic retrograde cholangiopancreatography (ERCP), in which a side-viewing endoscope is passed into the duodenum and a catheter introduces a radiopaque contrast medium into the pancreatic duct. Certain viral, parasitic, and bacterial infections may also precipitate acute attacks. Other causes of acute pancreatitis include penetrating duodenal ulcer, vascular compromise, hypertriglyceridemia, and various toxins.[3,6,21]

TABLE 51.2	Causes of Acute Pancreatitis

Obstruction
  Gallstones
  Sphincter of Oddi spasm or stenosis
  Periampullary or pancreatic tumors
  Periampullary duodenal diverticula
  Pancreas divisum with accessory duct obstruction
Infection
  Parasitic: ascariasis, clonorchiasis
  Viral: Coxsackie B virus, mumps, rubella, Epstein-Barr virus, cytomegalovirus, varicella, hepatitis A, hepatitis B
  Bacterial: *Mycoplasma* sp, *Legionella* sp, *Salmonella* sp, *Shigella* sp, *Mycobacterium tuberculosis*, *Campylobacter* sp
Toxins
  Alcohol
  Drugs (see Table 51.3)
  Scorpion venom
  Organophosphate insecticides
Trauma
  Postoperative
  Endoscopic retrograde cholangiopancreatography
  Endoscopic sphincterotomy
  Coronary artery bypass
  Blunt abdominal trauma
Metabolic
  Hypertriglyceridemia
  Hypercalcemia
Vascular
  Vasculitis
  Atherosclerotic emboli
  Hypoperfusion
Miscellaneous
  Idiopathic
  Hereditary pancreatitis
  Cystic fibrosis
  Penetrating duodenal ulcer
  Inflammatory bowel disease
  Hypothermia

(Data from Mitchell RMS, Byrne MF, Baille J. Pancreatitis. Lancet 361:1447–1455, 2003; Steer ML, Waxman I, Freedman S. Chronic pancreatitis. N Engl J Med 332:1482–1490, 1995; and Owyang C, Levitt MD. Chronic pancreatitis. In: Yamada T. Textbook of Gastroenterology. 2nd ed. Philadelphia: JB Lippincott, 1995:2061.)

Debate continues about the association of acute pancreatitis with pancreas divisum, a congenital abnormality in which the dorsal and ventral pancreatic ducts fail to fuse. Because pancreas divisum is a common anatomic abnormality with an overall incidence of about 7%, it may be an incidental finding in many patients with idiopathic pancreatitis.[6,21]

More than 85 drugs have been associated with acute pancreatitis, although the frequency of drug-induced disease generally is low.[24–36] Because scattered case reports make up the bulk of the literature on drug-induced pancreatic disease, it usually is difficult to link drugs with pancreatic inflammation conclusively. Mallory and Kern[25] classified drugs into three categories based on the clinical evidence implicating them in the development of acute pancreatitis: definite, probable, and questionable. The association is considered definite when drug therapy results in abdominal pain combined with hyperamylasemia that resolves when therapy is discontinued or recurs when the drug is reintroduced (Table 51.3). Because drug-induced acute pancreatitis cannot be distinguished clinically from that induced by other causes, it should be considered when other causes of disease have been ruled out.

PATHOPHYSIOLOGY

The inflammation and necrosis of acute pancreatitis begin as an autodigestive process initiated by the inappropriate activation and release of proteolytic and lipolytic enzymes into the interstitium of the organ. The activation of trypsinogen to trypsin within the acinar cells is the initial step in the pathogenesis of acute pancreatitis.[3] Trypsin can then activate other pancreatic proteases, including elastase, chymotrypsin, and carboxypeptidase, and phospholipase A_2, which then contribute to acinar cell inflammation. Elastase causes vascular damage by dissolving the elastic fibers of blood vessels. Chymotrypsin augments this vascular damage and the resulting edema, and phospholipase A_2 destroys acinar cell membranes. These pancreatic enzymes, after damaging acinar cells, leak into the interstitium, causing local inflammation. Lipase is also liberated from peripheral acinar cells, resulting in peripancreatic fat necrosis. The kinin and complement systems are activated by trypsin, leading to the release of vasoactive peptides, which cause vasodilation, increased vascular permeability, and accumulation of leukocytes.[17] In severe disease, pancreatic enzymes, vasoactive peptides, and other toxic factors extravasate from the pancreas into peripancreatic spaces and the peritoneal cavity, causing a widespread chemical irritation.[18] These materials may also reach the systemic circulation through retroperitoneal lymphatic and venous circulation to contribute to systemic complications, including shock, respiratory failure, and renal failure.[18]

Factors in acute pancreatitis that contribute to the transformation from a local inflammatory process into a multiorgan illness are not entirely understood. The contribution of

TABLE 51.3	Agents Associated with Acute Pancreatitis
Definite Association	Salicylates
Amiodarone	Sulfasalazine
Angiotensin-converting enzyme inhibitors	Zalcitabine
Asparaginase	**Questionable Association**
Azathioprine	Acetaminophen
Codeine	Ampicillin
Cytarabine	Carbamazepine
Didanosine	Cholestyramine
Estrogens	Cisplatin
Furosemide	Clonidine
Isoniazid	Colchicine
Losartan	Cyclosporine
Mercaptopurine	Cyproheptadine
Mesalamine	Diazoxide
Metronidazole	Diphenoxylate
Pentamidine	Ergotamine
Sulfonamides	Erythromycin
Sulindac	Gold compounds
Tetracycline	Indomethacin
Thiazides	Interleukin-2
Valproic acid	Isotretinoin
Probable Association	Ketoprofen
Bumetanide	Mefenamic acid
Chlorthalidone	Metolazone
Cimetidine	Naproxen
Clarithromycin	Nitrofurantoin
Clozapine	Opiates
Corticosteroids	Oxyphenbutazone
Ethacrynic acid	Phenolphthalein
Ifosfamide	Piroxicam
Ketorolac	Propoxyphene
Methyldopa	Ranitidine
Phenformin	Tryptophan
Procainamide	

Data from references 25–35.

leukocytes and their products in amplifying pancreatic inflammation into a generalized systemic inflammatory response has been recognized.[3,37] Neutrophils, macrophages, and monocytes invade the inflamed pancreas and release destructive mediators such as elastase, phospholipase A_2, platelet activating factor, nitric oxide, oxygen free radicals, and cytokines.[3] The inflammatory cytokines, particularly interleukin-1, interleukin-6, and tumor necrosis factor, appear to be important systemic mediators of acute pancreatitis.[37] Cytokines are produced not only locally, but also systemically in sites such as the spleen, liver, and lung, where they have been linked to organ dysfunction. Circulating levels of cytokines are higher in patients with severe acute pancreatitis, and these levels can be predictive of disease severity, end-organ failure, and mortality.[38,39] Consequently, cytokine antagonism may prove beneficial in treating patients with acute pancreatitis. Furthermore, impairment of the pancreatic microcirculation by the deleterious effects of leukocyte products on the vascular endothelium appears to be an important mechanism in pancreatic necrosis.[40]

The mechanism by which pancreatic enzymes become prematurely activated within the gland to initiate the cascade of events that causes acute pancreatitis is unknown. Proposed mechanisms focus on biliary tract stone disease, postulating that reflux of hepatic bile or duodenal contents into the pancreatic ductal system may activate enzymes within the pancreatic parenchyma.[3,6] More recently, investigators have proposed that activation of trypsin may occur within the pancreatic acinar cell rather than in the ductal or intercellular space.[3,21] Obstruction in the pancreatic duct could disturb the normal events that maintain segregation of lysosomal enzymes, including cathepsin B, from digestive enzymes, thus allowing them to mix intracellularly. Cathepsin B can convert trypsinogen to trypsin, which could then activate the remaining digestive zymogens. The mechanism of ethanol-induced pancreatitis is not understood but may include relaxation or spasm of the sphincter of Oddi, obstruction of small pancreatic ductules with proteinaceous plugs, or direct toxic effects of ethanol or one of its metabolites.[3,6,20]

The pathogenesis of drug-induced pancreatic injury has not been elucidated, but it does not appear to differ substantially from that of acute pancreatitis induced by other causes. Possible mechanisms include pancreatic ductal constriction, immune suppression, arteriolar thromboses, direct cellular toxicity, hepatic production of free radicals, and osmotic or metabolic effects.[26]

CLINICAL PRESENTATION AND DIAGNOSIS

SIGNS AND SYMPTOMS

The classic presentation of acute pancreatitis consists of abdominal pain, nausea, and vomiting; however, a patient's symptoms and physical findings may vary with the severity of disease.[15] The abdominal pain is usually located in the epigastrium or diffusely throughout the upper abdomen.[3] Pain is usually sudden in onset and peaks within 10 to 30 minutes.[41] Pain may be severe, and it is most commonly described as a steady, dull, or boring pain that often radiates to the back. Patients may move about continually in search of a comfortable position, with little relief.[6,15] Pain resolves over 1 to 3 days in mild cases but may last many days to weeks during severe attacks. Painless pancreatitis has been

reported infrequently. Nausea and vomiting are almost invariably present and are usually preceded by the onset of pain. Epigastric tenderness is a consistent finding on abdominal examination, as is abdominal distention. Bowel sounds often are diminished but not absent. Fever in the range of 100° to 102°F is seen in most patients as the pyrogenic products of pancreatic injury enter the circulation. Tachycardia and hypotension progressing to circulatory shock can occur in severe cases as a result of hypovolemia caused by vomiting, hemorrhage, and fluid sequestration within the retroperitoneal space. Circulating kinins and cytokines contribute to this circulatory instability through vasodilatory effects and increased vascular permeability.[17] Disorientation, delirium, or hallucinations are sometimes observed, although most patients present without changes in mental status.[3]

DIAGNOSIS AND CLINICAL FINDINGS

The diagnosis of acute pancreatitis is based on careful clinical evaluation of the patient, laboratory tests, and radiographic imaging. Mild cases of acute pancreatitis often represent a diagnostic dilemma because symptoms may be nonspecific and pancreatic enzyme levels and imaging studies are often virtually normal.[17] Occasionally, acute pancreatitis must be distinguished from other processes that present with abdominal pain and hyperamylasemia, such as acute cholecystitis or appendicitis, intestinal ischemia or infarction, perforated gastric or duodenal ulcer, intestinal obstruction, ectopic pregnancy, and common bile duct obstruction.[41]

LABORATORY TESTS

Leukocytosis, ranging from 10,000 to 25,000 cells per cubic millimeter, is a common finding during routine laboratory evaluation of patients with acute pancreatitis.[3,17] Hyperglycemia, transient hypertriglyceridemia, and hypoalbuminemia also are common. Liver function tests often reveal mild hyperbilirubinemia and elevated serum alkaline phosphatase and transaminase levels, which tend to be more pronounced with biliary pancreatitis. Hypovolemia may result in hemoconcentration, as evidenced by elevated hematocrit, blood urea nitrogen, and serum creatinine levels.

PANCREATIC ENZYMES

Elevation of the serum amylase level has remained central to the diagnosis of acute pancreatitis since its first association with the disease in 1929.[17,21] The pancreas and salivary glands account for most of the serum amylase activity in healthy people. The serum amylase level typically rises rapidly (from the normal range of 35 to 118 IU per liter) during the initial hours of an attack and then declines over the following 3 to 10 days.[3,6] The sensitivity of the test may be compromised if patients do not present early in the course of the disease. Furthermore, the test lacks specificity because hyperamylasemia is associated with a variety of nonpancreatic conditions, including diseases of the biliary tract, intestines, female genitourinary tract, lungs, prostate, and salivary glands.[42] Generally, patients with biliary pancreatitis present with a more marked hyperamylasemia than do patients with alcohol-related disease.[17,42] The measurement of serum amylase isoenzymes has been largely abandoned because most nonpancreatic abdominal diseases that simulate pancreatitis are associated with increased pancreatic rather than nonpancreatic amylase levels.[42]

In contrast, serum lipase is derived almost exclusively from the pancreas (normal range 2.3 to 20 IU per deciliter). Thus, it is more specific for acute pancreatitis and remains normal in a variety of conditions associated with elevations of serum amylase, including salivary gland disease, gynecologic disorders, and macroamylasemia associated with renal insufficiency.[3] However, hyperlipasemia may also occur in nonpancreatic acute abdominal conditions.[6,42] Although serum lipase typically parallels amylase in onset of elevation, lipase elevation persists longer, thus enhancing its diagnostic utility in patients who present several days after the onset of symptoms.

In summary, elevations in serum amylase and lipase activity support the diagnosis of acute pancreatitis. The assays are widely available and can be performed rapidly and reliably at low cost.[42] Values of serum amylase and lipase greater than three times the upper limit of normal are characteristic of acute pancreatitis and rarely occur in nonpancreatic conditions.[3] The magnitude of increase in serum amylase and lipase activity has no prognostic value and does not correlate with the severity of the acute attack.[41] Furthermore, daily measurement of pancreatic enzymes has little value in assessing a patient's progress or prognosis.[3] The use of other pancreatic enzymes, such as immunoreactive trypsinogen, chymotrypsin, elastase, and phospholipase A_2, as markers for acute pancreatitis does not appear to provide any diagnostic advantage over the determination of serum amylase and lipase activity. In addition, measuring the urinary amylase level and the amylase:creatinine clearance ratio offers little benefit in improving diagnostic accuracy. However, a rapid assay of urinary trypsinogen 2 may prove to be a reliable test in the future.[17,20,42]

IMAGING

Radiographic studies play an important role in confirming the diagnosis of pancreatitis and provide important etiologic and prognostic information. Although abdominal radiography is not considered diagnostic, it has several uses in this setting.[42] Most importantly, it may help to exclude nonpancreatic diseases that may mimic pancreatitis, including bowel obstruction and perforated viscus. The primary role of ultrasonography is in evaluating the biliary tract for stones, dilation, or obstruction.[42] Guidelines from the American College of Gastroenterology recommend performing an abdominal ultrasound within 24 to 48 hours of hospitalization for the initial episode of acute pancreatitis.[41] Computed tomography (CT) is useful for excluding other serious intra-abdominal conditions, but its utility early in an acute attack is controversial.[41] Dynamic contrast-enhanced CT scan, the best test for identi-

fying pancreatic necrosis, should be performed after the first 3 days in patients with severe acute pancreatitis to distinguish interstitial from necrotizing disease.[41]

ASSESSING SEVERITY

Multiple clinical criteria systems have been developed to assess the severity and prognosis of acute pancreatitis. Predictors of severity allow early identification of patients with the greatest likelihood of developing severe pancreatitis.[16,17,41] Ranson et al developed 11 prognostic criteria that can be measured 48 hours after hospital admission to assess the severity of an acute attack (Table 51.4).[41,43] The Acute Physiology and Chronic Health Evaluation II (APACHE II) is another list of clinical and laboratory values used to assess patients with acute pancreatitis that can be calculated within hours of admission and at daily intervals thereafter[6,21,44] (Table 51.5). Severe acute pancreatitis is characterized by three or more Ranson criteria or at least eight APACHE II points.[16] According to recent guidelines, the APACHE II score should be generated on the day of admission.[41] After 48 hours, the APACHE II or Ranson score may be used to follow the course of the patient with pancreatitis.[41]

COMPLICATIONS

The clinical course of acute pancreatitis is uncomplicated in approximately 80% of attacks. Thus, most patients with acute pancreatitis have mild disease that resolves promptly with conservative therapy.[17–19] The remaining patients de-

TABLE 51.4	Ranson's Prognostic Criteria	
	Nonbiliary Pancreatitis	Biliary Pancreatitis
On Admission		
Age (years)	>55	>70
White cells/mL	>16,000	>18,000
Glucose (mg/dL)	>200	>220
Lactate dehydrogenase (LDH) (IU/L)	>350	>400
Aspartate aminotransferase (AST) (IU/L)	>250	>250
Within 48 Hours of Admission		
Decrease in hematocrit (points)	>10	>10
Increase in blood urea nitrogen (mg/dL)	>5	>2
Calcium (mg/dL)	<8	<8
PaO_2 (mm Hg)	<60	—
Base deficit (mEq/L)	>4	>5
Fluid deficit (L)[a]	>6	>4

[a] Input minus output.
(From Ranson JHC. Etiological and prognostic factors in human acute pancreatitis: a review. Am J Gastroenterol 77:633–638, 1982.)

TABLE 51.5	APACHE II Variables
Temperature	Serum sodium
Heart rate	Serum potassium
Mean arterial pressure	Serum creatinine
Respiratory rate	Hematocrit
Oxygenation	White blood count
Arterial pH	Glasgow Coma Scale score
Age points	Chronic health assessment points

(Adapted from Agarwal N, Pitchumoni CS. Assessment of severity in acute pancreatitis. Am J Gastroenterol 86:1385–1391, 1991.)

velop severe disease that is usually the clinical expression of pancreatic necrosis.[16] Although the mortality of interstitial pancreatitis remains low (<less than 2%), necrotizing pancreatitis has a mortality ranging from 10% (sterile necrosis) to 30% (infected necrosis).[18]

Acute pancreatitis may be complicated by either local or systemic events (Table 51.6). Local events include the development of acute fluid collections in or near the pancreas, occurring early in the course of 30% to 50% of attacks.[45] Acute fluid collections lack a well-defined wall and

TABLE 51.6	Complications of Acute Pancreatitis

Local

  Necrosis (sterile or infected)

  Pancreatic fluid collection (sterile or infected)

  Pseudocyst

  Abscess

  Pancreatic ascites

  Blood vessel rupture or thrombosis

  Bowel necrosis, obstruction, perforation

  Ileus

  Fistula

Systemic

  Shock

  Renal failure

  Pulmonary insufficiency (including adult respiratory distress syndrome)

  Coagulopathy

  Gastrointestinal hemorrhage

  Encephalopathy

  Retinopathy

  Hypocalcemia

  Hyperglycemia

(Compiled from Steer ML, Waxman I, Freedman S. Chronic pancreatitis. N Engl J Med 332:1482–1490, 1995; and Owyang C, Levitt MD. Chronic pancreatitis. In: Yamada T. Textbook of Gastroenterology. 2nd ed. Philadelphia: JB Lippincott, 1995:2061.)

regress spontaneously in 50% of cases.[45] Fluid collections may also progress to become pseudocysts or abscesses. A pseudocyst is a collection of pancreatic juice enclosed by a well-defined wall of fibrous tissue forming 4 or more weeks after the onset of an acute attack.[45] Approximately 40% of these acute pseudocysts resolve within 6 weeks.[45] Pseudocysts may be clinically silent or they may cause severe abdominal pain and elevation of pancreatic enzymes. Pancreatic abscess, another late-developing complication, is a circumscribed intra-abdominal collection of pus containing little or no pancreatic necrosis.[45] The term *pancreatic abscess* is also used to describe infection within a pseudocyst. In contrast, the development of pancreatic necrosis is an early event appearing within the first 4 days of an acute attack. Necrosis can be found in approximately 20% of acute pancreatitis cases and is necessary for the subsequent development of infection. Pancreatic infection, which occurs in 30% to 50% of patients, usually develops in the second to third week of illness.[41] Infectious complications account for 80% of deaths from acute pancreatitis.[6,16,17]

Severe acute pancreatitis may be complicated by multiple organ system failure, which most commonly involves the cardiovascular, renal, and pulmonary systems.[6,21] Organ failure is the most important indicator of the severity of acute pancreatitis.[16,18] Cardiovascular decompensation, the result of hypovolemia and vasodilation caused by circulating vasoactive peptides and cytokines, is associated with morbidity and mortality. Acute renal failure is a consequence of hypovolemia and decreased renal perfusion. Pulmonary complications vary from mild arterial hypoxemia, usually detected during the first 2 days of an attack, to adult respiratory distress syndrome, the result of pulmonary parenchymal injury caused by circulating inflammatory mediators.[3] Systemic complications related to organ failure are responsible for death early in the course of acute pancreatitis.

PSYCHOSOCIAL ASPECTS

There have been few studies evaluating the psychosocial aspects of acute pancreatitis. These studies have primarily assessed patients with severe disease, whose quality of life is most likely to be affected. Even patients who recover from an acute attack can have long-term complications, such as diabetes, recurrent disease, and continued abdominal pain.[46] Another important factor in quality of life after severe pancreatitis is the role of alcohol, which can affect quality of life and mortality beyond the disease state. Up to 72% of those patients who had alcohol-induced pancreatitis will decrease their alcohol intake after their disease episode. This type of positive change could improve a patient's quality of life overall. When compared with population control groups, most patients who have recovered from an attack of severe acute pancreatitis rate their physical and mental health equivalent to that of the controls.[47]

THERAPEUTIC PLAN

In the absence of effective specific therapy for the underlying disease process, the treatment of acute pancreatitis remains largely supportive. In patients with mild disease, principles of management include eliminating oral intake, maintaining adequate hydration with intravenous fluid, and providing parenteral analgesia.[21,41] With standard conservative therapy, the majority of cases of acute pancreatitis subside within 3 to 10 days.[17] In contrast, severe acute pancreatitis almost invariably warrants treatment in an intensive care unit. Quantification of the attack severity with the APACHE II system or Ranson's criteria is an important early step.[22,41] A dynamic contrast-enhanced CT scan should be performed in patients with severe acute pancreatitis, as evidenced by the development of organ failure, to detect necrotizing pancreatitis (Fig. 51.3).[41] In the absence of clinical improvement, a CT-guided percutaneous aspiration should be performed to detect infected necrosis, which necessitates surgical débridement.[41] Patients must be reassessed and monitored throughout the attack for the development of complications, particularly organ failure and infection. In addition, eliminating factors that precipitated the acute attack may improve the patient's course and prevent recurrence of disease.[17,21]

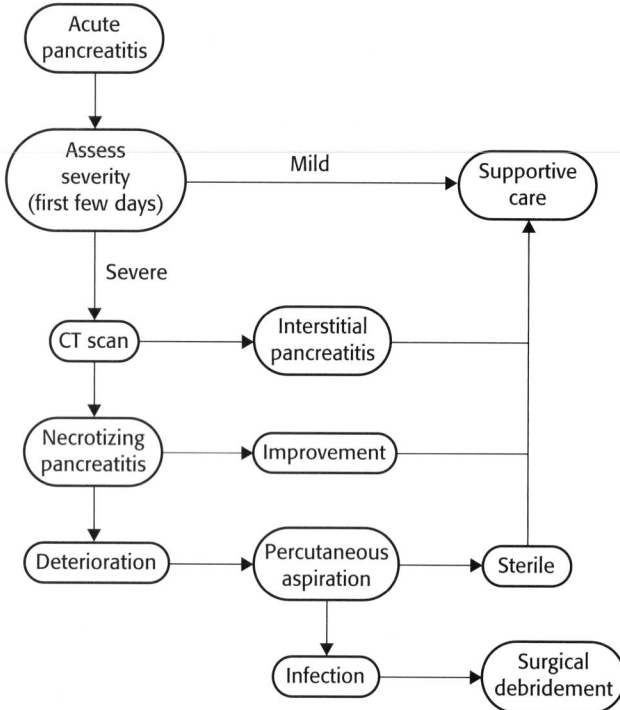

FIGURE 51.3 Algorithm for the management of acute pancreatitis. (Adapted with permission from Banks PA. Practice guidelines in acute pancreatitis. Am J Gastroenterol 92:384, 1997.)

TREATMENT GOALS: ACUTE PANCREATITIS

- Correct any underlying predisposing factors
- Correct biliary tract disease
- Discontinue any possible causative drugs
- Provide supportive care
- Maintain adequate hydration with intravenous fluids
- Provide parenteral analgesia to relieve pain
- Provide adequate nutritional intake
- Evaluate the need for antibiotics in the setting of necrotizing pancreatitis

TREATMENT

GENERAL SUPPORTIVE MEASURES

Acute pancreatitis may be associated with severe intravascular volume contraction and hypovolemia that result from exudation of protein-rich fluid into the inflamed peripancreatic retroperitoneum and peritoneal cavity. In addition, volume losses are incurred through vomiting, hemorrhage, and nasogastric suction. The primary goal of therapy early in the course of acute pancreatitis is to replace intravascular volume and electrolytes to avoid cardiovascular compromise and renal failure. Aggressive fluid resuscitation may also support the pancreatic microcirculation, limiting the development of necrosis. Volume replacement with crystalloid solutions is adequate for most patients, but intravenous colloids may be needed if protein-rich fluid losses are massive.

Potassium, calcium, and magnesium losses may also necessitate intravenous replacement. Hyperglycemia should be managed with insulin as needed. Clinical status, vital signs, and appropriate laboratory and radiographic studies should be reassessed frequently. Severe acute pancreatitis for which aggressive fluid resuscitation and maximal supportive care are needed should be managed in the intensive care setting. The complicated course of severe disease often necessitates continuous hemodynamic and arterial blood gas monitoring, as well as intensive management of cardiovascular, pulmonary, renal, and septic complications.

Traditionally, it has been standard practice to eliminate oral intake of food and liquids early in an acute attack to minimize pancreatic exocrine secretion and halt the autodigestive process. Nasojejunal feedings have been shown to be equally effective compared to total parenteral nutrition

(TPN) without some of the more serious complications seen with TPN and are preferred over TPN. Although it may be reasonable to restrict fat and protein intake to limit pancreatic stimulation, there is little evidence to support the benefit of a low-fat, low-protein diet.[3] Nasogastric suction has not been shown to improve the clinical course of mild to moderate pancreatitis,[47,48] but it is appropriate therapy for patients with severe nausea and vomiting or significant abdominal distention and ileus.[6,17,19,21]

NUTRITION

In 2002 the European Society for Clinical Nutrition and Metabolism (ESPEN) published a consensus article on the use of nutritional strategies in acute pancreatitis.[49] There are several risks from parenteral nutrition in a patient with acute pancreatitis, such as catheter-related sepsis, hyperglycemia, suppression of the immune system, and bacterial translocation resulting from a breakdown of the barrier the intestinal mucosa provides. There was no difference in outcomes in patients with acute pancreatitis who received either nasojejunal feedings or TPN. Disadvantages of TPN include sepsis and hyperglycemia, which can be a result of overfeeding. In addition, TPN costs four times more than nasojejunal feedings.[49]

An important part of therapy for acute pancreatitis is enteral nutrition early in the disease. Not only does this help to preserve body mass, but it also maintains the integrity of the structure and prevents the loss of function of the gastrointestinal tract. Even hypocaloric feedings can be beneficial, as noted by McClave et al.[49] Eighty-two percent of patients in this study who received nasojejunal feedings met their caloric goal, in contrast with 96% of TPN patients. Despite the number of patients not receiving adequate caloric intake, the patients receiving nasojejunal feedings showed no difference in terms of infections or length of stay compared to TPN patients.

Similar results have been seen in patients with severe pancreatitis. Improvements in systemic inflammatory responses were seen in patients who received nasojejunal feedings, compared to patients receiving TPN, who showed little improvement.[50]

Oral feedings may be restarted once pain is under control and the pancreatic enzymes have returned to normal levels. The initial diet should consist mainly of carbohydrates and protein, with fats being instituted gradually over 3 to 6 days.[49]

ANALGESIA

Narcotic analgesics are usually needed to control the severe abdominal pain that often accompanies acute pancreatitis. Transient elevations in serum amylase and lipase that often follow the administration of opiates should not preclude their use, because these effects do not appear to be detrimental to the disease course. Therapy is commonly initiated with meperidine administered parenterally at regular intervals in doses of 50 to 100 mg because it reportedly causes less spasm of the sphincter of Oddi than morphine and its derivatives.[17] However, because there is little evidence to suggest a clinically significant difference in the degree of sphincter spasm produced by any particular opiate, efficacy should be the primary guide for analgesic treatment of these patients.[3]

ANTIBIOTICS

Infection is a serious complication in severe acute necrotizing pancreatitis: mortality rates are reported to be approximately 20% to 30% in this patient population.[51] Even though infection has emerged as an important cause of death in acute pancreatitis, the role of prophylactic antibiotics remains to be firmly established. Early studies evaluating the use of antibiotics in patients with mild disease failed to show any clinical benefit; therefore, they are not recommended.[52] One study suggested that imipenem reduced the incidence of pancreatic infections, but the incidence of organ failure and the mortality rate were not affected.[53] Prophylactic cefuroxime has been shown to reduce mortality but not to decrease the incidence of infection.[54] It is appropriate to initiate empiric antibiotic therapy in patients with pancreatic necrosis confirmed by dynamic contrast-enhanced CT scan and clinical evidence of infection or a deteriorating clinical condition. The presence of infected necrosis should be confirmed with a CT-guided percutaneous needle aspiration of fluid from necrotic areas for Gram stain and culture (Fig. 51.3).[18,41] Pathogens most often isolated from infected necrosis include *Escherichia coli*, *Klebsiella pneumoniae*, *Enterococcus* sp, *Staphylococcus aureus*, *Pseudomonas aeruginosa*, *Proteus mirabilis*, *Enterobacter aerogenes*, and *Bacteroides fragilis*, presumably originating in the colon.[55] The possibility that infection results from a fungal source cannot be ruled out, as fungi are found in the intestine as normal flora and the opportunity for superinfection exists with prophylactic antibiotics.[56] An estimated 10% of cases of acute necrotic pancreatitis are thought to involve fungal organisms. There are no clear recommendations for prophylactic antifungal therapy in severe acute pancreatitis. Antibiotics that can achieve bactericidal concentrations in pancreatic tissue, such as the fluoroquinolones, metronidazole, and imipenem, should be used.[18,52,55] Once infection develops in the necrotic pancreas, surgical débridement is mandatory.[41]

CORRECTING BILIARY TRACT DISEASE

Virtually all clinicians agree that removing residual biliary tract stones is necessary to prevent recurrent attacks of biliary pancreatitis. However, the optimal timing of stone removal and the choice between endoscopic and surgical treatment are subjects of continuing debate. Early ERCP (within 72 hours of admission) is recommended for patients with gallstone pancreatitis who have evidence of biliary sepsis or organ failure.[3,41] Stones in the common bile duct should be removed and a sphincterotomy performed.[41] Otherwise, it appears that either surgical or endoscopic procedures for biliary duct clearance should be performed before discharge from the hospital once pancreatic inflammation has resolved.[6,17]

ALTERNATIVE THERAPIES

There are few studies of alternative therapies in acute pancreatitis. Based on the observation that serum antioxidants are depleted in acute pancreatitis and the correlation between the amount of depletion and severity of pancreatitis, antioxidant therapy (N-acetylcysteine, ascorbic acid, and sodium selenite given intravenously along with alpha-tocopherol and β-carotene given via a nasogastric tube) in patients with severe acute pancreatitis has been investigated. Although antioxidant levels returned to normal, there did not appear to be any additional benefit from this therapy.[57] Some benefit has been shown from including glutamine in TPN formulations for acute pancreatitis; however, TPN is no longer a preferred therapy.[58]

FUTURE THERAPIES

Although medical treatment of acute pancreatitis is currently supportive, major goals in the future should include limiting systemic complications and preventing pancreatic necrosis.[41] Attempts at inflammatory mediator antagonism have focused on activated pancreatic enzymes; however, the destructive products of leukocytes, including elastase, phospholipase A_2, platelet activating factor, nitric oxide, and cytokines, have not been addressed in prospective, randomized trials. Preliminary studies with the platelet activating factor antagonist lexipafant have demonstrated that a therapeutic window exists for cytokine antagonism.[59,60] Animal studies have also shown that colloidal hemodilution may improve the pancreatic microcirculation and minimize necrosis.[3] Well-designed, controlled, prospective studies are warranted to establish the value of these medical therapies. Additional studies are also needed to determine the optimal use of prophylactic antibiotics for improving mortality in patients with pancreatic necrosis.

IMPROVING OUTCOMES

Early identification of severe acute pancreatitis should enhance patient outcomes.[41] Formalized scoring systems and clinical evidence of organ failure can assist the clinician in this regard. Severe disease almost invariably warrants management in an intensive care unit for aggressive cardiovascular and pulmonary support. Patients must be reassessed and monitored throughout the attack for complications, particularly organ failure and infection. When infection is suspected, pharmacists should assist in selecting and monitoring appropriate antibiotic therapy. Invasive procedures such as surgical débridement of infected necrosis and endoscopic or surgical removal of gallstones also are important for optimizing patient outcome.[41] Cytokine antagonism may eventually have a role in reducing the morbidity and mortality of severe acute pancreatitis.[37]

In addition, eliminating factors that precipitated the acute attack may improve the patient's course and prevent recurrence of disease.[17,21] Pharmacists can assist in identifying drug-induced pancreatitis and recommend therapeutic alternatives for the offending agent. Because alcoholic pancreatitis is associated with chronic pancreatic damage, substance abuse counseling should be offered to support the patient's efforts to abstain.[6,21]

PHARMACOECONOMICS

Although data about the economic impact of acute pancreatitis are sparse, experts have recognized the resource demands of intensive care management in severe disease.[61] Because survivors of severe acute pancreatitis report excellent quality of life, these substantial costs may be justified.[61] As disease-specific therapies, such as cytokine antagonists, become available, their contribution to cost containment must be analyzed.

CHRONIC PANCREATITIS

DEFINITION

Chronic pancreatitis is generally defined as an inflammatory disease process leading to irreversible damage to pancreatic structure and function. All patients experience fibrosis and loss of exocrine tissue, and many lose endocrine function as well. The clinical course may consist of recurrent acute attacks, which are difficult to distinguish from acute pancreatitis, or chronic symptoms that usually, but not inevitably, progress. Students of medical history are referred to Pitchu-

moni's review of chronic pancreatitis from the first description of the pancreas in 300 BC to the present.[62]

ETIOLOGY

Subclassification of chronic pancreatitis based on etiologic, pathologic, radiologic, or other criteria has proved difficult. One classification system that has been used is the Marseilles-Rome system, which distinguishes three types.[63] The first type, chronic calcifying pancreatitis, is the most common, accounting for more than 95% of cases.[64] It usually results from alcohol abuse and is characterized by intraductal protein plugs and, often, calcified stones. The second type, chronic obstructive pancreatitis, is relatively uncommon and occurs as a result of obstruction of the main pancreatic duct by tumor, stricture, or congenital abnormalities. This type is notable in that protein plugs and stones are absent, and damage may be reversible in part when the obstruction is alleviated. The third type, chronic inflammatory pancreatitis, is characterized by fibrosis, infiltration by monocytes, and atrophy of exocrine tissue. This form has been associated with autoimmune disease.

A more recent classification is the TIGAR-O system.[2,65] This system proposes that there are several risk factors that may interact with each other to predispose patients to pancreatic disease. As a result, this system better addresses the complexity and heterogeneity of chronic pancreatitis.

Toxic-metabolic. This classification includes alcohol, the most common etiology of chronic pancreatitis in the United States and other developed countries. However, only 10% to 20% of alcoholics develop chronic pancreatitis.[66]

Idiopathic. Up to 30% of patients have no identifiable risk factors for the development of chronic pancreatitis.

Genetic. Several genes have been identified that seem to predispose patients to developing pancreatic disease.

Autoimmune. Although this has been thought to be rare, it may account for some of the cases of "idiopathic" chronic pancreatitis.

Recurrent and severe acute pancreatitis. Although historically acute pancreatitis and chronic pancreatitis have been regarded as discrete clinical entities, it is now thought that severe acute pancreatitis may cause permanent damage to the gland.

Obstructive. Obstruction of the main pancreatic duct by neoplasms, stenosis, or other mechanisms can cause chronic pancreatic damage.

In summary, the precise etiology of chronic pancreatitis is poorly understood and the subject of ongoing debate.[2] Multiple factors may be involved. The role of genetic predisposition has not yet been elucidated, although several genetic mutations have been associated with some forms of chronic pancreatitis. Ethanol abuse is involved in most cases of chronic pancreatitis, particularly in Western countries, accounting for approximately 70% of reported cases. Although a relatively small percentage of alcoholics actually develop clinical symptoms of chronic pancreatitis, as many as 45% show evidence of the disease at autopsy (approximately 50 times the incidence in nondrinkers).[5] A tropical form also exists in some Afro-Asian countries; malnutrition and perhaps dietary toxins are presumed to play a role.[67,68] Other potential etiologic factors include trauma, hyperparathyroidism/hypercalcemia, hyperlipidemia, autoimmune disease, and tobacco use.[2,3,5,69] Up to 30% of cases are classified as idiopathic, and this form appears to have two subsets: early and late onset. Although gallstone disease may coexist with chronic pancreatitis, cholelithiasis does not appear to predispose a patient to this disease.[3–5,62,70–72]

EPIDEMIOLOGY

As mentioned previously, the incidence and prevalence data are meager and specific to geographic area. Prevalence estimates range from 0.03% to 5%, and the incidence may approximate 3 to 9 per 100,000 inhabitants per year. Men are substantially more likely to be affected than women.[3–5,62]

PATHOPHYSIOLOGY

Over the past several decades, numerous theories have been advanced in an attempt to explain the complex pathogenesis of chronic pancreatitis. Although each may describe a piece of the puzzle, none adequately accounts for all findings. This may be due in part to the heterogeneity of the disease, as evidenced by the classification systems discussed previously.[2,3]

Alcohol-related injury to the pancreas is perhaps the best understood process. Ethanol is metabolized in pancreatic acinar cells by both oxidative and nonoxidative pathways. Ethanol, its metabolites, and the resulting increase in oxidative stress may all contribute to increased local levels of digestive enzymes and an increased risk of autodigestion. This results in inflammation and the release of proinflammatory cytokines. Although transforming growth factor-β has received much attention in recent years, other mediators may include platelet-derived growth factor, interleukin-1 and interleukin-6, and tumor necrosis factor-α. These mediators in turn activate pancreatic stellate cells that synthesize collagen and fibronectin, leading to fibrosis.[2,73,74]

A related theory that has been widely accepted in the past proposes that alcohol changes the nature of pancreatic secretions, predisposing to the formation of protein plugs and stones, leading to ductal obstruction. In the presence of alcohol, the absolute amount of protein in pancreatic secretions increases, facilitating the formation of protein plugs, particularly in the smaller ductules. GP2, a 97-kilodalton protein that is analogous to the renal cast protein uromodulin, has been isolated from ductal plugs and may play a role in their formation.[75] The resulting obstruction can lead to inflammation and fibrosis, and protein plugs act as a nidus for the formation of calcium carbonate stones.[3–5] In addition, there is decreased secretion of lithostatine, also known as pancreatic stone protein, which normally inhibits the formation of insoluble calcium salts in the ductules. Hence, a deficiency of this protein may allow increased precipitation of calcium salts, exacerbating obstruction, inflammation, and fibrosis.[3–5,76] Stones, however, are not found in all cases of alcoholic pancreatitis, and this process may not play a central role in the pathogenesis.[2]

However, alcohol-related injury is only one piece of the puzzle. A better understanding of the pathogenesis of chronic pancreatitis may lead to strategies for disease mitigation or prevention.

CLINICAL PRESENTATION AND DIAGNOSIS

SIGNS AND SYMPTOMS

Pain and maldigestion are the hallmarks of chronic pancreatitis, although a significant number of patients also develop diabetes mellitus, pseudocysts, or jaundice.[3,5,70,77] The causes of pain have not been delineated, but increased intraductal and parenchymal pressure, ischemia, pseudocyst, obstruction of the bile duct, or inflammation, especially in and around the pancreatic nerves, may be involved.[3,5,78–84] Pain may also be caused by extrapancreatic complications such as biliary stricture or duodenal stenosis.[3,5,84] This pain, sometimes accompanied by nausea and vomiting, is similar to that of acute pancreatitis. It is epigastric and often described as deep and penetrating, with a characteristic radiation to the back. Relief may be obtained by leaning forward from a sitting position, and pain is usually aggravated by eating. This pain with eating, in addition to maldigestion and malabsorption, contributes to the weight loss often observed in these patients.[3,5,82] Up to 20% of patients may be pain-free, but this is more commonly the case with idiopathic rather than alcoholic pancreatitis.[4,5,62,73,85]

Loss of exocrine function occurs in all cases of chronic pancreatitis, but it may remain subclinical until fairly late in the disease. Malabsorption does not manifest itself until less than 10% of pancreatic secretory function remains.[1,84] Lipase activity decreases relatively more than protease activity; therefore, steatorrhea presents earlier and is usually more severe than azotorrhea.[3,5,84,86,87] Although some decrease in absorption of carbohydrates and fat-soluble vitamins does occur, symptoms rarely develop.[5,84,87] Bicarbonate secretion also declines with disease progression.[64,84,88]

The following scenario summarizes the clinical course of a representative patient. He is an alcoholic who began to drink heavily at age 20 and who started to experience attacks of pain by age 30. Abdominal radiographs showed calcification of the pancreas. At 40 years of age, pancreatic insufficiency had progressed to the point that steatorrhea was troublesome, and he developed glucose intolerance. He was dead at 50, probably from complications of alcoholism rather than pancreatitis per se.[3,4,84,89] Major predictors of mortality appear to be the age at diagnosis (the older the patient, the worse the prognosis), smoking, and drinking.[90] Chronic pancreatitis is also associated with an increased risk of pancreatic cancer.[91–93]

DIAGNOSIS AND CLINICAL FINDINGS

A diagnosis of chronic pancreatitis is generally straightforward in an alcoholic patient with recurrent bouts of epigastric pain and evidence of calcification of the pancreas by radiography. The diagnosis is made more difficult, however, if the patient is without pain, or if a distinction is sought between chronic pancreatitis and either recurring acute pancreatitis or pancreatic cancer. Physical examination and routine laboratory tests are of limited utility, since the results are usually within normal limits. Even serum amylase and lipase levels are generally normal, although they may be elevated during acute exacerbations or decreased late in the disease. Imaging techniques and pancreatic function tests provide the most useful diagnostic tools.[3–5] They are presented below in approximately the order in which they should be considered based on effectiveness, invasiveness, and expense. A review of diagnostic criteria and methodologies has been recently published.[91]

Imaging Studies. Radiography can reveal calcifications (usually diagnostic for chronic pancreatitis) and displacement of the stomach or duodenum, indicating the presence of a pseudocyst. Ultrasonography usually shows calcifications, pancreatic enlargement, and pseudocysts, although CT is superior at detecting pseudocysts and can reveal dilated pancreatic ducts as well as pancreatic enlargement and calcifications. ERCP is the most sensitive procedure for viewing changes in the ductal system and is currently considered the gold standard of imaging; however, there is the risk of causing pancreatitis.[1,3,5,94,95] Newer techniques such as magnetic resonance cholangiopancreatography (MR-CP) and endoscopic ultrasonography (EUS) are gaining popularity.[3,94]

Pancreatic Function Tests. Pancreatic function tests may be used if imaging studies are inconclusive. These tests, which can be classified as direct or indirect, have been reviewed extensively.[3,5,96–99] Direct tests, including the secretin-pancreozymin and Lundh tests, are invasive, requiring intubation of the duodenum. In the secretin-pancreozymin test, usually considered the gold standard for measuring pancreatic secretory function, a patient is given intravenous secretin and CCK, and the subsequent increase in secretion is measured. The Lundh test is similar, with pancreatic secretion measured after the ingestion of a test meal.

Indirect tests measure markers of pancreatic function in the blood, urine, breath, or stool. Indirect tests are of limited usefulness due to their relative lack of sensitivity early in the course of chronic pancreatitis. Examples of indirect tests include measurement of fat or chymotrypsin in stool samples and measuring urinary excretion of para-aminobenzoic acid (PABA) after hydrolytic cleaving of PABA from NBT-PABA by chymotrypsin in the intestine (bentiromide test).

A combination of imaging studies and pancreatic function tests may be necessary for a definitive diagnosis of chronic pancreatitis, particularly early in the disease (Table 51.7).

PSYCHOSOCIAL ASPECTS

Many patients develop chronic pancreatitis as a result of alcoholism. This patient population can be very difficult to manage. If the patient is still actively drinking, every effort should be made to convince him or her to abstain. Unfortunately, however, this may not slow the course of the disease.[4] Alcoholics may also be at increased risk for addiction to opioid analgesic agents, complicating pain management. Treatment regimens and follow-up need to be tailored to individual patient profiles.

THERAPEUTIC PLAN

Chronic pancreatitis is usually progressive and, with the possible exception of the obstructive form, irreversible. Treatment, therefore, is directed at managing the pain, maldigestion, and other complications that arise from this disease. When a patient presents for medical treatment, assessment of

TABLE 51.7	Selected Diagnostic Tests for Chronic Pancreatitis

Imaging Techniques
- Plain abdominal radiography
- Ultrasonography
- Computed tomography
- Magnetic resonance cholangiopancreatography
- Endoscopic retrograde cholangiopancreatography[a]

Pancreatic Function Tests
- Direct tests: measurement of pancreatic exocrine secretions
  - Secretin-pancreozymin test[a]
  - Lundh test
- Indirect tests: measurement of enzyme action
  - Bentiromide (NBT-PABA) test
  - Fecal chymotrypsin concentration
  - Fecal fat analysis

[a] Currently considered gold standards. (1,3,69)

symptoms and prior medication use is an important starting point. In particular, narcotic use and potential for addiction should be evaluated.

TREATMENT GOALS: CHRONIC PANCREATITIS

Pain is the symptom that commonly brings patients to the attention of the medical community. Alleviation of this pain is an important goal of therapy. In addition, both exocrine and endocrine insufficiency must be appropriately managed. Treating exocrine insufficiency will be discussed in this chapter, while insulin insufficiency is covered in Chapter 40. Diabetes develops in 40% to 80% of chronic pancreatitis patients, usually late in the course of the disease.[3,5] One key difference between type 1 diabetes mellitus and pancreatic diabetes should be mentioned, however: in chronic pancreatitis, there is loss of glucagon as well as insulin secretion, leading to diabetes that is very hard to control, or ''brittle.''[3]

- Control pain using analgesics, enzyme replacement, and endoscopic and surgical treatment
- Manage maldigestion and malabsorption through enzyme replacement
- Manage diabetes

TREATMENT

PHARMACOTHERAPY

Pain. The pain of chronic pancreatitis, which may be episodic or persistent, is a poorly understood phenomenon, complicating decisions about therapy. The lack of controlled clinical trials makes it difficult to define treatment strategies. As a result, there has not been a universally accepted standard of care for these patients. Warshaw et al sought to address this in their review of pain management,[98] and they

proposed an algorithm for the treatment of pain in chronic pancreatitis (Fig. 51.4).[99]

Abstinence from alcohol may reduce pain in up to 50% of patients, but the majority will require some form of analgesia.[79,82,85,87] Having patients keep a log of their pain may aid in assessment.[98] Salicylates, nonsteroidal anti-inflammatory drugs, or acetaminophen should be tried initially, perhaps in conjunction with a low-fat diet.[98] Adjunctive therapy with tricyclic antidepressants or selective serotonin reuptake inhibitors may prove beneficial in some patients, although evidence of efficacy is merely anecdotal.[81,83,85,98]

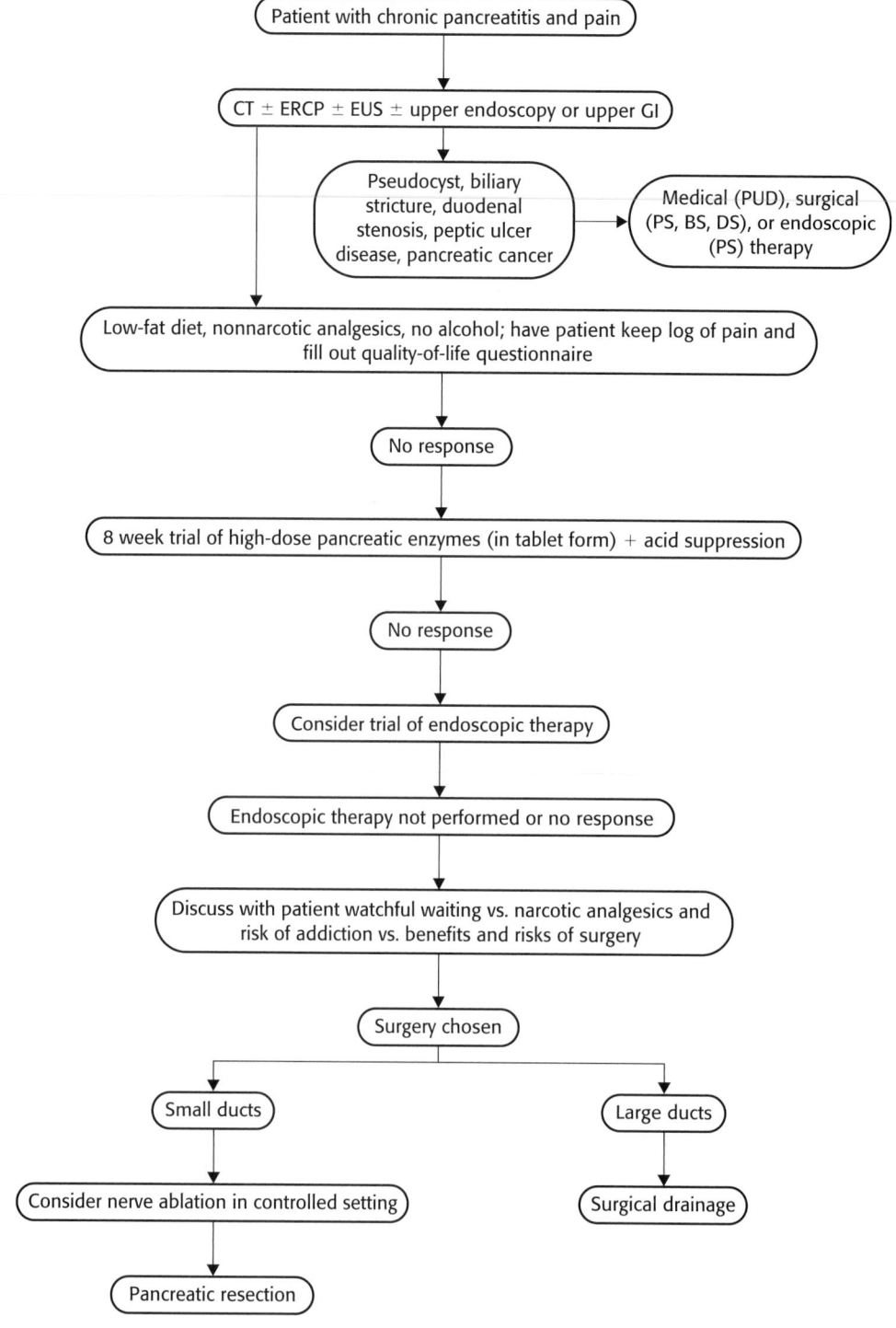

FIGURE 51.4 Guideline for treatment of pain in chronic pancreatitis. BS, biliary stricture; CT, computed tomography; DS, duodenal stenosis; ERCP, endoscopic retrograde cholangiopancreatography; EUS, endoscopic ultrasonography; PS, pseudocyst; PUD, peptic ulcer disease. (Reprinted with permission from Warshaw AL, Banks PA, Fernandez-del Castillo C. AGA technical review on treatment of pain in chronic pancreatitis. Gastroenterology 115:763–764, 1998.)

Enzyme replacement therapy, which will also be discussed for the treatment of maldigestion, may help to alleviate pain, especially in patients with nonalcoholic chronic pancreatitis.[3,7,72,82–84,98] Clinical trial data have not always shown effectiveness, however.[3,73,84,98,100] It is presumed that the presence of exogenous proteases in the duodenum suppresses pancreatic function through a negative feedback mechanism. This mechanism involves degradation of a CCK-releasing peptide by trypsin in the duodenum, inhibiting the release of CCK.[3,14,98,101] Enzymes contained in nonenteric-coated preparations may be more reliably delivered to the duodenum than enzymes from enteric-coated dosage forms, since the latter are sometimes released in more distal portions of the small intestine. This is due to the relatively low duodenal pH caused by decreased bicarbonate secretion in chronic pancreatitis.[63,88] As a result, nonenteric preparations may be more effective at suppressing CCK release and reducing pain.[1,3,72,98] In theory, the addition of an H_2-receptor antagonist or a proton pump inhibitor could decrease acid-stimulated pancreatic secretion and diminish pain, but this has not been demonstrated. These agents are frequently tried due to their ease of use and relative safety.[84,98]

Other agents may also have utility in the control of pain. Octreotide, a somatostatin analogue, has not consistently demonstrated efficacy in chronic disease,[1,84,98] but it may have a role in the management of pancreatic pseudocysts[102,103] and in decreasing complications after pancreatic surgery.[104] Antioxidant therapy may also prove beneficial, since patients with chronic pancreatitis seem to be deficient in endogenous antioxidants.[3,84,98] Further study is required before specific recommendations can be made, however.

For patients still experiencing pain, the choices remaining are opioid analgesics and interventional therapy. Unfortunately, there are no well-defined criteria for making this decision. Opioid analgesics may prove very effective, although there is a very real risk of addiction, particularly in this patient population.[73,84,98,105] Refer to Chapter 64 for a discussion of these agents.

Despite maximum medical management, up to 30% of patients still experience pain.[89] This pain may diminish, or "burn out," over time as the pancreas becomes progressively more fibrotic, but this phenomenon may not occur in as many patients as was once thought.[3,73,98] Approximately half of chronic pancreatitis patients will require endoscopic or surgical intervention to control pain, although this may not reliably improve qualify of life.[1]

Endoscopic treatment may be effective for stenosis, strictures, or stones. Stent placement relieves intraductal pressure and pain in many patients, although there is a risk of ductal injury. Patients may also experience pain relief with the elimination of intraductal pancreatic stones by lithotripsy or pancreatic duct sphincterotomy. Improvement is reported in 50% to 85% of patients undergoing endoscopic therapy, but many questions remain.[3,95,98,106]

Surgery is usually reserved for the patients with intractable pain. The procedure of choice for patients with dilated ducts (larger than 6 or 7 mm) is surgical drainage with a procedure called lateral pancreaticojejunostomy. For patients with small duct disease, surgical denervation and pancreatic resection are options. These procedures have been reviewed extensively.[3,72,98,107–109]

Maldigestion/Malabsorption. Patients with documented weight loss and steatorrhea should receive treatment for maldigestion. Two types of pancreatic enzyme replacement preparations are currently available. Pancreatin is derived from freeze-dried porcine or bovine pancreases and contains at least 2 USP units of lipase and 25 USP units each of protease and amylase per milligram. Pancrelipase, extracted from porcine pancreases, is more potent, containing at least 24, 100, and 100 USP units of lipase, protease, and amylase per milligram, respectively (Table 51.8).[108]

Rapid-release and enteric-coated dosage forms are available. While rapid-release forms more reliably deliver proteases to the upper duodenum, where they may exert a negative feedback inhibitory effect, they expose lipase to the acid environment of the stomach. Lipase is pH labile, maximally active at pH 8 and irreversibly inactivated at pH less than 4. Enteric-coated microspheres, which dissolve at approximately pH 5.6 to 6.0, better protect lipase from gastric acidity, but enzyme release may be delayed. While rapid-release forms are preferable for pain control, enteric-coated products are more effective in the treatment of steatorrhea.[1,72,84]

Since lipid malabsorption and steatorrhea are the primary clinical problems associated with pancreatic insufficiency, the dose of lipase to be delivered to the duodenum is a paramount concern. Maximal postprandial delivery of lipase from a normal pancreas is 140,000 units per hour for 4 hours. Supplying 5% to 10% of this will significantly decrease steatorrhea; therefore, the enzyme supplement should usually provide approximately 30,000 (25,000 to 40,000) units over a 4-hour period, although regimens should be individualized for each patient.[3,70,84,109–111]

Efficacy of therapy can be assessed by monitoring the fat content of stools. If steatorrhea persists, another agent can be added to increase gastric pH in an attempt to increase the delivery of active lipase to the duodenum. Agents that may be useful include H_2-receptor antagonists and proton pump inhibitors.[12,73,84,108,112]

Even with careful management of supplements, however, the elimination of steatorrhea is very difficult.[12,109] Research into other forms of enzyme replacement therapies, including bacterial lipase and bioengineered human gastric lipase, are ongoing.[109,110] Figure 51.5 presents one possible approach to enzyme replacement therapy for steatorrhea.

Patients should be counseled to take supplements just before or with meals. The microspheres/microtablets contained in capsules should not be crushed, but they may be mixed with soft food such as applesauce, if necessary. The pH of the food should be below 5 to avoid premature dissolu-

TABLE 51.8	Some Commercial Pancreatic Enzyme Preparations

Product[a]	Formulation[b]	Dosage Form[c]	Enzyme Content (USP Units)		
			Lipase	Protease	Amylase
Rapid Release					
Cotazym	PL	C	8,000	30,000	30,000
Donnazyme	PC	T	1,000	12,500	12,500
Ku-Zyme HP	PL	C	8,000	30,000	30,000
Panokase	PL	T	8,000	30,000	30,000
Pancreatin 4x USP	PC	T	12,000	60,000	60,000
8x USP	PC	T	22,500	180,000	180,000
Viokase	PL	P	16,800	70,000	70,000
Viokase 8	PL	T	8,000	30,000	30,000
Viokase 16	PL	T	16,000	60,000	60,000
Delayed-Release Capsules					
Cotazym-S	PL	MS	5,000	20,000	20,000
Creon 5 Minimicrospheres	PL	MS	5,000	18,750	16,600
Creon 10 Minimicrospheres	PL	MS	10,000	37,500	33,200
Creon 20 Minimicrospheres	PL	MS	20,000	75,000	66,400
Encron 10	PL	MS	10,000	37,500	33,200
Lipram 4500	PL	MS	4,500	25,000	20,000
Lipram-PN10	PL	MS	10,000	30,000	30,000
Lipram-CR10	PL	MS	10,000	37,500	33,200
Lipram-UL12	PL	MS	12,000	39,000	39,000
Lipram-PN16	PL	MS	16,000	48,000	48,000
Lipram-UL18	PL	MS	18,000	58,500	58,500
Lipram-UL20	PL	MS	20,000	65,000	65,000
Lipram-CR20	PL	MS	20,000	75,000	66,400
Pancrebarb MS-8	PL	MS	8,000	45,000	40,000
Pancrease	PL	MS	4,500	25,000	20,000
Pancrease MT-4	PL	MT	4,000	12,000	12,000
Pancrease MT-10	PL	MT	10,000	30,000	30,000
Pancrease MT-16	PL	MT	16,000	48,000	48,000
Pancrease MT-20	PL	MT	20,000	44,000	56,600
Pancron 10	PL	MS	10,000	37,500	33,200
Pancron 20	PL	MS	20,000	75,000	66,400
Ultrase	PL	MS	4,500	25,000	20,000
Ultrase MT12	PL	MT	12,000	39,000	39,000
Ultrase MT18	PL	MT	18,000	58,500	58,500
Ultrase MT20	PL	MT	20,000	65,000	65,000
Zymase	PL	MS	12,000	24,000	24,000

[a] These products, available before passage of the 1938 Food, Drug, and Cosmetic Act, are not approved by the FDA and cannot be considered pharmaceutically or therapeutically equivalent.[11]
[b] PC, pancreatin; PL, pancrelipase.
[c] C, capsule; MS, enteric-coated microspheres; MT, enteric-coated microtablets; P, powder; T, tablet.

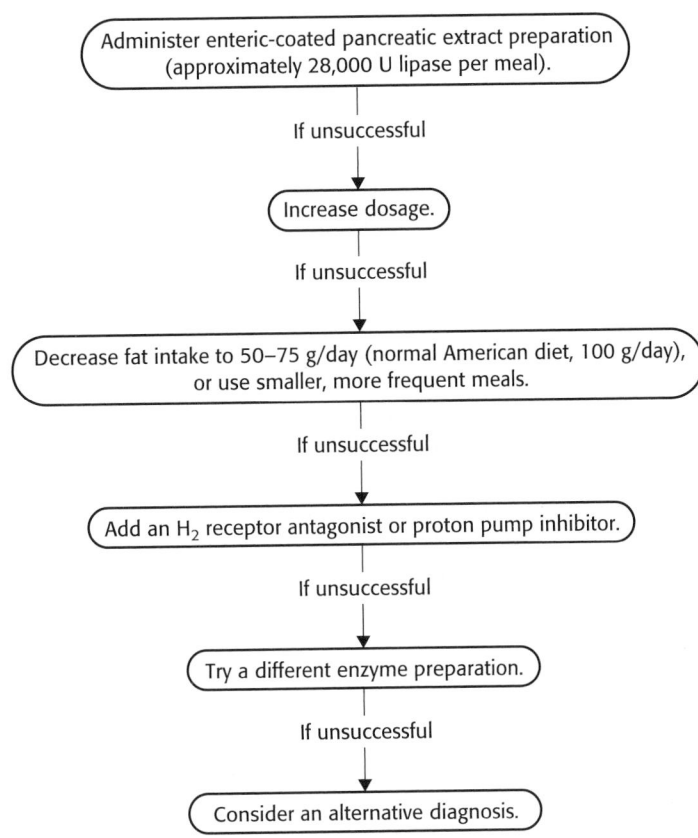

FIGURE 51.5 Treatment of steatorrhea.

tion of the enteric coating. Different products may not be bioequivalent, and changes in regimen should not be made without consulting a physician or pharmacist.[84]

Problems that may be encountered with enzyme-replacement therapy, especially at high doses, include abdominal pain, oral and perianal irritation, nausea, vomiting, diarrhea, and rare hypersensitivity. There have also been reports of hyperuricosuria, although this appears to be more common in cystic fibrosis patients receiving very high doses of pancreatic enzymes. Finally, patient compliance is often less than optimal due to the administration of large numbers of capsules, gastrointestinal distress, and expense.[13,70] The overall safety and tolerability of pancreatic extracts, however, appears to be good.[113]

FUTURE THERAPIES

Chronic pancreatitis is a heterogeneous disease state, and it is likely that response to a therapeutic modality depends, at least in part, upon the etiology and clinical course of the disease in a particular patient. This has not been addressed to date in clinical trials, since the study populations generally reflect the heterogeneity of the population at large. Defining which patient subgroup may benefit from a particular therapy will help to guide treatment. Gene therapy, although years from clinical application, may prevent or reverse pancreatic damage in certain patients.[1,111,114]

IMPROVING OUTCOMES

This patient population presents challenges, particularly if there is continued alcohol consumption. Substance abuse programs may help to establish and maintain abstinence, and referral to a pain clinic may be warranted. A multidisciplinary team approach should improve patient outcomes, although evidence for this approach is only anecdotal. One physician should manage narcotic analgesics.[83]

Quality of life data are sparse, and much of the data has been collected in patients who have undergone surgical intervention.[3,85,115] A more global study was recently conducted in Germany.[116] In this study, patients with chronic pancreatitis reported lower quality of life in all areas surveyed. As one might expect, chronic pain, pancreatic diarrhea, and unemployment were particularly problematic. There are also data to suggest that the development of insulin-requiring diabetes has a significant negative impact on quality of life.[115] Improving therapeutic outcomes will almost certainly contribute to improved quality of life for patients with chronic pancreatitis.

PHARMACOECONOMICS

To date, no studies have been published evaluating the economic impact of chronic pancreatitis or its therapy. This information will be needed to refine emerging therapeutic algorithms.

KEY POINTS

- Acute and chronic pancreatitis have historically been considered distinct clinical entities that are often, although not always, alcohol-related. Acute pancreatitis is an autodigestive process characterized by inflammation, edema, and necrosis, while chronic pancreatitis is the result of poorly understood processes leading to irreversible loss of functional tissue. In acute pancreatitis, it is important to establish the severity of the attack so that appropriate therapy can be instituted and the patient's risk for developing complications evaluated. With chronic pancreatitis, care is directed toward pain relief and managing declining endocrine and exocrine function. In both, therapy remains almost exclusively supportive. Although there have been recent advances in our understanding of pathophysiology and treatment, much remains unclear

- Controlled clinical trials are needed to assess the role of medical therapy directed at the underlying pathogenesis of acute and chronic pancreatic disease.
  Acute Pancreatitis:
  - The mortality associated with acute pancreatitis ranges from 5% to 10%
  - The most common causes of acute pancreatitis are alcohol and gallstones
  - Patients with severe acute pancreatitis should be identified early in the course of the disease and will likely require intensive care, including fluid replacement and nasojejunal feeding. Pain management with an opioid analgesic is usually required
  - Antibiotic prophylaxis is not recommended in cases of acute pancreatitis
  - Patients should be assessed throughout the course of an acute attack for the development of complications such as organ failure and infection
  - Therapy for acute pancreatitis is supportive. Future therapies will be directed at curtailing the inflammatory process
  Chronic Pancreatitis:
  - Most cases of chronic pancreatitis are alcohol-related and are usually progressive and irreversible
  - The clinical course of chronic pancreatitis varies widely, complicating the diagnosis and therapy
  - Treatment of chronic pancreatitis is directed at managing pain, steatorrhea, diabetes, and other complications
  - Future trials of chronic pancreatitis should stratify patients by etiology or clinical course, compare treatment regimens, determine the cost-effectiveness of therapy, and assess patients' quality of life

SUGGESTED READINGS

Meier R, Beglinger C, Layer P, et al. Consensus statement: ESPEN guidelines on nutrition in acute pancreatitis. Clin Nutr 21:173–183, 2002.

Mitchell RMS, Byrne MF, Baillie J. Pancreatitis. Lancet 361: 1447–1455, 2003.

Nathens AB, Curtis JR, Beale RJ, et al. Management of the critically ill patient with severe acute pancreatitis. Crit Care Med 32:2524–2536, 2004.

REFERENCES

1. Mitchell RMS, Byrne MF, Baille J. Pancreatitis. Lancet 361: 1447–1455, 2003.
2. Stevens T, Conwell DL, Auccaro G. Pathogenesis of chronic pancreatitis: an evident-based review of past theories and recent developments. Am J Gastroenterol 90:2256–2270, 2004.
3. Fosmark CE. Chronic pancreatitis. In: Feldman M, Sleisenger MH, Scharschmidt BF. Gastrointestinal and Liver Disease: Pathophysiology, Diagnosis, Management. 6th ed. Philadelphia: WB Saunders, 1998:809.
4. Steer ML, Waxman I, Freedman S. Chronic pancreatitis. N Engl J Med 332:1482–1490, 1995.
5. Owyang C, Levitt MD. Chronic pancreatitis. In: Yamada T. Textbook of Gastroenterology. 2nd ed. Philadelphia: JB Lippincott, 1995:2061.
6. Gorelick FS. Acute pancreatitis. In: Yamada T. Textbook of Gastroenterology. 2nd ed. Philadelphia: JB Lippincott, 1995:2064.
7. Magee DJ, Burdick JS. Anatomy, histology, embryology, and developmental anomalies of the pancreas. In: Feldman M, Sleisenger MH, Scharschmidt BF. Gastrointestinal and Liver Disease: Pathophysiology, Diagnosis, Management. 6th ed. Philadelphia: WB Saunders, 1998:871.
8. Simeone DM, Mulholland MW. Pancreas: anatomy and structural anomalies. In: Yamada T, ed. Textbook of Gastroenterology. 4th ed. Philadelphia: Lippincott Williams & Wilkins, 2003:2013–2026.
9. Pandol SJ. Pancreatic physiology and secretory testing. In: Feldman M, Sleisenger MH, Scharschmidt BF. Gastrointestinal and Liver Disease: Pathophysiology, Diagnosis, Management. 6th ed. Philadelphia: WB Saunders, 1998:871.
10. Owyang C, Williams JA. Pancreatic secretion. In: Yamada T. Textbook of Gastroenterology. 2nd ed. Philadelphia: JB Lippincott, 1995:361.
11. Valenzuela JE, Pancreatic physiology. In: Valenzuela JE, Reber HA, Ribet A. Medical and Surgical Diseases of the Pancreas. New York: Igaku-Shoin, 1991:1.
12. Lebenthal E, Rolston DDK, Holsclaw DS. Enzyme therapy for pancreatic insufficiency: present status and future needs. Pancreas 9: 1–12, 1994.
13. Chey WY. Regulation of pancreatic exocrine secretion. Int J Pancreatol 9:7–20, 1991.
14. Owyang C, Louie DS, Tatum D. Feedback regulation of pancreatic enzyme secretion: suppression of cholecystokinin release by trypsin. J Clin Invest 77:2042–2047, 1986.
15. DiMagno EP, Chari S. Acute pancreatitis. In: Feldman M, Sleisenger MH, Scharschmidt BF. Gastrointestinal and Liver Disease: Pathophysiology, Diagnosis, Management. 6th ed. Philadelphia: WB Saunders, 1998:913.
16. Bradley EL. A clinically based classification system for acute pancreatitis. Arch Surg 128:586–590, 1993.
17. Marshall JB. Acute pancreatitis: a review with an emphasis on new developments. Arch Intern Med 153:1185–1198, 1993.
18. Banks PA. Acute pancreatitis: medical and surgical management. Am J Gastroenterol 89(Suppl):S78–85, 1994.
19. DiMagno EP. Treatment of mild acute pancreatitis. In: Bradley EL. Acute pancreatitis: diagnosis and therapy. New York: Raven, 1994: 261–263.
20. Topazian M, Gorelick FS. Acute pancreatitis. In: Yamada T. Textbook of Gastroenterology. 2nd ed. Philadelphia: JB Lippincott, 1995:2026.
21. Steinberg W, Tenner S. Acute pancreatitis. N Engl J Med 330: 1198–2010, 1994.

22. Gupta PK, Al-Kawas FH. Acute pancreatitis: diagnosis and management. Am Fam Physician 52:435–443, 1995.
23. Moreau JA, Zinsmeister AR, Melton LJ, Dimagno EP. Gallstone pancreatitis and the effect of cholecystectomy: a population-based cohort study. Mayo Clin Proc 63:466, 1988.
24. Underwood TW, Frye CB. Drug-induced pancreatitis. Clin Pharm 12:440–448, 1993.
25. Mallory A, Kern F. Drug-induced pancreatitis: a critical review. Gastroenterology 78:813–820, 1980.
26. Runzi M, Layer P. Drug-associated pancreatitis: facts and fiction. Pancreas 13:100–109, 1996.
27. Goyal SB, Goyal RS. Ketorolac tromethamine-induced acute pancreatitis. Arch Intern Med 158:411, 1998.
28. Bosch X. Losartan-induced acute pancreatitis. Ann Intern Med 127:1043–1044, 1997.
29. Gerson R, Serrano A, Villalobos A, et al. Acute pancreatitis secondary to ifosfamide. J Emerg Med 15:645–647, 1997.
30. Bosch X, Bernadich O. Acute pancreatitis during treatment with amiodarone. Lancet 350:1300, 1997.
31. Liviu L, Yair L, Yehuda S. Pancreatitis induced by clarithromycin. Ann Intern Med 125:701, 1996.
32. Hastier P, Longo F, Buckley M, et al. Pancreatitis induced by codeine: a case report with positive rechallenge. Gut 41:705–706, 1997.
33. Fernandez J, Sala M, Panes J, et al. Acute pancreatitis after long-term 5-aminosalicyclic acid therapy. Am J Gastroenterol 92:2302–2303, 1997.
34. McBride CE, Yavorski RT, Moses FM, et al. Acute pancreatitis associated with continuous infusion cytarabine therapy: a case report. Cancer 77:2588–2591, 1996.
35. Madsen JS, Jacobsen IA. Angiotensin-converting enzyme inhibitor therapy and acute pancreatitis. Blood Pressure 4:369–371, 1995.
36. Castiella A, Lopez P, Bujanda L, Arenas J. Possible association of acute pancreatitis with naproxen. J Clin Gastroenterology 21:258, 1995.
37. Norman J. The role of cytokines in the pathogenesis of acute pancreatitis. Am J Surg 175:76–83, 1998.
38. Leser HG, Gross V, Scheibenbogen B. Elevations of serum interleukin-6 concentration precedes acute-phase response and reflects severity in acute pancreatitis. Gastroenterology 101:782–785, 1991.
39. Exley AR, Leese T, Holliday MP. Endotoxemia and serum tumor necrosis factor as prognostic markers in severe acute pancreatitis. Gut 33:1126–1128, 1992.
40. Bassi D, Kollias M, Fernandez-del Castillo C. Impairment of pancreatic microcirculation correlates with the severity of acute experimental pancreatitis. J Am Coll Surg 179:257, 1994.
41. Banks PA. Practice guidelines in acute pancreatitis. Am J Gastroenterol 92:377–386, 1997.
42. Agarwal N, Pitchumoni CS, Sivaprasad AV. Evaluating tests for acute pancreatitis. Am J Gastroenterol 85:356–365, 1990.
43. Ranson JHC. Etiological and prognostic factors in human acute pancreatitis: a review. Am J Gastroenterol 77:633–638, 1982.
44. Agarwal N, Pitchumoni CS. Assessment of severity in acute pancreatitis. Am J Gastroenterol 86:1385–1391, 1991.
45. Baron TH, Morgan DE. The diagnosis and management of fluid collections associated with pancreatitis. Am J Med 102:555–563, 1997.
46. Halonen KI, Pettila V, Leppaniemi AK, et al. Long-term health-related quality of life in survivors of severe acute pancreatitis. Intensive Care Med 29:782–786, 2003.
47. Soran A, Chelluri L, Lee KKW, et al. Outcome and quality of life of patients with acute pancreatitis requiring intensive care. J Surg Res 91:89–94, 2000.
48. McClave SA, Snider H, Owens N, et al. Clinical nutrition in pancreatitis. Dig Dis Sci 42:2035–2044, 1997.
49. Meier R, Beglinger C, Layer P, et al. Consensus statement: ESPEN guidelines on nutrition in acute pancreatitis. Clin Nutr 21:173–183, 2002.
50. Imrie CW, Carter CR, McKay CJ. Enteral and parenteral nutrition in acute pancreatitis. Best Pract Res Clin Gastroenterol 16:391–397, 2002.
51. Isenmann R, Runzi M, Kron M, et al. The German antibiotics in severe acute pancreatitis (ASAP) study group. Gastroenterology 126:997–1004, 2004.
52. Barie PS. A critical review of antibiotic prophylaxis in severe acute pancreatitis. Am J Surg 172(Suppl 6A):38S–43S, 1996.
53. Pederzoli P, Bassi C, Vesentini S, Campedelli A. A randomized multicenter clinical trial of antibiotic prophylaxis of septic complications in acute necrotizing pancreatitis with imipenem. Surg Gynecol Obstet 176:480–483, 1993.
54. Sainio V, Kemppainen E, Puolakkainen, et al. Early antibiotic treatment in acute necrotising pancreatitis. Lancet 346:663–667, 1995.
55. Buchler M, Malfertheiner P, Frie H, et al. Human pancreatic tissue concentration of bactericidal antibiotics. Gastroenterology 103:1902–1908, 1992.
56. De Waele JJ, Vogelaers D, Blot S, et al. Fungal infections in patients with severe acute pancreatitis and the use of prophylactic therapy. Clin Infect Dis 37:208–213, 2003.
57. Virlos IT, Mason J, Schofield RF, et al. Intravenous n-acetylcysteine, ascorbic acid and selenium-based anti-oxidant therapy in severe acute pancreatitis. Scand J Gastroenterol 38:1262–1267, 2003.
58. Ockenga J, Borchert K, Rifai K, et al. Effect of glutamine-enriched total parenteral nutrition in patients with acute pancreatitis. Clin Nutr 21:409–416, 2002.
59. McKay CJ, Curran F, Sharples C, et al. Prospective placebo-controlled randomized trial of lexipafant in predicted severe acute pancreatitis. Br J Surg 84:1239–1243, 1997.
60. Kingsnorth AN. Early treatment with lexipafant, a platelet activating factor antagonist reduces mortality in acute pancreatitis: a double-blind, randomized, placebo-controlled study. Gastroenterology 112:A453, 1997.
61. Neoptolemos JP, Raraty M, Finch M, et al. Acute pancreatitis: the substantial human and financial costs. Gut 42:886–890, 1998.
62. Pitchumoni CS. Chronic pancreatitis: a historical and clinical sketch of the pancreas and pancreatitis. Gastroenterologist 6:24–33, 1998.
63. Sarles H, Adler G, Dani R, et al. The pancreatitis classification of Marseilles-Rome, 1988. Scand J Gastroenterol 24:641–642, 1989.
64. Sarles H, Bernard JP, Johnson C. Pathogenesis and epidemiology of chronic pancreatitis. Ann Rev Med 40:453–468, 1989.
65. Etemad B, Whitcomb DC. Chronic pancreatitis: diagnosis, classification and new genetic developments. Gastroenterology 120:682–707, 2001.
66. Corrao G, Bagnardi V, Zambon A, et al. Exploring the dose–response relationship between alcohol consumption and the risk of several alcohol-related conditions: a meta-analysis. Addiction 94:1551–1673, 1999.
67. Barman KK, Premalatha G, Mohan V. Tropical chronic pancreatitis. Postgrad Med J 79:606–615, 2003.
68. Mohan V, Premalatha A, Pitchumoni CS. Tropical chronic pancreatitis: an update. J Clin Gastroenterol 36:337–346, 2003.
69. Kim K, Kim M, Song MH, et al. Autoimmune chronic pancreatitis. Am J Gastroenterol 99:1605–1616, 2004.
70. Mergener K, Baillie J. Chronic pancreatitis. Lancet 350:1379, 1997.
71. Ito T, Nakano I, Koyanagi S. Autoimmune pancreatitis as a new clinical entity: three cases of autoimmune pancreatitis with effective steroid therapy. Dig Dis Sci 42:1458–1468, 1997.
72. Toskes PP. Medical management of chronic pancreatitis. Scand J Gasteroenterol 30:74–80, 1995.
73. Apte MV, Wilkson JS. Alcohol-induced pancreatic injury. Best Pract Res Clin Gastoenterol 17:593–612, 2003.
74. Pandol SJ, Gukovsky I, Satoh A, et al. Emerging concepts for the mechanism of alcoholic pancreatitis from experimental models. J Gastroenterol 38:623–628, 2003.
75. Freedman SD, Sakamoto K, Venu RP. GP2, the homologue to the renal cast protein uromodulin, is a major component of intraductal plugs in chronic pancreatitis. J Clin Invest 29:83–90, 1993.
76. Yamadera K, Moriyama T, Makino I. Identification of immunoreactive pancreatic stone protein in pancreatic stone, pancreatic tissue, and pancreatic juice. Pancreas 5:255–260, 1990.
77. Larsen S. Diabetes mellitus secondary to chronic pancreatitis. Danish Med Bull 40:153–162, 1993.
78. Ebbehoj N. Pancreatic tissue fluid pressure and pain in chronic pancreatitis. Danish Med Bull 39:128–133, 1992.
79. Karanjia ND, Rever HA. The cause and management of the pain of chronic pancreatitis. Gastroenterol Clin North Am 19:895–904, 1990.

80. Tenner S, Levine RS, Steinberg WM. Drug treatment of acute and chronic pancreatitis. In: Lewis JH. A Pharmacologic Approach to Gastrointestinal Disorders. Baltimore: Williams & Wilkins, 1994: 311.

81. Bornman PC, Marks IN, Girdwood AW, et al. Pathogenesis of pain in chronic pancreatitis: ongoing enigma. World J Surg 27: 1175–1182, 2003.

82. Andren-Sandberg A, Hoem D, Gislason H. Pain management in chronic pancreatitis. Eur J Gastroenterol Hepatol 14:957–970, 2002.

83. Seastiano PD, di Mola FF, Bockman DE, et al. Chronic pancreatitis: the perspective of pain generation by neuroimmune interaction. Gut 52:907–911, 2003.

84. Khalid, Whitcomb DC. Conservative treatment of chronic pancreatitis. Eur J Gastroenterol Hepatol 14:943–949, 2002.

85. Glasbrenner B, Adler G. Evaluating pain and the quality of life in chronic pancreatitis. Int J Pancreatol 22:163–170, 1997.

86. Layer P, Holtmann G. Pancreatic enzymes in chronic pancreatitis. Int J Pancreatol 15:1–11, 1994.

87. Ladas SD, Giorgiotis K, Raptis SA. Complex carbohydrate malabsorption in exocrine pancreatic insufficiency. Gut 34:984–987, 1993.

88. Beglinger C. Relevant aspects of physiology in chronic pancreatitis. Dig Dis 10:326–329, 1992.

89. Young HS. V. Diseases of the pancreas. Sci Am 4:1–17, 1994.

90. Lowenfels AB, Maisonneuve P, Cavallini G, et al. Prognosis of chronic pancreatitis: an international multicenter study. Am J Gastroenterol 89:1467–1471, 1994.

91. Otsuki M. Chronic pancreatitis. Pancreatology 4:28–41, 2004.

92. Lowenfels AB, Maisonneuve P, Cavallini G, et al. Pancreatitis and the risk of pancreatic cancer. N Eng J Med 328:1433–1437, 1993.

93. Whitcomb DC. Inflammation and cancer V. Chronic pancreatitis and pancreatic cancer. Am J Physiol Gastrointest Liver Physiol 287:G315–G319, 2004.

94. Outwater EK, Siegelman ES. MR imaging of pancreatic disorders. Top Magn Reson Imag 8:265–289, 1996.

95. Bolen PJ, Fink AS. Endoscopic retrograde cholangiopancreatography in chronic pancreatitis. World J Surg 27:1183–1191, 2003.

96. Goldberg DM, Durie PR. Biochemical tests in the diagnosis of chronic pancreatitis and in the evaluation of pancreatic insufficiency. Clin Biochem 26:253–275, 1993.

97. Ribet A, Moreau J, Valenzuela JE. Diagnosis of chronic pancreatitis. In: Valenzuela JE, Reber HA, Ribet A. Medical and Surgical Diseases of the Pancreas. New York: Igaku-Shoin, 1991:113.

98. Chowdhury RS, Forsmark CE. Pancreatic function testing. Alimen Pharmacol Therap 17:733–750, 2003.

99. Chowdhury RS, Forsmark CE. Review article: pancreatic function testing. Aliment Pharmacol Ther 17:733–750, 2003.

100. Warshaw AL, Banks PA, Fernandez-Del Castillo C. AGA technical review: treatment of pain in chronic pancreatitis. Gastroenterology 115:765–776, 1998.

101. American Gastroenterological Association. American Gastroenterological Association medical position statement: treatment of pain in chronic pancreatitis. Gastroenterology 115:763–764, 1998.

102. Brown A, Hughes M, Tenner S. Does pancreatic enzyme supplementation reduce pain in patients with chronic pancreatitis? A meta-analysis. Am J Gastroenterol 92:2032, 1997.

103. Garces MC, Gomez-Cerozo J, Condoceo R. Postprandial cholecystokinin response in patients with chronic pancreatitis in treatment with oral substitutive pancreatic enzymes. Dig Dis Sci 43:562–566, 1998.

104. Malfertheiner P, Dominguez-Munoz JE, Buchler MW. Chronic pancreatitis: management of pain. Digestion 55(Suppl 1):29–34, 1994.

105. Buchler MW, Binder M, Friess H. Role of somatostatin and its analogues in the treatment of acute and chronic pancreatitis. Gut Suppl 3:S15–S19, 1994.

106. Friess H, Klempa I, Hermanek P, et al. Prophylaxis of complications after pancreatic surgery: results of a multicenter trial in Germany. Digestion 55(Suppl 1):35–50, 1994.

107. Isenhower HL, Mueller BA. Selection of narcotic analgesics for pain associated with pancreatitis. Am J Health-Syst Pharm 55:480, 1998.

108. Waxman I, Freedman SD, Zeroogian JM. Endoscopic therapy of chronic and recurrent pancreatitis. Dig Dis 16:134–143, 1998.

109. Ho HS, Frey CF. Current approach to the surgical management of chronic pancreatitis. Gastroenterologist 5:128–136, 1997.

110. Saakorafas GH, Anagnostopoulos G. Surgical management of chronic pancreatitis: current concepts and future perspectives. Int Surg 88:211–218, 2003.

111. Bradley EL, Bem J. Nerve blocks and neuroablative surgery for chronic pancreatitis. World J Surg 27:1241–1248, 2003.

112. Kraisinger M, Hochhaus G, Stecenko A, et al. Clinical pharmacology of pancreatic enzymes in patients with cystic fibrosis and in vitro performance of microencapsulated formulations. J Clin Pharmacol 34:158–166, 1994.

113. Layer P, Keller J, Lankisch PG. Pancreatic enzyme replacement therapy. Curr Gastroenterol Rep 3:101–108, 2001.

114. Layer P, Keller J. Lipase supplementation therapy: standards, alternatives, and perspectives. Pancreas 26:1–7, 2003.

115. Layer P, Keller J. Pancreatic enzymes: secretion and luminal nutrient digestion in health and disease. J Clin Gastroenterol 28:3–10, 1999.

116. Bruno MJ, Rauws EAJ, Hoek FJ, et al. Comparative effects of adjuvant cimetidine and omeprazole during pancreatic enzyme replacement therapy. Dig Dis Sci 39:988, 1994.

CASE STUDIES

CASE 21

TOPIC: Viral Hepatitis

THERAPEUTIC DIFFICULTY: Level 3
Helen E. Smith

Chapter 49: Hepatitis: Viral and Drug-Induced

■ Scenario

Patient and Setting: YZ, a 65-year-old Alaskan native female; physical exam at 8 weeks after starting interferon alpha-2b treatment

Chief Complaint: Increasing fatigue and depression

■ History of Present Illness

YZ presented at physical exam complaining of increasing fatigue and depression, which started 3 weeks after starting interferon. YZ describes feelings of irritability, hopelessness, helplessness, decreased motivation, guilt, and some thoughts of death but no suicidal thoughts or plan. YZ reports inability to perform activities such as gardening or housework without extreme fatigue. She has no pleasure in daily activities that she usually enjoys. She is easily irritated by everyone, including her grandchildren, which leaves her feeling frustrated and guilty. Patient also reports side effects from interferon therapy, including fever, headache, chills, fatigue, and a rash. The patient uses acetaminophen to treat the side effects of the interferon. She has slight edema of her extremities.

Medical History: Initial infection: Patient received blood transfusion in Anchorage due to complications of delivering her second child in 1960. Patient does not recall any symptoms that would indicate acute infection at that time.
Diagnosis of chronic HBV: Patient was diagnosed with chronic hepatitis B infection 8 weeks ago after presenting with complaints of extreme fatigue, weakness, malaise, and joint pain. Blood test at that time revealed elevated aminotransferases. Alkaline phosphatase, gamma-glutamyltransferase, bilirubin, albumin, platelets, prothrombin time, and white blood cell counts were normal. Hepatic encephalopathy, variceal bleeding, and ascites were not present. The liver was palpable, but less than 10 cm below the right costal margin

and with a rounded edge. Chronic hepatitis B was diagnosed following serology indicating the presence of HBsAg, HBeAg, anit-HBc (IgG), and HBV DNA. Anti-HBs, anti-HBe, anti-HVC, and anti-HVD were negative. Suspected infection was due to blood transfusion years ago during postpartum complications. Interferon alpha 2b treatment was initiated.
Laboratory values and clinical findings at 1 and 2 weeks after the initiation of interferon alpha 2b indicated aminotransferases were falling. Other values remained stable.
Patient cancelled her clinic appointment and laboratory tests scheduled 4 weeks after initiation of interferon alpha 2b therapy.

Surgical History: C-section in 1960

Family/Social History: Patient has no past history of drug abuse. The patient admits to "social" alcohol consumption (a few beers when with friends once or twice a month); patient claims she has not drunk alcohol since her diagnosis with HBV. History of "social" smoking in the past (1 pack per month), but patient has not smoked in years. Patient has children living in the area.

Medications:
Interferon alpha-2b, 5 million IU SQ daily for 16 weeks (patient is 8 weeks into the course of therapy)
Acetaminophen, patient estimates dose to be 2 to 6 extra-strength (500 mg) tablets 4 to 5 days a week for a total daily dose ranging from 1,000 mg to 3,000 mg
St. John's Wort, 300 mg three times daily

Allergies: Sulfas

■ Physical Examination

GEN: Well-developed, well-nourished woman with depressed affect and tearful
VS: BP 125/85, HR 80 beats/min, RR 12 breaths/min, T 37.5°C, Wt 72 kg, (Wt 6 weeks ago, 70 kg) Ht 150 cm
HEENT: WNL
COR: RRR without murmurs
CHEST: Clear
ABD: Soft, nontender, no ascites
GU: Deferred
RECT: Deferred
EXT: 1+ edema half-way up calf

NEURO: No encephalopathy, no asterixis, depressed affect

■ Results of Pertinent Laboratory Tests, Serum Drug Concentrations, and Diagnostic Tests Test Results

Sodium	142 (142)
Potassium	4.4 (4.4)
Chloride	107 (107)
Carbon dioxide	29 (29)
Ion gap	6
Glucose	6.38 (115)
Blood urea nitrogen	5.7 (16)
Creatinine	62 (0.7)
Protein (total)	70 (7)
Albumin	20 (2)
Bilirubin (total)	27.4 (1.6)
Calcium	2.2 (8.8)
Aspartate aminotransferase (AST)	1.5 (90)
Alkaline phosphatase (total)	21.7 (130)
Alanine aminotransferase (ALT)	1.2 (70)
Gamma glutamyl transferase	0.75 (45)
Magnesium	1.0 (2.0)
Phosphate	0.97 (3.0)
Prothrombin time patient	16.2 s
WBC	4×10^9/L (4×10^3)
Hemoglobin	90 (9.0)
Hematocrit	0.32 (32)
MCV	90 (90)
MCH	30 (30)
MCHC	336 (33.6)
Platelet count	200×10^9/L (200×10^3)
HBsAg	Positive
HBeAg	Positive
HBV DNA	183 pg/mL

■ Problem List

Identify principal problems from the scenario in priority order (see Answers in back of book for correct list of problems).

■ SOAP Note

To be completed by the student (see Answers in back of book for correct SOAP Note).

■ QUESTIONS

(See Answers in back of book for correct responses.)

1. Which parameter differentiates this patient's HBV infection as chronic rather than acute? (EO-2 and 5)
   a. HBsAb
   b. HBeAg
   c. HBc IgM
   d. HBc IgG

2. Which of the following is the most appropriate prescription for analgesia for this patient? (EO-10, 11)
   a. Aspirin 325–650 mg PO every 4 hours PRN (not to exceed 4 g/day)
   b. Anaprox 1,000 mg PO once a day
   c. Two Extra-strength Tylenol (1,000 mg) PO every 6 hours PRN
   d. Acetaminophen 650 mg PO every 6 hours PRN

3. Which interferon is the only FDA-approved interferon for the treatment of chronic HBV infection? (EO-11)
   a. Interferon alfa-2a
   b. Natural interferon alfa-n3
   c. Consensus interferon
   d. Interferon alfa-2b

4. Which of the following dosing regimens of Epivir-HBV is appropriate for a patient with a creatinine clearance between 15–29 mL/min? (EO-11)
   a. 35 mg first dose, then 10 mg once daily
   b. 100 mg first dose, then 50 mg once daily
   c. 100 mg first dose, then 25 mg once daily
   d. 100 mg once daily

5. Which of the following is the most important reason to discontinue interferon therapy in this patient? (EO-11, 10)
   a. Anemia
   b. Elevated LFTs
   c. Depression
   d. Inadequate decrease in HBV DNA

6. Which of the following medications is not an FDA-approved agent for treating HBV? (EO-11)
   a. Lamivudine
   b. Interferon alpha-2b
   c. Adefovir
   d. Ribavirin

7. If this patient were eligible to remain on interferon, what measures could be taken to reduce the flulike side effects she is experiencing?
   a. Take the interferon before bed
   b. Increase her acetaminophen dose
   c. Dose the interferon 3 times a week rather than once a day
   d. Give the interferon IM rather than SQ

8. Identify the risk factors for HBV infection in this patient.

9. Explain the rationale for the use of lamivudine in the treatment of HBV. (EO-7)

10. Discuss the difference between Epivir-HBV and Epivir and the reason why these medications are not interchangeable. (EO-8)

11. List findings that would support the decision to initiate interferon alpha-2b treatment at the time of chronic HBV diagnosis. (EO-2, 5)

12. List the parameters that indicate that interferon alph2b treatment is no longer appropriate for this patient at the time of her current exam. (EO-5)

13. Summarize concepts for drug therapy used to treat chronic HBV utilizing a key points format. (EO-18)

Anxiety Disorders

52

Talia Puzantian

DEFINITIONS

"Man is the only animal that blushes. Or needs to."

Mark Twain, *Following the Equator* (1897)

Anxiety is a commonly experienced emotion. It is an uncomfortable feeling of apprehension or fear coupled with sensations of physical arousal. It may be a normal response to some situations, allowing a person to prepare for and respond to the environment. If anxiety is excessive or interferes with functioning, it is considered a pathologic anxiety disorder.[1] An anxiety disorder may be a primary disorder or it may occur secondary to medical causes or substances (e.g., medications or illicit substances); it may occur as a response to acute stressors or it may be associated with another psychiatric disorder. An accurate diagnosis is essential in treating patients with anxiety appropriately. Primary anxiety disorders classified in the *Diagnostic and Statistical Manual of Mental Disorders, Fourth Edition Text Revision* (DSM-IV-TR) and discussed in this chapter include generalized anxiety disorder (GAD), panic disorder, obsessive-compulsive disorder (OCD), post-traumatic stress disorder (PTSD), and phobic disorders such as social anxiety disorder. Each of these disorders is distinct, with different presentations, diagnostic criteria, and treatment approaches.[1]

TREATMENT GOALS

- Treatment for anxiety disorders should focus on eliminating or decreasing associated symptoms with the goal of improving patient functioning and quality of life.
- Appropriate management of anxiety disorders includes minimizing adverse effects resulting from pharmacotherapy.
- Treatment should be based on the chronic and recurring nature of anxiety disorders, and the aim should be to prevent relapse or recurrence.
- Comorbid conditions should be identified and treatment should target these conditions, as well as the primary anxiety disorder.
- Consider combination (pharmacologic and nonpharmacologic) treatment approaches.
- Treatment for GAD should focus on reducing psychic feelings of anxiety and worry, as well as associated somatic symptoms.
- Treatment for panic disorder should decrease the frequency and severity of panic attacks, while reducing anticipatory anxiety and phobic avoidance.
- OCD treatment should reduce the time consumed by obsessions or compulsions and alleviate the distress and impairment caused by them.

■ The aim of PTSD treatment is to reduce reexperiencing of the traumatic event, avoidance, and numbing, as well as hyperarousal. Treatment should relieve distress and improve functioning and quality of life.

■ Patients in treatment for social phobia or social anxiety disorder should experience less fear of social or performance situations and reduce avoidance of such situations.

EPIDEMIOLOGY

Grouped together, anxiety disorders represent the most commonly occurring psychiatric illnesses. The most recent comprehensive information on the epidemiology of anxiety disorders was compiled by the US Alcohol, Drug Abuse, and Mental Health Administration (now Substance Abuse and Mental Health Services Administration, or SAMHSA) in the National Comorbidity Survey (NCS) of 8,098 adults.[2] This survey found the lifetime incidence of anxiety disorders to be 24.9%, occurring in nearly one in four Americans; it was also found that, in a given year, 17.2% of the US population will experience an anxiety disorder.[2] Even taken individually, the rates for the various anxiety disorders are remarkable (Table 52.1).[2–5] GAD occurs commonly, with a 5.1% lifetime prevalence and a 1-year prevalence of 3.1%.[2] The lifetime prevalence rate of panic disorder is 5% in women and 2% in men.[2] In the general population, although all will not meet criteria for panic disorder, 12.7% of American adults will experience a single panic attack during their lifetime.[6] Lifetime prevalence rates reported for OCD have ranged from 1% to 3% in various populations worldwide.[1,4] The estimated lifetime prevalence for PTSD is 7.8%, with much higher rates reported in traumatized populations such as combat veterans.[3,5] The most commonly occurring anxiety disorder seems to be social phobia, with a lifetime prevalence of 13.3% and a 12-month prevalence of 7.9%.[7] Although anxiety disorders are the most prevalent of psychiatric disorders and effective treatments are available, less than 30% of individuals who suffer from anxiety disorders seek treatment.[8]

PATHOPHYSIOLOGY

The pathophysiologic mechanisms of anxiety disorders have yet to be fully elucidated. Along with biologic theories that center on functional anatomy and the neurochemistry of anxiety, psychological, behavioral, and genetic theories have been proposed. It is clear that these are heterogeneous disorders that have no single causative mechanism.

Several neurotransmitters mediate anxiety. These include inhibitory amino acids such as γ-aminobutyric acid (GABA) and monoaminergic neurotransmitters such as serotonin (5-HT) and norepinephrine (NE). Corticotropin-releasing factor (CRF), cholecystokinin (CCK), and glutamate are also thought to contribute to anxiety. Various aspects of an anxiety response are mediated by neurotransmitters in anatomically distinct areas. Data from neuroimaging studies indicate that several key brain structures are involved in mediating the fear/anxiety response.

GABA SYSTEM

The GABA circuits are integrally involved in anxiety.[9] Evidence has pointed to the role of GABA dysfunction, as well as clinical experience with benzodiazepines, in various functional brain imaging studies. The role of the GABA–benzodiazepine receptor complex in anxiety disorders has not been fully characterized; however, a potential role has been implicated in panic disorder, GAD, and PTSD.[9] In GAD, reduced temporal lobe benzodiazepine receptors are observed; in PTSD, cortical benzodiazepine receptors are reduced, and in panic disorder, decreased GABA$_A$ binding is noted.[9] GABA is a ubiquitous system, with about 70% of synapses

TABLE 52.1	Anxiety Disorders Prevalence: National Comorbidity Survey (N=8,098)	
	12-Month Prevalence, %	Lifetime Prevalence, %
Generalized anxiety disorder	3.1	5.1
Panic disorder	2.3	3.5
Obsessive-compulsive disorder	0.6–1.3	2.5
Post-traumatic stress disorder	2.0–3.2	7.8
Social phobia	7.9	13.3

(From Kessler RC, McGonagle KA, Zhao S, et al. Lifetime and 12-month prevalence of DSM-III-R psychiatric disorders in the United States. Arch Gen Psychiatry 51:8–19, 1994; Kessler RC, Sonnega A, Bromet E, et al. Posttraumatic stress disorder in the National Comorbidity Survey. Arch Gen Psychiatry 52:1048–1060, 1994; Stein MB, Forde DR, Anderson G, et al. Obsessive-compulsive disorder in the community: an epidemiologic survey with clinical reappraisal. Am J Psychiatry 154:1120–1126, 1997; Stein MB, Walker JR, Haxen AL, et al. Full and partial posttraumatic stress disorder: findings from a community survey. Am J Psychiatry 154:1114–1119, 1997.)

in the brain providing GABAergic neurotransmission. It is the predominant inhibitory neurotransmitter system of the brain.

Postsynaptic GABA receptors include the $GABA_A$, $GABA_B$, and $GABA_C$ receptors.[10] Although no evidence has been found for the involvement of the $GABA_B$ and $GABA_C$ receptors in anxiety, considerable evidence links $GABA_A$ receptor dysfunction and the pathophysiology of anxiety disorders.[9] $GABA_A$ receptors act as gatekeepers for chloride channels and have multiple modulatory sites such as benzodiazepine (BZD) receptors, as well as binding sites for anticonvulsants and alcohol.[9,11] When GABA binds to the $GABA_A$ receptor, the chloride ion channel opens and more chloride enters the cell, resulting in hyperpolarization of the cell membrane and decreased nerve cell excitability (inhibitory neurotransmission).[9] BZDs facilitate the actions of GABA by binding to $GABA_A$ receptors and inducing conformational changes in the GABA binding site, thereby increasing the affinity of the receptor for GABA. This results in increased frequency of chloride channel opening, further hyperpolarization of the cell, and a more pronounced decrease in cellular excitability (Fig. 52.1; *see color insert*).[9]

$GABA_A$ receptors are members of the superfamily of ligand-gated ion channel receptors. Each $GABA_A$ receptor is an oligomeric transmembrane glycoprotein composed of a combination of five of the various 18 subunits thus far identified (α_{1-6}, β_{1-3}, γ_{1-3}, δ, ϵ, θ, and ρ_{1-3}), arranged around a central chloride channel.[12] Specific pharmacologic effects of receptors are determined by the various combinations of subunits that compose the $GABA_A$ receptors in different brain regions. Most $GABA_A$ receptor subtypes are believed to be composed of α, β, and γ subunits; the roles of the δ,

ϵ, and θ subunits, which have very limited expression in the brain, remain to be determined.[12] Only recently was the pharmacologic relevance of $GABA_A$ receptor subtypes identified for BZDs. Sedation, anterograde amnesia, and part of the seizure protection was found to be mediated by α_1-receptors, whereas anxiolysis was mediated by α_2-receptors.[12] Thus, the ideal anxiolytic agent may have preferential affinity at the α_2-receptor subtypes and limited activity at the α_1-subtypes, thereby achieving anxiolytic effects without sedation and cognitive impairment. Further dissection of the pharmacologic functions of $GABA_A$ receptor subtypes will open up new strategies in novel drug development.

SEROTONIN SYSTEM

The clinical observation that many anxiolytic agents affect serotonin neurotransmission has led to the postulation that 5-HT is involved in the pathophysiology of anxiety disorders. Serotonin is found primarily in neurons that originate in the dorsal and median raphe nucleus of the brainstem, innervating various brain regions such as the amygdala, basal ganglia, thalamus, and hypothalamus.[11] A variety of processes have been proposed for serotonergic dysfunction in anxiety, including deficient or excessive innervation to key structures and cellular mechanisms, such as abnormal regulation of 5-HT release or reuptake or abnormal responsiveness to 5-HT signals, which may lead to abnormal neurotransmission.[13] The serotonin reuptake transporter site (SERT) is the primary target of the selective serotonin reuptake inhibitors (SSRIs); by blocking SERT, the SSRIs acutely increase the concentration of extracellular serotonin in the synapse, resulting in greater activation of postsynaptic 5-HT receptors. At least 14 different postsynaptic 5-HT receptor subtypes have been discovered, several of which are believed to be potentially important in mood and anxiety regulation (5-HT$_{1A}$, 5-HT$_{1B}$, 5-HT$_{2A}$, 5-HT$_{2C}$, 5-HT$_3$).[13-15] Modulation of serotonergic systems has proved to be a successful approach in the pharmacologic treatment of anxiety disorders, with several SSRI agents approved for use in various anxiety disorders (i.e., panic disorder, GAD, OCD, PTSD, social anxiety disorder).

The amygdala, which is located in the anterior part of the medial temporal lobe, is a key structure involved in coordinating the fear response.[16] Its role includes detecting, coordinating, and maintaining fearful emotions; it is also important in vigilance, preliminary threat assessment, and determination of the meaning and importance of diverse stimuli.[17] The amygdala integrates information from multiple sensory areas to assess for threats, with consideration of input regarding the context of the presenting stimulus.[13] Once a threat has been detected by the amygdala, a rapid response is coordinated via ascending projections to motor areas and descending projections to brainstem nuclei that control autonomic responses and arousal.[13] Serotonin is the neurotransmitter that is found predominantly in the amygdala and frontal cortex; it has thus been proposed to play a role in anxiety disorders.

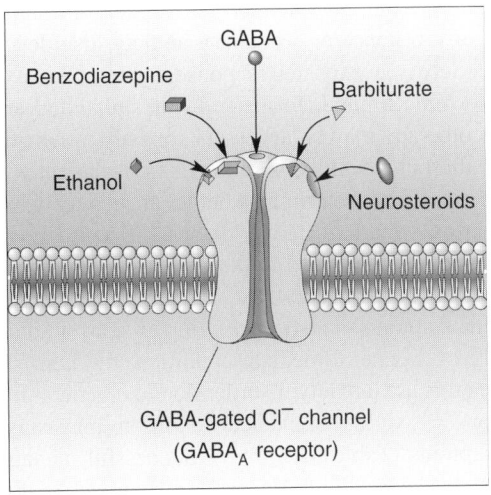

FIGURE 52.1 GABA-A receptor complex (*see color insert*). Drugs and their binding sites on the $GABA_A$ receptor. Binding of these drugs facilitates GABA binding, which in turn opens the channel, allowing high influx of chloride ions, cell membrane stabilization, and decreased neuronal firing. (From Bear MF, Connors BW, Parasido MA. Neuroscience—exploring the brain. 2nd edition. Philadelphia: Lippincott Williams & Wilkins, 2001.)

NORADRENERGIC SYSTEM

The locus ceruleus (LC), which is located in the brainstem, has extensive projections to the limbic system, cerebral cortex, and cerebellar cortex. The LC is the primary norepinephrine (NE)-containing area of the brain. According to the noradrenergic theory of anxiety, in the presence of perceived threat, the LC serves as an alarm center, releases NE, and stimulates the sympathetic and parasympathetic nervous systems. Substances that stimulate LC activity (e.g., caffeine, yohimbine, and isoproterenol) are usually anxiogenic; anxiolytic medications (e.g., antidepressants, benzodiazepines, and clonidine) decrease neuronal firing in the LC.[11,18] It is clear that the serotonergic and noradrenergic systems do not act independently; associations between these systems play a prominent role in the regulation of mood and anxiety. Serotonergic projections from the dorsal raphe nucleus inhibit firing of the LC, whereas noradrenergic projections from the LC have excitatory effects on cell bodies in the dorsal raphe, suggesting that the balance between 5-HT and NE affects the rate of discharge of the LC.[13]

CORTICOTROPIN-RELEASING FACTOR SYSTEM

Corticotropin-releasing factor is a stress-responsive neuropeptide that increases firing of LC noradrenergic neurons.[19] Pharmacologic, physiologic, and neuroanatomic evidence supports an important role for a CRF–NE interaction in the region of the LC in response to stressors.[13,19] Preclinical studies suggest that brain CRF systems mediate anxiety-like behavioral and somatic responses, and that CRF_1 antagonists block the anxiogenic-like effects of CRF and stress in animal models.[13,20] Cerebrospinal fluid levels of CRF are elevated in some anxiety disorders and normalize with effective treatment; hypersecretion of CRF has also been proposed in PTSD. On the basis of these preliminary data, selective CRF_1 antagonists are currently being explored as novel therapies in the treatment of patients with anxiety disorder.[13,20]

CHOLECYSTOKININ SYSTEM

Cholecystokinin is a regulatory peptide hormone predominantly found in the gastrointestinal tract and a neurotransmitter present throughout the nervous system. In the nervous system, CCK is involved in anxiogenesis.[21] Research has suggested that abnormalities in CCK functioning have been associated with some anxiety disorders and that systemic administration of CCK fragments produces anxiogenic effects.[21] The biologic effects of CCK are mediated by two specific G-protein–coupled receptor subtypes—CCK_1 and CCK_2. Research over the past 15 years has resulted in a broad assortment of potent and selective CCK_1 and CCK_2 antagonists. CCK_2 antagonists may have a role in the treatment of patients with anxiety disorder; further research is necessary to define their role.[21]

GLUTAMATE SYSTEM

Glutamate, the major excitatory amino acid in the central nervous system (CNS), is the single neurotransmitter that is integral to the functioning of up to 40% of all brain synapses.[22] The decarboxylation of glutamate forms GABA, the predominant inhibitory neurotransmitter in the CNS (described earlier). Growing preclinical data suggest that glutamatergic neurotransmission is heightened in several brain regions during stress.[13] Glutamate receptors have great functional and regional diversity, making the discovery of appropriate pharmacologic targets a challenge. Inotropic glutamate receptors, which comprise N-methyl-D-aspartate (NMDA), alpha-amino-3-hydroxy-5-methylisoxazole propionate (AMPA), and kainite, as well as metabotropic glutamate receptors, have been characterized. Although the neuropharmacology of glutamate is complex, pharmacologic targets that modulate glutamatergic activity, with both inotropic and metabotropic receptors as targets, are under development.[13] For example, the role of inotropic glutamate antagonists (e.g., lamotrigine, topiramate, riluzole) and metabotropic glutamate agonists (e.g., LY354740) in the treatment of anxiety disorders is currently under investigation.[13,23,24]

CLINICAL PRESENTATION AND DIAGNOSIS

Although anxiety disorders are classified together and comorbidities among the various anxiety disorders are not uncommon, it is important for the clinician to understand their differences, so the appropriate diagnosis can be made. The evaluation of a patient with an anxiety disorder should include consideration of medical and psychiatric illnesses and medications or substances used, as well as a thorough physical examination, mental status examination, laboratory testing, and social history. Such a workup will assist the practitioner in determining whether the anxiety is situational anxiety or a primary or secondary anxiety disorder. Situational anxiety is an expected response to stressful events that is usually time limited. In general, for situational anxiety, pharmacotherapy may be necessary for only a short time, if at all. A thorough evaluation of the anxious patient will also help the provider to determine whether an anxiety disorder is a primary or secondary anxiety disorder. Secondary anxiety disorders are characterized in the DSM-IV-TR as those due to a medical condition and those that are substance induced.

When symptoms of anxiety develop as a physiologic consequence of a general medical condition, the DSM-IV-TR classifies this as "anxiety disorder due to a general medical condition."[1] A variety of medical conditions may cause anxiety symptoms (Table 52.2).[1,25,26] Successful management of the medical condition is the primary approach to this type of anxiety; however, in some cases, pharmacologic or nonpharmacologic treatment for anxiety, or a combination of these, may be necessary.

During the evaluation of the patient with anxiety, if evidence of recent or prolonged substance use is observed, including medications with psychoactive effects, withdrawal

TABLE 52.2	Anxiety Secondary to Medical Conditions

Endocrine
  Addison disease
  Cushing disease
  Hyperadrenocorticism
  Hyperthyroidism
  Hypoglycemia
  Hypothyroidism
  Pheochromocytoma
Cardiovascular
  Angina pectoris
  Arrhythmia
  Congestive heart failure
  Mitral valve prolapse
  Myocardial infarction
Respiratory
  Asthma
  Chronic obstructive pulmonary disease
  Hyperventilation
  Pneumonia
  Pulmonary embolism
Metabolic
  Porphyria
  Vitamin B_{12} deficiency
Neurologic
  Central nervous system (CNS) neoplasms
  Chronic pain
  Encephalitis
  Parkinson disease
  Seizure disorder
  Vestibular dysfunction
Gastrointestinal
  Crohn disease
  Irritable bowel syndrome
  Peptic ulcer disease
  Ulcerative colitis
Inflammatory
  Rheumatoid arthritis
  Systemic lupus erythematosus
Miscellaneous
  Chronic infection, including human immunodeficiency
    virus (HIV)
  Malignancy

(From American Psychiatric Association. Diagnostic and statistical manual of mental disorders, DSM-IV-TR. Washington, DC: American Psychiatric Association, 2000:429–484; Arikian SR, Gorman JM. A review of the diagnosis, pharmacologic treatment, and economic aspects of anxiety disorders. Primary Care Companion J Clin Psychiatry 3:110–117, 2001; Harter MC, Conway KP, Merikangas KR. Associations between anxiety disorders and physical illness. Eur Arch Psychiatry Clin Neurosci 253:313–320, 2003.)

from a substance, or exposure to a toxin, a "substance-induced anxiety disorder" should be considered (Table 52.3).[1,27] Once the cause of substance-induced anxiety is eliminated, anxiety symptoms usually improve markedly or remit within days to weeks; if symptoms persist beyond 4 weeks, other causes for anxiety should be considered.[1]

Symptoms of anxiety may result from another underlying primary psychiatric disorder. Many psychiatric illnesses, including schizophrenia, major depression, dysthymia, mania, delirium, and dementia, may be associated with symptoms of anxiety. As with anxiety due to a general medical condition, treatment of the underlying cause of anxiety and, in some cases, short-term anxiolytic treatment is indicated. In many cases, however, patients with other psychiatric illnesses may also have a primary anxiety disorder. Comorbidity, particularly with major depression, occurs frequently with anxiety disorders.[28] Such patients should be treated aggressively for both illnesses, as those with comorbid anxiety and depression do not respond as well to therapy, have a more protracted course of illness, and experience less positive treatment outcomes than do patients with either noncomorbid psychiatric illness.[29]

The DSM-IV-TR classifies anxiety disorders (Table 52.4) and specifies the diagnostic criteria and clinical features for each anxiety disorder.[1] Panic attacks and agoraphobia are classified separately because each may occur in the context of several of the primary anxiety disorders. A panic attack is a discrete period characterized by a sudden onset of symptoms that generally subside within 10 minutes. During a panic attack, patients often report intense apprehension, fearfulness, or terror, often associated with feelings of impending doom. Symptoms such as shortness of breath, palpitations, chest pain, choking, and fear of "going crazy" or losing control are common (Table 52.5).[1] Agoraphobia describes anxiety about, or avoidance of, places or situations from which escape may be difficult or embarrassing.[1]

GENERALIZED ANXIETY DISORDER

GAD is characterized by excessive and pervasive anxiety and worry about multiple life circumstances, with symptoms occurring more days than not for a period of at least 6 months.[1] Patients with GAD experience significant distress and impairment of functioning, find it difficult to control the worry, and exhibit at least three of the somatic or psychological symptoms listed in the DSM-IV-TR diagnostic criteria, including restlessness, fatigue, difficulty concentrating, irritability, muscle tension, and sleep disturbance.[1] GAD occurs commonly and has the distinction of being the second most frequent psychiatric disorder after depression (Table 52.1).[30] Persons with GAD may have endured their symptoms for many years, without recognizing that such symptoms are out of the ordinary.

The pattern of onset of GAD differs from that of other anxiety disorders. Whereas most anxiety disorders have their onset before the age of 20 years, rates of GAD in the young are usually low, with substantially increasing prevalence

TABLE 52.3	**Substance-Induced Anxiety Disorder**
Central nervous system (CNS) stimulants	Procainamide
Amphetamines	Reserpine
Caffeine	Miscellaneous medications
Cannabis	Albuterol
Cocaine (and withdrawal)	Aminophylline
Ecstasy	Bromocriptine
Ephedrine	Dapsone
Hallucinogens	Dronabinol
Inhalants	Efavirenz
Methylphenidate	Fluoroquinolones
Nicotine (and withdrawal)	Interferons
Phencyclidine (PCP)	Isoniazid
Phenylephrine	Isoproterenol
Pseudoephedrine	Levodopa
CNS depressant withdrawal	Lidocaine
Barbiturates	Mefloquine
Benzodiazepines	Metoclopramide
Ethanol	Nicotinic acid
Opiates	Nonsteroidal anti-inflammatory drugs (NSAIDs)
Psychotropic medications	Sibutramine
Antipsychotics (akathisia)	Steroids
Bupropion	Theophylline
Buspirone	Thyroid hormone
Selective serotonin reuptake inhibitors (SSRIs)	Heavy metals and toxins
Tricyclic antidepressants (TCAs)	Carbon dioxide
Venlafaxine	Carbon monoxide
Cardiovascular medications	Gasoline
Angiotensin-converting enzyme (ACE) inhibitors	Nerve gases
Digoxin	Organophosphate insecticides
Hydralazine	Paint

From American Psychiatric Association. Diagnostic and statistical manual of mental disorders, DSM-IV-TR. Washington, DC: American Psychiatric Association, 2000:429–484; Anonymous. Drugs that may cause psychiatric symptoms. Med Lett Drugs Ther 44:59–62, 2002.)

observed with advancing age.[30–33] Women are approximately twice as likely as men to have GAD.[31,32] The natural course of GAD can be characterized as chronic with few complete remissions, a waxing and waning course of symptoms over time, and the occurrence of substantial comorbidity, particularly with depression.[1,34] Current comorbidity is estimated at 65% and lifetime comorbidity at 90%.[8] Psychiatric illnesses other than depression that occur comorbidly with GAD are substance use disorders and other anxiety disorders.[35] Often, patients do not seek treatment until additional psychiatric illnesses, and further functional impairments, have developed.

PANIC DISORDER

Panic disorder is characterized by recurrent unexpected panic attacks, the key features of which include intense car-diac and nervous system symptoms, fear of losing control, fear of dying, and feelings of unreality (Table 52.5). Panic attacks are not necessarily associated with panic disorder. Panic attacks may occur in the early stages of other psychiatric disorders, particularly major depression, or may be part of another anxiety disorder.[36] In panic disorder, the attacks are triggered randomly and are followed by at least 1 month of persistent concern about the possibility of additional panic attacks, worry about the consequences of the attacks, or significant behavioral changes related to the attacks (Table 52.6).[1] Two or more panic attacks must occur before a diagnosis of panic disorder is made; most persons with panic disorder have considerably more than two attacks. The frequency and severity of panic attacks vary widely, with some persons having moderately frequent attacks (e.g., once

TABLE 52.4	DSM-IV-TR Classification of Anxiety Disorders

Panic disorder

   Without agoraphobia

   With agoraphobia

Agoraphobia without history of panic disorder

Specific phobia

Social phobia (social anxiety disorder)

Obsessive-compulsive disorder

Post-traumatic stress disorder

Acute stress disorder

Generalized anxiety disorder

Anxiety disorder due to general medical condition

Substance-induced anxiety disorder

Anxiety disorder not otherwise specified

(From American Psychiatric Association. Diagnostic and statistical manual of mental disorders, DSM-IV-TR. Washington, DC: American Psychiatric Association, 2000:429–484.)

weekly for months at a time), others reporting short bursts of attacks (e.g., daily for a week), and still others reporting infrequent attacks (e.g., two per month over many years).[1]

Patients with panic disorder may or may not have agoraphobia, or anxiety about being in situations in which escape may be difficult or embarrassing, or in which help may not be available should a panic attack occur. Quality of life can

TABLE 52.5	DSM-IV-TR Diagnostic Criteria for Panic Attack

Discrete period of intense fear or discomfort, in which four or more of the following symptoms developed abruptly and reached a peak within 10 minutes:

Palpitations

Sweating

Trembling or shaking

Shortness of breath or smothering sensation

Feeling of choking

Chest pain or discomfort

Nausea or abdominal distress

Feeling dizzy, lightheaded, or faint

Feelings of unreality or being detached from oneself

Fear of losing control or going crazy

Fear of dying

Paresthesias (numbness or tingling sensations)

Chills or hot flushes

(From American Psychiatric Association. Diagnostic and statistical manual of mental disorders, DSM-IV-TR. Washington, DC: American Psychiatric Association, 2000:429–484.)

TABLE 52.6	DSM-IV-TR Diagnostic Criteria for Panic Disorder

Recurrent unexpected panic attacks (see Table 52.5)

At least one of the attacks has been followed by at least 1 month of one or more of the following:

   Persistent concern about having additional attacks

   Worry about the implications of the attack or its consequences

   Significant change in behavior related to attacks

Agoraphobia may or may not be present

Panic attacks are not due to substances used, medication taken, or a general medical or psychiatric condition

(From American Psychiatric Association. Diagnostic and statistical manual of mental disorders, DSM-IV-TR. Washington, DC: American Psychiatric Association, 2000:429–484.)

be markedly impaired by this phobic avoidance of places and things thought to trigger the attacks. Typically, patients with agoraphobia avoid places such as shopping centers, theaters, elevators, bridges, and trains, among others. In moderately severe cases, patients may venture out only with a companion; in severe cases, patients may become housebound.[1] The age of onset for panic disorder varies considerably but has typically been described as between late adolescence and the mid-30s.[1] Women have a twofold to threefold increased risk of developing panic disorder compared with men and are more likely to develop agoraphobia.[37] The usual course of illness is chronic, with waxing and waning of symptoms.

As with other anxiety disorders, comorbidity is common; up to 50% to 60% of patients with panic disorder will experience a major depressive episode during their lifetime. Comorbidity with other anxiety disorders is also common. Patients with comorbidities seem to exhibit greater symptom severity and persistence, role impairment, suicidality, and help-seeking behavior than do those with panic disorder alone.[38] The somatic symptoms of panic disorder increase the likelihood that these patients will consult primary care physicians and use emergency medical services; among psychiatric illnesses, panic disorder is associated with the highest rate of use of medical services.[39,40] One study showed that health care costs were approximately 11 times higher for patients with panic disorder than they were for controls.[41] Inadequate recognition and treatment of panic disorder has been observed in studies; early detection and intervention can serve to alleviate patient suffering, improve patient functioning, and reduce unnecessary health care costs.[40]

OBSESSIVE-COMPULSIVE DISORDER

The essential features of OCD are recurrent obsessions or compulsions that are severe enough to take longer than 1 hour per day or to cause significant impairment (Table

TABLE 52.7	DSM-IV-TR Diagnostic Criteria for Obsessive-Compulsive Disorder

Either obsessions or compulsions are present

Obsessions

    Recurrent and persistent thoughts, impulses, or images occur that are intrusive and inappropriate and that cause marked anxiety

    Thoughts, impulses, or images are not simply excessive worries about real-life problems

    Attempts are made to ignore, suppress, or neutralize the thoughts, impulses, or images

    It is recognized that thoughts, impulses, or images are a product of own mind

Compulsions

    Repetitive behaviors or mental acts occur that a person feels driven to perform in response to an obsession

    Behaviors or mental acts are aimed at preventing or reducing distress; however, behaviors or mental acts are not connected in a realistic way with what they are designed to prevent, or they are clearly excessive

It is recognized that the obsessions or compulsions are excessive or unreasonable (this criterion does not apply to children)

(From American Psychiatric Association. Diagnostic and statistical manual of mental disorders, DSM-IV-TR. Washington, DC: American Psychiatric Association, 2000:429–484.)

52.7).[1] Obsessions are persistent thoughts, impulses, or images that are experienced as intrusive and that cause anxiety or distress. Most commonly, obsessions are repeated thoughts about contamination (e.g., becoming contaminated by shaking hands), repeated doubts (e.g., wondering whether one turned the stove off or locked the door), a need to have things in a particular order (e.g., feeling distress when objects are disordered or asymmetrical), and aggressive or sexual thoughts or imagery.[1] Compulsions are repetitive behaviors (e.g., hand washing, checking, ordering or arranging symmetrically) or mental acts (e.g., counting, repeating words silently) that prevent or reduce anxiety. Patients with OCD recognize that the obsessions and compulsions are excessive or unreasonable; however, attempts at resisting them result in increasing anxiety, which is relieved only by yielding to the compulsion.[1] In contrast to behaviors that might be termed "compulsive," such as eating or gambling, patients with OCD do not derive pleasure from their compulsions. Often, patients are embarrassed by symptoms and go to great lengths to hide them; patients who present to health care providers generally do so because of severity of symptoms or complications of compulsions (e.g., dermatologic complications of repeated hand washing).[42]

OCD affects 2.5% of the population. Although OCD usually begins in adolescence or early adulthood, it may begin in childhood. Male patients tend to have an earlier onset (between ages 6 and 15 years) but females eventually catch up (onset between ages 20 and 29 years), with OCD rates in adults similar between the sexes. Onset of OCD is gradual; it is a chronic disorder with a waxing and waning course, with symptom exacerbation in times of stress.[1,43] As with other anxiety disorders, psychiatric comorbidity with OCD is common. Major depressive disorder is the most frequent comorbid condition, and early age at onset of OCD increases the risk of depressive disorder in persons with OCD.[44] Other comorbidities seen with OCD include social anxiety disorder, generalized anxiety disorder, panic disorder, schizophrenia, and schizoaffective disorder. Tics occur in 20% to 30% of patients with OCD, and 5% to 7% meet criteria for Tourette disorder.[1]

POST-TRAUMATIC STRESS DISORDER

PTSD has been referred to by various terms, including "shell shock," "combat fatigue," and "post-Vietnam" syndrome, and it has long been accepted as an adverse outcome of combat exposure.[45] Recently, PTSD has increasingly been recognized in civilians who have been exposed to traumatic events. PTSD is characterized by the development of symptoms after a person experiences or witnesses a traumatic event in which actual or threatened death or serious injury occurs (Table 52.8). Examples of traumatic events experienced directly by patients with PTSD include, but are not limited to, military combat, sexual or physical assault, being kidnapped or taken hostage, terrorist attack, torture, incarceration in a concentration camp or as a prisoner of war, natural or manmade disasters, severe accidents, or being diagnosed with a life-threatening illness. Response to the event involves intense fear, helplessness, or horror. Core symptoms of PTSD are grouped into three domains: reexperiencing the traumatic event (e.g., nightmares or flashbacks), avoidance of associated stimuli or an emotional numbing of general responsiveness, and hyperarousal (e.g., sleep difficulties, hypervigilance, exaggerated startle response, irritability or anger outbursts).[1] For the diagnosis of PTSD to be made, symptoms must be present for at least 1 month and must cause significant functional impairment.

Community-based studies in the United States have found the lifetime prevalence of PTSD to be approximately 8%. As would be expected, rates are much higher in selected samples. For example, in a group of 4,008 women, those who had been raped had a lifetime PTSD prevalence rate of 32%.[46] Sex differences have been recorded in rates of exposure to traumatic stressors, as well as to the subsequent development of PTSD. Although men are more likely to experience trauma, women seem to be twice as likely as men to develop PTSD.[3] This finding may not necessarily indicate that women are more vulnerable to developing PTSD, but rather that women experience a greater number of severe traumas that are associated with a higher likelihood of developing illness.[3]

Rates of PTSD are expected to increase as the frequency of exposure to traumatic events in the world continues to rise. It is interesting to note that of members of the popula-

TABLE 52.8	DSM-IV-TR Diagnostic Criteria for Post-traumatic Stress Disorder

A traumatic event was experienced in which the individual witnessed, experienced, or was confronted with actual or threatened death or serious injury and to which the person responded with intense fear, helplessness, or horror

Traumatic event is reexperienced persistently in some way (e.g., nightmares, flashbacks), or intense distress is experienced on exposure to stimuli associated with the traumatic event

The individual persistently avoids stimuli associated with the event and numbing of general responsiveness occurs, involving at least three of the following:

 Efforts to avoid thoughts, feelings, or conversations associated with the trauma

 Efforts to avoid activities, places, or people that are reminders of the trauma

 Inability to recall an important aspect of the trauma

 Markedly diminished interest in significant activities

 Feeling of detachment or estrangement from others

 Restricted range of affect

 Sense of foreshortened future

Persistent symptoms of increased arousal occur, involving at least two of the following:

 Difficulty falling or staying asleep

 Irritability or angry outbursts

 Difficulty concentrating

 Hypervigilance

 Exaggerated startle response

Above symptoms endure for at least 1 month

Symptoms cause clinically significant impairment in social, occupational, or other important area of functioning

(From American Psychiatric Association. Diagnostic and statistical manual of mental disorders, DSM-IV-TR. Washington, DC: American Psychiatric Association, 2000:429–484.)

tion who experience traumatic events, only a subset will ultimately develop illness. Risk research suggests that the most important factors may be the nature of the trauma, genetics, and the recovery environment.[47] The terrorist attacks of September 11, 2001, represent the largest act of terrorism and an unprecedented exposure to trauma in the United States. Surveys conducted following the event have detected a major burden of PTSD among adults exposed to the day's events. Direct exposure to the attacks or its consequences, amount of time spent viewing television coverage of the attacks, female sex, Hispanic ethnicity, and low level of social support were shown to be related to PTSD.[48,49]

PTSD has the distinction of being the disorder with the highest comorbidity, with reported rates of 88% of men and 79% of women with a history of PTSD having at least one comorbid psychiatric diagnosis.[3] Most often, the comorbid

illness is major depression, another anxiety disorder, or a substance abuse disorder. Suicide rates are strikingly high in patients with PTSD, who are six times more likely to attempt suicide than are those without the diagnosis.[50] The course of PTSD is highly variable, although data suggest that it is a persistent illness, with at least one third of patients never remitting independent of treatment and many patients continuing to suffer from subthreshold symptoms.[3,51]

PHOBIC DISORDERS

The DSM-IV-TR classifies phobic disorders into two categories: specific phobia (formerly simple phobia) and social phobia (also, more commonly, called social anxiety disorder).[1] Phobic disorders are characterized by excessive and unrealistic fears that are excessive or unreasonable and lead to avoidance behavior in attempts to minimize anxiety.

Specific phobia is the marked and persistent fear and avoidance of specific objects or situations. The DSM-IV-TR classifies specific phobias into five subtypes: animal type (e.g., snakes, dogs, spiders), natural environment type (e.g., storms, heights, water), blood/injection type (e.g., seeing blood or injury, receiving injection, other medical procedures), situational type (e.g., flying, driving, bridges, elevators), and others.[1] Exposure to the phobic object or situation results in intense anxiety, including panic attacks in some cases. Although it is recognized that the fear is excessive or unreasonable, avoidance of the object or situation follows. Although phobias are common, they rarely result in sufficient impairment of functioning or distress to warrant a diagnosis. Impairment or distress is required for diagnostic criteria to be met (e.g., career promotion may be threatened by avoidance of air travel).

The essential feature of social anxiety disorder is the marked and persistent fear and avoidance of social situations in which embarrassment or humiliation may occur. Although the line between social anxiety disorder and shyness is not perfectly clear, the former causes the sufferer marked distress and interferes with relationships and functioning, and the latter is far less disruptive.[52] Social anxiety disorder may be specified as generalized or specific. Generalized type refers to social anxiety in which fears are related to most social situations (e.g., conversations, dating, attending parties), whereas specific type refers to social anxiety in which fears are related to specific situations (e.g., public speaking, musical performance). Common symptoms that occur in social anxiety disorder include sweating, shaking, garbled speech, blushing, palpitations, and gastrointestinal distress.[52]

Social anxiety disorder occurs commonly, with a prevalence rate of 13%.[7] Symptoms usually begin in childhood or adolescence, with a mean age of onset of 10 to 13 years.[52] In community samples, women have twice the representation of men, but in clinical settings, the sex distribution is more even.[52] The course of illness is chronic, and symptoms are persistent and debilitating. Social anxiety disorder may have an enormous and detrimental effect on quality of life; studies show marked negative impact on earning ability, educational level, and vocational achievement.[53] Comorbidity, particularly with major depression, another anxiety disorder, or a substance use disorder, occurs commonly.[54] Because the comorbid condition is often the reason for medical or psychiatric evaluation, the diagnosis of social anxiety disorder and its treatment are often overlooked.

PSYCHOSOCIAL ASPECTS

Overcoming barriers to treatment, such as patients' lack of understanding that anxiety is a treatable illness or stigma attached to mental illness, is of foremost importance. Once patients are engaged in treatment, pharmacotherapy can be very effective in reducing symptoms and improving function. However, medications do not directly affect coping skills and relational skills with which patients may have difficulty as a result of their anxiety. Appropriately identifying and addressing such issues will improve patient outcomes. In addition, the recognition and management of comorbid psychiatric disorders, including substance use disorders, is critical in ensuring optimal response and reducing associated risks, such as suicidality.

THERAPEUTIC PLAN

Practice guidelines and consensus statements have been published for some of the anxiety disorders [e.g., American Psychiatric Association's guidelines for panic disorder (1998), Expert Consensus Guidelines for PTSD (1999) and for OCD (1997), and American Academy of Child and Adolescent Psychiatry's guidelines for treatment of children and adolescents with anxiety disorder (1997)]. Although these are comprehensive and may be of assistance in formulating a treatment plan for patients, they were composed several years ago and therefore do not incorporate recent data. In using these guidelines, one must consider this limitation, which could ultimately alter treatment decisions.

TREATMENT

Medications can be very effective for reducing symptoms of anxiety and improving patient function. Nonpharmacologic approaches can be very effective when used alone for mild anxiety or adjunctively with medications in more moderate to severe anxiety.

PHARMACOTHERAPY
Medications used to treat patients with anxiety disorders include BZDs, buspirone, β-blockers, and antidepressants, including monoamine oxidase inhibitors (MAOIs), tricyclic antidepressants (TCAs), SSRIs, and others. These various classes of medications are not equally effective across the spectrum of anxiety disorders; their uses are summarized in Table 52.9.

TABLE 52.9 Summary of Effective Pharmacologic Treatments for Patients With Anxiety Disorders

	GAD	Panic Disorder	OCD	PTSD	Social Phobias
BZDs	X	X[a]			
Buspirone	X				
β-Blockers					X[c]
MAOIs		X			X
TCAs	X	X	X[b]		
SSRIs	X	X	X	X	X[d]
Venlafaxine	X				X[d]

X indicates efficacy.
[a]High potency (e.g., alprazolam, clonazepam).
[b]Clomipramine.
[c]Performance anxiety.
[d]Social anxiety disorder.
BZD, benzodiazepine; GAD, generalized anxiety disorder; OCD, obsessive-compulsive disorder; PTSD, posttraumatic stress disorder; MAOI, monoamine oxidase inhibitor; TCA, tricyclic antidepressant; SSRI, selective serotonin reuptake inhibitor.

Benzodiazepines. BZDs are widely prescribed; four of them (alprazolam, clonazepam, diazepam, and lorazepam) are listed among the top 200 most commonly prescribed medications.[55] All BZDs currently marketed in the United States are Schedule IV agents. Some of these agents have not been approved by the US Food and Drug Administration (FDA) for anxiety; however, they all exert anxiolytic effects. In addition to anxiolytic properties, BZDs exert sedative-hypnotic, muscle relaxant, and anticonvulsant effects. They are prescribed for anxiety disorders, as well as for muscle spasticity, convulsive disorders, presurgical sedation, involuntary movement disorders, detoxification from alcohol and other substances, and anxiety associated with medical or psychiatric illness. Generally, pharmacokinetic differences, clinical trial data, and clinical experience dictate which agent should be used in which context.

BZDs likely exert their anxiolytic effects by binding to a specific site on the $GABA_A$ receptor and inducing a subtle change in its shape, increasing the affinity of the GABA receptor for GABA and increasing the movement of chloride ions into the neuron.[56] The net effect is potentiation of GABA effects, resulting in hyperpolarization and inhibition of neuronal firing.

The pharmacokinetic properties of BZDs are summarized in Table 52.10. Subtle differences in absorption, distribution (lipid solubility), and elimination determine clinical properties such as onset and duration of effect and can help clinicians to select the appropriate agent for a patient's individual needs. Administered orally, BZDs are generally well absorbed, usually within 1 to 2 hours.[57] The agents with the fastest absorption are diazepam and clorazepate; these agents are highly lipid soluble, thereby allowing easy and rapid

TABLE 52.10	Pharmacokinetic Summary of Benzodiazepines

Agent	Time to Peak Plasma Concentration (oral), hr	Metabolic Pathway	Major Active Metabolites	Half-life, hr[a]	Dose Range, mg/d	Approximate Dosage Equivalencies
Alprazolam (Xanax)	1–2	Oxidation (CYP3A4), glucuronidation	None	10–14	0.5–10	1
Chlordiazepoxide (Librium)	1–4	Oxidation, glucuronidation	Desmethylchlordiazepoxide; demoxepam; N-desmethyldiazepam; oxazepam	>100	10–200	50
Clonazepam (Klonopin)	1–4	Oxidation (CYP3A4), nitroreduction	None	20–80	0.5–12	0.5
Clorazepate (Tranxene)	1–2	Oxidation	N-desmethyldiazepam; oxazepam	>100	15–60	15
Diazepam (Valium)	0.5–2	Oxidation (CYP3A4, CYP2C19), glucuronidation	N-desmethyldiazepam; 3-hydroxydiazepam; oxazepam; temazepam	>100	2–40	10
Estazolam (ProSom)	2	Oxidation, glucuronidation	None	15–17	1–2	2
Flurazepam (Dalmane)	0.5–1	Oxidation, glucuronidation	N–1-hydroxyethylflurazepam; N-desalkylflurazepam	>100	15–30	30
Halazepam (Paxipam)	1–3	Oxidation, glucuronidation	N-desmethyldiazepam, oxazepam	>100	60–160	
Lorazepam (Ativan)	2–3	Glucuronidation	None	10–20	2–6	2
Oxazepam (Serax)	2–4	Glucuronidation	None	5–14	30–120	30
Quazepam (Doral)	2	Oxidation, glucuronidation	2–oxoquazepam; desalkyloxoquazepam	75	7.5–30	30
Temazepam (Restoril)	1–2	Glucuronidation	None	4–18	15–30	30
Triazolam (Halcion)	1–2	Oxidation (CYP3A4), glucuronidation	None	1.5–5	0.125–0.5	0.5

[a]Parent + metabolite(s).
(From Ballenger JC. Benzodiazepines. In: Schatzberg AF, Nemeroff CB, eds. Essentials of clinical psychopharmacology. Washington, DC: American Psychiatric Publishing, 2001:75–92; Greenblatt DJ, Divoll M, Abernety DR, et al. Clinical pharmacokinetics of the newer benzodiazepines. Clin Pharmacokinet 8:233–253, 1983; Wang JS, DeVane CL. Pharmacokinetics and drug interactions of the sedative hypnotics.Psychopharmacol Bull 37:10–29, 2003.)

passage into the CNS. High lipid solubility is also responsible for the rapid distribution from the CNS into peripheral inactive storage sites (e.g., adipose tissue). This rapid distribution into and out of the CNS may explain the ''rush'' experienced by some patients and may contribute to the abuse of these agents; it also explains the short duration of action with single dosing of these agents. Clorazepate is a prodrug that is converted rapidly through a pH-dependent process in the acidic gastric environment to N-desmethyldiazepam, the pharmacologically active entity. Temazepam, which has a slow dissolution rate, and oxazepam, which is the most hydrophilic, are the least rapidly absorbed. Chlordiazepoxide, diazepam, and lorazepam are available as injectable formulations. Lorazepam has the most predictable intramuscular absorption, whereas chlordiazepoxide and diazepam have slow and erratic absorption, respectively, and can induce pain with injection.[57]

Benzodiazepines generally produce nearly immediate therapeutic effects; thus, they may be prescribed for short-term, intermittent, ''as-needed'' use. After such single oral doses, the onset of action depends largely on absorption rate and lipid solubility; the duration of action after single doses depends on distribution (lipid solubility) and rate of elimination. After multiple doses (e.g., routine or scheduled dosing), pharmacologic effects vary according to rate and extent of drug accumulation, elimination half-life, and clearance. The duration of clinical effects of the benzodiazepines is not always predictable from the elimination half-life alone.

BZDs are biotransformed by two primary metabolic processes: hepatic microsomal oxidation (phase I metabolism) and glucuronide conjugation (phase II metabolism).[57] Oxidation may be impaired by aging, liver disease, or concurrent administration of medications that inhibit or induce oxidative processes; glucuronidation is not affected by these factors. Impaired oxidation due to one of the factors above leads to prolonged half-life and increased accumulation; this may result in excessive sedation and ataxia in some patients. Chlordiazepoxide, clorazepate, diazepam, flurazepam, and quazepam are BZDs with long half-lives, mostly caused by extensive metabolism to active metabolites that prolong the effects of the administered agent. During repeated dosing with these long-half-life benzodiazepines, accumulation of the parent compound and its pharmacologically active metabolites occurs. Following discontinuation of these long-half-life BZDs, elimination is slow because active metabolites may remain in the blood for several days or weeks, possibly resulting in persistent effects. The short- to intermediate-acting BZDs include alprazolam, clonazepam, estazolam, lorazepam, oxazepam, temazepam, and triazolam. These agents do not have significantly active metabolites that would prolong their half-lives. Lorazepam, oxazepam, and temazepam have the distinction of being metabolized through direct

conjugation with glucuronic acid (glucuronidated) and are thereby the least likely to be involved in pharmacokinetic drug interactions; these are the most appropriate BZDs for use in the context of impaired oxidative processes.

The dosing of BZDs should be highly individualized; some very general dosing guidelines are summarized in Table 52.11. Starting dose should be based on the patient's clinical experience with BZDs, and the lowest dose should be determined on the basis of age, weight, sex, and body size. Although BZDs with long half-lives may be dosed once daily at bedtime, they are often used in divided daily doses to minimize adverse effects. BZDs with shorter half-lives (e.g., alprazolam, lorazepam, oxazepam) are usually administered in divided daily doses (BID to QID). Alprazolam XR is a new, extended-release formulation that allows QD dosing and may be associated with fewer CNS adverse effects than the immediate-release preparation because of lower peak serum levels.[58] Additionally, with the extended-release formulation, less fluctuation of serum drug concen-

TABLE 52.11	General Dosing Guidelines for Adults of Antianxiety Medications[a]		
Medication	Initial Dosage and Schedule[b]	Titration Schedule	Maximum Dosage[c]
Benzodiazepines			
Alprazolam	0.25 mg TID	0.25–0.5 mg/d q2–4d	1 mg QID
Clonazepam	0.5 mg BID	0.5–1 mg/d q2–4d	3 mg BID
Diazepam	5 mg BID	2–5 mg/d q2–4d	40 mg QHS
Lorazepam	1 mg TID	0.5–1 mg/d q2–4d	5 mg BID
Oxazepam	10 mg TID	10–15 mg/d q2–4d	30 mg TID
Buspirone	5 mg TID	5 mg/d q2–3d	20 mg TID
β-Blockers			
Propranolol	10 mg TID	20–40 mg/d q2–3d	120 mg TID
Monoamine oxidase inhibitors			
Phenelzine	15 mg QAM	15 mg/d q3–4d	45 mg BID
Tranylcypromine	10 mg QAM		30 mg BID
Tricyclic antidepressants			
Clomipramine	25 mg QHS	25 mg/d q2–4d	250 mg QHS
Imipramine	25–50 mg QHS	10 mg/d q 1week	300 mg QHS
Nortriptyline	25 mg QHS	10 mg/d q1 week	150 mg QHS
Selective serotonin reuptake inhibitors			
Citalopram	20 mg QAM	20 mg/d q2–4 weeks	40 mg QAM
Escitalopram	10 mg QAM	50 mg/d q1 week	20 mg QAM
Fluoxetine	20 mg QAM	10 mg/d q1 week	80 mg QAM
Fluvoxamine	50 mg QHS	50 mg/d q1 week	150 mg BID
Paroxetine	20 mg QD		50 mg QD
Sertraline	50 mg QAM		200 mg QAM
Venlafaxine XR	37.5 mg QAM	37.5 mg/d q1 week	225 mg QAM

[a]Doses for geriatric patients should be reduced by 30% to 50%.
[b]Initial doses of antidepressants for treating panic disorder should be lower, and titration should be slower.
[c]Patients with panic disorder may need higher doses of benzodiazepine.

trations occurs, which may reduce the potential for breakthrough anxiety symptoms.[59]

Overall, BZDs are safe and well tolerated by most patients. The most common adverse effect is sedation. This may be a beneficial effect for patients with anxiety who also experience insomnia; however, physiologic tolerance to the sedative effects usually occurs within 1 to 2 weeks.[60] Tolerance to the anxiolytic effects of BZDs does not occur, and patients with anxiety can continue to experience therapeutic effects with long-term use.[61] Other adverse effects of BZDs include fatigue, ataxia, slurred speech, confusion, and anterograde amnesia (loss of memory for new information after medication ingestion). Anterograde amnesia seems to be dose related and reverses upon dose reduction or medication discontinuation.[62,63] Significant adverse effects, including falls, cognitive impairment, sedation, and impairment of driving skills, may be associated with benzodiazepine use in the elderly.[64] Falls in the elderly can have significant consequences (e.g., fractures, nursing home placement); therefore, the use of BZDs in the elderly should be avoided if possible or should be approached with great caution.[65–67] Paradoxical disinhibition involving excitement, agitation, or aggressiveness may occur rarely (in less than 1% of patients) with BZD use; patients at greater risk for this effect include the elderly, those with head injury, and those with developmental delays.[68,69] Respiratory depression may occur with BZDs, but this rarely occurs at therapeutic doses. Patients in whom respiratory depression may be significant include those with severe respiratory disease, including sleep apnea, and those who have ingested an overdose or who have combined BZDs with other respiratory depressants.

Drug interactions with BZDs can be categorized as pharmacodynamic or pharmacokinetic. Significant pharmacodynamic interactions occur with the coadministration of other CNS depressants, including alcohol, barbiturates, and opiates, which may potentiate effects. Pharmacokinetic interactions of clinical relevance may occur when BZDs that require oxidation are coadministered with other agents that have inhibitory or inductive effects on oxidative enzymes.[70] Some potent inhibitors include, but are not limited to, cimetidine, nefazodone, fluoxetine, fluvoxamine, erythromycin, ketoconazole, oral contraceptives, protease inhibitors, delavirdine, grapefruit juice, and isoniazid; use of these in combination with certain BZDs may lead to prolonged and increased effects. It is also important to consider that discontinuation of an enzyme inhibitor given concurrently with some BZDs may lead to offset of the drug interaction and, specifically, to BZD withdrawal.[71] Enzyme inducers such as nevirapine, efavirenz, carbamazepine, phenytoin, phenobarbital, and rifampin may reduce levels of benzodiazepine with the potential of breakthrough symptoms or withdrawal. Lorazepam, oxazepam, and temazepam pose the lowest risk with regard to pharmacokinetic interactions because they are not oxidatively metabolized.

Physiologic dependence, defined as emergence of withdrawal symptoms upon discontinuation of therapy, occurs with BZDs. The onset, duration, and severity of the withdrawal syndrome varies according to the dosage and duration of treatment, as well as the half-life of the agent and speed of discontinuation.[72] With short-half-life agents, withdrawal may begin within 1 to 2 days of discontinuation (or dosage reduction) and may be shorter in duration but more intense than withdrawal from longer-half-life agents, which may appear 5 to 10 days after discontinuation and may last a few weeks. Withdrawal is more likely to occur and to be more severe with longer duration of use, high dosage, and use of short-half-life agents. The characteristic symptoms of mild withdrawal are anxiety, insomnia, irritability, nausea, diaphoresis, systolic hypertension, tachycardia, and tremor. In more severe cases, confusion, delirium, psychosis, and seizures may occur.[72] Various strategies for BZD discontinuation have been proposed, including BZD tapering schedules, pharmacologic agents, and psychological interventions. The rate and schedule of BZD dosage reduction and discontinuation should be individualized. A 10% to 25% reduction in dose can be provided every 1 to 2 weeks, along with careful monitoring of withdrawal symptoms and symptoms of breakthrough anxiety, which often present similarly. Because withdrawal from short-acting BZDs may be more difficult, the patient's regimen may be converted to a longer-acting BZD such as clonazepam (equivalencies listed in Table 52.10) before dose is reduced.[73] Adjunctive medications, such as carbamazepine, valproic acid, and propranolol, among others, have also been used with varying degrees of success.[73] Although psychological interventions during BZD discontinuation may be supportive and may aid in dealing with exacerbations of anxiety, controlled clinical trial data have been conflicting regarding the role of formal psychological interventions in facilitating BZD discontinuation.[74–76] The most recent and best designed study showed that the role of cognitive-behavioral therapy is likely of limited value.[76]

Although physiologic dependence occurs routinely with BZDs, this is not synonymous with abuse. BZD abuse is defined as the inappropriate use of these agents that is inconsistent with acceptable medical practice, recreational in nature, or continued despite negative consequences. Patients with a history of or current substance use disorder, particularly involving alcohol, are more likely to abuse BZDs, and most benzodiazepine abusers concurrently abuse other substances.[77,78] Data suggest that patients without a history of substance use disorder who are taking BZDs for the treatment of an anxiety disorder are unlikely to escalate doses or abuse these agents.[79,80] Highly lipophilic benzodiazepines, such as diazepam, and agents with a short half-life and high potency, such as lorazepam or alprazolam, seem to be the most reinforcing benzodiazepines and, therefore, the ones most likely to be abused.[81]

Buspirone. Buspirone, an azapirone, is a structurally distinct anxiolytic agent. It is mechanistically unrelated to BZDs, has no CNS depressant effects, is not cross tolerant with BZDs, and lacks hypnotic, muscle relaxant, and anti-convulsant properties.[82,83] Dependence and withdrawal are not likely to occur with buspirone use, nor is abuse likely to be a problem.[84] These properties make buspirone an appealing choice, particularly over BZDs, for the treatment of patients with anxiety. However, because buspirone has not demonstrated efficacy across the spectrum of anxiety disorders, its use is limited. In several double-blind studies, buspirone, a 5-HT$_{1A}$ partial agonist, has demonstrated efficacy superior to placebo and equal to BZDs for the treatment of GAD.[85-92] However, in contrast to BZDs, which exert anxiolytic effects immediately, the initial therapeutic effects of buspirone are delayed by 1 to 2 weeks, with full effects occurring over several weeks; buspirone is not effective when taken intermittently or "as needed." Data suggest that buspirone may be ineffective in patients with GAD who previously responded to BZDs.[93] This finding may, at least in part, be related to BZD withdrawal symptoms, which are not treated with buspirone therapy alone.[94] Buspirone does not appear to be effective in treating patients with panic disorder or social anxiety disorder.[95,96] Although efficacy studies have been mixed in OCD, controlled studies have, for the most part, been negative.[97] It has been proposed that buspirone may be effective in alleviating symptoms of PTSD; however, no controlled trials to date have confirmed the preliminary results of an open trial.[98] Buspirone has been evaluated for the treatment of patients with numerous disorders other than anxiety; however, the only supportive data thus far may be those related to its use as augmentation to antidepressants in treatment-resistant depression and in controlling agitation in patients with dementia.[99]

Adverse effects of buspirone are generally mild and include dizziness, headache, nausea, and jitteriness.[100] The short plasma half-life of buspirone (2–3 hours) necessitates dosing of the medication three times daily. The initial dosage is 5 mg and the maximum daily dose is 60 mg (Table 52.11). Buspirone is metabolized by CYP3A4, and inducers of this enzyme (carbamazepine, phenytoin, modafinil, nevirapine, and rifampin, among others) may reduce serum levels, leading to decreased therapeutic effect. Inhibitors of this enzyme (e.g., erythromycin, fluoxetine, fluvoxamine, grapefruit juice, ketoconazole, nefazodone, and protease inhibitors, among others) may increase levels of buspirone; however, these types of interactions have not been deemed clinically significant because of the large therapeutic window of buspirone. The use of MAOIs should be avoided with buspirone because of the possibility that serotonin syndrome (described in the following section) may occur.

Antidepressants

Monoamine Oxidase Inhibitors. In addition to being effective in the treatment of patients with depressive disorders, MAOIs have been shown, in controlled trials, to be effective in panic disorder with agoraphobia, social phobia, and PTSD.[101] Among the available MAOIs, phenelzine is the agent most intensively studied in panic disorder. Although

several studies support its efficacy in panic disorder, it is generally regarded as an option of last resort for resistant cases because of its adverse effects, dietary restrictions, and potential drug interactions.[102-104] Similarly, phenelzine demonstrated substantial efficacy and was the first-line treatment for patients with social anxiety disorder before the discovery of newer antidepressants. Tranylcypromine, as well as phenelzine, has demonstrated efficacy in social anxiety disorder; however, MAOIs, are now used only when newer agents have failed.[105,106] MAOIs have shown efficacy in PTSD in controlled trials; however, in one 4-week study, phenelzine was not more effective than placebo.[107-109] Only uncontrolled case reports have noted MAOI efficacy in OCD.[101]

MAOIs present some limitations in terms of ease of use. They are usually administered in divided doses (BID or TID) owing to their short half-lives. The most common adverse effects include weight gain, sexual dysfunction, orthostatic hypotension, and edema. A severe and potentially fatal hypertensive crisis (severe hypertension, occipital headache, stiff neck, nausea, and vomiting) may occur when MAOIs are administered with sympathomimetic agents or foods high in tyramine content.[110] Recent publications have revised previous, excessively restrictive diets so as to refine restrictions and enhance dietary compliance.[111,112] A rare but potentially fatal serotonin syndrome (confusion, restlessness, myoclonus, hyperreflexia, diaphoresis, tremor, diarrhea, and fever) may occur when MAOIs are combined with other serotonergic agents.[113] In summary, despite controlled clinical data and early experience demonstrating the established efficacy of MAOIs for some anxiety disorders, the adverse effect profiles, dietary restrictions, and drug interaction potential of these agents preclude their routine use. These agents are best reserved for refractory cases that are unresponsive to safer alternatives.

Tricyclic Antidepressants. TCAs have been shown to be effective in a number of anxiety disorders. TCAs, particularly imipramine, have demonstrated efficacy in patients diagnosed with GAD with or without comorbid depression.[114] In controlled studies, TCAs have shown at least equivalent efficacy compared with BZDs and may be superior in long-term therapy, although BZDs have a faster onset of action.[115,116] In GAD, somatic symptoms seem most responsive to BZDs, whereas psychic symptoms of tension, apprehension, and worry have been more responsive to TCAs.[115,116] Patients taking TCAs have reported higher rates of adverse effects than BZD-treated patients.[116] Another study suggested that discontinuation of long-term BZD use in GAD can be facilitated significantly by coprescribing of imipramine before and during the BZD taper.[117]

TCAs, particularly imipramine and clomipramine, are well studied in panic disorder and were used regularly through the early 1990s, when SSRIs became more commonly used.[118-125] In one study in which 63% reported at least moderate improvement with TCA treatment, adverse effects were often difficult to tolerate, and 35% discontinued for this reason. Overstimulation, which occurred in 20%, was the most common reason for early discontinuation, and weight gain, which occurred in 34%, was the most common reason for stopping the drug later on.[121] The APA guidelines recommend reserving the use of TCAs for panic disorder after two failed trials of SSRIs.[102]

Clomipramine was the first agent approved by the FDA for the treatment of patients with OCD; its efficacy has been well documented in several controlled trials. Clomipramine is unique among the TCAs in its effectiveness in OCD; this may be due to its more specific and potent effects at inhibiting the reuptake of serotonin compared with other agents in the class. Direct comparisons have shown that clomipramine is equal in efficacy to various SSRIs; however, meta-analyses have suggested that clomipramine may be more effective than SSRIs.[97,126–130] Regardless of this potential, clomipramine is recommended as a second-line agent after SSRIs because of its less favorable tolerability profile.

A number of controlled studies, although small and limited to combat veteran populations, have evaluated the efficacy of TCAs in PTSD. Results range from modest symptom improvement with imipramine and moderate improvement with amitriptyline to no benefit with desipramine.[131–133] TCAs were not found to alleviate avoidance and numbing associated with PTSD.[134] Because of the high risk of suicide in patients with PTSD and the lethality of TCAs in overdose, these agents are best avoided. TCAs do not appear particularly useful for the treatment of patients with social anxiety disorder and are not recommended.[52]

Although a significant quantity of data exist to support the use of TCAs in some anxiety disorders, important limitations to their routine use must be noted. When first initiated for the treatment of patients with anxiety disorders, particularly GAD or panic disorder, TCAs may cause worsening anxiety or jitteriness; therefore, treatment should be initiated at one-quarter or one-half the usual dose, which should be titrated slowly. Other adverse effects associated with TCAs include sedation, orthostatic hypotension, dry mouth, blurred vision, constipation, sexual dysfunction, and weight gain. These adverse effects may interfere with patients' adherence to treatment and may thereby reduce their long-term utility. Also of concern is the potential for lethal overdose with TCAs, particularly in light of of the high rates of comorbid depression observed in patients with anxiety.

Selective Serotonin Reuptake Inhibitors. SSRIs are currently considered first-line agents for the treatment of patients with all five of the primary anxiety disorders. In GAD, paroxetine is the best studied SSRI, and it was the first in its class to receive FDA approval for this indication.[135–138] Although escitalopram is the only other SSRI with FDA approval for the treatment of patients with GAD, studies have also shown fluvoxamine, sertraline, and citalopram to be efficacious in reducing symptoms of GAD. SSRIs seem to be superior to placebo and as effective as TCAs, although

they are much better tolerated.[114,135] As with TCAs, an initial increase in anxiety has been noted when SSRIs are given to patients with GAD.[114] Initiation of lower doses (e.g., paroxetine 10 mg/day, sertraline 25 mg/day) and slow titration can effectively assist the clinician in managing this effect. Fluoxetine may be more likely than other SSRIs to induce anxiety when initiated, and no controlled data support its efficacy in GAD; therefore, it is best avoided. Also similar to TCAs, and different from BZDs, a delay in onset of therapeutic effect has been noted with SSRIs in GAD.[135] Only one long-term study published thus far has demonstrated that continued treatment with SSRI (paroxetine) significantly reduces the potential for relapse in GAD.[139]

Although only fluoxetine, paroxetine, and sertraline have received FDA approval for the indication of panic disorder, all SSRIs have been shown to be effective.[140–146] SSRIs reduce panic attack frequency and severity, anticipatory anxiety, and associated depression. A lack of direct comparator studies between TCAs and SSRIs led investigators to conduct an effect size analysis comparing efficacy trials with these agents.[147] No differences in effect size were found, indicating that both groups of antidepressants are equally effective in reducing panic symptoms, agoraphobic avoidance, depressive symptoms, and general anxiety. As might be expected, the number of dropouts was significantly lower in the group of patients treated with SSRIs (18%) than TCAs (31%). Patients with panic disorder are exquisitely sensitive to adverse effects; therefore, low initial doses are recommended (e.g., paroxetine 10 mg/day, sertraline 25 mg/day, fluoxetine 5 mg/day).

SSRIs are first-line treatment for patients with OCD; fluoxetine, fluvoxamine, paroxetine, and sertraline are the agents with FDA-approved indications.[127,148–154] Limited data support the efficacy of citalopram and escitalopram.[155] Only one published controlled study compared one SSRI with another; sertraline was shown to be more effective than fluoxetine for treating patients with OCD, although both groups improved significantly.[156] Given the relative paucity of comparative studies within the class, no one agent can be considered more effective than another. Unlike patients with GAD or panic disorder, patients with OCD can tolerate the usual SSRI starting dosages used in the treatment of patients with depression. In contrast to depression, however, therapeutic response in OCD may require a dose at the higher end of the dosage range and may not occur for 10 to 12 weeks.

The only FDA-approved medications for the treatment of PTSD are sertraline and paroxetine. Controlled studies in combat as well as civilian populations with PTSD have shown that these agents are effective for reducing all three core PTSD symptom clusters.[157–160] SSRIs also treat patients with comorbid depression and anxiety, which occur frequently with PTSD. Efficacy data for fluoxetine in PTSD are conflicting, and only uncontrolled data are available for the other SSRIs.[161–167] Therapeutic response to SSRIs in patients with PTSD may begin within the first 2 weeks of treatment, but full effects may take 2 to 3 months or longer.

Paroxetine and sertraline have received FDA approval for the indication of social anxiety disorder.[168-174] Fluvoxamine and escitalopram have shown good efficacy for social anxiety disorder in controlled trials.[175-177] Open trial data and case reports suggest a role for citalopram in social anxiety disorder, and one negative controlled pilot study with fluoxetine did not show a significant difference from placebo.[178-180] Unlike patients with panic disorder or GAD, patients with social anxiety disorder can tolerate the standard SSRI starting dose. Dosing of SSRIs for the treatment of patients with social anxiety disorder is similar to that used for treating those with major depression.

Adverse effects of SSRIs observed in patients with anxiety disorders are similar to those experienced in patients treated for depression. These include nausea, diarrhea, headache, insomnia, nervousness, and sexual dysfunction.

Venlafaxine. The serotonin and norepinephrine reuptake inhibitor, venlafaxine, was the first antidepressant to receive FDA approval for the indication of GAD. Controlled clinical trials have demonstrated the anxiolytic effects of venlafaxine noted in the short-term and long-term treatment of patients with GAD.[181-184] Although depression is a common comorbidity with GAD, venlafaxine has shown anxiolytic effects independent of antidepressant effects in outpatients with GAD without major depressive disorder.[182,184] In patients with comorbid depression, venlafaxine may be effective for both disorders. Venlafaxine is also indicated for the treatment of patients with social anxiety disorder. The efficacy of venlafaxine in social anxiety disorder has been established as superior to placebo and equal to paroxetine in two 12-week controlled studies in which patients received 75 to 225 mg per day.[185,186] The recommended starting dose for venlafaxine XR (extended-release formulation) is 37.5 mg per day, with an effective dosage range of 75 to 225 mg per day. The adverse effects of venlafaxine are very similar to those of SSRIs; the most common effect is nausea. Patients usually develop tolerance to this adverse effect within 1 to 2 weeks of continued treatment. Increases in supine diastolic blood pressure may occur, but usually not at doses less than 225 mg per day. Thus far, data on venlafaxine for the treatment of panic disorder, PTSD, and OCD are only preliminary and limited in nature; therefore, its use in these anxiety disorders cannot currently be recommended.[187-191]

β-Adrenergic Blockers. β-Adrenergic receptor blockers such as propranolol can be effective in reducing some of the somatic anxiety symptoms associated with acute stress reactions, adjustment disorders, generalized anxiety, panic disorder, and agoraphobia.[192,193] These agents act primarily by blocking peripheral adrenergic β-receptors; symptoms that are mediated through β-stimulation, such as tremor, sweating, flushing, and tachycardia, are helped most. Cognitive symptoms of anxiety do not seem to improve with β-blockers; therefore, these agents are not recommended as

a primary treatment option in GAD or panic disorder.[102,194] Single-dose β-blocker treatment is most effective in preventing performance anxiety (social phobia, specific type), with improvement noted within 1 to 2 hours and at relatively low doses (e.g., propranolol 10 to 40 mg or atenolol 25 to 100 mg).[52,193,195] β-Blockers are not recommended for the treatment of patients with generalized social phobia (social anxiety disorder) or OCD, although pindolol was shown to augment the therapeutic effects of paroxetine in patients with treatment-resistant OCD.[52,196] Propranolol may decrease the intrusive thoughts, nightmares, hypervigilance, and explosiveness associated with PTSD.[197] Emerging data also demonstrate that propranolol may be useful for mitigating PTSD symptoms, or perhaps even for preventing the development of PTSD, when prescribed shortly after trauma exposure.[198,199] In general, the role of β-blockers in the treatment of patients with anxiety disorders is extremely limited. However, in appropriate patients, they are well tolerated and lack abuse potential. Common adverse effects include dizziness, fatigue, bradycardia, and hypotension; careful monitoring of patients' vital signs is warranted. β-Blockers should be avoided in patients with medical contraindications.

NONPHARMACOLOGIC THERAPY

Nonpharmacologic treatment approaches in anxiety disorders include supportive or dynamic psychotherapy, cognitive therapy, behavioral therapy, and relaxation training. Relaxation training was previously central to the nonpharmacologic treatment of a variety of anxiety disorders but is now less routinely applied to disorders other than GAD.[200,201] Cognitive and behavioral therapies are the most studied and are often combined (cognitive-behavioral therapy, or CBT) to treat patients with various anxiety disorders.

CBT focuses directly on eliminating the exaggerated fears and associated avoidance responses that maintain the anxiety disorder. CBT may be exposure based, in which case patients are repeatedly confronted with the feared stimuli under controlled conditions with the goal of extinguishing fears as patients acquire a sense of safety. Through psychoeducational interventions, patients learn a new model for interpreting their anxiety experiences (cognitive restructuring). This aids patients in eliminating catastrophic thoughts that intensify anxiety. Many of the studies examining the strength of CBT interventions relative to pharmacologic therapies in the various anxiety disorders have been summarized in meta-analytic reviews.[202-206] These data provide consistent evidence that CBT offers equivalent efficacy to medications, with evidence for superiority over medications ranging from a subtle edge (panic disorder) to more pronounced (PTSD).[200] Although psychotherapeutic interventions such as CBT clearly have a role in the treatment of patients with anxiety disorders, they are underutilized.[207] This may be correlated with the increasing popularity of pharmacologic interventions. CBT should not be discounted when one is managing a patient with an anxiety disorder. Evidence supports the use of CBT as an effective first-line

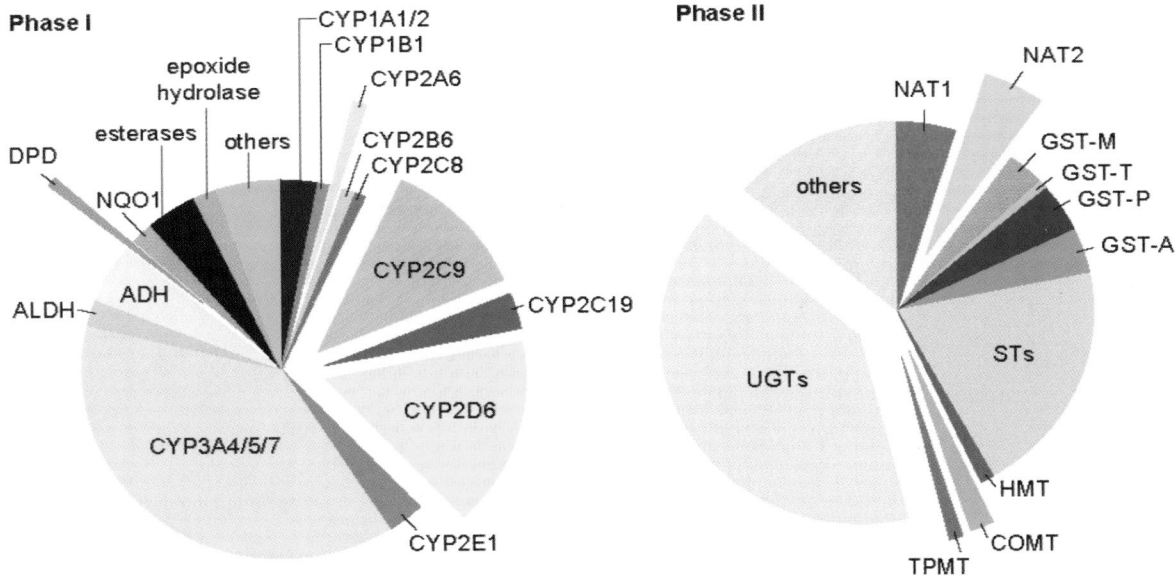

FIGURE 1.11 Major drug metabolizing enzymes. The percentage of phase I and phase II metabolism of drugs that each enzyme contributes is estimated by the relative size of each section of the corresponding chart.

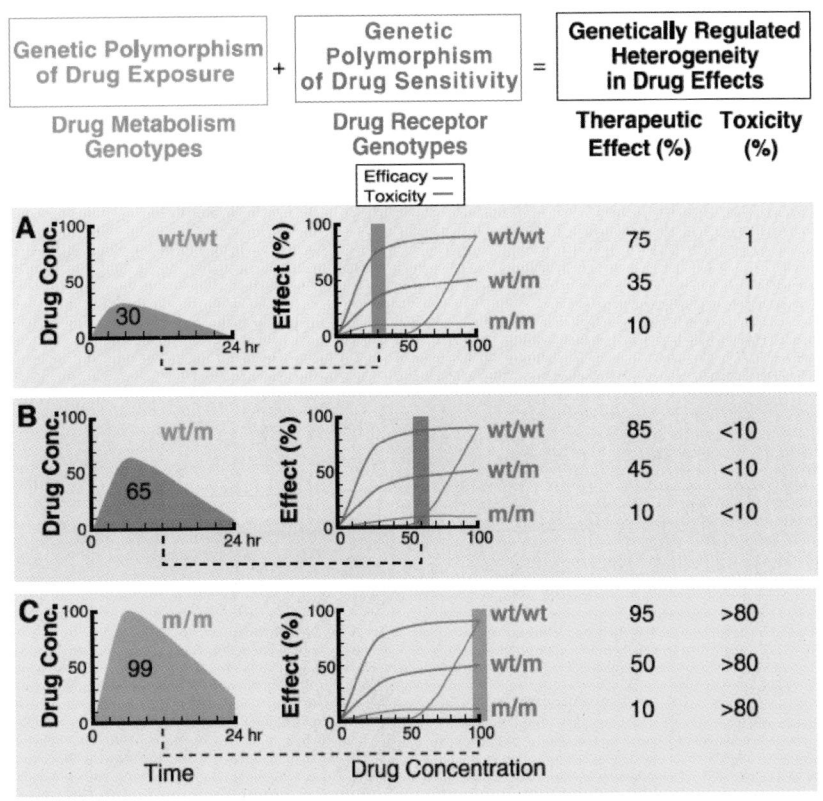

FIGURE 1.21 Polygenic determinants of drug effects. The potential consequences of administering the same dose of a medication to individuals with different drug metabolism genotypes and different drug-receptor genotypes is illustrated.

See images in the text for complete legend and credit lines.

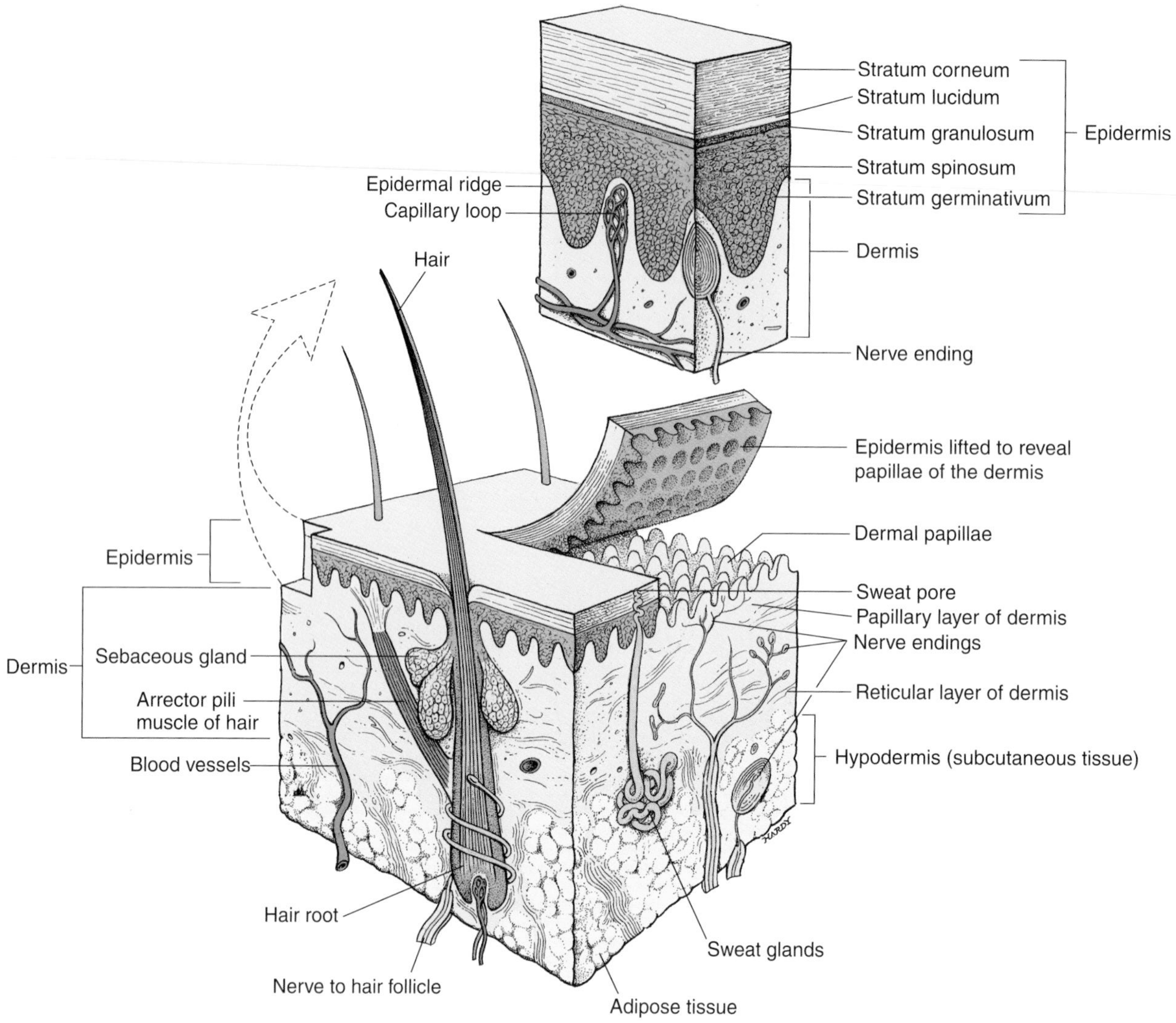

Stratum corneum
Stratum lucidum
Stratum granulosum ⎤
Stratum spinosum   ⎥ Epidermis
Stratum germinativum ⎦

Epidermal ridge
Capillary loop

Dermis

Hair

Nerve ending

Epidermis lifted to reveal papillae of the dermis

Dermal papillae

Epidermis

Sweat pore
Papillary layer of dermis
Nerve endings

Dermis

Sebaceous gland

Arrector pili muscle of hair

Blood vessels

Reticular layer of dermis

Hypodermis (subcutaneous tissue)

Hair root

Sweat glands

Nerve to hair follicle

Adipose tissue

FIGURE 9.1 Skin structure and components.

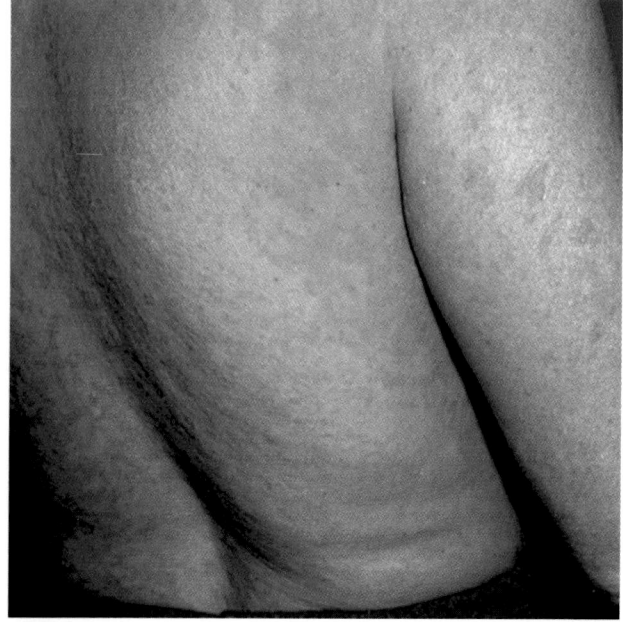

FIGURE 9.2 Atopic Dermatitis.

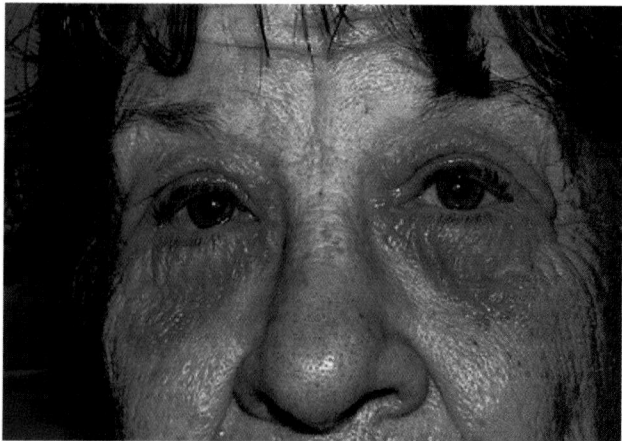

FIGURE 9.3 Allergic dermatitis following use of neomycin ophthalmic ointment.

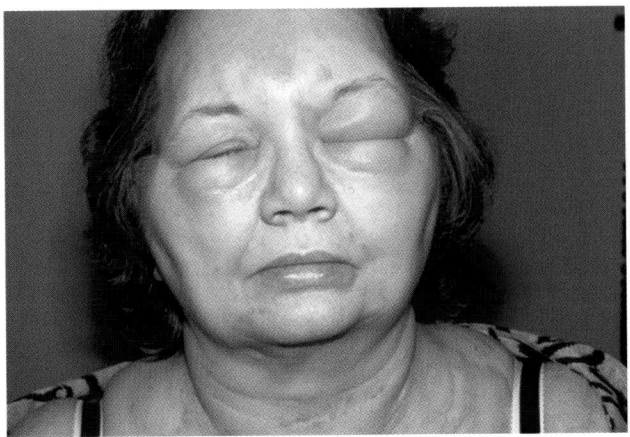

FIGURE 9.4 Urticaria with angioedema of the face and eyelids.

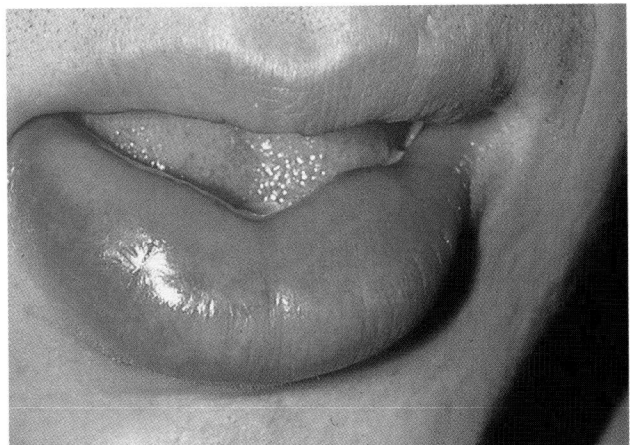

FIGURE 9.6 Angioedema. Note swelling of the lower lip and protruding tongue.

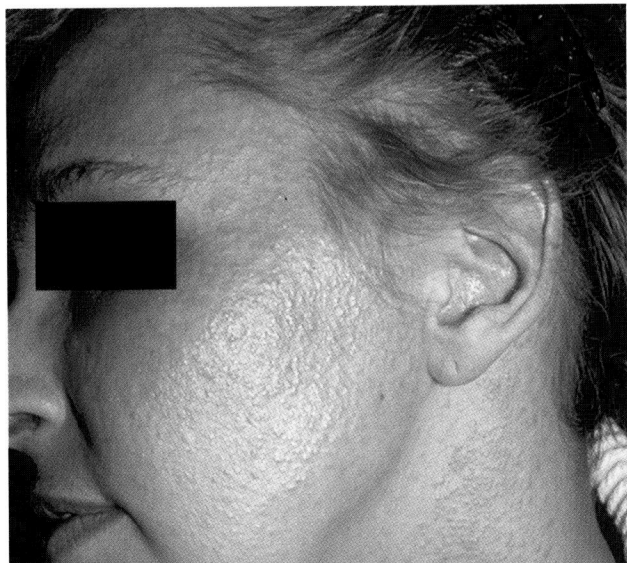

FIGURE 9.8 Photoallergic reaction to nonsteroidal anti-inflammatory drug. Two days after initiating piroxicam, patient developed eruption after sun exposure at beach. Note the lack of involvement of unprotected area under the jaw.

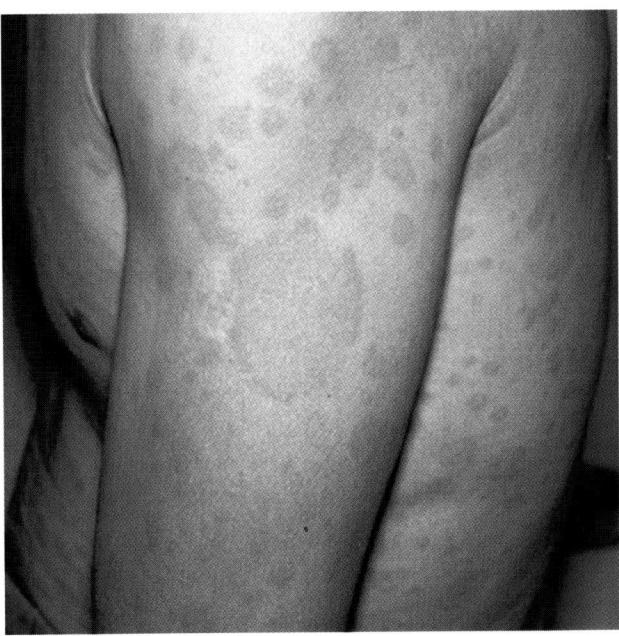

FIGURE 9.5 Urticarial drug eruption.

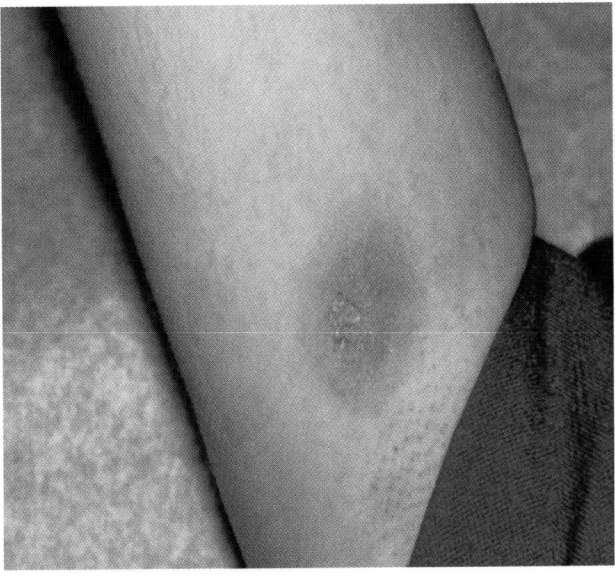

FIGURE 9.7 Fixed drug eruption. Lesion reappeared at original site after subsequent exposure to sulfonamide antibiotic.

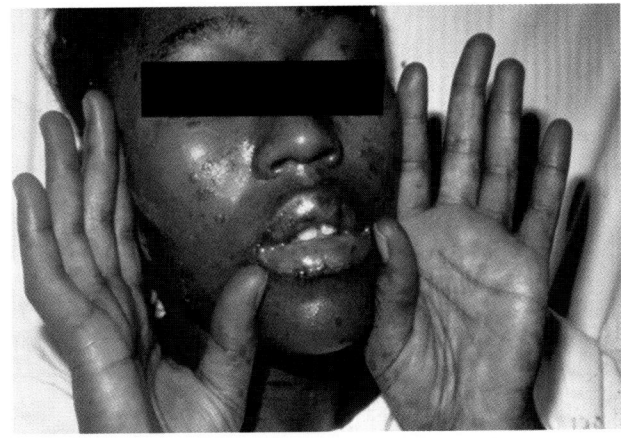

FIGURE 9.9 Erythema multiforme major. Extensive hemorrhagic crusting of mucous membranes and erythematous lesions were accompanied by fever.

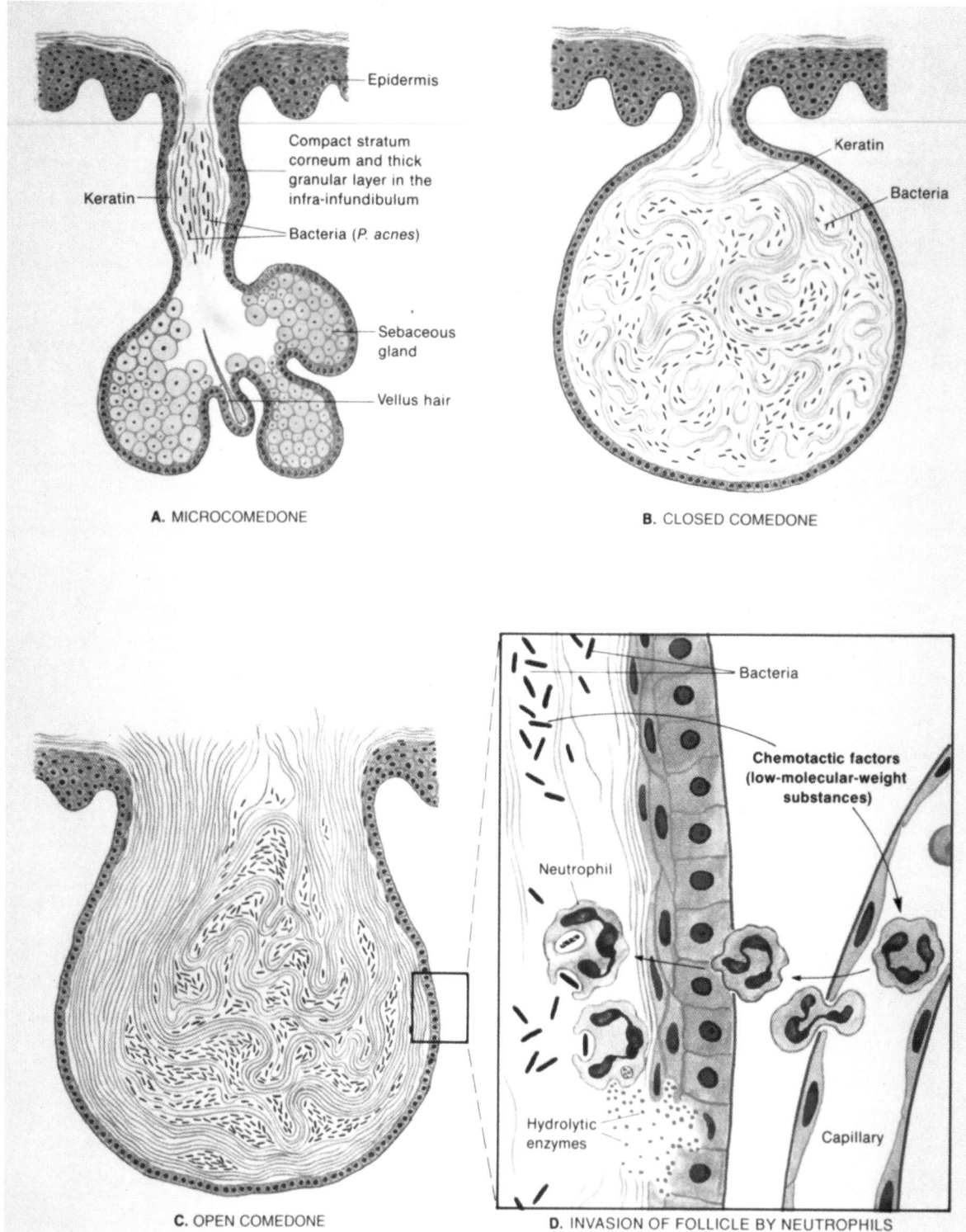

FIGURE 10.1 Pathogenesis of follicular distention, rupture, and inflammation in acne vulgaris. Acne is a disease of the follicular canal of a sebaceous follicle. A compact stratum corneum and a thickened granular layer in the infrainfundibulum are the beginning of the formation of a comedone. Microcomedones **(A)** and closed **(B)** and open **(C)** comedones form. Excessive sebum secretion occurs, and the bacterium *P. acnes* proliferates. The organism produces chemotactic factors, leading to neutrophil migration into the intact comedone. Neutrophilic enzymes are released and the comedone ruptures, inducing a cycle of chemotaxis and intense neutrophilic inflammation **(D)**.

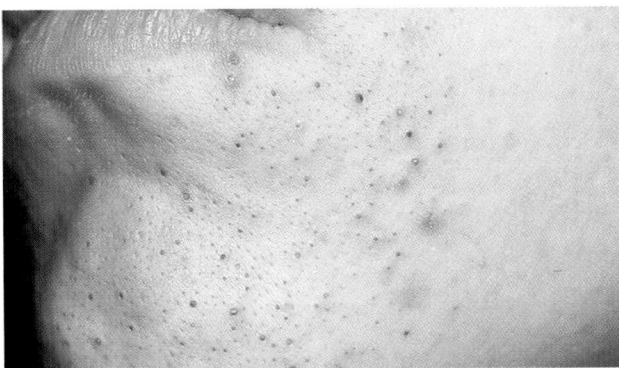

FIGURE 10.2 Noninflammatory lesions. The combination of open and closed comedones, as seen here, is most common in younger patients.

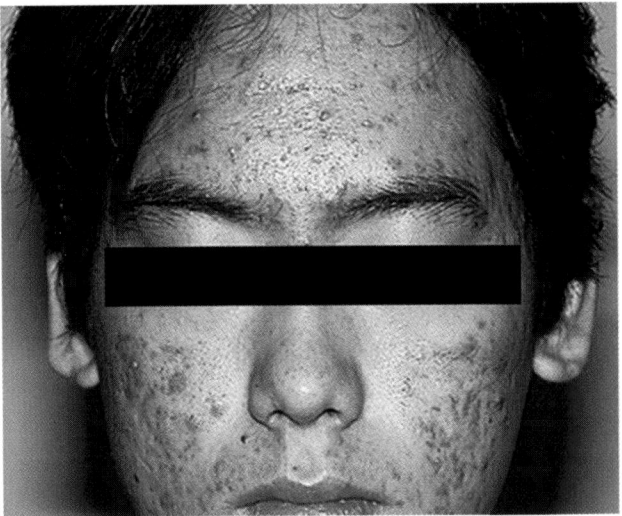

FIGURE 10.3 Severe cystic acne. This patient was subsequently treated with isotretinoin (Accutane).

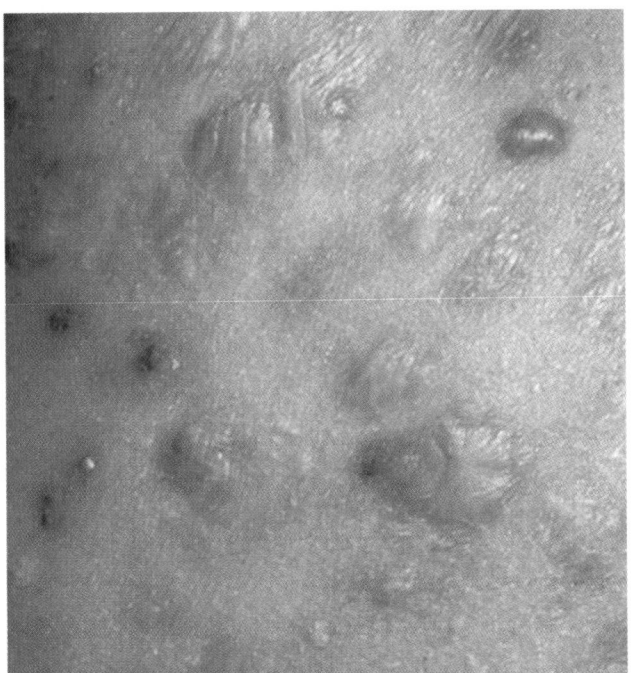

FIGURE 10.4 Acne scars. Hypertrophic scars. These lesions are characteristic of acne scars that occur on the trunk.

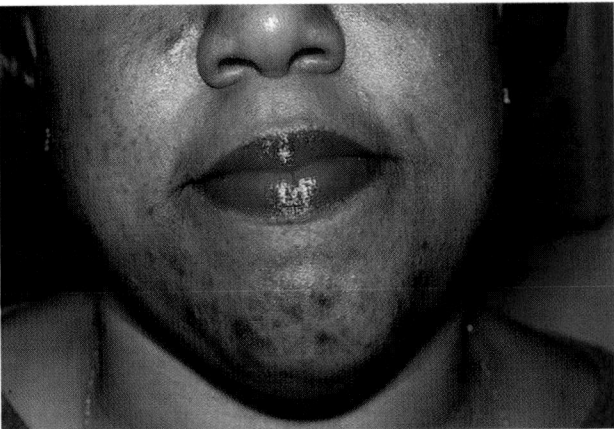

FIGURE 10.5 Postinflammatory hyperpigmentation is seen in this African-American patient.

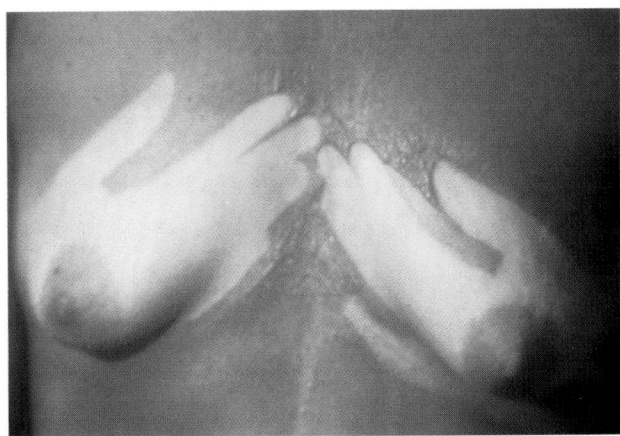

FIGURE 10.7 Drug photosensitivity eruption. Erythematous (exaggerated sunburn) reaction in a person who was taking demeclocycline (Declomycin) and fell asleep on the beach.

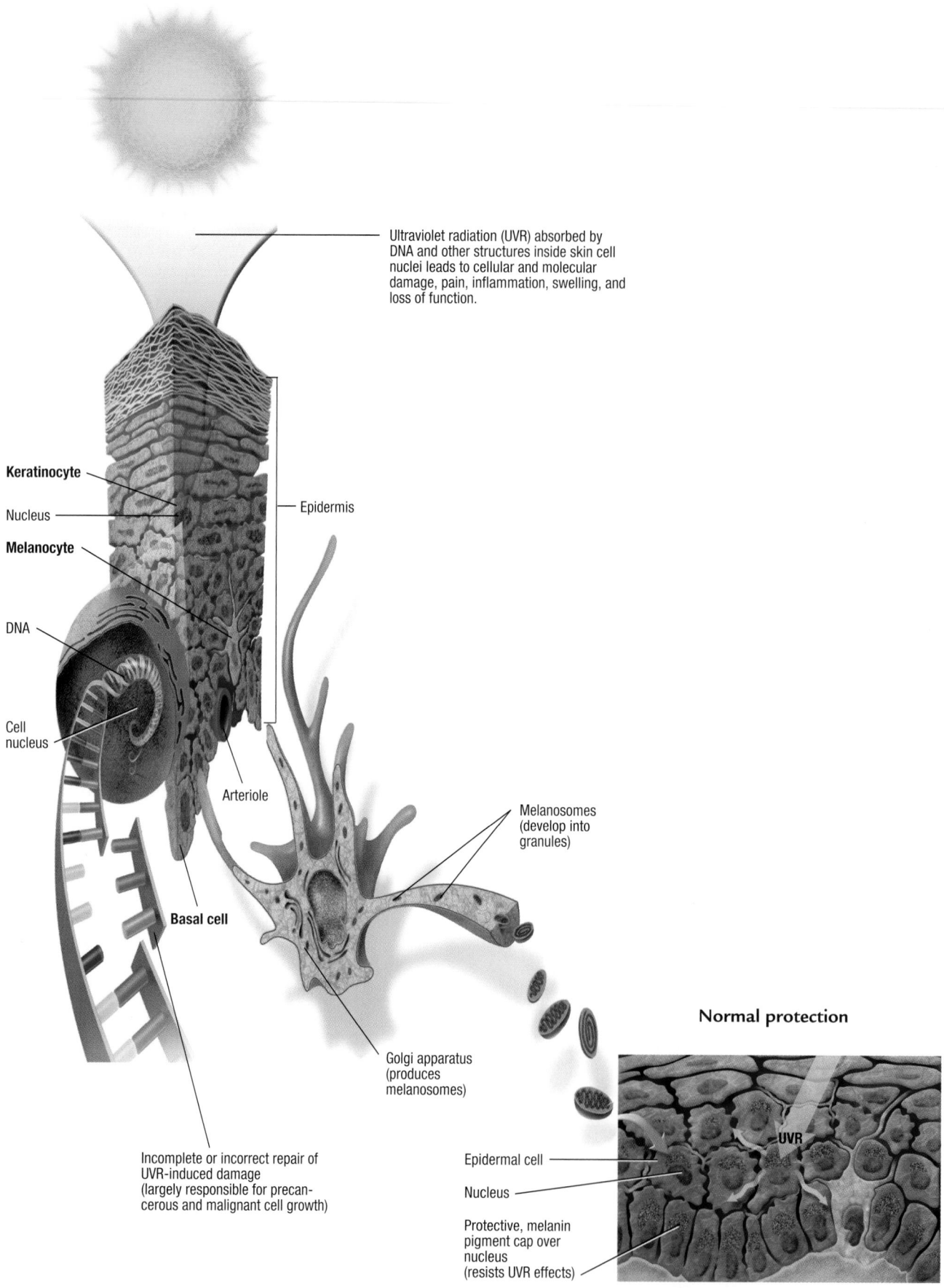

Ultraviolet radiation (UVR) absorbed by DNA and other structures inside skin cell nuclei leads to cellular and molecular damage, pain, inflammation, swelling, and loss of function.

Keratinocyte

Nucleus

Melanocyte

Epidermis

DNA

Cell nucleus

Arteriole

Melanosomes (develop into granules)

Basal cell

Golgi apparatus (produces melanosomes)

Incomplete or incorrect repair of UVR-induced damage (largely responsible for precancerous and malignant cell growth)

Normal protection

UVR

Epidermal cell

Nucleus

Protective, melanin pigment cap over nucleus (resists UVR effects)

FIGURE 10.6 Skin response to ultraviolet radiation.

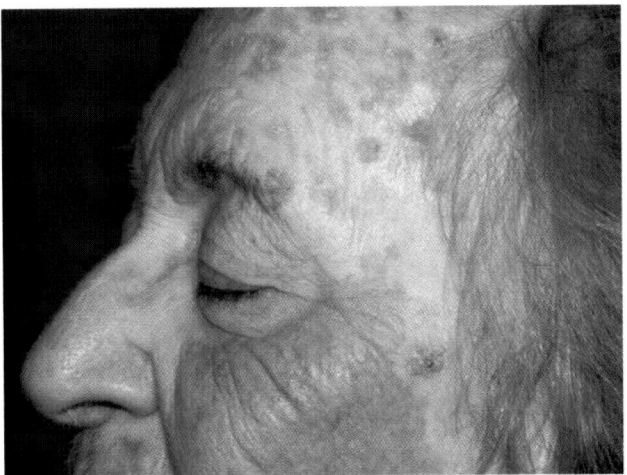

FIGURE 10.9 Actinic keratoses. This elderly woman has vitiligo. The solar keratoses occur primarily in areas of unprotected, melanocytes-poor, vitiliginous skin.

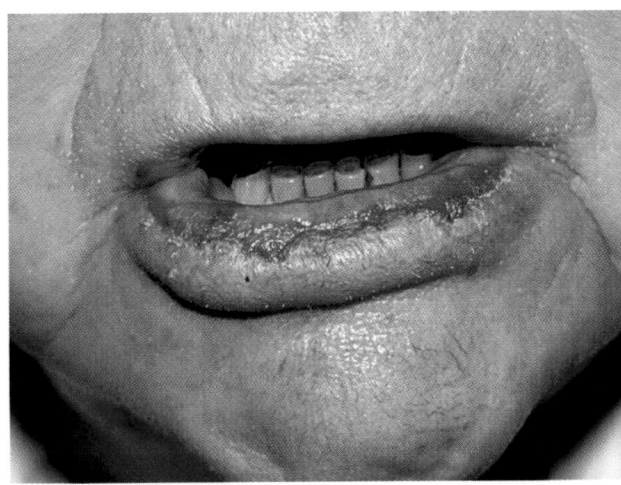

FIGURE 10.10 Actinic cheilitis. This patient is undergoing treatment with topical 5-fluorouracil for multiple solar keratoses of his lower lip.

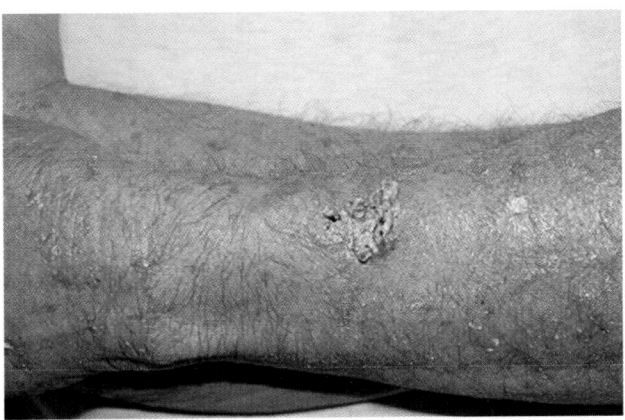

FIGURE 10.11 Nodular squamous cell carcinoma. The surrounding, smaller lesions are actinic keratoses.

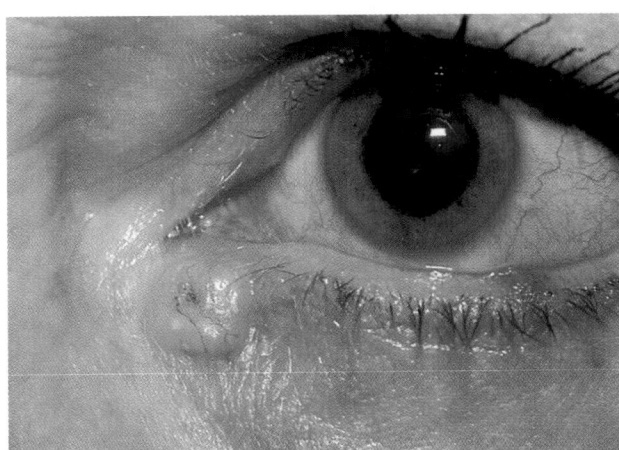

FIGURE 10.12 Basal cell carcinoma. Well-circumscribed, pearly gray tumor of the epithelium, with raised, rolled edges and central ulceration. An independent vascular pattern is also visible.

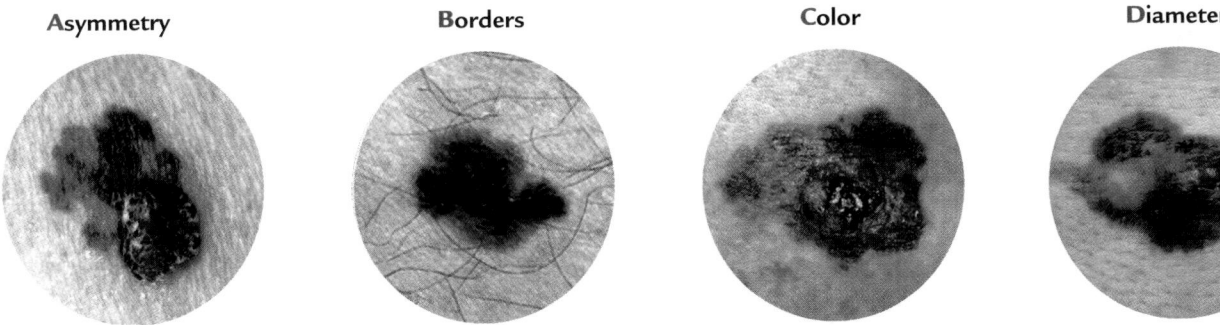

Asymmetry   Borders   Color   Diameter

FIGURE 10.13 Skin cancer: the ABCD's of malignant melanoma. A, asymmetry; B, borders; C, colors; D, diameter.

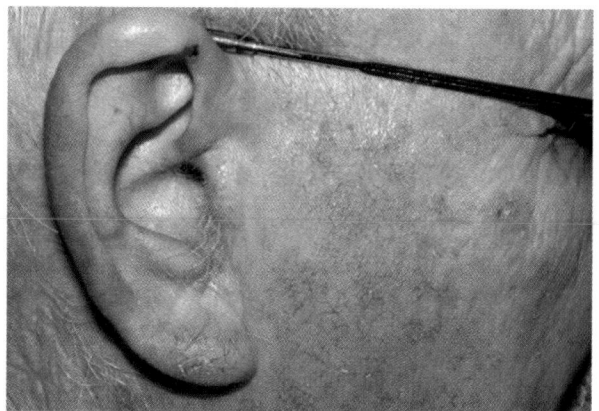

FIGURE 10.14 Actinic Keratoses. **A.** Before treatment, few lesions are clinically visible.

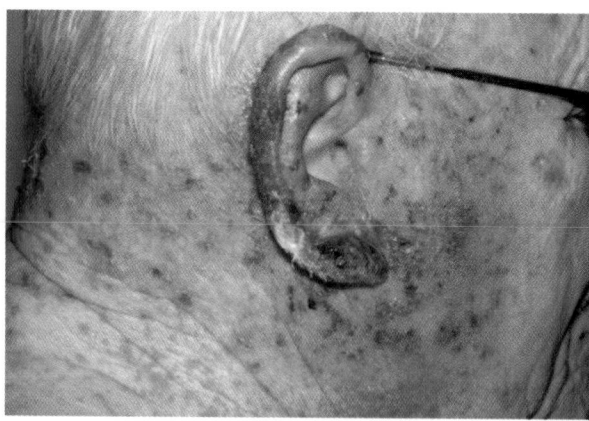

FIGURE 10.15 Actinic Keratoses. **B.** Two weeks after treatment with topical 5-fluorouracil, crusting and erythema are evident in areas that had lesions that were not initially apparent.

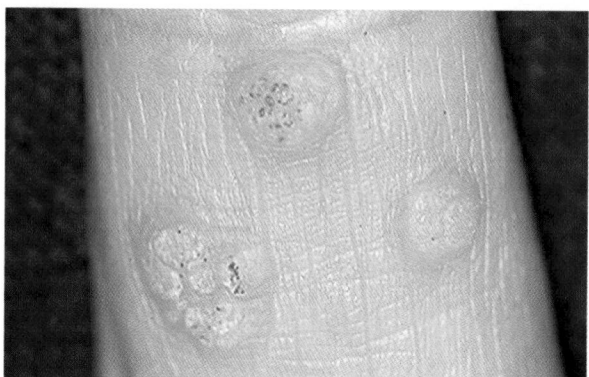

FIGURE 10.16 Common wart (verruca vulgaris).

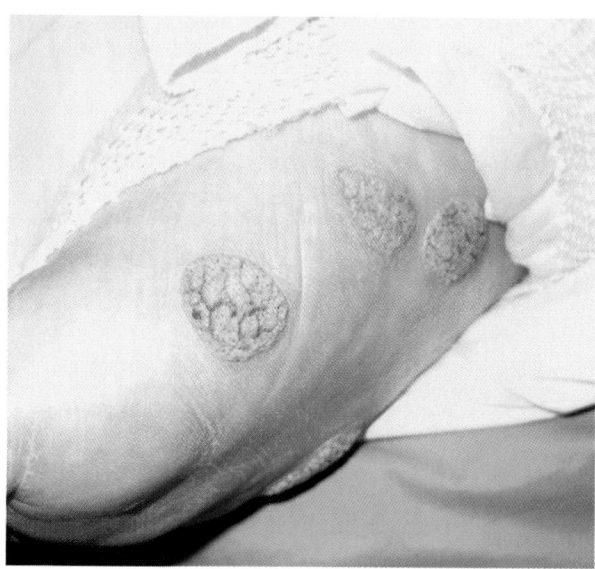

FIGURE 10.17 Plantar wart (verruca plantaris).

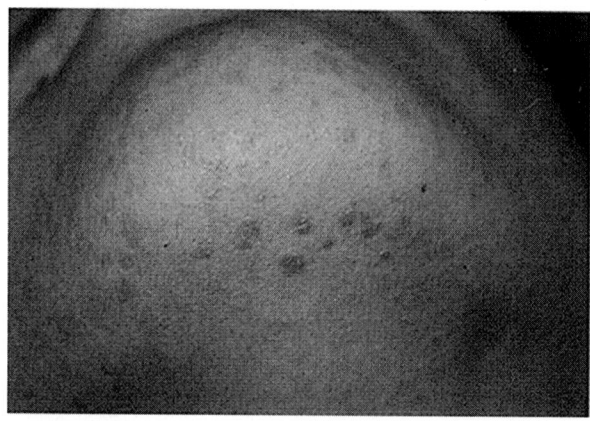

FIGURE 10.18 Flat warts (verruca plana).

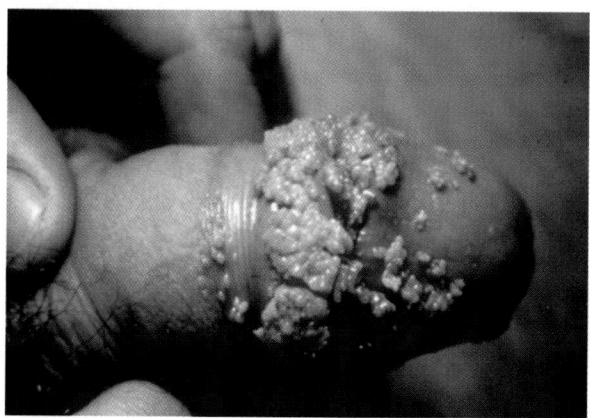

FIGURE 10.20 Condyloma acuminatum.

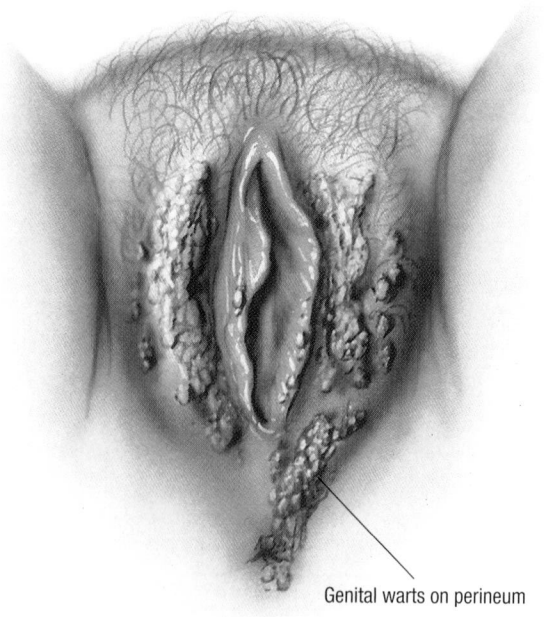

Genital warts on perineum

FIGURE 10.19 Vaginal warts.

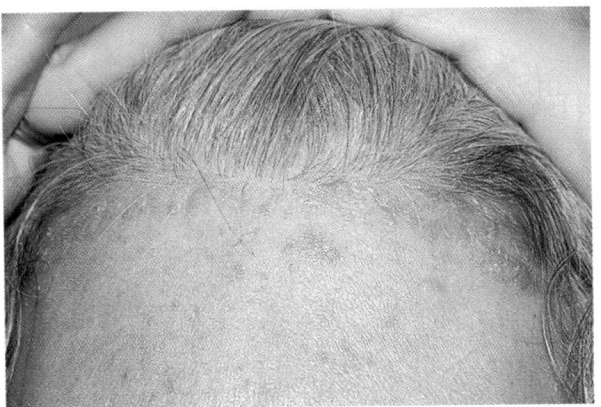

FIGURE 10.21 Seborrheic dermatitis. Scale and erythema are evident along the frontal hairline.

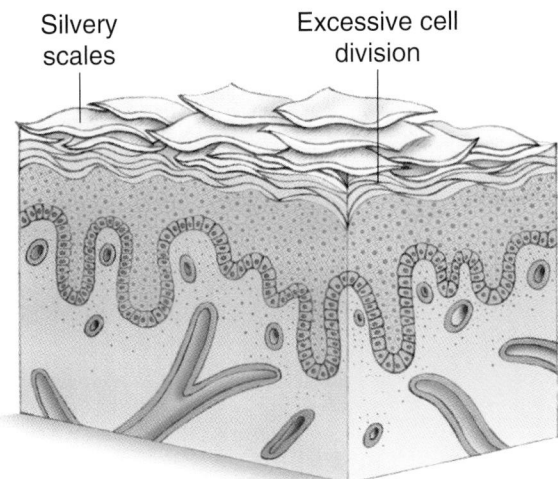

Silvery scales   Excessive cell division

Psoriasis

FIGURE 10.24 Psoriasis: silvery scales and excess cell division.

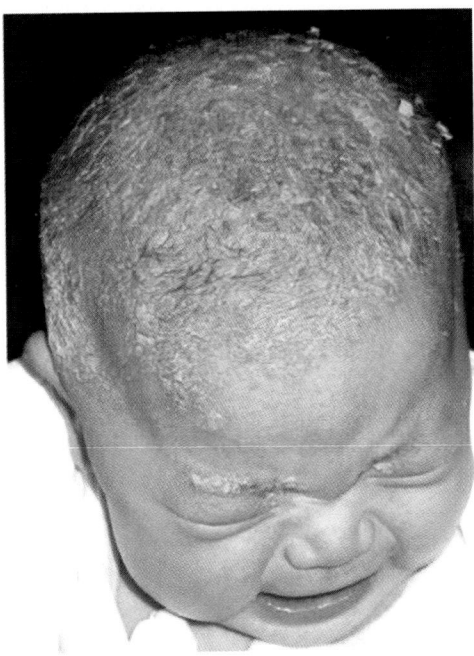

FIGURE 10.22 Infantile seborrheic dermatitis also known as cradle cap.

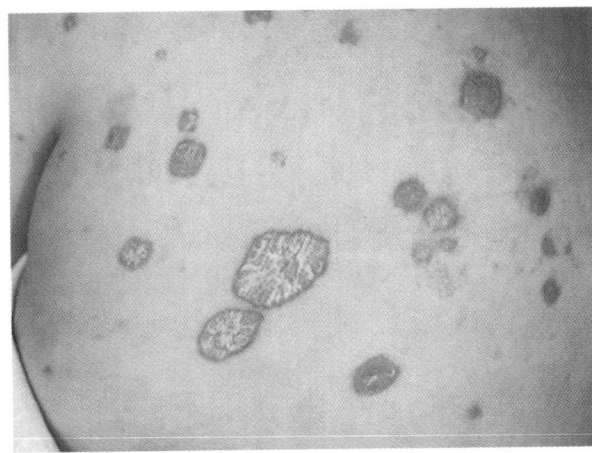

FIGURE 10.25 Typical lesions of plaque psoriasis on skin of the back.

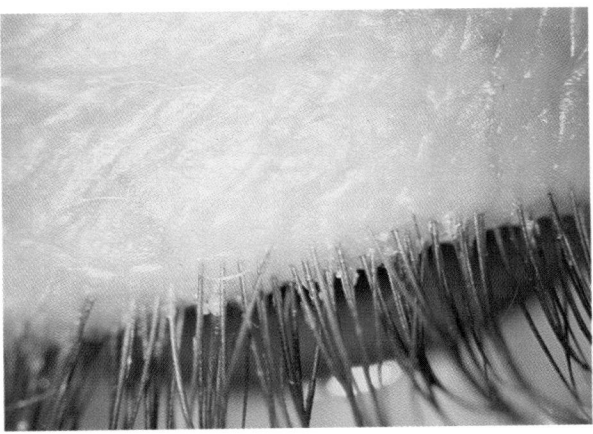

FIGURE 10.23 Seborrheic blepharitis is associated with crusting of the eyelids without meibomian gland inflammation and with seborrheic dermatitis of the eyebrows and scalp.

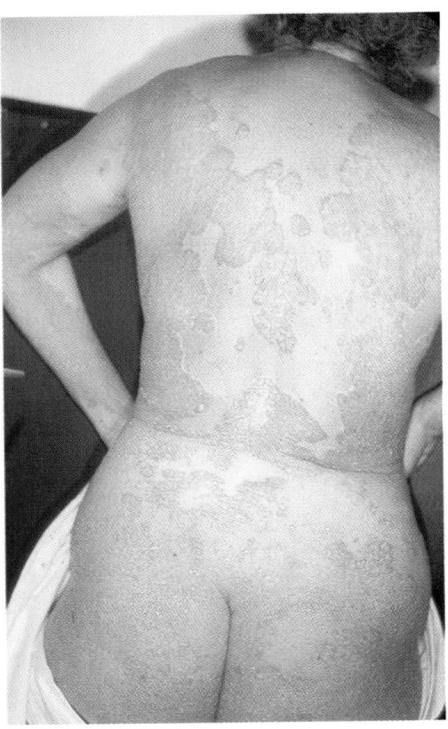

FIGURE 10.26 Psoriasis. Extensive, large plaques are evident on this patient.

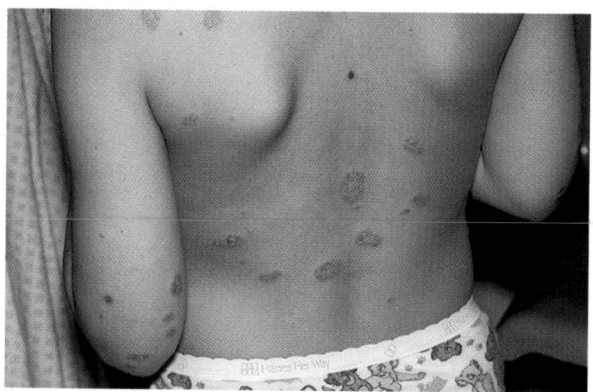

FIGURE 10.27 Guttate psoriasis.

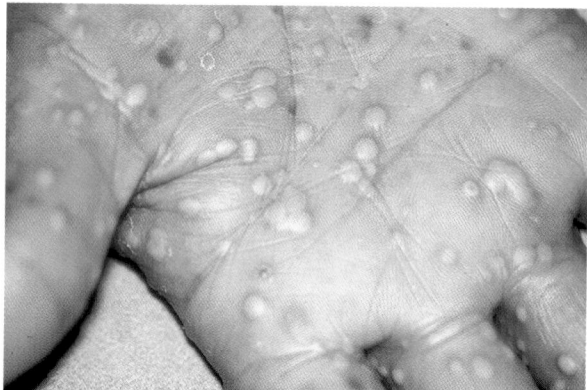

FIGURE 10.29 Pustular psoriasis.

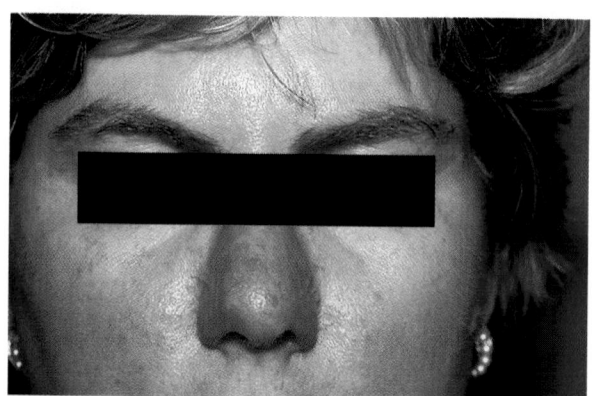

FIGURE 10.32 Prerosacea. This woman has "rosy cheeks" and telangiectasias.

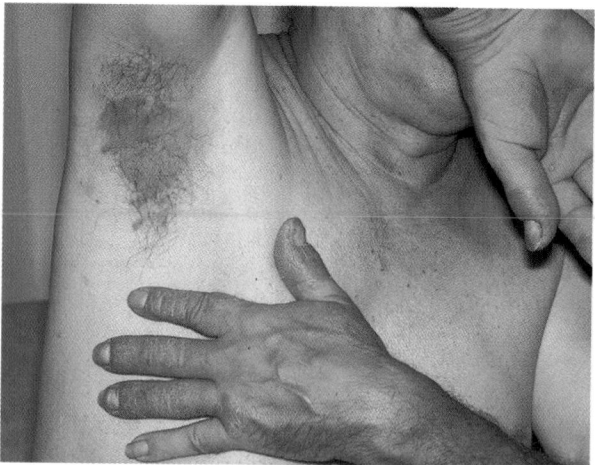

FIGURE 10.28 Inverse psoriasis.

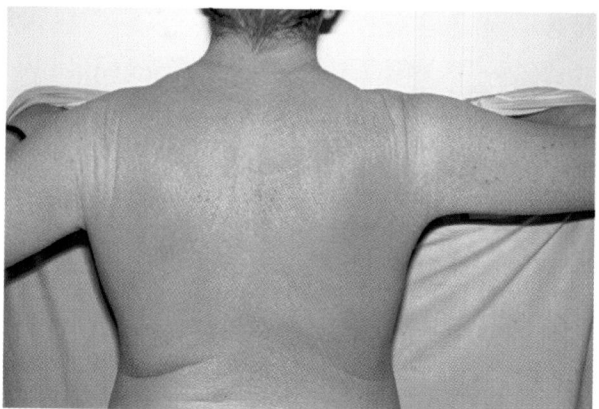

FIGURE 10.30 Erythrodermic psoriasis.

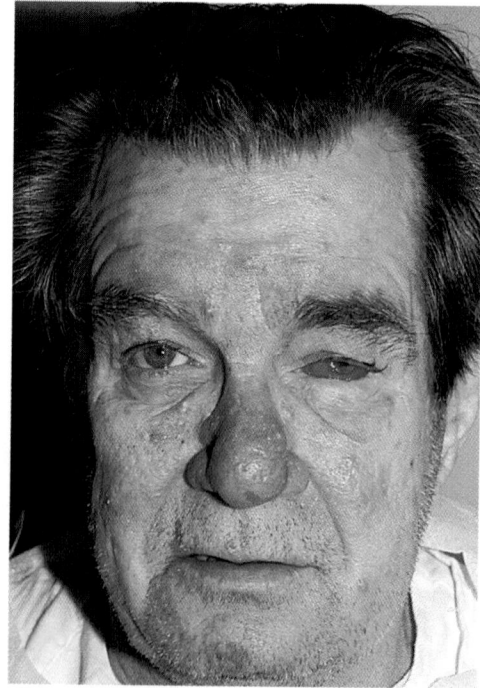

FIGURE 10.33 Rosacea is manifested by telangiectatic vessels on the skin—advanced case of rhinophyma. Blepharitis may also be associated.

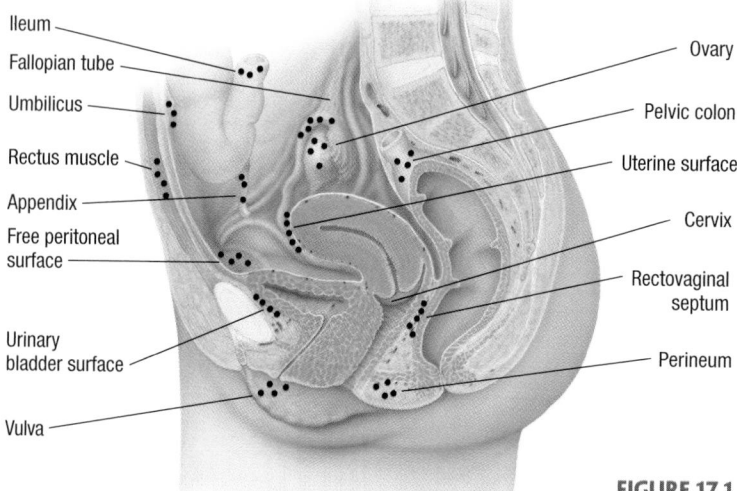

Ileum

Fallopian tube

Umbilicus

Rectus muscle

Appendix

Free peritoneal surface

Urinary bladder surface

Vulva

Ovary

Pelvic colon

Uterine surface

Cervix

Rectovaginal septum

Perineum

FIGURE 17.1 Common anatomic locations of endometriosis within the pelvic cavity.

MyPyramid
STEPS TO A HEALTHIER YOU
MyPyramid.gov
GRAINS
VEGETABLES
FRUITS
MILK
MEAT & BEANS

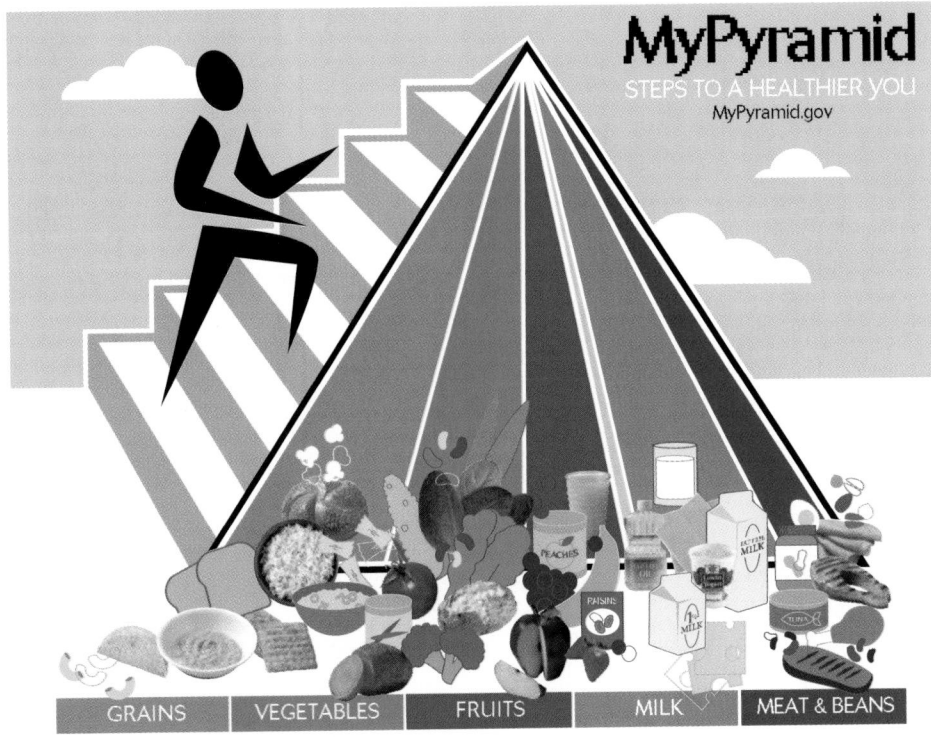

FIGURE 29.1 The USDA Food Guide Pyramid.

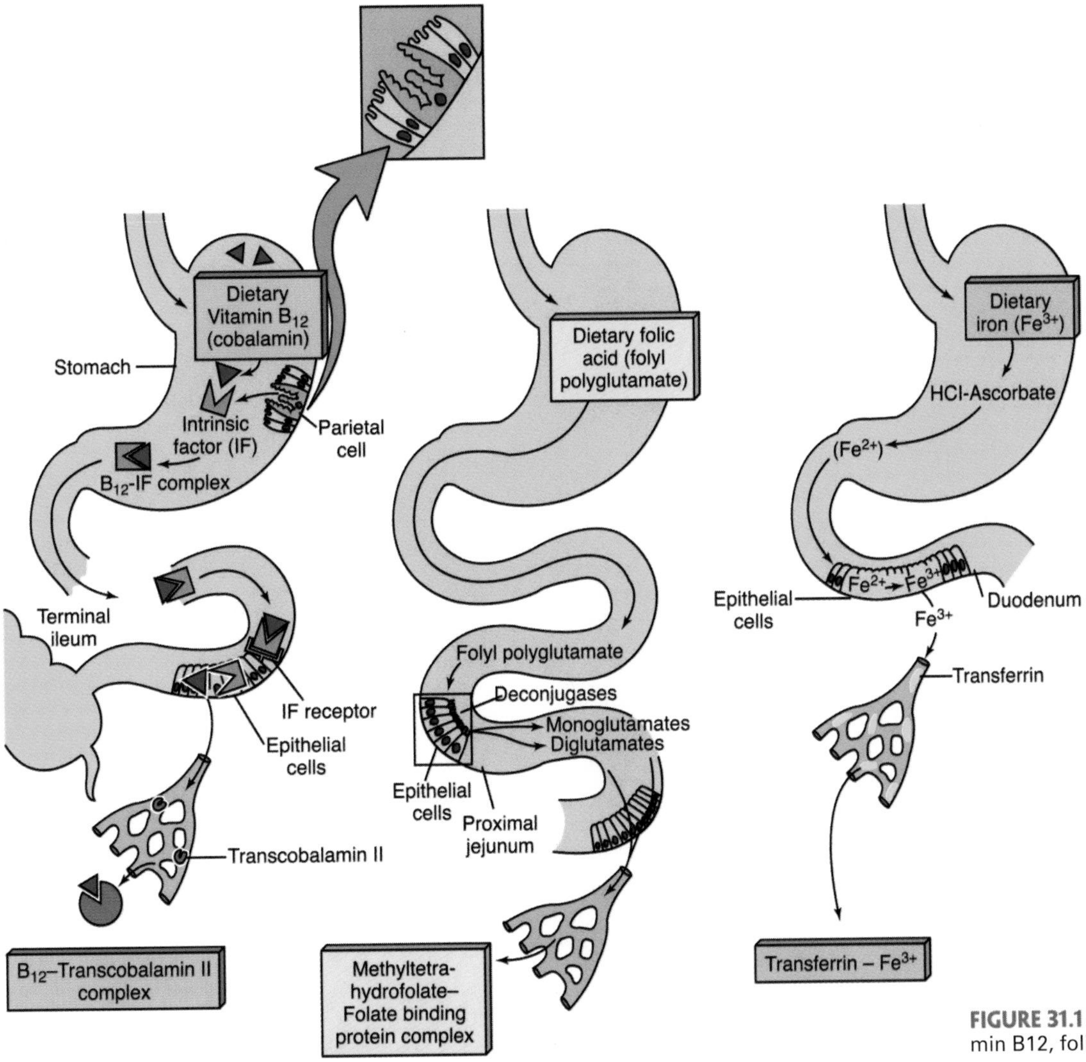
Dietary Vitamin B_{12} (cobalamin)
Stomach
Intrinsic factor (IF)
Parietal cell
B_{12}-IF complex
Terminal ileum
IF receptor
Epithelial cells
Transcobalamin II
B_{12}–Transcobalamin II complex
Dietary folic acid (folyl polyglutamate)
Folyl polyglutamate
Deconjugases
Monoglutamates
Diglutamates
Epithelial cells
Proximal jejunum
Methyltetra-hydrofolate–Folate binding protein complex
Dietary iron (Fe^{3+})
HCl-Ascorbate
(Fe^{2+})
Epithelial cells
Fe^{2+} → Fe^{3+}
Duodenum
Fe^{3+}
Transferrin
Transferrin – Fe^{3+}

FIGURE 31.1 Absorption of vitamin B12, folic acid, and iron.

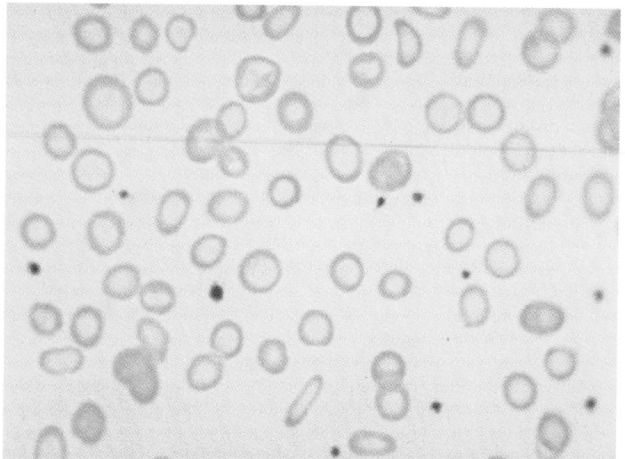

FIGURE 31.2 Iron deficient erythrocyte (hypochromic, microcytic). Pink central pallor greater than one-third of cell.

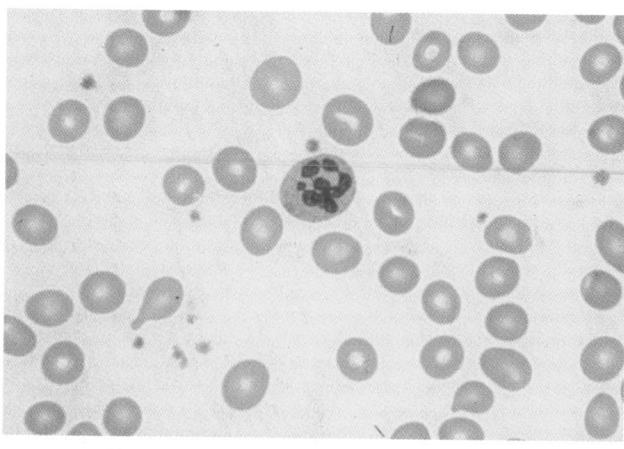

FIGURE 31.3 Vitamin B$_{12}$ deficiency. Macrocytic, normochromic anemia, thrombocytopenia with large platelets and hypersegmented neutrophils.

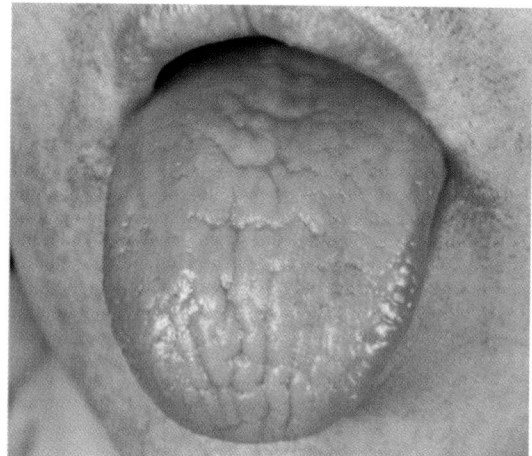

FIGURE 31.4 Smooth, reddish, shiny tongue without papillae due to vitamin B$_{12}$ deficiency.

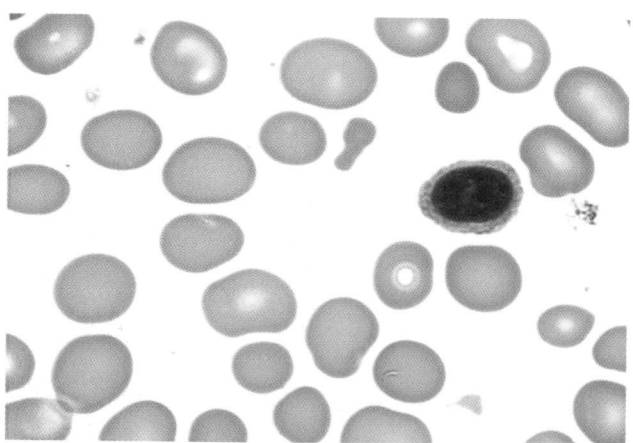

FIGURE 31.6 Folate deficiency. Peripheral blood smear showing macrocytic, normochromic anemia.

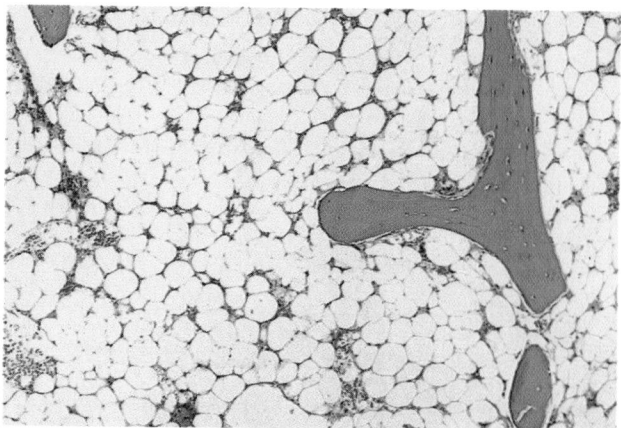

FIGURE 32.1 Aplastic anemia. The bone marrow consists largely of fat cells and lacks normal hemopoietic activity.

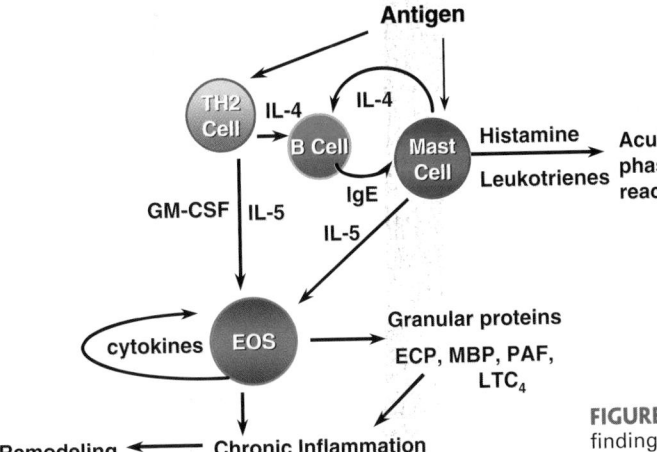

Airway lumen narrowing

Mucous gland hypertrophy and hyperplasia

Epithelial damage

Edema

Airway smooth-muscle hypertrophy, hyperplasia, and bronchoconstriction

Mucus hypersecretion

Inflammatory cell infiltration

Thickening of basement membrane

Vascular dilation

Goblet cell hyperplasia

FIGURE 34.1 Diagram illustrating the changes present in a fully contracted small airway.

Antigen

TH2 Cell — IL-4 → B Cell ← IL-4 → Mast Cell — **Histamine** → **Acute phase reaction**
Leukotrienes

GM-CSF IL-5 — IgE — IL-5

EOS ← cytokines

Granular proteins ECP, MBP, PAF, LTC₄

Remodeling ← **Chronic Inflammation**

FIGURE 34.2 Pathophysiologic findings in the asthmatic airway.

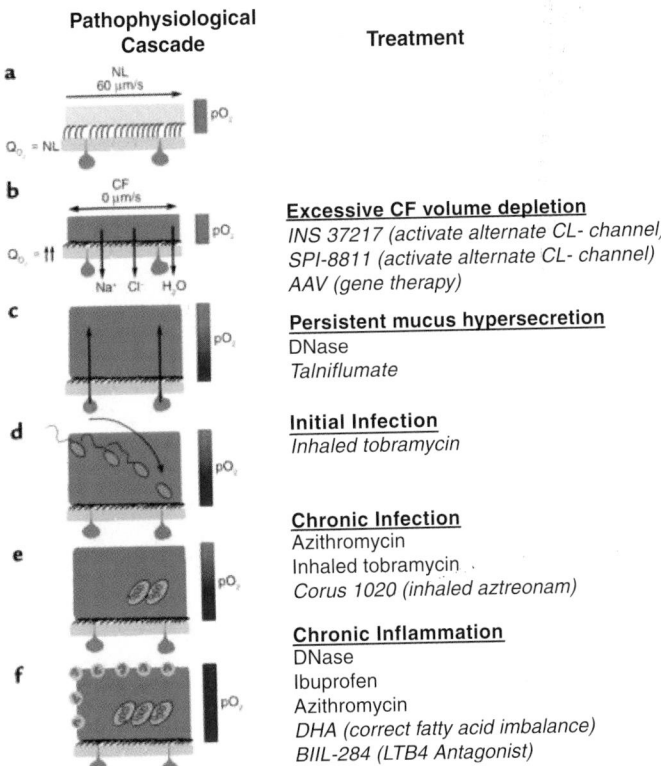

Pathophysiological Cascade   **Treatment**

a   NL 60 µm/s   pO₂
Q₀ = NL

b   CF 0 µm/s   pO₂
Q₀ = ↑↑   Na⁺ Cl⁻ H₂O

Excessive CF volume depletion
INS 37217 (activate alternate CL- channel)
SPI-8811 (activate alternate CL- channel)
AAV (gene therapy)

c   pO₂

Persistent mucus hypersecretion
DNase
Talniflumate

d   pO₂

Initial Infection
Inhaled tobramycin

e   pO₂

Chronic Infection
Azithromycin
Inhaled tobramycin
Corus 1020 (inhaled aztreonam)

f   pO₂

Chronic Inflammation
DNase
Ibuprofen
Azithromycin
DHA (correct fatty acid imbalance)
BIIL-284 (LTB4 Antagonist)

FIGURE 36.2 Proposed pathophysiologic cascade for cystic fibrosis (CF) lung disease and the therapeutic interventions targeted at each step.

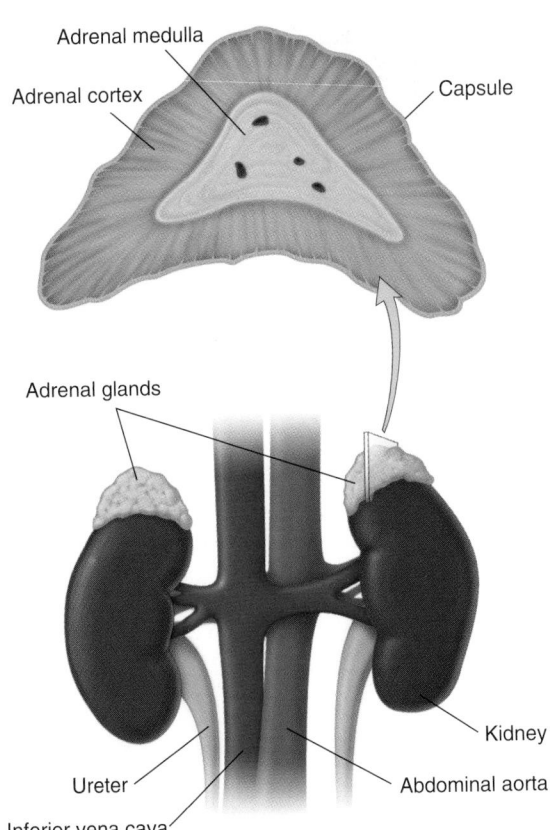

Adrenal medulla
Adrenal cortex
Capsule
Adrenal glands
Kidney
Ureter
Abdominal aorta
Inferior vena cava

FIGURE 37.1 Location and structure of the adrenal glands.

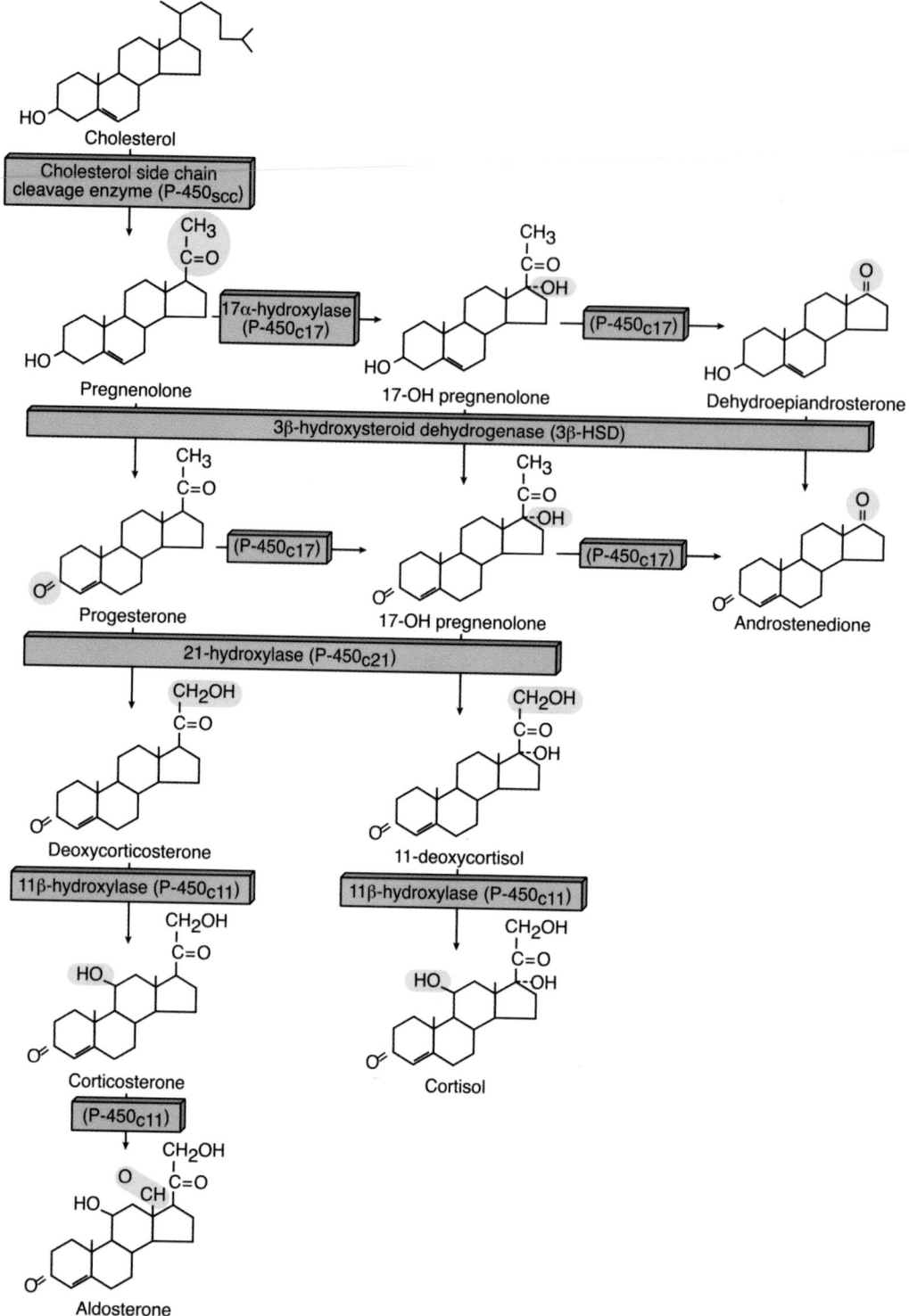

FIGURE 37.2 Biosynthetic pathways in the synthesis of adrenal corticosteroids.

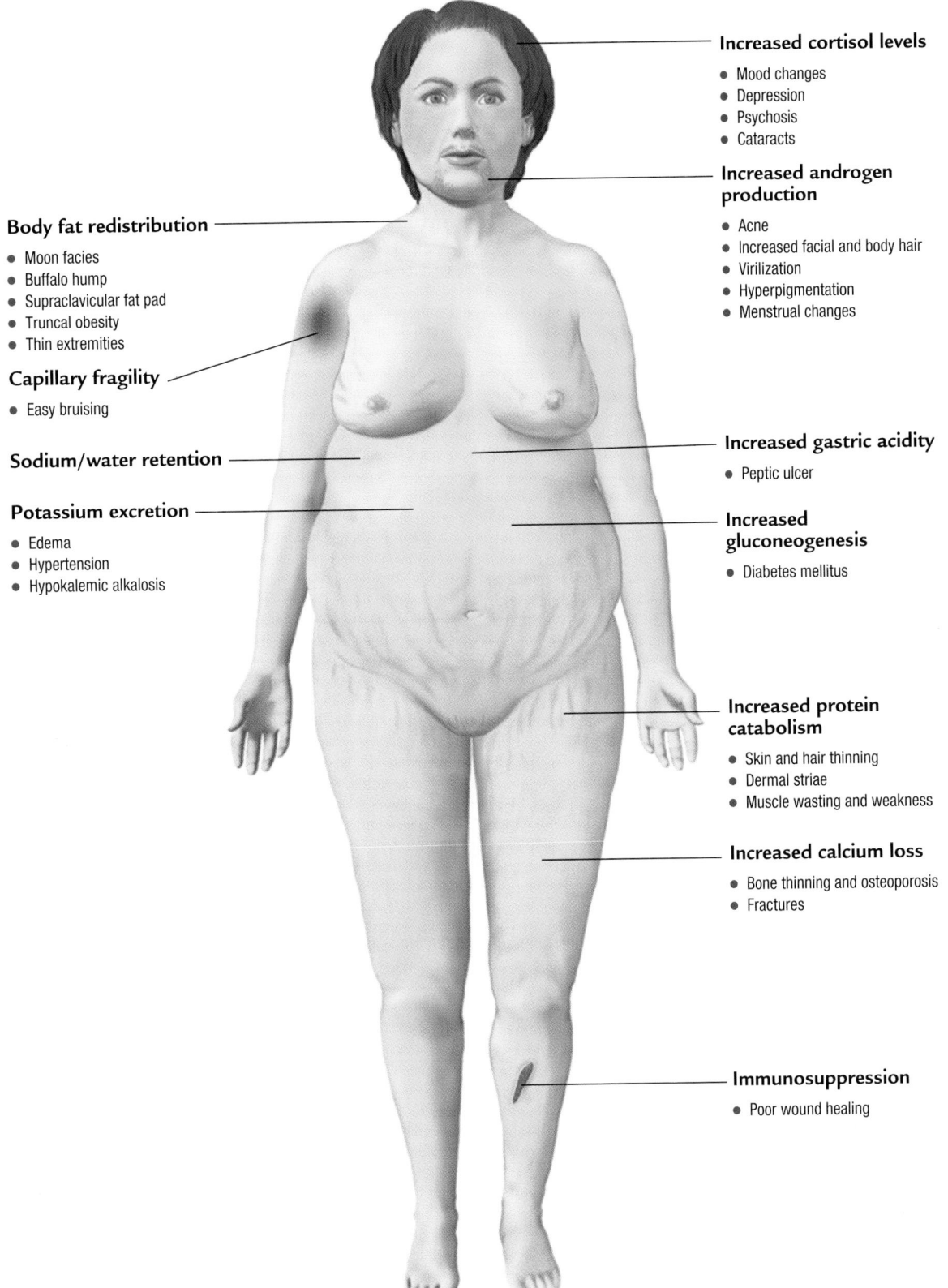

Increased cortisol levels

- Mood changes
- Depression
- Psychosis
- Cataracts

Increased androgen production

- Acne
- Increased facial and body hair
- Virilization
- Hyperpigmentation
- Menstrual changes

Body fat redistribution

- Moon facies
- Buffalo hump
- Supraclavicular fat pad
- Truncal obesity
- Thin extremities

Capillary fragility

- Easy bruising

Sodium/water retention

Potassium excretion

- Edema
- Hypertension
- Hypokalemic alkalosis

Increased gastric acidity

- Peptic ulcer

Increased gluconeogenesis

- Diabetes mellitus

Increased protein catabolism

- Skin and hair thinning
- Dermal striae
- Muscle wasting and weakness

Increased calcium loss

- Bone thinning and osteoporosis
- Fractures

Immunosuppression

- Poor wound healing

FIGURE 37.3 Manifestations of Cushing's syndrome.

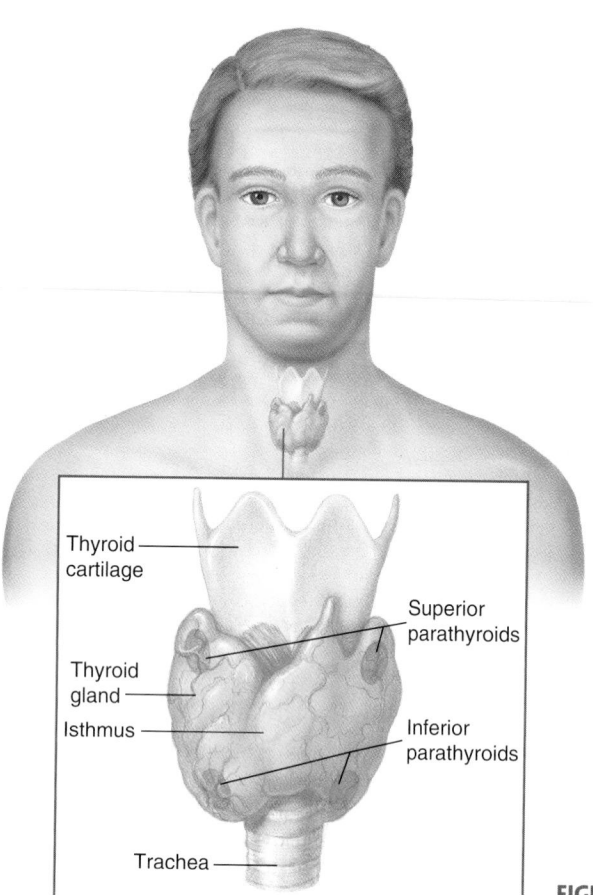

Thyroid
cartilage

Superior
parathyroids

Thyroid
gland

Isthmus

Inferior
parathyroids

Trachea

FIGURE 39.3 The thyroid and parathyroid glands.

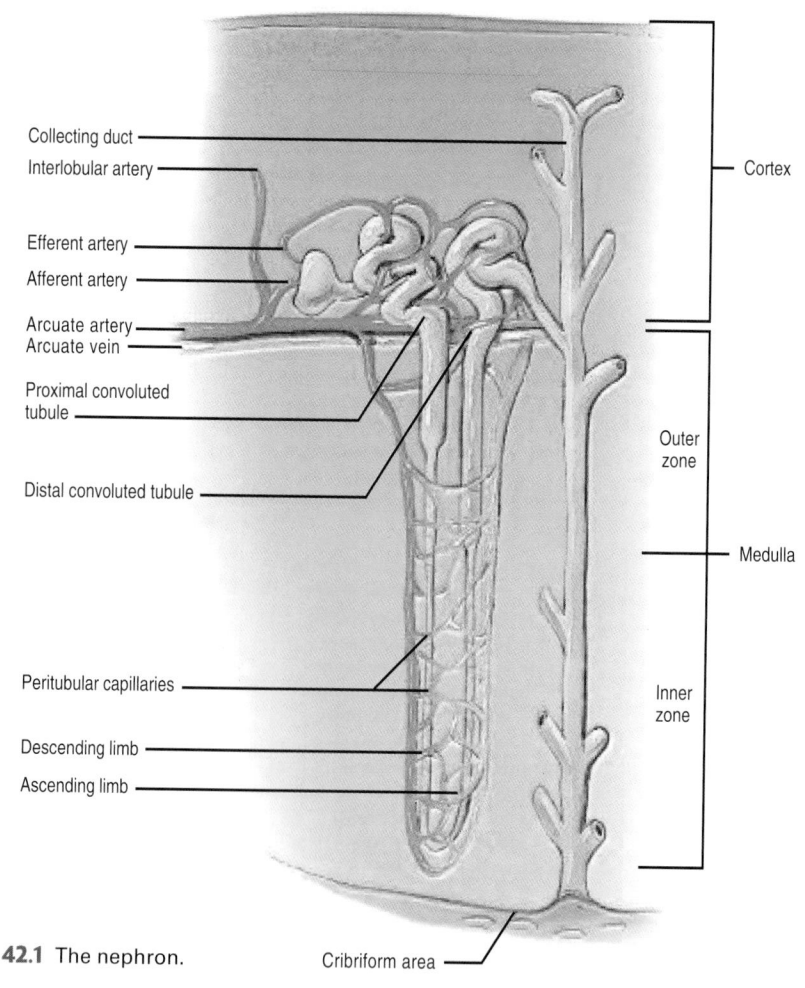

Collecting duct

Interlobular artery

Efferent artery

Afferent artery

Arcuate artery

Arcuate vein

Proximal convoluted
tubule

Distal convoluted tubule

Peritubular capillaries

Descending limb

Ascending limb

Cortex

Outer
zone

Medulla

Inner
zone

Cribriform area

FIGURE 42.1 The nephron.

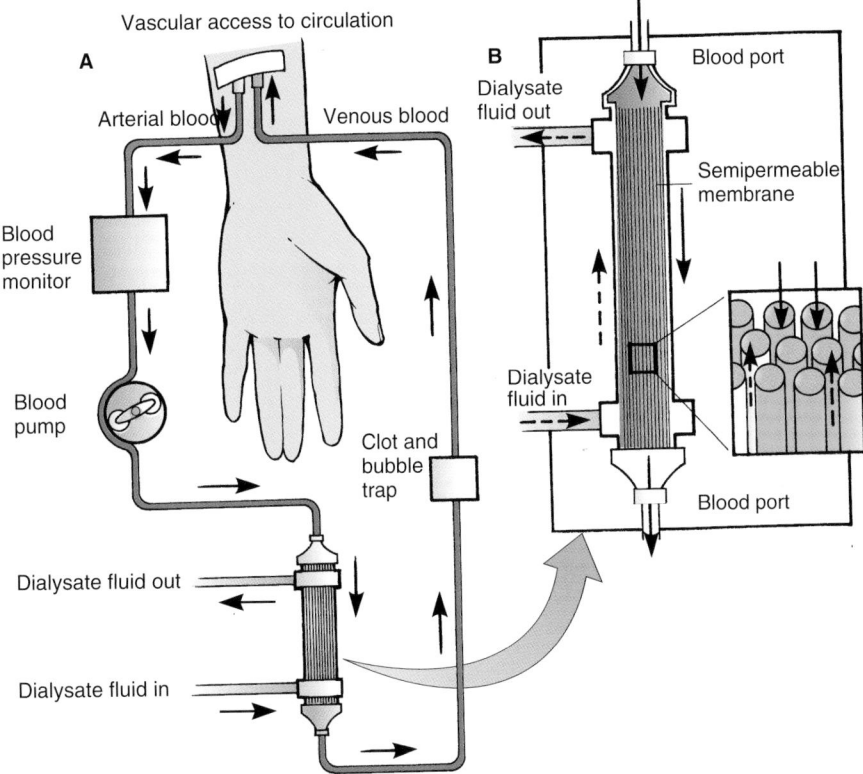

FIGURE 44.1 Hemodialysis schematic. An external pump provides the driving force for blood flow from the patient's arterial access site **(A)** through the dialyzer **(B)** where diffusion and ultrafiltration occur. Filtered blood is pumped back to the patient through the venous access. Dialysate flow moves in the opposite direction across the semipermeable membrane (dialyzer).

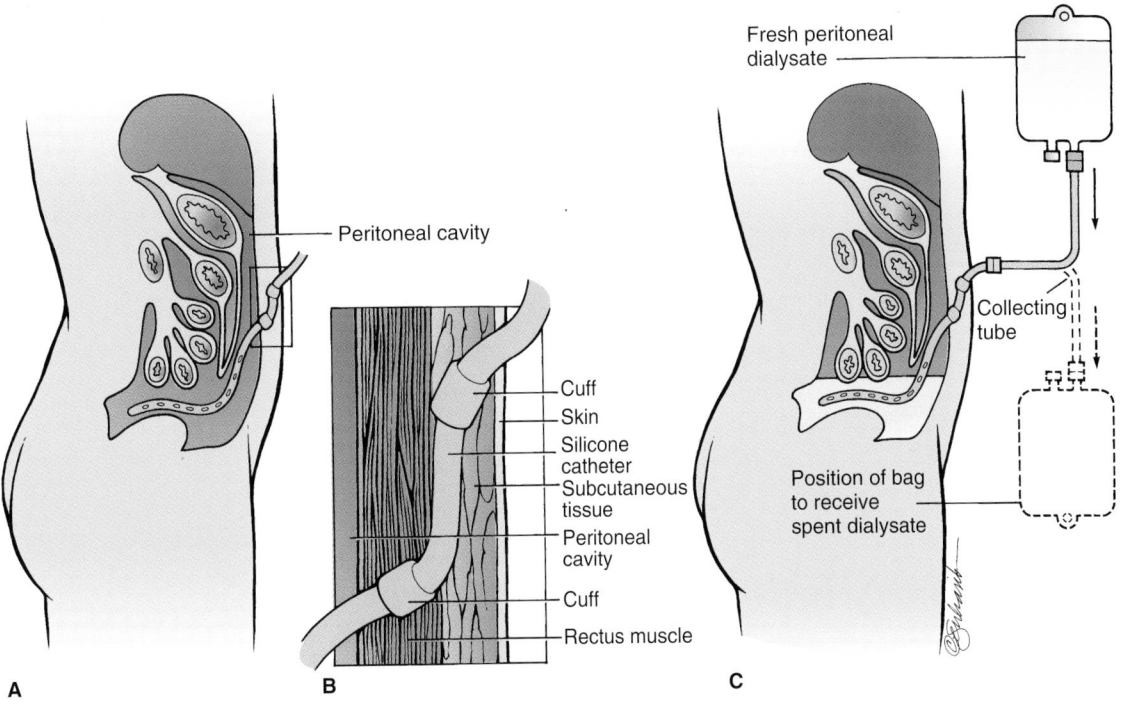

FIGURE 44.3 Peritoneal dialysis schematic and catheter placement.

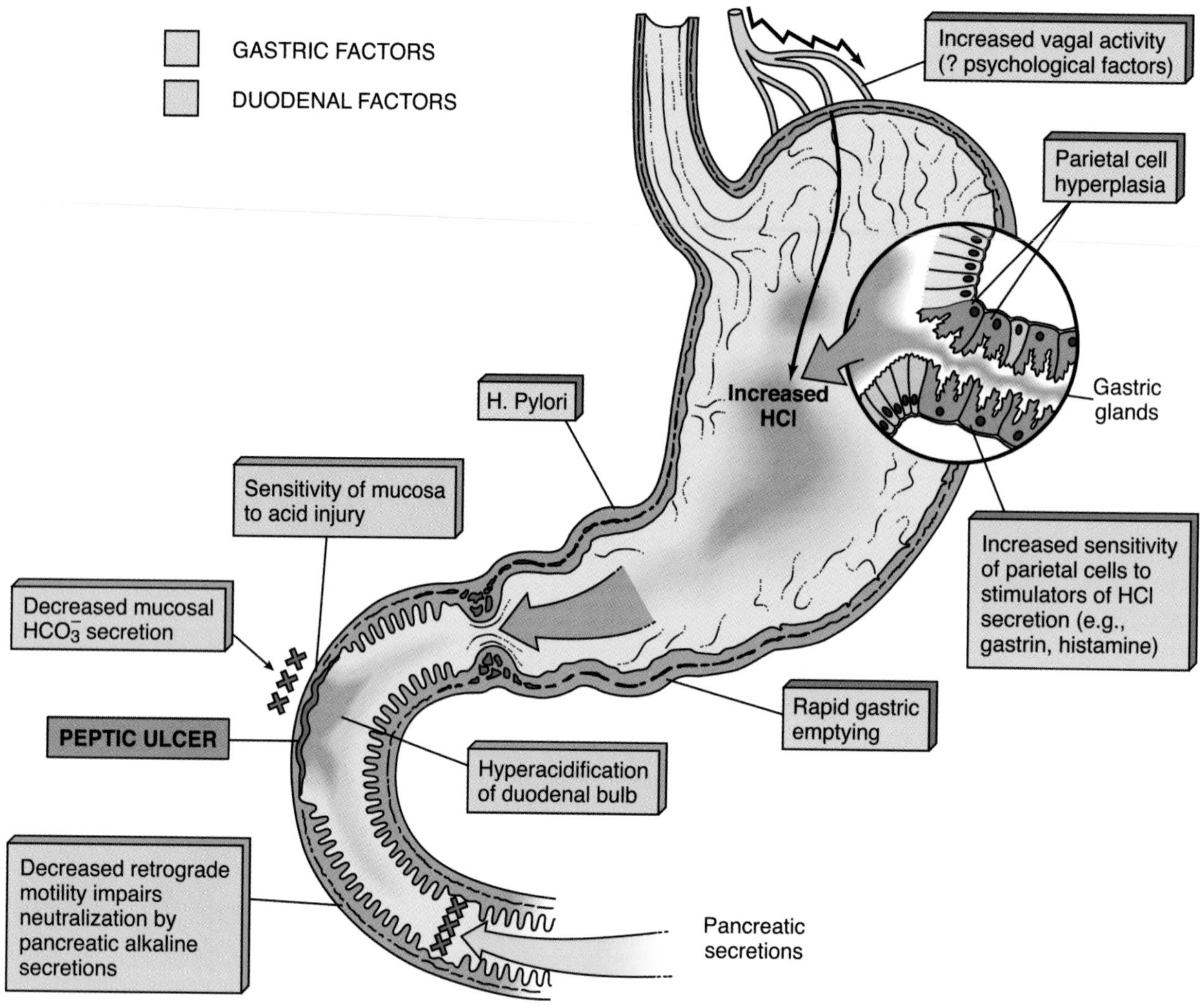

GASTRIC FACTORS

DUODENAL FACTORS

Increased vagal activity
(? psychological factors)

Parietal cell
hyperplasia

H. Pylori

Sensitivity of mucosa
to acid injury

Decreased mucosal
HCO_3^- secretion

PEPTIC ULCER

Increased
HCl

Gastric
glands

Increased sensitivity
of parietal cells to
stimulators of HCl
secretion (e.g.,
gastrin, histamine)

Rapid gastric
emptying

Hyperacidification
of duodenal bulb

Decreased retrograde
motility impairs
neutralization by
pancreatic alkaline
secretions

Pancreatic
secretions

FIGURE 45.1 Gastric and duodenal factors in the pathogenesis of duodenal peptic ulcers.

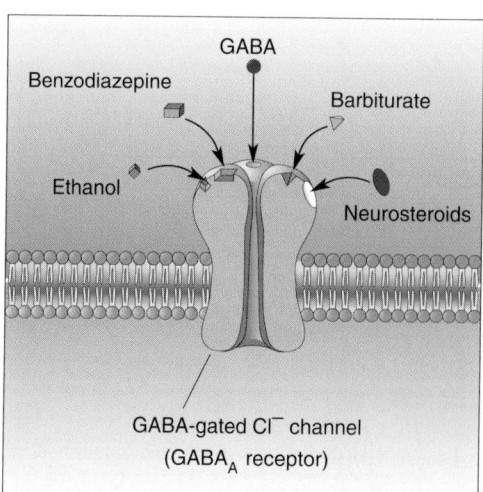

GABA

Benzodiazepine

Barbiturate

Ethanol

Neurosteroids

GABA-gated Cl⁻ channel
(GABA$_A$ receptor)

FIGURE 52.1 GABA$_A$ receptor complex. Drugs and
their binding sites on the GABA$_A$ receptor.
Binding of these drugs facilitates GABA binding
which in turn opens the channel, allowing high
influx of chloride ions, cell membrane
stabilization, and decreased neuronal firing.

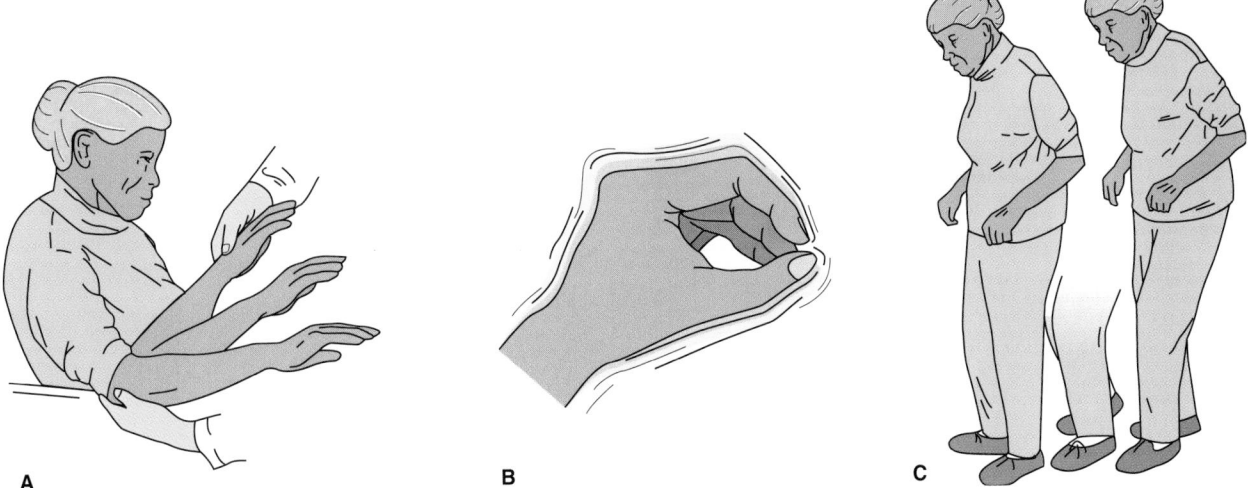

FIGURE 63.1 Parkinson's disease is manifested by **(A)** rigidity that accompanies passive flexion of extremities. "Cogwheeling" may be present; **(B)** "pill-rolling" tremor at rest; **(C)** slowness of movement characterized by a slow, shuffling gait and lack of arm swing.

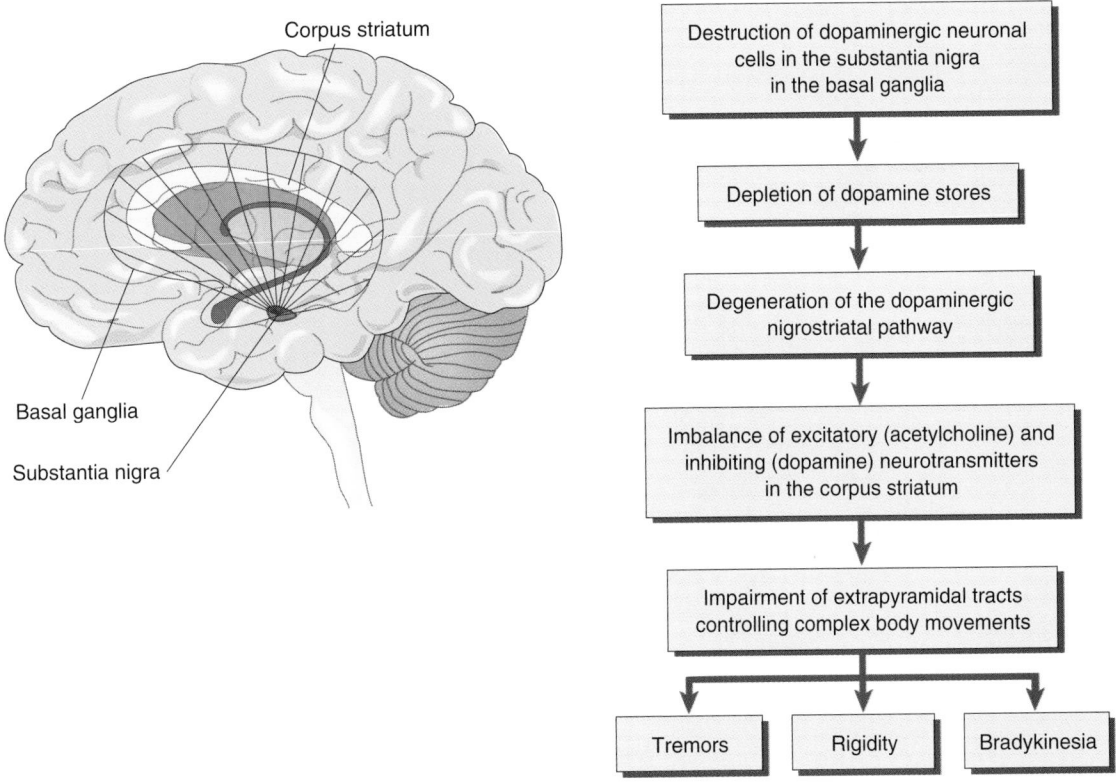

FIGURE 63.2 Etiology and pathophysiology of Parkinson's disease. **B.** The nuclei in the substantia nigra project neurons to the corpus striatum. The neurons transport dopamine to the corpus striatum. The loss of dopaminergic neurons in the substantia nigra result in subsequent development of the cardinal motor features of Parkinson's disease.

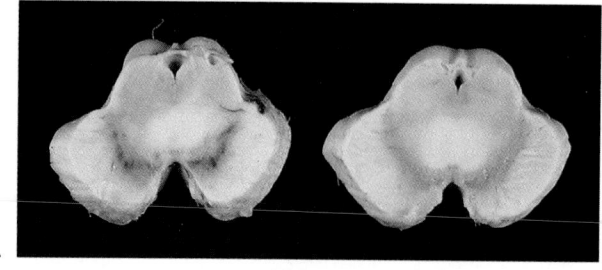

A

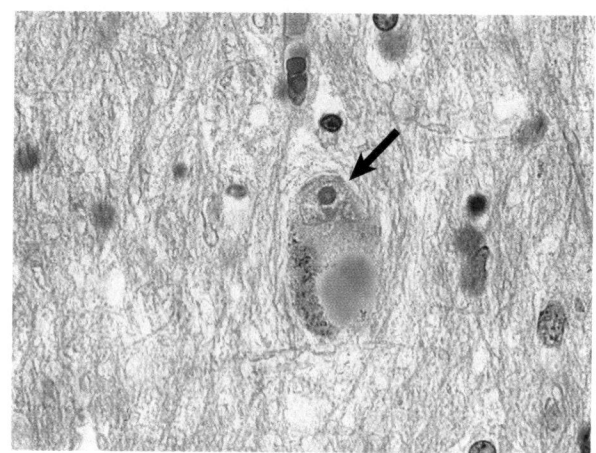

B

FIGURE 63.4 Pathology of Parkinson's disease. **A.** Normal substantia nigra of the midbrain (*left*) is heavily pigmented with neuromelanin; whereas the same region from a patient with Parkinson's disease (*right*) demonstrates depigmentation. **B.** Microscopic section of the substantia nigra pars compacta from a patient with Parkinson's disease shows a spherical eosinophilic inclusion (*arrow*) within the cytoplasm of a pigmented dopaminergic neuron. This inclusion body is termed a Lewy body.

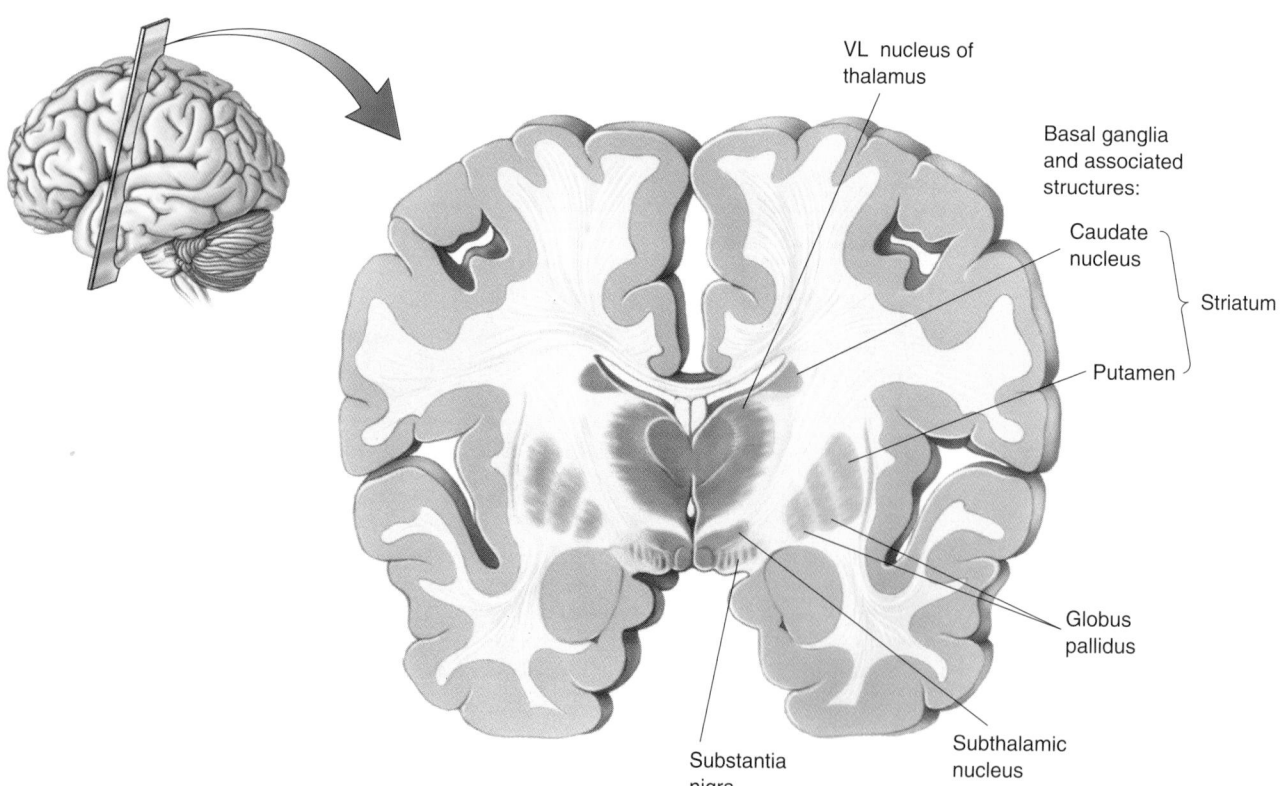

FIGURE 63.8 A coronal slice of the basal ganglia highlighting structures involved with movement.

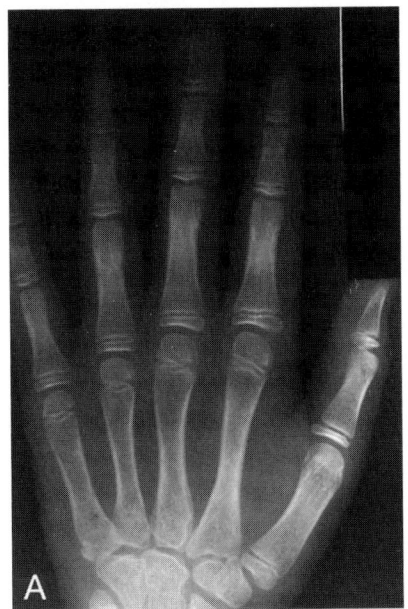

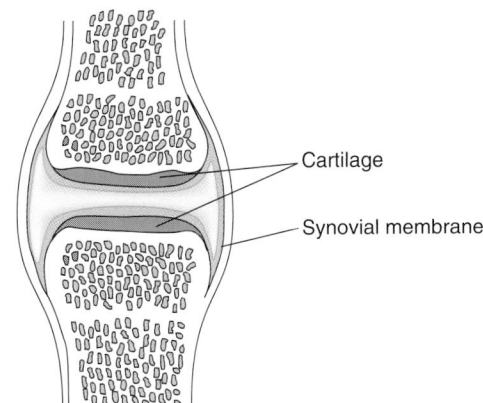

Cartilage

Synovial membrane

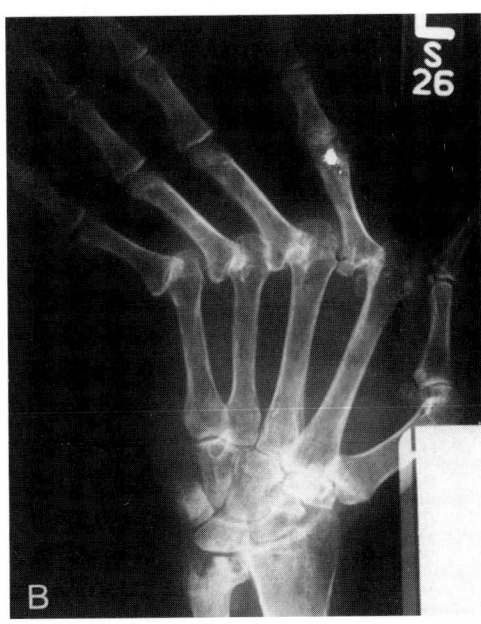

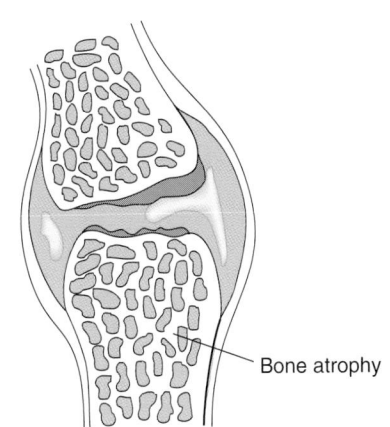

Bone atrophy

FIGURE 65.1 Joints of the hand affected by rheumatoid arthritis. **A.** X-ray of a normal hand. **B.** X-ray of hand with rheumatoid arthritis.

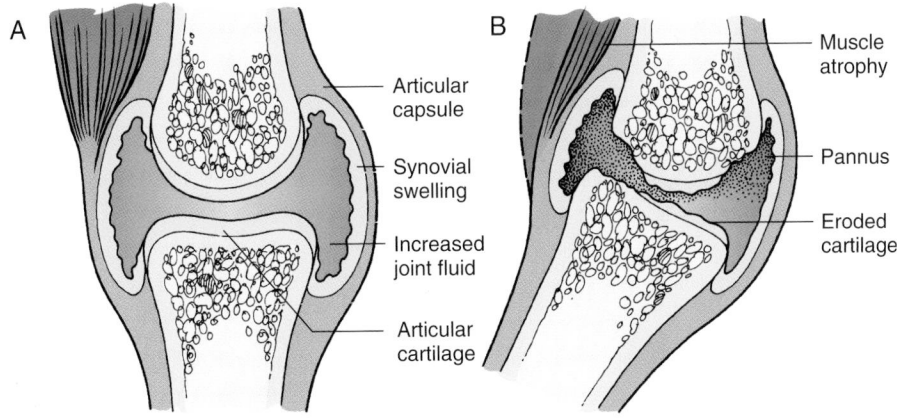

A

Articular capsule

Synovial swelling

Increased joint fluid

Articular cartilage

B

Muscle atrophy

Pannus

Eroded cartilage

FIGURE 65.2 Pathophysiology of rheumatoid arthritis. **A.** Joint structure with synovial swelling and fluid accumulation in joint. **B.** Pannus, eroded articular cartilage with joint space narrowing, muscle atrophy, and ankylosis.

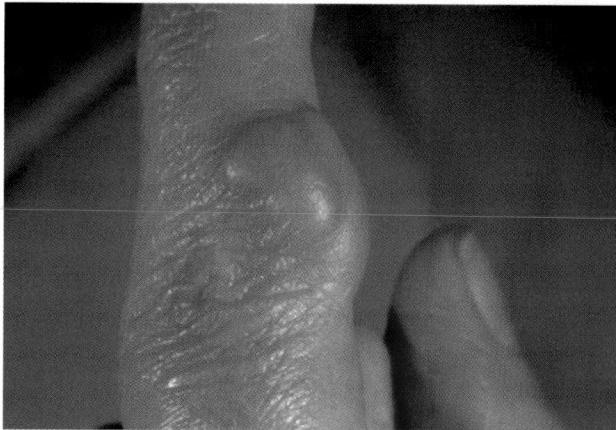

FIGURE 65.5 Rheumatoid nodule. A patient with rheumatoid arthritis has a mass on a digit.

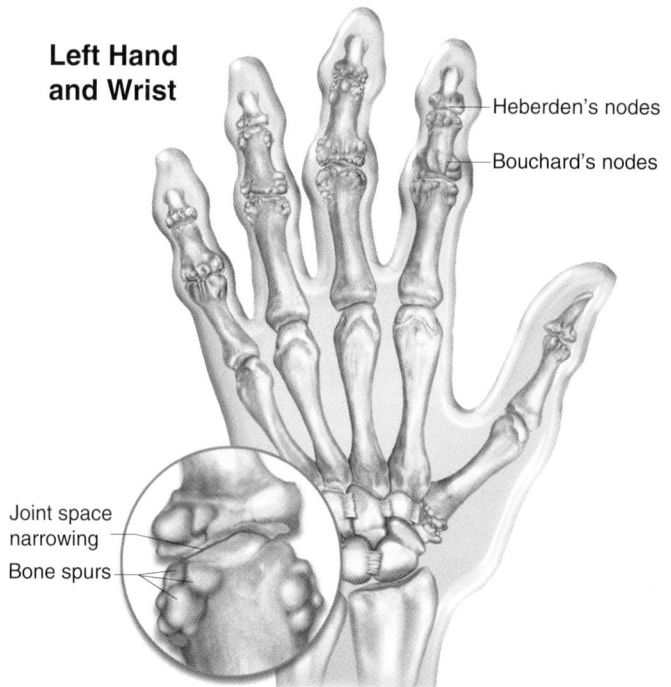

Left Hand and Wrist

Heberden's nodes

Bouchard's nodes

Joint space narrowing

Bone spurs

FIGURE 66.1 Joints affected by osteoarthritis: left hand and wrist.

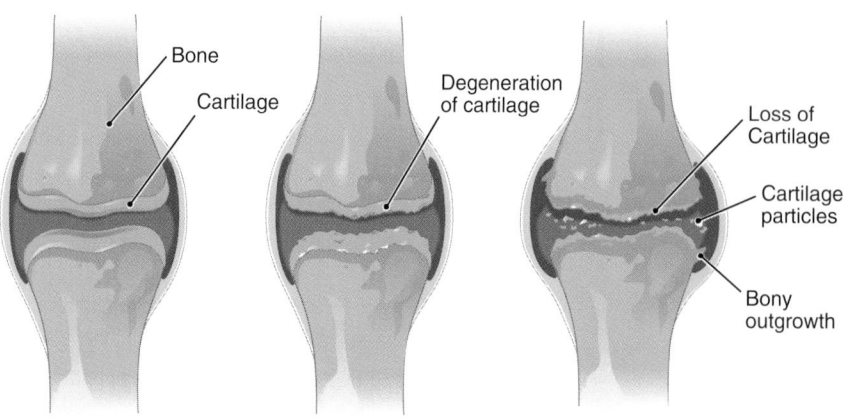

Bone

Cartilage

Degeneration of cartilage

Loss of Cartilage

Cartilage particles

Bony outgrowth

FIGURE 66.2 Osteoarthritis. **A.** Normal joint. **B.** Early stage of osteoarthritis. **C.** Late stage of disease.

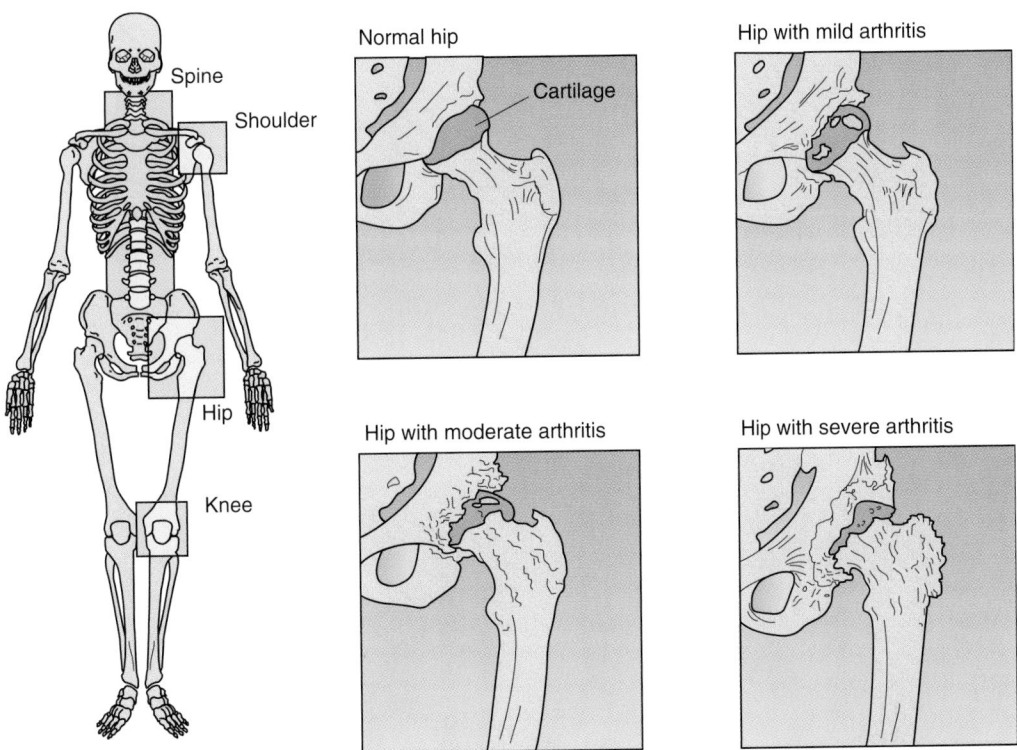

FIGURE 66.3 Osteoarthritis. **A.** Common sites of osteoarthritis. **B.** How osteoarthritis affects the hip.

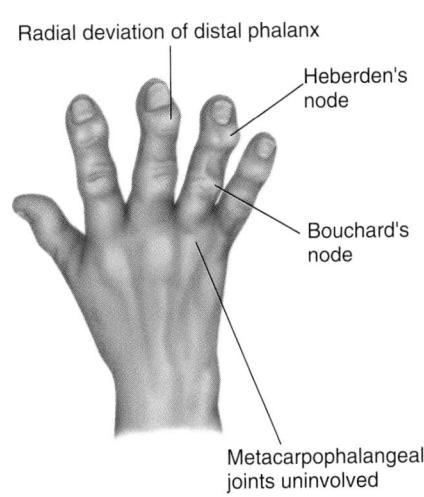

FIGURE 66.4 Osteoarthritis (degenerative joint disease). Nodules on the dorsolateral aspects of the distal interphalangeal joints (Heberden's nodes) are due to the bony overgrowth of osteoarthritis. Usually hard and painless, they affect the middle-aged or elderly and often, although not always, are associated with arthritic changes in other joints. Flexion and deviation deformities may develop. Similar nodules on the proximal interphalangeal joints (Bouchard's nodes) are less common. The metacarpophalangeal joints are spared.

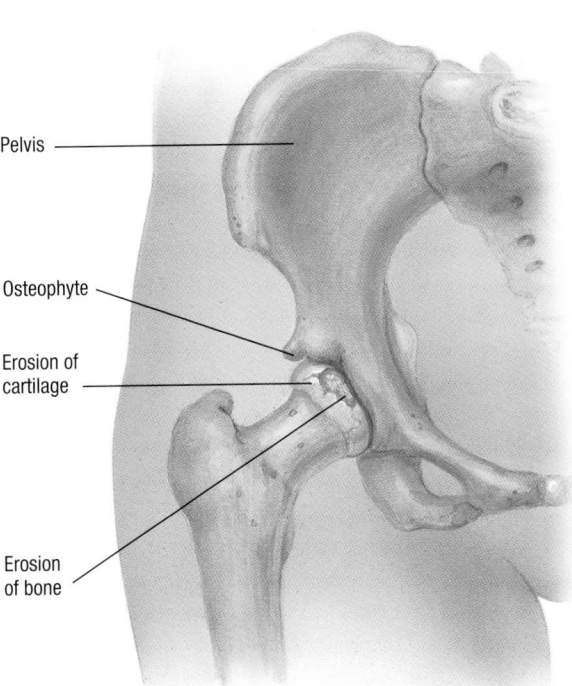

FIGURE 66.5 Hip joints affected by osteoarthritis.

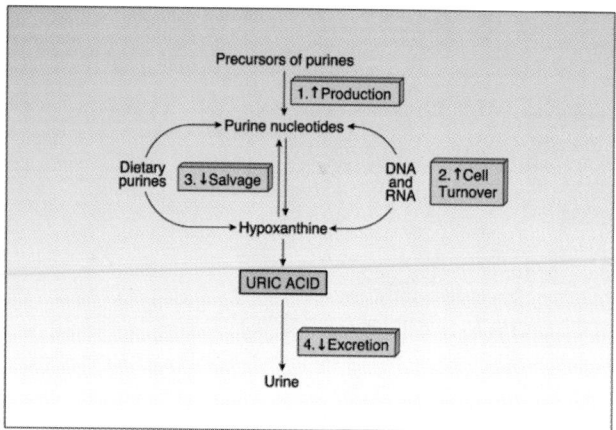

FIGURE 67.1 Pathogenesis of hyperuricemia and gout.

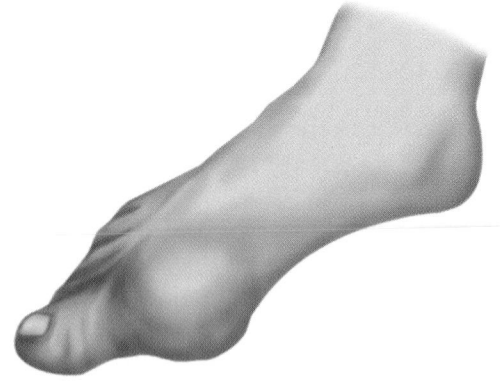

FIGURE 67.2 Acute gouty arthritis (metatarsophalangeal joint of the big toe).

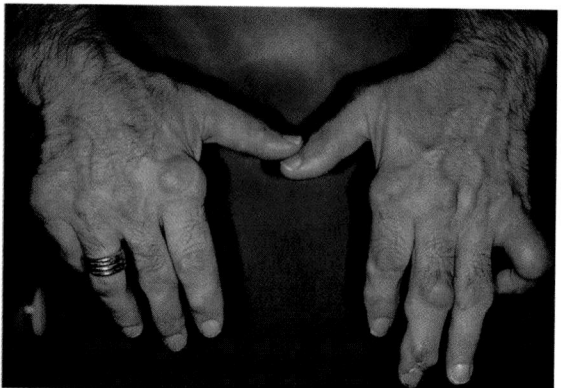

FIGURE 67.3 Chronic tophaceous gout involving hands and wrist.

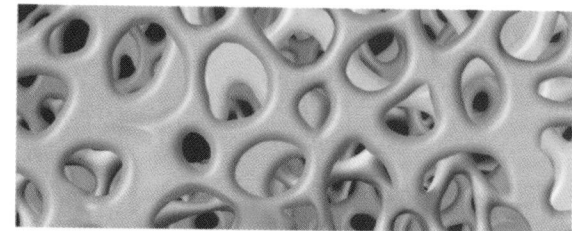

A

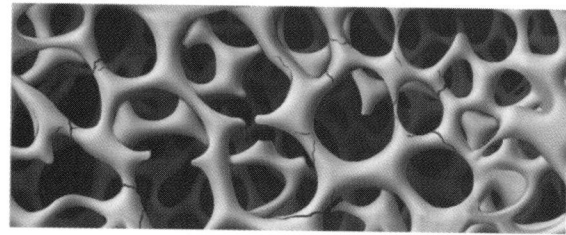

B

FIGURE 69.1 Comparison of healthy trabecular bone **(A)** and osteoporotic trabecular bone **(B)**. In addition to an overall decrease in bone tissue, there is a decrease in trabecular size and connectivity.

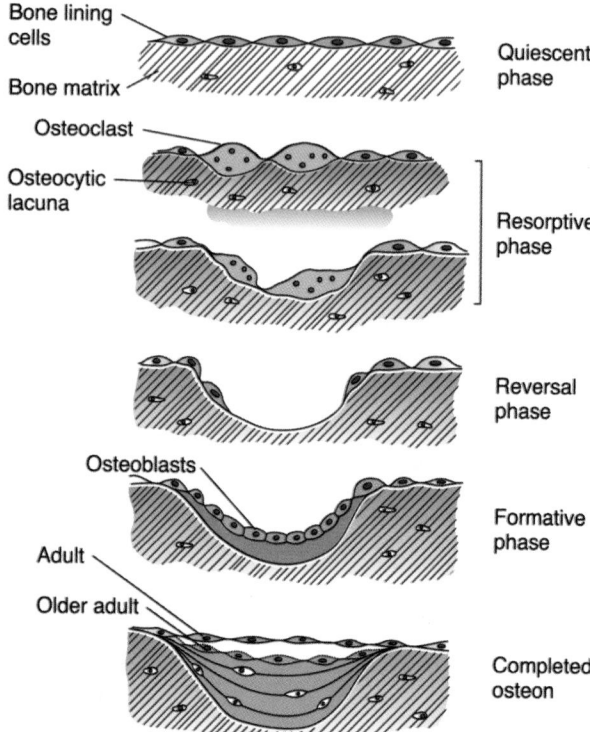

FIGURE 69.2 Bone remodeling sequence. Bone remodeling is initiated by the appearance of osteoclasts on a bone surface previously lined by fusiform cells. After development of a resorption bay, osteoclasts are replaced by osteoblasts which deposit new bone. The bone loss that attends aging (senile osteoporosis) is due to incomplete filling of resorption bays.

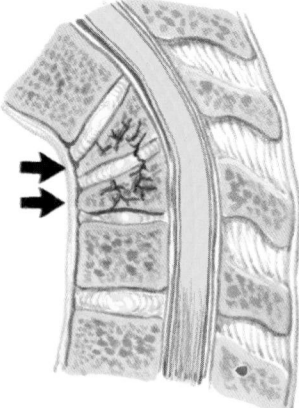

FIGURE 69.3 Vertebral fracture.

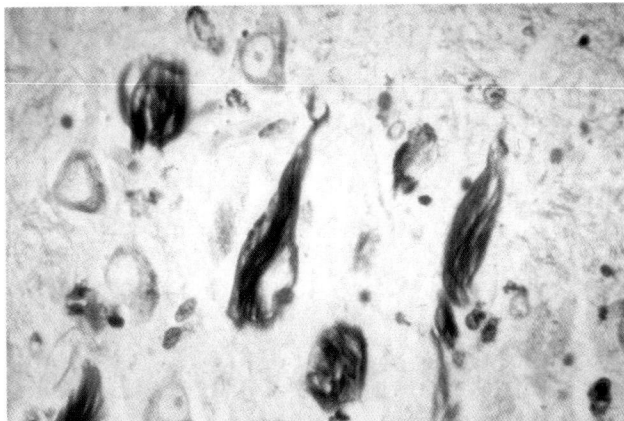

FIGURE 70.1 The cytoplasm of neurons distended by neurofibrillary tangles.

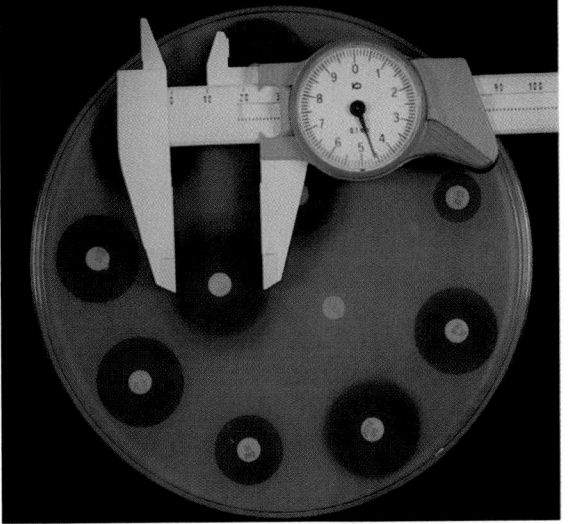

FIGURE 72.2 Photograph of a disk diffusion susceptibility test.

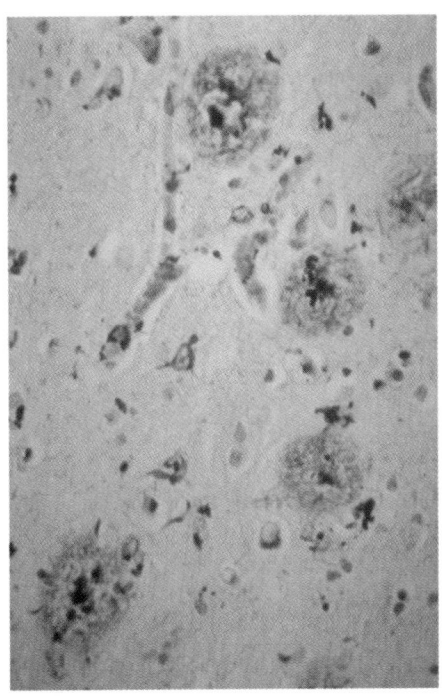

FIGURE 70.2 Neuritic plaques in the cerebral cortex, showing a dense core of amyloid.

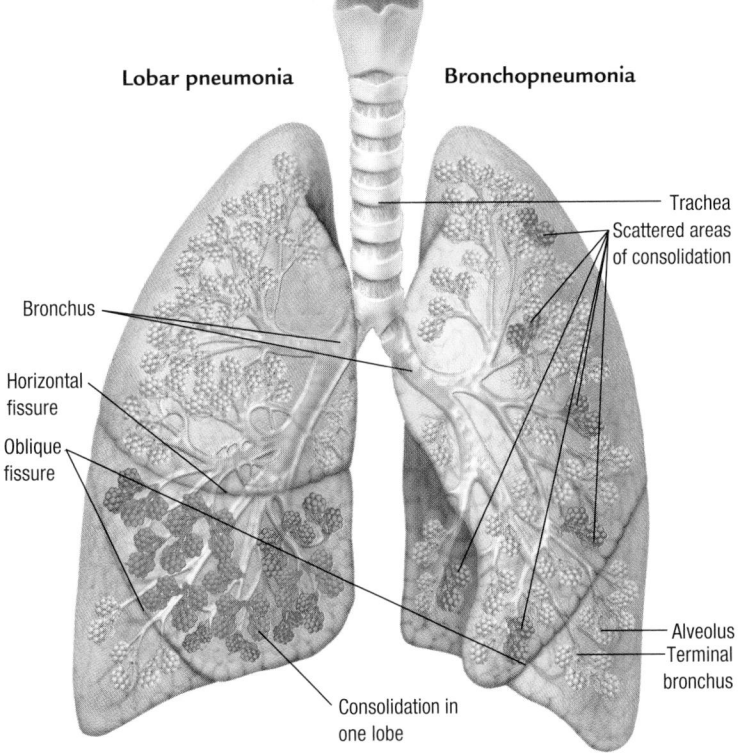

FIGURE 75.1 Types of pneumonia.

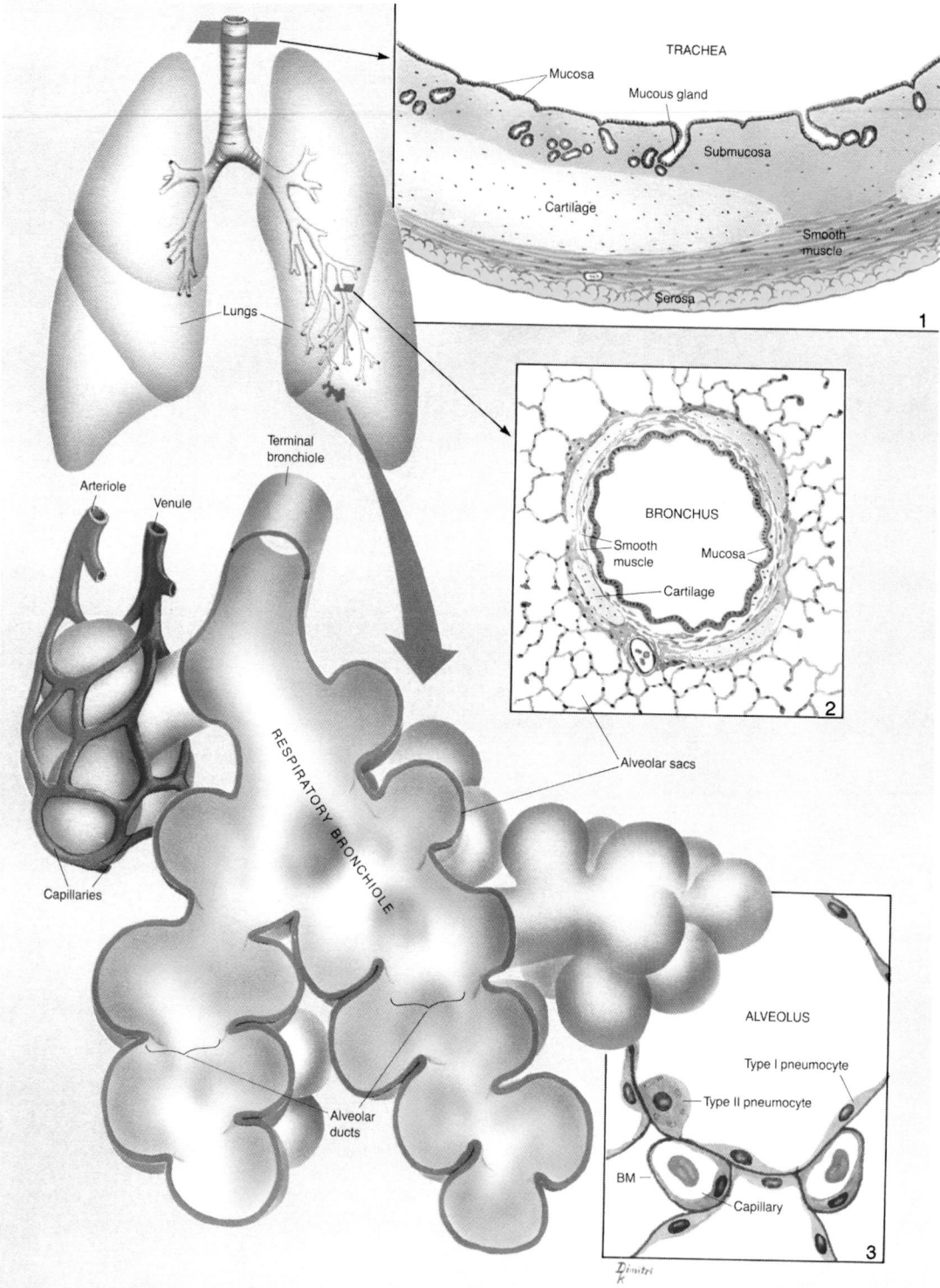

FIGURE 75.3 Anatomy of the lung.

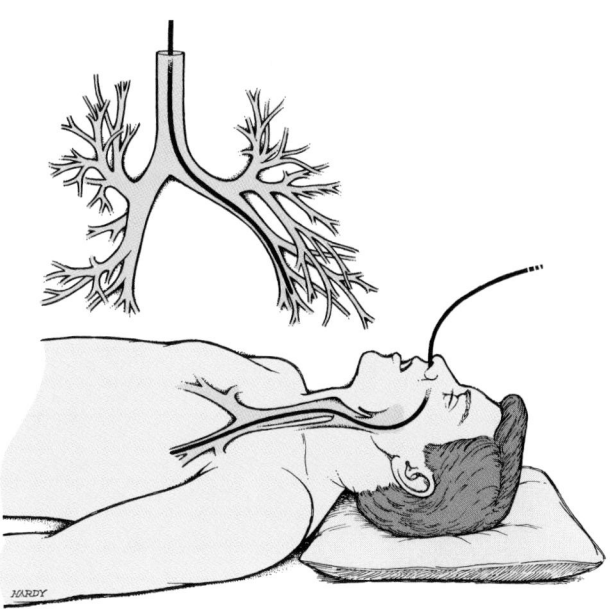

FIGURE 75.5 Fiber optic bronchoscope.

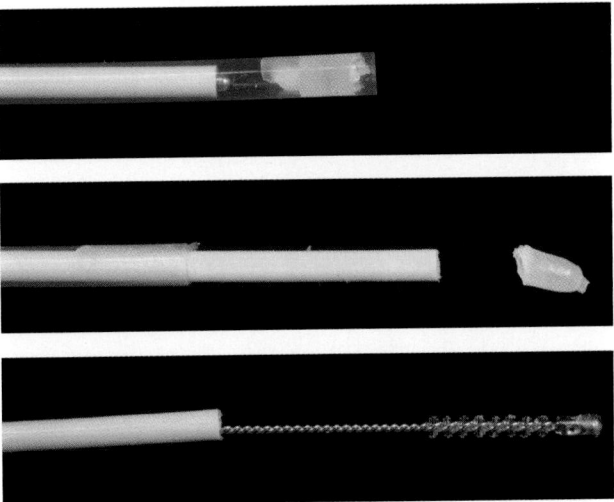

FIGURE 75.6 Protected specimen brush. **A.** Outer sheath with carbon-wax-plug intact; inner sheath can be seen inside the outer one. **B.** the inner catheter comes out of the sheath. **C.** the microbiological brush comes out of the inner catheter to collect specimens.

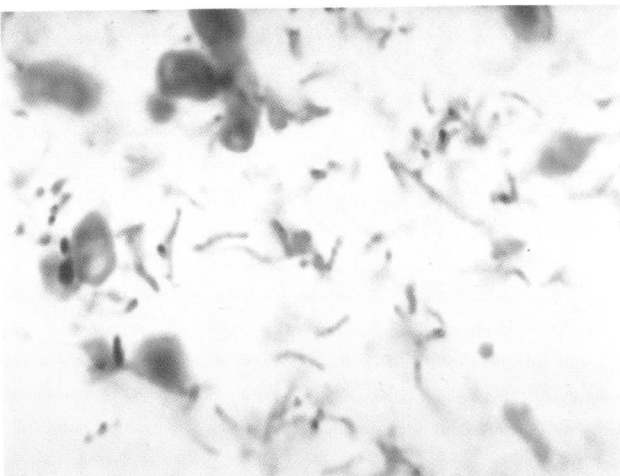

FIGURE 76.1. *Mycobacterium tuberculosis*. A smear of a pulmonary lesion shows slender, beaded, acid-fast bacilli.

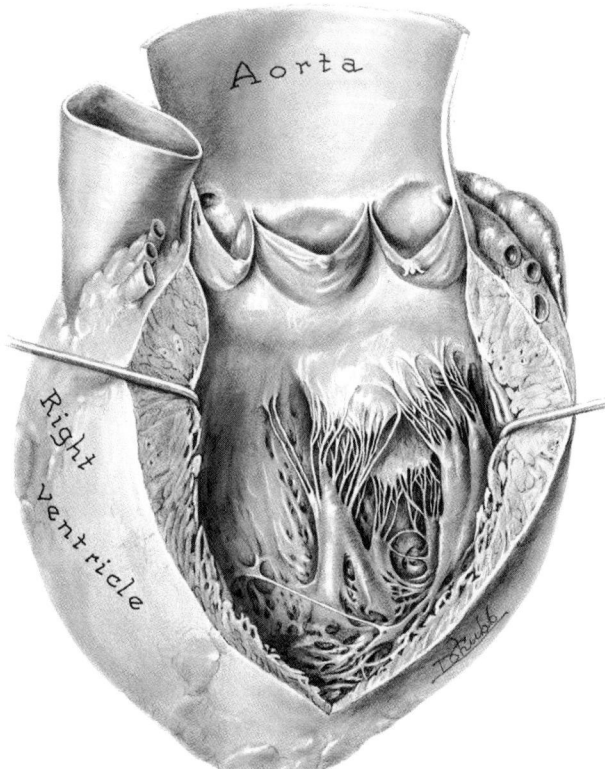

FIGURE 80.1 Schematic of normal aortic valve.

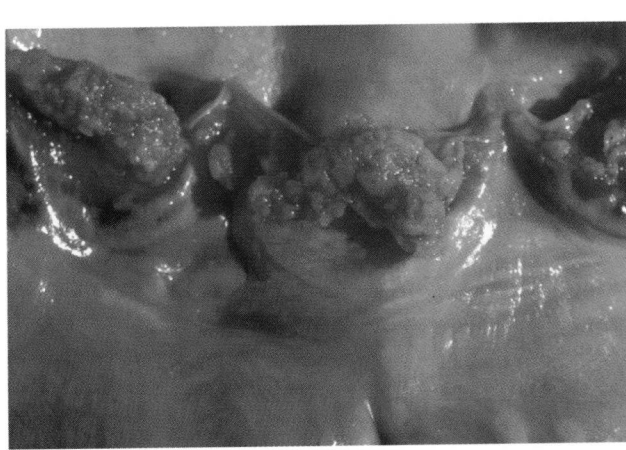

FIGURE 80.2 Picture of vegetations on aortic valve in an intra-venous drug abuser.

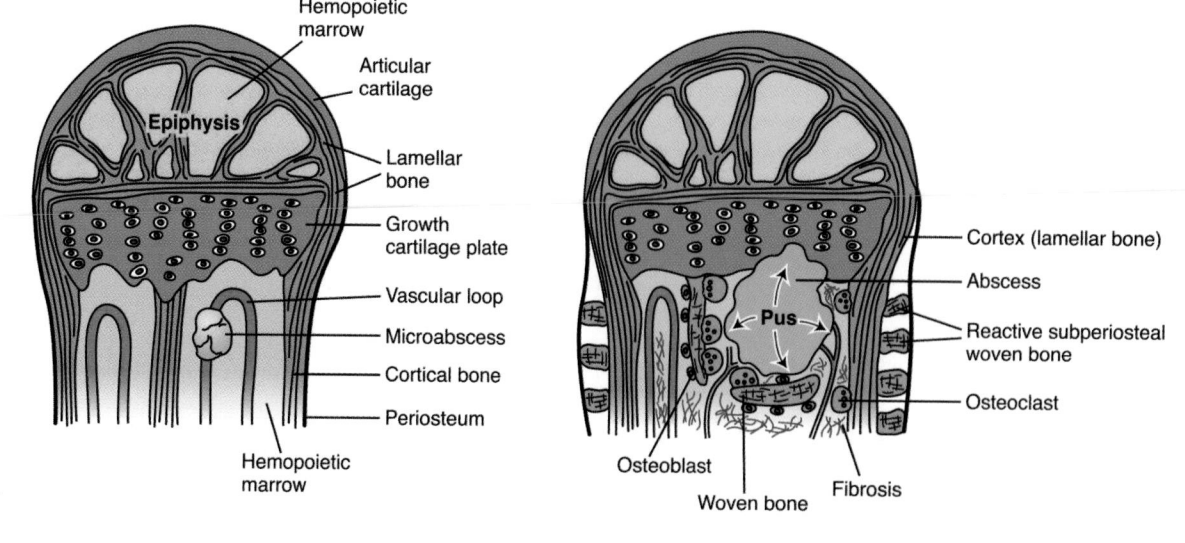

A

B

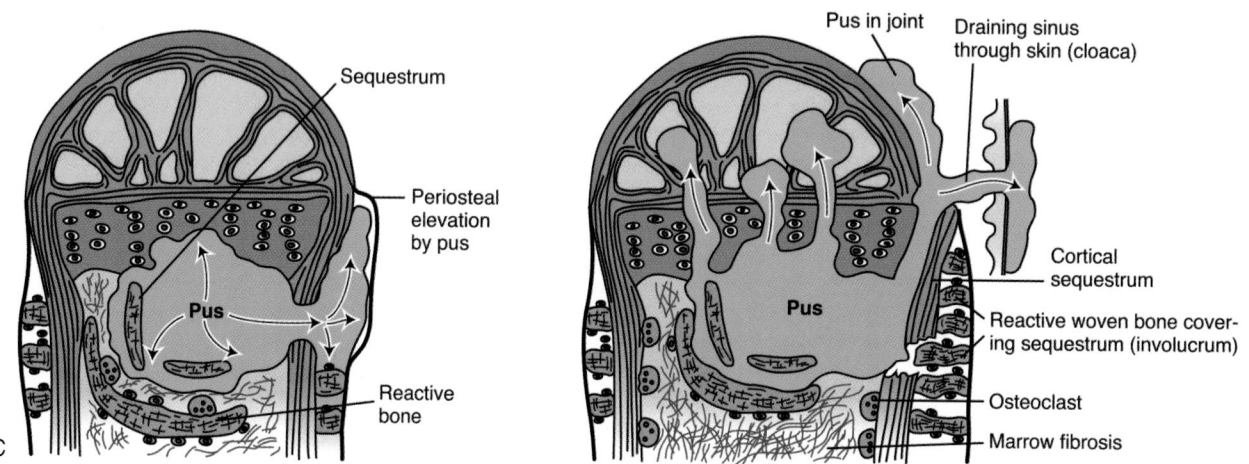

C

D

FIGURE 82.1 Pathogenesis of hematogenous osteomyelitis. **A.** The epiphysis, metaphysis, and growth plate are normal. A small, septic microabscess is forming at the capillary loop. **B.** The expansion of the septic focus stimulates resorption of adjacent bony trabeculae. Woven bone begins to surround this focus. The abscess expands into the cartilage and stimulates reactive bone formation by the periosteum. **C.** The abscess, which continues to expand through the cortex into the subperiosteal tissue, shears off the perforating arteries that supply the cortex with blood, thereby leading to necrosis of the cortex. **D.** The extension of this process into the joint space, the epiphysis, and the skin produces a draining sinus. The necrotic bone is called a sequestrum. The viable bone surrounding a sequestrum is termed the involucrum.

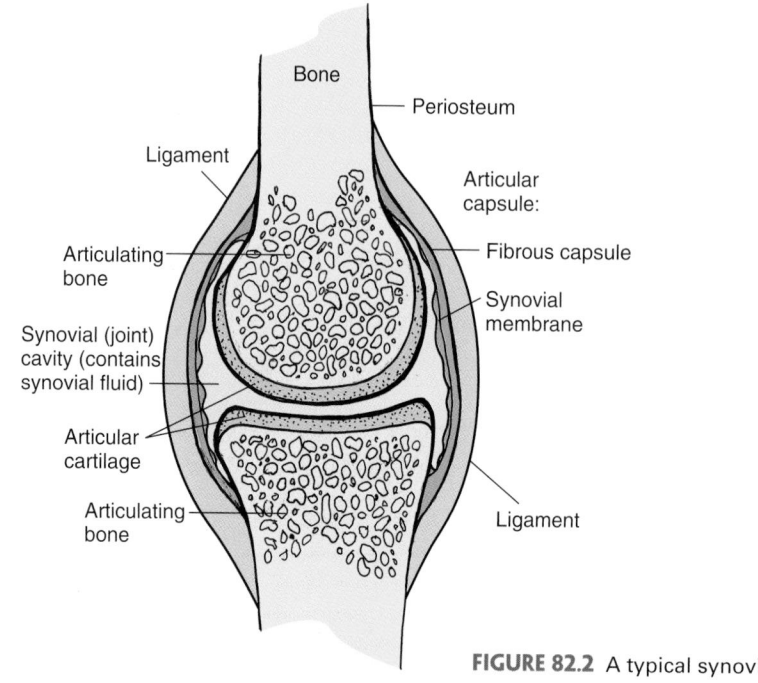

FIGURE 82.2 A typical synovial joint.

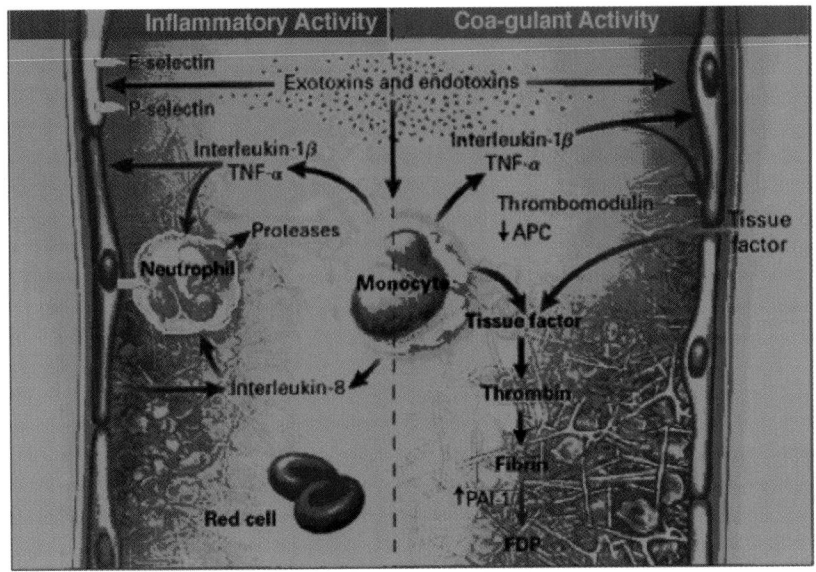

FIGURE 86.2 Mechanisms of injury to the microcirculation in severe sepsis.

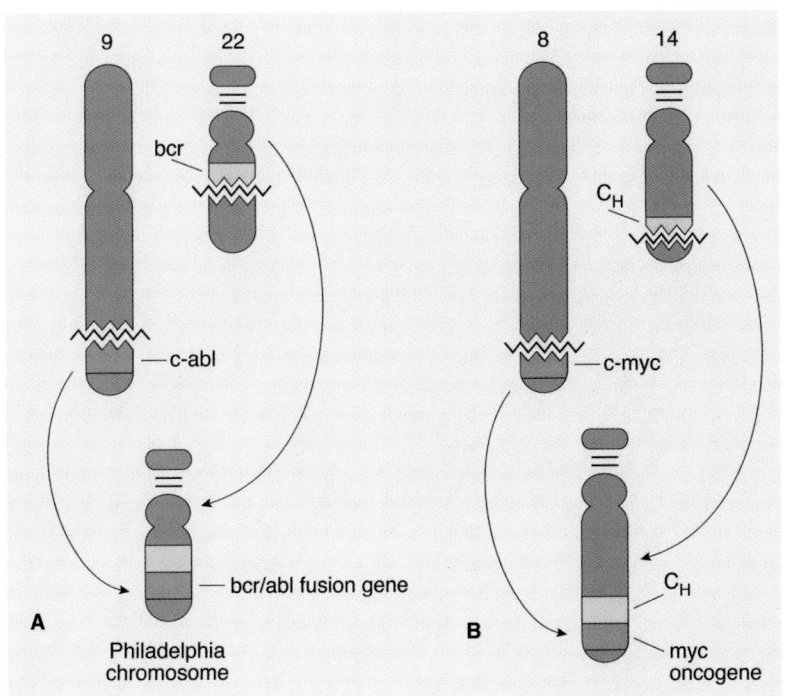

FIGURE 93.1 Oncogene activation by chromosomal relocation. **A**. Chronic myelogenous leukemia. Breaks at the ends of the long arms of chromosomes 9 and 22 allow reciprocal translocations to occur. The c-abl proto-oncogene on chromosome 9 is translocated to the breakpoint region (bcr) of chromosome 22. The result is the Philadelphia chromosome, which contains a new fusion gene coding for a hybrid oncogenic protein (bcr-abl), presumably involved in the pathogenesis of chronic myelogenous leukemia. **B**. Burkitt lymphoma. In this disorder, chromosomal breaks involve the long arms of chromosomes 8 and 14. The c-myc gene on chromosome 8 is translocated to a region on chromosome 14 adjacent to the gene coding for the constant region of an immunoglobulin heavy chain (CH). The expression of c-myc is enhanced by its association with the promoter/enhancer regions of the actively transcribed immunoglobulin genes.

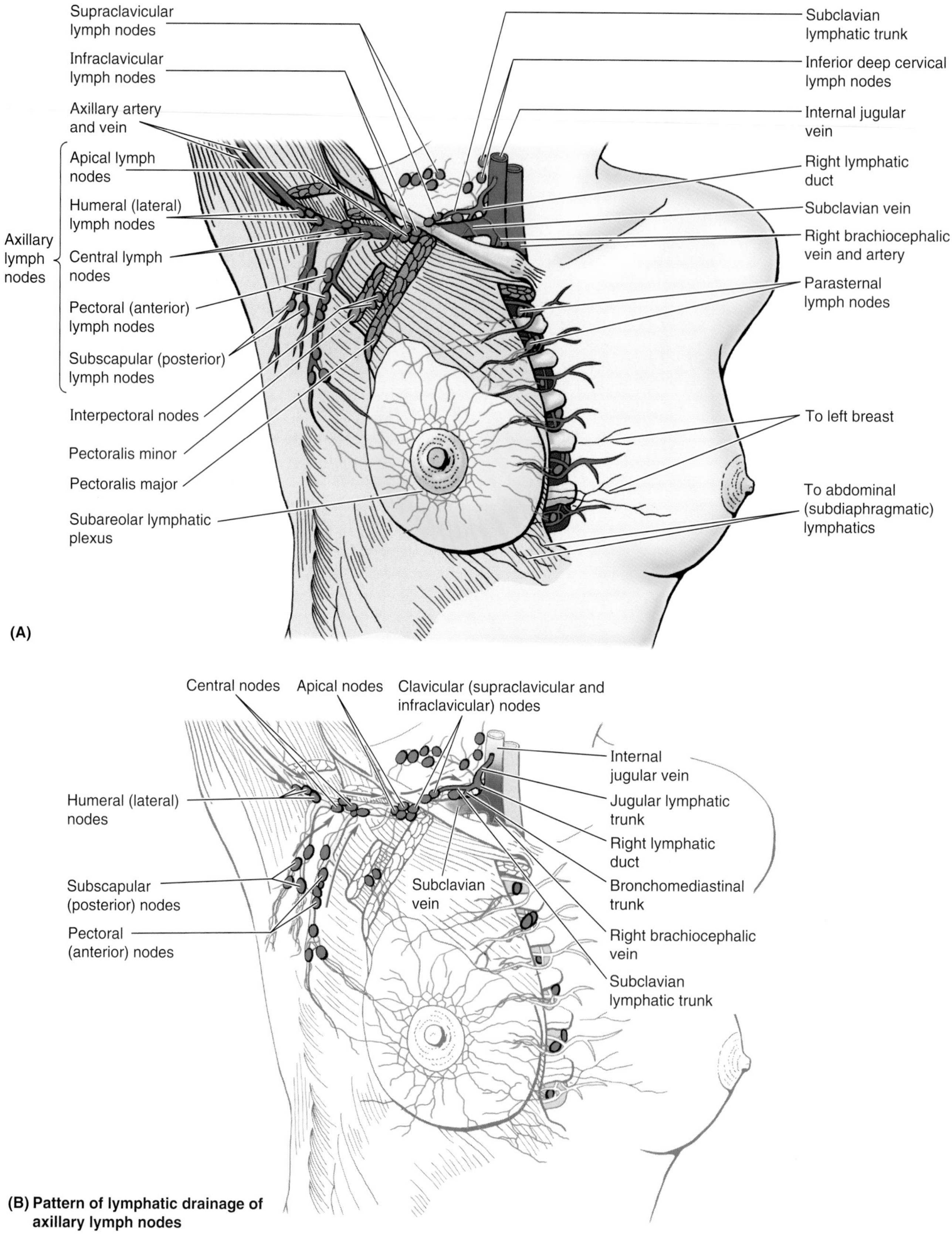

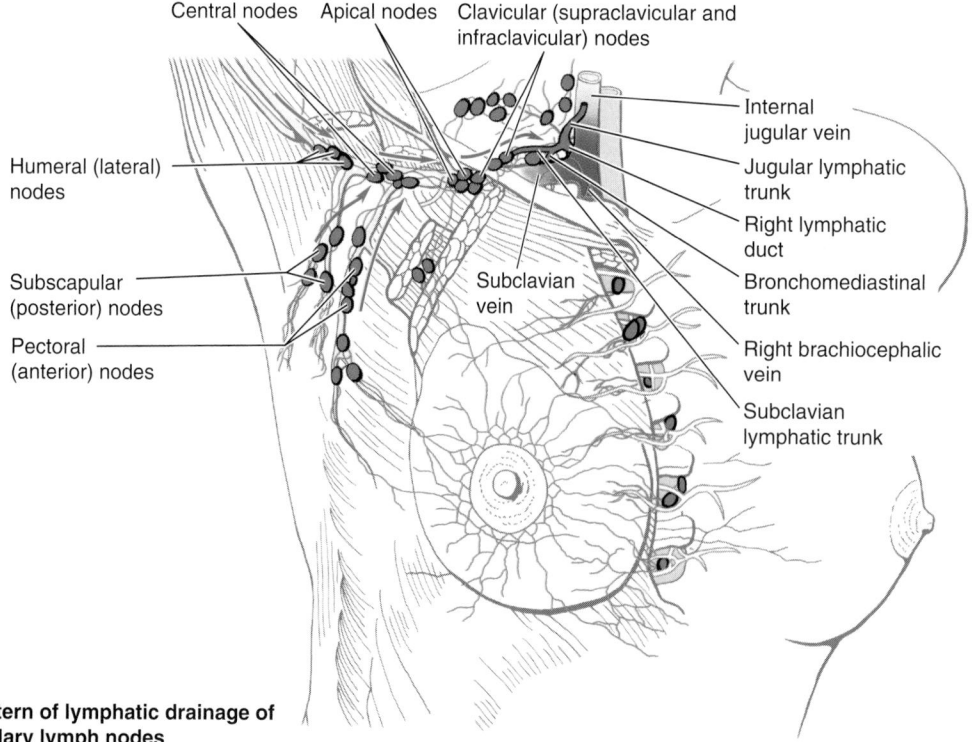

Supraclavicular lymph nodes

Infraclavicular lymph nodes

Axillary artery and vein

Axillary lymph nodes

Apical lymph nodes

Humeral (lateral) lymph nodes

Central lymph nodes

Pectoral (anterior) lymph nodes

Subscapular (posterior) lymph nodes

Interpectoral nodes

Pectoralis minor

Pectoralis major

Subareolar lymphatic plexus

Subclavian lymphatic trunk

Inferior deep cervical lymph nodes

Internal jugular vein

Right lymphatic duct

Subclavian vein

Right brachiocephalic vein and artery

Parasternal lymph nodes

To left breast

To abdominal (subdiaphragmatic) lymphatics

(A)

Central nodes   Apical nodes   Clavicular (supraclavicular and infraclavicular) nodes

Humeral (lateral) nodes

Subscapular (posterior) nodes

Pectoral (anterior) nodes

Subclavian vein

Internal jugular vein

Jugular lymphatic trunk

Right lymphatic duct

Bronchomediastinal trunk

Right brachiocephalic vein

Subclavian lymphatic trunk

(B) Pattern of lymphatic drainage of axillary lymph nodes

FIGURE 96.1 Breast tissue drainage and its relationship to tumor metastases.

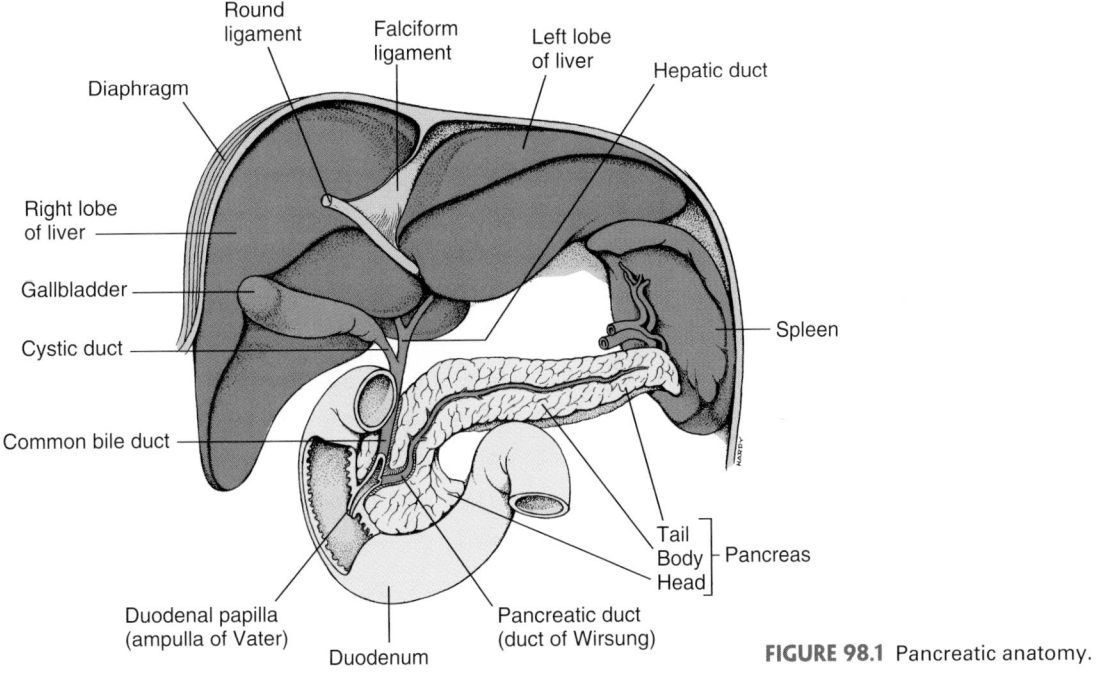

FIGURE 98.1 Pancreatic anatomy.

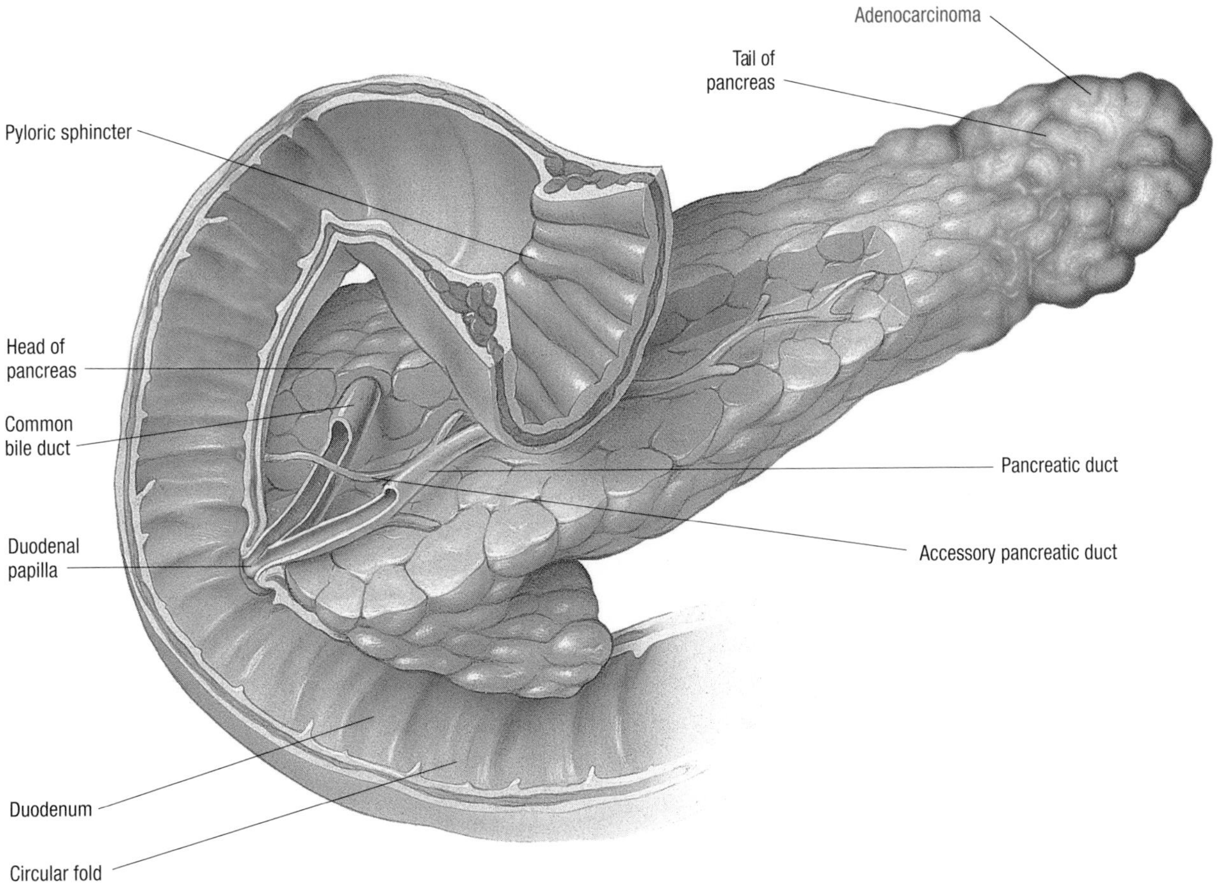

Round ligament
Falciform ligament
Left lobe of liver
Hepatic duct
Diaphragm
Right lobe of liver
Gallbladder
Cystic duct
Common bile duct
Spleen
Tail
Body — Pancreas
Head
Duodenal papilla (ampulla of Vater)
Duodenum
Pancreatic duct (duct of Wirsung)

Adenocarcinoma
Tail of pancreas
Pyloric sphincter
Head of pancreas
Common bile duct
Pancreatic duct
Duodenal papilla
Accessory pancreatic duct
Duodenum
Circular fold

FIGURE 98.2 Pancreatic tail lesion.

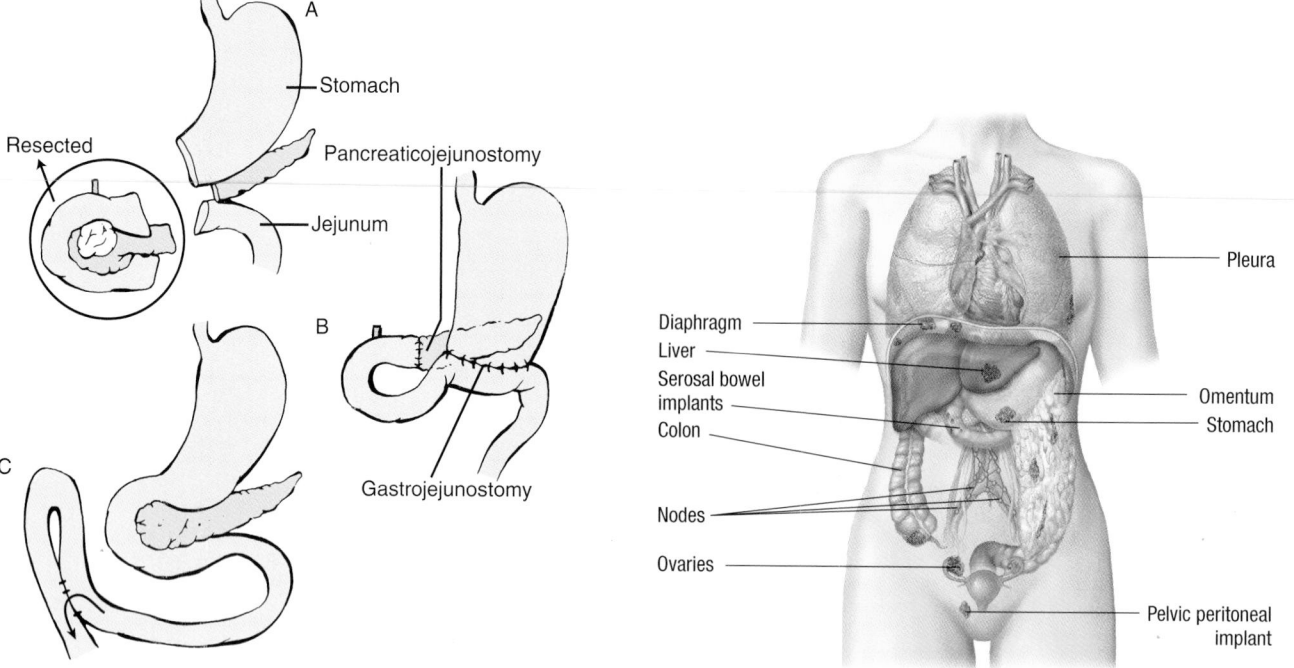

FIGURE 98.3 Whipple procedure.

FIGURE 102.1 Ovarian cancer.

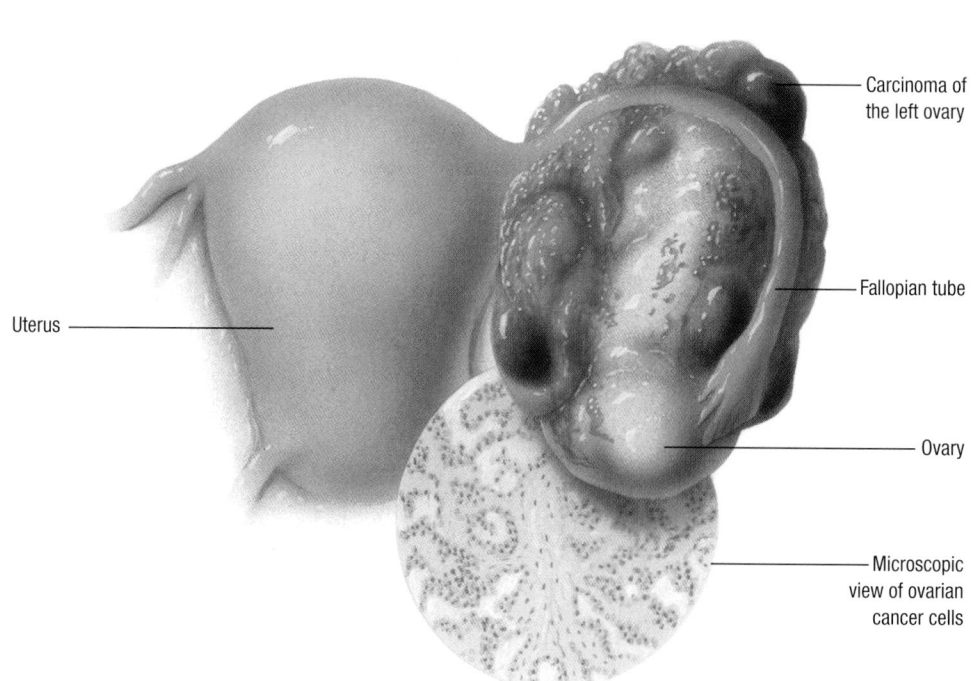

FIGURE 102.2 Likely metastatic sites for ovarian cancer.

treatment that offers longer-term maintenance of response, an augmentation to pharmacotherapy, and an alternative to medication nonresponders.[200] In many patients, pharmacotherapy provided in combination with CBT allows the patient to engage in psychological interventions, particularly exposure therapy.

ALTERNATIVE THERAPIES

Given their frequent use, it is imperative that the role of complementary treatments for anxiety disorders be evaluated. Unfortunately, very few alternative therapies have been studied systematically. Treatments with the best evidence of effectiveness in anxiety disorders include kava, exercise, relaxation training, and bibliotherapy; limited data suggest a role for meditation and inositol.[208] A Cochrane review of 11 randomized controlled trials concluded that kava, a member of the pepper family, was superior to placebo for treating patients with GAD and was well tolerated.[209] However, rare cases of liver failure, particularly at high doses, have been reported; additional safety data are needed.[210] Exercise has been shown to be as effective for mild to moderate anxiety, in the long term, as clomipramine is for panic disorder.[208,211-213] In multiple controlled trials, relaxation training demonstrated efficacy for dental phobia, panic disorder, and GAD; it may be less effective than other psychosocial interventions for social anxiety disorder, PTSD, and OCD.[208] The use of written materials, computer programs, audiotapes or videotapes for gaining problem-solving skills, or bibliotherapy has been successful in reducing anxiety with specific phobias in highly motivated individuals.[214] Bibliotherapy was not effective for panic disorder or OCD.[214] Several randomized controlled trials have found meditation to be an effective intervention in GAD; meditation has not been studied in other anxiety disorders.[208] Inositol is an isomer of glucose involved in a second messenger process used by serotonin and noradrenergic receptors. It has been shown to be effective in treating patients with panic disorder and OCD in randomized controlled trials; however, it was not effective in PTSD.[215-219] Larger and longer-term trials are now being conducted to better define the role of inositol in anxiety disorders. A useful resource comes from the Office of Dietary Supplements within the National Institutes of Health, which offers the International Bibliographic Information on Dietary Supplements (IBIDS) database. This database provides access to bibliographic citations and abstracts from published international and scientific literature on dietary supplements (http://dietary-supplements.info.nih.gov/Health_Information/IBIDS.aspx).

FUTURE THERAPIES

Recent findings in neuroscience are furthering our understanding of the pathophysiology of anxiety disorders and are leading to new molecular targets for the pharmacotherapy of anxiety.[23] Pagoclone is a partial benzodiazepine-GABA receptor agonist under development for the treatment of patients with panic disorder and generalized anxiety disorder. Its specific actions at the GABA receptor may provide anxiolytic effects without the usual adverse effects of benzodiazepines.[12,23,220] Manipulation of GABA levels achieved by selective inhibition of the transporter responsible for the reuptake of GABA in the CNS may be an effective treatment for patients with anxiety. Preclinical and preliminary clinical trials with the anticonvulsant tiagabine suggest that it may exert anxiolytic effects through such reuptake inhibition.[9,10,23,221] Calcium ion channel modulators such as pregabalin are also under investigation for the treatment of patients with GAD and social anxiety disorder.[23,222] Other potential pharmacotherapeutic strategies in development include selective 5-HT$_{1A}$ agonists, CRF antagonists, substance P antagonists, ionotropic glutamate receptor antagonists (e.g., the NMDA receptor antagonist lamotrigine), metabotropic glutamate receptor (mGluR) agonists, and brain-derived neurotrophic factor (BDNF).[23]

IMPROVING OUTCOMES

PATIENT EDUCATION

Patients with anxiety disorders benefit from education regarding their illness. This should include information regarding the biologic nature of their illness so that stigma, shame, and guilt can be eliminated. Patients should also be assured that effective treatments are available for their illness, although expectations should be realistic regarding which symptoms will improve and the time course over which improvement will occur. Patients should be educated regarding the course of their illness, as many anxiety disorders are chronic in nature with waxing and waning of symptoms and exacerbations of illness, particularly in times of stress. Patients can also be referred to support and resource organizations such as the National Alliance for the Mentally Ill (NAMI, http://www.nami.org), the Anxiety Disorders Association of America (ADAA, http://www.adaa.org), the Obsessive-Compulsive Foundation (OCF, http://www.ocfoundation.org), the Post-traumatic Stress Disorder Alliance Resource Center (http://www.ptsdalliance.org), and the Social Phobia/Social Anxiety Association (SP/SAA, http://www.socialphobia.org).

Patients taking BZDs should be told about the sedation that can occur, particularly early in therapy. Patients should also be cautioned regarding the potential for incoordination and impaired memory and cognition and should avoid using alcohol, which may intensify these effects. Patients should be warned to be particularly careful when driving or performing other tasks that require concentration and intact psychomotor skills, especially when the BZD is initiated. Patients should be educated regarding the potential for a withdrawal reaction if their BZD is abruptly discontinued or significantly decreased. For this reason, they should have refills ready in a timely manner and should talk with their prescriber before decreasing dose or discontinuing medication.

Patients should be given clear information regarding the therapeutic effects of buspirone so that their expectations are reasonable. They should expect buspirone to work only if taken routinely (as opposed to "as needed"); initial therapeutic effects may not be seen for 1 to 2 weeks and full effects may take several weeks. Setting appropriate expectations can help reduce patient self-discontinuation early in therapy, especially in patients who have previously experienced immediate anxiolytic effects with BZDs. Patients should also be assured regarding the lack of potential of buspirone for physical dependence, withdrawal, or abuse.

Patients receiving antidepressant therapy for an anxiety disorder should be counseled regarding the delay in onset of response. Although they may experience adverse effects with the first few doses, therapeutic effects may not be seen for weeks; given this information, they may be less likely to discontinue medication early on from perceived lack of efficacy. Patients, particularly those with panic disorder or GAD, should be cautioned regarding the potential for worsening anxiety when antidepressant therapy is initiated. Counseling of patients taking MAOIs should include a thorough discussion regarding the potential for drug and food interactions; patients should be given written materials with this information to use as a resource. Patients should be advised to tell all of their health care providers that they are taking MAOIs so that potential interactions can be prevented when new medications (including over-the-counter medications, herbals, and supplements) are initiated. Patients taking TCAs should be educated on how to manage adverse effects (e.g., use fiber, exercise, and hydration for constipation). Patients who are prescribed SSRIs should be educated regarding the early, but transient, effects of nausea, headache, and restlessness. They should be counseled on the adverse effects that may persist, including sexual dysfunction, and should be urged to report such effects to their prescriber. It should be made clear to patients that they should not abruptly discontinue SSRI treatment, as this may lead to a discontinuation syndrome characterized by paresthesias, irritability, vivid dreams, headache, and dizziness.[223] Patients on β-adrenergic blocking agents should be cautioned regarding the potential for dizziness secondary to orthostatic hypotension. Patients should be advised to support themselves and stand up slowly from a sitting or lying position to prevent a fall.

Women of childbearing potential should be educated about risks to the fetus of anxiolytic medication exposure. Most BZDs are classified as pregnancy category D because some evidence of risk to the fetus has been noted; however, the benefits of treatment may outweigh the risks in certain individual patients. In arriving at a decision whether to use these agents in pregnancy, one must consider evidence that untreated anxiety disorders can affect pregnancy outcomes.[224] Evidence has implicated BZD exposure during the first trimester in birth deformities, most often cleft lip or palate and limb or digit malformations.[225] Although this risk is elevated compared with that of nonexposed fetuses, the absolute risk remains small (<1%).[226] In general, first-trimester exposure should be avoided, if possible. However, many pregnancies are unplanned; thus, first-trimester exposure may inadvertently occur. In such cases, patients should be reminded of the potential dangers of abrupt discontinuation and should be referred to their prescriber to discuss gradual discontinuation. If the benefit of BZD is deemed greater than the risk in certain individual patients, treatment should be conservative. The lowest dose and the shortest duration can help minimize risks to the fetus and newborn.[227] Large doses, particularly of long-acting BZDs, may accumulate in the fetus. Newborns exposed to BZD in utero have demonstrated withdrawal symptoms, oversedation, muscle weakness, hypotonia, apnea, poor feeding, and impaired temperature regulation.[226]

DISEASE STATE MANAGEMENT STRATEGIES TO IMPROVE PATIENT OUTCOMES

The treatment of patients with anxiety disorders of all types should be comprehensive. Nonpharmacologic approaches should be combined with medications when appropriate, acceptable, and available to patients.

Generalized Anxiety Disorder. Therapeutic goals in the management of GAD include decreasing anxiety, improving function, and preventing relapse or recurrence. In treating patients with GAD, BZDs, buspirone, TCAs, SSRIs, and venlafaxine are all effective agents. Buspirone and antidepressants have a delay in onset of effect, and in moderate to severe cases of GAD, BZD augmentation of an antidepressant may be indicated for the short term. Antidepressants have several advantages over BZDs over the long term in that they may also be effective for comorbid depression, lack issues of dependence, withdrawal, and abuse, and lack adverse effects on memory and cognition. Although TCAs are at least as effective as BZDs in GAD, they carry a substantial liability in terms of adverse effects and toxicity in overdose; therefore, they are reserved for use after other agents have failed. Of the antidepressants, the SSRIs paroxetine and venlafaxine are the best studied agents and are considered first-line therapy. Buspirone is an effective first-line alternative, although, similar to antidepressants, it has a delay in onset of effect and is not effective for as-needed use. Buspirone may be a good choice for patients in whom BZDs are not appropriate (e.g., substance use history, fall risk, cognitive impairment) and for those who wish to avoid adverse effects of antidepressants. GAD is a chronic illness that requires long-term treatment, as relapse after medication discontinuation occurs commonly. The optimal duration of medication treatment is at least 6 to 12 months, with assessment and, if appropriate, gradual discontinuation of medication at that time; monitoring for relapse and need for reinstitution of treatment should be provided.

Panic Disorder. The goals of panic disorder treatment are to decrease the frequency and severity of panic attacks, reduce phobic avoidance behaviors, and improve functioning. High-potency BZDs and SSRIs are first-line treatments for patients with panic disorder and are often used in combination. Although TCAs and MAOIs have also shown efficacy, they are reserved as second- or third-line agents because of their adverse effect, toxicity, and drug interaction profiles. Patients with panic disorder are extremely sensitive to the initial effects of antidepressant therapy and may experience an increase in anxiety or panic. This can be minimized or avoided with low initial dosages or concurrent BZD therapy. Although BZDs have an immediate onset of effect and have shown long-term efficacy for the treatment of patients with panic disorder, SSRIs offer several clinical advantages over the long term. SSRIs can effectively treat patients with comorbid depression; in addition, they lack dependence, withdrawal, or abuse issues, as well as adverse effects on memory and cognition. However, it should be noted, of course, that SSRIs are not without adverse effects. SSRIs may be most appropriate in patients with panic disorder who have comorbid depression or substance use histories, or in whom other contraindications to BZD use exist. Given the chronic nature of panic disorder, patients should continue treatment for at least 6 to 12 months following response. Maintenance treatment has been shown to reduce relapse; if discontinuation of medication is deemed appropriate, it should be done in a gradual manner with continued monitoring for relapse and potential need for medication reinstitution.

Obsessive-compulsive Disorder. Pharmacotherapy used alone for the treatment of patients with OCD can result in 40% to 60% of patients responding, with mean improvement in symptoms of 20% to 40%.[42] Cognitive-behavioral therapy is very effective for OCD, particularly when combined with pharmacotherapy.[42] Managing patients through both modalities is ideal in that response rates are increased and symptomatology is reduced to a greater degree. Medications that potently inhibit reuptake of serotonin, such as SSRIs and clomipramine, are the drugs of choice in the treatment of patients with OCD. Because patients may be more likely to discontinue treatment with clomipramine secondary to adverse effects, it is considered a second-line agent after the SSRIs. Of the SSRIs, fluoxetine, fluvoxamine, paroxetine, and sertraline have the greatest quantity of available efficacy and safety data for this indication. More limited data have indicated that citalopram, escitalopram, and venlafaxine are likely also effective.[155,190,191] An adequate trial of medication requires at least 10 to 12 weeks of treatment, and optimal doses for treating patients with OCD may exceed those typically used to treat those with major depression.[42] For partial responders to SSRI or clomipramine therapy, augmentation therapy with antipsychotics, including the newer atypical antipsychotic agents, has been supported by clinical data.[228] Combination clomipramine and SSRI has also been shown to be an effective strategy in refractory

patients, although care must be taken to avoid serotonin syndrome due to a pharmacodynamic drug interaction or TCA toxicity secondary to a pharmacokinetic drug interaction.[229] A number of other augmentation strategies have been explored; however, in these trials, data were limited by size or design of the study, or results were negative.[42] Similar to other anxiety disorders, OCD is chronic, and duration of therapy should extend to at least 1 year after response. Maintenance pharmacotherapy is extremely effective for preventing relapse. If medication is discontinued after that time, it should be done in a gradual manner, and careful monitoring for relapse should be provided.

Post-traumatic Stress Disorder. For patients with mild PTSD, CBT may be adequate. For more moderate to severe cases, a combination of CBT and pharmacotherapy is ideal. SSRIs are the first-line pharmacotherapy for PTSD. Response to pharmacotherapy is very gradual and takes 8 to 12 weeks, or longer. Patients with PTSD may need to continue treatment for years. Data on other antidepressants are limited; however, it should be considered that medications that may be lethal in overdose should be avoided owing to the high suicide rates noted in patients with PTSD. Other medications have been studied, with varying efficacy. Carbamazepine, valproic acid, and other anticonvulsants may be beneficial for mood lability, aggression, intrusiveness, and hyperarousal symptoms. Antiadrenergic agents, including propranolol, clonidine, and prazosin, may be effective in countering adrenergic hyperactivity in patients with PTSD. Antipsychotics, although not effective for core symptoms of PTSD, are effective for psychotic symptoms that may occur in some patients with PTSD. Only a few studies have examined the role of BZDs in PTSD; it has been found that they are of limited value in addressing core symptoms. The added limitation is the risk of abuse in patients with PTSD, in whom comorbid substance use disorders are common. Oftentimes, the choice of medication is dictated by the prominence of specific PTSD symptoms and comorbid psychiatric illnesses.

Social Anxiety Disorder. For many patients with social anxiety disorder, symptoms emerged early in life and persisted for many years; therefore, symptoms may have become accepted as an immutable part of their personalities.[52] Treatment for patients with social anxiety disorder can be extremely effective and can have profound and striking effects on the lives of patients. Nonpharmacologic therapies, including social skills training, exposure therapy, and CBT, are very effective.[52] SSRIs are considered first-line pharmacotherapy for social anxiety disorder. SSRIs are dosed at typical antidepressant doses in patients with social anxiety disorder who don't seem to be as sensitive to their initial effects as patients with GAD or panic disorder. Therapeutic response generally occurs in 8 to 10 weeks; an adequate duration of treatment is thought to be at least 1 year.[52]

PHARMACOECONOMICS

Because of the somatic symptoms—such as heart palpitations, gastrointestinal problems, sweating, and feeling faint—that frequently accompany anxiety disorders, patients with anxiety often present to primary care physicians with their physical complaints, rather than to a psychiatrist. The primary care physician is challenged to detect anxiety in patients with physical complaints; delays in diagnosis, unnecessary tests, and inappropriate treatments are not uncommon.[25] These significantly contribute to increased costs to health care systems and prolonged impairment to the patient. Early and effective diagnosis and treatment of anxiety can significantly reduce symptoms, improve patient functioning, and lower the economic impact on health care systems and society. Simple screening tools used in the physician's office can quickly and accurately detect anxiety disorders. These often consist of short questionnaires that may be completed in the waiting room,[230] as well as physician-rated instruments such as the SWIKIR Anxiety Scale (Somatic complaints, Worries, Irritability, Keyed up, Initial insomnia, Relaxation difficulties),[231] the Primary Care Evaluation of Mental Disorders (PRIME-MD),[232] and the Well-Being Life Chart (WBLC).[233]

The higher prevalence rates of GAD, panic disorder, and PTSD in primary care outpatients compared with those reported in the general population suggest that patients with these anxiety disorders are high users of primary care resources.[45,234-236] Anxiety has also been reported to be associated with increased costs and reduced health-related quality of life in general medical inpatients.[237] The economic costs of anxiety disorders include not only psychiatric, non-psychiatric, and emergency care, hospitalization, and prescription medications, but also reduced productivity, absenteeism from work, and suicide.[8] Anxiety disorders rank among the top ten most costly mental health disorders affecting employers.[235,238] Most of the costs to employers are attributed to absence from work, disability losses, and decreased productivity. The burden of anxiety disorders on society cannot be discounted; unemployment, costs of public assistance programs, and impact of alcohol abuse and other substance use disorders are significant to society.

In 1990, the annual cost of anxiety disorders in the United States was estimated to be approximately $42.3 billion. This total cost comprises $23 billion in nonpsychiatric medical treatment costs, $13.3 billion in psychiatric treatment costs, $4.1 billion in indirect workplace costs, $1.2 billion in mortality costs, and $0.8 billion (or roughly, 2% of the total cost) in prescription pharmaceutical costs.[239] A similar study estimated the total cost of anxiety, also in 1990, to be $46.6 billion; this estimate included costs associated with crime, incarceration, social welfare administration, and family caregiving.[240] The estimates related to anxiety disorders in the United States represent substantial costs; more widespread awareness, appropriate diagnosis, and timely intervention may help to reduce the total burden of anxiety on individual persons and on society.

KEY POINTS

- Anxiety disorders are the most common psychiatric illnesses, with 1 in 4 Americans experiencing an anxiety disorder in their lifetime[2]
- As many as 75% of patients with anxiety disorders will also experience comorbid disorders, including major depression and substance use disorders[239]
- The costs of anxiety disorders to society and to health care systems are enormous, as are the effects of impairment on functioning and quality of life for those who suffer from anxiety
- Although anxiety may be detected with the use of simple screening tools and effectively treated, less than 30% of persons with these disorders seek treatment for anxiety; instead, they tend to be high users of general medical care[241,242]
- Nonpharmacologic interventions can be as effective as pharmacologic ones and may be more effective in preventing relapse. Patients must be motivated to participate if they are to obtain benefits from nonpharmacologic treatment modalities
- BZDs are considered first-line therapy for patients with GAD and panic disorder. Pharmacokinetic profiles that dictate onset of action, duration of effect, and potential for drug interactions can aid in agent selection
- For patients in whom a BZD is not appropriate (e.g., those with substance use disorder, sedation, cognitive impairment), buspirone should be considered for the treatment of GAD
- SSRIs are first-line agents in the treatment of social anxiety disorder, panic disorder, OCD, GAD, and PTSD. Venlafaxine can also be used as a first-line agent for GAD. Antidepressants are more likely than BZDs to be used to treat the common comorbid depression that occurs with these anxiety disorders. Because of the delay in onset of effect with antidepressants, a role for short-term BZD has been observed in the initial treatment phase, particularly in panic disorder
- Patients with PTSD may benefit from mood stabilizers, β-blockers, or antipsychotics, particularly for the treatment of persistent symptoms such as impulsivity, aggression, hyperarousal, and psychosis

SUGGESTED READINGS

Culpepper L. Identifying and treating panic disorder in primary care. J Clin Psychiatry 65 (Suppl 5):19–23, 2004.
Fricchione G. Clinical practice. Generalized anxiety disorder. N Engl J Med 351:675–682, 2004.

Jefferson JW. Social anxiety disorder: more than just a little shyness. Primary Care Companion J Clin Psychiatry 3:4–9, 2001.

Jenike MA. Obsessive-compulsive disorder. N Engl J Med 350: 259–265, 2004.

Schoenfeld FB, Marmar CR, Neylan TC. Current concepts in pharmacotherapy for posttraumatic stress disorder. Psychiatr Serv 55:519–531, 2004.

REFERENCES

1. American Psychiatric Association. Diagnostic and statistical manual of mental disorders, DSM-IV-TR. Washington, DC: American Psychiatric Association, 2000:429–484.
2. Kessler RC, McGonagle KA, Zhao S, et al. Lifetime and 12-month prevalence of DSM-III-R psychiatric disorders in the United States. Arch Gen Psychiatry 51:8–19, 1994.
3. Kessler RC, Sonnega A, Bromet E, et al. Posttraumatic stress disorder in the National Comorbidity Survey. Arch Gen Psychiatry 52:1048–1060, 1994.
4. Stein MB, Forde DR, Anderson G, et al. Obsessive-compulsive disorder in the community: an epidemiologic survey with clinical reappraisal. Am J Psychiatry 154:1120–1126, 1997.
5. Stein MB, Walker JR, Haxen AL, et al. Full and partial posttraumatic stress disorder: findings from a community survey. Am J Psychiatry 154:1114–1119, 1997.
6. Goodwin RD. The prevalence of panic attacks in the United States: 1980 to 1995. J Clin Epidemiol 56:914–916, 2003.
7. Kessler RC, Stein MB, Berglund P. Social phobia subtypes in the National Comorbidity Survey. Am J Psychiatry 155:613–619, 1998.
8. Lepine JP. The epidemiology of anxiety disorders: prevalence and societal costs. J Clin Psychiatry 63 (Suppl 14):4–8, 2002.
9. Nemeroff CB. The role of GABA in the pathophysiology and treatment of anxiety disorders. Psychopharmacol Bull 37:133–146, 2003.
10. Lydiard RB. The role of GABA in anxiety disorders. J Clin Psychiatry 64 (Suppl 3):21–27, 2003.
11. Ninan PT. The functional anatomy, neurochemistry, and pharmacology of anxiety. J Clin Psychiatry 60 (Suppl 22):12–17, 1999.
12. Mohler H, Fritschy JM, Rudolph U. A new benzodiazepine pharmacology. J Pharmacol Exp Ther 300:2–8, 2002.
13. Kent JM, Mathew SJ, Gorman JM. Molecular targets in the treatment of anxiety. Biol Psychiatry 52:1008–1030, 2002.
14. Hoyer D, Hannon J, Martin G. Molecular, pharmacological and functional diversity of 5-HT receptors. Pharmacol Biochem Behav 71:533–554, 2002.
15. Roth B, Lopez E, Patel S, et al. The multiplicity of serotonin receptors: uselessly diverse molecules or an embarrassment of riches? The Neuroscientist 6:252–262, 2000.
16. Davis M. The role of the amygdala in fear and anxiety. Annu Rev Neurosci 15:353–375, 1992.
17. Davis M, Whalen P. The amygdala: vigilance and emotion. Mol Psychiatry 6:13–34, 2001.
18. Gorman JM, Kent JM, Sullivan GM, et al. Neuroanatomical hypothesis of panic disorder, revised. Am J Psychiatry 157:493–505, 2000.
19. Koob GF. Corticotropin-releasing factor, norepinephrine, and stress. Biol Psychiatry 46:1167–1180, 1999.
20. Zorrilla EP, Koob GF. The therapeutic potential of CRF1 antagonists for anxiety. Expert Opin Investig Drugs 13:799–828, 2004.
21. Herranz R. Cholecystokinin antagonists: pharmacological and therapeutic potential. Med Res Rev 23:559–605, 2003.
22. Coyle J, Leski M, Morrison J. The diverse roles of L-glutamic acid in brain signal transduction. In: Davis K, Charney D, Coyle J, et al, eds. Neuropsychopharmacology: the fifth generation of progress. Philadelphia: Lippincott Williams & Wilkins, 2002:71–90.
23. Gorman JM. New molecular targets for antianxiety interventions. J Clin Psychiatry 64 (Suppl 3):28–35, 2003.
24. Bergink V, van Megen HJ, Westenberg HG. Glutamate and anxiety. Eur Neuropsychopharmacol 14:175–183, 2004.
25. Arikian SR, Gorman JM. A review of the diagnosis, pharmacologic treatment, and economic aspects of anxiety disorders. Primary Care Companion J Clin Psychiatry 3:110–117, 2001.
26. Harter MC, Conway KP, Merikangas KR. Associations between anxiety disorders and physical illness. Eur Arch Psychiatry Clin Neurosci 253:313–320, 2003.
27. Anonymous. Drugs that may cause psychiatric symptoms. Med Lett Drugs Ther 44:59–62, 2002.
28. Levine J, Cole DP, Chengappa KN, et al. Anxiety disorders and major depression, together or apart. Depress Anxiety 14:94–104, 2001.
29. Gorman JM. Comorbid depression and anxiety spectrum disorders. Depress Anxiety 4:160–168, 1996–1997.
30. Wittchen HU, Hoyer J. Generalized anxiety disorder: nature and course. J Clin Psychiatry 62 (Suppl 11):15–19, 2001.
31. Wittchen HU, Zhao S, Kessler RC, et al. DSM-III-R generalized anxiety disorder in the National Comorbidity Survey. Arch Gen Psychiatry 51:355–364, 1994.
32. Carter RM, Wittchen HU, Pfister H, et al. One-year prevalence of sub-threshold and threshold DSM-IV generalized anxiety disorder in a nationally representative sample. Depress Anxiety 3:78–88, 2001.
33. Kessler RC, Wittchen HU. Patterns and correlates of generalized anxiety disorder in community samples. J Clin Psychiatry 63 (Suppl 8):4–10, 2002.
34. Keller MB. The long-term clinical course of generalized anxiety disorder. J Clin Psychiatry 63 (Suppl 8):11–16, 2002.
35. Stein DJ. Comorbidity in generalized anxiety disorder: impact and implications. J Clin Psychiatry 62 (Suppl 11):29–34, 2001.
36. Culpepper L. Identifying and treating panic disorder in primary care. J Clin Psychiatry 65 (Suppl 5):19–23, 2004.
37. Pigott TA. Gender differences in the epidemiology and treatment of anxiety disorders. J Clin Psychiatry 60 (Suppl 18):4–15, 1999.
38. Roy-Byrne PP, Stang P, Wittchen HU, et al. Lifetime panic-depression comorbidity in the National Comorbidity Survey. Association with symptoms, impairment, course and help-seeking. Br J Psychiatry 176:229–235, 2000.
39. Zane RD, McAfee AT, Sherburne S, et al. Panic disorder and emergency services utilization. Acad Emerg Med 10:1065–1069, 2003.
40. Roy-Byrne PP, Stein MB, Russo J, et al. Panic disorder in the primary care setting: comorbidity, disability, service utilization, and treatment. J Clin Psychiatry 60:492–499, 1999.
41. Rees CS, Richards JC, Smith LM. Medical utilization and costs in panic disorder: a comparison with social phobia. J Anxiety Disord 12:421–435, 1998.
42. Jenike MA. Obsessive-compulsive disorder. N Engl J Med 350:259–265, 2004.
43. Maj M, Sartorius N, Okasha A, et al, eds. Obsessive-compulsive disorder. 2nd ed. Chichester, England: John Wiley, 2002.
44. Hong JP, Samuels J, Bienvenu OJ 3rd, et al. Clinical correlates of recurrent major depression in obsessive-compulsive disorder. Depress Anxiety 20:86–91, 2004.
45. Lecrubier Y. Posttraumatic stress disorder in primary care: a hidden diagnosis. J Clin Psychiatry 65 (Suppl 1):49–54, 2004.
46. Resnick H, Kilpatrick DG, Dansky BS, et al. Prevalence of civilian trauma and posttraumatic stress disorder in a representative national sample of women. J Consult Clin Psychol 61:984–991, 1993.
47. Ballenger JC, Davidson JRT, Lecrubier Y, et al. Consensus statement update on posttraumatic stress disorder from the International Consensus Group on Depression and Anxiety. J Clin Psychiatry 65 (Suppl 1):55–62, 2004.
48. Galea S, Ahern J, Resnick H, et al. Psychological sequelae of the September 11 terrorist attacks in New York City. N Engl J Med 346:982–987, 2002.
49. Schlenger WE, Caddell JM, Ebert L, et al. Psychological reactions to terrorist attacks: findings from the National Study of Americans' Reactions to September 11. JAMA 288:581–588, 2002.
50. Kessler RC, Borges G, Walters EE. Prevalence of and risk factors for lifetime suicide attempts in the National Comorbidity Survey. Arch Gen Psychiatry 56:617–626, 1999.
51. Zlotnick C, Rodriguez BF, Weisberg RB, et al. Chronicity in posttraumatic stress disorder and predictors of the course of posttraumatic stress disorder among primary care patients. J Nerv Ment Dis 192:153–159, 2004.
52. Jefferson JW. Social anxiety disorder: more than just a little shyness. Primary Care Companion J Clin Psychiatry 3:4–9, 2001.

53. Katzelnick DJ, Greist JH. Social anxiety disorder: an unrecognized problem in primary care. J Clin Psychiatry 62 (Suppl 1):11–15, 2001.

54. Belzer K, Schneier FR. Comorbidity of anxiety and depressive disorders: issues in conceptualization, assessment, and treatment. J Psychiatr Pract 10:296–306, 2004.

55. Anonymous. American druggist. Top 200 drugs of 2003. New York, NY: Hearst Corp, 2004.

56. Ballenger JC. Benzodiazepines. In: Schatzberg AF, Nemeroff CB, eds. Essentials of clinical psychopharmacology. Washington, DC: American Psychiatric Publishing, 2001:75–92.

57. Greenblatt DJ, Divoll M, Abernety DR, et al. Clinical pharmacokinetics of the newer benzodiazepines. Clin Pharmacokinet 8: 233–253, 1983.

58. Klein E. The role of extended-release benzodiazepines in the treatment of anxiety: a risk-benefit evaluation with a focus on extended-release alprazolam. J Clin Psychiatry 63 (Suppl 14):27–33, 2002.

59. Moroz G. High-potency benzodiazepines: recent clinical results. J Clin Psychiatry 65 (Suppl 5):13–18, 2004.

60. Miller LG, Greenblatt DJ, Barnhill JG, et al. Chronic benzodiazepine administration. I: Tolerance is associated with benzodiazepine receptor down regulation and decreased α-aminobutyric acid$_A$ receptor function. J Pharmacol Exp Ther 246:170–176, 1988.

61. Soumerai SB, Simoni-Wastila L, Singer C, et al. Lack of relationship between long-term use of benzodiazepines and escalation to high dosages. Psychiatr Serv 54:1006–1011, 2003.

62. Rickels K, Lucki I, Schweizer E, et al. Psychomotor performance of long-term benzodiazepine users before, during, and after benzodiazepine discontinuation. J Clin Psychopharmacol 19:107–113, 1999.

63. Buffett-Jerrott SE, Stewart SH. Cognitive and sedative effects of benzodiazepine use. Curr Pharm Des 8:45–58, 2002.

64. Madhusoodanan S, Bogunovic OJ. Safety of benzodiazepines in the geriatric population. Expert Opin Drug Saf 3:485–493, 2004.

65. Cumming RG, Le Couteur DG. Benzodiazepines and risk of hip fractures in older people: a review of the evidence. CNS Drugs 17: 825–837, 2003.

66. Petrovic M, Mariman A, Warie H, et al. Is there a rationale for prescription of benzodiazepines in the elderly? Review of the literature. Acta Clin Belg 58:27–36, 2003.

67. Wang PS, Bohn RL, Glynn RJ, et al. Hazardous benzodiazepine regimens in the elderly: effects of half-life, dosage, and duration on risk of hip fracture. Am J Psychiatry 158:892–898, 2001.

68. Mancuso CE, Tanzi MG, Gabay M. Paradoxical reactions to benzodiazepines: literature review and treatment options. Pharmacotherapy 24:1177–1185, 2004.

69. Kalachnik JE, Hanzel TE, Sevenich R, et al. Benzodiazepine behavioral side effects: review and implications for individuals with mental retardation. Am J Ment Retard 107:376–410, 2002.

70. Wang JS, DeVane CL. Pharmacokinetics and drug interactions of the sedative hypnotics. Psychopharmacol Bull 37:10–29, 2003.

71. Ninan PT. Pharmacokinetically induced benzodiazepine withdrawal. Psychopharmacol Bull 35:94–100, 2001.

72. Chouinard G. Issues in the clinical use of benzodiazepines: potency, withdrawal, and rebound. J Clin Psychiatry 65 (Suppl 5): 7–12, 2004.

73. Rickels K, DeMartinis N, Rynn M, et al. Pharmacologic strategies for discontinuing benzodiazepine treatment. J Clin Psychopharmacol 19 (6 Suppl 2):12S–16S, 1999.

74. Spiegel DA, Bruce TJ, Gregg SF, et al. Does cognitive behavior therapy assist slow-taper alprazolam discontinuation in panic disorder? Am J Psychiatry 151:876–881, 1994.

75. Otto MW, Pollack MH, Sachs GS, et al. Discontinuation of benzodiazepine treatment: efficacy of cognitive-behavioral therapy for patients with panic disorder. Am J Psychiatry 150:1485–1490, 1993.

76. Voshaar RC, Gorgels WJ, Mol AJ, et al. Tapering off long-term benzodiazepine use with or without group cognitive-behavioural therapy: three-condition, randomised controlled trial. Br J Psychiatry 182:498–504, 2003.

77. Fraser AD. Use and abuse of the benzodiazepines. Ther Drug Monit 20:481–489, 1998.

78. Roth SM. Anxiety disorders and the use and abuse of drugs. J Clin Psychiatry 50 (Suppl):30–35, 1989.

79. Busto U, Sellers EM, Naranjo CA, et al. Patterns of benzodiazepine abuse and dependence. Br J Addict 81:87–94, 1986.

80. Pollack MH. Long-term management of panic disorder. J Clin Psychiatry 51 (Suppl):11–13, 1990.

81. Roache JD, Meisch RA. Findings from self-administration research on the addiction potential of benzodiazepines. Psychiatr Ann 25: 153–157, 1995.

82. Cadieux RJ. Azapirones: an alternative to benzodiazepines for anxiety. Am Fam Physician 53:2349–2353, 1996.

83. Mahmood I, Sahajwalla C. Clinical pharmacokinetics and pharmacodynamics of buspirone, an anxiolytic drug. Clin Pharmacokinet 36:277–287, 1999.

84. Lader M. Can buspirone induce rebound, dependence or abuse? Br J Psychiatry 12 (Suppl):45–51, 1991.

85. Jacobson AF, Dominguez RA, Goldstein BJ, et al. Comparison of buspirone and diazepam in generalized anxiety disorder. Pharmacotherapy 5:290–296, 1985.

86. Feighner JP. Buspirone in the long-term treatment of generalized anxiety disorder. J Clin Psychiatry 48 (Suppl):3–6, 1987.

87. Pecknold JC, Matas M, Howarth BG, et al. Evaluation of buspirone as an antianxiety agent: buspirone and diazepam versus placebo. Can J Psychiatry 34:766–771, 1989.

88. Ansseau M, Papart P, Gerard MA, et al. Controlled comparison of buspirone and oxazepam in generalized anxiety. Neuropsychobiology 24:74–7, 1990–1991.

89. Strand M, Hetta J, Rosen A, et al. A double-blind, controlled trial in primary care patients with generalized anxiety: a comparison between buspirone and oxazepam. J Clin Psychiatry 51 (Suppl 9): 40–45, 1990.

90. Enkelmann R. Alprazolam versus buspirone in the treatment of outpatients with generalized anxiety disorder. Psychopharmacology 105:428–432, 1991.

91. Sramek JJ, Frackiewicz EJ, Cutler NR. Efficacy and safety of two dosing regimens of buspirone in the treatment of outpatients with persistent anxiety. Clin Ther 19:498–506, 1997.

92. Laakmann G, Schule C, Lorkowski G, et al. Buspirone and lorazepam in the treatment of generalized anxiety disorder in outpatients. Psychopharmacology 136:357–366, 1998.

93. Schweizer E, Rickels K, Lucki I. Resistance to the anti-anxiety effect of buspirone in patients with a history of benzodiazepine use. N Engl J Med 314:719–720, 1986.

94. Delle Chiaie R, Pancheri P, Casacchia M, et al. Assessment of the efficacy of buspirone in patients affected by generalized anxiety disorder, shifting to buspirone from prior treatment with lorazepam: a placebo-controlled, double-blind study. J Clin Psychopharmacol 15: 12–19, 1995.

95. Sheehan DV, Raj AB, Harnett-Sheehan K, et al. The relative efficacy of high-dose buspirone and alprazolam in the treatment of panic disorder: a double-blind placebo-controlled study. Acta Psychiatr Scand 88:1–11, 1993.

96. Davidson JR. Pharmacotherapy of social phobia. Acta Psychiatr Scand 417 (Suppl):65–71, 2003.

97. Hollander E, Kaplan A, Allen A, et al. Pharmacotherapy for obsessive-compulsive disorder. Psychiatr Clin North Am 23:643–656, 2000.

98. Duffy JD, Malloy PF. Efficacy of buspirone in the treatment of posttraumatic stress disorder: an open trial. Ann Clin Psychiatry 6: 33–37, 1994.

99. Apter JT, Allen LA. Buspirone: future directions. J Clin Psychopharmacol 19:86–93, 1999.

100. Pecknold JC. A risk-benefit assessment of buspirone in the treatment of anxiety disorders. Drug Saf 16:118–132, 1997.

101. Liebowitz MR, Hollander E, Schneier F, et al. Reversible and irreversible monoamine oxidase inhibitors in other psychiatric disorders. Acta Psychiatr Scand 360 (Suppl):29–34, 1990.

102. American Psychiatric Association. Practice guideline for the treatment of patients with panic disorder. Am J Psychiatry 155 (Suppl 5):1–34, 1998.

103. Norman TR, Burrows GD. Monoamine oxidase, monoamine oxidase inhibitors, and panic disorder. J Neural Transm 28 (Suppl): 53–63, 1989.

104. Sheehan DV. Monoamine oxidase inhibitors and alprazolam in the treatment of panic disorder and agoraphobia. Psychiatr Clin North Am 8:49–62, 1985.

105. Versiani M, Mundim FD, Nardi AE, et al. Tranylcypromine in social phobia. J Clin Psychopharmacol 8:279–283, 1988.

106. Aarre TF. Phenelzine efficacy in refractory social anxiety disorder: a case series. Nord J Psychiatry 57:313–315, 1993.

107. Southwick SM, Yehuda R, Giller E, et al. Use of tricyclics and monoamine oxidase inhibitors in the treatment of post traumatic stress disorder: a quantitative review. In: Murburg MM, ed. Catecholamine function in post-traumatic stress disorder: emerging concepts. Washington, DC: American Psychiatric Press, 1994.

108. Kosten TR, Frank JB, Dan E, et al. Pharmacotherapy for posttraumatic stress disorder using phenelzine or imipramine. J Nerv Ment Dis 179:366–370, 1991.

109. Shestatzky M, Greenberg D, Lerer B. A controlled trial of phenelzine in posttraumatic stress disorder. Psychiatry Res 24:149–155, 1988.

110. Lippman SB, Nash K. Monoamine oxidase inhibitor update. Potential adverse food and drug interactions. Drug Saf 5:195–204, 1990.

111. Gardner DM, Shulman KI, Walker SE, et al. The making of a user friendly MAOI diet. J Clin Psychiatry 57:99–104, 1996.

112. Walker SE, Shulman KI, Tailor SA, et al. Tyramine content of previously restricted foods in monoamine oxidase inhibitor diets. J Clin Psychopharmacol 16:383–388, 1996.

113. Radomski JW, Dursun SM, Reveley MA, et al. An exploratory approach to the serotonin syndrome: an update of clinical phenomenology and revised diagnostic criteria. Med Hypotheses 55:218–224, 2000.

114. Fricchione G. Clinical practice. Generalized anxiety disorder. N Engl J Med 351:675–682, 2004.

115. Hoehn-Saric R, McLeod DR, Zimmerli WD. Differential effects of alprazolam and imipramine in generalized anxiety disorder: somatic versus psychic symptoms. J Clin Psychiatry 49:293–301, 1988.

116. Rickels K, Downing R, Schweizer E, et al. Antidepressants for the treatment of generalized anxiety disorder. A placebo-controlled comparison of imipramine, trazodone, and diazepam. Arch Gen Psychiatry 50:884–895, 1993.

117. Rickels K, DeMartinis N, Garcia-Espana F, et al. Imipramine and buspirone in treatment of patients with generalized anxiety disorder who are discontinuing long-term benzodiazepine therapy. Am J Psychiatry 157:1973–1979, 2004.

118. Doyle A, Pollack MH. Long-term management of panic disorder. J Clin Psychiatry 65 (Suppl 5):24–28, 2004.

119. Rickels K, Schweizer E. Panic disorder: long-term pharmacotherapy and discontinuation. J Clin Psychopharmacol 18(6 Suppl 2):12S–18S, 1998.

120. Noyes R Jr, Garvey MJ, Cook BL. Follow-up study of patients with panic disorder and agoraphobia with panic attacks treated with tricyclic antidepressants. J Affect Disord 16:249–257, 1989.

121. Noyes R Jr, Garvey MJ, Cook BL, et al. Problems with tricyclic antidepressant use in patients with panic disorder or agoraphobia: results of a naturalistic follow-up study. J Clin Psychiatry 50:163–169, 1989.

122. Nagy LM, Krystal JH, Charney DS, et al. Long-term outcome of panic disorder after short-term imipramine and behavioral group treatment: 2.9-year naturalistic follow-up study. J Clin Psychopharmacol 13:16–24, 1993.

123. Lepola U, Arato M, Zhu Y, et al. Sertraline versus imipramine treatment of comorbid panic disorder and major depressive disorder. J Clin Psychiatry 64:654–662, 2003.

124. Cross-National Collaborative Panic Study, Second Phase Investigators. Drug treatment of panic disorder. Comparative efficacy of alprazolam, imipramine, and placebo. Br J Psychiatry 160:191–202, 1992.

125. Caillard V, Rouillon F, Viel JF, et al. Comparative effects of low and high doses of clomipramine and placebo in panic disorder: a double-blind controlled study. French University Antidepressant Group. Acta Psychiatr Scand 99:51–58, 1999.

126. The Clomipramine Collaborative Study Group. Clomipramine in the treatment of patients with obsessive-compulsive disorder. Arch Gen Psychiatry 48:730–738, 1991.

127. Flament MF, Bisserbe JC. Pharmacologic treatment of obsessive-compulsive disorder: comparative studies. J Clin Psychiatry 58 (Suppl 12):18–22, 1997.

128. Ackerman DL, Greenland S. Multivariate meta-analysis of controlled drug studies for obsessive-compulsive disorder. J Clin Psychopharmacol 22:309–317, 2002.

129. Piccinelli M, Pini S, Bellantuono C, et al. Efficacy of drug treatment in obsessive-compulsive disorder. A meta-analytic review. Br J Psychiatry 166:424–443, 1995.

130. McDonough M, Kennedy N. Pharmacological management of obsessive-compulsive disorder: a review for clinicians. Harv Rev Psychiatry 10:127–137, 2002.

131. Frank JB, Kosten TR, Giller EL Jr, et al. A randomized clinical trial of phenelzine and imipramine for posttraumatic stress disorder. Am J Psychiatry 145:1289–1291, 1988.

132. Davidson J, Kudler H, Smith R, et al. Treatment of posttraumatic stress disorder with amitriptyline and placebo. Arch Gen Psychiatry 47:259–266, 1990.

133. Reist C, Kauffmann CD, Haier RJ, et al. A controlled trial of desipramine in 18 men with posttraumatic stress disorder. Am J Psychiatry 146:513–516, 1989.

134. Schoenfeld FB, Marmar CR, Neylan TC. Current concepts in pharmacotherapy for posttraumatic stress disorder. Psychiatr Serv 55:519–531, 2004.

135. Gorman JM. Treatment of generalized anxiety disorder. J Clin Psychiatry 63 (Suppl 8):17–23, 2002.

136. Rocca P, Fonzo V, Scotta M, et al. Paroxetine efficacy in the treatment of generalized anxiety disorder. Acta Psychiatr Scand 95:444–450, 1997.

137. Rickels K, Zaninelli R, McCafferty J, et al. Paroxetine treatment of generalized anxiety disorder: a double-blind, placebo-controlled study. Am J Psychiatry 160:749–756, 2003.

138. Pollack MH, Zaninelli R, Goddard A, et al. Paroxetine in the treatment of generalized anxiety disorder: results of a placebo-controlled, flexible-dosage trial. J Clin Psychiatry 62:350–357, 2001.

139. Stocchi F, Nordera G, Jokinen RH, et al. Efficacy and tolerability of paroxetine for the long-term treatment of generalized anxiety disorder. J Clin Psychiatry 64:250–258, 2003.

140. Otto MW, Tuby KS, Gould RA, et al. An effect-size analysis of the relative efficacy and tolerability of serotonin selective reuptake inhibitors for panic disorder. Am J Psychiatry 158:1989–1992, 2001.

141. Michelson D, Lydiard RB, Pollack MH, et al. Outcome assessment and clinical improvement in panic disorder: evidence from a randomized controlled trial of fluoxetine and placebo. The Fluoxetine Panic Disorder Study Group. Am J Psychiatry 155:1570–1577, 1998.

142. Perna G, Bertani A, Caldirola D, et al. A comparison of citalopram and paroxetine in the treatment of panic disorder: a randomized, single-blind study. Pharmacopsychiatry 34:85–90, 2001.

143. Ballenger JC, Wheadon DE, Steiner M, et al. Double-blind, fixed-dose, placebo-controlled study of paroxetine in the treatment of panic disorder. Am J Psychiatry 155:36–42, 1998.

144. Asnis GM, Hameedi FA, Goddard AW, et al. Fluvoxamine in the treatment of panic disorder: a multi-center, double-blind, placebo-controlled study in outpatients. Psychiatry Res 103:1–14, 2001.

145. Pollack MH, Otto MW, Worthington JJ, et al. Sertraline in the treatment of panic disorder: a flexible-dose multicenter trial. Arch Gen Psychiatry 55:1010–1016, 1998.

146. Lecrubier Y, Bakker A, Dunbar G, et al. A comparison of paroxetine, clomipramine and placebo in the treatment of panic disorder. Collaborative Paroxetine Panic Study Investigators. Acta Psychiatr Scand 95:145–152, 1997.

147. Bakker A, van Balkom AJ, Spinhoven P. SSRIs vs. TCAs in the treatment of panic disorder: a meta-analysis. Acta Psychiatr Scand 106:163–167, 2002.

148. Mundo E, Bianchi L, Bellodi L. Efficacy of fluvoxamine, paroxetine, and citalopram in the treatment of obsessive-compulsive disorder: a single-blind study. J Clin Psychopharmacol 17:267–271, 1997.

149. Greist J, Chouinard G, DuBoff E, et al. Double-blind parallel comparison of three dosages of sertraline and placebo in outpatients with obsessive-compulsive disorder. Arch Gen Psychiatry 52:289–295, 1995.

150. Jenike MA, Baer L, Summergrad P, et al. Sertraline in obsessive-compulsive disorder: a double-blind comparison with placebo. Am J Psychiatry 147:923–928, 1990.

151. Goodman WK, Price LH, Delgado PL, et al. Specificity of seroto-nin reuptake inhibitors in the treatment of obsessive-compulsive dis-order. Comparison of fluvoxamine and desipramine. Arch Gen Psy-chiatry 47:577–585, 1990.

152. Dominguez RA. Serotonergic antidepressants and their efficacy in obsessive compulsive disorder. J Clin Psychiatry 53 (Suppl):56–59, 1992.

153. Jenike MA, Hyman S, Baer L, et al. A controlled trial of fluvoxa-mine in obsessive-compulsive disorder: implications for a serotoner-gic theory. Am J Psychiatry 147:1209–1215, 1990.

154. Pigott TA, Pato MT, Bernstein SE, et al. Controlled comparisons of clomipramine and fluoxetine in the treatment of obsessive-com-pulsive disorder. Behavioral and biological results. Arch Gen Psy-chiatry 47:926–932, 1990.

155. Montgomery SA, Kasper S, Stein DJ, et al. Citalopram 20 mg, 40 mg and 60 mg are all effective and well tolerated compared with placebo in obsessive-compulsive disorder. Int Clin Psychopharma-col 16:75–86, 2001.

156. Bergeron R, Ravindran AV, Chaput Y, et al. Sertraline and fluoxe-tine treatment of obsessive-compulsive disorder: results of a dou-ble-blind, 6-month treatment study. J Clin Psychopharmacol 22:148–154, 2002.

157. Marshall RD, Beebe KL, Oldham M, et al. Efficacy and safety of paroxetine treatment for chronic PTSD: a fixed-dose, placebo-con-trolled study. Am J Psychiatry 158:1982–1988, 2001.

158. Tucker P, Zaninelli R, Yehuda R, et al. Paroxetine in the treatment of chronic posttraumatic stress disorder: results of a placebo-con-trolled, flexible-dosage trial. J Clin Psychiatry 62:860–868, 2001.

159. Davidson J, Pearlstein T, Londborg P, et al. Efficacy of sertraline in preventing relapse of posttraumatic stress disorder: results of a 28-week double-blind, placebo-controlled study. Am J Psychiatry 158:1974–1981, 2001.

160. Brady K, Pearlstein T, Asnis GM, et al. Efficacy and safety of ser-traline treatment of posttraumatic stress disorder: a randomized con-trolled trial. JAMA 283:1837–1844, 2000.

161. Martenyi F, Brown EB, Zhang H, et al. Fluoxetine versus placebo in posttraumatic stress disorder. J Clin Psychiatry 63:199–206, 2002.

162. Hertzberg MA, Feldman ME, Beckham JC, et al. Lack of efficacy for fluoxetine in PTSD: a placebo controlled trial in combat veter-ans. Ann Clin Psychiatry 12:101–105, 2000.

163. Connor KM, Sutherland SM, Tupler LA, et al. Fluoxetine in post-traumatic stress disorder. Randomised, double-blind study. Br J Psy-chiatry 175:17–22, 1999.

164. Khouzam HR, el-Gabalawi F, Donnelly NJ. The clinical experience of citalopram in the treatment of post-traumatic stress disorder: a re-port of two Persian Gulf War veterans. Mil Med 166:921–923, 2001.

165. Seedat S, Stein DJ, Emsley RA. Open trial of citalopram in adults with post-traumatic stress disorder. Int J Neuropsychopharmacol 3:135–140, 2000.

166. Escalona R, Canive JM, Calais LA, et al. Fluvoxamine treatment in veterans with combat-related post-traumatic stress disorder. De-press Anxiety 15:29–33, 2002.

167. Davidson JR, Weisler RH, Malik M, et al. Fluvoxamine in civil-ians with posttraumatic stress disorder. J Clin Psychopharmacol 18:93–95, 1998.

168. Stein MB, Liebowitz MR, Lydiard RB, et al. Paroxetine treatment of generalized social phobia (social anxiety disorder): a randomized controlled trial. JAMA 280:708–713, 1998.

169. Baldwin D, Bobes J, Stein DJ, et al. Paroxetine in social phobia/so-cial anxiety disorder. Randomised, double-blind, placebo-controlled study. Paroxetine Study Group. Br J Psychiatry 175:120–126, 1999.

170. Liebowitz MR, Stein MB, Tancer M, et al. A randomized, double-blind, fixed-dose comparison of paroxetine and placebo in the treat-ment of generalized social anxiety disorder. J Clin Psychiatry 63:66–74, 2002.

171. Allgulander C. Paroxetine in social anxiety disorder: a randomized placebo-controlled study. Acta Psychiatr Scand 100:193–198, 1999.

172. Liebowitz MR, DeMartinis NA, Weihs K, et al. Efficacy of sertra-line in severe generalized social anxiety disorder: results of a dou-

ble-blind, placebo-controlled study. J Clin Psychiatry 64:785–792, 2003.

173. Van Ameringen MA, Lane RM, Walker JR, et al. Sertraline treat-ment of generalized social phobia: a 20-week, double-blind, pla-cebo-controlled study. Am J Psychiatry 158:275–281, 2001.

174. Katzelnick DJ, Kobak KA, Greist JH, et al. Sertraline for social phobia: a double-blind, placebo-controlled crossover study. Am J Psychiatry 152:1368–1371, 1995.

175. Westenberg HG, Stein DJ, Yang H, et al. A double-blind placebo-controlled study of controlled release fluvoxamine for the treatment of generalized social anxiety disorder. J Clin Psychopharmacol 24:49–55, 2004.

176. Davidson J, Yaryura-Tobias J, DuPont R, et al. Fluvoxamine-controlled release formulation for the treatment of generalized so-cial anxiety disorder. J Clin Psychopharmacol 24:118–125, 2004.

177. Lader M, Stender K, Burger V, et al. Efficacy and tolerability of es-citalopram in 12- and 24-week treatment of social anxiety disorder: randomised, double-blind, placebo-controlled, fixed-dose study. De-press Anxiety 19:241–248, 2004.

178. Simon NM, Sharma SG, Worthington JJ, et al. Citalopram for so-cial phobia: a clinical case series. Prog Neuropsychopharmacol Biol Psychiatry 25:1469–1474, 2001.

179. Simon NM, Korbly NB, Worthington JJ, et al. Citalopram for So-cial Anxiety Disorder: An Open-label Pilot Study in Refractory and Nonrefractory Patients. CNS Spectr 7:655–657, 2002.

180. Kobak KA, Greist JH, Jefferson JW, et al. Fluoxetine in social pho-bia: a double-blind, placebo-controlled pilot study. J Clin Psycho-pharmacol 22:257–262, 2002.

181. Sheehan DV. Venlafaxine extended release (XR) in the treatment of generalized anxiety disorder. J Clin Psychiatry 60 (Suppl 22):23–28, 1999.

182. Rickels K, Pollack MH, Sheehan DV, et al. Efficacy of extended-release venlafaxine in nondepressed outpatients with generalized anxiety disorder. Am J Psychiatry 157:968–974, 2000.

183. Allgulander C, Hackett D, Salinas E. Venlafaxine extended release (ER) in the treatment of generalised anxiety disorder: twenty-four-week placebo-controlled dose-ranging study. Br J Psychiatry 179:15–22, 2001.

184. Gelenberg AJ, Lydiard RB, Rudolph RL, et al. Efficacy of venla-faxine extended-release capsules in nondepressed outpatients with generalized anxiety disorder: a 6-month randomized controlled trial. JAMA 283:3082–3088, 2000.

185. Rickels K, Mangano R, Khan A. A double-blind, placebo-con-trolled study of a flexible dose of venlafaxine ER in adult outpa-tients with generalized social anxiety disorder. J Clin Psychophar-macol 24:488–496, 2004.

186. Allgulander C, Mangano R, Zhang J, et al. Efficacy of venlafaxine ER in patients with social anxiety disorder: a double-blind, pla-cebo-controlled, parallel-group comparison with paroxetine. Hum Psychopharmacol 19:387–396, 2004.

187. Bandelow B, Ruther E. Treatment-resistant panic disorder. CNS Spectr 9:725–739, 2004.

188. Smajkic A, Weine S, Djuric-Bijedic Z, et al. Sertraline, paroxetine, and venlafaxine in refugee posttraumatic stress disorder with depression symptoms. J Trauma Stress 14:445–452, 2001.

189. Hollander E, Friedberg J, Wasserman S, et al. Venlafaxine in treat-ment-resistant obsessive-compulsive disorder. J Clin Psychiatry 64:546–550, 2003.

190. Albert U, Aguglia E, Maina G, et al. Venlafaxine versus clomi-pramine in the treatment of obsessive-compulsive disorder: a pre-liminary single-blind, 12-week, controlled study. J Clin Psychiatry 63:1004–1009, 2002.

191. Denys D, van der Wee N, van Megen HJ, et al. A double blind comparison of venlafaxine and paroxetine in obsessive-compulsive disorder. J Clin Psychopharmacol 23:568–575, 2003.

192. Emilien G, Maloteaux JM. Current therapeutic uses and potential of beta-adrenoceptor agonists and antagonists. Eur J Clin Pharma-col 53:389–404, 1998.

193. Tyrer P. Current status of beta-blocking drugs in the treatment of anxiety disorders. Drugs 36:773–783, 1988.

194. Rouillon F. Long term therapy of generalized anxiety disorder. Eur Psychiatry 19:96–101, 2004.

195. Jefferson JW. Social phobia: a pharmacologic treatment overview. J Clin Psychiatry 56 (Suppl 5):18–24, 1995.

196. Dannon PN, Sasson Y, Hirschmann S, et al. Pindolol augmentation in treatment-resistant obsessive compulsive disorder: a double-blind placebo controlled trial. Eur Neuropsychopharmacol 10:165–169, 2000.

197. Kolb LC, Burris BC, Griffiths S. Propranolol and clonidine in the treatment of the chronic post traumatic stress disorders of war. In: van der Kolk BA, ed. Post-traumatic stress disorder: psychological and biological sequelae. Washington, DC: American Psychiatric Press, 1984.

198. Vaiva G, Ducrocq F, Jezequel K, et al. Immediate treatment with propranolol decreases posttraumatic stress disorder two months after trauma. Biol Psychiatry 54:947–949, 2003.

199. Pitman RK, Sanders KM, Zusman RM, et al. Pilot study of secondary prevention of posttraumatic stress disorder with propranolol. Biol Psychiatry 51:189–192, 2002.

200. Otto MW, Smits JA, Reese HE. Cognitive-behavioral therapy for the treatment of anxiety disorders. J Clin Psychiatry 65 (Suppl 5): 34–41, 2004.

201. Schmidt NB, Woolaway-Bickel K, Trakowski J, et al. Dismantling cognitive-behavioral treatment for panic disorder: questioning the utility of breathing retraining. J Consult Clin Psychol 68:417–424, 2000.

202. Kobak KA, Greist JH, Jefferson JW, et al. Behavioral versus pharmacological treatments of obsessive compulsive disorder: a meta-analysis. Psychopharmacology 136:205–216, 1993.

203. Gould RA, Otto MW, Pollack MH. A meta-analysis of treatment outcome for panic disorder. Clin Psychol Rev 15:819–844, 1995.

204. Gould RA, Otto MW, Pollack MH, et al. Cognitive-behavioral and pharmacological treatment of generalized anxiety disorder: a preliminary meta-analysis. Behav Therapy 28:285–305, 1997.

205. Gould R, Buckminster S, Pollack M, et al. Cognitive-behavioral and pharmacological treatment for social phobia: a meta-analysis. Clin Psychol Sci Pract 4:291–306, 1997.

206. Otto MW, Penava SJ, Pollack MH. Cognitive-behavioral and pharmacologic perspectives on the treatment of post-traumatic stress disorder. In: Pollack MH, Otto MW, Rosenbaum JF, eds. Challenges in clinical practice: pharmacologic and psychosocial strategies. New York, NY: Guilford Press, 1996:218–260.

207. Goisman RM, Warshaw MG, Keller MB. Psychosocial treatment prescriptions for generalized anxiety disorder, panic disorder, and social phobia, 1991–1996. Am J Psychiatry 156:1819–1821, 1999.

208. Jorm AF, Christensen H, Griffiths KM, et al. Effectiveness of complementary and self-help treatments for anxiety disorders. Med J Aust 181:S29–S46, 2004.

209. Pittler MH, Ernst E. Kava extract for treating anxiety. Cochrane Database Syst Rev (issue 1), 2003.

210. Bilia AR, Gallon S, Vincieri FF. Kava-kava and anxiety: growing knowledge about the efficacy and safety. Life Sci 70:2581–2597, 2002.

211. Broman-Fulks JJ, Berman ME, Rabian BA, et al. Effects of aerobic exercise on anxiety sensitivity. Behav Res Ther 42:125–136, 2004.

212. Broocks A, Bandelow B, Pekrun G, et al. Comparison of aerobic exercise, clomipramine, and placebo in the treatment of panic disorder. Am J Psychiatry 155:603–609, 1998.

213. Salmon P. Effects of physical exercise on anxiety, depression, and sensitivity to stress: a unifying theory. Clin Psychol Rev 21:33–61, 2001.

214. Newman MG, Erickson T, Przeworski A, et al. Self-help and minimal-contact therapies for anxiety disorders: is human contact necessary for therapeutic efficacy? J Clin Psychol 59:251–274, 2003.

215. Benjamin J, Levine J, Fux M, et al. Double-blind, placebo-controlled, crossover trial of inositol treatment for panic disorder. Am J Psychiatry 152:1084–1086, 1995.

216. Palatnik A, Frolov K, Fux M, et al. Double-blind, controlled, crossover trial of inositol versus fluvoxamine for the treatment of panic disorder. J Clin Psychopharmacol 21:335–339, 2001.

217. Fux M, Levine J, Aviv A, et al. Inositol treatment of obsessive-compulsive disorder. Am J Psychiatry 153:1219–1221, 1996.

218. Fux M, Benjamin J, Belmaker RH. Inositol versus placebo augmentation of serotonin reuptake inhibitors in the treatment of obses-sive-compulsive disorder: a double-blind cross-over study. Int J Neuropsychopharmacol 2:193–195, 1999.

219. Kaplan Z, Amir M, Swartz M, et al. Inositol treatment of post-traumatic stress disorder. Anxiety 2:51–52, 1996.

220. Sandford JJ, Forshall S, Bell C, et al. Crossover trial of pagoclone and placebo in patients with DSM-IV panic disorder. J Psychopharmacol 15:205–208, 2001.

221. Stahl SM. Anticonvulsants as anxiolytics, part 1: tiagabine and other anticonvulsants with actions on GABA. J Clin Psychiatry 65: 291–292, 2004.

222. Stahl SM. Anticonvulsants as anxiolytics, part 2: pregabalin and gabapentin as alpha(2)delta ligands at voltage-gated calcium channels. J Clin Psychiatry 65:460–461, 2004.

223. Black K, Shea C, Dursun S, et al. Selective serotonin reuptake inhibitor discontinuation syndrome: proposed diagnostic criteria. J Psychiatry Neurosci 25:255–261, 2000.

224. Levine RE, Oandasan AP, Primeau LA, et al. Anxiety disorders during pregnancy and postpartum. Am J Perinatol 20:239–248, 2003.

225. Iqbal MM, Sobhan T, Ryals T. Effects of commonly used benzodiazepines on the fetus, the neonate, and the nursing infant. Psychiatr Serv 53:39–49, 2002.

226. Committee on Drugs. American Academy of Pediatrics. Use of psychoactive medication during pregnancy and possible effects on the fetus and newborn. Pediatrics 105(4 Pt 1):880–887, 2000.

227. Craig M, Abel K. Drugs in pregnancy. Prescribing for psychiatric disorders in pregnancy and lactation. Best Pract Res Clin Obstet Gynaecol 15:1013–1030, 2001.

228. Walsh KH, McDougle CJ. Pharmacological augmentation strategies for treatment-resistant obsessive-compulsive disorder. Expert Opin Pharmacother 5:2059–2067, 2004.

229. Figueroa Y, Rosenberg DR, Birmaher B, et al. Combination treatment with clomipramine and selective serotonin reuptake inhibitors for obsessive-compulsive disorder in children and adolescents. J Child Adolesc Psychopharmacol 8:61–67, 1998.

230. Goldberg D, Bridges K, Duncan-Jones P, et al. Detecting anxiety and depression in general medical settings. BMJ 297:897–899, 1988.

231. Baughman OL III. Rapid diagnosis and treatment of anxiety and depression in primary care: the somatizing patient. J Fam Pract 39: 373–378, 1994.

232. Spitzer RL, Williams JBW, Kroenke K, et al. Utility of a new procedure for diagnosing mental disorders in primary care: the PRIME-MD 1000 Study. JAMA 272:1749–1756, 1994.

233. Zajecka J. Importance of establishing the diagnosis of persistent anxiety. J Clin Psychiatry 58 (Suppl 3):9–13, 1997.

234. Wittchen HU. Generalized anxiety disorder: prevalence, burden and cost to society. Depress Anxiety 16:162–171, 2002.

235. Lecrubier Y. The burden of depression and anxiety in general medicine. J Clin Psychiatry 62 (Suppl 8):4–9, 2001.

236. Walker EA, Katon W, Russo J, et al. Health care costs associated with posttraumatic stress disorder symptoms in women. Arch Gen Psychiatry 60:369–374, 2003.

237. Creed F, Morgan R, Fiddler M, et al. Depression and anxiety impair health-related quality of life and are associated with increased costs in general medical inpatients. Psychosomatics 43:302–309, 2002.

238. Goetzel RZ, Hawkins K, Ozminkowski RJ, et al. The health and productivity cost burden of the "top 10" physical and mental health conditions affecting six large U.S. employers in 1999. J Occup Environ Med 45:5–14, 2003.

239. Greenberg PE, Sisitsky T, Kessler RC, et al. The economic burden of anxiety disorders in the 1990s. J Clin Psychiatry 60:427–435, 1999.

240. DuPont RL, Rice DP, Miller LS, et al. Economic costs of anxiety disorders. Anxiety 2:167–172, 1996.

241. Leon AC, Portera L, Weissman MM, et al. The social costs of anxiety disorders. Br J Psychiatry 166 (Suppl 27):19–22, 1995.

242. Stein MB. Attending to anxiety disorders in primary care. J Clin Psychiatry 64 (Suppl 15):35–39, 2003.

Mood Disorders

53

Mary A. Gutierrez and Glen L. Stimmel

DEFINITION

The most prominent feature of the four primary mood disorders is a disturbance in mood, but they must be distinguished from the more brief syndromes of sadness that may be part of many other conditions or temporary reactions to life stressors and bereavement in response to a major loss. The primary mood disorders include major depression, dysthymia, bipolar disorders, and cyclothymia.

TREATMENT GOALS

For most patients, mood disorders are characterized by chronicity and recurrent episodes, so the goals of treatment necessarily focus on the elimination of acute symptoms in manic and depressive episodes and maintenance therapy to prevent relapse (return of original symptoms) and recurrence (future manic or depressive episodes).

EPIDEMIOLOGY

The lifetime prevalence of major depression is 17%, spread fairly evenly over the age groups from 15 to 54 years, and twice as common in women than in men.[1] Among elderly living in the community, the prevalence of major depression is 3%, but 15% to 25% for those living in nursing homes have a 13% annual incidence of new episodes.[2] Dysthymia has a lifetime prevalence of 6% and is two to three times more common in women. Bipolar disorders appear in 1.3% of the population (0.8% bipolar I and 0.5% bipolar II), and cyclothymia occurs in 0.4% to 1.0%. Bipolar I and cyclothymia are equally common in men and women, whereas bipolar II is more common in women.[3]

PATHOPHYSIOLOGY

Although much is known about the mechanism of action of various antidepressant drugs and mood stabilizing drugs, the exact etiology of mood disorders is not known. The most clearly established biologic fact regarding mood disorders is the existence of a genetic substrate, with genetic loading greatest in bipolar illness. At least two thirds of bipolar patients have a positive family history of mood disorder. A compelling convergence of information from computed tomography (CT), magnetic resonance imaging (MRI), positron emission tomography (PET), and single photon emission computed tomography (SPECT) studies of patients with depression suggest this disorder is associated with regional brain dysfunction, particularly changes in blood flow and/or metabolism in the frontal-temporal cortex and caudate nucleus.[4]

There are many drugs reported to cause depression, but establishing a direct causative relationship is very difficult. No drug has been shown to be causally related to depression with as high a frequency as that which occurs naturally. These drugs include many antihypertensives (reserpine, propranolol, methyldopa, clonidine), hormones (estrogen, progesterone), corticosteroids, and anti-Parkinson drugs (levodopa, amantadine).[5]

CLINICAL PRESENTATION AND DIAGNOSIS

The diagnostic criteria and symptoms of the four major mood disorders are listed in Table 53.1.[3]

MAJOR DEPRESSIVE DISORDER

Major depressive disorder includes patients who have experienced one episode of depression and those who have recurrent depressive episodes. This disorder is commonly referred to as unipolar. The frequency of episodes is quite variable; some patients have episodes separated by many years of normal functioning, whereas others have frequent clusters of episodes. Most patients with one major depressive episode will have more in the future. Of patients who recover from one depressive episode, 28% will experience a recurrence within one year, 62% within 5 years, and 75% within 10 years. Only 18% who recover from the index episode remain free of depressive episodes throughout the subsequent 10 years.[6] The risk of completed suicide in patients with major depression is 15%, which is about 30 times the risk in the general population. Several subtypes of major depression, each requiring somewhat different treatment approaches, are listed in Table 53.2.[3] Double depressions present clinically as major depression, and only a careful history will detect the preexisting dysthymia. Successful treatment of psychotic depression requires use of an antipsychotic drug for several weeks to months in combination with the antidepressant drug. Electroconvulsive therapy (ECT) remains the most effective treatment for psychotic depression.[7] Atypical depression presents with a reversal of the usual depressive symptoms, such as increased sleep and appetite. Monoamine oxidase inhibitors (MAOIs) have been shown to be more effective than tricyclic antidepressants (TCAs) for atypical depression. The newer antidepressants have not yet been compared to MAOIs for these depressions.[8] Seasonal affective disorder is unique in being responsive to sessions of bright light (2,500 lux), given 1 to 2 hours each day.[9]

DYSTHYMIA

Dysthymia is different from the other three primary mood disorders in that it is characterized by chronic depressive symptoms rather than episodes of mood disturbance. As a

TABLE 53.1	Symptoms and Diagnostic Criteria for Mood Disorders

Major Depressive Episode

Five or more of the following symptoms present nearly every day for 2 weeks:

Depressed mood most of every day[a]

Marked decreased interest or pleasure in most all activities (anhedonia)*

Appetite or weight change (>5% body weight in 1 month)

Insomnia or hypersomnia

Psychomotor agitation or retardation

Fatigue or loss of energy

Worthlessness, excessive guilt

Decreased ability to think or concentrate, indecisiveness

Recurrent thoughts of death, suicidal ideation or attempt

Dysthymia

Depressed mood most of the day, more days than not, for 2 years

When depressed, two or more of the following symptoms cause significant distress or impaired social or occupational functioning:

Poor appetite or overeating

Insomnia or hypersomnia

Low energy or fatigue

Low self-esteem

Poor concentration or indecisiveness

Feelings of hopelessness

Manic Episode

Distinct period of persistently elevated, expansive, or irritable mood lasting at least one week characterized by at least three of the following:

Inflated self-esteem or grandiosity

Decreased need for sleep

More talkative than usual; pressure to keep talking

Flight of ideas; subjective experience that thoughts are racing

Distractibility

Increase in goal-directed activities; psychomotor agitation

Excessive involvement in pleasurable activities which have a high potential for painful consequences (sexual, illegal, financial)

Marked impairment in occupational functioning or usual social activities; or necessity to hospitalize to prevent harm to self or others; or psychotic symptoms

Hypomania

Same symptoms as mania but last at least 4 days without impaired social or occupational functioning and no psychotic symptoms or need to hospitalize.

Cyclothymia

For at least 2 years, the presence of numerous periods of hypomanic symptoms and numerous periods of depressive symptoms that do not meet full criteria for mania or major depression

[a] one of these two symptoms must be present.

TABLE 53.2	Subtypes of Major Depression

Double Depression: dysthymia with a superimposed major depressive episode

Major Depression with psychotic features: most common psychotic symptom is delusions

Major Depression with Atypical Features: depression characterized by mood reactivity, in which mood brightens in response to a positive event, plus two of the following:

    Increased appetite and weight gain

    Hypersomnia

    Leaden paralysis (heavy leaden feeling of arms and legs)

    Interpersonal rejection sensitivity (long-standing)

Major Depression with Seasonal Pattern: episodes begin in fall or winter, remit in spring; 2 years of seasonal pattern necessary

chronic mild depression, dysthymia is most commonly encountered in primary care settings, is less often diagnosed and treated, yet causes significant social and occupational dysfunction. Antidepressant drugs now have established efficacy in the treatment of dysthymia. A common clinical mistake is to give dysthymic patients a lower dose of antidepressant because their depressive symptoms are less severe. For antidepressant drug treatment of dysthymia to be successful, full doses are necessary, just as if a major depression were being treated.[10,11]

BIPOLAR DISORDER

Two types of bipolar disorder have been described which depend on the severity of the manic episode. Bipolar I disorder is characterized by full manic episodes and major depressive episodes, whereas bipolar II disorder has hypomanic and major depressive episodes (Table 53.1). The diagnosis of bipolar disorder requires only one episode of mania. Depression is not necessary for the diagnosis, but is inevitable later in the course of the illness. After experiencing one manic episode, more than 90% of patients will have future episodes. The onset of mania is usually sudden and dramatic. Frequently manic patients do not recognize they are ill and resist treatment. Lability of mood is common, in which the mood can rapidly shift from one mood state to another. Many bipolar patients have an excellent work history between episodes, making prevention of relapse of critical importance. Mixed mania is a common type of bipolar illness in which manic and major depressive symptoms are present simultaneously. "Rapid cycling" is a term given to patients who experience four or more mood episodes in 1 year. "Secondary mania" is a term used to describe other causes for mania or hypomanic symptoms. Antidepressant drugs can switch bipolar patients into a manic or hypomanic episode, particularly when mood stabilizing medication is not used in combination with the antidepressant. Glucocorticoids, such as prednisone, stimulant drugs, and hyperthyroidism are other

examples of causal factors in secondary mania. Suicide attempts occur in about 25% of bipolar patients, with suicide completion rates of about 15%.[12]

CYCLOTHYMIA

Cyclothymia is a milder form of bipolar illness. It is a chronic mood disturbance of greater than 2 years characterized by numerous episodes of hypomania and depressions that are not severe enough to meet criteria for major depression (Table 53.1). Cyclothymia differs from bipolar type II disorder in that the depressive episodes in cyclothymia never meet criteria for major depression. Cyclothymia is frequently found in relatives of patients with bipolar disorder, as if the cyclothymic patient has the genetics for bipolar disorder but the full syndrome never develops. Cyclothymic patients may require mood stabilizers if their mood instability causes significant distress in their social and occupational functioning.

PSYCHOSOCIAL ASPECTS

Despite the primary role pharmacotherapy plays in the treatment of mood disorders, the psychosocial aspects of mood disorders must be identified and incorporated into a total treatment plan. At best, pharmacotherapy will eliminate symptoms of a manic or depressive episode, but the day-to-day coping skills, and strained relationships with family, friends, and work colleagues that result from the disorder must be supported and treated.

THERAPEUTIC PLAN

There are two recent practice guidelines for treatment of major depression,[13,14] and the latest revision by the American Psychiatric Association for practice guidelines for bipolar disorder was updated in 2002.[15] Two key concepts continue to be fostered in the revised practice guidelines for major depression. First is the need for continuation therapy for all patients and lifelong maintenance therapy for some patients (Table 53.3) and second, doses for continuation and

TABLE 53.3	Ideal Dose and Duration of Antidepressant Therapy for Major Depression

Acute Phase: 6–8 weeks at full therapeutic doses with the aim to reduce and eliminate symptoms

Continuation Phase: all patients receive 4–9 months more at full therapeutic dose with the aim to prevent relapse and return of depressive symptoms

Maintenance Phase: for patients with history of three or more depressive episodes, maintain at full therapeutic dose for an additional 1–2 years; for patients with a history of more than two episodes within 5 years, maintain at full therapeutic dose lifelong.

Aim is to prevent recurrence of future depressive episodes

maintenance therapy must be the same as the acute dose effective in eliminating depressive symptoms. When patients are given lower maintenance doses, their risk of relapse is much greater than when doses are maintained at acute dose levels. For example, patients successfully treated with paroxetine 40 mg daily given a 20 mg maintenance dose had a 52% recurrence of depression over 2 years compared to 24% recurrence with a maintenance dose of 40 mg daily.[16]

A growing concern is the undertreatment of major depression, both in its recognition in primary care settings, and the often inadequate dose and duration of treatment when recognized.[17] Undertreatment of depression is due to many factors, involving the patient, the provider, and health care systems. The shift toward primary care management of depression and away from specialty treatment raises concerns about quality of care and patient outcomes. Although the ideal pharmacotherapy of depression (Table 53.3) suggests antidepressants can be effective in at least 70% of patients, the reality of care actually falls far short of that ideal. It is estimated that only 5% to 10% of patients with depression are effectively treated over the course of their lifetime.[18]

The key concept of the bipolar treatment guidelines is to decrease the frequency, severity, and psychosocial consequences of episodes and to improve psychosocial functioning between episodes. Inadequate treatment or delay in treatment of manic episodes may lead to substantial and prolonged financial, legal, and social consequences.

TREATMENT OF DEPRESSIVE DISORDERS

PHARMACOTHERAPY

The many drug treatment options and effective dose ranges for depression in nonelderly adults are listed in Table 53.4. After three decades of use of TCAs, the last decade has seen a continuing evolution in the development of unique drug treatment options that have virtually eliminated TCAs as first-line therapy.

Clinical Relevance of Antidepressant Mechanisms.
Selecting an antidepressant drug for a patient, and rational combination drug therapy, can now be based on the unique differences in mechanism offered by the available antidepressants. Antidepressants began as pharmacologically "dirty" drugs, with the TCAs blocking reuptake of norepinephrine and to some extent serotonin (5-HT), but also having prominent antagonistic effects on muscarinic, histaminic, and adrenergic receptors. These latter effects caused the many adverse effects and toxicity of TCAs, and led to frequent noncompliance with therapy. More recently, the TCAs have mostly been replaced by the "cleaner" more specific selective serotonin reuptake inhibitors (SSRIs), which selectively enhance serotonin. Thus SSRIs have little to no cardiovascular, anticholinergic, and sedative effects so common with TCAs. However, by increasing serotonin in

TABLE 53.4 | Effective Dosage Ranges of Antidepressant Drugs

Drug	DoseRange (mg/day)
Selective Serotonin Reuptake Inhibitors (SSRIs)	
fluoxetine (Prozac)	10–60
sertraline (Zoloft)	50–200
paroxetine (Paxil)	20–50
fluvoxamine (Luvox)	100–200
citalopram (Celexa)	20–60
escitalopram (Lexapro)	10–20
Serotonin Norepinephrine Reuptake Inhibitor	
venlafaxine (Effexor)	225–375
duloxetine (Cymbalta)	40–60
Serotonin Antagonist Reuptake Inhibitors	
trazodone (Desyrel)	200–600
nefazodone (Serzone)	300–600
Norepinephrine Dopamine Reuptake Inhibitor	
bupropion (Wellbutrin)	300–450
Noradrenergic and Specific Serotonergic Antidepressant	
mirtazapine (Remeron)	15–45
Tricyclic Antidepressants (TCAs)	
amitriptyline (Elavil)	150–300
clomipramine (Anafranil)	150–250
desipramine (Norpramin)	150–300
doxepin (Sinequan)	150–300
imipramine (Tofranil)	150–300
nortriptyline (Pamelor)	50–150
protriptyline (Vivactil)	20–60
trimipramine (Surmontil)	150–300
Monoamine Oxidase Inhibitors (MAOIs)	
phenelzine (Nardil)	45–90
tranylcypromine (Parnate)	20–50

every serotonin pathway and at each of the dozen or more receptor subtypes, the therapeutic benefits are accompanied by unwanted anxiety, insomnia, sexual dysfunction, and gastrointestinal disturbances. The most recent phase in the evolution of antidepressants was the return to multiple mechanisms but ones which are selected to reduce unwanted effects while maintaining efficacy. Venlafaxine is a potent SSRI, but also blocks reuptake of norepinephrine. Though venlafaxine's adverse effect profile is similar to that of the SSRIs, its dual neurotransmitter effect at higher doses is suggested to offer enhanced efficacy.[19,20] Nefazodone has selective serotonergic effects, but has an added mechanism of blocking postsynaptic 5-HT-2 receptors preventing the sexual dysfunction so common with SSRIs. Since the 2001 black box warning regarding rare cases of life-threatening hepatic failure reported in patients treated with nefazodone, the use of nefazodone has greatly diminished. Patients should be advised to be alert for signs and symptoms of liver dysfunction (e.g., jaundice, anorexia, malaise) and to report them immediately.[21] Finally mirtazapine, by α-2 adrenergic blockade, has the dual effect of enhancing norepinephrine and serotonin, plus postsynaptically blocking the 5-HT-2 and 5-HT-3 receptors, preventing the sexual dysfunction, anxiogenic, and gastrointestinal adverse effects. This continuing evolution in antidepressant mechanisms allows the clinician to select and modify drug regimens to meet the needs of individual patients.[19]

Tricyclic Antidepressants. TCAs are very effective antidepressants but with an adverse effect profile that limits their use in the acute and maintenance phases of treatment (Table 53.5). One advantage TCAs have over newer antidepressants is the ability to use plasma levels to determine an effective TCA dose. TCAs with a well-established correlation of plasma level range with antidepressant efficacy include nortriptyline (50–150 ng/mL), desipramine (100–160 ng/mL),

amitriptyline (75–175 ng/mL), and imipramine (>200 ng/mL).[22] Nortriptyline is unique in having a curvilinear response, or therapeutic window, in which clinical efficacy declines as the level exceeds 150 ng/mL. Plasma level monitoring is not routine, but indicated when there is lack of response at therapeutic doses, significant adverse effects at lower doses, suspected noncompliance, the stopping or starting of known enzyme inhibitors or inducers, and in the elderly. Initial common, dose-related adverse effects include sedation, anticholinergic effects, and orthostatic hypotension. With maintenance therapy, weight gain is the most common adverse effect and is often responsible for discontinuation of therapy. A major disadvantage of TCAs is their lethality in overdose. Overdoses of more than 1,000 mg (a 5- to 10-day supply) of a TCA alone can be fatal.

Monoamine Oxidase Inhibitors. MAOIs are effective antidepressants with particular indication for atypical depression and treatment-resistant depression. Phenelzine and tranylcypromine are equal in efficacy with similar adverse effects such as orthostasis, dry mouth, insomnia, and sexual dysfunction. It is their orthostatic hypotensive effects that limit the initial dose and rate of dose titration. Severe hypertensive reactions following ingestion of foods containing high concentrations of tyramine is rare, and the risk can be minimized by careful monitoring and individually targeted dietary assessment and education. The severity of the reaction depends on many factors. Six milligrams of tyramine produces mild elevation of blood pressure, 10 mg has a marked pressor effect, and 25 mg can result in severe hypertensive crisis. The patient will first become aware of a sudden onset painful, throbbing occipital headache, and if severe, may progress to profuse sweating and palpitation. The foods to absolutely restrict include all aged cheeses and meats, concentrated yeast extracts, sauerkraut, and broad bean pods (fava beans). Most patients can safely continue their MAOI drug and eat many foods in moderation that are listed on MAOI diets. Although foods have received most of the attention, several drugs are more dangerous than foods in combination with MAOIs. They include sympathomimetics (e.g., pseudoephedrine), stimulants (amphetamines, cocaine), levodopa and meperidine, buspirone, venlafaxine, and SSRIs.[23]

Stimulants. Controversy continues whether psychostimulant drugs have any value in the treatment of mood disorders. Nine of ten placebo-control trials do not support their use in outpatients with mild to moderate depression. Stimulants have no place in the treatment of major depression. The best evidence for their efficacy is brief, low-dose therapy in apathetic institutionalized geriatric patients, with an expectation that depressed mood may improve partially at best. Methylphenidate (20–30 mg/day) for 2 to 4 weeks is usually tolerated well, with exacerbation of preexisting anxiety the only consistent adverse effect.[24]

Selective Serotonin Reuptake Inhibitors. The widespread acceptance and prescribing of SSRIs coupled with

TABLE 53.5	Common Adverse Effect Profiles of Antidepressants		
Drug	**Sedation**	**Anticholinergic**	**Orthostatic Hypotension**
Amitriptyline	high	high	high
Imipramine	moderate	moderate	high
Clomipramine	high	high	high
Doxepin	high	high	high
Nortriptyline	moderate	moderate	moderate
Desipramine	low	low	high
Phenelzine	moderate	low	very high
Tranylcypromine	low	low	very high
	Activation	**GI**	**Sexual Dysfunction**
Fluoxetine	high	high	high
Sertraline	low	high	high
Paroxetine	low	high	high
Fluvoxamine	sedation	high	high
Citalopram	low	high	high
Escitalopram	low	high	high
Venlafaxine	moderate	high	moderate
Bupropion	high	moderate	very low
Nefazodone	sedation	low	very low
Mirtazapine	sedation	very low	very low
Duloxetine	low	high	unknown

GI, gastrointestinal.

the declining use of TCAs in the 1990s are a result of the SSRI's greater safety in overdose, relative lack of cardiovascular and anticholinergic effects, and convenience because dosage titration is often unnecessary. An effective SSRI dose for depression is generally lower than that necessary to treat other disorders such as obsessive-compulsive disorder, panic disorder, and bulimia. The initial dose of fluoxetine should be 10 to 20 mg once daily in the mornings, most patients will require 20 mg daily, with 40 mg occasionally necessary. Sertraline's initial dose of 50 mg is followed by dose titration in most patients to an effective dose of 50 to 200 mg daily. Paroxetine can be initiated at either 10 or 20 mg usually given in the morning, with most patients requiring 20 to 40 mg.[25] Fluvoxamine should begin at 50 mg at bedtime and increased to 100 to 150 mg daily. Citalopram can begin at its minimally effective dose of 20 mg, with some patients requiring 30 to 40 mg daily. Escitalopram can be started at 10 mg in the morning or afternoon, and titration to 20 mg daily can be done after a week.[26] All six SSRIs can be given once daily.

As a group, the SSRIs cause the same common adverse effects, namely gastrointestinal (GI) distress and sexual dysfunction, but the drugs differ in their degree of risk for activation and insomnia or mild sedation (Table 53.5). There is no consistent evidence that the likelihood of GI effects or sexual dysfunction will differ among the five SSRIs if given in equivalent doses.[26–31] The expected degree of activation versus sedation does differ, with fluoxetine most likely to be activating, whereas paroxetine and fluvoxamine are likely to be the least activating with some patients experiencing some sedation. These differences suggest a recommendation of morning or bedtime daily dosing. Extrapyramidallike movement disorders have been reported with SSRIs, likely due to increased serotonergic input to dopaminergic pathways.[32] Fluoxetine has been associated with 75% of all reported cases, though it has been the most commonly prescribed SSRI, and in half of the reported cases, use of other medication may have played a causative role in the movement disorders.

Many antidepressants have the potential for sexual adverse effects. The incidence of sexual adverse drug reactions (ADRs) of individual antidepressants has been reported with a wide range. All phases of sexual functioning can be affected, but the most likely problem associated with antidepressants is delayed ejaculation in men and anorgasmia in men and women. It is difficult to ascertain the true incidence because the methodology of the studies is highly varied. The general consensus among clinician experts is that the serotonergic agonists are the most offending, with approximately 30% to 60% of patients taking SSRIs experiencing sexual adverse effects. The most offending serotonergic agent with higher sexual adverse effects is clomipramine, with some reports indicating prevalence as high as 96%.[33] Venlafaxine, TCAs, and MAOIs have a relative lower frequency but can still commonly cause sexual dysfunction. Bupropion, nefazodone, and mirtazapine have the lowest rates of sexual dysfunction, and represent the best alternative antidepressants when treatment must be changed.[34] For patients who are responding well to their SSRI but sexual dysfunction threatens compliance, nefazodone (150 mg) or mirtazapine (15 mg) adjunctively due to their 5-HT-2 blockade, may treat the sexual dysfunction and allow continuation of the effective antidepressant.[35] Though a dose-related effect, sexual dysfunction should not be managed by decreasing the dose of the antidepressant because continuation and maintenance doses should be the same as the acute dose. Serotonin antagonists such as cyproheptadine have also been used, but these may interfere with the antidepressant effect of the SSRI. Sildenafil is not directly effective for SSRI-induced delayed ejaculation or anorgasmia, but can be useful when erectile dysfunction is also present.

When SSRIs are discontinued, they must be gradually tapered rather than abruptly stopped. A gradual taper allows monitoring for signs of relapse, with a prompt resumption of drug therapy if seen. A discontinuation syndrome has been defined that includes symptoms of dizziness, problems with balance, insomnia, fatigue, nausea, irritability, anxiety/agitation, mild shocklike sensations, and headache.[36] It is more common with the shorter half-life SSRIs, especially paroxetine, and other serotonergic agents such as venlafaxine. Symptoms can be reversed within 24 hours on resumption of the original medication.

All SSRIs must be used cautiously in patients receiving other serotonin agonists, because fatalities have been reported from a serotonin syndrome. Serotonin syndrome is the result of overstimulation of 5-HT$_{1A}$ receptors. The drugs of greatest concern are the MAOIs, with caution also necessary with the SSRIs and other serotonergic antidepressants. Serotonin syndrome is characterized by a triad of mental, autonomic, and neurological disorders including symptoms of confusion, agitation, insomnia, fever, diaphoresis, myoclonus, tremor, and hyperreflexia.[37] Common symptoms of serotonergic syndrome include fever, agitation, diaphoresis, myoclonus, tremor, confusion, and diarrhea. Cardiovascular collapse, coma, and death are rare but possible.

Four of the SSRIs are inhibitors of cytochrome P-450 (CYP-450) isoenzymes, creating the potential for drug interactions with other drugs that rely on these isoenzymes for their metabolism. Citalopram and escitalopram do not have significant effects on P-450 isoenzymes, whereas the other four SSRIs, nefazodone, bupropion, and duloxetine are inhibitors. Venlafaxine and mirtazapine also have no clinically important effects on these isoenzymes. Table 53.6 lists a representative sample of potential drug-drug interactions of concern in which inhibition of the metabolism of substrate drugs may lead to increased blood levels and adverse effects.[38,39] The inhibitory properties of bupropion on the cytochrome isoenzyme 2D6 was not shown until years later in the market when cases and studies showed its 2D6 inhibition.[40] Information on drug-drug interactions as listed in Table 53.6 is constantly changing, so it should be not be viewed as comprehensive and completely accurate. The clinical signifi-

TABLE 53.6	Antidepressants and Cytochrome P-450 Drug Interactions	
CYP Isoenzyme	**Inhibitors**	**Substrate Drugs of Concern**
1A2 2D6	fluvoxamine paroxetine, fluoxetine, sertraline, bupropion,	theophylline, caffeine, tacrine, haloperidol, acetaminophen, TCAs, clozapine, olanzapine, duloxetine propranolol, timolol, metoprolol, desipramine, nortriptyline, risperidone, codeine, dextromethorphan, phenothiazines, type 1C antiarrhythmics (encainide, flecainide), duloxetine venlafaxine
2C9/19	fluvoxamine, fluoxetine	warfarin, phenytoin, benzodiazepines nonsteroidal anti-inflammatory agents
3A4	fluvoxamine, nefazodone	terfenadine, cyclosporine, steroids, triazolobenzodiazepines (alprazolam, triazolam, midazolam), erythromycin, nifedipine, diltiazem, verapamil, zolpidem, zaleplon, tamoxifen, indinavir, ritonavir, saquinavir

TCAs, tricyclic antidepressants.

cance of such interactions is highly variable and unpredictable; some interacting drugs may be used together if there is adequate monitoring and adjustment of dosage.

Venlafaxine. Venlafaxine is a potent serotonin SSRI inhibitor, and at the higher end of its dosing range (generally described as >150 mg/d) it is also a potent inhibitor of norepinephrine reuptake. Unlike SSRIs, it requires dose titration and must be given in divided doses unless the extended release formulation is used.[34] Initial recommended doses of 37.5 mg twice daily (bid) results in many patients experiencing nausea, so 18.75 mg bid is a better tolerated initial dose.[25] Most patients will require 225 mg daily, with some needing up to 375 mg. The extended release formulation allows once daily dosing, but offers no distinct advantage in terms of GI adverse effects.[41] Venlafaxine has an adverse effect profile similar to SSRIs (Table 53.5) with a unique effect of sustained increased diastolic pressure at higher doses. The incidence of elevated blood pressure is clinically significant only at dosages above 300 mg/day.[34,42] Regular blood pressure monitoring is necessary for patients on higher therapeutic daily doses of venlafaxine. It has no clinically important inhibitory effect on P-450 isoenzymes.

Nefazodone and Trazodone. Nefazodone has SSRI activity coupled with potent postsynaptic 5-HT-2A antagonism. Its more common adverse effects include initial sedation and orthostatic hypotension, so initial doses must be lower and divided. An initial dose of 50 mg in the morning and 50 mg at bedtime can be titrated upward to the minimum effective dose of 150 mg bid as quickly as tolerated by the patient. When an effective dose is established, nefazodone can be given once daily at bedtime.[25] The 5-HT-2A blocking effect is responsible for nefazodone not causing sexual dysfunction so commonly seen with other serotonergic antidepressants. Patients should be advised to be alert for signs

and symptoms of liver dysfunction (e.g., jaundice, anorexia, malaise, etc.) and to report them immediately because there is black box warning of rare cases of life-threatening hepatic failure reported in patients treated with nefazodone.[21] Nefazodone is a potent inhibitor of cytochrome P-450 3A4, giving it the potential for different drug interactions as compared to SSRIs (Table 53.6).

Trazodone is an effective antidepressant, but its sedative and orthostatic hypotensive effects make it difficult for most patients to achieve a therapeutic daily dose of 300 to 600 mg. Trazodone has undergone a resurgence of use as an adjunctive treatment with SSRIs or bupropion and is currently mostly used as a hypnotic drug in doses of 50 to 200 mg at bedtime. A rare but serious adverse effect of trazodone requiring patient counseling is priapism. Trazodone is responsible for more than 80% of all drug-induced cases of priapism, and its mechanism is thought to be related to potent α-adrenergic blockade with minimal anticholinergic properties, activating the sympathetic nervous system more than the parasympathetic nervous system. Sustained painful penile erection, if untreated, leads to permanent impotence in most cases. Immediate treatment is required, involving intracavernosal α-adrenergic agonists. Priapism is not dose-related, and has occurred with single doses of trazodone as low as 50 mg, so all male patients receiving trazodone must be counseled about this rare but potentially serious adverse effect. Nefazodone, though similar in mechanism, has only 5% of trazodone's α-adrenergic blocking effect, and has only been associated with causing priapism in a few case reports so far.[43]

Bupropion. Bupropion is an activating antidepressant with a unique mechanism of action essentially lacking cardiovascular, anticholinergic, and sexual dysfunction effects.[44] The finding of high seizure rates among bulimic patients treated with bupropion resulted in eventual marketing with limitations on the rate of dose escalation and maximum dosage. This complex dosing schedule, coupled with concern regarding seizures, limited the use of bupropion as a first-line agent. Development of a subsequent sustained release preparation has simplified the dosing schedule. Although daily doses of up to 450 mg are associated with a risk of 0.4% seizures, the risk dropped with the sustained release bupropion up to 300 mg daily to 0.1%.[25] Bupropion sustained release can be given in a maximum single dose of 200 mg, so its therapeutically effective dose of 300 mg/day must be given in a bid schedule. Immediate release bupropion can be given in a maximum of 150 mg per dose, so TID dosing is necessary if the dose exceeds 300 mg/day.[45] Bupropion has a mild dopamine agonist effect, meaning it may worsen preexisting psychotic symptoms. Bupropion has developed a reputation that it is less likely to cause bipolar depressed patients to switch into mania, so it has become a commonly used antidepressant in bipolar patients.[46]

Mirtazapine. Mirtazapine provides serotonin and norepinephrine agonist effects coupled with postsynaptic blockade of 5-HT-2 and 5-HT-3 receptors. This unique mechanism maintains clinical efficacy for depression while minimizing the activating, GI, and sexual dysfunction effects so common with SSRIs.[47] Its common adverse effects include sedation and weight gain, both of which are inversely related to dose. Thus, in contrast to what would normally be expected, if these symptoms occur, the dose should be increased rather than lowered. The initial dose is 15 mg at bedtime with an effective dose range of 15 to 45 mg. To minimize sedation and increased appetite, it is possible to begin therapy with 30 mg at bedtime.[25] In addition to its use as a single agent for depression, mirtazapine has been used as an adjunct to SSRIs to treat the GI and sexual dysfunction effects.

Duloxetine. Duloxetine, introduced in the United States in 2004, continues the evolution toward multiple mechanism antidepressants. Duloxetine has potent and balanced serotonin and norepinephrine reuptake inhibition.[48] In clinical trials thus far, duloxetine has demonstrated high remission rates in major depression. In an 8-week double-blind study, duloxetine 20 mg bid titrated up to a maximum of 60 mg bid was compared to placebo and fluoxetine 20 mg as an active control. Duloxetine demonstrated response and remission rates of 64% and 56%, respectively, compared to 52% and 30% for fluoxetine and 48% and 32% for placebo.[49] The only duloxetine adverse effects occurring statistically more frequently than placebo were insomnia (20%) and asthenia (17%). Duloxetine 60 mg, with once daily dosing, has been shown to have significantly greater clinical efficacy for depression compared to placebo.[50] Response and remission rates for duloxetine were 65% and 43%, respectively, compared to 42% and 28% for placebo. Duloxetine is a CYP1A2 substrate, so its levels may increase when given with CYP1A2 inhibitors, and its levels may decrease in smokers. Duloxetine has moderate CYP2D6 inhibitory ef-

fects, though it is too early to compare directly to the SSRIs (Table 53.6).

NONPHARMACOLOGIC THERAPY

Electroconvulsive Therapy. ECT remains the most effective treatment available for psychotic depression and treatment resistant depressions. It is more effective and more rapid in onset of effect compared to drug therapy. Disadvantages of ECT include frequent relapse after treatment termination, temporary cognitive impairment, a significant social stigma concerning its use, and in many states, legal barriers to its use. Following a successful course of ECT, there is a 50% risk of relapse within the next 12 months unless maintenance antidepressant drug therapy is given. Although ECT has a history of misuse and overuse before the 1970s, drug modification of ECT by anesthesia and neuromuscular blocking drugs make it a safe and humane treatment option. A series of two to three ECT treatments weekly for 2 to 3 weeks is usually effective. Although ECT often is more of a political or legal issue than a therapeutic issue, it should be viewed as a treatment option that can be lifesaving for patients who otherwise would not recover from their depressive illness.[51,52]

PSYCHOTHERAPY

A variety of psychotherapies are available as a sole treatment or adjunctive to antidepressant medication. Interpersonal psychotherapy, cognitive-behavioral therapy, behavioral therapy, brief dynamic therapy, and marital therapy have all been used in the treatment of depression. These psychotherapies have been shown to often be effective for mild to moderate depression, but studies in continuation or maintenance therapy are lacking. Medication can eliminate symptoms of depression, whereas psychotherapy is best at assisting the patient in day-to-day coping skills that can prevent relapse. Thus, a combination of medication and psychotherapy yields the best results.[53]

ALTERNATIVE THERAPIES

It is often assumed that herbal medicines are effective and completely safe or completely ineffective. Neither is true regarding St. John's wort (hypericum perforatum). A meta analysis of 23 randomized trials in mild to moderate depression found St. John's wort to be more effective than placebo. A comparison to standard antidepressants in fewer trials found an equal reduction of symptoms, but antidepressant doses were inadequate, and no information is available regarding efficacy in more severe depression.[54,55] Hypericin, a reddish pigment has been the focus of attention as the likely active antidepressant compound in St. John's wort. Though initially thought to have MAO inhibitor activity, pure hypericin lacks MAO activity, and other flavinoid components may be responsible for antidepressant activity. Doses of hypericin have ranged from 0.2 to 1.0 mg, or total plant extract of 2 to 4 g. Thus, there is no established effective dose range, and standardization of hypericum extracts on hypericin content is no guarantee of pharmacological equivalence.[56] In the meta analysis, 20% of patients taking St. John's wort reported side effects that included GI symptoms, photosensitivity and allergy, and fatigue. St. John's wort has been shown to lower the plasma concentration and/or the pharmacological effect of a number of drugs including alprazolam, cyclosporine, digoxin, fexofenadine, indinavir, methadone, simvastatin, theophylline, warfarin, and oral contraceptives. Proposed mechanism of this drug interaction are induction of P-glycoprotein and/or CYP-450 enzymes (particularly CYP 3A4) by St. John's wort. When St. John's wort is combined with SSRIs and other serotonergic agents, there is a risk of serotonergic syndrome.[57]

TREATMENT OF BIPOLAR DISORDERS

PHARMACOTHERAPY

The goal of treatment of bipolar disorders is to reestablish euthymia by treating acute episodes of mania, hypomania, or depression, and further, to prevent future episodes with maintenance drug therapy. At any one time, a bipolar patient may be manic, hypomanic, depressed, or euthymic. Mood stabilizers, including lithium and several anticonvulsant drugs, are used in all phases of the disorder in the acute and maintenance phase of therapy. Treatment of bipolar disorder is characterized by a frequent need to use multiple medications rather than monotherapy. Mood stabilizers are very commonly used in combination with antipsychotic drugs or benzodiazepines for manic episodes and in combination with antidepressants for depressive episodes.[58] Treating a depressive episode in a bipolar patient is the same as treatment of major depressive disorder as discussed earlier, with the exception that a mood stabilizer at adequate daily doses should be used along with the antidepressant. Use of an antidepressant alone carries a risk of pharmacologically switching the patient abruptly from depression to mania. An expert consensus guideline for treatment of depression in bipolar disorder suggests bupropion or SSRIs are preferred antidepressants in combination with a mood stabilizer. A common belief is that bupropion is least likely among antidepressants to cause a switch into mania based on its unique mechanism of action,[59] and that TCAs have a greater risk than SSRIs. A number of cases of induction of mania with bupropion and SSRIs have been reported, however, suggesting the need for a mood stabilizer even with these antidepressants.[60,61]

Lithium. The fact that a simple chemical element of nature can have such a profound clinical effect in treating bipolar disorder is amazing. The introduction of lithium in the United States in 1970 provided, for the first time, an effective treatment for mania, replacing the marginally effective use of chlorpromazine in 2,000 to 6,000 mg per day or excessive doses of sedative-hypnotics. Lithium was also the first drug with proven prophylactic value as maintenance therapy for patients with bipolar disorder. Lithium was very slow to gain acceptance, however, since lithium chloride was used in the 1940s as a salt substitute in cardiac patients, resulting in many cases of serious toxicity and deaths.

Lithium has proven efficacy for acute treatment of manic episodes and in the prevention of recurrent manic and depressive episodes in bipolar patients.[15] In addition, lithium is equal to antidepressants for maintenance therapy to prevent recurrence in unipolar major depression. Finally, lithium is the most effective of all adjunctive treatments to add to an antidepressant for treatment-resistant depression.[62] Lithium is effective in 60% to 90% of patients with an acute manic episode, but much less effective for mixed mania and rapid cycling patients.[63] Lithium's mechanism of action is still unknown despite many hypotheses. Current investigations are focusing on lithium's subcellular effects of decreasing the increased G protein activity observed in bipolar patients and lithium's ability to decrease second messenger activity, including cyclic adenosine monophosphate (AMP-c) and phosphatidylinositol.[64]

Lithium Pharmacokinetics. Lithium carbonate is almost completely absorbed from the GI tract within 8 hours of oral administration with peak blood levels achieved in 2 to 4 hours. Peak concentration from a single 600 mg dose is 0.45 to 0.85 mEq per liter. Initial distribution volume corresponds to the extracellular fluid space with a final volume of distribution of 0.8 to 1.2 L per kilogram. Lithium is not bound to proteins or metabolized, but it is excreted unchanged in the urine. Lithium is freely filtered through the glomerulus, about 80% being reabsorbed in the proximal tubule, competing with sodium. The average plasma elimination half-life is 18 to 24 hours.[65,66] Compared to younger patients, elderly eliminate lithium more slowly from a smaller volume of distribution. Elimination half-life of lithium in the elderly is about 25% longer than in younger patients, typically ranging up to 36 hours. The elderly require one third to one half less lithium doses than younger patients.[67]

There is a good correlation of clinical response and adverse effects to lithium levels. For acute mania, levels of 0.9 to 1.2 mEq per liter are often adequate, although levels as high as 1.5 mEq per liter are occasionally necessary. Maintenance levels of 0.6 to 0.8 mEq per liter are effective for most patients, but relapse rates are lower if levels are maintained at 0.6 to 1.2 mEq per liter (Table 53.7).[68] Levels above 1.5 mEq per liter are regularly associated with signs of toxicity, and levels above 2.0 mEq per liter result in serious toxicity. The narrow range between therapeutic and toxic levels makes plasma level monitoring mandatory for all patients receiving lithium. A 12-hour interval between the last dose and drawing the blood sample in a patient receiving the same divided daily dose for at least 1 week will yield a standardized lithium level which is reproducible.

TABLE 53.7	Therapeutic Dose and Levels of Mood Stabilizers	
Drug	**Oral Dose Range**	**Plasma Level**
Lithium	(mg/day)	
Acute	1,500–2,400	0.8–1.2 mEq/L
Maintenance	900–1,500	0.6–0.8 mEq/L
Valproate	750–4,000	50–125 mg/L

Lithium Dosing. For acute manic episodes, a daily dose of 1,500 to 2,400 mg is usually necessary to achieve a plasma level near 1.0 mEq per liter. The initial dose must be smaller and divided to assess tolerance of initial adverse effects. A typical starting dose of 300 mg three times daily (tid) is conservative, and can be increased by 300 mg increments every 2 to 3 days. More aggressive dosing titration may be necessary for some inpatients whose manic symptoms are severe and whose past history indicates the need for higher doses. A plasma level drawn 2 to 3 days after initiation of therapy can be used to calculate the steady-state level at that dose, with subsequent 300-mg dose increments yielding a plasma level increase of 0.15 to 0.35 mEq per liter (Table 53.8).[69] A loading dose of 30 mg per kilogram of slow-release lithium given in three divided doses over 6 hours has been shown to accurately predict a 12-hour level of 1.0 mEq per liter without adverse effects.[70] When a patient has reproducible blood levels on the same dose and is on maintenance therapy, annual blood levels are sufficient. Initiation of lithium for outpatient prophylaxis should be done very conservatively because the patient is not symptomatic and adverse effects may affect compliance. A reasonable starting dose is 300 mg bid, with weekly 300-mg dose increments. An oral daily dose of 900 to 1,500 mg will usually yield lithium plasma levels within the maintenance range of 0.6 to 0.8 mEq per liter. For most patients, the acute phase dose and blood level can be reduced by about one third for maintenance therapy.[71] Before lithium is begun, a physical examination and history should focus on detection of cardiovascular, endocrine, and renal disease. Baseline tests should include serum creatinine, blood urea nitrogen, complete blood count, urinalysis, thyroid function tests, electrolytes, serum calcium, pregnancy test in women of child-bearing age, and an electrocardiograph (ECG) if the patient is over 40 years of age or has cardiovascular disease.

Lithium Adverse Effects. Adverse effects and their relationship to therapeutic or toxic lithium levels and nondose-related adverse effects are listed in Table 53.9. Although the list is long, many patients with a carefully monitored and adjusted plasma level will experience few if any significant adverse effects. The most common adverse effects are polyuria, polydipsia, and weight gain. The most bothersome effects that lead to noncompliance, however, are weight gain, confusion, and mental slowness.[72] Most of the dose-related effects are related to peak plasma levels, so use of a slow-release preparation or bedtime dosing will often minimize these effects. The most common renal effect of lithium is impaired concentrating capacity due to reduced renal response to antidiuretic hormone (ADH), manifested as polyuria and secondary polydipsia. The mild polyuria seen early in treatment resolves in most patients with few patients troubled by persistent polyuria. Persistent polyuria can be mild and well tolerated but may progress to nephrogenic diabetes insipidus, characterized by urine output of greater than 3 L per day and urine-specific gravity as low as 1.002 to 1.005. Polyuria may be managed by changing to once daily dosing and lowering the dose as low as clinically possible, and in severe cases, addition of hydrochlorthiazide 25 to 50 mg or amiloride 5 to 20 mg per day. Use of amiloride is preferred because it does not affect lithium levels or potassium levels.[15] Much concern has been raised about the long-term renal effects of lithium. Although 10% to 20% of patients

TABLE 53.8	Lithium Steady-State Prediction	
Day	**Lithium Received**	**Plasma Level (mEq/L)**
1	900	—
2	900	—
3	900	0.51

Blood drawn on morning of day 3 prior to lithium administration, so 0.51 represents 2 days of 900 mg. Assume 24-hour half-life, 0.51 represents 75% of steady-state (ss) level

Estimated ss level at 900 mg/day = $100/75 \times 0.51 = 0.68$ mEq/L

For each 300-mg/day added, the new ss level will increase 0.15–0.35 mEq/L. Thus, to reach desired level of 1.0 mEq/L, should increase dose by 300 mg:

Estimated ss level at 1200 mg/day = $(0.68 + 0.15)$ to $(0.68 + 0.35) = 0.83$ to 1.03 mEq/L.

TABLE 53.9	Lithium Adverse Effects
Dose-related	
Therapeutic levels	nausea, diarrhea, polyuria, polydipsia, cognitive impairment, fine hand tremor (intention tremor), muscle weakness
Signs of toxicity	coarse hand tremor, persistent nausea, diarrhea, slurred speech, confusion, seizures, increased deep tendon reflexes, irregular pulse, hypotension coma
Nondose-related	nephrogenic diabetes, insipidus goiter, hypothyroidism, hypercalcemia, weight gain, macropapular or acneiform reactions, benign leukocytosis

display morphologic renal changes, there is no reduction in glomerular filtration rate or development of renal insufficiency. There are reports of a few patients developing a rising serum creatinine after 10 years of lithium therapy.[15]

GI effects are most apparent during the first week of therapy or after a dosage increase, and are directly related to peak plasma levels. Taking lithium with food and switching to the slow release formulation will successfully manage the nausea. Cognitive impairment is usually manifest as dulling, impaired memory, poor concentration, confusion, and mental slowness. It is difficult to detect while a patient manifests manic or depressive symptoms but it becomes more problematic during maintenance therapy. A fine hand tremor is seen in up to 50% of patients initially and may persist. Lithium tremor is not a resting tremor, not extrapyramidal based, but one which is noticeable on voluntary movement. Most patients are unaware of the tremor, becoming noticeable only when delicate movements are attempted such as drinking coffee or eating soup. Management of tremor includes dose reduction if possible, reduction of caffeine intake, and as a last resort, addition of a β-blocker. Propranolol (40–80 mg/day) or metoprolol (50–100 mg/day) are effective treatment options.

Lithium toxicity is usually seen when plasma levels exceed 1.5 mEq per liter, though signs of toxicity have been frequently reported with therapeutic levels in the elderly. Signs and symptoms of toxicity include worsening of many of the effects seen at therapeutic levels (marked tremor, severe nausea, and diarrhea), plus central effects of slurred speech, vertigo, and increased confusion. Patients and family members should be counseled about recognizing signs of toxicity, and they should be instructed to contact their prescriber immediately if these effects are seen. Lithium intoxication represents a serious medical emergency. Mild intoxication can quickly become severe if the patient continues lithium but stops eating due to worsening GI effects. Several days of fasting coupled with diarrhea means significant sodium loss, leading to increased lithium reabsorption and even higher levels. Hemodialysis is indicated when the lithium levels exceed 4.0 mEq per liter, the patient has renal failure, or if electrolyte and fluid balance cannot be maintained. Fatalities are uncommon and usually due to renal failure or cardiovascular collapse. Persistent neurologic and renal sequelae are more common.[15,73]

Lithium's endocrine and metabolic effects include the potential for a diffuse nontender goiter in 5% of patients with an equal number becoming hypothyroid. Lithium inhibits the synthesis and release of thyroid hormone, and inhibits the action of thyroid-stimulating hormone (TSH). The most consistent laboratory finding is an elevated TSH seen in about 30% of patients. A persistent elevated TSH for more than 3 months indicates replacement therapy with L-thyroxine. Thyroid function should be evaluated every 6 to 12 months, along with regular examination of the patient's neck for signs of goiter and eyes for exophthalmos. In the first year of lithium therapy, patients gain an average of 4 kg, with 20%

gaining more than 10 kg. Intake of high caloric fluids is common due to polydipsia, so patients should be counseled to drink water rather than sodas or juices.

Lithium may aggravate preexisting dermatologic conditions, especially acne and psoriasis. Leukocytosis during lithium therapy is secondary to neutrophilia accompanied by lymphocytopenia. The mean white blood cell count (WBC) increase is 3,000 to 4,000 per cubic millimeter, and is without the shift to the left seen in an infectious process. Although a benign effect, it is useful to obtain a baseline complete blood count before starting lithium.

Lithium Drug Interactions. There are relatively few drug-drug interactions of concern, but even a small increase in a lithium level can lead to severe adverse effects and toxicity. Thiazide diuretics will reduce lithium clearance within several days, causing lithium levels to rise as much as 50%. The combination of drugs can be used together, but lithium dosage must be reduced and plasma level monitoring increased. Nonsteroidal anti-inflammatory drugs, particularly indomethacin, naproxen, and ibuprofen decrease lithium clearance and may increase lithium levels by 20% to 60% after 3 to 7 days of concurrent use. Sulindac and aspirin do not significantly affect lithium levels. Angiotension-converting enzyme inhibitors may also substantially increase lithium levels by as much as 100% to 200%. Although all of these combinations may be used together, adjustment of lithium dose and closer plasma level monitoring is indicated.[74]

Lithium and Pregnancy. Any woman of child-bearing age should be using a contraceptive method while taking lithium, and a pregnancy test is mandatory before starting lithium therapy. The teratogenicity of lithium is well established with demonstrated malformations of the heart and large vessels in 4% to 12% of lithium babies versus 2% to 4% in untreated comparison groups.[75,76] Because the cardiovascular system is formed during weeks 3 to 9 after conception, lithium is contraindicated during the first trimester of pregnancy. Because other mood stabilizers, such as valproate, are also best avoided in the first trimester, symptomatic treatment with antipsychotic or antidepressant drugs is preferred if any drug treatment is necessary. Lithium may be used if absolutely necessary during the second and third trimester, but should be discontinued or the dosage reduced by 50% several weeks prior to the due date. The dehydration associated with labor and fluid shifts during delivery may lead to toxicity in the mother otherwise. Lithium should be resumed a few days after delivery with a reduced dose to counteract the increased risk of postpartum mania and depression. Infants breast fed by mothers taking lithium have serum concentrations of 10% to 50% of the mother's level, causing most clinicians to advise against breast feeding while on lithium.[15,76]

Valproate. Only valproate's use as a mood stabilizer is reviewed in this chapter. Valproate is now considered an equally effective first-line mood stabilizer when compared to lithium. Valproate is equal in efficacy to lithium for classic mania, and more effective than lithium for rapid cyclers, bipolar patients with comorbid substance abuse, and mixed mania.[62] Because mixed mania represents 40% to 50% of acutely manic patients, these efficacy differences suggest that valproate will supplant lithium as the most commonly used mood stabilizer. Valproate has minimal antidepressant activity, and it is more effective in preventing manic than depressive episodes.[15,77]

Valproate may be initiated in low divided doses to minimize initial GI adverse effects, such as 250 mg tid. The dose can be titrated upward by 250 to 500 mg daily every several days based on tolerance of adverse effects to reach the target level of 50 to 125 mg per liter (Table 53.7).[15,58] For acute manic patients, valproate can be safely given in a loading dose of 20 mg/kg/day in a divided schedule to achieve levels of at least 50 mg per liter within 24 hours.[78] In patients responsive to valproate, onset of clinical effect occurred within the first 3 days of therapy. Because lithium typically requires 7 to 10 days for onset of clinical response, this difference may be of clinical and pharmacoeconomic importance.[79] When an optimal dose has been achieved, the total daily dose may be given at bedtime to maximize compliance and convenience.

Other Mood Stabilizers. Because some patients may not respond to or tolerate lithium and valproate, there is a need for alternatives to these two first-line mood stabilizers. Carbamazepine has a long history of evaluation and use as a mood stabilizer, but is best considered an adjunctive treatment rather than an effective single agent mood stabilizer.[15] Newer anticonvulsants have recently become more commonly used as alternatives to lithium and valproate. Lamotrigine was approved by the Food and Drug Administration (FDA) in 2004 for maintenance treatment of bipolar I disorder to delay the time in occurrence of mood episodes in patients stabilized for acute mood episodes.[80] The proposed mechanism of action of the drug in patients with bipolar disorder is the inhibition of sodium and calcium channels in presynaptic neurons and subsequent stabilization of the neuronal membrane. Lamotrigine has not demonstrated efficacy in the treatment of acute mania, but has shown efficacy in significantly delaying time to intervention for a depressive episode, and limited efficacy in delaying time to intervention for a manic/hypomanic episode, compared with placebo. The dosage of lamotrigine has to be slowly titrated over a 6-week period to 200 mg daily to minimize the incidence of serious rash. Also, adjustments in the initial and target doses has to be observed when used with valproic acid with no more than 100 mg per dalton as the target dose in 6 weeks, whereas concurrent use with carbamazepine needs higher target doses with no more than 400 mg per dalton in 6 weeks.[81,82] Gabapentin has been prescribed off label and was used extensively in the late 1990s for bipolar disorders based on numerous open trial reports of its potential efficacy. Recent double-blinded studies and increased clinical experi-

ence have shown that gabapentin in not effective nor recommended for the treatment of bipolar disorder, and the FDA issued a warning letter to its manufacturer regarding their promotion of off-label uses of gabapentin without solid evidence.[83,84]

Symbyax is a combination formulation of olanzapine and fluoxetine approved in late 2003 for the treatment of depressive episodes associated with bipolar disorder. Olanzapine is an antipsychotic for preventing switching into mania secondary to the antidepressant therapy. The efficacy was established in two 8-week randomized, double-blind control studies. Clinicians who elect to use Symbyax for extended periods should reevaluate the risks and benefits of this combination medication for the individual patient. Common side effects include weight gain and sedation. Consideration with long-term use should also be placed on potential hyperglycemia effects associated with olanzapine and the enzyme inhibition interaction potential with fluoxetine.[85]

Acute Manic Episode. The decision to use lithium or valproate depends on presenting symptomatology as discussed above, and past history of response or adverse effects, and concurrent medical problems. Lithium is usually initiated in divided doses of 15 mg/kg/day, increased every 3 to 4 days up to a target plasma level of 1.0 mEq per liter. Because lithium has a lag time in onset of clinical effect, adjunctive medication is often necessary. If the patient is psychotic then an antipsychotic drug is indicated, but patients whose symptoms include only psychomotor agitation and sleep difficulty will benefit most from an adjunctive benzodiazepine. High-potency antipsychotic drugs are preferred to minimize concerns of excessive sedation and cardiovascular effects commonly seen with low-potency antipsychotic drugs. Haloperidol has been shown to be an effective adjunct, and doses seldom should exceed 10 mg per day.[86] Clonazepam and lorazepam, both in divided daily doses of 2 to 6 mg, are the preferred benzodiazepine adjuncts to lithium.[58] After symptoms have stabilized for 2 to 6 weeks, an attempt to taper and discontinue the adjunctive antipsychotic or benzodiazepine should begin so the patient eventually remains only on their mood stabilizer.

Valproate can be given in a loading dose as described above with the potential of an earlier onset of effect and decreased need for adjunctive medication. A target level of 45 to 60 mg per liter is often effective without significant adverse effects. Vomiting, nausea, and weakness are all more likely if levels are above 125 mg per liter.[87]

Maintenance Therapy with Mood Stabilizers. Bipolar disorder is usually recurrent, with a mean episode frequency of about four episodes in 10 years. Because this is highly variable, some patients may not have a second episode for years after their first. Patients with one manic episode, with good insight and a good support system, should be treated with a mood stabilizer for at least 1 year with consideration to attempt discontinuation of drug therapy. For patients with one manic episode with an acute onset, psychotic symptoms, or very disruptive symptoms, long-term maintenance therapy is recommended.[88] Bipolar patients with two episodes should receive long-term maintenance therapy.

Lithium has a well-established long-term efficacy in preventing manic and depressive episodes, though a high dropout from maintenance therapy limits its long-term value.[88-90] Valproate does not yet have controlled studies for maintenance therapy. Patients who are responsive to valproate acutely, however, are best continued in maintenance therapy on valproate. Discontinuation of lithium maintenance returns the patient to their underlying episode frequency, whereas continuing lithium reduces the frequency and severity of bipolar episodes. There is some evidence suggestive of lithium discontinuation refractoriness, in which patients who discontinue effective lithium prophylaxis develop a more severe and subsequent treatment resistance to lithium.[88] The occurrence of an episode of mania or depression during maintenance therapy does not suggest treatment failure. No mood stabilizer is effective in preventing all future episodes. Severe or repeated breakthrough episodes, however, suggests the need to reevaluate the drug regimen and consider alternative treatment options.[15]

IMPROVING OUTCOMES

PATIENT EDUCATION TO IMPROVE PATIENT ADHERENCE TO ANTIDEPRESSANTS

The ideal drug therapy for depression described in Table 53.3 is rarely achieved but should form the basis for counseling patients about proper use, dose, and duration of treatment. The delay of several weeks in onset of effect must be understood by patients. Because adverse effects may begin on the first day, and noticeable improvement in mood may take 1 to 2 weeks, patients may reasonably conclude that the drug is not working, only making them feel worse, leading to premature discontinuation. Likewise, patients must understand the need to continue drug therapy for at least 4 to 9 months after symptoms resolve to prevent recurrence of symptoms. Counseling regarding adverse effects should be guided by Table 53.5 so the common expectable effects are discussed, including comments about management of each adverse effect mentioned. Use of alcohol should be discouraged primarily due to concern that alcohol may worsen their mood. With the newer antidepressants essentially lacking sedative and orthostatic hypotensive effects, there are no significant pharmacologic-based interaction concerns. Telling a patient never to drink while taking an antidepressant is more likely to result in noncompliance with the medication because most patients will continue to drink. A focus on warning of the potential consequences of drinking, rather than instructions for abstinence, will allow the informed patient to make reasonable decisions.[91]

PATIENT EDUCATION TO IMPROVE PATIENT ADHERENCE TO MOOD STABILIZERS

The nature of manic episodes, characterized by euphoria, inflated self-esteem, and lack of insight often interferes with mood stabilizer medication compliance. Few patients choose to take medication that will eliminate their hypomania or manic symptoms unless they understand the negative consequences of their illness. Patient counseling that focuses on the medication's ability to prevent future episodes, especially the unwanted depressive episodes, and the negative financial, legal, and social consequences of manic episodes, is more effective than trying to convince a patient that a mood stabilizer will treat their euphoria, excessive optimism, and decreased need for sleep. Few patients are bothered by their manic or hypomanic symptoms. In a 5-year follow-up study in a lithium clinic, about one fourth of patients discontinued lithium on their own initiative. The most common reasons for patients to stop lithium included perceived inefficacy, adverse effects, and the conviction that medication was no longer required because the symptoms were gone.[90] Other studies in bipolar patients report medication noncompliance due to denial of illness and lack of control over one's life.[92] Patient counseling can address these reasons for discontinuation. An evaluation of a lithium education program using a videotape, written handout, and follow-up visit was found to increase the patients' knowledge about bipolar disorder and treatment and compliance with lithium therapy.[93] An eight-page education guide for patients and families has been published that provides educational material about bipolar illness, mood stabilizers, management of adverse effects, support groups, and a reading list of books by people with bipolar disorder or depression.[94] One comparison of compliance with lithium and valproate found full compliance with valproate to be significantly better.[92]

PHARMACOECONOMICS

Since the introduction of SSRIs, there have been a number of studies suggesting that effective treatment of depression lowers overall cost of care for depressed patients, and that SSRIs are less costly due to greater compliance and fewer dropouts due to adverse effects when compared to TCAs.[95] Failure to complete acute and continuation therapy is more costly overall than a completed course of antidepressant therapy.[96] SSRIs and nefazodone have been shown to decrease the total cost of care compared to TCAs despite their higher drug cost due to fewer hospitalizations, the much higher cost of treating TCA overdose, and a greater TCA discontinuation rate.[97,98]

FUTURE THERAPIES

There are currently no major advances in pharmacotherapy of depressive disorders on the near horizon. For mood stabilizers, the success of valproate has led to evaluation of many other anticonvulsants for mood disorders whose role has yet to be established.

KEY POINTS

- Mood disorders are characterized by episodes of mood disturbance, and for most patients they are recurrent, necessitating long-term maintenance drug therapy
- All patients with major depression require a minimum of 6 to 12 months of drug therapy at the full acute dose, and patients with a history of three or more episodes will benefit from lifelong maintenance drug therapy
- An understanding of the unique differences of antidepressants' mechanisms allows the most rational drug selection and rational combination drug therapy to maximize therapeutic benefit and minimize adverse effects
- TCAs are no longer the first-line antidepressants due to their significant adverse effect profile, lethality in overdose, and a high discontinuation rate by patients
- SSRIs have supplanted TCAs as first-line agents due to their greater tolerability and safety in overdose
- Venlafaxine, nefazodone, bupropion, mirtazapine, and duloxetine each have unique advantages and disadvantages compared to SSRIs that allow an individualization of drug selection
- St. John's wort is an effective treatment only for mild to moderate depression, but its efficacy for major depression and dose range remain to be established
- ECT remains an effective treatment option for severe depression when drug therapy fails
- Patient counseling regarding antidepressants must include discussion of their delayed onset of effect, the need for a minimum of 4 to 9 months of treatment after symptoms resolve, and common expectable adverse effects and their management
- SSRIs have demonstrated superiority in reducing total cost of care when compared to TCAs
- Valproate has equivalent efficacy compared to lithium for bipolar disorder, superior efficacy for rapid cyclers and mixed mania, but minimal antidepressant activity
- Use of loading doses of valproate for acute mania allows more rapid onset of clinical effect
- All mood stabilizers are commonly used in combination with antipsychotic drugs or benzodiazepines for acute mania, and antidepressants for bipolar depression

SUGGESTED READINGS

American Psychiatric Association. Practice guidelines for the treatment of patients with major depression disorder [revision]. Am J Psychiatry 157:1–45, 2004.

American Psychiatric Association. Practice guideline for the treatment of patients with bipolar disorder (revision). Am J Psychiatry 159:1–50, 2002.

Stahl SM. Essential psychopharmacology: neuroscientific basic and practical applications. 2nd ed. Cambridge: Cambridge University Press, 2000.

REFERENCES

1. Blazer DG, Kessler RC, McGonagle KA, et al. The prevalence and distribution of major depression in a national community sample: the national comorbidity survey. Am J Psychiatry 151:979–986, 1994.
2. Reynolds CF. Treatment of depression in late life. Am J Med 97 (Suppl 6A):39S–46S, 1994.
3. American Psychiatric Association. Diagnostic and statistical manual of mental disorders. 4th ed. Washington DC: American Psychiatric Association, 1994:317–391.
4. Cummings JL. The neuroanatomy of depression. J Clin Psychiatry 54 (Suppl 11):14–20, 1993.
5. Rush DR, Stimmel GL. When drugs cause psychiatric symptoms. Patient Care 23:57–75, 1989.
6. Hirschfeld RMA. Guidelines for the long-term treatment of depression. J Clin Psychiatry 55 (Suppl 12):61–69, 1994.
7. Schatzberg AF, Rothschild AJ. Psychotic (delusional) major depression: should it be included as a distinct syndrome in DSMIV? Am J Psychiatry 149:733–745, 1992.
8. Stewart JW, Tricamo E, McGrath PJ, et al. Prophylactic efficacy of phenelzine and imipramine in chronic atypical depression: likelihood of recurrence on discontinuation after 6 months' remission. Am J Psychiatry 154:31–36, 1997.
9. Lafer B, Sachs GS, Labbate LA, et al. Phototherapy for seasonal affective disorder: a blind comparison of three different schedules. Am J Psychiatry 151:1081–1083, 1994.
10. Shelton RC, Davidson J, Yonkers KA, et al. The undertreatment of dysthymia. J Clin Psychiatry 58:59–65, 1997.
11. Lapierre YD. Pharmacological therapy of dysthymia. Acta Psychiatr Scand 89 (Suppl 383):42–48, 1994.
12. Schatzberg AF. Bipolar disorder: recent issues in diagnosis and classification. J Clin Psychiatry 59 (Suppl 6):5–10, 1998.
13. Trivedi MH. Remission of depression and the Texas Medication Algorithm Project. Manag Care Interface (Suppl B):9–13, 2003.
14. American Psychiatric Association. Practice guidelines for the treatment of patients with major depression disorder [revision]. Am J Psychiatry 157:1–45, 2004.
15. American Psychiatric Association. Practice guideline for the treatment of patients with bipolar disorder [revision]. Am J Psychiatry 159:1–50, 2002.
16. Franchini L, Gasperini M, Perez J, et al. Dose-response efficacy of paroxetine in preventing depressive recurrences: a randomized, double-blind study. J Clin Psychiatry 59:229–232, 1998.
17. Hirschfeld RMA, Keller MB, Panico S, et al. The national depressive and manic-depressive association consensus statement on the undertreatment of depression. JAMA 277:333–340, 1997.
18. Docherty JP. Barriers to the diagnosis of depression in primary care. J Clin Psychiatry 58 (Suppl 1):5–10, 1997.
19. Stahl SM. Essential psychopharmacology: neuroscientific basic and practical applications. 2nd ed. Cambridge: Cambridge University Press, 2000.
20. Gutierrez MA, Stimmel GL, Aiso JY. Venlafaxine: a 2003 update. Clin Ther 25:2138–2154, 2003.
21. Serzone[R]. Product information. Princeton, NJ: Bristol-Myers Squibb Company, 2001.
22. Preskorn SH. Pharmacokinetics of antidepressants. J Clin Psychiatry 54 (Suppl 9):14–34, 1993.
23. Sweet RA, Brown EJ, Heimberg RG. Monoamine oxidase inhibitor dietary restrictions: what are we asking patients to give up? J Clin Psychiatry 56:196–201, 1995.
24. Satel SL, Nelson JC. Stimulants in the treatment of depression: a critical overview. J Clin Psychiatry 50:241–249, 1989.
25. Sussman N, Stimmel GL. New dosing strategies for psychotropic drugs. Primary Psychiatry 4:24–30, 1998.
26. Escitalopram®. Product information, Princeton, NJ: Bristol-Myers Squibb Company, 2001.

27. Stokes PE. Fluoxetine: a five-year review. Clin Ther 15:216–243, 1993.

28. Murdoch D, McTavish D. Sertraline: a review of its pharmacodynamic and pharmacokinetic properties. Drugs 44:604–624, 1992.

29. Nemeroff CB. The clinical pharmacology and use of paroxetine, a new selective serotonin reuptake inhibitor. Pharmacotherapy 14:127–138, 1994.

30. Kiev A, Feiger A. A double-blind comparison of fluvoxamine and paroxetine in the treatment of depressed outpatients. J Clin Psychiatry 58:146–152, 1997.

31. Noble S, Benfield P. Citalopram. CNS Drugs 8:410–431, 1997.

32. Leo RJ. Movement disorders associated with the serotonin reuptake inhibitors. J Clin Psychiatry 57:449–454, 1996.

33. Segraves RT. Antidepressant-induced sexual dysfunction. J Clin Psychiatry 59 (Suppl 4):48–54, 1998.

34. Gutierrez MA, Stimmel GL. Management of and counseling for psychotropic drug-induced sexual dysfunction. Pharmacotherapy 19:823–831, 1999.

35. Reynolds RD. Sertraline-induced anorgasmia treated with intermittent nefazodone [letter]. J Clin Psychiatry 58:89, 1997.

36. Haddad PM. Antidepressant discontinuation syndromes: clinical relevance, prevention and management. Drug Saf 23:183–97, 2001.

37. Birmes P, Coppin D, Schmitt L, et al. Serotonin syndrome: a brief review. CMAJ 168:1439–1442, 2003.

38. Jefferson JW. Drug interactions - friend or foe? J Clin Psychiatry 59 (Suppl 4):37–47, 1998.

39. Ereshefsky L. Drug-drug interactions involving antidepressants: focus on venlafaxine. J Clin Psychopharmacol 16 (Suppl 2):37S–53S, 1996.

40. Wellbutrin[R]. Product information. Greenville, NC: GlaxoSmithKline, 2004.

41. Cunningham LA. Once-daily venlafaxine extended release (XR) and venlafaxine immediate release (IR) in outpatients with major depression. Ann Clin Psychiatry 9:157–164, 1997.

42. Thase ME. Effects of venlafaxine on blood pressure: a meta-analysis of original data from 3744 depressed patients. J Clin Psychiatry 59:502–508, 1998.

43. Banos JE, Bosch F, Farre M. Drug-induced priapism. Med Toxicol 4:46–58, 1989.

44. Preskorn SH. Comparison of the tolerability of bupropion, fluoxetine, imipramine, nefazodone, paroxetine, sertraline, and venlafaxine. J Clin Psychiatry 56 (Suppl 6):12–21, 1995.

45. Davidson JRT, Connor KM. Bupropion sustained release: a therapeutic overview. J Clin Psychiatry 59 (Suppl 4):25–31, 1998.

46. Zarate CA, Tohen M, Baraibar G, et al. Prescribing trends of antidepressants in bipolar depression. J Clin Psychiatry 56:260–264, 1995.

47. Stimmel GL, Dopheide JA, Stahl SM. Mirtazapine: an antidepressant with noradrenergic and specific serotonergic effects. Pharmacotherapy 17:10–21, 1997.

48. Kirwin JL, Goren JL. Focus on duloxetine. Formulary 38:29–37, 2003.

49. Goldstein DJ, Mallinckrodt C, et al. Duloxetine in the treatment of major depressive disorder: a double-blind clinical trial. J Clin Psychiatry 63:225–231, 2002.

50. Detke M, Lu Y, et al. Duloxetine 60 mg once daily, for major depressive disorder: a randomized double-blind placebo-controlled trial. J Clin Psychiatry 63:308–315, 2002.

51. Lerer B, Shapiraa B, Calev A. et al. Antidepressant and cognitive effects of twice versus three times weekly ECT. Am J Psychiatry 152:564–570, 1995.

52. Welch CA. Electroconvulsive therapy. In: Treatment of psychiatric disorders. vol 3. Washington DC: American Psychiatric Association, 1989:1803–1813.

53. Arnow BA. Constantino MJ. Effectiveness of psychotherapy and combination treatment for chronic depression. J Clin Psychology 59:893–905, 2003.

54. Linde K, Ramirez G, Mulrow CD, et al. St John's wort for depression - an overview and meta-analysis of randomised clinical trials. Br Med J 313:253–258, 1996.

55. Volz HP. Controlled clinical trials of hypericum extracts in depressed patients - an overview. Pharmacopsychiatry 30 (Suppl 2):72–76, 1997.

56. deSmet PAGM, Nolen WA. St John's wort as an antidepressant: longer term studies are needed before it can be recommended in major depression [editorial]. Br Med J 313:241–242, 1996.

57. Izzo AA. Drug interactions with St. John's Wort (Hypericum perforatum): a review of the clinical evidence. Int J Clin Pharmacol Therapeutics 42:139–48, 2004.

58. Sachs GS. Bipolar mood disorder: practical strategies for acute and maintenance phase treatment. J Clin Psychopharmacol 16 (Suppl 1):32S–47S, 1996.

59. Frances AJ, Kahn DA, Carpenter D, et al. The expert consensus guidelines for treating depression in bipolar disorder. J Clin Psychiatry 59 (Suppl 4):73–79, 1998.

60. Fogelson DL, Bystritsky A, Pasnau R. Bupropion in the treatment of bipolar disorders: the same old story? J Clin Psychiatry 53:443–446, 1992.

61. Howland RH. Induction of mania with serotonin reuptake inhibitors. J Clin Psychopharmacol 16:425–427, 1996.

62. Rouillon F, Gorwood P. The use of lithium to augment antidepressant medication. J Clin Psychiatry 59 (Suppl 5):32–39, 1998.

63. Bowden CL. Predictors of response to divalproex and lithium. J Clin Psychiatry 56 (Suppl 3):25–30, 1995.

64. Ownby RL, Goodnick PJ. Lithium. In Goodnick PJ: Mania: clinical and research perspectives. Washington DC: American Psychiatric Press, 1998:241–262.

65. Amdisen A. Serum level monitoring and clinical pharmacokinetics of lithium. Clin Pharmacokinet 2:73–92, 1977.

66. Ward ME, Musa MN, Bailey L. Clinical pharmacokinetics of lithium. J Clin Pharmacol 34:280–285, 1994.

67. Hardy BG, Shulman KI, Mackenzie SE, et al. Pharmacokinetics of lithium in the elderly. J Clin Psychopharmacol 7:153–158, 1987.

68. Gelenberg AJ, Kane JM, Keller MB, et al. Comparison of standard and low serum levels of lithium for maintenance treatment of bipolar disorder. N Engl J Med 321:1489–1493, 1989.

69. Gutierrez MA, Walker NR, Kramer BA. Evaluation of a new steady-state lithium prediction method. Lithium 2:57–59, 1991.

70. Kook KA, Stimmel GL, Wilkins JN, et al. Accuracy and safety of a priori lithium loading. J Clin Psychiatry 46:49–51, 1985.

71. Bowden CL. Key treatment studies of lithium in manic-depressive illness: efficacy and side effects. J Clin Psychiatry 59 (Suppl 6):13–19, 1998.

72. Gitlin MJ, Cochran SD, Jamison KR. Maintenance lithium treatment: side effects and compliance. J Clin Psychiatry 50:127–131, 1989.

73. Rose SR, Klein-Schwartz, Oderda GM, et al. Lithium intoxication with acute renal failure and death. Drug Intell Clin Pharm 22:691–694, 1988.

74. Sarid-Segal O, Creelman WL, Ciraulo DA, et al. In: Ciraulo DA, Shader RI, Greenblatt DJ, Creelman WL. Drug interactions in psychiatry. 2nd ed. Baltimore: Williams & Wilkins, 1995:175–213.

75. Cohen LS, Friedman JM, Jefferson JW, et al. A reevaluation of risk of in utero exposure to lithium. JAMA 271:146–150, 1994.

76. Llewellyn A, Stowe ZN, Strader JR. The use of lithium and management of women with bipolar disorder during pregnancy and lactation. J Clin Psychiatry 59 (Suppl 6):57–64, 1998.

77. McElroy SL, Keck PE, Pope HG, et al. Valproate in the treatment of bipolar disorder: literature review and clinical guidelines. J Clin Psychopharmacol 12 (Suppl 1):42S–52S, 1992.

78. Keck PE, McElroy SL, Tugrul KC, et al. Valproate oral loading in the treatment of acute mania. J Clin Psychiatry 54:305–308, 1993.

79. Keck PE, Nabulsi AA, Taylor JL, et al. A pharmacoeconomic model of divalproex vs lithium in the acute and prophylactic treatment of bipolar I disorder. J Clin Psychiatry 57:213–222, 1996.

80. Lamictal® Product information. Greenville, NC: GlaxoSmithKline, 2004.

81. Bowden CL, Calabrese JR, Sachs G, et al. A placebo-controlled 18-month trial of lamotrigine and lithium maintenance treatment in recently manic or hypomanic patients with bipolar I disorder. Arch Gen Psychiatry 60:392–400, 2003.

82. Goldsmith DR, Wagstaff AJ, IbbotsonT, et al.. Spotlight on lamotrigine in bipolar disorder. CNS Drugs 18:63–67, 2004.

83. Mack A. Examination of the evidence for off-label use of gabapentin. J Managed Care Pharm 9:559–568, 2003.

84. Obrocea GV, Dunn RM, Frye MA, et al. Clinical predictors of response to lamotrigine and gabapentin monotherapy in refractory affective disorders. Biol Psychiatry 51:253–260, 2002.

85. Symbyax[R] product information. Indianapolis, IL: Eli Lilly and Company, 2004.

86. Rifkin A, Doddi S, Karajgi B, et al. Dosage of haloperidol for mania. Br J Psychiatry 165:113–116, 1994.

87. Bowden CL. Dosing strategies and time course of response to antimanic drugs. J Clin Psychiatry 57 (Suppl 13):4–9, 1996.

88. Dunner DL. Lithium carbonate: maintenance studies and consequences of withdrawal. J Clin Psychiatry 59 (Suppl 6):48–55, 1998.

89. Tondo L, Baldessarini RJ, Hennen J, et al. Lithium maintenance treatment of depression and mania in bipolar I and bipolar II disorders. Am J Psychiatry 155:638–645, 1998.

90. Maj M, Pirozzi R, Magliano L, et al. Long-term outcome of lithium prophylaxis in bipolar disorders: a 5 year prospective study of 402 patients at a lithium clinic. Am J Psychiatry 155:30–35, 1998.

91. Stimmel GL. How to counsel patients about depression and its treatment. Pharmacotherapy 15:100S–104S, 1995.

92. Weiss RD, Greenfield SF, Najavits LM, et al. Medication compliance among patients with bipolar disorder and substance use disorder. J Clin Psychiatry 59:172–174, 1998.

93. Peet M, Harvey NS. Lithium maintenance: a standard education programme for patients. Br J Psychiatry 158:197–200, 1991.

94. Kahn DA, Ross R, Rush J, Panico S. Expert consensus treatment guidelines for bipolar disorder: a guide for patients and families. J Clin Psychiatry 57(Suppl 12A):81–88, 1996.

95. Saklad SR. Pharmacoeconomic issues in the treatment of depression. Pharmacotherapy 15:76S–83S, 1995.

96. McCombs JS, Nichol MB, Stimmel GL, et al. The cost of antidepressant drug therapy failure: a study of antidepressant use patterns in a Medicaid population. J Clin Psychiatry 51(Suppl 6):60–69, 1990.

97. Revicki DA, Brown RE, Keller MB, et al. Cost-effectiveness of newer antidepressants compared with tricyclic antidepressants in managed care settings. J Clin Psychiatry 58:47–58, 1997.

98. Sclar DA, Robison LM, Skaer TL, et al. Antidepressant pharmacotherapy: economic evaluation of fluoxetine, paroxetine, and sertraline in a health maintenance organization. J Int Med Res 23:395–412, 1995.

Schizophrenia

Mary A. Gutierrez and Glen L. Stimmel

DEFINITION

Schizophrenia is a chronic thought disorder in which characteristic psychotic symptoms are seen during the acute phase of the illness with partial or full resolution of symptoms between psychotic episodes, coupled with deterioration from a previous level of social and occupational functioning. Schizophrenia is not synonymous with psychosis. The term "psychosis" is broader, inclusive of infectious, metabolic, endocrine, and drug-induced causes for psychotic symptoms such as delusions and hallucinations. Many psychiatric and neurologic disorders also may include psychotic symptoms, such as mania, major depression, and the dementias. Schizophrenia is not a split personality, Dr. Jekyll/Mr. Hyde syndrome, or multiple personality disorder. Although patients with schizophrenia may at times be psychotic and exhibit bizarre behavior, the long-term outcome of schizophrenia varies along a continuum between recovery and total incapacity with the majority displaying exacerbations and remissions.

TREATMENT GOALS

The goals and strategies of treating a patient with schizophrenia vary according to the phase and severity of illness. In the acute phase, the goal is to reduce or eliminate psychotic symptoms and improve functioning. During stabilization, the goal is to provide support to decrease the risk of relapse, increase the patient's adaptation to life in the community, and consolidate remission of symptoms. In the stable phase, the goal is to ensure that the patient maintains and improves his or her level of functioning and quality of life, and to treat any reemerging psychotic symptoms, while adverse-effect monitoring and management continues.[1]

EPIDEMIOLOGY

Schizophrenia affects an estimated 1% of the U.S. population with about 300,000 acute episodes occurring annually. The prevalence rate appears to be very constant across different countries and cultures. The age of onset typically occurs between the late teens and mid-30s, with males and females affected in roughly equal numbers. A later age of onset is more common in females, and is associated with less cognitive impairment and better outcome. Both genetic and environmental factors are important in the etiology of schizophrenia. Whereas the risk in the general population is about 1%, the risk for first-degree relatives is 10%. Substantial discordance rates in monozygotic twin studies (only 40%–50% risk) indicate that environmental factors are also important.[2]

PATHOPHYSIOLOGY

Schizophrenia is best viewed as a syndrome with a large continuum of pathophysiologic disruptions. The older hypothesis of overactive dopaminergic pathways is much too simplistic to explain schizophrenia. Thus far, the pathophysiology of dopaminergic and serotonergic systems is best understood. Overactivity of mesolimbic and mesocortical dopaminergic pathways to the temporolimbic region and frontal cortex are believed to explain the positive symptoms of schizophrenia, whereas the relative lack of dopaminergic function in the prefrontal cortex has been suggested to explain the negative symptoms of schizophrenia. Much of this work is based on an understanding of the mechanisms of action of antipsychotic drugs and their relative efficacy for specific symptoms. Dopamine blockade is associated with efficacy for positive symptoms. Serotonergic blockade enhances dopaminergic activity in the prefrontal cortex to decrease negative symptoms. Furthermore, dopaminergic systems can be modulated by a variety of other systems (adrenergic, cholinergic, and peptidergic). Although the clinical effects of drugs with well-known neurotransmitter mechanisms is evident, understanding the exact pathophysiology of schizophrenia remains indirect and undetermined.[3,4]

CLINICAL PRESENTATION AND DIAGNOSIS

SIGNS AND SYMPTOMS

Symptoms are classified as positive (excess or distortion of normal function) or negative (diminution or loss of normal function), correlating with differences in pathophysiology and responsiveness to drug therapy (Table 54.1).[2,5] The positive symptoms are most likely to lead to hospitalization and family disruption, but the negative symptoms interfere with patients being able to have close friends, maintain employment, relate to their families, and become integrated into their community. Negative symptoms contribute the most to the morbidity and economic costs of schizophrenia.

Positive Symptoms. A disturbance in perception is termed a hallucination in which one has a sensory awareness

TABLE 54.1	Symptoms of Schizophrenia

Positive Symptoms (distorted functions)
  hallucinations (e.g., hearing voices, seeing things)
  delusions (fixed false belief not shared by culture)
  disorganized speech, thought, language
  disorganized bizarre behavior
Negative Symptoms (diminished functions)
  alogia (decreased fluency of thought or speech)
  affective blunting of emotional expression
  avolition (lack of drive, motivation)
  anhedonia/asociality (decreased ability to feel pleasure/ form relationships)
  attention impairment (decreased ability to focus attention)

in the absence of an external stimulus. The most common example is an auditory hallucination in which voices or noises are perceived as coming from outside one's head when in fact no voices are present. Visual and tactile hallucinations are possible in schizophrenia, but are more characteristic of drug-induced psychoses. Delusions represent the most common disturbance in thought content, defined as a fixed-false belief. Delusions can vary in theme and content but are typically bizarre or terrifying. Persecutory or paranoid delusions are most common, in which the person believes he or she is being followed, spied on, or tormented. Referential delusions are also common, in which a person believes song lyrics, another's gesture, or television reports are specifically directed at him or her. A belief that one's thoughts are being inserted or withdrawn by an outside force, one's thoughts are being broadcast aloud, or one's body or actions are being controlled by an outside force are additional common delusions. False beliefs or concerns that are not firmly held are termed ideation (e.g., paranoid ideation, ideas of reference). Disorganized thinking and speech is described as ''loose associations'' or ''derailment'' in which the patient may shift from one topic to another with no awareness that the topics are unrelated. More severe thought disorder can be manifest as ''word salad'' in which unrelated words or phrases are strung together in speech. ''Concrete thinking'' is the loss of an ability to think in abstract terms. Bizarre behavior may be manifest as disheveled or unusual dress or grooming, poor hygiene, inappropriate sexual behavior, and odd mannerisms.

Negative Symptoms. Alogia, or poverty of speech, is manifest by very brief empty responses to questions related to a lack of thoughts, not a resistance to speak. Affective blunting is typically described as constricted affect, or at its worst, flat affect. There is an unchanging facial expression, decreased spontaneous movements, poverty of gestures, poor eye contact, and lack of vocal inflection. These symptoms may be interpreted by family as apathy, laziness, or indifference, and must also be distinguished from drug-induced pseudoparkinsonism and depressed mood. Avolition, or the lack of self-initiated goal-directed activity, directly interferes with psychosocial training programs and the potential for adequate social and occupational functioning.

DIAGNOSIS

In addition to the presence of the characteristic symptoms described above, the diagnosis of schizophrenia requires continuous signs of the disturbance for at least 6 months with at least 1 month of active symptoms, plus a marked decline in social or occupational functioning. Diagnostic criteria require two or more of the following symptoms during the 1 month of active symptoms: delusions, hallucinations, disorganized speech, grossly disorganized behavior, and negative symptoms. When all criteria are met except symptoms have been present for only 1 to 6 months, a diagnosis of schizophreniform disorder is given. Acute onset of psychotic symptoms lasting less than 1 month is termed brief psychotic disorder. Schizoaffective disorder is a distinct and separate psychotic mood disorder that meets diagnostic criteria for schizophrenia and a manic episode or major depressive episode. Although many acutely psychotic patients will often exhibit some mood disturbance, on follow-up, most will be found to have schizophrenia or a primary mood disorder. Schizoaffective disorder is a diagnosis that must be validated over time, because precision in diagnosis is needed to ensure patients receive the most appropriate pharmacotherapy for their disorder.[2]

THERAPEUTIC PLAN

The American Psychiatric Association (APA) published practice guidelines for schizophrenia in 1997,[1] with the second edition published as continuing medical education in their web site in 2004.[5] In the 7 years between the two editions of the APA practice guidelines, the atypical antipsychotic agents have emerged as the first line treatments. This trend is also reflected in several treatment algorithms, for example, the Texas Implementation Medication Algorithms (TIMA) Antipsychotic Algorithm 2003.[6]

TREATMENT

PHARMACOTHERAPY

Once referred to as major tranquilizers, antipsychotic drugs have a selective specific effect in eliminating or at least mini-mizing psychotic symptoms. They are not supersedatives or tranquilizers, however, and are most properly called antipsychotic drugs. The newer atypical antipsychotic drugs, with minimal potential for causing extrapyramidal side effects (EPS), have led to the abandonment of the term ''neuroleptic'' to refer to antipsychotic drugs.

Available Antipsychotic Drugs. Antipsychotic drugs can be classified chemically or pharmacologically, the latter having the most clinical relevance. Table 54.2 lists commonly used drugs using a classification of low- and high-potency, typical and atypical antipsychotic drugs. This classification groups the drugs based on similar adverse effect profiles and therapeutic efficacy. The typical drugs are potent dopamine-2 receptor blockers, while the atypical drugs have less dopaminergic blockade but greater serotonin-2 receptor blockade. The low-potency typical antipsychotic agents additionally have potent antihistaminic, antimuscarinic, and α-1 adrenergic blockade, leading to increased sedation and anticholinergic and cardiovascular effects with less EPS; while the high-potency typical antipsychotic agents' primary adverse effect is EPS. In general, the typical drugs effectively treat positive symptoms while the atypicals treat positive and negative symptoms and have minimal risk for EPS.[7]

Treatment of Acute Psychotic Episode. When a patient presents to an emergency room acutely psychotic, the many medical and drug-induced causes for psychosis must first be ruled out. Assuming a patient is experiencing an

TABLE 54.2	Oral Dosage Ranges and Potency		
Drug (generic/Trade name)	Acute Dose (mg/day)	Maintenance Dose (mg/day)	Potency[a]
chlorpromazine (Thorazine)	400–1500	200–600	low
thioridazine (Mellaril)	400–800[b]	200–600	low
fluphenazine (Prolixin)	10–60	3–20	high
perphenazine (Trilafon)	8–96	8–64	high
trifluoperazine (Stelazine)	20–80	5–20	high
thiothixene (Navane)	20–80	5–30	high
haloperidol (Haldol)	10–60	3–20	high
loxapine (Loxitane)	40–225	20–100	mid
molindone (Moban)	50–400	20–100	mid
clozapine (Clozapine)	300–600	150–400	[c]
risperidone (Risperdal)	4–8	2–6	[c]
olanzapine (Zyprexa)	10–20	5–20	[c]
quetiapine (Seroquel)	300–800	300–800	[c]
ziprasidone (Geodon)	80–160	40–160	[c]
aripiprazole (Abilify)	10–30	10–15	[c]

[a] Potency of the typical antipsychotic is based on dopaminergic blockade.
[b] absolute ceiling dose of 800 mg daily due to risk of pigmentary retinopathy;
[c] potency of atypicals cannot be compared to typicals.

acute exacerbation of their schizophrenia, the degree of agitation and hostility versus psychotic symptomatology dictates the pharmacotherapy decisions. Acute agitation and hostility are best treated by talking with the patient and use of physical restraints first, then use of a benzodiazepine and/or antipsychotic drug. Benzodiazepines, such as lorazepam 2 mg orally (PO) or intramuscularly (IM) every 30 minutes for three doses, can effectively reduce agitated behavior, reducing the dosage of antipsychotic drug necessary for the psychotic symptoms, and thus reducing the potential for adverse effects. Benzodiazepines are not recommended in the elderly, brain damaged, patients intoxicated with sedative-hypnotics, or those with a history of a paradoxical reaction to benzodiazepines. The psychotic symptoms will require an antipsychotic drug, which can safely be given in combination with the benzodiazepine. High-potency antipsychotic drugs (e.g., haloperidol) are preferred, and low-potency drugs should be avoided due to their sedative and cardiovascular effects.[8] The atypical antipsychotics are also starting to have a place in the acute treatment of psychotic agitation. The PO dose of risperidone plus lorazepam was shown to be as effective as intramuscular haloperidol plus lorazepam for the rapid control of agitation and psychosis.[9] Accelerated PO dose titration of olanzapine has also been shown to be as effective as PO haloperidol in reducing acute agitation in patients with schizophrenia.[10] Prior to 2003, only the conventional agents were available in IM formulation; however, IM ziprasidone and IM olanzapine have now been approved by the Food and Drug Administration (FDA) for the treatment of acute agitation associated with schizophrenia[11] and Bipolar I mania.[12] Dosing for IM ziprasidone for acute agitation is 10 mg every 2 hours or 20 mg every 4 hours up to 40 mg daily for up to 3 days, while IM olanzapine dose ranges from 2.5 to 10 mg, with not more than three doses of 10 mg every 2 to 4 hours. The introduction of these IM atypical antipsychotics preparations provides new treatment options for acute agitation.[13]

Maintenance Therapy. Many different strategies have been evaluated to minimize the risk of relapse in patients with schizophrenia. When patients discontinue their antipsychotic drug, they are at substantial risk for relapse. The efficacy of maintenance antipsychotic drugs in preventing relapse is well established. The clinical decisions regarding maintenance dose and length of therapy involve how to minimize the risk of relapse and adverse effects while maximizing treatment adherence. Virtually all patients with schizophrenia not treated with antipsychotic medication will relapse within about 3 years.[14] Across studies, the 1-year relapse rate after drug discontinuation averages 70%, while continuous use of antipsychotic maintenance therapy reduces the relapse rate to 23%.[15] The most effective method to prevent relapse is continuous drug therapy at minimal effective maintenance doses (Table 54.2), watching for relapse factors such as medication noncompliance, stress, inadequate social support, and substance abuse.[15,16] The atypi-

cal drugs offer minimal risk of extrapyramidal effects and tardive dyskinesia (TD) with maintenance therapy, which should enhance treatment adherence. Use of depot antipsychotic drugs has also been shown to significantly decrease relapse compared to use of PO medication, though those studies did not include the newer atypical antipsychotic drugs.[14] Risperidone became the first atypical long-acting injectable formulation available in the United States in 2004.[17]

Dosing Strategies. After an effective dose is found after upward titration of dosage, most patients will benefit from once daily dosing. For sedating drugs, bedtime dosing minimizes daytime sedation and minimizes the need for an additional hypnotic drug. Once daily dosing increases medication compliance and simplifies drug regimens. Only those patients unable to tolerate the adverse effects of once daily dosing should remain on divided dosing schedules.

Depot Formulations. The use of fluphenazine decanoate (FD) or haloperidol decanoate (HD) represents a unique option for maintenance drug therapy. The advantages of these formulations is that a patient can be given an IM injection every 2 to 4 weeks rather than ingesting daily PO medication. A depot antipsychotic is indicated for patients who respond well to acute PO drug therapy but are consistently non-compliant or refuse PO medication. Depot therapy should not be used acutely, due to variable and delayed onset of effect compared to PO medication. Treatment of acute symptoms requires the flexibility of dose titration offered by PO or nondepot IM preparations. Depot therapy should be given only after the PO dose has stabilized at an effective level, and the patient can be converted to the depot formulation. Studies of relapse rates find an average difference of 15% favoring depot to PO maintenance medication. Whereas depot therapy is used in 40% to 60% of European countries, estimates in the United States are only 10% to 20% of patients.[18] FD and HD are equally effective and have virtually identical adverse effect profiles.[19] HD can be given once monthly whereas FD requires twice monthly administration. The effective dose range for FD is 12.5 to 50 mg IM every 2 weeks, and HD is 100 to 450 mg IM every month. To convert a patient from PO haloperidol, the usual monthly maintenance dose range is 10 to 15 times the PO daily dose. With HD, peak haloperidol concentrations occur between 3 to 9 days, with an apparent elimination half-life of 3 weeks, and steady-state level with multiple dosing is reached after 12 to 16 weeks.[20]

In 2004, the long-acting injectable formulation of risperidone was approved for the treatment of schizophrenia. After the initial injection of risperidone has been administered, the patient should be continued on a PO antipsychotic for at least 3 weeks. Each long-acting risperidone dose begins to release risperidone 3 weeks after injection with an initial release of less than 1% of the dose, and drug release continues for 4 to 6 weeks. Steady state is reached after 4 consecutive injections when given at 2-week intervals. Most patients will require long-acting risperidone 25 mg every 2 weeks. Some refractory patients may require an initial dose of 37.5 mg. If, after four injections, the patient remains symptomatic, a dose of 50 mg may be warranted. Higher doses are associated with increased adverse effects, such as extrapyramidal symptoms.[17]

Adverse Effects and Their Management

Extrapyramidal Side Effects. EPS represent the most common and troublesome adverse effects of antipsychotic drugs, being the primary cause of noncompliance. There are three categories of EPS: (a) acute dystonias, (b) pseudoparkinsonism, and (c) akathisia. The definitions and symptoms are listed in Table 54.3. EPS are commonly caused by the typical antipsychotic drugs with dopaminergic blocking properties, but uncommonly seen with the atypical drugs with dopaminergic and serotonergic blocking effects.[21]

TABLE 54.3 Manifestations of Extrapyramidal Effects and Tardive Dyskinesia

Dsytonic Reactions (painful spasm of a muscle or muscle group)

oculogyric crisis – fixed upward stare

torticollis – neck twisting

trismus – clenched jaw

opisthotonus – arching of back

laryngospasm – difficulty breathing, speaking, swallowing

Pseudoparkinsonism

akinesia – rigidity and immobility

stiffness and slowness of voluntary movement

mask-like facial expression

drooling (sialorrhea)

stooped posture

shuffling, festinating gait

slow, monotone speech

tremor – regular rhythmic oscillations of extremities, especially hands and feet; pill-rolling movement of fingers

Akathisia (subjective inner feeling of restlessness, anxiety plus motor restlessness)

inability to sit still, constant pacing

continuous agitation and restless movements

rocking and shifting of weight while standing

shifting of legs, tapping of feet while sitting

Tardive Dyskinesia

mouth – rhythmical involuntary movements of tongue, lips, jaw; protrusion of tongue, puckering of mouth, chewing movements

choreiform – involuntary irregular purposeless quick movements of arms/legs; jerky, flailing movements

athethoid – continuous wormlike slow movements of arms

axial hyperkinesis – to and fro clonic movements of spine

Dystonic reactions are usually seen within the first 72 hours of treatment with a dopamine blocking drug, and are most frequent in young males. High potency drugs are most likely to cause dystonia (e.g., 65% of patients given haloperidol).[22] Fortunately, dystonic reactions are usually brief, and among all EPS, are most responsive to treatment. Anticholinergic agents, such as benztropine (2 mg IM) or diphenhydramine (50 mg IM), will usually be effective within 10 to 30 minutes. Because laryngospasm can represent a medical emergency, intravenous (IV) benztropine or diphenhydramine should be used. After acute treatment of any dystonic reaction, PO benztropine should be continued with the antipsychotic drug. Controversy remains regarding automatic use of anticholinergic agents prophylactically when antipsychotic drugs are begun in an attempt to prevent EPS. A decision regarding prophylaxis should be based on the relative risk factors present for EPS. Prophylaxis is indicated when one or more of the following risk factors is present: patients with a past history of EPS (particularly if noncompliant), patients given a high potency antipsychotic drug, and young males. Use of benztropine 1 mg PO twice daily (bid) prophylactically is effective and can be tapered and discontinued after 1 to 2 months if no EPS occur.[21]

Pseudoparkinsonism, resulting from dopaminergic blockade in the striatum, mimics Parkinson disease in its symptomatology. Symptoms may develop weeks to several months after starting an antipsychotic drug. Benztropine (1–6 mg PO daily) is preferred over trihexyphenidyl (5–15 mg daily) because its longer half-life allows once daily dosing. Because EPS movements disappear during sleep, benztropine is best dosed in the morning. Amantadine (100–400 mg daily) offers a second-line choice for patients not responsive to anticholinergic drugs or who cannot tolerate their adverse effects (dry mouth, blurry near vision, constipation, urinary retention, memory impairment).[21,23]

Akathisia is the most common EPS and is least responsive to treatment. It is often difficult to distinguish akathisia from psychotic agitation, which is crucial because treatment of each is very different. Akathisia is rarely responsive to anticholinergic agents, but is best treated with propranolol (40–160 mg daily) or benzodiazepines (e.g., lorazepam 1.5–5 mg daily or clonazepam 0.5–2 mg daily).[21,24] The severity of akathisia is often greater with the depot drugs; discontinuing depot fluphenazine or haloperidol due to intolerable and untreatable akathisia and switch to an atypical antipsychotic is common.

The approximate frequency of EPS caused in patients receiving thioridazine is 10% to 15%, chlorpromazine 20% to 25%, and fluphenazine and haloperidol 40% to 50% (Table 54.4). One of the major advantages of atypical drugs is their relative lack of EPS compared to typical antipsychotic drugs. Clozapine is the least likely antipsychotic drug to cause EPS, risperidone more than clozapine but much less than the typical antipsychotic drugs.[25,26]

Tardive Dyskinesia. TD is a late appearing antipsychotic drug-induced movement disorder that looks like an EPS but

Drug	Sedation	EPS	Anti-cholinergic	Postural Hypotension	Weight Gain	Hyper prolactinemia
Haloperidol	1	5	1	1	2	5
Fluphenazine	1	5	1	1	2	5
Thiothixene	2	4	2	1	2	4
Trifluoperazine	2	4	2	1	2	4
Molindone	1	3	1	1	0	3
Loxapine	2	3	2	2	2	3
Chlorpromazine	4	2	3	4	3	3
Thioridazine	4	2	4	4	4	3
Clozapine	4	0–1	4	5	5	0–1
Risperidone	1	1–2	1	3	3	3
Olanzapine	3	1	2	1	5	1
Quetiapine	3	0–1	1	3	3	0–1
Ziprasidone	1	1	1	1	0–1	1
Aripiprazole	1	1	1	1	0–1	0–1

TABLE 54.4 | Relative Adverse Effect Profiles

1, low; 5, high.

whose etiology and treatment are very different. For most patients, the movements of TD are restricted to the mouth area, are mild, and are not bothersome. Unlike EPS, TD typically appears on antipsychotic dosage reduction or discontinuation, improves when antipsychotic dose is increased, worsens with administration of anticholinergic drugs, and may persist for months or years after antipsychotic drugs are discontinued. All typical antipsychotic drugs are capable of causing TD due to their prominent dopaminergic blockade in the striatum. Though somewhat too early to be certain, the atypical antipsychotic drugs are believed to have a much lower risk of TD due to their serotonergic effects and much less striatal dopaminergic blocking effect. The risk of persistent TD based on prospective studies in all age groups suggest 20% after 5 years of cumulative typical antipsychotic drug exposure with an incidence of about 4% per year for the first 5 years. In older populations the rate is even higher.[27] TD is believed to result from long-term blockade of striatal dopaminergic receptors with resultant hypersensitivity of those receptors. There are no drug treatment options effective for TD despite case reports and open trials of over 60 different agents. Management of a patient with TD should consist of discontinuing any anticholinergic agent, and lowering the antipsychotic dose as low as clinically possible. Because the risk of TD is significantly lower with the atypical antipsychotics,[28] patients are rationally being switched to atypical drugs to spare the striatal dopaminergic system. Because treatment is so disappointing, prevention of TD is of greatest importance. All patients given antipsychotic drugs should be regularly monitored for early signs of TD (movements on the surface of the tongue,

facial tics such as frequent blinking, and choreoathetoid finger or toe movements). The Abnormal Involuntary Movement Scale (AIMS) is the most commonly used screening tool for TD.

Anticholinergic Effects. Peripheral anticholinergic effects are commonly experienced by patients taking chlorpromazine, thioridazine, and clozapine. In addition, patients taking high potency drugs often require anticholinergic agents for EPS, so they too are often bothered by dry mouth, blurred near vision, and constipation. These effects are dose-related and additive. Anticholinergic effects can be minimized by switching to once daily bedtime dosing or by decreasing dosage when possible. Constipation can be a more serious concern if left untreated, leading to impaction and ileus. The reduction in gastrointestinal (GI) motility and secretions results in a hard, dry stool that is best treated with increasing fluid intake, diet and exercise counseling, and stool softeners. Docusate (100–500 mg daily) will usually be effective within 2 to 3 days, and treatment can be on an interrupted basis for 4 to 7 days at a time.

More serious anticholinergic effects include urinary hesitancy and retention and cognitive impairment. Either effect requires immediate dosage reduction or switch to a less anticholinergic drug regimen. These two effects are magnified in intensity and severity in patients with prostatic hypertrophy, the elderly, or patients with dementia.

Cardiovascular Effects. The most frequent cardiovascular effect caused by typical and atypical drugs is orthostatic hypotension (Table 54.4). It is dose-related, and is most prominent in the first 2 weeks of therapy or after a dose increase. After several weeks, there is usually tolerance to the subjective dizziness, while the actual postural drop in blood pressure persists. The elderly and patients taking other drugs with hypotensive effects are at most risk for orthostatic hypotensive effects. Although easily prevented with patient education, orthostatic hypotension in the uncounseled can lead to falls, fractures, and subsequent noncompliance.

Thioridazine in doses above 300 mg daily, and to a lesser extent chlorpromazine, may induce electrocardiographic (ECG) changes, T-wave abnormalities in particular. A black box warning of possible QTc (QT interval corrected for heart rate) prolongation was added to its package insert in 2000 after studies with ziprasidone and typical antipsychotics found the highest risk with thioridazine. Months later a black box warning was also given to mesoridazine due to dose-dependent prolongation of the QT interval and three published reports of ventricular tachycardia.[29] The warning for these two agents is prolongation of QTc interval reported in a dose-related manner, associated with torsades de pointes and sudden death; reserve for patients not responding to or cannot tolerate other antipsychotics.[30,31] High-potency antipsychotic drugs have the potential for ECG changes only with parenteral administration. Haloperidol and droperidol parenterally in doses over 50 mg per 24 hours should be monitored because the QT_c interval may be increased by 25% over baseline.[26,32] Droperidol injections also got the addition of the new black box warning of QTc prolongation in 2003.[33]

Neuroleptic Malignant Syndrome. Neuroleptic malignant syndrome (NMS) is an uncommon but serious adverse effect that occurs in 1% to 2% of patients receiving antipsychotic drugs. NMS is characterized by (a) fever; (b) severe EPS such as lead pipe rigidity, trismus, and other dystonias; (c) signs of autonomic instability such as tachycardia, labile hypertension, diaphoresis, and incontinence; and (d) fluctuating levels of consciousness. In the 1980s, the mortality rate was 22%, which has now dropped to less than 5% due to earlier recognition and treatment. NMS typically occurs after 3 to 9 days of antipsychotic therapy with symptoms rapidly progressing over 24 to 72 hours, persisting 5 to 10 days after the antipsychotic drug is discontinued.[34] The etiology was once thought to be due to overwhelming dopaminergic blockade effects, because most NMS cases were seen in patients receiving high doses of high-potency drugs. This has been challenged by the reports of NMS cases with clozapine, risperidone, olanzapine, and quetiapine.[35] Treatment of NMS consists of discontinuation of the antipsychotic drug, parenteral hydration, and control of fever. Only if no marked improvement is seen after 1 to 2 days, dantrolene (240–600 mg/day) and/or bromocriptine (7.5–30 mg/day) can be considered, because recovery times have been reported to be longer with drug treated cases than those receiving only supportive care.[36]

Endocrine and Sexual Function Effects. The most common endocrine effects of antipsychotic drugs include menstrual irregularities and galactorrhea in up to 30% of women, and gynecomastia in men.[37,38] These effects are due to dopaminergic blockade causing prolactin levels to increase. No specific treatment is necessary beyond assuring the patient it is a reversible benign effect. Because ovulation may continue despite irregular or missed menstrual periods, continued contraception must be encouraged. Increased prolactin levels in men and women will decrease libido. Both decreased libido and erectile dysfunction are commonly reported in men with antipsychotic drugs. The atypical antipsychotics (particularly clozapine, quetiapine, and aripiprazole) are least likely to cause elevation in prolactin levels. Ejaculatory and orgasm difficulty is also a common complaint in 30% to 40% of men, most likely due to α-adrenergic blockade effect.[38] Retrograde ejaculation, in which semen flows backward into the bladder on ejaculation, is most often reported with thioridazine due to its α-adrenergic blockade.

The potential increased risk of hyperglycemia and worsening of glucose control with diabetes mellitus is the latest endocrine concern that caused the FDA to request all manufacturers of the atypical antipsychotic medications to add warning statements to drug labeling. All patients should be monitored for fasting blood sugar for diabetic risk. Although all the atypical antipsychotics have the potential for increased glucose, the most reports have been associated with clozapine and olanzapine.[39]

Seizures. Clozapine is the most likely antipsychotic drug to cause a seizure, followed by chlorpromazine, with haloperidol least likely.[40] Seizures are dose related, being more likely with rapid rate of upward dose titration and higher doses. With usual doses, seizures with antipsychotic drugs except clozapine occur in less than 0.5% of patients. Seizures occur in 1% to 2% of patients given clozapine in doses below 300 mg daily, but reach 5% when doses exceed 600 mg daily.[41]

Weight Gain. With the exception of molindone, all antipsychotic drugs may cause weight gain of as much as 5% to 15% of body weight. Clozapine and olanzapine are associated with the most weight gain, followed by quetiapine and risperidone. Ziprasidone and aripiprazole have the least potential for causing weight gain. Long-term studies report weight gain averages of about 7 kg for clozapine and olanzapine, 2 to 3 kg for risperidone, and 3 to 5 kg for quetiapine over 12 months. The exact mechanism of weight gain is unknown, but involves antihistaminic and serotonergic blockade effects. Molindone is unique in having a central anorexigenic effect via serotonin agonist activity coupled with its low affinity for histamine receptors. No effective treatment for weight gain has been identified beyond nutrition counseling, exercise, and dietary modification.[42]

Hyperlipidemia. Atypical antipsychotics, particularly clozapine and olanzapine, and less frequently with quetiapine and risperidone, are associated with elevated triglycerides.[39] Ziprasidone and aripiprazole are not associated with increased triglycerides to date. It is recommended that lipid panels should be obtained at baseline and routinely while a patient is on an atypical agent.

Drug Interactions. Most all drug interactions with antipsychotic drugs are predictable based on known pharmacologic and pharmacokinetic information. Common drug interactions include additive sedative, hypotensive, and anticholinergic effects. For example, alcohol will enhance the sedative and hypotensive effects of chlorpromazine and clozapine. All antipsychotics are extensively hepatically metabolized through microsomal oxidation and conjugation reactions, making them susceptible to enzyme inducers and inhibitors. The major cytochrome P-450 (CYP-450) enzyme(s) responsible for metabolism of antipsychotic drugs are clozapine 1A2, phenothiazines 2D6 and 1A2, haloperidol 1A2 and 2D6 (minor), risperidone 2D6, olanzapine 1A2, quetiapine 3A4, and aripiprazole 2D6 and 3A4. Clinicians should watch for altered effects when used with enzyme inducers and inhibitors. Cigarette smoking has been shown to increase clearance of many antipsychotic drugs metabolized by 1A2 isoenzymes by 50% to 150%.[3]

Unique Features of Atypical Antipsychotic Drugs. The atypical antipsychotic drugs as a group offer major advantages to patients compared to the typical antipsychotic drugs. The atypical drugs only infrequently cause EPS, should carry a much lower risk of TD, offer unique efficacy for negative symptoms and cognitive dysfunction, provide efficacy for some patients whose positive symptoms are refractory to typical antipsychotics, have shown cost-effectiveness for total cost of care despite their higher drug cost, and have very different and complex receptor binding profiles. These differences revolutionized the treatment of schizophrenia in the mid-1990s, with atypicals virtually replacing the typical drugs except for those patients already stabilized and doing well on the typical drugs and for treatment of agitated acute psychotic episodes.[43,44]

It has been more recently recognized that cognitive dysfunction may be a core symptom of schizophrenia for some patients, and that the degree of cognitive impairment predicts outcome better than other symptoms. It has long been recognized that anticholinergic agents (e.g., benztropine) have a profound negative effect on learning and memory functions. EPS from high-potency drugs means patients must often be given doses of anticholinergic drugs that will impair cognition. Likewise, the low potency drugs, along with clozapine and to a lesser extent olanzapine, have potent anticholinergic effects that may also impair learning and memory functions. Quetiapine, ziprasidone, and aripiprazole offer a low risk of EPS coupled with the least inherent anticholinergic effects.

Clozapine. Clozapine was the first marketed atypical antipsychotic offering major advantages but unique and serious adverse effects as well. Its unique efficacy for treatment-resistant patients and negative symptoms, and rarely causing EPS is related to its greater affinity to block serotonergic and dopamine-4 receptors than dopamine-2 receptors.[45] Frequent adverse effects include sedation, orthostatic hypotension, anticholinergic effects, and excessive salivation. Persistent sedation and prominent weight gain complicate long-term therapy. Seizures, as discussed above, are dose related and are 5 to 10 times more likely to occur than with other antipsychotic drugs. Agranulocytosis is the major adverse effect of concern, occurring in 0.4% to 2% of patients. Clozapine agranulocytosis is characterized by a white blood cell (WBC) count of less than 2,000 cells/mm³, a polymorphonuclear leukocyte count of less than 500 cells/mm³, and relative lymphopenia. WBC monitoring is a mandatory component of treatment, and despite weekly monitoring, 12 deaths (3.1% of cases) have been reported due to complications of clozapine agranulocytosis.[46] Early presenting symptoms of agranulocytosis include lethargy, weakness, fever, and sore throat. Because most cases occur within the first 6 months of therapy, weekly WBC monitoring is required for 6 months, then biweekly thereafter. If the WBC count falls below 3,000/mm³ or the absolute neutrophil count (ANC) is below 1,500/mm³, clozapine therapy should be immediately interrupted, and never rechallenged if the WBC falls below 2,000/mm³ and ANC less than 1,000/mm³. Initial dosing of clozapine must be very low and titrated upward slowly due to its significant adverse effect profile: 12.5 to 25 mg daily increased by 25 to 50 mg daily over 2 weeks. Most patients who respond will require 200 to 400 mg daily, though doses up to 900 mg daily may be necessary, especially for smokers.[41,47] An adequate trial with clozapine should be at least 8 weeks with plasma trough level above 350 to 400 ng per milliliter.[48] Because several other atypical antipsychotic drugs are now available offering the benefits of efficacy for negative symptoms and rare EPS without the concern of seizures and agranulocytosis, clozapine is now reserved only for the most treatment-resistant patients. Recently clozapine has also received an FDA indication for reducing the risk of recurrent suicidal behavior for patients with schizophrenia or schizoaffective disorders.[49]

Risperidone. Risperidone is a potent serotonin-2 (5-HT-2) receptor blocking agent with weaker but dose-dependent dopamine-2 (D-2) blockade. This mechanism supports its efficacy for negative symptoms and a lower risk of causing EPS.[50] The effective dose range for most patients is 2 to 6 mg daily. Risperidone is usually mildly sedating for most patients, and may be given at divided during the day or at bedtime. Common adverse effects include anxiety, somnolence, and EPS. Risk of EPS is dose-related (rare at 1–2 mg/day), but increasing as the dose exceeds 6 mg per day.[51] Risperidone is also available as a 1 mg per milliliter PO solution, an orally disintegrating tablet, and a long-acting, injectable formulation.

Olanzapine. Olanzapine is a serotonin and dopamine receptor antagonist with receptor effects similar to clozapine. It is effective for negative symptoms of schizophrenia, EPS are rare, and seizures and blood dyscrasias have not been reported. Common adverse effects include sedation and weight gain. Orthostatic hypotensive and anticholinergic effects are possible. Over several months of therapy, 56% of patients will gain more than 7% of their baseline weight. The initial dose is 5 or 10 mg once daily at bedtime. Efficacy in schizophrenia was demonstrated in a dose range of 10 to 15 mg per day in clinical trials.[52,53] However, doses above 20 mg per day are sometimes used in clinical practice, especially in smokers due to altered metabolism. Olanzapine is also available as an orally disintegrating tablet.

Quetiapine. Among the four atypical antipsychotic drugs discussed, quetiapine has the least affinity for dopamine receptors and thus should be least likely to cause EPS and elevations in prolactin levels. Its metabolism relies primarily on CYP 3A4, and can be affected by 3A4 inducers and inhibitors. Common adverse effects include sedation, orthostatic hypotension, and weight gain. Initial dose is 25 mg bid, increasing by 25 to 50 mg every 1 to 2 days up to a target range of 300 to 800 mg per day in a bid schedule.[54,55]

Ziprasidone. Ziprasidone acts as an antagonist at the D2, 5HT2A, and 5HT1D receptors, and as an agonist at the 5HT1A receptor. Ziprasidone also inhibits synaptic reuptake of serotonin and norepinephrine. Administration with food is recommended because absorption of ziprasidone is increased up to twofold in the presence of food. Less than one third of ziprasidone metabolic clearance is mediated by CYP 3A4 isenzymes, and approximately two thirds via reduction by aldehyde oxidase. Usual doses used are 40 to 160 mg per day on a bid schedule. Ziprasidone is also available as ziprasidone mesylate for intramuscular injection. In premarketing trials with ziprasidone, about 5% of patients developed rash and/or urticaria with discontinuation of treatment in about one sixth of these cases. Other common adverse effects reported with ziprasidone during these clinical trials were somnolence, extrapyramidal side effects (EPSEs), and respiratory disorder. Interestingly, most of the common side effects seen with the atypical antipsychotics, for example, weight gain and metabolic adverse drug reactions (ADRs) are minimal for ziprasidone. However, ziprasidone should be avoided in patients with histories of significant cardiovascular illness, (e.g., QT prolongation, recent acute myocardial infarction, or uncompensated heart failure). Ziprasidone should be discontinued in patients who are found to have persistent QTc measurements >500 ms. Patients should report any dizziness, palpitations, or syncope.[11]

Aripiprazole. Aripiprazole functions as a partial agonist at the D2 and the 5HT1A receptors, and as an antagonist at 5HT2A receptors. It has been proposed that the efficacy of aripiprazole is mediated through a combination of partial agonist activity at D2 and 5HT1A receptors and antagonist activity at 5HT2A receptors. Its metabolism is via the 3A4 and CYP 2D6 isoenzymes. Aripiprazole was effective in a dose range of 10 to 30 mg per day in acute clinical trials with the usual dose at 10 to 15 mg daily. Doses have to be reduced by half with concurrent use of 2D6 and 3A4 indu-

cers, and the doses have to be doubled to 20 to 30 mg when used with enzyme inhibitors. Common adverse effects reported with aripiprazole in clinical trials were headache, asthenia, constipation, anxiety, insomnia, lightheadedness, somnolence, akathisia, and rash.[12,56] The true incidence of ADRs will become clear with increased use and experience with this newest agent.

NONPHARMACOLOGIC THERAPY

Although antipsychotic drugs can eliminate or minimize psychotic symptoms, psychological, vocational, and social therapies are necessary to facilitate day-to-day coping skills and improve the long-term outcome of patients with schizophrenia. Prior to the availability of atypical antipsychotics, many patients remained socially isolated and dysfunctional due to their negative symptoms. Now that positive and negative symptoms can often be successfully treated, psychosocial treatment programs are even more necessary to assist patients in achieving their full social and occupational potential. If a patient with schizophrenia only receives medication, their treatment is inadequate.

PATIENT EDUCATION TO IMPROVE PATIENT ADHERENCE TO DRUG THERAPY

A principal reason to counsel patients taking antipsychotic drugs is to increase the likelihood of their compliance with maintenance therapy. The prevalence of medication noncompliance among patients with schizophrenia is 50% 1 year after discharge and 75% at 2 years. The factors most responsible for noncompliance with antipsychotic drugs include adverse effects (especially EPS), forgetfulness and cognitive deficits of schizophrenia, lack of insight, denial of illness, complexity of the drug regimen, and unsupportive family beliefs.[57] Patient and family education about the illness and appropriate expectations regarding treatment response, coupled with adequate monitoring and management of adverse effects can increase compliance and outcome.[58,59] It is critical for patients and family members to understand that antipsychotic drugs are primarily useful in preventing return of symptoms, so maintenance therapy is necessary after symptoms are gone. Support groups such as the National Alliance for the Mentally Ill (NAMI), with numerous local chapters, are very effective sources of information about schizophrenia for family members. Antipsychotic drugs are best described to patients and family members as medicine for "thinking," useful in treating such symptoms as hearing voices, confused or frightening thoughts, or fears of being around other people. After mentioning some positive aspects of the medication, then common adverse effects should be mentioned along with what to do if one occurs. Merely listing the possible adverse effects alone may scare the patient and provides no help in their knowing what to do about adverse effects that do occur. Table 54.4 suggests which adverse effects should be mentioned in counseling. For example, haloperidol counseling should focus on EPS (''muscle side effects''), whereas quetiapine counseling should focus on initial orthostatic hypotension and sedation.

PHARMACOECONOMICS

A survey in the United Kingdom found that 75% of the cost of treating schizophrenia was hospital-based and community-based care, whereas only 5% was drug cost, and 97% of the total direct cost of treating schizophrenia is incurred by less than half the patients.[60] Use of drug treatment, though initially expensive, which can successfully treat this subgroup of patients and reduce total cost of care will be a rational and cost-effective decision. Cost-effective studies with clozapine and risperidone have shown their higher drug costs are easily offset after 1 to 2 years due to a decreased rate of rehospitalization or less time spent in hospital.[61] An unknown cost factor involving improved outcome with atypical antipsychotic drugs, however, is the fact that as more patients' negative symptoms are successfully treated, there will be an increased need for psychosocial treatment programs to build or restore social and occupational skills.

ALTERNATIVE THERAPIES

For such significant psychotic disorders as schizophrenia, there are no alternative therapies or herbal remedies.

FUTURE THERAPIES

The success of the first few atypical antipsychotic drugs is leading to the development of additional antipsychotic drugs with complex mechanisms involving many neurotransmitter systems. Strategies to treat schizophrenia include the development of dopamine antagonists with high selectivity for different subtypes of dopamine receptors, dopamine partial agonists, antagonists at different serotonin receptor subtypes, drugs with mixed pharmacological profiles, supplementation with glutamatergic agents, and drugs which modify transmission via amino acids or peptides in the brain.[62]

KEY POINTS

- Schizophrenia is a chronic disorder requiring maintenance treatment to prevent relapse
- Atypical antipsychotics have revolutionized the treatment of schizophrenia in the mid-1990s, and negative symptoms can be effectively treated, EPS is a rare effect, and approximately 50% of previously treatment-

resistant patients hospitalized for decades can now be successfully treated and discharged to the community
- Clozapine opened the door to this new era, but its use is severely limited due to the risk of agranulocytosis and seizures
- Risperidone, olanzapine, quetiapine, ziprasidone, and aripiprazole represent the beginning of a new generation of atypical drugs which have become the first-line treatment for schizophrenia
- Effective treatment of negative symptoms has allowed many more patients to be able to benefit from occupational and psychosocial skills training programs
- Prudent use of a combination of a benzodiazepine with an antipsychotic drug is preferred over high-dose antipsychotic drug therapy when treating acute episodes
- Without maintenance medication, 70% of patients will relapse within 1 year
- Use of depot antipsychotic drugs is underutilized in the United States despite the fact that use of depot formulations lowers the relapse rate when compared to PO medication
- EPS and TD represent the most common and serious adverse effects from typical antipsychotic drugs, and are the primary cause of noncompliance with their treatment
- Weight gain is the most troublesome long-term adverse effect, and hyperglycemia and worsening of glucose control in diabetes mellitus is of most concern with some atypical antipsychotic drugs

SUGGESTED READINGS

Herz MI, Liberman RP, Lieberman JA, et al. APA practice guideline for the treatment of patients with schizophrenia. Am J Psychiatry 154 (Suppl 4):1–63, 1997.

Miller AL, Hall CS, Buchanan RW, et al. The Texas Medication Algorithm Project antipsychotic algorithm for schizophrenia: 2003 update. J Clin Psychiatry 65:500–508, 2004.

Stahl SM. Psychosis and schizophrenia. In: Stahl SM. Essential psychopharmacology of antipsychotics and mood stabilizers. Cambridge: Cambridge University Press, 2002:1–37.

REFERENCES

1. Herz MI, Liberman RP, Lieberman JA, et al. APA Practice guideline for the treatment of patients with schizophrenia. Am J Psychiatry 154 (Suppl 4):1–63, 1997.
2. American Psychiatric Association: Diagnostic and statistical manual of mental disorders. 4th ed. Text Revision. Washington DC: American Psychiatric Association, 2000:297–343.
3. Stahl SM. Psychosis and schizophrenia. In Stahl SM: Essential psychopharmacology of antipsychotics and mood stabilizers. Cambridge: Cambridge University Press, 2002:1–37.
4. Buchanan RW, Brandes M, Breier A. Treating negative symptoms: pharmacological strategies. In: Breier A. The new pharmacotherapy of schizophrenia. Washington DC: American Psychiatric Press, 1996:179–204.
5. Available at: http://www.psych.org/psych_pract/treatg/pg/SchizPG-Complete-Feb04.pdf. Accessed Sept. 4, 2004.

6. Miller AL, Hall CS, Buchanan RW, et al. The Texas Medication Algorithm Project antipsychotic algorithm for schizophrenia: 2003 update. J Clin Psychiatry 65:500–508, 2004.
7. Zavodnick S. A pharmacological and theoretical comparison of high and low potency neuroleptics. J Clin Psychiatry 39:332–336, 1978.
8. Hillard JR. Emergency treatment of acute psychosis. J Clin Psychiatry 59 (Suppl 1):57–60, 1998.
9. Currier GW, Chou JC, Feifel D, et al. Acute treatment of psychotic agitation: a randomized comparison of PO treatment with risperidone and lorazepam versus intramuscular treatment with haloperidol and lorazepam. J Clin Psychiatry 65:386–394, 2004.
10. Kinon BJ, Ahl J, Rotelli MD, et al. Efficacy of accelerated dose titration of olanzapine with adjunctive lorazepam to treat acute agitation in schizophrenia. Am J Emerg Med 22:181–186, 2004.
11. Geodon®. Product information. New York, NY: Pfizer Inc., 2003.
12. Zyprexa®. Product information. Indianapolis, IN: Eli Lilly and Company, 2004.
13. Citrome L. Atypical antipsychotics for acute agitation. New intramuscular options offer advantages. Postgrad Med 112:85–96, 2002.
14. Davis JM, Kane JM, Marder SR, et al. Dose response of prophylactic antipsychotics. J Clin Psychiatry 54 (Suppl 3):24–30, 1993.
15. Carpenter WT. Maintenance therapy of persons with schizophrenia. J Clin Psychiatry 57 (Suppl 9):10–18, 1996.
16. Bergen J, Hunt G, Armitage P, et al. Six-month outcome following a relapse of schizophrenia. Aust N Z J Psychiatry 32:815–22, 1998.
17. Risperdal® Consta. Product information. Titusville, NJ: Jassen Pharmaceutical Ltd., 2004.
18. Glazer WM, Kane JM. Depot neuroleptic therapy: an underutilized option. J Clin Psychiatry 53:426–433, 1992.
19. Chouinard G, Annable L, Campbell W. A randomized clinical trial of haloperidol decanoate and fluphenazine decanoate in the outpatient treatment of schizophrenia. J Clin Psychopharmacol 9:247–253, 1989.
20. Ereshefsky L, Toney G, Saklad SR, et al. A loading-dose strategy for converting from oral to depot haloperidol. Hosp Community Psychiatry 44:1155–1161, 1993.
21. Holloman LC, Marder SR. Management of acute extrapyramidal effects induced by antipsychotic drugs. Am J Health-Syst Pharm 54:2461–2477, 1997.
22. Remington GJ, Voineskos G, Pollock B, et al. Prevalence of neuroleptic-induced dystonia in mania and schizophrenia. Am J Psychiatry 147:1231–1233, 1990.
23. Tonda ME, Guthrie SK. Treatment of acute neuroleptic-induced movement disorders. Pharmacotherapy 14:543–560, 1994.
24. Sachdev P, Kruk J. Clinical characteristics and predisposing factors in acute drug-induced akathisia. Arch Gen Psychiatry 51:963–974, 1994.
25. Miller CH, Mohr R, Umbricht D, et al. The prevalence of acute extrapyramidal signs and symptoms in patients treated with clozapine, risperidone, and conventional antipsychotics. J Clin Psychiatry 59:69–75, 1998.
26. Leucht S, Pitschel-Walz G, Abraham D, et al. Efficacy and extrapyramidal side effects of the new antipsychotics olanzapine, quetiapine, risperidone, and sertindole compared to conventional antipsychotics and placebo. A meta-analysis of randomized controlled trials. Schizophr Res 35:51–68, 1999.
27. Morgenstern H, Glazer WM. Identifying risk factors for tardive dyskinesia among long-term outpatients maintained with neuroleptic medications. Arch Gen Psychiatry 50:723–773, 1993.
28. Dolder CR, Jeste DV. Incidence of tardive dyskinesia with typical versus atypical antipsychotics in very high risk patients. Biol Psychiatry 53:1142–1145, 2003.
29. Glassman AH, Bigger JT. Antipsychotic drugs: prolonged QTc interval, torsades de pointes, and sudden death. Am J Psychiatry 158:1774–1782, 2001.
30. Mellaril®. Product information, East Hanover, NJ: Norvartis Pharmaceutical Corporation, 2000.
31. Serentil®. Product information, East Hanover, NJ: Norvartis Pharmaceutical Corporation, 2000.
32. Lawrence KR, Nasraway SA. Conduction disturbances associated with administration of butyrophenone antipsychotics in the critically ill: a review of the literature. Pharmacotherapy 17:531–537, 1997.
33. Inapsine®. Product information. Buffalo Grove, IL: Akorn Pharmaceuticals Ltd, 2001.
34. Gurrera RJ, Chang SS, Romero JA. A comparison of diagnostic criteria for neuroleptic malignant syndrome. J Clin Psychiatry 53:56–62, 1992.
35. Ananth J, Parameswaran S, Gunatilake S, et al. Neuroleptic malignant syndrome and atypical antipsychotic drugs. J Clin Psychiatry 65:464–470, 2004.
36. Gelenberg AJ. The best treatment for NMS is: (A) dantrolene (B) bromocriptine (C) the combination (D) none of the above. Biol Ther Psychiatry News 15:13,16, 1992.
37. Zito JM, Sofair JB, Jaeger J. Self-reported neuroendocrine effects of antipsychotics in women: a pilot study. DICP Ann Pharmacother 24:176–180, 1990.
38. Segraves RT. The effects of minor tranquilizers, mood stabilizers, and antipsychotics on sexual function. Prim Psychiatry 4:46–48, 1997.
39. Wirshing DA, Boyd JA, Meng LR, et al. The effects of novel antipsychotics on glucose and lipid levels. J Clin Psychiatry 63:856–865, 2002.
40. Stimmel GL, Dopheide JA. Psychotropic drug-induced reductions in seizure threshold. CNS Drugs 1:37–50, 1996.
41. Lieberman JA. Maximizing clozapine therapy: managing side effects. J Clin Psychiatry 59 (Suppl 3):38–43, 1998.
42. Wirshing DA, Pierre JM, Erhart SM, et al. Understanding the new and evolving profile of adverse drug effects in schizophrenia. Psychiatr Clin North Am 26:165–190, 2003.
43. Stahl SM. Awakening from schizophrenia: intramolecular polypharmacy and the atypical antipsychotics. J Clin Psychiatry 58:381–382, 1997.
44. Lieberman JA. Understanding the mechanism of action of atypical antipsychotic drugs. Br J Psychiatry 163 (Suppl 22):7–18, 1993.
45. Meltzer HY. An overview of the mechanism of action of clozapine. J Clin Psychiatry 55 (Suppl 9B):47–52, 1994.
46. Honigfeld G, Arellano F, Sethi J, et al. Reducing clozapine-related morbidity and mortality: 5 years of experience with the Clozaril national registry. J Clin Psychiatry 59 (Suppl 3):3–7, 1998.
47. Conley RR. Optimizing treatment with clozapine. J Clin Psychiatry 59 (Suppl 3):44–48, 1998.
48. Schulte P. What is an adequate trial with clozapine? Therapeutic drug monitoring and time to response in treatment-refractory schizophrenia. Clin Pharmacokinet 42:607–618, 2003.
49. Clozaril®. Product information. East Hanover, NJ: Norvartis Pharmaceuticals Corporation, 2003.
50. Cohen LJ. Risperidone. Pharmacotherapy 14:253–265, 1994.
51. Curtis VA, Kerwin RW. A risk-benefit assessment of risperidone in schizophrenia. Drug Saf 12:139–145, 1995.
52. Bever KA, Perry PJ. Olanzapine: a serotonin-dopamine receptor antagonist for antipsychotic therapy. Am J Health-Syst Pharm 55:1003–1016, 1998.
53. Nemeroff CB. Dosing the antipsychotic medication olanzapine. J Clin Psychiatry 58 (Suppl 10):45–49, 1997.
54. Casey DE. Seroquel (quetiapine): preclinical and clinical findings of a new atypical antipsychotic. Exp Opin Invest Drugs 5:939–957, 1996.
55. Small JG, Hirsch SR, Arvanitis LA, et al. Quetiapine in patients with schizophrenia. Arch Gen Psychiatry 54:549–557, 1997.
56. Marder SR, McQuade RD, Stock E, et al. Aripiprazole in the treatment of schizophrenia: safety and tolerability in short-term, placebo-controlled trials. Schizophr Res 61:123–136, 2003.
57. Marder SR. Facilitating compliance with antipsychotic medication. J Clin Psychiatry 59 (Suppl 3):21–25, 1998.
58. Kemp R, Kirov G, Everitt B, et al. Randomised controlled trial of compliance therapy. Br J Psychiatry 172:413–419, 1998.
59. Fleischhacker WW, Meise U, Gunther V, et al. Compliance with antipsychotic drug treatment: influence of side effects. Acta Psychiatr Scand 89 (Suppl 382):11–15, 1994.
60. Davies LM, Drummond MF. Economics and schizophrenia: the real cost. Br J Psychiatry 165 (Suppl 25):18–21, 1994.
61. Hargreaves WA, Shumway M. Pharmacoeconomics of antipsychotic drug therapy. J Clin Psychiatry 57 (Suppl 9):66–76, 1996.
62. Fleischhacker WW. New developments in the pharmacotherapy of schizophrenia. J Neural Transm 64 (Suppl):105–17, 2003.

Sleep Disorders

55

Michael Z. Wincor

DEFINITION

On average, we spend one third of our lives sleeping, yet many of us take this psychophysiologic phenomenon for granted. Only when it becomes disturbed, do we pay some attention to it; even then, we probably heed the warnings of daytime fatigue less than we should, resulting in decreased productivity and increased accidents, work-related injuries, and medical errors.[1,2] We do not know why, but we definitely need to sleep, and the exact sleep need varies a great deal among individuals. It has been found in various national surveys that during the course of a year, 30% to 40% of members of the adult population have some complaint concerning sleep.[3–5] Up to 15% of the population experience a sleep problem as serious or chronic. Serious insomniacs tend to be older women with high levels of psychic distress and somatic anxiety, as well as multiple health problems. Between 2% and 4% of those surveyed use hypnotics or other psychotherapeutic agents to promote sleep. The vast majority of hypnotic users take these drugs for short periods (1 day to 2 weeks); only 11% (0.3% of all adults) report using the drugs regularly for a year or longer.[6] An additional 3% to 4% use nonprescription sleep aids. However, a small survey of community pharmacists indicated little involvement in counseling patients about over-the-counter sleep aids.[7] Although insomnia and daytime sleepiness are two of the most common human complaints, most seriously insomniac persons (85%) are untreated by prescription or nonprescription hypnotics. With a fundamental understanding of sleep disorders, the clinician can make an important contribution not only in encouraging patients to seek proper evaluation, but also in educating patients about prescription medications and nonpharmacologic treatment approaches, and advising them on selection of over-the-counter sleep aids as well.

TREATMENT GOALS

- Treat patients with any of the sleep disorders by normalizing sleep and, perhaps more important, improving daytime functioning and preventing the adverse consequences of disturbed sleep.
- Give any sleep complaint the same meticulous attention as that afforded a complaint of chest pain, flank pain, or coughing up blood.
- When you are assessing the sleep complaint, make a distinction between excessive daytime sleepiness, insomnia, and phenomena associated with specific sleep stages or sleep–wake transitions.
- For excessive daytime sleepiness, consider obstructive sleep apnea and narcolepsy, as well as self-imposed sleep deprivation.

- Avoid all central nervous system (CNS) depressants in the management of sleep apnea.
- For pharmacologic treatment of patients with narcolepsy, focus on the excessive daytime sleepiness (e.g., CNS stimulants, modafinil) and the cataplexy [e.g., protriptyline, selective serotonin reuptake inhibitors (SSRIs), sodium oxybate].
- For insomnia, distinguish between short-term and chronic types and identify the cause; both drug (e.g., CNS stimulants, CNS depressant withdrawal, ethanol) and nondrug factors (e.g., psychiatric disorders, medical disorders, circadian rhythm disorders, poor sleep hygiene) must be considered.
- If a treatable cause of insomnia is identified (e.g., major depression), give specific treatment that is appropriate for that problem (e.g., antidepressant).
- Aim for improved sleep and improved daytime functioning in the treatment of patients with insomnia; consider nondrug approaches (e.g., improved sleep hygiene).
- In general, treat patients with short-term, not persistent, insomnia with hypnotics. Drugs of choice are the benzodiazepines (BZDs) (e.g., flurazepam, temazepam, triazolam, quazepam, estazolam) and the BZD_1 receptor–specific nonbenzodiazepines (e.g., zolpidem, zaleplon, eszopiclone); selection of an agent is based on differences in pharmacokinetic profiles and the needs of the individual patient.
- Use antihistamines (e.g., hydroxyzine, diphenhydramine, doxylamine) for mild, short-term insomnia, with due caution in light of their strong anticholinergic properties and high incidence of "morning hangover."
- Consider trazodone and other sedating antidepressants to improve sleep in patients with major depression who are being treated with stimulating SSRIs; patients must be monitored for possible orthostatic hypotension and, when tricyclics are used, anticholinergic adverse effects.
- Consider melatonin for patients with circadian rhythm disorders (e.g., jet lag).
- Use kava kava and valerian only with recognition that quality assurance is sometimes less than adequate and that more information is needed with respect to appropriate indications, optimal dosing, short- and long-term adverse effects, and potential interactions; discourage use of kava kava in cases of potential hepatotoxicity.

EPIDEMIOLOGY

PARASOMNIAS

Of the more than 20 parasomnias, only sleepwalking (somnambulism), sleep terrors (pavor nocturnus), and nightmares are discussed in detail here. Both sleepwalking, or somnambulism, and sleep terrors are phenomena that occur in delta sleep, with peak prevalence at between 4 and 12 years of age. At least one episode of sleepwalking is seen in about 15% of children, and in 2% to 5% of adults. Sleep terrors (pavor nocturnus or night terrors) are seen in approximately 3% of children and less than 1% of adults, as they typically resolve during adolescence. It is estimated that 10% to 50% of children between 3 and 6 years of age suffer enough from nightmares to disturb their parents. Approximately 50% of members of the adult population admit to having at least an occasional nightmare, and perhaps 1% experience frequent nightmares (one or more per week).[8,9]

SLEEP APNEA

Sleep apnea generally first occurs in adulthood, usually over the age of 30, probably with a prevalence of 1% to 4% of the population; obstructive sleep apnea is at least eight times more prevalent in men than in women. Although the incidence of sleep apnea is high in the elderly, many are asymptomatic (i.e., they have no complaints that would have brought this condition to the attention of a physician or sleep-disorder specialist).[10,11]

NARCOLEPSY

Narcolepsy, along with obstructive sleep apnea, is a major cause of excessive daytime sleepiness and occurs in approximately 0.1% of the population. Its onset often is noted during adolescence.[12]

INSOMNIA

As stated earlier, up to 40% of all adults are afflicted with insomnia in a given year. Some surveys estimate that this percentage is not much higher than that of people who have a sleep problem at any given time.[3] The results of a prevalence study of randomly selected elderly (age 65 and older) individuals indicate that sleep apnea occurs in 24% and periodic limb movements during sleep are noted in 45%, with 10% showing both.[13,14]

The largest analysis of patients studied objectively in sleep disorder centers found that the most prevalent diagnosis for a complaint of insomnia was insomnia associated with psychiatric disorders (35%). Approximately half of patients had a major affective disorder and half had personality disorders; less than 5% had major psychoses. Psychophysiologic insomnia (15%) was the second most frequent diagnosis, followed by drug and alcohol dependence (12.4%). Nearly 9% of people with complaints of insomnia had no significant sleep pathology. Sleep apnea syndromes accounted for 6.2% of insomnia. Circadian rhythm disorders were diagnosed in only 2.9% of patients; however, this category may be underrepresented because of a lesser awareness at that time.[15]

The results, unfortunately, may not be representative of the population at large in that they represent findings in sleep disorder centers. Most persons with a sleep problem probably do not seek medical attention. Clinical practice surveys indicate that about two thirds of insomnia cases are associated with a psychiatric or medical disorder.[16] The most common sleep disorders may be adjustment sleep disorder (i.e., transient situational insomnia), insomnia associated with anxiety disorders, psychophysiologic insomnia, inadequate sleep hygiene, insomnia associated with mood disorders, obstructive sleep apnea syndrome, delayed or advanced sleep phase syndromes, shift work sleep disorders, alcohol/hypnotic/stimulant-dependent sleep disorders, and periodic limb movement disorder.

PATHOPHYSIOLOGY

SLEEP PHYSIOLOGY

Sleep has been studied in various ways. Behaviorally, one can observe changes in body position, decreased responsiveness to external stimuli, and eyelid closure. Anatomically, sleep-regulating centers in the brainstem have been identified. Neurochemically, various neurotransmitters are involved in sleep mechanisms. Not long ago, we simply pointed to norepinephrine as being involved in wakefulness and dreaming sleep and serotonin as involved in nondreaming sleep. Then, it became clear that an interaction occurs between the cholinergic systems and the noradrenergic systems. In the future, contributions of other neurotransmitters and various endogenous peptides will likely be elucidated.[17]

Electrophysiology and Sleep Stages. Currently, the standard method for observing and measuring sleep is through electrophysiology.[18] In the laboratory, sleep is recorded polygraphically, with electroencephalograms (EEGs), electro-oculograms (EOGs) from each of the two eyes, and electromyograms (EMGs), generally of the mentalis and submentalis muscles. Two EOGs, one EEG, and one EMG are the minimal recordings used for scoring sleep stages. A number of other physiologic variables may be needed to identify specific sleep disorders, as will be discussed. The entire recording process is often referred to as *polysomnography*. Today, by means of portable devices, such recordings may be obtained in the patient's home.

By means of these recordings, sleep can be divided into nonrapid eye movement (NREM) sleep, which is further subdivided into stages 1 through 4, and rapid eye movement (REM) sleep. Wakefulness is characterized by a low-voltage, fast EEG, high muscle tone, and various types of eye movement, including blinks. Stage 1 sleep is characterized by a low-voltage, mixed-frequency EEG; slightly decreased muscle tone; and slow, rolling eye movements. The subjective experience of this transition stage varies widely among individuals, some experiencing it as wakefulness, others as drowsiness, and yet others as sleep. Stage 2 is characterized by sleep spindles and K-complexes in the EEG and is recognized as unequivocal sleep. Stages 3 and 4 are characterized by high-amplitude, slow activity in the EEG known as delta waves; hence, these two stages together are often referred to as delta sleep. Delta sleep appears to be the deep, restorative sleep that most people (especially patients with insomnia) think of when they visualize sleep.

REM sleep is characterized by a low-voltage, mixed-frequency EEG, in many ways quite similar to that seen in Stage 1, but with very low muscle tone and bursts of bilaterally conjugate rapid eye movements. It appears as though the sleeper is watching a movie or actively observing some activity. Classical dreaming occurs in REM sleep; dream reports can be obtained 80% to 90% of the times that subjects are awakened during or at the end of REM periods. Brain and autonomic activity may be greater and more variable than during relaxed wakefulness.

Physiologic Changes During Sleep. Physiologically, much activity occurs during sleep. Although heart rate and respiratory rate are slow and regular during NREM sleep, they, along with blood pressure, become irregular with rapid changes in REM sleep. In the male, erections occur regularly during REM sleep. In fact, this phenomenon of nocturnal penile tumescence is often used in attempts to distinguish between psychological and physiologic causes of impotence. Body temperature descends to its lowest in the early morning; however, during REM sleep, the sleeper is poikilothermic (cold-blooded). Cortisol levels are lowest at sleep onset, and growth hormone is released during delta sleep. Melatonin secretion increases in sleep and can be suppressed by bright light.

Function of Sleep. Although the function of sleep is not clearly understood, it is believed that NREM sleep serves to restore, rejuvenate, and revitalize the body. Slow-wave sleep seems to play an important role in thermoregulation and tissue repair. Metabolic rate decreases during sleep, with not only a fall in body temperature, but also a decrease in glucose consumption and production of catabolic hormones. On the other hand, along with the increase in growth hormone that is seen in delta sleep, an increase in skeletal muscle protein synthesis is noted during sleep. Slow-wave sleep may have a role in maintaining immune function. It would appear, then, that adequate sleep is critical for growing children and persons with healing wounds or infections.

REM sleep may be needed to sort through short-term memory stores, delete unnecessary data, and lay down important information in long-term memory. REM sleep may also play a role in maintenance of noradrenergic receptor sensitivity. Whatever its role, REM sleep appears to be of vital physiologic importance in that REM deprivation leads to a dramatic REM rebound during recovery sleep.[19]

Sleep Cycle. The architecture of sleep in the normal young adult is cyclic. The sleeper quickly passes from wakefulness through stages 1 and 2, spending a moderate block of time in delta sleep. Some 90 minutes after sleep onset, the sleeper enters the first REM period of the night, which may last only 5 to 7 minutes. The cycle is repeated four to five times each night. As the night progresses, less time is spent in delta sleep, with most delta sleep occurring in the first half of the night. REM periods become longer and more intense, both physiologically and psychologically, as the night goes on. The final REM period of the night may last as long as 30 to 60 minutes. Most persons who recall a dream in the morning are waking from this REM period and remembering the dream's content. In general, one spends approximately 75% of the night in NREM sleep and the remaining 25% of the night in REM sleep.

In older adults, however, the typical sleep architecture described here may be quite different, with a considerable decrease in delta sleep, an increase in light sleep, an increase in awakenings during the night, and a generally more disrupted night of sleep. Total sleep time during the night may be slightly decreased, compared with that of young adults, but how much daytime napping and specific sleep pathologic conditions (e.g., sleep apnea with periodic limb movements) contribute to this apparent decrease is unclear. Even in randomly selected, noncomplaining, elderly persons, the incidence of sleep apnea with periodic limb movements is as high as 58%.[13,14,20]

Parameters that can be measured objectively in the sleep laboratory that are of particular interest with respect to insomnia and effects of medication on sleep are listed in Table 55.1. Latency to sleep onset (or sleep latency) is defined as the length of time a person takes to fall asleep after getting

TABLE 55.1	Sleep Parameters
Latency to sleep onset	
Total sleep time	
Sleep stage durations	
Sleep stage percentages of total sleep time	
Number of awakenings during the night	
Number of stage shifts during the night	
Rapid eye movement intensity	
Other physiologic measurements	

into bed. The number of awakenings and the number of stage shifts during the night are indications of how disrupted sleep has been. REM intensity, or the frequency of bursts of rapid eye movements, at times may be a more subtle indicator of changes in REM sleep than simply the total number of minutes spent in REM sleep during the night. Finally, other physiologic measurements may include electrocardiogram, respiration, oxygen saturation, and activity of the anterior tibialis muscles.

SLEEP APNEA

Sleep apnea is often described as obstructive, central, or mixed. Obstructive sleep apnea is caused by something obstructing the airway. The problem may be the tongue falling back across the airway, enlarged tonsils, or some other craniofacial abnormality. Respiratory effort continues, as is demonstrated by strain gauge recordings around the thorax and abdomen in the absence of nasal/oral airflow (measured by a device attached to the face below the nostrils). In central sleep apnea, respiratory effort ceases, indicating a problem in the respiratory centers of the brain, with resultant absence of nasal and oral airflow. Mixed sleep apnea seems to involve cessation of central respiratory effort, followed by an obstructive event; then, even when respiratory effort resumes, no airflow is present. In any of these cases, as oxygen saturation falls (which can be measured with an ear lobe oximeter) and carbon dioxide levels rise, the brain automatically produces a ''mini-arousal,'' resulting in resumption of breathing. Whether the patient complains of insomnia or of excessive daytime sleepiness is subjective, but obstructive sleep apnea seems to be highly associated with complaints of excessive daytime sleepiness.[10,11]

NARCOLEPSY

Sleep laboratory findings strongly suggest that narcolepsy involves a dysregulation of REM sleep. In addition to cataplexy and sleep paralysis (which represent the loss of muscle tone in REM sleep), narcoleptics have sleep-onset REM periods (i.e., instead of the normal latency of 90 minutes following sleep onset to the first REM period, they can make a transition from wakefulness immediately to REM sleep). Two HLA class II antigens, DR2 and DQ1, were believed to be important in the pathophysiology of narcolepsy. However, even when the DQ1 subtype DQB1*0602 was strongly linked with idiopathic narcolepsy, the specificity of this allele was disappointingly low. Recently, excitement has been generated over the role of hypocretin in the promotion of wakefulness and the inhibition of REM sleep. At this point, it seems likely that at least a subgroup of narcoleptics display a significant deficit in hypocretin.[12,21]

CLINICAL PRESENTATION AND DIAGNOSIS

HISTORICAL PERSPECTIVE

In the 1970s, a group of clinically oriented sleep researchers developed an organization, the Association of Sleep Disorders Centers, as well as a scheme for classifying sleep disorders.[22] Simply stated, disorders of initiating and maintaining sleep (DIMS) were equivalent to insomnia, disorders of excessive somnolence (DOES) were equivalent to excessive daytime sleepiness, disorders of the sleep–wake schedule involved disturbances of biologic rhythms, and parasomnias included a number of miscellaneous disorders associated with sleep, sleep stages, or partial arousals. A considerable amount of overlap in possible causes was noted among the major categories of disorders, with the exception of the parasomnias. In fact, the determining factor in applying a label to the patient was often the nature of the subjective complaint (e.g., ''Doctor, I'm not sleeping well at night'' vs. ''Doctor, I'm always sleepy'').

As sleep disorders clinicians worked with this classification scheme over the years, an international effort for revision and modification began. The result was *The International Classification of Sleep Disorders* (ICSD), an extensive listing and description of sleep disorders (as outlined in Table 55.2), which has subsequently been revised.[23] It was published by what was called the American Sleep Disorders Association, in cooperation with the European Sleep Research Society, the Japanese Society of Sleep Research, and the Latin American Sleep Society. Concurrently, but separately, a committee of the American Psychiatric Association was revising its official *Diagnostic and Statistical Manual of Mental Disorders* (DSM-IV). The result, subsequently revised, was a somewhat abbreviated nomenclature for the sleep disorders most likely to be encountered in a psychiatric practice.[24] It is outlined in Table 55.3 for the sake of completeness; however, because the ICSD is the more exhaustive, international classification, it will serve as the basis of this discussion. Eighty-four specific sleep disorders are described in the ICSD. It is beyond the scope of this chapter to cover each of them in detail; however, examples from each of the major categories are listed in Table 55.2 to provide the reader with an idea of the progress made over the past 30 years in identifying and classifying sleep disorders.

The entire field of sleep disorders medicine is still relatively young. For many of the sleep disorders, both cause and prevalence are as yet unclear (in instances where these are established or even postulated, such information will be mentioned). The remaining discussion is focused on the disorders that have been best studied, are seen most often, or are most likely to have a pharmacotherapeutic component to treatment. Particular emphasis is placed on insomnia and the use of hypnotics.

PARASOMNIAS

Somnambulism. Typically, the sleepwalker sits up, gets out of bed, walks around, and returns to bed. The person appears to be navigating well, but critical skills and reactivity are impaired (e.g., if you were to rearrange the furniture in the house, the sleepwalker would probably stumble over it).[8]

Sleep Terrors. Sleep terrors are characterized by extreme vocalizations, motility, and autonomic variability. Recall of

TABLE 55.2	International Classification of Sleep Disorders (ICSD): Framework and Examples

1. Dyssomnias

   Disorders that are characterized by difficulty in initiating or maintaining sleep, or by excessive sleepiness

   A. Intrinsic sleep disorders

   Developing within the body or from causes within the body

307.42–0	Psychophysiologic insomnia
347	Narcolepsy
780.53–0	Obstructive sleep apnea syndrome
780.51–0	Central sleep apnea syndrome
780.52–4	Periodic limb movement disorder
780.52–5	Restless legs syndrome

   B. Extrinsic sleep disorders

   Developing from causes outside of the body

307.41–1	Inadequate sleep hygiene
780.52–6	Environmental sleep disorder
780.52–0	Hypnotic-dependent sleep disorder
780.52–1	Stimulant-dependent sleep disorder
780.52–3	Alcohol-dependent sleep disorder

   C. Circadian rhythm sleep disorders

   Related to the timing of sleep in the 24-hour day

307.45–0	Time zone change (jet lag) syndrome
307.45–1	Shift work sleep disorder
780.55–0	Delayed sleep phase syndrome

2. Parasomnias

   Undesirable physical phenomena occurring predominantly during sleep, including disorders of arousal, partial arousal, and sleep stage transition

   A. Arousal disorders

   Disorders of impaired arousal from slow wave (delta) sleep

307.46–0	Sleepwalking
307.46–1	Sleep terrors

   B. Sleep–wake transition disorders

307.47–2	Sleep starts
307.47–3	Sleepwalking
729.82	Nocturnal leg cramps

   C. Parasomnias usually associated with REM sleep

307.47–0	Nightmares
780.56–2	Sleep paralysis
780.59–0	REM sleep behavior disorder

   D. Other parasomnias

306.8	Sleep bruxism
780.36–0	Sleep enuresis
786.09–1	Primary snoring

(continued)

TABLE 55.2	continued

3. Medical/psychiatric sleep disorders

A. Associated with mental disorders

290–299	Psychoses
296–301, 311	Mood disorders
300, 308, 309	Anxiety disorders
300	Panic disorder
303, 305	Alcoholism

B. Associated with neurologic disorders

331	Dementia
332	Parkinsonism

C. Associated with other medical disorders

490–496	Chronic obstructive pulmonary disease
493	Sleep-related asthma
530.81	Sleep-related gastroesophageal reflux
531–534	Peptic ulcer disease
729.1	Fibromyalgia

4. Proposed sleep disorders

Disorders for which insufficient or inadequate information is available to substantiate their unequivocal existence

780.54.3	Menstruation-associated sleep disorder
780.59–6	Pregnancy-associated sleep disorder
307.47–4	Terrifying hypnagogic hallucinations

(From American Academy of Sleep Medicine. International classification of sleep disorders, revised: diagnostic and coding manual. Chicago, IL: American Academy of Sleep Medicine, 2001.)

TABLE 55.3	DSM-IV Classification of Sleep Disorders

Primary Sleep Disorders

Dyssomnias

307.42	Primary insomnia
307.44	Primary hypersomnia
347	Narcolepsy
780.59	Breathing-related sleep disorder
307.45	Circadian rhythm sleep disorder
307.47	Dyssomnia not otherwise specified

Parasomnias

307.47	Nightmare disorder
307.46	Sleep terror disorder
307.46	Sleepwalking disorder
307.47	Parasomnia not otherwise specified

Sleep Disorders Related to Another Mental Disorder

307.42	Insomnia related to ...
307.44	Hypersomnia related to ...

Other Sleep Disorders

780.xx	Sleep disorder due to ... (a medical condition)
—	Substance-induced sleep disorder

(From American Psychiatric Association. Diagnostic and statistical manual of mental disorders, 4th edition, text revised. Washington DC: American Psychiatric Association, 2000.)

frightening content is minimal or absent. Hence, the phenomenon may be more disturbing to others in the house than to the child who is experiencing it. The parents of the child may hear a "blood-curdling" scream, run into the sleeper's bedroom, and find the child wet from perspiration, breathing forcefully, and experiencing tachycardia. Fortunately, the absence of frightening content results in nothing psychological with which to associate the event. Generally, amnesia for the event follows.[8]

Nightmares. Unlike sleep terrors, nightmares ("bad dreams") occur in REM sleep (in about 5% of the general population) and are associated with elaborate and frightening content. Less motility and autonomic variability are noted than in sleep terrors.[8]

SLEEP APNEA

Sleep apnea, a sleep-induced respiratory impairment, is a condition characterized by episodes of cessation of breath-ing.[10,11] Each apneic episode, often lasting 20 to 30 seconds, is terminated by a brief arousal from sleep during which breathing resumes. As many as several hundred of these "mini-arousals" may occur during a single night, but the patient may not be aware of their occurrence. The patient may instead complain of morning headache, irritability, and general difficulty with daytime functioning. Often, the bed partner is the best source of information, reporting that the patient snores very loudly or has periods during which breathing stops followed by gasps for air. Often, a recent history of weight gain is associated with onset of symptoms. Common complications of sleep apnea include arrhythmias, systolic or diastolic hypertension, and signs of pulmonary arterial hypertension and right-sided heart failure.

NARCOLEPSY

Patients with narcolepsy are extremely sleepy throughout the day and find themselves falling asleep at inopportune moments. Narcolepsy has four classic features: excessive daytime sleepiness, cataplexy, sleep paralysis, and hypnagogic hallucinations. Cataplexy is described as brief (lasting only seconds to minutes) episodes of muscle weakness that may result in the patient's collapsing. They are often precipitated by emotionally charged stimuli (e.g., laughter, anger, excitement). Sleep paralysis, which occurs during the transition between wakefulness and sleep, or between sleep and wakefulness, involves inhibition of the musculature. This is particularly frightening because the patient is aware of the paralysis. Hypnagogic hallucinations, which occur during the transition between wakefulness and sleep, are brief, dreamlike events, but they are perhaps more fragmented and bizarre than a typical dream.[12]

INSOMNIA

Insomnia is a problem that 95% of all adults have experienced at least once in their lives. It must be defined in terms of both amount of sleep and its perceived quality. No absolute number of hours of sleep per se constitutes insomnia because sleep need among persons is highly variable. The person who sleeps 5 hours per night, needs only 5 hours per night, and functions in his or her daily activities at peak performance does not have insomnia. However, the person who needs 8 hours per night, sleeps only 7 with a perception of fragmented sleep, and complains of daytime impairment may indeed be suffering from insomnia. Hence, insomnia must be seen as a perceived relative decrease in the quantity and/or quality of sleep, along with some perceived consequences in waking life. These perceptions take the form of a subjective complaint by the patient. In many respects, the sleep of patients with insomnia is not that dramatically different from that of good sleepers, but they perceive it as poor sleep. Unfortunately, at present, there is no definitive way to measure the quality of sleep in the sleep laboratory; however, it appears likely that fragmentation of sleep (as indicated by arousals, stage shifts, and perhaps, subtle findings in EEG frequencies) is most closely associated with perceived poor quality.[8,25]

Insomnia can be viewed from various perspectives. The severity (i.e., from mild to severe) clearly has implications with respect to treatment decisions. Whether insomnia is transient or chronic is important in both diagnosis and treatment. Finally, the pattern of a typical night may be characterized by difficulty falling sleep, difficulty staying asleep (numerous awakenings during the night), early morning awakening (3 to 4 hours earlier than expected, with an inability to return to sleep), or some combination of these problems.

The actual neurochemical or pathophysiologic bases for the various types of insomnia are, in general, unknown. Insomnia has numerous "causes." Many of the drug and nondrug factors associated with insomnia are listed in Tables 55.4 and 55.5. Medical causes include pain of various types (e.g., arthritis, pruritus, duodenal ulcer). Pain not only interferes with the ability to fall asleep but also may lead to increased nocturnal arousals and a generally "lighter" sleep. Nocturia may be part of a medical disorder or may result from a dose of a diuretic taken too late; the result in either case is fragmentation of sleep. Psychological or psychiatric causes of insomnia can be as common as worry or excitement (e.g., over an important examination or job interview).

TABLE 55.4	Nondrug Factors Associated With Long-Term Insomnia
Psychiatric disorders	Medical/neurologic disorders (*continued*)
Mood disorders	Asthma
Anxiety disorders	Bronchitis
Somatoform disorders	Chronic obstructive pulmonary disease
Eating disorders	Chronic liver failure
Personality disorders	Chronic renal failure
Chronic pain	Congestive heart failure
Alcohol/substance abuse	Cystic fibrosis
Sleep disorders	Dementia
Sleep apnea	Epilepsy
Periodic limb movement disorder	Gastroesophageal reflux
Restless legs syndrome	Head injury
Delayed sleep phase syndrome	Hyperthyroidism
Psychophysiologic conditioning	Hypoglycemia
Shift work	Malignancy
Medical/neurologic disorders	Menopause
Angina	Parkinson disease
Arthritis	Peptic ulcer disease

Almost everyone is familiar with an occasional bout of insomnia associated with emotional arousal. In addition, it is almost certain that some type of sleep disturbance will accompany an acute episode of any of the major psychiatric disorders (e.g., schizophrenia, major depression, mania), and often, the sleep disturbance is one of the diagnostic criteria. Other causes of sleep disturbance may include disruption of circadian rhythms (e.g., jet lag, work shift change), change in environment (e.g., sleeping for the first night or two in a hotel room in a strange city), sleep apnea, periodic limb movements, use of stimulant drugs, drug dependence, and drug withdrawal.

Often, it is useful to classify insomnia as transient, short-term, or persistent (also called *long-term* or *chronic*). This distinction is valuable for diagnosis and for treatment decisions. Transient insomnia occurs in an otherwise normal sleeper, lasts only for several days, and is often associated with acute stress or disruption of the biologic clock (e.g., jet lag, change in work schedule). Short-term insomnia is very similar to transient insomnia, except that its duration is several weeks. It too is often associated with some situational stress (e.g., loss of a loved one, family conflict, work conflict) or serious medical illness.

Persistent insomnia has a duration longer than several weeks and is often associated with psychiatric or medical conditions. Sleep apnea syndrome and the association of

TABLE 55.5	Drugs Associated With Insomnia		
• Alcohol	• Corticosteroids	• Oral contraceptives
• Amphetamines	• Decongestants	• Phenytoin
• Antipsychotics	• Diuretics	• Quinidine
• Appetite suppressants	• Hypnotics (long-term use)	• Reserpine
• β-Agonists/blockers	• Levodopa	• Selective and mixed serotonin and norepinephrine reuptake inhibitors
• Bupropion	• Methyldopa	
• Caffeine	• Methysergide	
• Clonidine	• MAO inhibitors	• Theophylline
• Cocaine	• Nicotine	• Thyroid preparations

MAO, monoamine oxidase.

insomnia with psychiatric disorders have already been discussed. Periodic limb movement disorder [also called *periodic leg movements*, *nocturnal myoclonus*, or *PMS (periodic movements during sleep)*] is characterized by periodic (every 20–40 seconds), stereotypic, myoclonic movements of the anterior tibialis or other limb muscles during sleep, resulting in arousals. As with the arousals of sleep apnea, the patient may experience several hundred per night and yet may not be aware of them the following day. Often, as with sleep apnea, the bed partner will voice the complaint, in this case about the sleeper's "kicking" throughout the night. The condition is age related, showing a marked increase in incidence in persons older than 40 years of age. A related condition that can affect the ability to fall asleep is restless legs syndrome. This is characterized by uncomfortable sensations in the legs at rest, which can be relieved by movement; hence, the patient feels the need to get out of bed and move around.

A number of biologic rhythm disorders may be associated with a complaint of persistent insomnia, for example, delayed sleep phase syndrome.[26] Patients want to fall asleep at 11:00 PM and awaken at 7:00 AM. They get into bed at 11:00 PM and find that they cannot fall asleep for 4 or 5 hours. When they wake up (usually with the help of an alarm or two) at 7:00 AM to meet their own and society's daily demands, they feel unrefreshed and tired. This pattern is repeated night after night. If patients are asked how late they would sleep if they did not have to get out of bed at 7:00 AM, they would probably say 11:00 AM or Noon; hence, they could indeed sleep 8 hours. The patient's ability to sleep simply does not coincide with the period set aside for sleep; the body (i.e., his or her internal biologic clock) is not sleepy at the time that he or she wants to be sleeping.

Drugs and alcohol may be associated with insomnia in numerous ways. Any drug with stimulant properties can disrupt sleep, especially if taken late in the day. The use of CNS depressants, including alcohol, can lead to dependence; then, on withdrawal, sleep that is more disturbed and restless is common. Even within a single night, alcohol can disrupt sleep. Although it may make the person feel more relaxed

and able to fall asleep, the short duration of action may allow a mild withdrawal in the middle of the night, associated with more disrupted sleep and increased dreaming caused by an REM rebound (i.e., early in the night, the alcohol suppresses REM sleep and, as the effect of the alcohol wears off, the tendency is to make up the lost REM sleep later in the night).

Psychophysiologic insomnia may be transient, short-term, or persistent. It is a conditioned or learned insomnia that the sleeper has associated with the bed, bedroom, or sleep process. The harder the patient tries, the more difficult it becomes to sleep. The patient becomes more and more focused on the inability to sleep and resultant daytime impairment. It is interesting to note that such persons sleep remarkably well in the laboratory or in a strange hotel room, away from the conditions with which insomnia is associated, or at times when they are not thinking about trying to fall asleep (e.g., while watching TV or reading).

Finally, sleep-related gastroesophageal reflux, characterized by regurgitation of gastric contents or fluid into the esophagus during sleep, can awaken the patient from sleep with heartburn or a sour taste in the mouth.

PSYCHOSOCIAL ASPECTS

Insomnia and other sleep disorders can be crippling for many people. As life becomes more complex, it is not unusual for the incidence of transient insomnia to increase. Seventy percent of persons who have difficulty sleeping never discuss the problem with a physician. Another 24% discuss their problem, but only as a secondary issue during a physician visit. Only 6% seek the help of a physician as a primary reason for their office visit.[5] To what extent this represents embarrassment, denial, stoicism, or underestimation of the significance of the problem on the part of patients versus inadequate exploration on the part of clinicians is uncertain. Nonetheless, impaired cognitive functioning, decreased job performance, increased absenteeism, and impaired quality of life have all been associated with insomnia.[27]

TREATMENT

PHARMACOTHERAPY

Parasomnias. Medications that may exacerbate or induce sleepwalking (e.g., thioridazine, chloral hydrate, lithium, fluphenazine, perphenazine, desipramine) should be discontinued if possible. Theoretically, sleepwalking can be reduced through suppression of delta sleep. Most BZDs suppress delta sleep, and in an adult with frequent episodes of sleepwalking, especially with a history of injury to self or others, a BZD may be a highly appropriate and efficacious intervention. However, in the treatment of a child who is sleepwalking, the benefit of treatment over simple protection of the child from injury is questionable in light of the unknown risks of long-term exposure of the child's developing CNS to BZDs. The same reservations about use of delta sleep suppressants apply to the treatment of children with sleep terrors.[8]

Sleep Apnea. The single most important pharmacologic intervention in the treatment of patients with any type of sleep apnea is careful avoidance of all drugs that have CNS depressant activity. These include anxiolytics, hypnotics, narcotics, and alcohol. Any agent that can interfere with the ability of the brain to produce an apnea-terminating miniarousal is potentially lethal. Even CNS depressants that appear to have little or no effect on respiration during wakefulness must be avoided because evidence suggests differential effects during sleep. Although some data indicate that a subset of patients with central sleep apnea, given triazolam, may experience improved sleep quality, increased total sleep time, and decreased apneic episodes,[28] it remains safest to avoid CNS depressants in all patients with sleep apnea. Active pharmacologic intervention in the treatment of patients with sleep apnea has met with mixed, fairly unimpressive results. Tricyclic antidepressants (TCAs), particularly protriptyline, have been used in both obstructive and central sleep apnea. Protriptyline may act by decreasing REM sleep or by increasing oropharyngeal muscle tone.[29] Respiratory stimulants, such as medroxyprogesterone[30] and acetazolamide,[31] show limited efficacy, and no studies demonstrate long-term effectiveness.

Narcolepsy. Pharmacologic treatment of patients with narcolepsy is directed toward excessive daytime sleepiness on the one hand and cataplexy on the other.[32,33] CNS stimulants are used to reduce sleepiness. Hesitation in prescribing amphetamines (due to concerns over abuse, tolerance, and dependence) has led to the more common use of methylphenidate, starting at 2.5 mg twice daily. Rarely, pemoline is started at a dose of 18.75 mg per day. Modafinil, which is not an amphetamine, was approved by the US Food and Drug Administration (FDA) for the treatment of patients with excessive daytime sleepiness associated with narcolepsy. Given as a single 200-mg dose each morning, modafinil produces increased alertness. Although modafinil is less

likely to be abused, it may not be as effective as methylphenidate or D-amphetamine.[34] In 2004, modafinil was approved by the FDA for two additional indications: (1) residual excessive daytime sleepiness associated with obstructive sleep apnea that is not fully responsive to traditional, nonpharmacologic treatment; and (2) sleepiness associated with shift work sleep disorder.[35]

To manage cataplexy, imipramine (in the past) and, more recently, the less sedating protriptyline (at an initial dose of 5 mg titrated up to 60 mg daily) have been used; in addition, selective serotonin reuptake inhibitors (SSRIs) are being prescribed increasingly. Recently, sodium oxybate (also known as gamma-hydroxybutyrate, or GHB) was approved by the FDA for the treatment of patients with cataplexy associated with narcolepsy. Not only does it significantly decrease the number of cataplectic attacks, it also appears to consolidate the fragmented nocturnal sleep seen in many patients with narcolepsy, while improving overall sleep quality. Most patients are stabilized by taking 6 g per night, although some may require as much as 9 g. Its short duration of action requires dosing at bedtime and again in the middle of the night. In contrast to the TCAs, which, when abruptly discontinued, are associated with a rebound in cataplexy, sodium oxybate can be discontinued with the cataplectic attacks returning only gradually. The most common adverse effects are dizziness, headache, nausea, and somnolence (as it is pharmacologically a CNS depressant). Because of the potential for abuse, this agent is highly controlled and is distributed by only one central pharmacy in the United States.[36,37]

General principles of pharmacologic management recommend using the lowest effective dose possible, with gradual titration and careful monitoring for therapeutic and adverse effects (particularly the anticholinergic and hypotensive effects of the TCA), and temporarily withdrawing the stimulant when tolerance has developed. It is ideal if the temporary withdrawal can be scheduled at a time when a return of daytime sleepiness will have the least impact on the general functioning of the patient (e.g., during a vacation break from work or school).

Insomnia. Treatment of patients with insomnia varies considerably according to the type of insomnia that is occurring. Again, an extremely important distinction exists between persistent or chronic and transient or short-term insomnia. Hypnotics are reserved primarily for use in patients with transient or short-term insomnia. The persistent insomnias often call for other specific interventions of choice. The persistent insomnias associated with major psychiatric disorders are most appropriately treated with the specific class of agents targeted for that particular disorder. For example, the patient with a major depressive disorder should be receiving an antidepressant as the primary drug treatment. Sleep disturbance, one symptom of the depressive episode, will be one of the first targeted symptoms to respond to the treatment. For the psychotic patient, selection and titration of an antipsychotic is the most appropriate treatment. If insomnia is associated with drug dependence or drug withdrawal, gradual tapering of the offending agent or administration of the equivalent amount of a cross-tolerant long-acting agent is the primary treatment. If insomnia is associated with a stimulant, in many cases the agent should simply be discontinued abruptly.

In cases of insomnia associated with medical disorders, adjunctive, short-term use of a hypnotic to promote sleep may be reasonable, while a specific treatment is given for the primary problem. Further, at times, a patient is best served by education. The elderly patient whose sleep has become fragmented or the "short sleeper" whose sleep need is small and who shows no daytime impairment may simply need assurance that he or she is sleeping normally.

Treatment of patients with periodic limb movement during sleep, one type of persistent insomnia, requires that an exception be made to the general rule of not using hypnotics for chronic insomnias, because it is occasionally treated with these agents. Originally, treatment was provided with clonazepam; however, it appears that an equivalent response can be obtained with any BZD.[38] The BZDs do not significantly reduce the number of movements, but patients report an improved quality of sleep and feeling more refreshed in the morning. For restless legs syndrome, after it has been determined that serum ferritin concentrations are adequate (>50 μg/mL), codeine and related compounds (e.g., oxycodone) or carbamazepine (typically one Percodan® tablet or 200 mg of carbamazepine given at bedtime) has helped some patients. Recently, considerable success has resulted from the use of carbidopa/levodopa at bedtime in both periodic limb movements and restless legs syndrome.[39,40] However, continued use has been associated with augmentation (i.e., symptoms occurring earlier in the day and with increasing severity); as a result, carbidopa/levodopa treatment has been replaced by dopamine agonist therapy (e.g., pramipexole, ropinirole).[41]

Hypnotics

The Ideal Hypnotic. At this point, a description of the ideal hypnotic may be helpful to the Reader. Although such an agent does not exist, keeping the ideal characteristics in mind can help one to put the existing agents into perspective. The ideal hypnotic should induce sleep rapidly after ingestion. It should maintain sleep for the entire duration expected, without lasting so long that it produces a "morning hangover" and impaired daytime performance. It should not induce development of tolerance or dependence when used over a number of consecutive nights, and abrupt discontinuation should not result in drug withdrawal or rebound insomnia. This agent should have a wide margin of safety, and it should make abnormal sleep normal, while not making the sleep of a normal sleeper abnormal. Finally, it should offer no potential for drug–drug interactions.

Classification and Pharmacology of Selected Agents. Many of the more commonly used hypnotic agents are presented

in Table 55.6. It should be noted that for older adults, dosing should begin at or below the low end of the dosage ranges shown. The older barbiturates have lost popularity as a result of their narrow margin of safety, moderately high abuse potential, possible drug–drug interactions caused by liver enzyme induction, suppression of delta and REM sleep with REM rebound following abrupt discontinuation, and loss of efficacy in inducing and maintaining sleep within 14 consecutive nights of use at a consistent dose.[42]

The older nonbarbiturate nonbenzodiazepines were once thought to be superior to the barbiturates because of their lack of barbiturate structure. However, with the exception of chloral hydrate, they share many of the disadvantages of the barbiturates, and they have additional ones as well. For instance, methaqualone, which is no longer available, was found to have an even higher abuse potential than the barbiturates. Glutethimide used in an overdose has presented emergency department staff not only with a CNS depressant overdose but also with anticholinergic toxicity. In many other countries, agents such as ethchlorvynol and glutethimide have not been available for decades. Although controversy has been expressed for the past 35 years about their availability in the United States, withdrawal from the market has been slow. Chloral hydrate, an exception, lacks some of these disadvantages, but it does displace other protein-bound drugs (e.g., warfarin); it also causes gastrointestinal irritation in some patients, and at the higher doses (1–2 g) needed for some patients, it may lose its effectiveness in inducing and maintaining sleep at least as rapidly as the barbiturates.[43]

The antihistamines, primarily diphenhydramine and doxylamine, are used for their sedative adverse effects. Some would argue that this drug class is a good choice for patients with high potential for abusing the BZDs (i.e., those with a history of or current problem with substance abuse). Unfortunately, little research into the hypnotic efficacy of these drugs has been done in the sleep laboratory. By subjective report, patients have assessed the soporific effect of diphenhydramine 50 mg to be equivalent to 60 mg of pentobarbital.[44]

Increasing the dose of diphenhydramine does not produce a linear increase in hypnotic effect, but it does cause greater anticholinergic adverse effects, which can be particularly troublesome in elderly patients. Not only are these patients bothered by constipation, urinary retention, dry mouth, and blurred near vision, they are also particularly sensitive to the central anticholinergic effects of confusion, disorientation, impaired short-term memory, and, at times, visual and tactile hallucinations. In addition, morning hangover is often experienced. Hence, the patient should be monitored for and counseled about these adverse effects, as well as about drug interactions with other CNS depressants.

In recent years, the more sedating antidepressants—amitriptyline, doxepin, and trazodone—have been used in relatively low doses as hypnotics. Similar to the antihistamines, they are used in a way that puts to good use their sedative adverse effects. All three of these agents may produce signif-

TABLE 55.6	Hypnotics—Classification and Dosages	
Generic Name	**Trade Name**	**Dosage Range**
Barbiturates		
Pentobarbital	Nembutal	100–200 mg
Secobarbital	Seconal	100–200 mg
Amobarbital	Amytal	100–200 mg
Nonbarbiturate Nonbenzodiazepines		
Ethchlorvynol	Placidyl	0.5–1.0 g
Chloral hydrate	Noctec	0.5–2.0 g
Antihistamines		
Amitriptyline	Elavil	10–50 mg
Trazodone	Desyrel	25–150 mg
Antihistamines		
Diphenhydramine	Benadryl, Sominex-2	25–100 mg
Doxylamine	Unisom	25–100 mg
"Natural" Products		
L-Tryptophan		1.0–4.0 g
Melatonin		0.3–5.0 mg
Valerian, kava kava		
Benzodiazepines		
Flurazepam	Dalmane	15–30 mg
Temazepam	Restoril	15–30 mg
Triazolam	Halcion	0.125–0.25 mg
Quazepam	Doral	7.5–15 mg
Estazolam	ProSom	1.0–2.0 mg
BZD$_1$ Receptor–Specific Nonbenzodiazepines		
Zolpidem	Ambien	5–10 mg
Zaleplon	Sonata	5–10 mg
Eszopiclone	Lunesta	2–3 mg

icant orthostatic hypotension; in addition, amitriptyline and doxepin are highly anticholinergic. No systematic studies have been conducted to assess efficacy in nondepressed patients with insomnia. On the other hand, trazodone given in doses of 50 to 150 mg at bedtime has been shown to improve sleep in patients with major depression who are treated in the morning with SSRIs[45]; there is no indication, however, that depression is relieved more quickly in this way than with the SSRI alone.

BZDs and other BZD agonists have come closest to being regarded as the ideal hypnotic. Indeed, this was one of several major conclusions of the Consensus Development Conference on Drugs and Insomnia, which was held at the National Institutes of Mental Health in November of 1983.[46] Three conclusions of significance to this discussion were that (1) hypnotics should be used primarily in the treatment of patients with transient or short-term insomnia (e.g., situational, jet lag, work shift change); (2) when pharmacotherapy

is indicated, a BZD is generally the drug of choice (although if this conference were held at present, other BZD agonists would most likely be included as well); and (3) selection of the specific agent should be made on the basis of its pharmacokinetic and pharmacodynamic characteristics in relation to the individual patient and situation.

Flurazepam was the first of the BZDs to be marketed as a hypnotic. Its favorable profile, as compared with those of barbiturates and nonbarbiturate nonbenzodiazepines, includes a wider margin of safety, lower abuse potential, and fewer drug–drug interactions. In addition, it produces little or no REM suppression at lower doses (15 mg), and even at higher doses (30 mg), REM suppression is not followed by REM rebound upon abrupt discontinuation of the drug, probably because of the slow elimination of its long-acting active metabolite, N-desalkylflurazepam. Whether flurazepam demonstrates withdrawal is unclear; one may need to look at sleep patterns several weeks beyond discontinuation of the drug. It offers the advantage of remaining effective at a consistent dose for at least 28 consecutive nights of use. It does suppress delta sleep, and the long-acting metabolite (with an elimination half-life of 47 to 100 hours) accumulates over time. This can cause impaired daytime functioning, especially in the elderly, leading to falls that result in injuries.[47] Peak plasma levels are achieved within 30 to 60 minutes.

Temazepam offers the advantage of a short to intermediate elimination half-life of 9.5 to 12.4 hours. However, the elimination half-life may be as long 20 to 30 hours in elderly patients, so one must watch for possible accumulation and morning hangover with repeated use. It shares many of the properties of flurazepam with respect to effects on sleep. In doses of 15 to 30 mg, it increases total sleep time and decreases the frequency and duration of nocturnal awakenings in patients with insomnia. It suppresses delta sleep, and, although REM sleep is decreased during the first half of the night, a corresponding increase occurs in the second half. Because it can take 1 to 2 hours for this agent to work, some question has arisen about its ability to significantly shorten sleep latency in the patient who has difficulty falling asleep. Initial studies of the drug included two dosage forms: a hard gelatin capsule with powder inside (available in the United States) and a soft gelatin capsule that contains a solution of the drug in polyethylene glycol. When given in the soft gelatin capsule formulation, the drug appears to be absorbed more quickly. This issue has yet to be adequately addressed by the manufacturers.

Triazolam, a triazolobenzodiazepine, is unique in that it is ultrashort to short acting, with an elimination half-life of 2 to 3 hours (5.5 hours at the most). Peak plasma levels are achieved within 30 to 80 minutes. Triazolam appears to be absorbed about as quickly as flurazepam, but it is eliminated much more rapidly. Although it suppresses REM sleep during the first half of the night, compensation for this has been noted in the second half (probably as drug levels are decreasing). It seems to have little effect on delta sleep, which distinguishes it from flurazepam, temazepam, and other benzodiazepines. It is the least likely of the BZDs to produce morning hangover. Indeed, at the 0.25-mg dose, its effect is equal to that achieved by placebo. Similar to flurazepam and temazepam, triazolam improves the general quality of sleep, decreases nocturnal awakenings, and increases total sleep time.[48–52]

Some concern has been expressed among clinicians and members of the general public that triazolam is more likely than other benzodiazepines to produce psychomotor impairment, psychological adverse effects, and anterograde amnesia. However, this may not be a unique risk of triazolam, but rather, a function of dose and pattern of use, potency, effect of combination with other CNS depressants, and mechanism of adverse drug reaction.[53]

Some of the concern that has been expressed regarding triazolam has been associated with ''traveler's amnesia.'' This is the situation that results when an individual who is flying across a number of time zones decides to force sleep during the flight by taking a short-acting hypnotic, perhaps having ingested some ethanol on the plane as well. Later, the traveler has little or no recall for a number of hours following ingestion of the drug (e.g., during arrival at the airport and subsequent activities). Until this form of anterograde amnesia is more fully understood, it may simply be safer for a traveler to readjust the internal biologic clock after arriving at his or her destination. Whatever the actual incidences of psychomotor impairment, psychological adverse affects, and anterograde amnesia may be (as yet unclear), especially at the lower doses currently being recommended and used, it is prudent for clinicians to carefully monitor and counsel patients who use triazolam.

Quazepam and estazolam are the last two BZDs that are marketed as hypnotics in the United States. Estazolam, the second triazolobenzodiazepine hypnotic, appears to decrease sleep latency and nocturnal awakenings, while increasing total sleep time and improving depth of sleep and sleep quality.[54] Peak plasma levels are achieved within 0.5 to 4 hours, although with doses that are generally used, onset of action appears to be similar to that seen with flurazepam and triazolam. The half-life of elimination is 8 to 28 hours. On the basis of its onset of action and elimination half-life, estazolam may be regarded as a ''faster-acting temazepam.'' This would characterize it as an agent that can significantly decrease sleep latency (a distinct advantage over temazepam) with duration of action that is intermediate between flurazepam and triazolam. However, results of objective sleep laboratory studies are mixed with respect to estazolam's ability to significantly decrease latency to sleep onset.

Although quazepam has an intriguing specificity for the BZD$_1$ receptor subtype, the clinical significance of this property is unclear. Indeed, although the parent compound has a 39-hour half-life of elimination, one of its metabolites, N-desalkyl-2-oxoquazepam, is identical to N-desalkylflurazepam, which is the long-acting active metabolite of flurazepam. Therefore, one would expect that, clinically, its properties would be very similar to those of flurazepam. It is doubtful that it offers any advantages over flurazepam. Peak plasma levels are achieved in 1 to 2 hours.[55]

Zolpidem is an imidazopyridine compound with a number of intriguing characteristics. It is not a benzodiazepine; however, the molecule is designed in such a way that it binds selectively to the BZD$_1$ receptor. Its specificity distinguishes it from all other currently marketed BZD hypnotics except quazepam, and the fact that it has no nonspecific BZD receptor binding metabolites distinguishes it from quazepam.

Pharmacologically, the BZD$_1$ receptor specificity of zolpidem seems to account for its strong hypnotic activity, with minimal anxiolytic, muscle relaxant, and anticonvulsant activity even at doses higher than those recommended for insomnia (although at extremely high doses, the specificity appears to be lost). This is certainly advantageous in a hypnotic agent; however, theoretically, one would exercise extreme caution in attempting to switch a patient from long-term and/or high-dose use of a BZD to zolpidem. Zolpidem would not be expected to protect the patient from withdrawal symptoms of increased anxiety, muscle disturbances, or convulsions. In addition, in patients for whom a single bedtime dose of a sedative-hypnotic is desired to help the patient sleep at night and to provide a carryover anxiolytic effect throughout the day, zolpidem would not appear to be appropriate.

Zolpidem is rapidly absorbed, resulting in a rapid onset of action. It has a mean plasma elimination half-life of 2.3 hours in healthy subjects, 2.9 hours in elderly patients, and close to 10 hours in patients with hepatic cirrhosis. It is metabolized to three major pharmacologically inactive metabolites.

With respect to specific effects on sleep, zolpidem reduces latency to sleep onset (sleep occurring within 20 to 30 minutes following ingestion), increases total sleep time, decreases the number of awakenings during the night, and subjectively improves the quality of sleep. Although some evidence exists for a slight suppression of REM sleep when higher-than-recommended doses are used, in most studies, the drug appears to have little effect on this stage of sleep. Different from most BZDs, zolpidem does not suppress delta sleep; in fact, in one study, delta sleep was increased in healthy, young adults to whom zolpidem was administered.

Zolpidem given in lower doses (5–10 mg) appears to provide a full night of sleep with little or no daytime impairment and few effects on memory. It appears to have a lower abuse potential than the BZDs. In fact, at very high doses, it produces nausea, dizziness, anxiety, and dysphoria; such effects would discourage many recreational drug users. Rebound insomnia has been minimal or absent following abrupt discontinuation of zolpidem. In a sleep laboratory study that lasted 4 weeks, no evidence of tolerance was seen polysomnographically. Subjectively, patients given zolpidem for 5 weeks or longer have reported no significant changes in efficacy over time.

Adverse effects associated with zolpidem (in doses ≤10 mg) have primarily been headache, drowsiness, dizziness, lethargy, nausea, myalgia, and sinusitis. Incidences of headache and drowsiness seem to be age related, and drowsiness, nausea, and anterograde amnesia appear to occur in a dose-related manner, increasing significantly at a dose of 20 mg. Falls and confusion may occur in elderly patients if they are treated with doses in excess of 10 mg (which is twice the recommended starting dose for this population). Except for apparently additive CNS depressant effects when zolpidem is used in combination with chlorpromazine or imipramine, no drug interactions have been noted with haloperidol, cimetidine, ranitidine, warfarin, or digoxin.[56]

Zaleplon, a BZD$_1$ receptor–specific pyrazolopyrimidine, appears to be similar to zolpidem in its dosing, onset of action, effects on sleep stages, and profile of adverse effects. The major difference between these agents is duration of action, in that zaleplon has an elimination half-life of about 1 hour. This property may make it most useful for sleep

initiation problems, with less likelihood that it will significantly increase total sleep time or decrease nocturnal awakenings. Whether it has lower incidences of psychomotor impairment, amnesia, and rebound insomnia than zolpidem has yet to be established.[57]

Eszopiclone, the most recently FDA-approved BZD agonist, is a BZD$_1$ receptor–specific pyrrolopyrazine; it is the S-isomer of zopiclone, which has been available in other countries for over 15 years. It is rapidly absorbed, reaching peak serum concentrations in 1 hour, or in 2 hours after a high-fat meal. The half-life of elimination is about 6 hours but may extend up to 9 hours in elderly patients. Adverse effects include drowsiness, dizziness, headache, dry mouth, and unpleasant taste, as well as mild and transient rebound insomnia and memory and psychomotor impairment. Effects on sleep stages appear similar to those seen with zolpidem and zaleplon. Although it may lie somewhere between the traditional benzodiazepines and zolpidem and zopiclone with respect to BZD$_1$ receptor specificity, a unique feature of eszopiclone is that FDA-approved labeling does not limit use to short-term treatment. This broad indication is based on the results of a double-blind, placebo-controlled study of 788 adults in which eszopiclone, at a dose of 3 mg, sustained its ability to induce and maintain sleep consistently for 6 months, with no evidence of tolerance, dependence, or abuse.[58]

Drug Withdrawal Insomnia and Rebound Insomnia. When barbiturates were used more commonly for the treatment of patients with insomnia, drug withdrawal insomnia was described as a phenomenon associated with abrupt discontinuation of the hypnotic after long-term use.[59] After long-term REM suppression, discontinuation led to REM rebound, which accounted for as much as 40% of total sleep time. This REM rebound was accompanied by very intense and frightening dreams, as well as a generally disrupted night of sleep. The patient generally did not understand the nature of the phenomenon and therefore was likely to return immediately to long-term, high-dose use. With gradual tapering of the drug or administration of an equivalent amount of a longer-acting agent and patient education regarding the possibility of temporarily increased dreaming and reduced quality of sleep, patients are better able to tolerate discontinuation of their hypnotics.

Recently, rebound insomnia has been described as a phenomenon associated with abrupt discontinuation of the shorter-acting BZDs (e.g., temazepam, triazolam)[60] and, to a lesser extent, other BZD agonists (e.g., zolpidem, zaleplon, eszopiclone). It involves worsening of sleep, even to levels beyond those noted before the patient was started on the drug. The exact incidence of this phenomenon is unclear, but it is prudent for the clinician to warn the patient about possible transient worsening of sleep immediately after the drug is stopped. Gradual tapering of the drug, rather than abrupt discontinuation, may lessen the severity of these withdrawal symptoms.[61] As an example, a patient who is taking

0.25 mg of triazolam every night for several weeks could reduce the dose by half (to 0.125 mg) for 3 nights, by half again (to one half of a 0.125-mg tablet) for the next 3 nights, and finally, discontinue the medication.

Problems and Controversies. Two important issues with insomnia and hypnotics are (1) that no one drug is ideal for every patient with insomnia, and (2) that not all patients with insomnia should be treated with hypnotics. As was previously stated, it is recommended that hypnotics be used primarily for the treatment of patients with transient or short-term insomnia. The implication is that a thorough assessment will be made of every patient with a complaint of insomnia. Although hypnotic-induced sleep may be unnatural in some respects, the ultimate measure of efficacy must be seen as optimal daytime performance.[62,63]

Some prescribers and patients believe that all hypnotics should be avoided because of the possibility that dependence may ensue. If hypnotics are used appropriately, that is, for brief periods and at low doses, the risk is low. Also, drug dependence insomnia, in which sleep worsens with long-term use of hypnotics even while the patient continues to take the drug, should not be a problem. In many respects, our society has been responsible for many of the transient insomnias (e.g., jet lag, work shift change, situational insomnia) and must take responsibility, either pharmacologically or nonpharmacologically, for assisting with the problem.

General Clinical Guidelines. A careful diagnostic assessment is necessary before any patient with insomnia is treated. See Table 55.7 for ideas on what types of questions clinicians

TABLE 55.7	Important Questions to Ask in Assessing a Sleep Complaint

How long have you had this problem?

What is your normal bedtime/sleep pattern and has it changed recently?

How long do you usually sleep? Do you go to sleep at about the same time each night? Do you take daytime naps?

How long does it take you to fall asleep? How often do you wake up during the night? What time do you wake up? Are you able to fall back to sleep?

Have you been experiencing pain, worry, stress, or work or family problems recently that could be associated with your sleep problem?

Do you suffer from any emotional or physical illness?

Do you consume any drugs, alcohol, or caffeine-containing foods or beverages?

Has your bed partner observed any snoring or unusual movements?

How do you feel upon awakening and during the day: tired, depressed, sleepy, irritable?

Do any of your relatives suffer from poor sleep?

Does anything help your sleep: sleeping pills, exercise, or sleeping in another room?

should ask when screening a patient with sleep complaints. The clinician should do the following: Do not allow your own experiences to interfere with your assessment. Unfortunately, because most of us have had at least an occasional bout of insomnia, we may too easily assume that everyone else's problems are similar to our own. Clarify the complaint and do a drug history. Assess the possibility that the problem is drug induced. Ask about stimulating drugs such as sympathomimetic decongestants or caffeine. Look for CNS depressant withdrawal such as moderate to heavy ethanol intake at dinner time. Assess the contribution of street drugs. In addition, consider sedating drugs and self-induced sleep deprivation as causes of excessive daytime sleepiness. Finally, find out what, if anything, has worked for the same problem in the past. Ask whether the problem is one of insomnia or excessive daytime sleepiness. Patients may be excessively sleepy if they have obstructive sleep apnea or narcolepsy. If it is a case of self-induced sleep deprivation (e.g., studying for examinations), caffeine tablets may be appropriate for short-term use, but evaluate possible drug–disease interactions (e.g., hypertension), and tell the patient about sleep hygiene. If the complaint is of insomnia, determine whether it is transient or chronic. If transient, a nonprescription sleep aid containing doxylamine or diphenhydramine may be worth a try for a few nights, but tell the patient about anticholinergic effects and possible morning hangover, and consider alternatives if the antihistamine is ineffective or intolerable. If insomnia is chronic, the patient deserves as meticulous an evaluation as the patient who comes in with a complaint of chronic stomach pain or unremitting, chronic headache. There are many reasons for chronic insomnia, and a number of them are treatable. Finally, be prepared for appreciation and praise. If treatable and responsive insomnia is identified in only one patient a year, the change in quality of life will make that patient forever grateful.

Until recently, when a decision was made to treat patients with insomnia pharmacologically, BZDs have been the treatment of choice; pharmacokinetic differences play a major role in the decision of which benzodiazepine should be used. Zolpidem, zaleplon, and eszopiclone offer even more options. In drug selection, the clinician must take into account onset of action and duration with respect to single versus multiple dosing and past history of response. If possible daytime impairment associated with accumulation of long-acting active metabolites (especially in elderly patients) is a concern, flurazepam and quazepam should be avoided; instead, one of the shorter-acting BZDs, zolpidem, or zaleplon should be chosen. Also, the clinician must recall that accumulation becomes a much greater concern with continuous use over several nights than with infrequent use as needed (in which drug action is terminated as quickly as it can be redistributed out of brain tissue). If the possible delayed onset of action of temazepam is a concern, one should choose the more rapidly acting flurazepam, triazolam, zolpidem, zaleplon, eszopiclone, or, perhaps, estazolam. If possible anterograde amnesia is a concern, the clinician should use very low doses, caution the patient, and consider avoiding hypnotic use in situations in which drug effects may not have worn off by the time the patient needs to be awake, alert, and fully functioning. Choices do not always have to be limited to the agents specifically marketed as hypnotics. For instance, diazepam is superior to flurazepam in onset of action, and yet, it shares the property of accumulation of a long-acting active metabolite under multiple-dosing conditions. In general, the choice of drug is based on pharmacokinetic profile and benefits sought.

Hypnotics should be avoided in patients with sleep apnea, patients who use alcohol or other CNS depressants heavily, pregnant patients, and patients in whom alert nighttime performance is mandatory (e.g., firemen, pilots). Although the BZD agonists are relatively safe, one must be cautious in giving them to patients with a high suicidal risk. Patients who overdose often use combinations of agents, frequently washing down everything with alcohol. The combination of BZD agonists with alcohol can be fatal. Most likely, an additive or synergistic mechanism is the basis for these interactions, resulting in impaired psychomotor functioning and excess sedation. Acute ethanol ingestion appears to enhance BZD absorption, decrease the volume of distribution, and impair elimination (as a result of hepatic enzyme inhibition). Zolpidem, zaleplon, and eszopiclone appear to have additive, not synergistic, effects when combined with alcohol, and it is recommended that these agents not be taken in combination with alcohol.

The benefit that the patient is seeking must be determined. Ideally, the patient is looking for outcomes of both improved sleep and improved daytime functioning. Simply increasing the number of hours of sleep is generally not a sufficient goal when one is prescribing hypnotics. When a particular hypnotic has been chosen, the lowest effective dose needed to achieve clear-cut benefit is used. This requires periodic follow-up with the patient, quantification of results, and education of the patient about the need to begin with a low dose and give it an adequate trial. For flurazepam, this is 15 mg; with triazolam in an elderly patient, the dose is 0.125 mg, or perhaps even half of a 0.125-mg tablet; for zolpidem, the dose is 5 mg in the elderly and 10 mg in the healthy adult. The importance of starting with a low dose cannot be overstated. For instance, with flurazepam, the optimal effect may not be experienced for 2 to 3 days, possibly because of slow accumulation of N-desalkylflurazepam. In addition, especially in elderly patients, daytime sequelae must be monitored. These are important educational and monitoring roles for the pharmacist. Questions that should be asked of patients when one is monitoring hypnotic effects and adverse effects are listed in Table 55.8. Drug–drug and drug–disease interactions should be identified and avoided. Examples of drug–drug interactions include additive CNS depression when hypnotics are combined with other CNS depressants, and accumulation of flurazepam, quazepam, and their long-acting metabolite N-desalkylflurazepam in the presence of cimetidine (which interferes with oxidative metabolic pro-

TABLE 55.8	Important Questions to Ask in Monitoring Hypnotic Therapy

Is your sleep improved?

Are you taking the medication as it was prescribed?

Have you increased your dose or taken a second dose at night?

Are you experiencing undesirable sleepiness in the morning or during the day?

Are you awakening early?

Have you noticed changes in your mood, behavior, or memory?

Are you more nervous, irritable, or anxious than usual?

Are you having problems with dizziness, unsteadiness, or light-headedness?

cesses) or other enzyme inhibitors. A primary drug–disease interaction is seen with the use of an agent that requires oxidative metabolic transformation (e.g., flurazepam, quazepam) in the presence of liver disease or old age. If one of the older nonbenzodiazepines is prescribed, the effect of liver enzyme induction must be kept in mind, as should the additive effects associated with other CNS depressants. With zolpidem, one must recall that the elimination half-life is increased approximately fourfold in the presence of hepatic cirrhosis. Potent CYP3A4 inhibitors (e.g., itraconazole, clarithromycin, ritonavir) can decrease serum concentrations of eszopiclone and prolong its duration of action; conversely, 3A4 inducers (e.g., rifampin) may decrease serum concentrations and reduce the effectiveness of eszopiclone. In either case, appropriate dosage adjustments must be made.

The issue of hypnotic use in patients with chronic insomnia is complex. With the exception of eszopiclone, few data are available regarding the efficacy and safety of hypnotics when taken for longer than 1 to 2 months. In addition, no evidence indicates that long-term hypnotic use produces lasting, objective improvement in sleep and daytime function in patients with many of the persistent insomnias. Therefore, if hypnotics are prescribed, the goals with chronic insomnia should generally consist of pulsed, intermittent treatment and periodic medical reevaluation. Indeed, for many patients with chronic insomnia, the underlying problem is a psychiatric condition, drug or alcohol dependence, sleep apnea, or delayed sleep phase syndrome. Treatments specific to the disorder and nonpharmacologic approaches should be tried first. If psychiatric and medical disorders have been ruled out and nonpharmacologic approaches have failed, referral to a sleep disorders center would be appropriate. In the rare instances in which a thorough sleep evaluation has been done and a hypnotic is used to treat chronic insomnia (e.g., periodic limb movement disorder), the patient should be evaluated often so that improvement in both sleep and daytime functioning can be detected and the persistence of therapeutic effect at a constant dose assessed. The reason for this, at least with the typical BZDs, is that longer-term use carries an increased risk of dependence, tolerance with resulting escalation of dose, and difficult withdrawal.

Patient education should include emphasis on short-term use, discussion of possible daytime sedation and impairment with longer-acting agents, the importance of avoiding other CNS depressants, and again, at least with the typical BZDs, the risks of tolerance and dependence if used for too long and/or at excessively high doses. If hypnotics are to be used for extended periods, it may be useful to suggest that a night or two be skipped occasionally. This allows the patient to see whether the drug is still really needed and may reduce the development of tolerance. When the drug is discontinued—ideally in a gradual, tapered way—the patient must be told about possible temporary withdrawal phenomena.

NONPHARMACOLOGIC THERAPY

Parasomnias. Fortunately, both somnambulism and sleep terrors are usually "outgrown." Treatment of a person who sleepwalks consists primarily of protecting him or her from harm. Interventions may include locking doors and windows at night and giving the sleepwalker a first floor bedroom. Again, for sleep terrors, treatment consists primarily of waiting for the disorder to be "outgrown." With respect to nightmares, after REM suppressant drug withdrawal is ruled out as the cause, psychological intervention is the usual treatment. Therapy may be as simple as a parent providing comfort and reassurance to a child with an occasional nightmare, or as complex as intensive psychotherapy provided for an adult with frequent, highly disturbing nightmares.[8]

Sleep Apnea. Treatment of patients with sleep apnea varies according to the type of sleep apnea that is under consideration. Sometimes, for obstructive sleep apnea, simple weight loss or removal of enlarged tonsils may solve the problem. At times, preventing the patient from sleeping on his or her back by sewing a tennis ball to the back of the nightshirt can lead to a significant decrease in apneic episodes. When life-threatening complications of repeated episodes of hypoxemia (e.g., arrhythmias, pulmonary hypertension, right ventricular failure) occur, aggressive intervention should be considered. A rather elegant plastic surgical procedure performed in some patients is the uvulopalatopharyngoplasty; it involves major reconstruction of the pharyngeal airspace. Unfortunately, in many cases, long-term follow-up has been lacking. Other, less dramatic surgical procedures—some involving laser surgery—have been performed recently. A helpful and commonly used approach is continuous positive airway pressure.[10,11] A small device is placed beside the bed and is connected by a tube to a facial mask worn by the patient throughout the night. This device, which is initially calibrated during one or two nights in a sleep disorders center, provides a continuous flow of air, which keeps the airway open. For many patients who are appropriately counseled and learn to tolerate the noise, mucosal drying, and minor discomfort of the facial mask, the

technique can have a major impact on the quality of sleep and resultant daytime functioning. Adhesive strips designed to spread open the nostrils may be of benefit, but probably only to those patients whose primary problem is characterized by constricted nasal passages that have the potential for such mechanical opening. Finally, various dental appliances designed to pull the tongue forward and maintain an open airway can be used.

Narcolepsy. Nonpharmacologic treatment of patients with narcolepsy includes several interventions. The patient and family members must be educated about the disorder to dispel the misconception that the patient is simply a lazy, unmotivated, nonproductive person. Local and national support groups are available. In addition, careful scheduling of daytime naps can be particularly helpful. The patient may feel fairly refreshed for up to several hours following a 15- or 20-minute nap.

Insomnia. Some general rules of sleep hygiene that can be recommended for both persistent and transient insomnias are presented in Table 55.9. In addition, other nonpharmacologic approaches are available. These include desensitization, meditation, biofeedback, and stimulus control, among others.[64] Indeed, in one small, randomized, placebo-controlled trial, cognitive behavioral therapy was found to be superior to zolpidem in patients with sleep-onset insomnia.[65] Patients with delayed sleep phase syndrome can be treated by chronotherapy or light therapy.[26,66] Because the patient with delayed sleep phase syndrome can sleep but is sleepy at the wrong time of the 24-hour day, chronotherapy provides a means of adjusting the internal clock by 2- to 3-hour blocks each day until sleep occurs at the desired time.

ALTERNATIVE THERAPIES

One amino acid, L-tryptophan, became popular as a natural hypnotic because it is a precursor to serotonin, a neurotransmitter that seems to be significantly involved in the regulation of sleep and wakefulness. L-Tryptophan had never been approved by the FDA as a hypnotic, but it was sold as a food supplement. The overall efficacy of this agent is unclear. Positive response is unpredictable because the predictors of response have never been clearly identified.[67] Some 1,500 cases (including 24 fatalities) of eosinophilia-myalgia syndrome associated with the use of L-tryptophan have been reported to the US Centers for Disease Control (CDC) in Atlanta.[68] The CDC defines this L-tryptophan–associated eosinophilia-myalgia syndrome as (1) an increase in eosinophils to counts above $1,000/mm^3$; (2) myalgia that interferes with daily activities; and (3) the absence of some other identifiable cause (e.g., parasites, leukemia). Although the nature of this association is unclear (e.g., there has been strong speculation that some contaminant was accidentally introduced into the bulk supplies shipped from overseas through use of a new strain of bacillus in the production process),

TABLE 55.9	Sleep Hygiene: Suggestions for Improved Sleep

1. Set a regular time to go to bed and a regular time to wake up. Regularity is a key component to improving sleep. You must set these times and adhere to them as diligently as possible. At least as important as a regular bedtime is the establishment of a regular wake-up time. No matter how long it took to fall asleep, no matter how little sleep you have had, and no matter how flexible your morning schedule is, there should be no "sleeping in." This would only further confuse and disorganize the internal biologic clock (i.e., the circadian pacemaker).

2. Engage in regular, moderate exercise early in the day; do not exercise vigorously in the evening. Heavy exercise too late in the evening can lead to a worsening of sleep in all but the best-conditioned athlete; therefore, for most of us, heavy exercise should be scheduled earlier in the day.

3. Generally avoid daytime naps. The idea is to consolidate sound, solid sleep through the night. Satisfying some of your sleep need during the day may prevent this. The exception is the person who routinely takes a daytime nap (e.g., the "siesta"); such a person generally has a somewhat shorter than average night of sleep.

4. Eat a light snack or beverage before bedtime if hungry; do not eat heavy or spicy food in the evening and do not eat late evening meals or drink large quantities of liquids in the evening. A heavy meal late in the evening can severely disrupt sleep in the patient with gastroesophageal reflux (e.g., "heartburn"). Too much liquid can result in multiple awakenings to go to the bathroom.

5. Make the bedroom as comfortable and secure as possible. You should attempt to see that the bedroom is dark and quiet and is neither too hot nor too cold. Although minor fluctuations in room temperature and firmness of the mattress probably have little impact on sleep, extremes can be disturbing. A sense of security can also be quite important.

6. Use the bedroom only for activities associated with sleep. Although many of us, while in bed, use the bedroom for watching television, preparing work for the following day, eating snacks, and paying bills, the individual with a sleep problem needs to set the bedroom aside for sleep only. (Sexual activity may be an exception.) In addition, just as warm milk and cookies become a ritual for some children before bedtime, some adults must develop a similar relaxing ritual that can be a part of the stimulus for a sleep response.

7. If not asleep within 30 minutes, move to another room and engage in a boring or relaxing activity. Get out of bed, leave the bedroom, and do something nonstimulating; for some this would be watching a late night talk show on television and for others it might be reading one's professional journals. After some 20 to 60 minutes, another attempt should be made to fall asleep. The idea is to not spend too much time in bed awake; an association between the bed and an inability to fall asleep can simply compound the problem.

8. Sleep only as much as needed to feel refreshed and alert during the day. Sleep need varies considerably among individuals. Discover for yourself what your sleep need is and satisfy it. Spending extra time in bed awake, thinking that you need to sleep more, may associate the bedroom with wakefulness rather than sleep.

9. Avoid or minimize use of caffeine (coffee, tea, and soft drinks), alcohol, and tobacco. Each person must discover how late such use can be tolerated. However, for the very sensitive, caffeine intake may need to be discontinued each day by noon. Although alcohol is often used as a self-treatment for relaxation and sleep induction, its rapid elimination during the first half of the night may result in some degree of withdrawal characterized by increased dreaming and nightmares as well as a general disruption of sleep during the latter half. In addition, nicotine may be stimulating in some persons.

10. Avoid routine use of hypnotics. Although hypnotics can be very effective for short-term treatment of a variety of insomnias, long-term use may result in a type of drug dependence insomnia characterized by sleep that is even worse than it was before use of the drug. If the sleep difficulty persists despite following the preceding suggestions and perhaps even a brief trial of nonprescription hypnotics, discuss the problem with a physician or pharmacist. Consider learning relaxation techniques or hypnosis. Some people simply need to be able to relax sufficiently to allow sleep to occur. Consider psychotherapy; because at least 35% of all patients seen in sleep disorders centers for complaints of insomnia have an identifiable psychiatric or psychological cause, some form of psychotherapy or psychiatric treatment may be helpful.

the FDA and the CDC have recommended that people should stop using this agent and that physicians should stop prescribing it. If L-tryptophan should come back into use, it should be noted that it is not a totally innocuous substance. Most commonly, people are bothered by its gastrointestinal irritation, which women who have been pregnant have compared with morning sickness. In addition, long-term use has been associated with niacin and pyridoxine deficiencies. The combination of L-tryptophan and a monoamine oxidase inhibitor (e.g., phenelzine, isocarboxazid, tranylcypromine) or fluoxetine may produce a ''serotonin syndrome,'' characterized by disorientation, agitation, hyperthermia, hyperreflexia, diaphoresis, ocular oscillations, and myoclonic jerking. Finally, low doses have been associated with changes in liver ultrastructure in normal rats and have been lethal in rats with adrenal insufficiency.

Melatonin, which is endogenously synthesized from serotonin and is secreted by the pineal gland, has recently become a popular ''natural'' self-treatment for patients with a variety of disorders. Exogenous melatonin products have not been approved by the FDA but are available in health food stores. Limited studies of doses generally ranging from 0.3 to 5 mg have demonstrated efficacy in the treatment of patients with insomnia, especially that associated with jet lag.[69]

However, it remains unclear what the optimal dose and administration times are, and a 2004 evidence-based report published by the Agency for Healthcare Research and Quality demonstrated overall lack of efficacy in the treatment of patients with all sleep disorders, with the possible exception of delayed sleep phase syndrome.[70] Large, controlled trials are needed because long-term efficacy is unclear and little is known about adverse effects, particularly long-term effects. In addition, the sources and purity of products sold in health food stores are uncertain. Synthetic melatonin agonists have recently been developed and are undergoing study.

Other natural products include valerian and kava kava. Similar to BZDs, both have been used in the treatment of patients with anxiety and insomnia, appear to act through central γ-aminobutyric acid (GABA) systems, and, at least in the case of kava kava, can interact with other CNS depressants (e.g., ethanol, alprazolam).[57,71] Both have been associated with hepatotoxicity. Until additional systematic studies have been conducted, as is also true for melatonin, patients should be cautioned with respect to what we do not know regarding safety, efficacy, purity, and sources.

IMPROVING OUTCOMES

As was discussed earlier (see the section on general clinical guidelines), clinicians can improve outcomes in patients with sleep disorders by first assuring that a careful and thorough assessment of the sleep complaint is completed. When this has been accomplished, therapy should be as specific as possible for the disorder identified. In all cases, it should be remembered that insomnia is a symptom, not a disorder. Helping the patient understand the nature of the disorder, the goals of treatment, and the importance of adhering to therapy and practicing good sleep hygiene all contribute to positive outcomes. Lastly, monitoring of therapeutic and adverse effects should be frequent and comprehensive.

PHARMACOECONOMICS

The significant impact of sleep disturbances on the many aspects of our lives is becoming increasingly clear. The US Department of Transportation estimates that up to 10% of automobile accidents are directly related to sleepiness, accounting for costs of $29 billion in fatalities and disabling injuries.[72] It is estimated that of the 25% of Americans who perform shift work, at least 60% have a chronic sleep disorder. Sleep disorders have been estimated to be responsible for 52% of work-related accidents, at a cost of $24 billion.[73] The relatively small cost of treatment far outweighs the cost of not treating patients with insomnia and other sleep disorders.

CONCLUSION

Sleep is a fascinating psychophysiologic phenomenon that is cyclic and can be measured electrophysiologically. Much is now known about sleep and its disorders, but sleep disorders medicine is young. Millions of patients have a variety of sleep disorders. They are a heterogeneous group of disorders capable of producing major social and/or occupational disability; disturbed sleep can be crippling for many people. With appropriate assessment and treatment, the transient insomnias can be managed to improve both nighttime sleep and daytime performance. Although there may be no cures for many of the persistent insomnias such as sleep apnea, enhanced understanding of these disorders is leading to prevention of harm to patients caused by inadequate assessment or inappropriate use of hypnotics. Further, with better assessment and increased referral by pharmacists, many patients with some of the persistent insomnias (e.g., psychiatric disorders, delayed sleep phase syndrome) can be helped significantly.

Sleep complaints deserve the same meticulous assessment and concern as complaints of chest pain, flank pain, or coughing up of blood. Disorders of excessive daytime sleepiness (obstructive sleep apnea and narcolepsy), problems with insomnia (transient and persistent types), and unusual behaviors and mental activity during sleep (sleepwalking, sleep terrors, and nightmares) have been described. Not all patients with sleep complaints should be treated with hypnotics; indeed, some sleep disorders may be worsened through the use of hypnotics or other drugs.

Use of hypnotics is generally most appropriately reserved for the treatment of patients with transient or short-term insomnia. Although a number of hypnotics are available, the BZDs and BZD$_1$ receptor–specific nonbenzodiazepines are currently accepted as the drugs of choice; selection within these groups is based primarily on differences in pharmacokinetic profiles. The clinician has the opportunity to play an important role in assessing the disorder, recommending treatment, or recommending further evaluation for the many patients with complaints of insomnia or excessive daytime sleepiness. The pharmacist can play a major role in educating the patient about therapy and monitoring for therapeutic and adverse effects. With careful diagnosis and treatment tailored to the patient and his or her particular problem, more people will be sleeping better and performing considerably better in their daily activities.

KEY POINTS

■ Treatment of patients with any of the sleep disorders is focused on normalizing sleep and, perhaps more important, improving daytime functioning and preventing the adverse consequences of disturbed sleep

- Any sleep complaint deserves the same meticulous attention as that afforded a complaint of chest pain, flank pain, or coughing up of blood; in assessing the sleep complaint, a distinction should be made between excessive daytime sleepiness, insomnia, and phenomena associated with specific sleep stages or sleep–wake transitions
- Sleep is an active, cyclic, psychophysiologic phenomenon the function of which is unclear, but the need for which is certain
- Parasomnias include delta sleep phenomena (e.g., sleepwalking, sleep terrors) and REM sleep phenomena (e.g., nightmares)
- In the case of excessive daytime sleepiness, consideration should be given to obstructive sleep apnea (characterized by repeated episodes of cessation of breathing, each terminated by a brief arousal, and often associated with loud snoring) and narcolepsy (characterized by excessive daytime sleepiness, cataplexy, sleep paralysis, and hypnagogic hallucinations), as well as self-imposed sleep deprivation
- A key guideline in the management of sleep apnea is to avoid use of all CNS depressants
- Pharmacologic treatment of patients with narcolepsy is directed toward the excessive daytime sleepiness (e.g., CNS stimulants, modafinil) and the cataplexy (e.g., protriptyline, SSRIs, sodium oxybate)
- Insomnia is a symptom, not a disease. Attempts must be made to distinguish between acute and chronic types and to identify the causes; both drug (e.g., CNS stimulants, CNS depressant withdrawal, use of ethanol) and nondrug factors (e.g., psychiatric disorders, medical disorders, circadian rhythm disorders, poor sleep hygiene) must be considered. If a treatable cause is identified (e.g., major depression), the specific treatment appropriate for that problem (e.g., antidepressant) should be primary
- The goal of treatment of patients with insomnia, including use of nondrug approaches (e.g., improved sleep hygiene), should be to improve both sleep and daytime functioning
- In general, patients with short-term insomnia are most appropriately treated with hypnotics, and the drugs of choice are the BZDs (e.g., flurazepam, temazepam, triazolam, quazepam, estazolam) and the BZD_1 receptor–specific nonbenzodiazepines (e.g., zolpidem, zaleplon, eszopiclone); selection of an agent is based on differences in pharmacokinetic profiles and the needs of the individual patient
- Antihistamines (e.g., hydroxyzine, diphenhydramine, doxylamine) may be used for mild, short-term insomnia, with due caution in light of their strong anticholinergic properties and high incidence of ''morning hangover''

- Trazodone and other sedating antidepressants may improve sleep in patients with major depression who are being treated with stimulating SSRIs; patients must be monitored for possible orthostatic hypotension and, in the case of TCAs, for anticholinergic adverse effects
- Melatonin may be considered in patients with circadian rhythm disorders (e.g., jet lag)
- Kava kava and valerian, similar to BZDs, appear to act upon central γ-aminobutyric acid systems; however, similar to melatonin, they should be used only with recognition that quality assurance is sometimes less than adequate; that more information is needed with respect to appropriate indications, optimal dosing, short- and long-term adverse effects, and potential interactions; and that kava kava has been associated with hepatotoxicity

REFERENCES

1. Lockley SW, Cronin JW, Evans EE, et al. Effect of reducing interns' weekly work hours on sleep and attentional failures. N Engl J Med 351:1829–1837, 2004.
2. Landrigan CP, Rothschild JM, Cronin JW, et al. Effect of reducing interns' work hours on serious medical errors in intensive care units. N Engl J Med; 351:1838–1848, 2004.
3. Bixler EO, Kales A, Soldatos CR, et al. Prevalence of sleep disorders in the Los Angeles metropolitan area. Am J Psychiatry 136:1257–1262, 1979.
4. Ohayon MM, Caulet M, Guilleminault C. How a general population perceives its sleep and how this relates to the complaint of insomnia. Sleep 20:715–723, 1997.
5. The Gallup Organization for the National Sleep Foundation. Sleep in America: 1995. Princeton, NJ: The Gallup Organization, 1995.
6. Mellinger GD, Balter MB, Uhlenhuth EH. Insomnia and its treatments. ArchGen Psychiatry 42:225–232, 1985.
7. Wincor MZ, Johnson KA. Non-prescription hypnotics: purchase and pharmacist-patient interaction in the community pharmacy. Presented to: 14th European Symposium on Clinical Pharmacy; October 1985; Stockholm, Sweden.
8. Kales A, Soldatos CR, Kales JD. Sleep disorders: insomnia, sleepwalking, night terrors, nightmares, and enuresis. Ann Intern Med 106:582–592, 1987.
9. Ohayon M, Guilleminault C, Priest RG. Night terrors, sleepwalking, and confusional arousal in the general population: their frequency and relationship to other sleep and mental disorders. J Clin Psychiatry 60:268–276, 1999.
10. Flemons W. Obstructive sleep apnea. N Engl J Med 347:498–504, 2002.
11. Caples SM, Garni A, Aboud F, et al. Obstructive sleep apnea. Ann Intern Med 142:187–197, 2005.
12. Overeem S, Mignot E, GirtvanDijk J, et al. Narcolepsy: clinical features, new pathophysiologic insights, and future perspectives. J Clin Neurophysiol 18:78–105, 2001.
13. Ancoli-Israel S, Kripke DF, Klauber MR, et al. Sleep-disordered breathing in community-dwelling elderly. Sleep 14:486–495, 1991.
14. Ancoli-Israel S, Kripke DF, Klauber MR, et al. Periodic limb movements in sleep in community-dwelling elderly. Sleep 14:496–500, 1991.
15. Coleman R, Roffwarg H, Kennedy S, et al. Sleep-wake disorders based on a polysomnographic diagnosis: a national cooperative study. JAMA 247:997–1003, 1982.
16. Radecki SE, Brunton SA. Management of insomnia in office-based practice: national prevalence and therapeutic patterns. Arch Fam Med 2:1129–1134, 1993.

17. España RA, Scammell TE. Sleep neurobiology for the clinician. Sleep 27:811–820, 2004.

18. Rechtschaffen A, Kales A, eds. A manual of standardized terminology, techniques and scoring system for sleep stages of human subjects. Washington DC: US Government Printing Office, 1968. Publication no. 204.

19. Karni A, Tanne D, Rubenstein BS, et al. Dependence on REM sleep of overnight improvement of a perceptual skill. Science 265: 679–682, 1994.

20. Bliwise DL. Sleep in normal aging and dementia. Sleep 16:40–81, 1993.

21. Mignot E. Sleep, sleep disorders and hypocretin (orexin). Sleep Medicine 5 (Suppl 1):S2–S8, 2004.

22. Sleep Disorders Classification Committee, Association of Sleep Disorders Centers. Diagnostic classification of sleep and arousal disorders. Sleep 2:1–137, 1979.

23. American Academy of Sleep Medicine. International classification of sleep disorders, revised: diagnostic and coding manual. Chicago, Ill: American Academy of Sleep Medicine, 2001.

24. American Psychiatric Association. Diagnostic and statistical manual of mental disorders, 4th edition, text revised. Washington DC: American Psychiatric Association, 2000.

25. Carskadon MA, Dement WC, Mitler MM, et al. Self reports versus sleep laboratory findings in 122 drug-free subjects with complaints of chronic insomnia. Am J Psychiatry 133:1382–1388, 1976.

26. Wyatt K. Delayed sleep phase syndrome: pathophysiology and treatment options. Sleep 27:1195–1203, 2004.

27. Zammit GK, Weiner J, Damato N, et al. Quality of life in people with insomnia. Sleep 22 (Suppl 2):S379–S385, 1999.

28. Bonnet MH, Dexter JR, Arand DL. The effect of triazolam on arousal and respiration in central sleep apnea patients. Sleep 13: 31–41, 1990.

29. Whyte KF, Gould GA, Airlie MA. Role of protriptyline and acetazolamide in the sleep apnea/hypopnea syndrome. Sleep 11: 463–472, 1988.

30. Strohl KP, Hensley MJ, Saunders NA, et al. Progesterone administration and progressive sleep apneas. JAMA 245:1230–1232, 1981.

31. Tojima H, Kunitomo F, Kimura H, et al. Effects of acetazolamide in patients with the sleep apnea syndrome. Thorax 43:113–118, 1988.

32. Mitler M, Hayduk R. Benefits and risks of pharmacotherapy for narcolepsy. Drug Safety 25:791–809, 2002.

33. Littner M, Johnson SF, McCall V, et al. Practice parameters for the treatment of narcolepsy: an update for 2000. Sleep 24:451–456, 2001.

34. US Modafinil in Narcolepsy Study Group. Randomized trial of modafinil for the treatment of pathological somnolence in narcolepsy. Ann Neurol 43:88–97, 1998.

35. Schwartz JRL, Hirshkowitz M, Erman MK, et al. Modafinil as adjunct therapy for daytime sleepiness in obstructive sleep apnea: a 12-week, open-label study. Chest 124:2192–2199, 2003.

36. US Xyrem® Multicenter Study Group. A randomized, double blind, placebo-controlled multicenter trial comparing the effects of three doses of orally administered sodium oxybate with placebo for the treatment of narcolepsy. Sleep 25:42–49, 2002.

37. US Xyrem® Multicenter Study Group. A 12-month, open-label, multicenter extension trial of orally administered sodium oxybate for the treatment of narcolepsy. Sleep 1:31–35, 2003.

38. Mitler MM, Browman CP, Menn SJ, et al. Nocturnal myoclonus: treatment efficacy of clonazepam and temazepam. Sleep 9:385–392, 1986.

39. Trenkwalder C, Walters AS, Hening WA. Periodic limb movements and restless legs syndrome. Neurol Clin 14:629–650, 1996.

40. Hening W, Allen R, Earley C, et al. The treatment of restless legs syndrome and periodic limb movement disorder. Sleep 22:970–999, 1999.

41. Bliwise DL, Freeman A, Ingram CD, et al. Randomized, double-blind, placebo-controlled, short-term trial of ropinirole in restless legs syndrome. Sleep Medicine 6:141–147, 2005.

42. Kales AK, Bixler EO, Kales JD, et al. Comparative effectiveness of nine hypnotic drugs: sleep laboratory studies. J Clin Pharmacol 17: 207–213,1977.

43. Kales A, Allen C, Scharf MB, et al. Hypnotic drugs and their effectiveness: all night EEG studies of insomniac subjects. Arch Gen Psychiatry 23:226–232, 1970.

44. Teutach G, Mahler DL, Brown CR, et al. Hypnotic efficacy of diphenhydramine, methapyrilene, and pentobarbital for nighttime sedation. Clin Pharmacol Ther 17:195–201, 1975.

45. Nierenberg AA, Adler LA, Peselow E, et al. Trazodone for antidepressant-associated insomnia. Am J Psychiatry 151:1069–1072, 1994.

46. National Institute of Mental Health, Consensus Development Conference. Drugs and insomnia: the use of medications to promote sleep. JAMA251:2410–2414, 1984.

47. Ray WA, Griffin MR, Downey W. Benzodiazepines of short and long elimination half-life and the risk of hip fracture. JAMA 262: 3303–3307,1989.

48. Ashton H. Guidelines for the rational use of benzodiazepines: when and what to use. Drugs 48:25–40, 1994.

49. Wincor MZ. Insomnia and the new benzodiazepines. Clin Pharm 1: 425–432, 1982.

50. Kales A, Kales JD. Sleep laboratory studies of hypnotic drugs: efficacy and withdrawal effects. J Clin Psychopharmacol 3:140–150, 1983.

51. Rickels K. Clinical trials of hypnotics. J Clin Psychopharmacol 3: 133, 1983.

52. Greenblatt DJ, Harmatz JS, Englehardt N, et al. Pharmacokinetic determinants of dynamic differences among three benzodiazepine hypnotics. Arch Gen Psychiatry 46:326–332, 1989.

53. Bunney WE, Azarnoff DL, Brown BW, et al. Report of the Institute of Medicine committee on the efficacy and safety of Halcion. Arch Gen Psychiatry 56:349–352, 1999.

54. Pierce MW, Shu VS. Efficacy of estazolam: the United States clinical experience. Am J Med 88 (Suppl 3A):6–11, 1990.

55. Kales A. Quazepam: hypnotic efficacy and side effects. Pharmacotherapy 10:1–12, 1990.

56. Langtry HD, Benfield P. Zolpidem: a review of its pharmacodynamic and pharmacokinetic properties and therapeutic potential. Drugs 40:291–313,1990.

57. Wagner J, Wagner ML, Hening WA. Beyond benzodiazepines: alternative pharmacologic agents for the treatment of insomnia. Ann Pharmacother 32:680–691, 1998.

58. Krystal AD, Walsh JK, Laska E, et al. Sustained efficacy of eszopiclone over six months of nightly treatment: results of a randomized, double-blind, placebo-controlled study in adults with chronic insomnia. Sleep 26:795–799, 2003.

59. Kales A, Bixler E, Tan T, et al. Chronic hypnotic-drug use: ineffectiveness, drug-withdrawal insomnia, and dependence. JAMA 227: 513–517, 1974.

60. Kales A, Scharf M, Kales J. Rebound insomnia: a new clinical syndrome. Science 201:1039–1041, 1978.

61. Schweizer E, Rickels K, Case G, et al. Long-term therapeutic use of benzodiazepines—II. Effects of gradual taper. Arch Gen Psychiatry 47:908–915, 1990.

62. Gillin JC, Byerley WF. The diagnosis and management of insomnia. N Engl J Med 322:239–247, 1990.

63. Everett DE, Avorn J, Baker MW. Clinical decision-making in the evaluation and treatment of insomnia. Am J Med 89:357–362, 1990.

64. Morin CM, Culbert JP, Schwartz SM: Nonpharmacological interventions for insomnia: a meta-analysis of treatment efficacy. Am J Psychiatry 151:1172–1180, 1994.

65. Jacobs GD, Pace-Schott EF, Stickgold R, et al. Cognitive behavior therapy and pharmacotherapy for insomnia: a randomized controlled trial and direct comparison. Arch Intern Med 164:1888–1896, 2004.

66. Czeisler CA, Kronauer RE, Allan JS, et al. Bright light induction of strong (type O) resetting of the human circadian pacemaker. Science 244:1328–1333, 1989.

67. Schneider-Helmert D, Spinweber CL Evaluation of L-tryptophan for treatment of insomnia: a review. Psychopharmacology 89:1–7, 1986.

68. Raphals P. Disease puzzle nears solution. Science 249:619, 1990.

69. Turek FW, Gillette MU. Melatonin, sleep and circadian rhythms: rationale for development of specific melatonin agonists. Sleep Medicine 5:523–532, 2004.

70. Buscemi N, Vandermeer B, Pandya R, et al. Melatonin for treatment of sleep disorders. Summary, evidence report/technology assessment (No. 108). Rockville, Md: Agency for Healthcare Research and Quality, November 2004. AHRQ Publication No. 05-E002-1.

71. Almeida JC, Grimsley EW. Coma from the health food store: interaction between kava and alprazolam. Ann Intern Med 125:940–941, 1996.

72. US Department of Transportation, National Highway Traffic Safety Administration (NHTSA). The involvement of sleep in motor vehicle crashes. NHTSA memorandum. Washington DC: US Department of Transportation, NHTSA, US Government Printing Office, November 22, 1995.

73. Leger D. The cost of sleep-related accidents: a report of the national commission on sleep disorders research. Sleep 17:84–93, 1994.

Attention Deficit Hyperactivity Disorder

56

Stephanie J. Phelps

TREATMENT GOALS

- Ensure an accurate diagnosis of Attention Deficit Hyperactivity Disorder (ADHD) in a child or an adult, using DMS-IV criteria.
- Establish treatment goals jointly with the patient and the family.
- Address patient concerns and misconceptions about ADHD with emphasis on how the disorder has an impact on a person's behaviors, academic performance, and social interactions.
- Identify core symptoms that can be used to monitor positive and negative responses to therapy.
- Select optimal drug therapy after consideration of any preexisting comorbidities.
- Improve the person's academic or work performance and enhance his or her social skills without producing intolerable or significant adverse effects.
- Educate and counsel patients, parents, and teachers about ADHD and drug therapy.
- Tailor drug therapy (dose and interval) based on patient response and tolerance.
- Monitor for clinical or laboratory evidence of side effects.
- Recognize when and how to discontinue therapy.

DEFINITION

Attention-deficit/hyperactivity disorder (ADHD) is characterized by persistent patterns of inattention, hyperactivity, and impulsivity.[1] Although all children may occasionally exhibit inattentive and restless behavior, a person with ADHD displays inattention and/or hyperactivity to a degree that is debilitating and more pronounced than that seen in other persons at a similar level of development.

The first official diagnostic criteria, for what we now call ADHD, were published in 1980. Like most psychiatric disorders, ADHD is a clinical diagnosis that relies on patient history, physical assessment, neurologic examination, and behavioral evaluation. Unfortunately, the diagnosis does not currently involve laboratory assessment or radiologic confir-

mation. While early *Diagnostic and Statistical Manual of Mental Disorders* (DSM) criteria focused on hyperactivity,[2] the revised criteria were broadened to include and emphasize inattention and impulsivity.[3] The current DSM-IV criteria allow a clinician to subtype a child's disorder as predominantly hyperactive, predominantly inattentive, or a combination of both.[1] The DSM-IV diagnostic criteria are limited because they fail to consider the developmental nature of the disorder; hence ADHD may go undetected in many adults.

Approximately 65% of children with ADHD also have at least one comorbid disorder. These include learning disabilities, behavioral disorders, and/or psychiatric conditions. Each of these may impair a child's academic performance, affect the child's self-image, and alter the ability to interact with peers and family members. When left untreated, these comorbid factors may increase a person's risk of a serious psychopathologic disorder later in life.[4] Overall, children with ADHD have a 25-fold greater risk of institutionalization for delinquent behaviors, a 10-fold greater risk of developing antisocial personality disorders, and a 5-fold greater risk of drug abuse.[5]

During the 1970s and 1980s, media debates focused on the "labeling" of children with ADHD and on the use of stimulants to treat this disorder. Allegations by some suggested that the diagnosis of ADHD was either a "myth" or was merely applied to control children who displayed unwanted behaviors. Most now agree that ADHD is one of the best-studied disorders in medicine, and the data on its validity are more compelling than those for many other disorders.[4,6] To date, more than 170 studies involving more than 6,000 school-aged children with ADHD have been published.[4]

Whereas most believe that ADHD has a neurobiologic foundation, its pathophysiology remains elusive. Recent advances in molecular biology have given us a better understanding of the genetic basis for ADHD. Likewise, a new imaging technique (i.e., functional magnetic resonance imaging [fMRI]) has suggested a possible neuroanatomic basis for the disorder. Obviously, there has been increased interest in these areas and their possible use in the diagnosis and treatment of ADHD.

The management of ADHD is complex and requires a multimodal approach that uses nonpharmacologic and pharmacologic therapies. Once comorbid factors are considered, optimal treatment is individualized based on the clinician's recommendation and the family's preferences.

Pharmacotherapy for ADHD originated approximately 60 years ago. Today the ability of medications to ameliorate the core effects of ADHD is well established. Certain drugs including stimulants (i.e., methylphenidate, dextroamphetamine, pemoline, and Adderall), tricyclic antidepressants (TCAs), and clonidine are used more frequently. Other agents (i.e., monoamine oxidase inhibitors, bupropion, venlafaxine, fluoxetine, and carbamazepine) are reserved for patients with more refractory disorders.

PREVALENCE

Today, ADHD is the most common neurobehavioral disorder of childhood.[4] Although reports of its occurrence in children range from as low as 1.7% to as high as 16%,[4] the DSM-IV notes that prevalence rates in the United States are approximately 3% to 5% (i.e., greater than 2 million children).[1] However, these figures probably underestimate the true incidence because they do not include preschool, adolescent, or adult patients. Historically, the incidence in males has been four to nine times higher than that noted in females[4,5]; however, the disorder is now being diagnosed more frequently in girls so that the male to female ratio is 2:1.[7] ADHD accounts for 50% of referrals to child neurologists, neuropsychologists, behavioral pediatricians, and child

psychiatrists.[8] Although one usually associates ADHD with preschool or school-aged children, 70% to 80% of children with ADHD will continue to exhibit some symptoms into adolescence or will qualify for the diagnosis of a full disorder.[6] Approximately 65% to 80% will have the full disorder in late adolescence (16–19 years of age). Only a small percentage (3%–8%) of hyperactive children will retain the disorder into adulthood when the DSM-IV criteria are applied.[6] However, when developmentally referenced and empirically based definitions are used and parents serve as a source of information, 68% of subjects continue to exhibit symptoms of the disorder into adulthood.[6]

ETIOLOGY

Although many factors correlate with an increased risk of ADHD, most relationships are extremely weak and nonspecific. Several items including dietary (i.e., sugar consumption, food additives and dyes, vitamin deficiencies, or food allergies), environmental factors (i.e., lead poisoning or high voltage wiring), poor prenatal care (i.e., alcohol and nicotine exposure), birth complications (i.e., brain damage), and poor parenting have been considered in the etiology of ADHD. For years, there has been speculation that minimal brain damage or minimal brain dysfunction may be associated with ADHD. Recently, it was suggested that hypoxia and hypotension in utero could selectively damage neurons located in anatomic regions important in ADHD.[9] The above causes are supported largely by anecdotal information. Hence, there is little if any controlled evidence to support their role and they have been largely discounted.

Many family, twin, and adoption studies have suggested a genetic link in ADHD.[10] Studies in adopted children show that siblings of children with ADHD have two to three times the risk of developing ADHD than normal control subjects. Furthermore, the diagnosis of ADHD is more frequently shared in full siblings than in half siblings. The strongest support for a familial link for the disorder comes from the finding that twins sharing the same genetic material (monozygotic twins) have a higher probability of experiencing ADHD than nonidentical (dizygotic) twins.

Recently, molecular biologic techniques have attempted to define a specific DNA sequence associated with ADHD. Although a causative gene has not been definitively identified, two possible candidates have been proposed. Current hypotheses suggest that specific alleles of either the dopamine transporter (*DAT1*) gene[11] and/or the dopamine receptor D_4 (*DRD4*) gene[12] may result in altered dopamine transmission.

PATHOPHYSIOLOGY

Few patients with ADHD undergo invasive studies that allow for any direct examination of neuropathology. Likewise, noninvasive studies (i.e., routine neuroimaging and electroencephalogram [EEG]) are usually normal and are, therefore, noncontributory. Hence, many indirect lines of evidence (i.e., fMRI) have led to our current understanding of the pathophysiology of ADHD. The indirect approach begins with the observed inability of the child with ADHD to maintain attention and compares this to what is currently speculated about attention mechanisms in the brain.

One current theory maintains that the posterior regions of the brain allow a person to switch from one activity to another, whereas the frontal regions of the brain allow a person to maintain a specific activity. The posterior brain regions (i.e., parietal cortex, a region of the brain where sensory stimuli converge) switch attention to a new activity and then "hand off" to the frontal brain regions (i.e., anterior cingulate gyrus and prefrontal cortex) that maintain the attention to the new activity. In particular, the region of the frontal lobes of the brain referred to as the "prefrontal cortex" seems to be important in maintaining attention and "working memory." Working memory is felt to be a person's ability to maintain subject matter in the mind continuously and to manipulate the subject matter intellectually. Examples of working memory include adding or subtracting numbers in one's head or naming all the states that begin with the letter "M."

Indirect evidence suggests that children with ADHD may have problems activating the frontal lobe regions that manage working memory. Persons with documented neuroanatomic damage to the frontal lobes, and particularly to the right frontal lobe, demonstrate behavior that is similar to that of children with ADHD (e.g., short attention span, impulsivity, and hyperactivity). Damage to the inferior right frontal lobe (orbitofrontal cortex) seems to be associated more with impulsivity and hyperactivity, whereas damage to the lateral right frontal lobe (laterofrontal cortex) seems to be associated with difficulties in maintaining attention. A magnetic resonance imaging (MRI) study noted that children with ADHD have 10% smaller right frontal lobes than do matched-control children.[13] Likewise, Filipek et al.[14] reported that a group of children with ADHD had brain volumes about 10% smaller than normal in the anterior superior and anterior inferior regions.[14]

Neuropsychologic tests have been developed that are sensitive to neuroanatomic damage in the frontal lobes and to damage in the parietal lobes. These same tests suggest that children with ADHD have problems with measures of frontal lobe function, but perform normally on measures of parietal lobe function. Positron emission tomography (PET) scans of normal adults given tasks that should require use of working memory show a relative increase in metabolism in the frontal lobes during the task. Adults with ADHD persisting from childhood, but not currently on medication, show a relative decrease in frontal lobe metabolism by PET scan on the same tasks. Those adults, when given stimulant medication, show a "normalization" of the PET scan with increased frontal lobe activity during the tasks.

Animal studies support the contention that the attention mechanisms are modulated by neurotransmitter input from several regions of the brainstem. The ventral tegmental area of the upper brainstem supplies dopaminergic and noradrenergic neurotransmitter input to the orbitofrontal and laterofrontal cortex (prefrontal cortex). The dorsal raphe in the brainstem activates the ventral tegmental gray and also provides serotonergic neurotransmission diffusely to the cerebral hemispheres, especially to the anterior cingulate gyrus. The locus ceruleus in the brainstem inhibits the dorsal raphe and provides noradrenergic neurotransmitter input to the parietal cortex and laterofrontal cortex (prefrontal cortex). The noradrenergic receptors in the prefrontal cortex are primarily α_2-adrenergic.

One hypothesis is that the locus ceruleus may periodically activate the parietal cortex and allow for a change of attention to a new stimulus. When the activity of the locus ceruleus subsides, the dorsal raphe is able to activate the ventral tegmental gray, which then releases dopamine to the prefrontal cortex to maintain attention. Animal studies have shown that the activation of the prefrontal cortex inhibits the parietal cortex and the locus ceruleus, thus decreasing the effect of new, but distracting, sensory stimuli. Another hypothesis is that in children with ADHD, the locus ceruleus activates the parietal cortex, allowing the child to change attention to new stimuli, but that the transition to activation of the ventral tegmental gray and prefrontal cortex is deficient. Thus, the child with ADHD does not properly activate frontal lobe working memory and does not inhibit new sensory information arriving by way of the parietal cortex.

Stimulant medications such as methylphenidate and amphetamine are thought to improve attention in children with ADHD by increasing dopamine and noradrenaline in the prefrontal cortex by activating working memory and inhibiting distraction from new stimuli. Clonidine, an α_2-adrenergic stimulant, is thought to improve attention primarily by action at the α_2-adrenergic postsynaptic receptors of the laterofrontal regions in prefrontal cortex.

Current studies do not clearly elucidate what role the dorsal raphe and serotonin may play in disorders of attention. However, there is a subset of children with ADHD and obsessive compulsive behavioral features that seem to improve when given serotonergic medications and become worse with dopaminergic/adrenergic medications.

CLINICAL PRESENTATION AND DIAGNOSIS

SIGNS AND SYMPTOMS

Patients with ADHD display persistent patterns of inattention, hyperactivity, and impulsivity. The inattention associated with ADHD can manifest in various ways. Although these patients are physically present during a school lesson, their minds seem to be elsewhere, making them literally unavailable to learn. Homework, if done or not lost, is often messy and incomplete, and appears to have been done in a haphazard manner. These patients lack organizational ability and poorly grasp time/task management skills. It is common for them to fail to follow through on requests and to partially complete or ignore chores. They often make careless mistakes, pay little attention to details or instruction, and give partial effort to many tasks instead of completing one entire assignment. Patients with ADHD are easily distracted and quickly abandon current tasks to focus on even the most trivial stimuli. This is especially true as the complexity or difficulty of a task increases. In social settings, they appear bored, quickly lose interest in conversation and switch from one topic to the next. They have difficulty following prescribed rules of conduct, as well as game rules during play time.

The hyperactive person appears to have an endless source of energy that can seldom be repressed. Generally, an active curious child is considered healthy in our society; however, the child with ADHD exhibits hyperactivity to a degree that is problematic. Children with ADHD are often described as being constantly ''on the go'' or ''driven by a motor.'' They have trouble remaining seated for any length of time and constantly squirm and fidget. Hyperactivity is also manifested by an inability to play quietly when expected, by running or playing raucously when inappropriate, and by excessive talking. These children are often unable to get through ''quiet time'' without incident. Their disruptive classroom behavior frequently draws disciplinary actions. As a child with ADHD develops, the presentation of hyperactivity changes. Before 3 years of age, activity increases. After 3 years of age, activity begins a downward trend, so that hyperactivity is generally not present by adolescence. Awareness of this pattern is important for successful therapy because one might wrongfully assume that a patient who is no longer hyperactive does not need continued treatment.

Impulsivity often causes a child to be labeled disruptive or disrespectful. It can manifest itself as impatience and the immediate expression of thought without regard to setting (e.g., blurting out answers, comments, and emotions). Impulsive children often interrupt conversations and show extreme frustration when they are not allowed to talk. These patients grab inappropriate objects (e.g., a hot skillet or fragile items), intrude into other people's space or tamper with others' possessions, and act without regard for consequences.

Because the presentation varies with age, it is important to consider age when assessing clinical presentation. Most parents describe their ''normal'' preschool children as inattentive and hyperactive, therefore a diagnosis of ADHD is difficult in this age group. The preschool child with ADHD generally has additional symptoms such as temper tantrums, argumentative behavior, and aggressive or fearless behavior. They may also exhibit sleep disturbances.

During the school-age years cognitive work becomes increasingly difficult. Although they may have above average intelligence, they may seem immature for their age. Their school performance is affected by difficulty concentrating or focusing on assigned tasks. Hence, these children have greater school failure and grade-repeating rates. A combination of low self-esteem and impulsivity, hyperactivity, and/or inattention may lead to difficulty in peer relationships. During this time, elementary school children may also begin to exhibit comorbid symptoms (i.e., reading difficulty).

Previously, it was thought that children with ADHD outgrew the disorder by puberty; however, we now know that this is not true. The presentation of ADHD in adolescents has not been well established. Symptoms may change with increasing age such that fewer symptoms are considered indicative of ADHD. Symptoms may go unnoticed because students no longer have one teacher for all subjects or are not in one class all day. Their inattention and cognitive difficulties may lead to poorly organized approaches to schoolwork. Failing to complete independent academic work is a hallmark of ADHD in the adolescent. These adolescents are generally 2 academic years behind their contemporaries.[15] Unfortunately, there is no evidence that early treatment with psychostimulants alters their later academic achievement. During these years, adolescents want greater independence and desire same-sex and opposite-sex peer relationships. However, patients with antisocial behaviors secondary to ADHD may have difficulty developing and maintaining relationships. These patients may also begin to display risky behaviors including higher rates of accidents (e.g., auto and bike), suicide attempts, teen pregnancy, violence, and substance abuse.[6]

It is now known that 30% to 70% of children with ADHD will continue to display some symptoms as adults.[3] On average, symptoms diminish by about 50% every 5 years between the ages of 10 and 25 years. Hyperactivity declines more quickly than impulsivity or inattentiveness.[16] The presence of disorganization continues to have an impact in the workplace and frequently requires the person to keep an extensive list of activities as reminders. These persons may feel that they ''never get their act together.'' Poor concentration and procrastination may persist into adulthood, leading to shifting activities (e.g., moving from one activity to another), endless unfinished projects, and frequent job changes. They may also have problems sustaining long-term relationships. The presence of intermittent explosive outbursts may be related to comorbid symptomatology or may be a special type of ADHD associated with labile mood. Perhaps because the early diagnostic criteria focused on hyperactivity, a vast majority of adult patients with no childhood evaluation or treatment are women. Women in whom ADHD was undiagnosed in childhood may display a high incidence of mood disorders (e.g., anxiety).

Prospective studies have described three potential outcomes in children with ADHD.[17] The first outcome, ''developmental delay,'' occurs in 30% of subjects. These persons no longer manifest any functional impairment. The second outcome is called ''continual display'' and occurs in 40% of subjects. These persons continue to have functionally impairing symptoms into adulthood. In addition, they may have a variety of different types of social and emotional difficulties. The third outcome occurs in 30% of patients and is called "developmental decay." Although these persons continue to exhibit the core symptoms of ADHD, they also develop serious psychopathologic disorders such as alcoholism, substance abuse, and antisocial personality disorder.

COMORBID DISORDERS

For years clinicians have noted an association between certain comorbid disorders and ADHD. In fact, approximately 65% of children with ADHD have at least one comorbid disorder that includes a learning disability (i.e., reading disability or dyslexia) and/or psychiatric conditions.[4] Estimates of reading disability in patients with ADHD range from as low as 9%[18] to as high as 92%.[19] Children with ADHD are also more likely to perform below expectations in reading and arithmetic.[20]

Although we do not currently understand why these comorbid disorders are associated with ADHD, several theories have been suggested. Some believe that ADHD is actually a consequence of a learning disability, reflecting the cumulative effects of a lack of motivation and disinterest in school.[21] Other groups believe that a reading disorder does not reflect a true comorbidity. They feel that an attention disorder is a cognitive problem that many children with reading disorders have and that inattention does not represent the symptom complex associated with ADHD.[22] A third group contends that there are separate cognitive deficits in reading disorders and ADHD. For example, children with reading disorders had difficulty with tasks involving confrontation naming and rapid automatized naming, while children with ADHD had difficulty with word list learning and recall.[23] The fourth group simply postulates that reading disorders and ADHD represent separate diagnostic entities that frequently occur in the same patient.[24]

A number of psychiatric conditions occur with ADHD. Between 10% and 20% of children in community and clinical studies have mood disorders, 20% have conduct disorders, and up to 40% have oppositional defiant disorders.[25] Bipolar disorder is being increasingly recognized in patients with ADHD.[26] Only about 7% of those with ADHD have tics or Tourette's syndrome, but 60% of those with Tourette's syndrome have ADHD.[4]

DIAGNOSIS

Table 56.1 outlines the current diagnostic criteria for ADHD.[1] Over the years, an evolving understanding of the disorder has contributed to the dynamic nature of the criteria. The DSM-II characterized "hyperkinetic reactions of childhood" as a disorder caused by suppression or internalization of interpersonal problems.[27] Ten years later, the DSM-III classified the disease as "attention deficit disorder" (ADD), with or without hyperactivity.[2] In the DSM-III-R the symptom criteria were further modified to stress the importance and core inclusion of hyperactivity. The qualifier with or without hyperactivity was deleted and the term "attention-

TABLE 56.1	DSM-IV Diagnostic Criteria for Attention-Deficit/Hyperactivity Disorder

Symptoms Present Before Age 7

Impairment from symptoms is present in two or more distinct settings (e.g., school, home, work)

Clear evidence of significant impairment in social, academic, or occupational functioning

Six (or more) symptoms of inattention or hyperactivity for longer than 6 months

Inattention

Often fails to give close attention to details or makes careless mistakes in schoolwork, work, or other activities

Often has difficulty sustaining attention in tasks or play activities

Often does not seem to listen when spoken to directly

Often does not follow through on instructions and fails to finish assignments

Often has difficulty organizing task and activities

Often avoids or dislikes tasks that require sustained mental effort

Often loses things necessary for tasks or activities (e.g., toys, books, assignments)

Is often forgetful in daily activities

Hyperactivity–Impulsivity

Often fidgets with hands or feet or squirms in seat

Often leaves seat in classroom or situations in which remaining seated is expected

Often runs or climbs about excessively when inappropriate

Often has difficulty playing quietly

Is often on the go or acts as if "driven by a motor"

Often talks excessively

Often blurts out answers before questions have been completed

Often has difficulty waiting turn

Often interrupts or intrudes on others

(From American Psychiatric Association. Diagnostic and statistical manual of mental disorders. 4th ed. (DSM-IV). Washington, DC: American Psychiatric Association, 1994, with permission.)

deficit/hyperactivity disorder" (ADHD) was born.[3] In addition, the new criteria broadened the definition to provide an increased emphasis on attention problems.[1,4] To reduce the number of false-positive diagnoses, the current DSM-IV criteria require that symptoms begin before the age of 7, be present in at least two settings (e.g., home and school), and be continuously present for at least 6 months.[1] When applied correctly, the criteria result in high interrater reliability, good validity, and high predictability of prognosis and medication effectiveness. Unfortunately, the current criteria fail to address the developmental nature of this disorder. ADHD remains undiagnosed in many adults because a patient's clinical presentation changes with age.

The essential feature for diagnosis is a consistent and persistent pattern of hyperactivity, impulsivity, and/or inat-

label study in children and adolescents reported positive effects on hyperactivity and attention.[113]

Anticonvulsants. Although carbamazepine is extensively used in Europe for the treatment of ADHD, it is not approved by the FDA for this indication; hence, its use in the United States is limited. However, because carbamazepine has a tricyclic structure and is used as a mood-stabilizing agent, intuitively one might expect it to have some efficacy in ADHD. Overall, some therapeutic effects have been noted in approximately 70% of children.[118] Although rare, the hematologic and hepatotoxic effects of carbamazepine make it less ideal than the TCAs. No studies have evaluated the effects of phenytoin or valproate in patients with ADHD.

Other Agents. Antipsychotics (e.g., chlorpromazine, haloperidol, and thioridazine) reduce hyperactivity; however, they do not improve cognition or attention span.[119] They are less effective than the stimulants or TCAs and are associated with significant adverse reactions including extrapyramidal effects and tardive dyskinesia. In larger doses the antipsychotics decrease cognitive function and impair learning. For these reasons, this class of medications should be given in the lowest possible doses, and use should be limited to patients with severe ADHD unresponsive to other agents.

Benzodiazepines and barbiturates are ineffective and worsen ADHD by causing paradoxical excitement and agitation.[28,120] Amantadine,[121] caffeine,[122] fenfluramine,[123] and lithium[124] are also ineffective.

NONPHARMACOLOGIC THERAPY

Psychosocial treatment of ADHD originated from the belief that it may overcome the limitations associated with pharmacologically based therapy. Although medications have been shown to improve the core symptoms of ADHD, they fail to result in normalization of a person's functioning.[38,40,41] The benefits of medication tend to be short-lived and reverse on drug withdrawal. In addition, medications may produce unpleasant side effects and lower self-esteem.[69,71] Psychosocial interventions focus on the development of functional skills (academic/social) and adaptive behaviors that patients with ADHD lack. These therapies come in a variety of forms, which may be combined to meet the specific needs of the individual patient. Generally, greater success has been observed using more intensely structured programs (clinical behavioral or summer treatment programs), which encompass various environments (home, classroom, and play) and involve parents, teachers, and children.[125] Unfortunately, these modalities have consistently proven less effective than medications when used alone.[5,126]

Cognitive-behavioral therapy (self-instructional training, cognitive modeling, cognitive/interpersonal problem solving, self-monitoring, and self-reinforcement) may be taught to an individual patient or in groups. These interventions attempt to teach ADHD patients self-control skills and internal problem-solving techniques that will ultimately decrease impulsivity and improve behavior and academic perfor-

mance.[126] Although mechanistically attractive, this modality has proven ineffective in children with ADHD. Although initial improvements are noted, they quickly subside because of a lack of generalization to new environments and because the child is not motivated to apply the newly learned techniques.

Behavioral therapies (behavior modification, contingency management, and operant conditioning) involve the identification of a patient's undesirable behaviors and the environmental conditions that elicit and maintain them.[5] Ultimately, behavioral changes are produced using positive or negative reinforcers. One example is the token economy, in which children earn or lose stars, points, etc., for displaying appropriate or inappropriate behaviors. These tokens may be traded for things the child likes (toys or privileges). Time out is a similar approach in which negative behaviors are discouraged by putting the child in a nonstimulating environment. These tools may be used by parents and teachers to encourage positive behaviors at home and at school. Although behavioral therapies are generally considered more efficacious than cognitive treatments, they suffer from the same inability to be generalized to new situations. Despite the short-term academic and social improvements, normalization in inattention, hyperactivity, and impulsivity rarely occurs.[5,127]

Patients with ADHD often require additional interventions tailored to their specific needs. Social skills training helps facilitate interactions between parents, siblings, students, and peers. Group social training is preferred because patients with ADHD lack self-monitoring skills. In addition, this setting allows practice and modeling of newly learned behaviors. Academic skills training involves instruction in proper study habits, note and test taking, organizational/time management skills, and the ability to follow directions. It is particularly important that education occur in an environment with minimal distractions where careful attention can be paid to any specific learning disabilities. Individual psychotherapy may be a useful adjunct for patients with ADHD who have low self-esteem, comorbid depression, or in those with difficulty coping with the ADHD symptoms. Therapists may also assist in increasing medication compliance using contingency-contracting. Family psychotherapy is indicated for families with prior dysfunction or for those with problems stemming from raising a child with ADHD. This may also serve as a means to reinforce or implement behavioral interventions. Therapeutic recreation uses participation in sports or play activities to improve peer interactions and self-image.

The concept of multimodal therapy has become popular because no single treatment modality (medication or psychosocial) has succeeded in producing long-term normalization across all areas affected by ADHD. Although combined therapy and medication-only treatments perform similarly for most measures, this is not a universal finding.[6,49,128] Some studies suggest combined therapy may produce additional clinical gains in selected patients.[128] Likewise, it may prevent the reappearance of certain ADHD-associated behaviors once medications are discontinued.[129] In other studies, multimodal therapy has permitted the use of lower doses of medications.[130] Although the conclusions drawn from these studies are limited due to sample size, design flaws, or short duration, multimodal treatment may be an attractive option for some patients (e.g., those with dose-related side effects, incomplete responses to medications, or certain comorbid conditions).

ALTERNATIVE THERAPIES

Alternative therapies include any nonprescription or behavior therapies. Over the years elimination diets, macronutritional and micronutritional supplements, antifungal and thyroid treatments, deleading procedures, and herbal therapies have been administered. In addition, acupuncture and EEG and electromyogram biofeedback have been performed.

Elimination Diets. The simple elimination of sugar and candy from the diet of children does not appear to affect symptoms in children with ADHD. Several controlled studies have reported significant improvement compared with placebo or deterioration of condition with a placebo substituted for the offending substance. At this time it is not known what percentage of the ADHD population has diet-associated ADHD. Preliminary evidence suggests that these patients are middle or upper class preschool-aged patients with atopy and prominent irritability and sleep disturbances. They also have physical and behavioral symptoms. If an offending agent can be identified, it may be possible to successfully desensitize the patient.

Nutritional Supplements. A variety of nutritional supplements have been used to treat ADHD. Macronutrients (amino acids, essential fatty acids, and carbohydrates) and micronutrients (vitamins and minerals) have been used. Although patients with ADHD may have low levels of amino acids including serotonin, supplementation with tryptophan, tyrosine, or phenylalanine has not produced long-term benefits.[6]

Children with ADHD have lower total serum free fatty acid concentrations. Specifically, both the *n*-3 and *n*-6 series of fatty acids are lower in children with ADHD than in control patients. Neuronal membranes are composed of polyunsaturated fatty acids (i.e., *n*-3 and *n*-6 series), therefore a deficiency of these essential nutrients may affect development. Likewise, aggression has been inhibited in young adults given docosahexaenoic acid of the *n*-3 series. Two double-blind placebo-control studies involving administration of a *n*-6 series fatty acid had varied results.[6]

Several studies have evaluated the supplementation of vitamins and minerals in patients with ADHD. Megavitamin cocktails and megadoses of select vitamins have proven ineffective.[6] Studies have also investigated the supplementation of iron, zinc, and magnesium in patients with ADHD. Supplementation of iron to nonanemic patients with ADHD resulted in improved parent scores but not teacher ratings on the Conners Parent and Teacher Rating Scales. Furthermore, improvements in verbal learning and memory, and a decrease in hyperactivity have been noted. Although several animal studies and anecdotal human experience suggest that zinc deficiency is associated with hyperactivity, no prospective studies have been performed to support routine zinc supplementation in patients with ADHD. However, one group of investigators did suggest that response to stimulants may be dependent on adequate intake of zinc.[6] Another report noted that 95% of children with ADHD are deficient in magnesium.[6] While no placebo-control trials have been conducted, one study reported that Conners ratings were significantly decreased in patients receiving magnesium.[6]

Deleading. Animal and human data suggest that lead toxicity can cause neuropsychiatric symptoms. Lead serum concentrations as low as 10 µg per deciliter have been associated with behavioral and cognitive problems. Some have advocated that patients with ADHD and elevations in serum lead concentrations should be treated with penicillamine (calcium disodium edetate, if allergic to penicillin).[6]

Herbal Treatments. A few open label studies have been conducted in China using combinations of Chinese herbs or herbal liquors or syrups.[6] Although these reports have noted positive results, placebo-control double-blind studies are warranted. To date, no studies have been reported on gingko biloba, Calmplex, or Defendol.

FUTURE THERAPIES

Although the stimulants have proven their short-term effectiveness in numerous studies of ADHD, future research is attempting to develop new, safe, effective, and nonaddictive medications. The discoveries of the potential site of action of stimulants and a genetic loci possibly responsible for ADHD symptoms have directed focus on agents that modulate the dopaminergic and noradrenergic systems. New diagnostic techniques, such as fMRI, may better define the neurologic basis of ADHD, assist in objective diagnosis, and provide additional directions in which to target new therapies.

IMPROVING OUTCOMES

PATIENT EDUCATION

There are a variety of drug classes used in the treatment of ADHD, each with various side effects and monitoring parameters. Faced with managed care cost containment and increased patient loads, physicians often do not discuss issues related to drug therapy with patients. This leaves unanswered questions that may result in patient frustration and unsuccessful therapy. Unlike many medical conditions, patient counseling must address the proper use of the medications (Table 56.5) and the social stigma tied to many of the agents (i.e., stimulants and antidepressants) used to treat

TABLE 56.5	Attention-Deficit/Hyperactivity Disorder (ADHD) Medication Counseling Tips
Medication	**Counseling Advice**
Stimulants	This medication is the most common medication used to treat ADHD. It is very effective with rapidly noticeable benefits (increased attention, decreased impulsivity/hyperactivity).
	Take this medication with meals to avoid upset stomach. If weight loss is noted, then the dose may need to be decreased. Some ADHD patients perform unusual behaviors while taking this medication, if this occurs the dose may need to be lowered or the medication stopped.
	This medication may worsen certain health conditions. Consult your doctor/pharmacist if you have a history of heart disease, another mental disorder (psychosis or mania), or a movement/tic disorder (Tourette's syndrome).
	This medication may increase the blood levels/effects of some other medications (warfarin, phenobarbital, phenytoin, primidone, tricyclic antidepressants, and clonidine). This is why it is important to notify your pharmacist/doctor of any current (or changes in your) medications (over-the-counter/prescription).
	If your doctor has prescribed pemoline, your doctor may have to do routine blood tests. Contact your doctor/pharmacist if you experience unusual tiredness, upper abdominal pain (2 weeks), nausea, vomiting, or dark-colored urine.
	Sustained-release products should not be crushed or chewed. If your doctor has prescribed Dexadrine Spansules, the capsules may be opened and the contents placed in food (applesauce) to ease swallowing.
Tricyclic antidepressants (TCAs)	Although this medication is used for depression, it does not mean you have the diagnosis of depression. This drug is also used to improve symptoms associated with ADHD.
	The most common side effects of this drug include dry mouth, constipation, urinary retention, weight gain, changes in blood pressure, and sedation. Occasionally, this medication worsens behaviors. Doses should be taken at bedtime to decrease their sedative effect. Regular dental visits and good dental hygiene are particularly important while taking this medication. In general, these side effects decrease while taking the medication or respond to dose reduction; if not contact your doctor/pharmacist.
	It is important that you do not stop taking this medication abruptly. Slow tapering is necessary to prevent withdrawal symptoms (flu-like symptoms).
	The effects of this medication may be increased by some other medications (cimetidine, phenothiazines, phenytoin, oral contraceptives, quinidine, selective serotonin reuptake inhibitors, and stimulants). Other medications/habits decrease their effect (phenobarbital and smoking). This is why it is important to tell your pharmacist/doctor of any current (or changes in your) medications (over-the-counter/prescription).
	This medication may worsen some medical conditions; tell your doctor if you have a history of heart disease, glaucoma, or seizure disorder/epilepsy.
	Your doctor may routinely monitor your heart while on this medication. Contact your doctor/pharmacist if you notice any unusual changes in heart rate, shortness of breath, or pain/tightening in the chest.
Monoamine oxidase Inhibitors (MAOIs)	Although this medication is used for depression, it does not mean you have the diagnosis of depression. This drug is also used to improve symptoms associated with ADHD.
	The effects of this medication may take time to appear. Some patients do not notice rapid improvements in ADHD symptoms.
	The most common side effects of this medication include weight gain, drowsiness, or insomnia. Taking initial doses at bedtime and eating smaller, more frequent meals may help minimize these effects.
	This medication may result in toxicity when used with some other medications (merperidine, antidepressants, stimulants, sympathomimetics). This is why it is important to notify your pharmacist/doctor of any current (or changes in your) medications (over-the-counter/prescription).

(continued)

TABLE 56.5	continued
Medication	**Counseling Advice**
	While taking this medication you need to be on a tyramine-free diet. This means avoiding eating certain foods (aged cheeses, wine, and certain processed meats). Consult your doctor/dietician for a comprehensive list of these foods.
	This medication may worsen some medical conditions; tell your doctor if you have a history of heart disease or pheochromocytoma (norepinephrine-secreting tumor).
	This medication has significantly increased blood pressures (hypertensive crisis) in some individuals. Contact your doctor/pharmacist if you experience any increase in heart rate, heartbeat pounding of the chest (palpitations), unusual sweating, or dizziness.
Bupropion	Although this medication is used for depression, it does not mean you have the diagnosis of depression. This drug is also used to improve symptoms associated with ADHD.
	The most common side effects of this medication are mild and include dry mouth, stomach upset, rash, and headache. Rarely do seizures occur. Tell your doctor if you have a history of a seizure disorder/epilepsy or an eating disorder. If one dose of medication is missed, contact your doctor/pharmacist before taking two doses.
	Although this medication has been used safely in patients with a tic disorder, it may increase the severity of tics in certain predisposed persons. Tell your doctor if you have a history of a tic disorder, Tourette's syndrome, or if while on this medication you experience a change in the frequency/severity of tic symptoms.
	Notify your doctor/pharmacist if you are taking or have recently taken (within 14 days) a monoamine oxidase inhibitor. Concurrent use has been associated with a sudden increase in blood pressure.
Clonidine	The effects of this medication may take time to appear. Some patients do not notice rapid improvements in ADHD symptoms.
	The most common side effects include sedation, dry mouth, nightmares, and decreases in blood pressure. These effects should decrease while on the medication. Taking the first dose at bedtime will help minimize its sedative effect.
	Some individuals become increasingly sad (depressed) while taking this medication. Contact your doctor/pharmacist if this occurs.
	It is important that this medication is not stopped abruptly because sudden increases in blood pressure may occur.
	If your doctor has prescribed the clonidine patch for you, you need to (a) wash and dry the area before application, (b) change the patch every 3 to 5 days, and (c) alternate the site of application to prevent a rash from occurring. Notify your doctor/pharmacist if one appears.
	This medication may worsen symptoms of heart disease. Tell your doctor/pharmacist if you have a heart condition or are taking any heart/blood pressure medications.

ADHD. Teaching about medication and treatment follow-up may include the patient, parent, and teacher. Many patients with ADHD have reading and/or learning impairments; thus counseling should include both easy-to-understand verbal and written instructions. In addition, the health care professional should provide a phone number for questions that may arise once the patient has left the clinic or pharmacy. This is particularly important for patients who are unable to pay attention while discussing their medications.

Patients may receive multiple medications, which may prove confusing to the patient or parent. Polytherapy also provides increased probability of drug interactions. The health care practitioner should inquire about use of any concurrent medications (prescription, over-the-counter, or herbal substances). In addition to potential interactions, responses may identify untreated comorbid conditions, drug contraindications (i.e., TCA with cardiac disease), or drug effects that may mimic the symptoms of ADHD.

In initial counseling and in follow-up, a side effect questionnaire (i.e., the BSEQ) should be used. This enables the health care professional to discern whether a side effect is drug-related or an effect of the disorder itself. As with all medications, patients and parents should be cautioned on the proper and safe storage of medications. This is particularly true for patients with prescriptions for agents with abuse or overdose potential (stimulants and TCAs). Next, the frequency of administration should be discussed. For example, typically methylphenidate is administered at breakfast, lunch, and possibly late afternoon. In contrast, the TCAs and pemoline can be administered once daily. Many patients with ADHD cannot be relied on to take their own medications. Careful coordination with multiple caregivers may be necessary to ensure that each dose is given. The health care provider may need to provide reminders or easy routines for the patient, parent, or teacher to follow (pill boxes, dose alarms, administration of medications at meals or after school). Some schools require that medication be kept in a professionally labeled bottle. This may require the clinician to provide a second labeled bottle for this purpose. Various members of the health care team may also need to inform the patient or parent or initiate any clinical or laboratory monitoring needed for a particular agent.

PATIENT ADHERENCE TO DRUG THERAPY

Adherence to drug therapy may be a particular problem with patients who have ADHD. Both clinical symptoms and environmental influences may decrease compliance. For example, a patient's inattention may result in forgotten doses. Patients with ADHD/oppositional disorder may refuse to take medications. In addition, patients with ADHD may have dysfunctional families in which the parent cannot be relied upon to administer medications either because of the primary dysfunction or the diversion of medications to other family members. ADHD does not produce physical morbidity, therefore patients may fail to realize the importance of taking their medications. Other patients may dread being labeled with a mental disorder (ADHD) or being perceived as a drug abuser. In addition, patients may worry about potential adverse effects. These concerns may make the patient hesitant to take medications in certain environments, if at all.

In addition to the above-mentioned medication reminders, the health care practitioner may need to dispel any patient concerns (i.e., stimulants used for ADHD rarely produce addiction, or growth suppression). Further assurance can be gained by mentioning means in which therapy will be monitored and implementation of ways to minimize side effects (i.e., slow dosage titration, taking initial doses at bedtime [TCAs or clonidine], or after meals [stimulants]). In skeptical or oppositional patients, the health care provider may need to discuss the importance of ADHD medications or contact parents or other health care workers about the need to incorporate medication compliance into behavioral modification programs. In patients reluctant to take medications at school or work or for those who frequently forget, a sustained-release product or an agent with a longer half-life (TCAs, clonidine, pemoline, or the dextro- and levoamphetamine product) may prove beneficial.

Many children and some adults cannot swallow pills. Selection of an appropriate dosage form may make adherence to therapy more likely. Many of the ADHD medications can be crushed or opened and placed in food or are chewable. Older patients may find the clonidine patch an attractive option.

DISEASE MANAGEMENT STRATEGIES

Once the diagnosis of ADHD is made, successful treatment hinges on tailoring therapy to a patient's preexisting conditions and impairments (Fig. 56.1). Specific or troublesome symptoms should be identified and used as guides or end points in therapy. Establishing these references may require input from the patient, parent, teachers, and other health care professionals. However, because medication effects are often short-lived and fail to improve all the manifestations of ADHD, nonpharmacologic interventions (behavioral modification, individual/family psychotherapy, and/or academic/social skills training) are essential for positive patient outcomes. This is particularly important for younger patients (<6 years) in whom therapy may prove less effective, in patients predisposed to medication-induced adverse effects, and in those with severe academic, social, or functional deficits.

If a patient's ADHD symptoms are severe enough to warrant pharmacotherapy, comorbid diseases should guide selection of an initial ADHD medication. Methylphenidate is the first medication tried in the majority (those without specific comorbidities) of patients with ADHD because of its proven efficacy, rapid onset, and lower severity of side effects (less than amphetamine-containing products). After an adequate trial (~1 month) with appropriate maintenance dosing, an alternative stimulant (dextroamphetamine or the dextro- and levoamphetamine combination) may be tried. If the next agent fails, second-line agents (TCAs, clonidine, or pemoline) may be considered. In patients with refractory ADHD, bupropion or an MAOI may prove effective.

Although stimulants are most commonly used, these agents may not be optimal for certain patients with ADHD. For example, clonidine has proven effective in decreasing both tics and ADHD symptoms making it the drug of choice in patients with Tourette's syndrome or tic disorders. Bupropion and the stimulants are avoided in those with movement disorders because of their potential (actual or perceived) ability to increase tic severity. Initial treatment in patients with comorbid depression or enuresis should be a TCA or possibly bupropion. Both drugs have the ability to decrease the seizure threshold and should be avoided in patients with epilepsy. The ability of stimulants (e.g., methylphenidate, dextroamphetamine, and the dextro- and levoamphetamine combination) to produce euphoria makes them a possible source of abuse; hence, if substance abuse is suspected (patient or family) pemoline or another class of medications is preferred. Combination therapy is an attractive option for patients with refractory ADHD and those prone to troublesome side effects. Polypharmacy may permit the use of lower doses of both medications or counteract the adverse effects of either agent. One example is the use of methylphenidate and clonidine for patients with persistent insomnia.

Because the severity of ADHD symptoms is influenced by multiple factors, a variety of measurement tools should be used to determine dosage titration and clinical response. Initially, drugs should be administered daily. Once a given patient's target symptoms show consistent improvement, the dose is held constant and drug holidays (i.e., weekends, summer time, and holidays) are encouraged. This assesses the further need for continued drug therapy, minimizes adverse effects, and may improve self-esteem.

PHARMACOECONOMICS

Although ADHD is frequently diagnosed, there is limited information about the amount of services received and the actual expense required for its treatment. Current data suggest that ADHD has a significant effect on the nation's economy and that the monetary demands of the disorder are growing. Many factors seem to contribute to the observed increase in expenditures. The use of diagnostic, mental health, and counseling services has consistently increased from 1989 to 1996. Children with ADHD seem to require a greater number of outpatient services (primary care and mental health) than children with or without other psychosocial problems.[6] As a result of these clinical visits, a greater percentage of patients with ADHD receive prescription medications. Medicaid studies note that polypharmacy has increased 7.5% each year over a 7-year period. Interestingly, family practitioners seem more likely to prescribe stimulants than pediatricians or psychiatrists.

Children and Adults With Attention Deficit Disorders (CHADD)[6] has conducted a survey evaluating the health care coverage for patients with ADHD. Results suggest that the majority of patients with ADHD have health care coverage with the greatest percentages belonging to preferred provider organizations (PPOs) and health maintenance organizations (HMOs). Despite this coverage, half of patients with ADHD felt that their health care plan did not offer the necessary access to professionals required to ensure proper treatment of the disorder. Approximately 62% of patients had to pay out-of-pocket expenses to receive this care. Among the 90% of patients receiving medications for ADHD, approximately 80% had to pay some amount for these medications. The cost of medications for ADHD can also result in a significant financial burden for families already paying for other health-related expenses.

- Most randomized clinical trials have assessed short-term (i.e., up to 3 months) use of stimulants. There are no long-term studies evaluating stimulants or psychosocial therapy use over several years. Likewise, there are no long-term outcome studies assessing the effect of medication-treated ADHD on educational and occupational achievements, involvement with the judicial system, or other areas of social dysfunction
- Treatment with stimulants does not ''normalize'' behavior problems. Although there is improvement in core symptoms there is little improvement in long-term academic performance or social skills
- Decreased appetite, insomnia, and irritability are common with the stimulants. High doses of stimulants may cause CNS damage, cardiovascular damage, hypertension, and possibly motor disorders
- The TCAs are the drugs of choice for the 30% of patients who fail to respond to stimulant medications or who cannot tolerate the side effects associated with stimulants. There is some evidence to suggest that patients who display greater anxiety, depression, or mood disturbances in conjunction with their ADHD may respond better to TCAs than to stimulants. Likewise, some believe that the condition of patients who exhibit aggression may deteriorate with TCAs
- Medically unexplained sudden death has been reported in children receiving normal doses of desipramine. For this reason, imipramine is preferred over desipramine in children and adults with ADHD. Although the American Academy of Pediatrics does not recommend routine ECG monitoring at this time, the American Academy of Child and Adolescent Psychiatry recommends a baseline ECG, one within days of a dosage increase, and another once steady state at maximal doses is achieved. Although the benefits of ECG monitoring are questionable, it would seem advisable to follow the more conservative guidelines

KEY POINTS

- The optimal management of ADHD is contingent on a reliable and accurate diagnosis using DSM-IV criteria
- Treatment goals should be established jointly with the patient and the family
- Treatment of ADHD must address multiple aspects of the child's disorder and should not be reduced to the use of medication alone
- The majority of patients will respond to one of the available stimulants (i.e., methylphenidate, dexamphetamine, dextro- and levoamphetamine combination or pemoline). Although few differences have been found among the stimulants, methylphenidate is the most studied and most used drug

REFERENCES

1. American Psychiatric Association. Diagnostic and statistical manual of mental disorders. 4th ed. (DSM IV). Washington, DC: American Psychiatric Association, 1994.
2. American Psychiatric Association. Diagnostic and statistical manual of mental disorders. 3rd ed. (DSM III). Washington, DC: American Psychiatric Association, 1982.
3. American Psychiatric Association. Diagnostic and statistical manual of mental disorders. 3rd ed. (DSM III-R). Washington, DC: American Psychiatric Association, 1987.
4. Goldman LS, Genel M, Bezman RJ, et al. Diagnosis and treatment of attention-deficit/hyperactivity disorder in children and adolescents. JAMA 279:1100–1107, 1998.
5. American Academy of Child and Adolescent Psychiatry. Practice parameters for the assessment and treatment of children, adolescents, and adults with attention-deficit/hyperactivity disorder. J Am Acad Child Adolesc Psychiatry 36:85S–121S, 1997.
6. NIH Consensus Development Conference. Attention deficit hyperactivity disorder. National Institutes of Health Continuing Medical Education. November 16–18, 1998.

7. Swanson JM, Lerner M, Williams L. More frequent diagnosis of attention deficit hyperactivity disorder. N Engl J Med 333:944, 1995.

8. Cantwell DP. Attention deficit disorder: a review of the past 10 years. J Am Acad Child Adolesc Psychiatry 35:978–987, 1996.

9. Lou HC. Etiology and pathogenesis of attention-deficit hyperactivity disorder (ADHD): significance of prematurity and perinatal hypoxic-hemodynamic encephalopathy. Acta Paediatr 85:1266–1271, 1996.

10. Working Group on Quality Issues. American Academy of Child and Adolescent Psychiatry. Summary of the pediatric parameters for the assessment and treatment of children, adolescents, and adults with ADHD. J Am Acad Child Adolesc Psychiatry 36: 1311–1317, 1997.

11. Cook EH, Stein MA, Krasowski CD, et al. Association of attention deficit disorder and the dopamine transporter gene. Am J Hum Genet 56:993–998, 1995.

12. LaHoste GJ, Swanson JM, Wigal SB, et al. Dopamine D4 receptor gene polymorphism is associated with attention deficit hyperactivity disorder. Mol Psychiatry 1:121–124, 1996.

13. Castellanos FX, Giedd JN, March WI, et al. Quantitative brain magnetic resonance imaging in attention-deficit hyperactivity disorder. Arch Gen Psychiatry 53:607–616, 1996.

14. Filipek PA, Semrud-Clikeman M, Steingard RJ, et al. Volumetric MRI analysis comparing subjects having attention-deficit hyperactivity disorder with normal controls. Neurology 48:589–601, 1997.

15. Woolf AD, Suckermann BS. Adolescence and its discontents: attentional disorders among teenagers and young adults. Pediatrician 13: 119–127, 1986.

16. Hill JC, Schoener EP. Age dependent decline of attention deficit hyperactivity disorder. Am J Psychiatry 153:1143–1146, 1996.

17. Cantwell DP. Hyperactive children have grown up. What have we learned about what happened to them? Arch Gen Psychiatry 42: 1026–1028, 1985.

18. Halperin JM, Gittelman R, Klein DF, et al. Reading disability hyperactive children: a distinct subgroup of attention deficit disorder with hyperactivity? J Abnorm Child Psychol 12:1–14, 1984.

19. Silver L. The relationship between learning disabilities, hyperactivity, distractibility, and behavioral problems. J Am Acad Child Adolesc Psychiatry 20:385–397, 1981.

20. Cantwell DP, Satterfield JH. The prevalence of academic underachievement in hyperactive children. J Pediatr Psychol 3:168–171, 1978.

21. McGee R, Share DL. Attention deficit disorder-hyperactivity and academic failure: which comes first and what should be treated? J Am Acad Child Adolesc Psychiatry 27:318–325, 1988.

22. Pennington BF, Groddirt D, Welsh MC. Contrasting cognitive deficits in attention deficit hyperactivity disorder versus reading disability. Dev Psychol 29:511–523, 1993.

23. Felton RH, Wood FB, Brown IS, et al. Separate verbal memory and naming deficits in attention disorder and reading disability. Brain Lung 31:171–184, 1987.

24. Shaywitz BA, Fletcher JM, Holahan JM, et al. Cognitive profiles of reading disability: interrelationships between reading disability and attention deficit-hyperactivity disorder. Child Neuropsychol 1: 170–186, 1995.

25. Wilens TE. Update on attention deficit hyperactivity disorder, I. Curr Affect Illness 15:5–12, 1996.

26. Biederman J, Faerone SV, Mick E, et al. Attention deficit hyperactivity disorder and juvenile mania an overlooked comorbidity? J Am Acad Child Adolesc Psychiatry 35:997–1008, 1996.

27. American Psychiatric Association. Diagnostic and statistical manual of mental disorders. 2nd ed. (DSM II). Washington, DC: American Psychiatric Association, 1968.

28. American Academy of Pediatrics. Committee on Drugs. Behavioral and cognitive effects of anticonvulsants therapy. Pediatrics 96: 538–540, 1995.

29. Diener MB, Milich R. Effects of positive feedback on the social interactions of boys with attention deficit hyperactivity disorder: a test of self-protective hypothesis. J Clin Child Psychol 26: 256–265, 1997.

30. Kwasman A, Tinsley BJ, Lepper HS. Pediatricians' knowledge and attitudes concerning diagnosis and treatment of attention deficit and hyperactivity disorder. A national survey approach. Arch Pediatr Adolesc Med 149:1211–1216, 1995.

31. Diller LH. The run on Ritalin: attention deficit disorder and stimulant treatment in the 1990's. Hastings Center Report 26:12–18, 1996.

32. Bradley C. The behavior of children receiving Benzedrine. Am J Psychiatry 94:577–585, 1937.

33. Safer DJ, Zito JM, Fine EM. Increased methylphenidate usage for attention deficit disorder in the 1990's. Pediatrics 98:1084–1088, 1996.

34. Zametkin AJ, Rapoport JL. Neurobiology of attention deficit disorder with hyperactivity: where have we come in 50 years? J Am Acad Child Adolesc Psychiatry 26:676–686, 1987.

35. Volkow ND, Ding Y, Fowler JS, et al. Is methylphenidate like cocaine? Arch Gen Psychiatry 52:456–463, 1995.

36. Elia J. Drug treatment for hyperactive children: therapeutic guidelines. Drugs 46:863–871, 1993.

37. Spencer T, Biederman J, Wilens T, et al. Pharmacotherapy of attention-deficit hyperactivity disorder across the life-cycle. J Am Acad Child Adolesc Psychiatry 35:409–432, 1996.

38. Barkley RA. A review of stimulant drug research with hyperactive children. J Child Psychol Psychiatry 18:137–165, 1977.

39. Rapport MD, Denny C, DuPaul GJ, et al. Attention deficit disorder and methylphenidate: normalized rates, clinical effectiveness, and response prediction in 76 children. J Am Acad Child Adolesc Psychiatry 33:882–893, 1994.

40. Jacobvitz D, Sroute LA, Stewart M, et al. Treatment of attentional and hyperactivity problems in children with sympathomimetic drugs: a comprehensive review. J Am Acad Child Adolesc Psychiatry 29:677–688, 1990.

41. Whalen CK, Henker B, Buhrmester D, et al. Does stimulant medication improve the peer status of hyperactive children? J Consult Clin Psychol 57:545–549, 1989.

42. Pelham WE, Walker JL, Sturges J, et al. Comparative effects of methylphenidate on ADD girls and boys. J Am Acad Child Adolesc Psychiatry 28:773–776, 1989.

43. Spencer T, Wilens T, Biederman J, et al. A double-blind, crossover comparison of methylphenidate and placebo in adults with childhood-onset attention deficit hyperactivity disorder. Arch Gen Psychiatry 52:434–443, 1995.

44. Buitelaar JK, Vander Gaag RJ, Swaab-Barneveld H, et al. Prediction of clinical response to methylphenidate in children with attention-deficit hyperactivity disorder. J Am Acad Child Adolesc Psychiatry 34:1025–1032, 1995.

45. Pelham WE, Swanson JM, Bender Furman M, et al. Pemoline effects on children with ADHD. a time-response by dose-response analysis on classroom measures. J Am Acad Child Adolesc Psychiatry 34:1504–1513, 1995.

46. Pelham WE, Aronoff H, Midlam J, et al. A comparison of Ritalin and Adderall: efficacy and time-course in children with attention-deficit/hyperactivity disorder. Pediatrics 103:e43, 1999.

47. Rapoport JL, Buchsbaum MS, Zahn TP, et al. Dextroamphetamine: cognitive and behavioral effects in normal prepubertal boys. Science 199:560–563, 1978.

48. Peloquin LJ, Klorman R. Effects of methylphenidate on normal children's mood, event-related potentials, and performance in memory scanning and vigilance. J Abnorm Psychol 95:88–98, 1986.

49. Satterfield JH, Satterfield BT, Schell AM. Therapeutic interventions to prevent delinquency in hyperactive boys. J Am Acad Child Adolesc Psychiatry 26:56–64, 1987.

50. Rapoport JL, Quinn PO, Bradbard G, et al. Imipramine and methylphenidate treatments of hyperactive boys. Arch Gen Psychiatry 30: 789–793, 1974.

51. Hunt RD. Treatment effects of oral and transdermal clonidine in relation to methylphenidate: an open pilot study in ADD-H. Psychopharmacol Bull 23:111–114, 1987.

52. Rapport MD, Carlson GA, Kelly KL, et al. Methylphenidate and desipramine in hospitalized children: I. Separate and combined effects on cognitive function. J Am Acad Child Adolesc Psychiatry 32:333–342, 1993.

53. Rapport MD, Stoner G, DuPaul GJ, et al. Methylphenidate in hyperactive children: differential effects of dose on academic, learning, and social behavior. J Abnorm Child Psychol 13:227–244, 1985.

54. Rapport MD, DuPaul GJ, Kelly KL. Attention deficit hyperactivity disorder and methylphenidate: the relationship between gross body

weight and drug response in children. Psychopharmacol Bulletin 25:285–290, 1989.

55. Rapport MD, Denny C. Titrating methylphenidate in children with attention deficit/hyperactivity disorder: is body mass predictive of clinical response? J Am Acad Child Adolesc Psychiatry 36: 523–530, 1997.

56. Brown GL, Ebert MH, Mikkelsen EJ, et al. Behavior and motor activity response in hyperactive children and plasma amphetamine levels following a sustained release preparation. J Am Acad Child Psychiatry 19:225–239, 1980.

57. Sprague RL, Sleator EK. Methylphenidate in hyperkinetic children: differences in dose effects on learning and social behavior. Science 198:1274–1276, 1977.

58. Pelham WE, Bender ME, Caddell J, et al. Methylphenidate and children with attention deficit disorder. Arch Gen Psychiatry 42: 948–952, 1985.

59. Swanson JM, Wigal S, Greenhill LL, et al. Analog classroom assessment of Adderall in children with ADHD. J Am Acad Child Adolesc Psychiatry 37:519–526, 1998.

60. McEvoy GK, ed. American Hospital Formulary Service drug information 98. Bethesda, MD: American Society of Hospital Pharmacists, 1998.

61. Sallee FR, Stiller RL, Perel JM. Pharmacodynamics of pemoline in attention deficit disorder with hyperactivity. J Am Acad Child Adolesc Psychiatry 31:244–251, 1992.

62. Sallee FR, Perel J, Bates T. Oral pemoline kinetics in hyperactive children. Clin Pharmacol Ther 37:606–609, 1985.

63. Collier CP, Soldin SJ, Swanson JM, et al. Pemoline pharmacokinetics and long term therapy in children with attention deficit disorder and hyperactivity. Clin Pharmacokinet 10:269–278, 1985.

64. Pelham WE, Greenslade KE, Vodde-Hamilton M, et al. Relative efficacy of long-acting stimulants on children with attention deficit-hyperactivity disorder: a comparison of standard methylphenidate, sustained-release methylphenidate, sustained-release dextroamphetamine, and pemoline. Pediatrics 86:226–237, 1990.

65. Safer DJ, Allen RP. Absence of tolerance to the behavioral effects of methylphenidate in hyperactive and inattentive children. Pediatric Pharmacol 115:1003–1008, 1989.

66. Stein MA, Blondis TA, Schnitzler ER, et al. Methylphenidate dosing: twice daily versus three times daily. Pediatrics 98:748–756, 1996.

67. Pelham WE, Sturges J, Hoza J, et al. Sustained release and standard methylphenidate effects on cognitive and social behavior in children with attention deficit disorder. Pediatrics 80:491–501, 1987.

68. Fitzpatrick PA, Klorman R, Brumaghim JT, et al. Effects of sustained release and standard preparations of methylphenidate on attention deficit disorder. J Am Acad Child Adolesc Psychiatry 31: 226–234, 1992.

69. Barkley RA, McMurray MB, Edelbrock CS, et al. Side effects of methylphenidate in children with attention deficit hyperactivity disorder: a systemic, placebo-controlled evaluation. Pediatrics 86: 184–192, 1990.

70. Ahmann PA, Waltonen SJ, Olson KA, et al. Placebo controlled evaluation of ritalin side effects. Pediatrics 91:1101–1106, 1993.

71. Efron D, Jarman F, Barker M. Side effects of methylphenidate and dexamphetamine in children with attention deficit hyperactivity disorder: a double-blind, crossover trial. Pediatrics 100:662–666, 1997.

72. Safer DJ, Allen R, Barr E. Depression of growth in hyperactive children on stimulant drugs. N Engl J Med 287:217–220, 1972.

73. Safer DJ, Allen RP. Factors influencing the suppressant effects of two stimulant drugs on the growth of hyperactive children. Pediatrics 51:660–667, 1973.

74. Gittelman Klein R, Landa B, Mattes JA, et al. Methylphenidate and growth in hyperactive children: a controlled withdrawal study. Arch Gen Psychiatry 45:1127–1130, 1988.

75. Spencer TJ, Biederman J, Harding M, et al. Growth deficits in ADHD children revisited: evidence for disorder-associated growth delays? J Am Acad Child Adolesc Psychiatry 35:1460–1469, 1996.

76. Lowe TL, Cohen DJ, Detlor J, et al. Stimulant medications precipitate Tourette's syndrome. JAMA 247:1168–1169, 1982.

77. Castellanos FX, Giedd JN, Elia J, et al. Controlled stimulant treatment of ADHD and comorbid Tourette's syndrome: effects of stimulant and dose. J Am Acad Child Adolesc Psychiatry 36:589–596, 1997.

78. Gadow KD, Nolan EE, Sverd J. Methylphenidate in hyperactive boys with comorbid tic disorder: II. Short-term behavioral effects in school settings. J Am Acad Child Adolesc Psychiatry 31: 462–471, 1992.

79. Jaffe SL. Intranasal abuse of prescribed methylphenidate by an alcohol and drug abusing adolescent with ADHD. J Am Acad Child Adolesc Psychiatry 30:773–775, 1991.

80. Goyer PF, Davis GC, Rapoport JL. Abuse of prescribed stimulant medication by a 13 year-old hyperactive boy. J Am Acad Child Adolesc Psychiatry 18:170–175, 1979.

81. Horner BR, Scheibe KE. Prevalence and implications of attention-deficit hyperactivity disorder among adolescents in treatment for substance abuse. J Am Acad Child Adolesc Phsychiatry 36:30–36, 1997.

82. Biederman J, Wilens T, Mick E, et al. Psychoactive substance use disorders in adults with attention deficit hyperactivity disorder (ADHD): effects of ADHD and psychiatric comorbidity. Am J Psychiatry 152:1652–1658, 1995.

83. Drug Enforcement Administration, Office of Diversion Control. Conference report: stimulant use in the treatment of ADHD. Washington DC, 1996.

84. Berkovitch M, Pope E, Phillips J, et al. Pemoline-associated fulminant liver failure: testing the evidence for causation. Clin Pharmacol Ther 57:696–698, 1995.

85. Christman AK, Fermo JD, Markowitz JS. Atomoxetine, a novel treatment for attention-deficit-hyperactivity disorder. Pharmacotherapy 24:1020–1036, 2004.

86. Corman SL, Fedutes BA, Culley CM. Atomoxetine: the first non-stimulant for the management of attention-deficiet/hyperactivity disorder. Am J Health Syst Pharm 61:2391–2399, 2004.

87. Eiland LS, Guest AL. Atomoxetine treatment of attention-deficit/hyperactivity disorder. Ann Pharmacother 38:86–90, 2004.

88. Barton J. Atomoxetine: a new pharmacotherapeutic approach in the management of attention deiffcet/hyperactivity disorder. Arch Dis Child 90 (Suppl 1):i26–i29, 2005.

89. Sauer JM, Witcher JW. Clinical pharmacokinetics of atomoxetine. Clin Pharmacokinet 44:571–590, 2005.

90. Witcher JW, Long AJ, Sauer JM, et al. Atomoxetine pharmacokinetics in children with attention deficit hyperactivity disorder. J Child Adolesc Psychopharmacol 13:53–64, 2003.

91. Product information. Strattera (atomoxetine). Indianapolis: Eli Lilly, December 2002.

92. Pliszka SR. Tricyclic antidepressants in the treatment of children with attention deficit disorder. J Am Acad Child Adolesc Psychiatry 26:127–132, 1987.

93. Biederman J, Baldessarini RJ, Wright V, et al. A double-blind controlled study of desipramine in the treatment of ADD: I. Efficacy. J Am Acad Child Adolesc Psychiatry 28:777–784, 1989.

94. Popper CW. Antidepressants in the treatment of attention-deficit/hyperactivity disorder. J Clin Psychiatry 58:14–29, 1997.

95. Biederman J, Baldessarini RJ, Wright V, et al. A double-blind placebo controlled study of desipramine in the treatment of ADD: II. Serum drug levels and cardiovascular findings. J Am Acad Child Adolesc Psychiatry 28:903–911, 1989.

96. Daly JM, Wilens T. The use of tricyclic antidepressants in children and adolescents. Pediatr Clin North Am 45:1123–1135, 1998.

97. Biederman J, Thisted RA, Greenhill L, et al. Estimation of the association between desipramine and the risk of sudden death in 5- to 14-year-old children. J Clin Psychiatry 56:87–93, 1995.

98. Committee on Children with Disabilities and Committee on Drugs. American Academy of Pediatrics. Medication for children with attentional disorders. Pediatrics 98:301–304, 1996.

99. Zametkin A, Rapoport JL, Murphy DL, et al. Treatment of hyperactive children with monoamine oxidase inhibitors: I. Clinical efficacy. Arch Gen Psychiatry 42:962–966, 1985.

100. Feigin A, Kurlan R, McDermott MP, et al. A controlled trial of deprenyl in children with Tourette's syndrome and attention deficit hyperactivity disorder. Neurology 46:965–968, 1996.

101. Casat CD, Pleasants DZ, Schroeder DH, et al. Bupropion in children with attention deficit disorder. Psychopharmacol Bull 25: 198–201, 1989.

102. Spencer T, Biederman J, Steingard R, et al. Bupropion exacerbates tics in children with attention-deficit hyperactivity disorder and Tourette's syndrome. J Am Acad Child Adolesc Psychiatry 32: 211–214, 1993.

103. Conners CK, Casat CD Gualtieri CT, et al. Bupropion hydrochloride in attention deficit disorder with hyperactivity. J Am Acad Child Adolesc Psychiatry 35:1314–1321, 1996.

104. Wender PH, Reimherr FW. Bupropion treatment of attention-deficit hyperactivity disorder in adults. Am J Psychiatry 148: 1018–1020, 1990.

105. Adler LA, Resnick S, Kunk M, et al. Open-label trial of venlafaxine in adults with ADD. Psychopharmacol Bull 31:785–788, 1995.

106. Hedges D, Reoherr FW, Rogers A, et al. An open trial of venlafaxine in adult patients with attention deficit hyperactivity disorder. Psychopharmacol Bull 31:779–783, 1995.

107. Findling RL, Schwartz MA, Flannery DL, et al. Venlafaxine in adults with attention-deficit/hyperactivity disorder. J Cln Psychiatry 57:184–189, 1996.

108. Olvera RL, Pliszka SR, Luh J, et al. An open trial of venlafaxine in the treatment of attention-deficit/hyperactivity disorder in children and adolescents. J Child Adolesc Psychiatry 6:241–250, 1996.

109. Pleak RR, Gormly LJ. Effects of venlafaxine for treatment of ADHD in a child [letter]. Am J Psychiatry 152:1099, 1995.

110. Barrickman L, Noyes R, Kuperman S, et al. Treatment of ADHD with fluoxetine: a preliminary trial J Am Acad Child Adolesc Psychiatry 30:762–767, 1991.

111. Campbell NB, Tamburrino MB, Evans CL, et al. Fluoxetine for ADHD in a young child. J Am Acad Child Adolesc Psychiatry 34: 1259–1260, 1995.

112. Frankenburg FR, Kando JC. Sertraline treatment of ADHD and Tourette's syndrome. J Clin Psychopharmacol 14:359–360, 1994.

113. Hunt RD, Mineraa RB, Cohen DJ. Clonidine benefits children with attention deficit disorder and hyperactivity: report of a double-blind placebo-crossover therapeutic trial. J Am Acad Child Psychiatry 24:617–629, 1985.

114. Wilens TE, Beiderman J, Spencer T. Clonidine for sleep disturbances associated with attention-deficit hyperactivity disorder. J Am Acad Child Adolesc Psychiatry 33:424–426, 1994.

115. Steingard R, Biederman J, Spencer T, et al. Comparison of clonidine response in the treatment of attention-deficit hyperactivity disorder with and without comorbid tic disorders. J Am Acad Child Adolesc Psychiatry 32:350–353, 1993.

116. Singer HS, Brown J, Quaskey S, et al. The treatment of attention-deficit hyperactivity disorder in Tourette's syndrome: a double-blind placebo-controlled study with clonidine and desipramine. Pediatrics 95:75–81, 1995.

117. Clonidine for treatment of attention-deficit/hyperactivity disorder. Med Lett Drug Ther 38:109–110, 1996.

118. Silva RR, Munoz DM, Alpert M. Carbamazepine use in children and adolescents with features of attention-deficit hyperactivity disorder: a meta-analysis. J Am Acad Child Adolesc Psychiatry 35: 352–358, 1996.

119. Winsberg BG, Yepes LE. Antipsychotic (major tranquilizers, neuroleptics). In: Werry JS, ed. Pediatric psychopharmacology: the use of behavior modifying drugs in children. New York: Brunner Mazel, 1978:234–274.

120. Millichap J. Drugs in the management of minimal brain dysfunction. Ann NY Acad Sci 205:321–324, 1973.

121. Mattes J, Gittelman R. A pilot trial of amantadine in hyperactive children. Presented at the New Clinical Drug Evaluations Unit (NCDEU) meeting. Key Biscayne, FL, May 1979.

122. Firestone P, Davey J, Goodman JT, et al. The effects of caffeine and methylphenidate on hyperactive children. J Am Acad Child Adolesc Psychiatry 17:445–456, 1978.

123. Donnelly M, Rapoport JL, Potter WZ, et al. Fenfluramine and dextroamphetamine treatment of childhood hyperactivity; clinical and biochemical findings. Arch Gen Psychiatry 46:205–212, 1989.

124. Greenhill LL, Reider RO, Wender PH, et al. Lithium carbonite in the treatment of hyperactive children. Arch Gen Psychiatry 28: 636–640, 1973.

125. Pelham WE, Wheeler T, Chronis A. Empirically supported psychosocial treatments for ADHD. J Clin Child Psychol 27:189–204, 1998.

126. Abikoff H. Cognitive training in ADHD children: less to it than meets the eye. J Learn Disabil 24:205–209, 1991.

127. Abikoff H, Gittelman R. Does behavior therapy normalize the classroom behavior of hyperactive children? Arch Gen Psychiatry 41: 449–454, 1984.

128. Klein RG, Abikoff H. Behavior therapy and methylphenidate in the treatment of children with ADHD. J Atten Disord 2:89, 1997.

129. Ialongo NS, Horn WF, Pascoe JM, et al. The effects of a multimodal intervention with attention-deficit hyperactivity disorder children: a 9-month follow-up. J Am Acad Child Adolesc Psychiatry 32:182–189, 1993.

130. Carlson CL. Pelham WE, Milich R, et al. Single and combined effects of methylphenidate and behavior therapy on the classroom performance of children with ADHD. J Abnorm Child Psychol 20: 213–231, 1992.

Obesity and Eating Disorders

57

Amy Heck Sheehan and Jacob P. Gettig

OBESITY

Obesity is a chronic disease with a worldwide prevalence that has increased at an alarming rate over the past three decades.[1] Obesity serves as a primary risk factor for the development of hypertension, dyslipidemia, type 2 diabetes, and coronary heart disease and contributes to the development of several other conditions, such as gallbladder disease, degenerative joint disease, sleep apnea, infertility, and certain types of cancers.[2,3] Because of these consequences, obesity has recently been identified as the second most common factor contributing to preventable death in the United States.[4] In addition to these health risks, obesity imparts significant economic burdens to society.[5]

DEFINITION

Obesity is generally defined as an accumulation of excess body fat to an extent that impairs health. Body mass index (BMI) is the preferred method for defining and measuring the degree of obesity and overweight, as it has been shown to correlate with total body fat and morbidity and mortality.[6] BMI is calculated by dividing body weight (measured in kilograms) by the square of height (measured in meters). Using nonmetric measurements, BMI is calculated by dividing body weight (measured in pounds) by the square of height (measured in inches) and multiplying the quotient by 704.5. A table of selected height and weight measurements categorized by BMI is shown in Figure 57.1. Epidemiologic research suggests that morbidity and mortality begin to increase with BMI values above 25 kg/m^2 and below 20 kg/m^2, suggesting a J-shaped curve relationship between body weight and total mortality.[6] The most recent National Institutes of Health (NIH) guidelines for the identification, evaluation, and treatment of overweight and obesity define overweight as a BMI of at least 25 kg/m^2 and obesity as a BMI of at least 30 kg/m^2.[6] Table 57.1 depicts the classification of overweight and obesity according to BMI as set forth by the NIH.

Height (inches)	19	20	21	22	23	24	25[a]	26	27	28	29	30[b]	31	32	33	34	35	36
	Body Weight (pounds)																	
58	90.7	95.5	100	105	110	115	119	124	129	134	138	143	148	153	158	162	167	172
59	93.9	98.8	104	109	114	119	124	128	133	138	143	148	153	158	163	168	173	178
60	97.1	102	107	112	118	123	128	133	138	143	148	153	158	164	169	174	179	184
61	100	106	111	116	121	127	132	137	143	148	153	158	164	169	174	180	185	190
62	104	109	115	120	125	131	136	142	147	153	158	164	169	175	180	186	191	196
63	107	113	118	124	130	135	141	146	152	158	163	169	175	180	186	192	197	203
64	110	116	122	128	134	140	145	151	157	163	169	174	180	186	192	198	203	209
65	114	120	126	132	138	144	150	156	162	168	174	180	186	192	198	204	210	216
66	117	124	130	136	142	148	155	161	167	173	179	185	192	198	204	210	216	223
67	121	127	134	140	147	153	159	166	172	178	185	191	198	204	210	217	223	229
68	125	131	138	144	151	158	164	171	177	184	190	197	203	210	217	223	230	236
69	128	135	142	149	155	162	169	176	182	189	196	203	209	216	223	230	237	243
70	132	139	146	153	160	167	174	181	188	195	202	209	216	223	230	236	243	250
71	136	143	150	157	165	172	179	186	193	200	207	215	222	229	236	243	250	258
72	140	147	155	162	169	177	184	191	199	206	213	221	228	235	243	250	258	265
73	144	151	159	166	174	182	189	197	204	212	219	227	234	242	250	257	265	272
74	148	155	163	171	179	187	194	202	210	218	225	233	241	249	256	264	272	280
75	152	160	168	176	184	192	200	208	216	224	232	240	247	255	263	271	279	287
76	156	164	172	180	189	197	205	213	221	230	238	246	254	262	271	279	287	295

aBMI ≥ 25: overweight
bBMI ≥ 30: obesity

FIGURE 57.1 Selected BMI units categorized by inches and pounds.

TREATMENT GOALS

- Reduce body weight.
- Maintain body weight.
- Prevent weight regain.
- Improve obesity-related comorbidities.[6]

TABLE 57.1	Classification of Overweight and Obesity by BMI
Classification	**BMI (kg/m^2)**
Underweight	<18.5
Normal	18.5–24.9
Overweight	25.0–29.9
Obesity	30.0–39.9
Extreme obesity	≥40

(Adapted from Preventing and managing the global epidemic of obesity. Report of the World Health Organization Consultation of Obesity. WHO, Geneva, June 1997; and Clinical Guidelines on the Identification, Evaluation, and Treatment of Overweight and Obesity in Adults, National Institutes of Health, National Heart, Lung and Blood Institute.)

Small decreases in weight of 5% to 10% can result in significant improvements in obesity-related cardiovascular risk factors such as hypertension, hyperlipidemia, and type 2 diabetes.[7,8] Therefore, an appropriate and realistic initial treatment goal for obesity is a reduction of 10% in total body weight over 6 months.[6] This equates to a loss of approximately 1 to 2 pounds per week. A treatment goal that emphasizes slow and consistent weight loss is preferred, because rapid weight loss will likely be accompanied by swift weight regain. Healthcare professionals can make a significant impact by providing appropriate counseling to encourage slow and consistent weight loss, as obese patients typically have weight loss goals in mind that are significantly greater than 10% of baseline. Once the patient achieves his or her desired weight loss goal, additional goals at the same slow and consistent rate should be developed. After the patient reaches his or her ultimate goal, weight maintenance and prevention of weight regain become life-long goals.

ETIOLOGY

In a few patients, obesity has an identifiable organic cause.[9] Weight gain in excess of 1 kg per day invariably implies fluid retention and is frequently a signal of cardiovascular, renal, or hepatic disorders. Certain medications, including corticosteroids, antipsychotics, antidepressants, and antiepileptics, may also contribute to weight gain.[10] Only rarely is obesity a symptom of a specific endocrinopathy, such as insulinoma, Cushing's disease, or hypothyroidism. More commonly, the development of idiopathic obesity is a complex process involving multiple factors such as environmental, genetic, cultural, socioeconomic, and psychological influences. In most cases, no single influence is solely responsible, but rather a combination of several influences contributes to the development of obesity.

ENVIRONMENTAL FACTORS

Modern environmental influences have played a significant role in the increased prevalence of overweight and obesity. Over the past 20 years, there has been a marked increase in the availability of appetizing, high-fat foods. These food choices are aggressively marketed through various advertising strategies and are often less expensive and more convenient than healthier food options. In addition, the average portion size for most items served in restaurants and in the home has increased significantly.[11,12] A recent food consumption survey reported that the average portion size of salty snacks, sugar-containing soft drinks, hamburgers, french fries, and Mexican food has increased significantly between 1977 and 1996.[12] At the same time, the advances in technology afforded by a Westernized society have resulted in decreased physical activity and a relatively sedentary lifestyle for most Americans. It is highly likely that increased caloric consumption and decreased physical activity are major contributors to the obesity epidemic in Western countries.

GENETIC FACTORS

The role of genetic influences on the development of obesity is a topic of extensive research. Environmental influences affecting caloric consumption can greatly confound this issue, making it difficult to determine the true impact of genetics on obesity. However, several familial studies have suggested that approximately 40% to 70% of individual variations in BMI may be attributed to genetic differences.[13–16] Twin studies have also reported that body weights of twin siblings appear to correlate well, even when the siblings were raised in separate households.[15,16] It has also been reported that when both parents are of normal weight, the incidence of having an obese child is approximately 9%. However, if one or both parents are obese, there is a 50% and 80% incidence of having an obese child, respectively.[17] Scientists have also identified numerous genetic polymorphisms that may predispose particular individuals to weight gain.[18]

CULTURAL, SOCIOECONOMIC, AND PSYCHOLOGICAL FACTORS

Eating habits are highly dependent on cultural, social, and religious beliefs. Socially acceptable or attractive body weights can vary substantially among different ethnic groups. Differences in socioeconomic status also appear to influence body weight: persons in lower socioeconomic classes tend to have a higher rate of obesity compared to their middle- and upper-class counterparts.[19] This relationship holds true particularly in females and does not appear as pronounced in males. Possible reasons for this disparity may include decreased access to inexpensive low-fat foods or fewer opportunities for physical activity. An individual's choice of physical leisure time activities can also play a significant role in body weight maintenance. In addition, psychological disorders such as binge eating disorder, depression, and schizophrenia are also associated with weight gain.

EPIDEMIOLOGY

It is currently estimated that approximately 65% of adults over the age of 20 living in the United States are overweight or obese.[20] By gender, 68.8% of men and 61.6% of women are overweight or obese. The prevalence of overweight and obesity has risen significantly over the past three decades. When epidemiologic data collected from 1976 to 1980 are compared to data collected from 1999 to 2000, the prevalence of overweight is noted to have increased by 40% (46% to 64.5%), while the prevalence of obesity increased by an astounding 110% (14.5% to 30.5%).[1] Figure 57.2 shows the increasing prevalence of overweight and obesity among U.S. adults as reported by the National Health and Nutrition Examination Survey (NHANES) conducted between 1976 and 2002.

Although this problem affects all ethnic groups and genders, the increased prevalence of overweight and obesity is most notable in African-American women (affecting 77.2%) and Mexican-American men (affecting 73.1%).[20] Finally, obesity is not only a problem in adults, but is also becoming prominent in children and adolescents. Recent data collected by the Centers for Disease Control and Prevention (CDC) estimate that 16% of children aged 6 to 19 years in the United States are overweight, suggesting that obesity trends will continue to worsen in the future.[20]

CLINICAL PRESENTATION

Most obese patients present with many serious comorbid conditions, including hypertension, type 2 diabetes, dyslipi-

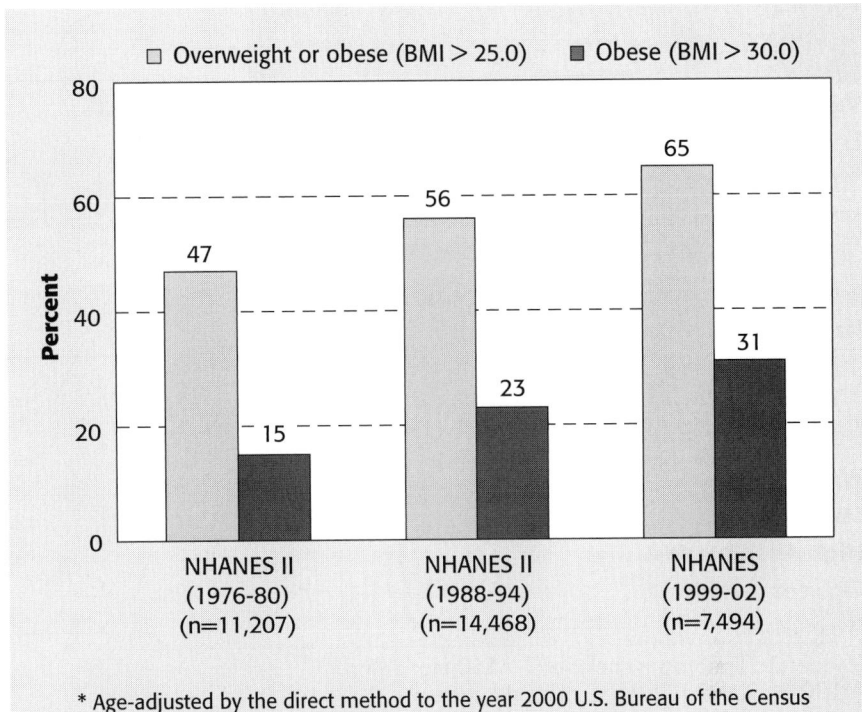

FIGURE 57.2 Age-adjusted prevalence of overweight and obesity among U.S. adults. (Adapted from the centers for Disease Control and Prevention and The National Center for Health Statistics, 1976–2002.

demia, coronary heart disease, stroke, sleep apnea, and certain cancers.[6] The most common obesity-related comorbidity is hypertension. A large international study involving approximately 10,000 men and women reported a systolic blood pressure increase of 3.0 mm Hg and a diastolic blood pressure increase of 2.3 mm Hg for every 10 kg of increased body weight.[21] In addition to hypertension, obesity is associated with other comorbidities that are known to significantly increase cardiovascular risk, such as high total cholesterol, elevated triglycerides, decreased high-density lipoprotein (HDL) cholesterol, and elevated low-density lipoprotein (LDL) cholesterol.[6] Type 2 diabetes and insulin resistance are also very common comorbidities associated with obesity. Epidemiologic studies have reported that approximately 27% of all new cases of type 2 diabetes may be directly linked to an adulthood weight gain as small as 5 kg.[22] Obese patients are also more likely to develop osteoarthritis, gallbladder disease, and infertility.

These associations emphasize the major role that obesity plays in morbidity and mortality. Significant excess weight is clearly detrimental to longevity, and a definite association exists between obesity and hypertension, diabetes, cardiovascular disease, and gastrointestinal disorders. This link pertains primarily to moderate and severe obesity, because the longevity of marginally or slightly obese persons compares favorably to that of nonobese persons. Risk factors associated with morbidity and mortality in obese patients are listed in Table 57.2.

As mentioned above, psychological problems are also associated with obesity. Obese and overweight individuals are often viewed as lazy, sloppy, unintelligent, or lacking will power. Therefore, low self-esteem, mental depression, or eating disorders such as anorexia, bulimia, or binge eating disorder may also be present in obese individuals.

DIAGNOSIS

Patients with massive obesity, peculiar fat distribution, or sudden, rapid weight gain require extensive evaluation. However, common idiopathic obesity does not usually demand elaborate evaluation techniques. Overweight and obesity are easily diagnosed by measuring height and weight and calculating BMI. However, it is important to note that BMI may not be an accurate measure of the degree of obesity in certain individuals, including athletes, body builders, or elderly patients, as it can overestimate body fat in muscular persons and underestimate body fat in older adults who have lost muscle mass. Other possibly more accurate methods to determine total body fat, such as bioelectrical impedance and dual-energy x-ray absorptiometry, offer no significant advantage over BMI and are expensive.

In addition to BMI, waist circumference should be measured to assist in determining the degree of obesity, associated risks, and morbidity. Observational studies indicate that the risk of obesity-related comorbidities is increased when body fat is concentrated in the abdominal region. A high risk of developing concomitant disease states is associated with a waist circumference of 102 cm (40 inches) in men and 88 cm (35 inches) in women.[6] The appropriate method

TABLE 57.2	Risk Factors for Obesity-Related Morbidity and Mortality

Very High Absolute Risk

Established coronary heart disease

   History of myocardial infarction

   History of angina pectoris (stable or unstable)

   History of coronary artery surgery

   History of coronary artery procedure (e.g., angioplasty)

Presence of other atherosclerotic diseases

   Peripheral arterial disease

   Abdominal aortic aneurysm

   Symptomatic carotid artery disease

Type 2 diabetes

Sleep apnea

High Absolute Risk

Cigarette smoking

Hypertension

Low-density lipoprotein cholesterol >160 mg/dL (or 130–159 mg/dL with ≥2 other risk factors)

High-density lipoprotein cholesterol <35 mg/dL

Impaired fasting glucose

Family history of premature cardiovascular disease

Male ≥45 years of age

Female ≥55 years of age (or postmenopausal)

Other Contributing Risk Factors

Serum triglycerides >200 mg/dL

Physical inactivity

(Adapted from Clinical Guidelines on the Identification, Evaluation, and Treatment of Overweight and Obesity in Adults, National Institutes of Health, National Heart, Lung and Blood Institute.)

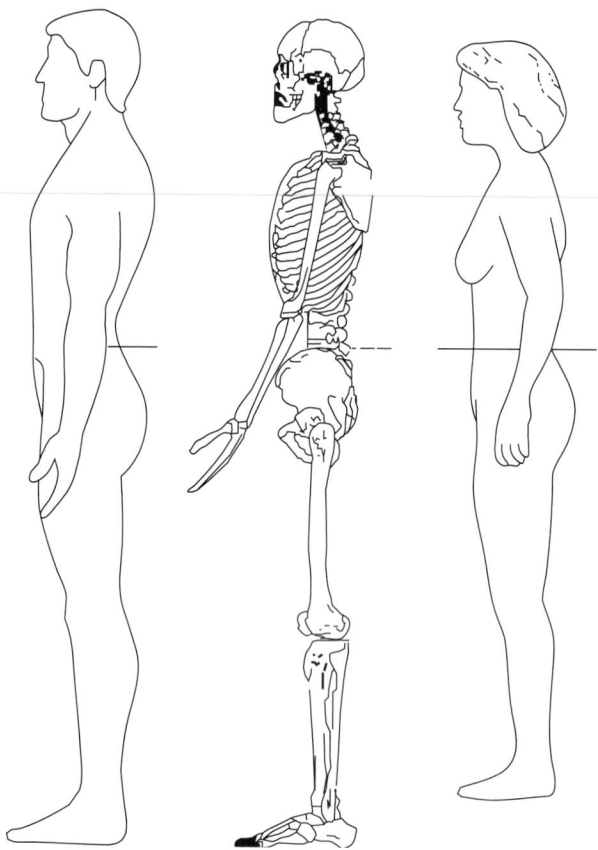

FIGURE 57.3 Appropriate method for measuring waist circumference. (Adapted from Clinical Guidelines on the Identification, Evaluation, and Treatment of Overweight and Obesity in Adults, National Institutes of Health, National Heart, Lung, and Blood Institute.)

for measuring waist circumference is illustrated in Figure 57.3. Although abdominal fat content is more accurately measured by magnetic resonance imaging and computed tomography, practicality and expense limit the clinical usefulness of these methods.

THERAPEUTIC PLAN

Weight loss therapy is indicated for all obese patients (BMI above 30 kg/m^2) and for overweight patients (BMI 25 to 29.9 kg/m^2) or patients with elevated waist circumferences (more than 102 cm in men and more than 88 cm in women) who have two or more risk factors. The mainstay of obesity management includes reduced calorie intake, increased physical activity, and behavioral modification. This combination has proven to be the safest and most effective therapeutic strategy for weight loss and long-term weight maintenance.[6] Unfortunately, overall clinical effectiveness is limited due to problems with patient adherence to the dietary modifications and increased physical activity. Pharmacotherapy may be considered in select patients who have failed to lose sufficient weight following a 6-month trial of diet, exercise, and behavioral modification. Successful weight management involves permanent lifestyle modifications and must include all components of this triad.

Guidelines released by the most recent NIH consensus panel suggest that the first step to obesity treatment is to assess the individual's weight status and risk factors for morbidity and mortality. Figure 57.4 depicts the treatment algorithm established by this group to provide a systematic process for the identification and treatment of overweight and obesity, recognizing that treatment for this condition also encompasses treatment of cardiovascular risk factors.[6]

TREATMENT

NONPHARMACOLOGIC TREATMENTS

Low-Calorie Diet. Current guidelines set forth by the NIH recommend caloric reduction by adherence to a low-calorie

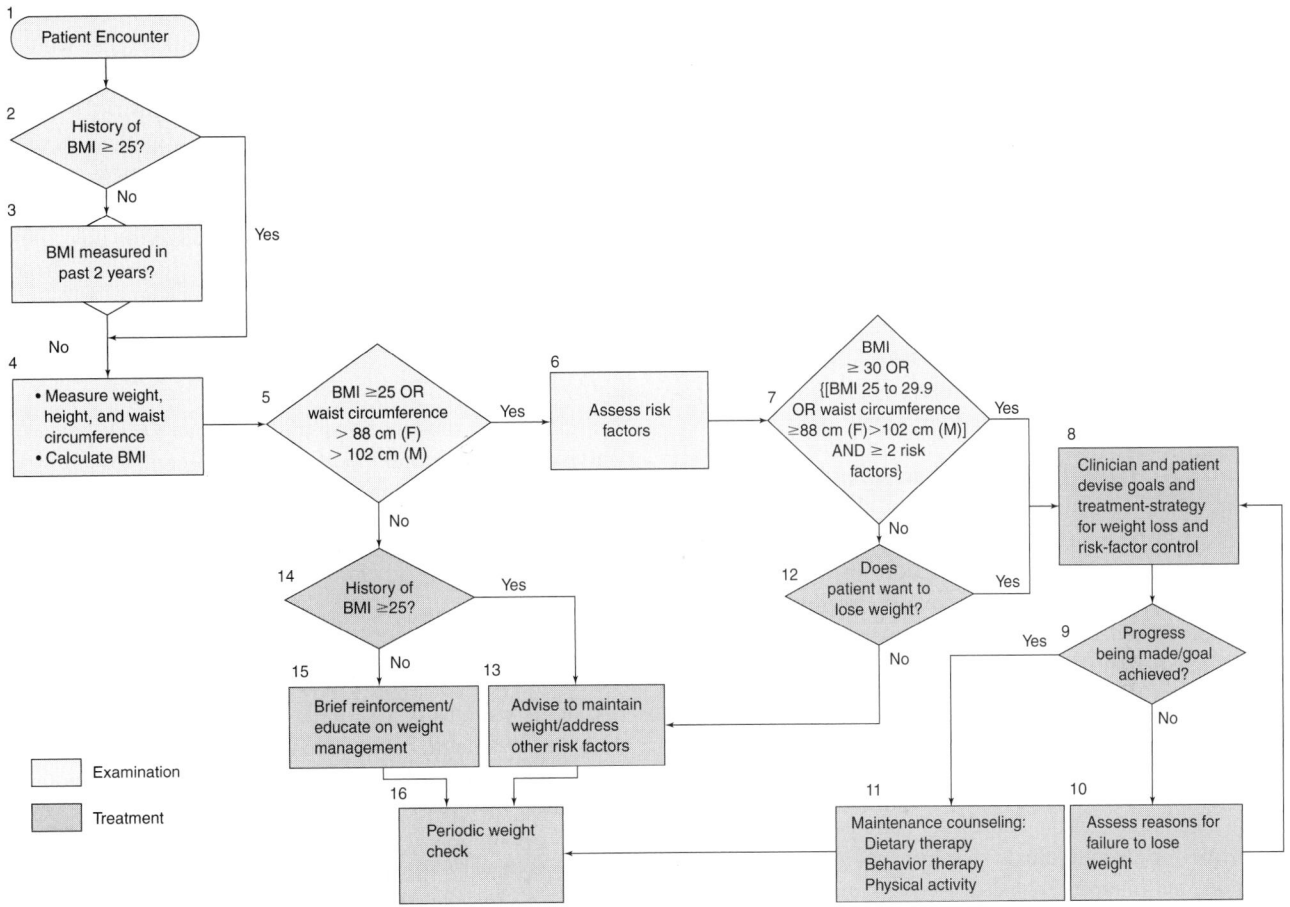

FIGURE 57.4 Obesity treatment algorithm. (Adapted from Clinical Guidelines on the Identification, Evaluation, and Treatment of Overweight and Obesity in Adults, National Institutes of Health, National Heart, Lung, and Blood Institute.)

diet (LCD), defined as a daily caloric deficit of 500 to 1,000 kilocalories (kcal), to provide approximately 800 to 1,200 kcal per day.[6] Clinical trials evaluating the efficacy of the LCD have reported a total weight loss of approximately 8% over a 6-month period of time. The composition of the LCD diet should follow the Step I Diet outlined by the Third Report of the Expert Panel on the Detection, Evaluation, and Treatment of High Blood Cholesterol in Adults (ATP III), as shown in Table 57.3.[23] The use of a very low-calorie diet (VLCD), defined as 250 to 800 kcal/day, is not recommended.[6,24] Although these diets appear very effective initially, overall weight loss after 1 year of treatment does not differ from that observed from the LCD.[25] Patient adherence to the VLCD is also particularly difficult, and the VLCD has been associated with complications such as hypokalemia, dehydration, and the development of gallstones.

The use of a low-carbohydrate, high-protein diet (e.g., the Atkins diet) has become very popular in recent years. Clinical studies evaluating the comparative efficacy of these diets to the conventional LCD have reported significantly greater weight loss at 3 and 6 months with the low-carbohydrate diet, but long-term weight loss at 1 year did not differ

TABLE 57.3	Recommended Composition of the Low-Calorie Diet
Nutrient	**Recommended Intake**
Calories	Approx. 500 to 1,000 kcal/day reduction
Total fat	25% to 35% or less of total calories
Saturated fat	<7% of total calories
Monounsaturated fat	≤20% of total calories
Polyunsaturated fat	≤10% of total calories
Cholesterol	<200 mg/day
Protein	~ 15% of total calories
Carbohydrate	50% to 60% or more of total calories
Fiber	20 to 30 g

(Adapted from Third Report of the National Cholesterol Education Program (NCEP) Expert Panel on Detection, Evaluation, and Treatment of High Blood Cholesterol in Adults (Adult Treatment Panel III). National Institutes of Health, National Heart, Lung and Blood Institute.)

significantly between the two diets.[26,27] Weight loss from low-carbohydrate diets has been associated with improvements in serum triglycerides and HDL cholesterol. However, it is not yet known whether these benefits translate into overall long-term mortality benefits.

Many patients may be tempted to try several types of "fad" diets. Diets involving limited foods, such as the grapefruit juice diet, the cabbage soup diet, and the Beverly Hills diet, promote nutritional misinformation and can result in severe health problems. These programs are not designed to achieve sustained weight loss over the long term and can promote weight cycling, which has been associated with increased mortality.[6] Healthcare professionals should warn patients about the risks associated with these diets.

Physical Activity. Exercise is an important component of weight loss therapy. Physical activity alone has not been shown to provide significant weight loss, but when used in combination with caloric restriction, increased physical activity can promote weight loss, reduce cardiovascular risk, and improve self-esteem and body image. Overweight and obese patients should be evaluated by a physician before beginning an exercise program and should be advised to start slowly and progressively increase the length and intensity of their exercise routine. Thirty to 45 minutes of moderate physical activity on 3 to 5 days per week is an appropriate initial recommendation for these patients. The ultimate objective for all individuals should be 30 minutes or more of moderate-intensity physical activity every day of the week.[6,28]

Behavioral Modification. Behavioral modification can also facilitate weight reduction. The primary goal of behavioral treatment is to modify behaviors that are associated with or promote overconsumption of calories and decreased physical activity. The addition of appropriate behavioral modification therapy to other weight loss strategies has been proven to improve the overall success of weight loss therapy.[6] Common components of behavioral modification include self-monitoring of eating habits, stress management, and social support, among others. Self-monitoring forces patients to record the type of food items eaten daily and when and where they were eaten. The purpose of daily record keeping is to increase the individual's awareness and identify specific eating patterns or behaviors. Once these patterns are identified, the second phase of behavioral therapy focuses on breaking the relationship between repetitive patterns and the actual ingestion of the meal. A number of self-help programs such as Weight Watchers, NutriSystem, Overeaters Anonymous, and Take Off Pounds Sensibly (TOPS), provide obese persons with important psychological support and motivation to bring about permanent weight control measures. These programs are enormously popular, with Weight Watchers alone claiming several million active members.

Surgical Intervention. Surgical intervention for weight loss should be reserved for severe cases of morbid obesity in patients with BMIs of at least 40 kg/m², or at least 35 kg/m² with comorbid conditions, who have failed other weight loss methods.[6] Common surgical techniques used to induce weight loss include gastric restriction or gastric bypass. These procedures can result in substantial weight loss, ranging from 110 to 200 pounds, and significant improvement in obesity-related comorbidities.[6,29] However, these techniques are not without risk: common complications include incisional hernias, gastritis, depression, and cholecystitis. Therefore, surgical intervention for weight loss should be limited to the most severe cases of obesity.

PHARMACOLOGIC TREATMENT

Pharmacologic therapy as an adjunct to an LCD, physical activity, and behavioral modification for weight loss therapy may be considered in patients who have a BMI of at least 30 kg/m², or a BMI of at least 27 kg/m² with concomitant obesity-related risk factors or comorbidities.[6] Obesity-related risk factors or comorbidities that justify drug therapy in patients with BMIs between 27 and 29.9 kg/m² include hypertension, dyslipidemia, coronary heart disease, type 2 diabetes, and sleep apnea. Pharmacologic therapy should not be used in patients who are mildly overweight. In addition, drug therapy should be instituted only after at least 6 months of adherence to an LCD, increased physical activity, and behavioral therapy. If a patient has failed to lose approximately 1 pound per week during this time, then the addition of pharmacologic therapy may be considered (Table 57.4). The need for continued adherence to an LCD, increased physical activity, and behavioral modification should also be emphasized, because drug therapy is effective only when used as an adjunct to these lifestyle modifications.

Sympathomimetic Agents. Several sympathomimetic agents are currently indicated for the short-term management of obesity, such as dextroamphetamine, diethylpropion, phendimetrazine, and phentermine, and mazindol. However, the clinical efficacy of these agents is limited because of the need for long-term dietary changes in combination with increased physical activity and behavioral modification for

TABLE 57.4	Criteria for Consideration of Pharmacologic Therapy for Obesity

BMI ≥30 kg/m²

OR

BMI ≥27 kg/m² with hypertension, dyslipidemia, coronary heart disease, type 2 diabetes, or sleep apnea

AND

Failure to lose at least 1 lb/week during 6 months of a low-calorie diet, increased physical activity, and behavior therapy

(Adapted from Clinical Guidelines on the Identification, Evaluation, and Treatment of Overweight and Obesity in Adults, National Institutes of Health, National Heart, Lung and Blood Institute.)

successful obesity management. Therefore, short-term treatment with a sympathomimetic agent is of limited value. The mechanism of action of these agents involves increasing the concentration of catecholamines to stimulate receptors in the hypothalamus, resulting in appetite suppression. Clinical studies evaluating the efficacy of sympathomimetic agents have reported small weight losses accompanied by weight regain, sometimes in excess of original weight lost, following discontinuation of drug therapy.[6,30] These agents may cause adverse events such as tachycardia and increased blood pressure, nervousness, sweating, headache, and constipation. For some agents, particularly the amphetamine derivatives, a significant potential for abuse and addiction also exists. For these reasons, sympathomimetic agents have no role in the long-term management of obesity.

Sibutramine. Sibutramine (Meridia) was the first antiobesity medication approved by the U.S. Food and Drug Administration (FDA) for the long-term management of obesity. Sibutramine exerts its pharmacologic effect by inhibiting the neuronal reuptake of serotonin, norepinephrine, and dopamine. Combined noradrenergic and serotonergic effects promote an early feeling of fullness and an overall decrease in caloric intake. The initial recommended dose of sibutramine for weight loss therapy is 10 mg daily, which may be increased to 15 mg daily after 4 weeks of therapy.

The efficacy of sibutramine as a weight loss treatment has been evaluated in numerous clinical studies lasting from 6 months to 2 years. Most studies evaluated the efficacy of sibutramine when used as an adjuvant to an LCD, increased exercise, and behavioral modification. The average weight loss reported after 1 year of treatment with sibutramine is approximately 4.5 kg (10 pounds).[31] Most weight loss associated with sibutramine treatment is observed during the first 6 months of therapy. Interestingly, the amount of weight loss a patient achieves after the first 4 weeks of therapy has been found to be highly predictive of overall weight loss success with sibutramine. Therefore, the manufacturer recommends that if a patient has not experienced adequate weight loss (about 4 pounds) during the first 4 weeks of therapy, the sibutramine dose may be increased (to 15 mg daily) or therapy may be discontinued.[32]

The most common adverse effects reported with sibutramine are dry mouth, headache, constipation, insomnia, nervousness, dizziness, nausea, and dyspepsia.[32] Importantly, sibutramine has been reported to cause small increases in blood pressure (1 to 3 mm Hg) and heart rate (4 or 5 beats per minute).[31] However, a few patients have experienced much higher and potentially dangerous increases in blood pressure (approximately 10 to 15 mm Hg).[32] Therefore, patients with uncontrolled hypertension should not receive sibutramine. Increases in blood pressure and heart rate have been shown to be dose-dependent; therefore, patients with controlled hypertension should receive the lowest dose of sibutramine (i.e., 5 mg daily), with close monitoring of blood pressure and heart rate before the dose is increased.[33] Blood pressure should be monitored closely in all patients starting sibutramine therapy and should be routinely monitored throughout therapy. The drug should be discontinued in any patient who experiences substantial increases in heart rate or blood pressure.[34] Accordingly, sibutramine should not be used in patients with a history of coronary heart disease, congestive heart failure, arrhythmias, or stroke.[32] Although sibutramine does have serotonergic effects, cardiac valvular disease associated with the drug has not been reported.[35,36]

Sibutramine is classified as a controlled substance because of the perceived potential for abuse of weight loss drugs. However, studies have shown that the abuse liability of sibutramine is low.[37]

Orlistat. Orlistat (Xenical) was the first antiobesity agent approved by the FDA that does not alter central nervous system neurotransmitters. Orlistat exerts its pharmacologic effect by irreversible inhibition of pancreatic and gastric lipases, which ultimately prevents the breakdown of dietary fat (in the form of triglycerides) into absorbable free fatty acids.[38] Undigested triglycerides are eliminated through the feces, decreasing the absorption of dietary fat. The recommended dose of orlistat for adults and adolescents is 120 mg administered three times daily during or up to 1 hour after each fat-containing meal.[39] Patients should be advised that consuming a high-fat meal along with orlistat may result in increased gastrointestinal adverse effects.

The efficacy of orlistat as a weight loss treatment has been evaluated in numerous clinical studies lasting from 6 months to 4 years. Most studies evaluated the efficacy of orlistat when used as an adjuvant to an LCD, increased exercise, and behavioral modification. The average weight loss reported after 1 year of treatment with orlistat is approximately 5 to 10 kg (10 to 20 pounds).[38] Orlistat has also been shown to improve the lipid profile, glycemic control, and blood pressure in obese patients.[38,40]

The most common adverse effects associated with orlistat include oily rectal spotting, flatulence and flatus with discharge, fecal urgency, fatty or oily stools, increased defecation, and fecal incontinence.[39] Patients should be advised that these adverse effects are generally mild and transient. Although orlistat appears to be slightly more efficacious than sibutramine, these adverse effects may be embarrassing or intolerable for some patients. Orlistat also inhibits the pancreatic enzyme responsible for the breakdown of vitamin esters, thereby decreasing absorption of fat-soluble vitamins. Therefore, the manufacturer recommends that patients receiving orlistat therapy also take a daily multiple-vitamin supplement.[39]

ALTERNATIVE THERAPIES

Common alternative therapy products promoted for weight loss include chromium picolinate, chitosan, guarana (caffeine), spirulina (also known as blue-green algae), ginseng, glucomannan, garcinia (hydroxycitric acid), pyruvate, ma huang (ephedra), and bitter orange (*Citrus aurantium*). Healthcare professionals should be aware that the efficacy and safety of these products have not been scientifically evaluated. In addition, some products can be very dangerous, particularly if taken by patients with underlying cardiovascular disorders. For example, several reports of serious adverse events, including death, have been associated with dietary supplements containing ephedra and caffeine combinations.[41] Because of these reports, the FDA banned all dietary supplements containing ephedrine alkaloids in early 2004.[42] Many weight loss products now promoted as "ephedra-free" contain bitter orange, which contains synephrine, a sympathomimetic amine that is structurally related to epinephrine.[43] When combined with caffeine, bitter orange may have the same potential to cause serious cardiovascular effects as ephedra alkaloids. Healthcare professionals are responsible for educating patients about the potential risks of these products and emphasizing the role of a reduced-calorie diet, increased physical activity, and behavioral modification for the long-term management of obesity.

FUTURE THERAPIES

Many new areas of drug development are being pursued as a result of the recognition of the morbidity and costs associated with overweight and obesity-related conditions. The first major breakthrough was with the discovery of the *ob* (obesity) gene and leptin.[44] Leptin is a hormone secreted by adipose cells in quantities directly proportional to their size and acts on neuronal targets in the hypothalamus to decrease appetite and increase energy expenditure.[44] Recent evidence suggests that leptin may also regulate several metabolic processes, such as insulin and glucocorticoid secretion, reproduction, and glucose transport within the small intestine.[45] Early research conducted in leptin-deficient mice suggested that leptin replacement therapy may induce significant weight loss. Unfortunately, treatment with recombinant leptin has not proved useful in human obesity, as obese humans have been found to be leptin-resistant. Nevertheless, leptin remains a primary focus in the search for new obesity treatments, and several leptin-analogues are in development. Axokine, a variant of ciliary neurotrophic factor (CNTF), is one such peptide in phase III development. Clinical trials indicate that Axokine activates leptin pathways in the hypothalamus to decrease appetite and increase energy expenditure, while at the same time bypassing leptin resistance in obese subjects.[46] Another agent in the final stages of testing for obesity treatment is rimonabant (Acomplia), a cannabinoid receptor antagonist. Antagonism of cannabinoid receptors located in the brain suppresses appetite and increases the metabolic rate. Results of initial clinical studies evaluat-

ing the efficacy of rimonabant have reported that the drug induces significant weight loss in obese patients and may also provide beneficial effects on serum lipid concentrations.[44] Other investigational agents being studied for obesity management include amylin, cholecystokinin A (CCK-A) agonists, neuropeptide Y (NPY) antagonists, and β3-adrenergic agonists, among others.

IMPROVING OUTCOMES

Information about improving outcomes for management of obesity is limited.[47] A multidisciplinary treatment approach—including the involvement of dietitians, exercise physiologists, psychologists, pharmacists, nurses, and physicians—appears to be the most effective method for improving weight loss outcomes in obese patients. Communication among the different healthcare professionals involved to maintain continuity of care is very important. Because many patients may not realize the significant health risks associated with obesity, healthcare professionals must help patients recognize when weight loss therapy should be instituted and must help them set realistic weight loss goals. Therefore, assessment of BMI and obesity risk status should be routinely conducted.

According to the 2002 Surgeon's General Call to Action to Prevent and Decrease Overweight and Obesity, several activities are recommended to improve the management of obesity in the United States. These include educating the public about the health risks associated with obesity, promoting healthy dietary habits and increased physical activity throughout society, and actively investing in research to facilitate understanding of the causes, prevention, and treatment of obesity.[48]

PATIENT EDUCATION

Healthcare professionals who are directly involved in the care of obese patients should provide appropriate educational instruction to help patients make appropriate dietary choices. Many obese patients may not be educated about the differences in caloric content of various foods. Without proper education, these patients will be unable to adhere to the recommended dietary modifications. In addition, patients receiving orlistat or sibutramine should be educated about the potential adverse effects of drug therapy. These patients should also be informed that drug therapy is successful only if it is used as an adjunct to a reduced-calorie diet, increased physical activity, and proper behavioral modifications.

Unfortunately, obese patients are often identified by society as being lazy, sloppy, or undisciplined. Because of this stereotype, many obese individuals may be embarrassed to seek medical care for their condition. Healthcare professionals should treat obese patients with the proper respect and support to promote long-term weight loss.

PHARMACOECONOMICS

The economic impact of obesity on society is staggering. According to one analysis, medical expenses for overweight and obesity accounted for 9.1% of total U.S. healthcare expenditures in 1998, approximately $78.5 billion.[49] Although modest decreases in weight can significantly improve the management of obesity-related risk factors and illnesses, long-term cost analyses of treatment to document overall economic benefit are limited. A few studies have evaluated the economic benefit of drug therapy with sibutramine and orlistat. These studies have concluded that both treatments are cost-effective methods for the management of obesity when they are used in combination with a reduced-calorie diet, exercise, and appropriate behavioral modification.[50–52] However, a number of third-party insurance plans do not cover the expenses associated with pharmacologic weight loss therapies or behavioral modification programs. The direct cost to patients for these treatment strategies can be quite large. Until pharmacoeconomic studies prove that significant long-term cost savings are associated with the use of these drugs and behavioral modification programs, patients will carry the primary responsibility for these costs.

EATING DISORDERS

TREATMENT GOALS

- Recognize the typical signs, symptoms, and behaviors often manifested by patients with eating disorders.
- Prevent, treat, and delay the progression of various secondary complications associated with eating disorders.
- Use behavioral therapy to increase the level of patient cooperation with treatment, assist patients in changing misperceptions about their eating disorder, enhance patients' ability to socialize comfortably with others, and combat other ill-formed psychologies that disrupt appropriate weight maintenance.
- In the anorexic patient, restore ideal body weight first, then proceed to maintain the patient at that weight.
- In certain circumstances, use pharmacotherapy to maintain weight and/or diminish or eliminate the characteristic anorectic or binge-and-purge behaviors associated with eating disorders. Overall treatment should aim at improving long-term patient outcomes and preventing nonadherence and relapse.

DEFINITION

The two classic eating disorders are anorexia nervosa and bulimia nervosa. Historical accounts of anorexia nervosa date back to 1684, when a young woman was described as a "skeleton clad only in skin."[53] The first modern account of anorexia nervosa was by Sir William Gull in the late 19th century.[54] Bulimia nervosa has only recently been recognized as a psychiatric problem, with the first scientific citation appearing in 1979.[55] Specific criteria for anorexia and bulimia are summarized in the American Psychiatric Association's *Diagnostic and Statistical Manual of Mental Disorders* (DSM-IV) and are presented in Table 57.5.[56]

In general, anorexia nervosa is a syndrome characterized by self-starvation, extreme weight loss, excessive exercise, body image disturbance, and an intense fear of becoming obese, despite being grossly underweight.[57] "Anorexia" is, however, a misnomer, because patients usually do not lose their appetites.

Bulimia nervosa is characterized by binge eating usually followed by some form of purging, such as self-induced vomiting, medication-induced vomiting (often with ipecac), laxative abuse, or associated behaviors such as diuretic use, diet pill use, or compulsive exercising.[58] Some bulimic patients with type 1 diabetes have even been known to omit the use of insulin as a purging strategy.[59]

The main characteristic difference between anorexia and bulimia is that anorexic patients are typically under ideal body weight, whereas bulimic patients are often normal weight. The two subtypes of anorexia are restrictive and binge/purge: the former patient prevents weight gain strictly by restricting intake, the latter patient by using binge/purge behaviors.[56] The two subtypes of bulimia are bingeing/purging and strictly purging: the former patient will binge eat and follow up with purging, and the latter patient will not binge eat but will still attempt to purge.[60] Most patients with eating disorders lie on a continuum between strictly restrictive and strictly binge/purge: about 50% of patients origi-

TABLE 57.5	DSM-IV Criteria for Anorexia Nervosa and Bulimia Nervosa

Anorexia nervosa

A. Refusal to maintain body weight at or above a minimal normal weight for age and height (e.g., weight loss leading to maintenance of body weight 15% below that expected or failure to make expected weight gain during period of growth, leading to body weight 15% below that expected).

B. Intense fear of gaining weight or becoming fat, even though underweight.

C. Disturbance in the way in which one's body weight, size, or shape is experienced; undue influence of body weight or shape on self-evaluation or denial of the seriousness of the current low body weight.

D. In females, absence of at least three consecutive menstrual cycles when otherwise expected to occur (primary or secondary amenorrhea). (A woman is considered to have amenorrhea if her periods occur only after hormone [e.g., estrogen] administration.)

Specify type

Restricting type: During the episode of anorexia nervosa the person does not regularly engage in binge eating or purging behavior (i.e., self-induced vomiting or the misuse of laxatives or diuretics).

Binge eating/purging type: During the episode of anorexia nervosa, the person regularly engages in binge-eating or purging behavior (i.e., self-induced vomiting or the misuse of laxatives or diuretics).

Bulimia nervosa

A. Recurrent episodes of binge eating. An episode of binge eating is characterized by both of the following:

　i. Eating, in a discrete period of time (e.g., within any 2-hour period), an amount of food that is definitely larger than most people would eat during a similar period of time and under similar circumstances.

　ii. A sense of lack of control over eating during the episode (e.g., a feeling that one cannot stop eating or control what or how much one is eating).

B. Recurrent inappropriate compensatory behavior to prevent weight gain, such as self-induced vomiting; misuse of laxatives, diuretics, or other medications; fasting; or excessive exercise.

C. The binge-eating and inappropriate compensatory behaviors both occur, on average, at least twice a week for 3 months. Self-evaluation is unduly influenced by body shape and weight. The disturbance does not occur exclusively during episodes of anorexia nervosa.

Specify Type

Purging type: The person regularly engages in self-induced vomiting or the misuse of laxatives or diuretics.

Nonpurging type: The person uses other inappropriate compensatory behaviors, such as fasting or excessive exercise, but does not regularly engage in self-induced vomiting or the misuse of laxatives or diuretics.

nally with anorexia develop binge/purge behaviors of bulimia, and about 5% of patients originally with bulimia develop restrictive behaviors of anorexia.[60,61]

ETIOLOGY

The exact precipitating factors of eating disorders are unknown, but genetic, chemical, cultural, and physiological influences may play a role in their development. It is proposed that in 50% to 83% of cases, genetics are a determining factor of disease progression. In fact, it was found that identical twins have a higher coupled incidence of eating disorders than do fraternal twins.[59] Similarly, higher rates of eating disorders are seen in the first-degree female relatives of patients diagnosed with eating disorders than in the general population.[60] Lower levels of serotonin may also be partly to blame. Abnormally low levels of serotonin were detected in the cerebrospinal fluid of bulimic patients. Dysregulation of serotonin may contribute to the two to three-and-a-half times higher prevalence of unipolar depression or bipolar disorder seen in patients with eating disorders.[59]

The preoccupation with food and eating seen in these patients stems partly from the cultural value that Western society places on thinness.[62] In early beauty pageants in the United States, models weighed 91% of the average woman's weight; models in similar pageants today weigh 82.5% of the average woman's weight.[53] However, current societal pressures cannot be fully to blame, because accounts of eating disorders date back to the mid-19th century and perhaps as far back as the 17th century.[53,61]

Premature birth and birth trauma have been also linked to the eventual development of eating disorders.[59]

Finally, there may be a critical weight under which death may be inevitable. A study found that rats deprived of food would keep running on a wheel until they died, but rats that were fed would continue to thrive. The conclusions of this experiment are telling and somewhat disturbing.[63]

EPIDEMIOLOGY

The overall prevalence for women meeting the diagnostic criteria from the DSM-IV for anorexia or bulimia is approximately 0.25% to 4%.[59] The prevalence of anorexia in women is 0.5% to 3.7%; the prevalence of bulimia in women is slightly higher, at 1.1% to 4.2%.[60] It is estimated that the incidence of anorexia and bulimia has doubled over the past two decades.

The typical eating disorder patient is female, white, and from a middle- to upper-class socioeconomic background.[60,61] The prevalence of eating disorders in males is much lower: about 5% to 10% of all cases in the United States are reported in males.[60,64] Although the United States is commonly targeted as having an above-average prevalence of eating disorders, other countries, such as Japan, China, Spain, Argentina, and Fiji, have seen escalating incidences of eating disorders over the past few years.[60]

Eating disorders may manifest as early as childhood but typically begin in adolescence, with a peak age of onset at 18 years of age.[60,62] Statistics in younger children are staggering. Approximately 42% of first- to third-grade girls would like to lose weight, and about 81% of 10-year-old girls fear weight gain. This progresses into adolescence, as it is estimated that 5% to 10% of postpubescent females have an eating disorder and that 25% to 35% of college women display binge/purge behaviors.[59]

Greater than 50% of all children and adolescents have eating disorders "not otherwise specified" (NOS), which may not meet all DSM-IV criteria for anorexia and bulimia and thus go undiagnosed. Healthcare professionals should be able to recognize these patients and, depending on the severity of the symptoms, may need to initiate therapy similar to that of a more clearly characterized eating disorder.[64]

Signs of eating disorders may not manifest until adulthood. In fact, it is estimated that a quarter of American men and slightly less than half of American women are dieting on any given day; one third of these dieters may progress to pathologic dieting.[65]

Perhaps the most disturbing statistic is that anorexia is the most common cause of death in females ages 15 to 24 years.[59] The estimated 10-year mortality rate of anorexia is 5.6%. Overall, data regarding psychiatric illnesses suggest that eating disorders and substance abuse disorders are the leading cause of excess mortality; in fact, research suggests that the two disorders are often interrelated.[59,60] In addition, a 6-year follow-up study of bulimic patients found that 1% had died by the end of the study period.[60]

CLINICAL PRESENTATION AND DIAGNOSIS

At diagnosis, healthcare professionals need to know when an anorexic or bulimic patient needs to be admitted to a hospital or inpatient rehabilitation program. The Society for Adolescent Medicine, consistently with the American Psychiatric Association, has developed criteria for admission for children, adolescents, and young adults to such programs, as outlined in Table 57.6. Some of the criteria for anorexia include less than 75% of ideal body weight, refusal to eat, body fat less than 10% of total body composition, and systolic blood pressure below 90 mm Hg. The criteria for bulimia include syncope, serum potassium level below 3.2 mEq per L, serum chloride below 88 mEq per L, hypothermia, and suicide risk.[64]

SIGNS AND SYMPTOMS

The generalized secretiveness and denial of signs and symptoms associated with eating disorders often make these ill-

TABLE 57.6	Criteria for Hospitalization of Children, Adolescents, or Young Adults with Eating Disorders

Anorexia Nervosa

- <75% ideal body weight, or ongoing weight loss despite intensive management
- Refusal to eat
- Body fat <10%
- Heart rate <50 beats per minute daytime, <45 beats per minute nighttime
- Systolic pressure <90
- Orthostatic changes in pulse (>20 beats per minute) or blood pressure (>10 mm Hg)
- Temperature <96°F
- Arrhythmia

Bulimia Nervosa

- Syncope
- Serum potassium concentration <3.2 mmol/L
- Serum chloride concentration <88 mmol/L
- Esophageal tears
- Cardiac arrhythmias, including prolonged QT_c
- Hypothermia
- Suicide risk
- Intractable vomiting
- Hematemesis
- Failure to respond to outpatient treatment

(Adapted from Committee on Adolescence. American Academy of Pediatrics Policy Statement: identifying and treating eating disorders. Pediatrics 111:204–211, 2003.)

nesses difficult to detect. Most patients with eating disorders do not come forward voluntarily to healthcare professionals; instead, they are often referred by external sources such as friends, teachers, coaches, companions, or family members.[60] Once referred, the patient usually denies symptoms and is petulant, highly secretive, deeply distrustful, and unwilling to reveal personal thoughts, behaviors, or routines. Some children even go so far as to put items in their clothes or drink excessive fluids prior to weighing to deceive healthcare professionals. Persons suspected of having an eating disorder should have a urine specific gravity assessed prior to weighing and should wear a hospital gown during weighing for the aforementioned reasons.[64,66]

If a patient is not self-referred or referred by external sources, healthcare professionals may need to recognize psychological comorbidities that aid in the detection of these elusive disorders. First, a number of affective or personality disorders may be present in patients with eating disorders. About 50% to 75% of patients with eating disorders may present as dysthymic or depressed, 25% may present as obsessive-compulsive, and 4% to 13% may present as bipolar.[60] Approximately 20% to 45% of patients may have some degree of social anxiety disorder,[53] and 42% to 75% of patients may have some form of personality disorder (e.g., narcissistic, borderline, histrionic).[60]

Patients with eating disorders are prone to engage in substance abuse. Substance abuse is consistently associated with binge/purge behaviors and is prevalent in about 12% to 18% of anorexics and 30% to 70% of bulimics.[59,60]

In addition to psychological signs, there are also physical signs, both morphologic and physiologic, that may aid in the detection of eating disorders. Anorexia is usually easier to detect than bulimia because of the underweight, gaunt appearance of many anorexic patients.[60] Also, patients with anorexia often appear younger than they actually are and may present with lethargy; constipation; orthostatic hypotension; dry, scaly skin; or brittle hair and nails.[53] Bulimic patients, on the other hand, are often at or above ideal body weight.[60] Russell's sign (ulcerous sores on the dorsal side of the patient's hand) is an effective way to identify patients who chronically induce vomiting.[62] Laboratory abnormalities found in patients with eating disorders include iron-deficiency anemia, magnesium deficiency, and elevated blood urea nitrogen (BUN).[53,59] Urine sodium to chloride content may be an accurate laboratory predictor for bulimia.[59] A complete list of signs and symptoms of eating disorders can be found in Table 57.7.

Pharmacists can play an important role in the detection of eating disorders by monitoring suspicious use of laxatives (e.g., senna or bisacodyl), enemas, diuretics, appetite suppressants, and syrup of ipecac and by educating patients on their appropriate use.[53,62] In fact, one small study noted a 50% reduction in patients' laxative use after 6 months of participation in a laxative taper protocol supervised solely by pharmacists.[67] The frequent use of loop or thiazide prescription diuretics by otherwise healthy young female patients should be cause for suspicion, because a study of 275 bulimic patients found that 34% admitted to using a prescription diuretic for weight control. Also, the particularly dangerous practice of chronically inducing vomiting with syrup of ipecac can lead to potentially fatal cardiac, gastrointestinal, or neuromuscular toxicities.[62,68]

Pharmacists should take an active role in the detection of eating disorders, because they are in an ideal position to monitor the over-the-counter and prescription drugs most often abused by such patients. Appropriate referrals to other healthcare professionals and regional or local support groups can be extremely helpful for getting these patients the proper and necessary care.

DIAGNOSIS AND CLINICAL FINDINGS

Upon diagnosis of an eating disorder, it is important for healthcare professionals to be able to estimate a patient's prognosis. Characteristics associated with a poor prognosis in anorexic patients include vomiting, initial low weight, and a history of family disturbances and marital problems.

TABLE 57.7 | Recognizing Patients with Eating Disorders

- Female in early to late teens who (a) exhibits weight loss or no significant weight gain during development (anorexia) or (b) exhibits frequent significant weight fluctuations (bulimia)

- Young women fitting the eating disorder stereotype who repeatedly purchase laxatives, enemas, appetite suppressants, syrup of ipecac, or diuretics and who typically cover themselves with baggy, nonconforming clothing to conceal their illness

- Complaints of irregular menstrual cycles or amenorrhea

- History of depression or alcohol/other drug use or abuse

- Other nonspecific complaints, such as swollen parotid glands, constipation, frequent sore throats from vomiting, abdominal complaints from laxative abuse

- Physical characteristics: Russell's sign, hypertrophied salivary glands, poor dentition, dehydration, edema, decreased subcutaneous fat, atrophic breasts, dry skin with lanugo, yellowing of skin due to carotenemia, sunken eyes, possible alopecia, bradycardia, hypotension, hypothermia, and abdominal bloating

- Laboratory screening: electrolyte imbalances, acidosis or alkalosis, anemia, leukopenia, thrombocytopenia, low plasma protein, hypoglycemia, and elevated liver enzymes; urine and stool samples to detect diuretic or laxative abuse

- Other signs: impulsivity (shoplifting, promiscuity), poor self-esteem, post-trauma symptoms, personality disorders, cognitive distortions, suicidal ideation/attempts, self-destructive or self-mutilating behaviors

---

Characteristics associated with a poor prognosis in bulimic patients include excessive vomiting and required hospitalization.[60]

The complications of anorexia are mainly those of starvation and result in nutritional deficiencies and, consequently, morphologic changes. For example, zinc deficiency, a common sequela of anorexia, can contribute to cachexia, decreased appetite, and amenorrhea.[59] Hypothalamic-pituitary gonadal dysfunction may also contribute to amenorrhea.[59] Thiamine deficiency, with an eventual sequela of Wernicke's encephalopathy, occurs in over one third of anorexic patients.[59] Patients with anorexia often have abnormally low levels of T3, although their thyroid-stimulating hormone and T4 levels are usually within normal limits.[59] Cortisol serum levels, which are implicated in the worsening of depression, are increased in patients with anorexia.[59] This overproduction of cortisol, in addition to lower levels of estrogen and deficient calcium intake, is thought to contribute to the osteoporosis seen in more than 50% of anorexic patients.[59] Externally, the growth of lanugo, a fine, primitive hair, indicates progression of anorexia and the body's natural attempt to combat hypothermia. Carotinemia, evidenced by a yellowish tint to the skin, is also indicative of the progression of anorexia.[66] Cardiac complications such as sinus bradycardia and cardiac arrhythmias are the most common cause of death.[69]

Digestive disturbances and laboratory abnormalities are the most prevalent complications associated with bulimia. In general, complications from bulimia tend to be less severe and are the consequences of chronic bingeing and purging. Most visibly noticeable of persons who purge excessively is the characteristic "chipmunk face" secondary to parotid gland swelling.[70] This painless enlargement of the salivary glands is known as sialadenosis.[62] Chronic bulimic patients often have poor enamel on their teeth, and upon inspection of the esophagus, Mallory–Weiss tears may be evident from constant exposure to acidic gastric contents.[62] Continual bingeing and purging can result in gastric dilation that ultimately may inhibit gastric motility.[59] About 5% of bulimic patients present with hypokalemia or hypomagnesiumia.[59,62] Hypokalemia from excessive vomiting or diuretic use can lead to pseudo-Bartter's syndrome, a condition in which the patient is normotensive yet alkalotic.[62] Cardiac complications such as arrhythmias can occur from prolonged hypovolemia and hypokalemia. In severe bulimia, the patient eventually loses the gag reflex and no longer needs stimulation to induce emesis. These patients are at increased risk for aspiration pneumonia, especially if under the influence of alcohol.[68]

Complications associated with anorexia and bulimia are reviewed and compared in Table 57.8.

PSYCHOSOCIAL ASPECTS

Psychosocial influences play a major role in the development, sustenance, and eventual recovery from eating disorders. Societal influences and personal experiences, especially at particularly vulnerable times, may shape the way a person views his or her body. For example, it is estimated that 20% to 30% of bulimic patients have a history of sexual abuse. It is noted that anorexic patients have difficulty with separation, expressing anger, and negotiating sexual behaviors; bulimic patients have difficulty with impulse control and often seem dissociated. Upon recovery, psychological changes should be expected. Although lethargy and malnutrition may cease, patients may become more anxious, depressed, or even suicidal as weight is restored. Unfortunately, this irrational and distorted view is one of the last perceptions to change after recovery.[60]

TREATMENT

Treatment of anorexia and bulimia requires a multidisciplinary approach, often incorporating psychotherapy and pharmacotherapy. Healthcare professionals should rarely embark on the task of treating patients single-handedly; instead, clinicians with expertise in specialty areas and the treatment of eating disorders should be consulted. Multidisciplinary teams often consist of the primary care physician, a specialized physician, psychiatrist, dietitian, and mental health professional (e.g., psychologist, social worker, or nurse). Clinical pharmacy specialists also play a major role in patient education and in the recommendation, selection, and monitoring of prescription and nonprescription medication. Treating eating disorders is virtually always a long-term process and requires considerable clinical skill, patience, and compassion to build an effective, trusting relationship with the patient.

PHARMACOTHERAPY

Anorexia. Despite several trials with a number of different pharmacologic agents, optimal and overwhelmingly successful drug therapies have not been identified for the treatment of anorexia. To complicate matters, anorectic patients and their families tend to deny the existence and severity of the illness and fail to obtain adequate medical and psychiatric care.[55] In general, studies show that using antidepressants such as fluoxetine during the early refeeding/hospitalization phase of anorexia is generally not effective.[60] It is proposed that anorexic patients may already have a relative lack of circulating serotonin, and therefore selective serotonin reuptake inhibitors (SSRIs) offer little added benefit by blocking the reuptake of an already deficient neurotransmitter.

However, patients who achieve ideal body weight and recover past the refeeding stage may have less future weight loss, less depression, and fewer rehospitalizations if started on an average of 40 mg fluoxetine daily.[60] In fact, a 52-week, double-blind placebo-controlled trial of fluoxetine use in restrictive anorexic females being treated as outpatients was conducted to examine if fluoxetine better prevented relapse after hospital discharge.[71] Patients received anywhere from 20 to 60 mg of fluoxetine or placebo daily and were evaluated every 4 weeks after discharge. Although only a few women completed the trial (19 fluoxetine, 20 placebo), statistically significant differences were found between the groups. Patients taking placebo relapsed significantly faster than patients taking fluoxetine. Also, patients taking fluoxetine had significant increases in weight, reduction in symptoms of anorexia, and overall improvement in mood compared to placebo patients. The authors concluded that fluoxetine therapy after discharge helps prevent relapse to anorexic symptoms.

Researchers also studied the addition of tryptophan, fish oils, and vitamin/mineral supplements to outpatient treatment with fluoxetine, and the results suggested that their addition conferred no additional benefit.[72]

Other antidepressants have been studied for the prevention of relapse and overall improvement in symptoms of anorexic patients after refeeding. Citalopram, another SSRI, was associated with additional weight loss compared to placebo in the outpatient treatment of anorexia and consequently did not prove to be a sound choice for pharmacotherapy.[73] However, a recent pilot study of citalopram for the treatment of anorexia showed significant improvement in

TABLE 57.8	Complications of Anorexia Nervosa and Bulimia Nervosa	
Organ System	**Anorexia Nervosa**	**Bulimia Nervosa**
Endocrine/Metabolic	Amenorrhea	Menstrual irregularities
	Decreased norepinephrine secretion	Metabolic acidosis
	Decreased somatomedin C	Electrolyte disturbances
	Low or erratic vasopressin secretion	
	Hypercarotenemia	
	Low gonadotropins, estrogens, testosterone	
	Sick euthyroid syndrome	
	Raised cortisol and positive dexamethasone suppression test	
	Raised growth hormone	
	Abnormal temperature regulation (hypothermia)	
	Dehydration, electrolyte disturbances (hypokalemia, hypomagnesemia, hypocalcemia, hyponatremia, hypophosphatemia)	
	Hypercholesterolemia	
	Hypoglycemia	
	Raised liver enzymes	
	Refeeding syndrome	
Cardiovascular	Bradycardia	Ipecac toxicity
	Hypotension	Arrhythmia
	Arrhythmia	Cardiomyopathy
	Prolonged QT interval	Orthostatic hypotension
	Decreased heart mass	
	Attenuated response to exercise	
	Pericardial effusion	
	Superior mesenteric artery syndrome	
Renal	Acute and chronic renal failure	Electrolyte disturbances (hypokalemia, diuretic-induced)
	Increased blood urea nitrogen	
	Partial diabetes insipidus	Renal failure
	Polyuria	Proteinuria
	Peripheral edema	Hematuria
Gastrointestinal	Decreased gastric emptying and motility	Sore throat
	Decreased lipase, lactose	Swelling of parotid gland (chipmunk face)
	Constipation	Acute gastric dilation, rupture, tearing
	Bowel obstruction	
	Elevated amylase	Esophagitis
	Pancreatitis	Stomatitis
	Irritable bowel syndrome	Hematemesis
	Elevated hepatic enzymes	Diarrhea
		Constipation
		Steatorrhea
		Dental carries, erosion of tooth enamel

(continued)

Organ System	Anorexia Nervosa	Bulimia Nervosa
		Decreased gastric emptying and motility
		Laxative dependence
		Hypokalemia (diuretic-induced)
		Rectal bleeding
		Gastric/duodenal ulcer
		Ipecac toxicity
Hematologic	Anemia	
	Leukopenia	
	Thrombocytopenia	
	Hypocellular bone marrow	
	Low plasma protein	
Pulmonary		Aspiration pneumonia
Musculoskeletal	Cramps, tetany	Muscle weakness
	Muscle weakness	Fasciculations
	Stress fractures	
	Osteopenia	
	Osteoporosis	
Immunologic	Impaired immune function	
	Low complement levels	
	Impaired T cells	
	Granulocyte abnormalities	
	Bacterial infections	
Neurologic	Impaired autonomic activity	Ipecac toxicity
	Seizures	
	Abnormal electroencephalogram	
	Nerve compressions	
	Peripheral neuritis	
	Cerebral atrophy	
Skin	Dry, scaly skin	Russell's sign
	Brittle hair and nails	Easy bruising
	Increased lanugo-like body hair	
	Easy bruising	

TABLE 57.8 continued

psychometric scales and BMI from baseline, but citalopram and placebo groups did not have significantly different BMIs at the end of the study.[74]

Although tricyclic antidepressants (TCAs) may be just as effective as SSRIs at the correct doses for the outpatient treatment of anorexia, their safety profiles are not desirable, especially considering the common adverse effects seen in anorexic patients. For example, TCAs can be detrimental in malnourished patients, as they can potentiate hypotension or arrhythmias in such patients.[60] In overdose TCAs pose a great threat to patients who are already depressed and at a high risk for suicide. Given the availability of safer drugs such as SSRIs, TCAs should not be used in the treatment of anorexia.

Although other antidepressants have been researched for their benefits in anorexic patients, the current literature suggests that fluoxetine is the antidepressant treatment of choice in anorexic patients after refeeding.[60] The unlabeled dosage range for fluoxetine in the treatment of anorexia is 20 to 80 mg daily. Slow upward dose titration over several days is advisable in these patients to decrease the severity and incidence of adverse effects. Other SSRIs have been investigated, but their use is limited to case reports.[60]

Because of the attention that some antipsychotic medications have received for suspected weight gain, research is beginning to focus on the benefit of using such medications for the treatment of anorexia. Some of the newer atypical antipsychotics may be especially useful in combination with SSRIs in patients with highly obsessive behaviors.[60]

Although no large, double-blind, placebo-controlled trials of antipsychotics in anorexia have been published, case reports, retrospective studies, and open-label trials suggest benefits of use. To date, olanzapine has been the most highly researched of the atypical antipsychotics for the treatment of anorexia. For example, a 10-question survey that asked 18 anorexic patients to assess different aspects of their disease before and during treatment with olanzapine showed that patients had significant reductions from baseline in obsessions about weight, reduced concern with body image, and reduced meal-related anxiety during treatment.[75] Patients in the study had been taking an average of 4.7 mg olanzapine daily. An open-label trial in 18 anorexic patients was designed to determine whether 10 mg olanzapine would result in significant weight gain over a 10-week period.[76] Patients were required to attend weekly study and adherence visits. A mean weight gain of 5 pounds from baseline was noted at the end of the trial (P <0.0138). Thirteen patients experienced sedation while taking olanzapine. A case series of two patients who received 1 to 1.5 mg daily of risperidone for the treatment of anorexia showed a significant improvement in weight and decreased delusional thinking.[77] Another open-label trial involving low doses of the older antipsychotic haloperidol was conducted in 13 outpatients with restrictive anorexia over 6 months.[78] At the end of the study, patients had experienced significant improvements in BMI (15.7 to 18.1 kg/m^2, P = 0.03) and eating disorder psychological tests such as the Eating Disorder Inventory (EDI).

Although trial design has not been ideal in this area of research, preliminary studies suggest that antipsychotic medications may be effective in decreasing delusional thinking about food while increasing weight as an added benefit. Finally, the American Psychiatric Association recommends that only patients with other psychological dysfunctions and anorexia should be treated with psychotropics such as antidepressants or antipsychotics.[60]

Other miscellaneous drugs have been researched for the treatment of anorexia. In a double-blind study of 72 patients with anorexia, high doses (32 mg/day) of the antihistamine cyproheptadine produced modest weight gain compared to amitriptyline and placebo.[79] Drugs such as clomipramine, lithium carbonate, and pimozide have also been studied but have shown little to no effect on improving symptoms of anorexia.[60]

A number of medications have been researched to allay the adverse effects and complications of anorexia. For example, metoclopramide has been used for bloating secondary to gastroparesis and premature satiety. Estrogen has been shown to increase bone mineral density in patients who have achieved near-normal weight, but it should not be offered until the patient's menstrual cycle is restored and significant weight gain has been achieved.[60] Finally, a small study of 15 patients sought to determine the effect of human growth hormone (HGH) on the cardiac stability of hospitalized anorexic patients.[80] In this 28-day, randomized, placebo-controlled trial, HGH patients achieved cardiac stability, defined as two consecutive mornings without orthostasis, significantly sooner than placebo patients (17 days vs. 37 days, P <0.02). However, no significant differences were seen in weight or overall length of stay between the groups.

Bulimia. Bulimic patients are often more likely to seek treatment than anorexic patients, but they have a low tolerance for extended adherence, leading to a high relapse rate.[81] Compared to anorexia, bulimia is more likely to respond to pharmacotherapy. In fact, pharmacotherapy alone will arrest bulimic symptoms in 30% to 40% of patients.[62]

Similar to anorexic patients, the most highly researched pharmacotherapeutic option for bulimic patients is antidepressants. Antidepressants have been shown to be effective in the treatment of bulimia even if the patient is not depressed.[60] Perhaps the most telling study performed in this area to date is a meta-analysis of 19 trials of 1,436 patients.[82] Only trials that compared antidepressants to placebo in bulimic patients were included, and the primary outcome objective was to see if antidepressants led to greater remission and clinical improvement rates (defined as 100% binge/purge behavior cessation and at least 50% of binge/purge behavior cessation, respectively) compared to placebo. Overall, patients taking any antidepressant had a significantly greater rate of remission or clinical improvement compared to placebo. As expected, patients taking any antidepressant also had a significantly greater rate of dropouts due to adverse events compared to placebo; however, no significant differences were found between the patient acceptability of antidepressant or placebo treatments.

Similar to the treatment of anorexia, one of the most studied medications for bulimia is fluoxetine. In fact, fluoxetine is the only antidepressant with an FDA-approved indication for the treatment of bulimia.[83] In a 16-week, multicenter, double-blind, placebo-controlled trial, 296 patients receiving fluoxetine 60 mg daily experienced significantly fewer mean purging episodes and binge-eating episodes than 102 patients receiving placebo.[84] In fact, 34.1% of the fluoxetine-treated patients had a 75% to 100% reduction in vomiting episodes at endpoint, compared to only 23% of the placebo patients. Adverse effects were mild with fluoxetine, but patients on fluoxetine experienced significantly more nausea, insomnia, anxiety, and dizziness than patients on placebo.

Other researchers set out to determine fluoxetine's long-term effect on maintenance therapy of bulimia. In a 52-week, multicenter, double-blind, placebo-controlled trial, 150 initial responders to fluoxetine were either continued at 60 mg daily (76 patients) or randomized to receive placebo (74 patients).[85] The primary outcome measure was the number of vomiting episodes per week, and patients were assessed every 4 weeks. At 3 months, the relapse rate was significantly lower in the fluoxetine group (19% in the fluoxetine group vs. 37% in the placebo group; $p <0.04$). Patients receiving fluoxetine had significantly fewer bingeing episodes and purging episodes and scored better on a number of psychometric scales than patients receiving placebo. The only adverse effect experienced significantly more often by fluoxetine patients than placebo patients was rhinitis.

Fluoxetine 60 to 80 mg daily for at least 6 months is typically used for the treatment of bulimia, as opposed to the average 20-mg daily dose used for depression.[60] Although fluoxetine is the only SSRI with an indication for bulimia nervosa, virtually all SSRIs have been used in clinical practice. SSRIs are usually given once daily and are well tolerated. Starting and maintenance doses for the other available SSRIs have not been agreed upon in clinical practice but are generally higher than those recommended for the treatment of depressive disorders. Persistent side effects of which patients complain most include dry mouth, increased sweating, decreased libido, and sexual dysfunction.

Various classes of antidepressants other than SSRIs have shown short-term (up to 3 months) efficacy in abating the symptoms of bulimia.[62] In fact, most antidepressants can decrease the frequency of bulimic symptoms by 50% to 60% in the first 6 to 8 weeks of treatment; however, other antidepressants have resulted in worsening of symptoms or introduce safety concerns that are not experienced with SSRIs.[62] For example, the doses of TCAs for the treatment of bulimia are essentially the same as those used for major depressive disorders and are administered for at least 6 to 8 weeks; however, TCAs should be chosen with caution because of their potential for unwanted adverse events. TCAs may increase the risk of cardiac arrhythmia and severe hypotension, especially in those in whom purging and vomiting has led to dehydration and cardiac dysfunction.[64] Other potential side effects include worsened constipation, increased risk of seizures, dry mouth, blurred vision, nausea, and sedation.

Open-label studies of trazodone, another serotonergic antidepressant, produced mixed results and worsening of bulimic behaviors.[86,87] As with its use in major depressive episodes, therapeutic doses of trazodone can rarely be achieved because of unwanted side effects such as orthostasis, arrhythmia, palpitations, dizziness, and blurred vision.

In general, bupropion should not be used in purging patients due to an increased risk for seizures.[60] In fact, in 1986 a trial of bupropion in a bulimic population resulted in a relatively high incidence of seizures, forcing the temporary withdrawal of bupropion from the market.[88]

Finally, a double-blind controlled study with phenelzine, a monoamine oxidase inhibitor (MAOI), produced a striking reduction in bingeing behavior in bulimic patients.[89] Phenelzine has an unlabeled indication for the treatment of bulimic patients who show characteristics of atypical depression, but the use of an MAOI in the treatment of bulimia is usually not warranted due to the availability of safer drugs. An SSRI

such as fluoxetine should be first choice for the treatment of bulimia unless directly contraindicated.

A variety of other medications have been used to treat bulimia, with mixed results. The anticonvulsants phenytoin, carbamazepine, and valproic acid have all been studied in the treatment of bulimia.[90–92] Results have been generally disappointing, but there have been isolated patients with symptomatic improvement. A subgroup of binge eaters whose behavior is secondary to a neurologic disorder analogous to epilepsy may be more likely to respond to an anticonvulsant agent.[93] Lithium and valproic acid, however, should not be the drug of choice for the treatment of bulimia because lithium serum levels can change with the patient's blood volume, and both drugs can contribute to weight gain. Although weight gain is usually desired in the treatment of anorexia, it is not as desirable in the treatment of bulimia because most patients are already near ideal body weight, and additional weight gain from drug therapy can lead to an overall worsening of delusional thinking about food. For example, a 12-year-old girl with schizophrenia being treated with risperidone at a maximum daily dose of 5 mg experienced a 20-kg weight gain within 3 months of starting medication; the girl became preoccupied with her weight and began engaging in binge/purge behaviors.[94] This suggests that patients at risk for initiating or worsening of bulimic symptoms upon weight gain might best be suited for weight-neutral pharmacotherapy.

Other prescription medications such as ondansetron and topiramate have shown promise for the treatment of bulimia, but data are lacking.[62,95–97] Likewise, there is a paucity of information about nonprescription supplements such as L-tryptophan and inositol that suggests that they could improve bulimic symptoms.[59]

Because of the number of complications that may accompany bulimia, healthcare professionals should be familiar with various treatment options. For example, sialadenosis can be reversed by applying heat to the glands or instructing the patient to suck on tart candies; pilocarpine 5 mg orally three times daily may work if these recommendations do not. Proton-pump inhibitors such as omeprazole, rabeprazole, esomeprazole, lansoprazole, or pantoprazole are used to combat reflux seen in bulimic patients. To arrest bone loss, 1,200 to 1,500 mg calcium and 400 to 800 IU vitamin D are recommended daily.[62] Some data suggest that DHEA can also help prevent bone loss.[59] Metoclopramide is often used as an antiemetic in patients with bulimia. Patients with laxative tolerance due to laxative abuse may require hydration, a higher-fiber diet, or glycerin suppositories or osmotic laxatives. To prevent cavities, patients should be encouraged to brush or rinse with fluoride every time after vomiting (although quitting vomiting would be ideal).

Finally, to correct the hypokalemia seen in severe cases of bulimia, volume should be repleted with normal saline and potassium supplementation should be provided with 40 to 80 mEq oral KCl. Practitioners may choose to keep the patient on a KCl supplement if purging is expected to continue.[62]

NONPHARMACOLOGIC THERAPY

Severe cases of anorexia requiring hospitalization as outlined in Table 57.6 will initially require refeeding at a rate that promotes safe weight gain. Oral feeding is preferred over nasogastric and parenteral feeding, because part of the refeeding process is to encourage nonpathologic thoughts about food ingestion.[60] A reasonable inpatient weight gain for adult anorexic patients is 2 to 3 pounds per week. Initially, adult patients should receive about 30 to 40 kcal/kg/day, but this can be adjusted up to 70 to 100 kcal/kg/day, depending on patient tolerance and the severity of the case.[60] A reasonable inpatient weight gain for pediatric anorexic patients is 0.5 to 2 pounds per week, with a recommended daily intake of 2,000 to 3,000 kcal during refeeding.[64] Adolescents may have higher nutritional requirements than adults, but established guidelines do not exist.[66] It may also be prudent to replete vitamins and minerals in addition to calories during refeeding (e.g., B vitamins, folate, magnesium, potassium, copper, and zinc).[59]

Healthcare professionals must practice caution while refeeding. Severely underweight patients can experience fluid retention, cardiac arrhythmias, seizures, and even heart failure if fed too quickly.[60] A ''refeeding syndrome'' that starts as severe hypophosphatemia and can progress to respiratory distress, cardiomyopathy, or neuropathy can occur from extracellular phosphorus being abruptly shifted intracellularly after rapid feeding. Practitioners should determine serum phosphorus level before initiating weight restoration.[59,64]

As the anorexic patient approaches ideal body weight, the focus should shift from weight restoration to the promotion of healthy attitudes toward eating and body image. Because most bulimic patients are already at normal weight, they will usually start treatment at this later phase. Dietitians should be involved with assisting patients to make healthy food choices. Exercise can be incorporated into the recovery program as long as the focus of exercise is placed on physical fitness and not caloric burning. The closer a patient is to ideal body weight upon discharge, the less chance of relapse. If a patient requires additional weight gain after discharge, a reasonable gain of 0.5 to 1 pound per week should be encouraged.[60]

During and after hospitalization, patients with eating disorders should participate in behavioral therapy, as it is an integral part of recovery. A large meta-analysis determined that behavioral therapy in combination with pharmacotherapy was more successful than pharmacotherapy alone for promoting weight gain and reducing hospital stay in anorexic patients.[60] Cognitive behavioral therapy (CBT) is the best studied of the different types of behavioral therapy for patients with eating disorders. CBT is documented to result in a 30% to 50% remission rate in 60% to 70% of the patients in whom it is used.[61] CBT is thought to be better at changing attitudes toward behaviors such as bingeing and purging,

whereas pharmacotherapy is thought to be better for reducing anxiety and improving mood.[60] Another technique known as interpersonal therapy has been used in patients with eating disorder, but evidence suggests that CBT is the superior technique. However, many psychiatrists are not trained in CBT and so lack the skills necessary to engage patients in CBT.[98] Behavioral therapy can be individual, group, family, supportive, or otherwise. Other approaches to counseling are being investigated.[99] Regardless of type, it is recommended that patients with eating disorders receive some form of behavioral therapy, because it is a mainstay of treatment.

Preventing eating disorders could become a focus of study, but little research has been published. One Australian study sought to determine the safety and efficacy of a self-esteem–focused school-based program on children's attitudes toward their bodies and food.[100] Four hundred seventy students (173 boys, 297 girls) ages 11.1 to 14.5 attended a weekly lesson about self-esteem and healthy lifestyle topics for 9 consecutive weeks. Students were administered validated questionnaires at baseline, at 3 months (at the conclusion of the program), and at 12 months (as follow-up). The desire for social acceptance and the importance of physical appearance were still significantly below baseline measures after 12 months. Of the students labeled as at high risk for developing eating disorders, 24.7% had significantly improved Body Dissatisfaction scores (both boys and girls), even at 12 months. The authors believed this program was successful because of its interactive approach and focus on self-esteem as opposed to eating disorders. Similar programs that focus on education about eating disorders may unwittingly portray them as glamorous, which may entice impressionable youths.[63] Although a few additional programs have been established and evaluated, more research is needed in this area to target the prevention of eating disorders, especially in children and adolescents.[101,102]

COMBINATION THERAPY

Because behavioral therapy and pharmacotherapy are two of the most common approaches to combating eating disorders, especially bulimia, it is important to know whether the combination of the two approaches results in faster or more effective symptom resolution. A meta-analysis was performed to determine if a combination of behavioral therapy and antidepressant therapy was more effective for the treatment of purging-type bulimia than behavioral therapy alone or antidepressant therapy alone.[103] Only randomized controlled trials lasting more than 4 weeks were assessed. One part of the analysis compared combination treatment to antidepressant therapy by evaluating the results of 247 patients in five trials. Combination therapy proved more effective than antidepressants alone for alleviation of short-term bingeing; absolute risk was reduced by 19% in patients receiving combination therapy. The second part of the analysis compared combination treatment to behavioral therapy by evaluating 343 patients in seven trials. Similarly, combination treatment proved more effective than behavioral therapy alone for alleviation of short-term bingeing ($p = 0.03$). However, 30% of patients dropped out of the combination treatment group as opposed to 16% of patients in the behavioral therapy group ($p = 0.01$). The data suggest that although combination therapy may increase the speed of recovery, patients may be more likely to relapse, probably due to the side effects from medications. Healthcare professionals should be certain that a patient is an appropriate candidate before initiating antidepressant therapy.

Some practical recommendations for the combination of antidepressant and behavioral therapy for the treatment of bulimia include the following[98]:

- Recommend behavioral therapy, especially CBT, if a psychiatrist trained in this technique is available.
- Start an SSRI such as fluoxetine, unless directly contraindicated, if:
  - The patient is severely depressed or has a family history of depression
  - The patient is mildly depressed or not depressed, but has not reduced vomiting frequency by 70% after the sixth session of behavioral therapy
  - The patient is mildly depressed or not depressed, has reduced vomiting frequency by 70% after the sixth session of behavioral therapy, but vomiting frequency begins to rise, even after significant behavioral therapy

Unfortunately, not enough data about combination treatment of anorexia are available to make analogous recommendations.

ALTERNATIVE THERAPIES

St. John's wort, an over-the-counter herbal antidepressant product, may be useful in patients with eating disorders owing to its reuptake inhibition of serotonin and norepinephrine. Although no clinical studies regarding its use in patients with eating disorders have been identified, it is an option for patients who prefer herbal supplements rather than prescription products.[104]

FUTURE THERAPIES

Future pharmacotherapeutic options for the treatment of eating disorders are being investigated, albeit not as extensively as they could be for these seemingly overlooked patients. Dronabinol has an FDA-approved indication for AIDS-related anorexia due to its effect on appetite stimulation, but research on its use in anorexia is lacking.[105] PH284, the first member of a new family of drugs known as vomeropherins, is currently in phase II trials for the treatment of anorexia and has recently shown promise by increasing the energy consumption and quality of life of cachectic cancer patients

who were administered the drug intranasally in a double-blind, placebo-controlled clinical trial.[106] Another drug in early clinical trials that may eventually prove useful for treating anorexia is AVR118, a novel peptide nucleic acid that has immunomodulator activity.[107]

In general, the pipeline of drugs specifically dedicated to treat anorexia or bulimia is not extensive; however, it is estimated that future research will seek to determine the effect of antipsychotics on anorexia and to further delineate the best pharmacotherapeutic options for bulimia.

Unfortunately, researching eating disorders is difficult. Trials designed to determine optimal therapy often have scant enrollment and high dropout rates. A comparison of recruitment rates between a study of partially recovered anorexic patients and two studies of bulimic patients found that the bulimic patients were recruited at a relatively constant rate, but the anorexic patients were more resistant to recruitment.[108] The authors of the report noted that a better approach to recruiting anorexic patients is to enroll many patients at different sites (multicenter) for a shorter time period instead of fewer patients at one site (single-center) for a longer time period. Appropriate patient-recruitment techniques should be a focus for clinical trial designers to ensure the future of this area of research.

IMPROVING OUTCOMES

Outcomes are generally better for bulimic patients than anorexic patients.[60] In an outcome analysis of 119 studies of 5,590 anorexic patients, about 45% of patients recovered from anorexia, 34% of patients with anorexia improved, and 21% of patients had chronic anorexia and did not improve.[109] It estimated that 5% to 10% of anorexic patients die from early mortality.[60,61] Conversely, in a 6-year follow-up study of bulimic patients, 60% of patients had a good outcome, 29% of patients had an intermediate outcome, 10% of patients had a poor outcome, and 1% of patients had died by study end.[60] Regardless of diagnosis, both anorexia and bulimia have significant margins for improvement of patient outcomes, but this can be achieved only by using a multidisciplinary approach to treatment, by developing the current body of published primary research, and by educating patients on the dangers of eating disorders.

SUMMARY

Anorexia and bulimia are serious, potentially fatal eating disorders found most commonly during adolescence. Female patients outnumber male patients by an incidence of 10:1. Current evidence suggests a relationship between depression or other neurotransmitter abnormalities and eating disorders, particularly bulimia. Recognition of eating disorders is often very difficult because of the highly secretive nature of the patient's illness. Early detection and diagnosis often help facilitate treatment and can prevent many of the serious and life-threatening complications often associated with eating disorders.

Successful treatment involves a multidisciplinary approach, often incorporating psychotherapy and pharmacotherapy. Although psychotherapy remains the cornerstone of treatment for both anorexia and bulimia, pharmacotherapy is commonly used. In general, bulimia responds more favorably to pharmacotherapy than does anorexia. Antidepressants, specifically SSRIs, have been used successfully in the treatment of eating disorders and appear to provide symptomatic relief regardless of a concomitant diagnosis of depression. A trial of antidepressants is considered appropriate in patients with eating disorders if behavioral therapy needs augmentation or is proving unsuccessful, or if severe depression is evident. In all cases, medication should complement psychotherapy rather than take its place.

These patients are often noncompliant and tend to misuse and overuse drugs. Relapses are heralded by excessive purchases of laxatives, syrup of ipecac, over-the-counter weight loss products, and surreptitious diuretic use. Through vigilant monitoring of patient adherence, keen observation for evidence of relapses, and continued research into eating disorders and their treatments, healthcare professionals can play an important role in the multidisciplinary management of these patients and the relentless pursuit to improve patient outcomes.

KEY POINTS

OBESITY

- Obesity is a chronic disease that affects approximately 65% of adults over the age of 20 living in the United States
- Body mass index (BMI) is the preferred method for defining and measuring the degree of obesity and overweight. The most recent National Institutes of Health (NIH) guidelines for the identification, evaluation, and treatment of overweight and obesity define overweight as a BMI of at least 25 kg/m^2 and obesity as a BMI of at least 30 kg/m^2
- Weight loss therapy is indicated for all obese patients (BMI >30 kg/m^2) and for overweight patients (BMI 25 to 29.9 kg/m^2) or patients with elevated waist circumferences (more than 102 cm in men and more than 88 cm in women) who have two or more risk factors
- An appropriate and realistic initial treatment goal for obesity is a reduction of 10% in total body weight over 6 months, which equates to a loss of approximately 1 to 2 pounds per week
- The mainstay of obesity management includes reduced caloric intake, increased physical activity, and behavioral modification. Pharmacotherapy may be considered

in select patients who have failed to lose sufficient weight following a 6-month trial of diet, exercise, and behavioral modification. Surgical intervention for weight loss should be reserved for severe cases of morbid obesity in patients with BMIs of at least 40 kg/m^2, or at least 35 kg/m^2 with comorbid conditions who have failed other weight loss methods
- Future goals for improving obesity management include educating the public about the health risks associated with obesity, promoting healthy dietary habits and increased physical activity throughout society, and actively investing in research to uncover the causes, prevention, and treatment of obesity

EATING DISORDERS

- The two classic eating disorders are anorexia bulimia and bulimia nervosa. Anorexia is a syndrome characterized by self-starvation, extreme weight loss, excessive exercise, body image disturbance, and an intense fear of becoming obese, despite being grossly underweight. Bulimia nervosa is characterized by binge eating usually followed by some form of purging, such as self-induced vomiting, medication-induced vomiting (ipecac), laxative abuse, or associated behaviors such as diuretic use, diet pill use, or compulsive exercising
- The most common type of eating disorder is normal-weight bulimia; these patients are within 10% of ideal weight despite purging
- Eating disorders are classified as psychiatric illnesses. Diagnosis is based on criteria from the fourth edition of the American Psychiatric Association's *Diagnostic and Statistical Manual of Mental Disorder* (DSM-IV)
- Complications associated with anorexia can affect virtually every physiologic organ system
- A particularly dangerous practice is the repeated induction of vomiting with syrup of ipecac. Chronic absorption of ipecac can lead to potentially fatal cardiac, gastrointestinal, and neuromuscular toxicity
- Treatment of anorexia and bulimia requires a multidisciplinary approach, often incorporating psychotherapy and pharmacotherapy. Psychotherapy is the mainstay of treatment and should not be replaced, overlooked, or downplayed when medication therapy is chosen. In general, bulimia responds more favorably to medication therapy than does anorexia
- Antidepressants, specifically SSRIs and TCAs, have been successful in the treatment of eating disorders and appear to provide symptomatic relief in patients who are not clinically depressed. SSRIs are preferred over TCAs because of their safer therapeutic profile. Other pharmacotherapeutic modalities such as cyproheptadine, anticonvulsants, and opiate antagonists have also been studied

SUGGESTED READINGS

American Psychiatric Association. Diagnostic and statistical manual of mental disorders, 4th ed., revised. Washington, DC: American Psychiatric Association, 1994.

American Psychiatric Association. Practice guideline for the treatment of patients with eating disorders. Am J Psychiatry (Suppl) 157:1–39, 2000.

Arterburn DE, Crane PK, Veenstra DL. The efficacy and safety of sibutramine for weight loss: a systematic review. Arch Intern Med 164: 994–1003, 2004.

Bacaltchuk J, Hay P. Antidepressants versus placebo for people with bulimia nervosa. Cochrane Database Syst Rev (4):CD003391, 2003.

Bacaltchuk J, Trefiglio RP, Oliveira IR, et al. Combination of antidepressants and psychological treatments for bulimia nervosa: a systematic review. Acta Psychiatr Scand 101:256–267, 2000.

Committee on Adolescence. American Academy of Pediatrics Policy Statement: identifying and treating eating disorders. Pediatrics 111: 204–211, 2003.

Curran MP, Scott LJ. Orlistat: a review of its use in the management of patients with obesity. Drugs 64:2845–2864, 2004.

U.S. Department of Health and Human Services. National Heart Lung and Blood Institute Obesity Initiative Expert Panel on the Identification, Evaluation, and Treatment of Overweight and Obesity in Adults. Washington, DC: U.S. Public Health Service, 1998.

REFERENCES

1. Stein CJ, Colditz GA. The epidemic of obesity. J Clin Endocrinol Metab 89:2522–2525, 2004.
2. Bray GA. Medical consequences of obesity. J Clin Endocrinol Metab 89:2583–2589, 2004.
3. Grundy SM. Obesity metabolic syndrome, and cardiovascular disease. J Clin Endocrinol Metab 89:2595–2600, 2004.
4. Mokdad AH, Marks, JS, Stroup DF, et al. Actual causes of death in the United States, 2000. JAMA 291:1238–1245, 2004.
5. Thompson D, Wolf AM. The medical-care cost burden of obesity. Obes Rev 2:189–197, 2001.
6. U.S. Department of Health and Human Services. National Heart Lung and Blood Institute Obesity Initiative Expert Panel on the Identification, Evaluation, and Treatment of Overweight and Obesity in Adults. Washington, DC: U.S. Public Health Service, 1998.
7. Goldstein DJ. Beneficial health effects of modest weight loss. Int J Obes Relat Metab Disord 16:397–415, 1992.
8. Mertens IL, Van Gaal LF. Overweight, obesity, and blood pressure: the effects of modest weight reduction. Obes Res 8:270–278, 2000.
9. Bray GA, Gray DS. Obesity. Part 1: pathogenesis. West J Med 149:429–441, 1988.
10. Pijl H, Meinders AE. Bodyweight change as an adverse effect of drug treatment. Drug Safe 14:329–342, 1996.
11. Diliberti N, Bordi PL, Conklin MT, et al. Increased portion size leads to increased energy intake in a restaurant meal. Obes Res 12: 562–568, 2004.
12. Nielsen SJ, Popkin BM. Patterns and trends in food portion sizes, 1977–1998. JAMA 289:450–453, 2003.
13. Bouchard C, Perusse L, Leblanc C, et al. Inheritance of the amount and distribution of human body fat. Int J Obes 12:205–215, 1988.
14. Tambs K, Moum T, Eaves L, et al. Genetics and environmental contributions to the variance of the body mass index in a Norwegian sample of first-degree and second-degree relatives. Am J Hum Biol 3:257–268, 1991.
15. Stunkard AJ, Harris JR, Pedersen NL, et al. The body-mass index of twins who have been reared apart. N Engl J Med 322: 1483–1487, 1990.
16. Allison DB, Kaprio J, Korkeila M, et al. The heritability of body mass index among an international sample of monozygotic twins reared apart. Int J Obes Relat Metab Disord 20:501–506, 1996.
17. Price RA, Cadoret RJ, Stunkard AJ, et al. Genetic contributions to human fatness: an adoption study. Am J Psychiatry 144: 1003–1008, 1987.
18. Loktionov A. Common gene polymorphisms and nutrition: emerging links with pathogenesis of multifactorial chronic diseases. J Nutr Biochem 14:426–451, 2003.
19. Leigh JP, Fries JF, Hubert HB. Gender and race differences in the correlation between body mass and education in the 1971–1975 NHANES I. J Epidemiol Community Health 46:191–196, 1992.
20. Hedley AA, Ogden CL, Johnson CL, et al. Prevalence of overweight and obesity amount US children, adolescents, and adults, 1999–2002. JAMA 291:2847–2850, 2004.
21. Dyer AR, Elliott P. The INTERSALT study: relations of body mass index to blood pressure. INTERSALT Co-operative Research Group. J Hum Hypertens 3:299–308, 1989.
22. Ford ES, Williamson DF, Liu S. Weight change and diabetes incidence: findings from a national cohort of US adults. Am J Epidemiol 146:214–222, 1997.
23. National Cholesterol Education Program (NCEP) Expert Panel on Detection, Evaluation, and Treatment of High Blood Cholesterol in Adults (Adult Treatment Panel III). Third Report of the National Cholesterol Education Program (NCEP) Expert Panel on Detection, Evaluation, and Treatment of High Blood Cholesterol in Adults final report. Circulation 106:3143–3421, 2002.
24. Klein S, Burke LE, Bray GA, et al. Clinical implications of obesity with specific focus on cardiovascular disease: a statement for professionals from the American Heart Association Council on Nutrition, Physical Activity, and Metabolism. Circulation 110: 2952–2967, 2004.
25. Wadden TA, Foster GD, Letizia KA. One-year behavioral treatment of obesity: comparison of moderate and severe caloric restriction and the effects of weight maintenance therapy. J Consult Clin Psychol 62:165–171, 1994.
26. Foster GD, Wyatt H, Hill JO, et al. A randomized trial of a low-carbohydrate diet for obesity. N Engl J Med 348:2082–2090, 2003.
27. Stern L, Iqbal N, Seshadri P, et al. The effects of a low-carbohydrate versus conventional weight loss diets in severely obese adults: one-year follow-up of a randomized trial. Ann Intern Med 140:778–785, 2004.
28. Thompson PD, Buchner D, Pina IL, et al. Exercise and physical activity in the prevention and treatment of atherosclerotic cardiovascular disease: a statement from the Council on Clinical Cardiology. Circulation 107:3109–3116, 2003.
29. Livingston EH. Obesity and its surgical management. Am J Surg 184:103–113, 2002.
30. Campbell ML, Mathys ML. Pharmacologic options for the treatment of obesity. Am J Health Syst Pharm 58:1301–1308, 2001.
31. Arterburn DE, Crane PK, Veenstra DL. The efficacy and safety of sibutramine for weight loss: a systematic review. Arch Intern Med 164:994–1003, 2004.
32. Meridia (sibutramine) product information. Abbott Laboratories, North Chicago, IL: December 2004.
33. Hazenberg BP. Randomized, double-blind, placebo-controlled multicenter study of sibutramine in obese hypertensive patients. Cardiology 94:152–158, 2000.
34. Jordan J, Scholze J, Matiba B, et al. Influence of sibutramine on blood pressure: evidence from placebo-controlled trials. Int J Obes Relat Metab Disord 2:1–8, 2005.
35. Bach DS, Rissanene AM, Mendel CM, et al. Absences of cardiac valve dysfunction in obese patients treated with sibutramine. Obes Res 7:363–369, 1999.
36. Zannad F, Gille B, Grentzinger A, et al. Effects of sibutramine on ventricular dimensions and heart valves in obese patients during weight reduction. Am Heart J 144:508–515, 2002.
37. Arfken CL, Schuster CR, Johanson CE. Postmarketing surveillance of abuse liability of sibutramine. Drug Alcohol Depend 69: 169–173, 2003.
38. Curran MP, Scott LJ. Orlistat: a review of its use in the management of patients with obesity. Drugs 64:2845–2864, 2004.
39. Xenical (orlistat) product information. Roche Pharmaceuticals; Nutley, NJ; October 2004.
40. Hutton B, Fergusson D. Changes in body weight and serum lipid profile in obese patients treated with orlistat in addition to a hypocaloric diet: a systematic review of randomized clinical trials. Am J Clin Nutr 80:1461–1468, 2004.
41. Haller CA, Benowitz NL. Adverse cardiovascular and central nervous system events associated with dietary supplements containing ephedra alkaloids. N Engl J Med 343:1833–1838, 2000.
42. Thompson CA. Ephedrine alkaloids banned from dietary supplements. Am J Health Syst Pharm 61:750–756, 2004.

43. Fugh-Berman A, Myers A. *Citrus aurantium*, an ingredient of dietary supplements marketed for weight loss: current status of clinical and basic research. Exp Biol Med 229:698–704, 2004.

44. Bays HE. Current and investigational antiobesity agents and obesity therapeutic treatment targets. Obes Res 12:1197–1211, 2004.

45. Bjorbaek C, Kahn BB. Leptin signaling in the central nervous system and the periphery. Recent Prog Horm Res 59:305–331, 2004.

46. Duff E, Baile CA. Ciliary neurotrophic factor: a role in obesity? Nutr Rev 61:423–426, 2003.

47. Harvey EL, Glenny AM, Kirk SF, et al. An updated systematic review of interventions to improve health professionals' management of obesity. Obes Rev 3:45–55, 2002.

48. The Surgeon's General Call to Action to Prevent and Decrease Overweight and Obesity. United States Department of Health and Human Services. Available at http://www.surgeongeneral.gov/topics/obesity/calltoaction/fact_vision.htm. Accessed Feb. 21, 2005.

49. Finkelstein EA, Fiebelkorn IC, Wang G. National medical spending attributable to overweight and obesity: how much, and who's paying? Health Affairs W3:219–226, 2003.

50. O'Meara S, Riemsma R, Shirran L, et al. The clinical effectiveness and cost-effectiveness of sibutramine in the management of obesity: a technology assessment. Health Technol Assess 6:1–97, 2002.

51. Lamotte M, Annemans L, Lefever A, et al. A health economic model to assess the long-term effects and cost-effectiveness of orlistat in obese type 2 diabetic patients. Diabetes Care 25:303–308, 2002.

52. Maetzel A, Ruof J, Covington M, et al. Economic evaluation of orlistat in overweight and obese patients with type 2 diabetes mellitus. Pharmacoeconomics 21:501–512, 2003.

53. Maddox RW, Long MA. Eating disorders: current concepts. J Am Pharm Assoc 39:378–387, 1999.

54. Mehler PS, Gray MC, Schulte M. Medical complications of anorexia nervosa. J Womens Health 6:533–541, 1997.

55. Russell G. Bulimia: an ominous variant of anorexia nervosa. Psychol Med 9:429, 1979.

56. American Psychiatric Association. Diagnostic and statistical manual of mental disorders, 4th ed. revised. Washington, DC: American Psychiatric Association, 1994.

57. Beresin EV. Anorexia nervosa. Compr Ther 23:664–671, 1997.

58. Muscari ME. Primary care of adolescents with bulimia nervosa. J Pediatr Health Care 10:17–25, 1996.

59. Patrick L. Eating disorders: a review of the literature with emphasis on medical complications and clinical nutrition. Altern Med Rev 7:184–202, 2002.

60. American Psychiatric Association. Practice guideline for the treatment of patients with eating disorders. Am J Psychiatry (Suppl) 157:1–39, 2000.

61. Kaye WH, Klump KL, Frank KW, et al. Anorexia and bulimia nervosa. Annu Rev Med 51:299–313, 2000.

62. Mehler PS. Bulimia nervosa. N Engl J Med 349:875–881, 2003.

63. Abraham SF. Dieting, body weight, body image and self-esteem in young women: doctors' dilemmas. Med J Aust 178:607–611, 2003.

64. Committee on Adolescence. American Academy of Pediatrics Policy Statement: identifying and treating eating disorders. Pediatrics 111:204–211, 2003.

65. National Eating Disorders Association. Statistics: eating disorders and their precursors. Available at http://www.nationaleatingdisorders.org (accessed October 2004).

66. Kaplan Seidenfeld ME, Sosin E, Rickert VI. Nutrition and eating disorders in adolescents. Mt Sinai J Med 71:155–161, 2004.

67. Harper J, Leung M, Birmingham CL. A blinded laxative taper for patients with eating disorders. Eating Weight Disord 9:147–150, 2004.

68. Adler AG, Walinsky P, Krall RA, et al. Death resulting from ipecac syrup poisoning. JAMA 243:1927–1928, 1980.

69. Herzog DB, Copeland PM. Eating disorders. N Engl J Med 313:295, 1985.

70. Daluiski A, Rahbar B, Meals RA. Russell's sign: subtle hand changes in patients with bulimia nervosa. Clin Orthop 343:107–109, 1997.

71. Kaye WH, Nagata T, Weltzin TE, et al. Double-blind placebo-controlled administration of fluoxetine in restricting- and restricting-purging type anorexia nervosa. Biol Psychiatry 49:644–652, 2001.

72. Barbarich NC, McConaha CW, Halmi KA, et al. Use of nutritional supplements to increase the efficacy of fluoxetine in the treatment of anorexia nervosa. Int J Eat Disord 35:10–15, 2004.

73. Bergh C, Eriksson M, Lindberg G, et al. Selective serotonin reuptake inhibitors in anorexia. Lancet 348:1459–1460, 1996.

74. Fassino S, Leombruni P, Abbate Daga G, et al. Efficacy of citalopram in anorexia nervosa: a pilot study. Eur Neuropsychopharmacol 12:453–459, 2002.

75. Malina A, Gaskill J, McConaha C, et al. Olanzapine treatment of anorexia nervosa: a retrospective study. Int J Eat Disord 33:234–237, 2003.

76. Powers PS, Santana CA, Bannon YS. Olanzapine in the treatment of anorexia nervosa: an open-label trial. Int J Eat Disord 32:146–154, 2002.

77. Newman-Toker J. Risperidone in anorexia nervosa. J Am Acad Child Adolesc Psychiatry 39:941–942, 2000.

78. Cassano GB, Miniati M, Pini S, et al. Six-month open trial of haloperidol as an adjunctive treatment for anorexia nervosa: a preliminary report. Int J Eat Disord 33:172–177, 2003.

79. Halmi KA, Eckert E, LaDu TJ, et al. Anorexia nervosa: treatment efficacy of cyproheptadine and amitriptyline. Arch Gen Psychiatry 43:177–181, 1986.

80. Hill K, Bucuvalas J, McClain C, et al. Pilot study of growth hormone administration during the refeeding of malnourished anorexia nervosa patients. J Child Adolesc Psychopharmacol 10:3–8, 2000.

81. Mitchell JE, Davis L, Goff G. The process of relapse in patients with bulimia. Int J Eat Disord 4:457, 1985.

82. Bacaltchuk J, Hay P. Antidepressants versus placebo for people with bulimia nervosa. Cochrane Database Syst Rev (4):CD003391, 2003.

83. Prozac (fluoxetine) [product information]. Indianapolis, IN: Eli Lilly and Company, August 2004.

84. Goldstein DJ, Wilson MG, Thompson VL, et al. Long-term fluoxetine treatment of bulimia nervosa. Br J Psychiatry 166:660–666, 1995.

85. Romano SJ, Halmi KA, Sarkar NP, et al. A placebo-controlled study of fluoxetine in continued treatment of bulimia nervosa after successful acute fluoxetine treatment. Am J Psychiatry 159:96–102, 2002.

86. Wold P. Trazodone in the treatment of bulimia. J Clin Psychiatry 44:275–276, 1983.

87. Pope HG, Hudson JI, Jonas JM. Antidepressant treatment of bulimia: preliminary experience and practical recommendations. J Clin Psychopharmacol 3:274–281, 1983.

88. Carson SW. Bupropion, is it here to stay? DICP Ann Pharmacother 23:704–705, 1989.

89. Walsh BT, Stewart JW, Roose SP, et al. Treatment of bulimia with phenelzine; a double-blind, placebo-controlled study. Arch Gen Psychiatry 41:1105–1109, 1984.

90. Wermuth BM, Davis KL, Hollister L, et al. Phenytoin treatment of the binge-eating syndrome. Am J Psychiatry 134:1249–1253, 1977.

91. Kaplan AS, Garfinkle PE, Darby PL, et al. Carbamazepine in the treatment of bulimia. Am J Psychiatry 140:1225–1229, 1983.

92. Herridge PL, Pope HG Jr. Treatment of bulimia and rapid cycling bipolar disorder with sodium valproate: a case report. J Clin Psychopharmacol 5:229–230, 1985.

93. Moore SL, Rakes SM. Binge eating: therapeutic response to diphenylhydantoin: case report. J Clin Psychiatry 43:385–386, 1982.

94. Crockford DN, Fisher G, Barker P. Risperidone, weight gain, and bulimia nervosa. Can J Psychiatry 42:326–327, 1997.

95. Hoopes SP, Reimherr FW, Hedges DW, et al. Treatment of bulimia nervosa with topiramate in a randomized, double-blind, placebo-controlled, part 1: improvement in binge and purge measures. J Clin Psychiatry 64:1335–1341, 2003.

96. Hedges DW, Reimherr FW, Hoopes SP, et al. Treatment of bulimia nervosa with topiramate in a randomized, double-blind, placebo-controlled, part 2: improvement in psychiatric measures. J Clin Psychiatry 64:1449–1454, 2003.

97. Fung SM, Ferrill MJ. Treatment of bulimia nervosa with ondansetron. Ann Pharmacother 35:1270–1273, 2001.

98. Mitchell JE, Peterson CB, Myers T, et al. Combining pharmacotherapy and psychotherapy in the treatment of patients with eating disorders. Psychiatr Clin North Am 24:315–323, 2001.

99. Thomson Centerwatch. Study Posting(10): Trial #56626, Anorexia, Ann Arbor, MI. http://www.centerwatch.com/patient/studies/stu56626.html (accessed November 2004).

100. O'Dea JA, Abraham S. Improving the body image, eating attitudes, and behaviors of young male and female adolescents: a new, educational approach that focuses on self-esteem. Int J Eat Disord 28: 43–57, 2000.

101. Zechowski C, Namyslowska I, Korolczuk A, et al. Eating disorder prevention program: pilot study. Psychiatr Pol 38:51–63, 2004.

102. Tilgner L, Wertheim EH, Paxton SJ. Effect of social desirability on adolescent girls' responses to an eating disorders prevention program. Int J Eat Disord 35:211–216, 2004.

103. Bacaltchuk J, Trefiglio RP, Oliveira IR, et al. Combination of antidepressants and psychological treatments for bulimia nervosa: a systematic review. Acta Psychiatr Scand 101:256–267, 2000.

104. Monograph. *Hypericum perforatum*. Altern Med Rev 9:318–325, 2004.

105. Thomson Centerwatch. CenterWatch Drugs in Clinical Trials Database: Marinol. http://www.centerwatch.com/professional/cwpipeline/details.asp?i = 1374&nav = &n = (accessed November 2004).

106. Pherin Pharmaceuticals. Product Pipeline. http://www.pherin.com/pipeline.html (accessed December 2004).

107. Advanced Viral Research Corporation. AVR118. http://www.adviral.com/ADVR/thisis/prodr.htm (accessed December 2004).

108. McDermott C, Agras WS, Crow SJ, et al. Participant recruitment for an anorexia nervosa treatment study. Int J Eat Disord 35: 33–41, 2004.

109. Steinhausen HC. The outcome of anorexia nervosa in the 20th century. Am J Psychiatry 159:1284–1293, 2002.

Alcoholism

Jeffrey N. Baldwin and Paul W. Jungnickel

58

DEFINITION

Alcoholism is a primary, chronic disease with genetic, psychosocial, and environmental factors that influence its development and manifestations. Alcoholism is often progressive and fatal and may be characterized by continuous or periodic impaired control over drinking, preoccupation with the drug alcohol, use of alcohol despite adverse consequences, and distortions in thinking, most notably denial.[1]

Alcohol abuse involves persistent patterns of heavy alcohol consumption with associated health or social consequences. Alcoholism is differentiated from abuse by the presence of craving, tolerance, and physical dependence, which result in behavioral changes and loss of control over drinking. Persons who are alcoholic experience both psychological and physical dependency and tolerance. Psychological dependency, which is perhaps the single most important factor, involves the compulsive use of and craving for a drug. Physical dependency is characterized by a series of physiologic events that occur when the drug is discontinued, including withdrawal or abstinence syndrome. Tolerance develops when continued use of a drug is required and increasing doses are needed to produce the same effect.

Although psychological dependency is the most important feature of addictive disorders, it is also the least understood. A person may be made physically dependent on alcohol, but abuse may not be recognized or diagnosed as such until behavioral effects secondary to psychological dependency are noted. Many persons consume alcoholic beverages, but relatively few develop physical and psychological dependency on the drug. A commonly held belief is that if someone does not drink daily or drinks only alcoholic beverages with relatively low alcohol content, such as wine or beer, he or she cannot be an alcoholic. The quantity, type, and frequency of alcohol consumption are relatively unimportant; loss of control over consumption once initiated and continued use of alcohol despite clear evidence of adverse consequences (social, physical, or legal) are more important in the diagnosis of alcoholism.

TREATMENT GOALS

- Describe the treatment of alcohol abuse and alcoholism both acutely and chronically.
- Establish treatment goals jointly with the patient.
- Maintain and support vital functions in patients with acute alcohol intoxication.
- Through drug therapy, convert the acutely agitated and alcohol-impaired patient with symptoms of toxic psychosis to a calm but arousable and responsive patient.
- Rule out alternative illnesses or causes of intoxication in the unconscious patient, including hypoglycemia, physical injury, and other drugs.

- Avoid pharmacologic attempts to accelerate the metabolism or clearance of alcohol from the body of the intoxicated patient.
- Ensure withdrawal from and detoxification of ethanol followed by subsequent interventions to maintain abstinence.
- Ensure detoxification from alcohol by substitution with, and slow withdrawing of, a longer-acting sedative-hypnotic medication.
- Individualize patient-specific drug regimens and doses in the treatment of patients with acute alcohol withdrawal, with consideration given to underlying conditions and concurrent polydrug abuse.
- Use nonpharmacologic therapy as appropriate to enhance the treatment of patients with clinical problems that accompany acute detoxification from alcohol.
- Encourage patient motivation to stop drinking; avoidance of psychoactive substances, including alcohol, whenever possible; and participation in recovery support programs.

EPIDEMIOLOGY

Alcohol is the most misused drug in the United States today. In 2002, approximately 9% of Americans older than 11 years of age; 9% of those 12 to 17 years old; 22% of those aged 18 to 25; and 7% of those older than age 25 were estimated to have had past-year dependence on, or abuse of, illicit drugs or alcohol. Illicit drugs included psychoactive prescription medications used nonmedicinally. Past-year alcohol dependence and past-year alcohol abuse or dependence, respectively, were estimated in approximately 4% and 8% of those older than 11 years of age; 2% and 6% of those 12 to 17 years old; 7% and 18% of those aged 18 to 25; and 3% and 4% of those older than age 25.[2] This does not include those recovering from alcoholism who did not drink during the year of the survey. The lifetime prevalence of alcohol dependence was estimated in a survey conducted from 1980 to 1984 to be approximately 14% for males and 3% for females.[3] Alcoholism risk is approximately 50% to 60% genetically determined.[4] A threefold to fourfold increase in alcoholism prevalence has been noted in first-degree relatives of persons with alcoholism (PWA).[5] Alcoholism is one of America's major health problems; it contributed to 85,000 deaths in the year 2000, making it the third leading cause of preventable mortality in the United States after tobacco (435,000 deaths that year) and poor diet and physical inactivity (400,000 deaths that year).[6] A meta-analysis found that women who consumed two or more drinks per day and men who consumed four or more drinks per day had higher mortality rates than nondrinkers.[7]

Alcoholism is a condition that is far more common than is generally perceived; only 3% to 5% of the country's population of PWA are classified as the "skid row" or public inebriate type. PWA come from all levels of our society; most are found in the working and homemaking populations. However, within industrialized countries, the prevalence of excessive drinking is higher among men from lower socioeconomic groups, whereas women do not demonstrate a direct relationship between socioeconomic standing and alcohol consumption.[8] The largest percentage of PWA in the United States are between the ages of 35 and 50 years. Professionals and business people have high rates of alcohol consumption and alcoholism. Alcohol use in the younger, school-aged population and "problem drinking" among women have increased, and these appear to be continuing trends.[9,10] Although the prevalence of alcohol misuse among older adults is low, detection of the problem is difficult, and it is often unrecognized. Vulnerability of the older PWA to the harmful effects of alcohol is much greater.[11]

Alcoholism is an illness that can shorten a person's life span considerably, and this has an impact on our entire society. About 40% of medical and surgery patients have an alcohol-related problem, and 15% of the total national health expenditure for hospital care is spent on alcohol-related illness.[12,13] In a 1996 analysis on the prevalence of alcohol involvement in crime, alcohol was involved in 40% of all traffic fatalities and homicides, as well as 30% of sexual assaults.[14]

Alcoholism is a treatable illness when it is diagnosed in its early stages. However, death rates from alcohol abuse in the major risk age groups, such as young men, are more than twice those of the general population. Unfortunately, a serious deficit in accessible and high-quality alcoholism treatment services has occurred because most available services are designed to deal with only the later stages of alcoholism. Alcoholism, similar to other diseases such as hypertension and diabetes mellitus, can be considered a biologic disease with a genetic predisposition that is activated by environmental factors.[15,16] Thus, a "biopsychosocial" approach is usually used in the identification, treatment, and ongoing recovery support systems for PWA. Difficulty in differentiating between alcohol abuse and alcoholism (alcohol dependence) may be cited by some as a reason for questioning the disease concept. However, other diseases such as hypertension may be equally difficult to define when borderline. A telephone survey found that about 89% of the surveyed population considered PWA to be ill, yet 47% also felt that the alcoholic person was morally weak[17]; this reveals a fairly strong public sentiment that alcoholism represents ''willful misconduct'' and is an important societal impediment to the identification and treatment of patients with the disease.

PATHOPHYSIOLOGY

Alcohol is a psychoactive agent that can be characterized pharmacologically as a sedative-hypnotic drug. At low doses, the action of alcohol is excitatory and stimulatory as a result of its depression of inhibitory centers in the brain. In a dose-response relationship, at sufficient doses, alcohol produces a depressant action. Although alcohol may provide relief of anxiety and sedation at one dose level, it may produce sleep and more profound depression of the central nervous system and respiratory system at higher levels.

Alcohol is present in a variety of popular beverages: beer and ale are products of the fermentation of cereal grains and contain 3% to 6% alcohol; wine, which results from the fermentation of yeast on sugars that are present in fruits, contains 11% to 20% alcohol; brandy is produced from the distillation of wine products and usually contains 40% alcohol; hard liquors, which are the distillates of fermented products such as grain (e.g., gin, rye, bourbon, scotch, rum, vodka), contain approximately 40% to 50% alcohol. Hard liquors are commonly labeled with a proof number that is twice the alcohol percent concentration by volume. Nonalcoholic (''NA'') beers and wines rarely are alcohol free; they often contain up to 1% alcohol.

Alcohol is efficiently and rapidly absorbed by the stomach and small intestine within 30 to 120 minutes after ingestion. Absorption is direct and is completed by simple (passive) diffusion; alcohol distributes freely in body tissues and fluids. Its reported volume of distribution ranges from 0.58 to 0.70 L per kg of body weight. The concentration of alcohol in the brain rapidly approaches that in the blood.

Factors that modify alcohol absorption are volume, dilution, rate of ingestion, and presence of food in the stomach. Protein and water both slow absorption of alcohol, whereas carbonation facilitates it. Both gastric and hepatic alcohol dehydrogenase (ADH) contribute to the first-pass metabolism of alcohol, resulting in its conversion to acetaldehyde. Gastric ADH has a lower affinity for alcohol and influences first-pass metabolism to a lesser extent than does hepatic ADH; however, it may play a significant role after consumption of one or two alcohol-containing drinks. The level of gastric ADH, which is involved in gastric metabolism of alcohol, is about 80% higher in nonalcoholic males than in females, whereas chronic alcoholism results in a decrease of about 40% in men and 15% in women. This may help to explain why blood alcohol levels in females, corrected for size, are relatively higher than in males; it also may partially explain the greater susceptibility to early onset of liver and brain damage in female PWA.[18] First-pass metabolism of alcohol tends to decrease as the volume consumed increases

and ADH, regardless of source, becomes saturated. Consumption of alcohol with food tends to increase first-pass metabolism by delaying gastric emptying and allowing for increased gastric metabolism.[19] Alcohol crosses the placenta and may be found in the milk of lactating mothers.

The liver is the main site of the first step in the oxidation of ethyl alcohol. Alcohol is oxidized by ADH to acetaldehyde, which subsequently is oxidized by acetaldehyde dehydrogenase to acetate. These reactions convert nicotinamide adenine dinucleotide (NAD) to reduced NAD (NADH). Excess NADH causes metabolic disorders such as hyperlactacidemia, hyperuricemia, hypoglycemia, and hyperlipidemia.[20] Acetaldehyde inhibits repair of alkylated nucleoproteins, reduces mitochondrial oxygen use, and promotes cell death through depletion of reduced glutathione, increased lipid peroxidation, and increased toxic effects of free radicals.[21–23] Long-term consumption of alcohol induces the microsomal ethanol-oxidizing system (MEOS), particularly cytochrome P-4502E1.[24] This induction contributes to metabolic tolerance to alcohol in PWA and increases the metabolism of a number of drugs, such as pentobarbital, propranolol, warfarin, and diazepam.[20] Unfortunately, cytochrome P-4502E1 converts many foreign substances into highly toxic metabolites; most notable among these are metabolites of cocaine and acetaminophen. Therapeutic amounts (e.g., 2.5 to 4 g/day) of acetaminophen can cause hepatic injury in heavy consumers of alcohol.[21] Conversely, short-term use of alcohol may inhibit metabolism of such drugs by direct competition for cytochrome P-4502E1.[20]

Most of the ingested dose of alcohol is eliminated by liver metabolism. Although most drugs are known to be metabolized or cleared from the body in a fixed percentage (''first order'') of the dose taken, alcohol is eliminated via nonlinear or saturation elimination kinetics and, therefore, is removed from the blood in a fixed amount (''zero order'') over time after hepatic ADH becomes saturated. In a 70-kg (approximately 150-lb) person, the rate of alcohol metabolism is approximately 7 g per hour, although this rate varies greatly according to genetics and other factors.[25] At this rate of metabolism, the blood alcohol level will decline at a rate of approximately 15 mg/dL/hr (3.3 mmol/L/hr). An average drink (1.5 oz of 80-proof distilled spirits, 5 oz of wine, or 12 oz of beer) contains about 15 g of ethyl alcohol. Because body water is approximately 65% of body weight, in a 70-kg person the expected blood ethyl alcohol content after one drink will be 15 g per 50 L, or 30 mg per dL (6.5 mmol/dL), with 50 L being the approximate volume of total body water calculated from the percentage of weight. Assuming alcohol metabolism at a rate of 7 g per hour, it would take approximately 2 hours for the blood ethyl alcohol level to return to zero after rapid consumption of a single drink. Within 1 hour after consumption of four typical drinks over a 1-hour period, a 70-kg person would have a blood ethanol concentration of at least 80 mg per dL (17.4 mmol/L), which is the legal level of intoxication in most states. However, as previously mentioned, wide variability in individual ethanol metabolism has been observed, so blood ethanol concentrations may vary considerably among persons who consume these amounts. Ethanol elimination by the kidneys and lungs and through sweat is minimal, with approximately 2% to 10% cleared by these routes, depending on the amount of alcohol ingested.

Alcohol affects almost every organ system in the body. Selected known medical complications and pathologic consequences from excessive alcohol consumption are summarized in Table 58.1.[26] Some of the most important complications are discussed in the following sections.

CARDIOVASCULAR SYSTEM

Modest to moderate consumption of alcohol (up to two drinks per day—particularly wine) has generally been shown to reduce the risk for myocardial infarction, possibly by increasing the levels of high-density lipoprotein cholesterol and antithrombotic activity.[27,28] However, consumption of alcohol in excess of two drinks per day is associated with increased health risks, including an increasing incidence of various cardiovascular diseases. It therefore seems unwise to encourage a nondrinker to begin consuming alcohol for the modest cardiovascular benefits that might be gained.

Cardiomyopathies are commonly seen in patients with chronic alcoholism, likely resulting from alterations in cardiac muscular contractile function.[29] These disorders present as low-output cardiac failure that cannot be differentiated from cardiomyopathies of other causes. Alcohol-related cardiomyopathies generally occur at 30 to 60 years of age, with individuals who consume 90 g or more of alcohol per day being at increased risk.

Heavy alcohol consumption is also related to other types of cardiovascular disease. For example, alcohol consumption of three or more drinks per day has been associated with an increased incidence of hypertension, and the alcohol consumption needed to induce hypertension may be even less in older individuals.[30] Heavy consumption of alcohol has been shown to increase the risk of various forms of stroke and to induce various types of cardiac arrhythmia.[31,32]

HEMATOPOIETIC SYSTEM

The association of anemia, macrocytosis, and alcoholism was long held to be attributable to nutritional deficiencies. Studies have shown that alcohol has a direct role in suppression of folate metabolism, depletion of folate from body stores, and malabsorption of folate. The direct toxicity of alcohol on erythropoiesis is demonstrated by vacuolation of erythroid and myeloid precursors.[33,34] A sideroblastic, or ''iron-loading,'' anemia can result from the impairment by alcohol of iron incorporation and metabolism in the red blood cell. Alcohol increases jejunal absorption of iron, as reflected in hemochromatosis and a rise in serum iron levels. Iron deficiency anemia due to gastritis and gastrointestinal bleeding also may occur. Alcoholic thrombocytopenia occurs in 25% to 30% of acutely ill PWA; platelets often have shorter than normal life spans, and thrombopoiesis is ineffective because of marrow suppression and folate deficiency.

HEPATIC SYSTEM

Three distinct histologic patterns of alcohol-induced liver disease have been identified: alcoholic steatosis, also known as fatty liver disease; alcoholic hepatitis; and alcoholic cirrhosis. All three may coexist simultaneously and do not represent a single progression. Cirrhosis may occur in the absence of clinically evident previous hepatitis.[35] The risk of developing alcoholic liver disease is related to the quantity and duration of alcohol consumption. Factors such as genetics, nutritional state, and environment also predispose to the development of alcoholic liver disease.[36] Alcoholic ''fatty liver'' disease is the most common alcohol-induced hepatic abnormality, occurring in 90% to 100% of PWA.

The postulated mechanism for fatty accumulation in the liver is that an increase in the NADH:NAD ratio during ethanol oxidation is responsible for accumulation of hepatic triglycerides. Uncomplicated fatty liver disease is usually asymptomatic or presents as nausea, vomiting, and right upper quadrant abdominal pain, rarely manifesting with the usual signs of liver disease, such as ascites, jaundice, or splenomegaly. Mild, usually reversible, elevation of liver enzymes is the most frequent laboratory finding. Not as relatively benign as once believed, fatty liver disease may progress to liver failure and occasionally death.

Alcoholic hepatitis is a much more serious disorder; 10% to 30% of PWA develop this complication, usually after years of excessive drinking or after an abrupt increase in alcohol intake. Liver injury results from the degenerative effects of alcohol on subcellular structures. The clinical course of alcoholic hepatitis includes acute or chronic asymptomatic, mild, severe, and fulminant forms. It is often an incidental diagnosis when hepatomegaly and mild elevations in liver function study results are detected during a physical examination. Some patients who develop the fulminant course will rapidly develop liver failure. The death rate in patients with severe alcoholic hepatitis is substantial.

The pathogenesis of alcoholic cirrhosis has not been completely determined. Although approximately half of survivors of alcoholic hepatitis subsequently experience cirrhosis of the liver, this condition may develop in the absence of any previously documented hepatitis. The liver is characterized as being finely nodular or grossly deformed, and it may be smaller or larger than normal. Laboratory findings include hyperbilirubinemia and hypoalbuminemia. Prolonged prothrombin time frequently occurs, with cirrhotic patients being at greatly increased risk of bleeding complications. Other complications from cirrhosis include hepatic encephalopathy; portal hypertension, ascites, and bleeding esophageal varices; portal vein thrombosis; and hepatorenal syndrome.

PANCREAS

Pancreatitis develops in approximately 5% of all PWA, with heavy alcohol use accounting for 35% of all cases of acute

TABLE 58.1	Complications of Excessive Alcohol Use	
Complication	**Usual Onset**	**Comments**
Increased morbidity and mortality	Chronic	Most common causes are hepatic cirrhosis, cancers of respiratory and gastrointestinal tracts, accidents, suicide, and cardiovascular diseases.
Fluid and electrolyte abnormalities	Acute	Alcohol has diuretic action as blood alcohol concentration increases. Stable or decreasing blood alcohol concentrations result in antidiuresis.
		Hyperosmolarity, hypokalemia, hypophosphatemia, and hypomagnesemia are common. Mild lactic acidemia may contribute to asymptomatic elevation of uric acid owing to interference with renal secretion of uric acid.
Hypoglycemia	Acute or chronic	Alcohol depletes liver glycogen stores and decreases gluconeogenesis; blood glucose may drop precipitously. Stupor and coma, apart from the direct effects of alcohol on the nervous system, are experienced. This is a dramatic but relatively uncommon complication.
Hyperglycemia	Acute	During early phases of alcohol withdrawal, blood glucose may be elevated because of increased release of catecholamines. Alcoholic pancreatitis and decreased peripheral glucose use are contributing factors.
Hyperketonemia	Acute	Persons with alcoholism (PWA) often develop hyperketonemia and metabolic acidosis in the absence of hyperglycemia. Often, the patient is hypoglycemic and without glycosuria. This is presumably caused by alcohol-induced starvation ketosis. Insulin should not be administered.
Hypothermia	Acute	Occurs often as a result of prolonged exposure to cold (not uncommon in unconscious or stuporous state); pancreatitis and meningitis may contribute.
Liver disease		Best known sequela of chronic alcoholism and a leading cause of morbidity and mortality. Three common liver diseases are often associated with alcoholism: acute fatty liver, alcoholic hepatitis, and alcoholic cirrhosis. Individual sensitivity is variable and the degree of liver dysfunction does not appear to be related only to the amount of alcohol ingested. Nutritional status, genetic composition, and immunologic factors appear to interact in the development of alcoholic liver disease.
Acute fatty liver	Acute or chronic	Develops in nearly all who ingest alcohol excessively (defined by some as an intake of at least 70 g of ethyl alcohol daily) even for only a few days. Treatment: stop drinking and give a diet with adequate vitamin and protein replacement.
Alcoholic hepatitis	Acute or chronic	Apparently, a toxic inflammatory response of the liver in 10% to 30% of PWA. A high percentage of those with alcoholic hepatitis who continue to drink develop cirrhosis within 5 to 10 years. Most patients require 8 to 12 weeks to show improvement from acute hepatitis. Treatment is supportive: an adequate diet, vitamin supplements, bed rest, and stopping drinking. Acute liver failure, accompanied by hepatic encephalopathy, bleeding esophageal varices, and hepatorenal syndrome, is often present in severe cases. Clinical features are similar to those of other forms of toxic or viral liver injury. Hepatomegaly, jaundice, splenomegaly, fever, and ascites are common. Corticosteroids may be of benefit in fulminant cases, but their exact role in treatment of patients with this disorder is still undetermined. Some studies have failed to show any benefit from their use.
Alcoholic or Laennec cirrhosis	Chronic	Symptoms are often nonspecific in character (e.g., fatigue, weight loss, lethargy). Other physical signs include slight hepatomegaly, splenomegaly, ascites, gynecomastia, spider angiomas, and palmar erythema. About 10% to 30% of PWA develop alcoholic cirrhosis, usually after drinking heavily for 10 to 15 years.

(continued)

TABLE 58.1	continued	
Complication	**Usual Onset**	**Comments**
		The three most common causes of death with alcoholic cirrhosis are bleeding esophageal varices, liver failure accompanied by encephalopathy and coma, and infection. Abstinence from alcohol and supportive care are the primary modes of treatment. Transplantation may be considered, particularly for those patients with a documented period of abstinence.
Portal hypertension	Acute or chronic	A sequela of hepatitis and cirrhosis. Return of blood from abdominal viscera to the heart is impaired as pressure rises and collateral blood vessels enlarge. Primary cause is increased resistance to hepatic blood flow due to fibrosis and nodular regeneration of the liver. All abdominal organs become congested; splenomegaly and ascites result.
Ascites	Acute or chronic	Seen often in patients with portal hypertension and may be worsened by a low serum albumin level. Treatment may include a low sodium diet, fluid restriction, spironolactone and other diuretics, and abdominal paracentesis. As liver disease improves, ascites often resolves. Careful monitoring of electrolytes must be done when diuretics and aldosterone antagonists are used.
Esophageal varices	Acute or chronic	These thin-walled, collateral blood vessels of the portal system are prone to hemorrhaging. Hemorrhage usually occurs when the portal pressure rises because of expanded plasma volume, worsening liver involvement, or increased intra-abdominal pressure. Thin vessel walls and accompanying esophagitis are contributing causes.
Hepatic encephalopathy	Acute or chronic	The central nervous system is depressed by toxins, which appear to be nitrogen-containing catabolic products of protein metabolism (e.g., ammonia) that cannot be eliminated by the diseased liver. This is the reason that hepatic encephalopathy is frequently precipitated by high intake of dietary protein or gastrointestinal bleeding, with digested blood being the contributing source of protein. The patient is usually lethargic, has "flapping tremor" and deterioration of fine movement, and can subsequently become unresponsive and comatose. The central nervous system is more sensitive than usual to anoxia, sedative-hypnotics, opiates, or tranquilizers; these factors may precipitate or exacerbate hepatic encephalopathy. Hepatic encephalopathy is reversible, and some patients return to normal mental functioning.
Pancreatitis	Acute or chronic	Acute pancreatitis occurs commonly in PWA and is most often seen in persons who have been drinking heavily for 8 to 10 years or longer. Often, no characteristic clinical picture except for abdominal pain is present. Nausea and vomiting are common. It is one of the more frequent causes for hospitalization of PWA after a drinking bout. Other manifestations of this condition include shock, hypocalcemia, hyperglycemia, marked fluid loss, and dehydration.
Upper GI ulcerative diseases	Acute or chronic	Acute gastritis, often hemorrhagic, is common in PWA and is worsened by the long-term use of aspirin or other nonsteroidal anti-inflammatory drugs (NSAIDs). The incidence of peptic ulcer is probably higher in PWA than in those who do not have alcoholism. Tearing of the gastroesophageal mucosa (Mallory-Weiss syndrome) with severe bleeding may occur as a consequence of vomiting; this should be considered a medical and surgical emergency. Gastroesophageal reflux disease (GERD) is common among heavy alcohol users because alcohol relaxes the lower esophageal sphincter, and ascites may contribute to GERD by increasing intra-abdominal pressure.

(continued)

TABLE 58.1	continued	
Complication	**Usual Onset**	**Comments**
Malabsorption	Chronic	Changes in gastrointestinal morphology and decreased enzyme activity in the intestinal tract have been observed in chronic alcoholic patients, even with an adequate diet. Thiamine, vitamin B_{12}, folate, xylose, iron, and fat malabsorption occur. Alcohol consumption and poor diet are major contributors to malabsorption.
Hyperlipidemia	Acute or chronic	Alcohol ingestion can induce an elevation of serum triglycerides, particularly in persons with preexisting hypertriglyceridemia. Hypertriglyceridemia may be a contributory factor to the hepatic and cardiovascular disorders related to alcohol, as well as to pancreatitis.
Cardiovascular disorders	Acute or chronic	Heavy alcohol use is related to a variety of cardiovascular disorders, including hypertension, various arrhythmias, stroke, and cardiomyopathies.
Myopathy	Acute or chronic	Generalized and occasionally focal muscle weakness develops during or after a heavy drinking bout. Muscle edema, pain, and cramps are common and may be accompanied by tenderness and edema. Elevated muscle enzymes (creatine phosphokinase and aldolase) may be present. In severe cases, myoglobulinuria can occur. Mortality is high (50%) when alcoholic myopathy occurs concomitantly with hyperkalemia and renal failure.
Infection	Acute or chronic	Acute and chronic alcohol ingestion decreases resistance to bacterial infection, especially in the respiratory tract. Most pulmonary infections in PWA are caused by *Pneumococcus*. Susceptibility to *Klebsiella* and *Haemophilus* organisms is also greater. Because they are debilitated, PWA have a higher risk of reactivated tuberculosis; it has been claimed that 20% of patients with active tuberculosis are PWA. Aspiration pneumonia is also a major complication. Spontaneous bacterial peritonitis is common in patients who have cirrhosis with ascites. Absence of elevation of white blood cell counts or temperature should not preclude the possibility of infection in a PWA.
Hematologic disorders (e.g., anemia, leukopenia, thrombocytopenia)	Chronic	Four major factors contribute to hematologic disorders: poor diet, blood loss, liver disease, and alcohol itself. Folate deficiency is probably the most important hematologic abnormality in PWA. Good diet alone cannot protect against bone marrow toxicity of alcohol if a major portion of calories are ingested as ethanol. Stopping of alcohol, intake of a nutritious diet that includes folic acid and multivitamins, and treatment of other medical complications nearly always reverse hematologic abnormalities.
Neurologic disorders, polyneuropathy	Chronic	A degenerative process of nerve and brain tissues secondary to nutritional deficiency is common with a long history of alcoholism. Clinical and pathologic features of polyneuropathy are almost identical to those of beriberi. Subjective sensory disturbances and loss of reflexes and motor activity occur. Recovery is slow and often incomplete, even with complete alcohol abstinence.
Wernicke encephalopathy	Acute	Clinical presentation includes ocular disturbances (e.g., nystagmus), muscle weakness or paralysis, diplopia, ataxia, disorientation, and confusion, often accompanying signs of thiamine deficiency. Patients with the condition can be treated with thiamine.
Korsakoff psychosis	Acute or chronic	More apparent disturbances in this disorder are cognitive defect and personality change. Memory may be affected to the exclusion of other components of mental function. Recent memory is affected to the greatest extent. Other clinical features often include confusion and confabulation. Recovery is slow and usually incomplete, despite treatment with thiamine and other vitamins, and cessation of drinking.

(continued)

TABLE 58.1	continued	
Complication	**Usual Onset**	**Comments**
Teratogenesis	Chronic	Multiple congenital defects, prenatal growth retardation, and delay in development are fetal abnormalities that result from heavy alcohol abuse during pregnancy.
Neonatal intoxication and withdrawal	Acute	Ethanol freely crosses the placental barrier. The clearance rate of alcohol is reduced in premature infants. Substantial impairment of motor activity, alertness, and respiration is reported in neonates after ethanol infusion just before delivery.
Sexual impotence, loss of libido	Chronic	Experienced often by male PWA. Endocrine effects of alcohol, characteristics of hypogonadism (e.g., gynecomastia), loss of facial hair, spider angiomata, testicular atrophy, and testosterone deficiency are seen.
Cancer	Chronic	Excessive use of alcohol combined with tobacco has been implicated in greater risks for cancers, particularly of the head, neck, mouth, pharynx, larynx, esophagus, colon, and liver. Alcohol may activate cocarcinogens through induction of cytochrome P-4502E1.

pancreatitis.[37] The initial presenting symptom is usually abdominal pain, which may be severe, that radiates from the upper abdomen to the back or both flanks. Both serum amylase and lipase levels are generally elevated, although lipase levels tend to be more sensitive and specific in the diagnosis of pancreatitis.

NEUROLOGIC SYSTEM

Wernicke encephalopathy and Korsakoff psychosis are two classic neurologic abnormalities associated with chronic alcoholism.[38] Both are caused by deficiencies in thiamine, a nutritional deficiency not uncommon in PWA. Because thiamine is a cofactor in glucose metabolism, Wernicke encephalopathy can be precipitated by administration of a large glucose load, as might typically occur in patients being managed for alcohol withdrawal. Thus, patients who are known or suspected to be alcoholic should be administered parenteral thiamine before or concurrently with the administration of dextrose-containing intravenous fluids.

Although classic Wernicke encephalopathy is not frequently encountered in clinical practice, it carries an estimated 10% to 20% mortality rate. Therefore, suspected cases represent medical emergencies, and patients must be promptly treated. Symptoms that include central nervous system (CNS) depression, ambulatory difficulties, and ocular abnormalities develop abruptly and evolve over several days. Other clinical features include hypothermia, hypotension, and polyneuropathy. Treatment is supportive in nature and includes the administration of thiamine.

About 80% of patients with Wernicke encephalopathy who do not recover in the first 48 to 72 hours will develop Korsakoff psychosis. These patients will develop both retrograde and anterograde amnesia. Memory of recent and current events is particularly affected. Fabrication of stories is

typical, particularly in the early stages of the disease. Many patients with Korsakoff psychosis do not recover completely and will require long-term care.

CLINICAL PRESENTATION AND DIAGNOSIS

SIGNS AND SYMPTOMS

Acute Alcohol Intoxication. The relation between blood ethyl alcohol concentration and clinical signs and symptoms of intoxication are variable and depend on rate of ingestion; amount consumed; alterations in absorption, metabolism, and excretion; and chronicity of exposure (Table 58.2). The correlation of blood alcohol concentration to behavioral effects has obvious medical and legal importance. As a consequence of tolerance, higher blood alcohol concentrations may be required to produce clinical effects in PWA than in occasional drinkers. Some drinkers exhibit such extreme degrees of tolerance to alcohol that they appear sober even with blood alcohol concentrations two to three times higher than the limit permitted by law for driving an automobile. The lethal blood alcohol level is variable but falls in the range of 400 to 700 mg per dL (86.8 to 151.9 mmol/L). The lethal level may be substantially lowered when opiates, neuroleptics, or other sedative-hypnotics are taken along with an excessive amount of alcohol.

Chronic Alcohol Abuse/Alcoholism. A myriad of medical complications can accompany alcoholism. Common early physical signs and symptoms of alcoholism include hypertension, gastritis, diarrhea or irritable colon, burns, bruises, red face, puffy face and eyes, enlarged nose with prominent veins, reddened conjunctiva, obesity, insomnia, and impotence.

TABLE 58.2	Blood Ethanol Concentrations and Clinical Effects in the Nontolerant Adult Drinker
Blood Ethanol Level in mg/dL (mmol/L)	**Clinical Effects**
20–99 (4.3–21.6)	Slight changes in mood and feelings progressing to muscular incoordination, impaired sensory function, and personality and behavioral changes (talkative, noisy, morose)
100–199 (21.7–43.3)	Marked mental impairment, incoordination, clumsiness, and unsteadiness in standing or walking, ataxia, prolonged reaction time, gross intoxication
200–299 (43.4–65)	Nausea, vomiting, diplopia, marked ataxia
300–399 (65.1–86.7)	Hypothermia, severe dysarthria, amnesia, stage 1 anesthesia
400–700 (86.8–151.9)	Coma, respiratory failure, and death

Malnutrition is commonplace among PWA.[39] Chronic alcohol consumption results in impaired digestion and absorption of essential nutrients. Nearly all PWA have diminished food intake while drinking because alcohol presumably suppresses appetite. Alcohol represents ''empty calories'' that lack nutritive value. Taken in excess, alcohol also prevents adequate gastrointestinal absorption of nutrients and contributes to debilitated and malnourished conditions. Nutritional problems that PWA are most susceptible to are deficiencies of protein, water-soluble vitamins, and some minerals. Identification and management of nutritional deficiencies is an important component of the overall treatment program for PWA.

Accumulation of fluids with resultant ascites is a frequent complication of alcoholic cirrhosis. It is secondary to portal hypertension and reduced plasma albumin concentrations, which reduce intravascular oncotic pressure. Reduced dietary protein intake and decreased hepatic synthetic function both contribute to reductions in albumin production. The focus of management is to supply a protein-restricted diet (no more than 40 g/day) to prevent the development of hepatic encephalopathy while attempting to replenish protein stores. Sodium and water intake must be carefully restricted so that only daily losses are replaced. It is important to remember that ''hidden sources'' of sodium, such as intravenously administered fluids that include plasma and drugs, may be responsible for unexpected reaccumulation of fluids in these patients.

In PWA, deficiencies in potassium and magnesium are often responsible for patients who present with lethargy and weakness. As was previously mentioned, thiamine deficiency can contribute to the development of Wernicke encephalopathy and Korsakoff psychosis. Folic acid deficiency is common in PWA and may result in macrocytic anemia.

Acute Alcohol Abstinence (Withdrawal) Syndrome.

An acute abstinence, or withdrawal, syndrome is a common problem experienced by the PWA when alcohol is discontinued abruptly; delirium tremens (DTs) is the most severe form. The severity of the withdrawal syndrome cannot always be predicted on the basis of the quantity or duration of alcohol ingestion. Although most patients experience only minor and moderate symptoms, described often as a ''hangover,'' it is difficult to rule out the possibility that progressively more severe and even life-threatening withdrawal reactions may occur. Wide variability in the severity and duration of this syndrome has been reported; in 5% to 6% of those who undergo this experience, it will progress to the most severe stage—delirium tremens.

The early physiologic and behavioral effects of acute alcohol abstinence (8 to 36 hours after cessation of drinking) include anorexia; tremors (''shakes''); flushing; increased blood pressure, pulse, respiration rate, and temperature; intermittent hallucinations; seizures (''rum fits''); sleep disturbance; and sweating. Mild to moderate withdrawal may stimulate PWA to resume drinking to reverse the symptoms. A common finding in the later progression of alcoholism is the use of morning drinks (''eye openers'') to reduce these effects occurring as a result of drinking the previous night. Late effects, experienced 2 to 6 days after cessation of drinking, may include severe tremors, marked agitation, profound disorientation, excitation, persistent visual and auditory hallucinations, marked sleep disturbances, fever, tachycardia, seizures, and other life-threatening complications. Patients who experience major alcohol withdrawal symptoms or DTs, which are estimated to occur in 5% of untreated withdrawing PWA, are seriously ill. Patients with DTs are febrile, disoriented, and agitated and often have an accompanying concurrent medical problem, such as infection or coma. Although the mortality rate for this condition has decreased during the past 50 years, deaths from DTs still occur (variously estimated at 5% to 20%), particularly in patients with underlying or alcohol-associated conditions such as pancreatitis, cirrhosis, gastrointestinal bleeding, pneumonia, or sepsis. It should not be taken for granted that the intoxicated or bizarre behavior of the PWA is an effect of alcohol; hypoxia, hyperosmolarity, hypomagnesemia, or hypoglycemia may be contributing to it.[40]

The exact pathophysiologic mechanism for the acute alcohol withdrawal syndrome is uncertain, and multiple mechanisms are likely involved. Chronic alcohol consumption results in a decrease in the γ-aminobutyric acid A (GABA-A) receptor response to GABA, a neuroreceptor that decreases brain excitability. Alcohol also inhibits the excitatory N-methyl-D-aspartate (NMDA) neuroreceptors, diminishing the brain's response to stimulation by glutamine. However, chronic alcohol use also upregulates the NMDA receptors. Thus, when patients stop the consumption of alcohol after chronic heavy use, a state of brain hyperexcitability may occur, caused by increased stimulation of the already upregulated NMDA receptors at a time when the brain's response to GABA is diminished.[41] This explains the CNS excitability that occurs as the blood alcohol concentration falls.

Fetal Alcohol Syndrome. The relation between heavy alcohol consumption in pregnancy and fetal abnormalities has been suspected since antiquity. Clarren and Smith[42] characterized this pattern of malformation known as fetal alcohol syndrome, or FAS, as follows: (a) prenatal and postnatal growth deficiency; (b) central nervous system dysfunction, including microcephaly, hypotonia, irritability and jitteriness, mental retardation, and poor coordination and hyperactivity during childhood; (c) craniofacial abnormalities, including short palpebral fissures, short upturned nose, hypoplastic philtrum, flat midface, and thinned upper lip; and (d) other major organ system defects, such as abnormalities of the eyes, ears, and mouth, heart murmurs, septal defects, genitourinary abnormalities, hemangiomas, and musculoskeletal problems such as hernias. Longitudinal studies show that these children experience immunodeficiency. No "catch-up" seems to occur in terms of either behavior or intellect in the impaired child with fetal alcohol syndrome.

A survey of pregnant women conducted in 1999 found that about 3% reported frequent drinking (i.e., more than 7 drinks/week, or drinking 5 or more drinks per occasion) during pregnancy.[43] The estimated prevalence of FAS in the United States is 0.5 to 2 per 1000 live births.[44]

Many factors may influence the phenotypic outcome of pregnancy in the alcoholic mother, including variable dose exposure at different gestational periods and the genetic background of the individual fetus. Alcohol, like other teratogens, does not uniformly affect all those exposed to it. Rather, there seems to be a continuum of effects of alcohol on the fetus, with increasingly severe outcomes generally associated with higher intakes of alcohol by the mother.[42] It should also be noted that alcohol readily enters breast milk, thereby providing alcohol to the nursing infant. There appears to be no established safe amount of alcohol or safe time to drink it during pregnancy and lactation.

DIAGNOSIS

Acute Intoxication. The severity of acute intoxication depends on a person's blood alcohol level and individual tolerance. Levels below 50 mg per dL (10.9 mmol/L), or 0.05%,

rarely produce significant effects in adults. In children, signs of alcohol intoxication are often prominent at this level. The presence or absence of the odor of alcohol on a patient's breath cannot be used to establish a diagnosis of alcohol intoxication. However, unique odors should still be noted because they may offer a diagnostic clue as to the overall clinical condition of an intoxicated patient. Plasma osmolality can be a useful indicator in that the relationship of osmolality to plasma alcohol is linear. A rise of approximately 25 to 30 mOsmol per kg (or mmol/kg) of water (H$_2$O) reflects a 100 mg per dL (21.8 mmol/L), or 0.1%, increase in plasma alcohol. Concomitant conditions such as trauma, blood loss, infection, multiple drug use, and hypoglycemia often complicate the recognition and assessment of an intoxicated patient; therefore, the measurement or estimate of the blood alcohol level or comparable analysis of urine, saliva, and expired air is valuable for confirming alcohol intoxication and for establishing an appropriate treatment plan.[40]

Other toxicologic tests, particularly for sedative drugs and for salicylates, may be indicated to detect suspected commonly occurring polydrug toxicity. In addition, specific laboratory studies for liver function; renal function; serum electrolytes with particular attention to the potassium, magnesium, and phosphate levels and the anion gap; arterial blood gases; and blood ketones and glucose should be performed routinely. After a prolonged drinking binge, myoglobinuria, hyperkalemia, and increased serum creatine kinase levels secondary to alcohol myopathy may occur. Electrocardiography should be performed, and changes characteristic of abnormal calcium, magnesium, and potassium levels or the presence of hypoxia or hypothermia should be recognized. An abdominal x-ray examination (of the kidney, ureters, and bladder) may offer useful clues to the identity of materials ingested in any possible multiple overdose involving an acutely alcohol-intoxicated patient. Some common drugs that are often taken in suicide attempts, such as phenothiazines; tricyclic antidepressants; heavy metals, including iron, arsenic, and halides; iodides and bromides; chloral hydrate; and enteric-coated tablets, are radiopaque. Comatose patients may require a computed tomography (CT) scan to rule out intracranial pathology. Chest radiographs may be indicated if aspiration is suspected.

Alcohol Abuse and Alcoholism. The diagnosis of alcoholism is difficult because of the societal stigmatization of the disease, denial, and imprecise diagnostic criteria. Clinical signs and subtleties of the condition are varied, elusive, and without reliable parameters. For chronic alcoholism, laboratory markers such as γ-glutamyl transferase (GGT), carbohydrate-deficient transferrin (CDT), or mean corpuscular volume (MCV) may provide clues but not a definitive diagnosis. Objective laboratory verification of the diagnosis is often unavailable or incomplete. Although a specific genetic marker for alcoholism had been suggested, recent research has failed to verify this; data derived from mapping of the human genome suggest that alcoholism is genetically heterogeneous, reflecting different predisposing genes in different families. Genetics likely represents only one of a number of factors (e.g., multiple gene loci, environment, sex, ethnicity) that affect predisposition.[45] Reliable biochemical or genetic markers for diagnosing alcoholism are not available. Much depends on the experience and motivation of the observer in deciding whether a patient is suffering from alcoholism or not. Unfortunately, many physicians and other health care professionals are poorly educated concerning the diagnosis of alcoholism, resulting in the underdiagnosis and mismanagement of alcohol-related problems. The first recognition of alcoholism often occurs during a hospitalization when an advanced manifestation of alcoholism, such as ascites or cirrhosis, is being treated. Many patients with unrecognized alcoholism probably experience minor withdrawal symptoms, such as agitation and insomnia, during the course of hospital stays or when admitted to nursing homes.

Early identification of an existing alcohol problem is important because the prognosis with treatment is much more promising when the difficulty is recognized early in its course. Clues that provide early recognition are found in the demographic, social, familial, and cultural characteristics of those who consume alcohol. Frequent episodes of drinking to the point of intoxication, an inability to control the intake of alcohol, alcoholic ''blackout'' periods (loss of memory while intoxicated, not passing out), drinking despite strong social contraindications such as job loss, legal problems such as drunk driving arrests, and family or marital discord resulting from pathologic drinking are signs of the presence of this condition. Several alcoholism screening tests are commonly used: [SMAST (*s*hort *M*ichigan *a*lcoholism *s*creening *t*est, CAGE (*c*ut down drinking, *a*nnoyed by criticism of drinking, *g*uilty about drinking, and *e*ye openers), AUDIT (*a*lcohol *u*se *d*isorders *i*dentification *t*est), and TWEAK (*t*olerance, others *w*orry about your drinking, *e*ye opener, *a*mnesia, c(*k*)ut down drinking)]; the CAGE, sometimes combined with drinking quantity and frequency questions, is applied most often because of its brevity, relative reliability, and ease of administration.[45]

Diagnostic criteria for alcohol abuse and alcoholism are often difficult and subjective; however, criteria from the *Diagnostic and Statistical Manual of Mental Disorders, 4th edition, Text Revision* (DSM-IV-TR), established by the American Psychiatric Association, can serve as a convenient starting point for the diagnosis of alcohol dependence.[46] Alcohol abuse is characterized by a maladaptive pattern of alcohol use that leads to clinically significant impairment. Within a 2-month period, one or more of the following criteria must be met: (a) negative effects on school or job performance, (b) neglect of household or child care responsibilities, (c) alcohol-related absences from school or work, (d) use of alcohol in physically hazardous conditions, and (e) legal difficulties as a result of alcohol use.[46] Persons may continue to consume alcohol despite knowing that continuation may result in social or interpersonal problems. Therefore, a single situation can fulfill several of the diagnostic

criteria for alcohol abuse. For example, a person who is arrested for the second instance of driving under the influence (DUI) of alcohol after consuming alcohol to the extent of intoxication fulfills several of the criteria. At minimum, the person has used alcohol in physically hazardous conditions by operating an automobile and will face legal difficulties as a result of the DUI arrest. Moreover, the person would not be able to return to work that afternoon and may not be able to fulfill child care responsibilities such as picking up a child at day care.

In alcohol dependence, the maladaptive pattern of alcohol use is manifested by at least three of the following during a 1-year period: (a) tolerance, (b) withdrawal, (c) alcohol is consumed in larger amounts or for a longer period than intended, (d) persistent desire or unsuccessful attempts to increase control or decrease consumption of alcohol, (e) much time spent to obtain or drink alcohol or recover from its effects, (f) social, occupational, or recreational activities discontinued or reduced as a result of drinking alcohol, and (g) alcohol use continued despite the knowledge of having a physical or psychological problem resulting from alcohol use. Tolerance can be manifested by the need for increased amounts of alcohol to achieve intoxication or the desired effect, or by diminished effect with continued use of the same amount of alcohol. Withdrawal is characterized by either of the following categories: (a) two or more of the following are present: autonomic hyperactivity (i.e., tachycardia or diaphoresis), hand tremor, insomnia, nausea or vomiting, hallucinations, psychomotor agitation, anxiety, or grand mal seizures; or (b) alcohol or other substances are taken to relieve or avoid withdrawal.[46]

PSYCHOSOCIAL ASPECTS

Alcoholism affects every aspect of the personal life and family life of the alcoholic. Employment, financial problems, family problems, and social isolation are only a few effects of chronic alcohol abuse. Specific psychosocial attributes are not easily identified as positive indicators of alcoholism. In an evaluation of Danish patients, lower educational levels were associated with an increased incidence of excessive alcohol consumption in men.[8] Among people 65 years or older, a positive association has been shown between volume of alcohol consumed and psychosocial well-being; however, drinking frequency was not related to psychosocial status.[11]

The challenge for the PWA and the clinician is to identify a cause-effect relationship between the psychosocial effects and alcoholism. For example, the PWA states that he or she drinks as a result of financial problems. However, the alcoholism then exacerbates the financial problems through the direct cost of alcohol and indirect effects such as missed work. The resultant potentiation of financial difficulty places the alcoholic in a vicious cycle. Parental alcoholism often disrupts family life; therefore, the effects of alcoholism on the children of PWA should also be addressed. A prominent negative effect of alcoholism is the disturbance of family rituals such as holidays, vacations, and school events. These disruptions can result in the children's perception of themselves as the cause of the disruption or as abnormal compared with their peers. The effects of such feelings of inadequacy can present social challenges for the child, such as problematic family rituals when the child reaches adulthood. However, the maintenance of family rituals even with heavy periods of drinking in an alcoholic parent is correlated with a lower incidence of alcoholism in the children of PWA.[47]

Higher levels of family conflict have been reported in families of PWA.[48] Families of PWA have been characterized by a lack of parenting, poor home management, and a lack of family communication skills.[49] Moreover, a multitude of problems have been associated with alcoholism, including emotional or physical violence, decreased family cohesion, decreased family organization, marital strain, financial problems, and frequent family relocations.[47] Each of these, along with other family problems, has consequences that expand the scope of involvement with alcohol and result in additional family dysfunction, which adds to the complexity of alcoholism.

THERAPEUTIC PLAN

The consensus diagnosis and treatment plans for patients with alcoholism are summarized and explained in this chapter. However, the criteria found in DSM-IV-TR, established by the American Psychiatric Association, serve as the gold standard for the diagnosis of alcoholism and other mental disorders.[46] The Agency for Health Care Policy and Research has published an evidence-based report entitled, "Pharmacotherapy of Alcohol Dependence," which addresses drug therapy for alcoholism.[50]

TREATMENT

PHARMACOTHERAPY

Acute Intoxication. The basic treatment for acute alcohol intoxication is to maintain and support vital functions (i.e., maintain a patent airway and adequate blood pressure, and avoid aspiration) during the detoxification process until support is no longer needed; this may take from 7 to 10 days.[51,52] In the comatose patient, particularly in cases of accidental ingestion of alcohol by a child, acute alcoholic hypoglycemia and other possible causes of coma such as subdural hematoma should be ruled out. CNS stimulants should not be used. Major problems encountered in the management of acute alcohol intoxication include (a) pneumonia, a leading cause of morbidity, (b) overhydration, and (c) complications from unnecessary therapeutic maneuvers.

The possible presence of alcohol should not be overlooked when the clinician is evaluating a suspected acute case of drug intoxication. One study revealed that almost one of every five patients with an acute drug overdose, in whom the presence of alcohol was unsuspected or thought to be irrelevant, was found to have high blood levels of alcohol. The notion that acute alcohol intoxication is benign should be dispelled. Diagnosis of any drug intoxication should include a blood ethanol determination, in addition to other laboratory tests.

Alcoholic coma is a life-threatening situation in which patients usually respond well to supportive treatment. Establishment of a clear airway and assisted ventilation are essential in patients with this condition. Oxygenation and volume replacement with intravenous fluids generally alleviate the hypotension. Patients who are experiencing protracted vomiting may have substantial fluid deficits. If alcoholic hypoglycemia is suspected, or if the blood glucose level is at 70 mg per dL (3.9 mmol/L) or lower, 50 to 100 mL of 50% glucose should be given intravenously. Parenteral thiamine 100 mg should be administered [either intramuscularly (IM) or by slow push intravenously (IV)] before or along with the glucose to prevent possible development or exacerbation of the Wernicke-Korsakoff syndrome. If recent ingestion of drugs is suspected, gastric lavage can be carefully performed in the unconscious patient, with appropriate guarding of the airway to avoid the risk of aspiration. Emetics, such as syrup of ipecac, should be used with great caution in any acutely intoxicated conscious alcoholic patient because tearing of the gastroesophageal mucosa may occur as a life-threatening consequence of ipecac-induced protracted vomiting.

The use of 10% and 40% solutions of fructose given orally or intravenously in attempts to accelerate the metabolism of ethanol is not recommended. The minimal benefits derived from such an effort are outweighed by the disadvantages. Adverse effects from fructose include nausea, vomiting, hyperuricemia, worsening of metabolic acidosis, and volume depletion. Increasing the rate of clearance of alcohol from the body leads to more rapid development of alcohol withdrawal symptoms.[53]

Administration of naloxone to reverse alcohol-induced coma has been reported to produce some beneficial effects in patients with acute alcohol intoxication. In cases described in the literature, responses were variable; in some patients, improvement was only slight. Difficulties encountered when attempts were made to exclude concomitant opiate use in those patients reported to have responded, as well as failed attempts to reproduce these findings in the laboratory, have left unresolved the issue of naloxone use as an antagonist to alcohol-induced coma.[54,55] Thus, it seems wise for clinicians to administer naloxone only to those patients in whom concomitant opiate use is suspected.

Patients who present with acute alcohol intoxication or alcohol withdrawal often suffer from alcohol-induced liver disease that requires immediate treatment. Alcohol and digested blood from bleeding esophageal varices can often precipitate or exacerbate hepatic encephalopathy. Appropriate treatment includes dietary protein restriction and administration of lactulose, both of which lower serum ammonia levels. The immediate approach to bleeding esophageal varices includes blood replacement and administration of intravenous octreotide to reduce intravariceal pressure. Bleeding esophageal varices should also be treated locally with endoscopically applied band ligation or injection sclerotherapy, with the goal of achieving rapid hemostasis. For patients who do not respond adequately, more invasive treatment may be needed to decompress varices. Options include balloon tamponade with a Sengstaken-Blakemore tube, a transjugular intrahepatic portosystemic shunt (TIPS), and various surgical shunting procedures.[56]

Toxic psychosis associated with acute alcohol intoxication occasionally presents as an emergency situation. It is characterized by a markedly impaired sensorium with confusion, amnesia, and disorientation. Often, a sudden onset of aggressive and hostile behavior occurs with associated psychotic symptoms, including hallucinations and delusions. Treatment of patients in this agitated phase can be accomplished with sedation to produce a calm, but still arousable, patient. Benzodiazepines and haloperidol can be used judiciously in these circumstances.

A number of considerations should be kept in mind when one is treating and caring for the patient who is acutely intoxicated or overdosed with alcohol. Symptoms of acute alcohol intoxication and response to treatment vary among patients. Factors such as age, weight, tolerance, and concomitant ingestion of other drugs must be considered. Polydrug abuse in the adult with alcohol intoxication should be suspected, and withdrawal from barbiturates or opiates may be a further complication. In children, the toxicologic effects of ingredients contained in alcoholic solutions that are used for cough and colds, for pain and allergic symptoms, or for sleep should be considered. Medical and surgical illnesses may contribute to the toxicologic problems of acute alcohol poisoning. The goals of treatment should be to maintain and support vital functions and to individualize all aspects of care and treatment.[40]

Acute Alcohol Abstinence (Withdrawal) Syndrome.

The primary objective of detoxification is to facilitate removal of alcohol from the body with as few withdrawal symptoms as possible.[57] This process involves the substitution and slow withdrawing of a long-acting sedative-hypnotic drug for the shorter-acting one, alcohol. Some patients in mild withdrawal may not require drugs for relief. In the past 30 years, many different drugs and drug combinations have been described in the medical literature for the treatment of patients in acute alcohol withdrawal. In like manner, a 1995 national survey of 176 inpatient treatment facilities reported great diversity in pharmacologic management of alcohol withdrawal. The most common drugs used in decreasing order were chlordiazepoxide, diazepam, barbiturates, phenytoin, clonidine, and oxazepam.[58] A review of the studies that investigated the effectiveness of drugs in treating patients with withdrawal syndrome suggests that many such studies were poorly controlled and lacked objective comparisons of effects. In carefully conducted studies, some drugs have not been shown to be much more effective than placebo. In many instances, the major benefit associated with antianxiety agents may be experienced by the nursing and medical staff, in that the patient is made more manageable.

Benzodiazepines. Benzodiazepines, such as diazepam, chlordiazepoxide, clorazepate, oxazepam, and lorazepam, are longer-acting and safer agents compared with other sedative-hypnotics, and they have anticonvulsant activity. They are used often because of the convenient dosage forms that are available. Diazepam, chlordiazepoxide, and lorezepam can be administered by oral and intravenous routes, often in gradually tapering doses. Clorazepate and oxazepam are available only in oral dosage forms. The usual therapeutic end point in the management of acute alcohol withdrawal symptoms is to produce a calm but awake patient, with the use of whatever doses are required to achieve this goal.[51,59]

The pharmacokinetics of these drugs in patients undergoing alcohol withdrawal and in patients with liver impairment has aroused a great deal of clinical and research interest. The elimination half-lives of oxazepam, lorazepam, chlordiazepoxide, clorazepate, and diazepam are 8, 16, 16, 24, and 32 hours, respectively, with wide individual variation noted. In patients with alcohol-induced cirrhosis, the elimination of benzodiazepines from the body is presumably decreased because of reduced clearance by the liver. Because the major metabolites of benzodiazepines (with the exception of oxazepam and lorazepam) are psychoactive, accumulation of effects during long-term administration of these drugs should be evaluated carefully in patients with cirrhosis. No evidence suggests that any one of the benzodiazepines is better than another for use in acute alcohol detoxification. However, when benzodiazepines are used in patients with hepatic dysfunction, careful monitoring of patient response is essential to ensure efficacy while preventing excessive CNS depression.

Dose requirements of these drugs when used for detoxification are variable. The usual range for diazepam is 30 to 200 mg during the first 24 hours, but occasionally, patients may require higher doses. It should be remembered that a withdrawing PWA may require higher doses of sedative-hypnotic drugs than are required by other agitated patients, probably because of tolerance and decreased sensitivity.[60] Some alcoholic patients are calmed only by doses that would be severely depressive in nonalcoholic patients. Because dose requirements are variable, no specific dosage schedule can be predicted for a given patient. In a patient who is undergoing a mild to moderate withdrawal syndrome, an initial dose of diazepam 20 mg can be administered orally, followed by 10 to 20 mg every 2 to 3 hours. However, elderly patients should receive only 10 mg initially, followed by doses every 4 to 6 hours, if needed. A comparable regimen for chlordiazepoxide would be 25 to 100 mg given every 2 to 6 hours, depending on symptoms. A total daily dose of

400 to 600 mg may be needed by extremely tolerant patients with severe symptoms. In the elderly patient, 50 mg two to four times a day should be sufficient for symptom relief. Reduced doses of benzodiazepines are generally sufficient for outpatients who experience mild withdrawal symptoms.[61]

For severe withdrawal, intravenous diazepam can be cautiously administered in a dose of 10 to 30 mg every 30 or more minutes until the patient is calm. Then, a maintenance regimen of 10 to 20 mg can be given intravenously or orally as needed during the day and in the evening to enable sleep. Comparable parenteral dosing regimens of chlordiazepoxide or lorazepam may also be used. Because of the risks of hypotension and respiratory depression, the patient should be assessed before and periodically after every intravenous dose of a sedative-hypnotic drug. Intramuscular administration of chlordiazepoxide and diazepam should be avoided because of their slow and erratic absorption, although intramuscular lorazepam does appear to be reliably absorbed. With the shorter-acting benzodiazepines, loading doses are not required; however, to maintain blood levels that are sufficient to sustain relief from withdrawal symptoms, doses of oxazepam and lorazepam at 15 to 30 mg and 1 to 4 mg, respectively, must be given at 6- to 8-hour intervals. Withdrawing these drugs during the detoxification process should be accomplished by lowering their dose rather than by lengthening their administration interval beyond 8 hours.

Every patient should be reevaluated and drug requirements reassessed every few hours until initial symptom control is achieved, and then at least daily during the maintenance phase. Predetermined, fixed dosing regimens have frequently been used, but they often contribute to unnecessary oversedation of patients who are undergoing withdrawal. Recently, studies have demonstrated that individualized therapy, triggered by patient symptoms, resulted in equivalent control of alcohol withdrawal (vs. fixed-dosing regimens) with lower total benzodiazepine doses and shortened duration of therapy.[62,63] Thus, the symptom-triggered approach is preferred, provided that patient care staff are sufficiently trained in its use.

Antipsychotics. Phenothiazine neuroleptics have not been shown to be any more effective than the sedative-hypnotic drugs and should not be used. Their use can result in increased seizures, impaired thermoregulation, extrapyramidal effects, and postural hypotension. The syncope and arrhythmias that can result from these drugs can produce serious consequences in the acutely withdrawing patient. At high doses, delirium may occur as a result of their anticholinergic effects.

Haloperidol in oral doses of 5 to 10 mg, or 5 mg IM, has been advocated for use in treating patients with hallucinations and acute agitation associated with alcohol. Although it produces less sedation, hypotension, and hypothermia compared with the phenothiazines, haloperidol, like other dopamine antagonists, may cause extrapyramidal and centrally mediated anticholinergic reactions. Extreme caution should be exercised with the use of this drug because CNS depression caused by the concomitant alcohol may be additive or potentiated.

Few data are available from which the newer atypical antipsychotic drugs can be evaluated for use in alcohol withdrawal; therefore, the use of these agents cannot currently be recommended.

Clonidine. Clonidine, a centrally acting inhibitor of adrenergic vasomotor centers used in the treatment of hypertension, has been compared with benzodiazepines in the management of acute alcohol withdrawal. Used successfully to treat patients in opiate withdrawal, clonidine can also relieve the tremors, tachycardia, systolic hypertension, and diaphoresis secondary to alcohol withdrawal, and it appears to be as effective as chlordiazepoxide. Because the ability of clonidine to protect against withdrawal seizures is uncertain, the role of the drug should remain limited to situations wherein the risks of seizures and serious medical or psychiatric complications are minimal.[59]

Carbamazepine. Carbamazepine has been shown to prevent alcohol withdrawal in animal studies, and it does not potentiate CNS or respiratory depression caused by alcohol. It has been widely used for alcohol withdrawal in Europe and has been shown to be comparable with oxazepam in treating patients in mild to moderate withdrawal. Currently, it is not widely used in the United States for the treatment of patients who are undergoing alcohol withdrawal.[57]

Divalproex Sodium. Recent small studies have suggested that divalproex sodium may be effective in the management of alcohol withdrawal, with efficacy that is similar to that of benzodiazepines.[64,65] Additional studies are needed to confirm or refute these findings. Divalproex sodium may have advantages over benzodiazepines in that it has less abuse potential, fewer CNS depressant effects, and lower potential synergy with alcohol.

Phenytoin. The routine use of phenytoin has not been shown to be effective in preventing seizures in patients undergoing alcohol withdrawal.[66] Seizures associated with acute alcohol withdrawal (''rum fits'') are usually self-limiting and often do not require anticonvulsant medication. Episodes are brief, consisting usually of a single grand mal–like seizure and only occasionally appearing as repeated seizures. Properly administered benzodiazepine therapy provides some protection from seizures during alcohol withdrawal.[67] Patients with focal neurologic deficits, head trauma, and underlying seizure disorders are at increased risk of seizures during alcohol withdrawal, and prophylactic phenytoin may be advisable in select patients. In the acute situation during status epilepticus, intravenous diazepam or phenytoin can be administered.

β-Blockers. Theoretically, a β-adrenergic blocking drug such as propranolol should be beneficial in preventing the adrenergic overactivity that occurs during alcohol withdrawal, as the alcohol withdrawal syndrome is likely to be mediated in part by the autonomic system. Propranolol has been shown to be effective in reducing tremor, blood pressure, heart rate, and urinary and total catecholamine levels in patients who are withdrawing from alcohol.[68]

Few clinical studies on the use of β-blockers in alcohol withdrawal have been published. A trial comparing atenolol with placebo in a large group of hospitalized patients withdrawing from alcohol showed that the drug had an ameliorating effect on the symptoms experienced. Because β-blockers lack anticonvulsant activity, both groups also received oxazepam 15 or 30 mg QID. Results showed a shorter duration of hospital stay, a reduced need for benzodiazepines during hospitalization, and a more rapid return of vital signs to normal in the atenolol-treated patients.[69]

Ethanol. The use of alcohol in the management of acute alcohol withdrawal symptoms is hazardous because of its short duration of action and the risk that metabolic, endocrine, and neurologic disturbances and pathologic changes will be sustained.

Thiamine (Vitamin B$_1$). The most serious consequences of thiamine deficiency experienced by PWA are neuromuscular effects. Wernicke encephalopathy and Korsakoff psychosis, characterized by ophthalmoplegia, ataxia, peripheral neuropathy, and progressive confusion, are manifestations of this deficiency.[70,71] Thiamine is routinely administered IM or IV in daily doses of 100 to 200 mg to withdrawing PWA as a preventative measure. Because glucose solutions are invariably administered to such patients, deficient stores of thiamine may be further depleted as a result. After several days of parenteral therapy, thiamine should be continued orally at a dose of 50 to 100 mg per day. Long-term oral thiamine is inexpensive and should be continued in PWA, particularly those who have a high likelihood of continuing to drink.

Vitamin K. Vitamin K is used particularly in patients with alcoholic hepatitis or cirrhosis because prothrombin production is often impaired owing to hepatic dysfunction. Although deficient vitamin K stores may be replenished, coagulation parameters may not be normalized in patients who lack sufficient hepatic synthetic function to produce adequate quantities of clotting factors.

Folic Acid. The moderate to severe anemia seen in PWA is usually of the megaloblastic type caused by folic acid deficiency. A combined megaloblastic and microcytic anemia indicating iron deficiency usually results from blood loss combined with nutritional deficits.[72] Folic acid supplementation should be provided as a component of the total nutritional intake of patients who are withdrawing from alcohol.

Fluids, Glucose, and Electrolytes. It is important to correct fluid and electrolyte imbalances, particularly of sodium, po-

tassium, and magnesium, that accompany acute withdrawal.[73,74] In some patients, water is retained and renal resorption of sodium, potassium, and chloride is increased, contrary to the notion that all acutely withdrawing PWA are dehydrated from the diuresis produced by alcohol.[75] An observation common in patients with severe alcohol withdrawal is hypomagnesemia, with serum levels ranging from 0.7 to 1.4 mEq per L (0.4 to 0.7 mmol/L). Because symptoms of withdrawal such as tremor, hyperreflexia, and seizures are similar to those associated with this condition, the administration of magnesium is thought to aid in reducing the severity of, and even preventing, some of these symptoms.

Summary. The following considerations should be kept in mind when one is treating and caring for the alcoholic patient in the acute withdrawal phase. The acute alcohol withdrawal syndrome and response to treatment vary among alcoholic patients. Polydrug abuse occurs in chronic alcoholism, and withdrawal from barbiturates or opiates can further complicate therapy. An opiate-dependent person who is also dependent on alcohol may be detoxified from the alcohol while being maintained on methadone. Benzodiazepines are the drugs of choice for treating patients with the acute alcohol withdrawal syndrome because they are clinically effective and distinctly safer than other medications. Patient variables may influence the pharmacokinetics of benzodiazepines, the dose, and the route of administration. Doses of medication used to treat patients with withdrawal symptoms should be tapered, rather than abruptly discontinued, to avoid delayed withdrawal symptoms. Complete eradication of withdrawal symptoms may indicate overmedication. Medical and surgical illness may worsen the acute withdrawal syndrome. Nonpharmacologic factors such as staff attitude and ward environment can be effective in helping with the anxiety, insomnia, depression, and other problems that often occur during acute detoxification. No evidence indicates that drug therapy during acute alcohol detoxification modifies the outcome of long-term treatment of alcoholism. Detoxification is the first—not the final—step in therapy for alcoholism. The most important factors in successful treatment of and ongoing recovery from alcoholism are the motivation of the patient to stop drinking and ongoing participation in recovery support programs, such as Alcoholics Anonymous (AA).

Chronic Alcoholism. Although the period of detoxification is relatively short, it may take months for the physiologic processes to return to normal. Maintaining a prolonged alcohol-free period after detoxification enhances treatment of the chronic alcoholic. It is commonly thought that alcoholism is primarily a manifestation of underlying psychiatric problems, and most methods of treatment and dealing with those problems will not succeed while the patient continues to drink. A variety of pharmacotherapeutic approaches are available for management of chronic alcoholism, including use of medications alone or in combination with behavioral modification techniques. Successful recovery maintenance for some individuals recovering from alcoholism depends upon pharmacotherapy provided under the direction of a physician or pharmacist who is experienced in addiction disorders.

Disulfiram. Disulfiram is best used in the context of a close physician–patient or therapist–patient relationship with attempts to modify behavior.[76] Only those committed to avoiding alcohol should normally receive this medication. A meta-analysis of the literature reported that study results involving oral disulfiram were variable; however, modest evidence of a reduction in drinking frequencies were noted, without a significant increase in abstinence. Positive evidence exists that disulfiram decreases the number of drinking days.[77]

When administered alone, disulfiram is relatively nontoxic, but in the presence of alcohol, it alters alcohol metabolism. Disulfiram causes an increase in blood acetaldehyde levels by interfering with acetaldehyde dehydrogenase action, producing an acetaldehyde syndrome. It also inhibits dopamine β-hydroxylase, leading to the release and depletion of norepinephrine stores. The patient becomes flushed and develops a scarlet appearance; as the vasodilation continues, palpitations, chest pain, hyperventilation, headache, tachycardia, weakness, hypotension, and syncope occur. Respiratory difficulty, nausea, vomiting, blurred vision, and vertigo may also occur. The reaction may be produced by as little as a few milliliters of alcohol and can last from 30 minutes to several hours. The action of disulfiram may last up to 10 days after the patient's last dose. At higher blood alcohol levels, more marked symptoms, including cardiac arrhythmias, heart failure, and death, are experienced.

The usual initial dosage of disulfiram is 250 to 500 mg per day for 5 to 7 days. The dosage may then be reduced to 125 to 250 mg per day. Disulfiram is rapidly absorbed from the gastrointestinal tract; it achieves full pharmacologic action in approximately 12 hours. Disulfiram is eliminated slowly; approximately 20% still remains in the body after a week. Although disulfiram is relatively safe for most patients, it can cause acneiform eruptions, fatigue, tremor, restlessness, impotence, and a garlicky or metallic taste in the mouth. With large doses, psychological depression occurs, probably as a result of interference in dopamine β-hydroxylase activity in the brain. Disulfiram has also been shown to retard the metabolism of oral anticoagulants, isoniazid, and other drugs. Any patient who receives disulfiram should be warned to avoid medications that contain alcohol, particularly over-the-counter preparations such as some cough and cold medicines, antihistamines, body and after-shave lotions, colognes, mouthwashes, and alcohol sponges.

The intensity and duration of disulfiram-alcohol reaction symptoms are related to the disulfiram dosage, the amount of alcohol consumed, and individual sensitivity. Blood alcohol levels as low as 5 to 10 mg per dL (1.1 to 2.2 mmol/L) can cause a mild reaction. Although the disulfiram-alcohol reaction is usually short-lived and without major sequelae, death can occur. In many fatalities, the disulfiram dose was excessive, but in others, no explanation was apparent. In these inexplicable fatalities, the causes of death were intracranial hemorrhage, acute myocardial infarction, pulmonary edema, and cerebral edema.[78] Table 59.3 summarizes special factors to be considered in the use of disulfiram.

Naltrexone. In 1994, naltrexone, an opiate antagonist, was approved for use in the treatment of patients with alcohol dependence. It attenuates the reinforcing but not the negative effects of alcohol consumption; feelings of intoxication and craving are reduced when alcohol is consumed by patients who are receiving naltrexone. It appears to be most effective when combined with support counseling in patients who experience heightened craving and high levels of somatic distress.[79] Patients must be motivated to comply with the once-daily oral regimen of this drug. Product cost may be a major deterrent to its wider use.

Naltrexone can precipitate narcotic withdrawal syndromes in patients who are dependent on opiates. It is also contraindicated in patients with active hepatitis or liver failure because high doses have caused hepatotoxicity. Baseline and every 3 month follow-up determinations of transaminase and bilirubin levels are recommended. Nausea is the most frequent side effect, coinciding with peak levels, which occur 90 minutes after administration. This attenuates over time. The recommended oral dose is 50 mg daily taken in the morning.[80]

Acamprosate. Acamprosate (calcium acetylhomotaurine), a structural analog of GABA, has been used in the treatment of patients with alcoholism in many countries for a number of years and was approved for use in the United States in 2004. Its mechanism, although unclear, appears to involve mainly the glutamate and GABA systems, possibly through restoration of balance in these neurotransmitter systems. A recent meta-analysis found a significant beneficial effect in maintaining abstinence in early alcoholism recovery.[81] Acamprosate, when combined with psychosocial support, improved the health-related quality-of-life profile in those recovering from alcoholism to levels comparable with healthy individuals.[82] It is indicated for the maintenance of those who are abstinent from alcohol at treatment initiation.

In studies, adverse events reported more frequently than placebo included slightly higher rates of suicide and diarrhea. Acamprosate has been classified as pregnancy category C because of fetal malformations reported in rats and rabbits; effects in children have not been evaluated. The usual dose is 666 mg (two 333-mg acamprosate calcium delayed-release tablets) given three times daily. Dosage adjustment may be necessary in renal, but not hepatic, impairment.[83]

Sedative-hypnotic Drugs. Anxiety and insomnia are common in PWA. Under most circumstances, these symptoms can be treated supportively, without psychotropic medications. The indiscriminate prescribing of antianxiety agents is all too frequent, and they have a high potential for abuse in the alcoholic population. No evidence supports outpatient

TABLE 58.3	Considerations in the Use of Disulfiram	
Issue	**Intervention/Patient Education**	**Monitoring**
Interview and counsel patient. Assess for informed consent, motivation, social stability.	Tell patient to avoid alcohol; give list of over-the-counter drugs and foods that contain alcohol. Give with caution concurrently with central nervous system depressants; it may potentiate their effects. Metallic taste may cause anorexia; good oral hygiene may reduce taste. Patient should carry appropriate medical alert identification with this drug. Adequate blood level may take up to 4 days, although effect begins within 12 hours. The effect may last up to a week after discontinuation of disulfiram.	Check for other medications that are being taken (e.g., phenytoin, diazepam, isoniazid, metronidazole, warfarin). Disulfiram can potentiate their therapeutic or toxic effects. Nausea and vomiting, dizziness, hypotension, headache, syncope, and flushed face in disulfiram–alcohol reaction are seen. Check for adverse effects (usually transient, lasting 2 weeks), drowsiness, fatigue, impotence, acneform eruption, and metallic taste.
Persons with moderate to severe hypertension, psychiatric problems, or suicidal ideation should not receive this drug.	Contact prescriber if these conditions exist in a patient who is prescribed disulfiram.	Provide ongoing monitoring when any medications are prescribed for these conditions.

use of psychotropic drugs in the long-term treatment of alcoholism. The use of placebos for relief of anxiety may be worthwhile when basic behavioral problems are dealt with concomitantly.

Antidepressants. Depression frequently occurs concurrently with alcoholism; antidepressant therapy is an increasingly accepted component of treatment for those so affected. Selective serotonin reuptake inhibitors (SSRIs) often represent the least toxic, best tolerated approach to antidepressant therapy.[84] Fluoxetine was reported to reduce heavy drinking in those with alcoholism who are depressed.[85] Sertraline was demonstrated to reduce drinking in those whose alcoholism is classified as of late onset.[86]

NONPHARMACOLOGIC THERAPY

Equally important in obtaining assistance for PWA is getting them to agree to be evaluated for the problem. Denial is a common characteristic of chemical dependency and is often associated with alcoholism. Although some patients may respond to a personal expression of concern from a friend, employer, or physician, many patients require a formal intervention to get help. A formal intervention is a carefully planned confrontation during which those who have observed alcohol-related behaviors report these in objective terms and present an ultimatum that the person get help or suffer consequences such as loss of job, family, friends, or

other significant support. A person such as a counselor normally coordinates interventions, and some professions provide trained interveners from within the profession to facilitate interventions. Usually, the person is encouraged to obtain formal evaluation or to enter treatment as soon as possible, preferably that day. The initial goal is to break through denial systems and help the person realize that alcoholism is a disease that can be treated. Recovery from alcoholism is a lifelong process. Relapse is only one drink away for PWA; they usually consider themselves "recovering" rather than "recovered" alcoholics.

Several techniques for behavioral modification are used with the chronic alcoholic. Individual psychotherapy is useful in those patients who are intelligent, well motivated, and financially secure. Group psychotherapy allows for interaction among PWA in dealing with difficulties that they have in common. An estimated success rate of 80% to 90% among health care professionals and 70% of employed people who participate in a full recovery program for at least 2 years can be contrasted with a 4-year sobriety rate of less than 5% for "skid row" PWA. In managing the chronic alcoholic, the goal is to achieve and maintain sobriety or prolong the periods of sobriety to give the patient time to learn to identify and avoid factors that may promote drinking, or so-called "slips."

The preferred full recovery program includes (a) education about the disease of alcoholism, (b) abstinence from alcohol and other psychoactive substances (not forever, but "one day at a time," as is recommended by AA), and (c) group therapy (regular attendance at AA meetings or the equivalent; formal, interactive group therapy, preferably for at least 2 years; and family therapy, including participation of family members in Al-Anon or similar support group meetings). Initially, treatment usually involves intensive outpatient therapy for a number of weeks, then regular "aftercare" meetings, usually accessed through the treatment provider. Difficult cases may require inpatient therapy.

Employee assistance programs are available through most major employers; these programs often require employees to sign a recovery agreement. Such agreements ensure understanding of the terms of continued employment, encourage ongoing sobriety, and provide employers with assurance of compliance. Random drug screening at employee expense is often a stated condition of the agreement.

For patients who have inadequate support systems in place at home to ensure sobriety during outpatient therapy or early in the recovery process after such therapy, "halfway" houses may be used. These provide a community living environment with fairly rigid rules, ongoing group therapy, and requirements, such as maintaining employment, that encourage responsibility and social adaptation during sobriety. Half-way houses are most often used by persons who are recovering from drug addictions other than alcohol and by those with multiple addictions.

The group support approach of AA takes a more structured and spiritually based approach to helping PWA and is reported to have returned many PWA to sobriety and maintenance of ongoing recovery. The basic tenets of AA's 12 steps are acceptance of the disease nature of alcoholism, acceptance of an external locus of control in life, "cleaning house" (guilt reduction through the process of confession and maintenance of ongoing honesty), and helping other PWA. AA is a private organization whose members offer mutual support to each other to remain free of alcohol. Meetings occur regularly in most communities and, globally, in most countries. PWA in early recovery are often encouraged to attend 90 AA meetings in 90 days; this encourages PWA to maintain frequent contact with a support system and forces them to attend a number of different meetings. Because AA meetings vary in format and character, the recovering alcoholic can eventually identify meetings that meet his or her specific needs and schedules. Other similar groups such as the Salvation Army also have help groups for assisting in the recovery of PWA. Alcoholism resources listed in the yellow pages of telephone books can identify these and other treatment and support resources in the community. Many support groups exist for specific populations, such as lawyers, physicians, pharmacists, and nurses. These exist to provide support for problems unique to recovery for each group and are not intended to replace participation in other support groups, such as AA.

ALTERNATIVE THERAPIES

St. John's Wort as an herbal treatment for depression and kudzu for the treatment of alcoholism have long-established histories of use. Although animal studies of these plant products and their derivatives in the treatment of alcoholism are promising, their place in therapy has yet to be established by well-controlled clinical trials.[87]

The prevailing notion is that alcohol may have some usefulness in the treatment of a variety of disorders and conditions. Clinical evidence, however, is not encouraging about the role of alcohol in therapy, and it may actually worsen many conditions for which its use has been suggested (Table 58.4).

FUTURE THERAPIES

Major advances in the treatment of patients with alcoholism have involved identification of the disease by health care professionals and psychological treatment. Although a number of medications are being investigated for alcoholism treatment, the following show the greatest promise. Topiramate may reduce alcohol craving and anxiety, possibly by reducing brain levels of dopamine.[88] It may be useful in treating PWA who are not abstinent.[89] Ondansetron may be useful in reducing cravings and drinking in those whose alcoholism is classified as of early onset.[90]

IMPROVING OUTCOMES

PATIENT EDUCATION

The health care professional is presented with a variety of unique patient education opportunities related to alcohol use. Because approximately two thirds of adults consume alcoholic beverages, it is not uncommon for medications that are prescribed by a physician or bought over-the-counter to be taken concomitantly with alcohol or while alcohol is still in the body. Alcohol may be present in some preparations and may interact with prescribed medications to produce untoward effects in the unsuspecting patient. Those consuming alcohol in any form should be encouraged to seek advice before taking any medications and to avoid taking psychoactive substances concurrently with alcohol.

In general, a practitioner who is experienced in addiction medicine should manage therapy with any psychoactive medication that is being received by those recovering from alcoholism and other drug dependencies. This does not mean that a recovering alcoholic or addict cannot receive controlled substances for specific, short-term uses, such as severe pain; however, the physician must limit the amount prescribed to no more than the amount required by most patients. The experienced practitioner must recognize the possibility that the recovering alcoholic may lose control

TABLE 58.4	"Therapeutic" Use of Alcohol
Proposed Use	**Actual Effect**
Relief of anxiety	Anxiety often worsens when blood alcohol level falls, as in withdrawal.
Bedtime sedation	Sleeplessness is less common as blood alcohol level declines.
Improved nutrition	Blood glucose levels become more labile; although each gram of alcohol = 7.1 calories on oxidation, "empty" calories are gained. Overall nutrition is not improved with alcohol because vitamins, minerals, or other essential dietary materials are absent in alcoholic beverages.
Diuresis of edema	Diuretic response to alcohol occurs when blood alcohol level is on the rise; antidiuresis, hyperosmolarity, and fluid retention occur as blood alcohol concentration falls.
Anemia	Iron metabolism and bone marrow function are affected, and folate antagonism contributes to anemia.
Lowering of blood glucose in diabetic patients	Lowering of blood glucose is negligible. In fact, alcohol produces more labile blood glucose levels.
Heart disease	The alcohol metabolite acetaldehyde is toxic to myocardium and is not effective as a coronary vasodilator. Alcohol is a myocardial depressant. Although alcohol enhances coronary blood flow, myocardial oxygen consumption simultaneously increases. Although small reductions in coronary heart disease occur in patients who are moderate consumers of alcohol (1–2 drinks per day), this does not justify a recommendation for any patient to begin drinking.
Anti-infective	Chronic alcoholism predisposes to systemic infection.

fairly rapidly and may attempt to obtain additional medication beyond the normal period of use.

PREVENTING DRUG–ALCOHOL INTERACTIONS

Alcohol administration in high concentrations results in increased metabolism by MEOS, with concurrent inhibition of metabolism of drugs that undergo microsomal degradation. The repeated administration of alcohol has been shown to cause nonspecific hepatic microsomal enzyme induction, resulting in increased clearance of alcohol and microsomally metabolized drugs, such as barbiturates.[91–93] After withdrawal of alcohol, enhanced hepatic metabolism of drugs may persist for some time, requiring higher doses of affected drugs. Metabolic pathways such as N-desmethylation of the longer-acting benzodiazepines and oxidation and glucuronidation are inhibited by acute alcohol intake. With long-term use, however, metabolism increases. This explains partially the "tolerance" to the action of sedatives that is observed in some PWA. Warfarin, phenytoin, and tolbutamide are nonpsychoactive drugs that are subject to hepatic microsomal enzyme activity. The plasma half-lives of these drugs are markedly decreased in some chronic and heavy users of alcohol as a result of their increased rate of clearance. Clinical reports of problems from such interactions, however, are few. Variable and unpredictable response to drugs in the

alcoholic should suggest the possibility of some metabolic alteration of drug kinetics. It has become increasingly evident that toxicity to certain drugs and chemicals is enhanced in PWA as a result of this mechanism. Although it is suggested that the risk of developing acetaminophen-induced hepatotoxicity is greater in those with alcoholism, recent reviews suggest that metabolism may actually be reduced through the MEOS system. Until this controversy is resolved, caution is recommended in the use of larger therapeutic doses of acetaminophen in PWA.[94]

Alcohol is primarily a CNS depressant. When it is combined with other drugs with similar depressing action on the CNS, an additive or synergistic effect occurs. This is the most important type of interaction between alcohol and other drugs.

PWA taking tolbutamide, griseofulvin, or metronidazole have reported a mild "disulfiram-like" reaction. Alcohol consumption during ceforanide, cefotetan, or cefoperazone therapy may precipitate a disulfiram-like reaction. Some alcoholic beverages such as Chianti wines contain appreciable amounts of tyramine, so that when they are ingested by patients using monoamine oxidase (MAO)-inhibiting drugs (e.g., procarbazine, pargyline), they cause an acute hypertensive episode. Interference with tyramine metabolism by MAO inhibitors results in the release of norepinephrine from

TABLE 58.5	Summary of Selected Drug–Alcohol Interactions		
Drugs Interacting with Alcohol	**Mechanism**	**Effect**	**Significance**
Anticoagulants (oral): warfarin	Metabolism enhanced with chronic alcohol abuse	Diminished anticoagulant effect	Moderate
	Metabolism reduced with acute alcohol intoxication	Increased anticoagulant effect	Moderate
Antihistamines and other CNS depressants	Additive	Increased CNS depression	Moderate
Aspirin (and other salicylates)	Additive	Increased occult blood loss and damage to gastric mucosa	Moderate
Anticonvulsants: phenytoin (e.g., Dilantin) and others	Metabolism enhanced with chronic alcohol abuse	Diminished anticonvulsant effect	Moderate
	Metabolism reduced with acute alcohol intoxication	Increased anticonvulsant effect	Moderate
Antimicrobials			
Isoniazid	Metabolism enhanced in chronic alcohol abuse	Diminished isoniazid effect	Moderate
		Increased incidence of isoniazid hepatitis	Not established
Cefoperazone, Metronidazole, Griseofulvin	Metabolism of alcohol reduced	Disulfiram-like reaction	Minor/moderate

CNS, central nervous system.

the sympathetic nerve terminal. A summary of selected drug–alcohol interactions is presented in Table 58.5.

DISEASE MANAGEMENT STRATEGIES TO IMPROVE PATIENT OUTCOMES

To improve patient outcomes, a therapeutic alliance should be formed with the patient. If at any time in the treatment process the patient feels as though the provider is judgmental, that alliance may be broken, resulting in a decrease in trust and a possible therapeutic setback. Therefore, it is imperative that the provider set goals with the patient at the initiation of treatment and assist the patient in attaining these goals. If therapeutic goals are agreed upon at the onset and trust is built, then the provider is given greater flexibility in straightforward discussions that are necessary. In addition, the practitioner should always remain cognizant of the psychosocial and patient confidentiality issues that accompany alcoholism.

PHARMACOECONOMICS

Estimates of the cost of alcohol abuse and alcoholism in the United States increased from $148 billion in 1992 to more than $184 billion in 1998. Of these costs, alcohol-related treatment cost estimates exceeded $26 billion, with alcohol-related comorbid conditions accounting for nearly $19 billion of this total. Estimates for 1998 of lost earnings due to premature death, lost productivity due to alcohol-related illness, including FAS, and lost earnings due to alcohol-related crimes or violence were, respectively, more than $36 billion, $87 billion, and $10 billion dollars.[95]

Total health care costs of PWA are significantly higher than those for persons who do not have alcoholism. Average 4-year family monthly medical costs were reported to be twice those of families with no apparent alcoholic members. However, the increase in costs was not totally due to alcoholic treatment. Monthly medical costs for PWA began to rise 6 months before detoxification, peaking at 13 times the average on the month before treatment.[96] No difference in cost of care has been noted between men and women. For PWA younger than 51 years of age, medical costs have been reported to return to average for those who do not have alcoholism after initiation of alcoholism treatment; however, patients older than 50 years of age continued to have elevated health care costs after cessation of treatment.[97] The increased cost of care in older patients emphasizes the importance of early detection and treatment.

CONCLUSION

A primary treatment goal for the PWA is long-term abstinence from alcohol. Much confusion has arisen in the midst of a widely publicized 1976 report by the Rand Corporation on alcoholism, which seems to imply that some PWA can return to social drinking.[98] Nevertheless, the professions of medicine and psychology have long advocated the opposing viewpoint. For instance, AA considers abstinence as the only goal for anyone with an alcohol problem. Careful evaluation of data from the Rand Report does not support the notion that PWA can safely return to drinking. What it does point out is that after an 18-month period, relatively few PWA were practicing long-term abstinence despite an impressive improvement rate (70%). Most had intermittent periods of abstinence interspersed with ''controlled'' drinking. Relapses to uncontrolled drinking by those who continued to drink in a controlled manner and by those who continued abstinence were found to be no different. Major methodologic problems are suggested by the large number (more than 80%) of subjects lost to follow-up at the end of the 18-month study period. The same investigators in a 1980 follow-up report sharply modified their original claims; however, this has accomplished little to discourage the many and vocal advocates of ''controlled drinking'' for PWA.[99]

The use of pharmacotherapy and chemical intervention to enhance efforts to abstain from alcohol use and prevent relapse has been receiving considerable attention as reports of promising experience with opiate antagonists, serotonergic drugs, and agents such as acamprosate emerge from the treatment community.[77] Effectiveness studies involving these and other prospects have been undergoing careful systematic and comparative review for assessment of evidence and outcomes.

Abstinence from alcohol is a primary goal of treatment and a means to an end. The treatment of patients with alcoholism is best accomplished when it is conducted with others in a relationship of understanding and trust. This may involve a concerned and interested friend or spouse; a professional person such as a pharmacist, therapist, or physician; or a member of a therapeutic or rehabilitative group. Dependency on alcohol is no different in any significant way from dependency on other addictive drugs such as opiates and benzodiazepines. Although differences in social attitudes toward drinking and drug abuse have been observed, many features of alcohol and ''hard drug'' addiction are remarkably similar. Similarities and differences should be appreciated and understood by those who are involved in the treatment, care, and rehabilitation of alcohol-dependent patients.

KEY POINTS

- The treatment of patients with alcohol dependency relies on a two-step approach that deals with withdrawal and detoxification followed by subsequent interventions to maintain abstinence
- Maintenance and support of vital functions are basic to the treatment strategy for acute alcohol intoxication
- Causes such as alcohol-induced hypoglycemia, physical events (subdural or head trauma), and other chemicals (drugs) should be ruled out in the unconscious alcohol-intoxicated or poisoned patient
- Pharmacologic attempts to accelerate the metabolism or clearance of alcohol from the body of the intoxicated patient are not recommended
- The goal of treatment for an acutely agitated and alcohol-impaired patient with toxic psychosis symptoms is to produce a calm, but still arousable, patient
- Detoxification from alcohol involves a process of substitution with and slow withdrawing of a longer-acting sedative-hypnotic medication for ethanol
- Doses and regimens of medications used to treat patients with acute alcohol withdrawal should be tailored to response, the presence of underlying conditions, and concurrent polydrug abuse
- Successful treatment for and recovery from chronic alcoholism is dependent on the patient's motivation to stop drinking; avoidance of psychoactive substances, including alcohol, except when therapeutically essential; and participation in recovery support programs

ACKNOWLEDGMENTS

The authors acknowledge the contributions of Jerry R. Phipps, Jr., and Theodore G. Tong, who coauthored the corresponding chapter in the Seventh Edition. Portions of that chapter have been used in this edition.

SUGGESTED READINGS

Dole EJ, Baldwin JN, Murawski MM, et al. American Association of Colleges of Pharmacy guidelines for the development of psychoactive substance use disorder policies for colleges of pharmacy. Am J Pharm Educ 63:28S–34S, 1999.

Hanson GR, Venturelli PJ, Fleckenstein AE. Drugs and society. 8th ed. Sudbury, Mass: Jones and Bartlett, 2004.

Hogue MD, McCormick DD, eds. Points of light: A guide for assisting chemically dependent health professional students. Washington, DC: American Pharmaceutical Association, 1996.

Inaba DS, Cohen WE. Uppers, downers, all arounders. 5th ed. Ashland, Ore: CNS Publications, 2004.

National Clearinghouse for Alcohol and Drug Information (NCADI). Available at: http://www.nida.nih.gov/PubCat/ or http://store.health.org/catalog/ Accessibility verified November 3, 2004 (accesses numerous, usually free and often online, substance abuse prevention, education, and assistance-related resources and current survey results).

REFERENCES

1. Morse RM, Flavin DK, for The Joint Committee of the National Council on Alcoholism and Drug Dependence and the American Society of Addiction Medicine to Study the Definition and Criteria for the Diagnosis of Alcoholism. The definition of alcoholism. JAMA 268:1012–1014, 1992.
2. Wright D. State estimates of substance use from the 2002 National Household Survey on Drug Abuse and Health (DHHS Publication No. SMA 04-3907, NSDUH Series H-23). Rockville, Md: Substance Abuse and Mental Health Services Administration, Office of Applied Studies, 2004.
3. Robins LN, Regier DA. Psychiatric disorders in America: The Epidemiologic Catchment Area Study. New York: Free Press/Macmillan, 1991.
4. Enoch M, Goldman D. Genetics of alcoholism and substance abuse. Psychiatr Clin North Am 22:289–299, 1999.
5. Schuckit MA. New findings in the genetics of alcoholism. JAMA 281:1875–1876, 1999.
6. Mokdad AH, Marks JS, Stroup DF, et al. Actual causes of death in the United States, 2000. JAMA 291:1238–1245, 2004.
7. Holman CD, English DR, Milne E, et al. Meta-analysis of alcohol and all-cause mortality: a validation of NHMRC recommendations. Med J Aust 164:141–145, 1996.
8. Droomers M, Schrijvers CT, Stronks K, et al. Educational differences in excessive alcohol consumption: the role of psychosocial and material stressors. Prev Med 29:1–10, 1999.
9. American Academy of Pediatrics Committee on Substance Abuse. Alcohol use and abuse: a pediatric concern. Pediatrics 95:439–442, 1995.
10. Blume LN, Nielsen NH, Riggs JA. Alcoholism and alcohol abuse among women: report of the council on scientific affairs. J Womens Health 7:861–871, 1998.
11. Graham K, Schmidt G. Alcohol use and psychosocial well-being among older adults. J Stud Alcohol 60:345–351, 1999.
12. US Department of Health and Human Services. Ninth special report to the US Congress on Alcohol and Health. Washington, DC: US Department of Health and Human Services, 1997.
13. Broadening the base of treatment for alcohol problems: report of a study by a committee of the Institute of Medicine. Washington, DC: National Academy Press, 1990.
14. US Department of Justice. Alcohol and crime: an analysis of national data on the prevalence of alcohol involvement in crime. Washington, DC: US Department of Justice, 1998.
15. US Department of Health and Human Services. Seventh special report to the US Congress on alcohol and health. Rockville, Md: US Department of Health and Human Services, 1990.
16. Wallace J. The new disease model of alcoholism. West J Med 152:502–505, 1990.
17. Blum TC, Roman PM, Bennett N. Public images of alcoholism: data from a Georgia survey. J Stud Alcohol 50:5–14, 1989.
18. Frezza M, di Padora C, Pozzata G, et al. High blood alcohol levels in women. N Engl J Med 322:95–99, 1990.
19. Oneta CM, Simanowski UA, Martinez M, et al. First pass metabolism of ethanol is strikingly influenced by the speed of gastric emptying. Gut 43:612–619, 1998.
20. Lieber CS, ed. Medical and nutritional complications of alcoholism: Mechanisms and management. New York: Plenum, 1992.
21. Espina N, Lima V, Lieber CS, et al. In vitro and in vivo inhibitory effect of ethanol and acetaldehyde on O-methylguanine transferase. Carcinogenesis 9:761–766, 1988.
22. Lieber CS, Baraona E, Hernandez-Munoz R, et al. Impaired oxygen utilization: a new mechanism for the hepatotoxicity of ethanol in sub-human primates. J Clin Invest 83:1682–1690, 1989.
23. Lieber CS. Medical disorders of alcoholism. N Engl J Med 333:1058–1065, 1995.
24. Lieber CS, DeCarli LM. Hepatic microsomal ethanol-oxidizing system: in vitro characteristics and adaptive properties in vivo. J Biol Chem 245:2505–2512, 1970.
25. Crabb DW, Dipple KM, Thomasson HR. Alcohol sensitivity, alcohol metabolism, risk of alcoholism, and the role of alcohol and aldehyde dehydrogenase genotypes. J Lab Clin Med 122:234–240, 1993.
26. Eckardt MJ, Harford TC, Kaelbar CT, et al. Health hazards associated with alcohol consumption. JAMA 246:648–666, 1981.
27. Mukamal KJ, Conigrave KM, Mittleman MA, et al. Roles of drinking pattern and type of alcohol consumed in coronary heart disease in men. N Engl J Med 348:109–118, 2003.
28. Goldberg IJ, Mosca L, Piano MR, et al. Wine and your heart: a science advisory for healthcare professionals from the Nutrition Committee, Council on Epidemiology and Prevention, and Council on Cardiovascular Nursing of the American Heart Association. Circulation 103:472–475, 2001.
29. Piano M. Alcoholic cardiomyopathy: incidence, clinical characteristics, and pathophysiology. Chest 121:1638–1650, 2002.
30. Wakabayashi I, Kobaba-Wakabayashi R. Effects of age on the relationship between drinking and atherosclerotic risk factors. Gerontology 48:151–156, 2002.
31. Segel LD, Klausner SC, Harney-Gnadt JJ, et al. Alcohol and the heart. Med Clin North Am 68:147–161, 1984.
32. Hillbom M, Haapaniemi H, Juvela S, et al. Recent alcohol consumption, cigarette smoking, and cerebral infarction in young adults. Stroke 26:40–45, 1995.
33. Eichner ER. The hematologic disorder of alcoholism. Am J Med 54:621–630, 1973.
34. Larkin EC, Watson-Williams EJ. Alcohol and blood. Med Clin North Am 68:105–120, 1984.
35. Lieber CS. Alcohol and the liver: 1984 update. Hepatology 4:1243–1260, 1984.
36. Pimstone NR, French SW. Alcoholic liver disease. Med Clin North Am 68:39–56, 1984.
37. Klatsky Steinberg W, Tenner S. Acute pancreatitis. N Engl J Med 330:1198–1210, 1994.
38. Reuler JB, Girard DE, Cooney TG. Wernicke's encephalopathy. N Engl J Med 312:1035–1039, 1985.
39. Leevy C, Baker H. Vitamins and alcoholism. Am J Clin Nutr 21:1325–1328, 1968.
40. Purdie FR, Honigman B, Rosen P. Acute organic brain syndrome: a review of 100 cases. Ann Emerg Med 10:455–461, 1981.
41. Bayard M, McIntyre J, Hill KR, et al. Alcohol withdrawal syndrome. Am Fam Physician 69:1443–1450, 2004.
42. Clarren SK, Smith DW. The fetal alcohol syndrome. N Engl J Med 298:1063–1067, 1978.
43. Centers for Disease Control and Prevention. Alcohol use among women of childbearing age–United States, 1991–1999. MMWR 51:273–276, 2002.
44. May PA, Gossage JP. Estimating the prevalence of fetal alcohol syndrome: a summary. Alcohol Res Health 25:159–167, 2001.
45. US Department of Health and Human Services. Recent progress in the genetics of alcoholism. In: 10th Special Report to the US Congress on Alcohol and Health. Washington, DC: US Department of Health and Human Services, 2000.
46. American Psychiatric Association. Diagnostic and statistical manual of mental disorders. 4th ed, text revision (DSM-IV-TR). Arlington, Va: American Psychiatric Publishing, 2000.
47. Johnson JL, Leff M. Children of substance abusers: overview of research findings. Pediatrics 103:1085–1099, 1999.
48. Moos RH, Billings AG. Children of alcoholics during the recovery process: alcohol and matched control families. Addict Behav 7:155–164, 1982.
49. Patterson GR, Stoughamer-Loeber M. The correlation of family management practices and delinquency. Child Dev 33:1299–1307, 1984.
50. Pharmacotherapy for alcohol dependence. Summary, evidence report/technology assessment, number 3. Rockville, Md: Agency for Health Care Policy and Research, 1999.
51. Sellers EM, Kalant H. Alcohol intoxication and withdrawal. N Engl J Med 294:757–762, 1976.
52. Khantzian EJ, McKenna GJ. Acute toxic withdrawal reactions associated with drug use and abuse. Ann Intern Med 90:361–372, 1979.
53. Thompson WL, Johnson AD, Maddrey WC. Diazepam and paraldehyde for treatment of severe delirium tremens. Ann Intern Med 82:175–180, 1975.
54. Lyon LJ, Antony J. Reversal of alcoholic coma by naloxone. Ann Intern Med 96:464–465, 1982.

55. Mattila MJ, Nuotto E, Seppala T. Naloxone is not an effective antagonist of ethanol. Lancet 1:775–776, 1981.

56. Sharaba AI, Rockey DC. Gastroesophageal variceal hemorrhage. N Engl J Med 345:669–681, 2001.

57. Mayo-Smith MF. Pharmacological management of alcohol withdrawal: a meta-analysis and evidence-based practice guideline: American Society of Addiction Medicine Working Group on Pharmacological Management of Alcohol Withdrawal. JAMA 278: 144–151, 1997.

58. Saitz R, Friedman LA, Mayo-Smith MF. Alcohol withdrawal: a nationwide survey of inpatient treatment practices. J Gen Intern Med 10:479–487, 1995.

59. Baumgartner GR, Rowen RC. Clonidine versus chlordiazepoxide in the management of acute alcohol withdrawal syndrome. Arch Intern Med 147:1223–1226, 1987.

60. Klotz UA, Avant GR, Hoyumpia A, et al. The effects of age and liver disease on the disposition and elimination of diazepam in an adult man. J Clin Invest 55:347–359, 1975.

61. Hayashida M, Alterman AL, McClellan AT, et al. Comparative effectiveness and cost of inpatient and outpatient detoxification of patients with mild to moderate alcohol withdrawal syndrome. N Engl J Med 320:358–365, 1989.

62. Saitz R, Mayo-Smith MF, Roberts MS, et al. Individualized treatment for alcohol withdrawal: a randomized double-blind controlled trial. JAMA 272:519–523, 1994.

63. Daeppen JB, Gache P, Landry U, et al. Symptom-triggered vs fixed-schedule doses of benzodiazepine for alcohol withdrawal. Arch Intern Med 162:1117–1121, 2002.

64. Longo LP, Campbell T, Hubatch S. Divalproex sodium (Depakote) for alcohol withdrawal and relapse prevention. J Addict Dis 21: 55–64, 2002.

65. Reoux JP, Saxon AJ, Malte CA, et al. Divalproex sodium in alcohol withdrawal: a randomized double-blind placebo-controlled clinical trial. Alcohol Clin Exp Res 25:1324–1329, 2001.

66. Rathev NK, D'Onofrio G, Fish SS, et al. The lack of efficacy of phenytoin in the prevention of recurrent alcohol-induced seizures. Ann Emerg Med 23:513–518, 1994.

67. Brown CG. The alcohol-withdrawal syndrome. West J Med 138: 579–581, 1983.

68. Mendelson JH. Propranolol and behavior of alcohol addicts after acute alcohol ingestion. Clin Pharmacol Ther 15:571–578, 1974.

69. Kraus ML, Gottlieb LD, Horwitz RI, et al. Randomized clinical trial of atenolol in patients with alcohol withdrawal. N Engl J Med 313:905–909, 1985.

70. Nakada T, Knight RT. Alcohol and the central nervous system. Med Clin North Am 68:121–131, 1984.

71. Victor M, Adams RD. On the etiology of the alcoholic neurologic diseases with special reference in the role of nutrition. Am J Clin Nutr 9:379–397, 1961.

72. Segel LD, Klausner SC, Harney-Gnadt JJ, et al. Alcohol and the heart. Med Clin North Am 68:147–161, 1984.

73. Vetter WR, Cohn LH, Reichgott M. Hypokalemia and electrocardiographic abnormalities during acute alcohol withdrawal. Arch Intern Med 120:536–541, 1967.

74. Beard JD, Knott DH. Fluid and electrolyte balance during acute withdrawal in chronic alcoholic patients. JAMA 204:135–139, 1968.

75. Kaysen G, Noth RH. The effects of alcohol on blood pressure and electrolytes. Med Clin North Am 68:221–246, 1984.

76. Fuller RK, Branchey L, Brightwell DR, et al. Disulfiram treatment of alcoholism: a Veterans Administration Cooperative study. JAMA 256:1449–1455, 1986.

77. Garbutt JC, West SL, Carety TS, et al. Pharmacological treatment of alcohol dependence. JAMA 281:1318–1325, 1999.

78. Elenbaas RM, Ryan JL, Robinson WA, et al. On the disulfiram-like activity of moxalactam. Clin Pharmacol Ther 32:347–355, 1982.

79. O'Malley SS, Jaffe A, Chang G, et al. Naltrexone and coping skills therapy for alcohol dependence: a controlled study. Arch Gen Psychiatry 49:881–887, 1992.

80. Saitz R, O'Malley SS. Pharmacotherapies for alcohol abuse. Med Clin North Am 81:881–907, 1997.

81. Mann K, Lehert P, Morgan MY. The efficacy of acamprosate in the maintenance of abstinence in alcohol-dependent individuals: results of a meta-analysis. Alcohol Clin Exp Res 28:51–63, 2004.

82. Morgan MY, Landron F, Lehert P. Improvement in quality of life after treatment for alcohol dependence with acamprosate and psychosocial support. Alcohol Clin Exp Res 28:64–77, 2004.

83. Campral® (acamprosate calcium) Delayed-Release Tablets insert. NDA 21-431, pages 5–19. Available at: http://www.fda.gov/cder/foi/label/2004/21431lbl.pdf. Accessed August 2, 2004.

84. Nunes EV, Levin FR. Treatment of depression in patients with alcohol and other drug dependence. A meta-analysis. JAMA 291: 1887–1896, 2004.

85. Cornelius JR, Salloum IM, Ehler JG, et al. Fluoxetine in depressed alcoholics. A double-blind placebo controlled trial. Arch Gen Psychiatry 54:700–705, 1997.

86. Pettinati HM, Volpicelli JR, Kranzler HR, et al. Sertraline treatment for alcohol dependence. Interactive efforts of medication and alcoholic subtype. Alcohol Clin Exp Res 24:1041–1049, 2000.

87. Overstreet DH, Keung W, Rezvanil AH, et al. Herbal remedies for alcoholism: promises and possible pitfalls. Alcohol Clin Exp Res 27:177–185, 2003.

88. Johnson BA, Ait-Daoud N, Bowden CL, et al. Oral topiramate for treatment of alcohol dependence: a randomized controlled trial. Lancet 361:1677–1685, 2003.

89. Johnson BA, Swift RM, Ait-Daoud N, et al. Development of novel pharmacotherapies for the treatment of alcohol dependence: focus on antiepileptics. Alcohol Clin Exp Res 28:295–301, 2004.

90. Kranzler HR, Pierucci-Lagha A, Feinn R, et al. Effects of ondansetron on early- versus late-onset alcoholics: a prospective, open-label study. Alcohol Clin Exp Res 27:1150–1155, 2003.

91. Lane EA, Guthrie S, Linnoila M. Effects of ethanol on drug and metabolite pharmacokinetics. Clin Pharmacokinet 10:228–247, 1985.

92. Hoyumpa AM, Schenker S. Ethanol-drug interaction. Annu Rev Med 33:113–149, 1982.

93. Lieber CS. Interaction of ethanol with drugs, hepatotoxic agents, carcinogens and vitamins. Alcohol Alcohol 25:157–176, 1990.

94. Hersh EV, Moore PA. Drug interactions in dentistry. The importance of knowing your CYPs. JADA 135:298–311, 2004.

95. Harwood H. Updating estimates of the economic costs of alcohol abuse in the United States: Estimates, update methods, and data. Falls Church, Va: The Lewin Group for the National Institute on Alcohol Abuse and Alcoholism, 2000. Available at: http://www.niaaa.nih.gov/publications/economic-2000/. Accessibility verified November 3, 2004.

96. Holder HD. The cost offsets of alcoholism treatment. Recent Dev Alcohol 14:361–374, 1998.

97. Blose JO, Holder HD. The utilization of medical care by treated alcoholics: longitudinal patterns by age, gender, and type of care. J Subst Abuse 3:13–27, 1991.

98. Armour DJ, Polich JM, Stambul HB. Alcoholism and treatment. The Rand Corporation, R-1739-NIAAA. New York: Wiley, 1978.

99. Polich JM, Armour DJ, Braiker HV. The course of alcoholism four years after treatment. The Rand Corporation, R-2433-NIAAA. New York: Wiley, 1980.

100. Nakada T, Knight RT. Alcohol and the central nervous system. Med Clin North Am 68:121–131, 1984.

101. Haller RG, Knochel JP. Skeletal muscle disease in alcoholism. Med Clin North Am 68:91–103, 1984.

102. Adams HG, Jordan C. Infections in the alcoholic. Med Clin North Am 68:179–201, 1984.

103. Kaysen G, Noth RH. The effects of alcohol on blood pressure and electrolytes. Med Clin North Am 68:221–246, 1984.

104. Williams HE. Alcoholic hypoglycemia and ketoacidosis. Med Clin North Am 68:33–38, 1984.

105. Altura BM. Introduction to the symposium and overview. Alcoholism (NY) 10:557–559, 1986.

Drug Addiction

59

S. Casey Laizure, John F. Weaver,

Richard P. Johnson, and Lamar E. Bailey

TREATMENT GOALS

- Identify specific drug abuse problems in the patient.
- Determine the need for drug detoxification and recommend appropriate therapy based on drug use history.
- Assess the patient's insight into his or her drug abuse problem.
- Provide patient education about both pharmacologic and nonpharmacologic treatment options to maintain long-term abstinence.
- Continue to monitor and reassess the treatment regimen, as drug addiction is a chronic relapsing disease.

DEFINITION

Drug addiction is a compulsion to use a drug of abuse even when the continued use interferes with work responsibilities, social activities, or family relationships or results in significant health problems. Perceptions and beliefs about drug addiction are shaped, perhaps more than any other medical illness, by personal experience. Whether through our own difficulties with drug use, or by observation of family members or friends, almost everyone has been exposed to the problems associated with drug addiction. This provides a common frame of reference that is helpful in understanding drug addiction, but it is also detrimental in that it makes it difficult to accept that drug addiction is a disease of the mind rather than a behavioral problem brought on by mental weakness and a lack of willpower. Addiction does not originate from cognitive centers in the cortex of the brain, but in the subcortical area known as the mesolimbic system. Thus, the driving force in the development and maintenance of addiction is not in the "thinking" part of the brain, but the midbrain, a more primitive area associated with emotions. When one consumes a drug of abuse and experiences euphoria, it is not the cortex that determines through reasoning that the experience was pleasurable; rather, subcortical structures are stimulated and in turn stimulate or essentially tell the cortex that it just experienced a pleasurable event. A pleasurable event, the driving force that leads to addiction, is thus anything that stimulates the proper subcortical structures in the mesolimbic system, a specific pathway known as the reward pathway.

Table 59.1 defines the terms used in this chapter.

THE REWARD PATHWAY

The reward pathway is a well-conserved system crucial for survival. It provides the drive for the basic functions required for survival of a species, including food, water, sex, and nurturing. Though the reward pathway did not evolve for the purpose of drug abuse, drug addiction is essentially a state in which the preferred drug has usurped the reward pathway. The power of addiction to alter an addict's behavior becomes more understandable when we realize that the mechanism of addiction uses the same neurologic structures that provide the basic drive necessary for survival.

1537

TABLE 59.1	Definitions of Common Terms

Addiction (substance dependence): uncontrollable, compulsive drug seeking and use, even in the face of negative health and social consequences

Cue: anything in the environment associated with drug use (e.g., drug paraphernalia, specific location)

Drug abuse: continued use of a drug even though it has negative effects on work, creates legal problems or family problems, or is physically hazardous

Extinction: in animal models, the elimination of a learned action such as lever-pressing to get a drug with rewarding effects after the drug is replaced with a placebo such as saline injection

Hedonic set point: the point at which pleasure is achieved

Place preference: in animal models, a specific location that the animal has learned to prefer because it is associated with drug administration that provides rewarding effects

Priming: in animal models, administration of a drug or other agent that results in reinstatement

Reinstatement: in animal models, the resuming of a previously learned action such as lever-pressing to get a drug after extinction

A simplified schematic of the reward pathway (Fig. 59.1) shows the three major components of this neural circuit: the ventral tegmental area (VTA), the nucleus accumbens (NAc), and the prefrontal cortex. A stimulus is interpreted as rewarding if it increases firing of impulses from the NAc to the prefrontal cortex. The specificity of this pathway has been demonstrated in rats with the implantation of an electrode into the NAc.[1] A rat will repeatedly press a lever to get an electrical stimulus into the NAc. If the electrode is moved even a few millimeters adjacent to the NAc, then the rat will no longer press the lever to receive an electrical impulse. All euphoria-inducing drugs of abuse stimulate this reward pathway, causing euphoria by increasing synaptic dopamine concentrations in the NAc, which result in increased firing of the dopaminergic neurons that are abundant in this pathway.

The vast majority of drug addictions involve alcohol, nicotine, opiates, central nervous system (CNS) stimulants, and marijuana. All of these drugs ultimately produce pleasure upon administration through their actions on the reward pathway, but the mechanisms preceding the final common event, increasing dopamine concentration in the NAc, differ significantly from each other.

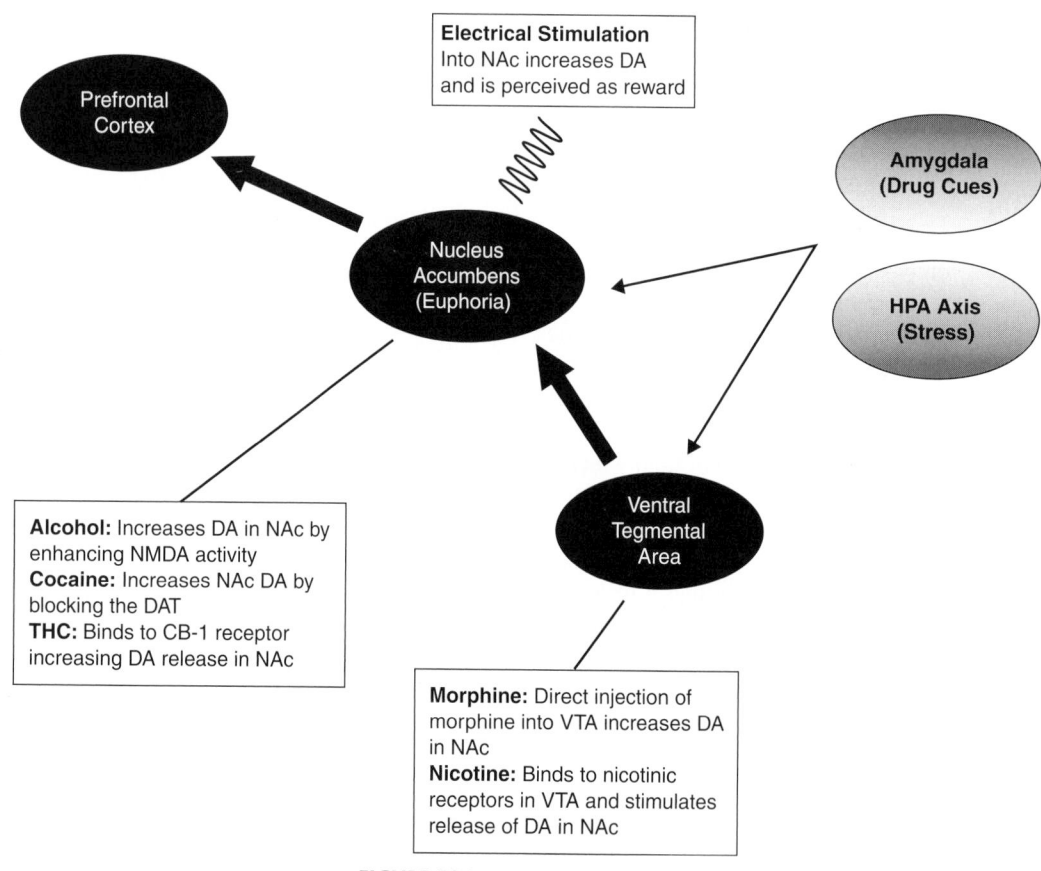

FIGURE 59.1 The reward pathway.

NEUROPATHOLOGY OF DRUG ADDICTION

Cocaine has the most direct effect on the reward pathway, increasing synaptic dopamine concentrations in the NAc by blocking the dopamine transporter. The NAc is rich in dopaminergic neurons, and the actions of released dopamine from the presynaptic neurons are normally terminated by the reuptake of dopamine into the presynaptic neuron by the dopamine transporter. Cocaine binds to the dopamine transporter, preventing dopamine reuptake into the presynaptic neuron and thereby increasing dopamine synaptic concentrations.

Opiates and tetrahydrocannabinol (THC) also increase synaptic dopamine concentrations in the NAc, though through indirect stimulation of dopamine activity in the NAc. Opiates bind to endogenous opiate receptors in the VTA, which reduces activity of the gamma-aminobutyric acid (GABA) system.[2] The decrease in GABA activity increases dopaminergic activity and leads to increased dopaminergic activity in the NAc.[3] THC binds to the type 1 cannabinoid receptor (CB-1) in the VTA, which increases VTA stimulation of the NAc, again manifest as an increase in dopamine synaptic concentrations.

The mechanism of alcohol is not as well understood, but it is believed to have N-methyl-D-aspartate (NMDA) agonist activity that indirectly stimulates dopamine activity in the NAc. Nicotine binds to nicotinic receptors in the VTA, stimulating release of dopamine in the NAc.

Thus, despite the different receptor systems affected by different drugs of abuse, they appear to have the same final common pathway of increasing synaptic dopamine concentrations in the NAc, which is ultimately perceived as a rewarding stimulus.

The neuropharmacology of benzodiazepine abuse tends to support the primary role of the reward pathway in the development of addiction, though it also demonstrates inconsistencies in the simplistic view of dopamine stimulation in the NAc as the mechanism of addiction. Benzodiazepines are generally regarded as having a high potential for physical dependence and abuse but a relatively low potential for addiction.[4,5] They are usually secondary drugs of abuse in many individuals who are dependent on alcohol or cocaine but are relatively uncommon as the primary drug of abuse. This is consistent with animal studies that, though documenting that benzodiazepines are self-injected, also show that initiating self-injection is more difficult and the strength of the desire to self-inject is weaker compared to drugs such as alcohol and cocaine.[6]

Neuropharmacologically, benzodiazepines do not cause increases in the synaptic dopamine levels in the NAc,[7,8] but act as an allosteric-receptor agonist on the GABA receptor. This lends credence to the theory that the major determinant of chronic benzodiazepine abuse is due to physical dependence rather than addiction. However, benzodiazepines have been shown to increase hedonic reactivity in the reward pathway even in dopamine-depleted rats, and, though uncommon, there are documented cases of benzodiazepine addiction.[9,10]

Although the increase in NAc dopamine concentrations explains the rewarding effects of drugs of abuse, it does not provide a complete explanation for drug addiction. All people who abuse drugs with the potential for addiction are susceptible to the euphoric or rewarding effects of drugs, but only a very small minority become addicted to drugs. In some way individuals who become addicted to drugs are different from those who abuse drugs and do not become addicted, though the specific neurochemical differences between the casual user and the addicted user remain elusive.

In addition, stimulation of reward centers is an immediate effect of drug use, but addiction develops over an extended period of drug use, so the temporal relationship between stimulation of the reward center and the development of addiction is incongruent. Other changes are occurring in the CNS that are far more complex than just stimulation of the reward center. Ahmed and Koob[11] postulate that the hedonic set point is elevated during the development of addiction. Drug use increases gradually to the point of uncontrolled use due to a need for a higher level of stimulation of the reward pathway. The increased drug use is not due to tolerance of the reward pathway to the drug, but rather a drive to achieve higher levels of intoxication due to an increase in the hedonic set point. This leads to a vicious cycle in which drug use increases the hedonic set point, which in turn leads to an increase in drug use until consumption becomes uncontrollable.[12] Thus, addiction is conceptualized as a dysregulation of the reward pathway caused by complex interactions with other neuroanatomic areas.

ETIOLOGY

References to drug taking for mind-altering or euphoric effects appear in the earliest known written records. An ancient Sumerian text from 3000 BC refers to poppy as the "joy plant," and alcoholism is identified as a specific problem in the Bible. Given the mechanism of addictive drugs in the CNS, it would be expected that the initiation of drug addiction in humans was determined by the availability of an addictive drug in society. Despite this long history of drug use and a basic understanding of the problems associated with drug addiction, our understanding of the specific causes of alcoholism and other drug addictions remains limited.

THEORIES OF DRUG ADDICTION

A large body of literature on the etiology of addiction focuses on adolescent drug use and the initiation of drug use that potentially leads to addiction. Thus, it focuses on peer pressure and other family and societal influences that increase the risk of drug experimentation, and not specifically on the causes of drug addiction. The motivation for this tactic is the assumption that reducing drug initiation in adolescents will result in a reduction in the development of drug addiction later in life, and there is good evidence that delaying drug initiation does, in fact, decrease the risk for the development of addiction later in life.[13,14]

Others have emphasized the development of drug addiction as a result of self-treatment in an attempt to relieve symptoms of anxiety, depression, and psychic distress associated with some other Axis I disorder such as major depression, schizophrenia, or bipolar disorder. Drug use is higher in patients with mental disorders, but this association does not prove the "self-treatment" hypothesis. Patients with mental disorders have lower socioeconomic status, increased unemployment rates, more interpersonal strife, and other stressors compared to the general population. Increased drug use can be explained by the increased stress associated with their illness rather than specific pathophysiology linking the occurrence of drug addiction with mental disorders.

Stress appears to be a very important factor in the development of drug addiction, as demonstrated by drug use in Vietnam veterans. Many servicemen became addicted to heroin while serving in Vietnam but stopped their drug use after returning from the war.[15] The increase in environmental stress resulted in an increase in the occurrence of drug addiction, but once the stress was relieved by their return home, most of the servicemen stopped using heroin despite its potent physical and psychological addictive properties.

GENETIC BASIS OF DRUG ADDICTION

Although the predilection for drug use to occur within families has been recognized since ancient times, the systematic study of genetics as a causative factor is a recent undertaking. Much of the evidence is derived from twin studies. By examining differences in drug use between monozygotic (identical) and dizygotic (fraternal) twins, the genetic predisposition toward drug use can be estimated. The results from numerous twin studies have shown that the initiation of drug use, reported to be as high as 80% in adolescent boys and 54% in adolescent girls,[16] is determined mostly by environmental factors, and long-term problem drug use is more dependent on genetic predisposition.[17] It is now widely accepted that genetic effects account for 40% to 60% of the variance in problem drug use.[13,18] Still, identifying specific genetic variants associated with drug use has been difficult, though some significant associations have been discovered.

Aldehyde dehydrogenase catalyzes the formation of acetaldehyde to acetate and is the primary pathway for the oxidation of acetaldehyde produced from ethanol by alcohol dehydrogenase. A single base pair difference referred to as the ALDH2*2 allele results in an enzyme with little activity. Inactivity of this enzyme results in a buildup of acetaldehyde in the blood when alcohol is consumed, resulting in the same symptoms that are seen with inhibition of this enzyme by disulfiram (i.e., flushing, nausea, and tachycardia). The ALDH2*2 allele is common in Asians and occurs in approximately 50% of Chinese and Japanese but is found in only 10% of Chinese and Japanese alcoholics. The explanation

for the reduced prevalence in the ALDH2*2 allele in Chinese and Japanese alcoholics is the occurrence of the unpleasant effects that result when alcohol is consumed in individuals with this allele. This genetic variation also demonstrates the strong drive in some individuals to consume alcohol, because even the unpleasant side effects associated with this allele do not stop all individuals from becoming alcoholics.[19]

The addictive substance in tobacco smoke, nicotine, is primarily metabolized to the inactive metabolite cotinine by the CYP2A6 hepatic isoenzyme. Individuals who have a defective CYP2A6 allele smoke fewer cigarettes than individuals with a fully functional allele, and individuals with duplicated forms of the CYP2A6 allele are at higher risk of becoming smokers and tend to smoke more cigarettes. In addition, methoxsalen, an inhibitor of the CYP2A6 isoenzyme, has been shown to decrease the number of cigarettes consumed in tobacco-addicted individuals.[20]

These genetic variants affect drug use by increasing the aversive effects of drug consumption and increasing the duration of activity of the addictive component, respectively. Thus, although they have demonstrable affects on drug consumption, they do not affect the underlying pathologic mechanisms associated with craving or the reward pathway.

The identification of specific genetic polymorphism affecting drug addiction is a relatively new area in drug addiction research that has produced some interesting discoveries. Chen et al[21] hypothesized that a 68 base-pair repeat in the promoter region of prodynorphin that modulates transcription was associated with vulnerability to cocaine addiction. This hypothesis was derived from their previous investigation showing that cocaine administration in rats increased mRNA levels of dynorphin, an endogenous opiate agonist. Their clinical studies showed that cocaine-addicted individuals were less likely to have a three or four 68 base-pair repeat than a nonaddicted control group. The greater the number of 68 base-pair repeats, the greater the transcription rate of prodynorphin, which results in an increased production of dynorphin mRNA. Stated another way, cocaine addicts tend to produce less dynorphin, and cocaine use may be a way of overcoming an intrinsic dynorphin deficiency. However, such associations between polymorphisms and addiction must be interpreted cautiously, because many nonaddicted controls did not have multiple 68 base-pair repeats, and many cocaine addicts did.

A more common genetic technique is the search for disease associations with single nucleotide polymorphisms (SNPs). Shi et al[22] identified two SNPs in the μ-opioid receptor gene in which guanine is replaced by adenine at one location and adenine by guanine at another that was associated with higher levels of drug use in heroin addicts. The authors concluded that this genetic variation may directly contribute to opioid drug-seeking behavior. However, another interpretation could be that having both SNPs decreases the pharmacologic response to heroin, thus requiring higher doses in the addict to get the same effect. This would affect the potency of the administered heroin but would have no effect on the underlying addiction.

The genetic determinants of drug addiction are a developing area of important research, but it suffers from our deficiency in the basic understanding of how addiction develops in the human brain. Until better models of addiction are developed that incorporate broader pathophysiologic mechanisms, genetic research will be limited to identifying specific genetic variations associated with addictions. Whether the genetic variation is a cause of or a result of the addiction will always be a question. Despite these shortcomings, each study contributes to the overall understanding of the addiction process, and in aggregate they will lead to an improved understanding and new therapies in the treatment of addiction. Our present understanding of the genetic basis of addiction confirms its importance in the development of addiction but does not allow the identification of specific causative factors.

Drug addiction in a specific individual is not an all-or-none process but exists as a potential risk on a continuum from low to high risk for the development of addiction. An individual's susceptibility to addiction depends on his or her inherent predilection based on genetic and environmental factors. Whether the individual manifests drug addiction will depend on his or her inherent susceptibility, availability of drugs, and environmental influences and stressors. Thus, the risk of addiction will increase as the availability of drugs and environmental stress increases and cultural influences develop that are conducive to drug use.

EPIDEMIOLOGY

The Substance Abuse and Mental Health Services Administration (SAMHSA) maintains yearly statistics on tobacco, alcohol, and illicit drug use. In the most recent report[23] there were an estimated 120 million Americans who were current alcohol users and 19.5 million Americans who were current illicit drug users. "Current drug use" was defined as drug use within the last 30 days preceding the survey interview. In addition to illegal street drugs, the nonmedical use of psychotherapeutic agents such as OxyContin was categorized as illicit drug use.

The prevalence of drug use, both alcohol and illicit, was lowest in 12-year-olds (the youngest age group included in the report) and increased with age until it peaked with the highest rates of alcohol and illicit drug use in 18- to 25-year-olds. The prevalence gradually declined after this peak as age increased.

An estimated 71.5 million Americans used tobacco products; of these, 61.1 million smoked cigarettes, 12.8 million smoked cigars, 7.8 million used smokeless tobacco, and 1.8 million smoked tobacco in pipes. The age-related prevalence of tobacco use followed a similar pattern, with the lowest prevalence in 12- to 17-year-olds, the highest prevalence in

18- to 25-year-olds, and a modest decline with increasing age.

These estimates of prevalence describe the extent and pattern of use during 2002. Changing patterns of drug use have important implications on drug policy, which can significantly affect the practice of pharmacy. The SAMHSA report on incidence or initiation of new drug users describes emerging patterns of drug use that will predict corresponding changes in the prevalence of use. The incidence of alcohol use steadily increased during the 1990s from 3.3 million new users in 1990 to 5.6 million in 2000, with youths under 18 accounting for most of the increase, doubling from 2.2 million in 1990 to 4.1 million in 2000. This increase was equally divided between boys and girls and suggests that future alcohol prevalence may have a more equal gender distribution. The most commonly used illicit drug, marijuana, had 2.6 million new users in 2001, a number that has been stable for the past 6 years. Cocaine use increased during the 1970s, peaking in 1981 with 1.8 million new users, and then declined during the 1990s, reaching 1.2 million new users in 2001. The annual number of new heroin users peaked at 246,000 in 1974 and was between 28,000 and 80,000 between 1988 and 1994, but the incidence has increased in recent years, with consistently greater than 100,000 new users in 1995 to 2001. The incidence of hallucinogen use increased from 168,000 to 956,000 between 1966 and 1970, primarily due to the widespread availability of LSD. A more recent increase that began in 1992, when there were approximately 706,000 new users, to 2001, when there were approximately 1.8 million new users, has been due to the introduction of Ecstasy (MDMA, 3-4 methylenedioxymethamphetamine).

The nonmedical use of psychotherapeutic agents, including pain relievers, tranquilizers, stimulants, and sedatives, has increased substantially in recent years (Fig. 59.2), a pattern particularly pertinent to pharmacists, as the most common methods of drug diversion involve pharmacies.

PATHOPHYSIOLOGY

The discovery of dopamine as the primary neurotransmitter in the reward pathway and the association between euphoric effects and increases in dopamine concentrations in this pathway, particularly in the NAc, led to the dopamine hypothesis of drug addiction. This theory held that drug use resulted in large transient increases in dopamine release in the reward pathway, but caused a depletion of dopamine with chronic use. The development of addiction was the result of insufficient dopamine levels in the reward pathway, and the continued use of drugs leading to addiction was the result of a vicious cycle in which the dopamine depletion was temporarily relieved by drug consumption, but this resulted in the continued depletion of dopamine, leading to more drug use.

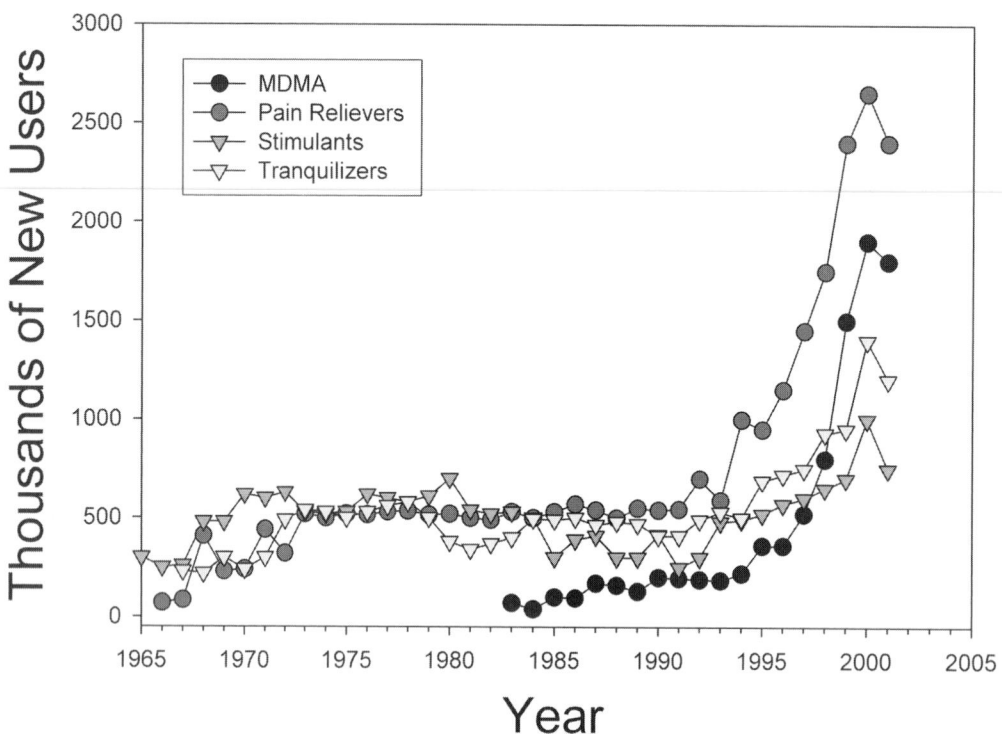

FIGURE 59.2 The number of new users by year from 1964 to 2001 by drug class. MDMA (3,4-methylenedioxymethamphetamine) is a stimulant and hallucinogen commonly known on the street as Ecstasy. The category "pain relievers" mainly consists of narcotic analgesics, the category "tranquilizers" mainly consists of benzodiazepines, and the category "stimulants" mainly consists of cocaine and methamphetamine. The largest increases in drug use in the past 10 years have involved prescription drugs,[23] which make up the bulk of the drug use categorized as pain relievers and tranquilizers.

Investigators studied cocaine as a model of this theory, as it dramatically increases dopamine concentration in the NAc and leads to an overall dopamine deficit with chronic use.[24] Treating this dopamine deficit with dopaminergic agents such as bromocriptine, amantadine, and pergolide was theorized to alleviate the dopamine deficit and reduce the craving for cocaine, reducing relapse in cocaine addicts. In a review of 17 studies with 1,224 total subjects, these agents were shown to provide no benefit in the treatment of cocaine dependence.[25]

It is now apparent that drug addiction is a complex disease, and the neuroanatomic underpinnings of addiction are equally complex. Recent research in animal models of addiction is beginning to reveal the extent of this complexity.

Every drug identified as addictive in humans is self-injected by animals. An animal, usually the rat, is fitted with a catheter to deliver the drug intravenously or directly into the reward center in the brain whenever a lever is pressed. The rat will quickly learn that pressing the lever provides a reward and willingly presses it repeatedly whenever allowed access to the lever. Over time, depending on how long access is allowed to the lever, the rat's drug self-administration will increase. If the drug solution is replaced by saline, the rat will initially keep pressing the lever, but without the subsequent reward, it will ultimately stop. This is referred to as extinc-

tion. If the rat is given a single dose of the drug after extinction, it will reinitiate lever pressing. This is referred to as priming, and the subsequent return of lever pressing as reinstatement.

Initiating self-injection followed by extinction, priming, and reinstatement is analogous to relapse in humans following a period of abstinence. A hallmark of reinstatement is that the rat will escalate drug self-injection much more rapidly compared to its initial exposure when it was drug-naïve. Human addiction follows the same pattern, with a long period of time required for establishing dependence, and a rapid escalation to uncontrolled drug use after a period of abstinence, even if abstinence was maintained for years.

Animal models have also been developed to better understand the mechanisms leading to relapse. Place preference is a model of craving or wanting a preferred drug. A rat learns to prefer a particular location because it is associated with drug administration. A rat in a cage with half the floor smooth and the other textured will tend to remain on the side with the textured floor if it is administered the drug while on that side only. Drug cues in humans such as exposure to drug paraphernalia cause relapse and have been modeled in animals by associating drug exposure with a cue such as a pulse of light or sound. When the rat presses the lever to self-inject drug, a light is activated while the lever is pressed. If the light is then inactivated and the drug replaced with saline, extinction occurs. Lever pressing can be reinstated by flashing the light.

Stress is recognized as an important cause of drug relapse in humans.[26] In rats, stress produced by a mild electric shock such as from a grid on the floor of the cage will reinstate lever pressing after extinction. Using animal models such as these, an evolving understanding of the pathophysiology of drug addiction has shed new light on its neuroanatomic basis and identified potential therapeutic targets for the treatment of drug addiction.

The reward pathway depicted in Figure 59.1, made up of the VTA, the NAc, and the prefrontal cortex, is necessary for the maintenance of drug self-injection. If this pathway is destroyed, then animals will not self-inject drugs of abuse. Two other important areas are the amygdala and the hypothalamic-pituitary-adrenal axis. Lesioning of the basolateral amygdala after extinction in the rat attenuates reinstatement of cocaine self-injection by cues but has no effect on reinstatement produced by a priming dose of cocaine; if the basolateral amygdala is destroyed prior to training to respond to a drug cue, then the rat cannot learn to respond to drug cues at all.[27] If the NAc is lesioned, then the rat will not self-inject cocaine but will still respond to a previously learned drug cue. Thus, the amygdala is not necessary for cocaine-primed reinstatement but is necessary for the learning of drug-associated cues and to some extent the response to previously learned drug-associated cues.[28] In addition, electrical stimulation of the basolateral amygdala increases dopamine release in the NAc and causes reinstatement of cocaine self-injection.[29] These animal findings are supported by human brain imaging studies that show increased activity in the amygdala of addicts exposed to drug cues.[30]

Stress is considered an important determinant of drug relapse in addicts,[26] and in rats stress induced by foot shock has been shown to result in reinstatement of both cocaine and heroin seeking.[31] This implicates the hypothalamic-pituitary-adrenal axis in drug relapse. However, Lee et al showed in squirrel monkeys that neither corticotropin releasing factor, adrenocorticotropic hormone, nor cortisol have any significant effect on cocaine reinstatement, and that the corticotropin releasing hormone antagonist, CP-154-526, did not inhibit priming-induced reinstatement.[32] However, corticotrophin releasing factor antagonists have been shown to reverse the anxiogenic effects of ethanol withdrawal, reverse opiate withdrawal,[33] and attenuate stress-induced ethanol reinstatement.[34]

Other investigators have focused on the molecular mechanism of drug addiction. Because drug addiction develops gradually, researchers have tried to identify long-term perturbations produced by repeated drug administration to animals. Two well-studied pathways associated with drug addiction are the second messenger adenosine $3',5'$-cyclic monophosphate (cAMP) transduction cascade and the ΔFosB protein. The rise in dopamine concentrations in the NAc stimulates dopamine postsynaptic receptors, which in-

creases cAMP levels intracellularly. The transcription factor, cAMP response element-binding protein (CREB), is induced by the increased cAMP levels and stimulates the activity of specific genes that lead to drug tolerance. Once drug use ceases, CREB activity quickly returns to normal. Its activity probably plays a role in drug tolerance and the negative reinforcing effects of drugs, but drug relapse, which can occur after years of abstinence, does not correlate with CREB activity. The protein ΔFosB increases with chronic drug use and remains elevated for a much longer period than CREB after drug use stops. Mutant mice with enhanced ΔFosB activity are hypersensitive to drugs of abuse and more likely to relapse following extinction. The ΔFosB protein also induces changes in dopamine neurons' dendritic structure that persist after ΔFosB levels return to normal, making it a better candidate for the pathophysiology of relapse than CREB.

CLINICAL PRESENTATION AND DIAGNOSIS

There are three separate phases of drug abuse treatment: intoxication, detoxification, and long-term abstinence. Intoxication is an acute medical problem associated with the excessive consumption of a drug of abuse, detoxification is the weaning of the patient off a drug of abuse so that the patient is drug-free, and long-term abstinence is the chronic treatment of the patient to prevent relapse.

Treating drug intoxication usually involves supportive care to maintain breathing and cardiovascular stability, the administration of anticonvulsants for seizure activity, and the administration of an antipsychotic/benzodiazepine combination such as haloperidol and lorazepam to control drug-induced psychosis and severe agitation. Because the pharmacologic activity of various drugs of abuse differs greatly, so does the treatment of intoxication. For CNS depressants such as heroin, alcohol, and benzodiazepines, the main concern are respiratory depression and drug-induced coma, while for CNS stimulants such as cocaine and methamphetamine, hypertension, cardiac arrhythmias, acute myocardial infarction, seizures, and drug-induced psychosis are the major concerns.

A specific pharmacologic antagonist for the treatment of drug intoxication is available only for the opiates and benzodiazepines. Naloxone is an opiate receptor antagonist that reverses the effects of opiate drugs by displacing the opiate from its receptor binding sites. Administration of naloxone will quickly reverse the effects of opiate intoxication; however, naloxone has a shorter half-life than most opiates, so intoxication can recur, necessitating additional administration of naloxone. Flumazenil is a specific benzodiazepine receptor antagonist and will reverse the effects of intoxication with a benzodiazepine. It also has a relatively short half-life, so additional doses may be required in the treatment of benzodiazepine intoxication.

For most drugs there is no specific antagonist available, and treatment is supportive to maintain respiratory and cardiovascular stability until the drug concentration falls below intoxicating levels.

Drug detoxification is limited to drugs with associated physical withdrawal symptoms that are either potentially fatal or extremely uncomfortable. The most common drugs requiring detoxification are alcohol, opiates, and benzodiazepines. Acute cessation of alcohol consumption in a person addicted is often associated with clinically significant symptoms such as hypertension, tremors, and agitation. The most severe form of alcohol withdrawal is referred to as delirium tremens and if untreated can be fatal.

Abrupt cessation of opiates in a dependent individual results in a very uncomfortable constellation of symptoms including abdominal cramps, muscle aches, lacrimation, piloerection, sweating, and rhinorrhea; however, this withdrawal syndrome is unlikely to be fatal unless the person has some underlying disorder such as cardiovascular disease. Benzodiazepines have a protracted withdrawal manifest mainly by anxiety symptoms.

The goal of detoxification is to avoid withdrawal symptoms while making the person drug-free. For any drug this can be done by giving a tapering dose of the drug. However, because receiving their drug of preference is likely to be a trigger for drug craving and drug seeking, the normal course is to use another drug with cross-tolerance if possible. In the case of alcohol withdrawal, either a benzodiazepine or phenobarbital is used in a tapering dose. Some have proposed the use of antipsychotics such as haloperidol, but agents that do not have GABA-ergic activity are not effective in preventing alcohol withdrawal and should be avoided. The use of the anticonvulsants valproic acid and carbamazepine has also been proposed, and there is some evidence that they may help in reducing alcohol withdrawal symptoms,[35,36] but more study needs to be done before these agents could be considered for widespread clinical use for alcohol withdrawal.

For opiate withdrawal, a great part of the symptomology associated with withdrawal is due to excessive sympathetic outflow from the CNS, especially the locus ceruleus. Given this mechanism, clonidine, a centrally acting alpha-2 agonist that reduces blood pressure by reducing sympathetic outflow from the locus ceruleus, has been used to treat opiate withdrawal. One drawback of clonidine is the decrease it produces in blood pressure and heart rate, which is often a dose-limiting effect in its use in controlling opiate withdrawal symptoms. Lofexidine, a new alpha-2 agonist, has less effect on blood pressure,[37] but it is not available in the United States. For individuals who have withdrawal symptoms not controlled by clonidine, it may be necessary to use a tapering dose of methadone, a long-acting μ-opiate receptor agonist. The extremely potent partial μ-opiate agonist buprenorphine may be used, but it can induce opiate withdrawal in heavy opiate users.[38]

In patients undergoing benzodiazepine withdrawal, giving a tapering dose of a long-acting benzodiazepine such as clonazepam can be used. Carbamazepine may be a more appropriate choice to assist in preventing long-term relapse, as tapering patients off benzodiazepines has been notoriously unsuccessful.[39]

Whatever the method chosen, the goal of detoxification is to make the person drug-free without the occurrence of significant medical complications or uncomfortable withdrawal symptoms, so that the patient can enter a long-term program for the treatment of the addiction.

Drug addiction and abuse are diagnosed using the criteria set forth by the Diagnostic and Statistical Manual for Mental Disorders, fourth edition, text revision (DSM-IV-TR).[40] The DSM-IV-TR refers to addiction as "substance dependence" and to drug abuse as "substance abuse." There are four criteria for drug abuse, but the patient needs to meet only one of them to satisfy the diagnosis. For addiction there are seven criteria; the patient must meet three within the past 12 months to be diagnosed with drug addiction (Table 59.2). If drug use involves more than one substance, then each diagnosis is listed separately.

The diagnoses of abuse and addiction are mutually exclusive; that is, a patient cannot be diagnosed with both alcohol abuse and addiction, but he can have multiple drug problems (e.g., alcohol addiction and cocaine abuse or addiction). The

---

TABLE 59.2	Diagnostic Criteria for Addiction (Substance Dependence) and Abuse (Substance Abuse)

Addiction (substance dependence)

1 Tolerance: need for increased amounts to achieve desired effect or diminished effect with use of the same amount of substance

2 Withdrawal: symptom complex associated with abrupt cessation of drug use

3 Drug is taken in larger amounts or over a longer period than was intended

4 A persistent desire or failed attempts to decrease drug use

5 A great deal of time is spent obtaining, using, and recovering from drug use

6 Social, occupational, and recreational activities are reduced due to drug use

7 Drug use is continued despite persistent negative consequences

Drug abuse (substance abuse)

1 Recurrent drug use resulting in failure to fulfill obligations at work, school, or home

2 Recurrent drug use in physically hazardous situations

3 Recurrent drug-related legal problems

4 Recurrent drug use despite drug-related interpersonal or social problems

(From American Psychiatric Association. Diagnostic and statistical manual of mental disorders, 4th ed., text revision, 2000.)

TABLE 59.3	Common Drugs of Abuse	
Agent	**Chemical Name**	**Class**
Ecstasy	3,4-methylenedioxymethamphetamine	Hallucinogenic
GHB	Gamma-hydroxybutyrate	Sedative
AMT	Alpha-methyltryptamine	Hallucinogenic
2C-B	4-bromo–2,5-dimethoxyphenethylamine	Hallucinogenic
DXM	Dextromethorphan hydrobromide	Cough suppressant
Ketamine	2-(2-chlorophenyl)–2-(methylamine)-cyclohexanone	Hallucinogenic
Butyl nitrite	3-methylbutylnitrite	Nitrite
Nitrous oxide	N_2O	Inhaled anesthetic
Inhalants	Various	Volatile gas

These are some common drugs of abuse that tend to be used specifically for their mind-altering effects. Inhalants include almost any volatile gas (e.g., gasoline, benzene, ether, chloroform, mineral spirits, acetone, and toluene).

diagnosis of drug abuse may be removed if the person stops abusing drugs, but the diagnosis of addiction is a lifetime diagnosis that once attained is never lost. If, for example, an alcohol addict remains drug-free even for years, then the diagnosis is alcohol addiction in full remission. The diagnosis of alcohol addiction is never removed from the record.

It is tempting to view drug abuse as the initial phase presaging the development of addiction. Although abuse of a drug often precedes addiction, there are many drugs that are abused but infrequently if ever evolve into addiction. Abuse of drugs and other substances seems to be a common occurrence in teens and young adults and usually involves substances that have euphoric, hallucinogenic, dissociative, or other reality-altering effects. Thus, unlike the classic description of the addict who says that he feels normal only when using drugs, drugs of abuse tend to be mind-altering and used with the specific intent to alter reality. The drugs most often abused listed in Table 59.3 tend to be associated with high risks of drug toxicity, and morbidity and mortality due to traumatic events associated with psychoactive drug effects.

PSYCHOSOCIAL ASPECTS

Drug abuse and addiction to specific drugs tends to wax and wane over time. The determinants of the prevalence of a particular drug at a particular time in a particular population are rooted in sociocultural acceptance of the drug, psychosocial stressors within the population, and economic factors. The trends in cocaine use from the early 1960s to the present day present a good model of the psychosocial aspects of drug abuse and addiction.

Cocaine appeared in the U.S. drug-using population in the late 1960s, and use gradually increased during the 1970s and into the 1980s. During this period cocaine in the form of cocaine hydrochloride was primarily snorted and was used as a recreational drug by a relatively small, affluent population.

In the early 1980s a new form of cocaine appeared, called freebase cocaine. Freebasing was a process that involved the use of volatile solvents to convert the cocaine hydrochloride salt to cocaine base. The salt is water-soluble and can be snorted or injected, while the base is water-insoluble and can be smoked, as it will pyrolize at a relatively low temperature. By converting cocaine from the salt to the base, it could be smoked, which greatly increased the efficiency of cocaine delivery compared to snorting. This made cocaine freebasing far more addictive than snorting, but the difficulty and cost of freebasing was a deterrent to its widespread use.

In the mid-1980s crack cocaine appeared in the marketplace. Crack cocaine is a convenient solid dosage form of the cocaine freebase. The name comes from the ''cracking'' sound it makes when heated. The cocaine does not burn, but vaporizes and is inhaled into the lungs. The lungs, with a surface area approximately equivalent to a football field, provide nearly complete and rapid absorption of the inhaled dose into the body. In fact, this method of administration is pharmacokinetically equivalent to an intravenous injection of cocaine, producing a cocaine plasma concentration-time profile that is superimposable to intravenous cocaine. Both the extent and rapid peak of cocaine concentration achieved with smoking increase its pharmacologic effects and addiction risk.

Crack overcame several barriers to the development of a larger cocaine market. It provided a ''high'' equivalent to intravenous use without the social stigma of being branded an IV drug user. It lowered the economic barrier, because a relatively small quantity of cocaine was required, making a ''high'' affordable to lower-income groups. It was much easier to store, transport, and use than intravenous cocaine. Cocaine suppliers were thus able to reach a lower socioeconomic population with more psychosocial stressors and an increased probability of drug use. Crack cocaine has subsequently become the predominant illicit drug use problem in poor inner-city populations.

The evolution of crack cocaine use demonstrates the importance of psychosocial and economic influences on the prevalence of drug use. The same influences are at play for legal drugs of abuse. Low-quality alcohol products with high alcohol content are widely marketed in low-income areas to tap into the same market as the cocaine suppliers—that is, the same market forces apply to both legal drugs of abuse and illicit drugs.

It is inconceivable that drug abuse and addiction will ever be eliminated, as the pathophysiology of addiction is an integral part of the basic drive to survive, and the economic structure in the United States limits our control of the marketplace. However, the opportunity for reducing psychosocial stressors through economic development does provide a feasible long-term strategy for reducing drug abuse and addiction in our society.

THERAPEUTIC PLAN

The goal of treatment is total abstinence from drug use. The first phase of the therapeutic plan is to get the patient to a drug-free state (i.e., detoxification). Once the patient can adequately participate in recovery, then a long-term plan for maintaining abstinence can be undertaken. This should include an integrated approach that involves cognitive, behavioral, and drug therapy. Adjunctive pharmacotherapy is available only for the treatment of alcohol and opiate addiction, but new drug therapies with a broader spectrum are being developed based on our increased understanding of the pathophysiology of drug addiction. Though progress is being made, addiction remains a chronic relapsing disease, and treatment should not be discontinued after long-term abstinence or if relapse occurs.

TREATMENT

NONPHARMACOLOGIC TREATMENT

Twelve-Step Program. The various 12-step recovery programs all stem from the original Alcoholics Anonymous (AA) model founded in 1935 by a group of alcoholics, including the widely known Dr. Bob and Bill W. AA is a model that remains widely available today. One of the unique aspects of the 12-step recovery process is the self-help nature of the program. There is no professional or clinical staff in charge, but rather recovering alcoholics offer support, direction, and reassurance to other alcoholics in recovery or wishing to be so.

The program is based on 12 steps of recovery work, which is designed to bring about behavioral, emotional, and spiritual changes in a manner of perpetual self-maintenance. The first step emphasizes one's "powerlessness" over alcohol. A paradoxical notion is implied in that admitting powerless-

ness in effect empowers the individual to recognize the magnitude of the problem and move away from the "denial" that often accompanies this disease model of addiction. Later steps include recognizing and admitting past wrongs made against others, making amends to others when appropriate, recognizing one's own defects and working toward resolution, and restoring a spiritual presence as an all-powerful source of guidance. AA members meet in various meeting places in communities all over the world. Meeting times and places are generally published in local brochures, and meetings generally occur at regularly scheduled times during all hours of the day and night. In many places, programs to assist family members of the alcoholic are also available (e.g., Al-Anon, Ala-teen) and are conducted in a similar format.

Since the advent of AA, sufferers of addictions other than alcohol have emulated the 12-step model. Narcotics Anonymous is an identical program for addicts who use any type of narcotic, whether illegally obtained or prescribed. Cocaine Anonymous follows the same model, but exclusively for cocaine addicts. The 12-step model's popularity and apparent success have resulted in its being adopted and modified by various church-oriented recovery programs. Finally, the model is widely used for individuals with gambling addictions (Gamblers Anonymous), eating disorders (Overeaters Anonymous), and addictions of a sexual nature (Sex Addicts Anonymous).

Cognitive, Behavioral, and Cognitive–Behavioral Therapies. Traditional psychotherapies have been used for treating addiction with mixed success. Although primarily used to treat behaviors classically deemed as "neurotic," cognitive and behavioral therapies are often used in the treatment of addiction as well. Cognitive therapies approach addictive behavior from the standpoint of an individual's erroneous processing of information. Specifically, individuals are believed to interpret life experiences in a distorted or biased manner. These cognitive distortions are viewed as the primary cause of failure in self-fulfillment and/or personal problem-solving. It is believed that as a result, people may suffer the emotional and biological consequences of the distortions, and therefore turn to drugs or alcohol for relief.

The strategy of cognitive therapy involves building a collaborative relationship between the addict and the therapist. A relationship is often developed in which the therapist is afforded the freedom to point out and interpret the maladaptive thinking patterns, a process known as "collaborative empiricism." Further therapy may attempt to find common themes or links across an individual's misperceptions ("guided discovery"). In the treatment of addiction, not only are the misperceptions made obvious to the patient, but the resulting behavior of substance abuse is also addressed as a component of maladaptive coping mechanisms. Emphasis is placed on the erroneous belief that one needs a substance to feel relief from an unwanted thought or emotion, and one can shift an uncomfortable cognitive experience to a frame of self-efficacy and success.

Behavioral strategies are less interested with initial thoughts and more interested in carrying out behaviors that will later change one's thoughts. Pure behavioral strategies focus exclusively on observable behaviors. In essence, the individual will carry out a behavior or series of behaviors to experience the reinforcement. Other behavioral theories believe behavior is a function of its consequences, rather than the consequences being the result of the behavior, a process B. F. Skinner named "operant conditioning." From an addictive perspective, Skinner would view the euphoric state of drug or alcohol intoxication as the cause of one's substance use, rather than the linear perspective of substance use causing the intoxicated state. By removing the behavior of substance use, one never experiences the cause of it, or in essence the euphoria.

Regardless of the behavioral perspective applied, the remaining notion is that once the maladaptive behavior is removed, the thought process will be affected as well. This principle is not far removed from the "acting as if" philosophy of AA, which emphasizes that regular meeting attendance and abstinence will ultimately remove one's sense of denial and increase one's desire for sobriety.

A variety of strategies combine both cognitive and behavioral perspectives and are generally regarded as cognitive-behavioral theories.

PHARMACOLOGIC TREATMENT
Alcohol Addiction
Aldehyde Dehydrogenase Inhibitors. Disulfiram was the first drug used in the treatment of alcohol addiction. It was a serendipitous discovery by Dr. Jacobsen resulting from coincidental exposure to alcohol during a study of disulfiram for the treatment of parasitic intestinal worms. Dr. Jacobsen had a policy of testing new drug entities on himself before giving them to his patients. He was attending a dinner party only hours after having taken a small dose of disulfiram and became violently ill after only a few sips of beer. Further investigation lead to the seminal paper on the disulfiram–alcohol reaction in humans.[41] This reaction occurs when alcohol is converted to acetaldehyde, and the conversion of acetaldehyde to acetate is blocked by disulfiram. This causes a rapid increase in blood acetaldehyde levels that results in dizziness, throbbing headache, chest pain, sweating, and vomiting. The severity of the reaction depends on individual susceptibility and on the amount of alcohol consumed and varies from mild nausea to, in rare cases, death. The mechanism of action of calcium carbamide is identical to the mechanism of action of disulfiram, but it is a much weaker inhibitor of aldehyde dehydrogenase, the enzyme responsible for the conversion of acetaldehyde to acetate. Both drugs are considered aversive therapy, preventing alcohol consumption by making the risk of severe negative consequences so great that alcohol consumption is inhibited.

It may seem obvious that disulfiram therapy would be effective in deterring alcohol consumption, but evidence from double-blind studies has been unable to demonstrate any substantial beneficial effect on maintaining alcohol abstinence.[42,43] It appears that those wishing to return to previous alcohol use simply stop taking the disulfiram and resume drinking. The failure of aversive therapy is predictable because it relies on negative reinforcement and does nothing to treat the underlying addiction.

Naltrexone and Acamprosate. Naltrexone and acamprosate have both been approved for use in the United States to treat alcohol addiction. Though chemically unrelated, they share the property of decreasing alcohol craving.

Naltrexone is a potent opiate μ-receptor antagonist that is theorized to decrease the craving for alcohol by blocking opiate receptors in the reward pathway, thereby decreasing the rewarding effects of alcohol. Its use in the treatment of alcohol addiction was investigated because naltrexone had been previously shown to cause a dose-dependent decrease in alcohol consumption in alcohol-preferring rats.[44,45] Both studies providing evidence of the efficacy of naltrexone in humans that are cited in support of its FDA-approved indication for alcohol addiction showed that naltrexone reduced relapse to heavy drinking but did not improve absolute abstinence from alcohol consumption.[46,47] In addition, studies of longer duration than the 12-week period of the two studies supporting FDA approval have reported conflicting results of the benefits of naltrexone on alcohol consumption.[48–51]

Acamprosate was approved for the treatment of alcohol addiction in the United States in late 2004, but it has been used for many years in Europe. Like naltrexone, it is theorized that acamprosate decreases the craving for alcohol, though the mechanism is unknown. The overwhelming majority of studies, conducted mostly outside the United States, show a modest but consistent increase in the duration of alcohol abstinence in patients receiving acamprosate compared to those receiving placebo.[52]

Opiate Addiction
Methadone Maintenance. Naltrexone has been used in the treatment of opiate addicts, but not with any significant degree of success. The idea is to completely detoxify the user off opiates and then give a daily oral naltrexone dose to block the effects of any administered opiate agonist. However, analogous to disulfiram, many users simply stop taking the naltrexone in order to re-experience the effects of exogenously administered opiates. Opiate addicts unable to stop their drug use can choose to enter a methadone or levo-alpha-acetyl methadol (LAAM) maintenance program, which is essentially a legalized form of controlled opiate addiction. Both of these drugs are full μ-receptor agonists with a much longer duration of activity than morphine and other commonly abused opiates. Chronic administration of a long-acting cross-tolerant agent reduces craving for the abused drug and reduces euphoric effects through the development of pharmacologic tolerance. These programs were

developed to remove opiate addicts from the criminal environments associated with drug acquisition and get them into treatment programs, with the ultimate goal of weaning them completely off opiates. However, many opiate addicts remain in maintenance programs indefinitely. Even so, the benefits of maintenance programs have been documented, with participants less likely to be involved in criminal activity, more likely to be employed, and suffering fewer medical problems.[53–55] Many users in maintenance programs are able to lead normal, productive lives. More opiate addicts could benefit from a maintenance program, but the requirement to visit a federally controlled maintenance program on a daily basis is a major barrier for many users.

Buprenorphine Maintenance. Recently the federal government has approved the use of buprenorphine for opiate maintenance that can be administered by primary care physicians from their office in an effort to improve access to maintenance programs.

Unlike methadone, which is a μ-receptor opiate agonist like morphine, buprenorphine, though extremely potent, is a partial agonist at the μ-receptor. It binds very tightly to the opiate receptor but has a ceiling effect. It causes less euphoria and less respiratory depression than full μ-receptor agonists. This makes it less likely to be abused and safer to use than methadone. If an exogenously administered opiate agonist like heroin is administered, the euphoric and other pharmacologic effects will be diminished, as buprenorphine is not easily displaced from the μ-receptor. Because of this partial agonist activity, implementing buprenorphine maintenance in a heavy opiate user can actually induce opiate withdrawal symptoms and should be done carefully.

Buprenorphine is not effective when taken orally because it is a CYP3A4 substrate that undergoes first-pass metabolism. It must be administered sublingually or intravenously. To further decrease its abuse potential, recent dosage formulations include naloxone. When taken sublingually the buprenorphine is rapidly absorbed but naloxone is poorly absorbed and has no significant effect, but if the tablet is dissolved and injected intravenously, then the naloxone will block the effects of the buprenorphine. It is hoped that removing the tight federal control on opiate maintenance will increase the number of opiate addicts entering maintenance programs.

The availability of pharmacotherapy for the treatment of drug addictions remains limited, and the agents that are available have at best modest efficacy with respect to maintaining long-term abstinence from drug use. Because of this, adjunctive pharmacotherapy is inconsistently used in the treatment of drug addictions. Some treatment programs use specific agents such as naltrexone routinely, while other programs use it rarely if at all. Until effective therapies are available with a more robust response, the overall impact of pharmacotherapy on the treatment of addiction will be minimal. Fortunately, significant progress is being made in our understanding of the mechanisms responsible for addiction, which will lead to better adjunctive pharmacotherapies that will improve long-term outcomes.

ALTERNATIVE THERAPIES

The most widely used and documented alternative therapy for the treatment of drug addiction is acupuncture. An ancient Oriental medical practice dating back more than 5,000 years, the use of acupuncture in the treatment of addiction started in the early 1970s, when it was used in the treatment of opiate withdrawal by Dr. Wen in Hong Kong. The discovery occurred when an opiate-addicted patient preparing to undergo a surgical procedure using acupuncture anesthesia noted complete resolution of opiate withdrawal symptoms. Subsequent investigations using acupuncture have been reported for the treatment of obesity,[56] smoking cessation, cocaine addiction,[57] and alcoholism,[58] and acupuncture techniques are used extensively by some clinics such as the Substance Abuse Division of the Lincoln Hospital in the South Bronx.[59,60] The effectiveness of acupuncture in producing analgesia is well documented and supported by empirical data showing that needle placement and stimulation results in the release of endorphins and enkephalins. This mechanism is also consistent with the beneficial effects of acupuncture in the treatment of opiate withdrawal. However, as previous discussions on the pathophysiology of addiction would predict, the neuroanatomical mechanisms of addiction, physical dependence, and tolerance are separate, so efficacy in the treatment of opiate withdrawal does not necessarily have any bearing on effectiveness in the treatment of opiate or any other type of addiction.

The efficacy of acupuncture for various medical conditions has been studied quite extensively. The use of acupuncture for surgical anesthesia, acute pain relief, and chemotherapy-induced nausea and vomiting is well accepted. In chronic conditions, such as fibromyalgia, osteoarthritis, and chronic back pain, the evidence is equivocal, and for acupuncture-based drug addiction treatment the evidence is inconclusive. The largest number of clinical studies using acupuncture for the treatment of a drug addiction have assessed its efficacy in smoking cessation. A recent review identified 22 studies adequate for analysis and found that acupuncture was not effective in improving smoking abstinence at any point. These findings cast doubt on the benefits of acupuncture in the treatment of addiction.[61] The review conceded that methodologic weaknesses in the studies make any firm conclusion for or against the use of acupuncture impossible, and concluded that further study is needed to define the role of acupuncture in the treatment of various drug addictions.

FUTURE THERAPIES

The long-term outlook on improving the success of drug addiction treatment depends on an increased understanding of the pathophysiology of addiction, and the development of pharmacotherapeutic agents directed at the mechanism underlying addiction in the CNS. Other therapies relying on aversive effects, blocking euphoric effects, or blocking the development of physical dependence will not contribute significantly to the treatment of drug addiction. For example, despite great interest in the use of vaccines for the treatment of drug addiction,[62] these agents will have a limited impact on drug addiction and its treatment because they do not actually treat addiction. Much more successful therapies will be developed that are derived from understanding the molecular mechanisms of craving and relapse.

Recent progress in the ability of investigators to manipulate the genome of animals such as mice is adding greatly to our understanding of the importance of specific neurochemical pathways in addiction (Table 59.4) and has the potential to identify new targets for pharmacotherapeutic agents. However, addiction is a complex behavior whose antecedents are not easily identified, and making inferences about addictive behavior in humans from studies conducted in animals is perilous, as evidenced by the initial misinterpretation of studies in mice without dopamine transporters (DAT knockout mice). Cocaine increases dopamine concentrations in the synaptic cleft by blocking the dopamine transporter, and its pharmacologic effects and addictive properties are believed to be the result of increased dopamine activity

brought about by blockade of this transporter. Giros et al[63] produced a strain of mice in which the dopamine transporter was nonfunctional. As predicted, the mice had increased locomotor activity and failed to respond to cocaine administration. However, the DAT knockout mice still self-injected cocaine, and this was seen as contradictory to the belief that dopamine release was necessary for the development of addiction. Further study revealed that DAT knockout mice still had increased levels of dopamine in the NAc following cocaine administration. Apparently, dopamine reuptake still occurred in knockout mice via norepinephrine transporters in the NAc. Thus, cocaine administration still resulted in increased dopamine concentrations in the NAc in the knockout mice because cocaine also blocks the norepinephrine transporter, and cocaine self-administration still occurred.[64]

New, sophisticated techniques such as knockout mice are crucial to increasing our understanding of the molecular basis of addiction, but our understanding of the pathophysiology of addiction remains rudimentary, and interpretation of these very specific manipulations to human addiction remains speculative. If addiction were a jigsaw puzzle, we are beginning to identify the pieces to the puzzle, but we have no idea how they fit together. Despite this limitation, promising new agents with unique mechanisms of action such as rimonabant are being studied in humans for the treatment of addiction (Table 59.5).

TABLE 59.4	Receptor Systems and Addiction		
Receptor	**Condition**	**Effect**	**Reference**
Dopamine	DAT knockout mice	Increased locomotor activity, still will self-inject cocaine	64
	D1, D2, and D3 agonist	D1 has no effect, D2 causes reinstatement of cocaine seeking, D3 decreased cocaine-seeking in response to cues	67
	D2 receptor knockout mice	Alcohol and morphine are no longer rewarding, but physical dependence still occurs	68,69
	DARPP-32 knockout mice	Decreased self-administration of ethanol, unable to establish ethanol place preference	70
Serotonin	5HT-1B knockout mice	Increased locomotor response to cocaine, more avidly self-inject	71
CREB	CREB$^{\alpha\Delta}$ (deficient activity)	Attenuated opiate withdrawal, no place preference for morphine, but still place preference for cocaine	2
Cannabinoid	CB1 knockout mice	Reduced stress-induced ethanol self-administration and reduced ethanol withdrawal	72

These are some of the animal studies that have used genetic techniques to identify important receptor systems associated with drug addiction. These studies reveal that multiple neurotransmitters and neural pathways have important roles in the development of addiction. Evidence from these and other studies indicates that separate pathways are responsible for euphoria, craving, response to drug cues, and physical dependence.

TABLE 59.5	Current Clinical Studies of Potential Therapeutic Agents for Addiction	
Agent	**Drug Class**	**Addiction**
Vanoxerine	Long-acting, high-affinity inhibitor of dopamine reuptake	Cocaine
Rimonabant	CB-1 receptor antagonist	Alcohol
Bupropion	Antidepressant	Methamphetamine
Baclofen	Skeletal muscle relaxant	Cocaine
Ondansetron	Antiemetic (5HT3 antagonist)	Alcohol
Selegiline	Monoamine type B inhibitor	Methamphetamine
Disulfiram	Aldehyde dehydrogenase inhibitor	Cocaine

These are some of the current ongoing clinical studies of potential therapeutic agents for the treatment of addiction. Studies include new indications for old agents such as bupropion, and the study of new classes of therapeutic agents such as rimonabant, a cannabinoid receptor antagonist.

IMPROVING OUTCOMES

Improving treatment outcomes is both an issue for individual treatment plans and a global issue of our health care system. On an individual basis it is crucial to tailor an addiction treatment plan to the individual, and to incorporate a combination of cognitive and behavioral therapy, pharmacotherapy, and a 12-step program or similar long-term treatment program. In addition, family members and significant others must also be included in the treatment plan. The success of an addiction treatment program is dependent on the individual's willingness to accept treatment, and on the development of a broad-based program that incorporates all facets of the individual's life (Fig. 59.3). One consistent predictor of improved outcome is the individual's retention in a treatment program. Treatment begins with detoxification, followed by a treatment program, and maintenance of abstinence through long-term participation in an aftercare program. The key to

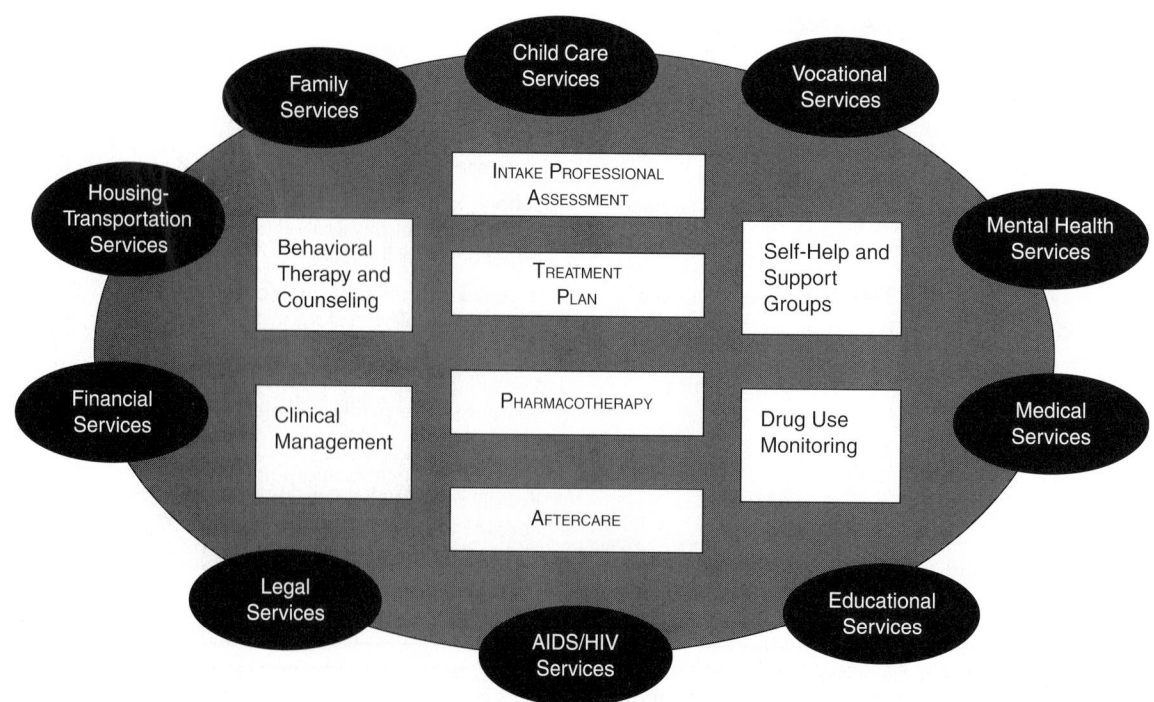

FIGURE 59.3 Components of a comprehensive drug addiction treatment program. (Adapted from National Institute on Drug Abuse slide series: Understanding drug abuse and addiction.)

TABLE 59.6	Economic Cost of Drug Use in the United States[a]	
	1992	**1998**
Alcohol Use		
Health expenditures	$18.8	$26.3
Lost productivity	107	134.2
Other	22.2	24.1
Total	$148	$184.6
Illicit Drug Use		
Premature death	$14.6	$16.6
Illnesses related to drug use	14.2	23.1
Hospitalizations/ institutionalization	1.5	1.8
Victims of crime	2.1	2.2
Lost productivity due to incarceration	37.1	54.8
Other	32.7	44.9
Total	$102.2	$143.4

The greatest economic cost to society is in lost productivity.
[a]The numbers in the table represent billions of dollars.

maintaining abstinence is active participation in a treatment program.

PHARMACOECONOMICS

The economic costs of drug addiction and abuse are staggering and growing at a rate greater than the combined population and inflation rate. Legalized drugs have the greatest societal costs due to the much larger proportion of the population exposed. Alcohol-associated problems affect some 100,000 people in the United States and cost over $184 billion a year. In comparison, all illicit drug use combined costs approximately $143.4 billion per year.[65,66] Table 59.6 breaks down the economic costs of alcohol and illicit drug use by category. The majority of societal costs are due to lost productivity and increased morbidity and mortality associated with drug use. The majority of lost productivity with alcohol use is due to the direct detrimental effects of alcohol, but with illicit drugs the majority of lost productivity is due to incarceration for drug offenses. In addition to lost productivity, the cost of incarceration (Table 59.6, Other) is a significant economic burden. These are only quantifiable costs; the true cost would include harm to children and other family members, but these cannot be easily quantified.

Improving outcomes over the entire population of addicted individuals involves issues of access to treatment programs, and the ability to encourage individuals to seek treatment. The vast majority of addicted individuals needing treatment do not receive it (Table 59.7). Impediments to individuals seeking treatment include lack of insurance coverage for treatment, poor family support structure, and stigma associated with seeking treatment. Government programs devoted to abolishing drug abuse are disproportionately devoted to attempting to control access and punish users at the expense of addiction treatment programs. This philosophy is inconsistent with the widely held belief in the medical community that addiction is a disease.

KEY POINTS

- Drug addiction is a disease resulting from the dysregulation of activity in the reward pathway of the brain
- Physical dependence to a drug is not addiction, though it is often a component of the patient's disease of addiction
- There are three phases of drug addiction treatment: intoxication, detoxification, and maintaining long-term abstinence
- Maintaining long-term abstinence requires persistent participation in a drug treatment program such as Alcoholics Anonymous

TABLE 59.7	Number of People 12 Years and Older in 2002 With Substance Abuse or Dependence, by Substance		
	Addiction or Abuse (millions)	**Number Receiving Treatment**	**% Receiving Treatment**
Alcohol only	14.9	2,222,000	14.9
Alcohol + illicit drug	3.2	709,000	22.2
Illicit drug only	3.9	429,000	11.0
Marijuana	4.3	326,800	7.6
Heroin	1.0	277,000	27.7
Cocaine	1.5	364,500	24.3
Pain relievers	1.5	270,000	18.0
Tobacco	38.7		

National Survey on Drug Use and Health: National Findings. Department of Health and Human Services Substance Abuse and Mental Health Services Administration, Washington DC, 2002.

- Drug therapies for the treatment of addiction have demonstrated only modest beneficial activity and are inconsistently used in the treatment of drug addiction
- Aversive therapies such as disulfiram are not effective in the long-term treatment of addiction
- Increasing knowledge of the neural mechanisms of drug addiction will lead to more effective therapies in the future

SUGGESTED READINGS

Colvin, R. Prescription drug addiction: a hidden epidemic. Omaha, Nebraska: Addicus Books, Inc., 2002.

Lowinson JH, Ruiz P, Millman RB, et al, eds. Substance abuse: a comprehensive textbook, 4th ed. Philadelphia: Lippincott Williams & Wilkins, 2005.

The Vaults of Erowid: Documenting the complex relationship between humans and psychoactive substances. Available at www.erowid.org.

U.S. Drug Enforcement Administration: Available at www.usdoj.gov/dea.

REFERENCES

1. Olds J, Milner, P. Positive reinforcement produced by electrical stimulation of septal area and other regions of the rat brain. J Comp Physiol Psychol 47:419–427, 1954.
2. Walters CL, Blendy JA. Different requirements for cAMP response element binding protein in positive and negative reinforcing properties of drugs of abuse. J Neurosci 21:9438–9444, 2001.
3. van den Brink W, van Ree JM. Pharmacological treatments for heroin and cocaine addiction. Eur Neuropsychopharmacol 13:476–487, 2003.
4. Juergens S. Alprazolam and diazepam: addiction potential. J Subst Abuse Treat 8:43–51, 1991.
5. O'Brien CP. Benzodiazepine use, abuse, and dependence. J Clin Psychiatry 66 (Suppl 2):28–33, 2005.
6. Weerts EM, Kaminski BJ, Griffiths RR. Stable low-rate midazolam self-injection with concurrent physical dependence under conditions of long-term continuous availability in baboons. Psychopharmacology (Berl) 135:70–81, 1998.
7. Finlay JM, Damsma G, Fibiger HC. Benzodiazepine-induced decreases in extracellular concentrations of dopamine in the nucleus accumbens after acute and repeated administration. Psychopharmacology (Berl) 106:202–208, 1992.
8. Rada P, Hoebel BG. Acetylcholine in the accumbens is decreased by diazepam and increased by benzodiazepine withdrawal: a possible mechanism for dependency. Eur J Pharmacol 508:131–138, 2005.
9. Berridge KC, Robinson TE. What is the role of dopamine in reward: hedonic impact, reward learning, or incentive salience? Brain Res Brain Res Rev 28:309–369, 1998.
10. Juergens SM, Morse RM. Alprazolam dependence in seven patients. Am J Psychiatry 145:625–627, 1988.
11. Ahmed SH, Koob GF. Transition from moderate to excessive drug intake: change in hedonic set point. Science 282:298–300, 1998.
12. Cami J, Farre M. Drug addiction. N Engl J Med 349:975–986, 2003.
13. Jacob T, Waterman B, Heath A, et al. Genetic and environmental effects on offspring alcoholism: new insights using an offspring-of-twins design. Arch Gen Psychiatry 60:1265–1272, 2003.
14. Robins LN. The natural history of adolescent drug use. Am J Public Health 74:656–657, 1984.
15. Robins LN, Slobodyan S. Post-Vietnam heroin use and injection by returning US veterans: clues to preventing injection today. Addiction 98:1053–1060, 2003.
16. Johnston CA, Watts VJ. Sensitization of adenylate cyclase: a general mechanism of neuroadaptation to persistent activation of Galpha(i/o)-coupled receptors? Life Sci 73:2913–2925, 2003.
17. Rhee SH, Hewitt JK, Young SE, et al. Genetic and environmental influences on substance initiation, use, and problem use in adolescents. Arch Gen Psychiatry 60:1256–1264, 2003.
18. Nestler EJ, Landsman D. Learning about addiction from the genome. Nature 409:834–835, 2001.
19. Matsushita S, Muramatsu T, Murayama M, et al. Alcoholism, ALDH2*2 allele and the A1 allele of the dopamine D2 receptor gene: an association study. Psychiatry Res 104:19–26, 2001.
20. Tyndale RF, Sellers EM. Variable CYP2A6-mediated nicotine metabolism alters smoking behavior and risk. Drug Metab Dispos 29:548–552, 2001.
21. Chen AC, LaForge KS, Ho A, et al. Potentially functional polymorphism in the promoter region of prodynorphin gene may be associated with protection against cocaine dependence or abuse. Am J Med Genet 114:429–435, 2002.
22. Shi J, Hui L, Xu Y, et al. Sequence variations in the mu-opioid receptor gene (OPRM1) associated with human addiction to heroin. Hum Mutat 19:459–460, 2002.
23. National Survey on Drug Use and Health: National Findings. Department of Health and Human Services (Substance Abuse and Mental Health Services Administration, Washington DC, 2002.
24. Ritz MC, Kuhar MJ. Psychostimulant drugs and a dopamine hypothesis regarding addiction: update on recent research. Biochem Soc Symp 59:51–64, 1993.
25. Soares BG, Lima MS, Reisser AA, et al. Dopamine agonists for cocaine dependence. Cochrane Database Syst Rev CD003352, 2003.
26. Kreek MJ, Koob GF. Drug dependence: stress and dysregulation of brain reward pathways. Drug Alcohol Depend 51:23–47, 1998.
27. See RE, Fuchs RA, Ledford CC, et al. Drug addiction, relapse, and the amygdala. Ann NY Acad Sci 985:294–307, 2003.
28. McLaughlin J, See RE. Selective inactivation of the dorsomedial prefrontal cortex and the basolateral amygdala attenuates conditioned-cued reinstatement of extinguished cocaine-seeking behavior in rats. Psychopharmacology (Berl) 168:57–65, 2003.
29. Hayes RJ, Vorel SR, Spector J, et al. Electrical and chemical stimulation of the basolateral complex of the amygdala reinstates cocaine-seeking behavior in the rat. Psychopharmacology (Berl) 168:75–83, 2003.
30. Childress AR, et al. Limbic activation during cue-induced cocaine craving. Am J Psychiatry 156:11–18, 1999.
31. Erb S, Shaham Y, Stewart J. The role of corticotropin-releasing factor and corticosterone in stress- and cocaine-induced relapse to cocaine seeking in rats. J Neurosci 18:5529–5536, 1998.
32. Lee B, Tiefenbacher S, Platt DM, et al. Role of the hypothalamic-pituitary-adrenal axis in reinstatement of cocaine-seeking behavior in squirrel monkeys. Psychopharmacology (Berl) 168:177–183, 2003.
33. Koob GF. The role of the striatopallidal and extended amygdala systems in drug addiction. Ann NY Acad Sci 877:445–460, 1999.
34. Valdez GR, Robert AJ, Chan K, et al. Increased ethanol self-administration and anxiety-like behavior during acute ethanol withdrawal and protracted abstinence: regulation by corticotropin-releasing factor. Alcohol Clin Exp Res 26:1494–1501, 2002.
35. Malcolm R, Myrick H, Roberts J, et al. The effects of carbamazepine and lorazepam on single versus multiple previous alcohol withdrawals in an outpatient randomized trial. J Gen Intern Med 17:349–355, 2002.
36. Reoux JP, Saxon AJ, Malte CA, et al. Divalproex sodium in alcohol withdrawal: a randomized double-blind placebo-controlled clinical trial. Alcohol Clin Exp Res 25:1324–1329, 2001.
37. Gowing L, Farrell M, Ali R, et al. Alpha-2 adrenergic agonists for the management of opioid withdrawal. Cochrane Database Syst Rev CD002024, 2003.
38. Clark NC, Lintzeris N, Muhleisen PJ. Severe opiate withdrawal in a heroin user precipitated by a massive buprenorphine dose. Med J Aust 176:166–167, 2002.
39. Rickels K, DeMartinis N, Rynn M, et al. Pharmacologic strategies for discontinuing benzodiazepine treatment. J Clin Psychopharmacol 19:12S–16S, 1999.
40. Diagnostic and Statistical Manual of Mental Disorders, 4th ed., text revision. Washington DC: American Psychiatric Association, 2000.
41. Asmussen E, Hald J, Jacobsen E. Studies of the effect of tetraethylthiuramdisulphide (Antabuse) and alcohol on respiration and circula-

tion in normal human subjects. Acta Pharmacol Toxicol 4:297–304, 1948.
42. Garbutt JC, West SL, Carey TS, et al. Pharmacological treatment of alcohol dependence: a review of the evidence. JAMA 281:1318–1325, 1999.
43. Kranzler HR. Pharmacotherapy of alcoholism: gaps in knowledge and opportunities for research. Alcohol Alcoholism 35:537–547, 2000.
44. Altshuler HL, Phillips PE, Feinhandler DA. Alteration of ethanol self-administration by naltrexone. Life Sci 26:679–688, 1980.
45. Krishnan-Sarin S, Wand GS, Li XW, et al. Effect of mu opioid receptor blockade on alcohol intake in rats bred for high alcohol drinking. Pharmacol Biochem Behav 59:627–635, 1998.
46. Volpicelli JR, Alterman AI, Hayashida M, et al. Naltrexone in the treatment of alcohol dependence. Arch Gen Psychiatry 49:876–880, 1992.
47. O'Malley SS, Jaffe AJ, Chang G, et al. Naltrexone and coping skills therapy for alcohol dependence. A controlled study. Arch Gen Psychiatry 49:881–887, 1992.
48. O'Malley SS, Jaffe AJ, Chang G, et al. Six-month follow-up of naltrexone and psychotherapy for alcohol dependence. Arch Gen Psychiatry 53:217–224, 1996.
49. Gastpar M, Bonnet U, Boning J, et al. Lack of efficacy of naltrexone in the prevention of alcohol relapse: results from a German multicenter study. J Clin Psychopharmacol 22:592–598, 2002.
50. Guardia J, Caso C, Arias F, et al. A double-blind, placebo-controlled study of naltrexone in the treatment of alcohol-dependence disorder: results from a multicenter clinical trial. Alcohol Clin Exp Res 26:1381–1387, 2002.
51. Krystal JH, Cramer JA, Krol WF, et al. Naltrexone in the treatment of alcohol dependence. N Engl J Med 345:1734–1739, 2001.
52. Mann K, Lehert P, Morgan MY. The efficacy of acamprosate in the maintenance of abstinence in alcohol-dependent individuals: results of a meta-analysis. Alcohol Clin Exp Res 28:51–63, 2004.
53. Dore GM, Walker JD, Paice JR, et al. Methadone maintenance treatment: outcomes from the Otago methadone programme. NZ Med J 112:442–445, 1999.
54. Sees KL, Delucchi KL, Masson C, et al. Methadone maintenance vs. 180-day psychosocially enriched detoxification for treatment of opioid dependence: a randomized controlled trial. JAMA 283:1303–1310, 2000.
55. Sees KL, Delucchi KL, Masson C, et al. Methadone maintenance for opioid dependence. JAMA 284:694–695, 2000.
56. Lacey JM, Tershakovec AM, Foster GD. Acupuncture for the treatment of obesity: a review of the evidence. Int J Obes Relat Metab Disord 27:419–427, 2003.
57. Margolin A, Kleber HD, Avants SK, et al. Acupuncture for the treatment of cocaine addiction: a randomized controlled trial. JAMA 287:55–63, 2002.
58. Sapir-Weise R, Berglund M, Frank A, et al. Acupuncture in alcoholism treatment: a randomized outpatient study. Alcohol Alcoholism 34:629–635, 1999.
59. Otto KC. Acupuncture and substance abuse: a synopsis, with indications for further research. Am J Addict 12:43–51, 2003.
60. Kolenda J. Detoxification. Acupuncture Today, www.acupunctureto-day.com, 2000.
61. White AR, Rampes H, Ernst E. Acupuncture for smoking cessation. Cochrane Database Syst Rev CD000009, 2002.
62. Haney M, Kosten TR. Therapeutic vaccines for substance dependence. Expert Rev Vaccines 3:11–18, 2004.
63. Giros B, Jaber M, Jones SR, et al. Hyperlocomotion and indifference to cocaine and amphetamine in mice lacking the dopamine transporter. Nature 379:606–612, 1996.
64. Carboni E, Spielewoy C, Vacca C, et al. Cocaine and amphetamine increase extracellular dopamine in the nucleus accumbens of mice lacking the dopamine transporter gene. J Neurosci 21(RC141):1–4, 2001.
65. The economic costs of drug abuse in the United States, 1992–1998. Office of National Drug Control Policy, 2001. Washington DC: Executive Office of the President, Publication No. NCJ-190636.
66. Shalala DE. The Tenth Special Report to the U.S. Congress on Alcohol and Health. U.S. Department of Health and Human Services, National Institute of Alcohol Abuse and Alcoholism, Washington DC, 2000.
67. Self DW, Barnhart WJ, Lehman DA, et al. Opposite modulation of cocaine-seeking behavior by D1- and D2-like dopamine receptor agonists. Science 271:1586–1589, 1996.
68. Risinger FO, Freeman PA, Rubinstein M, et al. Lack of operant ethanol self-administration in dopamine D2 receptor knockout mice. Psychopharmacology (Berl) 152:343–350, 2000.
69. Nestler EJ, Aghajanian GK. Molecular and cellular basis of addiction. Science 278:58–63, 1997.
70. Risinger FO, Freeman PA, Greengard P, et al. Motivational effects of ethanol in DARPP-32 knock-out mice. J Neurosci 21:340–348, 2001.
71. Rocha BA, Scearce-Levie K, Lucas JJ, et al. Increased vulnerability to cocaine in mice lacking the serotonin-1B receptor. Nature 393:175–178, 1998.
72. Racz I, Bilkei-Gorzo A, Toth ZE, et al. A critical role for the cannabinoid CB1 receptors in alcohol dependence and stress-stimulated ethanol drinking. J Neurosci 23:2453–2458, 2003.

Tobacco Use and Dependence

60

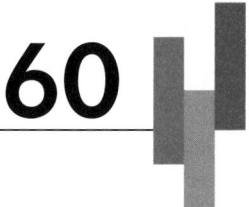

Andrea S. Franks

TREATMENT GOALS

The ultimate treatment goal for any patient who smokes or uses other tobacco products is complete, long-term abstinence from all tobacco products, achieved by the combination of behavioral and pharmacotherapeutic interventions.

DEFINITION

Tobacco dependence is a complex, chronic disease process that is characterized by multiple unsuccessful attempts to quit before sustained abstinence is achieved. While cigarettes are the most commonly used form of tobacco in the United States, other forms of tobacco are becoming increasingly popular and may be associated with similar health risks. These products include chewing tobacco, snuff, pipes, cigars, clove cigarettes (kreteks), and bidis.

MORTALITY

Tobacco use is the primary preventable cause of death. Globally, tobacco use is responsible for over 4.8 million premature deaths annually.[1] The World Health Organization (WHO) projects that by 2030, annual smoking-related deaths will increase to 10 million, with 7 million of those in developing countries.[2] One half of adolescents who regularly smoke will die from tobacco use, half of those dying during middle age, with a 20- to 25-year decrease in life expectancy compared to nonsmokers.[3]

In the United States, smoking results in more than 440,000 premature deaths annually, making it the nation's primary known preventable cause of death.[4] Smoking is responsible for one in five U.S. deaths overall, and one third of deaths due to cancer and heart disease.[5] During the period 1995 to 1999, almost 125,000 of the 153,000 lung cancer deaths could be attributed to tobacco use.[4] Cigarette smoking is responsible for 140,000 premature deaths from cardiovascular disease annually in the United States.[6]

MORBIDITY

In 2000, 8.6 million individuals in the United States had at least one smoking-related illness. Chronic bronchitis (49%) and emphysema (24%) were the most prevalent conditions among current smokers, with former smokers experiencing chronic bronchitis (26%), emphysema (24%), and heart attack (24%).[7]

Cigarette smoking contributes to coronary heart disease, peripheral vascular disease, and aortic aneurysm[8] and triples the risk of stroke.[5] In addition to being an independent risk factor for cardiovascular disease, smoking acts synergistically with and has an adverse impact on other risk factors, such as hyperlipidemia and hypertension.[8,9] Smoking contributes to cardiovascular disease by causing more atherogenic lipid profiles, promoting the development of atherosclerotic plaque, producing endothelial injury, causing vasoconstriction, increasing platelet aggregation with resultant thrombosis, increasing myocardial oxygen demand by increasing heart rate, and decreasing oxygen supply due to carbon monoxide.[8,9]

Smoking is the primary risk factor for chronic obstructive pulmonary disease (COPD), including chronic bronchitis and emphysema.[10,11] Tobacco use is responsible for 80% to

90% of COPD cases, although only 10% to 15% of smokers will develop COPD.[11] Cigarette smoke irritates the lungs, resulting in irreversible damage to the lung tissue that eventually leads to disability and death.[10,11]

According to the most recent Surgeon General's Report,[6] cigarette smoking adversely affects almost every organ in the human body. In addition to lung cancer, cigarette smoking has been conclusively linked to other malignancies, including leukemia and cancer of the stomach, pancreas, kidney, and cervix.[6] Smoking is also a risk factor for peptic ulcer disease, Crohn's disease, cataracts, macular degeneration, and osteoporosis.[5,6] Table 60.1 lists the established health consequences of smoking.

TABLE 60.1	Diseases and Adverse Effects Caused by Smoking

Cancer
Bladder cancer
Cervical cancer
Esophageal, gastric cancer
Kidney cancer
Laryngeal, oral cancer
Leukemia
Lung cancer
Pancreatic cancer
Cardiovascular disease
Abdominal aortic aneurysm
Cerebrovascular disease
Coronary heart disease
Respiratory disease
Chronic obstructive pulmonary disease
Pneumonia
Accelerated decline in lung function
Cough, wheeze, dyspnea
Asthma
Reproductive effects
Reduced fertility
Fetal growth restriction, low birthweight
Preterm delivery
Sudden infant death syndrome (SIDS)
Other
Low bone density, hip fracture
Peptic ulcer disease
Adverse surgical outcomes (poor wound healing, respiratory complications)

(U.S. Department of Health and Human Services. The health consequences of smoking: a report of the Surgeon General. Atlanta, Georgia: U.S. Department of Health and Human Services, CDC, National Center for Chronic Disease Prevention and Health Promotion, Office on Smoking and Health, 2004.)

PREGNANCY

Cigarette smoking during pregnancy has adverse consequences for both the child and mother. Several components of cigarette smoke have a negative impact on pregnancy. Nicotine acts as a vasoconstrictor and cellular toxin, while carbon monoxide binds to hemoglobin, causing a functional maternal anemia and reducing oxygen transfer to the fetus.[12]

Smoking impairs fertility, delays conception,[13] and may increase risk of miscarriage.[6] Additional risks include preterm delivery, stillbirth, and neonatal mortality.[12,13] Low birthweight is a key predictor of infant mortality.[14] Smoking has a dose-related effect on fetal growth[12] and is responsible for one third of the cases of intrauterine growth retardation in developing countries.[12]

Maternal smoking during and after pregnancy increases the risk of sudden infant death syndrome (SIDS)[6,12,13] and childhood asthma.[15] Additionally, smoking during pregnancy may have a negative impact on behavior in toddlers and childhood cognition and academic performance, as well as increasing the likelihood of that child becoming a smoker.[5]

ENVIRONMENTAL TOBACCO SMOKE

Secondhand smoke or environmental tobacco smoke consists of smoke diffused into the air directly from the burning cigarette, pipe, or cigar (sidestream smoke) and that exhaled from the lungs of the smoker (mainstream smoke).[16] Environmental tobacco smoke contains more than 4,000 chemicals, with more than 50 known carcinogens.[16] Environmental tobacco smoke results in 35,000 to 62,000 ischemic heart disease deaths and 3,000 lung cancer deaths annually in U.S. nonsmokers.[16] Nonsmokers with spouses who smoke experience an average 30% excess risk of ischemic heart disease death and nonfatal myocardial infarction.[9] Children's developing lungs are especially susceptible to the effects of environmental tobacco smoke. Environmental tobacco smoke exposure increases a child's risk of SIDS, asthma (induction and exacerbations), lower respiratory tract infection (bronchitis, pneumonia), and otitis media.[16]

EPIDEMIOLOGY

According to WHO estimates, 1.1 billion people worldwide smoke tobacco, one third of the entire population over age 15. Globally, these estimates include 47% of all men and 12% of all women. If the current trends continue, this number will have grown to 1.64 billion by 2030.[5]

In the United States in 2002, approximately 45.8 million adults (22.5%) were current smokers, with a higher prevalence in men (25.2%) than in women (20%). Among various racial/ethnic groups, American Indians had the highest rates of smoking (40.8%), while Hispanics (16.7%) and Asians (13.3%) had the lowest. Socioeconomic status is inversely related to smoking, with a prevalence of 32.9% in those living below the poverty level compared to 22.2% of those living above the poverty level. Educational attainment is also inversely related to smoking prevalence. The gaps in smoking status both by socioeconomic status and educational level are widening.[17] Individuals with psychiatric disorders are more likely to smoke, with an 80% smoking prevalence in schizophrenia and 50% to 60% in depression.[2,18] Substance abuse is associated with increased rates of smoking, with 55% to 80% of alcoholics smoking.[2]

The Centers for Disease Control and Prevention (CDC) reports that the prevalence of current cigarette use in U.S. high-school students increased from 27.5% in 1991 to a peak of 36.4% in 1997, then trended downward to 21.9% in 2003.[19] These trends appear to be related to significant increases in cigarette prices and educational efforts targeting adolescents. Although adolescent smoking rates have declined over the past few years, approximately 5,500 young people age 11 to 20 years experiment with cigarettes for the first time each day in the United States, with almost 3,000 becoming regular smokers each day.[20] Although U.S. smoking rates are decreasing overall and in high-school students, smoking rates are increasing in young adults (ages 18 to 24).[17]

Of the 4 million babies born annually in the United States, 0.8 to 1 million are born to mothers who smoked during pregnancy.[12] Smoking during pregnancy was reported by 11.4% of all women giving birth in the United States in 2002, down from 18.4% in 1990.[14] Most women resume smoking after delivery, with up to two thirds relapsing within 12 months.[21] In the United Kingdom, 25% of pregnant women smoke.[22]

Although 70% of smokers want to quit,[23] each year fewer than 5% are successful in their quit attempt.[24]

BENEFITS OF SMOKING CESSATION

Many adverse effects of smoking are at least partially reversible after smoking cessation. The benefits of smoking cessation are described in the 1990 Surgeon General's Report.[25] Immediate health benefits include improved pulmonary function and circulation. Within 1 to 9 months of cessation, former smokers regain ciliary function, facilitating the clearing of tar and secretions from the lungs and possibly causing a temporary increase in coughing.[25]

One year after a smoker quits, coronary heart disease risk decreases to half that of a current smoker.[25] Ten years after quitting, cancer risk is reduced by 30% to 50%.[5] Smoking cessation also improves survival rates in cancer patients.[5] Fifteen years after quitting, the individual's coronary heart disease risk is reduced to that of someone who has never smoked.[25]

PSYCHOSOCIAL ASPECTS OF TOBACCO DEPENDENCE

Tobacco addiction is complex and is influenced by nicotine pharmacology as well as environmental and psychosocial factors, conditioning, and heredity.[18] Cigarette smoking results in psychological and physiologic characteristics of dependence and addiction. These effects increase the compulsion to smoke by producing positive and negative reinforcement. The effects of positive reinforcement include pleasure, arousal, relaxation, reduced stress, enhanced vigilance, improved cognitive function, elevated mood, and decreased body weight. The effects of negative reinforcement include the relief of withdrawal symptoms such as irritability, restlessness, drowsiness, anxiety, hunger, weight gain, sleep disturbances, and difficulty concentrating.

The 1988 U.S. Surgeon General's Report, *The Health Consequences of Smoking: Nicotine Addiction*, concluded that tobacco products may result in chemical dependence and described nicotine as an addictive substance based on its psychoactive effects, highly controlled or compulsive use, and reinforcing pharmacologic effects.[26] The *Diagnostic and Statistical Manual of Mental Disorders* (DSM-IV) published by the American Psychiatric Association includes diagnostic criteria for substance dependence.[27] A patient is considered dependent if he or she reports experiencing at least three of the seven criteria listed in Table 60.2. Although the DSM-IV criteria are not nicotine-specific, they may be useful in this setting.

The Fagerström Test for Nicotine Dependence (FTND) is a six-item questionnaire designed to determine nicotine dependence (Table 60.3).[28] Number of cigarettes per day and time to first cigarette of the day are the most important indicators of dependence. A score of 5 or greater (range 0 to 10) on the FTND indicates a significant level of nicotine dependence. The FTND, along with a history of prior attempts to quit, is a valuable tool in determining a course of action for smoking cessation.[28]

PATHOPHYSIOLOGY OF TOBACCO USE AND DEPENDENCE

Tobacco smoke contains over 4,800 compounds, 500 in the gaseous vapor phase (carbon monoxide, cyanide, benzene) and others, most importantly nicotine, in the particulate phase. Tobacco smoke contains many known carcinogens, including nitrosamines, polycyclic aromatic hydrocarbons (PAH), benzene, and formaldehyde.[29]

Nicotine, the addictive component of cigarette smoke, is a tertiary amine. It activates nicotinic receptors in the peripheral and central nervous systems, with a variety of pharmacologic effects. It stimulates the release of neurotransmitters, including norepinephrine, acetylcholine, and dopamine, resulting in a stimulatory effect on the central nervous system. The release of dopamine and norepinephrine may result in feelings of arousal, pleasure, and reduced appetite, while acetylcholine may improve concentration and enhance cognitive function. Additionally, nicotine stimulates the mesolimbic dopaminergic system in the midbrain, activating the dopamine reward pathway and reinforcing the

TABLE 60.4	Drug Interactions with Smoking

Drug/Class	Mechanism and Effects of Interaction
Pharmacokinetic Interactions	
Caffeine	Induction of CYP1A2 increases metabolism, clearance increased 56%. Caffeine levels may increase with cessation.
Chlorpromazine	Decrease in area under the curve (36%) and serum concentrations (24%). Smokers may require higher doses than nonsmokers and may experience less sedation and hypotension.
Clozapine	Induction of CYP1A2 increases metabolism, plasma concentrations decreased by 28%.
Flecainide	Clearance increased 61%, trough serum concentration decreased by 25%. Smokers may require higher dosages.
Fluvoxamine	Induction of CYP1A2 increases metabolism, clearance increased by 25%, plasma concentrations decreased 47%. Smokers may require higher dosages, but dosage adjustments not recommended routinely.
Haloperidol	Clearance increased by 44%, serum concentrations decreased 70%.
Insulin	Smoking-induced vasoconstriction may decrease insulin absorption. Smoking may release endogenous substances that antagonize insulin. Smokers may require higher dosages.
Mexiletine	Clearance increased by 25%, half-life decreased 36%.
Olanzapine	Induction of CYP1A2 increases metabolism, clearance increased 40%–98%. Smokers may require higher dosages, but dosage adjustments not recommended routinely.
Tacrine	Induction of CYP1A2 increases metabolism, half-life decreased 50%, serum concentrations 3-fold lower. Smokers may require higher dosages.
Theophylline	Induction of CYP1A2 increases metabolism, clearance increased 58%–100%. Theophylline levels should be closely monitored if smoking initiated, discontinued, or changed. Smokers generally require higher maintenance doses.
Pharmacodynamic Interactions	
Benzodiazepines (chlordiazepoxide, diazepam)	Central nervous system stimulation by nicotine may decrease sedative effects.
β-Blockers	Nicotine-induced stimulation of sympathetic nervous system may blunt effects on lowering heart rate and blood pressure.
Opioids (propoxyphene, pentazocine)	Decreased analgesic effect by unknown mechanism. Smokers may require higher dosages.
Oral contraceptives	Increased risk of cardiovascular disease (stroke, myocardial infarction, thromboembolism) in women who smoke and use oral contraceptives concurrently. Risk significantly higher in women more than 35 years old who smoke ≥15 cigarettes daily.

(Table adapted with permission from Rx for change: clinician-assisted tobacco cessation. San Francisco: The Regents of the University of California, University of Southern California, and Western University of Health Sciences, 1999–2005. Copyright ©1999–2005 The Regents of the University of California, University of Southern California, and Western University of Health Sciences. All rights reserved.)

clude specific behavioral counseling strategies, a supportive clinical environment, and in most cases pharmacotherapy.

5. *Arrange:* Follow-up contact for relapse prevention should be *arranged*. This can be accomplished either in person or by telephone, with the first follow-up scheduled within the first week after a patient's quit date, followed by a second contact sometime during the first month. During these follow-up interventions, patients should be pro-

vided with encouragement, a pharmacotherapy evaluation, and relapse assessment. Counseling for relapse prevention is described in detail later in this chapter.

Counseling Patients Who Are *Not* Ready to Quit: The 5Rs. The initial goal for patients who are not ready to quit using tobacco is to motivate them to start thinking about quitting in the near future. Patients who are not ready to make a quit attempt may lack understanding of the adverse effects of tobacco, may feel they lack the commitment to quit, or may feel demoralized because of previous relapse. The clinical practice guidelines[24] recommend a brief motivational intervention that allows the clinician to educate, reassure, and motivate using the "5 R's": (a) relevance; (b) risks; (c) rewards; (d) roadblocks; (e) repetition (Table 60.5). This approach helps patients identify personal reasons for smoking, benefits of cessation, and barriers they may anticipate. At this point, the clinician should be empathetic and supportive while avoiding "cheerleading," arguing, or designing a specific treatment plan. The motivational interventions should be repeated at every visit.[24]

Counseling Patients Who *Are* Ready to Quit. The goals for patients who are ready to quit using tobacco in the next month are to address key issues for a quit attempt and to design and facilitate a treatment plan (Fig. 60.1). Clinicians should obtain a detailed tobacco use history, including how long the patient has smoked, how many cigarettes are smoked daily, and the details of previous quit attempts and reasons for relapse. Discussions should cover key issues involving tobacco cessation, including the patient's confidence in his or her ability to quit, social support system, and triggers and routines that are associated with tobacco use.[37]

The next step is to develop an individualized treatment plan. The clinical practice guidelines recommend the STAR quit plan: Set a quit date; Tell family, friends, and coworkers and solicit their support; Anticipate challenges; and Remove tobacco from the environment. The quit date should be set more than 3 days but less than 2 weeks away. This allows the patient time to establish support, to prepare for anticipated challenges, and to eliminate all tobacco products from the home, vehicle, and workplace.[24]

An important aspect of facilitating the quitting process is preparing the patient for withdrawal symptoms, which generally peak 1 to 2 days after cessation and then gradually decrease over a 2-week period (Table 60.6). Clinicians should inform their patients that using pharmacotherapy during a quit attempt could reduce their withdrawal symptoms and significantly increase their chances of quitting.[24,37]

Counseling Patients Who Have Recently Quit: Relapse Prevention. Because tobacco dependence is a chronic disease, relapse is common, especially during the first 3 months after quitting.[24] Relapse prevention interventions should be provided to all former smokers, particularly those who quit within the past 6 months. During these interventions, the tobacco user should be congratulated on any success and encouraged to remain abstinent, and should discuss personal benefits, successes, and barriers to continued abstinence, including withdrawal symptoms, cravings, or triggers. Problems and barriers should be addressed, and coping strategies for either a slip or full relapse should be identified.[24,37] If a patient has relapsed, he or she should be reminded that relapse can be used as a learning experience, and that the average smoker attempts to quit several times before attaining sustained abstinence.[24,35]

OTHER NONPHARMACOLOGIC METHODS OF SMOKING CESSATION

"Cold turkey" may be considered as a method of cessation, particularly in patients who smoke 10 cigarettes or fewer daily, or who are pregnant or breastfeeding.[24] Although cold turkey is the least costly method of cessation, patients are more likely to experience withdrawal symptoms, and 1-year abstinence rates are only 5%.

Nicotine fading is an attempt to gradually taper the amount of nicotine a smoker absorbs by either switching to cigarettes with less nicotine or decreasing the number of cigarettes smoked per day. The efficacy of this method is limited, however, because patients often compensate for the decrease in the amount of nicotine by their inhalation technique.

Aversion techniques have also been used as a method for smoking cessation, although they are usually ineffective. The theory behind this method is that exposure to the unpleasant effects of high, quick doses of nicotine prevent patients from returning to smoking. The process involves a

TABLE 60.5	Promoting Motivation to Quit: The Five R's
Relevance	The clinician should encourage the patient to think about the personal relevance of tobacco cessation, being as specific as possible. Use patient's health status, family situation, and history to personalize as possible.
Risks	The clinician should ask the patient to identify some negative consequences of smoking. These could include personal acute and long-term health risks as well as environmental tobacco smoke risks to family members.
Rewards	The clinician should ask the patient to describe some potential benefits of quitting tobacco use. Examples include improving health, providing a healthier environment for family members, and saving money.
Roadblocks	The clinician should ask the patient to identify potential barriers to stopping tobacco use, suggesting elements of treatment (problem-solving skills, pharmacotherapy) that could address those barriers. Examples may include withdrawal symptoms, weight gain, or depression.
Repetition	The motivational intervention should be repeated every time an unmotivated patient is in the clinical setting.

(From Fiore MC, Bailey WC, Cohen SJ, et al. Treating tobacco use and dependence: clinical practice guidelines. Rockville, MS: US Department of Health and Human Services, Public Health Service, 2000.)

STEP One: ASK about Tobacco Use

➲ Suggested Dialogue

✓ Do you ever smoke or use any type of tobacco?

– I take time to talk with all of my patients about tobacco use—because it's important.

STEP Two: Strongly ADVISE to Quit

It is important to be sensitive, because patients might be defensive of their smoking. Project empathy in your voice; be understanding, not reprimanding.

➲ Suggested Dialogue

– It's important that you quit as soon as possible, and I can help you.

– I realize that quitting is difficult. It is the most important thing you can do to protect your health now and in the future. I have training to help my patients quit, and when you are ready I will work with you to design a specialized treatment plan.

STEP Three: ASSESS Readiness to Quit

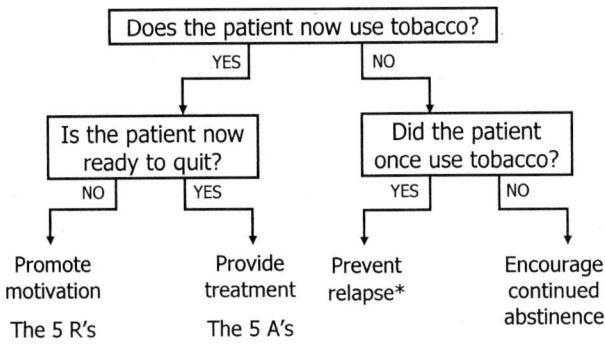

Promote motivation

The 5 R's

Provide treatment

The 5 A's

Prevent relapse*

Encourage continued abstinence

* Relapse prevention interventions not necessary if patient has not used tobacco for many years and is not at risk for re-initiation.

Fiore MC, Bailey WC, Cohen SJ, et al. *Treating Tobacco Use and Dependence. Clinical Practice Guideline.* Rockville, MD: U.S. Department of Health and Human Services, Public Health Service, 2000.

STEP Four: ASSIST with Quitting

✓ **Assess Tobacco Use History**
- Current use: type(s) of tobacco used, brand, amount
- Past use:
  – Duration of tobacco use
  – Changes in levels of use recently
- Past quit attempts:
  – Number of attempts, date of most recent attempt, duration
  – Methods used previously—What did or didn't work? Why or why not?
  – Prior medication administration, dose, compliance, duration of treatment
  – Reasons for relapse

✓ **Discuss Key Issues** (for the upcoming or current quit attempt)
- Reasons/motivation for wanting to quit (or avoid relapse)
- Confidence in ability to quit (or avoid relapse)
- Triggers for tobacco use
- Routines and situations associated with tobacco use
- Stress-related tobacco use
- Social support for quitting
- Concerns about weight gain
- Concerns about withdrawal symptoms

✓ **Facilitate Quitting Process**
- Discuss methods for quitting: pros and cons of the different methods
- Set a quit date: more than 2–3 days away but less than 2 weeks away
- Recommend Tobacco Use Log
- Discuss coping strategies (cognitive, behavioral)
- Discuss withdrawal symptoms
- Discuss concept of "slip" versus relapse
- Provide medication counseling: compliance, proper use, with demonstration
- Offer to assist throughout the quit attempt

✓ **Evaluate the Quit Attempt** (at follow-up)
- Status of attempt
- Inquire about "slips" and relapse
- Medication compliance and plans for discontinuation

STEP Five: ARRANGE Follow-up Counseling

✓ Monitor patients' progress throughout the quit attempt. Follow-up contact should occur during the first week after quitting. A second follow-up contact is recommended in the first month. Additional contacts should be scheduled as needed. Counseling contacts can occur face-to-face, by telephone, or by e-mail. Keep patient progress notes.
✓ Address temptations and triggers; discuss relapse prevention strategies.
✓ Congratulate patients for continued success.

FIGURE 60.1 Tobacco cessation counseling guidesheet. (Reprinted with permission. From Rx for change: clinician-assisted tobacco cessation. San Francisco: The Regents of the University of California, University of Southern California, and Western University of Health Sciences, 1999–2005. Copyright © 1999–2005 The Regents of the University of California, University of Southern California, and Western University of Health Sciences. All rights reserved.)

patient smoking intensely to the point of discomfort, nausea, and/or vomiting.[24]

The guidelines suggest that when time does not permit the clinician to provide comprehensive smoking cessation counseling, an abbreviated application of the 5 A's should be considered: Ask about tobacco use, Advise the patient to quit, Assess readiness to quit, then refer those who are willing to quit to a telephone counseling program or "quit line."[24] Clinical trials have demonstrated the effectiveness of telephone smoking cessation counseling.[38–40] A national network of toll-free smoking cessation quit lines is being established in the United States, with details available at Department of Health and Human Services website (http://www.smokefree.gov).

PHARMACOTHERAPY FOR SMOKING CESSATION

Pharmacotherapy is an important component of the treatment of tobacco dependence, doubling the likelihood of success with a smoking cessation attempt. The patient with a

high level of nicotine dependence who is attempting smoking cessation may have difficulty overcoming the initial withdrawal symptoms and may greatly benefit from pharmacotherapy. Clinical practice guidelines recommend that pharmacotherapy be considered for anyone without contraindications to its use.[24] The guidelines classify nicotine replacement therapy (NRT) and sustained-release bupropion as first-line therapy for tobacco cessation. Second-line pharmacotherapy options include clonidine and nortriptyline.[24]

Nicotine Replacement Therapy. NRT facilitates smoking cessation through both physical and behavioral mechanisms. NRT reduces the physical symptoms of nicotine withdrawal without exposing the patient to the carcinogens in smoke, and with lower and less variable plasma nicotine concentrations. Secondly, by addressing the physiologic component of the addiction, NRT allows the smoker to concentrate on coping strategies for the behavioral aspects of the condition.[30,41–43] Depending on the specific dosage

TABLE 60.6	Tobacco Withdrawal Symptoms and Management			
Symptoms	**Cause**	**Duration**	**Relief**
Chest tightness	Tension created by body's need for nicotine, muscle soreness from coughing	Few days	• Relaxation techniques • Deep breathing • Chew nicotine gum
Constipation, stomach pain, gas	Decreased intestinal movement	1–2 weeks	• Increase fluid intake • Increase dietary fiber
Cough, dry throat, nasal drip	Body ridding itself of mucus	Few days	• Increase fluid intake • Minimize stress during the first few weeks
Craving for a cigarette	Nicotine is highly addictive, and withdrawal causes cravings	Frequent for 2–3 days, can last months or years	• Let the urge pass (a few minutes) • Distract yourself • Exercise
Difficulty concentrating	Body adjusting to lack of stimulation from nicotine	Few weeks	• Plan work accordingly • Minimize stress during first few weeks
Dizziness	Body is receiving extra oxygen	1–2 days	• Move cautiously • Change positions slowly
Fatigue	Body is adjusting to lack of stimulation from nicotine	2–4 weeks	• Nap • Use nicotine replacement therapy
Hunger	Cigarette cravings can be confused with hunger; may be an oral craving for something in the mouth	Up to several weeks	• Drink water or low-calorie liquids • Low-calorie snacks
Insomnia	Nicotine affects sleep patterns, common to dream about smoking	1 week	• Avoid caffeine • Relaxation techniques
Irritability	Body craving nicotine	2–4 weeks	• Exercise • Hot bath • Relaxation techniques

(Table adapted with permission from Rx for change: clinician-assisted tobacco cessation. San Francisco: The Regents of the University of California, University of Southern California, and Western University of Health Sciences, 1999–2005. Copyright ©1999-2005 The Regents of the University of California, University of Southern California, and Western University of Health Sciences. All rights reserved.)

form, NRT results in a 1.5- to 2-fold increase in the odds of long-term success with a smoking cessation attempt.[44]

In the United States, three NRT products are currently available without a prescription (gum, patch, lozenge), while the oral inhaler and nasal spray are by prescription only. The pharmacokinetic properties of the different NRT products vary, but none delivers nicotine to the systemic circulation as quickly as inhaled cigarette smoke.[42,45] Product-specific details, dosage regimen, duration of therapy, and adverse effects of all first-line pharmacotherapies are described in Table 60.7.

Guidelines and product labeling include specific precautions regarding NRT in patients with cardiovascular disease, pregnant and breastfeeding women, and adolescents.[24] Although the benefits of cessation are thought to outweigh the risks of NRT, the guidelines recommend that these patients use NRT only under the supervision of their medical provider.

Despite the fact that smoking is an established, preventable risk factor for cardiovascular disease, 20% of patients with cardiovascular disease smoke.[46] Although nicotine has hemodynamic effects that may increase myocardial oxygen demand and cardiovascular risk acutely, medicinal nicotine results in lower nicotine levels than cigarettes and does not contain the other toxins that have prothrombotic and inflammatory effects.[42,46] Soon after the nicotine patch was marketed, the media reported a possible link between NRT and cardiovascular risk, based on anecdotal reports.[24,46] Since that time, studies have documented that there is no association between NRT and cardiovascular events, even in patients who continue to smoke on the patch.[24,46] However, NRT package inserts state that NRT should be used with caution within 2 weeks after a myocardial infarction, in patients with serious arrhythmias, and in those with angina pectoris.[24]

None of the NRT products are approved by the U.S. Food and Drug Administration (FDA) for use in pregnancy. NRT

TABLE 60.7	Pharmacotherapy		
Product	**Dosing**	**Duration**	**Adverse Effects**
Nicotine Gum			
Nicorette Generic Gum 2 mg, 4 mg; regular, mint, orange *OTC*	≥25 cigarettes/day: 4 mg <25 cigarettes/day: 2 mg Week 1–6: 1 piece q1-2h Week 7–9: 1 piece q2-4h Week 10–12: 1 piece q4-8h	Up to 12 weeks	Mouth/jaw soreness, hiccups, dyspepsia, hypersalivation Effects associated with incorrect chewing technique: lightheadedness, nausea and vomiting, throat and mouth irritation
Nicotine Lozenge			
Commit 2 mg, 4 mg *OTC*	*1st cigarette ≤30 min after* *waking: 4 mg* *1st cigarette >30 min after* *waking: 2 mg* Week 1–6: 1 lozenge q1-2h Week 7–9: 1 lozenge q2-4h Week 10–12: 1 lozenge q4-8h	Up to 12 weeks	Nausea, hiccups, cough, heartburn, headache, flatulence, insomnia
Nicotine Transdermal Patch			
Nicotrol Patch 5 mg, 10 mg, 15 mg 16-hour release *OTC*	>10 cigarettes/day: 15 mg/day for 6 weeks 10 mg/day for 2 weeks 5 mg/day for 2 weeks Not recommended for patients smoking ≤10 cigarettes per day	10 weeks	Local skin reactions (erythema, pruritus, burning), headache
Nicoderm CQ 7 mg, 14 mg, 21 mg 24-hour release *OTC*	>10 cigarettes/day: 21 mg/day for 6 weeks 14 mg/day for 2 weeks 7 mg/day for 2 weeks ≤10 cigarettes/day: 14 mg/day for 6 weeks 7 mg/day for 2 weeks	8–10 weeks	Local skin reactions (erythema, pruritus, burning), headache, sleep disturbances (insomnia) or abnormal/vivid dreams (associated with nocturnal nicotine absorption)
Generic Patch (formerly Habitrol) 7 mg, 14 mg, 21 mg 24-hour release *OTC*	>10 cigarettes/day: 21 mg/day for 4 weeks 14 mg/day for 2 weeks 7 mg/day for 2 weeks ≤10 cigarettes/day: 14 mg/day for 6 weeks 7 mg/day for 2 weeks	8 weeks	May wear patch for 16 hours (remove at bedtime) if patient experiences sleep disturbances
Nicotine Nasal Spray			
Nicotrol NS Metered spray 0.5 mg nicotine in 50 μL aqueous nicotine solution *Rx*	1 or 2 doses/hour (8–40 doses/day) One dose = 2 sprays (one in **each** nostril); each spray delivers 0.5 mg of nicotine to the nasal mucosa For best results, initially use at least 8 doses/day. Do not exceed 5 doses/ hour or 40 doses/day.	3–6 months Gradually decrease usage over 3–6 months	Nasal and/or throat irritation (hot, peppery, or burning sensation) rhinitis, tearing, sneezing, cough, headache

(continued)

TABLE 60.7	continued		
Product	**Dosing**	**Duration**	**Adverse Effects**
Nicotine Oral Inhaler			
Nicotrol Inhaler 10-mg cartridge delivers 4 mg inhaled nicotine vapor *Rx*	6–16 cartridges/day; individualized dosing Initially, use at least 6 cartridges/day. Nicotine depleted after 20 minutes of puffing. Open cartridge retains potency for 24 hours.	12 weeks, then taper over 6–12 weeks Up to 6 months	Mouth and/or throat irritation, unpleasant taste, cough, rhinitis, dyspepsia, hiccups, headache
Bupropion SR			
Zyban, generic Sustained-release tablet *Rx*	150 mg q AM for 3 days, then increase to 150 mg BID Set quit date 1–2 weeks **after** initiation of therapy. Allow at least 8 hours between doses. Avoid bedtime dosing to minimize insomnia.	7–12 weeks Maintenance up to 6 months	Insomnia, dry mouth, nervousness, difficulty concentrating, rash, constipation, seizures (risk is 0.1%)

(Adapted with permission from Rx for change: clinician-assisted tobacco cessation. San Francisco: The Regents of the University of California, University of Southern California, and Western University of Health Sciences, 1999–2005. Copyright ©1999-2005 The Regents of the University of California, University of Southern California, and Western University of Health Sciences. All rights reserved, 2000.)

products are classified as Pregnancy Category D, indicating evidence of risk to the human fetus.[12,24] The goal should be complete avoidance of all forms of nicotine during pregnancy; however, the risk of NRT is most likely lower than the risk of continued smoking, since the patient and fetus are exposed to lower levels of nicotine and avoid the other toxins in tobacco smoke, including carbon monoxide.[12,22,42] The use of NRT in pregnancy should be restricted to women who cannot quit without pharmacotherapy. If a pregnant or breastfeeding woman makes an informed decision to use NRT, she should use the lowest dose possible of a short-acting formulation (gum, lozenge) to provide intermittent rather than continuous nicotine exposure (patch).[24,42]

Transdermal Nicotine Replacement Therapy. Transdermal NRT has been shown to approximately double cessation rates compared to placebo.[24,44,47] Fiore et al[47] performed a meta-analysis evaluating nicotine patch studies with over 5,000 total participants and concluded that patients who use the nicotine patch are twice as likely to abstain from smoking as those who use placebo. The authors also concluded that the 16-hour and the 24-hour nicotine patches were equally efficacious, that extending the duration of therapy beyond 8 weeks did not increase efficacy, and that tapering off the nicotine patch did not demonstrate greater efficacy.[47] The clinical practice guidelines' analysis of transdermal nicotine compared to placebo supported earlier findings with an odds ratio of 1.9 versus placebo,[24] as did a more recent meta-analysis that found an odds ratio of 1.81.[44]

Nicotine patches consist of a disposable liner covering a layer of adhesive, a reservoir of nicotine, and an outer impermeable surface layer. There are currently four nicotine patches marketed in the United States. These delivery systems provide continuous, low levels of nicotine for either 16 hours or 24 hours and have slightly different recommended dosage regimens. The dosage schedules for the different transdermal nicotine products are described in Table 60.7. In general, heavy smokers require higher-dosage NRT patches for a longer duration of therapy than lighter smokers.[24] Conversely, individuals who smoke fewer than 10 cigarettes daily should consider initiating therapy with a lower-dose product.[24] NRT therapy dosage, duration of therapy, and tapering regimen must be individualized based on the patient's smoking habits and the development of either withdrawal symptoms or NRT side effects.

Because transdermal nicotine achieves much lower plasma levels than smoking, it is theorized that the standard doses may be insufficient for heavy smokers. Studies evaluating the safety and effectiveness of high-dose NRT have shown mixed results, with a potential increase in adverse effects.[43,44] High-dose NRT may be an option for smokers who are highly dependent or those who have been refractory to several quit attempts using standard therapy.

Although studies have shown that the 24-hour and 16-hour nicotine patches are equally efficacious,[47] individuals who describe a strong craving for the first cigarette of the morning may have a higher likelihood of success with the 24-hour patch.[48] The 16-hour patch may be useful for patients who experience vivid dreams or sleep disturbances with the 24-hour patch.[24]

The most common adverse effect reported with the patches is skin irritation, which occurs in up to 50% of patients.[24,30] These reactions are generally mild and self-limiting, may be caused by either occlusion or the adhesive, and can be minimized by rotating the application site.[24] Skin irritation may be treated with topical hydrocortisone (1%) or triamcinolone (0.5%) cream.[24,30] The 16-hour patch has a lower incidence of skin irritation than the 24-hour patch.[41] Fewer than 5% of patients have dermatologic reactions that require discontinuation of the patch. Individuals with dermatologic conditions such as psoriasis and eczema are more likely to develop skin irritation and should therefore avoid using the nicotine patch.[24]

Sleep disturbances, including insomnia and vivid dreams, have also been experienced by individuals using the nicotine patch.[24,30] These effects are associated with nocturnal nicotine absorption, are more common with the 24-hour patch versus the 16-hour patch, and can be minimized by removing the nicotine patch before bedtime.[24,30,41] Other less frequent adverse effects include headache (4%), nausea (4%), and vertigo (4%).[30]

Patients should be instructed to apply the nicotine patch to a relatively hairless area between the neck and waist immediately upon awakening, beginning on their quit day.[24,30] The 16-hour patch should be removed at bedtime, while the 24-hour patch is left on until the next patch is applied the following morning. After removal, the nicotine patch should be disposed of properly to prevent ingestion by pets or small children. Patients should be encouraged to continue their normal activities while wearing the patch, including bathing or swimming.[24]

Nicotine Gum. A recent meta-analysis evaluating the effectiveness of nicotine gum versus placebo for smoking cessation found an odds ratio of 1.66.[44] This is consistent with the clinical practice guidelines' analysis of 13 studies that found an odds ratio of 1.5 in cessation rates with gum compared to placebo.[24]

Nicotine polacrilex gum is available without a prescription in doses of 2 mg and 4 mg per piece. Nicotine gum is a buffered gum bound to an ion exchange resin that allows for the slow release of nicotine as the gum is chewed. The buffering agents increase the salivary pH to allow for rapid absorption through the oral mucosa.[30] Approximately half the dose is absorbed systemically from a piece of nicotine gum,[41] although absorption is decreased at a lower pH.[24,30] Because nicotine plasma concentrations peak about 30 minutes after the patient starts to chew the gum, it should be used on a scheduled basis rather than as needed.[30] Advantages of the nicotine gum include the ability of the patient to self-titrate the dosage as needed, and the gum's potential to attenuate weight gain.[24]

The 4-mg dose of nicotine gum has been shown to produce higher cessation rates and a longer time to relapse than the 2-mg dose in highly dependent smokers.[43,44] Therefore, the 4-mg dose is recommended for those smoking 25 or more cigarettes daily, the 2-mg dose for patients smoking fewer than 25 cigarettes per day.[24,49] Table 60.7 describes

the recommended dosage regimen. Although the dosage and duration of therapy can be tailored for each patient, gum should generally be used for up to 12 weeks, with a maximum of 24 pieces per day.[24]

Adverse effects with nicotine gum include jaw aches or fatigue, hiccups, dyspepsia, belching, mouth or throat irritation, and nausea.[24,30,41] These effects are generally mild and can be relieved with appropriate chewing technique. Because nicotine gum is harder than regular chewing gum, it may stick to or damage dental work. Therefore, patients with dentures, braces, recent dental work, or temporomandibular joint disease should use nicotine gum cautiously.

Patients should be reminded that nicotine gum should not be chewed like regular chewing gum. Instead, the ''chew and park'' technique should be used. Nicotine gum should be chewed slowly until a tingle or peppery (original flavor), minty, or orange taste is detected, usually after about 15 chews. The gum should then be ''parked'' between the cheek and gum until the flavor dissipates or the tingling subsides.[24,49] This routine should be repeated over a period of about 30 minutes, or until the flavor completely dissipates.[24] Additionally, because of decreased absorption at a low pH, patients should be instructed to avoid acidic beverages such as coffee, soda, and juices 15 minutes before and while chewing nicotine gum.[24,30]

Nasal Spray. Recent analyses of the smoking cessation literature have concluded that nicotine nasal spray more than doubles the chances of successful smoking cessation, with odds ratios of 2.35[44] and 2.7.[24]

Nicotine nasal spray (Nicotrol NS) is an aqueous, metered-dose fine mist spray available in the United States only by prescription.[30] Following nicotine nasal spray administration, approximately 50% of the dose of nicotine is absorbed rapidly across the nasal mucosa, faster than with any other NRT, with peak plasma concentrations within 5 to 15 minutes.[30] This rapid dosage delivery formulation was designed to mimic the nicotine delivery of cigarette smoking.[50]

Table 60.7 describes the nicotine nasal spray dosage regimen. Once an optimal dose is achieved, the patient should maintain this scheduled dose for up to 8 weeks and then gradually decrease over 4 to 6 weeks, for a total duration of therapy of 3 to 6 months.[24] Tapering strategies include decreasing the frequency of the nicotine nasal spray or decreasing the dose to half the usual dose by spraying into only one nostril.

The majority of patients (95%) will experience moderate to severe nasal irritation during the first few days of treatment. Although frequency and severity diminish with continued use, most patients (81%) experience mild to moderate nasal irritation after 3 weeks of therapy.[50] Other common adverse effects include sneezing, watery eyes, throat irritation, and coughing.[50] Nicotine nasal spray should be avoided in individuals with asthma, allergies, or sinus problems.[30] Due to its rapid onset of action and patient control of dosage delivery, nicotine nasal spray has the highest potential for dependence of all the NRT products.[24,30]

Clinicians should instruct the patient to prime the nasal spray pump prior to the first use. Patients should also be educated regarding administration technique. The patient should tilt the head back slightly and insert the bottle tip into the nostril. Patients should not sniff or inhale through the nose but should breathe through the mouth to enhance absorption via the nasal mucosa and to minimize irritant effects. Patients should be made aware of the dependence potential with this formulation and should be instructed not to use nicotine nasal spray for longer than 6 months.

Nicotine Lozenge. A recent meta-analysis of studies comparing either the nicotine lozenge or sublingual tablet (not available in the United States) to placebo concluded that the lozenge/tablet doubled the rates of abstinence.[44] A study evaluating the 2-mg and 4-mg lozenges versus placebo found that even after 1 year, the odds of abstinence were more than doubled in the treatment groups compared to placebo.[51]

The nicotine polacrilex lozenge, a sugar-free, mint-flavored lozenge, is available in 2-mg and 4-mg strengths without a prescription in the United States. Pharmacokinetically, the nicotine lozenge is similar to the gum, although it dissolves completely, delivering approximately 25% more nicotine than a comparable dose of gum, with peak nicotine levels 30 to 60 minutes after administration.[43] Like the gum, the nicotine lozenge contains buffers to enhance buccal absorption. Advantages of the nicotine lozenge include the ability to use this product more discreetly than the gum. Like the gum, the lozenge gives the patient the ability to adjust the dosage as needed.

The nicotine lozenge is unique in that its dosage regimen is determined by the amount of time before the first cigarette of the day is consumed. The ''time to first cigarette'' has been shown to correlate closely with the FTND score and is a simple way to assess a patient's level of nicotine dependence.[51] Patients who normally smoke their first cigarette of the day within 30 minutes of awakening should use the 4-mg lozenge, while those who wait longer than 30 minutes should use the 2-mg lozenge. Table 60.7 describes the lozenge dosage schedule.

The most commonly reported adverse effects of the lozenge include gastrointestinal complaints (nausea, hiccups, heartburn, flatulence) and cough. They are usually mild to moderate and transient,[51] although patients who chew lozenges or use excessive doses are more likely to experience gastrointestinal complaints.

Patients should be instructed to allow the lozenge to dissolve slowly in the mouth. The lozenge should occasionally be moved around the mouth until it is completely absorbed (20 to 30 minutes) and should not be bitten or chewed. Patients may notice a warm, tingling sensation as nicotine is absorbed. As with other oral forms of NRT, patients should have nothing to eat or drink 15 minutes before or during lozenge dissolution.

Nicotine Inhalation System. Use of the nicotine inhalation system more than doubles long-term abstinence rates, according to an evidence-based literature analysis (odds ratio 2.14)[44] and the clinical practice guidelines (odds ratio 2.5).[24] The nicotine inhaler is available by prescription and consists of a mouthpiece and a plastic cartridge delivering nicotine from a porous plug. The cartridge is inserted into the mouthpiece prior to use, and vaporized nicotine is released when air is inhaled through the device. Patients control the rate and depth of inhalation by puffing on the device; however, optimal effects are achieved in patients who inhale continuously over a 20-minute period.[52] Most of the nicotine released from the inhaler is absorbed across the oral mucosa, with less than 5% reaching the lower respiratory tract. Each cartridge delivers 4 mg of nicotine, but only half is systemically absorbed. Nicotine absorption across the buccal mucosa is relatively slow, with peak plasma concentrations occurring within about 15 minutes of inhalation.

The nicotine inhaler is unique in that it mimics the hand-to-mouth ritual of smoking to assist with the behavioral aspects of smoking cessation, while delivering a low dose of nicotine to attenuate physiologic withdrawal symptoms. This formulation may be particularly useful for patients who cannot forego the physical manipulation of the cigarette.[52]

Doses should be individualized for the patient. While patients may self-titrate to the level of nicotine they require, they should be instructed to use one cartridge every 1 to 2 hours while awake for the first 3 to 6 weeks. The highest abstinence rates are seen in patients using between 6 and 16 cartridges per day with frequent, continuous puffing for 20 minutes.[41,52] Treatment should be continued for a period of up to 12 weeks, followed by gradual tapering over the following 6 to 12 weeks, for a total duration of therapy less than 6 months.[52]

Up to 40% of patients experience local irritation of the mouth and throat with the nicotine inhaler.[24,52] Additionally, mild coughing (32%) and rhinitis (23%) may occur. These effects of local irritation generally subside with continued use. Other adverse effects include dyspepsia, hiccups, nausea, diarrhea, and taste disturbances. Because nicotine is an airway irritant and could cause bronchospasm, patients with asthma or COPD should use the nicotine inhaler with caution under direct supervision of a healthcare professional. Other forms of nicotine replacement might be preferable in patients with severe bronchospastic airway disease.[52]

There are several key points for patient education regarding the use of the nicotine inhaler. Prior to use, the nicotine cartridge is pushed into the mouthpiece, piercing the protective foil covering on the nicotine cartridge. Patients should be instructed to puff lightly on the cartridge, to minimize throat irritation. Once the cartridge is placed into the mouthpiece, it is effective for up to 24 hours. After using the nicotine inhaler, patients should separate the mouthpiece, remove the used cartridge, and discard it out of the reach of children and pets. The reusable mouthpiece should be cleaned regularly with soap and water.[52] Because acidic beverages decrease the buccal absorption of nicotine, patients should avoid eating or drinking anything except water for 15 minutes before and during inhalation.[24] Nicotine delivery from the inhaler is temperature-dependent and declines significantly at lower temperatures; therefore, patients should be instructed to keep the inhaler and cartridges in a warm area during cold weather.[24,52]

Because the current literature shows no significant difference in efficacy between the various NRT products,[44] patient preference currently determines which product should be used. Preliminary research describes subgroups of patients who may be more likely to respond to different formulations of NRT,[43] although further research is needed in this area. While the decision ultimately lies with the patient, clinicians can play a key role in selecting an NRT product, providing the patient with the education that each product requires, and providing professional support in the patient's smoking cessation attempt.

Bupropion. Bupropion SR is the first FDA-approved non-nicotine drug therapy with demonstrated effectiveness in smoking cessation.[24,53] Bupropion is an antidepressant with both noradrenergic and dopaminergic activity that decreases nicotine craving and minimizes withdrawal symptoms, and it has been shown to double abstinence rates compared to placebo.[24] Bupropion is currently available only with a prescription, with indications for depression and smoking cessation.

Because bupropion has a long half-life (21 hours), it can take up to a week to reach steady state. Therefore, bupropion should be initiated while the patient is still smoking with a target quit date after at least 1 week of treatment, generally in the second week.[53] The dosage regimen is described in Table 60.7.

Potential adverse effects with bupropion include insomnia, dry mouth, tremor, rash, and rarely seizures.[53] Insomnia (35% to 40%) and dry mouth (10%) are the most common side effects and generally decrease in severity with continued treatment. Seizures occur in 0.1% of patients without a history of seizure.[53] While bupropion is classified as Pregnancy Category B, there are no data on its use for smoking cessation in pregnancy.[12,53]

Bupropion is extensively metabolized to three active metabolites. Bupropion is converted to the active metabolite hydroxybupropion by cytochrome P450 CYP2B6. Therefore, the potential exists for a drug interaction between bupropion and drugs that affect the CYP2B6 isoenzyme (orphenadrine and cyclophosphamide). Because both bupropion and hydroxybupropion are inhibitors of the CYP2D6 isoenzyme, bupropion should be used cautiously with drugs that are metabolized by CYP2D6 isoenzyme, including some antidepressants, antipsychotics, β-blockers, and antiarrhythmics.[53]

Carbamazepine, phenobarbital, and phenytoin may induce bupropion metabolism, while cimetidine may inhibit its metabolism. Bupropion should be used cautiously with other medications that may lower seizure threshold. Concomitant use of bupropion and monoamine oxidase inhibitors is contraindicated.[53]

Because of bupropion's potential to decrease the seizure threshold, there are several contraindications to its use. Bupropion should not be used in patients with seizure disorders, bulimia, or anorexia nervosa because of increased seizure risk. Likewise, bupropion should be avoided in patients undergoing abrupt discontinuation of sedatives, including benzodiazepines, or alcohol.[53]

A recent evidence-based review of 19 trials evaluating the efficacy of bupropion versus placebo in smoking cessation with at least 6 months of follow-up concluded that bupropion doubles the odds of cessation.[54] Hurt et al[55] conducted a trial comparing abstinence rates in nondepressed smokers with 7 weeks of sustained-released bupropion compared to placebo. Results showed that 1-year abstinence rates were significantly higher in the bupropion groups (23%) compared to placebo (12%). Initially, weight gain was inversely related to bupropion dose, although after 6 months there was no difference in weight gain between groups.[55]

Hays et al[56] evaluated long-term therapy with sustained-release (SR) bupropion for relapse prevention. SR bupropion was compared to placebo in subjects who achieved initial abstinence after 7 weeks of open-label treatment with bupropion SR. After 12 months of medication, 55% of the bupropion SR group were abstinent versus 42% of the placebo group, and the active drug group gained less weight than the placebo group. One year after the drug was discontinued, however, abstinence rates were similar in the bupropion and placebo groups.[56] While bupropion may be useful to delay relapse and decrease weight gain in selected patients, it does not appear to provide significant benefit when used long term.

Combination Therapy
Bupropion Plus Nicotine Replacement Therapy. Jorenby et al[57] compared bupropion SR, nicotine patch, combination therapy with bupropion SR and nicotine patch, or placebo for smoking cessation. The placebo group had a 1-year abstinence rate of 16% compared to 16% in the nicotine group, 30% in the bupropion group, and 36% in the combination therapy group.[57] Bupropion alone or in combination with the nicotine patch resulted in higher rates of cessation than placebo or the patch alone. The difference between bupropion alone and combination therapy was not statistically significant. Additionally, the findings of this study are inconsistent with other literature regarding the efficacy of NRT versus placebo.

Simon et al[58] evaluated a 7-week course of bupropion SR or placebo added to NRT and counseling. While a nonsignificant trend favored bupropion at 3 months of follow-up, this effect was not sustained, as no significant difference in abstinence was observed at 6 and 12 months.

Combination Nicotine Replacement Therapy. Combination NRT may be an option for some patients who have been unsuccessful in their quit attempts using standard pharmacotherapy. Combination NRT includes two different delivery systems: a long-acting formulation (patch) to provide constant delivery of nicotine, and a short-acting product (gum, spray, inhaler) for use as needed, allowing the patient to self-adjust nicotine intake.[24] Several small studies have shown higher long-term abstinence rates with combination NRT compared to monotherapy.[44] However, because there are few safety data with this regimen, the clinical practice guidelines recommend combination NRT only in patients who cannot quit using a single type of first-line pharmacotherapy.[24]

OTHER POTENTIAL THERAPIES

The clinical practice guidelines classify clonidine and nortriptyline as second-line therapies for smoking cessation. Although they are considerably less expensive than first-line pharmacotherapies, these agents have a more limited role in tobacco cessation due to their adverse effect profiles and lack of FDA approval for this indication. Second-line therapies may be used after consideration of first-line treatments.[24]

Clonidine is an antihypertensive agent that may be used orally or transdermally for smoking cessation. While there is no established dosage regimen for this indication, clonidine doses in clinical trials have ranged from 0.1 to 0.75 mg per day.[24] In six trials of clonidine for at least 12 weeks (three oral, three transdermal), the pooled odds ratio for abstinence versus placebo was 1.89.[59] Clonidine's role in smoking cessation is limited by its dose-related side effects, including sedation, dry mouth, and the potential for rebound hypertension if discontinued abruptly.[24,59]

Nortriptyline, a tricyclic antidepressant, has been shown to increase rates of smoking cessation both as monotherapy[60] and in combination with the NRT patch.[61] In one small trial, 6-month smoking cessation rates with nortriptyline were similar to those with bupropion SR and superior to those with placebo.[62] When used as monotherapy, nortriptyline doubles[54] or triples[24] smoking cessation rates. In smoking cessation trials, nortriptyline is usually initiated at 25 mg per day and titrated to 75 to 100 mg per day.[24] Nortriptyline should be initiated 10 to 28 days prior to the quit date to reach steady-state levels, and should be continued for 12 weeks. Anticholinergic adverse effects are a common cause of nonadherence with nortriptyline.[24,61] These, along with the potential for cardiac arrhythmias and postural hypotension, limit the use of nortriptyline for this indication.[24]

Although nortriptyline and bupropion SR may be effective in smoking cessation, other antidepressants have failed to show benefit in clinic trials. Antidepressants that have shown no benefit for smoking cessation include the selective serotonin reuptake inhibitors fluoxetine, sertraline, and paroxetine, the atypical antidepressant venlafaxine, and the monoamine oxidase inhibitor moclobemide.[24,54]

The clinical practice guidelines[24] state that insufficient evidence is available to support the use of antidepressants other than bupropion SR and nortriptyline. Likewise, evidence is inadequate to support the use of silver acetate, anxiolytics (benzodiazepines, buspirone, β-antagonists), or the nicotine receptor antagonist mecamylamine[40] for smoking cessation. Opioid antagonists have failed to show benefit in this setting.[63]

ALTERNATIVE THERAPIES

While there is anecdotal evidence regarding the use of hypnosis and acupuncture for smoking cessation, there are insufficient data to support the use of these methods in this setting.[24,64] Lobeline is a nicotine-like alkaloid that is included in many herbal products marketed to assist with smoking cessation. While lobeline appears to have some nicotine agonist activity, there is no evidence to support its safety or efficacy in this setting.[40,65]

FUTURE THERAPIES

Recent discoveries in the neurobiology of nicotine addiction have identified other neurotransmitter systems that may be involved in tobacco dependence. This research is leading to the investigation of treatments targeting γ-aminobutyric acid (GABA), glutamate, endogenous opioids, and dopamine. Rimonabant, the first selective cannabinoid-1 receptor antagonist, has promise in the areas of smoking cessation and obesity.[66] Small, preliminary trials of the selective monoamine oxidase B inhibitor selegiline suggest that it may have a role in smoking cessation both as monotherapy[67] and in combination with NRT.[68] Other potential treatments include the cytochrome P-450 2A6 inhibitor methoxsalen, which exerts its effect by inhibiting nicotine metabolism, and anti-nicotine antibody-producing vaccines.[69]

The field of pharmacogenetics is making advances in smoking cessation, identifying genetic factors that influence response to treatment.[43] Additionally, researchers are starting to identify subgroups of patients who may respond to different pharmacotherapies based on gender, race, comorbid conditions, or other variables.[24,43,69]

IMPROVING OUTCOMES

Assisting patients in smoking cessation is one of the most important contributions clinicians can make to their patients' health. A meta-analysis of 29 trials evaluating the impact of smoking cessation interventions by healthcare professionals concluded that the likelihood of successful abstinence is increased 1.7 and 2.2 times in individuals who receive an intervention from either a non-physician or physician clinician.[24] Healthcare professionals in all practice settings can contribute to meeting the Healthy People 2010 goals regarding tobacco use.[21,34]

PHARMACOECONOMICS

The economic impact of tobacco-related illness is a world-wide problem with considerable direct and indirect costs.[70] In the United States, the economic toll of tobacco use is greater than $157 billion annually ($75 billion in direct medical costs, $82 billion in lost productivity), almost $3,400 per smoker.[4] In one year, $366 million was spent in the United States on neonatal care attributable to smoking.[6] For each pack of cigarettes sold in the United States in 1999, $3.45 was spent on smoking-attributable medical care and $3.73 was lost in productivity, for a total cost to society per pack of $7.18.[4] It is estimated that 6% to 15% of healthcare dollars in developed countries are spent on smoking-related illness each year.[70] According to the Federal Trade Commission, the tobacco industry spent $9.6 billion marketing its products in 2001, compared to total funding for tobacco control activities of $883 million.[21] Pharmacoeconomic studies have concluded that smoking cessation interventions, including counseling and pharmacotherapy, are highly cost-effective.[70,71]

KEY POINTS

- The impact of smoking and environmental tobacco smoke (secondhand smoke) on illness and premature death is well documented in the literature
- Smoking cessation has immediate and long-lasting benefits and is a major public health initiative
- A smoking cessation plan must be individualized for each patient through assessing his or her readiness to quit/stage of change, previous quit attempts, and potential drug–drug and drug–disease interactions with pharmacotherapies for smoking cessation

SUGGESTED READINGS

Fiore MC, Bailey WC, Cohen SJ, et al. Treating tobacco use and dependence: clinical practice guidelines. Rockville, MD: US Department of Health and Human Services, Public Health Service, 2000.
www.lungusa.org
www.smokefree.gov

REFERENCES

1. Ezzati M, Lopez AD. Estimates of global mortality attributable to smoking in 2000. Lancet 362:847–852, 2003.
2. Schroeder SA. Tobacco control in the wake of the 1998 master settlement agreement. N Engl J Med 350:294–301, 2004.
3. Peto R. Smoking and death: the past 40 years and the next 40. Br Med J 309:937–939, 1994.
4. Centers for Disease Control. Annual smoking-attributable mortality, years of potential life lost, and economic costs—United States, 1995–1999. MMWR 51:300–303, 2002.
5. Fagerstrom K. The epidemiology of smoking: health consequences and benefits of cessation. Drugs 62 (Suppl 2):1–9, 2002.
6. U.S. Department of Health and Human Services. The health consequences of smoking: a report of the Surgeon General. Atlanta, Geor-

gia: U.S. Department of Health and Human Services, CDC, National Center for Chronic Disease Prevention and Health Promotion, Office on Smoking and Health, 2004.
7. Centers for Disease Control. Cigarette smoking—attributable morbidity—United States, 2000. MMWR 52:842–844, 2003.
8. Burns DM. Epidemiology of smoking-induced cardiovascular disease. Progr Cardiovasc Dis 46:11–29, 2003.
9. Benowitz NL. Cigarette smoking and cardiovascular disease: pathophysiology and implications for treatment. Progr Cardiovasc Dis 46:91–111, 2003.
10. Pauwels RA, Buist AS, Calverley PM, et al. Global strategy for the diagnosis, management, and prevention of chronic obstructive pulmonary disease. NHLBI/WHO Global Initiative for Chronic Obstructive Lung Disease (GOLD) Workshop Summary. Am J Resp Critical Care Med 163:1256–1276, 2001.
11. Barnes PJ. Chronic obstructive pulmonary disease. N Engl J Med 343:269–280, 2000.
12. Benowitz NL, Dempsey DA, Goldenberg RL, et al. The use of pharmacotherapies for smoking cessation during pregnancy. Tobacco Control 9 (Suppl 3):iii91–iii94, 2000.
13. U.S. Department of Health and Human Services. Women and smoking. A report of the Surgeon General. Atlanta, Georgia: U.S. Department of Health and Human Services, Centers for Disease Control and Prevention, National Center for Chronic Disease Prevention and Health Promotion, Office on Smoking and Health, 2001.
14. Centers for Disease Control. Smoking during pregnancy—United States, 1990–2002. MMWR 53:911–915, 2004.
15. Li YF, Langholz B, Salam MT, et al. Maternal and grandmaternal smoking patterns are associated with early childhood asthma. Chest 127:1232–1241, 2005.
16. National Cancer Institute. Health effects of exposure to environmental tobacco smoke: the report of the California Environmental Protection Agency. Smoking and Tobacco Control Monograph No. 10. Bethesda, MD: U.S. Department of Health and Human Services, National Institutes of Health, National Cancer Institute, NIH Publication No. 99-4645, 1999.
17. Centers for Disease Control. Cigarette smoking among adults—United States, 2002. MMWR 53:427–431, 2004.
18. Benowitz NL. Nicotine addiction. Primary Care Clinics in Office Practice 26:611–631, 1999.
19. Centers for Disease Control. Cigarette use among high school students—United States, 1991–2003. MMWR 53:499–502, 2004.
20. Gilpin EA, Choi WS, Berry C, et al. How many adolescents start smoking each day in the United States? J Adolesc Health 25:248–255, 1999.
21. U.S. Department of Health and Human Services. Healthy People 2010: understanding and improving health, 2nd ed. Washington, DC: U.S. Government Printing Office, November 2000.
22. Coleman T, Britton J, Thornton J. Nicotine replacement therapy in pregnancy. Br Med J 328:965–966, 2004.
23. Centers for Disease Control. Cigarette smoking among adults—United States, 2000. MMWR 51:642–645, 2002.
24. Fiore MC, Bailey WC, Cohen SJ, et al. Treating tobacco use and dependence: clinical practice guidelines. Rockville, MS: US Department of Health and Human Services, Public Health Service, 2000.
25. U.S. Department of Health and Human Services. The health benefits of smoking cessation. A report of the Surgeon General. Washington, DC: US Department of Health and Human Services, Public Health Service, Centers for Disease Control and Prevention and Health Promotion, Office on Smoking and Health, 1990. DHHS Publication No. (CDC) 90-8416.
26. U.S. Department of Health and Human Services. The health consequences of smoking: nicotine addiction. A report of the Surgeon General. Washington, DC: Government Printing Office, 1988. DHHS Publication No. (PHS) 88-8406.
27. American Psychiatric Association. Diagnostic and statistical manual of mental disorders, 4th ed. (DSM-IV). Washington, DC, 2000.
28. Heatherton TF, Kozlowski LT, Frecker RC, et al. The Fagerstrom Test for Nicotine Dependence: a revision of the Fagerstrom Tolerance Questionnaire. Br J Addiction 86:1119–1127, 1991.
29. National Cancer Institute. Risks associated with low machine-measured yields of tar and nicotine. Smoking and Tobacco Control Monograph No. 13. Bethesda, MD: U.S. Department of Health and

Human Services, National Institutes of Health, National Cancer Institute, NIH Publication No. 02-5074, 2001.

30. Thompson GH, Hunter DA. Nicotine replacement therapy. Ann Pharmacother 32:1067–1075, 1998.

31. Zevin S, Benowitz NL. Drug interactions with tobacco smoking: an update. Clin Pharmacokinetics 36:425–438, 1999.

32. Seibert C, Barbouche E, Fagan J, et al. Prescribing oral contraceptives for women older than 35 years of age. Ann Intern Med 138:54–64, 2003.

33. Schiff I, Bell WR, Davis V, et al. Oral contraceptives and smoking, current considerations: recommendations of a consensus panel. Am J Obstet Gynecol 180:S383–384, 1999.

34. Calis KA, Hutchison LC, Elliott ME, et al. Healthy People 2010: challenges, opportunities, and a call to action for America's pharmacists ACCP White Paper. Pharmacotherapy 24:1241–1294, 2004.

35. Hudmon KS, Berger BA. Pharmacy applications of the transtheoretical model in smoking cessation. Am J Hospital Pharm 52:282–287, 1995.

36. Berger BA, Hudmon KS. Readiness for change: implications for patient care. J Am Pharm Assoc NS37:321–329, 1997.

37. Rx for change: clinician-assisted tobacco cessation. San Francisco: The Regents of the University of California, University of Southern California, and Western University of Health Sciences, 1999–2005.

38. Ossip-Klein DJ, McIntosh S. Quitlines in North America: evidence base and applications. Am J Med Sci 326:201–205, 2003.

39. Zhu SH Anderson CM, Tedeschi GJ, et al. Evidence of real-world effectiveness of a telephone quitline for smokers. N Engl J Med 347:1087–1093, 2002.

40. Sutherland G. Current approaches to the management of smoking cessation. Drugs 62 (Suppl 2):53–61, 2002.

41. Fant RV, Owen LL, Henningfield JE. Tobacco use and cessation: nicotine replacement therapy. Primary Care Clinics Office Practice 26:633–652, 1999.

42. Molyneux A. ABC of smoking cessation: nicotine replacement therapy. Br Med J 328:454–456, 2004.

43. Lerman C, Patterson F, Berrettini W. Treating tobacco dependence: state of the science and new directions. J Clin Oncol 23:311–323, 2005.

44. Silagy C, Lancaster T, Stead L, et al. Nicotine replacement therapy for smoking cessation. Cochrane Database of Systematic Reviews 3: CD000146, 2004.

45. Rigotti NA. Treatment of tobacco use and dependence. N Engl J Med 346:506–512, 2002.

46. Joseph AM, Fu SS. Safety issues in pharmacotherapy for smoking in patients with cardiovascular disease. Progr Cardiovasc Dis 45:429–441, 2003.

47. Fiore MC, Smith SS, Jorenby DE, et al. The effectiveness of the nicotine patch for smoking cessation: a meta-analysis. JAMA 271:1940–1947, 1994.

48. Shiffman S, Elash CA, Paton SM, et al. Comparative efficacy of 24-hour and 16-hour nicotine patches for relief of morning craving. Addiction 95:1185–1195, 2000.

49. Nicorette Package Insert. Research Triangle Park, NC: GlaxoSmithKline, 2004.

50. Nicotrol Nasal Spray Package Insert. New York: Pfizer, 2003.

51. Shiffman S, Dresler CM, Hajek P, et al. Efficacy of a nicotine lozenge of smoking cessation. Arch Intern Med 162:1267–1276, 2002.

52. Nicotrol Inhalation System Package Insert. New York: Pfizer, 2003.

53. Zyban Package Insert. Research Triangle Park, NC: GlaxoSmith Kline, January 2005.

54. Hughes JR, Stead LF, Lancaster T. Antidepressants for smoking cessation. Cochrane Database of Systematic Reviews 3:CD000031, 2004.

55. Hurt RD, Sachs DPL, Glover ED, et al. A comparison of sustained-release bupropion and placebo for smoking cessation. N Engl J Med 337:1195–1202, 1997.

56. Hays JT, Hurt RD, Rigotti NA, et al. Sustained-release bupropion for pharmacologic relapse prevention after smoking cessation. Ann Intern Med 135:423–433, 2001.

57. Jorenby DE, Leischow SJ, Nides MA, et al. A controlled trial of sustained-release bupropion, a nicotine patch, or both for smoking cessation. N Engl J Med 340:685–691, 1999.

58. Simon JA, Duncan C, Carmody TP, et al. Bupropion for smoking cessation: a randomized trial. Arch Intern Med 164:1797–1803, 2004.

59. Gourlay SG, Stead LF, Benowitz NL. Clonidine for smoking cessation. Cochrane Database of Systematic Reviews 3:CD000058, 2004.

60. daCosta CL, Younes RN, Cruz Lourenco MT. Stopping smoking: a prospective, randomized, double-blind study comparing nortriptyline to placebo. Chest 122:403–408, 2002.

61. Prochazka AV, Kick S, Steinbrunn C, et al. A randomized trial of nortriptyline combined with transdermal nicotine for smoking cessation. Arch Intern Med 164:2229–2233, 2004.

62. Hall SM, Humfleet GL, Reus VI, et al. Psychological intervention and antidepressant treatment in smoking cessation. Arch General Psychiatry 59:930–936, 2002.

63. David S, Lancaster T, Stead LF. Opioid antagonists for smoking cessation. Cochrane Database of Systematic Reviews 3:CD003086, 2001.

64. Villano LM, White AR. Alternative therapies for tobacco dependence. Med Clin North Am 88:1607–1621, 2004.

65. Stead LF, Hughes JR. Lobeline for smoking cessation. Cochrane Database Systematic Reviews 2:CD000124, 2000.

66. Boyd ST, Fremming BA. Rimonabant, a selective CB1 antagonist. Ann Pharmacother 39:684–690, 2005.

67. George TP, Vessicchio JC, Termine A, et al. A preliminary placebo-controlled trial of selegiline hydrochloride for smoking cessation. Biol Psychiatry 53:136–143, 2003.

68. Biberman R, Neumann R, Katzir I, et al. A randomized controlled trial of oral selegiline plus nicotine skin patch compared with placebo plus nicotine skin patch for smoking cessation. Addiction 98:1403–1407, 2003.

69. George TP, O'Malley SS. Current pharmacological treatments for nicotine dependence. Trends Pharmacol Sci 25:42–48, 2004.

70. Godfrey C, Fowler G. Pharmacoeconomic considerations in the management of smoking cessation. Drugs 62 (Suppl 2):63–70, 2002.

71. Parrott S, Godfrey C. ABC of smoking cessation: economics of smoking cessation. Br Med J 328:947–949, 2004.

CASE STUDIES

CASE 22

TOPIC: Bipolar Disorder

THERAPEUTIC DIFFICULTY: Level 3
Michael Angelini

Chapter 53: Mood Disorders

■ Scenario

Patient and Setting: SM, a 54-year-old black male; clinic appointment

Chief Complaint: Patient states that he is more fatigued and less motivated on sertraline 200 mg QAM than when he was taking sertraline 250 mg QAM.

■ History of Present Illness

SM is a 54-year-old married black male. He is being treated for bipolar I disorder, which he claims he has had since at least his 20s. He has tried divalproex in the past with some success on maintaining control over his mood but was not fully compliant with this medication. Serum levels were frequently in the 50 to 60 μg/mL range. He had recently been on a regimen of olanzapine 25 mg QHS and sertraline 250 mg QAM but gained approximately 30 lbs and requested a change. For the last 6 months, he has been maintained on sertraline 250 mg QAM and risperidone 5 mg QHS. He had run out of sertraline about 2 months ago and was off of the antidepressant for 3 weeks. He felt that depressive symptoms were returning because he was tired, isolating, and felt sad. SM was restarted on sertraline at 200 mg and noted some response, but he was still depressed and felt he was not back to baseline. SM's cycling phases occur about 4 times a year—mostly depressed mood although some manic periods do occur.

Medical History: History of opiate dependence, hypertension, benign prostatic hypertrophy (BPH), degenerative joint disease (DJD) of hips, right hip replacement in 2000, hepatitis C, seasonal allergies, bipolar I disorder

Surgical History: Total right hip replacement in 2000

Family/Social History: Family History: Father died of MI at 60 years of age, 12-year-old son has ADHD, mother has type 2 diabetes mellitus

Social History: Opiate dependence, last use was 10 years ago; denies tobacco use; lives with wife, an 18-year-old son, and a 12-year-old son

Medications:
Lisinopril, 10 mg BID
HCTZ, 12.5 mg QAM
Sertraline, 200 mg QAM
Risperidone, 5 mg QHS
Gabapentin, 600 mg BID
Terazosin, 2 mg QHS
APAP/cod, 1 tab BID PRN
Ibuprofen, 600 mg TID PRN

Allergies: Seasonal, no known medical allergies

■ Physical Examination

GEN: 54-year-old male in no acute distress. The patient's affect is sad with decreased range. Speech is slowed.
VS: BP 104/65, P 84, R 22, temp 37°C
SKIN: Darkening of skin over nasal bridge
HEENT: PERRLA, EOMI, mucosa moist, neck supple, no adenopathy
COR: RRR, no M/R/G
CHEST: CTA bilaterally
ABD: Soft, norm BS, nontender, nondistended, no hepatomegaly
GU: Deferred
EXT: No C/C/E
NEURO: CN II-XII intact, no focal deficits, motor strength 5/5 in all four extremities, sensation intact

■ Results of pertinent Laboratory Tests, Serum Drug Concentrations, and Diagnostic Tests

Na 137 (137)	WBC 4.6 × 10⁹	AST 0.90 (54)	Chol 4.19 (162)
K-3.6 (3.6)	(4.6 × 10³)	ALT 1.0 (60)	TG 2.81 (249)
Cl 103 (103)	PLT 162 × 10⁹	Alk Phos 2.2	HDL 0.72 (28)
CO2 26 (26)	(162 × 10³)	(130)	LDL 2.2 (84)
BUN 5.71 (16)	HGB 142 (14.2)	T.Bili 6.8 (0.4)	TSH 1.25 (1.25)
SCr 88.4 (1.0)	HCT 0.42 (42)	Alb 46 (4.6)	HbA₁C 0.05 (5.0)
	RBC 4.92 × 10¹²	Total Protein	
	(4.92 × 10⁶)	78 (7.8)	
	MCV-85.8		
	(85.8)		

INR-1.1
HCVRNQt >500,000 IU/mL (Hep C viral RNA load per mL of blood)

■ **Problem List**

Identify principal problems from the scenario in priority order (see Answers in back of book for correct list of problems).

■ **SOAP Note**

To be completed by the student (see Answers in back of book for correct SOAP Note).

■ **QUESTIONS**

(See Answers in back of book for correct responses.)

1. A combination of an atypical antipsychotic and an SSRI antidepressant is commonly used to treat bipolar disorder. Paroxetine should not be used in this patient because it: (EO-8, 9, 10)
   a. Is associated with a high risk of switching a bipolar patient into mania
   b. Is likely to worsen the patient's blood pressure
   c. Has a significant risk of causing hepatitis
   d. Will dramatically increase risperidone serum levels

2. Which of the following conditions present in SM is associated with a drug/disease interaction with valproic acid? (EO-8, 9)
   a. DJD
   b. HTN
   c. BPH
   d. Hepatitis C

3. Which of the following medications could cause a toxic episode if administered to a person who is stabilized on lithium? (EO-9, 10)
   a. Risperidone
   b. Lisinopril
   c. Sertraline
   d. Terazosin

4. SM uses ibuprofen irregularly but for about a week at a time. Which of the following medications is associated with a potentially fatal drug interaction with ibuprofen when used in this pattern? (EO-9)
   a. Lithium
   b. Carbamazepine
   c. Valproate
   d. Olanzapine

5. When initiating lamotrigine for the treatment of bipolar II disorder one must perform a slow upward titration. Which of the following potential effects of lamotrigine explains why this titration schedule is necessary? (EO-10)
   a. Arrhythmias
   b. Pancreatitis
   c. Thyroid dysfunction
   d. Rash

6. If SM's risperidone were switched to carbamazepine for treatment of his bipolar I disorder, which of the following medications would require a dose adjustment? (EO-8, 9)
   a. Sertraline
   b. HCTZ
   c. Gabapentin
   d. Lisinopril

7. Which of the following statements best describes the data regarding the use of gabapentin for bipolar disorder? (EO-11)
   a. Some open-label studies show efficacy, but more controlled studies have shown no efficacy in bipolar I disorder.
   b. Gabapentin is effective for maintenance therapy of bipolar disorder, but ineffective for acute manic episodes.
   c. Gabapentin has shown better efficacy than placebo in preventing depressed episodes from recurring.
   d. Gabapentin is FDA-approved for acute manic episodes, but is not approved for maintenance therapy.

8. A 47-year-old male patient is taking theophylline 200 mg BID for COPD, atenolol for HTN, and lithium 300 mg BID for bipolar I disorder. Which of the following introduces the greatest risk of causing a manic episode for this bipolar I patient stabilized on lithium? (EO-8, 9)
   a. A sustained increase in theophylline dose
   b. The addition of losartan to the patient's antihypertensive therapy
   c. As needed use of acetaminophen for new onset mild arthritic pain
   d. The addition of carbamazepine to treat new onset neuralgic pain

9. Concomitant use of clozapine and carbamazepine is not recommended due to the increased risk of which of the following? (EO-8, 9, 10)
   a. Seizures
   b. Weight gain
   c. Agranulocytosis
   d. Mania

10. Describe the mechanism by which hydrochlorothiazide causes changes in lithium serum levels. (EO-6, 7, 9)

11. Divalproex sodium (Depakote) is the most effective medication for mixed episodes and rapid cycling patients. Define a mixed state and describe a rapid cycling. (EO-2, 12)

12. List the monitoring parameters and the recommended frequency of monitoring for divalproex-induced pancreatitis. (EO-5, 10)

13. Describe the diagnostic differences between bipolar I and bipolar II disorder. (EO-2)

14. Identify factors that should be discussed with the patient regarding the use of medications to treat bipolar disorder that may help to improve adherence to the treatment plan. (EO-12, 14, 15, 16)

15. Summarize therapeutic, pathophysiologic, and disease management concepts for bipolar disorder utilizing a key points format. (EO-18)

CASE 23

TOPIC: Schizophrenia

THERAPEUTIC DIFFICULTY: Level 2
Richard Silvia

Chapter 54: Schizophrenia

■ Scenario

Patient and Setting: JD, a 43-year-old male; inpatient psychiatric unit

Chief Complaint: Auditory hallucinations and paranoid delusions of the FBI tracking him around the city, believe they want to arrest him in a plot to assassinate the Russian president, agitated and aggressive toward staff and other patients (believes they are part of FBI plot to frame him); has been drinking excessive amounts of colas and coffee over previous week or so

■ History of Present Illness

Stopped taking his olanzapine as an outpatient approximately 3 weeks ago due to weight gain (~10 kg in 3 weeks), was admitted to unit 3 weeks ago with current chief complaint, has history of akathisia to antipsychotics (including olanzapine) in the past

Medical History: Hepatitis C positive, HTN

Surgical History: None

Psychiatric History: Schizophrenia with multiple hospitalizations over past 22 years, history of noncompliance with medications as outpatient, previous antipsychotic trials of olanzapine, risperidone, perphenazine, aripiprazole, quetiapine, loxapine, haloperidol, chlorpromazine, and thioridazine

Family/Social History: Family History: Father was diagnosed with bipolar disorder, paternal grandmother had unknown mental illness
Social History: Patient has mother and two sisters that visit him regularly; prior history of IV heroin use—none in more than 5 years, current cigarette smoker 2 packs/day for 20 to 25 years; no reported alcohol intake

Medications:
Clozapine, 50 mg QAM and 100 mg QHS (started 5 days ago and being titrated upward)
Haloperidol, 10 mg BID
Clonazepam, 1 mg BID
Benztropine, 0.5 mg BID
Propranolol, 10 mg BID
Lisinopril, 40 mg PO QD
HCTZ, 50 mg QD
Docusate sodium, 100 mg BID
Multiple vitamin (MVI), QD
Lorazepam, 0.5–1 mg PO q8h PRN agitation
Haloperidol, 5 mg IV q8h PRN extreme agitation/ psychosis
Benztropine, 2 mg IV q8h PRN extreme agitation/ psychosis
Lorazepam, 1 mg IV q8h PRN extreme agitation/ psychosis
APAP, 325–650 q4–6h PRN pain
MOM, 30 mL QD PRN

Allergies: No known medication allergies

■ Physical Examination

GEN: Obese, poorly kept, acutely psychotic male
VS: BP 148/92, HR 96, RR 23, T 37.8°C, Wt 88 kg (Wt 1 month earlier, 76 kg), Ht 178 cm
HEENT: WNL
COR: WNL
CHEST: WNL
ABD: Mildly enlarged liver noted, no tenderness
GU: Deferred
RECT: Deferred
EXT: WNL
NEURO: Alert but inattentive, oriented to person and time only, believes he is in an FBI jail

■ Results of pertinent Laboratory Tests, Serum Drug Concentrations, and Diagnostic Tests

Drawn this morning (7:45 AM)

Na 132 (132)	Hgb 135 (13.5)		Glu 5.94 (107)
K 3.7 (3.7)	Lkcs 6.8 × 10⁹	AST 1.42 (85)	Ca 2.2 (4.4)
Cl 99 (99)	(6.8 × 10³)	ALT 1.53 (92)	PO₄ 0.97 (3.0)
HCO₃ 25 (25)	Plts 223 × 10⁹	LDH 4.50 (270)	Mg 1.0 (2.0)
BUN 6.4 (18)	(223 × 10³)	Alk Phos 2.25	Uric Acid 309
CR 97.2 (1.1)	MCV 103 (103)	(135)	(5.2)
	HgbA1C 0.065	Alb 35 (3.5)	
	(6.5%)	T Bili 34.2 (2.0)	

Hct 0.37 (37)

Hepatitis Panel (drawn upon admission): anti-HAV-negative, anti-HBc-negative, anti-HCV-positive

Hepatitis C labs (drawn 2 weeks ago): HCV RNA-positive, genotype-3A

Urine toxicology screen (drawn at admission): negative for cocaine, opiates, barbiturates, and amphetamines; positive for benzodiazepines

■ Problem List

Identify principal problems from the scenario in priority order (see Answers in back of book for correct list of problems).

■ SOAP Note

To be completed by the student (see Answers in back of book for correct SOAP Note).

■ QUESTIONS

(See Answers in back of book for correct responses.)

1. The two neurotransmitters that are believed to be predominantly affected in schizophrenia are: (EO-1)
   a. Dopamine and norepinephrine
   b. Acetylcholine and serotonin
   c. Serotonin and dopamine
   d. Acetylcholine and dopamine

2. List the two main symptom clusters in schizophrenia and the signs and symptoms of those symptom clusters seen in JD. (EO-2)

3. Describe what effect JD quitting smoking might have on his pharmacotherapy, and how you would correct any potential problems. (EO-4, 9)

4. Describe several common adverse effects of clozapine therapy. (EO-10)

5. Describe how to appropriately educate JD regarding the adverse effects of clozapine you listed in the previous question. (EO-14)

6. What is the main reason that clozapine must be titrated slowly to therapeutic dose? (EO-10, 11)
   a. Orthostasis
   b. Seizures
   c. Agranulocytosis
   d. Drooling

7. List and describe the various pharmacologic actions of the psychiatric medications JD is taking and separate these actions into beneficial (i.e., help treat the patient's illness) and detrimental (i.e., induce adverse effects) groups. (EO-7, 10, 11)

8. Which of the following are appropriate lab monitoring parameters for the use of clozapine in JD at this time? (EO-5)
   a. Complete blood count (every other week), serum prolactin (every 3 months), fasting serum glucose (monthly)
   b. Complete blood count (weekly), fasting serum glucose (monthly), serum lipid panel (every 3 months)
   c. Fasting serum glucose (monthly), serum lipid panel (every 3 months), serum prolactin (every 3 months)
   d. Complete blood count (weekly), fasting serum glucose (monthly), serum prolactin (every 3 months)

9. The state Medicaid office is questioning whether JD really needs to be on clozapine since it is rather expensive and has extra lab monitoring costs associated with its use. They would rather see JD treated with an older, less expensive antipsychotic such as loxapine. Which of the following is a valid reason why JD should be treated with clozapine? (EO-17)
   a. Clozapine should not be used in this patient as it is not appropriate.
   b. Clozapine has been shown to increase functionality, including ability to find employment.
   c. Clozapine has not been shown to be cost effective but since JD has failed other agents this is the only remaining option.
   d. Clozapine has been shown to reduce hospitalization rates and costs, a major component of total illness costs.

10. JD has developed a slight tremor in his hands. What type of medication-related problem might JD be developing? (EO-5, 10)
    a. Tardive dyskinesia
    b. Pseudoparkinsonism

c. Neuroleptic malignant syndrome
d. Akathisia

11. JD has "hinted" that he will not take any medications that might make him gain weight. Describe how you would intervene in JD's treatment to help prevent or minimize any weight gain from his current regimen. (EO-10, 14, 15)

12. Which of the following might potentially help aid in JD's compliance as an outpatient? (EO-15, 16)
   a. Describing all the possible adverse effects of JD's medication regimen
   b. Meeting with JD's family to discuss his illness and how it is being treated
   c. Sending JD home with printed medication information to read on his own
   d. Utilize maximum doses of JD's medications to ensure regimen effectiveness

13. Is JD appropriate for the use of a long-acting injection at this time? If so, recommend an agent and starting dose for this agent. (EO-8, 12)

14. Synthesize etiology, pathophysiology, epidemiology, therapeutic, and disease management concepts for schizophrenia utilizing a key points format. (EO-18)

CASE 24

TOPIC: Attention Deficit Hyperactivity Disorder

THERAPEUTIC DIFFICULTY: Level 1
Collin A. Hovinga

Chapter 56: Attention Deficit Hyperactivity Disorder

■ Scenario

Patient and Setting: JP, an active 9-year-old male; pediatrician's office

Chief Complaint: "He never listens or sits down and disrupts class regularly . . . What do we do to get him to behave?"

■ History of Present Illness

JP presents to the pediatrician's office with his parents and he is running around repeatedly singing "Row, Row, Row, Your Boat." His parents say

that his activity keeps getting worse around the house and he cannot sit for dinner. It first became noticeable when he started preschool. He has episodes where he withdraws and cries about every other week. His preschool teacher told JP's parents he would likely have trouble with the structure of grade school and has been struggling in both math and reading. His grades have been consistently poor because he is generally "spacey" in the classroom and does not finish his work. He routinely bothers and interrupts other students in class. JP's homework is messy and generally not done. He does not have many friends because of his behavior and he was unable to play baseball this year because of not paying attention at practice and during games.

Medical History: Born premature with intrauterine growth retardation secondary to maternal preclampsia at 32 weeks; asthma (nocturnal only) 4 years ago; complex partial epilepsy × 1.5 years (seizures 1/month)

Surgical History: None

Family/Social History: Lives with parents and two siblings; father describes his being active in childhood with poor school performance and in adulthood has had many jobs; mother and siblings are healthy without any significant health problems; mother recently quit smoking (was 2 pack/day smoker × 12 years); JP has difficulty making friends and has routine visits to the principal's office for disrupting class.

Medications:
Gabapentin, 300 mg TID
Theophylline Extended Release, 300 mg at HS

Allergies: None

■ Physical Examination

GEN: Active, talkative, healthy appearing but thin boy uncooperative with exam
VS: BP 110/60, HR 76, RR 20, T 37°C, Wt 24 kg (40th percentile)), Ht 132 cm (75th percentile)
HEENT: WNL
COR: WNL
CHEST: Clear to auscultation, no rhales or rhonci
ABD: WNL
GU: Deferred
RECT: Deferred
EXT: Occasional bruises on the extremities, minor abrasions
NEURO: Alert and oriented × 4

■ Results of pertinent Laboratory Tests, Serum Drug Concentrations, and Diagnostic Tests

Na 137 (137)	Cl 110 (110)	K 4.0 (4.0)
HCO_3 24 (24)	BUN 6.4 (18)	SCr 88.4 (1.0)
Hct 0.040 (40)	Hgb 120 (12)	WBC 12.0×10^9 (12.0×10^3)
Plts 300×10^9 (300×10^3)	Glu 6.2 (112)	
AST 33 (0.55)		
ALT 24 (0.40)		
Theophylline 11 (61)		
Lead (blood) <10 μg/dL		

■ Problem List

Identify principal problems from the scenario in priority order (see Answers in back of book for correct list of problems).

■ SOAP Note

To be completed by the student (see Answers in back of book for correct SOAP Note).

■ QUESTIONS

(See Answers in back of book for correct responses.)

1. The probable cause for JP's behavioral symptoms is: (EO-1, EO-2, EO-5)
   a. Anxiety disorder
   b. Medication toxicity
   c. Post-ictal confusion
   d. ADHD

2. Which of the following signs and symptoms does JP report that supports the primary diagnosis? (EO-2)
   a. Complex partial seizures
   b. Behavioral symptoms before the age of 4 years
   c. Sadness and withdrawal tendencies
   d. Behavioral symptoms occurring in more than one setting

3. Describe the common signs and symptoms of ADHD and factors to consider when diagnosing this disorder. (EO-2)

4. Which of the following factors is the most predictive of ADHD diagnosis? (EO-3)
   a. Poor parenting skills
   b. Medication toxicity
   c. Genetic heritability
   d. In-utero nicotine exposure

5. JP's behavioral symptoms failed to respond to methylphenidate; which of the following medications is most appropriate to treat JP? (EO-7, EO-8, EO-12)
   a. Adderall XR
   b. Imipramine
   c. Buproprion
   d. Clonidine

6. How do the principal mechanisms of action of the stimulants and atomoxetine in treating ADHD differ? (EO-7)
   a. Stimulants decrease norepinephrine, while atomoxetine increases dopamine
   b. Stimulants increase norepinephrine, while atomoxetine increases serotonin
   c. Stimulants increase dopamine, while atomoxetine increases norepinephrine
   d. Stimulants increase dopamine, while atomoxetine decreases norepinephrine

7. Identify which stimulants are longer-acting and may help prevent the need to give JP's dose during school hours. Which ones can be used if JP cannot swallow whole tablets? (EO-8, EO-14)

8. Which of the following methods might a community pharmacist best use to determine compliance with JP's ADHD therapy? (EO-16)
   a. Look at improvements in academic scores and teacher and parent rating scales
   b. Determine appropriateness of frequency of medication refills
   c. Question patient and parents regarding sleep patterns
   d. Ask classmates about their social interactions with JP

9. Which of the following is not an appropriate recommendation with regard to JP's ADHD treatment? (EO-8)
   a. JP's father should see a psychologist or psychiatrist for adulthood ADHD.
   b. JP's classmates should all be informed he has ADHD so as to help him.
   c. JP should receive medication and behavioral therapy.
   d. JP should receive antidepressant therapy.

10. Describe psychosocial factors that should be discussed when a patient presents to the pharmacy with therapy for newly diagnosed ADHD. (EO-16)

11. Which of the following is not a comorbid factor typically found in patients with ADHD? (EO-1)
    a. Aggression
    b. Tic disorder
    c. Sleep disturbances
    d. Schizophrenia

12. Synthesize etiology, pathophysiology, epidemiology, therapeutic, and disease management concepts for ADHD utilizing a key points format. (EO-18)

Headache

Mary L. Wagner and Stephen D. Silberstein

DEFINITION

In 1988, the International Headache Society (IHS) developed a headache classification system, which was revised in 2004. The system divides headaches into primary and secondary headache disorders, which are further subdivided into 14 subcategories (Table 61.1). The primary headache disorders include migraine headache, tension-type headache (TTH), cluster headache or other trigeminal autonomic cephalgia, and miscellaneous headaches not associated with structural lesions. Migraine is subdivided into six subtypes. TTH and cluster-type headaches are divided into episodic and chronic varieties. Chronic migraine, chronic TTH, hemicrania continua, and new daily persistent headache are subtypes of chronic daily headache. Chronic migraine is classified as a complication of migraine. Headaches that are a symptom of another disease are known as secondary headaches; they will not be discussed in this chapter, as they occur in less than 10% of younger patients and may require specialized treatment. However, these types of headaches are more prevalent in elderly patients[1] and should be considered as part of a thorough evaluation. Further information can be obtained from the IHS classification.[2]

TREATMENT GOALS

- Secondary causes for headaches are ruled out.
- Acute treatment alleviates headache pain and associated symptoms.
- Preventive treatment reduces the frequency and severity of anticipated attacks and improves the patient's quality of life.
- Lifestyle adjustments and behavior modification reduce the need for medication.
- Headache treatment takes into account any comorbid conditions and achieves maximum efficacy with minimal side effects.

EPIDEMIOLOGY

MIGRAINE HEADACHE

Migraine occurs in 18% of women, 6% of men, and 4% of children in the United States. Migraine prevalence increases most rapidly between puberty and age 40 and then declines. Organic, or secondary, causes of headaches must be considered in patients with onset after age 50. Most migraineurs have a family history of migraine, and most also have TTH. The lowest prevalence of headache in the United States is in people of Asian heritage and the highest is in Caucasians.

TABLE 61.1	**International Headache Society Classification of Headache**

A. Primary headache disorders

  1. Migraine

    1.1. Migraine without aura

    1.2. Migraine with aura

    1.3. Childhood periodic syndromes (often a precursor to migraine)

    1.4. Retinal migraine

    1.5. Complications of migraine

    1.6. Probable migraine

  2. Tension-type headache (TTH)

    2.1. Infrequent TTH (at least 10 episodes occurring <1 day per month; on average <12 days per year)

    2.2. Frequent TTH (at least 10 episodes occurring ≥1 day but <15 days per month)

    2.3. Chronic TTH (≥15 days per month, on average >3 months)

    2.4. Probable TTH

  3. Cluster headache and other trigeminal autonomic cephalgia

    3.1. Cluster

    3.2. Paroxysmal hemicrania

    3.3. Short-lasting unilateral neuralgiform headache attacks with conjunctional injections and tearing

    3.4. Probable trigeminal autonomic cephalgia

  4. Miscellaneous headaches not associated with structural lesions

B. Secondary headache disorders

  5. Headache attributed to head trauma

  6. Headache attributed to cranial, cervical, or vascular disorders

  7. Headache attributed to nonvascular intracranial disorders

  8. Headache attributed to substances or their withdrawal

  9. Headache attributed to infection

  10. Headache attributed to disorders of homeostasis

  11. Headache or facial pain attributed to disorders of the cranium, neck, eyes, ears, nose, sinuses, teeth, mouth, or other facial or cranial structures

  12. Headache attributed to a psychiatric disorder

  13. Cranial neuralgias and central causes of facial pain

  14. Other headache, cranial neuralgia, central or primary facial pain

(From Headache Classification Committee of the International Headache Society. Classification and diagnostic criteria for headache disorders, 2nd ed. Cephalgia 24 (Suppl 1):1–160, 2004.

The prevalence increases as household income decreases. Despite 10 million physician visits each year, migraine is still underdiagnosed and undertreated, because most persons with migraines do not see a physician. Medications are prescribed for only about a third of patients with headaches, and about half of these will discontinue their medications because of dissatisfaction with treatment results.[3–5]

TENSION-TYPE HEADACHE

TTH is the most common headache type, with a lifetime prevalence up to 80%. This form of headache is divided into infrequent episodic TTH, frequent episodic TTH, and chronic TTH. The episodic TTHs are further divided into headaches associated or not associated with pericranial tenderness. Only patients with more severe or chronic headaches that are unresponsive to over-the-counter preparations seek medical attention. TTH can begin at any age, but onset during adolescence or young adulthood is most common. Forty percent of patients have a family history of TTH. Headache prevalence declines with increasing age; severity decreases in women who continue to report headaches but does not change in men. Twenty-five percent of patients with TTH also have migraine. Patients with episodic TTH are no different from control subjects in terms of stress, depression, anxiety, emotional conflicts, sleeping problems, and fatigue, but chronic TTH is often complicated by coexisting conditions, such as migraine, depression, and drug overuse.[2,6,7]

CLUSTER HEADACHE

Cluster headache is less common than migraine or TTH, with a prevalence of 0.08% of women and 0.4% of men in the United States. Five percent of patients have a family history of cluster headache. Cluster headaches are divided into episodic and chronic varieties. Episodic headaches last 7 days to 1 year, with pain-free periods of 1 month or longer. Chronic headaches occur for more than 1 year, with remissions lasting less than 1 month. Ninety percent of patients have episodic cluster headaches. Cluster headaches can begin at any age, but they most commonly begin in the late 20s; only 10% of patients develop cluster headaches in their 60s. Cluster events may be associated with high altitude, sleep apnea, seasonal changes, or rapid eye movement sleep. They are often precipitated by alcohol, histamine, or vasodilators (e.g., nitroglycerin). These headaches may last throughout the patient's lifetime. Drug therapy may help change a patient's headaches from chronic to episodic cluster, but cure is rare.[2,7–9]

CHRONIC DAILY HEADACHE

''Chronic daily headache'' now refers to the headache disorders experienced very frequently (15 or more days a month), including headaches associated with medication overuse. Chronic daily headache can be divided into primary and secondary varieties.[3] The major primary disorders to consider are chronic migraine, hemicrania continua, chronic TTH, and new daily persistent headache.[10] Chronic TTH was included in the first IHS classification and inappropriately equated to chronic daily headache. Chronic migraine, new daily persistent headache, and hemicrania continua are primary chronic daily headache disorders that are included in the second IHS classification.[2] Many studies have described the process and associated features of chronic migraine,[3] which used to be called transformed or evolutive migraine or mixed headache. Patients with chronic migraine often have a past history of episodic migraine that began in their teens or 20s.[3,11] Most patients with this disorder are women, 90% of whom have a history of migraine without aura. Patients often report a process of transformation characterized by headaches that become more frequent over months to years, with the associated symptoms of photophobia, phonophobia, and nausea becoming less severe and less frequent.[3] Patients often develop (or transform into) a pattern of daily or nearly daily headaches that phenomenologically resemble a mixture of TTH and migraine—that is, the pain is often mild to moderate and is not always associated with photophobia, phonophobia, or gastrointestinal (GI) features. Other features of migraine, including unilaterality, GI symptoms, and aggravation by menstruation and other trigger factors, may persist. Attacks of full-blown migraine superimposed on a background of less severe headaches occur in many patients.[3]

New daily persistent headache is characterized by the relatively abrupt onset of an unremitting primary chronic daily headache. New daily persistent headache is likely to be a heterogeneous disorder and may reflect a postviral syndrome in some individuals. The daily headache develops abruptly, over less than 3 days. Patients with new daily persistent headache are generally younger than those with chronic migraine. Since new daily persistent headache and chronic TTH have similar characteristics, the presence or absence of a past history of headache distinguishes the disorders. A diagnosis of new daily persistent headache requires the absence of a history of evolution from migraine or episodic TTH. A diagnosis of new daily persistent headache takes precedence over chronic migraine and chronic TTH.[12]

Hemicrania continua is a rare, indomethacin-responsive headache disorder characterized by a continuous, moderately severe, unilateral headache that varies in intensity, waxing and waning without disappearing completely. Exacerbations of pain are often associated with autonomic disturbances, such as ptosis, miosis, tearing, and excessive sweating. Some patients experience photophobia, phonophobia, and nausea.[13] Although the disorder has a prompt and enduring response to indomethacin, the requirement of a therapeutic response is not absolute as a diagnostic criterion. Hemicrania continua exists in both continuous and remitting forms. In the remitting variety, headache phases last weeks to months, with prolonged pain-free remissions, while in the continuous variety,[14] headaches occur on a daily, continuous basis, sometimes for years. Both forms meet the criteria cited in Table 61.2. If the required dosage of indomethacin escalates or if indomethacin's efficacy is lost, the diagnosis should be questioned.

TABLE 61.2	Diagnostic Criteria: Hemicrania Continua

A. Headache for >3 months fulfilling criteria B–D

B. All of the following characteristics:
1. Unilateral pain without side-shift
2. Daily and continuous, without pain-free periods
3. Moderate intensity, but with exacerbations of severe pain

C. At least one of the following autonomic features occurs during exacerbations and ipsilateral to the side of pain:
1. Conjunctival injection and/or lacrimation
2. Nasal congestion and/or rhinorrhea
3. Ptosis and/or miosis

D. Complete response to therapeutic doses of indomethacin

E. Not attributed to another disorder

(From Headache Classification Committee of the International Headache Society. Classification and diagnostic criteria for headache disorders, 2nd ed. Cephalgia 24 (Suppl 1):1–160, 2004.)

Medication overuse headache was previously called rebound headache, drug-induced headache, and medication-misuse headache. Patients with frequent headaches often overuse analgesics, opioids, ergotamine, and triptans. Medication overuse can make headaches refractory to preventive medication. Although stopping the acute medication may result in the development of withdrawal symptoms and a period of increased headache, subsequent headache improvement usually occurs.[3] Overuse is now defined in terms of treatment days per month. It is crucial that treatment occur both frequently and regularly (i.e., several days each week). For example, the diagnostic criterion of use on 10 or more days a month (15 for simple analgesics) translates into 2 to 3 treatment days every week. Ergotamine-overuse headache requires intake on 10 or more days a month on a regular basis for 3 or more months. The headache is often daily and constant. Triptan-overuse headache is usually frequent, intermittent, and migrainous. Triptan intake (any formulation) on 10 or more days a month may increase migraine frequency to that of chronic migraine. Evidence suggests that this occurs sooner with triptan overuse than with ergotamine overuse (Table 61.3).[15,16]

PATHOPHYSIOLOGY

GENERAL PAIN THEORY

Pain control systems are involved in all headache types and play an important role in the perception of headaches. Peripheral pain receptors transmit sharp, localized pain via myelinated A-fibers and aching, burning pain via unmyelinated C-fibers to the dorsal horn of the spinal cord. Substance P and excitatory amino acids are believed to be the neurotransmitters for the peripheral pain transmission system. In the spinal cord, enkephalins and γ-aminobutyric acid (GABA) modulate pain transmission. From the dorsal horn, two ascending pathways carry pain sensations to the somatosensory cortex (neothalamic pathway) and to the limbic forebrain and other areas (paleothalamic pathway).[17]

The brain stem sites responsible for craniovascular pain are being mapped using fos-immunohistochemistry, a method for investigating activated cells. The trigeminal nucleus extends beyond the traditional nucleus caudalis to the dorsal horn of the high cervical region in a functional continuum that could be called the trigeminal nucleus cervicalis. This group of cells is the site for referral of head pain and may account for the pain distribution in migraine and other forms of headache. Information is transmitted to the trigeminocervical neurons in the caudal brain stem and high cervical spinal cord and then relayed to the thalamus. The thalamus passes information on to the cortex. Pain localization occurs in the somatosensory cortex, and emotional or affective responses occur in the frontal cortex, anterior cingulate, and insula cortex.

The central nervous system (CNS) modulates pain in part by the serotonergic and adrenergic pain-control systems. The

TABLE 61.3	**Pharmacologic Causes of Headache**

Antiarrhythmics (ajmaline, digitalis, disopyramide, quinidine)

Antidepressants (TCAs and SSRIs [fluoxetine, paroxetine])[a]

Antimicrobials (amantadine, chloroquine, didanosine, griseofulvin, isoniazid, metronidazole, nitrofurantoin, rifampin, tetracycline, trimethoprim)

Antithyroid agents (carbimazole, thiamazole)

Acetazolamide

Analgesics including NSAIDs[a,b,c]

Barbiturates

Bromocriptine

Caffeine[a,b,c]

Cannabis

Carbon monoxide[c]

Clofibrate

Corticosteroids[a]

Disulfiram

Ergot alkaloids[a,b,c]

Ethanol[a,c]

Etofibrate

GI agents (histamine H_1 antagonists, ondansetron)

Histamine H_2 antagonists

Hormonal agents[a,c] (estrogens, progestins, oral contraceptives)

Immunoglobulins

Interferons

Octreotide

Pentoxifylline

Prostacyclines

Triptans[a,c]

Sympathomimetics (amphetamines, cocaine,[c] dopamine, fenfluramine, isometheptene,[b] theophylline[c])

Vasodilators (calcium antagonists, captopril, dipyridamole, guanethidine, hydralazine, nifedipine, nitrates,[a,c] prazosin, reserpine, sildenafil[c])

Vitamin A

[a]Withdrawal may cause headaches.
[b]May cause rebound headaches when overused.
[c]Greater level of evidence indicating acute or chronic exposure causally related to headache.
GI, gastrointestinal; NSAID, nonsteroidal anti-inflammatory drug; SSRI, selective serotonin reuptake inhibitor; TCA, tricyclic antidepressant.
(From Headache Classification Committee of the International Headache Society. Classification and diagnostic criteria for headache disorders, 2nd ed. Cephalgia 24 (Suppl 1):1–160, 2004.)

descending serotonergic system originates in the periaqueductal gray of the midbrain and, via the raphe magnus in the medulla, connects with the dorsal horn of the spinal cord. Analgesia is produced in part by serotonin (5-hydroxytryptamine or 5-HT) interacting with enkephalin-containing neurons. The ascending serotonergic system innervates the cerebral blood vessels, the thalamus, the hypothalamus, and the cortex. It is involved in the regulation of cerebral blood flow (CBF), sleep, and neuroendocrine control. Both ascending and descending noradrenergic pathways originate in the locus ceruleus of the pons. The ascending noradrenergic pathway innervates the microcirculation and the cerebral cortex. The descending noradrenergic pathway terminates in the dorsal horn of the spinal cord. Analgesia may be produced by interaction with GABA-containing interneurons.[17]

The brain itself is insensitive to pain, but other structures, such as the skin of the scalp, the head and neck muscles, the great venous sinuses, the meningeal and cerebral arteries, parts of the fifth, ninth, and tenth cranial nerves, and parts of the dura mater, are pain sensitive. Pain impulses from these sites are transmitted to the spinal cord and brain stem. Direct connections between the primary sensory neurons (e.g., the trigeminal nerve) and the cerebral blood vessels have been detected.[17]

The trigeminal nerve contains calcitonin gene-related peptide (CGRP), substance P, and neurokinin A. Stimulation of the trigeminal nerve leads to release of these mediators from unmyelinated sensory fibers in the dural vasculature. CGRP mediates vasodilation, whereas substance P and neurokinin A induce vascular leakage with plasma protein extravasation (PPE), platelet aggregation, and mast cell degranulation, resulting in neurogenic inflammation (inflammation and dilation of cephalic vessels) and pain. Ergots and triptans block the release of these substances by stimulating 5-HT$_{1B/D}$ heteroreceptors on the trigeminal nerve endings.[7,18]

GENETICS

Migraine is a group of familial disorders with a genetic component. An epidemiologic survey found that first-degree relatives of migraineurs had a 1.5- to 1.9-fold greater risk of developing migraine.[19] Familial hemiplegic migraine is an autosomal dominant disorder associated with attacks of migraine, with and without aura, and hemiparesis. The gene has been mapped to chromosome 19p13 in approximately two thirds of cases.[20,21] The defect is due to at least 10 different missense mutations in the CACNA1A gene, which codes for the γ_1-subunit of a voltage dependent P/Q Ca^{2+} channel.[22] The same gene is associated with episodic ataxia and atrophy of the cerebellar vermis.[20] P-type neuronal Ca^{2+} channels mediate 5-HT and excitatory neurotransmitter release. Dysfunction may impair 5-HT release and predispose patients to migraine attacks or impair their self-aborting mechanism. Voltage-gated P/Q-type calcium channels mediate glutamate release, are involved in cortical spreading depression, and may be integral in initiating the migraine

aura.[23] A second gene has been mapped to chromosome 1q 21–23. The defect is a new mutation in the α2 subunit of the Na/K pump.[24]

MIGRAINE HEADACHE

Any migraine theory must explain the prodrome, aura, headache, and associated symptoms. Migraine is a neurovascular disorder: neuronal dysfunction, with subsequent vascular changes, is responsible for the onset and propagation of migraine headaches (Fig. 61.1).[7,18]

The hypothalamus and limbic system affect both afferent and efferent 5-HT and adrenergic pathways. Disturbances here may hasten the onset of the migraine prodrome. It is now believed that the migraine aura is due to neuronal dysfunction, not ischemia; ischemia rarely, if ever, occurs. Headache often begins while CBF is reduced;[25–27] thus, headache is not due to simple reflex vasodilation.[28] The migrainous fortification spectrum corresponds to an event moving across the cortex at 2 to 3 mm per minute.[29] Noxious stimulation of the rodent cerebral cortex produced a spreading decrease in electrical activity that moved at 2 to 3 mm per minute (cortical spreading depression).[30] Cortical spreading depression is characterized by shifts in cortical steady-state potential, transient increases in potassium, nitric oxide, and glutamate, and transient increases in CBF, followed by sustained decreases in neural activity.[25]

The aura is associated with an initial hyperemic (increased blood in the vessels) phase followed by reduced CBF, which moves across the cortex (spreading oligemia).[31] The rates of progression of spreading oligemia are similar to those of migrainous scotoma and cortical spreading depression, suggesting that they are related.[30,32–34] This has been confirmed by additional studies.[26,27,33,35–38] Blood oxygenation level-dependent (BOLD) functional MRI studies showed a wave of increased and then decreased BOLD signal propagated into the contiguous occipital cortex at 3 to 6 mm per minute.[28]

A link exists between the migraine aura and headache. Cortical spreading depression activates trigeminovascular afferents, causing a long-lasting increase in middle meningeal artery blood flow and PPE within the dura mater. Cortical spreading depression results in upregulation of inducible nitric oxide synthetase and inflammatory cytokines. This mechanism couples meningeal blood flow and neurogenic inflammation to cortical spreading depression but does not explain headache ipsilateral to the aura.[39]

Migraine headache probably results from the activation of meningeal nociceptors. Headache and its associated neurovascular changes are subserved by the trigeminal system. Reflex connections to the cranial parasympathetics form the trigeminoautonomic reflex. Activation results in vasoactive intestinal polypeptide release and vasodilation. Trigeminal sensory neurons contain substance P, CGRP, and neurokinin A. Stimulation results in substance P and CGRP release from sensory C-fiber terminals and neurogenic inflammation. The neuropeptides interact with the blood vessel wall, producing

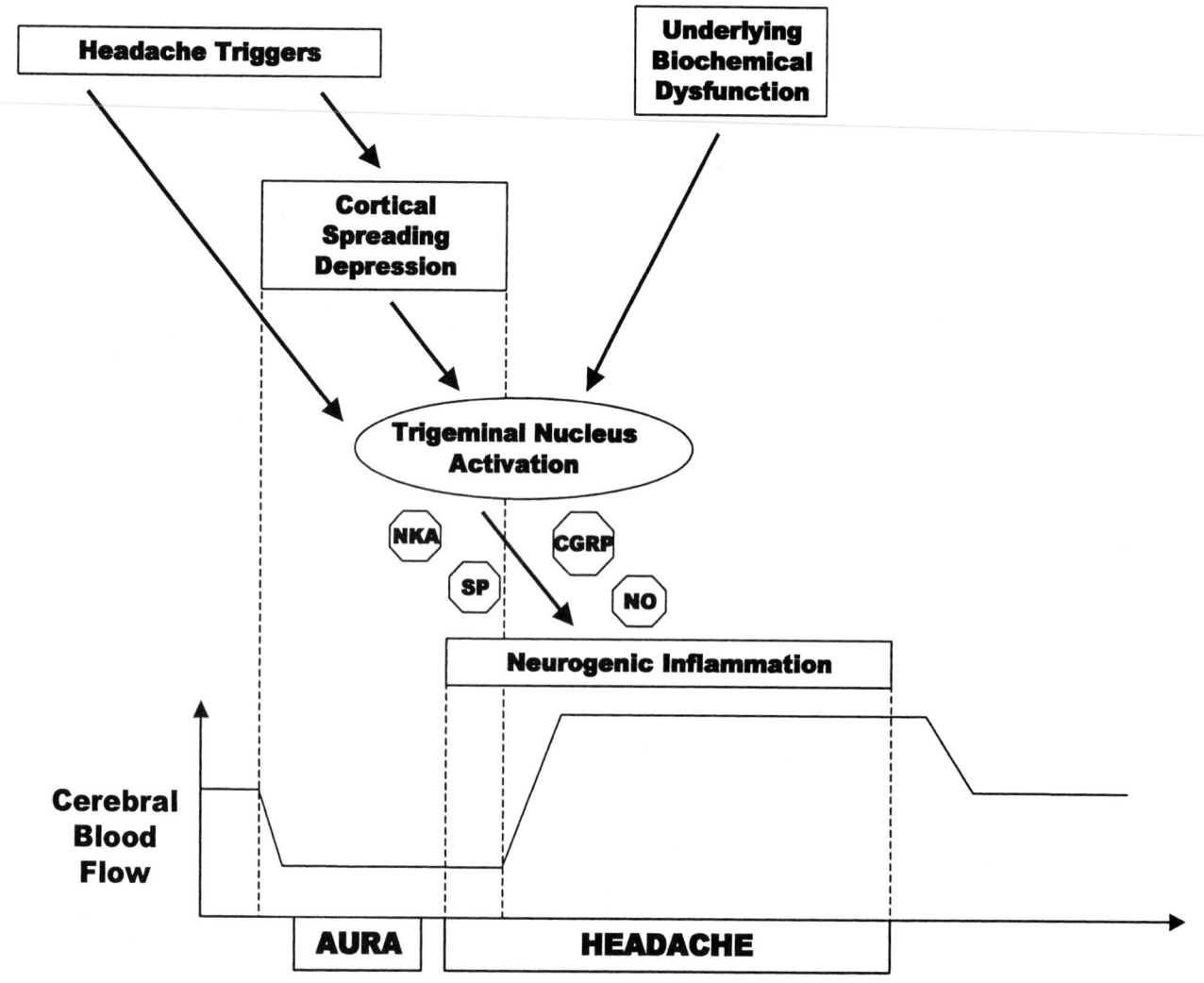

FIGURE 61.1 Pathophysiology of migraine headaches. The comprehensive neurovascular theory predicts relationships between neuronal events and cerebrovascular changes. Activation of the trigeminal nucleus complex results in the release of substance P (SP), neurokinin A (NKA), calcitonin gene-related peptide (CGRP), and nitric oxide (NO), which initiate neurogenic inflammation, alter cerebral blood flow, and propagate headache.

dilation, PPE and platelet activation. One study suggests that neurogenic inflammation occurs in humans. Neurogenic inflammation sensitizes nerve fibers (peripheral sensitization) that now respond to previously innocuous stimuli, such as blood vessel pulsations, causing, in part, the pain of migraine. Central sensitization can also occur. After meningeal irritation, c-fos expression (a marker for neuronal activation) occurs in the trigeminal nucleus caudalis and in the dorsal horn at the C_1 and C_2 levels.[4,18] CGRP, not substance P, is elevated in external jugular venous blood during migraine. Sumatriptan reduced elevated CGRP levels in a migraine attack and in experimental animals during trigeminal ganglion stimulation.[18] A potent specific CGRP antagonist[42] has

been reported to be effective in acute migraine treatment,[43] indicating CGRP may play a role in migraine headache.[40,41]

Patients often develop cutaneous allodynia (nonpainful skin stimuli are perceived as painful) during migraine attacks due to trigeminal sensitization.[44] Triptans can prevent, but not reverse, cutaneous allodynia.[45] Cutaneous allodynia can be used to predict the effectiveness of triptans.[44] Without allodynia, triptans completely relieved the headache and blocked the development of allodynia. In 90% of attacks with established allodynia, triptans provided little or no headache relief and did not suppress allodynia. However, late triptan therapy eliminated peripheral sensitization (throbbing pain aggravated by movement) even when pain relief was incomplete and allodynia was not suppressed.[44] Early intervention may work by preventing cutaneous allodynia and central sensitization.

Brain stem activation occurs in migraine. Using positron emission tomography, patients with right-sided migraine headache showed increased regional CBF in the left brain stem. Sumatriptan relieved the headache and associated symptoms but did not normalize brain stem regional CBF. This suggests that activation is due to factors other than, or in addition to, increased activity of the endogenous antinociceptive system.[46] A second report corroborates these findings.[47]

Serotonin may play an important role in the pathogenesis of migraine headaches. Increased 5-HT metabolism and decreased platelet 5-HT concentrations are associated with migraines. Reserpine, which depletes brain stores of 5-HT and catecholamines, promotes migraine headaches, whereas intravenous (IV) 5-HT aborts migraine headaches.[7,48] Interestingly, migraine headaches may decrease with age, possibly due to a decrease of 5-HT receptors in the brain. In addition, platelet concentrations of 5-HT are lower in patients with migraines who abuse analgesics versus those who do not abuse analgesics or people without headaches, possibly explaining chronic daily headache.[49] There are seven classes of 5-HT receptors: $5\text{-}HT_1$, $5\text{-}HT_2$, $5\text{-}HT_3$, $5\text{-}HT_4$, $5\text{-}HT_5$, $5\text{-}HT_6$, and $5\text{-}HT_7$. In humans, there are five $5\text{-}HT_1$ receptor subtypes: $5\text{-}HT_{1A}$, $5\text{-}HT_{1B}$, $5\text{-}HT_{1D}$, $5\text{-}HT_{1E}$, and $5\text{-}HT_{1F}$.[50] The $5\text{-}HT_{1B}$ receptor is located on intracranial blood vessels and CNS neurons. The $5\text{-}HT_{1D}$ receptor is located on CNS neurons and trigeminal nerve endings. $5\text{-}HT_{1F}$ receptors are located on trigeminal nerve endings.[51] It is believed that activation of the $5\text{-}HT_{1A}$ receptor causes nausea, while activation of the $5\text{-}HT_{1B}$ receptor produces vasoconstriction. Activation of $5\text{-}HT_{1D}$ receptors decreases the release of 5-HT, norepinephrine, acetylcholine, CGRP, and substance P. The inhibitory $5\text{-}HT_{1D}$ and perhaps the $5\text{-}HT_{1F}$ heteroreceptor on trigeminal nerve terminals block neurogenic inflammation by inhibiting the release of neuroactive peptides.

Ergots and triptans act at the $5\text{-}HT_{1B}$, $5\text{-}HT_{1D}$, and, in part, $5\text{-}HT_{1F}$ receptors. They constrict extracerebral intracranial vessels, inhibit trigeminal neurons, and block transmission in the trigeminal nucleus. They minimally constrict human coronary arteries. They block PPE[52] by activating prejunctional trigeminal $5\text{-}HT_{1D}$ and $5\text{-}HT_{1F}$ heteroreceptors, blocking neuropeptide release. PPE can be also be blocked by nonsteroidal anti-inflammatory drugs (NSAIDs), GABA agonists, neurosteroids, substance P antagonists, and the endothelin antagonist bosentan. Dihydroergotamine and the centrally penetrant triptans label nuclei in the brain stem and spinal cord that are involved in pain transmission and modulation.[18] The caudal trigeminal nucleus is activated by stimulation of the sagittal sinus, and this activity is transmitted to the thalamus. Ergots and triptans suppress this activation.

$5\text{-}HT_2$ stimulation results in bronchoconstriction, platelet aggregation, GI smooth muscle contraction, and neuronal depolarization in the CNS. Most drugs that prevent migraines are $5\text{-}HT_2$ antagonists. $5\text{-}HT_3$ stimulation causes nausea, vomiting, and activation of autonomic reflexes. Metoclopramide, a $5\text{-}HT_3$ antagonist, is useful in the treatment of migraine-induced nausea.[7,48]

Other neurotransmitters and mediators, such as histamine, catecholamines, vasoactive peptides, endogenous opioids, prostaglandins, free fatty acids, and steroid hormones, are also implicated in the pathogenesis of migraine. Migraineurs have increased plasma catecholamine levels before and during migraine attacks. Norepinephrine produces vasoconstriction via the postsynaptic α_1-receptors and promotes the release of serotonin from platelets. Dopaminergic hyperactivity may also play a major role in migraine pathogenesis.[53] Increased dopamine concentrations may be partially responsible for the nausea and other symptoms that occur during a migraine attack. Estrogens modulate $5\text{-}HT_1$ and $5\text{-}HT_2$ receptors and are implicated in the development of menstrual migraine. A rapid fall in estrogen, which increases prostaglandin and prolactin levels, may be responsible for the initiation of the migraine attack. Migraine often worsens during the first trimester of pregnancy but then remits thereafter due to sustained high estrogen levels.[7,54]

Migraineurs may have an altered blood–brain barrier during the headache phase. The locus ceruleus, a noradrenaline-containing cell group, may affect brain blood flow and blood–brain barrier permeability.[48] The efficacy of antimigraine drugs is dependent on access to the receptor site, but an altered blood–brain barrier may inhibit the delivery of drug to the site of action, thus diminishing its efficacy.

TENSION-TYPE HEADACHE

Physical or psychological stress or nonphysiologic working conditions may trigger episodic TTH. Chronic TTH may be associated with a perceived increase in stressful life events. TTH may also be precipitated by menstruation. Diminished sympathetic activity, decreased 5-HT concentration, and elevated substance P concentrations have been observed in the plasma of patients with TTH. Reduced CNS 5-HT levels may be responsible for abnormal pain modulation, producing the decreased pain thresholds observed in most patients with chronic TTH. Serotonin levels vary above or below normal in patients with episodic TTH.[6] Although many patients with TTH have muscle tenderness, TTH is not the result of sustained pericranial muscle contraction. Muscle ischemia is not present during headache, and muscle blood flow is normal. Increased nociception from strained muscles or reduced antinociception from emotional stress may modulate TTH. Central pain facilitatory neurons in the ventromedial medulla may produce supraspinal facilitation of the trigeminal nucleus caudalis, which also receives peripheral input from the cephalic blood vessels and the pericranial muscles. An imbalance between the facilitatory and inhibitory neurons to the trigeminal nucleus caudalis may produce central sensitization. Similar to migraine, chronic TTH may present with a neuron hypersensitivity in the trigeminal nucleus caudalis neurons secondary to supraspinal facilitation and a general increase in nociception.[3]

CLUSTER HEADACHE

The pathogenesis of cluster headaches has not been well defined. Any pathogenesis theory must explain the unilateral periorbital pain distribution, the severity, the autonomic symptoms, and the circadian rhythm of the attack. Cluster headache had been attributed to an inflammatory process in the cavernous sinus, which injures the pericarotid sympathetic nerves. This theory cannot explain the circadian rhythms of the attack, and in fact recent positron emission tomographic data have established that blood flow changes in the cavernous sinus region are not limited to cluster headache. Positron emission tomographic studies of a provoked attack of cluster headache have shown activation of the ipsilateral hypothalamus. Unlike migraine, there was no brain stem activation. This suggests that the pathophysiology of cluster and migraine headaches is driven from different areas of the CNS.[7,8,18]

Cluster events may be related to alterations in the circadian pacemaker. Attacks increase after time changes or when there is a loss of circadian rhythm for blood pressure, temperature, and hormones, including prolactin, melatonin, cortisol, and endorphins. The remarkable half-yearly, yearly, or even biennial cycling of the bouts is one of the most fascinating processes of human biology. Cluster headache may be regarded as a dysfunction of neurons in the pacemaker or clock regions of the brain (posterior hypothalamus), which allows activation of a trigeminal-autonomic loop in the brain stem. Migraine and cluster headaches may share a final common pathway: the trigeminal vascular system. Activation results in the release of vasoactive peptides and neurogenic inflammation. The hypothalamus projects to the triennial motor, but not sensory, nuclei. It could directly activate brain stem autonomic nuclei, which could lead to changes in the cavernous sinus. The hypothalamus could also have a direct effect on the descending pain control system. Plasma 5-HT metabolism may also be increased.[7,8,18]

CLINICAL PRESENTATION AND DIAGNOSIS

The 2004 IHS criteria for headache should be used to distinguish between the various primary headache disorders and those due to a secondary cause (see Table 61.1). Medical and pharmacologic causes of headache (see Table 61.3) should be considered. A complete history is needed for diagnosis and should include the following information: (1) age at headache onset; (2) time of headache onset (day or season); (3) description of the pain (location, severity, and type); (4) attack frequency (including any change in frequency); (5) associated symptoms; (6) precipitating factors; (7) methods of palliation used; (8) the patient's sleep habits; and (9) family history. In addition, a complete medication history

should be taken to evaluate the dose, duration of use, and effectiveness of previous headache medications and to determine whether any medications that could exacerbate headaches are being used. The diagnostic characteristics of headache disorders are summarized in Table 61.4.

MIGRAINE HEADACHE

The IHS subdivides migraine into migraine with aura and migraine without aura. A diagnosis of migraine without aura requires the patient to have at least five headache attacks, each lasting 4 to 72 hours, and two of the following characteristics: unilateral location, pulsating quality, moderate or severe intensity, or aggravation by routine physical activity. At least one of the following should occur during the attack: nausea/vomiting or photophobia and phonophobia.[2]

A diagnosis of migraine with aura requires the patient to have at least two attacks with one of the following: fully reversible visual (e.g., flickering lights, spots, lines, or loss of vision), sensory (e.g., pins and needles, numbness), or speech symptoms. Motor weakness should not occur. At least two of the following should also occur: (1) bilateral visual symptoms or unilateral sensory symptoms; (2) at least one symptom develops gradually over a period more than 5 minutes, different symptoms occur in succession, or both; (3) each symptom lasts more than 5 minutes but less than 60 minutes. The headache also needs to meet the same criteria as migraine without aura. The headache begins during the aura and follows the aura within 60 minutes. If the aura lasts longer than 1 hour but less than 1 week, the migraine is called migraine with prolonged aura.[2,7]

Migraine may consist of premonitory, aura, headache, and resolution phases (Table 61-5). Premonitory symptoms (prodrome) occur in up to 60% of patients. Symptoms begin hours to days before the headache and can continue into the aura and headache phases. During this time, patients may experience various psychological, neurologic, constitutional, or autonomic symptoms. These symptoms may be hard to diagnose because they may occur by themselves or with mild headaches.[4]

The aura, which occurs in about 20% of migraineurs, consists of visual, sensory, motor, or brain stem symptoms, or language disturbances. It develops over 5 to 20 minutes and lasts less than 1 hour. Symptoms may accompany the headache or occur up to an hour before the headache. Sometimes the aura may occur without the headache.[4]

The headache can begin at any time during the day. The pain usually develops gradually and then subsides after 4 to 72 hours in adults and 2 to 48 hours in children. If the headache lasts longer than 72 hours, it is labeled status migrainosus. The pain is usually located in the temples, but it can occur anywhere in the face or head and may radiate down the neck and shoulder. The pain is moderate to severe in intensity and usually described as throbbing or pulsating with a unilateral distribution; however, the symptoms may begin as, or become, bilateral. Most patients experience associated GI and neuropsychological symptoms, with nausea

TABLE 61.4	Differential Diagnosis by Presentation of Selected Headache Disorders						
Headache Type	Age of Onset (years)	Location	Duration	Frequency/ Timing	Severity	Quality	Associated Features
Migraine	10–40	Hemicranial	Several hours to 3 days	Variable	Moderate to severe	Throbbing > steady ache	Nausea, vomiting, photo/phono/ osmophobia, scotomata, neurologic deficits.
Tension type	20–50	Bilateral	30 min to ≥7 days	Variable	Dull ache may wax/wane	Vise-like, band-like pressure	Generally none
Cluster	15–40	Unilateral, peri/ retro-orbital	30–120 min	1–8 times per day, nocturnal attacks	Excruciating	Boring piercing	Ipsilateral conjunctival injection, lacrimation, nasal congestion, rhinorrhea, miosis, facial sweating
Mass lesion	Any	Any	Variable	Intermittent, nocturnal, upon arising	Moderate	Dull steady/ throbbing	Vomiting, nuchal rigidity, neurologic deficits
Subarachnoid hemorrhage	Adult	Global, often occipitonuchal	Variable	Acute onset	Excruciating	Explosive	Nausea, vomiting, nuchal rigidity, loss of consciousness, neurological deficits
Trigeminal neuralgia	50–70	2nd–3rd > 1st division's trigeminal nerve	Seconds, occur in volleys	Paroxysmal	Excruciating	Electric shock-like	Facial trigger facial points, spasm of muscles ipsilaterally (Tic)
Giant cell arteritis	>55	Temporal, any region	Intermittent, then continuous	Constant, can be worse at night	Variable	Variable	Tender scalp arteries, polymyalgia rheumatica, jaw claudication

(From Silberstein SD, Lipton RB, Goadsby PJ. Headache in clinical practice. Oxford: Isis Medical Media, 1998.)

being the most common. Nausea and vomiting occur in 90% and 30% of patients, respectively. Photophobia and phonophobia cause patients to seek relief in a dark, quiet room to decrease sensory stimulation. Most patients experience between one and four headaches a month.[4,7]

After the headache phase, the postdrome, or recovery phase, may occur and last up to 24 hours. During this phase, some patients may feel alert or tired, euphoric or depressed, or refreshed or worn out. Some may complain of poor concentration, food intolerance, or scalp tenderness.[4]

TENSION-TYPE HEADACHE

The diagnosis of TTH requires that patients experience at least 10 previous headaches over a period of less than 3 months, each lasting 30 minutes to 7 days, with at least two of the following characteristics: a pressing or tightening (nonpulsating) quality, mild to moderate intensity, bilateral location, and no aggravation with physical activity. In addition, patients should not have nausea or vomiting. They may have either photophobia or phonophobia but not both. Patients with chronic TTH may have one of the following:

mild nausea (not moderate or severe), photophobia, or phonophobia.[2,6,7]

Patients describe the onset of TTH as gradual, often occurring during or after stress. Headaches last 30 minutes to a week, with a median of 12 hours. The headache is typically worse later in the day. The pain is usually bilateral, may be located in the forehead, the temples, or the back of the head, and may radiate to the neck and shoulders. Patients describe the steady, nagging, persistent, dull, aching pain as a tightness, a soreness, a squeezing sensation, or a constricting, vise-like pressure. They may say, ''It's as if a band were wrapped around my head,'' or complain of scalp tenderness, rigid neck muscles, and jaw discomfort. Unlike migraine, there is no prodrome or associated autonomic or GI symptoms. Some patients complain of anorexia.[2,6,7]

CLUSTER HEADACHE

The diagnosis of cluster headache requires the patient to have at least five untreated attacks of severe, unilateral, orbital, supraorbital, and/or temporal pain lasting 15 to 180 minutes. At least one of the following associated symptoms

TABLE 61.5	Migraine Headache Symptoms

Premonitory Phase (Prodrome)

Psychological	Neurologic	General
Depression	Photophobia	Stiff neck
Euphoria and hyperactivity	Phonophobia	Cold feeling
Irritability	Hyperosmia	Sluggishness
Restlessness	Dysphasia	Thirst
Fatigue and drowsiness	Yawning	Polyuria
	Mental slowness or poor concentration	Anorexia or food cravings
		Diarrhea or constipation
		Fluid retention

Aura

Visual disturbances	Sensory	Language	Motor disturbance
Scotomata (partial loss of sight)	Paresthesias (numbness or tingling in the extremities and face, often migrating)	Difficulty speaking	Weakness
Photopsia (flashing lights)		Difficulty understanding language	Ataxia
See geometric shapes, rotating or shimmering objects			Monoparesis or hemiparesis
Scintillations (fluorescent light flashes)			Chorea
Teichopsia or fortification spectra (zig-zag banding of light and dark lines)			
Visual distortions or hallucinations			

Attack: Headache (Pain Description and Associated Symptoms)

Headache	Gastrointestinal	Neuropsychological	Other
Location (bilateral 40%, unilateral 60%)	Anorexia	Persistance of prodromal symptoms	Edema
Throbbing quality (40%–60%)	Food cravings	Photophobia (90%)	Polyuria
Scalp tenderness (66%)	Nausea (86%)	Phonophobia	Nasal stuffiness (10%–20%)
Short-lived "ice-pick" pain jabs (40%)	Vomiting (33%)	Osmophobia	Rhinorrhea
	Constipation	Lightheadedness	Sensations of heat, cold, sweating
	Diarrhea (16%)	Mood and mental changes	
	Gastroparesis		

Resolution or Postdrome Phase

Neuropsychological	Others
Fatigue or listlessness	Muscle weakness and aching
Irritability or mood changes	Anorexia or food cravings
Impaired concentration	Scalp tenderness

(From Silberstein SD, Lipton RB. Chronic daily headache, including transformed migraine, chronic tension-type headache, and medication overuse. In: Silberstein SD, Lipton RB, Dalessio DJ, eds. Wolff's headache and other head pain, 7th ed. New York: Oxford University Press, 2001:247–282; Silberstein SD. Migraine. Lancet 363:381–391, 2004; Olesen J, Tfelt-Hansen P, Welch KMA, eds. The headaches, 2nd ed. Philadelphia: Lippincott Williams & Wilkins, 2000.)

must occur: conjunctival injection, lacrimation, nasal congestion, rhinorrhea, facial sweating, miosis, ptosis, or eyelid edema. Headache frequency during a cluster attack varies from one every other day to eight per day. Episodic cluster headaches are distinguished by headache periods of 1 week to 1 year with remission periods lasting at least 14 days, whereas chronic cluster headaches have no remission periods or remissions lasting less than 14 days. Episodic cluster headaches can evolve into chronic cluster headaches.[2,8]

Cluster attacks may begin with slight discomfort that rapidly increases (within 15 minutes) to excruciating pain. The attacks often occur at the same time each day and frequently awaken patients from sleep. Untreated, attacks generally last for 30 to 90 minutes but can persist up to 180 minutes. The pain is described as unilateral, deep, constant, boring, pressing, piercing, or burning in nature and located behind or around the eye. It may radiate to the forehead, temples, jaws, nostrils, ears, neck, or shoulder. Patients may say, ''It's like driving a hot poker into my eye.'' Some patients cannot describe the pain, and 30% describe it as throbbing or pulsating. Patients are usually pain-free between cluster periods, with remissions lasting 6 months to 2 years; however, isolated, mild, brief attacks may occur between cluster periods. During an attack, patients often feel agitated or restless and feel the need to isolate themselves and move around. Associated symptoms of autonomic dysfunction, such as nasal obstruction, bradycardia, or lacrimation, may be present. Of these, lacrimation is reported by about 80% of patients. GI symptoms are uncommon. Most patients have one or two cluster periods a year that last 2 to 3 months, with one to two attacks per day.[2,7,8]

PSYCHOSOCIAL ASPECTS

Migraine has a substantial impact on health-related quality of life and impairs work, social activities, and family life. The World Health Organization ranks migraine among the world's most disabling medical illnesses.[55] Children and adults with headaches experience more physical complaints, stress, psychological symptoms, and decreased quality of life than do those without headaches. They also exhibit more absenteeism from school and work.[56,57] Some studies say headache patients are more likely to experience depression and anxiety.[58] Some patients live in fear that their headaches will affect their ability to meet obligations to family, coworkers, and friends. People who express resentment over having to make sacrifices to accommodate the needs of headache patients may reinforce these feelings.

THERAPEUTIC PLAN

MIGRAINE HEADACHE

Pharmacologic treatments should be added when nonpharmacologic treatments alone fail to provide adequate head-

ache relief. Avoiding headache triggers augments the efficacy of all medications for achieving pain relief. Pharmacologic therapy is divided into acute (abortive) and preventive treatment. The aim of acute treatment is to relieve headache pain and associated symptoms. It should be limited to two or three times a week. Preventive therapy should reduce the frequency and severity of anticipated attacks, but acute treatment is still needed for breakthrough attacks. Patients who think they are developing a headache should minimize sensory stimulation by resting in a dark, quiet place, apply an ice pack and pressure over the superficial temporal artery on the affected side, and use medication for acute headaches as soon as possible.[4,7,57,59]

The treatment algorithm is based on the patient's headache severity, concurrent symptoms, and comorbid conditions and the efficacy/adverse effect ratio and cost of the medications (Fig. 61.2). Generally, the agents with the highest efficacy/adverse effect ratio and lowest cost are used first. The route of administration depends on patient preference, prior response to that route of administration, and the presence of certain migraine-associated symptoms. For example, patients with severe nausea and vomiting or fast onset of symptoms should be treated with subcutaneous (SC), intramuscular (IM), IV, rectal (PR), or intranasal (IN) rather than oral medications. Patients with mild to moderate headache pain should be treated with analgesics, with or without caffeine. If these fail in the same or prior attacks, then triptans, dihydroergotamine, mixed analgesics, or opioids may be used. Patients with severe pain should start treatment with combination analgesics, opioids, triptans, or dihydroergotamine. Nonpharmacologic and adjunctive medications for associated headache symptoms may also be used concurrently. When the attacks are severe enough for the patient to go to an emergency department, IV forms of metoclopramide, dihydroergotamine, prochlorperazine, or chlormazine are often used. Sometimes IM ketorolac or IV valproic acid is used.[4,7,57,59]

After the acute attack is treated, patients should be educated about their disease, their medications, the use of a diary, and the possible need for preventive therapy. Nonpharmacologic treatments may minimize the need for medications. The U.S. Headache Consortium participants divided medications for preventive treatment into five groups, with group 1 being agents with proven high efficacy and mild to moderate adverse events and group 5 being medications proven to have limited or no efficacy. Practitioners should first select agents from group 1 or 2. Group 1 agents include amitriptyline, divalproex sodium, propranolol, and timolol. Group 2 agents include other β-blockers, nimodipine, verapamil, NSAIDs, fluoxetine, gabapentin, feverfew, magnesium, and vitamin B_2.[59] Topiramate was approved for migraine prevention after the publication of these guidelines and should also be included in group 1.

TENSION-TYPE HEADACHE

Patients with TTH usually self-medicate with over-the-counter analgesics, rarely seek medical attention, and may be at

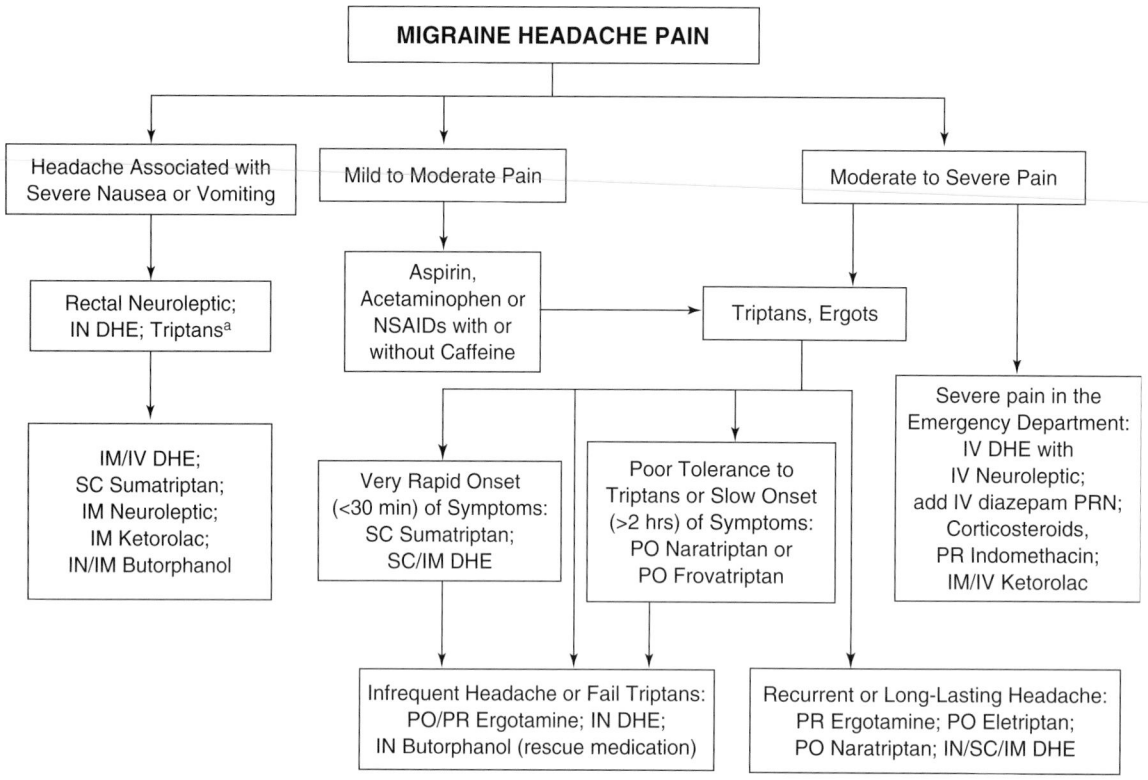

ᵃ Early onset of headache and gastrointestinal symptoms (15–60 min): IN zolmitriptan or sumatriptan; add antiemetic. Rizatriptan or zolmitriptan wafer formulations may be useful for patients who cannot swallow tablets.

FIGURE 61.2 Algorithm for the pharmacologic treatment of migraine headaches. Pharmacologic treatment is based on the headache's severity, the patient's concurrent symptoms and comorbid conditions, and the efficacy/adverse effect ratio and cost of medications. Parenteral, intranasal, or rectal preparations are also preferred when the pain intensifies in less than 1 hour. DHE, dihydroergotamine; NSAID, nonsteroidal anti-inflammatory drug. (Adapted from Wolf-Silberstein 2003; Olesen J, Tfelt-Hansen P, Welch KMA, eds. The headaches, 2nd ed. Philadelphia: Lippincott Williams & Wilkins, 2000; and Diamond S, Wenzel R. Practical approaches to migraine management. CNS Drugs 16:385–403, 2002.)

increased risk for chronic daily headache from medication overuse. First-line treatment consists of nonpharmacologic treatments followed by over-the-counter analgesics. Prescription analgesics may be used if the former fail. Preventive therapy is rarely needed but should be administered when a patient has frequent (>15 days per month) or long (>3 hours) headaches that produce disability or the need for frequent acute therapy. As patients with chronic TTH often have comorbid depression and anxiety, antidepressants are often used. Nonpharmacologic treatments and behavioral modification are important in minimizing the need for medication.[6,60]

CLUSTER HEADACHE

Since the oral absorption of most agents is generally slow, oral acute cluster headache treatment is ineffective. Effective acute treatments that provide rapid onset of action include oxygen inhalation, SC sumatriptan, IM/IV dihydroergotamine, or PO zolmitriptan (which is more lipophilic than sumatriptan). IN lidocaine is helpful as an adjunct. Although portable oxygen canisters are available, they are cumbersome.

Sumatriptan IN is not as effective as the SC form. Both IM and IV dihydroergotamine are used in a clinic setting. Although IN dihydroergotamine 1 mg decreased headache intensity, it did not prove effective in a double-blind trial. Higher doses may be needed, however, as another study found that 2 and 3 mg of IN dihydroergotamine were effective in reducing migraine headaches. Opioids are not usually indicated in the acute treatment of cluster headache because their efficacy is limited and frequent use may lead to addiction. Trials of zolmitriptan NS are ongoing.[7–10]

Ergotamine derivatives and corticosteroids are used as transitional treatment to break a cluster cycle before maintenance drugs take effect or to treat a refractory chronic cluster headache. Ergotamine products cannot be used within a 24-hour period after sumatriptan administration, one of the first choice options for acute treatment of cluster headaches, and should be given with caution, if at all, with methysergide, a preventive treatment, because of synergistic vasoconstriction. Corticosteroids work very quickly and do not aggravate side effects of other cluster treatments. To maximize effectiveness, they should be started early in a cluster period, continued until the patient is headache free for 2 weeks, and discontinued as a slow taper until they are needed for the next cluster period.[8,9]

Preventive treatment is usually started at the same time as the corticosteroid or ergotamine product. Most patients with cluster headaches require preventive treatment because each attack is too short in duration and too severe in intensity to be treated adequately with acute medication. Furthermore, failure to stop the headache quickly may result in months of suffering or medication overuse. Preventive therapies for cluster headaches include verapamil, methysergide, lithium, valproic acid, topiramate, melatonin, and topical capsaicin. If single-drug therapy fails, dual therapy with two of these agents may help. Refractory patients may benefit from repetitive IV dihydroergotamine in an inpatient setting over 3 days. Surgical options are reserved for patients who fail to respond to inpatient and outpatient treatments.[7–9]

Patients should be told to avoid naps, alcohol, prolonged exposure to volatile substances (i.e., solvents, gasoline, oil-based paint), excessive physical activity, and prolonged negative emotions (i.e., anger, hurt, anxiety). Patients should maintain a constant sleep–wake pattern. Patients who know that an attack will occur with high altitude may be able to prevent an attack by taking acetazolamide 250 mg twice daily 2 days prior to the exposure to high altitudes and for an additional 2 days.[7,8]

TREATMENT

PHARMACOTHERAPY

Drugs used for acute headache treatment include analgesics (alone or in combination with caffeine or barbiturates), opioids (alone or in combination with other drugs), isometheptene combinations, selective serotonin agonists (triptans), ergotamine derivatives, corticosteroids, neuroleptics, and antiemetics. Drugs used for preventive treatment include β-blockers, antidepressants, calcium channel blockers, serotonin antagonists, anticonvulsants, and lithium.[54] Practice guidelines were developed by the U.S. Headache Consortium (see the American Academy of Neurology website[59]) as well as by the American Academy of Family Physicians with the American College of Physicians-American Society of Internal Medicine.[61] Guidelines for acute and preventive headache treatment are described in Tables 61.6 and 61.7, respectively.

Some acute agents only provide analgesia, while others directly stop the migraine process. Patients should be treated as early as possible to improve treatment effectiveness. Acute agents are available in various routes of administration, and the choice of an agent should be individualized. A nonoral route of administration is a more appropriate choice if the time between headache onset and peak intensity is less than 1 hour or nausea and vomiting are present. A medication should be used for at least two attacks before deciding it is a failure, as the dose, formulation, or route may need to be

adjusted. Acute treatment should be restricted to 2 or 3 days a week to minimize the risk of drug overuse headache. The clinician should consider preventive treatments if excessive acute drug use occurs. Opioids or neuroleptics can be used as a rescue medication when other medications fail, and their use may prevent a visit to the physician.[4,54]

The criteria for preventive treatment include (1) more than two attacks a week (because of increased risk of drug overuse headache); (2) acute medication overuse; (3) contraindication to, ineffectiveness of, or troublesome adverse events with acute treatment; (4) migraine that interferes with a patient's daily routine despite acute treatment; (5) special circumstances, such as hemiplegic migraine or rare headache attacks that produce profound disruption or risk of permanent neurologic injury; or (6) patient preference. Preventive medication is usually given daily for months or years; however, treatment can be episodic, subacute, or chronic. It may be administered episodically when there is a known headache trigger, such as exercise or sexual activity. In such situations, patients are instructed to pretreat before exposure or activity. Patients who are undergoing a time-limited exposure to a trigger (high altitude ascent) or a reduced migraine threshold (menstruation) can be treated subacutely by medicating before and during the exposure. Patients with infrequent attacks are unlikely to receive sufficient benefit to justify the cost, side effects, and inconvenience of preventive treatment. When selecting a medication for preventive treatment, allow at least a 2- to 6-month trial of the medication. Combination therapy may be helpful for patients with refractory headaches. Combinations that work well together include (1) an antidepressant with a β-blocker, calcium channel blocker, valproic acid, or topiramate; (2) methysergide with a β-blocker or calcium channel blocker; or (3) a selective serotonin reuptake inhibitor (SSRI) with a tricyclic antidepressant (TCA).[4,54]

Drug choice depends on several factors, including the patient's headache type, comorbid conditions, and medication history, as well as each drug's pharmacologic profile. The medication selected should be started at a low dose and gradually increased to the dose necessary to achieve headache control or to the maximum recommended dose. Patients with migraine often respond to a lower dose of a drug than that recommended for other conditions, but they may also be more sensitive to the drug's adverse events. An adequate trial of preventive treatment may require 2 to 3 months before any relief is noticed. Once headache control has been achieved for 6 to 12 months, attempts should be made to slowly taper the drug over weeks and discontinue it if possible. Patients may continue to experience relief after discontinuing treatment; however, if they need to restart therapy, headache relief may be achieved with lower doses.[7,54]

Nonopioid Analgesics. Aspirin, acetaminophen, and other NSAIDs are used for acute treatment of migraines and TTH. They are indicated as first-line agents for the treatment

TABLE 61.6 | Acute Pharmacotherapy

Agent	Usual Adult Dose with Possible Repeat Dose prn	Maximum Daily Dose[a]	Time to Onset of Action	Headache	Comments
Ergot Alkaloids					
Dihydroergotamine					
IV	0.5–1 mg q8h	3 mg, 20 mg/week	<10 min	M,C	Useful for those who have early vomiting or headache recurrence. Do not use in pregnancy or patients with CAD, uncontrolled HTN, CVD, or PVD. Check for many drug interactions (i.e., triptans, β-blockers, methysergide, SSRIs).
IM	1 mg hourly	3 mg	30 min		
SC	1 mg hourly	3 mg	45 min		
IN	1 spray (0.5 mg) each nostril and repeat in 15 min. Can repeat again in 2 hrs	3 mg	<10 min		
Ergotamine				M,C	Onset of effect is variable. Onset is faster when given during the prodrome.
PO	2 mg	6 mg; 10 mg/week	30 min		
PR	2 mg	4 mg, 10 mg/week	<15 min		
SL	2 mg	6 mg; 10 mg/week	<30 min		
Selective Serotonin Agonists					
Sumatriptan				M	Triptans first line after analgesics fail. SC triptans are good for patients with early symptoms or vomiting. Triptans should be avoided in patients with pregnancy, CAD, CVD, or severe HTN. Do not use with ergots and space 2 weeks from MAOI if triptan metabolized by MAO. Check drug interactions if metabolized by CYP450.
SC	6 mg	12 mg	10–15 min	M,C	
PO	50–100 mg	300 mg	30–90 min	M	
IN	5–20 mg	40 mg	15–20 min	M	
Zolmitriptan				M,C	Oral disintegrating tablet helpful in patients with nausea.
PO	2.5–5.0 mg	10 mg	45–60 min		
IN	5 mg	10 mg	15–30 min		
Naratriptan PO	1–2.5 mg, may repeat once in 4 hrs	5 mg, or 2.5 mg in renal dysfunction	60–180 min	M	Prevention of menstrual migraine. Slower effect but better tolerability. Good for patients who have headache recurrence.
Rizatriptan PO	5–10 mg, may repeat twice, each time separated by 2 hours	30 mg	30–120 min	M	Disintegrating tablet formulation may benefit patients with nausea and vomiting. Reduce dose in patients taking propranolol.
Frovatriptan PO	2.5–5 mg, may repeat in 4 hrs	7.5 mg	120–180 min	M	Slower effect but better tolerability.
Almotriptan PO	6.25–12.5 mg, may repeat in 2 hrs	25 mg	60–180 min	M	
Eletriptan PO	20–40 mg, may repeat in 2 hours	80 mg	30–60 min	M	Good for patients who have headache recurrence.

Drug / Route	Dose	Maximum dose	Peak analgesia	Category	Comments
Opioid Analgesics					
Butorphanol					
IN	1 mg	8 mg	15 min	M	Opioids are good as rescue medication. Avoid in patients with risk of abuse. Less abuse potential with butorphanol than other opioids.
IM	2 mg	4 mg	10 min	M	
Hydromorphone PO	2–4 mg	16 mg	15–30 min	M	
Meperidine			*Peak analgesia*		
IV	75–100 mg	400 mg	20 min		
IM	75–100 mg	400 mg	30–50 min		
PO	300 mg	400 mg	60 min	M	
Morphine			*Peak analgesia*		
IV	5–10 mg q4h	b	20 min		
IM	5–10 mg q4h	b	30–60 min		
PR	10 mg q4h	b	20–60 min		
PO	30–60 mg q4h	60 mg	60 min	M	
Nonopioid Analgesics					
Aspirin PO	325–1000 mg, repeat 4 hrs	4	30 min	M,T	Avoid all analgesics in patients with bleeding disorders, kidney disease, gastritis, or PUD. Good in patients with CAD or TIA.
PR	300–600 mg	4	5 min		
Acetaminophen PO, PR	325–1000 mg, repeat q4h prn	4000 mg	60 min	M,T	Not effective alone. Avoid in patients with liver disease.
Ibuprofen PO	400–600 mg, repeat in 1–2 hrs	2400 mg	60 min	M,T	Ibuprofen may have fewer GI side effects than other NSAIDs.
Naproxen sodium PO	825 mg, may repeat 500 mg in 1 hour	1375 mg	<1 hr	M,T	Need to monitor renal function. Limit use to 5 days total. As good as chlorpromazine 25 mg IV. Inferior to meperidine. IM reserved for physician-supervised setting.
Ketorolac PO	10 mg, repeat q6h	40 mg	60 min	M,T	
IM	30–60 mg	90 mg	45–60 min		
Celecoxib PO	100–400 mg	800 mg		M,T	Potential CV safety issues only with long-term daily use.
Neuroleptics					
Chlorpromazine PO	10–50 mg TID	150 mg	60 min	M,T	Good for antiemetic and additive analgesic effect and rescue. Monitor for orthostatic hypotension and cardiac rhythm changes. Avoid neuroleptics in patients with Parkinson's disease or prolonged QTc.
IV	2.5–10 mg, repeat q6h	300 mg	15–30 min		

(continued)

TABLE 61.6	continued				
Agent	Usual Adult Dose with Possible Repeat Dose prn	Maximum Daily Dose[a]	Time to Onset of Action	Headache	Comments
IM	25–100 mg, repeat q6h	300 mg	15–30 min		
PR	25–100 mg	400 mg	15–30 min		
Prochlorperazine					
IV/IM	5–10 mg	40 mg	10–20 min	M,T	Antiemetic effect. Monitor for dizziness and drowsiness.
PR	25 mg	75 mg	60 min	M	
Thiothixene					
PO	5 mg	20 mg			
IM	5 mg	20 mg			
Corticosteroids					
Dexamethasone PO	4–8 mg; repeat in 60 min	32 mg		M,C	Used for intractable migraines
Prednisone PO	40–100 mg	200 mg		M,C	Short courses, then rapidly taper over 2 to 3 weeks
Miscellaneous Agents					
Lidocaine IN	1 mL of 4% solution every 15–30 min × 2 doses		15–30 min	M,C	Proper administration is imperative to get full benefit. Head must be lower than body >45 degrees.
Oxygen	7–10 L/min for 15–30 min IH		5–10 min	C	More effective when given at maximum pain intensity
Clonidine PO	0.2 mg	0.6 mg		M	Adjunct for drug detoxification
Metoclopramide					
PO	10 mg 5–10 min before or with simple analgesics		30 min	M	Gastrokinetic agent. Limit use to no more than 3 days/week.
IV			30 min		

[a] To prevent drug overuse headaches, patients should not use abortive agents more than 2–3 days per week.
[b] Depends on individual.

C, cluster headaches; CAD, coronary heart disease; CVD, cerebral vascular disease; GI, gastrointestinal; HTN, hypertension; IH, inhalation; IM, intramuscular; IN, intranasal; IV, intravenous; M, migraine headaches; MAOI, monoamine oxidase inhibitor; NSAID, nonsteroidal antiinflammatory agent; PO, oral; PR, rectal; PUD, peptic ulcer disease; PVD, peripheral vascular disease; SC, subcutaneous; SL, sublingual; SSRI, selective serotonin reuptake inhibitor; T, tension-type headaches; TIA, transient ischemic attack; TID, three times daily.

(From Silberstein SD, Lipton RB. Chronic daily headache, including transformed migraine, chronic tension-type headache, and medication overuse. In: Silberstein SD, Lipton RB, Dalessio DJ, eds. Wolff's headache and other head pain, 7th ed. New York: Oxford University Press, 2001:247–282; Silberstein SD. Migraine. Lancet 363:381–391, 2004; Olesen J, Tfelt-Hansen P, Welch KMA, eds. The headaches, 2nd ed. Philadelphia: Lippincott Williams & Wilkins, 2000.)

TABLE 61.7	Preventive Pharmacotherapy				
Drug	Starting Dose (mg/day)	Maximum Dose (mg/day)	Headache	Clinical Efficacy/ ADR Ratio[a]	Comments
β-Blockers					
Atenolol	25	200	M, T	2/2	β-Blockers are useful for patients with anxiety, HTN, and angina. Avoid blockers in patients with asthma, depression, CHF, diabetes, or Raynaud's disease. Maximal benefit may be delayed for 2–3 months. Begin with low doses and increase gradually. Monitor BP, pulse, lipids, and heart function.
Metoprolol	50	300	M, T	3/2	
Nadolol	20	240	M, T	3/2	
Propranolol[b]	40	320	M, T	3/2	
Timolol	10	30	M, T	1/2	
Calcium Channel Blockers					
Verapamil	120	720	M, T, C	2/2	Calcium channel blockers are useful for patients with prolonged aura, HTN, or angina. Monitor BP, pulse, lipids, constipation, and heart function. Higher doses needed for cluster headaches.
Nimodipine	120	360	C	2/2	
Diltiazem	90	360	M, C	0/2	
Serotonin Antagonists					
Cyproheptadine	2	16	M	1/5	Very commonly used in children. Antihistamine activity. Monitor for weight gain, sedation, and urinary retention. Fibrotic changes, requires drug holidays. Avoid in patients with angina or PVD.
Methysergide	1 mg q3d	12	M, T, C	3/5	
Antidepressants[2]					
Amitriptyline	10	300	M, T	3/5	TCAs useful for patients with depression, insomnia, OCD, anxiety, and pain syndromes. Monitor for anticholinergic effects and weight gain. Amitriptyline has the most and nortriptyline has the fewest anticholinergic effects.
Doxepin	10	150	M, T	1/5	
Imipramine	10	200	M, T	1/5	
Nortriptyline	10	125	M, T	3/5	
Protriptyline	10	60	M, T	2/5	MAOIs require close medical supervision and dietary restrictions.
Phenelzine	30	90	M, T	3/5	
Fluoxetine	10	80	M, T	1/3	SSRIs have fewer anticholinergic effects but more insomnia than TCAs.
Sertraline	25	100	M, T	1/3	
Venlafaxine	37.5	225	M	1/3	SNRI
Anticonvulsants					
Valproic acid/ divalproex[b]	250	3000	M, T, C	3/4	Valproic acid is useful in patients with mania, epilepsy, and anxiety. Avoid in liver disease and bleeding disorders. Divalproex has fewer GI effects than valproic acid. Monitor weight gain, LFTs, platelets, and bleeding time.
Topiramate	15	200	M, C	2/4	Topiramate is useful in patients with mania, epilepsy, and anxiety. Avoid in patients at risk for kidney stones, problems with cognitive impairment, intolerant of weight loss.
Nonopioid Analgesics					
Ibuprofen	800	2400	M	1/1	NSAIDs useful for patients with menstrual migraine or other pain disorders. Avoid in patients with PUD, bleeding, disorders, or kidney disease.
Naproxen	500	1500	M	1/1	
Corticosteroids					
Prednisone	40	100	C		For episodic cluster headaches and migraine status. Taper dose over 1–2 weeks.
Ergot Alkaloids					
Ergotamine	2	4	C		Avoid in M and chronic C because of rebound headache risk.
Methylergonovine	0.6	2	M,C		Preventive treatment in place of methysergide.

(continued)

| TABLE 61.7 | continued | | | | |

Drug	Starting Dose (mg/day)	Maximum Dose (mg/day)	Headache	Clinical Efficacy/ ADR Ratio[a]	Comments
Miscellaneous Agents with Promise					
Magnesium	400	600	M, T	1/1	Preventive treatment, questionable efficacy.
Riboflavin	400	400	M, T	2/1	Preventive treatment, some evidence for efficacy.
Botulinum toxin A (IM)	50 units	150 units	M, T		Injection-site discomfort, muscle weakness, and skin rash.

[a] Efficacy rating (0, ineffective, 1, somewhat effective, 2, effective, 3, very effective). ADR (adverse effect rating) (1, infrequent, 2, infrequent to occasional, 3, occasional, 4, occasional to frequent, 5, frequent).

[b] These agents are grouped under medications with the high efficacy and mild to moderate severity of ADRs based on the experience of the U.S. Headache Consortium.

BP, blood pressure; C, cluster headaches; CHF, congestive heart failure; GI, gastrointestinal; HTN, hypertension; IM, intramuscular; M, migraine headaches; MAOIs, monoamine oxidase inhibitors; NSAIDs, nonsteroidal antiinflammatory agents; OCD, obsessive-compulsive disorder; PUD, peptic ulcer disease; PVD, peripheral vascular disease; SNRI, selective norepinephrine reuptake inhibitors; SSRI, selective serotonin reuptake inhibitor; T, tension-type headaches; TCA, tricyclic antidepressant; LFTs, liver function tests.

(Adapted from Silberstein SD, Lipton RB. Chronic daily headache, including transformed migraine, chronic tension-type headache, and medication overuse. In: Silberstein SD, Lipton RB, Dalessio DJ, eds. Wolff's headache and other head pain, 7th ed. New York: Oxford University Press, 2001:247–282; Silberstein SD. Migraine. Lancet 363:381–391, 2004; Olesen J, Tfelt-Hansen P, Welch KMA, eds. The headaches, 2nd ed. Philadelphia: Lippincott Williams & Wilkins, 2000; and Silberstein SD. American Academy of Neurology practice parameter: evidence-based guidelines for migraine headache (an evidence-based review). Report of the quality standards subcommittee of the American Academy of Neurology, http://www.aan.com/professionals/practice/guideline/index.cfm.)

of mild to moderate migraine and are also helpful for menstrual migraine. Patients not responding to one agent may respond to another.

Nonopioid analgesics most likely decrease neurogenic inflammation and headaches by inhibiting prostaglandin synthesis or cyclooxygenase (COX-1 and COX-2 subtypes). Some NSAIDs (ketoprofen, indomethacin, diclofenac) also decrease leukotriene synthesis by inhibiting 5-lipo-oxygenase. In addition, NSAIDs interfere with several membrane-associated processes and cell adhesion molecules and have a direct desensitization effect on neurons.[54]

Aspirin, ibuprofen, naproxen, tolfenamic acid, and rofecoxib were more effective than placebo in the treatment of migraine headaches. Aspirin alone was inferior to ergotamine but in combination with metoclopramide was equivalent to PO sumatriptan in the treatment of migraine headaches. Rofecoxib was approved by the Food and Drug Administration for the treatment of migraine with or without aura, but it was withdrawn from the market in September 2004 because the drug had an increased risk of heart attack and stroke. Anecdotal evidence indicates that the other COX-2-specific NSAIDs, celecoxib and valdecoxib, may also be helpful in the treatment of migraine. Ketoprofen, naproxen, and tolfenamic acid have been shown to be equivalent to ergots in the treatment of migraine headaches. The more lipid-soluble NSAIDs, such as indomethacin or ketoprofen, may be more efficacious owing to greater CNS penetration.[62] Long-acting NSAIDs may have less risk of rebound headaches[62] and may be useful for treating patients who abuse ergotamine. Indomethacin and aspirin suppositories or ketorolac injections may be helpful for patients with nausea or vomiting. Ketoprofen IM may be useful in a clinic

setting. If needed, patients can repeat their analgesic dose in 1 to 2 hours as long as the maximum dose has not been reached. NSAIDs should not be taken continuously for more than 1 week for menstrual migraine (ketorolac must be limited to 5 days in any situation), and otherwise they should be limited to three times per week.[7,54]

Adverse reactions to nonopioid analgesics include GI upset, GI bleeding, peptic ulcers, abdominal pain, dizziness, fluid retention, sedation, and tinnitus. Aspirin should be avoided by patients with peptic ulcer disease or hematologic disorders, and by children less than 15 years of age. NSAIDs should be avoided by patients experiencing nausea and vomiting and are relatively contraindicated for patients with gastritis, peptic ulcer disease, or kidney disease. Patients should be told to take NSAIDs with meals to minimize adverse GI effects. They should be monitored for potential GI blood loss, renal dysfunction, hepatic dysfunction, worsening of hypertension, and aggravation of colitis.[54]

Opioid Analgesics. Opioids are useful for patients who have intractable menstrual migraine, have contraindications to other migraine medications (i.e., pregnancy), require rescue medication (failed ergot or triptan), or suffer from severe nightly headaches. Although these agents are not first-line agents for acute cluster headache therapy, nonparenteral opioid analgesics play a role in relieving cluster headaches, particularly in patients who cannot use ergots or sumatriptan. Opioids should not be used more than an average of 2 days per week. Dependence and the risk of rebound headaches after abrupt opioid discontinuation occur within 2 to 3 weeks of regular use; therefore, doses should be slowly reduced when therapy is discontinued. Combination preparations containing nonopioid analgesics, caffeine, and intermediate-acting barbiturates possess a similar abuse and rebound potential.[63,64]

The analgesic action of opioids is related to their action at the mu, kappa, and sigma opioid receptors that are located on neurons at supraspinal and spinal levels. Opioids may also produce peripheral analgesia by modulating neuropeptide release from receptor endings.

The efficacy of opioid analgesics in migraine headache treatment is poorly documented in the literature. Meperidine with hydroxyzine was no better than butorphanol IM or ketorolac IM but was less effective than dihydroergotamine with metoclopramide. Meperidine with dimenhydrinate was less effective than chlorpromazine IV. Meperidine with promethazine was no better than ketorolac or dihydroergotamine with metoclopramide. The nasal formulation of butorphanol is more effective than placebo and has a faster onset of action than IM methadone in patients with moderate to severe migraine. Although butorphanol (IN) was originally marketed for patient self-treatment of migraines, many physicians now feel that it should be reserved for refractory cases, as patients have developed physical and emotional dependence to this agent.[7,54]

The most common adverse events of opioids are sedation, nausea, and vomiting; however, psychiatric reactions have been reported. Butorphanol has an adverse event profile similar to that of most other opioids, but it is extremely sedating. In general, opioids should not be used when patients have a history of abuse potential. Opioids should be used only if the risk of abuse and sedation has been assessed.[7,54]

Combination Analgesic Preparations.

Combination products are used when patients do not respond to simple analgesics. Combination analgesics may have some advantages, as they can enhance efficacy and lessen adverse events. Prudent use of combination analgesics is very effective in stopping or reducing the severity of TTH. Patients with a history of coronary artery disease or transient ischemic attacks have limited choices for migraine relief, and combination analgesics are a good choice for them.[54]

Aspirin and acetaminophen are often combined with butalbital, caffeine, isometheptene mucate, and other opioids (codeine, propoxyphene, dihydrocodeine, hydrocodone, or oxycodone). Butalbital helps reduce anxiety and aids in sleep; however, some feel that the potential additive benefit of barbiturates is outweighed by its adverse events. Caffeine enhances drug absorption and may enhance analgesia,[65] but overuse may lead to chronic daily headache. Isometheptene mucate is a sympathomimetic amine that constricts blood vessels and it is combined with acetaminophen and dichloralphenazone, a tranquilizer (Midrin). A combination product containing acetaminophen, aspirin, and caffeine was superior to placebo in the treatment of migraine headaches.[66] Acute use of acetaminophen should be limited to 4000 mg per day for less than 10 days, and chronic use should be limited to less than 2600 mg per day. Combination product

use should be limited to two or three times per week to minimize drug overuse headaches.[54]

Selective Serotonin Agonists (Triptans).

There are currently seven triptan agents available in the United States: sumatriptan, zolmitriptan, naratriptan, rizatriptan, eletriptan, almotriptan, and frovatriptan. These are indicated for the acute treatment of moderate to severe migraine when analgesics have failed. They are not indicated during the aura phase. Sumatriptan SC and zolmitriptan PO are also indicated for the treatment of cluster headaches. All triptans are available in tablet formulations. Zolmitriptan and sumatriptan are available in an IN formulation that works within 15 minutes, more quickly than the standard tablets. Sumatriptan is also available in SC injection, and a rectal form is marketed in Europe. Rizatriptan and zolmitriptan are also available as a rapidly dissolving oral wafer tablet, which is helpful for those who are nauseated and do not want to drink water, but they do not work any faster than the tablets.[54,67]

Triptans relieve headaches by causing vasoconstriction of the pain-producing intracranial blood vessels by activation of 5-HT_{1B} receptors, inhibiting vasoactive neuropeptide release from trigeminal perivascular nerves by activation of 5-HT_{1D} receptors, and interrupting pain signal transmission through the trigeminocervical complex within the brain stem and upper cervical spinal cord by either 5-HT_{1B} or 5-HT_{1D} receptors.[68–70]

The pharmacokinetic properties of triptans are shown in Table 61.8. Triptans exhibit variable oral absorption, with almotriptan being the most bioavailable. The contents of rizatriptan and zolmitriptan wafers are not absorbed through the buccal cavity, but rather swallowed with the saliva and absorbed later in the GI system, so their onset time is similar to the tablet formulations. Zolmitriptan nasal spray is absorbed in the nasopharynx and is detected in the blood within 5 minutes following administration. The triptans are not highly protein bound. All triptans undergo hepatic biotransformation. Naratriptan, frovatriptan, and eletriptan are metabolized via cytochrome P-450, while the rest of the triptans undergo some monoamine oxidase (MAO_A) metabolism. More than half of the triptan metabolites are excreted into the urine, with 50% of the naratriptan dose being excreted unchanged in the urine. The half-life of naratriptan is approximately twice that of the other agents.

Some drugs, but not food, affect the pharmacokinetic properties of oral triptans. Oral contraceptives increase plasma naratriptan concentrations, whereas smoking decreases plasma naratriptan concentrations. Propranolol increases the plasma concentrations of rizatriptan (limiting the dose) and zolmitriptan. Cimetidine increases zolmitriptan concentrations. Eletriptan interacts with CYP3A4 inhibitors. Pharmacodynamic drug interactions with triptans are also important. Triptans should not be administered within 24 hours of treatment with an ergot alkaloid, methysergide, or another triptan. Serotonin syndrome (weakness, hyperreflexia, and poor coordination) may rarely occur when trip-

TABLE 61.8	Comparisons of Oral Triptans						
	Sumatriptan	**Naratriptan**	**Zolmitriptan**	**Rizatriptan**	**Frovatriptan**	**Almotriptan**	**Eletriptan**
Bioavailability (%)	14	60–70	40–50	45	20–30	70–80	50 (increased with fatty meal)
T_{max} during headache (hrs)	2.0–2.5[a]	2–4[a]	2–3[a]	1–1.5[b]	2–4[c]	1–4[c]	1–2.8[a]
Volume of distribution (L/kg)	2.4	2.5	7.0	2.0	3–4	2.5	2.0
Lipophilicity	Low	High	Moderate	Moderate	Low	Moderate	High
Half-life (hrs)	2.5	6	3	2–3	26	3–4	4, 6 in elderly
Metabolism	MAO$_A$	CYP450	MAO$_A$ CYP1A2	MAO$_A$	CYP1A2	MAO$_A$ CYP3A4, CYP2D6,	CYP3A4
Active metabolite	No	No	Yes	Yes	No	No	Yes
Renally excreted unchanged (%)	3	50	8	14	30	40–65	10
Therapeutic gain at 2 hrs (%)[d]	24–43	17–27	27–47	23–40	27–44	14–36	27–48
Pain-free therapeutic gain at 2 hours (%)[d]	12–24	11–17	14–33	20–33	NA	17–25	18–33
Headache recurrence in 24 hrs (%)	27–33	13–28	25–43	35–42	7–25	22–30	12–28

[a] The range indicates a shorter Tmax for patients without acute pain and a longer Tmax in patients with acute pain.

[b] Longer peak (1.6–2.5 hr) with wafer form of rizatriptan, but Tmax is not different with pain status.

[c] Food increased frovatriptan peak at 1 hr; pain status not discussed for frovatriptan and almotriptan.

[d] Difference between active drug and placebo. Range using all dose forms, with slightly higher response rates at higher doses.

NA, not available; T_{max}, Time to maximum concentration.

(Adapted from Olesen J, Tfelt-Hansen P, Welch KMA, eds. The headaches, 2nd ed. Philadelphia: Lippincott Williams & Wilkins, 2000; Silberstein SD. American Academy of Neurology practice parameter: evidence-based guidelines for migraine headache (an evidence-based review). Report of the quality standards subcommittee of the American Academy of Neurology, http://www.aan.com/professionals/practice/guideline/index.cfm; Rapaport AM, Tepper SJ, Bigal ME, et al. The triptan formulation. How to match patients and products. CNS Drugs 17:431–447, 2003; Diamond S, Wenzel R. Practical approaches to migraine management. CNS Drugs 16:385–403, 2002; and Adelman JU, Belsey J. Meta-analysis of oral triptan therapy for acute migraine: number needed to treat and relative cost to achieve relief within 2 hours. J Manag Care Pharm 9:483–90, 2003.)

tans and SSRIs are coadministered (some experts doubt that this syndrome ever occurs). Triptan therapy (except naratriptan) should not commence sooner than 2 weeks after MAO$_A$ inhibitor treatment discontinuation.[4,7,67]

SC sumatriptan offers the fastest onset of pain relief. Headache relief starts within 10 minutes of injection, and migraine pain is reduced or completely relieved in 70% of patients within 1 hour and in 86% of patients within 2 hours. PO sumatriptan is not as effective at relieving headache pain as SC sumatriptan. SC sumatriptan also ameliorates nausea, vomiting, photophobia, and phonophobia and is effective in the treatment of perioperative migraine, menstrual migraine, and early morning migraine. Smaller doses (2 to 4 mg) provide headache relief in 70% of patients with TTH and coexistent migraine, albeit with a slower onset of action (60 minutes). SC sumatriptan also effectively relieves cluster headaches, often producing benefit 5 to 7 minutes after administration. Headache relief at 1 and 2 hours was better with SC sumatriptan than with SC dihydroergotamine or IN dihydroergotamine. Recurrence rates, however, were lower with dihydroergotamine. Patients who received SC sumatriptan reported more side effects than those on IN dihydroergotamine but fewer side effects than SC dihydroergotamine.[67,71]

Sumatriptan administered SC has a faster onset of action than when given IN, with PO administration providing the slowest onset of action. Two hours after sumatriptan administration, the efficacy of a 20-mg nasal spray (62% to 78%) is slightly better than that of a 100-mg oral tablet (51% to 69%), comparable to that of a 25-mg suppository (68%), and equivalent to that of a 6-mg SC injection (62% to 85%).[71]

Although sumatriptan has the advantage of the fast-acting SC form, the newer oral triptans have some advantages over sumatriptan. Oral sumatriptan was inferior to oral eletriptan and oral rizatriptan in relieving headaches at 2 hours. Because rizatriptan has a faster onset of action, 15% to 30% more patients receiving rizatriptan than those taking sumatriptan are expected to reach headache relief at 2 hours. Oral eletriptan was more effective in relieving migraine headaches than ergotamine with caffeine (Cafergot). A meta-analysis indicated that almotriptan, eletriptan, and rizatriptan were the most cost-effective options in relieving headache pain. Naratriptan, frovatriptan, or eletriptan may be a good choice for those with recurring headaches, as these triptans have a lower headache recurrence rate, perhaps because of their longer half-life. The benefit of naratriptan and frovatriptan's lower risk of recurrence may be outweighed by its slower onset and the fact that a second dose of the triptan can be administered during the 8 to 12 hours that a recurrent headache is most likely to occur. If one triptan does not work, another may. Adding an NSAID to the triptan may improve response.[4,5,54,67]

Many patients who initially respond to sumatriptan report that headache symptoms return within 24 to 48 hours after dosing. In addition, approximately half of patients who take an oral triptan for migraine may require an additional dose or other relief medication 24 hours after the initial dose. Repeated administration of SC sumatriptan is not recommended for those with no response, although those with a partial response may receive an additional dose within a 24-hour interval. An IN sumatriptan dose may be repeated once in 2 hours if the headache persists. A dose-related increase in migraine relief is seen with doses up to 40 mg, suggesting a ceiling effect or saturation of the nasal mucosa.[67,71]

SC sumatriptan has the highest incidence of adverse events, while all oral triptans have a similar incidence of adverse events. Sumatriptan resulted in more adverse events than aspirin with metoclopramide. Less than 10% of patients receiving zolmitriptan, naratriptan, or rizatriptan discontinue treatment after a year as a result of adverse events. Triptans can cause coronary artery vasospasm and should be used cautiously by patients with coronary artery disease, peripheral vascular disease, or uncontrolled hypertension, patients at risk for these disorders, or those older than 40 years of age. Chest pressure is reported in about 4% of patients. A pretreatment electrocardiogram is suggested in patients over 40 or those with cardiac risk factors. Administering the first dose in the doctor's office may be helpful. Other adverse events include atypical sensations (paresthesia or warm feelings), pain sensations (neck, jaw, or chest pressure, pain, or tightness), GI symptoms (dry mouth and nausea), and neurologic symptoms (dizziness or somnolence). Administration of sumatriptan IN may lead to taste disturbances, nausea, and nasal discomfort, while SC sumatriptan causes injection-site pain, flushing, dizziness, and paresthesia. Triptans should be avoided by patients with coronary artery disease, diabetes, vascular disease, cerebrovascular disease, uncontrolled hypertension, prolonged aura, basilar migraine, or hemiplegic migraine.[7,54,67]

Nonselective Serotonin Agonists. Ergots are used for both acute and preventive treatment of migraine and cluster headaches. These agents effectively reduce the intensity and duration of attacks and are used to treat moderate to severe migraines when simple analgesics fail. Preventive ergot use, however, should be reserved for patients with menstrual migraine and cluster headaches and should be used at the beginning of a cycle. Ergotamine is available as sublingual, oral, or suppository dosage forms. The sublingual route of administration is the least effective, and the rectal route is the most effective. Ergotamine is also available in combination with caffeine.

Dihydroergotamine, an ergot derivative, is generally preferred over ergotamine because it causes less nausea (except when given IV) and rarely causes rebound headaches. It can be administered SC, IM, IV, or IN. Although the parenteral forms of dihydroergotamine are slightly more effective than the IN formulation, they cause more adverse events and are

limited to a clinic setting and should be administered with an antiemetic. Combining dihydroergotamine with prochlorperazine or metoclopramide improves efficacy.[7,54] Repetitive IV dihydroergotamine with metoclopramide or a neuroleptic is highly effective in treating chronic daily headache, status migrainosus, and cluster headache.

In contrast to the triptans, ergot alkaloids are nonspecific serotonergic ($5-HT_{1A}$, $5-HT_{1B}$, $5-HT_{1C}$, $5-HT_{1D}$, and $5-HT_{1F}$), adrenergic (α agonist and antagonist), and dopaminergic receptor agonists. Ergots also cause arterial and venous vasoconstriction, decrease platelet aggregation, and decrease neurogenic inflammation. Dihydroergotamine, a less potent vasoconstrictor, has a greater effect on venous capacitance vessels than on arterial resistance vessels and is a more potent α-adrenergic agonist.[7,54]

Ergotamine has been available for many years and is used as a reference standard in controlled trials of newer agents. Oral ergotamine (1 to 6 mg) was equivalent or superior to placebo, aspirin, isometheptene, and various NSAIDs, but not as good as oral sumatriptan. Likewise, ergotamine with caffeine was less effective than eletriptan.[7,72,73]

IV dihydroergotamine with metoclopramide was superior to placebo, meperidine with hydroxyzine, and butorphanol. Another study found that dihydroergotamine was superior to lidocaine but inferior to chlorpromazine. Dihydroergotamine can also be self-administered via SC injection, and 45% of patients interviewed after 2 to 3 years of self-administered IM dihydroergotamine had at least a 50% response. SC dihydroergotamine has a slower onset of action but is as effective as SC sumatriptan, with less headache recurrence, as headaches recur in fewer than 20% of patients treated with dihydroergotamine.[7,72–74]

Dihydroergotamine IN is as effective as oral ergotamine tartrate with caffeine but inferior to SC and IN sumatriptan in relieving migraine attacks. Dihydroergotamine nasal spray may not be as good as IV dihydroergotamine in relieving acute cluster headache. After 2 mg of IN dihydroergotamine, patients reported 65% headache relief at 2 hours and 70% relief at 4 hours. About 14% of responders report headache recurrence. Increasing the dose beyond 2 mg does not increase efficacy.[72,73,75]

Rectal ergotamine absorption is more complete and less erratic than oral. Dihydroergotamine absorption is most erratic with SC injection. The bioavailability of dihydroergotamine is 100% after IM administration, but only 40% after IN administration and less than 1% after oral, owing to extensive first-pass hepatic metabolism.[7,76] Ergotamine and dihydroergotamine are primarily metabolized in the liver, with a clearance about equal to hepatic blood flow. Ergotamine's elimination half-life is 3 hours, with a terminal half-life of approximately 21 hours. Dihydroergotamine's half-life is approximately 10 hours, and it has an active metabolite that is present at plasma concentrations five to seven times higher than those of the parent drug. Dosage schemes are individualized for each patient, starting with the lowest dose and increasing to the highest dose that does not cause nausea.[7]

Oral or rectal administration of antiemetics 15 to 30 minutes before ergotamine administration decreases the associated nausea.

Ergotamine's adverse events include nausea, vomiting, abdominal discomfort, peripheral vasoconstriction, thirst, pruritus, vertigo, muscle cramps, and paresthesias. Chronic ergotamine use can lead to vasospasm, anorectal ulcers, ischemic neuropathy, fibrotic disorders, and drug-induced headache. Ergotamine overuse can also cause medication overuse headaches in migraineurs, and clinicians often restrict its use to less than two doses a week, except in patients with cluster headache, who may use ergots nightly at the beginning of a cycle as a preventive measure. Overdose or prolonged use can cause ergotism and cyanosis, claudication, or gangrene of limbs. Symptoms of ergotism include nausea, confusion, drowsiness, postural hypotension, vasospasm, distal paresthesias, and coldness of the extremities. Ergotism should be treated with a vasodilator for 24 hours. Both ergotamine and dihydroergotamine should be used with caution in patients with coronary artery disease, peripheral vascular disease, or uncontrolled hypertension. They are contraindicated for pregnant patients or patients with sepsis, renal failure, or hepatic failure. Ergots are associated with higher rates of adverse events (nausea and vomiting) than sumatriptan, isometheptene, and NSAIDs.[7,54,72]

Dihydroergotamine's adverse events include burning at the injection site, dizziness, paresthesias, abdominal cramps, and chest tightness. Administration of IN dihydroergotamine may cause nausea (less than ergotamine), a bitter taste, and local irritation of the nose and throat. Patients who have cardiac risk factors or are older than 40 years of age should have an electrocardiogram before receiving the first ergot dose. Some feel that ergots should not be given to patients who have an aura lasting more than 30 minutes, because patients have decreased CBF during the aura and ergots can cause constriction of small cerebral arteries that could lead to arterial vasospasm.[7,53,72]

The risk of ergot-induced adverse events may be increased with concurrent use of CYP3A4 inhibitors, methysergide, β-blockers, dopamine, erythromycin derivatives, and sumatriptan. Coadministration with CYP3A4 inhibitors is contraindicated as it increases dihydroergotamine concentrations and increases the risk of life-threatening vasospasm and peripheral ischemia. To avoid excessive vasoconstriction, patients should wait at least 6 hours after a sumatriptan dose before taking an ergot preparation. Use should be limited to 2 days a week. Contraindications to ergots include renal or hepatic failure, pregnancy, hypertension, sepsis, and vascular disease (coronary, cerebral, or peripheral).[7,54,72]

Corticosteroids. Corticosteroids may decrease perivascular inflammation or affect the hypothalamic-pituitary axis. They are used in episodic and chronic cluster headaches as well as status migrainosus. IV corticosteroids may be used in combination with neuroleptics, opioids, metoclopramide, or dihydroergotamine to treat refractory migraine headaches. Parenteral corticosteroids may be beneficial as monotherapy when ergot preparations are contraindicated or have failed. Steroids are believed to be effective even when patients have had symptoms for a few days and have not responded to other migraine medications.[7,54]

Corticosteroids are the fastest acting of the cluster headache therapies, with responses occurring in 1 to 2 days. They are only used as initial therapy for less than a month to break the cluster headache cycle until other medications with slower onset of action can take effect. The most commonly used steroids for episodic cluster headaches are prednisone (up to 100 mg/day) and dexamethasone (4 mg twice daily) administered for 2 to 3 weeks in tapering doses. Prednisone produces marked relief in 77% of episodic cluster headache patients and partial improvement in another 12%. Steroids improve chronic cluster headaches in 40% of patients.[8,9,77]

Adverse events include insomnia, mood changes, hyponatremia, hyperglycemia, osteoporosis, and gastric ulcers. Episodic and chronic cluster headaches may recur when steroids are discontinued. Steroids are relatively contraindicated in patients with hypertension, peptic ulcer disease, diabetes, and diverticulosis.[9,77] Additional information regarding corticosteroid pharmacotherapy and monitoring is given in Chapter 65.

Neuroleptics. Phenothiazines are the neuroleptics most commonly used to treat acute migraine, TTH, and status migrainosus. These agents antagonize dopamine, decrease 5-HT reuptake, produce anticholinergic events, and block α-adrenergic receptors (which induces orthostatic hypotension). The dopaminergic blockade is responsible for the drug's beneficial antiemetic effect and undesirable extrapyramidal symptoms. IV injections of chlorpromazine or prochlorperazine are 50% to 80% effective in relieving migraine headaches.[7] Although this route of administration is more effective than the IM or rectal route, it carries a greater risk for orthostatic hypotension.[78] The pharmacokinetics of neuroleptic agents are very similar to those of the antidepressants, and some (chlorpromazine, thioridazine, and haloperidol) also have active metabolites. Droperidol, a neuroleptic related to haloperidol, had been shown in open trials to be an effective antimigraine agent when given IM or IV.[79] Placebo-controlled double-blind trials have now proven it to be effective.[80]

Patients may experience adverse events after parenteral injections of phenothiazines. Effects include drowsiness, postural hypotension, and akathisia.[7] Additional information regarding neuroleptic pharmacotherapy and monitoring is described in Chapter 54.

β-Blockers. β-Blockers are approximately 50% effective in producing a 50% reduction in migraine attack frequency and severity. Their action is most likely related to the inhibition of β1-receptors, with secondary effects on serotonin. β-Blockers with intrinsic sympathomimetic activity (ISA), such as pindolol, alprenolol, or acebutolol, are less effective in the treatment of migraine. β-Blockers are particularly useful for patients with anxiety, hypertension, or angina. The relative efficacy between the agents in this class (propranolol, metoprolol, timolol, nadolol, and atenolol) has not been clearly established, so the choice should be based on β1-selectivity, lack of ISA and idiosyncratic adverse events, and comorbid conditions. The use of long-acting formulations may improve compliance, and if one agent does not work, the patient may respond to a different β-blocker.[7,54]

β-Blockers are contraindicated when patients are pregnant or have asthma, depression, hypotension, congestive heart failure, Raynaud's disease, or diabetes. Approximately 10% to 15% of patients experience adverse events; the most common involve the CNS (fatigue, sedation, sleep abnormalities, depression, memory impairment, and hallucinations), but patients may also complain of GI upset, impotence, and cardiovascular effects (orthostasis, bradycardia, and decreased exercise tolerance). β-Blockers may precipitate ergotism when taken with an ergot preparation.[7,54,81] Additional information regarding β-blocker pharmacotherapy and monitoring is described in Section VI of this text.

Antidepressants. Some antidepressants are effective in reducing the frequency of migraine and TTH. Available agents include TCAs, which inhibit norepinephrine and serotonin reuptake; SSRIs; monoamine oxidase inhibitors (MAOIs), which block the degradation of catecholamines; and monoamine receptor-targeted drugs, such as trazodone (serotonin), mirtazapine (α2 antagonist), and bupropion (dopamine and norepinephrine). The antinociceptive activity of antidepressants may be related to decreases in β-receptor density and norepinephrine-mediated cyclic AMP response, upregulation of $GABA_B$-receptors, downregulation of $5\text{-}HT_2$ receptors, or downregulation of histamine receptors. Of these, inhibition of the $5\text{-}HT_2$ receptors and 5-HT reuptake inhibition may be the most important. Antidepressants are useful for patients with concurrent depression, anxiety, insomnia, or pain disorders. Generally the TCAs are much more effective than the SSRIs, but they have a greater risk of adverse events.[7,54]

Amitriptyline, nortriptyline, and doxepin are the most commonly used TCAs, but only amitriptyline has been extensively studied. Dosing should be individualized, as there is much variability in defining the therapeutic window. Low doses of TCAs, administered at bedtime, are usually sufficient and help patients tolerate the sedative effects. SSRIs have gained popularity due to their positive theoretical effect on migraine and their good safety profile. Fluoxetine has varying results in preventing migraine but improves chronic daily headache. Generally, the remaining antidepressants are reserved for those who fail to respond to the TCAs or SSRIs. Venlafaxine may be effective but also can cause severe withdrawal headaches.[82] Trazodone, a serotonin-specific antidepressant, should be avoided because it is metabolized to m-chlorophenylpiperazine, a $5\text{-}HT_{1A}$ and $5\text{-}HT_{2A/C}$ receptor agonist and migraine precipitant.[3,54]

Adverse events occur in 10% to 20% of patients taking TCAs and include anticholinergic effects, cardiovascular effects, sexual dysfunction, sedation, mental confusion, and weight gain. TCAs are contraindicated for patients with narrow-angle glaucoma, benign prostatic hyperplasia, or urinary retention and should be used with caution by patients with cardiac disease or seizure disorders. Although SSRIs are less likely to produce sedation, weight gain, and cardiovascular changes, they may induce headaches, anxiety, nervousness, insomnia, and sexual dysfunction. The adverse event profile of the MAOIs is similar to that of the TCAs, but concurrent ingestion of tyramine-containing foods, meperidine, or sympathomimetic agents, including isometheptene, may precipitate a hypertensive crisis. The concurrent use of fluoxetine and MAOIs has resulted in fatalities, and several weeks must elapse before one agent can be initiated after discontinuation of the other.[54] Additional information regarding antidepressant pharmacotherapy and monitoring is given in Chapter 53.

Calcium Channel Blockers. Calcium channel blockers are used primarily in migraine and cluster headache prevention, but some parenteral or sublingual formulations may be used acutely. Calcium channel blockers decrease the frequency of the attacks; they have minimal effect on headache severity and are generally not as effective as other agents. In addition, the vasodilatory action of some calcium channel blockers may induce or worsen migraine attacks. They are particularly useful in patients who have a prolonged aura phase or a migrainous infarction, cannot take β-blockers, or have hypertension or angina.[54]

The mechanism of action of calcium channel blockers is unclear. Calcium channel blockers affect slow voltage-sensitive calcium channels, of which there are three subtypes, L, T, and N. L-type calcium channels are present in cardiovascular smooth muscle, as well as endocrine cells and some neurons. T-type channels are also found in cardiac tissue, whereas N-type channels only affect neurons and mediate system neurotransmitter release. Most calcium channel blockers used for headache treatment affect the L-type channel.[83] Flunarizine exhibits nonspecific antagonism to sodium as well as primarily T- and N-type calcium channels and may therefore have an advantage in terms of cerebral cell protection and lack of cardiovascular effects.[84] It has been suggested that calcium channel blockers prevent hypoxia of cerebral neurons, contract vascular smooth muscles, and inhibit the calcium-dependent enzymes involved in prostaglandin formation. They may block 5-HT release, interfere with neurovascular inflammation, or interfere with the initiation and propagation of cortical spreading depression.[54]

Studies of calcium channel blockers in headache have focused primarily on three agents: verapamil, nimodipine, and flunarizine. Parenteral (20 mg) or sublingual (10 mg) flunarizine may be useful in treating acute migraine attacks. Oral verapamil prophylaxis is only 40% effective in reducing migraine frequency by 50%.[85] Nifedipine is not considered effective in migraine prophylaxis, usually causing a dull persistent headache, and nimodipine shows limited efficacy only in the prevention of migraine with aura. Small uncontrolled studies with diltiazem and nicardipine support their use in preventive migraine treatment.[86] Flunarizine appears to be the most efficacious and is comparable to β-blockers in this respect. Nimodipine and verapamil are 50% to 75% effective in reducing cluster headache symptoms. An adequate trial of therapy may require at least 2 months because of a delayed onset of action, which can increase a patient's frustration and decrease compliance.[7,8]

The most common adverse events associated with calcium channel blockers include dizziness, headache, depression, tremor, constipation, peripheral edema, hypotension, and bradycardia. Flunarizine may cause weight gain, sedation, extrapyramidal symptoms, and depression. Calcium channel blockers are relatively contraindicated in patients with significant heart block, congestive heart failure, hypotension, and sick sinus syndrome.[54] Additional information regarding calcium channel blocker pharmacotherapy and monitoring is described in Section VI of this text.

Serotonin Antagonists.

Methysergide. Methysergide is a semisynthetic ergot 5-HT$_{1B/D}$ receptor agonist and 5-HT$_2$ receptor antagonist used to prevent migraine and cluster headaches. It is no longer available in the United States. Methylergonovine (methylergometrine) is effective in migraine prophylaxis, but it has not been well studied. Several controlled trials have shown methysergide (3 to 6 mg/day) to be superior to cyproheptadine and comparable to pizotifen, lisuride, propranolol, and flunarizine in migraine prevention.[7,54,73]

Methysergide is about 70% effective in cluster headache prevention. It is less effective in chronic cluster headaches. Cluster cycles are usually less than 3 months in duration, and the development of long-term adverse events is less of a concern.[8,9,77]

Methysergide is used as a last resort in headache prevention because the risk of serious adverse events is greater than that of other medications. Initial adverse events, which often decrease with time, include muscle aches, hallucinations, abdominal discomfort, and nausea/vomiting. Concomitant administration of food or antacids or dividing the daily dose decreases GI effects. Other adverse events include peripheral arterial insufficiency, peripheral edema, and weight gain. Of most concern is retroperitoneal, pulmonary, or endocardial fibrosis, a rare and chronic complication with an incidence of 1 in 5,000. A 1-month drug holiday every 6 months to minimize these adverse events has been suggested, but this approach has not proven useful. When a drug holiday is initiated, the dose should be tapered down over at least a week to minimize rebound headaches. Fibrotic changes may be detected with auscultation of the heart, a chest radiograph, an echocardiogram, or magnetic resonance imaging of the abdomen. Methysergide use is contraindicated in patients with cardiovascular disease, cerebrovascular disease, severe

hypertension, peripheral vascular disease, peptic ulcer disease, pregnancy, and familial fibrotic disorders. Methysergide, combined with ergotamine or sumatriptan, can cause severe vasoconstriction.[7,54,73]

Cyproheptadine. Cyproheptadine is a 5-HT$_{2A}$, 5-HT$_{2B}$, and 5-HT$_{2C}$ antagonist with antihistaminic and anticholinergic activity. It is often used for migraine prophylaxis in childhood migraine or hormonally mediated migraines. Open-label studies indicate that cyproheptadine improves migraine in 43% to 65% of patients, but comparative trials indicate that it is inferior to methysergide. Adverse drug reactions are fewer than with methysergide and include drowsiness, dizziness, dry mouth, increased appetite, weight gain, and inhibition of childhood growth. Cyproheptadine is contraindicated for patients with glaucoma and prostatic hypertrophy. Administering the majority of the dose at bedtime may minimize daytime drowsiness. It may also reverse the positive effects of SSRIs.[7,49,54]

Anticonvulsants. Valproic acid and topiramate are both proven effective in preventing headache pain and are both approved by the Food and Drug Administration for this indication. Both are helpful in patients with migraine, chronic daily headache, and cluster headaches. Carbamazepine, phenytoin, vigabatrin, lamotrigine, zonisamide, and levetiracetam have limited studies, open-label trials, or inconsistent results. Antiepileptic medications may prevent headaches by stabilizing membranes or by inhibiting serotonergic neurons on the dorsal raphe nuclei. Valproic acid is the drug of choice for migraine patients with concurrent manic-depressive disorders, epilepsy, or anxiety disorders.[7,54,79] Topiramate is the drug of choice for migraine patients with epilepsy, essential tremor, or obesity.

Valproic acid has decreased migraine frequency by 39% to 43% over placebo. Headache frequency decreased by 50% in 48% of migrainures.[87-89] Valproic acid's efficacy is comparable to that of β-blockers and flunarizine.[87] The most common adverse events reported in these trials were nausea, dyspepsia, fatigue, increased appetite, and weight gain. Other adverse events include sedation, tremor, transient hair loss, increased bleeding time, and thrombocytopenia. Hepatotoxicity is rare, but baseline liver function tests should be obtained. Divalproex, a delayed-release valproic acid derivative, may minimize nausea. Valproic acid is relatively contraindicated for patients with liver disease or bleeding disorders and children younger than 10 years of age.

Gabapentin (1,800 to 2,400 mg) was less impressive, as it decreased migraine frequency by 50% in about 30% of patients in a placebo-controlled, double-blind trial, when a modified intent-to-treat analysis was used.[90] The most common adverse events were dizziness or giddiness and drowsiness.

Topiramate, a D-fructose derivative, has been associated with weight loss, not weight gain. In two large, double-blind, placebo-controlled, multicenter trials, topiramate, both 100 and 200 mg, was effective in reducing migraine attack frequency by 50% in half of the patients.[91,92] Dropouts due to adverse events were common in the topiramate groups but did not affect statistical significance. Topiramate is associated with weight loss, peripheral paresthesias, cognitive dysfunction, and kidney stones. To minimize adverse events, the dose should titrated up slowly, and there is rarely a need to increase the dose beyond 100 mg for migraine. Topiramate is better tolerated in patients with migraine than patients with epilepsy, who use higher doses.

Levetiracetam, lamotrigine, and gabapentin do not alter the metabolism of other drugs. Almost all other antiepileptic agents have drug interactions; therefore, one must assess for potential drug interactions whenever adding or discontinuing these agents. Valproic acid decreases the metabolism of many drugs. Topiramate at doses over 200 mg (above what is needed for migraine) decreases the effects of birth control pills. Thus, the efficacy and toxicity of any concomitant therapy should be evaluated when these antiepileptic drugs are added or discontinued. These agents should be avoided in pregnancy. Additional information regarding anticonvulsant pharmacotherapy and monitoring is given in Chapter 62.

Lithium Carbonate. Lithium is used in the treatment of both cyclic migraine and cluster headaches. The mechanism of action of lithium is unclear, but it may alter circadian rhythms, reduce rapid eye movement sleep, or decrease neuronal activity by depleting inositol. More patients with chronic (78%) than episodic (63%) cluster headache respond to preventive lithium, and in nearly 20% of patients receiving lithium, chronic cluster headaches change to episodic cluster headaches. Lithium improves headaches by 60% to 90% in 42% of patients with episodic cluster headaches and by more than 90% in 54% of patients with chronic cluster headaches. Triple therapy (lithium, verapamil, and ergotamine) has improved episodic cluster headaches in 90% of patients. Lithium has a half-life of approximately 24 hours, and a therapeutic response onset may take 1 to 2 weeks. Some patients may develop tolerance to lithium's effects. Serum concentrations should be monitored weekly during the titration phase and every 3 months thereafter.[5,7,9]

Common adverse events include tremor, polyuria, nausea, muscle weakness, and ankle edema. Long-term adverse events include hypothyroidism, renal failure, electrocardiogram changes, leukocytosis, and diabetes insipidus. Therefore, baseline monitoring should include thyroid function, urinalysis, electrocardiogram, leukocyte measurements, and electrolytes. Adverse events can be minimized by maintaining lithium serum concentrations at less than 1 mEq per liter. Caution should be used when lithium is administered in conjunction with verapamil, because lithium doses will most likely need to be reduced. Changes in the patient's dietary salt intake or initiation of diuretic therapy will affect renal lithium elimination.[7,9,54,77] Additional information on lithium pharmacotherapy and monitoring is found in Chapter 53.

Oxygen. Oxygen inhalation provides acute relief from cluster headaches, although it sometimes delays rather than aborts the attack. The key to a successful response is high oxygen flow and content as well as sufficient time for inhalation. Administered through a mask, hyperbaric oxygen effectively relieved cluster attacks within 5 minutes in nearly 70% of patients. Another trial with hyperbaric oxygen relieved cluster attacks in 86% of patients. In a preliminary report, 90% of patients treated with hyperbaric oxygen for 40 minutes had near-total migraine relief. Patients should maintain a canister at work and one at home and have an alternative therapy on hand when they are not at home or work. It may work well as an adjunct with other treatments.[9,8,77]

Miscellaneous Agents. Other agents that have been evaluated in small sample sizes or have shown inconsistent results include clonidine, calcitonin, capsaicin, captopril, lisinopril, candesartan, quetiapine, and papaverine for migraine headache. Clonidine may be helpful in patients being detoxified from drug abuse headaches, as it relieves withdrawal symptoms. Miscellaneous agents used in cluster headaches that have limited data include methylphenidate, antispasticity drugs, clonidine, histamine, and somatostatin.[54,77]

Adjunctive Therapy. Adjunctive medications relieve associated symptoms and provide synergistic analgesia. Many acute migraine medications relieve headache pain, but some have minimal or no effect on the associated symptoms of nausea, vomiting, and delayed GI emptying (gastric stasis). Gastric stasis may interfere with drug absorption. Metoclopramide decreases nausea and vomiting but also enhances drug absorption by decreasing gastric stasis. Adjunctive therapy is most effective when administered at symptom onset. Drowsiness and dizziness are the most common adverse events, but dystonic reactions may occur rarely. If patients cannot tolerate the side effects of metoclopramide, neuroleptics or ondansetron (a selective $5-HT_3$ receptor antagonist) will relieve associated symptoms. Caffeine coadministration may also improve drug absorption and analgesia; however, overuse can lead to chronic daily headache. Clonidine decreases autonomic withdrawal symptoms in patients who discontinue chronic or high opioid doses. The patch formulation may be helpful as adjunctive therapy for detoxification in patients who have headaches from medication overuse.[5,7,54,93]

NONPHARMACOLOGIC THERAPY

Nonpharmacologic treatments include reducing headache triggers, behavioral modifications, and various supportive therapies. Some patients may have an inherited predisposition to headaches triggered by various habits, foods, hormones, or environmental factors (Table 61.9). Identifying the trigger can be a difficult task for patients, as lists of migraine triggers have been based on anecdotal data, premonitory symptoms may be mistaken as a trigger, and a trigger may not consistently cause a migraine attack. Patients, however, should keep a diary of headache incidences

TABLE 61.9	Headache Triggers		
Habits/Mood	**Food**	**Hormonal**	**Environmental**
Irregular exercise	Alcohol	Pregnancy	Visual stimulation
Irregular meals	Caffeine[a]	Menopause	Altitude changes
Smoking	Monosodium glutamate	Ovulation	Extreme cold/heat
Alcohol	Tyramine		Loud noises
Stress/anxiety			Odors
Depression			

[a] Caffeine worsens headaches by causing rebound and withdrawal headaches.
(Adapted from Silberstein SD, Lipton RB. Chronic daily headache, including transformed migraine, chronic tension-type headache, and medication overuse. In: Silberstein SD, Lipton RB, Dalessio DJ, eds. Wolff's headache and other head pain, 7th ed. New York: Oxford University Press, 2001:247–282; Olesen J, Tfelt-Hansen P, Welch KMA, eds. The headaches, 2nd ed. Philadelphia: Lippincott Williams & Wilkins, 2000; and Diamond S, Wenzel R. Practical approaches to migraine management. CNS Drugs 16:385–403, 2002.)

and record the time, place, meals, weather, presence of menses, amount of sleep, or related habits that may be associated with the attack. Once a somewhat reproducible trigger has been determined, avoidance of the trigger may lessen attacks.[54]

Behavioral modification includes normalizing the patient's routine so that he or she minimizes variability in sleeping, eating, activities of daily living, and exercise times. Patients with migraine have been theorized to have a defect in chronobiologic synchronizing and thus have a harder time adjusting to changes in expected external stimuli.[54] Other behavioral modifications include biofeedback training, relaxation training, and cognitive-behavioral therapy (stress management). Biofeedback teaches patients to control bodily functions, including heart rate, blood pressure, and muscle tension, by receiving feedback by visual, auditory, or electromyographic instruments. Examples of relaxation training include progressive muscle relaxation, autogenic training, and meditation. Learning methods to release muscle tension, induce relaxation, and regulate breathing during daily activities helps alleviate headache pain. Cognitive-behavioral therapy has patients recognize how their thoughts play a role in generating a stress response and learn how to develop strategies to better cope with stress that results in headaches. Patients are asked to integrate 20 to 30 minutes of relaxation and/or biofeedback therapy into their daily activities. Conservative estimates from meta-analysis reviews have resulted in at least a 40% reduction in TTH and migraine headaches.[5,94,95]

Supportive treatments for migraine and TTH include hypnosis, psychotherapy, and physical therapy. These techniques may be used alone or in combination with drug therapy. Physical therapy helps patients relieve stress and muscle tension via massage, stretching exercises, aerobic exercises, ultrasound treatments, electric stimulation, and hot or cold pack therapy. Cold compresses to the affected area provided relief in 65% to 70% of TTH patients. Examples of over-the-counter supportive products include Migraine Ice or TheraPatch Headache Cool Gel Patch; these products are applied to the head or neck region and cool the skin for about 4 hours.[60,96]

ALTERNATIVE THERAPIES

Alternative therapies, such as acupuncture, chiropractic manipulation, herbal medicine, and aromatherapy, may be used alone or as adjunctive treatment.[97] Patients should consult a physician or pharmacist before trying these therapies, because some of them may present more risk than benefit. Most of these treatments induce relaxation and alleviate stress, and may be more beneficial for TTH or stress-related migraines.

Acupuncture is recognized by the World Health Organization as a treatment for more than 100 conditions, and acupuncturists are licensed in more than 30 states across the United States. Special needles are placed at acupuncture pressure points to restore a balance in the flow of energy within the body and prevent headaches. Several studies have reported a decrease in the frequency and severity of headaches after acupuncture treatments.[97]

Chiropractic treatment of headaches focuses on spinal manipulation to correct subluxations and reduce muscle tension. Spinal manipulation probably provides little benefit,[98] and patients who report no headache relief after 6 weeks should be reevaluated.[97]

Herbal or vitamin therapy includes St. John's wort, feverfew, magnesium, and riboflavin. St. John's wort (*Hypericum perforatum*) upregulates 5-HT$_{1A}$ and 5-HT$_{2A}$ receptors.[99] Feverfew (*Tanacetum parthenium*) may inhibit platelet aggregation and serotonin secretion.[100] Efficacy reports are conflicting and adverse events include mouth ulceration, oral inflammation, and loss of taste. Butterbur (*Petasites hybridus*) has shown promise in a double-blind, placebo-controlled study. Magnesium was effective in decreasing the number of migraine days and headache severity and shows promise in patients who have low levels of magnesium. Low magnesium concentrations can lead to a cascade of events that trigger migraine attacks. Adverse events include diarrhea and gastric irritation. Riboflavin (vitamin B_2) was effective in nearly 60% of patients reporting at least a 50% reduction in headache days with only minor adverse events; however, the analysis only used the last month of treatment. Eating foods that are rich in these vitamins may help, but some migraine experts recommend that patients take both magnesium and riboflavin supplements.[54]

The unique scent of essential oils used in aromatherapy may induce relaxation and relieve TTH or stress-related migraines. Patients inhale the vapors of chamomile, cardamom, lavender, marjoram, peppermint, and rosemary arising from a bowl of water or a bath. Many chiropractors, acupuncturists, and masseuses incorporate aromatherapy in their practice.

FUTURE THERAPIES

Antiepileptic medications, CGRP antagonists, angiotensin II receptor blockers, botulinim toxin injections, and $5-HT_{1F}$ receptor agonists are being evaluated for migraine. CGRP has a causative role in migraine. An international, multicenter, double-blind, randomized clinical trial of IV BIBN 4096 BS, a highly specific and potent nonpeptide CGRP-receptor antagonist, found that the 2.5-mg dose had a response rate of 66%, compared with 27% for placebo ($P = 0.001$). There were no serious adverse events. The CGRP antagonist was effective in treating acute attacks of migraine. It is no more effective than the triptans but does not appear to have any cardiovascular adverse events.[43]

Glutamatergic hyperactivity is implicated in migraine pathogenesis. LY293558, an AMPA/kainate (KA) receptor antagonist, was effective in preclinical models of migraine. Sang et al tested LY293558 in acute migraine in a randomized, triple-blind, parallel-group, double-dummy, multicenter trial. They gave 1.2 mg per kg IV LY293558, 6 mg SC sumatriptan, or placebo. Response rates were 69% for LY293558 ($P = 0.017$ vs. placebo), 86% for sumatriptan ($P < 0.01$ vs. placebo), and 25% for placebo. The results of this small migraine trial provide evidence for a potential role of nonvasoactive AMPA/KA antagonists in treating migraine.[101]

A recent placebo-controlled study evaluated the efficacy of candesartan, an angiotensin II type 1 receptor blocker, and found it to be effective in migraine prevention. It may be valuable for patients with coexisting hypertension.[102]

Currently, botulinum toxin type A, N-methyl-D-aspartate–receptor antagonists including magnesium, and nitric oxide synthase inhibitor are being evaluated for TTH.[103] Botulinum toxin type A is showing promise in both migraine and TTH. It is injected into the glabellar, temporal, frontal, and/or suboccipital regions of the head and neck. Side effects include injection-site pain, muscle weakness, and rash.[6,54] IN zolmitriptan is being evaluated for cluster headache.

IMPORVING OUTCOMES

PATIENT EDUCATION

Patients should be educated about their headaches, their medications, and how to monitor their progress. They should be reassured that headaches are not life-threatening and that headache frequency may be controlled but headaches may not completely disappear with treatment. Good sources of information for patient education include the National Headache Foundation (800-843-2256 or http://www.headaches. org) and the American Council for Headache Education (800-255-ACHE or http://www.achenet.org). Copies of patient guidelines for tracking headache triggers and maintaining a headache diary can be obtained at www.aan.com/ professionals/practice/guidelines.cfm under the headache encounter kit.

Counseling is imperative, as response to medications is often idiosyncratic. A medication that provides some patients relief without side effects may not be tolerated by other patients. Medication counseling should focus on the appropriate administration and monitoring of the prescribed medication. Patients should not adjust doses without consulting their physician or pharmacist. Medication overuse (excessive increases in dose or administration frequency) may be a sign of ineffective treatment, addiction, or tolerance and may lead to chronic daily headache. Patients need to be aware of common medication-related adverse events and the need to let their physician know when they occur.

If specific instructions are important for using the medication properly, the health care practitioner should make sure that the patient understands how to use the product. For example, patients receiving IN dihydroergotamine should be told how to assemble the applicator and administer the spray. The unused portions of the spray should be discarded after 8 hours. Those receiving IN sumatriptan or zolmitriptan should be told that they do not need to prime the applicator because each canister delivers only one dose. Patients receiving SC sumatriptan should be taught how to load the autoinjector and how to discard the empty syringes. When using the autoinjector syringe, the patient should inject the contents into the deltoid muscle or the lateral part of the thigh. However, the upper lateral quadrant of the gluteal area is a more appropriate injection site for muscular patients who lack adipose tissue in the thigh.[104]

Patients should be told that they need to take an active role in their treatment to ensure resolution and relief of headaches. They should use a headache diary, in which they should record the date and time of day that an attack occurs, as well as possible precipitating and relieving factors. Patients should also document the medications they take and any positive or negative effects of these medications. Personal feelings that they experience during headache attacks should also be recorded in the diary to help monitor changes in quality of life. They should try to maintain a regular sleeping, eating, and exercise schedule, as it may decrease headache frequency. Patients who smoke should enter a smoking cessation program. They should eat a well-balanced diet with foods rich in magnesium (e.g., nuts, wheat germ, buckwheat) and B vitamins (e.g., nuts, rice, bread products).

DISEASE MANAGEMENT STRATEGIES

Strategies that include using patient diaries, administering patient questionnaires for monitoring, improving patient adherence, and providing frequent patient education may improve outcomes. Maintaining a patient headache diary is helpful, as the health care provider can pick up patterns in headache triggers or frequency as well as assess medication compliance, effectiveness, and adverse events. This allows the physician to make more informed decisions with less trial and error. It helps patients be more aware of their disease process, as they are more aware of what triggers and controls their headaches. In addition, it helps patients be more accurate in recalling headache frequency and medication usage. The patient's diary should be reviewed at each visit.

Additional monitoring tools that are available online include the Migraine Disability Assessment questionnaire (MIDAS), available at http://www.midas-migraine.net/, and the Headache Impact Test (HIT), available at http://www.amihealthy.com/. MIDAS measures disability in the areas of paid work or school, household work and family activities, and social and leisure activities by assessing the number of days missed in these activity areas due to migraine. The HIT is a questionnaire that helps patients communicate the severity of their headache pain to their physician. It assesses the impact of the headaches and helps patients track their headache history and medication effectiveness over time.

Adherence should be improved by developing a good patient–physician partnership in which the patient learns to take ownership of his or her condition. Engaging the patient in the treatment plan and tailoring the treatment to meet the patient's individual needs based on headache severity, medication response history, and comorbid conditions enhances treatment success and results in continued adherence to the drug therapy plan. Patients need to be educated about their disease process and proper use of their medications at each visit.

PHARMACOECONOMICS

Approximately 28 million U.S. residents have severe migraine headaches. Nearly one in four U.S. households includes someone with migraine. In the United States, 25% of women who have migraine experience four or more severe attacks a month and 35% experience one to four severe attacks a month. In the same study, 92% of women and 89% of men with severe migraine had some headache-related disability.[105]

The economic burden of headaches includes both direct and indirect costs. Direct costs include the costs of diagnos-

ing and treating headaches. In a study comparing health care resource utilization in a managed care organization, migraineurs spent 64% more on health care resources and incurred greater direct costs, such as physician or emergency department visits, additional medications (2.8 times more), hospitalizations (2 times more), and diagnostic procedures (6 times more) than nonmigraineurs. The annual treatment cost for patients with migraine is over $1 billion per year.[106,107]

Although the direct costs are alarming, the indirect costs are even greater. The indirect costs include the economic costs society incurs due to loss of productivity and wages. In a 3-month period, patients with migraine miss 1.1 days of work, and those who continued to work reported that their work performance was reduced by 41%. Adults spend 3 million days bedridden each month and children miss 3.2 million days per school year. This results in American employers losing $13 billion per year from decreased productivity and missed workdays because of migraines. There is also a substantial impact on the family, as the headache patient's ability to take care of home issues is decreased.[106,108,109]

About 65% of patients suffering from headaches do not receive proper medical care and often self-medicate their condition with poor results.[57] Prescription drugs are expensive, and proper monitoring involves use of health care resources. Nevertheless, cost-effective care can significantly decrease the financial impact of headaches on society. Although preventive treatment increases treatment cost, it can decrease headache frequency and the cost of acute treatment and emergency department visits. Thus, cost-effective management of migraine headaches consists of appropriate use of nonpharmacologic and pharmacologic treatments to improve the patient's quality of life while minimizing overall cost. Proper management should optimize drug efficacy while reducing inappropriate drug usage and adverse effects.

Analgesics are the least expensive acute treatment option. Enteric-coated sustained-release or nasal formulations cost more. Generally, the ergots are less expensive than the triptans, but this benefit is offset by the cost of adjunctive medications for nausea. The cost of all the oral triptans is comparable; however, almotriptan was more cost-effective than sumatriptan in a meta-analysis of 53 studies using sustained pain-free and side-effect-free outcome points.[110] Another meta-analysis of triptan trials assessing pain relief within 2 hours found that almotriptan and rizatriptan were the most cost-effective triptans.[111] Nasal sprays are more expensive than oral formulations but less expensive than injectable formulations. The costs of the first-line agents (β-blockers and antidepressants) for preventive headache treatment are comparable.

Health-related quality-of-life scores improved and workplace productivity increased by 12.1 to 89.8 hours per year for patients receiving sumatriptan, which was greater than for other antimigraine therapies (aspirin, NSAIDs, opioids, barbiturates, caffeine, and ergot alkaloids).[71]

KEY POINTS

- Proper headache classification is essential in choosing the appropriate therapy.
- All secondary causes of headache must be ruled out.
- Inappropriate management of headaches has a significant economic impact on worker productivity, quality of life, and health care costs.
- The goal of treatment is to reduce the frequency and severity of attacks and improve quality of life.
- Treatment involves both pharmacologic and nonpharmacologic measures, and their effects may be synergistic.
- Acute treatment should be limited to two or three times a week to avoid the development of rebound or chronic daily headache.
- Preventive therapy may not eliminate all headaches, and acute treatment may still be needed for breakthrough attacks.

SUGGESTED READINGS

Diamond S, Wenzel R. Practical approaches to migraine management. CNS Drugs 16:385–403, 2002.
Ekbom K, Hardebo JE. Cluster headache: aetiology, diagnosis, and management. Drugs 62:61–69, 2002.
Headache Classification Committee of the International Headache Society. Classification and diagnostic criteria for headache disorders, 2nd ed. Cephalgia 24 (Suppl 1):1–160, 2004.
Markley HG. Topical agents in the treatment of cluster headache. Current Pain & Headache Reports 7:139–143, 2003.
Zhao C, Stillman MJ. New developments in the pharmacotherapy of tension-type headaches. Expert Opin Pharmacother 4:2229–2237, 2003.

REFERENCES

1. Evans RW. Geriatric headache. Ann Long-Term Care 10:28–35, 2002.
2. Headache Classification Committee of the International Headache Society. Classification and diagnostic criteria for headache disorders, 2nd ed. Cephalgia 24 (Suppl 1):1–160, 2004.
3. Silberstein SD, Lipton RB. Chronic daily headache, including transformed migraine, chronic tension-type headache, and medication overuse. In: Silberstein SD, Lipton RB, Dalessio DJ, eds. Wolff's headache and other head pain, 7th ed. New York: Oxford University Press, 2001:247–282.
4. Silberstein SD. Migraine. Lancet 363:381–391, 2004.
5. Aukerman G, Knutson D, Miser W. Management of acute migraine headache. American Family Physician 66:2123–2130, 2002.
6. Solomon S, Newman LC. Episodic tension-type headaches. In: Silberstein SD, Lipton RB, Dalessio DJ, eds. Wolff's headache and other head pain, 7th ed. New York: Oxford University Press, 2001: 238–246.
7. Olesen J, Tfelt-Hansen P, Welch KMA, eds. The headaches, 2nd ed. Philadelphia: Lippincott Williams & Wilkins, 2000.
8. Dodick DW, Campbell JK.Cluster headache: diagnosis, management, and treatment. In: Silberstein SD, Lipton RB, Dalessio DJ, eds. Wolff's headache and other head pain, 7th ed. New York: Oxford University Press, 2001:283–309.
9. Ekbom K, Hardebo JE. Cluster headache: aetiology, diagnosis, and management. Drugs 62:61–69, 2002.
10. Markley HG. Topical agents in the treatment of cluster headache. Current Pain & Headache Reports 7:139–143, 2003.
11. Silberstein SD, Lipton RB, Sliwinski M. Classification of daily and near-daily headaches: field trial of revised IHS criteria. Neurology 47:871–875, 1996.
12. Li D, Rozen TD. The clinical characteristics of new daily persistent headache. Cephalalgia 22:66–69, 2002.
13. Peres MF, Silberstein SD, Nahmias S, et al. Hemicrania continua is not that rare. Neurology 57:948–951, 2001.
14. Iordanidis T, Sjaastad O. Hemicrania continua: a case report. Cephalalgia 9:301–303, 1989.
15. Diener HC, Dahlof CG. Headache associated with chronic use of substances. In: Olesen J, Tfelt-Hansen P, Welch KMA, eds. The headaches, 2nd ed. Philadelphia: Lippincott Williams & Wilkins, 1999:871–878.
16. Limmroth V, Katsarava Z, Fritsche G, et al. Features of medication overuse headache following overuse of different acute headache drugs. Neurology 59:1011–1014, 2002.
17. Bonica JJ. The management of pain, 2nd ed. Philadelphia: Lea & Febiger, 1990.
18. Goadsby PJ. Pathophysiology of headache. In: Silberstein SD, Lipton RB, Dalessio DJ, eds. Wolff's headache and other head pain, 7th ed. New York: Oxford University Press, 2001:57–72.
19. Russell MB, Iselius L, Olesen J. Migraine without aura and migraine with aura are inherited disorders. Cephalalgia 16:305–309, 1996.
20. Ophoff RA, Terwindt GM, Vergouwe MN. Familial hemiplegic migraine and episodic ataxia type-2 are caused by mutations in the Ca2+ channel gene CACNLA4. Cell Tiss Res 87:543–552, 1996.
21. Joutel A, Bousser MG, Biousee V. A gene for familial hemiplegic migraine maps to chromosome 19. Nature Genetics 5:40–45, 1993.
22. Ducros A, Deiner C, Joutel A, et al. The clinical spectrum of familial hemiplegic migraine associated with mutations in a neuronal calcium channel. N Engl J Med 345:17–24, 2001.
23. Ferrari MD, Haan J. Genetics of headache. In: Silberstein SD, Lipton RB, Dalessio DJ, eds. Wolff's headache and other head pain, 7th ed. New York: Oxford University Press, 2001:73–84.
24. De Fusco M, Marconi R, Silvestri L, et al. Haploinsufficiency of ATP1A2 encoding the Na(+)/K(+) pump alpha2 subunit associated with familial hemiplegic migraine type 2. Nat Genet 33: 192–196, 2003.
25. Olesen J, Friberg L, Skyhoj-Olsen T. Timing and topography of cerebral blood flow, aura and headache during migraine attacks. Ann Neurol 28:791–798, 1990.
26. Sanchez-del Rio M, Bakker D, Wu O, et al. Perfusion weighted imaging during migraine: spontaneous visual aura and headache. Cephalalgia 19:701–707, 1999.
27. Cutrer FM, Sorenson AG, Weisskoff RM, et al. Perfusion-weighted imaging defects during spontaneous migrainous aura. Ann Neurol 43:25–31, 1998.
28. Hadjikhani N, Sanchez delRio M, Wu O, et al. Mechanisms of migraine aura revealed by functional MRI in human visual cortex. Proc Nat Acad Sci USA 98:4687–4692, 2001.
29. Lashley KS. Patterns of cerebral integration indicated by the scotomas of migraine. Arch Neurol 46:331–339, 1941.
30. Leão AAP. Spreading depression of activity in cerebral cortex. J Neurophysiol 7:359–390, 1944.
31. Olesen J, Larsen B, Lauritzen M. Focal hyperemia followed by spreading oligemia and impaired activation of RCBF in classic migraine. Ann Neurol 9:344–352, 1981.
32. Milner PM. Note on a possible correspondence between the scotomas of migraine and spreading depression of Leão. Electroencephalography Clin Neurophysiol 10:705, 1958.
33. Olesen J, Lauritzen M, Tfelt-Hansen PK, Henriksen L, et al. Spreading cerebral oligemia in classical and normal cerebral blood flow in common migraine. Headache 22:242–248, 1982.
34. Lauritzen M, Olesen J. Regional cerebral blood flow during migraine attacks by xenon-133 inhalation and emission tomography. Brain 107:447–461, 1984.
35. Cao Y, Welch KM, Aurora S, et al. Functional MRI-BOLD of visually triggered headache in patients with migraine. Arch Neurol 56:548–554, 1999.
36. Andersen AR, Friberg L, Skyloj-Olsen T, et al. Delayed hyperemia following hypoperfusion in classic migraine. Single photon emission tomographic demonstration. Arch Neurol 45:154–159, 1988.
37. Seto H, Shimizu M, Futatsuya R, et al. Basilar artery migraine. Reversible ischemia demonstrated by Tc-99m HMPAO brain SPECT. Clin Nucl Med 19:215–218, 1994.

38. Woods RP, Iacoboni M, Mazziotta JC. Bilateral spreading cerebral hypoperfusion during spontaneous migraine headaches. N Engl J Med 331:1689–1692, 1994.

39. Bolay H, Reuter U, Dunn AK, et al. Intrinsic brain activity triggers trigeminal meningeal afferents in a migraine model. Nat Med 8: 136–142, 2002.

40. O'Connor TP, Van der Kooy D. Enrichment of vasoactive neuropeptide (calcitonin gene related peptide) in trigeminal sensory projection to the intracranial arteries. J Neurosci 8:2468–2476, 1988.

41. O'Connor TP, vanderKooy D. Pattern of intracranial and extracranial projections of trigeminal ganglion cells. J Neurosci 6: 2200–2207, 1986.

42. Doods H, Hallermayer G, Wu D, et al. Pharmacological profile of BIBN-4096BS, the first selective small molecule CGRP antagonist. Br J Pharmacol 129:420–423, 2000.

43. Olesen J, Diener HC, Husstedt IW, et al. Calcitonin gene–related peptide receptor antagonist BIBN 4096 BS for the acute treatment of migraine. N Engl J Med 350:1104–1110, 2004.

44. Burstein R, Collins B, Bajwa Z, Jakubowski M. Triptan therapy can abort migraine attacks if given before the establishment or in the absence of cutaneous allodynia and central sensitization: clinical and preclinical evidence [abstract]. Headache 42:390–391, 2002.

45. Burstein R, Cutrer MF, Yarnitsky D. The development of cutaneous allodynia during a migraine attack: clinical evidence for the sequential recruitment of spinal and supraspinal nociceptive neurons in migraine. Brain 123:1703–1709, 2001.

46. Weiller C, May A, Limmroth V, et al. Brainstem activation in spontaneous human migraine attacks. Nat Med 1:658–660, 1995.

47. Bahra A, Matharu MS, Buchel C, et al. Brainstem activation specific to migraine headache. Lancet 357:1016–1017, 2001.

48. Silberstein SD, Lipton RB, Goadsby PJ. Headache in clinical practice. Oxford: Isis Medical Media, 1998.

49. Srikiatkhachorn A, Maneesri S, Govitrapong P, et al. Derangement of serotonin system in migrainous patients with analgesic abuse headache: clues from platelets. Headache 38:43–49, 1998.

50. Hartig PR, Hoyer D, Humphrey PPA, et al. Alignment of receptor nomenclature with the human genome: classification of 5HT-1B and 5HT1D receptor subtypes. Trends Pharmacol Sci 17:103–105, 1996.

51. Longmore J, Shaw D, Smith D, et al. Differential distribution of 5HT(1D)- and 5HT(1B)-immunoreactivity within the human trigeminocerebrovascular system: implications for the discovery of new antimigraine drugs. Cephalalgia 17:833–842, 1997.

52. Markowitz S, Saito K, Moskowitz MA. Neurogenically mediated plasma extravasation in dura mater: effect of ergot alkaloids. A possible mechanism of action in vascular headache. Cephalalgia 8: 83–91, 1988.

53. Peroutka SJ. Dopamine and migraine. Neurology 49:650–656, 1997.

54. Silberstein SD, Saper JR, Freitag FG. Migraine: diagnosis and treatment. In: Silberstein SD, Lipton RB, Dalessio DJ, ed. Wolff's headache and other head pain, 7th ed. New York: Oxford University Press, 2001:121–237.

55. Mathew NT, Kurman R, Perez F. Drug-induced refractory headache: clinical features and management. Headache 30:634–638, 1990.

56. Carlsson J, Larsson B, Mark A. Psychosocial functioning in schoolchildren with recurrent headaches. Headache 36:77–82, 1996.

57. Rapoport AM, Adelman JU. Cost of migraine management: a pharmacoeconomic overview. Am J Manag Care 4:531–545, 1998.

58. Spierings ELH, van Hoof MJ. Anxiety and depression in chronic headache sufferers. Headache Q 7:235–238, 1996.

59. Silberstein SD. American Academy of Neurology practice parameter: evidence-based guidelines for migraine headache (an evidence-based review). Report of the quality standards subcommittee of the American Academy of Neurology, http://www.aan.com/professionals/practice/guideline/index.cfm. Accessed August 2004.

60. Millea PJ, Brodie JJ. Tension-type headaches. American Physician 66:797–804, 2002.

61. Snow V, Weiss K, Wall EM, et al. Clinical guidelines: pharmacological management of acute attacks of migraine and prevention of migraine headaches. Ann Intern Med 137:840–849, 2002.

62. Bannwarth B, Netter P, Pourel J, et al. Clinical pharmacokinetics of nonsteroidal anti-inflammatory drugs in the cerebrospinal fluid. Biomed Pharmacother 43:121–126, 1989.

63. Baumel B. Migraine: a pharmacological review with newer options and delivery modalities. Neurology 44 (Suppl 3):S13–S17, 1994.

64. Markley HG. Chronic headache: appropriate use of opiate analgesics. Neurology 44 (Suppl 3):S18–S24, 1994.

65. Migliardi JR, Armellino JJ, Friedman M, et al. Caffeine as an analgesic adjuvant in tension headache. Clin Pharmacol Ther 56: 576–586, 1994.

66. Lipton RB, Stewart WF, Ryan RE, et al. Efficacy and safety of acetaminophen, aspirin, and caffeine in alleviating migraine headache pain. Arch Neurol 55:210–217, 1998.

67. Rapoport AM, Tepper SJ, Bigal ME, et al. The triptan formulation. How to match patients and products. CNS Drugs 17:431–447, 2003.

68. Longmore J, Shaw D, Smith D, et al. Differential distribution of 5HT1D and 5HT1B immunoreactivity within the human trigeminocerbrovascular system: implications for the discovery of new antimigraine drugs. Cephalagia 17:833–842, 1997.

69. Moskowitz MA, Cutrer FM. Sumatriptan: a receptor-targeted treatment for migraine. Annu Rev Med 44:145–154, 1993.

70. Goadsby PJ. 5-HT$_{1B/1D}$ agonists in migraine: comparative pharmacology and its therapeutic implications. CNS Drugs 10:271–286, 1998.

71. Perry CM, Markham A. Sumatriptan. An updated review of its use in migraine. Drugs 55:889–922, 1998.

72. Bigal ME, Tepper SJ. Ergotamine and dihydroergotamine: a review. Current Pain and Headache Reports 7:55–62, 2003.

73. Diamond S, Wenzel R. Practical approaches to migraine management. CNS Drugs 16:385–403, 2002.

74. Winner P, Ricalde O, Le Force B, et al. A double-blind study of subcutaneous dihydroergotamine vs. subcutaneous sumatriptan in the treatment of acute migraine. Arch Neurol 53:180–184, 1996.

75. Gallagher RM. Acute treatment of migraine with dihydroergotamine nasal spray. Dihydroergotamine Working Group. Arch Neurol 53:1285–1291, 1996.

76. Silberstein SD. The pharmacology of ergotamine and dihydroergotamine. Headache 37 (Suppl 1):S15–S25, 1997.

77. Dodick DW, Rozen TD, Goadsby PJ, et al. Cluster headache. Cephalgia 20:787–803, 2000.

78. Thomas SH, Stone CK, Ray VG, et al. Intravenous versus rectal prochlorperazine in the treatment of benign vascular or tension headache: a randomized, prospective, double-blind trial. Ann Emerg Med 24:923–927, 1994.

79. Wang SJ, Silberstein SD, Young WB. Droperidol treatment of acute refractory migraine and status migrainosus. Headache 37: 377–382, 1997.

80. Silberstein SD, Young WB, Mendizabal JE, et al. Acute migraine treatment with droperidol: a randomized, double-blind, placebo-controlled trial. Neurology 60:315–321, 2003.

81. Venter CP, Joubert PH, Buys AC. Severe peripheral ischaemia during concomitant use of β blockers and ergot alkaloids. Br Med J 289:288–289, 1984.

82. Mayr B. Bonelli R. Severe headache with venlafaxine withdrawal. Ann Pharmacother 37:1145–1146, 2003.

83. Triggle DJ. Calcium antagonists. History and perspective. Stroke 21 (Suppl 12):IV49–IV58, 1990.

84. Pauwels PJ, Leysen JE, Janssen PA. Ca + + and Na + channels involved in neuronal cell death. Protection by flunarizine. Life Sci 48:1881–1893, 1991.

85. Solomon GD. Verapamil in migraine prophylaxis: a five-year review. Headache 29:425–427, 1989.

86. Roumeau BJ. Nicardipine in the prevention of migraine headaches. Clin Ther 14:672–677, 1992.

87. Jensen R, Brinck T, Olesen J. Sodium valproate has a prophylactic effect in migraine without aura: a triple-blind, placebo-controlled, crossover study. Neurology 44:647–651, 1994.

88. Hering R, Kuritzky A. Sodium valproate has a prophylactic effect in migraine: a double-blind study vs placebo. Cephalalgia 12: 81–84, 1992.

89. Rothrock JF, Kelly NM, Brody ML, et al. A differential response to treatment with divalproex sodium in patients with intractable headache. Cephalalgia 14:241–244, 1994.

90. Mathew NT, Rapoport A, Saper J, et al. Efficacy of gabapentin in migraine prophylaxis. Headache 41:119–128, 2001.

91. Brandes JL, Jacobs DJ, Neto W, et al. Topiramate in the prevention of migraine headache: a randomized, double-blind, placebo-controlled, parallel study (MIGR-002) [abstract]. Neurology 60: A238, 2003.

92. Silberstein SD, Neto W, Schmitt J, et al. Topiramate in the prevention of migraine headache: a randomized, double-blind, placebo-controlled, multiple-dose study. For the MIGR001 Study Group. Arch Neurol 61:490–495, 2004.

93. Albibi R, McCallum RW. Metoclopramide: pharmacology and clinical application. Ann Intern Med 98:86–95, 1983.

94. Adler CS, Adler SM. Biofeedback psychotherapy for the treatment of headache. Headache 16:189–191, 1976.

95. Holroyd KA, Penzien DB, Lipchick GL. Behavioral management of headaches. In: Silberstein SD, Lipton RB, Dalessio DJ, ed. Wolff's headache and other head pain, 7th ed. New York: Oxford University Press, 2001:562–599.

96. Terrie Y. Taking the pain out of making choices for treating headaches and migraines. Pharmacy Times, October:78–82, 2003.

97. Fox A, Fox B. Alternative healing: headaches. Franklin Lakes, NJ: Career Press, 1996.

98. Bove G, Nilsson N. Spinal manipulation in the treatment of episodic tension-type headache: a randomized controlled trial. JAMA 280:1576–1579, 1998.

99. Teufel-Mayer R, Gleitz J. Effects of long-term administration of hypericum extracts on the affinity and density of the central serotonergic 5-HT1A and 5-HT2A receptors. Pharmacopsychiatry 30 (Suppl 2):113–116, 1997.

100. Groenwegen WA, Heptinstall S. A comparison of the effects of an extract of feverfew and parthenolide, a component of feverfew, on human platelet activity in-vitro. J Pharm Pharmacol 42:553–557, 1990.

101. Sang CN, Ramadan NM, Wallihan RG, et al. LY293558, a novel AMPA/GluR5 antagonist, is efficacious and well-tolerated in acute migraine. Cephalalgia 24:596–602, 2004.

102. Tronvik E, Stovner LJ, Helde G, et al. Prophylactic treatment of migraine with an angiotensin II receptor blocker; a randomized controlled trial. JAMA 289:65–69, 2003.

103. Zhao C, Stillman MJ. New developments in the pharmacotherapy of tension-type headaches. Expert Opinion Pharmacother 4: 2229–2237, 2003.

104. Frid A, Hardebo JE. The thigh may not be suitable as an injection site for patients self-injecting sumatriptan. Neurology 49:559–561, 1997.

105. Clouse JC, Osterhaus JT. Healthcare resource use and costs associated with migraine in a managed healthcare setting. Ann Pharmacother 28:659–664, 1994.

106. Lipton RB, Hamelsky SW, Stewart WF. Epidemiology and impact of headache. In: Silberstein SD, Lipton RB, Dalessio DJ, ed. Wolff's headache and other head pain, 7th ed. New York: Oxford University Press, 2001:562–599.

107. Mathew NT. Transformed migraine. Cephalalgia 13:78–83, 1993.

108. Stang PE, Osterhaus JT. Impact of migraine in the United States: data from the National Health Interview Survey. Headache 33: 29–35, 1993.

109. Osterhaus JT, Gutterman DG, Plachetka JR. Healthcare resource and lost labor costs of migraine headache in the United States. Pharmacoeconomics 2:67–76, 1992.

110. Adelman JU, Belsey J. Meta-analysis of oral triptan therapy for acute migraine: number needed to treat and relative cost to achieve relief within 2 hours. J Manag Care Pharm 9:483–90, 2003.

111. Williams P, Reeder CE. A comparison of the cost-effectiveness of almotriptan and sumatriptanin the treatment of acute migraine using a composite efficacy/tolerability end point. J Manage Care Pharm 19:259–265, 2004.

Seizure Disorders

Stephanie J. Phelps, James W. Wheless, and Brian K. Alldredge

SEIZURE DISORDERS

TREATMENT GOALS: SEIZURE DISORDERS

- Accurately diagnose the patient's seizure type and epilepsy syndrome and determine the etiology.
- Identify and eliminate patient-specific seizure precipitants.
- Select optimal anticonvulsant therapy based on seizure type, epilepsy syndrome, patient age, sex, and concomitant medical conditions.
- Complete control of seizures is always desirable, but it may not be realistic given the magnitude and severity of the seizure type. Therapy should be individualized to attain best possible seizure control.

- Monitor for clinical and laboratory evidence of adverse effects of drug therapy.
- Minimize the use of poly-drug therapy and sedating antiepileptic drugs whenever possible.
- Identify and address patient concerns regarding the effect of epilepsy and its management on daily activities, employment, and social interactions.
- Recognize when patients should be referred to a comprehensive epilepsy center for diagnostic evaluation or consideration of other modalities, such as surgery, vagus nerve stimulation, or the ketogenic diet.

DEFINITION

A "seizure" is defined as the clinical manifestation of excessive or hypersynchronous activity of neurons within the cerebral cortex.[1] Although the term often connotes an event characterized by an abrupt loss of consciousness with generalized muscle contraction and jerking (i.e., generalized tonic-clonic or grand mal seizure), the clinical manifestations of various seizure types are quite heterogeneous. The specific signs and symptoms that accompany the event depend on the functional area of the brain that is involved and may include various degrees of motor, sensory, or cognitive dysfunction. The word "epilepsy" comes from the Greek word meaning "to seize" and is used to describe a disorder of recurrent seizures due to a chronic, underlying cause. Patients who experience isolated seizures due to a correctable cause (e.g., drug toxicity, alcohol abuse, or metabolic abnormalities) do not necessarily have epilepsy.

EPIDEMIOLOGY

The lifetime prevalence of epilepsy is approximately 3%.[2] The incidence is highest in the first 10 years of life and declines thereafter to the age of 50 when the incidence increases again. Epilepsy begins before the age of 18 in more than 75% of individuals.[1] It is estimated that 1 of every 11 people in the United States will experience a seizure at some time during life.[2] This does not infer that 1 in 11 individuals develop epilepsy.

Seizures may result from primary or acquired disturbances of central nervous system (CNS) function, metabolic derangements, or a variety of systemic disorders. Some of the common causes of new-onset seizures are listed in Table 62.1. Common causes of seizures vary according to patient age. For example, fever is only a precipitant of seizures during late infancy and early childhood. Similarly, inherited forms of epilepsy usually begin in childhood or adolescence. In adulthood, acquired causes of seizures and epilepsy (e.g., stroke, CNS tumor, CNS infection, and drug and alcohol toxicity) are more common, and are referred to as symptomatic epilepsy.

Identification of the cause of seizures is of primary importance in the determination of subsequent management. If precipitating factors are identified that are amenable to intervention (e.g., metabolic disorders or CNS infection), then specific treatment modalities should be instituted to correct the underlying cause. Rarely is there a need for chronic antiepileptic drug (AED) therapy. Conversely, when no cause of seizures can be identified by history, physical examination, laboratory investigation, or neuroimaging studies, the seizure disorder is termed "cryptogenic," and if seizures recur, long-term AED therapy is warranted. Seizures that are felt to have a genetic basis (e.g., Juvenile Myoclonic Epilepsy) are termed "idiopathic."

Prescription, over-the-counter, and recreational drugs are particularly common causes of new-onset seizures. In most instances, drug-induced seizures are dose-related and occur with an overdose or when doses are not adjusted in patients

TABLE 62.1 | Common Causes of New-Onset Seizures

Primary or Acquired Neurological Disorders
Alzheimer's disease or other neurodegenerative diseases
Brain tumor
Central nervous system infection
Cerebrovascular disease
Febrile seizures of childhood
Genetic or developmental disorders
Head trauma
Idiopathic/genetic

Systemic or Metabolic Disorders
Alcohol abuse and withdrawal
Anoxia or ischemia
Drug overdose or toxicity
Eclampsia
Hepatic failure
Hypocalcemia
Hypoglycemia
Hypomagnesemia
Hyponatremia
Porphyria
Renal failure

TABLE 62.2	Drugs That Have Been Associated With Provoking or Drugs That May Exacerbate Seizures

Antiarrhythmic agents (class 1B)

Antimicrobials

β-Lactams and related compounds

Isoniazid

Quinolones

Antivirals

Acyclovir

Ganciclovir

Drugs of abuse

Amphetamine

Cocaine

Ephedra

Methylphenidate

Psychotropic agents

Antidepressants

Antipsychotics

Lithium

Sedative-hypnotic drug withdrawal

Alcohol

Barbiturates (short-acting)

Benzodiazepines (short-acting)

Miscellaneous

Cyclosporine

Lindane

Flumazenil

Metoclopramide

Normeperidine (accumulation in renal failure)

OKT3

Radiographic contrast agents

Theophylline

Tramadol

with impaired drug elimination capacity.[3] Persons with a history of seizures, epilepsy, or organic brain disease are more susceptible to drug-induced seizures. Table 62.2 lists drugs that have been associated with seizures. Individuals with epilepsy may also experience a worsening of their seizures or emergence of a new seizure type due to AED therapy.

PATHOPHYSIOLOGY

Seizures are caused by a perturbation in the normal balance of excitatory and inhibitory influences within the brain. Synchronized, high-frequency bursts of action potentials are the initiating event of a seizure. These bursts are caused by an influx of extracellular calcium followed by opening of voltage-dependent sodium channels. This depolarization phase is followed by a hyperpolarization phase that is mediated by the inhibitory neurotransmitter γ-aminobutyric acid (GABA) or by potassium channels. Most AEDs suppress seizures by altering ion flux through membrane channels or by altering neurotransmitter activity within the CNS.

CLINICAL PRESENTATION AND DIAGNOSIS

The classification of epileptic seizures by their clinical and electrophysiologic manifestations is needed to determine which AED is most likely to be effective. In most circumstances the seizure can be classified after a complete patient history in which the patient (or observer) describes the events that occurred during the attack. This should include questions about any symptoms that warn the patient of an impending seizure (i.e., the aura), the specific ictal manifestations, and any postictal abnormalities. Throughout this process, individual(s) should be discouraged from labeling the attacks, but rather they should be guided to relate the events as they were experienced or as they were described by others. The current scheme that is used for the classification of epileptic seizures and syndromes was established by the International League Against Epilepsy.[4,5] A modified version of this classification is presented in Table 62.3.

CLASSIFICATION OF SEIZURE AND EPILEPSY TYPES

Seizures are classified as generalized or partial on the basis of their clinical features and findings on electroencephalogram (EEG). Generalized seizures are those that begin in both hemispheres of the brain and are subdivided into convulsive and nonconvulsive generalized seizures according to the severity of associated motor disturbances. Nonconvulsive generalized seizures included absence (petit mal), myoclonic, and atonic seizures. Clonic and tonic-clonic seizures were previously referred to as grand mal seizures.

GENERALIZED SEIZURES

Generalized Tonic-Clonic Seizures. Generalized tonic-clonic seizures are characteristic of maximal involvement of neurons of both hemispheres of the brain. Typically, these seizures begin with tonic (rigid) flexion of the extremities followed by extension. During this phase, contraction of the diaphragm forces air from the lungs across the larynx to produce an audible cry. The tonic phase of the seizure usually lasts 15 to 20 seconds and is quickly followed by the clonic (jerking) phase, during which there are spasms of the trunk and extremities and often biting of the tongue. The

TABLE 62.3	International Classification of Epileptic Seizures and Syndromes

Partial seizures (focal, local)

Simple partial seizures (consciousness preserved)

With motor signs (jacksonian)

With somatosensory or special sensory symptoms

With autonomic symptoms or signs

With psychic symptoms

Complex partial seizures (consciousness impaired)

Simple partial onset followed by impaired consciousness

Impaired consciousness at onset

Secondarily generalized seizures

Simple partial seizures evolving to generalized tonic-clonic seizures

Complex partial seizures evolving to generalized tonic-clonic seizures

Simple partial seizures evolving to complex partial seizures evolving to generalized tonic-clonic seizures

Generalized-onset seizures (convulsive or nonconvulsive)

Tonic-clonic seizures

Absence seizures

Typical absence seizures

Atypical absence seizures

Myoclonic seizures

Tonic seizures

Atonic seizures

Localization-related (focal) epilepsies

Idiopathic

Benign epilepsy of childhood

Symptomatic

Temporal lobe epilepsy

Extratemporal epilepsy

Generalized epilepsy

Idiopathic

Benign neonatal convulsions

Childhood absence epilepsy

Juvenile myoclonic epilepsy

Other

Idiopathic and/or symptomatic

Infantile spasms (West syndrome)

Lennox-Gastaut syndrome

Myoclonic epilepsies

Special syndromes

Febrile seizures

(From Commission on Classification and Terminology of the International League Against Epilepsy. Proposal for revised clinical and electroencephalographic classification of epileptic seizures. Epilepsia 22:489–501, 1981; Commission on Classification and Terminology of the International League Against Epilepsy. Proposal for classification of epilepsies and epileptic syndromes. Epilepsia 26:268–278, 1985, with permission.)

clonic phase usually lasts 20 to 30 seconds and is followed by a postictal state, during which the patient may sleep or awaken confused and disoriented. There is then a gradual return of consciousness and orientation over a period of 15 to 30 minutes, after which the patient has no recall of the event. Increases in blood pressure and heart rate, incontinence of urine or feces, and a brief interruption of normal breathing with cyanosis commonly accompany this type of seizure. Generalized tonic-clonic seizures may begin in both hemispheres of the brain (referred to as primarily generalized seizures) or begin in a localized area of the cortex (a partial seizure) and subsequently spread to involve both hemispheres (referred to as secondarily generalized tonic-clonic seizures).

Absence Seizures. Absence (petit mal) seizures occur primarily during childhood and are characterized by an abrupt interruption of consciousness followed by a fixed stare. Automatisms (coordinated involuntary movements such as lip smacking, chewing, or grimacing) or mild clonic movements may also occur. During the seizure there is no loss of postural tone. The seizure usually lasts several seconds and ends as abruptly as it begins with the patient immediately regaining full alertness. Absence seizures may also cluster and occur as frequently as hundreds of times a day. When this happens the seizures are often initially perceived by family or teachers as daydreaming. This seizure type is characterized by a classic pattern on the EEG of bilateral 3-Hz spike and slow-wave discharges. Absence seizures usually have their onset between the ages of 4 and 12 years and remit during adolescence or early adulthood in 60% to 70% of patients. In the remainder, generalized tonic-clonic seizures usually develop. Atypical absence seizures differ from traditional absence seizures in having a longer duration, focal motor manifestations, different EEG pattern (<2.5-Hz spike and slow-wave), and a greater association with developmental delay.

Other Types of Generalized Seizures. Atonic seizures are characterized by a sudden loss of muscle tone. Because the patient may fall abruptly, injuries are common, and it is often necessary to protect the patient's head by prescribing the use of a helmet during the daytime. Myoclonic seizures are characterized by jerking movements of a single or multiple muscle groups. Tonic seizures are similar to generalized tonic-clonic seizures except that they lack the usual clonic phase.

PARTIAL SEIZURES

Partial seizures begin in one hemisphere of the brain and are often indicative of some underlying focal brain lesion (e.g., perinatal injury, trauma, injury due to bacterial or viral CNS infections, stroke, or brain tumor). Partial seizures are differentiated according to whether or not consciousness is impaired during the event. Complex partial seizures are associated with impairment of consciousness; simple partial seizures are not.

Simple Partial Seizures. Simple partial seizures or auras are characterized by motor manifestations (e.g., clonic jerking of one limb) or sensory symptoms (e.g., a foul odor or visual distortions). In some patients with motor symptoms the seizure may spread to contiguous areas of the cortex, resulting in the recruitment of additional muscle groups ("jacksonian march"). Autonomic symptoms such as piloerection or pupillary dilatation or psychic symptoms such as feelings of déjà vu or fear may also accompany simple partial seizures; however, they are less common. In all cases, patients can respond to their environment throughout the attack.

Complex Partial Seizures. Complex partial seizures (previously referred to as psychomotor or temporal lobe seizures) are characterized by impaired consciousness and a heterogeneous group of abnormal symptoms or behaviors. Although the variety of symptoms associated with complex partial seizures is wide, each individual usually reports stereotypical attacks. Auras precede complex partial seizures in many patients. Unusual epigastric sensations are the most common, although various motor, sensory, or psychic symptoms (as described for simple partial seizures) may occur. Consciousness is then impaired for an average of about 2 minutes. During this time, patients may exhibit automatisms such as lip smacking, buttoning or unbuttoning of clothing, or wandering behavior. Less often, the behavioral abnormalities include violent outbursts, crying, or sexual actions. Simple or partial complex seizures may spread to involve both hemispheres of the brain (usually as a generalized tonic-clonic seizure). These events are termed "partial seizures with secondary generalization."

EPILEPSY SYNDROMES

In some cases the seizure classification, etiologic diagnosis, patient age, and coexistent medical conditions can be used to define a specific epileptic syndrome. An epileptic syndrome is a constellation of signs and symptoms that tend to occur together. Identification of epileptic syndromes may provide useful information that is not necessarily implied by the etiologic diagnosis or the seizure classification, such as a specific choice of AED, the anticipated duration of AED therapy, natural history, and patient prognosis. Not all patients who have epilepsy can be classified as having an epileptic syndrome. Examples of epileptic syndromes include childhood absence epilepsy, juvenile myoclonic epilepsy, and Lennox-Gastaut syndrome.

FEBRILE SEIZURES

Febrile seizures are defined as seizures that occur in association with a febrile illness. The seizure typically occurs in otherwise neurologically and developmentally normal children who do not have any evidence of a CNS infection or other identifiable causes for a seizure. Febrile seizures are the most common form of epilepsy in children and represent 40% of all first seizures. They occur in 2% to 5% of children

less than 5 years of age with a peak onset at 14 to 18 months of age. A third of children will have a second febrile seizure before they outgrow the tendency to have febrile seizures. Febrile seizures are classified as simple or complex. Simple febrile seizures are usually benign, self-limiting, and associated with only a 2% to 3% risk of recurrent, nonfebrile seizures in later life.[6] They last less than 15 minutes and do not recur within 24 hours. Complex febrile seizures are prolonged (>15 minutes), occur in series (two or more in 24 hours), or have associated focal features. Febrile seizures do not cause brain damage, nervous system problems, paralysis, mental retardation, or death. Although most parents are concerned about the development of epilepsy, children with a history of complex febrile seizures are at only a slightly higher risk (3%) of developing epilepsy by age 7 than children who have not had febrile seizures.

Most febrile seizures are self-limited and are not associated with acute or long-term neurological sequelae, therefore treatment with an AED is generally not required. The majority of febrile seizures occur within 24 hours of the onset of a febrile episode; however, most parents are not aware that their child has a fever until a seizure occurs. Parents should be instructed to contact their physician as the child may need evaluation, and specific treatment for the febrile illness. Given the risks and benefits of the effective therapies, neither continuous nor intermittent AED therapy is recommended for children with one or more simple febrile seizures. Although intermittent anticonvulsants (phenobarbital) may prevent recurrences, the likelihood of adverse effect (e.g., ataxia, lethargy, irritability) usually outweighs any benefit.

Children with complex febrile seizures, preexisting neurologic abnormalities, or a family history of nonfebrile epilepsy are at greater risk for the development of epilepsy in later life. Although there is no evidence that the risk of nonfebrile epilepsy is reduced, drug therapy for the prevention of febrile seizures may be considered for these patients.

Phenobarbital is effective for the treatment of febrile seizures; however, it may cause serious adverse effects and must be administered continuously to ensure adequate drug concentrations at the onset of a febrile episode. For these reasons, many clinicians prefer intermittent treatment with rectal diazepam. Rectal administration of diazepam (using the parenteral solution or Diastat) results in rapid absorption and quickly provides protection from recurrent febrile seizures.[6] Although valproic acid is also effective as prophylactic therapy, it is not used because of the risk of hepatotoxicity in this age group. Carbamazepine and phenytoin are not effective, and none of the newer AEDs have been evaluated for efficacy in febrile seizures.

DIAGNOSIS

Table 62.4 outlines the features of a comprehensive evaluation for patients with new-onset seizures. The diagnosis of epilepsy and proper classification of epileptic seizures are

TABLE 62.4	Evaluation of the Patient with New-onset Seizures

Patient history
Perinatal and developmental history
History of febrile seizures
History of central nervous system infection, trauma
Family history of epilepsy

Physical examination

Seizure description
Preictal phenomena (aura)
Ictal manifestations (including level of consciousness)
Postictal state
Provocative factors

Laboratory assessment
Blood urea nitrogen
Cerebrospinal fluid profile (only if meningitis is suspected)
Complete blood count
Electrolytes and glucose
Osmolality
Toxicology screen (if indicated)

Neurological examination
Electroencephalogram
Computed tomography (only for trauma)
Magnetic resonance imaging

based primarily on the patient's history and witnessed accounts of the events. Although a complete evaluation usually includes other laboratory and diagnostic studies, a diagnosis of epilepsy can be clearly established only when an accurate and unambiguous history is obtained. Most patients and witnesses can give a clear account of generalized tonic-clonic seizures. However, more careful questioning is often necessary to elicit the subtle manifestations that accompany partial, absence, and other less dramatic seizure types.

Once it is apparent that a seizure has occurred, subsequent efforts should be directed toward establishing the cause. A thorough evaluation including a medical history and physical and laboratory examinations should focus on the variety of primary, metabolic, and systemic factors that may cause new-onset seizures (Table 62.1). Seizures that are a result of a reversible cause (e.g., acute metabolic or systemic disorder) must be differentiated from those that are related to a primary CNS disorder. Even with extensive workup, the etiology of epilepsy remains unidentified in 60% to 70% of patients. A genetic cause is suggested when the age at seizure onset is less than 25 years and there is a family history of epilepsy.[7] To date, genes associated with an increased risk for the development of epilepsy have been identified for a small number of epilepsy syndromes, such as benign familial neonatal seizures (chromosome 20), juvenile myoclonic epi-

lepsy (chromosomes 6, 8, or 15) and Baltic myoclonic seizures (chromosome 21). The EEG is a useful tool for the diagnosis and classification of seizures. Epileptiform discharges on the EEG in conjunction with a clinical history of spontaneously recurring seizures can usually help establish the diagnosis of epilepsy. Although epileptiform abnormalities on the EEG are usually seen during a seizure, most EEG recordings are made between seizures (interictal EEG). The lack of EEG abnormalities on an interictal recording rarely rules out the diagnosis of epilepsy. Epileptiform abnormalities are found in only about 50% of epileptic patients after a single interictal recording. The yield can be improved with repeated recordings; however, in 15% of epileptic patients no interictal EEG abnormalities are ever found.[7] Patients with absence seizures have a characteristic 3-Hz spike and slow-wave discharge on EEG, which may be precipitated by hyperventilation. Recording the EEG after sleep deprivation may increase the diagnostic yield of the study. Just as the diagnosis of epilepsy is rarely excluded on the basis of a normal interictal EEG, the presence of EEG abnormalities, in and of itself, is not diagnostic for epilepsy. EEG abnormalities are seen in 10% to 15% of the nonepileptic population and are not indicative of epilepsy unless strong evidence from the patient history supports the diagnosis.[7]

Regardless of seizure type, computed tomography (CT) and magnetic resonance imaging (MRI) scans are often used in the initial evaluation of patients with new-onset seizures. These tests are particularly useful when evidence from the history or neurological examination suggests a structural lesion of the brain (e.g., focal neurologic abnormalities or a history that is suggestive of partial seizures). MRI is more likely to detect lesions that are associated with partial epilepsy and is preferred over CT.[1] Positron emission tomography (PET), an advanced imaging technique that allows more precise localization of areas of abnormal blood flow or metabolism, is useful for evaluation of patients for whom surgical intervention is considered. However, its availability is limited by high equipment costs.

Finally, in some patients, seizure-like activity may be a manifestation of some other condition (Table 62.5). The misdiagnosis of these events as seizures can result in unnecessary and potentially harmful therapy. Accordingly, the diagnosis of epilepsy should be reevaluated whenever the seizure-like events fail to respond to the usual treatments.

PSYCHOSOCIAL ISSUES

In addition to the medical issues that accompany the diagnosis of epilepsy, patients and/or parents often experience anxiety and fear with the confirmation that they or their child have a disorder that is chronic, affects the brain, and is accompanied by a loss of control over their body and consciousness. Patients may experience an impaired sense of independence owing to the necessity for regular interactions with the health care system and the need for chronic, daily

TABLE 62.5	Disorders That May Mimic Epilepsy

Gastroesophageal reflux
Breath-holding spells
Migraine
Confusional
Basilar
With recurrent abdominal pain and cyclic vomiting
Sleep disorders (especially parasomnias)
Cardiovascular events
Pallid infantile syncope
Vasovagal attacks
Vasomotor syncope
Cardiac arrhythmias
Movement disorders
Shuddering attacks
Paroxysmal choreoathetosis
Nonepileptic myoclonus
Tics and habit spasms
Psychological disorders
Panic disorder
Hyperventilation attacks
Pseudoseizures
Rage attacks

(From Scheuer ML, Pedley TA. The evaluation and treatment of seizures. N Engl J Med 323:1468–1474, 1990, with permission.)

medication. In addition, persons with epilepsy are often subject to driving restrictions and a need to report their condition on applications for insurance and employment. Epilepsy also affects the lives of adolescents during years important to socialization. A comprehensive approach to the treatment of persons with epilepsy should include attention to medical, psychosocial, and environmental (or behavioral) factors because these issues significantly affect the patient's and their family's quality of life.

When a diagnosis of epilepsy is made, some alteration of the patient's usual activities may be required depending on the timing and clinical manifestation of seizures. For example, patients who are affected by seizures associated with loss of consciousness or normal muscle control should restrict activities that place them or others at risk of injury. This may include partial or complete restriction of driving privileges and avoidance of activities such as swimming unattended, working at heights, and operating potentially dangerous machinery. Common sense should be the ultimate guide in the determination of specific lifestyle limitations that the epileptic condition necessitates.

Certain changes in daily activities may reduce the occurrence of seizures by avoiding patient-specific risk factors. Conditions that are occasionally identified as seizure precipitants include stress, exercise, alcohol or caffeine consumption, altered sleep schedules, and missed meals. When these

or other precipitating conditions are identified, the patient and health care provider should work cooperatively to establish guidelines that minimize these risks yet do not unnecessarily encumber the patient's daily routine.

PRINCIPLES OF ANTIEPILEPTIC DRUG SELECTION AND USAGE

AED pharmacotherapy is the mainstay of epilepsy treatment and the likelihood of seizure recurrence informs the decision to initiate treatment. The goals of AED treatment are to completely control seizures and to minimize drug-related adverse effects. Specific end points must be individualized for each patient. The choice of AED should be based on the seizure type, the age and sex of the patient, concurrent medical conditions, available dosage formulation, potential adverse effects, likelihood for clinical important drug-drug or drug-nutrient interactions, and the pharmacokinetic and pharmacodynamic features of the individual drugs. When these factors are considered and the guiding principles of AED therapy are followed, good to excellent seizure control can be attained in most patients. However, some patients may continue to suffer from recurrent seizures despite appropriate drug treatment.

PREFERENCE FOR MONOTHERAPY WITH NONSEDATING AGENTS
Monotherapy is preferred to polytherapy with AEDs because of lower costs associated with medications and laboratory monitoring, reduced potential for adverse reactions and undesirable drug interactions, and improved medication compliance with a more simplified drug administration schedule. Furthermore, evidence indicates that polytherapy offers no advantage over monotherapy for the majority of patients. For patients in whom single-drug therapy does not provide sufficient seizure control, polytherapy may be necessary to achieve the goals of treatment.

In addition to selecting the minimum effective number of AEDs, it is important to choose agents on the basis of their adverse-effect profile. The specific adverse effects of each drug are discussed later; however, the use of sedating AEDs should be minimized or avoided. Phenobarbital, primidone, and benzodiazepines are examples of sedating AEDs; other drugs covered in this chapter are not. Although phenobarbital is as effective as phenytoin and carbamazepine for the treatment of secondarily generalized tonic-clonic seizures, the latter agents are preferred because of their relative lack of CNS depressant effects.

Sedation and decreased mentation are particularly common on initiation of therapy with barbiturate and benzodiazepines. However, over time an adaptive process occurs during which these effects become less noticeable. Despite the development of tolerance to the overt sedative effect of these drugs, evidence suggests that subtle effects on intelligence, memory, complex motor skills, and behavior often persist during treatment. These undesirable effects may be especially concerning in infants and young children during periods of neurological development and acquisition of learning skills. In some cases these changes are noted by patients or their families only after the drug is discontinued.[8] Although it infrequently requires discontinuation of phenobarbital, the AED can cause paradoxical hyperactivity in children.

When possible, therapy should begin with one of the nonsedating AEDs such as phenytoin, carbamazepine, valproate, ethosuximide, or any of the newer AEDs. Phenobarbital and benzodiazepines should be reserved until nonsedating alternatives have failed. Although not available in the United States, nitrazepam and clobazam are associated with less sedation than clonazepam. In summary, sedating AEDs should be avoided when possible, and in many cases, the substitution of nonsedating alternatives can result in noticeable improvement in cognitive, motor, and behavioral function.

DRUG SELECTION BASED ON SEIZURE CLASSIFICATION

Once the diagnosis of epilepsy has been made, the choice of AED therapy should be guided by the relative efficacy and toxicity of each agent. Proper classification of the patient's seizure type or epilepsy syndrome is the most important step in choosing the appropriate agent. Table 62.6 lists the preferred AEDs for the treatment of different seizure types and Table 62.7 summarizes the recommendations of the Quality Standards Subcommittee of the American Academy of Neurology and American Epilepsy Society (AAN Quality Standards Subcommittee) published guidelines for use of the new

AED in the treatment of children and adults with new onset[9] or refractory partial and generalized epilepsies.[10] The guidelines were constructed using an evidence-based assessment of the efficacy, tolerability, and safety of gabapentin, lamotrigine, topiramate, tiagabine, oxcarbazepine, levetiracetam, and zonisamide.

Partial Seizures. Overall, partial seizures do not respond to treatment as well as seizures that are generalized from their onset. Carbamazepine, phenytoin, phenobarbital, and primidone are equally effective for the treatment of partial seizures, including simple-partial, complex-partial, and secondarily generalized partial seizures.[11] However, carbamazepine and phenytoin are usually tolerated better. Phenytoin has a long half-life that allows for once-daily dosing and carbamazepine is available in two extended-release dosage forms, which allow for twice-daily dosing. However, phenytoin is associated with cosmetic changes that make it less desirable for the treatment of epilepsy in children, adolescents, and women. Valproate is also useful for the treatment of partial seizures, but carbamazepine provides better seizure control and fewer long-term adverse effects.[12]

Felbamate, gabapentin, lamotrigine, tiagabine, topiramate, levetiracetam, oxcarbazepine, zonisamide, and pregabalin are also effective for treating partial seizures. Lamotrigine and topiramate are effective as monotherapy and appear to be better tolerated than carbamazepine monotherapy.[13] The other new agents are primarily used as adjunctive therapy if monotherapy has failed or for patients who are intolerant of standard AEDs (e.g., carbamazepine, phenytoin, and valproate). Prospective clinical trials have not compared the relative efficacy of the new AEDs. Approximately 65% of patients with partial seizures attain complete control

TABLE 62.6	Antiepileptic Drugs of Choice Based on Seizure Classification			
		Generalized Seizures		
Partial Seizures[a]		**Generalized Tonic-Clonic**	**Absence**	**Myoclonic, Atonic, Atypical Absence**
Drugs of choice	Carbamazepine	Valproate	Ethosuximide	Valproate
	Phenytoin	Carbamazepine	Lamotrigine	Lamotrigine
	Lamotrigine	Phenytoin	Valproate	
	Oxcarbazepine	Topiramate		
	Topiramate[b]	Lamotrigine		
Alternatives	Gabapentin[b]	Levetiracetam	Clonazepam	Clonazepam
	Levetiracetam	Phenobarbital		Topiramate
	Phenobarbital	Phenytoin		Felbamate
	Pregabalin	Primidone		
	Primidone			
	Tiagabine[b]			
	Valproate			

[a] Simple-partial, complex-partial, and secondarily generalized tonic-clonic seizures.
[b] Used primarily as adjunctive therapy.

TABLE 62.7	FDA-Labeled Indications and Recommendations of the Practice Parameter Guidelines Working Group

| | Newly Diagnosed Epilepsy[9] | | | Refractory Epilepsy[10] | | |
| | | | | Complex Partial | | |
AED	Absence (FDA)	Primary/Gen (FDA)	Mono-tx[a] (FDA)	Mono-tx (FDA)	Adjunctive (FDA)	Primary Gen (FDA)
GBP	IE (NO)	IE (NO)	YES (NO)	IE (NO)	YES[b] (YES >3 years)	NO (YES >12 years)
LEV	IE (NO)	IE (NO)	IE (NO)	IE* (NO)	YES (YES >16 years)	IE (NO)
LTG	YES (NO)	IE (NO; YES for LGS)	YES (NO)	YES* (NO)	YES[b] (YES >2 years)	IE (NO)
OXC	IE (NO)	IE (NO)	YES (YES)	YES (YES)	YES[b] (YES >4 years)	IE (NO)
TGB	IE (NO)	IE (NO)	IE (NO)	IE (NO)	YES (YES >16 years)	IE (NO)
TMP	IE (NO)	IE (YES[c, d]; YES for LGS)	YES (YES)	YES (NO)	YES[b] (YES >2 years)	YES[b,d] (YES >2 years)
ZNS	IE (NO)	IE (NO)	IE (NO)	IE (NO)	YES (YES >16 years)	IE (NO)

[a]partial or mixed; [b]pediatric; [c]>10 years of age; [d]generalized tonic-clonic only.
FDA, Food and Drug Administration; AED, antiepileptic drug; GBP, gabapentin; IE, insufficient evidence; LEV, levetiracetam; LGS, Lennox-Gastaut syndrome; LTG, lamotrigine; OXC, oxcarbazepine; TGB, tiagabine; TMP, topiramate; ZNS, zonisamide.
(From French JA, Kanner AM, Bautista J, et al. Efficacy and tolerability of the new antiepileptic drugs I: treatment of new onset epilepsy: report of the Therapeutics and Technology Assessment Subcommittee and Quality Standards Subcommittee of the American Academy of Neurology and the American Epilepsy Society. Neurology 62:1252–1260, 2004; French JA, Kanner AM, Bautista J, et al. Efficacy and tolerability of the new antiepileptic drugs I: treatment of new onset epilepsy: report of the Therapeutics and Technology Assessment Subcommittee and Quality Standards Subcommittee of the American Academy of Neurology and the American Epilepsy Society. Neurology 62:1252–1260, 2004, with permission.)

of seizures with AED monotherapy.[14] In the remaining patients, a trial of adjunctive therapy is warranted.

Primary Generalized Tonic-Clonic Seizures. Valproate, lamotrigine, and topiramate are the drugs of choice for the treatment of primary generalized tonic-clonic seizures. At the time the AAN Quality Standards Subcommittee guidelines were published,[9] the members concluded that there were insufficient data to support the use of any of the new AEDs as monotherapy in newly diagnosed primary generalized tonic-clonic seizures; however, topiramate was recently approved as initial monotherapy for primary generalized seizures in those older than 10 years of age.

Valproate is often considered the drug of choice for the treatment of primarily generalized tonic-clonic seizures. Approximately 75% to 85% of patients achieve complete seizure control during monotherapy with this agent.[2] Lamotrigine and topiramate are emerging as more often used therapies in children younger than 2 years of age because of the higher risk of valproate-associated hepatotoxicity in this population. Phenobarbital and primidone are also effective against generalized tonic-clonic seizures, but because of their potential for adverse effects, they are usually reserved for use as alternative second-line or third-line agents. Carbamazepine, phenytoin, and oxcarbazepine can rarely exacerbate seizures in patients with primary generalized epilepsy syndromes. These children should be monitored closely for worsened seizures or the emergence of a new seizure type.

Absence Seizures. Ethosuximide, valproate, and lamotrigine are effective for the treatment of absence seizures. Ethosuximide may be preferred over valproate when only absence seizures are involved because of the potential for fewer serious adverse effects. The AAN Quality Standards Subcommittee concluded that sufficient data existed to support the use of lamotrigine as monotherapy for absence seizures.[9] Ethosuximide is not effective against generalize tonic-clonic seizures; therefore, valproate and lamotrigine are preferred if this seizure type is also present.[1] The response to these agents is usually dramatic. In controlled trials, 70% to 90% of patients who were treated with ethosuximide or valproate experienced cessation or a dramatic reduction in absence seizures.[15] The combination of ethosuximide and valproate is often effective when monotherapy fails to yield adequate results. Clonazepam is also effective against absence seizures. However, because of frequent dose-related adverse effects and the development of tolerance to the antiepileptic effect of this drug, it should be reserved for patients in whom ethosuximide and valproate fail. Carbamazepine and phenytoin are ineffective for the treatment of absence seizures and may even exacerbate these and other seizure types when used for the treatment of children with mixed seizure disorders.[3] Levetiracetam, zonisamide, and felbamate have some evidence of efficacy in absence epilepsy, but formal studies have not been performed.

Myoclonic, Atonic, and Atypical Absence Seizures. Valproate is effective for the treatment of myoclonic, atonic, and atypical absence seizures and is the initial drug of choice for patients with mixed seizure types. Valproate effectively controls myoclonic seizures in 75% to 90% of patients with generalized idiopathic and juvenile myoclonic epilepsy. Myoclonic seizures after anoxic encephalopathy are more resistant to treatment. Clonazepam is also effective as monotherapy or in combination with valproate when either drug alone does not provide adequate seizure control. Lamotrigine, topiramate, zonisamide, and felbamate are also effective against myoclonic, atonic, and atypical absence seizures.

INITIATING ANTIEPILEPTIC DRUG THERAPY

AEDs are more frequently associated with adverse effects during initiation of therapy; therefore, treatment should begin with low doses and the dose should be gradually escalated according to the patient's clinical status. When therapy is initiated too aggressively, patients may experience uncomfortable adverse effects and are often unwilling to continue treatment with that agent despite a reduction in dosage. Patients should be told to monitor for and report adverse effects so that an adjustment in therapy can be made as soon as possible. Phenytoin, phenobarbital, and levetiracetam are usually tolerated well when they are initiated near the usual maintenance dosage. Upon initiation of therapy, patients should understand the goal of treatment and the time course over which response is anticipated. The importance of strict compliance with the prescribed regimen should also be emphasized and the practitioner should attempt to identify any obstacles to adherence.

ADJUSTING AND MONITORING ANTIEPILEPTIC DRUG THERAPY

There is great interpatient variability in the dose-response relationship for all of the AEDs that are in common use. Therefore, after therapy is initiated, the optimal drug dose for each patient should be determined. This necessitates the titration of therapy until the desired clinical response is achieved or the patient experiences unacceptable adverse effects.

The determination of acceptable seizure control requires input from the patient and clinician. Although complete control of seizures is always desirable, it may not be realistic

given the magnitude and severity of the seizure type. Patients or parents may also choose to continue therapy that allows minimal interruption of their lifestyle even though seizures occasionally recur. The clinician must assess the temporary disability and potential for harm (to the patient and others) that may accompany a seizure. Use of this information, with input from the patient, should be used to determine if dosage adjustments should be made.

If the first agent does not achieve the desired goal, then an alternative AED that is appropriate for the patient's seizure type should be gradually substituted rather than added. Typically, after monotherapy has failed (usually with two or three agents) polytherapy should be tried. The first drug is usually removed once a successful dose or desired plasma concentration of the new agent is attained.

AED therapy fails for many reasons. Although various drugs may demonstrate equal efficacy in large populations of patients, an individual may respond better to one agent than to others. Additional factors that should be considered include poor medication compliance, erroneous diagnosis or seizure classification, progressive neurological disease, and lifestyle factors that compromise the efficacy of treatment (e.g., recreational drug or alcohol abuse, sleep deprivation). Noncompliance with treatment is a common cause of AED therapy failure, and this possibility should be carefully investigated. It is essential that the clinician create a culture that encourages the patient/family to discuss their compliance, or lack thereof, without fear of judgment. Common reasons for noncompliance include complicated dosing regimens, fear about chronic adverse effects of AED therapy or teratogenicity, and denial of the need for treatment. Patients who report a change in the character of their seizures (e.g., seizures are now preceded by an aura, whereas previously there was no warning) or frequent seizures after a long period of complete control should be referred for a thorough medical evaluation to rule out other neurological disease.

Plasma Antiepileptic Drug Monitoring. The widespread availability of blood concentration monitoring of AED therapy has had a dramatic effect on the use of these agents. For example, combination AED regimens were frequently begun (e.g., phenytoin and phenobarbital) before clinicians had the ability to individualize the doses for either agent. On the basis of past experience in which a single drug was occasionally ineffective and above-average doses sometimes led to toxicity, it was assumed that most patients would benefit if multiple drugs were used. Blood concentration monitoring and knowledge of the pharmacokinetic properties of AEDs are now used to maximize efficacy, minimize adverse effects, and evaluate compliance.

The "therapeutic" range of plasma concentrations is a useful guide for titrating therapy. Within this range, many patients achieve seizure control without unacceptable side effects. However, it is also common to observe an adequate response at concentrations below the lower end of the defined therapeutic range, and some patients tolerate and indeed require plasma concentrations above the upper limit of the range to maintain seizure control. Thus, although these limits are useful as guides to therapy, the clinician should strive to determine the optimum AED plasma concentration for each individual patient rather than relying on published ranges.[16] While a therapeutic range is available for the new AEDs, these reflect concentrations achieved during clinical trials and do not necessarily correspond with efficacy or toxicity. However, they may still be helpful in defining the optimum AED concentration for a given patient, evaluating compliance, and making adjustments in patients with altered renal function. Assays for the new AED are generally not available in clinical laboratories; hence, it may require weeks to obtain results.

When indicated, plasma concentration monitoring of AEDs is most useful under the following conditions: (a) to document the plasma concentration associated with good seizure control or failures, (b) to guide subsequent dosage adjustments that are required on a clinical basis, (c) to evaluate noncompliance, (d) to evaluate alterations in pharmacokinetics that are due to patient diversity, disease, or drug-drug interactions, and (e) to evaluate possible concentration-related adverse effects. The timing of blood sampling for drug concentration determination is important, particularly during therapy with AEDs that have a short half-life (e.g., carbamazepine and valproate). For these agents, blood concentrations can fluctuate significantly over the course of the dosing interval. Comparisons between drug concentrations may be inaccurate unless the blood is sampled at a consistent time relative to the dose. For most patients it is recommended that blood samples be taken in the morning, before the first daily dose of medication. An exception is patients with repeated, transient symptoms that are suggestive of dose-related drug toxicity or individuals who experience "break through" seizures at the end of a dosing interval. For these patients, blood sampling should coincide with the event so that the contribution of the drug can be assessed.

Plasma concentration monitoring of AEDs is often overused and misused.[16] It is common (and arguably appropriate) to document drug concentrations on an occasional basis in patients whose epileptic condition is well controlled (e.g., every 12 months). However, other drug concentration determinations should not be done unless there is clinical indication of their necessity. Likewise, there is often a tendency to adjust AED therapy on the basis of the concentration without considering the patient's clinical status. For example, it may be tempting to decrease the drug dose when the reported blood concentration is above the usual therapeutic range. However, some patients require higher concentrations than usual to achieve the desired pharmacological effect. Likewise, patients whose seizures are controlled with concentrations less than the therapeutic range neither need a dose increase nor should be assumed to no longer require AED treatment. In his editorial regarding the use of AED blood concentration monitoring, W. Edwin Dodson wrote that "changing an antiepileptic drug dose based only on the drug concentration is like driving a car looking only at the speedometer and not out the window. Wrecks are inevitable and frequent."[16]

WITHDRAWAL OF ANTIEPILEPTIC DRUG THERAPY

Several community-based studies have shown that among patients with epilepsy who are followed for more than 10 years, more than half attain a 2-year to 5-year remission from seizures during drug therapy. Remission rates tend to be highest for patients who have primary generalized seizures and range from 60% for those with tonic-clonic seizures to 80% for children with typical absence attacks.

In general, patients who remain free of seizures for 2 years or more may be considered candidates for AED withdrawal. The potential benefits of drug withdrawal include avoidance of the cognitive and behavioral effects of AED therapy, reduction in the risk of adverse drug reactions and drug interactions, and a return by the patient to a lifestyle that is unencumbered by the need for chronic medication. However, the decision to withdraw AED therapy is complex, medically and socially, and requires a clear explanation to the patient of the risks and benefits.

Medical factors that appear to affect the risk of seizure recurrence after AED drug withdrawal are summarized in Table 62.8. In particular, it is important to consider the age at onset of epilepsy, seizure type, EEG abnormalities, and rate of drug withdrawal in assessing the risk of seizure recurrence. Relapse rates after AED withdrawal in patients who have been free of seizures for 2 years or more are approximately 30% for children and 40% for adults with epilepsy.[17] Thus, 60% to 70% of patients will remain free of seizures when AED therapy is withdrawn after a 2-year remission.

TABLE 62.8	Factors That Affect the Risk of Seizure Recurrence After Antiepileptic Drug Withdrawal
Favorable Prognosis	**Unfavorable Prognosis**
Childhood-onset epilepsy	Adult-onset epilepsy
Longer seizure-free interval before drug withdrawal	Frequent seizures before remission
Absence seizures	Partial-onset seizures
Primary generalized tonic-clonic seizures	EEG abnormalities at time of drug withdrawal
Normal or improved EEG at time of drug withdrawal	Abnormal neurological examination and subnormal IQ
Normal neurological examination and normal IQ	Abrupt withdrawal of benzodiazepine or barbiturate antiepileptic drugs
	Atypical febrile seizures
	Juvenile myoclonic epilepsy

EEG, electroencephalogram.

The risk of seizure recurrence is highest during the period of AED reduction and within the first year after drug withdrawal.

The rate of AED withdrawal may also affect seizure recurrence. Gradual withdrawal is preferred and most practitioners discontinue therapy over a period of 1 to 3 months, depending on the patient and the drug. Abrupt withdrawal is a risk factor for status epilepticus. Furthermore, rapid removal of AED therapy itself may precipitate seizures due to drug withdrawal (as distinct from a recurrence of seizures due to the underlying epileptic condition). Seizures during withdrawal are most common with benzodiazepine or barbiturates. However, because there are no means to determine reliably whether recurrent seizures are related to a withdrawal phenomenon or the lack of a beneficial effect, the need for continued drug therapy is unclear unless the rate of taper is long enough to effectively rule out a drug withdrawal phenomenon.

Any decision to withdraw AED therapy on the basis of a favorable medical prognosis must also include a careful assessment of the patient's work and social environments. Not only should patients clearly understand the risks and benefits of drug withdrawal, they must also be encouraged to participate actively in the decision. Patients who have been seizure-free for long intervals, often have valid concerns about the possible recurrence of seizures at home, at work, or while driving. During AED withdrawal it is often recommended that the patient not drive for several months. Furthermore, in some areas a recurrent seizure during this period may result in the suspension of driving privileges until AED therapy is restarted and adequate control is demonstrated. These and other patient-specific social factors should be discussed with each individual for whom AED withdrawal is considered.

TREATING THE PREGNANT WOMAN WHO HAS EPILEPSY

Considerable controversy continues to surround the treatment of pregnant women who have epilepsy. Central issues are the risk of fetal malformations that are attributable to individual seizures and to the epileptic diathesis, the degree of additional risk that is attributable to AED therapy, and the antiepileptic agent of choice for minimizing the risk of fetal malformations. Although a detailed discussion of these issues is beyond the scope of this chapter, several important principles should be considered. The reader is referred to other reviews for additional discussion of this topic.[18,19]

Considerations that are unique during pregnancy include (a) changes in maternal seizure control, (b) the choice of antiepileptic agents, (c) alteration of AED pharmacokinetics, and (d) the potential for AED-associated coagulopathy in the newborn. Approximately 60% of women with epilepsy will have no change in seizure frequency during pregnancy.[18] Among the remaining patients, worsening of seizures occurs in approximately one third of pregnant women.[19] This may be attributable to several factors, including reduced medication compliance caused by fears that the medication may injure the developing fetus, pharmacokinetic changes in AED disposition, and sleep deprivation.

Overall, the incidence of fetal abnormalities in children of epileptic mothers is approximately 6%, roughly twice that found in the general population. Although there is considerable controversy about which AED has the lowest teratogenic risk, there is a clear association between some AEDs and fetal malformations. Currently, there is no conclusive evidence on which to base a preference for the use of carbamazepine, phenobarbital, phenytoin, or valproate during pregnancy.[19] No AED is clearly less teratogenic than the others, therefore the preferred AED during pregnancy is the drug that best controls the patient's seizures. The North American AED Pregnancy Registry does suggest that monotherapy with valproate and monotherapy with phenobarbital have higher rates of major malformations than other AED. Phenytoin has been associated with a constellation of anomalies including craniofacial malformations, mental retardation, deficiencies in growth, mental or motor performance, and limb defects that have been grouped as the fetal hydantoin syndrome. However, similar abnormalities have been associated with other AEDs.

It is clear that AED polytherapy is associated with a greater risk of fetal malformations. When possible, it is recommended that monotherapy (with the lowest effective dose) be used and that a dosage formulation that minimizes plasma peak to trough AED concentrations be used. The safety of newer AEDs (gabapentin, lamotrigine, oxcarbazepine topiramate, and tiagabine) has yet to be established; however, all of the newer AEDs are Food and Drug Administration (FDA) category C while the older AED are classified as category D.

Neural tube defects (specifically, with spina bifida) have been associated with maternal use of valproate (1%–2%) and carbamazepine (0.5%–1%) during pregnancy. The mechanism of teratogenesis caused by AEDs is unknown but may be related to folic acid deficiencies or to arene oxide intermediates that are generated during the metabolism of aromatic AEDs. Deficiencies of folate have been implicated in the development of neural tube defects. For this reason, all women with childbearing potential who have epilepsy should receive folic acid supplementation. The optimal dose is unknown but most practitioners use 1 to 2 mg daily. Although folic acid supplementation in women of childbearing years has become a standard recommendation, it is unclear if folic acid supplementation protects against the embryotoxic and teratogenic effects of AEDs. Despite supplementary folic acid, women taking valproate or carbamazepine should undergo perinatal diagnostic ultrasound to rule out neural tube defects.

Pregnancy is associated with significant changes in the pharmacokinetic properties of AEDs. These changes include acceleration of hepatic drug metabolism, increased apparent volume of distribution, and alterations in plasma protein binding. The result is a decline in plasma AED concentrations and, in some patients, loss of seizure control. Consequently, AED plasma concentrations and the clinical status of the patient should be monitored regularly during pregnancy. When assays are available, monitoring of unbound plasma concentrations of phenytoin, valproate, and carbamazepine is recommended due to protein binding changes associated with pregnancy. Plasma concentrations with these AEDs and with lamotrigine should be determined approximately every 3 months during pregnancy. After delivery, AED plasma concentrations should be determined weekly, and appropriate dosage adjustments should be made.

Approximately 50% of the infants who are born to mothers taking phenytoin, phenobarbital, and primidone during pregnancy are deficient in vitamin K-dependent clotting factors at birth. Although neonatal hemorrhage is uncommon, infants should be treated with 1 mg vitamin K intramuscularly immediately at birth. Clotting should then be monitored every 2 to 4 hours, and repeat doses of vitamin K should be administered as needed. Preferably, coagulopathy can be prevented by treating the mother with vitamin K 10 mg orally each day for 4 weeks before delivery.

All AEDs are excreted in breast milk to some degree. The ratio of breast milk to plasma concentration is 80% to 100% for ethosuximide, 40% to 50% for phenobarbital, 40% for carbamazepine, 18% to 20% for phenytoin, and 1% to 10% for valproic acid.[19] Although most epileptic mothers may safely breastfeed their infants, the potential effect of drug transfer to the baby should be considered, especially if the infant appears to be lethargic or irritable, or feeds poorly.

Despite the concern of parents and clinicians about the risks of epilepsy and AED therapy during pregnancy, it is important to realize that more than 90% of epileptic women have normal children. However, women with epilepsy must understand the value of prepregnancy planning and the risks for fetal abnormalities. They must also understand the potential consequences of medication noncompliance and the need for close monitoring of plasma concentrations during pregnancy and for several weeks after childbirth.

ANTIEPILEPTIC DRUGS

PHENOBARBITAL

All barbiturates have anticonvulsant activity but only phenobarbital and primidone are used commonly for the chronic treatment of epilepsy because they are effective at subhypnotic doses. Phenobarbital was first used for the treatment of seizures in 1912, and it continues to be prescribed widely. However, because of adverse effects on the CNS, this agent is now used primarily as an alternative when monotherapy with first-line agents has failed. Phenobarbital is most useful for the treatment of partial and generalized tonic-clonic seizures. It elevates the seizure threshold and prevents the spread of electrical seizure activity. Phenobarbital modulates the inhibitory action of GABA by increasing its binding to the $GABA_A$ receptor. The $GABA_A$ receptor forms a gated

CL^- channel by activating binding to the receptor and prolonging the time the channel is open. Phenobarbital also attenuates the postsynaptic effects of excitatory neurotransmitters such as glutamate.

Formulation and Dosage. Phenobarbital is available as the sodium salt in a variety of dosage forms, including oral capsules and tablets, elixir, and injectable preparations (Table 62.9). The usual maintenance dose of phenobarbital for adults is 90 mg every day (qd) and 3 to 5 mg per kilogram in neonates and children. Phenobarbital is usually given as a single daily dose at bedtime to avoid peak sedative effects during the day. Its long half-life causes significant delays in the achievement of steady-state concentrations; hence, a loading dose should be administered when a prompt effect is needed. The usual loading dose of phenobarbital is 15 mg per kilogram. When it is given intravenously, the rate of administration should not exceed 100 or 30 mg per minute in adults and children, respectively. Oral loading doses may also be used; however, the dose is usually divided into three equal increments and given over 24 hours. Patients should be monitored for the attendant sedation and lack of coordination that may occur with either route of administration.

Pharmacokinetics. The clinical pharmacokinetic features of phenobarbital are summarized in Table 62.10.

Phenobarbital is nearly completely absorbed after oral and intramuscular administration, with peak concentrations occurring in less than 4 hours. Neonates have delayed and incomplete absorption of oral phenobarbital. Although food may delay absorption, the absolute bioavailability is unchanged. Phenobarbital is 45% to 60% bound to plasma proteins, and for this reason, clinically significant protein binding interactions are rare. Phenobarbital is eliminated by a first-order process. Thirty percent to 50% of phenobarbital is metabolized by the liver to inactive products that are glucuronidated or sulfated and excreted in the urine. The half-life of phenobarbital ranges from 3 to 6 days in adults but varies significantly with age. The longest half-lives occur in newborns while the shortest occur in infants and children. Approximately 25% of the dose is excreted in the urine unchanged. Excretion of phenobarbital is enhanced significantly in alkaline urine and during forced diuresis.

Adverse Effects. CNS adverse effects during phenobarbital therapy are generally dose-related and include sedation, nystagmus, dizziness, and ataxia. Mild drowsiness is common on initiation of therapy, but tolerance to this effect usually develops within the first several weeks. Occasionally, sedation will persist during chronic treatment and for these patients the dose should be reduced. Reversible paradoxical hyperactivity may also occur in up to 40% of children who are treated with phenobarbital but this rarely requires discontinuation of therapy. Of greater concern are the subtle effects of phenobarbital on behavior, mood, and cognition. These behavioral changes usually occur within the first few months of therapy and are more prevalent in patients with organic

TABLE 62.9	Dosage Forms, Normal Maintenance Dose, and Interval for the Older Anticonvulsants

Generic (trade)	Dosage Form	Initial Dosage[a]	Maintenance Dose[b] (maximum dose)	Interval[b]
Carbamazepine (Tegretol and generic); Carbitrol Tegretol XR	suspension (100 mg/5 mL) tablet (100 mg) chewable (200 mg) capsule (200, 300) tablet (100, 200, 400 mg)	10–20 mg/kg/day (P) 100–200 mg bid (A)	20–40 mg/kg/day (P) (1,000 mg/day) 1,200 mg/day (1,600 mg/day) (A)	bid-tid qid (if suspension)
Ethosuximide (Zarotin and generics)	solution/syrup (250 mg/ 5 mL) capsule (250 mg)	250 mg qd (P) 500 mg qd (A)	20 mg/kg/day (P) (1.5 gm/day) 1,000–2,000 mg (A)	bid-tid
Fosphenytoin (Cerebyx)	parenteral (50 PE/1 mL)	15–20 PE/kg (loading dose)	4–6 PE/kg	q 6 or 8
Phenobarbital (generic)	elixir (various) tablet (various) parenteral (various)	3–5 mg/kg/day (P) 90 mg qd (A)	3–8 mg/kg/day (P) 100–300 mg/day (A)	qd (oral adults) qd-bid (pediatrics) IV (30–100 mg/min)
Phenytoin (Dilantin, Phenytek, and generics)	suspension (125 mg/5 mL) chewable (50 mg capsule (30, 100, 200, 300 mg) parenteral (50 mg/mL)	3–5 mg/kg/day (P) 100–300 mg/day (A)	5–10 mg/kg/day (P) 300–400 mg/day (A)	qd (Kapseals) bid tid-qid (if suspension)
Primidone (Mysoline)	tablet (50, 250 mg) suspension (250 mg/5 mL)	50–100 mg/day (P) 125–250 mg/day (A)	125–250 mg/day (10-25 mg/kg) (P) 125–250 (A)	tid

[a] See manufacturer information for titration scheme. With the exception of gabapentin, these anticonvulsants are begun at low doses and slowly titrated over weeks to a dose that will control the patients, seizures. [b] Dose and interval may decrease or increase in the presence of medication that induce or inhibit metabolism, respectively. See product information for maximum dosage.
A, adult; P, pediatric; bid, twice a day; tid, three times daily; qid, four times daily; qd, every day; PE, phenytoin equivalents; q, each, every; IV, intravenously; HS, half strength.

brain disease. A noticeable improvement in behavior may be seen when phenobarbital is replaced with valproate or carbamazepine. Phenobarbital may also cause depression and lack of interest or ambition that are recognized by others or appreciated only after discontinuation of the drug. Although the cognitive effects of phenobarbital are not well characterized, several investigations have found a dose-related impairment of memory, performance on intelligence and vigilance tests, work performance, and performance of complex verbal and nonverbal tasks. Alterations in cognition are particularly concerning in young children. These changes may persist despite the development of tolerance to the sedative effects of the drug.

Serious adverse effects of phenobarbital are uncommon, and, in general, this drug is associated with fewer idiosyncratic adverse effects than is phenytoin or carbamazepine.[11] Morbilliform rash is the most common idiosyncratic reaction, occurring in 1% to 3% of patients. Rarely, the rash may progress to Stevens-Johnson syndrome or exfoliative dermatitis or may occur in conjunction with symptoms of hepatitis or bone marrow suppression. The potential for cross-reactivity between phenobarbital and other aromatic AEDs (i.e., phenobarbital, carbamazepine, primidone) and lamotrigine should be considered in changing therapy for these patients. Patients who experience a moderate to severe dermatological reaction generally should avoid these agents. Megaloblastic anemia with folic acid deficiency occurs in less than 1% of phenobarbital-treated patients and responds to folic acid supplementation. Like phenytoin, phenobarbital is associated with bone disorders (e.g., osteomalacia) during chronic therapy.

Drug Interactions. Although many drug-drug interactions have been reported between phenobarbital and other drugs, a mechanistic approach to interactions should be considered whenever a medication is added to a patient's regimen.[20] Most drug interactions with phenobarbital are characterized by alterations of metabolism. By increasing the synthesis and retarding the degradation of hepatic enzymes, phenobarbital accelerates the metabolism of many agents that are metabolized by the mixed-function oxidase system (Table 62.11) including theophylline, warfarin, cyclosporine, chloramphenicol, chlorpromazine, haloperidol, oral contraceptives, and tricyclic antidepressants. It also affects the clearance of valproate, felbamate, lamotrigine, oxcarbazepine, topiramate, and zonisamide. The degree of enzyme induction and alteration of drug metabolism varies greatly among patients and is to some extent under genetic control. Enzyme induction usually last for 2 to 3 weeks after phenobarbital is discontinued. Carbamazepine concentrations may remain un-

TABLE 62.10 | Clinical Pharmacokinetics of Antiepileptic Drugs in Adults

AED	Bioavailability, % (time to peak, hours)	Volume of Distribution (L/kg)	Protein Binding (%)	Plasma Half-Life (hours)	Elimination (primary route)	CYP Isoenzymes Involved	Reference Range mg/L (μMol/L)
Carbamazepine	75–85 (4–8)	0.8–1.6	75–78	24–45	65% (hepatic); 15% UTG	3A4, 2C8, 1A2	4–12 (16–48)
Clonazepam	80–90 (1–4)	2.1–4.3	80–90	30–40	98% (hepatic)	3A	5–70 (16–220)
Clorazepate[a]	(0.5–2)	1–1.9	95–98	55–100	hepatic/renal	Unknown	Not determined
Ethosuximide	(1–7)	0.6–0.9	0	20–60	65% (hepatic)	Unknown	40–100 (283–708)
Felbamate	90 (2–4)	0.75–0.85	25	14–23	50% (hepatic); 15% UTG	3A4, 2E1	Not determined
Gabapentin[b]	60 (2–3)	0.7–0.8	0	5–7	100% (renal)	None	Not determined
Lamotrigine	98 (2–4)	0.9–1.2	55	14–27	65% UTG	Unknown	Not determined
Levetiracetam	100 (1)	0.55–0.7	<10	6–8	66% (renal)	None	Not determined
Oxcarbazepine	100 (4–6)	0.7[c]	40[c]	2 (9[c])	95% (renal)	Unknown	Not determined
Phenobarbital	95–100 (1–4)	0.50–0.57	48–54	72–144	30%–50% (hepatic)	2C9	10–40 (43–172)
Phenytoin	85–95 (4–8)	0.5–0.7	90–93	9–40	90% (hepatic)	2C9, MORE	10–20 (40–80)
Primidone	90–100 (1–3)	0.4–0.8	20–30	5–18	20%–30% (hepatic)	Unknown	5–15 (23–69)
Tiagabine	90 (1–1.5)	0.8–1.2	96	7–9	30% (hepatic)	3A4	Not determined
Topiramate	80 (3–4)	0.6–0.8	15	22–24	70% (renal)	Unknown	Not determined
Valproate	100 (2–8)	0.09–1.7	88–92	6–16	50%–70% (hepatic); 40% UTG	2C9, 2C19, 2A6	50–150 (200–400)
Zonisamide	100 (2–6)	1.45	40	63 (105 RBCs)	62% (renal)	3A4, CA5, 2C1	Not determined

[a] Pharmacokinetic values for N-desmethyldiazepam, the active metabolite of clorazepate.
[b] Half-life in newborns may be as long as 400 hours.
[c] Reported for MHD, the active metabolite of oxcarbazepine.
AED, antiepileptic drug; CYP, cytochrome; UGT, uridine diphosphate glucuronosyltransferase; RBCs, red blood cells

TABLE 62.11	Effects of Antiepileptic Drugs on Hepatic Metabolism

Drug[a]	Effect	Isoenzyme Involved
Carbamazepine	Inducer	CYP3A4, CYP2C9, CYP2C19
Ethosuximide	Inducer	CYP3A4
Felbamate	Inhibitor	CYP2C19, epoxide hydroxylase, β-oxidation
	Inducer	CYP3A4
Lamotrigine	Weak Inducer	UGT
Oxcarbazepine/MHD	Inhibitor	CYP2C19
	Inducer	CYP3A45
Phenobarbital	Inducer	CYP1A2, CYP2B6, CYP2C8, CYP2C9, CYP2C19, CYP3A4, UGT
Phenytoin	Inducer	CYP2C19, CYP3A4, UGT
	Inhibitor	CYP2C9
Topiramate	Inducer	β-oxidation
	Inhibitor	CYP2C19
Valproate	Inhibitor	CYP2C9, UGT, epoxide hydroxylase, β-oxidation
	Inhibitor	CYP2C19

[a]gabapentin, levetiracetam, tiagabine, zonisamide do not affect hepatic isoenzyme.
CYP, cytochrome; UGT, uridine diphosphate glucuronosyltransferase; MHD, 10-monohydroxy metabolite.

changed or decline during phenobarbital coadministration. Phenobarbital can also inhibit the metabolism of some drugs, presumably by competition for similar metabolic pathways. The effect of phenobarbital on plasma concentrations of phenytoin is unpredictable because induction and inhibition of metabolism probably occur (phenytoin and phenobarbital are substrates for CYP2C9). Phenytoin concentrations may modestly rise, decline, or (as in most cases) show no change. The effect of phenytoin on phenobarbital plasma concentrations is unpredictable, and in most cases, clinically important alterations are not seen. Valproate may inhibit CYP2C9 to cause a clinically important reduction in the metabolism of phenobarbital, with resultant symptoms of phenobarbital toxicity.

PRIMIDONE

Primidone is structurally related to the barbiturates, and like phenobarbital, it is effective for the treatment of partial and generalized tonic-clonic seizures. Primidone is an active anticonvulsant, as are its two major metabolites, phenobarbital and phenylethylmalonamide. Although the clinical use of primidone is similar to that of phenobarbital, adverse effects are more commonly a limiting factor during long-term primidone therapy. Some patients may respond to primidone therapy despite the failure of phenobarbital to control seizures.

Formulation and Dosage. Primidone (Mysoline and generic) is available as oral tablets and suspension (Table 62.9). Primidone should be initiated slowly, to allow the development of tolerance to the acute gastrointestinal and sedative effects of the parent drug. For those older than 8 years of age, therapy is started at a dose of 100 to 125 mg with gradual dosage increases every 4 to 7 days in 125-mg to 250-mg increments until the effective dose is reached. Children younger than 8 years are begun on 50 mg and are titrated by 50-mg to 100-mg increments. Doses are given twice a day (bid) or three times daily (tid).

Pharmacokinetics. Pharmacokinetic parameters of primidone are summarized in Table 62.10. Metabolic transformation of primidone to phenobarbital and phenylethylmalonamide occurs by oxidative metabolism and pyrimidine ring cleavage, respectively. Primidone and its metabolites are also excreted by the kidney to a significant extent. The half-life of primidone is relatively short, therefore the drug is usually given in divided doses to maintain more consistent plasma concentrations of the parent drug and reduce the likelihood of transient side effects at times of peak primidone concentrations. Pharmacokinetic monitoring of primidone therapy includes routine assessment of primidone and phenobarbital concentrations. Whereas primidone reaches steady-state concentrations quickly, there is usually a delay of 2 to 3 weeks before plateau concentrations of phenobarbital are attained. During chronic treatment, plasma concentrations of phenobarbital are approximately one to three times higher than those of primidone. This fact is sometimes useful in monitoring compliance.

Adverse Effects. The adverse effects of primidone are similar to those of phenobarbital. Thus, the potential for primidone-related neurotoxicity is of concern during long-term therapy. In addition, primidone itself is frequently associated with initial dose-related adverse effects, including sedation, dizziness, and nausea. Decreased libido and impotence appear to be more common during primidone therapy than with other AEDs. Serious adverse effects during primidone therapy are rare.

Drug Interactions. The metabolism of primidone or its metabolites can be affected by other AEDs, including phenytoin and valproate. Phenytoin increases phenobarbital concentrations during coadministration with primidone. The result is an approximate doubling of the phenobarbital: primidone concentration ratio. Valproate can reduce the hepatic clearance of metabolically derived phenobarbital and produce signs of barbiturate intoxication during primidone therapy. Conversely, valproate has a negligible effect on the plasma concentrations of primidone. Carbamazepine may increase the metabolism of primidone, although in many patients this interaction is not clinically important. Primidone concentrations are not significantly affected during phenytoin therapy.

ETHOSUXIMIDE

Ethosuximide is a member of the succinimide class of AEDs, which includes phensuximide and methsuximide. The latter agents share similar antiepileptic effects with ethosuximide, but they are rarely used in the treatment of seizures because they are less effective and their use is associated with more significant adverse effects. Ethosuximide is effective for the treatment of absence seizures, and is often preferred for young children because of the potential for valproate-associated hepatotoxicity. Ethosuximide has no activity against partial and generalized tonic-clonic seizures. Although the mechanism of ethosuximide's antiepileptic effect is unknown, the drug may suppress seizures by alteration of calcium flux in the thalamus or by the depletion of excitatory neurotransmitter stores within the CNS.

Formulation and Dosage. Ethosuximide is available as a capsule and syrup for oral use (Table 62.8). The initial dose of ethosuximide is 250 mg daily for children 3 to 6 years of age and 500 mg for children 6 years and older. The dose should be increased at weekly intervals in 250-mg increments as necessary. Infants require larger doses on a weight basis than adolescents and adults. Despite the long half-life of ethosuximide, the drug is often given in divided doses to minimize gastrointestinal distress.

Pharmacokinetics. Clinical pharmacokinetics of ethosuximide are summarized in Table 62.10. Ethosuximide is metabolized hepatically to inactive hydroxylated products that are then excreted. Approximately 20% of a given dose is excreted in the urine unchanged. Plasma concentration monitoring helps to guide therapy, but the upper end of the therapeutic range is loosely defined. Many patients tolerate concentrations greater than 100 mg per milliliter, and plasma concentrations of 150 mg per milliliter or greater are occasionally required for optimal treatment.

Adverse Effects. Sedation, nausea, anorexia, and headache are the most common adverse effects reported on initiation of ethosuximide therapy. Tolerance to these symptoms usually develops within the first weeks of treatment and can be minimized by reducing the dose or by introducing the drug gradually as outlined above. Behavioral disturbances, including irritability, depression, and frank psychosis, occur independent of the drug dose. These symptoms are rare and usually occur in children or adolescents who have a history

of behavioral or psychiatric problems. Discontinuation of the drug is usually required. In most patients, ethosuximide has no detrimental effect on intellectual function. Idiosyncratic reactions include mild, transient leukopenia, rare pancytopenia, rash, and systemic lupus erythematosus (SLE). Periodic complete blood counts should be performed during the first 6 to 12 months of therapy, and the patient should be observed for the development of clinical symptoms that suggest serious bone marrow suppression.

Drug Interactions. Ethosuximide is not an enzyme inducer or inhibitor and has no important effect on the disposition of most other AEDs. Ethosuximide concentrations may be reduced by carbamazepine and increased by valproate, presumably by enzyme induction and inhibition, respectively. Phenytoin, phenobarbital, and primidone have no clinical effect on ethosuximide concentrations.

CARBAMAZEPINE

Carbamazepine is a highly lipophilic iminostilbene compound that is structurally related to the tricyclic antidepressant imipramine. Carbamazepine is very effective for the treatment of partial and secondarily generalized tonic-clonic seizures, but it is not effective against myoclonic, absence, or febrile seizures. The antiepileptic effect of carbamazepine is attributed to the drug's ability to affect sodium channels to limit sustained, repetitive firing and alter synaptic transmission.

Formulation and Dosage. Carbamazepine (Tegretol, Carbatrol, and generic) is available as oral and chewable tablets, as a suspension, and as a controlled-release oral dosage form (Table 62.9). Advantages of these products include twice daily dosing and reduced fluctuations between peak and trough plasma concentrations (compared with immediate release products). The extended-release characteristics of Tegretol-XR are lost if the tablet is broken or chewed; hence, patients should be counseled to swallow the tablet whole. Carbatrol is formulated in a bead-filled capsule that can be emptied onto food. Patients and parents should be told that the bead shell may appear in the stool. No parenteral formulation of carbamazepine is available for commercial use. Initial and maintenance dose of carbamazepine are depicted in Table 62.9. The initial adult dose is gradually titrated, in 200-mg increments, every 3 to 7 days. Although the manufacturer recommends that daily doses of carbamazepine not exceed 1,200 mg, doses of 2,000 mg and above are occasionally required for optimal therapy. Children should be started on carbamazepine in doses ranging from 5 to 10 mg/kg/day divided bid or tid as tablets, or four times daily (qid) as suspension. Maintenance dose above 35 mg/kg/day are rarely needed. Loading doses of carbamazepine are not recommended for usual outpatient therapy because of gastric disturbances. However, single carbamazepine doses of 8 mg per kilogram (using tablets or suspension) are useful in patients for which rapid attainment of a therapeutic concentration is desired.[21]

Pharmacokinetics. A summary of the pharmacokinetic profile for carbamazepine can be found in Table 62.10. Absorption of carbamazepine from the gastrointestinal tract is slow and erratic and often does not follow first-order pharmacokinetics. The time to peak plasma concentrations after oral administration may vary from an average of 4 to 8 hours to as long as 24 hours. Although prolonged absorption of the drug may be due to slow dissolution of the drug from tablet form, the suspension is also absorbed erratically. Food has no consistent effect on the bioavailability of carbamazepine.

Carbamazepine is almost exclusively cleared by hepatic metabolism. The major metabolic pathway for elimination involves hepatic oxidation to the 10, 11-epoxide (CBZ-E), which possesses anticonvulsant activity. The remainder is glucuronidated, sulfur-conjugated, or oxidatively metabolized by other routes. Only 2% of the dose is recovered unchanged in the urine. The half-life of the drug after a single dose may range from 24 to 45 hours. With chronic administration the half-life of carbamazepine is reduced, and interindividual differences in clearance are enhanced. Increased clearance of carbamazepine occurs during the first few weeks of therapy because of autoinduction of the CYP3A4 isoenzyme of the cytochrome P-450 system. This causes an increase in oxidation to CBZ-E. Steady-state concentrations of carbamazepine are reached within several days after therapy is initiated; however, autoinduction may cause concentrations to decline by as much as 50% during the first 4 weeks of therapy. After 1 month, autoinduction is complete, and plasma concentrations vary predictably with changes in dosage. Thus, the metabolic clearance and half-life may vary significantly, depending on the duration of treatment and concomitant drug therapy. It is not uncommon to observe a reduction in the half-life of carbamazepine from 30 hours after a single dose to 12 hours with chronic therapy and a further reduction to 8 hours during polytherapy with other AEDs. Larger daily doses (>1,200 mg), more frequent administration (three or four times a day), or use of extended release formulations of carbamazepine are often necessary to minimize plasma concentration fluctuations and the attendant risk of breakthrough seizures or transient adverse effects (e.g., dizziness). In this situation, extended-release carbamazepine products are useful to simplify the dosing regimen and enhance compliance.

Because of the large interindividual variability in carbamazepine absorption and clearance, the time-dependent alterations in metabolism, and the potential for fluctuations in drug concentrations over a dosage interval, careful plasma concentration monitoring of carbamazepine is often needed to determine optimal therapy. Although plasma concentrations of CBZ-E are not routinely monitored, they generally account for 10% to 20% of the parent compound.

Adverse Effects. Initial, dose-related adverse effects of carbamazepine are common and include dizziness, drowsiness, anorexia, and nausea. Although tolerance to these effects develops within the first few weeks of therapy, their occurrence can be minimized or avoided by gradual dose titration. Persistent gastrointestinal upset may be relieved by giving the drug with meals. Reversible, dose-related symptoms of toxicity include diplopia (commonly the initial manifestation of toxicity), nausea, headache, dizziness, and ataxia. Dose-related toxicities may occur transiently at times of peak drug plasma concentrations because of fluctuations in the blood concentration of carbamazepine over the course of a usual dosage interval. Extended-release carbamazepine products are often useful for ameliorating these symptoms.

Other dose-related neuropsychiatric adverse effects include depression, irritability, mental sluggishness, and impairment of concentration and short-term memory.[22] However, these adverse effects are less common than with phenobarbital and primidone. Furthermore, in several clinical epilepsy trials, patients with personality and behavioral disorders who were treated with carbamazepine had significant improvement during therapy. Based on these observations and subsequent clinical trials this compound has been approved as a treatment of bipolar disorder. When dose-related adverse effects persist throughout the day, the total daily dose of carbamazepine should be decreased; when they are transient and occur 2 to 4 hours after a dose, an adjustment in the dosing schedule or a change to an extended release product may suffice. Unusual movement disorders and carbamazepine-induced seizures can occur acutely after an overdose.

Rash occurs between the first and second week of therapy in approximately 5% of those treated with carbamazepine. Benign, maculopapular, urticarial, and morbilliform reactions are the most common adverse effects and are generally managed with symptomatic measures (e.g., diphenhydramine). Although rare, exfoliative dermatitis and Stevens-Johnson syndrome may also occur. In some cases, rash may be accompanied by fever, generalized lymphadenopathy, hepatomegaly, splenomegaly, and, less commonly, nephritis and vasculitis. Symptoms are reversible on drug discontinuation, and corticosteroids may hasten recovery. Patients who experience a moderate to severe dermatologial reaction generally should avoid lamotrigine or other aromatic AEDs.[23] Other idiosyncratic adverse reactions include hepatitis and SLE. Carbamazepine-induced SLE is delayed, usually occurring after 6 to 12 months of therapy and generally resolves within weeks or months of withdrawing the drugs. Hepatitis usually occurs within the first few weeks of therapy and may coincide with eosinophilia and other symptoms of drug hypersensitivity. Carbamazepine may also cause a mild elevation of liver enzymes in fewer than 10% of patients, which appears to have no adverse clinical consequence.

Among the most worrisome of idiosyncratic adverse reactions is aplastic anemia. Although rare, this condition is fatal in about one half of affected patients. The incidence of carbamazepine-associated aplastic anemia is estimated to be 0.5 per 100,000 treatment-years.[24] Neither patient age nor daily or total dosage significantly affects this risk. Carbamazepine is also associated with a dose-independent transient leucopenia, which occurs in about 10% of patients. In most cases the leukopenia is mild and resolves, despite continuation of treatment. However, in about 2% of patients, leukopenia persists until the drug is removed.[24] Carbamazepine-induced leukopenia does not appear to be a risk factor for aplastic anemia. While aplastic anemia can develop at any time during the first year of carbamazepine treatment, leukopenia is most commonly seen within the first month. The risk of serious hematological reactions to carbamazepine can be minimized by patient education and laboratory monitoring. When therapy is initiated, patients should be counseled to seek immediate medical attention for abrupt onset of high fever, infection, petechiae, or unusual fatigue. If the diagnosis of aplastic anemia is confirmed, carbamazepine should be discontinued immediately, and the patient should not be given the drug again. Suggested laboratory monitoring should include complete blood counts before initiation of treatment and every 2 weeks for the first 2 months of therapy. If no abnormalities are detected, hematological monitoring should continue at intervals of 3 months or when the patient develops signs or symptoms of myelosuppression. If mild leukopenia develops, complete blood counts should be evaluated at 2-week intervals until they return to baseline values. Therapy should be discontinued if the absolute neutrophil count drops below 1,500/mm[3] or if infection occurs.

Carbamazepine may also cause hyponatremia and water retention, probably by increasing antidiuretic hormone secretion (syndrome of inappropriate antidiuretic hormone secretion [SIADH]). This effect appears to be dose-related and is most often associated with plasma concentrations above the therapeutic range. At low serum sodium concentrations (<120 mEq/L), patients may report headache, confusion, dizziness, or loss of seizure control. Treatment consists of water restriction and/or reduction or discontinuation of carbamazepine therapy. Treatment with demeclocycline may be effective for patients who require continued carbamazepine. Carbamazepine can cause cardiac conduction disturbances, primarily in older patients. Cardiotoxicity may be more common with larger doses and in patients with an underlying cardiac abnormality. A thorough history and baseline electrocardiogram should precede the initiation of carbamazepine therapy in older patients.

Drug Interactions. Carbamazepine enhances the clearance of drugs metabolized by uridine diphosphate glucuronosyltransferase (UGT) as well as the CYP2C and CYP3A isoenzymes of the cytochrome P-450 system (Table 62.11).[20] Protein binding is low and drug interactions due to this mechanism are not clinically important. Although multiple interactions have been reported between carbamazepine and other drugs, a mechanistic approach to interactions should be considered whenever a medication is added to a patient's regimen.[17] Increased elimination has been demonstrated for theophylline, doxycycline, haloperidol, warfarin, corticosteroids, and various hormones. The clearance of valproate, clonazepam, ethosuximide, lamotrigine, felbamate,

oxcarbazepine, zonisamide, and topiramate are also increased. Thus, the potential for reduced effectiveness of these agents should be considered when carbamazepine is begun. The failure rate of oral contraceptives is increased fourfold to fivefold during coadministration with carbamazepine and other enzyme-inducing AEDs (e.g., phenytoin, phenobarbital, and primidone), therefore patients should be monitored for breakthrough bleeding. An oral contraceptive with a higher estrogen content or an alternative form of birth control should be considered. The effect of carbamazepine on plasma concentrations of phenytoin, phenobarbital, and primidone is inconsistent and probably reflects various degrees of enzyme induction and inhibition. Routine monitoring of blood concentrations is recommended when carbamazepine is added to the regimen of any patient who is receiving AED therapy.

Drug interactions that affect CYP3A4 are common. Danazol, dextropropoxyphene, erythromycin, clarithromycin, isoniazid, verapamil, and diltiazem can inhibit carbamazepine metabolism and induce clinical symptoms of toxicity. Cimetidine may inhibit the metabolism of carbamazepine, but ranitidine has no effect. Carbamazepine concentrations can also be affected by concomitant therapy with other AEDs. Phenytoin, phenobarbital, and primidone may increase the metabolism of carbamazepine and lead to a reduction in the steady-state plasma concentration. However, in some patients, addition of phenytoin can result in an increase in carbamazepine concentrations. Carbamazepine blood concentrations may increase, decrease, or remain the same when valproate is added. This may occur due to valproate-mediated inhibition of carbamazepine metabolism via epoxide hydroxylase and the variable effects of valproate displacement of carbamazepine from protein-binding sites.

HYDANTOINS (PHENYTOIN AND FOSPHENYTOIN)

Phenytoin, a diphenyl-substituted hydantoin derivative, was introduced for the treatment of epilepsy in 1938. It soon became and continues to be one of the most widely prescribed AEDs because it possessed anticonvulsant activity at nonsedative doses. Phenytoin is effective for the treatment of partial and secondarily generalized tonic-clonic seizures, but it has no activity against absence and febrile seizures. Other hydantoin derivatives, including ethotoin and mephenytoin, also have anticonvulsant activity, but their clinical utility is limited. The specific mechanism of the anticonvulsant effect is unknown. Phenytoin blocks neuronal sodium and calcium conductance, and calcium-mediated excitatory neurotransmission, which probably is involved in its ability to regulate neuronal excitability under abnormal conditions.

Formulation and Dosage. Phenytoin (Dilantin, Phenytek, and generic) is available as the free acid in suspension and chewable tablets (Table 62.9). The sodium salt of phenytoin is contained in phenytoin capsules and phenytoin injectable; for these dosage forms, phenytoin content is expressed in milligrams of sodium phenytoin. Because of the difference in molecular weight between the acid and salt forms of the drug, the capsule and parenteral dosage forms contain 8% fewer phenytoin acid equivalents than the suspension and chewable tablets do. This difference in drug content should be accounted for when changing products. To solubilize the sodium salt of phenytoin into a parenteral dosage form 40% propylene glycol is added as a diluent.

Fosphenytoin (Cerebyx), a water-soluble prodrug of phenytoin for intravenous or intramuscular administration, is available for the acute treatment of seizures and for the treatment or prevention of seizures in patients unable to take medication by the oral route. Fosphenytoin is less hydrophobic than phenytoin, therefore it does not require propylene glycol as a diluent, and it is compatible with most common intravenous solutions (including those containing dextrose). Fosphenytoin is rapidly converted to phenytoin by circulating phosphatases with a half-life of 15 minutes.

Doses of fosphenytoin are expressed as phenytoin equivalents (PE), which are the milligram amounts of phenytoin released by the action of phosphatases on the parent drug. For example, a fosphenytoin dose of 500 mg PE releases 500 mg of phenytoin in the presence of phosphatases. Doses of fosphenytoin should be checked carefully to ensure that they are written as intended. Only extended-release phenytoin capsules (e.g., Dilantin Kapseals, Phenytek), are approved for once daily maintenance dosing. Although the suspension has been given successfully once a day, it is generally given in divided doses. The parenteral dosage form should be given in divided daily doses.

Loading doses of phenytoin or fosphenytoin help patients who require rapid attainment of a concentration within the therapeutic range for the drug. The usual loading dose of phenytoin is 15 to 18 mg per kilogram. Oral loading doses of phenytoin can be given as a single dose or divided into individual increments of 200 to 400 mg separated by 2 to 4 hours. Previously, it was recommended that oral loading doses be administered in small increments separated by several hours to enhance the rate of drug absorption. However, recent evidence suggests that oral administration of a single dose loading with phenytoin is well tolerated and results in a shorter delay in the attainment of a therapeutic plasma concentration than the split-dose technique.[25] By either method, phenytoin is absorbed slowly after oral administration, and the resultant peak plasma concentration is approximately half that achieved after an equivalent intravenous loading dose. When given by the intravenous route, phenytoin should be administered at a maximal rate of 50 mg per minute (1 mg/kg/min in pediatrics) to reduce the risk of hypotension and cardiac arrhythmias. These adverse effects are at least partially related to the 40% propylene glycol diluent that is used in the parenteral formulation of the drug; however, phenytoin itself also has active cardiovascular effects. Blood pressure, heart rate, and the electrocardiogram should be monitored periodically when large doses of phenytoin are administered intravenously. Fosphenytoin does not contain propylene glycol, and can therefore be administered intravenously at infusion rates up to 150 mg PE per minute and 3 mg PE/kg/min in adults and children, respectively.[26] When necessary phenytoin has been given intraosseously.

Pharmacokinetics. The pharmacokinetic parameters of phenytoin in adults are summarized in Table 62.10. Phenytoin is poorly water-soluble at acidic pH. Very little drug exists in solution in the stomach, and its absorption takes place primarily in the proximal part of the small intestine. The time to peak drug concentration after an oral loading dose of phenytoin may be delayed, because the rate of drug dissolution in intestinal fluid is dose-dependent. The bioavailability of phenytoin approaches 100% for most well-formulated products, but it is prudent to avoid changing dosage forms and products because small changes in bioavailability can result in large changes in plasma concentration (and seizure control). For reasons not fully understood, phenytoin suspension is poorly absorbed in infants and young children. In fact, plasma phenytoin concentration within the therapeutic range on intravenous therapy may become nondetectable following conversion to the same or increasing doses of the suspension.

Under normal conditions, phenytoin is approximately 90% bound to plasma proteins, primarily albumin. Conditions that can alter protein binding include renal failure, a lowered plasma albumin concentration or the presence of fetal albumin, and concomitant administration of displacing drugs. In each case these factors result in a decrease in phenytoin binding and an increase in the free fraction and volume of distribution. However, despite alterations in the free fraction, the free concentration of phenytoin is not changed significantly. The free drug exerts pharmacologic and toxic effects at receptor sites, so the clinical response to a given dose of phenytoin is unchanged by altered protein binding. However, careful interpretation of the total (bound and unbound) phenytoin concentration is warranted. Equation 62.1 approximates the concentration of phenytoin that would be observed if the albumin concentration were normal ($Cp_{adjusted}$) from the total (bound and unbound) concentration ($Cp_{measured}$) and the patient's albumin concentration (Alb) in grams per deciliter[24]:

$$Cp_{adjusted} = Cp_{measured} \div [(0.2 \times Alb) + 0.1] \quad (62.1)$$

In patients with end-stage renal disease (creatinine clearance <10 mL/min), the affinity of albumin for phenytoin is reduced by approximately 50%, and Equation 62.2 should be used[27]:

$$Cp_{adjusted} = Cp_{measured} \div [(0.1 \times Alb) + 0.1] \quad (62.2)$$

These equations were created for use in adults and have not proven as helpful in children. Free (unbound) concentrations are also available from many clinical laboratories. This assay requires 1 mL of serum, which may prohibit its use in neonates. Patients receiving a loading dose of fosphenytoin should have plasma phenytoin concentrations collected 2 hours or 4 hours after an intravenous (IV) or intramuscular (IM) dose, respectively.

Phenytoin is eliminated primarily by hepatic metabolism. The major metabolic route involves *para*-hydroxylation of the parent compound to yield 5-(*p*-hydroxyphenyl)-5-phenylhydantoin. This metabolite is then glucuronidated and excreted primarily in the urine. Other hydroxylated metabolites are also generated during phenytoin metabolism, and all metabolites are inactive. Less than 5% of the drug is eliminated unchanged in the urine.

Unlike many drugs that are cleared from the body by a first-order elimination process, the clearance of phenytoin varies over the range of plasma concentrations that are clinically useful for the treatment of seizures. At very low plasma concentrations, phenytoin clearance is first-order, and small dosage changes result in a proportional change in the concentration. However, as the phenytoin concentration approaches the upper end of the therapeutic range, the maximal capacity for phenytoin metabolism is approached (zero-order pharmacokinetics), and a change in dosage can result in a disproportionately large change in the steady-state concentration. Thus, phenytoin dosage adjustments must be made cautiously. Also, the time required to attain a steady-state concentration of phenytoin can vary from several days to several weeks. The Michaelis-Menten model of saturable enzyme kinetics has been used to characterize the relationship between phenytoin dose and plasma concentration at steady-state. By using Equation 62.3, the rate of phenytoin administration (in milligrams per day) can be calculated from the desired steady-state plasma concentration. Population estimates of V_{max} (maximal rate of phenytoin metabolism) and K_m (phenytoin concentration at which V_{max} is half-maximum) can be used if patient-specific data are not available.[24] Both V_{max} and K_m are influenced by age. Population estimates for V_{max} is 7 mg per liter (adults), 10 to 13 mg per liter (age 6 months–6 years), and 8 to 10 mg per liter (7–16 years). Population estimates for K_m are poorly defined for the pediatric population, but is 4 mg/kg/day in adults.

$$Ri = Vmax \cdot CpssKm \% Cpss \qquad (62.3)$$

Adverse Effects. Acute, dose-related adverse effects of phenytoin include ataxia, diplopia, dizziness, drowsiness, encephalopathy, and involuntary movements. These symptoms usually occur at phenytoin concentrations greater than 30 mg per milliliter and are reversible when phenytoin is discontinued or the dose is reduced. Involuntary movements during phenytoin intoxication may include dyskinesias of the limbs, trunk, or face and are completely reversible upon drug discontinuation. Phenytoin has also been reported to exacerbate seizures at high concentrations, but this is rare. Horizontal nystagmus is a dose-related effect that may occur at plasma concentrations within the therapeutic range and does not necessitate a reduction in dosage.

Adverse effects associated with long-term therapy include gingival hyperplasia, facial coarsening, peripheral neu-

ropathy, and vitamin deficiencies. Gingival hyperplasia is a dose-related effect that occurs in roughly 50% of patients taking phenytoin. Although there is no racial, sex, or age predilection for gingival hyperplasia it appears to be more frequent in young patients with epilepsy who are on polytherapy with AEDs. The exact mechanism for this adverse effect is unknown; however, when gingival macrophages are exposed to phenytoin they secrete increased amounts of platelet derived growth factor B, which may increase the proliferation of gingival cells. Phenytoin may also cause a deficiency of salivary immunoglobulin A (IgA) that can increase susceptibility to gingival inflammation.

Gingival hyperplasia usually begins within the first 3 months and may progress during the first year of therapy. Patients who are at risk for gingival hyperplasia include children and those with poor oral hygiene. Mild gum hyperplasia may respond to improved dental and periodontal hygiene or a reduction in phenytoin dosage. In advanced cases, gum resection surgery may be required. Alternative AED therapy should be considered for these patients. The presence of inflammation and dental plaque increases a patient's susceptibility, therefore they should be counseled to brush and floss their teeth on a regular basis and to have frequent dental checkups. Systemic administration of folic acid has been reported to delay the onset and reduce the incidence and severity of gingival hyperplasia.

Chronic phenytoin therapy is also associated with dysmorphic changes in the lips, nose, brow, and other facial structures as well as other cosmetic changes, including hirsutism and acne. These adverse effects are a major limitation to the use of phenytoin for the treatment of children, adolescents, and young women. Peripheral neuropathy with decreased deep tendon reflexes and sensory deficits may also occur during long-term phenytoin therapy. These symptoms are most common during polytherapy with phenytoin and phenobarbital and are not reversible. Phenytoin-induced megaloblastic anemia with folic acid deficiency occurs in fewer than 1% of patients and responds to folic acid supplementation.

Alterations of bone density, mass, and mineral content have been associated with phenytoin, usually when it is given in combination with other enzyme-inducing AEDs (e.g., carbamazepine and phenobarbital). Although most patients with AED-related bone disease are asymptomatic, clinically apparent osteomalacia and osteoporosis may occur and requires appropriate treatment. Whether patients without clinical evidence of bone disease benefit from prophylactic vitamin D and calcium supplementation is not known. Certainly, patients with known risk factors for metabolic bone disease (e.g., inadequate diet, sunlight, or exercise) should be monitored closely. AED-induced acceleration in vitamin D metabolism to less active products and impaired absorption of calcium may cause or contribute to this complication of chronic therapy.

Idiosyncratic adverse reactions usually occur within the first 8 weeks of therapy and include rash, hepatitis, lymphadenopathy, and hematologic alterations. Skin rashes, which occur in fewer than 10% of patients, usually manifest within the first 14 days of treatment and may be accompanied by hepatitis, lymphadenopathy, and fever. The rash is usually morbilliform but may progress to Stevens-Johnson syndrome, erythema multiforme, or toxic epidermal necrolysis. Phenytoin should be discontinued if the rash involves mucous membranes or is accompanied by fever or pain. Hepatitis occurs rarely and usually in the presence of fever, rash, and lymphadenopathy. It usually occurs during the first 3 weeks of therapy (but may be delayed by 1 year from initiation) and necessitates the immediate discontinuation of phenytoin. Although drug discontinuation optimizes the chance of recovery, some patients' conditions continue to deteriorate, and (rarely) phenytoin-induced hepatic injury leads to encephalopathy, coma, and death. Hematologic adverse reactions during phenytoin therapy include a modest, transient depression in leukocytes and, very rarely, aplastic anemia or agranulocytosis. Patients with severe idiosyncratic reactions to phenytoin should not be given the drug again. Also, the potential for cross-reactivity with other aromatic AEDs and lamotrigine should be considered.

The low water solubility of the parenteral dosage form causes phenytoin to crystallize when it is injected into muscle. This results in a depot of drug that is potentially damaging to local tissue and slowly and erratically absorbed from the injection site. For these reasons, phenytoin should not be given intramuscularly. Major advantages of fosphenytoin over phenytoin include less venous irritation and discomfort after intravenous administration, lack of tissue necrosis on infiltration, more reliable absorption after intramuscular administration, and improved admixture compatibility. For these reasons many consider fosphenytoin to be the preferred hydantoin for parenteral administration. However, fosphenytoin is significantly more expensive than parenteral phenytoin, and it can cause burning, itching, or paresthesias in groin and facial areas during intravenous administration. These symptoms are usually mild and resolve by stopping the infusion or reducing the infusion rate.

Drug Interactions. Although multiple drug-drug interactions have been reported between phenytoin and other medications a mechanistic approach to interactions should be considered whenever a drug is added to a patient's regimen.[20] Phenytoin is a potent inducer of hepatic microsomal enzymes and increases the metabolism of many medications (Table 62.11). Phenytoin can reduce the effectiveness of oral contraceptives, warfarin, corticosteroids, cyclosporine, and theophylline. It increases the metabolism of carbamazepine, valproate, felbamate, lamotrigine, topiramate, tiagabine, oxcarbazepine, zonisamide, and clonazepam, resulting in a decrease in plasma concentrations and a potential reduction in the clinical anticonvulsant effect. Phenytoin also may increase the ratio of primidone to phenobarbital concentrations when it is administered to patients whose conditions are stabilized with primidone. Although phenytoin may enhance

warfarin metabolism with long-term use, the effect is complicated, particularly early after the addition of phenytoin. Phenytoin can enhance the effect of warfarin initially, an effect probably caused by displacement of warfarin from protein binding sites and competition between the two drugs for metabolism. Phenytoin and the S-isomer of warfarin are metabolized by CYP2C9 isoenzymes. After 1 to 2 weeks, the metabolic induction properties of phenytoin predominate, and the clinical effect of warfarin may decline.[20] An increase in warfarin dosage may be needed to maintain a consistent anticoagulant effect. For these reasons, warfarin therapy should be monitored closely during phenytoin coadministration.

Drug interactions affecting phenytoin may involve alterations in phenytoin absorption, metabolism, or protein binding. Antacids and nutritional formulas have been shown to reduce plasma concentrations of phenytoin, but in neither case is the interaction predictable. Steady-state phenytoin concentrations may fall during coadministration with aluminum-containing and magnesium-containing antacids, but the magnitude of the effect is variable. Given the potential for an interaction, it is reasonable to space antacid and phenytoin doses by 2 to 3 hours. Phenytoin concentrations drop after institution of nasogastric feedings, but the mechanism of this interaction is unclear. With flushing of the nasogastric tube, phenytoin adsorption to the apparatus is probably minimal. Concurrent administration with Isocal and Osmolite, but not Ensure, may reduce phenytoin concentrations.[28] Patients' phenytoin concentrations should be monitored closely when enteral feedings are initiated or stopped, or if the formula is changed.

Heparin, phenylbutazone, tolbutamide, and valproate displace phenytoin from plasma protein-binding sites. Many drugs alter the metabolism of phenytoin. It is important to be aware of these interactions, because small changes in phenytoin clearance can have a large effect on the steady-state plasma concentration. Folic acid, alcohol, and rifampin can increase the metabolism of phenytoin. Drugs that can reduce the metabolism of phenytoin include several AEDs (felbamate, valproate, topiramate, oxcarbazepine) and other medication such as isoniazid, amiodarone, cimetidine, fluconazole, ketoconazole, omeprazole, fluoxetine, ticlopidine, disulfiram, sulfonamides, and chloramphenicol.[20]

VALPROATE

Valproate is a unique AED because of its chemical structure and broad activity against partial and generalized seizures. Unlike most other AEDs, which have a substituted heterocyclic ring structure, valproate is a short, branched-chain fatty acid. Many clinicians consider valproate to be the drug of choice for the treatment of primary generalized epilepsies including tonic-clonic and absence seizures.[29] Ethosuximide and valproate are each effective against absence seizures. Valproate is as effective as carbamazepine for the treatment of secondarily generalized tonic-clonic seizures, but carbamazepine appears to be more effective against complex partial seizures.[12] Valproate is also effective as monotherapy for treating patients who have a combination of generalized tonic-clonic seizures and absence or myoclonic seizures. The mechanism of action of valproate has not been completely elucidated but probably involves blockade of voltage-dependent sodium channels as well as potentiation of GABA, the primary inhibitory neurotransmitter within the CNS.

Formulation and Dosage. Valproate is available as valproic acid in soft gelatin capsule and syrup form, and as divalproex sodium in enteric-coated tablets, extended-release tablet, sprinkle capsule, and parenteral dosage form (Table 62.9). The sprinkle product may be emptied onto food. Divalproex sodium dissociates into valproate in the gastrointestinal tract. The parenteral product is available as an alternative for patients who cannot take medication by the oral route. Although it is not approved for status epileptics, it has been used for this purpose. Product labeling indicates that the administration rate for the IV product should not exceed 20 mg per minute; however, it has been given over 5 to 10 minutes (1.5–6 mg/kg/min) without problems. IM administration of parenteral valproate is not recommended as it has been associated with muscle necrosis in animals. Table 62.9 depicts initiation and maintenance doses of valproate. Once started the medication should be gradual titrated every 3 to 7 days to an effective dose. Twice-daily dosing of the delayed release (enteric coated) formulation can be used in some patients; however, three times daily dosing is recommended when valproate is given concomitantly with enzyme-inducing AEDs. Extended release valproate (Depakote ER) can be give once or twice daily.

Pharmacokinetics. Clinical pharmacokinetic features of the common AEDs are summarized in Table 62.10. The bioavailability of valproate is close to 100% for all oral dosage forms, but the rate of absorption may vary. Peak concentrations occur within 2 hours after administration of valproate syrup and capsules. Enteric-coated tablets were developed to minimize the gastric distress associated with the plain capsule by prolonging the rate of drug dissolution. Consequently, the time to peak concentration is delayed and may vary from 3 to 8 hours. Although food has no significant effect on the absorption of the soft gelatin capsules, the rate of valproate absorption from enteric-coated tablets is delayed.

Valproate is highly bound to plasma proteins, so the volume of distribution is small. The extent of protein binding varies and depends largely on the dose and plasma concentration of the drug. At concentrations less than 75 mg per liter, valproate is approximately 90% bound to plasma proteins, primarily albumin. As the total concentration of valproate increases greater than 100 mg per liter, albumin binding sites become saturated, and the free fraction of the drug may increase by up to 50%. The distribution and protein binding of valproate can be affected by a variety of other factors, including albumin and free fatty acid concentrations,

pregnancy, age, and the presence of displacing drugs (e.g., phenytoin).

The relationship between the dose and steady-state plasma concentrations of valproate is curvilinear. Thus, with increasing dosage, a less-than-proportional change in the plasma concentration occurs. Because only the unbound fraction of drug is available for metabolic transformation, this curvilinear relationship may be explained by the increase in valproate clearance that would be expected when free valproate concentrations increase as a consequence of saturable protein binding. Valproate is eliminated almost exclusively by hepatic metabolism with a half-life of 12 to 16 hours in healthy volunteers. The half-life may be reduced during concomitant therapy with other AEDs. Oxidation of valproate at the β and γ positions and glucuronide conjugation of the parent and metabolites are the primary routes of metabolism. The major metabolites of valproate are eliminated slowly and may also be active. This may explain the fact that the maximal response to valproate can be delayed by several weeks beyond the time required to achieve steady-state plasma concentrations of the parent drug. Also, the anticonvulsant effect during valproate therapy outlasts its presence in plasma, further supporting the hypothesis that metabolites contribute to the antiepileptic effect of the drug.

Adverse Effects. The most common adverse effects during valproate therapy are gastrointestinal. Nausea, vomiting, anorexia, or other symptoms of gastrointestinal discomfort are reported by as many as 35% of patients treated with capsules or syrup. Patient tolerance can be improved by using the enteric-coated (tablets or sprinkles) or extended release products, and most patients prefer them. The dose-related neurologic adverse effects that are seen with valproate are like those seen with other AEDs. A fine, rapid intention tremor (reversible, dose-related adverse effect) occurs frequently. When tremor occurs transiently during the day, adjustment of the drug regimen to minimize plasma concentration fluctuations may alleviate the problem. Otherwise, a reduction in the total daily dose of valproate or concomitant treatment with a low dose of propranolol or primidone may be necessary. Cognitive adverse effects of valproate are similar to those of phenytoin.[30]

Other dose-related adverse effects include weight gain, loss or thinning of hair, altered platelet function, and increases in hepatic enzymes. Weight gain occurs in up to 50% of individuals and is more common in adult women. The average weight gain for adults is 15 pounds and may require that the medication be discontinued. Changes in weight are probably due to a reduction in energy use, coupled with an increased appetite. A reduction in caloric intake and exercise can be very helpful. It remains uncertain if weight gain is greater when larger doses are given. Hair thinning or alopecia is transient and usually occurs on initiation of therapy in 5% to 12% of patients. The adverse effect is thought to exhibit a dose-dependent relationship with incidences up to 28% being reported following high valproate plasma concentrations. Reduction of valproate dosage may help. The hair almost always grows back after discontinuation of the medication; however, it often has a different texture. There is also evidence that zinc (25–50 mg/day) and selenium (10–20 μg/day) supplementation may improve hair loss. Valproate causes a dose-related reduction in platelet count and impairment of function leading to an increase in bleeding time.[31] These effects may be significant for patients with high plasma concentrations of valproate or those undergoing surgical procedures.

Approximately 40% of patients will experience a dose-related increase in serum transaminases during valproate therapy. This abnormality is usually asymptomatic and rapidly responds to a reduction in dose or discontinuation of the drug. Practitioners should discontinue valproate in the following instances: (a) an elevation in hepatic enzymes three times above baseline; (b) abnormalities in laboratory tests of hepatic synthesis or metabolism (e.g., elevated bilirubin or prothrombin time or decreased serum albumin concentration); or (c) the development of clinical signs or symptoms of hepatitis. Baseline laboratory values, including liver enzymes and hepatic function tests, should be determined before therapy is initiated.

Valproate has also been associated with fulminant hepatotoxicity leading to coma and death. Although the overall incidence of fatal hepatotoxicity is very low (1 in 50,000), certain patients are particularly at risk. Specific risk factors include age less than 2 years, AED polytherapy, and developmental delay.[32] The risk of fatal hepatotoxicity is exceedingly low in patients older than 10 years of age who are receiving monotherapy. When it occurs, fulminant hepatotoxicity is usually seen during the first 6 to 12 months of therapy. Gastrointestinal distress, anorexia, or sudden loss of seizure control may precede the development of fulminant hepatic failure, so patients should be counseled at the start of therapy to report these or other clinical signs or symptoms of hepatitis as soon as they develop. The prognosis may be improved if therapy is discontinued quickly.

Dreifuss et al[32] suggest the following guidelines for minimizing the risk of fatal valproate hepatotoxicity: (a) avoid administering valproate as part of AED polytherapy in children younger than age 3 years, unless monotherapy has failed or the potential benefits of polypharmacy outweigh the risks; (b) avoid administering valproate to those with preexisting liver disease or a family history of childhood hepatic disease; (c) administer valproate in the lowest possible dose that is consistent with seizure control; (d) avoid concomitant administration of valproate and salicylates, and avoid fasting in children with intercurrent illnesses; (e) monitor clinically for such symptoms as nausea, vomiting, headache, lethargy, edema, jaundice, or seizure breakthrough, especially after febrile illness. Greater recognition of patients who are at risk for valproate hepatotoxicity is probably responsible for the significant decrease in the number of hepatic fatalities despite the overall increased use of the drug.[1]

Acute pancreatitis is a rare, but a potentially life-threatening adverse effect, which occasionally progresses to bleeding and death.[33] This reaction may occur in children and adults and can present after several years of uneventful therapy. Although rare, valproate has been associated with polycystic ovarian disease in women.[34] The mechanism for this event remains elusive, but symptoms include irregular or no menstrual periods, facial and other hair growth, acne, changes in body shape and obesity.

Drug Interactions. Although multiple drug-drug interactions have been reported between valproate and other drugs, a mechanistic approach to interactions should be considered whenever a medication is added to a patient's regimen.[20] Metabolic interactions between valproate and other AEDs are common. Unlike phenytoin, carbamazepine, phenobarbital, and primidone, valproate is not an enzyme-inducing drug. Conversely, valproate inhibits the metabolism of drugs that are biotransformed by CYP2C9, epoxide hydrolase, and UGT enzymes (Table 62.11). This inhibition has been implicated in valproate interactions with phenobarbital and phenytoin (both metabolized by CYP2C9), and lamotrigine and lorazepam (both metabolized by glucuronidation).[20] Valproate inhibits the oxidative metabolism of phenobarbital, leading to an average increase in phenobarbital concentrations of 80% (0%–200%). The variability in this increase requires that blood concentrations of phenobarbital be monitored and that appropriate adjustment of phenobarbital be made as necessary. The interaction between phenytoin and valproate is complex and probably involves enzyme inhibition and protein binding displacement. Phenytoin concentrations commonly fall after initiation of valproate therapy, probably owing to displacement of phenytoin from protein-binding sites and an attendant increase in phenytoin clearance and volume of distribution. The free fraction of phenytoin may increase further with subsequent increases in valproate dosage. During continued therapy with valproate, phenytoin concentrations may remain low or rise to or above the preadministration concentration. Regardless of the subsequent change in phenytoin concentrations, the free fraction of phenytoin probably remains elevated during polytherapy and may increase further with increasing doses of valproate. Thus, total plasma concentrations of phenytoin should be interpreted cautiously. Monitoring of unbound phenytoin concentrations may be useful during concomitant valproate therapy.

The metabolism of valproate is susceptible to induction by other AEDs, including phenobarbital, carbamazepine, phenytoin, and primidone. Plasma concentrations of valproate decrease by an average of 30% to 40%, and the half-life is reduced to 6 to 9 hours. Monotherapy with valproate is highly recommended because of the difficulty of maintaining consistent therapeutic concentrations of valproate in individuals who are taking other AEDs. Antipyretic doses of aspirin may displace valproate from protein-binding sites and competitively inhibit β-oxidation. Unlike other AEDs, valproate does not increase the failure rate of oral contraceptives. However, because of potential neural tube effects, women of childbearing age should use this agent cautiously and routine supplementation of folic acid is recommended.

GABAPENTIN

Gabapentin is a chemically unique cyclohexane derivative of GABA that was synthesized to cross the blood-brain barrier and mimic the inhibitory effects of this neurotransmitter on the CNS. Gabapentin increases occipital lobe brain GABA concentrations; however, it is not known if this contributes to the drug's anticonvulsant effect.[35] Gabapentin is effective as adjunctive (add-on) therapy for patients with partial and secondarily generalized tonic-clonic seizures. In clinical trials, gabapentin reduces the frequency of these seizures by 50% or more in 25% of patients. By comparison, only 10% of placebo-treated patients experienced a similar reduction in seizures. Gabapentin is FDA approved as adjunctive therapy for partial seizures in patients older than 3 years of age and for adjunctive therapy for partial seizures with and without secondary generalization in those over 12 years of age. The AAN Quality Standards Subcommittee concluded that sufficient evidence exist to support the use of gabapentin in newly diagnosed partial seizures.[9] The drug has little or no activity against primarily generalized tonic-clonic and absence seizures. In addition to its use for epilepsy, gabapentin is primarily prescribed for the treatment of pain and psychiatric disorders.

Formulation and Dosage. Gabapentin (Neurontin) is available as capsules, tablets, and as an oral solution (Table 62.12). Therapy with gabapentin can be titrated to an effective dose rapidly, giving 300 mg on the first day, 300 mg twice on the second day, and 300 mg three times on the third day. Many practitioners now initiate gabapentin at a dose of 300 mg tid and find this to be well tolerated. Thereafter, therapy should be titrated according to patient response. Daily doses of 3,600 mg and above have been well tolerated and are sometimes required. Daily doses of 3,600 mg or less tid should be given. Daily doses above 3,600 mg should be divided into four doses to improve absorption. The starting dose in children ranges from 10 to 15 mg/kg/day divided into three daily doses. The dose is titrated over approximately 3 days to a maintenance dose of 25 to 40 mg/kg/day. Dosages up to 50 mg/kg/day have been well tolerated in a long-term clinical study.

Pharmacokinetics. The pharmacokinetic features of gabapentin are summarized in Table 62.10. Bioavailability is approximately 60% after oral administration of doses between 900 and 1,800 mg daily in adults and is significantly lower in children (30%). Further dosage increases result in less than proportional increases in plasma concentrations.

TABLE 62.12	Dosage Forms, Normal Maintenance Dose, and Interval for the Newer Anticonvulsants			
Generic (trade)	**Dosage Form**	**Initial Dosage**[a]	**Maintenance Dose**[b]	**Interval**[b]
Felbamate (Felbatol)	suspension (500 mg/5 mL) tablet (400, 600 mg)	15 mg/kg/day (P) 1,200 mg/day (A)	45 mg/kg/day (P) 1,200–3,600 mg/day (A)	tid-qid
Gabapentin (Neurontin)	capsules (100, 300, 400 mg) suspension (50 mg/mL)	10–15 mg/kg/day (P) 300 mg/day (A)	25–40 mg/kg/day (P) 900–3,600 mg/day (A)	tid
Lamotrigine (Lamictal)	tablet-chewable (5, 25 mg) tablet (25, 100, 150, 200 mg)	See Tables 62.13 and 62.14	5–15 mg/kg/day (P) 100–200 mg/day with VPA 300–500 mg/day without VPA (A)	qd-bid
Levetiracetam (Keppra)	tablet (250, 500, 750 mg)	5–10 mg/kg/day (P) 1,000 mg/day (A)	20–40 mg/kg/day 3,000 mg/day (A)	bid
Oxcarbazepine (Trileptal)	tablet (150, 300, 600 mg)	8–10 mg/kg/day (P) 600 mg/day (A)	900–1,800 mg/day[c] (P) 2,400 mg/day (A)	bid
Tiagabine (Gabitril)	tablet (2, 4, 16 mg)	0.1 mg/kg/day (P) 4 mg/day (A)	4–56 mg/day (A) 32 mg/day (A)	bid-qid
Topiramate (Topamax)	capsule-sprinkle (15, 25 mg) tablet (25, 100, 200 mg)	1 mg/kg/day (P) 25–50 mg/day (A)	5–10 mg/kg/day (P) 400 mg/day[d] (A)	bid
Zonisamide (Zonegran)	capsule (100 mg)	2–4 mg/kg/day (P) 100 mg/day (A)	12 mg/kg/day (P) 100–600 mg/day[d] (A)	qd

[a] See manufacturer information for titration scheme. With the exception of gabapentin, these anticonvulsants are begun at low doses and slowly titrated over weeks to a dose that will control the patient's seizures. [b] Dose and interval may decrease or increase in the presence of medication that induce or inhibit metabolism, respectively. See product information for maximum dosage. [c] 20–29 kg = 900 mg/day; 29.1–39 kg = 1200 mg/day; >39 kg = 1,800 mg/day. [d] no greater efficacy in treatment of CPS with doses >400 mg/day. A, adult; P, pediatric; tid, three times daily; qid, four times daily; qd, every day; bid, twice a day; VPA, valproate; CPS, complex partial seizures.

This lack of dose proportionality appears to be caused by saturation of the large neutral amino acid transport mechanism (system L transporter) that is responsible for gabapentin absorption across the intestinal membrane. The time to peak absorption is 2 to 3 hours. Food does not have an effect on the rate and extent of absorption; however, one study found an increase in peak plasma concentrations when gabapentin was given with a high-protein meal.[36]

Unlike other AEDs, gabapentin is neither metabolized nor bound to plasma proteins. The drug is excreted unchanged in the urine at a rate that is directly proportional to creatinine clearance. Reduction of gabapentin dosage is indicated when creatinine clearance is less than 60 mL per minute. In patients with normal renal function, the half-life of gabapentin is about 5 hours and does not change with chronic dosing. Although some studies have suggested that gabapentin is more effective at higher plasma concentrations, a therapeutic range of plasma concentrations has not yet been defined.

Adverse Effects. Overall, gabapentin is well tolerated and is associated with mild adverse effects, primarily affecting the CNS. In premarketing studies of gabapentin as adjunctive therapy, adverse effects included somnolence (19%), dizziness (17%), ataxia (12%), and fatigue (11%). Although infrequent, there have also been reports of CNS-related adverse events in children 3 to 12 years of age. These include emotional ability (6%), hostility and aggressive behaviors (5.2%), thought disorder (including concentration problems and change in school performance) (1.7%), and hyperkinesia (4.7%). These adverse effects appear to be dose-related and can be managed by adjustments of gabapentin dosage or the doses of concomitant agents. Rash appears in less than 1% of patients, a rate that compares favorably with those of other AEDs. Gabapentin has a nonaromatic structure, therefore the likelihood of a significant dermatological reaction is low when it is given to an individual who has experienced a major skin adverse event on another AED. Additional adverse effects may include weight gain (usually <10% of the baseline weight), movement disorders (dystonia or myoclonus), and lower extremity edema. Routine laboratory monitoring is not required during gabapentin therapy.

Drug Interactions. Gabapentin is neither metabolized nor bound to plasma proteins, therefore it has a much lower potential than other AEDs to interact with other drugs. Gabapentin does not affect the plasma concentrations of carbamazepine (including its epoxide metabolite), phenytoin, phenobarbital, or valproate. Likewise, these AEDs do not alter the disposition of gabapentin. Aluminum/magnesium hydroxide antacids (given concomitantly or 2 hours after gabapentin) and cimetidine have been shown to reduce gabapentin plasma concentrations by 12% to 20%, but these interactions are not likely to be clinically significant.

LAMOTRIGINE

Lamotrigine was originally synthesized in a drug development program to exploit the antiepileptic effect of novel antifolate agents. It has weak antifolate properties, but its anticonvulsant activity is unrelated to this property. Rather, lamotrigine inhibits voltage-dependent sodium channels, resulting in a decreased presynaptic release of excitatory neurotransmitters such as aspartate and glutamate. In this regard, its mechanism of action is similar to that of carbamazepine and phenytoin. Lamotrigine is FDA approved as monotherapy for partial seizures in adults and as adjunctive therapy in adults and children (≥2 years of age). Approximately 25% of patients experience a 50% or greater reduction in partial-onset seizures when lamotrigine is added to existing AED therapy. It is also approved for seizures associated with the Lennox-Gastaut syndrome and for conversion to monotherapy in those older than 16 years of age.

The goal of transition to a single agent is to successfully convert a patient while ensuring adequate seizure control without the risk of serious rash associated with the rapid titration of lamotrigine. Conversion dosing is influenced by the concomitant therapy with enzyme-inducing AEDs, and the presence of valproate. The AAN Quality Standards Subcommittee concluded that sufficient evidence exists to support the use of lamotrigine as monotherapy in absence, newly diagnosed partial or mixed seizures, and refractory partial epilepsy. Preliminary evidence suggests that lamotrigine also has activity against primary generalized epilepsies (including juvenile myoclonic epilepsy).

Formulation and Dosage. Lamotrigine (Lamictal) is available as an oral tablet and a chewable dispersible tablet. The dispersible tablet can be chewed, swallowed, or dissolved in liquid (Table 62.12). The smallest available strength is a 2-mg tablet, and only whole tablets should be administered. If the calculated dose cannot be achieved using whole tablets, the dose should be rounded down to the nearest whole tablet. Lamotrigine disposition is significantly affected by other AEDs, requiring sophisticated and complicated dosing regimens (Tables 62.13 and 62.14). When administered in combination with enzyme-inducing AEDs (carbamazepine, phenytoin, phenobarbital, and primidone) the dose should be larger than that given to patients receiving lamotrigine alone. When given with valproate alone, lamotrigine doses should be reduced further.

Pharmacokinetics. Clinical pharmacokinetic features of lamotrigine are summarized in Table 62.10. The oral bioavailability of lamotrigine is excellent and food has no significant effect on absorption. It is poorly bound to plasma proteins, making clinically significant interactions from this mechanism unlikely. Lamotrigine is metabolized by glucuronic acid conjugation to an inactive product. Its half-life is about a day during monotherapy, but other AEDs significantly affect the rate of elimination. Concomitant therapy with enzyme-inducing AEDs enhances lamotrigine metabolism and reduces the half-life to approximately 14 hours. The half-life is approximately 27 hours in those taking valproate and enzyme-inducing AEDs, but is increased to 59 hours in those given valproate without enzyme-inducing

TABLE 62.13	Initiation and Titration of Lamotrigine in Pediatric and Adult Patients

AED		Pediatric Dose	Adult Dose
LTG	Weeks 1 and 2	0.3mg/kg/day qd or divided bid	25 mg/day
	Weeks 3 and 4	0.6 mg/kg/day divided bid	50 mg/day
	Titration	add 0.6 mg/kg/day to the previously administered daily dose weekly	Increase 50 mg/day every 1 to 2 weeks
LTG + VPA[a]	Weeks 1 and 2	0.15 mg/kg/day qd or divided bid	25 mg every other day
	Weeks 3 and 4	0.3 mg/kg/day qd or bid	25 mg qd
	Titration	add 0.3 mg/kg/day to the previously administered daily dose weekly	Increase 25 to 50 mg/day every 1 to 2 weeks
LTG + INDUCERS[b]	Weeks 1 and 2	0.6 mg/kg/day divided bid	50 mg/day
	Weeks 3 and 4	1.2 mg/kg/day divided bid	100 mg/day divided bid
	Titration	add 1.2 mg/kg/day to the previously administered daily dose weekly	Increase 100 mg/day every week

[a] Valproate has been shown to decrease the apparent clearance of lamotrigine.
[b] Carbamazepine, phenytoin, phenobarbital, primidone, and rifampin have been shown to increase the apparent clearance of lamotrigine.
AED, antiepileptic drug; LTG, lamotrigine; VPA, valproate; qd, every day; bid, twice a day.

AEDs. No clear relationship exists between plasma concentrations of lamotrigine and clinical effect.

Adverse Effects. Adverse effects during lamotrigine therapy are usually mild or moderate and resolve with dosage reduction. Pooled data from placebo-control add-on studies found that the most common side effects involved the CNS and included dizziness (38%), headache (29%), diplopia (28%), ataxia (22%), and somnolence (14%). Approximately 10% of patients who received lamotrigine developed a skin rash, which is the most common reason for drug discontinuation (3%). Potentially life-threatening skin rashes, including Stevens-Johnson syndrome and toxic epidermal necrolysis, have been reported in as many as 1 of 50 to 1 of 100 children and 1 of 1,000 adults.[37] The rash usually develops in the first 2 to 8 weeks of therapy and is more common in patients receiving an AED regimen that includes valproate. However, cases have been reported after prolonged treatment (e.g., 6 months) and duration of therapy should not be used to predict the potential risk at the first appearance of a rash. The incidence of rash also increases with larger starting doses and a faster rate of dosage escalation. Patients should be counseled to report the occurrence of a skin rash to their health care provider immediately, and lamotrigine should be discontinued at the first sign of rash.

Drug Interactions. Lamotrigine metabolism can be affected by other AEDs; hence, these interactions may be clini-

TABLE 62.14	Conversion to Lamotrigine Monotherapy from Adjunctive Therapy with Valproate or other AED

Step	Lamotrigine	From valproate	From CBZ, PHT, PB, or PRM
1	Achieve a dose of 200 mg/day per Table 62-12	Maintain previous stable dose	
2	Maintain at 200 mg/day	↓ to 500 mg/day by decrements ≤ 500 mg/day per week and then maintain the dose of 500 mg/day for 1 week	
3	↑ to 300 mg/day and maintain for 1 week.	Simultaneously ↓ to 250 mg/day and maintain for 1 week.	
4	↑ by 100 mg/day every week to achieve a maintenance dose of 500 mg/day		Once titrated to 500 mg/day of lamotrigine begin to taper the above AED by ↓ 20% per week over a 4-week period

AED, antiepileptic drug; CBZ, carbamazepine; PHT, phenytoin; PB, phenobarbital; PRM, primidone.

cally significant and should be considered during the initiation and titration of lamotrigine. The addition of valproate increases lamotrigine plasma concentrations by more than twofold. Carbamazepine, phenytoin, phenobarbital, or primidone can decrease lamotrigine steady-state concentrations by approximately 40%. Acetaminophen can increase the clearance of lamotrigine, but the mechanism of this interaction is unknown. Lamotrigine is a weak inducer of UGT and causes a small increase in its own metabolism; however, it does not have a significant effect on the elimination of carbamazepine, phenytoin, phenobarbital, primidone, or oral contraceptives. Lamotrigine causes a modest decrease in valproate concentrations. There are conflicting reports on the effect of lamotrigine on CBZ-E concentrations. One study reported that lamotrigine had no effect on CBZ-E concentrations; however, another study reported that CBZ-E concentrations increased by a mean of 45%. After addition of lamotrigine to carbamazepine, some patients experience diplopia, dizziness, or somnolence without any evident change in carbamazepine or CBZ-E concentrations, suggesting a pharmacodynamic interaction between these agents.[20] Oral contraceptives lower the plasma concentration of lamotrigine by 40% to 60%.

TOPIRAMATE

Topiramate is a sulfamate-substituted monosaccharide derivative that is distinct from other AEDs in terms of chemical structure and mechanism of action. Although it is a sulfamate, it does not have a sulfa structure; hence, there should not be any cross reactivity in those with a sulfa allergy. The drug has several pharmacologic properties that may contribute to its anticonvulsant effect. It inhibits voltage-sensitive sodium channels; enhances GABA-mediated chloride flux across neuronal membranes; augments the activity of the neurotransmitter gamma-aminobutyrate at some subtypes of the GABA-A receptor and inhibits binding of kainate to a specific subtype of the excitotoxic glutamate receptor. Topiramate is also a weak inhibitor of carbonic anhydrase II and IV although this probably does not contribute to the drug's anticonvulsant properties.

Topiramate is approved as adjunctive treatment for partial, primary generalized tonic-clonic seizures and Lennox-Gastaut syndrome in adults and children ($\geq$2 years of age).[38] Topiramate is also FDA approved for initial monotherapy in those older than 10 years of age who have partial and primary generalized tonic-clonic seizures. Approximately 45% of patients with refractory partial epilepsy experience a 50% or greater reduction in seizures when topiramate is used as an adjunctive treatment. The AAN Quality Standards Subcommittee concluded that sufficient evidence exists to support the use of topiramate as monotherapy in new onset seizures[9] and as monotherapy for refractory partial seizures[10] (Table 62.7).

Formulation and Dosage. Topiramate (Topamax) is available as an oral tablet and sprinkle capsule that can be poured onto food (Table 62.12). Adult and pediatric doses can be found in Table 62.12. The initial dose should be increased at weekly intervals until maintenance doses are achieved. Some patients may experience improved tolerability (with regard to CNS adverse effects) when topiramate is introduced at a slower rate. For example, some practitioners prefer to begin topiramate at 25 mg daily, increase weekly by 25 mg per day until a dose of 50 mg bid is reached, and then continue by escalating the dose in 50 mg per day increments at weekly intervals. Most patients do not experience additional benefit from doses larger than 400 mg per day; however, occasionally larger doses (1,000 mg/day) may be required for optimal treatment.

Pharmacokinetics. Pharmacokinetic parameters of topiramate are summarized in Table 62.10. The oral bioavailability of topiramate is 80%, and peak plasma concentrations occur 3 to 4 hours after administration. Food delays the absorption, but the extent of absorption is unaffected. Topiramate has very low protein binding; therefore, interactions via this mechanism would not be expected. Urinary excretion of the unchanged drug is the predominant route of elimination; hence, dosage should be adjusted in those with a creatinine clearance less than 70 mL/min/1.73 m^2. The half-life of topiramate is 24 hours after a single dose to healthy adults. There is not a consistent correlation between topiramate plasma concentrations and clinical effect. Although it may help define an individual's optimal plasma concentration and evaluate compliance, routine monitoring of topiramate concentrations is not necessary.

Adverse Effects. Common adverse effects during topiramate therapy are usually mild or moderate and are minimized by using a conservative dose-escalation schedule. Pooled data from placebo-control trials of topiramate as adjunctive therapy indicate that the most common adverse effects are somnolence (30%), dizziness (28%), ataxia (21%), psychomotor slowing (17%), and problems with speech, such as word-finding difficulty (17%). Other adverse effects include difficulty with concentration or attention, confusion, weight loss, and tremor. Difficulty concentrating and psychomotor slowing are the most common reasons for discontinuation. A recent comparative study in healthy adults found more significant cognitive effects associated with topiramate than with gabapentin and lamotrigine.[39] Topiramate was discontinued due to adverse events in 11% of patients receiving 200 to 400 mg daily. This rate appeared to increase at dosages above 400 mg daily. Kidney stones occur in 1.5% of patients and those given topiramate should be counseled to maintain adequate fluid intake during topiramate treatment. Hyperchloremic, nonanion gap, and metabolic acidosis have been reported and are caused by renal bicarbonate loss due to the inhibitory effect of topiramate on carbonic anhydrase. Generally, this adverse effect occurs early in treatment although cases can occur at any time during treatment. Decreased sweating (oligohidrosis) and hyperthermia have been associated with topiramate. The majority of the reports have occurred in children. Individuals should be monitored closely for evidence of decreased sweating and increased body temperature, especially in hot weather. Topiramate is a carbonic anhydrase inhibitor and may also cause paresthesia.

Drug Interactions. Although topiramate is primarily renally eliminated, enzyme-inducing AEDs (e.g., carbamazepine, phenytoin, and phenobarbital) increase the proportion of topiramate clearance due to metabolism and cause a 40% to 50% decrease in topiramate concentrations. Topiramate can reduce the clearance of phenytoin. However, the magnitude of the effect is variable with phenytoin concentrations, increasing from 0% to 25%. Topiramate has no significant effect on the metabolism of other AEDs. Ethinyl estradiol concentrations are reduced during concomitant therapy with topiramate at doses larger that 200 mg daily and women should be monitored closely for breakthrough bleeding. Consideration should be given to using an oral contraceptive with a higher estrogen content (e.g., >35 μg of ethinyl estradiol).[20]

ZONISAMIDE

Zonisamide is chemically classified as a sulfonamide and should not be given to someone who is allergic to sulfa-type medications. The mechanism of action is unknown, but it does block sodium channels and reduce voltage-dependent, transient inward currents (T-type Ca^{2+} currents), consequently stabilizing neuronal membranes and suppressing neuronal hypersynchronization. It does not appear to potentiate the synaptic or postsynaptic activity of GABA or glutamate responses. Zonisamide also has weak carbonic anhydrase inhibiting activity, but this pharmacologic effect is not thought to be a major contributing factor to its antiseizure activity.

Formulation and Dosage. Zonisamide (Zonogran) is available for oral administration as a capsule (Table 62.12) and is indicated as adjunctive therapy in the treatment of partial seizures in those older than 16 years of age. The AAN Quality Standards Subcommittee concluded that insufficient evidence exists to support the use of zonisamide for any other indication.[9,10] Therapy should be initiated at a dose of 50 to100 mg daily. After two weeks, the dose may be increased to 200 mg per day for at least two weeks. It can then be increased to 300 to 400 mg per day. It may take up to 2 weeks to achieve steady-state concentrations because of its long half-life. A greater response has been noted at doses above 100 to 200 mg daily; however, the increase appears small. There is no evidence of an increased response at doses greater than 400 mg per day. Dosage should be adjusted in those with a creatinine clearance less than 70 mL/min/1.73 m².

Pharmacokinetics. Clinical pharmacokinetic features of zonisamide are summarized in Table 62.10. The absorption of zonisamide is excellent. Although food has no effect on its bioavailability, the time to maximum concentration is delayed. Zonisamide extensively binds to erythrocytes, resulting in an eightfold higher concentration in red blood cells (RBCs) than in plasma. The pharmacokinetics of zonisamide are proportional in doses ranging from 200 to 400 mg, but

becomes increasingly disproportionate at larger doses (i.e., 800 mg), perhaps due to saturable binding to RBCs. The elimination half-life of zonisamide is about 63 and 105 hours in plasma and RBCs, respectively. The apparent volume of distribution is about 1.45 L per kilogram with approximately 40% bound to plasma proteins. Zonisamide is excreted primarily in urine (62%) as parent drug and as the glucuronide of a metabolite. It is hepatically metabolized by CYP3A4, but it does not induce its own metabolism.

Adverse Effects. The adverse effect profile of zonisamide is very similar to that of topiramate. The most common adverse events were somnolence, fatigue and/or ataxia (6%), anorexia (3%), difficulty concentrating (2%), difficulty with memory, mental slowing, nausea/vomiting (2%), and weight loss (1%). The most serious adverse effect is a potentially fatal dermatological reaction that includes Stevens-Johnson syndrome and toxic epidermal necrolysis; hence, zonisamide should be discontinued in anyone who develops an unexplained rash. Decreased sweating (oligohidrosis) and hyperthermia have been associated with zonisamide. The majority of the reports have occurred in children. Individuals should be monitored closely for evidence of decreased sweating and increased body temperature, especially in hot weather. CNS-related adverse events include depression and psychosis, psychomotor slowing, difficulty with concentration, and speech or language problems, in particular, word-finding difficulties. Rare cases of reversible and irreversible psychosis have been described. Kidney stones composed of calcium or urate salts have been reported. In general, increasing fluid intake and urine output can help reduce the risk of stone formation.

Drug Interactions. Zonisamide does not affect steady-state plasma concentrations of phenytoin, carbamazepine, or valproate nor does it inhibit the clearance of other drugs that are metabolized by cytochrome P-450 isozymes. Concurrent medication with drugs that induce or inhibit CYP3A4 would be expected to alter plasma concentrations of zonisamide. Drugs that induce liver enzymes (phenytoin, carbamazepine, or phenobarbital) increase the metabolism and clearance of zonisamide and decrease its half-life. Protein binding of zonisamide is unaffected in the presence of therapeutic concentrations of phenytoin, phenobarbital, or carbamazepine.

TIAGABINE

Tiagabine, a nipecotic acid derivative with a chemical structure unique among AEDs, inhibits the reuptake of GABA into presynaptic neurons and glial cells. This is thought to be the mechanism of its anticonvulsant effect. The drug is approved as adjunctive therapy in adults with partial and secondarily generalized tonic-clonic seizures. In clinical trials, approximately 25% of patients treated with tiagabine demonstrate a 50% or greater reduction in partial-onset seizures. The AAN Quality Standards Subcommittee concluded that insufficient evidence exists to support the use of tiagabine for any other indication.[9,10]

Tiagabine (Gabatril) is available as oral tablets (Table 62.12). When administered with enzyme-inducing AEDs, it should be initiated at a dose of 4 mg daily and increased in 4 mg daily increments at weekly intervals. Usual maintenance dosages of tiagabine are 32 to 56 mg daily given in two to four divided doses. With doses larger than 32 mg daily, tid or qid dosing is often necessary to minimize transient adverse effects associated with peak blood concentrations. More conservative dose titration is usually needed when tiagabine is used with noninducing AEDs (e.g., valproate, gabapentin, or lamotrigine).

Pharmacokinetics. The oral bioavailability of tiagabine is 90% (Table 62.10). It is absorbed quickly with peak blood concentrations occurring 1 hour after administration. The extent of drug absorption is not affected by food. Tiagabine is highly bound to plasma proteins, primarily albumin and α_1-acid glycoprotein. Drug elimination is primarily by metabolism via CYP3A4 and glucuronidation enzymes. The half-life of tiagabine is 7 to 9 hours in healthy volunteers after a single dose, and it is shortened by 50% to 65% when coadministered with enzyme-inducing AEDs. There is no clear relationship between tiagabine blood concentrations and clinical response.

Adverse Effects. Common adverse effects reported during placebo-control, adjunctive therapy trials with tiagabine include dizziness (27%), lack of energy (20%), somnolence (18%), nausea (11%), and nervousness (10%). These adverse effects are usually dose-related and respond to a reduction in dosage or slowing of the rate of dose escalation. Other adverse effects that occur occasionally include tremor, generalized muscle weakness, and difficulty with concentration or attention. Toxic encephalopathy and nonconvulsive status epilepticus have been reported in patients taking doses larger than 56 mg per day.

Drug Interactions. Tiagabine does not induce or inhibit the metabolism of other AEDs. Although it is highly protein-bound, tiagabine does not appear to displace other highly protein-bound drugs such as phenytoin, valproate, or warfarin; however, tiagabine itself is displaced from protein binding sites by naproxen, valproate, and salicylates. The clinical significance of tiagabine displacement interactions is unknown. Drugs that inhibit CYP3A4 would be expected to reduce its metabolism. However, the effect of erythromycin (a CYP3A4 inhibitor) on tiagabine metabolism is inconsistent. Until further data are available, erythromycin, ketoconazole, and other inhibitors of CYP3A4 should be used cautiously with tiagabine.[20] Enzyme-inducing AEDs enhance the metabolism of tiagabine by 50% to 65%.

LEVETIRACETAM

Levetiracetam is a single enantiomer that is chemically unrelated to existing AEDs. Mechanism(s) by which it exerts its anticonvulsant effect are related to its effects on zinc and glycine binding sites to beta-carboline and by binding to a synaptic vessel protein. It does not affect the binding affinity for a variety of known receptors [(e.g., benzodiazepines, GABA, glycine, NMDA (N-methyl-D-aspartate)], reuptake

sites, and second messenger systems. It also does not appear to affect voltage-gated sodium or T-type calcium currents or to directly facilitate GABAnergic neurotransmission. It has been reported to oppose the activity of negative modulators of GABA-gated and glycine-gated currents in neuronal cell culture. Levetiracetam is indicated as adjunctive treatment of partial onset seizures in adults with epilepsy. The AAN Quality Standards Subcommittee concluded that insufficient evidence exists to support the use of levetiracetam for any other indication (Table 62.7).

Formulation and Dosage. Levetiracetam (Keppra) is available as a tablet and solution. (Table 62.12). Treatment should be initiated with a daily dose of 500 to 1,000 mg per day, given as twice daily dosing. Additional dosing increments may be given (1,000 mg/day additional every 2 weeks) to a maximum recommended daily dose of 3,000 mg. Although there is a tendency toward greater response with larger doses, a consistent increase in response to increased doses has not been shown. Dosing should be individualized in those with a CrCl less than 80 mL/min/1.73 m^2.

Pharmacokinetics. Clinical pharmacokinetic features of levetiracetam are summarized in Table 62.10. Levetiracetam is rapidly and completely absorbed after oral administration with peak plasma concentrations occurring in about an hour following oral administration. The tablets and oral solution are bioequivalent in rate and extent of absorption. Although food does not affect the extent of absorption, it may decrease the maximum concentration by 20% and delays the time to that concentration by 1.5 hours. The pharmacokinetics is linear and time-invariant, with low intrasubject and intersubject variability. More than half of a dose is renally excreted unchanged via glomerular filtration with subsequent partial tubular reabsorption. The major metabolic pathway of levetiracetam is an enzymatic hydrolysis of the acetamide group, and not dependent on any hepatic cytochrome P-450 isoenzyme. The metabolites have no known pharmacologic activity and are renally excreted. Studies have shown plasma half-life of levetiracetam is relatively short and is increased in the elderly and in those with renal impairment.

Adverse Effects. Levetiracetam has not been associated with significant adverse effects. It has been noted to cause somnolence and fatigue, coordination difficulties (i.e., ataxia, abnormal gait, or incoordination), and behavioral abnormalities. Somnolence, asthenia, and coordination difficulnbties occurred most frequently within the first month of treatment. Although extremely rare, mood disorder, psychosis, and hallucinations have been reported. These generally occur during the first weeks of therapy and resolve after a reduction or dose or discontinuation levetiracetam. Other behavioral symptoms (e.g., aggression, agitation, anxiety, depression, emotional lability) have been reported and generally resolve when the dose is reduced or the drug is discontinued.

Drug Interactions. Levetiracetam is unlikely to produce, or be subject to, pharmacokinetic drug interactions. Levetiracetam and its major metabolite are neither inhibitors of, nor high affinity substrates for, hepatic cytochrome P-450 isoenzymes, epoxide hydrolase, or uridine diphosphate (UDP)-glucuronidation enzymes. Levetiracetam and its major metabolite are less than 10% bound to plasma proteins; hence, clinically significant interactions with other drugs through competition for protein binding sites are unlikely.

OXCARBAZEPINE

Oxcarbazepine is a 10-keto analog of carbamazepine with a similar spectrum of anticonvulsant effect and an improved tolerability profile over carbamazepine. The precise mechanism by which oxcarbazepine exerts its effect is thought to occur via the 10-monohydroxy metabolite (MHD) of oxcarbazepine. Both moieties block voltage-sensitive sodium channels to prevent seizure spread by stabilizing hyperexcited neural membranes and by inhibition of repetitive neuronal firing. Oxcarbazepine is indicated as monotherapy or adjunctive therapy for the treatment of partial seizures in adults and children ages 4 to 16.

Formulation and Dosage. Oxcarbazepine (Trileptal) is available as an oral tablet and suspension, which may be interchanged at equal doses (Table 62.12). Treatment should be initiated with 300 to 600 mg per day (5–10 mg/kg/day) given twice a day. The dose may be increased at weekly intervals until desired control is obtained. The target maintenance doses should be achieved over 2 weeks. Patients receiving other AEDs may be converted to oxcarbazepine monotherapy. These patients should be started on oxcarbazepine (600 mg/day) while concurrently reducing the dose of the other AEDs. The concomitant AEDs should be completely withdrawn over 3 to 6 weeks, while the maximum dose of oxcarbazepine should be achieved in about 2 to 4 weeks. When oxcarbazepine is substituted for carbamazepine, the oxcarbazepine replacement dose should be 1.2 to 1.5 times the carbamazepine dose, using the lower conversion factor for those on larger baseline doses and in elderly patients.

Pharmacokinetics. Oxcarbazepine is completely absorbed and can be taken with or without food. Time to peak concentration ranges from 2 to 4 hours. Oxcarbazepine is metabolized by reductase enzymes to MDH, which is pharmacologically active; no epoxide metabolites of oxcarbazepine are formed. The half-life of the parent compound is 2 hours, while the half-life of MHD is about 9 hours. Steady-state plasma concentrations of MHD are reached within 2 to 3 days following twice daily dosing. At steady-state the pharmacokinetics of MHD are linear and show dose proportionality up to 2,400 mg/day. Patients with mild to moderate hepatic impairment do not require dosage adjustment, but patients with a creatinine clearance less than 30 mL per minute should receive one half the usual starting dosage, which is then increased slowly to achieve the desired clinical response.

Adverse Effects. Reports of adverse effects due to oxcarbazepine are rare. The most frequent side effect involves the CNS and includes headache, somnolence, dizziness, and nausea, all of which resolve following an adjustment in dosage. Rash has been reported with oxcarbazepine (3%), but the occurrence is less than that reported for carbamazepine. Cross-reactivity does exist between oxcarbazepine and carbamazepine, with allergic reactions reported in up to 30% of patients with a documented allergy to carbamazepine. Asymptomatic hyponatremia (serum sodium <125 mEq/L) has been noted in about 3% of patients and occurs more often than with carbamazepine. No clinically significant hematologic, renal, or liver changes have been reported.

Drug Interactions. An advantage of oxcarbazepine is that the drug is less likely to induce hepatic drug metabolism than carbamazepine. In patients receiving carbamazepine (or other enzyme-inducing AEDs), substitution with oxcarbazepine can result in induction of hepatic enzyme systems with subsequent increase in plasma concentrations of the remaining AEDs. Dosage adjustments may be needed in patients who are switched to oxcarbazepine from other AEDs with enzyme-inducing properties.

FELBAMATE

Felbamate is a chemically unique carbamate derivative that is structurally related to the sedative-hypnotic meprobamate. It was approved by the FDA in August 1993 and rapidly became a popular agent for several reasons: (a) it was the first new AED to be marketed in the United States since 1978; (b) it was the first drug that was brought to the market through the Antiepileptic Drug Development Program, a program established by the National Institutes for Neurological Disease and Stroke to facilitate the preclinical and clinical evaluation of new chemical entities for the treatment of epilepsy; (c) the drug was shown to be effective as monotherapy and adjunctive therapy for adults with partial seizures (with and without secondary generalization) and as adjunctive therapy for children with partial or generalized seizures associated with the Lennox-Gastaut syndrome; and (d) the drug seemed to be very well tolerated in clinical trials. In other preliminary studies, felbamate also was shown to have activity against absence, atypical absence, and juvenile myoclonic seizures. The mechanism of felbamate's antiepileptic effects is unknown. Felbamate is indicated as adjunctive therapy in adults when seizures are so severe as to warrant use despite risk of potentially life-threatening adverse effects. It is also indicated in children with uncontrolled Lennox-Gastaut syndrome.

Formulation and Dosage. Felbamate (Felbatol) is available as an oral tablet and oral suspension. Adult and pediatric doses are contained in Table 62.12. Some patients may require larger doses for maximal benefit. The dosages of concomitant AEDs are often reduced by 20% to 30% on initiation of felbamate therapy. Further reductions may be required during titration of therapy.

Pharmacokinetics. Pharmacokinetic features of felbamate are summarized in Table 62.10. Felbamate is well absorbed after oral administration and its bioavailability is un-affected by food or antacids. The drug is poorly bound to plasma proteins. Felbamate is eliminated by hydrolysis and cytochrome P–450-mediated metabolism to inactive prod-ucts and by renal excretion of unchanged drug (Table 62.11). The half-life is about one day and is not affected by chronic administration.

Adverse Effects. At the time of FDA approval, felbamate was shown to be well tolerated in many premarketing clinical trials. When administered as adjunctive therapy to adults with partial seizures, felbamate was associated with head-ache (37%), nausea (34%), somnolence (19%), anorexia (19%), dizziness (18%), insomnia (17%), and fatigue (17%). The incidence of these adverse effects was reduced by ap-proximately one half when felbamate was used as monother-apy. This suggests that concomitant AEDs were at least partly responsible for these symptoms. Weight loss was re-ported in 4% of adults and 6% of children receiving felba-mate.

One year after the introduction of felbamate, an associa-tion with potentially life-threatening hematologic and he-patic adverse effects was reported. These reports have caused reconsideration of the relative risks and benefits of felbamate therapy and the drug is currently recommended only for ''patients who respond inadequately to alternative treatments and whose epilepsy is so severe that a substantial risk of aplastic anemia and/or liver failure is deemed accept-able in light of the benefits conferred by its use.''[40]

A total of 34 cases of felbamate-associated aplastic ane-mia have been reported worldwide. It is estimated that the risk is more than 100-fold greater than that seen in the un-treated population. The estimated incidence of aplastic ane-mia is approximately 1 in 4,000.[40] For comparison, the risk of aplastic anemia with chloramphenicol is approximately 1 of 40,000. The risk of aplastic anemia is highest within the first year of therapy and does not appear to be related to felbamate dosage. Mortality has been approximately 30%.

Felbamate has also been associated with 23 cases of acute hepatic failure worldwide.[40] The period of highest risk ap-pears to be during the first year of therapy, and there is no clear correlation with felbamate dosage. The estimated incidence of felbamate-associated hepatotoxicity is 1 of 26,000 to 34,000. For comparison, the incidence of fulmi-nant hepatic failure associated with valproate is 1 of 10,000 to 49,000 exposures.[41]

In addition to amending the prescribing information for felbamate, the manufacturer has included a patient information/consent form with the package insert. The use of this or some other consent forms and the interpretation of the appropriate criteria for felbamate use vary widely among dif-ferent centers and individual prescribers. The use of labora-tory monitoring of hematological and hepatic function also varies. The manufacturer recommends that liver function tests be performed at baseline and at 1-week to 2-week intervals while treatment continues. No guidelines for hematological

monitoring are given. Practitioners at the University of Cali-fornia San Francisco (UCSF) Epilepsy Center order a com-plete blood count with differential, platelet count, serum iron, reticulocyte count, alanine transaminase, aspartate transami-nase, and bilirubin concentrations at baseline, every 2 weeks for months 1 and 2 of felbamate therapy, every month for months 3 to 12, and every 6 months thereafter. However, the value of these monitoring guidelines has not been established. Felbamate should probably be avoided for patients with a his-tory of autoimmune disorders, previous blood dyscrasias or AED drug allergy or hepatic abnormalities.

Drug Interactions. Felbamate is an inhibitor of β-oxida-tion and CYP2C19 metabolism (Table 62.11). Thus, the ad-dition of felbamate requires a reduction in the dosages of phenytoin, phenobarbital (both CYP2C19 substrates), and valproate (metabolized by β-oxidation). The effect of felba-mate on steady-state plasma concentrations of phenytoin and valproate is dose-related. At felbamate doses of 1,200 mg per day, phenytoin concentrations increase by an average of 23%. Felbamate doses of 1,800 mg per day increase phenyt-oin concentrations by an average of 47% above baseline. A reduction in phenytoin dosage of 20% to 30% on initiation of felbamate is usually sufficient to prevent symptoms of phenytoin toxicity. However, further phenytoin dosage re-ductions may be required as the dosage of felbamate is in-creased. Valproate dosages should be reduced by approxi-mately 30% on initiation of felbamate, and further dose reductions may be required during the titration of felbamate therapy. Felbamate is poorly bound to plasma proteins (pri-marily to albumin), so clinically significant protein-binding interactions are unlikely. Felbamate induces CYP3A4 me-tabolism, causing a decrease in mean carbamazepine concen-trations by 20% to 30%; however, CBZ-E concentrations increase by 30% to 55%. To prevent dose-related symptoms of toxicity such as diplopia, drowsiness, and ataxia, carba-mazepine doses should be reduced by approximately 30% when felbamate therapy is begun. Felbamate concentrations can also be affected by other AEDs. Phenytoin and carba-mazepine reduce steady-state concentrations of felbamate by 40% to 50%. However, because there is no consistent correlation between felbamate concentrations and clinical effect, no adjustment in felbamate dosage is required.

BENZODIAZEPINES–CLONAZEPAM

Diazepam, lorazepam, clonazepam, and clorazepate are the only benzodiazepine agents that are FDA-approved for the treatment of seizures. Diazepam and lorazepam have little utility in the chronic treatment of epilepsy, but are frequently used intravenously for the termination of status epilepticus. In general, benzodiazepines are more effective in suppress-ing generalized epileptiform activity than focal discharges and these agents limit the spread of epileptic discharges with-out suppressing the primary seizure focus. Nonetheless, clin-ical use of clonazepam and clorazepate for the chronic treat-ment of epilepsy includes generalized and partial seizure types. Although the precise mechanism of the anticonvulsant effect of these agents is unknown, the benzodiazepines are thought to facilitate inhibitory neurotransmission in the CNS by enhancing the postsynaptic effects of GABA.

Clonazepam is useful, alone or as an adjunct to other agents, for the treatment of Lennox-Gastaut syndrome and akinetic and myoclonic seizures. It is also useful for the treatment of absence seizures that fail to respond to valproate or ethosuximide. Clonazepam is not FDA approved for the treatment of partial or generalized tonic-clonic seizures, and experience in its use for the treatment of these seizure types is limited.

Formulation and Dosage. Clonazepam (Klonopin) is available as oral tablets in strengths of 0.5, 1, and 2 mg. An intravenous preparation is available for use in Europe, but it is not available in the United States. Clonazepam should be initiated at low doses (0.5 mg tid for adults; 0.01–0.03 mg/kg divided bid or tid a day for infants and children) and gradually titrated upward at 3 to 7-day intervals. The maximum recommended daily dose is 20 mg for adults and 0.1 to 0.2 mg per kilogram for infants and children. Although the half-life of clonazepam allows for once daily dosing for many patients, the drug is often administered in divided doses. This is particularly important for those who are intolerant of the transient sedative effects that occur after peak absorption and for infants and children, in whom the drug's half-life may be shortened.

Pharmacokinetics. Clonazepam is eliminated primarily by reduction of the nitro group to form 7-amino clonazepam, an inactive metabolite. Although loss of efficacy may occur during chronic therapy, clonazepam does not induce its own metabolism. There is wide variation in the relationship between the dose and plasma concentrations of clonazepam. There is also significant overlap between the plasma concentrations that are associated with the antiepileptic effect of the drug and those that are associated with dose-related adverse effects. For these reasons the therapeutic range of clonazepam concentrations is imprecisely defined, though many references cite a therapeutic range of 13 to 72 µg/mL. Monitoring of clonazepam concentrations during routine therapy is not often used.

Adverse Effects. Adverse effects are common during clonazepam treatment and necessitate drug discontinuation in up to one third of patients. Dose-related adverse effects are particularly common and include drowsiness and ataxia. Although tolerance of the overt sedative effects of clonazepam and other benzodiazepines usually develops during the first few weeks of therapy, mild impairment of cognitive and motor skills may persist throughout treatment. In others, dose-related adverse effects may require clonazepam to be discontinued. Clonazepam may also cause behavioral disturbances, including hyperactivity, irritability, restlessness, and aggressive or violent behavior. Children are affected more frequently than adults. Dosage reduction may be attempted but it does not always alleviate behavioral changes. Other adverse effects include excessive salivation, bronchial hypersecretion, and weight gain. In rare cases, exacerbation of seizures has been reported. Abrupt discontinuation of clonazepam may precipitate seizures or status epilepticus; therefore, it should be gradually withdrawn when treatment is to be terminated.

The long-term clinical use of clonazepam is limited by the development of tolerance to the antiepileptic effect. Approximately one third of patients who initially benefit from clonazepam therapy experience some loss of efficacy, usually within the first 6 months of treatment. Although the antiepileptic effect may be restored by increasing the dose, as many as 30% of patients who develop tolerance do not regain adequate seizure control.

Drug Interactions. Clinically important drug interactions with clonazepam are uncommon. Clonazepam has no significant effect on the pharmacokinetic disposition of phenytoin, carbamazepine, or primidone. However, phenytoin, carbamazepine, and phenobarbital can reduce the steady-state concentrations of clonazepam, presumably by the induction of hepatic metabolism. The combined use of clonazepam and valproate has been reported to exacerbate absence seizures. Although the simultaneous use of these agents is not a strict contraindication, caution should be observed.

BENZODIAZEPINES–CLORAZEPATE

Clorazepate dipotassium is approved for use as an adjunct to other agents for the treatment of partial seizures. Clorazepate is a prodrug that is rapidly decarboxylated in the acidic medium of the stomach to yield N-desmethyldiazepam (DMD), the primary active metabolite. This metabolite is responsible for the antiepileptic effect of the parent compound.

Formulation and Dosage. Clorazepate (Tranxene) is available as a prompt-release oral tablet (3.75, 7.5, and 15 mg) and as an extended-release oral tablet (11.5 and 22.5 mg) for once-daily dosing. Therapy with clorazepate should be initiated with the prompt-release form at a dose of 7.5 mg tid for adults and 7.5 mg bid for children (ages 9–12 years). The dose should be increased at 7-day intervals, in increments of 7.5 mg or less, to a maximum daily dose of 90 mg for adults and 60 mg for children. Transient dose-related adverse effects may be minimized and compliance may be improved by a change to the extended-released dosage form for patients whose seizures are controlled with clorazepate.

Pharmacokinetics. DMD and its hydroxylated metabolites (including oxazepam) are conjugated and excreted in the urine. Plasma concentration monitoring is of little use in the management of patients who are taking clorazepate.

Adverse Effects. Adverse effects of clorazepate are similar to those of clonazepam and include sedation, dizziness, hypersalivation, and behavioral changes. Tolerance to the antiepileptic effect of clorazepate has been reported, but it does not seem to be as common or to develop as quickly, as with clonazepam.

Drug Interactions. Concurrent antacid administration may significantly slow the rate of conversion from clorazepate to DMD, as can other disease states that are characterized by an increase in gastric pH. However, during prolonged administration, steady-state DMD concentrations are not significantly reduced. Smoking and concurrent AED therapy with enzyme-inducing agents can accelerate the metabolism of clorazepate. Clorazepate has no known effect on the disposition of other AEDs.

NONPHARMACOLOGIC THERAPIES

VAGUS NERVE STIMULATION

The vagus nerve stimulator is the first device approved for the treatment of epilepsy. It consists of a fully implantable pulse generator and an electrode that attaches to the left vagus nerve. Stimulation parameters are adjusted according to patient tolerance and seizure control. The device is usually programmed for stimulations lasting 30 seconds, followed by 5 minutes of off time, with this pattern repeating continuously while the device is in operation. There is also a hand-held magnet that can be used to manually activate the device to deliver a stimulus. This latter feature is used by some patients to abort seizures at the time their aura begins. The vagus nerve stimulator is approved for use in adults and adolescents as adjunctive treatment (with AED therapy) for partial-onset seizures that do not respond to drug therapy. In clinical trials, use of the vagus nerve stimulator reduces the frequency of seizures by 50% or more in 25% of patients. This response is comparable to many of the newer AEDs. The benefits from vagus nerve stimulation are maintained for up to 5 years (and possibly longer) with continued use of the device. Preliminary evidence also supports the efficacy of vagus nerve stimulation in children and in patients with medically refractory generalized-onset seizures; however, more study is needed to confirm these observations. The most common adverse effects associated with use of the vagus nerve stimulator are hoarseness, coughing, and throat discomfort during the stimulation burst.[42]

SURGERY

Approximately 20% to 35% of persons with epilepsy will have persistent seizures despite treatment with AEDs. Many of these patients may benefit from surgical intervention; however, only a small percentage of candidates are referred for evaluation at one of the many epilepsy-surgery centers that exist in the United States.[43] Patients who are most likely to benefit from surgery are those with partial-onset seizures whose symptoms remain intractable despite optimal medical therapy. The degree to which seizures and drug toxicity impair the functional abilities of the patient must also be con-

sidered. Presurgical evaluation includes intensive medical and neurological testing to localize the lesion. MRI, PET, and single-photon emission CT scans, as well as simultaneous EEG and video telemetry monitoring, are very useful in this regard. Neuropsychological testing is used to assess the potential effects of epilepsy surgery on memory and language function. Resection of a seizure focus from the anterior temporal lobe is the most common surgical procedure performed. After temporal lobectomy, approximately 65% of patients are rendered free of seizures for at least 2 years and 20% to 25% experience a significant reduction.[43]

KETOGENIC DIET

The ketogenic diet, introduced in the 1920s, is a high-fat, low-carbohydrate, low-protein diet that has recently experienced resurgence in popularity because of enhanced public interest.[44,45] The mechanism of the diet's benefit is unknown but is thought to be related to ketosis and its effect on brain neurochemistry. Children younger than 10 years of age are most likely to benefit for two reasons: (a) their brain may better use ketones as an energy source; (b) because the diet is unpalatable, children are more likely to comply with the diet when they depend on a parent or caregiver to prepare their meals. The diet has been used to treat patients with both partial-onset and generalized-onset seizures and 33% to 67% of patients experience a benefit in terms of reduced seizure frequency or intensity.[44] A 3-month trial is usually sufficient to determine if the diet will benefit the patient. The effect of the ketogenic diet on the clearance of AEDs has not been adequately studied; therefore, drug concentrations should be monitored during implementation of the diet. Also, acetazolamide (occasionally used for its anticonvulsant effects) should be discontinued when the diet is initiated to prevent the development of metabolic acidosis. Acetazolamide may be reintroduced several weeks after ketosis has been established.

BEHAVIORAL THERAPIES

Psychologic techniques for control of epileptic seizures are often successful for patients with seizures triggered by flashing lights or visual patterns, reading, or listening to music (referred to as reflex epilepsies). In these patients, behavioral conditioning has been used with success. The role of behavioral therapies in other types of epilepsy remains limited; however, some patients report benefit from relaxation and biofeedback therapies.

FUTURE THERAPIES

Several novel drugs are currently under investigation for possible use as AEDs in the United States. Vigabatrin (Sabril) is an investigational AED that has been extensively evaluated in the United States. The drug irreversibly inhibits GABA transaminase, resulting in an increase in brain and cerebrospinal fluid GABA concentrations. Although this drug is effective for adjunctive treatment of partial-onset seizures, recent reports of vigabatrin-related visual field defects (primarily loss of peripheral vision) are of concern and have delayed the approval of this drug in the United States. The cause of these visual disturbances is unknown. Recently, pregabalin (Lynca) has been approved for epilepsy and the package insert is being finalized. Several AEDs are in preclinical and clinical stages of development, some of which have novel mechanisms of action. In addition, new device therapies are being evaluated for patients with pharmacoresistant epilepsy.

IMPROVING OUTCOMES

In addition to pharmacological and nonpharmacologic therapies, patients with epilepsy (and their families) often benefit from education regarding their condition and reinforcement of the importance of compliance to prescribed regimens. Psychiatric comorbidity (such as anxiety, mood, or thought disorders) also may complicate the treatment of patients with epilepsy. These conditions may arise as a consequence of the psychosocial issues related to epilepsy or can be caused by neurochemical features related to epilepsy itself. When present, these problems require detection and proper management.

PATIENT EDUCATION

The Epilepsy Foundation of America (Landover, Maryland) and its local affiliates also have available a wide range of client services and brochures to help patients (and their families) understand epilepsy and its treatment and to deal with the problems and psychosocial implications of seizures. Advocacy information is also available, including legal rights as they relate to employment, insurance, and education, as well as information on driving restrictions by state. The Epilepsy Foundation of America can also be reached by telephone (1-800- EFA-1000) or via the Internet (http://www.efa.org). An excellent website for families, patients, or caregivers is www.epilepsy.com.

METHODS TO IMPROVE PATIENT ADHERENCE TO DRUG THERAPY

Noncompliance with AED therapy is a common cause for recurrent seizures in patients with epilepsy. Reasons for noncompliance include high drug costs, adverse effects, fears regarding potential medical or psychological effects of medication, memory deficit, and various lifestyle issues. An understanding of the factors that affect adherence to drug therapy is necessary to develop effective strategies to improve compliance. Patients should be questioned about these and other factors that affect their ability to take medication as prescribed. Education is often the most important intervention to improve adherence, as long as it is targeted appropriately to the patient's specific problems or concerns. Materials available from the Epilepsy Foundation of America (see

above) are often useful as educational aids. Reducing the number of divided daily doses that must be remembered by the patient may also improve compliance. Consistency in medication plasma concentrations is important for maintaining seizure control. Therefore, extended-release or sustained-release products help in this regard. Various other compliance aids are available, including medication alarms and pill containers divided into daily compartments.

DISEASE MANAGEMENT STRATEGIES TO IMPROVE PATIENT OUTCOMES

Given the high costs associated with epilepsy care and the complexity of care as it relates to diagnosis, treatment selection, and therapy adjustment, some facilities have instituted disease management strategies to improve the quality and cost efficiency of care. Patients with uncontrolled seizures and those who are high users of health care resources are often the target of such programs that focus on confirmation of a correct diagnosis, patient education, compliance education, and evaluation of appropriate drug selection and dosing. However, the utility of such disease-management programs has yet to be validated.

PHARMACOECONOMICS

It is estimated that the total cost of epilepsy to the United States, including direct and indirect costs, is approximately $12.5 billion per year.[46] Indirect costs of epilepsy associated with lost productivity is responsible for approximately 60% of total costs. AED treatment accounts for 40% of the total direct costs associated with treatment, making it the single most costly component of direct patient care and exceeding the costs of emergency services, inpatient hospital costs, and outpatient physician visits combined.[47] However, there have been very few cost-effectiveness studies on AED therapy, and most of the research in this regard has been sponsored by pharmaceutical companies with a vested interest in the study results.

Despite the lack of good pharmacoeconomic studies in epilepsy treatment, it is likely that patient-specific considerations in drug selection, monitoring, and therapy adjustments will improve seizure control and reduce the total costs of epilepsy care. Use of the least expensive AED may not equate to optimally cost-effective care. For example, in the treatment of a patient with medically refractory epilepsy, addition of an expensive, new AED as adjunctive therapy may well result in a reduction in total costs by reducing either direct costs (e.g., clinic or emergency room visits), indirect costs (e.g., missed work days), or both. Nonetheless, additional pharmacoeconomic studies are required to distinguish the relative cost-effectiveness of various treatment alternatives for patients with easily controlled and treatment-resistant seizures.

STATUS EPILEPTICUS

There are two types of status epileptics: (a) generalized convulsive and (b) nonconvulsive.[48] Generalized convulsive status epileptics (GCSE), accounts for 75% of all status epileptics and is a medical emergency that requires prompt, effective treatment to minimize permanent neurological damage and death. Although there is no consensus on its definition, the International Classification of Epileptic Seizures defines status epilepticus as: (a) any continuous seizure lasting longer than 5 minutes whether or not consciousness is impaired or (b) two or more seizures without full recovery of consciousness between events.[5] Morbidity and mortality after GCSE are related primarily to the condition that precipitated the episode and to neuronal injury from continuous electrical and convulsive seizure activity. Patient prognosis is more likely to be poor when seizures last longer than 90 minutes and when the event is caused by acute CNS injury such as stroke, anoxia, CNS infection, or head injury. The mortality associated with status epileptics (SEs) is approximately 10% in children, 20% in adults, and 38% in the elderly, even with aggressive anticonvulsant drug therapy.

The most common cause of GCSE in patients with a history of epilepsy is noncompliance with AED therapy. In addition, the various factors listed in Table 62.1 can cause seizures and are also potential causes of GCSE. The initial workup for patients should include a thorough medical and neurological evaluation to identify the cause of the patient's seizures. Potentially treatable causes of GCSE, such as CNS infection and metabolic abnormalities, should be identified and treated as soon as possible.

During GCSE, patients should receive oxygen supplementation and should be monitored for hyperthermia. Passive cooling measures should be used to minimize the potentially damaging effects of fever during prolonged convulsions. The EEG should be monitored in any patient who receives a paralytic agent and in patients who remain unconscious after the seizures have been controlled. In these situations, seizures may continue even in the absence of convulsive muscle movements.

Figure 62.1 outlines the timeline, sequence of drug administration, and dosing for drugs commonly used in the management of GCSE in adults.[49] Lorazepam is the agent of choice for the initial treatment of GCSE. Benzodiazepines, such as diazepam and lorazepam terminate GCSE in 80% to 90% of patients, usually within 3 to 5 minutes after intravenous administration. The usefulness of diazepam is limited by its short duration of anticonvulsant effect (15 minutes–2 hours). This drug is highly lipophilic and quickly redistributes out of the brain to other fat stores in the body. Lorazepam has a longer duration of action and is preferred over diazepam for this reason. Phenytoin and fosphenytoin are effective for the treatment of GCSE; however, the peak anticonvulsant effects of both drugs are delayed by approximately 20 minutes from the start of drug administration and they are usually administered after lorazepam. Phenytoin (and fosphenytoin) provides additional long-lasting protection from recurrent seizures. Phenobarbital is usually reserved for GCSE that does not stop after lorazepam and phenytoin. Like phenytoin, the peak effect of phenobarbital is delayed and because of the drug's sedative effect, phenobarbital can confound the assessment of mental status after seizures are terminated. High-dose, continuous infusions with anesthetic doses of either propofol or midazolam are the treatments of choice for GCSE that does not respond to the drugs discussed above.[49] Patients with refractory GCSE usually require admission to an intensive care unit for ventilatory support and continuous monitoring of the EEG and vascular hemodynamics.

TREATMENT GOALS: STATUS EPILEPTICUS

- Terminate seizures as quickly as possible.
- Identify and treat any potentially reversible causes.
- Medically manage systemic complications that arise from prolonged convulsive seizures (e.g., hyperthermia or hypoxia).

KEY POINTS

- An accurate diagnosis of the patient's seizure type and epilepsy syndrome is required for successful management
- Patient-specific seizure precipitants should be identified and eliminated

- Select optimal AED therapy based on seizure type, epilepsy syndrome, patient age, sex, and concomitant medical conditions
- Adjust AED therapy to attain complete control of seizures with minimal or no adverse effects
- Monitor for clinical and laboratory evidence of adverse effects of drug therapy

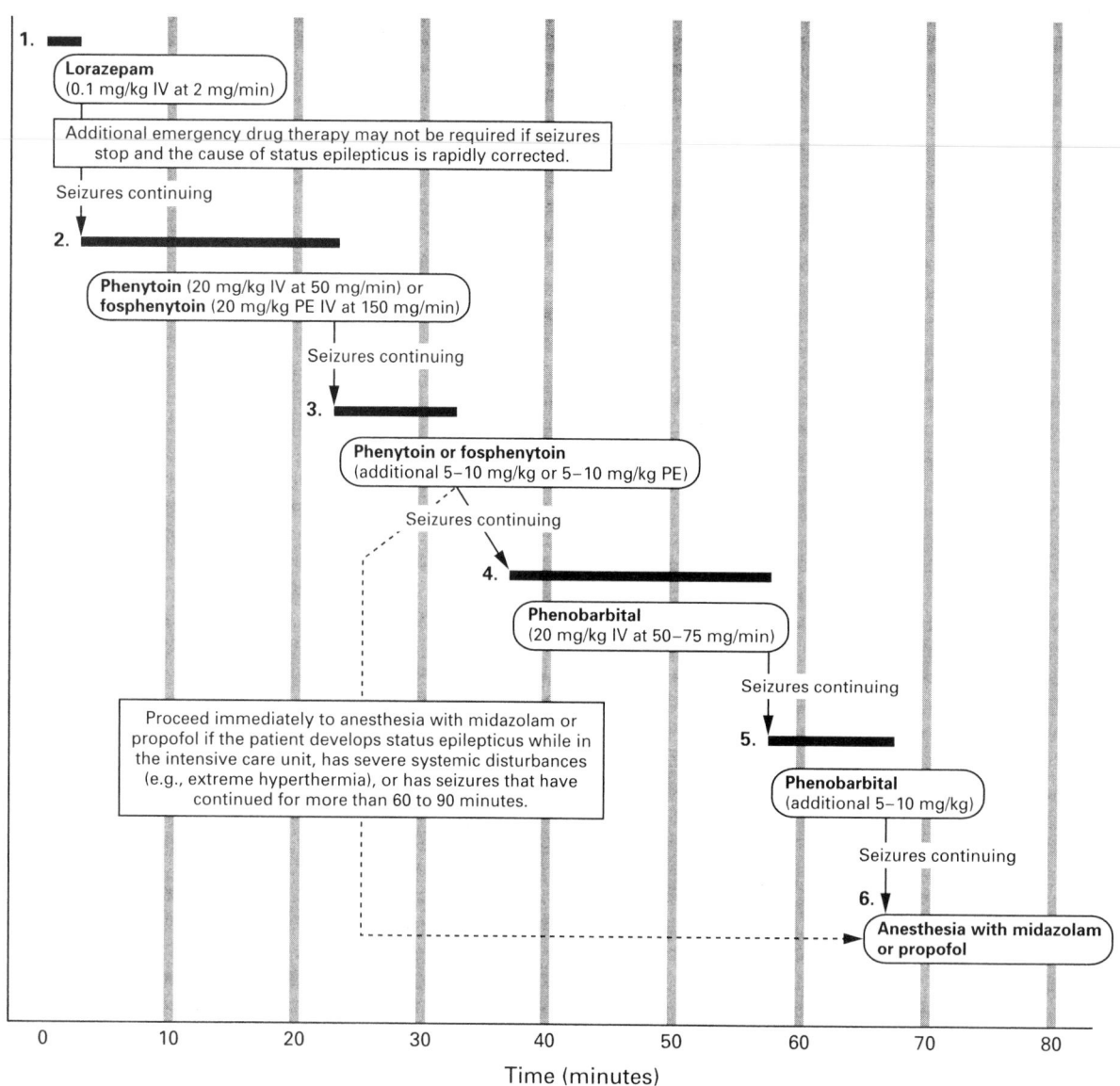

FIGURE 62.1 Antiepileptic drug therapy for status epilepticus. IV, intravenous; PE, phenytoin equivalents. The horizontal bars indicate the approximate duration of drug infusions. (From Lowenstein DH, Alldredge BK. Status epilepticus. N Engl J Med 338:970–976, 1998, with permission.)

- Minimize the use of poly-drug therapy and sedating AEDs whenever possible
- Periodic monitoring of AED blood concentrations may be useful for guiding subsequent dosage adjustments (for phenytoin in particular), and for monitoring medication compliance, adverse effects, and the effects of drugs or conditions that alter AED clearance
- The clinical status of the patient should be the ultimate guide regarding the necessity for dosage adjustment
- In patients who have persistent seizures despite titration of therapy to the maximal tolerated dosage, another AED should be gradually substituted for the original medication
- When sequential monotherapy with two or three AEDs fails to control seizures, consideration should then be given to adjunctive therapy with one of the new AEDs
- Recognize when patients should be referred to a comprehensive epilepsy center for diagnostic evaluation or initiation of other modalities (e.g., surgery, vagus nerve stimulation, or ketogenic diet)
- Patients and their families require education and support regarding epilepsy, its treatment, and its effect on daily activities

REFERENCES

1. Theodore WH, Porter RJ. Epilepsy: 100 elementary principles. 3rd ed. London: WB Saunders, 1995.
2. Scheuer ML, Pedley TA. The evaluation and treatment of seizures. N Engl J Med 323:1468–1474, 1990.
3. Alldredge BK, Simon RP. Drugs that can precipitate seizures. In: Resor SR, Kutt H, eds. The medical treatment of epilepsy. New York: Marcel Dekker, 1992:497–523.
4. Commission on Classification and Terminology of the International League Against Epilepsy. Proposal for revised clinical and electroencephalographic classification of epileptic seizures. Epilepsia 22: 489–501, 1981.
5. Commission on Classification and Terminology of the International League Against Epilepsy. Proposal for classification of epilepsies and epileptic syndromes. Epilepsia 26:268–278, 1985.
6. Knudsen FU. Febrile seizures–treatment and outcome. Brain Dev 18:438–449, 1996.
7. Chadwick D. Diagnosis of epilepsy. Lancet 336:291–295, 1990.
8. Theodore WH, Porter RJ. Removal of sedative-hypnotic antiepileptic drugs from the regimens of patients with intractable epilepsy. Ann Neurol 13:320–324, 1983.
9. French JA, Kanner AM, Bautista J, et al. Efficacy and tolerability of the new antiepileptic drugs I: treatment of new onset epilepsy: report of the Therapeutics and Technology Assessment Subcommittee and Quality Standards Subcommittee of the American Academy of Neurology and the American Epilepsy Society. Neurology 62: 1252–1260, 2004.
10. French JA, Kanner AM, Bautista J, et al. Efficacy and tolerability of the new antiepileptic drugs I: treatment of new onset epilepsy: report of the Therapeutics and Technology Assessment Subcommittee and Quality Standards Subcommittee of the American Academy of Neurology and the American Epilepsy Society. Neurology 62: 1252–1260, 2004.
11. Mattson RH, Cramer JA, Collins JF, et al. Comparison of carbamazepine, phenobarbital, phenytoin, and primidone in partial and secondarily generalized tonic-clonic seizures. N Engl J Med 313:145–151, 1985.
12. Mattson RH, Cramer JA, Collins JF, et al. A comparison of valproate with carbamazepine for the treatment of complex partial seizures and secondarily generalized tonic-clonic seizures in adults. N Engl J Med 327:765–771, 1992.
13. Marson AG, Chadwick DW. New antiepileptic drugs: a systematic review of their efficacy and tolerability. Br Med J 313:1169–1174, 1996.
14. Devinsky O. Patients with refractory seizures. N Engl J Med 340: 1565–1570, 1999.
15. Sato S, White BG, Penry JK, et al. Valproic acid versus ethosuximide in the treatment of absence seizures. Neurology 32:157–163, 1982.
16. Dodson WE. Level off. Neurology 39:1009–1010, 1989.
17. Report of the Quality Standards Subcommittee of the American Academy of Neurology. Practice parameter: a guideline for discontinuing antiepileptic drugs in seizure-free patients-summary statement. Neurology 47:600–602, 1996.
18. Zahn CA, Morrell MJ, Collins SD, et al. Management issues for women with epilepsy: a review of the literature. Neurology 51: 949–956, 1998.
19. Morrell MJ. Guidelines for the care of women with epilepsy. Neurology 51 (Suppl 4):S21–S27, 1998.
20. Anderson GD. A mechanistic approach to antiepileptic drug interactions. Ann Pharmacother 32:554–563, 1998.
21. Cohen H, Howland MA, Luciano DJ, et al. Feasibility and pharmacokinetics of carbamazepine oral loading doses. Am J Health-Syst Pharm 55:1134–1140, 1998.
22. Dalby MA. Behavioral effects of carbamazepine. In: Penry JK, Dalby DD, eds. Advances in neurology. New York: Raven Press, 1975:331–343.
23. Alldredge BK, Knutsen AP, Ferriero D. Antiepileptic drug hypersensitivity syndrome: in vitro and clinical observations. Pediatr Neurol 10:169–171, 1994.
24. Hart RG, Easton JD. Carbamazepine and hematological monitoring. Ann Neurol 11:309–312, 1982.
25. Tuchman AJ, Zisfein J, Paccione M, et al. Single-versus divided-dose oral phenytoin loading: a controlled study [Abstract]. Neurology 44 (Suppl 2):A295, 1994.
26. Boucher BA. Fosphenytoin: a novel phenytoin prodrug. Pharmacotherapy 16:777–791, 1996.
27. Winter ME, Tozer TN. Phenytoin. In: Evans WE, Schentag JJ, Jusko WJ, eds. Applied pharmacokinetics: principles of therapeutic drug monitoring. 3rd ed. Vancouver: Applied Therapeutics, 1992: 25.1–44.
28. Nation RL, Evans AM, Milne RW. Pharmacokinetic drug interactions with phenytoin (part II). Clin Pharmacokinet 18:131–150, 1990.
29. Brodie MJ, Dichter MA. Antiepileptic drugs. N Engl J Med 334: 168–175, 1996.
30. Meador KJ, Loring DW, Moore EE, et al. Comparative cognitive effects of phenobarbital, phenytoin, and valproate in healthy adults. Neurology 45:1494–1499, 1995.
31. Gidal B, Spencer N, Maly M, et al. Valproate-mediated disturbances of hemostasis: relationship to dose and plasma concentration. Neurology 44:1418–1422, 1994.
32. Dreifuss FE, Langer DH, Moline KA, et al. Valproic acid hepatic fatalities. II: US experience since 1984. Neurology 39:201–207, 1989.
33. Chapman SA, Wacksman GP, Patterson BD. Pancreatitis associated with valproic acid: A review of the literature. Pharmacotherapy 21: 1549–1560, 2001.
34. Ragson N. The relationship between polycystic ovary syndrome and antiepileptic drugs: a review of the evidence. J Clin Psychopharmacol 24:322–334, 2004.
35. Petroff OAC, Rothman DL, Behar KL, et al. The effect of gabapentin on brain gamma-aminobutyric acid in patients with epilepsy. Ann Neurol 39:95–99, 1996.
36. Gidal BE, Maly MM, Budde J, et al. Effect of a high-protein meal on gabapentin pharmacokinetics. Epilepsy Res 23:71–76, 1996.
37. Schlienger RG, Shapiro LE, Shear NH. Lamotrigine-induced severe cutaneous adverse reactions. Epilepsia 39 (Suppl 7):S22–26, 1998.
38. Sachdeo RC. Topiramate. Clinical profile in epilepsy. Clin Pharmacokinet 34:335–346, 1998.
39. Martin R, Kuzniecky R, Ho S, et al. Cognitive effects of topiramate, gabapentin, and lamotrigine in healthy young adults. Neurology 52: 321–327, 1999.
40. Felbatol product information. Cranbury, NJ: Wallace Laboratories, February 1999.
41. Pellock JM, Brodie MJ. Felbamate: 1997 update. Epilepsia 38: 1261–1264, 1997.
42. Schachter SC, Saper CB. Vagus nerve stimulation. Epilepsia 39: 677–686, 1998.
43. Engel J. Surgery for seizures. N Engl J Med 334:647–652, 1996.
44. Bainbridge JL, Gidal BE, Ryan M. The ketogenic diet. Pharmacotherapy 19:782–786, 1999.
45. Phelps SJ, Rose, DF, Hovinga C, et al. The Ketogenic Diet in intractable epilepsy of childhood: A review. Nutr Clin Prac 13: 267–282, 1998.
46. Epilepsy: a report to the nation. Landover, MD: Epilepsy Foundation of America, 1999.
47. Begley CE, Annegers JF, Lairson DR, et al. Cost of epilepsy in the United States: a model based on incidence and prognosis. Epilepsia 35:1230–1243, 1994.
48. Lowenstein DH, Alldredge BK. Status epilepticus. N Engl J Med 338:970–976, 1998.
49. Alldredge BK, Lowenstein DH. Status epilepticus: new concepts. Curr Opin Neurol 12:183–190, 1999.

Parkinsonism

63

Jack J. Chen and Sam K. Shimomura

*"Some turn this sickness yet might take,
Ev'n yet." But he: "What drug can make
. A wither'd palsy cease to shake?"
"The Two Voices," 1842*

—Alfred Lord Tennyson

DEFINITION

Parkinsonism is a movement disorder. In 1817, Dr. James Parkinson published a case series describing six patients afflicted with the ''shaking palsy'' (paralysis agitans), a chronic and progressive neurologic disorder[1] (Table 63.1). Since then, the term parkinsonism has been used to describe any clinical syndrome associated with the three cardinal clinical features of tremor, rigidity, and bradykinesia (Fig. 63.1; *see color insert*). Even today, very little can be added to Parkinson's keen observation of ''involuntary tremulous motion, with lessened muscular power, in parts not in action and even when supported; with a propensity to bend the trunk forwards, and to pass from a walking to a running pace.''[1] Parkinson also noted the development of several nonmotor symptoms (e.g., constipation, drooling, dysphagia, speech and sleep disturbances), the profound adverse impact on quality of life, and the importance of caregiver support.

The majority of parkinsonism cases are of the idiopathic type, in which the cause is unknown; it is commonly referred to as Parkinson disease (PD). Less common forms of parkinsonism are classified under secondary parkinsonisms (e.g., drug-induced), multisystem Parkinson plus syndromes, or hereditary parkinsonisms (Table 63.2).

Since the 1950s, drug-induced parkinsonism has been the second most common form of parkinsonism[9,10]. The two major types of parkinsonism-inducing agents are those that deplete central stores of dopamine (e.g., reserpine, methyldopa, tetrabenazine) and those that antagonize central dopamine receptors (e.g., chlorpromazine, haloperidol, metoclopramide). For all patients who present with signs and symptoms of parkinsonism, an inquiry should be made to assess for current use of the agents listed in Table 63.3. If drug-induced parkinsonism is suspected, discontinuation of the offending agent will result in improvement within 3 months; complete resolution usually occurs within 1 year. In a case-controlled study, older adults on metoclopramide were three times more likely to be on the antiparkinson drug levodopa than those not on metoclopramide.[11] This observation suggests that drug-induced parkinsonism is often misdiagnosed and treated as idiopathic PD.

Multisystem Parkinson plus syndromes are uncommon and characterized by the presence of parkinsonian motor features along with other unique autonomic, neurologic, and psychiatric abnormalities. Several variants have been characterized, such as corticobasal degeneration, multiple-system atrophies, and progressive supranuclear palsy. In general, these atypical parkinsonisms are unresponsive or at best transiently responsive to antiparkinson therapy.

TABLE 63.1	Historical Landmarks in Parkinson Disease
1817	James Parkinson publishes "An Essay on the Shaking Palsy"[1]
1860s	Belladonna alkaloids recognized for antiparkinson activity
1912	First published neurosurgical operation for relief of parkinsonism[2]
1912	Lewy bodies described[3]
1919	Depigmentation of the substantia nigra pars compacta described[4]
1951	First published trial of apomorphine for treatment of Parkinson disease[5]
1960	Parkinsonism attributed to striatal dopamine depletion[6]
1970	Levodopa approved by the U.S. Food and Drug Administration (FDA)
1973	Amantadine approved by the FDA
1975	Carbidopa/levodopa and carbidopa approved by the FDA
1978	Bromocriptine approved by the FDA for parkinsonism
1983	MPTP-induced parkinsonism (the "frozen addicts") reported[7]
1988	Pergolide approved by the FDA
1988	First fetal nigral tissue transplant for Parkinson disease[8]
1989	Selegiline approved by the FDA
1991	Carbidopa/levodopa sustained-release tablets introduced
1997	Pramipexole and ropinirole approved by the FDA
1997	Chronic deep brain stimulation device approved by the FDA for tremor associated with Parkinson disease
1998	Tolcapone approved by the FDA
1999	Entacapone approved by the FDA
2002	Chronic deep brain stimulation device approved by the FDA for Parkinson disease
2004	Apomorphine approved by the FDA

TREATMENT GOALS

- Improve motor function
- Maintain ability to complete daily activities independently
- Minimize development of treatment-emergent motor fluctuations and dyskinesias
- Minimize development of treatment-emergent hallucinations and psychosis
- Improve nonmotor symptoms
- Maintain quality of life

EPIDEMIOLOGY

In the United States, approximately 1 million people have PD, with a slight predominance towards men and Caucasians. The mean age at diagnosis is approximately 60 years and the crude annual incidence ranges from 16 to 19 individuals per 100,000.[12] When stratified according to age, the annual incidence increases dramatically to 115 individuals per 100,000 (65 to 74 years) and 255 individuals per 100,000 (75 to 84 years).[9] Similarly, the prevalence estimate also increases with age.[13] Less than 30% of cases are diagnosed before age 55 and less than 10% before age 40. The term juvenile parkinsonism refers to onset before age 21 years; the term young onset is used if the onset of parkinsonism occurs between 21 and 40 years of age.[14] Patients with PD can live a long life; however, epidemiologic data report a mortality risk of up to five times expected rates.[12,15] This risk is strongly related to the concomitant presence of gait disturbance and dementia.

ETIOLOGY

Parkinsonism is a disorder with a complex etiology combining varying contributions of genetic and environmental fac-

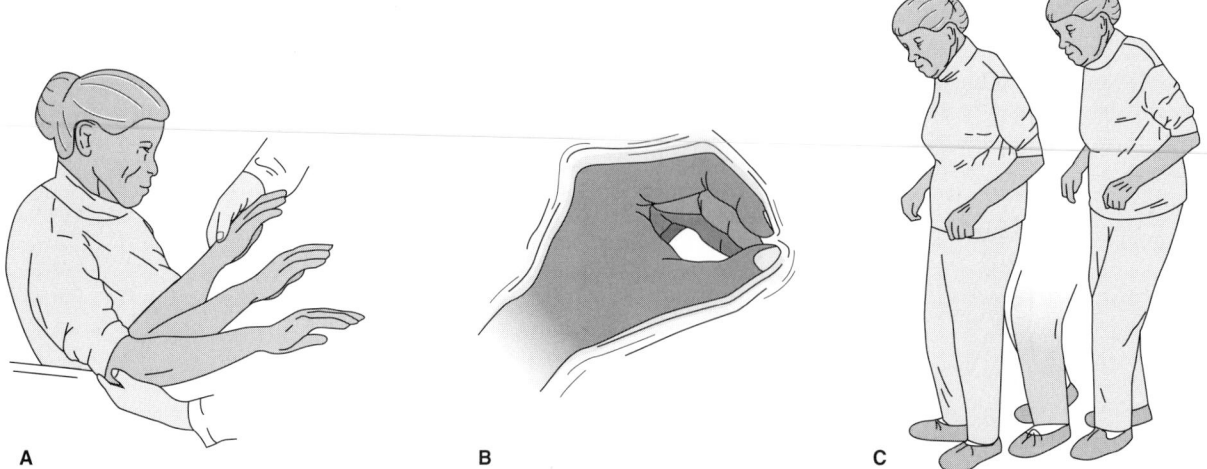

FIGURE 63.1 A. Parkinson's disease is manifested by rigidity that accompanies passive flexion of extremities. "Cogwheeling" may be present. **B.** "Pill-rolling" tremor at rest. **C.** Slowness of movement characterized by a slow, shuffling gait and lack of arm swing (*see color insert*). (From Smeltzer SC, Bare BG. Textbook of medical-surgical nursing, 9th ed. Philadelphia: Lippincott Williams & Wilkins, 2000.)

tors over time. Although the precise contribution of genetic and environmental factors remains to be determined, several sources provide clues. Case-controlled studies have reported a hereditary pattern in approximately 10% of cases and a two to three times greater risk of PD in first-degree relatives.[16–20] However, for individuals who develop PD at a younger age (before age 50 years), a greater potential for a hereditary basis exists.[17,18] Several forms of familial parkinsonism have been identified and linked to specific gene mutations (see Table 63.2). Results from a large twin study suggests that an as yet unidentified genetic mechanism plays a greater role in early-onset PD (when symptoms begin at or before age 50 years).[17] In patients with autosomal recessive juvenile parkinsonism, a mutation of the parkin gene can be found in approximately 50% of cases.[21] In late-onset parkinsonism, a mutation in the LRRK2 (leucine-rich repeat kinase 2) gene may underlie a significant percentage of cases in which parkinsonism is transmitted in an autosomal dominant manner.[22]

In the early 1980s, young addicts were developing severe parkinsonism within 24 hours after injecting a designer meperidine analogue. After much investigative effort, Langston et al discovered that the drug samples had been heavily contaminated with 1-methyl-4-phenyl-1,2,3,6-tetrahydropyridine (MPTP), a byproduct of the synthetic process.[7] MPTP was soon characterized as a protoxin converted by monoamine oxidase type B (MAO_B) to MPP^+ (1-methyl-4-phenylpyridine), a potent neurotoxin. Interestingly, MPP^+ is chemically related to the herbicide paraquat. Subsequently, population-based, case-controlled studies have demonstrated a higher risk of parkinsonism associated with occupational exposure to various herbicides and insecticides.[23] Ingestion of naturally occurring neurotoxins, such as herbal tea and fruits from the Annonaceae family (e.g., Annona muricata), have also been linked to parkinsonism.[24,25] All

of these substances are mitochondrial toxins. Mitochondrial poisoning results from a depletion of ATP and an increase in the production of damaging oxygen and nitrogen free radicals, leading to oxidative stress. Both processes are cytotoxic. Occupational exposure to high levels of manganese (e.g., arc welding fumes, manganese mines) has also been associated with parkinsonism, as has proximity to wood mills and drinking of well water in some communities.[26,27]

As far as protective factors, epidemiologic studies have consistently identified tobacco smoking and coffee consumption as protective for the development of PD.[28–31] Moderate to high intake of dietary vitamin E may also be protective.[32] However, it is not clear whether vitamin E supplements confer the same benefits.

Overall, on one end of the etiology spectrum, there are cases of parkinsonism inherited in an autosomal dominant or recessive Mendelian pattern; on the other end, there are cases of toxin-induced parkinsonism. Idiopathic PD, which represents the vast majority of cases, falls somewhere in between.

PATHOPHYSIOLOGY

The pathophysiology underlying the motor and nonmotor features of PD is complex. A major pathologic process is neuronal degeneration of the pigmented substantia nigra pars compacta (SNpc), a region of the basal ganglia that produces dopamine and is intrinsically involved in motor control (Fig. 63.2; *see color insert*). Dopamine modulates the direct and indirect pathways of the extrapyramidal motor circuit, which are mediated by γ-aminobutyric acid (GABA) and glutamate (Fig. 63.3). Inhibitory GABA-ergic pathways contribute to the major outflow pathways in the basal ganglia and striatum; as a result of dopamine depletion, the thalamus is over-

TABLE 63.2	Classification of Parkinsonism

Primary Parkinsonism

Idiopathic Parkinson disease

Secondary Parkinsonisms

Brain neoplasm

Drugs (e.g., haloperidol, metoclopramide, phenothiazines)

Infections (e.g., postencephalitic, human immunodeficiency virus associated, subacute sclerosing panencephalitis)

Metabolic (e.g., hypothyroidism, hepatocerebral degeneration, parathyroid abnormalities)

Normal-pressure hydrocephalus

Toxins (e.g., carbon monoxide, manganese, methanol, MPTP, organophosphate insecticides)

Head trauma (e.g., "punch drunk" syndrome)

Vascular (e.g., multi-infarct, Binswanger disease)

Multisystem Parkinson plus Syndromes

Corticobasal degeneration

Multiple-system atrophies (e.g., olivopontocerebellar atrophy, Shy-Drager syndrome, striatonigral degeneration)

Progressive supranuclear palsy (i.e., Steele-Richardson-Olszewski syndrome)

Dementia/Parkinsonism Syndromes

Alzheimer's disease with parkinsonism

Creutzfeldt-Jakob disease

Guamanian amyotrophic lateral sclerosis-parkinsonism dementia ("Lytico-Bodig")

Dementia with Lewy bodies

Frontotemporal dementia

Hereditary Parkinsonisms

Autosomal Dominant

α-synuclein gene mutation (PARK1)

Frontotemporal dementia parkinsonism (FTDP–17)

Huntington disease (juvenile form or Westphal variant)

Levodopa-responsive dystonia

LRRK2 (dardarin) mutation

Rapid-onset dystonia parkinsonism (DYT12)

Spinocerebellar ataxias (SCA2, SCA3)

Autosomal Recessive

Hallervorden-Spatz disease

Neuroacanthocytes

Niemann Pick type C

Wilson disease

Young-onset parkinsonism (DJ–1, parkin, PINK1)

X-linked Recessive

Fragile X tremor/ataxia syndrome (FXTAS)

Lubag (DYT3 or Filipino dystonia parkinsonism)

Waisman syndrome (X-linked parkinsonism with mental retardation)

TABLE 63.3	Drugs Commonly Associated with Parkinsonism

Cinnarizine and flunarizine[a]

Haloperidol

α-Methyldopa

Metoclopramide

Phenothiazines (e.g., chlorpromazine, mesoridazine, perphenazine, thioridazine)

Reserpine (Rauwolfia serpentina)

Tetrabenazine[a]

[a] Not marketed in the United States.

inhibited and movement becomes abnormal. It is estimated that parkinsonian features are not clinically apparent until a critical threshold of 80% loss of dopamine concentration has occurred.[33]

In addition to depigmentation of the SNpc, another defining histopathologic hallmark is the presence of Lewy bodies (LBs) (Fig. 63.4; *see color insert*). LBs are spherical, intracytoplasmic aggregates found in the remaining neurons of the SNpc and are composed of ubiquitin-positive proteinaceous aggregates of α-synuclein (a substance also found in amyloid plaques of Alzheimer's disease) and other misfolded proteins. Previously, LBs were believed to be detrimental; however, current evidence suggests that they may be a protective mechanism whereby intracellular neurotoxic products are isolated and prevented from causing further damage.[34] Lewy pathology has been proposed to develop in a predictable anatomic distribution within the parkinsonian brain.[35] In the preclinical stages of PD, LBs are initially found in the medulla oblongata, locus ceruleus, raphe nuclei, and olfactory bulb. This may correlate with observations that anxiety, depression, and impaired olfaction occur in preclinical stages of PD. As PD progresses to clinical stages, Lewy pathology ascends to the midbrain (particularly the SNpc), accounting for motor features. In advanced stages, Lewy pathology spreads to the cortex and may account for behavioral and cognitive changes. Thus, the pathology in PD affects not only dopaminergic SNpc cells but also nonnigral cell bodies that are involved in regulating acetylcholine, GABA, glutamate, norepinephrine, serotonin, and a range of other neuropeptides. The presence of nonnigral cell pathology may correlate with the development of various autonomic, behavioral, and cognitive symptoms in PD.

Normally, the SNpc is endowed with a variety of protective mechanisms, as it is a region inherently subjected to high levels of oxidant stress. Whether triggered by toxin exposure or genetic susceptibility or a combination of factors, the available evidence suggests that intracellular redox potential is altered due to a cascade of events involving mitochondrial complex I dysfunction, free radical generation, oxidant stress, and dysfunction of the ubiquitin-proteasome system (UPS) that ultimately results in cell death (see Fig.

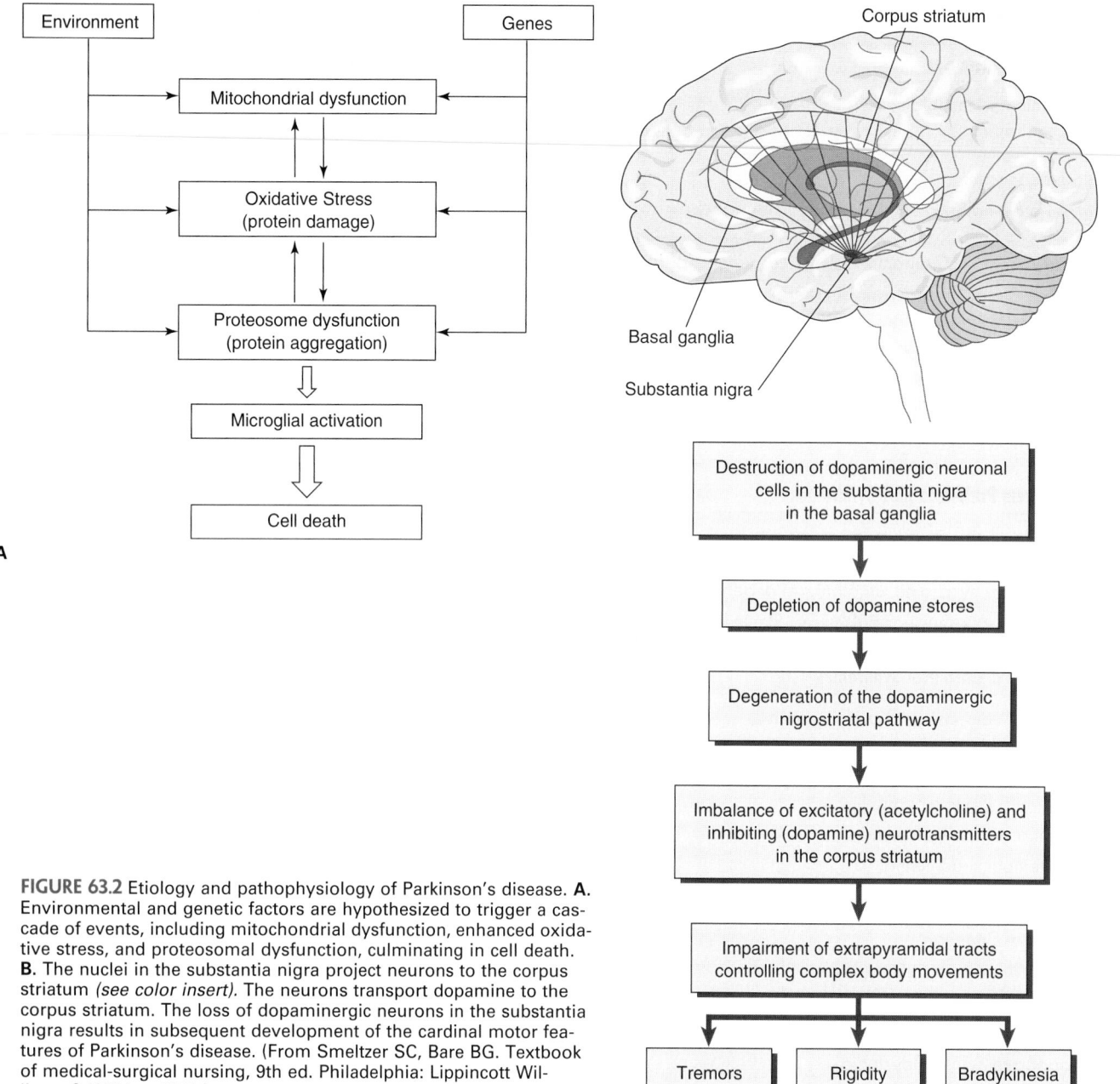

FIGURE 63.2 Etiology and pathophysiology of Parkinson's disease. **A.** Environmental and genetic factors are hypothesized to trigger a cascade of events, including mitochondrial dysfunction, enhanced oxidative stress, and proteosomal dysfunction, culminating in cell death. **B.** The nuclei in the substantia nigra project neurons to the corpus striatum *(see color insert)*. The neurons transport dopamine to the corpus striatum. The loss of dopaminergic neurons in the substantia nigra results in subsequent development of the cardinal motor features of Parkinson's disease. (From Smeltzer SC, Bare BG. Textbook of medical-surgical nursing, 9th ed. Philadelphia: Lippincott Williams & Wilkins, 2000.)

63.2).[34,36,37] Other events including excitotoxicity, inflammation, and toxic effects of nitric oxide have also been implicated. In the SNpc of patients with PD, concentrations of protective antioxidants (e.g., glutathione) are reduced and reactive oxidants (e.g., peroxynitrite, O_2^-, ^-OH, Fe^{3+}) are elevated. This results in a change in the redox state to a more oxidizing environment. Glutathione is a major antioxidant, and depleted levels are consistently found in patients with PD. The cause of glutathione depletion is unknown, but it renders the dopaminergic neurons more vulnerable to oxidant stress induced by reactive nitrogen and oxygen species. The neurons of the SNpc possess disproportionately long

dendrites that are poorly myelinated; this also enhances vulnerability to toxic factors.

In addition to oxidant stress and altered redox potential, accumulation of intracellular protein aggregates occurs. Within the brain, misfolded proteins are normally tagged by ubiquitin and targeted for degradation by the UPS. The UPS is the major route through which intracellular proteolysis is regulated. However, in PD, a malfunction or overload of the UPS system results in accumulation of unfolded or mutated proteins that are toxic. Ultimately, disruption of the intracellular milieu results in activation of surrounding microglia, which release cytokines, glutamate, and reactive nitrogen

Direct Pathway. In the normal brain, dopamine activates the D_1 receptor which results in activation of the striatum. The activated striatum inhibits the GPi/SNpr which disinhibits the thalamus. Disinhibition of the thalamus results in excitatory stimulus to the motor cortex. In Parkinson's disease, denervation of the striatal D_1 pathway ultimately results in excessive GABA outflow to the thalamus and reduced outflow to the motor cortex.

$$SNpc\ (D_1) — (+) \longrightarrow Striatum — (GABA) \longrightarrow GPi\ /\ SNpr — (GABA) \longrightarrow Thalamus — (glutamate) \longrightarrow Motor\ Cortex$$

Indirect Pathway. In the normal brain, dopamine activates the D_2 receptor which results in inhibition of the striatum. The inhibited striatum disinhibits the GPe. The disinhibited GPe results in more GABAergic activity to the STN and subsequently less activation of the GPi/SNpr. The reduced GABAergic outflow from the GPi/SNpr results in disinhibition of the thalamus and an increase in excitatory stimulus to the motor cortex. In Parkinson's disease, denervation of the striatal D_2 pathway also ultimately results in excessive GABA outflow to the thalamus and reduced outflow to the motor cortex.

$$SNpc\ (D_2) — (-) \longrightarrow Striatum \qquad GPi/SNpr — (GABA) \longrightarrow Thalamus — (glutamate) \longrightarrow Motor\ Cortex$$

GABA = γ-aminobutyric acid; GPi = globus pallidus interna; GPe = globus pallidus externa; SNpc = substantia nigra pars compacta; SNpr = substantia nigra pars reticularis; STN = subthalamic nucleus

FIGURE 63.3 Learned movement is regulated by a complex motor circuit involving the extrapyramidal motor system, which is composed of the basal ganglia (caudate nucleus, putamen, and globus pallidus) and the substantia nigra. The caudate nucleus and putamen are also known collectively as the striatum. The substantia nigra, which contains about 80% of the dopamine-producing cells in the brain, has two regions—the pars compacta (SNpc), which produces dopamine, and the pars reticulata (SNpr), which produces the inhibitory transmitter γ-aminobutyric acid (GABA). The SNpc neurons synthesize, store, and transport dopamine to the striatum. Striatal neurons then communicate with neurons of the thalamocortical pathway (subthalamic nucleus, thalamus, and cerebral cortex) via direct and indirect pathways. The direct pathway is linked to striatal D_1 receptors and the indirect pathway to striatal D_2 receptors. The internal capsule of the globus pallidus (GPi) and the GABA-ergic SNpr exert an inhibitory influence and act as the final common gateway to the thalamus.

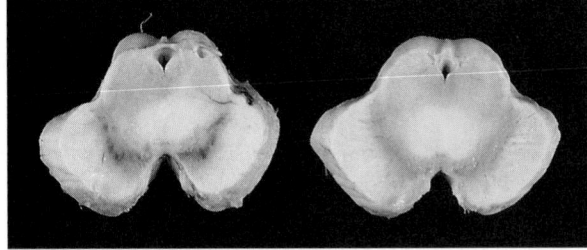
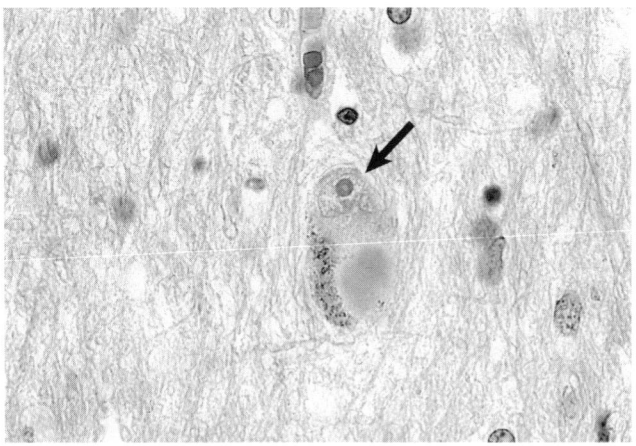

FIGURE 63.4 Pathology of Parkinson's disease. **A.** Normal substantia nigra of the midbrain (**left**) is heavily pigmented with neuromelanin, whereas the same region from a patient with Parkinson's disease (**right**) demonstrates depigmentation. **B.** Microscopic section of the substantia nigra pars compacta from a patient with Parkinson's disease shows a spherical eosinophilic inclusion (*arrow*) within the cytoplasm of a pigmented dopaminergic neuron. This inclusion body is termed a Lewy body *(see color insert)*. (From Rubin E, Farber JL. Pathology, 3rd ed. Philadelphia: Lippincott Williams & Wilkins, 1999.)

and oxygen species that induce apoptotic and necrotic cell death.

CLINICAL PRESENTATION AND DIAGNOSIS

The initial cardinal motor features of PD are tremor at rest, rigidity, and bradykinesia (see Fig. 63.1). Initially these motor features develop unilaterally and then spread to contralateral extremities.[38] As the disease progresses, postural instability (i.e., balance problem) develops. In addition to the primary motor features, nonmotor symptoms are also very common and significantly impair the patient's quality of life. Examples include bladder incontinence, constipation, dementia, drooling, dysphagia, erectile dysfunction, olfactory deficit, orthostatic hypotension, pain, paresthesias, seborrheic dermatitis, sleep disturbances, sweating, and temperature intolerances. Anxiety and depressive syndromes are also very common, and periodic screening for these conditions should be conducted.[39]

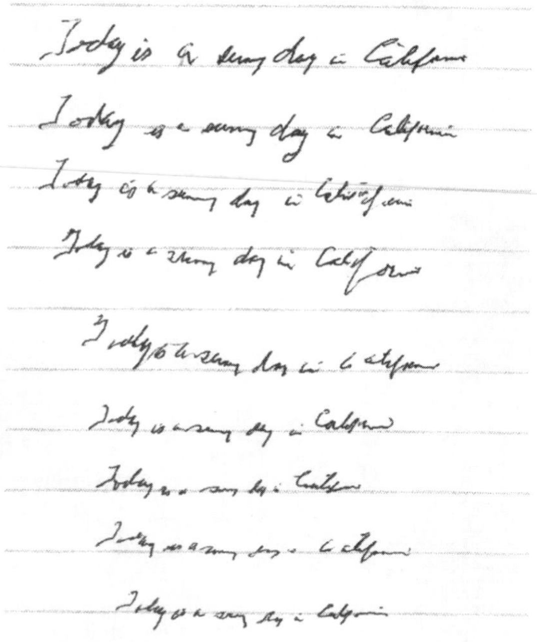

SIGNS AND SYMPTOMS

A rhythmic, pill-rolling tremor of the hand and upper extremities is often the most visible yet least disabling symptom. This tremor generally occurs at rest and is of slower frequency (3 to 6 Hz) than the tremor associated with alcoholism, essential tremor, hyperthyroidism, or nervousness. Patients will commonly report that the tremor disappears during sleep and is worsened by stress or excitement. In addition to rest tremor, a postural tremor (observable when arms are outstretched in front of the patient) is also common. Action tremor (e.g., tremor during writing) is uncommon. In contrast to the other cardinal features, tremor severity generally remains stable over time.[40]

Muscular rigidity or stiffness commonly affects the upper and lower extremities and axial regions such as the face and trunk. Rigidity of the extremities interferes with range of motion and is detected upon passive flexion at the elbow, wrist, or knee with the patient in a seated position. In the presence of tremor, the rigidity is associated with a cogwheel or ratchet-like quality upon examination. Rigidity of the face and trunk is often observable as a lack of facial expression (masked facies) and stooped posture. The masking of facial expression may be misinterpreted as apathy, unfriendliness, or depression.

Bradykinesia is defined as slowness of movement. On neurologic examination, bradykinesia is often assessed by finger taps performed with each hand separately (patient taps thumb with index finger in rapid succession with widest amplitude possible). Hand movements (patient opens and closes hands in rapid succession with widest amplitude possible) and leg agility (patient taps heel on ground in rapid succession, picking up entire leg; amplitude should be about 3 inches) are also assessed. Difficulty in initiating and executing learned movements contributes substantially to func-

FIGURE 63.5 Handwriting sample from a patient with Parkinson's disease demonstrates progressive micrographia. As the sentence "Today is a sunny day in California" is repeatedly handwritten, the letters get progressively smaller. The height of each lined row is approximately 5/16 inch (8 mm). (Courtesy of Jack J. Chen, PharmD, and David M. Swope, MD.)

tional impairment (e.g., significant interference with performing activities of daily living and walking). The combination of bradykinesia and rigidity often contributes to a characteristic slow, shuffling gait and reduced arm swing. Patients commonly report a worsening of handwriting, with small and illegible letters (micrographia; Fig. 63.5).

Postural instability or poor balance is a disabling symptom of advanced disease. Often a slow, shuffling gait is transformed into a rapid, festinating gait with a tendency to fall forward. Retropulsion with a tendency to fall backward also occurs. As a result, patients are at greater risk for falls and injuries and are less able to ambulate without assistance. This symptom is difficult to treat and is often resistant to pharmacotherapy.

Although not considered a cardinal feature, "freezing," or a sudden, episodic inhibition of lower extremity motor function, may occur and interferes with ambulation. Patients may report that their "feet are stuck to the floor" and that they have difficulty initiating steps (start hesitation) or turns (turn hesitation). Freezing often is exacerbated by anxiety or when perceived obstacles (e.g., doorways, turnstiles) are encountered. This symptom is also difficult to treat pharmacologically.

DIAGNOSIS

Universally applicable preclinical tests or screens for PD remain an unmet need. Neuroimaging techniques, such as magnetic resonance imaging, positron emission tomography, and single photon emission computed tomography, in combination with various radiotracers as biomarkers for PD, have emerged as promising diagnostic and screening tools. However, these techniques require refinement before they can be used widely in the assessment of PD.[41,42] Screening for impaired olfaction has been suggested for detection of increased PD risk later in life, but this method also requires additional validation.

Currently, the diagnosis of PD depends on clinical findings based on neurologic assessment. A definitive diagnosis of PD is possible only upon postmortem confirmation of LBs and depigmentation of the SNpc. A careful clinical diagnosis is essential because the treatment and prognosis of idiopathic PD differ markedly from that of drug-induced parkinsonism or multisystem Parkinson plus syndromes. Even when drug-induced parkinsonism is ruled out, misdiagnosis occurs in up to 25% of cases.[43] However, a clinical diagnosis of PD can be made with high probability if the patient presents with bradykinesia and either rest tremor or rigidity; motor features are initially unilateral; motor features are progressive; and there is an absence of early falls, dementia, or cerebellar (e.g., ataxia) or pyramidal (e.g., spasticity) signs.[44] The diagnosis is confirmed if there is an excellent and sustained symptomatic response to dopaminergic therapy. In the early stages of PD, telltale features are slight and may be difficult to detect, but as the disease progresses, the signs and symptoms become unmistakable. If action tremor is present in the absence of bradykinesia or rigidity, the diagnosis of essential tremor should be considered.[45]

Once a clinical diagnosis of PD is made, assessment scales are useful for monitoring disease progression. The Hoehn and Yahr scale is a user-friendly, multistaging system based essentially on the presence and severity of postural instability[46] (Table 63.4). The Unified Parkinson's Disease Rating Scale (UPDRS) is a sensitive method for evaluating functional status, disease progression, and effectiveness of antiparkinson therapy.[47] Neurologists specializing in PD often include portions of the UPDRS in the neurologic examination. Currently, the UPDRS is undergoing revision, particularly in assessment of nonmotor features. The Schwab &

England Activities of Daily Living scale and the Parkinson's Disease Quality of Life scale (PDQUALIF) are useful tools for assessing quality-of-life parameters specific to the disease (e.g., independence, personal hygiene, physical function, self-image, sexuality, sleep, and social function).[48]

PSYCHOSOCIAL ASPECTS

As PD progresses, the psychosocial impact on patients and family members becomes evident. Over time, patients who are employed will no longer be productive in the workforce; they will begin to require assistance with activities of daily living, and eventually loss of mobility results in dependence on a wheelchair. Significant cognitive impairment may also occur in advanced PD and, because of excessive caregiver burden, often results in nursing home placement. Behavioral changes, such as anxiety and depression, are common due to underlying disease-related biochemical imbalances, but they may also arise as a maladaptive psychological reaction. Social avoidance may arise from personal embarrassment or from a fear of falling outside the house. Because tremor is made worse by excitement or stress, patients may avoid public areas such as restaurants and theaters. Patients may have difficulty adjusting to gradual loss of autonomy (e.g., loss of employment or driving privileges). Likewise, family caregivers may experience greater levels of stress, frustration, anxiety, and depression, especially as the patient becomes increasingly dependent for assistance with activities of daily living.[49] Respite care or in-home services may be beneficial and can include a wide range of options, such as household maintenance, meal preparation, supervision of the client, and assistance with therapeutic activities. These short-term or temporary services enable caregivers to take a break from the daily routine of caregiving.

The adverse psychosocial impact of PD can be minimized by fostering a positive attitude and initiating psychoeducational interventions. Toward this end, interaction with clinicians and support groups can be a source of educational, emotional, and social support for patients and caregivers.

THERAPEUTIC PLAN

A simplified outline for the management of PD is provided in Figure 63.6. Therapy is lifelong and indicated when the patient expresses a desire for treatment to improve symptoms that are interfering with daily function. In early-stage PD, therapy is relatively straightforward, but with advancing disease and duration of levodopa treatment, the development of motor fluctuations and levodopa-related dyskinesias adds complexity to the therapeutic plan, and surgical interventions may be appropriate for qualified candidates. The development of concomitant autonomic (e.g., orthostatic hypotension) and psychiatric conditions (e.g., dementia, depression,

TABLE 63.4	Hoehn and Yahr Staging of Parkinson's Disease
Stage 1	Unilateral disease
Stage 2	Bilateral disease without balance impairment
Stage 3	Mild to moderate bilateral disease, some postural instability; physically independent
Stage 4	Severe disability; unable to live alone independently
Stage 5	Unable to walk or stand without assistance

(Adapted from Hoehn MM, Yahr MD. Parkinsonism: onset, progression and mortality. Neurology 17:427–442, 1967.)

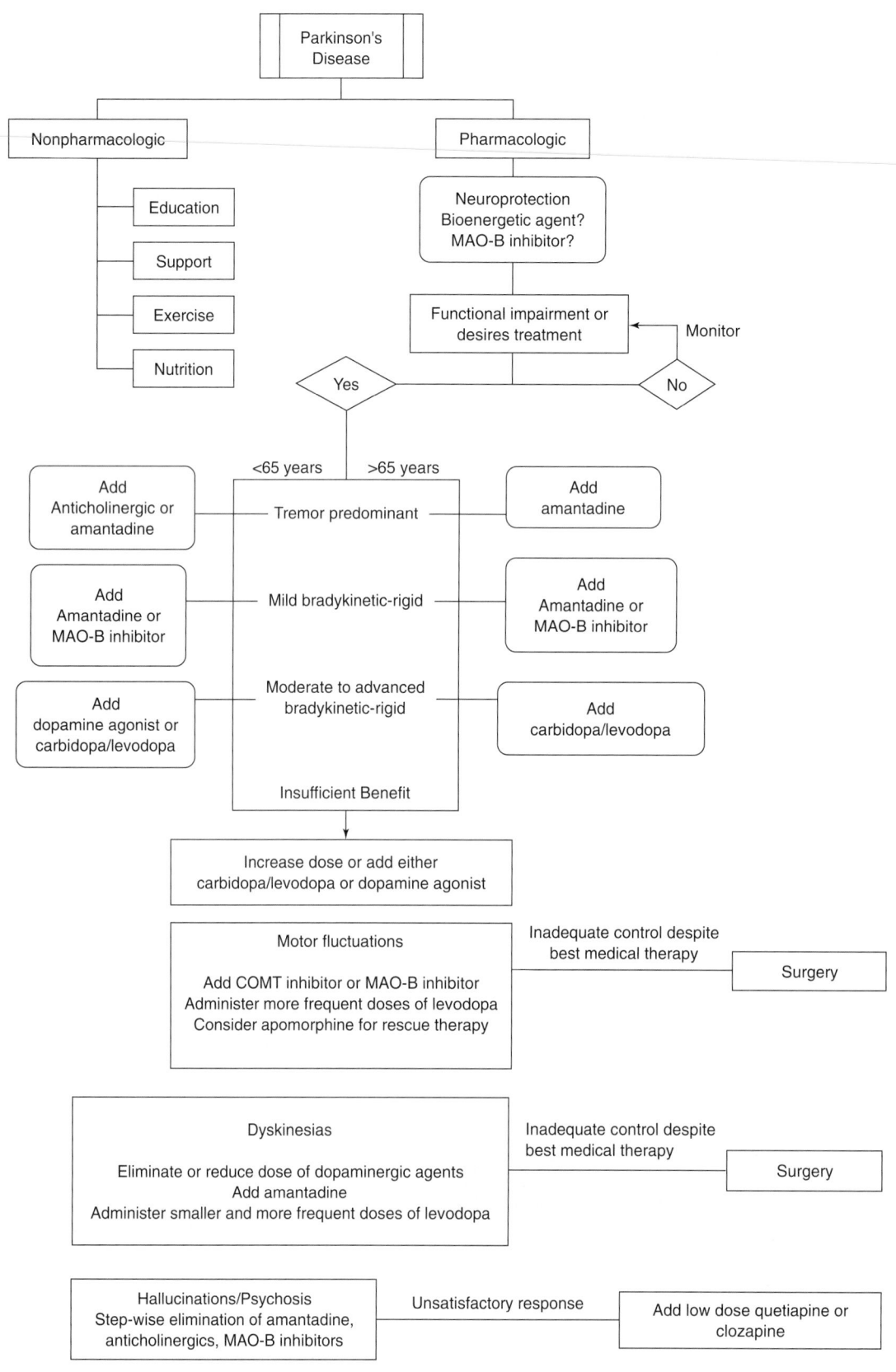

COMT = Catechol-O-methyltransferase; MAO-B = Monoamine oxidase type B

FIGURE 63.6 Simplified outline for management of early to advanced Parkinson's disease.

psychosis) adds yet another dimension of complexity to the therapeutic plan.

TREATMENT

PHARMACOTHERAPY

Antiparkinson agents and dosing regimens are listed in Table 63.5. Once a pharmacologic agent is chosen, the basic tenets of therapy are as follows: initiate therapy with dosage titration ("start low and go slow"), titrate the dosage up until the desired effect is achieved, and if intolerable side effects emerge, reduce the dosage or discontinue therapy. As the disease progresses, dosages will inevitably be adjusted and other antiparkinson agents will be added. In the absence of troublesome side effects, antiparkinson agents are continued indefinitely.

Anticholinergics. Before the advent of levodopa, centrally acting anticholinergic agents such as benztropine, biperiden, procyclidine, and trihexyphenidyl were mainstays of therapy. Symptomatic improvement with these agents is modest and favors tremor control. The most suitable candidates for the anticholinergics are younger patients with tremor-predominant disease. Common side effects include blurred vision, dry eyes, dry mouth, drowsiness, confusion, memory impairment, tachycardia, constipation, and urinary retention. Because of side effects, therapy generally is short-lived, particularly in older adults. However, in the absence of troublesome side effects, anticholinergic agents can be helpful. If therapy is to be discontinued after prolonged treatment, a downward dosage titration is recommended because abrupt withdrawal may result in severe agitation and confusion.

Amantadine. Amantadine hydrochloride is an antiviral agent that was serendipitously found to have antiparkinson activity.[50] The mechanism of antiparkinson activity remains unknown but may involve potentiation of neuronal dopamine release, blockade of dopamine reuptake, or antagonism of cholinergic or glutamatergic receptors.[51]

For patients with mild signs and symptoms, amantadine monotherapy may be considered. Within days of initiation, modest improvements in bradykinesia, rigidity, and tremor can be expected. With prolonged amantadine monotherapy, tachyphylaxis has been reported to occur, but discontinuation for a few weeks often restores responsiveness. Amantadine also demonstrates antidyskinesia effects and is useful for managing levodopa-induced dyskinesias.[52]

In general, side effects are mild. Central side effects include confusion, hallucinations, hyperexcitability, insomnia, and nightmares. These side effects often remit with a dosage reduction. If insomnia occurs, late-evening doses should be avoided. Other side effects include dizziness, nausea, orthostatic hypotension, and dry skin or eczema. Patients may also develop a benign form of livedo reticularis, a vascular cutaneous reaction characterized by a reddish-purple, fish-net-patterned mottling of the upper or lower extremities,

often accompanied by ankle edema. This condition resolves upon discontinuation of amantadine.

Abrupt discontinuation of therapy after prolonged treatment should be avoided due to the risk of withdrawal encephalopathy.[53] Because amantadine is renally excreted as unchanged drug and high plasma levels may precipitate toxic delirium, a dosage reduction is recommended for patients with creatinine clearance less than 50 mL/minute/1.73 m.[2,54]

Selective Monoamine Oxidase Type B Inhibitors. Inhibition of MAO_B is associated with reduced synaptic degradation of dopamine and prolonged dopaminergic activity. Two selective MAO_B inhibitors, rasagiline and selegiline, are available in the United States for management of PD. Both contain a propargylamine moiety, which is essential for conferring irreversible inhibition of MAO_B. At therapeutic doses, these agents preferentially inhibit MAO_B over MAO_A. Unlike the nonselective $MAO_{A/B}$ inhibitors, these agents do not require tyramine restriction when administered at therapeutic dosages.

Because of the risk of serotonin syndrome, concomitant use of either rasagiline or selegiline with meperidine is contraindicated. Caution is urged with concomitant use of selective serotonin reuptake inhibitors (SSRIs), imipramine, clomipramine, lithium, sibutramine, and high-dose dextromethorphan. However, SSRIs are commonly used in selegiline-treated patients, and serious serotonin syndrome is rare.[55] When combined with carbidopa/levodopa, dyskinesias may emerge or become worse and may require reduction of the levodopa dose.

Selegiline. Selegiline or L-deprenyl is a first-generation irreversible MAO_B inhibitor that is administered once or twice daily. Laboratory experiments demonstrate that selegiline and its metabolite, N-desmethylselegiline, also protect against apoptosis and free radical-induced neurotoxicity.[56] Unfortunately, the DATATOP trial, designed to evaluate the neuroprotective effect of selegiline in as yet untreated PD patients, yielded inconclusive results.[57] However, the trial did demonstrate that monotherapy with selegiline in early PD is associated with modest symptomatic benefits, a delay in the need for levodopa, and extended employability.

In moderate to advanced disease, adjunctive selegiline can be used to treat wearing-off symptoms. However, the role of selegiline is complicated by clinical data suggesting that cumulative exposure increases the risk of mortality (when used in combination with levodopa), especially in patients with a history of dementia, frequent falls, and postural hypotension.[58] Subsequent studies have failed to confirm an adverse effect of selegiline on mortality.[59–61]

Selegiline is metabolized to the amphetamine derivatives L-amphetamine and L-methamphetamine, which have been implicated in producing side effects such as insomnia and vivid dreaming. Some patients also report an increased sense of well-being. Other side effects include confusion, dizziness, dry mouth, hallucinations, nausea, and orthostatic hypotension. If insomnia occurs, patients should be instructed to take doses no later than noon. Uncommonly, exacerbation of pep-

TABLE 63.5	Antiparkinson Drugs and Dosage Titration
Drug	**Dosage Titration**
Amantadine (Symmetrel) 100-mg capsules or tablets, 50-mg/5 mL syrup	100 mg with breakfast; increase by 100 mg every 3 to 5 days to 100 mg 3 or 4 times daily. Reduce dosage for renal impairment.[a] Not to exceed 400 mg/day.
Anticholinergics	
Benztropine (Cogentin) 0.5-, 1-, 2-mg tablets	0.5 mg at bedtime; increase by 0.5 mg every 3 to 5 days to 1–2 mg twice daily
Trihexyphenidyl (Artane) 2- and 5-mg tablets, 2-mg/5 mL elixir	1 mg at bedtime; increase by 1 mg every 3 to 5 days to 1 mg 3 times daily
Monoamine Oxidase Type B Inhibitors	
Rasagiline (Agilect) 0.5- and 1-mg tablets*	0.5 to 1 mg once daily
Selegiline (Eldepryl) 5-mg tablets or capsules	5 mg in the morning for 1 week, then may increase to 5 mg twice daily (breakfast and lunch).
Dopamine Receptor Agonists	
Apomorphine (Apokyn) 10-mg/mL solution for injection in 3-mL cartridges	Test dose and dose titration performed under medical supervision. 0.2–0.6 mL (2–6 mg) subcutaneously as needed for intermittent "off" episodes. Reduce dose in renal impairment.[b] See notes on premedication.[c] Not to exceed 20 mg/day.
Bromocriptine (Parlodel) 2.5-mg tablets and 5-mg capsules	1.25 mg at bedtime; increase by 1.25 mg every 3 to 5 days to 5 mg 3 or 4 times daily. May increase to 40 mg/day.
Pergolide (Permax) 0.05-, 0.25-, 1-mg tablets	0.05 mg at bedtime; increase by 0.05 every 3 days to 0.2 mg 3 times daily; then change to 0.25 mg 3 times daily and increase by 0.25 mg every week to 1 mg 3 times daily. May increase to 6 mg/day.
Pramipexole (Mirapex) 0.125-, 0.25-, 1-, 1.5-mg tablets	0.125 mg at bedtime; increase by 0.125 mg every week to 0.5 mg 3 times daily.[d] May increase to 4.5 mg/day.
Ropinirole (Requip) 0.25-, 0.5-, 1-, 2-, 4-, 5-mg tablets	0.25 mg three times daily; increase by 0.25 mg every week to 1 mg 3 times daily; then increase by 0.5 mg every week to 3 mg 3 times daily. May increase to 24 mg/day.
Levodopa	
Carbidopa/levodopa (Sinemet, Parcopa) 10/100-, 25/100-, 25/250-mg tablets and orally disintegrating tablets	25/100 mg in the morning; increase by 25/100 mg every 3 to 5 days to 25/100 mg 3 times daily. Over time, increase dosage for additional symptomatic relief and increase dosing frequency if "end-of-dose wearing off" effect develops.
Carbidopa/levodopa sustained-release (Sinemet CR) 25/100-, 50/200-mg tablets	25/100 mg in the morning; increase by 25/100 mg every 3 to 5 days to 50/200 mg twice daily. Over time, increase dosage for additional symptomatic relief and increase dosing frequency if "end-of-dose wearing off" effect develops.
Carbidopa/levodopa/entacapone (Stalevo) 12.5/50/200-, 25/100/200-, 37.5/150/200-mg tablets	If taking carbidopa/levodopa (up to 600 mg/day) and experiencing wearing off (with no dyskinesia), convert to Stalevo at corresponding preexisting levodopa dose. For example, carbidopa/levodopa 25/100 mg 3 times daily converts to Stalevo 100 3 times daily.
Carbidopa (Lodosyn) 25-mg tablets	25 mg to be taken 30 minutes before carbidopa/levodopa doses
COMT Inhibitors	
Entacapone (Comtan) 200-mg tablets	200 mg with each dose of carbidopa/levodopa. May administer up to 8 times daily.
Tolcapone (Tasmar) 100- and 200-mg tablets	100 mg with the first dose of carbidopa/levodopa in the morning. Increase to 100 or 200 mg 3 times daily (at 6-hour intervals).

[a] Amantadine: 100 mg once daily if creatinine clearance (CrCl) = 40–50 mL/min/1.73 m^2; 200 mg twice weekly if CrCl = 30–40 mL/min/1.73 m^2.

[b] Apomorphine: For patients with mild to moderate renal impairment, the starting dose should be 0.1 mL (1 mg).

[c] Trimethobenzamide (300 mg orally 3 times daily) should be started 3 days prior to the test dose of apomorphine and continued for up to 2 months with therapy.

[d] Pramipexole: Twice-daily dosing if CrCl = 35–59 mL/min; once-daily dosing if CrCl = 15–34 mL/min.

COMT, catechol-O-methyltransferase.

*Not available in the United States at time of writing.

tic ulcer disease and elevations in liver enzymes may occur. An orally disintegrating formulation of selegiline that undergoes orobuccal absorption with reduced metabolism to amphetamine derivatives may be available in the near future.[62]

Rasagiline. Rasagiline is a second-generation, irreversible MAO_B inhibitor that is more potent than selegiline.[63] Rasagiline is administered once daily and is effective as monotherapy in early PD. In the TEMPO trial, rasagiline treatment was associated with improvements in motor function and activities of daily living scores.[64] Patients who started rasagiline early in PD had less functional decline than those whose treatment was delayed for 6 months.[65] These results suggest that treatment should be initiated early (perhaps even before the onset of functional disability) to maximize outcomes and that rasagiline may slow disease progression. Results from various preclinical studies also suggest that rasagiline possesses neuroprotective properties; clinical trials are under way to further evaluate its neuroprotective effects.

Once-daily rasagiline is also effective as adjunctive therapy in patients with advanced PD who are experiencing wearing-off fluctuations.[66,67] In one study of levodopa-treated patients with motor fluctuations, the efficacy of adding once-daily rasagiline was similar to that of adding entacapone to each levodopa dose.[67]

Rasagiline is metabolized by hepatic CYP-450 1A2, and concurrent use of potent CYP1A2 inhibitors (e.g., ciproflox-

acin) may increase rasagiline levels significantly. The major metabolite of rasagiline is aminoindan, which is devoid of amphetamine-like properties. Caution should be used when initiating treatment with rasagiline in patients with mild hepatic insufficiency. Rasagiline administered once daily is well tolerated, with an incidence of side effects similar to placebo in clinical studies.

Carbidopa/Levodopa. For more than 35 years, levodopa has been the most effective and enduring form of antiparkinson therapy. Levodopa, the L-isomer of the amino acid dihydroxyphenylalanine, is a natural precursor for all catecholamine neurotransmitters. Levodopa crosses the blood–brain barrier, where it is taken up by the neurons of the SNpc and converted to dopamine by the enzyme dopa decarboxylase (Fig. 63.7). The dopamine is then stored, transported, and eventually released to act on dopamine receptors in the striatum. In essence, levodopa therapy is a form of dopamine replacement analogous to estrogen as a form of hormone replacement therapy. Laboratory experiments have demonstrated that levodopa can be either neurotoxic or neurotrophic, depending on the experimental conditions.[68,69] However, the results of the ELLDOPA study demonstrated that levodopa does not hasten the clinical progression of PD, and it remains a mainstay of current PD therapy.[70]

Carbidopa (α-methyldopa hydrazine) is a reversible, peripheral dopa decarboxylase inhibitor that does not cross the

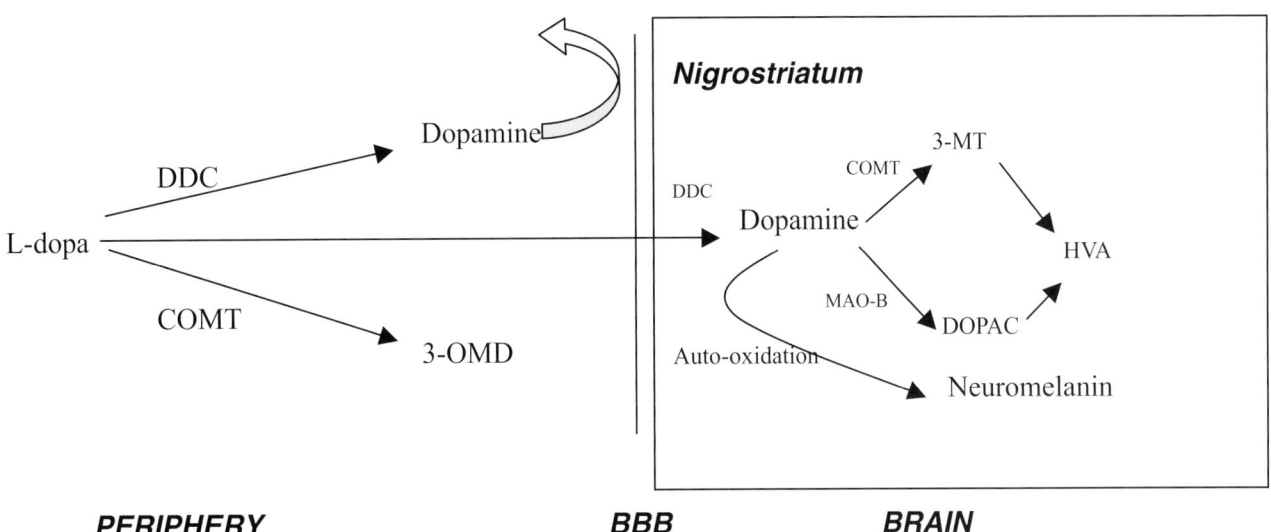

BBB = blood brain barrier; COMT = catechol-O-methyltransferase; DDC = dopa decarboxylase; MAO-B = monoamine oxidase B; 3-OMD = 3-O-methyldopa; 3-MT = 3-methoxytyramine; DOPAC = dihydroxyphenylacetic acid; HVA = homovanillic acid

FIGURE 63.7 Levodopa metabolic pathways.

blood–brain barrier. When administered in the absence of carbidopa, levodopa undergoes significant gastrointestinal and peripheral metabolism to dopamine. This is therapeutically undesirable because dopamine cannot cross the blood–brain barrier; it is also highly emetogenic because it stimulates the chemoreceptor trigger zone, which is outside the blood–brain barrier. With the addition of carbidopa, levodopa's bioavailability is doubled from 50% to almost 100% and levodopa's elimination half-life (normally 45 minutes) is extended considerably (Table 63.6). In addition, levodopa side effects, such as nausea and orthostatic hypotension, are significantly reduced, which allows for more rapid induction of therapy. Traditionally, it has been stated that 75 to 100 mg per day of carbidopa is needed for maximal enzyme inhibition. There is limited experience with total daily doses of greater than 200 mg carbidopa. The carbidopa and levodopa combination product is marketed under the name Sinemet (''without emesis''). Carbidopa is also available as a single-drug product. In some countries, a different peripheral dopa decarboxylase inhibitor, benserazide, is combined with levodopa and marketed under the name Madopar.

The effects of levodopa are immediate. Within days, improvement in bradykinesia and rigidity can be expected. Tremor improvement is less predictable, and improvements in postural instability should not be expected. Overall, motor function can be improved more than 50% in about two thirds of patients.

Dosage titration recommendations for carbidopa/levodopa products are listed in Table 63.5. Carbidopa/levodopa tablets are available in ratios of 1:4 (25/100 mg carbidopa/levodopa) or 1:10 (10/100 or 25/250 mg carbidopa/levodopa). For patients with swallowing difficulties, an orally disintegrating carbidopa/levodopa tablet is available. Therapy is initiated with the 25/100-mg carbidopa/levodopa tablets. Because approximately 75 mg of carbidopa is required to provide adequate inhibition of dopa decarboxylase, the initial maintenance dose is carbidopa/levodopa 25/100 mg three times daily. Patients should achieve this minimum daily dosage to determine the agent's effectiveness. Thereafter, the dosage or frequency can be increased.

The 10/100-mg tablet has a limited role in the modern management of PD. Initiation of therapy with the 10/100-mg tablet is undesirable because it will not provide an adequate amount of carbidopa for most patients. However, the 10/100-mg tablet can be used in patients who are already receiving close to 200 mg per day of carbidopa but who require additional levodopa for symptom control. There is no maximum therapeutic dosage for levodopa; however, most pa-

TABLE 63.6	Summary Characteristics of Levodopa and Dopamine Receptor Agonists					
	Carbidopa/Levodopa[a]	Apomorphine	Bromocriptine	Pergolide	Pramipexole	Ropinirole
Structure	Catecholamine	Aporphine	Ergot derivative	Ergot derivative	Non-ergot derivative	Non-ergot derivative
Receptor affinity	D_1 ++	D_1 +	D_1 −	D_1 +	D_1 0	D_1 0
	D_2 ++++	D_2 +++	D_2 +	D_2 ++	D_2 ++	D_2 ++
	D_3 ++++	D_3 +++	D_3 +	D_3 ++	D_3 +++	D_3 ++
	5-HT 0	5-HT +	5-HT +	5-HT +	5-HT 0	5-HT 0
	$\alpha 1$ 0	$\alpha 1$ +	$\alpha 1$ +	$\alpha 1$ +	$\alpha 1$ 0	$\alpha 1$ 0
	$\alpha 2$ 0	$\alpha 2$ +	$\alpha 2$ +	$\alpha 2$ +	$\alpha 2$ +	$\alpha 2$ 0
Route of administration	Oral	Subcutaneous	Oral	Oral	Oral	Oral
Oral bioavailability	99%	<5 (100%[b])	6%–8%	20%	>90%	55%
T_{max} (minutes)	45	10–20	70–100	60–120	60–180	60–90
Protein binding	20%–40%	>90%	>90%	90%	15%–20%	30%–40%
Elimination half-life	2–3 hours	40 minutes	6 hours	7–16 hours	8–12 hours	6 hours
Duration of action	1–4 hours	60–100 minutes	3–6 hours	4–6 hours	4–6 hours	4–6 hours
Elimination route	Plasma/tissue degradation	Hepatic	Hepatic	Hepatic/renal	Renal	Hepatic
Equivalent dose	NA	NA	10 mg	1 mg	1 mg	4 mg

[a] Characteristics for levodopa (when combined with carbidopa).
[b] Subcutaneous bioavailability.
+, mild affinity; ++, moderate affinity; +++, strong affinity; ++++, very strong affinity; 0, no affinity; −, mild antagonist; 5-HT, serotonin (5-hydroxytryptamine) receptor; $\alpha 1$, $\alpha 2$, alpha adrenergic receptors; T_{max}, time to peak plasma concentration.

tients do not require more than 800 to 1,000 mg per day. At this dosage, if effectiveness is minimal, an alternative diagnosis must be considered.

The latency time from dose administration to the onset of motor improvement is approximately 30 to 45 minutes. However, several factors can prolong the onset of effect, including delayed gastric motility (e.g., due to anticholinergic drugs or other medical conditions) and food. Because diet-derived large neutral amino acids compete with levodopa for transport across the blood–brain barrier, carbidopa/levodopa should be taken on an empty stomach (i.e., 30 minutes before or 1 to 2 hours after a meal) and with a glass of water to improve bioavailability.[71] However, in early disease, this drug–food interaction may not be clinically significant, and patients often need to take the drug with food to help alleviate gastrointestinal discomfort. Periodic dosage adjustment, either up or down, is expected and determined by the rate of disease progression, development of motor fluctuations, addition of other antiparkinson drugs, and emergence of dyskinesias, hallucinations, and other side effects. Levodopa is contraindicated in patients with narrow-angle glaucoma but may be used safely in wide-angle glaucoma if intraocular pressure is monitored carefully. Because dopamine is a melanin intermediate, levodopa is contraindicated in patients with malignant melanoma, but critical reviews of the literature suggest that melanoma progression is not influenced by levodopa.[72] Abrupt levodopa withdrawal after prolonged treatment should be avoided due to a risk for neuroleptic malignant-like syndrome characterized by confusion, fever, rigidity, and respiratory arrest.

Carbidopa/levodopa is also available as the proprietary product Sinemet CR, a sustained-release tablet designed to maintain more consistent plasma levels. In mild to moderate disease, Sinemet CR compares favorably with standard Sinemet, and less frequent dosing is needed.[73,74] The 25/100-mg CR tablet is intended to be used while titrating the dose to the initial maintenance dosage of 50/200 mg twice daily. Peripheral levodopa bioavailability with the CR formulation is less than that of standard Sinemet (71% vs. 99%, respectively).[75] Accordingly, a 30% higher total daily levodopa dosage may be needed for comparable therapeutic effects. Levodopa absorption occurs gradually over 4 to 5 hours and results in sustained plasma levels. Patients must be advised that Sinemet CR should not be chewed, crushed, or liquefied. Unlike the standard formulation, Sinemet CR should be taken with food to improve bioavailability. Food increases gastric retention and allows greater tablet erosion and thus more release of levodopa from the CR matrix. The latency time from dose administration to the onset of motor improvement is approximately 60 to 90 minutes. Patients with moderate to advanced disease may need a small booster dose of standard Sinemet in the morning. The limitations of the CR formulation include the potential to prolong dyskinesias, and some patients experience an unpredictable and erratic onset of effect.

Levodopa Side Effects. Common side effects associated with levodopa involve the gastrointestinal, cardiovascular, behavioral, and motor systems.

Gastrointestinal. Nausea is a common side effect that occurs during therapy initiation or a dosage increase. Administration with food may minimize nausea; in some cases, addition of supplemental carbidopa is required. Antiemetics that can be used include trimethobenzamide, serotonin (5HT$_3$)-receptor blockers (e.g., ondansetron), and the peripheral dopamine receptor blocker domperidone. Antiemetic agents with central antidopaminergic activity (e.g., droperidol, metoclopramide, prochlorperazine) will worsen PD and should be avoided. Less common side effects include abdominal pain, constipation, diarrhea, and dry mouth. Rarely, mild elevations of liver function tests, peptic ulcer, and gastrointestinal bleeding have been reported.

Cardiovascular. Orthostatic hypotension is a side effect of levodopa but can also be an autonomic dysfunction of underlying PD. Symptoms include syncope, dizziness, light-headedness, and fatigue. When severe, orthostatic hypotension significantly impairs ambulation and balance, resulting in falls. Pharmacologic interventions include supplementation with additional carbidopa, addition of fludrocortisone with salt supplementation, or addition of midodrine, an α-receptor agonist. Dosages of other drugs that exacerbate orthostatic hypotension, including amantadine, antihypertensive agents, diuretics, dopamine receptor agonists, and selegiline, should be reduced or eliminated. A variety of nonpharmacologic interventions also are available (e.g., elastic stockings).

Behavioral and Neuropsychiatric. Sedation resulting in excessive daytime somnolence may occur and compounds the underlying fatigue of PD. Patients may also experience confusion, hallucinations, psychosis, and, uncommonly, hypersexuality.

Hallucinations can occur in up to 50% and psychosis in up to 15% of patients with PD.[39] All antiparkinson agents can cause hallucinations, with levodopa or dopamine agonists commonly implicated. Hallucinations are a disturbance of sensory perception that may be perceived as real or recognized as unreal by patients. Unlike hallucinations in schizophrenia, hallucinations in PD are predominantly visual and less commonly auditory, gustatory, olfactory, tactile, or visceral. Psychosis in PD is a serious condition characterized by delusions, hallucinations, and impaired reality testing. Delusions with themes of home intrusion, personal harm, spousal infidelity, and theft of personal property are common. If untreated, psychotic symptomatology will result in significant anxiety, communication and social impairments, enhanced caregiver distress, and an increased risk of nursing home placement.[76]

Management of troublesome hallucinations or psychosis in PD consists of reducing dosages of antiparkinson agents in a stepwise manner (i.e., one drug at a time) until psychiatric symptoms improve or motor symptoms worsen, whichever

TABLE 63.7	Atypical Antipsychotics for Hallucinations/Psychosis in Parkinson's Disease

Drug	Dosage	Expected Net Benefit[a]
Clozapine	12.5–150 mg qhs	+++
Quetiapine	25–200 mg qhs	+++
Risperidone	0.25–2 mg/d	+
Olanzapine	2.5–5 mg qd	–
Aripiprazole	1–5 mg qd	–
Ziprasidone	Insufficient data in PD	Insufficient data in PD

[a] Expected net benefit = antipsychotic benefit relative to risk of exacerbating parkinsonism.
(Modified from Chen JJ. Anxiety, depression, and psychosis in Parkinson's disease: unmet needs and treatment challenges. Neurol Clin 22 (3 Suppl) :S63–90, 2004.)

occurs first. Generally, doses of amantadine, anticholinergics, or MAO_B inhibitors are reduced or discontinued first. Low doses of atypical antipsychotics, such as clozapine and quetiapine, are well tolerated and effective (Table 63.7).[39] Haloperidol and phenothiazine antipsychotics exacerbate parkinsonism and should be avoided (see Table 63.3). Cholinesterase inhibitors or memantine should be considered to treat concurrent underlying dementia.

Motor Complications. In levodopa-treated patients, up to 10% will develop associated motor complications within 1 year of treatment, 50% after 5 years, and 80% after 10 years.[77,78] Motor complications can be divided into two categories: fluctuations and dyskinesias. Motor fluctuations involve the so-called end-of-dose wearing off, which contributes to alternating periods of good mobility ("on") and hypomobility ("off") during the day. Motor "off" times interrupt the performance of daily activities, increase caregiver time, and are also associated with recurrence of various nonmotor features (e.g., anxiety, bladder and bowel problems, cognitive changes, pain, and speech and swallowing difficulties). Dyskinesias are periods of involuntary, choreiform movements associated with peak levels of levodopa and predominantly affect the extremities and trunk. Patients are generally not disabled by mild to moderate dyskinesias, but they can be embarrassing when in public. Younger patients are particularly susceptible to the fluctuations and dyskinesias.[79] The exact mechanism of motor complications is unknown, but the "unnatural" pulsatile pattern of peak and trough levodopa levels (due to its short elimination half-life and intermittent administration), changes of the dopamine receptors, and alterations of the motor output pathways within the basal ganglia are believed to play major roles.[80] Experimental studies demonstrate that maintaining continuous levodopa plasma levels, as opposed to the fluctuating levels associated with intermittent administration, minimizes the development of motor complications.

Initially, attempts to smooth out fluctuations and manage dyskinesias are straightforward, but over time these motor complications become more severe and management becomes challenging. Because motor fluctuations and dyskinesias arise in the presence of levodopa therapy, the issue of when to initiate carbidopa/levodopa, as compared to other antiparkinson agents, is paramount. Treatment with carbidopa/levodopa early in PD may speed up the development of motor complications; therefore, initial treatment with a dopamine receptor agonist or other antiparkinson agent, delaying the use of carbidopa/levodopa for as long as possible, is favored, especially in younger patients. For older patients, the long-term consequences of motor complications are less of a concern, and the initiation of carbidopa/levodopa is preferred.

Initially, a single given dose of carbidopa/levodopa may provide motor benefit for several hours. With advancing PD, however, the same given dose may provide benefit for only 1 to 2 hours. Most fluctuations are predictable and related to the waning of interdose levodopa levels. However, random "on/off" switches, "no on," and "delayed on" also occur and are difficult to treat. General management strategies include more frequent administration of carbidopa/levodopa, addition of a catechol-O-methyltransferase (COMT) inhibitor or selective MAO_B inhibitor, use of sustained-release carbidopa/levodopa, or addition of an oral dopamine agonist. Intermittent subcutaneous administration of apomorphine is recommended as "rescue" therapy for "off" episodes occurring despite optimized oral therapy. Compounded carbidopa/levodopa liquid formulations can be given every 1 to 2 hours or by continuous enteral infusion.[81,82] Some patients are more sensitive to dietary protein–levodopa interactions, and elimination of excess protein or a trial of protein redistribution may be worthwhile.[83,84] Nocturnal or early-morning "off" symptoms such as painful calf or foot dystonias are common and relieved either by clonazepam administered at bedtime or small dosages of carbidopa/levodopa in the morning.

Peak-dose dyskinesias and dystonias are predictable and are correlated with peak levodopa levels in the brain. Over time, the dose of levodopa that initially provided good mobility becomes the dose threshold associated with dyskinesias. During the day, patients may alternate between "off" and "on with dyskinesias," with few normal "on" periods in between. Less common forms of dyskinesias include square wave dyskinesia and diphasic dyskinesia.[85] Pharmacologic management consists of a trial of amantadine, which has proven antidyskinesia effects.[52] Alternatively, a reduction in the levodopa dose can help smooth out peak levels, but this may result in worsening of mobility and require supplementation with another antiparkinson agent. For patients with severe dyskinesias despite optimized medical management, surgery may be considered.

Drug Interactions. Several drugs interact with levodopa to produce undesirable effects (Table 63.8). Many of these

TABLE 63.8	Levodopa Drug Interactions
Drug	**Mechanism**
Butyrophenones	
Droperidol	Antagonistic at central dopamine receptors
Haloperidol	Antagonistic at central dopamine receptors
Inhalational Anesthesia	
Cyclopropane	Sensitizes myocardium and increases risk of levodopa-induced tachyarrhythmias
Halothane	Sensitizes myocardium and increases risk of levodopa-induced tachyarrhythmias
Iron supplements	Binds to levodopa in the stomach. Administer at least 2 hours apart.
Nonselective Monoamine Oxidase Inhibitors	
Phenelzine	Risk of "cheese" effect. Discontinue 2 weeks before initiating levodopa.
Tranylcypromine	Risk of "cheese" effect. Discontinue 2 weeks before initiating levodopa.
Methyldopa	Inhibits central conversion of levodopa to dopamine.
Phenothiazines	
Chlorpromazine	Antagonistic at central dopamine receptors
Fluphenazine	Antagonistic at central dopamine receptors
Mesoridazine	Antagonistic at central dopamine receptors
Perphenazine	Antagonistic at central dopamine receptors
Prochlorperazine	Antagonistic at central dopamine receptors
Thioridazine	Antagonistic at central dopamine receptors
Thiothixene	Antagonistic at central dopamine receptors
Trifluoperazine	Antagonistic at central dopamine receptors
Triflupromazine	Antagonistic at central dopamine receptors
Miscellaneous	
Amoxapine	Antagonistic at central dopamine receptors
Metoclopramide	Antagonistic at central dopamine receptors
Pimozide	Antagonistic at central dopamine receptors
Iron supplements	Binds to levodopa in gastrointestinal tract

drugs are still used in modern medicine. Drugs that block central dopamine receptors not only reduce the effectiveness of levodopa but also worsen underlying parkinsonism.

Laboratory Abnormalities and Assay Interference. Chronic treatment with carbidopa/levodopa has been associated with elevations in plasma homocysteine levels.[86,87] The mechanism by which carbidopa/levodopa might produce hyperhomocystinemia lies in its methylation by COMT (see Fig. 63.7), which uses S-adenosylmethionine as a methyl donor and yields S-adenosylhomocysteine. This last compound is rapidly converted to homocysteine. Epidemiologic evidence has linked hyperhomocystinemia to an increased risk of coronary artery disease, stroke, and dementia. Therefore, there are reasons to suggest that long-term treatment with carbidopa/levodopa may render patients at increased risk of stroke, heart disease, and dementia. At present, no controlled prospective studies have evaluated this phenomenon. Agents that reduce homocysteine levels (e.g., folic acid, vitamin B_{12}, COMT inhibitors) may lower homocysteine levels in PD, but consensus on routine supplementation is lacking.

Levodopa may interfere with the following laboratory tests, producing false-positive results: serum and urine uric acid readings measured by the colorimetric method (but not by the more specific ultraviolet uricase method)[88]; urine catecholamine, metanephrine, and vanillylmandelic acid; Labstix or Ketostix (used to detect urine ketones)[89]; and Phenistix (used to test for phenylketonuria).

Drug Holidays. In patients with severe levodopa-induced dyskinesias or psychosis, drug holidays (complete withdrawal of carbidopa/levodopa for up to 2 weeks) were previously recommended. However, drug holidays predispose patients to complications of immobility such as aspiration, deep vein thrombosis, and pulmonary embolism. The benefits of a drug holiday do not outweigh the risks, and this practice is not generally recommended.[90]

Catechol-O-Methyltransferase Inhibitors. The highly selective, reversible, nitrocatechol-structured COMT inhibitors (entacapone and tolcapone) extend the therapeutic activity of carbidopa/levodopa and are indicated for the management of wearing-off episodes. In the presence of carbidopa, levodopa metabolism is shifted toward the COMT pathway (see Fig. 63.7). With the coadministration of a COMT inhibitor, the levodopa area under the concentration time curve (AUC) and elimination half-life are increased. For most patients experiencing wearing off, up to 2 hours or more of additional ''on'' time per day can be achieved with the addition of a COMT inhibitor.[91,92] This extra ''on'' time is valued by patients and analogous to a sleep-deprived person getting an extra 2 hours of sleep per night. In general, COMT inhibitors do not significantly alter levodopa's absorption pharmacokinetics, peak plasma concentrations (C_{max}), and the time of peak occurrence (T_{max}).

Upon addition of a COMT inhibitor, patients should be informed that levodopa-related side effects (e.g., dyskinesias, dizziness, hallucinations, nausea) may be enhanced. These side effects can be alleviated by reducing the levodopa dose. Other side effects include dry mouth, intensification of urine coloration (caused by nitrocatechol metabolites), and diarrhea. The diarrhea may occur after 1 to 3 months of therapy initiation; it is usually self-limiting and responds to antidiarrheal agents. COMT inhibitors may inhibit the metabolism of other drugs with catechol structures, such as dobutamine, epinephrine, fenoldopam, isoproterenol, methyldopa, and nadolol. Overall, COMT inhibitors are preferred adjunctive agents to carbidopa/levodopa to improve duration of ''on'' time in patients experiencing wearing off.

Tolcapone. Tolcapone is a broad-spectrum (i.e., centrally and peripherally acting) COMT inhibitor with an elimination half-life of approximately 2 hours.[92] As such, it is administered 100 to 200 mg three times a day (at 6-hour intervals). As an adjunct to carbidopa/levodopa, tolcapone can double the half-life and AUC of levodopa and is associated with significant improvements in ''on'' time and reductions in ''off'' time in patients experiencing wearing-off motor fluctuations.[92] However, tolcapone use is associated with hepatocellular injury, and its use requires frequent assessment of liver function enzymes.

Entacapone. Entacapone is a peripherally acting COMT with an elimination half-life of approximately 30 to 45 minutes. As such, the drug is administered in conjunction with each dose of carbidopa/levodopa, up to a maximum of eight times per day. Entacapone increases levodopa's half-life and AUC by up to 50%.[91] Entacapone is also available in combi-

nation with carbidopa/levodopa as a three-drug-in-one tablet formulation marketed under the proprietary name Stalevo; this may offer a more convenient method of administration.

Entacapone is eliminated primarily via biliary excretion, and mild to moderate hepatic impairment increases bioavailability twofold. In patients with hepatic insufficiency, the dosage should be halved.[91] Entacapone is associated with few specific laboratory abnormalities. In clinical studies, the occurrence of significant liver enzyme elevations was low (<1%). Entacapone chelates iron, and administration with oral pharmaceutical iron preparations should be separated by at least 2 hours.[91]

Dopamine Agonists. Worldwide, many dopamine receptor agonists are available for managing PD: apomorphine, bromocriptine, cabergoline, lisuride, pergolide, piribedil, pramipexole, and ropinirole. Unlike levodopa, these agents directly stimulate striatal dopamine receptors and do not require enzymatic conversion to dopamine. Lisuride and piribedil are currently not marketed in the United States. Cabergoline (Dostinex), a synthetic, long-acting agonist, is available in the United States but does not have a Food and Drug Administration (FDA)-approved indication for treating parkinsonism. The remaining agonists (apomorphine, bromocriptine, pergolide, pramipexole, ropinirole) are available in the United States for the treatment of PD (see Table 63.5). Of the oral dopamine agonists, pramipexole and ropinirole are favored due to an improved risk–benefit profile.

Due to concerns about the development of levodopa-associated motor complications, the use of dopamine agonists in patients with early-stage PD is often preferred. When initiated in early-stage PD, dopamine agonists are similarly effective to carbidopa/levodopa, well tolerated, and associated with a reduced development of motor complications over time.[93,94] For younger patients, levodopa-sparing management strategies are particularly prudent because the emergence of disabling motor complications can have profound adverse effects on economic and social productivity. Eventually, as PD progresses, the addition of carbidopa/levodopa will become essential.

Preclinical studies also suggest that dopamine agonists may be neuroprotective. The mechanism of this neuroprotective effect may be due to attenuation of oxidant stress activity, enhancement of neurotrophic activity, or prevention of apoptosis.[95] However, to date, clinical neuroprotection studies have yielded inconclusive results.[96]

Dosing guidelines for the dopamine agonists are listed in Table 63.5. Slow dosage titration to a therapeutic dose is critical for successful therapy. One of the most common reasons for dopamine agonist failure is insufficient dosing. If needed, patients can be switched from one agonist to another via a rapid conversion to an equivalent therapeutic dose (see Table 63.6).[97] Abrupt discontinuation of therapy after prolonged treatment should be avoided due to the risk of neuroleptic malignant syndrome.

As a class, the common side effects of dopamine agonists are lower extremity edema, nausea, orthostatic hypotension, somnolence, and hallucinations/psychosis.[98] Unlike treatment with carbidopa/levodopa, monotherapy with dopamine agonists uncommonly induces dyskinesias. However, agonists have a greater tendency to cause confusion and hallucinations/psychosis and should be used with caution in patients with dementia or psychosis. Dopamine agonists have also been associated with infrequent episodes of sudden-onset sleep ("sleep attacks"), which may prove hazardous, especially while driving or operating heavy equipment.[99] Other side effects that differentiate each agonist are described in the following sections.

Apomorphine. Apomorphine is the only injectable antiparkinson agent available in the United States; it was the first dopamine agonist to be evaluated for the treatment of PD.[5] It is an aporphine alkaloid originally derived from morphine but lacks the narcotic properties of the parent compound. Apomorphine is considered the most potent agent in the dopamine agonist class. Due to extensive first-pass metabolism, apomorphine is commonly administered via subcutaneous injection.

Apomorphine is an effective "rescue" drug for rapid relief of intermittent "off" episodes in advanced PD. For patients with advanced PD experiencing intermittent "off" episodes despite optimized therapy, administration of subcutaneous apomorphine consistently and effectively triggers an "on" response within 20 minutes.[100] The effective dose ranges from 2 to 6 mg per injection; most patients require approximately 0.06 mg per kg. Sites of injection (abdomen, upper arm, and upper thigh) should be rotated to avoid the development of subcutaneous nodules. In some countries, apomorphine is also available for continuous subcutaneous injection with mini-pumps. Apomorphine should not be injected intravenously. Upon exposure to air, apomorphine rapidly oxidizes and will discolor fabrics a greenish color.

The route of apomorphine metabolism is unknown. Its elimination half-life is approximately 40 minutes, and the duration of benefit is up to 100 minutes.[101] These pharmacokinetic properties make apomorphine a suitable drug for intermittent "rescue" administration.

Apomorphine should be initiated in a clinic or office setting for test dose administration, monitoring of blood pressure, determination of therapeutic dose, and patient/caregiver education. A test dose is administered, and if orthostatic hypotension develops, the patient should not receive outpatient apomorphine therapy. Otherwise, a therapeutic dose is determined, and the patient or caregiver administers the drug as needed for "rescue" therapy during "off" episodes. Nausea and vomiting are common side effects; prior to apomorphine initiation, the patient should be premedicated with an antiemetic such as trimethobenzamide for 3 days. The antiemetic may be continued for up to 2 months. Other side effects include dizziness, dyskinesia, hallucinations, injection site irritation, rhinorrhea, somnolence,

and yawning at the onset of effect. Due to reports of severe hypotension and syncope, apomorphine is contraindicated with drugs in the serotonin (5HT$_3$)-receptor blocker class, including dolasetron, granisetron, and ondansetron.

Bromocriptine. Bromocriptine is an ergot-derived agonist that stimulates D$_2$ receptors and mildly antagonizes D$_1$ sites. The drug possesses poor oral bioavailability and is highly protein bound. Although originally indicated for disorders of hyperprolactinemia, bromocriptine was the first oral dopamine agonist to receive an FDA-approved indication for PD management (see Table 63.1). Overall, bromocriptine is generally considered to be less effective than pergolide, pramipexole, and ropinirole.[98] This may be due, in part, to mild D$_1$ antagonism.

Because of its ergotlike structure, bromocriptine also exerts agonist activity at α-receptors and serotonin receptors. This may contribute to other side effects such as vasoconstriction, rhinitis, erythromelalgia (a painful, reddish skin rash), pleuropulmonary disease, and retroperitoneal fibrosis. Bromocriptine-induced pleuropulmonary disease is reversible and occurs in about 2% to 5% of patients after 5 years of therapy. Patients receiving dosages greater than 20 mg per day for more than 6 months may be at increased risk.[102] A baseline chest radiograph is recommended before initial therapy.

Drugs that are potent inhibitors of the cytochrome P-450 3A4 enzyme (e.g., erythromycin, clarithromycin, nefazodone) may increase plasma bromocriptine levels by severalfold.[103]

Pergolide. Pergolide was the second oral agonist to receive an FDA-approved indication for treating PD. Pergolide is a semisynthetic ergot derivative with strong D$_2$ receptor agonism.[98] Unlike bromocriptine, pergolide also stimulates D$_1$ receptors. The therapeutic equivalency ratio of pergolide to bromocriptine is about 1:10.[97] In early PD, pergolide is effective as monotherapy, but with more advanced disease, symptomatic benefit is best when combined with levodopa.

Although pergolide has a long half-life, the duration of clinical activity is about 6 hours, and multiple daily doses are needed. Side effects are common but generally less frequent than with bromocriptine. As with bromocriptine, retroperitoneal fibrosis and other ergotamine-like side effects may occur. Pergolide use has been associated with the development of restrictive valvular heart disease, and monitoring for cardiac valvular dysfunction should be instituted.[104]

Pramipexole. Pramipexole is a second-generation dopamine receptor agonist. Pharmacologically, pramipexole differs from the first-generation agonists, bromocriptine and pergolide, in several respects. Pramipexole is a nonergot agonist, and ergotamine-related side effects, such as retroperitoneal fibrosis, are not to be expected. Pramipexole is very specific for the D$_3$-subtype receptor (which belongs to the D$_2$ receptor family).[98] The clinical effects associated with D$_3$-receptor specificity remain speculative, but they may include improved efficacy and antidepressant or mood-elevating activity. In a clinical study of depressed patients with PD receiving either pramipexole or pergolide, a significant improvement in depressive symptoms was observed only in the pramipexole-treated patients.[105] Pramipexole is excreted renally as unchanged drug and exhibits no significant inhibition of hepatic cytochrome P-450 enzymes. In patients with a creatinine clearance less than 60 mL per minute, elimination of pramipexole is reduced.

In early PD, pramipexole is effective as monotherapy, but with more advanced disease, symptomatic benefit is best when combined with levodopa.

Ropinirole. Ropinirole is a nonergot second-generation agonist that exhibits high affinity for D_2 and D_3 receptor subtypes, with minimal activity at nondopaminergic receptor sites (i.e., α, histaminic, cholinergic, serotonergic).[98]

Side effects are similar to those of pramipexole. Unlike pramipexole, ropinirole elimination is not affected by renal function. Ropinirole is metabolized in part by the CYP-450 1A2 isoenzyme, and inhibitors of this enzyme may increase ropinirole levels.

In early PD, ropinirole is effective as monotherapy, but with more advanced disease, symptomatic benefit is best when combined with levodopa. A sustained-release formulation of ropinirole is under development.

NONPHARMACOLOGIC THERAPY

Surgery. An enhanced understanding of the neuroanatomy of PD, coupled with developments in neuroimaging and surgical techniques, has revived the use of surgical interventions for PD. Surgery should be considered when patients are experiencing frequent motor fluctuations or disabling dyskinesia or tremor despite best medical therapy. Anatomic targets include the ventrointermediate thalamic nucleus (Vim), the globus pallidus internus (GPi), and the subthalamic nucleus (STN) (Fig. 63.8; *see color insert*). Once the target is localized, either electrothermal tissue ablation or chronic, high-frequency deep brain stimulation (DBS) is performed. Ablative techniques include pallidotomy, thalamotomy, and, recently, subthalamotomy. However, bilateral ablative procedures are associated with a high rate of side effects, and bilateral DBS has become the favored technique.[106] DBS has proven to be one of the best treatments to come along since levodopa and effectively increases "on" time. DBS does not cure PD, does not allow the patient to be free from medication, and does not provide symptomatic benefit more than the patient's best medicated "on" time. DBS does not improve mental function, postural instability, or voice quality. Demented patients are not candidates for surgery.

Unilateral and bilateral DBS procedures are well tolerated and are associated with advantages such as preservation of

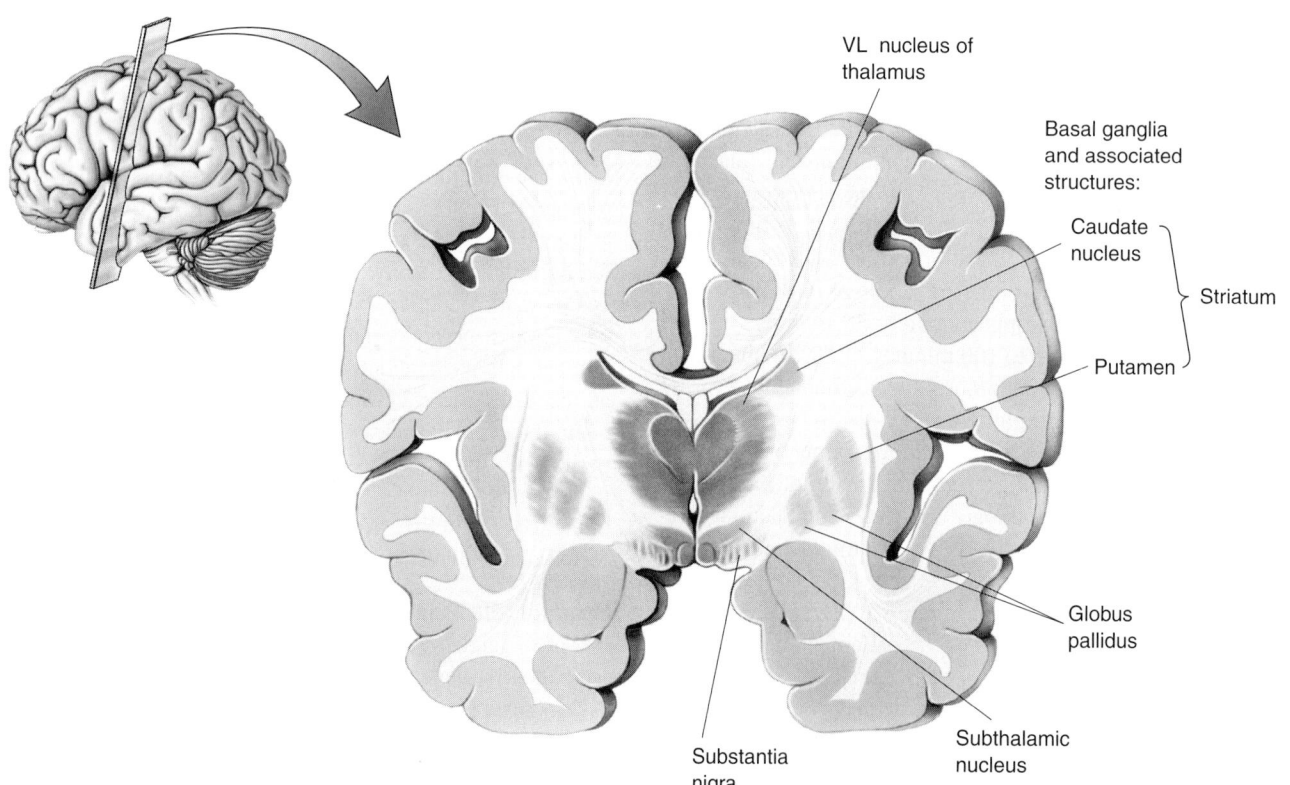

VL nucleus of thalamus

Basal ganglia and associated structures:

Caudate nucleus

Striatum

Putamen

Globus pallidus

Subthalamic nucleus

Substantia nigra

FIGURE 63.8 A coronal slice of the basal ganglia highlighting structures involved with movement (*see color insert*). (From Bear MF, Connors BW, Parasido MA. Neuroscience—exploring the brain, 2nd ed. Philadelphia: Lippincott Williams & Wilkins, 2001.)

neural tissue and ease of adjusting electrical stimulation to achieve optimal control while minimizing side effects. With DBS, a battery-powered neurostimulator (pacemaker-like device) is implanted subcutaneously near the clavicle and provides constant electrical stimulation, via electrode wires, to the targeted structure deep within the brain. The voltage, frequency, and pulse width of the electrical stimulation can be noninvasively adjusted to meet each patient's needs. For patients with disabling tremors, DBS of the Vim is the preferred procedure. For patients with advanced PD and significant motor fluctuations or disabling levodopa-induced dyskinesias despite optimized pharmacologic therapy, DBS of the STN or GPi is the preferred method and results in long-lasting benefits. Afterward, medication is still needed to manage bradykinesia and rigidity. With proper patient selection, electrode placement, and DBS programming, the procedure is very effective and, in combination with antiparkinson agents, allows for improved management of advanced PD.

Transcranial cortical magnetic stimulation (TMS) may offer a less invasive and less expensive alternative to DBS. Results of TMS in patients with PD are preliminary, and much work remains to refine this form of treatment.[107]

Grafting or transplantation of human fetal mesencephalon tissue into the striatum has received much attention. The transplantation strategy is based on the idea that dopaminergic neurons or neuroblasts can be used to replace or "restock" the dopaminergic neurons that are lost in patients with PD. Recent trials have demonstrated that grafted fetal tissue remains viable and improves dopamine uptake.[108,109] However, functional improvements were only marginal, and severe "off phase" dyskinesias were observed in a significant proportion of the transplanted patients. The fetal cell transplantation approach is promising, but several therapeutic and social issues surround this approach, and alternative sources of dopaminergic neurons based on stem cell technology and in vitro cell expansion techniques are under investigation.

ALTERNATIVE THERAPIES

Preparations of the legume Mucuna pruriens ("cowhage," "velvet bean," or "atmagupta" in India) have been used in India for the treatment of PD.[110] The seeds of M. pruriens contain larger amounts of levodopa than any other natural source.[111] In one study, the quality of motor improvement associated with 30 g of standardized Mucuna seed powder was equivalent to that of carbidopa/levodopa 50/200 mg.[112] The seeds of M. pruriens also contain coenzyme Q10 and nicotine adenine dinucleotide (NADH), which may contribute to the neuroprotective properties observed in animal models of PD.[113] The pods of the broad bean, Vicia faba, are another source of naturally occurring levodopa, and ingestion of V. faba pods has been shown to improve parkinsonian symptoms.[114] A 100-g serving of V. faba pods contains approximately 250 mg of levodopa. Ingestion of

large amounts of V. faba pods by persons with glucose-6-phosphate dehydrogenase deficiency may result in favism, a hemolytic anemia.

FUTURE THERAPIES

Therapies for PD under development include agents that may be neuroprotective or neurorestorative, agents designed to manage motor fluctuations and dyskinesias, and agents with novel delivery formulations. The search for a neuroprotective agent (i.e., an intervention that alters the underlying pathogenesis of PD and results in forestalling disease progression) is a particularly high priority research item.

Based on evidence suggesting that mitochondrial dysfunction and oxidative damage play a role in the pathogenesis of PD, bioenergetic compounds, such as coenzyme Q10 and creatine, are undergoing clinical screening for putative neuroprotective activity. These agents modulate mitochondrial energy metabolism and may exert antioxidative effects. In a pilot study of patients with early untreated PD, treatment with high-dose coenzyme Q10 1200 mg per day (with 1200 IU vitamin E per day) was associated with a reduction in functional decline.[115] In addition to coenzyme Q10 and creatine, minocycline and GPI-1485 are undergoing clinical screening studies for putative neuroprotection in PD.[116] Minocycline is a tetracycline derivative that has demonstrated benefit in some models of neurodegeneration (e.g., Huntington disease). The drug has several properties, including protection of mitochondrial membrane potential, prevention of inflammation, and inhibition of several toxic pathways, including apoptosis, microglial activation, and nitric oxide activity. GPI-1485 is a neuroimmunophilin ligand with neurotrophic properties.[117]

Istradefylline (KW-6002) is a novel selective adenosine A$_{2A}$ receptor antagonist that may provide a nondopaminergic approach to the treatment of PD. The adenosine A$_{2A}$ receptor is located almost exclusively in the basal ganglia, and blockade is believed to normalize GABA overactivity in the D$_2$ (indirect) pathway and improve PD symptoms and motor complications. Preliminary clinical data are encouraging.[118]

Rotigotine is a dopamine agonist under development as a transdermal delivery patch for once-daily administration. The patch will provide sustained levels of rotigotine over a 24-hour period to provide symptom control in patients with early PD or motor fluctuations.[119] Lisuride, another dopamine agonist, is also under investigation for transdermal and subcutaneous administration.

Other novel agents under investigation for PD include fipamezole (α2 adrenergic receptor antagonist), CEP 1437 (antiapoptotic agent), safinamide (ion channel modulator and MAO$_B$ inhibitor), sarizotan (serotonin 1A receptor agonist and D2 receptor partial agonist), and talampanel (AMPA receptor antagonist).[116]

Therapy with trophic or growth factors, such as intraputamenal infusion of glial cell-derived neurotrophic factor

(GDNF), to promote the restoration and maintenance of degenerating dopaminergic cells has been investigated in clinical trials. Efficacy and safety results are preliminary and much work remains to be done with these substances.[120,121]

IMPROVING OUTCOMES

Multidisciplinary education and intervention are vital and should also involve family members and caregivers. Educational pamphlets are readily available from various nonprofit organizations.

PATIENT EDUCATION

Patient-centered consultation styles are associated with higher patient satisfaction and improved health outcomes. Education should be appropriately selective and problem-oriented because disease progression and severity, presence of motor and nonmotor symptoms, and response to drug therapy differ for each patient. Patients and family members should understand what can be realistically expected from treatment. Support groups specific to the patient's demographic characteristics (e.g., age, ethnicity, gender) may offer greater appeal to some patients.

Additional information can be obtained from organizations such as the American Parkinson Disease Association (800-223-2732, www.apdaparkinson.org), the National Parkinson Foundation (800-327-4545, www.parkinson.org), Young Parkinson's Information and Referral Center (800-223-9776, www.youngparkinsons.org), and the Worldwide Education and Awareness for Movement Disorders organization (www.wemove.org). International associations can be contacted through the World Parkinson Disease Association (www.wpda.org).

METHODS TO IMPROVE ADHERENCE TO DRUG THERAPY

In outpatient neurology, dissatisfaction with communication relates significantly to nonadherence.[122] Sufficient time should be allocated to ensure that patients and caregivers understand the therapeutic plan and the purpose of their antiparkinson drugs. During initiation of a new antiparkinson drug, the titration schedule should be explained verbally and also provided in writing. The majority of antiparkinson agents are administered multiple times daily, and opportunities to simplify the dosing regimen or improve ease of administration should be considered when appropriate. Compliance aids such as calendar pill boxes may be recommended. Because of their close contact with patients when dispensing or providing clinical services, pharmacists can also play an important role in ensuring drug adherence and addressing barriers to adherence. Frequent inquiry about the effectiveness and tolerability of medications should be performed, as patients may choose not to adhere to medication (intentional nonadherence) to avoid adverse effects.

DISEASE MANAGEMENT STRATEGIES TO IMPROVE PATIENT OUTCOMES

Referral to a neurologist specializing in parkinsonism should be considered when the diagnosis of PD is in doubt, when patients are not responding to pharmacotherapy as expected, or when the patient has developed disabling motor complications. As the disease progresses, multidisciplinary intervention becomes vital for optimal and comprehensive care.

Consultation with a physical or occupational therapist is often very helpful for developing exercise routines and for improving the safety of work and living quarters. In addition to improving task performance, other benefits of exercise include improvements in balance, functional status, mood, quality of mobility provided by drugs, and mortality.[123-125]

Speech therapy can improve dysarthria, articulation, vocal loudness, and voice quality. Several forms of speech treatment are available, but not all produce long-lasting results. However, an intensive outpatient program known as the Lee Silverman Voice Treatment can provide long-term benefits.[126]

Consultation with a dietitian is recommended to minimize malnutrition and unwanted weight loss. Preventive nutrition is also important. For example, adequate calcium intake can help reduce the long-term risk of osteoporosis and bone fractures.

PHARMACOECONOMICS

Because it is a relatively common disorder, PD places a high economic burden on society.[127] Annual direct costs (e.g., drugs, medical equipment, hospitalizations) per patient, reported in U.S. dollars for the mid-1990s, ranges between $3,733 and $8,576 without home care and up to $12,256 when home care is included.[128-130] Overall, based on an estimated 1 million cases of PD in the United States, the direct costs associated with PD are in the range of $4 to $8 billion per year. To provide perspective, the estimated annual direct costs (in 1998 U.S. dollars) for dementing illness, stroke, and epilepsy are approximately $136 billion, $23.2 billion, and $820 million, respectively. If indirect costs such as lost productivity are included, the economic burden of PD balloons to $25 billion. Patient-specific factors that influence the cost of illness include age of symptom onset; level of disability; presence of motor complications, falls, and dementia; and nursing home placement.[131,132] For example, the total cost associated with Hoehn and Yahr stage 4 disease is up to 10 times that of patients with stage 2 disease.[131] The mean cost of patients with motor fluctuations is more than three times that of patients without motor fluctuations. A similar trend applies for patients with hallucinations and psychosis, who incur greater costs associated with nursing home placement.

Treatments that reduce the development of motor complications appear to be cost-effective, and the added cost of using a dopamine agonist in early PD instead of carbidopa/

levodopa is offset by savings due to avoided cases of dyskinesia.[133-135] Interventions or treatment approaches that slow disease progression (e.g., neuroprotection) are also likely to be cost-effective.

KEY POINTS

■ PD is a common neurodegenerative movement disorder characterized by tremor, rigidity, bradykinesia, and postural instability as well as autonomic and mental changes. The disease results in a reduction of quality of life for both patients and caregivers.

■ Depigmentation of the SNpc and presence of nigral LBs are core pathologic features of PD.

■ The cause of PD remains obscure. However, environmental and genetic factors are believed to play a role in promoting a cascade of events, including oxidant stress and accumulation of intracellular toxic proteins. Cell death occurs in several brain regions, particularly the SNpc, and is associated with depletion of nigrostriatal dopamine.

■ When available, neuroprotective therapy should be initiated as early as possible.

■ The initiation of symptomatic therapy should be based on the patient's level of functional impairment and quality of life. For example, hand tremor in a retiree, although a nuisance, may not interfere with daily activities, but it could endanger the livelihood of a dentist.

■ Anticholinergic agents should be considered for younger patients (<65 years of age) if tremor is the predominant symptom. Anticholinergic agents should be avoided in the elderly or in the presence of memory problems.

■ For mild bradykinesia and rigidity, amantadine or selective MAO_B inhibitors should be considered. As signs and symptoms worsen, a dopamine receptor agonist or carbidopa/levodopa is added.

■ Carbidopa/levodopa is the most effective oral agent for treatment of PD.

■ If cognitive or memory impairment is present, carbidopa/levodopa is preferred over amantadine, anticholinergics, dopamine receptor agonists, or selective MAO_B inhibitors because these latter agents tend to exacerbate underlying memory problems more than levodopa.

■ Younger patients are more likely to develop levodopa-related motor complications. For initial therapy, agents other than levodopa (e.g., amantadine, dopamine receptor agonists, selective MAO_B inhibitors) are preferred. As the disease progresses, all patients will eventually require carbidopa/levodopa.

■ Addition of a COMT inhibitor or a selective MAO_B inhibitor should be considered for managing motor fluctuations (i.e., "wearing off" effect).

■ Subcutaneous apomorphine provides a consistent and rapid onset of "on" time in patients experiencing frequent "off" episodes despite optimized pharmacotherapy.

■ Amantadine is useful for the management of levodopa-related dyskinesias.

■ Low doses of an atypical antipsychotic, such as quetiapine, are well tolerated and effective for managing hallucinations and psychosis in PD.

■ Surgery should be considered for patients with idiopathic PD and disabling dyskinesias, motor fluctuations, or tremors despite optimized medical therapy.

■ Ultimately, as stated by Schwab and England almost 50 years ago, "the secret to success with [PD] is complete adaptability to it."[136] Toward this end, education and multidisciplinary involvement are essential.

SUGGESTED READINGS

Chen JJ, Swope DM. Drug-induced movement disorders. In: Tisdale J, Miller D, eds. Drug-induced disease: prevention, detection, and management. Bethesda: American Society of Health-System Pharmacists, 2005.

Chen JJ. Anxiety, depression, and psychosis in Parkinson's disease: unmet needs and treatment challenges. Neurol Clin 22 (3 Suppl): S63–S90, 2004.

Drugs for Parkinson's Disease. Treat Guidel Med Lett 2:41–46, 2004.

Litvan I. Parkinsonian features: when are they Parkinson disease? JAMA 280:1654–1655, 1998.

Pahwa R, Lyons KE. Options in the treatment of motor fluctuations and dyskinesias in Parkinson's disease: a brief review. Neurol Clin 22 (3 Suppl):S35–S52, 2004.

REFERENCES

1. Parkinson J. An essay on the shaking palsy. London: Sherwood, Neely, and Jones, 1817.
2. Speelman JD, Bosch DA. Resurgence of functional neurosurgery for Parkinson's disease: a historical perspective. Mov Disord 13: 582–588, 1998.
3. Lewy FH. Paralysis agitans. I. Pathologische anatomie. In: Lewandowsky M, ed. Handbuch der neurologie. Berlin: Springer-Verlag, 1912:920–933.
4. Tretiakoff C. Contribution a l'etude de l'anatomie pathologique du locus niger de soemmering avec quelques deductions relatives a la pathogenie des troubles de tonus musculaire et de la maladie de Parkinson. Paris: Thesis, 1919.
5. Schwab RS, Amador LV, Littvin JY. Apomorphine in Parkinson's disease. Trans Am Neurol Assoc 56:251–253, 1951.
6. Ehringer H, Hornykiewicz O. Verteilung von Noradrenalin und Dopamin (3-Hydroxytyramin) im Gehirn des Menschen und ihr Verhalten bei Erkrankungen des extrapyramidalen Systems. Klin Wschr 38:1236–1239, 1960. Republished in English translation in Parkinsonism and Related Disorders 4:53–57, 1998.
7. Langston JW, Ballard P, Tetrud JW, et al. Chronic parkinsonism in humans due to a product of meperidine-analog synthesis. Science 219:979–980, 1983.
8. Lindvall O, Rehncrona S, Brundin P, et al. Human fetal dopamine neurons grafted into the striatum in two patients with severe Parkinson's disease. A detailed account of methodology and a 6-month follow-up. Arch Neurol 46:615–631, 1989.
9. Rajput AH, Offord KP, Beard CM, et al. Epidemiology of parkinsonism: incidence, classification, and mortality. Ann Neurol 16: 278–282, 1984.

10. Bower JH, Maraganore DM, McDonnell SK, et al. Incidence and distribution of parkinsonism in Olmstead County, Minnesota, 1976–1990. Neurology 52:1214–1220, 1999.

11. Avorn J, Gurwitz JH, Bohn RL, et al. Increased incidence of levodopa therapy following metoclopramide use. JAMA 274:1780–1782, 1995.

12. Twelves D, Perkins KS, Counsell C. Systematic review of incidence studies of Parkinson's disease. Mov Disord 18:19–31, 2003.

13. Bennett DA, Beckett LA, Murray AM, et al. Prevalence of parkinsonian signs and associated mortality in a community population of older people. N Engl J Med 334:71–76, 1996.

14. Quinn N, Critchley P, Mardsen CD. Young onset Parkinson's disease. Mov Disord 2:73–91, 1987.

15. Louis ED, Marder K, Cote L, et al. Mortality from Parkinson's disease. Arch Neurol 54:260–264, 1997.

16. McInerney-Leo A, Hadley DW, Gwinn-Hardy K, et al. Genetic testing in Parkinson's disease. Mov Disord 20:1–10, 2005.

17. Tanner CM, Ottman R, Goldman SM, et al. Parkinson disease in twins. An etiologic study. JAMA 281:341–346, 1999.

18. Hofer A, Gasser T. New aspects of genetic contributions to Parkinson's disease. J Mol Neurosci 24:417–424, 2004.

19. Golbe LI. The genetics of Parkinson's disease: a reconsideration. Neurology 40 (Suppl 3):7–14, 1990.

20. Marder K, Tang MX, Mejia H, et al. Risk of Parkinson's disease among first-degree relatives: a community-based study. Neurology 47:155–160, 1996.

21. Lucking CB, Durr A, Bonfati V, et al. Association between early-onset Parkinson's disease and mutations in the parkin gene. French Parkinson's Disease Genetics Study Group. N Engl J Med 342:1560–1570, 2000.

22. Kachergus J, Mata IF, Hulihan M, et al. Identification of a novel LRRK2 mutation linked to autosomal dominant parkinsonism: evidence of a common founder across European populations. Am J Hum Genet 76:672–80, 2005.

23. Firestone JA, Smith-Weller T, Franklin G, et al. Pesticides and risk of Parkinson disease: a population-based case-control study. Arch Neurol 62:91–95, 2005.

24. Spencer PS, Nunn PB, Hugon J, et al. Guam amyotrophic lateral sclerosis-parkinsonism with dementia linked to a plant excitant neurotoxin. Science 237:517–522, 1987.

25. Angibaud G, Gaultier C, Rascol O. Atypical parkinsonism and Annonaceae consumption in New Caledonia. Mov Disord 19:603–604, 2004.

26. Tanner CM, Chen B, Wang WZ, et al. Environmental factors in the etiology of Parkinson's disease. Can J Neurol Sci 14 (3 suppl):419–423, 1987.

27. Racette BA, Tabbal SD, Jennings D, et al. Prevalence of parkinsonism and relationship to exposure in a large sample of Alabama welders. Neurology 64:230–235, 2005.

28. Hernan MA, Takkouche B, Caamano-Isorna F, et al. A meta-analysis of coffee drinking, cigarette smoking, and the risk of Parkinson's disease. Ann Neurol 52:276–284, 2002.

29. Allam MF, Campbell MJ, Hofman A, et al. Smoking and Parkinson's disease: systematic review of prospective studies. Mov Disord 19:614–621, 2004.

30. Ascherio A, Weisskopf MG, O'Reilly EJ, et al. Coffee consumption, gender, and Parkinson's disease mortality in the cancer prevention study II cohort: the modifying effects of estrogen. Am J Epidemiol 160:977–984, 2004.

31. Wirdefeldt K, Gatz M, Pawitan Y, et al. Risk and protective factors for Parkinson's disease: a study in Swedish twins. Ann Neurol 57:27–33, 2005.

32. Etminan M, Gill SS, Samii A. Intake of vitamin E, vitamin C, and carotenoids and the risk of Parkinson's disease: a meta-analysis. Lancet Neurol 4:362–365, 2005.

33. Bernheimer H, Birkmayer W, Hornykiewicz O, et al. Brain dopamine and the syndromes of Parkinson and Huntington. Clinical, morphological and neurochemical correlations. J Neurol Sci 20:415–455, 1973.

34. Olanow CW, Perl DP, DeMartino GN, et al. Lewy-body formation is an aggresome-related process: a hypothesis. Lancet Neurol 3:496–503, 2004.

35. Braak H, Ghebremedhin E, Rub U, et al. Stages in the development of Parkinson's disease-related pathology. Cell Tissue Res 318:121–134, 2004.

36. Swerdlow RH, Parks JK, Miller SW, et al. Origin and functional consequences of the complex I defect in Parkinson's disease. Ann Neurol 40:663–671, 1996.

37. Jenner P. Oxidative stress in Parkinson's disease. Ann Neurol 53 (Suppl 3):S26–S38, 2003.

38. Poewe WH, Wenning GK. The natural history of Parkinson's disease. Ann Neurol 44 (Suppl 1):S1–S9, 1998.

39. Chen JJ. Anxiety, depression, and psychosis in Parkinson's disease: unmet needs and treatment challenges. Neurol Clin 22 (3 Suppl):S63–S90, 2004.

40. Louis ED, Tang MX, Cote L, et al. Progression of parkinsonian signs in Parkinson's disease. Arch Neurol 56:334–337, 1999.

41. Piccini P, Whone A. Functional brain imaging in the differential diagnosis of Parkinson's disease. Lancet Neurol 3:284–290, 2004.

42. Ravina B, Eidelberg D, Ahlskog JE, et al. The role of radiotracer imaging in Parkinson's disease. Neurology 64:208–215, 2005.

43. Hughes AJ, Daniel SE, Kilford L, et al. Accuracy of clinical diagnosis of idiopathic Parkinson's disease: a clinico-pathological study of 100 cases. J Neurol Neurosurg Psychiatry 55:181–184, 1992.

44. Litvan I. Parkinsonian features. When are they Parkinson's disease? JAMA 280:1654–1655, 1998.

45. Chen JJ, Swope D. Essential tremor: diagnosis and treatment. Pharmacotherapy 23:1105–1122, 2003.

46. Hoehn MM, Yahr MD. Parkinsonism: onset, progression and mortality. Neurology 17:427–442, 1967.

47. Fahn S, Elton RL, UPDRS Committee. Unified Parkinson's disease rating scale. In: Fahn S, Marsden CD, Calne DB, et al., eds. Recent developments in Parkinson's disease. Florham Park, NJ: Macmillan Health Care Information, 1987;2:153–164.

48. Welsh M, McDermott MP, Holloway RG, et al. Development and testing of the Parkinson's Disease Quality of Life Scale. Mov Disord 18:637–645, 2003.

49. Dura JR, Haywood-Niler E, Kiecolt-Glaser JK. Spousal caregivers of persons with Alzheimer's and Parkinson's disease dementia: a preliminary comparison. Gerontologist 30:332–336, 1990.

50. Schwab RS, England AC, Poskanzer DC, et al. Amantadine in the treatment of Parkinson's disease. JAMA 208:1168–1170, 1969.

51. Danysz W, Parsons CG, Kornhuber J, et al. Aminoadamantines as NMDA receptor antagonists and antiparkinsonian agents: preclinical studies. Neurosci Biobehav Rev 21:455–468, 1997.

52. Metman LV, Del Dotto P, LePoole K, et al. Amantadine for levodopa-induced dyskinesias: a 1-year follow-up study. Arch Neurol 56:1383–1386, 1999.

53. Factor SA, Molho ES, Brown DL. Acute delirium after withdrawal of amantadine in Parkinson's disease. Neurology 50:1456–1458, 1998.

54. Horadam VW, Sharp JG, Smilack JD, et al. Pharmacokinetics of amantadine hydrochloride in subjects with normal and impaired renal function. Ann Intern Med 94:454–458, 1981.

55. Richard IH, Kurlan R, Tanner C, et al. Serotonin syndrome and the combined use of deprenyl and an antidepressant in Parkinson's disease. Neurology 48:1070–1077, 1997.

56. Olanow CW, Mytilineou C, Tatton W. Current status of selegiline as a neuroprotective agent in Parkinson's disease. Mov Disord 13:55–58, 1988.

57. Parkinson Study Group. Effects of tocopherol and deprenyl on the progression of disability in early Parkinson's disease. N Engl J Med 328:176–183, 1993.

58. Ben-Shlomo Y, Churchyard A, Head J, et al. Investigation by Parkinson's Disease Research Group of the United Kingdom into excess mortality seen with combined levodopa and selegiline treatment in patients with early, mild Parkinson's disease: further results of randomised trial and confidential inquiry. Br J Med 316:1191–1196, 1998.

59. Heinonen EH, Myllyla V. Safety of selegiline (deprenyl) in the treatment of Parkinson's disease. Drug Saf 19:11–22, 1998.

60. Olanow CW, Myllyla VV, Sotaniemi KA, et al. Effect of selegiline on mortality in patients with Parkinson's disease. A meta-analysis. Neurology 825–830, 1998.

61. Marras C, McDermott MP, Rochon PA, et al. Survival in Parkinson disease: thirteen-year follow-up of the DATATOP cohort. Neurology 64:87–93, 2005.

62. Waters CH, Sethi KD, Hauser RA, et al. Zydis selegiline reduces off time in Parkinson's disease patients with motor fluctuations: a

3-month, randomized, placebo-controlled study. Mov Disord 19: 426–432, 2004.

63. Chen JJ, Swope DM. Clinical pharmacology of rasagiline. J Clin Pharmacol 45:878–894, 2005.

64. Parkinson Study Group. A controlled trial of rasagiline in early Parkinson disease: the TEMPO Study. Arch Neurol 59:1110–1118, 2002.

65. Parkinson Study Group. A controlled, randomized, delayed-start study of rasagiline in early Parkinson disease. Arch Neurol 61: 561–566, 2004.

66. Parkinson Study Group. A randomized placebo-controlled trial of rasagiline in levodopa-treated patients with Parkinson disease and motor fluctuations: the PRESTO Study. Arch Neurol 62:241–248, 2005.

67. Rascol O, Brooks DJ, Melamed E, et al. Rasagiline as an adjunct to levodopa in patients with Parkinson's disease and motor fluctuations (LARGO, Lasting effect in Adjunct therapy with Rasagiline Given Once daily, study): a randomised, double-blind, parallel-group trial. Lancet 365:947–954, 2005.

68. Mena MA, Davila V, Sulzer. Neurotrophic effects of l-dopa in postnatal midbrain dopamine neuron/cortical astrocyte cocultures. J Neurochem 69:1398–1408, 1997.

69. Melamed E, Offen D, Shirvan A, et al. Levodopa toxicity and apoptosis. Ann Neurol 44 (Suppl 1):S149–S154, 1998.

70. Parkinson Study Group. Levodopa and the progression of Parkinson's disease. N Engl J Med 351:2498–2508, 2004.

71. Leenders KL, Poewe WH, Palmer AJ, et al. Inhibition of l-[^{18}F]fluorodopa uptake into human brain by amino acids demonstrated by positron emission tomography. Ann Neurol 20:258–262, 1986.

72. Fiala KH, Whetteckey J, Manyam BV. Malignant melanoma and levodopa in Parkinson's disease: causality or coincidence? Parkinsonism Relat Disord 9:321–327, 2003.

73. Block G, Liss C, Reines S, et al. Comparison of immediate-release and controlled release carbidopa/levodopa in Parkinson's disease. A multicenter 5-year study. Eur Neurol 37:23–27, 1997.

74. Linazasoro G, Grandas F, Martinez-Martin PM, et al. Controlled-release levodopa in Parkinson's disease: influence of selection criteria and conversion recommendations in the clinical outcome of 450 patients. Clin Neuropharmacol 22:74–79, 1999.

75. Yeh KC, August TF, Bush DF, et al. Pharmacokinetics and bioavailability of Sinemet CR: a summary of human studies. Neurology 39 (Suppl 2):25–38, 1989.

76. Factor SA, Feustel PJ, Friedman JH, et al. Longitudinal outcome of Parkinson's disease patients with psychosis. Neurology 60: 1756–1761, 2003.

77. Stocchi F. Prevention and treatment of motor complications. Parkinsonism Relat Disord 9 (Suppl 2):S73–S81, 2003.

78. Pahwa R, Lyons KE. Options in the treatment of motor fluctuations and dyskinesias in Parkinson's disease: a brief review. Neurol Clin 22 (3 suppl):S35–S52, 2004.

79. Kostic V, Przedborski S, Flaster E, et al. Early development of levodopa-induced dyskinesias and response fluctuations in young-onset Parkinson's disease. Neurology 41:202–205, 1991.

80. Sage JI, Mark MH. Basic mechanisms of motor fluctuations. Neurology 44 (Suppl 6):S10–14, 1994.

81. Pappert EJ, Goetz CG, Niederman F, et al. Liquid levodopa/carbidopa produces significant improvement in motor function without dyskinesia exacerbation. Neurology 47:1493–1495, 1996.

82. Syed N, Murphy J, Zimmerman T, et al. Ten years' experience with enteral levodopa infusions for motor fluctuations in Parkinson's disease. Mov Disord 13:336–338, 1998.

83. Juncos JL, Fabbrini G, Mouradian MM, et al. Dietary influences on the antiparkinsonian response to levodopa. Arch Neurol 44: 1003–1005, 1987.

84. Riley D, Lang AE. Practical application of a low-protein diet for Parkinson's disease. Neurology 38:1026–1031, 1998.

85. Djaldetti R, Melamed E. Management of response fluctuations: practical guidelines. Neurology 51 (Suppl 2):S36–S40, 1998.

86. O'Suilleabhain PE, Bottiglieri T, Dewey RB Jr, et al. Modest increase in plasma homocysteine follows levodopa initiation in Parkinson's disease. Mov Disord 19:1403–1408, 2004.

87. Rogers JD, Sanchez-Saffon A, Frol AB, et al. Elevated plasma homocysteine levels in patients treated with levodopa. Arch Neurol 60:59–64, 2003.

88. Cawein MJ, Hewins JP. False rise in serum uric acid after l-dopa. N Engl J Med 28:1489–1490, 1969.

89. Cawein MJ, Williamson MA, Ebenezer C, et al. Levodopa and tests for ketonuria. N Engl J Med 283:659, 1970.

90. Mayeux R, Stern Y, Mulvey K, et al. Reappraisal of temporary levodopa withdrawal (''drug holiday'') in Parkinson's disease. N Engl J Med 313:724–728, 1985.

91. Holm KJ, Spencer CM. Entacapone: a review of its use in Parkinson's disease. Drugs 58:159–177, 1999.

92. Keating GM, Lyseng-Williamson KA. Tolcapone. A review of its use in the management of Parkinson's disease. CNS Drugs 19: 165–184, 2005.

93. Rascol O, Brooks DJ, Korczyn AD, et al. A five-year study of the incidence of dyskinesia in patients with early Parkinson's disease who were treated with ropinirole or levodopa. 056 Study Group. N Engl J Med 342:1484–1491, 2000.

94. Parkinson Study Group. Pramipexole vs. levodopa as initial treatment for Parkinson disease: a 4-year randomized controlled trial. Arch Neurol 61:1044–1053, 2004.

95. Le WD, Jankovic J. Are dopamine receptor agonists neuroprotective in Parkinson's disease? Drugs Aging 18:389–396, 2001.

96. Ahlskog JE. Slowing Parkinson's disease progression: recent dopamine agonist trials. Neurology 60:381–389, 2003.

97. Grosset K, Needleman F, Macphee G, et al. Switching from ergot to nonergot dopamine agonists in Parkinson's disease: a clinical series and five-drug dose conversion table. Mov Disord 19: 1370–1374, 2004.

98. Tuite P, Ebbitt B. Dopamine agonists. Semin Neurol 21:9–14, 2001.

99. Frucht S, Rogers JD, Greene PE, et al. Falling asleep at the wheel: motor vehicle mishaps in persons taking pramipexole and ropinirole. Neurology 52:1908–1910, 1999.

100. Dewey RB Jr, Hutton JT, LeWitt PA, et al. A randomized, double-blind, placebo-controlled trial of subcutaneously injected apomorphine for parkinsonian off-state events. Arch Neurol 58: 1385–1392, 2001.

101. Swope DM. Rapid treatment of ''wearing off'' in Parkinson's disease. Neurology 62 (Suppl 4):S27–S31, 2004.

102. McElvaney NG, Wilcox PG, Churg A, et al. Pleuropulmonary disease during bromocriptine treatment of Parkinson's disease. Arch Intern Med 148:2231–2236, 1998.

103. Nelson MV, Berchou RC, Kareti D, et al. Pharmacokinetic evaluation of erythromycin and caffeine administered with bromocriptine. Clin Pharmacol Ther 47:694–697, 1990.

104. Baseman DG, O'Suilleabhain PE, Reimold SC, et al. Pergolide use in Parkinson disease is associated with cardiac valve regurgitation. Neurology 63:301–304, 2004.

105. Rektorova I, Rektor I, Bares M, et al. Pramipexole and pergolide in the treatment of depression in Parkinson's disease: a national multicentre prospective randomized study. Eur J Neurol 10: 399–406, 2003.

106. Walter BL, Vitek JL. Surgical treatment for Parkinson's disease. Lancet Neurol 3:719–728, 2004.

107. Mally J, Farkas R, Tothfalusi L, et al. Long-term follow-up study with repetitive transcranial magnetic stimulation (rTMS) in Parkinson's disease. Brain Res Bull 64:259–263, 2004.

108. Freed CR, Green PE, Breeze RE, et al. Transplantation of embryonic dopamine neurons for severe Parkinson's disease. N Engl J Med 344:710–719, 2001.

109. Olanow CW, Goetz CG, Kordower JH, et al. A double-blind controlled trial of bilateral fetal nigral transplantation in Parkinson's disease. Ann Neurol 54:403–414, 2003.

110. Manyam B. Paralysis agitans and levodopa in ''Ayurveda'': ancient Indian medical treatise. Mov Disord 5:47–48, 1990.

111. Melvin E, Daxenbichler CH, Etten V, et al. L-dopa recovery from mucuna seed. J Agric Food Chem 20:1046–1048, 1972.

112. Katzenschlager R, Evans A, Manson A, et al. Mucuna pruriens in Parkinson's disease: a double-blind clinical and pharmacological study. J Neurol Neurosurg Psychiatry 75:1672–1677, 2004.

113. Manyam BV, Dhanasekaran M, Hare TA. Neuroprotective effects of the antiparkinson drug Mucuna pruriens. Phytother Res 18: 706–712, 2004.

114. Rabey JM, Vered Y, Shabtai H, et al. Improvement of parkinsonian features correlate with high plasma levodopa values after

broad bean (Vicia faba) consumption. J Neurol Neurosurg Psychiatry 55:725–727, 1992.

115. Shults CW, Oakes D, Kieburtz K, et al. Effects of coenzyme Q10 in early Parkinson's disease: evidence of slowing of the functional decline. Arch Neurol 59:1541–1550, 2002.

116. Hauser RA, Lyons KE. Future therapies for Parkinson's disease. Neurol Clin 22 (3 Suppl):S149–66, 2004.

117. Marshall VL, Grosset DG. GPI-1485. Curr Opin Investig Drugs 5: 107–112, 2004.

118. Hauser RA, Hubble JP, Truong DD, the Istradefylline US-001 Study Group. Randomized trial of the adenosine A(2A) receptor antagonist istradefylline in advanced PD. Neurology 61:297–303, 2003.

119. Parkinson Study Group. A controlled trial of rotigotine monotherapy in early Parkinson's disease. Arch Neurol 60:1721–1728, 2003.

120. Patel NK, Bunnage M, Plaha P, et al. Intraputamenal infusion of glial cell line-derived neurotrophic factor in PD: a two-year outcome study. Ann Neurol 57:298–302, 2005.

121. Amgen Inc. Following complete review of phase 2 trial data Amgen confirms decision to halt GDNF study; comprehensive review of scientific findings, patient safety, drove decision. http://www.amgen.com/media/media_pr_detail.jsp?year=2005&releaseID=673490 (accessed Nov. 10, 2005).

122. Grosset KA, Grosset DG. Patient-perceived involvement and satisfaction in Parkinson's disease: effect on therapy decisions and quality of life. Mov Disord 20:616–619, 2005.

123. Schenkman M, Donovan J, Tsubota J, et al. Management of individuals with Parkinson's disease: rationale and case studies. Phys Ther 69:944–955, 1989.

124. Bergen JL, Toole T, Elliott RG 3rd, et al. Aerobic exercise intervention improves aerobic capacity and movement initiation in Parkinson's disease patients. NeuroRehabilitation 17:161–168, 2002.

125. Hirsch MA, Toole T, Maitland CG, et al. The effects of balance training and high-intensity resistance training on persons with idiopathic Parkinson's disease. Arch Phys Med Rehabil 84:1109–1117, 2003.

126. Ramig LO, Countryman S, O'Brien C, et al. Intensive speech treatment for patients with Parkinson's disease: short- and long-term comparison of two techniques. Neurology 47:1496–1504, 1996.

127. Siderowf AD, Holloway RG, Stern MB. Cost-effectiveness analysis in Parkinson's disease: determining the value of interventions. Mov Disord 15:439–445, 2000.

128. Whetten-Goldstein K, Sloan F, Kulas E, et al. The burden of Parkinson's disease on society, family, and the individual. J Am Geriatr Soc 45:844–849, 1997.

129. Rubenstein LM, Chrischilles EA, Voelker MD. The impact of Parkinson's disease on health status, health expenditures, and productivity. Estimates from the National Medical Expenditure Survey. Pharmacoeconomics 12:486–498, 1997.

130. Dodel RC, Singer M, Kohne-Volland R, et al. The economic impact of Parkinson's disease. An estimation based on a 3-month prospective analysis. Pharmacoeconomics 14:299–312, 1998.

131. Keranen T, Kaakkola S, Sotaniemi K, et al. Economic burden and quality of life impairment increase with severity of PD. Parkinsonism Relat Disord 9:163–168, 2003.

132. Pressley JC, Louis ED, Tang MX, et al. The impact of comorbid disease and injuries on resource use and expenditures in parkinsonism. Neurology 60:87–93, 2003.

133. Iskedjian M, Einarson TR. Cost analysis of ropinirole versus levodopa in the treatment of Parkinson's disease. Pharmacoeconomics 21:115–127, 2003.

134. Lindgren P, Jonsson B, Duchane J. The cost-effectiveness of early cabergoline treatment compared to levodopa in Sweden. Eur J Health Econ 4:37–42, 2003.

135. Noyes K, Dick AW, Holloway RG; the Parkinson Study Group. Pramipexole vs. levodopa as initial treatment for Parkinson's disease: a randomized clinical-economic trial. Med Decis Making 24: 472–485, 2004.

136. Schwab RS, England AC. Parkinson's disease. J Chron Dis 8: 488–509, 1958.

Pain Management

64

Lori A. Reisner

Divinum est opus sedare dolorem. (Divine is the effort to conquer pain.)

—Hippocrates

DEFINITION

Pain is defined as "an unpleasant sensory and emotional experience associated with actual or potential tissue damage, or described in terms of such damage."[1] Pain is always subjective, and there are only a few validated tests that can quantitatively or qualitatively measure pain. Many are impractical in clinical settings, though simple tools such as pain scales are available to the clinician. Observations of pain behaviors such as grimacing or limping are crude methods at best, and can only be used to support rather than identify a patient's report of pain. Experimental models to more accurately measure pain in research trials include quantitative sensory testing (QST) of hot and cold pain thresholds and a capsaicin sensitivity test.

Acute pain arises from an injury, trauma, spasm, or disease of the skin, muscles, somatic structures, or viscera, and is limited in duration. It is perceived and communicated via the peripheral mechanisms identified as classic pain pathways (i.e., the A-δ and C fibers (see discussion in Pathophysiology section). The intensity of acute pain is usually proportional to the degree of damage, and it serves a biological purpose by inducing an organism to withdraw from or avoid a noxious stimulus. Diagnosis is usually straightforward with an identifiable cause. Acute pain decreases in intensity as the damaged area heals and tissue repair takes place.[2]

Chronic pain persists beyond what would be expected from a precipitating injury or tissue insult, and it is separated into malignant and nonmalignant categories. Malignant pain is related to terminal disease such as cancer. Nonmalignant pain was formerly called "benign"; a misnomer, as persons with nonmalignant pain often suffer a great deal of physical and psychological damage. Chronic pain is further characterized by its location: it may arise from visceral or myofascial (muscle and connective tissue) locations or from neurologic causes such as herpes zoster infection or diabetic neuropathy.

TREATMENT GOALS: PAIN

Treatment of acute pain focuses on superficial or deep location of pain and its origin and is directed toward the underlying etiology. Effective management involves the use of agents that target short-term symptomatic relief, and the goal is to mollify pain impulses during the period of tissue healing. Opiates such as morphine, hydromorphone, or fentanyl are used acutely in postsurgical pain treatment, but other important agents are the nonsteroidal anti-inflammatory drugs, since they can limit pain, swelling, and erythema at the site of trauma, enhancing patient comfort and possibly shortening the duration of the pain syndrome.

Treatment of chronic pain is directed not only toward symptoms but also to the suffering and disability produced. Symptoms of depression (hopelessness, helplessness, and sleep disturbance) may accompany chronic pain and must be treated concomitantly.[2]

Pain arising from cancer or other malignant disease exhibits characteristics of acute and chronic pain. It may be constant or intermittent in nature. A definable etiology, such as tumor recurrence, is usually present. Similar to chronic nonmalignant pain, therapy is composed of psychological and nonpharmacological interventions along with analgesics in effective and tolerable doses.

In the treatment of chronic pain, opioid or nonopioid analgesics should be dosed on an around-the-clock basis as there is no evidence that such pain will abate abruptly. Pain initially perceived as minor can progress to intolerable levels within a few hours. Once this phenomenon occurs, a larger dose of analgesic will be required to overcome pain-associated anxiety and bring the pain below the threshold of patient tolerance. For severe pain, habituation is not a concern as pain modulates the body's response to opioids and tolerance is slow to develop.

- Decrease subjective intensity and duration of the pain complaint.
- Decrease the potential for conversion of acute pain to chronic persistent pain syndromes.
- Decrease suffering and disability associated with pain.
- Decrease psychological and socioeconomic sequelae associated with undertreatment of pain.
- Minimize adverse reactions or intolerance to pain management therapies.
- Minimize inappropriate use of analgesic and adjunctive pain medications.
- Optimize drug therapy to take advantage of synergy and to avoid drug–drug interactions.
- Improve the patient's quality of life and optimize ability to perform activities of daily living.

EPIDEMIOLOGY

Pain is the most common symptom that provokes people to seek medical attention. Despite this, the epidemiology of pain is not as well documented as is the incidence of many chronic diseases. Comparatively little research has been done on the rate of occurrence of acute pain, since it is a natural consequence of trauma or surgery, and by definition is self-limiting. Studies evaluating the prevalence of pain in the community offer ranges of 7% to 64%, and the variation is due to sampling methods.[3] One survey estimated recurrent pain as affecting 37% of persons sampled, while 8% of these reported severe and persistent pain, and fewer than 3% had severe and persistent pain lasting longer than 6 days.[4] Backache is an example of a common pain complaint with a point prevalence of 15% to 30%, a 1-month prevalence of 30% to 40%, and a lifetime prevalence of about 60% to 80%.[5] Pain from osteoarthritis is thought to affect approximately half of the U.S. population over the age of 70 and increases with advancing age,[6] and headache is also a relatively common pain phenomenon. Both of these syndromes may be underreported due to the availability of over the counter analgesics. Though epidemiological studies are scarce and variable in their conclusions, chronic pain has a significant number of societal implications, and estimates of its economic impact due to medical treatments, disability, and lost work days have been attempted. Such estimates yield a cost to the U.S. economy of approximately $100 billion annually. Back pain, arthritis, and fibromyalgia are believed to be the greatest contributors to the economic burden of chronic pain. However, economic figures suffer the same statistical problems that plague prevalence estimates, and therefore, should be evaluated critically.

PATHOPHYSIOLOGY

During the 1960s, Melzack and Wall proposed the "gate control" theory of pain, in which it was thought that a painful stimulus acted on pain-sensitive receptors and caused an electrochemical nerve impulse to travel to the brain, which then initiated the physical and psychological responses to pain. Though certain key details of the gate control theory have since been revised, it is still widely accepted to explain the way pain signals are collected, transmitted, and interpreted within the central nervous system (CNS), as it allows for the existence of specific pain receptors and for the role of the ner-

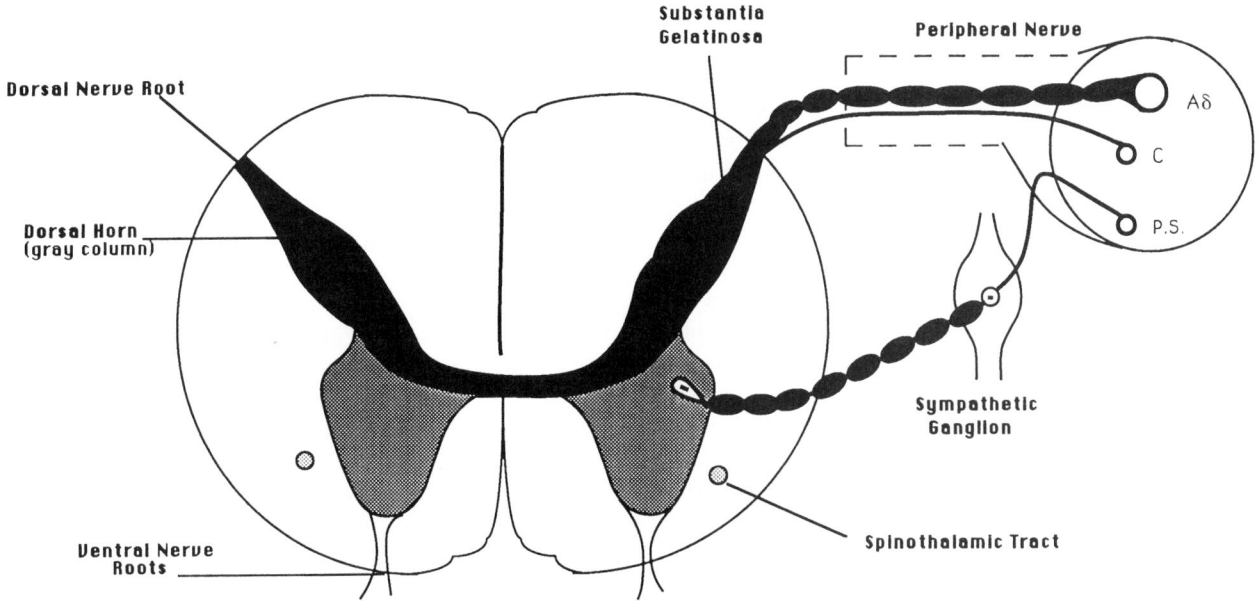

FIGURE 64.1 Transverse section of the spinal cord with peripheral nerve section illustrating two different types of axons: A-δ fibers and C fibers with cell bodies in the dorsal root and sympathetic fibers with cell bodies in the sympathetic ganglion. A-δ fibers and preganglionic sympathetic fibers are myelinated, whereas both C fibers and postganglionic sympathetic (PS) fibers are unmyelinated. The myelinated fibers carry impulses at a faster rate. Sympathetic fibers are thought to mediate some of the body's response to pain signals traveling along the peripheral nerve to the spinal cord and may also be involved in neurogenic inflammation. (From Fields HL. Pain. New York: McGraw-Hill, 1987; Clemente CD. Gray's Anatomy. 30th ed. Philadelphia: Lea & Febiger, 1985, with permission.)

vous system in pain mediation. Essentially, the gate control mechanism occurs as follows: afferent C fibers and A-delta (A-δ) nerve fibers transmit pain signals to an area known as the substantia gelatinosa, located in the dorsal horn of the spinal cord (Fig. 64.1). Cells within the dorsal horn collect and interpret these signals and send them to transmission cells with terminals projecting to distant sites outside of the dorsal horn. Some of the C fibers and the A-δ fibers terminate in the dorsal root horn, whereas others form a complex known as the lateral spinothalamic tract. Pain impulses travel upward along this tract to the thalamus and from there to the cerebral cortex of the brain.[7] Competing nerve impulses (i.e., stimulus from a different nerve branch) can block pain signals at the nervous system "gates," diminishing the intensity of the pain-relaying messages. Other controls exist that descend from the brain to inhibit firing of responsive neurons in the dorsal horn and, therefore, blunt or halt pain signals.[8]

PERIPHERAL PAIN SENSORY SYSTEM

When a painful (noxious) stimulus is applied to a sensitive area such as the skin, a series of events occur that are ultimately identified as a painful sensation. Sensitive tissues are those that contain pain receptors, also called "nociceptors." Nociceptors are primary afferent nerves with terminals outside of the spinal cord that respond to noxious stimuli. Two phenomena occur via the nociceptors.[9] The first is receptor activation or transduction in which chemical, thermal, or

mechanical energy is translated to an electrochemical nerve impulse in the primary afferent nerve. The second event is transmission of the impulse as coded electrochemical information to structures in the CNS that interpret the signal as pain. Transmission occurs initially in the spinal cord where neurons relay messages from the nociceptors to the brain. The messages elicit many responses such as a withdrawal reflex or a subjective perceptual event (for example, exclaiming "Ouch!"). The majority of nociceptors conduct their signals in two velocity ranges. Larger diameter, myelinated A-δ or rapid-firing fibers that include muscle receptors, among other primary afferents, constitute most of the known myelinated nociceptors. These A-δ fibers are most sensitive to stimulation by heat and by sharp, pointed instruments, hence they are known as mechanothermal or mechanical nociceptors. A third type of A-δ fiber may exist that is sensitive to irritant chemicals. A-δ fibers have the property of *sensitization*, that is, repeated application of a noxious stimulus produces increased sensitivity of these receptors.[10]

The unmyelinated axons are known as "C," or slow-firing fibers, and make up about 75% of the primary afferents in peripheral nerves. They have a smaller diameter than their fast-conducting counterparts and are sensitive to noxious thermal, mechanical, and chemical stimuli. As with the A-δ fibers, C fibers also sensitize with repeated application of painful stimuli, although they may be less sensitive immediately after a stimulus.[9]

Evidence of the role of A-δ and C fibers in pain perception is found in observations that brief, intense stimuli applied to a limb produce two distinct sensations: an early sharp, localized "pricking" pain of brief duration followed by a dull, diffuse, and prolonged unpleasant sensation.[11] By using compression to selectively block A-δ fibers, the initial sharp pain is abolished. Likewise, blockade of the C fibers by local anesthetics like lidocaine will lead to abolition of dull prolonged pain.[12,13]

How a pain sensation is perceived depends on the size of the area stimulated, the frequency of stimulus application, and the duration and location of the stimulus.[14] Although pain is a definite and singular experience based on activity in specific receptors, any single nociceptor's activity is influenced by simultaneous activity at nearby nociceptors. Thus, the pain experience is a composite of concurrent inputs at multiple receptors.[9]

When tissue injury occurs, the nociceptors undergo depolarization, leading to generation (transduction) of a nerve impulse. Depolarization is followed by pain and hypersensitivity lasting from minutes to days. Persistent pain can result from ongoing tissue damage or lingering chemical irritants released by cells during the initial insult. Other possibilities include a lasting change in the integrity of the receptor itself or even in the CNS.[9] Such changes are examples of neuroplasticity, which has garnered great interest in recent pain research. Neuroplasticity likely explains the transformation of acute to more chronic pain states following some injuries or traumatic events.

Stimulus intensity that exceeds the pain threshold of a nociceptor will result in visible signs of tissue damage. More extensive injuries lead to local increased sensitivity to mild stimuli, or hyperesthesia (hyperalgesia). Hyperesthesia causes injured tissues to develop tenderness so that normally innocuous stimuli produce pain. This hyperalgesia is paralleled by changes in the activity of the nociceptors, including sensitization. After superficial injury to the skin, an intense vasodilation occurs at the injury site (Fig. 64.2). This is rapidly followed by edema (a wheal) and secondary vasodilation that produces reddening (flare) that spreads into adjacent, uninjured skin. The hypersensitive region progressively enlarges with time and depends mainly on the activity of the C fibers as the flare and remote sensitization are blocked by local anesthetics. Thus, activity in C fibers causes vasodilation and sensitizes adjacent C fibers. The long-lasting changes that occur after injurious stimuli may play a major role in determining the intensity and quality of clinically important pain.[9]

CENTRAL PAIN TRANSMISSION

The cell bodies of the nociceptors are located in the dorsal root ganglion, and most of their axons terminate in the dorsal horn of the spinal cord. Some afferents project to the spinal cord through a ventral root as well, and both roots are thought to be important for pain transmission.

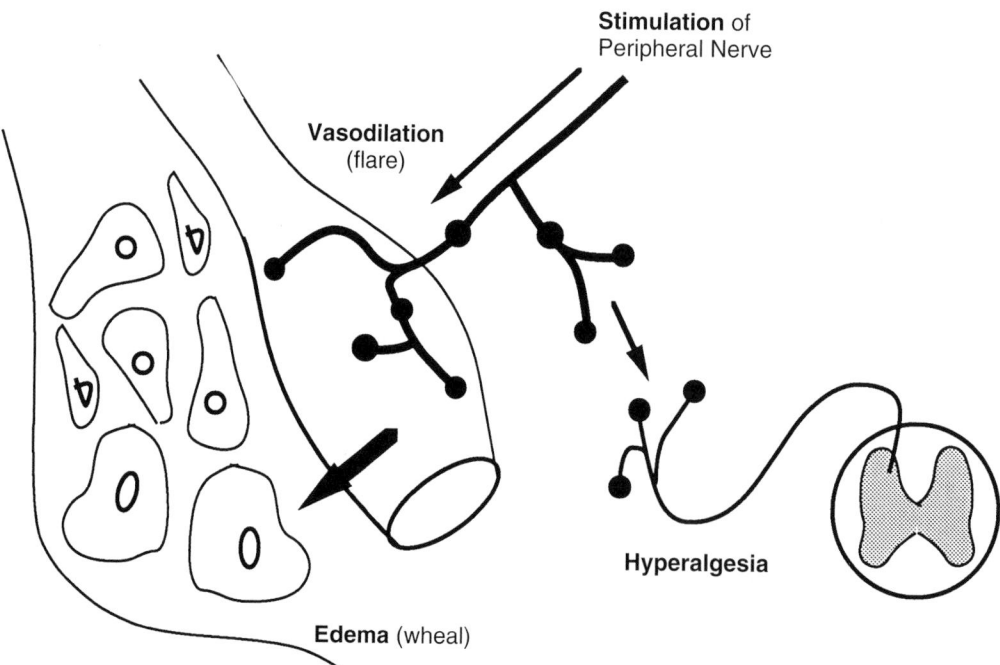

FIGURE 64.2 Events occurring after an insult to the peripheral nerve. Stimulation of the nerve ending produces a stimulus to vessel walls at the site of injury or trauma. Histamine, bradykinin, and other chemical mediators lead to vasodilation, then edema. Electrochemical signals across nociceptive synapses transmit the pain sensation to pathways in the spinal cord and ultimately to the brain, specifically the thalamus. (From Fields HL. Pain. New York: McGraw-Hill, 1997, with permission.)

Different pain-transmitting pathways may exist, including the spinothalamic, spinoreticular, spinocervical, and dorsal column tracts. Animal models of pain transmission have failed to precisely define the human pain pathways because of species differences, but it is understood that the various nociceptive pathways of the human, primate, cat, and rat reach their destination in the thalamus of the brain.[15]

The lateral spinothalamic tract is thought to be the dominant spinal cord pathway for signaling pain in humans, as lesions of this tract result in the absence of pain below the lesion. In addition, stimulation of this tract will induce pain in humans.[16] The termination zone of the spinothalamic tract and that of some dorsal column nuclei appear to overlap in the thalamus, and low-threshold stimulation of the dorsal column by electrical or chemical means can interrupt the flow of pain signal transmission. This ''gating'' provides the basis for the use of transcutaneous electrical nerve stimulation (TENS) and dorsal column electrical stimulators in the treatment of chronic pain.[17]

CNS opioid receptors have been identified in high concentration in the dorsal horn. They have also been localized in the brainstem, medulla, pons, amygdale, and cerebrum, including the limbic system. In man, administration of morphine into the ventricles of the brain produces potent pain relief in terminal cancer patients.[18] The mechanism of opioid analgesia is detailed later in this chapter.

PAIN-PRODUCING SUBSTANCES

Several chemical compounds accumulate near nociceptors after tissue injury. They may arise from cell leakage, from synthesis by local substrates released via enzymes induced by damage, or from release by the nociceptor itself (Table 64.1).[9]

Histamine from mast cells and potassium are among the substances released by tissue damage, both of which excite nociceptors and produce pain on injection into human skin.

Adenosine triphosphate (ATP) may also exhibit this effect. These compounds act alone or in combination to sensitize nociceptors.[19]

One substance known to produce pain is bradykinin, a polypeptide produced by cleavage of plasma proteins following tissue injury. Actions of bradykinin include low-concentration indirect production of hyperalgesia and high-concentration direct stimulation of nociceptors.[20]

Other compounds synthesized in the area of tissue damage are the by-products of arachidonic acid metabolism, including prostaglandins and leukotrienes. These chemicals are present in high concentrations in inflammatory fluids and are potent mediators of inflammation. Prostaglandins are formed from arachidonic acid via the enzyme cyclooxygenase; of these, prostaglandin E_2 (PGE_2) is the most potent. Prostacyclin (PGI_2) is also a potent inducer of pain and hyperalgesia. PGE_2 is thought to produce hyperalgesia by direct action on the nociceptors, but prostaglandins also sensitize nociceptors via coupling to a cyclic AMP system.[21] Other prostaglandins contribute to nociceptor activation by their interaction with additional chemical mediators. For example, prostaglandin E_1 produces pain only when injected with bradykinin or histamine. Similarly, norepinephrine may produce peripheral hyperalgesia via enhanced production of prostacyclin. Aspirin and other nonsteroidal anti-inflammatory drugs (NSAIDs) have analgesic activity due to their inhibition of cyclooxygenase.[22] Bradykinin-induced hyperalgesia may occur by stimulation of specific PGE_2 production, and can be blocked by the NSAIDs.[23]

Leukotrienes are produced from arachidonic acid by the enzyme lipoxygenase. Like prostaglandins, these agents produce hyperalgesia. However, leukotrienes are not notably blocked by cyclooxygenase inhibitors, but by the depletion of polymorphonuclear (PMN) leukocytes. Prostaglandins and leukotrienes may exert their hyperalgesic effects by mediation of other pain-eliciting compounds.[24]

TABLE 64.1	Chemicals That Are Active in Nociceptive Transduction		
Substance	Source	Enzyme Mediator	Producing Pain
Nociceptor Activators:			
Histamine	Released from mast cells	None known	+
Potassium	Released from damaged cells	None known	++
Bradykinin	Plasma proteins	Kallikrein	+++
Nociceptor Sensitizers:			
Prostaglandins	Arachidonic acid released by damaged cells	Cyclooxygenase	+/−
Leukotrienes	Arachidonic acid released by damaged cells	Lipoxygenase	+/−
Substance P	Primary afferent	None known	+/−
Glutamate, aspartate (excitatory amino acids)	Primary afferents	None known	+/−

(From Fields HL. Pain. New York: McGraw-Hill, 1987:32, with permission.)

In contrast to substrates released in the region of injury, nociceptors themselves discharge pain-enhancing substances. Substance P, a polypeptide, is liberated from some C fibers and excites pain transmission pathways in the dorsal horn. In experimental arthritis, intramuscular gold sodium thiomalate, a neurotoxin, causes substance P depletion by decreasing the number of C fibers in adjacent peripheral nerves. Substance P is a potent vasodilator and leads to release of histamine from mast cells, explaining its role in the immunomodulation and the pain of arthritis. Histamine itself also activates nociceptors and produces vasodilation.[25]

MODULATION AND INTERRUPTION OF CENTRAL PAIN PROCESSING

Opioid Receptors. Opioids administered into the spinal fluid reduce nearly all manifestations of clinical pain in humans. Subpopulations of these receptors are characterized by their sensitivity to selective opioid agonists.[26] Specific receptors in the CNS and peripheral tissues are responsible for modulating the effects of opioids and they are subdivided into four types: the mu (μ), delta (δ), kappa (κ), and epsilon (ϵ) receptors. Sigma (σ) receptors were once considered part of the class of opioid receptors, but are now classified as a distinct receptor type. The μ-receptors and κ-receptors produce analgesia, while the μ-receptor is responsible for the habituating and withdrawal effects of the opioids. μ-Receptors, located primarily in pain-modulating areas of the CNS, induce central analgesia and respiratory depression.[27] κ-Receptors are responsible for analgesia at the levels of the spinal cord and the brain and are found in greatest concentration in the cerebral cortex and in the substantia gelatinosa of the dorsal horn. They are thought to produce analgesia without inducing opioid habituation, therefore, there is great interest in the development of κ-specific receptor agonists. Though experimental κ-agonists such as spiradoline have shown low dependence and abuse liability, they are not ideal analgesics due to their psychotomimetic (hallucinogenic) and dysphoric effects. New evidence suggests that sex differences may exist with regard to receptor sensitivity. It has been suggested experimentally that males may derive better analgesia from μ-receptor activation, while κ-agonists may produce a greater analgesic response in women.[28] Δ-Receptors are located in the limbic area of the brain and in the spinal cord, and they may play a role in the euphoria that selected opioids produce. Evidence also exists implicating them in analgesia at the spinal cord level. Some researchers consider δ-receptors to be a subpopulation of the μ-receptors, or as mediators of μ-receptors. The function of ϵ-receptors has not yet been elucidated, while σ-receptors, though not true opioid receptors, are believed to produce the psychotomimetic and dysphoric effects of some opioid agonists and partial agonists such as butorphanol and pentazocine.[29]

Endogenous opioids, known as endorphins, enkephalins, and dynorphins, are found in varying concentrations in the CNS.[30] Dynorphins and enkephalins appear to be responsible for intrinsic regulation of pain perception within the me-dulla, while endorphins and enkephalins probably serve this function within the substantia gelatinosa. Each of the endogenous opioids has greater preference for a particular receptor type: β-endorphin and enkephalins are potent at μ-receptors and δ-receptors, respectively, while the κ-receptor is the target site for the dynorphins.[31]

The site of action of opioids depends on the method of administration. Systemically injected or ingested opioids will produce high brain opioid concentrations with relatively low spinal concentrations. The reverse occurs with spinal administration of the drug, that is, intrathecal (into the subarachnoid space) or epidural injection. At the spinal level, opioids are thought to inhibit pain signals carried by the A-δ and C fibers at their synapses in the substantia gelatinosa.

Opioids exert at least part of their analgesic action by inhibiting substance P release in the central and peripheral nervous systems. They also interfere with the actions of prostaglandins at peripheral sites, particularly μ-receptor-specific opioids that inhibit PGE_2 hyperalgesia in a dose-dependent fashion.[32] It is speculated that opioids produce analgesia by causing adenosine release, since methylxanthines such as caffeine can antagonize the effects of morphine.[33,34]

Opioids may exert their inhibitory actions via hyperpolarization of neurons by altered conductance of potassium or calcium. However, evidence exists that they also cause in vitro excitatory actions at the nerve terminals. This bimodal action is dose-dependent and helps explain the mechanisms of opioid tolerance and dependence.[35]

Tolerance and tachyphylaxis probably result from repeated exposure of receptors to high doses of opioid analgesics.[27] Continuously administered low-dose opioids can slow the development of tolerance. Patient-controlled analgesia (PCA), in which a controlled amount of drug is infused continuously, with bolus or "rescue" doses for breakthrough pain, produces less tolerance than intermittent high doses of an opioid. A second potential approach to delay tolerance is use of agents that are analgesic at a specific receptor; thus far, however, κ-specific or δ-specific agents are investigational only. Because of varying degrees of affinity for different receptors, opioids do not produce complete cross-tolerance. In general, greater cross-tolerance exists among opioids with high affinity to the same receptor, but less cross-tolerance is seen between opioids acting at different receptors. Since most available opioids have some affinity for each receptor type, the extent of cross-tolerance is variable and unpredictable.[36] When changing from one opioid agonist to another, half the calculated equianalgesic dose may be used initially and then the dose titrated upward as required.[37] Glutamate-sensitive receptor complexes in the CNS also play a role in the development of opioid tolerance. Blockade of one such receptor complex, known as the N-methyl-d-aspartate (NMDA) receptor, can attenuate opioid tolerance. Known antagonists of NMDA include dextromethorphan and ketamine, but these drugs are limited commercially because of dose-related side effects.

Beside their analgesic effects, opioids produce drowsiness, sedation, mood changes, disorientation, and memory impairment. Respiratory depression occurs by a direct action on the medullary respiratory and ventilation centers to reduce their responsiveness to carbon dioxide tension (Pco_2) and by depression of brain centers responsible for the rate and rhythm of respirations. Studies comparing morphine to other opioids have shown that equianalgesic doses of these agents do not differ significantly in their ability to depress respiration. Nausea and vomiting occur by opioid stimulation of dopamine release in the chemoreceptor trigger zone of the medulla. Opioid-induced emesis is treated with antiemetics that exert dopamine-blocking action (e.g., droperidol or prochlorperazine). Dopaminergic actions are also involved in the euphoria experienced with opioids.[38] Miosis occurs through a stimulatory effect on the oculomotor nerve, and pinpoint pupils are pathognomonic for opioid toxicity. Central stimulation by opioids can also induce skeletal muscle rigidity or convulsions, which may not be suppressed by anticonvulsant agents.[39]

Opioid receptors have been localized outside of the nervous system. In the gastrointestinal (GI) tract, opioids increase smooth muscle tone in portions of the stomach, duodenum, ileum, and large intestine, leading to decreased motility and spasm. Morphine reduces secretion of hydrochloric acid and pancreatic enzymes and inhibits mucosal transfer of fluids and electrolytes across the intestinal epithelium. Digestion and propulsion of food is delayed, and the absorption of oral drugs may be slowed. These properties have led to the development of the piperidine opioid congeners diphenoxylate and loperamide to treat hypersecretory diarrhea.

Therapeutic doses of morphine, codeine, or their analogs can lead to increased pressure in the common bile duct with elevations of serum lipase or amylase. Spasm and constriction of the sphincter of Oddi are probably responsible for this effect. Morphine appears to raise biliary pressure more than other opioids, but can still be used to treat pain from biliary colic or pancreatitis.[40] Muscarinic-anticholinergic drugs have been shown to block opioid-induced increases in sphincter of Oddi pressure,[41] which can also be blocked by naloxone. Ketorolac, a nonopioid analgesic, can also be used for biliary colic pain, without sphincter of Oddi dysfunction normally associated with opioids.[42]

In the cardiovascular system, opioids produce orthostatic hypotension by peripheral arteriolar and venous dilation. This is a direct effect and/or the result of opioid-stimulated histamine release. Vasodilation can be reversed partially by histamine-receptor (H_1) blocking agents and completely by opioid antagonists such as naloxone. Patients with coronary artery disease or evolving myocardial infarction may experience reduced myocardial oxygen consumption, but effects on the normal heart are insignificant. Opioid-induced respiratory depression can result in cerebrovascular dilation and increased intracranial pressure, effects that are hazardous in patients with cor pulmonale or in persons with cerebrovascular compromise who may suffer further damage from increased cerebrospinal fluid (CSF) pressure. A second factor that discourages use of opioids is depression of cognitive function and masking of cerebral damage secondary to pathophysiologies such as stroke.

In the smooth muscle of the bladder and ureter, opioids increase tone of the ureter and the vesical sphincter, leading to urinary hesitancy or retention. Such bladder effects can be reduced by administration of prazosin or similar α_1-adrenergic antagonists. In the uterus, morphine reverses oxytocin-stimulated hyperactivity, leading to prolonged labor. Opiates also depress respiration in the infant, as all opioids cross the placenta. Epidurally administered opioids are often used during parturition to reduce systemic effects. Preferred intravenous agents in obstetrics are the opioid agonist-antagonists butorphanol and nalbuphine because of their "ceiling effect" on respiration (i.e., higher doses do not increase the degree of neonatal respiratory depression).[43]

Cutaneous blood vessels dilate with opioids making the skin flushed and warm. Histamine release is partly responsible for these effects and for the pruritus and sweating that often follow opioid administration. Urticaria is particularly problematic following spinal administration of opioids, but it can be relieved with low doses of naloxone.[38]

Other Pain-Responsive Receptors. Table 64.2 lists the receptors that are involved in modulation of pain pathways. The adrenergic agonists norepinephrine and clonidine, an α_1-agonist, produce significant analgesia in man when administered into the spinal fluid, highlighting the role of adrenergic modulation of pain. Although it can produce peripheral hyperalgesia by enhancing prostacyclin production, norepinephrine acts centrally on the dorsal horn via descending impulses from the brain to inhibit pain. The antinociceptive actions of clonidine and norepinephrine can be reversed in a dose-dependent manner with adrenergic antagonists such as yohimbine.[44,45]

Serotonin receptors are found along the spinothalamic tract. Serotonin appears to reduce pain centrally by modulating descending impulses from the brain. This forms the basis of treatment of neuropathic pain syndromes with antidepressants that block presynaptic reuptake of serotonin.[46] However, noradrenergic systems are also involved in this phenomenon, since selective serotonin reuptake inhibitors (SSRIs) (e.g., fluoxetine) do not appear to be as effective in treating neurogenic pain as the tricyclic antidepressants that block reuptake of serotonin and norepinephrine.[47] In addition, studies with the noradrenergic agent desipramine demonstrate a pain-reducing effect despite negligible serotonergic activity.[48] Thus, descending modulatory pathways appear to be more dependent on noradrenergic effect than serotonergic activity, at least with currently available compounds. However, the mechanism of analgesic activity of antidepressants is complex and appears to be due in large part to local anesthetic (i.e., sodium channel blocking) effects in addition to monoaminergic effects.[49]

Receptor	Subtypes	Agonist	Action	Location	Antagonist
Opioid	μ, δ, κ	Morphine	Analgesia	Brain and spinal cord	Naloxone
Adrenergic	α₁	N/A	Reduced sympathetic outflow	Dorsal column	Prazosin
	α₂	Clonidine		Dorsal column	Yohimbine
	α and β	Norepinephrine		Dorsal column	Yohimbine
Serotonergic	multiple	Tricyclic antidepressants		Spinothalamic tract	Cyprohepatadine
		Sumatriptan	Antinociception		
Cholinergic	muscarinic, nicotinic	Acetylcholine	Antinociception	Dorsal horn	Atropine
GABAergic	A	N/A	Inhibition of nociceptor Activity	Peripheral	N/A
	B			Dorsal horn	N/A

TABLE 64.2 | Receptors Involved in Modulation of Pain Pathways

Cholinergic binding sites have been discovered in the dorsal horn. Application of the muscarinic agonist acetylcholine will produce analgesia that can be reversed by atropine. Opioid antagonists do not reduce such antinociceptive effects.[50]

GABAergic receptors are divided into two types: GABAₐ receptors are sensitive to muscimol and GABAᵦ receptors to baclofen. Of known GABAergic compounds, baclofen has been shown to produce analgesia, though nonspecific GABA agonists such as clonazepam may also be useful for some painful conditions.[51] GABAᵦ agonists inhibit firing of the nociceptors, particularly the C fibers. Unlike opioids, baclofen does not inhibit substance P release in the spinal cord. Baclofen is administered orally or intrathecally to treat central pain syndromes resulting from injury to the spinal cord, especially if consequent muscle spasms are involved.[52,53] Anticonvulsant medications with GABAergic activity (e.g., valproate) are also effective in certain painful conditions, such as migraine. However, analgesia may also be due to other mechanisms of valproate, such as antagonism of excitatory neurotransmitters.

CLINICAL PRESENTATION AND DIAGNOSIS

SIGNS AND SYMPTOMS
Acute pain may be accompanied by signs of autonomic nervous system activity (tachycardia, hypertension, diaphoresis, mydriasis, and pallor) that mimic those of anxiety, which often coexists with acute pain. Chronic pain is rarely accompanied by autonomic symptoms. Persons who report chronic pain often fail to show objective evidence of an ongoing pathological event on physical or radiologic examination, although patients who have undergone multiple surgeries can develop fibrotic (scar) tissue that may be apparent in imaging studies.

Superficial pain is derived from the skin or underlying subcutaneous and mucous tissues. It is characterized by local throbbing, burning, or pricking. It may be associated with tenderness, allodynia (pain from a stimulus which normally does not provoke pain), or hyperalgesia. Visceral pain presents as diffuse, dull, aching pain that is poorly localized and is noticed at the onset or early stages of disease. It may be associated with nausea and other autonomic symptoms. Deep somatic pain is dull and aching in nature, and can be localized, though there may be radiating components. Injury or disease of deep somatic structures produces the same response as does injury to the skin or viscera.[54]

DIAGNOSIS AND EVALUATION OF PAIN
In addition to physical examination, a simple "PQRST" mnemonic can aid the practitioner in evaluating pain. P represents the *palliative* or *precipitating* factors associated with the pain, such as diet, stress, or physical exertion. Q represents the *quality* of the pain, i.e., if it is sharp, dull, constant, aching, shooting, etc. R stands for *region* or *radiation* and is used to locate the pain. S is the *subjective* description by the patient of the pain's *severity* and its effects on daily activities and lifestyle. For example, does pain cause waking or appetite loss? Finally, T represents the *temporal*, or *time-related*, nature of the pain. It is useful to ask the patient whether the pain is worse in the evening or the morning, if it is related to any habitual daily activity, or other questions designed to detect diurnal, weekly, or monthly patterns. Women may experience differences in pain at various points in their menstrual cycles, as estrogen induces hyperalgesia.[55]

In addition to knowing how, where, and when the pain

began and what leads to its continuation, other pertinent facts about a patient's lifestyle are germane to accurate pain assessment. A pain questionnaire will aid in the evaluation and treatment of the chronic pain patient in the ambulatory care setting.[56]

Detailed information about the pain should be gathered to supplement the more general PQRST scale. It is necessary to determine what help the patient requests and if his or her goals are consistent with the treatment offered. Patients with chronic pain cannot always expect to be pain-free, as underlying degenerative pathophysiology or neuroplastic changes in the CNS may be permanent. Changes in aspects of lifestyle such as exercise and exertion, employment, and emotional approaches to living with chronic pain may reduce its dominance in one's life, however.

Location of the pain is ascertained with anatomic drawings on which the patient marks areas where it is worse. Colors can be used to demarcate different pain sensations, e.g., burning pain from aching pain. For pain intensity, a visual analog scale (VAS) is a reproducible method to measure and quantify pain. The VAS is a 10-cm line without subdivision marks. On the left extreme of the line "no pain" is written. On the rightmost extreme of the line, "worst pain I've ever had" is written (Fig. 64.3). A subject is asked to draw a hash mark on the line at the point best corresponding to his or her pain. Successive VAS scales are compared over time to evaluate response to therapy or changes in pain symptoms over time.

An important portion of any questionnaire involves the past medication history and current pain medication and other treatments. From this part of the evaluation, proper selection of analgesics, analgesic adjuncts, and patient compliance can be assessed. Patients who are compulsive in their consumption of pain medications, or those taking subtherapeutic doses of appropriate medication, can be identified. Potential interactions between prescription medications and over-the-counter products can also be assessed.

Finally, a checklist of problems related to major organ systems should be included. Patients who complain of multiple somatic symptoms along with pain may be experiencing depression or another affective disorder. Correction of the underlying depression may lead to remission of somatic complaints and improvement in pain scores.

Assessing pediatric pain is more difficult than with adults, as young children are often unable to adequately verbalize descriptors of pain intensity and quality. In children, a modi-

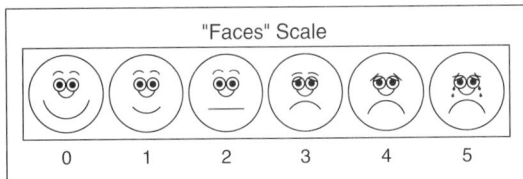

FIGURE 64.4 The Faces Pain Scale can be used to assess pain in children and adults with cognitive impairments or learning disabilities. (From Bieri D, Reeve RA, Champion GD, et al. The faces pain scale for the self-assessment of the severity of pain experienced by children: development, initial validation, and preliminary investigation for ratio scale properties. Pain 41: 139–150, 1990, with permission.)

fied visual scale, the Faces Pain Scale (Fig. 64.4) can be used.[57] Color scales, where red represents severe pain and blue represents no pain, can also be used in older children and adults with compromised cognitive ability (e.g., dementia).

Some researchers believe that human pain response can be divided into two categories: pain-sensitive (PS) or pain-tolerant (PT) subjects, who differ in aspects of pain behavior. PS subjects experience pain with qualitative differences that depend more on psychological variables than with PT subjects. These experiences can be measured by electroencephalography (EEG) devices. PS subjects demonstrate a lower pain threshold because of the role stress plays in pain responsivity and their higher observed stress level.[58] Further research will determine additional criteria for classifying pain response and if these two categories can be generalized to include a broad range of painful stimuli.

PSYCHOSOCIAL ASPECTS

Intensity of pain varies with each individual, with pain perception being determined by physiologic factors and a person's psychosocial background and pain experiences. Since pain is multifactorial in nature, it can be viewed in emotional, social, spiritual, and physical spheres (Fig. 64.5). Emotional pain consists of isolation, depression, and fear; factors which can reinforce each other. Social pain is comprised of strained or broken relationships and financial problems resulting from disability. Spiritual pain includes feelings of guilt, regret, or worthlessness, while physical pain encompasses disease and debilitation. Chronic pain can dull normal autonomic responses to stress (e.g., hypertension and sweating). Signs of depression most often manifest as sleep disturbance

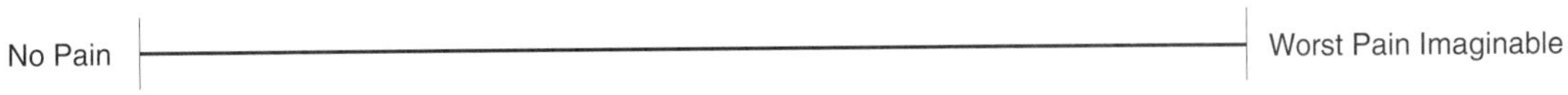

No Pain |——| Worst Pain Imaginable

FIGURE 64.3 Visual Analog Scale (VAS). The subject is asked to draw a hash mark at a point on the line corresponding to his or her pain. The line is usually 100 cm in length, and a ruler is used to measure the placement of the mark, with a corresponding number value (i.e., centimeters) assigned to the measurement. Subsequent VAS measurements can indicate improvement or worsening of pain severity.

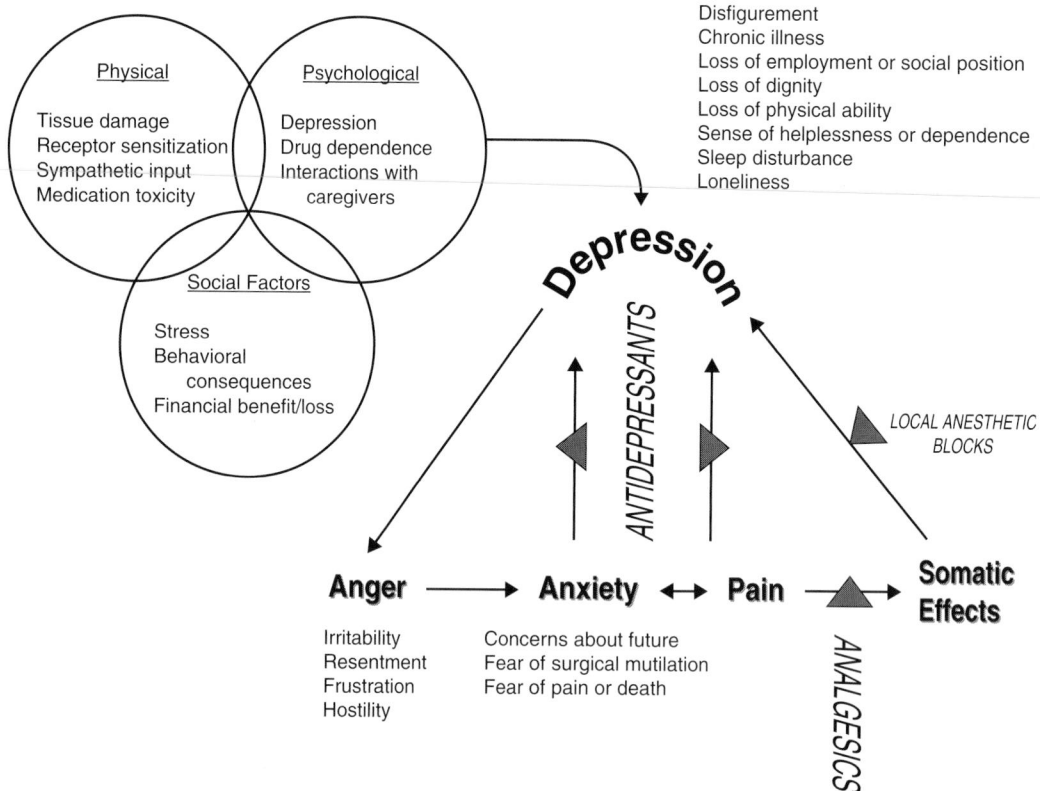

FIGURE 64.5 Determinants and modifiers of pain response and behavior. Portions of the pain, depression, and anger relationships can be interrupted by the pharmacological interventions shown.

and irritability. Delayed sleep onset and frequent waking may occur with patients reporting exhaustion from lack of sleep and from inability to tolerate the stresses imposed by continuous pain. Chronic pain often leads to anxiety and depression that in turn exacerbate the pain. This cycle can ultimately induce adoption of a ''pain lifestyle'' in which polypharmacy and polysurgery become over-represented in a patient's medical history. If secondary gain such as increased attention from family members or financial reward becomes an issue, there is less incentive to recover from a pain syndrome. Pain may also mask underlying psychological or physical abuse and can present itself as a symptom of emotional need.[59]

A distinction can usually be made between the ''pain patient'' and the patient in pain. The patient in pain may exhibit findings seen more often with acute pain such as pacing, grimacing, or alterations in heart rate and blood pressure. These persons will likely recover psychologically from the painful episode once adequate pain control is achieved. Even in many such patients with chronic pain, reliance on medications is stable at a minimal level, and the patient demonstrates a high degree of self-dependence in overcoming pain-related disability. Interaction with health care providers is not extensive, and the patient exhibits self-motivation in returning to a premorbid lifestyle.

The pain patient, however, is an individual who has suffered pain for a period of time long enough to produce notable changes in lifestyle, such as a discharge from employment and heavy reliance on family members or the health care system to offer relief. These patients may be tearful and anxious, and may also exhibit symptoms of acute pain that abate when the patient is distracted. In fact, distraction can be a useful technique used by the patient to retreat from intrusive thoughts about the pain. Patients with extreme pain behaviors will visit and/or call their health care providers often, and they may manipulate their medication regimens without the advice of a health care provider. Patients who use their medications more often than directed may be required to adhere to a treatment agreement with their provider(s), in which specific behaviors and rules for medication use are defined. The agreement may include the names and doses of medications, prohibitions on obtaining medications from other prescribers, expectations from the treatment course, steps to take in an emergency, etc. Such agreements need not be punitive and may help patients better understand what they can expect from the health care system and what they are empowered to undertake on their own. Pain patients may have difficulty establishing realistic goals for their therapy, such as longer periods of physical activity, and will repeatedly request a ''cure'' for their pain syndrome, even when none is likely to exist.

THERAPEUTIC PLAN

Pain therapy is begun with nonopioid analgesics where possible, followed by the step-wise addition of opioids and analgesic adjuncts (Fig. 64.6).

An algorithm for medication selection in various pain syndromes is illustrated in Figure 64.7. Cancer pain arises at the primary site as a result of tumor expansion, nerve compression or infiltration by the tumor, malignant obstruction, or infection of malignant ulcers. It may also occur at distant metastatic sites. Furthermore, treatment for tumors, such as radiation therapy, may lead to mucositis and subsequent pain. Some of the more commonly encountered symptoms of cancer pain occur in the musculoskeletal tissue and in the nervous system. Although the majority of bony metastases do not produce pain, infiltration of bone is the most common cause of cancer pain. A constant, unpleasant, burning sensation often indicates compression of somatic nerves by tumor. This pain can also be accompanied by an intermittent lancinating pain.[60]

For cancer pain, analgesics should be given at regular intervals and in adequate doses (Table 64.3). Medication should never be prescribed on an as required (prn) basis, as the objective is to maintain maximum possible patient comfort at all times by maintenance of therapeutic levels. Oral medication is preferred, especially long-acting drugs, unless factors prohibit such administration. These include malignant bowel obstruction or severe nausea from emetogenic chemotherapeutic agents. Sublingual opioid administration has also been studied, with the more lipophilic agents providing better analgesia than the less lipophilic morphine, presumably caused by improved absorption. An alkaline pH also enhances the sublingual absorption of most opioids. Rectal administration of suppositories may suffice, although this method is less reliable due to variable absorption of drugs from the rectal mucosa. Parenteral infusion is a dependable method of analgesic delivery, and can be used in the home setting and the hospital environment with portable, programmable infusion pumps. Many such pumps are now available with syringe drivers or medication cassettes that require infrequent refills. Medication can thus be prepared by a home health care agency and supplied to the patient on a regular basis.[61,62]

Treatment of mild to moderate cancer pain should begin with nonopioid analgesics; when these drugs alone are ineffective, they are combined with intermediate potency opioid agonists such as codeine or its derivatives. Nonsteroidal anti-inflammatory agents are effective in relieving many symptoms of bone-associated cancer pain, as are corticosteroids. However, the extensive adverse effect profile of the corticosteroids should be considered. Bony metastases release PGE_2, which sensitizes peripheral nociceptors. NSAIDs and corticosteroids act by inhibiting the elaboration of PGE_2. In addition to relieving pain, these drugs reduce stiffness, swelling, and tenderness.[63] Other effective treatments for bony metastatic pain include bisphosphonates such as pamidronate, bone-seeking isotopes such as strontium-99, and radiation therapy.[64,65]

Finally, potent opioid agonists such as morphine or methadone should be used in the pain management regimen.[66] A common agent for treatment of advanced cancer pain is morphine, due to its potency and dosing flexibility. It is generally well tolerated by patients with a terminal illness but may cause excess sedation or constipation. Alternatives include hydromorphone, methadone, fentanyl, and levorphanol. Diacetylmorphine (heroin) is not available in the United States and does not possess any advantages in treating pain, since it is hepatically metabolized in vivo to morphine, its active analgesic component. Heroin has a slightly faster onset of action but a shorter duration of analgesia than mor-

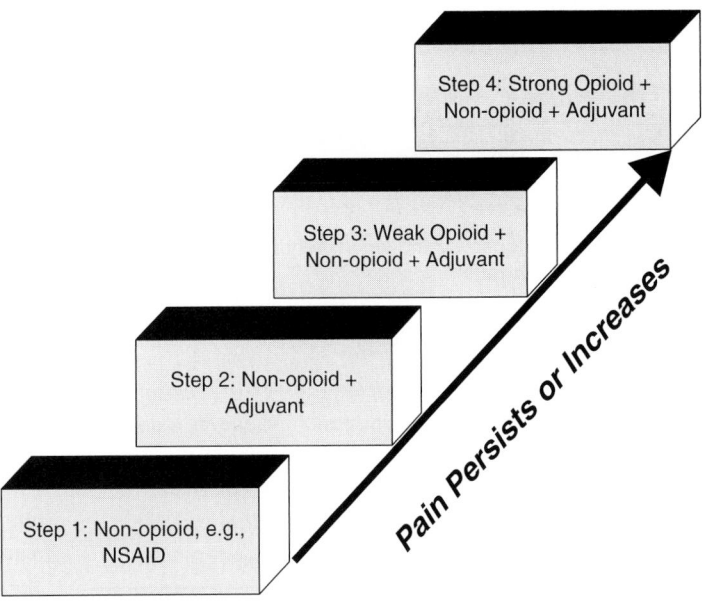

FIGURE 64.6 Analgesic stepladder for chronic pain management. Some pain specialists prefer to use a more aggressive approach, introducing an opioid analgesic earlier in the course of treatment. (From World Health Organization. Cancer Pain Relief. Geneva: World Health Organization, 1986, with permission).

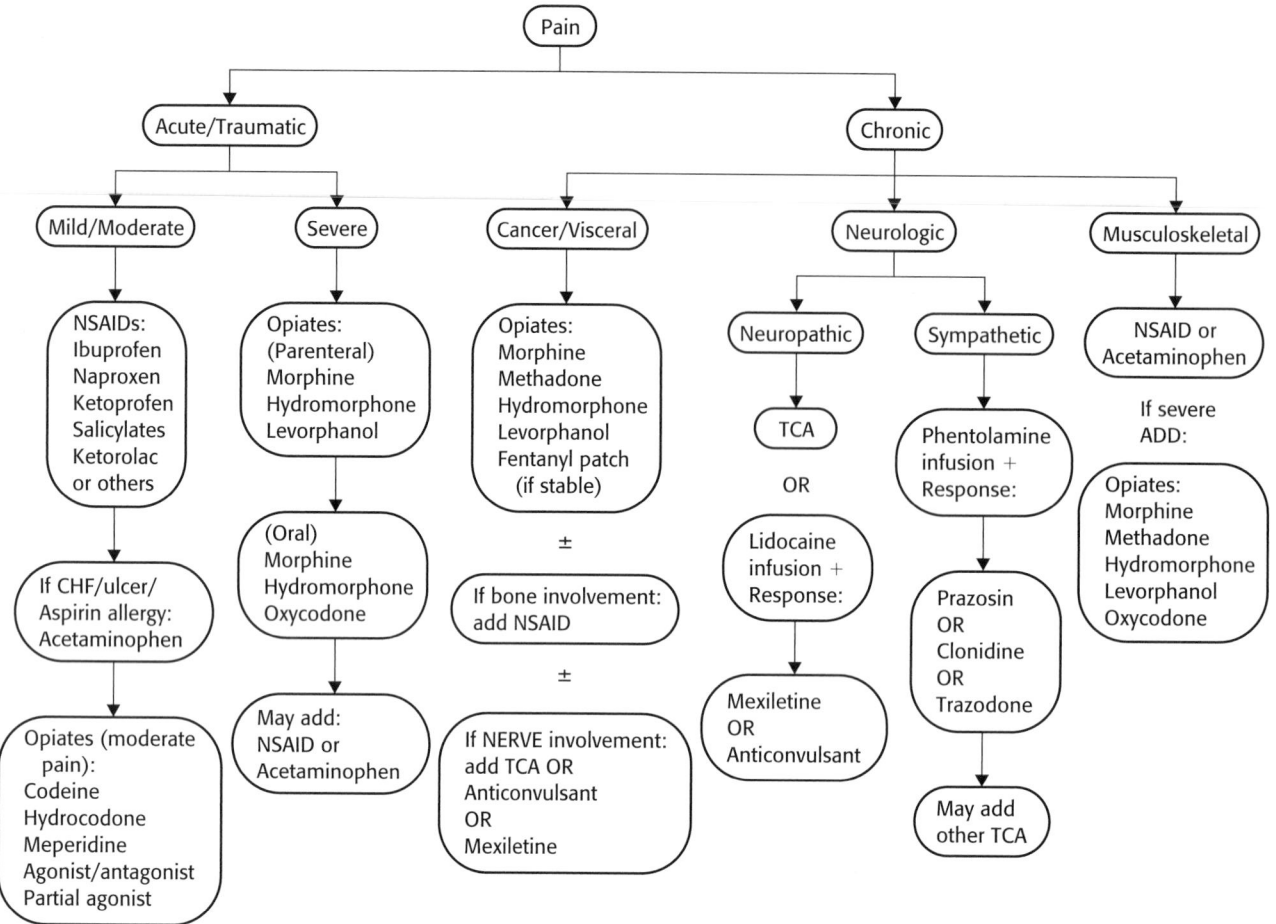

FIGURE 64.7 Algorithm for medication selection in the treatment of pain. CHF, congestive heart failure; NSAIDs, nonsteroidal anti-inflammatory drugs; TCA, tricyclic antidepressant.

TABLE 64.3	Principles of Analgesia for Cancer-Related Pain

1. Choose appropriate analgesic(s) for the source of pain, e.g., bone or nerve.
2. Determine the dose by individual requirement for optimal comfort or pain relief.
3. Schedule doses regularly (not prn)
4. Anticipate pain—do not "chase it"
5. Minimize sedation or other untoward effects
6. Utilize the oral route of administration whenever feasible
7. Treat nausea and constipation early with regular bowel regimen
8. Use adjunct medications whenever necessary
9. Tolerance and dependence are not problems

phine. It is more soluble, allowing use via the intramuscular route; however, methadone is an appropriate alternative to morphine.[67]

Analgesic adjuvants, such as tricyclic antidepressants, may be added to the drug regimen for cancer pain, particularly if neural involvement occurs. The benefits of analgesia may be enhanced by the psychotropic effects of the drugs on depression. Other adjuncts include antihistamines, phenothiazines, anticonvulsants, and amphetamines.[66,68]

Neuropathic pain can arise from discrete or generalized sites of nerve injury or may be idiopathic in nature. Two common neuropathic pain syndromes are postherpetic neuralgia ("shingles") and peripheral neuropathies arising from various causes such as diabetes mellitus or acquired immune deficiency syndrome; less common are neuropathies induced by agents such as the antiretroviral drugs zidovudine (AZT), didanosine (ddI), and zalcitabine (ddC) or the vinca alkaloids. Neuropathic pains are most often sharp, lancinating, burning, hot, electrical, shocking, or searing. They can be intermittent or constant, and they may involve paresthesias manifested by tingling or numbness of a limb. Neuropathic pain is relatively unresponsive to opioids, but this may be a function of inadequate dosing and underlying patient variables rather than due to the pharmacology of the opioids.[69,70]

Postherpetic neuralgia (PHN) is a persistent pain syndrome resulting from infection with varicella zoster virus (herpes zoster). The infection is initially manifested by fever, headache, lymphadenopathy, and malaise. It is followed by increasing pain or itching over a local area known as a dermatome, which is innervated by a specific nerve branch. Treatments for acute herpes zoster infection include systemic corticosteroids, antiviral agents, interferon, adenine arabinoside, and cimetidine. More invasive procedures, including somatic and sympathetic nerve blocks with local anesthetics and/or corticosteroids have proven efficacious.[71] Rarely, herpes zoster can leave an elderly or immunocompromised patient with permanent nerve damage resulting in persistent pain characterized as lancinating, burning, or itching. Common dermatomes affected by postherpetic neuralgia include cervical, cranial/trigeminal, thoracic, and lumbar regions. Herpes zoster is a reactivation of a latent virus originally acquired by acute varicella ("chickenpox") infection. The afferent nerve pathways undergo degeneration and interruption, causing deafferentation followed by nerve reorganization.[72] Tricyclic antidepressants are effective for the management of PHN, but they may be poorly tolerated. In addition to their pain remitting effects, tricyclic antidepressants can also treat the vegetative signs of depression such as sleep disturbance or anorexia.[73] Anticonvulsants are also used: carbamazepine and valproic acid have been used in doses of 600 to 1,200 mg per day or 500 to 1,500 mg per day, respectively. Gabapentin, in doses ranging from 2,400 to 4,800 mg per day or more, has also been used.[74] The anticonvulsants reduce complaints of lancinating pain. They are gradually adjusted upward from low starting doses, particularly in elderly patients.[75] Topical local anesthetics, such as lidocaine patch or other preparations, also help reduce pain of the affected dermatome.[76] A cream containing capsaicin, a purified derivative of the red chili pepper, can be applied directly to the area of itching and inflammation. Studies comparing this agent to placebo show a favorable response; however, its use is accompanied by one or more days of intense burning, since it acts as a nerve ending counterirritant by stimulating and then desensitizing afferent C fibers.[77] Other topical agents, such as aspirin and clonidine, may also prove useful.[78,79] Intravenous administration of lidocaine (5 mg/kg) has also been beneficial in PHN, as has its oral congener mexiletine.[80] Sympatholytic agents such as systemically administered clonidine may prove beneficial as well. Baclofen is also useful for refractory PHN pain of the trigeminal distribution.[81]

Diabetic neuropathy is usually reported as distal sensorimotor loss and is a long-term complication of diabetes mellitus. Like PHN, diabetic neuropathies respond well to the tricyclic antidepressants or anticonvulsants. Intravenous lidocaine has been administered with encouraging results, and mexiletine may also prove useful for this condition. Aldose reductase inhibitors that counteract hyperglycemia-induced metabolic changes at peripheral nerve sites show future promise for reversing early changes associated with functional nerve loss.[82,83]

Phantom limb pain has been described variously as burning, tingling, throbbing, shooting, and stabbing. Neurosurgical procedures are not permanently successful in reducing pain. Biofeedback has a role in increasing temperature and blood perfusion and in reducing discomfort at the amputation site. Anticonvulsants are helpful in reducing paroxysms of pain, as are tricyclic antidepressants.[84] Calcitonin may also play a role in the treatment of phantom limb pain.[85]

A syndrome known as sympathetically maintained pain, reflex sympathetic dystrophy (RSD), causalgia, complex regional pain syndrome (CRPS), or posttraumatic spreading neuralgia, predominates in areas of the extremities innervated by thoracolumbar branches of the nervous system. It may coexist with other forms of neuropathic pain. Causalgia is marked by burning pain, allodynia, and hyperpathia, and occurs in a hand or foot following nerve injury. RSD is continuous pain in a portion of an extremity following injury and is associated with sympathetic hyperactivity.[1] Causes include multiple fractures or surgery to a localized area without involvement of a major nerve. Manifestations of CRPS, in addition to burning pain stimulated by activity of the extremity, include vascular phenomena of coldness, numbness, or pain with changes in skin color. Trophic changes such as shiny, hairless skin, or loss of bone mass may occur later. The condition may be lifelong. Treatment involves vasoactive agents as well as analgesic medications. Initial episodes usually respond to local corticosteroid injections; more refractory cases respond to regional sympathetic blockade with local anesthetics or instillation of a sympatholytic agent such as guanethidine. Topical application of clonidine or capsaicin and systemic administration of alpha-adrenergic antagonists or calcium channel antagonists have been attempted.[86,87] A better understanding of this complex of syndromes is hoped to improve treatments. Recently, it has been suggested that immune modulators such as tumor necrosis factor (TNF-alpha) inhibitors may have some effect on treating this condition.

Myofascial pain arises from the muscles (myalgias), bones, joints (arthralgias), or connective tissue. Like a neuropathy, it can be idiopathic, iatrogenic, or injurious in origin. Muscle pain arising from exertion or strain is easily treated with the nonsteroidal anti-inflammatory agents, as is bone pain following dental or orthopedic procedures. Idiopathic musculoskeletal pain includes myositis and fasciitis, which are treated with local injections of anesthetics. Inflammatory diseases of muscle include polymyositis, dermatomyositis, and polymyalgia rheumatica. Flares may respond to low-dose intermittent steroids (e.g., prednisone 10–60 mg/day tapered over a 2-week period.[88] Fibromyalgia is a condition characterized by diffuse musculoskeletal aching with tender points and is often accompanied by poor sleep and symptoms of depression. Current theories about its pathogenesis involve CNS sensitization and hyperexcitability following persistent peripheral input from nociceptors in muscle.[89] Though standard treatments for fibromyalgia do not exist, tricyclic antidepressants, tramadol, muscle relaxants, and gabapentin have been used with variable results. SSRIs appear to be less useful.[90]

Examples of iatrogenic, or drug-induced musculoskeletal pains include those arising from the use of zidovudine, an agent used in treatment of acquired immune deficiency syndrome, muscle pain from the use of 3-hydroxy-3-methylglutaryl coenzyme A (HMG-CoA) reductase inhibitors to lower cholesterol, and amphetamine or phencyclidine overdose leading to rhabdomyolysis and myoglobinuria.[91] In 1989, an illness associated with consumption of L-tryptophan for insomnia was reported that included myalgia, eosinophilia, weakness, fever, arthralgia, dyspnea, rash, extremity edema, and pneumonia. The acute phase was notable for severe myalgia followed by proximal muscular weakness. Sensory and motor neuropathy were late complications and mimicked rheumatic diseases such as systemic sclerosis, polymyalgia rheumatica, or fibrositis. A contaminant of L-tryptophan was suspected. Patients did not respond adequately to nonsteroidal anti-inflammatory agents, hydroxychloroquine sulfate, or penicillamine. High-dose corticosteroids produced a modicum of success, though these drugs were often discontinued due to severe muscle cramping. Intramuscular injections of local anesthetic and steroid combinations (e.g., lidocaine/triamcinolone or bupivacaine/hydrocortisone) produced short-term reduction of myalgic pain. In extreme cases, the pain was opioid-responsive.[92]

Sickle cell disease results in acute infarctions and necrosis of organs secondary to vaso-occlusive episodes or "crises." Painful episodes are attributed to tissue injury from obstruction of blood flow by the deformed erythrocytes; however, a small population of persons affected with sickle cell disease report constant pain that persists between such episodes. Similarly, hemophilia may cause spontaneous bleeding into joints (hemarthroses) during flares of the disorder. Nonsteroidal anti-inflammatory agents and acetaminophen are the mainstay of therapy for mild to moderate pain of sickle cell crisis. Opiate analgesics, such as meperidine, morphine, or hydromorphone, are reserved for severe acute episodes and are dosed according to duration of action and relative potency. Consideration of hepatic or renal dysfunction due to veno-occlusion of these organs is required. When a crisis begins to abate, opioid tapering is instituted with pharmacologic emphasis placed on the nonopioid drugs.[93] Other treatments include vasodilators, such as dihydropyridine calcium-channel blockers.[94] Hydroxyurea is also being used to manage the disease with the goal of reducing crisis severity and frequency.[94]

TREATMENT

PHARMACOTHERAPY

Opioid Analgesics. Opioids include natural and synthetic agents. They reduce moderate to severe pain, and are unique in their ability to do this without producing loss of consciousness. All opioids have the potential for tolerance, habituation, and addiction. There are three classes of opioids: (a) the phenanthrene derivatives that include morphine, codeine, hydromorphone, levorphanol, oxymorphone, oxycodone, hydrocodone, dihydrocodeine, and opium; (b) the phenylpiperidine derivatives that include meperidine (pethidine), fentanyl, sufentanil, alfentanil, and remifentanil; (c) and the diphenylheptane derivatives that include methadone, levomethadyl, and propoxyphene (Table 64.4). Several agonist/antagonist combinations and partial opioid agonists are also available that are weaker than their pure agonist counterparts and are, thus, purported to be less habituating.

Potent Opiates. Morphine and other potent opioids are used to treat severe acute, chronic, or terminal malignant pain. They can be given orally, rectally, as continuous subcutaneous or intravenous infusions, parenterally, or directly into the CNS via epidural or intrathecal administration. The CNS route allows minute doses without sensory, motor, or sympathetic dysfunction. Other methods of administration include transdermal, intranasal, and buccal routes.

Required doses of opioids vary according to a patient's prior exposure, severity of pain, hepatic or renal function, and route of administration. The oral to parenteral morphine ratio is approximately 5:1, owing to a large first pass effect. Oral preparations include short acting tablets and elixirs and extended-release tablets. Conversion from short acting to longer duration formulations requires consideration of active drug and metabolite accumulation. One approach is to reduce the total daily dose by 25%, and divide this amount by three or four, then administer the resulting amount every 8 or 6 hours, respectively. When increasing the dose, an extra tablet is initially added at night to eliminate daytime somnolence, followed by the addition of subsequent tablets until effective analgesia is noted.

Morphine and hydromorphone exert major pharmacodynamic effects on μ-receptors and κ-receptors. Large doses of morphine can reduce systemic vascular resistance, producing a transient fall in blood pressure. Hydromorphone has less potential to produce nausea, vomiting, constipation, sedation, or euphoria than morphine, and it can be used as a substitute when these adverse effects warrant a therapeutic alternative. Concentrated parenteral preparations are useful for opioid-tolerant cancer patients in whom high opioid requirements have posed a problem because of the volume of drug required for administration. Though high-dose infusions of morphine or hydromorphone are associated with muscle rigidity and spasm, all opioids can cause muscular rigidity, presumably by accumulation in the sensitive regions of the brain.[95]

Oral morphine is variably absorbed with a bioavailability of approximately 20% to 30%. It is also absorbed rectally. Peak analgesia occurs about 20 to 60 minutes after a dose and lasts longer in opioid-naive individuals. The major metabolite of morphine is morphine-3-glucuronide, which is

TABLE 64.4	Centrally Acting Analgesic Characteristics						
	IM Dose (mg)	Oral Equivalent	Routes	Onset (minute)	Duration (hour)	t1/2 (hour)	Notes
Opioid agonists for severe pain							
Phenanthrenes:							
Morphine (various)	10	30	PO, SC, IV, IM, PR	IV: 5, PO: 60	3–6	2–3	
Hydromorphone (various)	1.5	7.5	PO, SC, IV, IM, PR	See morphine	3–6	2–4	
Levorphanol	2	4	PO, SC, IM	30–90	4–6	4–12	Accumulates
Oxymorphone	1.5	6	PO, SC, IV, IM	10–90	3–6	3–4	
Phenylpiperidines:							
Fentanyl (Sublimaze)	0.1	N/A	IV, spinal, buccal, patch	10	1–2	3–4	
Sufentanil (Sufenta)	10 µg	N/A	IV, IM, SC, intraspinal	10	2–4		Duration dose-related?
Diphenylheptanes:							
Methadone	5	5	PO, SC, IM	60	6–8	21–25	Accumulates
Opiods for mild to moderate pain							
Phenanthrenes:							
Codeine (various)	120	200	PO, SC, IV, IM	See morphine	3–6		
Hydrocodone (various)	N/A	30	PO	30–60	3–4		
Oxycodone (various)	N/A	20	PO	30–60	4–6		
Dihydrocodeine (various)	N/A	30	PO	30–60	4–6		
Phenylpiperidines:							
Meperidine (various)	100	400	PO, SC, IV, IM	15–60	1–3	3–4	Can provoke seizures
Pentazocine (Talwin)	30–60	150	PO, SC, IV, IM	10	3–4	2–4	Dysphoria common
Diphenylheptanes:							
Propoxyphene (Darvon)	N/A	65–130	PO	60–90	4–6	6–12	Hepatotoxic
Partial agonists/antagonists							
Buprenorphine (Buprenex, Subutex)	0.3	4	SC, IV, IM, sublingual	15	4–6	2–3	Not naloxone reversible
Butorphanol (Stadol)	2	N/A	SC, IV, IM, intranasal	15–45	3–4		Dysphoria can occur
Nalbuphine (Nubain)	10	N/A	SC, IV, IM	15	4–6	2–3	Respiratory ceiling
Opioid antagonists							
Naloxone (Narcan)	0.4–0.8	N/A	IV	10	2–3	1–1.5	
Naltrexone (Trexan)	N/A	50	PO	30–60	24–72	9–17	Duration dose-dependent

PO, orally; SC, subcutaneous; IV, intravenous; IM, intramuscular; PR, by way of the rectum.

inactive. Minor active metabolites include morphine-6-glucuronide and normorphine with a small amount biotransformed to codeine. Approximately 90% of morphine is excreted unchanged by the kidneys with most of the remaining 10% excreted via biliary elimination.[96]

Parenteral hydromorphone and levorphanol are about five times as potent as morphine with oral to parenteral ratios of 5:1 and 2:1, respectively. Both are available as tablets and as parenteral formulations for intravenous, intramuscular, or subcutaneous use. Hydromorphone can also be administered intraspinally or rectally.[97] Hydromorphone, a semisynthetic opioid, has a more rapid onset and shorter duration of action than morphine. Hydromorphone is converted mainly to a glucuronide metabolite with urinary excretion.[98] Levorphanol is a potent, semisynthetic opioid agonist for moderate to severe pain, including intractable pain in terminally ill patients. It produces more sedation and smooth muscle stimulation than does morphine in equianalgesic doses and has the same potential for habituation or addiction as naturally occurring opioids. Like methadone, it has a long half-life and a longer duration of action than morphine, meperidine, or hydromorphone. Levorphanol is well absorbed and, like hydromorphone, undergoes hepatic metabolism to a glucuronide conjugate excreted by the kidneys. Peak analgesia occurs approximately 20 to 90 minutes after intravenous or subcutaneous injection, respectively. Duration of analgesia may be shorter in opioid-tolerant individuals.[99] It is often used as a substitute when large requirements lead to the need for frequent morphine dosing.

Meperidine is used in moderate traumatic or postoperative pain and, like morphine, is given for pain from myocardial infarction or for sedation in patients with pulmonary edema. However, caution is advised in patients with atrial flutter or supraventricular tachycardia as meperidine can increase systemic vascular resistance and heart rate. Parenteral meperidine reduces rigors associated with amphotericin-B administration, and it is used as a premedication for patients receiving this antifungal agent. Some preparations contain metabisulfite preservatives that produce anaphylaxis or hypersensitivity reactions, especially in asthmatic patients. Parenteral meperidine has one tenth the potency of morphine. Because it is so poorly absorbed, oral doses are 25% to 30% as effective as parenteral doses. Meperidine is available as tablets, an oral solution, and an injectable preparation. It is metabolized to meperidinic acid, which is excreted by the kidneys as a glucuronide metabolite. Of greater importance is normeperidine, which can accumulate with renal impairment to induce central nervous stimulation and tonic-clonic seizures. Approximately one third of meperidine is converted to this N-demethyl metabolite, which has twice the convulsant activity, a fraction of the analgesic potency of meperidine, and a half-life of 12 to 16 hours.[100] Meperidine is shorter acting than morphine and produces the same degree, but a shorter duration, of respiratory depression. It is often administered during labor, caused by less extensive placental penetration, which reduces respiratory and CNS

depression in the newborn infant. Oral combinations with promethazine or acetaminophen and parenteral combinations with promethazine or atropine also exist, though there is little rationale in using such fixed dose combinations because patient-specific dosing is preferred. Combination products are more expensive than individual constituents and can produce additive side effects without providing additional benefit.

Methadone is useful for treatment of terminal painful conditions, as the longer duration of action allows for less frequent dosing. Methadone has unique pharmacokinetic properties: oral absorption is nearly complete, and the half-life is 13 to 47 hours with an average of 25 hours. Analgesic duration increases from 4 to 6 hours for a single dose to 6 to 8 hours after repeated administration. However, CNS depression persists up to 36 hours following overdose, an important factor in reversing the effects with the opioid antagonist naloxone. The half-life of naloxone is about 60 to 90 minutes, so a patient will require naloxone by continuous infusion until the risk period has ended.[97] Recently, methadone has been associated with an increasing number of deaths as determined by state public assistance utilization data, and many of these have occurred by inadvertent overdose or by fatal ventricular arrhythmias. Such events have been attributed to a number of factors, including more widespread use of methadone to improve cost-effectiveness of pain management regimens. However, increased prescribing of this drug by clinicians who are unfamiliar with its unique kinetic properties may predispose patients to risk of accumulation and toxicity. In addition to its long half-life, methadone is also a substrate of cytochrome P-450 3A4 (CYP3A4) enzyme, and thus has potential drug to drug interactions with inducers or inhibitors of this enzyme. In contrast, most other opioids are substrates of CYP2D6. Thus, prescribers may not be aware of the distinctive drug to drug interactions that can increase the risk of methadone use.

Methadone is roughly equivalent in potency to morphine on a single dose basis; however, with repeated administration accumulation in CNS and lipid tissues occurs. Thus, steady-state is not attained for several days, and doses should not be adjusted at intervals shorter than 5 to 7 days. Methadone is often used to manage pain and to taper a patient off of opioids in the event that they are not determined to provide the best available therapy. In weaning opioid-dependent patients, the total dose can be decreased 10% per day until a stable analgesic regimen is reached or until the patient discontinues the medication, depending on the treatment goals. Methadone is available as tablets, oral solution, and parenterally for intramuscular use.

Fentanyl is a synthetic opioid derivative of the 4-anilino-phenyl-piperidine class and is approximately 100 times more potent than morphine. It is used clinically as an analgesic administered intraspinally or intravenously and as a preoperative anesthetic agent because of its potency, rapid onset, and short duration of action. A transdermal patch can provide relatively consistent doses of fentanyl. This promotes adherence and improves convenience to the patient. A buccal preparation of fentanyl (a lozenge on a stick, similar to a lollipop) is available for breakthrough pain with cancer-related pain syndromes when the parenteral route is impractical. Fentanyl is a highly lipophilic agent, leading to rapid uptake and elimination, but orally the drug undergoes extensive first-pass metabolism. Parenteral administration has, therefore, been the typical route, but large initial doses required to sustain analgesia lead to a risk of overdose. Stable levels can be achieved by continuous intravenous administration when the infusion rate matches the plasma elimination rate. Transdermal administration has widened the clinical use of this agent because it also supplies the drug at a stable rate. Transdermal fentanyl is available in four strengths with patches releasing 25, 50, 75, or 100 μg per hour. Each patch lasts approximately 72 hours, but requires several days to reach steady-state concentrations. Supplemental doses of a short acting analgesic should be used as needed during the initial 24 hours after application to relieve breakthrough pain until the patch reaches maximal effect. Similarly, the drug is not rapidly eliminated if the patch must be removed due to untoward effects. Transdermal patches are noninvasive and offer an advantage in facilitating patient mobility. However, the buccal and transdermal delivery systems must be securely stored and carefully discarded to prevent inadvertent exposure to children or pets. Even after use, residual opioid in these products can cause significant harm. Conversion to an oral opioid can be done easily if such conversion becomes feasible. Sufentanil, another synthetic phenylpiperidine derivative, which is approximately 10 times more potent than fentanyl and more lipophilic, may also find future use with this novel route of administration.[39] Unlike previous permeability studies with other drugs, percutaneous penetration of these weak bases depends on pH but not on the anatomic location of the patch.[101] Remifentanil is a potent piperidine derivative used for perioperative analgesia.

Opioid Analgesics for Mild to Moderate Pain.

Codeine (methylmorphine) is a natural opioid derivative related to morphine. It is a less potent analgesic as are its derivatives hydrocodone and dihydrocodeine. Oxycodone, a third codeine derivative, exhibits intermediate potency. Propoxyphene is also less potent than its structural analog methadone. All of these drugs are effective for mild to moderate pain. Codeine is biotransformed to morphine, and medications such as fluoxetine, which diminish this conversion via inhibition of cytochrome P-450 (2D6) pathways, will reduce the opioid's efficacy. Practitioners should carefully evaluate the response of a patient given concomitant codeine and fluoxetine who reports suboptimal analgesia and consider an alternative opiate.

Tramadol is a "bimodal" agent that possesses activity at opioid and monoaminergic (serotonergic and noradrenergic) pathways in the CNS. An active metabolite demonstrates weak opioid receptor affinity, particularly at the μ-receptors.

Tramadol has been used in place of more potent opioid analgesics for treatment of moderate to moderately severe acute pain,[102] and also has utility in treating chronic pain syndromes such as low back pain and neuropathic conditions. Advantages of tramadol include lower abuse liability and reduced potential for respiratory depression. Disadvantages include adverse effects like dizziness, dry mouth, sedation, and constipation. At high doses it may induce seizures, but this effect is rare and most often associated with inadvertent or intentional overdose.[103] Typical doses for tramadol are 50 to 100 mg orally every 6 hours to a maximum of 400 mg per day. Elderly patients should be started at lower doses as they may be more sensitive to dizziness and other untoward effects. Accumulation can occur in the elderly and in patients with renal or hepatic impairment; therefore, a recommended starting dose in such patients is 50 mg every 12 hours.[97]

Agonist/Antagonists.

Agonists and antagonists have varying effects at different opioid receptors, and their affinity for any particular receptor is dose related. A characteristic of agonist/antagonist combinations is a "ceiling" effect with regard to analgesia and respiratory depression.[27] This means that doses above the threshold or ceiling do not increase the degree of analgesia or the potential for respiratory failure. Butorphanol, a synthetic opioid agonist-antagonist, is available parenterally and as an intranasal spray. Pentazocine, a benzomorphan derivative, does not decrease propulsive activity of the intestines in therapeutic doses.[39] It is contraindicated in myocardial infarction because it may increase blood pressure and systemic vascular resistance, and it has been combined with naloxone in oral preparations to discourage its abuse. Nalbuphine may have less psychotomimetic effects than butorphanol or pentazocine.[104]

Partial Agonists.

Buprenorphine and dezocine have less reported abuse liability than morphine, but they can precipitate withdrawal in opioid-dependent patients. Dezocine is a parenteral opioid analgesic with high μ-receptor affinity, moderate δ-affinity and κ-affinity, and low σ-affinity. It is no longer available in the U.S. though it is still used elsewhere. Buprenorphine has been administered parenterally and sublingually for postoperative or posttraumatic acute pain and opioid tapering programs. Recently, buprenorphine troches were also approved for opioid "detoxification." Like other opioids, partial agonists are metabolized by glucuronidation. In addition, dezocine appears to have a sulfate metabolite. Side effects of these agents include constipation or diarrhea, hypertension or hypotension, nausea, vomiting, anxiety, and sedation.[105]

Opioid Antagonists.

Naloxone is a short-acting, specific opioid receptor antagonist used to reverse the untoward side effects of opioids, such as pruritus and respiratory depression. It is a competitive saturable inhibitor of the opioid receptor and is usually administered in doses of 0.1 to 0.2 mg as needed. Care should be taken not to administer an excessive amount, as large doses will also reverse opioid analgesia and may precipitate abstinence symptoms.[97] Naltrexone is an oral opioid antagonist, and because of its extended duration of action, may be dosed as infrequently as twice weekly. It is most often used in treatment of opioid habitués. Selective peripheral antagonists, such as methylnaltrexone and almivopan, are being developed to manage the side effects of opioids without attenuating analgesia, particular for the GI tract and other smooth muscle systems adversely affected by opioids.[106,107] Because they do not achieve significant central concentrations, they can exert their effects without interfering with analgesia.

Innovative Methods of Drug Delivery. PCA devices were designed in the 1980s to take advantage of intravenous bolus injections to produce rapid analgesia along with slower infusion to produce steady-state opioid concentrations for sustained pain control. Typical agents used include morphine, hydromorphone, and fentanyl and can be injected via a blood vessel or delivered subcutaneously. Since opioid kinetics vary greatly between patients, the rates of infusion must be tailored. Many computerized PCA devices are available that rely on the same principle of a baseline infusion plus optional bolus and ''rescue'' doses. Boluses are self-administered and can be controlled by a predetermined lockout period. PCA is popular for acute postoperative pain relief, owing to its wide dosing flexibility. PCA is also useful for patients with chronic malignant pain, allowing patient independence. Many PCA devices are compact enough to be worn on a belt or carried in a pocket.[108] Ambulatory PCA devices, which use electrophoresis to drive an opioid across the skin and into systemic circulation from a drug-impregnated patch, are also being developed. Likewise, the concept of PCA is also being used in patient-controlled epidural anesthesia devices, whereby analgesic drug is administered epidurally rather than through a parenteral needle or catheter.

Opiates administered into the spinal fluid can be used for patients with malignant pain, acquired tolerance to systemic opioids, sudden exacerbations of pain (e.g., surgical amputees) and for patients in whom neurolytic techniques have failed. Morphine was the first opioid used in this manner. Unfortunately, spinal opioids may produce a greater degree of urinary retention, biphasic respiratory depression, urticaria, pruritus, nausea, and vomiting than opioids administered parenterally or orally. Agents that undergo significant migration up the spinal column toward the brain are most often associated with these side effects, as drug polarity influences such cephalad migration. Morphine is more polar than meperidine and undergoes a greater degree of migration, leading to delayed respiratory depression. It reaches the respiratory center approximately 3 hours after administration. Because of this, efforts have been made to reduce the severe side effects with combinations of opioids and local anesthetics such as bupivacaine and combinations with clonidine. By taking advantage of analgesic synergism via different mechanisms of action, smaller doses of each drug

may be administered. Several other analgesic opioid and nonopioid drugs have been studied since the introduction of intraspinal morphine. Spinally infused opioids have the potential for precipitating abstinence syndrome when withdrawn, but it is not clear if intraspinal opioids produce differences in the development of opioid tolerance when compared to oral administration. Changes in the opioid receptor number and/or drug-receptor affinity due to chronic occupation of the opioid receptors is believed to account for the tolerance phenomenon, but removal of an opioid for a period of 7 to 14 days can result in recovery of drug efficacy. Long-term spinal infusion of opioids does not cause permanent sensory or motor functional loss or histophysiologic changes, though it may lead to mild dorsal column degeneration. Disadvantages include risk of infection or puncture of the dura mater and catheter displacement.[109,110]

The entire volume of CSF turns over approximately every 5 hours. Any drug placed into the CSF is rapidly distributed and eliminated into systemic circulation. Bulk flow of CSF toward the head will cause a lumbar injection of an opioid to reach the brainstem, leading to effects such as drowsiness and vomiting within 2 to 4 hours. A bolus will cause concentrated drug to reach the brainstem, whereas a continuous infusion pump will allow a steady-state to be reached after five drug half-lives. Distribution across the dura from epidural administration occurs within 10 to 40 minutes. More lipid-soluble agents, such as methadone or fentanyl, will distribute along the spinal cord in a very limited manner due to rapid crossing of the dura and consequent migration out of the CSF.[111]

The action of opioids in the spinal cord make them ideal for powerful and relatively selective inhibition of pain information processing. Repeated bolus administration and continuous infusion of opioids into the epidural space for terminal cancer pain have demonstrated utility and efficacy. An implantable pump allows continuous infusion of opioids or other agents into the spinal space without requiring an external port. Spinal morphine or fentanyl has the advantage of providing adequate pain relief in patients when other forms of these drugs are not tolerated. Cancer patients receiving highly emetogenic antineoplastic drugs, for example, may lose significant amounts of oral drug by vomiting. A third advantage of this method of drug delivery is facilitation of ambulation, allowing a patient to leave the hospital. Epidural administration of opioids or other analgesic agents has also found use in the postoperative and obstetrical settings for short-term pain relief (2–5 days) following surgical procedures.[112,113]

Intrathecal opioid administration has received widespread attention. In vitro and in vivo data suggest a strong inverse relationship between intrathecal potency and lipophilicity for morphine, normorphine, methadone, meperidine, fentanyl, and buprenorphine. This can be explained by the rapid migration of highly lipophilic agents out of the CSF. Generalizations about relative intravenous or intramuscular opioid efficacy do not correlate to intrathecal or epidural potency, and specific δ-receptor agonists may prove useful for spinal infusion with minimal μ-receptor cross-tolerance. Similarly, clonidine via intrathecal administration can produce analgesia without morphine cross-tolerance.[114] Hormones as diverse as somatostatin and calcitonin have been administered intraspinally for analgesia. Intrathecal baclofen is used for treatment of intractable pain and spasm due to spinal injury. Like clonidine, baclofen can potentiate morphine analgesia or produce analgesic effects alone. Intrathecal methadone 5, 10, and 20 mg has been used for patients following orthopedic surgery; however, because of its higher side effect profile and lower efficacy when compared with morphine, it is not widely used via the intraspinal routes.[115,116]

Morphine can be administered directly into the brain's cerebral ventricles for treatment of cancer pain. Morphine administered in this fashion is effective and naloxone-reversible. The disadvantages of this technique are risk of meningitis, nausea, vomiting, and pruritus.[117]

Emerging technologies for opioid administration include disposable electronic PCA devices for self-limited ambulatory use and a foam-emulsion form of morphine that can be implanted by trocanter, similar to systems for long-term administration of hormonal agents.[118]

NONOPIOID ANALGESICS

Nonsteroidal Anti-inflammatory Drugs and Acetaminophen. Aspirin and other NSAIDs are useful for the treatment of pain from injury, surgery, trauma, arthritis, or cancer. The NSAIDs are especially effective in the management of bone pain.[119] Acetaminophen, though not possessing anti-inflammatory properties, is the most commonly used nonprescription pain reliever. NSAIDs differ from opioid analgesics in several ways: an analgesic ceiling exists for these agents, they are antipyretics, and they do not induce tolerance and physical or psychological dependence. In addition, their actions occur partly by inhibition of cyclooxygenase. Cyclooxygenase acts as a catalyst in the formation of prostaglandins that sensitize nociceptors to the effects of pain-eliciting substances such as bradykinin. Because of predominant action in the peripheral nervous system, the NSAIDs and acetaminophen work synergistically with the centrally acting opioids. NSAIDs also have central effects that contribute to their analgesic activity, and they have demonstrated a reduction in C-fiber activity in the thalamus.[120,121]

The NSAIDs are approximately equipotent and no structure-activity relationship exists for these agents. Some of the NSAIDs have been studied more extensively with regard to the pharmacokinetics of synovial and joint penetration. Patient response varies considerably, so a patient who does not obtain therapeutic efficacy with one drug at a maximum dose should be tried on an alternative NSAID.[52]

Absorption of the NSAIDs occurs in the stomach and duodenum. The rate of absorption increases with slower gastric emptying, or decreases when food or antacids are present in the stomach, although the total amount of drug absorbed is unchanged. Extent of absorption can be affected by the salt formulation. Currently, two products are available in the salt form: naproxen sodium and diclofenac potassium. Both agents are rapidly absorbed, and thus, are believed to reduce dyspepsia associated with gastric residence time. In addition, they possess a rapid onset of action, making them useful for treatment of migraine headache and other acute pain syndromes in the ambulatory setting. NSAIDs are eliminated primarily through biotransformation in the liver with metabolites excreted by the kidney. Some may undergo enterohepatic recirculation.[122]

The propionic acid class of agents includes ibuprofen, naproxen, fenoprofen, flurbiprofen, ketoprofen, and oxaprozin. Ketoprofen is unique in that it also inhibits the lipoxygenase enzyme that results in decreased leukotriene production. Whether this has clinical relevance is unknown. Ketoprofen is as effective in treating cancer pain as an acetaminophen and codeine combination in single dose comparisons.[123]

Ketorolac is a pyrrolacetic acid structurally related to zomepirac, tolmetin, and indomethacin, and it possesses potent analgesic with moderate anti-inflammatory activity. In postoperative pain, ketorolac is as effective as morphine, meperidine, or pentazocine, although the onset of action occurs slightly later. Like other NSAIDs, it inhibits platelet aggregation and can prolong bleeding time, induce gastric ulceration, or decrease renal function. Thus, its use is limited to 5 days or less. The most common side effects of ketorolac are somnolence and other central effects such as nausea and dizziness. Available for intramuscular and intravenous administration, it is well absorbed with a time to maximum effect of approximately 45 minutes. The major metabolite is a glucuronide, and elimination is mostly renal with approximately 90% excreted in the urine. The usual intramuscular dose is 30 to 60 mg as a single dose or 30 mg every 6 hours as needed. The maximum daily dose should not exceed 120 mg per day. Doses should be reduced by half for intravenous administration, elderly patients, those with decreased creatinine clearance, or patients who weigh less than 110 pounds (50 kg). The major role of ketorolac is acute postoperative analgesia when opioids are undesirable, as it is nonhabituating and does not appear to decrease respiratory drive.[124] It has also proven effective in managing pain due to biliary or renal colic.[125] There is little rationale to support the use of ketorolac in a patient tolerating oral medications or in one for whom intramuscular opioids are appropriate, and conversion to an oral NSAID, such as ibuprofen or naproxen, is indicated. Oral ketorolac is also available for the treatment of acute pain with a recommended maximum therapeutic duration of 5 days.

Anthranilic acids are also called fenamates, and although mefenamic acid is reported to have greater prostaglandin inhibition at the myometrium, it does not provide greater analgesia than other NSAIDs. Frequently reported adverse effects, such as diarrhea and CNS impairment have limited its use.

Piroxicam and meloxicam have an extended plasma half-life and can thus be dosed once daily.[126] Other once daily NSAIDs include oxaprozin, nabumetone (a nonacidic prodrug that is metabolized to an acetic acid), and sustained-release ketoprofen. However, once daily regimens are unsuitable for treatment of acute pain or most chronic pain syndromes, as plasma levels drop below analgesic threshold before the end of the dosing interval. They are useful for the treatment of rheumatologic conditions, since anti-inflammatory action persists beyond the duration of analgesia, and once-daily dosing enhances patient compliance.

Newer "cyclooxygenase-2"-selective NSAIDs, such as celecoxib, are available. These drugs are promoted as NSAIDs that disrupt inflammatory prostaglandin synthesis via inhibition of a specific subtype of cyclooxygenase (COX-2), but not the production of prostaglandins required for "housekeeping" or homeostatic functions in the body such as GI mucosal protection. Therefore, they are believed to have minimal propensity to cause GI ulceration or interfere with platelet function and may represent a significant clinical advancement over traditional NSAIDs for pain associated with osteoarthritis flares or rheumatoid arthritis.[127] However, potent inhibition of PGI2 (prostacyclin) by these drugs has recently been implicated in increased risk of cardiovascular events, particularly myocardial infarction. Rofecoxib was withdrawn from the U.S. market in September 2004 after it was discovered to double the risk of a major event (e.g., myocardial infarction) with long-term use when compared to placebo or some other nonselective NSAIDs.[128] Shortly afterward, valdecoxib was also withdrawn from the U.S. market as it was also associated with rare but severe dermatological reactions.

ANALGESIC ADJUNCTS

Antidepressants. Human response to pain includes the "fight or flight" reaction mounted against physical or emotional stresses. Two simultaneous phenomena occur: (a) corticoadrenal and (b) sympathetic responses. The first results in production of endogenous glucocorticoid steroids to mobilize energy sources and inhibit prostaglandins. The sympathetic response induces an outpouring of norepinephrine (a catecholamine) and serotonin (an indoleamine) within neuronal synaptic junctions. Tricyclic antidepressants that inhibit the reuptake and storage of these neurogenic amines have analgesic properties related to their ability to increase pain tolerance (Table 64.5).[129,130] This effect occurs in the absence of depression and the onset of analgesia is often more rapid than the antidepressant effect.[131] Tricyclic antidepressants also possess local anesthetic properties by sodium channel blockade in the neurons, which explains the more rapid antinociceptive effect.[132] In addition, vegetative symptoms associated with chronic pain, such as sleep disturbance and depression, are reduced by central serotonin enhancement. Serotonergic processes are part of endogenous pain inhibitory mechanisms, so tricyclic antidepressants have proven useful as adjuncts in chronic pain management.[133] Patients should be instructed that 1 to 3 weeks or more are typically required before such antinociception occurs.[134]

The antidepressants include several classes of agents that can be organized into three categories: the tricyclic antidepressants (TCAs), the monoamine oxidase inhibitors (MAOIs), and newer heterocyclic compounds. Clinical effects include improvement in mood and sleep, anxiolysis, and a decreased perception of pain. The tricyclic agents are

TABLE 64.5 | Antidepressants That Are Used as Analgesic Adjuvants

Medication	Trade Name(s)	Daily Dose (mg)	Cholinergic (Dry Mouth Constipation)	Histaminergic (Weight Gain Sedation)	Adrenergic (Orthostatic Hypotension) α_1	α_2	Notes
Tricyclic Tertiary Amines							
Amitriptyline	Elavil	25–150	Very high	Very high	High—very high	Moderate	
Doxepin	Sinequan	25–150	Moderate	Very high	High—very high	Moderate	+ Sleep effects
Imipramine	Tofranil	25–150	Moderate—high	Moderate	High	Insignificant	↑ Cardiac risks
Tricyclic Secondary Amines							
Desipramine	Norpramin	25–150	Slight	Slight	Moderate	None—slight	Often activating
Nortriptyline	Pamelor	25–100	Moderate	Moderate	Slight—moderate	Insignificant	
Heterocyclic[a]							
Nefazodone	Serzone	100–200	None—slight	None—slight	Moderate	Insignificant	+ Sleep effects
Trazodone	Desyrel	50–300	None—slight	Moderate	Very high	Moderate	+ Sleep effects
Venlafaxine	Effexor	75–225	Slight	None—slight	Unknown	Unknown	

[a] Pain relief with these agents is unproven or controversial.

commonly used in the management of neurogenic pain conditions. The MAOIs have been used infrequently for treatment of migraine headache and are reserved for patients refractory to the TCAs. MAOIs are more difficult to use due to food and drug interactions, and their benefits in treating pain have not been well documented. Newer nontricyclic agents include SSRIs, venlafaxine, mirtazepine, and bupropion, an aminoketone. None of these have been thoroughly studied for their effects on chronic pain, though bupropion exhibited a reduction in neuropathic pain in a single study. A new mixed reuptake inhibitor, duloxetine, has been approved for diabetic neuropathic pain and depression, but its superiority over older agents is unproven.[135]

The most commonly used antidepressant for painful conditions is amitriptyline in doses of 50 to 150 mg per day. Persons with chronic pain usually have poor sleep habits, making this drug useful in overcoming insomnia or nighttime waking. Amitriptyline has been found to exert more potent local anesthetic effects than lidocaine. An agent with fewer anticholinergic effects, such as nortriptyline, may be substituted for amitriptyline. Desipramine, an active metabolite of imipramine, is also less sedating and has fewer anticholinergic effects than its parent compound.

Analogs of fluoxetine with shorter half-lives prevent their accumulation in slow metabolizers, such as the elderly. Paroxetine is an SSRI modeled after the prototype agent zimeldine. It decreased symptoms of painful diabetic neuropathy without withdrawal effects or changes in nerve function measurements. Paroxetine at 40 mg per day is also devoid of autonomic side effects which frequently limit the use of TCAs.[136] However, efficacy studies with SSRIs in neuropathic pain have conflicting results, and most do not show an analgesic effect for this class of medications. Thus, while they may be helpful in treating depression, the SSRIs are not commonly used as agents to reduce pain symptoms.

Neuroleptics. Of the neuroleptics, fluphenazine will potentiate the effects of amitriptyline in patients with diabetic neuropathies and central (after stroke) pain. It also aids sleep onset and can be given in small doses of 1 mg at bedtime, up to a maximum of 3 mg per day in divided doses or all at bedtime.[137] Methotrimeprazine is available as a treatment for mild to moderate pain. Its duration of action is equal to that of morphine, and it possesses analgesic equivalence to morphine or meperidine without the similar habituating or addictive potential or likelihood of respiratory depression. It has been underutilized in chronic pain management due to the sedative and anticholinergic effects that decrease patient tolerance. The use of neuroleptics is debatable because of risk of extrapyramidal adverse effects, and phenothiazine analgesia is controversial,[138] although there is evidentiary support in migraine headaches.[139]

Anticonvulsants. The mechanism of action of carbamazepine and valproate is suppression of spontaneous neuronal firing. Lancinating, burning pains are best treated by these drugs, which are typically long-acting but can induce their own metabolism. Carbamazepine and valproate are prescribed for tic douloureux (trigeminal neuralgia), cranial nerve disorders, neural invasion by cancerous tumor, radiation fibrosis, surgical scarring, deafferentation, and other neuralgic syndromes. Doses of carbamazepine and valproate are the same as those used for treatment of convulsive disorders. Plasma levels should be monitored, as side effects may include bone marrow suppression, ataxia, diplopia, nausea, lymphadenopathy, and hepatic dysfunction. Periodic liver function tests, blood counts, and serum drug levels should be obtained for patients on chronic therapy.[140] Gabapentin is indicated for PHN and has been used successfully in a broad range of pain states, including neuropathy, multiple sclerosis, and migraine headache.[141,142] The dose range varies by response and patient tolerance and may range from 1,200 to 4,800 mg or more per day. The safety profile of gabapentin renders it a popular agent but because of its cost, it is not always a first-line consideration. Except for PHN and peripheral diabetic neuropathy, most reports on the efficacy of gabapentin are based on anecdotal cases.[143] Newer anticonvulsants, such as lamotrigine, may offer some use in the treatment of chronic neurogenic pain states in patients whose treatment with antidepressants or other anticonvulsants is unsuccessful.[144]

Pregabalin was approved in 2004 for postherpetic neuralgia with a similar mechanism of action as gabapentin. It seems to have more predictable pharmacokinetics, as absorption is not limited by active transporter saturability that occurs with gabapentin at higher doses.[145]

Other Medications. Lidocaine is also given for neuropathic syndromes, and like all local anesthetics, enters the CNS after intravenous administration. Mexiletine has been used in lidocaine-responsive patients requiring a longer acting agent, as the effects of lidocaine are short-lived. Both agents reduce neuronal firing via stabilization of sodium-conducting channels in nerve cell membranes. When administered systemically, they diffuse into the peripheral nerves. Analgesic doses of mexiletine are the same as those needed for antiarrhythmic effects (i.e., approximately 10 mg/kg/day to produce plasma levels of 0.75–2.0 μg/mL). The use of tocainide, an oral lidocaine analog, is not advised due to a higher incidence of serious adverse effects such as aplastic anemia. Side effects of lidocaine and mexiletine include dizziness, lightheadedness, ataxia, nausea, and vomiting. High doses of these agents can lead to tremor and convulsions. GI effects of mexiletine can be reduced by taking the medication with food or antacids.[146] The systemic side effects of lidocaine can be avoided by use of the lidocaine 5% patches, which are indicated for postherpetic neuralgia pain. The patches are generally well tolerated when applied to intact skin and do not normally produce clinically significant serum drug levels.

Intrapleural administration of bupivacaine has been performed in patients with rib fractures, and in patients with abdominal and thoracic pain following surgery, and exemplifies the many newer modalities available to the practitioner.[147]

Ziconotide (formerly known as SNX-111) was approved in 2004 and represents a novel class of biological poisons under investigation for the control of pain. Ziconotide is a peptide toxin derived from cone snails (conidae) of tropical ocean regions that use the poisons in harpoon-like structures to paralyze and kill their piscine prey. Their venom contains 100 or more peptides that target numerous ion channels and receptors in mammals, including several that are involved in disease. Fish die rapidly from minute quantities, while doses of 0.10 mg per hour or more are delivered intrathecally to humans who suffer from intractable pain conditions.[148]

Originally approved only for blepharospasm and spastic torticolis, botulinum toxin (Botox) has found popularity as a cosmetic agent (e.g., wrinkle treatment), and has been studied for myalgias of the upper or lower spinal column, including cervicomyalgia and low back pain. It has also been investigated for migraine headache and other pain syndromes. Unfortunately, the strength of evidence for these purposes has not yet led to approval by the Food and Drug Administration (FDA) for most pain indications.[149] The mechanism of action of botulinum toxin is disruption of neuromuscular impulses at the neuromuscular junction causing a temporary paralysis of the injected muscle via blockade of acetylcholine (ACh) release.

Two centrally acting α_2-agonists, clonidine and guanethidine, are also used for pain management. They reduce sympathetic outflow from the CNS by presynaptic inhibition of norepinephrine release. Clonidine may interact with opioid receptors by inducing the release of the endogenous peptide dynorphin, and has been used with some success in suppressing the symptoms of opioid withdrawal attributed to a hyperadrenergic state, including agitation, diarrhea, and sweating. This drug may also be used during surgery to reduce inhalation and opioid anesthetic requirements as it potentiates morphine analgesia. Unlike morphine, however, clonidine is not reversed by naloxone, though its actions can be blocked by κ-specific antagonists. Clonidine may also prove useful in patients with spinal cord injury and neuropathic and sympathetically mediated pain syndromes. It is available as an oral tablet or as a patch that provides constant blood levels of the drug for 5 to 7 days, thus increasing compliance. It is also available for intrathecal administration. Clonidine may produce orthostatic hypotension, so a candidate for therapy should first receive a baseline evaluation of blood pressure.[150,151] With a mechanism of action similar to that of clonidine, guanethidine is also used in patients with sympathetic pain. Guanethidine produces significant vasodilation, counteracting the vasoconstriction due to sympathetic hyperactivity with resultant warming of an affected extremity and a reduction in pain. Guanethidine holds promise in the treatment of pain associated with rheumatoid arthritis, as patient response to regional guanethidine blockade has been favorable.[152]

Peripheral α_1-antagonists (e.g., prazosin) have been used for the relief of sympathetically mediated pains such as reflex sympathetic dystrophy. Like clonidine, they produce vasodilation with significant orthostasis and should be dosed initially at bedtime to reduce the risk of syncope due to a precipitous drop in blood pressure. Doses can be gradually increased according to patient response and tolerance of side effects. Other agents used to relieve sympathetically mediated pain include intravenous phentolamine and oral phenoxybenzamine. However, these agents are nonselective for the α_1-receptor and also produce α_2-adrenergic effects. A test infusion of phentolamine can be used to predict guanethidine or prazosin response.[153] Unfortunately, the development of tachyphylaxis is frequent, and these drugs are often poorly tolerated.

Benzodiazepines such as diazepam are used for skeletal muscle relaxation and anxiolysis in the treatment of acute pain, while clonazepam has been used in the management of neuropathic and atypical facial pain. Side effects include sedation, cognitive impairment, and sometimes profound depression, all of which decrease activity of the pain patient, while some researchers believe benzodiazepines may even exacerbate pain. In addition, they produce habituation and serious withdrawal reactions including seizures. The elderly are more susceptible to these effects. Therefore, tricyclic antidepressants are more rational choices for relieving the insomnia and anxiety that accompanies chronic pain.[154]

Antihistamines, such as hydroxyzine and promethazine, have been used to augment the sedative or anxiolytic effects and reduce the itching associated with opioids. They may have some analgesic activity, although this is controversial.

Dextroamphetamine (5–10 mg/day) can be used in patients with cancer pain to overcome the sedation of opioids. It also relieves some vegetative effects of depression that often accompany a terminal diagnosis.[155] Methylphenidate (5–10 mg/day) has also been used for these purposes.

Special Considerations in Analgesic Pharmacotherapy. Opioids exert anticholinergic effects that can be compounded by the concomitant use of anticholinergic agents such as diphenhydramine, hydroxyzine, tricyclic antidepressants, or atropine. The most serious consequence of combined use of these drugs is precipitation of an anticholinergic crisis, manifested by psychosis, tachycardia, cardiac conduction abnormalities with possible first, second-degree or third-degree heart block, coma, and death by cardiorespiratory failure.

Alcohol is often used by patients with chronic pain to decrease suffering. They may drink themselves into a stupor to achieve pain relief by decreased consciousness. Combining analgesics and ethanol produces additive CNS depression with mood changes, depression of respiratory drive, and the danger of lethal overdose. Alcohol in combination with NSAIDs can lead to increased CNS side effects of the NSAIDs, such as disorientation and dizziness, and increased gastric irritation and ulceration.

As with alcohol and antihistamines, opioids can potentiate the effects of barbiturates, meprobamate or benzodiazepines, including transient delirium and respiratory failure. Of particular concern is the interaction between fentanyl and midazolam, an ultrashort acting benzodiazepine used in preoperative anesthetic "cocktails." This combination produced a few deaths from cardiorespiratory failure until lower doses of midazolam with more judicious perioperative monitoring of the patient were instituted.[156]

Patients with obstructive respiratory diseases, such as asthma and emphysema, or structural abnormalities, like kyphoscoliosis, are at greater risk of respiratory-driven depression with opioids. Half of the usual starting dose should be prescribed, titrating upward with careful attention to respiratory rate and oxygen saturation. Opioid suppression of the cerebellar chemoreceptor response to carbon dioxide can have catastrophic consequences in patients whose response to carbon dioxide is already blunted from chronic respiratory disease.

Patients with hepatic failure are at potential risk for drug-induced sequelae when given opioids or NSAIDs due to the inability of the liver to glucuronidate these agents for renal excretion. In addition, many NSAIDs have been shown to induce hepatocellular damage.[157] Acetaminophen is an agent commonly combined with centrally acting opioids. In patients with hepatic dysfunction secondary to alcoholic cirrhosis or hepatitis, chronic doses can precipitate hepatic failure. Cirrhosis also affects the disposition of opioids, as meperidine, pentazocine, and propoxyphene all exhibit increased bioavailability and decreased clearance.[158,159]

Most of the opioids are conjugated and demethylated in the liver to form nor-metabolites and glucuronide metabolites, both of which are excreted by the kidneys. In renal impairment, these metabolites accumulate and produce side effects that last longer than the biological half-lives of the parent compounds. This is particularly true of morphine, dihydrocodeine, propoxyphene, and meperidine. Methadone appears safe to use in renal dysfunction when administered at 12-hour or 24-hour intervals.[160,161]

NONPHARMACOLOGIC THERAPY

Surgery. Cordotomy is a method of severing the sympathetic chains that emanate from the spinal cord. Indications for such intervention are short life expectancy and specific unilateral or focal pain. In percutaneous cordotomy, a lesion is produced in the spinothalamic tract, most often at level of the first or second cervical vertebrae. This method has virtually replaced open cordotomy in which a quadrant of the spinal cord is almost completely severed at the cervical or thoracic level. Pain relief by either technique is transient, rarely lasting more than 2 years. The advantage of cordotomy includes analgesia without significant loss of motor function or touch sensation.[162]

Neuroablative Blocks and Neurolysis. Chemical destruction of nerves (neurolysis) is used at spinal nerve roots, and it is a relatively simple and painless procedure that can be done with minimal equipment. It is shorter acting than cordotomy, but unlike this procedure, can be done in the elderly and those with poor general health. Agents used include absolute alcohol and phenol.

Central and Peripheral Nervous System Stimulators. Various types of central and peripheral nervous system stimulators are used for neurogenic, neuropathic, and ischemic pain syndromes. Dorsal column stimulators (DCS) operate on a principle similar to that of TENS, as both produce analgesia by inducing partial depolarization of neurons. DCS consists of an electrode placed in the epidural space and attached to a programmable continuous-pulse pacemaker implanted into a subcutaneous pocket in the abdomen. A sensory thalamic stimulator (STS) consists of an electrode placed into the thalamus of the brain. DCS and STS are used in cases of intractable neurogenic pain unresponsive to medications or other therapies. Peripheral nerve stimulators (PNSs) are implantable devices that are most successful in pain syndromes caused by injury to a peripheral nerve. Newer stimulators are taking the form of thermal, vibrotactile, and magnetic stimulators, though these methods have not evolved sufficiently for widespread use in pain management.[163]

Physical Therapy. Physical and rehabilitative therapies have been used to treat acute pain resulting from sports injuries and chronic pain. The goals of physical therapy exercises and training are increased mobility, strength, and function, and a decrease in symptoms of pain or discomfort. Often, an additional goal is a return to employment.

ALTERNATIVE THERAPIES

ACUPUNCTURE

Acupuncture is a technique of specialized needle insertion along specific nerve tracts to alter electrochemical flow in nerve pathways and to reduce pain. It has been practiced in China and other Asian countries for centuries, and has gained popularity in the United States during the past few decades. Systemic effects are extremely rare, making it an alternative for patients with medical contraindications to drug therapies such as tricyclic antidepressants. It can also be used in conjunction with pharmacological therapies to improve response. With increasing acceptance of this practice, many health insurance companies now offer acupuncture as a covered benefit for their members. However, response is variable and unpredictable.[164]

HERBAL MEDICATIONS AND DIETARY SUPPLEMENTS

A variety of herbal medications have been used to treat pain arising from different regions of the body. Many of these herbal medicines contain volatile oils, such as camphor, and other compounds, such as sesquiterpene lactones and flavonoids. Feverfew (*Tanacetum parthenium*) contains all of these chemical entities and has been used for headache and rheumatic diseases (e.g., arthritis). It is thought to impede platelet aggregation and prostaglandin synthesis and release of antihistamines and other inflammatory mediators. Comfrey (*Symphytum officinale*), marigold (*Calendula officinalis*), peppermint (*Mentha piperita*), and primrose (*Primula elatior*) are a few examples of other herbals used for relief of muscle and neurogenic pain syndromes. It is difficult to find controlled clinical trials of these agents in humans, although some have undergone animal trials to identify their active components and the pharmacology of these components. Opium poppy (*Papaver somniferum*) is used as a natural analgesic in other parts of the world and gave rise to modern-day opioids such as morphine.[165] Marijuana (*Cannabis sativa*) is currently under investigation for analgesic properties using methods to evaluate the effects of cannabinoid receptors in mammals, but definitive trials are not yet documented. Over the past few years, two types of endogenous cannabinoid receptors have been found in mammalian tissues, but the function of these remains to be elucidated. The reader is referred to more extensive references for a complete review of herbal medications used for pain symptom relief.

Glucosamine and chondroitin sulfates are dietary supplements under investigation in clinical trials for relief of symptoms of osteoarthritis in weight-bearing joints such as the knee. Both are components of glycosaminoglycans. Glucosamine is also required for biosynthesis of glycoproteins, proteoglycans, and hyaluronate, all structural components of joint connective tissue. Limited studies comparing their use to NSAIDs are available, but more extensive trials are as yet unpublished.[166] The National Institutes of Health is currently investigating these agents.

PSYCHOLOGICAL INTERVENTIONS

Counseling, biofeedback, stress management training, and cognitive and behavioral techniques have been used to assist patients in reducing their symptoms of chronic pain. Self-hypnosis and self-relaxation are other methods used for this objective. In addition, such interventions can enhance coping skills and reduce disability and social isolation associated with long-term or lifelong painful conditions.[164] Meditation can also be useful in decreasing pain symptoms.

FUTURE THERAPIES

NMDA is an excitatory amino acid in the CNS that has been discovered to produce hyperalgesia of CNS origin. Glutamate may play a similar role in activating pain systems. Research into NMDA receptor antagonists has offered an exciting hint at the future of pharmacological agents for pain management. Such antagonists may prevent acute pain from transforming into chronic pain, and they may also attenuate opioid receptor tolerance when administered concomitantly.[167,168] Amanta-

dine, an antiviral drug also used in the treatment of Parkinson's disease, may show efficacy in managing neuropathy.[169] Ketamine, a commercially available anesthetic, is one such NMDA antagonist. Unfortunately, it is only available parenterally and produces occasional adverse reactions, such as dysphoria and hallucination. Dextrorphan, the demethylated metabolite of dextromethorphan, though not yet commercially available, is another agent undergoing investigation. Studies with combinations of dextromethorphan and morphine are ongoing.[170,171] Memantine appears to hold promise as an analgesic for some neuropathic pain syndromes.[172]

Cholecystokinin antagonists have gained attention for their role in analgesia based on observations that morphine-induced analgesia can be antagonized in vivo by cholecystokinin. Administration of proglumide, an investigational agent, potentiates morphine-induced analgesia in animals and humans. Calcium channel blockers may also potentiate morphine analgesia by modulation of calcium availability to the cell. These drugs, like proglumide, are devoid of any analgesic activity when given alone. Tizanidine, an α_2-adrenergic agonist with muscle relaxant properties, also offers hope for treating pain associated with myofascial dysfunction. Though chemically similar to clonidine, it is less potent in lowering blood pressure.

Endogenous opioid peptides (endorphins, dynorphins, and enkephalins) have not proven superior to exogenous opioids in the management of pain. Their analgesic effects are short in duration, and they produce the same side effects as drugs like morphine. Other nonopioid endogenous peptides have been suggested for their roles in pain modulation. Specific delta receptor agonists have risen to the forefront of opioid research. Recent evidence suggests they may produce analgesia without inducing habituation. Opioid peptides also show promise as therapeutic agents since they differ from opioids in several ways. Peptide analogs of enkephalins undergo degradation by placental enzymes, inhibiting or preventing their transfer across placental membranes. This would make them ideal agents in obstetrics by placing the fetus at less risk. Moreover, no δ-receptors have yet been demonstrated in fetal brain tissue, increasing the safety margin of future δ-specific peptides. Another advantage the peptides may have over their opioid counterparts is degradation to constituent amino acids instead of active and possibly toxic metabolites. There is less potential for renal or hepatic damage with such peptides. Fourth, peptide δ-agonists, as mentioned, are likely to have less dependence and abuse liability than μ-agonists or κ-agonists. Patients who have become tolerant to mu agonists such as morphine may benefit from little or no analgesic cross-tolerance with the delta opioid peptides.[173]

IMPROVING OUTCOMES

PATIENT EDUCATION

The pharmacist has a unique role in developing useful medicinal tools to ease suffering brought on by acute or chronic pain. Through rational drug prescribing habits and education of patients and caregivers, effective regimens can be designed to increase pain control while decreasing untoward drug side effects. The pharmacist can assist in implementing such regimens to reduce drug dependence and overall drug use while increasing patient activity. A movement toward pharmacist involvement with pain management teams is gaining momentum, as government and third-party insurers seek ways to reduce the financial burden of chronic pain in terms of dollars spent and work days lost due to disability. Specific patient education points should include the expected benefit of the drug(s), appropriate dose and schedule for administration, potential adverse reactions, and drug to drug or drug-disease interactions, and self-monitoring techniques for assessing response to therapy. Patients can be encouraged to maintain pain diaries documenting their pain levels and medication use throughout the day to assist health care providers in designing the most effective regimens. Pharmacist education regarding tapering or titration schedules is fundamental to optimal pain management, and written instructions should be provided along with verbal explanations of dosing schedules. The consequences of nonadherence should be emphasized.

METHODS TO IMPROVE ADHERENCE TO DRUG THERAPY

In acute pain management, time contingent dosing should be used initially to prevent escalating pain with downward tapering of the analgesic doses as pain severity allows. This can usually take place 1 to 2 days after the precipitating event. As above, written instruction will prevent confusion and ensure appropriate analgesic use. Chronic pain management should also involve time-contingent dosing regimens, and patients will require education regarding expectations for nonopioid analgesics. In particular, patients should be instructed not to use medications with latency to onset (e.g., tricyclic antidepressants) on a prn basis. They should be informed of the delay in obtaining therapeutic efficacy to avoid premature discontinuation or escalation of medications. Patients should also have another caregiver, such as a family member, who understands the medication regimen and can assist in monitoring for beneficial and deleterious effects of drug therapy. This is particularly true of the elderly, who may become forgetful if prescribed medications that produce cognitive impairment (opioids, antidepressants, neuroleptics, benzodiazepines, or muscle relaxants) and lead to over or under compliance with the specified regimen. The pharmacist should offer himself as a source of information and instruction and encourage patients to return if any problems with drug therapy develop.

DISEASE MANAGEMENT STRATEGIES TO IMPROVE PATIENT OUTCOMES

Multidisciplinary methods of pain management are the focus of effective treatment for complex chronic pain syndromes. The goal of centers utilizing these methods is not to ''cure'' pain, as this is often unachievable, but to ease the suffering of chronic pain patients and to reduce their reliance on opioids and other analgesics. These centers strive to improve pain control and improve psychological and physical functioning and conditioning by involving specialists in the fields of anesthesia, neurology/neurosurgery, clinical pharmacy, physical therapy, physiatry, psychiatry, psychology, and nursing.

The pharmacist's role in researching nontraditional medicines for pain relief is also integral to providing optimal care. In studies involving the use of lidocaine, antidepressants, and anticonvulsants for relief of chronic pain, pharmacists have served as coinvestigators. Even in the areas of traditional pain management, they can monitor medication compliance and efficacy. In the multidisciplinary setting, the pharmacist can provide counseling and guidance to patients who are adjusting their intake of antidepressants, anticonvulsants, or other nonopioid medications and monitor rational opioid use. A lucid understanding of pharmacology and pharmacokinetics is invaluable in this setting, since opioid habituation, abstinence, or narcosis are highly undesirable and counterproductive. Many clinic settings allow the pharmacist to see patients on a regular basis, documenting pain relief scores, monitoring side effects, determining when and by how much medication doses should be increased or decreased, selecting alternatives to nontolerated medications, and obtaining pharmacokinetic data or other laboratory parameters. Using the pharmacist's knowledge of real or potential drug interactions can assist in designing regimens that will be most useful in treating patients with acute or chronic debilitating pain syndromes.

PHARMACOECONOMICS

NSAIDs account for about $500 million annually of U.S. drug expenditures, while opioids and adjunctive medication therapies are associated with lower expenditures. However, clinically significant GI events (e.g., GI hemorrhage) attributed to NSAIDs may cause as many as 15,000 or more deaths in the United States each year and account for large expenditures related to hospitalization. Addition of misoprostol or antiulcer therapies can also increase the therapeutic costs of using NSAIDs. It is unknown at this time if newer COX–2-specific NSAIDs will impact these expenditures, as long-term postmarketing surveillance is required to make such a determination. Controversy over cardiovascular risks of COX-2 drugs may also introduce countervaling pharmacoeconomic arguments against their use due to the costs associated with increased morbidity and mortality.

Lost work days, frequent contacts with medical personnel, disability insurance premiums, and disability payments due to chronic pain also have a significant effect on the economy, although the global impact can only be estimated. Intangible factors, such as diminished quality of life, psychological changes (e.g., depression), and social isolation produced by chronic pain cannot be adequately measured.

The pharmacist can play a key role in reducing such economic burdens by educating patients and caregivers of the potential for adverse drug reactions and drug to drug interactions and can assist in screening patients who are at high risk for such untoward events. In addition, the pharmacist can help design medication regimens that minimize pharmacological overlap and optimize synergistic or additive effects of analgesics with different mechanisms of action.

KEY POINTS

Pain continues to be an enigmatic entity, but advances in molecular biology research are providing clues to more specific mechanisms of pain generation and chronicity. With better targeted therapies, patients should be able to expect adequate pain relief with a minimum of adverse events.

- Therapy should be directed to decrease subjective intensity and duration of the pain complaint, decrease the potential for conversion of acute pain to chronic persistent pain syndromes, decrease suffering and disability associated with pain
- Decrease psychological and socioeconomic sequelae associated with undertreatment of pain
- Minimize adverse reactions or intolerance to pain management therapies
- Optimize drug therapy to avoid drug to drug interactions
- Improve the patient's overall quality of life and ability to perform activities of daily living
- The pharmacist should use his or her unique understanding of drug mechanisms to develop effective treatment regimens in collaboration with other members of the patient's health care team
- The pharmacist should provide relevent and specific knowledge about opioids, NSAIDs, and other medications for pain relief, and be willing to contrast the costs and benefits of any therapies under consideration
- The pharmacist should also function as the primary provider of patient and physician education, and should assist in monitoring the outcome of pharmacological interventions
- The pharmacist can provide comparative information on the pharmacoeconomics of various drug therapies to mimimize the cost burdens of pain to society and to the individual patient

SUGGESTED READINGS

AGS Panel on Persistent Pain in Older Persons. The Management of Persistent Pain in Older Persons. JAGS 50:S205–S224, 2002.
Argoff CE. Pharmacologic management of chronic pain. J Am Osteopath Assoc 102 (Suppl 3):S21–S27, 2002.
Backonja M. Neuromodulating drugs for the symptomatic treatment of neuropathic pain. Curr Pain Headache Rep 8:212–216, 2004.
Clinical Practice Guideline. Management of cancer pain in adults and children. American Pain Society, 2005.
Crofford LJ. Specific cyclooxygenase-2 inhibitors: what have we learned since they came into widespread clinical use? Curr Opin Rheumatol 14:225–230, 2002.
Dworkin RH, Backonja M, Rowbotham MC, et al. Advances in neuropathic pain: diagnosis, mechanisms, and treatment recommendations. Arch Neurol 60:1524–1534, 2003.

REFERENCES

1. Merskey H. IASP Committee on Taxonomy, Classification of chronic pain: descriptions of chronic pain syndromes and definitions of pain terms. Pain (Suppl 3):S28–S217, 1986.
2. American Pain Society. Principles of analgesic use in the treatment of acute pain and chronic cancer pain. 2nd ed. Clin Pharm 9: 601–611, 1990.
3. Crombie IK. Epidemiology of persistent pain. In Jensen TS, Turner JA, Wiesenfeld-Hallin Z: Proceedings of the Eighth World Congress on Pain, Progress in Pain Research and Management, Seattle, WA, IASP Press, 1997:53–55.
4. Von Korff M, Dworkin SF, Le Resche L. Graded chronic pain status: an epidemiologic evaluation. Pain 40:279–291, 1990.
5. Clinical Standards Advisory Group. Epidemiology review: the epidemiology and cost of back pain. Annex to the CSAG Report on Back Pain. London: HMSO, 1994:1–72.
6. Felson DT. An update on the pathogenesis and epidemiology of osteoarthritis. Radiol Clin North Am 42:1–9, 2004.
7. Ganong WF. Review of medical physiology. Los Altos, California: Lange Medical Publications, 1985:105.
8. Wall PD. Presynaptic control of impulses at the first central synapse in the cutaneous pathway. In: Physiology of Spinal Neurons. Progress in Brain Research 12. Amsterdam: Elsevier, 1964:92–118.
9. Fields HL. Pain. New York: McGraw-Hill Book Company, 1987: 13–28.
10. Pogatzki EM, Gebhart GF, Brennan TJ. Characterization of Adelta- and C-fibers innervating the plantar rat hindpaw one day after an incision. J Neurophysiol 87:721–731, 2002.
11. Price DD, McHaffie JG, Larson MA. Spatial summation of heat-induced pain: influence of stimulus area and spatial separation of stimuli on perceived pain sensation intensity and unpleasantness. J Neurophysiol 62:1270–1279, 1989.
12. Torebjork HE. Afferent C units responding to mechanical, thermal and chemical stimuli in human non-glabrous skin. Acta Physiol Scand 92:374–390, 1974.
13. Koltzenburg M, Torebjork HE, Wahren LK. Nociceptor modulated central sensitization causes mechanical hyperalgesia in acute chemogenic and chronic neuropathic pain. Brain 117:579–591, 1994.
14. Cook AJ, Woolf CJ, Wall PD, et al. Dynamic receptive field plasticity in rat spinal cord dorsal horn following C-primary afferent input. Nature 325:151–153, 1987.
15. Willis WD. The origin and destination of pathways involved in pain transmission. In: Wall PD, Melzack R, eds. Textbook of pain. 2nd ed. New York: Churchill Livingstone, 1989:112–123.
16. Vierck CJ Jr, Greenspan JD, Ritz LA. Long-term changes in purposive and reflexive responses to nociceptive stimulation following anterolateral chordotomy. J Neurosci 10:2077–2095, 1990.
17. Campbell JN. Examination of possible mechanisms by which stimulation of the spinal cord in man relieves pain. Appl Neurophysiol 44:181–186, 1981.
18. Yaksh TL, Aimone LD, The central pharmacology of pain transmission. In: Wall PD, Melzack R, eds. Textbook of pain. 2nd ed. New York: Churchill Livingstone, 1989:190.
19. Perl ER. Sensitization of nociceptors and its relation to sensation. In: Bonica JJ, Albe-Fessard D, eds. Advances in pain research and therapy. Vol I. New York: Raven Press, 1976:17–28.
20. Habelt C, Kessler F, Distler C, et al. Interactions of inflammatory mediators and low pH not influenced by capsazepine in rat cutaneous nociceptors. Neuroreport 11:973–976, 2000.
21. Taiwo YO, Bjerknes LK, Goetzl EJ, et al. Mediation of primary afferent peripheral hyperalgesia by the cAMP second messenger system. Neurosci 32:577–580, 1989.

22. Ferreira SH. Prostaglandins, aspirin-like drugs, and analgesia. Nature 240:200–203, 1972.

23. Taiwo YO, Heller PH, Levine JD. Characterization of distinct phospholipases mediating bradykinin and noradrenaline hyperalgesia. Neuroscience 39:523–531, 1990.

24. Cunha JM, Sachs D, Canetti CA, et al. The critical role of leukotriene B4 in antigen-induced mechanical hyperalgesia in immunised rats. Br J Pharmacol 139:1135–1145, 2003.

25. De Miguel E, Arnalich F, Tato E, et al. The effect of gold salts on substance P levels in rheumatoid arthritis. Neurosci Lett 174: 185–187, 1994.

26. Law PY, Wong YH, Loh HH. Molecular mechanisms and regulation of opioid receptor signaling. Annual Rev Pharmacol Toxicol 40:389–430, 2000.

27. Yaksh TL. Pharmacology and mechanisms of opioid analgesic activity. Acta Anaesthesiol Scand 41:94–111, 1997.

28. Harris JA, Chang PC, Drake CT. Kappa opioid receptors in rat spinal cord: sex-linked distribution differences. Neuroscience 124: 879–890, 2004.

29. Bie B, Pan ZZ. Presynaptic mechanism for anti-analgesic and anti-hyperalgesic actions of kappa-opioid receptors. J Neurosci 23: 7262–7268, 2003.

30. Chaturvedi K. Opioid peptides, opioid receptors and mechanism of down regulation. Indian J Exp Biol 41:5–13, 2003.

31. Goldstein A, James IF. Multiple opiate receptors: criteria for identification and classification. Trends Pharmacol Sci 5:503–505, 1984.

32. Taiwo YO, Levine JD. Prostaglandins inhibit endogenous pain control mechanisms by blocking transmission at spinal noradrenergic synapses. J Neurosci 8:1346–1349, 1988.

33. Levine JD, Taiwo YO. Involvement of the mu-opiate receptor in peripheral analgesia. Neurosci 32:571–575, 1989.

34. Sollevi A. Adenosine for pain control. Acta Anaesthesiol Scand 110 (Suppl):135–136, 1997.

35. Sarne Y, Fields A, Keren O, et al. Stimulatory effects of opioids on transmitter release and possible cellular mechanisms: overview and original results. Neurochem Res 21:1353–1361, 1996.

36. Crain SM, Shen KF. Modulatory effects of Gs-coupled excitatory opioid receptor functions on opioid analgesia, tolerance, and dependence. Neurochem Res 21:1347–1351, 1996.

37. Anderson R, Saiers JH, Abram S, et al. Accuracy in equianalgesic dosing. Conversion dilemmas. J Pain Symptom Manage 21: 397–406, 2001.

38. Fundytus ME. Glutamate receptors and nociception: implications for the drug treatment of pain. CNS Drugs 15:29–58, 2001.

39. Jaffe JH, Martin WR. Opioid analgesics and antagonists. In: Gilman AG, Goodman LS, Rall TW, Murad F, eds. The pharmacological basis of therapeutics. 10th ed. New York: Macmillan, 2001: 491–531.

40. Thompson DR. Narcotic analgesic effects on the sphincter of Oddi: a review of the data and therapeutic implications in treating pancreatitis. Am J Gastroenterol 96:1266–1272, 2001.

41. Wu SD, Kong J, Wang W, et al. Effect of morphine and M-cholinoceptor blocking drugs on human sphincter of Oddi during choledochofiberscopy manometry. Hepatobiliary Pancreat Dis Int 2: 121–125, 2003.

42. Henderson SO, Swadron S, Newton E. Comparison of intravenous ketorolac and meperidine in the treatment of biliary colic. J Emerg Med 23:237–241, 2002.

43. Romagnoli A, Keats AS. Ceiling effect for respiratory depression by nalbuphine. Clin Pharmacol Ther 27:478–485, 1980.

44. Eisenach JC, De Kock M, Klimscha W. Alpha(2)-adrenergic agonists for regional anesthesia. A clinical review of clonidine (1984–1995). Anesthesiology 85:655–674, 1996.

45. Howe JR, Wang JY, Yaksh TL. Selective antagonism of the antinociceptive effect of intrathecally applied alpha-adrenergic agonists by intrathecal prazosin and intrathecal yohimbine. J Pharmacol Exp Ther 224:552–558, 1983.

46. Sawynok J. The 1988 Merck Frosst Award. The role of ascending and descending noradrenergic and serotonergic pathways in opioid and non-opioid antinociception as revealed by lesion studies. Can J Physiol Pharmacol 67:975–988, 1989.

47. Max MB, Lynch SA, Muir J, et al. Effects of desipramine, amitriptyline, and fluoxetine on pain in diabetic neuropathy. N Engl J Med 326:1250–1256, 1992.

48. Watkins LR, Mayer DJ. Multiple endogenous opiate and non-opiate analgesia systems: evidence of their existence and clinical implications.Ann N Y Acad Sci 467:273–299, 1986.

49. Gerner P. Tricyclic antidepressants and their local anesthetic properties: from bench to bedside and back again. Reg Anesth Pain Med 29:286–289, 2004.

50. Hartvig P, Gillberg PG, Gordh T Jr, et al. Cholinergic mechanisms in pain and analgesia. Trends Pharmacol Sci (Suppl):75–79, 1989.

51. Bartusch SL, Sanders BJ, D'Alessio JG, et al. Clonazepam for the treatment of lancinating phantom limb pain. Clin J Pain 12:59–62, 1996.

52. Panerai AE, Sacerdote P, Bianchi M, et al. Neuropharmacological approach to nociception. In: Lipton S, Tunks E, Zoppi M, eds. Advances in pain research and therapy. Vol. 13. The Pain Clinic. New York: Raven Press, 1990:41–44.

53. Zieglgansberger W. Dorsal horn neuropharmacology: baclofen and morphine. Ann N Y Acad Sci 531:150–156, 1988.

54. Bonica JJ. The management of pain. 2nd ed. Philadelphia: Lea & Febiger, 1990.

55. Dina OA, Aley KO, Isenberg W, et al. Sex hormones regulate the contribution of PKCepsilon and PKA signaling in inflammatory pain in the rat. Eur J Neurosci 13:2227–2233, 2001.

56. Fields HL. The Medical Center at the University of California, San Francisco Pain Questionnaire, copyright 1988.

57. Bieri D, Reeve RA, Champion GD, et al. The faces pain scale for the self-assessment of the severity of pain experienced by children: development, initial validation, and preliminary investigation for ratio scale properties. Pain 41:139–150, 1990.

58. Peters ML, Schmidt AJ. Human pain responsivity. Pain 41: 117–121, 1990.

59. Sternbach RA. Clinical aspects of pain. In: Sternbach RA, ed. The psychology of pain. 2nd ed. New York: Raven Press, 1986: 223–239.

60. Foley KM. Cancer pain syndromes. J Pain Symp Manag 2:T3–T7, 1987.

61. Portenoy R. Drug therapy for cancer pain. Am J Hosp Palliat Care 7:10–19, 1990.

62. Inturrisi CE. Newer methods of opioid drug delivery. In: IASP refresher course on pain management: book of abstracts. Hamburg, West Germany: International Association for the Study of Pain, 1987:27–39.

63. McDonnell FJ, Sloan JW, Hamann SR. Advances in cancer pain management. Curr Pain Headache Rep 5:265–271, 2001.

64. Vinholes JJ, Purohit OP, Abbey ME, et al. Relationships between biochemical and symptomatic response in a double-blind randomised trial of pamidronate for metastatic bone disease. Annals of Oncology 8:1243–1250, 1997.

65. Janjan N. Bone metastases: approaches to management. Semin Oncol 28 (Suppl 11):28–34, 2001.

66. World Health Organization. Cancer Pain Relief. Geneva: World Health Organization, 1986.

67. Inturrisi CE, Max MB, Foley KM, et al. The pharmacokinetics of heroin in patients with chronic pain. N Engl J Med 210: 1213–1217, 1984.

68. Farrar JT, Portenoy RK. Neuropathic cancer pain: the role of adjuvant analgesics. Oncology (Huntingt) 15:1435–1453, 2001.

69. Portenoy RK, Foley KM, Inturrisi CE. The nature of opioid responsiveness and its implications for neuropathic pain: new hypotheses derived from studies of opioid infusions. Pain 43:273–286, 1990.

70. Rowbotham MC, Twilling L, Davies PS, et al. Oral opioid therapy for chronic peripheral and central neuropathic pain. N Engl J Med 348:1223–1232, 2003.

71. Satterthwaite JR. Acute herpes zoster: Diagnosis and treatment. Pain Management 3:17–28, 1990.

72. Portenoy RK, Duma C, Foley KM. Acute herpetic and postherpetic neuralgia: clinical review and current management. Ann Neurol 20: 651–664, 1986.

73. Loeser JD. Postherpetic neuralgia: a review of pathophysiology and treatment. Presented at: Annual Meeting of the American Pain Society; November 8, 1986; Washington, DC.

74. Rowbotham M, Harden N, Stacey B, et al. Gabapentin for the treatment of postherpetic neuralgia: a randomized controlled trial. JAMA 280:1837–1842, 1998.

75. Backonja M. Neuromodulating drugs for the symptomatic treatment of neuropathic pain. Curr Pain Headache Rep 8:212–216, 2004.

76. Argoff CE, Katz N, Backonja M. Treatment of postherpetic neuralgia: a review of therapeutic options. J Pain Symptom Manage 28:396–411, 2004.

77. Bernstein JE, Korman NJ, Bickers DR, et al. Topical capsaicin treatment of chronic postherpetic neuralgia. J Am Acad Dermatol 21:265–270, 1989.

78. De Benedittis G, Lorenzetti A. Topical aspirin/diethyl ether mixture versus indomethacin and diclofenac/diethyl ether mixtures for acute herpetic neuralgia and postherpetic neuralgia: a double-blind crossover placebo-controlled study. Pain 65:45–51, 1996.

79. Abadir AR, Kraynack BJ, Mayda J II, et al. Postherpetic neuralgia: response to topical clonidine. Proc West Pharmacol Soc 39:47–48, 1996.

80. Galer BS, Harle J, Rowbotham MC. Response to intravenous lidocaine infusion predicts subsequent response to oral mexiletine: a prospective study. J Pain Symptom Manage 12:161–167, 1996.

81. Max MB, Schafer SC, Culnane M, et al. Association of pain relief with drug side effects in postherpetic neuralgia: a single-dose study of clonidine, codeine, ibuprofen, and placebo. Clin Pharmacol Ther 43:363–371, 1988.

82. Bach FW, Jensen TS, Kastrup J, et al. The effect of intravenous lidocaine on nociceptive processing in diabetic neuropathy. Pain 40:29–34, 1990.

83. Masson EA, Boulton AJ. Aldose reductase inhibitors in the treatment of diabetic neuropathy. A review of the rationale and clinical evidence. Drugs 39:190–202, 1990.

84. Halbert J, Crotty M, Cameron ID. Evidence for the optimal management of acute and chronic phantom pain: a systematic review. Clin J Pain 18:84–92, 2002.

85. Nikolajsen L, Jensen TS. Phantom limb pain. Br J Anaesth 87:107–116, 2001.

86. Fine PG. The pharmacologic management of sympathetically maintained pain. Hosp Formu 23:796–808, 1988.

87. Stanton-Hicks M. Complex regional pain syndrome. Anesthesiol Clin North Am 21:733–744, 2003.

88. Currie S. Inflammatory myopathies. Polymyositis and related disorders. In: Walton JN, ed. Disorders of voluntary muscle. 4th ed. Edinburgh: Churchill Livingstone, 1981:525–568.

89. Sorenson J, Graven-Nielsen T, Henriksson KG, et al. Hyperexcitability in fibromyalgia. J Rheumatol 25:152–155, 1998.

90. Wolfe F, Cathey MA, Hawley DJ. A double-blind placebo controlled trial of fluoxetine in fibramyalgia. Scand J Rheumatol 23:255–259, 1994.

91. Guis S, Mattei JP, Liote F. Drug-induced and toxic myopathies. Best Pract Res Clin Rheumatol 17:877–907, 2003.

92. Criswell LA, Sack KE. Tryptophan-induced eosinophilia myalgia syndrome. West J Med 153:269–274, 1990.

93. Claster S, Vichinsky EP. Managing sickle cell disease. BMJ 327:1151–1155, 2003.

94. Ellory JC, Culliford SJ, Smith PA, et al. Specific inhibition of Ca-activated K channels in red cells by selected dihydropyridine derivatives. Br J Pharmacol 111:903–905, 1994.

95. Andersen G, Christrup L, Sjogren P. Relationships among morphine metabolism, pain and side effects during long-term treatment: an update. J Pain Symptom Manage 25:74–91, 2003.

96. Hoskin PJ, Hanks GW, Aherne GW, et al. The bioavailability and pharmacokinetics of morphine after intravenous, oral and buccal administration in healthy volunteers. Br J Clin Pharmacol 27:499–505, 1989.

97. AHFS Drug Information. Bethesda, MD: American Society of Hospital Pharmacists, 2004:1671–1720.

98. Reidenberg MM, Goodman H, Erle H, et al. Hydromorphone levels and pain control in patients with severe chronic pain. Clin Pharmacol Ther 44:376–382, 1988.

99. Foley KM. Controversies in cancer pain: medical perspectives. Cancer 63:2257–2265, 1989.

100. Kaiko RF, Foley KM, Grabinsky PY, et al. Central nervous system excitatory effects of meperidine in cancer patients. Ann Neurol 13:180–185, 1983.

101. Roy SD, Flynn GL. Transdermal delivery of narcotic analgesics: pH, anatomical, and subject influences on cutaneous permeability of fentanyl and sufentanil. Pharmaceut Res 7:842–847, 1990.

102. Stamer UM, Maier C, Grond S, et al. Tramadol in the management of post-operative pain: a double-blind, placebo- and active drug-controlled study. Eur Acad Anaesth 14:646–654, 1997.

103. Lee RC, McTavish D, Sorkin EM. Tramadol—A preliminary review of its pharmacodynamic and pharmacokinetic properties, and therapeutic potential in acute and chronic pain states. Drugs 46:313–340, 1993.

104. Meyers FJ, Meyers FH. Management of chronic pain. Am Fam Physician 36:139–146, 1987.

105. O'Brien JJ, Benfield P. Dezocine: a preliminary review of its pharmacokinetic properties, and therapeutic efficacy. Drugs 38:226–248, 1989.

106. Yuan CS. Clinical status of methylnaltrexone, a new agent to prevent and manage opioid-induced side effects. J Support Oncol 2:111–122, 2004.

107. Kurz A, Sessler DI. Opioid-induced bowel dysfunction: pathophysiology and potential new therapies. Drugs 63:649–671, 2003.

108. Macintyre PE. Safety and efficacy of patient-controlled analgesia. Br J Anaesth 87:36–46, 2001.

109. Magora F. The spinal route. In: Lipton S, Tunks E, Zoppi M, eds. Advances in pain research and therapy. Vol. 13. The Pain Clinic. New York: Raven Press, 1990:309–314.

110. Max MB, Inturrisi CE, Kaiko RF, et al. Epidural and intrathecal opiates: cerebrospinal fluid and plasma profiles in patients with chronic cancer pain. Clin Pharmacol Ther 38:631–641, 1985.

111. Gourlay GK, Cherry DA, Plummer JL, et al. The influence of drug polarity on the absorption of opioid drugs into CSF and subsequent cephalad migration following lumbar epidural administration: application to morphine and pethidine. Pain 31:297–305, 1987.

112. Rawal N, Arner S, Gustaffson LL, et al. Present state of extradural and intradural opioid analgesia in Sweden. A nationwide follow-up survey. Br J Anaesth 59:791–799, 1987.

113. Onofrio BM, Yaksh TL. Long-term pain relief produced by intrathecal morphine infusion in 53 patients. J Neurosurg 72:200–209, 1990.

114. Coombs DW, Saunders RL, Fratkin JD, et al. Continuous intrathecal hydromorphone and clonidine for intractable cancer pain. J Neurosurg 64:890–894, 1986.

115. Dickinson AH, Sullivan AF, McQuay HJ. Intrathecal etorphine, fentanyl and buprenorphine on spinal nociceptive neurones in the rat. Pain 42:227–234, 1990.

116. Jacobson L, Chabal C, Brody MC, et al. Intrathecal methadone: a dose-response study and comparison with intrathecal morphine 0.5 mg. Pain 43:141–148, 1990.

117. Yaksh TL, Stevens CW. Properties of the modulation of spinal nociceptive transmission by receptor-selective agents. In: Dubner R, Gebhart GF, Bond MR, eds. Proceedings of the fifth world congress on pain. Amsterdam: Elsevier, 1988:417–435.

118. Viscusi ER. Emerging techniques for postoperative analgesia in orthopedic surgery. Am J Orthop 33 (5 Suppl):13–16, 2004.

119. McDonnell FJ, Sloan JW, Hamann SR. Advances in cancer pain management. Curr Oncol Rep 2:351–357, 2000.

120. McCormack K. The spinal actions of nonsteroidal anti-inflammatory drugs and the dissociation between their anti-inflammatory and analgesic effects. Drugs 47 (Suppl 5):28–45, 1994.

121. Jurna I, Brune K. Central effect of the non-steroid anti-inflammatory agents, indomethacin, ibuprofen, and diclofenac, determined in C fibre-evoked activity in single neurones of the rat thalamus. Pain 41:71–80, 1990.

122. Harris RH, Vavra I. Ketoprofen. In: Rainsford KD, ed. Anti-inflammatory and anti-rheumatic drugs. Vol II. Newer anti-inflammatory drugs. Boca Raton, Florida: CRC Press, 1985:151–170.

123. Sunshine A, Olson NZ. Analgesic efficacy of ketoprofen in postpartum, general surgery, and chronic cancer pain. J Clin Pharmacol 28:S47–S54, 1988.

124. Buckley MMT, Brogden RN. Ketorolac. A review of its pharmacodynamic and pharmacokinetic properties, and therapeutic potential. Drugs 39:86–109, 1990.

125. Gillis JC, Brogden RN. Ketorolac. A reappraisal of its pharmacodynamic and pharmacokinetic properties and therapeutic use in pain management. Drugs 53:139–88, 1997.

126. Wiseman EH. Pharmacologic studies with a new class of nonsteroidal anti-inflammatory agents—the oxicams—with special reference to piroxicam (Feldene). Am J Med 72:2–8, 1982.

127. Masferrer JL, Isakson PC, Seibert K. Cyclooxygenase-2 inhibitors: a new class of anti-inflammatory agents that spare the gastrointestinal tract. Gastroenterol Clin North Am 25:363–372, 1996.
128. FitzGerald GA. Coxibs and cardiovascular disease. N Engl J Med 351:1709–1711, 2004.
129. Lynch ME. Antidepressants as analgesics: a review of randomized controlled trials. J Psychiatry Neurosci 26:30–36, 2001.
130. Lee R, Spencer PS. Antidepressants and pain a review of the pharmacological data supporting the use of certain tricyclics in chronic pain. J Int Med Res 5 (1 Suppl):146–156, 1977.
131. Feinmann C. Pain relief by antidepressants: possible modes of action. Pain 23:1–8, 1985.
132. Bryson HM, Wilde MI. Amitriptyline. A review of its pharmacological properties and therapeutic use in chronic pain states. Drugs Aging 8:459–76, 1996.
133. Messing RB, Lytle LD. Serotonin-containing neurons: their possible role in pain and analgesia. Pain 4:1–21, 1977.
134. Magi G. The use of antidepressants in the treatment of chronic pain. Drugs 42:730–748, 1991.
135. Food and Drug Administration. Cymbalta (duloxetine) [package insert]. Available at: http://www.fda.gov/medwatch/SAFETY/2004/sep_PI/Cymbalta_PI.pdf. Accessed December 2004.
136. Sindrup SH, Gram LF, Brosen K, et al. The selective serotonin reuptake inhibitor paroxetine is effective in the treatment of diabetic neuropathy syndromes. Pain 42:135–145, 1990.
137. Davis JL, Lewis SB, Gerich JE, et al. Peripheral diabetic neuropathy treated with amitriptyline and fluphenazine. JAMA 238:2291–2292, 1977.
138. McGee JL, Alexander MR. Phenothiazine analgesia: fact or fantasy. Am J Hosp Pharm 36:633–650, 1979.
139. Bigal ME, Bordini CA, Speciali JG. Intravenous chlorpromazine in the emergency department treatment of migraines: a randomized controlled trial. J Emerg Med 23:141–148, 2002.
140. Spina E, Perugi G. Antiepileptic drugs: indications other than epilepsy. Epileptic Disord 6:57–75, 2004.
141. Backonja M, Beydoun A, Edwards KR, et al. Gabapentin for the symptomatic treatment of painful neuropathy in patients with diabetes mellitus: a randomized controlled trial. JAMA 280:1831–1836, 1998.
142. Rowbotham M, Harden N, Stacey B, et al. Gabapentin for the treatment of postherpetic neuralgia: a randomized controlled trial. JAMA 280:1837–1842, 1998.
143. Rosenberg JM, Harrell C, Ristic H, et al. The effect of gabapentin on neuropathic pain. Clin J Pain 13:251–255, 1997.
144. Dworkin RH, Backonja M, Rowbotham MC, et al. Advances in neuropathic pain: diagnosis, mechanisms, and treatment recommendations. Arch Neurol 60:1524–1534, 2003.
145. Bockbrader HN, Hunt T, Strand J, et al. Pregabalin pharmacokinetics and safety in healthy volunteers: results from two phase 1 studies. Neurology 54 (Suppl. 3):A421, 2000.
146. Chabal C, Russell LC, Burchiel KJ. The effects of intravenous lidocaine, tocainide and mexiletine on spontaneously active fibers originating in rat sciatic neuromas. Pain 38:333–338, 1989.
147. Rocco A, Reiestad F, Gudman J, et al. Intrapleural administration of local anesthetics for pain relief in patients with multiple rib fractures. Reg Anaesth 12:10–14, 1987.
148. Schroeder CI, Smythe ML, Lewis RJ. Development of small molecules that mimic the binding of omega-conotoxins at the N-type voltage-gated calcium channel. Mol Divers 8:127–134, 2004.
149. Aoki KR. Evidence for antinociceptive activity of botulinum toxin type A in pain management. Headache 43 (Suppl 1):S9–S15, 2003.
150. Crawley JN, Laverty R, Roth RH. Clonidine reversal of increased norepinephrine metabolite levels during morphine withdrawal. Eur J Pharmacol 57:247–250, 1979.
151. Maze M, Segal IS, Bloor BC. Clonidine and other alpha₂ adrenergic agonists: strategies for the rational use of these novel anesthetic agents. J Clin Anesth 1:146–157, 1988.
152. Levine JD, Fye K, Heller P, et al. Clinical response to regional intravenous guanethidine in patients with rheumatoid arthritis. J Rheumatol 13:1040–1043, 1986.
153. Exton JH. Mechanisms involved in α-adrenergic phenomena. Am J Physiol 248:E633–E647, 1985.
154. King SA, Strain JJ. Benzodiazepines and chronic pain. Pain 40:3–4, 1990.
155. Forrest WH, Brown BW, Brown CR, et al. Dextroamphetamine with morphine for the treatment of postoperative pain. New Engl J Med 296:712–715, 1977.
156. Forster A, Morel D, Bachmann M, et al. Respiratory depressant effects of different doses of midazolam and lack of reversal with naloxone -a double-blind randomized study. Anesth Analg 62:920–924, 1983.
157. Masubuchi Y, Saito H, Horie T. Structural requirements for the hepatotoxicity of nonsteroidal anti-inflammatory drugs in isolated rat hepatocytes. J Pharmacol Exper Ther 287:208–213, 1998.
158. Seeff LB, Cuccherini BA, Zimmerman HJ, et al. Acetaminophen hepatotoxicity in alcoholics. Ann Int Med 104:399–404, 1986.
159. Neal EA, Meffin PJ, Gregory PB, et al. Enhanced bioavailability and decreased clearance of analgesics in patients with cirrhosis. Gastroenterol 77:96–102, 1979.
160. Wolfert AI, Sica DA. Narcotic usage in renal failure [editorial]. Int J Artif Organs 11:411–415, 1988.
161. Kreek MJ, Schecter AJ, Gutjahr CL, et al. Methadone use in patients with chronic renal disease. Drug Alcohol Depend 5:197–205, 1980.
162. Siegfried J. Neurosurgical treatment of neurogenic pain. In: Lipton S, Tunks E, Zoppi M, eds. Advances in pain research and therapy. Vol. 13. The Pain Clinic. New York: Raven Press, 1990:207–215.
163. McGlone FP, Marsh D. Stimulators for treatment of pain. In: Lipton S, Tunks E, Zoppi M, eds. Advances in pain research and therapy. Vol. 13. The Pain Clinic. New York: Raven Press, 1990:79–82.
164. Justins DM. Management strategies for chronic pain. Ann Rheum Dis 55:588–596, 1996.
165. Gruenwald J, Brendler T, Jaenicke C (eds). PDR for Herbal Medicines. Montvale, NJ: Medical Economics Company, Inc., 1998:704, 712, 971, 1064, 1163, 1171.
166. Kelly GS. The role of glucosamine sulfate and chondroitin sulfates in the treatment of degenerative joint disease. Alt Med Rev 3:27–39, 1998.
167. Kolkehar R, Meller ST, Gebhart GF. Characterization of the role of spinal N-methyl-D-aspartate receptors in the nociceptor in the rat. Neurosci 57:385–395, 1993.
168. Øye I, Paulsen O, Maurset A. Effects of ketamine on sensory perception: evidence of a role of N-methyl-D-aspartate receptors. J Pharmacol Exp Ther 260:1209–1213, 1992.
169. Pud D, Eisenberg E, Spitzer A, et al. The NMDA receptor antagonist amantadine reduces surgical neuropathic pain in cancer patients: a double-blind, randomized, placebo-controlled trial. Pain 75:349–354, 1998.
170. Wiesenfeld-Hallin Z. Combined opioid-NMDA antagonist therapies. What advantages do they offer for the control of pain syndromes? Drugs 55:1–4, 1998.
171. Elliott KJ, Brodsky BS, Hyanansky BA, et al. Dextromethorphan shows efficacy in experimental pain (nociception) and opioid tolerance. Neurology 45 (Suppl 8):S66–S68, 1995.
172. Villetti G, Bergamaschi M, Bassani F, et al. Antinociceptive activity of the N-methyl-D-aspartate receptor antagonist N-(2-Indanyl)-glycinamide hydrochloride (CHF3381) in experimental models of inflammatory and neuropathic pain. J Pharmacol Exp Ther 306:804–814, 2003.
173. Rapaka RS, Porreca F. Development of delta opioid peptides as nonaddicting analgesics. Pharmaceut Res 8:1–8, 1991.

CASE STUDIES

CASE 25

TOPIC: Epilepsy

THERAPEUTIC DIFFICULTY: Level 3
Collin A. Hovinga

Chapter 62: Seizure Disorders

■ Scenario

Patient and Setting: JA, a 68-year-old male; hospitalized with mild confusion, acute distress

Chief Complaint: Dizziness, nausea, blurred vision with possible acute seizure

■ History of Present Illness

JA presented to the hospital with a productive cough lasting 1.5 months. "I can't seem to get over this cold." This is his third course of antibiotics for the same infection without clear resolution of symptoms. He reports a recent fall that occurred after complaining of dizziness, blurred vision, and acute nausea. "I felt woozy and then I don't remember much. This happened last week four times . . . can happen more or less; it depends on my sleep." Before this fall he was said to have right-sided head and eye deviation with repetitive right-sided arm movements.

Medical History: Motor vehicle accident (MVA) with a depressed skull fracture at 37 years of age. CT at the time showed that the injury was more on the left side than the right. Seizures occurred almost immediately following the accident then continued. JA presented soon after the accident and was started on phenytoin which initially controlled the seizures, but they soon recurred. His typical seizures present early in the morning, begin as an arrest of activity with motionless staring or some picking at his face, then progress to involve right-sided arm motion. The episodes often result in perioral cyanosis and pallor that are alarming to his daughter. These seizures occur sporadically, in that they may appear 2 to 3 times a week for a few weeks then remit for 1 to 2 months before reappearing. Typically, they last 5 to 7 minutes and during this time JA remains unresponsive. Depression × 10 years; congestive heart failure × 5 years; hypertension × 20 years; obesity

Surgical History: Status post-total surgical decompression of trauma site

Family/Social History: Retired with disability. Adopted, no known family history. Smokes 2 packs per day and drinks alcohol 2 to 3 times a week. Denies illicit drug use. His wife passed away last year and he now lives alone. Daughter visits 1 to 2 times a week to check on him.

Medications:
Carbamazepine (generic), 300 mg PO QID*
Lamotrigine, 200 mg PO BID*
Oxcarbazepine, 1,200 mg PO TID*
Citalopram, 30 mg PO HS
Amitriptyline, 150 mg PO HS
Hydrochlorothiazide, 50 mg PO HS
Aspirin, 325 mg PO QD
Metoprolol (Toprolol XL), 300 mg PO QD
Erythromycin, 400 mg PO BID

*In the last year, carbamazepine and then lamotrigine were added because of lack of incomplete response. Most recently his phenytoin has been discontinued and oxcarbazepine added. He reports that he sometimes is forgetful, but thinks he took all of his medications this morning

Allergies: Penicillin—rash

■ Physical Examination

GEN: Overweight man with mild confusion and productive cough (green sputum)
VS: T 40°C, BP 140/90, HR 104, RR 25, O$_2$ sat 92% nasal canula, Wt 105 kg, Ht 170 cm
SKIN: Warm, clammy
HEENT: MC/AT; EOMI; PERRLA; grossly intact bilaterally posterior oropharyngeal erythema petichiae with tenderness; gingival hypertrophy
NECK: Supple, mild LAD
LUNGS: Dyspnea, tachypnea, right side has diminished breath sounds throughout; left side CTA
CV: +S3, occasional tachycardia
ABD: Soft, NT/ND, no HSM, normal bowel sounds
EXT: 2+ edema in the lower extremities, mild bruising on arms and legs
NEURO: A and O × 2, CN II-CXII intact, motor 4/5 muscle strength on right and left. DTR 1+RUE, +1 LUE, 0 RLE, 0 LLE. Sensation to pin prick (+)

■ Results of Pertinent Laboratory Tests, Serum Drug Concentrations, and Diagnostic Tests

Na 115 (115)   Cl 104 (104)   K 4.0 (4.0)   Glu 5.9 (107)

HCO₃ 28 (28)   BUN 12.5 (35)   SCr 106 (1.2)

WBC 2.1×10^3 (2.1×10^3) diff: Lymphs 65; PMN 15; Mono 15; Bands 5

Hct 0.40 (40)   Hgb 130 (13)   Plts 300×10^9 (300×10^3)

Serum osmolarity 248 (248)

Urine Na 30 (30)

Urine osmolality 150 (150)

Carbamazepine 80.4 (19) — (6-hour postdose concentration)

EEG: Mild diffuse encephalopathy with spikes arising from the temporoparietal regions independently bilaterally

Chest x-ray: Consolidation of right superior and inferior lobes, mild cardiac enlargement

Sputum and blood culture: pending

■ Problem List

Identify principal problems from the scenario in priority order (see Answers in back of book for correct list of problems).

■ SOAP Note

To be completed by the student (see Answers in back of book for correct SOAP Note).

■ QUESTIONS

(See Answers in back of book for correct responses.)

1. What is the most likely cause of JA's productive cough, chest x-ray findings, and lack of response to antibiotic therapy? (EO-2, EO-5, EO-10)
   a. Citalopram-induced neutropenia with secondary pneumonia
   b. Carbamazepine-induced neutropenia with secondary pneumonia
   c. Oxcarbazepine-induced agranulocytosis with secondary upper respiratory tract infection
   d. Lamotrigine-induced agranulocytosis with secondary upper respiratory tract infection

2. Which of the following findings is associated with refractory epilepsy in patients diagnosed with epilepsy? (EO-1, E-15)
   a. Primary generalized seizures
   b. Failure to respond to two or more anticonvulsants
   c. Partial onset seizures
   d. Idiopathic or genetic cause for epilepsy

3. Which of the following macrolide antibiotics is least likely to inhibit carbamazepine's metabolism and is the most proper choice for JA? (EO-5, EO-9, EO-12)
   a. Troladomycin
   b. Clarithromycin
   c. Azithromycin
   d. Erythromycin

4. Describe the risk factors for lamotrigine-induced rash and the role of discontinuing either carbamazepine or oxcarbazepine in JA. How would the addition of valproic acid affect JA's lamotrigine therapy? (EO-4, EO-6, EO-8)

5. Which of the following changes in JA's drug therapy would be most appropriate? (EO-9, EO-10, EO-11, EO-12)
   a. Discontinue oxcarbamazpine, start topiramate
   b. Discontinue carbamazepine, start levetiracetam
   c. Load phenytoin, start phenytoin
   d. Load phenobarbital, start phenobarbital

6. What is the mechanism of action shared among JA's anticonvulsants? (EO-7)
   a. AMPA receptor antagonism
   b. Voltage-gated Ca+2-channel inhibition
   c. Voltage-gated Na-channel inhibition
   d. GABA agonism

7. Which of the following signs and symptoms is not consistent with SIADH? (EO-1, EO-10)
   a. Urine Na >20 mEq/L
   b. Urine Osmolarity >100 mOsm/kg
   c. Plasma Osmolarity >280 mOsm
   d. Dizziness, nausea, confusion, plasma Na <125 mEq/L

8. List measures needed to correct hyponatremia in JA. (EO-5, EO-9, EO-12)

9. Outline patient/family education that is necessary in this case. (EO-12, EO-17)

10. Based on JA's signs and symptoms, which of the following seizure types does he most likely have? (EO-1, EO-2)
    a. Generalized tonic-clonic
    b. Tonic
    c. Simple partial seizure
    d. Complex partial seizure

11. Which of the following medications is least likely to undergo a drug–drug interaction with carbamazepine? (EO-9, EO-2)
    a. Citalopram
    b. Paroxetine
    c. Fluoxetine
    d. Valproic acid

12. Describe factors that guide the selection of anti-convulsants in elderly patients with epilepsy. (EO-3, EO- 4, EO-15, EO-18)

13. List key points.

CASE 26

TOPIC: Parkinson's Disease

LEVEL OF THERAPEUTIC DIFFICULTY: Level 1
*Rowena S. Gascon, Jack J. Chen, and
Sam K. Shimomura*

Chapter 63: Parkinson's Disease

■ Scenario

Patient and Setting: AC, a right-handed 70-year-old white male; accompanied by his spouse at the neurology clinic

Chief Complaint: Symptom relief doesn't seem to last until the next dose of carbidopa/levodopa; rash on both legs

■ History of Present Illness

Diagnosed with Parkinson's disease (PD) 5 years ago; no history of head trauma, recent CT/MRI scans normal; currently Hoehn and Yahr Stage 2; patient reports past use of controlled-release carbidopa/levodopa was "not as effective"; no history of dopamine-receptor blocker use

Medical History: Hypertension (HTN) for 12 years; PD for 5 years

Surgical History: None

Family/Social History: Family History: No family history of parkinsonism or movement disorders; mother living with HTN and gout; father died of a myocardial infarction at age 83
Social History: No smoking history; occasional alcohol consumption; retired machine operator

Medications:
Atenolol, 50 mg PO QD
Rasagiline, 1 mg PO QD (receiving rasagiline as part of a clinical trial)
Amantadine, 100 mg PO TID
Multivitamins, 1 tablet PO QD
Hydrochlorothiazide, 25 mg PO QD
Carbidopa/levodopa, 25/100 mg PO TID

Allergies: PCN

■ Physical Examination

GEN: Well-developed, well-nourished male in no apparent distress; slow, shuffling gait; educed arm swing (right greater than left); no postural instability
VS: BP 137/88, HR 77, Wt 80 kg, Ht 177.8 cm
HEENT: Monotone speech with low volume; masked facies
COR: Deferred
CHEST: Deferred
ABD: Deferred
RECT: Deferred
EXT: Mild rest tremor in bilateral upper extremities (BUE) with right greater than left; "cogwheel" or "ratchet" motion in BUE with right > left; bradykinetic movement in BUE and bilateral lower extremities (BLE); micrographia; reddish-purple, fishnet patterned mottling in BLE; bilateral ankle edema
NEURO: Alert and oriented × 4; no weakness; remainder of neuro examination WNL except as noted above

■ Results of Pertinent Laboratory Tests, Serum Drug Concentrations, and Diagnostic Tests

Na 137 (137)	WBC 5.0 × 10⁹	AST 0.28 (17)	Gluc 5.8 (104)
K 3.8 (3.8)	(5.0 × 10³)	ALT 0.42 (25)	Ca 2.4 (9.5)
Cl 99 (99)	Hct 0.42 (42)	Alk Phos 0.69 (40)	PO₄ 1.2 (3.8)
HCO₃ 25 (25)	Hgb 160 (16)	Alb 42 (4.2)	Mg 1.1 (2.2)
BUN 5.3 (15)	Plts 350 × 10⁹	T Bili 5 (0.3)	
SCr 97 (1.1)	(350 × 10³)		
	MCV 80 (80)		

■ Problem List

Identify principal problems from the scenario in priority order (see Answers in back of book for correct list of problems).

■ SOAP Note

To be completed by the student (see Answers in back of book for correct SOAP Note).

■ QUESTIONS

(See Answers in back of book for correct responses.)

1. What is the probable cause of PD in AC? (EO-1)
   a. Familial
   b. Atenolol
   c. Idiopathic
   d. Brain neoplasm

2. Which classic motor features of PD does AC exhibit? (EO-2)

3. In AC, which of the following is a cause of his masked facies? (EO-5)
   a. Apathy
   b. Hostility
   c. Depression
   d. Facial rigidity

4. What is the mechanism of action of levodopa? (EO-7)
   a. Inhibits MAO-B
   b. Acts as a dopamine precursor
   c. Inhibits reuptake of dopamine
   d. Directly binds to dopamine receptors

5. Which of the following PD treatment procedures uses a pacemaker-type device that sends electrical impulses to the brain? (EO-7)
   a. Surgical ablation
   b. Stem cell therapy
   c. Deep brain stimulation
   d. Fetal cell transplantation

6. What are five key differences between immediate-release and controlled-release carbidopa/levodopa? (EO-6, 8)

7. Which of the following is most appropriate for the treatment of levodopa-associated nausea? (EO-8)
   a. Droperidol
   b. Promethazine
   c. Prochlorperazine
   d. Trimethobenzamide

8. Which of the following statements is true regarding rasagiline? (EO-8)
   a. A selective MAO-B inhibitor
   b. Requires a tyramine-restricted diet
   c. Recommended dose is 5 mg PO BID
   d. Metabolizes to amphetamine derivatives

9. If AC were to develop hallucinations and psychosis, which of the following antipsychotic agents would be most appropriate? (EO-8, 9)
   a. Quetiapine
   b. Amoxapine
   c. Haloperidol
   d. Chlorpromazine

10. Which of the following drugs is most likely to be associated with drug-induced parkinsonism? (EO-9)
    a. Sertraline
    b. Ondansetron
    c. Amitriptyline
    d. Metoclopramide

11. Describe the mechanism by which levodopa causes nausea. (EO-7, 10)

12. Which of the following describes the wearing-off phenomenon? (EO-10)
    a. A shortening of levodopa half-life as a result of prolonged chronic use
    b. A predictable waning of levodopa benefit resulting in return of symptoms prior to the next dose
    c. Involuntary choreiform movements involving the head, neck, torso, and extremities associated with levodopa peak levels
    d. Sudden transitions between "on" and "off" states that occur randomly and without relationship to timing of levodopa dose

13. Several years later, while on carbidopa/levodopa, AC develops involuntary writhing movements. Which of the following terms indicates this type of abnormal movements? (EO-10)
    a. Dystonia
    b. Dyskinesia
    c. Wearing-off
    d. Parkinsonism

14. Amantadine can be described as which of the following? (EO-8, 11)
    a. Antifungal agent
    b. Antipsychotic agent
    c. Antidyskinetic agent
    d. A hepatically cleared agent

15. A COMT inhibitor, such as entacapone, is used in the management of PD as an adjunct therapy to which of the following? (EO-8, 12)
    a. Carbidopa/levodopa to treat dyskinesia
    b. Dopamine receptor agonist to treat dyskinesia
    c. Carbidopa/levodopa to reduce wearing-off symptoms
    d. A direct dopamine agonist to reduce wearing-off symptoms

16. Summarize pathophysiologic, therapeutic, and disease management concepts for Parkinson's disease utilizing a key points format. (EO-18)

Rheumatoid Arthritis

65

Eric G. Boyce

TREATMENT GOALS

The goals of drug and nondrug therapy are to provide safe, effective, and cost-effective treatment that will diminish pain, improve well-being and functionality, prevent or slow disease progression, reverse joint deformities, and reduce the need for health care and disability services.

Future goals include the continued development of (1) more specific and safer therapies, (2) reliable predictors of those who will or will not have progressive disease or respond to therapies, and (3) preventive and curative therapies.

DEFINITION

Rheumatoid arthritis (RA) is a highly variable, chronic inflammatory condition of unknown etiology that affects mostly diarthrodial (hingelike) joints, but often with periarticular and systemic involvement. The word *rheuma* was defined by ancient Greek physicians to mean "flowing," which fit well with their humoral theory of disease. The term *rheumatism* was used in the 1600s by a French physician as an inexact label for a systemic condition associated with joint ailments. *Rheumatoid arthritis* was coined in 1858 as a label for cases reported in 1800 by a French medical student.[1]

ETIOLOGY

The etiology of rheumatoid arthritis is unknown but is most likely multifactorial, involving endogenous and exogenous factors. Genetic predisposition most likely interacts with endocrinologic, gastrointestinal, infectious, atmospheric, environmental, and other etiologic factors. The autoimmune nature of RA is documented by the presence of immune cell reactivity and the production of antibodies to endogenous elements such as immunoglobulins, collagen, and cellular components.

The etiologic role of genetic predisposition in RA is supported by the increased incidence of RA in certain families and monozygote twins (30% concordance), but genetics accounts for only 50% of the risk, according to current knowledge.[2] An immunogenetic etiology is suggested by the association of RA with genetically determined immunologic factors, including specific major histocompatibility complex (MHC) antigens and subtypes, the homozygous C-kappa genotype [constant region of immunoglobulin G (IgG)], T-lymphocyte receptor chains, defects in T-cell proliferation, corticotropin-releasing hormone genetic locus, tumor necrosis factor (TNF) receptor alleles, interferon-γ alleles, and complement C4 allotypes.[2–4] MHC class I antigens [human leukocyte antigen (HLA)-A, HLA-B, and HLA-C] are expressed on the surfaces of all nucleated cells and red blood cells, and are markers for cytotoxic T-cell (CD8+) and natural killer (NK) cell activation for removal of abnormal cells. MHC class II antigens (HLA-DR, HLA-DP, HLA-DQ) are expressed on the surfaces of macrophages and helper T-lymphocytes (CD4+) to assist in activation and regulation of the immune response to an antigen. MHC class III antigens are involved in innate immunity.

The onset of RA and the development of more severe RA are associated with MHC class II antigens [HLA-DR4 and HLA-DR1 (odds ratios of 2 to 4), HLA-DRB1 (HLA-DRB1*09, *0404 and others), HLA-DQA1[5]]; MHC class I antigens (HLA-A2 and HLA-B40 in Asian Indians, HLA-A23 and HLA-Aw33 in African-Americans); and possibly MHC III antigens (T-allele of a single nucleotide polymorphism in the promoter region). The HLA-DRB1 locus is a major determinant in the predisposition to RA, with up to 75% concordance and accounting for 40% to 50% of overall risk for the development of RA in some populations.[2,3,6] The HLA-DRB1 shared epitope region associated with increased risk for RA involves amino acid substitutions in eight contiguous positions (positions 67–74) on the molecule.[7] A single nucleotide substitution on the HLA-DRB1 gene will predict whether a patient has rheumatoid factor positive, worse prognosis RA, or rheumatoid factor negative, better prognosis RA, and two alleles may be associated with organ involvement in RA.[8,9] Evidence that supports the shared epitope theory of RA has led to findings of amino acid substitutions at the HLA-DRB1 molecule. The shared epitope of HLA-DRB1 is associated with younger age of onset, joint tenderness and swelling, joint erosions and deformities, increased erythrocyte sedimentation rate (ESR), and positive rheumatoid factor (RF) in patients with RA.[10] Many endogenous elements (e.g., collagen, cartilage glycoprotein, rheumatoid factor, bacterial products) have affinity for the shared epitope on HLA-DRB1 and may serve as activators of an immune response in RA. HLA-DR4 and a specific TNF receptor allele have demonstrated synergy in association with more severe RA in Taiwanese patients.[3] Conversely, select HLA types, subtypes, and epitopes (specific HLA-DRB1 genotypes such as HLA-DRBI*1036, *07, *1201, *1301, and HLA-DQA1 5), select TNF receptor alleles, and a specific interleukin (IL)-18 (proinflammatory) genotype appear to be less commonly associated with or protective against RA.[3,11,12] Differences in specific genotypes associated with RA are based on ethnicity. A functional haplotype of the peptidylarginine deiminase 4 (PADI4) gene is associated with an increased incidence of RA in Japanese patients, but not in those from the United Kingdom.[13] HLA-DRB1 alleles were not associated with RA in African Colombians. However, HLA typing was not useful in predicting which patients with RA would go into remission.[14]

These associations provide strong evidence that immunogenetics plays an important role in RA. Conversely, bone marrow transplantation from a patient with RA did not lead to development of RA in the recipient, who was also the donor's sibling.[15] This case raises many questions and illustrates the complexity and limits of current knowledge in the pathogenesis of RA. Proving that specific genetic sequences cause a specific disease is difficult because of difficulty in identifying whether the gene is strongly or loosely linked to the disease, the presence of multiple gene foci in complex diseases (such as rheumatoid arthritis), genetic predisposition that varies (e.g., by sex, by ethnicity), and accuracy of the diagnosis.[16]

Infectious etiologies of RA are supported by a number of findings,[2] many of which overlap with genetic and autoimmune etiologies. Patients with RA demonstrate hyperreactivity and/or increased antibody titers to Epstein-Barr virus, human T-cell lymphotropic virus (HTLV) I/II, *Mycobacterium tuberculosis*, *Proteus mirabilis*, possibly *Escherichia coli* and *Klebsiella pneumoniae*, normal human gut flora antigen, and the superantigen staphylococcal enterotoxin B. The shared epitope amino acid sequence in the hypervariable region of HLA-DRB1 that predisposes patients to RA is similar to the amino acid sequence of proteins produced by *E. coli*, *Brucella ovis*, *Lactobacillus lactis*, and Epstein-Barr virus. HTLV I has been associated with an increased incidence of RA. Single or chronic exposure to one of these organisms could trigger the expression of HLA antigens and subsequent activation of the immune system, resulting in a chronic immunologic and inflammatory reaction to an endogenous antigen. Treatment of patients with chronic infection in rare cases has led to improved responses to other therapies among those with refractory RA. However, only a few antimicrobial agents have demonstrated efficacy against RA, and the action of those drugs in RA is more likely due to immunologic effects.[17–20]

Endocrinologic etiologic links to RA are supported by increased risk for onset of RA in women and after breastfeeding, reduced risk associated with a history of pregnancy, and decreased severity in patients who used oral contraceptives before the onset of RA.[2,21] Oral contraceptive use, but not hormone replacement therapy, has been associated with a decreased risk of RA,[22] which may indicate the importance of the reason for the use of those therapies or of the patient's age. Other hormonal genes that are associated with RA are those of corticotropin-releasing hormone and estrogen synthase.[2,3] Studies have revealed no differences in cortisol or estrogen levels in patients with RA, but such patients do have a suppressed cortisol response to inflammation.[23,24] During pregnancy in women with RA, approximately 75% experience a decrease in the activity of RA, but increases and no change can also be seen. Decreases in RA activity during pregnancy may be due to decreased production of certain inflammatory cytokines or abnormal immunoglobulins. Both prolactin, which has proinflammatory effects, and arginine vasopressin are increased in patients with RA. Breast-feeding after first pregnancy is associated with the development of RA.[2] Additionally, a weak association has been noted between thyroid disorders and RA.

Other factors provide evidence of alternative etiologic factors. Gastrointestinal etiologic factors include the presence of hyperreactivity or antibodies to enteric organisms and to gluten. In general, however, food antigens are unlikely to be responsible for the activation of T-cells in RA. Changes in the atmosphere, particularly changes in barometric pressure, are associated with acute worsening of the disease. Smoking may be associated with an increased risk of RA, particularly in men.[2,25] Neuroendocrinologic etiologies or pathogeneses are supported by a decrease in RA in a limb affected by a stroke. Age may be a factor; elderly-onset RA in Japanese patients was more strongly associated with a different shared epitope amino acid sequence than was non–elderly-onset RA in patients or control subjects.

Some dietary products or supplements may be associated with a decreased risk of RA. Intake of dietary and supplemental vitamin D, supplemental zinc, or β-cryptoxanthin was inversely associated with the occurrence of RA.[26,27] Products with a possible trend for decreasing the risk of RA include supplemental vitamin C, vitamin E, copper and manganese, and dietary fruits and cruciferous vegetables.[27] In women, decaffeinated coffee was associated with an increased risk, and tea with a decreased risk, of RA.[28]

The etiology of RA remains a mystery. Differences among various populations with respect to association with HLA allele, clinical presentation, and severity complicate the clinician's ability to determine causation. However, genetic, other endogenous, and exogenous factors all appear to be important in the etiology of RA.

EPIDEMIOLOGY

RA, the most common chronic arthritis, affects 0.3% to 2.3% of the population. It is two to three times more common in women than in men.[29,30] Recent reports have demonstrated a decrease in the incidence of RA in the United States and other countries.[29] It can be seen in any culture or race. An increased incidence has been reported among Chippewa Indians (6.8%), Pima Indians (5.3%), and Mexican Americans, but a decreased incidence or prevalence is seen in Chinese, Japanese, African Colombians, and those in developing countries.[2] RA occurs at any age, with the peak incidence in women occurring between 30 and 60 years of age. However, a recent study in Norway has found a peak incidence in those older than 60 years of age.[31] Epidemiologic factors not associated with the development of RA include geographic latitude and hepatitis C.

PATHOPHYSIOLOGY

The precise pathophysiology of rheumatoid arthritis remains unknown but appears to involve a complex series of events involving T-lymphocytes, B-lymphocytes, macrophages, and a number of cytokines and enzymes, leading to inflammation and destruction of bone and cartilage. TNF-α and IL-1 appear to be intimately involved in this process, but numerous other cytokines, inflammatory mediators, and enzymes also seem to play an important role. Continued advances in our understanding of the pathogenesis of RA have led and will continue to lead to the development of more specific and more effective therapies.

IMMUNE DYSFUNCTION IN RHEUMATOID ARTHRITIS

Activation or lack of control of an immune response, growth of an invasive synovial membrane, and activation of inflammatory cells and release of inflammatory and enzymatic substances result in the sustained, progressive inflammation and destruction of cartilage, bone, and other tissues seen in RA.[1,32] The chronic inflammation, synovial proliferation, and bone and cartilage destruction observed in RA appear to be associated with abnormalities in immune, inflammatory, and repair responses that result from secretions and other activities of macrophages, fibroblasts (which may be specialized macrophages), lymphocytes, neutrophils, mast cells, and other immune cells.

A normal immune reaction to an antigen begins with nonspecific phagocytosis, followed by the development and activation of specific, adaptive processes, removal of the antigen, formation of memory immune cells, and, finally, a decrease in the reaction. Macrophages initially engulf and process the antigen, present the antigen to helper T-lymphocytes (T$_H$-cells, CD4+) and B-lymphocytes (B-cells), and secrete IL-1 to activate T$_H$-cells. Type 1 T$_H$-cells (Th1) are activated by IL-12, produce select cytokines (i.e., IL-2, lymphotoxin, and interferon-γ), and appear to be proinflammatory. Type 2 T$_H$-cells (Th2) are activated by IL-4, produce select cytokines (i.e., IL-4, IL-5, IL-10, and IL-13), may enhance B-cell activity, and appear to have anti-inflammatory actions. B-lymphocytes secrete IL-10, which may regulate antigen-processing cell secretion and subsequent activation of Th1 and Th2 cells. MHC class II antigens and cellular adhesion molecules are expressed on the surfaces of macrophages and other antigen-processing cells in association with processed antigen and regulate the interaction with activated helper T-cells. When activated, Th1 cells secrete IL-2, which, in turn, activates and enhances proliferation of T$_H$-cells, cytotoxic T-cells (T$_C$-cells, CD8+), suppressor T-cells (T$_S$-cells, CD8+), B-cells, NK cells, memory T- and B-cells, macrophages, and other phagocytes. Activated Th1 cells also secrete IFN-γ, which enhances the expression of MHC class II antigens and the function of macrophages. Through genetic rearrangement, B-cells and T-cells assist in the development of reactive regions that are more specific for the antigen, resulting in secretion of more specific immunoglobulins by B-cells and enhanced binding by T-cells. Immunoglobulins (or antibodies) bind to the antigen and facilitate its removal by macrophages and other phagocytes.

The stimulation of numerous cells and the development of antigen-specific binding sites greatly enhance the rate and specificity of the reaction to the antigen. As the antigen is removed and suppressor T-cells become more important, the immune reaction eventually diminishes. Specific memory B- and T-lymphocytes remain dormant until subsequent exposure to that antigen occurs, at which time they initiate a rapid, specific response to the antigen. The normal immune reaction is much more complicated than is indicated in this overview, and it involves numerous other cytokines. No or little tissue destruction is expected in a normal immune response, but abnormalities in the immune response associated with RA result in inflammation and damage both within and outside the joint.

The antigen responsible for initiating the immunologic events in RA is unknown. Potential candidates include the Fc (constant) region of IgG, collagen (from cartilage, synovium, blood vessels, etc.), cartilage components, numerous infectious agents or their products, and superantigens. Synovial macrophages appear to be in a hyperactive state in patients with RA, possibly activated by immune complexes, complement, interferon (IFN)-γ, and the antigens listed below (Table 65.1). Hyperreactivity to antigens may be linked to MHC class II antigens, adhesion molecules, or chronic exposure to the antigen. The expression of MHC class I antigens, which is associated with cytotoxicity, and the increased expression of adhesion molecules on the surfaces of rheumatoid synovial fibroblasts are enhanced by IL-1, TNF-α, and IFN-γ.

Macrophages release a number of factors that are important in the pathophysiology of RA, including IL-1, TNF, destructive enzymes (collagenase, proteases), inflammatory prostaglandins [prostaglandin E_2 (PGE_2)] and leukotrienes (LTB_4), and other factors [granulocyte-macrophage colony-stimulating factor (GM-CSF)]. IL-1 stimulates the activation and proliferation of helper T-cells (CD4+) and secretion of tissue growth factor. IL-1 and TNF are chemotactic, enhance the expression of adhesion and MHC class antigens, and stimulate the secretion of PGE_2, destructive enzymes (collagenase, proteases), substance P (a mediator of pain), and other cytokines (e.g., GM-CSF, IL-6). TNF-α is secreted with IL-1 and correlates with rheumatoid cachexia. Levels

TABLE 65.1	Actions of Immunologic Mediators in Rheumatoid Arthritis	
Substance	**Source**	**Stimulates (Inhibits)**
IL-1, TNF	Macrophages	MHC-I expression, chemotaxis
		Release of PGE_2, IL-6, GM-CSF, collagenase, metalloprotease, substance P
IL-1	Macrophages	Lymphocyte proliferation and activation
		Growth factor release
IL-6	Fibroblasts	T-cell and B-cell function
	T-lymphocytes	GM-CSF release
IL-10	Synovial cells	IgM and IgG release
	B-cells	(Inhibits TNF-α action)
	Memory CD4+ T-cells	(Inhibits activation of antigen-processing cells and T-cells)
IL-13	Synovial macrophages	(Inhibits production of IL-1-β, TNF-α) HLA-DR expression
IL-15	Synovial	T-cell migration and activation
	Endothelial cells	TNF production by T-cells and macrophages
IFN-γ	T-lymphocytes	MHC-I and MHC-II expression
		(Inhibits collagenase and PGE_2 release)
GM-CSF	Macrophages	Bone marrow cell formation, IL-1 production
	Lymphocytes	PMN activation, monocyte attraction
PGE_2	Fibroblasts	Growth factor release, cartilage degradation, inflammation, pain
Collagenase	Fibroblasts	Cartilage degradation
Growth factors		Synovial tissue proliferation
Transforming growth factor		Synovial tissue proliferation, IL-1 production, monocyte chemotaxis (Inhibits lymphokine and protease secretion, synoviocyte growth, and HLA-DR expression)

GM-CSF, granulocyte-macrophage colony-stimulating factor; IFN, interferon; IL, interleukin; MHC, major histocompatibility complex; PG, prostaglandin; PMN, neutrophils; TNF, tumor necrosis factor.

of IL-1, TNF-α, GM-CSF, and soluble IL-2 receptors are increased in the blood, synovial fluid, and synovial tissue in patients with RA and may correlate with disease activity. Secretion of IL-1 and/or TNF is inhibited by IFN-γ,[33] IL-4, IL-10, and IL-13. Natural inhibitors of the action of IL-1 and TNF include receptor antagonists (IL-1Ra), soluble receptors (soluble TNF receptors), and IL-10. IL-10 also inhibits the secretion of GM-CSF and the proliferation of synovial monocytes.

Helper T-cell (CD4 +) dysregulation plays a key role in the pathophysiology of RA. TNF-α appears to stimulate helper T-cell (CD4 +) proliferation.[34] T-lymphocytes are activated by IL-1, IL-2, enhanced HLA-DR antigen expression, other interleukins (IL-12, IL-15), and numerous antigens, including chondrocyte membrane, synovial cell antigen, superantigen, human collagen (types I, II, IV, and V), cartilage proteoglycans and metalloproteases, *Mycobacterium tuberculosis*, *M. bovis* heat-shock protein, tetanus toxoid, and a synovial protein similar to the Fc portion of IgG. Relatively few antigens appear to be primarily responsible for T-cell activation, and those antigens appear to change over time. IL-15 and soluble adhesion molecules from synovial endothelial cells mediate T-cell migration into the synovial capsule. T-cells appear to accumulate in RA synovium, seeming to be autoreactive and displaying atypical proliferation and differentiation. In RA synovium, Th1 cells predominate over Th2 cells and helper T-lymphocytes (CD4 +) may occur in greater number than suppressor/cytotoxic (CD8 +) T-cells. T-cells from patients with RA demonstrate markers for activated (CD3 +) and suppressor/cytotoxic (CD8 +) T-cells, increased activation of surface adhesion and signaling lymphocytic activation molecules, and mature and hyperreactive memory T-cells. Synovial T-cells and peripheral CD8 + T-cells have decreased β-adrenergic receptors, which may lead to a decreased inhibitor effect of catecholamines on T-cell activity. Patients with RA have gone into remission when infected with the human immunodeficiency virus.[35] Lymphotoxin B, which is secreted by T- and B-lymphocytes, stimulates fibroblasts to secrete inflammatory mediators, upregulated adhesion molecules, and cytokines that attract and retain lymphocytes in the synovium.[36] Lymphotoxin B also appears to be involved in the formation of lymphoid tissue in the synovial tissue of patients with RA.

Despite the role of T-cells in RA and the accumulation of T-cells in RA synovium, T-cell function in RA synovium is actually suppressed. This suppression has been documented by low numbers of activated T_H-cells, hyporesponsive T-cells, diminished expression of activation receptors, and T_H-cell defects in proliferation and production of IL-2, IL-4, TNF-α, IFN-γ, and IL-6 in RA synovium. The activation of T-cells appears to be suppressed by suppressor T-cells, IL-4, IL-10, soluble vascular cell adhesion molecules (sVCAM), selective antigen–MHC class II activation, site-specific alterations in activation, and TNF-α. The suppressed T-cell state may explain the accumulation of T-cells

and continued inflammatory activity in synovial tissue resulting from direct activation by antigens.

B-cells (B-lymphocytes) become activated plasma cells; they then produce and secrete specific antibody and IL-10. Stimuli for this activation include IL-2, IL-10, and select synovial antigens such as mitochondria resulting from destruction of synovial cells and/or cartilage. Plasma cells (activated B-cells) are the most prevalent, highly active monocytes found in synovial tissue and blood vessels of patients with RA. Normal and mutated clonal rearrangement patterns for the hypervariable region of the secreted immunoglobulins have been found. Memory B-cells appear to accumulate and reside for long periods in synovial membrane in those with RA.

Antibodies and the consequences of antibody release (immune complexes and complement activation) also increase in patients with RA. RF is an autoantibody directed against the Fc portion of IgG that is positive in 80% of patients with RA. RF from patients with RA has a higher affinity for antigens and is a more potent activator of complement compared with RF from people without RA. Hyaluronic acid, a normal component of synovial fluid, appears to facilitate the formation of immune complexes of rheumatoid factor and IgG. RF may also bind native and inactivate C1q, part of the complement cascade, possibly because of the similarity in antigenicity of C1q to type II collagen. IgG antibody to collagen chains is seen early in the course of erosive RA but decreases over the first year of the disease. Immune complexes containing n-acetylglucosamine, a cartilage glycoprotein, are higher in RA than in other inflammatory disorders. IgG lacking galactose in the Fc portion is increased in patients with RA and in those with more active disease and is decreased during pregnancy. Other autoantibodies are also seen in RA (see later). The expression of Fc receptors on peripheral monocytes (which assist in the removal of immune complexes) correlated with RA disease activity,[37] indicating the importance of the immune complexes in RA. The increased secretion of antibody and enhanced formation of immune complexes in RA appear to sustain the immune reaction and may be responsible for joint and extra-articular manifestations of the disease.

Phagocytes and immune cells found in synovial fluid and/or tissue include macrophages, NK cells (found in early rheumatoid synovial tissue), neutrophils (activated by IFN-γ), and mast cells. Macrophages may also be the target of destruction by activated cytotoxic T-cells. In RA, programmed cell death, or apoptosis, is decreased in fibroblasts of proliferating synovium fibroblasts and is increased in bone marrow precursor cells. Neutrophils may remain in a primed, semiactivated state in RA. Mast cells are found in invasive synovial tissue and may be important in the destruction of cartilage and inflammatory edema because of an association with increases in IL-1, TNF, stromelysin-1, and collagenase; they may also enhance production of PGE_2 and proteases. Phagocytic cells are responsible for removal of damaged cells and debris, and they initiate repair. However, immune dysregulation in RA leads to damage caused by these cells. Macrophages, similar to helper T-lymphocytes, play a key role in the pathophysiology of RA.

In RA, a large number of cytokines contribute to inflammatory and/or destructive processes. Helper T-cells are responsible for the secretion of IL-2, IL-6, IL-8, IL-10, IFN-γ, and GM-CSF. IL-6 is increased in patients with RA, possibly because of an antibody against an IL-6 signal-controlling protein.[38] IL-6 increases production of GM-CSF, immunoglobulins, and acute-phase reactants following secretion from monocytes, T-cells, and fibroblasts (Table 65.1). IL-6 production is stimulated by IL-1-β, GM-CSF, IFN-γ, and TNF-α but is inhibited by IL-10, IL-4, IL-13, IL-1Ra, and anti-CD14 monoclonal antibody. GM-CSF, secreted from numerous sources, promotes the growth of certain bone marrow cell lines, increases MHC class II expression on synovial macrophages, stimulates IL-1 production, activates neutrophils, and attracts monocytes (Table 65.1). IL-8 is secreted by T-cell–stimulated synoviocytes in RA and appears to be a chemoattractant for neutrophils. IFN-γ increases MHC class I/II antigen expression and macrophage activation. A large number of proinflammatory mediators have been noted, including IL-17 and IL-18. Further research on the importance of these mediators will assist investigators in the development of specific therapies.

PATHOPHYSIOLOGIC CHANGES IN JOINTS AND ASSOCIATED STRUCTURES

A normal diarthrodial joint is a functional interface that supports and limits the relative movement of two or more bones over defined ranges. The joint capsule surrounds the joint space and connects to the surrounding bones (Fig. 65.1). The synovium, or synovial tissue, is the internal structure of the joint capsule that secretes synovial fluid and contains many blood vessels and immunologically active cells. Connective tissue surrounds the synovial tissue and provides stability to the joint capsule and the synovial lining membrane. Tendons, ligaments, and muscles also serve to support and stabilize the joint. Cartilage, which is composed of a proteoglycan matrix and 70% water, is bathed in synovial fluid and acts to cushion the forces between opposing bones during movement or compression. Synovial fluid provides nutrients to the cartilage, removes wastes from the cartilage, and helps maintain the structure of the cartilage through hydration. This normal anatomy and physiology are altered in RA through changes in bone, cartilage, supporting tissues, and synovial tissue and fluid that are mediated immunologically and through inflammation.

Synovial tissue proliferates in RA, becomes hypervascular, and develops into an invasive tissue known as the pannus (Fig. 65.2). Growth factors (platelet-derived, epidermal, transforming, basic fibroblast) and receptors for these growth factors in synovial fluid and tissue may produce an autocrine, tumorlike growth of synovial tissue and synovial blood vessels in RA. IL-1 and PGE$_2$ (Table 65.1) regulate platelet-derived growth factor. Transforming growth factor

decreases lymphokine and protease secretion, synoviocyte growth, and HLA-DR expression but enhances collagen and fibronectin gene transcription, protease inhibitor and IL-1 production, monocyte chemotaxis, and immunosuppression. Endothelial precursor cells are found in RA synovium; these may assist in the development of vasculature to support the pannus. Migrating circulatory macrophages may also help maintain the hyperplastic, invasive synovium. Lymphatic vessels increase in number in inflammatory synovial membranes.

Bone resorption and cartilage destruction that occur in RA are due to cellular activities and secretions and generally progress over time. Collagenase, PGE$_2$, plasminogen activator, and stromelysin are able to degrade cartilage or collagen and are produced by synovial fibroblasts or chondrocytes after stimulation by IL-1 or TNF.[33] The effects of IL-1 and TNF on collagenase and PGE$_2$ production are diminished by IFN-γ (Table 65.1).[33] Decreased secretion of IFN-γ may be associated with increased joint destruction. Erosive disease is also associated with increased secretion of IgG to collagen early in the course of the disease, induction of osteoclastogenesis by IL-6 and soluble IL-6 receptors, stimulation of osteoclast differentiation by IL-11, hyperreactivity of T-cells to chondrocyte membrane, and phagocytosis of cartilage and type II collagen. Cartilage repair may be reduced by a decrease in the formation of cartilage precursors by synovial cells. Plasma parathyroid hormone and calcitriol levels may also correlate with periarticular bone loss in patients with RA. Improved imaging techniques have enabled clinicians to identify the destruction of bone and cartilage in more than 50% of patients with RA.

Changes in synovial fluid, synovial tissue, cartilage, and bone result from chronic inflammation, synovial proliferation, and collagen destruction of RA. Pressure within the joint increases from vacuum or subatmospheric pressures in the normal joint to supra-atmospheric pressure in the inflamed joint. Rheumatoid synovial fluid is similar to that seen in other inflammatory joint diseases with respect to leukocytosis (mostly polymorphonuclear cells) and decreased viscosity. The synovial tissue becomes hypervascular and blood flow increases with vasodilation, but this may not be enough to meet the metabolic demands resulting from the inflammation. Lactate levels are high in inflamed synovial fluid. Increased synovial fluid, synovial tissue proliferation, and cartilage destruction lead to discomfort and limitation of movement. Destruction of cartilage and bone, in addition to disruption of positioning and functioning of tendons and ligaments, further destabilizes the joint.

CLINICAL PRESENTATION AND DIAGNOSIS

SIGNS AND SYMPTOMS

The onset of RA varies from slow and insidious to rapidly progressive. The course of the disease is also highly variable: 10% to 20% of patients have a relatively short course with

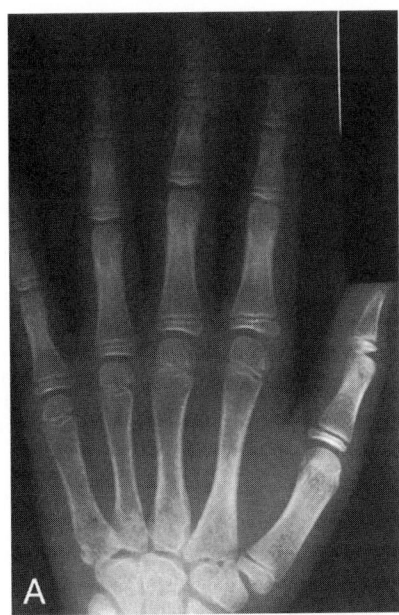

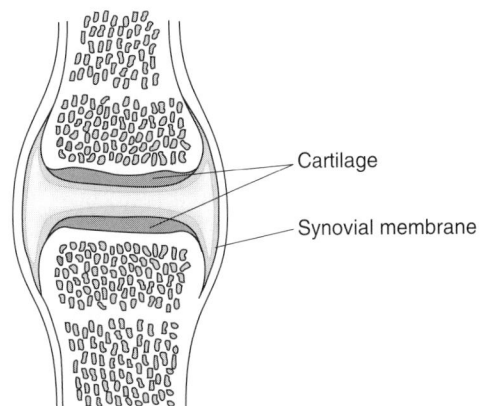

Cartilage

Synovial membrane

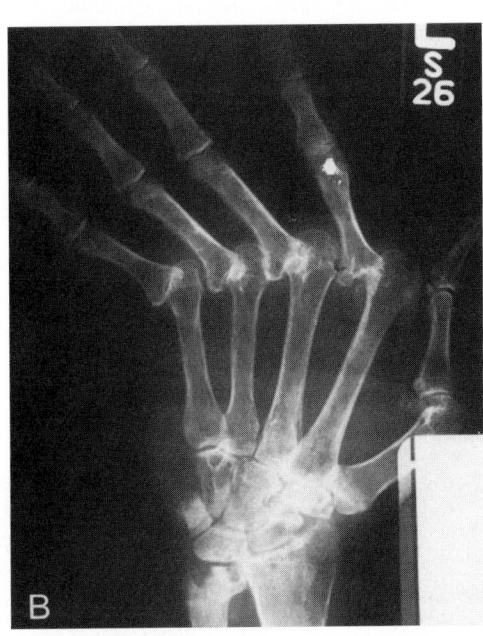

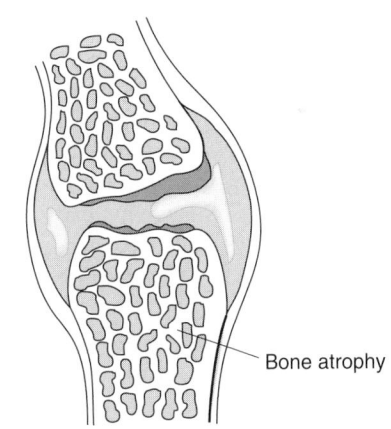

Bone atrophy

FIGURE 65.1. Joints of the hand affected by rheumatoid arthritis. A. Radiograph of normal hand. B. Radiograph of hand with rheumatoid arthritis. (From Harris JH, Harris WH, Novelline RA. The radiology of emergency medicine. 3rd edition. Baltimore: Williams & Wilkins, 1995: 440, 467.)

subsequent remission; 70% to 80% have mild to moderate disease with cyclic exacerbation; and 10% to 20% develop progressive, overtly destructive disease. More severe disease at onset and follow-up may be seen in those patients from poor socioeconomic settings.[39] Severity at onset may or may not be worse in women than in men but appeared in some studies to be milder in younger women than in older women.[40,41] Restricted activity is noted in 70% of patients with RA and 89% of patients with RA plus at least one comorbid disorder.[42] Proper assessment of the patient's abilities is needed as part of an adequate assessment of disease. Functional classification serves as a means to classify a patient's global ability to perform daily living activities (Table 65.2). Functional limitations were more likely in those with increased function at baseline, delayed time to diagnosis, and recent erythrocyte sedimentation rate.[43] More specific activities of daily living questionnaires and quality-of-life surveys are also useful but are not widely used clinically.

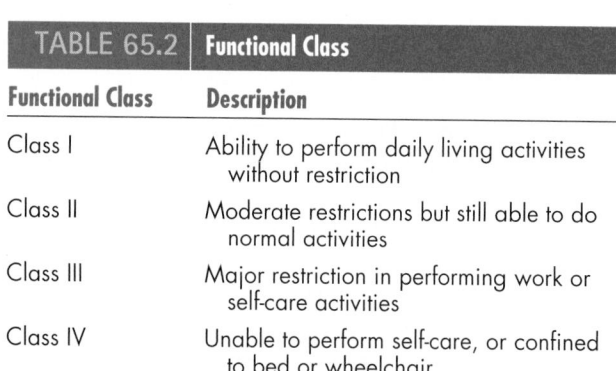

FIGURE 65.2. Pathophysiology of rheumatoid arthritis. A. Joint structure with synovial swelling and fluid accumulation in joint. B. Pannus, eroded articular cartilage with joint space narrowing, muscle atrophy, and ankylosis. (From Nettina SM. The Lippincott manual of nursing practice. 7th edition. Baltimore: Lippincott Williams & Wilkins, 2001.)

Joints are the primary areas of involvement in RA; disorders range from quiescent or mild synovitis to severe synovitis, considerable synovial thickening and/or proliferation, detectable synovial fluid, and obvious bone deformity. RA usually affects diarthrodial joints, including the joints of the hands (Figs. 65.1 to 65.4) and feet such as the proximal interphalangeal (PIP) joints, metacarpophalangeal (MCP) joints, metatarsophalangeal (MTP) joints, wrists, and/or ankles. Elbows, shoulders, sternoclavicular joints, temporomandibular joints, knees, and hips are commonly involved. Cervical spine involvement may lead to severe pain, subluxation, and destabilization.

Stiffness is a gel-like sensation experienced in the joints or more generally in patients with RA when they attempt to move after waking in the morning or after a period of inactivity. Patients are likely to describe it as pain or discomfort. The degree of stiffness diminishes with movement, usually over the first few hours after awakening in the morning or after moving about after a period of inactivity. Plasma levels of keratan sulfate, a large cartilage proteoglycan degradation product, are inversely proportionate to the duration of morning stiffness.

Erosive joint disease, mostly in the hands, is seen within the first 2 years of RA in 67% to 73% of those patients with progressive destructive RA; it progresses most rapidly over the first 5 years and continues to progress over at least 20 years.[44,45] Joint destruction in RA has been correlated or associated with a baseline number of swollen and tender joints, radiographic joint score, disability, rheumatoid factor titers (total, IgA, IgM), rheumatoid nodules, HLA-DR4, specific shared epitopes of HLA-DRB1, IgG lacking galactose, memory T-cells, ESR, C-reactive protein (CRP), and anti–keratin antibody titers. Conversely, select epitopes of HLA-DP and HLA-DR are associated with nonerosive disease. Bone erosions and joint deformities are due to the destruction of periarticular bone by inflammatory mediators, enzymes, phagocytosis, and physical stress. Common deformities seen in RA include subluxations, ulnar deviation, swan neck deformities, boutonniere deformities, hammer or cock-up toe formation, and ankylosis (Figs. 65.1 to 65.4).

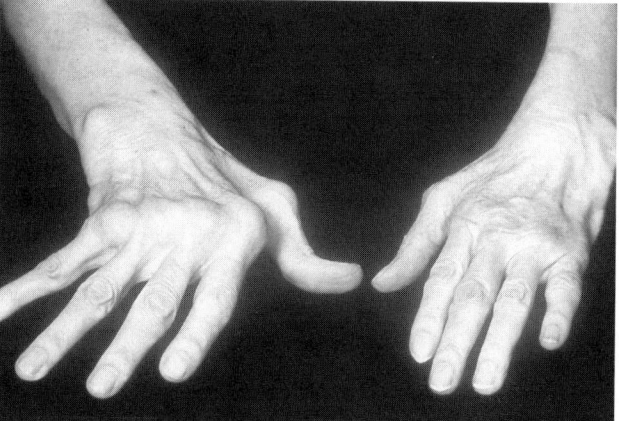

FIGURE 65.3. Ulnar deviation with volar subluxation of the MCP joints. Ulnar deviation with volar subluxation of the MCP joints of the fingers in an individual with rheumatoid arthritis occurs when swelling destabilizes the joints and the tendons of the fingers migrate and exert a deforming force. (From Oatis CA. Kinesiology—The mechanics and pathomechanics of human movement. Baltimore: Lippincott Williams & Wilkins, 2004.)

TABLE 65.2	Functional Class
Functional Class	**Description**
Class I	Ability to perform daily living activities without restriction
Class II	Moderate restrictions but still able to do normal activities
Class III	Major restriction in performing work or self-care activities
Class IV	Unable to perform self-care, or confined to bed or wheelchair

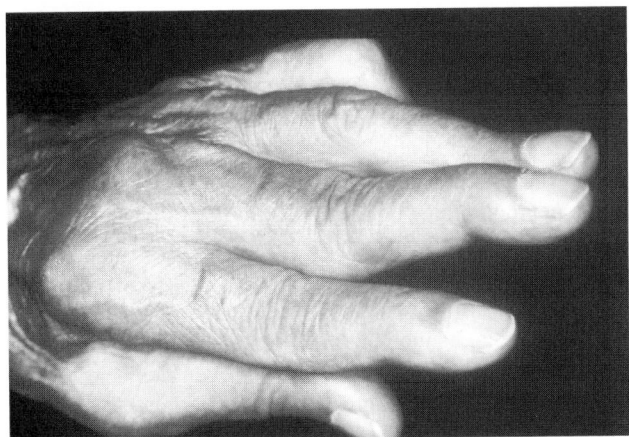

FIGURE 65.4 A swan neck deformity in an individual with rheumatoid arthritis. A swan neck deformity in an individual with rheumatoid arthritis consists of hyperextension of the PIP joint with flexion of the DIP joint. (Reprinted from the ARHP Assessment and Management of Rheumatic Diseases: The Teaching Slide Collection for Clinicians and Educators. Copyright 1997. Used with permission of the American College of Rheumatology.)

Cervical spine subluxations are more likely to develop in patients with severe peripheral arthritis and older age. Opposing or compensating forces lead to a zigzag pattern of deformity. In the late stages of progressive disease, bony deformities may predominate and acute inflammation may be absent or minimal. Joints become destabilized owing to bone, muscle, tendon, ligament, or joint capsule changes. The amount of joint destruction can be quantified by three techniques (Steinbrocker stage, Larsen score, modified Sharp score), but these measures have only fair correlation with patient function. Advances in the prevention of these deformities are likely to progress considerably if the use of HLA typing and other clinical variables are found to have reasonable sensitivity, specificity, availability, and affordability in determining which patients are at high risk.

The generalized osteopenia seen in patients with RA is related to or worsened by inflammatory mediators, relative immobility, corticosteroids, hormonal changes in postmenopausal women, and age-related effects in elderly men and women. Patients with RA have a twofold increase in osteoporosis. Both RA and corticosteroid use are independently associated with the development of osteoporosis and vertebral fractures.[46] Osteoporosis in patients with RA is both peripheral and vertebral and worsens with duration and severity of RA and low lean body mass.[47]

General constitutional symptoms are common in RA. Fatigue, which occurs in many patients, particularly during active RA, may be related to abnormal sleep patterns, anemia, depression, muscle weakness, and/or neuropeptides. The cachexia and muscle weakness that occur in RA are associated with inactivity, catabolic effects of inflammatory mediators (TNF), use of corticosteroids, and other factors but are not associated with a decrease in growth hormone.

Extra-articular involvement in RA is more likely to be seen in those patients who have a positive rheumatoid factor, IgA rheumatoid factor, HLA-DR4, HLA-DR1, HLA-DR3, select shared epitopes for HLA-DRB1 chain sequences, higher proportions of a specific helper T-cell, circulating immune complexes, male sex, and/or more severe arthritis. Extra-articular features include rheumatoid nodules, vasculitis, vital organ effects, anemia, thrombocytopenia, Felty syndrome, Sjögren syndrome, and ocular inflammation, in addition to generalized constitutional symptoms. Extra-articular manifestations demonstrate the systemic immune effects associated with RA.

Rheumatoid nodules (Fig. 65.5), which contain monocytes and macrophages surrounding a necrotic area, occur in 25% of patients with RA, almost all of whom are rheumatoid factor positive. Other risk factors for the development of rheumatoid nodules include longer duration of RA, more severe RA, other extra-articular manifestations, and a specific shared epitope of the HLA-DRB1 chain sequence. Methotrexate may increase the number of rheumatoid nodules in some patients.[48] Rheumatoid nodules generally occur subcutaneously over bone in pressure point areas but may be found in other tissues and organs.

Vasculitis is most likely to be found in patients with severe, nodular, rheumatoid factor positive RA and also in those with a specific shared epitope of the HLA-DRB1 chain sequence, perinuclear antineutrophilic cytoplasmic antibody (pANCA), and/or a high ESR. The incidence of vasculitis appears to be decreasing, possibly because of the more aggressive use of anti-inflammatory–immunosuppressive therapies. Vasculitis varies from minor skin lesions to major organ vascular involvement. Clues to the presence of vascular inflammation include the presence of the spectrum of skin manifestations from palpable purpura to digital infarcts, ischemic ulcers, and progression to gangrene and necrosis. Larger vessel involvement with major organ compromise is seen on rare occasions.

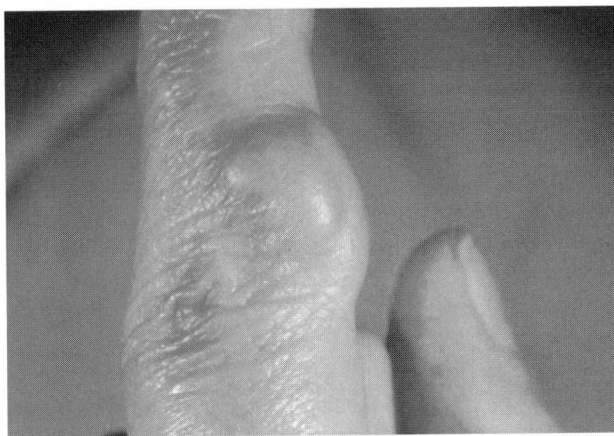

FIGURE 65.5. Rheumatoid nodule. A patient with rheumatoid arthritis has a mass on a digit. (From Rubin E, Farber JL. Pathology. 3rd edition. Philadelphia: Lippincott Williams & Wilkins, 1999.)

Anemia of chronic inflammatory disease is seen in patients with RA; it worsens as the arthritis worsens. Mild anemia is seen in 33% to 60% of patients with RA.[49] This anemia is related to the inability to utilize iron stores and responds poorly to iron therapy. Anemia of chronic disease may occur in conjunction with iron deficiency. Improvements in clinical symptoms of RA and anemia appear related. Hemolytic anemia and autoimmune thrombocytopenia are rare features of RA. Anemia may also be caused by the drugs used to treat patients with RA, gastrointestinal ulcers with bleeding [caused by nonsteroidal anti-inflammatory drugs (NSAIDs), systemic corticosteroids], bone marrow suppression (due to methotrexate, azathioprine, gold salts, cyclophosphamide), hemolytic/immune anemia (due to sulfasalazine, antimalarials, gold salts, penicillamine, sulfasalazine), and numerous other nonrelated disorders. Drug-associated thrombocytopenia has also been noted.

Immunologically associated disorders may be seen in association with RA. The combination of RA, splenomegaly, and leukopenia (sometimes in association with thrombocytopenia, lymphadenopathy, leg ulcers, and infections) defines Felty syndrome. Felty syndrome is more common in patients with severe, rheumatoid factor–positive, nodular RA and with HLA-DRB1*04. Large granular lymphocyte leukemia may be associated with RA and may be confused with Felty syndrome. Joint infections may occur more commonly in patients with RA, particularly in those with prosthetic joints. Tuberculosis is more common among patients with RA in some studies but not in others[50]; however, it is more common in those on infliximab and possibly other immunosuppressive therapies.[50] Amyloidosis may be more common in RA because of inflammatory mediator–induced production of amyloid protein by the liver. Amyloidosis is seen in 7% of those with RA and may affect the GI tract and kidneys. Leukopenia and/or immunosuppression is seen with many drugs used to treat patients with RA. Infection in patients with RA is associated with older age, comorbidities (e.g., chronic lung disease, alcoholism, organic brain disease, diabetes mellitus), extra-articular manifestations of RA, use of corticosteroids, and leukopenia—but not with disease severity or use of disease-modifying antirheumatic drugs (DMARDs) in general (except TNF-α and IL-1 inhibitors).[51] Patients with RA have increased risks for bone, joint, skin, soft tissue, and respiratory tract infections.

Vital organs are also affected in RA. Rheumatoid lung disease occurs in up to 20% of patients with RA and is characterized by pulmonary effusions, pleuritis, bronchiolitis, interstitial pneumonitis, obstruction, and possibly fibrosis. Rheumatoid lung may be associated with pANCA. Other causes of lung disorders include the therapy for RA (e.g., methotrexate, gold salts, penicillamine, cyclophosphamide), rheumatoid nodules, and genetic and environmental factors. Renal disease secondary to RA is presumed to be rare, but a study in 143 Japanese patients with RA revealed that 21 (15%) had mesangial proliferation glomerulonephritis (12 of whom had IgA-related nephritis), 7 had membranous ne-

phropathy, 7 had amyloid nephropathy, and 6 had minor abnormalities.[52] Rarely, renal disease in patients with RA has been associated with pANCA. However, subclinical renal dysfunction is found, particularly in patients with progressive RA. Renal abnormalities in RA may be more commonly due to medications (e.g., NSAIDs, cyclosporine, gold salts, penicillamine) or amyloidosis. Serositis (pericarditis and pleuritis) may occur more commonly in male patients.

The most common cardiac manifestation in RA is asymptomatic pericarditis with or without effusions. Ventricular hypertrophy and subclinical left ventricular dysfunction are common and may progress to clinical ventricular dysfunction in patients with progressive RA. Arterial elasticity and endothelium-dependent vasodilation are decreased and systemic vascular resistance and arterial wall thickness are increased in RA.[53–55] Patients with RA have increased risk for myocardial infarction and congestive heart failure. Carotid and peripheral vascular disease was found to be more common in RA.[56] Risk of stroke was higher in patients with RA, but not at a statistically significant level in a large prospective study.[57] The increased risks for myocardial infarction and other cardiovascular events are above those predicted by cardiovascular risk determinants in the general population. Corticosteroids appear to play a role in some patients. Mitral valve regurgitation was seen in 80% of patients with RA compared with 37% of controls. Heart valve dysfunction, embolic phenomena, conduction defects, aortitis, mild primary pulmonary hypertension, and cardiomyopathy occur infrequently.

Keratoconjunctivitis sicca with complaints of dry eyes (xerophthalmia) and dry mouth (xerostomia) is a clue to the presence of secondary Sjögren syndrome. Keratoconjunctivitis sicca is associated with a higher proportion of specific B-cell and IgA RF. Other ocular abnormalities in patients with RA include episcleritis, scleritis, and scleromalacia perforans.

Neurologic complications are frequently seen in RA. Their pathogenesis is usually related to myelopathies associated with cervical spine instability, entrapment of peripheral nerves through confined compartments (such as carpal tunnel syndrome), or ischemic neuropathies related to vasculitis often presenting as a mononeuritis multiplex. A peripheral neuropathy commonly associated with ganglioside antibodies is seen in patients with severe RA. Cyclosporine, gold salts, and penicillamine may also cause neurologic disorders.

RFs are autoantibodies (IgM, IgG, and/or IgA) that are directed against the Fc portion of IgG and found in blood and synovial fluid. Plasma titers of RF are positive in approximately 80% of patients with RA, but also in up to 5% of the population at large and of patients with a variety of inflammatory or infectious disorders such as endocarditis, tuberculosis, and systemic lupus erythematosus. The incidence of positive RF is associated with age of onset in women, with 85% of those having positive RF younger than 40 years of age at onset compared with 66% older than 60 years of age; however, the rate was 86% in men with no age association.[58] RF is measured in both titers and units. Titers that define a positive RF may vary but in general are 1:32 or greater. In patients with RA who have a positive rheumatoid factor (RF +), higher plasma titers of RF are usually associated with more active RA. IgM RF and IgA RF are associated with more severe disease. Numerous factors are associated with the presence or absence of RF in patients with RA, as noted earlier, but HLA-DR4 is associated with RF + RA and HLA-DR1 with RF − RA. Does seronegative (RF negative) RA exist? The answer is unclear. It is more likely that secretion of RF is on a continuum, with all patients having B-cells that can secrete RF but only 80% of those patients secreting an amount of RF that is sufficiently large to be detected. Additionally, fractionation has revealed ''hidden'' IgM RF in seronegative patients with RA.

Other antibodies found in patients with RA include antinuclear antibodies, antifilaggrin antibodies (antikeratin antibodies and antiperinuclear antibodies), anti–RA 33 antibodies, and antithyroid antibodies. Antinuclear antibodies, which are autoantibodies against nuclear proteins in patients with systemic lupus erythematosus and other autoimmune disorders, are found in low titers in patients with RA. The incidence of a positive ANA is associated with age of onset in women, with 63% of those having positive RF younger than 40 years of age at onset compared with 31% older than 60 years of age; however, the incidence was 35% in men with no age association.[58] Antifilaggrin antibodies, such as antiperinuclear antibodies and antikeratin antibodies, may be more specific for the diagnosis of RA than RF, but they are not yet used clinically. Antiperinuclear antibodies are found in 45% to 60% of patients with RA. Antikeratin antibodies are found in 16% of Greek patients with RA and may be associated with positive RF, HLA-DR1, male sex, and radiographic progression of RA. ANCA is seen in 5% to 20% of patients with RA but globally is unrelated to serology and severity, except for some clinical features, as noted earlier. Also as noted earlier, IgG lacking galactose on the Fc component is found in RA, more commonly with active disease.

ESR is a nonspecific, clinically useful indicator of inflammation that correlates with synovial tissue inflammation and vasculitis. ESR is measured by placing anticoagulated whole blood in a small tube for 1 hour, allowing red blood cells to fall to the bottom of the tube, then measuring the number of millimeters that the red blood cells have vacated. Normal ESRs are generally 0 to 15 mm per hour, but may vary according to method and sex of the patient. CRP concentrations and platelet counts are nonspecific acute-phase reactants that are elevated in patients with active RA and may assist in the clinical assessment of disease. Plasma hyaluronic acid levels correlate with the number of tender or swollen joints but are not used clinically.

Joint x-rays are helpful in working up and following patients with RA. Early x-ray findings include soft tissue swelling. Periarticular bone loss may occur within 3 to 4 months of onset of RA. Bone erosions, bone cysts, and deformities may become evident as the disease progresses (Figs. 65.1 to 65.4). Radiographic classification is useful in following patients over time. Joint scintigraphy may be useful in detecting soft tissue swelling in early RA but adds nothing to the clinical examination. Magnetic resonance imaging (MRI) scans are well suited for use in the evaluation of early erosive disease, soft tissue (such as synovial tissue), cartilage, ligaments, and changes in bone marrow, but these are not used as commonly as joint x-rays. The evaluation of synovial proliferation by MRI scans is more sensitive and correlates better with clinical deterioration or improvement than does an evaluation performed with joint x-rays. Echography has also been used.

COMORBIDITIES

Patients with RA appear to be at higher risk for subclinical atherosclerosis,[59] cardiovascular events, lymphomas, preeclampsia and preterm delivery,[60] depression, and anxiety.[61] Increased inflammation, as measured by CRP, is associated with hypertension, increased triglycerides and homocysteine, and decreased high-density lipoprotein (HDL) cholesterol and insulin sensitivity.[62] Comorbidities that may be associated with RA and its therapy include peptic ulcer disease, osteoporosis, and infection. Males with RA have a higher risk for hypogonadism, possibly secondary to a central mechanism that controls hormonal synthesis or secretion.[63] However, patients with RA are less likely to have atopic diseases (e.g., hay fever, allergies).[64]

PROGNOSIS

The prognosis in most patients with rheumatoid arthritis is expected to be good, but is dependent on the course of the disease. Approximately 10% to 20% of patients with RA have a mild single cycle of the disease that remits spontaneously, 70% to 80% have multiple cycles of mild to moderate arthritis, and 10% to 15% have multiple cycles of progressive, severe disease. Patients with RA may experience temporary or permanent disability, considerable morbidity from medications or the systemic features of the disease, and some decrease in survival, particularly those with more severe disease. Quality of life, which can be assessed through a number of questionnaires, is affected in many patients at some time during the course of the disease. A very small number of patients will become confined to a wheelchair or bed because of RA. Overall survival is estimated to be 5% to 10% less among patients with RA than in the general population.

DIAGNOSIS AND CLINICAL FINDINGS

The American College of Rheumatology revised its criteria for the classification of rheumatoid arthritis in 1988.[65] These criteria (Table 65.3) are intended to serve as the standard in research and in the clinical setting, but they are not intended to impede the clinician's ability to make a diagnosis of RA on the basis of clinical findings and impressions. These classification criteria emphasize the chronic, symmetrical, and

TABLE 65.3	Classification of Rheumatoid Arthritis Based on the 1987 Revised "Traditional" Method

The patient must meet four of the following seven criteria to be classified as having rheumatoid arthritis:

1. Morning stiffness of or near joints, lasting 1 hour before maximum benefit.
2. Arthritis, as demonstrated by soft tissue swelling or fluid, in three or more joint areas, including right or left PIP, MCP, wrist, elbow, MTP, ankle, or knee joints.[a,b]
3. Arthritis, as demonstrated by soft tissue swelling or fluid, in the hand joints (PIP, MCP, or wrist).[a,b]
4. Symmetrical arthritis in the areas noted in criteria #2. PIP, MCP, and MTP joint area symmetry does not need to be absolute for this criterion to be met.[a,b]
5. Rheumatoid nodules as noted by subcutaneous nodules near bones or joints or on extensor surfaces.[b]
6. Positive rheumatoid factor determined by a test that is positive in less than 5% of normal subjects.
7. Radiologic changes of the hands or wrists, including erosions or bone decalcification in or next to involved joints.

[a] Present for at least 6 weeks.
[b] Must be observed by physician.
PIP, proximal interphalangeal joint(s); MCP, metacarpophalangeal joint(s); MTP, metatarsophalangeal joint(s).
(From Tilley BC, Alarcon GS, Heyse SP, et al. Minocycline in rheumatoid arthritis: a 48-week, double-blind, placebo-controlled trial. Ann Intern Med 122:81–89, 1995.)

small peripheral joint involvement associated with RA, as well as signs of its underlying pathophysiology. Despite these revised criteria and extensive educational efforts, the diagnosis of RA may be delayed by 36 weeks (median range, 4 weeks to 10+ years) after onset of symptoms and up to 18 weeks after the first medical encounter.[66] Children with chronic arthritis who meet certain diagnostic criteria are given a diagnosis of juvenile rheumatoid arthritis, which is not the same as a diagnosis of RA.

PSYCHOSOCIAL ASPECTS

Anxiety and depression are commonly seen in patients with RA, appear to be associated with disease activity, and may affect patients' perceptions of their arthritis activity.[61] Depression is associated with loss of valued activities.[67] Social stress and lack of social support are important features in the development of anxiety and depression in patients with RA. In patients with RA in the United States, depression is more common in women and Hispanics, particularly among those who have not been acculturated.[68] Antidepressants appear to be the major therapy for depression in these patients, with few additional benefits noted with the addition of cognitive-behavioral therapy.[69] Falls or fear of falling are

more common among patients with RA with more severe disease and other of comorbid conditions. Social problems also occur commonly in patients with RA. The healthcare professional should evaluate the impact of RA by assessing not only the physical limitations of the patient, but also the influence of those limitations on the patient's perceptions of expectations and living. The risk of schizophrenia is lower in patients with RA, and the risk of RA appears lower among patients with schizophrenia.[70]

As noted earlier, more severe disease at onset and follow-up may be noted in those patients from poor socioeconomic settings.[39] However, those with lower socioeconomic status use fewer health resources than do those with higher socioeconomic status.[71] RA can also influence patients' socioeconomic status or future by limiting their ability to work fully, thereby diminishing income.

THERAPEUTIC PLAN

The goals of therapy in rheumatoid arthritis are to improve or maintain current function in the patient's daily living activities, diminish progression of the patient's joint and extra-articular disease, and minimize adverse drug effects through beneficial, safe, and cost-effective means.[72,73] Therapy should be individualized for each patient according to the course of RA, the degree of articular and extra-articular disease, concurrent diseases and therapies, age, the need for relief, and a host of other factors. Very few patients will achieve a cure. Specific measures, such as surgery, are useful in correcting deformities and enhancing the ability to perform certain tasks.

Many treatment approaches and algorithms have been used in RA.[72,73] Therapy generally includes a series of levels of therapy to be administered according to the patient's level of disease. A basic level of therapy provides the fundamental first-line therapies that include proper amounts of rest and exercise, appropriate diet and education, and, possibly, the long-term administration of NSAIDs. The current approach used by experts is to aggressively add DMARDs to this basic therapy early in the disease, or as soon as progressive or sustained disease is seen or expected. This therapy is usually initiated with a single DMARD (usually methotrexate), but a very aggressive stepdown approach with a combination of DMARDs and high doses of systemic corticosteroids (with eventual decrease in dose of the corticoid and discontinuation of one of the DMARDs) has been used.[74] Patients may be sequentially treated with different DMARDs if lack of efficacy, loss of effect, or onset of adverse effects occurs. Physical and occupational devices to assist with ambulation and daily living activities, intra-articular injections of anti-inflammatory agents, surgery, and the treatment of extra-articular manifestations of RA are added to the program when they are needed at any level.

TREATMENT

PHARMACOTHERAPY

Pharmacogenomics. The association of drug efficacy with safety may be dependent on genetic factors, but few studies have been conducted in patients with RA. The three-drug combination of methotrexate, sulfasalazine, and hydroxychloroquine appears to be superior to those individual agents, particularly in patients with the shared HLA-DR1 epitope.[75] Of historical interest, injectable gold–induced proteinuria is associated with HLA-DRw3 or HLA-B8, and gold-induced skin toxicity is associated with the presence of anti-Ro (SSA) autoantibody.[76]

Disease-Modifying Antirheumatic Drugs. Disease-modifying antirheumatic drugs, also known as second-line agents, or disease-controlling or slow-acting antirheumatic drugs (SAARDs) include biologic response modifiers, other specific immunotherapies, antiproliferative agents, and miscellaneous agents. These agents differ in terms of their action on the immune system, onset of effect, adverse effects, and costs. Biologic response modifiers include TNF inhibitors (adalimumab, etanercept, infliximab) and an IL-1 inhibitor (anakinra). Biologic response modifiers are defined in this chapter as normally occurring or modified immune system components, including soluble receptors, immunoglobulins, and antigens that modify the immune response in RA. Other specific immunotherapies include calcineuron inhibitors, which act to modify the immunologic and/or inflammatory response of RA in a relatively specific manner. The antiproliferative drugs used in RA inhibit the proliferation of lymphocytes and other white blood cells in the bone marrow as a major part of their action in RA, but they have other effects on the immune system and on the proliferation of other cells, including perhaps the proliferating synovium of RA. These agents are mostly anticancer drugs with antimetabolite or alkylator activity, and they inhibit DNA replication. Methotrexate is the most widely used antiproliferative agent in RA, but leflunomide, mycophenolate mofetil, and azathioprine have also demonstrated benefits in patients with RA. Other antiproliferative drugs (cyclophosphamide, chlorambucil, mechlorethamine, paclitaxel) have demonstrated efficacy in RA, but their routine use is limited by toxicity. The group of miscellaneous immunotherapies includes modalities that do not fall into the other groups because of nonspecific or other effects on the immune system. This group includes commonly used drugs such as sulfasalazine, antimalarials, tetracyclines, gold salts, and penicillamine.

The use of DMARDs in RA is increasing, with probably well over 50% of patients with RA now receiving these drugs. DMARDs should be used as early as possible in patients with progressive, persistent, or potentially progressive RA. These agents are able to diminish the inflammation and slow the progression of joint destruction. A small case control study revealed that patients who did not use DMARDs had damage in 57% more joints and a 122% higher overall radiographic score compared with those who received DMARDs.[77] DMARDs may lead to remission in up to 5% of patients.

In patients with recently diagnosed RA without progressive disease, the use of DMARDs is somewhat controversial because it is difficult to predict which patients will go on to progressive, erosive disease, and whether toxicity and cost will be offset by potential benefits. Factors that predict which patients are at high risk for progressive joint destruction include specific HLA-DRB1 chain sequences, higher baseline ESR, first year progression, female sex, and a combination of positive rheumatoid factor, involvement of at least two large joints, and disease lasting longer than 3 months.[77,78] Aggressive therapy with DMARDs appears to be more effective if initiated early in the course of the disease than if initiated later. A number of DMARDs have proved useful in early RA.[74] In patients with early progressive disease, initiation of intramuscular gold was associated with improvement in overall health only when started within the first 2 years of disease onset.

Choosing among DMARDs has become somewhat difficult because of the growing number of available agents and the complexity of evaluating relative efficacy, safety, and costs. The onset of action of the DMARDs varies from days or weeks to weeks or months. In general, the biologic response modifiers (TNF-α inhibitors and IL-1 inhibitors) appear to be among the most effective and rapidly acting DMARDs, with some effects seen in days. Antiproliferative DMARDs appear to be moderately to highly effective but may take 6 to 8 weeks to work. Methotrexate and leflunomide appear to be among the most efficacious of the commonly used antiproliferative DMARDs, and they have reasonable safety profiles. Hydroxychloroquine is reasonably safe but is among the least effective of the DMARDs; it is most useful when given in combination with other DMARDs. Sulfasalazine and azathioprine have good safety profiles and appear to be intermediate in efficacy. The high risks of adverse effects associated with injectable gold salts, penicillamine, and cyclophosphamide and the low efficacy-to-safety ratio of auranofin (an oral gold salt) limit the use of these agents in the routine treatment of patients. Despite the need for long-term therapy with DMARDs, only 50% of those starting the drug will be taking oral gold (auranofin) after 10 months; taking hydroxychloroquine, penicillamine, injectable gold, or azathioprine after 20 to 27 months; and taking methotrexate after 60 months.[79] Other reports have found that 70% of patients are able to continue methotrexate for 5 years or longer. No direct comparisons of TNF-α inhibitors with IL-1 inhibitors have been conducted in patients with RA, making it difficult to validate the animal model findings that TNF-α had stronger proinflammatory effects and IL-1 had stronger effects on the destruction of cartilage and bone. However, a small study found no response to anakinra (IL-1 inhibitor) in those who had not responded to a TNF inhibitor.[80] On the basis of those data and the data that indicated that combination etanercept-anakinra was no more effective than etanercept alone, TNF and IL-1 inhibitors may act through or on a common pathway. Currently, many experts prefer to use TNF inhibitors before they try IL-1 inhibitors, possibly because experience with TNF inhibitors is more extensive.

The use of DMARDs continues to evolve through increased experience with an expanding number of selective biologic response modifiers. It is also controversial whether a single DMARD or a combination of two or three DMARDs should be added to basic therapy. Currently, on the basis of efficacy, safety, and cost, methotrexate is widely considered the initial DMARD of choice in moderate to severe RA, whether it is given as the only DMARD or is used in combination with other DMARDs. Leflunomide or sulfasalazine may also be used initially. Biologic response modifiers may eventually become the initial drugs of choice in moderate to severe RA, but their use is currently limited by concerns about cost and long-term adverse effects. Methotrexate, azathioprine, cyclophosphamide, cyclosporine, and tumor necrosis factor-α inhibitors are useful in treating patients with extra-articular manifestations such as steroid-resistant rheumatoid lung or vasculitis.

Combinations of Disease-Modifying Antirheumatic Drugs. Combinations of DMARDs can be used as the initial DMARD regimen, but they are definitely indicated with RA that is refractory to single-agent DMARD therapy. The goal of using DMARD combinations is to increase efficacy without increasing adverse effects through the use of drugs with different mechanisms of action. A few combination regimens have been associated with reversal of bony erosions. In patients who have lost the response or have had incomplete response to methotrexate, the addition of etanercept, infliximab, adalimumab, anakinra, cyclosporine, sulfasalazine, leflunomide, auranofin, or azathioprine is likely to be of benefit.[74,75,81–86] Leflunomide may also be combined with sulfasalazine, but little research has investigated the use of leflunomide with tumor necrosis factor inhibitors or interleukin-1 inhibitors. A number of three-drug combinations have been used effectively, including methotrexate-sulfasalazine-hydroxychloroquine, methotrexate-cyclosporine-sulfasalazine, and methotrexate-cyclosporine-infliximab.[75,87,88] DMARD

therapy may be initiated with an aggressive regimen that is then scaled back. A step-down approach in early RA involves starting with the combination of sulfasalazine, methotrexate, and prednisolone (60 mg/day), then slowly decreasing the doses of methotrexate and the corticoid until stopping them at 28 and 40 weeks, respectively.[74] Another approach is to initiate therapy with methotrexate and hydroxychloroquine, then discontinue one of them when a response has stabilized.[86] In a 10-year study, a very aggressive combination of 3 days of intravenous methylprednisolone and cyclophosphamide followed by methotrexate, cyclosporine, and mycophenolate mofetil was very effective in diminishing mortality, disability, and the overall burden of RA.[89] Cyclophosphamide is very effective when used in DMARD combinations, but it is not routinely used because of the potential for development of secondary tumors and other serious adverse effects. Although animal models demonstrated that blockage of both IL-1 and TNF-α reduced the inflammation and destruction in an arthritis model over each type of blockade alone,[90] the combination of etanercept and anakinra did not appear to be more efficacious than etanercept alone and was associated with an increased risk of serious infection, injection site reaction, and neutropenia.[91] Combinations of DMARDs can be very effective in RA; this option may eventually become the DMARD treatment of choice in patient with progressive RA.

Tumor Necrosis Factor-α Inhibitors. The TNF-α inhibitors that are currently available (adalimumab, etanercept, and infliximab, Table 65.4) are very effective in the treatment of patients with RA and appear to have similar efficacy in RA when added to methotrexate therapy.[92–97] These agents bind TNF-α and then are removed by phagocytic cells, leading to a decrease in TNF-α concentrations, binding to receptors, and subsequent actions. TNF-α blockade decreases neutrophil migration into inflamed joints, diminishes the secretion of IL-1, IL-6, and IL-8, and inhibits cartilage destruction in an animal model of RA.[90] Additionally, TNF-α inhibitors reverse the inhibition of endothelium-dependent vasodilation in RA, thereby having the potential to diminish risks for cardiovascular events.[55] These agents have an onset of effect in days to 1 month and can improve quality of life

TABLE 65.4	Characteristics of Tumor Necrosis Factor-α Inhibitors and the Interleukin-1 Inhibitor	
Drug	**Description**	**Usual Dosage and Administration**
Adalimumab	Recombinant humanized anti-TNF monoclonal antibody	40 mg every other week subcutaneously
Etanercept	Soluble TNF-α receptors (p-75) attached to the Fc portion of human IgG₁	16 mg two times per week subcutaneously
Infliximab	Murine TNF-α binding region chimerized to human IgG₁	3 mg/kg at weeks 2 and 6, then every 8 weeks intravenously over 2 hours. Use with methotrexate
Anakinra	Recombinant human IL-1 receptor antagonist	100 mg per day subcutaneously

Ig, immunoglobulin; IL, interleukin; TNF, tumor necrosis factor.

and delay joint destruction alone or when added to methotrexate.[94–96]

Infliximab must be used with methotrexate to prevent the development of neutralizing antibodies, but cyclosporine can be used in patients who cannot tolerate MTX.[98] TNF-α inhibitors may also be useful in treating patients with select extra-articular manifestations of RA such as rheumatoid lung and refractory vasculitis. Adverse effects include injection site reactions, minor upper respiratory tract symptoms, and allergic reactions. Adalimumab has been used successfully in a patient with an anaphylactic reaction to infliximab.[99] TNF inhibitors have been associated with leukopenia and an increase in infections, most commonly mycobacterial and histoplasmosis infections, but also listeriosis, *Pneumocystis*, and fungal (coccidiomycosis) infections.[100–102] The risk of infections may be higher with infliximab (plus methotrexate).[101]

Infections with *Staphylococcus aureus* or *E. coli* in patients on TNF inhibitors appear to induce anticardiolipin and anti-DNA antibodies, an action that is reversed by eradication of bacteria.[103] TNF inhibitors appear to increase the risks for lymphoma[104] drug-induced lupus, seizures, demyelinating syndromes, and worsening of multiple sclerosis and congestive heart failure in patients with RA.[100,102] However, heart failure was not more common in those on TNF-α inhibitors.[105] In a large retrospective study, serious and nonserious liver toxicity was higher in those taking biologic modifiers than in those on leflunomide or methotrexate.[106] No evidence suggests that TNF-α inhibitors are teratogenic or harmful to fetuses.[102] Absolute or relative contraindications to the use of TNF-α inhibitors include active or recurrent infection, moderate heart failure, and the presence of cancer. It may be best to avoid the use of live vaccines in patients receiving TNF-α inhibitors.

Interleukin-1 Inhibitors. IL-1 inhibitors are also effective in decreasing signs, symptoms, disease progression, and dysfunction in patients with RA.[107,108] IL-1 blockade blocks macrophage infiltration in the synovium in patients with RA[109] but does not inhibit cartilage destruction in an animal model of RA.[90] Anakinra, the only IL-1 inhibitor that is currently available, is a recombinant IL-1 receptor antagonist that binds to the IL-1 receptor and blocks the effects of IL-1 at the receptor without activating the receptor itself. Anakinra has an onset of anti-inflammatory effect within 1 month in many patients and has demonstrated a decrease in progressive joint destruction in RA after 24 and 48 weeks of therapy.[110] The adverse effects of anakinra are similar to those seen with TNF-α inhibitors, including injection site reaction (in up to 71% of patients), increased risk of serious infection (1 to 2% incidence), headache (14%), and hypersensitivity. Injection site reactions are self-limiting in some patients. Comorbidities (history of cardiovascular event, pulmonary disease, renal disease, infection, diabetes, cancer, or central nervous system event) did not increase the risk of infection in patients on anakinra.[111] Antianakinra antibodies

have also been detected, but the significance of those antibodies is unclear.

Calcineuron Inhibitors. Cyclosporine (CyA, cyclosporin A, Neoral, Sandimmune) is effective in RA, possibly because it causes decreases in helper T-cell secretion of IL-2, T-cell recruitment into rheumatoid synovial tissue, and IL-10, IL-15, and TNF-α concentrations in RA. Initial doses are 2.5 mg/kg/day, given in two doses; this may be increased to a recommended maximum of 4 mg/kg/day, but doses up to 10 mg/kg/day have been used. It is indicated for use in patients who have failed methotrexate and may be used alone or in combination with methotrexate.[81] The efficacy of cyclosporine in refractory RA may be partly due to its binding to p-glycoprotein and its ability to reverse the effects of a multidrug resistance gene. Cyclosporine plus an oral corticosteroid may also be beneficial in the treatment of patients with rheumatoid lung and other inflammatory extra-articular manifestations of RA.

Cyclosporine has complicated, variable pharmacokinetics, including variable absorption, binding to lipoproteins and red blood cells, and extensive hepatic metabolism via the cytochrome P450 system. Measurement of cyclosporine concentrations is not a commonly used approach for monitoring patients with RA because relatively low doses are used compared with those given to prevent transplant rejection. If this approach is used, interpretation of the measured value requires knowledge of the type of sample (blood vs. plasma or serum) and assay, as well as of timing relative to the dose.

The use of cyclosporine in RA is somewhat limited by adverse effects and the need for monitoring every 2 to 6 weeks. Nephrotoxicity, hypertension, infection, gingival hyperplasia, hypertrichosis, fatigue, and gastrointestinal and neurologic complaints (paresthesias) are frequent in patients with transplants, but they are less frequent with the lower doses used in patients with RA. The mean decrease in renal function of 16% in patients taking cyclosporine for RA rarely leads to irreversible, structural damage. Infections associated with cyclosporine include *Pneumocystis carinii* and fungal, viral, and bacterial infections.

Drug interactions with cyclosporine are numerous and involve both pharmacokinetic and pharmacodynamic mechanisms. Drugs that enhance (e.g., rifampin, phenytoin) or inhibit (e.g., cimetidine, ketoconazole, ciprofloxacin) CYP3A4 will alter the clearance of cyclosporine. Drugs with renal toxicity may also enhance the renal toxicity of cyclosporine. The use of NSAIDs with cyclosporine in the treatment of patients with RA does not usually lead to renal toxicity,[112] probably in part because of the lower doses of cyclosporine used in RA compared with the doses used in prevention of transplant rejection. Cyclosporine increases the serum concentrations of diclofenac and serum creatinine. Cyclosporine inhibits the metabolism of methotrexate and decreases its clearance by 18%.[113]

Tacrolimus (Prograf, FK-506) is similar to cyclosporine in many respects. Tacrolimus also inhibits secretion of

IL-2 by helper T-cells, results in immunosuppression and prophylaxis against rejection of transplants, and inhibits IL-6 release. Additionally, the pharmacokinetic and adverse effect profiles of tacrolimus are very similar to those of cyclosporine. It can be anticipated to have effects in RA that are similar to those of cyclosporine.

Methotrexate. Methotrexate (MTX, Rheumatrex) is effective in RA at doses ranging from 7.5 to 20 mg administered weekly, orally, intramuscularly, or subcutaneously,[114] in one dose or in three equal doses every 12 hours. An oral solution of 10 mg of injectable MTX mixed in 8 ounces of water may be substituted for oral tablets,[115] resulting in less expensive drug acquisition costs. High-dose MTX (500 mg/m^2) followed by leucovorin rescue every 2 weeks has been of some use in patients with refractory RA.[116] MTX inhibits leukotriene synthesis, decreases TNF-α concentrations, and inhibits dihydrofolate reductase, which results in decreases in proliferation of T-lymphocytes, B-lymphocytes, and rapidly dividing (but not slowly dividing) synoviocytes, along with apoptosis of activated peripheral blood T-lymphocytes[117] (but not resting lymphocytes). MTX differs from other non–biologic response modifier DMARDs in its rapid response (as early as 4 to 6 weeks), the arthritis flare seen soon after withdrawal of MTX,[118] and the increase in rheumatoid nodules noted during its use.[48] MTX was most effective in decreasing tender joint counts in a meta-analysis of DMARDs. Patients who initially respond to MTX, then have a worsening in RA, are likely to respond to an increase in the dose of MTX. MTX is contraindicated in pregnant women.

MTX oral absorption averages 70% but is highly variable, diminishes following cholecystectomy, and reportedly decreases by 13.5% over time in patients with RA. Oral tablets and diluted intravenous MTX used orally appear to have equal bioavailability.[115] MTX is found in high levels in synovial membrane and bone even after serum levels have diminished. Approximately 10% of MTX is metabolized to an active metabolite, 7-hydroxy-methotrexate. Biliary excretion may account for 9% to 26% of MTX elimination and 2% to 5% of 7-hydroxy metabolite elimination after low doses of MTX. MTX clearance is decreased in patients who are elderly or who have decreased renal function, is increased by hemodialysis, and is not altered by peritoneal dialysis.

Patients are monitored every 2 weeks initially, then eventually every 6 weeks, for adverse effects from MTX. Pooled clinical studies have revealed that withdrawals from MTX are due to hepatic effects (10.3%), mucous membrane effects (2.6%), nausea and/or vomiting (2.1%), gastrointestinal effects (2.1%), leukopenia (1%), blood effects (1.5%), and diarrhea (0.5%). Most liver effects were seen as elevations of liver enzyme levels rather than as abnormalities on liver biopsy. Liver biopsies are the definitive method used to detect hepatotoxicity, but they are not routinely recommended in patients with RA who are receiving MTX, because of the low incidence of hepatotoxicity and the morbidity, mortality,

and costs associated with liver biopsy. An increased incidence of abnormalities in liver enzymes is seen in patients taking MTX plus aspirin,[119] and in those with alcoholism, diabetes, or obesity. Although usually irreversible, severe liver toxicity is occasionally reversible. Many clinicians believe that monitoring of liver enzymes could be performed every 3 to 4 months because of the low risk of alterations in MTX therapy caused by liver toxicity in patients with RA.[120] Sustained elevation of mean corpuscular volume in a patient treated with MTX may indicate folate deficiency and may predict MTX hematologic toxicity. Severe neutropenia, thrombocytopenia, anemia, and pancytopenia may develop with low doses of MTX, especially in those patients with old age, renal disease, hypoalbuminemia, and concomitant antiproliferative agents. MTX-induced pancytopenia may respond to pulse methylprednisolone and granulocyte colony-stimulating factor (G-CSF).[121] MTX causes immunosuppression and possibly an increase in postsurgical infections,[122] but no consensus has been reached about whether or not it should be stopped before major surgery is performed. MTX induces or reactivates infections such as herpes zoster or Epstein-Barr, which may be followed by complications such as shingles or Epstein-Barr virus–associated lymphoma, respectively. Patients with RA have an increased incidence of MTX-induced pulmonary toxicity, particularly those patients with increased age, smoking history, preexisting interstitial pulmonary disorders, rheumatoid lung, diabetes, hypoalbuminemia, and previous adverse effects to disease-modifying drugs, and possibly those with previous pulmonary disorders.[123–125] The incidence is reportedly low but has been as high as 2%. MTX-induced lung toxicity begins as a pneumonitis with symptoms of cough, shortness of breath, and/or fever; it then may progress to pulmonary fibrosis and possibly death.[126] Pulmonary problems recur upon rechallenge with MTX, with an increased risk of mortality.[126] Methotrexate was associated with increased mortality in patients with preexisting cardiovascular disease, but not in those without cardiovascular disease, possibly because of increases in homocysteine blood levels.[127] Hypersensitivity, rashes, and vasculitis are rarely associated with MTX.

Concurrent folic acid and leucovorin administration may diminish MTX-induced stomatitis and macrocytic anemia, but leucovorin use can diminish MTX efficacy.[128] Folic acid is usually administered at doses of 1 mg per day for 4 days per week; this is done by omitting the day before, the day of, and the day after MTX administration. Folic acid doses up to 27.5 mg per week have been used. Folic acid also diminishes the risk of hyperhomocysteinemia and therefore may decrease the risk of cardiovascular disease.[129] Severe MTX toxicity is reversed by leucovorin. Allopurinol mouthwashes (5-mg/mL suspension in water) have been useful in the treatment of patients with MTX-induced stomatitis,[130] but patients should be discouraged from swallowing the suspension.

Drug interactions involving MTX may have serious consequences. As was noted earlier, aspirin is associated with increases in MTX hepatotoxicity. Salicylate and probenecid inhibit MTX excretion. However, no clinically relevant effects of NSAIDs (aspirin, diclofenac, ibuprofen, indomethacin, and naproxen) on MTX pharmacokinetics have been observed.[131] Cholestyramine binds to MTX and enhances its excretion. Trimethoprim and antiproliferative drugs increase the toxicity of MTX. Folinic acid may reverse the efficacy of MTX, depending on the dose and timing of administration.

Leflunomide. Leflunomide (Arava) is effective in RA when given as a loading dose of 100 mg daily for 3 days followed by 10 to 20 mg per day.[132] Leflunomide 100 mg once weekly appeared to be as effective and safe as 20 mg daily, and the 100-mg regimen improved compliance.[133] Leflunomide is rapidly metabolized to an active metabolite (A77 1726), a malononitrilamide with a half-life of 11 to 16 days that is more than 99% plasma protein bound.[132] This metabolite inhibits B- and T-cell proliferation, antibody secretion, and cellular adhesion. Leflunomide's active metabolite inhibits nucleotide (pyrimidine) synthesis through inhibition of dihydroorotate dehydrogenase. Major adverse effects of leflunomide include gastrointestinal disturbances, weight loss, allergic reactions, transient elevations of liver transaminases, and reversible alopecia. Liver toxicity has been a concern with leflunomide, but the rate of leflunomide-associated serious and nonserious liver toxicity was similar to that seen with methotrexate and lower than those noted with biological modifiers.[106] Decreases in hematocrit, hemoglobin, and platelets are seen less often but do not usually require discontinuation of the drug. Leflunomide is contraindicated in pregnancy. Both efficacy and adverse effects are more common with higher doses of leflunomide. Cholestyramine and activated charcoal decrease plasma levels of the active metabolite by 40% to 50%.

Azathioprine. Azathioprine (Imuran) has demonstrated efficacy in treating patients with RA at doses of 1.0 to 2.5 mg/kg/day, or 50 to 200 mg per day. Azathioprine has a half-life of 0.2 to 1 hour, is removed by hemodialysis, and is converted to 6-mercaptopurine, its active form. Purine inhibition by 6-mercaptopurine inhibits proliferation of lymphocytes and other white blood cells. Allopurinol inhibits the metabolism of azathioprine, which requires that the dose of azathioprine should be decreased by 67% to 75%.

Azathioprine and MTX have common adverse effects. The risk of adverse effects from azathioprine has been a matter of concern, but a postmarketing surveillance study has revealed a relatively safe adverse effect profile in RA.[134] Monitoring of complete blood counts, administration of liver function tests, and examination of mucous membranes every 2 to 6 weeks are necessary for evaluation of azathioprine-induced gastrointestinal distress, leukopenia, anemia, stomatitis, pancreatitis, pneumonitis, and liver toxicity. Infection and pulmonary toxicity have also been reported. Severe bone marrow suppression is rarely seen and may be associated with deficiencies in purine metabolic enzymes. Azathioprine may be associated with the development of tumors, but this is seen only in case reports.

Mycophenolate Mofetil. Mycophenolate mofetil (MMF, CellCept) has been used and approved for use in the prevention of transplant rejection, but it has also been used in the treatment of patients with RA at doses of 2,000 mg per day.[1,135] Mycophenolate mofetil is a prodrug for mycophenolic acid, which is a noncompetitive, reversible inhibitor of inosine monophosphate dehydrogenase that disrupts the synthesis of guanine nucleotides. MMF appears to inhibit the proliferation of lymphocytes to a greater extent than the proliferation of other cells. In patients with RA, MMF decreased rheumatoid factor, swelling, and pain. However, only 8 of 28 patients responded in one study.[1] The drug is well tolerated in patients with RA; reversible gastrointestinal effects, including nausea, vomiting, abdominal pain, and diarrhea, are the most common adverse effects. However, bone marrow suppression and liver toxicity have been reported in transplant patients.

Sulfasalazine. Sulfasalazine (Azulfidine) was designed in the 1940s to treat patients with RA, but it has only recently been used widely in the treatment of those with RA following promising study findings. Sulfasalazine is broken down to sulfapyridine and aminosalicylate in the gut. Both sulfasalazine and its sulfapyridine metabolite have effects against RA. Sulfasalazine decreases secretion of IL-6, immunoglobulins, and rheumatoid factors in RA. It is often used in patients with mild RA but is also effective in patients with moderate to severe disease.

The adverse effect withdrawal rate from sulfasalazine is intermediate compared with those of other DMARDs, but the occurrence of serious adverse effects with sulfasalazine is low. Sulfasalazine was withdrawn for nausea and/or vomiting (12.5%), skin rash (3.8%), liver effects (1.6%), leukopenia (1.1%), mucous membrane effects (1.1%), fever (1.1%), anemia (0.5%), and lung effects (0.5%). Folate deficiency may be commonly seen in patients on sulfasalazine and may be associated with chronic hemolytic anemia in some patients. Toxic epidermal necrolysis and drug-induced lupus are rarely seen with sulfasalazine. Monitoring for toxicity is mostly based upon clinical presentation of the patient.

Antimalarials. Antimalarials have been used in RA since a 1951 report described a patient whose RA improved after mepacrine was used to treat the patient's discoid lupus.[136] Chloroquine (Aralen) was used most often for a time, but it has been widely replaced by hydroxychloroquine in the treatment of patients with RA, although chloroquine may be more effective. Hydroxychloroquine diminishes the functions of macrophages but also increases pain thresholds. Hydroxychloroquine is used at doses of 2 to 4 mg per kg or 200 to 400 mg per day orally. Antimalarials are used in milder disease or in combination with other DMARDs.

Hydroxychloroquine (Plaquenil) is readily absorbed following oral administration, with peak levels attained in 1 to 3 hours. Hydroxychloroquine is 45% bound to serum albumin, distributes into red blood cells and other tissues, and has a half-life of approximately 40 days. Dosage adjustments are not needed in renal dysfunction because only 22% to 34% of hydroxychloroquine is excreted unchanged in urine.

Pooled data from clinical studies reveal that hydroxychloroquine is among the least toxic of the DMARDs. Adverse effects include gastrointestinal tract effects (4.6%), rash (2.3%), ocular problems (0.7%), and, less commonly, leukopenia and central nervous system, neuromuscular, and cardiac effects. Hydroxychloroquine is rarely discontinued because of retinopathy at the dosage ranges listed above; this has caused experts to question the need for a complete ophthalmic examination performed by an ophthalmologist every 6 to 12 months during therapy. However, hydroxychloroquine may also exacerbate psoriasis and cause allergic rashes, hemolytic anemia, and gastrointestinal and neurologic effects. Chloroquine has decreased the normal response to intradermal rabies vaccine in normal subjects and may induce heart block.

Tetracyclines. Tetracyclines, minocycline (Minocin), and doxycycline (Doryx, Vibramycin, Vibra-Tabs) may be of benefit in treating patients with RA in a pattern similar to that seen with other DMARDs, with a slow onset of effect and no loss of effect shortly after discontinuation of the drug.[17-19] Tetracyclines have decreased IL-6 and rheumatoid factor, and they are postulated to decrease the production of collagenase, thereby reducing the inflammation and destruction caused by those enzymes.[19] Minocycline 100 mg given twice daily was effective as early as after 1 month of therapy in open-label and placebo-controlled studies.[18] The major adverse effects caused by tetracyclines include gastrointestinal effects, dizziness, and photosensitivity reactions.

Other DMARDs. A number of disease-modifying antirheumatic drugs have considerable historical significance but are now used only rarely because of the low benefit-to-risk ratio. Drugs with considerable efficacy but high in risk for adverse effects include injectable gold salts and penicillamine. Serious adverse effects resulting from gold salts and penicillamine include renal, dermatologic, and hematologic toxicities. Oral gold—auranofin—is associated with a lower incidence of the same serious adverse effects than injectable gold salts but is less effective.

Nonsteroidal Anti-Inflammatory Drugs. NSAIDs are considered to be an integral part of the treatment of patients with RA. However, data indicate that NSAID use has dropped to the extent that only 76% of patients with RA are taking an NSAID.[79,137] NSAIDs inhibit prostaglandin synthesis, as well as membrane-related enzyme activities, membrane anion transport, arachidonate precursor uptake and insertion into monocyte membranes, collagenase release, T-cell responses to IL-2, and neutrophil function.

NSAIDs also enhance cytotoxic and suppressor T-cell activities, which may result in inhibition of B-cell activity. Most currently available NSAIDs increase or do not alter leukotriene levels, but ketoprofen and investigational agents inhibit leukotriene synthesis and bradykinin activity. Glycosaminoglycan synthesis in joint cartilage is inhibited by sodium salicylate, but other NSAIDs are noted to inhibit cartilage destruction. The clinical significance of many of these differences is unclear. The D-isomer (S[+] isomer) of the propionate derivatives demonstrates anti-inflammatory activity.

NSAID-induced inhibition of cyclooxygenase-mediated prostaglandin synthesis appears to be responsible for many of the beneficial and harmful effects of NSAIDs. Prostaglandins are locally active components derived from phospholipids that have two major activities: regulation of organ function and reaction to damage. Cyclooxygenase-1 (COX-1) is involved in the synthesis of prostaglandins that regulate organ function (e.g., vasodilation, vasoconstriction, bronchoconstriction, bronchodilation, gastric secretion, insulin secretion). Cyclooxygenase-2 (COX-2) is involved in the synthesis of prostaglandins that react to damage, resulting in inflammation and pain.[138] COX-2 selectivity is determined by the ratio of the concentration needed to inhibit COX-2 to the concentration needed to inhibit COX-1. In general, NSAIDs can be classified as nonselective, intermediately COX-2 selective, and highly COX-2 selective (Table 65.5).[138-140] Nonselective NSAIDs include ibuprofen, naproxen, indomethacin, and numerous older NSAIDs. Those with intermediate COX-2 selectivity include etodolac, nabumetone, and meloxicam. Highly selective COX-2–inhibiting NSAIDs include celecoxib, valdecoxib, and currently unap-

TABLE 65.5	COX-2 Selectivity: Ratios of COX-1:COX-2 Inhibitory Concentrations	
Drug	**Whole Blood**	**In Vitro**
Lumiracoxib		400
Etoricoxib	106	344
Rofecoxib	35	272
Valdecoxib	30	60–61.5
Celecoxib	7.6	29.6–30
Diclofenac	3.0	
Etodolac	2.4	
Meloxicam	2.0	
Parecoxib		
Indomethacin	0.4	
Ibuprofen	0.2–0.5	
Naproxen and metabolite	0.7–1.5	
Piroxicam	0.08	
Acetaminophen	1.6	

proved agents such as etoricoxib and lumiracoxib. The potential decrease in adverse effects of gastrointestinal ulceration and bleeding, renal dysfunction, and inhibition of platelet aggregation by COX-2–specific NSAIDs may be offset by an increase in cardiovascular events.

All NSAIDs are essentially equivalent in the treatment of patients with RA, although some patients appear to be helped more by certain NSAIDs than by others. The impression that nonacetylated salicylates are less effective is not documented by clinical studies.[141] The anti-inflammatory effects of NSAIDs in RA are seen within a few days to a week (longer for agents with longer half-lives), with maximum effects seen in 1 to 4 weeks. Analgesic and antipyretic effects of NSAIDs are seen within hours. NSAIDs decrease ESR, CRP, RF, and the number of circulating activated T-cells in patients with RA. Hemoglobin and hematocrit, if decreased because of an anemia of the chronic inflammatory process of RA, may not increase even if the patient has had a good response to the NSAID. This minimal response is due to increased bleeding or limited effects on the underlying disease process.

NSAIDs are traditionally considered to be part of the background therapy for patients with mild to late and early to advanced RA, but long-term toxicity limits their use so that many patients decrease the dose or stop the NSAID when the response to DMARDs is evident. Adverse effects, cost, and ease of administration are major factors to be considered when one chooses an NSAID. If a patient does not tolerate or respond to maximum anti-inflammatory doses after 2 weeks, or if the patient loses response, then subsequent selections can be taken from a different or the same chemical class. Less than 50% of those starting an NSAID will be taking that agent after 12 months.[79] Aspirin is inexpensive and may be safer than was previously thought,[142] but it is still reserved for use in those who are not responding to other NSAIDs. The high doses of NSAIDs needed to treat patients with RA increase the likelihood of toxicity.

NSAIDs are generally well absorbed following oral administration and are highly bound to albumin. Plasma protein binding of salicylates is greater than 95% at low levels, but it diminishes as the salicylate level increases and as binding sites become saturated. The half-lives and dosing of NSAIDs vary considerably (Table 65.6).[141] Synovial fluid levels of NSAIDs rise and fall at slower rates than their serum levels do, with synovial fluid levels becoming greater than serum levels at times proportionate to their half-lives.[143] This may explain in part why ibuprofen, which has a half-life of 2.1 hours, is effective when given two to four times daily.[141] Synovial fluid levels of NSAIDs with longer half-lives generally do not exceed serum levels during the dosing interval.[143] Most NSAIDs undergo hepatic metabolism, but appreciable amounts are excreted unchanged in urine. Glucuronidation of ketoprofen and possibly other NSAIDs may be reversed in patients with renal failure.[141] Aspirin is rapidly deacetylated in plasma to salicylic acid, which then displays nonlinear pharmacokinetics at anti-inflammatory

plasma levels of 150 to 250 mg per L. Sulindac is metabolized to an inactive, renally excreted metabolite and its active metabolite. Nabumetone is metabolized to its active component. At high doses, naproxen is unusual in that its excretion is increased and serum levels are lower than expected for the increase in dose. End-stage renal disease prolongs the half-life of diflunisal (Table 65.6). Dosage adjustments may be needed in patients with end-stage renal or hepatic disease, depending upon the specific drug that is used.

Adverse effects from NSAIDs involve many organ systems, demonstrate considerable interpatient variability, and require careful monitoring.[144] Indomethacin and meclofenamate are frequently associated with severe adverse effects. Older studies demonstrated that aspirin was associated with a greater number of adverse effects than were other NSAIDs; however, recent studies have demonstrated a safer profile for aspirin probably because of the current use of lower doses of aspirin (2,665 mg/day on average) compared with previous higher doses (2,600 to 5,000 mg/day), or possibly as the result of patient selection.[142]

Gastrointestinal effects, the most common problem associated with NSAIDs, include discomfort, distress, nausea, vomiting, diarrhea, bleeding, and ulceration. COX-2 selective and nonselective NSAIDs appear to cause similar incidences of minor gastrointestinal adverse effects. Meclofenamate has a high incidence of diarrhea. Microbleeding is greater from aspirin than from other NSAIDs. Gastric ulceration or bleeding occurs in 0.5% to 3% of patients on nonselective NSAIDs, but mucosal damage is found in up to 75% of patients taking long-term NSAIDs. COX-2 selective NSAIDs cause gastric or duodenal ulceration, but at a rate that is 50% to 70% lower than the rate seen with nonselective NSAIDs.[145] However, when low-dose aspirin is added to the COX-2 selective NSAID, the risk of ulceration or hemorrhage is similar to that seen with nonselective NSAIDs. Nabumetone and etodolac also cause less gastric or duodenal ulceration than is caused by nonselective NSAIDs.

The ulcerogenic effects of NSAIDs are due in part to an increase in gastric acidity that may occur after 1 month of NSAID therapy.[146] Patients at high risk for peptic ulceration or bleeding include the elderly, smokers, and those with a history of peptic ulcer disease, gastrointestinal bleeding, or liver or renal disease; those on high doses of NSAIDs or on nonselective NSAIDs; and those who receive corticosteroids on a long-term basis. No apparent association has been observed between NSAID-induced ulceration and *Helicobacter pylori* infection.[147] It is unclear whether it is more beneficial and cost-effective to use a COX-2 selective NSAID or a nonselective NSAID plus a gastroprotective agent (proton pump inhibitor, histamine-2 antagonist, PGE_1 analog) in a patient at high risk for NSAID-induced ulceration or hemorrhage. Proton pump inhibitors such as omeprazole are effective in protecting against gastrointestinal ulceration. Histamine-2 receptor antagonists are less effective in preventing NSAID-associated gastric ulceration or bleeding but are useful in preventing duodenal ulceration or bleeding

TABLE 65.6	Nonsteroidal Anti-Inflammatory Drugs Used in Rheumatoid Arthritis

Drug (active metabolite)	Half-life, hours		Daily Dose in RA, mg/day	Doses per Day
	Normal	In ESRD		
Acetic Acids				
Diclofenac	1–2	1–2	150–200	3–4
Etodolac	7	NC[a]	800–1,200	3–4
Indomethacin	1–16	NC	100–200	3–4
Indomethacin SR	1–16	NC	150	1–2
Nabumetone (acetic acid)	22–30[b]	39	1,000–2,000	1–2
Sulindac	8	NC	300–400	2
(sulfide)	16–18			
Tolmetin	1–5		1,600–2,000	3–4
Fenamates				
Meclofenamate	1–3		300–400	3–4
Oxicams				
Meloxicam				
Piroxicam	30–86	44	10–20	1
Propionates				
Fenoprofen	1.5–4		1,600–3,200	3–4
Flurbiprofen	3–6		200–300	2–4
Ibuprofen	1–2.5	2.5	1,600–3,200	3–4
Ketoprofen	1–4	3.2	150–300	3–4
Ketoprofen SR[c]	1–4	3.2	200	1
Naproxen	9–17	15	500–1,500	2–3
Oxaprozin	42–50		1,200–1,800	1
Salicylates				
Aspirin	0.2–0.3	NC	2,400–6,500	3–5
(Salicylate)	2–30	NC		
Diflunisal	5–20	15–138	500–1,500	2–3
Salsalate	2–30	NC	2,000–3,000	3–4
Other salicylates	2–30	NC	2,400–6,500	3–5
COX–2 Selective				
Celecoxib	11	NC	200–400	1–2
Valdecoxib	8	NC	20	1–2

[a] No change in half-life.
[b] Longer half-life in elderly patients.
ESRD, end-stage renal disease; SR, sustained-release.

in high-risk patients. Misoprostol, a PGE_1 analog, protects against gastric and duodenal ulceration associated with long-term NSAID use, but it is also associated with considerable diarrhea and gastrointestinal cramping and is contraindicated in pregnancy because of its ability to induce abortions. A misoprostol-diclofenac combination product (Arthrotec) provides a convenient method of drug administration in those patients at risk for ulceration. Sucralfate has little protective effect against NSAID-induced ulceration. Histamine-2 antagonists and sulcralfate diminish the dyspepsia associated with NSAIDs. Treatment of patients with NSAID-induced gastric or duodenal ulcers includes histamine-2 antagonists and proton pump inhibitors. Proton pump inhibitors or high dose histamine-2 antagonists may lead to a higher ulcer healing rate in patients who remain on an NSAID, or who smoke cigarettes.

Commonly occurring central nervous effects from NSAIDs include dizziness, fussiness, and headache. These occur more commonly in the elderly. The use of indomethacin is limited by the high percentage of resultant central nervous system effects, including hallucinations, dizziness, headaches, confusion, disorientation, and nightmares. Aseptic meningitis occurs rarely, most often in patients with systemic lupus erythematosus who take ibuprofen, but it has occurred with the use of other NSAIDs and with other disorders such as RA.

The most common NSAID-induced renal disorder is a decrease in renal blood flow that is due to prostaglandin inhibition, but interstitial nephritis, tubular necrosis, and papillary necrosis are also observed. Patients with cardiovascular conditions or cirrhosis and those who are elderly, elderly on loop diuretics, on high doses of NSAIDs, or renally insufficient are at higher risk of NSAID-induced renal disease. These patients need increased levels of vasodilating renal prostaglandins to maintain sufficient renal blood flow and glomerular filtration. Nabumetone, etodolac, sulindac, and nonacetylated salicylates have less of an effect on renal prostaglandins than do other NSAIDs and may be preferred for use in high-risk patients. COX-2 selective NSAIDs cause renal dysfunction, but the rate and/or magnitude of the renal dysfunction is similar to or less than that seen with nonselective NSAIDs. NSAID-induced prostaglandin-mediated renal dysfunction is generally reversible, but chronic renal failure has been reported.

NSAIDs inhibit platelet aggregation due to concentration-dependent inhibition of platelet thromboxane production. Production of vascular prostacyclin, an antithrombotic prostaglandin, may also be inhibited. Nabumetone, etodolac, and nonacetylated salicylates and intermediate and highly COX-2 selective NSAIDs have minimal effects on thromboxane production and do not inhibit platelet aggregation. Highly COX-2 selective NSAIDs decreased prostacyclin production by 58% and thromboxane production by up to 17%, compared with decreases of 75% in prostacyclin production and 85% in thromboxane production following use of a nonselective NSAID.[148] Rofecoxib, a highly COX-2 selective NSAID, was recently withdrawn from the market following research that demonstrated an increased risk of cardiovascular events. It is unclear whether that risk is a class effect of highly COX-2 selective NSAIDs or is specific to select agents. A slightly increased risk of cardiovascular events in patients on highly COX-2 selective NSAIDs compared with nonselective NSAIDs has been seen for other agents, but not in all comparisons.[149] Aspirin causes irreversible inhibition of platelet aggregation that persists for 3 to 7 days, but the effect is reversible with other NSAIDs. A nonacetylated salicylate, an NSAID with a short half-life, or, possibly, a COX-2 selective NSAID is preferred in patients who are about to undergo surgery. The antiplatelet effect generally disappears within 24 hours of cessation of a nonselective NSAID with a short half-life. Ibuprofen can block the antiplatelet effects of aspirin through competitive interaction at the site of action in platelets. Severe aspirin toxicity is associated with hypoprothrombinemia. Agranulocytosis and aplas-

tic anemia are rarely associated with NSAIDs. Infertility is a rare complication of NSAID use.[150]

NSAIDs are associated with cholestatic and/or cellular hepatotoxicity. Aspirin, diclofenac, or sulindac may cause a higher incidence of liver toxicity.[141] Aspirin-induced hepatotoxicity has been associated with more active arthritis. NSAID-associated hepatotoxicity is generally reversible but may lead to chronic liver failure, the need for a liver transplant, or death.

Hypersensitivity reactions to NSAIDs include bronchoconstriction, nasal polyps, urticaria, rhinitis, angioedema, and anaphylaxis. Bronchospasm and nasal polyps may be due to the inhibition of prostaglandin synthesis, which is consistent with the cross-sensitivity among these drugs.[151] The most widely recognized disorder is aspirin-induced asthmatic attacks. Nonacetylated salicylates have been suggested as safe alternatives in sensitive patients, but cross-sensitivity with nonacetylated salicylates has occurred.[152] Highly selective COX-2 inhibitors have not been associated with cross-reactivity and may prove to be the NSAIDs of choice in those with NSAID-induced bronchospasm. Celecoxib has a sulfa moiety and therefore may be associated with allergic reactions in patients with a history of "sulfa" allergy. Photosensitivity may also be associated with NSAIDs.

Drug interactions associated with NSAIDs are generally mediated by pharmacodynamic or pharmacokinetic effects. NSAIDs may diminish the effectiveness of antihypertensives (β-blockers, ACE inhibitors) and loop diuretics through effects on renal prostaglandins, but this effect ranges from serious to minor. Inhibition of renal function may alter the pharmacokinetics of renally excreted drugs. Celecoxib inhibits CYP2D6; valdecoxib inhibits CYP2C19 and CYP2C9 (cytochrome P-450 isoenzymes) and may decrease the metabolism of select drugs metabolized by those enzymes (e.g., warfarin, diazepam). With many NSAIDs, lithium levels increase after use, but this is not the case with aspirin or sulindac. Salicylates inhibit the action of uricosurics. Aspirin interacts pharmacokinetically with warfarin, but all NSAIDs that exhibit antiplatelet effects increase the bleeding potential in patients on warfarin. High-dose methotrexate may be much more toxic when used with NSAIDs, but the low doses of methotrexate used to treat patients with RA are usually safely administered with most NSAIDs. Aspirin plus methotrexate may increase the incidence of increased liver enzymes to a level over that seen with each drug alone.[119] Acetazolamide levels are increased by use of aspirin, which displaces protein binding and decreases renal clearance of azetazolamide. NSAIDs may increase the renal toxicity of nephrotoxic drugs such as cyclosporine and tacrolimus.

NSAIDs may be the target of pharmacokinetic or pharmacodynamic interactions. Salicylate levels are decreased by magnesium–aluminum hydroxide combination antacids, which increase urine pH and enhance salicylate renal excretion, and by corticosteroids, which enhance liver metabolism and renal clearance. Celecoxib and valdecoxib are metabolized by cytochrome P-450 isoenzymes, which may lead to decreased concentrations when coadministered with phenytoin (for valdecoxib) and increased concentrations with fluconazole. Other drugs that induce or inhibit those enzymes can also be expected to interact. Cyclosporine markedly increases the serum concentrations of diclofenac, leading to the need for a decreased dose of diclofenac when the two drugs are used concomitantly. Drugs that cause gastrointestinal or renal toxicity may increase NSAID toxicity. NSAIDs may interact with each other pharmacokinetically and pharmacodynamically, but only the additive toxicity is of clinical relevance.

The selection of an NSAID to be used in a patient with RA is based mostly on the adverse effect profiles and costs of the agents, but dosing convenience can also be an important factor. Many patients prefer a drug that can be taken once or twice daily, instead of more frequently. Newer agents and those without generic equivalents are more expensive. That cost can be justified in patients who are at high risk for NSAID-induced gastrointestinal ulceration or renal dysfunction, for whom the more expensive agent diminishes that risk. Patients who have been switched to COX-2 selective NSAIDs have experienced more previous adverse drug reactions, GI complaints, severe arthritis, disability, and use of health care resources compared with those who were not switched and stayed on a nonselective NSAID.[153] Further epidemiologic and economic research is needed for more accurate determination of the impact of using nonselective or COX-2 selective NSAIDs on a long-term basis in patients with RA.

Miscellaneous Drugs. A number of other miscellaneous therapies have been tested or tried in patients with RA but can be considered to be of little use or are not approved at this time. Dapsone is used in a variety of autoimmune disorders but should be reserved for highly refractory RA because of the occurrence of adverse effects.[154] Metronidazole (Flagyl) was effective in those patients with RA who could tolerate it, but the level of toxicity was unacceptable.[20] Inhibitors of the synthesis or action of leukotrienes have been approved for the treatment of patients with asthma and may be of benefit in RA. Zileuton (Zyflo), an inhibitor of 5-lipoxygenase and leukotriene B4 synthesis, at doses of 2,400 mg per day, was found to be superior to placebo and ibuprofen 2,400 mg per day in patients with RA.[155] Montelukast (Singulair) and zafirlukast (Accolate) are leukotriene receptor antagonists that may also be of benefit. Hydroxymethyl glutaryl coenzyme A (HMG Co-A) reductase inhibitors (''statins'') have demonstrated efficacy in RA.

Corticosteroids. Corticosteroids have been used to treat patients with RA through low oral daily doses in at least 30% of patients, intra-articular injections in less than 10% of patients, and intravenous pulses of high doses rarely.[137] Iontophoresis has also been used to administer corticosteroids.[156] Corticosteroids inhibit T- and B-cell activity, chemotaxis and migration of leukocytes, number of mast cells

in rheumatoid synovium, and release of collagenase and lysosomal enzymes.

Low-dose oral corticosteroids given at prednisone-equivalent doses of 2.5 to 15 mg per day can dramatically decrease swelling and tenderness and improve the sense of well-being in patients treated with NSAIDs, just started on DMARDs, or not responding to a DMARD.[157] Low-dose oral corticosteroids may reduce bone turnover, but not cartilage turnover. Long-term systemic corticosteroid use is probably not associated with an increase in bony erosions. However, risks of cumulative toxic effects on the skeleton, metabolism, and other organ systems limit the long-term use and dose of corticosteroids. Each 1 mg per day of prednisone is associated with a 5% increase in the risk of vertebral fracture or deformity.[158] Long-term low-dose or intermittent-pulse corticosteroids are associated with decreased insulin sensitivity. MTX may enhance corticoid-induced demineralization in the lumbar spine, but not in the femoral neck. A small number of patients who are taking systemic corticosteroids are also taking calcium, estrogens, or other prophylactive therapy. Bisphosphonates (e.g., alendronate), calcitonin, and supplementation with calcium and vitamin D are helpful in treating patients with corticosteroid-induced osteoporosis or in prevention. Corticosteroids may increase the incidences of peptic ulcer and gastrointestinal hemorrhage, particularly in patients receiving NSAIDs. Hypothalamic-pituitary-adrenal suppression may be seen, even with the use of low-dose corticosteroids. Low-dose oral corticosteroids are superior to placebo and to NSAIDs in RA and appear to be acceptable if used intermittently.[159] The use of low-dose corticosteroids early in the course of progressive RA can diminish inflammation with no long-term consequences. An unconventional use of corticosteroids in RA includes an approach similar to patient-controlled analgesia, and may result in lower average daily doses. High-dose corticosteroids are the initial drugs of choice for severe extra-articular features of RA such as vasculitis and rheumatoid lung. Pulse corticosteroids (methylprednisolone 250–1,000 mg for 1–3 days once or at 4- to 6-week intervals) do not provide sustained benefit in the management of RA and are associated with vertebral fractures. Systemic acute and cumulative adverse effects of corticosteroids require that they be used only when other therapies are not effective.

Intra-articular injections of corticosteroids should be used judiciously, preferably in only a few joints that are inflamed to the point of considerably limiting a patient's ability to function or rehabilitate. Intra-articular injections of corticosteroids include compounds that are relatively insoluble salts of active corticosteroids. A needle with attached syringe is inserted into a joint space under aseptic conditions. Synovial fluid is removed and should be analyzed further for white blood cells and differential, bacteria, crystals, and other features. With the needle still in place, the syringe is changed and the corticosteroid is injected. A dose of 2.5 to 10 mg of prednisolone tebutate equivalents would be used in a small joint such as a PIP, MCP, or MTP joint of a hand or foot; 10 to 25 mg in a wrist, ankle, or elbow; and 20 to 50 mg in a shoulder, ankle, knee, or hip. These insoluble corticosteroid salts may also benefit patients with tenosynovitis, bursitis, and carpal tunnel syndrome. Following injection of the joint or other structure, brief passive range of motion or activity can be used to enhance spread of the drug; this should be followed by a period of joint rest that lasts 24 to 48 hours. Intra-articular corticosteroids may cause a crystal synovitis because of their insoluble nature. Joint infections are rare, but multiple injections to the same joint may result in breakdown of articular cartilage. However, joint replacement was not more common in those joints receiving the highest number of corticoid injections.[160] The effects of this modality can be dramatic and may last for months to years.

Iontophoresis techniques of administering corticosteroids involve the use of electrically charged ions to assist in the transport of drug through the skin. Application of the active, soluble corticosteroids occurs on the skin near the joint over a series of treatments given three times weekly. A 1-week series of iontophoresis treatments to the knee with dexamethasone (4 mg in 1:1 water solution per treatment) led to improvements in pain and range of motion.[156] However, long-term efficacy and toxicity have not been well documented.

Pulsed, high-dose methylprednisolone (1 g daily intravenously for 1 to 3 days) may produce short-term benefits in the treatment of patients with refractory RA or those with severe extra-articular disease. It does not appear to have long-term effects or retard disease progression. Pulsed methylprednisolone has been able to decrease synovial fluid in polymorphonuclear cells, lymphocytes, immune complexes, and CRP. Severe adverse effects with high-dose, pulsed corticosteroids include short-term dose-related effects of corticosteroids (e.g., hyperglycemia, immunosuppression, sodium and fluid retention), dysgeusia in more than 50% of patients, hypotension, and the rare occurrence of seizures, cardiac arrhythmias, sudden death, and gastrointestinal ulceration or perforation.[161]

Other Pharmacotherapy. Systemic and topical analgesics may benefit selected patients with RA. Systemic analgesics, such as acetaminophen and opioid analgesics, are generally considered to be of limited benefit because of the inflammatory nature of this disease, but they may help occasionally as adjuncts to anti-inflammatory medications. Topical ointments, creams, and liniments provide some local relief. Although these may be designated as topical, systemic absorption is possible and may lead to toxicity or drug interactions, such as the increased effect of warfarin in patients who use topical salicylates.[162] Capsaicin cream inhibits substance P and relieves the pain associated with joint inflammation, but its effects are not anti-inflammatory.

Adjunctive Therapy. Adjunctive therapy is needed for the treatment of patients with general and extra-articular manifestations of RA. Antidepressant, antianxiety, and sedative-hypnotic agents should be used when needed. The bedtime use of benzodiazepines results in improved sleep, diminished morning stiffness, and less sleepiness during the daytime.[163] Patients with Sjögren syndrome are treated with methylcel-

lulose eyedrops and glycerol oral solutions to enhance lubrication of the eyes and mouth, respectively. Cholinergic agonists such as pilocarpine (Salagen) and cevimeline (Exovac) may help relieve dry mouth by stimulating the secretion of saliva. The anemia of chronic inflammatory disease responds to decreases in the inflammation of RA or to epoetin alfa administration, as long as iron stores are adequate.[164] RA-associated hemolytic anemia, autoimmune thrombocytopenia, pulmonary disease, and vasculitis generally respond to moderate to high doses of systemic corticosteroids (0.5 to 2.0 mg/kg/day of prednisone or equivalent). The addition of cyclophosphamide (oral or pulsed intravenous), methotrexate, azathioprine, cyclosporine, TNF inhibitors, or pulse methylprednisolone (0.25 to 1 g/day for 3 days) may be needed in refractory cases. Refractory thrombocytopenia may also respond to the addition of danazol. Therapy for patients with extra-articular manifestations of RA is based on the nature and severity of the disorder. Many of these manifestations will improve as the RA is relieved.

NONPHARMACOLOGIC THERAPY

Emotional support appears to provide only short-term benefit in relieving depression in patients with RA, but functional support for daily living activities appears to have long-term benefits in diminishing depression.[165] Passive coping strategies can be effective in diminishing pain.

Rest and exercise need to be balanced. Rest serves to spare joints and decrease inflammation which may lead to repair of damaged tissues. Patients with RA and fatigue should not diminish activity completely but should be encouraged to rest on a routine basis each day. Prolonged immobility may lead to increased stiffness and diminished mobility of joints and strength. For selected patients, hospitalization with rest and possibly minor revisions in drug therapy may have dramatic results. Intensive hospitalization for 14 days resulted in a threefold improvement in RA at a 2.5-fold increase in cost over no hospitalization, but the effects of hospitalization may last for at least 2 years.

Exercise has an important role in the treatment of patients with RA. Physical therapists assist patients by developing appropriate exercise programs that decrease joint inflammation, maintain range of motion, and increase overall well-being through range of motion, cardiovascular fitness, or strength-building programs that do not cause too much stress on joints and muscles. Such exercise programs may also diminish the development of osteoporosis in those with severe RA, on corticosteroids, or otherwise prone to develop osteoporosis. Exercise has been shown to improve physical function in patients with RA, but it does not change the number or activity of immune cells or mediators, except that it may cause a decrease in peripheral CD4+ T-cell count. A sustained program of weight bearing and aerobic exercise to build strength and cardiovascular fitness was effective in diminishing the loss of bone mineral density in the hips, but not in the spine.[166]

Occupational therapists assist in the design and use of special eating utensils, grooming aids, working aids, and other self-help aids that are useful in maintaining patients' self-reliance. Splints may be useful in stabilizing a weak joint, resting an active joint, or possibly diminishing the rate of joint destruction. Walking aids or wheelchairs may dramatically improve a patient's mobility and stability when mobile. Cold packs, hot packs, and hot paraffin wax treatments may decrease inflammation and discomfort.

Surgery is very useful in RA to repair or replace damaged joints, fuse joints for stability, correct tendon or ligament instability, release carpal tunnel syndrome, remove rheumatoid nodules, or remove invasive synovium. Radical surgical synovectomy may be beneficial in patients with refractory disease, particularly in those who are HLA-DRB1*0405 negative. Initial studies on the use of photodynamic laser therapy, which uses photosensitizing agents followed by laser ablation of synovial tissue, have been beneficial in RA.

Proper nutrition is important in helping patients lose weight if overweight, but patients must have sufficient protein intake to maintain or enhance muscle mass and sufficient calcium intake to potentially diminish the periarticular osteopenia that may occur. Many patients with severe RA lose weight, so maintenance of adequate nutrition is vital. Sodium fluoride can diminish the spinal bone loss associated with RA. After study findings revealed that patients with RA who were taking DMARDs had lower levels of selenium compared with normal subjects, selenium supplementation in patients with RA led to the use of lower doses of NSAIDs and systemic corticosteroids.[167] Vitamin E supplementation (α-tocopherol 1,200 mg/day) provides a small amount of pain relief that is additive to the anti-inflammatory drug effects noted in patients with RA.[168]

Removal or replacement of lymphocytes may be of benefit in patients with RA. A commercially available immunoabsorbent column containing staphylococcal protein A bound to a silica matrix (Prosorba) used with a plasmapheresis device was effective in refractory RA, probably because of removal of immunoglobulins.[169] Stem cell (bone marrow) transplantation has been found to induce sustained remission in some patients with RA, and an initial remission followed by an attenuated relapse in others.[15] Total lymphoid irradiation and thoracic duct drainage have been of benefit in patients with RA. Autologous stem cell transplantation was effective in a small trial, but the effects lasted only 1.5 to 9 months.[170]

ALTERNATIVE THERAPIES

Altering the fatty acid precursors of prostanoids and leukotrienes has also shown some benefit through the use of γ-linolenic acid (GLA),[171,172] eicosapentaenoic acid (EPA), and docosahexaenoic acid (DHA),[173] as well as vegetarian and elemental diets.[174–176] GLA (n-9 or omega-9 fatty acids found in borage seed oil, evening primrose oil, and black currant seed oil) and EPA and DHA (n-3 or omega-3 fatty acids found in fish oil) lead to the formation of prostaglan-

dins and leukotrienes that are anti-inflammatory or less inflammatory than PGE_2 or LTB_4, which are derived from arachidonic acid (n-6 or omega-6 fatty acid). Fish oil supplementation also decreases IL-1 concentrations and may provide sufficient relief for patients to be able to stop taking NSAIDs.[173] However, α-linolenic acid, a precursor of n-3 fatty acids found in flaxseed oil, was of no benefit in RA. Vegetarian diets lead to decreases in rheumatoid factor and other inflammatory measures.[175] An uncooked vegetarian diet rich in lactobacilli alters gut bacteria[177] and may be of benefit in RA, but it is difficult to tolerate. An elemental diet is a hypoallergenic diet that is composed of amino acids, glucose, trace elements, and vitamins. Use of an elemental diet followed by careful reintroduction of regular foods may decrease the activity of RA but is difficult to tolerate.[176] The effects of supplementation or special diets generally lead to modest benefits. Supplementation with fatty acid precursors may lead to some gastrointestinal intolerance (e.g., nausea, diarrhea). Vegetarian and elemental diets may be difficult for some patients to tolerate and may lead to deficiencies of vitamins or minerals. For patients who are unwilling or unable to take supplements or dramatically change their diet, increasing the quantities of vegetables and deep sea fish and decreasing the quantities of other animal fats in their diets may provide some benefit for their arthritis and their health in general.

Nontraditional therapies abound. Patients must be cautioned regarding the use of anecdotal or unproven therapies, including copper bracelets, herbal remedies, megadose vitamins, bee venom, snake venom, and others. Such remedies may provide relief in anecdotal reports, but few stand up to the rigor of controlled clinical study. Static magnetic fields have demonstrated efficacy in pain relief in RA knees, but they have little effect on inflammation.[178] Acupuncture, which provides pain relief, has been shown to decrease serum concentrations of IgG, IgM, and IgA, but not of IgE. Herbal remedies, such as Chinese thunder god vine,[179] and antioxidants, such as N-acetylcysteine,[180] have immunologic actions that may prove useful in RA.

Oral type II collagen, derived from chicks, when given in low doses has been found to be of some benefit in treating patients with RA,[181] particularly in patients with higher concentrations of antibody to collagen. A low dose of 20 μg per day proved to be superior to higher doses and to placebo.[181] Other formulations of type II collagen have been effective in RA.[182] This follows the hypothesis that low oral doses of an autoantigen (in this case, collagen) can desensitize patients to that autoantigen, lead to a decrease in antibodies to the autoantigen collagen, and decrease the manifestations of autoimmune disease. Adverse effects to the oral collagen were rare or were not seen.

FUTURE THERAPIES

Advances in the understanding and assessment of rheumatoid arthritis, immunology, molecular biology, and the effects of currently used and investigational therapies should lead to advances in therapy for patients with RA. It appears that goals include designing therapies that specifically act against possible defects in the HLA-DR4 antigen, macrophages, lymphocytes, mast cells, or other components of the immune system in patients with RA. Investigational drugs that inhibit TNF-α include a monoclonal antibody (CDP571), pegylated molecules (CDP870 and PEG-r-Hu-sTNF-RI), and a soluble p55 TNF receptor agent (lenercept). The CD20 inhibitor rituximab, which selectively depletes B-lymphocytes, has been shown to be effective in RA.[183] A costimulation blocker, which interferes with the interaction between antigen-presenting cells and T_H-cells, has also been effective in RA.[184] Selective p38 mitogen–activated protein kinase inhibitors may also be useful. Another target of therapy may be angiogenesis, that is, the development of blood vessels that assist in the proliferation of pannus. Advances have also been made in the understanding and treatment of patients with extra-articular manifestations of RA. Nerve growth factor has been an effective therapy in a small study of vasculitis ulcers.[185] Inhibitors of plasminogen activation, for example, may decrease the bony destruction seen in RA.[186]

IMPROVING OUTCOMES

PATIENT EDUCATION

Education and other nondrug therapies are widely used at all stages of RA. Patients should be well informed of the nature and possible progression of their disease with the goal of promoting self-awareness, self-determination, and self-reliance, as well as the knowledge of when to seek help from others. Family support is essential, especially because of negative attitudes toward the patient's disease that may lead to less coping and adaptation and more stress. Education programs can lead to improved knowledge, compliance, exercise, rest, and joint protection, but they have little effect on health status.[187] Psychoeducational programs improve coping over the short term, but their long-term effects on physical and psychological health may or may not evident.

METHODS FOR IMPROVING ADHERENCE TO DRUG THERAPY

Adherence to drug therapy in RA is influenced by the level of understanding of the benefits and risks of therapy and the disease, the availability of support or assistance with therapy, the design of the therapeutic regimen (some may be complicated), the immediate consequences of missed doses, functional disability, quality of life, age, and sex. Patient education programs on the benefits and risks of drugs in RA may result in improved adherence, but they do not necessarily enhance control of the disease.[187,188] Returning patients may be more compliant than new patients. When exercise programs are prescribed in RA, one-on-one and supervised group exercise sessions appear to promote better adherence

than is observed with unsupervised home-based exercise programs. Drug regimen and support personnel may also influence compliance. Patients were more compliant with infliximab (administered every 8 weeks by intravenous injection, usually through an infusion service) than with etanercept (administered twice weekly by subcutaneous injection) or methotrexate (administered once weekly by mouth).[189] Complicated regimens include loading doses of leflunomide, followed by dosing at the frequency of etanercept. In general, when leflunomide is started, a loading dose of 100 mg daily for 3 days is recommended, but patients can be started on routine maintenance doses of 10 or 20 mg daily if adherence or misunderstanding is a potential issue. Additionally, a once-weekly dosing regimen of leflunomide (100 mg in one dose) improved adherence compared with daily dosing of leflunomide (20 mg per day).[133]

The level of adherence in patients with RA is not well studied. On the basis of the data discussed previously, adherence can be improved by enhancing the patient's understanding of the drugs and the disease, decreasing the complexity of the dosage regimen, and ensuring effective patient–health care professional interactions and support.

DISEASE MANAGEMENT STRATEGIES FOR IMPROVING PATIENT OUTCOMES

The overall quality of care for patients with RA is suboptimal, including that of care provided for those with RA and comorbidities, and those who require health care maintenance.[190] A number of strategies can be used to address specific problems and issues. Delays in diagnosis and treatment, as well as undertreatment and delayed use of DMARDs in patients with aggressive disease, may worsen prognosis. The quality of care is improved when the appropriate medical specialists are involved in the care of patients.[190] Rheumatologists are more likely to use DMARDs than are general practitioners, and they tend to use those drugs earlier in the disease in an attempt to diminish long-term joint destruction. Enhancing the provision of functional assistance with daily living activities is likely to diminish the depressive symptoms associated with rheumatoid arthritis.[165] Management of fatigue can enhance a patient's quality of life.[191]

The perioperative use of therapies for rheumatoid arthritis has not been fully developed.[192] It would appear that it is prudent to discontinue aspirin and other nonselective, platelet-active NSAIDs 3 to 5 days before surgery to prevent excessive bleeding. Although the risk of postoperative infection may be increased, evidence supports the safe use of systemic corticosteroids following surgery. Methotrexate use may be associated with an increased risk of postoperative infection,[122] but it may still be used perioperatively. Infliximab has been used safely perioperatively in patients with inflammatory bowel disease.[192]

Finally, efforts should be initiated to prevent, minimize, and manage comorbidities. Effective management of the inflammation associated with RA is likely to diminish the development of extra-articular manifestations and improve cardiovascular outcomes. Appropriate selection of therapy can be used to minimize therapy-induced comorbidities, such NSAID-induced gastrointestinal ulceration and renal dysfunction, corticosteroid-induced osteoporosis and glucose intolerance, and increased risk or activation of infection by a number of agents.

PHARMACOECONOMICS

A comprehensive pharmacoeconomic analysis of patients with RA would include the costs of drug acquisition and administration, adverse effect monitoring and treatment, changes in functional disability and productivity, and overall survival and comorbidities. The costs to the patient, insurer, employer, and society are all important, but some are more difficult to measure than others. Depending on the study, major costs may be associated with decreased productivity or sick leave, monitoring and treatment for adverse effects of drugs, or drug acquisition (for biologic response modifiers). Patients with RA are extensive users of the health care system, with usage rates and costs that are two to three times greater than those of the general population or of patients with hypertension.[42] Employer costs for medical, pharmaceutical, and disability claims may also be two to three times higher for patients with RA.[193] Patients with lower socioeconomic status use fewer health care resources than do those with higher socioeconomic status.[71] Annual direct costs (in 2001 US dollars) were $19,016 in patients on biologic response modifiers and $6,160 in patients who were not receiving biologic response modifiers.[194] Direct costs for patients with low functional ability were $5,000 higher than costs for patients who were functioning well.[194] Approximately 29% of patients stop working after the onset of RA because of the disorder.[195] Patients who work miss an average of 3 to 30 days per year because of their disease. The costs of joint replacement are substantial and are estimated to be higher in patients with RA than in those with osteoarthritis. These facts point out the need for assessment of indirect costs associated with disease activity and progression, as well as assessment of the direct costs of medical care.

Biologic response modifiers are expensive but may have cost-effectiveness or cost-utility benefits. Etanercept and infliximab (plus methotrexate) have been cost-effective compared with other DMARDs.[196–198] Long-term therapy with etanercept has improved the patient's ability to work and has decreased utilization of health care resources.[199] Long-term therapy with infliximab (plus methotrexate) has improved the ability to work.[199] Etanercept was estimated to be more cost-effective than infliximab plus methotrexate in a European study.[200] The cost-effectiveness of anakinra was above generally accepted limits and appeared to be higher than that of etanercept or infliximab in a United Kingdom–based analysis of worldwide data.[201] An analysis performed in Europe found that anakinra was associated with an increase in days worked and in productivity at work and at home.[202]

Non–biologic response modifier DMARD drug therapy costs (drug, monitoring, toxicity) differed among agents, with per-patient per-month estimates of $227 for hydroxychloroquine, $233 for sulfasalazine, $340 for methotrexate, and $425 for other drugs or combinations in a study published in 2000.[203] Methotrexate and sulfasalazine have similar cost-effectiveness.[196] The direct costs of leflunomide are 42% to 53% lower than those of etanercept and infliximab (plus methotrexate),[204] but indirect costs were not determined. Leflunomide may provide reasonable cost-effectiveness and cost-utility benefits in RA,[205] but it may not be as cost-effective as methotrexate or sulfasalazine.[196] Cyclosporine was not as cost-effective as azathioprine, when equal efficacy is assumed.[206] Combination DMARDs (methotrexate, sulfasalazine, and hydroxychloroquine) plus a corticosteroid improved productivity over single-DMARD therapy with or without a corticosteroid in patients with early RA.[207]

The cost of NSAIDs is also an important consideration in RA. A number of studies have estimated or documented that the addition of gastroprotective agents to NSAIDs, or the use of COX-2 selective NSAIDs, is generally cost-effective in patients at high risk for NSAID-induced ulceration, but not in patients at lower risk. The use of COX-2 selective NSAIDs prevents one gastrointestinal ulcer or bleed for every 10 to 12 high-risk patients, for every 17 to 33 patients with lower risk, and for every 42 to 106 patients with a low risk of NSAID-induced ulceration or bleeding.[145] An economic study from Hong Kong of those at high risk for ulceration revealed that therapy with a nonselective NSAID plus a histamine-2 antagonist or with a COX-2 selective NSAID was less costly than therapy with a nonselective NSAID plus misoprostol or a proton pump inhibitor.[208] However, adding a gastroprotective agent to a nonselective NSAID may be more cost-effective than using a COX-2 selective NSAID if COX-2 selective NSAIDs increase the risk of cardiovascular events, or if low-dose aspirin or a gastroprotective agent is continued or added to the COX-2 selective NSAID. Proton pump inhibitors have been used in 40% of patients on a COX-2 selective NSAID. The costs and morbidity of increasing blood pressure in patients with RA are noteworthy,[209] but these have not been adequately studied.

The overall cost-effectiveness of low-dose oral corticosteroids is difficult to determine. A pharmacoeconomic analysis of osteoporosis prevention in patients with RA determined that it is more cost-effective to initiate bisphosphonate (e.g., alendronate) therapy when the bone mineral density T-score is −2.5 than with a T-score of −1.0.[210]

KEY POINTS

- Rheumatoid arthritis is a chronic, autoimmune disease of unknown etiology that affects joints and other tissues and organs

- Alterations in the immune, inflammatory, and related systems result in the tumorlike proliferation of synovial tissue and the destruction of bone and cartilage
- The variable course of rheumatoid arthritis may or may not be altered by the drug and nondrug therapies used
- Nondrug therapies are used to help the patient cope and to maintain solutions or correct the problems associated with rheumatoid arthritis
- NSAIDs are used as one of the first-line treatments for patients with acute inflammation, but they may also have effects on the immune system and on cartilage formation and destruction
- COX-2 selective NSAIDs appear to have a lower potential to cause gastrointestinal ulceration but are more costly than nonselective NSAIDs and may be associated with other adverse effects
- In patients with progressive or probable progressive disease, the aggressive use of DMARDs is supported by evidence
- Currently, methotrexate is the initial DMARD to be used, but biologic response modifiers and combinations of DMARDs are used in refractory disease
- Extra-articular manifestations require appropriate management
- Systemic corticosteroids are efficacious but are also associated with considerable long-term toxicity
- Pharmacoeconomic studies have provided initial information on the cost-effectiveness and cost-utility of new and expensive therapies
- The major goals of therapy should be to minimize functional disability and suffering, which will result in better patient and economic outcomes

SUGGESTED READINGS

American College of Rheumatology Subcommittee on Rheumatoid Arthritis Guidelines. Guidelines for the management of rheumatoid arthritis: 2002 update. Arthritis Rheum 46:328–346, 2002.

Anonymous. Guidelines for monitoring drug therapy in rheumatoid arthritis. Arthritis Rheum 39:723–731, 1996.

Choi HK, Seeger JD, Kuntz KM. A cost effectiveness analysis of treatment options for methotrexate-naive rheumatoid arthritis. J Rheumatol 29:1156–1165, 2002.

Choy EH, Panayi GS. Cytokine pathways and joint inflammation in rheumatoid arthritis. N Engl J Med 344:907–916, 2001.

O'Dell JR. Therapeutic strategies for rheumatoid arthritis. N Engl J Med 350:2591–2602, 2004.

Saag KG, Criswell LA, Sems KM, et al. Low-dose corticosteroids in rheumatoid arthritis. A meta-analysis of their moderate-term effectiveness. Arthritis Rheum 39:1818–1825, 1996.

REFERENCES

1. Schiff M. Emerging treatments for rheumatoid arthritis. Am J Med 102 (1 Suppl):11S–15S, 1997.
2. Silman AJ, Pearson JE. Epidemiology and genetics of rheumatoid arthritis. Arthritis Res 4 (Suppl 3):S265–S272, 2002.
3. Yen JH, Tsai WC, Chen CJ, et al. Tumor necrosis factor receptor 2 microsatellite and exon 6 polymorphisms in rheumatoid arthritis in Taiwan. J Rheumatol 30:438–442, 2003.
4. Silman AJ, Pearson JE. Epidemiology and genetics of rheumatoid arthritis. Arthritis Res 4 (Suppl 3):S265–S272, 2002.
5. Yen JH, Chen CJ, Tsai WC, et al. HLA-DQA1 genotyping in patients with rheumatoid arthritis in Taiwan. Kaohsiung J Med Sci 17:183–189, 2001.
6. Milicic A, Lee D, Brown MA, et al. HLA-DR/DQ haplotype in rheumatoid arthritis: novel allelic associations in UK Caucasians. J Rheumatol 29:1821–1826, 2002.
7. de Vries N, Tijssen H, van Riel PL, et al. Reshaping the shared epitope hypothesis: HLA-associated risk for rheumatoid arthritis is encoded by amino acid substitutions at positions 67-74 of the HLA-DRB1 molecule. Arthritis Rheum 46:921–928, 2002.
8. Weyand CM, McCarthy TG, Goronzy JJ. Correlation between disease phenotype and genetic heterogeneity in rheumatoid arthritis. J Clin Invest 95:2120–2126, 1995.
9. Weyand CM, Goronzy JJ. Inherited and noninherited risk factors in rheumatoid arthritis. Curr Opin Rheumatol 7:206–213, 1995.
10. del Rincon I, Battafarano DF, Arroyo RA, et al. Heterogeneity between men and women in the influence of the HLA-DRB1 shared epitope on the clinical expression of rheumatoid arthritis. Arthritis Rheum 46:1480–1488, 2002.
11. Shibue T, Tsuchiya N, Komata T, et al. Tumor necrosis factor alpha 5′-flanking region, tumor necrosis factor receptor II, and HLA-DRB1 polymorphisms in Japanese patients with rheumatoid arthritis. Arthritis Rheum 43:753–757, 2000.
12. Sivalingam SP, Yoon KH, Koh DR, et al. Single-nucleotide polymorphisms of the interleukin-18 gene promoter region in rheumatoid arthritis patients: protective effect of AA genotype. Tissue Antigens 62:498–504, 2003.
13. Barton A, Bowes J, Eyre S, et al. A functional haplotype of the PADI4 gene associated with rheumatoid arthritis in a Japanese population is not associated in a United Kingdom population. Arthritis Rheum 50:1117–1121, 2004.
14. Molenaar ET, Voskuyl AE, van der Horst-Bruinsma IE, et al. Influence of HLA polymorphism on persistent remission in rheumatoid arthritis. Ann Rheum Dis 61:351–353, 2002.
15. Snowden JA, Kearney P, Kearney A, et al. Long-term outcome of autoimmune disease following allogeneic bone marrow transplantation. Arthritis Rheum 41:453–459, 1998.
16. Risch N. Searching for genes in complex diseases: lessons from systemic lupus erythematosus. J Clin Invest 105:1503–1506, 2000.
17. Tilley BC, Alarcon GS, Heyse SP, et al. Minocycline in rheumatoid arthritis: a 48-week, double-blind, placebo-controlled trial. Ann Intern Med 122:81–89, 1995.
18. O'Dell JR, Haire CE, Palmer W, et al. Treatment of early rheumatoid arthritis with minocycline or placebo: results of a randomized, double-blind, placebo-controlled trial. Arthritis Rheum 40:842–848, 1997.
19. Nordstrom D, Lindy O, Lauhio A, et al. Anti-collagenolytic mechanism of action of doxycycline treatment in rheumatoid arthritis. Rheum Int 17:175–180, 1998.
20. Marshall DA, Hunter JA, Capell HA. Double blind, placebo controlled study of metronidazole as a disease modifying agent in the treatment of rheumatoid arthritis. Ann Rheum Dis 51:758–760, 1992.
21. Brennan P, Silman A. Breast-feeding and the onset of rheumatoid arthritis. Arthritis Rheum 37:808–813, 1994.
22. Doran MF, Crowson CS, O'Fallon WM, et al. The effect of oral contraceptives and estrogen replacement therapy on the risk of rheumatoid arthritis: a population based study. J Rheumatol 31:207–213, 2004.
23. Gudbjornsson B, Skogseid B, Oberg K, et al. Intact adrenocorticotropic hormone secretion but impaired cortisol response in patients with active rheumatoid arthritis. Effect of glucocorticoids. J Rheumatol 23:596–602, 1996.
24. Straub RH, Paimela L, Peltomaa R, et al. Inadequately low serum levels of steroid hormones in relation to interleukin-6 and tumor necrosis factor in untreated patients with early rheumatoid arthritis and reactive arthritis. Arthritis Rheum 46:654–662, 2002.
25. Krishnan E. Smoking, gender and rheumatoid arthritis—epidemiological clues to etiology. Results from the behavioral risk factor surveillance system. Joint Bone Spine 70:496–502, 2002.
26. Merlino LA, Curtis J, Mikuls TR, et al, for the Iowa Women's Health Study. Vitamin D intake is inversely associated with rheu-

matoid arthritis: results from the Iowa Women's Health Study. Arthritis Rheum 50:72–77, 2004.

27. Cerhan JR, Saag KG, Merlino LA, et al. Antioxidant micronutrients and risk of rheumatoid arthritis in a cohort of older women. Am J Epidemiol 157:345–354, 2003.

28. Mikuls TR, Cerhan JR, Criswell LA, et al. Coffee, tea, and caffeine consumption and risk of rheumatoid arthritis: results from the Iowa Women's Health Study. Arthritis Rheum 46:83–91, 2002.

29. Kvien TK. Epidemiology and burden of illness of rheumatoid arthritis. Pharmacoeconomics 22 (2 Suppl):1–12, 2004.

30. Rasch EK, Hirsch R, Paulose-Ram R, et al. Prevalence of rheumatoid arthritis in persons 60 years of age and older in the United States: effect of different methods of case classification. Arthritis Rheum 48:917–926, 2003.

31. Kvien TK, Uhlig T. The Oslo experience with arthritis registries. Clin Exp Rheumatol 21 (5 Suppl 31):S118–S122, 2003.

32. Choy EH. Panayi GS. Cytokine pathways and joint inflammation in rheumatoid arthritis. N Engl J Med 344:907–916, 2001.

33. Meyer FA, Yaron I, Yaron M. Synergistic, additive, and antagonistic effects of interleukin-1β, tumor necrosis factor α, and δ-interferon on prostaglandin E, hyaluronic acid, and collagenase production by cultured synovial fibroblasts. Arthritis Rheum 33: 1518–1525, 2000.

34. Wagner U, Pierer M, Wahle M, et al. Ex vivo homeostatic proliferation of CD4+ T cells in rheumatoid arthritis is dysregulated and driven by membrane-anchored TNF alpha. J Immunol 173: 2825–2833, 2004.

35. Calabrese LH, Wilke WS, Perkins AD, et al. Rheumatoid arthritis complicated by infection with the human immunodeficiency virus and the development of Sjogren's syndrome. Arthritis Rheum 32: 1453–1457, 1989.

36. Braun A, Takemura S, Vallejo AN, et al. Lymphotoxin beta-mediated stimulation of synoviocytes in rheumatoid arthritis. Arthritis Rheum 50:2140–2150, 2004.

37. Hepburn AL, Mason JC, Davies KA. Expression of Fc gamma and complement receptors on peripheral blood monocytes in systemic lupus erythematosus and rheumatoid arthritis. Rheumatology 43: 547–554, 2004.

38. Tanaka M, Kishimura M, Ozaki S, et al. Cloning of novel soluble gp130 and detection of its neutralizing autoantibodies in rheumatoid arthritis. J Clin Invest 106:137–144, 2000.

39. McEntegart A, Morrison E, Capell HA, et al. Effect of social deprivation on disease severity and outcome in patients with rheumatoid arthritis. Ann Rheum Dis 56:410–413, 1997.

40. Voulgari PV, Papadopoulos IA, Alamanos Y, et al. Early rheumatoid arthritis: does gender influence disease expression? Clin Exp Rheumatol 22:165–170, 2004.

41. Tengstrand B, Ahlmen M, Hafstrom I. The influence of sex on rheumatoid arthritis: a prospective study of onset and outcome after 2 years. J Rheumatol 31:214–222, 2004.

42. Yelin EH, Felts WR. A summary of the impact of musculoskeletal conditions in the United States. Arthritis Rheum 33:750–755, 1990.

43. Tikly M, Zannettou N, Hopley M. A longitudinal study of rheumatoid arthritis in South Africans. Medgenmed [Computer File]. Medscape General Medicine 5:2, 2003.

44. Pincus T, Fuchs HA, Callahan LF, et al. Early radiographic joint space narrowing and erosion and later malalignment in rheumatoid arthritis: a longitudinal analysis. J Rheumatol 25:636–640, 1998.

45. Kaarela K, Kautiainen H. Continuous progression of radiological destruction in seropositive rheumatoid arthritis. J Rheumatol 24: 1285–1287, 1997.

46. Orstavik RE, Haugeberg G, Mowinckel P, et al. Vertebral deformities in rheumatoid arthritis: a comparison with population-based controls. Arch Intern Med 164:420–425, 2004.

47. Shibuya K, Hagino H, Morio Y, et al. Cross-sectional and longitudinal study of osteoporosis in patients with rheumatoid arthritis. Clin Rheumatol 21:150–158, 2002.

48. Bautista BB, Boyce E, Koronkowski M, et al. Effects of second line drugs on progression or regression of rheumatoid nodules. J Clin Rheumatol 1:213–218, 1995.

49. Wilson A, Yu HT, Goodnough LT, et al. Prevalence and outcomes of anemia in rheumatoid arthritis: a systematic review of the literature. Am J Med 116 (Suppl 7A):50S–57S, 2004.

50. Wolfe F, Michaud K, Anderson J, et al. Tuberculosis infection in patients with rheumatoid arthritis and the effect of infliximab therapy. Arthritis Rheum 50:372–379, 2004.

51. Doran MF, Crowson CS, Pond GR, et al. Predictors of infection in rheumatoid arthritis. Arthritis Rheum 46:2294–2300, 2002.

52. Nakano M, Ueno M, Nishi S, et al. Determination of IgA- and IgM-rheumatoid factors in patients with rheumatoid arthritis with and without nephropathy. Ann Rheum Dis 55:520–524, 1996.

53. Wong M, Toh L, Wilson A, et al. Reduced arterial elasticity in rheumatoid arthritis and the relationship to vascular disease risk factors and inflammation. Arthritis Rheum 48:81–89, 2003.

54. Kumeda Y, Inaba M, Goto H, et al. Increased thickness of the arterial intima-media detected by ultrasonography in patients with rheumatoid arthritis. Arthritis Rheum 46:1489–1497, 2002.

55. Gonzalez-Juanatey C, Testa A, Garcia-Castelo A, et al. Active but transient improvement of endothelial function in rheumatoid arthritis patients undergoing long-term treatment with anti-tumor necrosis factor alpha antibody. Arthritis Rheum 51:447–450, 2004.

56. Alkaabi JK, Ho M, Levison R, et al. Rheumatoid arthritis and macrovascular disease. Rheumatology 42:292–297, 2003.

57. Solomon DH, Karlson EW, Rimm EB, et al. Cardiovascular morbidity and mortality in women diagnosed with rheumatoid arthritis. Circulation 107:1303–1307, 2003.

58. Jacobsen S. Young age of onset is associated with increased prevalence of circulating IgM rheumatoid factor and antinuclear antibodies at presentation in women with rheumatoid arthritis. Clin Rheumatol 23:121–122, 2004.

59. Gonzalez-Juanatey C, Llorca J, Testa A, et al. Increased prevalence of severe subclinical atherosclerotic findings in long-term treated rheumatoid arthritis patients without clinically evident atherosclerotic disease. Medicine 82:407–413, 2003.

60. Wolfberg AJ, Lee-Parritz A, Peller AJ, et al. Association of rheumatologic disease with preeclampsia. Obstet Gynecol 103: 1190–1193, 2004.

61. el-Miedany YM, el-Rasheed AH. Is anxiety a more common disorder than depression in rheumatoid arthritis? Joint Bone Spine 69: 300–306, 2002.

62. Dessein PH, Stanwix AE, Joffe BI. Cardiovascular risk in rheumatoid arthritis versus osteoarthritis: acute phase response related decreased insulin sensitivity and high-density lipoprotein cholesterol as well as clustering of metabolic syndrome features in rheumatoid arthritis. Arthritis Res 4:R5, 2002.

63. Tengstrand B, Carlstrom K, Hafstrom I. Bioavailable testosterone in men with rheumatoid arthritis—high frequency of hypogonadism. Rheumatology 41:285–289, 2002.

64. Hartung AD, Bohnert A, Hackstein H, et al. Th2-mediated atopic disease protection in Th1-mediated rheumatoid arthritis. Clin Exp Rheumatol 21:481–484, 2003.

65. Arnett FC, Edworthy SM, Bloch DA, et al. The American Rheumatism Association 1987 revised criteria for the classification of rheumatoid arthritis. Arthritis Rheum 31:315–324, 1988.

66. Chan KA, Felson DT, Yood RA, et al. The lag time between onset of symptoms and diagnosis of rheumatoid arthritis. Arthritis Rheum 37:814–820, 1994.

67. Katz PP, Yelin EH. The development of depressive symptoms among women with rheumatoid arthritis. Arthritis Rheum 38: 49–56, 1995.

68. Escalante A, del Rincon I, Mulrow CD. Symptoms of depression and psychological distress among Hispanics with rheumatoid arthritis. Arthritis Care Res 13:156–167, 2000.

69. Parker JC, Smarr KL, Slaughter JR, et al. Management of depression in rheumatoid arthritis: a combined pharmacologic and cognitive-behavioral approach. Arthritis Rheum 49:766–777, 2003.

70. Gorwood P, Pouchot J, Vinceneux P, et al. Rheumatoid arthritis and schizophrenia: a negative association at a dimensional level. Schizophrenia Res 66:21–29, 2004.

71. Jacobi CE, Mol GD, Boshuizen HC, et al. Impact of socioeconomic status on the course of rheumatoid arthritis and on related use of health care services. Arthritis Rheum 49:567–573, 2003.

72. American College of Rheumatology Subcommittee on Rheumatoid Arthritis Guidelines. Guidelines for the management of rheumatoid arthritis: 2002 update. Arthritis Rheum 46:328–346, 2002.

73. O'Dell JR. Therapeutic strategies for rheumatoid arthritis. N Engl J Med 350:2591–2602, 2004.

74. Boers M, Verhoeven AC, Markusse HM, et al. Randomised comparison of combined step-down prednisolone, methotrexate and sulphasalazine with sulphasalazine alone in early rheumatoid arthritis. Lancet 350:309–318, 1997.

75. O'Dell JR, Nepom BS, Haire C, et al. HLA-DRB1 typing in rheumatoid arthritis: predicting response to specific treatments. Ann Rheum Dis 57:209–213, 1998.

76. Tishler M, Nyman J, Wahren M, et al. Anti-Ro (SSA) antibodies in rheumatoid arthritis patients with gold-induced side effects. Rheumatol Int 17:133–135, 1997.

77. Brennan P, Harrison B, Barrett E, et al. A simple algorithm to predict the development of radiological erosions in patients with early rheumatoid arthritis: prospective cohort study. BMJ 313:471–476, 1996.

78. Fex E, Jonsson K, Johnson U, et al. Development of radiographic damage during the first 5-6 yr of rheumatoid arthritis. A prospective follow-up study of a Swedish cohort. Br J Rheumatol 35: 1106–1115, 1996.

79. Pincus T, Callahan LF. Variability in individual responses of 532 patients with rheumatoid arthritis to first-line and second-line drugs. Agents Actions 44 (Suppl):67–75, 1993.

80. Buch MH, Bingham SJ, Seto Y, et al. Lack of response to anakinra in rheumatoid arthritis following failure of tumor necrosis factor alpha blockade. Arthritis Rheum 50:725–728, 2004.

81. Weinblatt ME, Keystone EC, Furst DE, et al. Adalimumab, a fully human anti-tumor necrosis factor alpha monoclonal antibody, for the treatment of rheumatoid arthritis in patients taking concomitant methotrexate: the ARMADA trial. Arthritis Rheum 48:35–45, 2003.

82. Cohen SB, Moreland LW, Cush JJ, et al, for the 990145 Study Group. A multicentre, double blind, randomised, placebo controlled trial of anakinra (Kineret), a recombinant interleukin 1 receptor antagonist, in patients with rheumatoid arthritis treated with background methotrexate. Ann Rheum Dis 63:1062–1068, 2004.

83. Stein CM, Pincus T, Yocum D, et al. Combination treatment of severe rheumatoid arthritis with cyclosporine and methotrexate for forty-eight weeks: an open-label extension study. The Methotrexate-Cyclosporine Combination Study Group. Arthritis Rheum 40: 1843–1851, 1997.

84. Felson DT, Anderson JJ, Meenan RF. The efficacy and toxicity of combination therapy in rheumatoid arthritis: a meta-analysis. Arthritis Rheum 37:1487–1491, 1994.

85. Verhoeven AC, Boers M, Tugwell P. Combination therapy in rheumatoid arthritis: updated systematic review. Br J Rheumatol 37: 612–619, 1998.

86. Clegg DO, Dietz F, Duffy J, et al. Safety and efficacy of hydroxychloroquine as maintenance therapy for rheumatoid arthritis after combination therapy with methotrexate and hydroxychloroquine. J Rheumatol 24:1896–1902, 1997.

87. Ferraccioli GF, Assaloni R, Di Poi E, et al. Rescue of combination therapy failures using infliximab, while maintaining the combination or monotherapy with methotrexate: results of an open trial. Rheumatology 41:1109–1112, 2002.

88. Ferraccioli GF, Gremese E, Tomietto P, et al. Analysis of improvements, full responses, remission and toxicity in rheumatoid patients treated with step-up combination therapy (methotrexate, cyclosporin A, sulphasalazine) or monotherapy for three years. Rheumatology 41:892–898, 2002.

89. Darmawan J, Rasker JJ, Nuralim H. Reduced burden of disease and improved outcome of patients with rheumatoid factor positive rheumatoid arthritis compared with dropouts. A 10 year observational study. J Rheumatol Suppl 67:50–53, 2003.

90. Zwerina J, Hayer S, Tohidast-Akrad M, et al. Single and combined inhibition of tumor necrosis factor, interleukin-1, and RANKL pathways in tumor necrosis factor-induced arthritis: effects on synovial inflammation, bone erosion, and cartilage destruction. Arthritis Rheum 50:277–290, 2004.

91. Genovese MC, Cohen S, Moreland L, et al, for the 20000223 Study Group. Combination therapy with etanercept and anakinra in the treatment of patients with rheumatoid arthritis who have been treated unsuccessfully with methotrexate. Arthritis Rheum 50: 1412–1419, 2004.

92. Moreland LW, Baumgartner SW, Schiff MH, et al. Treatment of rheumatoid arthritis with a recombinant human tumor necrosis factor receptor (p75)-Fc fusion protein. N Engl J Med 337:141–147, 1997.

93. Hochberg MC, Tracy JK, Hawkins-Holt M, et al. Comparison of the efficacy of the tumour necrosis factor alpha blocking agents adalimumab, etanercept, and infliximab when added to methotrexate in patients with active rheumatoid arthritis. Ann Rheum Dis 62 (Suppl 2):ii13–ii6, 2003.

94. Torrance GW, Tugwell P, Amorosi S, et al. Improvement in health utility among patients with rheumatoid arthritis treated with adalimumab (a human anti-TNF monoclonal antibody) plus methotrexate. Rheumatology 43:712–718, 2004.

95. Keystone EC, Kavanaugh AF, Sharp JT, et al. Radiographic, clinical, and functional outcomes of treatment with adalimumab (a human anti-tumor necrosis factor monoclonal antibody) in patients with active rheumatoid arthritis receiving concomitant methotrexate therapy: a randomized, placebo-controlled, 52-week trial. Arthritis Rheum 50:1400–1411, 2004.

96. Weinblatt ME, Keystone EC, Furst DE, et al. Adalimumab, a fully human anti-tumor necrosis factor alpha monoclonal antibody, for the treatment of rheumatoid arthritis in patients taking concomitant methotrexate: the ARMADA trial. Arthritis Rheum 48:35–45, 2003.

97. Lipsky PE, van der Heijde DM, St Clair EW, et al. Anti-Tumor Necrosis Factor Trial in Rheumatoid Arthritis With Concomitant Therapy Study Group. Infliximab and methotrexate in the treatment of rheumatoid arthritis. N Engl J Med 343:1594–1602, 2000.

98. Temekonidis TI, Georgiadis AN, Alamanos Y, et al. Infliximab treatment in combination with cyclosporin A in patients with severe refractory rheumatoid arthritis. Ann Rheum Dis 61:822–825, 2002.

99. Stallmach A, Giese T, Schmidt C, et al. Severe anaphylactic reaction to infliximab: successful treatment with adalimumab—report of a case. Eur J Gastroenterol Hepatol 16:627–630, 2004.

100. Weisman MH. What are the risks of biologic therapy in rheumatoid arthritis? An update on safety. J Rheumatol Suppl 65:33–38, 2002.

101. Hamilton CD. Infectious complications of treatment with biologic agents. Curr Opin Rheumatol 16:393–398, 2004.

102. Khanna D, McMahon M, Furst DE. Safety of tumour necrosis factor-alpha antagonists. Drug Saf 27:307–324, 2004.

103. Ferraccioli G, Mecchia F, Di Poi E, et al. Anticardiolipin antibodies in rheumatoid patients treated with etanercept or conventional combination therapy: direct and indirect evidence for a possible association with infections. Ann Rheum Dis 61:358–361, 2002.

104. Wolfe F, Michaud K. Lymphoma in rheumatoid arthritis: the effect of methotrexate and anti-tumor necrosis factor therapy in 18,572 patients. Arthritis Rheum 50:1740–1751, 2004.

105. Wolfe F, Michaud K. Heart failure in rheumatoid arthritis: rates, predictors, and the effect of anti-tumor necrosis factor therapy. Am J Med 116:305–311, 2004.

106. Suissa S, Ernst P, Hudson M, et al. Newer disease-modifying antirheumatic drugs and the risk of serious hepatic adverse events in patients with rheumatoid arthritis. Am J Med 117:87–92, 2004.

107. Fleischmann RM, Schechtman J, Bennett R, et al. Anakinra, a recombinant human interleukin-1 receptor antagonist (r-metHuIL-1ra), in patients with rheumatoid arthritis: a large, international, multicenter, placebo-controlled trial. Arthritis Rheum 48:927–934, 2003.

108. Nuki G, Bresnihan B, Bear MB, et al, for the European Group of Clinical Investigators. Long-term safety and maintenance of clinical improvement following treatment with anakinra (recombinant human interleukin-1 receptor antagonist) in patients with rheumatoid arthritis: extension phase of a randomized, double-blind, placebo-controlled trial. Arthritis Rheum 46:2838–2846, 2002.

109. Cunnane G, Madigan A, Murphy E, et al. The effects of treatment with interleukin-1 receptor antagonist on the inflamed synovial membrane in rheumatoid arthritis. Rheumatology 40:62–69, 2001.

110. Bresnihan B, Newmark R, Robbins S, et al. Effects of anakinra monotherapy on joint damage in patients with rheumatoid arthritis. Extension of a 24-week randomized, placebo-controlled trial. J Rheumatol 31:1103–1111, 2004.

111. Schiff MH, DiVittorio G, Tesser J, et al. The safety of anakinra in high-risk patients with active rheumatoid arthritis: six-month obser-

vations of patients with comorbid conditions. Arthritis Rheum 50: 1752–1760, 2004.

112. Kovarik JM, Mueller EA, Gerbeau C, et al. Cyclosporine and nonsteroidal antiinflammatory drugs: exploring potential drug interactions and their implications for the treatment of rheumatoid arthritis. J Clin Pharmacol 37:336–343, 1997.

113. Fox RI, Morgan SL, Smith HT, et al. Combined oral cyclosporin and methotrexate therapy in patients with rheumatoid arthritis elevates methotrexate levels and reduces 7-hydroxymethotrexate levels when compared with methotrexate alone. Rheumatology 42: 989–994, 2003.

114. Brooks PJ, Spruill WJ, Parish RC, et al. Pharmacokinetics of methotrexate administered by intramuscular and subcutaneous injections in patients with rheumatoid arthritis. Arthritis Rheum 33:91–94, 1990.

115. Marshall PS, Gertner E. Oral administration of an easily prepared solution of injectable methotrexate diluted in water: a comparison of serum concentrations vs methotrexate tablets and clinical utility. J Rheumatol 23:455–458, 1996.

116. Shiroky JB, Neville C, Skelton JD. High dose intravenous methotrexate for refractory rheumatoid arthritis. J Rheumatol 19: 247–251, 1992.

117. Genestier L, Paillot R, Fournel S, et al. Immunosuppressive properties of methotrexate: apoptosis and clonal deletion of activated peripheral T cells. J Clin Invest 102:322–328, 1998.

118. Kremer JM, Rynes RI, Bartholomew LE. Severe flare of rheumatoid arthritis after discontinuation of long-term methotrexate therapy: double-blind study. Am J Med 82:781–786, 1987.

119. Fries JF, Singh F, Lenert L, et al. Aspirin, hydroxychloroquine, and hepatic enzyme abnormalities with methotrexate in rheumatoid arthritis. Arthritis Rheum 33:1611–1619, 1990.

120. Yazici Y, Erkan D, Paget SA. Monitoring by rheumatologists for methotrexate-, etanercept-, infliximab-, and anakinra-associated adverse events. Arthritis Rheum 48:2769–2772, 2003.

121. Kondo H, Date Y. Benefit of simultaneous rhG-CSF and methylprednisolone 'pulse' therapy for methotrexate-induced bone marrow failure in rheumatoid arthritis. Int J Hematol 65:159–163, 1997.

122. Carpenter MT, West SG, Vogelgesang SA, et al. Postoperative joint infections in rheumatoid arthritis patients on methotrexate therapy. Orthopedics 19:207–210, 1996.

123. Ohosone Y, Okano Y, Kameda H, et al. Clinical characteristics of patients with rheumatoid arthritis and methotrexate induced pneumonitis. J Rheumatol 24:2299–2303, 1997.

124. Alarcon GS, Kremer JM, Macaluso M, et al. Risk factors for methotrexate-induced lung injury in patients with rheumatoid arthritis. A multicenter, case-control study. Methotrexate-Lung Study Group. Ann Intern Med 127:356–364, 1997.

125. Saag KG, Kolluri S, Koehnke RK, et al. Rheumatoid arthritis lung disease. Determinants of radiographic and physiologic abnormalities. Arthritis Rheum 39:1711–1719, 1996.

126. Kremer JM, Alarcon GS, Weinblatt ME, et al. Clinical, laboratory, radiographic, and histopathologic features of methotrexate-associated lung injury in patients with rheumatoid arthritis: a multicenter study with literature review. Arthritis Rheum 40:1829–1837, 1997.

127. Landewe RBM, van den Borne BEEM, Breedveld FC, et al. Methotrexate effects in patients with rheumatoid arthritis with cardiovascular comorbidity [letter]. Lancet 355:1616–1617, 2000.

128. Ortiz Z, Shea B, Suarez-Almazor ME, et al. The efficacy of folic acid and folinic acid in reducing methotrexate gastrointestinal toxicity in rheumatoid arthritis. A metaanalysis of randomized controlled trials. J Rheumatol 25:36–43, 1998.

129. Morgan SL, Baggott JE, Lee JY, et al. Folic acid supplementation prevents deficient blood folate levels and hyperhomocysteinemia during long term, low dose methotrexate therapy for rheumatoid arthritis: implications for cardiovascular disease prevention. J Rheumatol 25:441–446, 1998.

130. Montecucco C, Caporali R, Rossi S, et al. Allopurinol mouthwashes in methotrexate-induced stomatitis [letter]. Arthritis Rheum 37:777–778, 1994.

131. Iqbal MP, Baig JA, Ali AA, et al. The effects of non-steroidal antiinflammatory drugs on the disposition of methotrexate in patients with rheumatoid arthritis. Biopharm Drug Dispos 19:163–167, 1998.

132. Mladenovic V, Domljan Z, Rozman B, et al. Safety and effectiveness of leflunomide in the treatment of patients with active rheumatoid arthritis. Results of a randomized, placebo-controlled, phase II study. Arthritis Rheum 38:1595–1603, 1995.

133. Jaimes-Hernandez J, Robles-San Roman M, Suarez-Otero R, et al. Rheumatoid arthritis treatment with weekly leflunomide: an open-label study. J Rheumatol 31:235–237, 2004.

134. Singh G, Fries JF, Spitz P, et al. Toxic effects of azathioprine in rheumatoid arthritis: a national post-marketing perspective. Arthritis Rheum 32:837–843, 1989.

135. Goldblum R. Therapy of rheumatoid arthritis with mycophenolate mofetil. Clin Exp Rheumatol 11 (Suppl 8):S117–S119, 1993.

136. Page F. Treatment of lupus erythematosus with mepacrine. Lancet 2:755–758, 1951.

137. Ward MM, Fries JF. Trends in antirheumatic medication use among patients with rheumatoid arthritis, 1981-1996. J Rheumatol 25:408–416, 1998.

138. Jouzeau JY, Terlain B, Abi D, et al. Cyclo-oxygenase isoenzymes: how recent findings affect thinking about nonsteroidal anti-inflammatory drugs. Drugs 53:563–582, 1997.

139. Capone ML, Tacconelli S, Sciulli MG, et al. Clinical pharmacology of selective COX-2 inhibitors. Int J Immunopathol Pharmacol 16 (2 Suppl):49–58, 2003.

140. Tacconelli S, Capone ML, Sciulli MG, et al. The biochemical selectivity of novel COX-2 inhibitors in whole blood assays of COX-isozyme activity. Curr Med Res Opin 18:503–511, 2002.

141. Furst DE. Review: are there differences among nonsteroidal antiinflammatory drugs? Comparing acetylated salicylates, nonacetylated salicylates, and nonacetylated nonsteroidal antiinflammatory drugs. Arthritis Rheum 37:1–9, 1994.

142. Fries JF, Ramey DR, Singh G, et al. A reevaluation of aspirin therapy in rheumatoid arthritis. Arch Intern Med 153:2465–2471, 1993.

143. Netter P, Bannwarth B, Royer-Morrot MJ. Recent findings on the pharmacokinetics of non-steroidal anti-inflammatory drugs in synovial fluid. Clin Pharmacokinet 17:145–162, 1989.

144. Anonymous. Guideline for monitoring drug therapy in rheumatoid arthritis. Arthritis Rheum 39:723–731, 1996.

145. Laine L, Bombardier C, Hawkey CJ, et al. Stratifying the risk of NSAID-related upper gastrointestinal clinical events: results of a double-blind outcomes study in patients with rheumatoid arthritis. Gastroenterology 123:1006–1012, 2002.

146. Savarino V, Mela GS, Zentilin P, et al. Effect of one-month treatment with nonsteroidal antiinflammatory drugs (NSAIDs) on gastric pH of rheumatoid arthritis patients. Dig Dis Sci 43:459–463, 1998.

147. Gubbins GP, Schubert TT, Attaasio F, et al. *Helicobacter pylori* seroprevalence in patients with rheumatoid arthritis: effect of nonsteroidal anti-inflammatory drugs and gold compounds. Am J Med 93:412–418, 1992.

148. Schwartz JI, Vandormael K, Thach C, et al. Effect of rofecoxib, etoricoxib, celecoxib, and naproxen on urinary excretion of prostanoids in elderly volunteers [abstract]. Clin Pharmacol Ther 75:34, 2004.

149. Farkouh ME, Kirshner H, Harrington RA, et al. Comparison of lumiracoxib with naproxen and ibuprofen in the Therapeutic Arthritis Research and Gastrointestinal Event Trial (TARGET), cardiovascular outcomes: randomised controlled trial. Lancet. 364:675–684, 2004.

150. Akil M, Amos RS, Stewart P. Infertility may sometimes be associated with NSAID consumption. Br J Rheumatol 35:76–78, 1996.

151. Szczeklik A, Gryglewski RJ, Czerniawska-Mysik G. Relationship of inhibition of prostaglandin biosynthesis by analgesics to asthma attacks in aspirin-sensitive patients. BMJ 1:67–69, 1975.

152. Chudwin DS, Strub M, Golden HE, et al. Sensitivity to non-acetylated salicylates in a patient with asthma, nasal polyps, and rheumatoid arthritis. Ann Allergy 57:133–134, 1987.

153. Wolfe F, Flowers N, Burke TA, et al. Increase in lifetime adverse drug reactions, service utilization, and disease severity among patients who will start COX-2 specific inhibitors: quantitative assessment of channeling bias and confounding by indication in 6689 patients with rheumatoid arthritis and osteoarthritis. J Rheumatol 29: 1015–1022, 2002.

154. Chang DJ, Lamothe M, Stevens RM, et al. Dapsone in rheumatoid arthritis. Semin Arthritis Rheum 25:390–403, 1996.

155. Weinblatt ME, Kremer JM, Coblyn JS, et al. Zileutin, a 5-lipoxygenase inhibitor, in rheumatoid arthritis. J Rheumatol 19:1537–1541, 1992.

156. Li LC, Scudds RA, Heck CS, et al. The efficacy of dexamethasone iontophoresis for the treatment of rheumatoid arthritic knees: a pilot study. Arthritis Care Res 9:126–132, 1996.

157. Saag KG, Criswell LA, Sems KM, et al. Low-dose corticosteroids in rheumatoid arthritis. A meta-analysis of their moderate-term effectiveness. Arthritis Rheum 39:1818–1825, 1996.

158. de Nijs RN, Jacobs JW, Bijlsma JW, et al, for the Osteoporosis Working Group, Dutch Society for Rheumatology. Prevalence of vertebral deformities and symptomatic vertebral fractures in corticosteroid treated patients with rheumatoid arthritis. Rheumatology 40:1375–1383, 2001.

159. Gotzsche PC, Johansen HK. Meta-analysis of short-term low dose prednisolone versus placebo and non-steroidal anti-inflammatory drugs in rheumatoid arthritis. BMJ 316:811–818, 1998.

160. Roberts WN, Babcock EA, Breitbach SA, et al. Corticosteroid injection in rheumatoid arthritis does not increase rate of total joint arthroplasty. J Rheumatol 23:1001–1004, 1996.

161. Baethge BA, Lidsky MD, Goldberg JW. A study of adverse effects of high-dose intravenous (pulse) methylprednisolone therapy in patients with rheumatic disease. Ann Pharmacother 26:316–320, 1992.

162. Yip ASB, Chow WH, Tai YT, et al. Adverse effect of topical methylsalicylate ointment on warfarin anticoagulation: an unrecognized potential hazard. Postgrad Med J 66:367–369, 1990.

163. Walsh JK, Muehlbach MJ, Lauter SA, et al. Effects of triazolam on sleep, daytime sleepiness, and morning stiffness in patients with rheumatoid arthritis. J Rheumatol 23:245–252, 1996.

164. Pincus T, Olsen NJ, Russell IJ, et al. Multicenter study of recombinant human erythropoietin in correction of anemia in rheumatoid arthritis. Am J Med 89:161–168, 1990.

165. Neugebauer A, Katz PP. Impact of social support on valued activity disability and depressive symptoms in patients with rheumatoid arthritis. Arthritis Rheum 51:586–592, 2004.

166. de Jong Z, Munneke M, Lems WF, et al. Slowing of bone loss in patients with rheumatoid arthritis by long-term high-intensity exercise: results of a randomized, controlled trial. Arthritis Rheum 50:1066–1076, 2004.

167. Heinle K, Adam A, Gradl M, et al. [Selenium concentration in erythrocytes of patients with rheumatoid arthritis. Clinical and laboratory chemistry infection markers during administration of selenium] [German]. Med Klinik 92 (Suppl 3):29–31, 1997.

168. Edmonds SE, Winyard PG, Guo R, et al. Putative analgesic activity of repeated oral doses of vitamin E in the treatment of rheumatoid arthritis. Results of a prospective placebo controlled double blind trial. Ann Rheum Dis 56:649–655, 1997.

169. Felson DT, LaValley MP, Baldassare AR, et al. The Prosorba column for treatment of refractory rheumatoid arthritis: a randomized, double-blind, sham-controlled trial. Arthritis Rheum 42:2153–2159, 1999.

170. Bingham SJ, Snowden J, McGonagle D, et al. Autologous stem cell transplantation for rheumatoid arthritis—interim report of 6 patients. J Rheumatol Suppl 64:21–24, 2001.

171. Leventhal LJ, Boyce EG, Zurier RB. Treatment of rheumatoid arthritis with gamma-linolenic acid. Ann Intern Med 119:867–873, 1993.

172. Leventhal LJ, Boyce EG, Zurier RB. Treatment of rheumatoid arthritis with blackcurrant seed oil. Br J Rheumatol 33:847–852, 1994.

173. Ariza-Ariza R, Mestanza-Peralta M, Cardiel MH. Omega-3 fatty acids in rheumatoid arthritis: an overview. Semin Arthritis Rheum 27;366–370, 1998.

174. Haugen MA, Kjeldsen-Kragh J, Bjerve KS, et al. Changes in plasma phospholipid fatty acids and their relationship to disease activity in rheumatoid arthritis patients treated with a vegetarian diet. Br J Nutrition 72:555–566, 1994.

175. Kjeldsen-Kragh J, Mellbye OJ, Haugen M, et al. Changes in laboratory variables in rheumatoid arthritis patients during a trial of fast-

176. ing and one-year vegetarian diet. Scand J Rheumatol 24:85–93, 1995.

176. Kavanaghi R, Workman E, Nash P, et al. The effects of elemental diet and subsequent food reintroduction on rheumatoid arthritis. Br J Rheumatol 34:270–273, 1995.

177. Peltonen R, Nenonen M, Helve T, et al. Faecal microbial flora and disease activity in rheumatoid arthritis during a vegan diet. Br J Rheumatol 36:64–68, 1997.

178. Segal NA, Toda Y, Huston J, et al. Two configurations of static magnetic fields for treating rheumatoid arthritis of the knee: a double-blind clinical trial. Arch Phys Med Rehabil 82:1453–1460, 2001.

179. Lipsky PE, Tao XL. A potential new treatment for rheumatoid arthritis: thunder god vine. Semin Arthritis Rheum 26:713–723, 1997.

180. Sato M, Miyazaki T, Nagaya T, et al. Antioxidants inhibit tumor necrosis factor-alpha mediated stimulation of interleukin-8, monocyte chemoattractant protein-1, and collagenase expression in cultured human synovial cells. J Rheumatol 23:432–438, 1996.

181. Barnett ML, Kremer JM, St. Clair EW, et al. Treatment of rheumatoid arthritis with oral type II collagen. Results of a multicenter, double-blind, placebo-controlled trial. Arthritis Rheum 41:290–297, 1998.

182. Gimsa U, Sieper J, Braun J, et al. Type II collagen serology: a guide to clinical responsiveness to oral tolerance? Rheumatol Int 16:237–240, 1997.

183. Edwards JC, Szczepanski L, Szechinski J, et al. Efficacy of B-cell-targeted therapy with rituximab in patients with rheumatoid arthritis. N Engl J Med 350:2572–2581, 2004.

184. Kremer JM, Westhovens R, Leon M, et al. Treatment of rheumatoid arthritis by selective inhibition of T-cell activation with fusion protein CTLA4Ig. N Engl J Med 349:1907–1915, 2003.

185. Tuveri M, Generini S, Matucci-Cerinic M, et al. NGF, a useful tool in the treatment of chronic vasculitic ulcers in rheumatoid arthritis. Lancet 356:1739–1740, 2000.

186. Ronday HK, Te Koppele JM, Greenwald RA, et al. Tranexamic acid, an inhibitor of plasminogen activation, reduces urinary collagen cross-link excretion in both experimental and rheumatoid arthritis. Br J Rheumatol 37:34–38, 1998.

187. Niedermann K, Fransen J, Knols R, et al. Gap between short- and long-term effects of patient education in rheumatoid arthritis patients: a systematic review. Arthritis Rheum 51:388–398, 2004.

188. Hill J, Bird H, Johnson S. Effect of patient education on adherence to drug treatment for rheumatoid arthritis: a randomised controlled trial. Ann Rheum Dis 60:869–875, 2001.

189. Harley CR, Frytak JR, Tandon N. Treatment compliance and dosage administration among rheumatoid arthritis patients receiving infliximab, etanercept, or methotrexate. Am J Manag Care 9 (6 Suppl):S136–S143, 2003.

190. MacLean CH, Louie R, Leake B, et al. Quality of care for patients with rheumatoid arthritis. JAMA 284:984–992, 2000.

191. Rupp I, Boshuizen HC, Jacobi CE, et al. Impact of fatigue on health-related quality of life in rheumatoid arthritis. Arthritis Rheum 51:578–585, 2004.

192. Rosandich PA, Kelley JT 3rd, Conn DL. Perioperative management of patients with rheumatoid arthritis in the era of biologic response modifiers. Curr Opin Rheumatol 16:192–198, 2004.

193. Birnbaum HG, Barton M, Greenberg PE, et al. Direct and indirect costs of rheumatoid arthritis to an employer. J Occup Environ Med 42:588–596, 2000.

194. Michaud K, Messer J, Choi HK, et al. Direct medical costs and their predictors in patients with rheumatoid arthritis: a three-year study of 7,527 patients. Arthritis Rheum 48:2750–2762, 2003.

195. Young A, Dixey J, Kulinskaya E, et al. Which patients stop working because of rheumatoid arthritis? Results of five years' follow up in 732 patients from the Early RA Study (ERAS). Ann Rheum Dis 61:335–340, 2002.

196. Choi HK, Seeger JD, Kuntz KM. A cost effectiveness analysis of treatment options for methotrexate-naive rheumatoid arthritis. J Rheumatol 29:1156–1165, 2002.

197. Lyseng-Williamson KA, Foster RH. Infliximab: a pharmacoeconomic review of its use in rheumatoid arthritis. Pharmacoeconomics 22:107–132, 2004.

198. Wong JB, Singh G, Kavanaugh A. Estimating the cost-effectiveness of 54 weeks of infliximab for rheumatoid arthritis. Am J Med 113:400–408, 2002.
199. Moreland LW. Drugs that block tumour necrosis factor: experience in patients with rheumatoid arthritis. Pharmacoeconomics 22 (2 Suppl):39–53, 2004.
200. Nuijten MJ, Engelfriet P, Duijn K, et al. A cost-cost study comparing etanercept with infliximab in rheumatoid arthritis. Pharmacoeconomics 19:1051–1064, 2001.
201. Clark W, Jobanputra P, Barton P, et al. The clinical and cost-effectiveness of anakinra for the treatment of rheumatoid arthritis in adults: a systematic review and economic analysis. Health Technol Assess 8:iii–iv, ix–x, 1–105, 2004.
202. Bresnihan B. Anakinra as a new therapeutic option in rheumatoid arthritis: clinical results and perspectives. Clin Exp Rheumatol 20 (5 Suppl 27):S32–S34, 2002.
203. Griffiths RI, Bar-Din M, MacLean CH, et al. Medical resource use and costs among rheumatoid arthritis patients receiving disease-modifying antirheumatic drug therapy. Arthritis Care Res 13: 213–226, 2000.
204. Ollendorf DA, Peterson AN, Doyle J, et al. Impact of leflunomide versus biologic agents on the costs of care for rheumatoid arthritis in a managed care population. Am J Manag Care 8 (7 Suppl): S203–213, 2002.
205. Maetzel A, Strand V, Tugwell P, et al. Cost effectiveness of adding leflunomide to a 5-year strategy of conventional disease-modifying antirheumatic drugs in patients with rheumatoid arthritis. Arthritis Rheum 47:655–661, 2002.
206. Anis AH, Tugwell PX, Wells GA, et al. A cost effectiveness analysis of cyclosporine in rheumatoid arthritis. J Rheumatol 23: 609–616, 1996.
207. Puolakka K, Kautiainen H, Mottonen T, et al. Impact of initial aggressive drug treatment with a combination of disease-modifying antirheumatic drugs on the development of work disability in early rheumatoid arthritis: a five-year randomized followup trial. Arthritis Rheum 50:55–62, 2004.
208. You JH, Lee KK, Chan TY, et al. Arthritis treatment in Hong Kong—cost analysis of celecoxib versus conventional NSAIDs, with or without gastroprotective agents. Aliment Pharmacol Ther 16:2089–2096, 2002.
209. Singh G, Miller JD, Huse DM, et al. Consequences of increased systolic blood pressure in patients with osteoarthritis and rheumatoid arthritis. J Rheumatol 30:714–719, 2003.
210. Solomon DH, Kuntz KM. Should postmenopausal women with rheumatoid arthritis who are starting corticosteroid treatment be screened for osteoporosis? A cost-effectiveness analysis. Arthritis Rheum 43:1967–1975, 2000.

Osteoarthritis

Ralph E. Small

DEFINITION

Osteoarthritis (OA) is the most common form of arthritis, affecting about 12.1% of all people over the age of 25 years in the United States. It is a major cause of morbidity and disability, especially among the older population.[1] OA creates more dependency in walking, climbing stairs, and other activities involving the lower extremities than any other disease that affects older adults.[2] The management of OA is an economic burden on the healthcare system. The cost of managing OA in the United States is estimated to be $15.5 billion, three times the cost of managing rheumatoid arthritis.[3] More that half of these costs are indirect; they are due to chronic loss of work and severely reduced quality of life.[4]

OA is a disease that affects mainly the weight-bearing joints of the peripheral and axial skeleton. This leads to pain, decreased range of motion, deformities, and progressive disability in about 80% of people with osteoarthritis. Other terms often used to describe OA include degenerative joint disease, hypertrophic arthritis, or osteoarthrosis. OA is a group of overlapping distinct diseases that may have different etiologies but have similar biologic, morphologic, and clinical outcomes. The disease processes affect not only the articular cartilage but also the entire joint, including the subchondral bone, ligaments, capsule, synovial membrane, and periarticular muscles. Ultimately the articular cartilage deteriorates, with fibrillation, fissures, ulceration, and full-thickness loss of the joint surface.[5]

TREATMENT GOALS

Monitoring and goals of treatment for patients with OA are individualized. It is important to consider patient age, concurrent disease states, and the extent of joint involvement when establishing the patient's goals:[6,7]

- Control pain
- Minimize disability
- Decrease joint stiffness
- Maintain mobility and function
- Maintain or improve quality of life
- Educate patients and family members about OA and its therapies.

EPIDEMIOLOGY

The etiology of OA remains unknown, but several theories have been developed to explain its pathogenesis. Systemic and local factors have been identified that may contribute to the likelihood that a joint will develop OA.[8,9] Systemic factors include age, sex, and genetic predisposition. It is believed that these systemic factors make the cartilage more susceptible to daily injury and less efficient with respect to repair. Systemic factors may alter the effects of growth factor and cytokines that contribute to the development of cartilage matrix. An example of such a change would be the decreased responsiveness of chondrocytes to growth factor that stimulates repair as a person ages. Other factors may increase deterioration of cartilage through increased activity of matrix metalloproteinases and collagenolytic enzymes. With the systemic component in place, local factors such as repetitive joint injury, obesity, muscle weakness, and joint deformity begin to cause joint breakdown.

More than 80% of persons over 50 years of age have radiographic evidence of OA.[4] Many of these patients will experience significant pain and disability. The prevalence and incidence of OA increase with advancing age. Men have a higher prevalence and incidence of OA than women before the age of 55; however, after age 55, women are more likely to develop OA.[10] It is believed that the increased incidence of OA in older women is due to postmenopausal estrogen deficiency. The incidence and prevalence of OA plateau after age 80 for both men and women.[11]

The development of OA in one joint is associated strongly with the development of OA in other joints throughout the body.[12] In patients who have OA of the hand (Fig. 66.1; *see color insert*), involvement of various hand joints [distal interphalangeal (DIP), carpometacarpal (CMC), and wrist joints] is more likely than involvement in both the hands and knees, or in the hands and hips.

Children of parents with OA are at increased risk of developing OA themselves, especially if the onset of OA in the parent was in middle age or earlier, or the disease was polyarticular.[10] A mutation involving type II procollagen has been discovered in families with an extensive history of early-onset severe OA.[13] Inheritance plays an important role in the development of hand OA, with a greater than 50% occurrence associated with a family history. In OA of the knee the percentage is smaller, partially because OA develops more as a function of repeated mechanical injury to the joint.[14]

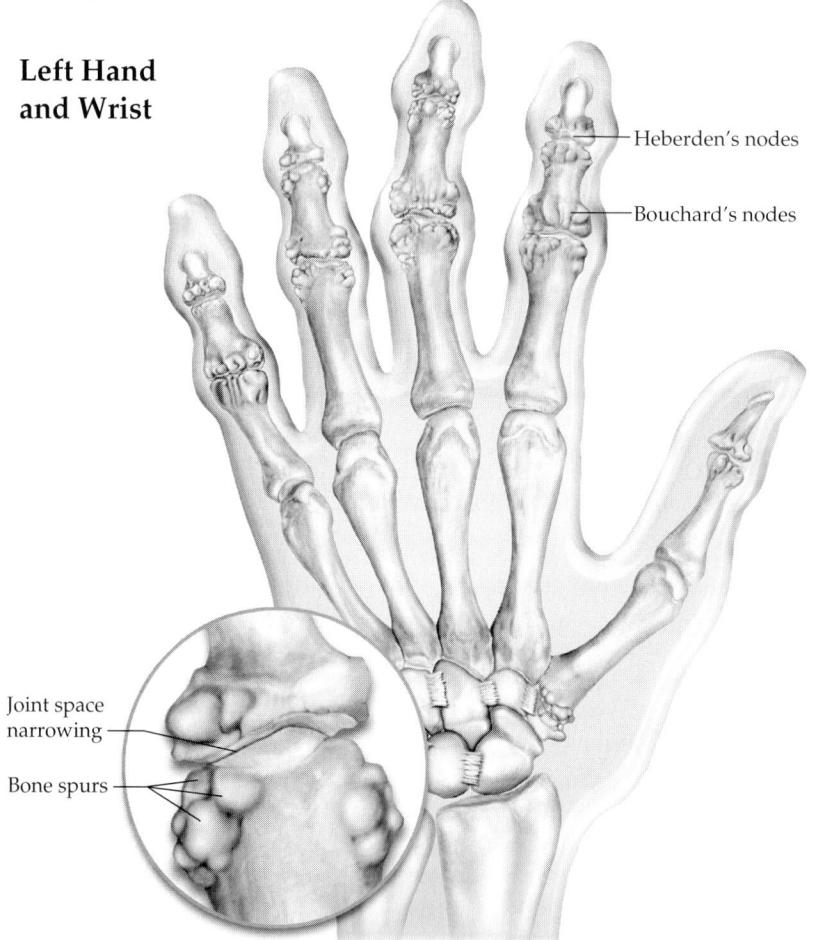

Left Hand and Wrist

Heberden's nodes

Bouchard's nodes

Joint space narrowing

Bone spurs

FIGURE 66.1 Joints affected by osteoarthritis: left hand and wrist (*see color insert*). (Asset provided by Anatomical Chart Co.)

Suggestions that subchondral bone deformations protect articular cartilage from damage during impact loading of the joint and findings that osteoporosis and OA were inversely related reveal a lower than expected rate of OA in patients with osteoporosis.[15,16] Also, patients with OA have a higher bone density than age-matched control subjects. Increased bone density and OA are both linked to obesity; however, the association of OA with high bone density is independent of body mass index (BMI).[17] This increase in bone density is believed to be linked to the presence of circulating bone growth factor and the formation of osteophytes.

Increased body weight has been closely associated with the development of OA of the knee.[10] A high BMI has been shown to contribute significantly to the overall risk of requiring total hip replacement due to primary osteoarthritis.[18,19] Weight is believed to act via two mechanisms to cause OA. First, increased body weight increases the amount of force across the weight-bearing joints, which may cause cartilage breakdown.[20] Second, excess adipose tissue may increase the presence of metabolic components such as hormones and growth factor, which affect cartilage or bone in such a way to predispose to OA development.[10] Weight change also affects the risk of developing OA. In women who were considered obese, a weight loss of 11 pounds was shown to decrease the risk of developing symptomatic OA of the knee by 50%.[21]

Major injury to the joint or surrounding tissue is a common cause of OA. Injury increases the stress on a joint and the surrounding cartilage and leads to the progressive changes associated with OA.[10] In the Framingham study, men with a history of major knee injury (cruciate ligament damage or meniscal tears) had a five to six times greater risk of developing OA of the knee than those without knee injury; for women, the risk was greater than threefold.[22] Overall, the cumulative incidence of OA of the knee by 65 years of age is 13.9% in patients who had a knee injury during adolescence and young adulthood and 6.0% in those who did not.[23] Development of OA has also been associated with repetitive joint use. Occupations such as farming, mill working, moving, and mining place repeated stress on the hips, hands, and knees. Several studies have indicated a high correlation and increased risk of developing OA in persons working in these professions.[10] Athletic activities have also been examined for the risk of developing OA. The effect of sports is difficult to assess, because major injury may occur to athletes during sporting events. The effects of endurance, high-intensity, and high-impact activity on the development of OA are difficult to establish; however, studies have shown that athletes are at increased risk of developing OA, especially in weight-bearing joints.[24,25] Soccer players and weight lifters have been identified as having an increased risk of developing premature OA of the knee.[26] This risk may be due to knee injuries associated with soccer or the increase in body mass seen in weight lifters. Participants in sports that involve repetitive nontraumatic loading (e.g.,

running, jogging, or shooting) have a small risk of developing premature OA.

PATHOPHYSIOLOGY

OA is no longer considered a disease of aging and wear and tear on the joint, but rather a condition that is dynamic in nature. It involves not only biomechanical forces, but also inflammatory, biochemical, and immunologic components. Changes seen in OA are visible not only in the articular cartilage and associated joint, but also in subchondral bone.[1] Pathologic changes within the joint may be reparative, rather than destructive, because normal function of the joint is trying to be maintained.[1]

Normal cartilage dissipates the force and stress caused by weight bearing due to the unique elasticity and compressibility of its molecular components.[27] Within the diarthrodial joint, cartilage provides a low-friction surface that covers both the concave and convex ends of the bone. Two essential roles of joint cartilage include the ability to promote joint stability during use and to distribute load across the joint, thereby preventing concentrations of stress within the joint. Upon weight bearing at the joint, cartilage is compressed (up to 40%), providing a large contact area that disperses the force uniformly to the underlying bone. Because of the relative thinness of the cartilage layer (1 to 4 mm), other shock-absorbing mechanisms must be in place to protect the joint.

Efficient functioning of the diarthrodial joint and its components is greatly impaired in OA. Changes that occur within the cartilage matrix include increased water and proteoglycan content. Although an exact mechanism is not known, this is related to a breakdown within the collagen fibers and release of proteoglycans. The cartilage then increases its hydration and thickens. Due to disruption of the cartilage matrix, metalloproteinases are released, which degrade proteoglycans and initiate the repair process within the joint. The increase in degradation stimulates chondrocyte activity; however, the capacity of chondrocyte proliferation is limited and proteoglycan degradation continues while water content increases. The resulting cartilage is thin and shows signs of softening, fibrillation, and ulceration on the surface.

Significant changes also occur within the subchondral bone as OA progresses. The destruction of protective cartilage leads to exposure of underlying bone and abrasion within the joint. As the cartilage layer is completely eroded away, dense, smooth bone is exposed. This grinding motion stimulates osteoclast/osteoblast activity, and bone resorption and vascular changes begin to occur. Without cartilage, dispersion of weight across the joint no longer occurs, thereby leading to microfractures and cysts in the subchondral plate. New bone is formed to help repair the fracture at the joint margin, thus leading to the formation of osteophytes. Formation of these bony projections may be an attempt by the body to repair and stabilize the joint; however, this leads to further

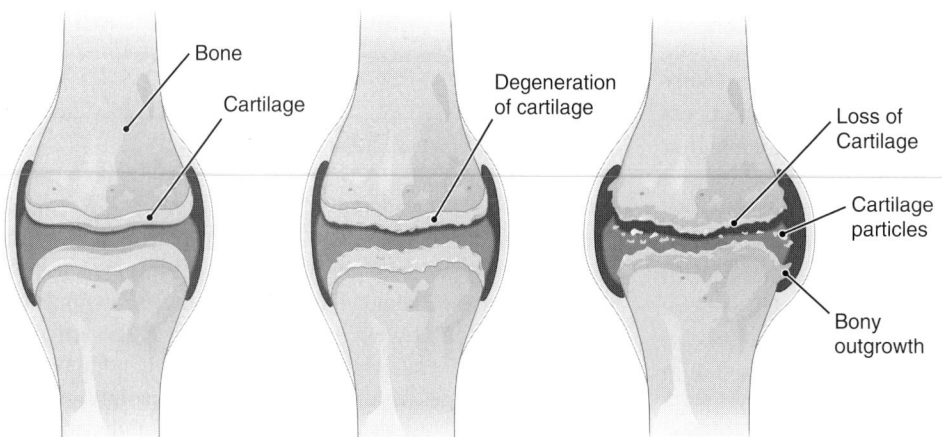

FIGURE 66.2 Osteoarthritis (*see color insert*). **A.** Normal joint. **B.** Early stage of osteoarthritis. **C.** Late stage of disease. (From Cohen BJ. Medical terminology, 4th ed. Philadelphia: Lippincott Williams & Wilkins, 2003.)

disfiguration and friction within the joint. This is illustrated in Figures 66.2 and 66.3 (*see color insert*).

Joint capsule and synovium changes occur secondary to OA. The release of matrix components, as well as bony formations, leads to inflammation within the synovium. This may be a prostaglandin-mediated process or an immune response to cartilage antigens. The degree of inflammation within the joint is significantly less than that seen in rheumatoid arthritis.

CLINICAL PRESENTATION AND DIAGNOSIS

SIGNS AND SYMPTOMS

The clinical presentation of OA depends on the duration of disease, the joints affected, and the severity of joint involvement. Pain is the predominant symptom among patients with OA and occurs early in the disease process. Initially, patients

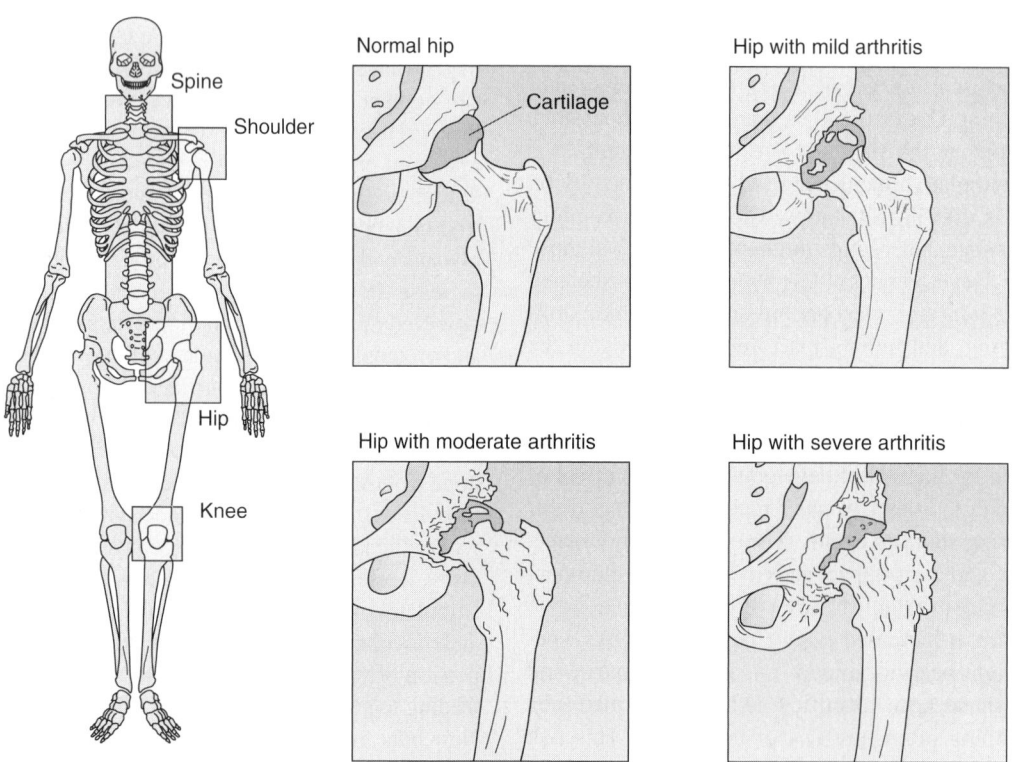

FIGURE 66.3 Osteoarthritis (*see color insert*). **A.** Common sites of osteoarthritis. **B.** How osteoarthritis affects the hip. (From Willis MC. Medical terminology: a programmed learning approach to the language of health care. Baltimore: Lippincott Williams & Wilkins, 2002.)

experience pain only upon use of the joint and describe it as deep, dull, and aching. Relief is achieved when the joint is at rest or when weight is removed. However, as OA progresses, the pain becomes constant and increases in severity. The pain may vary with changes in weather or barometric pressure. Because articular cartilage is aneural, pain arises from other structures such as microfractures in subchondral bone, synovitis, stretching of the joint capsule due to muscle spasm or joint instability, hypertension within the bone marrow related to thickening of subchondral bone, and stretched nerve endings around osteophytes.[28] Other factors such as anxiety, depression, muscle weakness, and physical demands (either occupational or physiologic) also contribute to pain in OA.[29] Vigorous exercise and increased physical activity at work seem to increase the chances of developing OA symptoms, whereas modest exercise may decrease the risk.

Joint stiffness is another complaint often expressed by patients with OA. This stiffness, unlike that in patients with rheumatoid arthritis, is relatively short in duration. Stiffness is related to periods of inactivity and resolves upon movement of the joint. In the morning, a patient with OA may awaken with joint stiffness, which resolves within 30 minutes, whereas a patient with rheumatoid arthritis may have stiffness that persists for several hours after awakening. As OA progresses, quick recovery from joint stiffness is slowed. Stiffness may also worsen with changes in weather or barometric pressure.

Crepitus, or joint "cracking" and "popping," is related to irregularities that develop on the joint surface and loss of cartilage within the joint. This is experienced when the joint is moved and most commonly occurs in OA of the knee. Crepitus may not only be felt by the patient but may also be heard at times. Development of bony proliferations leads to the development of joint enlargement.

Joint deformity is another common finding in OA, especially as the disease advances. Physical examination of a patient with OA provides more information about the physical presentation of disease and the extent of deformity. OA involvement in the hand typically affects the DIP, proximal interphalangeal (PIP), and first CMC joints. Advanced disease is associated with subluxation of the joint and gross deformity. In OA, Heberden's nodes are bony enlargements of the DIP joints with loss of joint space and osteophyte formation. A similar bony enlargement of the PIP joint is called a Bouchard's node (Fig. 66.4; *see color insert*). Isolation of knee pain and symptoms is important because it allows the practitioner to identify the specific area of the knee that is involved. Bowlegged deformities are associated with the medial region, whereas knock-knee deformities correspond to lateral involvement. In patients with OA of the hip, as well as the knee, the development of a limp is a source of concern. This may be caused by either changes within the joint or compensation of surrounding muscle due to instability or muscle atrophy (Fig. 66.5; *see color insert*).

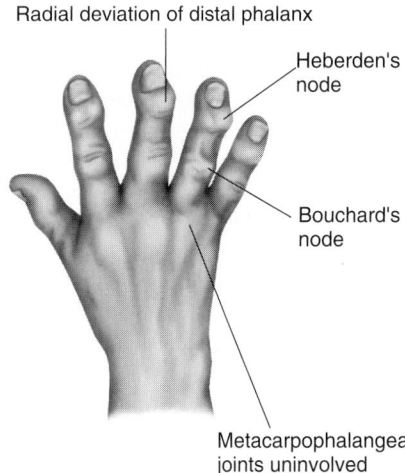

FIGURE 66.4 Osteoarthritis (degenerative joint disease; *see color insert*). Nodules on the dorsolateral aspects of the distal interphalangeal joints (Heberden's nodes) are due to the bony overgrowth of osteoarthritis. Usually hard and painless, they affect the middle-aged or elderly and often, although not always, are associated with arthritic changes in other joints. Flexion and deviation deformities may develop. Similar nodules on the proximal interphalangeal joints (Bouchard's nodes) are less common. The metacarpophalangeal joints are spared. (From Bickley LS, Szilagyi P. Bates' guide to physical examination and history taking, 8th ed. Philadelphia: Lippincott Williams & Wilkins, 2003.)

Hip

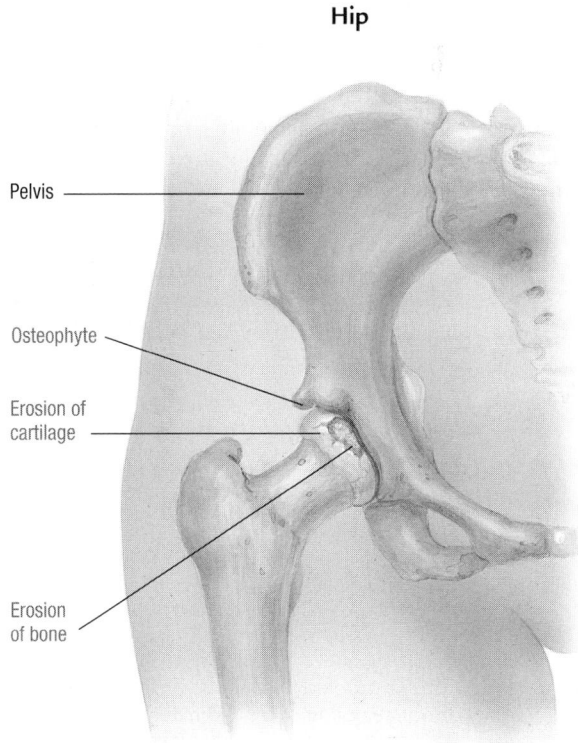

FIGURE 66.5 Hip joints affected by osteoarthritis (*see color insert*). (Asset provided by Anatomical Chart Co.)

Few laboratory changes occur in patients with OA. Erythrocyte sedimentation rate (ESR), C-reactive protein (CRP), electrolyte and hematologic markers, and urinalysis are generally found to be within normal limits. Patients will not have a positive test result for rheumatoid factor, and analysis of synovial fluid may indicate the presence of mild leukocytosis.

DIAGNOSIS

When diagnosing OA, many factors must be considered, including a careful evaluation of the patient's history, physical examination of affected joints, and radiographic findings. A complete evaluation of a patient with OA would include classification of the disease, identification of the joints involved, radiologic and clinical staging, notation of any physical deformities (contracture or atrophy), and assessment of the patient's functional capacity.[30]

A good history should include questions about the duration and severity of symptoms and the patient's ability to perform simple daily tasks.

Classification of OA clinically is beneficial for understanding the underlying pathogenesis of the disease. OA can be divided into either primary (idiopathic) or secondary forms. The cause of primary OA is not clearly understood. Development may be linked to either thickening of the cartilage and sclerosis of the subchondral bone, which damages the shock-absorbing capabilities of the joint, or imbalance of hormonal and metabolic control in cartilage formation/degradation, leading initially to cartilage hyperplasia and later to increased breakdown of cartilage.[31] Secondary OA may be caused by overuse or repetitive use of the joint, trauma, inflammatory joint disease, metabolic processes that may weaken cartilage, or congenital or acquired anatomic deformities.[32] To further aid in the classification of OA, the American College of Rheumatology (ACR) has developed criteria that review clinical, laboratory, and radiographic findings seen in OA, as well as the location of joint involvement[33–35] (Tables 66.1 and 66.2).

TABLE 66.1	American College of Rheumatology Classification Criteria for OA of the Hip

Traditional format

Hip pain **and** at least 2 of the following 3 items:

    Erythrocyte sedimentation rate <20 mm/hour

    Radiographic femoral or acetabular osteophytes

    Radiographic joint space narrowing

Classification tree

Hip pain **and** radiographic femoral or acetabular osteophytes

    Or

Hip pain **and** radiographic joint space narrowing **and** erythrocyte sedimentation rate <20 mm/hour

(From Kuettner K, Goldberg V. Introduction. In: Kuettner K, Goldberg V, eds. Osteoarthritic disorders. Rosemont, IL: American Academy of Orthopedic Surgeons; 1995:xxi–xxv.)

TABLE 66.2	American College of Rheumatology Classification Criteria for OA of the Knee

Traditional format

Knee pain **and** radiographic osteophytes **and** at least 1 of the following 3 items:

    Age >50 years

    Morning stiffness (≤30 minutes in duration)

    Crepitus on motion

Classification tree

Knee pain **and** radiographic osteophytes

    Or

Knee pain **and** age ≥40 years **and** morning stiffness ≤30 minutes in duration **and** crepitus on motion

(From Bradley J, Brandt K, Katz B, et al. Treatment of knee osteoarthritis: relationship of clinical features of joint inflammation to the response to a nonsteroidal anti-inflammatory drug or pure analgesic. J Rheumatol 19:1950–1954, 1992.)

Radiographic evaluation is a necessity for diagnosing OA; however, the need for comparative radiographs, as well as reference standards, imposes limitations on the interpretation of radiographs.[36] With disease progression, joint space narrowing due to cartilage degeneration, fractures in subchondral bone, and osteophytes (bone spurs) and cysts along the joint margin are visible. Arthroscopic evaluation of the joint may determine the extent of joint involvement in OA. This procedure is generally more prognostic than diagnostic. Quantitative magnetic resonance imaging can measure the progression of OA of the knee precisely and can help to identify patients with rapidly progressing disease.[37]

PSYCHOSOCIAL ASPECTS

Psychosocial factors play an important role in OA. Depression, anxiety, avoidance, and decreased quality of life are several factors that may influence the way patients perceive the pain and disability associated with their disease.[38] It is important to identify and address these factors to optimize patient therapy.

The degree of seriousness with which OA is initially viewed by patients is critical to their ability to cope with the disease.[39] Those who saw the disease as threatening were more likely to be depressed than those who accepted the diagnosis and strategies for treatment. Patients with increased pain often focused on activities and stressors in their lives, which led to avoidance of physical activity and anticipation about performance of activities of daily living (ADLs). Perceived quality-of-life is also important in managing OA. Using quality-of-life instruments, patients with OA were found to have lower life satisfaction than patients receiving dialysis; the more severe the symptoms of OA, the lower the quality-of-life rating.[40]

THERAPEUTIC PLAN

Current treatment of patients with OA focuses on symptom control because there are no disease-modifying agents available.[1] The effectiveness of therapy can be measured subjectively by lessening of pain and decreasing joint stiffness, or objectively by evaluation of joint range of motion and radiographic changes. Numerous clinical guidelines, including recently updated guidelines published by the American Pain Society and the ACR, emphasize the initial use of acetaminophen for the control of mild to moderate pain in patients with OA.[6,7] A therapeutic plan should be developed for each patient based on the extent and distribution of joint involvement, as well as other concurrent diseases that may be present.[1] Both nonpharmacologic and pharmacologic therapies should be used (Tables 66.3 and 66.4).

TREATMENT

PHARMACOTHERAPY

Pain relief is the primary indication for initiating drug therapy in patients with OA (Figs. 66.6 and 66.7).[5] Because there are no medications currently available that reverse or alter the structural and biochemical changes associated with OA, drug therapy is targeted at symptom control. Individualization of patient therapy is important when dealing with medications. Many patients with OA are older and have con-

TABLE 66.3	Nonpharmacologic Therapy for Patients With OA

Patient education

Self-management programs (e.g., Arthritis Foundation Self-Management Program)

Personalized social support through telephone contact

Weight loss (if overweight)

Aerobic exercise programs

Physical therapy

Range-of-motion exercises

Muscle strengthening exercises

Assistive devices for ambulation

Patellar taping

Appropriate footwear

Lateral-wedged insoles (for genu varum)

Bracing

Occupational therapy

Joint protection and energy conservation

Assistive devices for activities of daily living

(From American College of Rheumatology Subcommittee. Recommendations for the medical management of osteoarthritis of the hip and knee, 2000 update. Arthritis Rheum 43:1905–1915, 2002.)

TABLE 66.4	Pharmacologic Therapy for Patients With OA

Oral

  Acetaminophen 4 g/d

  COX-2-specific inhibitor: celecoxib 200 mg/d

  Nonselective NSAID (ibuprofen 1,600 mg/d, Arthrotec 150 mg/d, Voltaren 150 mg/d, naproxen 750 mg/d, sulindac 200 mg/d) plus misoprostol or a proton pump inhibitor

  Nonacetylated salicylate

  Other pure analgesics

    Tramadol (Ultram) 50 mg/dose (up to 400 mg/d), Ultracet 37.5 mg/dose (up to 300 mg/d)

    Opioids

Alternative therapy: glucosamine 1,500 mg/d (alone or in combination with chondroitin)

Intraarticular

  Glucocorticoids

  Hyaluronan

Topical

  Capsaicin

  Methyl salicylate

(Adapted from American College of Rheumatology Subcommittee. Recommendations for the medical management of osteoarthritis of the hip and knee, 2000 update. Arthritis Rheum 43:1905–1915, 2002.)

current diseases. Careful selection of agents and evaluation are important to minimize adverse effects and maximize efficacy.

Acetaminophen. Acetaminophen is the recommended initial drug of choice for treating symptomatic OA.[5] Doses of up to 4 g per day may be used with minimal occurrence

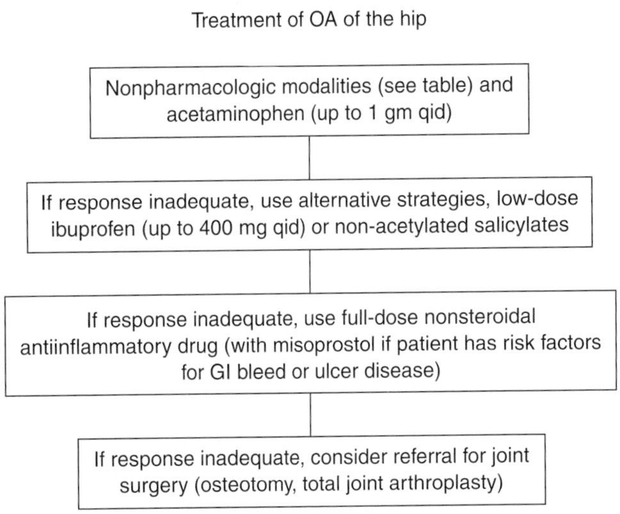

Treatment of OA of the hip

Nonpharmacologic modalities (see table) and acetaminophen (up to 1 gm qid)

If response inadequate, use alternative strategies, low-dose ibuprofen (up to 400 mg qid) or non-acetylated salicylates

If response inadequate, use full-dose nonsteroidal antiinflammatory drug (with misoprostol if patient has risk factors for GI bleed or ulcer disease)

If response inadequate, consider referral for joint surgery (osteotomy, total joint arthroplasty)

FIGURE 66.6 Treatment of OA of the hip.

Treatment of OA of the knee

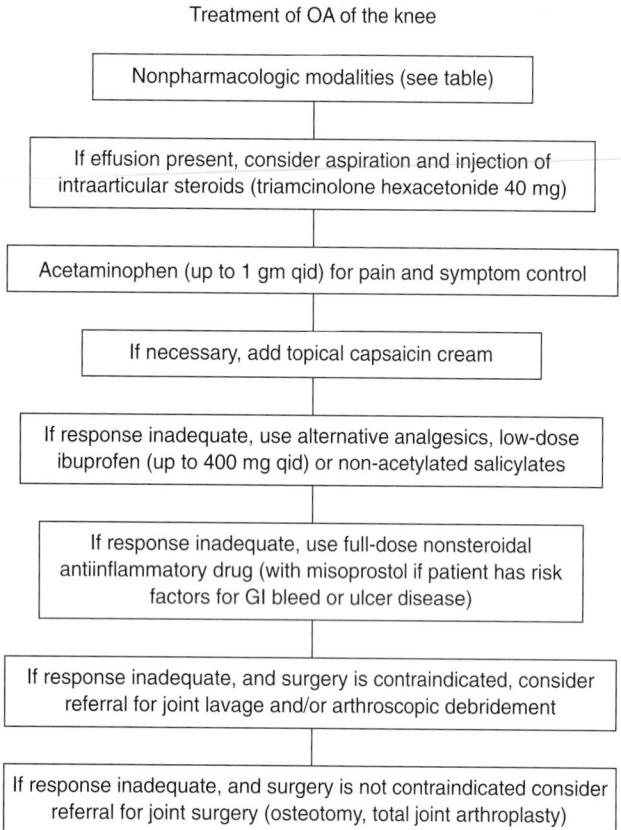

FIGURE 66.7 Treatment of OA of the knee.

of side effects. Early comparative studies between acetaminophen and nonsteroidal anti-inflammatory drugs (NSAIDs) showed no difference in efficacy, even in the presence of inflammatory symptoms such as synovitis and joint swelling.[41–43] Acetaminophen was associated with fewer adverse events. Low (analgesic) doses of NSAIDs may prove effective for patients who fail to achieve satisfactory or complete pain relief from maximal doses of acetaminophen.

Use of acetaminophen has been linked to the development of liver toxicity.[5] This side effect is rare and is generally seen in patients with underlying liver conditions, in patients who consume alcohol on a chronic basis, or in patients who take more than the maximum recommended daily dosage.[44,45] All patients should be cautioned against consuming other products (e.g., cold and flu medications) that contain acetaminophen. Acetaminophen may prolong the half-life of warfarin sodium, so International Normalized Ratio (INR) values should be monitored or a lower dose of acetaminophen used.

Tramadol. The new ACR guidelines include the non-NSAID, nonnarcotic drug tramadol for the treatment of pain associated with OA. Tramadol is a centrally acting synthetic analgesic indicated for the treatment of moderate to moderately severe pain. Tramadol has a dual mechanism of action, binding to the μ-opioid receptor and inhibiting the reuptake of norepinephrine (NE) and serotonin (5-HT).[46] Tramadol's

abuse potential is low (fewer than 1.5 cases per 100,000 exposed),[47] and tramadol is not a scheduled medication in the United States.

Alone[48,49] or in combination with other treatments,[50–52] tramadol has been shown to be effective in treating OA pain. Adding tramadol to acetaminophen may be an appropriate alternative to NSAIDs in many patients with OA. Tramadol can also be useful for OA breakthrough pain. Tramadol has been shown to allow for a reduction of the naproxen dose in patients taking naproxen for OA pain and is recommended as add-on therapy to NSAID treatment of OA.[6]

Tramadol is safe in combination with other analgesics and NSAIDs. Due to tramadol's inhibition of NE/5-HT reuptake, concomitant treatment with monoamine oxidase inhibitors and selective serotonin reuptake inhibitors has been reported to result in serotonin syndrome.[53]

The adverse effect profile of tramadol is distinct from those of NSAIDs and opioids, making it an attractive alternative for elderly persons, who make up the majority of OA patients. Adverse effects are usually mild and include nausea, vomiting, and dizziness. There have also been rare reports of seizures,[54] although the authors of a case-control study involving more than 11,000 patients concluded that all analgesics have a similar incidence of idiopathic seizures.[55]

Adverse effects of tramadol are usually reversible, and titrating the dose in select patients can improve tolerability.[56,57] Accordingly, its manufacturer revised the product information to recommend starting tramadol at 25 mg or 50 mg daily and titrating upward slowly when appropriate.[58] Final doses of 50 mg to 100 mg every 4 to 6 hours are recommended, with a maximum daily dose of 400 mg (300 mg/day in elderly patients).

Opioids. Opioids are recommended for chronic OA pain that has not responded well to other treatments.[6] Due to the development of tolerance, dependence, and adverse effects with chronic opioid treatment, however, opioids are best used in combination with other analgesics or supplementally during episodes of increased pain. One study has shown that in a subset of OA patients, there are occasions when the benefits of long-term opioid use for severe noncancer pain may outweigh the risks.[59]

Constipation is a common adverse effect of opioid treatment and should be treated prophylactically in most cases.[6] Respiratory depression and somnolence may also develop, limiting the use of opioids.[60] Agents such as naloxone can reverse respiratory depression.[61] Because the primary goal of treatment is to relieve pain and suffering in cases of severe exacerbation of joint pain, opioids should not be withheld from these patients, but long-term opioid therapy for OA should be conservatively prescribed and carefully monitored.[62]

Some of the more common opioids given for OA pain are morphine, methadone, codeine, hydromorphone, and oxycodone. The dose used varies with the drug, the route of administration, the patient, and the severity of the pain. Opioid-naïve patients should be started with a dose that is equivalent to 5 to 10 mg morphine (intramuscular) every 3 to 4 hours, titrated slowly to provide pain relief without severe adverse effects.

The fentanyl transdermal patch is often used for the treatment of chronic pain. Its safety and efficacy profiles are similar to those of other opioid treatments, and because of its ease of administration, adherence rates are believed to be higher.[63] Patients using the fentanyl patch still experience many of the adverse effects associated with opioids (e.g., dizziness, respiratory depression).[64] Opioid-naïve patients should be started on the patch at 25 mg every 72 hours, and titrated up as appropriate.

NSAIDs. Recent clinical trials have found NSAIDs to be more efficacious than acetaminophen in some groups of patients with OA.[65-67] Moreover, there is evidence suggesting OA patients prefer NSAIDs over acetaminophen. To assess this controversy, a recent meta-analysis was performed to compare the efficacy and safety of recommended dosages of NSAIDs, including cyclo-oxygenase-2 (COX-2) inhibitors, versus acetaminophen in the treatment of symptomatic hip and knee OA.[68] NSAIDs were found to be statistically superior in reducing rest and walking pain. Safety, measured by discontinuation due to adverse drug reactions, was not statistically different between the groups.

Principles of appropriate NSAID use for patients with OA include use of the minimum effective dose, use of no more than one NSAID simultaneously, assessment of benefit after a period of 1 month (change or discontinue therapy if no benefit seen), and patient education regarding not taking the medication during pain-free periods.[1]

Among people age 65 and older, as many as 30% of all hospitalizations and deaths related to peptic ulcer disease can be attributed to NSAID use.[69] In addition to age, other risk factors associated with NSAID-induced peptic ulcer disease include a history of peptic ulcer disease or upper gastrointestinal (GI) bleeding, concomitant use of corticosteroids or oral anticoagulants, high NSAID dose, and possibly smoking and alcohol consumption. NSAIDs may also increase the risk of developing chronic renal disease in patients who are over age 60 and have hypertension or congestive heart failure.[5] Serum creatinine levels should be monitored to detect changes in renal function.

Pharmacokinetic profiles of individual NSAIDs are generally similar, with the major difference being half-life. Absorption of NSAIDs is extensive and all are highly protein bound. Elimination is via hepatic metabolism to inactive metabolites, except for sulindac and nabumetone, which are converted to active metabolites. Analgesic effects are generally seen within 1 to 2 hours after taking the NSAID, whereas maximum anti-inflammatory effects are obtained after 2 to 3 weeks of continuous administration.

Selection of a NSAID should be based upon frequency of dosing, cost, efficacy, and toxicities. Aspirin, ibuprofen, naproxen, and ketoprofen are all available as nonprescription

products and may be available at a lower cost than prescription NSAIDs. The ACR suggests the use of low-dose ibuprofen (less than 1,600 mg/day) on an as-needed basis initially because of its lower cost, similar efficacy, and fewer GI toxicities.[6] Increased all-cause and cardiovascular mortality is the result when aspirin for cardioprotection is used concomitantly with ibuprofen or other NSAIDs for patients with OA.[70-73] This drug–drug interaction did not occur when aspirin was given concomitantly with acetaminophen, diclofenac, or selective COX-2 inhibitors. To overcome this potential problem, aspirin may be taken early in the morning and allowed a couple of hours to work before NSAIDs are taken. Monitoring patients for increased risk of GI bleeding should occur while they are on concomitant therapy.

The variation in GI side effect profiles of NSAIDs may be a result of the COX selectivity of individual drugs. COX serves as the rate-limiting enzyme in prostaglandin production. Inhibition of this enzyme decreases prostaglandin-induced initiation and maintenance of inflammatory responses.[74] COX has been identified to have two isoforms (COX-1 and COX-2). COX-1 is beneficial in helping to maintain normal cellular physiologic processes in the GI tract, kidneys, and blood. In the gut, COX-1 stimulates the secretion of bicarbonate and mucus and reduces stomach acid secretion.[75] All of these actions protect the lining of the stomach against irritants. COX-2 is involved in selectively activating proinflammatory cytokines and does not have a gastroprotective effect. Therefore, the ideal NSAID would selectively inhibit COX-2 to reduce the inflammatory response, but also maintain the GI and renal protective nature of COX-1. Several agents have been developed that are COX-2 selective, including valdecoxib, celecoxib, and rofecoxib. The clinical benefit of these selective COX-2 inhibitors for patients with OA has been proven, but the potential for adverse drug reactions is a concern. Rofecoxib and valdecoxib have been shown in studies to exhibit an increase in cardiovascular events, particularly acute myocardial infarction. Valdecoxib has been shown to increase cardiovascular events when used in coronary artery bypass graft patients. Due to the increased incidence of hypertension, congestive heart failure, and acute myocardial infarctions in patients taking rofecoxib or valdecoxib, they were voluntarily removed from the market. Whether rofecoxib and valdecoxib stay off the market remains to be determined, as a recent recommendation of an advisory committee of the U.S. Food and Drug Administration was re-entry to the market for rofecoxib with additional monitoring of its dose and potential adverse events. Celecoxib, in high doses over a long period of time, appears to increase the risk of cardiovascular events. Celecoxib could continue to be used with more rigorous monitoring.

Topical Agents. For patients who do not respond to oral analgesics, or those who refuse to take systemic therapy, the use of topical liniments, gels, and creams is appropriate.[6] Local application of agents avoids systemic side effects and allows the use of more potent agents. Topical products containing methyl salicylate may be helpful. Capsaicin is a topical rubefacient derived from the pepper plant. The primary effects of capsaicin are related to its activity in the peripheral portion of the sensory nervous system. It works to excite nociceptive C-afferent neurons, causing the release of substance P.[76] Substance P is an essential chemical mediator in the transmission of pain from the peripheral to central nervous system. Upon repeated application of capsaicin substance P is depleted, leading to inhibition of pain sensation.

Capsaicin should be applied to the affected joints four times a day.[6] After 2 weeks of continuous application, maximal pain relief is noted and the frequency of application may be reduced. Capsaicin may be used either as monotherapy or in combination with oral agents. Associated side effects include a mild stinging or burning sensation, but patients rarely discontinue therapy due to this reaction. Because capsaicin is safe and effective and does not have systemic side effects, it should be considered for the management of pain associated with OA.

Corticosteroids. The role of corticosteroids in the management of OA remains controversial. Systemic corticosteroids should be avoided, because prolonged use leads to the development of side effects that outweigh any benefits of therapy. On the other hand, intraarticular injections of corticosteroids may be beneficial.[77] For OA of the hip, the efficacy of such injections has not been determined, and they are not recommended as a part of routine medical management. For patients with OA of the knee, intraarticular injections of corticosteroids may be appropriate. Triamcinolone acetonide or hexacetonide at a dose of 40 mg is beneficial in reducing pain, especially when signs of effusion or local inflammation are present. It is recommended that injections not be performed more than three or four times per year, because there is concern that repeated injections into the joint may lead to progressive cartilage damage.[6] Patients may experience synovitis following an injection, which is due to a local reaction to the suspended steroid crystals. This reaction is mild and lasts for a short time.

Hyaluronic Acid Derivatives. High-molecular-weight hyaluronan, sodium hyaluronate, and hylan G-F 20 are three glycosaminoglycan polysaccharide compounds that have been approved by the U.S. Food and Drug Administration for the treatment of pain associated with OA of the knee. There are four products known as hyaluronic acid that are indicated for patients who have not responded adequately to nonpharmacologic therapy and treatment with analgesics. In patients with OA, both elasticity and viscosity within the synovial fluid are reduced.[6] Viscosupplementation by administration of hyaluronic acid and its derivatives is believed to restore the composition of synovial fluid such that normal tissue regeneration and function may occur. It has been shown that hyaluronan inhibits interleukin (IL)-1β-stimulated production of matrix metalloproteinases 1, 3, and 13 in human articular cartilage.[78] This supports the clinical use

of hyaluronan in the treatment of OA. The action of hyaluronan on IL-1β may involve direct interaction between hyaluronan and CD44 on chondrocytes. Researchers have found that any benefit of intraarticular treatment of knee OA with hyaluronic acid is small at best and possibly overstated because of the bias favoring publication of studies with positive results.[79] Approximately 80% of the treatment effect was accounted for by the placebo effect of an intraarticular injection. The highest-molecular-weight formulation of hyaluronan may have greater effects.[80]

The most common side effect reported with hyaluronic acid is pain at the injection site. Other side effects such as swelling, effusion, warmth, and redness at the injection site have also been reported. Hyaluronic acid should not be administered with anesthetics concurrently, because it may become diluted such that safety and efficacy may be compromised. Subcutaneous local anesthetics may be administered. Hyaluronan should be considered for patients not responding to other therapies, and prior to joint replacement.[81]

NONPHARMACOLOGIC THERAPY

Physical and occupational therapies play a crucial role in the management of patients with OA who have functional limitations.[5] Physical therapists assess muscle strength, range of motion, mobility, and ambulation. Instruction can then be provided about appropriate exercises and the use of modalities such as heat and cold to aid range of motion and mobility. Application of warm compresses or warm water soaks may be beneficial before exercise to help relieve joint pain and stiffness.[5] Occupational therapists assess ADLs and recommend devices such as splints, canes, wall bars, and raised toilet seats, which improve patient independence and accommodate functional disability. Appropriate assessment and intervention in ADLs, mobility, and ambulation have a significant impact on the patient's quality of life. Joint protection and hand exercises have been found to increase grip strength and global hand function in patients with OA.[82]

The goals of exercise for patients with OA should include reduction of joint impairment, improvement in joint function, protection of the joint from further damage, and prevention of disability. Before beginning an exercise program, complete cardiac assessment should be performed to identify any underlying disease and to establish a target heart rate. An exercise program should consist of both aerobic and range-of-motion and strengthening exercises. Aquatic aerobics programs target these areas and should be recommended to patients with OA.[6]

For overweight patients, weight reduction may reduce the symptoms of OA, especially in the weight-bearing joints.[1] Specific changes to the diet (restricted intake of meats; no preservatives; fish oil, alfalfa, and zinc) have not been shown to be beneficial for patients with OA and are not recommended.[83] The combination of modest weight loss plus moderate aerobic exercise provides better overall improvements in self-reported measures of function and pain and in performance measures of mobility in older overweight and obese adults with knee OA compared with either intervention alone.[84]

Traditional Chinese acupuncture has been shown to be an effective intervention for the relief of pain and improvement of function in patients with symptomatic knee OA. Tai chi, a marriage of martial art and dance, was shown to decrease self-reported pain scores by 50% in patients with OA. Tai chi also produces stronger muscles, increased joint range of motion, and enhanced flexibility. Yoga, which brings balance to the body, mind, and spirit, also builds strength and helps stabilize joints. It too has been shown to decrease pain by 50% among patients with knee OA.

Other measures that have been tried but for which additional research is needed are baths, energy, magnetic bracelets, cod-liver-oil supplements, ginger extract, avocado/soybean extract, and leech therapy.[85–87]

Surgical intervention is indicated for patients who have severe pain that has failed to respond to medical therapy and has progressively decreased their ADLs. Arthroscopic débridement and lavage of the joint space is beneficial for patients who refuse surgery or for whom surgery is not recommended. The removal of matrix debris and inflammatory mediators has been suggested as possible reasons for benefit from lavage. Osteotomy (the surgical cutting and repositioning of bone) may provide relief, because restructuring and repositioning of the bone places the joint back into normal alignment. This procedure may help to prevent disease progression in patients who are not candidates for arthroplasty (also known as joint replacement). Complete joint arthroplasty is responsible for a dramatic improvement in quality of life in patients with OA. Before arthroplasty is performed, careful consideration needs to be given to the patient's health status, the surgeon performing the procedure, the hospital where it will be performed, and postoperative management and rehabilitation.

ALTERNATIVE THERAPIES

The combination of glucosamine sulfate and chondroitin sulfate has been touted as a "miracle cure" for OA. Both compounds are found naturally in the body and are essential to the formation of cartilage. Glucosamine is a basic component of articular cartilage glycosaminoglycans and acts as a substrate in the synthesis of proteoglycans. With aging, the body decreases the synthesis of glucosamine, and the synovial fluid becomes thin and is no longer effective in lubricating the joint. The rationale for the use of glucosamine sulfate 1,500 mg daily in OA is to provide the building blocks for cartilage regeneration. Chondroitin is another constituent in the cartilage matrix. Because of its chemical nature, chondroitin has a strong ability to retain water and gives cartilage its shock-absorbing characteristics. The primary function of chondroitin is to prevent premature breakdown of existing cartilage by partially inhibiting the proteolytic enzyme elastase. Chondroitin also serves to stimulate RNA synthesis of chondrocytes. Whereas chondroitin may be used alone in the management of OA, the combination of glucosamine sulfate and chondroitin sulfate is believed to have a synergistic effect by stimulating cartilage production and inhibiting its destruction.

Recent studies involving glucosamine have shown relief of symptoms and slowing of the progression of OA when studied over a 3-year period.[88,89]

Side effects associated with the use of these agents include mild gastric discomfort, dyspepsia, nausea, and euphoria. Chondroitin sulfate does have potential anticoagulant activity; however, laboratory evaluation of patients before and after treatment suggested no significant hematologic changes with chondroitin use for 6 months.

FUTURE THERAPIES

Until recently, OA was considered an inevitable and irreversible part of aging. However, research has led to a better understanding of the disease and new ways to manage it. New therapies are being developed that one day may prevent, stop, reverse, or even cure OA. Development of safer NSAIDs, evaluation of gene therapy, application of currently available medications for new indications, and exploration into the role of cytokines in OA are just some of the areas of research and development.

Because OA may develop from genetic defects in collagen, researchers are targeting therapies to specifically block defective genes. Transfer of genes directly into the joint that stimulate cartilage formation or inhibit cartilage breakdown are being evaluated for therapeutic use.[90] Control of tissue inhibitors of metalloproteinases and metalloproteinase genes would provide an opportunity to control a patient's disease.[91] Doxycycline has been shown to inhibit collagenase activity in articular cartilage.[92] This activity prevented proteoglycan loss, cell death, and deposition of weak collagen matrix in vitro. Therapies that interact with cytokines are also in development. Administration of tumor growth factor-β via liposomes may induce repair of articular cartilage lesions. Although structure or disease-modifying agents for OA (SMOADs) are not yet available, research is underway to determine whether such agents are beneficial. Small collagen fragments, produced in the joint when collagen is degraded by proteases, stimulate the synthesis of collagen. Collagen hydrolysate introduced exogenously, which is absorbed by the intestine and accumulates in the joint cartilage, therefore has the potential to stimulate collagen production in the remaining chondrocytes in patients with OA.[93] This counteracts the degenerative processes and may prevent the development of OA. Antiresorptive agents, such as alendronate and risedronate, are being studied in OA of the knee.[94] Diacerein, an inhibitor of IL-1β synthesis in OA synovium, is also being studied. Colchicine has exhibited significantly greater symptomatic benefit for patients with acute OA of the knee when given with an NSAID.[95] Further study is needed.

IMPROVING OUTCOMES

The ultimate outcome for treating patients with OA is to have patients reach their therapeutic goals. Many interventions can help patients to reach these goals and have been proven to be beneficial for the management of patients with OA.

PATIENT EDUCATION

Patient education is the cornerstone of nonpharmacologic management of OA. Education of family members, friends, and caregivers is integral because they provide a support structure for the patient.[6] Patients should be encouraged to become involved in the Arthritis Self-Help Course available through the Arthritis Foundation. The Arthritis Foundation provides educational materials for patients and families, information about providers, identification of other agencies offering both physical and economic support to patients, and information on various drugs used to treat OA. The Arthritis Foundation may be reached at 1-800-283-7800 or www.arthritis.org.

Providing patients with social support emphasizes not only the importance of personal patient contact but also the significant impact that interventions can have in improving patient care and outcomes. Trained lay personnel can review such items as joint pain, medication and treatment adherence, drug toxicities, appointments with providers, and overall patient quality-of-life. This provides another source of information about treatment effectiveness and reinforces the collaborative effort needed for optimal patient care. Self-management and support groups for patients have led to decreased pain, decreased number of physician visits, and improved overall quality-of-life for participants.[96] Use of social support networks has been shown to improve the patient's pain and functional status while not significantly increasing costs.[97]

The benefits of aerobic exercise and weight reduction have also been shown by a decrease in symptoms and improvement in ambulation.[98,99] Development and execution of an appropriate therapeutic plan allows patients to receive maximal benefit and reach therapeutic goals.

Providing education has a positive impact on both the health and psychosocial status of patients dealing with OA.[100] Education should be offered not only to the patient but also to family, friends, and caregivers. Topics should include the development and progression of OA, pain control, appropriate use of medications, side effects or adverse events from medications, appropriate techniques for exercise and rest, weight reduction (if appropriate), modifications/adaptations for ADLs, and support services. It is also important for patients to understand the waxing-and-waning nature of their disease and the need to adjust their care plans accord-

ingly. Encouraging patients to become involved in self-management programs allows them to be active participants in their own care. The benefits of such programs include decreased pain, less frequent physician visits, and overall improvement in quality-of-life. Educational materials such as videos, pamphlets, and newsletters, as well as information regarding support services available, may be obtained from either local chapters or the national office of the Arthritis Foundation.

METHODS TO IMPROVE PATIENT ADHERENCE TO DRUG THERAPY

Adherence to both nonpharmacologic and pharmacologic treatment regimens is essential to ensure optimal patient outcomes. Many factors may contribute to nonadherence, such as failure to understand the importance of therapy, failure to understand the drug regimen instructions, multiple drug therapy, frequency of administration, lack of effect from therapy, adverse events, fear of becoming drug dependent, disappearance of symptoms, comorbid conditions, and cost of treatment. Recognizing and identifying these factors can aid in developing appropriate treatment plans.

Use of patient education and support groups greatly increases patients' understanding of the disease process and the role of therapy in improving their condition. With this understanding come improved outcomes and increased adherence. Evaluation of OA patients involved with self-management programs has shown significant improvement in medication and therapy (physical and occupational) adherence.[101] The frequency of medication administration also has an impact on adherence to therapy. Data show that as the frequency of administration increases, adherence decreases By choosing extended-release formulations or medications with longer half-lives, administration once or twice a day may be possible, leading to improved adherence and outcomes. Adherence may also be improved by the use of special packaging. Nonsafety tops on prescription bottles may ease opening of containers for patients with OA who have involvement in their hands or wrists. For patients with complicated medication regimens or those who are cognitively or visually impaired, the use of blister packaging may assist in appropriate medication usage.

To improve patient adherence, it is important to identify factors that may lead to nonadherence, to develop a treatment plan that correlates with the patient's normal activities, to educate the patient and family members, and to monitor therapy on a regular basis. These steps will allow both patient and practitioner to meet therapeutic goals and optimize care.

DISEASE MANAGEMENT STRATEGIES TO IMPROVE PATIENT OUTCOMES

An appropriately designed therapeutic plan focuses on both pain relief and minimization of disability, because as of yet there are no disease-modifying drugs for OA. Combination therapy with both pharmacologic and nonpharmacologic modalities has proven to be beneficial in improving patient outcomes. Data suggest that exercise programs should be recommended along with standard pharmacologic therapy. Occupational therapy may be beneficial in helping patients adapt to functional limitations imposed by OA.

Principles of pharmacologic therapy include selection of an appropriate agent, optimal therapeutic dosing, use of the minimal effective dose to minimize side effects, and appropriate duration of therapy with selected agents. Benefit should be assessed after 1 month of therapy, at which point either dosage adjustments or selection of another agent may be necessary if optimal results are not achieved. Analgesia is the cornerstone of pharmacologic therapy, and appropriate therapeutic agents should be chosen to meet this goal.

Other important components of disease management are monitoring and evaluation of therapy. Both subjective and objective parameters should be used to assess disease pro-

---

TABLE 66.5	The Arthritis Foundation's Quality Indicators for OA
Topic Area	**Quality Indicator**
Physical examination	1. IF a patient is begun on a drug treatment for "joint pain," "arthritis," or "arthralgia," THEN evidence that the affected joint was examined should be documented.
Pain and functional assessment	2. IF a patient is diagnosed with symptomatic osteoarthritis of the knee or hip, THEN his or her pain should be assessed annually and when new to a practice.
	3. IF a patient is diagnosed with symptomatic osteoarthritis of the knee or hip, THEN his or her functional status should be assessed annually and when new to a practice.
Education	4. IF a patient has had a diagnosis of symptomatic osteoarthritis of the knee or hip for >3 months, THEN education about the natural history, treatment, and self-management of osteoarthritis should have been given or recommended at least once.
Exercise	5. IF an ambulatory patient has had a diagnosis of symptomatic osteoarthritis of the knee or hip for >3 months, THEN a directed or supervised muscle strengthening or aerobic exercise program should have been prescribed at least once and reviewed at least once per year.
Weight loss	6. IF an individual is overweight (as defined by body mass index of $\geq$27 kg/m^2), THEN the individual should be advised to lose weight annually.
	7. IF a patient has symptomatic osteoarthritis of the knee or hip and is overweight (as defined by body mass index of $\geq$27 kg/m^2), THEN the patient should be advised to lose weight at least annually AND the benefit of weight loss on the symptoms of osteoarthritis should be explained to the patient.
	8. IF a patient has symptomatic osteoarthritis of the knee or hip and has been overweight (as defined by body mass index of $\geq$27 kg/m^2) for 3 years, THEN the patient should receive referral to a weight loss program.
Assistive devices	9. IF a patient has had symptomatic osteoarthritis of the knee or hip and reports difficulty walking to accomplish activities of daily living for >3 months, THEN the patient's walking ability should be assessed for need for ambulatory assistive devices.
	10. IF a patient has a diagnosis of osteoarthritis and reports difficulties with nonambulatory activities of daily living, THEN the patient's functional ability with problem tasks should be assessed for need of nonambulatory assistive devices to aid with problem tasks.
Pharmacologic therapy	11. IF a nonnarcotic pharmacologic therapy is initiated to treat osteoarthritis pain of mild or moderate severity, THEN acetaminophen should be the first drug used, unless there is a documented contraindication to use.
	12. IF oral pharmacologic therapy for osteoarthritis is changed from acetaminophen to a different oral agent, THEN there should be evidence that the patient has had a trial of maximum dose acetaminophen (suitable for age/comorbidities).
Surgery	13. IF a patient with severe symptomatic osteoarthritis of the knee or hip has failed to respond to nonpharmacologic and pharmacologic therapy, THEN the patient should be offered referral to an orthopedic surgeon.
Radiographs	14. IF a patient has hip or knee osteoarthritis AND has worsening complaints accompanied by a progressive decrease in activities AND no previous radiograph during the preceding 3 months, THEN a knee or hip radiograph should be performed within 3 months.

[From Pencharz J, MacLean C. Measuring quality in arthritis care: The Arthritis Foundation's quality indicator set for osteoarthritis. Arthritis Rheum (Arthritis Care and Research) 51:538–548, 2004.]

gression and patient outcomes. Quality-of-life indicators, walking distance, ACR criteria, pain ratings, and Western Ontario MacMaster University Osteoarthritis Index (WOMAC) scores are beneficial in completely assessing the patient with OA. The Arthritis Foundation's quality indicators for OA are listed in Table 66.5.[102] These explicit process measures can be used to compare the care provided by different healthcare providers and different healthcare delivery systems. In addition, they may be used to compare the changes in care over time and ultimately to document and improve the quality of care for patients with OA.

Because OA is a chronic disease with multiple etiologies and risk factors, it may be possible to look at prevention as a disease management strategy. Primary prevention measures include reduction of known risk factors such as obesity and preventing major joint injury. Secondary prevention has not been established but may include screenings for persons who may have early, asymptomatic disease. Tertiary prevention involves prevention of disability for those who already have active disease. Ongoing research in this area will provide practitioners with strategies to both prevent and more effectively treat OA in the future.

PHARMACOECONOMICS

The World Development Report estimates that there are 11.2 million disability-adjusted life-years lost each year due to OA.[103] Pain, the predominant symptom of OA, accounts for much of the disability and impaired quality-of-life associated with OA, as well as the increased use of healthcare resources by patients with OA.[50] Evaluating the pharmacoeconomics of OA not only provides a means to compare costs, but also examines the benefits and effectiveness associated with different therapies.

In an economic analysis comparing acetaminophen to NSAIDs either with or without misoprostol prophylaxis, the costs associated with treating patients with NSAIDs were significantly higher than the costs of treatment with acetaminophen.[104] This study examined not only drug costs but also the associated costs of treating adverse events and the costs of prophylaxis for patients receiving NSAIDs in a managed care organization. Using retrospective medical and prescription claims data, the investigators determined that the average expected treatment cost for NSAIDs was $61 per treatment month compared to acetaminophen at $19 per treatment month. The costs associated with treating adverse events in NSAID users were $106 in patients not receiving prophylaxis and $55 in patients who received prophylaxis compared to $12 in patients receiving acetaminophen. Acetaminophen was determined to be the most cost-effective choice of therapy for patients with mild to moderate OA due to its decreased cost and decreased incidence and cost of side effects. When acetaminophen was compared to low-cost NSAIDs (ibuprofen) at $18 per treatment month in drug costs, the costs of treating adverse effects associated with

NSAID use still made acetaminophen the least costly treatment alternative.

KEY POINTS

- Treatment goals are to control pain, minimize disability, decrease joint stiffness, maintain mobility and functioning, maintain or improve quality-of-life, and educate patients and family members about OA and its therapies
- Use nonpharmacologic modalities in conjunction with pharmacologic modalities in the management of patients with OA
- Acetaminophen is considered first-line therapy and is a cost-effective treatment for OA
- Psychosocial factors may influence the patient's perception of pain and disability associated with OA
- Future therapies in OA may include agents produced to target specific cytokines or disease-modifying drugs for OA
- Resources are available for patients and healthcare practitioners from the Arthritis Foundation

SUGGESTED READINGS

Felson D, Zhang Y. An update on the epidemiology of knee and hip osteoarthritis with a view to prevention. Arthritis Rheum 41: 1343–1355, 1998.

Lee C, Straus W, Balshaw R, et al. A comparison of the efficacy and safety of nonsteroidal anti-inflammatory agents versus acetaminophen in the treatment of osteoarthritis: a meta-analysis. Arthritis Rheum (Arthritis Care and Research) 51:746–754, 2004.

Pencharz J, MacLean C. Measuring quality in arthritis care: the Arthritis Foundation's quality indicator set for osteoarthritis. Arthritis Rheum (Arthritis Care and Research) 51:538–548, 2004.

Todd C. Meeting the therapeutic challenge of the patient with osteoarthritis. J Am Pharm Assoc 42:74–82, 2002.

REFERENCES

1. Creamer P, Hochberg M. Osteoarthritis. Lancet 350:503–509, 1997.
2. Guccione A, Felson D, Anderson J, et al. The effects of specific medical conditions on functional limitations of elders in the Framingham Study. Am J Public Health 84:351–358, 1994.
3. Dunlap D, Manheim L, Yelin E, et al. The costs of arthritis. Arthritis Rheum (Arthritis Care and Research) 49:101–113, 2003.
4. Todd C. Meeting the therapeutic challenge of the patient with osteoarthritis. J Am Pharm Assoc 42:74–82, 2002.
5. Kuettner K, Goldberg V. Introduction. In: Kuettner K, Goldberg V, eds. Osteoarthritic disorders. Rosemont, IL: American Academy of Orthopedic Surgeons; 1995:xxi–xxv.
6. American College of Rheumatology Subcommittee. Recommendations for the medical management of osteoarthritis of the hip and knee, 2000 update. Arthritis Rheum 43:1905–1915, 2002.
7. American Pain Society (APS). New clinical guideline for the treatment of arthritis pain, 2002. http://www.ampainsoc.org. APS, 470 W. Lake Ave., Glenview, IL 60025-1485.
8. Dieppe P, Cushnaghan J, Shepstone L. The Bristol "OA500" Study: progression of osteoarthritis (OA) over 3 years and the relationship between clinical and radiographic changes at the knee joint. Osteoarthritis Cartilage 5:57–97, 1997.

9. Rogers J, Shepstone L, Dieppe P. Is osteoarthritis a systemic disorder of bone? Arthritis Rheum 50:452–457, 2004.

10. Felson D, Zhang Y. An update on the epidemiology of knee and hip osteoarthritis with a view to prevention. Arthritis Rheum 41:1343–1355, 1998.

11. Oliveria S, Felson D, Reed J, et al. Incidence of symptomatic hand, hip, and knee osteoarthritis among patients in a health maintenance organization. Arthritis Rheum 38:1134–1141, 1995.

12. Hirsch R, Lethbridge-Cejku M, Scott W Jr., et al. Association of hand and knee osteoarthritis: evidence for a polyarticular disease subset. Ann Rheum Dis 55:25–29, 1996.

13. Ritvaniemi P, Korkko J, Bonaventure J, et al. Identification of COL2A1 gene mutations in patients with chondrodysplasias and familial osteoarthritis. Arthritis Rheum 38:999–1004, 1995.

14. Felson D, Couropmitree N, Chaisson C, et al. Evidence for a Mendelian gene in a segregation analysis of generalized radiographic osteoarthritis; the Framingham Study. Arthritis Rheum 41:1064–1071, 1998.

15. Dequeker J, Boonen S, Aerssens J, et al. Inverse relationship between osteoarthritis–osteoporosis: what is the evidence? What are the consequences? Br J Rheumatol 35:813–820, 1996.

16. Hart D, Mootoosamy I, Doyle D, et al. The relationship between osteoarthritis and osteoporosis in the general population: the Chingford Study. Ann Rheum Dis 53:158–162, 1994.

17. Hannan M, Anderson J, Zhang Y, et al. Bone mineral density and knee osteoarthritis in elderly men and women: the Framingham Study. Arthritis Rheum 36:1671–1680, 1993.

18. Flugsrud G, Nordsletten L, Espehaug B, et al. Risk factors for total hip replacement due to primary osteoarthritis. Arthritis Rheum 46:675–682, 2002.

19. Lane N, Nevitt M, Hochberg M, et al. Progression of radiographic hip osteoarthritis over eight years in a community sample of elderly white women. Arthritis Rheum 50:1477–1486, 2004.

20. Schipplein O, Andriacchi T. Interaction between active and passive knee stabilizers during level walking. J Orthop Res 9:113–119, 1991.

21. Felson D, Zhang Y, Anthony J, et al. Weight loss reduces the risk for symptomatic knee osteoarthritis in women. Ann Intern Med 116:535–539, 1992.

22. Zhang Y, Glynn R, Felson D. Musculoskeletal disease research: should we analyze the joint or the person? J Rheumatol 23:1130–1134, 1996.

23. Gelber A, Hochberg M, Mead L, et al. Joint injury in young adults and risk for subsequent knee and hip osteoarthritis. Ann Intern Med 133:321–328, 2000.

24. Spector T, Harris P, Hart D, et al. Risk of osteoarthritis associated with long term weight-bearing sports: a radiologic survey of the hips and knees in female ex-athletes and population controls. Arthritis Rheum 39:988–995, 1996.

25. Vingard E, Alfredsson L, Goldie I, et al. Sports and osteoarthrosis of the hip: an epidemiologic study. Am J Sports Med 21:195–200, 1993.

26. Kujala U, Kettunen J, Paananen H, et al. Knee osteoarthritis in former runners, soccer players, weight lifters, and shooters. Arthritis Rheum 38:539–546, 1995.

27. Pinals R. Mechanisms of joint destruction, pain and disability in osteoarthritis. Drugs 52 (Suppl 3):14–20, 1996.

28. Schaible H, Neugebauer V, Schmidt R. Osteoarthritis and pain. Semin Arthritis Rheum 18:30–34, 1989.

29. Hochberg M, Lawrence R, Everett D, et al. Epidemiologic association of pain in osteoarthritis of the knee; data from the National Health and Nutrition Examination survey and the National Health and Nutrition Examination I. Epidemiologic follow-up survey. Semin Arthritis Rheum 18:4–9, 1989.

30. Balint G, Szebenyi B. Diagnosis of osteoarthritis: guidelines and current pitfalls. Drugs 52 (Suppl 3):1–13, 1996.

31. Buckwalter J. Osteoarthritis and articular cartilage use, disuse and abuse: experimental studies. J Rheumatol 22 (Suppl 43):13–15, 1995.

32. Schumacher R Jr. Secondary osteoarthritis. In: Moskowitz R, Howell D, Goldberg V, et al, eds. Osteoarthritis. Diagnosis and medical/surgical management. 2nd ed. Philadelphia: WB Saunders, 1992:367–398.

33. Altman R, Asch E, Bloch D, et al. Development of criteria for the classification and reporting of osteoarthritis. Classification of osteoarthritis of the knee. Arthritis Rheum 29:1030–1049, 1986.

34. Altman R, Alarcon G, Appelrouth D, et al. The ACR criteria for the classification and reporting of osteoarthritis of the hand. Arthritis Rheum 33:1601–1610, 1990.

35. Altman R, Alarcon G, Appelrouth D, et al. The ACR criteria for the classification and reporting of osteoarthritis of the hip. Arthritis Rheum 34:505–514, 1991.

36. Hart D, Spector T. Radiographic criteria for epidemiologic studies of osteoarthritis. J Rheumatol 22 (Suppl 43):46–48, 1995.

37. Raynauld, J, Martel-Pelletier J, Berthiaume M, et al. Quantitative magnetic resonance imaging evaluation of knee osteoarthritis progression over two years and correlation with clinical symptoms and radiologic changes. Arthritis Rheum 50:476–487, 2004.

38. Creamer P, Hochberg M. The relationship between psychosocial variables and pain reporting in osteoarthritis of the knee. Arthritis Rheum (Arthritis Care and Research) 11:60–65, 1998.

39. Hampson S, Glasgow R, Zeiss A. Coping with osteoarthritis by older adults. Arthritis Rheum (Arthritis Care and Research) 9:133–141, 1996.

40. Kee C, Harris S, Booth L, et al. Perspectives on the nursing management of osteoarthritis. Geriatr Nurs 19:19–27, 1998.

41. Bradley J, Brandt K, Katz B, et al. Comparison of an anti-inflammatory dose of ibuprofen, an analgesic dose of ibuprofen, and acetaminophen in the treatment of patients with osteoarthritis of the knee. N Engl J Med 325:87–91, 1991.

42. Bradley J, Brandt K, Katz B, et al. Treatment of knee osteoarthritis: relationship of clinical features of joint inflammation to the response to a nonsteroidal anti-inflammatory drug or pure analgesic. J Rheumatol 19:1950–1954, 1992.

43. Dieppe P, Cushnaghan J, Hasani M, et al. A 2-year, placebo controlled trial of nonsteroidal anti-inflammatory therapy in osteoarthritis of the knee joint. Br J Rheumatol 32:595–600, 1993.

44. Acetaminophen, NSAIDs and alcohol. Med Lett Drugs Ther 38:55–56, 1996.

45. Benison H, Kaczynski J, Wallerstedt S. Paracetamol medication and alcohol abuse: a dangerous combination for the liver and kidney. Scand J Gastroenterol 22:701–704, 1987.

46. Raffa R, Friderichs E. The basic science aspect of tramadol hydrochloride. Pain Rev 3:271, 1996.

47. Cicero T, Adams E, Geller A, et al. A postmarketing surveillance program to monitor Ultram (tramadol hydrochloride) abuse in the United States. Drug Alcohol Depend 57:7–22, 1999.

48. Jensen E, Ginsberg F. Tramadol versus dextropropoxyphene in the treatment of osteoarthritis. Drug Invest 8:211–218, 1994.

49. Fleischmann R, Caldwell J, Roth S, et al. Tramadol for the treatment of joint pain associated with osteoarthritis: a randomized, double-blind, placebo-controlled trial. Curr Ther Res 113–128, 2001.

50. Katz W. Pharmacology and clinical experience with tramadol in osteoarthritis. Drugs 52 (Suppl 3):39–47, 1996.

51. Roth S. Efficacy and safety of tramadol HCl in breakthrough musculoskeletal pain attributed to osteoarthritis. J Rheumatol 25:1358–1363, 1998.

52. Schnitzer T, Kamin M, Olson W. Tramadol allows reduction of naproxen dose among patients with naproxen-responsive osteoarthritis pain: a randomized, double-blind, placebo-controlled study. Arthritis Rheum 42:1370–1377, 1999.

53. Mason B, Blackburn K. Possible serotonin syndrome associated with tramadol and sertraline coadministration. Ann Pharmacother 31:175–177, 1997.

54. Kahn L, Alderfer R, Graham D. Seizures reported with tramadol. JAMA 278:1661, 1997.

55. Gasse C, Derby L, Vasilakis-Scaramozza C, et al. Incidence of first-time idiopathic seizures in users of tramadol. Pharmacotherapy 20:629–634, 2000.

56. Ruoff G. Slowing the initial titration rate of tramadol improves tolerability. Pharmacotherapy 19:88–93, 1999.

57. Petrone D, Kamin M, Olson W. Slowing the titration rate of tramadol HCl reduces the incidence of discontinuation due to nausea and/or vomiting: a double-blind randomized trial. J Clin Pharm Ther 24:115–123, 1999.

58. Ortho-McNeil Pharmaceutical. Ultram (tramadol hydrochloride tablets) [prescribing information]. In: Physicians' Desk Reference. Montvale, NJ: Medical Economics Co, 2004:2398–2401.

59. Bannwarth B. Risk-benefit assessment of opioids in chronic noncancer pain. Drug Saf 21:283–296, 1999.
60. Lawlor P, Bruera E. Side-effects of opioids in chronic pain treatment. Curr Opin Anaesthesiol 11:539–545, 1998.
61. Cherny N. Opioid analgesics: comparative features and prescribing guidelines. Drugs 51:713–737, 1996.
62. Savage S. Opioid use in the management of chronic pain. Med Clin North Am 83:761–786, 1999.
63. Ahmedzai S, Brooks D. Transdermal fentanyl versus sustained-release oral morphine in cancer pain: preference, efficacy, and quality of life. The TTS-Fentanyl Comparative Trial Group. J Pain Symptom Manage 13:254–261, 1997.
64. Grond S, Zech D, Lehmann, K, et al. Transdermal fentanyl in the long-term treatment of cancer pain: a prospective study of 50 patients with advanced cancer of the gastrointestinal tract or the head and neck region. Pain 69:191–198, 1997.
65. Felson D. The verdict favors nonsteroidal anti-inflammatory drugs for treatment of osteoarthritis and a plea for more evidence on other treatments. Arthritis Rheum 44:1477–1480, 2001.
66. Pincus T, Koch G, Sokka T, et al. A randomized, double-blind, crossover clinical trial of diclofenac plus misoprostol versus acetaminophen in patients with osteoarthritis of the hip or knee. Arthritis Rheum 44:1587–1598, 2001.
67. Schiff M, Minic M. Comparison of the analgesic efficacy and safety of nonprescription doses of naproxen sodium and ibuprofen in the treatment of osteoarthritis of the knee. J Rheumatol 31:1373–1383, 2004.
68. Lee C, Straus W, Balshaw R, et al. A comparison of the efficacy and safety of nonsteroidal anti-inflammatory agents versus acetaminophen in the treatment of osteoarthritis: a meta-analysis. Arthritis Rheum (Arthritis Care and Research) 51:746–754, 2004.
69. Lichtenstein D, Syngal S, Wolfe M. Nonsteroidal anti-inflammatory drugs and the gastrointestinal tract: the double-edged sword. Arthritis Rheum 35:5–18, 1995.
70. Catella-Lawson F. Cyclooxygenase inhibitors and the antiplatelet effects of aspirin. N Engl J Med 345:1809–1817, 2001.
71. MacDonald T, Wei L. Effect of ibuprofen on cardioprotective effect of aspirin. Lancet 361:573–574, 2003.
72. Kurth T. Inhibition of clinical benefits of aspirin on first myocardial infarction by nonsteroidal anti-inflammatory drugs. Circulation 108:1191–1195, 2003.
73. Garcia Rodriquez L. Nonsteroidal anti-inflammatory drugs and the risk of myocardial infarction in the general population. Circulation 109:3000–3006, 2004.
74. Siebrerer K, Masferrer J. Role of inducible cyclo-oxygenase (COX-2) inflammation. Receptor 4:17–23, 1994.
75. Simon L. Nonsteroidal anti-inflammatory drugs and their effects: the importance of COX ''selectivity.'' J Clin Rheumatol 2:135–140, 1996.
76. Fusco B, Giacovazzo M. Peppers and pain: the promise of capsaicin. Drugs 53:909–914, 1997.
77. Raynauld J, Buckland-Wright C, Ward R, et al. Safety and efficacy of long-term intraarticular steroid injections in osteoarthritis of the knee. Arthritis Rheum 48:370–377, 2003.
78. Julovi S, Yasuda T, Shimizu M, et al. Inhibition of interleukin-1 β-stimulated production of matrix metalloproteinases by hyaluronan via CD44 in human articular cartilage. Arthritis Rheum 50:516–525, 2004.
79. Lo G, LaValley M, McAlindon T, et al. Intra-articular hyaluronic acid in treatment of knee osteoarthritis: a meta-analysis. JAMA 290:3115–3121, 2003.
80. Wang C, Lin J, Chang C, et al. Therapeutic effects of hyaluronic acid on osteoarthritis of the knee. J Bone Joint Surg [Am] 86:538–545, 2004.
81. Simon L. Viscosupplementation therapy with intra-articular hyaluronic acid: fact or fantasy? Rheum Dis Clin North Am 25:345–357, 1999.
82. Stamm T, Machold K, Smolen J, et al. Joint protection and home hand exercises improve hand function in patients with hand osteoarthritis: a randomized controlled trial. Arthritis Rheum (Arthritis Care and Research) 47:44–49, 2002.
83. Panush R. Is there a role for diet or other questionable therapies in managing rheumatic diseases? Bull Rheum Dis 42:1–4, 1993.
84. Messier S, Loeser R, Miller G, et al. Exercise and dietary weight loss in overweight and obese older adults with knee osteoarthritis. Arthritis Rheum 50:1501–1510, 2004.
85. Michalsen A, Klotz S, Ludtke R, et al. Effectiveness of leech therapy in osteoarthritis of the knee: a randomized, controlled trial. Ann Intern Med 139:724–730, 2003.
86. Altman R, Marcussen K. Effects of a ginger extract on knee pain in patients with osteoarthritis. Arthritis Rheum 44:2531–2538, 2001.
87. Pray W, Pray J. Self-care options for arthritis therapy. US Pharmacist 5:19–24, 2004.
88. Reginster J, Deroisy R, Rovati L, et al. Long-term effects of glucosamine sulphate on osteoarthritis progression: a randomised, placebo-controlled clinical trial. Lancet 357:251–256, 2001.
89. Pavelka K, Gatterova J, Olejarova M, et al. Glucosamine sulfate use and delay of progression of knee osteoarthritis. Arch Intern Med 162:2113–2123, 2002.
90. Evans C, Robbins P. Potential treatment of osteoarthritis by gene therapy. Rheum Dis Clin North Am 25:333–344, 1999.
91. Lozasa C, Altman R. Chondroprotection in osteoarthritis. Bull Rheum Dis 46:5–7, 1997.
92. Cole A, Chubinskaya S, Luchene L, et al. Doxycycline disrupts chondrocyte differentiation and inhibits cartilage matrix degradation. Arthritis Rheum 32:1727–1734, 1994.
93. Oesser S, Seifert J. Stimulation of type II collagen biosynthesis and secretion in bovine chondrocytes cultured with degraded collagen. Cell Tissue Res 311:393–399, 2003.
94. Carbone L, Nevitt M, Wildy K, et al. The relationship of antiresorptive drug use to structural findings and symptoms of knee osteoarthritis. Arthritis Rheum 50:3516–3525, 2004.
95. Das S, Ramakrishnan S, Mishra K, et al. A randomized controlled trial to evaluate the slow-acting symptom-modifying effects of colchicine in osteoarthritis of the knee: a preliminary report. Arthritis Rheum (Arthritis Care and Research) 47:280–284, 2002.
96. Lorig K, Lubeck D, Kraines T, et al. Outcomes of self-help education for patients with arthritis. Arthritis Rheum 28:680–685, 1985.
97. Weinberger M, Tierney W, Booher P, et al. Can the provision of information to patients with osteoarthritis improve functional status? A randomized, controlled trial. Arthritis Rheum 32:1577–1583, 1989.
98. Roddy E, Zhang W, Doherty M, et al. Evidence-based recommendations for the role of exercise in the management of osteoarthritis of the hip or knee—the MOVE consensus. Rheumatology 44:67–73, 2005.
99. Bijlsma J, Dekker J. A step forward for exercise in the management of osteoarthritis. Rheumatology 44:5–6, 2005.
100. Lorig K, Konkol L, Gonzalez V. Arthritis patient education: a review of the literature. Patient Educ Couns 10:207–252, 1987.
101. Barlow J, Turner A, Wright C. Long-term outcomes of an arthritis self-management programme. Br J Rheumatol 37:1315–1319, 1998.
102. Pencharz J, MacLean C. Measuring quality in arthritis care: The Arthritis Foundation's quality indicator set for osteoarthritis. Arthritis Rheum (Arthritis Care and Research) 51:538–548, 2004.
103. Tugwell P. Economic evaluation of the management of pain in osteoarthritis. Drugs 52 (Suppl 3):48–58, 1996.
104. Holzer S, Cuerdon T. Development of an economic model comparing acetaminophen to NSAIDs in the treatment of mild-to-moderate osteoarthritis. Am J Manag Care 2 (Suppl):S15–26, 1996.

Gout and Hyperuricemia

67

William W. McCloskey and Maria D. Kostka-Rokosz

DEFINITION

Gout, a chronic metabolic disease, most commonly afflicts men over 30 years old. It was recognized as an illness and treated before the ancient Greeks ruled the Mediterranean world. Gout was associated with wealthy intellectuals who were known to overindulge in food and drink. Despite such a long history, no specific cause was identified until 1848, when uric acid was identified as the cause of gout. One of the major therapeutic advances of the 19th century was the use of colchicine to treat symptoms of the disease. When the role of purines in the disease process was discovered, specific dietary recommendations were made for patients with gout. Currently, acute attacks of gout are treated with colchicine, nonselective nonsteroidal anti-inflammatory drugs (NSAIDs), various corticosteroids, and corticotropin. The role of selective cyclooxygenase-2 (COX-2) inhibitors in the treatment of acute attacks is being investigated. Therapy with uricosuric agents and allopurinol is reserved for the long-term management of hyperuricemia.

Uric acid is an end product of protein catabolism. Since humans lack the enzyme uricase, which degrades uric acid to the soluble excretion product allantoin, uric acid is the final product resulting from the breakdown of purines. DNA and RNA are degraded, yielding the nucleosides adenosine and guanosine. The enzyme xanthine oxidase converts guanosine directly to xanthine and converts adenosine first to hypoxanthine then to xanthine. Xanthine is then converted to uric acid (Fig. 67.1; *see color insert*).

Total body content of uric acid ranges from 1.0 to 1.2 g in normal men, with a daily turnover rate of 600 to 800 mg. These values are slightly lower for women. Normally, this turnover represents 50% to 60% of the daily urate pool. Approximately 70% of uric acid is excreted in the urine; the remainder is secreted by a passive process into the gastrointestinal (GI) tract and is degraded by intestinal microorganisms to ammonia and carbon dioxide.[1,2]

A four-component theory for urate handling by the kidney best explains the actions of drugs to increase or decrease uric acid levels. These four components are filtration, reabsorption, secretion, and postsecretory reabsorption, which occur in the later part of the proximal tubule or in the distal tubule. Approximately 95% of serum uric acid is filtered freely across the glomerulus; 5% is protein bound. Of the filtered urate, 98% to 100% is reabsorbed in the early part of the proximal tubule. A variable percentage of the filtered load is secreted back into the tubular lumen in a more distal part of the proximal tubule. The fourth component occurs in the distal part of the proximal tubule or in the distal tubule.[2]

Hyperuricemia is defined as a urate level greater than 7.0 mg per dL (450 μmol/L) in men and 6.0 mg per dL (350 μmol/L) in women.[3–5] These values are more than two standard deviations above mean population values. The lower value in women results from an estrogen-dependent sex difference. This difference, which manifests at puberty and is related to greater urate clearance, diminishes or disappears in women after menopause.[6]

Two laboratory methods are used to measure serum urate concentrations. The colorimetric method is used by most autoanalyzers. Since it is nonspecific, false elevations can result from uremia, amino acids in the test sample, high vitamin C dosages, levodopa, and xanthines such as caffeine, theobromine, and theophylline. The uricase method is more specific than the colorimetric method. Clinicians must be aware of the method used to analyze uric acid serum levels. The definitions of hyperuricemia given here are based on uricase determinations.[7,8]

TREATMENT GOALS

- Terminate the pain and inflammation associated with an acute gout attack.
- Limit and treat acute attack recurrences.
- Gradually reduce serum uric acid concentrations in patients with symptomatic hyperuricemia.

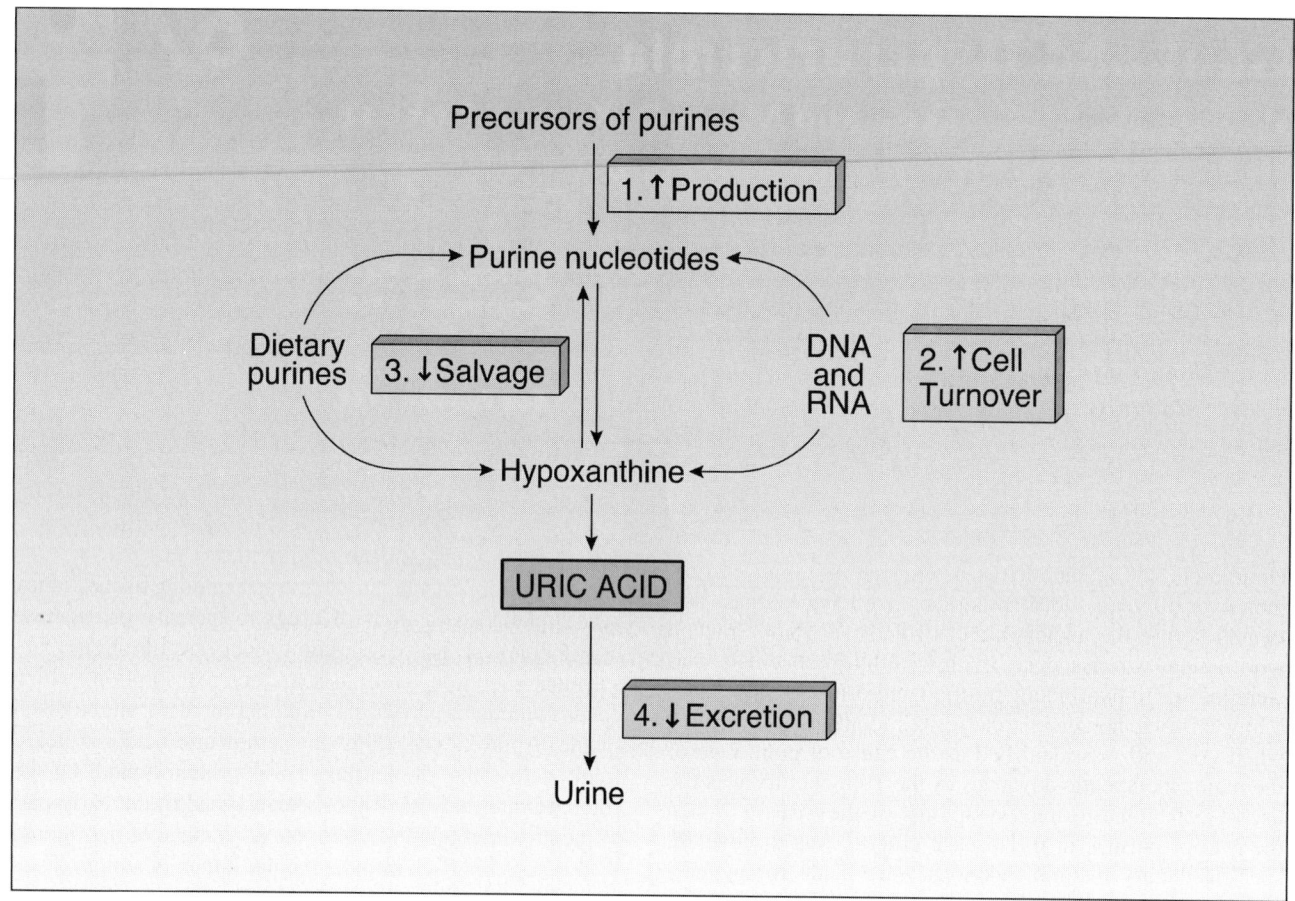

Precursors of purines

1. ↑ Production

Purine nucleotides

Dietary purines   3. ↓ Salvage   DNA and RNA   2. ↑ Cell Turnover

Hypoxanthine

URIC ACID

4. ↓ Excretion

Urine

FIGURE 67.1 Pathogenesis of hyperuricemia and gout (*see color insert*). (Image from Rubin E, Farber JL. Pathology, 3rd ed. Philadelphia: Lippincott Williams & Wilkins, 1999.)

EPIDEMIOLOGY

Hyperuricemia and gout have traditionally been classified as either primary or secondary. Primary gout refers to cases in which the basic metabolic defect is unknown or, if it is known, the main manifestation is that of hyperuricemia and gout. Secondary gout refers to cases in which hyperuricemia is part of some other acquired disorder or in which the basic metabolic defect underlying the hyperuricemia is known but the main clinical characteristics are not those of gout. Since the distinctions between primary and secondary gout may not always be clear,[2] the disease is currently described by four clinical phases: asymptomatic hyperuricemia, acute gouty arthritis, intercritical gout, and chronic tophaceous gout.[5,9,10]

Patients with hyperuricemia have elevated serum uric acid levels that are caused by an increased production of uric acid, an impaired clearance, or both. Most patients with gout are underexcreters of uric acid, with only 10% to 20% being overproducers.[3] Although high serum urate levels predispose patients to gout, many patients with hyperuricemia are asymptomatic and never develop the disease.

Increased urate production can result from a variety of factors. Nutritional indiscretions, such as excessive purine

and fructose intake, as well as alcohol use may contribute to hyperuricemia and gout.[3–5,10] Recent prospective cohort studies verify that there is an association between high intake of meat and seafood[11,12] and the use of various types of alcoholic beverages[13] and an increased risk of gout. Obesity may cause high serum urate levels due to increased urate production and decreased urate excretion.[3–5,10] Some patients with hyperuricemia and gout may suffer from syndrome X, which is characterized by insulin resistance, hyperinsulinemia, central obesity, and dyslipidemia and is associated with hypertension and atherosclerosis.[4,14]

Enzymatic defects such as hypoxanthine-guanine phosphoribosyltransferase deficiency (Lesch-Nyhan syndrome), phosphoribosyl-pyrophosphate synthetase hyperactivity (which converts purines to uric acid), aldolase-beta deficiency, and glucose-6-phosphate deficiency (glycogen storage disease) may cause hyperuricemia and gout.[5,9] Hyperuricemia may be associated with any condition that causes an increase in the cell proliferation rate, such as lymphoid and myeloid proliferative disorders, myeloid metaplasia, polycythemia vera, hematologic neoplastic diseases such as leukemias and lymphomas, and psoriasis.[5,9,10] Hyperuricemia may also occur with sickle cell anemia, hemolytic anemia with secondary erythrocytosis, and thalassemia, although it is not common in primary red blood cell disorders.[2] Cytotoxic agents are blamed for urate production due to tumor lysis syndrome.

Hyperuricemia may also be caused by impairment in the renal excretion of uric acid. Dehydration, renal disorders such as polycystic kidney disease, and renal insufficiency from hypertension and chronic renal failure play a role in the etiology of hyperuricemia. Chronic lead toxicity from contaminated ''moonshine'' or various trades such as painting is associated with gout and hyperuricemia. Increased ketoacids and lactic acid, due to exercise and uncontrolled diabetes and other conditions such as hypothyroidism, hyperparathyroidism, and hypoparathyroidism have all been associated with elevated uric acid levels, presumably because they reduce renal urate excretion.[5,10,14]

Pharmacologic agents are responsible for drug-induced hyperuricemia. Diuretics are often implicated; the mechanism, though not clear, may relate to an increased reabsorption of uric acid in the proximal tubule, a decreased tubular secretion, or an increased postsecretory reabsorption of uric acid. Spironolactone, a nonselective aldosterone antagonist, does not cause hyperuricemia.[15] Preliminary evidence suggests that eplerenone (Inspra), a new selective aldosterone antagonist, is rarely associated with hyperuricemia when used in combination with losartan.[16]

Aspirin can increase serum urate concentrations when used in dosages of less than 2 g per day by inhibiting tubular secretion. Salicylate dosages of more than 2 g cause a uricosuric effect by inhibiting reabsorption of uric acid.

Pyrazinamide inhibits renal urate secretion, and ethambutol, another antitubercular drug, is also associated with decreased renal clearance of uric acid. Other drugs that may increase serum levels of uric acid include nicotinic acid, levodopa, and didanosine.[3,5,9,10,14]

The immunosuppressant cyclosporine has been implicated as a cause of hyperuricemia. Although initial adverse event reports focused on cyclosporine-induced nephrotoxicity, the literature currently focuses on drug-induced hyperuricemia and gout in the renal,[17] liver,[18] and cardiac[19,20] transplant populations. Hyperuricemia occurs as a result of cyclosporine-induced renal insufficiency, which causes decreased uric acid clearance by the kidney.[17] Depending on how it is defined, hyperuricemia occurs independently from cyclosporine-induced nephrotoxicity in 30% to 60% of patients, and gouty arthritis develops in 4% to 10% of cyclosporine-treated patients. Lin et al[17] reported hyperuricemia in 84% of renal transplant patients treated with cyclosporine compared to 30% in an azathioprine-treated group; however, actual gout occurred in only 7% of these patients. A longitudinal study of the subgroup of the cyclosporine-treated patients revealed that hyperuricemia occurred within 3 months after transplantation, with the first attack of gout occurring in 24 months. The prevalence and onset of gout in cardiac transplant patients may be higher due to larger cyclosporine doses.[20]

Many studies have related gout to genetic, racial, geographic, dietary, and other socioeconomic factors. Although still controversial, a relationship appears to exist between hyperuricemia and gout and coronary heart disease. The one consistent marker is the relationship between elevated uric acid levels and gout. Although the prevalence of gout in the United States is estimated to be 8.4 per 1,000 individuals, the true prevalence is not known.[21] The epidemiology of gout was studied as a part of the Heart Disease Epidemiology Study in Framingham, Massachusetts. The study involved 5127 subjects aged 30 to 59 on initial evaluation. Before entry into the study, 13 subjects, 0.2% of the total population, had experienced a gouty attack. The mean age of the population at the beginning of the study was 44 years. Fourteen years later, when the mean age of the population was 58, 1.5% of the population (76 subjects) had experienced an attack of gout. Gout had occurred in 2.8% of the men and 0.4% of the women. The prevalence of gouty arthritis was found to increase with increasing uric acid levels. The frequency of gout was 0.6% in men with uric acid levels under 6 mg per dL (360 μmol/L), 1.9% with levels of 6 to 6.9 mg per dL (360 to 410 μmol/L), and 20% with uric acid levels above 7 mg per dL (420 μmol/L).[22] Ninety percent of men had gout when levels exceeded 9 mg per dL (530 μmol/L).

PATHOPHYSIOLOGY

Urate crystal formation in patients with gout is most likely due to a combination of factors. The degree of hyperuricemia, abrupt increases or decreases in serum uric acid levels, and the presence of certain protein polysaccharides play a role. The location of the joint, physical state, joint temperature, and resolution of joint effusions are also involved in urate crystal formation.[23]

Acute attacks of gout develop when monosodium urate (MSU) crystals deposit in the synovium of joints and in soft tissues. These crystals are derived from either preformed synovial deposits or de novo synthesis. Typically, acute attacks affect the peripheral joints; the most distal joints are more likely to be affected early in the course of a patient's gouty arthritis. A possible explanation for this involves joint temperature, because MSU solubility varies directly with temperature. The solubility of urate in physiologic saline is 6.8 mg per dL (400 μmol/L) at 37°C but only 4.5 mg per dL (270 μmol/L) at 30°C. Joint temperatures decrease distally. The average temperature of the knee is 33°C; that of the ankle is 29°C. Temperature alone, however, cannot explain why gout develops in some people and not in others with similar uric acid levels. Also involved may be the increased solubility of urate in proteoglycans, chondroitin sulfate, and hyaluronic acid, which are abundant in the synovial fluid and cartilage. Urate solubility may be affected by genetic or environmental alterations in these substances that predispose the patient to, or even initiate, attacks of gout.[2,23]

Simkin, who was concerned with the predisposition of gout in the first metatarsophalangeal joint, proposed another explanation. During the normal walking process, the base of the big toe is subjected to extreme forces. Shoes compound the problem by forcing the joint to endure these forces in an unnatural position. The joint that has experienced degenerative changes or recent trauma, including trauma that may have gone unnoticed, is likely to be the site of a synovial effusion. While the patient sleeps at night, the effusion resolves. Water leaves the joint faster than urate does, and the result is a transiently high intraarticular urate concentration that favors crystal formation. This explains the common nocturnal onset of gout in the big toe and may help to explain the occasional attack of gout that develops in a person with a normal urate serum concentration.[24]

Urate crystals in the synovial fluid or surrounding tissues and the reaction of the body's defense mechanisms to these crystals cause the typical gouty attack. MSU crystals have sharp, irregular crystal facets with multiple outward projections. These surface irregularities favor the adsorption of immunoglobulin and other polypeptides. Adsorption of these polypeptides increases crystal phagocytosis by polymorphonuclear leukocytes or neutrophils.[9,25,26] Phagocytosis of the crystal–protein complex causes cell destruction and release of intracellular enzymes. The neutrophils continue the inflammatory process by activating the prostaglandin, kinin, complement, and leukotriene cascades[25] and by releasing chemotactic factors that cause further inflammation due to neutrophil recruitment.[9,27] Cells of the synovial lining further the inflammatory process by producing interleukin-1, interleukin-6, interleukin-8, prostaglandin E2, tumor necrosis factor-α, and leukotriene B4. Although the extent of involvement of these other factors is unclear, the role of polymorphonuclear leukocytes is well established.

CLINICAL PRESENTATION AND DIAGNOSIS

SIGNS AND SYMPTOMS

The classic presentation of gout is that of a sudden onset of excruciating pain in a joint in the lower extremity, with approximately 50% of initial attacks involving the first metatarsophalangeal joint of the great toe (podagra) (Fig. 67.2; *see color insert*); however, other joints, such as the knee, ankle, and instep, may be involved as well.[3] Most patients are in previously good health without a clear underlying cause for the disease, but attacks may be precipitated by trauma, stress, excessive alcohol intake, certain medications, or diets high in purine content. Acute attacks generally occur at night, and the pain is usually severe enough that even the slightest pressure from bed sheets cannot be tolerated. The pain is generally accompanied within hours by inflammation, warmth and swelling of the joint, and in some instances a mild fever.[3,5]

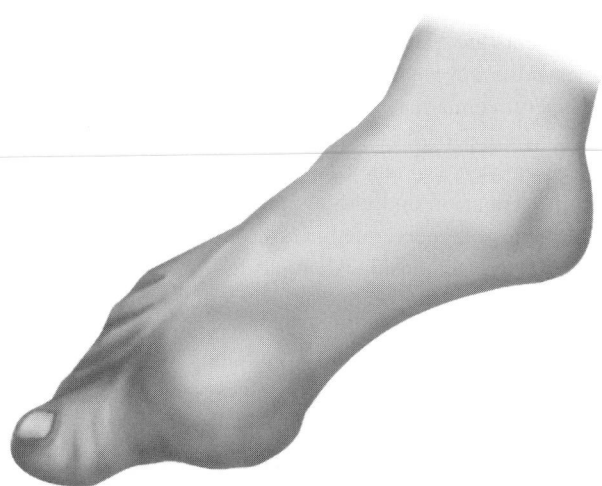

FIGURE 67.2 Acute gouty arthritis (metatarsophalangeal joint of the big toe) *(see color insert)*. (From Bickley LS, Szilagyi P. Bates' guide to physical examination and history taking, 8th ed. Philadelphia: Lippincott Williams & Wilkins, 2003.)

In approximately 80% of cases, the initial gout attack involves only one joint (monoarticular), although multiple joint involvement (polyarticular) may occur as well, particularly in elderly women.[1] It is estimated that 25% of older women present with hand involvement and polyarticular disease.[28] Less commonly involved sites for gout attacks are the shoulder, hip, spine, and sacroiliac, sternoclavicular, and temporomandibular joints.[24,29]

The course of acute gout is variable, and an untreated attack may last from a few hours to several days.[1] As the patient recovers, the skin over the affected joint often desquamates. Although a first gouty attack may be very severe, with marked swelling and incapacitation, recovery often is complete, and patients generally return to their previous state of health until the next episode.[30] Although some patients may never experience another attack, most untreated individuals will experience a second event within 1 to 2 years.[1] The asymptomatic periods between attacks are called "intercritical" periods, which become shorter as the disease progresses. Synovial fluid analysis of the first metatarsophalangeal and knee joints for the presence of MSU crystals during this intercritical period may assist with an earlier diagnosis of gout.[31] Over time, as the disease progresses in untreated or suboptimally treated patients, subsequent gout attacks are typically polyarticular and more severe, last longer, and are more likely to be accompanied by fever, leukocytosis, and an elevated erythrocyte sedimentation rate.[1]

Eventually, untreated patients may enter a chronic polyarticular phase without pain-free intercritical periods, during which the intervals between attacks become shorter and the symptoms of the attack do not resolve completely. Chronic joint symptoms may be mistaken for osteoarthritis, especially in the elderly, or rheumatoid arthritis, particularly in the presence of uric acid deposits in subcutaneous tissues, which may be confused with rheumatoid nodules. It is rare that a patient would have both gout and rheumatoid arthritis.[32,33]

Chronic tophaceous gout is an uncommon but relatively severe complication of long-standing, inadequately treated disease. This form of gout is characterized by visible deposits of urate crystals (tophi) in connective tissues and joint structures that result in a destructive arthropathy and secondary osteoarthritis.[10] Tophi are rubbery nodules that are commonly found on the hand, foot, knee, helix or antihelix of the ear, olecranon bursa (elbow), and Achilles tendon.[10] Figure 67.3 (*see color insert*) illustrates these characteristic urate deposits on the hands and wrists in a patient with chronic tophaceous gout. Tophaceous gout is a direct consequence of consistently elevated levels of uric acid. Levels of uric acid from 10 to 11 mg per dL (590 to 650 μmol/L) have been reported to be associated with minimal to moderate tophi, levels in excess of 11 mg per dL (650 μmol/L) with more widespread deposits.[34] Fortunately, the appropriate use of allopurinol and uricosurics has reduced the occurrence of chronic tophaceous gout overall, and tophi generally occur in less than 10% of gout patients.[35] Because cyclosporine therapy causes uric acid retention, tophi may be more common in posttransplant patients.[36]

Renal complications of hyperuricemia are of major concern and include uric acid nephrolithiasis (kidney stones), urate nephropathy, and acute uric acid nephropathy. It is estimated that approximately 20% of patients with gout will develop uric acid kidney stones at some point in their illness. Sometimes patients present with symptomatic uric acid kidney stones even before the development of gouty arthritis or tophi.[7] Recent data from a large cohort of male health professionals found that a history of gout doubled the multivariate relative risk of kidney stones in men, although a history of kidney stones did not increase the risk of gout.[37] This study suggests that patients with gout should be advised

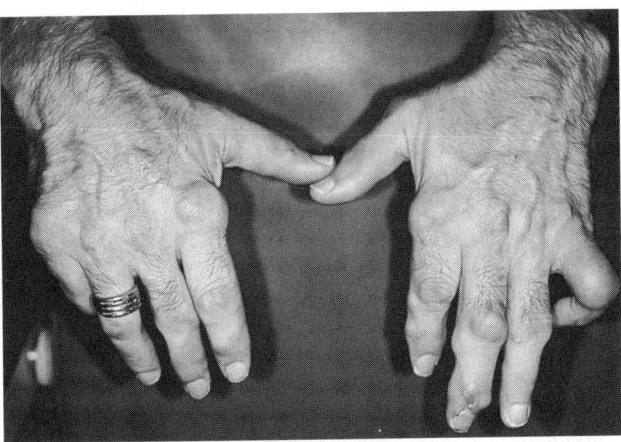

FIGURE 67.3 Chronic tophaceous gout involving hands and wrist (*see color insert*). (From Gold DH, Weingeist TA. Color atlas of the eye in systemic disease. Baltimore: Lippincott Williams & Wilkins, 2001.)

to increase their fluid intake and decrease their sodium consumption, especially if there is a family history of kidney stones, to reduce the risk of stone formation.

Urate nephropathy is a slowly progressive disease that results from the deposition of urate crystals in the renal interstitium. It is not clear whether chronic renal impairment in gout patients is a result of these urate deposits, or perhaps is due to concomitant diseases such as hypertension and diabetes or NSAID therapy. Conversely, uric acid nephropathy results from the large-scale deposition of uric acid crystals in the collecting tubules, resulting in acute renal failure. This is an uncommon problem but does occur in patients who overproduce and overexcrete uric acid as a result of aggressive chemotherapy, lymphoma, leukemia, or enzymatic defects. The renal failure correlates not with the serum urate concentration but with the total amount of uric acid excreted. Renal damage usually becomes present when there is coexisting diabetes, hypertension, renal vascular disease, glomerulonephritis, or some other primary cause of nephropathy that is not directly related to gout.[38-40] Patients with lymphoproliferative malignancies receiving chemotherapy should receive agents that lower uric acid levels, such as allopurinol or recombinant urate oxidase (rasburicase), to prevent uric acid nephropathy.[41]

DIAGNOSIS AND CLINICAL FINDINGS

Diagnosing gout is a challenge, but the diagnosis must be clearly established before expensive and potentially harmful drug therapy is initiated. The diagnosis should not be based only on serum uric acid levels, as treatment is generally not warranted for the majority of patients with asymptomatic hyperuricemia. Also, normal serum urate levels do not rule out the possibility of gout, as nearly 40% of patients have normal levels during an acute attack.[42]

Any assessment of a patient with gout should include a thorough history and physical examination. A family history may indicate a predisposition for gout, and any medications the patient is taking should be evaluated for their potential to induce hyperuricemia. Gout should be considered in someone with an acute onset of monoarticular or asymmetric polyarticular arthritis of the distal extremities. The diagnosis of acute gouty arthritis is most clearly established by aspirating and examining synovial fluid for the presence of MSU crystals. Urate crystals are characteristically needle-shaped and negatively birefringent when viewed under a polarized light microscope, but crystals may be seen under a standard light microscope as well.[10] As noted previously, MSU crystals are often detectable during asymptomatic intercritical periods, which can assist in making an earlier diagnosis and initiating treatment. During an acute gouty attack, synovial fluid has an elevated white blood cell count (5,000 to 50,000 cells/mm³), with a predominance of polymorphonuclear leukocytes.[3] A culture of the synovial fluid aspirate should also be performed to eliminate the possibility of infection, since infectious arthritis may be present in addition to gouty arthritis. Radiographic findings are generally normal in early stages of the disease and do not help make the diagnosis. With more chronic cases of gout, tophaceous deposits can be depicted on x-rays before they are visible on physical examination, and bony tophaceous lesions may be seen in joints that were previously asymptomatic. The characteristic radiographic finding of chronic gouty arthritis is a well-marginated erosion around the joint with overhanging edges or margins (Fig. 67.4).[9]

The American Rheumatism Association has established criteria that may assist in diagnosing gout, particularly if there is difficulty with aspirating fluid from affected joints (Table 67.1).[43] Rheumatoid arthritis, osteoarthritis, pseudogout (calcium pyrophosphate dehydrate deposition disease), and spondyloarthropathies all present similarly and may be mistaken for gout.[44] Consequently, if a patient's joint symptoms do not resolve over time despite normalization of uric acid levels, another diagnosis should be considered.[30]

Sometimes it is helpful to classify patients with hyperuricemia as either "overproducers" or "underexcretors" of uric acid to identify a possible underlying disorder or to

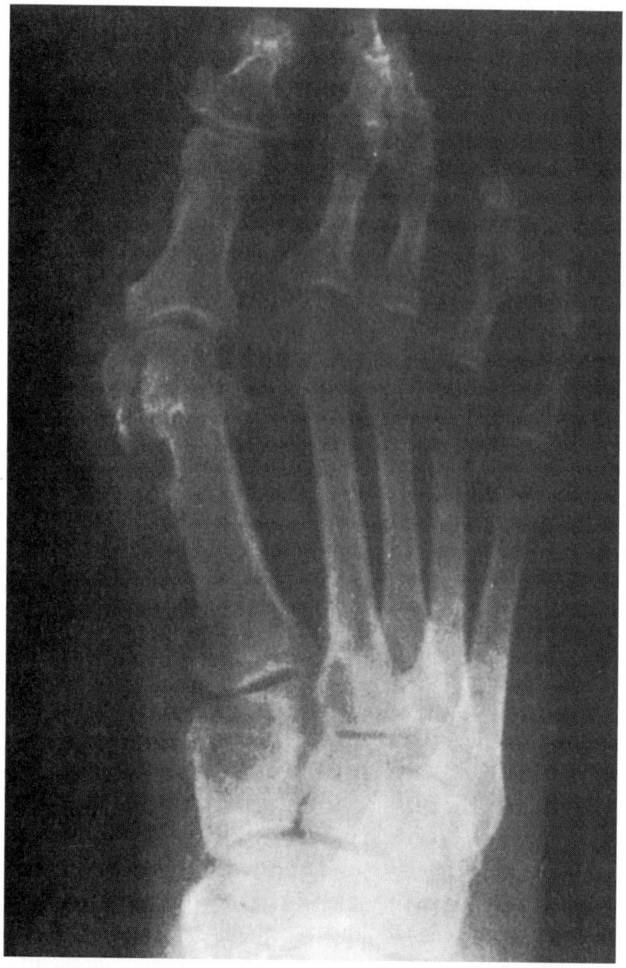

FIGURE 67.4 Radiograph of right foot of patient with gout. (From Barker LR, Burton JR, Zieve PD. Principles of ambulatory medicine, 4th ed. Baltimore: Lippincott Williams & Wilkins, 1995:935, with permission.)

TABLE 67.1	American Rheumatism Association Criteria for Diagnosis of Acute Gout

Definitive

Demonstration of sodium urate crystals in affected joint

Suggestive (six or more should be present)

One acute attack of arthritis

Development of maximum inflammation with 24 hours

Episode of monoarticular arthritis

Redness over joint area

Painful and swollen first metatarsophalangeal joint

Unilateral attack on first metatarsophalangeal joint

Unilateral attack on tarsal joint

Suspicion or presence of a tophus

Hyperuricemia

Asymptomatic swelling in a joint

Negative joint culture

Joint cysts with and/or erosions without osteopenia on x-ray

determine the type of chronic drug therapy to initiate. Overproducers have a urinary urate excretion greater than 600 mg in 24 hours on a purine-restricted diet or greater than 800 to 1,000 mg on a regular Western diet.[45,46] Approximately 75% of patients with primary gout have decreased uric acid excretion, so this is the predominant type of problem that exists in this population.[45] However, knowing whether the patient is an overproducer may alert the clinician to the possibility of a myeloproliferative disorder or another disease associated with increased uric acid production.[46] In addition, overproducers are more likely to develop kidney stones.[46] Unfortunately, maintaining dietary restrictions and obtaining 24-hour urine collections are not easily accomplished, especially in an ambulatory care setting. Consequently, alternative tests have been suggested to facilitate categorizing the patient type. One method is determining the ratio of uric acid to creatinine (Ua/Cr) in a spot urine sample; however, this test has not correlated very well with the 24-hour urine collection.[46] Another simple method that has been evaluated uses a combination of spot urine and blood samples to determine which patients may be candidates for uricosuric therapy.[47] This method incorporates a formula using serum creatinine (SCr × Ua/Cr) in addition to the spot urine Ua/Cr test. The rationale for the combination of tests was to reduce the influence that urinary creatinine excretion has on Ua/Cr and creatinine clearance has on the SCr × Ua/Cr. The study classified cutoffs for both tests (0.34 for the Ua/Cr and 28.1 for the Scr × Ua/Cr) to correlate with low 24-hour uric acid excretion ($<$2.84 mmol/m^2/day). Using a combination of both tests increased the specificity over the Ua/Cr alone without significantly altering sensitivity or diagnostic accuracy. It is suggested that using this combination of simple tests may help identify gout patients who have low uric acid excretion, for whom it would be appropriate to administer uricosuric agents. Because these drugs increase uric acid excretion, they can increase the risk of urolithiasis and should not be administered to individuals who are over-producers of uric acid.[47]

THERAPEUTIC PLAN

There are three primary objectives in treating patients with gout: to relieve acute symptoms, to prevent recurrent attacks, and to reduce serum uric acid concentrations in order to prevent long-term complications such as the development of tophi and urate nephropathy. Agents that are useful for acute attacks include NSAIDs, colchicine, corticosteroids, and corticotropin. Prophylaxis with NSAIDs or colchicine may be used for patients at risk for another attack, such as patients on diuretics or those with renal impairment. It is generally accepted that serum uric acid levels should not be reduced until the acute attack has been effectively treated since doing so could worsen the arthritis, although the over-all risk of this complication remains unclear.[45] In some cases, patients may be able to control their hyperuricemia with diet modification and weight reduction and uric acid-lowering therapy may not be necessary. If the decision is made to initiate uric acid-lowering therapy, the xanthine oxidase in-hibitor allopurinol or the uricosuric drugs probenecid and sulfinpyrazone are typically used. Hypouricemic therapy is used to decrease the body stores of urate in an attempt to prevent or reverse the complications of urate deposition. Be-cause these agents can precipitate an acute attack of gout when therapy is instituted, gradual dose increases and pro-phylactic anti-inflammatory drug therapy with NSAIDs or colchicine is suggested as a means to reduce the risk of this complication.[48]

TREATMENT

ACUTE GOUTY ARTHRITIS

Acute gout is characterized by being spontaneous and self-limiting, and treatment should be directed at rapidly reliev-ing pain and restoring joint mobility.[45] Selection of the most appropriate drug therapy regimen requires an understanding of the potential risks and benefits, especially in certain popu-lations that may be predisposed to side effects, such as the elderly. Adjunctive treatment with ice and resting the af-fected joint should be considered for acute attacks as well.[3] Anti-inflammatory medications should be started as soon as possible after the onset of pain and may need to be supple-mented with opiate analgesics in some cases. Once the attack resolves, patients should undertake appropriate lifestyle modifications such as reduction in alcohol consumption, weight reduction, and limiting dietary purine intake to pre-vent further episodes.[10]

Nonsteroidal Anti-inflammatory Drugs. For younger patients without major health issues, NSAIDs are considered the treatment of choice for acute gouty attacks. NSAIDs are highly effective and generally provide considerable im-provement in symptoms within 24 hours.[45] Most patients have complete resolution of the attack within 5 to 8 days after therapy is started.[49] The therapeutic success associated with NSAID therapy is dependent not so much on what spe-cific agent is selected, but how soon after the attack therapy is started.[10] Table 67.2 lists selected agents for the treatment of gout, but a number of NSAIDs may be used with compara-ble success, although only a few of them are actually FDA approved for this specific use. Indomethacin, a potent anti-inflammatory drug with antipyretic and analgesic properties, is commonly considered the agent of choice, although there is no clear evidence to show that any one NSAID is more effective than another.[3] Maximum doses of NSAIDs should be initiated immediately after the onset of symptoms and continued for 24 hours after the attack has resolved. Doses then should be tapered over 48 to 72 hours.[10]

Conventional NSAIDs work by nonselectively inhibiting both COX-1 and COX-2, isoenzymes that catalyze the con-version of arachidonic acid to proinflammatory mediators, especially prostaglandin E2. Recent clinical trials comparing indomethacin with the investigational COX-2-selective in-hibitor etoricoxib for the treatment of acute gouty arthritis have demonstrated that 120 mg once daily of etoricoxib is comparable to 50 mg of indomethacin three times a day.[50,51] The relative advantage of the COX-2-selective NSAIDs is that they are associated with fewer GI side effects than the nonselective agents, since GI toxicity is believed to be due to COX-1 inhibition. However, there are no clinical trials assessing those commercially available COX-2 inhibitors for treatment of acute gout. In addition, rofecoxib was voluntary recalled from the market by the manufacturer in September 2004 due to an increase in serious cardiovascular effects, including strokes and myocardial infarction, in long-term study patients taking it as compared to placebo. In April 2005, valdecoxib was also voluntarily withdrawn due to sim-ilar concerns of increased risk of cardiovascular events. There were reports of serious and potentially life-threatening skin reactions, including deaths, as well. At this time, cele-coxib is the only COX-2 inhibitor remaining on the U.S. market. Until further review of their safety can be conducted, the FDA is recommending limited use of COX-2 inhibi-tors.[52] Therefore, given their expense relative to generic NSAIDs, lack of clinical data on their use for acute gout, and safety questions that need to be resolved, COX-2 inhibitors should be reserved for short-term use in select patients who cannot tolerate other NSAIDs due to GI side effects.

Although they are effective for relieving pain, NSAIDs are associated with some significant adverse reactions that may limit their use in some patients, including GI, renal, and cardiac side effects. The GI side effects are dose related and can include bleeding and perforation; therefore, NSAIDs should be avoided in patients with active peptic ulcer dis-

TABLE 67.2	Selected Nonsteroidal Anti-inflammatory Agents Used for Acute Gouty Attacks		
Generic Name	**Brand Name(s)**	**Recommended Dosage**	**Comments**
Naproxen	Aleve (OTC) Anaprox Naprosyn Also available generically	750 mg initially followed by 250 mg q8h (naproxen); 825 mg followed by 275 mg q8h (sodium salt)[a]	Avoid in patients with GI disorders, renal impairment, congestive heart failure, or liver disease. Available as anion and sodium salt.
Indomethacin	Indocin Also available generically	100 mg initially, then 50 mg 3 times a day	Avoid in patients with GI disorders, renal impairment, congestive heart failure, or liver disease.
Sulindac	Clinoril Also available generically	200 mg twice daily	Avoid in patients with GI disorders, renal impairment, congestive heart failure, or liver disease. May be less nephrotoxic than other NSAIDs, although no clear evidence to support this claim.
Celecoxib	Celebrex	400 mg day 1, then 100 mg twice a day[b]	Selective COX-2 inhibitor; may have fewer GI side effects. Concern that this class of drug may be associated with an increased risk of cardiovascular side effects. More expensive than nonselective NSAIDs. Not FDA approved for gout. No published studies in gout to date.
Etoricoxib	Arcoxia	120 mg once daily	Selective COX-2 inhibitor; may have fewer GI side effects. Concern that this class of drug may be associated with an increased risk of cardiovascular side effects. Currently not available in the United States but has been studied for treatment of gout.

[a] 275 mg naproxen sodium = 250 mg Naprosyn.
[b] Doses based on recommendations for acute pain.

ease. Patients should be advised to take NSAIDs with food, milk, or an antacid to reduce GI upset. The routine use of NSAIDs can also lead to renal complications, including papillary necrosis, interstitial nephritis, and acute renal impairment, and NSAIDs should be used with caution and monitored closely in patients with preexisting kidney disease.[5] NSAIDs can also cause fluid retention, which is problematic for patients with congestive heart failure. NSAIDs should not be used in patients receiving oral anticoagulants since they can impair platelet function and increase the risk of bleeding.[10] Of particular concern is the use of NSAIDs in the elderly, as they are the drug class most commonly associated with hospitalization due to adverse drug reactions in this population.[53] Limiting NSAID use to 1 to 3 days and administering antacids or other gastroprotective agents is recommended to reduce complications in geriatric patients.[53]

Corticosteroids and Corticotropin. Short courses of systemic corticosteroids are effective for the treatment of gout and serve as suitable alternatives for patients who are not candidates for NSAIDs, particularly the elderly. Corticosteroids may be given via a variety of routes, including orally, intramuscularly, intra-articularly, or intravenously. Oral prednisone may be given in doses of 40 to 60 mg per day for 3 days, and then tapered by 10 to 15 mg every 3 days

until completion. Caution should be exercised in diabetic patients, but systemic steroid side effects are generally rare with this short-term dosing schedule. The tapering in dose may result in a symptom flare, which can be prevented with low dose colchicine (0.6 to 1.2 mg/day).[45] In a clinical study evaluating patients with acute gout, a single dose of intramuscular triamcinolone acetonide (60 mg) was shown to be as effective as indomethacin 50 mg three times a day.[54] A single dose of intravenous methylprednisolone (50 to 150 mg) may be considered an alternative to oral prednisone in certain situations as well.[1]

When only one or two joints are involved, an intra-articular injection of a long-acting corticosteroid is considered a reasonable treatment strategy, assuming infection as a cause of the inflammation has been ruled out. Depending on the size of the joint, a dose of triamcinolone acetonide, triamcinolone hexacetonide, or methylprednisolone may be administered. Typical doses of these agents range from 5 to 20 mg for small joints and 10 to 40 mg for larger joints.[10]

Another treatment option is the administration of corticotrophin (adrenocorticotropic hormone, ACTH), which stimulates the adrenal cortex to secrete cortisol, corticosterone, and other androgens. The exact mechanism of action for treatment of gout is not clear, but it is speculated that ACTH receptors on leukocytes may play a role in a regulatory pathway between the immune and neuroendocrine systems. Since T and B lymphocytes as well as macrophages can be modulated by ACTH, corticotrophin may work in gout by a mechanism different from its cortisol-releasing properties. Although studies evaluating corticotrophin for the treatment of gout are methodologically limited, it may be an option when other regimens are not appropriate.[55] Corticotropin is generally administered intramuscularly at a dose of 40 to 80 IU, and doses may be repeated every 6 to 12 hours if necessary. Corticotropin may also be administered subcutaneously or intravenously.[56]

Colchicine. Colchicine, an alkaloid of *Colchicum autumnale*, was isolated in 1820 and is the oldest available agent for treatment of gout. The drug is unique in that it has anti-inflammatory activity primarily limited to gout and some related disorders. It has no analgesic activity, and it has no effect on serum urate levels or urinary excretion of uric acid.

Colchicine is very effective in alleviating acute gouty attacks, especially when therapy is initiated within 24 hours after the onset of symptoms; it tends to be less effective after the first day of gouty arthritis. Unfortunately, its usefulness is somewhat limited by its dose-dependent side effects. For this reason, patients without contraindications should be treated first with an NSAID because NSAIDs are less toxic than colchicine when used in the short term.[10,30] It is estimated that 80% of patients receiving colchicine will experience GI side effects such as nausea, vomiting, or diarrhea at therapeutic doses.[10] In addition to treating acute attacks, colchicine is also used to prevent gouty attacks when uric acid-lowering therapy is being initiated. Since colchicine's pharmacologic action is rather selective for gout, it has been used as a diagnostic method because of the dramatic response in gout patients after therapy is initiated. Patients with gout will generally experience some relief within 12 hours, and the pain is usually gone within 24 to 48 hours. However, patients with pseudogout and calcific tendinitis may experience relief as well, so clinicians cannot rely on a therapeutic response to colchicine as a definitive diagnostic tool for gout.[3]

When administered orally, colchicine is rapidly absorbed from the GI tract and partially diacetylated in the liver. The parent compound and metabolites are found in high concentrations in the GI tract due to enterohepatic recycling. This may contribute to the acute GI toxicity associated with colchicine therapy. Colchicine is concentrated in leukocytes, and the drug may be detected for several days in circulating leukocytes after a single intravenous dose. Most of the drug and its metabolites are excreted in the feces, with smaller amounts excreted in the urine. The half-life of colchicine is prolonged in patients with severe renal impairment secondary to significant decreases in renal excretion, and therefore the recommended oral and intravenous doses should be reduced by 50% in patients with reduced creatinine clearance (10 to 50 mg/min). Colchicine should be avoided in patients with a creatinine clearance less than 10 mg per minute.[10,57]

Since colchicine has a very narrow therapeutic index, it is extremely important that both clinicians and patients are aware of appropriate dosing. The oral dose that provides relief is generally close to the dose that causes GI side effects. A typical oral dose is 0.5 to 0.6 mg every 1 to 2 hours until the pain is abated, adverse GI effects (nausea, vomiting, or diarrhea) develop, or a maximum dose of 6 to 8 mg has been administered. An interval of 3 days is suggested if a repeat course of therapy is needed. Patients should become familiar with the cumulative dose required to resolve an acute attack without causing diarrhea or GI discomfort as a reference point for subsequent attacks. Because of the GI side effects, patients with preexisting GI disorders such as inflammatory bowel disease, diverticulitis, peptic ulcer disease, or a history of GI bleeding should not be given oral colchicine.[5,48]

Colchicine may be administered intravenously for patients who cannot tolerate the oral route, although this route is associated with serious side effects, including bone marrow suppression, hepatic necrosis, disseminated intravascular coagulation, seizures, and death.[58] Because of the risks associated with intravenous colchicine, only clinicians very familiar with this method of administration are advised to use it. Fatalities associated with intravenous colchicine administration are generally a result of a lack of understanding of how to dose the drug appropriately.[59] Since colchicine causes severe local irritation to the skin and surrounding tissues, it must never be given subcutaneously or intramuscularly. When administered intravenously, colchicine should be mixed with preservative-free 0.9% sodium chloride for injection, because dextrose 5% in water or diluents with bacteriostatic agents may cause precipitation. To avoid extravasation, the dose should be administered slowly into the line of a freely flowing intravenous solution of normal saline, and care should be taken to ensure that the intravenous injection site is patent and not infiltrating. The initial dose of intravenous colchicine is generally 2 mg, followed by doses of 0.5 mg every 6 hours until a maximum of 4 mg per treatment course has been administered. Unlike oral administration, intravenous colchicine is not typically associated with GI symptoms, which are used as an early warning sign of colchicine toxicity and which help set parameters for the clinician on the amount of drug that should be given. If patients are receiving oral colchicine at the time of an acute attack, are elderly, or have renal impairment, it is recommended the intravenous dose be halved. In addition, patients receiving intravenous colchicine should not receive subsequent doses of colchicine by any route for at least 7 days.[10,48,57]

Low-dose colchicine may be used to reduce the frequency of gouty attacks, particularly in patients beginning uric acid-lowering therapy or in whom doses of corticosteroids are being tapered. Patients who experience less than one attack per year may be given 0.5 to 0.6 mg colchicine one to four times each week. If attacks are more frequent, the dosage usually is 0.5 to 0.6 mg each day. Some patients may need as much as three times this dosage each day to control the symptoms. Patients with a history of gout who are undergoing surgical procedures should receive 0.5 to 0.6 mg of colchicine three times daily for 3 days before and 3 days after surgery.[60] Because colchicine only alleviates symptoms and does not prevent the accumulation of MSU deposits and damage to joints, it should not be used as long-term monotherapy for chronic gout.[3]

In addition to GI toxicity, colchicine may cause bone marrow depression with agranulocytosis, thrombocytopenia, leukopenia, and aplastic anemia. These adverse effects are rare and usually occur only in patients who have received excessive dosages or who have decreased renal or hepatic function. Other uncommon side effects that may occur with chronic colchicine administration include alopecia, rashes, peripheral neuropathy, myopathy, vesicular dermatitis, anuria, renal damage, or hematuria. Increased serum concentrations of alkaline phosphatase and aspartate transaminase may also occur with colchicine administration.[61] A small number of cases of rhabdomyolysis have also been reported.[62,63]

HYPERURICEMIA

As noted previously, hyperuricemia is a result of either an overproduction or underexcretion of uric acid. Individuals are considered to have hyperuricemia when their serum uric acid concentration is greater than 7 mg per dL (420 μmol/L), measured by the automated enzymatic method (uricase).[64] Some institutions may normalize laboratory values within ±2 standard deviations of the average uric acid level for the specific population they serve, and therefore the upper limit of normal may be higher in these cases (8 mg/dL, 480 μmol/L).[7] Hyperuricemia itself is not a disease per se, so the decision to treat must be based on careful evaluation of the patient's specific clinical situation. Clinicians should investigate for any underlying causes of hyperuricemia, such as drugs, renal insufficiency, and myeloproliferative and lymphoproliferative disorders, before initiating uric acid-lowering therapy. For most patients who require treatment for hyperuricemia, therapy will need to be continued indefinitely. Consequently, the clinician must carefully consider the risk of drug interactions, adverse reactions, and costs associated with treatment when deciding to initiate therapy. In asymptomatic patients, treatment of hyperuricemia remains controversial. There is some concern that hyperuricemia may be a risk factor for hypertension, coronary artery disease, renal insufficiency, and metabolic syndrome X (insulin resistance, hyperinsulinemia, glucose intolerance, dyslipidemia, hypertension, and abdominal obesity).[64] However, whether it is only an associated finding in these conditions or an independent risk factor has not been clearly established. While some evidence from animal studies suggests that elevated uric acid levels may play a pathogenic

role in renal and cardiovascular disease, further studies in humans are needed to resolve this issue.[65,66] Therefore, based on available clinical evidence, there is currently no accepted indication for urate-lowering agents for patients with asymptomatic hyperuricemia.[67]

Since most patients never develop symptoms of gout, and its role as a risk factor for some diseases has not been definitively established, treatment of hyperuricemia is generally limited to select situations: patients undergoing chemotherapy or radiation therapy, when extensive cell lysis increases purine nucleic acids, which are metabolized into uric acid; patients with a history of gouty attacks or tophi; and patients with serum uric acid levels in excess of 12 mg per dL (720 μmol/L),[68] since high urate concentrations may be associated with joint changes and renal complications. One important consideration is that the patient must be willing to take uric acid-lowering therapy on a chronic schedule, as intermittent therapy has not been shown to be effective.[69]

Once the decision to treat has been made, the drug therapy options are either those agents that lower urate production (xanthine oxidase inhibitors) or those that increase excretion (uricosurics). There are two uricosuric agents, probenecid and sulfinpyrazone, available to increase renal elimination of uric acid. Benzbromarone, a promising potent uricosuric, was withdrawn from some foreign markets in 2003 due to serious liver toxicity, which could affect its future availability in the United States.[70,71] The angiotensin II receptor antagonist losartan and the fibric acid derivative fenofibrate have both been shown to increase the renal clearance of uric acid. These agents may prove useful in patients with gout who also have hypertension or hypertriglyceridemia.[72–74] The NSAID diflunisal also has some uricosuric properties in addition to its analgesic effects at doses of 500 to 1,000 mg per day,[7] but the clinical significance of this effect has not been clearly established. Currently, allopurinol is the only xanthine oxidase inhibitor available in the United States.

Establishing whether a patient is an "overproducer" or "underexcretor" can help determine what treatment option to select for a particular patient. However, most patients are empirically started on allopurinol since it works well in both types of patients and may be conveniently dosed once daily.[45] Uric acid-lowering therapies can potentially precipitate acute gouty attacks, possibly due to sudden changes in concentration of serum urate levels. Therefore, low-dose prophylactic colchicine or NSAIDs should be given until uric acid levels are reduced.[48] To avoid worsening an acute gouty attack, general practice is not to start urate-lowering therapy during the inflammatory phase of the disease, although this issue has not been completely resolved.[45] The goal of uric acid-lowering therapy is to reduce urate levels to below 6 mg per dL (360 μmol/L); a level below 5 mg per dL (300 μmol/L) may be necessary for resorption of tophi.[46,48]

Allopurinol. Allopurinol is currently the most commonly used agent for the long-term control of chronic gout. While it is the drug of choice in overproducers of uric acid, it is effective in patients who are underexcretors as well. Allopurinol works by inhibiting xanthine oxidase, the enzyme that catalyzes the conversion of xanthine to uric acid and hypoxanthine to xanthine; therefore, it decreases the concentrations of both serum and urinary uric acid. The major active metabolite of allopurinol is oxypurinol, also a xanthine oxidase inhibitor, and a drug that is being investigated for use in the treatment of allopurinol-intolerant hyperuricemia. The manufacturer (Cardiome Pharma) reports that oxypurinol may be a successful treatment in 70% of allopurinol-intolerant patients. Recently the FDA has requested that the manufacturer provide additional clinical and manufacturing data prior to approving the marketing of oxypurinol in the United States.[75] However, oxypurinol is available in the United States on a compassionate-use basis for patients who have experienced minor allergic reactions to allopurinol.

Allopurinol is well absorbed from the intestinal tract and has a half-life of only 1 to 2 hours. However, the half-life of oxypurinol is much longer than that of allopurinol: it is approximately 15 to 30 hours in patients with normal renal function. The longer half-life of this active metabolite may explain why most patients can be treated with once-daily doses of allopurinol.[57]

The use of allopurinol is generally recommended for patients with tophaceous gout, patients with increased uric acid production or nephrolithiasis, patients who cannot tolerate or do not respond to uricosuric agents, patients with renal insufficiency, and patients older than 60 years of age. Allopurinol is also used for the prevention of acute urate nephropathy in patients receiving cytotoxic therapy for malignancies, and it reduces the chances of the patient developing secondary uric acid nephropathy from myeloproliferative neoplastic diseases.[53,57]

Serum uric acid levels begin to decline within 1 to 2 days after starting allopurinol therapy and reach a nadir within 7 to 14 days. Along with this reduction in serum urate there is a decrease in urinary uric acid excretion. Allopurinol is generally dosed orally at 100 to 300 mg per day. The average dosage for an adult with normal renal function is 300 mg once per day, which results in a normalization of uric acid levels in approximately 85% of patients.[48] For some patients, 100 to 200 mg per day may be adequate. For moderately severe tophaceous gout, 400 to 600 mg/day in divided doses may be needed. In patients with impaired renal function, allopurinol and oxypurinol may accumulate, and the daily dose should be reduced. It is suggested that the dose of allopurinol be reduced to 200 mg daily if the creatinine clearance is 60 to 90 mL per minute, 100 mg daily if the creatinine clearance is 30 to 59 mL per minute, and 50 to 100 mg daily for patients with a creatinine clearance less than 30 mL per minute.[45] Some suggest doses of 100 mg every 2 to 3 days for a creatinine clearance less than 10 mL per minute.[76] To reduce the risk of precipitating an acute gouty attack,

allopurinol therapy should be started at 50 to 100 mg per day and slowly increased over 3 to 4 weeks until the recommended target dose is reached.[10]

Allopurinol is generally well tolerated, although the frequency of adverse effects increases in the presence of renal insufficiency. A mild pruritic maculopapular rash develops in approximately 2% of patients and will resolve when the drug is discontinued. In some cases the rash will not occur if the drug is restarted at lower doses. The frequency of rash is higher in patients receiving ampicillin or amoxicillin. A rare but more serious hypersensitivity reaction is manifested by exfoliative dermatitis, often associated with vasculitis, fever, eosinophilia, hepatic dysfunction, and renal failure. This reaction is more likely to occur in patients with renal impairment or in patients on diuretic therapy.[48] Approximately half of patients with mild hypersensitivity reactions may be successfully desensitized to the toxic effects of allopurinol. A standard regimen is to administer an initial dose of 10 to 25 μg per day as a diluted oral suspension, and then double the dose every 3 to 14 days until a desired target dose is reached.[45] Oxypurinol is one option for patients with minor hypersensitivity reactions in whom uricosurics are contraindicated, although cross-sensitivity may still occur.[7] For allopurinol-intolerant patients receiving cytotoxic therapy, rasburicase (Elitek) is an option. Rasburicase is a recombinant form of uricase, the enzyme that converts uric acid to allantoin, which is more soluble in the urine than uric acid. The drug is currently FDA approved only for the treatment of hyperuricemia secondary to chemotherapy and tumor lysis in children, although limited studies suggest that it may be effective in adults as well.[77] Rasburicase must be administered intravenously and is extremely expensive, so allopurinol remains the drug of choice in cancer patients if it is not contraindicated.

Since both azathioprine and 6-mercaptopurine are metabolized by xanthine oxidase, concomitant administration with allopurinol will impair their inactivation and increase their potential toxicity, including bone marrow suppression, nausea, and vomiting. Therefore, when they are administered with allopurinol, the dose of both these cytotoxic agents should be reduced to 25% to 33% of their usual dose.[78]

Uricosuric Agents. Uricosuric agents are generally recommended for younger patients with normal renal function who are underexcretors of uric acid. Both probenecid and sulfinpyrazone competitively inhibit the active reabsorption of uric acid at the proximal convoluted tubule. This tubular blocking action promotes the urinary excretion of uric acid, resulting in a decrease in serum urate concentrations. In the presence of renal dysfunction (creatinine clearance <50 mL/min), uricosurics are not effective and are contraindicated because of the increased risk of urolithiasis in these patients. Consequently, because elderly patients often have some degree of renal impairment, allopurinol is generally recommended for older individuals.[53] The primary concern associated with uricosuric therapy is the risk of urolithiasis and impairment of renal function. To reduce this risk, therapy should begin at a low dose that is slowly increased, and the patient should maintain a high volume of urine by drinking at least 2 liters of fluid per day. In addition, alkalinization of the urine to a pH above 6 will increase the solubility of uric acid and may reduce urate deposition in the renal tubules. Alkalinization may be achieved through the use of sodium bicarbonate (1 g three or four times a day) or potassium citrate solutions (30 to 80 mEq/day in divided doses),[7,48] but caution must be exercised to avoid systemic metabolic changes (e.g., sodium or potassium overload) when using this approach. Uricosuric drugs should not be used to treat hyperuricemia caused by cancer chemotherapy, myeloproliferative neoplastic diseases, or radiation because of greatly increased risks of uric acid nephropathy.

Both probenecid and sulfinpyrazone have rapid and complete absorption. Peak levels are achieved within 1 to 5 hours with probenecid and within 1 hour with sulfinpyrazone. The elimination half-life of probenecid is dose-dependent and ranges from 5 to 8 hours, and the half-life of sulfinpyrazone is approximately 3 hours after intravenous injection, although the uricosuric effect can last up to 10 hours after oral administration.[57] While allopurinol may be generally dosed once daily, both uricosuric agents are given in divided daily does.

Dosages of 1 to 2 g of probenecid can cause a fourfold to sixfold increase in uric acid elimination.[79] Therapy should begin with 250 mg twice a day during the first week of therapy and then be increased gradually in increments of 250 to 500 mg per week to reduce the risk of precipitating an acute gouty attack. Approximately 50% of patients will achieve an adequate lowering of urate with a dose of 1 g per day or less in two divided doses, and 85% of patients at a dose of 2 g per day or less.[7]

Probenecid is generally well tolerated, and the adverse effects most commonly reported with therapy are nausea and vomiting, headache, and anorexia. Patients can reduce the GI effects by taking probenecid with food, and it should be used cautiously in patients with a history of peptic ulcer disease. Rarely hypersensitivity reactions with fever, dermatitis, and urticaria and nephritic syndrome have been reported.[57] Since probenecid can increase the number of gouty attacks during the first few months of therapy, it is commercially available in a fixed combination with colchicine (Col-BENEMID). While this product may be a convenient alternative for patients who require prophylactic colchicine, to reduce the risk of colchicine toxicity, patients should be evaluated carefully to see if chronic anti-inflammatory administration is required.

Because probenecid inhibits the renal tubular secretion of many weak organic acids, it is associated with some significant drug interactions. Probenecid inhibits the secretion of many antimicrobials, including the penicillins, cephalosporins, nalidixic acid, rifampicin, and nitrofurantoin. This leads to higher levels of antibiotics for prolonged periods. This drug interaction has been used therapeutically to increase the duration and plasma concentrations of the penicillins and cephalosporins. Probenecid can also increase the

serum concentrations of fluoroquinolones that are primarily eliminated renally, including ciprofloxacin, levofloxacin, and gatifloxacin. While the interaction in not considered clinically significant, patients should be monitored for side effects if they are receiving any of these agents with probenecid.[80] Probenecid impairs the tubular secretion of cidofovir, but it is recommended for use in combination with cidofovir to offset cidofovir-induced nephrotoxicity.[81] The overall effects of the combination of probenecid and allopurinol are additive, even though probenecid enhances oxypurinol metabolism. However, the clinical advantage to the combination for refractory disease has not been clearly established.[45] Probenecid and sulfinpyrazone therapy should not be used in patients receiving even low doses of aspirin because aspirin blocks uric acid excretion, reducing the therapeutic effect of these uricosuric agents. A crossover study in a small group of patients with gouty arthritis concluded that low-dose (325 mg/day) enteric-coated aspirin did not significantly interfere with the uricosuric effects of probenecid.[82] However, it would still be advisable to avoid this combination if possible.

Sulfinpyrazone is an analogue of the NSAID phenylbutazone, but it does not possess any anti-inflammatory or analgesic effects. It is a more potent uricosuric than probenecid and also has antiplatelet properties. Therapy should be initiated at 50 mg twice a day for about the first week. The dosage is then increased by 100-mg increments each week until an effective maintenance dosage of 200 to 400 mg per day is achieved.[45] Like probenecid, sulfinpyrazone may increase the frequency of acute attacks during the first year of therapy, which can warrant the use of prophylactic colchicine or an NSAID.[5]

When used in recommended dosages, sulfinpyrazone usually is well tolerated, with a low rate of adverse effects. The most common adverse effects are those affecting the GI tract (nausea or peptic ulcer reactivation), reported in as many as 15% of patients. Bronchoconstriction may occur in patients who are aspirin-sensitive. In addition to these adverse effects, sulfinpyrazone has been noted to cause an immunoallergic acute interstitial nephritis. These changes are for the most part reversible. Periodic blood counts should be obtained during sulfinpyrazone therapy because of the rare occurrence of anemia, leukopenia, thrombocytopenia, and agranulocytosis. Because it inhibits platelets, there is an increased risk of bleeding, especially in patients receiving warfarin therapy.

Although sulfinpyrazone inhibits the renal tubular secretion of many weak organic acids, the elevation in plasma concentrations of penicillins and cephalosporins is not clinically useful.

KEY POINTS

■ Gout is characterized by hyperuricemia secondary to either an overproduction or an underexcretion of uric acid. It is an acute inflammatory joint disease in which uric acid crystals are deposited in the affected joints.

- Disease progression is variable and patient dependent. The risk of progression to a debilitating chronic disease is lower today because effective treatments have been developed.

- Acute gouty attacks may be treated with an NSAID, colchicine, corticosteroid, or corticotrophin.

- Treatment with hypouricemic agents for long-term control should be based on careful patient assessment, weighing the relative risks and benefits of drug therapy. If considered appropriate, therapy is life-long.

- It may not be necessary to initiate drug therapy for occasional gouty attacks or in patients with asymptomatic hyperuricemia. In these cases, alterations in diet and lifestyle may be enough to keep a patient symptom-free.

ACKNOWLEDGMENTS

The authors acknowledge the contributions of Pierre A. Maloley, PharmD, and Gina R. Westfall, PharmD, who wrote the corresponding chapter in the seventh edition. Portions of that chapter have been used in this edition.

SUGGESTED READINGS

Kim KY, Schumacher HR, Hunsche E, et al. A literature review of the epidemiology and treatment of acute gout. Clin Ther 25:1593–1617, 2003.

Monu JUV, Pope TL. Gout: a clinical and radiologic review. Radiol Clin North Am 42:169–184, 2004.

Rott KT, Agudelo CA. Gout. JAMA 289:2857–2860, 2003.

Terkeltaub RA. Gout. N Engl J Med 349:1647–1655, 2003.

Wade WE, Cooper JW. Managing hyperuricemia and gout in the geriatric patient. J Geriatric Drug Therapy 12:73–86, 1999.

Wortmann RL. Gout and hyperuricemia. Curr Opin Rheumatol 14: 281–286, 2002.

REFERENCES

1. Becker MA. Clinical gout and the pathogenesis of hyperuricemia. In: Koopman WJ, ed. Arthritis and allied conditions: a textbook of rheumatology, 14th ed, vol. 2. Philadelphia: Lippincott Williams & Wilkins, 2001:2281–2313.
2. Boss GR, Seegmiller JE. Hyperuricemia and gout: classification, complications and management. N Engl J Med 300:1459–1468, 1979.
3. Rott KT, Agudelo CA. Gout. JAMA 289:2857–2860, 2003.
4. Fam AG. Gout, diet, and the insulin resistance syndrome. J Rheumatol 29:1350–1355, 2002.
5. Kim KY, Schumacher HR, Hunsche E, et al. A literature review of the epidemiology and treatment of acute gout. Clin Ther 25: 1593–1617, 2003.
6. Lo B. Hyperuricemia and gout. West J Med 142:104–107, 1985.
7. Edwards NL. Management of hyperuricemia. In: Koopman WJ, ed. Arthritis and allied conditions: a textbook of rheumatology, 14th ed, vol 2. Philadelphia: Lippincott Williams & Wilkins, 2001: 2314–2328.
8. Schwinghammer TL. Rheumatic diseases. In: Lee M, ed. Basic skills in interpreting laboratory data, 3rd ed. Bethesda, MD: American Society of Health-System Pharmacists, 2004:563–592.
9. Monu JUV, Pope TL. Gout: a clinical and radiologic review. Radiol Clin North Am 42:169–184, 2004.
10. Harris MD, Siegel LB, Alloway JA. Gout and hyperuricemia. Am Fam Phys 59:925–934, 1999.
11. Choi HK, Atkinson K, Karlson EW, et al. Purine-rich foods, dairy and protein intake, and the risk of gout in men. N Engl J Med 350: 1093–1103, 2004.
12. Johnson RJ, Rideout BA. Uric acid and diet: insights into the epidemic of cardiovascular disease. N Engl J Med 350:1071–1073, 2004.
13. Choi HK, Atkinson K, Karlson EW, et al. Alcohol intake and risk of incident gout in men: a prospective study. Lancet 363: 1277–1281, 2004.
14. Terkeltaub R. Crystal deposition diseases. In: Goldman L, Ausiello D, eds. Cecil textbook of medicine, 22nd ed, vol. 2. Philadelphia: Saunders, 2004:1702–1710.
15. Bjornson DC, Overdiek HWPM, Editorial Staff. Spironolactone (drug monograph). In: Klasco RK, ed. DRUGDEX system. Greenwood Village, CO: Thomson MICROMEDEX (edition expires 9/2004).
16. Zillich AJ, Carter BL. Eplerenone: a novel selective aldosterone blocker. Ann Pharmacother 36:1567–1576, 2002.
17. Lin HY, Rocher LL, McQuillan MA, et al. Cyclosporine-induced hyperuricemia and gout. N Engl J Med 321:287–292, 1989.
18. Neal DA, Tom BDM, Gimson AES, et al. Hyperuricemia, gout, and renal function after liver transplantation. Transplantation 72: 1689–1691, 2001.
19. Burack DA, Griffith BP, Thompson ME. Hyperuricemia and gout among heart transplant recipients receiving cyclosporine. Am J Med 92:141–146, 1992.
20. Myers BD, Ross J, Newton L, et al. Cyclosporine-associated chronic nephropathy. N Engl J Med 311:699–705, 1984.
21. Lawrence RC, Helmick CG, Arnett FC, et al. Estimates of the prevalence of arthritis and selected musculoskeletal disorders in the United States. Arthritis Rheum 41:778–799, 1998.
22. Hall AP, Barry PE, Dawber TR, et al. Epidemiology of gout and hyperuricemia: a long-term population study. N Engl J Med 42: 27–37, 1967.
23. Terkeltaub RA. Pathogenesis and treatment of crystal-induced inflammation. In: Koopman WJ, ed. Arthritis and allied conditions: a textbook of rheumatology, 14th ed, vol. 2. Philadelphia: Lippincott Williams & Wilkins, 2001:2329–2347.
24. Simkin PA. The pathogenesis of podagra. Ann Intern Med 86: 230–233, 1977.
25. Ward MM. Crystal-induced synovitis. In: Kelley's textbook of internal medicine, 4th ed. Philadelphia: Lippincott Williams & Wilkins, 2000:1370–1375.
26. Kozin F, McCarty DJ. Protein adsorption to monosodium urate, pyrophosphate dehydrate and silica crystals. Arthritis Rheum 19 (Suppl):433–438, 1976.
27. Phelps P, Andrews R, Rosenbloom J. Demonstration of chemotactic factor in human gout: further characterization of occurrence and structure. J Rheumatol 8:889–894, 1981.
28. ter Borg EJ, Rasker J. Gout in the elderly; a separate entity? Ann Rheum Dis 46:72–76, 1987.
29. Hadler NM, Franck WA, Bress NM, et al. Acute polyarticular gout. Am J Med 56:715–719, 1974.
30. German DC, Holmes EW. Hyperuricemia and gout. Med Clin North Am 70:419–436, 1986.
31. Pascual E, Batlle-Gualda E, Martinez A, et al. Synovial fluid analysis for the diagnosis of intercritical gout. Ann Intern Med 131: 756–759, 1999.
32. Ginsberg MH, Genant HK, Yu T-F, et al. Rheumatoid nodulosis: an unusual variant of rheumatoid disease. Arthritis Rheum 18:49–58, 1975.
33. Schapira D, Stahl S, Izhak OB, et al. Chronic tophaceous gouty arthritis mimicking rheumatoid arthritis. Sem Arthritis Rheum 29: 56–63, 1999.
34. Gutman AB. The past four decades of progress in the knowledge of gout with an assessment of the present status. Arthritis Rheum 16: 431–445, 1973.
35. Davis JC. A practical approach to gout. Postgrad Med 106:115–123, 1999.
36. Clive DM. Renal transplant-associated hyperuricemia and gout. J Am Soc Nephrol 11:974–979, 2000.
37. Kramer HJ, Choi HK, Atkinson K, et al. The association between gout and nephrolithiasis in men: the Health Professionals' Follow-Up Study. Kidney Int 64:1022–1026, 2003.

38. Liang MH, Fries JF. Asymptomatic hyperuricemia: the case for conservative management. Ann Intern Med 88:666–670, 1978.

39. Yu TF, Berger L. Renal function in gout. IV: An analysis of 524 gouty subjects including long-term follow-up studies. Am J Med 1982;72:95–100, 1975.

40. Palella TD, Kelley WN. An approach to hyperuricemia and gout. Geriatrics 39:89–102, 1984.

41. Davidson MB, Thakkar S, Hix JK, et al. Pathophysiology, clinical consequences, and treatment of tumor lysis syndrome. Am J Med 116:546–554, 2004.

42. Logan JA, Morrison E, McGill P. Serum uric acid levels in acute gout. Ann Rheum Dis 56:696–697, 1997.

43. Wallace SL, Robinson H, Masi AT, et al. Preliminary criteria for the classification of the acute arthritis of primary gout. Arthritis Rheum 20:895–900, 1977.

44. Bomalaski JS, Schumacher HR. Podagra is more than gout. Bull Rheum Dis 34:1–8, 1984.

45. Terkeltaub RA. Gout. N Engl J Med 349:1647–1655, 2003.

46. Wortmann RL. Gout and hyperuricemia. Curr Opin Rheumatol 14:281–286, 2002.

47. Yamamoto T, Moriwaki Y, Takahashi S, et al. A simple method of selecting gout patients for treatment with uricosuric agents, using spot urine and blood samples. J Rheumatol 29:1937–1941, 2002.

48. Emmerson BT. The management of gout. N Engl J Med 334:445–451, 1996.

49. Agudelo CA. Gout and hyperuricemia. Curr Opin Rheumatol 1:286–293, 1989.

50. Rubin BR, Burton R, Navarra S, et al. Efficacy and safety profile of treatment with etoricoxib 120 mg once daily with indomethacin 50 mg three times daily in acute gout: a randomized controlled trial. Arthritis Rheum 50:598–606, 2004.

51. Schumacher HR Jr., Boice JA, Daikh DI, et al. Randomized double-blind trial of etoricoxib and indomethacin in treatment of acute gouty arthritis. Br Med J 324:1488–1492, 2002.

52. FDA Talk Paper. FDA issues public health advisory recommending limited use of COX-2 inhibitors. Available at: http://www.fda.gov/bbs/topics/ANSWERS/2004/ANS01336.html Accessed January 2005.

53. Wade WE, Cooper JW. Managing hyperuricemia and gout in the geriatric patient. J Geriatric Drug Therapy 12:73–86, 1999.

54. Alloway JA, Moriarty MJ, Hoogland YT, et al. Comparison of triamcinolone acetonide with indomethacin in the treatment of acute gouty arthritis. J Rheumatol 20:111–113, 1993.

55. Taylor CT, Brooks NC, Kelley KW. Corticotropin for acute management of gout. Ann Pharmacother 35:365–368, 2001.

56. Schlesinger N, Backer DG, Schumacher HR Jr. How well have diagnostic tests and therapies for gout been evaluated? Curr Opin Rheumatol 11:441–445, 1999.

57. Roberts LJ, Morrow JD. Analgesic-antipyretic and anti-inflammatory agents and drugs employed in the treatment of gout. In: Hardeman JG, Limbird LE, Goodman Gilman A, eds. Goodman and Gilman's the pharmacological basis of therapeutics, 10th ed. New York: McGraw-Hill, 2001:687–731.

58. Schlesinger N, Schumacher HR. Gout: can management be improved? Curr Opin Rheumatol 13:240–244, 2001.

59. Bonnel RA, Villalba ML, Karwoski CB. Deaths associated with inappropriate intravenous colchicine administration. J Emerg Med 22:385–387, 2002.

60. Simkin PA. Management of gout. Ann Intern Med 90:812–816, 1979.

61. Naidus RM, Rodvien R, Milke CH. Colchicine toxicity: a multisystem disease. Arch Intern Med 137:394–396, 1977.

62. Boomershine KH. Colchicine-induced rhabdomyolysis. Ann Pharmacother 36:824–826, 2002.

63. Phanish MK, Krishnamurthy S, Bloodworth LLO. Colchicine-induced rhabdomyolysis. Am J Med 114:166–167, 2003.

64. Mandell BF. Hyperuricemia and gout: a reign of complacency. Cleve Clin J Med 69:589–593, 2002.

65. Johnson RJ, Kang DH, Feig D, et al. Is there a pathogenetic role for uric acid in hypertension and cardiovascular and renal disease? Hypertension 41:1183–1190, 2003.

66. Johnson RJ, Kivlighn SD, Kim YG, et al. Reappraisal of the pathogenesis and consequences of hyperuricemia in hypertension, cardiovascular and renal disease. Am J Kidney Dis 33:225–234, 1999.

67. Mikuls TR, MacLean CH, Olivieri J, et al. Quality care indicators for gout management. Arthritis Rheum 50:937–943, 2004.

68. Dincer HE, Dincer AP, Levinson DJ. Asymptomatic hyperuricemia: to treat or not to treat. Cleve Clin J Med 69:594–608, 2002.

69. Bull PW, Scott JT. Intermittent control of hyperuricemia in the treatment of gout. J Rheumatol 16:1246–1448, 1989.

70. Myers OL, Cassim B, Mody GM. Hyperuricemia and gout: clinical guideline 2003. South African Med J 93:961–971, 2003.

71. Studds TW, Editorial Staff. Benzbromarone (drug monograph). In: Klasco RK, ed. DRUGDEX system. Greenwood Village, CO: Thomson MICROMEDEX (edition expires 9/2004).

72. Hepburn AL, Kaye SA, Feher MD. Long-term remission from gout associated with fenofibrate therapy. Clin Rheumatol 22:73–76, 2003.

73. Hepburn AL, Feher MD. Gout. N Engl J Med 350:519–520, 2004.

74. Takahashi S, Moriwaki Y, Yamamoto T, et al. Effects of combination treatment using anti-hyperuricaemic agents with fenofibrate and/or losartan on uric acid metabolism. Ann Rheum Dis 62:572–575, 2003.

75. Drugs.com. Oxypurinol regulatory filing accepted for review. Available at http://www.drugs.com/nda_oxypurinol_040309.html. Accessed July 2004.

76. Hande KR, Noone RM, Stone WJ. Severe allopurinol toxicity: description and guidelines for prevention in patients with renal insufficiency. Am J Med 76:47–56, 1984.

77. Pui C-H, Jeha S, Irwin D, et al. Recombinant urate oxidase (rasburicase) in the prevention and treatment of malignancy-associated hyperuricemia in pediatric and adult patients: results of a compassionate-use trial. Leukemia 15:1505–1509, 2001.

78. Klasco RK, ed. DRUG-REAX® system. Greenwood Village, CO: Thomson MICROMEDEX (edition expires 9/2004).

79. Bergman HD. Drug therapy in gout. US Pharm 2:58–64, 1977.

80. Fish DN. Fluoroquinolone adverse effects and drug interactions. Pharmacotherapy 21:253S–272S, 2001.

81. Cundy KC. Clinical pharmacokinetics of the antiviral nucleotide analogues cidovir and adefovir. Clin Pharmacokinetics 36:127–143, 1999.

82. Harris M, Bryant LR, Danaher, et al. Effect of low-dose aspirin on serum urate levels and urinary excretion in patients receiving probenecid for gouty arthritis. J Rheumatol 27:2873–2876, 2000.

Systemic Lupus Erythematosus

Susan Krikorian

68

DEFINITION

Systemic lupus erythematosus (SLE) is a chronic, nonspecific autoimmune inflammatory disease that typically affects multiple organs and systems, including the skin, joints, muscles, lungs, heart, kidneys, and the central nervous and circulatory systems.[1] Individuals with SLE are noted with production of antibodies and inflammatory responses that are mistakenly directed at their own tissues.[2,3] This abnormal reaction can occur in any organ system. The natural history of SLE is highly variable. SLE is characterized by periods of disease activity or flares followed by disease quiescence or remissions, particularly in the early stages of the disease.

The diagnosis of SLE can be difficult particularly in the early stages of the disease because signs and symptoms are often nonspecific.[2] Other autoimmune inflammatory diseases such as rheumatoid arthritis, Sjögren syndrome, scleroderma, Raynauds phenomenon, and systemic vasculitis often present with similar signs and symptoms and should be distinguished from SLE by careful clinical examination and laboratory testing. Overlap syndrome is coined when two different rheumatic autoimmune diseases such as SLE and rheumatoid arthritis coexist in the same individual.

The diagnosis is further complicated by the high degree of variability of the disease and one in which it is difficult to predict long-term progression and outcomes. For most people, SLE is a mild, chronic disease affecting mainly the mucocutaneous tissues, joints, and muscles characterized by rashes, arthritis, myalgias, and fatigue. For others, SLE may be rapidly progressive affecting internal organs and systems leading to early mortality from kidney failure secondary to glomerulonephritis, thromboembolic events from the antiphospholipid syndrome (APS), or severe infections from cytopenias. In patients with long-standing SLE, coronary artery disease has become the leading cause of death.

Five-year survival rates have dramatically improved since the 1950s from less than 50% to more than 95%, however, mortality rates in patients with SLE are still three to five times higher than the general population.[4]

Although the clinical manifestations of SLE are heterogeneous, SLE can be distinguished from a number of related cutaneous lupus syndromes (drug-induced lupus erythematosus, discoid lupus, subacute cutaneous lupus).[2,3] Systemic lupus is the most serious form as it can affect any organ in the body.

ETIOLOGY

The origin of SLE is unknown. It can occur at all ages, but is more common in young women. There is a strong genetic component associated with susceptibility and severity possibly triggered by immunologic, hormonal, and environmental factors.[5]

The disease tends to occur within families but without a clear pattern of inheritance. Familial aggregation has been reported as 2% to 5% among siblings of patients with SLE, 7% to 12% of first-degree and second-degree relatives with lupus, whereas concordance among monozygotic twins (identical twins) is 25% to 50%.[6] Dizygotic twins and other full siblings have only a 2% to 5% rate of concordance. This suggests an important role for genetic predisposition and susceptibility to SLE.

Familial (genetic) factors have been identified in SLE. Common genetic markers seen in SLE patients are the genes for human leukocyte antigen (HLA)-B8, DR-2, and DR3. Less common are the genes for HLA-DQw1 and DMA*0401. There may be other markers for this disease including complement deficiencies, and allelic variants or polymorphisms of the Fc portion of immunoglobulin G (IgG) (Fc receptors) genes.[7]

Overall, it is estimated that in less than 5% of patients with SLE a single susceptibility gene may be responsible, whereas for the remaining patients multiple genes are required.[6] Results from genome scans have identified eight chromosomal regions to date associated with linkage to SLE.

The genetic predisposition in SLE is supported by the high incidence of SLE in patients with certain complex deficiencies ($C1_q$, C2, and C4) and associations of disease and autoantibody production with certain HLA class II alleles (i.e., HLA-DR2 and HLA-DR3).[8,9] The most common genetic marker associated with SLE in many ethnic groups is a defective or deleted HLA class III allele (C3AQO). Polymorphisms in low-affinity IgG(Fc_γ) receptors, which are important for the clearance of immune complexes, are also implicated in the pathogenesis of SLE. Deficiency in mannose binding lecithin has also been implicated (Table 68.1).[10]

Most cases of SLE flares are sporadic without identifiable predisposing factors, with the exception of ultraviolet (UV)-B light. This finding suggests that multiple environmental or yet unknown factors may trigger the disease.[6] Chemicals such as hydrazine-containing hair dyes, foods containing L-canavanine such as alfalfa sprouts, and microorganisms have also been implicated to cause SLE in genetically susceptible individuals.[5,8]

Hormone levels can influence disease activity and expression via their immunomodulatory effects. A high-estrogen, low-androgen state has been implicated in the pathogenesis of SLE. In SLE patients, elevated plasma 16 α hydroxyestrone, low plasma testosterone, and raised plasma luteinizing hormone (LH) values, low progesterone, and low dihydroepiandrosterone (DHEA) have been observed.[5] Increasing endogenous estrogen concentration has also been shown to influence disease activity and prognosis in SLE.

Flares of SLE usually coincide with periods of rapid hormonal changes including pregnancy, peurperium, and ovulation stimulation during in vitro fertilization. The administration of large doses of exogenous estrogens in the form of high-dose estrogen containing oral contraceptives (OC) and hormone replacement therapy (HRT) may exacerbate the disease in patients with existing lupus. Low-dose estrogen containing OC are associated with less risk. It has also been noted that, in many women, disease flares are more common during the second half of the menstrual cycle, after the bicycle surge of estrogens. Improvement in lupus activity has been reported when patients had undergone oophorectomy or menopause.

Epidemiological studies also reveal a proportional increased risk of SLE associated with exogenous estrogens. It was shown that the past use of OC pills and HRT was associ-

---

TABLE 68.1	Examples of Genes That Increase Susceptibility to Systemic Lupus Erythematosus (SLE) in Humans

In the MHC region on chromosome 6:

C2, C4: Individuals with deficiencies in these complement components have increased risk for SLE (they are less rare than C1q deficiencies, but many individuals with deficiencies of C2 and C4 do not develop SLE)

DR2, DR3: Each predisposes to SLE, usually in different clinical subsets (e.g., nephritis more likely with DR2, dermatitis and Sjögren's more likely with DR3); vary in different ethnic groups

TNF-α polymorphisms: In some ethnic groups; may not be independent risk factor from extended haplotype containing allele that encodes synthesis of low quantities of TNF-α

In non-MHC regions:

C1q: The majority of individuals with homozygous deficiency of C1q (which is rare) have SLE (C1q is cleaved when activated by immune complexes; it also binds to apoptotic blebs and probably participates in clearing of apoptotic cells; its absence may also predispose to infection)

Region on chromosome 1; 1q41–42 (PARP is possible; agreement on the susceptibility gene in this region has not been reached)

Fc-γ RIIA and RIIIA (determines binding, phagocytosis, and ultimate disposal of immune complexes containing IgG2 for RIIA and IgG1 and IgG3 for RIIIA; particularly predisposing to lupus nephritis in African-American, European whites, and some South Korean populations)

IL-10 and Bcl polymorphisms inherited together (particularly in Hispanic Americans)

Polymorphisms in a region near IL-6

Several regions on chromosomes other than chromosome 1 found in genome scanning from multiple centers (genes not yet defined)

Polymorphism of mannose-binding protein

MHC, major histocompatibility complex; TNF, tumor necrosis factor; PARP, poly (ADP-ribose); Ig, Immunoglobulin; IL interleukin.
(From Wallace DJ, Hahn BH, eds. Dubois' lupus erythematosus, 6th ed. Philadelphia: Lippincott Williams & Wilkins, 2002; 89. With permission.)

ated with a slightly increased risk of SLE in a large cohort of nurses as part of the Nurses' Health Study.[11,12] An increased risk of SLE or discoid lupus in postmenopausal women receiving HRT for more than 2 years when compared to nonusers was also reported in another case-control study.[13] Late onset SLE, defined as first onset of disease after the age of 50 years, usually has a benign disease course with less serious organ involvement.

Patients with Klinefelter syndrome, a condition characterized by hypergonadotrophic hypogonadism, are prone to SLE and further suggest a role for endogenous sex hormones in disease predisposition.[5]

Hyperprolactinemia has been reported in some patients with SLE of both sexes. Serum prolactin concentrations have been shown to correlate with disease activity in some studies. The exact role of prolactin in SLE requires further investigation because a positive correlation between lupus activity and prolactin values cannot be demonstrated consistently.

Finally, there is preliminary evidence that a defective hypothalamic-pituitary-adrenal (HPA) is present in lupus. A study on a group of active, untreated female patients with SLE reports that the cortisol response to hypoglycemia is significantly lower than in healthy controls. A defective HPA may confer susceptibility to autoimmune disorders.

EPIDEMIOLOGY

SLE is predominantly a disease of younger women. Rarely, the first onset of SLE develops before puberty and after menopause.[1,2,5] The disease affects mostly females in their childbearing years between the ages of 15 and 55 years, approximately nine times more often than men in this age group. This group comprises 65% of all SLE cases. Female predilection is less pronounced outside the reproductive age range. In less commonly affected age groups, the female to male ratio is approximately 2:1 in children and in adults over

the age of 50 years. Drug-induced lupus (DIL) erythematosus, where the female to male ratio is equal, is the most common form of lupus affecting older individuals from drug exposure, and it is a self-limiting brief illness if the causative agent is identified and discontinued.

The worldwide prevalence rate of SLE is 1.2 per 1,000. In the United States, incidence rates range from 2 to 5 per 100,000 population per year. Estimates of SLE cases in the United States range from 270,000 to over 1 million. Prevalence, incidence, and severity of SLE vary across ethnicities and geographic areas. African-American women are three times as likely to be affected as European-Americans. SLE is also more common in women of Asian and Hispanic descent.[14]

The Centers for Disease Control and Prevention has reported that the lupus-associated death rate has risen from 879 in 1979 to 1,406 in 1998.[15] Lupus deaths in African-American women, who were 45–64 years of age, sharply rose 70% compared with a small increase in white women during the same time period.[16]

PATHOPHYSIOLOGY

The pathogenesis of SLE is unknown. The immune system plays a crucial role in the pathogenesis of active inflammatory and noninflammatory mechanisms of organ damage in SLE.[5,8,9] Multiple factors may play a role in this process such as defects in cell activation, tolerance, apoptosis, impaired immune complex clearance, idiopathic networks, and disruption of regulatory cell pathways (Fig. 68.1).

Pathogenic subsets of autoantibodies, directed at various self-antigens, and pathogenic immune complexes are responsible for inflammation of the skin and internal organs. Several immune system abnormalities involving excessive polyclonal B-cell activation by T cells have resulted in an increased number of antibody producing cells, autoantibody production, and immune complex formation.[17,18]

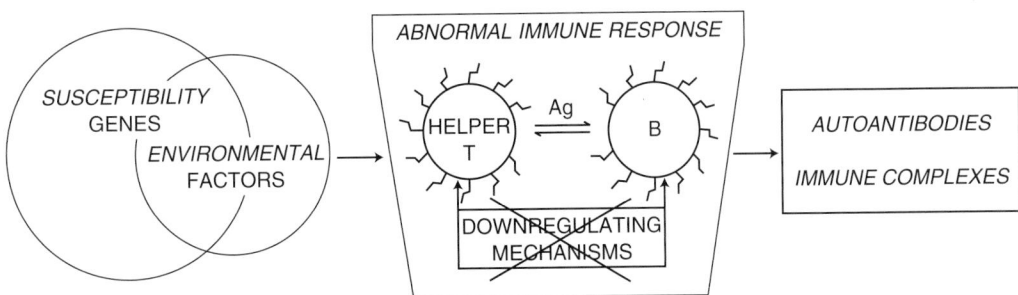

FIGURE 68.1 An overview of the pathogenesis of systemic lupus erythematosus (SLE). Interactions between susceptibility genes and environmental factors lead to abnormal immune responses. Those responses consist of hyperactive T-cell help for hyperactive B cells with polyclonal activation and specific antigenetic stimulation of both types of cell. Down-regulating mechanisms that shut off such hyperactive responses in normal individuals are impaired in patients with SLE. The result of the abnormal immune response is production of autoantibodies (autoAbs), some of which form immune complexes (ICs). Pathogenic subsets of the autoAb and the IC deposit in or on tissues and initiate the damage that is characteristic of SLE. (From Wallace DJ, Hahn BH, eds. Dubois' lupus erythematosus. 6th ed. Philadelphia: Lippincott Williams & Wilkins, 2002:88, with permission.)

B-cell hyperactivity and the production of pathogenic autoantibodies is thought to be caused by the loss of immune tolerance, increased antigenic load, excess T-cell help, defective B-cell suppression, and the shifting of T helper 1 (Th1) to Th2 immune responses.

Overproduction of interleukin (IL)-10 seems to play a role in SLE, involving an imbalance of IL-10 and IL-12. Other cytokines such as tumor necrosis factor α (TNF-α), interferon γ (INF-γ), transforming growth factor β (TGF-β), IL-1, IL-2, IL-4, IL-6, IL-16, IL-17, and IL-18 may be also be implicated. They exert their proinflammatory and antiinflammatory effects on the immune cells helper or CD4+ lymphocytes.

T-cell help is responsible in the development of full-blown disease, particularly by CD4+CD8−, CD4−CD8+, and CD4−CD8− phenotypes.[5] The synthesis and secretion of pathogenic autoantibodies in SLE is driven by the interaction of CD4+ and CD8+ helper T cells, and double negative T cells (CD4−CD8−) with B cells. This action may result from the inhibition of Th1 response and the enhancement of CD40L expression on lupus T cells may indirectly promote the Th2 response and lead to further B-cell hyperactivity.

It is believed that defective immune regulatory mechanisms such as the clearance of immune complexes by phagocytic cells also contribute to the development of SLE.[6] A recent study demonstrated that noninflammatory engulfment phagocytosis of apoptotic cells is impaired in patients with SLE. Persistently circulating apoptotic waste may serve as an immunogen for the induction of autoreactive lymphocytes and as an antigen for immune complex formation.

Antinuclear antibodies (ANAs) may be detected specific for SLE. When these antibodies form immune complexes with their specific antigen and fixed complement they could precipitate in the glomeruli, skin, lung, synovium, and mesothelium. Inflammation, vasculitis, immune complex deposition, and vasculopathy are the primary pathological findings in SLE.

The best characterized organ pathology is the kidney. Lupus nephritis is common with SLE because immune complexes are often deposited in the basement membrane of the glomeruli. Renal biopsies in patients with SLE reveal mesangial cell proliferation, inflammation, basement membrane abnormalities, and immune complex deposition (comprised of immunoglobulins and complement components) with light immunofluorescence microscopy.

Other organs systems affected by SLE usually are visualized with nonspecific inflammation or vascular abnormalities and are unremarkable. Arteriosclerosis is a complication of longstanding SLE associated with hypertension (BP>140/90), corticosteroids, and other drugs.

CLINICAL PRESENTATION AND DIAGNOSIS

SIGNS AND SYMPTOMS

Clinical features are diverse. The clinical presentation of SLE is variable, and the signs and symptoms may be very subtle especially early in the course of the disease leading to a delay in diagnosis because symptoms are not always initially associated with the disease. Symptomatic flares associated with disease activity followed by periods of remission are typical during the clinical course of the disease.[19]

Constitutional. Symptoms may not always appear concurrently. In the early stages, fatigue and general malaise, fever in the absence of infection, and weight loss are the usual chief complaints. Fatigue is often the earliest manifestation of SLE, clearly the most common and debilitating symptom in patients with SLE.[2,5]

Muscloskeletal. Arthritis, arthralgia, and myalgia are described in all patients with SLE. Intermittent symmetric arthritis and arthralgias can be confused with rheumatoid arthritis early in the course of the disease. Patients typically present with polyarticular joint involvement and complain of mild to moderate pain. It is nonerosive and nondeforming, usually affecting the joints of the hands, wrist, knees, and feet. Other symptomatology may include diffuse puffiness or tenderness, and a feeling of warmth in the affected joints. Tenosynovitis and bursitis may also be present. Myopathy may also occur during periods of active disease or secondary to treatment (e.g., corticosteroids, hydroxychloroquine). In approximately 10% to 30% of patients, muscle pain due to fibromyalgia has been reported.[1]

Cutaneous. Three main types of rash are associated with SLE. They can be distinguished by their mucocutaneous manifestations on sunlight exposed areas, such as acute cutaneous lupus, discoid lupus, subacute cutaneous lupus. Mucosal manifestations of the mouth and nose may be present.[5,8,19]

Acute cutaneous lupus is triggered by exposure to ultraviolet light or is associated with exacerbation of systemic disease. The classic "butterfly rash" occurs in approximately 56% of patients, which consists of an erythematous skin rash over the malar area of the cheeks and the bridge of the nose (sparing the nasolabial folds), oftentimes raised and very inflamed. The rash persists for weeks and resolves without scarring.

Approximately 27% of SLE patients develop discoid lupus erythematosus (DLE), characterized by circular rimmed, raised patches with keratotic scaling on the scalp, face, or neck. The lesions are usually associated with disfigurement from depigmentation and scarring of the skin. Permanent hair loss may develop if the rash is located on the scalp.

A distinct subset, subacute cutaneous lupus erythematosus (SCLE), is associated with symmetric, superficial, nonscarring, ring-shaped skin lesions with resultant alopecia. The lesions are located on the shoulders, upper arms, chest, back, and neck. DLE and SCLE usually have no other systemic involvement.

Mucosal manifestations are frequent in SLE. They present as painful, recurrent ulcers in the mouth, nose, and genital cavity. Vasculitic skin lesions such as purpura, subcutaneous nodules, nail fold infarcts, ulcers, vasculitic urticaria, panniculitis, and gangrene of the digits may also develop in patients with SLE, DLE, and SCLE. Livedo reticularis is a common feature of the APS.

DIAGNOSIS AND CLINICAL FEATURES

The diagnostic workup includes an assessment of the clinical presentation, physical examination, appropriate diagnostic tests, and consideration of an alternative diagnosis. Many autoimmune diseases have overlapping features so the exact classification may be difficult. Features of SLE, rheumatoid arthritis, polymyositis, and scleroderma may overlap. Drug-induced lupus erythematosus (DILE) should always be included on the differential list and will be discussed later (Table 68.2).[19]

The American College of Rheumatology (ACR) first developed diagnostic criteria for SLE in 1971 (revised in 1982 and 1997) that are highly specific and sensitive that has permitted classification of patients for purposes of research, epidemiology, and clinical trials (Table 68.3).[20,21] The classification is based on 11 criteria. A person shall be said to have SLE if 4 or more of the 11 criteria are present, serially or simultaneously during any interval of observation. The ACR revised criteria is reported to have an overall specificity of 95% and sensitivity of 85% in the diagnosis of SLE.

More than 95% of patients with symptomatic SLE have a positive ANA test with a very high concentration (titer >1:160) which supports the diagnosis of SLE but the test is not specific because it may indicate chronic liver or renal disease, infection, malignancy, or other autoimmune disease

TABLE 68.2 Prevalence of Clinical and Laboratory Abnormalities in Drug-Induced Lupus and Systemic Lupus Erythematosus

Feature	Hydralazine-Induced Lupus	Procainamide-Induced Lupus	Systemic Lupus Erythematosus
Symptoms			
Arthralgia	80%	85%	
Arthritis	50–100%	20%	80%
Pleuritis, pleural effusion	<5%	50%	44%
Fever, weight loss	40%–50%	45%	48%
Myalgia	<5%	35%	60%
Hepatosplenomegaly	15%	25%	5%–10%
Pericarditis	<5%	15%	20%
Rash	25%	<5%	71%
Glomerulonephritis	5%–10%	<5%	42%
CNS disease	>5%	>5%	32%
Signs			
ANA	>95%	>95%	97%
LE cell	>50%	80%	71%
Antihistone	>95%	>95%	54%
Anti-[(H2A-H2B)-DNA]	43%	96%	70%
Antidenatured DNA	50%–90%	50%	82%
Antinative DNA	<5%	<5%	28%–67%
Anticardiolipin	5%–15%	5%–20%	35%
Rheumatoid factor	20%	30%	25%–30%
Anemia	35%	20%	42%
Elevated ESR	60%	60%–80%	>50%
Leukopenia	5%–25%	15%	46%
+Coombs test	<5%	25%	25%
Elevated gammaglobulins	10%–50%	25%	32%
Hypocomplementemia	<5%	<5%	51%

Each prevalence represents a consensus value ±5 percentage points. Abnormalities occurring in fewer than 5% of patients are not listed.
ANA, antinuclear antibodies; LE, lupus erythematosus; ESR, erythrocyte sedimentation rate.
(From Wallace DJ, Hahn BH, eds. Dubois' lupus erythematosus. 6th ed. Philadelphia: Lippincott Williams & Wilkins, 2002: 891.)

TABLE 68.3	Revised American College of Rheumatology Criteria for Systemic Lupus Erythematosus
Criterion	**Definition**
1. Malar rash	Fixed malar erythema, flat or raised
2. Discoid rash	Erythematous raised patches with keratotic scaling and follicular plugging: atrophic scarring may occur in older lesions
3. Photosensitivity	Skin rash as an unusual reaction to sunlight, by patient history or physician observation
4. Oral ulcers	Oral or nasopharyngeal ulcers, usually painless, observed by physician
5. Arthritis	Nonerosive arthritis involving two or more peripheral joints, characterized by tenderness, swelling, or effusion
6. Serositis	a. Pleuritis (convincing history of pleuritic pain or rub heard by physician or evidence of pleural effusion) OR b. Pericarditis (documented by ECG or rub or evidence of pericardial effusion)
7. Renal disorder	a. Persistent proteinuria >0.5 g/day or >3+ OR b. Cellular casts of any type
8. Neurologic disorder	a. Seizures (in the absence of other causes) b. Psychosis (in the absence of other causes)
9. Hematologic disorder	a. Hemolytic anemia b. Leukopenia (<4,000/mm^3 on two or more occasions) c. Lymphopenia (<1,500/mm^3 on two or more occasions) d. Thrombocytopenia (<100,000/mm^3 in the absence of offending drugs)
10. Immunologic disorder	a. Anti-dsDNA OR b. Anti-Sm OR c. Positive finding of anti-phospholipid antibodies based on 1) An abnormal serum level of IgG or IgM anticardiolipin antibodies, OR 2) A positive test result for lupus anticoagulant using a standard method, OR 3) A false-positive serologic test for syphilis known to be positive for ≥6 months and confirmed by *Treponema pallidum* immobilization or fluorescent treponemal antibody absorption test
11. Antinuclear antibody	An abnormal titer of ANA by immunofluorescence or an equivalent assay at any time and in the absence of drugs known to be associated with "drug-induced lupus syndrome"

ECG, electrocardiograph; dsDNA, double-stranded DNA; Sm, Smith antibodies; IgG, immunoglobulin G; IgM, immunoglobulin M; ANA, antinuclear antibodies.

(From Koopman WJ, Moreland LW. Arthritis and allied conditions: a textbook of rheumatology. 14th ed. Philadelphia: Lippincott Williams & Wilkins, 2001: 1456.)

such as rheumatoid arthritis, scleroderma, or polymyositis.[22] In contrast, asymptomatic patients with SLE oftentimes have a low antibody titer (<1:80). However, no consistent correlation between disease activity and ANA titer has been established. Lastly, a negative ANA test makes the diagnosis unlikely, but not impossible.

After a repeat positive ANA screening test, more specific autoantibodies to SLE may be found (Table 68.4). The presence of atypical antibodies, characteristically against the cell nucleus nuclear components is a hallmark feature and associated with a diverse array of clinical manifestations in SLE. When more than one antibody is present in a patient with symptoms, the clinician may consider the diagnosis of SLE. The specific antibodies may predict the patient's prognosis and likelihood for organ damage.

Anti–double-stranded DNA (dsDNA) and anti-Smith (Sm) antibodies are unique to patients with SLE. A high titer of anti-dsDNA antibodies is the most helpful confirmatory test for SLE and increases the likelihood of lupus nephritis. Anti-Sm is very specific for SLE but is formed infrequently. Patients with pulmonary disease are more likely to present with a speckled ANA pattern, reflecting the presence of anti-Sm antibodies. Antiribosomal and antineuronal antibodies support the diagnosis of central nervous system (CNS) lupus. Antihistone antibodies are typically seen in DILE. Anti-Ro (SSA) and anti-La (SSB) antibodies are found in approximately 50% of patients with SLE and indicative of a higher likelihood of cutaneous manifestations, photosensitivity, and the neonatal lupus (see Table 68.8). Others are specific for the APS and include lupus anticoagu-

TABLE 68.4	Sensitivity, Specificity and Predictive Values of Autoantibodies in Patients with Systemic Lupus Erythematosus and Drug-Induced Lupus									
	ANA	**dsDNA**	**ssDNA**	**Histone**	**Nucleo-protein**	**Sm**	**RNP (U1-RNP)**	**Ro (SS-A)**	**La (SS-B)**	**PCNA**
SLE										
Sensitivity (%)	99	70	80	30–80	58	25	50	25–35	15	5
Specificity (%)	80	95	50	Mod.	Mod.	99	87–94	—	—	95
Predictive value (%)	15–35	95	50	Mod.	Mod.	97	46–85	—	—	95
DIL										
Sensitivity (%)	N/A		80	95	50					
Specificity (%)	N/A	1–5	50	Hi	Mod.					
Predictive value (%)	N/A	1–5	50	Hi	Mod.					

ANA, antinuclear antibodies; DIL, drug-induced lupus; dsDNA, double-stranded DNA; PCNA, proliferating cell nuclear antigen; RNP, ribonucleoprotein; SLE, systemic lupus erythematosus; sm, Smith antibodies; ssDNA, single-stranded DNA.

lant (LA) and antibodies to anticardiolipin (aCL), increasing the risk for thrombosis or spontaneous abortions during pregnancy.

Finally, increasing concentrations of anti-dsDNA bodies and decreasing levels of serum complement are associated with increased disease activity. The erythrocyte sedimentation rate (ESR) may be elevated, but does not correlate with disease activity.

Investigators have shown that serologic autoimmunity precedes clinical symptoms of autoimmunity in up to 90% of cases.[23] In one clinical trial analyzing blood specimens from approximately 5 million U.S. armed forces personnel, investigators identified 130 individuals with a diagnosis of SLE and were able to look at the natural history of SLE before the disease became apparent. At least one positive serologic autoantibody test was identified prior to the diagnosis of SLE in 88%. On average, serologic autoimmunity was detected on average 3.3 years prior (up to 9.4 years) before the diagnosis of SLE, and autoantibody formation evolved sequentially in a clearly defined pattern. Antinuclear, antiphospholipid, anti-Ro, and anti-La autoantibodies were seen earlier than anti-dsDNA, anti-Sm, and antiribononucleoprotein antibodies.

Experts in the field strongly recommend early referral of SLE patients to a rheumatologist by the primary care provider in cases of diagnostic uncertainty and for management advice, particularly when symptoms are mild to moderate.[24]

Ancillary diagnostic imaging tests include chest x-ray, x-rays of affected joints, echocardiography for evaluation of pericardial, myocardial, and endocardial involvement, chest computed tomography (CT) to define parenchymal lung disease, and brain magnetic resonance imaging (MRI) to evaluate patients with CNS lupus.

In addition to cutaneous, joint, and muscle manifestations seen in SLE, a number of major systemic manifestations may also be present, particularly pulmonary, cardiac, renal, neurological, hematological, and vascular (Table 68.5).

Pulmonary. Pleural involvement (SLE pleuritis) is the most common respiratory component in patients with SLE and has been found at autopsy in 38% of patients.[1,5,8] Small to moderate pleural effusions may be detected that are associated with pleural pain, cough, dyspnea, and fever. Bacterial pneumonia is first ruled out in all patients who present with fever and infiltrates.[25]

Rarely, patients develop acute pneumonitis that is detected by the presence of atelectasis on chest x-ray. Its occurrence is increased immediately postpartum and is usually a diagnosis of exclusion and highly responsive to steroids. Acute alveolar-capillary damage, probably mediated by immune complex deposition, is the cause. It occurs as a result of alveolar wall inflammation, alveolar wall necrosis, alveolar hemorrhage, edema, hyaline membrane formation, infiltration of the interstitium by inflammatory cells, and capillary thrombi. Alveolar hemorrhage, a common process in patients with SLE, is associated with similar clinical and pathologic findings as acute lupus pneumonitis.

In contrast, chronic diffuse interstitial lung disease and pulmonary arterial hypertension are rare. Finally, approximately 25% of SLE patients characteristically develop weakness of the diaphragm and other respiratory muscles with clinically significant, unexplained dyspnea (worse in the supine position). This is known as shrinking lung syndrome. It is characterized by low lung volume and the inability to generate a respiratory effort.

Cardiac. Cardiac complications involving the pericardium, valves, myocardium, and coronary arteries are frequently seen in SLE patients.[2,3,5,8]

In patients with mild pericarditis, pericardial effusions on presentation are usually small and no hemodynamic compromise is apparent. Severe restrictive pericarditis requiring treatment is responsive to high-dose steroids that may result in gradual, almost complete recovery.[26]

TABLE 68.5	Clinical Manifestations in Systemic Lupus Erythematosus by Organ Systems	
Manifestation	**Percent of Patients Positive During Course of Disease**	**Signs and Symptoms**
Systemic	95	Fever, malaise, fatigue
Musculoskeletal	95	Arthritis, arthralgias, myositis, tenosynovitis
Hematologic	85	Hemolytic anemia, leucopenia, lymphopenia, thrombocytopenia
Skin	80	Malar (butterfly) rash, discoid lesions, photosensitivity, maculopapular rash, alopecia, and oral, genital, or nasal ulcers
Neurologic	60	Psychosis, seizures, depression, cognitive impairment, headache, cerebritis, peripheral neuropathy
Cardiopulmonary	60	Pericarditis, myositis, Libman-Sachs endocarditis, pleuritis, pulmonary hypertension, alveolar hemorrhage, "shrinking lung" syndrome, interstitial lung disease, pulmonary emboli
Renal	50	Glomerulonephritis, membranous nephropathy, nephrotic syndrome
GI	45	Pancreatitis, peritoneal serositis, hepatitis, hepatomegaly
Vascular	15	Arterial or venous thrombosis

(From Petri MA. Systemic lupus erythematosus: clinical aspects. In: Koopman WJ, et al., eds. Arthritis and allied conditions – a textbook of rheumatology. 14th ed. Philadelphia: Lippincott Williams & Wilkins, 2001:1455–1492; Wallace DJ, Hahn BH, eds. Dubois' lupus erythematosus. 6th ed. Philadelphia: Lippincott Williams & Wilkins, 2002; Humes HD, ed. Kelley's Essentials of internal medicine. 2nd ed. Philadelphia: Lippincott Williams & Wilkins, 2001; Lahita RG, ed. Systemic lupus erythematosus. 4th ed. London: Elsevier Academic Press, 2004; Hahn BH. Systemic lupus erythematosus. In: Braunwald E, et al., eds. Harrison's principles of internal medicine. 15th ed. New York: McGraw–Hill, 2001: 1922–1928; Peterson KS, Winchester RJ. Systemic lupus erythematosus: pathogenesis. In: Koopman WJ, et al., eds. Arthritis and allied conditions – a textbook of rheumatology. 14th ed. Philadelphia: Lippincott Williams & Wilkins, 2001.)

Valvular heart disease is usually asymptomatic at onset. Further examination may reveal valve leaflet thickening with or without nonbacterial vegetations (Libman–Sacks endocarditis) that may be a risk factor for valve incompetence, congestive heart failure (CHF), or emboli formation.

Increased incidence of accelerated artherosclerosis in SLE has been shown. It is unclear if steroid use predisposes the SLE population. Investigators have reported that SLE in itself may predispose to accelerated artheroslceosis because traditional risk factors could not account for the increase in cardiovascular disease among SLE patients.[27]

The following traditional risk factors for heart disease should be screened and minimized in SLE: dyslipidemia, hypertension, hyperglycemia, tobacco use, and obesity. Potential disease-specific potential risk factors addressed in SLE patients include minimizing long-term steroid use, reducing homocysteine levels with folate supplementation, and preventing thrombosis with aspirin or warfarin in patients with APS.

Patients with SLE have an increased risk of myocardial infarction compared with the general population. Coronary artery disease (CAD) is an important risk factor for morbidity and MI is 50 times more common in women with SLE who are 35 to 44 years of age than their nonlupus counterparts.[28–30]

Neurologic. CNS manifestations are often nonspecific and diverse and may occur during the course of disease in 60% of patients with idiopathic SLE.[2,5,8] Depression is common and may affect patient compliance. In addition, anxiety, migraine headaches, memory loss, and seizures have been re-

ported as well. A host of less common manifestations may occur in SLE patients such as frank psychosis, acute confusional states, demyelinating disorders, cerebrovascular disease, movement disorders, aseptic meningitis, encephalopathy, myelopathy, monomyopathy or polymyopathy of cranial or peripheral nerves, autonomic dysfunction, acute demyelinating polyneuropathy (Guillain–Barré), mood disorders, optic neuritis, subarachnoid hemorrhage, pseudotumor cerebri, and hypothalamic dysfunction with inappropriate secretion of vasopressin. The most devastating complications are cerebrovascular accident and transverse myelitis.

The diagnosis of CNS lupus is difficult because laboratory and routine diagnostic tests sometimes do not reveal any abnormalities in patients with neurologic complaints. Of these patients, only 70% have abnormal electroencephalograms, 50% have elevated protein in the cerebrospinal fluid, and 30% have elevated mononuclear cells. Acute and chronic CNS lesions are best detected by MRI with contrast. CT is used to rule out bleeding or mass lesions.

Renal. Approximately 50% of patients develop renal disease from lupus nephritis,[2,5] a form of glomerulonephritis, which is a poor prognostic indicator.[31] African-Americans and Asians have an increased risk of lupus nephritis. Risk factors include the inheritance of HLA-DR2 and HLA-B8, and polymorphisms of Fc receptors for IgG.

Deposition of immune complexes consisting of anti-DNA deposit in the kidney leads to complement activation and chemotaxis of neutrophils resulting in local inflammation. In situ deposition of antibody and antigen complexes may also lead to complement activation and leukocyte mediated injury.

Antibodies against specific cellular targets (i.e., antiribosomal P) may produce renal injury. The presence of anti-dsDNA antibodies and hypocomplementemia, particularly decreasing C3, is diagnostic for lupus nephritis. The fall and rise of these parameters are used to monitor response to therapy and renal disease severity.

With therapeutic intervention, clinical manifestations of the disease should improve within days to weeks. Renal biopsies may help to differentiate mesangial, or mild, focal proliferative nephritis from diffuse proliferative nephritis and guide therapy.

According to the World Health Organization (WHO) classification, SLE nephritis is associated with six histologically distinct categories (Classes I–VI) (Table 68.6). Apart from close monitoring, Class I and Class II lesions have an excellent prognosis. Class III and Class IV lesions are associated with proliferative disease requiring aggressive immunosuppressive treatment to induce remission and delay the rapid progression to end-stage renal disease (ESRD) (Class VI).

An active urinary sediment including red blood cells, red blood cell casts, proteinuria, and a markedly reduced creatinine clearance is usually seen in active disease. (Classes III and VI). Nephropathy is a marker for lupus activity, but also for more aggressive immunosuppression and increased hypercoagulopathy, owing to nephritic or nephrotic syndrome.

The prognosis for lupus nephritis has improved, with the most recent survival rate being 75% to 85% over 10 years. This is the result of a better understanding of the disease, earlier recognition, and aggressive immunosuppressive treatment.

Hematologic. Normochromic, normocytic anemia is seen in 40% of SLE patients.[2,3,5,8] Hemolytic anemia, leukopenia,

lymphopenia, and thrombocytopenia may be present in up to 85% of SLE patients during the course of the disease and are all items in the ACR diagnostic criteria.

APS, a potentially hypercoagulable disorder, may occur in the presence of SLE. Three primary classes of antibodies are associated with the APS in SLE. They include antibodies to LA, aCL, and those directed at specific molecules, including β_2-glycoprotein. The female to male ratio is 2 to 1. APS may occur as a manifestation of lupus or may occur as an isolated discrete syndrome.

APS is characterized by recurrent venous or arterial thrombosis, spontaneous abortions or recurrent fetal loss, and thrombocytopenia from antiphospholipid antibodies. Spontaneous abortion and stillbirths occur in approximately 10% and 30% of patients with SLE, especially in women with LA and/or aCL antibodies.

Abrupt hormonal changes, the presence of antiphospholipid antibodies, and teratogenic immunosuppressive therapy are factors in pregnancy-related complications in SLE. However with careful planning, the majority of patients with SLE with or without APS can have a normal pregnancy without serious complications unless ovarian function has been altered by immunosuppressive therapy. In vitro fertilization, control of symptoms with hydroxychloroquine during pregnancy in place of immunosuppressive therapy, close monitoring of disease activity, and aggressive fetal monitoring are recommended.

Neonatal lupus syndrome is also seen in some neonates born to mothers with SLE. Transfer of certain maternal ANA to the fetus may lead to neonatal lupus, a condition characterized by congenital heart block, rash, or thrombocytopenia in the infant. In addition to antiphospholipid tests, tests for antibodies to Ro (SSA) and La (SSB) can help to predict neonatal lupus.[32]

Vasculitic. Vasculitis affecting small blood vessels in the skin, CNS, and coronary branch are seen in SLE.[5] Vasculitic

TABLE 68.6	World Health Organization (WHO) Histologic Classification of Lupus Nephritis
Class	**Brief description**
I. Normal	No histologic abnormalities
II. Mesangial lupus nephritis	Abnormalities limited to mesangium with mesangial deposition of immune complexes, hypercellularity, and increased matrix
III. Focal proliferative glomerulonephritis	Glomerular capillary hypercellularity and inflammatory lesions that involve >50% of glomeruli (usually in segmental pattern); mesangial and capillary loop immune complex deposits
IV. Diffuse, proliferative glomerulonephritis	Glomerular capillary hypercellularity and inflammatory lesions that involve >50% of glomeruli usually in a diffuse pattern; mesangial and diffuse (subendothelial and subepithelial) capillary loop immune complexes and complement
V. Membranous glomerulonephritis	Generalized thickening of the capillary loops; subepithelial and intramembranous immune complexes

(From Schrier RW, ed. Diseases of the kidney and urinary tract. 7th ed. Philadelphia: Lippincott Williams & Wilkins, 2001; 1842.)

skin lesions include petechiae, purpura, urticaria, nodules, atrophy of the finger pads, and livedo reticularis may occur. Other vascular processes found in the CNS and coronary vessels may be related to thrombosis or embolism. Because lupus vasculitis involves vessels smaller than 50 μm, angiograms may not be helpful in the detection of vasculitis and vascular occlusions or emboli.

Gastrointestinal. Gastrointestinal (GI) manifestations such as nausea, diarrhea, and vague discomfort are commonly reported in SLE patients and may occur in up to 45% of patients during the course of illness.[5,8] Esophageal dysmotility may also occur. Acute pancreatitis may be severe and is usually associated with flares or treatment with steroids or azathioprine.

PSYCHOSOCIAL ASPECTS

Clinicians should be aware of the psychosocial issues when treating patients with SLE. Some of the issues include patient frustration during the diagnostic process, to feelings of isolation and depression, and family stresses. Chronicity of disease, recurrent flares, and remissions present constant challenges for patients and clinicians. SLE shortens life expectancy, creates significant morbidity, and accounts for significant health care expenditures. Therefore, clinicians must be empathetic and help patients develop effective coping skills and identify support resources. Symptomatic control using conditioning exercises, applying heat to affected joints, weight loss if necessary, and relaxation techniques may help patients cope.

THERAPEUTIC PLAN

Of utmost importance is the active role undertaken by the patient or patient's caregiver in managing the SLE. A treatment plan is developed by health care providers based on the patient's age, sex, overall health status, symptoms, and lifestyle. Because the therapeutic plan is tailored to the patient's needs, it is likely to change during the clinical course of the disease depending on response to therapy, side effects of therapy, medication adherence, and severity of end-organ involvement.[2,3,5,8] As treatment progresses, additional specialty health care professionals often help in making nonpharmacologic and pharmacologic recommendations. The goals of therapy are to prevent flares, treat active disease, and to minimize organ damage and complications. Health care providers and patients should reevaluate the plan regularly to ensure its effectiveness.

Treatment is individualized according to disease activity and the organs affected. Clinicians often advise avoiding sulfa antibiotics, oral contraceptives, and estrogen products because they may induce flares. Patients are counseled on preventative care and regular monitoring by their physicians during follow-up appointments every 3 to 6 months.

General lifestyle measures should be encouraged in all patients with SLE. Consider the combination of a nonsteroidal anti-inflammatory drug (NSAID) or cyclooxygenase (COX)-2 inhibitor with or without hydroxychloroquine in patients with mild lupus. Hydroxychloroquine may be effective in controlling skin and joint manifestations of the disease in addition to its benefit as an adjunctive, steroid-sparing agent. Patients with inadequate response to this combination should be prescribed low-dose corticosteroids whereas, high-dose steroids are recommended in acute flares.

Corticosteroid regimens depend on the initial presentation, comorbidities, and response to prior treatment modalities. A lupus rash can be treated with topical steroids. Hydrocortisone topical may be effective in mild superficial involvement, whereas more potent steroids (i.e., fluorinated steroids) are used for thicker lesions. Steroid ointments and gels are more potent than creams and lotions. Ointments are used for dry lesions, whereas lotions are used for scalp lesions. In mild to moderate cases, oral prednisone (60 mg daily) is given initially until resolution of signs of active disease permits tapering the dose.

More intensive or induction therapy using immunosuppression with methylprednisolone (+) or (−) cyclophosphamide, azathioprine, or mycophenolate mofetil is used in patients with major organ or system involvement (e.g., active disease associated with lupus nephritis, CNS lupus, or APS).

Aggressive generalized management of comorbidities including hypertension, proteinuria, infections, hyperlipidemia, and thrombotic coagulopathy and prevention of osteoporosis and other potential drug-induced adverse effects will affect morbidity and long-term prognosis.

TREATMENT

PHARMACOTHERAPY

Nonselective Nonsteroidal Anti-Inflammatory Drugs and Selective Cyclooxygenase-2 Inhibitors. The mainstay of SLE treatment in mild disease is supportive with the use of antiinflammatory doses of NSAID for symptomatic relief of joint pain and serositis, and pain associated with pleurisy and pericarditis.[5,8] They are also used for systemic symptoms of fever and fatigue. Side effects and the risk of serious GI symptoms can limit their long-term use. When a NSAID is chosen, potential side effects and cost should be a consideration. The dose should be increased to the recommended maximum over 1 to 2 weeks. The drug should not be abandoned until the patient has been on the maximal dose for at least 2 weeks because NSAIDs may take this much time to reach maximal efficacy. If after 2 weeks of receiving the maximal dose the results are disappointing, an alternate NSAID should be tried. Naproxen (500 mg twice daily) and Ibuprofen (600 mg four times daily) are some of the least expensive NSAIDs. The use of a proton pump inhibitor (i.e., misoprostol) with NSAID reduces the incidence of gastric and duodenal ulcers.

Although COX-2 inhibitors may cause fewer GI side effects such as ulcers and bleeding than other NSAIDs, they may increase a person's risk of heart attack and stroke. The COX-2 inhibitor Rofecoxib (Vioxx) was voluntarily withdrawn from the market in 2004 after study results showed an increased risk of heart attack and stroke after 18 months of continuous use.[33]

Celecoxib, a COX-2 inhibitor, has the same efficacy as NSAIDs but fewer GI side effects and have no direct effect on platelets. However, up to 12% of patients on a COX-2 inhibitor can develop ulcers. Initial studies suggest that even one aspirin a day (e.g., cardiac or stroke prophylaxis) may negate any GI advantage of the COX-2 inhibitors. Thus, although celecoxib may be effective for decreasing GI complications, its usefulness for minimizing GI risk in aspirin users is questionable.[34] Nonselective NSAID therapy may be appropriate for chronic pain management in aspirin users given that suitable GI prophylactic measures are used in high-risk patients whereas COX-2 inhibitors are preferred in patients with thrombocytopenia because of their lack of effect on platelets.

Antimalarials. Combination therapy with an NSAID and hydroxychloroquine (Plaquenil) is used in patients with mild lupus whose overriding symptoms are fatigue, arthralgia, arthritis, and rash.[1–3,5,8] The addition of hydroxychloroquine, an antimalarial, has anti-inflammatory effects and may be used to control skin, fatigue, and joint symptoms, and reduce the time to flareups, as an adjunctive treatment for arthritic and cutaneous manifestations. In addition, hydroxychloroquine may have added benefit to SLE patients due to its antithrombotic and lipid-lowering properties, and steroid sparing effects.

Hydroxychloroquine is more commonly used than chloroquine because it is associated with less corneal deposition (opacities) and retinopathy.[35] This is a dose-dependent effect and the risk is low if the dose is less than 6.5 mg/kg/day and restricted to less than 600 mg per day with hydroxychloroquine. The dose should be reduced in patients weighing less than 61 kg. Ophthalmic symptoms include blurred vision, night blindness, missing or blanched out areas in the central or peripheral fields, light flashes and streaks, and photophobia, and is associated with a bull's-eye appearance in the macular region. Patients should be screened for the presence of ''premaculopathy'' antimalarial retinopathy during regularly scheduled eye examinations at 3- to 6-month intervals because this is a reversible stage.

In SLE, the usual oral hydroxychloroquine dose is 400 mg administered daily for 4 to 12 weeks, and tapered by 50% to the daily maintenance dose of 200 mg. Objective benefit usually becomes apparent within 8 weeks. If no benefit in disease activity occurs after 6 months, the agent should be withdrawn.

Relapse has been reported on discontinuation of hydroxychloroquine in patients with stable lupus.[36] A statistically significant increase in the incidence of flares that required corticosteroid treatment on discontinuation of hydroxychloroquine was seen in a randomized control trial in 47 patients with stable lupus.

Corticosteroids, Methotrexate in Mild to Moderate Disease. The addition of a short course of low-dose corticosteroid (e.g., prednisone) should be considered in patients poorly responsive to the combination of NSAIDs and hydroxychloroquine. When these agents are combined in mild to moderate disease activity, low corticosteroid doses may be effective thereby minimizing side effects.[1–3,5,8] If the symptoms are not well controlled, short tapered courses of corticosteroids may be required.

Cutaneous manifestations may be effectively controlled with topical corticosteroid formulations. Low-dose oral prednisone (10 mg/day) may be used for mild disease activity and limited to a duration of 4 to 6 weeks. If necessary, every other day maintenance therapy at the lowest effective dose is given. NSAIDs or COX-2 inhibitors may be combined with prednisone to lower the dose and minimize side effects or given on the off day of the alternate day therapy.

Prednisone can also be helpful for treating acute flares with or without systemic symptoms in initial adult doses of 1 mg/kg/day, up to 60 mg per day, and tapered over 8 weeks.

Methotrexate (MTX), a dihydrofolate reductase inhibitor, is an alternative agent to hydroxychloroquine, and may be used with or without low-dose corticosteroids in persistent arthritis, rash, or serositis. Weekly doses of 7.5 to 15 mg (maximum 25 mg) of MTX is effective and may control joint and skin manifestations, allowing a decrease in corticosteroid dose. It can be given orally or by subcutaneous injection. Parenteral administration is preferred in patients who experience drug-related nausea. Hepatotoxicity is a potential toxicity associated with MTX, therefore patients should be screened for preexisting liver disease from hepatitis B or C, excessive alcohol use, or diabetes, with baseline liver function tests and tests done periodically throughout therapy. Trimethoprim should be avoided because it may lead to toxic serum MTX levels.

Corticosteroids and Cytotoxic Agents in Severe Disease. Judicious use of high-dose oral corticosteroids, including large intravenous (IV) doses, particularly in severe disease is warranted. With treatment, symptomatic acute manifestations of the disease and laboratory parameters should improve within weeks to months.

More intensive immunosuppression may be necessary in patients with major organ involvement and life-threatening complications (e.g., severe flares of joint symptoms, lupus nephritis, or CNS lupus) who fail conventional corticosteroid therapy. In the acute management of these manifestations, combination therapy with high-dose corticosteroid (e.g., oral prednisone 40–60 mg/day or IV methylprednisolone 0.5–1.0 g/day) and pulse IV cyclophosphamide is recommended.

Lupus Nephritis Treatment. In patients diagnosed with diffuse proliferative glomerulonephritis (Class IV), the cytotoxic agent of choice, cyclophosphamide in combo with methylprednisolone, has been shown to slow down disease progression, decrease the frequency of relapse events, and reduce the risk of ESRD.[5,37] A similar trend in favor of IV cyclophosphamide and methylprednisolone induction therapy has been reported in patients with severe Class V disease activity. Monthly "pulse" IV cyclophosphamide (0.5–1.0 g/m^2 of body surface area) in combination with pulse IV methylprednisolone may effectively reduce kidney scarring compared with corticosteroids alone.

The most studied regimens involve treatment of lupus nephritis. An induction phase consisting of "pulse" IV methylprednisolone (0.5–1.0 g/day) for 3 days followed by oral prednisone (40–60 mg/day) for the first month only plus pulse IV cyclophosphamide (0.5–1.0 g/m^2) and continued for 6 months is given during active disease in patients with biopsy proven WHO Classes III and IV lesions. The combination of cyclophosphamide and steroids is superior to steroids or cyclophosphamide alone. After the first month, oral prednisone 0.5 mg/kg/day is given between monthly pulses of methylprednisolone and cyclophosphamide to avoid the cumulative effect of long-term daily prednisone.[38]

Because relapse rates are high after discontinuation of a 6-month course, many patients require maintenance therapy an additional 18 months with pulse IV cyclophosphamide every 3 months and oral prednisone 0.5 mg/kg/day (Fig. 68.2).[39]

Cyclophosphamide is an inhibitor of T-cell proliferation and the transcription of IL-2. It tends to be toxic with many patients having one or more side effects. Acute toxicity includes nausea or vomiting (58%), alopecia (26%), dysuria

(26%), hemorrhagic cystitis (14%), herpes zoster (5%). Other adverse reactions include leukopenia, thrombocytopenia, and amenorrhea in premenopausal women.

Intermittent monthly pulse therapy is preferred by many clinicians because patients receive a lower cumulative dose compared with oral cyclophosphamide regimen and are able to reduce dose-related toxicity. A reduction in the incidence rate of serious bladder complications (hemorrhagic cystitis, bladder fibrosis, and bladder transitional cell or squamous cell carcinoma) has been shown with IV cyclophosphamide.

Moreover, other predictable drug-related toxicities such as bone marrow suppression, nausea and vomiting (readily treated with antiemetics), reversible alopecia, and loss of fertility from ovarian failure in females or azoospermia in males are limitations of therapy. Also, whether daily oral cyclophosphamide is more efficacious than pulse cyclophosphamide remains uncertain. Vigilant monitoring of complete blood counts and platelets is required to avoid serious sequelae associated with neutropenia (infections), thrombocytopenia (bleeding), or anemia. The hematologic effects are dose-related and reversible on reduction of cyclophosphamide dose. Leukopenia, thrombocytopenia, and anemia in patients with acute SLE can reflect drug-induced bone marrow suppression and not represent hematologic manifestations of the disease itself. Herpes zoster is commonly seen in patients with SLE who receive cyclophosphamide or mycophenolate mofetil.

Other potent immunosuppressive drugs such as azathioprine, mycophenolate mofetil, and MTX have been used as second-line therapy, although their role in the management

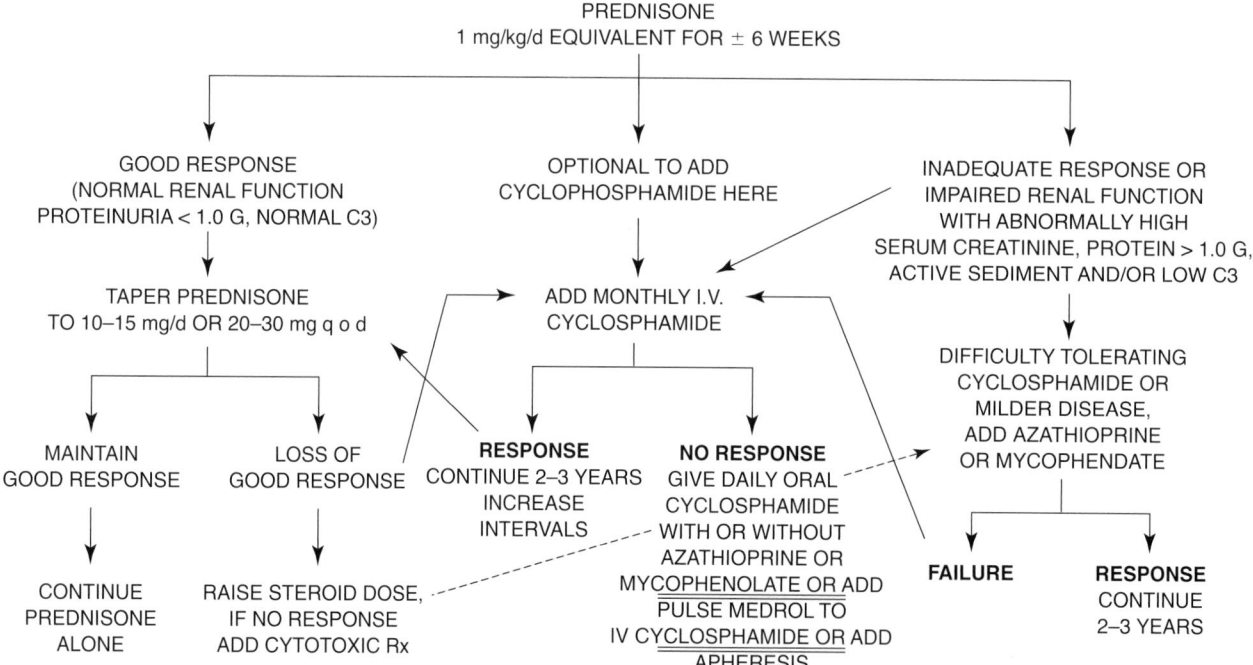

FIGURE 68.2 Algorithm for the treatment of proliferative (Class III or IV) nephritis. (From Wallace DJ, Hahn BH, eds. Dubois' lupus erythematosus, 6th ed. Philadelphia: Lippincott Williams & Wilkins, 2002:1082.)

of lupus nephritis is not well established. In the presence of worsening kidney function or severe nephritic syndrome associated with Classes I, II, or V lesions, cyclosporine A in combination with corticosteroids has been used to treat lupus nephritis.[31] Due to the unknown long-term risks in SLE, these agents are typically reserved for patients who fail or only partially respond to standard therapy.

After completion of induction therapy, alternate maintenance regimens consist of oral azathioprine (1–3 mg/kg/day) plus oral prednisone (0.5 mg/kg/day), or oral mycophenolate mofetil (0.5–3.0 g/day) plus oral prednisone (0.5 mg/kg/day) have been investigated. In a randomized, controlled trial following short-term cyclophosphamide therapy, maintenance therapy with azathioprine or mycophenolate mofetil appeared to be more efficacious and safer than long-term IV cyclophosphamide.[40,41]

However in some recent trials, some experts have suggested that sequential therapies using IV cyclophosphamide and steroid induction × 7 months followed by oral azathioprine or mycophenolate mofetil maintenance regimens are effective and offer better benefit-to-risk ratios than long-term IV cyclophosphamide in SLE patients with proliferative lupus nephritis.[42]

Adjunctive treatment of comorbid conditions in lupus nephritis is also necessary to delay disease progression.[2,5,8] Hypertension, often accompanies proliferative nephritis, and is associated with a poor prognosis. Angiotensin-converting enzyme (ACE) inhibitors are first-line antihypertensive treatment in lupus nephritis because they have antiproteinuric effects and considered renoprotective. In addition, patients should follow a renal low protein diet and salt restriction. Hypercholesterolemia may be a complication of lupus nephritis and a side effect of steroid treatment. Lifestyle modification and a restricted diet low in saturated and transaturated fat to maintain a normal body weight should be followed. The addition of cholesterol-lowering drugs according to the third report of the Expert Panel on Detection, Evaluation, and Treatment of High Blood Cholesterol in Adults Treatment Panel (ATP) III by the National Cholesterol Education Program (NCEP) offers guidelines to maintain high-density lipoprotein (HDL), low-density lipoprotein (LDL), and triglycerides at recommended levels.

Patients on long-term hemodialysis appear to tolerate it well. Although the clinical course of SLE may be more quiescent in hemodialyis patients because ESRD in itself is an immunocompromised state.[1,2,5] However, flares are not absent entirely, and hemodialysis patients may occasionally experience disease activity. Furthermore, although the rate of allograft loss is twice as high (approximately 50% at 5 years) in SLE patients compared to patients who undergo renal transplantation secondary to ESRD from all other causes, no increase in mortality rates (>90% patients survival at 5 years) is seen in SLE patients. Recurrence of SLE in the transplanted allograft has been reported rarely, most likely because patients take chronic immunosuppression to prevent allograft rejection, a maneuver that keeps SLE suppressed at same time.

Central Nervous System Lupus Treatment. Immunosuppressive therapy is helpful reversing neurologic problems, however, their recurrence has been reported to occur in one third of patients. Treatment options include cyclophosphamide and corticosteroids. There is no evidence to show that cyclophosphamide is more effective or safer than methylprednisolone in CNS lupus. Symptomatic treatment is dependent on the presence of specific neurologic symptoms. Anticonvulsants, antipsychotics, antidepressants, antianxiety medications, and antimigraine have all been used in the management of CNS lupus.

Management of Blood Disorders with Systemic Lupus Erythematosus. Patients with SLE may be prone to antibody-mediated destruction of peripheral blood cells resulting in thrombocytopenia, neutropenia, lymphopenia, or hemolytic anemia. Leukopenia with lymphopenia is often a measure of disease activity.[1,2,5] When it occurs in the absence of cytotoxic drug therapy in patients with SLE, it is not a significant risk for infection.

Treatment of Coombs-positive hemolytic anemia with an acute declining hematocrit and reticulocytosis requires treatment with high-dose steroids. When the hematocrit rises, steroids can be tapered. Pulse dose IV steroids, azathioprine, cyclophosphamide, or splenectomy may be used if unresponsive to high-dose oral steroids. In refractory cases, IV immune globulin and danazol have been used.

Even though mild thrombocytopenia is common in all patients with no serious sequelae, approximately 5% of patients experience severe thrombocytopenia with bleeding and purpura necessitating treatment with high dose corticosteroids.

Serious organ involvement such as neuropsychiatric manifestations, hemolytic anemia, APS, and renal disease in SLE is associated with thrombocytopenia. Thrombocytopenia can be categorized into two groups and forecasts a poor prognosis for SLE and increased mortality. Acute thrombocytopenia may occur with severe, multisystem SLE disease flares or is present even when the disease is otherwise quiescent.[43]

Management of Antiphospholipid Syndrome with Systemic Lupus Erythematosus. In nonpregnant patients with poor results to steroids, IV gamma globulin is indicated for short-term improvement. Immunosuppression is only given in APS in the presence of severe thrombocytopenia. Cytotoxic drugs such as vincristine, cyclosporine, danazole, and/or splenectomy may be necessary as adjunctive agents when conventional treatment measures are not effective in reversing low platelet counts within 2 weeks. Rituximab, an anti-CD20 chimeric monoclonal antibody, which effectively depletes B cells, may be considered when the patient is refractory to high-dose steroids, and before splenectomy if the patient is at risk of surgery (splenectomy) due to APS. Patients have shown to have a rapid and sustained effect resulting in a significant decrease in immunoglobulin M (IgM) cardiolipin titers after 4 weekly doses, allowing progressive tapering of daily prednisone doses to less than or equal to 5 mg.[44]

Prophylaxis heparin or low molecular weight (LMW) heparin therapy is used during pregnancy in women with antiphospholipid antibodies who have a history of thrombotic events or spontaneous abortions.[45] Although the use of low-dose aspirin during pregnancy has been reported effective in preventing thrombosis and fetal loss by some investigators, controlled, randomized clinical trials are needed to confirm these findings. Warfarin is contraindicated in the first trimester due to its teratogenicity. In the second and third trimesters, warfarin should be used with caution because it is associated with an increased risk of maternal and fetal bleeding.

Patients with persistent LA or aCL antibodies and a history of thrombosis are at increased risk of recurrent thrombosis. Life-long anticoagulation with warfarin has demonstrated benefit in decreasing the incidence of recurrent thrombosis.

Chronic anticoagulation with warfarin is indicated for the prevention of catastrophic thrombotic events, because arterial thrombosis can result in strokes, transient ischemic attacks, and gangrene of the extremities or digits.

Heparin may be needed to be substituted for warfarin during pregnancy. Patients with APS who are at risk for recurrent thrombosis are prescribed heparin, warfarin, LMW heparins or antiplatelet drug such as low-dose aspirin in patients with a contraindication or intolerance to heparin. Normal fertility rates occur in SLE patients, however, pregnancy has varied effects on SLE disease activity.

In the absence of SLE-related severe renal or cardiac disease and quiescent states, full-term pregnancy resulting in the delivery of normal infants is predicted. In case of severe disease activity during pregnancy, corticosteroids can be administered because they do not cause fetal abnormalities.

Another complication associated with APS is neonatal lupus. It occurs when maternal anti-Ro (SS-A) is transmitted across the placenta. The infant may develop a transient skin rash, thrombocytopenia, and rarely, permanent heart block.

Evidence supporting the use of low-dose aspirin, ticlopidine, or clopidrogel in the prevention of thrombosis in patients with positive antiphospholipid antibodies is lacking.

No difference in the overall risk of recurrent thrombosis was shown in randomized clinical trials evaluating standard [target international normalized ratio (INR) 2.0–3.0] or high intensity (target INR 3.0–4.0) warfarin in patients with APS. In fact, a lower rate of thrombosis was seen in the standard therapy group. Chronic standard warfarin therapy in doses to maintain INR at 2.0 to 3.0 has been shown effective in the prevention of venous and arterial thrombosis.[46,47]

Patients who develop recurrent thrombosis while maintaining a therapeutic INR of 2.0 to 3.0 may need to be switched to high intensity warfarin therapy or started on low-dose aspirin therapy.[48]

Furthermore, investigators have found no statistically significant difference in the risk of stroke in patients with APS as compared to patients without APS, or that warfarin was superior to aspirin for secondary prevention of stroke in a large, randomized clinical trial.

Steroids with or without immunosuppressive drugs with anticoagulation have been used for acute flares in nonpregnant patients with APS. Consideration for degenerative vascular changes in blood vessels (from hyperlipidemia and circulating immune complexes) from long-term steroid use may predispose them to cerebral and CAD, so in some patients, anticoagulation is more appropriate than immunosuppression.

Safety of prednisone and NSAIDs in pregnancy is not well established. No evidence exists for risks to the fetus of prednisone (<20 mg/da) or NSAIDs in the first two trimesters. Potential toxicities associated with prednisone include gestational diabetes and hypertension. NSAIDs should be avoided in the last trimester due to potential premature closure of the ductus, prolonged labor, and peripartum hemorrhage. Short-acting NSAIDs, such as ibuprofen and low-dose oral prednisone, have poor transfer into breast milk and are considered safe for breast-feeding mothers to use.[49]

NONPHARMACOLOGIC THERAPY

Because no cure for SLE has been found, pharmacologic and nonpharmacologic treatment are aimed at controlling symptoms, minimizing fatigue, and restoring activities of daily living.

Patient education and counseling is an important element of nonpharmacologic management of SLE and minimizing complications related to therapy. Clinicians should encourage general lifestyle measures to limit the onset and severity of disease exacerbations. Patients must be counseled about the avoidance of overexposure to sunlight and the use of high-factor sunscreen protection. Ideal body weight should be achieved and maintained because obesity stresses the musculoskeletal system. Vigorous activity should be avoided when the joints are tender and inflamed because of the danger of intensifying joint inflammation or causing injury to surrounding areas weakened by inflammation. However, modest physical activity will maintain good joint movement and prevent muscular atrophy. Dietary and lifestyle modifications should include a good balance of rest and moderate exercise, smoking cessation, appropriate nutritional food intake diet, and adherence to a diet low in saturated fat.

Weight-bearing exercises and oral calcium and vitamin D supplementation are the first steps in the prevention of osteoporosis. However most patients will also require bisphosphonate therapy.

ALTERNATIVE THERAPIES

SLE patients may seek other ways of treating the disease because of the nature, cost, and potential for serious adverse effects from conventional therapy. Randomized clinical trials using alternative methods of treatment in SLE such as special diets, nutritional supplements, fish oils, ointments and creams, chiropractic treatment, and homeopathy need to be further investigated to assess their effectiveness in stabilizing disease or preventing organ damage.[5] Some of these alternative or complementary approaches may not be harmful, and may be reasonable in some patients due to their symptomatic and psychological benefit. These approaches and support groups may also help patients cope with some of the stress associated with living with chronic illness if incorporated into the patient's treatment plan.

SLE patients must trust their health care providers and feel comfortable in asking questions about care because it will allow them to engage in an open dialogue, make informed choices about treatment options, seek medical help when needed, and keep appointments for regular health checkups and follow-up.

FUTURE THERAPIES

Clinical investigators are looking for newer agents to replace broad immunosuppression with early, selective, and individualized intervention. The U.S. Food and Drug Administration (FDA) is preparing new guidelines for drug companies developing lupus drugs to consider proxy biologic markers and other techniques that can show more clearly that new drugs are efficacious.[50,51]

The precise role of genetic and environmental factors in the development of SLE is unknown. Furthermore, there are clear differences in racial susceptibility to SLE and its complications such as lupus nephritis. Identification of susceptibility genes and their contribution to disease are also under investigation. Patient-specific genetic ''portfolios'' coupled with more understanding of environmental triggers could lead to more effective preventative therapy in the future.

Immunomodulation and better drug delivery resulting in antigen-specific gene tolerance induction, up regulation of anti-inflammatory or down regulation of inflammatory pathways, and the elimination of activated immune cells by advances in biotechnology are anticipated in the future.

Research into new targets for therapy is now underway including induction of tolerance to self-antigens, prevention of autoantibody production, interference with cytokines, and signaling pathways activated during the autoimmune antibody-mediated processes.

One such strategy using anti–B-cell therapy with Rituximab (anti-CD-20) has been shown to block the T–cell-mediated antibody production from B lymphocytes. Clinical trials investigating the efficacy and safety of rituximab in blocking autoantibodies are underway in SLE patients.[52]

Other T-cell inhibitors under investigation include anti-CD4 monoclonal antibodies, anti-CD40 ligand monoclonal antibodies, and cytotoxic T lymphocyte antigen (CTLA)-41g.[53] The safety and efficacy in SLE of other experimental biologic agents such as anticytokine monoclonal antibodies, particularly anti-IL-6 and anti-IL-10 monoclonal antibodies and anti–TNF-therapy, will be assessed in future clinical trials. Other experimental strategies that need further investigation include manipulation of apoptosis, suppression of

complement activation, suppression of anti-dsDNA production, gene therapy, and stem cell transplantations.

Investigation is also underway in the identification and treatment of microorganism triggers and stem cell therapy. The FDA is currently reviewing the hormone DHEA in SLE. If approved, it will be the first medication specifically approved for SLE in the last 30 years.[54]

The role of DHEA, a hormone produced primarily by the adrenal glands, and SLE has been investigated. Low levels of DHEA have been observed in patients with SLE. Corticosteroid administration may also decrease DHEA production. Several placebo-control studies with orally administered synthetic prasterone (200 mg/day) have shown it improves symptoms associated with mild to moderate, severe, and active SLE or it stabilizes disease activity better than placebo.[5]

After adrenal production, DHEA is believed to have mild intrinsic androgenic properties and is a precursor for the synthesis in peripheral tissues of various sex steroids. DHEA serum levels are low in patients with SLE irrespective of disease activity or treatment. DHEA may also have mild immunoregulatory properties. Its effects in humans have not been fully elucidated, although T-cell immunomodulation and an increase in IL-2, IL-5, and IL-6 have been observed in murine and in vitro experimental models. The likely benefits of DHEA reported in published and unpublished studies include the overall improvement of SLE symptomatology and decreased corticosteroid requirement. Potential benefits of DHEA therapy include decreased flares, bone-sparing effect, and improved cognitive function. Acne is the most frequent side effect reported in DHEA trials in SLE. Long-term safety and efficacy are not yet established, including the potential risks on lowering HDL cholesterol, unknown hormonal effects on the endometrium, ovaries, and breast in women with SLE. Also the risks and benefits of DHEA use in men with SLE are unknown. More importantly, patients should be advised to avoid over-the-counter DHEA preparations because the reliability and purity of such preparations is unregulated in the United States.

In a randomized double-blind clinical trial,[55] prasterone (200 mg/day) was shown to improve symptoms or stabilize symptoms of active disease in female patients with SLE and was generally well tolerated. Patients received standard treatment for 12 months (prednisone ≤10 mg/da, antimalarials, immunosuppressive agents with doses stable for 6 months prior to study entry and remain the same throughout trial). Acne and hirsuitism were reported as the main adverse drug reactions (ADRs) while taking prasterone. Serum levels of HDL cholesterol, triglycerides, and C3 complement significantly decreased during prasterone therapy. Serum testosterone increased and estradiol increased to a lesser extent.

Bromocriptine, a dopamine agonist that selectively inhibits prolactin secretion from the pituitary has been shown to be useful in nonlife-threatening SLE.[5] Gonadotrophin releasing hormone (GnRH) has been shown in mice to be immunostimulatory, however, its role in SLE needs to be determined.

Ways to prevent spontaneous abortions during pregnancy include the identification of gene activity patterns to help in diagnosis and in monitoring the disease. Interferon-α has potent effects on the immune system and may play a role in the development of SLE, thus investigators are trying to find ways to block it. To target B cells and block their destructive effects, drugs need to be found that would selectively eliminate disease-causing B-cells without harming normal infection-fighting B cells.

IMPROVING OUTCOMES

PATIENT EDUCATION

At the initial referral patients should be educated about the nature of their condition. They need to know that SLE usually is a lifelong disease. Current therapy can provide significant improvement, but complete relief is unlikely. Failure to follow a therapeutic plan can lead to unnecessary morbidity and mortality.[56]

Patients need to know that prognosis has improved over the years and survival in SLE patients is 90% to 95% at 2 years, 82% to 90% at 5 years, 71% to 80% at 10 years, and 63% to 75% at 20 years. In lupus nephritis patients, the overall survival rate in the first 10 years is approximately 75% to 85%.[15,57] Overall, the 10-year survival rate has increased from 50% in the 1950s to 90%.[58]

A multicenter observational study included 1,000 SLE patients followed by a team of physicians from 1990–2000 reported their findings. The mean age of participants at study entry was 37 years and mean age of death was 44 years. The mortality rate in this study was a modest 8% at 10 years. Deaths were attributed to active disease, infections, thrombosis, and malignancy; however, infections and active SLE were the leading cause of deaths in the first 5 years, whereas thrombosis was the leading cause of death in the second 5 years. The presence of lupus nephritis at time of diagnosis was the strongest predictor of death. It was shown that patients in the first 5 years tend to have more inflammatory manifestations and disease activity than those in the second 5 years of the disease. Patients also experience fewer infections, less nephropathy, less arthritis, and less disease activity in the second 5 years.[59]

African-Americans and Hispanics generally have severe disease and poor outcome.[16,60] Poor prognostic indicators include the presence of high serum creatinine levels, hypertension, nephritic syndrome, anemia, hypoalbuminemia, hypocomplementemia at time of diagnosis, and low socioeconomic status. Other factors leading to poor prognosis include thrombocytopenia, serious CNS lupus, antibodies to phospholipids, and African-American race. Infections, active renal disease activity, and thromboembolic events are the leading causes of death attributed to SLE in the first and second decades.

Prevention of disease-related and treatment-related long-term consequences of SLE is very important. Identify risk factors for arteriosclerotic disease and treat aggressively. Provide appropriate dietary advice and lipid-lowering therapy, if necessary. An elevated serum homocysteine level is an independent risk factor for arteriosclerosis and may be present or even higher in SLE patients.

Patients should be counseled to avoid taking over-the-counter NSAIDs unless they are under a physician's direction. They should be monitored for NSAID-related adverse effects associated with GI, hematologic, liver, and kidney findings. Patients taking high-dose steroids and cyclophosphamide have a higher risk of infection, thus patients should be counseled to practice good hygiene and hand washing techniques. Clinicians should consider prophylaxis against *Pneumocystis carinii* pneumonia and prescribe vaccinations against influenza and pneumococcus being mindful to also avoid live/attenuated vaccines in SLE patients receiving immunosuppression. Osteoporosis prevention with standard therapy is essential. Common respiratory infections can be prevented by frequent hand washing and other simple hygiene measures.

Fatigue is the most common complaint and an often debilitating symptom that may be controlled by energy conservation. Other potentially beneficial strategies include photoprotection by protective clothing and high-factor sunscreen use and avoidance of excess sun. Contraception control consisting of avoiding pregnancy during increased disease activity or while using immunosuppressive therapy is also advised. It is also important to rule out the presence of anti-Ro (SSA) in women because they are at risk of transferring antibodies to the fetus resulting in neonatal lupus, congenital heart block, or miscarriage. Pregnancy may lead to an increased risk of flareups. Breast-feeding may increase the risk of a postpartum flareup by the proinflammatory effects of prolactin.

METHODS TO IMPROVE ADHERENCE

Research literature addressing patient adherence issues for SLE treatment has identified several factors that influence adherence among adults. Patients requiring treatment may not experience symptoms of the disease, but may experience toxicity of the medication and may require additional education to convince the patient of the importance of medication adherence. Factors that may influence adherence include competing demand on time, knowledge of SLE and preventative therapy, intention to take medication, lack of social support, financial burden of medications and care, and reliance on alternative medications. Some programs use peers on a telephone hotline to provide emotional support for people with lupus or for family members with lupus.

Persons affected by lupus and their families need help in understanding SLE because it is a multisystem disease with no cure. A multidisciplinary support network should be in place as patients deal with depression, fear, and possible disability. Of utmost importance is the role of pharmacists in medication counseling and preventative care of long-term health consequences, joint protection principles, energy conservation, pain and stress management, and coping techniques in a multidisciplinary approach.

Some barriers to overcome to improve adherence have been identified. In one study, depression, medication concerns, physical symptoms, and the need for child and elder care were associated with nonadherence in African-American women. Perceived treatment inefficacy and lacking trust in physicians were associated with nonadherence in whites.[61]

Another study showed that a multidisciplinary approach using educational interventions designed to improve self-efficacy, couple communication about lupus, social support, and problem solving followed by monthly telephone calls significantly improved couple communication, self-efficacy, mental health status, and fatigue.[62]

DISEASE MANAGEMENT STRATEGIES TO IMPROVE PATIENT OUTCOMES

Pain, lifestyle changes, and emotional problems are the most difficult to cope with. Steroid-sparing protocols, prophylaxis for infections, and prevention of osteoporosis are recommended.[63] Prevention of lupus-related complications from lupus itself or its treatment such as hypertension, hypercholesterolemia, and osteoporosis should be undertaken. Regular checkups, preventative screening (pap smear, mammography for women and prostate exam for men) and an update on immunizations for influenza and pneumococcus are recommended in all patients.

The prognosis of SLE has improved largely due to the early recognition of milder forms of the disease, vigilant monitoring, preventive infection control measures, and the use of pulse dose corticosteroids and immunosuppressive agents in severe disease. However, patients with renal and CNS disease have the worst 5-year survival rates, and infection continues to be a major cause of death.

Safety of estrogens for birth control, regulating menstrual cycles for women, and as hormonal replacement therapy in SLE is under investigation by the National Institutes of Health.

Some outstanding issues to be resolved in the future regarding patients with SLE include the role of anticoagulation in patients with APS without previous thrombosis, therapy of neuropsychiatric SLE, uniform definition of clinical endpoints for clinical trials in SLE, accurate assessment of disease activity and predictors of flareups in lupus pregnancy, and identifying strategies in the management of patients with serologic markers before evidence of clinical disease.[64]

DRUG-INDUCED LUPUS

The etiology of DIL is unknown. Drugs may induce the antigenicity of nucleoproteins leading to the production of autoantibodies and the production of antihistone antibodies.

A number of drugs have been implicated in the induction of a lupuslike syndrome known as DIL erythematosus with manifestations ranging from an isolated positive ANA test result to a clinical lupus syndrome.[1–3,5]

Although more than 100 drugs have been reported to cause DIL, the drugs most commonly implicated are hydralazine and procainamide. Other drugs include quinidine, phenytoin, primidone, isoniazid, chlorpromazine, penicillamine, practolol, propylthiouracil, methylthiouracil, and methyldopa (Table 68.7).

The gender ratio for DIL is equal, whereas it is predominant in women in idiopathic SLE. DIL is reportedly more prevalent in whites. Clinical features tend to be milder in DIL and commonly include arthritis, arthralgias, myalgias, and fever. Pleural and pericardial effusions are prominent. A photosensitive skin rash, lymphadenopathy, splenomegaly, anemia, leucopenia are less likely to occur. CNS involvement and renal disease are usually absent. SLE patients with systemic or cutaneous disease are not at higher risk of developing flares if prescribed these agents for other conditions.

TABLE 68.7	Drug-Induced Lupus (DIL)

Definite

Procainamide, hydralazine, minocycline, diltiazem, penicillamine, isoniazid, infliximab, etanercept, interferon-alfa, methyldopa, chlorpromazine, practolol.

Probable

Phenytoin, trimethadione, ethosuximide, quinidine, antithyroid drugs, sulfonamides, rifampin, nitrofurantoin, β-blockers, lithium, paraaminosalicylate, captopril, interferon gamma, hydrochlorothiazide, glyburide, carbamazepine, sulfasalazine, terbinafine, amiodarone, ticlopidine, docetaxel

Possible

Gold salts, penicillin, tetracycline, reserpine, valproate, lovastatin, simvastatin, atorvastatin, griseofulvin, gemfibrozil, timolol ophthalmic

(From Petri MA. Systemic lupus erythematosus: clinical aspects. In: Koopman WJ, et al., eds. Arthritis and allied conditions—a textbook of rheumatology. 14th ed. Philadelphia: Lippincott Williams & Wilkins, 2001: 1455–1492; Wallace DJ, Hahn BH, eds. Dubois' lupus erythematosus. 6th ed. Philadelphia: Lippincott Williams & Wilkins, 2002; Humes HD, ed. Kelley's Essentials of internal medicine. 2nd ed. Philadelphia: Lippincott Williams & Wilkins, 2001; Lahita RG, ed. Systemic lupus erythematosus. 4th ed. London: Elsevier Academic Press, 2004; Hahn BH. Systemic lupus erythematosus. In: Braunwald E, et al., eds. Harrison's principles of internal medicine. 15th ed. New York: McGraw-Hill, 2001:1922–1928; Peterson KS, Winchester RJ. Systemic lupus erythematosus: pathogenesis. In: Koopman WJ, et al., eds. Arthritis and allied conditions—a textbook of rheumatology. 14th ed. Philadelphia: Lippincott Williams & Wilkins, 2001.)

Laboratory studies in patients may help distinguish the syndrome from spontaneous SLE. A positive ANA test result tends to have antibodies to single-stranded DNA (anti-dsDNA is typically not present) and antihistone-DNA complex. Antihistone antibodies are present in more than 90% of cases but are not specific for DIL. Serum complement is rarely reduced in DIL. Because there are no established criteria for the diagnosis of DIL by the ACR, clinicians should be aware that patients may present with fewer than four symptoms. Diagnosis of DIL is usually based on temporal association of clinical manifestations to drug ingestion and a positive ANA followed by a remission of symptoms following discontinuation of the offending agent (Table 68.8).

It has been estimated that 5% to 10% of all lupus cases in the United States may be drug related. Hydralazine and procainamide are the drugs most frequently reported to cause DIL. Typically, patients present with clinical manifestations of DIL after many months or years of chronic use. Up to 30% of patients taking procainamide who seroconvert from negative to positive ANA develop DIL. Even though clinical manifestations have been reported to develop as early after procainamide treatment as 1 week and as late after treatment as 12 years, they usually occur within a few months to a year. Up to 21% of patients taking high-dose hydralazine (200 mg/day) or a cumulative dose of 100 g develop DIL.

Risk factors in susceptible individuals are related to duration of hydralazine therapy and dose. Patients with the HLA-DR3 antigen are at risk of developing DIL. They are classified as ''slow acetylators'' and have a genetically determined inability to acetylate the amine or hydrazine moiety of these drugs. Nonacetylated metabolites accumulate, bind to nucleoprotein or cellular macromolecules, form an antigenic complex, and induce an immune reaction. Drugs chemically related to aromatic amine and hydrazines, such as procainamide and hydralazine, may lead to DIL in genetically slow acetylator phenotypes.[65]

The risk of developing DIL is substantially less with other reported drugs. Symptoms usually resolve in a few weeks when the offending agent is removed, although the ANA test may remain positive for several months after withdrawal of the agent.

NSAIDs may help to control symptoms of DIL associated with arthritis, myalgias, fever, and pleuritis. Although systemic manifestations are rare in DIL, corticosteroids and immunosuppressives may be indicated.

Clinicians should be aware of postmarketing surveillance and case reports of DIL reported with newer agents. Ticlopidine, rituximab, terbinafine, celecoxib, infliximab, etanercept, and ziprasidone have been associated anecdotally with SLE. The ANA was increased by 10% in all patients receiving the drugs.[66–69]

Cotrimazole has been known to trigger the onset of SLE in susceptible individuals, and in others with a prior diagnosis of SLE it has induced symptomatic flares. It is thought that sulfa drugs may be linked to lupus activity and clinicians ask patients to avoid them.

PHARMACOECONOMICS

Health care costs and patient outcomes are important considerations and considerable in SLE and lupus nephritis especially in cases when patients progress to ESRD end-stage renal disease requiring hemodialysis or renal transplantation. Long-term sequelae associated with cardiovascular and hematologic complications such as stroke and myocardial infarction (MI) in addition to those sequelae associated with steroid treatment such as osteoporosis or avascular necrosis,

---

TABLE 68.8	Guidelines for Identifying Drug-Induced Lupus

1. Continuous treatment with a known lupus-inducing drug for at least 1 month and usually much longer.

2. Presenting symptoms:

   Common: arthralgias, myalgias, malaise, fever, serositis (pleuropericarditis, especially with procainamide), polyarthritis (especially with quinidine and minicycline).

   Rare: rash or other dermatologic problems, glomerulonephritis (primarily with hydralazine).

3. Unrelated symptoms suggestive of SLE: multisystem involvement especially neurologic, renal, and skin symptoms.

4. Laboratory profile:

   Common: ANA that is due to antihistone antibodies especially IgG anti-[(H2A-H2B)-DNA], leukopenia, thrombocytopenia, and mild anemia, increased ESR.

   Absent or rare: antibodies to native DNA, 5m, RNP, Ro (SSA); Ila (SSB); hypocomplementemia.

5. Improvement and permanent resolution of symptoms generally within days or weeks after discontinuation of therapy. Serologic findings, especially autoantibody levels, often require months to resolve.

SLE, systemic lupus erythematosus; ANA, antinuclear antibodies; IgG, immunoglobulin G; ESR, erythrocyte sedimentation rate; Sm, Smith antibodies; RNP, ribonucleoprotein.
(From Wallace DJ, Hahn BH, eds. Dubois' Lupus erythematosus, 6th ed. Philadelphia: Lippincott Williams & Wilkins, 2002: 896.)

significantly affect quality of life and the rise in health care costs. Serious infections associated with immunosuppressive therapy are also important quality of life and health cost considerations.[70–72]

Inflated by the Medical Care consumer price index to 2000, the annual direct costs for SLE in the United States was reported at $15,733. The true financial burden of SLE on patients, payers, employers, and society is underestimated using annual direct costs. This is especially true for SLE because the disease inflicts young individuals at the prime of their productivity and subjects them to chronic disability.

A subsequent report was issued in 2002.[73] The average annual cost of lupus relating to medical and lost productivity has been estimated at $26,000 per person. In 2002, this translated into an annual cost of $7.3 billion dollars based on an estimate of 270,000 people with SLE in the United States.

KEY POINTS

- The etiology and pathogenesis of SLE involves complicated and multifactorial interactions among various genetic and environmental factors.
- Multiple genes contribute to disease susceptibility, including genes encoding complement and other components, of the immune response, and HLA Class I and Class II genes.
- The interaction of gender, hormonal milieu, environmental factors, and the hypothalamic-pituitary-adrenal (HPA) axis is probably required to precipitate the onset of disease.
- Defective immune regulatory mechanisms, such as the clearance of apoptotic cells and immune complexes, are important contributors to the development of SLE.
- The loss of immune tolerance, increased antigenic load, excess T-cell help, defective B-cell suppression, and the shifting of T helper 1 (Th1) to Th2 immune responses leads to B-cell hyperactivity and the production of pathogenic autoantibodies associated with SLE.
- Management of SLE is complicated by variability in clinical presentation and course of disease and response to therapy.
- NSAIDs and antimalarials may be effective in mild forms of the disease affecting the cutaneous and musculoskeletal systems
- Steroids and/or potent immunosuppressives may be used to manage moderate to severe SLE including lupus nephritis, CNS lupus, or APS.
- The risk of myocardial infarction, stroke, kidney failure, and osteoporosis is higher in SLE patients than in the general population.
- The goal of therapy is to suppress disease activity and progression to end-organ failure and minimize toxicity of treatment.
- Patient outcome in SLE is has been steadily improving but potential infections and drug-related adverse side effects are complications associated with immunosuppressive therapy.

SUGGESTED READINGS

Lahita RG, ed. Systemic lupus erythematosus. 4th ed. London: Elsevier Academic Press, 2004.

Petri MA. Systemic lupus erythematosus: clinical aspects. In: Koopman WJ, ed. Arthritis and allied conditions—A textbook of rheumatology. 14th ed. Philadelphia: Lippincott Williams & Wilkins, 2001: 1455–1492.

Wallace DJ, Hahn BH, eds. Dubois' lupus erythematosus. 6th ed. Philadelphia: Lippincott Williams & Wilkins, 2002.

REFERENCES

1. Petri MA. Systemic lupus erythematosus: clinical aspects. In: Koopman WJ, ed. Arthritis and allied conditions—a textbook of rheumatology. 14th ed. Philadelphia: Lippincott Williams & Wilkins, 2001: 1455–1492.
2. Wallace DJ, Hahn BH, eds. Dubois' lupus erythematous. 6th ed. Philadelphia: Lippincott Williams & Wilkins, 2002.
3. Humes HD, ed. Kelley's Essentials of internal medicine. 2nd ed. Philadelphia: Lippincott Williams & Wilkins, 2001.
4. Borchers AT, Keen CL, Shoenfeld Y, et al. Surviving the butterfly and the wolf: mortality trend in systemic erythematosus. Autoimmun Rev 3:423–453, 2004.
5. Lahita RG, ed. Systemic lupus erythematosus. 4th ed. London: Elsevier Academic Press, 2004.
6. Mok CC, Lau CS. Pathogenesis of systemic lupus erythematosus. J Clin Pathol 56:481–490, 2003.
7. Shen N, Tsao BP. Current advances in the human lupus genetics. Curr Rheumatol Rep 6:391–398, 2004.
8. Hahn BH. Systemic lupus erythematosus. In: Kasper DL, Braunwald E, Fauci AS, et al., eds. Harrison's principles of internal medicine. 15th ed. New York: McGraw-Hill, 2001:1922–1928.
9. Peterson KS, Winchester RJ. Systemic lupus erythematosus: pathogenesis. In: Koopman WJ, ed. Arthritis and allied conditions—a textbook of rheumatology. 14th ed. Philadelphia: Lippincott Williams & Wilkins, 2001.
10. Mok MY, Jack DL, Lau CS, et al. Antibodies to mannose binding lecithin in patients with systemic lupus erythematosus. Lupus 13: 522–528, 2004.
11. Sanchez-Guerrero J, Liang MH, Karlson EW, et al. Postmenopausal estrogen therapy and the risk of developing systemic lupus erythematosus. Ann Intern Med 122:430–433, 1995.
12. Sanchez-Guerrero J, Karlson EW, Liang MH, et al. Past use of oral contraceptives and the risk of developing systemic lupus erythematosus. Arthritis Rheum 40:804–808, 1997.
13. Meir CR, Sturkenboom NC, Cohen AS, et al. Postmenopausal estrogen replacement therapy and the risk of developing systemic erythematosus or discoid lupus. J Rheumatol 25:1515–1519, 1998.
14. McCarthy DJ, Manzi S, Medsger TA, et al. Incidence of systemic lupus erythematosus. Race and gender differences. Arthritis Rheum 38:1260–1270, 1995.
15. Uramoto KM, Michet CJ Jr, Thumboo J, et al. Trends in the incidence and mortality of systemic lupus erythematosus. 1950–1992. Arthritis Rheum 42:46–50, 1999.
16. Anon. Trends in deaths from systemic lupus erythematosus–United States, 1979–1998. MMWR 51:371–373, 2002.
17. Hahn B. Pathogenesis of systemic lupus erythematosus. In: Ruddy S, Harris ED Jr, Sledge CB, et al., eds. Kelley's textbook of rheumatology. 6th ed. Philadelphia: WB Saunders, 2001:1089–1103.
18. Shur P. Systemic lupus erythematosus. In: Goldman L, Bennett J, eds. Cecil textbook of medicine. 21st ed. Philadelphia: WB Saunders, 2000:1509–1517.
19. Gill JM, Quisel AM, Rocca PV, et al. Diagnosis of systemic lupus erythematosus. Am Fam Physician 68:2179–2186, 2003.

20. Tan EM, Cohen AS, Fries JF, et al. The 1982 revised criteria for the classification of systemic lupus erythematosus. Arthritis Rheum 25:1271–1277, 1982.

21. Hochberg MC. Updating the American College of Rheumatology revised criteria for the classification of systemic lupus erythematosus [Letter]. Arthritis Rheum 40:1725, 1997.

22. Reeves WH, Satoh M. Autoantibodies in systemic erythematosus. In: Koopman WJ, ed. Arthritis and allied conditions—a textbook of rheumatology. 14th ed. Philadelphia: Lippincott Williams & Wilkins, 2001.

23. Arbuckle MR, McClain MT, Rubertone MV, et al. Development of autoantibodies before the onset of systematic lupus erythematosus. N Engl J Med 348:1526–1533, 2003.

24. American College of Rheumatology. Guidelines for referral and management of systemic lupus erythematosus in adults. American College of Rheumatology Ad Hoc Committee on Systemic Lupus Erythematosus Guidelines. Arthritis Rheum 42:1785–1796, 1999.

25. Wiedemann H, Matthay R. Pulmonary manifestations of systemic lupus erythematosus. J Thorac Imaging 7:1–18, 1992.

26. Bijl M, Brouwer J, Kallenberg GG. Cardiac abnormalities in SLE: pancarditis (clinical conference) Lupus 9:236–240, 2000.

27. Karrar A, Aqueira W, Block JA. Coronary artery disease in systemic lupus erythematosus. Semin Arthritis Rheum 30:436–443, 2001.

28. Manzi S, Meilahn EN, Rairie JE, et al. Age-specific incidence rates of myocardial infarction and angina in women with systemic lupus erythematosus: comparison with the Framingham Study. Am J Epidemiol 145:408–415, 1997.

29. Roman MJ, Shanker B-A, Davis A, et al. Prevalence and correlated of accelerated atherosclerosis in systemic lupus erythematosus. N Engl J Med 349:2399–2406, 2003.

30. Asanuma Y, Oeser A, Shintani AK, et al. Premature coronary-artery atherosclerosis in systemic lupus erythematosus. N Engl J Med 349:2407–2415, 2003.

31. Kotzin BL, Achenbach GA, West SG. Renal involvement in systemic lupus erythematosus. In: Koopman WJ, ed. Arthritis and allied conditions—a textbook of rheumatology. 14th ed. Philadelphia: Lippincott Williams & Wilkins, 2001.

32. Lockshin MD, Sammaritano LR. Lupus pregnancy. Autoimmunity 36:33–40, 2003.

33. Available at: http://www.fda.gov/medwatch/SAFETY/2004/safety04.htm#vioxx. Accessed 10/05/2005.

34. The Celecoxib Long-term Arthritis Safety Study (CLASS) compared celecoxib with the non-selective NSAIDs ibuprofen and diclofenac with regard to the incidence of adverse GI events. JAMA 284:1247–1255, 2000.

35. Finbloom DS, Silver K, Newsome DA, et al. Comparison of hydroxychloroquine and chloroquine use and the development of retinal toxicity. J Rheumatol 12:692–694, 1985.

36. The Canadian Hydroxychloroquine Study Group. A randomized study of the effect of withdrawing hydroxychloroquine sulfate in systemic lupus erythematosus. N Engl J Med 324:150–154, 1991.

37. Hejaili FF, Moist LM, Clark WF. Treatment of lupus nephritis. Drugs 63:257–274, 2003.

38. Reveille JD. The treatment of systemic lupus erythematosus. In: Koopman WJ, ed. Arthritis and allied conditions—a textbook of rheumatology. 14th ed. Philadelphia: Lippincott Williams & Wilkins, 2001.

39. Flanc RS, Strippoli GF, Chadban SJ, et al. Treatment of diffuse proliferative lupus nephritis: a meta-analysis of randomized controlled trials. Am J Kidney Dis 43;197–208, 2004.

40. Balow JE, Austin HA. Maintenance therapy for lupus nephritis. N Engl J Med 350:1044–1046, 2004.

41. Badsha H, Edwards CJ. Intravenous pulses of methylprednisolone for systemic lupus erythematosus. Semin Arthritis Rheum 32:370–377, 2003.

42. Contreras G, Pardo V, Leclercq B, et al. Sequential therapies for proliferative lupus nephritis. N Engl J Med 350:971–980, 2004.

43. Levine JS, Branch DW, Rauch J. The antiphospholipid syndrome. N Engl J Med 346:752–763, 2002.

44. Erdozain JG, Ruiz-Irastorza G, Egurbide MV, et al. Sustained response to rituximab of autoimmune hemolytic anemia associated with antiphospholipid syndrome. Haematologica 89:34, 2004.

45. Petri M. Hopkins lupus cohort: 1999 update. Rheum Dis Clin North Am 26:199–213, 2000.

46. Crowther MA, Ginsberg JS, Julian J, et al. A comparison of two intensities of warfarin for the prevention of recurrent thrombosis in patients with the antiphospholipid antibody syndrome. N Engl J Med 349:1133–1138, 2003.

47. Finazzi G, Marchioli R, Barbui T. A randomized clinical trial of oral anticoagulant therapy in patients with antiphospholipid syndrome: the WAPS study [abstract]. J Thromb Haemost 1 (Suppl 1):OC365, 2003.

48. Levine SR, Brey RL, Tilley BC, et al. Antiphospholipid antibodies and subsequent thrombo-occlusive events in patients with ischemic stroke. APASS-WARSS STUDY. JAMA 291:576–584, 2004.

49. Spencer JP, Gonzalez LS, Barnhart DJ. Medications in the breast-feeding mother. Am Fam Physician 64:119–126, 2001.

50. Illei GG, Tackey E, Lapteva L, et al. Biomarkers in systemic lupus erythematosus. I. General overview of biomarkers and their applicability. Arthritis Rheum 50:1709–1720, 2004.

51. Mittleman BB. Biomarkers for systemic lupus erythematosus: has the time finally arrived? Arthritis Res Ther 6:223–244, 2004.

52. Kazkaz H, Isenberg D. Anti B-cell therapy (rituximab) in the treatment of autoimmune diseases. Curr Opin Pharmacol 4:398–402, 2004.

53. Kuiper-Geertsma DG, Derksen RH. Newer drugs for the treatment of lupus nephritis. Drugs 63:167–180, 2003.

54. van Vollenhoven RF. Dehyrdroepiandrosterone in systemic lupus erythematosus. Rheum Dis Clin North Am 26:349–362, 2000.

55. Petri MA, Mease PJ, Merrill JT, et al. Effects of prasterone on disease activity and symptoms in women with active systemic lupus erythematosus. Arthritis Rheum 50:2858–2868, 2004.

56. Bruce IN, Gladman DD, Urowitz MB. Factors associated with refractory renal disease in patients with systemic lupus erythematosus. Arthritis Care Res 13:406–408, 2000.

57. Urowitz MB, Gladman DD, Abu-Shakra M, et al. Evolving spectrum of mortality and morbidity in SLE. Lupus 8:253–255, 1999.

58. Cervera R, Khalashta MA, Font J, et al. Morbidity and mortality in systemic lupus erythematosus during a 10-year period: a comparison of early and late manifestations in a cohort of 1,000 patients. Medicine 82:299–308, 2003.

59. Alarcon GC, McGwin G Jr, Bastian HM, et al. Systemic lupus erythematosus in three ethnic groups. Predictors of early mortality in the LUMINA cohort. Arthritis Rheum 45:191–202, 2001.

60. Alarcon GC, McGwin G Jr, Petri M, et al. Baseline characteristics of a multiethnic lupus cohort: PROFILE. Lupus 11:95–101, 2002.

61. Mosley-Williams A, Lumley MA, Gillis M, et al. Barriers to treatment adherence among African American and white women with systemic lupus erythematosus. Arthritis Rheum 47:630–638, 2002.

62. Karslon EW, Liang MH, Eaton H, et al. A randomized clinical trial of a psychoeducational intervention to improve outcomes in systemic lupus erythematosus. Arthritis Rheum 50:1832–1841, 2004.

63. American College of Rheumatology Ad Hoc Committee on Glucocorticoid-Induced Osteoporosis. 2001 Update. Arthritis Rheum 44:1496–1503, 2001.

64. Ruiz-Irastorza G, Khamashta MA, Castellino G, et al. Systemic lupus erythematosus. Lancet 357:1027–1031, 2003.

65. Antonov D, Kazandjieva J, Etugov D, et al. Drug-induced lupus erythematosus. Clin Dermatol 22:157–166, 2004.

66. Shakoor N, Michalska M, Harrus CA. Drug-induced systemic lupus erythematosus associated with etanercept therapy. Lancet 359:579–581, 2002.

67. Elkayam O, Caspi D. Infliximab induced lupus in patients with rheumatoid arthritis. Clin Exp Rheumatol 22:502–503, 2004.

68. Charles PJ, Smeenk RTJ, DeJong J, et al. Assessment of antibodies to double-stranded DNA induced in rheumatoid arthritis patients following treatment with infliximab, a monoclonal antibody to tumor necrosis factor α. Arthritis Rheum 43:2383–90, 2000.

69. Swensen E, Ravasia S. Ziprasidone-induced lupus erythematosus. Can J Psychiatry 49:413–414, 2004.

70. Clarke AE, Petri MA, Manzi S, et al. An international perspective on the well being and health care costs for people with systemic lupus erythematosus. Tri-Nation Study Group. J Rheumatol 26:1500–1511, 1999.

71. Clarke AE, Penrod J, St.Pierre Y, et al. Underestimating the value of women: assessing the indirect costs of women with systemic

lupus erythematosus. Tri-Nation Study Group. J Rheumatol 27: 2597–2604, 2000.

72. Gironimi G, Clarke AE, Hamilton VH, et al. Comparing health care expenditures between systemic lupus erythematosus patients in Stanford and Montreal. Arthritis Rheum 39:979–987, 1996.

73. Williams JP, Meyers JA. Immune-mediated inflammatory disorders (I.M.I.D.s): the economic and clinical costs. Am J Manag Care 8: S664–S681, 2002.

Addendum. Complete agreement among clinicians does not exist with regard to the specific instruments that should be used to measure disease activity. For a complete discussion, reader is asked to refer to:

Isenberg D, Ramsey-Goldman R. Assessing patients with lupus: towards a drug responder index. Rheumatology 38:1045–1049, 1999.

Formal Assessment of Disease Activity in SLE.

SLAM Systemic Lupus Activity Measure[1]
SLEDAI Systemic Lupus Erythematosus Disease Activity Index[2]
ECLAM European Community Lupus Activity Measure[3]
BILAG British Isles Lupus Assessment Group[4]

Assessment of Organ Damage. SLICC/ACR Systemic Lupus International Collaborative Clinics/American College of Rheumatology[5]

Patient's Assessment of Health Status. SF-20 Medical Outcome Survey Short-Form-20[6]

1. Liang M, Socher SA, Roberts WN, et al. Measurement of systemic lupus erythematosus activity in clinical research. Arthritis Rheum 31: 817–825, 1988.

2. Bombardier Q, Gladman DD, Urowitz MB, et al. Derivation of the SLEDAI. A disease activity index for lupus patients. Arthritis Rheum 35:630–640, 1992.

3. Vitali C, Bencivelli W, Isenberg DA, et al. Disease activity in systemic lupus erythematosus: report of the European Workshop for Rheumatology Research II. Identification of the variables indicative of disease activity and their use in the development of an activity score. Clin Exp Rheumatol 10:541–547, 1992.

4. Symmons DPM, Coppock JS, Bacon PA, et al. Development of a computerised index of clinical disease activity in systemic lupus erythematosus. Q J Med 69:927–937, 1988.

5. Gladman DD, Ginzler E, Goldsmith C, et al. The development and initial validation of the Systemic Lupus International Collaborating Clinics/American College of Rheumatology damage index for systemic lupus erythematosus. Arthritis Rheum 39:363–369, 1996.

6. Stewart AL, Hays RD, Ware JE Jr. The MOS Short-form general health survey reliability and validity in a patient population. Med Care 26:724–735, 1988.

Osteoporosis and Osteomalacia

69

Louise Parent-Stevens

Osteoporosis and osteomalacia are two diseases of the calcified connective tissue (bone). The primary pathologic difference is that although both cause deficient mineralization of bone, osteoporosis also results in loss of bone matrix. These disorders may be silent for an extended period, resulting in a delay of diagnosis. Patients can have both disorders concomitantly. Typically, osteomalacia is diagnosed visually in children by the bending of long bones. Osteoporosis is often undetected until a fracture occurs. As the population

ages, these bone diseases, especially osteoporosis, become increasingly prevalent. More than $15 billion is spent annually on treatment of these potentially preventable disorders.[1] Therefore, prevention must become the cornerstone of therapy. This chapter addresses the pathophysiology and etiology of osteoporosis and osteomalacia, then focuses on the various diagnostic, therapeutic, and preventive modalities currently in use.

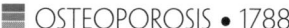

OSTEOPOROSIS

DEFINITION

Osteoporosis is defined as ''compromised bone strength predisposing a person to an increased risk of fracture''[2] (Fig. 69.1; *see color insert*). The World Health Organization

(WHO) has established general diagnostic categories of bone loss based on the degree of deviation from the mean bone mineral density (BMD) in normal young adults (T score; Table 69.1).[3]

TREATMENT GOALS

- Prevent disease by maximizing and maintaining bone mass.
- Prevent further bone loss in patients with disease
- Prevent fractures.

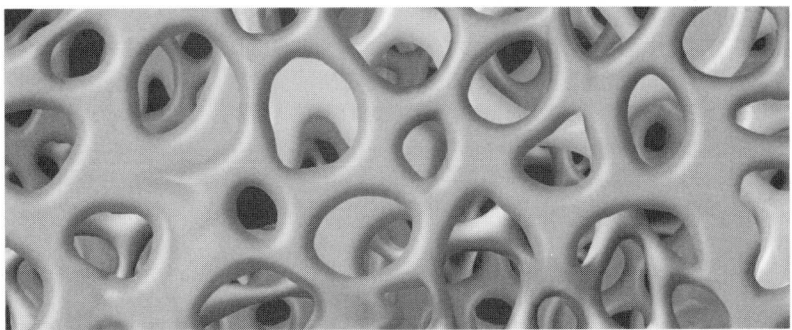
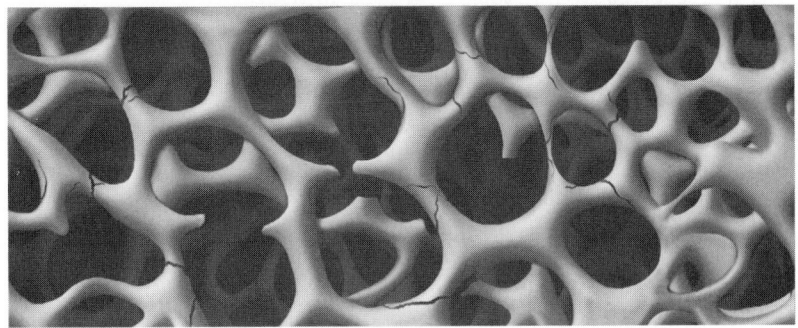

FIGURE 69.1 Comparison of healthy trabecular bone **(A)** and osteoporotic trabecular bone **(B)** (*see color insert*). In addition to an overall decrease in bone tissue, there is a decrease in trabecular size and connectivity. (Assets from Anatomical Chart Co., with permission.)

ETIOLOGY

Osteoporosis can be divided into several types. Type I (postmenopausal) osteoporosis is associated with accelerated bone loss (range 1%–5% of total bone/year) beginning with the onset of menopause and lasting approximately 10 years. This results in an increased risk of vertebral compression and distal forearm fractures in the 10 to 20 years after onset.[4,5] Type II (senile) osteoporosis is more insidious, causing progressive bone loss in both cortical and trabecular bone (approximately 0.5%–1% per year) over many years, resulting in hip and vertebral fractures (VFs) in both men and women over age 70. Type III (secondary) osteoporosis may be caused by disease, medications (Table 69.2), or immobilization due to accidents or serious illness. Secondary osteoporosis can occur at any age.

TYPE I (POSTMENOPAUSAL) OSTEOPOROSIS

Estrogen may modulate bone metabolism using multiple pathways. Binding of estrogen to receptors on osteoblasts may directly increase osteoblast activity. Estrogen binding to osteoblasts may also suppress the secretion of cytokine-

TABLE 69.1	World Health Organization Diagnostic Criteria for Osteoporosis and Osteopenia
	Bone Mineral Density (T Score[a])
Normal	<1 SD below normal
Osteopenia	1–2.5 SD below normal
Osteoporosis	≥2.5 SD below normal, no history of fractures
Severe (established) Osteoporosis	≥2.5 SD below normal, history of nonviolent fractures

[a] SD from mean of young adult bone mineral density.
(From U.S. Preventive Services Task Force. Screening for osteoporosis in postmenopausal women: recommendations and rationale. Available at: http:www.preventiveservices.ahrq.gov. Accessed Nov 9, 2005.)

TABLE 69.2	Causes of Type III (Secondary) Osteoporosis
Diseases	**Drugs**
Hyperadrenalism	Corticosteroids
Hyperthyroidism	Excessive thyroid hormone
Hyperparathyroidism	Heparin (>6 mo)
Inflammatory arthritis	Anticonvulsants
Hypogonadism	Furosemide
Chronic renal failure	Aluminum-containing antacids
Chronic liver disease	Cyclosporine A, Tacrolimus
Malabsorption syndromes	Medroxyprogesterone acetate
Alcoholism	Gonadotropin-releasing hormone agonists
Diabetes mellitus, type I	
Multiple myeloma	Aromatase inhibitors
Calcium or Vitamin D deficiency	Methotrexate

activating factors. The cessation of estrogen production associated with menopause triggers an increase in cytokine synthesis, including interleukins 1 and 6 and tumor necrosis factor (TNF), which in turn stimulates osteoclast activity.[4,6] In type I (postmenopausal) osteoporosis, this enhanced osteoclast activity in the presence of normal osteoblast function leads to accelerated bone loss. Bone loss is greater at trabecular sites than cortical sites.

TYPE II (SENILE) OSTEOPOROSIS

Although the precise cause of senile osteoporosis is not known, it is probably the result of several changes that occur during the aging process. These include an age-related decrease in gastrointestinal (GI) calcium absorption, a gradual increase in serum parathyroid hormone (PTH) concentration, and a decreased rate of vitamin D activation.[7] In men, a gradual decline in testosterone production seen with increasing age may also contribute to osteoporosis.[8]

TYPE III (SECONDARY) OSTEOPOROSIS
Drug-Induced Osteoporosis

Glucocorticoids. Corticosteroid-induced bone loss has been recognized since Cushing first described hypercortisolism in the 1930s, but the true incidence of osteoporosis in patients receiving steroids is not known. Fracture rates approaching 50% have been reported in patients receiving long-term glucocorticoid therapy.[9] Proposed mechanisms of this drug-induced side effect include an alteration in calcium absorption and elimination leading to secondary hyperparathyroidism, an inhibitory effect on sex hormone production, and direct inhibition of osteoblast function. The effect of glucocorticoids on bone appears to be dose-dependent and duration-dependent with the greatest loss occurring during the first 6–12 months of therapy. Prednisone at a dosage of 7.5 mg or more per day is associated with significant bone loss, with trabecular bone loss being greater than cortical bone loss. It is unclear if physiologic dosages have deleterious effects on bone, but alternate day dosing does not appear to be safer than daily dosing. Inhaled corticosteroids do not decrease bone density at low to moderate dosages, but may have some effect at higher dosages.[10] Men are equally affected, and no protection appears to be offered by race. Some bone mass restoration may occur on withdrawal of glucocorticoid therapy.[9] The recommendations developed by the American College of Rheumatology Task Force on Osteoporosis Guidelines for minimizing bone loss associated with corticosteroid therapy are summarized in Table 69.3.[11]

Anticoagulants. Long-term heparin therapy was first reported to cause osteoporosis in 1964.[9] It is estimated that one third of patients on chronic heparin will demonstrate bone loss, and approximately 2% will suffer a symptomatic fracture. Some studies suggest that the risk of developing osteoporosis with heparin is dose-dependent and duration-dependent (e.g., >15,000 U/day for >3 months).[9] Potential mechanisms include increased osteoclast activity and decreased osteoblast activity, a hypocalcemia-induced increase

TABLE 69.3	American College of Rheumatology Guidelines for the Prevention and Treatment of Glucocorticoid-Induced Osteoporosis

For all patients

Choose the corticosteroid regimen with the lowest risk
  Inhaled or topical
  Lowest possible dosage
  Alternate-day therapy not protective
Encourage appropriate lifestyle modifications
  Cessation of tobacco use
  Limited alcohol intake
  Regular exercise regimen
Prescribe dietary modifications and nutritional supplements
  Calcium 1,500 mg/day
  Vitamin D 400–800 IU/day or calcitriol 0.5–1.0 µg/day

For patients on long-term therapy (>6 months)

Evaluate
  Bone mineral density at baseline and every 6–12 months
  Gonadal function
  Calcium balance
Consider thiazide diuretic if otherwise indicated (e.g., patient is hypertensive)
Correct hypogonadal state if present
  Premenopausal women: oral contraception
  Postmenopausal women: hormone replacement therapy (estrogen ± progesterone)
  Men: testosterone
Consider alternative or additional therapy in hormone-replete patients, patients unable to take hormonal therapy, patients on high-dose corticosteroids, and patients who have established osteoporosis
  Bisphosphonates (alendronate, risedronate, etidronate)
  Reserve calcitonin for patients who cannot take bisphosphonates

(Adapted from American College of Rheumatology Ad Hoc Committee on Glucocorticoid-Induced Osteoporosis. Recommendations for the prevention and treatment of glucocorticoid-induced osteoporosis: 2001 update. Arthritis Rheum 44:1496–1503, 2001.)

in PTH activity, heparin-induced increase in collagenase activity, and a decrease in the production of 1,25-hydroxyvitamin D [1,25-$(OH)_2$-D] caused by decreased renal conversion enzyme activity. Bone loss has been shown to reverse after heparin is discontinued. Studies suggest that a risk of osteoporosis also exists with low molecular weight heparin but to a lesser degree than with heparin.[9,12] Oral anticoagulants may also increase the risk of osteoporosis by their antagonistic effect on vitamin K, a key factor in the synthesis of bone matrix proteins. Small but significant decreases in bone density and an increased relative risk of vertebral and rib fractures have been reported in patients on long-term oral anticoagulation[13,14] Whether calcium and vitamin D supplementation during anticoagulant therapy is beneficial is not known, but it is considered prudent.

Gonadotropin-Releasing Hormone Agonists. The gonadotropin-releasing hormone (GnRH) agonists, leuprolide, goserelin, and nafarelin, are associated with bone loss in men and women.[15,16] Initial stimulation of the hypothalamic-pituitary-ovarian or hypothalamic-pituitary-testicular axis is followed by shutdown of these axes via down-regulation of receptors. The net result is a hypogonadic state. Trabecular bone loss can be rapid with up to 7% of bone mass lost within 6 months. Increased fracture rates have been reported.[9,15,17] Although bone loss is at least partially reversible, especially in young women, it is recommended that use of these agents be limited to 6 months, unless a bone-protective agent is used concurrently. Therapy with low-dose estrogen and progesterone (called add-back therapy) or progesterone alone may minimize the osteoporotic effects of GnRH agonists, allowing longer use in women. However, hormone therapy (HT) may limit the therapeutic effects of the GnRH agonist in conditions such as endometriosis, leiomyomata, or premenstrual syndrome.[18,19] Bisphosphonates have been shown to prevent the bone density changes associated with GnRH agonist therapy in men and women.[15,20]

Antiepileptic Drugs. Antiepileptic drugs (AEDs) are well known to cause osteomalacia by their effects on vitamin D metabolism (see section on osteomalacia). However, there is also evidence that supports an increased risk of osteoporosis with chronic use of AEDs.[21] In addition to their effects on vitamin D, these agents may have direct effects on bone metabolism that contribute to the loss of bone density.

Other Substances. Furosemide and other loop diuretics are known to cause calciuria, as are caffeine and phosphorus-containing cola sodas. Conversely, thiazide diuretics, which decrease urinary calcium excretion and may inhibit bone resorption, appear to be protective of bone mass.[22] High phosphorus content in the GI tract inhibits calcium absorption, as does alcohol. Cigarette smoking appears to have an antiestrogenic effect.[23] Although these compounds are not known to result in overt bone loss, they are often prescribed and/or ingested by those at risk for osteoporosis. Minimizing ingestion of these compounds is prudent.

Psychotropic drugs do not directly affect bone density. However, older individuals using such agents, including benzodiazepines, antidepressants, and anticonvulsants, appear to have a greater risk of hip fracture related to an increased risk of falls.[24,25]

Other Causes of Osteoporosis. Anorexia nervosa can decrease bone density by two mechanisms: dietary calcium and vitamin D deficiency and pseudomenopause induction. Many anorexic women have estrogen deficiency and cease to have menstrual cycles. The bone loss associated with anorexia resembles that of menopause. Likewise, premature

ovarian failure and premenopausal surgical castration (oophorectomy) result in estrogen deficiency that will accelerate bone loss, unless hormone replacement is initiated.

In men, idiopathic or iatrogenic loss of or decrease in testosterone production results in accelerated bone loss. Because low serum testosterone may not impair sexual function, patients may be unaware of their increased risk. Other causes of osteoporosis in men include Cushing syndrome, hyperthyroidism, cancer, glucocorticoid therapy, chronic alcohol ingestion and other dietary factors, smoking, and prolonged immobilization. In one study of men with vertebral fractures, more than half had an underlying condition that contributed to bone loss, supporting evaluation for an underlying cause in men presenting with low bone density.[8]

Patients with quadriplegia or paraplegia and posttraumatic immobilization resulting in traction or prolonged bed rest are at risk for bone loss. Daily weight bearing activity improves bone density and is essential to good skeletal health.[26]

EPIDEMIOLOGY

Osteoporosis is primarily a disease of older adults. The Third National Health and Nutrition Examination Survey (NHANES III), which measured BMD of the proximal femur in a random, noninstitutionalized population of U.S. residents, documented an osteoporosis rate of 13% to 18% in women over age 50 and a 37% to 50% rate of osteopenia in this population. The rate of osteopenia in men 50 years or older was 38% to 47%, similar to that in women, but the rate of osteoporosis (4%–6%) was lower than in women. Based on this prevalence, an estimated 4 to 6 million women and 1 to 2 million men over 50 years of age in the United States have osteoporosis, and an additional 13 to 17 million women and 8 to 13 million men have osteopenia.[27] In the United States, 1.5 million fractures annually, including 250,000 hip fractures, are attributed to osteoporosis.[28] The prevalence of VFs in white women in the United States is approximately 5% in women 50–59 years of age but increases to 50% in women 80 years and older.[29] The risk of hip fractures also increases significantly with increasing age.[28] African-American women have a lower risk of fractures compared to white women due to a higher baseline bone density.[30] As the proportion of older adults in the United States increases, greater numbers of patients will be at risk for fractures related to low bone density.

PATHOPHYSIOLOGY

Skeletal formation begins during the sixth week of embryologic development. The skeletal mass of infants doubles in the first year of life, and 37% of the total skeletal mass is accumulated during adolescence. Skeletal growth continues until genetic height is attained, but bone mineralization continues until the third decade. Calcium, vitamin D, and weight bearing activity are the key components of bone growth. Other factors, including growth hormone, are involved in optimal bone production, but their roles have not been fully elucidated.

BONE REMODELING

Bone loss (resorption) and formation is a dynamic process that occurs throughout life. These two opposing processes are usually coupled in bone-remodeling units (BRUs). There are more than 1 million active BRUs, involving 15% to 20% of the bone surface at any given time.[31] This is shown schematically in Figure 69.2 (*see color insert*). BRUs serve two important functions: (a) to provide the serum with a readily available source of calcium for maintaining physiologic processes such as muscle contraction and nerve conduction and (b) to strengthen, revitalize, and rehydrate the bone matrix.

Bone resorption occurs on the bone surface. Trabecular (cancellous) bone is found primarily in the vertebrae and the metaphyses of long bones, and has a greater surface area than cortical bone. The long bone shafts are primarily cortical (compact) in structure. Approximately 25% of trabecular bone is remodeled each year, compared to approximately 2% to 3% of cortical bone.[32]

In normal bone, activation of the BRU by stimulation of osteoclasts can be triggered by multiple factors, including PTH, vitamin D, and locally produced cytokines, such as interleukins and TNF. During their average life span of 12 days, osteoclasts secrete collagenases and proteinases that solubilize bone matrix, releasing calcium into circulation for physiological functions. Once the osteoclast dies, osteoblast differentiation is stimulated by locally produced growth factors such as bone morphogenetic proteins and insulinlike growth factors. Over a 10-day period, osteoblasts lay down new bone matrix (osteoid) at the sites of previous resorption. Once bone formation is complete, the inactivated osteoblasts differentiate into flattened lining cells (surface osteocytes) on the new bone. The new bone is then mineralized with hydroxyapatite, a compound consisting primarily of calcium and phosphorus, having the chemical structure $Ca_{10}(PO_4)_6(OH)_2$. The complete mineralization and hardening process takes several months.[33]

BONE STRENGTH

Resistance to fracture is a function of bone strength. BMD is the major component of bone strength, accounting for 50% to 75% of fracture resistance. Other factors that contribute to bone strength include bone dimensions (external diameter and cortical thickness), microarchitecture (trabecular number, shape, and connectivity), and tissue quality. The degree of bone mineralization and rate of remodeling may also affect bone strength. Other than BMD, direct evaluation of the components of bone strength is difficult.[34]

CLINICAL PRESENTATION AND DIAGNOSIS

SIGNS AND SYMPTOMS

Osteoporosis is considered a silent disease in that loss of bone density is asymptomatic in the absence of a fracture.

VFs are the most common osteoporotic fracture (Fig. 69.3; *see color insert*). Most VFs are precipitated by normal

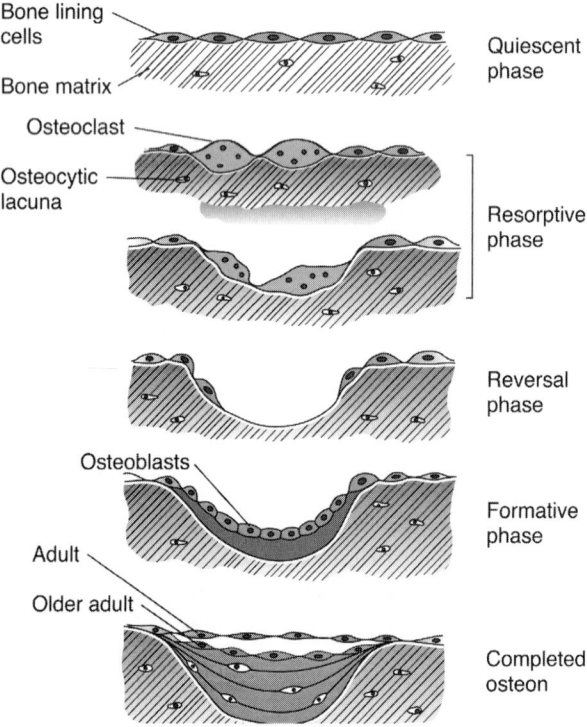

FIGURE 69.2 Bone remodeling sequence (*see color insert*). Bone remodeling is initiated by the appearance of osteoclasts on a bone surface previously lined by fusiform cells. After development of a resorption bay, osteoclasts are replaced by osteoblasts which deposit new bone. The bone loss that attends aging (senile osteoporosis) is due to incomplete filling of resorption bays. (Image from Rubin E, Farber JL Pathology. 3rd ed. Philadelphia: Lippincott, Williams & Wilkins, 1999, with permission.)

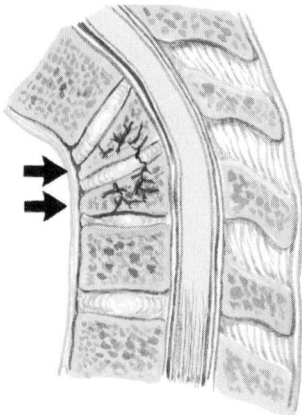

FIGURE 69.3 Vertebral fracture (*see color insert*). (Asset from Anatomical Chart Co., with permission.)

activities such as bending or lifting rather than by trauma. Back pain in the lumbar or thoracic spine is the primary symptom of a VF. This acute pain generally resolves over time. However, many patients are asymptomatic or do not recognize the pain as a symptom of VF. It is estimated that two thirds of all VFs go undiagnosed due to lack of acute symptoms.[29] The patient may notice a loss in height, or it may be identified during yearly physical examinations. Progressive kyphosis, or curvature of the spine, may develop as compression fractures worsen, resulting in the classic dowager's hump. In severe cases, the ribs rest on the iliac crest of the pelvis, causing abdominal protrusion due to the loss of truncal space. The presence of vertebral deformity is associated with chronic pain and decreased function. In addition, the presence of a VF increases the risk of subsequent fractures fourfold.[29] VFs are associated with an increased rate of morbidity in women and men that may be attributed, in part, to general poor health and concomitant diseases in the affected population.

Wrist fractures, primarily of the distal radius, may occur if the patient falls and lands on an instinctively outstretched hand. Although wrist fractures have not been associated with increased mortality, less than optimal functioning was reported in approximately half of patients 6 months after the event.[29]

Fracture of the hip at the proximal femur most often occurs secondary to a fall. Fracture of the proximal humerus or pelvis may also occur. Fractures necessitating surgery or prolonged hospitalization place the patient at risk for thromboembolic sequelae, pneumonia, infection, and worsening of disease caused by immobilization. Hip fractures are associated with a mortality rate of 10% to 20% within the first year postevent for women and the 1-year mortality rate is significantly greater for men than for women.[8,29] Approximately half of hip fracture patients are unable to ambulate independently after the fracture, and one third are no longer able to function without significant outside assistance.[29]

DIAGNOSIS AND CLINICAL FINDINGS

As noted, many cases of osteoporosis are not identified until a fracture occurs. However, osteoporosis and osteopenia can be diagnosed by measuring BMD. Early identification of bone loss can lead to intervention and prevention of subsequent osteoporotic fracture.

The presence of risk factors for osteoporosis (Table 69.4) is used as criteria for BMD screening. The U.S. Preventive Services Task Force recommends bone density screening for all women 65 years of age and older. They also recommend initiation of screening at age 60 years for women at increased risk for osteoporosis.[3] There are no guidelines regarding bone density screening for women under age 60 or for men, however, screening can be justified for patients with significant risk factors, such as hypogonadism, or long-term use of drugs associated with osteoporosis.

In the absence of a secondary cause of osteoporosis, routine serum or urine chemistries generally are not helpful in

TABLE 69.4	Factors That Increase or Decrease Risk of Developing Osteoporosis and Osteoporosis-Related Fractures
Risk Factors	**Protective Factors**
General	High normal body mass
Slender build (thin, small frame)	African or Mediterranean race
White or Asian race	Weight bearing exercise
Female sex	Estrogen replacement therapy
Menopause	Adequate lifetime calcium intake
Oophorectomy during reproductive years	Avoidance of risk factors
Positive family history	Thiazide diuretic use
Medical therapy (see Table 69.2)	Oral contraceptive use
Diet	
Chronic low calcium intake	
Chronic high phosphorus intake	
Personal habits	
Smoking	
Heavy caffeine/cola consumption	
Heavy alcohol consumption	
Inactivity	
Risk for falls	
Frailty	
Impaired vision or hearing	
Use of psychotropic medications	

diagnosis. Serum calcium, phosphorus, total alkaline phosphatase, PTH, 25-hydroxyvitamin D (25-OH-D), and 1,25-$(OH)_2$-D usually are within normal limits.

Biochemical Markers. Biochemical markers of bone remodeling reflect metabolic activity in bone. Markers of bone resorption, which may be measured in urine or serum, include byproducts of collagen catabolism, such as pyridinoline (PYD) and deoxypyridinoline (DPD), the collagen telopeptides, N-telopeptide-to-helix (NTX) and c-telopeptide-to-helix (CTX) and products of osteoclast function, such as bone sialoprotein (BSP) and tartrate-resistant acid phosphatase (TRACP). Markers of bone formation, which are measured in serum, include bone-specific alkaline phosphatase (BSAP), serum osteocalcin (bone Gla-protein), and the carboxy- and amino-terminal propeptides of Type I procollagen (PICP and PINP). Due to intersubject and intrasubject variability, biochemical markers are not diagnostic for osteoporosis and do not eliminate the need to measure BMD. However, studies suggest that biochemical markers can identify individuals with an accelerated rate of bone turnover, which has been correlated with an increased risk of fracture. Biochemical markers may also be used for rapid evaluation of response to and compliance with drug therapy; one study found that a significant change in biochemical markers at 6 and 12 weeks of therapy was associated with a decreased risk of fracture after 3 years of treatment.[35] Use of biochemical markers to monitor treatment response may lead to more timely adjustments in therapy.

Bone Mineral Density Testing. Several radiographic techniques are available for evaluation of BMD (Table 69.5). Although routine spinal radiograph may be performed to assess back pain in symptomatic patients, standard x-rays are not adequately sensitive to diagnose or monitor treatment of osteoporosis. Dual-energy x-ray absorptiometry (DEXA) of the hip and spine is considered the gold standard for diagnosis of osteoporosis. BMD, as measured by DEXA, has been well correlated with risk of fracture and is used as a surrogate end point for the assessment of treatment efficacy in osteoporosis.[36] However, cost and the lack of widespread availability limit the usefulness of DEXA as a screening method for the general population. Quantitative ultrasound (QUS), which uses sound waves to evaluate bone density, is more portable, less expensive, and does not use radiation, making it more practical than DEXA as a screening tool. However, QUS may be less accurate than DEXA at predicting fracture risk, therefore, it is recommended that abnormal BMD results on QUS be confirmed by DEXA.[37] Peripheral densitometry at the heel or distal forearm with single-energy x-ray absorptiometry (SXA) or DEXA is less expensive than central DEXA but may be less predictive of fractures. Radiographic absorptiometry compares density of bones in the hand with the known densities of a wedge of aluminum.

Quantitated computed tomography (QCT) is a good indicator of density of trabecular bone. However, it is the most expensive technique and exposes the patient to the greatest amount of radiation.

Use of BMD studies for evaluation of response to therapy is limited by the precision error of these technologies. For DEXA machines, a change in BMD of less than 3% to 5% is insignificant and does not necessarily indicate therapeutic failure. Depending on the estimated rate of bone loss, BMD may be repeated at 1 to 2 years for pharmacotherapeutic monitoring.

PSYCHOSOCIAL ASPECTS

Osteoporosis can have a significant psychosocial impact. Chronic back pain from VFs may lead to depression. Fear of falling and sustaining a fracture may lead individuals to restrict their activities, resulting in isolation. Loss of ability to ambulate after hip fracture can also lead to isolation and may require institutionalization because of inability to provide self-care. A higher degree of physical impairment from osteoporosis appears to be associated with a greater loss in quality of life.[38]

THERAPEUTIC PLAN

The goals of osteoporosis management include prevention and treatment. Preventive therapy includes maximizing bone mass during the formative years and then maintaining bone mass once peak bone mass has been achieved. For patients with established osteoporosis, the ideal treatment goal is to replenish bone mass. Unfortunately, there are limited thera-

TABLE 69.5	Bone Mineral Density Measurement Methods		
Method	**Evaluable Sites**	**Radiation Dosage**	**Comments**
Single-energy photon absorptiometry (SPA)	Forearm Calcaneus (heel)	Very low	10- to 15-min scan time Accurate and precise Limited to peripheral bone
Dual-energy x-ray absorptiometry (DEXA)	Spine Lateral lumbar spine Proximal femur Total body	Low	Scan time <5 min Correlated with fracture risk Accurate and precise High cost
Quantitative computed tomography (QCT)	Spine Radius	High Low	High cost Not well correlated with fracture risk
Quantitative ultrasonometry (QUS)	Calcaneus Patella	None	Inexpensive Portable Correlated with fracture risk

(Adapted from Hodgson SF, Watts NB, Bilezikian JP, et al. American Association of Clinical Endocrinologists medical guidelines for clinical practice for the prevention and treatment of postmenopausal osteoporosis: 2001 edition, with selected updates for 2003. Endocr Pract 9:544–564, 2003; Miller PD. Bone mineral density-clinical use and application. Endocrinol Metab Clin North Am 32:159–179, 2003.)

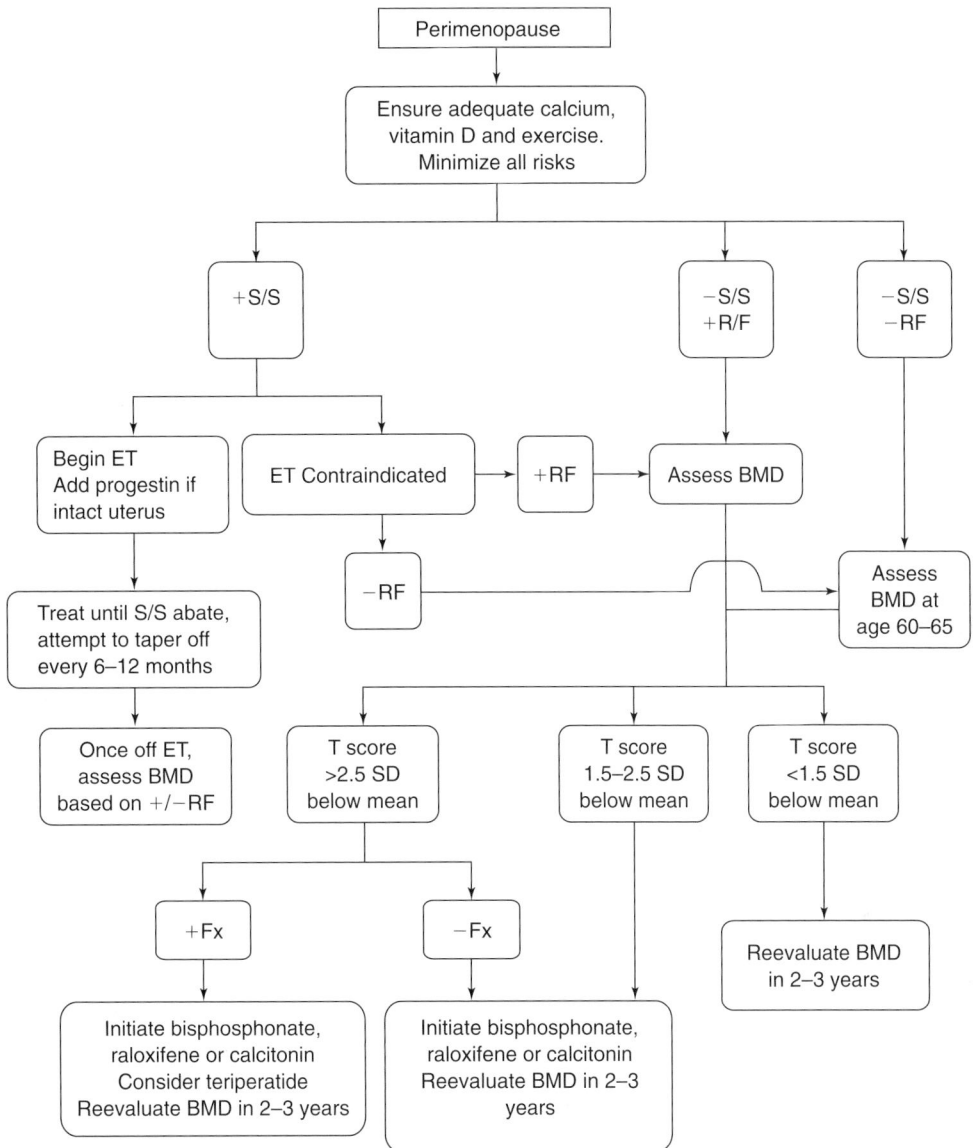

FIGURE 69.4 Decision algorithm for osteoporosis treatment and prevention in perimenopausal women. BMD, bone mineral density; ET, estrogen therapy; RF, risk factors; S/S, signs/symptoms (vasomotor, urogenital).

peutic options for replacing lost bone. Therefore, osteoporosis treatment focuses on preventing further bone loss and decreasing the risk of fractures. Figure 69.4 is a decision algorithm for osteoporosis prevention and treatment in postmenopausal women.

PREVENTION AND TREATMENT

PHARMACOLOGIC TREATMENT

Calcium. Calcium is a key element in the therapy of osteoporosis. Adequate calcium intake throughout life is essential for optimizing peak bone mass and may affect the rate at which bone is lost later in life. Calcium alone is inadequate to completely inhibit the rapid bone loss that occurs at meno-

pause but is necessary to optimize response to antiresorptive agents.[39] In older individuals, calcium supplementation has been shown to reduce the risk of VFs; however, its effect on hip fractures is less clear.[40] Calcium supplementation appears to be most beneficial in subjects with the lowest calcium intake.[41] Recommendations for calcium intake are listed in Table 69.6. The National Institutes of Health recommends higher calcium intakes for some age groups than the currently established recommended daily intakes (RDI).[42] As a general rule, when calculating dietary calcium intake, each full serving of a dietary source known to be high in calcium is estimated to contain 250 to 300 mg of calcium (Table 69.7).

Dietary calcium and supplements are equally efficacious if ingestion (in milligrams of elemental calcium) is equal.

TABLE 69.6	Recommended Calcium Intakes	
	Elemental Calcium (mg/day)	
Group	**Current RDI**	**NIH Consensus**
Infant		
Birth to 6 mo	400	400
6–12 mo	600	600
Children		
1–5 yr	800	800
6–10 yr	800	800–1,200
Adolescents		
11–18 yr	1,200	1,200–1,500
Men		
19–24 yr	1,200	1,200–1,000
25–65 yr	800	1,000
65 yr	800	1,500
Women		
19–24 yr	1,200	1,200–1,500
25–50 yr	800	1,000
50 yr on estrogen	800	1,000
50 yr not on estrogen	800	1,500
65 yr	800	1,500
Pregnant or lactating	1,200	1,200–1,500

RDI, recommended daily intake; NIH, National Institutes of Health.
(Adapted from NIH Consensus Development Panel on Optimal Calcium Intake. Optimal calcium intake. JAMA 272:1942–1947, 1994.)

Calcium carbonate and tribasic calcium phosphate have the greatest percentage of elemental calcium, 40% and 39%, respectively. Table 69.8 lists the variety of calcium supplements available. Calcium absorption is rate limited; divided doses are better absorbed than a large single daily dose. Calcium carbonate requires acid for optimal absorption and should be taken with a meal, whereas calcium citrate is not dependent on gastric pH for absorption and may be taken without regard to meals.

Calcium supplementation is generally well tolerated. The primary side effects from calcium supplements are GI, including nausea and constipation. Even when calcium intake is high, the risk for hypercalcemia (in the absence of excessive vitamin D) is rare because homeostatic mechanisms decrease intestinal absorption of calcium. The use of calcium supplements is rarely associated with hypercalciuria or renal calcium stones. Fiber impairs absorption, as does iron therapy. Patients should take tetracycline compounds and calcium at least 2 hours apart to avoid intestinal chelation.

Vitamin D. Vitamin D is a fat soluble vitamin that has many hormonelike functions. Vitamin D3 can be produced endogenously in the skin on exposure to ultraviolet light (UVB). The two exogenous sources of vitamin D are ergosterol (vitamin D_2) from plant sources and cholecalciferol (vitamin D_3) from animal sources, such as fish liver oils and fortified milk. These compounds first undergo hydroxylation in the liver to 25-OH-D, then are further hydroxylated in the kidney to result in the physiologically active compound 1,25-$(OH)_2$-D. The production of 1,25-$(OH)_2$-D is influenced by PTH, calcium, and phosphorus. Its presence enhances GI absorption of calcium. Optimal serum 25-OH-D serum concentrations range from 20 to 30 ng per milliliter.

TABLE 69.7	Calcium Content of Selected Foods				
Dairy Foods	**Serving Size**	**Calcium Content (mg)**	**Nondairy Foods**	**Serving Size**	**Calcium Content (mg)**
Ricotta cheese	1 cup	500–670	Collard greens, cooked	1 cup	350
Yogurt	1 cup	275–450	Sardines, canned with bones	3 oz	325
Milk, all types	1 cup	290–300	Soymilk, calcium fortified	1 cup	300
Hard cheeses	1 oz	205–275	Spinach, cooked	1 cup	250–275
Cottage cheese	1 cup	125–150	Kale, Turnip greens, cooked	1 cup	200–250
Frozen yogurt, soft serve	½ cup	100	Juice, calcium-fortified	1 cup	100–300
Ice cream	½ cup	80	Salmon, canned with bones	3 oz	180
Cream cheese	1 oz	20	Molasses, blackstrap	1 tablespoon	170
			Tofu, soft	4 oz	130
			Tofu, firm	2.6 oz	140
			Dry beans, cooked	1 cup	125
			Broccoli	1 cup	90
			Almonds	1 oz	70

TABLE 69.8	Selected Calcium Supplements					
Salt	Elemental Calcium (%)	Solubility	Selected Products	Calcium/ Tablet (mg)	Number of tablets needed to equal 1000 mg	Relative Cost/ 1000 mg
Calcium carbonate	40	Insoluble	Generic	600	2	$
			OsCal	500	2	$–$$
			Caltrate	600	2	$
			Tums	200, 300, 400, 500	5, 4, 3, 2	$–$$
Tribasic calcium phosphate	39	Insoluble	Posture	600	2	$$
Calcium citrate	21	Soluble	Generic	200, 250	5, 4	$
			Citracal	200	10 mL	$$
			Calcitrate	200, 225	5	$$
					5, 5	
Calcium lactate	18	Soluble	Generic,	84	12	$$$
			Cal-Lac	96	11	
				100	10	
Calcium gluconate	9	Soluble	Generic	45, 58	22, 18	$$–$$$$
			Calcionate	347/15 mL	45 mL	
Calcium glubionate	6.5	Soluble	Calcionate, Calciquid	117 mg/5 cc	42.5 mL	$$$–$$$$

Due to a decreased ability of aging skin to produce vitamin D3, the RDI for vitamin D increases with increasing age; 200 international units (IU) for persons 50 years of age and younger, 400 IU for those 51 to 70 years of age, and 800 IU for persons over 70 years of age.[43] Vitamin D deficiency appears to be more common than previously suspected; in one study, more than half of recently hospitalized individuals were vitamin D deficient. Risk factors for vitamin D deficiency include low dietary intake, limited exposure to UV light, being institutionalized or housebound, older age, use of anticonvulsant drugs or corticosteroids, renal disease, cirrhosis, and winter season.[44] Several studies have reported that osteoporotic patients are more likely to have deficient 25-OH-D serum concentrations than those without osteoporosis.[44]

A meta analysis of studies examining the use of vitamin D in the treatment of osteoporosis suggests a possible benefit of the agent on BMD and non-VFs.[45] A meta analysis of studies using calcitriol, (1,25 (OH)2-D), concluded that there was a decreased risk of VF but no significant effect on non-VFs when compared to placebo.[45] Baseline vitamin D status may be a confounding factor in evaluating the efficacy of vitamin D supplementation; patients who are vitamin D deficient may benefit more from supplementation than those who are vitamin D replete.

Patients at risk for vitamin D deficiency, such as older adults or patients on low-dose corticosteroids or anticonvulsant therapy, should be given vitamin D_2 or vitamin D_3 at dosages of 800 IU daily. Calcitriol, a prescription-only form of activated vitamin D, should be given at doses of 0.5 µg per day to patients on high-dose corticosteroids, patients

with renal failure, and patients with established osteoporosis. After calcitriol therapy is initiated, serum calcium and 24-hour urine calcium excretion should be assessed to ensure efficacy and the absence of hypercalcemia.[11] Concomitant use of thiazide diuretics and calcitriol may increase the risk of adverse effects. Patients exhibiting symptoms of anorexia, nausea, and weakness should be evaluated for possible hypercalcemia. For a comparison of vitamin D supplements see Table 69.9.

Estrogen. Postmenopausal estrogen therapy, taken with or without progestin, has been shown to significantly decrease the rate of bone turnover and reduce the risk of osteoporotic fractures, especially in women who initiate use early after onset of menopause.[40,46] In the recent past, many women were kept on hormone replacement therapy for osteoporosis prevention and possible cardioprotective benefits. However, in 2002, the Women's Health Initiative, a study of postmenopausal estrogen therapy, documented a lack of cardiovascular protection and an increased risk of breast cancer with long-term use (>5 years). Based on these outcomes, current recommendations advise against long-term use of HT solely for the prevention of osteoporosis.[47,48] (See Chapter 17 for more information on the use of estrogen/progestin therapy.) However, women who are using HT for management of menopausal symptoms will experience a delay in postmenopausal bone loss and may be able to postpone initiation of antiosteoporotic therapy until they discontinue HT (see Fig. 69.4).

Bisphosphonates. The bisphosphonates are compounds that adsorb onto hydroxyapatite crystals at sites of active bone resorption and inhibit osteoclastic activity without a

TABLE 69.9	Vitamin D Preparations[a]		
Product	**Component**	**Strength**	**Availability**
Ergocalciferol	D_2	8,000 IU/mL (drops)	OTC
		50,000 IU (tablets, capsules)	Rx
Cholecalciferol	D_3	400 IU (tablets)	OTC
		1,000 IU (tablets)	
Calcifediol	25-OH-D_3	20 µg, 50 µg (capsules)	Rx
Calcitriol (Rocaltrol)	1,25-(OH)$_2$-D_3	0.25 µg, 0.5 µg (capsules), 1 µg/mL (solution)	Rx
Dihydrotachysterol (DHT, Hytakerol)	Synthetic D_2	0.125 mg (tablets, capsules)	Rx
		0.2 mg, 0.4 mg (tablets)	
		0.2 mg/mL (solution)	
Paricalcitol (Zemplar)	Synthetic vitamin D analog	5 µg/mL (injection)	Rx
Doxercalciferol (Hectorol)	Synthetic vitamin D analog	2.5 µg (capsules	Rx

[a] 1 IU vitamin D activity = 0.025 µg vitamin D_3; 40,000 IU vitamin D activity = 1 mg vitamin D_3.
OTC, over-the-counter; Rx, prescription.

subsequent effect on osteoblastic activity. There are six bisphosphonates on the US market, however, only three are currently approved by the Food and Drug Administration (FDA) for the management of osteoporosis. These agents are considered by many to be first-line treatment for osteoporosis.

Alendronate and Risedronate. Alendronate is approved by the FDA for the prevention of osteoporosis in postmenopausal women and the treatment of osteoporosis in men, postmenopausal women, and those with corticosteroid-induced osteoporosis. In women with osteoporosis, with or without preexisting fractures, alendronate therapy results in small but significant increases in BMD and significantly decreased risk of vertebral, hip, and wrist fractures. The greatest benefit is seen in women with preexisting fractures.[49,50,51] Alendronate preserves bone mass in postmenopausal women with osteopenia compared to women taking placebo.[52] The drug has also increased bone density in patients receiving glucocorticoids.[53] Use of alendronate for up to 10 years has been shown to maintain therapeutic benefit with minimal risk of adverse effects.[54]

Risedronate carries an FDA-approved indication for the treatment and prevention of postmenopausal and corticosteroid-induced osteoporosis. In clinical trials it has been shown to increase BMD and decrease the risk of vertebral and non-VFs in women who have postmenopausal osteoporosis. In patients on corticosteroids, risedronate decreased the rate of bone loss and fractures.[55]

Neither alendronate nor risedronate are metabolized; drug not adsorbed onto bone is excreted unchanged in urine and feces. Oral bioavailability of these agents is less than 1% under ideal conditions. Alendronate is contraindicated in patients with creatinine clearance less than 35 mL per minute and risedronate is contraindicated when creatinine clearance is less than 30 mL per minute. Side effects of these drugs

are primarily GI in nature, including abdominal pain or distension, nausea, dyspepsia, constipation, flatulence, and dysphagia. Esophagitis has been reported and in many cases was felt to be caused by inappropriate drug administration; proper drug use should be reinforced at each visit. Both agents should be used cautiously in patients with a history of preexisting GI problems, especially gastroesophageal reflux or dysmotility disorders and should be avoided in pregnant women (FDA Pregnancy Category C).

Alendronate is available as once-daily or once-weekly tablets. The dose depends on the indication; 5 mg daily or 35 mg weekly for prevention and 10 mg daily or 70 mg weekly for treatment. The treatment and prevention dose of risedronate is 5 mg daily or 35 mg weekly. To optimize absorption, these agents should be taken on arising in the morning. Patients should be instructed to ingest the tablet with 6 to 8 oz of plain water at least 30 minutes before ingesting other medications (including calcium), foods, or beverages. The patient should not lie down for 30 minutes after ingesting the medication. Adequate calcium and vitamin D intake is also necessary to ensure optimal response to the bisphosphonates.

There is limited data comparing the efficacy and safety of the FDA-approved bisphosphonates. One study found that weekly alendronate resulted in significantly greater improvement in BMD and biochemical markers of bone turnover than daily administered risedronate. There was no significant difference in fracture rates, and the side effect profiles were similar.[56] However, an endoscopic study found that risedronate was associated with a lower risk for gastric ulcers.[57] Further comparison studies are needed to assist clinicians in making a choice for therapy.

Other bisphosphonates. Other currently available bisphosphonates were studied in the management of osteoporosis but are not approved by the FDA for this indication. The first-generation agent, etidronate, inhibits mineralization of newly formed bone at a dose similar to its antiresorptive dose. To minimize abnormal bone mineralization, the drug is administered cyclically: 400 mg by mouth daily for 2 weeks in 12- to 16-week cycles. Improved BMD in the spine and hip have been reported, but the data on fracture reduction is not conclusive.[58] Etidronate is well tolerated, the most common side effects being GI.

Intravenous administration of pamidronate or zoledronic acid at intervals ranging from 1 to 12 months has been shown to improve BMD in postmenopausal women and men receiving androgen deprivation therapy.[15,59,60] Ibandronate, recently FDA-approved for osteoporosis at an oral dose of 150 mg once monthly, has been shown to decrease VFs in postmenopausal women.[61]

Selective Estrogen Receptor Modulators.
Selective estrogen receptor modulators (SERMs) are synthetic compounds that exhibit estrogenic properties in some tissues while exerting antiestrogenic activities in other tissues. Raloxifene, the only SERM currently approved by the FDA for prevention and treatment of postmenopausal osteoporosis, is an estrogen agonist in bone and lipids, but an estrogen antagonist in breast and endometrial tissue. Tamoxifen, the first commercially available SERM, has antiestrogenic effects in breast tissue, but has estrogenic properties in bone, the lipoprotein system, and the uterus. Tamoxifen, approved for the treatment and prevention of breast cancer, demonstrates a protective effect on bone, but has not been studied prospectively for osteoporosis.

Raloxifene, like estrogen, inhibits bone resorption, but its effects on bone may not be as great as those seen with estrogen or the bisphosphonates.[62] Raloxifene decreases total cholesterol and low density lipoprotein (LDL) levels in a fashion similar to estrogen, but it has less marked effects on high density lipoprotein (HDL) and HDL_2 cholesterol and triglycerides.[62] Unlike estrogen, raloxifene does not stimulate endometrial tissue proliferation, and it appears to exert a protective effect on the breast.

Clinical trials in postmenopausal women have shown that raloxifene increases BMD at the spine and hip and significantly decreases the risk of VF. A significant decrease in non-VFs has not been documented.[63] In the postmenopausal osteoporosis studies of raloxifene, a decreased risk of breast cancer and cardiovascular disease was noted, which led to the development of trials specifically designed to evaluate these outcomes. The results of these ongoing studies will aid in determining the optimal use of raloxifene.[62]

Dosing of raloxifene is 60 mg daily without regard to meals, and 60% of the dose is absorbed. The drug has a high first-pass metabolism, and the major route of elimination is in the feces. Its half-life is approximately 25 hours. Use of raloxifene in patients with significant liver impairment has not been studied. Adverse effects include hot flashes and leg cramps. The risk of thromboembolism increases with raloxifene, especially during the first 4 months of therapy. Patients who will be immobilized for a prolonged period of time should have therapy discontinued 72 hours before the start of immobilization or as soon as possible thereafter.

Based on currently available information, raloxifene should be reserved for postmenopausal women at risk for osteoporosis who cannot take bisphosphonates or who are also at increased risk for breast cancer.

Calcitonin.
Calcitonin is an endogenous hormone secreted by the thyroid gland in response to dietary or elevated serum calcium. Salmon calcitonin is approved by the FDA for the prevention of postmenopausal osteoporosis. Calcitonin prevents bone resorption by inhibiting osteoclast activity and has been shown to significantly increase BMD. The decrease in VF rates is greater than would be predicted by the increase in BMD, suggesting that calcitonin may also affect components of bone strength other than BMD. The drug has its greatest effect on the spine and is most effective in patients who have high bone turnover rates. Clinical trials have not shown a significant decrease in non-VFs.[64] Calcitonin also has a significant analgesic effect on acute pain from VF that is independent of its effects on bone metabolism.[65]

Calcitonin is given by injection or intranasal spray. The recommended injectable dosage is 100 IU (subcutaneous or intramuscular) and the intranasal dosage is 200 IU (one spray) per day in alternate nostrils. An oral formulation is under investigation. Patients should ingest adequate calcium and vitamin D during calcitonin treatment. Studies up to 5 years in duration show evidence of continued benefit.

Side effects of injectable calcitonin include nausea and GI discomfort in approximately 8% to 10% of patients; this may be minimized by bedtime administration. Initially, facial flushing and dermatitis may occur in 2% to 5% of patients, but these effects usually abate with continued therapy. Pruritus at the injection site is also problematic. To minimize these side effects, patients should be instructed to administer calcitonin subcutaneously rather than intramuscularly. The intranasal formulation appears to be better tolerated; rhinitis is the most commonly reported side effect. Although antibodies have been reported in patients receiving salmon calcitonin, their impact on clinical response is unclear.

Although it is not considered a first-line agent, calcitonin is a viable therapeutic option for patients who cannot tolerate other antiosteoporotic agents. It may also be considered in patients with back pain caused by VF.

Teriparatide.
PTH, the primary regulator of calcium homeostasis, has a dual effect on bone. Continuous infusion of PTH stimulates bone resorption, whereas once-daily injections of PTH stimulate osteoblastic activity. Clinical trials of recombinant human PTH (teriparatide) have shown increases in BMD in men and postmenopausal women with osteoporosis. The increases in BMD were greater than those seen after treatment with antiresorptive agents. A significant decrease in VF was also seen. The greatest effect was seen in the lumbar spine, suggesting that PTH preferentially affects trabecular bone. However, increases in BMD have also been

seen at nonvertebral sites. Histologically, bone formed secondary to teriparatide use appears to be normal, and improvements in microarchitecture have been seen.[66]

Teriparatide has 95% bioavailability and a half-life of 1 hour after subcutaneous injection. Although elimination studies have not been done on teriparatide, it is believed that endogenous PTH is metabolized and renally eliminated.[66]

Teriparatide is approved by the FDA for the treatment of osteoporosis in men and postmenopausal women at high risk for fracture. The agent is available as a 3 mL (250 μg/mL) prefilled pen-injector containing a 28 day supply of medication. The drug must be kept refrigerated. The dose of teriparatide is 20 μg daily as a subcutaneous injection into the thigh or abdomen. Use of this agent is limited to 2-years' duration due to lack of long-term safety data.

Adverse effects of teriparatide include nausea and headache. Patients should be advised that orthostatic hypotension may occur. Transient, asymptomatic increases in serum calcium levels have been reported, peaking at 4 to 6 hours after injection and returning to baseline within 24 hours. The drug should not be used in persons with preexisting hypercalcemia and patients should be advised to report persistent symptoms consistent with hypercalcemia (nausea, muscle weakness). Teriparatide carries a black box warning about the occurrence of bone tumors in animal models after long-term use. Although bone tumors have not been reported in human subjects, the drug should not be used in individuals at increased risk for osteosarcoma, including those with Paget Disease, previous skeletal radiation, increases in serum alkaline phosphatase of unknown etiology, children or young adults with open epiphyses.

Although teriparatide is the only FDA-approved agent that significantly stimulates bone formation, its high cost and injectable route of administration dictate that it be reserved for individuals at high risk for fracture and those who have failed antiresorptive therapy.

Combination Therapy. The benefits of combination antiresorptive therapy for osteoporosis are not well established. Addition of a bisphosphonate (etidronate, risedronate, or alendronate) to HT in postmenopausal women results in greater increases in BMD at the spine and hip than with either agent alone. A similar result was seen with the combination of raloxifene and alendronate. Use of calcitonin in combination with HT or estrogen plus methyltestosterone resulted in significant improvements in BMD at the spine but not at the hip. No significant differences in fracture rates were reported in any of these studies.[67]

The combination of parathyroid hormone and antiresorptive agents is controversial. Concurrent use of estrogen replacement therapy and PTH may mitigate the initial loss in cortical bone seen with PTH.[68] Use of PTH and alendronate together increases BMD more than alendronate alone but less than PTH alone, suggesting an antagonistic effect of the combination on PTH efficacy.[69,70] However, one year of PTH followed by a year of alendronate therapy resulted in significant increases in trabecular bone density and maintenance of cortical bone mass, suggesting that sequential therapy may be useful.[71]

Until more data is available regarding the effect of combination therapy on fractures, its routine use cannot be recommended.

NONPHARMACOLOGIC THERAPY

Exercise. Mechanical stress, such as that achieved by weight bearing activity, is well known to increase bone density and strength, whereas immobilization and a sedentary life style promote bone loss. Both observational and intervention studies have shown that BMD is greater in active versus sedentary individuals. Low intensity exercise, such as walking and low impact aerobics, can slow or halt bone loss, while more intensive regimens, such as weight training and high impact aerobics, have been shown to increase BMD. The increased muscle strength and improved balance seen with regular exercise may also decrease the risk of falls and subsequent fractures. Epidemiologic studies support this concept, but a decreased risk of fractures with exercise has not been confirmed in controlled trials.[26]

The optimal duration, intensity, frequency, and type of exercise needed to maintain or increase BMD is not known. Patients should be encouraged to participate in a regimen that is convenient and comfortable because consistency is a key component of any exercise regimen designed to protect bone. If the exercise regimen is not maintained, bone loss resumes.

Protection Against Falls. Osteoporotic hip fractures often result from a fall. Strategies for minimizing this risk include modifying the home environment (e.g., installing handrails, using nonslip rugs), using assistive ambulatory devices for stability and minimizing use of central nervous system–active drugs. Hip protectors may also provide protection for high-risk patients in long-term care facilities.[72]

ALTERNATIVE THERAPY

Epidemiologic data suggests that diets high in soy products decrease the risk of osteoporosis. This protective effect has been attributed to phytoestrogens, which are plant-based compounds with weak estrogenic activity. Isoflavone, the phytoestrogen found in soy protein, has shown a dose-related bone protective effect in studies; however, its optimal dose and long-term safety are unknown. Patients desiring to use natural products should be encouraged to increase their intake of soy-based foods rather than supplement with isolated isoflavones.[73]

FUTURE THERAPIES

Fluoride. Fluoride is not approved by the FDA for treating osteoporosis in the United States but it is approved in many European countries. At doses of at least 30 mg daily, sodium fluoride increases osteoblastic activity, thus uncoupling the BRU in favor of anabolism. Fluoride also substitutes for the hydroxyl ion in the crystal lattice, resulting in fluoroapatite instead of the physiologic compound hydroxyapatite. Studies have consistently shown that fluoride increases spinal bone mass up to 5% per year for a period of up to 4 years without significant effects on appendicular bone. However, a corresponding decrease in fracture rate has not been seen, suggesting that the bone formed by fluoride is of poor quality.[74]

The most common side effect of fluoride therapy is GI; including pain, nausea, diarrhea, or constipation. Up to 20% of patients may experience painful lower extremity syndrome. This acute-onset leg pain may be caused by cortical bone stress fractures.[75]

Further studies may identify a role for fluoride in the management of osteoporosis but at this time, it cannot be recommended for routine use.

Ipriflavone. Ipriflavone is a synthetic derivative of naturally occurring phytoestrogens. Although it has no apparent estrogenic activity in humans, it has been shown to have an inhibitory effect on osteoclasts while stimulating osteoblasts.[76] Some but not all studies have shown that 600 mg daily of ipriflavone maintains or increases BMD in postmenopausal women.[76,77] The drug appears to be well tolerated; GI side effects are the most common. Further studies are needed to define the role of this agent in treating osteoporosis.

Strontium Ranelate. Strontium ranelate (SR), an investigational agent, appears to inhibit bone resorption via a direct effect on osteoclasts and stimulates bone formation by increasing osteoblast precursors and stimulating collagen synthesis. Studies of SR (2 gm daily) in postmenopausal women with osteoporosis have reported a significant increase in BMD (approximately 12% in the spine and 7% in the femur) after 2 years of therapy. There was a significant decrease in VF versus placebo, however, the difference in non-VFs was not significant. SR appears to be well tolerated, and diarrhea was the most common adverse reaction in the clinical trials. Transient increases in serum calcium and creatine kinase levels and decreases in serum phosphate levels were reported during the initial months of the trials but normalized in the majority of patients without drug discontinuation.[78]

IMPROVING OUTCOMES

PATIENT EDUCATION

Many women are unaware of the risks for osteoporosis and how they can protect themselves.[79] The pharmacist is in a key position to provide the counseling and education needed for successful prevention and treatment. Adolescents should be advised to increase their calcium intake and exercise so that they enter their adult years with optimal bone mass. Perimenopausal and postmenopausal women should be encouraged to ingest adequate calcium, participate in weight bearing exercise, have adequate exposure to sunlight for vi-

tamin D production, and minimize the risk factors listed in Table 69.4. Patients who have been prescribed antiosteoporotic agents should be thoroughly educated on correct use, especially with the bisphosphonates, calcitonin, and teriparatide.

METHODS TO IMPROVE ADHERENCE

Osteoporosis is a noncurable disease and optimal treatment requires ongoing adherence to the prescribed regimen. However, one study showed that 19% to 26% of patients stopped therapy within 1 year of initiation. Reasons for stopping therapy included side effects and lack of understanding of personal risk for osteoporosis.[80] To optimize compliance, patients should be educated about their personal risk of osteoporosis, including BMD test results. Choice of therapy should be individualized and patients should be thoroughly educated to minimize the risk of side effects. Follow-up evaluation of BMD or biochemical markers can reassure patients that the therapy is having its desired effect, which may also reinforce adherence.

DISEASE MANAGEMENT STRATEGIES TO IMPROVE PATIENT OUTCOMES

Individuals who are unaware of their risk for osteoporosis are unlikely to seek out BMD testing. The availability of osteoporosis screening programs based in community pharmacies can provide a valuable service by early identification of persons with osteopenia or osteoporosis.[81] Pharmacists should review patient profiles for use of drugs that increase risk for bone disorders and initiate discussion regarding appropriate preventive measures.

PHARMACOECONOMICS

The direct medical costs of osteoporotic fractures have been estimated at $2,000 for a VF and $11,000 for a hip fracture, based on health care costs in the early 1990s.[82] The cost of preventing or osteoporotic fractures can vary widely. The estimated annual cost of antiosteoporotic drugs is outlined in Table 69.10. Due to their therapeutic importance and low cost, calcium and vitamin D supplementation should be recommended for all patients at risk. Estrogen therapy, with or without progestin supplementation, is one of the least expensive options; however, it is not considered an appropriate choice for long-term prevention of osteoporosis because of its risks. For patients at moderate risk, the bisphosphonates, raloxifene or calcitonin are appropriate choices. Because of its greater expense, teriparatide should be reserved for patients at high risk of fracture.

CONCLUSION

The approach to osteoporosis management is threefold. The optimal approach is to maximize bone density by encourag-

TABLE 69.10	Annual Cost of Drug Therapy for Osteoporosis		
Agent	**Daily Dosage**	**Generic Available**	**Annual Cost**[a]
Calcium (carbonate or citrate)	1,000 mg	Yes	$20–$62
Vitamin D	800 IU	Yes	$7–$11
Calcitriol	0.25–0.5 µg	Yes (solution only)	$218–$349
Alendronate	5 mg (or 35 mg weekly)	No	$852–$912
Alendronate	10 mg (or 70 mg weekly)	No	$852–$888
Risedronate	5 mg (or 35 mg weekly)	No	$852–$912
Raloxifene	60 mg	No	$984
Calcitonin nasal spray	200 IU	No	$1,044
Calcitonin injection	100 IU	No	$3,639
Teriperatide	20 µg	No	$7,200

[a] Average wholesale price (2004).

ing healthy lifestyles, including adequate calcium intake and weight bearing activity in children and young adults. For older adults, prevention includes minimizing risk factors, optimizing bone-preserving interventions (calcium, vitamin D, weight bearing activity) and initiating antiresorptive agents in those with low bone density. A decision algorithm such as the one in Figure 69.4 can be used for therapeutic decision making. For those who have already sustained an osteoporotic fracture, antiresorptive agents or teriparatide may be appropriate. Therapy for osteoporosis is still in evolution, and it will take several generations to define the optimal protocol.

OSTEOMALACIA

DEFINITION

Osteomalacia is a bone disorder characterized by inadequate bone mineralization, resulting in bone deformities. Rickets, the childhood manifestation, involves the growth plate and formed bone. Osteomalacia does not involve the epiphyses and occurs in adults. Osteomalacia was first described in 1645 in northern Europe during the industrial revolution, when many children and adults worked long hours with very little exposure to sunlight. However, it was not until the 1800s that an association with lack of sunlight was suggested. The identification of vitamin D and its sources has prevented most cases of vitamin-D-deficient rickets (VDDR), but several circumstances may put patients at risk for osteomalacia today.

TREATMENT GOALS

■ Select treatment based on underlying disorder.
■ Once acute episode has been resolved, initiate appropriate preventive therapy.

ETIOLOGY

Osteomalacia develops when phosphorus and calcium are not available for production of hydroxyapatite, the mineralized compound of bone matrix. The causes vary and include inadequate dietary intake of calcium, phosphorus, or vitamin D; genetic or acquired deficiencies of enzymes; and neoplasia.[83] Table 69.11 lists types of osteomalacia, causes, and general treatment guidelines.

EPIDEMIOLOGY

The exact incidence of osteomalacia is unknown. There is concern regarding a possible resurgence of rickets precipi-

TABLE 69.11	Osteomalacia Causes and Treatments	
Type	**Cause**	**Treatment**
VDDR	Inadequate sunlight Inadequate dietary intake Unsupplemented breastfeeding	Ultraviolet lamp or increased sun exposure Vitamin D
Inadequate calcium absorption	Chelators in diet: phytates, oxalates, excess phosphate	Dietary changes Calcium supplements
Inadequate calcium intake	Lack of dietary calcium	Dietary changes Calcium supplements

Phosphorus deficiency	Aluminum ingestion
	Prematurity with prolonged feeding of low-
	  phosphorus formula or TPN
		Avoidance of aluminum antacids,
		  contaminated sources
		Increased phosphorus intake

Gastric rickets	Gastrectomy Achlorhydria	Calcium citrate or other highly soluble calcium salt
Biliary rickets	Abnormal fat metabolism	Injectable vitamin D

Enteric rickets	Injury to small bowel by diseases such as
	  Crohn, coeliac sprue, short bowel
	  syndrome
		Injectable vitamin D

Hypophosphatemic rickets
  (Albright syndrome)
	Genetic or acquired fault of phosphorus
	  reabsorption in proximal tubule
		Phosphate, $1,25\text{-}(OH)_2\text{-}D$

Type I VDDR	Genetic or acquired deficiency of 25-hydroxyvitamin D–1-hydroxylase	$1,25\text{-}(OH)_2\text{-}D$
Type II VDDR	Intracellular $1,25\text{-}(OH)_2\text{-}D$ receptor defect	$1,25\text{-}(OH)_2\text{-}D$ and calcium
Renal tubular acidosis	Varied, results in calcium wasting	Alkalinization with sodium bicarbonate

Oncogenic or tumor-induced
  osteomalacia
	Bone and soft tissue neoplasia	Tumor resection
		Bisphosphonates, vitamin D,
		  phosphorus

Osteomalacia caused by
  hepatic-enzyme inducers
  (phenytoin, phenobarbital,
  rifampin)
	Stimulation of cytochrome P–450 enzyme
	  pathway resulting in accelerated
	  metabolism and deficient 25-OH-D
		$1,25\text{-}(OH)_2\text{-}D$

TPN-induced rickets in
  premature infants
	Inadequate calcium and phosphorus in
	  TPN solution
		Increase calcium and phosphorus to
		  maximum solubility

TPN, total parenteral nutrition; $1,25\text{-}(OH)_2\text{-}D$, 1,25-hydroxyvitamin D; VDDR, vitamin D-deficient rickets.

tated by multiple factors.[84] The population at increased risk for rickets includes infants born to mothers with vitamin D deficiency, exclusively breast-fed infants who do not receive vitamin D supplementation, children with low intake of calcium or vitamin D fortified foods, consistent use of sunscreens, darker skin pigmentation, and habitation at higher latitudes. Risk factors for osteomalacia include chronic renal impairment, low calcium intake, vitamin D deficiency and chronic use of medications that affect vitamin D.

PATHOPHYSIOLOGY

In osteomalacia, the bone remodeling process proceeds normally by the deposition of osteoid tissue at the sites of previous bone resorption. Osteomalacia is characterized by the body's inability to fully mineralize the newly formed osteoid tissue, resulting in decreased bone strength.

CLINICAL PRESENTATION AND DIAGNOSIS

SIGNS AND SYMPTOMS

Although there are multiple pathogenic causes, manifestations are similar with all causes. The bone manifestations of rickets include bowed legs in ambulatory children, enlarged wrists, and swollen costochondral rib junctions. Dentition may be delayed and there is greater risk of dental caries. Children may be apathetic and irritable. In severe cases, nonosseous manifestations can include hypocalcemic convulsions, tetany, myopathy, and heart failure.[84]

Adult osteomalacia manifests more subtly; the most common complaint is diffuse bone pain. Fatigue and malaise may also be present. As the disease progresses muscle weakness and altered gait may occur.[83]

DIAGNOSIS AND CLINICAL FINDINGS

The diagnostic radiological finding in rickets is cupping, splaying, and fraying of the metaphyses.[84] In children and adults, cortical and trabecular mineralized bone are covered by a large osteoid seam, an area of unmineralized bone. Generalized osteopenia may be present. Looser's lines, also known as pseudofractures, are strongly suggestive of osteomalacia.[83]

On serum chemistry analysis, PTH and alkaline phosphatase are elevated. Serum calcium and phosphorus may be normal or low, depending on the etiology. Calcidiol (25-OH-D) is low. Urinary calcium typically is low, unless the patient has phosphorus deficiency. In hypophosphatemic rickets, urinary phosphate is elevated.[83]

Evaluation of tetracycline uptake in bone can be used diagnostically for osteomalacia. Typically, two short courses (2–3 days) of tetracycline are administered at a 10- to 11-day interval. Bone biopsy of the iliac crest is performed 3 to 5 days after the second course. This site is used because it contains cortical and trabecular bone. The distance between the two tetracycline bands is observed and measured via fluorescent microscopy. This test assesses the rate of bone mineralization and can also differentiate osteoporosis from osteomalacia.[85]

TREATMENT

The treatment of osteomalacia depends on the underlying disorder identified, as seen in Table 69.11. If the cause is vitamin D deficiency, large dosages may be needed for 2 to 4 months but can be reduced as healing ensues. Therapy with vitamin D can be monitored with serum alkaline phosphatase, which decreases as body stores of vitamin D are depleted and therapeutic action occurs. Adequate calcium must also be given. Table 69.9 lists the vitamin D preparations and typical dosages available. The success of treatment depends on the underlying disorder.

IMPROVING OUTCOMES

The best prognosis for osteomalacia is obtained by preventive measures. The American Academy of Pediatrics recently recommended that all infants, children, and adolescents receive supplementation with 200 IU of vitamin D daily to prevent vitamin D-deficiency rickets.[86] Early identification and treatment can prevent bone deformities; therefore, patients at risk, such as premature infants on total parental nutrition, patients on phenytoin therapy, patients who have undergone gastrectomy, and others with conditions

listed in Table 69.11 should be monitored closely. After acute disease resolves, dietary therapy may be adequate to prevent relapse, depending on the underlying cause.

KEY POINTS

- Osteoporosis is a disease characterized by loss of bone mass and is clinically silent until a fracture occurs.
- As the population ages, there will be a significant increase in the number of women and men at risk for osteoporotic fractures.
- Preventive measures, such as exercise and risk avoidance, are key to maximizing bone mass and reducing risk of fractures.
- Adequate calcium intake, via diet or supplementation, should be recommended for all patients.
- Screening for patients at risk, by risk assessment and BMD measurements, can lead to early intervention and decreased risk of fractures.
- Patients on medications that may cause bone loss, such as glucocorticoids, should institute preventive measures and be monitored closely for the development of osteoporosis.
- Estrogen therapy, with or without progestin, prevents postmenopausal bone loss but is not recommended for long-term use due to its risks.
- Alendronate, risedronate and raloxifene decrease the risk of VF in women with osteoporosis and prevent bone loss in osteopenic postmenopausal women.
- In addition to decreasing bone resorption, calcitonin provides significant analgesic benefit for patients who have back pain caused by VF.
- Teriparatide can significantly increase BMD and decrease the risk of additional fractures in patients with established osteoporosis.
- Osteomalacia and rickets, two disorders of bone mineralization, often are caused by diet, drug, or disease-induced deficiencies in vitamin D, calcium, or phosphorus.

SUGGESTED READINGS

AACE Osteoporosis Task Force. American Association of Clinical Endocrinologists medical guidelines for clinic practice for the prevention and treatment of postmenopausal osteoporosis: 2001 edition, with selected updates for 2003. Endocr Pract 9:545–64, 2003.

American College of Rheumatology Ad Hoc Committee on Glucocorticoid-Induced Osteoporosis. Recommendations for the prevention and treatment of glucocorticoid-induced osteoporosis: 2001 updates. Arthritis Rheum 44:1498–1503, 2001.

Prince RL, Glendenning P. Disorders of bone and mineral other than osteoporosis. MJA 180:354–359, 2004.

Tannirandorn P, Epstein S. Drug-induced bone loss. Osteoporos Int 11: 637–659, 2000.

REFERENCES

1. Melton LJ III. Adverse outcomes of osteoporotic fractures in the general population. J Bone Miner Res 18:1139–1141, 2003.

2. NIH Consensus Development Panel on Osteoporosis Prevention, Diagnosis and Therapy. Osteoporosis prevention, diagnosis and therapy. JAMA 285:785–796, 2001.
3. U.S. Preventive Services Task Force. Screening for osteoporosis in postmenopausal women: recommendations and rationale. Available at: http:www.preventiveservices.ahrq.gov. Accessed Nov. 9, 2005.
4. Rosen CJ, Kessenich CR. The pathophysiology and treatment of postmenopausal osteoporosis: an evidence-based approach to estrogen replacement therapy. Endocrinol Metab Clin North Am 26: 295–311, 1997.
5. Hodgson SF, Watts NB, Bilezikian JP, et al. American Association of Clinical Endocrinologists medical guidelines for clinical practice for the prevention and treatment of postmenopausal osteoporosis: 2001 edition, with selected updates for 2003. Endocr Pract 9: 544–564, 2003.
6. Raisz GA, Rodan GA. Pathogenesis of osteoporosis. Endocrinol Metab Clin North Am 32:15–24, 2003.
7. Resnick NM, Greenspan SL. ''Senile'' osteoporosis reconsidered. JAMA 261:1025–1029, 1989.
8. Olszynski WP, Davison KS, Adachi JD, et al. Osteoporosis in men: epidemiology, diagnosis, prevention and treatment. Clin Ther 26: 15–28, 2004.
9. Tannirandorn P, Epstein S. Drug-induced bone loss. Osteoporos Int 11:637–659, 2000.
10. Ip M, Lam K, Yam L, et al. Decreased bone mineral density in premenopausal asthma patients receiving long-term inhaled steroids. Chest 105:1722–1727, 1994.
11. American College of Rheumatology Ad Hoc Committee on Glucocorticoid-Induced Osteoporosis. Recommendations for the prevention and treatment of glucocorticoid-induced osteoporosis: 2001 update. Arthritis Rheum 44:1496–1503, 2001.
12. Nelson-Piercy C. Heparin-induced osteoporosis. Scand J Rheumatol 27:S68–S71, 1998.
13. Caraballo PJ, Heit JA, Atkinson EJ, et al. Long-term use of oral anticoagulants and the risk of fracture. Arch Intern Med 159: 1750–1756, 1999.
14. Wawrzynska L, Tomkowski WZ, Przedlacki J, et al. Changes in bone density during long-term administration of low-molecular-weight heparins or acenocoumarol for secondary prophylaxis of venous thromboembolism. Pathophysiol Haemoszt Thromb 33:64–67, 2003.
15. Smith MR. Management of treatment-related osteoporosis in men with prostate cancer. Cancer Treat Rev 29:211–218, 2003.
16. Uemura T, Mohri J, Osada H, et al. Effect of gonadotropin-releasing hormone agonist on the bone mineral density of patients with endometriosis. Fertil Steril 62:246–250, 1994.
17. Cann CE. Bone densitometry as an adjunct to GnRH agonist therapy. J Reprod Med 43 (Suppl):321, 1998.
18. Hornstein MD, Surrey ES, Weisberg GW, et al. Leuprolide acetate depot and hormonal add-back in endometriosis: a 12-month study. Obstet Gynecol 91:16–24, 1998.
19. Surrey ES. Add-back therapy and gonadotropin-releasing hormone agonists in the treatment of patients with endometriosis: can a consensus be reached? Fertil Steril 71:420, 1999.
20. Mukherjee T, Barad D, Turk R, et al. A randomized, placebo-controlled study on the effect of cyclic intermittent etidronate therapy on the bone mineral density changes associated with six months of gonadotropin-releasing hormone agonist treatment. Am J Obstet Gynecol 175:105–109, 1996.
21. Farhat G, Yamout B, Mikati MA, et al. Effect of antiepileptic drugs on bone density in ambulatory patients. Neurology 58:1348–1353, 2002.
22. Feskanich D, Willett WC, Stampfer MJ, et al. A prospective study of thiazide use and fractures in women. Osteoporos Int 7:79–84, 1997.
23. Kiel DP, Baron JA, Anderson JJ, et al. Smoking eliminates the protective effect of oral estrogens on the risk for hip fracture among women. Ann Intern Med 116:716–721, 1992.
24. Cumming RG, Le Couteur DG. Benzodiazepines and risk of hip fracture in older people: a review of the evidence. CNS Drugs 17: 825–837, 2003.
25. Ensrud KR, Blackwell TL, Mangione CM, et al. Central nervous system-active medications and risk for falls in older women. J Am Geriatr Soc 50:1629–1637, 2002.
26. Todd JA, Robinson RJ. Osteoporosis and exercise. Postgrad Med J 79:320–323, 2003.
27. Looker AC, Orwoll ES, Johnston CC Jr, et al. Prevalence of low femoral bone density in older U.S. adults from NHANES III. J Bone Miner Res 12:1761–1768, 1997.
28. Riggs BL, Melton LJ III. The worldwide problem of osteoporosis: Insights afforded by epidemiology. Bone 17:505S–11S, 1995.
29. Cummings SR, Melton LJ III. Epidemiology and outcomes of osteoporotic fractures. Lancet 359:1761–1767, 2002.
30. Bohannon AD. Osteoporosis and African-American women. J Women Health Gen Based Med 8:609–615, 1999.
31. Kanis JA. The restoration of skeletal mass: a theoretic overview. Am J Med 91 (Suppl 5B):29S–36S, 1991.
32. Silverberg SJ, Lindsay R. Postmenopausal osteoporosis. Med Clin North Am 71:41–57, 1987.
33. Jilka RL. Biology of the basic multicellular unit and the pathophysiology of osteoporosis. Med Pediatr Oncol 41:182–185, 2003.
34. Ammann P, Rizzoli R. Bone strength and its determinants. Osteoporos Int 14:S13–S18, 2003.
35. Seibel MJ. Biochemical markers of bone remodeling. Endocrinol Metab Clin North Am 32:83–113, 2003.
36. Miller PD. Bone mineral density-clinical use and application. Endocrinol Metab Clin North Am 32:159–179, 2003.
37. Cummings SR, Bates D, Black DM. Clinical use of bone densitometry. JAMA 288:1889–1897, 2002.
38. Martin AR, Sornay-Rendu E, Chandler JM, et al. The impact of osteoporosis on quality-of-life: the OFELY Cohort. Bone 31:32–36, 2002.
39. North American Menopause Society. The role of calcium in peri- and postmenopausal women: consensus opinion of The North American Menopause Society. Menopause 8:84–95, 2001.
40. National Osteoporosis Foundation. Osteoporosis: review of the evidence for prevention, diagnosis, and treatment and cost-effectiveness analysis. Osteoporos Int 4:S7–S80, 1998.
41. Dawson-Hughes B, Dallal GE, Krall EA, et al. A controlled trial of the effect of calcium supplementation on bone density in postmenopausal women. N Engl J Med 323:878–883, 1990.
42. NIH Consensus Development Panel on Optimal Calcium Intake. Optimal calcium intake. JAMA 272:1942–1947, 1994.
43. Meunier PJ. Calcium, vitamin D and vitamin K in the prevention of fractures due to osteoporosis. Osteoporos Int 2:S48–S52, 1999.
44. Thomas MK, Lloyd-Jones DM, Thadhani RI, et al. Hypovitaminosis D in medical inpatients. N Engl J Med 338:777–783, 1998.
45. Papadimitropoulos E, Wells G, Shea B, et al. Meta-analysis of the efficacy of vitamin D treatment in preventing osteoporosis in postmenopausal women. Endocrin Rev 23:560–569, 2002.
46. Torgerson DJ, Bell-Syer SEM. Hormone replacement therapy and prevention of nonvertebral fractures: a meta-analysis of randomized trials. JAMA 285:2891–2897, 2001.
47. US Preventive Services Task Force. Postmenopausal hormone replacement therapy for primary prevention of chronic conditions: recommendations and rationale. Ann Intern Med 137:834–839, 2002.
48. North American Menopause Society. Estrogen and progestogen use in peri- and postmenopausal women: September 2003 position statement of the North American Menopause Society. Menopause 10: 497–506, 2003.
49. Ensrud KE, Black DM, Palermo L, et al. Treatment with alendronate prevents fractures in women at highest risk: results from the Fracture Intervention Trial. Arch Intern Med 157:2617–2624, 1997.
50. Liberman UA, Weiss SR, Broll J, et al. Effect of oral alendronate on bone mineral density and the incidence of fractures in postmenopausal osteoporosis. N Engl J Med 333:1437–1443, 1995.
51. Black DM, Cummings SR, Karpf DB, et al. Randomised trial of effect of alendronate on risk of fracture in women with existing vertebral fractures. Lancet 348:1535–1541, 1996.
52. Cummings SR, Black DM, Thompson DE, et al. Effect of alendronate on risk of fracture in women with low bone density but without vertebral fractures: results from the Fracture Intervention Trial. JAMA 280:2077–2082, 1998.
53. Saag KG, Emkey R, Schnitzer TJ, et al. Alendronate for the prevention and treatment of glucocorticoid-induced osteoporosis. N Engl J Med 339:292–299, 1998.
54. Bone HG, Hosking D, Devogelaer J, et al. Ten years' experience with alendronate for osteoporosis in postmenopausal women. N Engl J Med 350:1189–1199, 2004.

55. Cranney A, Tugwell P, Adachi J, et al. Meta-analysis of risedronate for the treatment of postmenopausal osteoporosis. Endocrin Rev 23: 517–523, 2002.

56. Hosking D, Adami S, Felsenberg D, et al. Comparison of change in bone resorption and bone mineral density with once-weekly alendronate and daily risedronate: a randomized placebo-controlled study. Curr Med Res Opin 19:383–394, 2003.

57. Thomason AB, Marshall JK, Hunt RH, et al. 14 day endoscopy study comparing risedronate and alendronate in postmenopausal women stratified by Helicobacter pylori status. J Rheumatol 29: 1965–1974, 2002.

58. Cranney A, Guyatt G, Krolicki N, et al. A meta-analysis of etidronate for the treatment of postmenopausal osteoporosis. Osteoporos Int 12:140–151, 2001.

59. Reid IR, Brown JP, Burckhardt P, et al. Intravenous zoledronic acid in postmenopausal women with low bone mineral density. N Engl J Med 346:653–661, 2002.

60. Heijckmann AC, Juttmann JR, Wolffenbuttel BH. Intravenous pamidronate compared with oral alendronate for the treatment of postmenopausal osteoporosis. Neth J Med 60:307–309, 2002.

61. Chestnut CH III, Skag A, Christiansen C, et al. Effects of oral ibandronate administered daily or intermittently on fracture risk in postmenopausal osteoporosis. J Bone Miner Res 19:1241–1249, 2004.

62. Riggs BL, Hartmann LC. Selective estrogen-receptor modulators—mechanisms of action and application to clinical practice. N Engl J Med 348:618–629, 2003.

63. Cranney A, Tugwell P, Zytaruk N, et al. Meta-analysis of raloxifene for the prevention and treatment of postmenopausal osteoporosis. Endocrin Rev 23:524–528, 2002.

64. Body JJ. Calcitonin for the long-term prevention and treatment of postmenopausal osteoporosis. Bone 30:75S–79S, 2002.

65. Gennari C. Analgesic effect of calcitonin in osteoporosis. Bone 30: 67S–70S, 2002.

66. Cappuzzo KA, Delafuente JC. Teriparatide for severe osteoporosis. Ann Pharmacother 38:294–302, 2004.

67. Compston, JE, Watts NB. Combination therapy for postmenopausal osteoporosis. Clin Endocrinol 56:565–569, 2002.

68. Lindsay R, Nieves J, Formica C, et al. Randomised controlled study of effect of parathyroid hormone on vertebral-bone mass and fracture incidence among postmenopausal women on oestrogen with osteoporosis. Lancet 350:550–555, 1997.

69. Finkelstein JS, Hayes A, Hunzelman JL, et al. The effects of parathyroid hormone, alendronate, or both in men with osteoporosis. N Engl J Med 349:1215–1229, 2003.

70. Black DM, Greenspan SL, Ensrud KE, et al. The effects of parathyroid hormone and alendronate alone or in combination in postmenopausal osteoporosis. N Engl J Med 349:1207–1215, 2003.

71. Rittmaster RS, Bolognese M, Ettinger MP, et al. Enhancement of bone mass in osteoporotic women with parathyroid hormone followed by alendronate. J Clin Endocrinol Metab 85:2129–2134, 2000.

72. Parker MJ, Gillespie LD, Gillespie WJ. Hip protectors for preventing hip fractures in the elderly. Cochrane Database Syst Rev 3: CD001255, 2003.

73. North American Menopause Society. The role of isoflavones in menopausal health: Consensus opinion of the North American Menopause Society. Menopause 7:215–229, 2000.

74. Haguenauer D, Welch V, Shea B, et al. Anabolic agents to treat osteoporosis in older people: is there still place for fluoride? J Am Geriatr Soc 2001;49:1387–1389, 2001.

75. Meunier PJ, Sebert JL, Reginster JY, et al. Fluoride salts are no better at preventing new vertebral fractures than calcium–vitamin D in postmenopausal osteoporosis: the FAVO Study. Osteoporos Int 8: 4–12, 1998.

76. Anon. Ipriflavone. Alt Med Rev 5:260–263, 2000.

77. Alexandersen P, Toussaint A, Christiansen C, et al. Ipriflavone in the treatment of postmenopausal osteoporosis: A randomized controlled trial. JAMA 285:1482–1488, 2001.

78. Meunier PJ, Roux C, Seeman E, et al. The effects of strontium ranelate on the risk of vertebral fracture in women with postmenopausal osteoporosis. N Engl J Med 350:459–468, 2004.

79. Ailinger RL, Emerson J. Women's knowledge of osteoporosis. Appl Nurs Res 11:111–114, 1998.

80. Tosteson ANA, Grove MR, Hammond CS, et al. Early discontinuation of treatment for osteoporosis. Am J Med 115:209–216, 2003.

81. Cerulli J, Zeolla MM. Impact and feasibility of a community pharmacy bone mineral density screening and education program. J Am Pharm Assoc 44:161–167, 2004.

82. Gabriel SE, Tosteson ANA, Leibson CL, et al. Direct medical costs attributable to osteoporotic fractures. Osteoporos Int 13:323–330, 2002.

83. Prince RL, Glendenning P. Disorders of bone and mineral other than osteoporosis. Med J Aust 180:354–359, 2004.

84. Wharton B, Bishop N. Rickets. Lancet 362:1389–1400, 2003.

85. Recker RR. Bone biopsy and histomorphometry in clinical practice. In: Favus MJ, ed. Primer on the metabolic bone diseases and disorders of mineral metabolism. 3rd ed. Philadelphia: Lippincott-Raven, 1996:164–167.

86. Gartner LM, Greer FR. Prevention of rickets and vitamin D deficiency: New guidelines for vitamin D intake. Pediatrics 111: 908–909, 2003.

CASE STUDIES

CASE 27

TOPIC: Rheumatoid Arthritis

THERAPEUTIC DIFFICULTY: Level 2
Eric Boyce

Chapter 65: Rheumatoid Arthritis

■ Scenario

Patient and Setting: MB, a 45-year-old female; outpatient clinic

Chief Complaint: Routinely scheduled follow-up visit 6 months after diagnosis with rheumatoid arthritis; complains of fatigue, swelling of joints in hands, wrists, and feet

■ History of Present Illness

Diagnosed with rheumatoid arthritis 6 months ago following 1 year of fatigue, malaise, and increased swelling in joints of hands and feet. Ibuprofen 400 mg QID was initial therapy, but increased to 600 mg QID 3 months ago; some relief, but symptoms persist.

Medical History: Perennial seasonal rhinitis for 10 years, three normal pregnancies

Surgical History: None

Family/Social History: Family History: Mother alive, 65 years old, has arthritis in her knees and back, osteoporosis; father, 70 years old, with hypertension (HTN), diabetes mellitus Type 2, dyslipidemia, and congestive heart failure (CHF)
Social History: Alcohol: 1–2 glasses of wine nightly. Denies smoking cigarettes or illegal/recreational drug use

Medications:
Ibuprofen, 400 mg PO QID
One-a-Day Vitamins, 1 PO QAM
Ortho Tri-Cyclin, 1 PO QAM
Calcium carbonate, 500 mg 2 PO QAM
Loratidine, 10 mg PO QD PRN

Allergies: Documented allergy to "sulfa" drugs and penicillin—both caused minor rash, no anaphylaxis

Review of Symptoms/Systems: General: feels stiff each morning for 2 to 3 hours; able to perform all self-care and daily activities, but does so with discomfort; skin: developing some wrinkles, no other problems; headaches occasionally, particularly when her allergies are active; eyes: had to buy reading glasses to read small print, but no inflammation or discomfort; denies photosensitivity, urinary or bowel problems, vaginitis, SOB, perimenopausal symptoms.

■ Physical Examination

GEN: Well-developed, well-nourished woman appearing in some discomfort SOB
VS: BP 118/78, HR 82, RR 16, T 37.2°C, Wt 53 kg, Ht 160 cm, pain 5 out of 10
HEENT: PERRLA, EOMI, neck supple, no lymphadenopathy
DERM: A few minor bruises, olive complexion, no rashes or discoloration
COR: RRR, no murmurs/rubs/gallops
CHEST: CTAP, no wheezes/rhonchi/rales
ABD: Active bowel sounds, no tenderness or pain
GU: Deferred
RECT: Guaiac negative
EXT: Metacarpophalangeal joints (MCPs), proximal interphalangeal joints (PIPs), wrists, metatarsophalangeal joints (MTPs): 2+ swelling and 2+ tenderness bilaterally; strength 3/5; sensations and pulses WNL
NEURO: Alert and oriented X4, CN II-XII intact

■ Results of Pertinent Laboratory Tests, Serum Drug Concentrations, and Diagnostic Tests

Na 138 (138)	AST 0.37 (22)	Hct 0.33 (33)
K 4.1 (4.1)	ALT 0.47 (28)	Hgb 117 (11.7)
Cl 101 (101)	Plts 430 × 10⁹	Lkcs 6.0 × 10⁹
HCO₃ 25 (25)	(430 × 10⁹)	(6.0 × 10³)
BUN 4.6 (13)	MCV 88 (88)	LDH 1.5 (90)
Mg 1.2 (2.4)	Uric Acid 202 (34)	Alk Phos 1.7 (100)
Glu 5.0 (90)	Ca 2.2 (8.8)	PO₄ 0.95 (3.1)
Alb 42 (4.2)	CR 88 (1.0)	T Bili 6.8 (0.4)

ANA negative
RF positive, 1:640
ESR 45 mm/hour
X-ray of hands and wrists: soft tissue swelling of MCPs, PIPs, and carpals with small erosions of bone in MCPs 3, 4, and 5 bilaterally. No deformities noted

■ Problem List

Identify principal problems from the scenario in priority order (see Answers in back of book for correct list of problems).

1807

■ SOAP Note

To be completed by the student (see Answers in back of book for correct SOAP Note).

■ QUESTIONS

(See Answers in back of book for correct responses.)

1. List the extra-articular (nonjoint) signs and symptoms of rheumatoid arthritis seen in MB and others that are not evident. (EO-2)

2. What is the major adverse effect associated with the long-term use of high-dose ibuprofen in MB? (EO-8)
   a. Renal dysfunction
   b. Cardiac dysfunction
   c. Liver dysfunction
   d. Gastrointestinal ulceration

3. The major evidence that MB has progressive rheumatoid arthritis is/are her: (EO-4)
   a. High rheumatoid factor
   b. Elevated erythrocyte sedimentation rate
   c. Bony erosions seen on joint x-rays
   d. Prolonged morning stiffness

4. Folic acid is used in combination with methotrexate to prevent methotrexate-induced (EO-8, 10)
   a. Anemia and stomatitis
   b. Renal toxicity
   c. Rheumatoid nodulosis
   d. Infection

5. Describe the mechanisms of action of the renal, platelet, and gastrointestinal adverse effects of ibuprofen. (EO-5, 8)

6. Compare methotrexate to etanercept in the treatment of patients with rheumatoid arthritis and describe the most likely reasons why methotrexate was selected over etanercept as the initial disease-modifying antirheumatic drug in this patient. (EO-6, 8, 13)

7. Chronic therapy with low-dose oral prednisone is likely to (EO-8)
   a. Cause osteoporosis and hypothalamic-pituitary-adrenal axis suppression
   b. Crystal-induced arthritis and tendon rupture
   c. Bone marrow suppression and renal dysfunction
   d. Decrease serum cholesterol and glucose

8. Which of the following two drugs are most likely to cause an allergic reaction in MB based on her history? (EO-6, 8)
   a. Naproxen and nabumetone
   b. Hydroxychloroquine and sulindac
   c. Celecoxib and sulfasalazine
   d. Infliximab and leflunomide

9. Which of the following disease-modifying anti-rheumatic drugs is least likely to cause infection? (EO-8)
   a. Etanercept
   b. Methotrexate
   c. Anakinra
   d. Sulfasalazine

10. MB is still early in the course of her rheumatoid arthritis. If her disease continues to progress, she can be expected to experience a continued loss of function, diminished quality of life, joint deformities, and (EO-1, 2)
    a. Depression
    b. Schizophrenia
    c. Seizures
    d. Obsessive-compulsive disorder

11. Which of the following disease-modifying anti-rheumatic drugs is most likely to have the highest drug acquisition costs? (EO-13)
    a. Methotrexate
    b. Adalimumab
    c. Sulfasalazine
    d. Leflunomide

12. How would your therapeutic regimen change if MB had been on methotrexate already without adverse effects, but still had evidence of active disease (joint swelling and pain) and progressive disease (worsening of bony erosions)? (EO-9, 10)

13. Summarize therapeutic, pathophysiologic, and disease management concepts for the treatment of rheumatoid arthritis utilizing a key points format. (EO-18)

CASE 28

TOPIC: Osteoarthritis

THERAPEUTIC DIFFICULTY: Level 2
Ralph E. Small

Chapter 66: Osteoarthritis

■ Scenario

Patient and Setting: CD, a 78-year-old female; general medicine clinic

Chief Complaint: Nausea, right upper quadrant abdominal pain, and aching pain in left knee

■ History of Present Illness

Intermittent relief of osteoarthritis (OA) of the hips, knees, and hands with PRN acetaminophen, ibuprofen; orthopedic surgeon prescribed 7-day supply of propoxyphene apsylate/acetaminophen (100/650 mg) for recent increase in pain level 6 weeks ago; CD did not return for reevaluation as directed and obtained additional courses of propoxyphene napsylate/acetaminophen from internist, dentist, outpatient emergency center over past few weeks; recent increase in activity (weekly bowling, ballroom dance lessons), takes extra propoxyphene napsylate/acetaminophen after activities; new-onset joint swelling in past week; difficulty sleeping, increased irritability ("snapping" at family members often) for 6 weeks

Medical History: OA/degenerative joint disease (DJD) for 20 years; difficulty falling asleep for approximately 3 years (time of husband's death); osteoporosis for 4 years

Surgical History: Right knee replacement 1 year ago (left knee replacement recommended, CD reluctant)

Family/Social History: Family History: Lives alone, performs weight-bearing tasks regularly; refuses family assistance with chores; eats "fast food" 4–5 times per week
Social History: No tobacco use; drinks caffeinated tea daily and two glasses of sherry at night to fall asleep

Medications:
Acetaminophen, 325 mg PO q6h PRN pain × 15 years
Ibuprofen, 200 mg PO q6h PRN pain, occasionally × 2 years
Acetaminophen, 650 mg/propoxyphene napsylate 100 mg, 1 tab PO q4h PRN pain (per physician order) and 2 tabs PO PRN severe pain (self-initiated); 6 to 8 tablets daily × 6 weeks
Triazolam, 0.0625 to 0.125 mg PO QHS PRN for sleep × 3 years
Alendronate, 70 mg PO q week with water first thing in the morning and at least 30 minutes before first food, beverage, or other medication. Stand for at least 30 minutes
Calcium carbonate, 1,200 mg/day
Vitamin D, 400 IU/day

Allergies: No known drug allergies

■ Physical Examination

GEN: Elderly, fairly obese woman in moderate distress

VS: BP 125/80, HR 85, RR 20, T 37°C, Wt 60 kg, Ht 153 cm (decreased from past)
HEENT: WNL
COR: WNL
CHEST: Kyphosis, otherwise WNL
ABD: RUQ tenderness; mild guarding; moderately obese
GU: Deferred
RECT: Deferred
EXT: Limited range of motion of left knee with mild swelling, tenderness, warmth
NEURO: Alert, O × 3

■ Results of Pertinent Laboratory Tests, Serum Drug Concentrations, and Diagnostic Tests

Na 140 (140)	Lkcs 8.5 × 10^9 (8.5 × 10^3)	Alk Phos 2.0 (120)
K 3.9 (3.9)	Plts 180 × 10^9 (180 × 10^3)	Alb 33 (3.3)
Cl 103 (103)	MCV 91 (91)	T Bili 17.1 (1.0)
HCO_3 27 (27)	Cr 88.4 (1.0)	Glu 5.6 (100)
BUN 4.3 (12)	AST 0.33 (20)	Ca 4.5 (8.9)
ESR 15 (15)	ALT 0.50 (30)	PO_4 1.2 (3.7)
Hct 0.36 (36)	Mg 0.95 (2.3)	
Hgb 120 (12)	INR normal	

X-ray: Joint-space narrowing, left knee; chest-increased width of intervertebral spaces
DXA: T score −1.2 (± 1)

■ Problem List

Identify principal problems from the scenario in priority order (see Answers in back of book for correct list of problems).

■ SOAP Note

To be completed by the student (see Answers in back of book for correct SOAP Note).

■ QUESTIONS

(See Answers in back of book for correct responses.)

1. The most likely cause for CD's worsening pain associated with osteoarthritis is: (EO-1)
   a. Use of propoxyphene/acetaminophen for pain
   b. Frequent heavy, weight-bearing activities such as mowing the lawn, bowling, and vacuuming
   c. Use of ibuprofen PRN
   d. Elevated liver function tests

2. CD presents with many signs and symptoms of osteoarthritis. Which of the following is not present? (EO-2)
   a. Joint stiffness
   b. Crepitus
   c. Joint deformity
   d. Joint space narrowing on radiography

3. List potential causes for CD's chronic insomnia. (EO-1)

4. What psychosocial factors may adversely influence CD's perception of pain and disability associated with osteoarthritis? (EO-15)

5. CD is experiencing right upper quadrant abdominal pain. Results of CD's laboratory tests indicate normal levels of AST, ALT, and alkaline phosphatase. These laboratory tests were evaluated because an elevation could potentially occur from which of her medications? (EO-10)
   a. Triazolam
   b. Ibuprofen
   c. Acetaminophen
   d. Propoxyphene

6. Which of the following factors present in CD's history may make her more susceptible to drug-induced liver toxicity? (EO-4, 6, 8)
   a. Alcohol consumption
   b. Caffeine consumption
   c. Kyphosis
   d. Allergy to aspirin

7. Describe the mechanisms of action of the pharmacologic and nonpharmacologic interventions in this case. (EO-7)

8. Which of the following would be an appropriate principle to follow for appropriate NSAID use in CD? (EO-8)
   a. Use of minimum effective dose
   b. Assessment of benefit after 4 months
   c. Patient education regarding appropriate use after 2 weeks of therapy
   d. Use of more than one NSAID simultaneously

9. Which of the following pharmacologic treatment problems is present in CD's existing treatment plan? (EO-11)
   a. Inadequate trial of triazolam for insomnia
   b. Daily acetaminophen therapy exceeds recommended dose

   c. Propoxyphene dose inadequate for pain control
   d. Acetaminophen therapy is inadequate in the treatment of osteoarthritis

10. What risk factor does CD have that may predispose her to NSAID-induced peptic ulcer disease (PUD)? (EO-4, 6, 8, 10)
    a. History of upper GI bleed
    b. Concomitant use of corticosteroids
    c. Age
    d. High NSAID dose

11. After 1 month of therapy with acetaminophen 1 g and topical capsaicin, CD's response is inadequate and signs of effusion and increased inflammation are present in her left knee. Which of the following treatment modalities would be an appropriate option? (EO-8, 12)
    a. Prednisone 2 mg/kg PO QD
    b. Acetaminophen 1,000 mg PO QID, with additional doses PRN
    c. Ibuprofen 1,000 mg PO QID
    d. Triamcinolone acetonide 40 mg intra-articular injection

12. Evaluate the pharmacoeconomic considerations associated with CD's plan of care. (EO-17)

13. List the education points for CD with regards to the proper use of topical capsaicin. (EO-11, 12, 14, 15)

14. If CD's physician decided to initiate therapy with meloxicam 7.5 mg daily, given CD's complaints of nausea and right upper quadrant abdominal pain, what could be done to further reduce the risk of gastrointestinal complications? (EO-8, 10, 11, 12)
    a. Initiate concomitant therapy with a calcium/magnesium antacid four times daily (after meals and at bedtime)
    b. Initiate concomitant therapy with rabeprazole 20 mg daily 30 minutes before breakfast
    c. Initiate concomitant therapy with sucralfate 1 g QID (before meals and at bedtime)
    d. Initiate concomitant therapy with cimetidine 300 mg QID

15. Summarize pathophysiologic, therapeutic, and disease management concepts for osteoarthritis utilizing a key points format. (EO-18)

Alzheimer's Disease

70

Nathan Rawls

DEFINITION

In 1907 Alois Alzheimer, a neuropsychiatrist, first described a syndrome of clinical features characterized by a decline of memory and other cognitive functions in comparison with the patient's previous level of function.[1] Dr. Alzheimer described a specific patient, Auguste D., who over a prolonged period had worsening memory and loss of the ability to care for herself. The dementia he described is now called Alzheimer's disease (AD) or primary degenerative dementia of the Alzheimer's type (DAT).[2] Dementia is a general term used to characterize a progressive decline in cognition that results in impairment of occupational, social, and normal living activities. Cognition is defined as that operation of the mind process by which we become aware of objects of thought and perception, including all aspects of perceiving, thinking, and remembering.[3]

Disturbances in memory are the hallmark of AD, but other cognitive functions such as language use, visual-spatial perception, and the ability to learn, solve problems, perform mathematical calculations, think abstractly, and make appropriate judgments are also affected. This disease has an insidious onset, is progressive, and is differentiated by the exclusion of other diseases that would account for the cognitive deterioration and personality changes. AD is a chronic, degenerative neurologic disease with symptoms that are treatable but has no known cure.

TREATMENT GOALS

- Accurately diagnose the cause of dementia to provide appropriate treatment. For example, in dementia due to stroke, medications such as aspirin may prevent further stroke and impairment.
- Recognize that some depressed patients may present with symptoms similar to Alzheimer's disease and require careful diagnosis and a therapeutic trial of an antidepressant that may resolve the cognitive symptoms.
- Use medications to prevent progression of the disease. In Alzheimer's disease, new medications may slow the disease process and maintain the patient's function while sustaining the best quality of life.
- Treat other causes of dementia symptoms.
- Manage psychiatric symptoms if necessary.
- Provide a safe environment for the patient.

- Provide health maintenance and optimize sensory input (such as glasses for sight, hearing aids, walkers for ambulation).
- Maintain function: activities of daily living (ADLs) are self-maintenance skills such as dressing, bathing, eating, toileting, and ambulating; and ADLs are higher-order skills such as managing finances, driving a car, adhering to medication schedule, and using the telephone.
- Plan for future medical, financial, and legal decisions.
- Provide caregiver education and support.

ETIOLOGY

The etiology of AD is unknown, but the effect of the disease process leads to neuronal injury. Evidence suggests that a chronic inflammatory process may contribute to neuron pathogenesis. The major biochemical abnormality observed in AD is a 40% to 90% reduction in the enzyme choline acetyltransferase in the cerebral cortex and hippocampus. The deficiency of this enzyme causes decreased synthesis of acetylcholine in the brain. The loss of acetyltransferase in the brain appears to begin before the onset of clinical symptoms. There seems to be a strong correlation between the degree of enzyme reduction and the amount of acetylcholine and the decline of mental status scores and abnormal symptoms.

Although acetylcholine may be the primary neurotransmitter deficit associated with AD, other neurotransmitters have been implicated. Variable losses in the amount of norepinephrine and the biosynthetic enzyme dopamine β-hydroxylase and decreases of serotonin may account for noncognitive symptoms of depression and aggression. Clinical symptoms exhibited may be the result of a combination of neurotransmitter deficiencies in different individuals. There is evidence to support that the changes seen with AD is the result of β-amyloid (Aβ) accumulation in the brain. Aβ is a fragment of amyloid precursor protein (APP) and accumulates as amyloid plaques on neurons and may cause inflammation and cell death. The ''amyloid hypothesis'' is based on animal studies and the observation that individuals with Down syndrome have a genetic predisposition to develop amyloid plaques and usually develop symptoms of AD by middle age.[4]

EPIDEMIOLOGY

AD primarily affects the elderly and is the cause of a majority of dementia cases. It affects more than 4.5 million people in the United States. More than 100,000 people die of AD each year.[5] The prevalence of dementia doubles every 5 years from the ages of 60 to 90. A community-based study of elderly people found that 5% to 10% of the U.S. population over age 65 has AD. The prevalence increases with age and may reach nearly 30% to 50% in those more than 85

years old.[6] Although the dementia syndrome may be caused by more than 70 disorders (Table 70.1), more than 50% of the cases are attributed to AD; this is followed by dementia associated with cardiovascular disease, or a combination of the two. Other significant causes of dementia include Parkinson disease, neurodegenerative disorders such as Lewy body disease, toxins, and metabolic disorders. The putative risk factors for AD include advancing age, a history of dementia, and Down syndrome in a first-degree relative.[7] Other possible risk factors are previous head trauma, a family history of Down syndrome, and thyroid disease.

AD may be considered as familial (having a definite pattern of inheritance) or sporadic (occurring at random). Currently four genes are thought to be involved in the development of AD. One genetic risk factor on chromosome 19, apolipoprotein E-4 (APOE), is associated with late-onset (after age 60–65) AD.[8] At least three autosomal-dominant genes have been identified and account for about one half of early-onset symptoms (before age 60). These genes are presenilin 1 on chromosome 14,[9] rare ones such as presenilin 2 on chromosome 1, and APP on chromosome 21.[10]

PATHOPHYSIOLOGY

From brain autopsy studies, patients with AD have been found to have cortical atrophy and a significant loss of neurons. Two hallmark histopathologic features linked to AD are an increase in amyloid plaques and a high density of neurofibrillary tangles.[11] Within neuronal cells are microtubules which are bundles of paired helical filamentous structures that are necessary for normal cell function. These microtubules are connected by tau protein and in patients with AD, tau protein is damaged and allows neurons to twist into filaments that disrupt normal cell function (Fig. 70.1; *see color insert*). Neurofibrillary tangles are diagnostic for AD and were first reported by Dr. Alzheimer.

Amyloid plaques containing Aβ protein, accumulate with normal aging but occur in quantitative excess in AD. Aβ is the core of neuritic plaques and is a fragment from APP. APP is a larger transmembrane protein that is normally neuroprotective but in AD patients cleavage results in excessive Aβ. Aβ forms the central core of amyloid plaques, which are dense insoluble deposits that form around neurons and disrupt cell function (Fig. 70.2; *see color insert*). In autopsy

TABLE 70.1	Causes of Dementia Syndrome[a]

Psychiatric Disorders	**Infections**
Depression	AIDS
Delirium	Neurosyphilis
Paranoid states	Meningitis
Schizophrenia	Tuberculosis
Trauma	Pneumonia
Subdural hematoma	Creutzfeldt-Jakob (slow virus)
Dementia pugilistica	**Intracranial conditions**
Drugs and Toxins	Hydrocephalus
Anticholinergics	Neoplasms
Antidepressants	Strokes
Anticonvulsants	**Degenerative neurological disorders**
Alcohol	Alzheimer's disease
Benzodiazepines	Frontotemporal dementia
Barbiturates	Huntington chorea
Propranolol	Parkinson's disease
Methyldopa	Dementia with Lewy bodies
Reserpine	**Cardiovascular**
Heavy metal poisoning	Congestive heart failure
Organophosphates	Arrhythmia
Metabolic Disorders	Vascular occlusion
Renal failure	**Nutritional disorders**
Fluid/electrolyte imbalances	Vitamin B_{12} deficiency
Hypoglycemia/hyperglycemia	Folate deficiency
Hypothyroidism/hyperthyroidism	Thiamine deficiency
Hepatic failure	**Collagen vascular disorders**
Addison disease	Systemic lupus erythematosus
Cushing syndrome	Temporal arteritis
Hypopituitarism	
Severe anemia	
Hypoxia/anoxia	

[a] Table represents a partial list.
AIDS, acquired immunodeficiency disease.

studies, the degree of plaque formation has been highly correlated with the degree of clinical impairment observed when the patient was alive.

Mutations of APP gene on chromosomes 21 and 14 have been linked to familial AD.[12] Current research has shown a possible role for APOE in the pathogenesis of AD. The APOE gene occurs in three versions with APOE-4 being associated with an increased risk of AD. APOE-4 is a protein that binds to the Aβ and is present in neuritic plaques and tangles. Because it makes amyloid deposition in plaques more likely, it is considered a risk factor for developing late-onset AD.[13] APOE testing can be done and has been considered as a possible screening method for asymptomatic persons concerned about developing AD. The federal government has recommended against APOE blood testing because the presence of this gene is not diagnostic for AD and as there is no preventative action that can be taken, a positive result would not provide benefit.[14]

CLINICAL PRESENTATION AND DIAGNOSIS

SIGNS AND SYMPTOMS
The pathophysiology of AD may begin long before clinical symptoms are apparent. There is an extended time course

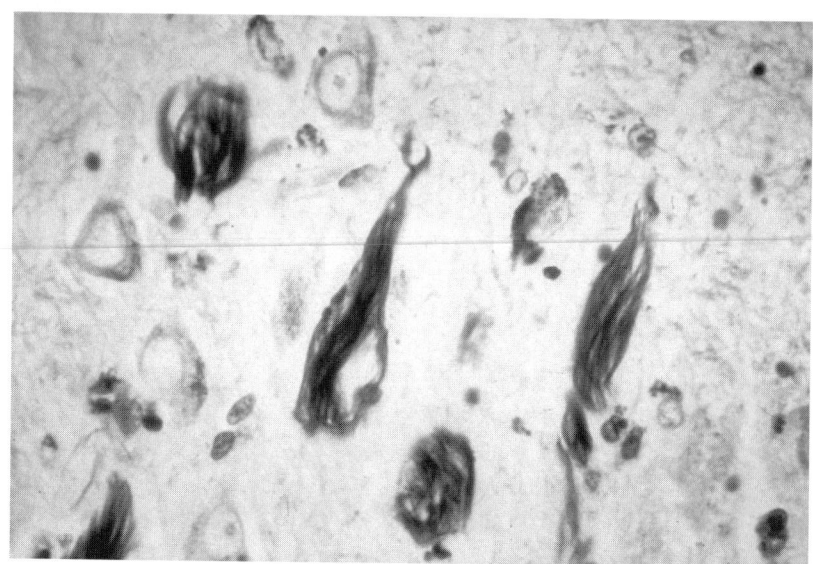

FIGURE 70.1 The cytoplasm of neurons distended by neurofibrillary tangles (*see color insert*). (From Rubin E, Faber JL. Pathology. 3rd ed. Philadelphia: Lippincott Williams & Wilkins, 1999.)

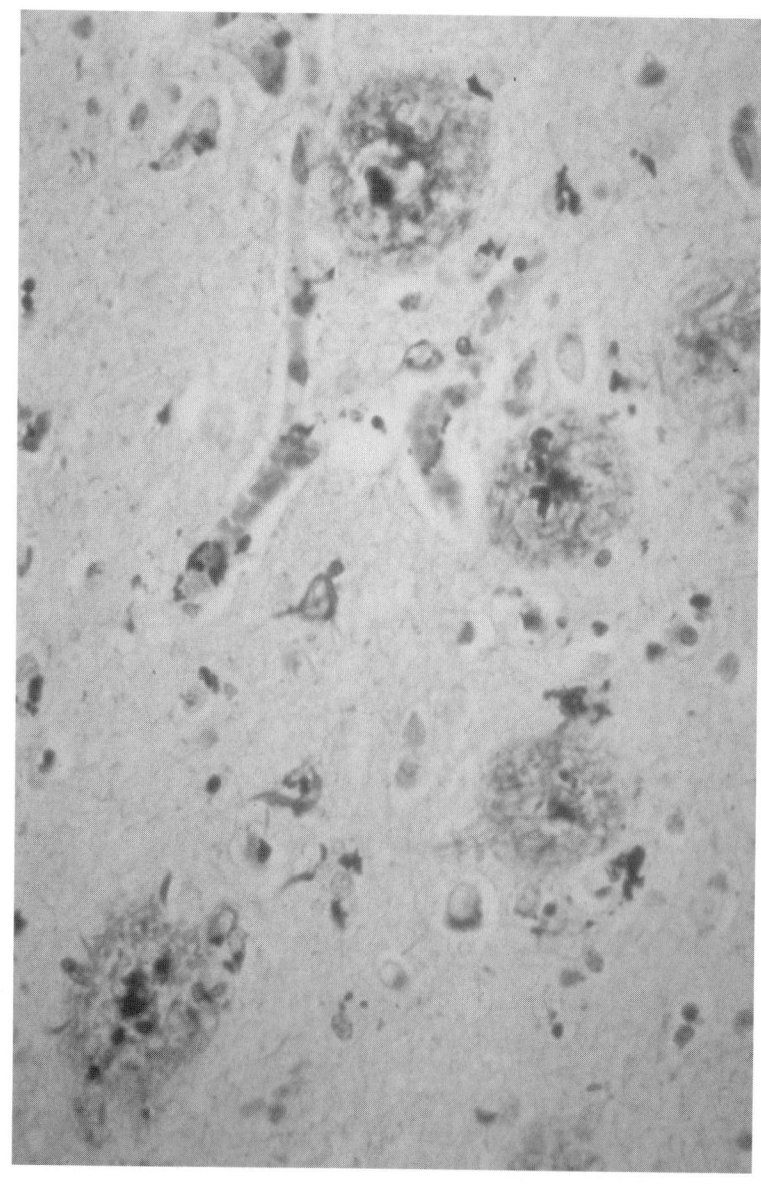

FIGURE 70.2 Neuritic plaques in the cerebral cortex, showing a dense core of amyloid (*see color insert*). (From Rubin E, Faber JL. Pathology. 3rd ed. Philadelphia: Lippincott Williams & Wilkins, 1999.)

with risk factors from genetic predisposition and environment in the clinical expression of the disease. AD causes a progressive deterioration in intellectual abilities such that it interferes with the person's ability to function in occupational or social situations. Several cognitive changes may occur, including: (a) progressive deterioration of short-term memory or the ability to learn and retain small amounts of information; (b) language dysfunction (aphasia) such as difficulty finding words and loss of auditory comprehension leading to inability to understand questions and follow directions; and (c) inability to draw and recognize two-dimensional and three-dimensional figures. In addition, patients may have difficulty balancing a checkbook, driving, using a telephone, and taking medications as prescribed. They may forget to turn off the stove while cooking, may become disoriented or lost, and may not be able to dress and feed themselves. Eventually the patient loses the ability to care for himself or herself. Behavioral disturbances are prevalent and may increase as the disease progresses.

The onset of symptoms often is overlooked or dismissed as a natural progression of aging. In early or mild dementia, the most common symptoms include signs of depression, personality changes, and misidentifications. As the disease progresses, there may be increases in agitation, psychiatric symptoms such as mood disturbances, and psychotic symptoms such as delusions, hallucinations, and paranoia. The average duration of illness from clinical onset of symptoms to death is said to be 8 to 11 years but current efforts to diagnose AD earlier will result in longer duration of illness being reported in the future.

Occasional difficulty remembering names or word finding may be associated with aging and should not be confused with AD. A syndrome of mild cognitive impairment (MCI) has been described with the chief complaint of memory loss and without the more pervasive symptoms normally associated with AD. There has been a report that up to 40% of MCI patients will develop AD within 3 years of being identified with this syndrome and some research suggest that MCI is often an early stage of AD.[15]

Medications may cause delirium or exacerbate an existing organic dementia. Delirium can also be caused by a variety of medical conditions which require immediate management to prevent morbidity and mortality. Delirium can be confused with worsening dementia in an AD patient and this could delay treatment of an underlying medical condition. Delirium tends to have an abrupt onset, a fluctuating course, and is associated with a decline in consciousness, disorientation, and perceptual disturbances (Table 70.2). In addition to causing delirium, many medications may cause memory impairment and confusion. Any medication the patient is taking should be evaluated for possible misadventures such as intoxication, drug interactions, and medication misuse.

The elderly use many medicines that are high in anticholinergic side effects; these effects are additive; therefore, more anticholinergic medications increase the likelihood that clinical symptoms will develop. It is critical to obtain

TABLE 70.2	Diagnostic Criteria for Delirium (DSM-IV)

A. Disturbance of consciousness (i.e., reduced clarity of awareness of the environment) with reduced ability to focus, sustain, or shift attention.

B. A change in cognition (such as memory deficit, disorientation, language disturbance, or the development of a perceptual disturbance that is not better accounted for by a preexisting, established, or evolving dementia).

C. The disturbance develops over a short period of time (usually hours to days) and tends to fluctuate during the course of the day.

D. There is evidence from the history, physical examination, or laboratory findings that the disturbance is caused by the direct physiological consequences of a general medical condition.

DSM-IV, Diagnostic and Statistical Manual of Mental Disorders. (From American Psychiatric Association. Diagnostic and Statistical Manual of Mental Disorders. 4th ed. Washington, DC: American Psychiatric Association, 1994:142–143, with permission.)

an accurate list of medications and dosages the patient is taking, including nonprescription drugs and supplements (Table 70.3). Discontinuing unnecessary medications, tapering to geriatric dosages, or changing the selection of medication to decrease side effects is an important process and may be a vital therapeutic intervention.

DIAGNOSIS

Much attention in recent years has been directed at the early diagnosis of AD. This not only would allow for the patient and caregiver/s to be better prepared but would also allow for newer treatments the opportunity to slow or prevent cognitive decline. Diagnostic criteria such as in the Diagnostic and Statistical Manual of Mental Disorders (DSM)-IV (Table 70.4) and a number of guidelines are available to assist clinicians.[17-21] Key elements of the clinical syndrome in mild AD are insidious onset, progressive course, impaired orientation, learning and recent speech, empty speech and anomia, visuospatial problems, apathy, poor self-awareness, and emotional withdrawal.

The diagnosis of AD should include a detailed medical history and evaluation using diagnostic criteria such as in DSM-IV (see Table 70.4), laboratories (Table 70.5), and physical examination along with an assessment of functional performance and a mental status examination.[22] The Mini-Mental State Examination (MMSE) is the most frequently used brief mental status examination in the United States.[23] The MMSE is simple and easy to administer and accepted by most practitioners as a practical method of evaluating cognitive functioning. With a maximum score of 30, scores of less than 20 indicate moderate impairment and less than 10 would indicate severe cognitive decline. Untreated AD patients have been reported to decline 2–4 points per year.[24] Visual, auditory, and physical functioning can adversely influence MMSE scores. Race, language, cultural background,

TABLE 70.3	Anticholinergic Agents
Class	**Agents**
Antidepressants	Highest effects: amitriptyline, amoxapine, clomipramine, protriptyline, Moderate effects: bupropion, doxepin, imipramine, maprotiline, trimipramine Minimal effects: nortriptyline, desipramine, trazodone, paroxetine
Antiparkinson agents	Benztropine, trihexyphenidyl
Antipsychotics	Highest effects: clozapine, mesoridazine, olanzapine, promazine, triflupromazine, thioridazine Moderate effects: chlorpromazine, chlorprothixene, pimozide
Antispasmodics	Atropine, belladonna alkaloids, dicyclomine, glycopyrrolate, hyoscyamine, methscopolamine, oxyphencyclimine, propantheline, oxybutynin, flavoxalate, terodiline
Antihistamines	Highest effects: carbinoxamine, clemastine, diphenhydramine, promethazine Moderate effects: azatadine, brompheniramine, chlorpheniramine, cyproheptadine, dexchlorpheniramine, triprolidine, hydroxyzine
Antiemetic/antivertigo agents	Meclizine, scopolamine, dimenhydrinate, trimethobenzamide, prochlorperazine

(From Pharmacy benefits management-medical advisory panel. The Management of Cognitive Changes in Alzheimer's Disease. VHA PBM-SHG Publication No. 99–0013. Hines, IL: Pharmacy Benefits Management Strategic Healthcare Group, Veterans Health Administration, Department of Veterans Affairs, August 1999,[28] with permission.)

TABLE 70.4	Diagnostic Criteria for Dementia of the Alzheimer's Type (DSM-IV)

A. The development of multiple cognitive deficits manifested by the following:

   (1) Memory impairment (impaired ability to learn new information or to recall previously learned information)

   (2) One (or more) of the following cognitive disturbances:

      (a) aphasia (language)

      (b) apraxia (impaired motor activities)

      (c) agnosia (failure to recognize or identify objects)

      (d) disturbance in executive functioning (i.e., planning, organizing, abstracting, sequencing).

B. The cognitive deficits in Criteria A1 and A2 each cause significant impairment in social or occupational functioning and represent a significant decline from a previous level of functioning.

C. The course is characterized by gradual onset and continuing cognitive decline.

D. The cognitive deficits in Criteria A1 and A2 are not due to any of the following:

   (1) Other central nervous system conditions that cause progressive deficits in memory and cognition (e.g., strokes, Parkinson's disease, subdural hematoma)

   (2) Systemic conditions that are known to cause dementia (e.g., hypothyroidism, vitamin B12 or folic acid deficiency, neurosyphilis, HIV, infection)

   (3) Substance-induced conditions.

E. The deficits do not occur exclusively during the course of a delirium.

F. The disturbance is not better accounted for by another Axis 1 disorder (e.g., major depressive disorder, schizophrenia).

DSM-IV, Diagnostic and Statistical Manual of Mental Disorders; HIV, human immunodeficiency virus.
(From the American Psychiatric Association. Diagnostic and Statistical Manual of Mental Disorders. 4th ed. Washington, DC: American Psychiatric Association, 1994:142–143, with permission.)

TABLE 70.5	Diagnostic Tests for Alzheimer's Disease

Mini-Mental State Examination (MMSE)

Patient history (to include medical, medications, course of current condition, family history, functional status)

Physical examination (to identify any medical conditions that could cause cognitive decline)

Laboratory tests (CBC, BUN, glucose, calcium, electrolytes, T4, TSH, B$_{12}$, liver function tests, syphilis serology)

CT or MRI scan

Neuropsychologic testing (when indicated)

BUN, blood urea nitrogen; CBC, complete blood cell count; CT, computed tomography; MRI, magnetic resonance imaging; T4, thyroxine; TSH, thyroid-stimulating hormone.

age, and education can also affect scores with dementia in well-educated persons being under diagnosed and the poorly educated appearing more impaired. A quick screening test used in clinical settings is the Clock Drawing Task.[25] Inability to draw a clock with numbers in place and to place the hands at a specific time would indicate possible cognitive impairment and the need for further evaluation.

Neuroimaging studies are not specific in AD and may be normal in the early stages of this disease. Computerized tomography (CT) and magnetic resonance imaging (MRI) can help to identify other conditions such as tumors or strokes that can cause cognitive impairment. In the absence of other causes, neuroimaging in AD patients shows cortical atrophy, a finding in many normal elderly, and it is not diagnostic. Confirmation of the diagnosis of AD requires postmortem examination or brain biopsy to identify characteristic neurofibrillary tangles and amyloid plaques. Therefore, the diagnosis of AD is based on clinical assessment. It is estimated that experienced clinicians can correctly diagnose AD in more than 80% of cases.[26]

PSYCHOSOCIAL ASPECTS

The diagnosis of AD can have a profound effect on the patient and the patient's family. During the early stages of the disease, while some memory remains intact, patients may experience anxiety, depression, and become hostile. Restrictions in activities such as driving, hobbies, and work can cause frustration and anger. As the dementia progresses, patients may be less upset by their losses while the caregiver's burden increases. The stress associated with caregiving for a patient with AD may result in anxiety, depression, and physical illness for the caregiver. Caregivers report social isolation, with fewer visits from friends and fewer opportunities to participate in normal daily activities. Caregivers often have poor sleep patterns and may neglect their own health needs due to the restrictions imposed by the continuous attention necessary to provide care for a patient with AD. The

progression of AD causes increased demands on caregivers and the health care system. Severe AD has a profound impact on family members, particularly those involved in caring for the affected individual. Patients will develop dependence on others for total care and will often develop medical problems associated with decreased mobility. Psychotic symptoms and agitation may become significant concerns and cause stress to family members. Issues involving institutionalization, resuscitative measures, and life-support measures require family members to make difficult and often traumatic decisions. Family support services are particularly important in helping family caregivers cope with the emotional and social consequences of AD.

THERAPEUTIC PLAN

Guidelines are available to assist in the early and accurate identification of AD. The Agency for Health Care Policy Research (AHCPR) has published early assessment guidelines for this disease because early recognition may allow for better care planning by the patient and family.[27] Early identification will allow the use of new therapies, which may slow or halt the progression of this progressive dementia. Other practice guidelines have been developed by government and professional organizations that provide similar approaches for the treatment of AD.[19–21]

Guidelines for the pharmacologic management of cognitive changes caused by AD have been developed by the Department of Veterans Affairs.[28] These guidelines provide a systematic approach to using medications in the treatment of AD. These guidelines are dynamic, with periodic revisions, and can be located on the internet at www.pbm.va.gov.

TREATMENT

Historically, a wide variety of medications have been proposed to treat AD; however, most early trials were undertaken without an understanding of the pathophysiology of the disease. While the current armamentarium does not offer unequivocally effective treatment, medications are palliative and may delay symptom progression. General guidelines for treating Alzheimer patients are outlined in Table 70.6. Health care professionals should be informed about current modalities to guide treatments, manage therapy, and determine when to discontinue ineffective medications.

In the last 10 years a number of medications have become available that are used to improve cognitive functioning though none have been able to prevent progression of this disease. Currently, four cholinesterase inhibitors have been approved to treat mild to moderate AD. They have demonstrated cognitive improvement, some stabilization of behaviors and mood, and may improve functioning during the course of the disease. An N-methyl-D-aspartate (NMDA)

TABLE 70.6 | Guidelines for Treating Patients with Alzheimer's Disease

1. The differential diagnosis of cognitive impairment is imperative.

2. Before treatment, rigorously pursue the diagnosis of any treatable states that may cause dementia symptoms, especially evaluate for depression.

3. Avoid any unnecessary use of medications. Many medications cause symptoms that may be mistaken for dementia. The elderly have little reserve capacity against side effects and are therefore more prone to additive, adverse effects.

4. Individualize therapy. Each patient exhibits different behavioral and cognitive manifestations. Optimum dosages of medications used in treating Alzheimer disease have not been established. Dosage must be individualized, monitored, and titrated frequently.

5. Because of the progressive nature of the disease, medications used to treat some symptoms may need to be adjusted and may be discontinued.

6. Carefully monitor patients on medications. Goals of therapy and evaluation for efficacy for drug therapy should be ongoing.

7. Discontinue ineffective or unnecessary medications.

receptor partial agonist is also approved for use in moderate to severe AD. In addition, some medications that may be protective against the development of Alzheimer's are being evaluated.[29] The most frequently used medications for AD patients are symptomatic and help to control unwanted behaviors and maintain patient function. They do not affect the outcome of the disease process, and patients continue to decline.

PHARMACOTHERAPY

Therapeutic Treatments. Therapeutic drugs that slow progression of brain failure or reverse or alleviate disease symptoms are being evaluated. When AD is further characterized, treatment will likely consist of a combination of medications. Drug therapy will probably affect the balance of cholinergic and other neurotransmitter systems because of the multiple neurochemical abnormalities and brain functions affected. Eventually, when more specific causes are known, therapies can be directed at reversing pathologic damage and disease progression. In addition, several medications are being studied for the possibility that they can prevent or slow the appearance of the clinical symptoms of AD. Currently all available medications used to treat AD provide modest symptomatic benefits and do not alter the eventual progression of this degenerative neurologic disorder.

Cholinergic Agents. At present the cholinergic deficit hypothesis provides the most viable and consistent explanation of the memory impairment that occurs in AD, but it does not

account for all the clinical deficits. Neurochemical studies of patients with AD consistently show a deficiency of the neurotransmitter acetylcholine and choline acetyltransferase, the enzyme that is responsible for synthesis of acetylcholine. A positive correlation has been reported between the degree of cognitive impairment of AD patients and decreases in choline acetyltransferase and acetylcholine.[30] Comparisons between patients with AD and age-matched controls have demonstrated neuron losses in the nucleus basalis of Meynert, an area that is thought to provide cholinergic input to the cortex and a major cholinergic pathway leading from the septum to the hippocampus, a structure that is critical to normal memory (and learning) functions.[31] Several pharmacologic efforts to augment cholinergic activity have focused on (a) increasing acetylcholine synthesis and release, (b) limiting acetylcholine breakdown by inhibiting acetylcholinesterase, and (c) directly stimulating acetylcholine receptors.[32,33]

Agents such as choline and lecithin (phosphatidylcholine) serve as precursors to acetylcholine, and large amounts have been shown to increase acetylcholine concentrations in the brain. Clinical trials of choline and lecithin have not shown convincing evidence that these substances improve cognition in patients with AD. This is probably because the enzyme choline acetyltransferase, which is required for these precursors to be synthesized to acetylcholine, is depleted in AD.

Two enzymes are responsible for the hydrolysis of acetylcholine (ACh): acetylcholinesterase (AChE) and butyrylcholinesterase (BChE). AChE is primarily responsible for ACh metabolism in the brain, and BChE has predominant activity in the periphery. A selective AChE agent without BChE effect may decrease side-effects such as gastrointestinal distress and hepatic effects.

Cholinesterase inhibitors (physostigmine, tacrine, donepezil, rivastigmine, galantamine) block AChE and increase the amount of available ACh in the synaptic cleft by limiting the breakdown of ACh. AChE inhibitors are currently the most extensively used and studied class of medications for the treatment of AD. They show mild benefits and slight improvements in mental status, slowing of progression, and minimizing of behaviors.

Intravenous doses of physostigmine have shown statistically significant and transient improvement in visual recognition memory tests.[34] Although several studies corroborate improvements,[35,36] physostigmine use is limited by the short duration of action and adverse effects such as nausea, vomiting, diarrhea, dizziness, and headache. The limitations of physostigmine led to the development of oral cholinesterase inhibitors.

Tacrine. Tacrine was approved in 1993 and was the first drug indicated to treat mild to moderate AD. Tacrine [tetrahydroaminoacridine (THA)] is a reversible cholinesterase inhibitor with a longer duration of action than physostigmine and is taken orally. Tacrine elevates ACh levels in the cerebral cortex and is a palliative treatment for AD when used in therapeutic dosages.[37] Tacrine has shown dose-related benefits in cognitive function and attention tasks and improved measures of quality of life.[38,39] Tacrine does not alter the course of the progress of dementia, and a slow decline in function will continue.

A high prevalence (30%) of abnormal liver function tests (elevated transaminase), which usually return to normal with decreases in dosage or discontinuance of drug therapy, has been observed in patients treated with tacrine. A few occurrences of liver necrosis and jaundice also have been reported.[40] Tacrine requires frequent liver function testing during treatment initiation and routine monitoring because of the concern of hepatotoxicity. With the introduction of other cholinesterase inhibitor agents that have a lower risk of toxicity, tacrine is rarely used.

Donepezil. Donepezil was the second AChE inhibitor approved in 1996 to treat AD. Donepezil is a reversible inhibitor of AChE indicated for the treatment of mild to moderate AD. It is well absorbed and is metabolized by cytochrome P-450 with renal excretion of unchanged drug. It has a long elimination half-life of approximately 72 hours, which is not altered in the elderly or in patients with renal or hepatic dysfunction. Both 5-mg and 10-mg daily doses have shown patient improvement in a variety of clinical trials.[41,42] The benefit of the 10-mg dose is not always clinically significant, but may provide additional benefit for some patients. The treatment course usually results in mild increases in cognitive testing using the AD Assessment Scale (ADAS-cog) and in caregiver impression scale, and a slowing of decline when compared to a placebo. Studies with a placebo washout period showed a decline in function within weeks until function declined to near baseline.[43] Donepezil has demonstrated efficacy in the treatment of neuropsychiatric symptoms in patients with mild to moderate AD.[44] In addition, clinical studies suggest that donepezil's benefits extend into more advanced AD.[45]

Adverse effects are usually mild. The most common are gastrointestinal, such as nausea and diarrhea, insomnia, fatigue, and muscle cramps. There is an increase in side effects from the 5-mg to the 10-mg dose, but over a 6-week titration period most side effects resolve and begin to approach the occurrence found in the 5-mg dose. Because of the relative ease of titration, starting at the 5-mg dose for 4 to 6 weeks and then increasing to 10 mg to evaluate for maximal benefit is recommended. If there are no side effects or mild effects, the patient should be left on the 10-mg dose given daily. Donepezil has the advantage of being dosed once daily and there is no change in absorption if given with food. Donepezil is metabolized by cytochrome P-450 (CYP) isoenzymes 2D6 and 3A4 but does not alter isoenzyme activity. Therefore, drugs that inhibit CYP2D6 and 3A4 will increase levels of donepezil, and donepezil does not alter other drug levels.[43]

Rivastigmine. Rivastigmine is an intermediate-acting, slowly reversible (pseudoirreversible) inhibitor of cholinesterases, with relative specificity for brain AChE and BuChE. While AChE activity decreases in advanced AD, BuChE activity remains fixed or may increase. The significance of this is unclear but some researchers feel that rivastigmine might have added benefit in advanced AD. Rivastigmine has a relatively short elimination half-life but clinical effects persist. Rivastigmine is not metabolized by cytochrome P450 and nicotine use increases clearance by 23%. Clinical trials of rivastigmine in mild to moderate AD patients indicated improvement over placebo in ADAS-Cog scores with both groups declining below baseline function by six months.[46,47]

Adverse effects associated with rivastigmine include nausea, vomiting, diarrhea, and anorexia. In controlled trials, weight loss of greater than 7% of baseline weight occurred in 26% of women and 18% of men on high rivastigmine doses (>9 mg/day) as compared those on placebo (6% of women, 4% of men).[48] Weight loss might be related to gastrointestinal complaints rather than a direct appetite suppression. Headache and dizziness were also frequently reported adverse effects.

Rivastigmine requires twice daily dosing with gradual increases to decrease the chance of adverse effects. Dosing begins with 1.5 mg twice daily, then 3 mg twice daily, 4.5 mg twice daily, 6 mg twice daily with a minimum of 2 weeks between dose increases. An increased interval may be necessary due to adverse effects and if therapy is interrupted for more than a few doses therapy should be restarted at the next lower dose level. Pharmacokinetic interactions are unlikely with CYP isoenzyme inducers or inhibitors because rivastigmine is only minimally metabolized by this mechanism and it does not alter other drugs.[48]

Galantamine. Galantamine is a reversible, competitive acetylcholinesterase inhibitor that also binds allosterically with nicotinic acetylcholine receptors. Nicotinic receptor stimulation results in increased ACh release and possible protection against $A\beta$ neurotoxicity, effects that might provide additional benefits in treating AD.[49] Galantamine is metabolized by cytochrome P450 enzymes (CYP2D6 and CYP3A4) in the liver so there is a risk of other drugs causing changes in drug levels. No liver toxicity has been reported but as with other AChE inhibitors, galantamine causes gastrointestinal side effects, more than caused by donepezil and less than rivastigmine. Other side effects include syncope, muscle cramps, and sleep disturbances. Double-blind, placebo-control studies have shown that galantamine provides benefits in AD similar to those seen with other AChE inhibitors.[50–52]

Galantamine has an elimination half life of 5 to 7 hours and requires twice daily dosing beginning with 4 mg twice daily, then 8 mg twice daily, followed by 12 mg twice daily with titration at 4-week intervals. Increases may be limited by dose related increased adverse effects and patients with severe renal or hepatic dysfunction should not receive more than 16 mg/day. Galantamine is metabolized primarily by CYP2D6 and 3A4 isoenzymes and drugs that inhibit these enzymes will increase galantamine activity. Galantamine does not affect the metabolism of other drugs.[53]

As a class, acetylcholinesterase inhibitors have been shown to have beneficial effects on cognitive, functional, and behavioral symptoms of AD in short-term use. With continued use treated patients have worsening symptoms but to a lesser extent than with untreated patients. The optimal duration of treatment has not been determined though trials lasting up to a year have shown benefits of active drug over placebo.[42] Most clinicians will continue treatment with a specific drug for at least 6 months to evaluate for benefits. In the absence of therapeutic response some clinicians will switch to a different acetylcholinesterase inhibitor. It has been reported that up to 50% of patients switched from one drug to another responded favorably.[54] Guidelines for switching drugs are limited, but care should be taken to assure that patients are not completely without inhibition during the switch process.[55] Cholinesterase inhibitors may increase gastric acid secretion and require caution in patients with active peptic ulcer disease. Like other drugs that can increase ACh activity, caution should also be taken in prescribing to patients with severe asthma or chronic obstructive pulmonary disease.[56] Table 70.7 is summary of prescribing information concerning cholinesterase inhibitors.

N-methyl-D-aspartate Receptor Partial Antagonist. Glutamate is an excitatory neurotransmitter that may play a role in the development and progression of neurodegenerative disease. A hypothesis for the role of glutamate is that excessive release of this neuroexcitatory transmitter leads to overstimulation of the major glutamate receptor NMDA causing damage to neurons.[57] Agents that block NMDA receptors would theoretically reduce degenerative changes to the brain. A variety of drugs block NMDA receptors, including amantadine, rimantadine, ketamine, memantine, and dextromethorphan.

Memantine. Memantine is the only drug in this class that is used to treat AD and is considered a noncompetitive, moderate affinity, NMDA antagonist that, due to moderate affinity to receptors, is unlikely to interfere with the physiologic activity of the receptor. In addition to AD, memantine has been investigated for the treatment of phantom limb pain, neurogenic bladder dysfunction, Parkinson disease, and as a vigilance enhancer in comatose patients.[58] Memantine has been commercially available outside the United States since 1982 and was approved for use in the United States in 2003 for moderate to severe AD.[59] A 28-week, double-blind, placebo controlled trial of 181 moderate to severe AD patients found statistically significant difference in favor of memantine with the Clinician's Interview Based Assessment of Change-Plus (CIBIC-Plus) and the AD Cooperative Study-Activities of Daily Living Inventory (ADCS/ADL).[60] A similar study was conducted comparing the addition of meman-

tine or placebo to ongoing donepezil therapy found a statistically significant difference in favor of memantine plus donepezil with the Severe Impairment Battery (SIB) and the ADCS/ADL measures.[61] In both studies memantine was well tolerated and side effects were similar to placebo. While statistically significant benefits on cognition and functioning have been reported with memantine, the clinical benefits may be less apparent to clinicians and caregivers. Though positive benefits have been reported, there is no evidence that memantine prevents or slows neurodegeneration in patients with AD.[59] A review of memantine studies reported that while memantine-treated patients had less cognitive deterioration the benefits were not clinically discernable.[62]

Memantine is well absorbed orally and readily crosses the blood-brain barrier. Memantine's absorption is not altered by food and there is minimal protein binding. It is primarily eliminated renally and does not affect liver enzyme activity. Though it has an elimination half-life of 60 to 80 hours, twice daily dosing is recommended. The recommended starting dose is 5 mg daily with a target dose of 20 mg daily. The dose should be increased in 5-mg increments with a minimum interval between dose increases of one week. Dose reduction should be considered in patients with mild to moderate renal impairment and it is not recommended for patients with severe renal impairment. Adverse effects are generally mild and include blood pressure elevations and headache. Memantine is not associated with alterations in drug levels related to CYP isoenzyme activity.[59]

While evidence supports the cholinergic hypothesis of memory and cognitive function, it is highly unlikely that this impairment is the sole disorder occurring in AD. The role of glutamate in AD and the impact of Aβ on this disease continues to be explored. AD represents multiple disorders and subtypes that share certain features and probably results from a combination of neuronal changes (such as a decrease in protein synthesis, production of abnormal proteins, and impaired energy production) and neurotransmitter deficits in the brain. With advancing knowledge of the causes of AD, new therapies can be developed. The pharmacologic efforts to treat AD have been based on various theories, and the list of therapies continues to grow.[63] Ultimately, therapy will probably consist of a combination of medications used to prevent clinical symptoms in those with a genetic predisposition and medications based on cause and specific symptoms. The optimal therapy will prevent or reverse the disease process itself.

Symptomatic Treatment. During the course of AD, patients experience memory dysfunction, progressive loss of cognitive ability, difficulties in the use of language, disorientation, confusion, disruption of the sleep-wake cycle, personality changes, and a lack of emotional control that often results in anxiety, agitation, and aggression. Pharmacotherapy is often used to alleviate some of these symptoms. All psychotropics should be used with caution; those with little or no anticholinergic side effects are usually preferred. They

TABLE 70.7 | Cholinesterase Inhibitors

Drug	Dose and Dosing	Time to Steady State	Elimination Half-life	Effects of Food	CYP450 Isoenzyme Metabolic Pathway	Adverse Effects[a]
Tacrine (Cognex)	40–160 mg/day qid dosing, titration necessary[b]	35 hours	1.3–7 hours	30%+ decrease in bioavailability	CYP1A2 CYP2D6 CYP3A4	Diarrhea Anorexia Dyspepsia Gastritis Nausea
Donepezil (Aricept)	5–10 mg/day once daily, begin with 5 mg	15 days	70 hours	None	CYP2D6 CYP3A4	Nausea[c] Diarrhea Vomiting Fatigue Anorexia
Rivastigmine (Exelon)	6–12 mg/day twice daily, titration necessary[b,d]	10 hours	1.5 hours	30% decrease of Cmax	Not by CYP450	Nausea Vomiting Anorexia Dyspepsia Asthenia
Galantamine (Razadyne)	16–32 mg/day twice daily, titration necessary[b]	35 hours	7 hours	None	CYP2D6 CYP3A4	Nausea Vomiting Anorexia Dyspepsia Anorexia Weight loss

[a] Greater than 5% of patients and twice the placebo rate. [b] If therapy interrupted for several days or longer, should restart at the lowest dose and titrate to the previous dose. [c] No difference from placebo if dose titrated at 6 weeks. [d] Take with meals to reduce side effects.
CYP, cytochrome P-450; qid, four times daily.
From Manufacturer's product information.

should be started at low dosages and titrated according to therapeutic response and side effects.[64]

Antidepressants. Early stages of AD are often accompanied by depressive symptoms that may respond to drug therapy. Depressive symptoms such as agitation, memory loss, and insomnia can be confused as dementia. Resolution of depression results in improvement of mood, functional abilities, and possibly cognitive abilities.[65] A therapeutic trial of antidepressants, preferably low in anticholinergic side effects, can be effective in treating "pseudodementia" or depressive symptoms. In general, antidepressants are encouraged and should be chosen for these patients as for other depressed patients by side-effect profiles and response to medication. Low dosages given once or twice a day are often beneficial. The sedating antidepressant, trazodone, can also be used as a sedative and to help decrease excessive excitation and agitation. The selective serotonin reuptake inhibitor (SSRI) antidepressants are effective for depression and offer a preferable side effect profile, although they do have the potential for increasing anxiety symptoms, agitation, and insomnia. The SSRIs, with the exception of paroxetine, are free of anticholinergic effects. Mirtazapine, a serotonin and α-2 NE receptor antagonist antidepressant, is associated with weight gain and may be used in patients who are underweight. Some

caution must be used since mirtazapine is a potent H-1 antagonist and causes sedation. Tricyclic antidepressants should be avoided in depressed AD patients due to anticholinergic and cardiac effects and their use limited to low dose desipramine or nortriptyline for treating peripheral neuropathy and pain syndromes.

Hypnotics. Insomnia is a common complaint of the elderly, and sleep disturbances are frequent with patients who have dementia. Sleep disturbance may be manifested by night awakening, pacing, trying to leave the environment, or searching for lost items. Sleep irregularities should be addressed initially with social interventions; regulating schedules, keeping patients active during the day, and preventing daytime napping all help to decrease nighttime insomnia. Sleep difficulties often distress patients and caregivers and can lead to exhaustion of caregivers. Sedating antidepressants such as trazodone or nortriptyline given at bedtime may be beneficial.

When a hypnotic is absolutely necessary, the lowest dosage for the shortest duration should be used. The short-acting agents such as zolpidem (5–10 mg) and temazepam (7.5 mg) may be helpful. Longer half-life benzodiazepines should be avoided because of their tendency to accumulate and cause over-sedation and an increased risk for falling. Diphenhydramine and other antihistamines have been used for sleep because of moderate sedating properties. However, the anticholinergic effects may increase confusion and psychotic symptoms and make them undesirable in this population.

Alcohol intake should be discontinued or kept to a minimum because of its effects on cognition, disruption of sleep pattern, and other side effects; furthermore, drug interactions and excessive intake can cause delirium or dementia.

All hypnotics should be used sparingly because of their widespread central nervous system depressant effects. They can increase confusion and memory impairment, worsen depressive symptoms, and aggravate most of the cognitive symptoms occurring in AD. The efficacy of long-term, routine use of hypnotics has not been proven. Maintaining daytime activity and nocturnal sleep, and giving other sedating medications at bedtime and hypnotics "as needed" can sufficiently control insomnia.

Anxiolytics. Anxiety frequently affects patients who are experiencing memory loss. The elderly may manifest their anxiety in somatic forms such as agitation, motor restlessness, and insomnia. Buspirone is sometimes effective for the anxiety and agitation in AD and has minimal side effects. Starting dosages such as 5 mg three times a day or 10 mg twice a day may be beneficial for anxiety and may benefit the patient with agitated symptoms occurring with dementia.[66] The effective dosage range is usually 15 to 30 mg daily with mild side effects of dizziness, drowsiness, and nausea. Buspirone should not be used "as needed" and takes several weeks for maximal effect.

The use of benzodiazepines for anxiety is limited by their side effects and possibility of worsening dementia symptoms. Short–half-life benzodiazepines in low dosages (e.g., lorazepam 0.5–1.0 mg) given once or twice a day may be useful. Because they act on the central nervous system, they may produce confusion, drowsiness, and amnesia, features that mimic and confound AD. They can also cause gait instability and have been correlated with an increased frequency of falls.

Antipsychotics. Antipsychotics are indicated for the treatment of specific psychotic symptoms. Delusions are common, especially with suspiciousness or persecution (e.g., false claims that people are stealing misplaced items, or feeling that someone is trying to harm them); visual hallucinations are more common than auditory hallucinations in this population. Paranoia and severe agitation, which may be distressful to the patient or interfere with the caregiver's ability to provide care, may need treatment with medication. The addition of a low-dose antipsychotic may be sufficient to control psychotic symptoms and allow a patient to remain in the home environment.

No single agent is always superior. Antipsychotics do not affect higher cortical functions such as memory, judgment, and problem solving. The high-potency antipsychotics (haloperidol, fluphenazine) leave the patient more prone to extrapyramidal side effects such as pseudoparkinsonism and tar-

dive dyskinesia. Low-potency agents (chlorpromazine, thioridazine) are anticholinergic and have cardiovascular side effects that make them undesirable in this population. The adverse effects may further impair the remaining physical and cognitive functions of patients with AD. Movement may be decreased, hypotension may cause more falls, and sedation may exacerbate confusion. Low dosages of high-potency antipsychotics (haloperidol or risperidone 0.5–1 mg) given daily or divided twice a day are usually sufficient. The newer atypical antipsychotic agents (risperidone, olanzapine, quetiapine, ziprasidone, aripiprazole), which affect dopamine and serotonin, may be beneficial and have a more desirable extrapyramidal side effect profile. Reports of increased cardiovascular events with risperidone and poor diabetic and blood pressure control with olanzapine would indicate that while less problematic than earlier antipsychotics, the newer agents still require monitoring.[5,6] The Food and Drug Administration has determined that the use of atypical antipsychotics to treat behavioral disorders in elderly patients with dementia is associated with increased mortality. A review of 17 placebo-control trials found there was a 1.6–1.7-fold increase in mortality for patients taking active drug as compared to placebo. Cardiac events such as heart failure and infections such as pneumonia accounted for most deaths. A warning of this risk will be included in product information for the atypical antipsychotics. Limited data suggest that older antipsychotics have a similar risk and labeling changes may also be required for these agents.[67]

It should be emphasized that antipsychotics should only be used for distressful, incapacitating symptoms. Brief hallucinations such as seeing children in their room or misperceptions that do not create distress to the patient are better left unmedicated. Caregivers should be educated about the temporary, benign nature of these episodes.

Agitation is a term that refers to a range of behavior disturbances that include verbal and physical aggression, combativeness, and disinhibition. Newly developed agitation may be a sign of a medical problem such as discomfort, pain, depression, delirium, constipation, lack of sleep, loneliness, and acute illness such as urinary tract infections. When these medical problems are controlled, the symptoms often resolve. The efficacy of antipsychotics in controlling agitation is modest. Antipsychotic use should be minimized and is indicated only for symptoms that are harmful and distressing to the patient that cannot be controlled by all other means. They have potentially severe and possibly permanent side effects, including tardive dyskinesia and pseudoparkinsonism. Lower doses than needed to treat schizophrenia are often effective, and as AD progresses patients may no longer need antipsychotic medications. Therefore, it is important to attempt a dosage reduction or trial off antipsychotic therapy to determine if the drug is still needed. Strict monitoring is imperative to prevent more harm than benefit from the use of these medications. Federal guidelines for nursing homes require that antipsychotic use be closely monitored for appropriate indications, correct dosing, and for adverse effects.[68]

Mood Stabilizers. Agitation often occurs in nursing home residents and includes physically aggressive (striking out, grabbing), nonaggressive (wandering, restlessness), and verbally aggressive (cursing, constant screaming) behaviors. The frequency of agitated behavior increases with the progression of AD.[69] Alternative drugs such as carbamazepine,[70,71] trazodone,[72] and β-blockers[73,74] have been suggested for controlling significant and possibly dangerous behavior. Benefits have been shown, but studies are preliminary and include small sample populations of patients.[75] Caution should be taken with the use of β-blockers in this population. These patients frequently suffer from concurrent problems such as diabetes, chronic obstructive pulmonary disease, and heart block, which are contraindications to their use.

Valproic acid, an anticonvulsant used for mood stabilization, has shown some efficacy in treating nonpsychotic agitation. Relatively low dosages may improve symptoms of restlessness, vegetative signs, and striking behaviors with minimal side effects. The primary side effect is gastrointestinal disturbance, which is minimized by using the coated formulation, starting at a low dosage (125 mg twice to three times daily) and titrating slowly.[76]

Benefits of psychotropic medications are variable, and responses to agents are highly individual and limited by adverse effects. Psychotropics are useful and can improve behavior and function, easing patients' distress, and lessening the burden of care. Because AD is progressive, therapy should be evaluated at least every 6 months to ensure that the fewest medications are being used in the lowest effective dosages. Tapering psychotropic medications in stabilized patients at regular intervals is an effective tool to assess the need for continued therapy.

Families and caregivers should be counseled. They must understand that psychotropic medications may improve some symptoms, but they will not prevent further deterioration of function or progression of the disease. The caregivers' understanding of the disease process and the effects of drug therapy will often lessen the need to use these types of medications.

NONPHARMACOLOGIC THERAPY

Managing the environment of the patient with AD is an important treatment consideration. A safe, stable, comfortable environment will minimize the strain of decreasing mental capacities and lessen confusion and agitation. Patients should be stimulated and helped to function, but choices that may overwhelm and confuse them should be limited. Providing a calendar to reinforce orientation and written directions to help find necessary items may improve functioning in early AD. Labeling items with names and laying out one change of clothes will help maintain the patient's ability to perform the activities of daily living. Alterations in sur-

roundings such as room changes should be minimized; they may cause an increase in confusion and disorientation. Physical and psychosocial stressors such as minor surgery, bereavement, or institutionalization can and often will aggravate intellectual deficits in a demented patient. Within reason, familiar furnishings, diet, and routines should be maintained. Providing regular exercise may reduce behaviors such as wandering and restlessness. Insomnia may benefit from keeping the patient active during the day and allowing adequate daylight in the living area to reinforce a normal wake-sleep cycle. Eating difficulties may require pureed or finger foods and simple verbal directions such as "pick up your spoon" remembering to use one-step instructions.

Providing a safe environment and avoiding activities that have a potential of harm is an important component of caring for an AD patient. Driving, operating machinery, and using potentially dangerous devices require normal cognitive functioning and AD patients should be monitored and prevented from causing harm to themselves or others. Patients with mild AD will often become lost while driving before they develop difficulty with operating a automobile and caregivers will often need to intervene to prevent operation of motor vehicles. The loss of these activities can often be the source of significant tension and anger that may be directed at the caregiver.

Caregiver training is important. Caregivers must understand the limitations of the patient's cognition and how that affects his or her behaviors and functioning. Patients are often confused and cannot process what is going on around them. Many of the interactions between patients and caregivers can be modified to best suit the patient and to prevent or minimize incidents that might lead to agitation and difficulty in caring for the individual.

ALTERNATIVE THERAPIES

VITAMIN E
Vitamin E (alpha-tocopherol) has demonstrated the ability to interact with cell membranes, trapping free radicals with the reduction of oxidative damage to cells. This has led to the investigation of vitamin E in AD with a randomized clinical trial at doses of 1,000 U twice daily resulting in an average delay of 230 days to institutionalization compared with placebo. Selegiline, a monoamine oxidase-B inhibitor which may act as an antioxidant, was also studied in this trial and resulted in a similar delay in progression compared to placebo.[77] While vitamin E has been recommended by some clinicians and included in The American Academy of Neurology practice parameter, the side effects of selegiline do not support its use in AD.[78] Vitamin E may interfere with vitamin K absorption and can result in increased risk of bleeding. Several other studies have not supported benefits of vitamin E in AD and at least one report has indicated increased risk associated with high doses.[79] A meta analysis of 19 randomized, controlled trials was performed to evalu-

ate the relationship between vitamin E supplements and total mortality. This study found a statistically significant relationship between vitamin E dosage and mortality and found an increased risk of death associated with doses greater than 150 U per day.[80] This indication of increased risk may outweigh any modest benefits and decrease the role of vitamin E supplementation in AD.

GINKGO BILOBA

Extracts of the ginkgo biloba leaf are widely available as nonprescription supplements and are used by many people for their cognitive effects. The extracts contain many constituents such as flavonoids and terpenoids. Neuroprotective effects may be caused by reduced capillary fragility, antioxidant effects, and inhibition of platelet aggregation. In Germany, ginkgo biloba has been approved for treating dementia and cerebral circulatory disturbances. Ginkgo biloba studies in the United States have shown modest benefits in short-term memory and caregiver behavior assessment. In 1997, researchers reported a clinical trial using 120 mg a day of ginkgo biloba in mild to moderately severe AD as compared to placebo. Because 60% of subjects did not complete this study, the findings are difficult to interpret. Although the difference in improvement between those taking ginkgo biloba and placebo was statistically significant, the clinical difference was negligible. Adverse effects are usually mild gastrointestinal symptoms, headache, dizziness, and vertigo.[81] Ginkgo biloba is considered a dietary supplement and not a drug, thus, there is little control over the contents in commercial preparations. Ginkgo biloba use has also been associated with increased risk of bleeding and hemorrhage.[56] Further research is necessary to establish if ginkgo biloba has a role in the treatment of AD.

FUTURE THERAPIES

AMYLOID ALTERATION

The role of $A\beta$ in AD has led to research directed at approaches to reduce the development of amyloid plaques. The "amyloid hypothesis" is based on the abnormal processing of APP leading to excessive production of $A\beta$. APP is cleaved into smaller protein segments by secretase enzymes with beta and gamma secretase being instrumental in $A\beta$ production. Currently secretase inhibitors are under development for the prevention and treatment of AD.[82] The impact of altering the biologic processing of APP by inhibiting enzyme activity is complicated by the fact that the function of APP is still unknown.

Another strategy for preventing and treating AD has been the development of a vaccine to reduce cortical deposits of $A\beta$. Such a vaccine would mobilize the immune system to produce antibodies against $A\beta$. Researchers have developed a vaccine that, in animal models, causes a significant reduction in cerebral amyloid deposition.[83–85] In 2002, a clinical trial of an AD vaccine in humans was halted when some patients developed meningoencephalitis.[86] Research continues to determine the future role of vaccination in treating AD. Research is also underway to explore the possibility of administering laboratory-produced antibodies rather than using the patient's immune system in an effort to reduce the potential adverse effects seen with the vaccine.

ESTROGEN THERAPY

Epidemiologic reviews have suggested a role for estrogens reducing the occurrence of AD in women taking hormone replacement therapy.[87,88] In response to these reports, well-controlled clinical trials were conducted showing no benefit in reducing AD and there is at least one study that indicates some increased risk of dementia among postmenopausal women taking hormone replacement therapy.[89–91] Based upon this evidence, hormone replacement therapy is not recommended in the treatment or prevention of AD.

ANTI-INFLAMMATORY DRUGS

A few studies postulate a possible role of nonsteroidal anti-inflammatory drugs (NSAIDs) in the prevention or slowing of decline due to AD based on the assumption that their use would reduce the inflammatory component in the formation of neuritic plaques. A retrospective evaluation of 1686 participants found the risk of AD was reduced by 50% in people who reported taking NSAIDs with a reduction to 60% with two or more years of NSAID use.[92] Although this evidence was encouraging, there have been several clinical trials that have reported no benefits from NSAIDs or from prednisone.[93–95] In addition to lack of support from clinical trials, the frequent occurrence of side effects such as ulcers, GI distress, and nephrotoxicity with these agents make the prescribing of NSAIDs not recommended for elderly patients solely to prevent AD.

CHOLESTEROL-LOWERING AGENTS

Retrospective epidemiological studies have suggested that the use of 3-hydroxy-3-methylglutaryl coenzyme A (HMG CoA) reductase inhibitors (statins) reduce the risk of developing AD.[96,97] Recent clinical trials with pravastatin and simvastatin have shown no cognitive benefits of either drug.[98,99] Of additional concern is a randomized double-blind clinical trial of 283 subjects which found those receiving the statin drug performed worse on certain neuropsychological tests than those on placebo.[100] Further investigation will be necessary to determine the role of cholesterol lowering drugs in AD.

IMPROVING OUTCOMES

Because of the lack of nursing home beds and their high costs, alternative care will become even more important in the future. Patients who are in early stages of AD need education and counseling. When family members become involved in care, their understanding of drug therapy and their ability to assist with medication adherence should be evaluated. Care for the caregivers is often as important as care of the patient. Remember that an aging spouse may be on the borderline of competency and function, and the added burden of caring for a demented mate may be too much for the person to handle properly. When the caregiver gives out, the care system suffers. Day care and home care services are offered by various local agencies and provide different levels of supervision and activities for patients with AD. Day care is especially important in providing much needed respite for the caregivers at home.

PATIENT EDUCATION

Persons diagnosed with mild, early AD may benefit from education concerning AD and be more likely to cooperate with treatment and experience less anxiety. Educational efforts may be hindered by AD patients who frequently deny having any memory problem and lack insight into their condition. As AD progresses education is directed at the family and caregivers. Caring for individuals with AD can be extremely stressful and require a great deal of time, energy, and understanding of how best to provide care and where to locate supportive services can greatly reduce this stress. Referring the family to supportive services and to books such as *The Thirty-Six-Hour Day*[101] will provide access to needed information and assistance with coping with AD. Relatives of an AD patient with changes in cognitive abilities and personality often experience a loss of relationship with the AD patient and grieve for their own losses.[102] Community support groups allow for families and caregivers to meet together and share their experiences in coping with difficult situations. Understanding issues such as advanced directives, durable power of attorney, and how to access support services is critical to helping the caregiver cope with the challenges associated with AD. Caregivers need to be educated on how to manage daily activities, the role of day care, respite care, and home support services. National organizations such as The Alzheimer's Association and government institutes such as the National Institute on Aging (NIA) and the Administration on Aging provide educational activities concerning these and other interventions that can reduce the stress and fatigue experienced by caregivers (Table 70.8).

METHODS TO IMPROVE ADHERENCE TO DRUG THERAPY

Due to the core symptom of memory decline, adherence to drug therapy is a ongoing challenge for individuals with AD. With the approval of more medications to treat AD, adherence with medications becomes more important. Patients in early stages may be able to manage a limited number of medications given once or twice a day but reminder systems and adherence evaluation should be performed periodically. Besides pharmacotherapy, a comprehensive plan should include adequate nutrition, correction of sensory deficits (e.g., glasses, hearing aid), and attention to the social environment.

TABLE 70.8 Caregiver Resources

The Alzheimer's Association: A national nonprofit organization that provides a wide range of information and services to patients with Alzheimer disease and their caregivers, friends, and families. Every state has at least one local chapter. Contact at: 800–272–3900

www.alz.org

Administration on Aging: Coordinates delivery of services specified by the Older Americans Act. Services are coordinated via Agencies on Aging and include nutrition services, access services, and related support. Contact at: 202–619–0724

www.aoa.gov

The National Institute of Aging (NIA): As a part of the federal government's National Institutes of Health, provides direction concerning research on aging and provides professional and public information. Contact at: 301–496–1752

www.nih.gov.nia

Alzheimer's Disease Education and Referral Center (ADEAR): A service of the National Institute on Aging, provides information and publications on Alzheimer's disease to health professionals and the public. ADEAR is a national resource for all aspects of Alzheimer's disease. Contact at: 800–438–4380

www.alzheimers.org/adear

The National Council on the Aging, Inc (NCOA): An association of organizations and individuals committed to promoting the dignity and well-being of older persons. It serves as a national resource for service providers and consumers. Contact at: 800–375–1014

www.ncoa.org

The National Family Caregiver Association (NFCA): A nonprofit organization directed at improving the quality of life for the caregiver. Services include educational materials and a nationwide peer support network. Contact at: 800–896–3650

www.nfcacares.org

Eldercare Locator: A nationwide directory assistance service designed to help older persons and caregivers locate local resources. They can refer you to the appropriate Area Agency on Aging. Contact at: 800–677–1116

www.n4a.org

DISEASE MANAGEMENT STRATEGIES TO IMPROVE PATIENT OUTCOMES

A therapeutic approach should provide adequate emotional support for family members and those who provide daily patient care. There are no medical cures, and the disease waxes and wanes but is progressive. Often a rational presentation of the course will minimize fears, allow rational expectations, and enhance the family's ability to provide support to the patient without dependence on excessive medication. It must be remembered that all medications have toxicities, and many may exacerbate the symptoms they are supposed to relieve. Medications are often used to maintain patients in the home. Caregivers must understand the dangers of overmedicating and the need to administer medications only as directed. Families and the caregivers closest to the patients should be included in therapeutic decisions and often provide the best monitoring information. It is also important that caregivers stay healthy by eating and resting properly and not neglecting their own medical needs.

PHARMACOECONOMICS

The economic impact of AD on health care is enormous and will be increasing as more people live longer. In 1994, the yearly direct and indirect monetary costs associated with AD were reported to exceed $100 billion in the United States. Total costs, direct and indirect, over the course of the illness have been estimated at $173,000 per patient.[103] Direct health care costs include clinic visits, medications, hospitalizations, and nursing home care. Nonmedical costs include social services, day care, home health services, and the cost of equipment for home care. Caregivers also have increased medical costs for the treatment of medical illness, depression, and increased hospitalizations associated with the stress of caregiving. Indirect costs include loss of productivity for both the patient and caregiver.[104]

The cost of care for patients with AD increases with the severity of the disease. Persons with dementia use emergency rooms, have acute hospital admissions, and have physician interventions two to three times more than persons without dementia.[105] Patients with advanced, severe dementias will usually require nursing home care, often for extended periods of time. Patients with AD have a median length of nursing home stay that is more than ten times the national average for all other diagnoses.[106] Efforts to slow the progression of the dementia and use of assisted living or home care programs should have a positive impact on the future cost of care for patients with AD. Drug therapies directed at stopping or slowing the progression of AD will allow patients to remain in a less restrictive and less costly environment.

KEY POINTS

- AD is a complex, progressive, degenerative disorder with no known cure.
- All potentially reversible dementias should be identified and treated before a diagnosis of AD can be made.
- Patients with AD may require pharmacologic treatment for depression, anxiety, and behavioral manifestations.
- A safe environment is essential for providing care for patients with AD.
- Caregiver education and support are necessary to assist in maintaining Alzheimer patients in the least restrictive environment.

- New drug therapies may prevent the progression of AD.
- When antipsychotics are used to control psychoses or disruptive behavior, the lowest dosage for the shortest period of time is recommended.
- Maintain the most appropriate level of care and to keep the patient as functional and comfortable for as long as possible.

SUGGESTED READINGS

Alva G, Potkin S. Alzheimer's disease and other dementias. Clinics in Geriatric Medicine 2003;19:141–53

Geldmacher DS. Differential diagnosis of dementia syndromes. Clin Geriatr Med 20:27–44, 2004.

Pharmacy benefits management–medical advisory panel. The Management of Cognitive Changes in Alzheimer disease. VHA PBM-SHG Publication No. 99-0013. Hines, IL: Pharmacy Benefits Management Strategic Healthcare Group, Veterans Health Administration, Department of Veterans Affairs, August 1999.

Scarpini E, Scheltens P, Feldman H. Treatment of Alzheimer's disease: current status and new perspectives. Lancet Neurol 9:539–547, 2003.

REFERENCES

1. Huppert FA, Tym E. Clinical and neuropsychological assessment of dementia. Br Med Bull 42:11–18, 1986.
2. Geldmacher DS. Differential diagnosis of dementia syndromes. Clin Geriatric Med 20:162–173, 2004.
3. Dorland's illustrated medical dictionary. 28th ed. Philadelphia: W.B Saunders, 1995.
4. US Department of Health and Human Services, Public Health Services, National Institute on Aging. Alzheimer's Disease Genetics: Fact Sheet. Silver Spring, MD: Alzheimer's Disease Education and Referral Center;1999. NIH publication 99–4664.
5. Advisory Panel on Alzheimer's Disease. Alzheimer's Disease and Related Dementias: Acute and Long-term Care Services. Washington, DC: U.S. Dept. of Health and Human Services, 1996, NIH publication 96-4136.
6. Evans DA, Funkenstein HH, Albert MS, et al. Prevalence of Alzheimer's disease in a community population of older persons higher than previously reported. JAMA 262:2551–2556, 1989.
7. Fox JH, Heston LL, Terry RD. Zeroing in on Alzheimer's disease. Patient Care 20:68–91, 1986.
8. Saunders AM, Schmader K, Breitner JC, et al. Apolipoprotein E4 allele distribution in late-onset Alzheimer's disease and in other amyloid-forming diseases. Lancet 342:710–711, 1993.
9. Schellenberg GD, Bird TD, Wijsman EM, et al. Genetic linkage evidence for a familial Alzheimer's disease locus on chromosome 14. Science 258:668–671, 1992.
10. Levy-Lahad E, Wijsman EM, Nemens E, et al. A familial Alzheimer's disease locus on chromosome 1. Science 269:970–973, 1995.
11. Caputo CB, Salama AI. The amyloid proteins of Alzheimer's disease as potential targets for drug therapy. Neurobiol Aging 1989; 10:451–461.
12. Liddell M, Williams J, Bayer A, et al. Confirmation of association between the e4 allele of apolipoprotein E and Alzheimer's disease. J Med Genet 31:197–200, 1994.
13. Mayeux R, Stern Y, Ottman R, et al. The apolipoprotein e4 allele in patients with Alzheimer's disease. Ann Neurol 34:752–754, 1993.
14. US Department of Health and Human Services, Public Health Services, National Institute on Aging. Alzheimer's disease Genetics: Fact Sheet. Silver Spring, MD: Alzheimer's Disease Education and Referral Center; August 5 1997. NIH publication 97-4012.
15. Morris JC, Storandt M, Miller JP, et al. Mild cognitive impairment represents early-stage AD, Arch Neurol 58:3, 397–405, 2001.

16. American Psychiatric Association. Diagnostic and Statistical Manual of Mental Disorders. 4th ed. Washington, DC: American Psychiatric Association, 1994:142–143.

17. Anonymous. Swedish consensus on dementia diseases. Acta Neurol Scand 157 (Suppl):1–31, 1994.

18. Anonymous. Recognition and Initial Assessment of Alzheimer's Disease and Related Dementias, Clinical Practice Guidelines: 19, AHCPR, Nov. 1996.

19. Patterson CJS, Gauthier S, Bergman H, et al. The recognition, assessment and management of dementing disorders: Conclusions from the Canadian Conference of Dementia. Can Med Assoc 160 (Suppl 12):S1–S15, 1999.

20. Small GW, Rabins PV, Barry PP, et al. Diagnosis and treatment of Alzheimer's disease and related disorders: Consensus statement of the American Association for Geriatric Psychiatry, the Alzheimer's Association, and the American Geriatrics Society. JAMA 278: 1363–1371, 1997.

21. Knopman DS, DeKosy ST, Cumming JL, et al. Practice parameter: diagnosis of dementia (an evidence-based review): report of the Quality Standards Subcommittee of the American Academy of Neurology. Neurology 56:1143–1153, 2001.

22. McKhann G, Drachman D, Folstein M, et al. Clinical diagnosis of Alzheimer's disease. Neurology 34:939–944, 1984.

23. Folstein MF, Folstein SE, McHugh PR. Mini-Mental State: A practical method for grading the cognitive state of patients for the clinician. Kidlington, UK: Elsevier Science, Ltd., 1974:196–198.

24. Doraiswamy PM, Bieber F, Kaiser L, et al. The Alzheimer's disease assessment scale: patterns and predictors of baseline cognitive performance in multicenter Alzheimer's disease trials. Neurology 48:1511–1517, 1997.

25. Tucoko H, Hadjistavropoulos T, Miller JA, et al. The Clock Test: a sensitive measure to differentiate normal elderly from those with Alzheimer's disease. J Am Geriatr Soc 40:579–584, 1992.

26. Becker JT, Boller F, Lopez OL, et al. Alzheimer research program. The natural history of Alzheimer's disease: description of study cohort and accuracy of diagnosis. Arch Neurol 51:585–594, 1994.

27. Early identification of Alzheimer's disease–type dementias. Clinical Guideline 19, Rockville, MD: Agency for Health Care Policy and Research, USHHS No. 96-0703, Sept. 1996.

28. Pharmacy benefits management–medical advisory panel. The Management of Cognitive Changes in Alzheimer's Disease. VHA PBM-SHG Publication No. 99-0013. Hines, IL: Pharmacy Benefits Management Strategic Healthcare Group, Veterans Health Administration, Department of Veterans Affairs, August 1999.

29. Van Reekum R, Black S, Conn D, et al. Cognition enhancing drugs in dementia: A guide to the near future. Can J Psych 42 (Suppl 1):35s–50s, 1997.

30. Bartus RT, Dean RL, Beer B, et al. The cholinergic hypothesis of geriatric memory dysfunction. Science 217:408–414, 1982.

31. Davis BM, Mohs RC, Greenwald BS, et al. Clinical studies of the cholinergic deficit in Alzheimer's disease. 1: neurochemical and neuroendocrine studies. J Am Ger Soc 33:741–748, 1985.

32. Hollander E, Mohs RC, Davis KL. Cholinergic approaches to the treatment of Alzheimer's disease. Br Med Bull 42:97–100, 1986.

33. Kumar V, Calache M. Treatment of Alzheimer's disease with cholinergic drugs. Int J Clin Pharmacol Ther Toxicol 29:23–37, 1993.

34. Davis KL, Mohs RC. Enhancement of memory processes in Alzheimer's disease with multiple dose intravenous physostigmine. Am J Psychol 139:1421–1424, 1982.

35. Christie JE, Shering A, Ferguson J, et al. Physostigmine and arecoline effects of intravenous infusions in Alzheimer presenile dementia. Br J Psychol 138:46–50, 1982.

36. Thal LJ, Masur DM, Blau AD, et al. Chronic oral physostigmine without lecithin improves memory in Alzheimer's disease. J Am Geriatr Soc 37:42–48, 1989.

37. Summer WK, Majovski LV, Marsh GM, et al. Oral tetrahydroaminoacridine in long-term treatment of senile dementia, Alzheimer type. N Engl J Med 315:1241–1245, 1986.

38. Knapp MJ, Knopman DS, Soloman PR, et al. A 30-week randomized controlled trial of high-dose tacrine in patients with Alzheimer's disease. JAMA 271:985–991, 1994.

39. Davis KL, Thal LJ, Ganzu ER, et al. A double blind, placebo controlled multicenter study of tacrine for Alzheimer's disease. N Engl J Med 327:1253–1259, 1992.

40. Gamzu ER, Thal LJ, Davis KL. Therapeutic trials using tacrine and other cholinesterase inhibitors. Adv Neurol 51:241–245, 1990.

41. Rogers SL, Farlow MR, Doody RS, et al. and the Donepezil Study Group. A 24-week, double-blind, placebo-controlled trial of donepezil in patients with Alzheimer's disease. Neurology 50:136–145, 1998.

42. Winblad B, Engedal K, Soininen H, et al. A 1-year, randomized, placebo-controlled study of donepezil in patient with mild to moderate AD. Neurology 57:489–495, 2001.

43. Aricept (donepezil) full prescribing information. Teaneck, NJ: Eisai Inc, February 2000.

44. Holmes C, Wilkinson D, Dean C, et al. The efficacy of donepezil in the treatment of neuropsychiatric symptoms in Alzheimer's disease. Neurology 63:214–219, 2004.

45. Feldman H, Gauthier S, Hecker J, et al. A 24-week, randomized, double-blind study of donepezil in moderate to severe Alzheimer's disease. Neurology 57:613–620, 2001.

46. Corey-Bloom J, Anand R, Veach J. A randomized trial evaluating the efficacy and safety of ENA 713 (rivastigmine tartrate), a new acetylcholinesterase inhibitor, in patients with mild to moderately severe Alzheimer's disease. Int J Geriatr Psychopharmacol 1: 55–65, 1998.

47. Rosler M, Anand R, Cicin-Sain A, et al. Efficacy and safety of rivastigmine in patients with Alzheimer's disease: international randomized controlled trial. BMJ 318:633–638, 1999.

48. Exelon (rivastigmine) full prescribing information. Morris Plains, NJ: Novartis Pharmaceuticals Corporation, April 2000.

49. Kihara T, Shimoharma S, Urushitani M, et al. Stimulation of $\alpha4\beta2$ nicotinic acetylcholine receptors inhibits β-amyloid toxicity. Brain Res 792:331–334, 1998.

50. Tariot PN, Solomon PR, Morris JC, et al. A 5-month, randomized, placebo-controlled trial of galantamine in AD. Neurology 54: 2269–2276, 2000.

51. Raskind MA, Perskin ER, Wessel T, et al. Galantamine in AD. A 6-month, randomized placebo-controlled trial with a 6-month extension Neurology 54:2261–2268, 2000.

52. Wilcock GK, Lilienfeld S, Galens E. Efficacy and safety of galantamine in patients with mild to moderate Alzheimer's disease: multicenter randomized controlled trial. BMJ 321:1445–1449, 2000.

53. Reminyl (galantamine) full prescribing information. Titusville, NJ: Janssen Pharmaceutica Products LP, August 2002.

54. Auriacombe S, Pere JJ, Loria-Kanza Y, et al. Efficacy and safety of rivastigmine in patients with Alzheimer's disease who failed to benefit from treatment with donepezil. Curr Med Res Opin 18: 129–138, 2002.

55. Emre E. Switching cholinesterase inhibitors in patients with Alzheimer's disease. Int J Clin Pract 127:64–72, 2002.

56. ASHF Drug Information. Bethesda, MD: American Society of Health-System Pharmacists, 2005.

57. Ackerly S, Grierson AJ, Brownless J, et al. Glutamate slow axonal transport of neurofilaments in transfected neurons. J Cell Biol 150: 165–176, 2000.

58. Parson CG, Danysz W, Quack G. Memantine is a clinically well tolerated N-methyl-D-aspartate (NMDA) receptor antagonist-a review of preclinical data. Neuropharmacology 38:735–767, 1999.

59. Namenda (memantine) full prescribing information. St. Louis, MO: Forest Pharmaceuticals, Inc., October 2003.

60. Reisber B, Doody MD, Stoffler A, et al. Memantine in moderate-to-severe Alzheimer's disease. N Engl J Med 348:1333–1341, 2003.

61. Tariot P, Farlow MR, Grossber GT, et al. Memantine treatment in patients with moderate to severe Alzheimer's disease already receiving donepezil. A randomized controlled trial. JAMA 291: 317–324, 2004.

62. Aresoa SA, Sherrif F. Memantine for dementia (Cochrane Review). In: The Cochrane Library. No.3. Chichester, UK: John Wiley & Sons, Ltd., 2004.

63. Hake AM, Farlow MR. On the horizon: pathways for drug development in Alzheimer's disease. Clin Geriatr Med 20:141–153, 2004.

64. American Psychiatric Association. Practice guideline for the treatment of patients with Alzheimer's disease and other dementias of late life. Am J Psychiatr 154 (Suppl 5):1–30, 1997.

65. Reifler BS, Larson E, Teri L, et al. Dementia of the Alzheimer's type and depression. J Am Geriatr Soc 34:855–859, 1986.

66. Sakauye DM, Camp CJ, Lord PA, et al. Effects of buspirone on agitation associated with dementia. Am J Geriatr Psychiatr 1:82–84, 1993.

67. U.S. Food and Drug Administration. Center for Drug Evaluation and Research: Atypical Antipsychotic Drugs Information. 4/11/05. Available at: www.fda.gov/cder/infopage/antipsychotics.htm. Accessed April 15, 2005.

68. Omnibus Budget Reconciliation Act (OBRA). U.S. Health Care Financing Administration, 1987.

69. Reisberg B, Franssen E, Sclan S, et al. Stage specific incidence of potentially remediable behavioral symptoms in aging and Alzheimer disease. Bull Clin Neurosci 54:95–112, 1989.

70. Lemke MR. Effect of carbamazepine on agitation in Alzheimer's inpatients refractory to neuroleptics. J Clin Psychiatry 56:354–357, 1995.

71. Tariot PN, Erb R, Podgprski CA, et al. Efficacy and tolerability of carbamazepine for agitation and aggression in dementia. Am J Psych 155:54–61, 1998.

72. Lebert F, Pasquier F, Petit H. Behavioral effects of trazodone in Alzheimer's disease. J Clin Psych 55:536–538, 1994.

73. Weiler PG, Mungas D, Bernick C, et al. Propranolol for the control of disruptive behavior in senile dementia. J Geriatr Psychiatry Neurol 1:226–230, 1988.

74. Greendyke RM, Kanter DR. Therapeutic effects of pindolol on behavioral disturbances associated with organic brain disease: a double-blind study. J Clin Psychiatry 47:423–426, 1986.

75. Schneider LS, Sobin PB. Non-neuroleptic treatment of behavior symptoms and agitation in Alzheimer's disease and other dementias. Psychopharmacol Bull 28:71–79, 1992.

76. Lott AD, McElroy SL, Keys MA, et al. Valproate in the treatment of behavioral agitation in elderly patients with dementia. J Neuropsychiatry Clin Neurosci 7:314–319, 1995.

77. Sano M, Ernesto C, Thomas RG, et al. A controlled trial of selegiline, alpha-tocopherol, or both as treatment for Alzheimer's disease. N Engl J Med 336:1216–1222, 1997.

78. Doody RS, Steven JC, Beck C, et al. Practice parameter: management of dementia (an evidence-based review). Report of the Quality Standards Subcommittee of the American Academy of Neurology. Neurology 56:1154–1166, 2001.

79. Laurin D, Maski KH, Foley DJ, et al. Midlife dietary intake of antioxidants and risk of late-life incident dementia: the Honolulu-Asia Aging Study. Am J Epidemiol 159:959–967, 2004.

80. Miller ER, Pastor-Barriuso R, Dalal D, et al. Meta-analysis: high-dose vitamin E supplementation may increase all-cause mortality. Ann Intern Med 142:37–46, 2005.

81. LeBars PL, Katz MM, Berman N, et al. A placebo-controlled, double-blind, randomized trial of an extract of ginkgo biloba for dementia. JAMA 278:1327–1332, 1997.

82. Dewachter I, Van Leuven F. Secretases as targets for the treatment of Alzheimer's disease: the prospects. Lancet Neurol 1:409–416, 2002.

83. Schenk D, barbour R, Dunn W, et al. Immunization with amyloid-β attenuates Alzheimer-disease-like pathology in the PDAOO mouse. Nature 400:173–177, 1999.

84. Janus C, Pearon J, McLaurin J, et al. A β-peptide immunization reduces behavioral impairment and plaques in a model of Alzheimer's disease. Nature 408:979–982, 2000.

85. Morgan D, Diamon DM, Gottschall PE, et al. A β-peptide vaccination prevents memory loss in an animal model of Alzheimer's disease. Nature 408:982–985, 2000.

86. Schenk D. Amyloid-beta immunotherapy for Alzheimer's disease: the end of the beginning. Nature 3:824–828, 2002.

87. Birge SJ. The role of estrogen in the treatment of Alzheimer's disease. Neurology 48(Suppl 7):S36–S41, 1997.

88. Kawas C, Resnick S, Morrison A, et al. A prospective study of estrogen replacement therapy and the risk of developing Alzheimer's disease: The Baltimore Longitudinal Study of Aging. Neurology 48:1517–1521, 1997.

89. Henderson VW, Paganini-Hill A, Miller BL, et al. Estrogen for Alzheimer's disease in women: randomized, double-blind, placebo-controlled trial. Neurology 54:295–301, 2000.

90. Mulnard RA, Cotman CW, Kasaw C, et al. Estrogen replacement therapy for treatment of mild to moderate Alzheimer disease: a randomized controlled trial. JAMA 283:1007–1015, 2000.

91. Shumaker SA, Legault C, Rapp SR, et al. Estrogen plus progestin and the incidence of dementia and mild cognitive impairment in postmenopausal women: the Women's Health Initiative Memory Study: a randomized controlled trial. JAMA 289:2651–2662, 2003.

92. Steward WF, Kawas C, Corrada M, et al. Risk of Alzheimer's disease and duration of NSAID use. Neurology 48:626–632, 1997.

93. Aisen PS, Davis Kl, Berg JD, et al. A randomized controlled trial of prednisone in Alzheimer's disease. Neurology 54:588–593, 2000.

94. Scharf S, Mander A, Ugoni A, et al. A double-blind, placebo-controlled trial of diclofenac/misoprostol in Alzheimer's disease. Neurology 53:197–201, 1999.

95. Aisen PS, Schafer KA, Grundman M, et al. Effect of rofecoxib or naproxen vs placebo on Alzheimer's disease progression: a randomized controlled trial. JAMA 289:2819–2826, 2003.

96. Jick H. Statins and the risk of dementia. Lancet 356:1627–1631, 2000.

97. Wolozin B. Decreased prevalence of Alzheimer's disease associated with 3-hydroxy-3-methylglutaryl coenzyme A reduce inhibitors. Arch Neurol 57:1439–1443, 2000.

98. Shepherd J, Blauw GJ, Murphy MB. Pravastatin in elderly individuals at risk of vascular disease (PROSPER) a randomized controlled trial. Lancet 360:1623–1630, 2002.

99. Collins R, Armitage J, Parish S. MRC/BHF Heart Protection Study of cholesterol lowering with simvastatin in 20536 high-risk individuals a randomized placebo-controlled trial. Lancet 360:7–22, 2002.

100. Muldoon MF, Ryan CM, Sereika SM, et al. Randomized trial of the effect of simvastatin on cognitive functioning in hypercholesterolemic adults. Am J Med 117:756–762, 2004.

101. Mace NL, Rabins PV. The thirty-six-hour day: a family guide to caring for persons with Alzheimer's disease, related dementing illness, and memory loss in later life. 2nd ed. New York: Warner Books, 1992.

102. Howell M. Caretakers' views on responsibilities for the care of the demented elderly. J Am Geriatr Soc 32:657–660, 1984.

103. Ernst RL, Hay JW. The U.S. economic and social costs of Alzheimer's disease revisited. Am J Public Health 84:1261–1264, 1994.

104. Hamdy RC, Turnbull RM, Clar W, et al. Alzheimer's disease–a handbook for caregivers. St. Louis: Mosby, 1994.

105. Torian L, Davidson E, Fulop G, et al. The effect of dementia on acute care in a geriatric medical unit. Int Psychogeriatr 4:231–239, 1993.

106. Welch HG, Walsh JS, Larson EB. The cost of institutional care in Alzheimer's disease: nursing home and hospital care in a prospective cohort. J Am Geriatr Soc 40:221–224, 1992.

Geriatric Drug Therapy

71

Susan W. Miller

TREATMENT GOALS

- Resolve the symptoms of a specific condition and slow progression of the negative outcomes of the condition.
- Avoid medication-related problems.
- Set an actual target clinical parameter for the problem being treated, such as a specific blood pressure, glucose level, or reduction in incidences of problematic behaviors.
- Set an appropriate duration of therapy and consider dosage reductions or discontinue drugs at the end of that time.
- Select the most appropriate pharmacologic alternative based on the patient's clinical status and comorbid conditions.
- Initiate therapy with a low dose (25% to 33% the usual recommended dose) and increase slowly to account for prolonged drug half-life.
- Use the fewest medications possible.
- Minimize the number and dose of medications with effects on the central nervous system.
- Consider the effect of the selected medication on the functional ability and quality of life of the patient.

DEMOGRAPHICS AND DRUG USE PATTERNS

More than 35 million people, or 12.6% of the population, in the United States are over 65 years of age. By the year 2030, it is projected that the older population will more than double to 70 million, with the largest increases in the 75- to 84-year age group and the frail or 85-years-and-over age group.[1] People reaching 65 years of age have an average life expectancy of an additional 17.9 years (19.2 years for women, 16.3 years for men).[2] Factors contributing to the growing numbers of elderly include the increased birth rate-

prior to 1920 and after World War II, the decrease in mortality associated with the development of antibiotics and vaccines, improvements in sanitation and technology, and a decline in midlife mortality from coronary artery disease.

The past 25 years have seen a revolution in our knowledge of how the processes of aging affect drug therapy. With this knowledge has come progress in caring for patients over 65 years of age. Advances in medical technology have enhanced studies of the physiologic changes of aging, and there is now a broader understanding of how physiologic changes affect the treatment of disease and the use of medications in older patients.[3]

Because older adults experience a higher rate of chronic conditions compared to the population at large, they are more likely to use healthcare services. The elderly (those over 65 years of age) represented 20% of hospital discharges and used a third of the days of care in 1970; in 2000, the elderly made up almost 40% of hospital discharges and used almost half of the hospital days. Many advances in medical care (including cardiovascular interventions and drug therapies) occurred during this time. These may have decreased death rates but also could have resulted in a heightened risk of hospitalization for the elderly.[4] Older patients are admitted to hospitals more than three times as often as younger patients, are hospitalized 50% longer, and use twice as many prescription medications as the general population. Although only 4% of the total elderly population lives in a nursing home at any one time, about 20% spend some time in a nursing home during their lifetime. Some important statistics concerning geriatrics and medications are the following:[5]

- Adverse drug reactions are among the top five greatest threats to the health of seniors.
- Twenty-eight percent of hospitalizations among seniors are due to adverse drug reactions.
- 32,000 seniors suffer hip fractures each year due to falls caused by medication-related problems.
- The elderly account for about 12.6% of the U.S. population but consume approximately 34% of total prescriptions.
- On average, individuals 65 to 69 years old take nearly 14 prescriptions per year, and individuals aged 80 to 84 years take an average of 18 prescriptions per year.
- One of the fastest-growing areas of healthcare delivery is personal care or assisted living facilities, which offer room, board, and limited supervision and provision of care for older residents.
- These demographic changes will continue to have a major impact on healthcare staffing, practice, and expenditures.

Landmark studies such as the following have established the rates of medication use among various groups of older patients:

1. The Dunedin Study, a longitudinal, epidemiologic study starting in 1978 examining the drug use patterns of an ambulatory, elderly population, showed that the number of prescribed and nonprescribed drugs increased from an average of 2.9 to 4.08 over a 10-year increase in age.[6]
2. The Boston Collaborative Drug Surveillance Program reported on drug use patterns in several hospitals and found that the average number of drug exposures increased with age, from 6.3 per patient in the 16- to 25-year-old category to 9.7 in patients over 65 years of age.[7]
3. Medication use in long-term care facilities has been reported to be high,[8,9] and the most recent investigations report an average of 6.69 (± 1.12) routinely scheduled general medication orders and 2.61 (± 1.35) as-needed medication orders per patient. Of a nationally surveyed group of nursing facility residents, 27.1% were reported

to have nine or more routinely scheduled medications. Among the regularly scheduled psychotherapeutic categories, antidepressants were the most commonly prescribed (34.5 ± 12.1%), followed by antipsychotics (16.9 ± 7.2%), anxiolytics (10.1 ± 5.4%) and hypnotics (2.3 ± 2.5%).[10] These numbers are affected by attention to compliance with regulations regarding medication use in these facilities and the role of the consultant pharmacist in the long-term care setting.[11]

PSYCHOSOCIAL ASPECTS

Geriatric patients use more medications than younger patients because they have more symptoms of disease. A second contributing factor to drug use in older patients is the psychosocial aspect of drug use. These psychosocial issues can cause either an increase or a decrease in medication use. Included in these psychosocial aspects is the attitude that medications are available that can cure almost any disease or alleviate any symptom; therefore, a patient should be prescribed a medication to manage any disease or symptom. Many older patients equate drugs (medications) with narcotics (''dope'') and therefore view them as something to be avoided. Research has shown an inverse correlation between the number of medications people take and their satisfaction with life and health. Increased consumption of medications has been reported in women who are not satisfied with their lives. Other opinions regarding medication use by geriatric patients include the following beliefs:

- Physicians would not prescribe any medication that could be harmful.
- The U.S. Food and Drug Administration (FDA) makes sure that all drugs are safe.
- Over-the-counter drugs are completely safe and are not really drugs.
- All drugs can be addicting.
- If a little bit of a drug is good, then more would be better.
- Vitamins and herbal products are harmless because they are ''natural'' products.

It is important for pharmacists and other healthcare professionals to listen to older patients' opinions about drug therapy and respond to them with the best interest of the patient in mind.

MEDICATION-RELATED PROBLEMS IN GERIATRIC PATIENTS

The Institute of Medicine (IOM)'s report on deaths from medical errors estimated that the cost to the U.S. economy was $8 billion annually.[12] In 2000, it was estimated that medication-related problems caused 106,000 deaths annually at a cost of $85 billion.[13] Other calculated costs of medication-related problems include $76.6 billion for ambulatory care,[14] $20 billion for hospitals,[15] and $4 billion for nursing homes.[16]

Problems with medication therapy in geriatric patients can be described in different ways. Several terms that often appear in the literature are polypharmacy, adverse drug reactions (ADRs), appropriateness of therapy, and compliance.

Polypharmacy (the use of multiple prescription and over-the-counter medications, especially by older people with chronic health problems) has been identified as the principal drug safety issue of the future.[17] Patient acuity may be the most important determinant of medication use in the elderly. Studies on drug use among geriatric patients have shown a wide variation in the number of drugs used by older people based on their relative independence or level of care. Other major factors influencing medication use in older patients, especially medication use in long-term care facilities, are (a) the initiation of diagnosis-related groups (DRGs), emphasizing shorter hospital stays and therefore discharging higher-acuity patients (potentially on more medications) to nursing facilities[18]; and (b) the effects of the HCFA [Health Care Financing Administration, now called Centers for Medicare and Medicaid Services (CMS)] regulations on stressing rational drug use in nursing facilities and subsequent monitoring of drug therapy by pharmacists.[19,20]

One fourth of nursing home admissions have been attributed to the inability of older patients to manage their medications,[21] and up to 17% of hospital admissions of patients above the age of 65 years are attributable to ADRs.[22,23] Much of the ADR reporting in elderly patients was documented primarily in the nursing facility setting,[24,25] but elderly patients living in the community have also been shown to be at risk for drug-related problems.[26]

Among other factors, the use of multiple prescription medications for the management of chronic diseases in the aging population increases the risk for medication-related problems. Other risk factors for medication-related problems are listed in Table 71.1.[27] Older patients are at increased risk for ADRs compared to younger patients and often have an atypical presentation of the ADR that may be confused with aging or disease progression. Cognitive impairment and behavioral changes frequently are the result of drug therapy; therefore, the medical evaluation of the older patient should include a thorough review of drug therapy to screen for possible drug effects (Table 71.2).[28] Additional factors contributing specifically to ADRs in geriatric patients are listed in Table 71.3.

More than one in six elderly Americans are taking prescription drugs that are not suited for geriatric patients and may lead to physical or mental deterioration and possibly death.[29] Recently, strategies have been developed in attempts to foster appropriate prescribing of medications in the geriatric population overall. Medications reported to be inappropriate for use in the elderly are listed in Table 71.4. Criteria describing inappropriate medications for use in older patients were originally developed by a consensus panel of experts in geriatric care, geriatric pharmacology, geriatric psychopharmacology, and nursing home care. These experts

TABLE 71.1	Potential Risk Factors for Drug-Related Problems in Elderly Nursing Facility Residents
Specific Medication	**Class of Medication**
Digoxin	Anticonvulsants
Warfarin	Antiarrhythmics
Lithium	Antipsychotics
Theophylline	Antidepressants
Chlorpropamide	Sedative–hypnotics
Glyburide	Benzodiazepines
	Histamine$_2$ antagonists
	Nonsteroidal anti-inflammatories
	Anticholinergics
	Angiotensin-converting enzyme inhibitors
	Diuretics
	New prescription for antibiotic
	Narcotic analgesics

Patient Characteristics

More than six active chronic medical diagnoses

More than 12 medication doses per day

Recent transfer from hospital

Advanced age (>85 years)

New prescription for antibiotic

Prior adverse drug reaction

Cancer

Depression

Low body weight or body mass index (<22 kg/m^2)

Six or more medications

Cognitive impairment (including dementia)

Decreased renal function (estimated creatinine clearance <50 mL/min)

(Adapted from Fouts M, Hanlon J, Pieper C, et al. Identification of elderly nursing facility residents at high risk for drug-related problems. Consult Pharm 12:1103–1111, 1997.)

agreed on criteria defining inappropriate medication use in nursing home residents. The criteria relate to certain medications that should not be used and doses and durations of therapy of some medications that should not be exceeded in the older, nursing facility patient.[30,31] The criteria have been updated to include two types of statements: (a) medications or medication classes that should generally be avoided in persons 65 years or older because they are either ineffective or they pose an unnecessarily high risk for older persons and a safer alternative is available; and (b) medications that should not be used in older persons known to have specific medical conditions.[32] The medications that should be avoided are listed in Table 71.4.

TABLE 71.2	Medications That Can Cause Mental Status Changes
Amantadine	Morphine
Anticholinergics and atropine	Narcotics
Barbiturates	Nonsteroidal anti-inflammatories
Benzodiazepines	Penicillin G procaine
Bromocriptine	Phenytoin
Buspirone	Pilocarpine
Caffeine	Propoxyphene
Calcium channel blockers	Propranolol
Captopril	Quinidine
Carbamazepine	Salicylates
Cephalosporins	Selective serotonin reuptake inhibitors
Corticosteroids	Selegiline
Digoxin	Sulfonamides
Estrogens	Theophylline
Fluoroquinolones	Thiazide diuretics
Histamine H_2receptor antagonists	Tricyclic antidepressants
HMG-CoA reductase inhibitors	Valproic acid
Levodopa	Vinblastine
Meperidine	Vincristine
Methyldopa	Zolpidem
Monoamine oxidase inhibitors	

(Adapted from Drugs that cause psychiatric symptoms. Med Lett Drugs Ther 40:21–24, 1998.)

The Medication Appropriateness Index (MAI) is a rating scale that provides parameters for the evaluation of 10 key elements of medication prescribing.[33] For each parameter, the index has operational definitions, explicit instructions, and an assigned weight. The evaluator rates the medication as appropriate, marginally appropriate, or inappropriate

TABLE 71.3	Reasons for High Frequencies of Adverse Drug Reactions (ADRs) in the Elderly

Multiple chronic diseases requiring treatment with potent medications

Several physicians prescribing therapy independently

Inappropriate identification of altered presentation of ADRs

Patient noncompliance with prescribed medications

Inappropriate self-medication

Inadequate patient education about prescribed or over-the-counter medications

Age-related physiologic changes that alter drug kinetics and pharmacologic response to drugs

based on the operational definitions and then calculates a medication appropriateness score. Higher scores indicate less appropriate prescribing. These parameters are listed in Table 71.5. Both the Beers criteria and MAI methods of prescribing and monitoring drug therapy stress the importance of considering the individual patient's clinical and health status and concomitant medications he or she is receiving before prescribing additional medications.

Despite these strategies for improving the prescribing of medications for geriatric patients, drug-related morbidity and mortality in nursing facilities still exists. It has been estimated that for every dollar spent on drugs in nursing facilities, two dollars in healthcare resources are consumed in the treatment of drug-related problems in this patient population.[16]

Compliance is defined as the extent to which a patient's behavior coincides with a prescriber's planned medical regimen. Noncompliance or nonadherence with drug therapy occurs in one half to one third of elderly patients.[34] Most of the time, too little medication is consumed.[35] Poor communication between healthcare professionals and patients, coupled with declining cognitive function, and complicated drug regimens are major reasons for noncompliance in older patients. Pharmacists should make a special effort to counsel these high-risk patients by providing both verbal reinforcement and written instructions to ensure an understanding of why the drug was prescribed, its correct use, the proper administration time consistent with lifestyle and activities, and the common side effects. Upon refill visits to the pharmacy, the pharmacist should ask the patient and caregiver subtle and open-ended questions related to side effects and potentially serious ADRs. Eliminating unnecessary or duplicative therapy in addition to simplifying the drug regimen will help minimize ADRs and maximize compliance. Pharmacists should be aware of the major risk factors for noncompliance and assess each patient for the presence of risk factors (Table 71.6).

EFFECTS OF AGING ON DRUG ACTIONS

It has been estimated that many of the ADRs encountered in the elderly are the result of dose-related pharmacokinetic changes and thus may be prevented if these changes are considered when prescribing drug therapy.[36] The aging process alone can influence drug response by interfering in various degrees with the fraction of drug absorbed (f), the plasma drug half-life ($T\frac{1}{2}$), the volume of drug distribution in the body (Vd), and the metabolic and renal clearance from the body (Cl). By predicting which drugs will be affected by age-related changes, the correct dose and dosing interval can be better estimated. In addition to alterations in drug kinetics, age can also influence the pharmacologic response of drugs.

TABLE 71.4	Potentially Inappropriate Medication Use in Older Adults

Propoxyphene and combination products

Nonsteroidal anti-inflammatory drugs

   Indomethacin

   Pentazocine

   Ketorolac

   Trimethobenzamide

Muscle relaxants or antispasmodic agents

   Methocarbamol

   Carisoprodol

   Chlorzoxazone

   Metaxalone

   Cyclobenzaprine

   Oxybutynin

   Orphenadrine

Antidepressants

   Amitriptyline

      Chlordiazepoxide/amitriptyline

      Perphenazine/amitriptyline

      Doxepin

      Daily fluoxetine

Meprobamate

Sedative or hypnotic agents

Short-acting benzodiazepines (total daily dosage limits)

      Lorazepam doses >3 mg

      Oxazepam doses >60 mg

      Alprazolam doses >2 mg

      Temazepam doses >15 mg

      Triazolam doses >0.25 mg

Long-acting benzodiazepines

Flurazepam

Chlordiazepoxide

Chlordiazepoxide/amitriptyline

Clidinium/chlordiazepoxide

Diazepam

Quazepam

Halazepam

Chlorazepate

Disopyramide

Amiodarone

Digoxin at doses >0.125 mg/d except when treating atrial arrhythmias

Platelet inhibitors

   Short-acting dipyridamole

      Ticlopidine

Antihypertensive agents

   Methyldopa and methyldopa-hydrochlorothiazide

   Reserpine at doses >0.25 mg

   Guanethidine

   Guanadrel

Doxazosin

Clonidine

Ethacrynic acid

Short-acting nifedipine

Chlorpropamide

Antipsychotics

   Thioridazine

   Mesoridazine

Analgesic agents

   Meperidine

Gastrointestinal antispasmodic agents

   Dicyclomine

   Hyoscyamine

   Propantheline

   Belladonna alkaloids

   Clidinium/chlordiazepoxide

Anticholinergics and antihistamines

   Chlorpheniramine

   Diphenhydramine

   Hydroxyzine

   Cyproheptadine

   Promethazine

   Tripelennamine

   Dexchlorpheniramine

   Diphenhydramine

Dementia treatments

   Ergot mesyloids

   Cyclandelate

   Isoxsuprine

Ferrous sulfate >325 mg/d

All barbiturates (except phenobarbital when used to control seizures)

Amphetamines and anorexic agents

Long term use of full-dosage, longer half-life non-COX-selective nonsteroidal antiinflammatory agents

Naproxen

Oxaprozin

Piroxicam

Long-term use of stimulant laxatives (except in the presence of opiate analgesic use)

   Bisacodyl

   Cascara sagrada

   Neoloid

Mineral oil

Methyltestosterone

Cimetidine

Desiccated thyroid

Estrogens only (oral)

Nitrofurantoin

(Adapted from Fick DM, Cooper JW, Wade WE, et al. Updating the Beers criteria for potentially inappropriate medication use in older adults. Arch Intern Med 163:2716–2724, 2003.)

TABLE 71.5	Criteria of Medication Appropriateness Index

1. Is there an indication for the drug?
2. Is the medication effective for the condition?
3. Is the dosage correct?
4. Are the directions correct?
5. Are the directions practical?
6. Are there clinically significant drug–drug interactions?
7. Are there clinically significant drug–disease interactions?
8. Is there unnecessary duplication with other drugs?
9. Is the duration of therapy acceptable?
10. Is this drug the least expensive alternative compared to others of equal utility?

(Adapted from Hanlon JT, Schmader KE, Samsa GP, et al. A method for assessing drug therapy appropriateness. J Clin Epidemiol 45:1045–1051, 1992.)

ABSORPTION

Product formulation, inherent drug properties, and patient variables can influence the rate, and in some cases the extent, of drug absorption in the elderly. In terms of product formulation, it is common for a geriatric patient to have difficulty swallowing a tablet or capsule, and it is frequently necessary to use a liquid dosage form or crush the tablet for administration with food or via a nasogastric tube. In general, extended-release, enteric-coated, and sublingual products should not be crushed because of adverse effects on absorption half-life and toxicity.

Age-related physiologic changes in the gastrointestinal tract include elevated gastric pH, delayed gastric emptying time, and decreases in both gastrointestinal motility and intestinal blood flow. These age-related physiologic changes alone do not seem to influence the passive transport mechanisms by which most drugs are absorbed. Medications that undergo first-pass metabolism are absorbed more completely in the older patient. This requires smaller initial and maintenance doses of these medications when used to man-

TABLE 71.6	Major Risk Factors for Noncompliance

Chronic disease or long-term therapy
Use of multiple pharmacies
Psychiatric illness
Cognitive impairment
Multiple physicians
Multiple medications
Multiple or complicated dosing schemes
Ineffective communication with healthcare professionals

TABLE 71.7	Medications Affected by Extensive First-Pass Hepatic Metabolism

Amitriptyline	Methylphenidate
Desipramine	Metoprolol
Dextropropoxyphene	Morphine
Dihydroergotamine	Nifedipine
Diltiazem	Nitroglycerin
5-Fluorouracil	Pentazocine
Hydralazine	Propranolol
Labetalol	Salicylamide
Lidocaine	Verapamil
6-Mercaptopurine	

age chronic diseases (Table 71.7). The age-related delay in gastric emptying allows more contact time in the stomach for potentially ulcerogenic drugs such as the nonsteroidal antiinflammatory drugs (NSAIDs), increases the frequency of drug interactions with antacids, provides more chance for binding, may increase the absorption of poorly soluble drugs, and may delay the onset of action of the weakly basic drugs.

Age reduces the active transport mechanisms involved in the absorption of sugars (galactose), vitamins (thiamine, folic acid), and minerals (calcium, iron). Because of these changes in absorption, as well as the fact that the elderly often do not consume a balanced diet due to food preferences or economic reasons, the use of a multivitamin and mineral supplement should be considered.

Problems with bioavailability and bioequivalency have been reported with many medications, and the issue of generic substitution is especially important to the geriatric patient because medication costs are so relevant to this population.[37] Studies have shown wide bioavailability and bioequivalency differences between various brands of generic tolbutamide, phenytoin, prednisone, furosemide, digoxin, and levothyroxine.[38] Indiscriminate switching among products should be avoided, especially for drugs in critical therapeutic categories such as cardiovascular or hormone replacement agents, and for medications prescribed for debilitated or frail patients.

Physiologic changes and diseases, such as heart failure, often necessitate the use of the intravenous route of administration because of incomplete absorption via the oral and intramuscular routes. There is also a decrease in absorption of intramuscularly administered drugs in bedridden elderly patients, probably due to changes in regional blood flow and reduced muscle mass.

In conclusion, although the potential for problems with absorption of medications exists in geriatric patients, practice has shown that these changes are of little clinical significance. Changes in gastric motility and blood flow can affect the extent of absorption (peak concentration) and the rate of absorption (time to peak concentration), but completeness of absorption of drugs in geriatric patients is similar to that in younger patients; however, delays in onset of activity may occur.

DISTRIBUTION

Increasing age can alter the distribution of a medication to the target organ. Although total protein is unaffected by aging, the plasma albumin portion often decreases in elderly, debilitated patients. Albumin acts as a drug carrier, binding the drug until it is needed. If albumin is decreased, there will be a resultant increase in active, unbound drug (free fraction). The importance of the increased free fraction is questionable because although more free drug is available for receptor binding, more free drug is also available for metabolism and elimination.[39]

In addition to age and diet, disease states such as cirrhosis, renal failure, and malnutrition can reduce albumin levels. Reduced protein binding is seen with phenytoin, but the drug is cleared from the plasma more rapidly, as described above. Initial doses of most highly protein-bound drugs (greater than 90% protein-bound) should be reduced and titrated slowly if there is evidence of decreased albumin. For extensively protein-bound drugs whose binding is reduced due to hypoproteinemia, practitioners should expect both therapeutic and toxic events at lower total serum concentrations.[40] If several highly protein-bound drugs are used together, the chance of the patient suffering a drug interaction increases. In the case of meperidine, there is a decrease in the binding to red blood cells with increasing age,[41] thus increasing the amount of free drug available systemically. This may result in an increased incidence of respiratory depression, or in the case of meperidine's active metabolite normeperidine, central nervous system (CNS) stimulation to the point of seizures.

Alpha-1-acid glycoprotein (AAG) is a protein that also binds to some medications. AAG is described as an acute-phase reactant and can increase with age, especially in acutely ill patients and those with inflammation. The release of AAG may increase the protein binding of basic drugs, such as lidocaine and propranolol, decreasing the amount of unbound or active drug and thus decreasing the pharmacologic effect.[42,43]

Changes in the ratio of lean body weight to fat can also alter medication distribution and thus pharmacologic response. With aging, total body water is decreased and total body fat is increased. These changes influence the onset and duration of action of highly tissue-bound drugs such as digoxin and water-soluble drugs such as alcohol, lithium, or morphine. The dosages of most water-soluble drugs are based on an estimation of lean body weight:[44]

$$\text{Men} = 50 \text{ kg} + 2.3(\text{inches in height} > 5 \text{ ft})$$

$$\text{Women} = 45 \text{ kg} + 2.3(\text{inches in height} > 5 \text{ ft})$$

If actual weight is less than estimated body weight, the actual weight should be used in dosage calculations.

Between the ages of 18 and 85 years, there is an increase in total body fat in both women and men; lean body mass will eventually decrease in both groups as well. With increasing age, the volume of distribution of lipophilic drugs increases as a result of an increase in the fat to lean muscle ratio, diminished protein binding, and a decrease in total body weight. Fat-soluble drugs, including many CNS active drugs, may have a delayed onset of action and subsequently accumulate in adipose tissue, prolonging their duration of action, sometimes with adverse effects on the patient.

ELIMINATION

Drugs are primarily cleared from the body by metabolism in the liver, excretion by the kidneys, or some combination of the two processes. With increasing age, a decrease in total body clearance results in higher average plasma drug concentrations and an enhanced pharmacologic response; both could lead to drug toxicity. Age-related physiologic changes in the kidney influence drug elimination and response in the geriatric patient to a greater extent than age-related physiologic changes that occur in the liver.

Hepatic Metabolism. Age-related physiologic changes, such as reductions in liver mass, hepatic metabolizing enzyme activity, and liver blood flow, may account for the decreased elimination of some hepatically metabolized medications in the elderly patient. Medications that are biotransformed in the liver may be affected by these changes. Drug metabolism can also be affected at all ages by gender, genetics, smoking, diet, concomitant drugs, and diseases. Hepatic metabolism is highly dependent on blood flow. From 25 years of age and up, there is a continual reduction in hepatic blood flow; in the presence of congestive heart failure, hepatic blood flow is further compromised. With drugs that are highly dependent on hepatic metabolism, such as most β-blockers, lidocaine, theophylline, and the narcotic analgesics, the decrease in hepatic clearance could increase the plasma concentrations of these drugs to toxic levels.

In addition to alterations of hepatic blood flow, age influences the rate of hepatic clearance of drugs by causing changes in the intrinsic activity of some liver enzymes. Hepatic metabolism occurs by two mechanisms: the microsomal enzyme mixed-function oxidase system (phase I), which includes the cytochrome P-450 systems; and conjugation of the drug molecule with a glucuronide, a sulfa, or an acetyl moiety (phase II). Phase I metabolism may produce compounds with pharmacologic activity, whereas phase II metabolism usually produces inactive metabolites. Reductions in phase I metabolism are often noted in the geriatric patient, and several enzymatic reactions of the cytochrome P-450 systems are slowed dramatically with advancing age. Of the more than 30 cytochrome P-450 isoenzymes identified, the major ones responsible for drug metabolism include CYP3A4, CYP2D6, CYP1A2, and the CYP2C subfamily.[45]

TABLE 71.8	Problematic Drugs Involving the Cytochrome P-450 Enzyme System

Antihistamines (selected nonsedating agents)

Antipsychotic agents (selected agents)

Azole antifungal agents

β-Blockers (selected agents)

Benzodiazepines (short- and intermediate-acting)

Carbamazepine

Cimetidine

Cisapride

HMG-CoA reductase inhibitors

Macrolide antibiotics

Narcotic analgesics

Phenobarbital

Phenytoin

Quinolones (selected agents)

Tricyclic antidepressants (selected agents)

Selective serotonin reuptake inhibitors (selected agents)

Warfarin

(Adapted from Michalets EL. Update; clinically significant cytochrome P-450 drug interactions. Pharmacotherapy 18:84–112, 1998.)

Vigilant monitoring of drug therapy is necessary to avoid life-threatening drug interactions among commonly prescribed medications (Table 71.8).

Phase II metabolism is usually unaffected by aging. The clinical effect of these changes results in slowed metabolism and prolonged duration of action for medications using phase I metabolic pathways but not for those using phase II metabolic pathways.[46,47] Studies seem to suggest that in elderly patients initial doses of hepatically metabolized drugs should be reduced by one-third to one-half the usual recommended starting dose, and then the dosage should be adjusted based on the clinical response.

Renal Elimination. The glomerular filtration rate (GFR) may decrease as much as 50% with increasing age, and this can directly affect the renal elimination of drugs or their active metabolites. Serum creatinine is frequently used to monitor renal function, but this test is of limited usefulness in monitoring the GFR in the older patient. Significant elevations of serum creatinine do not occur unless a majority of the kidney function has deteriorated. The production of creatinine, which depends on muscle mass, is decreased in the elderly; therefore, an apparently normal serum creatinine in an older patient may not be a valid predictor of drug elimination. Blood urea nitrogen (BUN) is also not a useful indicator of renal function because it can be affected by hydration status, diet, and blood loss.

The GFR is reduced due to age-related decreases in renal mass, loss of functional nephrons, and diminished renal ar-tery perfusion. A commonly used estimation of GFR in the geriatric population is the creatinine clearance (Cl_{Cr}), which correlates well with both GFR and tubular secretion. Cl_{Cr} can be estimated by a standard equation developed by Cockroft and Gault[48] that takes into consideration age, body weight, and serum creatinine in patients with stable renal function:

$$Cl_{Cr}\,(male) = \frac{lean\ body\ weight\,(kg) \times (140 - age\ in\ years)}{serum\ creatinine \times 72}$$

$$Cl_{Cr}\,(female) = 0.85 \times Cl_{Cr}\,(male)$$

This, as well as other Cl_{Cr}-estimating equations in common clinical use, have been reported to provide unacceptable predictions of creatinine clearance in a representative sample of healthy elderly persons.[49] An evaluation of several methods of calculations and nomograms used to estimate creatinine clearance in older patients determined that the use of published equations and rounding low serum creatinine values up to 1.0 mg per dL caused a significant underestimation of actual creatinine clearance in older patients. This study suggested that the practice of rounding up serum creatinine concentrations could lead to underdosing of certain medications such as aminoglycosides.[50]

Equations and nomograms are simply estimates of an individual's actual renal function, and although the estimates appear to be less accurate in the geriatric population, the difficulty in collecting 24-hour urine samples may preclude more accurate Cl_{Cr} determinations. In clinical practice the Cockroft and Gault equation is used routinely, with the knowledge that it is providing only an estimate of the renal function of the older patient.

To avoid drug toxicity, dosages of renally excreted drugs (or active metabolites) must be adjusted if the estimated Cl_{Cr} is less than 30 mL per minute (Table 71.9). Many drug monographs now contain dosing guidelines based on declining renal function, and practitioners should refer to these or similar references for dosing guidelines for renally excreted drugs in the presence of varying degrees of renal failure. Dosage or interval adjustments are necessary to prevent drug-related problems.

A summary of pharmacokinetic changes with aging is found in Table 71.10.

EFFECTS OF AGING ON DRUG RESPONSE

With increasing age, there is an increased intolerance to drugs as a result of altered pharmacodynamic response at the target organs. Altered response may be due to a reduction in receptor number and sensitivity, depletion of neurotransmitters, the presence of disease, or physiologic changes. With aging, there is evidence of a depletion in the neurotransmitters acetylcholine, dopamine, and serotonin; a depletion in several hormones; a decrease in the enzymatic degradation of monoamine oxidase; an impaired baroreceptor

TABLE 71.9	Examples of Medications Primarily Excreted by the Kidney

Acetazolamide	Lithium
Allopurinol	Methotrexate
Amiloride	Metoclopramide
Angiotensin-converting enzyme inhibitors	Nadolol
Amantadine	Norfloxacin
Aminoglycosides	Penicillins
Atenolol	Probenecid
Cephalosporins	Procainamide
Chlorpropamide	Quinidine
Ciprofloxacin	Spironolactone
Digoxin	Sulfamethoxazole
Disopyramide	Sulfinpyrazone
Ethambutol	Thiazides
Fluconazole	Trimethoprim
Furosemide	Vancomycin
Gentamicin	
Histamine2-receptor antagonists	

TABLE 71.10	Age-Related Physiologic Changes Affecting Pharmacokinetic Parameters

Parameter	Direction of Change
Absorption	
Gastric pH	Increase
Absorptive surface	Decrease
Splanchnic blood flow	Decrease
Gastrointestinal motility	Decrease
Gastric emptying rate	Decrease
Distribution	
Cardiac output	Decrease
Total body weight	Decrease
Lean body mass	Decrease
Serum albumin	Decrease[a]
Alpha$_1$-acid glycoprotein	Increase
Body fat	Increase
Relative tissue perfusion	Decrease
Metabolism	
Hepatic mass	Decrease
Hepatic blood flow	Decrease
Hepatic function	Decrease
Hepatic enzyme activity	Decrease
Phase 1 reactions	Decrease
Phase 2 reactions	No change
Excretion	
Renal mass	Decrease
Renal blood flow	Decrease
Glomerular filtration rate	Decrease
Tubular secretion	Decrease

[a] Potential to decrease in chronically ill, malnourished patients; otherwise is normal.

response to blood pressure changes; a decreased responsiveness to β-adrenergic receptors; and increased pain tolerance.[51] Each of these changes can affect the older patient's response to medications.

Many drugs routinely prescribed for geriatric patients have adverse effects on the CNS, such as cognitive impairment and memory loss. Careful monitoring of these agents is necessary in an effort to differentiate among drug effectiveness, adverse effects, or progression of a disease process. Altered end-organ sensitivity may result in exaggerated pharmacologic response, as seen with the barbiturates and benzodiazepines. Other drug classes affected include the narcotic analgesics, antihypertensive agents, anticholinergic agents, phenothiazines, and tricyclic antidepressants. It appears that with many of these agents, geriatric patients are more sensitive to both the therapeutic and adverse effects, so lower initial and maintenance doses are recommended. A diminished pharmacologic response is also possible and occurs with the β-blockers, β-agonists, and some calcium channel blockers.

Increased sensitivity to warfarin in the geriatric patient has been shown, and recommendations for warfarin prescribing are to reduce the average daily dosage by 30% to 40% and monitor carefully, keeping the International Normalized Ratio (INR) within the therapeutic range.[52] Elderly women have been reported to be more susceptible to the bleeding complications of heparin,[53] and hematuria has been shown

to be a useful and sensitive clinical parameter to monitor for heparin or warfarin toxicity.

Dosing adjustments of medications are often necessary, because many of these same drugs are also influenced by age-related physiologic changes, especially drug distribution and elimination. The net effect in an individual patient is often difficult to predict. For example, in elderly patients, there is an increased bioavailability of β-blockers but a decreased responsiveness at the receptor-site level. Another example is that the inotropic effect of theophylline is increased with age, but the bronchodilator effect is decreased. The homeostatic reserves in geriatric patients are less efficient and result in unpredictable drug effects and an impaired ability to recover from drug-induced problems (Fig. 71.1).

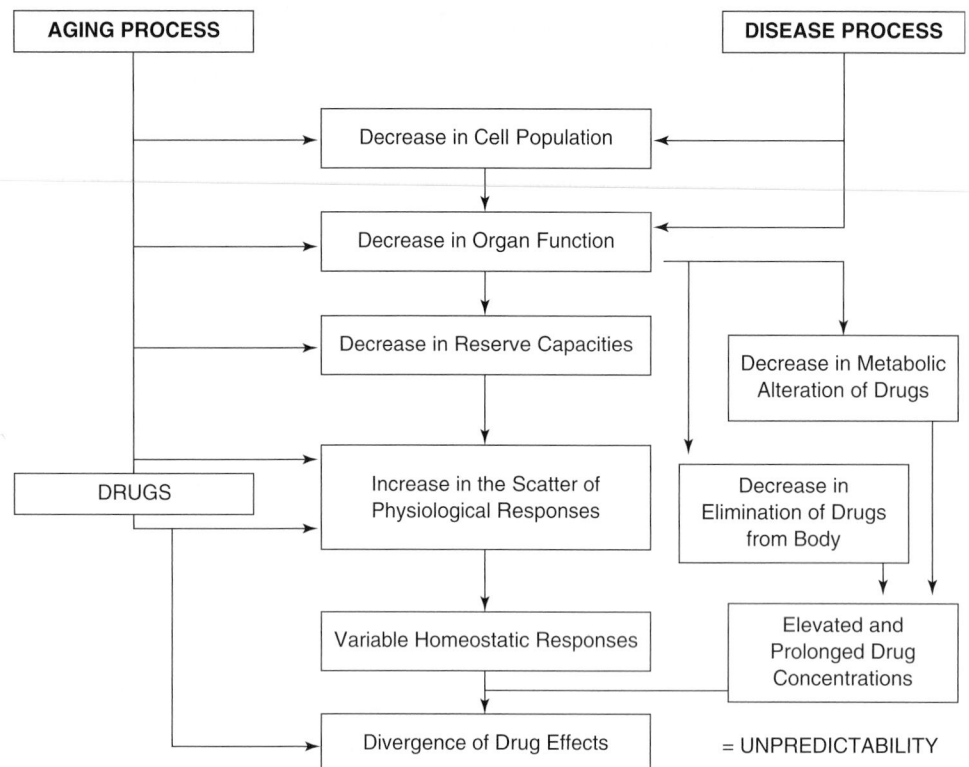

FIGURE 71.1 Unpredictability of drug effects in the aged.

Numerous drug therapies require special attention when prescribed to geriatric patients, and dosage titration should always be based on a balance between optimal clinical response and minimal adverse effects.

TREATMENT

DIABETES

The American Diabetes Association has established guidelines for the management of diabetes in geriatric patients.[54] Aging changes related to glucose metabolism include impaired pancreatic secretion of insulin, changes in the renal threshold for glucose, and impaired glucose tolerance. Goals of management for older patients include the following:

■ Patients with no associated problems or diabetes complications and with a reasonable life expectancy (10 years or more) should strive for the best possible glycemic control without causing hypoglycemia:
  ○ Fasting blood glucose (FBG) 100 to 120 mg per dL
  ○ Postprandial (pp) glucose 180 mg per dL or less
  ○ Hemoglobin (Hb) A1$_c$ within 1% of upper limits of normal (4.0% to 6.0%)[54]
■ Less aggressive management is acceptable in patients with advanced diabetes complications or impaired cognitive function, inability to comply with regimen, or neuropsychiatric disorders:
  ○ FBG less than 140 mg per dL
  ○ pp glucose less than 200 to 220 mg per dL

  ○ HbA1$_c$ less than 8%[54] (Patients who have an HbA1$_c$ >7% for any length of time have been shown to have an increase in complications associated with diabetes.)

Selection of treatment modalities for the elderly diabetic should take into consideration comorbid conditions, concomitant drug therapy, side effect profiles of the drug therapy, routes of drug elimination, and ease of monitoring. Blood glucose monitoring provides the best index of control for the elderly diabetic because urine glucose monitoring has been shown to be unreliable due to age-related increases in the renal threshold.

CARDIOVASCULAR DISEASE

Aging produces several hemodynamic changes that may influence the choice of cardiovascular agents, such as an increase in peripheral vascular resistance and decreases in renal blood flow, plasma volume, plasma renin, aldosterone, and cardiac output. With an increase in peripheral vascular resistance, elderly patients may exhibit an enhanced response to vasodilators, especially diuretics, calcium channel blockers, and angiotensin-converting enzyme (ACE) inhibitors.

Hypertension occurs in more than two thirds of individuals over 65 years of age. This is also the population with the lowest rates of blood pressure control. It has been shown that an elevated pulse pressure [systolic blood pressure

(SBP) minus diastolic blood pressure (DBP)], which indicates reduced vascular compliance in large arteries, may be a better marker of increased cardiovascular risk than either SBP or DBP alone.[55] In practice, pulse pressures greater than 50 mm Hg are indicative of elevated pulse pressures. This is particularly important to older patients, who often have an isolated elevation of SBP (140 mm Hg or greater, with a DBP below 90 mm Hg).

Although primary hypertension is the most common form of hypertension in older patients, other causes of hypertension such as atherosclerotic renovascular hypertension or primary aldosteronism, may occur more frequently in older persons, especially in those whose hypertension first presented after 60 years of age or is resistant to treatment.[56]

Large trials have shown that treatment of hypertension in older persons produces major benefits in the reduction of stroke, coronary heart disease, cardiovascular disease, heart failure, and mortality.[57–59] The Seventh Report of the Joint National Committee on Prevention, Detection, Evaluation, and Treatment of High Blood Pressure (JNC 7)[60] recommends the following regarding hypertension in older patients:

- The goal of treatment of hypertension in older patients should be the same as in younger patients (below 140/90 mm Hg, if possible), although an interim SBP goal of below 160 mm Hg may be necessary in patients with significant systolic hypertension.
- Initial therapy should address lifestyle modifications of modest salt reduction, weight loss, and exercise. Drug treatment should be initiated if lifestyle modifications are not successful in decreasing the blood pressure.
- Antihypertensive drug therapy should be implemented cautiously in older patients because they may be more sensitive to volume depletion and sympathetic inhibition than younger patients. Although all classes of antihypertensive medications have been shown to be effective in lowering blood pressure, thiazide diuretics or β-blockers in combination with thiazide diuretics are recommended because they have been shown to be effective in reducing mortality and morbidity as well.[61] Other initial therapy choices include the calcium channel blockers, ACE inhibitors, and α-blockers, and studies are underway to determine the effect of these classes of drugs on the mortality and morbidity of hypertension.

The JNC 7 also gives guidelines on drug therapy selection for hypertension in the presence of comorbid conditions and concomitant drug therapy. JNC 7 recommends that the same principles be followed for older patients as in younger patients. Initial dosages may be lower to avoid symptoms; however, most older patients achieve blood pressure control at standard doses and on multiple drug therapy.

With the age-related decline in renal function, the choice and dosage of a diuretic is important. Because older patients have a decreased plasma volume and lower levels of aldosterone, aggressive diuretic therapy to reduce blood pressure is generally not indicated. Therapy should be started with a small dose of hydrochlorothiazide (12.5 mg) or its equivalent, increasing to a maximum dose of 25 mg twice a day. With a creatinine clearance of less than 30 mL per minute, a loop diuretic such as furosemide, bumetanide, or metolazone is recommended, because thiazide agents will be ineffective. Diuretic combinations with a potassium-sparing agent can be useful, but hyperkalemia may develop from reduced potassium excretion, the concurrent use of potassium supplements, or concurrent use of ACE inhibitors.

Older patients often exhibit an impaired baroreceptor reflex response that makes them more susceptible to hypotension. Aggressive treatment of hypertension will often result in severe orthostasis, leading to falls and subsequent injuries. There is evidence of a drop in blood pressure of 20 mm Hg or greater in one fourth of healthy elderly patients undergoing positional changes. Drugs that interfere with the baroreceptor reflex, such as adrenergic-blocking agents, should be used cautiously because of the increased risk of falls and fractures.

Blood pressure should be measured in the standing as well as the sitting position, and antihypertensive treatments should be initiated with smaller dosages and in longer intervals than usual. Additional complications of aggressive antihypertensive therapy are cognitive dysfunction resulting from hypoperfusion to the brain and exaggerated side effects of the medications. In general, initial doses of antihypertensives for geriatric patients are reduced by one third to one half, with slow titration until the desired response is achieved.

According to the Heart Failure Society of America (HFSA) guidelines[62] and the American College of Cardiology/American Heart Association guidelines,[63] heart failure patients, after treatment of comorbid conditions such as hypertension, dyslipidemias, and contributing lifestyle habits, should be managed with ACE inhibitors, followed by the addition of β-receptor antagonists, diuretics, and lastly digoxin, depending on the type and degree of symptoms exhibited. In general, the geriatric population is at greater risk of adverse effects from the medications used to manage heart failure.[64] Older patients are more sensitive to the hypotensive effects of all vasodilators, the renal insufficiency and hyperkalemia resulting from ACE inhibitor use, digoxin toxicity resulting from reduced renal function and lean body weight, and cardiac conduction abnormalities resulting from digoxin and β-blocker use.

ANXIETY AND INSOMNIA

As many as half of the patients over 50 years of age report experiencing insomnia, and it has been shown that hypnotic drug use increases with increasing age. Due to age-related changes in the CNS, a general guideline for dosing anxiolytics and sedative–hypnotics is to start with one-third to one-half the usual recommended initial dose, or to extend the time interval between doses. Geriatric patients are more sensitive to the cortical depressant effects of the benzodiazepines and can appear to be cognitively impaired, depressed, or both as a result of chronic intoxication. In the older patient, benzodiazepines are effective in reducing sleep latency, but chronic or repeated use can lead to overmedication, additive side effects, or hypersomnolence. When used regularly in the elderly, they can cause significant toxicity, including dependence, hangover effect, dysphoria, and withdrawal symptoms on discontinuation. An increased risk of hip fracture has been correlated directly with the use of long-acting benzodiazepines; users of benzodiazepines with a short half-life had no significantly increased risk compared to controls.[65]

When selecting a benzodiazepine for use in geriatric patients, considerations should include the specific symptoms and needs of the patient (i.e., sleep latency, sleep maintenance, or early morning wakening anxiety) and the metabolic pathway of the drug. Shorter-acting agents such as oxazepam, lorazepam, temazepam, and triazolam may be preferable. Nonbenzodiazepine agents such as buspirone and zolpidem are useful therapeutic alternatives that lack the adverse effects of the benzodiazepines. Diphenhydramine is useful for occasional insomnia or anxiety in the geriatric patient, but the risk of anticholinergic delirium or worsening of the patient's cognitive state can occur if it is used too frequently, in excessive doses, or with other drugs that have anticholinergic properties. Recommended dosing information on anxiolytics and sedative–hypnotics is listed in Table 71.11.

PSYCHOSIS AND BEHAVIORAL PROBLEMS

In the geriatric population, antipsychotic agents are useful for the treatment of psychoses and severe behavioral manifestations associated with dementia. Behavioral symptoms occurring with dementia include anxiety, agitation, aggression, paranoia, hallucinations, and combativeness. When these symptoms occur, they are disturbing to both the patient and the caregiver. Guidelines that are a part of the Omnibus Budget Reconciliation Act (OBRA) require that before an antipsychotic agent is prescribed for the management of a dementia patient in a nursing facility, the clinical record must contain (in addition to the diagnosis of dementia) both quantitative and qualitative documentation of associated psychotic and/or agitated behaviors that present a danger to the patient or to others. Inappropriate use of antipsychotic agents in dementia patients includes use limited to the treatment of wandering, poor self-care, restlessness, impaired memory, anxiety, depression, insomnia, unsociability, indifference to surroundings, fidgeting, nervousness, uncooperativeness, or agitated behaviors that do not represent a danger to the resident or others. OBRA guidelines also require periodic (every 6 months) trial dosage reductions to determine the lowest effective dose for a particular patient.[66]

The phenothiazine antipsychotics (low-potency agents) have prominent sedative, cardiovascular, anticholinergic, and neurologic side effects that are often manifested in elderly patients, most likely as a result of a decreased ability of the hepatic enzymes to metabolize the drugs to inactive metabolites and/or to altered receptor sensitivity. Nonpheno-

TABLE 71.11	Recommended Maximum Doses of Anxiolytics, Sedatives, and Hypnotics

	Medication Usual Dose, Adults	
	<65 Years (mg/day) Usual Dose	Adults ≥65 (mg/day)
Benzodiazepine Anxiolytics		
Alprazolam	0.75–4	0.125–0.75
Chlordiazepoxide[a]	15–100	10–20
Chlorazepate[a]	15–60	7.5–15
Diazepam[a]	6–40	1–5
Halazepam[a]	60–100	20–40
Lorazepam	2–6	0.25–2
Oxazepam	30–120	10–30
Prazepam[a]	20–60	10–15
Benzodiazepine Sedative–Hypnotics		
Estazolam	1–2	0.5–1
Flurazepam[a]	15–30	15
Quazepam[a]	7.5–15	7.5
Temazepam	15–30	7.5–15
Triazolam	0.125–0.5	0.0625–0.125
Clonazepam[a]	1.5–20	0.5–1.5
Other Anxiolytics and Sedatives		
Buspirone	15–60	10–60
Chloral hydrate	250–1,000	250–500
Diphenhydramine[a]	25–200	25–50
Hydroxyzine[a]	25–600	10–50
Paroxetine	60	20
Venlafaxine XR	225–375	75–225
Zaleplon	20–40	5–10
Zolpidem	5–20	2.5–10

[a] Not recommended for use in geriatric patients.

thiazine antipsychotics (high-potency agents) are less sedating and cause less anticholinergic toxicity but can cause more adverse neurologic effects, such as tardive dyskinesia. The initial dose of either class of antipsychotic should be small and gradually increased according to the clinical response of the patient. Drugs may be given in divided doses or as a single daily dose, with small doses of "as-needed orders" for repeating the dose, to determine the lowest effective dose and to minimize size effects. Maximum daily doses should be approximately one-fourth those recommended in younger patients (Table 71.12).

The newer atypical antipsychotic agents such as clozapine, risperidone, olanzapine, and quetiapine are frequently prescribed to manage disruptive behaviors such as agitation, combativeness, or aggression in dementia patients. Smaller dosages (as compared to those useful for managing psy-

TABLE 71.12	Recommended Maximum Doses of Oral Antipsychotics and Other Medications for Behavioral Disturbances Associated With Dementia		
Medication	**Adult Age <65**	**Geriatric Age ≥65**	**Geriatric/Dementia Age ≥65**
Aripiprazole[a]	10–15		
Acetophenazine	300	150	20
Carbamazepine[b]			100–1,000
Chlorpromazine[c]	1,600	800	75
Chlorprothixene	1,600	800	75
Clozapine[c]	450	25	50
Divalproex sodium[b]			250–2,000
Fluphenazine	40	20	1–4
Haloperidol	100	50	0.25–4
Loxapine	250	125	5–10
Mesoridazine[c]	500	250	25
Molindone	225	112	5–10
Olanzapine	10–20	5–10	2.5–10
Perphenazine	64	32	2–8
Promazine	500	50	150
Quetiapine	750	400	50–200
Risperidone	16	4–8	0.5–2
Thioridazine[c]	800	400	75
Thiothixene	60	30	1–7
Trifluoperazine	80	40	2.5–8
Trifluopromazine	100	20	–
Valproic acid[b]	750–2,000	–	250–1,750

All doses are given as mg/day.
[a] Limited clinical experience in this population.
[b] Serum concentrations do not correlate with behavioral response.
[c] Not recommended for use in geriatric patients.

chosis) are usually prescribed to manage the associated behaviors of dementia patients, and clinical studies assessingspecific maximum and minimum doses are being conducted.Aripiprazole may also have a place in the management of the behavioral symptoms of dementia. Alternative therapies for problem behaviors associated with dementia include lithium and selected anticonvulsants such as carbamazepine and valproic acid.[67]

DEPRESSION

Clinical depression is common among geriatric patients and is often underdiagnosed and therefore undertreated in the nursing facility population (and the geriatric population in general).[68] The presentation of depression in an older patient can be atypical and dismissed as cognitive impairment, reaction to a chronic illness, or an understandable response to institutionalization. All antidepressants appear to be equally effective in the treatment of major depressive illness.[69,70] The choice of an antidepressant agent should be based on

factors such as adverse effects, prior response, concurrent nonpsychiatric medical illness, and concomitant medical illness. Dosing should be titrated upward and patients assessed at 6 weeks for response to therapy. For a full therapeutic response, patients should be treated for 4 to 9 months and then considered for maintenance therapy, which may be lifelong. Recommended dosing information on antidepressants is listed in Table 71.13.

MILD TO MODERATE PAIN

Many older patients suffer from some degree of chronic, nonmalignant pain from several sources, including rheumatoid arthritis, osteoarthritis, and irritable bowel syndrome. Agents recommended for mild to moderate pain include maximal dosages of acetaminophen, nonacetylated salicylates, and analgesic doses of COX-2 selective NSAIDs such as celecoxib or rofecoxib. (Rofecoxib was recently voluntarily recalled from the market as a result of concerns over an increased risk of cardiovascular events, including heart at-

TABLE 71.13	Recommended Dosage Ranges of Antidepressants	
Medication	**Adult Age <65**	**Geriatric Age ≥65**
Amitriptyline[c]	75–300	25–150
Amoxapine[c]	150–600	25–300
Bupropion	225–450	50–100
Citalopram	20–40	10–20
Desipramine	75–300	10–100
Doxepin	75–300	10–75
Escitalopram	10–20	5–10
Fluoxetine	20–80	10–40
Fluvoxamine	50–300	[a]
Imipramine	75–300	10–150
Maprotiline	75–300	25–75
Mirtazapine	15–45	15–45
Nefazodone	300–600	200–400
Nortriptyline	75–300	10–75
Paroxetine[b]	20–50	10–30
Protriptyline	15–60	15–20
Sertraline[b]	75–200	25–200
Trazodone	150–600	25–150
Trimipramine	75–300	25–100
Venlafaxine	75–375	[a]

All dosages are given as mg/day.
[a] Limited clinical experience in this population.
[b] Preferred agents in geriatric patients.
[c] Not recommended for use in geriatric patients.

tack and stroke in patients taking rofecoxib. At the time of this writing, celecoxib remains on the market.) If analgesic doses of COX-2 agents are not effective in relieving pain, higher doses may be used or the patient may be switched to a nonselective NSAID. When using nonselective NSAIDs, gastrointestinal protective agents may be necessary.[71,72]

Geriatric patients are significantly more sensitive to the pain-relieving effect of narcotics because of changes in receptor number and function, alterations in protein binding, and prolonged clearance of these agents. These changes allow narcotics to be more effective in smaller doses in geriatric patients compared to younger patients. The elderly, as a group, are more likely to develop narcotic side effects of constipation, respiratory depression, cough suppression, and cognitive impairment when compared to younger patients.[73]

No evidence yet shows the superiority of one narcotic over another on the basis of age alone. Meperidine is not recommended for chronic analgesic therapy due to toxicities associated with its metabolite, normeperidine. Meperidine is found on the Beers list and in the CMS (aka HCFA) Guide

to Surveyors and is considered a problematic analgesic choice for the geriatric patient.[32]

The dosing of narcotic analgesics in the older patient should be done cautiously by increasing the dose until the patient obtains pain relief for at least 4 hours. The dose should be administered prior to the pain occurring to avoid anticipatory anxiety and behavioral reinforcement of drug use, especially in terminally ill patients with chronic pain. Adjuvant analgesic relief may be provided by the use of tricyclic antidepressants, valproic acid, carbamazepine, or NSAIDs.

PREVENTIVE CARE

Mortality and morbidity from pneumococcal pneumonia, influenza, and tetanus infections is very high in the geriatric population. Older patients show a response to antibody formation from the polyvalent pneumococcal vaccine that is comparable to that in the younger population.[74] All persons 65 years of age and older should receive the pneumococcal vaccine, including previously unvaccinated persons and persons who have not received vaccine within 5 years (and were less than 65 years of age at the time of vaccination). All persons who have unknown vaccination status should receive one dose of pneumococcal vaccine.[75] A favorable antibody response is likewise elicited from an annual influenza vaccine administered to a geriatric patient, with an efficacy rate of 70% to 80% against the influenza strains of the season. It usually takes 4 to 8 weeks to elicit a full antibody response, so vaccinations must be given in advance of the anticipated flu season.

Although cases of tetanus have decreased dramatically as a result of mandatory pediatric vaccination programs, elderly individuals are a major at-risk population for this disease due to declining titers with increasing age. Adults who have completed a primary series of tetanus immunization should receive booster doses every 10 years. The majority of elderly patients, particularly those with chronic diseases, should be immunized with a documented dose of polyvalent pneumococcal vaccine, an annual influenza vaccine, and a tetanus booster every 10 years.

CONCLUSION

Because of the many possibilities for age-related changes and medication actions and adverse effects, designing therapeutic regimens for geriatric patients can be complicated. When providing care for geriatric patients, it is necessary to continually reevaluate the need for existing or new medications. Proper medication use by geriatric patients should include optimization of drug therapy to meet the patient's medical needs while avoiding ADRs; patient education to maximize adherence to drug therapy regimens; and regular review of the patient's drug therapy to screen for the following:

1. Is each medication necessary?
2. Are nonpharmacologic alternatives available?
3. Is the lowest effective dose being used?
4. Are there any unaddressed medical or drug-related problems?

Above all, communication among the pharmacist, the physician, the nurse, the patient, and the patient's caregiver is of utmost importance in meeting the goals of therapy.

KEY POINTS

- Elderly patients account for 30% of all medications prescribed in the United States, but they also consume substantial quantities of over-the-counter medications
- Polypharmacy, or the use of multiple prescription and over-the-counter medications, especially by older people with chronic health problems, has been identified as the principal drug safety issue of the future
- Older patients are at higher risk for ADRs compared to younger patients and often have an atypical presentation of the ADR that may be confused with aging or disease progression
- More than one in six elderly Americans are taking prescription drugs that are not suited for geriatric patients and that may lead to physical or mental deterioration and possibly death
- In both prescribing and monitoring medication therapy in geriatric patients, it is extremely important to consider the individual patient's clinical and health status and concomitant medications
- By predicting which drugs can be affected by age-related physiologic and pharmacokinetic changes, the correct dose and dosing interval can be more accurately estimated
- Changes in gastric motility and blood flow can affect the extent of absorption and the rate of absorption, but the completeness of absorption of medications in geriatric patients is similar to that in younger patients; however, a delay in the onset of activity may occur
- The importance of increased free fraction of a medication (due to a decrease in binding to albumin) is questionable because although additional free drug is available for receptor binding, more free drug is also available for metabolism and elimination
- Age-related physiologic changes in the kidney influence drug elimination and response in the geriatric patient to a greater extent than age-related physiologic changes that occur in the liver
- To avoid drug toxicity, the dosages of renally excreted drugs (or active metabolites) must be adjusted if the creatinine clearance is less than 30 mL per minute
- With increasing age, there is an increased intolerance to medications as a result of altered pharmacodynamic response at the target organs
- Due to the many possibilities for age-related change and medication actions and adverse effects, designing therapeutic regimens for geriatric patients can be complicated
- Regular review of the drug regimen of a geriatric patient should include asking the following questions:
  - Is each medication necessary?
  - Are nonpharmacologic alternatives available?
  - Is the lowest effective dose being used?
  - Are there any unaddressed medical or drug-related problems?

REFERENCES

1. U.S. Department of Health and Human Services, Administration on Aging. A profile of older Americans, 2002. Available at www.aoa.gov. Accessed May 8, 2004.
2. Abrams WB, Berkow R. The Merck manual of geriatrics. MSD Research Laboratories, Rahway, NJ, 1995:1115–1123.
3. Steiner JF. Pharmacotherapy problems in the elderly. J Am Pharm Assoc NS36:431–467;1996
4. Hall MJ, Owings MF. 2000 National Hospital Discharge Survey. Advance data from vital and health statistics No. 329, June 19, 2002. Available at www.cdc.gov/nchs. Accessed May 8, 2004.
5. Senior Care Pharmacy Facts. Available at www.ascp.com. Accessed May 8, 2004.
6. Stewart RB, Moore MT, May FE, et al. Changing patterns of therapeutic agents in the elderly: a ten-year overview. Age Aging 20:182–188, 1991.
7. Miller DR. Drug surveillance utilizing epidemiologic methods. Am J Hosp Pharm 30:584–592, 1973.
8. Tobias DE, Pulliam CC. General and psychotherapeutic medication use in 372 nursing facilities: a national survey. Consult Pharm 9:449–461, 1994.
9. Tobias DE, Pulliam CC. General and psychotherapeutic medication use in 878 nursing facilities: a 1997 national survey. Consult Pharm 12:1401–1408, 1997.
10. Tobias DE, Sey M. General and psychotherapeutic medication use in 878 nursing facilities: a year 2000 national survey. Consult Pharm 16:50–58, 2001.
11. Kidder SW. Cost-benefit of pharmacist-conducted drug-regimen reviews. Consult Pharm 2:394–398, 1987.
12. Kohn L, Corrigan J, Donaldson M, eds. To err is human: building a safer health system. Washington DC: National Academy Press, 1999. Available at http://books.nap.edu/htm/to__err__is__human/. Accessed May 9, 2004.
13. Perry DP. When medicine hurts instead of helps. Consult Pharm 14:1326–1330, 1999.
14. Johnson JA, Bootman JL. Drug-related morbidity and mortality: a cost-of-illness model. Arch Intern Med 155:1949–1956, 1995.
15. Bates DW, Spell N, Cullen DJ, et al. for the Adverse Drug Events Prevention Study Group. The costs of adverse drug events in hospitalized patients. JAMA 277:307–311, 1997.
16. Bootman JL, Harrison DL, Cox E. The health care cost of drug-related morbidity and mortality in nursing facilities. Arch Intern Med 157:2089–2096, 1997.
17. Healthy People 2000: national health promotion and disease prevention objectives. Washington DC: U.S. Department of Health and Human Services, 1990.
18. Tresch DD, Duthie EH, Newton M. Coping with diagnosis-related groups. Arch Intern Med 148:1393–1396, 1988.
19. Simonson W. Consultant pharmacy practice, 2d ed. Alexandria, VA: American Society of Consultant Pharmacists, 1991:13–26.
20. Health Care Financing Administration. State operations manual – provider certification transmittal #250, P139–P150, 1992.
21. Green LW, Mullen PD, Stainbrook GL. Programs to reduce drug errors in the elderly: direct and indirect evidence from patient education. J Geriatric Drug Ther 1:3–18, 1986.

22. Gurwitz JH, Avorn J. The ambiguous relation between aging and adverse drug reactions. Ann Intern Med 114:956–966, 1991.

23. Colley CA, Lucas LM. Polypharmacy: the cure becomes the disease. J Gen Intern Med 8:278–283, 1993.

24. Gurwitz JH, Soumerai SB, Avorn J. Improving medication prescribing and utilization in the nursing home. J Am Geriatric Soc 38:542–552, 1990.

25. Avorn J, Gurwitz JH. Drug use in the nursing home. Ann Intern Med 123:195–204, 1995.

26. Wilcox SM, Himmelstein DU, Woolhandler S. Inappropriate drug prescribing for the community-dwelling elderly. JAMA 272:292–296, 1994.

27. Fouts M, Hanlon J, Pieper C, et al. Identification of elderly nursing facility residents at high risk for drug-related problems. Consult Pharm 12:1103–1111, 1997.

28. Drugs that cause psychiatric symptoms. Med Lett Drugs Ther 40:21–24, 1998.

29. Hanlon JT, Schmader K, Ruby C, et al. Suboptimal prescribing in older inpatients and outpatients. J Am Geriatric Soc 49:200–209, 2001.

30. Beers MH, Ouslander JG, Fingold SF, et al. Inappropriate medication prescribing in skilled-nursing facilities. Ann Intern Med 117:684–689, 1992.

31. Beers MH. Explicit criteria for determining potentially inappropriate medication use by the elderly, an update. Arch Intern Med 157:1531–1536, 1997.

32. Fick DM, Cooper JW, Wade WE, et al. Updating the Beers criteria for potentially inappropriate medication use in older adults. Arch Intern Med 163:2716–2724, 2003.

33. Hanlon JT, Schmader KE, Samsa GP, et al. A method for assessing drug therapy appropriateness. J Clin Epidemiol 45:1045–1051, 1992.

34. Morrow D, Leirer V, Sheikh J. Adherence and medication instructions: review and recommendations. J Am Geriatric Soc 36:1147–1160, 1988.

35. Cooper JK, Love DW, Raffoul PR. Intentional prescription nonadherence (noncompliance) by the elderly. J Am Geriatric Soc 30:329–333, 1982.

36. Greenblatt DG, Sellers EM, Shader RI. Drug disposition in old age. N Engl J Med 306:1081–1088, 1982.

37. Miller SW, Strom JG. Drug-product selection: implications for the geriatric patient. Consult Pharm 5:30–37, 1990.

38. Riley TN, Ravis WS. Key concepts in drug bioequivalence. US Pharm 12:40–53, 1987.

39. Hayes MJ, Langman MJS, Short AH. Changes in drug metabolism with increasing age. Br J Clin Pharmacol 2:73–79, 1975.

40. Greenblatt DJ, Sellers EM, Koch-Weser J. Importance of protein binding for the interpretation of serum or plasma drug concentrations. J Clin Pharmacol 22:259–263, 1982.

41. Mather LE, Tucker GT, Pflug AE, et al. Meperidine kinetics in man. Clin Pharmacol Ther 17:21–30, 1975.

42. Lalonde RL, Tenero DM, Burlew BS, et al. Effects of age on protein binding and disposition of propranolol stereoisomer. Clin Pharmacol Ther 47:447–455,1990.

43. Davis D, Grossman SH, Kitchell BB, et al. Age-related changes in the plasma protein binding of lidocaine and diazepam. Clin Res 28:234A, 1980.

44. Devine B. Gentamicin therapy. Drug Intel Clin Pharm 8:650–655, 1974.

45. Michalets EL. Update; clinically significant cytochrome P-450 drug interactions. Pharmacotherapy 18:84–112, 1998.

46. Vestal RE, Norris AH, Tobin J, et al. Antipyrine metabolism in man: influence of age, alcohol, caffeine, and smoking. Clin Pharmacol Ther 18:425–432, 1975.

47. Greenblatt DJ, Divoll M, Harmatz JS, et al. Oxazepam kinetics: influence and effects of age and sex. J Pharmacol Exp Ther 215:86–91, 1980.

48. Cockroft DW, Gault MH. Prediction of creatinine clearance from serum creatinine. Nephron 16:31–41, 1976.

49. Malmrose LC, Gray SL, Peiper CF, et al. Measured versus estimated creatinine clearance in a high-functioning elderly sample: MacArthur Foundation study of successful aging. J Am Geriatric Soc 41:715–721, 1993.

50. Smythe M, Hoffman J, Kizy K, et al. Estimating creatinine clearance in elderly patient with low serum creatinine concentrations. Am J Hosp Pharm 51:198–204, 1994.

51. Feely J, Cloakley D. Altered pharmacodynamics in the elderly. Clin Geriatric Med 6:269–283, 1990.

52. Gurwitz JH, Avorn J, Ross-Degnan D, et al. Aging and the anticoagulant response to warfarin therapy. Ann Intern Med 116:901–904, 1992.

53. Jick H, Slone D, Borda IT, et al. Efficacy and toxicity of heparin in relation to age and sex. N Engl J Med 279:284–286, 1968.

54. Standards of medical care for patients with diabetes mellitus. Diabetes Care, American Diabetes Association. 26:3160–3167, 2003.

55. Madhaven S, Ooi WL, Cohen H, et al. Relation of pulse pressure and blood pressure reduction to the incidence of myocardial infarction. Hypertension 23:395–401, 1994.

56. Setaro JF, Black HR. Refractory hypertension N Engl J Med 69:997–999, 1994.

57. Staessen JA, Fagard R, Thijs L, et al. for the systolic hypertension (Syst-Eur) trial investigators. Morbidity and mortality in the placebo-controlled European trial on isolated systolic hypertension in the elderly. Lancet 350:757–764, 1997.

58. SHEP Cooperative Research Group. Prevention of stroke by antihypertensive drug treatment in older persons with isolated systolic hypertension: final results of the Systolic Hypertension in the Elderly Program (SHEP). JAMA 265:3255–3264, 1991.

59. National High Blood Pressure Education Program Working Group. Report on hypertension in the elderly. Hypertension 23:275–285, 1994.

60. The Seventh Report of the Joint National Committee on Prevention, Detection, Evaluation, and Treatment of High Blood Pressure (JNC VII). U.S. Department of Health and Human Services. NIH Pub No. 03–5233, May 2003. Available at www.nhlbi.nih.gov/guidelines. Accessed May 9, 2004.

61. MacMahon S, Rodgers A. The effects of blood pressure reduction in older patients: an overview of five randomized controlled trials in elderly hypertensives. Clin Exp Hypertens 15:967–978, 1993.

62. Heart Failure Society of America (HFSA) Practice Guidelines. HFSA guidelines for management of patients with heart failure caused by left ventricular systolic dysfunction: pharmacologic approaches. J Cardiac Failure 5:357–382, 1999. Available at www.hfsa.org. Accessed May 8, 2004.

63. Hunt SA, Chin MJ. ACC/AHA guidelines for the evaluation and management of chronic heart failure in the adult. J Heart Lung Transplant 21:189–203, 2002.

64. Cody RJ. Physiological changes due to age. Implications for drug therapy of congestive heart failure. Drugs Aging 3:320–334, 1993.

65. Ray WA, Griffin MR, Downey W. Benzodiazepines of long and short elimination half-life and the risk of hip fracture. JAMA 262:3303–3307, 1989.

66. Federal Register 56(187):483, 1991.

67. Yeager BR, Farnett LE, Ruzicka SA. Management of the behavioral manifestations of dementia. Arch Intern Med 155:250–260, 1995.

68. Rovner BW, German PS, Brant IJ, et al. Depression and mortality in nursing home elderly. JAMA 265:993–996, 1991.

69. Solai LK, Mulsant BH, Pollock BG. Selective serotonin reuptake inhibitors for late-life depression: a comparative review. Drugs Aging 18:355–368, 2001.

70. Williams JW, Jr., Mulrow CD, Chiquette E, et al. A systematic review of newer pharmacotherapies for depression in adults: evidence report summary. Ann Intern Med 132:741–756, 2000.

71. AGS Panel on Persistent Pain in Older Persons. The management of persistent pain in older persons. J Am Geriatric Soc 50:205–224S, 2002.

72. American College of Rheumatology Subcommittee on Osteoarthritis Guidelines. Recommendations for the medical management of osteoarthritis of the hip and knee: 2000 update. Arthritis Rheum 43:1905–1915, 2000.

73. Kaiko RF, Wallenstein SL, Rogers AG, et al. Narcotics in the elderly. Med Clin North Am 66:1079–1089, 1982.

74. Amman AJ, Schiffman G, Ausrian R. The antibody response to pneumococcal capsular polysaccharides in the aged individuals. Proc Soc Exp Biol Med 164:321, 1980.

75. Centers for Disease Control and Prevention. Prevention of pneumococcal disease: recommendations of the Advisory Committee on Immunization Practices (ACIP). MMWR 46(No. RR-8):1–10, 1997.

CASE STUDIES

TOPIC: Geriatric Drug Therapy/ Polypharmacy

THERAPEUTIC DIFFICULTY: Level 1
Susan W. Miller

Chapter 71: Geriatric Drug Therapy

■ Scenario

Patient and Setting: SM, an 86-year-old widowed female living with her daughter in the daughter's home presents to her primary physician for evaluation

Chief Complaint: New-onset confusion and lethargy; loss of appetite, and recent 3-lb weight loss

History of Present Illness: Daughter noticed memory loss and confusion in her mother over the previous 2-week period. The daughter also reports that her mother is unusually tired most of the time. During this time, the patient has not been eating her meals as usual and a weight loss is noted. Patient developed symptoms of a cold 2 weeks ago and has been taking Nyquil nightly for 14 days and acetaminophen as needed for the cold symptoms

Medical History: Hypertension (HTN) for 40 years; heart failure (HF) for 25 years; osteoarthritis (OA) for 25 years; insomnia for 20 years; anxiety; seborrhea; seasonal allergies; chronic constipation

Surgical History: Noncontributory

Family/Social History: Family History: Mother and father died of "old age"
Social History: No history of smoking or alcohol intake; childbirth × 3; widowed × 10 years

Medications:
Digoxin, 0.125 mg PO QD
HCTZ, 50 mg PO QD
KCl 10%, 20 mEq PO QD
Lisinopril, 10 mg PO QD
ASA, 81 mg PO QD
Diazepam, 2 mg PO BID
Nabumetone, 500 mg PO BID
Ferrous sulfate, 325 mg PO TID
Multivitamin with minerals, 1 tablet PO QD
Psyllium, 15 mL in fluids PO BID
Sertraline, 50 mg PO QD

Diphenhydramine, 50 mg PO PRN for allergy symptoms
Lorazepam, 0.5 mg PO Q 6 hours PRN nervousness
Trazodone, 100 mg PO Q HS for sleep
T-Gel Shampoo, 2 × weekly
Acetaminophen, 650 mg QID

Allergies: Penicillin (skin rash); codeine (stomach upset)

■ Physical Examination

GEN: Thin, pale female
VS: BP 110/70, HR 80, T 37°C, Wt 93.5 lb (42.5 kg), Ht 155 cm
HEENT: Cerumen in ear
COR: + S_3
CHEST: WNL, chest clear
ABD: Hypoactive bowel sounds
BACK: Kyphotic
GU: Deferred
RECT: Occult blood-positive
EXT: Skin tear on right forearm; 1+ pitting ankle edema
NEURO: Lethargic; O × 2
SKIN: Thin skin; poor skin turgor; seborrheic lesions present

■ Results of Pertinent Laboratory Tests, Serum Drug Concentrations, and Diagnostic Tests

Na 148 (148)	Hgb 118 (11.8)	Lkcs 10.8 × 10⁹ (10.8 × 10³)
K 4.8 (4.8)	Hct 0.36 (36)	Lkcs differential: WNL
Cl 115 (115)	Ca 2.4 (9.6)	Plts 240 × 10⁹ (240 × 10³)
HCO₃ 28 (28)	Mg 1.0 (2.0)	Glu (fasting) 7.8 (140)
BUN 10.5 (30)	CR 120 (1.4)	

Digoxin 3 months prior: 2.3 nmol/L (1.8 ng/dL)

■ Problem List

Identify principal problems from the scenario in priority order (see Answers in back of book for correct list of problems).

■ SOAP Note

To be completed by the student (see Answers in back of book for correct SOAP Note).

■ QUESTIONS

(See Answers in back of book for correct responses.)

1. All of the following factors present in SM that make her at risk for drug related problems except: (EO-1)
   a. Age greater than 85 years
   b. Living in the community
   c. Consuming more than six medications
   d. More than six medical diagnoses

2. All of the following can contribute to anorexia and weight loss in SM except: (EO-10)
   a. Digoxin
   b. Sertraline
   c. Nabumetone
   d. Acetaminophen

3. SM presents with all of the following signs and symptoms of anticholinergic toxicity except: (EO-2)
   a. Confusion
   b. Memory loss
   c. Anorexia
   d. Constipation

4. List nonpharmacologic and pharmacologic therapeutic options for treatment of seborrhea. (EO-11)

5. Which of the following is least likely to contribute to constipation in geriatric patients? (EO-1)
   a. Medications with anticholinergic activity
   b. Dehydration
   c. Low-fiber diet
   d. Regular exercise

6. All of the following are acceptable choices for management of SM's insomnia except: (EO-12)
   a. Trazodone 25 mg PO Q HS
   b. Zolpidem 5 mg PO Q HS
   c. Flurazepam 30 mg PO Q HS
   d. Zaleplon 5 mg PO Q H

7. Which of the following is an important consideration in determining the maintenance dose of digoxin? (EO-5, 6)
   a. Renal function
   b. Hepatic function
   c. Mental status
   d. Serum albumin level

8. Abnormalities (increased or decreased) in serum potassium will be evidenced by all of the following except: (EO-2, 5)
   a. Muscle cramps
   b. Cardiac arrhythmias
   c. Lethargy
   d. Bradycardia

9. Should medications be prescribed for SM's memory loss? Why? (EO-12)

10. Calculate the creatinine clearance for SM using the Cockroft-Gault formula. (EO-5, 6)

11. What are some therapies other than NSAIDs or COX-2 inhibitors that may be useful for the symptoms associated with osteoarthritis? (EO-12)

12. SM should be monitored for signs and symptoms of depression. List these signs and symptoms of depression that could manifest in a geriatric patient not receiving antidepressant therapy. (EO-1)

13. What psychosocial factors may affect SM's adherence to the nonpharmacologic and pharmacologic therapies? (EO-15)

14. Which of the following changes in body composition commonly found in geriatric patients can affect the pharmacokinetics of medications? (EO-4)
    a. Increased muscle mass
    b. Increased total body fat
    c. Increased total body water
    d. Increased albumin

15. Which of the following conditions present in the geriatric patient has the greatest effect on hepatic metabolism of medications? (EO-4, 5)
    a. Reduced hepatic blood flow
    b. Increased efficiency of phase I metabolism
    c. Increased efficiency of phase II metabolism
    d. Reduced glomerular filtration rate (GFR)

16. Geriatric patients exhibit an altered pharmacodynamic response to all of the following medications or classes of medications except? (EO-4, 8)
    a. Beta-blocking agents
    b. Benzodiazepines
    c. Narcotic analgesics
    d. Cephalosporins

17. Summarize therapeutic, pathophysiologic, and disease management concepts for gastric carcinoma utilizing a key points format. (EO-18)

Infectious Diseases: Introduction   **72**

Erika J. Ernst

Selecting and monitoring antimicrobial therapy require an understanding of the interrelations among the patient, microbiology laboratory, and pharmacologic factors (Fig. 72.1). Some patient factors, such as immune status, affect both potential pathogens (bug) and the antimicrobial agents selected to treat them (drug). The selection process for an appropriate antimicrobial regimen involves several steps (Table 72.1). First, the need for antimicrobial therapy must be established. Unfortunately, this important first step is not always accomplished, leading to inappropriate use of antimicrobials. It has been estimated that 50% to 75% of physician office visits for colds, bronchitis, and upper respiratory tract infections result in prescriptions for antibiotics. These prescriptions largely represent inappropriate use of antibiotics, because over 90% of these infections are caused by viruses, and antibiotics have little clinical impact on their resolution.[1]

ESTABLISHING INFECTION

Establishing the presence of a bacterial infection is not easy and requires piecing together clinical and laboratory clues of infection. Clinically, an infection is suspected when a patient displays the hallmark signs of inflammation, fever, pain, swelling, and redness. A fever, described as an increase in the body's temperature, which normally fluctuates between 36.2° and 37.2°C (97.5° to 98.9°F), is generally defined as an elevated body temperature of 37.7°C (99.9°F) or above.[2] This symptom can be misleading, however, because not all febrile responses are infectious in origin. For example, many collagen vascular disease manifestations also may include fever. There are many other clinical signs of infection, some of which may be more specific for a particular pathogen or site of infection. For example, a ''stiff neck'' is an important sign of meningitis. The disease-specific signs and symptoms of infection are discussed elsewhere in this volume.

The hallmark sign of infection on laboratory analysis is an increased white blood cell count. The body upregulates the release of white blood cells into the circulation in response to invasion of microbial pathogens, resulting in a higher-than-usual percentage of immature neutrophils called bands. This laboratory finding is sometimes referred to as a shift to the left. Other laboratory signs of infection include an increased erythrocyte sedimentation rate (ESR) and increased liver transaminase enzyme tests (LFTs). The elevated ESR and LFTs are nonspecific results and also may be the result of noninfectious medical problems. When the collection of clinical and laboratory signs and symptoms in a particular patient suggests infection, the next step in the antimicrobial selection process is to attempt to establish the causative pathogen.

IDENTIFYING THE PATHOGEN

In the case of suspected infection, culture specimens are obtained from the suspected site in an attempt to identify the pathogen(s) responsible. The type of specimen differs depending on the site of infection and patient characteristics. For example, one obtains sputum when pneumonia or a lung infection is suspected, a urine culture for cystitis (bladder) or pyelonephritis (kidney infection), and cerebrospinal fluid (CSF) for meningitis. The Gram stain is a useful test for rapid characterization of an organism by cell wall structure and cell morphology. It is performed on sputum, urine, CSF, and wound specimens; however, it is not performed on blood samples because of the large sample volume (approximately 20 mL) that is usually necessary for successful growth of organisms from the blood.[3] The Gram stain results are reported by the staining characteristics of the organism (gram-positive or gram-negative) and the cell morphology [cocci or bacilli (rods)]. Additional characterization using bacterial oxygen tolerance (i.e., aerobic versus anaerobic) also is useful (Table 72.2). Not all bacterial organisms can be seen or are distinguishable using Gram staining, particularly organisms that grow intracellularly or do not have peptidoglycan-containing cell walls (Table 72.3). Determining an organism's Gram staining characteristics narrows the list of potential pathogens and may assist in directing initial empiric therapy. For example, if a patient suspected of having pneumonia has gram-negative rods in his or her sputum,

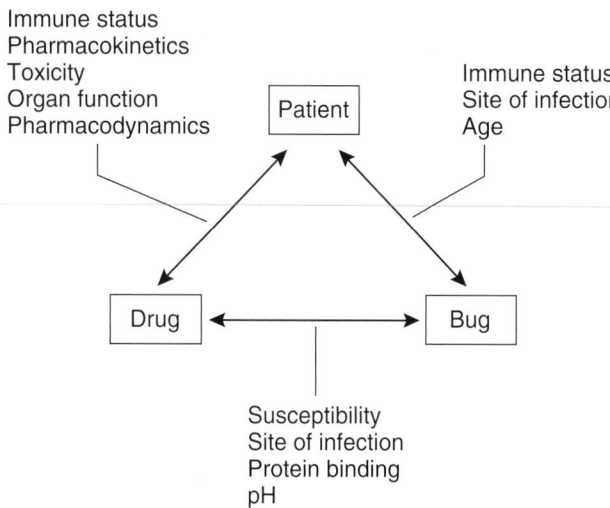

FIGURE 72.1 Interrelations of patient, microbiologic, and pharmacologic factors.

then doxycycline, which is sometimes used for treating pneumonia, is an inappropriate selection in this situation because it is not active against most gram-negative rods. In addition to Gram staining, other tests that are commonly used for rapid identification of organisms include the acid-fast bacilli (AFB) stain for mycobacteria, India ink for *Cryptococcus* sp, and potassium hydroxide (KOH) for other fungal pathogens. Antibody staining and detection methods are sometimes used, as well as DNA probes using polymerase chain reaction (PCR) amplification techniques, which are being widely developed.

Culture and sensitivity testing are the next steps after staining techniques. They are limited by the time required to complete the testing process, which varies depending on the organism but usually requires at least 48 hours. Four general types of susceptibility testing methods are used clinically: disk diffusion testing, broth microdilution testing, Etest methods, and automated systems. Other susceptibility testing methods exist, namely agar dilution and macrodilution; however, they are used mainly for drug development because they are more labor-intensive.

TABLE 72.1	Antimicrobial Drug Therapy Selection Process
Step 1	Establish the need for antimicrobial therapy.
Step 2	Attempt to identify the pathogen.
Step 3	Select empiric antimicrobial therapy.
Step 4	Monitor therapy for efficacy and toxicity.
Step 5	Refine antimicrobial therapy for definitive identification of pathogen or infection.

TABLE 72.2	Categorization of Organisms by Gram Staining Characteristics and Oxygen Tolerance
Gram-Positive Cocci	**Gram-Negative Cocci**
Aerobic	**Aerobic**
Staphylococcus aureus	Neisseria gonorrhoeae
Staphylococcus epidermidis	Neisseria meningitidis
Streptococcus pyogenes	Moraxella catarrhalis
Streptococcus pneumoniae	
Viridans streptococci	
Enterococcus faecalis	
Enterococcus faecium	
Anaerobic	
Peptostreptococcus sp	
Peptococcus sp	
Gram-Positive Bacilli	**Gram-Negative Bacilli**
Aerobic	**Aerobic**
Listeria monocytogenes	Escherichia coli
Bacillus anthracis	Klebsiella pneumoniae
Corynebacterium diphtheriae	Proteus mirabilis
Corynebacterium jeikeium (group JK)	Serratia marcescens
Rhodococcus sp	Pseudomonas aeruginosa
	Enterobacter sp
	Haemophilus influenzae
	Legionella pneumophila
Anaerobic	**Anaerobic**
Clostridium difficile	Bacteroides fragilis
Clostridium perfringens	Fusobacterium sp
Clostridium tetani	
Propionibacterium acnes	
Actinomyces sp	

The disk diffusion test is performed by placing disks, each impregnated with different antibiotics, on an agar plate that has been "streaked" or inoculated to completely cover the surface with organism. This test also is referred to as the Kirby-Bauer test after the authors who first described this method.[4] After a period of incubation, during which the antibiotic has diffused into the agar, the plates are inspected for growth in the circumference zone surrounding the disk. Zones of inhibition and results are reported as sensitive or resistant, depending on the size of the zone of inhibition (Fig. 72.2; *see color insert*).

Broth microdilution testing involves a microtiter tray with each row containing serial twofold dilutions of a particular

TABLE 72.3	Microorganisms Not Seen on Gram Stain

Bacterial Organisms

Chlamydia sp, including *C. pneumoniae*

Mycoplasma sp, including *M. pneumoniae*

Legionella pneumoniae

Listeria monocytogenes

Mycobacteria, such as *M. tuberculosis* and *M. avium intracellulare*

Rickettsiae, including *R. rickettsii* and *Coxiella burnetii*

Spirochetes, such as *Treponema pallidum*

Viral Organisms

Influenza A and B

Hepatitis viruses

Cytomegalovirus

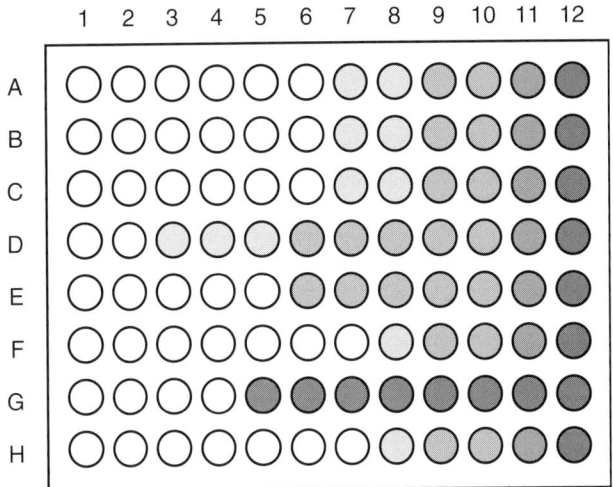

FIGURE 72.3 Schematic of microtiter tray for MIC testing. Individual antibiotics are tested in each row (A–H) at doubling concentrations in each well from high (column 1) to low (column 11), with a column containing no antibiotic (column 12) serving as a growth control. The MIC for each antibiotic is the concentration in the first well containing no visual growth. For example, the MIC for the drug in row D is the concentration in well 2, whereas the MIC for drugs F and H is the concentration in well 7, which may be different for each drug depending on the concentrations tested.

antibiotic. The organism under study is added to each well in the tray and allowed to incubate before it is inspected for growth. The minimum inhibitory concentration (MIC) is defined as the well containing the lowest concentration of antibiotic that inhibited growth of the organism as determined by visual inspection of the wells (Fig. 72.3).

The Etest (AB Biodisk Solna, Sweden) is a method that combines the disk diffusion and microdilution methods. A strip is impregnated with an antibiotic but contains a concentration gradient as opposed to a single concentration. This strip is placed on an agar plate containing a "lawn" of organism. The MIC is the point on the test strip at which the zone of inhibition intersects the test strip (Fig. 72.4).[5]

Automated systems for susceptibility testing, also referred to as "rapid" methods, may provide test results in as little as 8 hours, compared to 24 to 48 hours with more

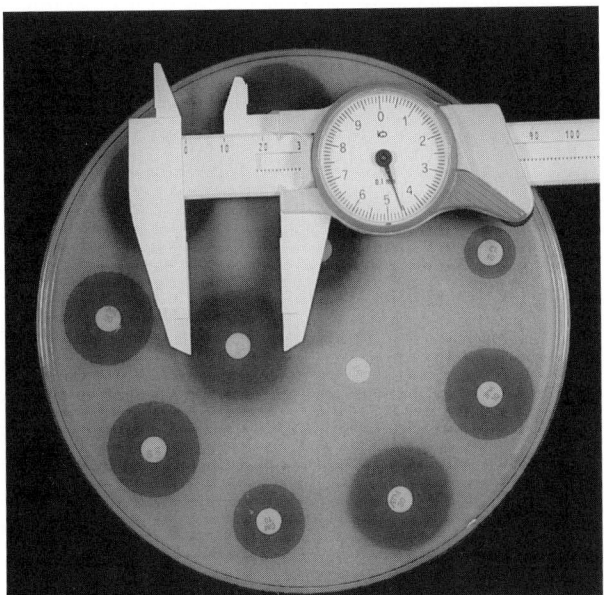

FIGURE 72.2 Photograph of a disk diffusion susceptibility test (see color insert). Antibiotic-containing disks are placed on a plate of media containing a "lawn" of organisms. Following a period of incubation, the plate is inspected and zones of inhibition are measured. Disks display varying zone sizes that may be sensitive or resistant, depending on the breakpoint value for each antibiotic. (From McClatchey KD. Clinical laboratory medicine, 2nd ed. Philadelphia: Lippincott Williams & Wilkins, 2002.)

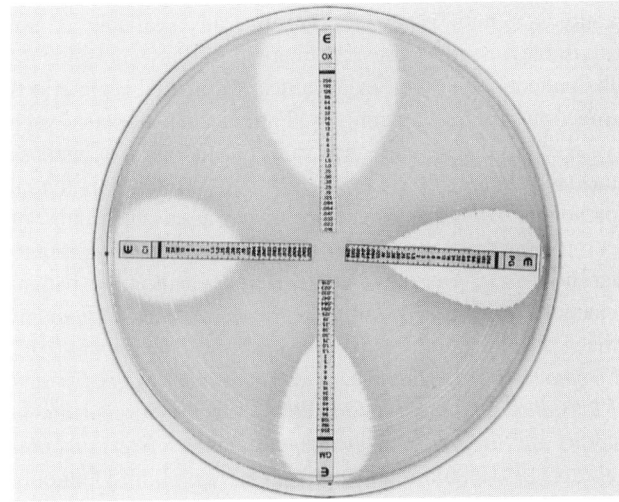

FIGURE 72.4 Photograph of Etest method. An Etest strip is placed on a media plate containing growing organism. After a period of incubation, the MIC is determined by the point at which the zone of inhibition intersects the test strip. The concentrations at each point are printed on the test strip. (From McClatchey KD. Clinical laboratory medicine, 2nd ed. Philadelphia: Lippincott Williams & Wilkins, 2002.)

traditional methods. However, sometimes confirmatory tests of rapid results are necessary, making them available closer to 24 hours after the specimen reaches the laboratory. This is still an improvement over other traditional methods. One limitation of the automated systems is their cost. Smaller laboratories may not be able to justify the cost of an expensive laboratory system, although while equipment cost is increased, personnel costs may be decreased. At least one study has shown that rapid testing may have a positive impact on patient care.[6]

An organism is considered susceptible or resistant to an antimicrobial based on standardized results of breakpoint values for the MIC or zone of inhibition, depending on the testing method and the particular microorganism as well as the drug. These breakpoint values are determined by the CLSI (Clinical and Laboratory Standards Institute, formerly referred to as the National Committee on Clinical Laboratory Standards (NCCLS)), an organization that develops and recommends laboratory testing methods.[7] Several criteria influence the breakpoint determinations, including a drug's pharmacokinetics, tissue penetration, and protein binding and the general susceptibility of a microorganism to antibiotics.

SELECTING ANTIMICROBIAL THERAPY

Establishing the causative pathogen through laboratory testing is not always possible because of limitations in specimen collection and handling. Generally, empiric antibiotics, directed at potential pathogens, are begun before the results of culture and sensitivity tests are available. Gram stain results may or may not be more quickly available in order to guide empiric therapy. Waiting to administer antibiotics until after these results are available is not advisable in most cases and may result in worsening of the patient's condition or even death in the case of serious infections such as meningitis. Patient characteristics such as age, immune status, and comorbid diseases, as well as the site of infection, are factors that influence potential pathogens. Infections generally are caused by groups of common pathogens that are specific colonizers of a particular body site, but they may differ depending on patient characteristics. For example, the most common organisms that cause meningitis in neonates are *Escherichia coli*, *Streptococcus agalactiae*, *Listeria monocytogenes*, and *Klebsiella* sp, whereas the likely infecting organisms in adults are *Streptococcus pneumoniae* and *Neisseria meningitidis*.[8–10] Cellulitis, an infection of the skin, commonly is caused by group A streptococci, which usually are found on the skin but do not cause infection unless the mucosal barrier is compromised. In contrast, patients with diabetes mellitus or peripheral vascular disease develop lower limb cellulitis, which more often is caused by enteric gram-negative bacilli or anaerobic organisms.[11]

It is often difficult to distinguish bacterial colonization from active infection. For example, patients with chronic obstructive pulmonary disease often are found to have large numbers of organisms in their sputum that may or may not be indicative of pneumonia. Likewise, some specimens may contain organisms that are not responsible for infection but rather are a result of contamination, such as a blood sample that grows coagulase-negative staphylococci. This organism is a common skin colonizer that may have contaminated the blood sample as it was being obtained. If the skin was not properly cleansed, the venipuncture needle can pick up organisms from the skin when it is pierced, resulting in bacterial contamination of the specimen.

Empiric therapy often is necessary before microbiologic information is available; it generally treats a broad spectrum of potential pathogens, because most infectious diseases may be caused by a variety of microorganisms. Definitive or directed therapy is determined for each patient when the pathogenic organisms have been identified and their antimicrobial susceptibility patterns are known. After the infecting organism has been identified and its susceptibility pattern determined, directed therapy is useful. Directed therapy is important because it is a more patient-specific regimen and is perhaps narrower in spectrum.

PATIENT FACTORS INFLUENCING EMPIRIC DRUG SELECTION

Antimicrobial therapy should be selected to maximize efficacy and minimize toxicity. To accomplish this, it is important to consider patient factors such as allergy, renal and hepatic function, site of infection, concomitant drug therapy, and underlying conditions such as chronic illness and pregnancy. Proper assessment of reported drug allergies is important because many undesirable side effects are often reported as an allergy that should not necessarily preclude treatment with a given antibiotic.[12] For example, erythromycin often causes gastrointestinal upset, which may be reported by the patient to be an allergy. Renal function and hepatic function are important patient characteristics to consider before drug selection, because these are the main routes of drug elimination; thus, toxicity may result if dosages are not adjusted for impaired organ function. Furthermore, preexisting organ impairment may influence the drug selection for drugs that are toxic to the kidney (e.g., the aminoglycosides) or liver (e.g., isoniazid).[13,14] Concomitant drugs may interact with some antimicrobial agents; fluconazole may be a better choice than ketoconazole in a patient taking an H_2-blocker such as ranitidine, because ketoconazole absorption is influenced by gastric pH, whereas fluconazole is not.[15,16] Pregnancy and other conditions may influence antibiotic selection. Sulfonamide antibiotics are not recommended in the last trimester of pregnancy because they can cause kernicterus (increased bilirubin leading to brain damage); suitable alternative agents should be selected for pregnant patients.[17]

PHARMACOLOGIC FACTORS INFLUENCING DRUG SELECTION

In addition to patient factors, drug factors such as pharmacokinetic and pharmacodynamic characteristics of antibiotics should be considered during the selection process. Pharmacokinetic factors such as maximal serum concentration (C_{max}), half-life ($t_{1/2}$), and area under the concentration–time curve (AUC) influence selection. A drug with a longer half-life may be selected to enhance compliance. Tissue penetration and protein binding are important factors because a drug cannot be effective if adequate concentration is not achieved at the site of infection. For example, many antimicrobial agents, β-lactams included, do not adequately penetrate the prostate to optimally treat prostatitis, even though they achieve high concentrations in the urine. Therefore, when selecting an antimicrobial agent for the treatment of prostatitis, the penetration of potential drug therapies into this tissue must be evaluated. Similarly, when treating meningitis, it is imperative to evaluate drug penetration into the CSF. Generally, drugs that are highly protein-bound do not penetrate well enough into the CSF to achieve adequate bactericidal concentration.[18] The area of antimicrobial pharmacodynamics (the relationship between drug concentration and the rate and extent of microbial killing) is becoming more important for drug therapy selection.

Antimicrobial pharmacodynamics generally investigates the pharmacokinetics of the drug (AUC, C_{max}) in relationship to the MIC of a pathogen. For the aminoglycoside and quinolone antibiotics, the factor associated with a successful outcome in animal models is maximizing the ratio of C_{max} or AUC relative to the MIC.[19,20] This means that achieving a higher peak concentration in the body relative to the MIC of the organism is associated with eradication of the organism. This is termed concentration-dependent activity, increasing activity with increasing concentrations.

Antibiotics also have a postantibiotic effect (PAE), which is the period of time an antibiotic continues to suppress growth of an organism after the antibiotic has been removed from the in vitro culture medium. PAE is generally an organism-specific effect. Most antimicrobials display a PAE against gram-positive cocci, whereas the aminoglycosides and fluoroquinolones also produce PAE in gram-negative bacilli. The clinical importance of PAE is not clearly defined, although animal studies suggest that antimicrobials, which produce PAE, may be administered to allow the serum drug concentration to fall below the MIC of the infecting organism.[21]

Antibiotics that display concentration-dependent activity and an extended PAE may be given less frequently than anticipated by their half-life.[22] To take advantage of the pharmacodynamic properties of the aminoglycosides, once-daily dosing instead of the traditional multiple daily doses has been studied extensively and shown to be effective and safe in many patient populations.[23] This application of the pharmacodynamic properties of the aminoglycosides may actually reduce the incidence of drug-induced renal toxicity

while maintaining positive clinical outcomes. By comparison, cell wall-active antibiotics such as the β-lactams do not display concentration-dependent activity or a prolonged PAE. Rather, they display concentration-independent (or time-dependent) microbiologic activity. This means that as long as the serum or tissue drug concentration remains at or above the MIC of the organism, the activity of the drug is maximized.[24] Therefore, a β-lactam may be given as small, frequent doses or as a continuous infusion (which may be impractical) to maximize its pharmacodynamic properties.[22,25] This area of research offers an opportunity for the application of the interrelations among the bug, drug, and patient factors associated with successful treatment.

SELECTING COMBINATION THERAPY

Combination therapy may be necessary on many occasions. First, more than one antimicrobial may be required to treat a number of potential pathogens. For example, aerobic and anaerobic coverage is needed in patients with peritonitis, and only a few antimicrobial agents have both aerobic and anaerobic activity. Second, combination therapy may be selected to take advantage of synergistic properties of the antimicrobials. Synergy occurs when two drugs given in combination are more active together than either drug alone.[26] β-lactam antibiotics in combination with aminoglycosides display synergy in vitro against a variety of pathogens, including *Enterococcus* sp and *Pseudomonas aeruginosa*, and are often given together.[27] Combination therapy may be selected to decrease the potential for resistance during therapy. This is the case with the treatment of tuberculosis, which is always treated with at least three drugs to prevent the development of resistance.[28] Some disadvantages of combination therapy include the increased cost associated with administering more than one antibiotic, the potential for increased frequency of side effects, and possible antagonistic combinations. In combination, the antifungal agents fluconazole and amphotericin B have been shown in vitro to display antagonism.[29,30] Other potentially antagonistic combinations include the induction of β-lactamases by double β-lactam therapy.[31] It is difficult to document antagonistic combinations in humans; however, combinations shown to be antagonistic in vitro generally are avoided in vivo to avoid the potential for therapeutic failure.

SELECTING MICROBICIDAL THERAPY

The selection of an antimicrobial that is able to kill an organism instead of simply inhibiting its growth is desirable in some clinical situations. Generally, these include infections where the site of infection is not easily penetrated. Examples include meningitis, endocarditis, and osteomyelitis. Also, patients who are immunosuppressed, in particular neutropenic patients, are more often considered for ''cidal'' therapy. While most of the clinical data support the use of microbicidal activity for bacterial infections, many serious infections in vulnerable patients are fungal infections, making selection of an antifungal agent with fungicidal activity desirable. Microbicidal activity is bug- and drug-specific. For example, the echinocandin antifungals exhibit concentration-dependent fungicidal activity against *Candida* but not *Aspergillus*. By comparison, some triazole antifungals are fungicidal against *Aspergillus* but not *Candida*.[32]

MONITORING RESPONSE

The next step in the drug selection process is monitoring therapy to determine if any changes are necessary. Monitoring antimicrobial drug therapy is important for ensuring successful and safe outcomes. Symptomatic improvement is a hallmark sign of effective antibiotic therapy and generally is considered a clinical cure if maintained after completion of therapy. Microbiologic cure is the documentation of eradication of the infecting organism. Microbiologic cure generally is used in research studies and is applicable outside this setting for certain severe infections such as endocarditis and meningitis. Interestingly, some patients judged to be cured clinically may represent a microbiologic failure—that is, they appear to be symptomatically improved, but the infecting organism was not completely eradicated with treatment, as is the case in many pulmonary or skin and soft tissue infections. Microbiologic cure, therefore, is not an expected treatment goal for many infections. Therapeutic (clinical) failure occurs when a patient fails to improve clinically on a given antibiotic. This may occur because of bacterial resistance, inadequate dosage, noncompliance, or superinfection with another organism. In certain cases, antibiotic administration alone is inadequate for cure and a surgical débridement or repair procedure is necessary for a successful outcome. For example, a person with an abscess may need to have it drained surgically, or infected devices such as a prosthetic joint may need to be removed for resolution of osteomyelitis.

Antibiotic toxicity is the other main area for therapy monitoring. Complications may be minimized if side effects are evaluated early and dosages are adjusted or medications are changed. A patient's renal function should be closely monitored because many antimicrobials are eliminated by the kidneys, and drug accumulation with resultant toxicities is possible. Changes in renal function may require alterations in the dosage or dosing schedule of the antibiotic. Serum levels of certain antibiotics, such as aminoglycosides, may be measured to ensure an adequate dosage regimen and to avoid potentially toxic levels.

For patients receiving antibiotics in the outpatient setting, patient and family education is important for successful treatment. Patients should be informed about food–drug and drug–drug interactions and proper storage and handling of their antibiotics. Some antibiotics, such as penicillin, should be taken on an empty stomach, whereas others need to be taken with food. Many antibiotic suspensions used for children need to be shaken well and stored in the refrigerator. The need for compliance and the importance of completing the entire course of antibiotics as prescribed should always be emphasized to avoid the emergence of bacterial resistance. Relapse may occur if the infection is not treated for an adequate length of time.

REFINING ANTIMICROBIAL THERAPY

The final step in the drug selection process is to refine empiric therapy based on the results of identification and susceptibility tests. The MIC results should be reviewed to ensure that the causative pathogen is sensitive to the antibiotic selected. Ideally, the least expensive yet effective agent is selected. A child with meningitis may be started on cefotaxime for empiric therapy. When the culture and sensitivity report results reveal S. pneumoniae to be sensitive to penicillin, therapy may be changed to the less-expensive and narrower-spectrum agent. Several factors other than the cost of the medication influence the cost-effectiveness of a selected regimen. Costs of therapy include not only nursing administration, pharmacy preparation, and storage costs, but also costs associated with monitoring therapy, such as laboratory tests to monitor for toxicities (e.g., serum creatinine, LFTs) or more expensive serum drug concentrations. An expensive medication that is given once daily and has relatively no monitoring expenses may be associated with a lower overall cost compared with an inexpensive antibiotic that is given multiple times a day or has expensive monitoring costs. The antimicrobial selection process requires careful consideration of several steps. At each step, the interrelations of patient, bug, and drug factors need to be fully evaluated to ensure a successful outcome.

REFERENCES

1. Gonzalez R, Steiner JF, Sande MA. Antibiotic prescribing for adults with colds, upper respiratory tract infections, and bronchitis by ambulatory care physicians. JAMA 278:901–904, 1997.
2. Gelfand JA, Dinarello CA, Wolff SM. Fever, including fever of unknown origin. In: Isselbacher KJ, Brawnwald E, Wilson JD, et al., eds. Harrison's principles of internal medicine, 13th ed. New York: McGraw-Hill, 1994:81.
3. Woods GL, Washington JA. The clinician and the microbiology laboratory. In: Mandel GL, Bennett JE, Dolin R, eds. Mandel, Douglas and Bennett's principles and practice of infectious diseases, 4th ed. New York: Churchill Livingstone, 1995:169.
4. Bauer AW, Kirby MM, Sherris JC, et al. Antibiotic susceptibility testing by a standardized, single-disk method. Am J Clin Pathol 45:493–496, 1966.
5. Thornsberry C. Forward to ETEST symposium. Diag Microbiol Infect Dis 15:459–463, 1992.
6. Doern GV, Vautour R, Gaudet M, et al. Clinical impact of rapid in vitro susceptibility testing and bacterial identification. J Clin Microbiol 32:1757–1762, 1994.
7. Clinical and Laboratory Standards Institute. Performance standards for antimicrobial susceptibility testing. In: Sixty informational supplement: CLSI document M100-S6. Wayne, PA: CLSI, 1995.
8. Schuchat A, Robinson K, Wenger JD, et al. Bacterial meningitis in the United States in 1995. N Engl J Med 337:970–976, 1997.
9. Durand ML, Calderwood SB, Weber DJ, et al. Acute bacterial meningitis in adults. A review of 493 episodes. N Engl J Med 328:21–28, 1993.

10. Rockowitz J, Tunkel AR. Bacterial meningitis. Practical guidelines for management. Drugs 50:838–853, 1995.
11. Fox HR, Karcmer AW. Management of diabetic foot infections, including the use of home intravenous antibiotic therapy. Clin Podiatr Med Surg 13:671–681, 1996.
12. Weiss ME. Drug allergy. Med Clin North Am 76:857–882, 1992.
13. Kahlmeter G, Dahlager JI. Aminoglycoside toxicity: a review of clinical studies published between 1975 and 1982. J Antimicrob Chemother 13 (Suppl A):9–23, 1984.
14. Salpeter SR. Fatal isoniazid-induced hepatitis: its risk during chemoprophylaxis. West J Med 159:560–564, 1993.
15. Van Der Meer JW, Keuning JJ, Scheijgrond HW, et al. The influence of gastric acidity on the bioavailability of ketoconazole. J Antimicrob Chemother 6:552–554, 1980.
16. Albengres E, Le Louet H, Tillement JP. Systemic antifungal agents. Drug interactions of clinical significance. Drug Safety 18:83–97, 1998.
17. Cockerill FR 3rd, Edson RS. Trimethoprim-sulfamethoxazole. Mayo Clin Proc 62:921–929, 1987.
18. Lutsar I, McCracken GH Jr, Friedland IR. Antibiotic pharmacodynamics in cerebrospinal fluid. Clin Infect Dis 27:1117–1127, 1998.
19. Lacy MK, Nicolau DP, Nightingale CH, et al. The pharmacodynamics of aminoglycosides. Clin Infect Dis 27:23–27, 1998.
20. Lode H, Borner K, Koeppe P. Pharmacodynamics of fluoroquinolones. Clin Infect Dis 27:33–39, 1998.
21. Shibl AM, Pechere JC, Ramadan MA. Postantibiotic effect and host–bacteria interactions. J Antimicrob Chemother 36:885–887, 1995.
22. Drusano GL. Role of pharmacokinetics in the outcome of infections. Antimicrob Agents Chemother 32:289–297, 1988.
23. Preston SL, Briceland LL. Single daily dosing of aminoglycosides. Pharmacotherapy 15:297–316, 1995.
24. Soriano F, Garcia-Corbeira P, Ponte C, et al. Correlation of pharmacodynamic parameters of five beta-lactam antibiotics with therapeutic efficacies in an animal model. Antimicrob Agents Chemother 40:2686–2690, 1996.
25. Eliopoulos GM, Moellering RC. Antimicrobial combinations. In: Lorian V. Antibiotics in laboratory medicine, 4th ed. Baltimore: Williams & Wilkins, 1996:330.
26. Drusano GL. Human pharmacodynamics of beta lactams, aminoglycosides and their combination. Scand J Infect Dis Suppl 74:235–248, 1990.
27. Craig WA, Ebert SC. Continuous infusion of beta-lactam antibiotics. Antimicrob Agents Chemother 36:2577–2583, 1992.
28. Iseman MD. Treatment of multidrug-resistant tuberculosis. N Engl J Med 329:784–791, 1993.
29. Lewis RE, Lund BC, Klepser ME, et al. Assessment of antifungal activities of fluconazole and amphotericin B administered alone and in combination against Candida albicans by using a dynamic in vitro mycotic infection model. Antimicrob Agents Chemother 42:1382–1386, 1998.
30. Sugar AM, Liu X. Interactions of itraconazole with amphotericin b in the treatment of murine invasive candidiasis. J Infect Dis 177:1660–1663, 1998.
31. Hopefl AW. Overview of synergy with reference to double beta-lactam combinations. DICP 25:972–977, 1991.
32. Pfaller MA, Sheehan DJ, Rex JH. Determination of fungicidal activities against yeast and molds: lessons learned from bactericidal testing and the need for standardization. Clin Microbiol Reviews 17:268–280, 2004.

Immunization Therapy

73

Stephan L. Foster and Michael D. Hogue

OVERVIEW

Immunization for disease prevention was used by the late 1790s, when inoculation with cowpox was used to provide immunity against smallpox. Using immunization-induced immunity has successfully controlled and even eliminated disease.[1] In 1972, the World Health Organization (WHO) declared that smallpox had been eradicated by the worldwide vaccination program. The last case of wild-type polio in the western hemisphere was reported in 1991, and the number of polio-endemic countries has decreased to 6 by 2003.[2] Certification of worldwide eradication of polio is planned for 2005.[3] As part of the Healthy People 2010 initiative, goals have been set to enhance the immunization status of people of all ages.[4]

To improve quality of life through disease prevention, immunizations are being offered in a variety of nontraditional settings, including pharmacies, businesses, and community settings. While pediatric immunization rates in the United States have been in the 90th percentile or better, adult immunization rates fall far behind. Many healthcare providers, including pharmacists, are beginning to focus their efforts on this underserved group.

The Centers for Disease Control and Prevention (CDC) publishes revised recommendations for the prevention and treatment of infectious disease. The Advisory Committee for Immunizations Practice (ACIP) is a group of respected scientists in the field of immunology that makes recommendations to the CDC. Other agencies involved in the development and approval of the current Recommended Childhood and Adolescent Immunization Schedule (Harmonized Schedule) include the American Academy of Pediatrics (AAP) and the American Association of Family Physicians (AAFP). Agencies that develop the Recommended Adult Immunization Schedule by Age Group and Medical Condition include the ACIP, AAFP, and the American College of Obstetricians and Gynecology. As changes occur, they are published in the *Morbidity and Mortality Weekly Review* (*MMWR-CDC*), in *Pediatrics,* and in various other medical journals. The CDC provides the most current online immunization information, including ACIP recommendations, at the National Immunization Program web site (www.cdc.gov/nip).

ACTIVE IMMUNIZATION

Immunization stimulates an endogenous immunologic response using an attenuated live or inactivated microorganism or antigenic products from a microorganism. A single injection may not be sufficient to stimulate the desired response, and a series of primary injections may be needed. In some cases, booster immunizations are provided at scheduled intervals throughout life to retain an adequate antibody response.

Passive or temporary immunity is provided by exogenous antibodies in the form of immunoglobulin G (IgG). In addition to antibody replacement, IgG is effective in other types of diseases, primarily those that are autoimmune. Many specific immune globulin products are now available, and more are being studied.

IMMUNE SYSTEM DEVELOPMENT

The immune system begins to develop early in fetal life. At 7 weeks' gestation, small lymphocytes appear in the circulation, and at 9 weeks, B cells primarily involved in the humoral immune response are seen in fetal liver. At term birth, all of the components of the immune system are present and functional, but immunoglobulin production is low. However, active transport of maternal IgG across the placenta results in IgG serum concentrations in term neonates that are 5% to 10% greater than in the mother. Although neonates can produce all classes of immunoglobulins, they cannot produce specific antibodies against all antigens. At birth, there is no immunologic memory, complement concentrations are low, opsonin activity is poor, and neutrophil chemotaxis and phagocytosis are reduced. By 1 year of age, complement concentrations in the classic and alternative pathways are at adult values. By 2 years of age, the memory response to polysaccharide antigen is present, immune-complex diseases begin to appear, and immunoglobulin M (IgM) concentrations reach adult values. Secretory immunoglobulin A (IgA) peaks by 2 to 4 years; however, the capacity for specific IgA antibody production slowly matures until puberty. Adult IgG concentrations are reached by 4 to 6 years of age.

The age at which an infant can respond appropriately to a specific immunization depends on the disappearance of transplacentally acquired antibodies and the maturity of the immune system to respond to specific antigens. The presence of maternally derived antibodies may prevent an appropriate response for the first year of life; therefore, immunization against these antigens is delayed. Children less than 2 years of age have a poor response to polysaccharide antigens due to the T-cell–independent response they produce.[5] Conjugation of polysaccharide vaccines with a protein carrier, such as a nontoxic diphtheria toxin in the case of pneumococcal conjugate vaccine, induces a T-cell–dependent response, to which children less than 2 years of age can then respond adequately. Immunity is not conferred against the carrier protein itself (e.g., diphtheria toxin), which has no relative antigenicity alone; rather, immunity is enhanced to the primary antigen to which the protein is being conjugated (i.e., pneumococcal or *Haemophilus influenzae* type B polysaccharides).[6] Furthermore, to overcome persistent maternal antibodies and immature cellular immunity, some vaccines require greater dosages of antigen in infants and young children than would be required for primary immunization in older children and adults. For example, the diphtheria toxoid dosage used to immunize those less than 7 years of age (DTaP, DT) is three times greater than the dosage used in older individuals. In fact, in individuals over age 7, the amount of diphtheria antigen present in DTaP significantly increases the incidence of vaccine side effects in older children and adults compared to Td, which contains one-third the amount of diphtheria antigen. The presence of disease, allergies, immunosuppression, dialysis, pregnancy, travel, and epidemics may require modification of an immunization schedule or dosage and consideration of the immunization type (live or inactivated) or other components. Travel to countries where a specific infectious disease is endemic may require immunization or prophylactic measures to prevent infection.

FACTORS AFFECTING IMMUNOGENICITY OF IMMUNIZING AGENTS

Vaccines are composed of antigenic components of microorganisms (bacteria and viruses). Vaccines are classified as live, attenuated, or inactivated (killed). Live vaccines must replicate to induce an immune response. Formaldehyde or hydrogen peroxide is commonly used in the process of attenuation, making live vaccines noninfectious yet immunogenic. Inactivated vaccines are produced from whole microorganisms (whole cell vaccines), immunogenic components of the microorganisms (e.g., viral particles, recombinant DNA, polysaccharide), or toxins produced by the microorganisms (toxoids). Whole cell vaccines have largely been removed from the U.S. market due to their propensity to cause more severe adverse effects; they have been replaced by acellular vaccines. Inactivated vaccines are produced using antigens from recombinant DNA technology, bacterial cell-wall components (polysaccharide vaccines), surface antigens of viruses, toxins that are rendered nontoxic, conjugation of polysaccharides to protein carriers, or other undefined processes. The response induced by many vaccines confers a long-lasting and, in many cases, permanent immunity. Attenuated live vaccines stimulate an immunologic response similar to natural infection, usually resulting in lifelong immunity. However, live vaccines carry the risk, albeit small, for the development of the disease it is designed to prevent. In general, polysaccharide vaccines are less immunogenic than other types of vaccines and elicit a minimal response in those less than 2 years of age due to the inability to respond to T-cell–independent stimulation. Conjugation of the polysaccharide to proteins improves immunogenicity even in infants as young as 6 weeks of age. The process of conjugation is effective in young children because of the production of peptides created by the recognition of the carrier protein, converting to a T-cell–dependent process.

OTHER IMMUNIZATION COMPONENTS

Immunizations contain products that are added to enhance immunogenicity, to preserve the product, or to stabilize the product or are residual from the antigenic detoxifying process. Aluminum phosphate, aluminum hydroxide, and calcium phosphate are used as adjuvants to delay absorption and increase antigenicity. Thimerosal, a mercury derivative, and 2-phenoxyethanol may be added as preservatives. Possible other ingredients include lactose, sucrose, gelatin, sorbitol, neomycin, and streptomycin. Residual proteins from the development process are present in several vaccines. Two vaccines produced in chick embryos (eggs) are influenza and yellow fever; therefore, allergies to eggs must be determined. The hepatitis B vaccine is developed using recombinant technology with *Saccharomyces cerevisiae* (baker's yeast), to which hypersensitivity reactions have been rarely observed.[7] Some vaccines are treated with formaldehyde during antigenic processing. Immunizations, their components, and their preferred route of administration are listed in Tables 73.1 through 73.3.

ROUTE OF ADMINISTRATION

Although a few vaccines are given orally or intranasally, most are given as subcutaneous (SC), intramuscular (IM), or intradermal injections. If immunizations are not administered according to the recommended route, the desired immunologic response may not occur. Products containing aluminum should be given intramuscularly because of the increased risk of tissue irritation with SC administration. IM injections should be given in the anterolateral aspect of the thigh in infants and the deltoid muscle in children or older individuals. Injections in the buttocks should be avoided because the presence of fat can interfere with absorption, there is potential for damaging the sciatic nerve, and the gluteal muscles are not developed in infants. SC immunizations should be given in the anterolateral aspect of the upper arm or thigh.

Patients at risk for bleeding, including those with hemophilia or those who are anticoagulated, are at increased risk for hematoma development following immunization. Recommendations for these patients when vaccination is deemed necessary include using a 23-gauge needle or smaller and applying direct pressure at the injection site for at least 2 minutes, without rubbing.[8]

ANTIBODY RESPONSE TO IMMUNIZATION

The antibody response begins soon after immunization, but adequate protection against disease may not be achieved for weeks. In some cases, the response to the first dose is insufficient to protect against disease or the initial response wanes with time; thus, complete vaccination may require a series of doses given at least 28 days apart. Immunization against several diseases can be accomplished at the same time, either with an approved combination product or with multiple injections at different sites. One live vaccine may interfere with the antibody response of another live vaccine if not given simultaneously. Live vaccines not given on the same day should be separated by 28 days if possible to maximize the antibody response.

DELAYED OR MISSED IMMUNIZATIONS

It is unnecessary to restart any vaccine series, even if the last dose administered in the series was a number of months or years earlier. Instead, the series should be resumed and immunizations that have not been given should be administered at the recommended intervals. The CDC publishes a catch-up schedule for all vaccines in *Epidemiology and Prevention of Vaccine Preventable Diseases*, a text that is revised every 2 to 3 years.[9] When it is impossible to verify a patient's vaccination history, it is better to restart the series and administer potentially "extra" doses than to risk inadequate protection against disease.

While many vaccines administered as a series are begun during childhood, immunization screening sometimes reveals adults who have not received the primary series of one or more routine vaccines. Vaccines administered to adults are identical to those used in children, with a few important exceptions. Children should receive DTaP, but individuals over age 7 should receive Td, which contains one third of the diphtheria antigen of DTaP and results in fewer adverse events in older children and adults. The primary series of Td is three doses, the first two administered at least 4 weeks apart and a third dose 6 to 12 months later. Booster doses of Td are then administered every 10 years. The primary series of varicella vaccine in adults who have not been immunized during childhood and have not had primary varicella infection (chickenpox) consists of two doses administered 4 to 8 weeks apart. One dose of MMR should be administered to any adult born after 1957 if the measles, mumps, or rubella (MMR) vaccination history is unreliable. Some adults at high risk of exposure may require a second dose. *H. influenzae* type b (Hib) vaccine should not be administered in any person over age 5; therefore, adults need not be screened for this vaccine. Pneumococcal vaccine is given in a series as the pneumococcal conjugate, 7-valent vaccine only to children younger than 5 years of age. Series dosing of pneumococcal vaccine after age 5 is unnecessary.[8]

VACCINE-RELATED ADVERSE EVENTS REPORTING

All immunizations can produce adverse effects, but they are predominantly mild and self-limiting. Although rare, certain adverse events temporally associated with immunization have resulted in severe permanent injury or death. Serious side effects temporally related to immunization must be reported to the U.S. Department of Health and Human Services through the Vaccine Adverse Event Reporting System (VAERS).[10] VAERS serves as the system for monitoring and tracking suspected serious adverse events after immunization.[11,12] VAERS forms can be completed online at www.vaers.hhs.gov.

(*text continues on page 1862*)

TABLE 73.1 | Routine Immunizations Available in the United States, 2004

Disease	Immunization Type	Antigenic Components and Amount	Other Components[a]	Route[b]	Brand Name	Marketed by
Hepatitis B	Inactivated virus vaccine	Hepatitis B surface antigen (HbsAg) adw subtype produced in yeast cells using recombinant DNA technology 5 µg/0.5 mL (pediatric), 10 µg/mL (adult), 40 µg/mL (dialysis)	A, YP	IM	Recombivax HB	Merck and Co.
		10 µg/0.5 mL (pediatric/adolescent) 20 µg/mL (adult)	A, T[c], YP	IM	Engerix B	GlaxoSmithKline
Tetanus + diphtheria	Toxoid + toxoid	Clostridium tetani + Corynebacterium diphtheriae endotoxins flocculating units (Lf)5 Lf (T) + 6.7 Lf (D)	A, T, F	IM	DT	Sanofi Pasteur
Tetanus + diphtheria + pertussis	Toxoid + toxoid + acellular vaccine	5 Lf (T) + 15 Lf (D) + 10 µg PT + 5 µg FHA + 3 µg PRN + 5 µg Fimbriae types 2 and 3	A, F, Pe	IM	Daptacel	Sanofi Pasteur
		10 Lf (T) + 25 Lf (D) + 25 µg PT + 25 µg FHA + 8 µg PRN	A, F, P, Pe	IM	Infanrix	GlaxoSmithKline
		5 Lf (T) + 25 Lf (D) + 23.4 µg PT + 23.4 µg FHA	A, T,[c,d] F, G, P	IM	Tripedia	Sanofi Pasteur
Haemophilus influenzae type b	Conjugated polysaccharide vaccine	10 µg Hib PRP conjugated to 24 µg tetanus toxoid		IM	ActHIB	Sanofi Pasteur
		10 µg Hib PRP conjugated to 25 µg diphtheria CRM_{125} protein		IM	HibTITER	Wyeth
		7.5 µg Hib PRP conjugated to 125 µg Neisseria meningitidis outer membrane protein complex	A	IM	PedvaxHIB	Merck and Co.
Hepatitis A	Inactivated virus vaccine	Hepatitis A viral strain HM175, 360 and 720 ELISA (EL) units (children); 1,440 EL units (adults)	A, F, Pe, N	M	Havrix	GlaxoSmithKline
Hepatitis B + Haemophilus influenzae type b	Inactivated virus vaccine + conjugated polysaccharide vaccine	7.5 µg Hib PRP conjugated to 125 µg Neisseria meningitidis outer membrane protein complex + 5 µg hepatitis B surface antigen (HbsAg) adw subtype produced in yeast cells using recombinant DNA technology	A, YP	IM	Comvax (Recombivax + PedvaxHIB)	Merck and Co.
Polio	Inactivated virus vaccine	Types 1, 2, 3 polio virus 40 D antigen units of type 1, 8 D antigen units of type 2, 34 D antigen units of type 3	F, Pe, N, St, Px	IM, SC	IPOL	Sanofi Pasteur

(continues)

TABLE 73.1 continued

Disease	Immunization Type	Antigenic Components and Amount	Other Components[a]	Route[b]	Brand Name	Marketed by
Tetanus + diphtheria + pertussis + polio + hepatitis B	Toxoid + toxoid + acellular vaccine + inactivated virus vaccine	10 Lf (T) + 25 Lf (D) + 25 μg PT + 25 μg FHA + 8 μg PRN + types 1, 2, 3 polio virus 40 D antigen units of type 1, 8 D antigen units of type 2, 34 D antigen units of type 3 + 10 μg Hepatitis B surface antigen (HbsAg) adw subtype produced in yeast cells using recombinant DNA technology	A, T,[c] F, P, Pe, N, St, Px YP	IM	Pediarix	GlaxoSmithKline
Streptococcus pneumoniae	Conjugated polysaccharide vaccine	16 μg capsular saccharides of Streptococcus pneumoniae serotypes 4, 6B, 9V, 14, 18C, 19F, and 23F conjugated to 20 μg diphtheria CRM_{125} protein	A	IM	Prevnar	Wyeth
	Polysaccharide vaccine	25 μg of each of 23 capsular saccharides of Streptococcus pneumoniae serotypes 1, 2, 3, 4, 5, 6B, 7F, 9N, 9V, 10A, 11A, 12F, 14, 15B, 17F, 18C, 19F, 19A, 20, 22F, 23F, 33F	Ph	IM, SC	Pneumovax 23	Merck and Co.
Measles + mumps + rubella	Attenuated live virus vaccine	1,000 tissue culture infectious doses ($TCID_{50}$) of Enders attenuated Edmonton measles strain + 20,000 $TCID_{50}$ of Jeryl Lynn mumps strain + 1,000 $TCID_{50}$ of Wistar RA 27/3 rubella strain	N, G, Ch	SC	M-M-R II	Merck and Co.
Varicella	Attenuated live virus vaccine	≥1,350 plaque-forming units (PFU) of Oka/Merck varicella virus	N, G	SC	Varivax	Merck and Co.
Influenza	Inactivated virus vaccine	Two type A viral antigens and one type B based upon epidemiologic data gathered 6 to 9 months prior to the next season	T,[c,d] F, G, Ch	IM	Fluzone	Sanofi Pasteur
		Two type A viral antigens and one type B based on epidemiologic data gathered 6 to 9 months prior to the next season	T, N, Px	IM	Fluvirin	Chiron
	Cold-adapted, live, attenuated virus vaccine	Two type A viral antigens and one type B based on epidemiologic data gathered 6 to 9 months prior to the next season	Gn, Ch	Intranasal	FluMist	MedImmune

[a] A, aluminum; T, thimerosal; F, formaldehyde; G, gelatin; P, polysorbate; Pe, 2-phenoxyethanol; N, neomycin; St, streptomycin; Px, polymyxin B; Gn, gentamicin; YP, yeast protein; Ch, produced in chick embryo cell line; Ph, phenol; MP, mouse serum protein.
[b] IM, intramuscular; SC, subcutaneous.
[c] Single-dose vial contains no preservatives, but it contains a trace amount of thimerosal (mercury) from the manufacturing process.
[d] Multidose vial contains thimerosal as a preservative.

TABLE 73.2 | **Nonroutine Immunizations**

Disease	Immunization Type	Antigenic Components and Amount	Other Components[a]	Route[b]	Brand Name	Marketed by
Hepatitis A + hepatitis B	Inactivated virus vaccine	Hepatitis A virus antigen, 50 unit/mL	A, F	IM	Vaqta	Merck and Co.
		Hepatitis A viral strain HM175 720 ELISA (EL) units combined with 20 μg hepatitis B surface antigen (HbsAg) adw subtype produced in yeast cells using recombinant DNA technology	A, F, Pe, N, T,[c] YP	IM	Twinrix	GlaxoSmithKline
Neisseria meningitidis	Polysaccharide vaccine	Polysaccharide (50 μg each) of groups A, C, Y, and W-135 meningococcus	T[d]	SC	Menomune	Sanofi Pasteur
	Conjugated polysaccharide vaccine	Polysaccharide (4 μg each) of groups A, C, Y, and W-135 meningococcus conjugated to 48 μg diphtheria toxoid protein carrier	F	IM	Menactra	Sanofi Pasteur
Tuberculosis	Live, attenuated virus	Bacillus of Calmette and Guerin (BCG strain of Mycobacterium bovis (TICE) 1 to 8 × 10^8 colony-forming units	gly, L	Per	BCG vaccine, USP	Organon Inc.
Japanese encephalitis	Inactivated virus vaccine	Nakayama-NIH strain of Japanese encephalitis virus	T, F, G, P	SC	JEVAX	Sanofi Pasteur
Typhoid (Salmonella typhi)	Polysaccharide vaccine	25 μg Vi polysaccharide extract	Ph	IM	Typhim Vi	Sanofi Pasteur
Yellow fever	Live virus vaccine	17D strain of yellow fever virus 4.74 log$_{10}$ plaque-forming units	S, G, Ch	SC	YF-VAX	Sanofi Pasteur

[a] A, aluminum; T, thimerosal; F, formaldehyde; G, gelatin; P, polysorbate; Pe, 2-phenoxyethanol; N, neomycin; St, streptomycin; Px, polymyxin B; Gn, gentamicin; YP, yeast protein; Ch, produced in chick embryo cell line; Ph, phenol; MP, mouse serum protein.

[b] IM, intramuscular; SC, subcutaneous; per, percutaneous using a multiple-puncture disc.

[c] Single-dose vial contains no preservatives, but it contains a trace amount of thimerosal (mercury) from the manufacturing process.

[d] Multidose vial contains thimerosal as a preservative.

TABLE 73.3	Immunizations for Special Groups and Travel					
Disease	**Immunization Type**	**Antigenic Components and Amount**	**Other Components**[a]	**Route**[b]	**Brand Name**	**Marketed By**
Cholera	Killed vaccine	Eight units each of Ogawa and Inaba serotypes of *Vibrio cholerae* per mL (dose 0.2–0.5 mL depending on age)	Ph	IM, SC, ID	Cholera vaccine	Wyeth Laboratories
Hepatitis A	Inactivated virus vaccine	Hepatitis A viral strain HM175, 360, and 720 ELISA (EL) units for children; 1,440 EL units for adults	A	IM	Harvix	SmithKline Beecham
		Hepatitis A virus antigen, 50 units/mL				
Influenza	Activated virus vaccine	Two type A viral antigens and one type B based on epidemiologic data 6 to 9 months before the next influenza season	A, F	IM	VAQTA	Merck and Co.
			T, F, P, Ch	IM	FluShield	Wyeth Laboratories
Japanese encephalitis	Inactivated virus vaccine	Japanese encephalitis virus	T, F, G, Ch	IM	Fluzone	Sanofi Pasteur
			S, T, G, F	SC	JE-VAX	Sanofi Pasteur
Lyme disease	Acellular	Nakayama-NIH strain	MP			
		30 mg outer surface lipoprotein (OspA) of *Borrelia burgdorferi*	A, Pe	IM	LYMErix	SmithKline Beecham
Neisseria meningitidis	Polysaccharide vaccine	Polysaccharide from 4 types (50 µg each) of groups A, C, Y, and W-135 meningococcus	T, L	SC	Menomune	Sanofi Pasteur

Disease	Type	Description	Additives	Route[b]	Brand	Manufacturer
Rabies	Inactivated virus vaccine	Wistar rabies virus strain	N, P, alb	IM	Imovax	Sanofi Pasteur
	Inactivated	PM-1503–3M, 2.5 IU of rabies antigen/mL	N, P, alb	ID	Imovax Rabies I.D.	Sanofi Pasteur
	Inactivated	Kissling strain of Challenge virus standard rabies virus	A	IM	Rabies Vaccine Adsorbed	BioPort Corp.
	Inactivated	Flury LEP grown in chicken fibroblast culture		IM	RabAvert	Chiron Corp.
Streptococcus pneumoniae	Polysaccharide vaccine	Polysaccharide from 23 types (25 µg each) of pneumococcus	T	IM	PNU-IMUNE 23	Lederle
			Ph	SC	PNEUMOVAX 23	Merck and Co.
Tuberculosis	Live, attenuated virus	Bacillus of Calmette and Guerin [BCG] strain of *Mycobacterium bovis* (TICE) 1 to 8×10^8 colony-forming units	gly, L	Per	BCG vaccine, USP	Organon Inc.
Typhoid	Killed vaccine	*Salmonella typhosa* (Ty-2 strain) #(1000) million/mL (dose is 0.25 or 0.5 mL)	Ph	SC	Typhoid vaccine	Wyeth Laboratories
	Polysaccharide vaccine	polysaccharide from *Salmonella typhi* Ty-2 strain, 25 mg/0.5 mL dose	Ph	IM	Typhim Vi	Sanofi Pasteur
	Live, attenuated virus	*Salmonella typhi* Ty 21a, 2 to 6×10^9 colony-forming units	S, L, As	Oral	Vivotif Berna	Berna Products Corp.
Yellow fever	Live virus vaccine	17 D strain of yellow fever virus 5.04 log10 plaque-forming units (PFU)	S, G, Ch	SC	YF-VAX	Sanofi Pasteur

[a]A, aluminum; T, thimerosal; F, 0.02% formaldehyde; G, gelatin; P, polysorbate; Pe, 2-phenoxyethanol; S, sorbitol; N, neomycin; St, streptomycin; Px, polymyxin B; YP, yeast protein; L, lactose; Ch, produced in chick embryo cell line; Ph, phenol; A, albumin; MP, mouse serum protein; As, ascorbic acid; gly, glycerin.

[b]IM, intramuscular; SC, subcutaneous; ID, intradermal; Per, percutaneous using a multiple-puncture disc.

NATIONAL VACCINE INJURY COMPENSATION PROGRAM

The National Vaccine Injury Compensation Program (VICP) was passed to provide financial assistance to individuals with serious adverse reactions that were temporally related to vaccination, in turn relieving manufacturers and providers of significant financial burden. A complete listing of adverse events that must be reported under VICP is available at www.hrsa.gov/osp/vicp. Funding for this program is provided by a tax on each vaccine.[13] As of 2004, any vaccine that contains at least one of the following antigens is covered by VICP regardless of the patient's age: diphtheria, tetanus, pertussis, measles, mumps, rubella, polio, hepatitis B, Hib, pneumococcal, influenza, and varicella. In addition, hepatitis A is covered in states where the CDC recommends routine immunization. Customarily, as vaccines are added to the recommended Childhood and Adolescent Immunization

Schedule they are also added to the VICP, even though valid claims filed under VICP are not age dependent. Funds are available to provide treatment and rehabilitation costs that are not covered by private insurance. If this route of compensation is used, the right to institute legal proceedings against the manufacturer or individuals who prescribed or administered the vaccine is relinquished.[14] Reportable adverse events are not necessarily eligible for compensation. For example, a febrile seizure should be reported but is not compensable unless encephalopathy occurs within 72 hours.

ROUTINE PEDIATRIC AND ADOLESCENT IMMUNIZATIONS

The harmonized schedule for routine pediatric and adolescent immunizations is updated at least annually, and often more frequently (Table 73.4). Individual states have immu-

TABLE 73.4	Recommended Childhood and Adolescent Immunization Schedule

Vaccine ▼ / Age ►	Birth	1 month	2 months	4 months	6 months	12 months	15 months	18 months	24 months	4–6 years	11–12 years	13–18 years
Hepatitis B[1]	HepB #1	HepB #2			HepB #3						HepB Series	
Diphtheria, Tetanus, Pertussis[2]			DTaP	DTaP	DTaP		DTaP			DTaP	Td	Td
Haemophilus influenzae type b[3]			Hib	Hib	Hib	Hib						
Inactivated Poliovirus			IPV	IPV		IPV				IPV		
Measles, Mumps, Rubella[4]						MMR #1				MMR #2	MMR #2	
Varicella[5]						Varicella				Varicella		
Pneumococcal[6]			PCV	PCV	PCV	PCV			PCV	PPV		
Influenza[7]						Influenza (Yearly)				Influenza (Yearly)		
Hepatitis A[8]										Hepatitis A Series		

Vaccines below red line are for selected populations

This schedule indicates the recommended ages for routine administration of currently licensed childhood vaccines, as of December 1, 2004, for children through age 18 years. Any dose not administered at the recommended age should be administered at any subsequent visit when indicated and feasible.

■ Indicates age groups that warrant special effort to administer those vaccines not previously administered. Additional vaccines may be licensed and recommended during the year. Licensed combination vaccines may be used whenever any components of the combination are indicated and other components of the vaccine are not contraindicated. Providers should consult the manufacturers' package inserts for detailed recommendations. Clinically significant adverse events that follow immunization should be reported to the Vaccine Adverse Event Reporting System (VAERS). Guidance about how to obtain and complete a VAERS form are available at www.vaers.org or by telephone, 800-822-7967.

▨ Range of recommended ages
▨ Preadolescent assessment
▨ Only if mother HBsAg(–)
■ Catch-up immunization

nization requirements for day care and school enrollment that may be more or less stringent than the CDC's recommendations, but most state requirements are consistent with federal standards.

Misconceptions regarding contraindications and precautions to immunization result in a significant number of missed opportunities for vaccination. Sound clinical judgment that appropriately considers precautions and absolute contraindications should minimize missed vaccination opportunities and avoidable adverse events. With the exception of hepatitis B vaccine, which is administered at birth, routine pediatric immunizations begin when an infant is 6 to 8 weeks of age. Vaccination of infants should begin from the time of birth, regardless of the length of gestation; no adjustment of the schedule should be made for preterm infants.[8,12,15]

Routine pediatric immunizations currently recommended by CDC for all U.S. children include DTaP, Hib, hepatitis B, polio, MMR, varicella, influenza, and pneumococcal conjugate. The etiologic agent, disease manifestations, and complications prevented by these vaccines are briefly reviewed in Table 73.5.

DIPHTHERIA, TETANUS, PERTUSSIS

In Africa in 1999, WHO estimated there were 164,000 cases of tetanus and 110,000 deaths. The number of reported cases of neonatal tetanus in this region in 1998 was 4,838.[16] In the United States, 130 cases of tetanus were reported between 1998 and 2000, or an average of 43 cases each year, occurring most frequently in inadequately immunized persons or those with an unknown history of vaccination.[17] The annual number of cases of diphtheria in the United States has been no more than two per year since 1980. Active infection with diphtheria or tetanus does not necessarily confer immunity, and immunization during convalescence is required. All individuals should receive a primary series of diphtheria and tetanus vaccine and should receive a booster dose every 10 years throughout life.[8,18]

In 1934, the incidence of pertussis was more than 250,000, with 7,500 deaths.[18] The number of cases of pertussis dramatically decreased with vaccination. However, recent epidemiologic data have shown that the number of cases of pertussis is increasing.[19] In 2001, 2002, 2003, and 2004, respectively, there were 5,396, 8,296, 11,647, and 18,957 cases in the United States. Several reasons account for the steady increase seen in the number of cases since 1980, including an increased incidence in infants who have not yet received their complete series and who have been exposed to adolescent and adult carriers whose immunity to the disease has waned. Pertussis in adolescents and adults often goes unrecognized because the symptoms are often milder, and a severe persistent cough may be the only overt symptom of infection.[20–23] Neither active infection with pertussis nor receipt of the vaccine series provides lifelong immunity.[20,21,24] A review of 1996 cases in Vermont found that 68% of those who had pertussis (most cases of which were confirmed by culture) had received four pertussis vaccina-

tions.[25] U.S. vaccine manufacturers have brought an adult formulation of the pertussis vaccine.

Immunization against diphtheria, tetanus, and pertussis (DTP) was originally formulated with a whole-cell pertussis vaccine (DTwP). The pertussis vaccine component, believed to be the cause of many of the adverse reactions, was the endotoxin produced by *Bordetella pertussis*. A febrile response to DTwP was common and resulted in an increased risk for seizures in children with a preexisting neurologic disorder or provided the first pyrogenic stimulus for a febrile seizure.[18] Because of these effects, an acellular formulation of the vaccine (DTaP) was first licensed in 1991 for the fourth and fifth doses of the vaccine series; it was subsequently licensed for the entire series in 1996. Because of the decreased rate of side effects with DTaP, DTwP is no longer recommended in the harmonized schedule and is not available on the U.S. market.

Anaphylactic reactions are rare. Contraindications to vaccination include severe allergic reactions to a prior dose and the development of encephalopathy within 7 days of vaccination that is not identifiable to another cause. In the absence of a community-wide outbreak of pertussis, certain previous adverse events following pertussis vaccination are generally considered contraindications. These include persistent, uncontrollable crying for 3 hours or more within 48 hours, hypotonic-hyporesponsive state, a fever above 40.5°C (104.9°F) not attributable to another cause, or a seizure occurring within 72 hours of immunization. These side effects are extremely rare, occurring at 25% to 50% the rate of DTwP.[26] DT can be given to complete the primary series for tetanus and diphtheria in these patients.[12]

Precautions for the use of DTaP include moderate or severe acute illness. In these patients, vaccination should be deferred until the illness is resolved. Parents should be questioned about reactions to previous vaccinations before repeat doses are given. In most cases of progressive or unstable neurologic status unrelated to vaccine administration, vaccination should be delayed until the disorder has been treated or defined.[8] Pretreatment with acetaminophen (10 to 15 mg/kg) at the time of and 4 to 8 hours after immunization decreases the risk of some adverse effects.[27]

POLIO

In 1954, Jonas Salk developed an inactivated polio vaccine (IPV) that did not confer long-term immunity, nor did it provide mucosal (IgA) immunity. In 1961, Albert Sabin developed a live, attenuated oral polio vaccine (OPV) that protects against polio and induces gastrointestinal (GI) immunity. OPV resulted in lifelong immunity and is inexpensive and easy to administer. Since 1979, the only cases of polio in the United States have been vaccine-associated or imported from other countries where polio remains endemic. OPV immunization has virtually eradicated naturally occurring polio from the United States, and its continued use worldwide is considered important in the global eradication

TABLE 73.5	Diseases Prevented by Routine Pediatric Immunizations		

Causative Agent	Disease Manifestations	Disease Complications or Long-Term Sequelae	Comments
Corynebacterium diphtheriae (diphtheria)	Local inflammation and necrosis of mucous membranes resulting in the formation of plaquelike membranes	Cardiomyopathy, neuropathy, hepatic necrosis	Treated with diphtheria antitoxin and antibiotics. Disease does not induce immunity. Vaccination is required.
Bordetella pertussis (whooping cough)	1- to 2-week catarrhal stage with upper respiratory tract symptoms, followed by 3 weeks of severe paroxysmal coughing (whoops). Recovery is weeks to months.	Severe coughing can produce asphyxia, cerebral anoxia, seizures, coma. Permanent neurological damage or death can occur.	Most severe in young. Adolescents and adults may only have persistent severe cough and may be a reservoir for infection. Immunity duration after disease is unknown.
Clostridium tetani tetanus (lockjaw)	Pain, generalized muscle rigidity, and spasm that can be progressive	Airway obstruction, cyanosis asphyxiation	Treatment is supportive with tetanus immunoglobulin, antitoxin, and tetanus toxoid. Disease does not result in immunity.
Poliomyelitis enterovirus (spinal or bulbar polio)	90% of cases are asymptomatic. Minor infection: fever, malaise, headache, nausea	Paralysis, neurologic weakness	Cases previously reported in the United States were associated with OPV.
Morbillivirus (measles)	Prodrome (1–2 weeks): Koplik spots on buccal/pharyngeal mucosa, fever, cough, conjunctivitis, photophobia, coryza. Later: high fever, maculopapular rash on face and neck that spreads downward.	Otitis media, croup, diarrhea, thrombocytopenic purpura, death (3 in 1,000 cases), encephalitis (1 in 1,000 cases)	Highly contagious; active infection results in lifelong immunity.
Paramyxovirus (mumps)	Fever, neck muscle pain, malaise, and headache, unilateral or bilateral parotid gland swelling	Orchitis or epididymitis (45% in postpubertal males that can result in sterility, 7% postpubertal girls), encephalitis (1 in 6,000)	Repeat cases can occur.
Rubivirus (rubella)	Mild catarrhal symptoms, erythematous discrete rash, low-grade fever, cervical lymphadenopathy	Congenital rubella (50%–80% during 1st trimester), 10%–20% (2nd trimester), arthritis and neuritis more common in older females	Congenital rubella may result in low birthweight, hepatomegaly, splenomegaly, congenital heart disease, cataracts, hearing loss, or mental retardation.
Haemophilus influenzae type b	Meningitis, epiglottitis, pneumonia, septic arthritis, osteomyelitis, cellulitis, otitis media, pericarditis	Hearing loss, mental retardation, death	Disease in those >2 years old results in permanent immunity. Index case and close contacts need rifampin prophylaxis.
Hepatitis B virus	Acute hepatitis, jaundice, fatigue, hepatomegaly	Chronic hepatitis, cirrhosis, hepatocellular carcinoma. Asymptomatic carriers are a reservoir and transmit disease.	Spread through direct contact with body fluids. 90% of infants born to infected mothers become carriers or develop infection.
Influenza	Fever, myalgias, headache, nonproductive cough, sore throat, rhinitis	Secondary bacterial pneumonia, encephalopathy, transverse myelitis, Reye syndrome, myositis, myocarditis, pericarditis, death	Spread through respiratory droplets. Annual change in virus requires yearly vaccination.

(continues)

TABLE 73.5 | **continued**

Causative Agent	Disease Manifestations	Disease Complications or Long-Term Sequelae	Comments
Pneumococcus	Pneumonia, bacteremia, sinusitis, acute otitis	Meningitis, death	Most common manifestation is invasive bacteremia without a site of infection.
Varicella virus (chickenpox)	Fever, maculopapular rash with characteristic vesicular pruritic lesions	Group A streptococcal secondary infection, necrotizing fasciitis, encephalopathy, pneumonia	Active infection usually results in permanent immunity. Reactivation of latent virus results in zoster or shingles.

of polio. Wild polio was identified in 9 countries in 2002 and 15 countries in 2001.[28]

OPV has been preferred since its introduction in the 1960s owing to its high efficacy, low cost, ease of use, and resultant mucosal immunity. After OPV is given, the virus replicates and is present in the oral pharynx and GI tract for 6 to 8 weeks. Because of this, OPV should not be given at intervals less than 8 weeks, and at least two OPV doses are needed to provide mucosal immunity. Also, live virus shed in stool from vaccinated individuals enhances immunization rates by exposing unimmunized persons to the vaccine virus, thereby resulting in indirect immunization.[29]

Rarely, vaccine-associated paralytic polio (VAPP) occurred with OPV, most commonly with the first dose, in approximately one case per 750,000.[30] Those at increased risk included individuals with unknown immunodeficiency disorders at the time of vaccination and close contacts who were underimmunized or immunocompromised. In 1988, an improved and enhanced-potency inactivated vaccine was licensed and replaced the Salk vaccine.[31] Because viral shedding does not occur with IPV and VAPP has not been attributed to its use, IPV is now the preferred vaccine for use in the United States. Disadvantages with this vaccine are that it is more expensive, is administered by injection, and does not provide mucosal immunity.

Because the only cases of polio in the United States since 1979 have been either imported or have been associated with OPV, the CDC no longer recommends use of OPV in the harmonized pediatric schedule. Accordingly, the manufacturer of OPV suspended U.S. distribution in 2001.

Children should receive four doses of IPV as a primary series at 2 months, 4 months, 6 to 18 months, and 4 to 6 years of age. It is unlikely that any adult in the United States would have failed to receive a primary polio vaccine series, and thus routine immunization of adults is not recommended. An additional booster dose of IPV is recommended for adults traveling to regions of the world where polio is endemic.

IPV has a very mild side effect profile, with only pain and erythema at the injection site being commonly seen. Mild fever following vaccination is less common. Unlike OPV, IPV is safe for use in immunocompromised patients and in patients with immunocompromised household contacts.[30] IPV is not recommended for use in pregnancy unless the mother has never received the primary series and travel to an endemic region cannot be avoided, in which case the vaccine may be administered in the second or third trimester of pregnancy.

HAEMOPHILUS INFLUENZAE TYPE B

Before availability of an effective vaccine, Hib was the leading cause of bacterial meningitis in the United States, with about 20,000 cases per year. As many as 30% of all cases of Hib meningitis resulted in hearing loss or other long-term neurologic sequelae; 3% to 6% of cases resulted in death.[32] Hib is a polysaccharide-encapsulated bacteria. Often the polysaccharide of *H. influenzae* organisms can be identified by type, with multiple typable and nontypeable strains occurring. However, 95% of all invasive illness caused by *H. influenzae* is from the type b polysaccharide, and thus the illness is often referred to only by its abbreviated name.[33] Polysaccharide vaccines are poorly immunogenic, particularly in infants younger than 2 years of age, the age at which over two thirds of Hib meningitis cases occur. This is due to elicitation of a T-cell–independent response by polysaccharide vaccines, a process that requires B-cell response without T-helper cells. Conjugation of Hib polysaccharide with a protein shifts the immune response to a T-cell–dependent process.

Multiple conjugated vaccines are currently available on the U.S. market and are all indicated for use in the primary, four-dose vaccine series of 2, 4, 6, and 12 to 15 months of age. All of the currently marketed vaccines contain the polyribosylribitol phosphate (PRP) capsule of Hib, which is the portion of the organism to which antibody is produced.[33] Three different protein conjugates are used: Diphtheria CRM 197 Protein Conjugate (HbOC), Meningococcal Protein Conjugate (PRP-OMP), and Tetanus Protein Conjugate (PRP-T). One multiple antigen vaccine containing HbOC and DTaP is also available on the market in an effort to reduce the total number of injections required in the crowded pediatric schedule. The combination HbOC-DTaP vaccine is indicated for use whenever both DTaP and Hib appear at the same time on the harmonized schedule (i.e., 2, 4, 6, and 12 to 15 months of age). The CDC currently recommends that, whenever possible, the conjugate vaccine used for the first dose should be continued for all doses in the series. However, there is no need to restart the series if a different conjugate vaccine must be used.[9,34]

As with other conjugate vaccines, immunity is not conferred against the protein conjugate (i.e., meningococcus, tetanus, or diphtheria), and active immunization with available diphtheria- and tetanus antigen-containing vaccines should still occur in all children. Otitis media and upper respiratory tract infections in children are frequently caused by nontypeable *H. influenzae*, and the vaccine is not effective against these organisms.

Because of rapidly declining rates of clinical infection after age 2 and virtually no cases of invasive Hib infection observed after age 5, immunization against Hib is not indicated for older children or adults. The only exception is that individuals of any age with asplenia (functional or anatomic) or immunosuppression (i.e., HIV infection, leukemia) may receive one dose of Hib vaccine, since these populations are at increased risk of morbidity from Hib infection.[35] Individuals with immunoglobulin deficiency or Hodgkin's disease and those who are recipients of a bone marrow transplant or who are receiving chemotherapy may have a decreased response to Hib conjugate vaccination. Children with solid tumors have a 50% response rate to HbOC vaccine compared to children with leukemia, who have an 80% response rate.[35] Reports have shown that individuals with sickle cell disease, those who have undergone splenectomy, and those with HIV infection have a good response to Hib vaccination.[36–38]

Few adverse effects are associated with Hib vaccines. Approximately 25% of recipients experience pain and local redness or swelling at the site of injection. These reactions generally are mild and resolve in 24 hours. Systemic effects such as fever or irritability occur infrequently. When Hib is administered at the same time as DTaP, the incidence of these effects is not greater than with DTaP alone.

HEPATITIS B

Infection with hepatitis B virus (HBV) is a significant cause of morbidity and mortality owing to acute and chronic hepatitis, cirrhosis, and hepatocellular carcinoma. Chronic carriers may be asymptomatic and provide a reservoir for viral transmission. Universal immunization against HBV must be achieved to decrease HBV transmission and eradicate the disease.[39]

The risk of becoming chronically infected is inversely related to age at the time of infection; the youngest patients are at highest risk. The initial dose of the three-dose hepatitis B vaccine series should be administered immediately after birth and before discharge to home. If not treated, 80% to 90% of infants born to hepatitis B surface antigen (HBsAg)-positive mothers will become infected. The carrier state can be prevented in approximately 90% of infants who are given

the vaccine and hepatitis B immune globulin (HBIG) within 12 hours of birth. Thus, identification of HBsAg-positive mothers is important. This measure also may identify other contacts of the mother who are at risk of infection so they can be treated. Other groups at high risk include hemodialysis patients, those who receive blood products frequently, or those exposed to infected body fluids, such as blood or semen.

Hepatitis B vaccine is recommended for all infants and children before starting school. Those on hemodialysis or who are immunosuppressed may require larger dosages to induce antibody concentrations that are considered protective. Long-term follow-up in children and adults indicates that immune memory remains for 5 to 9 years, even though antibody titers decline.[39] Booster doses of HBV vaccine are not currently recommended; however, the CDC surveillance of HBV infection will confirm that vaccine-induced immunity continues. There is no need to restart the vaccine series if a delay is encountered between any of the doses in the series.

Healthcare workers should undergo serologic testing 1 month after completion of the series. An anti-HBs test result of at least 10 mIU per mL indicates immunity, and no further serologic testing should be performed. If the results are negative, the three-dose series should be repeated in the healthcare worker and anti-HBs testing repeated 1 to 2 months following the final dose. If the results are still negative, the healthcare worker is considered a nonresponder, and further vaccine doses and testing are unnecessary.[40] Routine serologic testing of vaccine recipients who are not healthcare workers is not indicated. However, individuals receiving hemodialysis, immunosuppressed patients with HBV exposure risk, including those with HIV, and patients being treated after exposure should be tested as indicated above for healthcare workers using the same protocol in the event of negative titers.

Most people who become infected acquire the disease as adolescents or adults. Healthcare workers, hospital staff, clients or staff of institutions for the mentally retarded, recipients of clotting factors, household contacts of HBV carriers, hemodialysis patients, men who have sex with men, persons with multiple heterosexual partners, and intravenous drug abusers are at increased risk for HBV infection and require preexposure hepatitis B vaccine. Persons requiring postexposure hepatitis B vaccine include infants born to carrier mothers, people with accidental percutaneous or permucosal exposure to infected blood, sexual partners of persons with acute HBV infection, and household contacts of persons with acute HBV infection.[12]

Between 1% and 6% of patients report injection site pain and temperature greater than 37.7°C (99.9°F) following vaccination. Allergy to the vaccine is reported rarely, and anaphylaxis has been reported to occur in about one in 600,000 doses. There has been no evidence of an association with HBV vaccine and Guillain-Barré syndrome since the introduction of the recombinant HBV vaccines. Furthermore, recombinant HBV vaccines have no potential for contamination with HIV.

INFLUENZA

Influenza viruses are orthomyxoviruses of three primary antigenic types: A, B, and C. Types A and B cause infection in humans and animals, while type C viruses are confined to animal hosts. Historically, influenza A infections have caused the majority of illnesses in the United States. The most likely explanation for this pattern is the ability of surface antigens present on the type A virus to mutate, thereby creating slight variations in the virulence and antigenicity of the virus from one influenza season to the next. Influenza B viruses mutate more slowly than influenza A viruses. The two surface antigens of influenza type A are hemagglutinin (H) and neuraminidase (N). An antigenic shift is a major shift in circulating virus that occurs in either the H or the N surface antigens. Antigenic drifts are minor variations within the same subtype. Since identification of subtypes has been available, human influenza epidemics and pandemics due to type A viruses have been associated with type A(H1N1) and type A(H2N3) antigens. Other subtypes of A viruses have appeared due to genetic reassortment and antigenic changes, but widespread disease has not occurred.

Vaccination against influenza is the best mechanism of disease protection. Influenza is characterized by the sudden onset of fever, headache, malaise, muscle aches, and cough. Respiratory symptoms often become more prominent with progression of the illness. In certain populations (i.e., immunocompromised, older adults), influenza may result in hospitalization, with progression to a viral or secondary bacterial pneumonia, respiratory distress, and death. Influenza epidemics have been responsible for an average of 36,000 deaths per year in the United States between 1990 and 1999.[41] During years of inactivated vaccine shortage, those at highest risk should receive priority for vaccine as soon as it becomes available, with mass immunization clinics being delayed until November and December. In the absence of a shortage, anyone seeking vaccination should be immunized. The ACIP notifies providers via the National Immunization Program (NIP) web site (www.cdc.gov/nip) and through *Morbidity and Mortality Weekly Report* (MMWR) of the priority groups and procedures for the current influenza season. Because of higher rates of morbidity and mortality from infection, the ACIP recommends that the following individuals receive an annual inactivated influenza vaccination: persons aged at least 65 years; residents of nursing homes and other chronic-care facilities that house persons of any age who have chronic medical conditions; adults and children who have chronic disorders of the pulmonary or cardiovascular systems, including asthma; adults and children who required regular medical follow-up or hospitalization during the preceding year because of chronic metabolic diseases (including diabetes mellitus), renal dysfunction, hemoglobinopathies, or immunosuppression (including immunosuppression caused by medications or by HIV); children and

adolescents (aged 6 months to 18 years) who are receiving long-term aspirin therapy and therefore might be at risk for experiencing Reye syndrome after influenza infection; women who will be pregnant during the influenza season; and children aged 6 to 23 months.[42] In October 2003, routine influenza vaccination for healthy infants aged 6 to 23 months was made a full recommendation by the ACIP. This was added to the harmonized pediatric and adolescent schedule beginning with the 2004 influenza season due to the increased risk of complications from influenza.[42] Vaccination is also recommended for persons aged 50 to 64 years because this group (approximately 42 million U.S. citizens) has an increased prevalence of persons with high-risk conditions (approximately 12 million with at least one high-risk condition).[43] The other group in which influenza vaccination is highly recommended is persons who can transmit influenza to those at high risk. This includes healthcare workers; employees of nursing homes, chronic-care facilities, and assisted living facilities; persons who provide home care to high-risk people; and household contacts of high-risk individuals. Recommendations for influenza vaccine were also made to include household contacts and out-of-home caregivers of infants less than 23 months of age.[42]

Live, attenuated influenza vaccine (LAIV) administered by nasal spray was approved by the FDA in June 2003.[44] It is indicated only for persons aged 5 to 49 years who are otherwise healthy. While efficacy studies have been conducted on children as young as 15 months of age and the vaccine has been shown effective, LAIV has not been evaluated relative to the administration of other vaccines (including those in the pediatric schedule), and its coadministration effects are unknown at this time.[45] Because nasal flu vaccine is a live, attenuated vaccine, it does have at least the theoretical potential to cause a mild case of influenza, although this was not observed in premarketing research performed on the vaccine.[46] Studies that have evaluated viral shedding from the vaccine virus, which relates to the risk of transmitting influenza vaccine virus to recipient contacts, also found that there was only slight viral shedding in nasal secretions after LAIV administration.[47] Little or no viral shedding was observed in patients with HIV and in patients over age 65 with a chronic disease.[48,49]

The most common adverse events associated with LAIV include runny nose and sore throat. Despite early studies showing efficacy in high-risk populations, further research is needed, and the vaccine should not be used in high-risk individuals for whom the inactivated vaccine is indicated.

MEASLES, MUMPS, RUBELLA

The number of reported measles cases declined drastically from the previous low of 309 in 1995 to 44 in 2002.[50] The incidences of mumps and rubella have remained low and continue to decline.[51] The incidence of congenital rubella syndrome (CRS) parallels the incidence of rubella and is amplified when outbreaks occur in unvaccinated populations of women of child-bearing age.[52] There were no cases of

CRS in the United States in 2003. Even though the vaccine is a live, attenuated vaccine requiring replication in the host to produce an immune response, there is no risk of transmission to household or casual contacts from vaccine recipients.

Several factors related to the MMR vaccine must be considered before administration. People born before 1957 likely had the disease and do not require immunization. MMR and the individual vaccines are live virus vaccines and should not be administered to immunosuppressed individuals, with the exception of young children with HIV infection. Individuals who are to receive immunosuppressive doses of steroids, chemotherapy, or radiation should be immunized either 2 weeks before or 3 months after therapy.[8,53] For those who receive immune globulin for measles prophylaxis during outbreaks, MMR can be given 5 months after a dose of 0.25 mL per kg in healthy individuals, or 6 months after a dose of 0.5 mL per kg in immunosuppressed individuals.[54] Therefore, the length of time a patient should wait to receive MMR vaccine depends on the dose of immune globulin received. Current recommendations from the CDC should always be consulted prior to vaccine administration.[54] Because of the presence of maternal antibodies, MMR vaccine should not be given earlier than 12 months of age and is recommended for use between 12 and 15 months of age as a primary dose followed by a booster dose at 4 to 5 years of age. The receipt of blood transfusion is also a valid reason for deferral of vaccination due to the presence of donor antibodies. Single-antigen measles and single-antigen mumps vaccines, as well as dual-antigen measles-mumps (MM) vaccine, are available on the U.S. market but should be used only if the patient has an absolute contraindication to the rubella component of the MMR vaccine.

Adverse events related to these vaccines are primarily clinical symptoms of mild disease. Symptoms consistent with subclinical measles infection occur from 6 to 11 days after immunization and include a transient rash, fever up to 39.4°C (102.9°F), headache, cough, sore throat, photophobia, and malaise. Although rare, seizures have been reported during the febrile episode, particularly in children less than 2 years of age. Arthralgias and joint pain have been reported in up to 25% of susceptible adult women 2 to 6 weeks after receiving rubella vaccines. Self-limited thrombocytopenia occurring within 2 months of vaccination is rare (one case per 30,000 to 40,000 doses).

Measles and mumps viruses used in the vaccine are grown in chick embryo cell culture, which raises a concern for patients with hypersensitivity to eggs. One strategy to vaccinate these individuals has been to perform scratch-and-prick tests to determine sensitivity, and to vaccinate using a desensitization protocol. One study evaluated MMR vaccination in children with hypersensitivity to egg protein and found that a positive skin test occurred in only 3 of 17.[55] Subsequent administration of MMR resulted in no immediate or delayed hypersensitivity.[55] The chance of reaction is remote because of the small amounts of egg cross-reacting protein present in the vaccine. Furthermore, skin testing for reactivity to vaccine is not predictive of allergic reactions. Current recommendations are to observe MMR vaccinees with egg hypersensitivity for 90 minutes after vaccination with the standard dosage. The vaccine should be given to these patients only in an environment with emergency equipment and appropriate personnel to treat anaphylaxis.[12]

PNEUMOCOCCAL DISEASE

Streptococcus pneumoniae is the leading cause of community-acquired pneumonia and the second leading cause of bacterial meningitis in the United States. With an estimated 40,000 deaths or more occurring each year, it is the leading cause of vaccine-preventable death in the United States in many years, being outpaced only by influenza deaths during epidemic years. There are 80 identifiable pneumococcal serotypes, 23 of which are responsible for 85% to 90% of worldwide disease isolates.[56-58] Emerging pneumococcal resistance increases the importance of immunization in high-risk individuals.[59,60]

Because *S. pneumoniae* is an encapsulated bacterium, production of a polysaccharide vaccine provided initial protection against the disease. A 14-valent pneumococcal vaccine was available for many years and was replaced in 1984 by the 23-valent vaccine (PPV) used today. Like other polysaccharide vaccines, efficacy is relatively low compared to other types of vaccine. The vaccine is 48% to 70% effective, with greater protection against pneumococcal bacteremia and meningitis than against pneumococcal pneumonia. Factors decreasing immunogenicity to PPV include older patients, patients with alcoholic cirrhosis or insulin-dependent diabetes mellitus, children 2 years of age or less, and patients who are immunocompromised. The vaccine is recommended for all individuals aged 65 years and older regardless of health status; patients aged 2 years or more with functional or anatomic asplenia; immunocompetent individuals aged 2 years or more who are at increased risk for illness and death related to pneumococcal disease due to chronic illness (i.e., diabetes, chronic lung disease excluding asthma, cardiac disease, alcoholism, chronic liver disease, or cerebrospinal fluid leaks); persons aged 2 years or more receiving immunosuppressive chemotherapy, including long-term systemic corticosteroids; persons aged 2 years or more who are immunocompromised due to illness (i.e., Hodgkin disease, leukemia, multiple myeloma, generalized malignancy, HIV infection, chronic renal failure, nephritic syndrome, organ and bone marrow transplant recipients, or other immunocompromised condition).

PPV is not immunogenic in children under age 2 for reasons stated earlier in this chapter. However, because pneumococcal meningitis is a significant cause of pediatric morbidity and mortality, in 2000, a 7-valent conjugated pneumococcal vaccine (PCV) was introduced to the market specifically for children. The vaccine is conjugated with a diphtheria protein carrier, which improves the immunogenicity of the vaccine and converts the immune response to a T-cell–dependent response to which infants can adequately respond. PCV does not provide protection against diphtheria, as the protein carrier itself is not immunogenic. Efficacy of PCV is as high as 97% against invasive pneumococcal disease and 73% against pneumonia.[59] Current recommendations for use of PCV are for all children aged 2 to 23 months, as well as children aged 24 to 59 months with an increased risk of pneumococcal disease, such as immunocompromising conditions including sickle cell disease, HIV, diseases requiring radiation therapy or chemotherapy, and renal disease, as well as children with chronic illness such as cardiac disease, diabetes, chronic pulmonary disease (excluding asthma unless on high-dose steroids), and cerebrospinal fluid leaks.[59] In addition, for children of African American or Native American descent, as well as all children aged 24 to 59 months in group daycare, the clinician should consider use of the vaccine due to the increased rates of pneumococcal disease in these populations. The primary series consists of four doses at 2, 4, 6, and 12 to 15 months of age. Patients over age 5 years who are at high risk for pneumococcal disease should receive PPV, since the efficacy of PCV in children over age 5 and adults has not been studied. Children at the highest risk of infection aged 24 months and over may receive PPV as long as the dose is given at least 2 months after the last dose of PCV.

The issue of repeat or ''booster'' doses of PPV has been a topic of much debate over the years. Because PPV elicits a T-cell–independent response, immunologic memory is not produced to a great degree; therefore, certain groups should receive a second dose of PPV at least 5 years apart. There appears to be no benefit to administering more than two doses of PPV in a patient's lifetime. It is acceptable for children who received the PCV series during childhood to receive PPV during later childhood, adolescence, or adulthood if indications warrant. Individuals who should receive a second dose of PPV include those with functional or anatomic asplenia, HIV infection, lymphoma, multiple myeloma, Hodgkin disease, generalized malignancy, chronic renal failure, nephritic syndrome, or organ or bone marrow transplantation or persons on chronic systemic steroid therapy. Persons who are aged 65 and older and who received their first dose of pneumococcal vaccine at least 5 years earlier and were less than 65 at their first vaccination should also receive a second dose of PPV. A few very-high-risk children may be revaccinated with PCV 3 years after their initial dose so long as they are aged 10 years or less, including children with functional or anatomic asplenia, nephrotic syndrome, renal failure, or renal transplantation.[59,60]

Few serious adverse effects have been reported with either PPV or PCV. Because the vaccines are inactivated, they cannot cause the disease they are designed to prevent. Discomfort, induration, and erythema at the injection site occur in about half of all PPV or PCV vaccine recipients. Systemic effects such as fever, muscle aches, chills, headache, nausea, and photophobia have infrequently been reported. PCV administered concomitantly with DTaP and other routine pediatric vaccines results in an increased inci-

dence of fever 100.4°F or higher compared to controls; however, the benefits of vaccinating children with both vaccines outweighs the risk of fever, and children should receive all vaccines concomitantly in a fashion consistent with the pediatric immunization schedule.[61] A meta-analysis of nine randomized, controlled pneumococcal vaccine efficacy trials including over 7,000 patients found no occurrences of anaphylaxis.[62]

VARICELLA

Varicella-zoster virus (VZV) is a highly contagious, usually self-limiting infection that may affect susceptible adults or children. Primary infection of VZV is commonly known as chickenpox. The virus is spread via respiratory droplet transmission or by contact with the lesions of reactivated latent zoster infection. In the early 1990s, disease transmission followed the birth cohort, with an infection rate of approximately 90% of annual births, or about 4 million cases per year. This resulted in about 11,000 annual hospitalizations and 100 deaths.[63] The severity of varicella is greater in neonates, infants less than 1 year of age, immunocompromised persons of any age, and adults. Much of the societal cost associated with varicella is related to the time parents lose from work to care for children who are not allowed to go to school or day care while the lesions remain.[64] Reactivation of the latent virus results in herpes zoster (shingles), and it involves the thoracic, cervical, lumbar, or sacral nerves, typically appearing along a single dermatome during any one episode.

The vaccine was first developed from a virus isolated from a child in Japan in the early 1970s. It was licensed for use in the United States in 1995 and is indicated primarily for all children aged 12 to 18 months. It may also be used in adults who have never been infected with VZV or who have never been immunized. The vaccine is a live, attenuated vaccine, and a mild breakthrough rash may occur following vaccination. The vaccine should be avoided during pregnancy, primarily due to the theoretical risks associated with live vaccines in this population. Protective efficacy of the vaccine is about 86% for any infection and approaches 100% in preventing severe disease in immunocompetent individuals with close contact.[65] Vaccination should be avoided for at least 5 months following administration of immunoglobulin. The vaccine should also be avoided in immunocompromised individuals.

Adverse effects associated with varicella vaccination include transient pain, tenderness, or redness at the injection site in 20% to 35% of vaccinees. Within 1 month, 8% develop a mild maculopapular or varicelliform rash with a few lesions. Vaccinees who develop breakthrough varicella have milder cases and a shorter duration of lesions than those who contract varicella naturally. Vaccinated children with leukemia who develop a rash may transmit the vaccine virus to susceptible contacts; however, the virus rarely has been recovered from these lesions in immunocompetent individuals.[66] Viral transmission from vaccinees who develop a varicella rash to immunocompromised contacts is not a sufficient reason to withhold vaccination. The effects of varicella immunization on the later occurrence of zoster are of concern. The occurrence of zoster appears to be directly related to the number of lesions (or vesicles); thus, those who have few lesions are at less risk for zoster. The full effect of varicella vaccination on adult varicella infection and cases of zoster in the future remains to be seen.

ROTAVIRUS

Rotavirus is the leading cause of dehydrating diarrhea in children less than 5 years of age; transmission is fecal–oral. Each year, rotavirus infection accounts for 70,000 hospital admissions and 100 deaths in the United States.[67] Serotypes 1, 2, 3, and 4 are responsible for the majority of human disease.

A live, attenuated virus oral vaccine that relied upon GI replication was removed from the market shortly after its introduction due to a relationship between the vaccine and the development of intussusception. Because of the morbidity and mortality of rotavirus illness, vaccine manufacturers are studying possible recombinant technology for development of an inactivated vaccine to replace the previous live virus vaccine.

NONROUTINE VACCINES

Vaccines that do not appear as part of the routine immunization schedule for either adults or pediatrics are listed in Table 73.2.

HEPATITIS A

First isolated in 1979, hepatitis A is a picornavirus. Humans are the only known natural host of this highly contagious disease that is transmitted by the fecal–oral route. The virus then replicates in the liver, with virus present in the bloodstream within 10 to 12 days of infection. Blood titers peak approximately 14 days prior to the onset of symptoms. Virus is excreted in the feces from just before onset of symptoms through approximately the third week of clinical illness. The incubation period of hepatitis A ranges from 14 to 50 days, with an average incubation of 28 days. Onset of symptoms is abrupt and indistinguishable from other forms of viral hepatitis. While most individuals have clinical resolution within 2 months, approximately 10% to 15% of patients will have prolonged signs and symptoms for up to 6 months. Infants and children younger than 6 years of age are typically asymptomatic. Because of underreporting and asymptomatic infections, the CDC estimates that as many as 180,000 cases of hepatitis A occur in the United States each year, for an incidence of 10 cases per 100,000 population.[9] Worldwide, 1.4 million cases are reported each year; it is believed that the actual number of cases is several times that, making hepatitis A one of the most common vaccine-preventable diseases worldwide.

Hepatitis A vaccine was first available in the United States in 1995. The vaccine is produced by propagation of cell-culture-adapted virus in human fibroblasts, purification from cell lysates, inactivation with formalin, and adsorption to an aluminum hydroxide adjuvant. One of the two available vaccines (HAVRIX, GlaxoSmithKline), is also prepared with the preservative 2-phenoxy-ethanol.[68] The vaccine is recommended for individuals planning international travel to an endemic area, regardless of length of stay. In 1999, ACIP recommended that routine vaccination of children 2 years of age and older be implemented in communities where the average annual incidence of hepatitis A is 10 cases per 100,000 population, or twice the U.S. average incidence. ACIP also recommends that the vaccine be considered in communities where the average incidence is 10 to 20 cases per 100,000 population. Additional high-risk groups who should receive the vaccine include Native American, Alaskan Native, Pacific Islander, and selected Hispanic communities, as well as certain religious communities. Drug users (both injecting and noninjecting), as well as men who have sex with men, should also receive the vaccine. Persons with clotting-factor disorders may be at increased risk of hepatitis A.[68]

The vaccine should be given at least 2 weeks prior to expected hepatitis A exposure (i.e., travel to endemic area), and completion of the series prior to potential exposure is desirable. It appears that both vaccines currently available are interchangeable, although completion of the two-dose series with the same product is preferable.[69] Table 73.4 outlines the recommended doses of the available vaccines. The efficacy of hepatitis A vaccination was demonstrated in Thai children living in an area with an outbreak rate of 119 cases per 100,000 population.[70] Antibody titers were increased for 4 years, and the authors suggested that protection may last as long as 20 years.[70] Adverse effects include injection site pain, erythema, and swelling. Mild systemic complaints of malaise, fatigue, and low-grade fever are rarely reported, and there have never been any reported serious adverse reactions associated with this vaccine.[9,68]

During hepatitis A outbreaks or when the first dose of vaccine cannot be given at least 2 weeks prior to travel to an endemic area, standard immune globulin may be given concurrently with vaccination. Immune globulin is more than 85% effective in preventing hepatitis A in these situations.[68]

LYME DISEASE

The causative agent for Lyme disease is *Borrelia burgdorferi*, a spirochete that uses the hard tick as its primary vector. Most cases are reported in the mid-Atlantic, northeastern, and midwestern United States; however, cases have been reported from 45 states. An initial local reaction, termed erythema migrans, occurs at the site of the tick bite and may be accompanied by fever, headache, and arthralgia. The initial lesion can expand over days to weeks to include an area more than 5 cm in diameter with vesicular or necrotic areas. Multiple erythema migrans occurs 3 to 5 weeks later and includes multiple lesions that are smaller than the initial rash. During this period, cranial nerve palsies, meningitis, and conjunctivitis can occur, in addition to arthralgia, myalgia, headache, and fatigue. Later disease occurs up to 1 year after exposure and is characterized by chronic arthritis and, in certain cases, encephalopathy and neuropathy.

The vaccine consists of the *B. burgdorferi* outer surface lipoprotein A (OspA) and is manufactured using recombinant technology. Immunization stimulates the formation of endogenous antibodies that are transferred to the attached tick and kill the spirochetes present in the tick midgut, thus preventing transfer of the spirochete into the human. Susceptible individuals between the ages of 15 and 70 years of age should receive three doses, the second 1 month after the first and the third 1 year after the first. Vaccine efficacy after the first dose was 49% or 68%; after the third dose, it was 76% or 92%.[71,72] Adverse effects that occur within 30 days of immunization include local reactions at the injection site, chills, fever, muscle aches, and flulike symptoms. While the vaccine is still FDA approved for use in the United States, the manufacturer has withdrawn the vaccine from the market due to disappointing demand.

MENINGOCOCCAL DISEASE

Neisseria meningitidis is a gram-negative diplococcus that causes meningococcemia with or without meningitis. The onset of fever, chills, malaise, and the characteristic rash is abrupt, and progression to disseminated intravascular coagulation, shock, coma, and death can occur within a few hours. Infection occurs most often in children less than 5 years of age, with most disease occurring in those 6 to 12 months of age. Although nine serotypes have been identified, groups B, C, Y, and W-135 are the most common causes of disease in the United States. Disease transmission is by aerosolized droplets from close personal contact with symptomatic individuals or asymptomatic colonized carriers. Approximately 3% of households with an index case will have more than one secondary case.

Two vaccines are currently available. One vaccine contains polysaccharide antigens for serotypes A, C, Y, and W-135; therefore, the immunologic response is generally poor in those less than 2 years of age.[73] Recently, a conjugate meningococcal vaccine was approved for patients ages 11 to 55 years. The ACIP recommends routine vaccination of adolescents 11 or 12 years of age. Guidelines for use in special situations have not been developed for the meningococcal conjugate vaccine at this time. Serotype B, one of the major causes of disease, is not included in either vaccine. In addition, a patient with meningococcal disease requires rifampin prophylaxis to eradicate nasopharyngeal carriage.

Meningococcal vaccination is routinely performed in the military. People who have functional or anatomic asplenia or complement deficiency should be vaccinated. During an epidemic, infants 3 to 18 months of age should be given two doses 3 months apart. After vaccination, the duration of immunity for serotype A in children less than 4 years of age is probably less than 3 years.[12] Adverse effects seen with meningococcal vaccine include mild local and systemic effects. Fever is more common in younger children but is rarely greater than 38.5°C (101.3°F).[73]

RABIES

Rabies is caused by an RNA virus of the rhabdovirus group that affects the central nervous system. Known natural reservoirs include skunks, foxes, raccoons, coyotes, and bats, but all mammals can be infected. Transmission is primarily by infected secretions, usually saliva, that are transmitted by a bite. Initially, the virus remains close to the wound; however, migration along a neuronal pathway to the central nervous system ultimately occurs. The incubation period is between 20 and 60 days but may be more than 6 months. Rabies has occurred secondary to a corneal transplant from a donor who unknowingly had rabies. The clinical manifestations of rabies can be divided into three stages: nonspecific prodrome, acute encephalitis, and profound dysfunction of brain stem centers. Recovery without intervention is rare and occurs slowly.

The most effective means of decreasing rabies in humans is the extensive rabies vaccination program conducted in domestic animals.[74] From 1980 to 1997 in the United States, 36 cases of rabies were reported in humans; 58% of these cases were from wild animal exposure.[75] Although rabies among humans is rare in the United States, every year approximately 16,000 to 39,000 persons receive postexposure prophylaxis.[76]

There are currently four formulations of three distinct inactivated rabies vaccines approved by the FDA. The vaccines are considered equally efficacious. Human diploid cell vaccine can be administered intradermally or intramuscularly (two different formulations) and is prepared from the Pitman-Moore strain of rabies virus grown on MRC-5 human diploid cell culture, concentrated by ultrafiltration, and inactivated with β-propiolactone.[77] Rabies vaccine adsorbed (RVA) is distributed only in Michigan by BioPort Corporation and is prepared from the Kissling strain of Challenge Virus Standard (CVS) rabies virus adapted to fetal rhesus lung diploid cell culture.[78] Purified chick embryo cell vaccine (PCEC), available in the United States since 1997, is prepared from the fixed rabies virus strain Flury LEP grown in primary cultures of chicken fibroblasts. The virus is inactivated with β-propiolactone.[75] Table 73.6 lists the available vaccines, as well as available postexposure rabies immunoglobulins (RIG).

Individuals who have a high risk for exposure to rabies, such as veterinarians and dog catchers, should receive preexposure prophylaxis against rabies. For pre-exposure immunization, injections are given on days 0, 7, and 28 (three doses), and intradermal injections (HDCV) may be appropriate. Routine serologic testing is recommended only for those who are immunosuppressed. Administration should be IM for pre-exposure rabies prophylaxis in individuals receiving

TABLE 73.6	Rabies Biologics—United States, 2004	
Human Rabies Vaccine	**Product Name**	**Manufacturer**
Human diploid cell vaccine (HFCV) Intramuscular Intradermal	Imovax Imovax Rabies I.D.	Aventis Pasteur
Rabies vaccine adsorbed (RVA) Intramuscular	Rabies Vaccine Adsorbed (RVA)	BioPort Corp.
Purified chick embryo cell vaccine (PCEC) Intramuscular	RabAvert	Chiron Corp.
Rabies immune globulin (RIG)	Imogam Rabies-HT	Aventis Pasteur
Rabies immune globulin (RIG)	BayRab	Bayer Corp. Pharmaceutical Div.

(Adapted from Human Rabies Prevention—United States, 1999. Recommendations of the Advisory Committee on Immunization Practices (ACIP), 2000.)

chloroquine or mefloquine for malaria prophylaxis. In this situation, intradermal injection of rabies vaccine may not result in an appropriate antibody response.

Unimmunized individuals who are acutely exposed should be immunized with the appropriate product given IM on days 0, 3, 7, 14, and 28.[12] Intradermal injections should not be used. RIG 20 IU per kg should be given as soon as possible, but no longer than 8 days after exposure, infiltrating as much of the dose around the bite as possible, with the remainder given IM at a site distant to vaccine administration. Persons who are previously immunized should receive two IM doses of vaccine, one immediately and one 3 days later. RIG should not be given to individuals who have been immunized before exposure.

Vaccination causes local discomfort, swelling, erythema, and induration in up to 90% of individuals; it usually subsides in 1 to 3 days. Up to 10% of patients have systemic reactions that include nausea, vomiting, abdominal pain, headache, malaise, and low-grade fever. An immune complexlike reaction characterized by urticaria with or without arthralgia, arthritis, or angioedema has been reported in up to 7% of individuals receiving boosters.[12,75] Anaphylactic reactions have been reported rarely. Once initiated, rabies prophylaxis should not be discontinued because of local or mild systemic reactions to the vaccine.

TUBERCULOSIS

Tuberculosis (TB) is a necrotizing bacterial infection caused by *Mycobacterium tuberculosis*. Occasionally, *Mycobacterium bovis* has caused human disease in the United States. After many years of decline, the incidence of TB in the United States has increased because of patients with AIDS developing secondary TB. In addition to an increased incidence, there has been an increase in the number of cases of TB that are resistant to multiple drugs.[79] Screening for TB exposure and infection is done through skin testing. Children should receive either the multiple puncture or the Mantoux TB skin test at about 15 months of age (concurrent with first MMR), before school entry, and during adolescence (14 to 16 years of age). Individuals in high-risk groups, including those who are contacts of adults with TB or those with HIV, immunosuppression, Hodgkin's disease, lymphoma, diabetes mellitus, chronic renal failure, and malnutrition, should receive annual TB skin tests.[12] See Chapter 76 for a complete discussion of tuberculosis.

The TICE strain of bacillus Calmette–Guerin (BCG) of *M. bovis* is used for this live vaccine. Administration is percutaneous using a multiple-puncture disk. Small, red papules appear at the site within 10 to 14 days of immunization and reach maximum intensity after 4 to 6 weeks. A tuberculin skin test is given 2 to 3 months after immunization. If the response is negative, a second dose of the vaccine should be given. Usually the site has completely healed and faded by 6 months, but some persons have a residual scar. Because vaccination should result in a positive TB skin test, this test is not useful for identifying TB in BCG vaccinees. Adverse effects include skin ulceration at the site, regional adenitis, and, occasionally, lupoid reactions. Osteitis has been reported from 4 months to 2 years after BCG vaccination in neonates; the incidence varies according to country, which may relate to the product used.[80]

A meta-analysis evaluating the occurrence of TB in those vaccinated with BCG found that the incidence was decreased by 50%.[79] The duration of protection is not known, but sensitivity to tuberculin skin testing has persisted for 7 to 10 years. Routine vaccination with BCG vaccine is not recommended. Candidates for vaccination include children in close contact with infected patients who are untreated, ineffectively treated, or resistant to treatment, and may include other groups that have an excessive new infection rate.[81] Because of the risk for development of disease, BCG is contraindicated in patients who are immunosuppressed or who have burns, symptomatic HIV, or skin infections.[12]

VACCINATION FOR TRAVEL

Travel to developing countries may expose the traveler to diseases that are endemic in other areas of the world. Immunization or prophylactic measures decrease the likelihood of contracting these diseases (see Table 73.3). Before traveling to areas outside the United States, travelers and healthcare providers should consult the CDC web site for up-to-date, destination-specific information about immunizations recommended or required, as well as prophylactic medications and other measures that are advised. This should be done as early as possible before anticipated travel to allow adequate time to obtain all necessary vaccinations.[82,83] The vaccines discussed here are used almost exclusively for international travel. However, a number of vaccines previously discussed, including hepatitis A, hepatitis B, Td, MMR, IPV, meningococcal, and influenza vaccines, may also be indicated based on a variety of factors.

CHOLERA

Cholera is a food- and water-borne illness characterized by severe, dehydrating diarrhea; it may be fatal. Cholera is problematic in regions where conditions are unsanitary. The inactivated cholera vaccine previously available in the United States resulted in adequate immunity in only 40% to 60% of vaccinees, the duration of effect was relatively short, and the vaccine was not effective against the most common serotype responsible for disease. For these reasons, cholera vaccination is no longer recommended by the CDC, and no country requires documentation of cholera vaccination prior to entry. Experimental live, attenuated oral cholera vaccines appear to be more effective, with fewer side effects. Travelers should consult the CDC for food and water precautions before visiting regions where cholera is endemic.

JAPANESE ENCEPHALITIS

Japanese encephalitis is a mosquito-borne viral disease that frequently is fatal. The disease rarely occurs on the main islands of Japan or in Hong Kong but is common in rural Asian rice-growing areas, where the infected mosquitoes thrive. The vaccine (JE-VAX, Aventis Pasteur) can be used in individuals more than 1 year of age; a three-dose schedule is recommended, with the first two immunizations given 1 week apart and the third dose given 1 or 3 weeks (preferred) after the second. Length of immunity is likely more than 1 year. Allergic reactions, including urticaria and angioedema, have occurred as late as 17 days after vaccination, and individuals should remain in an area where there is easy access to medical care for 10 days after vaccination. Thus, the immunization series must be completed more than 10 days before travel. Regardless of vaccination status, travelers should follow mosquito precautions in endemic areas.[84]

TYPHOID

Typhoid fever is caused by ingestion of water and food contaminated by *Salmonella typhi*. Vaccination is recommended for individuals who travel to rural areas of tropical countries or to areas where there are unsanitary conditions and an increased risk for disease exposure. Although immunization results in antibody production in 50% to 90% of individuals, the degree of immunity is not great and can be readily overcome with a large inoculum.

Two vaccines are available, including one administered intramuscularly (inactivated polysaccharide) and one that is given orally (live, attenuated). A third vaccine is provided by the U.S. government for military use. A single dose of inactivated vaccine produces seroconversion in approximately 93% of healthy adults, but the effect is not long-lasting. A booster is required every 2 years if reexposure is expected. The vaccine is approved for use in persons aged 2 years and older.[85]

The primary immunization series with Vivotif Berna (Swiss Serum and Vaccine Institute), the oral typhoid vaccine, consists of one capsule every other day for four doses. Capsules are stored in the refrigerator and should be taken with cool water about 1 hour before a meal. If these conditions are not followed, the series must be restarted. The oral vaccine is indicated in persons aged 6 years and older. This vaccine is contraindicated in persons with an acute febrile illness or acute GI illness, and in individuals receiving sulfa drugs or antibiotics. The same dosage and schedule is repeated every 5 years if reexposure to typhoid is expected.[85]

Side effects following oral typhoid vaccine are rare and not statistically different from placebo but may include abdominal discomfort, nausea, vomiting, fever, headache, rash, or urticaria. Inactivated polysaccharide typhoid vaccine causes a greater degree of side effects than oral vaccine, but in only about 1% of recipients; side effects may include headache, fever, and erythema or induration (≥ 1 cm).[85]

YELLOW FEVER

Urban yellow fever is transmitted from infected humans by the *Aedes aegypti* mosquito, which has been controlled or eliminated in many African and South American countries. Jungle yellow fever also is transmitted by mosquito vectors, and it is responsible for most yellow fever cases reported today. Those who will be traveling to rural endemic areas or laboratory workers who may be exposed to the virus should be vaccinated.[83,86] A single dose induces immunity that persists for more than 10 years. Infants less than 4 months of age should not be vaccinated because of the increased risk of encephalitis, and vaccination of infants from 4 to 9 months of age should be based on estimates of risk of exposure to yellow fever.[82] The vaccine is available only in yellow fever vaccination centers, where yellow fever vaccination certificates, required for entrance into some countries, are issued.

Up to 10% of vaccinees have mild headaches, myalgia, or low-grade fever from 5 to 10 days after immunization. Immediate hypersensitivity reactions are rare. Cases of fever, jaundice, and multiple organ system failure have been reported.[87] Yellow fever vaccine is a live virus vaccine grown in chick embryo culture; it should not be given to those who are immunocompromised or experience anaphylactic reactions to eggs. In these cases, an immunization waiver stating the contraindication may be sufficient to gain entrance into countries that require yellow fever immunization certificates. If the risk for yellow fever is high and immunization necessary, skin testing may be performed to determine the vaccine allergic potential. If skin tests are positive, a desensitization protocol can be accomplished by subcutaneous injection of 0.05 mL of a 1:10 dilution of vaccine followed by increasing amounts of full-strength vaccine of 0.05, 0.1, 0.15, and 0.2 mL every 15 to 20 minutes, with appropriate emergency equipment and qualified personnel available.[88]

PASSIVE IMMUNIZATION

Direct administration of nonspecific (e.g., immunoglobulin) or specific (e.g., antitoxin) antibodies results in short-term immunity. After the exogenous antibodies are metabolized, the immunity disappears and reexposure can result in infection. This is a prophylactic measure, and the duration of protection is limited and dose-related.

Immune globulin can be given without regard to the timing and spacing of inactivated vaccines. It should be administered simultaneous to inactivated vaccine in the event of postexposure prophylaxis (e.g., rabies exposure, tetanus exposure, hepatitis exposure). In general, immunization with a live virus vaccine (e.g., MMR, varicella) should be delayed for 2 to 11 months, depending on the dose of immune globulin that has been administered. Clinicians can consult the manufacturer's labeling or the CDC for specific recommendations. When concomitant dosing of immune globulin and a live virus vaccine occurs, the immunization should be repeated at an appropriate interval unless seroconversion is documented. The exception to this rule is yellow fever vaccine administration, because there is no apparent interference with the antibody response.

IMMUNE GLOBULIN

Immune globulin is used to provide exogenous antibodies to individuals who have immunodeficiency or certain autoimmune or infectious diseases, or who are exposed to certain infectious diseases. Immune globulin products are prepared from more than 1,000 donors to ensure a broad spectrum of antibodies; however, this results in a potential for viral contamination. To minimize this potential, all donor units are tested for viral contamination before fractionation. Furthermore, newer fractionation techniques are effective in removing or inactivating HIV in donor units spiked with the virus. The risk for transmission of HIV from immune globulin remains theoretical, and no cases of HIV infection have been directly attributed to infusion of immune globulin. However, several cases of hepatitis C were associated with two brands of immunoglobulin for intravenous use (IGIV),

which were voluntarily withdrawn from the market.[89] The manufacturing process has since been modified to include a solvent detergent treatment designed to inactivate viruses. Other viral inactivation procedures being used now include incubation at low pH, enzyme addition, and pasteurization.

A different type of concern was the discovery that individuals who died of Creutzfeldt-Jakob disease, a rare, slowly progressive neurologic disease caused by prions, had donated blood that was used in the preparation of IGIV products. Although the risk of transmitting Creutzfeldt-Jakob disease through IGIV infusion is theoretical, the FDA recommended withdrawal of IGIV that contained plasma from donors (a) subsequently diagnosed with Creutzfeldt-Jakob disease; (b) with blood relatives who have Creutzfeldt-Jakob disease; (c) who received pituitary-derived human growth hormone; or (d) who received a dura mater transplant. This withdrawal resulted in a significant shortage of blood products, including IGIV.

Because IGIV is a purified immune globulin product that is infused intravenously, larger dosages of immune globulin can easily be given. IGIV is produced by a variety of manufacturers and varies in immune globulin concentrations, IgA content, manufacturing techniques, additives, product form, storage requirements, and FDA-approved indications.

IGIV is used primarily to treat immunodeficiency syndromes resulting from a lack of or impaired function of immunoglobulin. In patients with IgG subclass deficiency, IGIV is reserved for those who have recurrent infections. Other approved indications include infection prophylaxis in bone marrow transplant patients more than 17 years of age, children with HIV, and patients with chronic lymphocytic leukemia. IGIV treatment prevents or reduces the number of infections in people with immunodeficiency. An IgG concentration less than 200 mg per dL (normal $\geq$1,500 mg/dL) is associated with an increased risk for sudden, overwhelming bacterial infection. Increasing serum concentrations to more than 400 mg per dL is sufficient in most cases.[90] Although the lowest effective dosage is 150 mg per kg, an IGIV dosage of 200 to 400 mg per kg per month is used in most patients.[90] In addition to use in immunodeficiencies, IGIV is approved for use in treating idiopathic thrombocytopenic purpura and Kawasaki disease. Although the precise mechanism for efficacy in these diseases is not known, it is likely due to immunomodulation.

IGIV has been used to treat many other diseases. The University Hospital Consortium Expert Panel made recommendations for off-label use of IGIV that included patients with Guillain-Barré syndrome, severe posttransfusion purpura, and chronic inflammatory demyelinating polyneuropathy.[91] IGIV also has been used in patients with burns, multiple myeloma, cytomegalovirus infection, and neonatal sepsis, but its routine use in these conditions is not recommended.[90,91]

Up to 10% of patients who receive IGIV have nausea, vomiting, chills, fever, malaise, fatigue, dizziness, headache, urticaria, tightness in the chest, flushing, dyspnea, and pain in the chest, hip, or back. These effects are usually related to the rate of infusion and can be managed by stopping the infusion until the symptoms subside and restarting the infusion at a lower rate. Pretreatment with acetaminophen, diphenhydramine, or glucocorticoids can decrease side effects. Patients with IgA deficiency are at risk for developing anaphylaxis owing to anti-IgA antibody formation; they should receive products with the lowest IgA concentration.

The protein content of immune globulin for intramuscular use (IGIM) is about 165 mg per mL. IGIM is used to provide passive immunity to individuals within 2 weeks of exposure to hepatitis A, non-A non-B hepatitis, measles, and rubella. A dose of 0.02 mL per kg given before or within 2 weeks of exposure to hepatitis A is 80% to 90% successful in preventing infection.[12] For exposure to measles, a dose of 0.25 mL per kg in healthy individuals or 0.5 mL per kg in immunosuppressed or immunodeficient individuals, but not to exceed a total of 15 mL, given within 6 days of exposure can decrease morbidity or prevent the disease. Measles vaccination should be deferred 5 months in those who receive 0.25 mL per kg and 6 months in those receiving 0.5 mL per kg.[54] Because of the large volume, the dosage may need to be divided and administered at multiple sites. Associated adverse effects are primarily pain at the injection site and, less commonly, flushing, headache, chills, and nausea.[12] IGIM should not be infused intravenously.

HYPERIMMUNE GLOBULINS

Immune globulin products with high concentrations of specific antibodies are used to provide immunity against specific diseases. These products are made from the serum of individuals with increased concentrations of the specific antibody. All plasma used to prepare hyperimmune globulin products is negative for HBsAg. Hyperimmune globulin products include cytomegalovirus (CMVIG), hepatitis B (HBIG), tetanus (TIG), rabies (RIG), Rhesus (RhIG), varicella zoster (VZIG), and respiratory syncytial virus (RSV-IGIV).[12,39,92–98] CMVIG and RSV-IGIV are administered intravenously, whereas the other products are given IM. The use of these products is reviewed in Table 73.7. The usual adverse effects are local pain and tenderness at the site of injection for products given IM; fever, rash, and, rarely, anaphylactic shock may occur. Other hyperimmune globulin products are being studied and may find a place in therapy for specific indications such as *Pseudomonas aeruginosa* immune globulin in cystic fibrosis.

TABLE 73.7	Hyperimmune Globulins
Product	**Indication and Use**
Cytomegalovirus immune globulin (CMVIG)	Used in renal, liver, and bone marrow transplant patients. Some controversy remains as to whether the benefits of CMVIG outweigh the increased cost over IVIG.[92,93]
Hepatitis B immune globulin (HBIG)	Postexposure to hepatitis B. Should be given within 24 hours of percutaneous exposure and within 14 days of sexual contact. Neonates born to HBsAg-positive or unknown status mothers are given HBIG and the first dose of hepatitis B vaccine within 12 hours of birth.[39]
Rabies immune globulin (RIG)	Postexposure to rabies given concurrently with vaccine. RIG should be administered within 7 days of initiation of the vaccination schedule. Not to be used in individuals previously vaccinated.[75]
Rh (rhesus) immune globulin (RhIG)	Rh-negative mother following delivery of an Rh-positive fetus to prevent subsequent infant deaths from erythroblastosis fetalis.[91] Ideally, given within 72 hours of delivery but may given up to 28 days after. Should be given regardless of the duration of pregnancy.
	Rh-positive children with acute and chronic idiopathic thrombocytopenic purpura (ITP) and adults with chronic ITP. Doses vary depending on patient's hematocrit. In vivo hemolysis can occur and result in anemia.[95,96]
Respiratory syncytial virus immune globulin (RS IVIG)	Prevention of RSV infections in high-risk premature infants and children <24 months with bronchopulmonary dysplasia. Infusions are given once a month during RSV season. Fluid overload is problematic. Not indicated in those with congenital heart disease.[98]
Tetanus immune globulin (TIG)	Postexposure for tetanus-prone wounds and active tetanus infection. Administer with Td (a) if minor wound and >10 years since Td; (b) if major wound and >5 years since Td; and (c) if Td primary immunization series incomplete.[18]
Varicella zoster immune globulin (VZIG)	Postexposure to high-risk individuals including (a) children <15 years old who have not had varicella; (b) persons who are immunocompromised; (c) infants born to mothers who develop varicella 5 days before or 2 days after delivery; and (d) premature infants <28 weeks' gestation. Administer within 48 hours for maximum benefit and no later than 96 hours following exposure.[97]

ANTITOXINS

Antitoxins are derived from equine serum; therefore, the risk for severe allergic reactions including anaphylaxis is increased, and special precautions must be taken prior to administration. First, a careful history of past allergic responses (especially to animals) should be elicited because these individuals may be extremely sensitive to antitoxins. Then a scratch test or ''eye test'' should be performed to determine an individual's sensitivity; if the result is negative, a small amount of very dilute antitoxin is injected intradermally.[12] A negative response to the intradermal test dose does not rule out the possibility of a systemic reaction. Indications for the use of antitoxins are very limited, and these products should be used only in the presence of an appropriately trained individual with the necessary emergency equipment available. Usually antitoxin is given IM; however, in some cases, intravenous infusion may be used. The risk for a systemic reaction with intravenous infusion is increased; thus, doses should be dilute and infused very slowly, and the patient should be monitored closely. Antitoxins are available through the CDC for the treatment of diphtheria, tetanus, and botulism.

IMMUNOCOMPROMISED HOST

The antibody response to immunization in immunocompromised individuals is less than in healthy individuals, but usually the response is adequate. In some situations, as with hepatitis B vaccination, it is prudent to measure antibody concentrations and give boosters if antibody concentrations fall. Because endogenous immunity is not intact in these individuals, live vaccines may have enhanced or prolonged viral replication, resulting in systemic disease. Patients who are immunosuppressed because of disease (e.g., malignancy, immune deficiency syndromes) or who are receiving immunosuppressants (e.g., high-dose steroids, chemotherapy, irradiation) should not be given live virus vaccines (OPV, MMR, varicella, oral typhoid, BCG, and yellow fever) because of the risk for development of active disease, with the exception that children with HIV should receive MMR.[99]

Individuals with asymptomatic HIV infection should receive inactivated vaccines. The AAP and ACIP recommend that children with HIV receive routine pediatric immunizations (DTaP, IPV, MMR, Hib) regardless of symptoms.[12] In addition, the AAP and ACIP recommend immunizing children with symptomatic HIV infection against pneumococcal infection and influenza.[12,100] Varicella vaccination is not recommended in children with HIV.[12]

Cancer patients may be immunosuppressed owing to the malignancy, poor nutritional status, or anticancer therapy (e.g., irradiation, chemotherapy). Patients with active malignant disease should not be given live vaccines. Although killed vaccines and toxoids may be given, the degree of immune response to the immunization depends on the chemotherapeutic agent being used and may be inadequate to confer immunity. Whenever possible, vaccines should be given before radiation or chemotherapy. Patients more than 2 years old with Hodgkin lymphoma should be immunized with pneumococcal and Hib vaccines 10 to 14 days before therapy is started. Patients who have not received chemotherapy for 3 to 4 weeks may have an adequate antibody response to influenza vaccine. Live virus vaccines, such as varicella, can be given to patients who are in remission from leukemia when 3 months have elapsed since the last chemotherapy was administered.

After immunosuppressive therapy has been discontinued, a quantitatively normal immunologic response usually develops 3 to 12 months later. Corticosteroids given as replacement therapy (e.g., Addison's disease); topical steroid therapy; long-term alternate-day therapy with low to moderate doses of short-acting steroids; or single-dose intraarticular, bursal, or tendon injections are not usually immunosuppressive, and live virus vaccine administration is not contraindicated in patients receiving these.[12] Those who receive prednisone-equivalent dosages of 2 mg per kg or 20 mg or greater (in those >10 kg) a day or every other day for 14 days or less can be given a live virus vaccine immediately after discontinuation of the glucocorticoid; however, some clinicians advocate waiting 2 weeks. Patients receiving prednisone-equivalent dosages of 2 mg per kg or more than 20 mg (in those >10 kg) a day or every other day for more than 14 days should not receive live virus vaccine until they have been off glucocorticoids for at least 1 month.[12]

Individuals with functional (e.g., sickle cell disease) or anatomic asplenia have an increased risk of infection from encapsulated microorganisms; the risk appears to be greatest in children. Pneumococcus is the most common encapsulated pathogen in splenectomized individuals. Immunization with the pneumococcal, meningococcal, and Hib vaccines is recommended for all asplenic individuals more than 2 years of age.

PREGNANCY AND LACTATION

The consequences of natural infection and the likelihood of exposure must be balanced against the risk of immunization for both the mother and baby during pregnancy and lactation.[8,101] No vaccine has been shown to cause harm to either the mother or the fetus during pregnancy; however, it is generally recommended that vaccines be avoided during the first trimester and that live vaccines be deferred in the mother until after birth. Inactivated influenza vaccine is specifically indicated during pregnancy during influenza season.[42] In addition, Td is recommended in the third trimester in women who have not received a Td booster within the previous 10 years and in those previously unimmunized against tetanus and diphtheria.[18] In general, passive immunization with immune globulin is considered safe for pregnant women.[8,12]

Immunization with the MMR live, attenuated virus vaccine is contraindicated in pregnancy. Because of the potential risk of fetal rubella infection, women of child-bearing age who are vaccinated with these agents should be counseled to avoid conception for 28 days following immunization.[102] Although immunization with MMR should be avoided immediately before and during pregnancy, published findings of women who inadvertently received the rubella vaccine within 3 months of conception reported no evidence that the vaccination was responsible for congenital rubella syndrome.[51] Congenital varicella is associated with significant fetal abnormalities; therefore, varicella vaccine should not be given within 1 month of a planned pregnancy or during pregnancy.[12] Manufacturers of live vaccines (i.e., MMR and varicella) have established registries to track inadvertent pregnant vaccine recipients and the associated outcomes. The clinician can consult the manufacturer's labeling or the CDC web site for more information. Routine pregnancy testing prior to vaccination is not recommended. A pregnant mother is not a reason to defer vaccination (either live or inactivated) in children living in the household.

An unimmunized and pregnant woman who anticipates travel outside the United States and exposure to wild-type polio virus should be immunized with IPV, although due to decades of aggressive polio immunization initiatives in the United States, it is highly unlikely this situation would arise.[3] If travel to an area with a high risk for contracting yellow fever cannot be postponed, the yellow fever vaccine should be given.[8,86]

The postpartum period is thought to be a good time to review the woman's immunization status and update any necessary immunizations. Breast-feeding is not adversely affected by immunizations in the infant or mother, and lactation is not a contraindication to immunization with any agent.[8,12] Most live viruses from vaccines are not transferred to breast milk. Although there may be transfer of antibody to the infant who is fed with breast milk, this is not associated with any difficulties. Infants who are breast-fed should be immunized according to the usual schedule. Immunization should not be adjusted for gestation in preterm infants.

PHARMACY CONSIDERATIONS

Pharmacists, as drug therapy experts, should be up to date on current vaccines and immunoglobulin preparations, including indications for use, contraindications, adverse effects, vaccine composition, storage recommendations, and reconstitution if applicable. The primary goal should be to protect public health while minimizing adverse reactions and maximizing patient response. The package insert should be consulted for specific product information, and the CDC should be consulted regularly for current recommendations. Pharmacists should also be knowledgeable about the proven science of vaccines. A variety of myths exist in the lay press and public regarding vaccine adverse effects and contraindications. Many of these myths have been debunked in prominent scientific and governmental documents, most accessible from the Internet (www.vaccinesafety.edu). As of May 2004, the Institute of Medicine has published eight reports on immunization safety (www.iom.edu/reports).

Although rare, individuals who experience anaphylactic reactions to eggs may have a similar reaction to a vaccine grown in chick embryo culture. MMR, influenza vaccine (both inactivated and live, attenuated), and yellow fever vaccines are all grown in egg culture. MMR can generally be safely given to patients with an egg allergy. Desensitization or a graded protocol can be used for other vaccines grown in chick embryo cultures, but patients should generally be referred to an allergist/immunologist or primary care physician for immunization. Rather than administer influenza vaccine in egg-allergic patients, the use of antivirals (e.g., rimantadine, rinamivir) for prophylaxis is preferred.

Trace amounts of antibiotics (e.g., neomycin, streptomycin) or preservatives (e.g., thimerosal) added to immunobiologics may be responsible for hypersensitivity reactions. Delayed minor reactions attributed to neomycin or streptomycin have been reported between 48 and 96 hours after immunization with MMR. Anyone with a history of anaphylactic reaction to neomycin or streptomycin should not receive vaccines that contain these antibiotics. No vaccine contains penicillin or any antibiotic other than neomycin and streptomycin. Mercury, from thimerosal, may accumulate in individuals who receive repeated courses of IGIM; however, thimerosal in the minute quantities found in certain vaccines has never been proven to cause adverse events in infants or children.[103]

Antisera or antitoxins of animal origin are likely to cause allergic reactions. Horse serum is used to produce diphtheria, tetanus, and botulism antitoxins; equine antirabies serum; and antivenins. Biologicals of equine origin are inherently immunogenic; thus, all patients should undergo a scratch test or eye test using a dilution of the product before treatment to determine the intensity of precautions to be taken during administration.

Safe handling and storage of vaccines and immunobiologics are essential to ensure vaccine potency and to prevent vaccine failure.[104] Pharmacists should be familiar with the usual appearance of lyophilized and reconstituted products to help validate that product integrity was maintained during transport, and to ensure that product degradation did not occur during storage. The shelf-life should be validated and expiration dates noted, and the appropriate storage conditions should be maintained. Care must be taken to ensure timely reconstitution before immunization to maintain potency and prevent vaccine failure.

Pharmacist-administered immunization is a tremendous health service that can be offered in the community and ambulatory setting. Vaccine records must be perpetual and not purged with other pharmacy data. In addition, most systems are computerized; therefore, prescription data can be screened for identification of high-risk patients and information can easily be shared with other healthcare providers. Pharmacists involved in administering immunizations should receive advanced credentials in immunizations or complete advanced immunization training before graduation from pharmacy school. Pharmacists should also be certified in cardiopulmonary resuscitation (CPR) or basic cardiac life support in the unlikely event that anaphylaxis should occur in a vaccine recipient.

FUTURE IMMUNIZATION THERAPY

A renewed commitment to disease prevention has focused attention on developing safer and more efficacious immunizations, simplifying schedules, increasing vaccine supplies, developing more combination vaccines, expanding locations for vaccine administration, and producing new immunizations for diseases that currently are not preventable.[105] Several combination vaccines for pediatric use have been introduced to the U.S. market in recent years, as has a combination hepatitis A and hepatitis B vaccine for adolescents and adults. Additional combination vaccines are under development to further simplify the pediatric schedule. An adult pertussis vaccine will likely be approved by the FDA in the near future.

Vaccine development for HIV has been a slow and tedious process. Because of the ability of HIV to mutate, the creation of an effective vaccine has been elusive. However, international research, including phase 2 and 3 clinical trials, is ongoing to find a safe, effective HIV vaccine.

Immunizations of the future may be derived from a component of an organism that stimulates the immunologic response. They also may be an "empty" viral particle or they may be manufactured using recombinant DNA technology. Different administration routes are being explored, including further development of intranasal aerosols and development of time-release capsules. One manufacturer is researching hydrogen-propelled intradermal injection of particles attached to gold molecules for seroconversion of hepatitis B nonresponders. The further development of safer, more effective vaccines will have a positive impact on decreasing infectious diseases, provided that immunizations are administered to the appropriate target population.[106]

Finally, the use of "therapeutic" vaccines is an emerging area of research. Anticancer vaccines designed to either prevent, such as human papillomavirus vaccine development, or treat various tumors are the focus of a tremendous amount of financial and expert resources. Therapeutic vaccines are being explored to treat a host of conditions that have an immune component to their etiology. Certainly the next decade will prove pivotal as breakthroughs are made in immunology and vaccine development.

PHARMACOECONOMICS

The economic benefits of universal routine pediatric immunizations and immunizing targeted groups at increased risk for influenza and pneumococcal disease are unquestioned. Because of its preventative nature, vaccination is generally more cost-effective than treatment of the diseases. The decision to introduce a vaccine into the market must take into account the incidence of disease, the cost of treating the disease, and the budget available to support vaccination.[107] Politics can influence the decision as much as medical and economic factors. The quality of economic studies has been quite variable, but economics will play a larger role in future discussions as more immunizations are developed.[108]

KEY POINTS

- Immunization prevents potentially devastating diseases in infants, children, adolescents, and adults.
- To improve quality of life through disease prevention, immunizations are being offered in a variety of nontraditional settings, including pharmacies, businesses, and community settings.
- Adverse effects associated with immunizations are related to the type of immunization. In general, adverse effects associated with inactive or killed vaccines are related to the injection site and consist of redness and soreness. Fever also can occur soon after injection. Immunization with live vaccines results in subclinical infection in immunocompetent individuals, and the adverse effects mimic those seen with the disease. Individuals who are immunocompromised should not receive live vaccines.
- As changes in vaccination protocols occur, they are published in the *Morbidity and Mortality Weekly Review* (*MMWR-CDC*), in *Pediatrics,* and in various other medical journals. The CDC provides the most current online immunization information, including ACIP recommendations, at the National Immunization Program web site (www.cdc.gov/nip).
- Immune globulin is used to provide exogenous antibodies to individuals who have immunodeficiency or certain autoimmune or infectious diseases, or who are exposed to certain infectious diseases.
- Antitoxins are derived from equine serum; therefore, the risk for severe allergic reactions, including anaphylaxis, is increased, and special precautions must be taken prior to administration.

REFERENCES

1. Certification of poliomyelitis eradication—the Americas, 1994. MMWR 43:720–722, 1994.
2. Brief report: global polio eradication initiative strategic plan, 2004. MMWR 53:107–108, 2004.
3. CDC. Background on global polio eradication initiative. http://www.cdc.gov/nip/global/stopteam/backgrd.htm (accessed 6/14/04).
4. Healthy People 2010. http://www.healthypeople.gov (accessed 6/14/04).
5. Janeway CA, Travers P, Walport M, et al., eds. Immunobiology: the immune system in health and disease, 5th ed. New York: Garland Publishing, 2001.
6. van den Dobbelsteen GP, van Rees EP. Mucosal immune responses to pneumococcal polysaccharides: implications for vaccination. Trends Microbiol 3:155–159, 1995.
7. Offit PA, Jew RK. Addressing parents' concerns: do vaccines contain harmful preservatives, adjuvants, additives, or residuals? Pediatrics 112:1394–1401, 2003.

8. CDC. General recommendations on immunization. recommendations of the Advisory Committee on Immunization Practices (ACIP) and the American Academy of Family Physicians (AAFP). MMWR 51:1–35, 2002.
9. CDC. Epidemiology and prevention of vaccine-preventable diseases, the pink book, 8th ed. Atlanta: CDC Publications, 2004 http://www.cdc.gov/nip/publications/pink/default.htm (accessed 6/14/04).
10. Braun MM, Ellenberg SS. Descriptive epidemiology of adverse events after immunization: reports to the Vaccine Adverse Event Reporting System (VAERS), 1991–1994. J Pediatr 131:529–535, 1997.
11. Surveillance for safety after immunization: vaccine adverse event reporting system (VAERS), United States: 1991–2001. MMWR 52:1–23, 2003.
12. American Academy of Pediatrics. 2003 Red book report of the Committee on Infectious Diseases, 26th ed. AAP, 2003.
13. Bartell LA, Charney SA. National vaccine injury compensation act: a viable alternative to litigation? J Pharm Pract 2:36–44, 1989.
14. Clayton EW, Hickson GB. Compensation under the National Childhood Vaccine Injury Act. J Pediatr 116:508–513, 1990.
15. Bernbaum J, Draft A, Samuelson J, et al. Half-dose immunization for diphtheria, tetanus, pertussis: response of preterm infants. Pediatrics 83:471–476, 1989.
16. World Health Organization. Neonatal tetanus. http://www.afro.who.int/nnt/factsandfigures.html (accessed 6/14/04).
17. Tetanus surveillance, United States, 1998–2000. MMWR 52:1–8, 2003.
18. CDC. Diphtheria, tetanus, and pertussis: recommendations for vaccine use and other preventive measures. Recommendations of the ACIP. MMWR 40:1–28, 1991.
19. Bass JW, Wittler RR. Return of epidemic pertussis in the United States. Pediatr Infect Dis J 13:343–345, 19940.
20. Halperin SA, Bortolussi R, MacLean D, et al. Persistence of pertussis in an immunized population: results of the Nova Scotia enhanced pertussis surveillance program. J Pediatr 115:686–693, 1989.
21. Cromer BA, Goydos J, Hackell J, et al. Unrecognized pertussis infection in adolescents. Am J Dis Child 147:575–577, 1993.
22. Aoyama T, Takeuchi Y, Goto A, et al. Pertussis in adults. Am J Dis Child 146:163–166, 1992.
23. Nelson JD. The changing epidemiology of pertussis in young infants. The role of adults as reservoirs of infection. Am J Dis Child 132:371–373, 1978.
24. CDC. Pertussis vaccination: use of acellular pertussis vaccine among infants and young children. MMWR 46:1–25, 1997.
25. CDC. Pertussis outbreak—Vermont, 1996. MMWR 46:822–826, 1997.
26. Decker MD, Edwards KM, Steinhoff MC, et al. Comparison of 13 acellular pertussis vaccines: adverse reactions. Pediatrics 96(Suppl): 557–566, 1995.
27. Ipp MM, Gold R, Greenberg S, et al. Acetaminophen prophylaxis of adverse reactions following vaccination of infants with diphtheria-pertussis-tetanus toxoids-polio vaccine. Pediatr Infect Dis J 6: 721–725, 1987.
28. CDC. Laboratory surveillance for wild and vaccine-derived polioviruses, January 2002–June 2003. MMWR 53:913–916, 2003.
29. McBean AM, Modlin FJ. Rationale for the sequential use of inactivated poliovirus vaccine and live attenuated poliovirus vaccine for routine poliomyelitis immunization in the United States. Pediatr Infect Dis J 6:881–887, 1987.
30. CDC. Polio prevention in the United States. Updated recommendations of the Advisory Committee on Immunization Practices (ACIP). MMWR 49:1–22, 2000.
31. Adenyl-Jones SC, Faden H, Ferdon MB, et al. Systemic and local immune responses to enhanced-potency inactivated poliovirus vaccine in premature and term infants. J Pediatr 120:686–689, 1992.
32. Broome CV. Epidemiology of Haemophilus influenzae type b infections in the United States. Pediatr Infect Dis J 6:779–782, 1987.
33. CDC. Haemophilus b conjugate vaccines for prevention of Haemophilus influenzae type b disease among infants and children 2 months of age and older: recommendations of the ACIP. MMWR 40:1–7, 1991.
34. CDC. Recommendations for use of Haemophilus b conjugate vaccines and a combined diphtheria, tetanus, pertussis, and Haemophilus b vaccine: recommendations of the Advisory Committee on Immunization Practices (ACIP). MMWR 42:1–15, 1993.
35. Shenep JL, Feldman S, Gigliotti F, et al. Response of immunocompromised children with solid tumors to a conjugated vaccine for Haemophilus influenzae type b. J Pediatr 125:581–584, 1994.
36. Frank AL, Labotka RJ, Rao S, et al. Haemophilus influenzae type b immunization of children with sickle cell diseases. Pediatrics 82: 571–575, 1988.
37. Jakacki R, Luery N, McVerry P, et al. Haemophilus influenzae diphtheria protein conjugate immunization after therapy in splenectomized patients with Hodgkin disease. Ann Intern Med 112: 143–144, 1990.
38. Steinhoff MC, Auerbach BS, Nelson K, et al. Effect of protein conjugation on immune response of HIV-infected adults to H. influenzae type b (Hib) polysaccharide (PS) vaccine. In: Program and Abstracts of the 30th Interscience Conference on Antimicrobial Agents and Chemotherapy, Atlanta, GA, Oct. 21–24, 1990.
39. American Academy of Pediatrics Committee on Infectious Diseases. Universal hepatitis B immunization. Pediatrics 89;795–800, 1992.
40. Immunization Action coalition. Hepatitis B and the healthcare worker fact sheet (www.immunize.org, accessed 2/22/04).
41. Thompson WW, Shay DK, Weintraub E, et al. Mortality associated with influenza and respiratory syncytial virus in the United States. JAMA 289:179–186, 2003.
42. CDC. Prevention and control of influenza: recommendations of the Advisory Committee on Immunization Practices. MMWR 52:1–39, 2004.
43. Fukuda K, O'Mara D, Singleton JA. Drug shortages, part 4: how the delayed distribution of influenza vaccine created shortages in 2000 and 2001. Pharm Ther 27:235–242, 2002.
44. CDC. Using live, attenuated influenza vaccine for prevention and control of influenza. Supplemental recommendations of the Advisory Committee on Immunization Practices (ACIP). MMWR 53: 1–8, 2004.
45. Belshe RB, Mendelman PM, Treanor J, et al. The efficacy of live attenuated, cold-adapted, trivalent, intranasal influenza virus vaccine in children. N Engl J Med 338:1405–1412, 1998.
46. Nichol KL, Mendelman PM, Mallon KP, et al. Effectiveness of live, attenuated intranasal influenza virus vaccine in healthy, working adults. JAMA 282:137–144, 1999.
47. Zangwill KM, Droge J, Mendelman P, et al. Prospective, randomized, placebo-controlled evaluation of the safety and immunogenicity of three lots of intranasal trivalent influenza vaccine among young children. Pediatr Infect Dis J 20:740–746, 2001.
48. King JC, Treanor J, Fast PE, et al. Comparison of the safety, vaccine virus shedding, and immunogenicity of influenza virus vaccine, trivalent, types A and B, live cold-adapted, administered to human immunodeficiency virus (HIV)-infected and non-HIV-infected adults. J Infect Dis 181:725–728, 2000.
49. Jackson LA, Holmes SJ, Mendleman PM, et al. Safety of a trivalent live attenuated intranasal influenza vaccine, FluMist, administered in addition to parenteral trivalent inactivated influenza vaccine to seniors with chronic medical conditions. Vaccine 17: 1905–1909, 1999.
50. CDC. Summary of notifiable diseases, United States 2002. MMWR 51:1–84, 2004.
51. CDC. Measles, mumps, rubella-vaccine use and strategies for elimination of measles, rubella, and congenital rubella syndrome and control of mumps: recommendations of the Advisory Committee on Immunization Practices (ACIP). MMWR 47:1–57, 1998.
52. Rubella and congenital rubella syndrome—United States, January 1, 1992–May 7, 1994. MMWR 43:391–401, 1994.
53. CDC. Use of vaccines and immune globulins in persons with altered immunocompetence. Recommendations of the Advisory Committee on Immunization practices. MMWR 42:1–18, 1993.
54. American Academy of Pediatrics Committee on Infectious Diseases. Recommended timing of routine measles immunization for children who have recently received immune globulin preparations. Pediatrics 93:682–685, 1994.
55. James JM, Burks AW, Roberson P, et al. Safe administration of the measles vaccine to children allergic to eggs. N Engl J Med 332:1262–1266, 1995.

56. Butler JC, Breiman RF, Lipman HP, et al. Serotype distribution of *Streptococcus pneumoniae* infections among preschool children in the United States, 1978–1994: implications for development of a conjugate vaccine. J Infect Dis 171:885–9, 1995.

57. Robbins JB, Austrian R, Lee CJ, et al. Considerations for formulating the second-generation pneumococcal capsular vaccine with emphasis on the cross-reactive types within groups. J Infect Dis 148:1136–1159, 1983.

58. Butler JC, Breiman RF, Campbell JF, et al. Pneumococcal polysaccharide vaccine efficacy: an evaluation of current recommendations. JAMA 270:1826–1831, 1993.

59. Preventing pneumococcal disease among infants and young children: recommendations of the Advisory Committee on Immunization Practices (ACIP). MMWR 49:1–35, 2000.

60. Prevention of pneumococcal disease: recommendations of the Advisory Committee on Immunization Practices (ACIP). MMWR 46:1–24, 1997.

61. Black S, Shinefield H, Fireman B, et al. Efficacy, safety, and immunogenicity of heptavalent pneumococcal conjugate vaccine in children. Pediatr Infect Dis 19:187–195, 2000.

62. Fine MJ, Smith MA, Carson CA, et al. Efficacy of pneumococcal vaccination in adults: a meta-analysis of randomized controlled trials. Arch Intern Med 154:2666–77, 1994.

63. Jumaan A, Hughes H. Schmid S. Varicella. In: Vaccine-preventable diseases surveillance manual, 3rd ed. Atlanta, GA: Centers for Disease Control, 2002.

64. Lieu TA, Cochi SL, Black SB, et al. Cost-effectiveness of a routine varicella vaccination program for US children. JAMA 271:375–381, 1994.

65. Izurieta HS, Strebel PM, Blake PA. Postlicensure effectiveness of varicella vaccine during an outbreak in a child care center. JAMA 278:1495–1499, 1997.

66. Gershon AA, Steinberg SP, Gelb L, et al. Live attenuated varicella vaccine use in immunocompromised children and adults. Pediatrics 78(Suppl):757–762, 1986.

67. Ho M-S, Glass RI, Pinsky PF, et al. Rotavirus as a cause of diarrheal morbidity and mortality in the United States. J Infect Dis 158:1112–1116, 1988.

68. Prevention of hepatitis A through active or passive immunization: recommendations of the Advisory Committee on Immunization Practices. MMWR 48:1–37, 1999.

69. Feinstone S, Gust I. Hepatitis A vaccine. In: Plotkin S, Orenstein W, ed. Vaccines, 3rd ed. Philadelphia: WB Saunders, 1999:650–671.

70. Innis BL, Snitbhan R, Kunasol P, et al. Protection against hepatitis A by an inactivated vaccine. JAMA 271:1328–1334, 1994.

71. Steere AC, Sikand VK, Meurice F, et al. Vaccination against Lyme disease with recombinant *Borrelia burgdorferi* outer-surface lipoprotein A with adjuvant. N Engl J Med 339:209–215, 1998.

72. Sigal LH, Zahradnik JM, Lavin P, et al. A vaccine consisting of recombinant *Borrelia burgdorferi* outer-surface protein A to prevent Lyme disease. N Engl J Med 339:216–222, 1998.

73. Peltola H, Safary A, Kayhty H, et al. Evaluation of two tetravalent $(ACYW_{135})$ meningococcal vaccines in infants and small children: a clinical study comparing immunogenicity of O-acetyl-negative and O-acetyl-positive group C polysaccharide. Pediatrics 76:91–96, 1985.

74. Fishbein DB, Robinson LE. Rabies. N Engl J Med 329:1632–1638, 1993.

75. CDC. Human rabies prevention—United States, 1999, Recommendations of the Advisory Committee on Immunization Practices (ACIP). MMWR 48:1–21, 1999.

76. Krebs JW, Long-Marin SC, Childs JE. Causes, costs and estimates of rabies postexposure prophylaxis treatments in the United States. J Public Health Manage Pract 4:57–63, 1998.

77. Wiktor TJ, Plotkin SA, Koprowski H. Development and clinical trials of the new human rabies vaccine of tissue culture (human diploid cell) origin. Dev Biol Stand 40:3–9, 1978.

78. CDC. Rabies vaccine, adsorbed: a new rabies vaccine for use in humans. MMWR 37:217–218, 223, 1988.

79. Colditz GA, Brewer TF, Berkey CS, et al. Efficacy of BCG vaccine in the prevention of tuberculosis. JAMA 271:698–702, 1994.

80. Advisory Council for the Elimination of Tuberculosis and the ACIP. The role of BCG vaccine in the prevention and control of tuberculosis in the United States. MMWR 45:1–18, 1996.

81. Smith KC, Green HL. A case for Bacillus Calmette-Guerin vaccine in United States-born children. Pediatr Infect Dis J 18:15–17, 1999.

82. Hill DR, Pearson RD. Health advice for international travel. Ann Intern Med 108:839–852, 1988.

83. Wolfe MS. Vaccines for foreign travel. Pediatr Clin North Am 37:757–769, 1990.

84. CDC. Inactivated Japanese encephalitis vaccine. Recommendations of the Advisory Committee on Immunization Practices (ACIP). MMWR 42:1–15, 1993.

85. CDC. Typhoid immunization. Recommendations of the Advisory Committee on Immunization Practices (ACIP). MMWR 43:1–7, 1994.

86. CDC. Yellow fever vaccine: recommendations of the Advisory Committee on Immunization Practices (ACIP), 2002. MMWR 51:1–10, 2002.

87. Adverse events associated with 17D-derived yellow fever vaccination, United States 2001–2002. MMWR 51:989–993, 2002.

88. Aventis Pasteur, Inc. YF-VAX (product information). Swiftwater, PA: Aventis Pasteur, Inc, 2004.

89. Schneider L, Geha R, Magnuson WG. Outbreak of hepatitis C associated with intravenous immunoglobulin administration—United States, October 1993–June 1994. MMWR 43:505–509, 1994.

90. Phelps SJ, Reynolds MA, Tami JA, et al. ASHP therapeutic guidelines for intravenous immune globulin. ASHP Commission on Therapeutics. Clin Pharmacol 11:117–136, 1991.

91. Ratko TA, Burnett DA, Foulke GE, et al. Recommendations for off-label use of intravenously administered immunoglobulin preparations. JAMA 273:1865–1870, 1995.

92. Snydman DR, Werner BG, Dougherty NN, et al. A further analysis of the use of cytomegalovirus immune globulin in orthotopic liver transplant patients at risk for primary infection. Transplant Proc 26(Suppl 1):23–27, 1994.

93. Glowacki LS, Smaill FM. Meta-analysis of immune globulin prophylaxis in transplant recipients for the prevention of symptomatic cytomegalovirus disease. Transplant Proc 25:1408–1410, 1993.

94. Duerbeck NB, Seeds JW. Rhesus immunization in pregnancy: a review. Obstet Gynecol 48:801–810, 1993.

95. Andrew M, Blanchette VS, Adams M, et al. A multicenter study of the treatment of childhood chronic idiopathic thrombocytopenic purpura with anti-D. J Pediatr 120:522–527, 1992.

96. Blanchette V, Imbach P, Andrew M, et al. Randomised trial of intravenous immunoglobulin G, intravenous anti-D, and oral prednisone in childhood acute immune thrombocytopenic purpura. Lancet 344:703–707, 1994.

97. CDC. Advisory Committee on Immunization Practices. Recommendations on varicella-zoster immune globulin for the prevention of chickenpox. MMWR 33:84–100, 1984.

98. American Academy of Pediatrics Committee on Infectious Diseases. Respiratory syncytial virus immune globulin intravenous: indications for use. Pediatrics 99:645–650, 1997.

99. CDC. Recommendations of the Advisory Committee on Immunization Practices (ACIP): use of vaccines and immune globulins in persons with altered immunocompetence. MMWR 42:1–18, 1993.

100. Onorato IM, Markowitz LE, Oxtoby MJ. Childhood immunization, vaccine-preventable diseases, and infection with human immunodeficiency virus. Pediatr Infect Dis J 7:588–595, 1988.

101. Saballus MK, Lake KD, Wager GP. Immunizing the pregnant woman. Postgrad Med 81:103–113, 1987.

102. CDC. Revised ACIP recommendations for avoiding pregnancy after receiving a rubella-containing vaccine. MMWR 50:1117, 2001.

103. Institute of Medicine. Immunization safety review: thimerosal-containing vaccines and neurodevelopmental disorders. http://www.iom.edu/reports (accessed 6/14/04).

104. Casto DT, Brunell PA. Safe handling of vaccines. Pediatrics 87:108–112, 1991.

105. Ellis RW, Douglas RG. New vaccine technologies. JAMA 271:929–931, 1994.

106. Ada G. Vaccines and vaccination. N Engl J Med 345:1042–1053, 2001.

107. Kou U. More vaccines? Using economic analysis to decide. Bull World Health Org 80:263, 2002.

108. Walker D, Fox-Rushby JA. Economic evaluation of communicable disease interventions in developing countries: a critical review of the published literature. Health Economics 9:681–698, 2000.

Upper Respiratory Infections

74

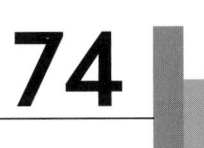

David E. Nix

THE COMMON COLD

TREATMENT GOALS: THE COMMON COLD

- Avoid use of antimicrobial agents.
- Relieve symptoms by treatment with acetaminophen and decongestants (adults) throughout the course of the illness.
- Symptoms should start improving within 5 to 7 days.

The common cold is not a single infectious disease, but rather a group of self-limiting viral upper respiratory infections (URIs) producing a similar clinical syndrome. The average preschool child contracts approximately 6 to 10 colds per year, and the average adult has 2 to 4 colds annually. Colds account for $25 billion in productivity loss, including $16.6 billion in on-job productivity loss, $8 billion in absenteeism, and $230 million in caregiver absenteeism. On average, adults with a cold lose 8.7 hours of work time due to absenteeism and reduced productivity.[1] Roughly 23 million lost work days and 26 million missed school days are the result of the common cold each year.[2] Many more people continue their usual activities with lower productivity and uncomfortable symptoms. Furthermore, expenditures for products used to treat cold symptoms exceed $2.5 billion annually after adjusting for inflation.[3,4]

The common cold is generally regarded as a mild condition that rarely causes significant morbidity. However, serious exacerbations of underlying disease may occur in patients with asthma or preexisting obstructive lung disease.[5] Patients with the common cold are also more susceptible to acquiring otitis media and sinusitis.[6–8]

EPIDEMIOLOGY

The common cold is caused by a number of viruses, including rhinovirus, coronaviruses, respiratory syncytial virus

(RSV), parainfluenza virus, adenovirus, enterovirus, influenza A virus, and influenza B virus. Rhinovirus is by far the most common: it is isolated in 52% to 53% of patients with cold-like symptoms.[9,10] There are more than 100 different antigenic types of rhinovirus.[11] Influenza A virus and coronaviruses were isolated from 5% to 9% of patients. Occasionally, more than one viral agent was isolated (5%) or viral agents were isolated along with potential bacterial pathogens (3%), including *Chlamydia pneumoniae*, *Mycoplasma pneumoniae*, *Streptococcus pneumoniae*, and *Haemophilus influenzae*.[10] With state-of-the-art diagnostic methods in one study, the etiology could not be established in 30% of patients with cold-like symptoms.

Rhinovirus is present year-round, but the incidence of infection peaks in the early spring (April and May) and autumn, reaching the highest incidence in the autumn.[10,12] The incidence of infection from coronaviruses, the second most common viral agents, peaks in the early summer and again in the autumn to early winter. Coronavirus has been detected in up to 30% of URIs.[13] The pattern of RSV infection is similar to that for rhinovirus, but the peak incidence is slightly later in the spring (April through June) and autumn (October through November). The isolation of influenza A virus from patients with cold-like symptoms is indicative of a mild influenza illness, and the incidence is expected to follow trends in influenza illness within a community. Parainfluenza virus type 3 is present in summer months and is associated with annual outbreaks or epidemics.[14] Isolation of adenovirus is fairly constant throughout the year.[10]

Transmission of the common cold may occur by direct contact with nasopharyngeal secretions or by inhalation of small and large airborne particles.[15,16] Viruses can be isolated from the hands of patients with the common cold. Transmission may occur with a simple touch or handshake.[17] Cold viruses can remain viable on hands for about 2 hours. In addition, nasal secretions after being deposited on inanimate objects (e.g., door handles or faucets) may harbor viable virus particles for several days.[18] The uninfected individual acquires the virus on his or her hands, then inoculates the mucosal surfaces by touching the face, nose, or eyes.[16] Transmission can be prevented by washing hands frequently with disinfectants, by using virucidal tissues, and perhaps by avoiding facial and eye contact with the hands, but these methods are not very practical. One study suggested that aerosol transmission is an important mode of transmission in adults.[17]

CLINICAL PRESENTATION AND DIAGNOSIS

SIGNS AND SYMPTOMS

The incubation period for the common cold after exposure varies by specific etiology. The symptoms of rhinovirus infection may begin as early as 16 hours after inoculation. The incubation period for coronaviruses is 24 to 48 hours,

whereas RSV and parainfluenza viruses have an incubation period of 72 hours. Signs and symptoms of the common cold include sore throat, nasal obstruction, nasal stuffiness, mild fever, sneezing, watery eyes, hoarseness, cough, headache, malaise, myalgia, sinus pain, and postnasal discharge. Tyrrell et al[19] reported signs and symptoms of volunteers who were infected experimentally with rhinovirus ($n = 71$), RSV ($n = 11$), or coronavirus ($n = 34$). The signs and symptoms were similar despite differences in the viral etiology, although cough and hoarseness were more prevalent and nasal obstruction less common with one of the three strains of rhinovirus. The average percentage of patients experiencing a particular symptom is given in Table 74.1.

Typically, the common cold begins as a sore "scratchy" throat and progresses to include nasal stuffiness and nasal obstruction. The pharynx may be slightly red, with signs of postnasal drainage; however, marked redness and exudate suggest pharyngitis rather than the common cold. With the common cold, sore throat generally resolves within 24 to 72 hours. The nasal discharge is initially thin but becomes thicker within a day or so. Infection caused by adenoviruses and enteroviruses is more often associated with fever, pharyngitis, and systemic symptomatology.[20] Usually, influenza presents with high fever (38.5°C or higher), pronounced malaise, prostration, and myalgia, but mild cases of influenza may mimic cold-like symptoms. The common cold may last 2 to 14 days; about 7 to 10 days is most common.

DIAGNOSIS

The common cold is diagnosed based on clinical signs and symptoms and exclusion of more serious illnesses. Because of the self-limiting nature of the common cold and the lack of effective treatment, there is no indication for performing viral cultures or other specific diagnostic testing. In very

TABLE 74.1	Average Percentage of 116 Volunteers Exhibiting Various Symptoms After Experimental Infection with Cold Viruses (Rhinovirus, Respiratory Syncytial Virus, or Coronavirus)		
Symptom	**%**	**Symptom**	**%**
Nasal stuffiness	95	Sinus pain	21
Nasal obstruction	91	Chills	18
Sore throat	80	Myalgia	14
Sneezing	72	Postnasal discharge	12
Headache	40	Evening fever	7
Malaise	39	Morning fever	6
Watery eyes	30	Cervical adenitis	3
Cough	25	Sputum production	3
Hoarseness	25		

(From Dick EC, Jennings LC, Mink KA, et al. Aerosol transmission of rhinovirus colds. J Infect Dis 156:442–448, 1987.)

TABLE 74.2	Symptomatic Differences Between the Common Cold and Influenza	
Symptom	**Common Cold**	**Influenza**
Fever	None to mild (<100.5° F)	102–104° F; lasts 3–4 days
Headache	None to mild	Prominent
General aches	None to slight	Usual; often severe
Fatigue and weakness	Mild	Usual; may last 2–3 weeks
Exhaustion	Rare	Early and prominent
Stuffy nose	Common	Sometimes
Sore throat	Common	Sometimes
Sneezing	Usual	Sometimes
Cough, chest discomfort	Mild	Common, can become severe

(Adapted with modifications from NIAID, http://www.vrc.nih.gov/publications/pdf/ColdAllergy.pdf, accessed 8/10/05.)

young children, common cold symptoms may precede croup or bronchiolitis. In young adults and children older than 4 years, the cold-like symptoms need only to be distinguished from allergies and vasomotor rhinitis. Because influenza results in more serious complications and carries a significant risk of mortality in elderly patients, this disease must be distinguished from the common cold. Table 74.2 lists general differences between the common cold and influenza. Knowing the patterns of URIs within a region is helpful to distinguish the common cold from influenza and other infections. The presence of lower respiratory symptoms such as wheezing can, in most cases, be used to exclude the common cold. However, infection with cold viruses in patients with asthma and underlying obstructive pulmonary disease may exacerbate the underlying illness.

After about 3 days of symptoms, the common cold should not progress further in terms of severity. Most patients will exhibit only rhinitis, nasal congestion and obstruction, and possibly mild cough. Significant worsening of symptoms after 3 days or the presence of conjunctivitis, laryngitis, pharyngitis, muscle aches, or lower respiratory signs should bring the diagnosis of the common cold into question.[20] Wheezing in patients without a history of asthma is also of concern. However, patients with asthma or airway hyperresponsiveness may experience increases in wheezing, particularly in response to exercise, for weeks after having the common cold.

TREATMENT

There is no widely accepted specific therapy for the common cold. Use of interferon nasal spray,[21] zinc gluconate loz-

enges,[22] high-dose vitamin C,[23] and investigational antiviral drugs[24–29] has shown limited or no benefit in shortening the duration of symptoms and/or reducing viral shedding. High-dose vitamin C (at least 1 g/day) may provide a small benefit, but this benefit is controversial.[23] In addition, several of the treatments (interferon, zinc gluconate, and antiviral drugs) are associated with significant side effects. Zinc gluconate lozenges are unpalatable. A nasal spray containing soluble intercellular adhesion molecule 1 (ICAM-1) was shown to reduce cold symptoms by almost 50% when used before or within 12 hours after experimental rhinovirus infection. ICAM-1 is responsible for binding of rhinovirus to susceptible nasopharyngeal cells, permitting virus entry. Soluble ICAM-1 is a competitive inhibitor of this binding. It is likely that this therapy will be expensive if it becomes available. Moreover, it is not clear whether treatment given beyond 12 hours after exposure to rhinovirus would be effective.[30]

Current therapy for the common cold focuses on symptomatic relief and includes analgesics, systemic and topical decongestants, and antihistamines. Aspirin and acetaminophen suppress the development of antibodies and prolong the duration of viral shedding.[31] These agents reduce fever, which may be a protective response to infection, but fever is present in only a small minority of patients. Aspirin and acetaminophen may be useful to reduce headache, malaise, and muscle aches if they are present. However, these agents should not be used routinely for the common cold. The association of aspirin use and Reye's syndrome in children with influenza warrants further caution in the routine use of aspirin.[32] This association has not been described in association with the common cold. However, influenza sometimes mimics the common cold and Reye's syndrome has been reported, although rarely, with adenoviruses and parainfluenza viruses. Ibuprofen and naproxen have no detrimental effect on serum antibody response and virus shedding and appear effective for relieving some cold symptoms.[31,33]

The use of antihistamines to relieve cold symptoms is controversial. Histamine does not appear to play a significant role in the pathogenesis of the common cold. First-generation antihistamines possess anticholinergic action, which may reduce nasal secretions. The use of a sustained-release formulation of brompheniramine was effective for reducing sneezing, rhinorrhea, and cough after experimentally induced rhinovirus colds.[34] In patients with natural colds, clemastine provided some symptomatic relief of rhinorrhea and sneezing, but the effects appeared less prominent.[35] A review of studies before 1996 concluded that antihistamines do not have major effects on overall cold symptoms, although some attenuation of sneezing and rhinorrhea may occur.[36] These minor benefits must be weighed against the potential for side effects, primarily somnolence and dry mouth and throat. In young children, benefits of antihistamines have not been demonstrated other than to induce somnolence.[18] These agents are not approved for use in children less than 6 years old, although use is common. Intranasal ipratropium bromide, an anticholinergic agent, is efficacious for reducing rhinorrhea and sneezing.[37]

Systemic and topical decongestants have been widely used to relieve nasal congestion. Topical solutions of oxymetazoline, xylometazoline, and phenylpropanolamine are rapidly effective in relieving congestion and improving nasal airflow.[38] With xylometazoline, this effect persists for 6 hours. These agents are indicated only for short-term use (3 days or less) because rebound congestion can occur with more prolonged use. Systemic decongestants, including pseudoephedrine and phenylpropanolamine, also are effective for symptomatic relief. Phenylpropanolamine was recently removed from the market due to increased risk of hemorrhagic stroke. A recent study showed that oral pseudoephedrine is more effective than placebo for relieving nasal congestion.[39] None of the decongestants have been shown to be effective in young children.[18]

Intranasal and inhalation formulations of sodium cromoglycate (cromolyn sodium), used every 2 hours for the first 2 days, then four times daily thereafter, provide symptomatic relief of cold symptoms compared to placebo. The duration of cold symptoms was significantly shortened and symptoms decreased in the final 3 days.[40]

Cough associated with the common cold is usually related to postnasal drainage and throat irritation and is under voluntary control. Antitussive agents such as codeine are not effective for this type of cough.[41,42] Codeine may be useful for chronic cough based on a reflex mechanism that occurs in some patients after resolution of the cold. Antihistamines and decongestants may be effective in relieving cough associated with acute URI.

Considerable interest in the effectiveness of Echinacea for prevention and treatment of the common cold has evolved in recent years. A systematic review conducted in 1990 concluded that the majority of studies show a modest benefit in prevention and treatment of the common cold.[43] Since then, a number of controlled studies have found no benefit, while two studies have shown benefit. Differences in the products used (root vs. aerial parts, Echinacea species, preparation, stability, and so forth) must be considered when interpreting the results of studies. Many of the negative studies have a low statistical power and design problems are also common. At this time, the use of Echinacea for prevention or treatment cannot be recommended, although the potential harm of using these products appears to be expense only.

There is no role for the use of antibacterial drugs in the treatment of the common cold.[44] Antibiotics may be required only to manage complications such as acute otitis media or acute rhinosinusitis.

ACUTE RHINOSINUSITIS

TREATMENT GOALS: ACUTE RHINOSINUSITIS

■ Provide optimal and appropriate antimicrobial therapy.
■ Symptoms should improve within 48 to 72 hours.

Acute rhinosinusitis is an extremely common URI, accounting for 16 to 25 million physician visits annually. Although the costs of managing acute rhinosinusitis are uncertain, expenditures of $200 million for prescription drugs and more than $2 billion for over-the-counter drugs have been estimated.[45,46] History and physical examination are the most practical methods used to diagnose acute rhinosinusitis, but the clinical presentation is nonspecific. A limited computed tomography (CT) scan provides the most definitive information for diagnosing sinusitis.[47] Since most cases of sinusitis are not serious and are self-limited, a CT scan is not cost-effective. Standard sinus radiographs are difficult to interpret and are not very sensitive or specific.

Antimicrobial therapy is considered appropriate for the treatment of acute rhinosinusitis,[48] but the benefits of such treatment have recently been questioned.[49-51]

EPIDEMIOLOGY

The most common bacterial pathogens isolated from sinus aspirates in adults are *S. pneumoniae* (41%), *H. influenzae* (35%), and *Moraxella catarrhalis* (4%). Various streptococcal species and anaerobes from oral flora represented 14% of the isolates, and *Staphylococcus aureus* accounted for 3%. The isolation of oral flora from the paranasal sinuses may be associated with periodontal disease. Bacteria were not isolated in 41% of the patients with presumed acute maxillary sinusitis.[52,53] Many of these patients with negative bacterial cultures are considered to have viral sinusitis associated with the common cold.[6] In children with acute maxillary sinusitis, *S. pneumoniae* (41%) is the most common cause, followed by *H. influenzae* (19%) and *M. catarrhalis* (19%). *M. catarrhalis* is isolated more frequently in children less than 5 years of age.[53,54] As in adults, no bacteria could be recovered in almost 40% of children with acute maxillary sinusitis. Causative agents in neonates include *Listeria monocytogenes* and gram-negative enteric bacteria in addition to the organisms listed for adults and children. The same is true for immunocompromised patients, in whom fungi and gram-negative bacteria are more likely present.

CLINICAL PRESENTATION AND DIAGNOSIS

SIGNS AND SYMPTOMS

Acute rhinosinusitis presents as sinus tenderness, cough, sinus pressure, nasal obstruction, headache, postnasal drainage, discolored nasal discharge, and sore throat. Halitosis, malaise, fever, chills, maxillary toothache, and periorbital swelling occur less commonly.[55] Signs and symptoms of acute sinusitis are nonspecific and also may occur with allergic rhinitis and viral URIs. Allergic rhinitis and viral URI often precede the development of acute rhinosinusitis. In fact, 39% to 87% of patients with the common cold have radiographic evidence of sinusitis on day 7 of their illness.[6,56] Obstruction of the nasal or sinus passages caused by septal spurs, nasal polyps, tumors, foreign bodies, and mucosal hypertrophy also predispose an individual to acute rhinosinusitis. Sinusitis can be classified according to the duration of symptoms: acute (2 to 4 weeks), subacute (2 to 4 weeks to 2 to 3 months), and chronic (2 to 3 months or longer).[57]

The most common presentation occurs in persons with initial cold-like symptoms. Colored nasal discharge, nasal obstruction, facial pressure, and cough persist or worsen by 8 to 10 days after the onset of symptoms. Although symptoms of the common cold may persist for 14 days or longer, improvement should occur by the end of the first week.[58] A lack of improvement or worsening after 1 week could indicate acute rhinosinusitis. A second presentation, occurring in fewer patients, includes fever (temperature 38°C or higher), chills, facial pain, and marked tenderness, erythema, or swelling.

The maxillary sinuses are most frequently involved in acute rhinosinusitis, followed by the frontal sinuses.[58] Infection involving the frontal, ethmoid, and sphenoid sinuses has been most commonly associated with intracranial complications, although such complications are rare.[59,60] Maxillary sinusitis is most often associated with pain over one cheekbone, under the eye, or resembling a maxillary toothache. Moderate to severe frontal headache and tenderness above the eyebrows and nose are consistent with frontal sinusitis. The ethmoid sinuses are located on each side of the nasal cavity. Ethmoid sinusitis is associated with pain at the inner corner of the eye, periorbital or temporal headache, and tenderness over the lacrimal fossa. The sphenoid sinuses are located posterior to the nasal pharynx just below the cranial cavity. Patients with sphenoid sinusitis may have multifocal headache involving the occipital, frontal, temporal, and retro-orbital regions.

DIAGNOSIS

It is not cost-effective to use radiologic and invasive procedures for the diagnosis of acute rhinosinusitis in most patients.[48] A careful history and physical examination are sufficient for presumptive diagnosis of acute rhinosinusitis. The nasal mucosa should be examined using an otoscope with nasal speculum after the use of a topical decongestant. The presence of thick, colored, mucopurulent secretions is consistent with acute rhinosinusitis. The presence of clear, watery secretions is more consistent with allergic rhinitis, particularly in patients with a history of seasonal allergic disorders. Sinus tenderness, sinus pressure, and postnasal discharge are often used as criteria for diagnosing sinusitis, but these findings have not been shown to be sensitive and specific for identifying acute rhinosinusitis.[55] Characteristics associated with greater than 70% sensitivity include colored nasal discharge, cough, and sneezing. The specificities of these three characteristics were only 52%, 44%, and 34%, respectively. The presence of a maxillary toothache and painful chewing were quite specific (93% and 84%, respectively), but they were present in only 11% to 15% of patients. Failure to improve after use of decongestants was 80% specific but was present in only 28% of patients.[61]

These data are often used to discredit the accuracy of clinical examination in diagnosing sinusitis.[58] It is important to use groups of characteristics rather than single characteristics. When maxillary toothache, colored nasal discharge, poor response to decongestants, abnormal transillumination, and purulent nasal secretions on examination are considered, the predicted probability of sinusitis was 9%, 21%, 40%, 63%, 81%, or 92% if 0 to 5 of the above factors are present, respectively.[61] The major problem with these data is that sinus radiographs were used as the gold standard to establish the diagnosis of sinusitis; clearly, the results would be more certain if CT was used. Transillumination is a technique in which a strong light source is directed toward the lacrimal area and the light transmitted through the sinus is observed. If there is normal transmission of light, the sinus is probably not infected. Transillumination has poor sensitivity and specificity when used by itself.[62,63]

From a therapeutic perspective, the ability to distinguish between acute bacterial sinusitis and acute viral sinusitis is relevant. The presence of unilateral nasal discharge and pain is the best predictor of bacterial infection. A history of purulent nasal discharge and the presence of maxillary tooth pain or purulent nasal secretions also suggest bacterial infection.[64] However, none of these signs provides definitive evidence. Culture obtained by sinus puncture and aspiration is the gold standard for differentiating bacterial from viral disease, but this procedure is generally reserved for clinical studies and patients with complicated or serious acute sinusitis.

Sinus radiography is the most common imaging technique used to evaluate patients with sinusitis. Opacification, mucosal thickening, polyps, or air-fluid levels in patients with a history compatible with acute rhinosinusitis are regarded as evidence for the diagnosis. The ethmoid sinuses cannot be evaluated using sinus radiographs. In addition, there is considerable controversy on the true value of sinus radiographs because of the high frequency of false-positive and false-negative results.[48]

A CT scan is considered the gold standard radiographic method for evaluating sinusitis. However, because of the limited availability and high expense, this procedure is most commonly used for immunocompromised patients, patients with suspected intracranial complications, patients with periorbital extension (swelling or edema), or patients with refractory disease. A limited CT scan of the sinuses is becoming more economical and more widely available, leading many specialists to recommend abandoning sinus radiographs in favor of a CT scan. Surgical decompression and sinus cultures also should be considered in these patients.[58] A CT scan may also be useful in patients with recurrent acute rhinosinusitis in whom structural abnormalities are suspected.

Magnetic resonance imaging (MRI) scans are comparable to CT scans for evaluating soft tissue abnormalities, but MRI is not useful for evaluating bony abnormalities. Neither CT or MRI should be used routinely due to cost, the frequency of abnormalities in asymptomatic patients, and inability to distinguish bacterial from viral infection.[64] Recent guidelines suggest reserving these procedures for patients who are surgical candidates.[65]

The definitive method for establishing the etiology of infection is sinus puncture, aspiration, and culture. This invasive technique is warranted only for neonates, immunocompromised patients, patients who fail to improve after treatment, and patients with suppurative complications such as periorbital cellulitis, meningitis, or intracranial abscess. Sinus cultures are also used in clinical trials of antimicrobial agents and in studies to examine the etiology of acute rhinosinusitis.

TREATMENT

The scope of this review is limited to the treatment of nonimmunocompromised children and adults. The management of patients with severe pain and/or focal neurologic signs or evidence of meningitis is also beyond the scope of this review. "Persistent symptoms" include symptoms lasting more than 10 to 14 days but less than 30 days. "Severe symptoms" include a fever of at least 39°C, with purulent nasal discharge present for 3 to 4 consecutive days, and ill appearance.[65] "Uncomplicated sinusitis" refers to acute (symptoms lasting less than 30 days) rhinosinusitis that does not meet the definition of persistent or severe.

The first question to be addressed is whether antimicrobial therapy is warranted for uncomplicated acute rhinosinus-

itis. Many studies have involved patients referred to ear-nose-and-throat specialists for evaluation and treatment. These patients are more likely to have severe or recurrent disease or failure to respond to initial treatment. Without any antimicrobial treatment, resolution of symptoms occurs in 70% to 80% of patients with presumed acute rhinosinusitis.[49–51] In a recent double-blind, randomized controlled trial, the efficacy of amoxicillin was not superior to that of placebo after a 7-day treatment period. Cure or substantial improvement was noted in 83% of patients given amoxicillin and 77% of patients given placebo ($p = 0.01$). Adverse effects, including gastrointestinal complaints and skin rash, were significantly more common in the treatment group (28% vs. 9%, respectively).[49] Patients eligible for entry into the study had to be previously referred for sinus radiographs. The radiographs were then used as part of the enrollment criteria. Sinus radiographs are not sensitive or specific for the diagnosis of acute rhinosinusitis. In addition, many clinicians do not regard amoxicillin as a first-line agent for treatment of acute rhinosinusitis. A similar study failed to show a significant benefit of doxycycline compared to placebo.[50] A review of all placebo-controlled trials between 1966 and 1996 revealed numerous methodologic problems and concluded that the effectiveness or lack thereof of antibiotics in acute rhinosinusitis is not based on sufficient evidence.[51]

Despite any controversy, antibiotic therapy is considered appropriate for acute rhinosinusitis that is persistent or severe.[48,58] Early therapy of acute rhinosinusitis may reduce mucosal damage and scarring that may lead to recurrent acute rhinosinusitis or chronic sinusitis. Antibacterial therapy is generally not needed for children at least 2 years of age or adults with uncomplicated acute sinusitis. In children younger than 2 years of age, antibacterial therapy should be considered if the child attends day care or has recently received antibacterial therapy.[65]

Resistance to antibacterial drugs in community-acquired respiratory pathogens is a major consideration that has evolved over the past two decades. Penicillin susceptibility among isolates of *S. pneumoniae* is classified as resistant [mean inhibitory concentration (MIC) > 1 μg/mL], intermediate (MIC 0.1 to 1 μg/mL), or susceptible (MIC < 0.1 μg/mL). Isolates that are not susceptible to penicillin represent approximately 52% of total isolates from children aged 0 to 2 years, 39% from children aged 3 to 14 years, and 31% to 32% from older children and adults. Up to two thirds of the nonsusceptible isolates are classified as resistant as opposed to intermediate.[66] The likelihood of penicillin resistance in children tends to increase during the winter as the respiratory infection season progresses.[67] Reduced susceptibility to penicillin is associated with increased resistance to several other antibacterial classes, including cephalosporins, macrolides, sulfonamides, tetracyclines, and lincomycins. Approximately 30% to 37% of isolates of *H. influenzae* are expected to be resistant to amoxicillin due to β-lactamase production.[68] This type of resistance is overcome by the use of the combination amoxicillin/clavulanate. Only 0.1% of strains are resistant to amoxicillin and are β-lactamase negative. Many strains are resistant to early-generation cephalosporins, including cephalexin, cephradine, cefaclor, and macrolides. Of the second-generation cephalosporins, cefuroxime axetil is active against at least 95% of *H. influenzae* isolates. The third-generation oral cephalosporins, including cefprozil, cefdinir, ceftibuten, cefixime, and cefpodoxime, are effective against essentially 100% of *H. influenzae* strains. Of the macrolides, azithromycin appears to be the most active, while erythromycin has minimal activity. Clarithromycin by itself also has very limited activity against *H. influenzae*; however, the active metabolite, 25-hydroxyclarithromycin, may increase the activity in vivo. There are also differences in the pharmacokinetics in that azithromycin undergoes extensive intracellular accumulation and has lower serum and interstitial fluid concentrations. These differences were counterbalancing, and the efficacies of azithromycin and clarithromycin were similar in an experimental model of lower respiratory infection.[68,69] More than 90% of *M. catarrhalis* isolates produce a penicillinase and are resistant to amoxicillin. These organisms are susceptible to all oral cephalosporins and amoxicillin/clavulanate.[63] Newer fluoroquinolones (levofloxacin, gatifloxacin, gemifloxacin, and moxifloxacin) are active against most *S. pneumoniae* and essentially all *H. influenzae* and *M. catarrhalis* isolates, irrespective of penicillin susceptibility.

Antibacterial therapy for acute rhinosinusitis will be discussed based on the American Academy of Pediatrics practice guidelines,[65] although these guidelines are also appropriate for adults. Amoxicillin is considered the first-line agent in doses of 45 or 80 to 90 mg/kg/day. In children this dose is typically given in two divided doses (every 12 hours). The higher dose is preferred in children with risk factors for penicillin-resistant *S. pneumoniae*, including attending day care, recent treatment with antibiotics, or failure to respond to the lower dose after 3 days. Cefdinir, cefuroxime, and cefpodoxime are alternatives that can be used in patients with penicillin allergy only if the reaction was not a type 1 hypersensitivity reaction and provided the reaction was not serious. In cases of type 1 allergy, clarithromycin, azithromycin, and clindamycin are alternatives. The use of trimethoprim/sulfamethoxazole or erythromycin/sulfasoxazole is no longer recommended due to substantial resistance.[65] Treatment should be continued until the patient is symptom-free for 7 days. For most patients, a 10-day course is sufficient.

Response to antibacterial therapy should be re-evaluated after 3 days. If the patient does not have a marked reduction in nasal discharge and cough and does not feel better in general, either the antibacterial agent is ineffective or the diagnosis may be wrong. The usual second-line therapy is high-dose amoxicillin/clavulanate.[65] If the patient had been treated initially with the lower dose of amoxicillin (45 mg/kg/day), an increase to 80 to 90 mg/kg/day may increase the eradication of *S. pneumoniae* with intermediate or low-level resistance to amoxicillin. Penicillin resistance in *S. pneu-*

moniae is not mediated through β-lactamase production; consequently, clavulanic acid adds no benefit for treatment of this pathogen. The clavulanic acid counteracts resistance in most strains of *H. influenzae* and *M. catarrhalis* that are resistant to amoxicillin. Oral cephalosporins (cefdinir, cefuroxime, or cefpodoxime) are also considered potential second-line therapies, although they are not more effective than high-dose amoxicillin for penicillin-resistant *S. pneumoniae* infection. Newer fluoroquinones can be considered in adult patients. Other options include intramuscular ceftriaxone (50 mg/kg) as a single dose or as three doses administered every 48 hours. The AAP guideline suggests giving a single dose to children in whom vomiting precludes administration of oral antibiotics, followed by oral antibiotics beginning 24 hours later.[65]

Other groups such as the Sinus and Allergy Health Partnership recommend that amoxicillin/clavulanate and the three oral cephalosporins listed above should be included as first-line antibiotics for treatment of acute sinusitis.

In patients who fail to respond to first- or second-line therapies, the options include intravenous ceftriaxone or cefotaxime, or consultation with an otolaryngologist to obtain a sinus culture by needle aspiration. Further therapy is then guided by the results of the culture and susceptibility testing.

Some general comments can be made about the selection of antimicrobial drugs for treatment of acute rhinosinusitis. First, comparative trials of different antimicrobial agents usually do not show superiority of one agent over another. Studies conducted before 1990 and even in the early 1990s probably had few cases of patients infected with penicillin-resistant *S. pneumoniae,* and this may affect the outcome of therapy. Sample sizes are typically planned without considering the rate of spontaneous resolution. If a study is conducted with 100 patients in each of two treatment groups and the spontaneous resolution rate is 70%, then one is effectively comparing 30 patients in each treatment group. This makes it more difficult to conclude that true differences exist.

The following drugs have been compared to amoxicillin/clavulanate (500 mg every 8 hours) in randomized trials: azithromycin (500 mg once daily 3 days), levofloxacin (500 mg once daily), cefprozil (500 mg every 12 hours), roxithromycin (150 mg every 12 hours), ceftibuten (400 mg every day), cefdinir (300 mg every 12 hours and 600 mg once daily), clarithromycin (500 mg every 12 hours), cefuroxime axetil (250 mg every 12 hours), and loracarbef (400 mg every 12 hours).[70-79] Amoxicillin 750 to 1,500 mg per day every 8 to 12 hours was the reference treatment for the following drugs: cefpodoxime axetil (200 mg every 12 hours), cefaclor (500 mg every 8 hours), clarithromycin (500 mg every 12 hours), cefixime (400 mg once daily), azithromycin (500 mg, then 250 mg once daily 4 days), cefuroxime axetil (250 mg every 12 hours), and minocycline (100 mg twice daily).[80-87] Finally, cefuroxime axetil (250 mg twice daily) served as the reference treatment in comparative trials including sparfloxacin (400 mg, then 200 mg/day for 5 days) and ciprofloxacin (500 mg twice daily).[88,89] All of the treatments were administered for 8 to 10 days unless otherwise stated. The clinical effectiveness was not significantly different between treatments in any of the studies; however, a few of the studies had sample sizes less than 100 patients. The only study concluding superiority of a treatment involved a comparison between cefpodoxime and cefaclor. Cefpodoxime was more effective, with cure in 84% compared to 68% with cefaclor.[90] Other trials were performed but are not discussed here due to the lack of a reference or use of a nonstandard reference drug. Better tolerance was concluded in eight studies in which amoxicillin/clavulanate served as the reference drug. Amoxicillin/clavulanate typically causes a greater frequency of gastrointestinal complaints, especially diarrhea. No comparative studies involving children younger than 12 years of age were found.

Adjunctive (symptomatic) treatment with topical and systemic decongestants is commonly used for acute rhinosinusitis. These agents relieve symptoms of nasal congestion, but there is no evidence that they promote sinus drainage. Oral phenylpropanolamine was shown not to improve maxillary sinus drainage assessed by CT scan in one study.[91] In another study, treatment with topical oxymetazoline and an oral antihistamine–decongestant combination (brompheniramine and phenylpropanolamine) was no more effective than placebo in children with acute rhinosinusitis.[92] Although documentation of efficacy is poor, decongestants may be used to provide symptomatic relief of nasal congestion.[58] Antihistamines may be useful in patients who have allergic rhinitis concurrently. Because allergic rhinitis is a predisposing condition for sinusitis, the effectiveness of intranasal corticosteroids as adjunctive therapy for acute rhinosinusitis has been studied. Intranasal flunisolide and budesonide provide some relief of symptoms (facial pain and tenderness, turbinate swelling, and global assessment) and somewhat faster resolution of abnormal radiographic findings.[93,94]

Rarely, surgical decompression using sinus puncture or fiberoptic rhinoscopy is required to manage an infected sinus and prevent suppurative complications.[48]

Table 74.3 lists antimicrobial drugs that are approved by the U.S. Food and Drug Administration (FDA) for the treatment of sinusitis. Antimicrobial drugs that are well-established treatments for acute sinusitis based on published studies but are not approved by the FDA are also included. Amoxicillin, for example, is not approved for the treatment of acute rhinosinusitis, but it is frequently used as a reference treatment. The fluoroquinolones are relatively contraindicated for use in children. These drugs should not be used except for serious infections for which other agents are believed to be inferior. Sinusitis, therefore, would not be an indication except in immunocompromised patients with a documented pathogen resistant to other readily available drugs. Many of the fluoroquinolones are FDA approved for the treatment of acute maxillary sinusitis in adults. Other

TABLE 74.3	Antimicrobial Agents Approved by the U.S. Food and Drug Administration for Treating Acute Sinusitis in Children and Adults	
Drug	**Approved Dosage for Children**	**Approved Dosage for Adults**
Amoxicillin	20 mg/kg q12h or 45 mg/kg q12h	500 mg q8h
Amoxicillin/ clavulanate (dosage based on amoxicillin)	13.3 mg/kg q8h or 22.5 mg/kg q12h or 90 mg/kg q24h (ES-600)	500 mg q8h or 875 mg q12h or 2000/125 mg q12h (XR)
Cefdinir	7 mg/kg q12h or 14 mg/kg q24h	300 mg q12h or 600 mg q24h
Cefpodoxime	5 mg/kg q12h	200 mg q12h
Cefprozil	7.5–15 mg/kg q12h	250–500 mg q12h
Cefuroxime axetil	15 mg/kg q12h	250 mg q12h
Loracarbef	15 mg/kg q12h	400 mg q12h
Azithromycin	10 mg/kg q24h (3 days)	500 mg q24h (3 days)
Clarithromycin	7.5 mg/kg q12h	500 mg q12h or 1000 mg q24h (XL)
Ciprofloxacin	Not approved[a]	500 mg q12h
Gatifloxacin	Not approved[a]	400 mg q24h
Levofloxacin	Not approved[a]	500 mg q24h or 750 mg q24h (5 days)
Moxifloxacin	Not approved[a]	400 mg q24h

Use and dosage should be confirmed in official references for children <2 years of age. Approved duration of treatment is 10 days unless otherwise noted.
[a] Fluoroquinolones are relatively contraindicated in children except in serious infections where alternative treatments are not available.

sources should be consulted for antibiotic use and dosing in children less than 2 years of age. Many of the manufacturers' dose recommendations do not cover children younger than 2 months to 2 years.

COMPLICATIONS

Serious complications resulting from acute rhinosinusitis are uncommon. In one large public hospital, 12 patients with suppurative intracranial infections with a sinogenic source were identified over a 10-year period.[95] Of patients requiring hospital admission for sinusitis, 3.7% had intracranial infection. The most common infectious complications included cerebral abscess, meningitis, epidural abscess, and subdural abscess. Other complications, including periorbital cellulites, are occasionally reported. It appears that intracranial complications are more common with chronic sinusitis than with acute rhinosinusitis.[96] In children, cerebral abscess, extra-axial abscess, and meningitis were reported, but only 13 cases were found over 10 years in a large pediatric hospital.[97] Clearly, surveillance for these infrequent complications is necessary to ensure that the risk is not substantially increased with more limited use of antimicrobial drugs.

OTITIS MEDIA

TREATMENT GOALS: OTITIS MEDIA

- Provide optimal and appropriate antimicrobial therapy.
- Symptoms should improve within 48 to 72 hours.

Infection of the middle ear may present as acute otitis media (AOM) or as otitis media with effusion (OME or serous otitis media). AOM is extremely prevalent in young children, occurring in most children at least once within the first 6 years of life. Many of these children also develop chronic OME, which may be associated with hearing impairment and learning disability. Care of otitis media is estimated to account for over 24.5 million physician office visits annually.[98] Tympanostomy for the management of OME is the most common surgical procedures involving children. From a population-based study in Calgary, the rate of tympanostomy tube insertion peaks at 54.2 per 1,000 children between 12 and 23 months of age.[99] Treatment of AOM also accounts for the largest single use of antibacterial drugs in children, and much of this use is considered overuse.[100]

EPIDEMIOLOGY

As early as 6 months of age, 48% of infants experience at least one episode of AOM. By 1 year of age, 62% to 79% of infants experience one or more episodes of otitis media, and almost 20% have had three or more episodes. The frequency of at least one occurrence of otitis media further increases to 83% to 92% by 2 to 3 years of age. The peak incidence for AOM is between the age of 6 months and 1 year.[101,102] The most important risk factors for development of otitis media are lower socioeconomic status and contact with a large number of other children (common in day-care settings).[102] The risk of AOM and OME appears to be higher in infants who are not breastfed, African-American children who live in urban environments, boys, and children exposed to secondhand smoke. Children who contract AOM early in life are more likely to have recurrent otitis media.

The eustachian tube connects to the middle ear at a 10-degree angle at birth, and the angle increases up to about 45 degrees in adulthood. The eustachian tube also lengthens to about double its original length by adulthood. Because of the acute angle in young children, there is a greater risk of obstruction, leading to fluid accumulation.[103] The presence of a viral respiratory tract infection or seasonal allergic rhinitis may also contribute to eustachian tube dysfunction. Once the eustachian tube is blocked, conditions are excellent for bacterial proliferation. Neonates and infants lack a fully mature immune system, and this contributes to the higher incidence of AOM. Breastfeeding reduces susceptibility to AOM, possibly by contributing passive immunity.

Increases in the incidence of AOM are noted throughout the autumn season. The incidence peaks in the winter and gradually decreases in the spring and summer, coinciding with the peak times for viral URIs.[103] Exposure to cigarette smoke and other irritants is a risk factor for developing AOM and OME. Many children develop OME after an episode of AOM; however, OME may occur in children without such history. OME may be associated with the same bacterial pathogens that are found with AOM.

The pathogens involved in otitis media are essentially the same as those involved in acute rhinosinusitis. *S. pneumoniae*, *H. influenzae*, and *M. catarrhalis* account for approximately 30% to 47%, 14% to 35%, and less than 14% of the identified pathogens, respectively.[104,105] About one third (26% to 43%) of the cultures are sterile, and some of these may involve viral agents. Penicillin-resistant *S. pneumoniae* is an increasing problem in children with AOM, particularly in children who attend day-care centers. Strains that are not susceptible to penicillin accounted for 43% of *S. pneumoniae* isolates from 2000 to 2003 compared to 20% for the prior 4 years at one center. The majority of the nonsusceptible isolates were classified as resistant (MIC >1 μg/mL). Infection with penicillin-resistant *S. pneumoniae* is a risk factor for recurrent otitis media and is associated with prior antimicrobial use.[106] Among children with recurrent or persistent

AOM, the frequency of *S. pneumoniae* and non–penicillin-susceptible *S. pneumoniae* may be stabilizing or even decreasing, while β-lactamase–producing *H. influenzae* appears to be increasingly important. This may be due to the use of high-dose amoxicillin and 7-valent pneumococcal conjugate vaccine.[107] Less frequently encountered pathogens include *Streptococcus pyogenes*, *S. aureus*, and *Peptostreptococcus* spp. In neonates, the list of potential pathogens also includes Enterobacteriaceae, group B streptococci, and *Pseudomonas aeruginosa*.[108]

CLINICAL PRESENTATION AND DIAGNOSIS

SIGNS AND SYMPTOMS

AOM is characterized by acute onset of ear pain, fever, and middle-ear effusion. Ear pulling, crying, irritability, anorexia, vomiting, and diarrhea are common in young children. These symptoms are nonspecific, though, as up to 72% of children without AOM present with these symptoms.[109] OME is associated with a more insidious onset and a relatively chronic course. This disease is characterized by excessive fluid in the middle ear, mild symptoms including ear pain and discomfort, and a hearing deficit. Spontaneous rupture of the tympanic membrane, discharge in the external ear canal, and vertigo may occur.[110] Many cases of OME are detected only after routine otologic examination or after a child fails a routine audiometric examination. However, OME can have substantial effects on quality of life.[111]

DIAGNOSIS

In infants, the most common symptoms are irritability/lethargy (69%), fever (52%), cough (36%), vomiting (21%), diarrhea (20%), tachypnea (20%), and anorexia (18%).[112] The most common symptoms associated with AOM in children include earache, sore throat, night restlessness, and fever.[110] The diagnosis of AOM is made on the basis of acute symptoms, middle ear effusion, and middle ear inflammation. Techniques used to demonstrate reduced tympanic membrane mobility are important to confirm diagnosis.[109] The pneumatic otoscope introduces a puff of air while the movement of the tympanic membrane is observed. If the membrane is resistant to movement, then the middle ear is considered to contain excess fluid. The tympanic membrane is typically bulging, and loss of the ossicular landmarks and light reflex is noted. Erythema and pronounced vascularity may also be observed.[113] Tympanometry is another technique that may be used.[114] The instrument produces sound waves, and the movement response of the tympanic membrane is recorded. Both techniques require that the patient remain still during the examination. Inflammation can be documented with prominent erythema of the tympanic membrane or otalgia with distinct localization.

Most patients with AOM are managed empirically based on the most probable pathogens. In certain patients, a culture may be obtained by puncturing the tympanic membrane and aspirating fluid. This procedure is known as a diagnostic tympanocentesis. Tympanocentesis is indicated for children who are critically ill or who have sepsis syndrome, patients who have a poor response to antimicrobial therapy, neonates, immunocompromised patients, and patients with suspected suppurative complications.[115]

OME is defined as fluid in the middle ear without signs and symptoms of acute ear infection. The presence of tympanic membrane erythema should not be used as the sole criterion to exclude OME because it is present in about 5% of cases of OME.[109] Middle ear fluid should be confirmed by pneumatic otoscopy or tympanometry.

TREATMENT

Early treatment of AOM with antimicrobial drugs has been routinely used in the United States; however, other countries (e.g., The Netherlands) have adopted a wait-for-3-days policy. There is no evidence that the outcomes differ between the early treatment and the more conservative approach. Recently, because of the increasing incidence of drug-resistant bacteria, delayed antimicrobial therapy is being implemented in the United States.[116] Untreated AOM is associated with a spontaneous resolution rate of approximately 81%. Antimicrobial therapy can increase the resolution rate, but only by about 14%. Thus, only 14 of 100 patients treated would benefit from antimicrobial therapy.[117] Antimicrobial therapy may cause adverse effects (e.g., diarrhea and skin rashes) that offset the potential benefits of therapy. The cost of therapy and potential promotion of drug-resistant bacteria must also be considered.

Guidelines for diagnosis and management of acute otitis media have been developed jointly by the American Academy of Pediatrics and the American Academy of Family Physicians. Infants less than 6 months of age with suspected AOM should receive antibacterial therapy. Children aged 6 months to 2 years with a certain diagnosis of AOM should also receive antibacterial therapy. Children at least 6 months of age who have an uncertain diagnosis of AOM or any child over 2 years of age with a certain or uncertain diagnosis of AOM should be considered for an observation option. For the observation option, symptomatic treatment is provided and antibacterial treatment is deferred for 48 to 72 hours. For this purpose, "certain diagnosis" is defined by rapid onset of symptoms, signs of middle ear effusion, and signs and symptoms of middle ear inflammation. The observation option should be limited to children who are otherwise healthy and have nonsevere illness (defined by mild otalgia and fever <39°C). There must also be a cooperative caregiver/parent with a ready means of communicating with the clinician. The observation option is designed to reduce unnecessary antibacterial drug use because 61% of children exhibit improvement within 24 hours irrespective of antibacterial therapy. Antibacterial therapy exhibits only a modest beneficial effect, with a number needed to treat of 8.[118]

Similar guidelines for diagnosis and management of OME are available. OME should be documented using pneumatic otoscopy and should be differentiated from AOM. Patients should be observed every 3 months initially. Since antibiotics do not show long-term efficacy, they should not be tried for at least 3 months. At this point, antibiotic use is optional and many physicians will observe for another 3 months. Once the decision to use antibiotics is made, the patient should be given a single course of amoxicillin (or an alternative agent). Repeating the treatment course and trials of different agents are not recommended.[119]

A meta-analysis to evaluate the role of antimicrobial therapy for the treatment of OME was performed using published studies from 1980 to 1990.[120] This study pooled data from 1,325 children from 10 different trials. Antimicrobial therapy resulted in an additional 22.8% increase in the resolution of middle ear effusion compared to no antimicrobial treatment. Studies that reported the lowest spontaneous resolution rate tended to have higher relative differences with antimicrobial treatment.

Amoxicillin is the drug of choice selected by consensus.[116] This therapy is inexpensive, and clinical trials have not shown any of the newer antimicrobial agents to be more effective. The same issues of antimicrobial resistance discussed for acute rhinosinusitis apply for AOM and OME. Because the incidence of penicillin-resistant S. pneumoniae has risen in recent years, studies performed more than 5 to 10 years earlier may not be representative of cases of AOM seen today. Meta-analyses were conducted in the early 1990s evaluating the efficacy of antimicrobial drugs for treating both AOM and OME. For OME, a meta-analysis included results from 5,400 children from 33 randomized controlled trials.[120] Antimicrobial therapy was marginally effective compared to placebo, with resolution occurring an average of 13.7% (95% confidence interval 8.2% to 19.2%) more often with treatment. There was no evidence that extended-spectrum drugs (amoxicillin/clavulanate, sulfamethoxazole/trimethoprim, erythromycin/sulfasoxazole, penicillin/sulfasoxazole, or any cephalosporin) performed better than standard-spectrum drugs (amoxicillin, penicillin, or erythromycin). The drugs grouped as extended-spectrum would be expected to have differing spectrums against H. influenzae and penicillin-resistant S. pneumoniae. Because of this grouping, this study fails to answer whether amoxicillin/clavulanate, cefuroxime axetil, or cefpodoxime, β-lactam drugs that provide the best overall time above the MIC,[121] are more effective than amoxicillin. Some dissent remains on the selection of amoxicillin as first-line therapy. Treatment with amoxicillin is associated with posttreatment colonization of nonsusceptible organisms to a greater extent than selected cephalosporins and azithromycin.[122] Oral cephalosporins (cefdinir, cefprozil, cefuroxime, and cefpodoxime) provide similar percentage time above the MIC in middle ear fluid. These agents may be better tolerated and more

convenient for some situations, but they are more expensive.[123]

Because of the increased prevalence of penicillin-resistant S. pneumoniae, higher doses of amoxicillin (80 to 90 mg/kg/day) are now recommended.[118] However, there is controversy over whether this dose is needed in communities that have a low prevalence of high-level penicillin resistance (MIC >2 μg/mL) among patients with treatment indications.[124] Cefdinir, cefuroxime, and cefpodoxime are alternatives that can be used in patients with penicillin allergy only if the reaction was not a type 1 hypersensitivity reaction and provided the reaction was not serious. In cases of type 1 allergy, clarithromycin, azithromycin, and clindamycin are alternatives.[118] Trimethoprim/sulfamethoxazole and erythromycin/sulfasoxazole are listed as alternative drugs in the AOM guideline; however, isolates of S. pneumoniae are increasingly resistant to these combinations. Consequently, these combinations are no longer recommended in the guideline for acute rhinosinusitis.[65] Thus, it is appropriate to avoid use of these agents in AOM as well. Antibacterial therapy should be administered for 10 days in children less than 6 years of age and in older children with severe symptoms. Otherwise, treatment for 5 to 7 days appears to provide similar outcomes.[118]

Forty-eight to 72 hours after starting antibacterial therapy, some improvement in symptoms should be apparent. If the patient is not improved, the diagnosis needs to be reevaluated and a change in the antibacterial therapy considered.

It is reasonable to use amoxicillin/clavulanate or a cephalosporin (cefuroxime, cefdinir, or cefpodoxime) in patients who fail to respond to amoxicillin. These agents are generally not active against strains of S. pneumoniae that are resistant to high-dose amoxicillin. However, they do add coverage for amoxicillin-resistant H. influenzae and M. catarrhalis. For patients with refractory disease where penicillin-resistant S. pneumoniae is proven or suspected, treatment with intramuscular ceftriaxone (50 mg/kg daily for 3 days) should be considered.[125] In adult patients, one of the newer fluoroquinolones (e.g., levofloxacin, moxifloxacin, gatifloxacin, or gemifloxacin) with improved S. pneumoniae coverage may be used.

The duration of treatment for AOM was investigated in a separate meta-analysis.[126] Several trials have evaluated short-course therapy (3 to 5 days) versus standard therapy (8 to 10 days). The results were affected by the time in which the outcome assessment was made. If the outcome assessment was performed at 8 to 19 days, an advantage was observed in favor of the standard treatment duration (odds ratio 1.52, 95% confidence interval 1.17 to 1.98). Stated another way, a child would be 1.52 times more likely to have continued symptoms on days 8 to 19 if treated with short-course therapy compared to 8 to 10 days. This small difference diminished when the assessment of efficacy was made at 20 to 30 days (odds ratio 1.22, 95% confidence interval 0.98 to 1.54) or 31 to 40 days (odds ratio 1.16, 95% confidence interval 0.87 to 1.55). Similar results were

TABLE 74.4	Oral Antimicrobial Agents Approved by the U.S. Food and Drug Administration for Treating Otitis Media in Children and Adults	
Drug	**Approved Dosage for Children**	**Approved Dosage for Adults**
Amoxicillin	20 mg/kg q12h or 45 mg/kg q12h	500 mg q8h or 500-750 mg q12h
Amoxicillin/ clavulanate (dosage based on amoxicillin)	13.3 mg/kg q8h or 22.5 mg/kg q12h or 45 mg/kg q12h 90 mg/kg q24h (ES-600)	500 mg q8h or 875 mg q12h or 2,000/125 mg q12h (XR)
Cefdinir	7 mg/kg q12h	Not approved
Cefixime	4 mg/kg q12h	400 mg q24h
Cefpodoxime	5 mg/kg q12h (5–10 days)	200 mg q12h
Cefprozil	15 mg/kg q12h	Not approved
Ceftibuten	9 mg/kg q24h (3 days)	400 mg q24h
Cefuroxime axetil	15 mg/kg q12h (suspension)	250 mg q12h
Loracarbef	15 mg/kg q12hr	Not approved
Azithromycin	10 mg/kg q24h or 10 mg/kg for 1 dose, then 5 mg/kg q24h for 4 doses	Not approved
Clarithromycin	7.5 mg/kg q12h	Not approved

Use and dosage should be confirmed in official references for children <6 months of age. Treatment duration is 10 days unless otherwise stated.
High-dose regimen is recommended in areas where *S. pneumoniae* strains that are not penicillin-susceptible are prevalent (see text).

obtained in a recent double-blind randomized clinical trial.[127] However, short-course therapy is not recommended for children younger than 2 years of age[98] and should be used with greater caution in children aged 2 to 5 years. Current guidelines suggest using a standard duration in patients under 6 years of age.[118]

Table 74.4 lists the drugs currently approved for the treatment of otitis media in children and adults. Although amoxicillin is considered the gold standard, agents that exhibit stability to β-lactamases are commonly used. When indicated, guidelines for selecting antibacterial therapy for OME are the same as for AOM.

COMPLICATIONS

Otogenic complications of AOM include tympanic membrane perforation, cholesteatoma (middle ear cyst), ossicular fixation or destruction, labyrinthitis, and chronic otitis media. Because of persistent hearing loss associated with OME, impairment of speech/language acquisition and delayed cognitive development may result. Additional complications include cervical abscess, temporal osteomyelitis, facial paralysis, mastoiditis, brain abscess, meningitis, subdural or epidural abscess, lateral sinus thrombosis, and hydrocephalus.[128] The incidence of intracranial complications after AOM is estimated to be 0.04% to 0.15%. Acute mastoiditis was the most common serious complication in the preantibiotic era. This infection is typically caused by *S. pneumoniae*, and more than 60% of patients require surgery (mastoidectomy) for management.[129] There has been concern that more restrictive use of antimicrobial agents may lead to an increased frequency of complications, but this has not been observed to date.

PHARYNGITIS

TREATMENT GOALS: PHARYNGITIS

■ Provide optimal and appropriate antimicrobial therapy when indicated.
■ Reduce symptoms by use of analgesics and local anesthetics.

Acute pharyngitis is a common infectious disease, particularly in children. This infection may be caused by a variety of viral and bacterial pathogens.[130] Most cases of acute pharyngitis are self-limited, and specific treatment is needed only for pharyngitis caused by group A β-hemolytic streptococci (*S. pyogenes*). Rare causes of bacterial pharyngitis that also require treatment include *Neisseria gonorrhoeae, Francisella tularensis, Yersinia pestis,* and *Corynebacterium diphtheriae.*[130] Identification of these latter pathogens necessitates special laboratory testing that is needed only in limited clinical settings.

EPIDEMIOLOGY

The most important cause of pharyngitis or tonsillitis in terms of the need for treatment and frequency of occurrence is *S. pyogenes*. Acute bacterial pharyngitis may also be caused by group C and G streptococci, *Arcanobacterium hemolyticum*, and possibly *M. pneumoniae* and *Chlamydia pneumoniae*. In addition, viral causes include rhinovirus, coronavirus, adenovirus, parainfluenza virus, herpes simplex virus, influenza virus, coxsackievirus, Epstein-Barr virus, and cytomegalovirus.[130,131] The presence of sore throat is associated with more than 10% of primary care physician visits, yet less than 20% of patients with a sore throat actually visit a heath care provider.[132]

Nearly all common causes of pharyngitis are self-limiting, with symptoms lasting from 2 to 7 days. Pharyngitis caused by group A β-hemolytic streptococci (GABHS) is sometimes associated with rheumatic fever, which is considered a nonsuppurative sequela. Because of the potential seriousness of rheumatic fever, identification of GABHS infection and appropriate therapy are warranted.[130] In the first half of the 20th century, acute rheumatic fever was a relatively common complication of GABHS infection. Many patients who developed rheumatic fever went on to develop rheumatic heart disease, requiring long-term antimicrobial prophylaxis and eventually heart valve replacements.[132] In a study of military recruits, rheumatic fever occurred in 4.1% of patients with group A β-hemolytic streptococcal pharyngitis who were not treated with an antimicrobial drug.[133] The endemic risk of rheumatic fever after untreated streptococcal pharyngitis in the second half of the 20th century ranged from 0.3% to 0.4%.[132] Epidemics or outbreaks of rheumatic fever have occurred sporadically, and its incidence may approach 3% during these outbreaks.

Cases of GABHS infection in the United States are most commonly associated with serotypes M1, M2, M4, and M12. Serotypes M1, M3, and M18 appear more commonly in patients with suppurative complications, and M3 and M18 appear to be more commonly associated with rheumatic fever.[134]

CLINICAL PRESENTATION AND DIAGNOSIS

SIGNS AND SYMPTOMS

Classically, group A β-hemolytic streptococcal GABHS is characterized by an acute-onset sore throat with fever, tonsillar exudate, and swollen, tender anterior cervical lymph nodes. Numerous studies have shown that GABHS cases are difficult to differentiate from other causes of acute pharyngitis based on symptoms alone, even by experienced clinicians. The throat is usually quite erythematous, with patches of purulent exudate (white to gray) on the tonsils and posterior pharynx. Erythema of the uvula and tongue is sometimes

present. Fever is typically greater than 38°C, although the clinical course is highly variable.[130]

DIAGNOSIS

The only reliable method of diagnosing GABHS infection is a throat culture or rapid antigen detection test (RADT). A throat culture is performed by swabbing the posterior pharynx and then plating the specimen on sheep blood agar, followed by incubation for at least 18 to 24 hours. Recovery may be higher if the plate is incubated for 36 to 48 hours before the final determination of the presence or absence of GABHS. GABHS colonies produce surrounding β-hemolysis, which is recognized earlier when they are incubated in an anaerobic environment. Routine cultures may be set up with a glass cover slip placed over the area of inoculation. Alternatively, a stab culture can be prepared by inoculating the specimen under the surface of the agar to create a reduced-oxygen environment. Culture is considered to be more than 90% sensitive and highly specific.[130]

RADT allows the immediate testing of patients during an office visit. A RADT is performed from a throat swab, and the test requires less than 5 minutes. Although a positive RADT result is very specific for GABHS, the sensitivity is only 60% to 90% compared with culture. For this reason, IDSA guidelines suggest performing a culture on any patient with a negative RADT.[130] Patients with a positive RADT should be treated with an antimicrobial agent without the need for a follow-up culture. A position paper endorsed by the Centers for Disease Control and Prevention, the American Academy of Family Physicians, and the American College of Physicians (CDC/AAFP/ACP) provides several options[135] that are based on the criteria described in the next paragraph. In this paper, throat cultures are not recommended for routine use. If patients have two or more criteria to support GABHS infection, the health care provider can follow one of the following three diagnostic/treatment strategies:

1. Test patients with two or more criteria using RADT, and limit therapy to those with a positive RADT.
2. Test patients with two or three criteria, and limit antibiotic use to patients with a positive RADT or those with four criteria.
3. Do not use any diagnostic test, and limit therapy to patients with three or four criteria.[135]

However, this strategy of empirically treating patients with three or four criteria would lead to a high rate of unnecessary antibiotic prescriptions in adults.[136]

There is controversy regarding who should have a culture or RADT performed. The extreme view is that a culture needs to be performed in any patient with pharyngitis because GABHS cannot be distinguished from other causes of acute pharyngitis on clinical grounds. Fewer than 10% to 20% of patients with pharyngitis actually seek medical care; however, the incidence of rheumatic fever remains low. This prompted a Canadian group to develop four criteria to establish the risk of GABHS infection:[137] absence of cough, history of temperature greater than 38°C, tonsillar exudate, and swollen, tender anterior cervical nodes. The probability of having GABHS infection was 2% to 3% if none of the criteria were present, 3% to 7% if one criterion was present, 8% to 16% if two criteria were present, 19% to 34% if three criteria were present, and 41% to 61% if all four criteria were present. The group suggested that no culture or therapy should be provided for low-risk patients with one or no criteria. Patients with two or three criteria should have throat cultures performed and then be treated only if the culture results are positive. In specific situations, patients with all four of the above criteria could be treated empirically, before culture results are obtained, to reduce the symptoms and potential transmission to others. The latter suggestion is most rational when there is evidence of a local epidemic. Epidemiologic factors should be considered when deciding to treat for GABHS. The presence of sore throat in patients who have been in close contact with an individual with known streptococcal pharyngitis suggests GABHS as the etiology. Increased probability of GABHS infection is also associated with the presence of sore throat in the winter and early spring in children between the ages of 5 and 15 years.

TREATMENT

Treatment for streptococcal pharyngitis may be initiated to reduce the duration of symptoms, limit spread, and prevent rheumatic fever. Because of the self-limited nature of streptococcal pharyngitis, the primary goal of treatment is not to hasten resolution of symptoms; however, if antimicrobial therapy is initiated within the first 24 to 36 hours of symptoms, some benefit in the resolution time may occur.[132,138] Occasionally, epidemics or clusters of pharyngitis caused by GABHS occur in military bases, schools, and other places where large groups congregate. If therapy is initiated early, within 24 to 36 hours of symptom onset, the time of contagiousness is shortened. The primary reason for treating patients with streptococcal pharyngitis is the prevention of acute rheumatic fever. Antimicrobial treatment appears effective in preventing rheumatic fever if administered as late as 7 to 9 days after the onset of symptoms.[128]

Only one study, conducted in 1950, assessed the effect of antibiotic treatment on the risk of rheumatic fever. Procaine penicillin G, 300,000 U given intramuscularly every other day for three doses, resulted in a reduction in the incidence of rheumatic fever from 4.1% with placebo to 0.39%.[133] Oral penicillin V, 250 mg two to four times daily for 10 days, was later substituted for procaine penicillin G. The risk of rheumatic fever after streptococcal pharyngitis appeared to be falling even before therapy was shown to be beneficial. Today, the true risk of rheumatic fever is unknown, but it appears to be much lower.[130]

Penicillin therapy in patients with streptococcal pharyngitis may be harmful because of the eradication of α-hemolytic streptococci and other bacteria that make up the normal pharyngeal flora. The presence of commensal organisms may provide some protection against infections with pathogenic bacteria. In addition, unnecessary use of antimicrobial drugs may contribute to the emergence of drug-resistant bacteria, cause adverse drug effects, and increase the risk of recurrent pharyngitis.[132] The latter observation may be a result of a dampened immune response to infection.

Penicillin treatment is associated with a 15% to 20% rate of failure to eradicate GABHS from the pharynx. The significance of this finding remains unclear, but some clinicians believe that this represents clinical failure in terms of the ability to prevent rheumatic fever.[133] Repeat throat cultures at the end of therapy are not recommended for asymptomatic patients.[130] The failure of penicillin to eradicate GABHS may be due to the presence of commensal organisms such as H. influenzae and M. catarrhalis. These organisms produce β-lactamase in the local environment, which may result in the destruction of penicillin.[133] Treatment with β-lactamase-stable antimicrobial agents such as amoxicillin/clavulanate, cephalosporins, and macrolides resulted in higher eradication rates of GABHS in some studies. However, it remains unproved whether the improved eradication rate translates to a lower risk of rheumatic fever.

Erythromycin is the recommended alternative for treating penicillin-allergic patients with GABHS pharyngitis.[130] Recommended regimens include 20 to 40 mg/kg/day of erythromycin estolate or 40 mg/kg/day of erythromycin ethylsuccinate administered in three or four divided doses per day for 10 days.[139] Although all strains of S. pyogenes are susceptible to penicillin, low rates of resistance to erythromycin have been noted in the United States; resistance is more frequent in Europe. Also, erythromycin is inactive against H. influenzae and M. catarrhalis, which may be copathogens in some patients with streptococcal pharyngitis. Many patients are unwilling to complete a 10-day regimen of erythromycin because of gastrointestinal adverse effects.[139] For this reason, clarithromycin or azithromycin is often used in place of erythromycin. Both of these agents have the benefit of less-frequent dosing (twice daily for clarithromycin and once daily for azithromycin). In addition, a shorter course (5 days) is recommended with azithromycin (12 mg/kg/day). Clarithromycin (15 mg/kg/day) and azithromycin achieve greater eradication rates of GABHS than the standard penicillin V treatment and cause fewer gastrointestinal effects than erythromycin.[139,140]

Amoxicillin/clavulanate contains an inhibitor of β-lactamases, and this agent would be expected to have advantages when β-lactamases are present, due to copathogens or commensal organisms. There is no evidence from clinical studies that amoxicillin/clavulanate is more effective than penicillin. Penicillin V therapy was associated with a 9.6% persistence rate of GABHS, whereas amoxicillin/clavulanate treatment was associated with a 3.8% persistence rate (difference not significant), although β-lactamase activity was detected in 74% of patients in whom the organism persisted at the end of treatment.[141]

Several oral cephalosporins have been studied for the treatment of streptococcal pharyngitis. Many of the studies concluded that higher eradication rates of GABHS were seen with oral cephalosporins than with penicillin V.[140] Cephalosporins appear to eradicate GABHS in chronic carriers much more effectively than penicillin V. Many patients may be chronic carriers of GABHS with infection due to a virus or other pathogen. It is not possible to distinguish colonization from infection in these patients. Thus, there is controversy whether the lower eradication rate for penicillin V is clinically important. Oral cephalosporins are better tolerated than amoxicillin/clavulanic acid and erythromycin, but they are considerably more expensive. A meta-analysis published in 2004 showed that cephalosporin treatment was associated with improved clinical and microbiologic outcomes compared to penicillin V.[142] However, others have discounted the higher GABHS persistence rate seen with penicillin as merely chronic carriage, which is not associated with adverse consequences. They, the IDSA guideline, and the CDC/AAFP/ACP position paper recommends continued use of penicillin V based on its low cost, narrow spectrum of activity, and good safety profile.[130,135,143]

Table 74.5 lists the antimicrobial agents that are approved for the treatment of acute streptococcal pharyngitis.

COMPLICATIONS

Complications of acute group A β-hemolytic streptococcal pharyngitis can be divided into suppurative complications, toxin-mediated complications, and nonsuppurative complications.

Suppurative complications involve contiguous spread of infection, including peritonsillar abscess, retropharyngeal abscess, cervical lymphadenitis, otitis media, sinusitis, and mastoiditis.[128,129] Recent reports include an apparent increase in streptococcal bacteremia, and some of these cases were related to primary pharyngitis.[144] Lemierre's syndrome, or postanginal sepsis, originates as acute pharyngitis that progresses to septic thrombophlebitis of the internal jugular vein. Septic thrombi then disseminate to the lung, liver, and other organs and usually involve *Fusobacterium* sp. This pathogen is present as normal pharyngeal flora and gains access to the bloodstream as a result of pharyngeal inflammation.[145]

Scarlet fever is the classic toxin-mediated complication; it resulted in substantial mortality in the preantibiotic era. This syndrome is currently termed streptococcal toxic shock-like syndrome (TSLS). TSLS typically occurs after necrotizing fasciitis or myositis with toxin-producing strains of *S. pyogenes*. Approximately 10% to 20% of cases resulted from primary pharyngitis. TSLS presents as hypotension, multisystem organ failure, and erythematous rash or desquamation. The incidence of TSLS appears to have increased since 1988.[144]

TABLE 74.5 Antimicrobial Agents Approved by the U.S. Food and Drug Administration for Treating Acute Group A β–Hemolytic Streptococci Pharyngitis in Children and Adults

Drug	Approved Dosage for Children	Approved Dosage for Adults
Penicillin V	20 mg/kg/day divided q8–12h (≤50 kg) 15 mg/kg/day divided q8–12h (≥50kg)	250 mg q8–12h
Benzathine penicillin G (single intramuscular dose)	300,000–600,000 U (≤27 kg) or 900,000 U (>27 kg)	1.2 million U
Amoxicillin	20–40 mg/kg/day divided q8h	250–500 mg q8h
Cefaclor	20 mg/kg/day divided q12h	375 mg q12h
Cefadroxil	30 mg/kg/day divided q12–24h	1 g/day divided q12–24h
Cefdinir	14 mg/kg q24h	600 mg/day divided q12–24h
Cefixime	8 mg/kg/day divided q12–24h	400 mg divided q12-24h
Cefpodoxime	10 mg/kg/day divided q12h	100 mg q12h
Cefprozil	15 mg/kg/day divided q12h	500 mg q24h
Ceftibuten	9 mg/kg q24h	400 mg q24h
Cefuroxime axetil	25 mg/kg/day divided q12h (suspension)	250 mg q12h
Cephalexin	25–50 mg/kg/day divided q12h	1 g/day divided q6h or q12h
Cephradine	25–50 mg/kg/day divided q6–12h	1 g/day divided q12–24h
Loracarbef	15 mg/kg/day divided q12h	200 mg q12h
Erythromycin (dosage of erythromycin base)	20–50 mg/kg/day divide q6h	250–500 mg q6h
Azithromycin	12 mg/kg q24h for 5 days	500 mg, 250 mg q24h for 4 days
Clarithromycin	15 mg/kg/day divided q12h	250 mg q12h

Use and dosage should be confirmed in official references for children < 6 months old.

Nonsuppurative complications of GABHS infection include rheumatic fever and acute glomerulonephritis. Rheumatic fever is an autoimmune disorder that results in carditis (heart valve destruction), polyarthritis, chorea, and less frequently erythema marginatum and subcutaneous nodules.[144,146] Several outbreaks of rheumatic fever have been reported since 1984. The most serious sequela of rheumatic fever is heart valve damage, which worsens with subsequent infections involving GABHS. Rheumatic heart disease is an important cause of cardiovascular mortality and morbidity in underdeveloped countries but is uncommon in developed regions.[144]

Acute glomerulonephritis is an inflammatory disorder that follows pharyngeal or cutaneous infection with nephrogenic strains of GABHS. Approximately 10% to 15% of patients infected with such strains develop acute glomerulonephritis. Glomerulonephritis typically occurs in young children, approximately 10 days after GABHS infection, and presents as edema, hypertension, acute renal failure, and rust-colored urine. The inflammation is believed to result from immune complex deposition in glomerular tissue. Most patients recover without serious sequelae.[128] The treatment of streptococcal pharyngitis with antimicrobial agents does not appear to prevent acute glomerulonephritis as it does acute rheumatic fever.

ACUTE LARYNGOTRACHEOBRONCHITIS (VIRAL CROUP)

TREATMENT GOALS: ACUTE LARYNGOTRACHEOBRONCHITIS (VIRAL CROUP)

- Maintain the airway.
- Reduce inflammation and airway complications by use of dexamethasone.
- Marked improvement should occur in 2 to 3 days.

Viral croup is a common, usually self-limiting illness of young children. The disease is characterized by noisy breathing (inspiratory stridor) and a dry bark-like cough. The cough and abnormal breathing sounds result from inflammation and edema of the tracheal walls and impaired mobility of the vocal cords. In the most severe forms, the inflammation is extensive enough to obstruct the airway.

EPIDEMIOLOGY

Viral croup occurs in children between 1 and 6 years of age, with the highest incidence during the second year of life.[147] Up to 5% of children contract viral croup between their first and second birthday. The peak incidence occurs in the late fall and winter, and boys are affected at a disproportionately higher rate than girls. Although most cases of viral croup are caused by the parainfluenza virus, croup may also be caused by adenovirus, respiratory syncytial virus, and influenza A virus.

CLINICAL PRESENTATION AND DIAGNOSIS

SIGNS AND SYMPTOMS

Viral croup usually begins with mild cold-like symptoms, including rhinorrhea, mild pharyngitis, cough, and low-grade fever. As inflammation and edema of the tracheal wall develop, the lumen narrows, thereby restricting airflow. Inspiratory stridor occurs due to air passing through the narrowed opening, and this is often audible from a distance. The child's speech is hoarse because of the swelling and altered mobility of the vocal cords. Expiratory stridor and wheezing may also be present, but lung breath sounds are normal. Most children show improvement after 1 to 2 days and resolution of symptoms by 3 to 7 days.

DIAGNOSIS

Viral croup must be differentiated from spasmodic croup, acute epiglottitis, bacterial tracheitis, and a variety of other conditions that lead to tracheal edema and obstruction. Foreign bodies lodged in the trachea must also be considered. Most children with viral croup have a normal oxygen saturation as determined by pulse oximetry. The presence of hypoxia and a low oxygen saturation indicates severe obstruction and the need for immediate treatment. Radiologic studies, including a radiograph of the neck and a limited CT scan, may support the clinical diagnosis. A CT scan provides the most sensitive and specific confirmation, but the procedure is not routinely necessary. Laryngoscopy is particularly helpful when a foreign body or acute epiglottitis is suspected. However, this procedure should not be performed in children with hypoxia or severe respiratory distress.

TREATMENT

The management of viral croup should focus on assessment of airway obstruction and maintenance of an open airway. Emergency airway management and hospital admission may be required in severe cases. Symptomatic treatment may include analgesics (acetaminophen or ibuprofen) and adequate hydration. Cool mist therapy has been used to elevate humidity, which is believed to decrease the viscosity of mucous secretions and soothe inflamed mucosa. Humidified air is not routinely recommended.[147]

Aerosolized epinephrine delivered by nebulizer should be used in children with severe airway narrowing as assessed by a decreased oxygen saturation and labored breathing.[147] The epinephrine decreases swelling and edema through α-receptor stimulation and constriction of small arterioles.

Caution is advised in children with tachycardia and underlying congenital heart disease. Children given this treatment should be observed during and for 2 hours after administration. Aerosolized epinephrine may reduce the need for intubation and tracheostomy.

Corticosteroids (e.g., dexamethasone 0.6 mg/kg) are recommended in children with croup. Most children can be managed with a single dose of oral dexamethasone. A one-time repeat dose is warranted if the child vomits after the first dose. Intramuscular dexamethasone may be used in children who cannot tolerate the oral dose.[148] Nebulized budesonide (2 mg) is equivalent to oral or intramuscular dexamethasone for moderate to severe viral croup.[149] Corticosteroids reduce the need for intubation, shorten the time to improvement and the duration of the emergency room or hospital stay, and reduce the need for repeated aerosol epinephrine administration.[147,148]

ACUTE EPIGLOTTITIS

TREATMENT GOALS: ACUTE EPIGLOTTITIS

- Maintain the airway.
- Provide optimal and appropriate antimicrobial therapy.
- Rapid improvement should occur within 24 to 48 hours.

Acute epiglottitis is a very serious condition involving cellulitis and swelling of the epiglottis. Children with acute epiglottis are at significant risk for acute airway obstruction and death if endotracheal intubation or emergency tracheostomy is not performed.

Acute epiglottitis is usually caused by infection with *H influenzae* type B. Fortunately, the availability and widespread use of *Haemophilus* type B vaccine in children has almost eliminated acute epiglottitis, and this topic will be discussed only briefly in this chapter. In addition to *H. influenzae* type B, acute epiglottitis may be caused by *S. pneumoniae*, β-hemolytic streptococci, *S aureus*, and aerobic gram-negative bacteria. Most cases of acute epiglottitis due to organisms other than GABHS and *H. influenzae* occur in immunocompromised individuals.[150] Two recent studies have documented the rare occurrence of acute epiglottitis in patients who have received *H. influenzae* type B vaccination; thus, vaccine failure does occur.[151,152]

KEY POINTS

THE COMMON COLD
- Symptoms may overlap with bacterial causes of URI
- Antimicrobial agents are not effective and should not be used
- Symptomatic treatment is with acetaminophen and/or a decongestant

ACUTE RHINOSINUSITIS
- Acute rhinosinusitis must be differentiated from viral URI (more severe or persistent symptoms)

- First-line treatment is amoxicillin. Alternatives include amoxicillin/clavulanate, selected oral cephalosporins, newer macrolides, and fluoroquinolones (adults only)
- Five-day treatment regimens are as effective as 10-day regimens for some agents in children older than 2 years of age (older than 6 years for severe illness) and adults

OTITIS MEDIA
- AOM must be differentiated from OME
- Antimicrobial treatment is indicated for AOM in children less than 2 years of age. The option of ''watchful waiting'' may be appropriate if the diagnosis is uncertain or the child is more than 2 years old

■ Antimicrobial treatment is optional for OME if symptoms persist for 3 to 6 months
■ First-line treatment with amoxicillin is recommended by consensus groups. Alternatives are the same as listed for acute rhinosinusitis

PHARYNGITIS

■ A definitive diagnosis is made by RADT and/or culture, but the need for culture is controversial
■ Patients with GABHS should be treated with oral penicillin V. An alternative treatment is oral erythromycin, but oral cephalosporins, newer macrolides, and amoxicillin/clavulanate are also effective

ACUTE LARYNGOTRACHEOBRONCHITIS (VIRAL CROUP)

■ Viral croup must be differentiated from other causes of acute airway obstruction
■ Most patients should receive a single dose of oral dexamethasone
■ Analgesics may be given for symptomatic relief
■ The use of nebulized epinephrine should be reserved for children with severe illness and respiratory distress
■ Anti-infective therapy is not recommended

ACUTE EPIGLOTTITIS

■ Acute epiglottitis is usually caused by type B *H. influenzae*
■ Acute epiglottitis is now rare due to widespread use of the *H. influenzae* type B vaccine in children

REFERENCES

1. Bramley TJ, Lerner D, Sarnes M. Productivity losses related to the common cold. J Occup Environ Med 44:822–829, 2002.
2. Turner RB. The treatment of the common cold. J Infect Dis Pharmacother 1:21–34, 1995.
3. Tompkins RK, Wood RW, Wolcott BW, et al. The effectiveness and cost of acute respiratory illness medical care provided by physicians and algorithm-assisted physicians' assistants. Med Care 15:991–1003, 1977.
4. Rosenthal I. Expense of physician care spurs OTC, self-care market. Drug Top 132:62–63, 1988.
5. Busse WW. The role of the common cold in asthma. J Clin Pharmacol 39:241–245, 1999.
6. Puhakka T, Mäkelä MJ, Alanen A, et al. Sinusitis in the common cold. J Allergy Clin Immunol 102:403–408, 1998.
7. Moody SA, Alper CM, Doyle WJ. Daily tympanometry in children during the cold season: association of otitis media with upper respiratory tract infections. Int J Pediatr Otorhinolaryngol 45:143–150, 1998.
8. Elkhatieb A, Hipskind G, Woerner D, et al. Middle ear abnormalities during natural rhinovirus colds in adults. J Infect Dis 168:618–621, 1993.
9. Monto AS, Sullivan KM. Acute respiratory illness in the community. Frequency of illness and the agents involved. Epidemiol Infect 110:145–160, 1993.
10. Mäkelä MJ, Puhakka T, Ruuskanen O, et al. Viruses and bacteria in the etiology of the common cold. J Clin Microbiol 36:539–542, 1998.
11. Pitkäranta A, Hayden FG. Rhinoviruses: important respiratory pathogens. Ann Med 30:529–537, 1998.
12. Arruda E, Pitkäranta A, Witek TJ Jr, et al. Frequency and natural history of rhinovirus infections in adults during autumn. J Clin Microbiol 35:2864–2868, 1997.
13. Isaacs D, Flowers D, Clarke JR, et al. Epidemiology of coronavirus respiratory infections. Arch Dis Child 58:500–503, 1983.
14. Easton AJ, Eglin RP. Epidemiology of parainfluenza virus type 3 in England and Wales over a 10-year period. Epidemiol Infect 102:531–535, 1989.
15. Gwaltney JM Jr, Moskalski PB, Hendley JO. Hand-to-hand transmission of rhinovirus. Ann Intern Med 88:463–467, 1978.
16. Gwaltney JM Jr, Hendley JO. Transmission of experimental rhinovirus by contaminated surfaces. Am J Epidemiol 116:828–833, 1982.
17. Dick EC, Jennings LC, Mink KA, et al. Aerosol transmission of rhinovirus colds. J Infect Dis 156:442–448, 1987.
18. Kelley LF. Pediatric cough and cold preparations. Pediatr Rev 2004;25:115–123.
19. Tyrrell DAJ, Cohen S, Schlarb JE. Signs and symptoms in common colds. Epidemiol Infect 111:143–156, 1993.
20. Kirkpatrick GL. The common cold. Primary Care 23:657–675, 1996.
21. Sperber SJ, Levine PA, Sorrentino JV, et al. Ineffectiveness of recombinant interferon-beta serine nasal drops for prophylaxis of natural colds. J Infect Dis 160:700–705, 1989.
22. Macknin ML, Piedmonte M, Calendine C, et al. Zinc gluconate lozenges for treating the common cold in children. JAMA 279:1962–1967, 1998.
23. Hemila H. Vitamin C supplementation and common cold symptoms: problems with inaccurate reviews. Nutrition 12:804–809, 1996.
24. Hayden F, Hipskind GJ, Woerner DH, et al. Intranasal pirodavir (R77,975) treatment of rhinovirus colds. Antimicrob Agents Chemother 39:290–294, 1995.
25. al Nakib W, Higgins PG, Barrow GI, et al. Suppression of colds in human volunteers challenged with rhinovirus by a new synthetic drug (R61837). Antimicrob Agents Chemother 33:522–525, 1989.
26. Zerial A, Werner GH, Phillpotts RJ, et al. Studies on 44 081 R.P., a new antirhinovirus compound, in cell cultures and in volunteers. Antimicrob Agents Chemother 27:846–850, 1985.
27. Miller FD, Monto AS, DeLong DC, et al. Controlled trial of enviroxime against natural rhinovirus infections in a community. Antimicrob Agents Chemother 27:102–106, 1985.
28. Phillpotts RJ, Higgins PG, Willman JS, et al. Evaluation of the antirhinovirus chalcone Ro 09-0415 given orally to volunteers. J Antimicrob Chemother 14:403–409, 1984.
29. Phillpotts RJ, Wallace J, Tyrrell DA, et al. Failure of oral 4′,6–dichloroflavan to protect against rhinovirus infection in man. Arch Virol 75:115–121, 1983.
30. Turner RB, Wecker MT, Pohl G, et al. Efficacy of tremacamra, a soluble intercellular adhesion molecule 1, for experimental rhinovirus infection: a randomized clinical trial. JAMA 281:1797–1804, 1999.
31. Graham NM, Burrell CJ, Douglas RM, et al. Adverse effects of aspirin, acetaminophen, and ibuprofen on immune function, viral shedding, and clinical status in rhinovirus-infected volunteers. J Infect Dis 162:1277–1282, 1990
32. Brown AK, Fikrig S, Finberg L. Aspirin and Reye syndrome. J Pediatr 102:157–158, 1983.
33. Sperber SJ, Hendley JO, Hayden FG, et al. Effects of naproxen on experimental rhinovirus colds. A randomized, double-blind, controlled trial. Ann Intern Med 117:37–41, 1992.
34. Gwaltner JM Jr, Druce HM. Efficacy of brompheniramine maleate for the treatment of rhinovirus colds. Clin Infect Dis 25:1188–1194, 1997.
35. Turner RB, Sperber SJ, Sorrentino JV, et al. Effectiveness of clemastine fumarate for treatment of rhinorrhea and sneezing associated with the common cold. Clin Infect Dis 25:824–830, 1997.
36. Luks D, Anderson MR. Antihistamines and the common cold. A review and critique of the literature. J Gen Intern Med 11:240–244, 1996.
37. Hayden FG, Diamond L, Wood PB, et al. Effectiveness and safety of intranasal ipratropium bromide in common colds. A randomized,

double-blind, placebo-controlled trial. Ann Intern Med 125:89–97, 1996.

38. Smith MB, Feldman W. Over-the-counter cold medications. A critical review of clinical trials between 1950 and 1991. JAMA 269: 2258–2263, 1993.

39. Taverner D, Danz C, Economos D. The effects of oral pseudoephedrine on nasal patency in the common cold: a double-blind single-dose placebo-controlled trial. Clin Otolaryngol Allied Sci 24:47–51, 1999.

40. Aberg N, Aberg B, Alestig K. The effect of inhaled and intranasal sodium cromoglycate on symptoms of upper respiratory tract infections. Clin Exp Allergy 26:1045–1050, 1996.

41. Freestone C, Eccles R. Assessment of the antitussive efficacy of codeine in cough associated with common cold. J Pharm Pharmacol 49:1045–1049, 1997.

42. Curley FJ, Irwin RS, Pratter MR, et al. Cough and the common cold. Am Rev Respir Dis 138:305–311, 1988.

43. Melchart D, Linde K, Fischer P, et al. Echinacea for preventing and treating the common cold. Cochrane Database of Systematic Reviews 2:CD000530, 2000.

44. Dowell SF, Schwartz B, Phillips WR. Appropriate use of antibiotics for URIs in children: part II. Cough, pharyngitis and the common cold. The Pediatric URI Consensus Team. Am Fam Physician 58:1335–1342, 45, 1998.

45. Kankam CG, Sallis R. Acute rhinosinusitis in adults: difficult to diagnose, essential to treat. Postgrad Med 102:253–258, 1997.

46. Josephson GD, Gross CW. Diagnosis and management of acute and chronic sinusitis. Compr Ther 23:708–714, 1997.

47. Duvoisin B, Landry M, Chapuis L, et al. Low-dose CT and inflammatory disease of the paranasal sinuses. Neuroradiology 33: 403–406, 1991.

48. Joint Council of Allergy, Asthma and Immunology. Sinusitis practice parameters. J Allergy Clin Immunol 102 (Suppl):S107–S144, 1998.

49. van Buchem FL, Knottnerus JA, Schrijnemaekers VJJ, et al. Primary-care based randomized placebo-controlled trial of antibiotic treatment in acute maxillary sinusitis. Lancet 349:683–687, 1997.

50. Stalman W, van Essen GA, van der Graaf Y, et al. The end of antibiotic treatment in adults with acute rhinosinusitis-like complaints in general practice? A placebo-controlled double-blind randomized doxycycline trial. Br J Gen Pract 47:794–799, 1997.

51. Stalman W, van Essen GA, van der Graaf Y, et al. Maxillary sinusitis in adults: an evaluation of placebo-controlled double-blind trials. Fam Pract 14:124–129, 1997.

52. Gwaltney JM, Scheld WM, Sande MA, et al. The microbial etiology and antimicrobial therapy of adults with acute community-acquired sinusitis: a 15-year experience at the University of Virginia and review of other selected studies. J Allergy Clin Immunol 90: 457–462, 1992.

53. Wald ER. Microbiology of acute and chronic sinusitis in children and adults. Am J Med Sci 316:13–20, 1998.

54. Wald ER. Microbiology of acute and chronic sinusitis in children. J Allergy Clin Immunol 90:452–460, 1992.

55. Hueston WJ, Ebertein C, Johnson D, et al. Criteria used by clinicians to differentiate sinusitis from viral upper respiratory tract infection. J Fam Pract 46:487–492, 1998.

56. Gwaltney JM Jr, Phillips CD, Miller RD, et al. Computer tomographic study of the common cold. N Engl J Med 330:25–30, 1994.

57. Wald ER, Byers C, Guerra N, et al. Subacute sinusitis in children. J Pediatr 115:28–32, 1989.

58. Gwaltney JM Jr. Acute community-acquired sinusitis. Clin Infect Dis 23:1209–1225, 1996.

59. Giannoni CM, Stewart MG, Alford EL. Intracranial complications of sinusitis. Laryngoscope 107:863–867, 1997.

60. Clayman GL, Adams GL, Paugh DR, et al. Intracranial complications of paranasal sinusitis: a combined institutional review. Laryngoscope 101:234–239, 1991.

61. Williams JW Jr, Simel DL, Roberts L, et al. Clinical evaluation for sinusitis. Making the diagnosis by history and physical examination. Ann Intern Med 117:705–710, 1992.

62. Otten FW, Grote JJ. The diagnostic value of transillumination for maxillary sinusitis in children. Int J Pediatr Otorhinolaryngol 18: 9–11, 1989.

63. Spector SL, Lotan A, English G, et al. Comparison between transillumination and the roentgenogram in diagnosing paranasal sinus disease. J Allergy Clin Immunol 67:22–26, 1981.

64. DeAlleaume L, Parker S. What findings distinguish acute bacterial sinusitis? J Fam Pract 52:563–564, 2003.

65. American Academy of Pediatrics. Clinical practice guideline: management of sinusitis. Pediatrics 108:798–808, 2001.

66. Brown SD, Farrell DJ. Antibacterial susceptibility among Streptococcus pneumoniae isolated from paediatric and adult patients as part of the PROTEKT US study in 2001–2002. J Antimicrob Chemother 54 (Suppl S1):i23–i29, 2004.

67. Hoberman A, Paradise JL, Greenberg DP, et al. Penicillin susceptibility of pneumococcal isolates causing acute otitis media in children: seasonal variation. Pediatr Infect Dis J 24:115–120, 2005.

68. Thornsberry C, Ogilvie P, Kahn J, et al. Surveillance of antimicrobial resistance in Streptococcus. pneumoniae, Haemophilus influenzae, and Moraxella catarrhalis in the United States in 1996–1997 respiratory season. Diagn Microbiol Infect Dis 29:249–257, 1997.

69. Alder JD, Ewing PJ, Nilius AM, et al. Dynamics of clarithromycin and azithromycin efficacies against experimental Haemophilus influenzae pulmonary infection. Antimicrob Agents Chemother 42: 2385–2390, 1998.

70. Klapan I, Culig J, Oreskovic K, et al. Azithromycin versus amoxicillin/clavulanate in the treatment of acute sinusitis. Am J Otolaryngol 20:7–11, 1999.

71. Adelglass J, DeAbate CA, McElvaine P, et al. Comparison of the effectiveness of levofloxacin and amoxicillin–clavulanate for the treatment of acute sinusitis in adults. Otolaryngol Head Neck Surg 120:320–327, 1999.

72. Adelglass J, Bundy JM, Woods R. Efficacy and tolerability of cefprozil versus amoxicillin/clavulanate for the treatment of adults with severe sinusitis. Clin Ther 20:1115–1129, 1998.

73. Chatzimanolis E, Marsan N, Lefatzis D, et al. Comparison of roxithromycin with co-amoxiclav in patients with sinusitis. J Antimicrob Chemother 41 (Suppl B):81–84, 1998.

74. Sterkers O. Efficacy and tolerability of ceftibuten versus amoxicillin/clavulanate in the treatment of acute sinusitis. Chemotherapy 43:352–357, 1997.

75. De Abate CA, Perrotta RJ, Dennington ML, et al. The efficacy and safety of once-daily ceftibuten compared with co-amoxiclav in the treatment of acute bacterial sinusitis. J Chemother 4:358–363, 1992.

76. Gwaltney JM Jr, Savolainen S, Rivas P, et al. Comparative effectiveness and safety of cefdinir and amoxicillin–clavulanate in treatment of acute community-acquired bacterial sinusitis. Cefdinir Sinusitis Study Group. Antimicrob Agents Chemother 41:1517–1520, 1997.

77. Dubois J, Saint-Pierre C, Tremblay C. Efficacy of clarithromycin vs. amoxicillin/clavulanate in the treatment of acute maxillary sinusitis. Ear Nose Throat J 72:804–810, 1993.

78. Camacho AE, Cobo R, Otte J, et al. Clinical comparison of cefuroxime axetil and amoxicillin/clavulanate in the treatment of patients with acute bacterial maxillary sinusitis. Am J Med 93:271–276, 1992.

79. Sydnor TA Jr, Scheld WM, Gwaltney J Jr, et al. Loracarbef (LY 163892) vs amoxicillin/clavulanate in bacterial maxillary sinusitis. Ear Nose Throat J 71:225–232, 1992.

80. von Sydow C, Savolainen S, Soderqvist A. Treatment of acute maxillary sinusitis: comparing cefpodoxime proxetil with amoxicillin. Scand J Infect Dis 27:229–234, 1995.

81. Huck W, Reed BD, Nielsen RW, et al. Cefaclor vs amoxicillin in the treatment of acute, recurrent, and chronic sinusitis. Arch Fam Med 2:497–503, 1993.

82. Wald ER, Reilly JS, Casselbrant M, et al. Treatment of acute maxillary sinusitis in childhood: a comparative study of amoxicillin and cefaclor. J Pediatr 104:297–302, 1984.

83. Calhoun KH, Hokanson JA. Multicenter comparison of clarithromycin and amoxicillin in the treatment of acute maxillary sinusitis. Arch Fam Med 2:837–840, 1993.

84. Edelstein DR, Avner SE, Chow JM, et al. Once-a-day therapy for sinusitis: a comparison study of cefixime and amoxicillin. Laryngoscope 103:33–41, 1993.

85. Casiano RR. Azithromycin and amoxicillin in the treatment of acute maxillary sinusitis. Am J Med 91 (Suppl 3A):27S–30S, 1991.

86. Brodie DP, Knight S, Cunningham K. Comparative study of cefuroxime axetil and amoxicillin in the treatment of acute sinusitis in general practice. J Intern Med Res 17:547–551, 1989.

87. Mattucci KF, Levin WJ, Habib MA. Acute bacterial sinusitis. Minocycline vs amoxicillin. Arch Otolaryngol Head Neck Surg 112: 73–76, 1986.

88. Klein GL, Whalen E, Echols RM, et al. Ciprofloxacin versus cefuroxime axetil in the treatment of adult patients with acute bacterial sinusitis. J Otolaryngol 27:10–16, 1998.

89. Gehanno P, Berche P. Sparfloxacin versus cefuroxime axetil in the treatment of acute purulent sinusitis. Sinusitis Study Group. J Antimicrob Chemother 37 (Suppl A):105–114, 1996.

90. Gehanno P, Depondt J, Barry B, et al. Comparison of cefpodoxime proxetil with cefaclor in the treatment of sinusitis. J Antimicrob Chemother 26 (Suppl E):87–91, 1990.

91. Aust R, Drettner B, Falck B. Studies of the effect of peroral fenyl-propanolamin on the functional size of the human maxillary ostium. Acta Otolaryngol 88:455–458, 1979.

92. McCormick DP, John SD, Swischuk LE, et al. A double-blind, placebo-controlled trial of decongestant-antihistamine for the treatment of sinusitis in children. Clin Pediatr 35:457–460, 1996.

93. Meltzer EO, Orgel HA, Backhaus JW, et al. Intranasal flunisolide spray as an adjunct to oral antibiotic therapy for sinusitis. J Allergy Clin Immunol 92:812–823, 1993.

94. Ovarnberg Y, Kantola O, Salo J, et al. Influence of topical steroid treatment on maxillary sinusitis. Rhinology 30:103–112, 1992.

95. Giannoni CM, Stewart MG, Alford EL. Intracranial complications of sinusitis. Laryngoscope 107:863–867, 1997.

96. Clayman GL, Adams GL, Paugh DR, et al. Intracranial complications of paranasal sinusitis: a combined institutional review. Laryngoscope 101:234–239, 1991.

97. Giannoni C, Sulek M, Friedman EM. Intracranial complications of sinusitis: a pediatric series. Am J Rhinol 12:173–178, 1998.

98. Dowell SF, Marcy SM, Phillips WR, et al. Otitis media: principles of judicious use of antimicrobial agents. Pediatrics 101 (Suppl): 165–171, 1998.

99. Desai SN, Kellner JD, Drummond D. Population-based, age-specific myringotomy with tympanostomy tube insertion rates in Calgary, Canada. Pediatr Infect Dis J 21:348–350, 2002.

100. Garbutt J, Jeffe DB, Shackelford P. Diagnosis and treatment of acute otitis media: an assessment. Pediatrics 112:143–149, 2003.

101. Teele DW, Klein JO, Rosner B. Epidemiology of otitis media during the first seven years of life in children in greater Boston: a prospective cohort study. J Infect Dis 160:83–94, 1989.

102. Paradise JL, Rochette HE, Colborn DK, et al. Otitis media in 2253 Pittsburgh-area infants: prevalence and risk factors during the first two years of life. Pediatrics 99:318–333, 1997.

103. Haddad J Jr. Treatment of acute otitis media and its complications. Otolaryngol Clin North Am 27:431–441, 1994.

104. Arguedas A, Loaiza C, Perez A, et al. Microbiology of acute otitis media in Costa Rican children. Pediatr Infect Dis J 17:680–689, 1998.

105. Brook I, Gober AE. Microbiologic characteristics of persistent otitis media. Arch Otolaryngol Head Neck Surg 124:1350–1352, 1998.

106. Hoberman A, Paradise JL, Greenberg DP, et al. Penicillin susceptibility of pneumococcal isolates causing acute otitis media in children. Pediatr Infect Dis J. 24: 115–120, 2005.

107. Casey JR, Pichichero ME. Changes in frequency and pathogens causing acute otitis media in 1995–2003. Pediatr Infect Dis J. 23: 824–828, 2004.

108. Shurin PA, Howie VM, Pelton SI, et al. Bacterial etiology of otitis media during the first six weeks of life. J Pediatr 92:893–896, 1978.

109. Rothman R, Owens T, Simel DL. Does this child have acute otitis media? JAMA 290:1633–1640, 2003.

110. Faden H, Duffy L, Boeve M. Otitis media: back to basics. Pediatr Infect Dis J 17:1105–1113, 1998.

111. Timmerman AA, Anteunis LJC, Meesters CMG. Response-shift bias and parent-reported quality of life in children with otitis media. Arch Otolaryngol Head Neck Surg. 129:987–991, 2005.

112. Tetzlaff TR, Ashworth C, Nelson JD. Otitis media in children less than 12 weeks of age. Pediatrics 59:827–832, 1977.

113. Pelton SI. Otoscopy for the diagnosis of otitis media. Pediatr Infect Dis J 17:540–543, 1998.

114. Brookhouser PE. Use of tympanometry in office practice for diagnosis of otitis media. Pediatr Infect Dis J 17:544–551, 1998.

115. Hoberman A, Paradise JL, Wald ER. Tympanocentesis technique revisited. Pediatr Infect Dis J 16 (Suppl 2):S25–S26, 1997.

116. Culpepper L, Froom J. Routine antimicrobial treatment of acute otitis media: is it necessary? JAMA 278:1643–1645, 1997.

117. Rosenfeld RM. What to expect from medical treatment of otitis media. Pediatr Infect Dis J 14:731–738, 1995.

118. Subcommittee on Management of Acute Otitis Media, American Academy of Pediatrics and American Academy of Family Physicians. Diagnosis and management of acute otitis media. Pediatrics 113:1451–1465, 2004.

119. American Academy of Family Physicians, American Academy of Otolaryngology-Head and Neck Surgery, and American Academy of Pediatrics Subcommittee on Otitis Media With Effusion. Otitis media with effusion. Pediatrics 113:1412–1429, 2004.

120. Rosenfeld RM, Vertrees JE, Carr J, et al. Clinical efficacy of antimicrobial drugs for acute otitis media: meta-analysis of 5400 children from thirty-three randomized trials. J Pediatr 124:355–367, 1994.

121. Craig WA, Andes D. Pharmacokinetics and pharmacodynamics of antibiotics in otitis media. Pediatr Infect Dis J 15:255–259, 1996.

122. Toltzis P, Dul M, O'Riordan AO, et al. Impact of amoxicillin on pneumococcal colonization compared with other therapies for acute otitis media. Pediatr Infect Dis J 24:24–28, 2005.

123. Brook I. Use of oral cephalosporins in the treatment of acute otitis media in children. Int J Antimicrob Agents 24:18–23, 2004.

124. Garbutt J, St. Geme JW III, May A, et al. Developing community-specific recommendations for first-line treatment of acute otitis media: is high-dose amoxicillin necessary? Pediatrics 114: 342–347, 2005.

125. Leibovitz E, Piglansky L, Raiz S, et al. Bacteriologic efficacy of a three-day intramuscular ceftriaxone regimen in nonresponsive acute otitis media. Pediatr Infect Dis J 17:1126–1131, 1998.

126. Kozyrskyj AL, Hildes-Ripstein E, Longstaffe SEA, et al. Treatment of acute otitis media with a shortened course of antibiotics: a meta-analysis. JAMA 279:1736–1742, 1998.

127. Cohen R, Levy C, Boucherat M, et al. A multicenter, randomized, double-blind trial of 5 versus 10 days of antibiotic therapy for acute otitis media in young children. J Pediatr 133:634–639, 1998.

128. Gooch WM III. Potential infectious disease complications of upper respiratory tract infections. Pediatr Infect Dis J 17 (Suppl): S79–S82, 1998.

129. Barry B, Delattre J, Vie F, et al. Otogenic intracranial infection in adults. Laryngoscope 109:483–487, 1999.

130. Bisno AL, Gerber MA, Gwaltney JM Jr, et al. Diagnosis and management of group A streptococcal pharyngitis: a practice guideline. Clin Infect Dis 25:574–583, 1997.

131. Espositio S, Blasi F, Bosis S, et al. Aetiology of acute pharyngitis: the role of atypical bacteria. J Med Microbiol. 53:645–651, 2004.

132. McIsaac WJ, Goel V, Slaughter PM, et al. Reconsidering sore throats. Part 1: problems with current clinical practice. Can Fam Physician 43:485–493, 1997.

133. Pichichero ME. Streptococcal pharyngitis: is penicillin still the right choice? Compr Ther 22:782–787, 1996.

134. Johnson DR, Stevens DL, Kaplan EL. Epidemiologic analysis of group A streptococcal serotypes associated with severe systemic infections, rheumatic fever, or uncomplicated pharyngitis. J Infect Dis 166:374–382, 1992.

135. Cooper RJ, Hoffman JR, Bartlett JG, et al. Principles of appropriate antibiotic use for acute pharyngitis in adults: background. Ann Intern Med 134:509–517, 2001.

136. McIsaac WJ, Kellner JD, Aufricht P, et al. Empirical validation of guidelines for the management of pharyngitis in children and adults. JAMA 291:1587–1595, 2004.

137. McIsaac WJ, Goel V, Slaughter PM, et al. Reconsidering sore throats. Part 2: alternative approach and practical office tool. Can Fam Physician 43:495–500, 1997.

138. Dagnelie CF, van der Garaaf Y, De Melker RA. Do patients with sore throat benefit from penicillin? A randomized double-blind placebo-controlled clinical trial with penicillin V in general practice. Br J Gen Pract 46:589–593, 1996.

139. Tarlow MJ. Macrolides in the management of streptococcal pharyngitis/tonsillitis. Pediatr Infect Dis 16:444–448, 1997.
140. Shulman ST. Evaluation of penicillins, cephalosporins, and macrolides for therapy of streptococcal pharyngitis. Pediatrics 97:955–959, 1996.
141. Dykhuizen RS, Golder D, Reid TMS, et al. Phenoxymethyl penicillin versus co-amoxiclav in the treatment of acute streptococcal pharyngitis, and the role of β-lactamase activity in saliva. J Antimicrob Chemother 37:133–138, 1996.
142. Casey JR, Pichichero ME. Meta-analysis of cephalosporin versus penicillin treatment of group A streptococcal tonsillopharyngitis in children. Pediatrics 113:866–882, 2005.
143. Shulman ST, Gerber MA. So what's wrong with penicillin for strep throat? Pediatrics 113:1816–1819, 2004.
144. Shulman ST. Complications of streptococcal pharyngitis. Pediatr Infect Dis J 13 (Suppl):S70–S74, 1994.
145. Williams A, Nagy M, Wingate J, et al. Lemierre syndrome: a complication of acute pharyngitis. Int J Pediatr Otorhinolaryngol 45:51–57, 1998.
146. Dajani AS. Current status of nonsuppurative complications of group A streptococci. Pediatr Infect Dis J 10 (Suppl):S25–S27, 1991.
147. Leung AKC, Kellner JD, Johnson DW. Viral croup: a current perspective. J Pediatr Health Care 18:297–301, 2004.
148. Bjornson CL, Klassen TP, Williamson J, et al. A randomized trial of a single dose of oral dexamethasone for mild croup. N Engl J Med 351:1306–1313, 2004.
149. Johnson DW, Jacobson S, Edney PC, et al. A comparison of nebulized budesonide, intramuscular dexamethasone, and placebo for moderately severe croup. N Engl J Med 339:498–503, 1998.
150. Stroud RH, Friedman NR. An update on inflammatory disorders of the pediatric airway: epiglottitis, croup, and tracheitis. Am J Otolaryngol. 22:268–275, 2001.
151. Shah RK, Roberson DW, Jones DT. Epiglottitis in the *Haemophilus influenzae* type B vaccine era: changing trends. Laryngoscope 114:557–560, 2004.
152. McEwan J, Giridharan W, Clarke RW, Shears P. Paediatric acute epiglottitis: not a disappearing entity. Pediatr Otorhinolaryngol 67:317–321, 2003.

Pneumonia

Douglas Slain

75

TREATMENT GOALS

- Optimize the use of diagnostic methods to ensure an accurate diagnosis of pneumonia.
- Recognize patients at risk for antibiotic-resistant organisms.
- Administer appropriate antibiotics as early as possible in severely ill patients.
- Select the most appropriate, safe, and cost-effective antibiotic, given the patient's specific situation.
- Limit the selection of antimicrobial resistance by avoiding indiscriminate antibiotic use and by observing optimal infection control practices.
- When possible, treat as outpatients, or with oral antibiotics, to limit complications and costs of care.

OVERVIEW

DEFINITION

Pneumonia is defined as an infection or inflammation of the lung parenchyma caused most often by microbial pathogens. Noninfectious pneumonia or pneumonitis results from exposure to drugs, fluids, or chemicals. The condition of pneumonia has been described in the earliest recorded descriptions of human diseases.[1] The word pneumonia is of Greek origin, meaning "a condition about the lung." Pneumonia was a common cause of death throughout antiquity and the preantibiotic era. Revered physician Sir William Osler (1849–1919) referred to pneumonia as "the captain of the men of death," highlighting the poor outcomes associated with this type of infection before the advent of antimicrobials and modern supportive care measures.[2] Despite major advances in diagnosis and treatment, however, mortality associated with pneumonia remains high, especially in the elderly.[3]

Pneumonia has often been classified by the environmental setting in which it developed. The three classic types of pneumonia are community-acquired pneumonia (CAP), hospital-acquired pneumonia (HAP), and nursing home-acquired pneumonia (NHAP).[4,5] The most frequent type of HAP is ventilator-associated pneumonia (VAP). The term "nosocomial pneumonia" is a broader term that incorporates HAP and VAP and the more recently established entity healthcare-associated pneumonia (HCAP). HCAP is included within the spectrum of HAP and VAP. HCAP was coined to include patients who may be at greater risk of being infected with resistant nosocomial organisms but who may have developed the infection by exposure to the healthcare system but outside of a hospital. By definition, HCAP includes patients hospitalized in an acute care hospital for 2 or more days within 90 days of the infection; those who lived in a nursing home or long-term care facility; those who received recent intravenous antibiotic therapy, chemotherapy, or wound care within the past 30 days of the current infection; or those who attended a hospital or hemodialysis clinic.[5,6]

Aspiration pneumonia can be a subtype of any of the above types of pneumonia. *Aspiration pneumonia* is defined as a pneumonia that results from the abnormal entry of endogenous secretions or exogenous substances into the lower airways.[7,8] Since most cases of pneumonia are associated with aspiration, many clinicians reserve the term "aspiration pneumonia" for pneumonia that arises from macroaspiration of large quantities of endogenous oropharyngeal or gastrointestinal secretions.

Pneumonia has also been classified by pattern of lung involvement. The term "bronchopneumonia" is used to describe a pneumonia that involves many relatively small areas of lung tissue, whereas "lobar pneumonia" is used to describe a pneumonia affecting one or more lobes of the lung (Fig. 75.1; *see color insert*).[9,10]

Diagnosing pneumonia is straightforward in many patients, but identifying the causative microorganisms remains difficult in most types of pneumonias. As such, antimicrobial therapy for pneumonia is often empiric.[5,11,12] Therefore, it is important for clinicians to be aware of the common pathogens encountered in the specific types of pneumonia.

This chapter will review pneumonia and its therapeutics in the general adult population. Readers are directed to more specific resources for a more in-depth discussion of pneumonia in children and in immunocompromised patients.

EPIDEMIOLOGY

In the United States, pneumonia is reported to be the sixth leading cause of death, and the most common infectious cause of death.[11,13] The elderly, the immunocompromised, those with preexisting cardiopulmonary disease, and the critically ill are at increased risk of mortality.

Approximately 5.6 million cases of CAP occur annually in the United States, with about a fourth of cases requiring hospitalization.[11,14] In the outpatient setting, the mortality rate remains low (less than 1% to 5%) for CAP patients not requiring hospital admission.[15,16] The mortality rate for CAP patients who require hospitalization averages about 14%.[17] For patients with CAP requiring admission to the intensive care unit (ICU), the mortality rate approaches 40%.[11]

Several reports state that the incidence of pneumonia appears to be greater in the winter, leading to the misnomer of a "pneumonia season."[5] In reality, pneumonia can happen year round.

Pneumonia is the second most common hospital-acquired infection, occurring in 0.5% to 3% of hospitalized patients.[18,19] However, it is the leading cause of death among patients with hospital-acquired infections. Mortality rates range from 10% to 40%, with the greatest risk of mortality in mechanically ventilated patients.[18] It is estimated that 8% to 28% of patients receiving mechanical ventilation will develop VAP.[20] Crude mortality rates for patients with VAP have ranged from 24% to 76%.[20] Recent case-matching studies suggest that the attributable mortality of VAP is in the range of 33% to 50%.[5]

Pneumonia is the leading cause of death among nursing home patients.[21] Estimates of NHAP range from 0.3 to 2.5 cases per 1,000 days of resident care.[22] This rate greatly exceeds that of elderly persons living in the community. Nursing home patients account for 10% to 20% of all patients hospitalized for pneumonia.[21]

The cost burden of pneumonia is astounding. Total costs of treating pneumonia have been estimated to be as high as $23 billion each year.[13] In the United States, 89% of the $8.4 billion spent annually for patients with CAP is spent on inpatient care.[23] Obviously, appreciable savings can be realized through early discharge of patients with low risk of death. When pneumonia develops in hospitalized patients, it can prolong their length of stay by an average of 7 to 9 days, which can increase the cost of their care by more than $40,000.[5] Efforts to prevent the development of nosocomial pneumonia reduce morbidity, mortality, and costs.

Pneumonia can be caused by a wide array of bacteria, viruses, fungi, parasites, and other microbes (Table 75.1).[24] However, there are about five to seven common organisms that are generally regarded as common causative pathogens for each type of pneumonia. It is important for clinicians to know the common causes so that they can identify prudent empiric therapy. In most cases, the causative organism is one that has colonized the patient's upper respiratory tract before the development of pneumonia.

PATHOPHYSIOLOGY

HOST DEFENSES AND PATHOGENESIS

The human respiratory system is constantly exposed to foreign material, chemicals, and potentially infectious microor-

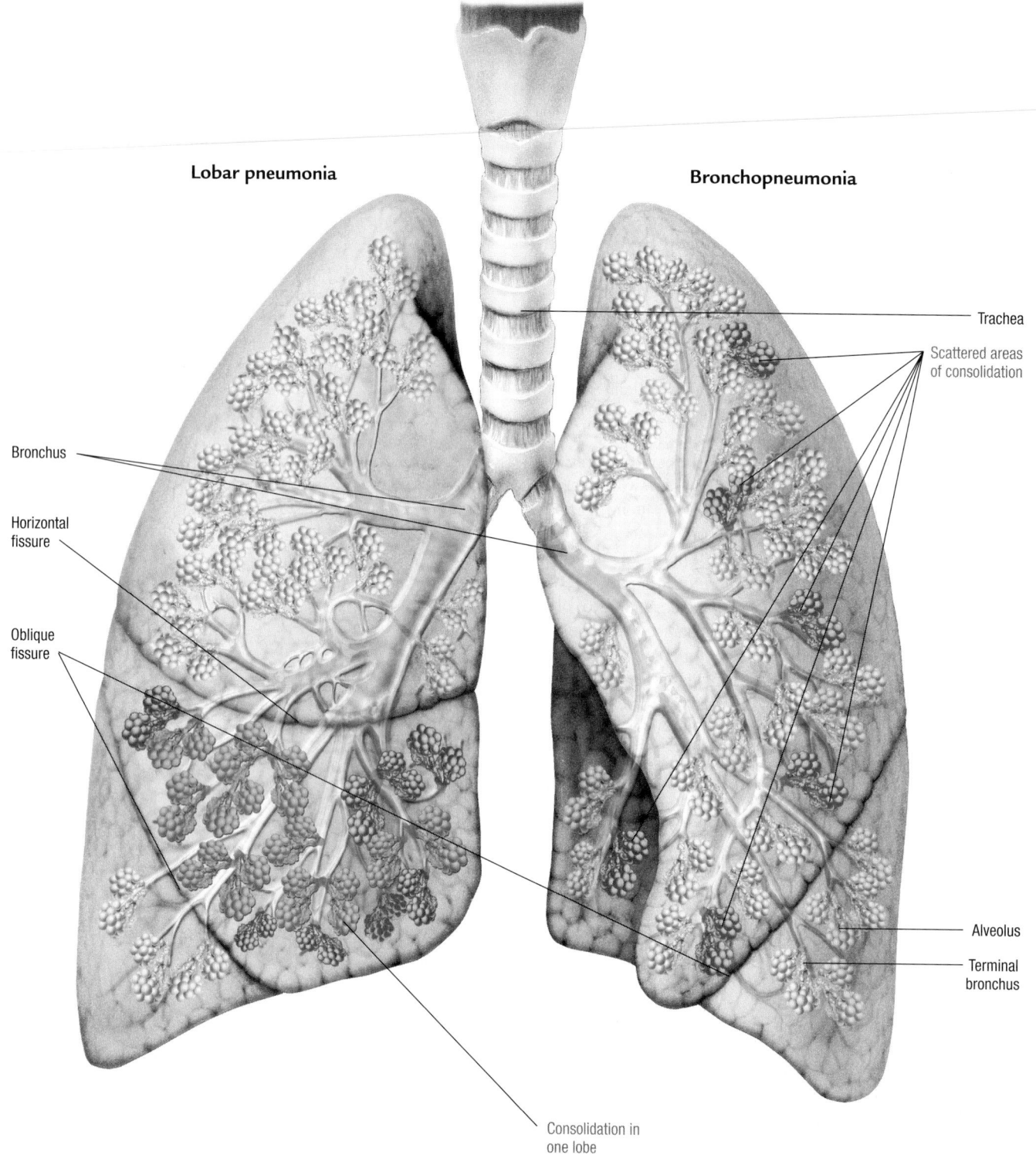

Lobar pneumonia

Bronchopneumonia

Trachea

Scattered areas
of consolidation

Bronchus

Horizontal
fissure

Oblique
fissure

Alveolus

Terminal
bronchus

Consolidation in
one lobe

FIGURE 75.1 Types of pneumonia (*see color insert*). (Asset provided by Anatomical Chart Co.)

ganisms. Pneumonia or pneumonitis can result when these substances accumulate in the lower respiratory tract. Fortunately, the body can maintain a nearly sterile lower respiratory tract through the efforts of an elaborate array of host defenses.[25,26] These respiratory defenses are largely com-

posed of anatomic barriers, mechanical barriers, humoral and cell-mediated immune cells, and phagocytic cells (Fig. 75.2). For pneumonia to develop, there typically has to be a defect in host defenses, exposure to a particularly virulent pathogen, and/or exposure to a large inoculum. Microorga-

TABLE 75.1   Microbial Agents That Cause Acute Pneumonia

Bacterial	Fungal	Viral
Common	*Aspergillus* spp	**Children**
Streptococcus pneumoniae	*Candida* spp	Common
Staphylococcus aureus	*Coccidioides immitis*	Respiratory syncytial virus
Haemophilus influenzae	*Cryptococcus neoformans*	Parainfluenza virus types 1, 2, 3
Mixed anaerobic bacteria (aspiration)	*Histoplasma capsulatum*	Influenza A virus
Bacteroides spp	Agents of mucormycosis	Uncommon
Fusobacterium spp	*Rhizopus* spp	Adenovirus types 1, 2, 3, 5
Peptostreptococcus spp	*Absidia* spp	Influenza B virus
Peptococcus spp	*Mucor* spp	Rhinovirus
Prevotella spp	*Cunninghamella* spp	Coxsackievirus
Enterobacteriaceae		Echovirus
Escherichia coli	Rickettsial	Measles virus
Klebsiella pneumoniae	*Coxiella burnetii*	Hantavirus
Enterobacter spp	*Rickettsia rickettsiae*	**Adults**
Serratia spp		Common
Pseudomonas aeruginosa	Mycoplasma and chlamydia	Influenza A virus
Legionella spp (including *L. pneumophila* and *L. micdadei*)	*Mycoplasma pneumoniae*	Influenza B virus
	Chlamydia psittaci	Adenovirus types 4 and 7 (in military recruits)
Uncommon	*Chlamydia trachomatis*	
Acinetobacter var. *anitratus*	*Chlamydophila pneumoniae*	Uncommon
Actinomyces and *Arachnia* spp	Mycobacterial	Rhinovirus
Aeromonas hydrophilia	*Mycobacterium tuberculosis*	Adenovirus types 1, 2, 3, 5
Bacillus spp	Nontuberculous mycobacteria	Enteroviruses
Moraxella catarrhalis		Echovirus
Campylobacter fetus	Parasitic	Coxsackievirus
Eikenella corrodens	*Ascaris lumbricoides*	Poliovirus
Francisella tularensis	*Pneumocystis carinii*	Epstein-Barr virus
Neisseria meningitidis	*Strongyloides stercoralis*	Cytomegalovirus
Nocardia spp	*Toxoplasma gondii*	Respiratory syncytial virus
Pasteurella multocida	*Paragonimus westermani*	Varicella-zoster virus
Proteus spp		Parainfluenza virus
Pseudomonas pseudomallei		Measles virus
Salmonella spp		Herpes simplex virus
Enterococcus faecalis		Hantavirus
Streptococcus pyogenes		Human herpesvirus 6
Yersinia pestis		

(Reprinted with permission from Donowitz GR, Mandell GL. Acute pneumonia. In: Mandell GL, Bennett JE, Dolin R, eds. Mandell, Douglas, and Bennett's principles and practice of infectious diseases, 6th ed. Philadelphia: Elsevier, 2005:819–845.)

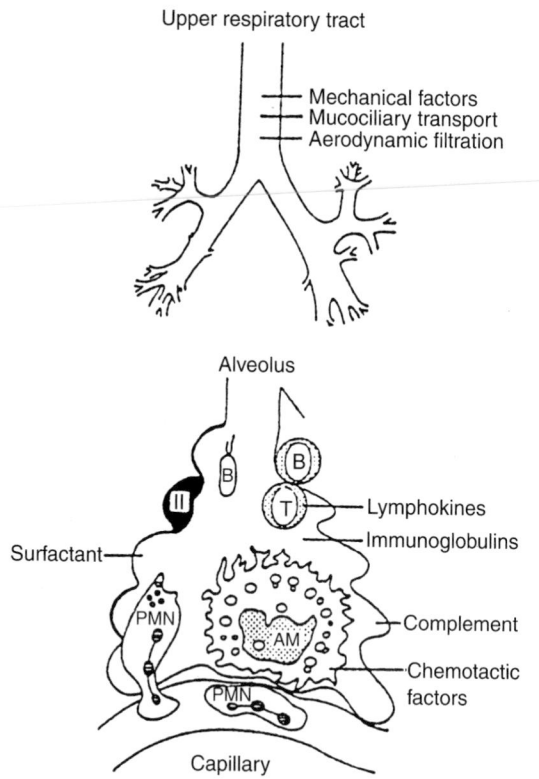

Upper respiratory tract

Mechanical factors
Mucociliary transport
Aerodynamic filtration

Alveolus

Lymphokines
Immunoglobulins

Surfactant

Complement

Chemotactic factors

Capillary

FIGURE 75.2 Defense mechanisms of the lung. (Reprinted with permission from Reynolds HY. Host defense impairments that may lead to respiratory infections. Clin Chest Med 8:344, 1987.)

nisms gain access to the lungs by three distinct mechanisms: hematogenous spread, inhalation of airborne pathogens, or aspiration of oropharyngeal (and possibly gastric) material. Of these mechanisms, aspiration is the major cause of most cases of pneumonia.[27] Otherwise healthy individuals can aspirate small amounts (microaspiration) of oropharyngeal material on a daily basis, especially while sleeping.[8] However, due to the low burden of virulent organisms and intact host defenses, pneumonic sequelae fail to develop. Microaspiration is different from the entity classically referred to as ''aspiration pneumonia'' or ''aspiration pneumonitis.'' The later processes refer to pneumonia that results from aspiration of larger volumes of oropharyngeal or gastric contents, respectively.[7]

In the upper respiratory tract, nasal hair and mucus-producing cells in the nasal mucosa serve as an initial mechanical filter against microorganisms entering through the nose.[28] Organisms present in the nasopharynx can be cleared from the respiratory tract by being expectorated through the nose or mouth or by being swallowed via the pharynx and esophagus. The oropharynx is an area rich with microbial flora. These commensal organisms limit the ability of other bacteria to colonize.[29,30] In addition, saliva and the constant sloughing of epithelial cells can further prevent colonization of the oropharynx by pathogens. The mucosal surfaces of the upper respiratory tract produce secretory immunoglobulin

A (IgA), which has antibacterial and antiviral activity.[28] In addition, other immunoglobulins, salivary proteases, fibronectin, and mucus are present in oropharyngeal secretions that interfere with bacterial adherence.[26,29] The epiglottis is a leaf-shaped flap of cartilage, covered with mucous membrane, situated behind the root of the tongue. It covers the entrance to the larynx and the lower respiratory tract during swallowing. If the epiglottis is breached by pharyngeal material, a cough reflex is usually triggered to promote retrograde clearance.[26] These two mechanisms keep most foreign material out of the lung.

The cells lining the central airways (trachea and bronchioles) consist of predominantly ciliated columnar epithelial cells interspersed with mucus-secreting cells. The ciliated cells beat in a coordinated fashion to clear material in a retrograde fashion from the lower airways toward the oropharynx. The sharp angles of the branching conducting airways of the trachea and bronchi allow particulate material to become trapped in tracheobronchial mucus. Trapped material can then be removed by the mucociliary transport system or via cough.

The branching airways (bronchi) lead distally to the alveoli, which are the thin-walled capillary-rich sacs where the exchange of oxygen and carbon dioxide takes place (Fig. 75.3; *see color insert*).[31] Mucociliary cells are not present at the level of the alveoli. Defenses in the alveolar region are primarily mediated by immune and phagocytic cells.

Alveolar lining fluid consists largely of surfactant (secreted by type II pneumocytes), fibronectin, immunoglobulin G (IgG), complement, free fatty acid, and iron-binding proteins. Each of these substances plays a role in host lung defenses. Surfactant may exert antibacterial activity against staphylococci and certain gram-negative pathogens.[26] Encapsulated bacteria are processed and opsonized by IgG, surfactant, fibronectin, and complement before phagocytic cells can recognize them.

Alveolar macrophages are the predominant resident phagocytic cells found in the alveoli and interstitial spaces and on surfaces of the airways. When faced with a serious bacterial insult, alveolar macrophages can release chemotactic factors, which attract the nearby phagocytic polymorphonuclear leukocytes marginating in the lung capillary. Phagocytic cells engulf bacteria and produce oxidative enzymes within lysosomes that usually destroy bacteria. Alveolar macrophages frequently require IgG to enhance their intracellular killing.[26] Bacteria can trigger immune lymphocytes to release effector substances called lymphokines, which can further enhance phagocytic activity.[26]

Phagocytic cells are mobile and can migrate to other alveoli. Phagocytes containing neutralized bacteria can move proximally in the respiratory tract, where they are eventually removed from the lung with the help of the mucociliary transport system.

MECHANISM OF PATHOGENESIS

In the pathogenesis of microaspiration-associated pneumonia, pathogenic organisms must first colonize the naso-

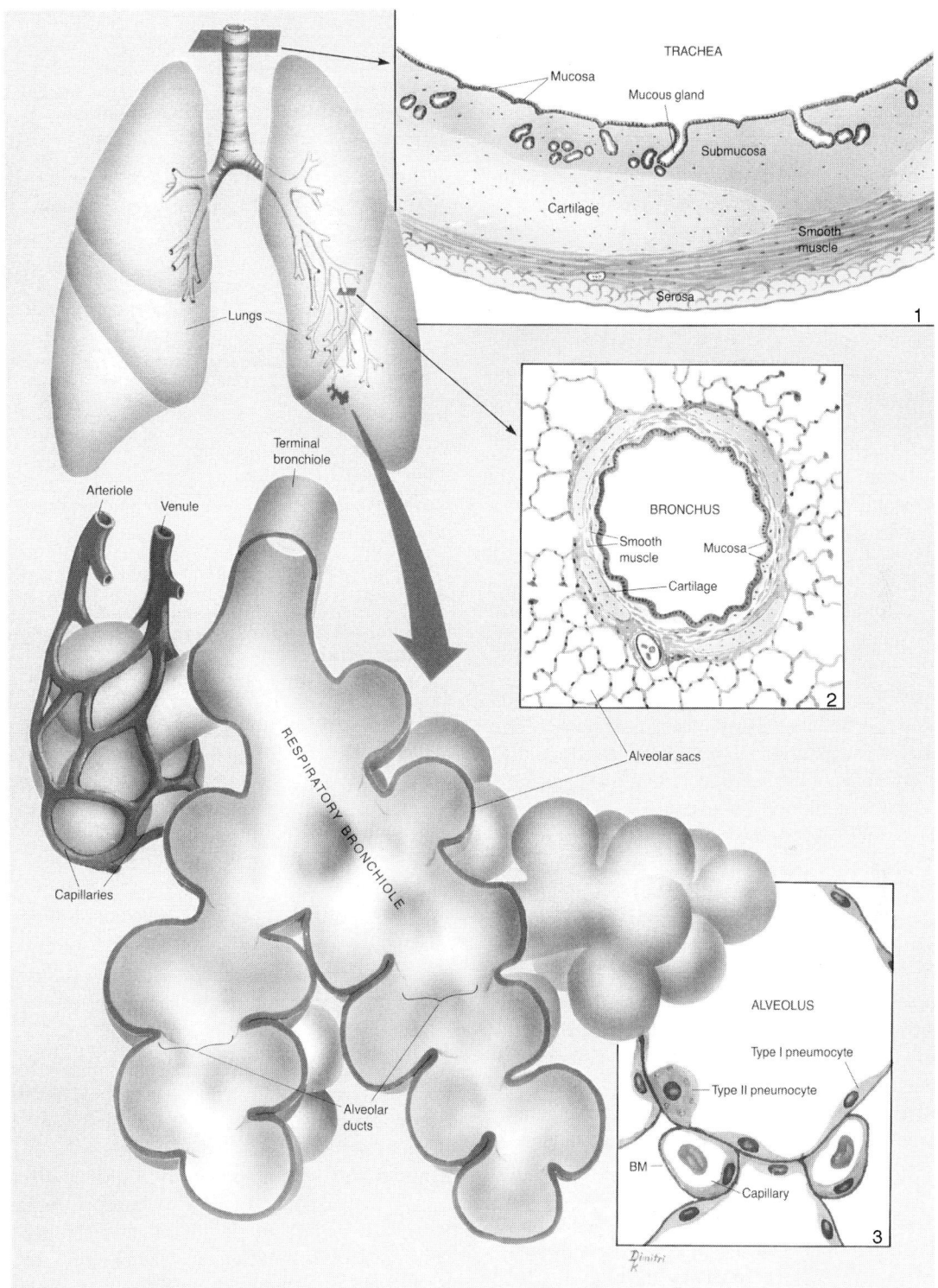

FIGURE 75.3 Anatomy of the lung (*see color insert*). (From Rubin E, Farber JL. Pathology, 3rd ed. Philadelphia: Lippincott Williams & Wilkins, 1999.)

oropharynx. Adherence of microorganisms to epithelial surfaces initiates the colonization process. Despite the many barriers to attachment described above, pathogenic organisms may still attach and colonize. A variety of aerobic and anaerobic bacteria may reside on the mucosal surfaces of the naso-oropharynx. Common organisms include *Neisseria* species, *Moraxella catarrhalis*, *Streptococcus* species (including *Streptococcus pneumoniae*), *Mycoplasma pneumoniae*, *Staphylococcus aureus*, and yeast.[26] Individuals with chronic airway disease may also harbor *Haemophilus influenzae*. A variety of anaerobic organisms inhabit the areas around the teeth and gums.

Enteric gram-negative agents are infrequent oropharyngeal colonizers in community-dwelling individuals, but colonization rates increase with advanced age and in nursing home residents.[32] Patients with nosocomial forms of pneumonia may be exposed to additional pathogens, including antibiotic-resistant bacteria. These organisms can be transferred from healthcare workers or other patients or from the healthcare environment (e.g., air, water, devices, equipment, fomites). Antecedent use of antibiotics can eliminate susceptible resident flora, permitting more pathogenic or resistant organisms to colonize the naso-oropharynx.

Impairment of host defenses is a key element in the pathogenesis of pneumonia. In many situations, bacteria-containing secretions overwhelm or bypass mechanical barriers, or the host has developed diminished mucociliary transport or diminished alveolar macrophage and chemotactic activity. Table 75.2 lists some of the many conditions that have been associated with these diminished host defenses.

A few key examples bear mentioning to highlight pathogenic processes. Factors that interfere with epiglottic closure and cough reflex may predispose individuals to aspiration.[26] Without a good cough response, secretions can accumulate in the airways. Poor cough reflex can be seen in patients who have received anesthesia and in individuals with impaired consciousness resulting from drugs or disease. Nasogastric and endotracheal tubes breach natural anatomic barriers and interfere with the cough reflex, which provides easier access to the lower respiratory tract for microorganisms. Defects in ciliary function or damage to cilia may result from cigarette smoking, genetic disorders, or infections with certain viruses or *M. pneumoniae*.[26] As a result, the ciliary clearance of mucus and trapped secretions is impaired. Viruses such as influenza can infect and destroy ciliated epithelial cells, often causing regions of denuded nonfunctioning cells along the conducting airways.[33] These airway changes can place patients at risk for post-influenza superinfections with virulent bacterial organisms such as *S. aureus*.[12] Patients with chronic lung disease often produce excessive mucus secretions that may overwhelm the mucociliary clearance mechanism.

Inhalation of aerosolized organisms is not as common a cause of pneumonia as microaspiration, but it is the major route for *Mycobacterium tuberculosis*, *Legionella pneumophila*, fungi, and viruses.[27] Inhaled pathogens will ob-

TABLE 75.2	Conditions That Diminish Key Host Defenses

Overwhelm or Bypass Mechanical Barriers, Predisposing Patients to Aspiration

Alcohol or drug abuse	Anesthesia
Seizures	Head trauma
Stroke	Parkinson's disease
Multiple sclerosis	Dysphagia
Neurologic disorders	Esophageal cancer
Vomiting	Gastroesophageal reflux disorder

Diminished Mucociliary Transport of Cellular and Bacterial Debris

Tracheostomy	Nasogastric or endotracheal tube
Bronchoscopy	
Smoking	Chronic lung diseases
Immotile cilia syndrome	Cystic fibrosis
Viral infections	Aging
Hyperoxia	Inhalation of toxic substances

Diminished Alveolar Macrophage Activity and Chemotaxis

Alcohol ingestion	Advanced age
Diabetes mellitus	Sickle cell diseases
Malnutrition	Immunosuppressive therapy
Hypogammaglobulinemia	Chronic obstructive pulmonary disease
Viral infection	
AIDS	Malignancy
Cystic fibrosis	Bacterial endotoxin
Hypoxemia	Metabolic acidosis
Pulmonary edema	Uremia
Hyperoxia	Mechanical obstruction

viously elude certain host defense mechanisms. Particle size, inoculum quantity, and airflow patterns will determine what defense mechanisms interact with inhaled organisms. Hematogenous seeding of the lungs may even be less common than inhalation, but it appears to be an important route for *S. aureus* pneumonia. Risks of pulmonary seeding may be particularly higher in right-sided endocarditis.[34] Urinary pathogens like *Escherichia coli* may also migrate to the lung in patients with uroseptic bacteremia.[35]

Many host defenses are compromised in patients receiving mechanical ventilation. The pathogenesis of VAP usually begins shortly after intubation.[36] Endotracheal tubes separate the vocal cords and push the epiglottis aside and allow direct access to the lower respiratory tract. A balloon cuff wedges the endotracheal tube into place in the trachea. Intubated patients are usually sedated and even medically paralyzed and cannot mount a cough reflex. Oropharyngeal secretions, often containing bacteria, pool on the outside of

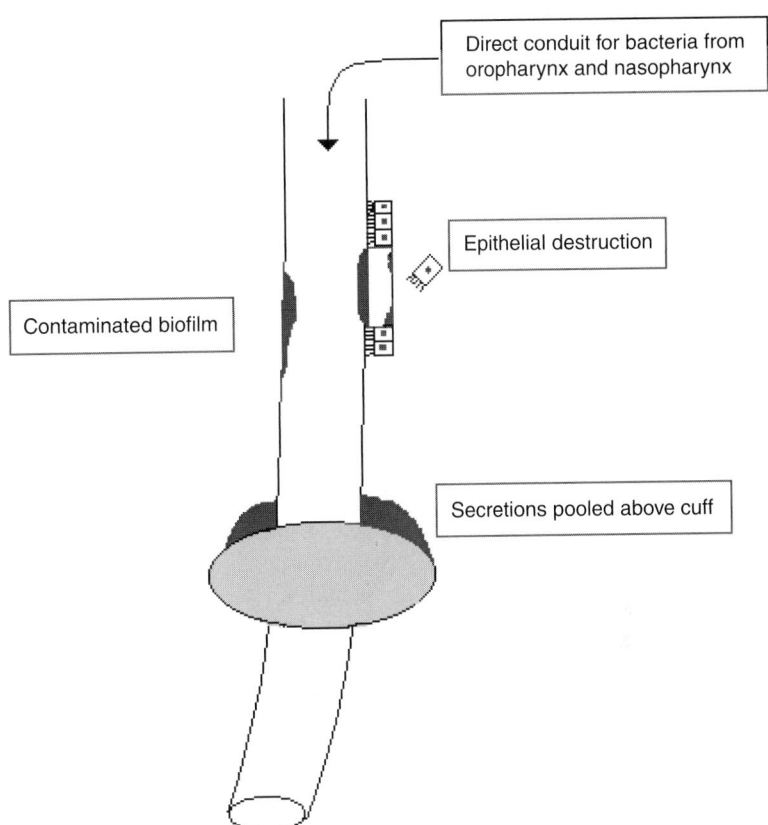

Direct conduit for bacteria from oropharynx and nasopharynx

Epithelial destruction

Contaminated biofilm

Secretions pooled above cuff

FIGURE 75.4 Potential ways by which the endotracheal tube may disrupt lung host defense mechanisms and lead to enhanced risk of lower respiratory tract infections. (From Mason CM, Nelson S Pulmonary host defenses: implications for therapy. Clin Chest Med 20:475–488, 1999.)

endotracheal tubes above the inflated cuff (Fig. 75.4).[37] These pooled secretions can traverse the cuff and seep into the lower lung during suctioning, manipulation of the tube or the patient, and even during periods of pressure changes of mechanical ventilation.[38] Multiple studies have identified formation of bacterial biofilm on the inside of endotracheal tubes with prolonged ventilation, which can serve as a continued nidus of infection if left in place.[39] Pooled secretions will also have the opportunity to enter the lungs when the cuff is deflated during tube removal. Patients requiring reintubation after being off ventilation are at increased risk of VAP, as the tube can forcibly introduce colonizing bacteria into the lower airways.[38] Intubation may further perpetuate pneumonia through destruction of epithelial tissue in the upper airway.[37] Improperly cleaned respiratory or ventilation devices have been reported to be a source of bacteria.[40] Bacterial spread associated with these devices is likely due to direct inoculation into the lower airway of infected condensate. The Centers for Disease Control and Prevention (CDC), along with the Healthcare Infection Control Practices Advisory Committee (HICPAC), recently published guidelines for the prevention of nosocomial pneumonia that include measures on disinfecting, sterilizing, and maintaining respiratory equipment.[40]

Once pathogens enter the alveoli (by any route), they must contend with immunoglobulins, complement, fibronectin, iron-containing proteins, surfactant, alveolar macrophages, and neutrophils. States of hypogammaglobulinemia can impair opsonization of encapsulated pathogens such as *S. pneumoniae* and certain types of *H. influenzae*.[26] Patients with neutropenia or other types of immunosuppression have diminished inflammatory and phagocytic responses. Certain "intracellular" pathogens, such as the atypical pathogens, can survive within phagocytes.[41] Drug therapy against these pathogens may not be very effective if the drugs cannot achieve therapeutic concentrations inside these cells.

As neutrophils and fluids migrate and fill the alveolar spaces, an exudative inflammatory reaction creates the local manifestations of pneumonitis and pulmonary consolidation (solidification). Systemic manifestations that include fever, chills, and myalgias often accompany these changes in the lung. The inflammatory reactions lead to a derangement of proper lung function and vital gas exchange, which in turn results in respiratory distress or failure. During a bout of pneumonia, patients can develop respiratory muscle fatigue, which can exacerbate the condition.[27] Bacteria may migrate to the bloodstream and even spread to other organs. Patients with transient or persistent bacteremia may even progress to septic shock and death.[27] In general, pneumonia with bacteremia may require a longer time to cure.[12,42,43] Bacteremic pneumonia has been associated with a higher rate of mortality.[41] Patients with pneumonia can go on to develop complications such as abscesses or pleural empyemas, which are collections of pus in the lung or pleural cavity.[11,44]

Clinical presentations of pneumonia can vary widely. Independent risk factors for poor outcomes include advanced age, presence of comorbidities, poor nutritional status, hyponatremia, azotemia, high fever, bacteremia, immunosuppression including asplenia, and alcoholism.[11] Pneumonias caused by *S. aureus* or gram-negative bacilli and aspiration pneumonia have been independently associated with higher mortality.[43,45]

RISK FACTORS FOR PNEUMONIA

The elderly, the immunosuppressed, smokers, and individuals with chronic medical conditions such as chronic obstructive lung disease, congestive heart failure, coronary artery disease, diabetes, alcoholism, renal failure, malignancy, dementia, chronic neurologic disease, seizure disorders, and chronic liver disease are all at increased risk for developing pneumonia.[46] Many of these conditions diminish alveolar macrophage activity, chemotaxis, cough reflex, or the mucociliary transport system. Patients who have previously had pneumonia or recently had influenza are also at increased risk for developing pneumonia.[8] Hospitalized patients receiving mechanical ventilation are 20 times more likely to develop pneumonia than nonventilated hospitalized patients.[20]

Other risk factors for nosocomial pneumonia in hospitalized patients include trauma, surgery, and medications or therapies that impair lung defenses. The role of the gastrointestinal tract in the pathogenesis of VAP has been studied and debated over the past few decades.[47] Retrograde movement of bacteria living in gastric contents into the upper respiratory tract, with eventual aspiration into the lung, may be an important cause of VAP. The fact that supine positioning seems to be a risk factor for aspiration pneumonia in susceptible patients appears to be consistent with this theory.

Growth of bacteria in the gastric environment is enhanced in situations of hypoacidity.[48] Medications such as H_2-receptor antagonists and proton-pump inhibitors (PPIs) reduce gastric acidity. Many ventilated patients receive these agents for stress-ulcer prophylaxis. Use of these agents has been identified as a risk factor for developing VAP.[5,48]

Enteral feeding of ventilated patients has also been associated with higher rates of VAP.[49] The increased risk may be explained by the fact that these formulations typically promote alkalinization of the gastric environment and may increase the risk of aspiration. The clinical importance of the gastric route as a cause of pneumonia is not well established.[20]

PREVENTIVE STRATEGIES

Efforts to prevent the development of CAP have primarily focused on vaccinations, smoking cessation, and treatment of underlying chronic diseases (e.g., chronic obstructive pulmonary disease). The most relevant vaccinations are the pneumococcal and influenza vaccines. Prevention of pneumonia through vaccination programs and influenza prophylaxis with antiviral drugs is of critical importance for elderly persons and nursing home residents.[50,51] The antiviral drugs amantadine and rimantadine can be used for treatment and prophylaxis against influenza.[51] The neuraminidase inhibitors oseltamivir and zanamivir are both approved to treat influenza A and B, but only oseltamivir is approved by the U.S. Food and Drug Administration (FDA) for prophylaxis. Vaccination with 23-valent pneumococcal polysaccharide vaccine is recommended for high-risk patients, including those 65 years of age and older.[50]

The effectiveness of the vaccines usually depends on the recipient's age and state of immunocompetence.[51] The effectiveness of the influenza vaccine has been estimated to be about 58% in individuals 65 years of age and older.[51] Estimates of preventive effectiveness from the pneumococcal vaccine range from 38% to 80%.[52,53]

More information about immunization therapy can be found in Chapter 73.

Given the high morbidity and mortality of VAP, many preventive strategies have been developed to address various modifiable risk factors of VAP. However, many of these interventions have not consistently proven to be beneficial in well-designed clinical trials.

One of the best ways to avoid VAP is by using noninvasive positive-pressure ventilation devices instead of invasive mechanical ventilation whenever possible.[54] If invasive ventilation is required, shortening the duration of ventilation may reduce the incidence of VAP. Draining the ventilator circuit of condensate and using heat and moisture exchangers may reduce the occurrence of VAP by limiting the possibility of introducing contaminated condensate into the lower airway.[54,55]

Endotracheal suctioning, which is often performed, has not been shown to reduce the risk of VAP.[56] Continuous aspiration or drainage of subglottic secretions can provide a reduction in VAP, but it may not always be available.

Semirecumbent positioning (45-degree angle) of patients has been shown to reduce the occurrence of VAP,[54,56] but in clinical practice it is often difficult to maintain this degree of elevation.

Use of the non-pH-altering drug sucralfate for stress ulcer prophylaxis has been associated with lower rates of VAP than with antacids or H_2 antagonists in some reports,[48,56,57] but sucralfate may not be as effective at preventing stress ulcer-associated bleeding.[48] VAP data from comparative studies between sucralfate and PPIs are not currently available.

Methods of reducing the risk of VAP due to enteral feeding have included acidifying the feeds, administering feeds postpylorically, or using parenteral nutrition.[48,58] The benefits of these measures are not known. Use of parenteral nutrition carries the additional risks of line infections and complications, higher costs, and loss of intestinal tract architecture, which may promote bacterial translocation.[48] As such, most experts recommend enteral feeding over parenteral nutrition when possible. Efforts to prevent gastric overdistention, such as administering the promotility agent metoclopramide and limiting use of narcotics or anticholinergic drugs, are routinely employed despite a lack of supportive data.[55]

The importance of preventive measures focused on limiting the gastropulmonary route of spread may not be that important, given that available data suggest a more important role for colonization of the oropharynx.[47]

The use of topical chlorhexidine or topical antibiotics within the oral cavity has demonstrated a reduction in VAP in cardiac surgery patients.[59,60] These topical agents may be combined with orally administered antibiotics to provide selective decontamination of the digestive tract. Selective decontamination has been studied in many prospective studies and meta-analyses and has been associated with reductions in VAP.[56,60] Despite the reported benefits of topical or selective decontamination preventive measures, study design limitations, a lack of effect on mortality, and increased potential for selecting resistant pathogens has left many clinicians wary of using them.

The benefit of prophylactic intravenous antibiotic therapy in critically ill patients has not been shown. This practice may increase the selection of resistant pathogens and has not been advocated for widespread use.[54]

Clinicians interested in successful preventive strategies must include proper infection control practices and surveillance of hospital and ICU infection rates.

CLINICAL PRESENTATION AND DIAGNOSIS

The diagnosis of pneumonia is usually based on clinical, radiographic, and laboratory findings. An accurate and complete medical history including pet exposure, travel history, and occupational exposures, and a physical examination are advised. Patients at risk for active tuberculosis infections will undergo additional assessment (see Chapter 76). Patients with more severe presentations typically go through more extensive diagnostic workups. When patients initially present for care, they are first assessed for severity of illness. This information can be determined from symptoms, vital signs, oxygenation status, functional status, and effects on comorbidities. Decisions about the site of care can then be made.

SIGNS AND SYMPTOMS

Common signs and symptoms of pneumonia include fever or hypothermia combined with cough, wheeze, dyspnea, increased sputum production, change in sputum consistency, and pleuritic chest pain. Some patients with pneumonia have fatigue, headache, diarrhea, nausea, vomiting, and night sweats. The most common laboratory abnormality in pneumonia is leukocytosis (elevated white blood cell count) with

an increase in immature forms of neutrophils (left shift). Patients with moderate to severe pneumonia may appear more ''septic,'' with altered vital signs. Septic patients often manifest with tachypnea, tachycardia, and hypotension. Patients with *Legionella* infection in particular have presented with bradycardia.[24] Patients with poor ventilation may appear hypoxic or cyanotic. Many of these clinical signs and symptoms are not specific to pneumonia in adults.

The clinical presentation may be more subtle in the elderly.[61] Patients over 65 years of age usually have a less effective cough reflex and immune system function.[62] As such, they are less likely to experience fever and chills. It is also not uncommon to see a change in mental status and functional capacity in elderly patients with pneumonia.[62,63] This vague presentation in elderly patients may lead to a delayed diagnosis of pneumonia. Unfortunately, the elderly have the highest rate of mortality and may benefit substantially from prompt antibiotic treatment.

Clinically, pneumonia has been described as being lobar pneumonia, bronchopneumonia, or interstitial pneumonia.[10] Lobar pneumonia involves the greater part of a particular lobe of the lung, whereas bronchopneumonia is manifested by a patchy pattern of consolidation that may involve one or several lobes of the lungs. Interstitial pneumonia may appear patchy or diffuse. Pneumonia may be manifested by unilateral or bilateral lung involvement.

These patterns are best seen on radiographic films but may be appreciated on physical chest examination. Inflammatory processes are usually confined to the interstitium, including the alveolar walls and bronchovascular connective tissue. ''Crackles'' or ''rales'' and diminished breath sounds are often heard on auscultation of the lung in patients with pneumonia.[63] Breath sounds may appear very diminished or even absent in patients with pleural effusion. Lobar consolidation is identified in about 30% of patients with pneumonia on physical examination.[8,63] ''Dullness'' on chest percussion is indicative of consolidation.[13,63] Likewise, a number of characteristic vocal resonance changes are associated with consolidation. Vowel tone changes (i.e., ''E'' to ''A'') on auscultation suggest consolidation.[64] *Whispered pectoriloquy* is when words whispered by the patient are heard through the stethoscope over a consolidated or cavitary portion of lung tissue.[64] *Bronchophony* is when the sound of certain spoken words (i.e., ''ninety-nine'') are heard better through the stethoscope over a consolidated portion of the lungs.

Patients should have arterial oxygen saturation measured to determine the need for supplemental oxygen. Arterial blood gas measurements should be obtained in patients likely to have metabolic or respiratory acidosis.

The differential diagnosis for a patient with pneumonia may include congestive heart failure, exacerbations of chronic bronchitis, and bronchiectasis.[65] It may be particularly difficult to determine whether a ventilated patient has developed pneumonia based on clinical signs and symptoms.

RADIOGRAPHIC FINDINGS

Chest x-rays are important diagnostic tools and are generally obtained for all patients being worked up for pneumonia.[24,66] Radiography not only helps to establish the diagnosis of pneumonia, but it also may identify complications (e.g., pleural effusions, abscesses), detect other diseases of the lung, help assess the severity of pneumonia, and serve as a baseline for the assessment of treatment response.[65,66] Patients with very mild clinical presentations of pneumonia may be empirically diagnosed by their physician and treated presumptively without a chest radiograph. In the pathophysiology of pneumonia, pus and exudates accumulate in the lungs, causing areas of increased density, which results in a corresponding opacity or "infiltrate" on the chest radiograph.

Overall, the use of chest radiography has not been that helpful for making a specific microbial etiologic diagnosis, but some findings are suggestive of certain types of infections.[65] Lobar consolidation, cavitation, and pleural effusions are most often associated with bacterial pneumonias.[24] Necrotizing pneumonia, cavitation, and empyema are most often associated with anaerobes, staphylococci, and gram-negative organisms.[24] Chest radiographs suggestive of aspiration pneumonia are characterized by infiltrates in dependent segments of the lungs.[67] These would include the superior segments of the lower lobes or posterior segments of the upper lobes in a patient in the recumbent position, or in the lower lobes of patients in the upright position. It has been reported that patients with pneumonia may fail to show infiltrates on chest radiographs if they cannot mount a sufficient inflammatory response, such as in dehydration, advanced age, neutropenia, or early in the pneumonia process.[13] These assertions remain controversial, as they have not been proven through formal studies.[8,68] The appearance of infiltrates on a chest x-ray may be associated with noninfectious causes such as congestive heart failure, atelectasis, pulmonary emboli with infarction, chemical pneumonitis, cancer, Wegener's granulomatosis, sarcoidosis, interstitial lung disease, and vasculitis.[8]

Although chest radiography is one of the most important tools in the diagnosis of pneumonia, it is subject to variability of interobserver interpretation. In addition, portable chest radiographs, which are frequently used in ICUs, are usually of lesser quality.[69] Computed tomography (CT) can provide additional information about detailed morphologic changes of the lung.[24] CT may be helpful if the lung is obscured by the diaphragm or masses or for differentiating infectious pneumonia from noninfectious infiltrates.[24,70] Chest x-rays and CT scans can identify lung abscesses and cavities. Due to the high cost, higher degree of radiation, and limited benefit over chest radiography in most cases of pneumonia, CT is usually reserved for more complicated cases.

EXAMINATION AND CULTURE OF RESPIRATORY SECRETIONS

Expectorated Sputum. Sputum and respiratory secretions may be collected for culture or Gram staining from patients likely to have pneumonia. As previously mentioned, one of the most challenging features of pneumonia is the identification of the responsible pathogens. Prospective studies in CAP have failed to identify a causative organism in 40% to 60% of cases using routine diagnostic methods.[12] Gram staining of expectorated sputum can be a very simple, quick, and inexpensive process. However, the value of Gram staining of sputum in pneumonia has been one of the most controversial aspects of pneumonia therapeutics. Even published CAP guidelines are split on the recommendation for routine Gram staining of expectorated sputum.[11,12]

Key limitations of Gram staining are (a) specimens are often contaminated during collection by bacteria colonizing the oropharynx; (b) not all pathogens can be visualized with the technique; (c) prior use of antibiotics can reduce the yield of organisms; (d) the technique is observer-dependent; (e) specimens are frequently of unacceptable quality; (f) fastidious organisms may not thrive during transport and processing; and (g) many patients cannot produce enough sputum.[24,71] The latter point is especially true for elderly patients. Nebulized albuterol, saline, or hypertonic saline has been used to promote the induction of sputum in individuals who have difficulty producing sputum, but this may not substantially improve the yield.

Despite these limitations, sputum Gram staining remains a primary tool for aiding in empiric therapeutic decisions. A good lower respiratory tract sputum specimen typically has fewer than 10 squamous epithelial cells and greater than 25 neutrophils per low-power field and evidence of a predominant bacterial morphotype on microscopy.[72] Specimens meeting these criteria are generally regarded as "good-quality specimens." Such a specimen is less likely to be contaminated with organisms colonizing the upper airways.

Unfortunately, most CAP patients cannot produce good-quality specimens. In one prospective study, only 41% (59) of 144 bacteremic CAP patients could produce a specimen with fewer than 10 squamous epithelial cells and greater than 25 neutrophils.[73] Of these 59 specimens, 79% (47) showed the predominance of a bacterial morphotype. Forty of the 47 (85%) good-quality specimens predicted the blood cultures, thus affirming the value of a good-quality specimen for guiding antibiotic therapy.

The sensitivity and specificity of Gram staining of expectorated sputum has ranged from 15% to 100% in different studies.[74] In general, sputum Gram staining of good-quality specimens is an insensitive but specific diagnostic tool for CAP.[72] Gram stain results are most reliable if they are corroborated with pathogens isolated later from the blood or pleural fluid.

S. pneumoniae (otherwise known as "the pneumococcus") has been the predominant organism identified by Gram staining of good-quality specimens from CAP patients. Gram staining is of little value in identifying atypical pathogens. Therefore, atypical pathogens should be considered when a good-quality specimen does not show bacteria. Sputum specimens that are deemed acceptable may be processed for culture and antibiotic sensitivity testing to better guide therapy.

Routine culturing of expectorated sputum lacks sensitivity and specificity.[12] Sputum culture may only identify the presence of the pneumococcus in about 50% to 60% of patients with pneumococcal bacteremia and signs of pneumonia.[24,75,76] The sensitivity of sputum Gram staining for identifying pneumococcal pneumonia is generally better than culture of sputum.[72] The yield of fastidious bacteria such as the pneumococcus and *H. influenzae* can be drastically reduced when a respiratory specimen is collected after a patient has received antibiotic therapy.[77] In addition, improper collection or transport or delays in specimen processing may result in failure of sputum culture to identify the presence of bacteria.[78,79]

Macroexamination of sputum may give clues as to the microbial etiology. Observers should note the color, amount, consistency, and odor of the sputum specimens.[24] Mucopurulent samples are associated more with bacteria, whereas watery or scant specimens may be more consistent with atypical organisms. Rusty-colored sputum has been associated more with *S. pneumoniae* and ''red currant jelly'' sputum has been more associated with *K. pneumoniae*. Anaerobes are said to produce putrid or foul-smelling sputum.[24,67] The predictability of these observations has not been established.

Blood Cultures. Collecting blood for culture remains an important part of the diagnostic work-up for patients hospitalized with pneumonia. Blood cultures are positive 4% to 18% of the time in CAP patients who are hospitalized; the rate is even higher in patients admitted to the ICU.[72,74] Patients with pneumonia may experience transient episodes of bacteremia, which may be missed with infrequent blood culturing. Bacteremia is rarely encountered in patients with milder cases of pneumonia. Therefore, routine collection of blood for culture in mild cases of pneumonia is not justified. The most common pathogen isolated from the bloodstream in patients with CAP has been the pneumococcus.[74]

The value of blood culture in the diagnosis of CAP has been recently questioned. Opponents argue that the cost and benefit of blood culturing is not justified due to the low yield of pathogens from the blood, and the observation that physicians rarely narrow the spectrum of antibiotic therapy to older, less costly drugs when a pathogen such as a penicillin-susceptible pneumococcus is identified.[80,81] Antecedent use of antibiotics can decrease the yield of bacteria in blood culture.[82] However, blood culturing is clearly justified in nosocomial pneumonia given the broad array of pathogens, including resistant species of certain pathogens.

Lower Tract Specimens. Noninvasive techniques for collecting respiratory specimens like sputum sampling are limited by frequent contamination by oropharyngeal flora, which may lead to overprescribing of antiinfectives. More invasive methods for collecting samples of lower respiratory tract specimens have been used as a way of avoiding contamination. They include endotracheal aspiration (minimally invasive), bronchoalveolar lavage (BAL), protected specimen brush collection, transtracheal aspiration, thoracentesis, and open lung biopsy.[83,84]

Although these invasive procedures are rarely used in the routine work-up for CAP, some are frequently used in the diagnostic work-up for VAP. Specimen collection by BAL or protected specimen brush is usually done via a fiberoptic bronchoscope, as an invasive procedure that requires conscious sedation.[83] BAL is performed by advancing a bronchoscope into distal segments of the lung and then instilling and aspirating aliquots of saline (Fig. 75.5; *see color insert*). Protected specimen brush collection is performed by introducing a brush from an inner cannula (Fig. 75.6) through a bronchoscope at a distal lung site. The BAL technique samples a much larger area of the lung than the protected specimen brush method.

Bronchoscopic BAL and protected specimen brush collection provide direct access to bronchial and parenchymal tissues at the site of lung inflammation. Unfortunately, even specimens collected via bronchoscopy are subject to contamination by upper airway flora.[83,85] Upper airway bacteria may be picked up as the bronchoscope or collection catheter passes through the naso-oropharynx or traverses the endotracheal tube (in intubated patients) during introduction. Consequently, clinicians struggle with distinguishing colonization from infection even with these more invasive methods.

Qualitative or semiquantitative (using ''light,'' ''moderate,'' or ''heavy'' to describe quantity) analysis of cultures from endotracheal aspirates may provide useful information for identifying causes of pneumonia, but they tend to lack specificity.[5] Therefore, the higher rate of false-positive results may lead to inappropriate antimicrobial use. Quantitative analysis of endotracheal aspirates or BAL or protected specimen brush specimens usually provides greater specificity for the diagnosis of VAP.[55,86] The traditional quantitative cutoff values for endotracheal aspirates are 10^5 to 10^6 colony-forming units (cfu) per mL or higher; the traditional cutoff is usually 10^4 cfu per mL or higher for BAL and 10^3 cfu/mL or higher for the protected specimen brush technique.

These criteria may be further confounded by prior administration of antimicrobials and differences in local bronchoscopic procedures.[5,87] Pathogen identification via bronchoscopic procedures is not a quick process. Cultures of specimens collected via BAL or protected specimen brush usually take an additional 48 to 72 hours. Bronchoscopy requires skilled personnel and is often not feasible or available at certain times or at certain facilities. Therefore, ''blind'' nonbronchoscopic sampling with mini-BAL, protected specimen brush, or bronchial suctioning has been performed.[83,84] These methods have not been as well studied but may provide clinicians with useful information through a less invasive method.

Transtracheal aspiration is an older method that involves the insertion of a 14-gauge needle through the cricothyroid membrane into the trachea.[72] Use of this technique has

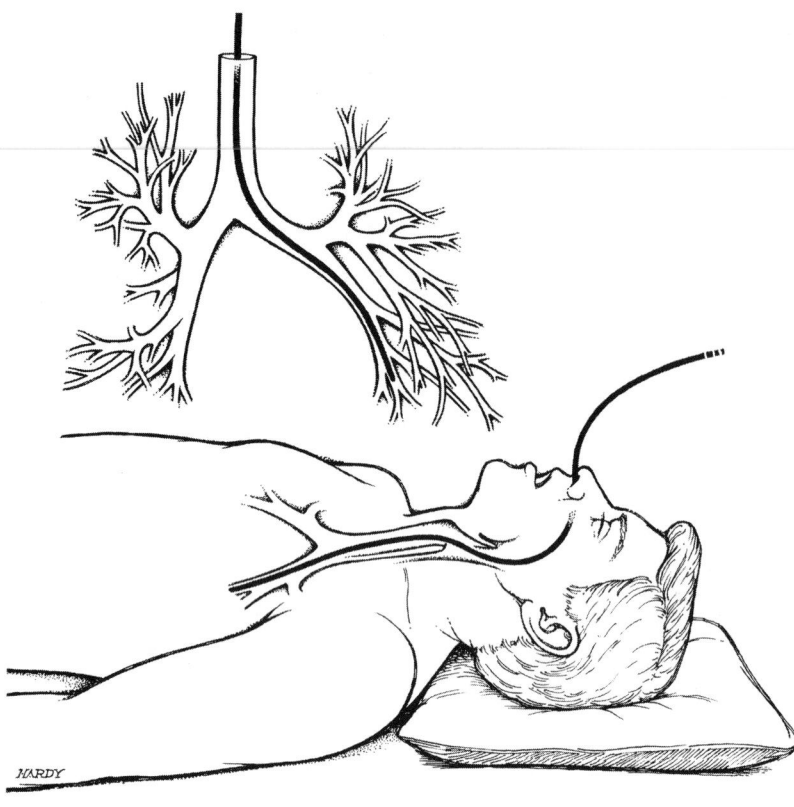

FIGURE 75.5 Fiberoptic bronchoscope (*see color insert*). (From Neil O. Hardy, West-point, CT.)

waned, probably due in part to safety concerns, lack of skilled proceduralists, and the availability of other diagnostic methods. Open-lung biopsy, the most invasive method, is typically reserved for difficult-to-diagnose immunocompro-mised patients.[83] Thoracentesis is usually performed to exclude empyema in patients showing pleural effusion on a chest radiograph.[72] Pleural fluid collected during thoracentesis may be sent for microbial examination.

TYPES OF PNEUMONIA

COMMUNITY-ACQUIRED PNEUMONIA

ETIOLOGY

The most common cause of CAP is *S. pneumoniae* or simply "the pneumococcus." It has been reported to cause 20% to 75% of cases of CAP (Table 75.3).[8] Other common causes of CAP are *H. influenzae* (3% to 12%) and the atypical respiratory pathogens. The "atypical" pathogens are *M. pneumoniae*, *Chlamydophila* (formerly classified as *Chlamydia*) *pneumoniae*, and *L. pneumophila*. Prevalence rates for these nonzoonotic atypical pathogens have varied widely from study to study. Rates generally range from 1% to 18% for *M. pneumoniae*, 1% to 6% for *C. pneumoniae*, and 2% to 8% for *Legionella* species.[8] *Legionella* exhibits greater geographic variability than the other two agents. Recent research suggests that coinfection with an atypical pathogen and traditional bacterial agents occurs with some regularity.[88] Organisms such as *S. pneumoniae* may have a symbiotic relationship with an atypical pathogen.

The likelihood of a patient having a resistant *S. pneumoniae* pneumonia may be greater in patients with the following risk factors: older than 65 years of age, received β-lactams within the past 3 months, alcoholism, immunosuppression, medical comorbidities, and exposure to a child in a day care.[11] Patients may be at greater risk for enteric gram-negative pathogens if they reside in nursing homes, have underlying cardiopulmonary comorbidities, or received recent antibiotic therapy.

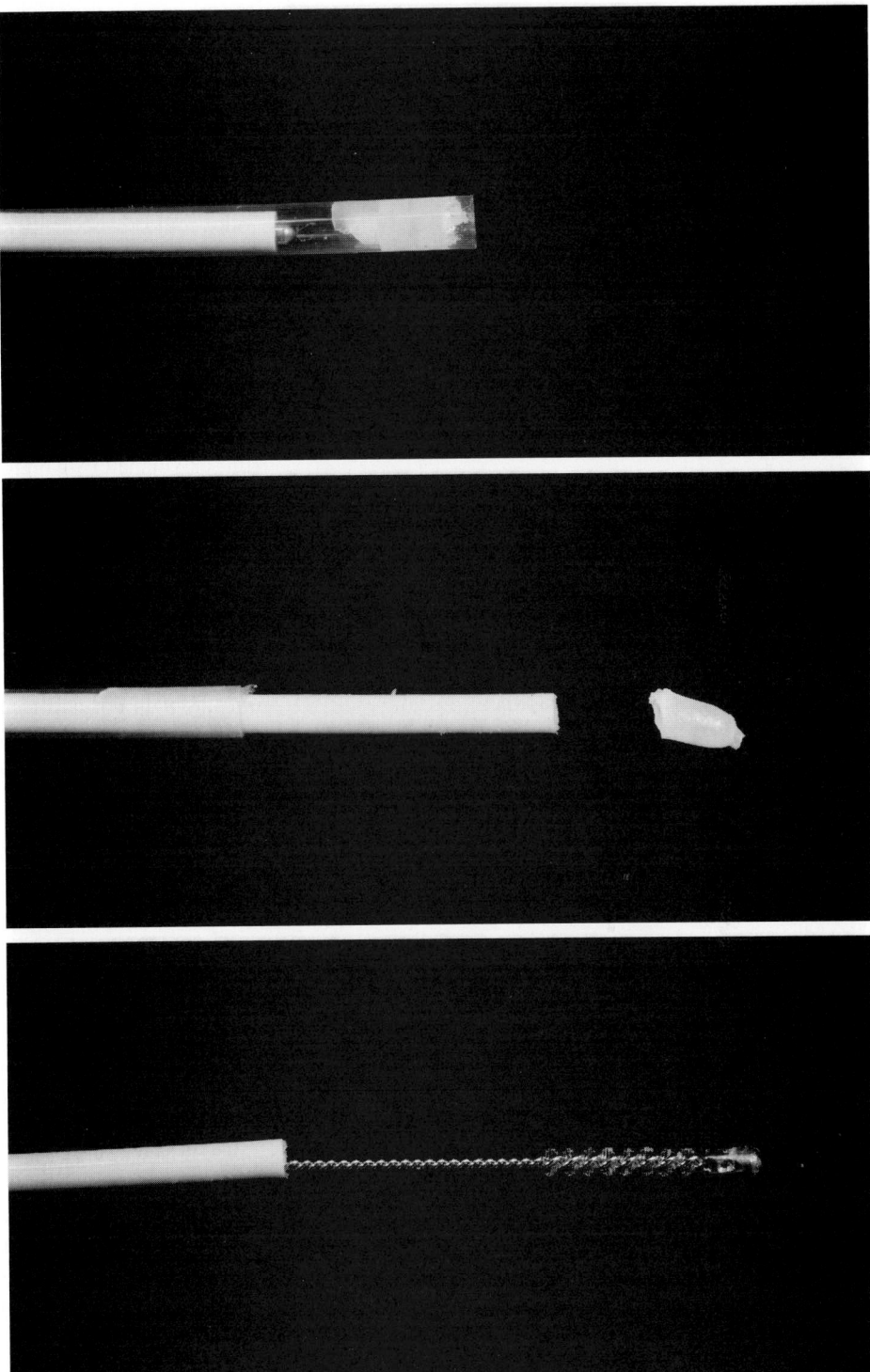

FIGURE 75.6 Protected specimen brush. **A.** Outer sheath with carbon-wax-plug intact; inner sheath can be seen inside the outer one. **B.** The inner catheter comes out of the sheath. **C.** The microbiologic brush comes out of the inner catheter to collect specimens.

Viral pathogens account for about 2% to 15% of cases of CAP.[89] Influenza virus is the most common cause, followed by parainfluenza virus, adenovirus, and respiratory syncytial virus (RSV). Other less common causative agents include *Moraxella catarrhalis*, *S. aureus*, Enterobacteriaceae, *Pseudomonas aeruginosa*, anaerobes, *Chlamydophila psittaci*, and *Coxiella burnetii*.[24]

KEY PATHOGENS

STREPTOCOCCUS PNEUMONIAE

This virulent, gram-positive diplococci should be considered as a potential pathogen in most cases of CAP, even if not identified by routine microbiologic testing. This fastidious

TABLE 75.3	Microbiology of Community-Acquired Pneumonia	
Streptococcus pneumoniae		20%–75%
Mycoplasma pneumoniae		1%–18%
Haemophilus influenzae		3%–12%
Chlamydophila pneumoniae		1%–6%
Legionella pneumophila		2%–8%
Gram-negative bacilli		3%–10%
Staphylococcus aureus		1%–5%
Viruses		2%–16%

(Adapted from Bartlett JG. Management of respiratory tract infections, 2nd ed. Philadelphia: Lippincott Williams & Wilkins, 1999, with permission.)

organism may not always be recovered from sputum collections. The pneumococcus can evade phagocytosis due to the presence of a polysaccharide capsule, which makes it difficult to clear from sites of infection. At least 80 different types of capsules have been identified.[90] The current 23-valent pneumococcal vaccine contains capsular polysaccharide from 23 of the most common types.

Until recently the pneumococcus was susceptible to many antibiotics, including penicillin.[91] Unfortunately, pneumococcal resistance to penicillin and other antimicrobials has increased in recent years, making empiric therapy decisions more difficult. Several clinical reports of lack of β-lactam susceptibility started surfacing in the early 1990s.[91]

Resistance to penicillins and cephalosporins is manifested by an alteration in key penicillin-binding proteins in the cell wall.[92] As a result, the affinity of β-lactams for their pharmacologic targets is diminished. The susceptibility of *S. pneumoniae* to penicillin is currently defined by the Clinical and Laboratory Standards Institute/National Committee for Clinical Laboratory Standards (NCCLS) as a minimum inhibitory concentration (MIC) of 0.06 μg per mL or less.[93] Isolates with reduced susceptibility (intermediate resistance) have an MIC of 0.1 to 1.0 μg per mL, and resistant isolates have an MIC of 2.0 μg per mL or more.

These breakpoints were largely based on drug levels achieved in the cerebrospinal fluid for meningitis treatment.[50] Their value for predicting clinical outcomes in pneumonia has been questioned, as most β-lactam antibiotics achieve higher concentrations in the lungs than in the meninges.

With these breakpoints, there is wide variability in the incidence of lack of penicillin susceptibility worldwide. In the United States, rates of penicillin resistance in pneumococci have varied from as high as 36% in Southeastern states to as low as 17% in Northwestern states.[94] The clinical significance of in vitro penicillin resistance on clinical outcomes remains unclear in nonmeningeal pneumococcal infections. A number of studies have shown that pneumonias caused by even intermediate-high level penicillin-resistant strains of pneumococci can be effectively treated with appropriate doses of β-lactams such as ampicillin, amoxicillin–clavulanate, cefotaxime, and ceftriaxone.[95,96] Mortality rates appear to be higher only in patients infected with organisms with an MIC of 4 μg per mL or higher.[95,97]

Given this, many experts recommend that the penicillin MIC breakpoints be raised so that traditional first-line antibiotics could be used, thus sparing the use of newer agents.[50,95] At present penicillin breakpoints remain unchanged, but newer NCCLS breakpoints have been raised for ceftriaxone and cefotaxime for nonmeningeal infections. Under these new definitions susceptibility is defined as MIC 1 μg per mL or less, intermediate resistance is defined as MIC of 2 μg per mL, and resistant is defined as 4 μg per mL or higher.[98] Breakpoint values for amoxicillin (including amoxicillin–clavulanate) are higher because these drugs are not used to treat meningeal infections.[99] *S. pneumoniae* isolates are reported as susceptible to amoxicillin if the MIC is 2 μg per mL or less, intermediate if MIC is 4 μg per mL, and resistant if MIC is 8 μg per mL or higher. Higher doses of amoxicillin (3 to 4 g/day) appear to be active against more than 90% of *S pneumoniae* isolates.[50] The addition of clavulanate to amoxicillin will not improve activity against *S. pneumonia*, as it is not a β-lactamase producer. It is not known whether the new pharmacokinetically enhanced formulation of amoxicillin–clavulanate (2,000 mg/125 mg) provides any additional clinical effectiveness over traditional forms of the drug in the treatment of CAP.[100]

Both β-lactam-susceptible and β-lactam-resistant strains of pneumococci can show resistance to other classes of antimicrobials, including macrolides, trimethoprim–sulfamethoxazole (TMP-SMZ), lincosamides (i.e., clindamycin), or tetracyclines.[95] Penicillin-resistant strains usually are resistant to multiple drugs.[92] Pneumococcal resistance to macrolides has increased worldwide. Across the United States, the national average of macrolide resistance in pneumococci is about 25% to 30%.[94] Resistance to macrolides is typically manifested by two mechanisms of resistance. The first is a *mef*A genetically encoded efflux pump that can expel macrolides from the bacteria.[101] This type of resistance produces low to moderate levels of resistance to macrolides. Advanced macrolides (azithromycin and clarithromycin) may still produce successful results. The other mechanism is an *erm*B-encoded mutation that causes a methylation of the 23S rRNA within the 50S ribosomal subunit. Alteration of this drug target will cause a high level of resistance that expresses an MLS_B phenotypic resistance affecting macrolides, lincosamides, and B-type streptogramins.

TMP-SMZ resistance is caused primarily by mutations to target-binding sites for the two drugs.[92] Rates of pneumococcal resistance to TMP-SMZ in the United States are about 35% to 40%. Pneumococcal resistance to tetracyclines has been estimated at about 20%.[92] Doxycycline susceptibility may not always be predicted by tetracycline in vitro testing.[102] About 90% to 95% of isolates of *S. pneumoniae* appear to be sensitive to doxycycline.[103]

Resistance to antipneumococcal fluoroquinolones remains very low but appears to be increasing with increased fluoroquinolone use in the community.[104] Many experts have suggested limiting the use of fluoroquinolones in situations where resistant *S. pneumoniae* is unlikely in order to preserve their utility.[11,95] Many papers have highlighted in vitro pharmacodynamic differences between the antipneumococcal fluoroquinolones, but no study has reported a true clinical advantage for any specific agent at this point.[105,106]

Pneumococci have not displayed in vitro resistance to vancomycin and linezolid.[103] These agents have typically been held in reserve for the treatment of resistant pneumococci.

A rapid pneumococcal urinary antigen test was recently approved by the FDA.[107] This test is an immunochromatographic membrane assay that detects pneumococcal cell wall polysaccharide in the urine. This test should be used in conjunction with other diagnostic methods. The sensitivity and the specificity of this test are reported to be 50% to 80% and about 90%, respectively.[50] The test may be useful in situations where prior antibiotics were administered. Therefore, this test may be useful when trying to administer antibiotics within the first few hours of presenting to the hospital. Some have questioned whether this test provides any quicker or more useful information than Gram staining of sputum.[50]

HAEMOPHILUS INFLUENZAE

H. influenzae is a small gram-negative, aerobic coccobacilli (pleomorphic rod).[108] There are six encapsulated types (a through f), and nonencapsulated or nontypeable serotypes. Type B has been widely responsible for invasive disease in young children. Widespread use of the vaccine against type B *H. influenzae* has dramatically reduced the occurrence of diseases from this organism. It is the nontypeable form of *H. influenzae* that is usually seen in adult pneumonia.

H. influenzae is a common commensal organism that colonizes the upper respiratory tract. The organism can be pathogenic, especially in patients with compromised immune systems and comorbidities. This organism may be particularly important as a cause of CAP in patients who have chronic obstructive pulmonary disease or who smoke.

Prior to the 1970s, most strains of *H. influenzae* were generally susceptible to ampicillin.[108] Now at least 25% to 30% of strains worldwide produce β-lactamase, making this agent nonsusceptible to agents such as ampicillin.[103] β-lactamase inhibitor (clavulanate, tazobactam, or sulbactam) combination products typically maintain activity against β-lactamase-producing strains of *H. influenzae*. Second- and third-generation cephalosporins typically maintain good activity against *H. influenzae*.[108] Erythromycin is not active against *H. influenzae*, but the advanced-generation macrolides can be effective. Clarithromycin does not have potent *H. influenzae* activity itself but when combined with its 14-OH-clarithromycin metabolite can display additive or synergistic effects against the organism.[108] Doxycycline and TMP-SMZ are active against *H. influenzae* but have displayed variable rates of resistance geographically. Fluoroquinolones appear to have very good activity against *H. influenzae*, with only rare reports of resistance at present.[103,108]

ATYPICAL PATHOGENS (*M. PNEUMONIAE, C. PNEUMONIAE,* AND *L. PNEUMOPHILA*)

The term "atypical" originated from the observation that these organisms were associated with pneumonic infections whose clinical presentation was different than that observed for the more classic pneumococcal pneumonia presentation of high fever, chills, pleuritic chest pain, lobar consolidation, purulent sputum, and often toxic appearance.[24] The "atypical pneumonia syndrome" was often associated with a more subacute or gradual illness, a nonproductive cough, and extrapulmonary symptoms such as headache, hoarseness, pharyngitis, myalgias, and gastrointestinal complaints.[109] Some clinicians have suggested that clinical presentation could differentiate between atypical and more typical pathogens.[110] Current treatment guidelines caution against using such predictive techniques, as this has never been validated.[11] Using clinical presentation to identify pathogens may be useful only if it corroborates with other diagnostic findings. *M. pneumoniae* and *C. pneumoniae* are most frequently associated with mild to moderate cases of pneumonia but can actually cause a wide range of clinical infection.

M. pneumoniae is a small aerobic organism now classified as a bacterium that lacks a true bacterial cell wall. It is a common cause of upper and lower respiratory tract infections among children and young adults and is an increasingly recognized cause of moderate to severe CAP in the elderly.[111] *M. pneumoniae* can be transmitted person to person through respiratory secretions. It has a long incubation period (about 2 to 4 weeks) and can spread easily within a family or closed environment.[111] Diagnosis of pneumonia caused by this organism is usually empiric due to the lack of reliable and practical diagnostic tests. Growth of the organism in culture requires special media, long periods of incubation, and special technical procedures that are not viable options in daily practice. *M. pneumoniae* will not take up Gram stain due to the lack of a cell wall. Serologic testing has been used to diagnose *M. pneumoniae* infection, but diagnostic criteria depend on a fourfold increase in antibody titer between acute and convalescent sera levels of IgG and IgM. Alternatively, a single titer greater than 1:64 has been used.[50] Unfortunately, it takes days to weeks to identify a positive test. Therefore, serology testing cannot help with initial diagnosis, but rather may be used to provide epidemiologic information. Because *M. pneumoniae* is devoid of a cell wall, β-lactam antibiotics lack activity against this organism.[111] In addition, *M. pneumoniae, C. pneumoniae,* and *Legionella* species all have developed the ability to survive within phagocytic immune cells. As such, these intracellular organisms can evade the antibacterial activity of antibiotics in the bloodstream. Therefore, antibiotics with good intracellular penetration and activity, such as macrolides, tetracyclines, fluoroquinolones, and ketolides, are recommended.

Newer advanced-generation macrolides tend to achieve higher intracellular concentrations than erythromycin.

C. pneumoniae (also called the TWAR agent) is an obligate intracellular gram-negative bacterium. Similar to *M. pneumoniae*, it is transmitted person to person and has a long incubation period. *C. pneumoniae* can cause upper or lower respiratory tract infections.[111] Rhinitis, sore throat, and hoarseness may precede cases of lower tract infection. Pneumonia caused by this organism is usually mild to moderate in severity, but it may cause more severe disease in the elderly or in individuals with chronic comorbidities. Seroprevalence is low during early childhood years but continues to increase to greater than 50% by early adult years.[111] *C. pneumoniae* may grow in cell culture, but the organism tends to be fastidious and slow-growing, which limits the value of cell culture in clinical practice. Gram staining is of little value in the diagnosis of *C. pneumoniae*. Similar to serologic testing with *M. pneumoniae,* a fourfold increase in antibody titer between acute and convalescent sera levels of IgG or a single IgM titer of more than 1:16 microimmunofluorescence may suggest a recent infection.[50] Treatment for *C. pneumoniae* pneumonia is empiric given the lack of a quick and reliable diagnostic method for identification and drug susceptibility. Macrolides, tetracyclines, fluoroquinolones, and ketolides usually provide effective therapy.

Legionella species are gram-negative, aerobic bacilli that can cause community- or institutional-acquired pneumonia. *L. pneumophila* species are responsible for about 85% of cases of legionellosis.[112] About 70% of cases are caused by *L. pneumophila* serogroup 1.[12] Still other species (e.g., *L. micdadei, L. bozemanii*) may be encountered. Legionnaires' disease can present with a broad spectrum of clinical presentations, ranging from mild cough to sepsis with multiple organ failure. *Legionella* pneumonia has been associated with a more critical presentation and higher mortality rate than *M. pneumoniae* or *C. pneumoniae*.[111] Mortality rates associated with *Legionella* pneumonia range from 5% to 25% in immunocompetent patients and are believed to be substantially higher in immunocompromised patients.[12] The incidence of Legionnaires' disease may peak between late summer and early fall.[113] *L. pneumophila* appears to thrive in fresh water environments. Outbreaks have been associated with contaminated water distribution systems, cooling towers, and ventilation systems.[114] It was after an outbreak at a hotel hosting an American Legion convention in 1976 that the organism was first recognized. The genus was named in response to this initial outbreak.[115] Risk factors for developing Legionnaires' disease include advanced age, smoking, chronic lung disease, alcoholism, use of immunosuppressant drugs, and compromised cell-mediated immunity.[50] In addition to classic pneumonia signs and symptoms, patients may present with high fevers (above 40°C), gastrointestinal symptoms including diarrhea, confusion, bradycardia, hyponatremia, and elevated liver enzymes. Unfortunately, studies have failed to find any pathognomonic signs or symptoms for *Legionella* pneumonia.[116]

Gram staining of Legionella has not proven widely useful, despite small reports of success.[117] However, clinicians should consider the agent if a sputum Gram stain shows the presence of small pleomorphic gram-negative rods, without any other gram-negative rod being detected on sputum or blood culture. *Legionella* can be cultured, but it usually requires special media and several days to grow.[118] The specificity of a positive *Legionella* sputum culture approaches 100%, but the estimated sensitivity for sputum culture to detect *Legionella* ranges from less than 10% to 80%. The value of blood culture is even more insensitive for diagnosing legionellosis. The *Legionella* direct fluorescent antibody (DFA) test is more rapid, producing results within 4 hours, but the sensitivity is estimated to be only 33% to 70%.[119] This test is used to detect *Legionella* antigens in sputum or BAL fluid. The sensitivity and specificity are typically higher with BAL specimens. Currently, the most useful routine test for Legionnaire's disease is the *Legionella* urine antigen assay. This rapid test detects the presence of soluble *L. pneumophila* serogroup type I antigen in urine.[118] The sensitivity of the test is reported to be 70% to 90% and the specificity is reported to exceed 99%. Unfortunately, the current assays do not reliably detect other less common species or serogroups of *Legionella*. Serologic and nucleic acid amplification (PCR) testing for *Legionella* have been developed but have limited practicality for clinical patient care at this time. All of the *Legionella* tests appear to have good specificity.[118] Therefore, a positive test with any of these tests is indicative of *Legionella* infection.

There has been controversy over the appropriate situations in which to employ specific testing for *Legionella*.[116] Recent guidelines by the Infectious Disease Society of America (IDSA) advocate specific testing for *Legionella* in any patient hospitalized with enigmatic pneumonia that requires ICU admission in the presence of an epidemic, or failure to respond to β-lactam regimens.[50] Practice guidelines recognize the high rate of mortality associated with *Legionella* pneumonia and note that delaying therapy can contribute to negative patient outcomes.[116] Thus, all recommended empiric regimens for moderate to severe CAP include an agent that has activity against *Legionella*.[11,12,50,119]

The mainstay of therapy for *Legionella* pneumonia has historically been high doses of intravenous erythromycin (2 to 4 grams/day, divided into four doses) with or without rifampin (600 mg/day).[120] Upon clinical improvement, patients were often switched to oral erythromycin. Newer, more potent agents such as azithromycin and fluoroquinolones have supplanted erythromycin as the agents of choice because they are better tolerated, produce superior concentrations in lung tissue, have less potential for drug interactions, and require less frequent administration and reduced intravenous fluid volumes.[50] In addition to their in vitro activity against *Legionella*, these newer drugs appear to provide higher intracellular concentrations. Although rifampin displays excellent in vitro activity against *Legionella*, it is not used alone due to concerns about rapid development of resistance.[121] In addition, rifampin is a potent cytochrome P-450 enzyme inducer and may interfere with other medications. The synergistic use of rifampin with advanced macrolides and fluoroquinolones has not been advocated.[50]

Other agents that have displayed clinical efficacy against *Legionella* include doxycycline, TMP-SMZ, and telithromycin.[50,122] Although many β-lactams appear to be active against *Legionella* in vitro, they do not display sufficient activity against intracellular *Legionella*.[120] Ten to 21 days of antibiotic therapy has been advocated for treatment of *Legionella* pneumonia.[86] Shorter courses in some patients may be effective,[123,124] especially with drugs with a long half-life, such as azithromycin. A few small studies have reported 100% cure rates with as few as 3 to 5 days of azithromycin therapy in less severe cases.[123] Nonetheless, longer courses are advised for immunocompromised or critically ill patients.

THERAPEUTIC PLAN

Over the past decade there have been a number of organizations or expert panels that have published practice guidelines for the management of CAP. These include IDSA, the American Thoracic Society (ATS), CDC Therapeutic Working Group, the Canadian Infectious Diseases Society/Canadian Thoracic Society, and the British Thoracic Society.[11,12,50,125,126] These guidelines were developed to assist clinicians in making prudent therapeutic decisions that promote effective treatment of CAP and that limit the occurrence of bacterial resistance. Many of the guidelines were developed using tiered evidence-based recommendations; however, different guidelines often make different recommendations. The recommendations presented in this chapter are largely derived from the most recent versions of the ATS and IDSA guidelines.[11,50]

One of the most difficult decisions that physicians face is whether to admit a patient with CAP to the hospital. Clinicians must take into consideration the age of the patient, vital signs, level of consciousness, comorbid diseases, laboratory abnormalities, and social support structure. Many experts believe that a great majority of patients with CAP can be safely treated as outpatients, either with oral medications or home infusion therapy.[50]

Clinical pathways, treatment algorithms, and prognostic scoring systems have been developed to aid clinicians in admission and treatment decisions. A pneumonia severity scoring system or "prediction rule" was developed from the Pneumonia Patient Outcomes Research Team study (PORT) to assess mortality risks among patients with CAP.[127] The PORT prediction rule (also referred to as Pneumonia Severity Index) stratifies patients into one of five risk classifications (Fig. 75.7). Patients are scored based on age, comorbid conditions, and physical and laboratory abnormalities. Patients in the lowest two risk classes (I and II) are predicted to have low rates of mortality and can usually be treated as outpatients. Patients in class III have a low mortality risk and can either be treated as outpatients or hospitalized briefly for observation and treatment before treatment on an outpatient basis. Patients in classes IV and V are at a higher risk of mortality and should be hospitalized for care. Although other investigators have independently validated the PORT prediction rule to some degree, it should serve as an aid for clinicians and researchers and should not take the place of sound clinician judgment.

Approximately 10% of patients with CAP are severely ill and require ICU admission with or without mechanical ventilation.[24] Although there are no standard guidelines for deciding when to admit a patient to the ICU, a number of publications[11,24] have provided the following criteria:

1. Respiratory rate above 30 breaths per minute
2. PaO_2/FiO_2 below 250 or PO_2 below 50 to 60 mm Hg breathing room air
3. Chest radiographs showing bilateral involvement, multilobar involvement, or significant progression of disease in the first 48 hours of admission
4. Hypotension (systolic blood pressure below 90 mm Hg or diastolic blood pressure below 60 mm Hg)
5. Need for vasopressors
6. Urine output less than 20 mL per hour or less than 80 mL over a 4-hour period
7. Blood urea nitrogen above 19.6 mg per dL
8. Abnormal mental status

Regardless of the site of care within the hospital, it is important to initiate antibiotic therapy in a timely fashion, especially in patients with a higher risk of mortality. Ideally sputum and blood culture specimens should be collected before administering antibiotics so as not to compromise microbial yield. A retrospective analysis of 14,000 patients showed that a delay of more than 8 hours from time of admission to receipt of first dose of antibiotic was associated with increased mortality.[128] Therefore, obtaining pretreatment specimens should not excessively delay the start of antibiotic therapy in elderly or severely ill patients.

TREATMENT

A list of antibacterial agents and dosages frequently used in the treatment of CAP can be found in Table 75.4. Antibiotic choices must be individualized, taking into account antimicrobial spectrum, resistance, pharmacokinetic and pharmacodynamic principles, potential for adverse effects, drug interactions, convenience, route of administration, and costs. Optimal treatment of CAP remains a challenge for clinicians, largely because of the empiric therapeutic nature of the disease. No single regimen can cover all potential pathogens. As a general rule, the ATS and IDSA guidelines recommend that empiric regimens for patients with CAP contain an agent that typically has activity against *S. pneumoniae*, *H. influenzae*, and atypical pathogens.[11,12,50] Multiple drug classes can

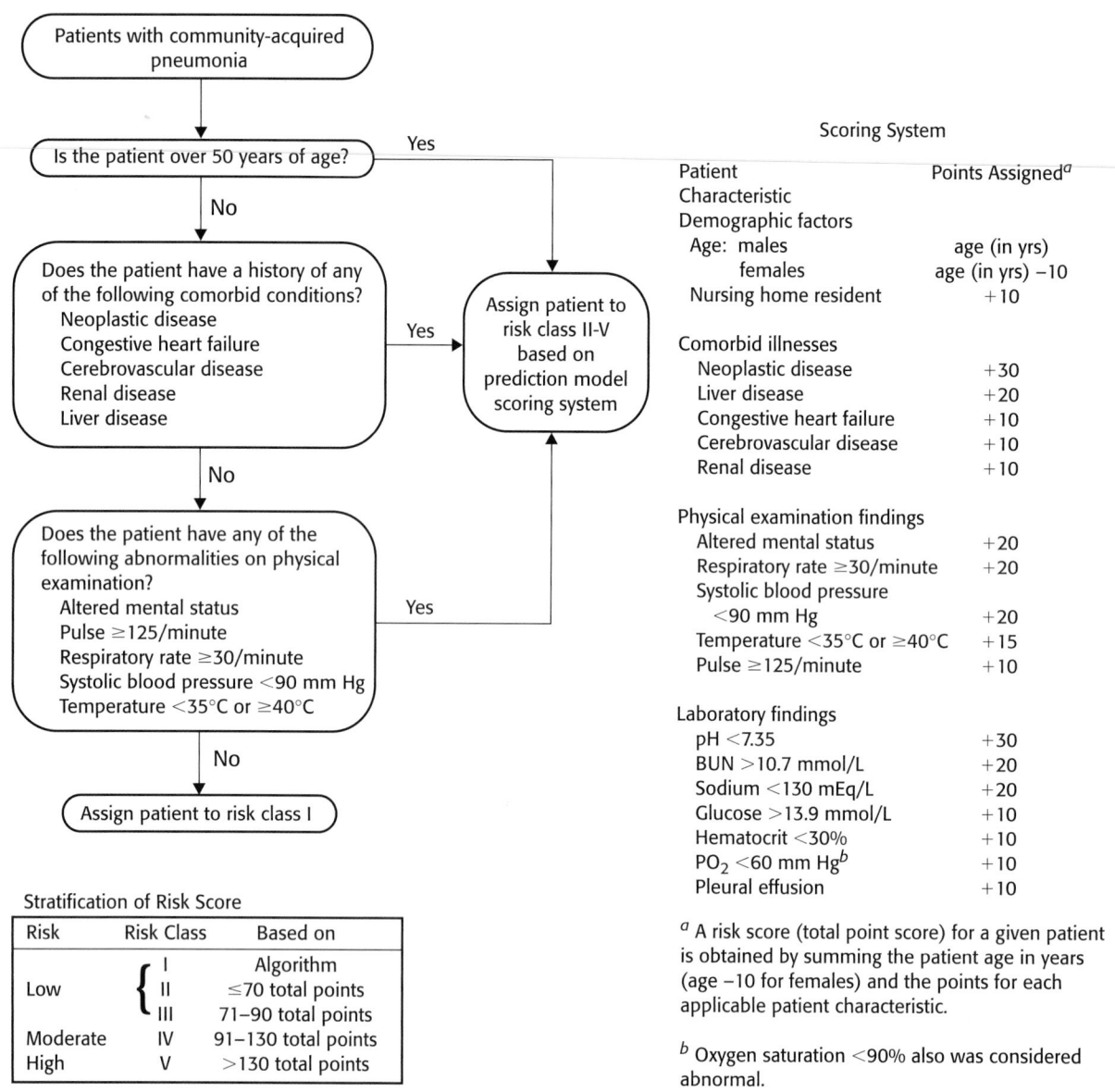

Scoring System

Patient Characteristic	Points Assigned[a]
Demographic factors	
Age: males	age (in yrs)
females	age (in yrs) −10
Nursing home resident	+10
Comorbid illnesses	
Neoplastic disease	+30
Liver disease	+20
Congestive heart failure	+10
Cerebrovascular disease	+10
Renal disease	+10
Physical examination findings	
Altered mental status	+20
Respiratory rate ≥30/minute	+20
Systolic blood pressure	
<90 mm Hg	+20
Temperature <35°C or ≥40°C	+15
Pulse ≥125/minute	+10
Laboratory findings	
pH <7.35	+30
BUN >10.7 mmol/L	+20
Sodium <130 mEq/L	+20
Glucose >13.9 mmol/L	+10
Hematocrit <30%	+10
PO_2 <60 mm Hg[b]	+10
Pleural effusion	+10

[a] A risk score (total point score) for a given patient is obtained by summing the patient age in years (age −10 for females) and the points for each applicable patient characteristic.

[b] Oxygen saturation <90% also was considered abnormal.

Stratification of Risk Score

Risk	Risk Class	Based on
	I	Algorithm
Low	II	≤70 total points
	III	71–90 total points
Moderate	IV	91–130 total points
High	V	>130 total points

FIGURE 75.7 Prediction model for identifying and stratifying patient risk for persons with community-acquired pneumonia. (Reprinted with permission from Barlett JG, Breiman RF, Mandell LA, et al. Community-acquired pneumonia in adults: guidelines for management. Clin Infect Dis 26:811–838, 1998.)

exert activity against nonresistant *S. pneumoniae* and *H. influenzae*. Only macrolides, doxycycline, fluoroquinolones, and ketolides cover the three atypical pathogens.[100] Therefore, according to the ATS and IDSA guidelines, all empiric regimens will contain one of these agents.

Contrary to this, recent research suggests that even β-lactam monotherapy may be adequate for mild to moderate CAP due to *M. pneumoniae* or *C. pneumoniae*.[129–131] British guidelines differ from the North American guidelines in that they do not always recommend agents with atypical coverage.[126] These observations highlight the lack of evidence-based information behind many of the recommendations. Clearly, more well-designed research is needed. Table

75.5 summarizes the empiric treatment recommendations adapted from the ATS and IDSA guidelines.[11,50]

Mild to moderate CAP in patients stable enough to be treated as outpatients will most likely be attributed to *S. pneumoniae*, atypical pathogens, viruses, and *H. influenzae* (especially in smokers and those with chronic obstructive pulmonary disease).[11] Oral administration of antibiotics is preferred in these milder cases if patients can tolerate them. If patients lack cardiopulmonary comorbidities and are at low risk for aspiration or drug-resistant *S. pneumoniae*, then monotherapy with an oral macrolide or doxycycline is advised. Advanced macrolides (clarithromycin or azithromycin) are preferred in most situations, as erythromycin

TABLE 75.4	Usual Dosages of Agents Used to Treat Community-Acquired Pneumonia	
Agent	**Oral**	**Parenteral**
Penicillins		
Penicillin V	500 mg QID	
Penicillin G		500,000–2 million units q4–6h
Ampicillin	500 mg QID	1–2 g q6h
Amoxicillin	500–1,000 mg TID	
Oxacillin/nafcillin	500 mg QID	1–3 g q6h
Ticarcillin		3–6 g q6h
Piperacillin		3–6 g q6h
β-Lactamase Inhibitors		
Amoxicillin/clavulanate	500 mg q8h or 875 mg q12h	
Amoxicillin/clavulanate XR	2,000 mg q12h	
Ampicillin/sulbactam		1.5–3 g q6h
Ticarcillin/clavulanate		3.1 g q4–6h
Piperacillin/tazobactam		3.375–4.5 g q6–8h
Cephalosporins		
Cefuroxime	500 mg q12h	750–1,500 mg q8h
Cefaclor	500 mg TID	
Cefdinir	300 mg q12h	
Cefprozil	500 mg q12h	
Cefotaxime		1–2 g q8h
Ceftriaxone		1 g q24h
Ceftazidime		1–2 g q8h
Cefixime	400 mg qd	
Cefpodoxime	400 mg q12h	
Cefepime		1–2 g q12h
Carbapenems		
Ertapenem		1,000 mg IM or IV q24h
Imipenem		500–1,000 mg q6–8h
Meropenem		500–1,000 mg q8h
Macrolides		
Erythromycin	250–500 mg QID	1 g q6h
Clarithromycin	500 mg q12h	
Azithromycin	500 mg qd	500 mg q24h
Fluoroquinolones		
Levofloxacin	500–750 mg qd	500–750 mg qd
Ciprofloxacin	500–750 mg q12h	200–400 mg q12h
Gatifloxacin	400 mg qd	400 mg qd
Moxifloxacin	400 mg qd	
Gemifloxacin	320 mg qd	
Miscellaneous		
Telithromycin	800 mg qd	
TMP-SMX	1 DS Tablet q12h	10 mg/kg daily in 2–4 divided doses
Doxycycline	100 mg q12h	100 mg q12h
Metronidazole	500 mg q8–12h	500 mg q8–12h
Vancomycin		1 g q12h (adjustments often made based on therapeutic drug monitoring)

| TABLE 75.5 | Guidelines for the Selection of Empiric Antimicrobial Therapy for Patients With Community-Acquired Pneumonia[a] |

Patient Type	Common Organisms	Therapy[b]

Outpatients with no cardiopulmonary disease and no modifying risk factors (i.e., resistant *Pneumococcus* or gram-negatives)	*Streptococcus pneumoniae*
	Mycoplasma pneumoniae
	Chlamydophila pneumoniae
	Haemophilus influenzae
	Respiratory viruses
		Oral advanced-generation macrolide
		  Azithromycin
		  Clarithromycin
		  or
		Oral doxycycline
		  or
		Oral Ketolide[c]
		  Telithromycin

Outpatients with cardiopulmonary disease and/or modifying risk factors (i.e., resistant *Pneumococcus* or Gram-negatives)	*Streptococcus pneumoniae*, including drug-resistant type
	Mycoplasma pneumoniae
	Chlamydophila pneumoniae
	Mixed (bacteria + atypical pathogen)
	Haemophilus influenzae
	Enteric gram-negatives
	Respiratory viruses
		Oral β-lactam antibiotic
		  Cefpodoxime
		  Cefuroxime
		  High-dose amoxicillin[d]
		  Amoxicillin/clavulanate
		  Parenteral ceftriaxone followed by oral cefpodoxime
		    plus
		  Oral macrolide or doxycycline
		    or
		Oral antipneumococcal fluoroquinolone alone
		or
		Oral telithromycin[c]

Non-ICU inpatients with no cardiopulmonary disease and no modifying risk factors (i.e., resistant *Pneumococcus* or gram-negatives)	*Streptococcus pneumoniae*
	Haemophilus influenzae
	Mycoplasma pneumoniae
	Chlamydia pneumoniae
	Mixed (bacteria + atypical pathogen)
	Respiratory virus
	Legionella spp
		IV azithromycin
		(If macrolide allergic or intolerant: doxycycline)
		    plus
		β-lactam antibiotic
		  Cefotaxime
		  Ceftriaxone
		  Ampicillin/sulbactam
		  High-dose ampicillin
		  Ertapenem
		    or
		Antipneumococcal fluoroquinolone alone

Non-ICU inpatients with cardiopulmonary disease and/or modifying risk factors (i.e., resistant *Pneumococcus* or gram-negatives), including nursing home patients	*Streptococcus pneumoniae*, including drug-resistant type
	Haemophilus influenzae
	Mycoplasma pneumoniae
	Chlamydophila pneumoniae
	Mixed (bacteria + atypical pathogen)
	Enteric gram-negatives
	Aspiration (anaerobes)
	Respiratory virus
		IV β-lactam antibiotic
		  Cefotaxime
		  Ceftriaxone
		  Ampicillin/sulbactam
		  High-dose ampicillin
		  Ertapenem
		    plus
		IV or oral macrolide or doxycycline

(continued)

TABLE 75.5	continued	
Patient Type	**Common Organisms**	**Therapy**[b]
	Legionella spp	or
		IV antipneumococcal fluoroquinolone alone
ICU Patients with no risks for *Pseudomonas*	*Streptococcus pneumoniae,* including drug-resistant type	IV β-lactam antibiotic
		plus either
	Legionella spp	IV macrolide (azithromycin) or IV fluoroquinolone
	Haemophilus influenzae	
	Enteric gram-negatives	
	Staphylococcus aureus	
	Mycoplasma pneumoniae	
	Respiratory virus	
ICU patients with risks for *Pseudomonas*	All of the above pathogens plus *Pseudomonas aeruginosa*	Selected IV antipseudomonal β-lactam antibiotics
		Cefepime
		Imipenem
		Meropenem
		Piperacillin/tazobactam
		plus
		IV antipseudomonal fluoroquinolone (ciprofloxacin) or
		IV aminoglycoside
		plus either
		IV macrolide
		or IV fluoroquinolone

[a] Excludes patients at risk for HIV.

[b] In no particular order.

[c] FDA approval occurred after most recent versions of IDSA or ATS CAP guidelines; therefore, use of this agent was not included in the published guidelines.

[d] High-dose amoxicillin = 1g q8h.

(Adapted with permission from Niederman MS, Mandell LA, Anzueto A, et al. Guidelines for the management of adults with community-acquired pneumonia. Diagnosis, assessment of severity, antimicrobial therapy, and prevention. Am J Respir Crit Care Med 163:1730–1754, 2001; and Mandell LA, Bartlett JG, Dowell SF, et al. Update of practice guidelines for the management of community-acquired pneumonia in immunocompetent adults. Clin Infect Dis 37:1405–33, 2003.)

lacks activity against *H. influenzae*.[108] General use of fluoroquinolones is not advocated in these otherwise healthy individuals so as to preserve their utility. Increased fluoroquinolone use in the community and in the hospital has been implicated as a cause of fluoroquinolone resistance.[104,132]

An oral β-lactam (cefuroxime, cefpodoxime, high-dose amoxicillin, or amoxicillin/clavulanate) plus a macrolide or doxycycline or monotherapy with an oral antipneumococcal fluoroquinolone is advised for patients with cardiopulmonary diseases, aspiration risks, or risks of having drug-resistant *S. pneumoniae* or enteric gram-negative infections. A single dose of intravenous or intramuscular ceftriaxone

can be substituted for the oral β-lactam as the initial dose in the physician's office or emergency department.[11]

Since the most recent IDSA and ATS guidelines were published, a new agent has been approved by the FDA. Telithromycin is the first drug approved from the ketolide class of antibiotics.[133] It was approved for mild to moderate CAP, including pneumonia caused by macrolide-resistant stains of pneumococcus.[134] Telithromycin's mechanism of action is similar to that of macrolides. The drug inhibits protein synthesis by binding to the bacterial 50S ribosomal subunit. However, the drug can maintain activity against *mef*A- and *erm*B-associated macrolide resistance in pneumococci. This agent is available only as an oral agent. It is acceptable for use in patients managed as outpatients, even if macrolide resistance is possible.

Empiric treatment of patients who require hospital admission but not ICU treatment is aimed at the same core CAP pathogens. However, infections caused by *L. pneumophila* may be more frequent in this patient population.[4] Therapy with an intravenous β-lactam (cefuroxime, ceftriaxone, high-dose amoxicillin, ampicillin/sulbactam, or ertapenem) plus a macrolide or doxycycline or monotherapy with an antipneumococcal fluoroquinolone is recommended.[11,50]

Treatment of severe CAP in patients requiring ICU admission should empirically provide coverage for the two most lethal pathogens, *S. pneumoniae* and *L. pneumophila*. Of course, atypical pathogens, viruses, and *H. influenzae* may still cause CAP in this setting. In addition, *S. aureus* and enteric gram-negative rods are encountered more frequently in CAP patients treated in this setting, but not often enough to warrant empiric coverage in all patients. An intravenous β-lactam (cefotaxime or ceftriaxone) plus either a macrolide or fluoroquinolone (even ciprofloxacin) is appropriate empiric therapy in this setting. The recommendation of combination therapy for patients treated in the ICU is based on limited data supporting monotherapy with fluoroquinolones in critically ill patients with pneumococcal pneumonia. Fluoroquinolones may be used as monotherapy in patients who cannot take β-lactams.[50] If *P. aeruginosa* is suspected, a regimen with two antipseudomonal agents should be initiated. An antipseudomonal β-lactam (cefepime, imipenem–cilastatin, meropenem, or piperacillin/tazobactam) can be used in combination with ciprofloxacin. Alternatively, an aminoglycoside with either a macrolide or fluoroquinolone may be combined with the antipseudomonal β-lactam. Aztreonam has been used in situations of β-lactam allergy. *P. aeruginosa* is a very rare cause of CAP. It is usually encountered in patients with immune deficiencies or structural lung diseases (e.g., bronchiectasis, cystic fibrosis).

Empiric antibiotic regimens can be changed or narrowed if the results of culture or in vitro sensitivity tests become available. Most patients will have a clinical response within 3 days of therapy.[11] Several studies have shown that oral antibiotic therapy can safely be administered to patients showing an initial response to intravenous antibiotics.[135,136] Many hospitals have adopted intravenous–oral switch programs for patients with CAP. Patients must be improving clinically and must be hemodynamically stable before switching to oral therapy. Oral therapy is not appropriate for patients with nausea or vomiting or those who have disorders that impair gastrointestinal absorption. Generally, patients showing clinical improvement are switched after at least 48 hours of intravenous antibiotics.

The use of early oral antibiotic therapy can substantially lower costs by shortening the hospital stay and by avoiding the higher cost of intravenous drugs. In addition, complications of intravenous therapy such as phlebitis and catheter-associated infections can be reduced.

Early discharge for patients with moderate CAP has been advocated by most experts.[11,136,137] Some clinicians even treat CAP patients who are not critically ill at home with intravenous therapy.[138] This option can be advocated only for patients who have dependable, supportive care at home. Such an approach can reduce costs and improve quality of life. CAP patients may return to activities of daily life quicker when treated at home with intravenous antibiotics compared to similar patients treated in the hospital.[138]

The optimal length of antibiotic therapy has never been well defined for CAP. Traditionally, therapy has been 7 to 14 days in uncomplicated courses.[11] Recent research with newer agents with longer serum or tissue half-lives may support treatments of 5 to 10 days. Ten to 14 days of antibiotic therapy has been advocated for treatment of immunosuppressed patients and those with *Legionella* pneumonia.[11]

ASSESSMENT OF RESPONSE TO TREATMENT

Defervescence usually occurs within 48 to 72 hours of appropriate antibiotic therapy.[11] Use of antipyretics may mask fever, and this must be considered in the assessment. Leukocytosis typically resolves within the first 4 to 5 days. Patients usually begin to feel better within the first 3 to 5 days of treatment. Abnormal findings on chest examination (e.g., crackles) resolve more slowly. Radiographic improvement may take weeks to resolve after effective therapy. Some individuals present with slowly resolving CAP in which radiographic abnormalities persist for more than 4 weeks. This is usually seen in patients who are elderly, have a history of alcoholism, who have significant comorbidities, or who were bacteremic.[11,24] Failure to respond to therapy should prompt clinicians to look for rare or unusual pathogens, resistant organisms, or noninfectious conditions.

NOSOCOMIAL PNEUMONIA

The term "nosocomial pneumonia" used to be synonymous with HAP, which is defined as a pneumonia that occurs 48 hours or more after admission. The most common type of HAP is VAP, defined as a pneumonia that develops more than 48 hours after intubation and mechanical ventilation. Nosocomial pneumonia now encompasses the newly identified HCAP, which includes pneumonia patients hospitalized in an acute care hospital for 2 or more days within 90 days of the infection; those who lived in a nursing home or long-term care facility; those who received recent intravenous antibiotic therapy, chemotherapy, or wound care within the past 30 days of the current infection; or those who attended a hospital or hemodialysis clinic.[5,6] Recently a joint ATS and IDSA guideline paper was published for the management of adults with HAP, VAP, and HCAP.[5] Recommendations from that guideline paper will serve as the backbone for the therapeutic approach and treatment of nosocomial pneumonia in this chapter.

ETIOLOGY

HAP is often referred to as being either "early" or "late" in onset. Early-onset HAP usually refers to pneumonia that develops within 4 days of admission. This type of nosocomial pneumonia is most often attributed to community-acquired organisms that were colonizing the patient around the time of hospital admission.[5,18,139] Common pathogens include *S. pneumoniae*, *H. influenzae*, methicillin-susceptible *S. aureus*, and enteric gram-negative bacilli (i.e., *Escherichia coli*, *Klebsiella pneumoniae*, *Serratia marcescens*, and *Proteus* species) (Table 75.6). Late-onset HAP (5 days or more) is more likely to be caused by more resistant gram-negative bacilli (e.g., *P. aeruginosa*, *Enterobacter* spp., *Acinetobacter* spp), *S. aureus* [including methicillin-resistant *S. aureus* (MRSA)], and *L. pneumophila*. Atypical pathogens are not generally regarded as common causes of nosocomial pneumonia. However, *L. pneumophila* has caused outbreaks of nosocomial pneumonia in hospitalized patients.[114] These outbreaks have largely been attributed to contaminated hospital water sources. Patients at greatest risk of *Legionella* infections are those with chronic medical conditions, cigarette smokers, and the immunosuppressed.[119]

| TABLE 75.6 | Spectrum and Crude Frequency of Pathogens Associated With Hospital-Acquired Pneumonia by Time of Onset |

Pathogen	Onset of Pneumonia	Crude Frequency (%)
Common pathogens		
Streptococcus pneumoniae	Early[a]	10–20
Haemophilus influenzae	Early	5–15
Anaerobic bacteria	Early	10–30[b]
Staphylococcus aureus	Early/Late	20–30
Gram-negative bacilli[c]	Late	30–60
Legionella pneumophila	Late	0–15
Uncommon pathogens	Late	<1
Influenza A and B	Late	<1
Respiratory syncytial virus	Late	0–15[d]
Aspergillus	Late	<1
Pneumocystis carinii	Late	<1
Mycobacterium tuberculosis	Late	<1

[a] First 4 days of hospitalization.
[b] Frequency is lower in late-onset ventilator-associated pneumonia.
[c] *Escherichia coli*, *Klebsiella pneumoniae*, *Enterobacter* spp, *Serratia marcescens*, *Acinetobacter* spp, *Pseudomonas aeruginosa*.
[d] May cause seasonal epidemics, especially in children.

(From Craven DE, Steger KA, Fleming CA. Hospital-acquired pneumonia. In: Wachter RM, Goldman L, Hollander H, eds. Hospital medicine. Philadelphia: Lippincott Williams & Wilkins, Philadelphia, 2000:491–498.)

The pathogenic role of anaerobes in nosocomial pneumonia is not well defined. Anaerobes have been reported as a cause of aspiration pneumonia in HAP and NHAP.[18] Although anaerobes frequently colonize the lower airways of ventilated patients, they are reported to be a very infrequent cause of VAP.[36,140–142] Clinical trials comparing drugs with anaerobic activity against regimens lacking anaerobic activity in VAP have not reported any difference in clinical efficacy.[143] Still, there has been speculation that anaerobes may play an important role in VAP.[140,141]

Organisms that have been associated with higher rates of mortality in nosocomial pneumonia are *P. aeruginosa*, *S. aureus*, *Acinetobacter* spp., and *Stenotrophomonas maltophilia*.[144] Rates of mortality are higher in bacteremic patients.[5,24] The risk of VAP being caused by pathogens that are resistant to multiple drugs is increased if the duration of mechanical ventilation has been longer than 6 days, or if prior broad-spectrum antibiotics had been used.[5] The relative frequency of nosocomial pneumonia caused by specific pathogens can vary considerably from hospital to hospital. Therefore, it is important for clinicians to be familiar with local hospital infection patterns, especially in the ICUs.

DIAGNOSIS

Diagnosing nosocomial pneumonia remains a challenge for clinicians, particularly in mechanically ventilated patients. Balancing the need to quickly administer antibiotics to patients who actually have pneumonia against not giving antibiotics to patients without pneumonia is a major dilemma in nosocomial pneumonia. Overtreatment for pneumonia in the hospital setting increases antibiotic resistance, the cost of care, and the incidence of side effects; therefore, indiscriminate use of antibiotics needs to be limited. On the other hand, delays in administering antibiotic therapy to patients with nosocomial pneumonia have been associated with increased mortality.[145] Therapy should be administered within 24 hours of diagnosis, if not sooner.

In the ICU setting, many patients appear as though they have pneumonia but actually do not. Most clinical signs of infection are not specific to pneumonia. Therefore, clinicians should evaluate other potential sites of infection as well. Likewise, not every patient receiving mechanical ventilation with pulmonary infiltrates has pneumonia.[146] Congestive heart failure, atelectasis, pulmonary thromboembolism, pulmonary edema, and pulmonary drug reactions are a few noninfectious conditions that may cause radiographic infiltrates.

Clinically, the findings of a new infiltrate with fever, leukocytosis or leukopenia, and purulent secretions suggest pneumonia. Unfortunately, clinical diagnosis with or without sputum examination often lacks diagnostic specificity. The isolation of organisms from ventilated patients with tracheal colonization or tracheobronchitis often leads to an overestimation of VAP and overuse of antibiotics.[5]

If it is apparent that a patient has pneumonia, identifying the actual organism causing the pneumonia remains difficult. More invasive quantitative bronchoscopic techniques have been used to provide clinicians with more specific information about the presence of bacteria in the distal regions of the lung.[83] Using these invasive procedures should not be taken lightly, as they are costly and carry the risk for complications such as bleeding or pneumothorax formation. Furthermore, the invasive methods have never been proven as a gold standard diagnostic method for VAP, although they are more specific than less invasive methods. At least one multicenter trial has reported that the use of quantitative, invasive BAL or protected sputum brush methods was associated with fewer deaths at 14 days, earlier improvement of organ dysfunction, and less antibiotic use compared to a clinical approach with nonquantitative, noninvasive diagnostic methods.[86] Other studies have not shown a mortality benefit from the use of the invasive techniques.[147,148] This may be due in part to the fact that microbiologic data obtained via bronchoscopic techniques may not provide quick enough information to guide antibiotic therapy.[47] Bronchoscopic collection of specimens via BAL or protected sputum brush requires skilled specialists and rigorous adherence to proper microbiologic procedures. Even with optimal performance, these invasive techniques can provide spurious results, especially in patients who have started or changed antibiotics within the preceding 24 to 72 hours. Recent studies have reported comparable results between quantitative culturing of endotracheal specimens and quantitative bronchoscopic procedures in VAP.[5,149]

All things considered, the use of quantitative evaluations of endotracheal or bronchoscopic collections are favored over qualitative or semiquantitative noninvasive evaluations, as they provide for a more conservative diagnosis of VAP.[5] Nonbronchoscopic "blind" BAL or protected sputum brush techniques may be useful when bronchoscopy is not available or not an option, but these methods are less specific than the bronchoscopic methods and have not been well studied.[83,84]

The Clinical Pulmonary Infection Score (CPIS) is a grading tool developed to aid clinicians in diagnosing VAP.[150] The original scoring system evaluated six different clinical, radiographic, physiologic, and microbiologic parameters (Table 75.7). A score of 6 or more has been associated with a high likelihood of pneumonia when validated by quantitative BAL cultures. Modified versions of the CPIS have been developed. Although the CPIS may provide useful information when combined with other diagnostic tools, it has not been proven to be very sensitive or specific by itself.

THERAPEUTIC PLAN

Given the many uncertainties of diagnosis and the benefit of early treatment, empiric therapy is often started as soon as pneumonia is deemed likely. Several studies have shown

TABLE 75.7	Clinical Pulmonary Infection Score, Used for the Diagnosis of Ventilator-Associated Pneumonia

Temperature (°C)

36.5–38.4 = 0 points

38.5–38.9 = 1 point

≥39.9 or ≤36.5 = 2 points

Blood Leukocytes/mm³

≥4,000 or ≤11,000 = 0 points

<4,000 or >11,000 = 1 point

≥500 band forms = +1 point

Tracheal Secretions

Purulent secretions = 1 point

Purulent tracheal secretions suctioned from patient <14 times/24 hours = 0 points

Purulent tracheal secretions suctioned from patient ≥14 times/24 hours = 1 point

Oxygenation (PaO$_2$/FiO$_2$, mm Hg)

>240 or acute respiratory distress syndrome (ARDS) = 0 points

≤240 and no evidence of ARDS = 2 points

Pulmonary Radiography

No infiltrate = 0 points

Diffused (or patchy) infiltrate = 1 point

Localized infiltrate = 2 points

Culture of Tracheal Aspirate (semiquantitative: 0, 1, 2, or 3+)

Pathogenic bacteria cultured ≤1+ or no growth = 0 points

Pathogenic bacteria cultured >1+ = 1 point

Pathogenic bacteria seen on Gram stain >1+ = +1 point

Total score >6 is consistent with ventilator-associated pneumonia. (From Pugin J, Auckentholer R, Mili N, et al. Diagnosis of ventilator-associated pneumonia by bacteriologic analysis of bronchoscopic and nonbronchoscopic blind bronchoalveolar lavage fluid. Am Rev Respir Dis 138:117–120, 1998.)

that mortality in VAP is higher when empiric coverage is subsequently found to be "inappropriate" for the organisms causing the pneumonia.[151] Switching to appropriate antibiotics later may not lessen the rate of increased mortality.[147] The main reason for inadequate therapy is the presence of pathogens that are resistant to multiple drugs. Therefore, when selecting an appropriate empiric antibiotic regimen for a patient with nosocomial pneumonia, clinicians must be familiar with local hospital resistance patterns and must determine the patient's risk for resistant organisms. Risk factors for pathogens resistant to multiple drugs as a cause of nosocomial pneumonia appear in Table 75.8.

The treatment of nosocomial pneumonia has changed considerably during the past decade. New treatment paradigms have been used at many institutions in an effort to

TABLE 75.8	Risk Factors for Multidrug-Resistant Pathogens Causing Hospital-Acquired Pneumonia, Healthcare-Associated Pneumonia, and Ventilator-Associated Pneumonia

- Antimicrobial therapy in preceding 90 days
- Current hospitalization of 5 days or more
- High frequency of antibiotic resistance in the community or in the specific hospital unit
- Presence of risk factors for healthcare-associated pneumonia
    - Hospitalization for 2 days or more in the preceding 90 days
    - Residence in a nursing home or extended care facility
    - Home infusion therapy (including antibiotics)
    - Chronic dialysis within 30 days
    - Home wound care
    - Family member with multidrug-resistant pathogen
- Immunosuppressive disease and/or therapy

(From Niederman MS, Craven DE, Bonten MJ, et al. American Thoracic Society, Infectious Diseases Society of America. Guidelines for the management of adults with hospital-acquired, ventilator-associated, and healthcare-associated pneumonia. Am J Respir Crit Care Med 171:388–416, 2005.)

maximize positive outcomes without increasing resistance or superinfection. To avoid the use of inappropriate empiric antibiotic regimens in patients with nosocomial pneumonia, one approach is to prescribe early broad-spectrum antibiotic agents, with a commitment to narrow the spectrum of coverage on the basis of serial clinical and quantitative microbiologic data.[151] This approach has been called "de-escalation." Selection of initial empiric broad-spectrum therapy should be based on local resistance patterns. The de-escalation approach has not been well studied through large prospective trials. Another component is to use shorter courses of antibiotics. The traditional duration of therapy for nosocomial pneumonia has been 10 to 21 days, despite the lack of studies determining appropriate length of therapy.[5] There are many indications that 10 to 21 days may be excessive in many situations.

A key determinant in the development of resistance and superinfection appears to be prolonged antibiotic therapy.[152–154] In the setting of VAP, colonization with resistant organisms does not typically occur until the second week of antibiotic therapy.[155] Clinical responses to therapy are typically apparent within the first 6 days of therapy. In addition, appropriate antibiotic therapy appears to rapidly eradicate endotracheal colonization by S. pneumoniae, H. influenzae, and S. aureus. Interestingly, colonization with gram-negative Enterobacteriaceae and P. aeruginosa may persist longer, despite clinical response.[155]

Short-course therapy has been evaluated in a number of studies. A prospective, randomized trial was conducted in

French ICUs comparing 8 days of therapy to the more traditional 15 days of therapy for VAP.[153] The diagnosis of VAP was confirmed by quantitative BAL or protected sputum brush culture. Clinical outcomes were equivalent between the groups, except that a higher rate of recurrence from nonfermentive gram-negative bacteria (e.g., P. aeruginosa, Acinetobacter species) was reported in the 8-day group.

In a small study at a single veterans' hospital a modified version of the CPIS was incorporated into a treatment protocol to assist in identifying patients with a low probability of difficult-to-treat VAP.[156] The researchers compared 10 to 21 days of standard therapy against ciprofloxacin for 3 days (in patients with a CPIS score of 6 or less) with a repeat CPIS-guided decision to continue dosing protocol. The investigators reported that in patients with CPIS scores of 6 or less, antibiotics could be discontinued after 3 days of therapy safely, without adversely affecting length of stay or mortality. These results suggest that patients with low CPIS scores are either capable of rapid clinical response or may not have VAP to begin with.

KEY PATHOGENS

Although initial therapy regimens for nosocomial pneumonia are usually empiric, sometimes definitive pathogen-directed therapy is needed for a specific organism as microbiology data become available. In either situation, special consideration needs to be given to antibiotic resistance and local resistance patterns. Four key nosocomial pneumonia pathogens or types of pathogens with potential for multiple-drug resistance need special attention.

STAPHYLOCOCCUS AUREUS

S aureus is a virulent gram-positive coccus that appears in clusters on Gram stain. It is reported to cause about 20% to 40% of cases of nosocomial pneumonia.[157] According to recent estimates in the United States, more than 50% of S. aureus in the ICU setting are MRSA.[158] This resistant type of S. aureus expresses a mecA gene-encoded altered penicillin-binding protein that has reduced affinity for all available β-lactam antibiotics.[159] MRSA usually carries resistant traits against many non-β-lactam antibiotics as well. As a result, vancomycin has been the drug of choice against MRSA for most serious infections. Unfortunately, vancomycin has not produced high cure rates in pneumonia even though it is bactericidal against essentially all clinical isolates when tested in vitro.[160] It has been speculated that failures may be a result of poor lung penetration of vancomycin with standard dosing regimens (targeting serum trough concentrations of 5 to 10 μg/mL).[5,161] New guidelines have recommend targeting trough concentrations of 15 to 20 μg per mL, despite a lack of sound evidence-based support.[5] The streptogramin combination quinupristin–dalfopristin was studied for MRSA nosocomial pneumonia but unfortunately displayed worse outcomes than vancomycin.[160]

Linezolid, a novel oxazolidinone with good epithelial lining fluid penetration, was compared with vancomycin in two prospective trials of nosocomial pneumonia.[162,163] Overall, linezolid and vancomycin were equally effective in treating nosocomial pneumonia with respect to clinical and microbiologic outcomes. Linezolid and vancomycin displayed similar rates of adverse drug events. When the two studies were combined and analyzed retrospectively, Kaplan-Meier survival analysis was significantly better for linezolid in patients believed to have MRSA pneumonia or MRSA VAP.[164,165] Bacterial eradication rates were significantly better in the intent-to-treat analysis of the MRSA VAP patient subset. Logistic regression also showed that linezolid was independent predictor of ''cure'' for all VAP subsets. The studies had many confounding variables to consider. No difference in mortality could be found in the VAP subset diagnosed with quantitative invasive techniques. The vancomycin group had about twice as many patients with cardiac disease, diabetes, and renal disease in the MRSA subset. In addition, vancomycin dosing was probably subtherapeutic for MRSA pneumonia. Nonetheless, the two drugs appear to be comparable for most patients with nosocomial pneumonia or VAP. Better studies are needed to elucidate whether linezolid is superior to vancomycin for patients with MRSA pneumonia.

PSEUDOMONAS AERUGINOSA

P. aeruginosa is a nonfermenting aerobic gram-negative bacilli that is a common cause of nosocomial pneumonia.[18,166] The organism thrives in moist environments and can live in slime-enclosed biofilms. Patients may be colonized with *P aeruginosa* without being infected, making a causative link difficult. Given the virulence and high mortality rate associated with the organism and its potential for developing resistance to multiple antibiotics via multiple mechanisms (i.e., reduced access to site of drug action, lack of porin channels, drug efflux pumps, β-lactamase production), many have advocated treating *P. aeruginosa* pneumonia with combination therapy.[36,166,167] Unfortunately there has never been a well-designed prospective trial comparing combination therapy versus monotherapy in patients with *P aeruginosa* pneumonia.[166]

When combination therapy is used clinically, an aminoglycoside or an antipseudomonal fluoroquinolone is usually added to an antipseudomonal β-lactam. Combination antipseudomonal therapy may be advisable for initial empiric regimens in patients at risk for *P aeruginosa* infection to better ensure ''appropriate'' coverage until sensitivities are known.[5,36] Patients responding to aminoglycoside combinations can drop the aminoglycoside after a few days to avoid added toxicity.

ENTEROBACTERIACEAE (*KLEBSIELLA, ENTEROBACTER, PROTEUS, AND SERRATIA* SPECIES)

These members of the family Enterobacteriaceae are among the most common causes of nosocomial pneumonia.[18] Although *K. pneumoniae* resists penicillins such as ampicillin, it has traditionally been susceptible to cephalosporins, extended-spectrum penicillins, carbapenems, β-lactamase-inhibitor combination products, fluoroquinolones, and aminoglycosides. *Proteus* species tend to display similar baseline susceptibility patterns. *Enterobacter* and *Serratia* species tend to express higher levels of baseline resistance to antibiotics. Treatment options for these organisms often include extended-spectrum penicillins, third- or fourth-generation cephalosporins, carbapenems, fluoroquinolones, and aminoglycosides.[5] Enterobacteriaceae can express a number of different resistance mechanisms, including β-lactamases, extended-spectrum β-lactamases, and *ampC* β-lactamases.[168,169] Extended-spectrum β-lactamases and *ampC* β-lactamases inactivate third-generation cephalosporins. These same organisms seldom maintain susceptibility to extended-spectrum penicillins or β-lactamase-inhibitor combination products. *Enterobacter* and *Serratia* species in particular can express a chromosomal *ampC* β-lactamase that is inducible. Carbapenems usually maintain activity against most multiple-drug-resistant strains of these organisms.[169] The fourth-generation cephalosporin cefepime may maintain activity against *ampC*-producing organisms, particularly *Enterobacter* species.[168] Enterobacteriaceae have displayed variable levels of resistance to fluoroquinolones and aminoglycosides.[169]

ACINETOBACTER SPECIES AND STENOTROPHOMONAS MALTOPHILIA

These multiple-drug-resistant nonfermentive gram-negative bacilli are less common causes of VAP. They typically express native resistance to most antibiotics. Treatment options for *Acinetobacter* species are often limited to carbapenems, ampicillin–sulbactam, and colistin or polymyxin B.[5,170] Most clinical *S. maltophilia* isolates are believed to represent colonization rather than infection. However, significant infections develop in immunocompromised and severely debilitated patients.[171] This organism produces a metallo-β-lactamase that causes resistance to even carbapenems. Agents of choice for *S. maltophilia* are sulfamethoxazole–trimethoprim, ticarcillin–clavulanate, or a fluoroquinolone. Currently, there are no data to support combination therapy over monotherapy for pneumonia caused by these organisms.[5,170,171]

TREATMENT

Treatment of nosocomial pneumonia varies widely from hospital to hospital. Treatment protocols depend on clinical and microbiologic diagnostic factors. Figures 75.8 and 75.9 highlight a modern approach to managing patients with nosocomial pneumonia.[5] Empiric antibiotic therapies are largely based on time of onset of pneumonia and risks for resistant bacteria.[5] Patients with early-onset HAP or VAP who are without risk factors for multiple-drug-resistant bacteria

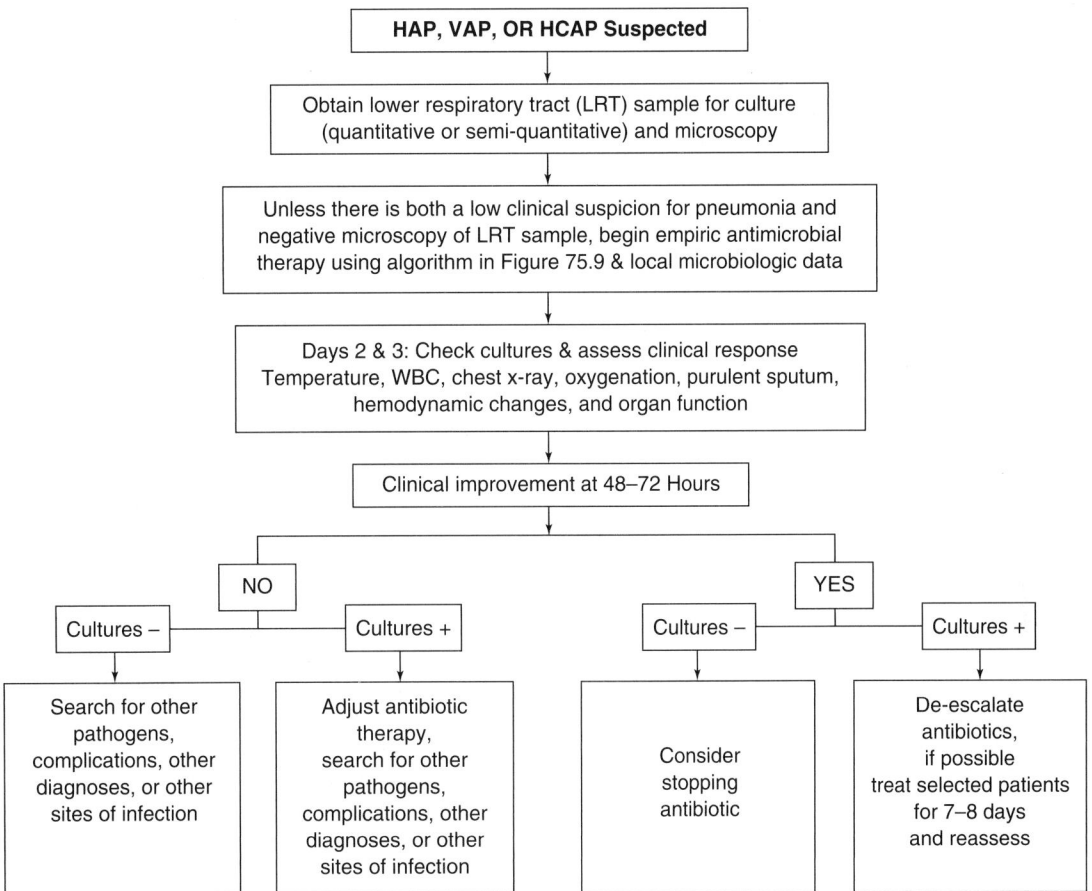

FIGURE 75.8 Management strategies for a patient with nosocomial pneumonia. (From Niederman MS, Craven DE, Bonten MJ, et al. American Thoracic Society, Infectious Diseases Society of America. Guidelines for the management of adults with hospital-acquired, ventilator-associated, and healthcare-associated pneumonia. Am J Respir Crit Care Med 171:388–416, 2005.)

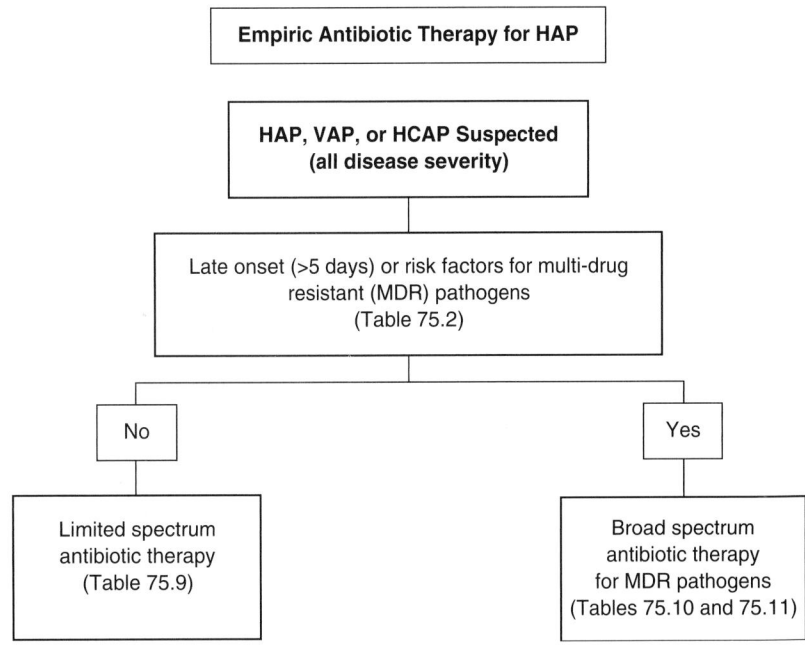

FIGURE 75.9 Algorithm for initiating empiric antibiotic therapy for nosocomial pneumonia. (From Niederman MS, Craven DE, Bonten MJ, et al. American Thoracic Society, Infectious Diseases Society of America. Guidelines for the management of adults with hospital-acquired, ventilator-associated, and healthcare-associated pneumonia. Am J Respir Crit Care Med 171:388–416, 2005.)

should receive therapy targeted at *S. pneumoniae, H. influenzae*, methicillin-susceptible *S. aureus*, and antibiotic-sensitive enteric gram-negative bacilli (i.e., *E. coli, K. pneumoniae, Enterobacter* spp., *Proteus* spp). The ATS/IDSA guidelines recommend using ceftriaxone, levofloxacin, moxifloxacin, ciprofloxacin, ampicillin–sulbactam, or ertapenem in this situation (Table 75.9).

Patients with late-onset nosocomial pneumonia should receive empiric regimens that cover the same core pathogens plus multiple-drug-resistant organisms. Coverage for resistant pathogens should be based on local infection rates and resistance patterns. Key resistant pathogens that cause nosocomial pneumonia include *P. aeruginosa, K. pneumonia* (extended-spectrum β-lactamase producers), *Acinetobacter* species, and potentially MRSA. Prudent empiric regimens for these patients include combinations of an antipseudomonal β-lactam (ceftazidime, cefepime, piperacillin/tazobactam, imipenem, or meropenem) plus an antipseudomonal fluoroquinolone (ciprofloxacin or levofloxacin) or aminoglycoside plus or minus linezolid or vancomycin for MRSA (Tables 75.10 and 75.11). If *L. pneumophila* is suspected, a macrolide or fluoroquinolone should be included in the empiric regimen.

The choice of particular antibiotic agents should also be based on side effects and recent antibiotic use. It is practical

to avoid the same drug or drug class that a patient may have recently received. Empiric regimens can be modified when the results of respiratory or blood cultures are known. Where possible, broad-spectrum empiric regimens should be narrowed or de-escalated. Patients with risk factors for multiple-drug-resistant pathogens, including those fulfilling the HCAP criteria, should be empirically treated for potentially resistant organisms regardless of day of onset. Ideally, empiric antibiotic therapy should be administered within 24 hours of diagnosis of VAP.[145]

Although combination regimens are listed as prudent empiric therapies for patients with possibly resistant nosocomial pneumonia, there are no data that documents superiority over monotherapy for susceptible organisms. The purpose of combination therapy in the empiric regimen is to cover organisms that may be resistant to one of the drugs. The addition of aminoglycosides to β-lactam antibiotics has displayed synergy in in vitro studies. Clinically, the beneficial effects of synergy have been proven only in neutropenic patients, not in pneumonia patients. Aminoglycosides do not penetrate well into respiratory secretions relative to serum.[36] Their usefulness is also limited by their ability to cause nephrotoxicity. A reduced rate of nephrotoxicity and enhanced lung penetration may be realized with the use of high-peak extended-interval dosing, but unfortunately data are lacking to document this. Nephrotoxicity may also be infrequent if aminoglycosides are used for only 5 to 7 days. In contrast to aminoglycosides, fluoroquinolones achieve good concentrations in bronchial secretions, have a broad-spectrum of activity, and rarely cause nephrotoxicity.

Clinical efficacy rates between fluoroquinolones and β-lactams appear to be comparable.[172] Unfortunately, fluoroquinolones have not displayed synergy with β-lactams or aminoglycosides in animal models of pneumonia.[36] The clinical utility of fluoroquinolones for nosocomial pneumonia is becoming limited by increasing rates of resistance.[167] At some institutions, the susceptibility of *P. aeruginosa* to ciprofloxacin is <50%. These trends are due in large part to increased fluoroquinolone use.[132,154]

The traditional length of therapy for patients with nosocomial pneumonia has been 10 to 21 days. The latest guidelines recommend shorter courses of antibiotic therapy (about 7 days) for patients with HAP or VAP who are responding clinically and who are not likely to be infected by *P. aeruginosa, L. pneumophila*, or *Acinetobacter* species.[5] Treatment of these agents may require 14 days of therapy. Stopping therapy after a critical evaluation at 3 days in patients with low suspicion of VAP may be appropriate.[5,156]

TABLE 75.9	Initial Empiric Antibiotic Therapy for Hospital-Acquired or Ventilator-Associated Pneumonia in Patients With No Known Risk Factors for Multidrug-Resistant Pathogens, Early Onset, and Any Disease Severity

Potential Pathogen	Recommended Antibiotic[a]
Streptococcus pneumoniae[b]	Ceftriaxone
Haemophilus influenzae	or
Methicillin-sensitive *Staphylococcus aureus*	Levofloxacin, moxifloxacin, or ciprofloxacin
Antibiotic-sensitive enteric gram-negative bacilli	or
Escherichia coli	Ampicillin/sulbactam
Klebsiella pneumoniae	or
Enterobacter spp	Ertapenem
Proteus spp	
Serratia marcescens	

[a] See Table 75.11 for proper initial doses.
[b] The frequency of penicillin-resistant *S. pneumoniae* and multidrug-resistant *S. pneumoniae* is increasing; levofloxacin or moxifloxacin is preferred to ciprofloxacin and the role of other new quinolones, such as gatifloxacin, has not been established.
(From Niederman MS, Craven DE, Bonten MJ, et al. American Thoracic Society, Infectious Diseases Society of America. Guidelines for the management of adults with hospital-acquired, ventilator-associated, and healthcare-associated pneumonia. Am J Respir Crit Care Med 171:388–416, 2005.)

NURSING HOME-ACQUIRED PNEUMONIA

NHAP is best discussed as an entity distinct from other types of pneumonia, even though many patients with NHAP may now fit under the diagnostic criteria of HCAP.[5]

TABLE 75.10	Initial Empiric Therapy or Hospital-Acquired, Ventilator-Associated, or Healthcare-Associated Pneumonia in Patients With Late-Onset Disease or Risk Factors for Multidrug-Resistant Pathogens and All Disease Severity
Potential Pathogens	**Combination Antibiotic Therapy**[a]
Pathogens listed in Table 75.3 and multidrug-resistant pathogens	Antipseudomonal cephalosporin (cefepime, ceftazidime)
Pseudomonas aeruginosa	or
Klebsiella pneumoniae (extended-spectrum β-lactamase-positive)[b]	Antipseudomonal carbapenem (imipenem or meropenem)
	or
Acinetobacter species	β-lactam/β-lactamase inhibitor (piperacillin-tazobactam)
	plus
	Antipseudomonal fluoroquinolone[b] (ciprofloxacin or levofloxacin)
	or
	Aminoglycoside (amikacin, gentamicin, or tobramycin)
	plus
Methicillin-resistant *Staphylococcus aureus*	Linezolid or vancomycin[c]
Legionella pneumophila[b]	

[a] See Table 75.5 for adequate initial dosing of antibiotics. Initial antibiotic therapy should be adjusted or streamlined on the basis of microbiologic data and clinical response to therapy.

[b] If an extended-spectrum β-lactamase-positive strain, such as *K. pneumoniae*, or an *Acinetobacter* species is suspected, a carbapenem is a reliable choice. If *L. pneumophila* is suspected, the combination antibiotic regimen should include a macrolide (e.g., azithromycin) or a fluoroquinolone (e.g., ciprofloxacin or levofloxacin) should be used rather than an aminoglycoside.

[c] If risk factors for methicillin-resistant *S aureus* are present or there is a high incidence locally.

(From Niederman MS, Craven DE, Bonten MJ, et al. American Thoracic Society, Infectious Diseases Society of America. Guidelines for the management of adults with hospital-acquired, ventilator-associated, and healthcare-associated pneumonia. Am J Respir Crit Care Med 171:388–416, 2005.)

Therapeutic decision making for NHAP is hindered by a lack of quality information about causative pathogens and a lack of well-designed treatment studies in this population. This is unfortunate, as mortality rates are higher in this population than in age-matched community-dwelling patients.[173] Nursing home residents with pneumonia may present differently than age-matched community-dwelling patients. In one small study, nursing home residents had lower rates of chills, pleuritic chest pain, headache, anorexia, myalgias, and productive cough compared to patients from the community.[62] In addition, many nursing home residents have dementia, which may mask certain symptoms of pneumonia and has been identified as a risk factor for aspiration.[174] A milder presentation and the presence of dementia may make it difficult to diagnose pneumonia in a timely manner. As a result, there is often a delay in starting therapy. Interestingly, mortality rates in NHAP appear to correlate with the degree of dementia.[175]

ETIOLOGY

The etiology of NHAP has been the subject of great debate. The value of sputum examination is limited in this population, as greater than 50% of elderly nursing home residents cannot produce sputum specimens adequate for analysis.[176]

The organisms most often reported to cause NHAP are *S. pneumoniae*, *H. influenzae*, *S. aureus*, and enteric gram-negative bacilli.[32,177] Nursing home patients are frequently colonized with enteric gram-negative bacilli. The rate of oropharyngeal colonization with gram-negative bacilli is higher in the elderly in general, but especially if they live in nursing homes.[27] Interestingly, studies using strict criteria for evaluation of quality sputum specimens isolated gram-negative bacilli only 0% to 12% of the time.[177] Therefore, the need to empirically cover nursing home patients for gram-negative bacilli (other than *H. influenzae*) is not well established. The general need to empirically cover for *S. aureus* has also not been established. Reports of *S. aureus* isolation from patients with NHAP may reflect colonization more than infection in a majority of patients. Asymptomatic carriage of *S. aureus*, including MRSA, is reported to be frequent among nursing home staff and residents.[178]

Antibiotic resistance is a particular concern in NHAP. The pattern of frequent admissions and discharges in this population, combined with frequent antibiotic use, may create a milieu of antibiotic-resistant "nursing home flora." Also, nursing home patients typically receive antibiotics more often than patients in the community.[179] There are many reasons for the increased antibiotic use. Rates of urinary tract infections and skin and soft tissue infections are very high in nursing homes. Also, nursing home patients

TABLE 75.11	Initial Intravenous, Adult Doses of Antibiotics for Empiric Therapy of Hospital-Acquired Pneumonia, Including Ventilator-Associated Pneumonia, and Healthcare-Associated Pneumonia in Patients with Late-Onset Disease or Risk Factors for Multidrug-Resistant Pathogens

Antibiotic	Dosage[a]
Antipseudomonal cephalosporin	
Cefepime	1–2 g q8–12h
Ceftazidime	2 g q8h
Carbapenems	
Imipenem	500 mg q6h or 1 g q8h
Meropenem	1 g q8h
β-Lactam/β-lactamase inhibitor	
Piperacillin–tazobactam	4.5 g q6h
Aminoglycosides	
Gentamicin	7 mg/kg qd[b]
Tobramycin	7 mg/kg qd[b]
Amikacin	20 mg/kg qd[b]
Antipseudomonal quinolones	
Levofloxacin	750 mg qd
Ciprofloxacin	400 mg q8h
Vancomycin	15 mg/kg q12h[c]
Linezolid	600 mg q12h

[a] Dosages are based on normal hepatic function.
[b] Trough levels for gentamicin and tobramycin should be <1 μg/mL; for amikacin they should be <4–5 μg/mL.
[c] Trough levels for vancomycin should be 15–20 μg/mL.
(From Niederman MS, Craven DE, Bonten MJ, et al. American Thoracic Society, Infectious Diseases Society of America. Guidelines for the management of adults with hospital-acquired, ventilator-associated, and healthcare-associated pneumonia. Am J Respir Crit Care Med 171:388–416, 2005.)

may receive unwarranted antibiotics for chronic bronchitis or chemical pneumonitis from aspiration of noninfectious gastric contents. The potential for cross-transmission of resistant microorganisms among residents and employees of nursing homes is great. Outbreaks of pneumonia caused by resistant bacteria have occurred in nursing homes.[180] Cases of MRSA have been reported to spread with relative ease.[181]

The high risk of aspiration in nursing home patients may put them at increased risk for anaerobic lung infections. Contrary to this long-held belief, at least one recent study has questioned the pathogenic role of anaerobes in NHAP.[182] These investigators identified a predominance of gram-negative bacilli isolated from elderly nursing home patients with aspiration pneumonia. Only to a lesser degree did they isolate anaerobic bacteria. These organisms were primarily *Pre-*

votella and *Fusobacterium* species. Although aspiration is common in long-term care facility residents, many develop aspiration pneumonitis rather than aspiration pneumonia.[183] Pneumonitis rarely requires the use of antibiotics.[7] Nursing home patients also experience pneumonia from *Mycobacterium tuberculosis*, adenovirus, influenza, and respiratory syncytial virus more often than individuals in the community.[11] Influenza is responsible for a substantial proportion of the high morbidity and mortality seen in NHAP.[32]

THERAPEUTIC PLAN

The decision to admit an NHAP patient to the hospital may be even more controversial than with CAP patients because it is not clear whether hospitalization improves patient outcomes.[21,184] Of course, the decision to admit a patient is often influenced by the clinical status of the patient, wishes of family members, third-party payers, and the capabilities of the nursing home staff. By avoiding unnecessary hospital admissions, patients may avoid higher healthcare costs, exposure to resistant bacteria, or further impairment of mental or functional status.[21] Since most nursing homes have support staff present 24 hours a day, it makes sense to treat nonseptic, ventilatory, and hemodynamically stable NHAP patients at the nursing home, if policy permits.[21] A number of small studies have shown that most patients with NHAP can be safely treated at nursing home facilities, often with oral antibiotics.[184,185] Given the high mortality rate associated with NHAP, efforts to administer early and appropriate therapy are critical.

TREATMENT

Evidence-based guidelines for the treatment of NHAP have not been developed, probably due to the lack of well-designed, randomized, controlled trials in this patient population. Nonetheless, the ATS and the IDSA guidelines do make certain non-evidence-based recommendations about nursing home patients that take into account comorbid diseases and risks for resistant or special pathogens.[11,12,50] The recent updated version of the IDSA CAP guidelines promotes the use of an antipneumococcal fluoroquinolone alone or amoxicillin–clavulanate plus an advanced macrolide for nursing home patients treated as outpatients.[50] They recommended that clinicians give consideration to an agent with antianaerobic activity such as amoxicillin–clavulanate or clindamycin in the empiric regimen for nursing home patients. The updated IDSA guideline paper recommended similar regimens for the treatment of patients requiring hospitalization regardless of nursing home residence status.[50] The newer joint ATS/IDSA guidelines for the management of nosocomial pneumonia highlight the higher risk for resistant bacteria in patients admitted from nursing homes.[5] According to this document, patients with HCAP at risk for resistant bacteria would be best treated with the same regimens advocated for other types of nosocomial pneumonia (Table 75.10).

ASPIRATION PNEUMONIA AND LUNG ABSCESS

As previously defined, aspiration pneumonia is a pneumonic process that results from abnormal entry of significant volumes (macroaspiration) of oropharyngeal or gastrointestinal contents into the lower respiratory tract. The term ''aspiration pneumonia'' is best applied to aspiration from an oropharyngeal source; the term ''aspiration pneumonitis'' is best applied to pulmonary sequelae that arise from aspiration of sterile gastric contents. This usually noninfectious inflammatory process results from chemical injury by gastric acid or from exposure to particulate material (e.g., food). Patients experiencing noninfectious or chemical pneumonitis may present clinically like those with infectious pneumonia. It is not uncommon for pneumonitis patients to have fever, hypoxemia, bronchospasm, and infiltrates on radiography. Some patients may even experience both types of aspiration syndromes simultaneously. Antimicrobial therapy is not generally advocated for a pneumonitis-type presentation unless the condition fails to respond to at least 48 hours of supportive treatment.[7]

Clinically, aspiration pneumonia can present like any other type of pneumonia. It may appear indolent initially but can progress into a very complicated pneumonia characterized by lung abscesses, empyema, or lung necrosis. Some patients are reported to manifest a productive cough with the production of foul-smelling sputum.[67] Chest radiographs that suggest aspiration pneumonia are characterized by infiltrates in dependent pulmonary segments of the lungs. These would include the superior segments of the lower lobes or posterior segments of the upper lobes in a patient in the recumbent position, or in the lower lobes of patients in the upright position.

There are many risk factors and conditions that can predispose a person to developing aspiration (macroaspiration) pneumonia. Conditions that cause a decrease in the level of consciousness (alcohol or drug abuse, seizure disorders, head trauma, sedation or anesthesia) can compromise cough reflex and glottic closure. Neurologic disorders such as stroke and Parkinson's disease can result in dysphagia.[186] Individuals experiencing gastroesophageal reflex or protracted vomiting are predisposed by virtue of overwhelming normal defense barriers and mechanisms. Instrumentation of the airway (e.g., endotracheal intubation, bronchoscopy) creates a mechanical disruption of the glottic closure and provides easy access to the lung.[7,8] Nasogastric tubes may provide a route from the naso-oropharynx and gastrointestinal tract to the upper airway.[8] Patients with any of these risks or conditions may have greater risk of aspiration when in a recumbent position.

Many clinicians believe that aspiration pneumonia is most commonly associated with anaerobic bacteria.[67] This belief was influenced by a number of studies from the 1970s that identified a preponderance of anaerobic organisms in the transtracheal aspirates and respiratory secretions of patients with aspiration pneumonia. Findings from these early studies are limited by the fact that they did not sample deeper respiratory specimens. Nonetheless, anaerobes represent a significant proportion of oral (primarily from the gingival crevice) and/or gastrointestinal flora. Therefore, they may gain access to the lower airways during aspiration. Periodontal disease in particular has been implicated as a key source of anaerobic pathogens that cause aspiration pneumonia.[7] The most frequently isolated anaerobes in aspiration pneumonia have been gram-positive peptostreptococci and gram-negative *Bacteroides*, *Prevotella*, and *Fusobacterium* species.[67]

The role of anaerobic bacteria in the pathogenesis of aspiration pneumonia continues to be a source of great controversy.[7] A number of recent microbiologic investigations of respiratory samples from patients with aspiration pneumonia have not identified significant proportions of anaerobic organisms.[7,182] Anaerobe identification in many institutional microbiology laboratories remains difficult. The need for proper specimen collection, specific media, and rapid transportation can affect the yield of responsible organisms. One small study using mini-BAL sample collection and specific methods to transport and isolate anaerobes in patients with aspiration pneumonia failed to identify any pathogenic anaerobes.[142] Using similar methods, a study in 95 nursing home residents with aspiration pneumonia reported the isolation of only 11 anaerobes, either alone or with other pathogens.[182] Likewise, similar studies in patients with VAP reported isolation of anaerobes in less than 2% of isolates.[187]

Regardless of the role of anaerobes in aspiration pneumonia, clinicians must not ignore the usual pneumonia-causing pathogens. Gram stains and culture of respiratory specimens in aspiration pneumonia will often suggest a polymicrobial infection. Anaerobes, which tend to have low intrinsic virulence, are often isolated along with more virulent aerobic pathogens. This may reflect either coinfection of two pathogenic agents or coexistence of colonizing anaerobes with a pneumonia-causing aerobic organism. The latter is supported by the fact that many patients with aspiration pneumonia resolve their infection with antibiotic regimens that lack significant antianaerobic activity.[182] Of course, it cannot be ruled out that antibiotics not thought to have significant anaerobic activity may have sufficient activity against anaerobes. Some experts recommend the use of standard pneumonia treatment regimens.[7]

Despite the controversy over anaerobic pathogens, references continue to recommend regimens that include agents with activity against anaerobic pathogens for aspiration pneumonia.[11,50] The ATS guidelines state that if a patient is suspected of having aspiration pneumonia and anaerobes are present in a specimen or if a lung abscess, empyema, or necrotizing pneumonia is present, antianaerobic coverage should be included in the antimicrobial regimen.[11]

Antianaerobic agents may be considered for patients with aspiration pneumonia in which no other pathogen has been isolated. All other pneumonia patients would not generally require antianaerobic agents as part of their antimicrobial regimen. Historically, Penicillin G has been efficacious in certain cases of community-acquired aspiration pneumonia.[8,67] The empiric use of this agent has fallen out of favor because a significant proportion of the gram-negative anaerobes produce β-lactamase.[67] Therefore, more stable antianaerobic agents are now used.[50,186] These include clindamycin, β-lactam/β-lactamase inhibitor combination agents, ertapenem, and metronidazole. High failure rates with metronidazole monotherapy may be attributed to its lack of activity against some common microaerophilic gram-positive anaerobes.[67] Therefore, penicillin G has been combined with metronidazole to cover a wider range of oral anaerobes.[67,86] The newer fluoroquinolone agents, moxifloxacin and gatifloxacin, have in vitro activity against a number of anaerobic organisms and may be useful against true anaerobic aspiration pneumonias.[12] Unfortunately, they have not been well studied clinically for aspiration pneumonia.

The decision to use antianaerobic agents should not be taken lightly. Unbridled use of antianaerobic agents can eliminate commensal organisms in a patient's normal gastrointestinal flora. Opportunists such as *Clostridium difficile* and enterococci, including vancomycin-resistant enterococci, can proliferate under the pressure of antianaerobic agents.[188,189]

Of course, alteration of intestinal flora is not just limited to antianaerobic drugs. In addition to antianaerobic coverage, empiric therapies targeted against *S. pneumoniae* and *H. influenzae* are advised in cases of community-acquired aspiration pneumonia. Additional coverage of *S. aureus* and gram-negative bacilli is advised in hospital-acquired aspiration pneumonia.[5]

Efforts to prevent aspiration in high-risk individuals include placing patients in a semirecumbent position, not allowing a patient to be placed supine until 1 to 2 hours after eating, maximizing oral hygiene, and closely managing feeding tubes.

Lung abscesses are a relatively uncommon complication of pneumonia.[190] Abscesses are usually associated with aspiration pneumonia when they do happen. The clinical presentation of pneumonia with lung abscesses is similar to pulmonary tuberculosis. Many cases have an indolent onset, are characterized by night sweats, weight loss, and tissue necrosis, and have cavitary-type lesions. Despite the controversy in aspiration pneumonia, anaerobic and microaerophilic organisms have been isolated frequently from lung abscesses. The current view of these infections is that they tend to be polymicrobial.[190,191] Lung abscesses often drain spontaneously, which can promote an abundance of purulent sputum. Antibiotics are the cornerstones of therapy for most lung abscesses. Postural drainage and physiotherapy will

often shorten the time to defervescence. Alternatively, bronchoscopy, percutaneous drains, and surgery can be used to promote drainage. Prolonged antibiotic therapy of up to 2 to 4 months is often required to prevent relapses.[24]

Empyema is another complication of aspiration pneumonia. A pleural empyema is defined as a collection of pus in the pleural cavity.[44] Since the development of potent antibiotics, empyema as a complication of pneumonia has become infrequent. Anaerobes are the predominant organism found on thoracentesis in the setting of empyema associated with pneumonia. The collections are often polymicrobial. Other common pathogens isolated in empyema are *S aureus*, gram-negative bacilli, and to a lesser extent streptococci. The treatment of empyemas should be surgical drainage and directed antibiotic therapy.[8]

KEY POINTS

- Pneumonia remains a significant cause of morbidity and mortality despite the availability of broad-spectrum antibiotics
- Diagnosing pneumonia is straightforward in many patients, but identifying the causative microorganism remains difficult
- Sputum Gram staining of ''good-quality'' specimens is an insensitive but specific diagnostic tool that can be useful for directing empiric CAP therapy
- Chest radiographs are important diagnostic tools and are generally obtained for all patients being worked up for pneumonia
- *Streptococcus pneumoniae* should be considered as a potential pathogen in most cases of CAP, even if not identified by routine microbiologic testing
- Regardless of site of care, it is important to initiate antibiotic therapy in a timely fashion, especially in patients with a higher risk of mortality
- Factors to take into consideration when selecting antibiotic therapy for pneumonia should include spectrum of activity, pharmacokinetics, pharmacodynamics, adverse effects, clinical efficacy, route of administration, and cost
- Once the causative organism is reliably identified through microbiologic testing, therapy may be streamlined to a narrow-spectrum and more cost-effective agent
- Many experts believe that a great majority of patients with CAP can be safely treated as outpatients, either with oral medications or home infusion therapy
- Widespread use of fluoroquinolones should be limited in otherwise healthy individuals with CAP so as to preserve their utility
- Not every patient receiving mechanical ventilation with pulmonary infiltrates has pneumonia
- ''Quantitative'' analysis of endotracheal aspirates or BAL or protected sputum brush specimens usually pro-

vides greater specificity for the diagnosis of VAP than ''qualitative'' methods

■ Mortality in VAP is higher when empiric coverage is subsequently found to be ''inappropriate'' for the organisms causing the pneumonia

■ Although combination regimens are listed as prudent empiric therapies for patients with possibly resistant nosocomial pneumonia, there are no data that documents superiority over monotherapy for susceptible organisms

■ Selection of antibiotic resistance pathogens or superinfections may be reduced by limiting courses of antibiotics to 1 week or less for VAP in select patients

■ The pattern of frequent admissions and discharges among nursing home patients, combined with frequent antibiotic use, may create a milieu of antibiotic resistance in this population

■ Although aspiration is common in long-term care facility residents, many develop aspiration pneumonitis rather than aspiration pneumonia. Pneumonitis rarely requires the use of antibiotics

■ The pathogenic role of anaerobic organisms in aspiration pneumonia may not be as important as more traditional respiratory pathogens

SUGGESTED READINGS

Bartlett JG, Dowell SF, Mandell LA, et al. Practice guidelines for the management of community-acquired pneumonia in adults. Infectious Diseases Society of America. Clin Infect Dis 31:347–382, 2000.

Mandell LA, Bartlett JG, Dowell SF, et al. Update of practice guidelines for the management of community-acquired pneumonia in immunocompetent adults. Clin Infect Dis 37:1405–1433, 2003.

Mylotte JM. Nursing home-acquired pneumonia. Clin Infect Dis 35: 1205–1211, 2002.

Niederman MS, Craven DE, Bonten MJ, et al. American Thoracic Society, Infectious Diseases Society of America. Guidelines for the management of adults with hospital-acquired, ventilator-associated, and healthcare-associated pneumonia. Am J Respir Crit Care Med 171: 388–416, 2005.

Niederman MS, Mandell LA, Anzueto A, et al. Guidelines for the management of adults with community-acquired pneumonia. Diagnosis, assessment of severity, antimicrobial therapy, and prevention. Am J Respir Crit Care Med 163:1730–1754, 2001.

REFERENCES

1. Murray J. The captain of the men of death. In: Marrie TJ, ed. Community-acquired pneumonia. New York: Kluwer Academic Publishers, 2001:1–12.
2. Osler W. The principles and practice of medicine. New York: D. Appleton and Co., 1892.
3. Ferrara AM, Fietta AM. New developments in antibacterial choice for lower respiratory tract infections in elderly patients. Drugs Aging 21:167–186, 2004.
4. File TM. Community-acquired pneumonia. Lancet 362:1991–2001, 2003.
5. Niederman MS, Craven DE, Bonten MJ, et al. American Thoracic Society, Infectious Diseases Society of America. Guidelines for the management of adults with hospital-acquired, ventilator-associated, and healthcare-associated pneumonia. Am J Respir Crit Care Med 171:388–416, 2005.
6. Craven DE, Palladino R, McQuillen DP. Healthcare-associated pneumonia in adults: management principles to improve outcomes. Infect Dis Clin North Am 18:939–962, 2004.
7. Marik PE. Aspiration pneumonitis and aspiration pneumonia. N Engl J Med 344:665–671, 2001.
8. Bartlett JG. Management of respiratory tract infections, 2nd ed. Philadelphia: Lippincott Williams & Wilkins, 1999.
9. Stedman TL, ed. Stedman's pathology and laboratory medicine words, 4th ed. Philadelphia: Lippincott Williams & Wilkins, 2005.
10. Molina C, Walker DH. The pathology of community-acquired pneumonia. In: Marrie TJ, ed. Community-acquired pneumonia. New York: Kluwer Academic Publishers, 2001:101–129.
11. Niederman MS, Mandell LA, Anzueto A, et al. Guidelines for the management of adults with community-acquired pneumonia. Diagnosis, assessment of severity, antimicrobial therapy, and prevention. Am J Respir Crit Care Med 163:1730–1754, 2001.
12. Bartlett JG, Dowell SF, Mandell LA, et al. Practice guidelines for the management of community-acquired pneumonia in adults. Infectious Diseases Society of America. Clin Infect Dis 31:347–382, 2000.
13. Marrie TJ. Community-acquired pneumonia. Clin Infct Dis 18: 501–513, 1994.
14. Garibaldi RA. Epidemiology of community-acquired respiratory tract infections in adults. Incidence, etiology, and impact. Am J Med 78 (Suppl 6B):32–37, 1985.
15. Gilbert K, Fine MJ. Assessing prognosis and predicting patient outcomes in community-acquired pneumonia. Semin Respir Infect 9: 140–152, 1994.
16. Koivula I, Sten M, Makela PH. Risk factors for pneumonia in elderly. Am J Med 96:313–320, 1994.
17. Fine MJ, Smith MA, Carson CA, et al. Prognosis and outcomes of patients with community-acquired pneumonia. A meta-analysis. JAMA 275:134–141, 1996.
18. Craven DE, Steger KA, Fleming CA. Hospital-acquired pneumonia. In: Wachter RM, Goldman L, Hollander H, eds. Hospital medicine. Philadephia: Lippincott Williams & Wilkins, 2000:491–498.
19. Alcon A, Fabregas N, Torres A. Hospital-acquired pneumonia: etiologic considerations. Infect Dis Clinic North Am 17:679–695, 2003.
20. Chastre J, Fagon JY. Ventilator-associated pneumonia. Am J Respir Crit Care Med 165:867–903, 2002.
21. Muder RR. Management of nursing home-acquired pneumonia: unresolved issues and priorities for future investigation. J Am Geriatr Soc 48:95–96, 2000.
22. Mylotte JM. Nursing home-acquired pneumonia. Clin Infect Dis 35:1205–1211, 2002.
23. Niederman MS, McComb JS, Unger AN, et al. The cost of treating community-acquired pneumonia. Clin Ther 20:820–837, 1998.
24. Donowitz GR, Mandell GL. Acute pneumonia. In: Mandell GL, Bennett JE, Dolin R, eds. Mandell, Douglas, and Bennett's principles and practice of infectious diseases, 6th ed. Philadelphia: Elsevier, 2005:819–845.
25. Reynolds HY. Host defense impairments that may lead to respiratory infections. Clin Chest Med 8:339–358, 1987.
26. Reynolds HY. Normal and defective respiratory host defenses. In: Pennington JE, ed. Respiratory infections: diagnosis and management, 3rd ed. New York: Raven Press, Ltd., 1994:1–34.
27. Patrick W. Pathophysiology of pneumonia and the clinical consequences. In: Marrie TJ, ed. Community-acquired pneumonia. New York: Kluwer Academic Publishers, 2001:179–192.
28. Mason CM, Nelson S Pulmonary host defenses: implications for therapy. Clin Chest Med 20:475–488, 1999.
29. Woods DE. Bacterial colonization of the respiratoy tract: clinical significance. In: Pennington JE, ed. Respiratory infections: diagnosis and management, 3rd ed. New York: Raven Press, Ltd., 1994: 1–34.
30. Thompson R. Prevention of nosocomial pneumonia. Med Clin North Am 78:1185–1198, 1994.
31. Rubin E, Farber JL. The respiratory system. In: Rubin E, Farber JL, eds. Pathology, 3rd ed. Hagerstown, MD: Lippincott-Raven, 1999:591–666.
32. Simor AE. Nursing home acquired pneumonia. In: Marrie TJ, ed. Community-acquired pneumonia. New York: Kluwer Academic Publishers, 2001:143–162.

33. Busse WW. Pathogenesis and sequelae of respiratory infections. Rev Infect Dis 13 (Suppl 6):S477–485, 1991.
34. al-Ujayli B, Nafziger DA, Saravolatz L. Pneumonia due to *Staphylococcus aureus* infection. Clin Chest Med 16:111–120, 1995.
35. Jonas M, Cunha BA. Bacteremic *Escherichia coli* pneumonia. Arch Intern Med 142:2157–2159, 1982.
36. Rello J, Paiva JA, Baraibar J, et al. International Conference for the Development of Consensus on the Diagnosis and Treatment of Ventilator-Associated Pneumonia. Chest 120:955–970, 2001.
37. Mason CM, Nelson S Pulmonary host defenses. Implications for therapy. Clin Chest Med 20:475–488, 1999.
38. Rumbak MJ. The pathogenesis of ventilator-associated pneumonia. Sem Resp Crit Care Med 23:427–434, 2002.
39. Feldman C, Kassel M, Cantrell J, et al. The presence and sequence of endotracheal tube colonization in patients undergoing mechanical ventilation. Eur Respir J 13:546–551, 1999.
40. Tablan OC, Anderson LJ, Besser R, et al. Guidelines for preventing health-care–associated pneumonia, 2003: recommendations of CDC and the Healthcare Infection Control Practices Advisory Committee. MMWR Recomm Rep 53(RR–3):1–36, 2004.
41. Butts JD. Intracellular concentrations of antibacterial agents and related clinical implications. Clin Pharmacokinet 27:63–84, 1994.
42. Brandenburg JA, Marrie TJ, Coley CM, et al. Clinical presentation, processes and outcomes of care for patients with pneumococcal pneumonia. J Gen Intern Med 15:638–646, 2000.
43. Fine MJ, Smith MA, Carson CA, et al. Prognosis and outcomes of patients with community-acquired pneumonia: a meta analysis. JAMA 275:134–141, 1996.
44. Bryant RE, Salmon CJ. Pleural empyema. Clin Infect Dis 22:747–764, 1996.
45. Fine MJ, Hough LJ, Medsger AR, et al. The hospital admission decision for patients with community-acquired pneumonia. Results from the Pneumonia Patient Outcomes Research Team cohort study. Arch Intern Med 157:36–44, 1997.
46. Lieberman D, Lieberman D. Community-acquired pneumonia in the elderly. Drugs Aging 17:93–105, 2000.
47. Mehta RM, Niederman MS Nosocomial pneumonia in the intensive care unit: controversies and dilemmas. J Intensive Care Med 18:175–188, 2003.
48. Bonten MJM, Kollef MH, Hall JB. Risk factors for ventilator-associated pneumonia: from epidemiology to patient management. Clin Infect Dis 38:1141–1149, 2004.
49. Pingleton SK, Hinthorn DR, Liu C, et al. Enteral nutrition in patients receiving mechanical ventilation. Multiple sources of tracheal colonization include the stomach. Am J Med 80:827–832, 1986.
50. Mandell LA, Bartlett, JG, Dowell SF, et al. Update of practice guidelines for the management of community-acquired pneumonia in immunocompetent adults.Clin Infect Dis 37:1405–1433, 2003.
51. Bridges CB, Harper SA, Fukuda K, et al. Prevention and control of influenza: recommendations of the Advisory Committee on Immunization Practices (ACIP). MMWR 52 (RR–8):1–34, 2003.
52. Conaty S, Watson L, Dinnes J, et al. The effectiveness of pneumococcal polysaccharide vaccines in adults: a systematic review of observational studies and comparison with results from randomised controlled trials. Vaccine 22:3214–3224, 2004.
53. Ortqvist A, Hedlund J, Burman LA, et al. Randomised trial of 23-valent pneumococcal capsular polysaccharide vaccine in prevention of pneumonia in middle-aged and elderly people. Swedish Pneumococcal Vaccination Study Group. Lancet 351:399–403, 1998.
54. Kollef MH. Prevention of hospital-associated pneumonia and ventilator-associated pneumonia. Crit Care Med 32:1396–1405, 2004.
55. Kollef MH. The prevention of ventilator-associated pneumonia. N Engl J Med 340:627–634, 1999.
56. Dodek P, Keenan S, Cook D, et al. Evidence-based clinical practice guideline for prevention of ventilator-associated pneumonia. Ann Intern Med 141:305–313, 2004.
57. Cook DJ, Reeve BK, Guyatt GH, et al. Stress ulcer prophylaxis in critically ill patients. Resolving discordant meta-analyses. JAMA 275:308–314, 1996.
58. Heyland DK, Cook DJ, Schoenfeld PS, et al. The effect of acidified enteral feeds on gastric colonization in critically ill patients: results of a multicenter randomized trial. Crit Care Med 27:2399–2406, 1999.
59. DeRiso AJ, Ladowski JS, Dillon TA, et al. Chlorhexidine gluconate 0.12% oral rinse reduces the incidence of total nosocomial respiratory infection and nonprophylactic systemic antibiotic use in patients undergoing heart surgery. Chest 109:1556–1561, 1996.
60. Bonten MJ. Strategies for prevention of hospital-acquired pneumonia: oral and selective decontamination of the gastrointestinal tract. Semin Respir Crit Care Med 23:481–488, 2002.
61. Marrie TJ, Haldane EV, Faulkner RS, et al. Community-acquired pneumonia requiring hospitalization: is it different in the elderly? J Am Geriatr Soc 33:671–680, 1985.
62. Marrie TJ. Community-acquired pneumonia in the elderly. Clin Infect Dis 31:1066–1078, 2000.
63. Mabie M, Wunderink RG. Use and limitations of clinical and radiologic diagnosis of pneumonia. Semin Resp Infect 18:72–79, 2003.
64. Bickley LS, Szilagyi PG, eds. Bates' guide to physical examination and history taking, 8th ed. Philadelphia: Lippincott Williams & Wilkins, 2003.
65. Ruiz M, Arosio C, Salman P, et al. Diagnosis of pneumonia and monitoring of infection eradication. Drugs 60:1289–1302, 2000.
66. Levy M, Dromer F, Brion N, et al. Community-acquired pneumonia. Importance of initial noninvasive bacteriologic and radiographic investigations. Chest 93:43–48, 1988.
67. Bartlett JG. Anaerobic bacterial infections of the lung and pleural space. Clin Infect Dis 16 (Suppl 4):S248–255, 1993.
68. Fein AM, Niederman MS Severe pneumonia in the elderly. Clin Geriatr Med 10:121–143, 1994.
69. Trotman-Dickenson B. Radiology in the intensive care unit (part 1). J Intensive Care Med 18:198–210, 2003.
70. Wheeler Jh, Fishman EK. Computed tomography in the management of chest infections. Clin Infect Dis 23:232–240, 1996.
71. Smith PR. What diagnostic tests are needed for community-acquired pneumonia? Med Clin North Am 85:1381–1396, 2001.
72. Skerrett SJ. Diagnostic testing for community-acquired pneumonia. Clin Chest Med 20:531–548, 1999.
73. Gleckman R, DeVita J, Hibert D, et al. Sputum Gram stain assessment in community-acquired bacteremic pneumonia. J Clin Microbiol 26:846–849, 1988.
74. Davidson RJ, MacDonald KS Laboratory diagnosis of community-acquired pneumonia. In: Marrie TJ, ed. Community-acquired pneumonia. New York: Kluwer Academic Publishers, 2001:35–43.
75. Barrett-Connor E. The nonvalue of sputum culture in the diagnosis of pneumococcal pneumonia. Am Rev Respir Dis 103:845–848, 1971.
76. Williams SG, Kauffman CA. Survival of *Streptococcus pneumoniae* in sputum from patients with pneumonia. J Clin Microb 7:3–5, 1978.
77. Musher DM, Montoya R, Wanahita A. Diagnostic value of microscopic examination of Gram-stained sputum and sputum cultures in patients with bacteremic pneumococcal pneumonia. Clin Infect Dis 39:165–169, 2004.
78. Plouffe JF, McNally C, File TM. Value of noninvasive studies in community-acquired pneumonia. Infect Dis Clin North Am 12:689–699, 1998.
79. Bartlett JG. Decline in microbial studies for patients with pulmonary infections. Clin Infect Dis 39:170–172, 2004.
80. Bryan CS Blood cultures for community-acquired pneumonia: no place to skimp. Chest 116:1153–1155, 1999.
81. Ewig S, Schlochtermeier M, Goke N, et al. Applying sputum as a diagnostic tool in pneumonia. Chest 121:1486–1492, 2002.
82. Glerant JC, Hellmuth D, Schmit JL, et al. Utility of blood cultures in community-acquired pneumonia requiring hospitalization: influence of antibiotic treatment before admission. Respir Med 93:208–212, 1999.
83. Torres A, El-Ebiary M. Invasive diagnostic techniques for pneumonia: protected specimen brush, bronchoalveolar lavage, and lung biopsy methods. Infect Dis Clin North Am 12:701–722, 1998.
84. Grossman RF, Fein A. Evidence-based assessment of diagnostic tests for ventilator-associated pneumonia: executive summary. Chest 117 (Suppl):177S–181S, 2000.
85. Johanson WG, Seidenfeld JJ, Gomez P, et al. Bacteriologic diagnosis of nosocomial pneumonia following prolonged mechanical ventilation. Am Rev Respir Dis 137:259–264, 1988.
86. Fagon JY, Chastre J, Wolff M, et al. Invasive and noninvasive strategies for management of suspected ventilator-associated pneumonia. Ann Intern Med 132:621–630, 2000.

87. Souweine B, Veber B, Bedos JP, et al. Diagnostic accuracy of protected specimen brush and bronchoalveolar lavage in nosocomial pneumonia: impact of previous antimicrobial treatments. Crit Care Med 26:236–244, 1998.

88. Lieberman D. Atypical pathogens in community-acquired pneumonia. Clin Chest Med 20:489–497, 1999.

89. Bartlett JG, Mundy LM. Community-acquired pneumonia. N Engl J Med 333:1618–1623, 1995.

90. Friedland IR, McCracken GH. Streptococcus pneumoniae. In: Yu VL, ed. Antimicrobial therapy and vaccines. Baltimore: Williams & Wilkins, 1999:433–443.

91. Campbell GD, Silberman R. Drug-resistant *Streptococcus pneumoniae*. Clin Infect Dis 26:1188–1195, 1998.

92. Jacobs MR. *Streptococcus pneumoniae*: epidemiology and patterns of resistance. Am J Med 117:3S–15S, 2004.

93. American Society of Health-System Pharmacists. ASHP therapeutic position statement on strategies for identifying and preventing pneumococcal resistance. Am J Health-Syst Pharm 61:2430–2435, 2004.

94. Karchmer AW. Increased antibiotic resistance in respiratory tract pathogens: PROTEKT US: An update. Clin Infect Dis 39 (Suppl 3):S142–150, 2004.

95. Heffelfinger JD, Dowell SF, Jorgensen JH, et al. Management of community-acquired pneumonia in the era of pneumococcal resistance: a report from the Drug-Resistant *Streptococcus pneumoniae* Therapeutic Working Group. Arch Intern Med 160:1399–1408, 2000.

96. Yu VL, Chiou CC, Feldman C, et al. An international prospective study of pneumococcal bacteremia: correlation with in vitro resistance, antibiotics administered, and clinical outcome. Clin Infect Dis 37:230–237, 2003.

97. Feikin DR, Schuchat A, Kolczak M, et al. Mortality from invasive pneumococcal pneumonia in the era of antibiotic resistance, 1995–1997. Am J Public Health 90:223–229, 2000.

98. Daily P, Farley M, Jorgensen JH, et al. Effect of new susceptibility breakpoints on reporting of resistance in *Streptococcus pneumoniae*, United States, 2003. MMWR 53:152–154, 2004.

99. Jones RN, Mutnick AH, Varnam DJ. Impact of modified nonmeningeal *Streptococcus pneumoniae* interpretive criteria (NCCLS M100-S12) on the susceptibility patterns of five parenteral cephalosporins: report from the SENTRY antimicrobial surveillance program (1997 to 2001). J Clin Microbiol 40:4332–4333, 2002.

100. File TM, Lode H, Kurz H, et al. Double-blind, randomized study of the efficacy and safety of oral pharmacokinetically enhanced amoxicillin-clavulanate (2,000/125 milligrams) versus those of amoxicillin-clavulanate (875/125 milligrams), both given twice daily for 7 days, in treatment of bacterial community-acquired pneumonia in adults. Antimicrob Agents Chemother 48:3323–3331, 2004.

101. Nuermberger E, Bishai WR. The clinical significance of macrolide-resistant *Streptococcus pneumoniae*: it's all relative. Clin Infect Dis 38:99–103, 2004.

102. Shea KW, Cunha BA. Doxycycline activity against *Streptococcus pneumoniae*. Chest 108:1775–1776, 1995.

103. Thornsberry C, Sahm DF, Kelly LJ, et al. Regional trends in antimicrobial resistance among clinical isolates of *Streptococcus pneumoniae*, *Haemophilus influenzae*, and *Moraxella catarrhalis* in the United States: results from the TRUST Surveillance Program, 1999–2000. Clin Infect Dis 34 (Suppl 1):S4–16, 2002.

104. Chen DK, McGeer A, de Azavedo JC, et al. Decreased susceptibility of Streptococcus pneumoniae to fluoroquinolones in Canada. N Engl J Med 34:341:233–239, 1999.

105. Scheld WM. Maintaining fluoroquinolone class efficacy: review of influencing factors. Emerg Infect Dis 9:1–9, 2003.

106. MacGowan AP, Bowker KE. Mechanism of fluoroquinolone resistance is an important factor in determining the antimicrobial effect of gemifloxacin against *Streptococcus pneumoniae* in an in vitro pharmacokinetic model. Antimicrob Agents Chemother 47:1096–1100, 2003.

107. Roson B, Fernandez-Sabe N, Carratala J, et al. Contribution of a urinary antigen assay (Binax NOW) to the early diagnosis of pneumococcal pneumonia. Clin Infect Dis 38:222–226, 2004.

108. Herbert MA, Moxon RE. *Haemophilus influenzae*. In: Yu VL, ed. Antimicrobial therapy and vaccines. Baltimore: Williams & Wilkins, 1999:213–227.

109. Reiman HA. An acute infection of the respiratory tract with atypical pneumonia. JAMA 111:2377–2384, 1938.

110. Gupta SK, Sarosi GA. The role of atypical pathogens in community-acquired pneumonia. Med Clin North Am 85:1349–1365, 2001.

111. File TM, Tan JS, Plouffe JF. The role of atypical pathogens: *Mycoplasma pneumoniae*, *Chlamydia pneumoniae*, and *Legionella pneumophila* in respiratory infection. Infect Dis Clin North Am 12:569–592, 1998.

112. Vergis EN, Yu VL. *Legionella* species. In: Yu VL, ed. Antimicrobial therapy and vaccines. Baltimore: Williams & Wilkins, 1999:257–272.

113. Cunha BA. Atypical pneumonias. Postgrad Med 90:89–101, 1991.

114. Berthelot P, Grattard F, Ros A, et al. Nosocomial legionellosis outbreak over a three-year period. Clin Microbiol Infect 4:385–391, 1998.

115. Brenner DJ. Classification of the Legionellae. Semin Respir Infect 2:190–205, 1987.

116. Yu VL, Ramirez J, Roig J, et al. Legionnaires' disease and the updated IDSA guidelines for community-acquired pneumonia. Clin Infect Dis 39:1734–1737, 2004.

117. Baptiste-Desruisseaux, Duperval R, Marcoux JA. Legionnaires' disease in immunocompromised host: usefulness of Gram's stain. Can Med Assoc J 133:117–118, 1985.

118. Murdoch DR. Diagnosis of *Legionella* infection. Clin Infect Dis 36:64–69, 2003.

119. Roig J, Rello J. Legionnaires' disease: a rational approach to therapy. J Antimicrob Chemother 51:1119–1129, 2003.

120. Edelstein PH. Antimicrobial chemotherapy for Legionnaires' disease: a review. Clin Infect Dis 21 (Suppl 3):S265–276, 1995.

121. Nielsen K, Bangsborg JM, Hoiby N. Susceptibility of *Legionella* species to five antibiotics and development of resistance by exposure to erythromycin, ciprofloxacin, and rifampicin. Diagn Microbiol Infect Dis 36:43–48, 2000.

122. Carbon C, Nusrat R. Efficacy of telithromycin in community-acquired pneumonia caused by *Legionella pneumophila*. Eur J Clin Microbiol Infect Dis 23:650–652, 2004.

123. Myburgh J, Nagel GJ, Petschel E. The efficacy and tolerance of a three-day course of azithromycin in the treatment of community-acquired pneumonia. J Antimicrob Chemother 31 (Suppl E):163–169, 1993.

124. Plouffe JF, Breiman RF, Fields BS, et al. Azithromycin in the treatment of *Legionella* pneumonia requiring hospitalization. Clin Infect Dis 37:1475–1480, 2003.

125. Mandell LA, Marrie TJ, Grossman RF, et al. Canadian guidelines for the initial management of community-acquired pneumonia: an evidence-based update by the Canadian Infectious Diseases Society and the Canadian Thoracic Society. Clin Infect Dis 31:383–421, 2000.

126. MacFarlane J, Boswell T, Douglas G, et al. BTS guidelines for the management of community-acquired pneumonia in adults. Thorax 56 (Suppl 4):1–64, 2001.

127. Fine MJ, Aubele TE, Yealy DM, et al. A prediction rule to identify low-risk patients with community-acquired pneumonia. N Engl J Med 336:243–250, 1997.

128. Meehan TP, Fine MJ, Krumhol HM, et al. Quality of care, process, and outcomes in elderly patients with pneumonia. JAMA 278:2080–2084, 1997.

129. Mills GD, Oehley MR, Arrol B. Effectiveness of β-lactam antibiotics compared with antibiotics active against atypical pathogens in non-severe community acquired pneumonia: meta-analysis. Br Med J 330:456–460, 2005.

130. Hedlund J, Ortqvist A. Management of patients with community-acquired pneumonia treated in hospital in Sweden. Scand J Infect Dis 34:887–892, 2002.

131. Ortiz-Ruiz G, Vetter N, Isaacs R, et al. Ertapenem versus ceftriaxone for the treatment of community-acquired pneumonia in adults: combined analysis of two multicentre randomized, double-blind studies. J Antimicrob Chemother 53 (Suppl 2):59–66, 2004.

132. Neuhauser MM, Weinstein RA, Rydman R, et al. Antibiotic resistance among gram-negative bacilli in U.S intensive care units: implications for fluoroquinolone use. JAMA 289:885–888, 2003.

133. Bearden DT, Neuhauser MM, Garey KW. Telithromycin: an oral ketolide for respiratory infections. Pharmacotherapy 21:1204–1222, 2001.

134. Aventis Pharmaceuticals. Ketek (telithromycin) prescribing information. Kansas City, MO, October 2004.

135. van der Eerden MM, de Graaff CS, Vlaspolder F, et al. Evaluation of an algorithm for switching from IV to PO therapy in clinical practice in patients with community-acquired pneumonia. Clin Ther 26:294–303, 2004.

136. Ramirez JA, Vargas S, Ritter GW, et al. Early switch from intravenous to oral antibiotics and early hospital discharge: a prospective observational study of 200 consecutive patients with community-acquired pneumonia. Arch Intern Med 159:2449–2454, 1999.

137. Cunha BA. Empiric therapy of community-acquired pneumonia: guidelines for the perplexed? Chest 125:1913–1919, 2004.

138. Eron LJ, Passos S Early discharge of infected patients through appropriate antibiotic use. Arch Intern Med 161:61–65, 2001.

139. Brun-Buisson C. Guidelines for treatment of hospital-acquired pneumonia. Semin Resp Crit Care Med 23:457–469, 2002.

140. Robert R, Grollier G, Frat JP, et al. Colonization of lower respiratory tract with anaerobic bacteria in mechanically ventilated patients. Intensive Care Med 29:1062–1068, 2003.

141. Robert R, Grollier C, Hira M, et al. A role for anaerobic bacteria in patients with ventilatory acquired pneumonia: yes or no? Chest 117:1214–1215, 2000.

142. Marik PE, Careau P. The role of anaerobes in patients with ventilator-associated pneumonia and aspiration pneumonia. Chest 115:178–183, 1999.

143. Brun-Buisson C, Sollet JP, Schweich H, et al. Treatment of ventilator-associated pneumonia with piperacillin-tazobactam/amikacin versus ceftazidime/amikacin: a multicenter, randomized controlled trial. VAP Study Group. Clin Infect Dis 26:346–354, 1998.

144. Luna CM, Niederman MS What is the natural history of resolution of nosocomial pneumonia? Semin Respir Crit Care Med 23:471–479, 2002.

145. Iregui M, Ward S, Sherman RN, et al. Clinical importance of delays in the initiation of appropriate antibiotic treatment for ventilator-associated pneumonia. Chest 122:262–268, 2002.

146. Meduri GU, Mauldin GL, Wunderink RG, et al. Causes of fever and pulmonary densities in patients with clinical manifestations of ventilator-associated pneumonia. Chest 106:221–235, 1994.

147. Luna CM, Vujacich P, Niederman MS, et al. Impact of BAL data on the therapy and outcome of ventilator-associated pneumonia. Chest 111:676–685, 1997.

148. Ruiz M, Torres A, Ewig S, et al. Noninvasive versus invasive microbial investigation in ventilator-associated pneumonia: evaluation of outcome. Am J Respir Crit Care Med 162:119–125, 2000.

149. Wu CL, Yang DI, Wang NY, et al. Quantitative culture of endotracheal aspirates in the diagnosis of ventilator-associated pneumonia in patients with treatment failure. Chest 122:662–668, 2002.

150. Pugin J, Auckenthaler R, Mili N, et al. Diagnosis of ventilator-associated pneumonia by bacteriologic analysis of bronchoscopic and nonbronchoscopic ''blind'' bronchoalveolar lavage fluid. Am Rev Respir Dis 143:1121–1129, 1991.

151. Kollef MH. Appropriate empirical antibacterial therapy for nosocomial infections. Drugs 63:2157–2168, 2003.

152. Yu VL, Singh N. Excessive antimicrobial usage causes measurable harm to patients with suspected ventilator-associated pneumonia. Intensive Care Med 30:735–738, 2004.

153. Chastre J, Wolff M, Fagon JY, et al. Comparison of 8 vs. 15 days of antibiotic therapy for ventilator-associated pneumonia in adults. JAMA 290:2588–2598, 2003.

154. Nseir S, DiPompeo CD, Soubrier S, et al. First-generation fluoroquinolone use and subsequent emergence of multiple drug-resistant bacteria in the intensive care unit. Crit Care Med 33:283–289, 2005.

155. Dennesen PJW, van der Ven AJ, Kessels AGH, et al. Resolution of infectious parameters after antimicrobial therapy in patients with ventilator-associated pneumonia. Am J Respir Crit Care Med 163:1371–1375, 2001.

156. Singh N, Rogers P, Atwood CW, et al. Short-course empiric antibiotic therapy for patients with pulmonary infiltrates in the intensive care unit. A proposed solution for indiscriminate antibiotic prescription. Am J Respir Crit Care Med 162:505–511, 2000.

157. Craven DE, Steger. Epidemiology of nosocomial pneumonia. Chest 108 (Suppl):1S–16S, 1995.

158. Streit JM, Jones RN, Sader HS, et al. Assessment of pathogen occurrences and resistance profiles among infected patients in the intensive care unit: report from the SENTRY Antimicrobial Surveillance Program (North America, 2001). Int J Antimicrob Agents 24:111–118, 2004.

159. Paradisi F, Corti G, Messeri D. Antistaphylococcal (MSSA, MRSA, MSSE, MRSE) antibiotics. Med Clin North Am 85:1–17, 2001.

160. Fagon JY, Patrick H, Haas DW, et al. Treatment of gram-positive nosocomial pneumonia: prospective randomized comparison of quinupristin/dalfopristin versus vancomycin. Am J Resp Crit Care Med 161:753–762, 2000.

161. Moise-Broder PA, Forrest A, Birmingham MC, et al. Pharmacodynamics of vancomycin and other antimicrobials in patients with *Staphylococcus aureus* lower respiratory tract infections. Clin Pharmacokinet 43:925–942, 2004.

162. Rubinstein E, Cammarata S, Oliphant T, et al. Linezolid (PNU–100766) versus vancomycin in the treatment of hospitalized patients with nosocomial pneumonia: a randomized, double-blind, multicenter study. Clin Infect Dis 32:402–412, 2001.

163. Wunderink RG, Cammarata SK, Oliphant TH, et al. Continuation of a randomized, double-blind, multicenter study of linezolid versus vancomycin in the treatment of patients with nosocomial pneumonia. Clin Ther 25:980–992, 2003.

164. Wunderink RG, Rello J, Cammarata SK, et al. Analysis of two double-blind studies of patients with methicillin-resistant *Staphylococcus aureus* nosocomial pneumonia. Chest 124:1789–1797, 2004.

165. Kollef MH, Rello J, Cammarata SK, et al. Clinical cure and survival in gram-positive ventilator-associated pneumonia: retrospective analysis of two double-blind studies comparing linezolid with vancomycin. Intensive Care Med 30:388–394, 2004.

166. Yu VL, Paterson DL. *Pseudomonas aeruginosa*. In: Yu VL, ed. Antimicrobial therapy and vaccines. Baltimore: Williams & Wilkins, 1999:348–358.

167. Livermore D. Of *Pseudomonas*, porins, pumps, and carbapenems. J Antimicrob Chemother 47:247–250, 2001.

168. Waterer GW, Wunderink RG. Increasing threat of gram-negative bacteria. Crit Care Med 29 (Suppl):N75–81, 2001.

169. Patterson JE. Extended-spectrum beta-lactamases. Semin Respir Crit Care Med 24:79–87, 2003.

170. Bergogne-Berezin E. *Acinetobacter* species. In: Yu VL, ed. Antimicrobial therapy and vaccines. Baltimore: Williams & Wilkins, 1999:3–9.

171. Muder RR. *Stenotrophomonas* (*Xanthomonas*) *maltophilia*. In: Yu VL, ed. Antimicrobial therapy and vaccines. Baltimore: Williams & Wilkins, 1999:417–419.

172. Shorr AF, Susia GB, Kollef MH. Quinolones for treatment of nosocomial pneumonia: a meta-analysis. Clin Infect Dis 40 (Suppl 2):S115–122, 2005.

173. Capitano B, Nicolau DP. Evolving epidemiology and cost of resistance to antimicrobial agents in long-term care facilities. J Am Med Dir Assoc 4 (3 Suppl):S90–99, 2003.

174. Low JA, Chan DK, Hung WT, et al. Treatment of recurrent aspiration pneumonia in end-stage dementia: preferences and choices of a group of elderly nursing home residents. Intern Med J 33:345–349, 2003.

175. van der Steen JT, Ooms ME, Mehr DR, et al. Severe dementia and adverse outcomes of nursing home-acquired pneumonia: evidence for mediation by functional and pathophysiological decline. J Am Geriatr Soc 50:439–448, 2002.

176. Loeb M. Pneumonia in older persons. Clin Infect Dis 37:1335–1339, 2003.

177. Muder RR. Pneumonia in residents of long-term care facilities: epidemiology, etiology, management, and prevention. Am J Med 105:319–330, 1998.

178. Bradley SF. Methicillin-resistant *Staphylococcus aureus*: long-term care concerns. Am J Med 106:2S–10S, 1999.

179. Loeb M, Brazil K, Lohfeld L, et al. Optimizing antibiotics in residents of nursing homes. BMC Health Serv Res 2:Article 17, 2002.

180. Nuorti JP, Butler JC, Crutcher JM, et al. An outbreak of multidrug-resistant pneumococcal pneumonia and bacteremia among unvaccinated nursing home residents. N Engl J Med 338:1861–1868, 1998.

181. Strausbaugh LJ, Jacobson C, Sewell DL, et al. Methicillin-resistant *Staphylococcus aureus* in extended-care facilities: experiences in a Veterans' Affairs nursing home and a review of the literature. Infect Control Hosp Epidemiol 12:36–45, 1991.

182. El-Solh AA, Pietrantoni C, Bhat A, et al. Microbiology of severe aspiration pneumonia in institutionalized elderly. Am J Resp Crit Care Med 167:1650–1654, 2003.

183. Mylotte JM, Goodnough S, Naughton BJ. Pneumonia versus aspiration pneumonitis in nursing home residents. J Am Geriatr Soc 51: 17–23, 2003.

184. Fried TR, Gillick MR, Lipsitz LA. Short-term functional outcomes of long-term care residents with pneumonia treated with and without hospital transfer. J Am Geriatr Soc 45:302–306, 1997.

185. Kruse RL, Mehr DR, Boles KE, et al. Does hospitalization impact survival after lower respiratory infection in nursing home residents? Med Care 42:860–870, 2004.

186. Finegold SM. Aspiration pneumonia. Rev Infect Dis 13 (Suppl 9): S737–742, 1991.

187. Marik P. Aliens, anaerobes and the lung! Intensive Care Med 29: 1035–1037, 2003.

188. Donskey CJ, Chowdhry TK, Hecker MT, et al. Effect of antibiotic therapy on the density of vancomycin-resistant enterococci in the stool of colonized patients. N Engl J Med 343:1952–1932, 2000.

189. Climo MW, Isreal DS, Wong ES, et al. Hospital-wide restriction of clindamycin: effect on the incidence of *Clostridium difficile*-associated diarrhea and cost. Ann Intern Med 128:989–995, 1998.

190. Davies CWH, Gleeson FV, Davies RJO. Lung abscess. In: Marrie TJ, ed. Community-acquired pneumonia. New York: Kluwer Academic Publishers, 2001:369–386.

191. Bartlett JG. The role of anaerobic bacteria in lung abscess. Clin Infect Dis 40:923–925, 2005.

Tuberculosis

Caroline S. Zeind, Helene Hardy, and Greta K. Gourley

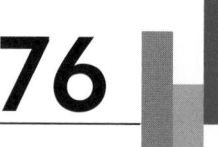

Tuberculosis (TB) is responsible for over 2 million deaths annually.[1] The human immunodeficiency virus type 1 (HIV-1) epidemic has significantly contributed to the resurgence of TB worldwide, with HIV-1 infection being the most potent risk factor for the development of active TB.[2,3] The emergence of multi–drug-resistant TB is a worldwide problem and threatens efforts to control the disease.[4,5] The bacterial organism can cause disease in virtually any organ, but the lungs are predominantly affected.[6] Effective chemotherapy is available to cure virtually all cases of TB. Global strategies are focused on halting the spread of TB and curing infectious cases.

HISTORY

TB is one of the oldest diseases known to man, as evidenced by findings of TB spinal disease within Egyptian mummies dating back to 4000 to 2000 BC.[7] During the time of Hippocrates, pulmonary TB was called phthisis by the Greeks (''consumption'') because the disease caused a general wasting.[8] During the industrialization and urbanization of the 17th and 18th centuries in Europe, the incidence of TB rose significantly to epidemic proportions. In the mid-19th century, mortality rates in eastern cities in the United States averaged 400 per 100,000 population.[8] TB proliferates in crowded, unsanitary, urban conditions, and improvements in these socioeconomic conditions have led to declining TB rates.

The infectious etiology of TB was debated until Robert Koch, in 1882, identified the tubercle bacillus as the cause of human TB.[8] This led to the development of basic TB disease control strategies[9]: the creation of the sanatorium movement in Europe (1854) and in the United States (1882) to isolate infectious individuals[10]; the use of pasteurization of cow's milk (virtually eliminating human disease caused by Mycobacterium bovis); the creation of bacille Calmette-Guérin (BCG) vaccine[11]; and, in the 1940s, the discovery of anti-TB drugs. Prior to the availability of anti-TB drugs, the number of TB cases began to decline with the improvement in socioeconomic conditions and the use of sanatoria to isolate infectious individuals. The discovery of chemotherapy that could cure established disease and prevent progression of infection to disease led to the closing of sanatoria.[11] Since then, curative chemotherapy and contact investigation for persons with infectious TB have remained the cornerstones of effective management of this disease.

ETIOLOGIC AGENT

M. tuberculosis, or the tubercle bacillus, is a member of the genus Mycobacteriaceae, order actinomycetales,[6,12] and is the etiologic agent of human TB. It belongs to the M. tuber-

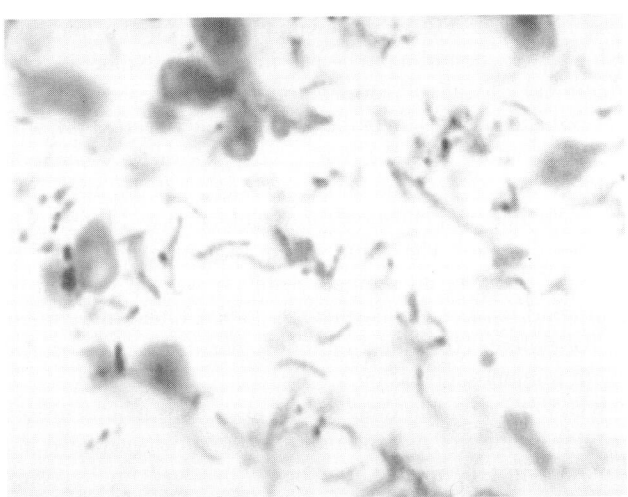

FIGURE 76.1 Mycobacterium tuberculosis (see color insert). A smear of a pulmonary lesion shows slender, beaded, acid-fast bacilli. (From Rubin E., Farber JL. Pathology, 3rd ed. Philadelphia: Lippincott Williams & Wilkins, 1999.)

culosis complex.[6] Other members of this complex are Mycobacterium africanum and *Mycobacterium ulcerans*, which are also primarily human pathogens, and *Mycobacterium bovis*, which causes TB primarily in cattle and other animals; however, *M. bovis* can cause human disease through extensive contact with infected animals or can be transmitted by unpasteurized milk.[6]

Mycobacteria are rod-shaped, non-spore-forming, slow-growing (4 to 6 weeks) aerobic bacteria.[12] The bacilli do not stain readily, but once stained they resist decolorization with acid alcohol, which has led to their classification as acid-fast bacilli (AFB) (Fig. 76.1; see color insert). The bacilli have a high content of mycolic acids, long-chain cross-linked fatty acids, and other cell wall lipids that are primarily responsible for the acid fastness. Heat or detergents are usually required for primary staining because of the lipid characteristics of these organisms.

M. tuberculosis contains many immunoreactive substances, such as surface lipids and water-soluble components of cell wall peptidoglycan, that appear to exert their effects through primary actions on host macrophages.[12] Mycobacteria contain several protein and polysaccharide antigens that are involved in the pathogenesis of disease.

EPIDEMIOLOGY

TUBERCULOSIS IN THE WORLD

TB remains one of the deadliest diseases in the world. Eight million new TB cases are estimated to occur each year in the world; most of them occur in developing countries where resources to treat infected individuals are limited and HIV infection is common. Within the past 10 years, it has become clear that the spread of HIV infection worldwide and the

immigration of persons have resulted in increased number of TB cases worldwide.

TUBERCULOSIS IN THE UNITED STATES: BETTER BUT NOT GONE

Eradication of TB, even in industrialized countries, remains a significant challenge. In the United States it is estimated that 15 million people are infected with *M tuberculosis*, while 20% to 40% of the world's population is estimated to be infected with this pathogen.[13] In the United States, the implementation of well-structured infection-control programs has resulted in the significant decrease in the number of TB cases identified over the past 10 years.[14] In 2002 in the United States there were 15,075 cases of active TB (5.2 cases per 100,000 people), representing a significant decrease from 1992 (10.5 cases per 100,000), when the number of cases peaked, marking the resurgence of TB in the United States (Fig. 76.2).[13] The 2002 rate represents the lowest number of TB cases since 1953, when national reporting was started.

DEMOGRAPHICS

Age Group and Gender. In persons older than 25 years and born in the United States, men are reported to contract the disease at a rate two times higher than that of women; a similar number of TB cases are reported between foreign-born men and women.[14] In 2002, the rate of TB infection remained the highest in persons older than 65 years (8.8 cases per 100,000), followed by persons 25 to 44 years old (6.2 cases per 100,000) and children 0 to 14 years old (1.5 cases per 100,000) (Fig. 76.3).

Ethnicity and Geographic Location. Case rates in 2002 were highest among Asian/Pacific Islanders (27.8 cases per 100,000), non-Hispanic blacks (12.6 cases per 100,000), and Hispanics (10.4 cases per 100,000), and lowest for non-Hispanic whites (1.5 cases per 100,000).[14] The TB case rate for foreign-born individuals remained at least 8 to 10 times higher than for U.S.-born individuals (2.9 cases per 100,000

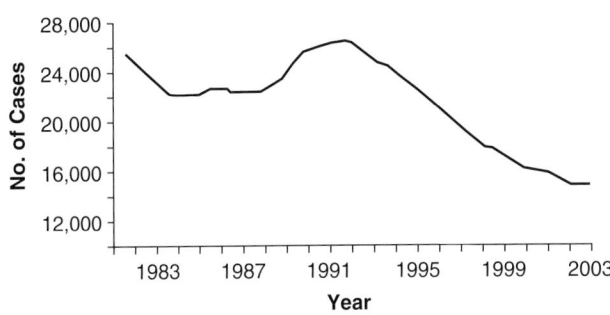

FIGURE 76.2 TB cases reported in the United States, 1982–2003. (From Centers for Disease Control and Prevention, National Center for HIV, STD, and TB Prevention, Division of Tuberculosis Elimination Web site. Available at http://www.cdc.gov/nchstp/tb/pub/slidesets/surv/surv2003/default.htm. Accessed July 18, 2005.)

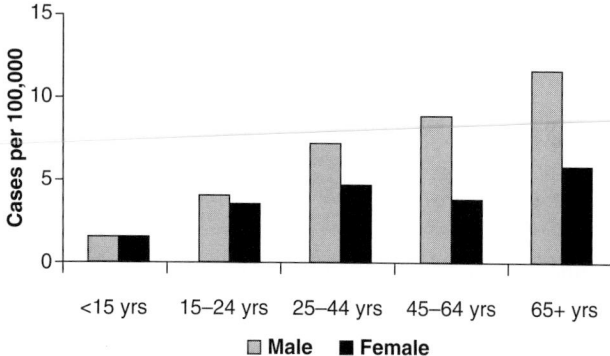

FIGURE 76.3 TB case rates in the United States (cases per 100,000) by age group and sex, 2003. (From Centers for Disease Control and Prevention, National Center for HIV, STD, and TB Prevention, Division of Tuberculosis Elimination Web site. Available at http://www.cdc.gov/nchstp/tb/pub/slidesets/surv/surv2003/default.htm. Accessed July 18, 2005.)

in U.S.-born persons versus 23.1 cases per 100,000 in foreign-born individuals). Immigrants from Mexico have the highest prevalence of TB cases reported in foreign-born individuals.

TRANSMISSION AND PATHOGENESIS

TRANSMISSION

From Exposure to Infection. *M. tuberculosis* is acquired by inhalation of infectious airborne particles, called droplet nuclei, that are small enough (1 to 5 μm) to reach the alveolar air spaces.[6] Patients with active pulmonary or laryngeal TB expel these airborne droplets primarily by coughing, sneezing, or vocalizing; the particles can remain suspended in the air for several hours, allowing exposure to a susceptible person (contact) and entry into the terminal air passages. Factors that determine the probability of infection are the intimacy and duration of that contact, the degree of infectiousness of the case, and host defenses. Crowded areas with poorly ventilated rooms favor the transmission of TB because of the greater intensity of the case and the contact.

From Infection to Disease. The risk of developing disease after being infected is primarily dependent on endogenous factors such as an individual's innate susceptibility to disease and level of function of cell-mediated immunity.[6] Clinical illness that results directly following infection is classified as primary TB and is common in young children and infants. This form of TB is often severe but is usually not transmissible. When infection is acquired later in life, there is a greater chance that the immune system will contain it, at least temporarily. The majority of infected individuals who will ultimately develop TB will do so within the first year or two after infection. Bacilli that are dormant, however, may persist for years before being reactivated to produce secondary tuberculosis, which is usually infectious. It is estimated that about 10% of infected persons will eventually develop active TB. In areas with high rates of TB transmission, reinfection of a previously infected individual is common and may also favor development of disease.

Several diseases favor the development of active TB, with HIV infection being the most potent risk factor.[2] The individual's degree of immunosuppression will directly affect the risk that latent *M. tuberculosis* infection will progress to active disease.[6] The ability of an individual to mount an intact cell-mediated immune response will be reduced by certain diseases such as silicosis, diabetes mellitus, chronic renal failure, HIV infection, and other diseases associated with immunosuppression.

HIV infection has dramatically altered the natural history of TB because of its profound effects on cell-mediated immunity. In HIV-infected persons with severe immunosuppression (CD4+ cell counts below 100), TB will develop rapidly after the initial infection with *M. tuberculosis*.[6] Up to 50% of HIV-infected persons with a CD4 count less than 100 will develop active TB within 2 years of the initial infection if they are not given preventive therapy.[15] This contrasts with 10% of individuals in the general population. Consequently, a person infected with latent TB (infected but not treated) who acquires HIV infection will develop TB at a rate of 5% to 12% per year.[16] As a result, pulmonary TB was added to the list of indicator diseases in the 1993 acquired immunodeficiency syndrome (AIDS) surveillance case definition. Table 76.1 highlights high-prevalence and high-risk groups.

PATHOGENESIS

Upon inhalation of droplet nuclei containing tubercle bacilli from an infectious individual, the interaction of *M. tubercu-*

TABLE 76.1	Populations at Risk	
High-Prevalence Groups	**High-Risk Groups**
Born in countries with high prevalence of TB	Children <4 years of age
	Persons with HIV infection/AIDS
Poor access to health care	Close contact with infectious TB (e.g., health care workers)
Living in a nursing home, shelter, drug treatment center, correctional facility	Tuberculin test converted to positive in the past 2 years
	Chest radiographs suggestive of old TB infection
Injection drug user	Certain medical conditions (diabetes mellitus, silicosis, long-term therapy with corticosteroids, immuno-suppressive therapy, Hodgkin's disease, head and neck cancer, severe kidney disease, malnutrition, solid organ transplantation)

(Adapted from Iademarco MF, Castro KG. Epidemiology of tuberculosis. Semin Resp Infect 18:225–240, 2003.)

losis with the human host begins.[6] The majority of inhaled microorganisms will be caught by the mucociliary mechanisms of the bronchial tree and expelled. However, a small fraction (generally less than 10%) will reach the alveoli. The development of an infection will depend on the virulence of the bacteria and the ability of the host macrophages to destroy the bacteria. If the bacilli survive they will multiply slowly, dividing approximately every 25 to 32 hours within the alveolar macrophages, and their growth will kill the macrophage, resulting in lysis. The bacilli released as a result of macrophage lysis will be ingested by monocytes that are stimulated by the release of chemotactic factors. Generally, little to no symptoms occurs at these initial stages of infection.

During the 2 to 4 weeks following infection, while bacilli continue to replicate within the intracellular environment, two additional host responses occur.[6] The first response is a tissue-damaging response that is a result of a delayed-type hypersensitivity (DTH) reaction. This reaction occurs in response to various bacilli antigens. The second response is a cell-mediated response that activates macrophages that can destroy and ingest the bacilli. Although both responses can inhibit the growth of the bacilli, the form of TB that develops is determined by the balance of these host immune responses.

With the development of specific immunity, the collection of lymphocytes and activated macrophages leads to the formation of granulomatous lesions (referred to as tubercles).[6] The tissue-damaging response limits mycobacterial multiplication within the macrophages and leads to the development of early solid necrosis at the center of the tubercle lesion. The bacilli can survive within the lesions, but a low oxygen tension and low pH exist within the necrotic environment of the lesion that inhibits mycobacterial growth. At this stage, some lesions may undergo fibrosis and calcification and heal, while others may undergo progression.

Cell-mediated immunity is crucial during this early stage because further multiplication and spread can ensue.[6] Activated macrophages gather around the center of the tubercle and neutralize the organism without causing further destruction of tissue. The necrotic center of the tubercle is transformed into a soft cheese-like formation referred to as "caseous necrosis." Even though healing occurs, the mycobacteria may persist within macrophages as dormant organisms for several years, and these lesions may later undergo calcification.

During the early stages of infection following ingestion of the tubercle bacilli by macrophages, the bacilli are transported to regional lymph nodes.[6] If the spread of the organism is not contained at the level of regional lymph nodes, the bacilli spread to many parts of the body through the bloodstream and lymphatic system. The bacilli divide well within tissues of the liver, spleen, kidneys, bone, meninges, and apices of the lungs. Widespread dissemination can occur as well as lesion formation. The majority of lesions of dis-

seminated TB heal, although they remain potential foci of later reactivation.

Cell-mediated immunity results in partial protection by macrophages, which phagocytize the bacilli, and T lymphocytes, which produce lymphokines.[6] A number of cytokines, such as interleukin (IL)-1, IL-6, and tumor necrosis factor α, are secreted by alveolar macrophages. In addition, macrophages have an important role in processing and presenting antigens to T lymphocytes, thus resulting in the proliferation of CD4+ lymphocytes, which are crucial to host's immune defenses against *M. tuberculosis*. CD4+ cells follow two maturation pathways that result in TH1 cells and TH2 cells, which produce different cytokines that influence the host's response to infection.

Concurrent with the appearance of immunity, DTH to *M. tuberculosis* develops and is revealed by the purified protein derivative (PPD) skin test. Most people who are infected with TB will have a positive reaction to the PPD skin test within 2 to 12 weeks from the initial contact, a condition known as latent infection. Because *M. tuberculosis* does not produce endotoxins or exotoxins, the host cellular immune response to the infection will not be detected by a reaction to the tuberculin skin test until a threshold of 10^3 to 10^4 in bacteria is reached. Only 5% to 10% of persons with latent TB ever progress to active TB, and it is most likely to happen within the first 2 years after infection.

Cell-mediated immunity effectively contains the infection in 90% to 95% of immunocompetent people, and no clinical disease develops. These individuals undergo complete healing of primary TB lesions with no subsequent evidence of disease. Of the remaining 5% to 10%, half will develop disease within the first year or two because of ineffective immunity and the other half will develop disease later in life. Clinical disease results from failure to control the mycobacterial replication that followed initial infection (progressive primary TB) or when latent organisms overcome immunologic control (reactivation TB).

CLINICAL MANIFESTATIONS

Before the recognition of HIV infection, the majority of cases of TB were pulmonary. However, extrapulmonary TB, either alone or in combination with pulmonary TB, occurs in up to two thirds of patients infected with HIV who have TB.[6]

PULMONARY TUBERCULOSIS

Pulmonary TB can be further categorized as primary or post-primary (secondary). Primary pulmonary disease results from initial infection with *M. tuberculosis* and occurs in areas of high TB prevalence.[6] This form of pulmonary disease often occurs in children, with localization in the middle and lower lung zones. Lesions form after infection, and in most cases the lesions heal spontaneously. Children with impaired immunity may progress to clinical illness.

Postprimary disease is also referred to as adult-type, reactivation, or secondary TB and occurs most frequently from reactivation of remotely acquired latent infection.[6] This form of pulmonary disease tends to be localized to the apical and posterior segments of the upper lobes. The extent of lung involvement varies considerably, from minimal clinical illness barely discernible on chest radiographs to major involvement with extensive cavitation and debilitating symptoms.

Early in the course of postprimary disease, nonspecific findings usually present insidiously with symptoms such as fever, chills, and night sweats, weight loss, anorexia, and general malaise.[6] Cough eventually develops in most patients; it may be nonproductive initially and then may become productive with purulent sputum. Although a less frequent finding, hemoptysis may occur.

EXTRAPULMONARY TUBERCULOSIS

Extrapulmonary and disseminated TB may occur at sites such as the lymph nodes, genitourinary tract, pleura, bone and joints, spine, peritoneum, or meninges. Infection at extrapulmonary sites is much more common in HIV-infected persons than in the non-HIV-infected population (30% to 50% versus 15%) because of immunosuppression and the failure of the immune system to contain *M. tuberculosis*. Clinical manifestations of disseminated disease depend on the predominant site of involvement; systemic symptoms include fever, night sweats, anorexia, and weight loss.

SCREENING AND DIAGNOSIS

Clinicians should use the following strategies to prevent and control TB[17]:

1. Identify and completely treat persons with active TB.
2. Conduct thorough contact investigations (find and evaluate persons who have had contact with TB patients, determine whether they have infection or active disease, and treat them appropriately).
3. Screen high-risk populations to identify persons with latent TB infection and provide appropriate therapy to prevent the infection from progressing to active TB.

TUBERCULIN SKIN TESTING

Tuberculin skin testing (TST) is a screening test that identifies persons at high risk for developing TB who would benefit from treatment of latent tuberculosis infection (LTBI) if detected (refer to the section on treatment of LTBI).[18] This skin test is of limited value in the diagnosis of active TB due to its low sensitivity and specificity. The focus on high-risk groups has led to the term ''targeted tuberculin testing'' to promote directed activities.

Administration and Reading Test. The TST is the only proven method for identifying infection with *M. tuberculosis*

in persons who do not have TB disease. The preferred skin test is the Mantoux method, which is an intradermal injection of 0.1 mL of 5 tuberculin units (TU) of purified protein derivative (PPD) into the dorsal or volar surface of the forearm. The reaction to the injected tuberculin is a DTH response, which should be examined and interpreted by a trained health care provider 48 to 72 hours after test administration. By gentle palpation of the indurated area, the transverse diameter of the induration is measured; erythema should be excluded from the measurement.

Interpretation of Skin Reactions. Three cut-off levels have been recommended for defining a positive TST: 5 mm or more for persons at highest risk for developing TB disease, 10 mm or more for persons at high risk, and 15 mm or more of induration for persons at low risk (Table 76.2). Routine TST is not recommended for persons at low risk for LTBI; however, if these persons are tested (e.g., at entry into a workplace where risk for exposure to TB exists), the higher cutoff of 15 mm is recommended. If a person has a negative TST reaction and upon a repeat TST within 2 years an increase in reaction size of at least 10 mm occurs, the result should be interpreted as skin conversion due to recent infection with *M. tuberculosis*.

No method can distinguish between tuberculin reactions caused by vaccination with the TB vaccine (BCG) and those caused by infection due to *M. tuberculosis*. Therefore, a positive TST in a person who has been vaccinated in the past with BCG indicates infection with *M. tuberculosis* when the person tested is at increased risk for infection or has medical conditions that increase the risk for disease.

Anergy. A negative TST does not rule out TB infection or disease, because about 10% of adults and children have anergy for tuberculin (the DTH response is delayed or absent owing to cell-mediated deficiency).[19] Host factors such as poor nutrition, young or old age, poor nutrition, and immunosuppression due to diseases such as HIV infection or drugs can lower tuberculin reactivity. Because an impaired DTH response is directly related to a decrease in CD4+ cell counts, the incidence of anergy increases in HIV-infected persons as well as those with other immunosuppressive conditions.[19]

Anergy skin testing assesses the response to skin-test antigens in which a cell-mediated DTH response is expected. Mumps and Candida antigens are approved by the U.S. Food and Drug Administration (FDA) for use in intradermal DTH testing to assess cell-mediated immunity. Both antigens are applied using the Mantoux method, with a cut-off measurement of 5 mm of induration. Factors limiting the usefulness of anergy testing include the variability in the available anergy testing methods, their lack of reproducibility, and the variability in absolute risk for TB among anergic groups.[20] Currently, anergy testing is not recommended for routine use in persons with HIV-1 infection or in other immunocompromised hosts.[20,21] However, in selected situations, DTH evaluation may be useful in guiding individual decisions.

TABLE 76.2	Interpretation of Tuberculin Skin Test Results
Reaction	**Criteria**
≥5 mm of induration: Considered positive for the highest-risk groups	• Recent close contacts of TB patients • HIV-positive persons • Fibrotic changes on chest radiograph consistent with previous TB • Persons with organ transplants and other immunosuppressed patients (receiving the equivalent of ≥15 mg/d of prednisone for 1 month or more)[a]
≥10 mm of induration: Considered positive for other high-risk groups	• Persons with medical conditions: diabetes mellitus, silicosis, chronic renal failure, some hematologic disorders (e.g., leukemias and lymphomas), other specific malignancies (e.g., carcinoma of the head or neck and lung), weight loss of ≥10% of ideal body weight, gastrectomy, and jejunoileal bypass • Recent immigrants (i.e., within the last 5 years) from high-prevalence countries • Injection drug users • Mycobacteriology laboratory personnel • Children <4 years old or infants, children, and adolescents exposed to adults at high risk
≥15 mm of induration: Considered positive for persons who do not meet criteria listed above	• Routine screening is not recommended for populations at low risk for infection with M tuberculosis.

[a] Risk of TB in persons treated with corticosteroids increases with higher doses and longer duration. (From CDC. Targeted tuberculin testing and treatment of latent tuberculosis infection. MMWR 49 (RR6):1–45, 2000.)

DIAGNOSIS OF TUBERCULOSIS

A high index of suspicion is necessary for proper identification of TB cases.[6,17] The patient evaluation should include a medical history, including assessing whether the patient has medical conditions, especially HIV infection, that increase the risk for TB. If symptoms suggestive of TB are present in an individual infected with HIV, the patient should undergo chest radiography and clinical evaluation.[17] If HIV infection is recognized in a patient for the first time, TST should be performed.[17] If the result is positive (at least 5 mm of induration), the patient should undergo chest radiography and clinical evaluation for the exclusion of active TB. If symptoms suggestive of TB are present in an individual infected with HIV, the patient should undergo chest radiography and clinical evaluation regardless of his or her TST status (Table 76.3).

AFB Microscopy. In patients with suspected pulmonary TB, three sputum specimens should be collected and submitted to the laboratory for microscopic examination for AFB smear and mycobacteriology culture.[6] Sputum induction with hypertonic saline may be necessary to obtain specimens in persons unable to produce sputum. Microscopic examination of specimens such as sputum or tissue that reveal AFB provides strong inferential evidence for the diagnosis of TB. A lack of positive acid-fast smears does not rule out presumptive TB, because smears may be negative.[17] For exam-

TABLE 76.3	Latent TB versus TB Disease
Latent TB infection[a]	Asymptomatic; does not feel sick
	Cannot spread TB to others
	Usually has a positive PPD
TB disease	Symptomatic: weakness or fatigue; weight loss, chills, fever, night sweats, cough (may contain blood)
	Can spread TB to others
	Usually has a positive PPD
	May have an abnormal chest x-ray and/or positive sputum smear and/or culture
	Examples of immunocompromised persons at risk of developing active disease include those with HIV infection, diabetes, cancer of the head or neck, leukemia, or Hodgkin's disease, or silicosis; and persons on medications such as corticosteroids and immunologic agents

[a] Most people with latent TB infection never develop TB disease. In these people, the TB bacteria remain inactive for a lifetime without causing disease. However, in others, especially immunocompromised individuals, the bacteria become active and cause TB disease.

ple, 40% to 67% of patients infected with HIV who have TB were found on microscopic examination of sputum specimens to be positive for AFB.[22-24] When extrapulmonary TB is suspected, a variety of clinical specimens other than sputum (e.g., urine, cerebrospinal fluid, pleural fluid, pus, or biopsy specimens) may be needed for examination.[6]

Mycobacterial Culture. The definitive diagnosis of TB relies upon the isolation and identification of *M. tuberculosis* obtained from a specimen, most commonly sputum.[6] Because *M. tuberculosis* is a slow-growing organism, the conventional culturing technique takes several weeks. Older systems that took about 4 weeks have been replaced by newer systems, such as the BACTEC radiometric system, which speed up the process, thus reducing culturing time by about 2 weeks. Antimicrobial susceptibility testing of initial *M. tuberculosis* isolates from all patients should be performed to test susceptibility to the primary drugs used for treatment.[17] In some cases, such as HIV infection, in which atypical findings occur, culture-negative findings do not rule out a diagnosis of TB and a clinical diagnosis will be supported by other findings.

A newer method of diagnosis, the Mycobacteria Growth Indicator Tube (MGIT), appears to be a rapid, easy-to-use system with a high accuracy for detecting mycobacteria directly from clinical specimens.[25] This system uses a tradi-tional broth medium and a novel fluorescent indicator for the recovery of mycobacteria from patient specimens. The fluorescence in the MGIT is readily visible without elaborate instrumentation, enabling large numbers of cultures to be read quickly. Other newer methods of diagnosis that appear promising include serologic tests that use enzyme-linked immunosorbent (ELISA) techniques and gene amplification by the polymerase chain reaction (PCR).[6]

Radiographic Procedures. As stated above, an individual presenting with respiratory symptoms and an abnormal chest radiograph supports an initial suspicion of pulmonary TB.[6] The extent of pulmonary disease varies from minimal clinical illness that is barely discernible on chest radiographs to major involvement with extensive cavitation and debilitating symptoms. Before HIV infection became common, most cases of TB were pulmonary. However, with the advent of AIDS, the finding of a normal chest radiograph does not rule out the diagnosis of pulmonary TB. Persons with HIV infection and TB may have a chest radiograph that shows a classic reactivation pattern, an "atypical" (i.e., pleural effusion) pattern, or evidence of past infection (i.e., calcified lymph node or lung nodule). It is important that all patients with TB receive counseling and testing for HIV infection as early in the diagnosis process as possible, at least by the time treatment for TB is initiated.[17]

TREATMENT GOALS

- Drug therapy goals include curing infected patients and impeding transmission to others.
- A primary aim is to provide the most efficacious anti-TB regimen with the least toxicity for the shortest period of time.
- Treatment of active TB requires combination therapy.
- Implementation of directly observed therapy is encouraged in all settings.

TREATMENT

The development of anti-TB agents revolutionized the prognosis of patients with TB.[26] Streptomycin was introduced for the management of TB during the 1940s, but it soon became apparent that streptomycin monotherapy frequently resulted in treatment failure associated with in vitro resistance to the drug.[27,28] In the 1950s and 1960s, isoniazid and paraaminosalicylic acid were combined with streptomycin in a regimen that cured TB in nearly all patients. Treatment programs were very successful because they were carried out in hospitals, where adherence to therapy could be ensured. As a consequence, acquired drug resistance was uncommon. During the late 1960s, therapy shifted to the outpatient setting. Unfortunately, reduced adherence to anti-TB regimens in the outpatient setting has led to rising rates of treatment failure, relapse, and acquired drug resistance.[29-34]

Most patients with TB can be cured with adherence to therapeutic regimens.[26] The goal of drug therapy of active TB is twofold: to cure the infection and to impede the transmission of tubercle bacilli in the community. On the basis of controlled clinical trials, three basic principles for the treatment of TB have evolved: (a) regimens for treatment of disease must contain multiple drugs to which the organisms are susceptible, (b) the drugs must be taken regularly, and (c) drug therapy must continue for a sufficient period of time.[17,35] The aim of therapy is to provide the most efficacious regimen with the least toxicity possible for the shortest period of time.

Three subpopulations of the tubercle bacilli can coexist during an infection.[12] Anti-TB agents are targeted toward various sites of mycobacterial growth in the body (Table 76.4).[36] The most numerous population consists of extracellular bacteria; these organisms are killed most readily by

TABLE 76.4	Principal Activity and Site of Action of the Major Anti-TB Agents	
Agent	**Activity**	**Site of Action**
Isoniazid (INH)	Bactericidal	Intracellular bacilli, extracellular bacilli, bacilli in caseous lesions
Rifampin	Bactericidal	Intracellular bacilli, extracellular bacilli, bacilli in caseous lesions
Pyrazinamide	Bactericidal	Intracellular bacilli
Streptomycin	Bactericidal	Extracellular bacilli
Ethambutol	Bacteriostatic	Intracellular bacilli, extracellular bacilli

(From Hooker KD, Jost PM. Tuberculosis. In: Herfindal ET, Gourley DR, Hart LL, eds. Clinical pharmacy and therapeutics, 5th ed. Baltimore: Williams & Wilkins, 1992:1092–1108.)

isoniazid and streptomycin and to a lesser extent by rifampin. The second population is composed of organisms that seek out the acidic environment of caseating granulomas; rifampin exhibits the greatest activity in killing these organisms. The final population of organisms exists within the activated macrophages (intracellular). Because of the acidic environment within macrophages, the activity of most anti-TB agents is inhibited. Pyrazinamide has the greatest activity against this population and augments the potency of isoniazid and rifampin.

Current anti-TB regimens use combinations of agents to eliminate extracellular organisms from the sputum, decrease infectivity, and destroy slowly dividing organisms within granulomas and macrophages.[37–39] By combining various agents, regimens as short as 6 months can be used while minimizing drug resistance.

First-line agents form the core of initial regimens for the treatment of TB. Currently, isoniazid, rifampin, pyrazinamide, and ethambutol are considered first-line agents. In specific situations, as described in a later section, rifabutin and rifapentine may be considered first-line agents. Streptomycin was previously considered a first-line agent; however, in many parts of the world, an increase in the prevalence of resistance to this agent has limited its overall usefulness. In some instances, this agent may be used as part of the initial treatment regimen, although it is no longer considered a first-line agent.[17]

Because of a higher degree of toxicity and a lower degree of efficacy, several agents are considered second-line agents. These agents are reserved for situations in which TB is resistant to first-line drugs or the patient cannot tolerate some of the first-line agents.

FIRST-LINE AGENTS

Isoniazid. Since its introduction in 1952, isonicotinicyl hydrazine (INH) has been the most widely used anti-TB agent; it is a first-line agent for treatment of all forms of TB caused by organisms known or presumed to be susceptible to the drug.[17] The drug exhibits many qualities of an ideal agent: it is bactericidal, relatively nontoxic, inexpensive, and well absorbed orally or parenterally. INH is available as tablets, syrup, and aqueous solution for intravenous or intramuscular injection.

INH interferes with the biosynthesis of mycolic acids that are produced by the cross-linking of fatty acid chains derived from acetyl coenzyme A (acetyl CoA). Mycolic acids are important constituents of the mycobacterial cell wall.[40] Isoniazid inhibits fatty acid synthetase 2 (FAS2), which catalyzes the linkages of long saturated hydrocarbon chains that are starting materials for the synthesis of the mycolic acid.[41] The drug is actively transported into the bacterium, where it kills rapidly multiplying extracellular bacteria and inhibits the growth of dormant organisms within macrophages and caseating granulomas.[42]

Pharmacokinetics. INH generally is administered in adults as a single maximum dose of 5 mg per kg (300 mg) and 15 mg per kg (900 mg) once, twice, or three times weekly. In children, dosing of INH is 10 to 15 mg per kg (maximum 300 mg) daily and 20 to 30 mg per kg (900 mg) twice weekly.[17] Rapid and complete absorption occurs following oral administration, achieving peak concentrations of 3 to 5 µg per mL after a dose of 3 to 5 mg per kg.[43] When INH is administered orally with food, a reduction in the extent of absorption and peak plasma concentration may occur. Although ingestion of food delays and decreases absorption of INH, given the wide therapeutic margin of INH as well as other first-line agents, the effects of food are of little clinical significance. If epigastric distress or nausea occurs, with INH alone or in combination with other first-line agents, patients can take INH and other first-line agents with food or change the hour of dosing. Aluminum-containing antacids may also decrease gastrointestinal (GI) absorption of INH.[44] The drug is widely distributed throughout the body; significant quantities have been detected in the pleural, ascitic, and cerebrospinal fluid; caseous material; saliva; skin; and muscle.[17,45]

Metabolism via the hepatic P-450 mixed oxidase system accounts for 70% to 90% of the elimination of INH. Several metabolic pathways are involved, with acetylation being the major one.[46,47] After acetylation by the liver, the drug is excreted as a metabolite by the kidneys; it appears unchanged in the urine, along with other metabolites, including hydrazones.[26] The relative fractions of INH, acetylisoniazid, and hydrazones in the urine differ considerably among patients. The rate of acetylation of INH is genetically controlled.[48] Individuals are categorized as either fast or slow acetylators, depending on the rate of acetylation of INH in the liver. Approximately 45% to 65% of the American and northern European populations are classified as slow acetylators. Inuit (Eskimos) and Asians primarily are rapid acetylators. The elimination rate of INH depends on acetylator phenotype; half-lives of approximately 0.5 to 2 hours are observed in fast acetylators and 2 to 5 hours in slow acetylators.[42] Patients who are slow acetylators may be more susceptible to the side effects related to higher concentrations, such as peripheral neuropathy.[26] It has been postulated that hepatotoxicity is more common in rapid acetylators, owing to the production of larger amounts of the metabolite acetylhydrazine.[49] The acetylhydrazine metabolite is thought to be involved in the development of INH-induced hepatotoxicity.[47] More recent data suggest that rapid acetylators are not at increased risk for hepatitis from INH and that the rate of acetylation is unlikely to be of therapeutic significance.[50,51]

Only a small amount of INH is eliminated unchanged by the kidneys. Therefore, dosage adjustments in patients with renal dysfunction are necessary only for individuals who are slow acetylators with a creatinine clearance less than 10 mL per minute.[52,53] A reduction of the daily dose by 50% is recommended for these individuals, as well as for those with severe hepatic disease, to prevent accumulation of the drug and to reduce the potential for hepatotoxicity. In patients who are undergoing dialysis, significant amounts of INH are removed from the blood by hemodialysis and peritoneal dialysis, so dosage adjustments may be necessary.

Adverse Effects. Approximately 10% to 20% of persons receiving INH alone for treatment of latent TB infection experience elevations in aminotransferases up to five times the normal limit. In most cases, transaminase values return to pretreatment values despite continuation of INH.

The incidence of clinical hepatitis occurring in 11,141 persons receiving INH alone as treatment for latent TB infection was 0.1% to 0.15%[54]; previous studies had suggested a higher rate.[55–57] When INH is administered in combination with rifampin, the risk of clinical hepatitis is increased, with an average of 2.7% in 19 reports.[57] The risk of hepatitis when INH is administered alone increases with increasing age. A U.S. Public Health Service Surveillance Study evaluated the toxicity of INH in 13,838 patients.[55] The results showed that the rate of hepatitis increased directly with increasing age to 65 years. The rate of hepatitis was 0% in patients less than 20 years old, 0.3% in patients 20 to 34 years old, 1.2% in patients 35 to 49 years old, and 2.3% in patients 50 to 64 years old. Other risk factors include excessive or chronic alcohol consumption, underlying liver disease, intravenous drug use, and, data suggest, the postpartum period, particularly among Hispanic women.[58–60] More recent data estimate that the rate of fatal hepatitis is lower than the previously reported rate of 0.023%. Cases of fatal hepatitis have been associated with continued administration of INH despite onset of symptoms.

Baseline measurement of liver enzyme levels should be performed for patients receiving INH, and levels should be monitored periodically.[6,17] In patients older than 35 years, a transaminase measurement, such as aspartate aminotransferase (AST, SGOT), should be obtained before initiation of therapy.[17] Patients should be questioned monthly about signs and symptoms of liver disease and should be instructed to report to their physician any of the prodromal symptoms of hepatitis (e.g., malaise, fatigue, weakness, anorexia, or nausea). Should these symptoms appear or if signs suggesting hepatic damage occur (e.g., liver enlargement with tenderness, jaundice, or dark urine), prompt discontinuation of INH is warranted; this usually prevents progression (Table 76.5).[17] Some clinicians recommend discontinuation of INH if transaminase values exceed three to five times the normal levels.[26]

Peripheral neuropathy appears to be a dose-dependent adverse effect of INH.[12,17] It is uncommon at a dose of 5 mg per kg, occurring in 2% of patients receiving INH. At higher dosages, peripheral neuropathy may develop in 10% to 20% of patients. Peripheral neuropathy is most likely caused by INH-induced depletion of pyridoxine stores or competitive inhibition with pyridoxine in its role as a cofactor in the synthesis of synaptic neurotransmitters.[60] Pyridoxine (25 mg/day) should be given with INH to patients who have conditions in which neuropathy is common (e.g., diabetes, uremia, alcoholism, or malnutrition).[17,42] Persons with HIV infection who are undergoing TB treatment with INH also should receive supplementation with pyridoxine to reduce the occurrence of INH-induced side effects in both the central and peripheral nervous systems.[17] For pregnant women and persons who have a seizure disorder, pyridoxine should be given with INH. As previously mentioned, patients with slow acetylation may be more susceptible to the development of peripheral neuropathy.[26]

Other rare adverse effects reported with INH administration include various central nervous system (CNS) toxicities (i.e., hallucinations, convulsions), dermatologic (i.e., acne, allergic rashes), hematologic (i.e., aplastic anemia), and GI effects.[12] A lupus-like syndrome characterized by the development of antinuclear antibodies occurs in approximately 20% of patients taking INH; however, clinical lupus erythematosus occurs in less than 1% of patients and requires drug discontinuation.

TABLE 76.5	Signs and Symptoms of Hepatic Damage or Other Adverse Effects

Unexplained anorexia

Nausea

Vomiting

Dark urine

Icterus

Rash

Persistent paresthesias of hands and feet

Persistent fatigue

Weakness or fever of 3 days or more

Abdominal tenderness (especially right upper quadrant)

(From American Thoracic Society, CDC, and Infectious Diseases Society of America. Treatment of tuberculosis. Am J Resp Crit Care Med 167:603–662, 2003.)

Drug Interactions. Several drug interactions have been reported with the use of INH in combination with other agents.[12,61] INH is a relatively potent inhibitor of several cytochrome P-450–dependent isozymes (CYP-2C9, CYP-2C19, and CYP-2E1).[62–64] INH inhibits the metabolism of several agents, including phenytoin, disulfiram, carbamazepine, warfarin, benzodiazepines, and vitamin D; increased serum concentrations may occur with concomitant use of INH.[61]

Studies examining the interaction between INH and phenytoin found that phenytoin intoxication occurs mainly in slow acetylators of INH.[63–65] Phenytoin serum levels must be monitored in patients taking INH and phenytoin concomitantly, especially slow acetylators of INH. A reduction in the dosage of phenytoin is warranted for patients exhibiting clinical symptoms of phenytoin intoxication or toxic serum phenytoin levels.

As mentioned previously, concomitant administration of INH and food results in impaired absorption of INH; the peak concentration, the mean concentration, and the total amount of drug are reduced.[66,67] Because aluminum-containing antacids may decrease GI absorption of INH, administering INH at least 1 hour before taking antacids is recommended.[43] More studies evaluating INH absorption with antacids and laxatives are necessary.[44,68]

INH is also an inhibitor of monoamine and diamine oxidase.[69] Adverse reactions such as skin flushing, palpitations, headache, nausea and vomiting, and itching have been reported rarely in patients who are taking INH and ingesting foods with high histamine or tyramine content.[69–79] These reactions were attributed to monoamine and diamine oxidase inhibition by INH. Patients should be counseled that if flushing occurs, they should avoid foods with high histamine or tyramine content (e.g., selected fishes, cheeses, and wines).[61]

INH may exhibit enzymatic induction of certain agents.[61] In patients taking INH, rifampin, and ketoconazole concomitantly, decreases in ketoconazole concentrations have been reported; this interaction appears to involve an additive affect of INH and rifampin to reduce ketoconazole concentrations.[80,81]

The potential interaction between INH and theophylline has been examined in various European and U.S. studies.[82–84] In studies using INH at dosages of 400 mg per day or 10 mg/kg/day, a reduction in theophylline clearance was observed.[82,83] A study in the United States that used INH at a dosage of 300 mg per day reported a mean 16% increase in theophylline clearance.[84] On the basis of these studies, it appears that INH at dosages of 300 mg per day does not cause clinically significant decreases in theophylline clearance.[85] In patients taking larger daily doses of INH (e.g., 400 or 600 mg), and possibly in underweight individuals taking 300 mg per day, this interaction may be significant. A summary of clinically significant INH interactions is provided in Table 76.6.[61] Included are INH interactions that require further study and should be considered in monitoring therapy.

Rifamycins: Rifampin, Rifabutin, and Rifapentine. Three rifamycins are FDA approved for the treatment of TB in the United States: rifampin, rifabutin, and rifapentine. Rifamycins are selective inhibitors of bacterial RNA polymerase, the enzyme responsible for DNA transcription, preventing chain initiation.[86] They exhibit a broad spectrum of activity that includes activity against Neisseria, Staphylococcus, Haemophilus, most streptococci, and several species of Enterobacteriaceae.[41] The drugs are bactericidal for *M. tuberculosis*, with most strains being inhibited in vitro by concentrations of 0.5 µg per mL. Rifamycins exhibit greater activity than INH against slower-growing or intermittently growing organisms that are present in macrophages.[87] Furthermore, rifamycins are unique in their ability to destroy the organisms in semisolid caseous material. When used in combination with INH, synergy is obtained, thus enabling the duration of treatment for TB to be shortened from 18 to 24 months to 6 to 9 months.[86]

As mentioned previously, rifampin has been a mainstay first-line anti-TB agent. Rifabutin is generally reserved as a substitute for rifampin if patients are taking a medication that has unacceptable interactions with rifampin or for those with intolerance to rifampin.

Rifapentine is generally used in the continuation phase of treatment for HIV-seronegative patients with noncavitary, drug-susceptible pulmonary TB who have negative sputum smears upon completion of the initial phase of treatment.[17] Because of the rifapentine's long half-life, dosing is less frequent; it may be administered once weekly, reducing the number of pills that a patient must take to cure pulmonary TB. In studies in South Africa, the use of this agent enabled patients to take their medications just once a week during the last 4 months of therapy. This simplification of the regimen holds promise for achieving higher adherence rates and lower drug resistance rates; however, the use of rifapentine is contraindicated in HIV-infected patients because of an unacceptably high rate of relapse, frequently with organisms that have acquired resistance to rifamycins.[88]

Rifampin is available as capsules and an aqueous solution for parenteral administration. In adults the recommended dose is 10 mg per kg (600 mg) maximum once daily, twice weekly, or three times weekly and in children 10 to 20 mg per kg (600 mg) maximum once daily or twice weekly. Rifabutin is available as 150-mg oral capsules, and the adult dosage is 5 mg per kg (300 mg) daily, twice, or three times daily. When used concomitantly with protease inhibitors or nonnucleoside reverse transcriptase inhibitors, the dose may require adjustment due to drug–drug interactions. Rifapentine is available as 150-mg tablets, and the adult dosage is 10 mg per kg (600 mg) once weekly during the continuation phase of treatment. A dose of 900 mg appears to be well tolerated, although the clinical efficacy of this dose has not been established.[89]

TABLE 76.6	Isoniazid (INH) Interactions	
Agent	**Comments**	**Clinical Management**
Acetaminophen[a]	Combined with INH, hepatotoxicity is more likely to occur.	Monitor for signs and symptoms of hepatotoxicity; periodically monitor liver enzymes.
Antacids (aluminum hydroxide)	May delay and decrease absorption of INH	Give INH at least 1 hour before antacids.
Anticoagulants	Increased effect reported at INH dose of 9 mg/kg/day; unlikely to occur at lower doses	Monitor INR; decrease in anticoagulant dosage may be necessary.
Benzodiazepines	Rifampin's effect if given concomitantly should be considered.	Decrease in dosage of select benzodiazepines may be necessary.
Carbamazepine[b]	Increased carbamazepine levels and toxicity possible	Monitor serum carbamazepine levels; decrease in carbamazepine dosage may be necessary.
Cheese, fish, wine[b]	Avoid foods with high histamine or tyramine content.	Monitor for flushing, palpitations, headache, itching, nausea, and vomiting.
Ketoconazole[b]	INH has an additive effect with rifampin to decrease ketoconazole concentrations.	Monitor; adjust dosage if necessary.
Phenytoin[b]	Mainly occurs in slow acetylators of INH. If rifampin is given concurrently, phenytoin levels are decreased (i.e., induction effects outweighs INH's inhibitory effect).	Monitor serum phenytoin levels; decrease in phenytoin dosage may be necessary.
Theophylline	Potential decrease in theophylline clearance appears to occur at INH doses >300 mg/day. If rifampin is given concurrently, theophylline levels are decreased (i.e., induction effect outweighs INH's inhibitory effect).	Monitor serum theophylline levels.
Vitamin D	Further study necessary	Monitor vitamin D levels as well as calcium and phosphate levels in select patients.

[a] O'Shea D, Kim RB, Wilkinson GR. Modulation of CYP 2E1 activity by Isoniazid in rapid and slow N-acetylators. Br J Clin Pharmacol 43:99–103, 1997; and Chien JY, Peter RM, Nolan CM, et al. Influence of polymorphic N-acetyltransferase phenotype on the inhibition of acetaminophen bioactivation with long-term isoniazid. Clin Pharm Ther 61:24–34, 1997.
[b] Clinical significance established.
(From Baciewicz AM, Self TH. Isoniazid interactions. South Med J 78:714–718, 1985.)

Pharmacokinetics. The pharmacokinetic properties of rifampin, rifabutin, and rifapentine are summarized in Table 76.7.

Adverse Effects. In recommended doses, the rifamycins are generally well tolerated.[90,91] The adverse effects of rifapentine are similar to those associated with rifampin; rifabutin is associated with both similar and unique adverse effects in comparison to the other rifamycins.

Severe, true hypersensitivity reactions are uncommon with the rifamycins. Pruritus with or without rash occurs in as many as 6% of patients receiving rifampin but is generally self-limited. More recent studies of patients receiving rifabutin report rash as an uncommon occurrence.

The incidence of GI reactions (nausea, anorexia, abdominal pain) is variable with rifamycins, but symptoms are rarely severe enough to necessitate discontinuation of the drug.

Although uncommon at recommended doses of rifampin, an influenza-like syndrome may occur with intermittent administration of doses greater than 10 mg per kg.[92] The patient may report fever, chills, malaise, arthralgias, and headache. The syndrome also may include interstitial nephritis, acute renal failure, eosinophilia, thrombocytopenia, hemolytic anemia, and shock. Patients taking rifampin should be monitored for changes in renal function and skin appearance. Adherence to the prescribed dosing regimen is important because interrupted therapy may cause an increase in the

TABLE 76.7	Pharmacokinetics of Rifamycins		
	Rifampin	**Rifabutin**	**Rifapentine**
Absorption	Well absorbed	Readily absorbed (53%)	Bioavailability: ~70%
	Food may delay or slightly reduce peak.	Food may delay or slightly reduce peak.	Food increases AUC and C_{max} by 43% and 44% respectively.
Distribution	Highly lipophilic; crosses blood–brain barrier well	V_d: 9.32 L/kg; distributes to body tissues including the lungs, liver, spleen, eyes, and kidneys	V_d: ~70.2 L; rifapentine and metabolite accumulate in human monocyte-derived macrophages with intracellular/extracellular ratios of 24:1 and 7:1 respectively.
	Protein binding: 80%	Protein binding: 85%	Protein binding: rifapentine and 25-desacetyl metabolite: 97.7% and 93.2%, primarily to albumin
Metabolism	Hepatic; undergoes enterohepatic recirculation	Hepatic; metabolized to active and inactive metabolites	Hepatic; hydrolyzed by an esterase and esterase enzyme to form the active metabolite 25-desacetyl rifapentine
	Substrate (major) of CYP2A6, 2C8/9, 3A4	Substrate (major) of CYP1A2, 3A4	Induces CYP2C8/9 (strong), 3A4 (strong)
	Induces CYP1A2 (strong), 2A6 (strong), 2B6 (strong), 2C8/9 (strong), 2C19 (strong), 3A4 (strong)	Induces CYP3A4 (strong)	
Elimination	Urine (~30%) as unchanged drug	Urine (10% as unchanged drug, 53% as metabolites)	Urine (17% primarily as metabolites)
	Feces (60% to 65%)	Feces (10% as unchanged drug, 30% as metabolites)	Dosing adjustment in renal or hepatic impairment: Unknown
	Hepatic impairment: Dose reductions may be necessary to reduce hepatotoxicity.	Dosage adjustment in renal impairment:	
	Hemodialysis or peritoneal dialysis: Plasma rifampin concentrations are not significantly affected by hemodialysis or peritoneal dialysis.	Cl_{cr} <30 mL/min: Reduce dose by 50%	
Terminal elimination half-life	3–4 hours; prolonged with hepatic impairment; end-stage renal disease: 1.8–11 hours	45 hours (range 16–69 hours)	14–17 hours; 25-desacetyl rifapentine: 13 hours

incidence of toxicity. The influenza-like syndrome is rare in patients taking rifabutin.

Elevations in hepatic enzymes occur in approximately 10% to 15% of patients when rifampin is administered alone.[93] In combination with INH, elevations in serum transaminases may occur in 20% to 30% of patients.[94] This usually occurs within the first 8 weeks of therapy. The development of hepatitis in patients with normal hepatic function who are taking rifampin is rare. Alcoholism, chronic liver disease, and advanced age may increase the risk of hepatotoxicity with the administration of rifampin alone or in combination with INH. Rifabutin exhibits a similar incidence of asymptomatic elevation of liver enzymes, and clinical hepatitis occurs in less than 1% of patients.

Rifampin, as well as rifabutin and rifapentine, may impart an orange discoloration to the urine, feces, sputum, tears, and sweat. Soft contact lenses may be permanently discolored and patients should be counseled accordingly.[41,95,96]

Neutropenia has been reported in a placebo-controlled, double-blind trial of patients with advanced AIDS taking rifabutin. Neutropenia appears to be a dose-related effect that occurs more frequently with daily administration as opposed to intermittent administration.[97] In other studies of patients with HIV and non-HIV infection, neutropenia was not associated with rifabutin.[97]

Uveitis is a rare complication (less than 0.01%) with the use of rifabutin alone at the standard 300-mg daily dose. When used in higher doses or in combination with drugs that can reduce its clearance, the occurrence is higher (8%).

Drug Interactions. The rifamycins are inducers of hepatic microsomal enzymes.[98] Of the three available rifamycins, rifampin is the most potent CYP-450 inducer, whereas rifabutin has significantly less activity as an inducer; rifapentine, the most recently approved rifamycin derivative, has intermediate activity as an inducer.[98] Rifampin may enhance the elimination of several drugs, including theophylline, warfarin, oral contraceptive agents, phenytoin, cyclosporine, glucocorticoids, methadone, ketoconazole, and oral sulfonylureas.[99–102] These interactions may result in decreased efficacy of these agents, such as reduced efficacy of oral contraceptives, including several reports of unplanned pregnancy.[102,103] Rifabutin and rifapentine also may enhance the elimination of various drugs; these agents, like rifampin, also may reduce the efficacy of oral contraceptives, and alternative forms of birth control should be recommended.[95,96] Potentially clinically significant rifampin drug interactions that have been reported more recently include interactions with haloperidol, several antiarrhythmics, diltiazem, fluconazole, and select benzodiazepines.[101]

Over the past few years several antiretroviral agents have been FDA approved for the management of HIV disease. Because mycobacterial infections such as TB are common in patients infected with HIV, drug interactions must be carefully assessed to ensure efficacy and to avoid toxicity.[17] Two major classes of antiretroviral agents, the HIV protease inhibitors (PIs) and the nonnucleoside reverse transcriptase inhibitors (NNRTIs), are extensively biotransformed via CYP-450 (oxidative) metabolism.[98] Among the NNRTIs, delavirdine inhibits CYP-3A4 as well as CYP-2C19. Efavirenz induces CYP-3A4 and CYP-2B6 while inhibiting CYP-2C19. Nevirapine induces CYP-3A4 and CYP-2B6. Antiretroviral agents within these classes exhibit substantial drug interactions with the rifamycins, often requiring dosing adjustment of rifamycins.

In 1996 the Centers for Disease Control and Prevention (CDC) established guidelines to assist clinicians in making therapeutic decisions regarding treatment of TB in patients with HIV infection.[104] Recently, the CDC revised these guidelines to include more recent data from studies that evaluated alternative therapies for managing patients infected with HIV with drug-susceptible TB and infection.[98] The updated guidelines no longer recommend discontinuation of all PI-containing therapies to allow the use of rifampin for TB treatment for patients with HIV-related TB. The revised guidelines and more recent studies provide treatment options for patients who are taking antiretroviral agents that are extensively metabolized via the cytochrome P450 system, thus enabling continued antiretroviral therapy during treatment of TB.[105–107] As mentioned previously, rifabutin exhibits fewer induction effects than rifampin and is a reasonable alternative to rifampin in TB treatment regimens in patients with HIV infection.[98] A Medwatch 2005 safety summary notified health care professionals that drug-induced hepatitis with elevated transaminase levels has been observed in healthy volunteers receiving rifampin 600 mg once daily in combination with ritonavir 100 mg/saquinavir 1000 mg twice daily (http://www.fda.gov/medwatch/SAFETY/2005/safety05.htm#Invirase). A summary of rifamycin–antiretroviral drug interactions and dosing adjustment is presented in Table 76.8.[98–101,108] Table 76.9 highlights other drug interactions with rifampin.[98–101,108]

Ethambutol. Ethambutol is a synthetic antimycobacterial agent that generally is considered to be tuberculostatic in the recommended doses.[41] Its precise mechanism of action is unknown, although it has been shown to inhibit the incorporation of mycolic acid into the mycobacterial cell wall.[109] Inhibition of mycobacterial growth requires approximately 24 hours. In vivo activity of ethambutol appears to be targeted toward actively dividing mycobacteria. Most strains of *M. tuberculosis* are inhibited in vitro by concentrations of 1 to 5 μg per mL.[17] The peak plasma concentration 2 to 4 hours after an oral dose of 15 mg per kg is approximately 5 μg per mL.[41]

Pharmacokinetics. Approximately 75% to 85% of ethambutol is absorbed from the GI tract.[41] Administering the drug with food does not interfere with absorption. Either single daily doses of 15 to 20 mg per kg or a twice-weekly regimen of 50 mg per kg may be chosen. Although ethambutol penetrates well into most tissues and fluids, concentrations in cerebrospinal fluid are low, even in the presence of meningeal inflammation. About two thirds of an oral dose of ethambutol is eliminated in the urine; approximately 50% is excreted unchanged via glomerular filtration and tubular secretion. Hepatic metabolism occurs through oxidation, and two inactive metabolites are formed. Up to 15% of the drug is excreted in the urine in the form of these inactive metabolites.[110] About 20% is excreted as unchanged drug in the feces. The serum half-life is approximately 4 hours in patients with normal renal function and may increase to 7 hours or longer in patients with renal failure.[65] Dosage adjustment is required for patients who have renal impairment.[111]

TABLE 76.8	Rifamycin–Antiretroviral Drug Interactions		
	Rifampin	**Rifabutin**	**Rifapentine[b]**
Protease inhibitors	Ritonavir: use standard dose of rifampin and ritonavir (600mg bid RTV)	Protease inhibitors can be used in combination with rifabutin, provided that rifabutin dose is adjusted.	Should not be used in combination with protease inhibitors[b]
	Dual protease inhibitor combinations:		
	LPV/r: 400/100 mg bid + 300 mg ritonavir bid + 600 mg rifampin	Ritonavir, atazanavir: use rifabutin 150 mg qod or 150 mg three times per week	
	Contraindicated combinations:	Amprenavir, fosamprenavir, indinavir, nelfinavir	
	Amprenavir ($\downarrow$AUC by 82%, $\downarrow$ C_{min} 92%), fosamprenavir, atazanavir, indinavir, nelfinavir, saquinavir, saquinavir/ritonavir (increased transaminases up to 20 times upper limit of normal)[a]	Contraindicated combinations: saquinavir ($\downarrow$AUC saquinavir by 43%)	
Nonnucleoside reverse transcriptase inhibitors	Efavirenz: No dose adjustment (600 mg efavirenz + 600 mg rifampin, once a day)	Efavirenz: increase rifabutin dose to 450 mg qd Nevirapine: no need for dose adjustment	Should not be used in combination with protease inhibitors[b]
	Nevirapine: use only if no other option exists, $\downarrow$ nevirapine (AUC) by up to 58% and C_{min} by 68%		

[a] http://www.rocheusa.com/products/invirase/Invirase_DrLetter.pdf; accessed February 2005.
[b] HIV-infected persons treated with rifapentine for TB have a higher rate of relapse.
(Adapted from Veldkamo A, Hoetelmans R, et al. Ritonavir enables combined therapy with rifampin and saquinavir. Clin Infect Disease 29:1586, 1999; La Porte C, Colbers E, Bertz R, et al. Pharmacokinetics of two adjusted dose regimens of lopinavir/ritonavir in combination with rifampin in healthy volunteers. 42nd Interscience Conference on Antimicrobial Agents and Chemotherapy, San Diego, 2002: Abstract #A-1823; Spradling O, Drociuk D, McLaughlin S, et al. Drug–drug interactions in inmates treated for HIV and Mycobacterium tuberculosis infection or disease: an institutional tuberculosis outbreak. Clin Infect Dis 35:1106–1112, 2002.)

Adverse Effects. Ethambutol is a relatively safe drug and produces few adverse effects at the recommended dosages.[41] The most toxic effect of ethambutol is retrobulbar neuritis, which is characterized by decreased visual acuity, decreased red–green color discrimination that may affect one or both eyes, or central scotomata.[112] This appears to be a dose-related phenomenon that is more common at doses above 50 mg/kg/day. The occurrence is reported to be 5% in patients taking daily doses of 25 mg per kg and less than 1% in patients taking 15 mg/kg/day.[41] In patients with renal impairment, the frequency of ocular toxicity is increased because of accumulation of the drug. Baseline examination of visual acuity should be performed as well as testing of color discrimination before initiation of ethambutol therapy. Monthly visits should include questions about visual disturbances, and monthly testing of visual acuity and color discrimination is recommended for patients taking doses greater than 15 to 25 mg per kg, those taking the drug for longer than 2 months, and any patient with renal insufficiency. Patients should be instructed to report any changes in visual acuity

and to seek medical attention immediately if changes do occur. This agent can be used safely in older children but should be used with caution in children who are too young for assessment of visual acuity and red–green color discrimination (generally less than 5 years of age). The use of alternative agents should be considered. If there is concern about resistance to INH or rifampin, ethambutol can be used with careful monitoring.

Other adverse effects of ethambutol include hypersensitivity reactions, neuritis, GI intolerance, headache, and hyperuricemia. Increased concentration of urate in the blood is most likely due to decreased clearance of renal urate.[113]

Pyrazinamide. Pyrazinamide, a synthetic pyrazine analogue of nicotinamide, exhibits bactericidal activity against mycobacteria in an acid environment.[41] Although its precise mechanism is unknown, the drug is slowly bactericidal against the slow-growing bacilli within the acidic pH of the macrophages.[114] The unique intracellular activity of the drug has led to the incorporation of pyrazinamide into the initial

TABLE 76.9	Rifampin Drug Interactions[a]	
Agent	**Comments***	**Clinical Management**
Antacids	Further study necessary	May need to separate doses of rifampin and aluminum hydroxide
Anticoagulants, oral[b]	Decreased effect may occur.	Increase anticoagulant dose based on monitoring of INR.
Atovaquone	Atovaquone concentration may be subtherapeutic.	Monitor clinical response; increased dosage may be required.
β-Blockers	Decreased effect may occur.	May need to increase propranolol or metoprolol dose
Chloramphenicol	Chloramphenicol concentration may be subtherapeutic.	Monitor serum chloramphenicol concentration; if necessary increase dosage.
Clarithromycin	Further study necessary	Monitor signs and symptoms of infection.
Contraceptives, oral[b]	Document patient counseling. Unplanned pregnancy may occur.	Use alternative forms of birth control.
Cyclosporine[b]	Cyclosporine levels may be subtherapeutic.	Monitor serum cyclosporine concentration; increase in dosage is likely.
Dapsone	Further study is necessary when used for *Pneumocystis carinii* prophylaxis.	Monitor for hematologic toxic effects.
Diazepam	A 300% increase in diazepam oral clearance has been reported.	Monitor clinical response; increase diazepam dose if necessary.
Digitoxin[b]	Decreased effect may occur.	Monitor serum digitoxin concentration; monitor for arrhythmia control and signs and symptoms of heart failure. Increase dose if necessary.
Digoxin	Interaction is most likely to be significant in patients with renal impairment.	Monitor serum digoxin concentrations; monitor for arrhythmia control and signs and symptoms of heart failure.
Diltiazem	Alternative agent recommended because even a very large increase in oral diltiazem dose may not be sufficient (similar interaction with verapamil).	Use an alternative agent if possible.
Disopyramide	Initial study reported a reduction in disopyramide serum half-life by about 50%.	Monitor arrhythmic control; increase dose if necessary.
Doxycycline	Doxycycline concentration may be subtherapeutic.	Monitor clinical response and serum doxycycline concentrations; increased dosage may be needed.
Fluconazole	A 22% decrease in fluconazole serum half-life was reported in one trial in healthy subjects.	May need to increase fluconazole dosage; monitor signs and symptoms of infection.
Glucocorticoids[b]	Decreased effect may occur.	Increase glucocorticoid dosage twofold to threefold.
Haloperidol	Initial study indicates that serum concentrations and half-life are decreased by about 50%.	Monitor serum haloperidol levels; change dosing regimen if necessary.
Itraconazole	Decreased effect may occur.	Monitor clinical response; dosage increase is likely.
Ketoconazole[b]	Avoid combination if possible.	If used, monitor serum ketoconazole concentrations; increase dosage if necessary.
Methadone[b]	Decreased effect may occur.	Increase methadone dose; control withdrawal symptoms.
Midazolam	Decreased effect may occur.	Monitor for decreased efficacy; increase dose as necessary.
Nifedipine	Alternative class of drugs should be considered.	Monitor clinical response; increase in dosage may be necessary.
Nortriptyline	Decreased effect may occur.	Monitor clinical response and serum nortriptyline concentrations.

(continued)

TABLE 76.9	continued	
Agent	**Comments***	**Clinical Management**
Pefloxacin	Awaiting further study	Moderate rifampin induction effect; no dosage adjustment recommended.
Phenytoin[b]	Phenytoin levels may be subtherapeutic.	Monitor phenytoin serum levels; increase dose if necessary.
Propafenone	Decreased effect may occur.	Monitor arrhythmic control and serum propafenone levels; increase dose if necessary.
Quinidine[b]	Quinidine levels may be subtherapeutic.	Monitor arrhythmic control and serum quinidine levels; increase dose if necessary.
Sulfonylureas	Monitor blood glucose on discontinuation of rifampin.	Monitor blood glucose control; increase sulfonylurea dose if necessary.
Tacrolimus	Decreased effect may occur.	Monitor serum tacrolimus concentrations and clinical response; increase in dosage may be necessary.
Theophylline[b]	Theophylline levels may be subtherapeutic.	Monitor serum theophylline levels; dosage increase is likely.
Tocainamide	Approximately 30% decrease in tocainamide serum half-life was reported in one trial in healthy subjects.	Monitor arrhythmic control; increase dose if necessary.
Triazolam	Decreased effect may occur.	Monitor for decreased efficacy; increase dosage as necessary.
Verapamil[b]	Alternative agent is recommended because even a very large increase in oral verapamil dose may not be sufficient.	If used, monitor serum verapamil levels; monitor clinical response.

[a] For each interaction, when rifampin is discontinued, enzyme induction effect is slowly reduced over 1 to 2 weeks.

[b] Major clinical significance is well established.

(From Borcherding SM, Baciewicz AM, Self TH. Update on rifampin drug interactions II. Arch Intern Med 152:711–715, 1992; and Strayhorn VA, Baciewicz AM, Self TH. Update on rifampin drug interactions, III. Arch Intern Med 157:2453–2458, 1997. See references 99 and 100 for further information.)

*Rifampin's effect on co-administered agent.

phase of therapy. The drug has been used recently in short-course regimens with INH and rifampin for the treatment of TB.[115] The minimum inhibitory concentration in an acid environment is 20 μg per mL against *M tuberculosis*, although the tubercle bacilli within the monocytes are killed by concentrations of 12.5 μg per mL.[41]

Pharmacokinetics. Pyrazinamide is well absorbed from the GI tract, with peak serum concentrations occurring approximately 2 hours after ingestion. Following doses of 20 to 25 mg per kg, peak serum concentrations range from 30 to 50 μg per mL. The drug is widely distributed throughout the body, including the cerebrospinal fluid. Pyrazinamide is primarily excreted by glomerular filtration, but it is also hydrolyzed and hydroxylated. In patients with normal renal function, the elimination half-life is 9 to 10 hours. In patients with renal impairment, minor dosage adjustments may be required. The usual dosage is 15 to 30 mg/kg/day (maximum 2 g), 50 to 70 mg per kg two times a week (maximum 4 g), or 50 to 70 mg per kg three times a week (maximum 3 g).

Adverse Effects. The most common and toxic effect of pyrazinamide is dose-dependent hepatotoxicity.[41] In early studies using high doses of 3 g per day (40 to 50 mg per kg), a 15% incidence of hepatotoxicity was reported. Transient, asymptomatic elevations of serum transaminase levels are the earliest abnormalities produced by the drug. Initial 2-month regimens consisting of INH, rifampin, and pyrazinamide, which use pyrazinamide at a dosage of 15 to 30 mg per kg, do not show a significant increase in hepatotoxicity.[116,117]

Other adverse effects include hypersensitivity reactions, photosensitivity, GI intolerance, dysuria, malaise, fever, and non-gouty polyarthralgias.[41] Although polyarthralgias occur in up to 40% of patients taking daily doses of pyrazinamide, this rarely requires discontinuation of the drug or adjustment of the dosage. Aspirin or other nonsteroidal anti-inflammatory agents usually provide symptomatic relief of pyrazinamide-related arthralgias.[17] Pyrazinamide may cause elevations in prothrombin time (by decreasing prothrombin concentration or activity) and serum bilirubin levels.[41] Because pyrazinamide inhibits renal tubular secretion of uric acid, hyperuricemia occurs frequently.[118] Acute gout is uncommon; however, acute gouty attacks may be problematic in individuals with a history of gout precipitation, and this is a general contraindication to the use of this drug.

SECOND-LINE AGENTS

Streptomycin. Streptomycin, an aminoglycoside antibiotic, was the first clinically effective drug to become available for the treatment of TB.[41] The drug is bactericidal in an alkaline environment and acts by inhibiting protein synthesis. It is highly effective within the extracellular environment, but it diffuses poorly into granulomas and macrophages and lacks activity in the intracellular environment. The majority of strains of *M. tuberculosis* are inhibited in vitro at a concentration of 8 μg per mL. The drug is available as an aqueous solution in vials of 1 g. The manufacturer recommends that streptomycin (and capreomycin) be administered only intramuscularly. Difficulty arises when patients require treatment but lack sufficient body mass to tolerate intramuscular injections. Because aminoglycosides are poorly absorbed from the GI tract, the intravenous route has been used as an alternative. The National Jewish Center for Immunology and Respiratory Medicine has published its policy for administering streptomycin and capreomycin by the intravenous route.[119]

Following an intramuscular dose of 15 mg per kg, peak serum concentrations averaging approximately 40 μg per mL are achieved. Excretion is primarily renal, with the majority of drug being excreted unchanged in the urine. The half-life in blood ranges from 2 to 5 hours in patients with normal renal function. In patients with renal insufficiency, the dosage should be reduced.[53] Streptomycin has moderate tissue penetration.

Ototoxicity, the major toxic effect of streptomycin,[17] usually results in vertigo and ataxia, although hearing loss also may occur. Other adverse effects include hypersensitivity and fever. Nephrotoxicity occasionally occurs, although streptomycin has fewer adverse effects on the kidneys than do kanamycin and capreomycin. The risk of nephrotoxicity increases with age and may be increased in patients taking other nephrotoxic drugs concomitantly or in patients with preexisting renal insufficiency. It is recommended that a total cumulative dose of no more than 120 g be given because the risk of ototoxicity increases with increasing single doses and with cumulative does, particularly above 100 to 120 g.

Nephrotoxicity is less common with streptomycin than with kanamycin and capreomycin. All patients taking streptomycin should have baseline hearing and renal function tests, as well as periodic monitoring for changes. Several drug interactions are possible with concomitant administration of streptomycin. As with other aminoglycosides, although rare, streptomycin interacts with neuromuscular blocking agents, which may result in prolonged respiratory depression.[120]

Capreomycin, Kanamycin, and Amikacin.

Capreomycin, kanamycin, and amikacin are injectable aminoglycoside antibiotics that may be used in combination with other effective anti-TB drugs.[17] Concurrent administration of more than one aminoglycoside should be avoided. Capreomycin and kanamycin both inhibit protein synthesis and are tuberculostatic. Amikacin is tuberculocidal against *M. tuberculosis* in vitro.[17] Although most streptomycin-resistant strains are susceptible to both amikacin and kanamycin, there appears to be cross-resistance between the two agents. Amikacin may be more accessible than the other aminoglycosides in some areas and serum drug concentrations may be more readily available.

The monitoring parameters for these aminoglycosides are similar to those of streptomycin (refer to the earlier section on streptomycin). The risk of ototoxicity increases in the elderly and with concurrent use of diuretics. Vestibular disturbances and deafness may occur, and careful monitoring is important. Nephrotoxic effects associated with these agents may be more frequent than with streptomycin. For patients with severe hepatic disease, caution should also be exercised because of the predisposition to hepatorenal syndrome.

Paraaminosalicylic Acid. Paraaminosalicylic acid is a tuberculostatic agent rarely used in current anti-TB regimens.[41] It is a structural analogue of paraaminobenzoic acid (PABA); thus, its mechanism of action appears to be similar to that of sulfonamides, competitive antagonism of PABA. Most strains of *M. tuberculosis* in vitro are inhibited at concentrations of 1 μg per mL. The usual dose in adults and children is 150 mg per kg by mouth (maximum 10 to 12 g/day), administered in divided doses. The drug is well absorbed from the GI tract and distributes throughout the total body water, achieving high concentrations in the pleural fluid and caseous tissue. However, concentration levels in the cerebrospinal fluid are low, possibly because of active transport outward.[121,122] Following a single 4-g oral dose, plasma concentrations ranging from 75 to 100 μg per mL are achieved within 1 to 2 hours. The high dosages are necessary because the drug has an elimination half-life of about 1 hour.[41] More than 80% of the drug is eliminated in the urine; approximately 50% is in the form of an acetylated compound. The dosage should be reduced in patients with renal dysfunction. A significant sodium load is present in a dose when the tablet preparation is used.[17] In the United States, the only available formulation is granules in 4-g packets. In some countries, tablets are still available, and a solution for intravenous administration is available in Europe.[17]

The frequency of adverse effects associated with the use of paraaminosalicylic acid ranges from 10% to 30%.[41] The most frequent complaint is GI upset (i.e., nausea, vomiting, anorexia, diarrhea, and epigastric pain), which may contribute to patient nonadherence to therapy. Other adverse effects include hypersensitivity reactions in 5% to 10% of patients, thrombocytopenia, and rarely hepatitis. Probenecid blocks the renal excretion of paraaminosalicylic acid, resulting in increased plasma concentrations of paraaminosalicylic acid; caution should be exercised with this combination because of the possibility of paraaminosalicylic acid toxicity. Patients should be counseled about the importance of adherence to therapy. The drug should be administered in two to four equally divided doses with meals to minimize gastric irritation.[41]

Ethionamide. Ethionamide is an oral agent that is structurally similar to INH but has less activity.[41] Although its exact mechanism is unknown, like INH, ethionamide targets the FAS2 complex and is mycocidal.[42] It is used as a second-line agent in combination with other anti-TB agents following failure with the primary regimens. Its precise mechanism of action is unknown, although it appears to involve protein synthesis inhibition. The majority of *M. tuberculosis* strains are inhibited by concentrations of 0.6 to 2.5 μg per mL. The activity of this agent may be either tuberculostatic or tuberculocidal, depending on the susceptibility of the organism and drug concentration at the site of infection. Rapid resistance occurs in vitro, and cross-resistance occurs between ethionamide and INH. The recommended daily dose is 15 to 20 mg per kg, with a maximum dosage of 1 g per day.[17] Absorption is rapid from the GI tract following oral administration.[41] Peak concentrations of approximately 20 μg per mL are achieved in 3 hours following a 1-g dose. The serum half-life is approximately 3 hours. Ethionamide is evenly distributed into the blood and various organs. Metabolism is predominantly hepatic.

The most common adverse effects of ethionamide are anorexia, nausea, and vomiting. For most patients it is necessary to gradually increase the dose to the full amount. A useful approach to maintaining treatment is administering ethionamide at bedtime with an antiemetic drug taken 30 minutes before the dose and occasionally a hypnotic.[17] Other adverse effects include arthralgias, impotence, photosensitivity dermatitis, gynecomastia, hypothyroidism, hepatitis, and a metallic taste in the mouth. The frequency of hepatitis associated with ethionamide has been reported to be around 2%.[122,123] Hepatic enzymes should be monitored monthly and the drug should be discontinued if the hepatic enzymes reach five times normal levels, even in the absence of symptoms.

Cycloserine. Cycloserine is an anti-TB agent that is an analogue of the amino acid d-alanine. Like ethionamide, use of the drug is limited to certain situations.[17] Most strains of *M. tuberculosis* are inhibited by concentrations of 5 to 20 μg per mL, and the drug is considered to be bacteriostatic.[41] Cycloserine inhibits the processes that incorporate d-alanine in bacterial cell wall synthesis. The drug is available in 250-mg capsules. Following the usual adult dose of 10 to 15 mg/kg/day (1,000 mg), usually 500 to 750 mg per day given in two doses, the drug is rapidly absorbed from the GI tract. Cycloserine distributes into most body fluids and tissue, including the cerebrospinal fluid.

The most common adverse effects of the drug involve the CNS and range from mild reactions such as headache to severe reactions, including psychosis and seizures. These reactions tend to appear within the first 2 weeks of therapy and usually disappear on discontinuation of the drug. CNS effects of cycloserine are more likely to occur in patients who have a history of psychological problems or a chronic psychiatric condition. The mental status of these patients should be assessed regularly to monitor for these adverse effects. Other adverse effects include peripheral neuropathy, especially when the drug is used in combination with INH; thus, 100 to 200 mg per day of pyridoxine is usually administered with cycloserine. Cycloserine inhibits the hepatic metabolism of phenytoin, especially when it is taken with INH.[9] If necessary, the dosage of phenytoin should be reduced. Cycloserine is contraindicated in individuals with a history of epilepsy, depression, or severe anxiety.[41] The risk of CNS effects may be increased with concurrent use with ethionamide, INH, and alcohol.

Fluoroquinolones. Although not FDA approved for the treatment of TB, several fluoroquinolones have demonstrated activity against TB. Levofloxacin, moxifloxacin, and gatifloxacin exhibit the greatest activity against *M. tuberculosis*.[124–127] Based upon experience and safety profile with levofloxacin, this agent is the preferred oral fluoroquinolone for treatment of drug-resistant TB caused by organisms known or presumed to be sensitive to this class of drugs, or when first-line agents cannot be used. Limited data are available about the long-term safety of moxifloxacin and gatifloxacin, especially at doses above 400 mg per day. Due to concerns about the effects of the fluoroquinolones on bone and cartilage growth in children and adolescents, the long-term use of these agents (more than several weeks) has not been approved. However, most experts agree that in situations of multi–drug-resistant TB, these agents should be considered.[17] Cross-resistance appears to be a class effect and has been demonstrated among ciprofloxacin, ofloxacin, and levofloxacin.[128]

OTHER AGENTS

Thiacetazone is an anti-TB agent that is biochemically related to INH.[17] The drug is not available in the United States. However, it is used in many resource-poor developing countries because limited funds have often forced administrators of TB control programs to use suboptimal treatment regimens. Its activity is bacteriostatic, and it is more toxic than INH. Standard therapy in a large part of sub-Saharan Africa has consisted of the use of INH, thiacetazone, and streptomycin for 2 months and then INH and thiacetazone for 10 months.[129] The failure rate of this regimen is more than 10% in fully adherent HIV-seronegative patients with TB, and it is even less effective for HIV-infected patients.[129–131] Moreover, cutaneous hypersensitivity reactions have occurred in 10% to 20% of patients infected with HIV; these reactions may be severe and occasionally have been fatal.[132,133] Consequently, the World Health Organization (WHO) is seeking resources that would enable the use of supervised short-course chemotherapy with rifampin, including regimens in countries in which the prevalence of HIV and TB is high.[134] The vestibular toxicity associated with the use of streptomycin may be potentiated by the concurrent use of thiacetazone.

Amoxicillin is an aminopenicillin with a broad spectrum of antibacterial activity against many gram-positive and gram-negative microorganisms. The in vitro activity against *M. tuberculosis* is greatly enhanced by the addition of a β-lactamase inhibitor to amoxicillin.[135] The β-lactamase inhibitors (e.g., clavulanic acid) lack intrinsic antimycobacterial activity; however, they inhibit the enzyme that is partially responsible for the resistance of *M. tuberculosis* to β-lactam antibiotics. A 7-day study compared the activity of amoxicillin/clavulanate, ofloxacin, and INH by measuring the effects on recovery of *M. tuberculosis* colony-forming units from sputum of patients with smear-positive TB.[136] The results of early bactericidal activity of amoxicillin/clavulanate was comparable to the activity reported for anti-TB agents other than INH. Further studies are necessary to define the role of β-lactam antibiotics as anti-TB agents.

Other agents under investigation include sulfonamides, macrolides, folate antagonists, and interferon-γ administered via aerosolization.[137]

INITIATING TREATMENT AND RECOMMENDED TREATMENT REGIMENS

Patients suspected of having TB should have the appropriate specimens collected for microscopic examination and culture prior to initiation of therapy. For pulmonary TB, three sputum specimens should be obtained 6 to 24 hours apart.

Susceptibility testing for INH, rifampin, and ethambutol should be performed on an initial positive culture. Patients should be placed in an AFB isolation room, which has negative pressure meeting appropriate criteria, to prevent transmission of *M. tuberculosis* to others.[17] All patients with TB should receive counseling and testing for HIV infection; patients with epidemiologic factors suggesting a risk for hepatitis B or C should also have serologic tests for these viruses.

Four basic regimens are available for the treatment of TB caused by organisms that are known or presumed to be susceptible to the first-line agents INH, rifampin, pyrazinamide, and ethambutol (Table 76.10).[17] A four-drug regimen is used initially for all patients based on the findings of the current proportion of TB cases that are caused by INH-resistant strains. For children the regimens used are the same, although depending on the circumstances, ethambutol may not be used in the initial phase of the regimen (refer to the ethambutol section). Several studies in children have shown a success rate greater than 95% with a three-drug combination of INH and rifampin, with pyrazinamide supplemented during the first 2 months of therapy. For adults, each regimen has a 2-month initial phase in which INH, rifampin, pyrazinamide, and ethambutol are given daily throughout, daily for 2 weeks followed by twice weekly for 6 weeks or three times a week, followed by a selection of several options for the continuation phase of either 4 or 7 months (Table 76.10).

TABLE 76.10	Drug Regimens for Culture-Positive Pulmonary TB Caused by Drug-Susceptible Organism			
Regimens	**Initial Phase Interval and Doses (minimum duration)**	**Continuation Phase Interval and Doses (minimum and doses)**		
Regimen 1: INH, rifampin, pyrazinamide, ethambutol	7 days/wk × 56 doses (8 weeks) or 5 days/wk × 40 doses (8 weeks)[a]	1a. INH/rifampin	7 days/wk × 126 doses (18 weeks) or 5 days/wk × 90 doses (18 weeks)	
		1b. INH/rifampin 1c. INH/RPT[b]	Twice weekly × 36 doses (18 weeks) Once weekly × 18 doses (18 weeks)	
Regimen 2: INH, rifampin, pyrazinamide, ethambutol	7 days/wk × 14 doses (2 weeks); then twice daily × 12 doses (6 weeks) or 5 days/wk × 10 doses (2 weeks),[a] then twice weekly × 12 doses (6 weeks)	2a. INH/rifampin 2b. INH/RPT[b]	Twice weekly × 36 doses (18 weeks) Once weekly × 18 doses (18 weeks)	
Regimen 3: INH, rifampin, pyrazinamide, ethambutol	Three times weekly × 24 doses (8 weeks)	3a. INH/rifampin	Three times weekly × 54 doses (18 wk)	
Regimen 4: INH, rifampin, ethambutol	7 days/wk × 56 doses (8 weeks) or 5 days/wk × 40 doses (8 weeks)[a]	4a. INH/rifampin 4b. INH/rifapentine	7 days/wk × 217 doses (31 weeks) or 5 days/wk × 155 doses (31 weeks) Twice weekly × 62 doses (31 weeks)	

[a] 5-day-a-week administration is always given by DOT.

[b] Options 1c and 2b should be used only in HIV-negative patients who have negative sputum smears at the time of completion of 2 months of therapy.

(Adapted from American Thoracic Society, CDC, and Infectious Diseases Society of America. Treatment of tuberculosis. Am J Resp Crit Care Med 167:603–662, 2003.)

Currently, the minimal duration of treatment for adults and children with culture-positive TB is 6 months (26 weeks).

Baseline measurements of AST, bilirubin, alkaline phosphatase, serum creatinine, a complete blood count, and a platelet count are required for adults who are treated for TB.[9] The serum uric acid level should be measured if pyrazinamide is used. Baseline examination of visual acuity and color vision is necessary for patients who are to be treated with ethambutol. Baseline tests are useful in detecting abnormalities that may complicate a regimen; adjustments in dosages may be necessary on the basis of these values. They also provide a means of comparison with measurements obtained during therapy if an adverse reaction is suspected.

For patients with HIV infection, the recommendations for the treatment of TB in adults are essentially the same as those for adults without HIV infection: a 6-month regimen consisting of an initial phase of INH, rifampin, pyrazinamide, and ethambutol given for 2 months followed by INH and rifampin for 4 months when TB is known or presumed to be susceptible to the first-line agents.[17] The regimen may be given as daily or intermittently (Table 76.10). However, data in patients with advanced HIV disease (CD4+ cell counts below 100) reveal an increased frequency of rifamycin resistance. Thus, patients with advanced HIV disease should be treated with daily or three-times-weekly therapy in the continuation phase and twice-weekly drug administration in the continuation phase should not be used in patients with CD4+ cell counts below 100. Patients with less advanced HIV disease may be considered for twice-weekly therapy. Once-weekly administration of INH and rifapentine in the continuation phase should be avoided in any patient with HIV infection. For management of children and adolescents with HIV infection and pulmonary TB, the American Academy of Pediatrics recommends that initial therapy should always include at least three drugs and the total duration of therapy should be at least 9 months, although data to support this recommendation are lacking.

Another important aspect to consider when selecting a TB treatment regimen in patients with HIV infection are the drug interactions between rifampin, a potent CYP-450 inducer (refer to the rifamycin section), and the antiretroviral classes PI or NNRTI. Because rifampin markedly lowers serum levels of PIs and NNRTIs due to induction of cytochrome P450 CYP-3, suboptimal antiretroviral activity and subsequently acquired drug resistance may occur. Rifabutin has a role in treating patients with HIV infection on antiretroviral agents with TB due to its clinical efficacy and because it has less of an effect on induction of hepatic enzymes than rifampin.[17]

DIRECTLY OBSERVED THERAPY

Patient adherence to anti-TB therapy is essential to achieve positive outcomes for both the patient and the community where he or she lives. Yet there are many factors that can interfere with adherence to these treatment regimens, such as cultural and linguistic barriers to cooperation, lifestyle differences, homelessness, substance abuse, and many other conditions that are competing priorities for the patient. When initiating an anti-TB regimen it is important to take a patient-centered approach and to determine an appropriate care plan.

Patient-centered TB treatment programs are important because they are designed to incorporate a broad range of approaches based on the needs and circumstances of individual patients. Directly observed therapy (DOT) is the preferred initial strategy recommended for all regimens to ensure patient adherence to anti-TB medications.[17,138,139] DOT can be provided daily or intermittently and can be administered in the clinical setting or any mutually agreeable site (e.g., patient's home, place of employment, school, street corner). In DOT the patient is observed by a health care provider or other responsible person as the patient ingests the anti-TB medications. In addition, DOT provides the opportunity for patient education and also enables earlier detection of adverse effects.[140] DOT has been used in both low-incidence and high-incidence areas of TB. The data from published studies of DOT in high incidence areas have yielded mixed results. In two studies DOT did not demonstrate benefit, and in one study there was a significant advantage for DOT.[140–142] The studies did show the importance of aggressive interventions when patients missed doses rather than merely limiting DOT to passive observation of medication ingestion. Clinical experience with different DOT regimens suggests that patients being managed by DOT administered 5 days a week have a rate of successful therapy similar to those being given drugs 7 days a week. Therefore, a practical approach may be for ''daily therapy'' to be given for 5 days a week, and the required number of doses can be adjusted accordingly.

The involvement of pharmacists in DOT programs will be beneficial for several reasons. Not only can pharmacists promote patient adherence to therapy, but they also can provide drug information to patients and monitor for drug-induced adverse effects.[139] It is important to keep in mind that DOT does not ensure adherence because it does not guarantee ingestion of all doses of every medication. For example, patients may miss appointments or may not actually swallow the pills. Thus, monitoring response to DOT is an important aspect of a patient-centered regimen.

The cost of implementing DOT is more than offset by the savings that result from the decreased risk of treatment failure, relapse, drug resistance, and secondary spread.[17,138] This patient-centered approach appears to be effective in a variety of high-risk groups such as the homeless, refugees, the unemployed, substance abusers, and patients with HIV infection.[143,144] In addition, this strategy appears effective regardless of the country or community where the program is implemented. DOT should be considered in all patients who are treated for TB and is strongly recommended in patients with HIV infection; there appears to be a reduced degree of safety in treating patients with HIV infection, and patient adherence to anti-TB therapy is crucial. The options available for administration with DOT are listed in Table

76.10.[17] DOT also should be used in children who are treated for TB.

Anti-TB regimens can be simplified by using fixed-dose combination preparations. Experts suggest that fixed-dose combination formulations should be used when DOT is given daily and when DOT is not possible.[17] The WHO and the International Union Against Tuberculosis and Lung Disease (IUATLD) strongly recommend use of the combination formulations as a means of simplifying regimens and improving patient adherence to therapy. A four-drug combination formulation is available in some countries. When DOT is not administered, combination preparations can decrease the risk of the patient taking only one drug and thus may help minimize the development of drug resistance. Two combination preparations are available in the United States: a combination of INH, rifampin, and pyrazinamide (Rifater) and a combination of INH and rifampin (Rifamate).

From a psychosocial perspective, treatment of TB should take into account several considerations. Health care workers should provide compassionate care and offer support services to patients, caregivers, and family members who will be involved with the care of the patient. Clinicians should identify whether depression, anxiety, fear, or feelings of isolation are present and refer the patient to a clinical specialist and support groups. Because TB may have negative connotations, clinicians should educate patients about the disease and assure them that having TB should not be viewed as shameful. It is also important for clinicians to provide information to the patient regarding infectivity that will allow the individual to know when he or she can return to daily activities.

DRUG-RESISTANT TUBERCULOSIS

Combination anti-TB therapy is necessary to prevent the emergence of a drug-resistant population as a result of the selection pressure from administration of a single agent.[17] Of the first-line agents, INH and rifampin have considerable ability to prevent the emergence of drug resistance when given with another drug. Ethambutol and streptomycin are also effective in preventing the emergence of drug resistance, but pyrazinamide is not very effective in this regard. Resistance to antimycobacterial agents in general is chromosomal.[42] INH resistance generally results from a mutation in the mycobacterial enzyme catalase-peroxidase, whose role is to activate INH, thus enabling the drug to exert its mycobacterial effect; ethambutol resistance typically results from mutations in, or overexpression of, target enzymes.

Multi–drug-resistant TB is defined as a case of TB caused by a strain of *M. tuberculosis* that exhibits resistance to at least INH and rifampin.[4,5] Microbial resistance to anti-TB agents may be classified as either primary or acquired.[4] Primary drug resistance occurs in patients without a history or other evidence of prior treatment. Various risk factors for primary resistance include coming from a country with a high prevalence of drug-resistant TB, exposure to a patient with drug-resistant TB, and greater than 4% primary resis-

tance to INH within the community.[17] Acquired drug resistance occurs in patients who have been treated with anti-TB agents for at least 1 month, including those with treatment failures and relapses.[4] The quality of TB treatment affects the development of both types of resistance. Inadequate treatment allows the emergence of resistant organisms, producing acquired drug resistance in patients who are inadequately treated. Once these organisms are transmitted and TB develops, the infected person has ''primary'' resistant disease. It is estimated that the average cost for treating a case of multi–drug-resistant is $180,000, which is much more costly than treating a case caused by a drug-susceptible strain ($12,000).[144,145]

Although the exact magnitude of worldwide drug resistance is unknown, surveillance of the prevalence of resistance in 35 countries suggests that this is a global problem.[4] ''Hot zones'' of ongoing transmission have been identified in several countries. In 1994 the Global Project on Anti-Tuberculosis Drug Resistance Surveillance was initiated by the WHO and the IUATLD. The purpose was to use standardized methods to measure the prevalence of resistance to anti-TB drugs in countries throughout the world.[4] The results of the first 4 years of the project were published and contained information on drug resistance to INH, rifampin, ethambutol, and streptomycin in 35 countries or regions on five continents. Results revealed that primary multidrug resistance was observed in every country surveyed except Kenya, and the median prevalence was 1.4% (range 0% to 14.4%). In persons with acquired drug resistance the median prevalence of multidrug resistance multi–drug was 13% (range 0% to 54%), much higher than the rate due to primary resistance. The overall prevalence of multi–drug-resistant TB was 2.2% (range 0% to 22.1%). Although the overall prevalence reported is low, the high prevalences in the former Soviet Union, Asia, the Dominican Republic, and Argentina are concerning. A recent reversal of previously declining rates of TB in Eastern Europe and in particular the former Soviet Union probably is due to an irregular supply of drugs and nonstandardized regimens; other contributing factors may include nosocomial infection and outbreaks in prisons.[4,146,147] The relationship between drug resistance and the quality of TB control programs is complex; however, there may be a link between the quality of TB control programs and levels of drug resistance.[4]

EXTRAPULMONARY TUBERCULOSIS

Extrapulmonary sites most commonly associated with TB include the lymph nodes, pleura, genitourinary tract, bones and joints, meninges, and peritoneum. The general treatment principles of pulmonary TB are also applied to extrapulmonary TB. Although the data evaluating the treatment of extrapulmonary TB are limited, increasing evidence suggests that 6- to 9-month regimens that include INH and rifampin are effective. As with pulmonary TB, a 6-month regimen is recommended for treating TB that includes any site with the exception of the meninges, for which a 9- to 12-month regimen is recommended. Response to therapy must be carefully monitored; for patients who are slow to respond, an extension of therapy should be considered. The addition of glucocorticoids for adjunctive therapy of TB is recommended in the management of TB pericarditis and TB meningitis. The potent anti-inflammatory activity of glucocorticoids is beneficial in a disease such as TB where the host response plays such an important role. The use of glucocorticoids can accelerate clinical improvement and reduce mortality in effusive-constrictive pericarditis and can decrease neurologic sequelae in meningitis. In general, prednisone may be administered at a daily dose of 20 to 60 mg for up to 6 weeks. Dexamethasone, in dosages up to 12 mg per day, is the preferred drug in TB meningitis. It is important to monitor the interaction of rifampin with glucocorticoids, which results in an accelerated metabolism and potential adrenal crises (Table 76.9).

MONITORING RESPONSE TO ANTITUBERCULOSIS THERAPY

During the treatment of patients with pulmonary TB, bacteriologic evaluation is the preferred method of monitoring response to therapy. A sputum specimen for AFB smear and culture should be obtained at monthly intervals until two consecutive specimens are negative on culture. More than 80% of patients with positive pretreatment cultures should convert to negative after 2 months of therapy with regimens consisting of INH and rifampin. If drug resistance is not demonstrated, the treatment should be continued with DOT. If resistant organisms are present, the treatment regimen should be modified and must include at least two drugs to which the organisms are susceptible (refer to the section on management of drug-resistant TB).

Patients whose sputum converts to negative following 2 months of therapy require at least one further sputum smear and culture performed at the completion of therapy.[9] Chest radiographs during therapy are not as useful as sputum examination; on completion of therapy, a chest radiograph provides a baseline for comparison with future radiographs. Routine follow-up is not necessary for patients with susceptible organisms who exhibit a prompt and adequate bacteriologic response following therapy with regimens containing INH and rifampin. Patients whose sputum cultures do not convert to negative following 3 months of therapy should have drug susceptibility testing repeated. Patients with positive cultures following 4 months of treatment should be considered as having failed treatment and managed accordingly. Monitoring patients with extrapulmonary TB is more difficult and many times not feasible. In such cases, patients should be assessed clinically.

All patients, adults and children, who are receiving anti-TB therapy should be monitored clinically for adverse drug effects and should be instructed to watch for common adverse effects of their medications.[9] Routine monitoring of liver or renal function or platelet count is not necessary unless there were abnormalities at baseline or there are clinical reasons for obtaining measurements. Patients with abnormalities of hepatic or renal function at baseline should have repeat measurements early in the course of treatment and regularly to ensure that there has not been any worsening. In general, routine laboratory monitoring for toxicity in patients with normal baseline tests is not necessary. Should symptoms suggest drug toxicity, appropriate laboratory testing should be performed to confirm or exclude such toxicity.

MANAGING TREATMENT FAILURE AND RELAPSE

Patients whose sputum does not convert to negative after 3 months of what should be effective treatment are suspected of treatment failure, and those whose sputum cultures remain positive after 4 months of treatment are considered treatment failures.[17] Treatment failure may be the result of nonadherence to the drug regimen, drug resistance, malabsorption of drugs, laboratory error, and extreme biologic variation in response.[17] A current sputum specimen should be obtained and susceptibility testing should be performed at this time. The currently used regimen may be continued while the results are pending, or at least three drugs that are not part of the current regimen can be added. Once the results of the susceptibility testing are available, the regimen should be adjusted accordingly and DOT should be used.

Unlike patients who are treatment failures, patients who relapse after completion of a regimen containing INH and rifampin with organisms that are susceptible to the drugs at the start of therapy usually maintain susceptibility to these agents.[17] Relapses generally occur within the first 6 to 12 months following completion of therapy. In general, the management of these patients involves reinstitution of the regimen previously used with DOT. If drug susceptibility testing reveals resistant organisms, the regimen must be modified and reinstituted.

MANAGEMENT OF TUBERCULOSIS CAUSED BY DRUG-RESISTANT ORGANISMS

Managing patients with TB caused by drug-resistant organisms is extremely challenging. These patients require specialized treatment because they are at high risk for treatment failure and further acquired resistance.[148] In several outbreaks of multi–drug-resistant TB, organisms were resistant to both INH and rifampin and frequently to ethambutol, as well as to other agents.[17] In these situations the response to treatment with standard initial regimens is poor. Because most cases of multi–drug-resistant TB have occurred among adults infected with HIV, there has been transmission of infection and progression to disease among their contacts.

When initiating therapy for TB, clinicians should be aware of the prevalence of drug resistance in their communities, as well as the epidemiologic features of the people who are most likely to be carrying these organisms.[17] Patients with newly diagnosed TB should have drug susceptibility testing performed in a competent laboratory on the organisms that were initially isolated. The earliest identification of growth can be achieved by radiometric or colorimetric detection techniques. If performance of full drug susceptibility studies is not possible, testing for resistance to rifampin can identify strains that are likely to have multiple drug resistance. Because controlled or randomized studies have not been performed among patients with various patterns of drug resistance, guidelines are available for the treatment of drug-resistant TB that are based upon general principles, extrapolations, and expert opinion.[17]

Good data are not available on the efficacy and duration of therapy of various regimens used for patients with organisms resistant to both INH and rifampin.[17] On discovery of drug resistance, it is likely that many patients will demonstrate resistance to other first-line agents. In managing patients who show resistance to one or more drugs, at least two drugs, preferably three, to which the organism is susceptible should be used, with continuation of this regimen until sputum conversion is documented. Patients with multi–drug-resistant TB in which there is resistance to first-line agents in addition to INH and rifampin should be placed on regimens that use four to six medications. Current treatment regimens for treatment of multi–drug-resistant TB use drugs that are less effective and more toxic and often must be administered for 12 to 18 months. For strains resistant to INH and rifampin, combinations of ethambutol, pyrazinamide, and streptomycin, in addition to another injectable agent (i.e., amikacin), and possibly a fluoroquinolone can be administered for 12 to 18 months and for at least 9 months after sputum conversion. Resistance to rifampin is nearly always associated with cross-resistance to rifabutin and rifapentine.

A strategy that includes DOT, along with specific provisions for treating multi–drug-resistant TB, has been proposed by a group of TB experts.[148] This approach has been termed ''DOTS-plus'' and is designed to triage patients to individualized treatment regimens or, if possible, into empirical retreatment schemes appropriate to the local epidemiology.[148] A community-based approach to treating multi–drug-resistant TB in Peru using ''DOTS-plus'' obtained successful results.[147] This recently introduced strategy holds great promise for use in other areas with outbreaks of multi–drug-resistant TB.

SPECIAL TREATMENT CIRCUMSTANCES

PREGNANT AND LACTATING PATIENTS

In pregnant women with TB, the benefits of treatment outweigh the risks. Treatment of a pregnant woman with suspected TB should be started if the probability of TB is moderate to high. The regimen should include INH, rifampin, and ethambutol (unless primary INH resistance is likely). Although these agents cross the placenta, they do not appear to have teratogenic effects. Pyridoxine is recommended when INH is used. Because of inadequate teratogenic data, pyrazinamide is not recommended, although it can probably

be used safely during pregnancy and is recommended by the WHO and the IUATLD. Treatment of TB during pregnancy should be for a minimum of 9 months if pyrazinamide is not used as part of the initial regimen. Other drugs that should be avoided include streptomycin, kanamycin, capreomycin, cycloserine, and ethionamide. Of these, streptomycin is the only one with documented teratogenic effects (interference with ear development and congenital deafness).[17,149,150]

Small concentrations of anti-TB drugs are present in breast milk. However, breast-feeding should not be discouraged in women being treated with first line-agents because the small concentrations of these agents in breast milk do not cause toxicity in the newborn. Breast-feeding is not considered an effective treatment for treatment of TB or latent TB infection in the nursing infant.[17,151] As with pregnancy, supplemental pyridoxine is recommended for the nursing mother receiving INH.

PREVENTION

The most effective way to prevent TB is to diagnose patients with TB rapidly and to initiate anti-TB therapy with the goal of achieving cure. Administration of preventive chemotherapy and BCG vaccination are additional strategies.

TREATMENT OF LATENT TUBERCULOSIS INFECTION

An important component of TB control is the treatment of LTBI to prevent active disease in individuals with a positive TST and who are at risk of reactivation of TB. This strategy, once termed ''preventive therapy,'' is based upon results of clinical studies that found a significant (over 90%) reduction in the risk of active TB in patients who received a 6- to 12-month course of INH. The benefits of treating LTBI outweigh the risk of adverse effects of INH.

Adherence to INH therapy for a 6- to 12-month period has been challenging due to the relatively long duration of therapy and concerns regarding toxicity. Therefore, there has been increasing interest in the development of shorter, rifampin-based regimens that could be used as alternatives to the mainstay of treatment for LTBI with INH. A randomized, open-label controlled trial in the United States compared an alternative short-course regimen consisting of daily rifampin and pyrazinamide for treatment of LTBI to a 6- to 12-month daily INH regimen in persons with HIV infection.[152] The study examined 1583 HIV-positive persons aged 13 years or older with a positive TST. Culture-confirmed TB was the primary endpoint and proven or probable TB, adverse events, and death, compared by treatment group, were secondary endpoints. The results showed a similar outcome in terms of safety and efficacy of the two regimens. The short-course regimen offers practical advantages over the INH regimen.

Specific evaluations must be completed before institution of treatment of LTBI for individuals with a positive TST (refer to Tuberculin Skin Testing section). These evaluations include determining whether therapy for LTBI is warranted, ruling out active disease, and identifying any contraindications to therapy.

Four regimens are recommended for the treatment of adults with LTBI. One of the regimens used for treatment of LTBI in non–HIV-infected persons is a 9-month course of INH daily (5 mg/kg, maximum 300 mg/day). A shorter regimen—INH daily for 6 months in HIV-negative adults—may provide a more favorable outcome from a cost-effectiveness standpoint. For HIV-positive persons, INH should be administered for 9 months. Shorter regimens for adults are 2 months of daily rifampin plus pyrazinamide or rifampin daily for 4 months. According to the American Academy of Pediatrics, children should receive 9 months of INH therapy either daily or twice weekly.

USE OF BACILLE CALMETTE-GUÉRIN VACCINE

BCG vaccines are live vaccines derived from an attenuated strain of *M. bovis*.[14,153] The vaccine was first administered to humans in the early 1920s. BCG vaccination is usually administered by the intradermal method and often results in local adverse effects; serious or long-term complications are rare.[154] The health care provider should refer to the package labeling prior to administration for the specified dosage and route indicated because there are many different BCG vaccines available worldwide that are derived from the original strain. The vaccines vary in efficacy; estimates of efficacy rates have ranged from 0% to 80% in randomized, placebo-controlled trials and in case-control studies.[14,153] Higher rates of efficacy in the protection of young children have been observed in prevention of more serious forms of TB, such as TB meningitis and miliary TB.[14,153]

In the United States, the risk for TB infection in the overall population is low and a national policy is not indicated for BCG vaccination.[153] Furthermore, the use of BCG vaccine is limited because its efficacy is uncertain in preventing infectious forms of TB, and the reactivity to tuberculin that occurs after vaccination interferes with the management of persons who are possibly infected with TB.[153] Therefore, the use of BCG vaccine in the United States is reserved for situations in which individuals meet the following specific criteria:

- Infants and children who live in high-risk settings if that no other options are available (i.e., removing the child from the source of infection)
- Health care providers who work in settings in which the likelihood of transmission and infection with multi–drug-resistant TB is high and the TB control precautions have failed.

Although BCG is an alternative to preventive therapy in cases discussed in the preceding section, it should not be used if there is other active infection, depressed host immunity (e.g., HIV infection, therapy with immunosuppressive drugs), or pregnancy.[14,153]

Because many developing countries lack the ability to diagnose HIV infection in newborns and because TB transmission to children is common in these countries, WHO recommends that all infants in Africa without symptomatic HIV infection continue to receive BCG vaccine.[154] The benefits of BCG outweigh the risk in infants without HIV infection and possibly infants infected with HIV who are not yet immunocompromised; however, as previously mentioned, the BCG vaccination is contraindicated in adults infected with HIV.

CONCLUSION

Unfortunately, TB is not a conquered disease of the past. The resurgence of TB and the rising prevalence of drug resistance worldwide indicate that the battle is being lost.[138] Several factors have been identified that are contributing to this deteriorating situation. Inadequate implementation of preventive TB measures delays the diagnosis of TB, which facilitates transmission to others. Other factors include the problems of homelessness, poverty, substance abuse, and the HIV epidemic.[138] In addition, insufficient funding of TB control programs, lack of accessibility to anti-TB medications, and counterfeit anti-TB agents in various countries are important issues that require exploration and commitment by government agencies, the pharmaceutical industry, and health care providers.

Drug therapy continues to be the cornerstone of an effective TB treatment plan, enabling TB to be a curable and preventable disease.[17] Advances in drug development, including a more effective vaccine, will assist in the elimination of TB. Of equal importance, rapid patient identification and isolation are necessary components of TB control programs. Various strategies have been developed to ensure effective therapy of TB.[17] DOT will eliminate patient nonadherence to therapy and can be administered two or three times a week. The overall clinical and social management of patients with TB and their contacts is the ultimate goal. In this setting, the success of therapy is achievable.

KEY POINTS

- TB is a global public health problem
- TB is transmitted by aerosolized droplet nuclei
- Transmission can be reduced by adequate ventilation and ultraviolet lighting
- Close contacts are highly susceptible
- Contact investigation is an important component of TB prevention and control

SUGGESTED READINGS

American Thoracic Society, CDC, and Infectious Diseases Society of America. Treatment of tuberculosis. Am J Resp Critical Care Med 167:603–662, 2003.

Notice to readers: updated guidelines for the use of rifamycins for the treatment of tuberculosis among HIV-infected patients taking protease inhibitors or nonnucleoside reverse transcriptase inhibitors. MMWR 53:37, 2004. (New guidelines regarding interactions among these agents with recommendations for their use from CDC and partners are available at http://www.cdc.gov/nchstp/tb/tb_hiv_drugs/toc.htm.)

Sterling TR, Lehmann HP, Frieden TR. Impact of DOTS compared with DOTS-plus on multidrug resistant tuberculosis and tuberculosis deaths: decision analysis. Br Med J 326: 574–79, 2003.

Transmission of Mycobacterium tuberculosis associated with failed completion of treatment of latent tuberculosis infection, Chickasaw County, Mississippi. MMWR 52:222–224, 2003.

Update: adverse event data and revised American Thoracic Society/CDC recommendations against the use of rifampin and pyrazinamide for treatment of latent tuberculosis infection. MMWR 52:735–739, 2003.

REFERENCES

1. WHO. Global tuberculosis control: surveillance, planning and financing report, 2004.
2. Cahn P, Perez H, Ben G, et al. Tuberculosis and HIV: a partnership against the most vulnerable. J Int Assoc Physicians ADIS Care 2:106–123, 2003.
3. Corbett EL, Watt CJ, Walker N, et al. The growing burden of tuberculosis: global trends and interactions with the HIV epidemic. Arch Intern Med 163:1009–1021, 2003.
4. Pablos-Mendez A, Raviglione MC, Laszlo A, et al. Global surveillance for antituberculosis drug resistance, 1994–1997. N Engl J Med 338:1641–1649, 1998.
5. Cohn DL, Bustreo F, Raviglione MC. Drug-resistant tuberculosis: review of the worldwide situation and the WHO/IUATLD global surveillance project. Clin Infect Dis 24:S121–130, 1997.
6. Raviglione MC, O'Brien RJ. Tuberculosis. In: Braunwald E, Fauci AS, Isslebacher KJ, et al, eds. Harrison's principles of internal medicine, 15th ed. New York: McGraw-Hill, 2001:1024–1034.
7. Morse D, Brothwell DR, Ucko PJ. Tuberculosis in ancient Egypt. Am Rev Resp Dis 90:524–541, 1964.
8. Smith KC, Starke JR. Bacille Calmette-Guérin vaccine. In Plotkin SA, Orenstein WA, eds. Vaccines, 4th ed. Philadelphia: Elsevier Inc., 2004:179–209.
9. Bloom BR, Murray CJL. Tuberculosis: commentary on a re-emergent killer. Science 257:1055–1064, 1992.
10. Nemir RL. Perspectives in adolescent tuberculosis: three decades of experience. Pediatrics 78:399–404, 1986.
11. Raviglione MC, Snider DE Jr, Kochi A. Global epidemiology of tuberculosis. Morbidity and Mortality of a worldwide epidemic. JAMA 273:220–226, 1995.
12. Haas DW. Mycobacterium tuberculosis. In Mandell GL, Bennett JE, Dolin R, eds. Mandell, Douglas, and Bennett's principles and practice of infectious diseases, 5th ed. New York: Churchill Livingston, 2000:2576–2607.
13. World Health Organization. Groups at risks: WHO report on the tuberculosis epidemic. Geneva. Switzerland, WHO, 1996.
14. CDC. Reported tuberculosis cases in the U.S., 2002. Atlanta: U.S. Department of Health and Human Services, CDC, September 2003.
15. Daley CL, Small M, Schecter F, et al. An outbreak of tuberculosis with accelerated progression among persons infected with the human immunodeficiency virus. N Engl J Med 326:231–235, 1992.
16. Selwyn P, Hartel D, Lewis V, et al. A prospective study of the risk of tuberculosis among intravenous drug users with human immunodeficiency virus infection. N Engl J Med 320:545–550, 1989.
17. American Thoracic Society, CDC, and Infectious Diseases Society of America. Treatment of tuberculosis. Am J Resp Crit Care Med 167:603–662, 2003.
18. CDC. Targeted tuberculin testing and treatment of latent tuberculosis infection. MMWR 49 (RR6):1–45, 2000.
19. Nelson KE, Solomon L, Bonds M, et al. Prevalence of tuberculin positivity and skin anergy in HIV-1 seropositive and seronegative intravenous drug users. JAMA 267: 369–373, 1992.
20. CDC. Anergy skin testing and preventive therapy for HIV-infected persons: revised recommendations. MMWR 46 (RR15):1–10, 1997.
21. CDC. Targeted tuberculin testing and treatment. MMWR 49 (RR06):1–54, 2000.
22. Klein NC, Duncanson FP, Lenox TH III. Use of mycobacterial smears in the diagnosis of pulmonary tuberculosis in AIDS/ARC patients. Chest 95:1190–1192, 1989.
23. Long R, Scalcini M, Manfreda J, et al. The impact of HIV on the usefulness of sputum smears for the diagnosis of tuberculosis. Am J Public Health 81:1326–1328, 1991.
24. Elliot AM, Namaambo K, Allen BW, et al. Negative sputum smear results in HIV-positive patients with pulmonary tuberculosis in Lusaka, Zambia. Tuber Lung Dis 74:191–194, 1993.
25. Casal M, Gutierrex J, Vaquero M. Comparative evaluation of the Mycobacteria Growth Indicator Tube with the BACTEC 460 TB system and Lowenstein-Jensen medium for isolation of mycobacteria from clinical specimens. Int J Tuberc Lung Dis 1:81–84, 1997.
26. Van Scog RE, Wilkowske CJ. Antituberculous agents. Mayo Clin Proc 67:179–187, 1992.
27. Mitchison DA. Development of streptomycin-resistant strains of tubercle bacilli in pulmonary tuberculosis: results of simultaneous sensitivity tests in liquid and on solid media. Thorax 5:144–146, 1950.
28. Canetti G. Present aspects of bacterial resistance in tuberculosis. Am Rev Resp Dis 92:687–703, 1965.
29. Hobby GL. Primary drug resistance in tuberculosis: a review. Am Rev Resp Dis 86:839–846, 1962.
30. Hobby GL. Primary drug resistance in tuberculosis: a review. Am Rev Resp Dis 87:29–36, 1963.
31. Doster B, Caras CJ, Snider DE. A continuing survey of primary drug resistance in tuberculosis, 1961 to 1968: a U.S. Public Health Service cooperative study. Am Rev Resp Dis 113:419–427, 1976.
32. Kopnoff C, Kilburn JO, Glassroth JL, et al. A continuing survey of tuberculosis primary drug resistance in the United States: March 1975 to November 1977: a United States Public Health Service cooperative study. Am Rev Respr Dis 118:835–842, 1978.
33. Snider DE, Cauthen GM, Farer LS, et al. Drug-resistant tuberculosis. Am Rev Resp Dis 144:732, 1991.
34. Iseman MD. Treatment of multidrug-resistant tuberculosis. N Engl J Med 329:784–791, 1993.
35. Perez-Stable EJ, Hopewell PC. Chemotherapy of tuberculosis. Semin Respir Med 9:459, 1988.
36. Hooker KD, Jost PM. Tuberculosis. In: Herfindal ET, Gourley DR, Hart LL, eds. Clinical pharmacy and therapeutics, 5th ed. Baltimore: Williams & Wilkins, 1992:1092–1108.
37. Aquinas SM. Short-course therapy for tuberculosis. Drugs 24: 118–132, 1982.
38. Angel JH. The case for short-course chemotherapy of pulmonary tuberculosis. Drugs 27:1–8, 1983.
39. Stratton MA, Reed MD. Short-course drug therapy for tuberculosis. Clin Pharm 5:977–987, 1986.
40. Takayama K, Schnoes HK, Armstrong EL, et al. Site of inhibitory action of isoniazid in the synthesis of mycolic acids in Mycobacterium tuberculosis. J Lipid Res 16:308–317, 1975.
41. Petri WA. Drugs used in the chemotherapy of tuberculosis, Mycobacterium avium complex disease, and leprosy. In Hardman JG, Limbird LE, eds. Goodman & Gilman's The pharmacological basis of therapeutics, 10th ed. New York: Macmillan, 1996:1273–1286.
42. Arnaout RA, Rando RR. Pharmacology of the bacterial cell wall. In Golan DE, Tashjian AH, Armstrong EJ, et al, eds. Principles of pharmacology, the pathophysiologic basis of drug therapy, 1st ed. Philadelphia: Lippincott Williams & Wilkins, 2005:569–576.
43. Dickinson JM, Aber VR, Mitchison DA. Bactericidal activity of streptomycin, isoniazid, rifampin, ethambutol, and pyrazinamide alone and in combination against Mycobacterium tuberculosis. Am Rev Resp Dis 116:627–635, 1977.
44. Hurwitz A, Schlozman DL. Effect of antacids on gastrointestinal absorption of isoniazid in rat and man. Am Rev Respr Dis 109: 41–47, 1974.
45. Holdiness MR. Cerebrospinal fluid pharmacokinetics of antituberculous antibiotics. Clin Pharmacokinet 10:532–534, 1985.

46. Maddrey WC, Boitnott JK. Isoniazid hepatitis. Ann Intern Med 79: 1–12, 1973.

47. Mitchell JR, Zimmerman HJ, Ishak KG. Isoniazid liver injury: clinical spectrum, pathology and probable pathogenesis. Ann Intern Med 84:181–192, 1976.

48. Evans D, Manley KA, McKusick VA. Genetic control of isoniazid metabolism in man. Br Med J 2:485–491, 1960.

49. Mitchell JR, Thorgeirsson UP, Black M, et al. Increased incidence of isoniazid hepatitis in rapid acetylators: possible relation in hydrazine metabolites. Clin Pharmacol Ther 18:70–79, 1975.

50. Alexander MR, Louie SG, Guernsy BG. Isoniazid-associated hepatitis. Clin Pharm 1:148–153, 1982.

51. Martinez-Roig A, Cami J, Llorens-Terol J, et al. Acetylation phenotype and hepatotoxicity in the treatment of tuberculosis in children. Pediatrics 77:912–915, 1986.

52. Anderson RJ, Gambertoglio JG, Schrier RW. Clinical use of drugs in renal failure. Springfield, IL: Charles C Thomas, 1976.

53. Bennett WM, Aronoff GR, Morrison G, et al. Drug prescribing in renal failure: dosing guidelines for adults. Am J Kidney Dis 3: 155–193, 1983.

54. Nolan CM, Goldberg SV, Buskin SE. Hepatotoxicity associated with isoniazid preventive therapy. JAMA 281:1014–1018, 1999.

55. Kopanoff DE, Snider DE, Caras GJ. Isoniazid-related hepatitis: a US Public Health Service cooperative surveillance study. Am Rev Resp Dis 117:991–1001, 1979.

56. Black M, Mitchell JR, Zimmerman HJ, et al. Isoniazid-associated hepatitis in 114 patients. Gastroenterology 69:289–302, 1975.

57. Steele MA, Burk RF, DesPrez RM. Toxic hepatitis with isoniazid and rifampin. Chest 99:465–471, 1991.

58. Franks AL, Binkin NJ, Snider DE Jr, et al. Isoniazid hepatitis among pregnant and postpartum Hispanic patients. Public Health Rep 104:151–155, 1989.

59. Snider DE, Caras GH. Isoniazid-associated hepatitis deaths: a review of available information. Am Rev Resp Dis 145:494–497, 1992.

60. Girling DJ. Adverse effects of antituberculous drugs. Drugs 23: 56–74, 1982.

61. Baciewicz AM, Self TH. Isoniazid interactions. South Med J 78: 714–718, 1985.

62. Maukkassah SF, Bidlack WF, Yang WCT. Mechanism of the inhibitory action of isoniazid on microsomal drug metabolism. Biochem Pharmacol 30:1651–1658, 1981.

63. Kutt H, Brennan R, Dehejia H, et al. Diphenylhydantoin intoxication. Am Rev Resp Dis 101:377–384, 1970.

64. Self TH, Chrisman CR, Baciewicz AM. Isoniazid drug and food interactions. Am J Med Sci 317:304–311, 1999.

65. Miller RR, Porter J, Greenblatt DJ. Clinical importance of the interaction of phenytoin and isoniazid. Chest 75:356–358, 1979.

66. Melander A, Danielson K, Hanson A, et al. Reduction of isoniazid bioavailability in normal men by concomitant intake of food. Acta Med Scand 200:93–97, 1976.

67. Mannistro P, Mantyla R, Klinge R, et al. Influence of various diets on the bioavailability of isoniazid. J Antimicrob Chemother 10: 427–434, 1982.

68. Mattila MJ, Takki S, Jussila J. Effects of sodium sulphate and castor oil on drug absorption from the human intestine. Ann Clin Res 6:19–24, 1974.

69. Hauser MJ, Baier H. Interactions of isoniazid with foods. Drug Intell Clin Pharmacol 16:617–618, 1982.

70. Smith CK, Durack DT. Isoniazid and reaction to cheese. Ann Intern Med 78:520–521, 1978.

71. Lejonc JL, Gusmini D, Brochard P. Isoniazid and reaction to cheese [letter]. Ann Intern Med 91:793, 1979.

72. Uragoda CG, Lodha SC. Histamine intoxication in a tuberculous patient after ingestion of cheese. Tubercle 60:59–61, 1979.

73. Lejonc JL, Schaeffer A, Brochard P, et al. Hypertension arterielle paroxystique provoquee sous isoniazide par l'ingestion de gruyere: deux cas. Ann Med Interne 131:346–348, 1980.

74. Uragoda CG, Kottegoda SR. Adverse reactions to isoniazid on ingestion of fish with a high histamine content. Tubercle 58:83–89, 1977.

75. Senanayake N, Vyravanathan S, Kanagasuriyam S. Cerebrovascular accident after a ''skipjack'' reaction in a patient taking isoniazid. Br Med J 2:1127–1128, 1978.

76. Uragoda CG. Histamine poisoning in tuberculous patients after ingestion of tuna fish. Am Rev Respir Dis 121:157–159, 1980.

77. Aloysius DJ, Uragoda CG. Histamine poisoning on ingestion of tuna fish. J Trop Med Hyg 86:13–15, 1983.

78. Uragoda CG. Histamine poisoning in tuberculosis patients on ingestion of tropical fish. J Trop Med Hyg 81:243–245, 1978.

79. Uragoda CG. Histamine intoxication with isoniazid and a species of fish. Ceylon Med J 23:109–110, 1978.

80. Brass C, Galgiani JN, Blaschke TF, et al. Disposition of ketoconazole, an oral antifungal in humans. Antimicrob Agents Chemother 21:151–158, 1982.

81. Englehard D, Stutman HR, Marks MI. Interaction of ketoconazole with rifampin and isoniazid. N Engl J Med 74:18–47, 1983.

82. Hoglund P, Nillson LG, Paulsen O. Interaction between isoniazid and theophylline. Eur J Resp Dis 70:110–116, 1987.

83. Samigun M, Santoso B. Lowering of theophylline clearance by isoniazid in slow and rapid acetylators. Br J Clin Pharmacol 29: 570–573, 1990.

84. Thompson JR, Buckart GJ, Self TH, et al. Isoniazid–induced alterations of theophylline pharmacokinetics. Curr Ther Res 32:921–925, 1982.

85. Thompson JR, Self TH. Theophylline and isoniazid. Br J Clin Pharmacol 30:909, 1990.

86. Wehrli W. Rifampin: mechanisms of action and resistance. Rev Infect Dis 5:S412–417, 1983.

87. Thornsberry C, Hill BC, Swenson JM, et al. Rifampin: spectrum of antibacterial activity. Rev Infect Dis 5:S412–417, 1983.

88. Vernon A, et al. Early report: acquired rifamycin monoresistance in patients with HIV-related tuberculosis treated with once-weekly rifapentine and isoniazid. Lancet 353:1843, 1999.

89. Bock NN, Sterling TR, Hamilton CD, et al. A prospective, randomized, double-blind study of tolerability of rifapentine 600, 900, and 1,200 mg plus isoniazid in the continuation phase of tuberculosis treatment. Am J Resp Crit Care Med 165:1526–1530, 2002.

90. Furesz S. Clinical and biological properties of rifampicin. Antibiot Chemother 16:316–351, 1970.

91. Grosset J, Leventis S. Adverse effects of rifampin. Rev Infec Dis 5:S440–446, 1983.

92. Flynn CT, Rainford DJ, Hope E. Acute renal failure and rifampicin: danger of unsuspected intermittent dosage. Br Med J 2:428, 1974.

93. Girling DJ, Hitze HL. Adverse reactions to rifampicin. Bull WHO 57:45–49, 1979.

94. Gronhagen-Riska C, Hellstrom PE, Froseth B. Predisposing factors in hepatitis induced by isoniazid-rifampin treatment of tuberculosis. Am Rev Respir Dis 118:461–466, 1978.

95. Pharmacia & Upjohn Company. Rifabutin (Mycobutin) product information, 1996.

96. Hoechst Marion Roussel. Rifapentine (Priftin) product information, 1998.

97. Griffith DE, Brown BA, Wallace RJ. Varying dosages of rifabutin affect white blood cell and platelet counts in human immunodeficiency virus-negative patients who are receiving multidrug regimens for pulmonary Mycobacterium avium complex disease. Clin Infect Dis 23:1321–1322, 1996.

98. Notice to readers: updated guidelines for the use of rifamycins for the treatment of tuberculosis among HIV-infected patients taking protease inhibitors or nonnucleoside reverse transcriptase inhibitors. MMWR 53:37, 2004. (New Guidelines regarding interactions among these agents with recommendations for their use from CDC and partners at available at http://www.cdc.gov/nchstp/tb/tb_hiv_drugs/toc.htm.)

99. Baciewicz AM, Self TH. Rifampin drug interactions. Arch Intern Med 144:1167, 1984.

100. Baciewicz AM, Self TH, Bakemeyer WB. Update on rifampin drug interactions. Arch Intern Med 147:565, 1987.

101. Borcherding SM, Baciewicz AM, Self TH. Update on rifampin drug interactions II. Arch Intern Med 152:711–715, 1992.

102. Gupta KC, Joshi JV, Anklesria PS, et al. Plasma rifampicin levels during oral contraception. J Assoc Phys India 36:365–366, 1988.

103. Skolnick, JL, Stoler BS, Katz DB, et al. Rifampin, oral contraceptives, and pregnancy. JAMA 236:1382, 1976.

104. CDC. Clinical update: impact of HIV protease inhibitors in the treatment of HIV-infected tuberculosis patients with rifampin. MMWR 45:921–925, 1996.

105. Veldkamo A, Hoetelmans R, et al. Ritonavir enables combined therapy with rifampin and saquinavir. Clin Infect Disease 29:1586, 1999.
106. La Porte C, Colbers E, Bertz R, et al. Pharmacokinetics of two adjusted dose regimens of lopinavir/ritonavir in combination with rifampin in healthy volunteers. 42nd Interscience Conference on Antimicrobial Agents and Chemotherapy, San Diego, 2002: Abstract #A-1823.
107. Spradling O, Drociuk D, McLaughlin S, et al. Drug–drug interactions in inmates treated for HIV and Mycobacterium tuberculosis infection or disease: an institutional tuberculosis outbreak. Clin Infect Dis 35:1106–1112, 2002.
108. Strayhorn VA, Baciewicz AM, Self TH. Update on rifampin drug interactions, III. Arch Intern Med 157:2453–2458, 1997.
109. Takayama K, Armstrong EL, Kunugi KA. Inhibition by ethambutol of mycolic acid transfer into the cell wall of Mycobacterium smegmatis. Antimicrob Agents Chemother 16:240, 1979.
110. Peets EA, Sweeney WM, Place VA. The absorption, excretion and metabolic fate of ethambutol in man. Am Rev Resp Dis 91:51–58, 1965.
111. Holdiness MR. Clinical pharmacokinetics of the antituberculous drugs. Clin Pharmacokinet 9:511–544, 1984.
112. Liebold JE. The ocular toxicity of ethambutol and its relation to dose. Ann NY Acad Sci 135:904–909, 1966.
113. Postlethwaite AE, Bartel AG, Kelly WN. Hyperuricemia due to ethambutol. N Engl J Med 286:761–762, 1972.
114. Mackandess GB. The intracellular activity of pyrazinamide and nicotinamide. Am Rev Tuberc 74:718–728, 1956.
115. Zierski M, Bek E. Side effects of drug regimens used in short course chemotherapy for pulmonary tuberculosis: a controlled study. Tubercle 61:41–49, 1980.
116. Pilheu JA, De Salvo MC, Koch O, et al. Liver alterations in antituberculosis regimens containing pyrazinamide. Chest 80:720–724, 1981.
117. Steele MA, Des Prez RM. The role of pyrazinamide in tuberculosis chemotherapy. Chest 94:845, 1988.
118. Cullen JH, Early LJA, Fiore JM. The occurrence of hyperuricemia during pyrazinamide-isoniazid therapy. Am Rev Tuberc Pulm Dis 74:289–292, 1956.
119. Peloquin CA. Comment: intravenous streptomycin. Ann Pharmaocother 27:1546–1547, 1993.
120. Hansten PD, Horn JR. Drug interactions analysis and management. Vancouver: Applied Therapeutics, 1997.
121. Spector R, Lorenza WV. The active transport of para-aminosalicylic acid from the cerebrospinal fluid. J Pharmacol Exp Ther 185:642–648, 1973.
122. Pernod J. Hepatic tolerance of ethionamide. Am Rev Resp Dis 92:39–42, 1965.
123. Phillips S, Tashman H. Ethionamide jaundice. Am Rev Resp Dis 87:896–898, 1963.
124. Gillespie SH, Kennedy N. Fluoroquinolones: a new treatment for tuberculosis? Int J Tuberc Lung Dis 2:265–271, 1998.
125. Kennedy N, Fox R, Kisyombe GM, et al. Early bactericidal and sterilizing activities of ciprofloxacin in pulmonary tuberculosis. Am Rev Resp Dis 148:1547–1551, 1993.
126. Kennedy N, Berger L, Curram J, et al. Randomized controlled trial of a drug regimen that includes ciprofloxacin for the treatment of pulmonary tuberculosis. Clin Infect Dis 22:827–833, 1996.
127. Fujiwara PI, ed. Clinical policies and protocols. New York: Bureau of Tuberculosis Control, New York City Department of Health, 1999.
128. Sander CC. Review of preclinical studies of ofloxacin. Clin Infect Dis 14:526–538, 1991.
129. Shafer RW, Edlin BR. Tuberculosis in patients infected with human immunodeficiency virus: perspective on the past decade. Clin Infect Dis 22:683–704, 1996.
130. Perriens JH, Colebunders RL, Karahunga C, et al. Increased mortality and tuberculosis treatment failure rate among human immunodeficiency virus (HIV) seronegative patients with pulmonary tuberculosis treated with "standard" chemotherapy in Kinshasa, Zaire. Am Rev Resp Dis 144:750–755, 1991.
131. Okwera A, Whalen C, Byekwaso F, et al. Randomized trial of thiacetazone and rifampicin-containing regimens for pulmonary tuberculosis in HIV-infected Ugandans. Lancet 344:1323–1328, 1994.
132. Nunn P, Kibuga D, Gathua S, et al. Cutaneous hypersensitivity reactions due to thiacetazone in HIV-1 seropositive patients treated for tuberculosis. Lancet 337:627–630, 1991.
133. Chintu C, Luo C, Bhat G, et al. Cutaneous hypersensitivity reactions due to thiacetazone in the treatment of tuberculosis in Zambian children infected with HIV-1. Arch Dis Child 68:665–668, 1993.
134. Raviglione MC, Narain JB, Kochi A. HIV-associated tuberculosis in developing countries: clinical features, diagnosis, and treatment. WHO 70:515–526, 1992.
135. Wong CS, Palmer GS, Cynamon MH. In vitro susceptibility of Mycobacterium tuberculosis, Mycobacterium bovis, and Mycobacterium kansasii to amoxicillin and ticarcillin in combination with clavulanic acid. J Antimicrob Chemother 22:863–866, 1988.
136. Chambers HF, Kocagoz T, Sipit T, et al. Activity of amoxicillin/clavulanate in patients with tuberculosis. Clin Infect Dis 26:874–877, 1998.
137. Condos R, Rom WN, Schluger NW. Treatment of multidrug-resistant pulmonary tuberculosis with interferon-γ via aerosol. Lancet 349:1513–1515, 1997.
138. Iseman MD, Cohn DL, Sbarbaro JA. Directly observed treatment of tuberculosis: we can't afford not to try it. N Engl J Med 328:576–578, 1993.
139. Ebert SC. ASHP Therapeutic position statement on strategies for preventing and treating multi-drug resistant tuberculosis. Am J Health Syst Pharm 54:428–431, 1997.
140. Zwarenstein M, Schoeman JH, Vundule C, et al. Randomised controlled trial of self-supervised and directly observed treatment of tuberculosis. Lancet 352:1340–1343, 1998.
141. Walley JD, Khan MR, Newell JN, et al. Effectivenss of the direct observation component of DOTS for tuberculosis: a randomized controlled trial in Pakistan. Lancet 357: 664–669, 2001.
142. Kamolratanakul P, Sawert H, Lertmaharit S, et al. Randomized controlled trial of directly observed treatment (DOT) for patients with pulmonary tuberculosis in Thailand. Trans R Soc Trop Med Hyg 5:552–557, 1999.
143. Mahmoudi A, Iseman MD. Pitfalls in the care of patients with tuberculosis: common errors and their association with the acquisition of drug resistance. JAMA 270:65–68, 1993.
144. Chaulk CP, Kazandjian VA for the Public Health Tuberculosis Guidelines Panel. Directly observed therapy for treatment completion of pulmonary tuberculosis. Consensus statement of the Public Health Tuberculosis Guidelines Panel. JAMA 279:943–947, 1988.
145. Cohen ML. Epidemiology of drug resistance: implications for a post-antibiotic era. Science 257:1050–1055, 1992.
146. Connix R, Pfyffer GE, Mathieu C, et al. Drug-resistant tuberculosis in prisons in Azerbaijan: case study. Br Med J 316:1423–1425, 1998.
147. Raviglione MC, Rieder HL, Styblo K, et al. Tuberculosis trends in Eastern Europe and the former USSR. Tuberc Lung Dis 75:400–416, 1994.
148. Farmer P, Kim JY. Community based approaches to the control of multidrug resistant tuberculosis: introducing "DOTS-plus." Br Med J 317:671–674, 1998.
149. Briggs GG, Freeman RK, Yaffeb SJ. Drugs in pregnancy and lactation. 6th ed. Baltimore: Lippincott, Williams & Wilkins, 2002: 509–510, 731–732, 1189, 1222–1223, 1280–1281.
150. Snider DE, Layde RM, Johnson MW, et al. Treatment of tuberculosis during pregnancy. Am Rev Resp Dis 122:65, 1980.
151. Snider DE, Powell KE. Should women taking antituberculosis drugs breastfeed? Arch Intern Med 144:589, 1984.
152. Gordon F, Chaisson RE, Matts JP, et al. Rifampin and pyrazinamide vs isoniazid for prevention of tuberculosis in HIV-infected persons. JAMA 283:1445–1458, 2000.
153. CDC. The role of BCG vaccine in the prevention and control of tuberculosis in the United States. MMWR 45 (RR-4):1–15, 1996.
154. World Health Organization. BCG immunization and paediatric HIV infection. Wkly Epidemiol Rec 67:129–132, 1992.

Urinary Tract Infections

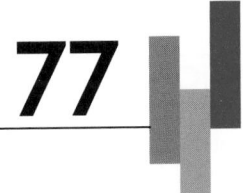

Cinda L. Christensen

DEFINITIONS

Any site or structure within the urinary tract can become infected, but the bladder (cystitis) and kidney (pyelonephritis) are most frequently involved. In men, the prostate, epididymis, and testis can also become infected by bacteria originating from the urinary tract.[1] The presence of bacteria or fungi in the urine is termed bacteriuria or funguria, respectively. However, the detection of bacteria or fungi in the urine does not always imply infection or a clinically significant condition. Bacteria in the urine without signs and symptoms of infection is termed asymptomatic bacteriuria.

Urinary tract infections (UTIs) are classified as either uncomplicated or complicated. This distinction is important since management strategies often differ between these two groups. Uncomplicated UTIs include acute cystitis and pyelonephritis in otherwise healthy individuals. These patients have the lowest risk of complications or treatment failure. Complicated infections can be acute or chronic and occur in a diverse mix of patients with metabolic, functional, or structural abnormalities of the urinary tract or kidneys.[2,3] Metabolic factors include diabetes mellitus, renal failure, and kidney transplantation. Examples of functional abnormalities are neurogenic bladder and vesicoureteral reflux. Structural abnormalities result from stones, tumors, strictures, or foreign objects such as catheters, stents, and other forms of instrumentation.[3]

Recurrent infection in a patient with a previous UTI can be due to either a relapse or reinfection. Relapses are caused by the same microorganism as in the preceding infection and usually occur within 2 to 4 weeks after treatment has ended.[4] Reinfections typically occur after a greater length of time and may be due to a new strain or species. Patients who never improve or who immediately relapse following completion of treatment have persistent infection.[5,6]

Urosepsis is a serious condition in which the bacterial species found within the urinary tract is also recovered from the patient's blood in conjunction with the clinical picture of sepsis. Patients who develop urosepsis are usually physically debilitated or have an underlying immunodeficiency.

TREATMENT GOALS

- Eradicate pathogenic strains of bacteria or fungi from the urinary tract (i.e., microbiologic cure).
- Resolve or alleviate associated symptoms (i.e., achieve clinical cure).
- Limit the extent and severity of infection so as to prevent significant morbidity or mortality.
- Achieve successful clinical outcome with a treatment regimen that is cost-effective, has minimal risk of adverse reactions, and is not prohibitive to patient compliance.
- Minimize alterations in normal microbial flora that may result in vaginal candidiasis, *Clostridium difficile* colitis, or the emergence of resistant organisms within the urinary tract or other body sites.
- Prevent recurrent infection by patient education, prophylaxis, or suppressive therapy.
- Ensure the patient comprehends how to take medications, what the possible side effects of therapy are, and how to avoid relevant drug–drug interactions.

ETIOLOGY/MICROBIOLOGY

Enteric bacteria are the most common organisms causing urinary tract infections. This is due to the anatomic proximity of bowel flora to the urethra, particularly in women. More important is the pathogenicity specific to the urinary tract that certain species of enteric organisms have acquired. Such organisms are called uropathogens for their ability to cause infection even in the healthy host. The most prevalent causative agent is *Escherichia coli* among all patient groups in both upper and lower tract infections (Table 77.1). Uropathogenic *E. coli* (UPEC) may possess one or more virulence factors that allow for colonization and persistence within the urinary tract. The number of factors expressed may correlate with the severity of infection.[7]

A key virulence factor is the presence of bacterial structures named adhesins, which mediate bacterial attachment to urinary epithelium.[7,8] UPEC strains with the greatest capacity for attachment to uroepithelial receptors succeed more frequently in establishing infection.[9,10] Close attachment to epithelial cells improves the chances for cellular invasion and results in higher exposure to cytotoxic or inflammatory compounds released by UPEC strains.[11] Strong affinity for urinary tract epithelium also correlates with bacterial persistence within the vagina and periurethral area in women. Subsequently, the same strain can be responsible for recurrent UTI in women if therapy is not effective against UPEC strains harbored outside the urinary tract.[4] The most pathogenic strains of *E. coli* are those that have filamentous adhesins termed p-pili or p-fimbriae. *E. coli* with p-pili are responsible for almost all cases of bacteremic pyelonephritis in previously healthy patients.[5,12] Other UPEC virulence factors include diminished susceptibility to phagocytosis, iron extraction from host sources, and adaptations to the nutrient-poor environment of the urine.[11]

In uncomplicated UTI in women, *Staphylococcus saprophyticus* is the next most common causative organism. *S. saprophyticus* is a coagulase-negative staphylococcus that does not originate from the bowel. This organism causes cystitis and pyelonephritis clinically similar to *E. coli*.[13] Risk factors for UTI due to *S. saprophyticus* include use of spermicide-coated condoms, young age, previous UTI, and multiple sexual partners.[14]

Other bacteria known to cause UTIs in a small but significant number of patients are *Klebsiella* spp. and *Proteus mirabilis*.[13,15] These enteric organisms are often difficult to eradicate from the urinary tract, particularly when the kidney is involved. Both organisms are capable of possessing various adhesins and other uropathogenic virulence factors. *Proteus mirabilis* often produces urease, which mediates the conversion of urea to ammonia. This raises urinary pH, which can then initiate the formation of urinary stones or encrustations on catheters. Stones can become a continuous nidus for infection and a cause of treatment failure by obstructing urine flow or by harboring organisms.[2,11,16]

In complicated UTIs, a broader spectrum of microbial species is encountered. A greater variety of organisms can cause infection because the required degree of microbial virulence is lower in patients with structural or functional abnormalities of the urinary tract. Many of these patients have received multiple courses of antimicrobial therapy and have become colonized with microorganisms that are intrinsically resistant or have acquired resistance to standard treatment regimens.[3] Also, recovery of more than one organism from culture is not uncommon. Although *E. coli* is most frequently identified as the causative agent in complicated UTI, other organisms such as *Candida* spp., *Pseudomonas aeruginosa*, enterococci, *Enterobacter* spp., and other gram-negative aerobic bacilli are common pathogens in this patient population.[6,17–19] Fungal UTIs

TABLE 77.1	Prevalence of Organisms Causing Urinary Tract Infections			
Causative Organism	**Cystitis**	**Pyelonephritis**	**Complicated**	**Catheterized**
E. coli	80	85	40	21
S. saprophyticus	9	5		
Coagulase-negative staphylococci			5	8
Klebsiella spp.	4	5	8	6
Proteus spp.	3	3	5	6
Candida spp.			1	20
P. aeruginosa			14	10
Enterococci			13	11
Enterobacter spp.			6	6
Other	4	2	8	12

Numbers are percentages.
(Data from references 3, 13, 15, 18, 34, 50, 64, 82, and 103.)

are common among hospitalized patients, particularly those with diabetes mellitus, urinary catheterization, malignancy, recent broad-spectrum antibacterial therapy, and kidney transplantation.[20] In addition to *Staphylococcus aureus* and *Candida* spp., *Mycobacterium tuberculosis* and *Salmonella* spp. can infect the urinary tract via dissemination from the bloodstream. Pseudomonal UTI may be acquired via the bloodstream or the urethra.[2]

Asymptomatic bacteriuria and funguria are usually due to a variety of relatively nonvirulent bacteria or fungi. Patients with functional or structural defects often harbor organisms intermittently or chronically. These nonpathogenic strains do not effectively invade or attach to uroepithelium, so a full immune response with subsequent clinical symptoms does not develop.[10] The presence of these nonpathogenic organisms may actually protect against infection by more virulent bacteria.[21,22]

EPIDEMIOLOGY

PREVALENCE

UTIs are responsible for over 7 million outpatient visits and 1 million hospitalizations in the United States annually.[6,23] As one of the most common infectious diseases, UTIs have a significant financial and human public health impact. Each year, an estimated $1.6 billion is spent in the United States diagnosing and treating acute bladder infections in women alone.[24] Such women will typically experience 6.1 days of symptoms and lose 1.2 days of work or school.[17] UTIs are also the most common hospital-acquired infection, accounting for up to 40% of nosocomial infections.[25]

In the general population, 3.5% of individuals have asymptomatic bacteriuria.[7] However, the prevalence patterns of bacteriuria vary for men and women and at different ages (Table 77.2).[1] In infancy, boys are five to eight times more likely to develop bacteriuria and UTIs than are girls, owing to the greater incidence of congenital genitourinary tract abnormalities in boys.[26] Among older children and throughout early and middle adulthood, women far outnumber men in the development of UTIs. UTIs are very rare in healthy younger men unless the urinary tract has undergone instrumentation. As men reach their older years, the prevalence of bacteriuria increases dramatically, almost equaling that of women. In women, the prevalence of bacteriuria rises more steadily with increasing age.[27] This increase is approximately 1% per decade of life.[7]

Symptomatic UTIs can occur in essentially all members of the population but are most prevalent among young and middle-aged women. Between the ages of 20 and 40 years, about a third of women will have experienced an UTI. Overall, over half of all women will develop an UTI at some point in their life.[24] Although most women have only a single episode, 25% to 50% will experience a recurrent infection, 12% within a year of the initial episode.[4,17,28] For women

TABLE 77.2	Prevalence of Bacteriuria in Various Populations	
Population	**Male (%)**	**Female (%)**
Community-Based		
Infants	2	0.5
Young children	0.1	1.5
College students	<0.01	5
Adults (30–65 years old)	0.1	10
Elderly persons		
65–85 years old	5	15
>85 years old	15	25
Patient-Based		
Adults (medical clinic)	4	6
Adults (urology clinic)	8	—
Adult inpatient		
<70 years old	7.5	30
>70 years old	25	30
Institutionalized elderly persons	>30	>30
Patients after instrumentation		
Urethral catheterization	5	5
Transurethral procedures	20	40

Percentages are approximations derived from a wide range of values from many studies in diverse settings; in these studies, specimens were obtained by various methods, and different definitions of bacteriuria were used.

(Adapted with permission from Lipsky BA. Urinary tract infections in men. Ann Intern Med 110:138–150, 1989.)

with two preceding UTIs, 47% will have another recurrence within a year.[4] In otherwise healthy women, most of these recurrences are reinfections.

MORBIDITY/MORTALITY

Although recurrent infections can significantly alter a patient's quality of life, most UTIs do not result in long-term morbidity or mortality. Studies have shown that chronic asymptomatic bacteriuria does not contribute to renal impairment, nor does frequent recurrent cystitis.[29–31] With effective treatment, acute uncomplicated pyelonephritis usually results in only minimal renal scarring that is clinically insignificant.[2,32]

There are notable exceptions to the usually benign course of most UTIs. UTIs can contribute to scarring and renal failure in infants and children with anatomic anomalies such as vesicoureteral reflux. The uncommon development of chronic pyelonephritis can also lead to irreversible renal dysfunction. Asymptomatic bacteriuria in pregnant women has been shown to increase the risk of infant mortality and low birthweight.[2,27] Patients at highest risk for UTI-associated mortality are bacteremic patients with multiple comorbidities or long-term catheterization.[33,34]

RISK FACTORS

Multiple risk factors can predispose an individual to the development of a UTI (Table 77.3). Among healthy young women, the most common risk factor is sexual activity, with the highest risk occurring within 48 hours of intercourse.[35] This increased risk is possibly due to the facilitated movement of organisms from the vaginal introitus into the urethra.[2] Also, the use of either a diaphragm with spermicide or a spermicide-coated condom results in a two- to three-fold increased risk of acquiring a UTI.[36,37] The spermicide, usually nonoxnol-9, appears to alter vaginal flora such that urinary pathogens can colonize the vaginal introitus more easily. Lower estrogen levels in postmenopausal women and recent antibiotic use can also alter vaginal flora and predispose to bacteriuria and UTI.[29,38]

Additional risk factors are associated with the development of pyelonephritis. Pregnancy-induced changes, such as decreased peristalsis and dilation of the ureters, allow bacteria easier access to the kidneys during the later stages of pregnancy.[27] Decreased neutrophil function, renal microangiopathy, neurogenic bladder, and glucosuria, which are often associated with diabetes, may contribute to the greater frequency of upper tract involvement in these patients.[39,40] Obstruction of the ureters by stones, strictures, or tumors also increases susceptibility to pyelonephritis. Fifteen percent of all stones are infectious and can be a cause of recurrent UTIs.[16]

TABLE 77.3	Risk Factors for Developing Bacteriuria and Urinary Tract Infections
Age Group	**Risk Factor**
Children	Congenital anomalies such as vesicoureteral reflux, male sex
Healthy young or middle-aged women	Sexual activity, diaphragm or condom use with spermicide, history of UTI in childhood, prior adult UTI, prior administration of antibiotics
Healthy young or middle-aged men	Instrumentation of urinary tract, lack of circumcision, anal intercourse
Elderly	Uterine prolapse and low estrogen level in women, prostatic hypertrophy, decreased antimicrobial activity of prostatic secretions in men, diabetes, functional debility (bedridden), bowel incontinence
All ages	Catheterization, other instrumentation, neurogenic bladder, nephrolithiasis, obstructive tumors and strictures, certain blood groups, renal failure, kidney transplantation

(Data from references 1, 6, 9, 23, 26, 36, 37, 38, 40, and 104.)

PATHOPHYSIOLOGY

Organisms enter the urinary tract primarily via an ascending route from the urethra. Less commonly, organisms from the blood infect one or both kidneys and then descend into the bladder with the flow of urine.[40] The organisms infecting via the ascending route originate almost exclusively from the bowel. These organisms spread to the perineum and, in women, colonize the vaginal introitus and vagina. Once the vaginal introitus and periurethral area are colonized, bacteria can readily gain entry into the urethra and bladder. Since vaginal colonization with potential urinary pathogens is an important intermediate step in pathogenesis, changes in vaginal flora or pH that promote colonization of urinary pathogens dramatically increase the risk of developing a UTI.[36,38] In healthy adult men, UTIs are very uncommon due to the greater distance organisms must travel from the perineum to urethra. Also, the longer urethra in males further discourages entry into the bladder.[1,2]

After bacteria (or fungi) reach the bladder, the balance between host defenses and bacterial virulence will determine whether the bacteria will be able to survive, replicate efficiently, and invade the bladder mucosa. Most bacteria introduced into the bladder of healthy individuals are normally cleared by host defenses within 2 to 3 days. However, if patients have high postvoid residuals, alterations in urine flow from stones or strictures, or prolonged urethral catheterization, bacteriuria may never spontaneously resolve. Chronic or intermittent bacteriuria may remain asymptomatic if the organisms are not able to adhere to and invade the bladder mucosa.[2] The presence of these nonpathogenic strains within the bladder may protect these high-risk individuals from infection by discouraging subsequent colonization with more uropathogenic organisms.[22]

UPEC strains, however, readily attach to and invade bladder epithelial cells, where the organisms may replicate intracellularly or become quiescent. The infected host cells may then respond by undergoing exfoliation or apoptosis such that the intracellular bacteria are mechanically removed with urination. Persistence of viable microbes harbored within epithelial cells may be a source of relapsing UTIs.[8]

Mucosal attachment and invasion also triggers a host immune response. The mucosal cells release chemokines that attract neutrophils to the affected tissues. Recruited neutrophils cross the mucosa and are released into the urine (pyuria) to phagocytose infecting organisms.[22] With the onset of this local inflammatory response, the patient may experience symptoms of infection. Systemic responses such as fever or leukocytosis rarely occur with uncomplicated cystitis. Spontaneous resolution of infection may occur in 70% of previously healthy females within 30 days.[2]

Pyelonephritis results when bacteria ascend the ureters and infect one or both kidneys. The entire kidney is rarely involved; instead, patchy areas of necrosis and scarring are found adjacent to normal tissue.[2] Local inflammation occurs with neutrophil recruitment, but in pyelonephritis, the host also experiences a systemic response resulting in leukocytosis, cytokine release, and immunoglobulin M (IgM) and immunoglobulin G (IgG) elevations. A significant number of patients will be bacteremic, and urosepsis may develop in those with comorbidities.[10] Full recovery and sterilization of the kidney tissue may take as long as 6 to 10 weeks, even in previously healthy patients.[2]

For both cystitis and pyelonephritis, neutrophil response is crucial to the successful clearance of organisms from the urinary tract. Genetically based variations in host response that result in suboptimal neutrophil recruitment, activation, and phagocytosis of uropathogens may predispose some seemingly healthy individuals to UTIs or frequent reinfections.[8,22,41]

Acquisition of a UTI from the descending route appears to account for only 3% of all UTIs. Bacteremia or fungemia from a non-urinary tract source rarely results in clinically significant kidney infection. The exception is for organisms with a special affinity for kidney tissue such as *S. aureus* or *Candida* spp.[2] Complete ureteral obstruction or preexisting renal injury substantially increases the risk of kidney infection in the presence of bacteremia.[40] Once the kidney is infected, bacteria or fungi can enter the urine stream and proceed to the bladder, where bacteriuria may then be detected.

HOST DEFENSES

The host defenses that deter bacteria from colonizing the urinary tract are primarily mechanical and not immunologic. Urination washes out microorganisms that have entered the urethra and bladder. Since normal postvoid bladder residuals are only 0.09 to 2.4 mL, the vast majority of colonizing organisms are physically removed with each void.[2] The peristaltic action of the ureters and the one-way vesicoureteral valve at the junction with the bladder dissuades pathogens from ascending from the bladder to the kidneys.[27]

Other host defenses discourage replication or attachment of microorganisms. Tamm-Horsfall protein, low-molecular-weight sugars, secretory immunoglobulin A (IgA), and uromucoid can act as false ligands for bacterial attachment, leaving fewer bacteria to attach to the mucosa.[8] In men, prostatic secretions contain compounds with antibacterial properties. The pH and osmolarity of urine can alter bacterial growth in that both very dilute urine and concentrated urine with low pH can inhibit growth.[40]

Individuals with abnormal urine dynamics are at greater risk of UTI. For example, patients with neurogenic bladder have higher postvoid residual urine volumes and so are less efficient at removing bacteria with urination. Also, the dilated ureters of women in the later stages of pregnancy cannot prevent organisms from reaching the kidneys. In healthy people, therefore, an uncomplicated UTI results when the virulence of the pathogen is sufficient to overcome normal host defenses. Conversely, a complicated UTI often results from the inadequacy of host defenses to prevent even low-

virulence organisms from establishing infection. The immune system has no significant role in preventing UTIs but is activated only after bladder mucosa or kidney tissue has been invaded. Therefore, immunocompromised patients do not have a greater incidence of UTIs but are at higher risk of severe forms of infection and treatment failure when they do occur.[42,43]

CLINICAL PRESENTATION AND DIAGNOSIS

SIGNS AND SYMPTOMS

Acute Uncomplicated Cystitis. The vast majority of patients diagnosed with acute uncomplicated cystitis are young to middle-aged women. The majority of women will experience the typical symptoms of pain or burning on urination (dysuria), frequent voiding of small amounts of urine (frequency), and needing to urinate immediately (urgency).[44] Suprapubic tenderness or low back pain may be reported in some individuals. Few patients experience systemic symptoms such as fever or chills, even though 20% to 30% will have "silent" involvement of the kidney.[15,17] On gross visual examination, the urine may look cloudy or blood-tinged. On urinalysis, nearly all patients will have pyuria and 40% will have hematuria.[6,17,45]

Making the diagnosis of acute cystitis is relatively straightforward in patients with typical symptoms and pyuria, especially if the patient reports sexual activity within the previous 24 to 48 hours.[15] However, only 65% of women presenting for medical care with symptoms possibly referable to the urinary tract actually have a UTI.[46] Infections of the vagina such as candidiasis, bacterial vaginosis, and trichomoniasis need to be ruled out.[17] Sexually transmitted infections such as chlamydial urethritis also can mimic bacterial cystitis. Patients with cystitis associated with sexual activity with a new partner should be screened for sexually transmitted diseases, since coinfection is not uncommon.[47]

The presence of the characteristic symptoms of dysuria, frequency, and urgency, in addition to a positive dipstick or microscopic urinalysis for pyuria, is usually sufficient to make the diagnosis of uncomplicated cystitis in otherwise healthy patients. These patients usually can be started on antimicrobial treatment without further workup.[6] To assist in making the diagnosis, individuals with unclear symptoms or a negative urinalysis should have a urine sample collected for culture and sensitivity testing. Due to the possibility of atypical or resistant organisms, a urine culture is also indicated for patients who recently received antimicrobial therapy. A microscopic urinalysis should be performed in any symptomatic patient when the less sensitive dipstick result is negative for pyuria. Older women, children (particularly infants), men of all ages, diabetics, and patients with early relapse of UTI are at risk for complicated or upper tract UTI and should have a more extensive history and physical examination performed. Also, these patients often have a broader range of possible pathogens and should have a urine culture performed.[1,17]

Many women with acute uncomplicated cystitis experience recurrent infections, the majority of which are reinfections with the same bacteria. A more extensive history and physical examination, along with a microscopic urinalysis and urine culture, is indicated at least once for these patients. If no complicating factors are uncovered, invasive diagnostic procedures rarely uncover abnormalities.[17] Future episodes are given minimal diagnostic workup and are treated with standard regimens.

Acute Uncomplicated Pyelonephritis.

Acute uncomplicated pyelonephritis can range from a relatively benign to a relatively severe, destructive infection of the kidney. At presentation, some patients complain merely of mild fever or flank pain, while others experience a full range of symptoms such as fever, chills, nausea, vomiting, flank pain, costovertebral angle tenderness, weakness, malaise, or headache.[48] Symptoms of cystitis may not always precede the development of pyelonephritis. Notably, patients at either age extreme may present with mild, nonspecific symptoms in the face of significant kidney involvement.[15]

The initial workup of the patient with presumptive pyelonephritis includes a complete blood count, urinalysis, urine Gram stain, and urine culture. Blood cultures should also be obtained in patients with severe symptoms because 20% to 30% of patients are bacteremic.[10] A uropathogen will be identified from blood culture in 10% of patients with no growth or mixed organisms on urine culture.[49] Most individuals will have a leukocytosis with increased band cells (often termed a left shift). On urinalysis, substantial pyuria is almost always present, and hematuria, proteinuria, and white blood cell casts may also be seen.[45] Urine bacterial counts of 10^5 colony-forming units (CFU) or more per mL are detected in 80% to 95% of patients. A higher cutoff of 10^4 CFU per mL is generally recommended for the diagnosis of acute pyelonephritis, because low bacterial counts are infrequently associated with pyelonephritis compared to cystitis.[17] For symptomatic patients with lower bacterial counts, urinary tract obstruction or a perinephric abscess should be considered. The Gram stain may be useful in directing initial treatment, while culture and antimicrobial susceptibilities are essential for the redirection of therapy in patients who are unresponsive to or intolerant of initial treatment.[45]

The decision to hospitalize the patient is primarily based on the severity of symptoms. Patients with persistent nausea and vomiting cannot take oral antimicrobials and will therefore require parenteral therapy. Adjunctive care, such as intravenous fluid replacement or parenteral pain medications, may also necessitate hospitalization. Patients who are deemed to be at high risk for noncompliance or who might fail to return for follow-up should also be hospitalized.

Most hospitalized patients improve significantly within 72 hours of starting treatment and can be discharged home within 3 to 4 days. Culture results are available by this time

and an appropriate oral home regimen can be selected. For both inpatients and outpatients, failure to improve on effective antimicrobials after 72 hours, or an early relapse, warrants further diagnostic testing to rule out a renal abscess or obstruction.[15] Approximately 12% of outpatients treated for pyelonephritis with standard regimens will return to medical care for persistent symptoms.[50]

Complicated Urinary Tract Infections.

Complicated UTIs occur in a diverse mix of patients who have an increased risk of either acquiring a UTI or experiencing a severe or persistent UTI. This category includes patients with mild lower tract disease as well as those with significant kidney infection and urosepsis. The clinical presentation may include the hallmark symptoms of dysuria, frequency, and urgency. However, vaguer symptoms of fatigue, headache, temperature instability, and irritability may be the only clues.[42] Immunocompromised persons may not exhibit the usual symptoms due to their dampened inflammatory response to infection. An important example of this is the debilitated elderly patient, who may have UTI-associated bacteremia in the absence of fever or leukocytosis.[33] Men with prostatic enlargement and UTI may complain only of obstructive symptoms, but further questioning can reveal symptoms referable to a UTI.[1] Therefore, the clinician must hold a greater degree of suspicion for possible UTI in these individuals, since treatment delays may lead to more serious infections.[51]

In the patient suspected of having urinary abnormalities, an extensive workup may be indicated to delineate the extent of the abnormality and to determine whether it is correctable. Without amelioration of the underlying problem, relapses or reinfections are to be expected.[3,7] Some infections may never be cured without corrective action, as in the presence of kidney stones or urinary stents.[42]

For patients with known or suspected complicated UTIs, a urinalysis, urine culture, blood count, and serum creatinine should be performed. For those who are sicker or are immunocompromised, blood culture and imaging studies of the upper tract may be indicated to determine the extent and severity of infection.[15] Diabetics in particular have an increased risk of perinephric abscess or emphysematous pyelonephritis.[52] Pyuria is expected but is less specific, since the primary urinary abnormality may be responsible for the presence of white blood cells.[15]

An appropriately obtained urine culture is crucial to effective treatment, since a multitude of non-uropathogens with varied antimicrobial susceptibilities can infect the urinary tract in individuals with hampered host defenses. Colony counts are usually 10^5 CFU or more per mL. Negative culture results may necessitate further testing for fastidious organisms. It may be reasonable to wait for culture and sensitivity results before initiating treatment in the stable patient with lower tract infection. Because persistence and relapse of infections are common, a repeat urine culture 1 or 2 weeks after therapy may be helpful.[6]

Hospitalization is indicated for patients who cannot take oral medications, need other intravenous therapy, or have probable kidney involvement or possible urosepsis. The diagnosis of urosepsis is made when bacteremia originating from a urinary source is associated with fever, tachycardia, hypotension, and general decompensation.[51] Urosepsis occurs most frequently in debilitated elderly patients, immunocompromised persons, and those with chronic urinary obstruction.[2]

Nosocomial and Catheter-Associated Urinary Tract Infection. The majority of nosocomial UTIs are associated with indwelling urinary catheters.[25] Other confounding factors in nosocomial UTI include the severity of the underlying illness causing hospitalization; antimicrobial therapy for other infections, which increases the risk for resistant or unusual organisms; multiple medications being administered, which may interact with UTI treatment; and possibly the inability of the patient to describe symptoms of UTI due to altered mental status. Management of catheter-associated UTI varies considerably depending on whether catheterization is short term or chronic.

Even with good insertion and maintenance techniques, the incidence of bacteriuria among catheterized patients increases with time at a rate of 3% to 10% per day of catheterization. Thus, a large percentage of patients will be bacteriuric after a week and virtually all will be bacteriuric after a month of catheterization. The organisms are believed to gain entry via the space between the catheter and the urethral mucosa. The biofilm that develops on catheters may allow organisms within it to elude leukocytes and antimicrobials.[6,53] Patients with long-term catheters often have polymicrobial bacteriuria.[53]

Differentiating between infection and colonization can be difficult because bacteriuria is present in almost all patients with prolonged catheterization. Among hospitalized patients, symptoms may not be clearly associated with the urinary tract, since they may have other reasons for lower abdominal discomfort, leukocytosis, and fevers. Also, the usual symptoms of dysuria, hesitancy, and urgency are not seen in catheterized patients. Often the only symptoms manifested are confusion or fever. In spinal cord-injured patients, symptoms may include fever, diaphoresis, abdominal pain, or increased muscle spasticity.[25] Overall, only 30% to 50% of infected patients undergoing short-term catheterization will experience symptoms.[53,54] For patients who have symptoms, a urinalysis and culture of urine and blood should be obtained. Screening for bacteriuria in asymptomatic individuals is generally discouraged because antimicrobial treatment in this situation can lead to recolonization with more resistant strains.[53]

Antimicrobial treatment of catheter-associated UTI has relatively high failure and relapse rates.[6] Removing the catheter increases cure rates, but for patients who require chronic catheterization, replacement with a new catheter does not always improve the odds for success. Recurrence rates in patients chronically catheterized may be improved with suprapubic bladder catheterization, because bacterial colonization on the abdominal wall is less than in the periurethral area.[25,39,53]

DIAGNOSIS

Diagnostic tests are used when the clinical presentation or physical examination does not yield a clear diagnosis. The most frequently used tests are dipstick urinalysis, urine microscopy with or without Gram stain, and quantitative urine culture with antimicrobial susceptibility. Such tests help to determine whether the patient's symptoms are consistent with UTI and to identify the infecting organism. Other diagnostic procedures include localization tests such as bilateral ureteral catheterization, bladder washout techniques, and antibody-coated bacteria assays.[45] These procedures are used to differentiate upper tract infections from lower tract ones, but they are rarely necessary in the management of most patients. Ultrasound and computed tomography (CT) studies may help to identify renal abscesses or structural abnormalities of the kidneys. Intravenous pyelograms are performed less frequently but may also help to assess possible structural defects and urine flow patterns.

Collecting the urine specimen correctly is important to ensure the accuracy of the results for both urinalysis and urine culture. In noncatheterized patients, urine is collected in a sterile container midway through urination. Using a midstream voided urine sample is preferred, although some data show that contamination rates are similar without this precaution.[55] Although rarely done in routine cases, specimens obtained via urethral catheterization or suprapubic bladder aspiration have the lowest risk of contamination.

Urinalysis. A complete urinalysis consists of biochemical dipstick testing of fresh urine and a microscopic examination of the urine sediment. Urine dipsticks have multiple reagent pads that undergo color changes when dipped in the urine sample. The pad colors are then compared to a standardized color reference. Most dipsticks can determine pH and can give a quantitative value for red blood cells, protein, nitrites, and leukocyte esterase.[45] Leukocyte esterase, an enzyme produced by activated leukocytes, is used as a marker for the presence of leukocytes in the urine sample.[21] The dipstick urinalysis is often the only diagnostic test used by the office- or clinic-based practitioner to confirm the clinical diagnosis of uncomplicated cystitis.[6] On microscopic examination of the urine sediment, the number of leukocytes, erythrocytes, bacteria, fungi, and other solid elements can be quantified.

The most important aspects of the urinalysis in diagnosing urinary tract infections are pH and the presence of nitrites, blood (hematuria), bacteria (bacteriuria), fungi (funguria), and particularly leukocytes (pyuria) or white blood cell casts.[17,45] A high pH may indicate the presence of urea-splitting organisms such as *Proteus* spp. The conversion of nitrates in urine to nitrites has been associated with the presence of enteric bacteria.[56] In patients who are not menstruating, the presence of hematuria can localize the problem to the urinary tract. Finding microorganisms on urinalysis may assist in making the diagnosis of UTI but may also represent contamination from organisms residing in the distal urethra or periurethral area.

The leukocyte count is of primary importance when determining the significance of bacteriuria and confirming UTI as the cause of dysuria.[45,57] Pyuria usually is defined as eight leukocytes or more per mm^3, which correlates to two to five leukocytes per high-power field.[6] However, most patients with UTIs have 20 or more leukocytes per mm^3. Pyuria in the absence of bacteriuria or a positive urine culture can occur in patients with vaginal infections or urethritis due to *Chlamydia* or other fastidious organisms.[57]

Urine Culture. Several culture techniques are available, but the biplate method is used most commonly. With the biplate method, a selective medium on one side of the culture dish is used to isolate possible gram-negative urinary pathogens, while the other side usually contains nonselective culture medium. Use of the selective culture medium often allows for more rapid identification of potential uropathogens. The microorganism colony count is determined using the nonselective side of the plate. The number of colonies can be correlated to the number of organisms or CFU per mL in the original urine sample. Using the standard inoculum size, this method can detect bacterial concentrations of 10^3 CFU or more per mL. Antibacterial susceptibility testing is then performed on the predominant organisms recovered from the biplate.

Traditionally, a single-species microorganism count of 10^5 CFU or more per mL from a midstream urine specimen was considered indicative of infection. Multiple studies have shown, however, that as few as 10^2 CFU per mL in a symptomatic patient with pyuria represents true infection.[57] Up to half of all young women with true uncomplicated cystitis will have bacterial counts of 10^2 to 10^4 CFU per mL.[46]

According to the Infectious Diseases Society of America guidelines, a midstream urine culture of 10^3 CFU or more per mL of a single uropathogen is indicative of cystitis in patients with pyuria and symptoms consistent with lower tract infection.[15] However, for unspeciated coagulase-negative staphylococci, 10^5 CFU per mL is used as a cutoff due to the potential for contamination by these organisms. In a symptomatic patient with pyuria, a midstream urine culture with less than 10^2 CFU per mL can be seen in patients with chlamydial urethritis, infections due to other fastidious organisms, early infection, partially treated infection, and candidal or bacterial vaginitis.[2,39] In symptomatic women without pyuria, 10^5 CFU or more per mL is still required for the diagnosis of UTI. However, any sample with 10^2 CFU or more per mL obtained by suprapubic bladder aspiration or urethral catheterization is considered significant.[58] For patients without risk factors for complicated UTI, any urine culture result with mixed organisms or with a nonuropathogen is probably due to contamination.

Urine cultures are not routinely done for presumed cases of uncomplicated lower UTI, because the causative agent is reliably *E. coli* and occasionally *S. saprophyticus*. The finding of typical clinical symptoms in patients with pyuria or hematuria is usually sufficient to make the diagnosis and start empiric treatment.[6,45] However, with unclear symptoms, complicated cases, treatment failure, or pyelonephritis, a urine culture should be done to confirm the diagnosis and to ensure effective treatment. Also, patients with urinary tract symptoms who do not demonstrate pyuria by urinalysis should have a urine culture performed.[3,23] A urine Gram stain may be useful to guide initial treatment for complicated UTIs.

THERAPEUTIC PLAN

Once the diagnosis and classification of UTI are made, a therapeutic plan is formed from a consideration of patient factors, microbiologic factors, and clinical outcome data. Table 77.4 summarizes the commonly recommended therapeutic regimens. These general recommendations are applicable in the majority of circumstances, but recognizing situations where the usual treatment is inappropriate is of considerable importance.

Standard guidelines for treatment may not be applicable when antimicrobial resistance patterns in the local community or in individual patients differ from national or regional patterns. This is most important for patients at risk for progressive or serious infection.

Published clinical outcome data can demonstrate superior or comparable efficacy between treatment regimens while controlling for patient and microbiologic factors. Such data are most usefully applied to individual cases when the study and treatment cases are similar.

For compliant patients who fail to respond to treatment or relapse quickly, a urine culture should be performed, if not done originally, to rule out unusual or resistant organisms. Otherwise, plans for a more extensive diagnostic workup should be considered.

TREATMENT

PHARMACOTHERAPY

Antimicrobial agents ideally suited for the treatment of cystitis should achieve relatively high concentrations in urine with oral administration, demonstrate activity against the most common uropathogens, eliminate uropathogens from the vagina and bowel with minimal impact on normal flora, and have a relatively benign adverse reaction profile. Agents for the treatment of pyelonephritis or prostatitis should also achieve significant concentrations in kidney and prostate tissues.

Table 77.5 offers a pharmacologic comparison of available agents. Antimicrobials currently considered first-line treatment, namely trimethoprim/sulfamethoxazole (TMP/

TABLE 77.4	Treatment Regimens for Bacterial Urinary Tract Infections		
Condition	**Usual Pathogens**	**Mitigating Circumstances**	**Recommended Empirical Treatment**
Acute uncomplicated cystitis in women	E. coli, S. saprophyticus, P. mirabilis, Klebsiella pneumoniae	None	3-day regimen: oral TMP/SMX, trimethoprim, fluoroquinolone; 7-day regimen: nitrofurantoin
		Locations with high TMP/SMX E. coli resistance	3-day regimen: oral ciprofloxacin, levofloxacin, gatifloxacin, ofloxacin, norfloxacin; 7-day regimen: nitrofurantoin
		Diabetes, symptoms for >7 days, recent UTI, age >65 yr	Consider 7-day regimen: oral TMP/SMX, trimethoprim, ciprofloxacin, levofloxacin, gatifloxacin, ofloxacin, or norfloxacin
		Pregnancy	Consider 7-day regimen: oral amoxicillin, nitrofurantoin, cefpodoxime proxetil, or trimethoprim
Acute uncomplicated pyelonephritis in women	E. coli, P. mirabilis, K. pneumoniae, S. saprophyticus	Mild to moderate illness, no nausea or vomiting—outpatient therapy	Oral TMP/SMX (if organism is susceptible), ciprofloxacin, ofloxacin for 7–10 days
		Severe illness–hospitalization required	Parenteral extended-spectrum cephalosporin, ciprofloxacin, levofloxacin, gatifloxacin, or gentamicin (with or without ampicillin) until fever is gone; then oral TMP/SMX or fluoroquinolone as per culture results for 10–14 days
		Pregnancy–hospitalization recommended	Parenteral extended-spectrum cephalosporin, gentamicin (with or without ampicillin), or aztreonam until fever is gone; then oral amoxicillin, a cephalosporin, or TMP/SMX (during second trimester only) for 14 days
Complicated UTI	E. coli, Proteus spp., Klebsiella spp., Pseudomonas spp., Serratia spp., enterococci, staphylococci	Mild to moderate illness, no nausea or vomiting—outpatient therapy	Oral ciprofloxacin, levofloxacin, gatifloxacin, or ofloxacin for 7–10 days
		Severe illness or possible urosepsis—hospitalization required	Parenteral ampicillin and gentamicin, fluoroquinolone, ceftriaxone, aztreonam until fever is gone; then oral TMP/SMX, ciprofloxacin, levofloxacin, gatifloxacin, ofloxacin as per culture results for 10–14 days

TMP/SMX, trimethoprim-sulfamethoxazole.
(Data from Stamm WE, Hooton TM. Management of urinary tract infections in adults. N Engl J Med 329:1328–1334, 1993; Fihn SD. Acute uncomplicated urinary tract infection in women. N Engl J Med 349:259–266, 2003; Hooton TM. The current management strategies for community-acquired urinary tract infection. Infect Dis Clin North Am 17:303–332, 2003; Raz R, Chazan B, Kennes Y, et al. Empiric use of trimethoprim-sulfamethoxazole (TMP-SMX) in the treatment of women with uncomplicated urinary tract infections, in a geographical area with a high prevalence of TMP-SMX-resistant uropathogens. Clin Infect Dis 34:1165–1169, 2002.)

SMX), trimethoprim, or the fluoroquinolones, have most of the preferred characteristics. TMP/SMX has been the drug of choice for most UTIs for many years because of these qualities, but decreasing antibacterial activity against E. coli and other gram-negative bacilli has led some clinicians to limit its use to low-risk patients or to those with pathogens with documented susceptibility.[6] Patients at higher risk for TMP/SMX-resistant strains include those with complicated UTI or recent prior exposure to TMP/SMX and those who live in areas with high endemic resistance rates (e.g., the western and south-central areas of the United States).[59]

Although clinically efficacious, fluoroquinolones are expensive, and excessive use has been shown to increase bacterial resistance to this valuable class of antimicrobials. Although E. coli resistance to fluoroquinolones is still relatively uncommon among outpatients with UTIs, resistance rates have increased to 2.5% in 2001 from less than 1% in 1997.[60]

| TABLE 77.5 | Pharmacologic Data and Oral Treatment Doses for Uncomplicated Cystitis | | | | | |

Drug	Adult Dose	Adjustment for Renal Failure[a]	Pediatric Dose (>2 mo of age)	Peak Urine Concentration (μg/mL)	Adverse Reactions (with Short-Term Use)	Significant Drug Interactions
TMP/SMX	1 DS BID × 3 days	Not recommended	4 mg TMP/kg BID	>30/>40	Allergic reaction, nausea, photosensitivity	Warfarin, cyclosporin, phenytoin, sulfonylureas, methotrexate
Trimethoprim	100 mg BID × 7–10 days	Not recommended	2–3 mg/kg BID	30–180	Rash, nausea	Phenytoin
Ciprofloxacin	250 mg BID × 3 days	250 mg QD	Not recommended	>200	Headache, rash, nausea, photosensitivity	Antacids, sucralfate, Ca, Mg, Fe, dairy products, warfarin, theophylline, caffeine
Ciprofloxacin extended-release	500 mg QD × 3 days	None	Not recommended	>300	Same as above	Same as above
Gatifloxacin	400 mg × 1 OR 200 mg QD × 3 days	None	Not recommended		Same as ciprofloxacin	
Levofloxacin	250 mg QD × 3 days	250 mg QOD	Not recommended	>100	Same as ciprofloxacin	Like ciprofloxacin, lesser effect of warfarin, methylxanthines
Norfloxacin	400 mg BID × 3–7 days	400 mg QD	Not recommended	>200	Same as ciprofloxacin	Like ciprofloxacin, lesser effect of warfarin, methylxanthines
Ofloxacin	200 mg BID × 3–7 days	100 mg QD	Not recommended	>200	Insomnia, same as ciprofloxacin	Like ciprofloxacin, lesser effect on warfarin, methylxanthines
Cephalexin/ Cephradine	500 mg BID × 7 days	250 mg BID	10 mg/kg TID	2000	Allergic reaction	
Nitrofurantoin (macrocrystal)	50–100 mg QID × 7 days	Not recommended	1.5 mg/kg QID	50–150	Nausea, headache	Urine alkalinizing agents, probenecid
Fosfomycin	3 g × 1 (mixed in water)	None	Not recommended if <12 years	>1000	Diarrhea, headache	Metoclopramide

TMP/SMX, trimethoprim-sulfamethoxazole.
[a] Creatinine clearance <10 mL/minute

Fluoroquinolones are relatively contraindicated in young children and pregnant women due to reports of cartilage abnormalities in studies on immature animals. Fluoroquinolones may be preferred in the treatment of prostatitis due to their excellent penetration into prostatic tissues.[61]

Although inexpensive, well tolerated, and active against most uropathogens in vitro, the oral first-generation cephalosporins and nitrofurantoin have higher relapse and reinfection rates. This is attributed to tissue concentrations inadequate to treat silent kidney infection or eliminate the reservoir of uropathogens in the vagina.[2,6] Also, the very rapid elimination of most β-lactams may result in insufficient urinary concentrations at the end of the dosing interval.[44] As a result of high resistance rates and low tissue concentrations, amoxicillin is considered unreliable except for the treatment of documented enterococcal UTI. β-Lactam antimicrobials also have been associated with higher rates of post-treatment candidal vaginitis.[17,62]

Single-agent trimethoprim meets most of the desired criteria, but antibacterial activity also has decreased over time. Gentamicin has long demonstrated clinical efficacy, but the risk of renal toxicity and ototoxicity and the need for parenteral administration have limited its use to upper tract or nosocomial UTIs.

Uncomplicated Cystitis. Most antimicrobials that are approved for use in women with uncomplicated UTI achieve a greater than 80% success rate with 7 or more days of therapy in clinical trials. Clinical outcome results may vary, however, due to differences in study population, patient exclusion criteria, and length of follow-up.[63] Overall susceptibility rates for organisms isolated from patients with uncomplicated UTI are greater than 90% for fluoroquinolones, nitrofurantoin, and fosfomycin. TMP/SMX and first-generation cephalosporins are active against 80% to 85% of isolates, whereas less than 60% remain susceptible to ampicillin or amoxicillin.[59,60,64] Some areas of the United States have reported *E. coli* resistance rates to TMP/SMX above 20%, and areas of southern Europe have rates close to 35%.[44] *E. coli* resistance results in a 50% failure rate among women treated with TMP/SMX.[59,65] Therefore, empiric treatment with TMP/SMX is not recommended in areas where *E. coli* resistance exceeds 20%.[24,66]

Interest in decreasing treatment duration has lead to studies of single-dose and 3-day regimens. Single-dose regimens have generally produced success rates lower than either 3-day or 7-day regimens. Although associated with fewer adverse reactions, single-dose treatment also results in higher relapse and reinfection rates.[63] These recurrences have been attributed to incomplete clearance of uropathogens from the vagina and inadequate treatment of silent upper tract disease.[2] UTIs due to *S. saprophyticus* and those in elderly women have significantly higher failure rates with single-dose therapy.[66–68]

Trimethoprim given as a large single dose yields long-term cure rates of 71% versus 87% for a 7-day regimen.[68] TMP/SMX given as a single dose (two DS tablets) versus 10 days of standard twice-daily dosing resulted in 76% and 95% success rates, respectively, at early follow-up.[69] Single-dose fluoroquinolone treatment has been associated with 78% to greater than 90% success rates, with norfloxacin producing the poorest results.[70–72] Single-dose treatment with 400 mg gatifloxacin has demonstrated a long-term cure rate of 90%, which was equivalent to a 3-day regimen of either gatifloxacin or ciprofloxacin. Greater success rates with single-dose gatifloxacin may be due to its prolonged half-life; urinary concentrations are greater than the mean inhibitory concentration (MIC) of most uropathogens for more than 48 hours.[73]

Fosfomycin, a drug approved only for single-dose treatment, has demonstrated a cure rate of approximately 80%.[66] Patients without a history of recurrent UTI and those ex-

pected to be poorly compliant with standard regimens are the best candidates for single-dose treatment.[69]

Success rates with 3-day courses of fluoroquinolones or TMP/SMX have been approximately 82% to 90% comparable to longer courses.[72,74–76] The efficacy of 3-day regimens has been shown in a broad range of patients, including infants and elderly women.[77,78] Thus, 3-day regimens are usually recommended when using a fluoroquinolone or TMP/SMX for treatment. Three-day regimens are also associated with fewer adverse reactions, a lower incidence of vaginitis, and a lower cost.[23] Short-course regimens of cephalosporins, amoxicillin, and nitrofurantoin are associated with significantly lower success rates and are therefore not recommended.[75]

Uncomplicated Pyelonephritis. The preferred antimicrobials for the treatment of pyelonephritis target the same uropathogens as in lower tract infection. Fluoroquinolones and TMP/SMX are the mainstays of treatment and can be given orally in stable outpatients. Oral β-lactam antimicrobials and nitrofurantoin attain inadequate kidney tissue concentrations and should not be used.[6] For patients requiring hospitalization, intravenously administered ciprofloxacin, levofloxacin, or gatifloxacin may be used empirically, but TMP/SMX should be avoided before culture and sensitivity data are known. Parenterally administered extended-spectrum cephalosporins are also appropriate and may be preferred for pregnant women.[44,66] The previously standard regimen of gentamicin with or without ampicillin is still used in many institutions.

Patients receiving parenteral therapy can be switched to an oral treatment regimen once clinical improvement is seen and nausea has resolved. Urine culture results should be available after 48 hours and should guide oral antimicrobial selection. Dosing for TMP/SMX is the same as for cystitis, but fluoroquinolone doses should be increased to systemic infection treatment doses.[6] Cure rates of 90% or higher have been demonstrated with fluoroquinolone treatment as short as 7 days, regardless of route of administration.[79–82] TMP/SMX treatment results in similar cure rates for infections due to susceptible *E. coli* strains, but when resistance rates near 20%, outcomes are significantly poorer compared to fluoroquinolones.[81]

A total of 7 to 10 days of therapy is sufficient in most cases; therapy beyond 14 days does not improve outcomes.[83]

Complicated Urinary Tract Infections. Making generalized recommendations for the treatment of complicated UTIs is difficult because of the diversity of underlying defects that give rise to these infections. Because of the wider range of possible causative agents and the higher risk of treatment failure or relapse, broad-spectrum antimicrobials with good tissue penetration are generally preferred for empiric therapy. Table 77.6 lists pooled susceptibility data for urinary isolates from hospitalized patients across North America. TMP/SMX should be used cautiously, or only after susceptibility results are available, in areas with known high

| TABLE 77.6 | In Vitro Antimicrobial Susceptibilities of Urinary Isolates From Hospitalized Patients in North America |

Organism	Ofloxacin	Ciprofloxacin	Norfloxacin	Ampicillin	Cefazolin	Ceftriaxone	Gentamicin	Nitrofurantoin	TMP/SMX
E. coli	>99*	96	100	58–66	71–91	>99	98	96	77
Klebsiella spp.	95	92–96	96	6	81–84	93–99	93–95	68	89
Enterococcus spp.	40–70	24–66	60	88	13	9	NT	92	NT
Pseudomonas spp.	69–73	66	91	0	1	15–44	84	1	93
Proteus spp.	98–100	94–100	99	89–94	91–94	98	94–97	0	100
Enterobacter spp.	94–100	93–100	100	5–12	9–12	70–82	94–97	43	100
Coagulase-negative staphylococci	70–81	69–80	80	17–57	52–72	46–61	60	99	NT

TMP/SMX, trimethoprim-sulfamethoxazole; NT, not tested.

*Numbers are given as percentage of strains susceptible.

(Data from Gordon KA, Jones RN. Susceptibility patterns of orally administered antimicrobials among urinary tract infection pathogens from hospitalized patients in North America: comparison report to Europe and Latin America. Results from the SENTRY Antimicrobial Surveillance Program (2000). Diag Micro Infect Dis 45:295–301, 2003; Jones RN, Kehrberg EN, Erwin ME, et al. Prevalence of important pathogens and antimicrobial activity of parenteral drugs at numerous medical centers in the United States. Study on the threat of emerging resistances: real or perceived? Diagn Microbiol Infect Dis 19:203–215, 1994; Hoban DJ, Jones RN. Canadian ofloxacin susceptibility study: a comparative study from 18 medical centers. Chemotherapy 41:34–38, 1995; Gillenwater JY, Clark M. Tentative direct antimicrobial susceptibility testing in urine. J Urol 156:149–153, 1996.

TMP/SMX resistance rates.[6,84] Most fluoroquinolones produce short-term cure rates of 65% to 90%, but recurrences are expectantly high.[84,85] Convincing data are lacking, however, that one drug or class of drugs is more effective than another for these patients, in whom relapse rates are often as high as 50%.[3,4,80]

Mild to moderate complicated UTIs usually can be treated with oral medications, but parenteral therapy with a fluoroquinolone or extended-spectrum cephalosporin may be needed for significantly ill hospitalized patients who cannot take oral medications.[82] For possible enterococcal infections, ampicillin, with or without low-dose gentamicin, is reasonable for most patients requiring intravenous therapy. Nitrofurantoin has been used in the treatment of cystitis due to both susceptible and vancomycin-resistant enterococci.[59] Fluoroquinolones that achieve high urinary concentrations have also cleared enterococcal UTI in 70% or more of cases.[79,82]

Empiric antipseudomonal therapy may be appropriate for some patients with nosocomial UTI, or those with prior history of pseudomonal UTI.[6] Antipseudomonal cephalosporins, aztreonam, extended-spectrum penicillins/β-lactamase inhibitors, carbapenems, aminoglycosides, and most fluoroquinolones could be used for these patients. Two drug regimens may be necessary for upper tract infection with P. aeruginosa. Once clinical improvement is accomplished, oral antimicrobials can be used to complete therapy in suitable patients.[6]

The recommended length of treatment for most complicated UTIs is usually 7 to 14 days, but patients with bacteremic complicated UTI or urosepsis should receive at least 14 days of treatment. Infections in men with prostatitis or patients with another persistent nidus of infection require

several weeks of treatment for cure. Patients with chronic indwelling urinary catheters are persistently colonized with microorganisms; therefore, the goal of therapy in these individuals should be resolution of symptoms and not absence of bacteriuria.[3] Success rates are improved when the catheter is replaced with the initiation of antimicrobial therapy.[86]

Fungal UTIs occur most frequently in hospitalized patients with urinary catheters. Removal of the catheter, improved control of blood sugar in diabetics, and discontinuance of antibacterial agents may improve outcomes.[87] Bladder irrigation with amphotericin B at 5 to 50 mg per liter for a few days has been shown to be effective for fungal cystitis in patients who require continued catheterization.[88] Fluconazole 100 mg orally or intravenously daily for at least 5 days eradicates Candida spp. from the bladder in 73% to 77% of patients.[20,89] However, some data suggest that no therapy may be appropriate in nondiabetic, lower-risk patients.[90]

Prophylactic and Suppressive Therapy. Patients with frequent recurrences of uncomplicated cystitis may benefit from either continuous or postcoital prophylaxis. Continuous prophylactic therapy is given either daily or a few days per week at doses lower than those used for treatment.[6] Table 77.7 lists the agents and doses used for continuous prophylaxis. In women whose recurrent infections are associated with sexual activity, single-dose postcoital prophylaxis may be appropriate. Postcoital prophylaxis with ciprofloxacin 125 mg has been shown to be as effective as daily prophylaxis.[91] Other effective regimens for postcoital prophylaxis include TMP/SMX 40 mg/200 mg, cephalexin 250 mg, and nitrofurantoin 50 mg as single doses.[3]

Reliable patients with less frequent recurrences may do well with self-initiated therapy. These patients keep a supply

TABLE 77.7	Continuous Antimicrobial Prophylactic Regimens for Recurrent Urinary Tract Infection		
Antimicrobial Agent	**Daily Dose**	**Infections/Patient-Year**	**Vaginal Flora Effect**
TMP/SMX	40 mg/200 mg	0–0.15	+
Trimethoprim	100 mg	0–0.15	+
Norfloxacin	200 mg	0–0.15	+
Nitrofurantoin	50–100 mg	0.1–0.8	−
Nitrofurantoin (macrodantin)	50–100 mg	0.3	−
Cephalexin	125–250 mg	Not assessed	−
Cefaclor	250 mg	0.3	−
Cephradine	250 mg	Not assessed	−

Agents are generally given at bedtime, daily or 3 times per week. Those that have an effect on reducing vaginal colonization with uropathogens are indicated: +, reduces vaginal colonization with uropathogens; −, no reduction in vaginal colonization with uropathogens. (Adapted with permission from Stapleton A, Stamm WE. Prevention of urinary tract infection. Infect Dis Clin North Am 11:719–733, 1997.)

of antimicrobials at home, and with recurrence of typical symptoms, they can begin treatment immediately. With this method, appropriate self-initiation of treatment occurs in 92% to 94% of episodes.[92] Treatment is usually a single dose or a 3-day regimen.[6] Figure 77.1 shows the usual management of recurrent cystitis in women.

Few patients with recurrent complicated UTIs benefit from long-term prophylactic therapy because treatment of patients with uncorrectable underlying abnormalities merely results in colonization with more resistant organisms.[2,3] This is particularly true of chronically catheterized patients.

Pregnant women with cystitis or pyelonephritis have been shown to benefit from antimicrobial prophylaxis to prevent bacteriuria and infection.[2,62] Pregnant women with significant bacteriuria have a higher incidence of pyelonephritis, premature delivery, low-birthweight infants, and infant mortality. Therefore, continuous prophylaxis is given to pregnant women with either asymptomatic bacteriuria or UTI.[93]

Antimicrobial prophylaxis is also indicated for infants with vesicoureteric reflux because recurrent infection is common in these patients, and at this age it has been associated with permanent renal damage.[2]

Approaches to lowering the frequency of recurrent infection may include changing the contraceptive method for patients using a diaphragm with spermicide, postcoital voiding, treatment of the partner in patients with recurrent *S. sapro-*

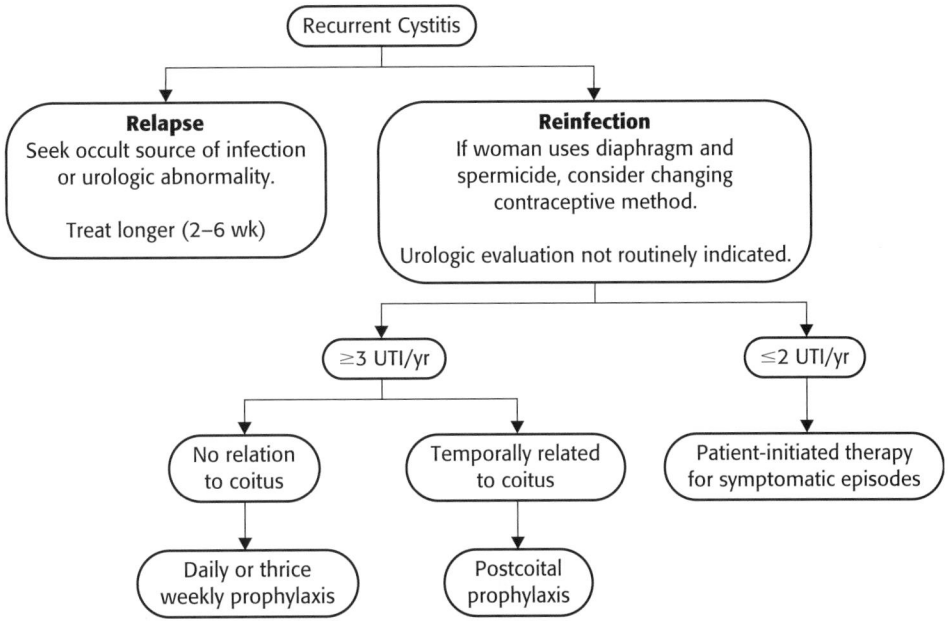

FIGURE 77.1 Algorithm for managing recurrent cystitis in women. (Adapted with permission from Stamm WE, Hooton TM. Management of urinary tract infections in adults. N Engl J Med 329:1331, 1993.)

phyticus infection, and systemic or topical estrogen replacement therapy in postmenopausal women.[35,94]

Adjunctive Therapy. Some patients benefit from adjunctive therapy with phenazopyridine, a urinary analgesic, to decrease the discomfort associated with bladder spasms. Acetaminophen or nonsteroidal anti-inflammatory agents can be used to alleviate fevers, aches, and pains.

Oral estrogen replacement therapy and intravaginally applied estrogen has been tried to reduce UTI recurrence rates among postmenopausal women. Studies have shown that estrogen can normalize the vaginal milieu, which then discourages colonization by uropathogens, but the results have been inconsistent.[29,95,96]

ALTERNATIVE THERAPIES

A few alternative therapies have shown promise in reducing UTI rates among patients with frequent recurrences. Most notably, cranberry juice consumption has been associated with decreased rates of UTI. Originally, the acidity of cranberry juice was believed to decrease recurrences, but studies have concluded that the volume of cranberry juice required to significantly decrease urinary pH would be prohibitive to patient compliance. It is now believed that the high level of fruit tannins called proanthocyanidins in cranberry juice inhibits P-fimbriated *E. coli* adherence to urinary epithelium. Several well-controlled trials have shown that cranberry juice or cranberry extract intake can significantly decrease the risk of UTI.[62,97]

The restoration of normal vaginal flora via the administration of probiotic formulations of lactobacilli has also been studied as a means to decrease UTI rates. However, various formulations given orally or topically have failed to produce convincing results thus far.[97,98]

FUTURE THERAPIES

Research is under way examining the efficacy of vaccination against uropathogenic strains of *E. coli* and other enteric organisms. Mucosal vaccination using multiple doses of a vaginal suppository comprising killed whole-cell uropathogenic strains has demonstrated significant improvement in the time to next UTI.[99] An orally administered vaccine containing immunostimulating fractions of *E. coli* also has reduced recurrence rates. Excellent results have been found thus far in animal studies of a parenterally administered *E. coli* fimbrial subunit vaccine.[97] More studies will be needed to prove the benefit of such vaccines.

IMPROVING OUTCOMES

For most UTIs, clinical cure is an obtainable goal. A multitude of regimens are effective, so the clinician must weigh the risks and benefits of a given regimen for each patient. Obtaining a complete drug history should identify possible risks for adverse drug and hypersensitivity reactions. Assessment of potential patient compliance is a major factor in improving outcomes. A drug regimen that requires multiple doses per day for 7 days or more is a setup for nonadherence.

Appropriate follow-up is also important so that patients who fail to respond to therapy or relapse early can be assessed quickly for possible complicating factors, some of which may be correctable. Any patient who fails to respond to therapy or experiences a relapse should be questioned about adherence to the prescribed treatment, as nonadherence is a common explanation for treatment failure.

PATIENT EDUCATION

All patients receiving antimicrobial therapy should be informed of possible adverse reactions and drug–drug interactions, and how best to avoid or manage them. Mild antimicrobial-associated diarrhea may be tolerable, but severe diarrhea requires a call to the prescriber. Photosensitivity reactions are common with TMP/SMX as well as with some fluoroquinolones, and patients should be cautioned about sun exposure and the use of sunscreens. Patients prescribed ciprofloxacin should be warned to decrease or eliminate caffeine from their diets, particularly if they are sensitive to the effects of caffeine. Patients should also be informed to avoid taking fluoroquinolones with iron or other mineral supplements, thereby preventing treatment failure from decreased absorption of the drug.

Self-initiated therapy for recurrent cystitis requires education about potential drug interactions, as the patient may be taking new medications the next time UTI treatment is started. The patient should also be warned not to self-initiate therapy if she suspects or knows she has become pregnant, as both TMP/SMX and fluoroquinolones are relatively contraindicated during pregnancy.

PHARMACOECONOMICS

A few studies have analyzed the cost-effectiveness of the commonly recommended approaches to UTI treatment. It has been recommended that diagnostic studies such as urine culture, urine microscopy, and even dipstick urinalysis should be reserved for complicated UTIs and pyelonephritis. Many practitioners treat empirically without any laboratory workup because most women with uncomplicated UTIs will experience pathognomonic symptoms. This practice has been found to be cost-effective in these patients, although one third may be treated unnecessarily.[100] Hypothetically, over-the-counter antibiotic treatment of UTIs may provide easier access to treatment, quicker symptom relief, and reduced physician office charges. However, this approach was not projected to be cost-effective due to the long-term costs associated with increased bacterial resistance.[101]

Antimicrobial choice and duration of treatment can significantly affect the overall cost of therapy. TMP/SMX has been used successfully and inexpensively for many years, but the trend toward increasing bacterial resistance with subsequent treatment failures may eventually make other options more cost-effective.[102] First-generation cephalosporins and nitrofurantoin are relatively inexpensive and active against most uropathogens, but higher relapse rates and poorer patient compliance with the required 7-day treatment regimen may lead to greater costs associated with retreatment. Fluoroquinolone success rates are excellent, but higher drug costs and the risk of eventual bacterial resistance have prevented fluoroquinolones from becoming the preferred agents for all patients.

Patients with severe UTIs have traditionally been given parenteral antimicrobials for initial treatment. However, oral administration of highly bioavailable antimicrobials, such as TMP/SMX and the fluoroquinolones, can achieve similar clinical outcomes at substantially lower cost. Ciprofloxacin has been shown to be equally efficacious, either intravenously or orally, with severe pyelonephritis or complicated UTI.[82]

KEY POINTS

■ UTIs can involve the bladder (cystitis), the kidney (pyelonephritis), or other urinary structures, and the severity can vary substantially between patients.

■ The highest prevalence is in young to middle-aged women.

■ Uncomplicated UTIs occur in otherwise healthy persons, while complicated UTIs occur in persons with structural, functional, or immunologic abnormalities.

■ Uropathogens originate primarily from the bowel, with *E. coli* the most prevalent pathogen.

■ The most common symptoms associated with cystitis are dysuria, frequency, and urgency.

■ Pyelonephritis is often associated with fever, chills, nausea, and leukocytosis.

■ Pyuria and bacteriuria with at least 10^3 CFU per mL is generally considered indicative of UTI in symptomatic patients.

■ Therapy with TMP/SMX or a fluoroquinolone is recommended for 3 days in healthy women with uncomplicated cystitis, 7 to 10 days for pyelonephritis, and 7 to 14 days for complicated UTIs.

■ Prostatitis treatment requires prolonged antimicrobial administration with an agent that achieves good concentrations in prostatic fluid (e.g., fluoroquinolones).

■ Recurrent uncomplicated UTIs may be managed with prophylactic or self-initiated therapy.

■ Individualization of therapy is dictated by illness severity, microbiologic susceptibility, allergy history, drug interactions, compliance potential, and cost.

SUGGESTED READINGS

Hooton TM. The current management strategies for community-acquired urinary tract infection. *Infect Dis Clin North Am* 17:303–332, 2003.

Lundstrom T, Sobel J. Nosocomial candiduria: a review. *Clin Infect Dis* 32:1602–1607, 2001.

Mulvey MA, Schilling JD, et al. Bad bugs and beleaguered bladders: interplay between uropathogenic *Escherichia coli* and innate host defenses. *PNAS* 97:8829–8835, 2000.

Wilson ML, Gaido L. Laboratory diagnosis of urinary tract infections in adult patients. *Clin Infect Dis* 38:1150–1158, 2004.

REFERENCES

1. Lipsky BA. Urinary tract infections in men: epidemiology, pathophysiology, diagnosis, and treatment. Ann Intern Med 110: 138–150, 1989.
2. Rubin RH, Cotran RS, Tolkoff-Rubin NE. Urinary tract infection, pyelonephritis, and reflux nephropathy. In: Brenner BM, ed. Brenner and Rector's the kidney, 5th ed. Philadelphia: WB Saunders, 1997:1597–1654.
3. Nicolle LE. A practical guide to the management of complicated urinary tract infection. Drugs 53:583–592, 1997.
4. Ikaheimo R, Slitonen A, Heiskanen T, et al. Recurrence of urinary tract infection in a primary care setting: analysis of a 1-year follow-up of 179 women. Clin Infect Dis 22:91–99, 1996.
5. Tolkoff-Rubin NE, Rubin RH. Urinary tract infection in the immunocompromised host. Lessons from kidney transplantation and the AIDS epidemic. Infect Dis Clin North Am 11:707–717, 1997.
6. Stamm WE, Hooton TM. Management of urinary tract infections in adults. N Engl J Med 329:1328–1334, 1993.
7. Krieger JN. Urinary tract infections: what's new? J Urol 168: 2351–2358, 2002.
8. Mulvey MA, Schilling JD, Martinez JJ, et al. Bad bugs and beleaguered bladders: interplay between uropathogenic *Escherichia coli* and innate host defenses. PNAS 97:8829–8835, 2000.
9. Lomberg H, Hanson LA, Jacobsson B, et al. Correlation of P blood group, vesicoureteral reflux, and bacterial attachment in patients with recurrent pyelonephritis. N Engl J Med 308:1189–1192, 1983.
10. Svanborg C, Godaly G. Bacterial virulence in urinary tract infection. Infect Dis Clin North Am 11:513–529, 1997.
11. Johnson JR. Microbial virulence determinants and the pathogenesis of urinary tract infection. Infect Dis Clin North Am 17:261–278, 2003.
12. Kantele A, Mottonen T, Ala-Kaila K, et al. P Fimbria-specific B cell responses in patients with urinary tract infection. J Infect Dis 188:1885–1891, 2003.
13. Latham RH, Running K, Stamm WE. Urinary tract infections in young adult women caused by *Staphylococcus saprophyticus*. JAMA 250:3063–3066, 1983.
14. Fihn SD, Boyko EJ, Chen CL, et al. Use of spermicide-coated condoms and other risk factors for urinary tract infection caused by *Staphylococcus saprophyticus*. Arch Intern Med 158:281–287, 1998.
15. Falagas ME, Gorbach SL. Practice guidelines: urinary tract infections. Infect Dis Clin Pract 4:241–257, 1995.
16. Abrahams HM, Stoller ML. Infection and urinary stones. Curr Opin Urol 13:63–67, 2003.
17. Hooton TM, Stamm WE. Diagnosis and treatment of uncomplicated urinary tract infection. Infect Dis Clin North Am 11: 551–581, 1997.

18. Kollef MH, Sharpless L, Vlasnik J, et al. The impact of nosocomial infections on patient outcomes following cardiac surgery. Chest 112:666–675, 1997.

19. Paick SH, Park HK, Oh S, et al. Characteristics of bacterial colonization and urinary tract infection after indwelling of double-J ureteral stent. Urology 62:214–217, 2003.

20. Jacobs LG. Fungal urinary tract infections in the elderly. Treatment guidelines. Drugs Aging 8:89–96, 1996.

21. Hoberman A, Wald ER. Urinary tract infections in young febrile children. Pediatr Infect Dis J 16:11–17, 1997.

22. Wullt B, Bergsten G, Fischer H, et al. The host response to urinary tract infection. Infect Dis Clin North Am 17:279–301, 2003.

23. Wisinger DB. Urinary tract infections. Current management strategies. Postgrad Med 100:229–236, 1996.

24. Fihn SD. Acute uncomplicated urinary tract infection in women. N Engl J Med 349:259–266, 2003.

25. Saint S, Chenoweth CE. Biofilms and catheter-associated urinary tract infections. Infect Dis Clin North Am 17:411–432, 2003.

26. Schlager TA. Urinary tract infections in infants and children. Infect Dis Clin North Am 17:353–365, 2003.

27. Patterson TF, Andriole VT. Detection, significance, and therapy of bacteriuria in pregnancy. Update in the managed health care era. Infect Dis Clin North Am 11:593–607, 1997.

28. Scholes D, Hooton TM, Roberts PL, et al. Risk factors for recurrent urinary tract infection in young women. J Infect Dis 182:1177–1182, 2000.

29. Nicolle LE. Asymptomatic bacteriuria in the elderly. Infect Dis Clin North Am 11:647–661, 1997.

30. Nicolle LE, Henderson E, Bjornson J, et al. The association of bacteriuria with resident characteristics and survival in elderly institutionalized men. Ann Intern Med 106:682–686, 1987.

31. Abrutyn E, Mossey J, Berlin JA, et al. Does asymptomatic bacteriuria predict mortality and does antimicrobial treatment reduce mortality in elderly ambulatory women? Ann Intern Med 120:827–833, 1994.

32. Raz R, Sakran W, Chazan B, et al. Long-term follow-up of women hospitalized for acute pyelonephritis. Clin Infect Dis 37:1014–1020, 2003.

33. Ackermann RJ, Monroe PW. Bacteremic urinary tract infection in older people. J Am Geriatr Soc 44:927–933, 1996.

34. Platt R, Polk BF, Murdock B, et al. Mortality associated with nosocomial urinary-tract infection. N Engl J Med 307:637–642, 1982.

35. Strom BL, Collins M, West SL, et al. Sexual activity, contraceptive use, and other risk factors for symptomatic and asymptomatic bacteriuria. A case control study. Ann Intern Med 107:816–823, 1987.

36. Fihn SD, Latham RH, Roberts P, et al. Association between diaphragm use and urinary tract infection. JAMA 254:240–245, 1985.

37. Fihn SD, Boyko EJ, Normand EH, et al. Association between use of spermicide-coated condoms and Escherichia coli urinary tract infections in young women. Am J Epidemiol 144:512–520, 1996.

38. Smith HS, Hughes JP, Hooton TM, et al. Antecedent antimicrobial use increases the risk of uncomplicated cystitis in young women. Clin Infect Dis 25:63–68, 1997.

39. Kunin C. Urinary tract infections: detection, prevention, and management, 5th ed. Baltimore: Williams & Wilkins, 1997.

40. Sobel JD. Pathogenesis of urinary tract infection. Role of host defenses. Infect Dis Clin North Am 11:531–549, 1997.

41. Condron C, Toomey D, Casey RG, et al. Neutrophil bactericidal function is defective in patients with recurrent urinary tract infections. Urol Res 17:329–334, 2003.

42. Ronald AR, Harding GKM. Complicated urinary tract infections. Infect Dis Clin North Am 11:583–591, 1997.

43. Gordon KA, Jones RN. Susceptibility patterns of orally administered antimicrobials among urinary tract infection pathogens from hospitalized patients in North America: comparison report to Europe and Latin America. Results from the SENTRY Antimicrobial Surveillance Program (2000). Diag Micro Infect Dis 45:295–301, 2003.

44. Hooton TM. The current management strategies for community-acquired urinary tract infection. Infect Dis Clin North Am 17:303–332, 2003.

45. Komaroff AL. Urinalysis and urine culture in women with dysuria. Ann Intern Med 104:212–218, 1986.

46. Stamm WE, Counts GW, Running KR, et al. Diagnosis of coliform infection in acutely dysuric women. N Engl J Med 307:463–468, 1982.

47. Berg E, Benson DM, Haraszkiewicz P, et al. High prevalence of sexually transmitted disease in women with urinary infections. Acad Emerg Med 3:1030–1043, 1996.

48. Johnson JR, Stamm WE. Urinary tract infections in women: diagnosis and treatment. Ann Intern Med 111:906–917, 1989.

49. Velasco M, Martinez JA, Moreno-Martinez A, et al. Blood cultures for women with uncomplicated acute pyelonephritis: are they necessary? Clin Infect Dis 37:1127–1130, 2003.

50. Pinson AG, Philbrick JT, Lindbeck GH, et al. ED management of acute pyelonephritis in women: a cohort study. Am J Emerg Med 12:271–278, 1994.

51. Pewitt EB, Schaeffner AJ. Urinary tract infection in urology, including acute and chronic prostatitis. Infect Dis Clin North Am 11:623–645, 1997.

52. Patterson JE, Andriole VT. Bacterial urinary tract infections in diabetes. Infect Dis Clin North Am 11:735–750, 1997.

53. Warren JW. Catheter-associated urinary tract infections. Infect Dis Clin North Am 11:609–621, 1997.

54. Beaujean DJMA, Blok HEM, Vandenbroucke-Grauls CMJE, et al. Surveillance of nosocomial infections in geriatric patients. J Hosp Infect 36:275–284, 1997.

55. Lifshitz E, Kramer L. Outpatient urine culture: does collection technique matter? Arch Intern Med 160:2537–2540, 2000.

56. Wilson ML, Gaido L. Laboratory diagnosis of urinary tract infections in adult patients. Clin Infect Dis 38:1150–1158, 2004.

57. Kunin CM, VanArsdale White L, Hua Hua T. A reassessment of the importance of ''low count'' bacteriuria in young women with acute urinary symptoms. Ann Intern Med 119:454–460, 1993.

58. Stark RP, Maki DG. Bacteriuria in the catheterized patient. What quantitative level of bacteriuria is relevant? N Engl J Med 311:560–564, 1984.

59. Gupta K. Emerging antibiotic resistance in urinary tract pathogens. Infect Dis Clin North Am 17:243–259, 2003.

60. Karlowsky JA, Kelly LJ, Thornsberry C, et al. Trends in antimicrobials resistance among urinary tract infection isolates of Escherichia coli from female outpatients in the United States. Antimicrob Agent Chemother 46:2540–2545, 2002.

61. Krieger JN. Prostatitis revisited. New definitions, new approaches. Infect Dis Clin North Am 17:395–409, 2003.

62. Stapleton A, Stamm WE. Prevention of urinary tract infection. Infect Dis Clin North Am 11:719–733, 1997.

63. Rubin RH, Shapiro ED, Andriole VT, et al. Evaluation of new anti-infective drugs for the treatment of urinary tract infection. Clin Infect Dis 15 (Suppl):S216, 1992.

64. Gupta K, Sahm DF, Mayfield D, et al. Antimicrobial resistance among uropathogens that cause community-acquired urinary tract infections in women: a national analysis. Clin Infect Dis 33:89–94, 2001.

65. Raz R, Chazan B, Kennes Y, et al. Empiric use of trimethoprim-sulfamethoxazole (TMP-SMX) in the treatment of women with uncomplicated urinary tract infections, in a geographical area with a high prevalence of TMP-SMX-resistant uropathogens. Clin Infect Dis 34:1165–1169, 2002.

66. Warren JW, Abrutyn E, Hebel JR, et al. Guidelines for antimicrobials treatment of uncomplicated acute bacterial cystitis and acute pyelonephritis in women. Clin Infect Dis 29:745–758, 1999.

67. Arav-Boger R, Leibovici L, Danon YL. Urinary tract infections with low and high colony counts in young women. Arch Intern Med 154:300–304, 1994.

68. Osterberg E, Aberg H, Hallander HO, et al. Efficacy of single-dose versus seven-day trimethoprim treatment of cystitis in women: a randomized double-blind study. J Infect Dis 161:942–947, 1990.

59. Fihn SD, Johnson C, Roberts PL, et al. Trimethoprim-sulfamethoxazole for acute dysuria in women: a single dose or 10-day course. A double-blind, randomized study. Ann Intern Med 108:350–357, 1988.

70. Jardin A, Cesana M, and the French Multicenter Urinary Tract Infection-Rufloxacin Group. Randomized, double-blind comparison of single-dose regimens of rufloxacin and pefloxacin for acute uncomplicated cystitis in women. Antimicrob Agents Chemother 39:215–220, 1995.

71. Hooton TM, Johnson C, Winter C, et al. Single-dose and three-day regimens of ofloxacin versus trimethoprim-sulfamethoxazole for acute cystitis in women. Antimicrob Agents Chemother 35: 1479–1483, 1991.

72. Saginur R, Nicolle LE, Canadian Infectious Diseases Society Clinical Trials Study Group. Single-dose compared with 3-day norfloxacin treatment of uncomplicated urinary tract infection in women. Arch Intern Med 152:1233–1237, 1992.

73. Richard GA, Mathew CP, Kirstein JM, et al. Single-dose fluoroquinolone therapy of acute uncomplicated urinary tract infection in women: results from a randomized, double-blind, multicenter trial comparing single-dose to 3-day fluoroquinolone regimens. Urology 59:334–339, 2002.

74. Iravani A, Tice AD, McCarty J, et al. Short-course ciprofloxacin treatment of acute uncomplicated urinary tract infection in women. The minimum effective dose. Arch Intern Med 155:485–494, 1995.

75. Hooton TM, Winter C, Tiu F, et al. Randomized comparative trial and cost analysis of 3-day antimicrobial regimens for treatment of acute cystitis in women. JAMA 273:41–45, 1995.

76. Henry DC, Bettis RB, Riffer E, et al. Comparison of once-daily extended-release ciprofloxacin and conventional twice-daily ciprofloxacin for the treatment of uncomplicated urinary tract infection in women. Clin Ther 24:2088–2104, 2002.

77. Michael M, Hodson EM, Craig JC, et al. Short compared with standard duration of antibiotic treatment for urinary tract infection: a systematic review of randomised controlled trials. Arch Dis Child 87:118–123, 2002.

78. Vogel T, Verreault R, Gourdeau M, et al. Optimal duration of antibiotic therapy for uncomplicated urinary tract infection in older women: a double-blind randomized controlled trial. CMAJ 170: 469–473, 2004.

79. Naber KG, Bartnicki A, Bischoff W, et al. Gatifloxacin 200mg or 400mg once daily is as effective as ciprofloxacin 500mg twice daily for the treatment of patients with acute pyelonephritis or complicated urinary tract infections. Intl J Antimicrob Agent 23S1: S41–S53, 2004.

80. Talan DA, Klimberg IW, Nicolle LE, et al. Once-daily, extended-release ciprofloxacin for complicated urinary tract infections and acute uncomplicated pyelonephritis. J Urol 171:734–739, 2004.

81. Talan DA, Stamm WE, Hooton TM, et al. Comparison of ciprofloxacin (7 days) and trimethoprim-sulfamethoxazole (14 days) for acute uncomplicated pyelonephritis in women. JAMA 283: 1583–1590, 2000.

82. Mombelli G, Pezzoli R, Pinoja-Lutz G, et al. Oral vs intravenous ciprofloxacin in the initial empirical management of severe pyelonephritis or complicated urinary tract infections. Arch Intern Med 159:53–58, 1999.

83. Stamm WE, McKevitt M, Counts GW. Acute renal infection in women: treatment with trimethoprim-sulfamethoxazole or ampicillin for two or six weeks. Ann Intern Med 106:341–345, 1987.

84. Nicolle LE, Louie TJ, Dubois J, et al. Treatment of complicated urinary tract infections with lomefloxacin compared with that with trimethoprim-sulfamethoxazole. Antimicrob Agents Chemother 38: 1368–1373, 1994.

85. Frankenschmidt A, Naber KG, Bischoff W, et al. Once-daily fleroxacin versus twice-daily ciprofloxacin in the treatment of complicated urinary tract infections. J Urol 158:1494–1499, 1997.

86. Raz R, Schiller D, Nicolle LE. Chronic indwelling catheter replacement before antimicrobials therapy for symptomatic urinary tract infection. J Urol 164:1254–1258, 2000.

87. Lundstrom T, Sobel J. Nosocomial candiduria: a review. Clin Infect Dis 32:1602–1607, 2001.

88. Jacobs LG, Skidmore EA, Cardoso LA, et al. Bladder irrigation with amphotericin B for treatment of fungal urinary tract infections. Clin Infect Dis 18:313–318, 1994.

89. Sobel JD, Kauffman CA, McKinsey D, et al. Candiduria: a randomized, double-blind study of treatment with fluconazole and placebo. Clin Infect Dis 30:19–24, 2000.

90. Kauffman CA, Vazquez JA, Sobel JD, et al. Prospective multicenter surveillance study of funguria in hospitalized patients. Clin Infect Dis 30:14–18, 2000.

91. Melekos MD, Werner Asbach H, Gerharz E, et al. Post-intercourse versus daily ciprofloxacin prophylaxis for recurrent urinary tract infections in premenopausal women. J Urol 157:935–939, 1997.

92. Gupta K, Hooton TM, Roberts PL, et al. Patient-initiated treatment of uncomplicated recurrent urinary tract infections in young women. Ann Intern Med 135:9–16, 2001.

93. Nicolle LE. Asymptomatic bacteriuria. When to screen and when to treat. Infect Dis Clin North Am 17:367–394, 2003.

94. Griebling TL, Nygaard IE. The role of estrogen replacement therapy in the management of urinary tract incontinence and urinary tract infection in postmenopausal women. Endocrin Metabol Clin North Am 26:347–360, 1997.

95. Brown JS, Vittinghoff E, Kanaya AM, et al. Urinary tract infections in postmenopausal women: effect of hormone therapy and risk factors. Obstet Gynecol 98:1045–1052, 2001.

96. Raz R, Colodner R, Rohana Y, et al. Effectiveness of estriol-containing vaginal pessaries and nitrofurantoin macrocrystal therapy in the prevention of recurrent urinary tract infection in postmenopausal women. Clin Infect Dis 36:1362–1368, 2003.

97. Stapleton A. Novel approaches to prevention of urinary tract infections. Infect Dis Clin North Am 17:457–471, 2003.

98. Kontiokari T, Sundqvist K, Nuutinen M, et al. Randomised trial of cranberry-lingonberry juice and Lactobacillus GG drink for the prevention of urinary tract infections in women. Br Med J 322:1–5, 2001.

99. Uehling DT, Hopkins WJ, Elkahwaji JE, et al. Phase 2 clinical trial of a vaginal mucosal vaccine for urinary tract infections. J Urol 170:867–869, 2003.

100. Barry HC, Ebell MH, Hickner J. Evaluation of suspected urinary tract infection in ambulatory women: a cost analysis of office-based strategies. J Fam Pract 44:49–60, 1997.

101. Rubin N, Foxman B. The cost-effectiveness of placing urinary tract infection treatment over the counter. J Clin Epidemiol 49: 1315–1321, 1996.

102. Plumridge RJ, Golledge CL. Treatment of urinary tract infection. Clinical and economic considerations. Pharmacoeconomics 9: 295–306, 1996.

103. National Nosocomial Infections Surveillance (NNIS) Report, data summary from October 1986–April 1997, issued May 1997. Am J Infect Control 25:477–487, 1997.

104. Hooton TM, Scholes D, Hughes JP, et al. A prospective study of risk factors for symptomatic urinary tract infection in young women. N Engl J Med 335:468–474, 1996.

105. Jones RN, Kehrberg EN, Erwin ME, et al. Prevalence of important pathogens and antimicrobial activity of parenteral drugs at numerous medical centers in the United States. Study on the threat of emerging resistances: real or perceived? Diagn Microbiol Infect Dis 19:203–215, 1994.

106. Hoban DJ, Jones RN. Canadian ofloxacin susceptibility study: a comparative study from 18 medical centers. Chemotherapy 41: 34–38, 1995.

107. Gillenwater JY, Clark M. Tentative direct antimicrobial susceptibility testing in urine. J Urol 156:149–153, 1996.

Intraabdominal Infections

78

Douglas N. Fish

DEFINITION

Intraabdominal infections are among the most common types of infections encountered in clinical practice, yet they remain among the most challenging to manage effectively. These infections present serious clinical problems because they are difficult to diagnose and successful treatment requires aggressive use of nonpharmacologic modalities as well as antibiotics. Such infections generally occur after bowel contents and bacteria leak from the gastrointestinal (GI) tract into the sterile environment of the peritoneal cavity or retroperitoneal space. The peritoneal cavity is the cavity extending from below the diaphragm to the floor of the pelvis; the retroperitoneal space lies posterior to the peritoneal cavity and just in front of the spine, with its associated musculature and tissues. Infections of these spaces may result in either diffuse peritonitis, an acute inflammation of the peritoneal cavity, or localized abscesses.

Intraabdominal infections are defined in this chapter as primary peritonitis, secondary peritonitis, tertiary peritonitis, and intraabdominal abscess. Primary peritonitis may seemingly occur spontaneously without any obvious source of peritoneal contamination; therefore, it is sometimes referred to as spontaneous bacterial peritonitis (SBP). Primary peritonitis may occur in children but most commonly occurs in adults who have a history of alcoholic cirrhosis and refractory ascites.[1–3] Primary peritonitis is also associated with postnecrotic liver disease, nephrosis, acute or chronic hepatitis, peritoneal dialysis, or other conditions associated with ascites or abnormal fluid collections in the peritoneum.[3] Secondary peritonitis is usually associated with one or more processes that result in introduction of fecal material or other contents from the lumen of the GI tract directly into the peritoneal cavity. These include such diverse processes as abdominal trauma; surgery; or intrinsic obstructive, neoplastic, or inflammatory GI diseases (Table 78.1). Tertiary peritonitis is defined as a later stage in the disease process, when apparently adequate management of secondary peritonitis is followed by clinical peritonitis and systemic signs of sepsis (e.g., fever, tachycardia, tachypnea, hypotension, elevated cardiac index, low systemic vascular resistance, leukopenia, leukocytosis, and/or multiorgan failure) that persist or recur at least 48 hours later.[3–5] Health care-associated intraabdominal infections, usually referred to as nosocomial intraabdominal infections, often occur after elective or emergent surgery. Intraabdominal abscess may be associated with any of these major types of intraabdominal infection.

TREATMENT GOALS

- Provide appropriate pharmacologic and nonpharmacologic therapies.
- Maintain general homeostatic support, including management of hemodynamic, respiratory, and intestinal integrity; analgesia; sedation; and fluid and nutritional support for the patient.
- Provide adequate source control in the form of surgical repair of intraabdominal injuries, drainage of contaminated fluids, and/or radiologically guided procedures to remove infected fluid collections.

■ Select an appropriate antimicrobial agent for pharmacologic treatment that targets the suspected organisms, including facultative gram-negative aerobes, obligate anaerobes, and gram-positive aerobes as necessary.
■ Eradicate infecting microorganisms to prevent bacteremia or extension of the infection to other internal organs and spaces, decrease the likelihood of recurrent infections, and shorten the time to resolution of clinical signs and symptoms.
■ Prevent treatment failures leading to the development of tertiary peritonitis, intraabdominal abscess, or other complications.[6]

TABLE 78.1	Etiology of Secondary Peritonitis
Primary infectious causes	Appendicitis (gangrenous, necrotizing, abscessed)
	Biliary tract infection (acute cholecystitis, ascending/necrotizing cholangitis)
	Diverticulitis (perforation)
	Gynecologic infections (salpingitis, severe endometritis)
	Pancreatitis (infectious, necrotizing)
	Pelvic inflammatory disease
	Ruptured abscess (hepatic, pancreatic, splenic)
	Typhlitis (neonates and children)
Iatrogenic and/or procedure-related	Colonoscopy or endoscopy
	Dehiscence or leakage of gastrointestinal anastomoses
	Intraoperative events
	Paracentesis
Inflammatory bowel disease	Crohn's disease, ulcerative colitis
Neoplasms	Bowel obstruction
	Perforation (gastric, intestinal)
Peptic ulcer disease	Gastric or duodenal perforation
Small bowel obstructions	
Trauma	Blunt trauma with intestinal rupture (motor vehicle accidents, other nonpenetrating traumas)
Vascular ischemia	Arterio- or veno-occlusive disorders/ events affecting mesenteric vessels (hypercoagulable disorders, atrial fibrillation/flutter with left ventricular clots, inflammatory bowel diseases)
	Severe ischemia without occlusion (severe atherosclerotic disease, severe cardiac dysfunction)

EPIDEMIOLOGY

Primary peritonitis (also frequently referred to as SBP) refers to an invasion of bacteria into the peritoneal cavity without obvious perforation of the bowel or other source of contamination. It occurs predominantly in infants and young children (10% to 20% of cases) and in adults with cirrhosis and large collections of ascitic fluid.[3] Secondary peritonitis refers to a peritoneal infection secondary to perforation, bowel necrosis, or some penetrating infectious process. Perforation of a hollow viscus accounts for 60% to 80% of cases of secondary peritonitis and may be due to a large variety of causes, including complications of peptic ulcer disease, trauma, severe diverticulitis, and many others (Table 78.1). Tertiary peritonitis refers to persistent or recurrent intraabdominal infections seen in critically ill and/or immunocompromised patients after management of secondary peritonitis.[5–8] Postoperative infections occurring after elective or emergent surgical procedures are considered to be health care-associated intraabdominal infections and are quite different from other types of infections in terms of their microbiology and associated pathogens.

The microbiology of intraabdominal infections is a critical factor in the epidemiology of this infection. The specific organisms involved in these infections are a major determinant of the extent and severity of infection as well as dictating the type of antimicrobial therapy used to treat them. Enterobacteriaceae (gram-negative aerobic bacterial flora) and anaerobes originating from the GI tract cause the great majority of intraabdominal infections. In general, however, the normal GI tract bacterial flora is of low virulence. The number of different bacterial species and the absolute quantity of bacterial load within the lumen of the gut increase as one travels down the GI tract from the mouth to the anus. This flora is stable early in childhood and for the most part does not differ with geographic location, race, diet, or increasing age. In the human stomach there are usually less than 10^4 colony-forming units (CFU) per mL of aerobic and anaerobic microflora. Acidity of gastric fluids and normal GI motility are important factors that inhibit bacterial growth in this region.[9] Trauma or diseases of the stomach and duodenal region may compromise these protective factors. Thus, medical conditions such as gastric or duodenal ulcerations, achlorhydria, obstructing gastric or duodenal malignancies, and upper GI hemorrhage may result in abnormal proliferation of the local flora (e.g., anaerobic streptococci, Viridans streptococci, lactobacilli, and yeast). Certain drug therapies may also cause changes in the types or numbers of bacteria present in the upper GI tract, particularly those that alter gastric pH (e.g., antacids, histamine$_2$-receptor antagonists, proton pump inhibitors).

The microflora of the proximal small bowel is similar to that in the stomach, although increased numbers of Enterobacteriaceae and *Bacteroides* spp. may be found. Peristalsis is most pronounced in the jejunum and upper ileum, which in part explains the low bacterial counts relative to the distal ileum. Injury or disease of this upper portion of the GI tract results in relatively low bacterial inocula into the peritoneal cavity. Thus, the number and severity of clinical infections related to such injuries would be fewer compared with injuries of the large bowel. Between the proximal and terminal ileum is a bacterial transition zone where the composition of organisms changes toward greater numbers of aerobic and anaerobic gram-negative bacilli, and bacterial loads increase up to 10^8 CFU per mL.

The highest concentration of microorganisms in the GI tract is in the colon. As many as 10^{11} CFU per mL organisms are present and account for roughly one third of the total weight of the GI contents. Anaerobes typically outnumber aerobes by a ratio of approximately 1,000 to 1, with *Bacteroides* spp. being the predominant bacteria.[10] Under the usual conditions within the lumen of the GI tract these anaerobic organisms behave as harmless commensals, but when introduced into surrounding host tissues and the peritoneal cavity they exhibit significant pathogenic potential. Certain underlying clinical conditions, such as compromised vascular supply or tissue necrosis, as well as perforations may predispose a patient to anaerobic infections. Such clinical situations are associated with confined tissue spaces with a low oxidation-reduction potential and hypoxia, and thus provide an environment favorable for uncontrolled anaerobic proliferation.

Although more than 400 species of anaerobes reside in the colon and 200 in the oral cavity, only a few are associated with most clinical anaerobic infections. *Bacteroides fragilis* accounts for only approximately 5% of the colonic microflora, yet it causes many times the incidence of clinical infection compared with any other *Bacteroides* spp.

Pathogens isolated from patients with various types of intraabdominal infection can be quite varied (Table 78.2).[3–5,11–14] By necessity, antimicrobial regimens for the treatment of intraabdominal infection are selected based, at least in part, on specific pathogens most likely to be found in these various types of infection as well as the probable source (i.e., anatomic site) of the infection. Thus, clinicians must be aware of the differences in the bacterial microflora in various portions of the GI tract.

The bacteria isolated from the ascitic fluid in patients with SBP are usually those of the normal intestinal flora. More than 90% of all cases of SBP are monomicrobial, with aerobic gram-negative bacilli being responsible for more than two thirds of all cases. *Escherichia coli* accounts for nearly half of these cases, followed by *Klebsiella* spp, *Enterobacter* spp, *Proteus mirabilis*, and other gram-negative aerobic bacteria.[3] Primary peritonitis in children is commonly caused by *Streptococcus pneumoniae* and group A streptococci. Anaerobes are quite unusual as a cause of primary peritonitis. In contrast, secondary peritonitis infections are classically "mixed" and involve both aerobic and anaerobic bacteria. Within this setting of mixed bacteria, there appears to be the potential for bacterial synergism. The aerobic Enterobacteriaceae have been demonstrated to lower oxygen tension or redox potential within the peritoneal cavity, thus promoting the growth of obligate anaerobes. Conversely, there is some evidence that the presence of anaerobic organisms enhances the pathogenicity of aerobic gram-negative bacilli. A variety of obligate anaerobes have been observed to interfere with intracellular bacterial killing by polymorphonuclear leukocytes (PMNs), as well as PMN chemotaxis and phagocytosis.[15] The bacteria of tertiary peritonitis often involves organisms with low intrinsic virulence, such as *Staphylococcus epidermidis* or *Enterococcus faecium*. However, more difficult gram-negative bacilli, including inducible β-lactamase producers such as *Enterobacter* spp, *Serratia* spp, *Citrobacter* spp, and *Pseudomonas aeruginosa*, as well as *Candida* spp, may also be seen in these infections.

Observations in humans and in animal models of intraabdominal infection reveal a biphasic disease process. After intraabdominal inoculation of intestinal flora, animals initially developed acute peritonitis, predominantly caused by aerobic gram-negative bacilli and less frequently by enterococci.[16] This phase is associated with an approximately 40% mortality rate. Surviving animals later developed intraabdominal abscesses that were culture-positive most often for obligate anaerobes. However, when large inocula (5×10^7 CFU/mL) of a single strain of bacteria were used, no strain alone, either aerobic or anaerobic, was able to induce abscesses. This evidence reaffirms the significance of bacterial synergism in the formation of abscesses.

The microbiology of peritonitis in patients receiving continuous ambulatory peritoneal dialysis (CAPD) reveals that most cases are caused by the aerobic organisms commonly residing on the skin. Most episodes (70% of cases) are caused by gram-positive cocci (*S. aureus*, *S. epidermidis*, and various streptococci). Enterobacteriaceae cause infection less frequently (25% of cases), and also occasionally anaerobes, mycobacteria, and fungi are the cause (total of <5% of cases). It is thought that anaerobic organisms rarely cause infection in this group of patients because of the high oxygen tension present in the dialysate.

TABLE 78.2	Isolation of Pathogens From Blood and Peritoneal Fluid Cultures in Patients with Secondary Peritonitis		

Aerobic Bacteria

Gram-negative bacilli		*Escherichia coli*	32–99%
		Klebsiella	2–30%
		Enterobacter	2–26%
		Proteus	4–23%
		Pseudomonas aeruginosa	2–15%
Gram-positive cocci		Enterococci	6–24%
		Streptococci	6–55%
		Staphylococci	6–24%
Miscellaneous aerobic bacteria			2–22%

Anaerobic Bacteria

		Bacteroides fragilis	23–100%
		Other *Bacteroides* spp	19–58%
		Clostridium	5–36%
		Fusobacterium	3–35%
		Streptococci	0–19%
		Miscellaneous anaerobes	0–25%

(Data from Johnson CC, Baldessarre J, Levison ME. Peritonitis: update on pathophysiology, clinical manifestations, and management. Clin Infect Dis 124:1035–1047, 1997; Marshall JC, Innes M. Intensive care unit management of intraabdominal infection. Crit Care Med 31:2228–2237, 2003; Levison ME, Bush LM. Peritonitis and other intraabdominal infections. In: Mandell GL, Bennett JE, Dolin R, eds. Mandell, Douglas and Bennett's Principles and Practice of Infectious Diseases. 5th ed. Philadelphia: Churchill Livingstone, 2000:821–856; Lau WY, Teoh-Chan CH, Fan ST, et al. The bacteriology and septic complication of patients with appendicitis. Ann Surg 200:576–581, 1984; Jones RC, Thal ER, Johnson NA, et al. Evaluation of antibiotic therapy following penetrating abdominal trauma. Ann Surg 201:576–585, 1985; Solomkin JS, Dellinger EP, Christou NV, et al. Results of a multicenter trial comparing imipenem/cilastatin to tobramycin/clindamycin for intraabdominal infections. Ann Surg 212:581–591, 1990; and Barie PS, Vogel SB, Patchen Dellinger EP, et al. A randomized, double-blind clinical trial comparing cefepime plus metronidazole with imipenem-cilastatin in the treatment of complicated intraabdominal infections. Arch Surg 132:1254–1302, 1997.)

PATHOPHYSIOLOGY

The pathogenesis of primary peritonitis is still not well understood. It may result from bacterial spread from hematogenous or lymphatic sources or from microperforation (e.g., intestinal transmural migration, or translocation) of an otherwise intact GI tract. Newer evidence indicates that direct translocation of bacteria is responsible for many infections, but other mechanisms such as mesenteric inflammation and splanchnic vasodilatation may also play important roles in the pathophysiology leading to primary peritonitis.[3] Secondary peritonitis from traumatic injury or GI disease results in the following situations when the first-line host defense mechanisms become overwhelmed: very large bacterial inocula, bacterial contamination caused by mixed aerobic and anaerobic flora that act synergistically to evade the first-line host defenses, and often the presence of foreign materials (e.g., CAPD catheters, organic fecal matter, soil or debris following traumatic injuries) that cause host defenses to be less efficient, and intraleukocytic sequestration of organisms to occur.[2,17]

The concept of mixed bacterial infection is especially relevant to secondary and tertiary peritonitis and intraabdominal abscesses.[18] As many as 400 to 500 anaerobic and aerobic species of microorganisms have been found to be present as part of the normal intestinal flora. Thus, when infection occurs after spillage of GI contents, multiple organisms may be responsible. However, the mere presence of an organism in the peritoneum does not guarantee its pathogenicity or true involvement in the infectious process. Enterobacteriaceae can produce endotoxins and thus can trigger septic shock. *Bacteroides* spp have a certain virulence factor, the polysaccharide capsule, that explains in part the observed pathogenicity of these organisms. The presence of other organisms, such as *Enterococcus* spp, has not reproducibly caused morbidity or mortality.

Even after identification of the pathogens, clinical outcome may be influenced by other factors. They include the bacterial load at the site of infection (i.e., the inoculum size) and immunologic variables relating to local host defenses, as well as the general systemic immune response and the severity of any underlying intrinsic GI disease. Most important are the success of surgical interventions performed, and whether administered antimicrobial agents penetrate to the site of infection and are pharmacologically active in that environment. All of these factors should be considered when selecting antimicrobial therapy, as well as when assessing clinical response.

A general understanding of the anatomic relationships within the peritoneal cavity is important for determining the possible sources of intraabdominal infection, as well as anticipating the extent and routes of spread of infection. The peritoneal cavity in males is a completely closed space, whereas in females the free ends of the fallopian tubes penetrate into it. This distinction is important because peritonitis often accompanies pelvic inflammatory disease, especially if infection of the fallopian tubes is severe. Organs found within the peritoneal cavity include the stomach, jejunum, ileum, transverse and sigmoid colon, cecum, liver, gallbladder, pancreas, spleen, and appendix. The peritoneal cavity has various pouches and recesses in which bacteria or infected exudate may collect and become loculated, potentially leading to the formation of abscesses. The peritoneal cavity is lined by a serous membrane that consists of a monolayer of mesothelial cells, beneath which are lymphatics, blood vessels, and nerve endings. The peritoneal space usually contains sufficient fluid to maintain surface moistness, which facilitates movement of the viscera. This moist peritoneal membrane is also highly permeable, so solutes and water are quickly transported in a bidirectional manner.

Host defense mechanisms generally combat bacterial invasion of the peritoneal cavity. Humoral and cellular immune defense mechanisms form the initial response to bacterial contamination, and the regional lymphatic circulation clears the bacterial debris. Intraabdominal infection results when these first-line host defenses are initially overwhelmed by the very large bacterial inoculum along with synergistically acting mixed bacterial flora and potentially foreign materials. The peritoneal membrane next responds by exuding a fluid containing opsonins, antibodies, complement, PMNs, and macrophages into the peritoneal cavity. This inflammatory response is presumably facilitated by local vasodilation and increased vascular permeability. Inflammation increases the membrane's permeability so that the transport of large molecules and protein is enhanced. This may also improve an antimicrobial agent's ability to penetrate into the peritoneal cavity during peritonitis.

CLINICAL PRESENTATION AND DIAGNOSIS

SIGNS AND SYMPTOMS
General malaise, prostration, nausea, vomiting, diarrhea, fever, dehydration, leukocytosis with a left shift, and electrolyte imbalance are common systemic symptoms that may be observed in patients with intraabdominal infections. Intraabdominal abscesses may often "smolder" for long periods of time without symptoms or with inconsistent symptoms.

Aerobic and anaerobic gram-negative bacteria may release endotoxin, a lipopolysaccharide from the bacterial cell wall, into the bloodstream, which is responsible at least in part for some of the serious clinical findings and complications observed in intraabdominal infections. These findings include sepsis and septic shock, acute respiratory distress syndrome, and disseminated intravascular coagulation. Although none of these clinical findings is specific to intraabdominal infections, the presence of such complications is an ominous clinical finding. Severe sepsis occurs in approximately 11% of patients with peritonitis and is associated with a 13-fold increased relative risk of death compared to patients without severe sepsis.[19] Factors associated with an increased risk of developing sepsis include the specific source of infection, extent of peritonitis, increasing age, and preexisting organ dysfunction.[19] Hypotension may also be exacerbated by reduced intravascular volume secondary to the massive influx of fluid from the vascular space into the peritoneum during peritonitis.

Abdominal pain and tenderness may be localized or general.[6] Specific abdominal pain associated with breathing or coughing, rebound tenderness, and tenderness to gentle abdominal percussion or exploration are additional signs of acute peritonitis. The musculature overlying the area of inflamed peritoneum may become spastic. Involuntary muscle rigidity of the entire abdominal wall ("guarding") may develop with diffuse peritonitis. This muscle rigidity, however, is frequently absent or difficult to elicit in patients in the latter stages of peritonitis, patients who are obese, or patients with significant extravasation or "third-spacing" of intravascular fluid (e.g., ascites).

DIAGNOSIS AND CLINICAL FINDINGS
The serous fluid in the peritoneal cavity is normally clear yellow, with a low specific gravity (<1.016) and a low protein concentration (usually <3 g/dL), with albumin being the predominant protein. Fibrinogen is not normally present. Solute concentrations are similar to those observed in plasma. A few leukocytes (<300/mL) and desquamated serosal cells also may be found.

Infected peritoneal fluid is often visibly cloudy. Measurements used for immediate diagnosis include pH less than 7.34 and a PMN count greater than 500 cells per mL in peritoneal fluid. Other positive predictive observations include a peritoneal fluid lactate concentration greater than 25 mg per dL and a fluid glucose concentration less than 60 mg per dL. Diagnostic sensitivity improves when multiple parameters are used to establish the diagnosis.[20]

Specimens from the infected tissue or fluid should be obtained during surgery or by needle aspirate and directly cultured for both anaerobic and aerobic bacteria. Gram stain of specimens also may help to identify potential pathogens more quickly so that empiric antimicrobial therapy can be tailored to the patient. The Gram staining procedure is especially important in situations where the patient has been on antibiotics before obtaining the specimen; in this situation the bacterial numbers may be suppressed to the point that no growth occurs on culture.

The diagnosis of intraabdominal abscesses has been greatly improved in recent years, particularly with the use of very sensitive computed tomography (CT) scans.[21] Isotope scans and ultrasonography are much less useful because of nonspecific and false-positive results. Also, CT-guided needle aspiration procedures or placement of percutaneous drains have been established in the last decade as important surgical adjuncts in the management of intraperitoneal infection.

PSYCHOSOCIAL ASPECTS

Patients with intraabdominal infections represent a broad cross-section of all psychological and social strata. Primary peritonitis in adults often occurs in patients with severe alcohol dependency.[22] Secondary peritonitis occurs in a broad range of patients. Infections are often related to perforations, ulcerations, and malignancies; therefore, patients may have received these injuries from motor vehicle or other accidents, domestic violence, or violent or crime-related activities. Tertiary peritonitis occurs in immunocompromised patients, such as those infected with the human immunodeficiency virus (HIV) or with cancer. The attitudes of patients toward pharmacotherapy and overall management schemes play a pivotal role in their acceptance of therapy.

THERAPEUTIC PLAN

Recommendations concerning the selection and use of antimicrobial therapy for the treatment of intraabdominal infections were published by the Surgical Infection Society (SIS) in 2002 and the Infectious Diseases Society of America (IDSA) in 2003.[23-25] These comprehensive and evidence-based guidelines address the epidemiology of intraabdominal infections, associated microbiology, and appropriate selection of antiinfective agents based on pharmacokinetics, mechanism of action, prevalence of microbial resistance, drug safety, and demonstrated clinical efficacy. These guidelines also address the timing of initiation of antibiotic therapy, modification of drug therapy based on culture results, and duration of therapy. These guidelines classify infections as complicated (requiring an operative procedure), uncomplicated (managed pharmacologically), and postoperative wound (operative procedure should be curative, but antiinfective drugs are used to prevent further infection at the site). Recommendations for the selection and use of antimicrobials for intraabdominal infections as further discussed in this

chapter are based on these recent guidelines published by the SIS and the IDSA.[23-25]

TREATMENT

PHARMACOTHERAPY

Certain types of intraabdominal infections do not require antimicrobial therapy for appropriate management.[3,23-25] Acute perforations of the upper GI tract (i.e., stomach, duodenum, and proximal jejunum) are associated with a low risk of peritonitis because the bacterial loads at these sites are relatively low. Therefore, specific antimicrobial therapy beyond customary perioperative antibiotic prophylaxis is not usually required if surgery occurs promptly. An exception to this general rule is patients who have underlying diseases or drug therapy that predispose to alterations in normal bacterial flora. Normal short-term perioperative antibiotic prophylaxis alone is also usually sufficient for acute appendicitis without evidence of gangrene, perforation, abscess, or generalized peritonitis. Finally, acute cholecystitis and pancreatitis are often noninfectious inflammatory processes that do not require specific antimicrobial therapy. Infectious cholecystitis or necrotizing pancreatitis, either documented or highly suspected based on clinical and radiologic findings, should be treated similar to other types of secondary peritonitis.[3,23-25]

Once an intraabdominal infection is suspected, appropriate antimicrobial therapy should be started immediately, even before the final diagnosis is made.[5,25] Fluid administration should be initiated before giving antibiotics to ensure adequate tissue perfusion and distribution of antibiotics to the site of infection. Antibiotics should be started before any surgical interventions to reduce the incidence of surgical wound infections. The proper sequence of events in the initial management of an intraabdominal infection should be as follows:

1. Careful clinical evaluation to establish high suspicion of infection
2. Administration of fluids to replenish intravascular volumes and maintain adequate tissue perfusion
3. Initiation of appropriate antimicrobial therapy
4. Surgical intervention as necessary[23,25]

Selection of empiric antimicrobial therapy should follow a careful thought process that considers first the suspected site and source of infection, along with the most likely pathogens (Table 78.3). Empiric therapy should be chosen to include, as narrowly as possible, only the most likely organisms. It is helpful to classify the infection as either community-acquired or health care–associated (i.e., nosocomial) to consider the types of organisms most commonly found in each, and appropriate susceptibility data should then be applied to the antibiotic selection process. Using antibiotics with the narrowest spectrum possible also reduces the incidence of secondary drug resistance, superinfection, and potential con-

TABLE 78.3	Common Pathogens That Should Be Considered During Empiric Therapy of Intraabdominal Infections		
Infection Type/Source	**Aerobic Bacteria**	**Anaerobic Bacteria**	**Other**
Primary peritonitis			
Adults	*Escherichia coli, Klebsiella, Streptococcus pneumoniae,* other streptococci	Rare	
Children	*Streptococcus pneumoniae,* group A streptococci, *E. coli*	Rare	
Secondary peritonitis			
Stomach, proximal small intestine	*E. coli, Klebsiella,* streptococci	Less common	
Biliary tract	*E. coli, Klebsiella, Enterobacter, Proteus, Enterococcus*	*Bacteroides fragilis* (less common)	
Distal small intestine, colon	*E. coli, Klebsiella, Enterobacter, Proteus*	*B. fragilis,* other *Bacteroides* species, *Clostridium, Fusobacterium,* gram-positive cocci	
Appendicitis (gangrenous, necrotic)	*E. coli, Klebsiella, Enterobacter, Proteus, Pseudomonas aeruginosa*	*B. fragilis,* other *Bacteroides* species, *Clostridium, Fusobacterium,* gram-positive cocci	
Tertiary peritonitis	*Staphylococcus aureus,* coagulase-negative staphylococci, *Enterococcus, P aeruginosa*	Less common	Candida
Health care-associated infections	*S. aureus* (including MRSA), *P. aeruginosa, E. coli, Klebsiella, Enterobacter, Proteus, Serratia,* other hospital-acquired gram-negative bacilli.	Less common	Candida
Abscesses	*E. coli, Klebsiella, Enterobacter, Enterococcus*	*B. fragilis,* other *Bacteroides* species, *Clostridium,* gram-positive cocci	
Peritonitis associated with continuous ambulatory peritoneal dialysis.	*S. aureus, Streptococcus, E. coli, Klebsiella*	Rare	

MRSA, methicillin-resistant *S. aureus.*

fusion when assessing clinical response or drug-related problems.

Next, the unique pharmacologic properties of each potential antimicrobial must be considered with regard to its ability to penetrate to the site of infection; lack or presence of a significant inoculum effect (alteration in drug activity caused by large bacterial numbers at the infection site); and its activity in various infection environments such as those with lower pH (as in abscesses) or more anaerobic conditions. Other factors that must be taken into consideration when selecting appropriate antimicrobial therapy include potential drug-related adverse reactions, convenience of dosing regimens, and cost of therapy. Table 78.4 lists antimicrobial agents that may be useful in the treatment of various intraabdominal infections, either as monotherapy or as part of regimens using combinations of drugs. The recommended adult

drug dosages are provided as well as a general description of the spectrum of antibacterial activity. Parenteral antibiotics are usually used initially, although subsequent conversion to oral regimens is possible in many patients.

Primary Peritonitis. Primary peritonitis associated with hepatic cirrhosis is usually caused by a single pathogen, and in 80% to 85% of cases three organisms are responsible: *E. coli,* streptococci such as *S. pneumoniae,* and *Klebsiella* spp. Monotherapy with an agent that provides adequate activity against gram-negative aerobic bacilli and streptococci is therefore a reasonable choice for treatment. Second- and third-generation cephalosporins are commonly used for this indication and have provided good clinical efficacy. Fluoroquinolones with good streptococcal activity (levofloxacin, gatifloxacin, moxifloxacin) are also effective, but concerns

TABLE 78.4	Antimicrobials for Empiric Therapy of Intraabdominal Infections: Usual Dosage and Spectrum of Activity			
Generic Name (Trade Name)	Usual Adult Daily Dosage	Activity Against *Bacteroides fragilis*	Activity Against Enterobacteriaceae	Activity Against *Enterococcus* spp
Metronidazole (Flagyl)	500 mg q8h	Yes	No	No
Clindamycin (Cleocin)	600–900 mg q8h	Yes	No	No
Cefuroxime (Zinacef, Kefurox)	750 mg or 1.5 g q8h	No	Yes	No
Cefotetan (Cefotan)	1–2 g q12h	Yes	Yes	No
Cefoxitin (Mefoxin)	1–2 g q6–8h	Yes	Yes	No
Cefotaxime (Claforan)	1–2 g q6–8h	Some	Yes	No
Ceftizoxime (Ceftizox)	1–2 g q6–8h	Yes	Yes	No
Ceftazidime (Fortaz, Tazidime, Tazicef)	1–2 g q8h	No	Yes	No
Ceftriaxone (Rocephin)	1–2 g q24h	No	Yes	No
Cefepime (Maxipime)	1–2 g q12h	No	Yes	No
Ampicillin/sulbactam (Unasyn)	1.5–3 g q6h	Yes	Yes	Yes
Ticarcillin/clavulanic acid (Timentin)	3.1 g q4h	Yes	Yes	Some
Piperacillin/tazobactam (Zosyn)	3.375–4.5 g q6h	Yes	Yes	Yes
Ertapenem (Invanz)	1 g q24h	Yes	Yes	No
Imipenem (Primaxin)	500 mg q6–8h	Yes	Yes	No
Meropenem (Merrem)	1 g q8h	Yes	Yes	No
Tigecycline (Tygacil)	100 mg × 1 dose, then 50 mg q12h	Yes	Yes	Yes
Ciprofloxacin (Cipro)	400 mg q8–12h	No	Yes	No
Levofloxacin (Levaquin)	500–750 mg q24h	No	Yes	No
Gatifloxacin (Tequin)	400 mg q24h	Some	Yes	No
Moxifloxacin (Avelox)	400 mg q24h	Yes	Yes	No
Gentamicin or Tobramycin	Peak 5–10 μg/mL, trough <2 μg/mL	No	Yes	No
Aztreonam (Azactam)	1 g q6–8h	No	Yes	No
Penicillin G[b]	1–2 million units q4–6h	No	No	Yes
Ampicillin[b]	1–2 g q4–6h	No	Some	Yes
Vancomycin (Vancocin)[c]	1 g q12h (trough 5–10 μg/mL)	No	No	Yes
Quinupristin/dalfopristin (Synercid)[d]	7.5 mg/kg q8h	No	No	Some
Linezolid (Zyvox)[d]	600 mg q12h	Some	No	Yes
Daptomycin (Cubicin)[d]	4 mg/kg q24h	No	No	Yes

[a]Not adjusted for renal impairment
[b]For *Enterococcus* spp when required
[c]For *Enterococcus* spp or methicillin-resistant *S. aureus*
[d]For vancomycin-resistant enterococci or methicillin-resistant *S. aureus* not responsive to vancomycin

regarding overuse of fluoroquinolones make these agents more suitable as alternatives to cephalosporins for this indication. Trimethoprim/sulfamethoxazole would also be a reasonable alternative for treatment of primary peritonitis in patients with cirrhosis. Ampicillin plus an aminoglycoside is often recommended for treatment of this infection. However, many physicians are hesitant to use aminoglycosides in pa-

tients with advanced cirrhosis due to the risk of drug-induced nephrotoxicity and potential association with hepatorenal syndrome, an irreversible and often fatal complication of end-stage liver disease. The risks and benefits of aminoglycoside-based therapy must be carefully evaluated in these patients, and other antibiotics are usually more preferable. Anaerobic bacteria are very uncommon as a cause of SBP, and the use of antibiotics with antianaerobic activity is not necessary. The presence of anaerobes such as *B. fragilis* should serve as a warning that a more complicated infection such as secondary peritonitis may be present. Agents with good antistaphylococcal activity are also not necessary, since *S. aureus* is also unusual as a cause of SBP. One exception to this is the occurrence of new infection in patients who have recently had pericentesis performed; antistaphylococcal antibiotics should be considered in these patients since *S aureus* or other skin flora may have been introduced into the peritoneal cavity during the procedure.

Administration of human serum albumin has been shown to significantly reduce mortality in patients with cirrhosis and primary peritonitis.[26] Administration of 1.5 g per kg of albumin on day 1 and 1 g per kg on day 3 of therapy reduced overall mortality to 10% in patients receiving albumin compared to 29% in those who received no albumin. The occurrence of renal impairment was also significantly reduced in patients receiving albumin compared to those who did not (10% vs. 33%, respectively). The benefits of albumin in this population are presumably related to increased plasma oncotic pressure, which helps prevent deleterious leakage of intravascular fluids into the abdominal cavity, thereby maintaining effective circulating blood volumes and preventing hemodynamic complications of infection. Although albumin may have important benefits in the treatment of SBP, it is considered to be adjunctive therapy and must be used together with prompt administration of antimicrobial agents.[26]

Prophylaxis of SBP through administration of antibiotics is common in high-risk cirrhotic patients (active GI bleeding, ascitic fluid protein levels of <1 g/dL, and patients with refractory ascites and a previous history of primary peritonitis). Selective decontamination of the gut with oral norfloxacin (400 mg daily) or trimethoprim/sulfamethoxazole (one double-strength tablet daily for 5 days every week) has been shown to be effective in reducing the incidence of primary peritonitis in such patients.[4,27]

Secondary Peritonitis. Effective treatment of secondary peritonitis is directed toward both aerobic gram-negative bacilli and *B fragilis* group anaerobes. The aerobic pathogens are responsible for early infectious morbidity and mortality, while anaerobes are the cause of late complications such as abscesses. Recommended regimens for empiric treatment of complicated intraabdominal infection, including community-acquired secondary peritonitis and health care-associated (i.e., nosocomial) infections, are shown in Figure 78.1. A wide range of monotherapy and combination therapy regimens are acceptable and recommended for the treatment of intraabdominal infections.[23–25] No antimicrobial regimen has been consistently shown to be superior to others in well-designed clinical trials. There are also no clear differences in efficacy between monotherapy versus combination regimens.[23,28,29] Therefore, recommended drugs and regimens are considered to be comparable in efficacy, and the choice of a specific regimen should be based on the other pharmacologic and clinical factors previously discussed. The following descriptions of various antibiotic therapies provide brief discussions of relative advantages and disadvantages and provide a framework for understanding the recommendations of the SIS and IDSA.

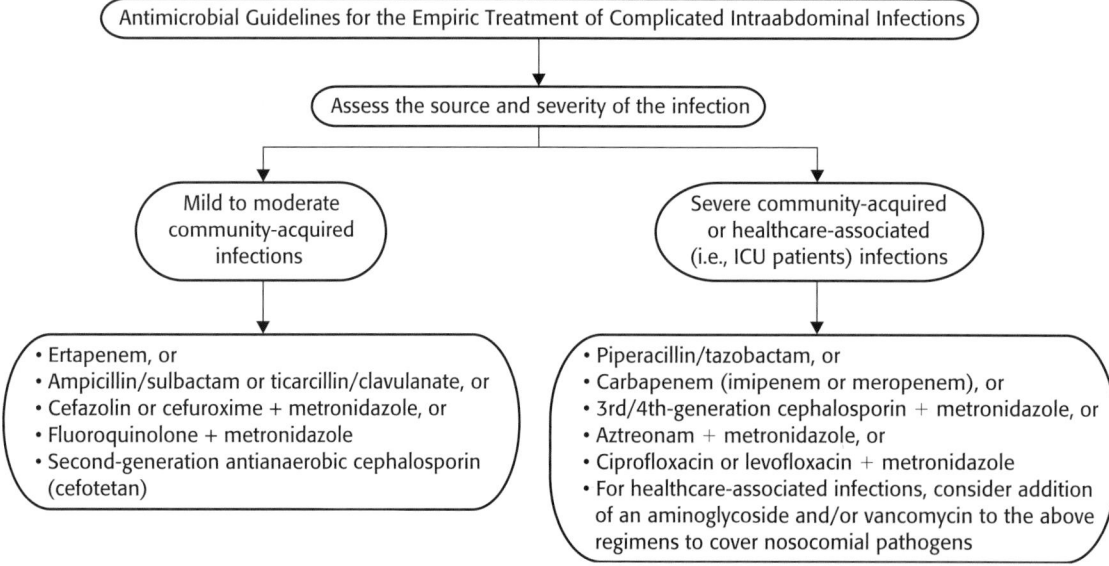

FIGURE 78.1 Recommendations for empiric antibiotic therapy for the treatment of community-acquired secondary peritonitis. (From Mazuski JE, Sawyer RG, Nathens AB, et al. The Surgical Infection Society guidelines on antimicrobial therapy for intraabdominal infections: an executive summary. Surg Infect 3:161–174, 2002; and Solomkin JS, Mazuski JE, Baron EJ, et al. Guidelines for the selection of anti-infective agents for complicated intraabdominal infections. Clin Infect Dis 37:997–1005, 2003.)

β-Lactam antibiotics, either as monotherapy or as part of combination regimens, are considered to be first-line agents in the treatment of both community-acquired and health care-associated intraabdominal infections. β-Lactam/β-lactamase inhibitor combination agents (specifically ampicillin/sulbactam and ticarcillin/clavulanate), and cefazolin or cefuroxime in combination with metronidazole are recommended by the SIS and IDSA as appropriate choices for community-acquired infections of mild to moderate severity.[23–25] These agents provide appropriate yet relatively narrow-spectrum activity against aerobic gram-negative bacilli and anaerobes, low risk of toxicity, and potential for cost-effective therapy. For more severe community-acquired infections, piperacillin/tazobactam and third-generation (ceftriaxone, cefotaxime, ceftizoxime, ceftazidime) or fourth-generation cephalosporins (cefepime) in combination with metronidazole are recommended due to their expanded spectrum of activity against gram-negative aerobic bacilli. β-Lactam/β-lactamase inhibitor combination agents provide excellent activity against anaerobes and may be used as monotherapy, but all of the cephalosporins listed above should be combined with metronidazole due to their relatively weak antianaerobic activity. Aztreonam plus metronidazole or clindamycin would also be an appropriate choice for empiric therapy of secondary peritonitis. Although antianaerobic second-generation cephalosporins (cefoxitin, cefotetan) have been extensively used for treatment of intraabdominal infections, their use is not uniformly recommended due to concerns regarding increasing resistance to these drugs among *B. fragilis* group organisms and the association of this resistance with poor patient outcomes.[25,30–32] Although the SIS and IDSA differ somewhat in their recommendations for use of the antianaerobic second-generation cephalosporins, these agents may be considered as alternative agents for the treatment of community-acquired infections of mild to moderate severity.

Piperacillin/tazobactam and antipseudomonal cephalosporins (ceftazidime and cefepime) are also potentially appropriate choices for empiric therapy of health care-associated intraabdominal infections due to their excellent activity against *P. aeruginosa* and other aerobic gram-negative nosocomial pathogens. These agents are often used in combination with aminoglycosides or fluoroquinolones for this indication. The choice of specific agents for empiric treatment of health care-associated infections, as well as the need for combination regimens, must be dictated by institution-specific susceptibility patterns and subsequently guided by culture results. Aztreonam also has an appropriate spectrum of gram-negative activity and may be useful for treatment of infections in patients with severe β-lactam allergies. Anaerobic organisms are not as commonly encountered in health care-associated intraabdominal infections, so the routine use of agents with antianaerobic activity is not recommended.[16,17] The use of metronidazole in combination with third- or fourth-generation cephalosporins is therefore not necessary for these infections.

The carbapenems are excellent agents that are stable against many types of β-lactamase enzymes and have excellent activity against gram-negative aerobic organisms, many gram-positive aerobes, and anaerobic bacteria. Ertapenem is a newer carbapenem that shares the excellent activity of the carbapenem class in most respects; however, unlike imipenem/cilastatin and meropenem, it has little activity against *P. aeruginosa*. Ertapenem has been shown to be as effective as piperacillin/tazobactam or ceftriaxone plus metronidazole in the treatment of complicated intraabdominal infections.[33,34] Lack of antipseudomonal activity makes ertapenem suitable for the treatment of mild to moderately severe community-acquired intraabdominal infections, and this agent is recommended as a first-line agent in these patients.[23,25] The broader spectrum of activity of imipenem/cilastatin and meropenem, particularly for *P. aeruginosa*, makes them most appropriate for the treatment of community-acquired infections in patients who are severely ill and at high risk of death or complications. Imipenem/cilastatin and meropenem are also recommended for the treatment of health care-associated infections, where *P. aeruginosa* or other more resistant pathogens are more common.

Aminoglycosides are often used to provide specific antimicrobial activity against aerobic gram-negative bacilli and have been extensively used as part of combination regimens (e.g., with metronidazole or clindamycin) in the treatment of intraabdominal infections for many years. However, these agents have a narrow therapeutic window, with the potential for nephrotoxicity and ototoxicity. Although the use of high-dose (5 to 7 mg/kg/day), extended-interval, or "once-daily" regimens may reduce the risk of toxicities and need for monitoring of serum concentrations, there is controversy as to whether the aminoglycosides should be routinely recommended for the treatment of community-acquired intraabdominal infections due to the availability of equally effective and less toxic agents.[23,25,35] Aminoglycoside-containing regimens may be considered for patients with allergies to β-lactam antibiotics, but fluoroquinolone-based regimens are currently recommended by some authorities as the drugs of choice in these patients.[25] The aminoglycosides are, however, still recommended as first-line agents for use in the treatment of health care-associated intraabdominal infections when local susceptibility patterns of nosocomial pathogens suggest that their use may be appropriate.[23,25] When aminoglycosides are to be used, either extended-interval (5 to 7 mg/kg/day) or traditional divided-dose regimens appear to be clinically equivalent.[36] When traditional regimens are used, peak serum concentrations for gentamicin or tobramycin of approximately 5 to 6 μg per mL are probably sufficient for most patients. The choice of a particular dosing method and regimen should be determined for each individual patient based on the patient's weight, renal function, suspected pathogens and associated aminoglycoside susceptibilities, and other factors specific to the patient. Individualization of dosing regimens based on serum concentration measurements is appropriate and should be routinely done in patients receiving traditional regimens.

Fluoroquinolones (e.g., ciprofloxacin, levofloxacin, gatifloxacin, moxifloxacin) have excellent abdominal penetration and often superior gram-negative aerobic activity compared with many cephalosporins. The favorable adverse-effect profile of the fluoroquinolones also makes them attractive for the treatment of intraabdominal infections. A potential disadvantage of the fluoroquinolones is that they must be used as part of combination regimens along with agents such as metronidazole that provide adequate activity against anaerobic pathogens. Although moxifloxacin has good in vitro activity against many anaerobic organisms and demonstrated efficacy in the treatment of intraabdominal infections through well-designed clinical trials, its routine use as monotherapy cannot be recommended at this time. In addition, increasing resistance among B. fragilis group isolates has led to specific recommendations that moxifloxacin and gatifloxacin should also be used in combination with metronidazole.[25] A final consideration in the use of the fluoroquinolones is that they may be administered orally to complete a course of antibiotic treatment in order to provide more cost-effective therapy.[37] Oral ciprofloxacin plus oral metronidazole has been shown to be as effective as intravenous piperacillin/tazobactam or imipenem/cilastatin in patients who have responded well to initial parenteral therapy and can be switched to oral therapy.[38,39] The other fluoroquinolones are probably also effective as part of oral regimens but have not been well studied in this regard, as has ciprofloxacin. Although the fluoroquinolones are generally most suited to community-acquired infections, ciprofloxacin and levofloxacin may also be considered for use in health care-associated infections due to their antipseudomonal activity. However, increasing fluoroquinolone resistance among P. aeruginosa makes it important to consider local susceptibility patterns when the use of these agents is being considered.

Clindamycin has been used successfully for treatment of intraabdominal infections and abscesses. The value of clindamycin has been reduced, however, by the emergence of clindamycin-resistant B. fragilis. The prevalence of clindamycin-resistant B. fragilis has been reported to exceed 20% in some regions.[40,41] Metronidazole is bactericidal for a wide range of anaerobic bacteria and is associated with little resistance after many years of use. Because of its excellent antianaerobic activity, little resistance, and very narrow overall spectrum of activity, metronidazole is usually favored over clindamycin as the antianaerobic drug of choice to be used as part of combination regimens for complicated intraabdominal infections.[25] Metronidazole should be avoided during pregnancy and lactation because of concerns of teratogenicity. β-Lactam/β-lactamase inhibitor combination agents would be appropriate choices in patients who should not receive metronidazole; clindamycin-containing combination regimens would also be considered acceptable and would be particularly appropriate in patients with severe β-lactam allergies.

Tigecycline is a new agent that was recently approved by the U.S. Food and Drug Administration for the treatment of complicated skin/skin structure and intraabdominal infections. Tigecycline is a tetracycline derivative with a broad spectrum of antibacterial activity that includes many gram-negative aerobes, gram-positive cocci including methicillin-resistant S. aureus (MRSA) and vancomycin-resistant enterococci (VRE), and anaerobes. A notable exception to tigecycline's excellent spectrum of activity is P. aeruginosa, against which tigecycline has relatively poor activity. Tigecycline has been shown to be equivalent to imipenem/cilastatin in the treatment of complicated intraabdominal infections and would be suitable for the treatment of mild, moderate, and severe community-acquired infections.[42] Lack of significant antipseudomonal activity makes tigecycline less appropriate for empiric treatment of health care-associated infections. Tigecycline is associated with significant GI adverse effects, which are primarily seen during infusion of the drug; the drug is otherwise well tolerated with no important toxicities.

Controversy still exists regarding the need for empiric coverage of Enterococcus spp. Current recommendations do not emphasize the need for routine empiric coverage of enterococci, and it is usually not necessary.[23–25] Exceptions to this recommendation are patients exhibiting signs of septic shock or situations in which cultures of blood or peritoneal fluid reveal the presence of enterococci.[25] Since immunocompromised patients also have a relatively increased risk of enterococcal infection, specific coverage for enterococci may also be considered empirically in these patients. Enterococci have also been reported as a cause of superinfection in patients who have previously received broad-spectrum antibiotics for treatment of intraabdominal infections, and coverage for enterococci could also be justified in such patients.[43] Ampicillin is considered the drug of choice for empiric treatment of enterococci due to its excellent in vitro activity, favorable adverse effect profile, and low cost. Vancomycin is also active against most enterococci, but the increasing prevalence of VRE and concerns regarding the potential development of staphylococcal resistance dictate that the routine empiric use of vancomycin should be discouraged for this indication. Other antibiotics with good activity against Enterococcus spp (e.g., daptomycin, linezolid) should be reserved for the treatment of documented enterococcal infections when first-line therapies cannot be used due to resistance, allergies, or clinical failure.

Tertiary peritonitis occurs in a subset of patients who have been treated for secondary peritonitis but who have persistent or recurrent signs of infection. The microbiology of tertiary peritonitis is strikingly different from that of secondary peritonitis and is very similar to that of nosocomial infections in critically ill patients.[5,8] Specifically, tertiary peritonitis is associated with a high rate of infection with staphylococci, enterococci, P. aeruginosa, and Candida, but the presence of anaerobic organisms is uncommon. The mortality for patients with tertiary peritonitis is typically in excess of 50%, but optimal therapeutic strategies are not well defined. The need for repeated surgeries is a predictor of poor patient outcomes, with multiple procedures often necessary and high associated operative mortality rates.[44] The exact benefits of systemic antibiotic therapy are also not well established.[5,8,45] Antimicrobial therapy for tertiary peritonitis should be guided by culture results and susceptibility testing, with regimens being kept as narrow in spectrum as possible and antianaerobic agents being avoided.[5]

Health Care-Associated Infections. Postoperative infections differ considerably from primary or secondary peritonitis, so the selection of appropriate antibiotics is much different. Health care-associated infections are generally similar in their microbiology to other types of nosocomial infections and are often associated with more resistant gram-negative organisms such as *Enterobacter* spp, *Serratia* spp, *Citrobacter* spp, and *P. aeruginosa*. Gram-positive cocci such as *S. aureus* (including MRSA) and enterococci are much more common in these infections compared to primary or secondary peritonitis, and *Candida* spp may also be associated with these infections. Because of the wide variety of pathogens that may be present, these patients must be empirically treated with broad-spectrum regimens that provide adequate coverage against many potential organisms. Failure to provide adequate empiric antimicrobial therapy is associated with poor patient outcomes.[46] Empiric antimicrobial regimens should at a minimum provide activity against gram-negative aerobes, including *P. aeruginosa*, and staphylococci. Combination regimens that include antipseudomonal carbapenems (imipenem/cilastatin, meropenem), piperacillin/tazobactam, or cefepime plus an aminoglycoside or fluoroquinolone are often recommended. The choice of specific antibiotics should be based on the antibiotic susceptibilities in the specific institution. Anaerobic organisms are not commonly isolated in these infections, so the use of antibiotics with antianaerobic activity is not specifically needed.

The increasing frequency of infection due to MRSA and VRE is of particular concern in the management of health care-associated infections.[47–49] Intraabdominal infection caused by MRSA or VRE is an indicator of poor patient prognosis and higher overall severity of illness and is associated with an increased length of hospital stay.[50] These pathogens are more likely to be associated with postoperative wound infections in institutions with high rates of other nosocomial infections caused by these organisms (e.g., 20% to 25% MRSA among *S. aureus* isolates), and patients with prior nasal colonization with MRSA may also be at higher risk.[51] Vancomycin is the drug of choice for the treatment of suspected or documented infections due to MRSA. Linezolid or daptomycin would be more appropriate in institutions with high rates of infection caused by VRE, or when this pathogen is documented to be present. Patients in whom

Candida is suspected or documented should be treated with high-dose fluconazole (400 to 800 mg/day in patients with good renal function). Amphotericin B is also appropriate for invasive *Candida* infections, but its use is often limited by the potential for nephrotoxicity. Newer agents such as caspofungin, micafungin, and voriconazole may be appropriate alternatives in institutions with high rates of infections due to organisms such as *Candida krusei, C. tropicalis,* and *C. glabrata*, which are less susceptible or resistant to fluconazole, but their use should be reserved for patients unable to tolerate amphotericin B or those who are at high risk for toxicities.

Infections Associated With Continuous Ambulatory Peritoneal Dialysis. Patients receiving CAPD have a relatively high incidence of peritonitis, often arising from bacterial contamination caused during the technical aspects of CAPD administration.[52] The potential advantages of efficiency of CAPD compared with conventional intermittent hemodialysis have been tempered by this constant risk of peritonitis. Peritonitis in patients receiving CAPD may be caused by a wide range of bacterial pathogens, and specific antimicrobial regimens should be selected based on culture and susceptibility information. For initial empiric therapy while awaiting culture results, or in patients in whom culture information is not available, a first-generation cephalosporin or penicillinase-resistant penicillin (e.g., nafcillin, oxacillin) plus an aminoglycoside is often recommended to provide activity against gram-negative enteric bacilli, streptococci, and staphylococci. *S. aureus* is a common cause of peritonitis in CAPD, and therapy with a first-generation cephalosporin or penicillinase-resistant penicillin is preferred. Vancomycin should be reserved for patients with allergies to β-lactam antibiotics or with infections caused by MRSA. Aerobic gram-negative enteric bacilli (e.g., *E. coli, Klebsiella*) are also common causes of infection during CAPD and are usually successfully treated with aminoglycosides or cephalosporins. Again, specific antibiotics for these and other pathogens should be selected based on culture and susceptibility testing.

Special considerations must be taken into account when considering intraperitoneal drug administration for the treatment of peritonitis in patients receiving CAPD.[52] Studies have shown a loss of activity of some antibiotics in dialysis fluid owing to the low pH and high osmolarity of the dialysate solution. Aminoglycosides specifically have shown to have reduced bactericidal activity when the test medium pH is lowered to pH 5.5, which simulates the pH of infected dialysate solution. Also, β-lactams and aminoglycosides should not be mixed in the same peritoneal dialysis bag because there may be significant inactivation of the aminoglycoside, depending on the β-lactam used. These are important considerations when CAPD patients treated with aminoglycosides do not clinically respond as expected.

Duration of Antimicrobial Therapy. The appropriate duration of treatment for intraabdominal infections has not been well defined. Patients with posttraumatic secondary peritonitis may be treated with as little as 24 hours of antibiotics if surgical repairs are performed promptly (within 12 hours of the injury) and adequately.[23–25,53,54] For established peritonitis, antimicrobial therapy should be continued until clinical signs and symptoms of infection have resolved.[23–25] Assessment of clinical resolution should include normalization of temperature and white blood cell count as well as return of normal GI function. A total duration of therapy of 5 to 7 days is recommended in most patients. Longer courses of therapy (>7 days) may be required in patients who have persistent or recurrent evidence of intraabdominal infection. However, in such patients with unresolved infection, source control is often found to have been inadequate, and appropriate diagnostic procedures should be performed to assess the need for additional interventions.[5,23–25,48] Complications such as abscess formation should also be suspected in these patients. If no actual evidence of active infection is discovered after careful evaluation, antimicrobial therapy should be discontinued and the patient closely monitored.[23–25]

NONPHARMACOLOGIC THERAPY

In the patient with secondary or tertiary intraabdominal infection, the crucial therapy modality is prompt, adequate surgical intervention. Such surgical intervention is referred to as "source control." Surgical management of intraabdominal infections is initially based on any operative procedures necessary to repair GI perforations or injury. The primary goal of surgical intervention is to repair the source of bacterial contamination of the peritoneal cavity and prevent additional contamination. Equally important are débridement procedures to remove any infected or necrotic tissue and infectious foci, and drainage of abscesses or infected peritoneal fluid or pus. Debulking of infected or devitalized tissue also allows antibiotics and host defenses to have an impact on the outcome of the infection. Effective source control is thus crucial for management of the initial infection as well as for prevention of recurrences. In fact, adequate source control is often considered to be as important, if not more so, than selection of appropriate antibiotics.[5,23–25,55] This is true in the management of intraabdominal abscess as well as in secondary and tertiary peritonitis. Antibiotics are used to control systemic complications of sepsis and are ineffective if appropriate drainage is not achieved. Deaths do occur from undrained intraabdominal abscesses.[56] Surgical intervention has little place in primary peritonitis, but exploratory laparotomy is sometimes used to achieve a definitive diagnosis.

Surgery may be a therapeutic plan in CAPD patients to remove an infected catheter. The indication for Tenckhoff catheter removal in CAPD patients with peritonitis has not been established. Some physicians believe continuing regular CAPD in patients with peritonitis improves outcome because infectious exudate can be physically removed by each dialysis. Others feel that it is important to remove the catheter (thus losing dialysis access) because curing an infection

that involves a foreign body (i.e., the catheter) is extremely difficult. If a patient has not responded to therapy alone within 5 days, a conservative recommendation would be to consider removing the Tenckhoff catheter. Experience with fungal and *Pseudomonas* peritonitis in CAPD suggests that early catheter removal is indicated.

Along with surgical interventions and adequate source control, aggressive repletion and management of fluids are critical to achieving optimal patient outcomes.[5,53,55] Shifts of fluid and protein into the abdominal cavity as a result of severe inflammation of the peritoneum may be very severe and result in significant decreases in intravascular fluid volume. Important loss of circulating blood volume may also be the result of traumatic injuries that cause significant hemorrhage. Aggressive fluid therapy is thus necessary to restore and maintain proper intravascular volume, which allows for adequate cardiac function and tissue perfusion. In patients with significant blood loss, infusions of packed red blood cells or whole blood are often necessary to maintain adequate oxygen-carrying capacity of the blood while also achieving sufficient intravascular volume. In intraabdominal infections not associated with trauma, administration of large volumes of crystalloid solutions (i.e., 0.9% sodium chloride, lactated Ringer's solution) are often necessary to restore and maintain adequate circulatory volume. Rates of administration and total volumes of crystalloid solutions and/or blood products should be based on assessment of blood pressure, heart rate, central venous pressures, hematocrit, urinary output, and any other clinical or laboratory parameters (e.g., observed or measured rates of continued hemorrhage).[5,53,55] As previously discussed, administration of human serum albumin in the treatment of primary peritonitis in cirrhotic patients exerts beneficial effects by preventing the extravascular leakage of fluid and maintaining effective intravascular volume.[26]

ALTERNATIVE THERAPIES

Alternative therapies are not recommended because of the high mortality rate (80%) for penetrating intraabdominal trauma before surgical and pharmacologic intervention. Adequate source control, prompt administration of appropriate antibiotics, and good supportive care will remain the critical modalities in achieving favorable patient outcomes.

FUTURE THERAPIES

Advances in the treatment of intraabdominal infections may involve development of new antimicrobial agents. These antibiotics should have excellent intraabdominal penetration, should be stable in the acidic medium of an abscess, and should provide activity against commonly encountered pathogens, including multidrug-resistant strains. Tigecycline has promise as a new agent for treatment of intraabdominal infections due to its activity against both gram-positive and gram-negative aerobic pathogens, including MRSA and VRE, as well as good anaerobic activity. However, the lack of potent antipseudomonal activity will probably limit its use as empiric monotherapy in many patients. Newer broad-spectrum fourth-generation cephalosporins including cefpirome and ceftobiprole may also offer promise as agents for these infections, as will new drugs such as oritavancin and dalbavancin with activity against multidrug-resistant gram-positive pathogens. However, as previously discussed, adequate source control and supportive care are often as important to favorable patient outcomes as the selection of specific antimicrobial therapy. The availability of newer agents will offer more flexibility in drug selection and administration and provide improved activity against some resistant organisms, but it is rather unlikely that these new drugs will significantly improve overall patient outcomes compared to currently available agents.

Monoclonal antibodies may enhance host response and help prevent tissue injury associated with the infection-related inflammatory process. The role of monoclonal antibodies or other types of biologic modifiers aimed at either blocking or enhancing mediators of host inflammatory responses has yet to be defined in the treatment of intraabdominal infections.[57] Intravenous immune globulin has also been reported to improve outcomes in patients with postsurgical intraabdominal infection, but its use cannot be routinely recommended at this time.[58] Future improvements in early diagnosis of intraabdominal infection, identification of the locations of septic foci including abscesses, and rapid identification of infecting pathogens offer perhaps the best hope for significantly improving patient outcomes.[5,48,59]

IMPROVING OUTCOMES

SBP in adults with cirrhosis and ascites is reported to occur in as many as 8% to 27% of patients and has a mortality rate of approximately 30% to 40%. The overall mortality rate in these patients may be as high as 60% to 70% because SBP is often accompanied by severe hepatic failure.

Most patients with secondary peritonitis can be placed in one of three categories: penetrating abdominal trauma, appendicitis, or other.[60] Generally, patients with posttraumatic infections are young men and have a very low rate of morbidity and mortality, although the prognosis of secondary peritonitis is closely associated with early diagnosis and prompt surgical intervention. Age, ostomy formation (performed for many left colonic injuries), shock, number of organs injured, and amount of blood or blood products required before surgery are all important factors in predicting the risk of infection in patients with penetrating abdominal trauma.[53,61] Postoperative complication rates have been associated with the extent of organ failure or numbers of organs affected, duration and stage of illness, adequacy of surgical procedures, and presence of other chronic underlying illnesses, including immunosuppression. An important outcome indicator is length of hospital stay; it is 7 to 14 days for most intraabdominal infections, although in patients with complications it can be a great deal longer.

PATIENT EDUCATION

Patients with intraabdominal infections must be educated on their disease presentation and treatment. Patients at high risk for primary peritonitis should be placed on prophylactic therapy and must be counseled on the benefits of prophylaxis. Patients who are alcoholic must be referred to treatment and support centers for abstinence from alcohol. In addition, patients should be educated on nutritional status and proper diet. All patients must be educated on the complications that can occur without medical and pharmacologic treatment.

Patients should be educated on potential adverse effects of their treatment, such as GI distress, headaches, and dizziness. Furthermore, patients need to be counseled on potential drug and food interactions with their medications prior to discharge. Fluoroquinolones should not be taken concomitantly with food or multivitamins, with iron supplements, or with divalent ions and products such as antacids.

METHODS TO IMPROVE PATIENT ADHERENCE TO DRUG THERAPY

Patients with intraabdominal infections are primarily treated in an acute hospital setting. On discharge, oral agents may be given; at this time steps should be taken to counsel patients on adherence.

Prevention of recurrence of primary peritonitis requires prophylactic therapy. Patients should be educated on the benefits of treatment. Lifestyle modifications can be made to assist patients in their adherence to regimens. Such modifications can involve marking on a calendar or using a pill box with daily markings, or the patient can try associating medication administration with performing a daily activity, such as brushing teeth.

DISEASE MANAGEMENT STRATEGIES TO IMPROVE PATIENT OUTCOMES

Support of intravascular volume with fluid therapy is essential to maintain adequate blood pressure and renal perfusion. The use of plasma volume expanders, such as albumin and hetastarch, has not been shown to be essential in this setting; in addition, they are expensive. Electrolyte imbalances and metabolic acidosis should be corrected with intravenous therapy.

Oral intake of foods should be temporarily discontinued and nasogastric (NG) suction started as soon as peritonitis is suspected to prevent GI distention. Suction should be continued until peristaltic activity returns and the patient begins to pass flatus. NG suction may contribute to the patient's overall fluid loss and dehydration, as well as acid–base and electrolyte problems.

Oral medications should be discontinued in patients receiving NG suctioning. The GI absorption of oral medications under such circumstances may be erratic owing to changes in pH and motility. The drug may also be inadvertently removed from the GI tract by the suctioning procedure.

Therapy of patients with paralytic ileus consists of GI tract rest, NG suction, and treatment of the underlying GI disease. Adynamic or paralytic ileus occurs to some extent with any peritoneal injury or surgery, including peritoneal inflammation. Early in the course of peritoneal irritation the intestine may have a transient period of hyperperistalsis, but soon after, motility decreases or is even absent to the point of obstruction. Severity and duration depend on the type of insult, but it usually lasts from 2 to 3 days, even in an uncomplicated surgical case. Studies indicate that the pathogenesis of this condition involves neurogenic, hormonal, and local factors. The adrenergic response to intraabdominal inflammation stimulates the sympathetic pathways of the intestine, resulting in the slowing of peristalsis. The accumulation of gas and fluids within the bowel lumen distends the intestinal wall to the point at which intraluminal pressure exceeds capillary perfusion pressure, causing bowel ischemia.

Symptoms of paralytic ileus include progressive abdominal distention and vomiting of pooled gastric contents and biliary secretions. Localized pain and profuse vomiting usually occur only if there is complete bowel obstruction and strangulation.

Patients with abdominal adhesions require surgical treatment to free these attachments. As a normal host defense, the body attempts to isolate infections of the abdomen into localized pockets. The peritoneum exudes large quantities of fibrin into the peritoneal fluid while fibrinolytic activity is reduced. The result is the formation of a network of fibrinous strands between the loops of bowel and the adjacent visceral surfaces. If the fibrin is not reabsorbed, the strands are invaded by fibroblasts and develop a blood supply. Fibrin strands transform into firm adhesive bands. The absence of peristalsis allows these adhesions to form more easily.

Surgical intervention also is required for patient improvement. Proper drainage is required to remove foreign and purulent masses from affected areas. Surgical correction of perforations as well as the underlying pathology of the infection is also required. Newer radiologic methods, ultrasonography, and CT scanning can be used for early diagnosis and greatly improve patient outcome. In addition, support of vital organs and proper nutrition have a great impact on the improvement of recovering patients. Patients requiring mechanical or other measures to support vital organs may have reduced nutritional intake.

Multiple complications that affect patient outcome also may arise. Organ failure may occur owing to shock and/or infections. These complications must be managed individually to improve patient outcome.

PHARMACOECONOMICS

The severity of intraabdominal infections can be stratified from mild to moderate infections (community-acquired) in which a single agent can be used, versus severe or nosocomial intraabdominal infections, in which two or more agents are often used. Various pharmacoeconomic studies have compared monotherapy versus combination regimens (e.g., second-generation cephalosporin or carbapenem vs. a β-lactam/β-lactamase inhibitor combination, carbapenem vs. cefepime plus metronidazole).[62-64] Treatment failures, clinical cure, number of adverse events, number of antibiotic doses, and duration of antibiotic therapy are all pharmacoeconomic outcome measures. The outcomes of such studies have not been entirely consistent, and specific agents cannot necessarily be recommended based on their results because methodologies and outcomes measures have differed between the studies. However, it is clear that monotherapy does not necessarily confer an automatic economic advantage compared to combination regimens. Also, the influence of specific types of infections has not been well characterized. Severe or nosocomial intraabdominal infections are inherently more expensive because of the complications that may arise in immunocompromised patients.[14,65] Furthermore, treatment cost increases with the number of laboratory tests ordered and the length of hospital stay (usually in the intensive care unit). Direct drug costs are outweighed by the cost of adverse drug effects and the cost of treatment failures. Length of hospital stay continues to be an important outcome indicator and is one of the determinants of treatment cost. The use of inappropriate empiric antibiotic therapy for community-acquired infections is associated with more days of parenteral antibiotic therapy and longer hospital stays.[66] Appropriate antibiotic selection is thus important in reducing costs of therapy as well as providing favorable clinical outcomes. Early switch from parenteral to oral antibiotic therapy is also an important and very feasible means of reducing the costs of therapy.[37-39]

KEY POINTS

- *Peritonitis* is a general term for infection and inflammation of the peritoneal cavity as a result of microbial contamination. Peritonitis can be very severe and is associated with a number of complications, including abscess formation, sepsis, and multiple organ dysfunction syndrome
- General supportive care of patients with severe peritonitis may include management of hemodynamic, respiratory, and intestinal integrity; analgesia; sedation; and fluid and nutritional support
- The goals of antimicrobial therapy in the treatment of intraabdominal infections are eradicating the infecting microorganisms, reducing the incidence of recurrent infections, and shortening the time to resolution of clinical signs and symptoms
- Antimicrobial therapy should be initiated as soon as an intraabdominal infection is suspected. Therapy should

not be delayed until the final diagnosis of infection is made

- Primary peritonitis occurs most commonly in adults with cirrhosis and refractory ascites and is usually caused by a single organism. *E. coli*, *Klebsiella*, and streptococci are the most common pathogens

- Appropriate antibiotics for empiric therapy of primary peritonitis usually consist of second- or third-generation cephalosporins. Fluoroquinolones or trimethoprim/sulfamethoxazole are suitable alternatives. Although traditionally recommended, ampicillin plus an aminoglycoside is now less frequently used due to concerns regarding nephrotoxicity in patients with cirrhosis

- Secondary peritonitis is caused by a variety of specific etiologies that result in perforation of bowel and/or introduction of large bacterial inocula directly into the abdominal cavity

- Surgical intervention to provide adequate source control, supportive care to maintain homeostatic support, and rapid initiation of appropriate antimicrobial therapy are the most important aspects of effective management of secondary peritonitis

- Adequate source control consists of surgical repair of intraabdominal injuries or other source of contamination, drainage of contaminated or infected fluids, and/or radiologically guided procedures to remove infected fluid collections

- Appropriate antimicrobial agents for empiric treatment of secondary peritonitis should include agents with good activity against aerobic gram-negative bacilli and anaerobes such as *B. fragilis*

- In the treatment of secondary peritonitis, monotherapy with a single antibibotic is considered to be as effective as combination therapy with two or more agents. Recommended regimens for mild to moderate community-acquired infections include ampicillin/sulbactam, ertapenem, cefazolin or cefuroxime plus metronidazole, or a fluoroquinolone plus metronidazole. Recommended therapy for more severe community-acquired infection consists of piperacillin/tazobactam, imipenem/cilastatin, meropenem, a third- or fourth-generation cephalosporin plus metronidazole, or ciprofloxacin or levofloxacin plus metronidazole

- The use of aminoglycosides for treatment of intraabdominal infections is controversial due to the availability of equally effective and less toxic alternatives. If used, aminoglycosides may be used in either extended-interval regimens (5 to 7 mg/kg/day) or in traditional divided-dose regimens, with individualization of dosing based on measured serum concentrations

- Clindamycin is an acceptable alternative to metronidazole in providing anaerobic coverage in combination regimens. However, resistance to clindamycin among *B. fragilis* and other anaerobes is increasing

- The use of antianaerobic second-generation cephalosporins (e.g., cefoxitin) in the treatment of secondary peritonitis is somewhat controversial due to increasing rates of resistance among anaerobic bacteria such as *B. fragilis*

- The appropriate duration of therapy for most cases of primary and secondary peritonitis is approximately 5 to 7 days

- Tertiary peritonitis is defined as clinical signs and symptoms of peritonitis that persist or recur more than 48 hours after apparently adequate management of secondary peritonitis. Management of tertiary peritonitis is extremely challenging, and the infection is associated with high (~50%) mortality rates. Common pathogens include staphylococci, *P. aeruginosa*, and *Candida*; antimicrobial therapy must be guided by culture and susceptibility test results

- Health care-associated (nosocomial) intraabdominal infections usually involve surgical wound infections and may be caused by a wide variety of gram-negative and gram-positive bacterial pathogens as well as *Candida*. Infections due to multidrug-resistant gram-positive pathogens such as methicillin-resistant *S. aureus* and vancomycin-resistant *Enterococcus* are becoming increasingly important in these infections. Antimicrobial therapy must be guided by culture and susceptibility test results

- Treatment of intraabdominal abscess is the same as that for secondary peritonitis. Anaerobes are commonly involved in abscess formation, and antimicrobial therapy is secondary to drainage

- Intraabdominal infections associated with CAPD are commonly caused by staphylococci, streptococci, and enteric gram-negative bacilli such as *E. coli*. Empiric therapy with an antistaphylococcal penicillin or cephalosporin plus an aminoglycoside is appropriate; subsequent therapy should be guided by culture and susceptibility test results

- Direct drug cost is outweighed by the cost of adverse drug effects and the cost of treatment failures

SUGGESTED READINGS

Cheadle WG, Spain DA. The continuing challenge of intraabdominal infection. Am J Surg 186(Suppl 5A):15S–22S, 2003.

Marshall JC, Innes M. Intensive care unit management of intraabdominal infection. Crit Care Med 31:2228–2237, 2003.

Mazuski JE, Sawyer RG, Nathens AB, et al. The Surgical Infection Society guidelines on antimicrobial therapy for intraabdominal infections: an executive summary. Surg Infect 3:161–234, 2002.

Solomkin JS, Mazuski JE, Baron EJ, et al. Guidelines for the selection of anti-infective agents for complicated intraabdominal infections. Clin Infect Dis 37:997–1005, 2003.

REFERENCES

1. Bhuva M, Ganger D, Jensen D. Spontaneous bacterial peritonitis: an update on evaluation, management, and prevention. Am J Med 97: 169–175, 1994.

2. Such J, Runyon BA. Spontaneous bacterial peritonitis. Clin Infect Dis 27:669–676, 1998.

3. Kramer L, Druml W. Ascites and intraabdominal infection. Curr Opinion Crit Care 10:146–151, 2004.

4. Johnson CC, Baldessarre J, Levison ME. Peritonitis: update on pathophysiology, clinical manifestations, and management. Clin Infect Dis 124:1035–1047, 1997.

5. Marshall JC, Innes M. Intensive care unit management of intraabdominal infection. Crit Care Med 31:2228–2237, 2003.

6. Levison ME, Bush LM. Peritonitis and other intraabdominal infections. In: Mandell GL, Bennett JE, Dolin R, eds. Mandell, Douglas and Bennett's Principles and Practice of Infectious Diseases. 5th ed. Philadelphia: Churchill Livingstone, 2000:821–856.

7. Farthmann EH, Schoffel U. Epidemiology and pathophysiology of intraabdominal infections (IAI). Infection 26:329–334, 1998.

8. Nathens AB, Rotstein OD, Marshall JC. Tertiary peritonitis: clinical features of a complex nosocomial infection. World J Surg 22:158–163, 1998.

9. Nichols RL. Intraabdominal sepsis: characterization and treatment. J Infect Dis 135(Suppl):S54–S57, 1977.

10. Hentges DJ. The anaerobic microflora of the human body. Clin Infect Dis 16(Suppl):S175–S180, 1993.

11. Lau WY, Teoh-Chan CH, Fan ST, et al. The bacteriology and septic complication of patients with appendicitis. Ann Surg 200:576–581, 1984.

12. Jones RC, Thal ER, Johnson NA, et al. Evaluation of antibiotic therapy following penetrating abdominal trauma. Ann Surg 201:576–585, 1985.

13. Solomkin JS, Dellinger EP, Christou NV, et al. Results of a multicenter trial comparing imipenem/cilastatin to tobramycin/clindamycin for intraabdominal infections. Ann Surg 212:581–591, 1990.

14. Barie PS, Vogel SB, Patchen Dellinger EP, et al. A randomized, double-blind clinical trial comparing cefepime plus metronidazole with imipenem-cilastatin in the treatment of complicated intraabdominal infections. Arch Surg 132:1254–1302, 1997.

15. Ingham HR, Tharagonnet D, Sisson PR, et al. Inhibition of phagocytosis in vitro by obligate anaerobes. Lancet 2:1252–1254, 1977.

16. Onderdonk AB, Shapiro ME, Finberg RW, et al. Use of a model of intraabdominal sepsis for studies of the pathogenicity of Bacteroides fragilis. Rev Infect Dis 6(Suppl):S91–S95, 1984.

17. Buggy BP, Schaberg DR, Swartz RD. Intraleukocytic sequestration as a cause of persistent Staphylococcus aureus peritonitis in continuous ambulatory dialysis. Am J Med 76:1035–1039, 1984.

18. Dougherty SH. Antimicrobial culture and susceptibility testing has little value for routine management of secondary bacterial peritonitis. Clin Infect Dis 25(Suppl 2):S258–S261, 1997.

19. Anaya DA, Nathens AB. Risk factors for severe sepsis in secondary peritonitis. Surg Infect 4:355–362, 2003.

20. Garcia-Tsao G, Conn HO, Lerner E. The diagnosis of bacterial peritonitis: comparison of pH, lactate concentration and leukocyte count. Hepatology 5:91–96, 1985.

21. Wilson SE. A critical analysis of recent innovations in the treatment of intraabdominal infection. Surg Gynecol Obstet 177(Suppl):11–17, 1993.

22. Peteet JR, Brenner S, Curtiss D, et al. A stage of change approach to addiction in the medical setting. Gen Hosp Psychiatry 20:267–273, 1998.

23. Mazuski JE, Sawyer RG, Nathens AB, et al. The Surgical Infection Society guidelines on antimicrobial therapy for intraabdominal infections: an executive summary. Surg Infec 3:161–174, 2002.

24. Mazuski JE, Sawyer RG, Nathens AB, et al. The Surgical Infection Society guidelines on antimicrobial therapy for intraabdominal infections: an executive summary. Surg Infect 3:175–234, 2002.

25. Solomkin JS, Mazuski JE, Baron EJ, et al. Guidelines for the selection of anti-infective agents for complicated intraabdominal infections. Clin Infect Dis 37:997–1005, 2003.

26. Sort P, Navasa M, Arroyo V, et al. Effect of intravenous albumin on renal impairment and mortality in patients with cirrhosis and spontaneous bacterial peritonitis. N Engl J Med 341:403–409, 1999.

27. Singh N, Gayowski T, Yu VL, et al. Trimethoprim-sulfamethoxazole for the prevention of spontaneous bacterial peritonitis in cirrhosis: a randomized trial. Ann Intern Med 122:595–598, 1995.

28. DiPiro JT, Cue JI. Single-agent versus combination antibiotic therapy in the management of intraabdominal infections. Pharmacotherapy 14:266–272, 1994.

29. Bohnen JM. Antibiotic therapy for abdominal infection. World J Surg 22:152–157, 1998.

30. Snydman DR, Cuchural GJ Jr, McDermott L, et al. Correlation of various in vitro testing methods with clinical outcomes in patients with Bacteroides fragilis group infections treated with cefoxitin: a retrospective analysis. Antimicrob Agents Chemother 36:540–544, 1992.

31. Johnson CC. Susceptibility of anaerobic bacteria to beta-lactam antibiotics in the United States. Clin Infect Dis 16(Suppl 4):S371–S376, 1993.

32. Nguyen MH, Yu VL, Morris AJ, et al. Antimicrobial resistance and clinical outcome of Bacteroides bacteremia: findings of a multicenter prospective observational trial. Clin Infect Dis 30:870–876, 2000.

33. Solomkin JS, Yellin AE, Rotstein OD, et al. Ertapenem versus piperacillin/tazobactam in the treatment of complicated intraabdominal infections: results of a double-blind, randomized comparative phase III trial. Ann Surg 235–245, 2003.

34. Yellin AE, Hassett JM, Fernandez A, et al. Ertapenem monotherapy versus combination therapy with ceftriaxone plus metronidazole for treatment of complicated intraabdominal infections in adults. Intl J Antimicrob Agents 20:165–173, 2002.

35. Bailey JA, Virgo KS, DiPiro JT. Aminoglycosides for intraabdominal infection: equal to the challenge? Surg Infect 3:315–335, 2002.

36. Gilbert DN. Once-daily aminoglycoside therapy. AntimicrobAgents Chemother 35:339–345, 1991.

37. Solomkin JS, Dellinger EP, Bohnen JM, et al. The role of oral antimicrobials for the management of intraabdominal infections. New Horizons 6(Suppl 2):S46–S52, 1998.

38. Cohn SM, Lipsett PA, Buchman TG, et al. Comparison of intravenous/oral ciprofloxacin plus metronidazole versus piperacillin/tazobactam in the treatment of complicated intraabdominal infections. Ann Surg 232:254–262, 2000.

39. Solomkin JS, Reinhart HH, Dellinger EP, et al. Results of a randomized trial comparing sequential intravenous/oral treatment with ciprofloxacin plus metronidazole to imipenem/cilastatin for intraabdominal infections. The Intraabdominal Infection Study Group. Ann Surg 223:303–315, 1996.

40. Rasmussen BA, Bush K, Tally FP. Antimicrobial resistance in Bacteroides. Clin Infect Dis 16(Suppl 4):S390–S400, 1993.

41. Aldridge K, Ashcraft D. Ertapenem (ETP), a new antimicrobial: comparative in vitro activity against clinically significant anaerobes. In: Abstracts of the 41st Interscience Conference on Antimicrobial Agents and Chemotherapy. Dec. 14–17, 2001, Chicago. Abstract E-806.

42. Dartois N, Gioud-Paquet M, Ellis-Grosse EJ, et al. Tigecycline vs imipenem/cilastatin for treatment of complicated intraabdominal infections. In: Abstracts of the 44th Interscience Conference on Antimicrobial Agents and Chemotherapy. Oct. 30–Nov. 2, 2004, Washington, DC. Abstract C2-1985.

43. Sitges-Serra A, Lopez MJ, Girvent M, et al. Postoperative enterococcal infection after treatment of complicated intraabdominal sepsis. Br J Surg 89:361–367, 2002.

44. Uggeri FR, Perego E, Franciosi C, et al. Surgical approach to the intraabdominal infections. Minerva Anestesiologica 70:175–179, 2004.

45. Sawyer RG, Rosenlof LK, Adams RB, et al. Peritonitis into the 1990s: changing pathogens and changing strategies in the critically ill. Am Surgeon 58:82–87, 1992.

46. Montravers P, Gauzit R, Muller C, et al. Emergence of antibiotic-resistant bacteria in cases of peritonitis after intraabdominal surgery affects the efficacy of empirical antimicrobial therapy. Clin Infect Dis 23:486–494, 1996.

47. Wilson MA. Skin and soft tissue infections: impact of resistant gram-positive bacteria. Am J Surg 186(Suppl 5A):35S–41S, 2003.

48. Cheadle WG, Spain DA. The continuing challenge of intraabdominal infection. Am J Surg 186(Suppl 5A):15S–22S, 2003.

49. Barie PS. Antibiotic-resistant gram-positive cocci: implications for surgical practice. World J Surg 22:118–126, 1998.

50. Pelletier SJ, Raymond DP, Crabtree TD, et al. Outcome analysis of intraabdominal infection with resistant gram-positive organisms. Surg Infect 3:11–19, 2002.

51. Fierobe L, Decre D, Muller C, et al. Methicillin-resistant Staphylococcus aureus as a causative agent of postoperative intraabdominal

infection: relation to nasal colonization. Clin Infect Dis 29: 1231–1238, 1999.

52. Horton MW, Deeter RG, Sherman RA. Treatment of peritonitis in patients undergoing continuous ambulatory peritoneal dialysis. Clin Pharmacol 9:102–118, 1990.

53. Morales CH, Villegas MI, Villavicencio R, et al. Intraabdominal infections in patients with abdominal trauma. Arch Surg 139: 1278–1285, 2004.

54. Bozorgzadeh A, Pizzi WF, Barie PS, et al. The duration of antibiotic administration in predicting abdominal trauma. Am J Surg 172: 125–135, 1999.

55. Barie PS, Hydo LJ, Eachempati SR. Longitudinal outcomes of intraabdominal infection complicated by critical illness. Surg Infect 5: 365–373, 2004.

56. Fry DE, Garrison RN, Heitsch RC, et al. Determinants of death in patients with intraabdominal abscess. Surgery 88:517–522, 1980.

57. Dellinger EP. Can one use biologic modifiers to prevent multiple organ dysfunction syndrome after abdominal infections? Surg Infect 1:239–247, 2000.

58. Reith HB, Rauchschwalbe SK, Mittelkotter U, et al. IgM-enriched immunoglobulin (pentaglobin) positively influences the course of post-surgical intraabdominal infections. Eur J Med Res 9:479–484, 2004.

59. Schein M, Wittman DH, Holzheimer R, et al. Hypothesis: compartmentalization of cytokines in intraabdominal infection. Surgery 119: 694–700, 1996.

60. DiPiro JT. Considerations for therapy of mixed infections: focus on intraabdominal infection. Pharmacotherapy 15(Suppl):15S–21S, 1995.

61. Nichols RL, Smith JW. Risk of infection, infecting flora and treatment considerations in penetrating abdominal trauma. Surg Gynecol Obstet 177(Suppl):50–54, 1993.

62. Messick CR, Mamdani M, McNicholl IR, et al. Pharmacoeconomic analysis of ampicillin-sulbactam versus cefoxitin in the treatment of intraabdominal infections. Pharmacotherapy 18:175–183, 1998.

63. Jaccard C, Troillet N, Harbarth S, et al. Prospective randomized comparison of imipenem-cilastatin and piperacillin-tazobactam in nosocomial pneumonia or peritonitis. Antimicrob Agents Chemother 42:2966–2972, 1998.

64. Barie PS, Rotstein OD, Dellinger EP, et al. The cost-effectiveness of cefepime plus metronidazole verus imipenem/cilastatin in the treatment of complicated intraabdominal infections. Surg Infect 5: 269–280, 2004.

65. Collins MD, Dajani AS, Kim KS, et al. Comparison of ampicillin/ sulbactam plus aminoglycoside vs. ampicillin plus clindamycin plus aminoglycoside in the treatment of intraabdominal infections in children. The Multicenter Group. Pediatr Infect Dis 17(Suppl 3): S15–S21, 1998.

66. Cattan P, Yin DD, Sarfati E, et al. Cost of care for inpatients with community-acquired intraabdominal infections. Eur J Clin Microbiol Infect Dis 21:787–793, 2002.

Gastrointestinal Infections

79

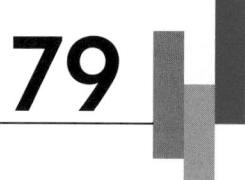

Kevin W. Garey and Laura N. Gerard

Diarrheal disease or gastroenteritis is the fourth leading cause of death worldwide, with more than 3 million deaths per year.[1,2] For children less than 5 years old, the median global estimates of diarrheal disease are 3.2 episodes per child-year, increasing to over 10.4 episodes per child-year in developing countries such as those in sub-Saharan Africa.[3] Between 1992 and 2000, diarrheal diseases accounted for 21% of all deaths in children less than 5 years old worldwide. In the United States, 211 million to 375 million cases of acute diarrhea are reported each year (1.4 episodes per person per year).[4] Acute diarrhea is responsible for more than 900,000 hospitalizations and 6,000 deaths annually. Viruses, bacteria, protozoa, and fungus are causative organisms for infectious diarrhea. In hospitalized patients, *Clostridium difficile* is an important nosocomial pathogen associated with antibiotic-related diarrhea. This chapter will focus on the pathophysiology, causative organisms, and treatment recommendations for infectious diarrhea in the community and hospital.

DEFINITIONS

Diarrhea is defined as the production of stool of abnormally loose consistency, usually associated with excessive frequency of defecation and excessive stool output.[5] Acute diarrhea lasts 14 days or less. Persistent diarrhea lasts more than 14 days. Chronic diarrhea lasts more than 30 days.

Dysentery is defined as frequent, small bowel movements accompanied by blood and mucus with tenesmus or pain on defecation.

Antibiotic-associated diarrhea is defined as unexplained diarrhea that occurs in association with the administration of antibiotics. The antimicrobials most frequently implicated include clindamycin, extended-spectrum penicillins, and cephalosporins, although almost all antibiotic classes have been reported to cause diarrhea.[6] *C. difficile*-associated diarrhea (CDAD) is caused by the spore-forming, gram-positive bacillus *C. difficile*.[7]

INFECTIOUS DIARRHEA NOT DUE TO CLOSTRIDIUM DIFFICILE

TREATMENT GOALS

■ Initial assessment should consist of an evaluation for dehydration, duration of illness, and inflammatory versus noninflammatory diarrhea.

■ Symptomatic therapy should be initiated, with further management dictated by key clinical and epidemiologic findings.

■ Fecal specimens should be obtained if a patient is experiencing severe, bloody, inflammatory, or persistent diarrhea or if an outbreak is suspected.

ETIOLOGY

Microbial causes of gastroenteritis include viruses, bacteria, fungus, and protozoa (Tables 79.1 and 79.2).[8–10] In the United States, data on enteropathogens responsible for gastroenteritis are collected through the Foodborne Disease Active Surveillance Network (FoodNet) of the Centers for Disease Control and Prevention (CDC).[4] Established in 1996, FoodNet is a collaboration between the CDC, the Food and Drug Administration, and selected state health departments. FoodNet conducts active surveillance for seven bacterial and two parasitic pathogens. Reports of other pathogens are recorded by the National Notifiable Disease Surveillance System and the Public Health Laboratory Information System.[11,12]

VIRUSES

Viruses that cause gastroenteritis include astrovirus, rotavirus, enteric adenoviruses, and caliciviruses.[13] Caliciviruses are generally categorized into two genera: ''Norwalk-like viruses'' (NLV) or small round structured virus and ''Sapporo-like virus'' (SLV) or typical calicivirus. Viruses are the most common cause of gastroenteritis.[9] It is estimated that 32% to 42% of foodborne enteric infections in the United States are caused by viruses.[14] Epidemiologic evidence has shown that calicivirus alone may cause gastroenteritis as frequently as the most common bacterial pathogens, such as *Salmonella*. Rotavirus is the main cause of severe diarrhea in children under 5 years of age. Rotavirus is responsible for more than 130 million episodes of diarrhea throughout the world and 20% to 60% of cases of gastroenteritis requiring hospitalization.[15–17] Enteric adenoviruses, astrovirus, and calicivirus are also frequently implicated in childhood diarrhea. In adults, caliciviruses are the main cause of viral gastroenteritis and generally occur in epidemic outbreaks.[18,19]

Unlike bacteria, viruses are strictly intracellular organisms and cannot replicate in food or water. Therefore, viral contamination is less likely than bacterial contamination during food processing. Viral infection of contaminated food generally depends on viral stability and virulence, the inoculum of virus present in the food, and host susceptibility. Generally, food will look, smell, and taste normal.

BACTERIA

In 2003, the most common bacteria responsible for foodborne illnesses was *Salmonella* (14.5 cases per 100,000), followed by *Campylobacter* (12.6 cases per 100,000), *Shigella* (7.3 cases per 100,000), and *Escherichia coli* O157 (1.1 cases per 100,000).[10] Less common bacterial causes of infectious diarrhea include *Vibrio*, *Yersinia*, *Clostridium perfringens*, *Staphylococcus aureus*, *Bacillus cereus*, *Chlamydia*, *Aeromonas*, and *Plesiomonas*.[5] In hospitalized patients, *C. difficile* accounts for approximately 30% of all cases of infectious diarrhea.[20]

Salmonella, Shigella, Campylobacter. *Salmonella* species are gram-negative bacilli known to cause infectious diarrhea. The most common serotypes are *S. enteritidis* and *S. typhimurium. S. enteritidis* causes an estimated 2.4 million cases of food poisoning every year.[21] Chicken grade A shell eggs are implicated in 82% of reported cases.[22] Alfalfa sprouts are also a recognized source of *Salmonella* poisoning.[22] Although rare in the United States, *S. typhi*, the causative organism for typhoid fever, is a significant cause of infectious diarrhea in developing nations.

Shigella, nonmotile, gram-negative bacilli, are classified into four major subgroups, *S. dysenteriae, S. flexneri, S. boydii*, and *S. sonnei. S. dysenteriae* and *S. flexneri* are the predominant species worldwide. Infections due to *Shigella* are highly contagious due to the low inoculum required for infection. All *Shigella* species are capable of producing a potent Shiga toxin with enterotoxic, cytotoxic, and neurotoxic properties. Person-to-person spread is the most common source of infections.

Campylobacter species are motile, gram-negative rods; *C. jejuni* accounts for the majority of cases of infectious diarrhea. Cases generally arise due to outbreaks in contaminated eggs or poultry or other meats.[23,24] Recent studies have shown that 88% of chickens in retail markets are culture-

TABLE 79.1	Causative Organisms of Infectious Diarrhea
Virus	**Bacteria**
Common	
Adenovirus	*Campylobacter*
Astrovirus	*Escherichia coli* O157
Calicivirus	*Salmonella*
Rotavirus	*Shigella*
Uncommon	
Aichivirus	*Aeromonas*
Coronavirus	*Bacillus cereus*
Cytomegalovirus	*Chlamydia*
Human immunodeficiency virus	*Clostridium perfringens*
	Plesiomonas
Picobirnavirus	*Staphylococcus aureus*
Torovirus	*Vibrio*
	Yersinia

TABLE 79.2	**Characteristics of Pathogens Known to Cause Infectious Diarrhea**				
Pathogen	**Microbiology**	**Modes of Transmission**	**Incubation Period**	**Most Common Species**	**Epidemiology**
Campylobacter	Motile, gram-negative rods	Contaminated milk, poultry, eggs, other animals	1–7 d	C jejuni	Peak incidence in early summer
Salmonella	Encapsulated, gram-negative bacilli	Chicken eggs, poultry,	6–72 h	S typhi	Causative organisms for typhoid fever
				S enteritidis, others	Sporadic occurrence with peak incidence during summer months
Shigella	Nonmotile, gram-negative bacilli. Produce potent Shiga toxins.	Person-to-person transmission	6 h–9 d	S dysenteriae S flexneri	Causative organism for dysentery Predominant in male homosexuals
				S boydii	More common in young (<15 years) children
				S sonnei	More common in older (>15 years) children
Escherichia coli	Gram-negative bacilli	Ground beef, traveler's diarrhea	1–3 d	ETEC	Common cause of traveler's diarrhea
				EHEC EAEC	O157:H7 most common in U.S. Emerging pathogen for traveler's diarrhea
Rotavirus	RNA virus	Person-to-person transmission, epidemics	1–3 d	ELISA kit available to detect rotavirus-specific antigen	Most common cause of gastroenteritis in infants and small children in developed nations
Calicivirus	RNA virus	Foodborne outbreaks	1–3 d	Norwalk-like virus	Generally short-lived illness (2–3 d) with vomiting a prominent symptom

ETEC, enterotoxigenic *E. coli*; EHEC, enterohemorrhagic *E. coli*; EAEC, enteroaggregative *E. coli*.

positive for *Campylobacter*. Exposure to sick pets, especially puppies, has been reported in outbreaks.[21] Due to the use of quinolones in chicken, fluoroquinolone-resistant *Campylobacter* has emerged as a significant pathogen in the United States.[24]

Diarrheagenic *Escherichia coli*. A number of cases of *E. coli* food poisoning have received national attention in the past two decades.[25] Six types of *E. coli* have specific characteristics that enable them to cause diarrhea in susceptible hosts.[26] These include enterotoxigenic *E. coli* (ETEC), enteroinvasive *E. coli* (EIEC), enterohemorrhagic *E. coli* (EHEC), enteropathogenic *E. coli* (EPEC), diffusely adherent *E. coli* (DAEC), and enteroaggregative *E. coli* (EAEC). Terminology for these pathogens is due to specific interaction with intestinal mucosa, certain virulence properties, or secretion of various toxins. ETEC, the most common cause of traveler's diarrhea, is characterized by adherence to the gastric mucosa and production of toxins. EHEC is characterized by bloody diarrhea that may be complicated by the hemolytic-uremic syndrome (HUS) or thrombotic thrombocytopenic purpura. *E coli* serotype O157:H7, the most common type of EHEC in the United States, is transmitted mainly through ground beef.[27] Recently, EAEC has emerged

as a significant enteric pathogen; it may be responsible for 9% to 26% of cases of adult traveler's diarrhea and 20% to 30% of cases of persistent diarrhea in developing countries.[26]

Giardia and Cryptosporidium. *Giardia*, a flagellated, enteric protozoan, and *Cryptosporidium*, an intracellular protozoan parasite, are common causes of endemic and epidemic diarrheal diseases throughout the world.[28] Infection is caused by ingestion of cysts or oocytes from infected patients. Although uncommon in the United States, infections from these parasites are common in developing nations.

PATHOPHYSIOLOGY

Infectious diarrhea involves a net fluid balance derangement in the gastrointestinal tract.[29] With a normal daily fluid intake of 1.5 L along with salivary, gastric, biliary, and pancreatic secretion, approximately 8.5 L of fluid enters the upper gastrointestinal tract each day. In addition, a bidirectional flux of fluids occurs in the small intestine, generally exceeding 50 L each day. Daily fecal fluid excretion is normally less than 150 mL per day, which indicates that the vast majority of fluids are reabsorbed, usually in the small intestine. Thus, even a small derangement in fluid reabsorption can overload the large intestine's ability to reabsorb fluids.

Enteric microbes can alter normal fluid reabsorption physiology in one of three ways (Table 79.3). First, noninflammatory diarrhea is characterized by a shift in the flux of bidirectional water and electrolytes and is generally caused by intraluminal toxins or minimally invasive bacteria. Second, inflammatory diarrhea is characterized by destruction of the ileus or colon, usually due to cytotoxin production or direct microbial invasion. Production of lipo-oxygenase or other host factors may also contribute to the diarrhea. Third, penetrating diarrhea is caused by organisms that penetrate intact intestinal mucosa, usually in the distal small intestine, to multiply in reticuloendothelial cells or the lymphatic system.

A number of host and microbial properties increase the risk for infectious diarrhea. Age-related susceptibility to certain pathogens is well documented. For example, rotavirus generally infects young children, whereas calicivirus is more commonly isolated from adults.[30,31] Age-related differences are likely due to differences in intestinal immunity as well as pathogen exposure. Other host factors include gastric acidity, intestinal motility, and normal enteric flora that limit the overgrowth of pathogenic organisms.[29] Microbial factors that increase the risk of diarrhea include a variety of toxins, including neurotoxins, enterotoxins, and cytotoxins. Neurotoxins, produced by *S. aureus* and *Bacillus cereus*, are exotoxins that affect the central nervous system and do not directly affect fluid secretion in the intestine. Enterotoxins have a direct effect on intestinal mucosa to increase fluid secretion and cause voluminous watery diarrhea. *Vibrio cholerae*, *E. coli*, *Salmonella*, *Shigella*, and *Clostridium per-*

fringens all produce a variety of enterotoxins. Cytotoxins are responsible for mucosal destruction, resulting in inflammatory colitis. Enterohemorrhagic *E. coli* or *E. coli* O157:H7 produces one or two cytotoxins that cause hemorrhagic colitis or HUS.[27] The ability of bacteria to attach and penetrate the gastrointestinal mucosa as well as invade and destroy epithelial cells also increases their virulence.

CLINICAL PRESENTATION AND DIAGNOSIS

Infectious diarrhea is generally classified into noninflammatory or inflammatory diarrhea.[32] Inflammatory diarrhea is characterized by bloody, purulent, mucoid stools and is often accompanied by tenesmus, fever, and abdominal pain. Noninflammatory diarrhea is generally less severe; typical signs and symptoms include watery diarrhea without fever, abdominal pain, fecal white blood cells, or occult blood.[33] Although there is considerable overlap, noninflammatory diarrhea is generally caused by viruses, *S. aureus*, *B. cereus*, or *C. perfringens*. Inflammatory bacterial diarrhea is generally caused by *Vibrio*, *Shigella*, certain strains of *E. coli*, *Campylobacter*, *Yersinia*, *Chlamydia*, and *C. difficile*. In the United States, most cases of watery, noninflammatory diarrhea are self-limited and last less than 1 day.[8] Typical signs and symptoms of infectious diarrhea based on specific pathogens are shown in Table 79.4. Microbiologic examination of the stool or antibiotic therapy is generally not necessary in these cases. In contrast, inflammatory diarrhea is more often accompanied by a specific pathogen, and patients may benefit from antibiotic therapy.

TYPHOID FEVER
Human typhoid fever is a severe systemic illness caused by *Salmonella typhi*. In the pre-antibiotic era, typhoid fever was

TABLE 79.3	Pathophysiology of Infectious Diarrhea		
Characteristic	Altered Fluid Absorption Capacity	Inflammatory Destruction of Colon or Ileus	Penetrating
Mechanism	Noninflammatory shift in bidirectional water and electrolyte flux	Bacterial invasion or cytotoxicity of organisms into colon or ileus	Penetration of a microbe through an intact mucosa into the reticuloendothelial system
Location in gastrointestinal tract	Proximal small intestine	Colon or ileus	Distal small intestine
Key features	No fecal leukocytes; minimally increased lactoferrin	Presence of fecal leukocytes; increased lactoferrin	Presence of fecal leukocytes
Pathogens	*Escherichia coli* ETEC *Vibrio cholerae* *Staphylococcus aureus* Rotavirus Norwalk-like virus	*Salmonella enteritidis* *Shigella* *Campylobacter jejuni* *Clostridium difficile*	*Salmonella typhi*

ETEC, enterotoxigenic *E coli*.

TABLE 79.4	Clinical Features of Infectious Diarrhea for Specific Pathogens				
Pathogen	**Abdominal Pain**	**Vomiting or Nausea**	**Fever**	**Inflammatory Cells**	**Heme-Positive Stools**
Campylobacter	Frequent	Frequent	Frequent	Present	Variable
Salmonella	Frequent	Frequent	Frequent	Present	Variable
Shigella	Frequent	Frequent	Frequent	Present	Variable
E coli O157:H7	Frequent	Frequent	Uncommon	Present	Frequent
S aureus	Frequent	Frequent	Uncommon	Uncommon	Uncommon
Vibrio	Variable	Frequent	Uncommon	Uncommon	Uncommon
Rotavirus	Mild	Frequent	Uncommon	Uncommon	Uncommon
Calicivirus	Mild	Frequent	Uncommon	Uncommon	Uncommon

associated with a 15% mortality rate, and in antibiotic-resistant strains mortality can range from 15% to 30%.[34] Clinical presentation varies, but hospitalizations most often occur in children or young adults. After an incubation period of 7 to 14 days, patients present with fever, malaise, and influenza-like symptoms. A relative bradycardia is often reported. Blanching, erythematous, maculopapular lesions approximately 2 to 4 mm in diameter are reported in 5% to 30% of cases. Complications of typhoid fever include gastrointestinal bleeding or perforation, central nervous system manifestations, and death.

E. COLI O157:H7 AND HEMOLYTIC-UREMIC SYNDROME

HUS is defined as the presence of microangiopathic hemolytic anemia, acute renal failure, and thrombocytopenia.[27] In the United States, the most common cause of HUS is Shiga-toxin-producing *E. coli* (STEC) serotype O157:H7. Cattle have been recognized as the main source of *E. coli* O157:H7, although other animals, including sheep, pigs, and deer, also can be reservoirs for the organism.

THERAPEUTIC PLAN

An approach to the evaluation and management of infectious diarrhea is presented in Figure 79.1. Initial assessment should consist of an evaluation for dehydration, duration of illness, and inflammatory versus noninflammatory diarrhea. Symptomatic therapy should be initiated, with further management dictated by key clinical and epidemiologic findings. Fecal specimens should be obtained if a patient is experiencing severe, bloody, inflammatory, or persistent diarrhea or if an outbreak is suspected.

PHARMACOTHERAPY

Oral Rehydration Therapy. The most common risks associated with diarrheal diseases are dehydration and malnutrition. Non-cola beverages, Gatorade, fruit juices, and

"Mom's chicken soup" are generally sufficient for patients with mild or moderate diarrhea.[5] For more severe diarrhea, rehydration with glucose-containing oral rehydration solution (ORS) should be instituted. Since its introduction in 1968, ORS has been hailed as "potentially the most important medical advance of this century."[35,36] In patients with diarrhea, nutrient-independent sodium absorption across the intestinal epithelial cells is impaired; however, the coupled transport of glucose and sodium is preserved.[37] The original ORS contained 90 mEq per L of sodium. This amount was chosen as a compromise between normal sodium loss due to cholera infections in adults (approximately 120 to 140 mEq/L of stool) and other enteropathogens (<80 mEq/L of stool). The original ORS solution was estimated to have saved millions of lives since its introduction but was associated with hypernatremia in patients without cholera. Due to this concern, a new ORS formulation was introduced in 2002. This solution preserves the 1:1 M ratio of sodium to glucose that is necessary for efficient transport, but it has a lower osmolarity and sodium content. The reduced-osmolarity ORS has been shown to decrease stool output, reduce vomiting, and reduce the need for supplemental intravenous therapy.[38,39] However, the reduced-osmolarity ORS has been associated with hyponatremia in patients with cholera, and some experts have advocated the creation of a cholera-specific ORS with a higher osmolarity and sodium content.[40] Regardless of formulation, initial treatment for severe dehydration must include administration of a rehydration solution; this can be accomplished with an oral glucose-containing electrolyte solution in the vast majority of cases.[7]

Antibiotics. Most cases of infectious diarrhea are self-limited and do not require therapy beyond adequate hydration and other supportive care. For certain pathogens, such as *Salmonella* or STEC, antibiotic therapy has been shown to either prolong the duration of shedding (*Salmonella*) or increase the risk of life-threatening complications (STEC). Treatment recommendations for specific pathogens are listed in Table 79.5.

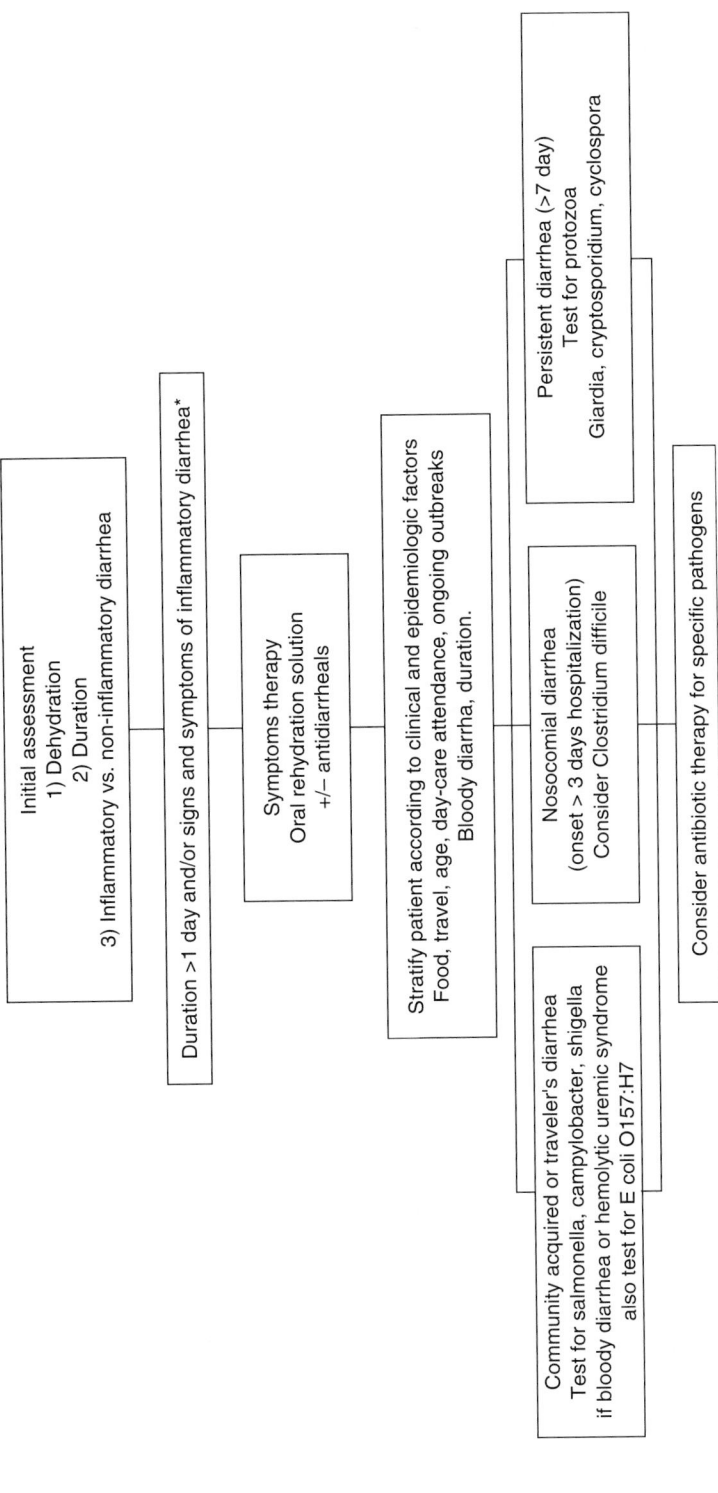

FIGURE 79.1 Evaluation and management of infectious diarrhea.

TABLE 79.5	Treatment Recommendations for Pathogens Known to Cause Infectious Diarrhea
Pathogen	**Adult Treatment Recommendation**
Salmonella	Antibiotics are generally not recommended for healthy patients with mild to moderate illness.
	Fluoroquinolones[a] may be used for persons at high risk for bacteremia or dissemination (<1 year, >50 years, or immunocompromised).
	TMP-SMX may be used if susceptibility known.
Shigella	Fluoroquinolones[a] for 1–3 days
	TMP-SMX may be used if susceptibility known
Campylobacter	Antibiotics are generally not recommended for healthy patients with mild to moderate illness.
	Erythromycin or azithromycin should be initiated within 4 days from the start of symptoms.
	Fluoroquinolone resistance is >80% in some areas of Southeast Asia.
E coli (enterotoxigenic, enteropathogenic, enteroinvasive)	Fluoroquinolones[a] for 1–3 days TMP-SMX may be used if susceptibility known.
E coli Shiga toxin producing (O157:H7)	Avoid antibiotics and antimotility agents, especially TMP-SMX and fluoroquinolones.
Giardia	Metronidazole 250–750 mg tid for 7–10 days
Cryptosporidium	Paromomycin + azithromycin or nitazoxanide in immunocompromised patients. Nitazoxanide has proven efficacy in children.

[a] Fluoroquinolones include ciprofloxacin 500 mg PO bid, levofloxacin 500 mg PO once daily, or norfloxacin 400 mg PO bid.
TMP-SMX, trimethoprim-sulfamethoxazole.

Shigella. Randomized controlled studies have shown that antibiotic therapy with ampicillin, azithromycin, or ciprofloxacin decreases the duration of diarrhea, fever, tenesmus, and organism shedding.[41,42] Increased resistance to ampicillin and trimethoprim–sulfamethoxazole has limited their use. However, recent studies have shown that fluoroquinolones are safe and effective in children with shigellosis.[43]

Campylobacter. Erythromycin has been shown to reduce organism shedding and reduce diarrhea if given within 4 days of the onset of symptoms.[43] Immunocompromised patients (especially AIDS patients) and pregnant women may especially benefit from therapy due to the increased risk of complications and persistent symptoms in these populations. The use of quinolones for *Campylobacter* infections is limited due to the widespread resistance secondary to fluoroquinolone use in poultry.[24]

Salmonella. Treatment of uncomplicated *Salmonella* gastroenteritis is generally not recommended, as antibiotic therapy has been shown to prolong bacterial shedding and increase person-to-person transmission and relapse.[21] However, persons at highest risk for bacteremia and dissemination of *Salmonella* should receive treatment with a quinolone or trimethoprim-sulfamethoxazole. These persons include infants 12 months or younger, the elderly (>50 years), patients with lymphoproliferative disorders or AIDS or other immunosuppressive disorders, transplant recipients, and those on long-term corticosteroids.

Escherichia coli O157:H7. Antibiotic agents such as trimethoprim-sulfamethoxazole and quinolones have been shown to induce the production of Shiga toxins associated with *E. coli* O157:H7 and increase a patient's risk for HUS.[44,45] For this reason, persons with suspected or proven diarrhea secondary to STEC should receive supportive care only; antibiotics should be avoided.

Traveler's Diarrhea. Most cases of traveler's diarrhea are self-limited and do not require antibiotic therapy. However, many trials involving multiple antibiotics, including quinolones, have shown that antibiotics decrease the duration of symptoms from 2 to 4 days to less than 1 day with a single dose.[46] Due to the rapid resolution of symptoms upon treatment, prophylaxis against traveler's diarrhea is generally not recommended. Recently, the nonabsorbable rifamycin rifaximin has been shown to have equal efficacy to ciprofloxacin for the treatment of traveler's diarrhea.[47]

Empirical Treatment for Community-Acquired Diarrheal Illness. Empiric antibiotic therapy in patients with severe, community-acquired diarrhea has been shown to reduce the duration of symptoms from 4 to 6 days to 1 to 2 days.[48] For patients with evidence of inflammatory diarrhea (fever, tenesmus, dysentery, or fecal leukocytes or lactoferrin), empiric therapy with a fluoroquinolone (for adults) or trimethoprim-sulfamethoxazole (for children) is often initiated pending the results of fecal testing. However, the decision to use an antibiotic must be weighed against the likelihood of a resistant organism (especially *Campylobacter*), prolonged shedding of an organism (*Salmonella*), or the risk of life-threatening complications (STEC).

Persistent Diarrhea. In the United States, protozoal pathogens such as *Giardia* and *Cryptosporidium* are the most frequent causes of persistent diarrhea lasting for more than 7 days.[8,49] *Giardia* infections generally respond to metronidazole. *Cryptosporidium* commonly affects immunocompromised patients (especially AIDS patients) and can be difficult to eradicate without immune reconstitution. Nitazoxanide, a broad-spectrum antiparasitic agent, has been shown in children to reduce oocyte shedding and hasten resolution of shedding.[50]

Antidiarrheals. Only loperamide, bismuth subsalicylate, and kaolin have been shown in clinical studies to reduce symptoms caused by infectious diarrhea. Loperamide inhibits peristalsis and possesses antisecretory properties without the potential for addiction, unlike other opiates. Loperamide has been shown to shorten the duration of diarrhea by 1 day in patients with traveler's diarrhea or dysentery.[51,52] However, it may prolong fever in patients with *Shigella*, may lead to toxic megacolon in patients with *C. difficile*, and may increase the risk of HUS in patients with STEC.[53] For this reason, loperamide should not be used in patients with bloody or suspected inflammatory diarrhea.

Bismuth subsalicylate has been shown to reduce the symptoms of traveler's diarrhea and decrease stool output in children.[54] It has also been shown to shorten the duration of symptoms in experimental models of nonviral illness.

FUTURE THERAPIES

Calmodulin inhibitors, chloride channel blockers, enkephalinase inhibitors, and prostaglandin blockers are under investigation as antisecretory agents.[8] Synthetic toxin binders, recombinant bacteria, and monoclonal antibodies that bind and inactivate STEC are in development.[55] Vaccines directed against rotavirus, diarrheogenic *E. coli*, *Shigella*, *Salmonella*, and *Campylobacter* are also under development.[56]

ANTIBIOTIC-ASSOCIATED DIARRHEA AND CLOSTRIDIUM DIFFICILE

TREATMENT GOALS

- Provide supportive care, such as correction of fluid and electrolyte imbalances.
- Discontinue the offending antibiotic if possible. If discontinuation of antibiotics is not appropriate, consider changing to an agent less frequently associated with CDAD.
- Avoid antiperistaltic agents and practice stringent infection control precautions.

ETIOLOGY

Antibiotic-associated diarrhea may cause symptoms ranging from colitis (more serious progressive disease) to "nuisance diarrhea" (frequent loose, watery stools with no other complications).[20] Infection with *C. difficile* accounts for only about 10% to 20% of cases of antibiotic-associated diarrhea, but it accounts for a majority of cases of colitis associated with antimicrobial use.[57–59] Antibiotic-associated diarrhea may also be caused by other enteric pathogens, by the direct effect of antimicrobial agents on the intestinal mucosa, and by other consequences of reduced concentrations of fecal flora.[20] CDAD is the major hospital-acquired gastrointestinal infection in the United States.[60] Infection with *C. difficile* may produce a spectrum of outcomes that range from asymptomatic colonization to acute diarrhea to pseudomembranous colitis, which can be life-threatening if left untreated.[61]

EPIDEMIOLOGY AND PATHOPHYSIOLOGY

The incidence of antibiotic-associated diarrhea varies greatly depending on the antibiotic implicated and its spectrum of activity. It is estimated that up to 15% of hospitalized patients receiving β-lactam antibiotics will experience diarrhea, and 10% to 25% of those receiving clindamycin will experience diarrhea.[20,62] Antibiotics may decrease the amount of anaerobes found in the gastrointestinal tract as a part of normal flora. The metabolism of carbohydrates may be altered, leading to osmotic diarrhea, or there may be a decrease in the rate of metabolism of primary bile acids, which act as secretory agents in the gastrointestinal tract.

Antibiotic-associated diarrhea may also be due to the effects that drugs have on the gastrointestinal tract other than antimicrobial activity. For example, erythromycin accelerates gastric emptying by acting as a motilin-receptor agonist, and clavulanate may stimulate small bowel activity.[63] Non-antimicrobial agents such as laxatives, antacids, and products containing lactose or sorbitol have also been implicated as causes of nosocomial diarrhea.[64]

C. difficile is recognized as a frequent cause of antibiotic-associated diarrhea and colitis.[65] It is implicated in approximately 20% of cases of antibiotic-associated diarrhea, in 50% to 75% of cases of antibiotic-associated colitis, and in more than 90% of cases of antibiotic-associated pseudo-membranous colitis.[20,66] Risk factors associated with CDAD include advanced age, hospitalization, and antimicrobial use.[59,67]

Development of CDAD is dependent on several factors. Treatment with antimicrobials and the acquisition of *C. difficile* are major contributing factors. All antimicrobials have the potential to cause CDAD or colitis, including vancomycin and metronidazole, agents used to treat the disorder itself. Although almost all antimicrobials have been associated with CDAD, clindamycin, cephalosporins, and extended-spectrum penicillins have been most commonly implicated.[20]

C. difficile is transmitted via the fecal–oral route. *C. difficile* spores and vegetative cells are ingested into the stomach; there, most of the vegetative cells are killed, but spores can survive gastric acidity. The spores then germinate in the small intestine and *C. difficile* passes into the large intestine, where they adhere to the epithelium of the colon. Here, pathogenic *C. difficile* produce two potent exotoxins, toxin A and toxin B, which are responsible for clinical manifestations such as diarrhea and colitis.[67] The toxins also induce the release of proinflammatory mediators and cytokines, causing activation of the enteric nervous system, leading to neutrophil chemotaxis and fluid secretion.[68] Toxin B is associated with tissue damage and fluid accumulation; toxin A displays enterotoxigenic properties.[67]

CLINICAL PRESENTATION AND DIAGNOSIS

Antibiotic-associated diarrhea typically begins after 5 to 10 days of antibiotic therapy. However, diarrhea has been reported as early as the first day of therapy and as late as 10 weeks after the cessation of therapy. Signs and symptoms typically include frequent, watery stools with or without abdominal cramping that occurs in association with the administration of antimicrobial agents. Evidence of colitis is usually not present.[61]

The spectrum of disease caused by *C. difficile* includes asymptomatic carrier state, antibiotic-associated diarrhea, pseudomembranous colitis, and fulminant colitis. The wide range of disease may be related to host immune response and virulence factors of the organism itself.[57] An asymptomatic carrier state persists for many patients infected with *C. difficile*. These patients serve as a reservoir and may perpetuate

contamination of the hospital environment. Treatment of asymptomatic carriers with antibiotics has not been shown to be beneficial and is not recommended.

Characteristic signs and symptoms of *C. difficile* include diarrhea, malaise, abdominal pain, nausea, fever, and peripheral leukocytosis.[61] Pseudomembranous enterocolitis is the characteristic marker for *C. difficile* colitis. Patients with pseudomembranous colitis have more serious disease than those with colitis and no pseudomembrane formation. Complications include perforation and peritonitis. Recurrent disease is observed in 5% to 40% of patients and is generally due to intraluminal persistence of *C. difficile* spores that germinate after discontinuation of therapy.[67]

DIAGNOSIS AND CLINICAL FINDINGS

CDAD should be considered in patients exposed to antimicrobial agents within 2 months or if diarrhea has started after 72 hours of hospitalization.[59] Various methods and assays are available for the detection of *C. difficile* infection. In most cases, toxin testing or *C. difficile* culture of a single stool specimen effectively establishes the diagnosis. Repeat testing or endoscopy or both may also be necessary.

The gold standard for diagnosis has been the cytotoxin assay that uses tissue culture. It is the most sensitive test, but results may not be available for 24 to 48 hours.[69] Enzyme immunoassays and toxin-culture assays are also available. Enzyme immunoassays have good specificity, but 100 to 1,000 pg of either toxin A or toxin B must be present for the test to be positive. Commercially available reagents will detect toxin A or toxins A and B. Those that detect toxin A and B are preferred, because 1% to 2% of cases involve strains of *C. difficile* that produce toxin B only.[70] The results of this test should be available within hours to 1 day. It may be useful to test more than one stool specimen for *C. difficile* toxin. Performing enzyme immunoassays on two to three specimens increases the diagnostic yield by 5% to 10% but also increases the cost.[71]

THERAPEUTIC PLAN

The decision to continue, change, or discontinue antibiotics depends on the severity of symptoms, the probability of *C. difficile* infection, and the need for continued antibiotic therapy. The therapeutic plan would also include supportive care, such as correction of fluid and electrolyte imbalances, if needed.[61] The therapeutic plan includes discontinuing the offending antibiotic if possible. If discontinuation of antibiotics is not appropriate, changing to an agent less frequently associated with CDAD should be attempted. Supportive care is also recommended to maintain adequate hydration and correct electrolyte imbalances. Other measures are avoiding antiperistaltic agents and placing the patient on isolation precautions.[7]

TREATMENT

PHARMACOTHERAPY

First-line oral agents for CDAD include vancomycin and metronidazole. Indications for treatment with these agents include positive assays for *C. difficile* toxin, with evidence of colitis (fever, leukocytosis, and characteristic findings on computed tomography or endoscopy), severe diarrhea, or persistent diarrhea despite discontinuation of the suspected offending agent.[20] Although oral metronidazole and vancomycin are considered equally efficacious, metronidazole is considered the drug of choice due to cost and concerns about increased rates of vancomycin-resistant enterococci due to vancomycin use.[59]

Oral metronidazole (500 mg three times a day or 250 mg four times a day) and oral vancomycin (125 to 500 mg four times a day) produce similar response rates of 90% to 97%.[72,73] The usual duration of therapy is 10 days. Ideally, treatment of CDAD should be oral because *C. difficile* is restricted to the lumen of the colon. If a patient cannot tolerate oral medications due to paralytic ileus, nasogastric suctioning, or intestinal obstruction, intravenous metronidazole is effective and produces moderate concentrations of the drug in the colon.[59] Vancomycin should not be given intravenously as the primary treatment of CDAD because effective concentrations cannot be achieved in the colon lumen. Indications for oral vancomycin include pregnancy, lactation, intolerance to metronidazole, or failure to respond to metronidazole after 3 to 5 days of therapy. The expected response to therapy is resolution of fever in 1 day and resolution of diarrhea in 4 to 5 days.[20] Lack of response to either metronidazole or vancomycin should elicit an assessment of adherence, an alternative diagnosis, or an evaluation for ileus or toxic megacolon, because these conditions may hinder the drugs from reaching their site of action.

As stated above, antiperistaltic agents such as loperamide and diphenoxylate with atropine should be avoided because there is a theoretical risk of damage and inflammation with prolonged mucosal exposure to *C. difficile* toxins.

Despite appropriate antimicrobial treatment, recurrent CDAD occurs in 20% to 25% of cases.[59,66] Symptoms may reappear 3 to 21 days after metronidazole or vancomycin has been discontinued. Most relapses respond to another 10-day course of either metronidazole or vancomycin, but 3% to 5% of patents have more than six relapses.[20,74] Relapse after antibiotic treatment does not appear to be related to whether metronidazole or vancomycin was used or by dose or duration of treatment. Recurrences occur due to persistence of the spore forms of *C. difficile* that are not eradicated by antibiotic treatment, or reinfection with a new strain.

The best treatment for relapsing CDAD has yet to be established. It has been proposed that for repeat relapses, treatment for 4 to 6 weeks may be needed to control *C. difficile* infection while the normal gut flora becomes reestab-lished. Other approaches included pulse-dosed vancomycin, administration of anion-exchange resins like cholestyramine to absorb *C. difficile* toxin, the use of agents to antagonize *C. difficile*, like *Saccaromyces boulardii*[62] or *Lactobacillus* GG,[75] vancomycin plus rifampin,[65] bacterial enemas incorporating aerobic and anaerobic bacteria,[76] and rectal infusion of donor feces.[77]

NONPHARMACOLOGIC THERAPY

Surgical intervention may be necessary in cases complicated by toxin megacolon or colon perforation. The overall mortality rate in cases requiring surgery is around 30% to 35%, although some case series describe up to 50% mortality rates.[78,79]

FUTURE THERAPIES

C. difficile colonization results from loss of protection by the intestinal flora after antimicrobial administration. One problem associated with *C. difficile* colitis is symptomatic relapse following a course of antibiotics. This is likely due to the disruption of normal gastrointestinal flora, which allows for the overgrowth of *C. difficile* and the subsequent production of toxins, causing the symptoms associated with CDAD. A study of 18 patients reported results following donor stool transplantation in patients with recurrent *C. difficile* colitis.[80] Stool samples were obtained and prepared 6 hours or less before the procedure. The recipient was treated with oral vancomycin for 4 days before the procedure. A nasogastric tube was placed and 25 mL of the stool suspension was instilled before removal of the tube. There was only one recurrence of *C. difficile* colitis during a 90-day follow-up, and no adverse effects were reported. Patients with recurrent *C. difficile* colitis may benefit from stool transplantation, but additional studies are needed to determine the role for this treatment option.

C. difficile-induced colitis is caused by the release of two exotoxins, toxins A and B. The generation of antibody response to toxin A through natural exposure may be associated with protection from disease. An inability to acquire immunity to toxin A puts patients at risk for recurrent disease. An active vaccine and immunologic approaches are under development and may prove effective against severe or relapsing *C. difficile* infection.[81] Although immunization against *C. difficile* toxins may provide patients with symptomatic relief, there are insufficient data to assess whether this will influence intestinal colonization rates.

IMPROVING OUTCOMES

Awareness and education of hospital personnel, caregivers, and patients are necessary to promote the prevention and control of diarrheal illnesses, including CDAD. The Society for Hospital Epidemiology for America recommends the following to control the spread of *C. difficile* infection:

- Personnel should wash their hands frequently with soap.
- Clinicians should wear vinyl gloves when caring for patients.
- Environmental surfaces should be cleaned with sporicidal agents.
- Symptomatic patients should be placed in private rooms, especially if incontinent of stool.
- The use of rectal thermometers should be avoided.
- Outbreaks may require antimicrobial restrictions.[60]

Limiting the use of unnecessary antimicrobials may also help to decrease resistance and adverse effects.

PATIENT EDUCATION

Many diarrheal diseases can be prevented by using good personal hygiene and safe food preparation habits. Handwashing with soap is an effective way to prevent the spread of disease and should be emphasized to caregivers of persons with diarrheal disease. Immunocompromised patients are more susceptible to enteric pathogens and may experience more severe diarrheal disease.[7]

Patients must be educated about the potential side effect of diarrhea, which may be due to almost any class of antimicrobial agent. Dehydration is a consequence of any diarrheal illness, and patients should be aware that severe dehydration may result in postural hypotension, reduced urination, and dry mucous membranes. Patients must also be aware that a healthcare provider should be alerted if these symptoms persist or are associated with severe abdominal cramping, fever, or blood in the stool.

Patients should be counseled on the common side effects of metronidazole, including metallic taste, nausea, vomiting, diarrhea, headache, and confusion. Patients should be cautioned against drinking alcohol while taking metronidazole due to the potential for disulfiram-like reactions.

PHARMACOECONOMICS

C. difficile is the most frequent cause of nosocomial infectious diarrhea and is responsible for an estimated $1 billion in healthcare costs in the United States alone.[66,74,82] A study of 271 patients was conducted to determine whether patients whose hospital stay is complicated by CDAD experienced differences in hospital length of stay, cost, and survival rates. Fifteen percent of patients experienced nosocomial CDAD. Those patients incurred adjusted hospital costs almost $4,000 higher than patients who did not develop CDAD, and they had an increased length of stay by 3.6 days.[82] The financial burden associated with CDAD may vary between institutions. Cost of single-room occupancy, infection control measures, increased length of stay, and staff time must all be taken into consideration.

KEY POINTS

- Gastroenteritis or infectious diarrhea is the fourth leading cause of death worldwide, with more than 3 million deaths
- The most common microbial causes of gastroenteritis include viruses (rotavirus and calicivirus) and bacteria (*Campylobacter*, *Salmonella*, *Shigella*, and certain strains of *E. coli*)
- Infectious diarrhea is generally classified into noninflammatory or inflammatory diarrhea. Inflammatory diarrhea is characterized by bloody, purulent, mucoid stools and is often accompanied by tenesmus, fever, and abdominal pain. Noninflammatory diarrhea is generally less severe; typical signs and symptoms include watery diarrhea without fever, abdominal pain, fecal white blood cells, or occult blood
- The most common risks associated with diarrheal diseases are dehydration and malnutrition. For severe diarrhea, rehydration with glucose-containing oral rehydration solution (ORS) should be instituted
- The vast majority of cases of infectious diarrhea are self-limited and do not require therapy beyond adequate hydration and other supportive care. For certain pathogens, such as *Salmonella* or STEC, antibiotic therapy has been shown to either prolong the duration of shedding (*Salmonella*) or increase the risk of life-threatening complications (STEC)
- Empiric antibiotic therapy in patients with severe, community-acquired diarrhea has been shown to reduce the duration of symptoms from 4 to 6 days to 1 to 2 days. For patients with evidence of inflammatory diarrhea (fever, tenesmus, dysentery, or fecal leukocytes or lactoferrin), empiric therapy with a fluoroquinolone (for adults) or trimethoprim-sulfamethoxazole (for children) is often initiated, pending results of fecal testing. However, the decision to use an antibiotic must be weighed against the likelihood of a resistant organism (especially *Campylobacter*), prolonged shedding of an organism (*Salmonella*), or risk of life-threatening complications (STEC)
- The prevention and control of infectious diarrhea can be accomplished by two major principles: proper personal hygiene and appropriate food preparation measures. Handwashing by healthcare providers, isolation precautions for patients with *C. difficile* infection, the use of gloves and disposable equipment when possible, and limited use of antimicrobials may offer means to control the spread of these illnesses
- Antibiotic-associated diarrhea may be an adverse effect associated with any class of antimicrobial agent, but it is most frequently seen with clindamycin, extended-spectrum penicillins, and cephalosporins. If possible, the offending agent should be removed, in addition to adequate rehydration and restoration of electrolyte imbalances if necessary

■ Patients with CDAD should be monitored closely for adequate rehydration and restoration of electrolyte imbalances. The drug of choice for CDAD is oral metronidazole for 10 days. Oral vancomycin is an alternative treatment. Many patients will experience relapses of CDAD despite appropriate antimicrobial therapy, and alternative treatment options may need to be considered for these patients

SUGGESTED READINGS

Bartlett JG. Clinical practice. Antibiotic-associated diarrhea. N Engl J Med 346:334–339, 2002.

Guerrant RL, VanGilder T, Steiner TS, et al. Practice guidelines for the management of infectious diarrhea. Clin Infect Dis 32:331–350, 2001.

Thielman NM, Guerrant RL. Acute infectious diarrhea. New Engl J Med 350:38–47, 2004.

REFERENCES

1. Murray CJ, Lopez AD. Alternative projections of mortality and disability by cause 1990–2020: Global Burden of Disease Study. Lancet 349:1498–1504, 1997.
2. Ilnyckyj A. Clinical evaluation and management of acute infectious diarrhea in adults. Gastroenterol Clin North Am 30:599–609, 2001.
3. Kosek M, Bern C, Guerrant RL. The global burden of diarrhoeal disease, as estimated from studies published between 1992 and 2000. Bull World Health Organ 81:197–204, 2003.
4. Mead PS, Slutsker L, Dietz V, et al. Food-related illness and death in the United States. Emerg Infect Dis 5:607–625, 1999.
5. Aranda-Michel J, Giannella RA. Acute diarrhea. a practical review. Am J Med 106:670–676, 1999.
6. Bartlett JG. Antibiotic-associated diarrhea. Clin Infect Dis 15:573–581, 1992.
7. Guerrant RL, Van Gilder T, Steiner TS, et al. Practice guidelines for the management of infectious diarrhea. Clin Infect Dis 32:331–351, 2001.
8. Thielman NM, Guerrant RL. Clinical practice. Acute infectious diarrhea. N Engl J Med 350:38–47, 2004.
9. Koopmans M, von Bonsdorff CH, Vinje J, et al. Foodborne viruses. FEMS Microbiol Rev 26:187–205, 2002.
10. Preliminary FoodNet data on the incidence of infection with pathogens transmitted commonly through food—selected sites, United States, 2003. MMWR Morb Mortal Wkly Rep 53:338–343, 2004.
11. Groseclose SL, Brathwaite WS, Hall PA, et al. Summary of notifiable diseases—United States, 2002. MMWR Morb Mortal Wkly Rep51:1–84, 2004.
12. Bean NH, Martin SM, Bradford H, Jr. PHLIS: an electronic system for reporting public health data from remote sites. Am J Public Health 82:1273–1276, 1992.
13. Wilhelmi I, Roman E, Sanchez-Fauquier A. Viruses causing gastroenteritis. Clin Microbiol Infect 9:247–262, 2003.
14. Hedberg CW, Osterholm MT. Outbreaks of food-borne and waterborne viral gastroenteritis. Clin Microbiol Rev 6:199–210, 1993.
15. Johansen K, Bennet R, Bondesson K, et al. Incidence and estimates of the disease burden of rotavirus in Sweden. Acta Paediatr Suppl 88:20–23, 1999.
16. Glass RI, Kilgore PE, Holman RC, et al. The epidemiology of rotavirus diarrhea in the United States: surveillance and estimates of disease burden. J Infect Dis 174 (Suppl 1):S5–11, 1996.
17. Jin S, Kilgore PE, Holman RC, et al. Trends in hospitalizations for diarrhea in United States children from 1979 through 1992. estimates of the morbidity associated with rotavirus. Pediatr Infect Dis J 15:397–404, 1996.
18. Hardy ME. Norwalk and ''Norwalk-like viruses'' in epidemic gastroenteritis. Clin Lab Med 19:675–690, 1999.
19. Goodgame RW. Viral causes of diarrhea. Gastroenterol Clin North Am 30:779–795, 2001.
20. Bartlett JG. Clinical practice. Antibiotic-associated diarrhea. N Engl J Med 346:334–339, 2002.
21. Oldfield EC, 3rd. Emerging foodborne pathogens: keeping your patients and your families safe. Rev Gastroenterol Disord 1:177–186, 2001.
22. Outbreaks of Salmonella serotype enteritidis infection associated with eating shell eggs—United States, 1999–2001. MMWR Morb Mortal Wkly Rep 51:1149–1152, 2003.
23. Altekruse SF, Stern NJ, Fields PI, et al. Campylobacter jejuni—an emerging foodborne pathogen. Emerg Infect Dis 5:28–35, 1999.
24. Smith KE, Besser JM, Hedberg CW, et al. Quinolone-resistant Campylobacter jejuni infections in Minnesota, 1992–1998. Investigation Team. N Engl J Med 340:1525–1532, 1999.
25. Riley LW, Remis RS, Helgerson SD, et al. Hemorrhagic colitis associated with a rare Escherichia coli serotype. N Engl J Med 308:681–685, 1983.
26. Huang DB, Koo H, DuPont HL. Enteroaggregative Escherichia coli. An emerging pathogen. Curr Infect Dis Rep 6:83–86, 2004.
27. Ochoa TJ, Cleary TG. Epidemiology and spectrum of disease of Escherichia coli O157. Curr Opin Infect Dis 16:259–263, 2003.
28. Leclerc H, Schwartzbrod L, Dei-Cas E. Microbial agents associated with waterborne diseases. Crit Rev Microbiol 28:371–409, 2002.
29. Guerrant RL, Steiner TS. Gastrointestinal infections and food poisoning. In Mandel GL, Bennet JE, Dolin R, eds. Principles and practice of infectious diseases. Philadelphia: Churchill Livingstone, 2000:1076.
30. Sobel J, Gomes TA, Ramos RT, et al. Pathogen-specific risk factors and protective factors for acute diarrheal illness in children aged 12–59 months in Sao Paulo, Brazil. Clin Infect Dis 38:1545–1551, 2004.
31. Rockx B, De Wit M, Vennema H, et al. Natural history of human calicivirus infection: a prospective cohort study. Clin Infect Dis 35:246–253, 2002.
32. Ina K, Kusugami K, Ohta M. Bacterial hemorrhagic enterocolitis. J Gastroenterol 38:111–120, 2003.
33. Turgeon DK, Fritsche TR. Laboratory approaches to infectious diarrhea. Gastroenterol Clin North Am 30:693–707, 2001.
34. Parry CM, Hien TT, Dougan G, et al. Typhoid fever. N Engl J Med 347:1770–1782, 2002.
35. Hirschhorn N, Kinzie JL, Sachar DB, et al. Decrease in net stool output in cholera during intestinal perfusion with glucose-containing solutions. N Engl J Med 279:176–181, 1968.
36. Water with sugar and salt. Lancet 2:300–301, 1978.
37. Duggan C, Fontaine O, Pierce NF, et al. Scientific rationale for a change in the composition of oral rehydration solution. JAMA 291:2628–2631, 2004.
38. Hahn S, Kim Y, Garner P. Reduced osmolarity oral rehydration solution for treating dehydration due to diarrhoea in children. systematic review. Br Med J 323:81–85, 2001.
39. Alam NH, Majumder RN, Fuchs GJ. Efficacy and safety of oral rehydration solution with reduced osmolarity in adults with cholera: a randomised double-blind clinical trial. CHOICE study group. Lancet 354:296–299, 1999.
40. Nalin DR, Hirschhorn N, Greenough W, 3rd, et al. Clinical concerns about reduced-osmolarity oral rehydration solution. JAMA 291:2632–2635, 2004.
41. Khan WA, Seas C, Dhar U, et al. Treatment of shigellosis. V. Comparison of azithromycin and ciprofloxacin. A double-blind, randomized, controlled trial. Ann Intern Med 126:697–703, 1997.
42. Bennish ML, Salam MA, Haider R, et al. Therapy for shigellosis. II. Randomized, double-blind comparison of ciprofloxacin and ampicillin. J Infect Dis 162:711–716, 1990.
43. Multicenter, randomized, double blind clinical trial of short course versus standard course oral ciprofloxacin for Shigella dysenteriae type 1 dysentery in children. Pediatr Infect Dis J 21:1136–1141, 2002.
44. Wong CS, Jelacic S, Habeeb RL, et al. The risk of the hemolytic–uremic syndrome after antibiotic treatment of Escherichia coli O157:H7 infections. N Engl J Med 342:1930–1936, 2000.
45. Safdar N, Said A, Gangnon RE, et al. Risk of hemolytic uremic syndrome after antibiotic treatment of Escherichia coli O157:H7 enteritis: a meta-analysis. JAMA 288:996–1001, 2002.

46. Adachi JA, Ostrosky-Zeichner L, DuPont HL, et al. Empirical antimicrobial therapy for traveler's diarrhea. Clin Infect Dis 31:1079–1083, 2000.

47. DuPont HL, Jiang ZD, Ericsson CD, et al. Rifaximin versus ciprofloxacin for the treatment of traveler's diarrhea: a randomized, double-blind clinical trial. Clin Infect Dis 33:1807–1815, 2001.

48. Dryden MS, Gabb RJ, Wright SK. Empirical treatment of severe acute community–acquired gastroenteritis with ciprofloxacin. Clin Infect Dis 22:1019–1025, 1996.

49. Kosek M, Alcantara C, Lima AA, et al. Cryptosporidiosis: an update. Lancet Infect Dis 1:262–269, 2001.

50. Rossignol JF, Ayoub A, Ayers MS. Treatment of diarrhea caused by *Cryptosporidium parvum*: a prospective randomized, double-blind, placebo-controlled study of nitazoxanide. J Infect Dis 184:103–106, 2001.

51. Ericsson CD, DuPont HL, Mathewson JJ, et al. Treatment of traveler's diarrhea with sulfamethoxazole and trimethoprim and loperamide. JAMA 263:257–261, 1990.

52. DuPont HL, Flores Sanchez J, Ericsson CD, et al. Comparative efficacy of loperamide hydrochloride and bismuth subsalicylate in the management of acute diarrhea. Am J Med 88:15S–19S, 1990.

53. DuPont HL, Hornick RB. Adverse effect of Lomotil therapy in shigellosis. JAMA 226:1525–1528, 1973.

54. DuPont HL, Ericsson CD, Johnson PC, et al. Use of bismuth subsalicylate for the prevention of travelers' diarrhea. Rev Infect Dis 12 (Suppl 1):S64–67, 1990.

55. MacConnachie AA, Todd WA. Potential therapeutic agents for the prevention and treatment of haemolytic uraemic syndrome in Shiga-toxin-producing *Escherichia coli* infection. Curr Opin Infect Dis 17:479–482, 2004.

56. Levine MM. Immunization against bacterial diseases of the intestine. J Pediatr Gastroenterol Nutr 31:336–355, 2000.

57. Kelly CP, LaMont JT. *Clostridium difficile* infection. Ann Rev Med 49:375–390, 1998.

58. Gerding DN. Disease associated with *Clostridium difficile* infection. Ann Intern Med 110:255–257, 1989.

59. Fekety R, Shah AB. Diagnosis and treatment of *Clostridium difficile* colitis. JAMA 269:71–75, 1993.

60. Gerding DN, Johnson S, Peterson LR, et al. *Clostridium difficile*–associated diarrhea and colitis. Infect Control Hosp Epidemiol 16:459–477, 1995.

61. Hurley BW, Nguyen CC. The spectrum of pseudomembranous enterocolitis and antibiotic-associated diarrhea. Arch Intern Med 162:2177–2184, 2002.

62. McFarland LV, Surawicz CM, Greenberg RN, et al. Prevention of beta-lactam–associated diarrhea by *Saccharomyces boulardii* compared with placebo. Am J Gastroenterol. 90:439–448, 1995.

63. Hogenauer C, Hammer HF, Krejs GJ, et al. Mechanisms and management of antibiotic-associated diarrhea. Clin Infect Dis 27:702–710, 1998.

64. Chassany O, Michaux A, Bergmann JF. Drug-induced diarrhoea. Drug Saf 22:53–72, 2000.

65. Johnson S, Gerding DN. *Clostridium difficile*-associated diarrhea. Clin Infect Dis 26:1027–1034, 1998.

66. Kelly CP, Pothoulakis C, LaMont JT. *Clostridium difficile* colitis. N Engl J Med 330:257–262, 1994.

67. Poutanen SM, Simor AE. *Clostridium difficile*–associated diarrhea in adults. CMAJ 171:51–58, 2004.

68. Jefferson KK, Smith MF Jr, Bobak DA. Roles of intracellular calcium and NF-kappa B in the *Clostridium difficile* toxin A–induced upregulation and secretion of IL-8 from human monocytes. J Immunol 163:5183–5191, 1999.

69. Mylonakis E, Ryan ET, Calderwood SB. *Clostridium difficile*–associated diarrhea. A review. Arch Intern Med 161:525–533, 2000.

70. Johnson S, Kent SA, O'Leary KJ, et al. Fatal pseudomembranous colitis associated with a variant *Clostridium difficile* strain not detected by toxin A immunoassay. Ann Intern Med 135:434–438, 2001.

71. Manabe YC, Vinetz JM, Moore RD, et al. *Clostridium difficile* colitis: an efficient clinical approach to diagnosis. Ann Intern Med 123:835–840, 1995.

72. Wenisch C, Parschalk B, Hasenhundl M, et al. Comparison of vancomycin, teicoplanin, metronidazole, and fusidic acid for the treatment of *Clostridium difficile*–associated diarrhea. Clin Infect Dis 22:813–818, 1996.

73. Teasley DG, Gerding DN, Olson MM, et al. Prospective randomised trial of metronidazole versus vancomycin for *Clostridium difficile*–associated diarrhoea and colitis. Lancet 2:1043–1046, 1983.

74. McFarland LV, Surawicz CM, Rubin M, et al. Recurrent *Clostridium difficile* disease: epidemiology and clinical characteristics. Infect Control Hosp Epidemiol 20:43–50, 1999.

75. Gorbach SL, Chang TW, Goldin B. Successful treatment of relapsing *Clostridium difficile* colitis with Lactobacillus GG. Lancet 2:1519, 1987.

76. Tvede M, Rask-Madsen J. Bacteriotherapy for *Clostridium difficile* diarrhoea. Lancet 1:1156–1160, 1989.

77. Schwan A, Sjolin S, Trottestam U, et al. Relapsing *Clostridium difficile* enterocolitis cured by rectal infusion of normal faeces. Scand J Infect Dis 16:211–215, 1984.

78. Synnott K, Mealy K, Merry C, et al. Timing of surgery for fulminating pseudomembranous colitis. Br J Surg 85:229–231, 1998.

79. Morris JB, Zollinger RM Jr, Stellato TA. Role of surgery in antibiotic-induced pseudomembranous enterocolitis. Am J Surg 160:535–539, 1990.

80. Aas J, Gessert CE, Bakken JS. Recurrent *Clostridium difficile* colitis: case series involving 18 patients treated with donor stool administered via a nasogastric tube. Clin Infect Dis 36:580–585, 2003.

81. Giannasca PJ, Warny M. Active and passive immunization against *Clostridium difficile* diarrhea and colitis. Vaccine 22:848–856, 2004.

82. Kyne L, Hamel MB, Polavaram R, et al. Health care costs and mortality associated with nosocomial diarrhea due to *Clostridium difficile*. Clin Infect Dis 34:346–353, 2002.

Infective Endocarditis

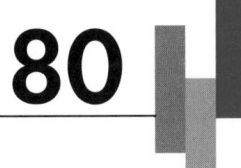

80

Diane M. Cappelletty and Shirley Palmer-Murrow

DEFINITION

Endocarditis is an infection of the inner lining of the heart and the mucosa that underlies it, but the term refers most commonly to an infection of a heart valve. The mural endocardium, papillary muscles, and chordae tendineae can be involved in the infection, but the complications and clinical manifestations usually arise from the involvement of the tricuspid, mitral, or aortic valves.[1,2]

Subacute disease is an indolent infection that may produce signs and symptoms over periods as long as several months before a diagnosis is made. Acute infection is of rapid onset, with fulminant symptoms. Traditionally, patients with subacute disease have all the "classic" manifestations of the disease. However, the diagnosis is now suspected in any febrile illness of unclear cause, so progression to chronicity is becoming less common.[2,3]

TREATMENT GOALS

The goal of treatment is to eradicate infection. This is accomplished by the use of antimicrobial therapy to sterilize the infected valve and surrounding structures, with adjunctive surgery, if necessary, for excision of infected tissue and repair or replacement of the affected valve. Once cure is achieved, prevention of recurrent episodes becomes a predominant concern.

- Antimicrobials used in the treatment of endocarditis should always be bactericidal.
- Antimicrobials must be given in high doses to penetrate the valvular vegetation at the site of infection.
- Therapy must be prolonged (2 to at least 6 weeks) to achieve complete sterilization.
- Combination therapy is sometimes required for adequate bactericidal activity.
- Adequate monitoring for toxicity of antimicrobials and complications of endocarditis is necessary.
- Surgery may be indicated to cure infection or restore cardiac function.
- Mortality may occur as a result of severe hemodynamic compromise or from complications arising from embolic phenomena.
- Recurrent episodes can be prevented by giving prophylactic antibiotics before procedures that result in transient bacteremic episodes.

EPIDEMIOLOGY

There are approximately 15,000 to 20,000 new cases of infective endocarditis each year in the United States.[4] The clinical spectrum of infective endocarditis has changed significantly in the past few decades. Infection due to *viridans* streptococci, which were responsible for 70% to 80% of all cases in the 1960s and 1970s, has declined to only 30% to 40% of cases.[2,3] Enterococci are the causative pathogens in approximately 5% to 18% of cases, and other streptococci account for an additional 15% to 25% of cases.[2] Staphylococci account for 20% to 35% of all cases and account for the majority of isolates among injection drug users.[2,5] The incidence of methicillin-resistant isolates has increased significantly, accounting for 40% of isolates of *Staphylococcus aureus* in injection drug users at one medical center and 84% to 87% of coagulase-negative staphylococci isolates in cases of prosthetic valve endocarditis occurring in the first year after surgery.[6,7] Gram-negative bacteria account for up to 10% of cases, most frequently in patients with prosthetic valves or in injection drug users.[2,6] Fungi, particularly *Candida albicans*, are seen in 5% of cases or less.[1,2] Anaerobic endocarditis is rare. Up to 20% of cases may be "culture-negative"; this could result from incorrect diagnosis, prior administration of antibiotics, failure to isolate slow-growing fastidious organisms [HACEK group (*Haemophilus* spp., *Actinobacillus actinomycetemcomitans*, *Cardiobacterium hominis*, *Eikenella corrodens*, *Kingella kingii*), nutritionally variant streptococci, or anaerobes], or a nonbacterial etiology.[2]

RISK FACTORS

Risk factors associated with the development of infective endocarditis include intravenous drug use, presence of intravascular devices, some types of underlying valvular heart disease, or the presence of a prosthetic heart valve. Injection drug users develop endocarditis more frequently than the general population, probably because of frequent nonsterile intravenous injections. The most common valve affected is the tricuspid valve, although other valves may be affected also. The bacteriology of infective endocarditis in this population is primarily composed of *S. aureus* (50% to 60%), streptococci (15%), and gram-negative bacilli and fungi (25% to 35%).[6]

The incidence of intravascular device-related infective endocarditis, once thought to be uncommon, is increasing. A group of investigators at Duke University Medical Center determined that approximately 51% of *S. aureus* infective endocarditis cases were presumed to be associated with intravascular devices, and 53% of these infections were community-acquired.[8] A review of all *S. aureus* infective endocarditis cases occurring in Denmark over a 10-year period found that 33% of cases were nosocomially acquired, and 25% of these were associated with infected intravascular devices.[9] In a prospective study by Fowler et al, the prevalence of endocarditis in patients with intravascular catheter-related *S. aureus* bacteremia was 23%, which has led to the suggestion that all such patients should routinely undergo transesophageal echocardiography (TEE) to assist in early detection of infective endocarditis and permit prompt institution of appropriate antimicrobial therapy.[10,11]

Certain congenital or acquired valvular heart defects predispose to the development of infective endocarditis. These include mitral valve prolapse, degenerative valvular lesions, rheumatic heart disease, ventricular septal defect, coarctation of the aorta, and congenital bicuspid aortic valve.[2] The risk of infection is greater with some conditions than others. For example, patients with mitral valve prolapse are approximately eight times more likely to develop infective endocarditis than patients in the general population.[3] Infective endo-

carditis in patients with preexisting valvular damage usually results from transient bacteremia with organisms that colonize mucosal surfaces and are considered normal flora. The most common sites of infection are the mitral and aortic valves. *Viridans* streptococci, which are found in the mouth, are responsible for the majority of cases of native valve endocarditis in patients who are not drug users.[12] The remainder of cases are due to enterococci, other streptococci, and gram-negative bacilli.

Patients with prosthetic cardiac valves are at risk for developing infective endocarditis, which is categorized as either early or late onset. Prosthetic valve endocarditis (PVE) occurring within the first 2 months after surgery (early PVE) is caused by organisms introduced during or shortly after surgery while the patient is still in the hospital. The most frequently cultured organisms are coagulase-negative staphylococci (35%), followed by *S. aureus* (17%), gram-negative bacilli (16%), and fungi (10%).[13] Infections occurring beyond 2 months (late PVE) are usually caused by the same organisms that produce diseases on native valves (i.e., primarily streptococci); however, endocarditis due to coagulase-negative staphylococci may not be detected until months after surgery due to its indolent course.[7] For this reason, some investigators have proposed changing the definition of early PVE to include infections occurring during the first year after valve replacement.[14,15] The rate of PVE ranges from 1% to 4% during the first year after surgery and is approximately 1% per year afterward.[3] Endocarditis is especially devastating in patients with prosthetic valves, since fatal complications can occur quickly. A recent study by the Department of Veterans Affairs found overall mortality rates of 46%, with no difference between early and late PVE. However, mortality was twice as high in patients with New York Heart Association class III or IV congestive heart failure compared with those in classes I and II.[16] Other factors associated with poor prognosis include onset within 12 months of implantation; gram-negative, fungal, or *S. aureus* etiology; or aortic valve involvement.[2,17]

There has been a significant trend in recent years toward an increase in the age of patients with infective endocarditis.[2,3,18] This is at least partly due to marked decreases in the prevalence of rheumatic heart disease, the longevity of persons in modern society (leading to degenerative valvular lesions), and increasing numbers of older patients with prosthetic cardiac valves.[3,18] Although increased age was associated with a poorer prognosis in previous years, a recent study found mortality in elderly patients to be similar to that of younger patients, which the authors attributed to improved diagnostic sensitivity of TEE, leading to earlier diagnosis.[18]

The overall mortality for all forms of infective endocarditis is approximately 25% to 30%. However, the mortality ranges from 10% to 15% in penicillin-sensitive streptococcal endocarditis to 90% or more in fungal infection.[2,19] Factors associated with a poor prognosis include heart failure, renal failure, left-sided (aortic or mitral valve) involvement, infection of a prosthetic valve, cerebral embolism, and infection with gram-negative bacilli or fungi.[2,20]

PATHOPHYSIOLOGY

As mentioned earlier, the tissues involved in infective endocarditis are primarily the tricuspid, mitral, and aortic valves; the valve of the pulmonary artery is rarely infected. The tricuspid valve is the most common site of infection in intravenous drug users. The mitral and aortic valves are also involved in this group of patients, as well as in patients with underlying valve pathology. Damage to the mitral and aortic valves leads to more severe hemodynamic alterations than tricuspid disease.[1,2] Lesions of the chordae, the atrial or ventricular walls, and the pulmonary artery or aorta are considered satellite infections to the primary valvular involvement.[1]

Four factors are necessary in the pathogenesis of the infection: (a) a previously damaged cardiac valve; (b) a platelet-fibrin thrombus; (c) bacteremia; and (d) bacterial adherence.[1] In a published series of patients with fatal infective endocarditis, autopsy revealed that the mitral valve was involved in 86%, the aortic valve in 55%, the tricuspid valve in 20%, and the pulmonic valve in only 1%.[2] Correlating the pressure gradient across these valves with the relative frequency of infection makes a strong argument for mechanical stress as an important factor in the pathogenesis of infective endocarditis. Similarly, the hemodynamic alterations that occur across an incompetent valve result in abnormal "jets" of blood that may damage the endocardium and provide a locus for infection. This change in hemodynamics also creates a low-pressure "sink," which sets up an additional site for infection. Consequently, vegetations in infective endocarditis are most commonly found on the low-pressure side of the valve: the atrial surfaces of the mitral and tricuspid valves and the ventricular surface of the aortic valve.[1,2]

Once the endothelial surface of the valve is damaged, collagen is exposed, and a sterile platelet-fibrin thrombus is formed. This is referred to as nonbacterial thrombotic endocarditis.[1,2] The next critical factor in the pathogenesis of the infection is the presence of bacteremia. Bacteremia or fungemia arises secondary to another focus of infection, colonization on intravascular catheters, or dental or surgical procedures. The procedures that can induce a transient bacteremia with the potential for producing endocarditis include tooth extraction, periodontal surgery, liver biopsy, endoscopy or sigmoidoscopy, and manipulations of the genitourinary tract. The organisms causing infective endocarditis in these cases can usually be traced to the site of the procedure. For example, *viridans* streptococci, nonenterococcal group D streptococci, and other facultative organisms are normal flora of the nasopharynx. Enterococci and gram-negative bacilli usually arise from the urinary or gastrointestinal tracts. Staphylococci are found on the skin and may colonize the nasopharynx. Fungi may arise from the bowel, as can certain gram-negative and anaerobic organisms. Bacteria and fungi may also colonize certain areas of skin and thus gain entrance to the circulation via intravenous catheters.[1,2]

The final step in the development of infective endocarditis occurs when organisms adhere to the thrombus. The adherence properties of an organism correlate directly with the ability of that organism to produce endocarditis.[1,2] For instance, some strains of streptococci and staphylococci produce virulence factors such as dextran or fibrinonectin that promote adherence to traumatized endothelial cells.[1] Production of an extracellular polysaccharide matrix, or slime, allows coagulase-negative staphylococci to adhere to prosthetic materials and resist phagocytosis.[7] Once organisms adhere to the thrombus, they begin to multiply. Within 24 hours, the bacteria undergo a period of exponential growth, reach a very high inoculum (approximately 10^9 colony-forming units/gram), and enter a "resting" stage of low metabolic activity.[21] Additional platelet-fibrin deposition occurs, resulting in sequestration from leukocytes and enlargement of the infected thrombus, which now is termed a vegetation.[1,21] Figures 80.1 and 80.2 (*see color insert*) depict a normal aortic valve and one with a vegetation on it. The vegetation is the source of prolonged and continuous bacteremia, the hallmark sign of infective endocarditis.

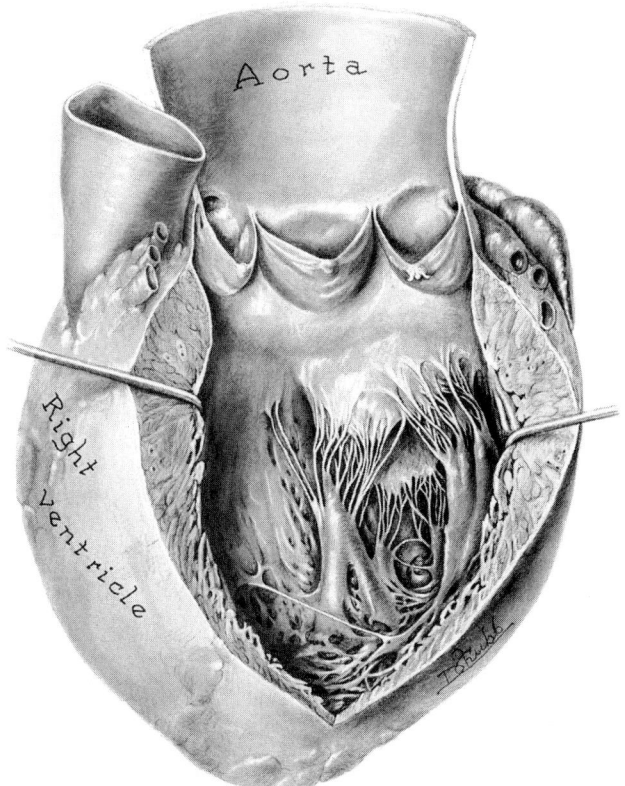

FIGURE 80.1 Schematic of normal aortic valve (*see color insert*). (From Grants Atlas of Anatomy.)

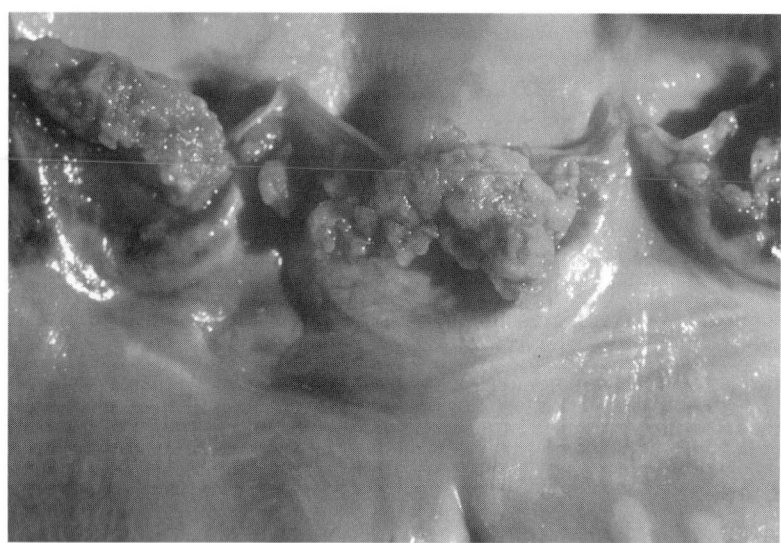

FIGURE 80.2 Vegetations on aortic valve in an intravenous drug abuser (*see color insert*). (From Rubin E, Farber JL. Pathology, 3rd ed. Philadelphia: Lippincott Williams & Wilkins, 1999.)

CLINICAL PRESENTATION AND DIAGNOSIS

SIGNS AND SYMPTOMS

The classic signs and symptoms of infective endocarditis such as Osler's nodes, Janeway lesions, clubbing of the fingers, splinter hemorrhages, and retinal lesions are now seen infrequently.[1,17] The primary reason for this is the high index of suspicion for the disease in a patient with fever of unknown origin, leading to a relatively earlier diagnosis before the development of these more chronic findings. The most common signs and symptoms are a heart murmur or a change in a previously noted murmur, fever, embolic episodes, splenomegaly, skin manifestations (primarily petechiae), weakness, dyspnea, night sweats, anorexia, weight loss, and malaise.[2,17] These are not present in all cases, but the key criterion for the diagnosis is a positive blood culture.

DIAGNOSIS

Two sets of criteria exist for diagnosing endocarditis, the Duke criteria (Tables 80.1 and 80.2) and the von Reyn (Beth Israel) criteria.[22,23] The Duke criteria are more recent than Beth Israel's and incorporate echocardiographic findings into the classification schemes. It has been found to be more sensitive (>80%) than the Beth Israel criteria (51%) and is the most cited and used (22).

Echocardiography is the technique of choice for identifying vegetations and is a very important tool for the diagnosis of infective endocarditis.[17,24] Transesophageal imaging allows higher-resolution imaging because the transducer is immediately adjacent to the heart. In contrast to the standard transthoracic echocardiography (TTE), TEE is much more sensitive (>86% detection of vegetations vs. only 58% for TTE).[4,24] TEE is superior to TTE for identifying small vege-

tations, vegetations on either pulmonic or prosthetic valves, and intracardiac abscesses.[4] If there is a low clinical suspicion or patient risk for infective endocarditis, then TTE is recommended; however, if there is a high clinical suspicion or patient risk, then TEE is preferred.[4]

TABLE 80.1	Duke Criteria for Diagnosis of Infective Endocarditis

Definite infective endocarditis

Pathologic criteria

    Microorganisms: demonstrated by culture or histology in a vegetation, *or* in a vegetation that has embolized, *or* in an intracardiac abscess, *or*

    Pathologic lesions: vegetation or intracardiac abscess present, confirmed by histology showing active endocarditis.

Clinical criteria (using definitions listed in Table 80.2)

    2 major criteria, *or*

    1 major criterion plus 3 minor criteria, *or*

    5 minor criteria

Possible infective endocarditis

Findings consistent with infective endocarditis that fall short of "Definitive" but not "Rejected."

Rejected

Firm alternative diagnosis explaining evidence of infective endocarditis, *or*

Resolution of manifestations of endocarditis, with antibiotic therapy for 4 days or less, *or*

No pathologic evidence of infective endocarditis at surgery or autopsy, after antibiotic therapy for 4 days or less.

(Reprinted from Durack DT, Lukes AS, Bright DK. New criteria for diagnosis of infective endocarditis: utilization of specific echocardiographic findings. Am J Med 96:200–209, 1994. Copyright 1994, with permission from Excerpta Medica Inc.)

TABLE 80.2	Definitions of Terminology Used in Duke Criteria

Major Criteria

Positive blood culture for infective endocarditis

Typical microorganism for infective endocarditis from 2 separate blood cultures:

   Viridans streptococci, *Streptococcus bovis*, HACEK group, *or*

   Community-acquired *S. aureus* or enterococci, in the absence of a primary focus, *or*

Persistently positive blood culture, defined as recovery of a microorganism consistent with infective endocarditis from:

   (i)   Blood cultures drawn more than 12 hours apart, *or*

   (ii) All of three or a majority of four or more separate blood cultures, with first and last drawn at least 1 hour apart

Evidence of endocardial involvement

   Positive echocardiogram for infective endocarditis

   (i)   Oscillating intracardiac mass, on valve or supporting structures, or in the path of regurgitant jets, or on implanted material, in the absence of an alternative anatomic explanation, *or*

   (ii) Abscess, *or*

   (iii) New partial dehiscence of prosthetic valve, *or*

   New valvular regurgitation (increase or change in preexisting murmur not sufficient)

Minor Criteria

Predisposition: predisposing heart condition or intravenous drug use Fever: ≥38°C (100.4°F)

Vascular phenomena: major arterial emboli, septic pulmonary infarcts, mycotic aneurysm, intracranial hemorrhage, conjunctival hemorrhages, Janeway lesions

Immunologic phenomena: glomerulonephritis, Osler's nodes, Roth spots, rheumatoid factor

Microbiologic evidence: positive blood culture[a] but not meeting major criterion as noted previously, or serologic evidence of active infection with organism consistent with infective endocarditis

Echocardiogram: consistent with infective endocarditis but not meeting major criterion as noted previously

---

HACEK, *Haemophilus* spp., *Actinobacillus actinomycetemcomitans*, *Cardiobacterium hominis*, *Eikenella* spp., and *Kingella kingae*.

[a] Excluding single positive cultures for coagulase-negative staphylococci or organisms that do not cause endocarditis.

(Reprinted from Durack DT, Lukes AS, Bright DK. New criteria for diagnosis of infective endocarditis: utilization of specific echocardiographic findings. Am J Med 96:200–209, 1994. Copyright 1994, with permission from Excerpta Medica Inc.)

The bacteremia in infective endocarditis is usually continuous but low grade.[2] In practice, three blood cultures taken over an extended period in a patient who is not critically ill should produce a very high yield. In acutely ill patients, two or three blood cultures should be taken rapidly from different sites before starting antibiotic therapy. Other criteria that support the diagnosis of endocarditis include fever, immunologic manifestations, and vascular phenomena (see Table 80.2).

Infective endocarditis in intravenous drug users is frequently heralded by neurologic dysfunction or pulmonary emboli.[2,6,17] This may misdirect diagnostic efforts, which again points to the importance of obtaining sufficient blood cultures in a febrile patient with a history of symptoms consistent with infective endocarditis.

COMPLICATIONS

Complications from infective endocarditis may be classified as cardiac or extracardiac. The most common cardiac com-plication is congestive heart failure, which is the leading cause of death in patients with infective endocarditis.[15,25–27] Less frequent complications include intracardiac abscesses, conduction defects, infection- or immune complex-mediated pericarditis, and myocardial infarction.[26,27]

Extracardiac complications are usually related to embolic events, which occur in at least one third of patients with infective endocarditis.[2] Patients with tricuspid valve infective endocarditis commonly have pulmonary emboli, while those with left-sided infective endocarditis are more likely to have systemic embolic events. Many patients develop renal insufficiency, which may be due to several factors such as metastatic abscesses within the kidney from infected emboli (predominantly staphylococcal infection), infarction of the kidney from compromised blood flow caused by aseptic emboli, immune-complex nephritis caused by deposition of immunoglobulins and complement on the glomerular basement membrane, or even nephrotoxicity of the antimicrobials used for treatment.[2] Splenic artery emboli may result in splenic infarction (44% incidence), splenomegaly, and abdominal pain.[2]

Involvement of the central nervous system (CNS) occurs in 20% to 40% of patients with infective endocarditis, most frequently in those with left-sided involvement and/or *S. aureus* etiology.[28] The predominant CNS manifestations are cerebral embolism, mycotic aneurysm, meningitis, brain abscess, encephalopathy, or seizures. Presenting symptoms differ depending on the type of manifestation or location of the emboli but almost always include headache. Various imaging techniques (computed tomography, magnetic resonance imaging) may be useful for diagnosis of CNS involvement; neurosurgery may be indicated in cases of aneurysm or intracranial hemorrhage.[28]

TREATMENT

PHARMACOTHERAPY

Curing infective endocarditis is difficult and requires sterilization of the vegetation. Sequestration of the infecting organisms within an avascular vegetation provides protection from the circulating antibodies and white blood cells. In the absence of humoral or cellular immune mechanisms, antibiotics must be capable of bactericidal activity. This fact has been proven clinically by the failure of bacteriostatic antibiotics such as the tetracyclines, erythromycin, and chloramphenicol to cure endocarditis. In addition, organisms in a vegetation exhibit reduced metabolic activity and are less susceptible to antimicrobials, which are primarily effective against rapidly dividing cells. The high organism load within the vegetation may also result in decreased effectiveness of drug therapy. Thus, organisms that appear to be susceptible to an antimicrobial in vitro using standard inocula (10^5/mL) may exhibit "tolerance" at the high inocula encountered in vivo (10^9 to 10^{10}/g).[29] Failure of antibiotics to penetrate in sufficient concentrations into the core of the vegetation also contributes to the difficulty of treatment.[30] All of these factors combined necessitate the use of high-dose, bactericidal antimicrobial therapy for a prolonged duration to achieve sterilization. Anticoagulant therapy for the treatment of endocarditis (other than that necessary for the management of a prosthetic valve) is contraindicated due to the risk of intracerebral hemorrhage.[31]

Empiric therapy is most often instituted before the culture results are known, especially in acutely ill patients. The choice of empiric therapy should be based on the most likely infecting organism, as well as the institution's or community's resistance patterns. For example, an elderly man with a history of enterococcal urinary tract infections should be treated for enterococcal infective endocarditis. Likewise, an intravenous drug user with acute disease should be treated for disease due to *S. aureus* until culture results are obtained; in a community where a high incidence of intravenous drug users are known to have methicillin-resistant *S. aureus*, empiric use of vancomycin may be warranted. Therapy should

be revised as soon as culture and susceptibility results are available and tailored to the pathogen, even if the patient is responding favorably to empiric therapy.

Clinical improvement usually occurs within 4 to 10 days, but it is not unusual for a patient to remain bacteremic for 5 to 7 days after therapy is instituted. Prolonged bacteremia (>7 days) may indicate emergence of resistant subpopulations, inadequate antimicrobial therapy, or the presence of abscesses or other foci of infection. The antibiotic regimen should be reevaluated, and imaging studies (i.e., TEE) may need to be conducted or repeated to assess the need for surgery. Due to the complexity of the pathophysiology of infective endocarditis, the duration of therapy is often 4 to 6 weeks in order to cure the disease with or without surgical intervention.

Table 80.3 lists the most recent recommendations of the American Heart Association for treatment of common types of endocarditis.[12]

Streptococcal Infection (*Viridans Streptococci, S. bovis*). Most streptococci (except enterococci) are highly susceptible to penicillin G [minimum inhibitory concentration (MIC) <0.1 µg/mL], and therapy with penicillin alone for 4 weeks is highly effective.[2,12] A 4-week regimen of ceftriaxone administered once daily has also been found to be as effective as penicillin and facilitates outpatient treatment.[32] Vancomycin is the drug of choice for patients with severe β-lactam allergy. A 2-week regimen of penicillin and an aminoglycoside is an appropriate alternative in patients with uncomplicated infective endocarditis but may be more toxic because of the aminoglycoside.[12] A 2-week regimen of ceftriaxone and netilmicin dosed once daily has also been found to be effective for uncomplicated streptococcal infective endocarditis.[33] Netilmicin is not commonly used in the United States; however, other aminoglycosides (i.e., gentamicin) may be substituted. When infective endocarditis is due to streptococci that are relatively resistant to penicillin (MIC >0.1 µg/mL and <0.5 µg/mL), combination therapy with penicillin (4 weeks) plus an aminoglycoside (2 weeks) is recommended. Infective endocarditis due to nutritionally variant streptococci or *viridans* streptococci with penicillin MICs of more than 0.5 µg per mL should be treated with a 4- to 6-week course of high-dose penicillin or ampicillin plus an aminoglycoside for the entire course. The same regimen is also recommended for streptococcal PVE, but a full 6-week course is required.[12]

Enterococcal Infection. Enterococcal infective endocarditis is difficult to treat because enterococci are relatively resistant to penicillin (MIC approximately 4 µg/mL) and vancomycin (MIC approximately 2 µg/mL) and are not killed by these drugs when used alone. Enterococci are also resistant to standard concentrations of aminoglycosides; however, adding aminoglycosides to penicillin, ampicillin, or vancomycin may result in synergistic killing of most organisms. This situation requires a special aminoglycoside susceptibility study in order to predict whether synergy will

TABLE 80.3 | Antimicrobial Therapy for Native Valve (NV) and Prosthetic Valve (PV) Endocarditis

Organism	Regimens (preferred regimen listed first)	Dosage and Route	Duration (weeks)
Streptococci, NV (penicillin MIC ≤0.1 μg/mL)	Penicillin G	12–18 MU/day IV	4
	Ceftriaxone	2 g IM/IV once daily	4
	"Short-course" regimen[a]	12–18 MU/day IV	2
	Penicillin G plus gentamicin[b]	1 mg/kg q8h IV[c]	2
	"Short-course" regimen[a]	2 g IM/IV once daily	2
	Ceftriaxone plus gentamicin	4 mg/kg IV once daily	2
	Vancomycin	15 mg/kg q12h IV[d]	4
		18 MU/day IV	4
Streptococci, NV (penicillin MIC >0.1 μg/mL but ≤0.5 μg/mL)	Penicillin G plus gentamicin[b]	1 mg/kg q8h IV[c]	2
	Vancomycin	15 mg/kg q12h IV[d]	4
		18–30 MU/day	4–6
Streptococci, NV, (penicillin MIC >0.5 μg/mL	Penicillin G plus gentamicin[b]	1 mg/kg q8h IV[c]	4–6
		2 g IV q4h	4–6
	Ampicillin plus gentamicin[b]	1 mg/kg q8h IV[c]	4–6
	Vancomycin	15 mg/kg q12h IV[d]	4–6
Streptococci, PV	Penicillin G plus gentamicin[b]	12–18 MU/day IV	6
		1 mg/kg q8h IV[c]	2
		18–30 MU/day	4–6
Enterococci, NV	Penicillin G plus gentamicin[b]	1 mg/kg q8h IV[c]	4–6
		2 g IV q4h	4–6
	Ampicillin plus gentamicin[b]	1 mg/kg q8h IV[c]	4–6
	Vancomycin plus gentamicin[b]	15 mg/kg q12h IV[d]	4–6
		1 mg/kg q8h IV[c]	4–6
		18–30 MU/day	≥6
Enterococci, PV	Penicillin G plus gentamicin[b]	1 mg/kg q8h IV[c]	≥6
		2 g IV q4h	≥6
	Ampicillin plus gentamicin[b]	1 mg/kg q8h IV[c]	≥6
	Vancomycin plus gentamicin[b]	15 mg/kg q12h IV[d]	≥6
		1 mg/kg q8h IV[c]	≥6
		2 g IV q4h	4–6
Staphylococci, NV methicillin-susceptible	Nafcillin or oxacillin +/− gentamicin	1 mg/kg q8h IV[c]	3–5 days
		2 g IV q8h	4–6
	Cefazolin +/− gentamicin	1 mg/kg q8h IV[c]	3–5 days
	"Short-course" regimen[e]	2 g IV q4h	2
	Nafcillin or oxacillin plus gentamicin	1 mg/kg q8h IV[c]	2
	Vancomycin +/− gentamicin	15 mg/kg q12h IV[d]	4–6
		1 mg/kg q8h IV[c]	3–5 days
Staphylococci, PV methicillin-susceptible	Nafcillin or oxacillin plus gentamicin plus rifampin	2 g IV q4h	≥6
		1 mg/kg q8h IV[c]	2
		300 mg PO q8h	≥6
Staphylococci, NV methicillin-resistant	Vancomycin +/− gentamicin	15 mg/kg q12h IV[d]	4–6
		1 mg/kg q8h IV[c]	3–5 days
Staphylococci, PV methicillin-resistant	Vancomycin plus gentamicin plus rifampin	15 mg/kg q12h IV[d]	≥6
		1 mg/kg q8h IV[c]	2
		300 mg PO q8h	≥6

(continued)

TABLE 80.3	continued			
Organism	Regimens (preferred regimen listed first)	Dosage and Route	Duration (weeks)
HACEK organisms	Ceftriaxone	2 g IM/IV once daily	4
	Ampicillin plus gentamicin	2 g IV q4h	4
		1 mg/kg q8h IV[c]	4

[a] Short-course regimens indicated in uncomplicated streptococcal infective endocarditis only.

[b] May substitute streptomycin (7.5 mg/kg q12h) for strains exhibiting high-level resistance to gentamicin (>500 μg/mL) and sensitivity to streptomycin (MIC <2000 μg/mL).

[c] Dosage must be adjusted for renal dysfunction (target peak approximately 3 μg/mL, trough <0.5 μg/mL).

[d] Dosage must be adjusted for renal dysfunction (target peak approximately 30 to 45 μg/mL, trough approximately 10 to 15 μg/mL).

[e] Short-course regimen indicated only for uncomplicated, right-sided infective endocarditis due to methicillin-sensitive strains of *S. aureus* in injection drug users.

(Adapted from Wilson WR, Karchmer AW, Dajani AD, et al. Antibiotic treatment of adults with infective endocarditis due to streptococci, enterococci, staphylococci, and HACEK microorganisms. JAMA 274:1706–1713, 1995. Copyright 1995, American Medical Association.)

be achieved. If the isolate is inhibited by less than 2000 μg per mL of streptomycin or less than 500 μg per mL of gentamicin, the organism exhibits only "low-level" resistance, and addition of the aminoglycoside to the β-lactam or vancomycin will likely result in synergy. For an organism exhibiting "high-level" resistance (MIC ≥2000 μg/mL of streptomycin and ≥500 μg/mL of gentamicin), synergy will not be obtained with penicillin or vancomycin.[12,34] High-level gentamicin resistance is common in some isolates of enterococci and is now being encountered in *viridans* streptococci.[2,34] In some centers, as many as 60% of *Enterococcus faecium* isolates exhibit high-level resistance to gentamicin.[2,17,34] Approximately 30% to 50% of these gentamicin-resistant strains are susceptible to streptomycin, and the penicillin/streptomycin combination will be bactericidal.[34] Due to intrinsic resistance of *E. faecium* to most other aminoglycosides, only gentamicin and streptomycin are routinely tested and used.[34]

The preferred regimen for the treatment of enterococcal infective endocarditis consists of penicillin or ampicillin plus an aminoglycoside for 6 weeks. Traditional dosing of aminoglycosides (i.e., 1 mg/kg at an interval appropriate for renal function) is recommended, as studies have shown that once-daily dosing regimens are suboptimal for enterococcal infective endocarditis.[35–37]

Increasing numbers of enterococci are highly resistant to multiple antimicrobials, including aminoglycosides, penicillins, and glycopeptides (e.g., vancomycin). Treatment options for these organisms are limited. In patients with ampicillin-sensitive, high-level aminoglycoside-resistant strains, the traditional penicillin/aminoglycoside combination is unlikely to be effective.[34,38] Therapy with high-dose penicillin G or ampicillin alone for 6 to 12 weeks may be effective, but adjunctive surgery may be required.[12,34,38] Experimental models of endocarditis suggest that continuous intravenous infusion of penicillin may be more effective than intermittent bolus administration of the same total daily dose.[34] However, experience with these regimens in

humans is limited, and it is not known whether continuous infusions will achieve adequate concentrations in endocardial vegetations.

Some isolates of enterococcus (especially *E. faecium*) are found to be resistant to penicillins by virtue of the production of β-lactamase or by alteration of penicillin-binding proteins (PBPs). The β-lactamase-producing strains are effectively treated with a β-lactam/β-lactamase inhibitor combination (e.g., ampicillin/sulbactam) plus an aminoglycoside (if the isolate is susceptible to an aminoglycoside). The presence of penicillin resistance mediated by PBP alteration necessitates the use of vancomycin plus an aminoglycoside. This latter regimen is considered suboptimal therapy because glycopeptides are less rapidly bactericidal than β-lactams.[2,17]

Finally, vancomycin-resistant enterococci (VRE) have also emerged as pathogens. Most VRE isolates in the United States are *E. faecium*, which are often resistant to all cell wall-active agents (i.e., penicillins, cephalosporins), aminoglycosides, and numerous other antibiotics.[39] Hence, therapy selection is extremely difficult. If the isolate is susceptible to ampicillin with an MIC of 32 mg per liter or less, then high-dose ampicillin therapy may be effective.[39] If it is resistant to ampicillin, additional susceptibility testing to other antimicrobial agents and possibly even time-kill curves with various combinations may help to guide therapy. In vitro and animal studies suggest that some isolates may be inhibited synergistically by combinations of β-lactams, glycopeptides, and aminoglycosides, despite resistance to one of the agents.[38] Combination therapy with fluoroquinolones and β-lactams or aminoglycosides has also been reported to be effective in vitro; however, animal studies have found conflicting results.[38] There are anecdotal reports of the effectiveness of minocycline, doxycycline, chloramphenicol, and rifampin/gentamicin/ciprofloxacin in the treatment of other systemic VRE infections, but these agents have not been studied prospectively in humans in a clinical trial.[39] One combination agent with good in vitro activity against vancomycin-resistant *E. faecium* is quinupristin-dalfopristin (Synercid), a pristinamycin derivative. This agent has been used for treatment of VRE infections with some success; however, in vitro data suggest it may not be bactericidal against enterococci, which is necessary for successful treatment of endocarditis. In addition, Synercid has little activity against *E. faecalis* isolates. Linezolid, the first of the oxazolidinone class of antibiotics, is bacteriostatic against enterococci but has been used with mixed success in treating infective endocarditis caused by VRE.[40,41] The most reliable management for endocarditis caused by multiply resistant strains of enterococci appears to be surgical replacement of the valve accompanied by the best available medical therapy for very prolonged periods.[2,12]

Staphylococcal Infection. Infective endocarditis may be due to coagulase-positive staphylococci (*S. aureus*) or coagulase-negative staphylococci (*S. epidermidis* is the species most often associated). *S. aureus* is an extremely virulent pathogen capable of infecting both native and prosthetic valves.

Almost all staphylococci produce β-lactamase (e.g., "penase"), which confers resistance to penicillins. Infective endocarditis due to penicillin-susceptible strains (approximately 2% of cases) may be treated with penicillin G. The drugs of choice for treatment of β-lactamase-producing, methicillin-susceptible strains of *S. aureus* (MSSA) are oxacillin and nafcillin. Addition of an aminoglycoside for the initial 2 weeks of therapy was not shown in clinical trials to improve overall outcomes; therefore, use of gentamicin is advocated only during the first 3 to 5 days of therapy to potentially achieve more rapid clearance of bacteremia and reduce the time patients are febrile.[3] First-generation cephalosporins such as cefazolin may be used in cases of mild penicillin allergy (i.e., mild rash), although experience with these agents is minimal and has been associated with reported failures. Thus, this may be a situation for penicillin (i.e., nafcillin) desensitization. Vancomycin may be substituted for nafcillin or oxacillin in patients with immediate hypersensitivity reactions to β-lactams. However, in numerous studies using time-kill curves, in animal models, and in clinical trials, vancomycin has been shown to be less rapidly bactericidal than β-lactam antibiotics, and suboptimal outcomes have been documented.[3,12,42,43] Based on such data, vancomycin should only be used when absolutely indicated. The standard duration of therapy for native valve infective endocarditis due to MSSA is 4 to 6 weeks. Shorter courses of therapy have been found to be effective only in intravenous drug users with uncomplicated right-sided disease; these patients may be treated with nafcillin plus an aminoglycoside for a full 2 weeks.[44] Intravenous drug users with evidence of left-sided or metastatic disease should receive the standard course of therapy, as should patients with β-lactam allergy, since a short 2-week course of vancomycin plus tobramycin was shown to be ineffective.[12,44]

Patients infected with methicillin-resistant *S. aureus* (MRSA) should receive vancomycin for 4 to 6 weeks; gentamicin may be added for at least the first 3 to 5 days. Few alternatives to vancomycin exist for MRSA. There have been studies assessing the efficacy of intravenous and oral ciprofloxacin for the treatment of *S. aureus* (particularly MRSA) endocarditis.[3,45] Rifampin added to ciprofloxacin appears to prevent the emergence of quinolone resistance. Unfortunately, widespread ciprofloxacin resistance among MRSA organisms may render this combination ineffective. In vitro studies, animal models, and small human studies have found imipenem to be effective for the treatment of infective endocarditis due to MSSA or MRSA.[46–48] An additional treatment alternative may be trimethoprim/sulfamethoxazole with or without rifampin. This agent was effective in the treatment of some cases of right-sided infective endocarditis due to MRSA, although failures occurred in some patients with MSSA.[49]

Patients with staphylococcal (*S. aureus* and *S. epidermidis*) PVE require at least 6 weeks of therapy with multiple antibiotics. High-dose rifampin (300 mg TID orally) is recommended in combination with nafcillin/oxacillin or vancomycin for the entire course, as it has been shown to improve sterilization of infected prosthetic material.[12] Gentamicin should be added during the first 2 weeks of therapy if the isolate is susceptible. If it is resistant to aminoglycosides, substitution of a fluoroquinolone may be considered.[12] Coagulase-negative staphylococci are often resistant to methicillin (>80% incidence). Endocarditis due to these organisms, usually found on prosthetic valves, should be treated with vancomycin plus rifampin for the entire 6 weeks, with an aminoglycoside added for the first 2 weeks of treatment.[12]

Gram-Negative Infection. Gram-negative bacillary endocarditis should be treated for at least 6 weeks with bactericidal antibiotics to which the infecting organisms are sensitive. The empiric treatment of gram-negative endocarditis should include an aminoglycoside at maximal doses (5 to 8 mg/kg/d) in combination with a β-lactam compound.[2,4,17] Third-generation cephalosporins (cefotaxime, ceftizoxime, ceftriaxone), extended-spectrum penicillins (piperacillin, mezlocillin), fluoroquinolones, and imipenem may provide adequate therapy for endocarditis caused by aerobic gram-negative bacilli.

Infective endocarditis due to *P. aeruginosa* is most frequently seen in intravenous drug users.[4,50] Combination therapy with high doses of an antipseudomonal β-lactam plus an aminoglycoside (5 to 8 mg/kg/d) is required, in conjunction with valve replacement in patients with left-sided disease, to achieve cure.[4,6,50] Despite "adequate" therapeutic regimens, morbidity and mortality rates from pseudomonal infective endocarditis remain high.[4,6]

HACEK organisms occur in 5% to 10% of cases of native valve endocarditis. Treatment with a third-generation cephalosporin or ampicillin plus gentamicin for 3 to 4 weeks for native valve infection and 6 weeks for prosthetic valve infection is recommended. Alternative therapy for penicillin-allergic patients includes trimethoprim/sulfamethoxazole or fluoroquinolones, though clinical data with these drugs are lacking.[12]

Other Organisms. The treatment of other forms of endocarditis is less well established. Infections due to anaerobes, although rare, are associated with a high mortality rate.[2] These infections tend to be very destructive and often require surgical intervention. Many anaerobic organisms, such as those found in the oropharynx, are highly susceptible to penicillin G. For penicillin-resistant organisms such as *Bacteroides fragilis* and related species, another bactericidal agent such as metronidazole should be chosen. β-lactam/β-lactamase inhibitor combinations (e.g., ampicillin/sulbactam, piperacillin/tazobactam, ticarcillin/clavulanate) and imipenem are also active in vitro against *B. fragilis* and most other anaerobes and may be considered. Clindamycin and chloramphenicol are bacteriostatic and should be avoided.[2]

Fungal endocarditis is virtually impossible to cure without surgery, and even with seemingly adequate fungicidal therapy, the mortality rate is very high. This is probably due to several reasons: the invasiveness of the organisms; the large friable vegetations produced on the valve causing a high rate of major embolic complications; the lack of fungicidal activity with available antifungal agents; and the negligible penetration of the antifungal agent into the vegetation.[2,51,52] Patients at risk for fungal endocarditis include injection drug users, recent prosthetic valve recipients, and patients recently hospitalized who had surgery, received broad-spectrum antibiotics, received hyperalimentation, or had long-term intravenous catheters.[52] Fungal species most frequently associated with infective endocarditis are *Aspergillus* and *Candida*.[19,51,52] The mainstay of therapy is amphotericin B given for a prolonged period of time, along with early valve replacement.[51] Use of liposomal amphotericin B formulations may be better tolerated, but efficacy studies are needed. The addition of 5-flucytosine (5-FC) for the treatment of *Candida* infections may be considered; however, toxicities include dose-related bone marrow suppression, which may be worsened due to drug accumulation secondary to amphotericin-induced impaired renal function. Fluconazole and itraconazole have in vitro activity against many fungi, but these agents are fungistatic and data to support use in fungal infective endocarditis are lacking.[2,51]

NONPHARMACOLOGIC THERAPY

Valve replacement is indicated for many intractable complications of endocarditis. Indications for surgery include severe hemodynamic compromise, valvular obstruction, evidence of intracardiac extension or abscess, persistent bacteremia, relapse following ''adequate'' therapy, an infecting organism that is resistant to available antimicrobials, fungal infective endocarditis, left-sided pseudomonal infec-

tive endocarditis, more than one major embolic event, and instability of an infected prosthetic valve.[4,50,53,54]

PREVENTION OF ENDOCARDITIS

Bacteremia from most sources is usually transient and nearly always inconsequential in the normal individual. However, in the patient with congenital or acquired heart disease or a prosthetic valve, any bacteremia may lead to endocarditis. In assessing the risk of a bacteremia to an individual patient, important considerations include the incidence of bacteremia with a given procedure, as well as the most likely organisms, the type of cardiac abnormality, and perhaps the concentration of the bacteria in the bloodstream.[55]

Only indirect evidence from animal studies demonstrates the effect of prophylactic systemic antibiotics in bacteremia-producing procedures. There are no prospective controlled trials of endocarditis prophylaxis in humans, and the recom-

TABLE 80.4	Cardiac Conditions

Endocarditis Prophylaxis Recommended

High-risk category

    Prosthetic cardiac valves, including bioprosthetic and homograph valves

    Previous bacterial endocarditis

    Complex cyanotic congenital heart disease (e.g., single ventricle states, transposition of the great arteries, tetralogy of Fallot)

    Surgically constructed systemic pulmonary shunts or conduits

Moderate-risk category

    Most other congenital cardiac malformations

    Acquired valvular dysfunction (e.g., rheumatic heart disease)

    Hypertrophic cardiomyopathy

    Mitral valve prolapse with valvular regurgitation and/or thickened leaflets

Endocarditis Prophylaxis Not Recommended

Isolated secundum atrial septal defect

Surgical repair of atrial septal defect, ventricular septal defect, or patent ductus arteriosis (without residua beyond 6 months)

Previous coronary artery bypass graft surgery

Mitral valve prolapse, without regurgitation

Physiologic, functional, or innocent heart murmurs

Previous Kawasaki disease without valvular dysfunction

Previous rheumatic fever without valvular dysfunction

Cardiac pacemakers and implanted defibrillators

(Adapted from Dajani AS, Taubert KA, Wilson W, et al. Prevention of bacterial endocarditis: recommendations by the American Heart Association. JAMA 277:1794–1801, 1997. Copyright 1997, American Medical Association.)

mended regimens are derived from experiments in the rabbit model. The American Heart Association recommends the use of prophylactic antimicrobials before, during, and after a procedure likely to produce bacteremia.[56] These include all dental procedures likely to induce gingival bleeding, tonsillectomy/adenoidectomy, surgical procedures or biopsy involving respiratory mucosa, bronchoscopy, incision and drainage of infected tissue, and various genitourinary and gastrointestinal procedures. Table 80.4 lists cardiac conditions for which prophylaxis is recommended and those where it is considered unnecessary.[56] Table 80.5 lists dental and other

procedures where prophylaxis is or is not recommended.[56] Patients who have a history of rheumatic fever with residual valvular disease should receive a prophylactic regimen recommended by the American Heart Association before specific surgical/dental procedures, as drug regimens used to prevent recurrence of acute rheumatic fever are not adequate for prevention of endocarditis.[57] If the patient is currently receiving a penicillin for secondary prevention of rheumatic fever, a regimen without penicillin should be used for endocarditis prophylaxis.[57] The American Heart Association guidelines for prophylaxis are summarized in Tables 80.6 and 80.7.[56]

TABLE 80.5	Dental or Surgical Procedures

Endocarditis Prophylaxis Recommended

Dental procedures

  Dental extractions

  Periodontal procedures including surgery, scaling and root planing, probing, and recall maintenance

  Dental implant placement and reimplantation of avulsed teeth

  Endodontic (root canal) instrumentation or surgery only beyond the apex

  Subgingival placement of antibiotic fibers or strips

  Initial placement of orthodontic bands but not brackets

  Intraligamentary local anesthetic injections

  Prophylactic cleaning of teeth or implants where bleeding is anticipated

Respiratory tract procedures

  Tonsillectomy and/or adenoidectomy

  Surgical operations that involve respiratory mucosa

  Bronchoscopy with rigid bronchoscope

Gastrointestinal tract procedures

  Sclerotherapy for esophageal varices

  Esophageal stricture dilation

  Endoscopic retrograde cholangiography with biliary obstruction

  Biliary tract surgery

  Surgical operations that involve intestinal mucosa

Genitourinary tract procedures

  Prostatic surgery

  Cystoscopy

  Urethral dilation

Endocarditis Prophylaxis Not Recommended

Dental procedures

  Restorative dentistry (operative and prosthodontic)

  Local anesthetic injections

Intracanal endodontic treatment; postplacement and buildup

Placement of rubber dams

Postoperative suture removal

Placement of removable prosthodontic or orthodontic appliances

Taking of oral impressions

Fluoride treatments

Orthodontic appliance adjustment

Shedding of primary teeth

Respiratory tract procedures

  Endotracheal intubation

  Bronchoscopy with a flexible bronchoscope

  Tympanostomy tube insertion

Gastrointestinal tract procedures

  Transesophageal echocardiography

  Endoscopy with/without gastrointestinal biopsy

Genitourinary tract procedures

  Vaginal hysterectomy

  Vaginal delivery

  Cesarean section

  In uninfected tissue: urethral catheterization, uterine dilatation and curettage, therapeutic abortion, sterilization procedures, or insertion/removal of intrauterine devices

Other procedures

  Cardiac catheterization, including balloon angioplasty

  Implanted cardiac pacemakers, implanted defibrillators, and coronary stents

  Incision or biopsy of surgically scrubbed skin

  Circumcision

(Adapted from Dajani AS, Taubert KA, Wilson W, et al. Prevention of bacterial endocarditis: recommendations by the American Heart Association. JAMA 277:1794–1801, 1997. Copyright 1997, American Medical Association.)

TABLE 80.6	Prophylactic Regimens for Dental, Oral, Respiratory Tract, or Esophageal Procedures	
Situation	**Agent**	**Adult Regimen**
Standard prophylaxis	Amoxicillin	2 g PO, 1 hour before procedure
Unable to take oral medications	Ampicillin	2 g IM/IV, within 30 minutes of procedure
Penicillin allergy	Clindamycin OR	600 mg PO, 1 hour before procedure
	Cephalexin or cefadroxil OR	2 g PO, 1 hour before procedure
	Azithromycin or clarithromycin	500 mg PO, 1 hour before procedure
Penicillin allergy, unable to take oral medications	Clindamycin OR	600 mg IV within 30 minutes of procedure
	Cefazolin	1 g IV within 30 minutes of procedure

(Adapted from Dajani AS, Taubert KA, Wilson W, et al. Prevention of bacterial endocarditis: recommendations by the American Heart Association. JAMA 277:1794–1801, 1997. Copyright 1997, American Medical Association.)

TABLE 80.7	Prophylactic Regimens for Genitourinary and Gastrointestinal (Excluding Esophageal) Procedures	
Situation	**Agent**	**Adult Regimen**
High-risk patients	Ampicillin PLUS	Ampicillin 2 g IM/IV PLUS
	Gentamicin	Gentamicin 1.5 mg/kg within 30 minutes of procedure, FOLLOWED BY Ampicillin 1 g IM/IV OR Amoxicillin 1 g PO 6 hours later.
High-risk patients, penicillin allergy	Vancomycin PLUS	Vancomycin 1 g IV over 1–2 hours PLUS
	Gentamicin	Gentamicin 1.5 mg/kg; infusions completed within 30 minutes of procedure
Moderate-risk patients	Amoxicillin OR	Amoxicillin 2 g PO 1 hour before procedure OR
	Ampicillin	Ampicillin 2 g IM/IV within 30 minutes before procedure
Moderate-risk patients, penicillin allergy	Vancomycin	Vancomycin 1 g IV over 1–2 hours; infusion completed within 30 minutes of procedure

(Adapted from Dajani AS, Taubert KA, Wilson W, et al. Prevention of bacterial endocarditis: recommendations by the American Heart Association. JAMA 277:1794–1801, 1997. Copyright 1997, American Medical Association.)

KEY POINTS

- Infective endocarditis is a potentially life-threatening infection that requires early recognition and aggressive and prolonged treatment for successful management
- High-dose antimicrobial therapy is needed, as infective endocarditis is difficult to treat because of an absence of host defenses, poor penetration of antibiotics into the vegetation, high organism burden, and reduced metabolic state of organisms at the site of infection
- Combination therapy is required for treatment of infective endocarditis due to *P. aeruginosa*, enterococci, or tolerant organisms
- Combination therapy may also be useful to shorten the duration of therapy for susceptible organisms (*S. aureus*, streptococci) as long as a penicillin is part of the regimen
- Infections due to pathogens that are resistant to multiple drugs, such as enterococci, are increasing in prevalence, and combinations of antibiotics are frequently used to achieve synergistic bactericidal effects
- Surgical removal of the infected valve is often necessary in patients with the following characteristics: severe hemodynamic compromise; intracardiac abscess; gram-negative, fungal, or other nonbacterial etiology; infection due to resistant organisms; PVE; relapse after "adequate" therapy; multiple embolic events
- Newer antimicrobials such as quinupristin/dalfopristin, linezolid, lipopeptides, glycylcyclines, and fluoroquinolones may have a role in the treatment of infective endocarditis
- A minimum of 6 weeks of therapy is required for successful treatment of PVE, and replacement of the infected prosthesis may be necessary
- Prevention of infection is best achieved by recognition of patients at risk, identification of clinical situations likely to produce bacteremia, and use of the recommended prophylactic regimens

REFERENCES

1. Sullam PM, Drake TA. Sande MA. Pathogenesis of endocarditis. Am J Med 78:110–115, 1985.
2. Scheld WM, Sande MA. Endocarditis and intravascular infections. In: Mandell GL, Bennett JE, Dolin R, eds. Principles and practice of infectious diseases, 4th ed. New York: Churchill Livingstone, 1995: 740–783.
3. Bayer AS. Infective endocarditis. Clin Infect Dis 17:313–322, 1993.
4. Bayer AS, Bolger AF, Taubert KA, et al. Diagnosis and management of infective endocarditis and its complications. Circulation 98: 2936–2948, 1998.
5. Chambers HF, Korzeniowski OM, Sande MA, et al. *Staphylococcus aureus* endocarditis: clinical manifestations in addicts and non-addicts. Medicine 62:170–177, 1983.
6. Levine DP, Crane LR, Zervos MJ. Bacteremia in narcotic addicts at the Detroit Medical Center. II. Infectious endocarditis: a prospective comparative study. Rev Infect Dis 8:374–396, 1986.
7. Whitener C, Caputo GM, Weitekamp MR, et al. Endocarditis due to coagulase-negative staphylococci. Infect Dis Clin North Am 7: 81–96, 1993.
8. Roder BL, Wandall DA, Frimodt-Meller N, et al. Clinical features of *Staphylococcus aureus* endocarditis: a 10-year experience in Denmark. Arch Intern Med 159:462–469, 1999.
9. Fowler VG Jr, Sanders LL, Kong LK, et al. Infective endocarditis due to *Staphylococcus aureus*: 59 prospectively identified cases with follow-up. Clin Infect Dis 28:106–114, 1999.
10. Fowler VG Jr, Li J, Corey GR, et al. Role of echocardiography in evaluation of patients with *Staphylococcus aureus* bacteremia: experience in 103 patients. J Am Coll Cardiol 30:1072–1078, 1997.
11. Watanakunakorn C. Editorial response: increasing importance of intravascular device-associated *Staphylococcus aureus* endocarditis. Clin Infect Dis 28:115–116, 1999.
12. Wilson WR, Karchmer AW, Dajani AD, et al. Antibiotic treatment of adults with infective endocarditis due to streptococci, enterococci, staphylococci, and HACEK microorganisms. JAMA 274: 1706–1713, 1995.
13. Threlkeld MB, Cobbs CG. Infectious disorders of prosthetic valves and intravascular devices. In: Mandell GL, Bennett JE, Dolin R, eds. Principles and practice of infectious diseases, 4th ed. New York: Churchill Livingstone, 1995:783–793.
14. Vlessis AA, KhakiA, Grunkemeier GL, et al. Risk, diagnosis and management of prosthetic valve endocarditis: a review. J Heart Valve Dis 6:443–465, 1997.
15. Caulderwood SB, Swinski LA, Karchmer AW, et al. Prosthetic valve endocarditis: analysis of factors affecting outcome of therapy. J Thorac Cardiovasc Surg 92:776–783, 1986.
16. Grover FL, Cohen DJ, Oprian C, et al. Determinants of the occurrence of and survival from prosthetic valve endocarditis. J Thorac Cardiovasc Surg 108:207–14, 1994.
17. Molavi A. Endocarditis: recognition, management, and prophylaxis. Cardiovasc Clin 23:139–174, 1993.
18. Werner GS, Schulz R, Fuchs JB, et al. Infective endocarditis in the elderly in the era of transesophageal echocardiography: clinical features and prognosis compared with younger patients. Am J Med 100:90–97, 1996.
19. Nassar RM, Melgar GR, Longworth DL, et al. Incidence and risk of developing fungal prosthetic valve endocarditis after nosocomial candidemia. Am J Med 103:25–32, 1997.
20. Siddiq S, Missri J, Silverman DI. Endocarditis in an urban hospital in the 1990s. Arch Intern Med 156:2454–2458, 1996.
21. Durack DT, Beeson PB. Experimental bacterial endocarditis. I. Colonization of a sterile vegetation. Br J Exp Pathol 53:44–49, 1972.
22. Durack DT, Lukes AS, Bright DK, et al. New criteria for diagnosis of infective endocarditis. Am J Med 96:200–209, 1994.
23. Von Reyn CF, Levy BS, Arbeit RD, et al. Infective endocarditis: analysis based on strict case definitions. Ann Intern Med 94: 505–511, 1981.
24. Daniel WG, Mugge A. Transesophageal echocardiography. N Engl J Med 332:1268–1279, 1995.
25. Murphy JG, Foster-Smith K. Management of complications of infective endocarditis with emphasis on echocardiographic findings. Infect Dis Clin North Am 7:153–165, 1993.
26. Wilson WR, Giuliani ER, Danielson GK, et al. Management of complications of infective endocarditis. Mayo Clin Proc 47:162–170, 1982.
27. Weinstein L. Life-threatening complications of infective endocarditis and their management. Arch Intern Med 146:953–957, 1986.
28. Tunkel AR, Kaye D. Neurologic complications of infective endocarditis. Neurol Clin 11:419–440, 1993.
29. Baldassarre JS, Kaye D. Principles and overview of antibiotic therapy. In: Kaye D, ed. Infective endocarditis. New York: Raven Press, 1992:169–190.
30. Carbon C, Cremieux AC, Fantin B. Pharmacokinetic and pharmacodynamic aspects of therapy of experimental endocarditis. Infect Dis Clin North Am 7:37–51, 1993.
31. Kanter MC, Hart RG. Neurologic complications of infective endocarditis. Neurology 41:1015–1020, 1991.
32. Francioli P, Etienne J, Hoigne R, et al. Treatment of streptococcal endocarditis with a single daily dose of ceftriaxone sodium for 4 weeks. JAMA 267:264–267, 1992.

33. Francioli P, Ruch W, Stamboulian, and the International Infective Endocarditis Study Group. Treatment of streptococcal endocarditis with a single daily dose of ceftriaxone and netilmicin for 14 days: a prospective multicenter study. Clin Infect Dis 21:1406–1410, 1995.

34. Eliopoulos GM. Aminoglycoside-resistant enterococcal endocarditis. Infect Dis Clin North Am 7:117–133, 1993.

35. Fantin B, Carbon C. Importance of the aminoglycoside dosing regimen in the penicillin-netilmicin combination for treatment of *Enterococcus faecalis*-induced experimental endocarditis. Antimicrob Agents Chemother 34:2387–2391, 1990.

36. Marangos MN, Nicolau DP, Quintiliani R, et al. Influence of gentamicin dosing interval on the efficacy of penicillin-containing regimens in experimental *Enterococcus faecalis* endocarditis. J Antimicrob Chemother 39:519–522, 1997.

37. Schwank S, Blaser J. Once- versus thrice-daily netilmicin combined with amoxicillin, penicillin, or vancomycin against *Enterococcus faecalis* in a pharmacodynamic in vitro model. Antimicrob Agents Chemother 40:2258–2261, 1996.

38. Landman D, Quale JM. Management of infections due to resistant enterococci: a review of therapeutic options. J Antimicrob Chemother 40:161–170, 1997.

39. Murray BE. Vancomycin-resistant enterococci. Am J Med 101:284–293, 1997.

40. Zimmer SM, Caliendo AM, Thigpen MC, et al. Failure of linezolid treatment for enterococcal endocarditis. Clin Infect Dis 37:3;e29–30, 2003.

41. Ang JY, Lua JL, Turner DR, Asmar BI. Vancomycin-resistant *Enterococcus faecium* endocarditis in a premature infant successfully treated with linezolid. Pediatr Infect Dis J 22:12;1101–1103, 2003.

42. Small PM, Chambers HF. Vancomycin for *Staphylococcus aureus* endocarditis in intravenous drug abusers. Antimicrob Agents Chemother 34:1227–1231, 1990.

43. Levine DP, Fromm BS, Reddy BR. Slow response to vancomycin or vancomycin plus rifampin therapy among patients with methicillin-resistant *Staphylococcus aureus* endocarditis. Ann Intern Med 115:674–680, 1991.

44. Chambers HF. Short-course combination and oral therapies of *Staphylococcus aureus* endocarditis. Infect Dis Clin North Am 7:69–79, 1993.

45. Heldman AW, Hartert TV, Ray SC, et al. Oral antibiotic treatment of right-sided staphylococcal endocarditis in injection drug users: prospective randomized comparison with parenteral therapy. Am J Med 101:68–76, 1996.

46. Palmer SM, Rybak MJ. An evaluation of the bactericidal activity of ampicillin/sulbactam, piperacillin/tazobactam, imipenem, or nafcillin alone and in combination with vancomycin against methicillin-resistant *Staphylococcus aureus* (MRSA) in time-kill curves with infected fibrin clots. J Antimicrob Chemother 39:515–518, 1997.

47. Chandrasekar PH, Levine DP, Price S, et al. Comparative efficacies of imipenem-cilastatin and vancomycin in experimental aortic valve endocarditis due to methicillin-resistant *Staphylococcus aureus*. J Antimicrob Chemother 21:461–469, 1988.

48. Dickinson G, Rodriguez K, Arcey S, et al. Efficacy of imipenem/cilastatin in endocarditis. Am J Med 78:117–121, 1985.

49. Markowitz N, Quinn EL, Saravolatz LD. Trimethoprim-sulfamethoxazole compared to vancomycin for the treatment of *Staphylococcus aureus* infection. Ann Intern Med 117:390–398, 1992.

50. Komshian SV, Tablan OC, Palutke W, et al. Characteristics of left-sided endocarditis due to *Pseudomonas aeruginosa* in the Detroit Medical Center. Rev Infect Dis 12:693–702, 1990.

51. Gilbert HM, Peters ED, Lang SJ, et al. Successful treatment of fungal prosthetic valve endocarditis: case report and review. Clin Infect Dis 22:348–354, 1996.

52. Rubinstein E, Lang R. Fungal endocarditis. Eur Heart J 16 (Suppl B):84–89, 1995.

53. Alsip SG, Blackstone EH, Kirklin JW, et al. Indications for cardiac surgery in patients with active infective endocarditis. Am J Med 78:138–148, 1985.

54. Moon MR, Stinson EB, Miller DC. Surgical treatment of endocarditis. Prog Cardiovasc Dis 40:239–264, 1997.

55. Durack DT. Prevention of infective endocarditis. N Engl J Med 332:38–44, 1995.

56. Dajani AS, Taubert KA, Wilson W, et al. Prevention of bacterial endocarditis: recommendations by the American Heart Association. JAMA 277:1794–1801, 1997.

57. Dajani A, Taubert K, Ferrieri P, et al. Treatment of acute streptococcal pharyngitis and prevention of rheumatic fever: a statement for health professionals. Pediatrics 96:758–764, 1995.

Central Nervous System Infections

81

Constance M. Pfeiffer, Lisa M. Avery, and Amy L. Pakyz

The central nervous system (CNS) is composed of the brain and the spinal cord. The brain is surrounded by membranes (the meninges) and is protected by the skull. CNS infections can occur in the membranes between the skull and the brain (meningitis) or within the brain itself (encephalitis or brain abscesses), or may be associated with an indwelling CNS device (e.g., shunt infections).

CNS infections are associated with significant morbidity and mortality. These infections are caused by a variety of pathogens, including bacteria, viruses, fungi, and parasites. Predisposing factors for the development of CNS infections include sinusitis, otitis media, head injury, and the presence of systemic infections.

TREATMENT GOALS: CENTRAL NERVOUS SYSTEM INFECTIONS

- Diagnose and initiate therapy promptly. A delay in therapy of a few hours may result in increased morbidity and mortality.
- Base treatment on the site or type of infection (e.g., meningitis, abscess vs. shunt infection), the suspected pathogens and their anticipated susceptibilities, and individual patient characteristics.
- Use only antimicrobials that have a bactericidal mechanism of action, and include all agents in a combination regimen.
- Select antimicrobials that have good penetration through the blood–brain barrier (BBB) and achieve adequate cerebrospinal fluid (CSF) drug concentrations.
- Ensure high-dose antimicrobial dosage regimens to ensure adequate CSF concentrations that should exceed the minimum bactericidal concentration (MBC) of the pathogen by at least eight to ten times.
- Note that because of the unidirectional flow of CSF, direct instillation of antibiotics into the CSF (via lumbar puncture or intraventricularly) will achieve only therapeutic antibiotic concentrations *below* the point of instillation.

EPIDEMIOLOGY

A variety of factors influence the suspected cause of meningitis. Age (Table 81.1), underlying risk factors (e.g., immunocompromised), and seasonal variations can be useful in directing empiric therapy. In adults, three organisms—*Neisseria meningitidis (N. meningitidis), Streptococcus pneumoniae (S. pneumoniae),* and *Haemophilus influenzae (H. influenzae)*—are most commonly responsible for meningitis. Gram-negative meningitis is extremely rare in adults, except when postneurosurgical meningitis occurs. However, meningitis due to enteric organisms, most frequently *Escherichia coli (E. coli),* is common in neonates. Geriatric patients are more likely to develop meningitis due to *Listeria monocytogenes,* although *S. pneumoniae* and *N. meningitidis* are still the most common pathogens in this age group.[1,2]

Age cannot be used as the only criterion for empiric antibiotic therapy selection. Several other factors should influence the decision-making process. Nosocomial meningitis or status post open head trauma increases the index of suspicion for gram-negative bacilli and staphylococcal infections. Specifically, patients with indwelling shunts may develop *Staphylococcus epidermidis* meningitis (frequently methicillin resistant). Other risk factors can also predispose patients to certain types of meningitis. Alcoholism, asplenia, bacterial pneumonia, sinusitis, head trauma, immunosuppression, and sickle cell disease increase the likelihood of *S. pneumoniae* meningitis. Lyme meningitis due to *Borrelia burgdorferi* (neuroborreliosis) is becoming more common in areas endemic for Lyme disease.

PATHOPHYSIOLOGY

Pathogens are thought to infect the meninges through three pathways: hematogenous seeding, direct inoculation (trauma, neurosurgery), or contiguous spread from a parameningeal focus (e.g., sinusitis, dental surgery). Virulence factors may also play a role for certain meningeal pathogens. Encapsulated organisms such as *S. pneumoniae* and *H. influenzae* type b are easily able to cross the BBB into the CNS, and they are also resistant to phagocytosis in the bloodstream; *N. meningitidis* use pili on their cell surface to breach and attach to the mucosal barrier.

When pathogens have entered the CNS, a cascade of events occurs. The presence of bacterial cell wall products triggers the production of cytokines, including interleukin-1, tumor necrosis factor, and prostaglandin E_2, which initially leads to increased blood flow to the brain. These cytokines also increase BBB permeability by interfering with the integrity of capillary tight junctions, allowing cerebral edema to occur. Cytotoxins released from neutrophils, and possibly bacteria themselves, also contribute to the development of cerebral edema.

Intracranial pressure rises secondary to increased blood flow and edema, resulting in decreased cerebral perfusion. The inflammatory process may cause vasculitis and throm-

TABLE 81.1	Common Pathogens That Cause Meningitis (Arranged by Patient Age Group)	
Age Group	**Common Pathogens**	**Empiric Treatment**
Neonates	Group B streptococcus	Ampicillin + cefotaxime or ampicillin + an aminoglycoside
	Listeria monocytogenes	
	Gram-negative bacilli	
	Gram-positive bacilli	
Infants (1–3 months)	*Streptococcus pneumoniae*	Ampicillin + cefotaxime or ceftriaxone + vancomycin ± dexamethasone
	Neisseria meningitidis	
	Rarely, *Haemophilus influenzae* pathogens seen in neonates	
3 months to 50 years	*Streptococcus pneumoniae*	Cefotaxime or ceftriaxone ± vancomycin
	Neisseria meningitidis	
	Rarely, *Haemophilus influenzae*	
Older adults (>50 years)	*Streptococcus pneumoniae*	Ampicillin + cefotaxime or ceftriaxone + vancomycin ± dexamethasone
	Listeria monocytogenes	
	Gram-negative bacilli	

botic events that contribute to overall cerebral ischemia, which may ultimately result in significant neurologic sequelae.

CLINICAL PRESENTATION AND DIAGNOSIS

SIGNS AND SYMPTOMS

Symptoms of meningitis may occur acutely, within 24 hours, or insidiously, over 1 to 7 days. Acute meningitis is associated with a higher fatality rate (50%) and is most commonly caused by bacteria. Subacute meningitis may be caused by viral, mycobacterial, fungal, or bacterial infection and is generally associated with a lower mortality rate (<25%).[3] A patient with acute or subacute meningitis may have symptoms of meningeal inflammation such as vomiting, headache, lethargy, confusion, or neck stiffness. Fever, rigors, myalgias, and photophobia are seen as well. Less commonly, patients experience focal symptoms such as seizures, cranial nerve palsies, or hemiparesis. The clinical presentation in neonates and in older adults is more insidious. Neonates and young infants lack the meningeal signs and symptoms but may display hypothermia or hyperthermia, listlessness, lethargy, high-pitched crying, nausea, vomiting, anorexia, poor eating habits, irritability, and seizures. Late clinical manifestations in infants include neck stiffness and a full fontanelle. Older adults may have only new-onset confusion and no other cardinal signs, such as fever or nuchal rigidity, so meningitis can easily be misdiagnosed. A prospective study conducted in the Netherlands evaluated 696 cases of community-acquired acute bacterial meningitis in adults, and found that the classic triad of fever, neck stiffness, and a change in mental status was found in only 44% of episodes. Two of the following symptoms of headache, fever, neck stiffness, and altered mental status were found in 95% of cases.[4]

On physical examination, patients may have nuchal rigidity or meningismus, a positive Kernig or Brudzinski sign, and papilledema. The Kernig sign is elicited by placing the patient in the supine position, then flexing the thigh perpendicular to the abdomen with the knee also in the flexed position. As the leg is extended, the patient with meningitis resists leg extension. The Brudzinski sign is evident when forward neck flexion results in flexion of the hips and knees. A petechial or purpuric rash predominantly on the extremities is consistent with *N. meningitidis*, although it may also occur with streptococci or *H. influenzae* infection.

DIAGNOSIS

It is imperative that a rapid diagnosis of meningitis be made to ensure prompt, appropriate therapy. A lumbar puncture (LP) is used to confirm the diagnosis and identify the pathogen. The goal is to obtain and evaluate the CSF within 30 minutes of presentation. However, it must first be deter-

mined whether it is safe to perform the LP (i.e., rule out contraindications to performing an LP, such as a mass lesion, brain abscess, or subdural empyema). This may be done by examining the patient for the presence of focal neurologic signs. The patient should also be evaluated for papilledema, hemiparesis, aphasia, ataxia, and visual field defects, which may suggest an extreme increase in intracranial pressure. If papilledema or neurologic signs are present, an LP is contraindicated because of the risk of brain herniation. Computed tomography (CT) or magnetic resonance imaging (MRI) may be performed before an LP is done, to help in the assessment process. Whether CT should be performed before all LPs is a topic of debate. Proponents believe that neurologic signs may be missed because of the patient's inability to participate in a complete neurologic examination. Papilledema or lack thereof is not a reliable marker of the presence or absence of increased intracranial pressure (ICP) and therefore should not be used as the sole safety indicator.

Guidelines published by the Infectious Diseases Society of America (IDSA) recommend that a CT be performed in patients who are immunocompromised, have a history of selected CNS diseases (infections associated with CSF shunts, hydrocephalus, or trauma; those occurring after neurosurgery; or various space-occupying lesions), new-onset seizure, papilledema, altered consciousness or focal neurologic deficit, or a delay in performance of diagnostic lumbar puncture. In infants and children, it is not recommended that lumbar puncture be delayed in those experiencing seizures because seizures can occur in up to 30% of children who present with bacterial meningitis.[5]

When an LP is delayed so that a CT scan can be obtained, blood cultures should be obtained for culture and empiric antibiotics should be initiated, along with any adjunctive therapy. A delay in the start of therapy can lead to increased morbidity and mortality.

Before the CSF is removed, opening pressure can be measured. In meningitis, pressures generally exceed 200 mm H_2O (normal: <150 mm H_2O in supine position). Pressures greater than 600 mm H_2O may be consistent with intracranial masses. A repeat LP may be necessary if treatment response is inadequate.

The CSF is also evaluated for gross visual turbidity, cell analysis, glucose and protein concentrations, and Gram stain and culture. A normal CSF sample should be colorless and clear. In bacterial meningitis, the CSF may be cloudy; however, in fungal and viral meningitis, the fluid is generally clear. A pleocytosis (increased number of white blood cells) with a predominance of neutrophils is consistent with bacterial meningitis; however, approximately 10% of patients present with a lymphocyte predominance, defined as greater than 50% lymphocytes or monocytes in the CSF.[5] A lymphocytic pleocytosis is consistent with fungal, mycobacterial, or viral infection, although viral meningitis may have an initial neutrophilic predominance. Characteristics of the CSF in adults with various types of meningitis are summarized

TABLE 81.2	Cerebrospinal Fluid Characteristics in Meningitis			
Pathogen	White Blood Cell Count (cells/m³)	Predominant Cell Type in Differential	Glucose Ratio (cerebrospinal fluid to blood)	Protein Concentration (mg/dL)
None (normal cerebrospinal fluid)	<5	Lymphocytes Monocytes	0.5–0.6	20–40
Bacterial	1,000–100,000	Neutrophils	<0.5	100–500
Fungal	10–1,000	Lymphocytic	<0.5	100–500
Mycobacteria	100–400	Lymphocytic	<0.5	100–500
Viral	10–1,000	Lymphocytic (polymorpho-nuclear leukocytes early)	0.5–0.6	50–100

in Table 81.2. In neonates, the total normal number of white blood cells in the CSF is higher than in adults (Table 81.3); by age 1 year, the normal values are the same as those in adults. The glucose concentration in normal CSF is 50% to 60% (or 0.5:1 ratio) of the simultaneous serum glucose—generally, 3 to 6.1 mmol per L (70–110 mg/dL). In bacterial, fungal, and mycobacterial infections, the CSF:blood glucose ratio is generally less than 0.4, whereas in viral meningitis, the CSF:blood glucose ratio is normal. For an accurate assessment of CSF glucose, a plasma glucose sample should be obtained before the LP. This is especially important in diabetic patients whose plasma glucose may be elevated; therefore, the relative glucose in the CSF may appear normal.

Another issue that should be considered is whether the patient received dextrose 50% (D50) in the emergency room before the lumbar puncture. The time for glucose to reach equilibrium between the blood and CSF after D50 administration is a minimum of 30 minutes, and it may take up to 4 hours. Effects on CSF glucose will not be seen if the D50 injection was given less than 30 minutes before the LP.[1–3,6,7]

An elevated protein concentration is a sign of disruption of the BBB. In adults, the normal protein concentration range is 20 to 40 mg per dL. Although protein elevation is a non-specific finding, it is generally noted in meningitis (100–500 mg/dL), except in viral meningitis, wherein the concentrations are somewhat lower (50–100 mg/dL). In neonates, the normal protein concentration is 20 to 150 mg per dL because of the immaturity of the BBB; by age 1 year, the upper limit of normal decreases to 45 mg per dL.[1–3,6,7]

Some clinicians advocate the measurement of lactate in the CSF to aid in the differential diagnosis of bacterial men-

ingitis in postoperative neurosurgical patients. Patients with a CSF lactate concentration of 4.0 mmol per L or greater should be considered for empiric antimicrobial therapy, pending other laboratory studies. This may aid clinicians in diagnosing postoperative meningitis when the usual CSF findings such as elevated white blood cell counts, positive Gram stain results, diminished glucose concentrations, and elevated protein concentrations are not sensitive or specific enough to distinguish a bacterial from a nonbacterial meningeal syndrome. Measurement of CSF lactate is not recommended for patients in whom community-acquired bacterial meningitis is a concern, as other factors such as cerebral hypoxia and ischemia, anaerobic glycolysis, vascular compromise, and CSF leukocyte metabolism may elevate CSF lactate concentrations.[5]

Other laboratory tests such as C-reactive protein and procalcitonin have been studied for their usefulness in the diagnosis of acute bacterial meningitis. These tests have not been established as diagnostic tools, however, and they cannot be used to determine whether patients should receive antimicrobial therapy.[5]

A Gram stain of the CSF provides another tool for rapid diagnosis of bacterial meningitis and can be used to guide empiric therapy.[8] A causative bacterial organism may be detected on Gram stain in up to 60% to 80% of untreated patients, and in 40% to 60% of those who have already received some antibiotic therapy.[7,8] The diagnostic accuracy of the Gram stain is related to the concentration of bacterial colonies and the particular microorganism involved. More than 10^5 colony-forming units (cfu) per milliliter of bacteria correlates with a positive Gram stain.[7] If tuberculosis or

TABLE 81.3	Normal Values for Cerebrospinal Fluid in Pediatric Populations		
	Full-Term Neonate	Infant	Child
White blood cell count	0–25 cells/mm³	0–8 cells/mm³	0–5 cells/mm³
Protein concentration	20–150 mg/dL	14–45 mg/dL	15–45 mg/dL
Glucose concentration	20–40 mg/dL	70–90 mg/dL	50–80 mg/dL

cryptococcal meningitis is suspected, acid-fast stain or India ink stain, respectively, is used.

CSF cultures are positive in 70% to 80% of cases of bacterial meningitis and can help direct antibiotic therapy. Blood cultures are positive in 40% to 60% of patients with *H. influenzae,* meningococcal, and pneumococcal meningitis.

Other cultures, such as respiratory and urinary tract cultures, may be of some use if systemic infection sources are identified as the potential cause of meningitis. As in other types of infection, the patient may have a peripheral leukocytosis (white blood cell count >10,000/mm^3). Other diagnostic tests include fungal cultures, cryptococcal antigen testing, and Venereal Disease Research Laboratory (VDRL) testing to rule out neurosyphilis.

Rapid diagnostic tests are available to assist in the identification of organisms present in bacterial meningitis. The latex agglutination test detects in CSF, serum, or urine the polysaccharide antigen of *H. influenzae* type b, *S. pneumoniae, N. meningitidis, E. coli* K1, and group B streptococci. The results are generally available in 20 to 30 minutes. The overall sensitivity of the latex agglutination test ranges from 50% to 100%; however, its sensitivity is lower for *N. meningitidis*.[9] A negative test does not rule out infection caused by a particular organism. Bacterial antigen tests should not be used to alter the decision to administer antibiotics; false positives have also been noted. The IDSA meningitis guidelines do not recommend routine use of antigen testing to determine the bacterial cause of meningitis; however, some experts would use it in cases in which a negative CSF Gram stain is obtained. Latex agglutination may play a role in identifying the causative organism for patients who received antibiotics before LP and have negative Gram stain or culture procedures.[5] Polymerase

chain reaction (PCR) techniques are currently being used in the rapid diagnosis of CNS infections such as herpesvirus. Identification of enterovirus using reverse transcriptase (RT)-PCR is now possible and is used in the clinical setting for rapid diagnosis of enteroviral meningitis. This may enable a shortened length of hospitalization and decreased use of antimicrobial therapy for empiric treatment of bacterial meningitis.

TREATMENT

PHARMACOKINETIC AND PHARMACODYNAMIC CONSIDERATIONS

The presence of the BBB and the unidirectional flow of CSF complicate the treatment of patients with CNS infections. Tightly joined endothelial cells of brain capillaries form the BBB, which acts as a semipermeable membrane, regulating drug concentrations that enter and exit the CSF. To ensure adequate CSF bactericidal activity, therapy must include only those antimicrobials that can penetrate the BBB and achieve adequate levels in the CSF. Factors that influence the ability of drugs to cross the BBB are lipophilicity, degree of ionization, molecular weight, and complexity of structure. Nonionized, lipophilic, low-molecular-weight molecules passively diffuse across the BBB more readily than do large, complex, hydrophilic, or ionized molecules. Because only free drug is capable of traversing the BBB, agents that are highly protein bound are at a potential disadvantage.

Meningeal inflammation that occurs along with meningitis actually enhances the penetration of certain antibiotics through the BBB (Table 81.4). Although the exact mechanism is unknown, it may be related to the impairment of

TABLE 81.4	Cerebrospinal Fluid (CSF) Penetration—Drug Characteristics	
Achieve Adequate CSF Concentration Without Meningeal Inflammation	**Achieve Adequate CSF Concentration Only if Meningeal Inflammation Exists**	**Do Not Achieve Adequate CSF Concentration**
Sulfonamides	Penicillins	Aminoglycosides
Trimethoprim	Penicillin G	Vancomycin
Chloramphenicol	Ampicillin	Polymyxin
Isoniazid	Nafcillin	Amphotericin B
Metronidazole	Antipseudomonal penicillins	
Fluconazole	Imipenem	
Flucytosine	Meropenem	
Pyrazinamide	Aztreonam	
	Third-generation cephalosporins	
	Quinolones	
	Ciprofloxacin	
	Ofloxacin	
	Rifampin	

active transport pumps and the disruption of tight junctions of the capillaries. For example, the penicillin class of drugs achieves low CSF concentrations when the meninges are normal, but in the presence of meningitis and inflamed meninges, much higher concentrations are achievable. Because the degree of inflammation correlates with the percentage of antibiotic penetration, when inflammation decreases, as occurs with the healing process, the percentage of antibiotic penetration also decreases. Additionally, concomitant corticosteroid use causes a decrease in inflammation, a decrease in BBB permeability, and thus a decrease in CSF antibiotic concentration. Adjuvant corticosteroid use has been advocated in several instances of bacterial meningitis treatment, so antibiotic dosages and CSF penetration must be assessed carefully.

To control the active secretion of substances, the BBB also has a series of transport pumps. These stereospecific carriers remove weak organic acids such as penicillin, ampicillin, nafcillin, and cefazolin from the CSF through the choroid plexus. These ''exit pumps'' are saturable and may be inhibited by weak organic acids such as probenecid.

To optimize antibiotic concentrations in the CNS and overcome the permeability and secretory problems of the BBB, the direct instillation of antibiotics into the CSF is also an option. CSF is produced by the choroid plexus at a rate of 0.5 mL per minute and flows unidirectionally from lateral ventricles to the third and fourth ventricles and then to the subarachnoid space. CSF then flows through the subarachnoid space into the spinal column. This unidirectional flow is important to remember when one is administering drugs directly into the CSF because therapeutic levels of antibiotic will be achieved below the site of injection, but not above.

Drugs can be introduced directly into the CSF at a variety of sites and routes. Intraventricular injection is the most invasive method; it consists of placement of a subcutaneous reservoir with a catheter that is placed directly into one of the lateral ventricles. Intrathecal administration requires that a needle be inserted into the subarachnoid space. Intracisternal administration is the injection of drug at the base of the skull, and intralumbar administration refers to an injection given via a lumbar puncture site. These administration methods are used as adjunctive therapy and never as a sole method of drug administration.

After the issue of drug penetration into the CSF has been addressed, the pharmacodynamic properties of the antimicrobial must be considered. As in endocarditis and osteomyelitis, the antibiotic chosen for the treatment of patients with CNS infection must be bactericidal. This is an important factor because, compared with blood, the CSF has decreased immunoglobulins, complement, and opsonic activity, which results in impaired phagocytic activity against encapsulated bacteria. Bactericidal antibiotics include agents such as penicillins, cephalosporins, vancomycin, quinolones, penems, and aminoglycosides. The concentrations of bactericidal agents must exceed the MBC of the organism by at least 8 to 10 times if the maximum rate of bacterial kill is to be achieved.[1]

Agents such as erythromycin, clindamycin, and tetracycline are bacteriostatic and should not be used for the treatment of patients with meningitis. Although chloramphenicol is considered to be bacteriostatic for most organisms, it does have bactericidal activity against certain bacteria (e.g., *S. pneumoniae, H. influenzae, N. meningitidis*); therefore, it is an option for the treatment of patients with meningitis due to these pathogens. Use of bacteriostatic agents in combination with bactericidal agents may result in antagonism and is thus not recommended.

Empiric treatment of suspected meningitis is guided by the age of the patient (Table 81.1), expected pathogens (Table 81.5), and results of the Gram stain of the CSF (Table 81.6), if available. Empiric therapy generally consists of a third-generation cephalosporin and sometimes one or more additional antibiotics, as indicated by patient-specific characteristics. Common regimens are ceftriaxone 2 g every 12 hours and cefotaxime 2 g every 4 to 6 hours.[3,6] The addition of vancomycin or ampicillin may be indicated in certain

TABLE 81.5	Common Pathogens That Cause Meningitis and Empiric Antibiotic Therapy in Patient Populations

Patient Type	Common Pathogens	Empiric Therapy
Alcoholic or debilitated patient (chronic illness)	*Streptococcus pneumoniae* *Listeria monocytogenes* Gram-negative bacilli	Ampicillin + ceftriaxone + vancomycin
Impaired cellular immunity (high-dose steroids, lymphoma, myeloma, etc.)	*Listeria monocytogenes* Gram-negative bacilli (*Pseudomonas aeruginosa*)	Ampicillin + ceftazidime or cefepime
Postneurosurgery or head trauma	*Streptococcus pneumoniae* *Staphylococcus aureus* Gram-negative bacilli (enteric gram-negative bacilli and *Pseudomonas aeruginosa*)	Vancomycin + ceftazidime or cefepime

TABLE 81.6	Empiric Antibiotic Therapy for Patients With Meningitis Using Cerebrospinal Fluid Gram Stain Morphologic Information

Gram Stain Result	Likely Pathogen	Empiric Therapy
Gram-negative bacilli	*Haemophilus influenzae* Enteric organisms *Pseudomonas aeruginosa*	Ceftazidime or cefepime and aminoglycoside (add dexamethasone if pediatric patient)
Gram-negative cocci	*Neisseria meningitidis*	Penicillin G or ceftriaxone or cefotaxime
Gram-positive bacilli	*Listeria monocytogenes*	Ampicillin and aminoglycoside IV
Gram-positive cocci	*Streptococcus pneumoniae*	Vancomycin and ceftriaxone or cefotaxime (consider dexamethasone)

patient populations. Pathogen-specific treatment is discussed in the following sections.

PHARMACOTHERAPY

Streptococcus pneumoniae Meningitis. *Streptococcus pneumoniae*, commonly called *pneumococcus*, is a gram-positive coccus seen on Gram stain in pairs or short chains. It is an encapsulated organism with 85 different serotypes. In 40% to 50% of cases, the patient has a concomitant pneumococcal pneumonia or otitis media infection.[10] In addition, patients may have a contiguous or distant focus of infection such as pneumonia, mastoiditis, sinusitis, or endocarditis.

In the past, empiric therapy for patients with *S. pneumoniae* included penicillin or ampicillin. Although penicillin has traditionally been the first-line agent, there has recently been an increase in the rate of resistance of pneumococci to penicillin therapy. Now, antibiotic resistance rates are as high as 35% in some areas of the United States.[11] Resistance to β-lactam antimicrobials results from alterations in the penicillin-binding proteins of the bacterial cell wall.[12] The Centers for Disease Control and Prevention (CDC) has standardized the classification of penicillin resistance. *S pneumoniae* is considered sensitive to penicillin if the minimum inhibitory concentration (MIC) is 0.1 μg/mL or less. If the MIC is 0.1 to 1.0 μg/mL, the isolate is classified as intermediate, and if the MIC is 2.0 μg/mL or greater, the strain is considered resistant, previously referred to as *high-level resistance*. Cephalosporins are not currently affected to the same degree as penicillins, possibly because cephalosporins bind to several different penicillin-binding proteins. Therefore, susceptibility testing should include ceftriaxone or cefotaxime even for known penicillin-resistant strains. Resistance to cephalosporins is defined as MIC greater than 0.5 μg/mL. Antibiotics that typically exhibit cross resistance include chloramphenicol, erythromycin, trimethoprim–sulfamethoxazole, aminoglycosides, and tetracycline. Risk factors for the development of penicillin resistance include age younger than 5 years, frequent antibiotic use, and the use of prophylactic antibiotics to prevent chronic infections, such as otitis media.[13]

Because of the high rate of penicillin resistance, empiric therapy for patients with proven or suspected pneumococcal meningitis should include vancomycin in addition to ceftriaxone or cefotaxime until sensitivity results are available. A less conservative approach would be to continue to use monotherapy with ceftriaxone or cefotaxime. However, the number of case reports of cephalosporin-resistant isolates has been increasing.[14]

Empiric therapy may sometimes include the use of adjuvant dexamethasone. Based on the results of a randomized, placebo-controlled, double-blind multicenter trial showing that unfavorable outcomes and death were lower in a group receiving dexamethasone, it is recommended that dexamethasone (0.15 mg/kg q6h for 2 to 4 days, with the first dose administered 10 to 20 minutes before, or at least with, the first dose of antibiotics) be started in adults with suspected or proven pneumococcal meningitis.[15] Dexamethasone can be discontinued if the CSF Gram stain does not show gram-positive diplococci, or if blood or CSF cultures are negative for *S. pneumoniae*. Additionally, if patients have already received antimicrobial therapy, dexamethasone should not be given because it is unlikely to be effective. No cases of high-level resistant pneumococci were reported in this trial, so it is not known whether dexamethasone is efficacious in this setting. Current IDSA guidelines recommend that dexamethasone be given to all adults with pneumococcal meningitis, even if culture results show high-level penicillin and cephalosporin resistance.[5] Furthermore, these guidelines recommend that the addition of rifampin PO to the combination of a third-generation cephalosporin and vancomycin may be considered pending culture and susceptibility testing, because of the possibility of pneumococcal meningitis caused by high-level penicillin- or cephalosporin-resistant strains. In children, dexamethasone has not been shown to decrease vancomycin penetration to a significant degree and should be included in the empiric regimen in combination with cefotaxime or ceftriaxone in children who are receiving steroids. It appears that timing of dexamethasone is important in pneumococcal meningitis; administration before or concurrently with antibiotics produces a better outcome. Short courses (i.e., first 2 days of therapy) of corticosteroid administration may be optimal.[16]

Monotherapy with vancomycin or rifampin is not appropriate because of the erratic CSF penetration of vancomycin and the rapid development of rifampin resistance during rifampin monotherapy. Empiric therapy for patients with severe penicillin allergies (i.e., anaphylaxis) should include vancomycin in addition to rifampin. Some clinicians would use rifampin with a third-generation cephalosporin, with or without vancomycin, in patients with high-level penicillin- or cephalosporin-resistant isolates. IDSA guidelines recommend that rifampin be added only after the clinician is certain whether the isolate shows susceptibility and that a delay is expected in the clinical or microbiologic response.[5] Cephalosporins and penems (meropenem and imipenem) should not be used in such patients because they may cause life-threatening allergic cross-sensitivity reactions.

As soon as sensitivity results are available, empiric therapy can be modified to provide narrower coverage. The treatment of choice in patients with penicillin-sensitive strains (MIC ≤0.1 μg/mL) is high-dose penicillin or ampicillin. Patients with intermediately sensitive strains of pneumococcus (MIC 0.1–1.0 μg/mL) that are susceptible to third-generation cephalosporins should be treated with either ceftriaxone or cefotaxime. Patients with isolates that display high-level resistance (MIC ≥2.0) should be treated with vancomycin plus either ceftriaxone or cefotaxime. In pediatric patients who are not responding after 24 to 48 hours of therapy with vancomycin plus cefotaxime or ceftriaxone, rifampin may be added or substituted for vancomycin.[17] The duration of therapy is 10 to 14 days.

Alternative therapies for treatment of patients with meningitis caused by *S. pneumoniae* include cefepime, a fourth-generation cephalosporin, chloramphenicol, and meropenem. Chloramphenicol has been used to treat meningitis in children with resistance to penicillin and cephalosporins. It has been associated with poor outcomes (death, serious neurologic deficits, and poor clinical response), despite the fact that MIC values suggested sensitivity to this drug.[8] Meropenem is a carbapenem that has activity similar to imipenem but differs in its stability against renal tubular dehydropeptidases; therefore, meropenem does not require the enzyme inhibitor cilastatin. Meropenem has also been shown to be associated with a lower incidence of seizures. Fluoroquinolones such as gatifloxacin or moxifloxacin have enhanced in vitro activity against *S. pneumoniae* and may be useful in cases of high-level penicillin *S. pneumoniae* resistance; however, their efficacy has not yet been established in clinical trials, and they should be used only in patients who are not responding to initial therapy.[5] A 23-valent polysaccharide vaccine to prevent systemic pneumococcal infection has been available since 1983. Because 90% of all pneumococcal isolates are covered, the vaccine should be highly recommended to patients at risk for infection. Proper vaccination should decrease the incidence of pneumococcal infections, including resistance strains, because six of the seven serotypes commonly associated with resistance are contained in the vaccine.[18] Recommendations for vaccination

with pneumococcal vaccine include (1) adults 65 years of age or older; (2) adults and children aged 2 to 64 years with chronic illnesses such as cardiovascular or pulmonary disease, diabetes mellitus, alcoholism, cirrhosis, CSF leaks, or functional or anatomic asplenia and those living in special environments or social settings (certain Native American populations and Alaskan natives); (3) immunocompromised patients 2 years of age or older, including those with hematologic or generalized malignancies, chronic renal failure, or nephrotic syndrome, those receiving immunosuppressive chemotherapy, patients with human immunodeficiency virus (HIV) infection, and those who have had a bone marrow or organ transplant; and (5) cochlear implant recipients.[11]

Efficacy has not been established in infants and very young children. The usual dose of the vaccine is 0.5 mL given intramuscularly or subcutaneously. Adverse effects include local reactions at the injection site, low-grade fever, weakness, myalgias, and rash, although the incidence is low. Chemoprophylaxis, in addition to vaccination, is recommended in children with functional or anatomic asplenia. Prophylaxis can be addressed with penicillin G or V given at a dose of 125 mg PO twice a day in children younger than age 5 years, and 250 mg PO twice a day in children age 5 years or older.[17,18]

In 2000, a seven-valent pneumococcal conjugate vaccine became available in the United States for use in infants and young children younger than 2 years of age and in high-risk children 2 through 4 years of age. This vaccine is projected to significantly decrease the incidence of childhood pneumococcal meningitis. According to data from the Active Bacterial Core Surveillance of the CDC, the vaccine has lowered rates of invasive disease from *S. pneumoniae* since it was introduced. The largest decline has been noted in children younger than 2 years of age (69%), and the vaccine is also possibly the cause of lower rates of disease in adults.[19] Additionally, a lowering of the rate of disease caused by strains that were not susceptible to penicillin was noted. The vaccine is given as a four-dose regimen to infants at 2, 4, 6, and 12 to 15 months of age.

Neisseria meningitidis Meningitis. *Neisseria meningitidis* is a gram-negative organism that causes both endemic and epidemic disease. Because of the success of *H. influenzae* type b vaccination programs, *N. meningitidis* has become the leading cause of bacterial meningitis in the United States, with an estimated 2,600 cases per year[2,20] and a fatality rate of approximately 10% despite antibiotic therapy to which strains remain clinically sensitive.[2,18,21] The incidence of endemic meningococcal disease increases in late winter to early spring. Children 3 to 12 months of age, asplenic patients, and patients with C3 and C5-9 complement deficiencies have increased incidences of meningococcal disease. Previously, military recruits had high rates of serogroup C meningococcal disease; however, since the advent of routine meningococcal vaccination of recruits, incidence has decreased substantially. HIV-infected persons do not appear to be at increased risk for epidemic serogroup A meningococcal disease; however, they may be at increased risk for sporadic meningococcal disease or disease caused by other serogroups.[22,23] Asymptomatic colonization of the upper respiratory tract is common, and transmission from person to person occurs through inhalation of droplets of respiratory secretions. Close contacts of *N. meningitidis*–infected patients are at increased risk for development of disease.

N. meningitidis has multiple serogroups known to cause invasive disease. According to population-based surveillance conducted from 1992 to 1996, serogroup C caused 35% of cases of meningococcal disease, serogroup B 32%, and serogroup Y 26%.[24] Serogroups W-135 and Y account for remaining cases. Serogroup A, an uncommon cause of endemic disease in the United States, is the most common cause of epidemic disease elsewhere in the world.[21,23] Statewide epidemics and localized community outbreaks in the United States have been due to serogroups B and C.[25,26]

Clinical features of *N. meningitidis* infection include rapid onset, with meningococcemia, of fever, chills, malaise, and rash. The rash may be maculopapular, petechial, or urticarial. In fulminant disease, the rash may become puerperal and is associated with a syndrome of disseminated intravascular coagulation, shock, coma, and death (Waterhouse-Friderichsen syndrome). This may occur within a few hours of presentation despite adequate antibiotic therapy. Other signs of meningococcal meningitis are common in infection with other pathogens.

When the CSF Gram stain reveals gram-negative cocci, meningococcal meningitis is assumed and empiric therapy can be directed toward that organism.[8] The drug of choice for the treatment of patients with meningococcal meningitis is penicillin G administered as 4 million units every 4 hours for 7 days for adults with normal renal function.[9,17,27,28] Penicillin dose adjustment should be considered in patients with an estimated creatinine clearance of less than 30 mL per minute. Rare strains of *N. meningitidis* are resistant or relatively resistant to penicillin. Surveillance for the development of resistance is necessary because in the future, the standard therapy for meningococcal meningitis may be third-generation cephalosporins. Cefotaxime (2 g every 4 to 6 hours) and ceftriaxone (2 g every 12 to 24 hours) are used as second-line agents for patients with penicillin allergy, although cross sensitivity is sometimes seen. Chloramphenicol may be used in patients with allergy to both penicillin and cephalosporins. Other alternatives include sulfonamides and fluoroquinolones. No data support the use of corticosteroids in the treatment of patients with meningococcal meningitis.[29] In fact, there is some concern that corticosteroids may adversely affect the ability of antibiotics to achieve adequate penetration of the CSF, leading to recrudescence and relapse.

Penicillin does not cure the carrier state and eradicate *N. meningitidis* from the nasopharynx; therefore, patients also must be treated with oral rifampin 10 mg per kg (maximum 600 mg) every 12 hours for 2 days.[27,30] Respiratory isolation should be instituted for 24 hours after therapy initiation to avoid transmission. Household, child care center, and nursery school contacts should be given antibiotic prophylaxis as soon as possible after exposure to the primary case is discovered. Prophylaxis of medical care workers is not recommended unless exposure to respiratory secretions resulting from doing mouth-to-mouth resuscitation, intubation, or suctioning occurs before adequate antibiotics are administered for 24 hours. The drug of choice for prophylaxis is rifampin, administered in the same dosing regimen as that used for nasopharynx eradication.[17,18,20] A 4-day regimen of 20 mg/kg/day (maximum 600 mg) is also effective.[17] Ceftriaxone (250 mg adults, 125 mg children younger than age 12 years) given as a single intramuscular dose has proved more effective than rifampin in eradicating serogroup A *N. meningitidis;* however, efficacy has not been confirmed for other strains.[31] Sulfisoxazole and ciprofloxacin (500 mg as a single dose) have also been used with some success.

A quadrivalent meningococcal vaccine is commercially available. This vaccine is active against serogroups A, C, Y, and W-135. Unfortunately, no vaccine is available with activity against serogroup B. The vaccine is given as a single 0.5-mL dose and consists of 50 µg of each of the purified bacterial capsular polysaccharides. Routine vaccination of children is not recommended because infants constitute the group at highest risk and generally exhibit a poor response to all but the serogroup A component.[17,31] Vaccination should be considered in children older than 2 years of age in high-risk groups, including functional or anatomically asplenic patients and those with terminal complement component deficiency. The vaccine may be considered as an adjunct to antibiotic prophylaxis and may be useful in containing outbreaks of meningococcal disease due to the represented serogroups. Military recruits are routinely vaccinated because of the frequency of serogroup C infection in this population.[17,18] Vaccination of college students who reside in dormitories is now recommended by the American College Health Association and the Advisory Committee on Immunization Practices (ACIP).

Haemophilus influenzae type b Meningitis. *Haemophilus influenzae* type b is an encapsulated gram-negative pleomorphic coccobacillus. Approximately 30% to 50% of children carry *Haemophilus* asymptomatically in the nasopharynx, generally as the avirulent, nonencapsulated species. These nonencapsulated strains are a common cause of otitis media, sinusitis, and bronchitis, and up to 80% of adults are carriers.[1] Colonization by the type b conjugate ranges from 2% to 5%. Children younger than 2 years old are at the highest risk of developing infection with this organism, as are adults with predisposing factors such as sickle cell disease, asplenia, immunodeficiency states, malignancy, head trauma, neurosurgery, sinusitis, otitis media, or CSF leak. Alaskan Eskimo, Apache, and Navajo Native Americans also are at increased risk owing to genetic factors. Patients commonly develop meningitis after an upper respiratory tract infection or otitis media. Complications of *H. influenzae* meningitis include deafness, blindness, seizure disorders, behavior disorders, and a decrease in school performance.

Previously, empiric therapy for patients with this pathogen was ampicillin. However, this has recently been revised because of the increase in frequency of plasmid-mediated β-lactamase production, now seen in up to 12% to 40% of isolates. Presently, ceftriaxone and cefotaxime are the first-line empiric agents. They also have excellent in vitro activity against the other most commonly encountered meningeal pathogens, cause few serious adverse reactions and drug interactions, and have been shown to rapidly sterilize CSF cultures. Disadvantages of chloramphenicol are the drug–drug interactions that affect the metabolism of other agents through cytochrome P-450, such as phenytoin, rifampin, carbamazepine, and phenobarbital, and the serum drug concentration monitoring that must be done to ensure adequate therapy. Cefuroxime was previously used in the treatment of those with bacterial meningitis, but clinical studies demonstrated an increase in hearing loss in cefuroxime-treated children compared with third-generation cephalosporins, possibly caused by delayed sterilization of CSF fluid.[32] Duration of therapy is 7 to 10 days in uncomplicated cases.

Similar to meningococcus, chemoprophylaxis is recommended to stop contact spread. Rifampin is used because it eradicates nasopharyngeal carriage of *H. influenzae* type b.[18] Minocycline is an alternative, although CNS adverse effects discourage its use. Rifampin prophylaxis is recommended for all household contacts—children and adults—if there is one unvaccinated contact younger than 4 years of age. The only exclusion is pregnancy, because of the unknown risk of rifampin exposure to the fetus. A *household contact* is defined as an individual who resides with the index patient, or a nonresident who spent 4 or more hours with the index patient for at least 5 of the 7 days preceding the day of hospital admission of the index patient.[17] In households with a fully vaccinated, immunocompromised child, all members should receive rifampin prophylaxis because of the possibility of inadequate immune response to the vaccine. Because most secondary cases occur the first week after the patient has been hospitalized, prophylactic therapy should be administered promptly. Some benefit may be gained through therapy that is instituted up to 7 days after the index case occurs. If the family does require prophylaxis and the index patient was treated with ampicillin or chloramphenicol before hospital discharge, the index patient should also receive rifampin prophylaxis.[18] Prophylaxis in the index case is not necessary if the patient received either cefotaxime or ceftriaxone, because these drugs eradicate *H. influenzae* from the nasopharynx.[17]

The recommendations are controversial for patients who attend a day care center or nursery school. Rifampin is indicated if one case of *H. influenzae* meningitis occurs at a day care facility that is attended by any unvaccinated child who is younger than 2 years of age and whose contact time is

greater than 25 hours per week. Unvaccinated children should receive a dose of conjugate vaccine and should then complete the vaccination series. If the children are older than 2 years of age, there is no need for rifampin. If two or more cases of invasive disease occur within 60 days, and unvaccinated or incompletely vaccinated children are exposed, all children and supervisory personnel should promptly receive rifampin therapy.[17]

The dose of rifampin is 20 mg per kg (maximum 600 mg) PO every day for 4 doses.[17] Formal dosing guidelines are not available for children younger than 1 month of age, but some experts recommend 10 mg per kg (maximum 600 mg) daily for 4 days.[18] If children cannot swallow the capsules, rifampin powder may be mixed in applesauce before administration, or a 1% suspension in simple syrup may be compounded. Adverse effects include an orange-red discoloration of the urine and other body fluids, gastrointestinal disturbances, headache, drowsiness, dizziness, and elevated liver enzymes. Patients who wear soft contact lenses should be counseled regarding the possibility of permanent staining of their lenses during therapy. Rifampin is also a potent inducer of hepatic microsomal cytochrome P-450 enzymes and may lower the concentrations of multiple drugs, including oral contraceptives, glucocorticoids, and oral anticoagulants.

Since the development of the vaccine, the incidence of *H. influenzae* type b meningitis has dramatically declined by more than 90%.[33] This effect has not been seen in developing countries, however, because of the decreased availability of the vaccine. *H. influenzae* type b conjugate vaccine contains antigenic capsular polysaccharide ribosylribitol phosphate (PRP). It is coupled with carrier proteins such as diphtheria toxoid (PRP-D), *N. meningitidis* protein (PRP-OMP), tetanus toxoid (PRP-T), or diphtheria CRM197 (mutant) protein (HbOC). Currently, three doses of either HbOC or PRP-T are recommended at 2, 4, and 6 months, or two doses given at 2 and 4 months for PRP-OMP. PRP-D is not recommended for children younger than 12 months. Booster doses of any of the four conjugate vaccines are given at 12 to 15 months. The vaccine does not affect nasopharyngeal carriage.

Listeria monocytogenes Meningitis. *Listeria monocytogenes* is a gram-positive aerobic bacillus that may be mistaken for the diphtheroids present in normal skin flora. Pregnant women, newborns, older adults, and immunocompromised persons are predisposed to *Listeria* infections. *Listeria* is the cause of 8% of cases of bacterial meningitis in the United States.[34] The incidence of *Listeria* infection is greatest in the summer and early fall. Contaminated coleslaw, milk, cheeses, raw vegetables, turkey franks, alfalfa tablets, and processed meats have been the source of outbreaks associated with food poisoning.[34] Antibiotics that have activity against *Listeria* include penicillin G, ampicillin, erythromycin, trimethoprim-sulfamethoxazole, chloramphenicol, rifampin, tetracyclines, and aminoglycosides. In bacterial meningitis, when *Listeria* is one of the suspected pathogens (i.e., Gram stain reveals gram-positive bacilli, or the patient is older than 50 years of age, debilitated, or an alcoholic), empiric therapy should consist of a third-generation cephalosporin combined with ampicillin, because cephalosporins have no activity against this organism. However, because only trimethoprim-sulfamethoxazole and aminoglycosides are bactericidal against *Listeria,* penicillin monotherapy of *Listeria* meningitis has led to mortality rates as high as 30%.[35] Therefore, the treatment of choice for patients with documented *Listeria* meningitis includes ampicillin in combination with an aminoglycoside, given either intravenously or intrathecally.[9,35] The aminoglycoside is added because of its documented in vitro synergy.[36–39] Trimethoprim-sulfamethoxazole is an alternative therapy for patients with penicillin allergy. Meropenem appears to have in vitro activity against *Listeria* and achieves adequate CSF drug concentrations.[39,40] Further study is necessary to evaluate the efficacy of meropenem in treating *Listeria* meningitis in humans.

Gram-Negative Bacillary Meningitis. Gram-negative bacilli are an uncommon cause of meningitis. Patients more likely to develop gram-negative meningitis include older adults, neonates, the immunocompromised, and those with a history of recent trauma or neurosurgery. Although *S. pneumoniae* is the most common pathogen when a CSF leak is present, *S. aureus* and gram-negative infections are also common in this setting. Enterobacteriaceae (especially *E. coli* and *Klebsiella* species) and *Pseudomonas* species are the most commonly implicated gram-negative pathogens. Gram-negative meningitis in the older adult generally has a poor prognosis and involves a protracted clinical course.

Before the introduction of third-generation cephalosporins such as ceftazidime and cefotaxime, aminoglycoside therapy with or without chloramphenicol resulted in gram-negative meningitis mortality rates of 40% to 90%.[41] Treatment of patients with gram-negative bacterial meningitis was revolutionized by the advent of third-generation cephalosporins, which result in cure rates of 78% to 94%.[9,42] These agents have excellent activity versus gram-negative organisms and achieve high levels in the CSF. The greatest experience in gram-negative infections is with cefotaxime[28,43,44] and ceftazidime.[45,46] The usual dosage of cefotaxime is 2 g every 4 hours. If *Pseudomonas* is implicated, ceftazidime 2 to 3 g every 6 to 8 hours or cefepime 2 g every 8 hours plus intrathecal and systemic aminoglycoside therapy may be used empirically.[28] When sensitivity to ceftazidime is established, the need for an aminoglycoside may be reassessed. Although aminoglycosides cover a wide range of gram-negative pathogens, they do not penetrate well into the CSF. Therefore, when these antibiotics are used, they are often delivered directly into the CSF through intrathecal administration. Preservative-free formulations of gentamicin or amikacin are used in doses of 8 mg and 20 to 30 mg daily, respectively.[28] However, even with intrathecal administration, therapeutic aminoglycoside levels are not obtained in the ventricles. Ventriculitis is commonly associated with gram-negative meningitis and may require intraventricular aminoglycoside administration through a reservoir. In resistant cases of coliform or *Pseudomonas* meningitis, direct instillation into the lateral ventricles of gentamicin 4 mg every 12 hours is sometimes used.

If initial therapy with cefotaxime or ceftazidime with or without an aminoglycoside fails or is contraindicated because of allergy, alternative agents with gram-negative activity may be used. Imipenem should be avoided because of its propensity to induce seizures (incidence of greater than 30% of treated patients in one series).[47,48] Meropenem may be a reasonable alternative, especially in cases of meningitis caused by gram-negative bacilli that produce extended-spectrum β-lactamases, or that have the possibility of hyper-producing β-lactamases such as *Enterobacter* species, *Citrobacter* species, or *Serratia marcescens*.[5,49] Trimethoprim-sulfamethoxazole is occasionally used when β-lactam antibiotics cannot be tolerated; however, recurrence with this regimen is common. Fluoroquinolones and aztreonam are other possible alternatives.

Treatment of patients with gram-negative bacterial meningitis should be guided by in vitro susceptibility patterns as soon as final identification of the organism is made, and therapy should be continued for 14 days after cultures become negative.

Fungal Meningitis. The two most common causes of fungal meningitis are *Cryptococcus neoformans* and coccidioidomycosis.[50] Bird droppings, rotten fruits and vegetables, wood rot, and soil contain cryptococcus. Infection occurs through inhalation of the aerosolized spores which results in primary pulmonary disease that disseminates to the central nervous system. The onset of disease is gradual, generally over 4 or more weeks, and it is most prevalent in the immunosuppressed.[51] Patients most commonly experience headache along with alteration in mental status, nuchal rigidity, fever, and papilledema. Examination of the CSF reveals a pleocytosis. Diagnosis is made by India ink stain, culture, and latex agglutination test, which identifies the circulating capsular antigen in the serum of CSF. With these three methods, the diagnosis can be made in 98% to 99% of cases.[51]

The preferred treatment regimen in persons who do not have HIV infection is amphotericin 0.5 to 1 mg/kg/day and flucytosine 100 to 150 mg/kg/day for 6 weeks. A total of 1 to 2 g of amphotericin should be administered. The combination of flucytosine and amphotericin has been found to be superior to amphotericin alone in patients who do not have HIV infection, leading to successful outcomes in 75% of treated patients.[52] A study in HIV-infected patients with cryptococcal meningitis found that the addition of flucytosine 100 mg/kg/day during the first 2 weeks of amphotericin therapy did not improve clinical response.[53] Fluconazole achieves good CSF concentration, is available as an oral agent, and is better tolerated than amphotericin. Studies have shown efficacy with fluconazole as primary therapy in HIV-infected patients who have good prognostic signs. There is a high rate of relapse, so long-term suppressive therapy is often given. The usual regimen for cryptococcal meningitis in HIV-infected patients is amphotericin B 0.7 to 1.0 mg/kg/day for 2 weeks followed by fluconazole 800 mg per day orally for 2 days, then 400 mg per day for 8 weeks and 200 mg per day indefinitely.[52,53] Lipid formulations of amphotericin B can by used for patients with impaired renal function, as these agents are associated with less nephrotoxicity than conventional amphotericin; however, their costs often preclude use of these agents as front-line therapy. Lipid formulations of amphotericin B have not been well studied in the treatment of patients with cryptococcal meningitis, but AmBisome has been given at doses of 4 mg/kg/day.

Therapy with amphotericin B may cause significant adverse drug reactions, including nephrotoxicity, electrolyte abnormalities, infusion-related toxicities, anemia, thrombocytopenia, and phlebitis. Not only is amphotericin toxic, it also achieves low CSF concentrations. Flucytosine (5-FC) is associated with bone marrow suppression, nausea and vomiting, and liver abnormalities.

Coccidioidomycosis is caused by *Coccidioides immitis*. This fungus is present in the soil of southwestern United States, Mexico, and Central America. Hyphal segment fragments release arthroconidia, the infectious particles, which are aerosolized and inhaled. When inhaled, the infection disseminates within 3 to 6 months to the skin, musculoskeletal system, and meninges. In tissues, the spherules develop and form endospores. People at increased risk for CNS infection include immunocompromised persons, infants, older adults, nonwhite persons (highest risk in black, Filipino, and Asian persons), males, and pregnant women. Headache is the most common symptom of fungal meningitis. Symptoms of meningeal irritation are usually absent. Approximately 90% of patients die within 12 months without active treatment.[54] Amphotericin given intrathecally, intracisternally, or intravenously is used. The azoles also have activity against coccidioidomycosis. Comparative trials with the azoles and amphotericin have not been conducted, but because of the advantages of azoles, fluconazole, itraconazole, and ketoconazole may be used. Similar to cryptococcus, maintenance therapy is required because the relapse rate is high.

Viral Meningitis. *Aseptic meningitis* is defined as the presence of meningeal signs and symptoms, as well as CSF abnormalities consistent with meningitis, with stains and cultures that are negative for bacteria or fungi. The most common causes of aseptic meningitis are viruses, particularly enterovirus, herpes, lymphocytic choriomeningitis, and mumps.[55,56] Drugs have also been implicated as a cause of aseptic meningitis (Table 81.7).[57] West Nile virus may cause aseptic meningitis or asymmetric flaccid paralysis, although encephalitis is more common.

Enteroviruses are members of the picornavirus family and consist of poliovirus, coxsackievirus A and B, and echovirus

TABLE 81.7	Aseptic Meningitis Syndrome—Drug-Related Causes
Ibuprofen	
Trimethoprim-sulfamethoxazole	
Sulindac	
Naproxen	
Tolmetin	
Diclofenac	
Muromonab-CD3 (Orthoclone OKT3)	
Carbamazepine	
Immune globulin	
Phenazopyridine	
Vaccines—mumps and rubella	

and are the most common causes of aseptic meningitis.[55] Transmission of these viruses occurs via fecal-oral and respiratory routes. Infants, children, and young adults (age younger than 40 years) are at risk for development of enteroviral infections. Symptoms are gradual or abrupt and are similar to bacterial meningitis. Focal neurologic symptoms are uncommon. An increased incidence of infections is usually seen in the late summer and early fall in temperate climates. Enteroviral infections are self-limited. Patients are given supportive care, including hydration and pain control.[57]

Herpes simplex virus types 1 and 2 have both been associated with CNS infections. Herpes simplex virus type 1 (HSV1) has been associated with meningoencephalitis, which is potentially fatal; herpes simplex virus type 2 (HSV2) is predominantly associated with meningitis, which is usually a self-limited syndrome. The diagnosis and treatment of herpes simplex CNS infections is reviewed during the discussion of encephalitis.

IMPROVING OUTCOMES

The use of corticosteroids as adjunctive therapy in meningitis remains controversial. The pathogenesis of meningitis, as reviewed earlier, consists of the release of cytokines that cause brain edema, increased intracranial pressure, and enhanced BBB permeability. Steroids inhibit the synthesis of these cytokines, thus blocking this cascade of events. CSF inflammation normalizes more rapidly with steroid therapy. Steroids may reduce the penetration of antibiotics into the CSF. A rabbit model of meningitis showed a decrease in CSF concentrations and a delay in CSF sterilization when ceftriaxone or vancomycin was combined with dexamethasone. This may be detrimental in cases where the MIC of the pathogen is increased and the achievable concentration at the site of infection is decreased. Adverse effects of steroids are also a concern; reports of secondary fevers and risk of gastrointestinal bleeding with 4-day steroid regimens are increased.[29,58,59]

Evidence of the beneficial effects of steroid therapy in meningitis has been found. The addition of dexamethasone to cephalosporin therapy has resulted in a reduction in neurologic sequelae, especially hearing loss, in children. A meta-analysis of clinical trials since 1988 confirms the benefit of corticosteroid treatment in *H. influenzae* type b infection, and the Infectious Diseases Committee of the American Academy of Pediatrics advocates the use of dexamethasone for the treatment of patients with meningitis caused by *H. influenzae*.[16,20]

The use of steroids in infants and children with meningitis due to *S. pneumoniae* is controversial. A statement from the Committee on Infectious Diseases of the American Academy of Pediatrics recommends weighing the risks/benefits of steroids in infants and children 6 weeks of age and older.[5]

The use of steroids in adults with pneumococcal meningitis was previously discussed in the *S. pneumoniae* section.

No evidence supports the efficacy of corticosteroids in minimizing neurologic sequelae from *N. meningitidis,* fungal, or viral meningitis. The administration of dexamethasone has been shown to improve survival but not reduce the incidence of severe disability in adolescents and adults with tuberculosis meningitis.[60]

ENCEPHALITIS

EPIDEMIOLOGY

Encephalitis is a direct infection of the brain parenchyma. Viruses are by far the most common pathogens associated with encephalitis (although fungi, rickettsiae, and protozoans have also been implicated), and viral encephalitis will be the main focus of the discussion here. Viruses associated with encephalitis include arboviruses, varicella-zoster virus, herpes simplex virus, measles, mumps, cytomegalovirus, HIV, and rabies.[61,62]

PATHOPHYSIOLOGY

Virus enters the CNS through hematogenous spread. The organism may enter the bloodstream through the respiratory or gastrointestinal tract or may be introduced through an insect or animal bite. Viral replication occurs at the site of entry, followed by spilling into the systemic circulation and, finally, infection of distant sites, including the CNS. In the CNS, cell dysfunction due to viral invasion and inflammatory changes similar to those seen in meningitis occur.

CLINICAL PRESENTATION AND DIAGNOSIS

SIGNS AND SYMPTOMS

Clinical manifestations include a prodrome for several days that may consist of myalgia, fever, malaise, rash, or mild upper respiratory symptoms. Following the prodromal period, headache, drowsiness, change in mental status, and meningismus signify the development of encephalitis. As the infection progresses, drowsiness and confusion increase and eventually may lead to coma. Seizures are common, and focal signs associated with the area of the brain where the infection is concentrated may appear. Intracranial pressure may be increased.[58]

DIAGNOSIS

The symptoms of viral encephalitis mimic a large range of other disease states, including bacterial meningitis, fungal or protozoan encephalitis, brain abscess, neoplasm, and drug overdose; these conditions should be ruled out quickly. Peripheral blood smear should be examined for parasites and blood cultures obtained. Increased intracranial pressure should be ruled out before lumbar puncture is obtained. CT, electroencephalogram (EEG), or radionuclide brain scan should be performed to identify any focal lesions, masses, or cerebral edema. Focal infarctions in the temporal lobes may indicate herpes simplex infection. The CSF exhibits leukocytosis, usually predominantly with lymphocytes, although polymorphonuclear neutrophils or leukocytes (PMNs) may be present in early stages. Red cells may be observed if a necrotizing component is present, as is seen in herpes simplex encephalitis. Glucose content is normal, protein is raised, and organisms are not found on Gram stain. HSV2 can be cultured from the CSF, but HSV1 cannot. Rapid diagnosis of herpesvirus encephalitis through brain biopsy or PCR assay[61] is imperative because a specific and effective therapy is available. The mortality rate of untreated herpes encephalitis is 60% to 80%.[62–66]

Symptoms are generally nonspecific for the different viruses; however, several organisms (e.g., herpes simplex, rabies) demonstrate tropism for certain areas of the brain, and the resulting focal signs may increase the index of suspicion for a particular pathogen. Because of the commonality of symptoms of encephalitis, patient history can be an important consideration in determining the probable causative pathogen. Signs of infection outside the CNS may be helpful in diagnosing cases of encephalitis secondary to varicella, measles, mumps, or herpes simplex. Cytomegalovirus encephalitis is generally seen in infants and the immunocompromised, including organ transplant patients and HIV-infected patients. Travel history, season, or evidence or history of insect or animal bite may also provide clues to pathogen identity. Japanese encephalitis is the most common arbovirus infection worldwide and is endemic in Japan, Southeast Asia, China, India, and the Philippines. Eastern equine encephalitis occurs in the Atlantic and Gulf coasts of the United States and is reported mainly in summer and autumn. Evidence of a dog, cat, or raccoon bite increases suspicion for rabies infection, especially in endemic areas. Brain biopsy has been used when herpes simplex virus is suspected; however, there is no guarantee that the biopsy specimen contains virus, so its yield may be low. Despite efforts to determine the causative organism, in approximately one third of cases, no identification is made.

TREATMENT

Treatment of patients with viral encephalitis is, with the exception of herpes simplex virus, primarily symptomatic. Anticonvulsants are used to control seizure activity; adequate nutrition, hydration, and oxygen are provided as needed; and those with cerebral edema are treated with intubation and hyperventilation, diuretics, or corticosteroids.[58] The use of dexamethasone in these patients is controversial because of the theoretical inhibition of interferon synthesis, which may impair host defense mechanisms against the virus.[62]

Comparative studies have found parenteral acyclovir to be superior to vidarabine for the treatment of herpes encephalitis.[63–66] Therefore, acyclovir is widely accepted as the drug of choice.[63–67] Herpes simplex virus should be treated with acyclovir 10 mg per kg IV infused over 1 hour every 8 hours for 14 to 21 days. Rapid institution of acyclovir treatment has been shown to decrease mortality rates to less than 30%.[67] Survival and recovery may be predicted by the patient's neurologic status at the time of presentation. Acyclovir resistance has been reported, especially in patients with a history of previous or long-term acyclovir treatment.[68] Therapy with foscarnet may be indicated in patients with herpes simplex virus that is resistant to acyclovir.

BRAIN ABSCESS

EPIDEMIOLOGY

Approximately 1 in 10,000 hospital admissions are due to a brain abscess, with males (2:1 vs. females) younger than 20 years of age having the highest incidence. Contiguous infection, hematogenous dissemination, or direct trauma may be the cause. Paranasal sinus, middle ear, mastoid, and dental infections result in contiguous spread by direct extension or through vascular channels. The result is generally a single abscess. Concurrent sinusitis or dental infections commonly cause frontal lobe brain abscesses. Temporal lobe or cerebellar abscesses may be the result of otitis media.[69]

Multiple metastatic abscesses are caused by hematogenous spread from pulmonary infection, osteomyelitis, dental abscess, endocarditis, and skin pustules. Diverse pathogens may be involved in this clinical situation, and their identity depends on the original source of the bacteremia. Table 81.8 outlines common sources of brain abscesses and associated pathogens. In approximately 25% of cases, no apparent source of infection can be identified.[70]

Certain patient populations are at increased risk for brain abscesses. Children with cyanotic congenital cardiac anomalies, such as tetralogy of Fallot (i.e., right-to-left shunts), are at increased risk for development of hematogenously spread brain lesions. Infants and neonates develop brain abscess caused by gram-negative organisms. Immunocompromised patients are at increased risk of fungal abscesses caused by *Candida*, *Aspergillus*, *C. neoformans*, *Blastomyces*, *Histoplasma*, *Mucor*, and *Rhizopus*. *L. monocytogenes* and *Nocardia asteroides* also cause infection in immunocompromised persons. *Toxoplasma gondii* causes brain abscess in patients with acquired immunodeficiency syndrome (AIDS).

PATHOPHYSIOLOGY

A brain abscess is a potentially life-threatening infection that is precipitated by a focal suppurative process within the brain parenchyma. Brain abscesses result from bacterial, fungal, or parasitic infections that seed an area of necrosis in the brain. Bone fragments and debris caused by neurosurgery and cranial trauma may serve as a nidus of infection in some cases. The pathology of brain abscess formation can be divided into four stages.[71] Stage 1 is an early cerebritis that occurs on day 1 to day 3. Day 4 to day 9 marks the beginning of stage 2, or the late cerebritis phase. Fibroblasts produce the reticulin network that is the framework for the collagen capsule. At this stage, maximal edema is seen. From day 10 through day 13 (stage 3), the capsule becomes more developed around the necrotic center (early encapsulation stage). The capsule serves as a protective structure by controlling

TABLE 81.8	Brain Abscess: Common Pathogens by Risk Factor	
Cause	**Pathogens**	**Recommended Therapy**
Sinusitis	Streptococci Staphylococci Anaerobes *Haemophilus influenzae*	Third-generation cephalosporin and metronidazole
Otitis media/ mastoiditis	Streptococci *Bacteroides* Gram-negative organisms	Third-generation cephalosporin and metronidazole
Dental infections	*Fusobacterium* *Bacteroides* Streptococci	Penicillin and metronidazole
Cranial trauma and neurosurgery	*Staphylococcus aureus* Streptococci	Nafcillin or vancomycin (MRSA)

MRSA, methicillin-resistant *Staphylococcus aureus*.

the spread of infection and limiting the destruction of brain parenchyma. Encapsulation is completed in stage 4, the late capsule stage.[71]

CLINICAL PRESENTATION AND DIAGNOSIS

SIGNS AND SYMPTOMS

The clinical symptoms of patients with brain abscesses are nonspecific and depend on size and location of the abscess, number of lesions, virulence of the organism, host response, and severity of cerebral edema that accompanies the abscess. Patients may have abrupt symptoms or insidious onset over weeks. Most patients develop a constant, progressively worsening headache that is not relieved with analgesics. Nausea and vomiting occur as a sign of increasing intracranial pressure. Patients may have a low-grade fever (<101.5°F), focal neurologic deficits, and changes in mentation. The spectrum of consciousness can range from mild confusion to coma. Obtunded or comatose individuals have a worse prognosis. In a study of 45 consecutive cases, the most common symptoms were headache (72%), fever (42%), seizure (35%), nausea and vomiting (35%), and confusion (26%).[72] Symptoms may also provide clues to the area of the brain that is infected. Parietal lobe abscesses are associated with the development of hemiparesis; ataxia, and nystagmus and are associated with cerebellar lesions. Symptoms common in infants include vomiting, irritability, seizures, poor feeding, enlarging head circumference, and bulging fontanelles.

DIAGNOSIS

Unlike meningitis, diagnosis of brain abscesses does not depend on CSF findings. Lumbar punctures are contraindicated because the diagnostic usefulness is poor and the risks are high. Blood and urine cultures are also rarely helpful. The peripheral white blood cell count may be mildly elevated (<15,000/mL^3), as may the erythrocyte sedimentation rate (45 to 50 mm/hr). CT and MRI aid the clinician in making an early diagnosis and in monitoring therapy. The sensitivity of these procedures exceeds 95%, and they confirm the exact location of the lesion. To identify the causative organism, aspiration of the abscess is performed. This sample is then stained and cultured for potential pathogens, including both aerobic and anaerobic organisms.

TREATMENT

When the diagnosis is confirmed, antibiotic therapy alone or combined with surgery is the cornerstone of treatment. Surgical procedures include excision or aspiration of the purulent material. These procedures not only remove the purulent material but also decrease mass effect and intracranial pressure. Generally, if CT suggests cerebritis and the abscess is smaller than 2.5 cm, antibiotics can be initiated and the patient observed for response.[70,71] Otherwise, the abscess should be surgically drained.

Antibiotics used for the treatment of patients with brain abscesses must be bactericidal and able to achieve high tissue concentrations in the brain. This does not always correlate with CSF concentrations. Antibiotics such as chloramphenicol, metronidazole, penicillin, nafcillin, vancomycin, and trimethoprim-sulfamethoxazole and third-generation cephalosporins achieve therapeutic concentrations (Table 81.9). Another consideration when one is choosing appropriate therapy is that agents should not be inactivated or rendered unstable by an acidic environment or purulent material because both exist within the abscess. Organisms that are sensitive to aminoglycosides have reduced susceptibility when the pH is low (i.e., acidic environment). A third-generation cephalosporin (cefotaxime 2 g every 4 hours or ceftriaxone 2 g every 12 hours) plus metronidazole (7.5 mg/kg every 6 hours or 15 mg/kg every 12 hours) are commonly used.[70]

TABLE 81.9	Antibiotics Used in Central Nervous System Infection		
Drug	**Dosing in Children**	**Dosing in Adults**	**Adverse Effects**
Penicillin G	250,000–400,000 U/kg/day divided in 6 doses (q4h)	3–4 million U q4h (up to 24 million U/day)	Leukopenia Anemia
Ampicillin	100–200 mg/kg/day divided in 4 doses	2 g q4h	Seizures in renal failure
Nafcillin/oxacillin	100 mg/kg/day divided in 4 doses	2 g q4h	Hepatotoxicity[b] Acute interstitial nephritis
Ceftriaxone	100 mg/kg/day divided q12–24h[a]	1–2 g q12–24h (up to 4 g/day)	Gastrointestinal upset Biliary sludging
Ceftazidime	225–300 mg/kg/day divided in 3 or 4 doses	2 g q6–8h	
Cefotaxime	225–300 mg/kg/day divided in 3 or 4 doses	2 g q4h	
Rifampin	20 mg/kg/day divided into 2 doses		
Aminoglycosides		Gentamicin/tobramycin:	Nephrotoxicity
Gentamicin			Ototoxicity
Tobramycin		IT: 8–10 mg QD	
Amikacin		IV: 2 mg/kg load	
		Maintenance dosing to follow per drug target levels Amikacin: IT: 20–30 mg QD IV: 15 mg/kg load Maintenance dosing to follow per drug target levels	
Vancomycin	60 mg/kg/day divided in 4 doses	IV: 1–2 g q8–12h Intraventricular: 10 mg/day Target peak serum concentration: 35–40 μg/mL Trough concentration: 15–20 μg/mL	Red-man (neck) syndrome Nephrotoxicity Ototoxicity Leukopenia
Chloramphenicol	75–100 mg/kg/day divided in 4 doses	IV: 75–100 mg/kg/day divided in 4 doses (up to 6 g/day)	Aplastic anemia Thrombocytopenia Leukopenia Gray baby syndrome
Amphotericin B	IV: 0.3–1.0 mg/kg/day	IT: 25–300 μg q48–72h (max 500 μg–1 mg) IV: 0.3–1.0 mg/kg/day	Fever Chills Nephrotoxicity Hypokalemia Hypomagnesemia
Fluconazole		400 mg loading dose on day 1, then 200 mg QD	Gastrointestinal upset Elevated liver enzymes
Flucytosine		150 mg/kg/day divided q6h	Myelosuppression Anemia Hepatitis Nausea Vomiting Diarrhea

IT, intrathecal.

[a] q24h dosing may be appropriate for penicillin-sensitive strains. Strains that are intermediate or resistant require q12h dosing.

[b] Oxacillin has a higher incidence of hepatotoxicity.

High-dose penicillin G (20 to 24 million units/day) has also been used in combination with metronidazole with good results.[70] The duration of therapy ranges from 6 to 8 weeks but is dependent on the patient's response. A course of oral antibiotics may be given following intravenous therapy, in some cases for 2 to 6 months. A total course of 3 to 4 weeks may be appropriate for some patients if the abscess was surgically excised.[73] Other appropriate empiric regimens, based on likely sources of infection and common pathogens, are listed in Table 81.8.

Corticosteroids have been used as adjuvant therapy, although no significant benefit has been observed in survival. Steroids reduce cerebral edema and mass effect, but they also decrease the host defense mechanism and antibiotic concentrations. This may cause a delay in killing of the organism.

Corticosteroids may be beneficial in patients with elevated intracranial pressure or significant mass effect causing neurologic deficits. In these cases, corticosteroids might prevent potentially life-threatening cerebral edema and hernia-tion. High-dose corticosteroids (dexamethasone 10 mg every 6 hours) are usually given until the patient is stabilized; they are then tapered over 3 to 7 days.[70] In severe cases of elevated intracranial pressure, mannitol and intubation with hyperventilation may be necessary.

Long-term neurologic sequelae may result from brain abscesses. These include seizures, cognitive dysfunction, focal neurologic deficits, and epilepsy. Mortality rates associated with this entity ranged from 40% to 60% in the preantibiotic era.[74,75] Now, with availability of CT, diagnosis is made earlier and mortality rates range from 0% to 24%.[76] Recurrence rate ranges from 5% to 10%, and recurrence usually occurs within 6 weeks of treatment. This may be due to inadequate antibiotic therapy, use of incorrect antibiotic, failure to aspirate a large abscess, presence of a foreign body, or failure to eradicate the underlying source of infection. Rupture of an intraventricular brain abscess is associated with an extremely high mortality rate (greater than 80%).[70] Craniotomy and debridement of the abscess site may be necessary.

SHUNT INFECTIONS

EPIDEMIOLOGY

Hydrocephalus is an abnormal increase in the amount of CSF that results in enlargement of the ventricles, which can cause brain atrophy. To relieve this pressure, ventriculoperitoneal (VP) and ventriculoatrial (VA) shunts are placed. A VP shunt relieves pressure by draining CSF into the peritoneal cavity; VA shunts drain into the right atrium. The shunts are composed of a proximal ventricular catheter, a one-way valve or subcutaneous reservoir, and a distal catheter inserted into the peritoneum or right atrium.[77] Because CSF shunts interfere with normal host defenses, they are associated with infection. Infection rates are between 2% and 40%.[78]

PATHOPHYSIOLOGY

Bacteria are introduced retrograde from the distal end of the shunt, through wound or skin infections, hematogenously, or, most commonly, by colonization at the time of shunt placement surgery.

Organisms that make up the skin flora are the most common pathogens in shunt-related infections. *Staphylococcus epidermidis* produces a ''slime layer'' that is composed of an exopolysaccharide substance that not only increases its adherence to the foreign body but also decreases the activity of the antibiotic. Second to *S. epidermidis*, *S. aureus* is isolated in most cases. Gram-negative organisms, such as *E. coli*, *Klebsiella* species, *Proteus* species, and *Pseudomonas* species, may cause infections. *Haemophilus influenzae*, *S. pneumoniae*, *N. meningitidis*, and fungal infections occur less commonly.[77,78]

CLINICAL PRESENTATION AND DIAGNOSIS

SIGNS AND SYMPTOMS

The symptoms of shunt infections are nonspecific. The most common problems experienced are related to the malfunctioning of the shunt, and these include headache, nausea, lethargy, and changes in mental status. Patients may have a low-grade fever (temperature <100°F). If a VP shunt is in place, abdominal symptoms may be noted. Infections of VA devices may result in chronic bacteremia and septic pulmonary emboli.[77]

DIAGNOSIS

Diagnosis of a shunt infection is made on the basis of blood cultures, CSF Gram stain, and cultures taken directly from the reservoir. In shunt infections, the CSF sample usually has increased protein and neutrophils, but the glucose concentration may be normal.

TREATMENT

Effective treatment consists of administration of antibiotics and removal of the shunt, either by externalization of the distal ends of the catheter or by complete removal.

Antibiotics may be given intraventricularly through the reservoir or intravenously. Treatment of *S. epidermidis* and methicillin-resistant *Staphylococcus aureus* (MRSA) includes vancomycin 2 g per day with the addition of rifampin 10 to 20 mg/kg/day. Vancomycin also may be given intraventricularly at a dose of 10 mg per day in adults. The goal is to maintain serum and CSF vancomycin trough concentrations at between 10 and 20 μg/mL. Elevated vancomycin concentrations may cause neurotoxicity; therefore, CSF levels are helpful in maintaining therapy within the therapeutic range.[77,78] An alternative therapy would be trimethoprim-sulfamethoxazole 10 to 20 mg/kg/day with or without rifampin. Methicillin-sensitive *S. aureus* is treated with penicillinase-resistant penicillins such as nafcillin at doses of at least 12 g per day.[78] Gram-negative enteric organisms other than *P. aeruginosa* respond to treatment with ceftriaxone or cefotaxime. Ceftazidime or cefepime 2 g IV every 8 hours, with the addition of an aminoglycoside in some cases, is used for the treatment of *P. aeruginosa*.[78]

PHARMACOECONOMICS OF CENTRAL NERVOUS SYSTEM INFECTIONS

Pharmacoeconomic considerations of central nervous system infections primarily concern chemoprophylaxis of meningitis and vaccination programs. Unfortunately, there is a paucity of pharmacoeconomic analyses of these measures. Adherence to the criteria set forth for the use of chemoprophylaxis and vaccination against *N. meningitidis* and *H. influenzae* infections should reduce the cost of these interventions to society, and their appropriate application should ensure reduction of disease. Obviously, these measures may lead to the avoidance of epidemics and endemic outbreaks, as evidenced by the success of meningococcal vaccine in decreasing meningitis incidence in military recruits. Widespread vaccination against *H. influenzae* infection in children has caused a dramatic decline in the frequency of meningitis caused by this organism, and the availability of the heptavalent conjugate pneumococcal vaccine since 2000 is expected to largely decrease the frequency of meningitis due to *S. pneumoniae*. Quantification of the cost-effectiveness of widespread vaccination against *N. meningitidis* and the further refinement of chemoprophylaxis guidelines may be necessary in the future.

KEY POINTS

- Initiate therapy promptly. A delay in therapy of a few hours may result in increased morbidity and mortality.
- Use antimicrobials that are bactericidal.
- Select antimicrobials that have good penetration into the CSF.
- Antimicrobials should be dosed appropriately to ensure adequate CSF penetration and should exceed the MBC by eight to ten times.
- When instilling antibiotics directly into the CSF, one must remember that therapeutic antibiotic levels are achieved *below* the point of instillation, but not above.

MENINGITIS

- Empiric antibiotic therapy should be directed by the Gram stain of CSF (if available) and the patient's age and underlying health status. Empiric regimens usually include a third-generation cephalosporin (e.g., ceftriaxone) with or without additional antibiotics (ampicillin, vancomycin).
- Corticosteroids should be used in childhood *H. influenzae* meningitis and should be considered in *S. pneumoniae* meningitis (pediatric or adult) to decrease the incidence of long-term neurologic deficits, specifically, hearing loss.
- Exposed contacts to meningitis index patients with *H. influenzae* and *N. meningitidis* may require chemoprophylaxis.
- Vaccines are available to decrease the incidence of disease and, therefore, perhaps meningitis due to *H. influenzae*, *N. meningitidis,* and *S. pneumoniae* in at-risk populations.

ENCEPHALITIS

- Treatment of patients with most types of viral encephalitis is symptomatic (e.g., anticonvulsants, nutritional support, reduction of increased intracranial pressure).
- Rapid diagnosis to rule out herpes simplex infection is imperative because directed therapy is available.
- Acyclovir is the drug of choice for herpes encephalitis and has been proved to significantly reduce morbidity and mortality.

BRAIN ABSCESS

- Antibiotic therapy may not be sufficient to cause resolution of brain abscesses larger than 2.5 cm; therefore, surgical drainage is often indicated.
- Antibiotic therapy is directed by the suspected source of infection (if identifiable) and the results of culture or Gram stain of the abscess aspirate. Empiric therapy should include a broad-spectrum agent that covers both aerobes and anaerobes.
- Duration of antibiotic therapy is generally 6 to 8 weeks, but it may be longer depending on clinical response.

SHUNT INFECTIONS

- Removal of the shunt is most often recommended
- Empiric therapy is directed toward nosocomial pathogens, including methicillin-resistant staphylococci (*S. aureus* and *S. epidermidis*) and nosocomial gram-negative bacilli.

REFERENCES

1. Tunkel AR, Scheld WM. Acute meningitis. In: Mandell GL, Bennett JE, Dolin R, eds. Principles and practice of infectious diseases. 4th ed. New York: Churchill Livingstone, 1995:831–864.
2. Jackson LA, Wenger JD. Laboratory-based surveillance for meningococcal disease in selected areas—United States, 1989–1991. CDC surveillance summaries (June). MMWR 42 (SS-2):21–30, 1993.
3. Durand ML, Calderwood SB, Weber DJ, et al. Acute bacterial meningitis in adults: a review of 493 episodes. N Engl J Med 328:21–28, 1993.
4. Van de Beek D, de Gans J, Spanjaard L, et al. Clinical features and prognostic factors in adults with bacterial meningitis. N Engl J Med 351:1849–1859, 2004.
5. Tunkel AR, Hartman BJ, Kaplan SL, et al. Practice guidelines for the management of bacterial meningitis. Clin Infect Dis 39:1267–1281, 2004.
6. Wispelwey B, Tunkel AR, Scheld WM. Bacterial meningitis in adults. Infect Dis Clin North Am 4:645–659, 1990.
7. Greenlee JE. Approach to diagnosis of meningitis, cerebrospinal fluid evaluation. Infect Dis Clin North Am 4:583–599, 1993.
8. Quagliariello VJ, Scheld WM. Treatment of bacterial meningitis. N Engl J Med 336:708–716, 1997.
9. Tunkel AR, Wispelwey B, Scheld WM. Bacterial meningitis: recent advances in pathophysiology and treatment. Ann Intern Med 112:610–623, 1990.
10. Miller LG, Choi C. Meningitis in older patients: how to diagnose and treat a deadly infection. Geriatrics 52:43–55, 1997.
11. Prevention of pneumococcal disease: Recommendations of the Advisory Committee on Immunization Practices (ACIP). MMWR 46 (RR-08):1–24,1997.
12. Coffey TJ, Daniels M, McDougal LK, et al. Genetic analysis of clinical isolates of *Streptococcus pneumoniae* with high-level resistance to expanded spectrum cephalosporins. Antimicrob Agents Chemother 39:1306–1313, 1995.
13. Breiman RF, Butler JC, Tenover FC, et al. Emergence of drug-resistant pneumococcal infections in the United States. JAMA 271:1831–1835, 1994.
14. Gold H, Moellering RC. Antimicrobial resistance. N Engl J Med 335:1445, 1996.
15. De Gans, van de Beek D. Dexamethasone in adults with bacterial meningitis. N Engl J Med 347:1549–1556, 2002.
16. McIntyre PB, Berkey CS, King SM. Dexamethasone as adjunctive therapy in bacterial meningitis: a meta analysis of randomized clinical trials since 1988. JAMA 278:925–931, 1997.
17. Committee on Infectious Diseases, American Academy of Pediatrics. In: Peter G, ed. 1997 red book: report of the committee on infectious diseases. 24th ed. Elk Grove Village, Ill: American Academy of Pediatrics, 1997:222, 357–363, 410–418.
18. Lieberman JM, Greenberg DP, Ward JI. Prevention of bacterial meningitis, vaccines and chemoprophylaxis. Infect Dis Clin North Am 4:703–729, 1990.
19. Whitney CG, Farley MM, Hadler J, et al. Decline in invasive pneumococcal disease after the introduction of protein-polysaccharide conjugate vaccine. N Engl J Med 348:1737–1746, 2003.
20. Control and prevention of meningococcal disease. Recommendations of the Advisory Committee on Immunization Practices (ACIP). MMWR 46 (RR-5):1–7, 1997.
21. Jackson LA, Tenover FC, Baker C, et al. Prevalence of *Neisseria meningitidis* relatively resistant to penicillin in the United States, 1991. J Infect Dis 169:438–441, 1994.
22. Pinner RW, Onyango F, Perkins BA, et al. Epidemic meningococcal disease in Nairobi, Kenya, 1989. J Infect Dis 166:359–364, 1992.
23. Stephens DS, Hajjeh RA, Baughman WS, et al. Sporadic meningococcal disease in adults: results of a 5-year population-based study. Ann Intern Med 123:937–940, 1995.
24. Rosenstein NE, Perkins BA, Stephens DS, et al. The changing epidemiology of meningococcal disease in the United States, 1992–1996. J Infect Dis 180:1894–1901, 1999.
25. Jackson LA, Schuchat A, Reeves MW, et al. Serogroup C meningococcal outbreaks in the United States: an emerging threat. JAMA 273:383–389, 1995.
26. Serogroup. B meningococcal disease—Oregon, 1994. MMWR 44:121–124, 1995.
27. Luby JP. Southwestern Internal Medicine Conference: infections in the central nervous system. Am J Med Sci 304:379–391, 1992.
28. Kaplan SL. New aspects of prevention and therapy of meningitis. Infect Dis Clin North Am 6:197–213, 1992.
29. Schaad UB, Kaplan SL, McCracken GH. Steroid therapy for bacterial meningitis. Clin Infect Dis 20:685–690, 1995.
30. Schwartz B, Al-Ruwais A, A'Ashi J, et al. Comparative efficacy of ceftriaxone and rifampin in eradicating pharyngeal carriage of group A *Neisseria meningitidis*. Lancet 1:1239–1242, 1988.
31. Goldschneider I, Lepow ML, Gotschlich EG, et al. Immunogenicity of group A and group C meningococcal polysaccharides in human infants. J Infect Dis 128:769–772, 1973.
32. Schaad UB, Suter S, Gianella-Borradori A, et al. A comparison of ceftriaxone and cefuroxime for the treatment of bacterial meningitis in children. N Engl J Med 322:141–147, 1990.
33. Adams WG, Deaver KA, Cochi SL, et al. Decline of childhood *Haemophilus influenzae* type b (Hib) disease in the Hib vaccine era. JAMA 269:221–226, 1993.
34. Tunkel AR, Scheld WM. Acute meningitis. In: Mandell GL, Bennett JE, Dolin R, eds. Principles and practice of infectious diseases. 6th ed. New York: Churchill Livingstone, 2004:1.
35. Skogberg K, Syrjanen J, Jahkola M, et al. Clinical presentation and outcome of listeriosis in patients with and without immunosuppressive therapy. Clin Infect Dis 14:815–821, 1992.
36. Trautmann M, Wagner J, Chahin M, et al. *Listeria* meningitis: report of ten recent cases and review of current therapeutic recommendations. J Infect 10:107–114, 1985.
37. Hansen PB, Jensen TH, Lykkegaard S, et al. *Listeria monocytogenes* meningitis in adults. Sixteen consecutive cases 1973–1982. Scand J Infect Dis 19:55–60, 1987.
38. Lorber B. Listeriosis. Clin Infect Dis 24:1, 1997.
39. Nairn K, Shepherd GL, Edwards JR. Efficacy of meropenem in experimental meningitis. J Antimicrob Chemother 36 (Suppl A):73–84, 1995.
40. Dagan R, Velghe L, Rodda JL, et al. Penetration of meropenem into the cerebrospinal fluid of patients with inflamed meninges. J Antimicrob Chemother 34:175–179, 1994.
41. Cherubin CE, Marr JS, Sierra MF, et al. *Listeria* and gram negative bacillary meningitis in New York City 1972–1979. Am J Med 71:199–209, 1981.
42. Cherubin CE, Corrado ML, Nair SR, et al. Treatment of gram negative bacillary meningitis. Role of new cephalosporin antibiotics. Rev Infect Dis 4 (Suppl):S453–S464, 1982.
43. Jacobs RF. Cefotaxime treatment of gram negative enteric meningitis in infants and children. Drugs 35 (Suppl 2):185–189, 1988.
44. Kaplan SL, Patrick CC. Cefotaxime and aminoglycoside treatment of meningitis caused by gram-negative enteric organisms. Pediatr Infect Dis J 9:810–814, 1990.
45. Fong IW, Tomkins KB. Review of *Pseudomonas aeruginosa* meningitis with special emphasis on treatment with ceftazidime. Rev Infect Dis 7:604–612, 1985.
46. Rodriguez WJ, Khan WN, Cocchetti DM, et al. Treatment of *Pseudomonas aeruginosa* meningitis with or without concurrent therapy. Pediatr Infect Dis J 9:83–87, 1990.
47. Calandra GB, Brown KR, Grad LC, et al. The efficacy results and safety profile of imipenem/cilastatin from the clinical research trials. J Clin Pharmacol 28:120–127, 1988.

48. Wong VK, Wright HT Jr, Ross LA, et al. Imipenem/cilastatin treatment of bacterial meningitis in children. Pediatr Infect Dis J 10: 122–125, 1991.
49. Donnelly JP, Horrevorts AM, Sauerwein RW, et al. High-dose meropenem in meningitis due to *Pseudomonas aeruginosa*. Lancet 339: 1117, 1992.
50. Medoff G, Kobayashi GS. Systemic fungal infections: an overview. Hosp Pract 2:41–52, 1991.
51. Bennett JE, Dismukes W, Duma R. A comparison of amphotericin B alone and combined with flucytosine in the treatment of cryptococcal meningitis. N Engl J Med 301:126–131, 1979.
52. Van Der Horst CM, Saag MS, Cloud GA, et al. Treatment of cryptococcal meningitis associated with acquired immune deficiency syndrome. N Engl J Med 337:15, 1997.
53. Stevens DA. Coccidiomycosis. N Engl J Med 332:1077–1082, 1995.
54. Nelson S, Sealy DP, Schneider EF. The aseptic meningitis syndrome. Am Fam Physician 48:809–815, 1993.
55. Marinac JS. Drug- and chemical-induced aseptic meningitis: a review of the literature. Ann Pharmacother 26:813–821, 1992.
56. Rubeiz H, Roos RP. Viral meningitis and encephalitis. Semin Neurol 12:165–177, 1992.
57. Lambert HP. Meningitis. J Neurol Neurosurg Psych 57:405–415, 1994.
58. Lebel MH, Frey BJ, Syrogrannopoulos GA. Dexamethasone therapy for bacterial meningitis. Results of two double-blind, placebo controlled trials. N Engl J Med 319:964–971, 1988.
59. Anderson M. Management of cerebral infection. J Neurol Neurosurg Psychiatry 56:1243–1258, 1993.
60. Thwaites GE, Duc Bang N, Huy N, et al. Dexamethasone for the treatment of tuberculosis meningitis in adolescents and adults. N Engl J Med 351:1741–1751, 2004.
61. Domingues RB, Tsanacles AM, Pannuti CS, et al. Evaluation of the range of clinical presentations of herpes simplex encephalitis by using polymerase chain reaction assay of cerebrospinal fluid samples. Clin Infect Dis 25:86–91, 1997.
62. Hirsch MS. Herpes simplex virus. In: Mandell GL, Bennett JE, Dolin R, eds. Principles and practice of infectious diseases. 4th ed. New York: Churchill Livingstone, 1995:1336–1345.
63. Whitley RJ, Alford CA, Hirsch MS, et al. Vidarabine versus acyclovir therapy of herpes simplex encephalitis. N Engl J Med 314: 144–149, 1986.
64. Skoldenberg B, Forsgren M. Acyclovir versus vidarabine in herpes simplex encephalitis. Scand Infect Dis 47:89–96, 1985.
65. Skoldenberg B, Forsgren M, Alestig K, et al. Acyclovir versus vidarabine in herpes simplex encephalitis. Randomised multicenter study in consecutive Swedish patients. Lancet 2:707–711, 1984.
66. Peterslund NA. Herpes zoster associated encephalitis: clinical findings and acyclovir treatment. Scand J Infect Dis 20:583–592, 1988.
67. O'Brien JJ, Campoli-Richards DM. Acyclovir: an updated review of its antiviral activity, pharmacokinetic properties and therapeutic efficacy. Drugs 37:233–309, 1989.
68. Gately A, Gander R, Johnson P. Herpes simplex virus type 2 meningoencephalitis resistant to acyclovir in a patient with AIDS. J Infect Dis 161:711, 1990.
69. Britt RH, Enzmann DR. Clinical stages of human brain abscesses on serial CT scans after contrast infusion. Computerized tomographic, neuropathological and clinical correlations. J Neurosurg 59: 972–989, 1983.
70. Mathisen GE, Johnson JP. Brain abscess. Clin Infect Dis 25: 763–781, 1997.
71. Chun CH, Johnson JD, Hofstetter M, et al. Brain abscess, a study of 45 consecutive cases. Medicine 65:415–431, 1986.
72. Garfield J. Management of supratentorial intracranial abscess: a review of 200 cases. Br Med J 2:7, 1969.
73. Tunkel AR. Brain Abscess. In: Mandell GL, Bennett JE, Dolin R, eds. Principles and practice of infectious diseases. 6th ed. New York: Churchill Livingstone, 2004:1.
74. Bellar AJ, Sahar A, Praiss I. Brain abscess. Review of 89 cases over 30 years. J Neurol Neurosurg Psychiatry 36:757, 1973.
75. Small M, Dale BAB. Intracranial suppuration 1969–1982—a 15 year review. Clin Otolaryngol 9:315, 1984.
76. Gorbach SL, Bartlett JG, Blacklow NR. Infectious diseases. 9th ed. Philadelphia: WB Saunders, 1992.
77. Luer MS, Halton J. Vancomycin administration into the cerebrospinal fluid: a review. Ann Pharmacother 27:912–921, 1993.
78. Kaufmann BA, Tunkel AR, Pryor JC, et al. Meningitis in the neurosurgical patient. Infect Dis Clin North Am 4:677–701, 1990.

Bone and Joint Infections

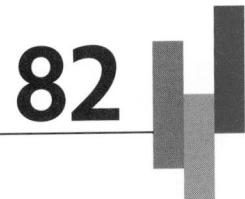

Gregory V. Stajich and Kalen B. Porter

OSTEOMYELITIS

TREATMENT GOALS: OSTEOMYELITIS

- Arrest the infectious process.
- Prevent permanent bone damage and deformity.
- Reverse all signs and symptoms of disease.
- Prevent chronic infection.

DEFINITION

Osteomyelitis is a microbial infection of the bone associated with bacteria, fungi, and rarely mycobacteria. The result of this invasion is an inflammatory destructive process.

Osteomyelitis can occur in any bone of the body. It begins as an acute infection and if left untreated may progress to a chronic disease. Factors such as the anatomic site of the bone involved, the chronicity and extent of infection, the patient's age, the presence of prosthetic devices, the causative agent, and concomitant host diseases influence the clinical manifestations, therapy, and prognosis of the disease. Despite the advent of more potent antimicrobial therapy and enhanced diagnostic procedures and surgical techniques, the treatment of osteomyelitis continues to pose a diagnostic and therapeutic challenge. The discussion in this chapter is limited to infections of bacterial origin.

EPIDEMIOLOGY

Osteomyelitis has been categorized using several different classification systems. Historically, the type of osteomyelitis was described as acute, subacute, or chronic depending on the stage of illness (i.e., onset of symptoms and duration of clinical manifestations). In 1970, the Waldvogel classification system was developed; it classifies osteomyelitis into hematogenous, contiguous, and chronic depending on pathogenesis.[1-3] The Waldvogel classification system is described in Table 82.1. A more recent system developed in the 1980s, the Cierny-Mader staging system, classifies osteomyelitis based on the status of the disease process, status of the host, and anatomic location.[4]

Acute hematogenous osteomyelitis describes an infection whose source of bacteria is the bloodstream. More than 85% of cases occur in children under 17 years of

TABLE 82.1	Categorization of Osteomyelitis			
Type	**Age Distribution**	**Bones Involved**	**Major Clinical Findings**	**Microbiology**
Hematogenous	1–20 years	Long bones	Initial episode:	Single pathogen
			Fever	
	>50 years	Vertebrae	Local tenderness	
			Local swelling	
			Decreased range of motion	
			Recurrent episode:	
			Exudative drainage	
Contiguous	>50 years	Femur	Initial episode:	Polymicrobial
		Tibia	Fever	
		Skull	Erythema	
		Mandible	Swelling	
			Sinus tract formation	
			Recurrent episode:	
			Exudative drainage	
			Sinus tract formation	
Contiguous with vascular insufficiency	>50 years	Feet	Initial and recurrent episode:	Polymicrobial
		Toes	Pain[a]	
			Swelling	
			Erythema	
			Exudative drainage	
			Ulceration	
Chronic	Adults	Any	Pain	Polymicrobial
			Erythema	
			Exudative drainage	
			Sinus tract formation	
			Decreased range of motion	

[a] May be blunted by concurrent neuropathy
(From Mader JT, Calhoun JH. Osteomyelitis. In: Mandell GL, Douglas RG, Bennett JE Jr., eds. Principles and practice of infectious diseases. New York: Churchill Livingstone, 1995:1039–1051.)

age. The long bones are usually affected in children; adults typically have involvement of the thoracic or lumbar vertebrae. At any age, males are more likely to acquire hematogenous osteomyelitis.[5] This type of infection typically has an onset of a few days to a week and is commonly caused by a single pathogen.

Contiguous osteomyelitis can result from direct bacterial inoculation of the bone from an exogenous source (trauma, surgery) or from extension of an adjacent soft tissue infection. Contiguous osteomyelitis has a biphasic age distribution. In younger individuals, the source tends to be trauma or surgery; in older adults, decubitus ulcers and infected joint prostheses are common sources of infection.[6] Contiguous osteomyelitis may also be associated with vascular insufficiency. This type of infection is usually seen in older individuals (50 to 70 years of age) with concomitant illnesses such

as diabetes mellitus or peripheral vascular disease. These infections, which are often polymicrobial, develop as an extension of an existing localized infection and can affect the toes, metatarsals, tarsals, or hindfoot.

Chronic osteomyelitis is seen predominantly in adults. A variety of factors have been used to define chronic osteomyelitis, including the chronicity of the disease, lack of response to antibiotic therapy, and the presence of necrotic bone or sinus tract. Any bone infection may progress to chronic osteomyelitis.

ETIOLOGY

Osteomyelitis is a purulent inflammation of bone caused most often by bacteria and only occasionally by other micro-

TABLE 82.2	Commonly Isolated Organisms in Bacterial Osteomyelitis Based on Patient Age			
Neonate (<1 month)	**Infants (1 month–1 year)**	**Children and Adolescents (1–16 years)**	**Adults (>16 years)**
S. aureus	S. aureus	S. aureus	S. aureus
Group B streptococci	Group A streptococci	Group A streptococci	Streptococci
			Enterococci
Enterobacteriaceae (particularly E. coli)	S. pneumoniae	S. pneumoniae	Gram-negative bacilli
			Pseudomonas aeruginosa
			E. coli
			Anaerobes

organisms. The most common bacterial causes of osteomyelitis categorized by patient age are listed in Table 82.2. *Staphylococcus aureus* is the most common causative organism in all categories of osteomyelitis. In children, *S. aureus* accounts for 60% to 90% of isolates in acute hematogenous osteomyelitis.[7] One reason for this high rate is due to the skeletal anatomy of a child, which favors entrapment of organisms.[8] *S. aureus* is isolated in adult osteomyelitis in up to 75% of cases.[9] *Staphylococcus epidermidis* (coagulase-negative *Staphylococcus*) is a common pathogen among patients with prosthetic joint infections.

Streptococcal species are also prevalent among all categories of osteomyelitis. In the neonatal period, infections are commonly caused by group B streptococci. Group A streptococci and *Streptococcus pneumoniae* are commonly isolated pathogens in infants, children, and adolescents. Enterococci (group D streptococci) can also be isolated in adult osteomyelitis.

Gram-negative organisms commonly isolated in osteomyelitis include Enterobacteriaceae, especially *Escherichia coli*, *Pseudomonas aeruginosa*, and *Salmonella* species. Neonates are at particularly high risk for osteomyelitis due to *E. coli*. In adults, gram-negative organisms are commonly isolated in nosocomial infections. *P. aeruginosa* has been reported to cause infection in intravenous drug users. Patients with sickle cell disease are often infected with *Salmonella* species.

In children older than 5 years of age, *Haemophilus influenzae* was once a prevalent pathogen, but its incidence has decreased due to the routine immunization of infants.[10]

Polymicrobial infections are common in adult osteomyelitis and may include three or more pathogens. Patients with diabetes are at increased risk for the development of polymicrobial osteomyelitis secondary to the presence of diabetic foot ulcers or infections. Anaerobes such as *Bacteroides fragilis*, other Bacteroides species, Fusobacterium, Clostridium, and microaerophilic cocci can also be significant pathogens in osteomyelitis, especially in patients with diabetes.[11]

The most commonly isolated microorganisms in osteomyelitis and their clinical associations are listed in Table 82.3.

RISK FACTORS

Risk factors for the development of osteomyelitis are outlined in Table 82.4. The identification and knowledge of specific risk factors can aid in the early diagnosis of osteomyelitis in some patients and perhaps prevention of the infection in others.

Hematogenous dissemination of bacteria is one of the most important risk factors for the development of acute hematogenous osteomyelitis. This infection is predominantly a disease of children. Identification of septic foci that are associated with the promotion of bacteremia is important for overall treatment and pathogen recognition. For example, acute pharyngitis, minor lacerations, cellulitis, and cuta-

TABLE 82.3	Microorganisms Commonly Isolated in Osteomyelitis
Microorganism	**Clinical Association**
Staphylococcus aureus	Most common organism among all types of osteomyelitis
Coagulase-negative staphylococci	Foreign-body infection
Enterobacteriaceae	Nosocomial infections
Pseudomonas aeruginosa	Nosocomial infections
	Intravenous drug users
Salmonella	Sickle cell disease
Pasteurella multocida or Eikenella corrodens	Human or animal bites
Anaerobic bacteria	Diabetic foot infections
Bartonella henselae	HIV infection

TABLE 82.4	**Risk Factors Associated with the Development of Osteomyelitis**

Hematogenous

Bacteremic foci

  Noninvasive

    Acute pharyngitis

    Minor laceration

    Cellulitis

    Cutaneous abscess

    Sickle cell anemia

    Respiratory/urinary tract infections

  Invasive

    IV catheter

    IV drug user

    Hemodialysis

    Heel stick

Nonpenetrating trauma

Contiguous

Direct inoculation

  Penetrating trauma

    Open reduction of fracture

    Gunshot wound

    Orthopedic procedure

    Diagnostic procedure

    Animal bite

    Puncture wound

    Adjacent foci

    Surgery

    Postoperative wound infection

    Soft tissue infection

    Poor oral hygiene

    Chronic tooth infection

Contiguous With Vascular Insufficiency

Diabetes mellitus

Peripheral vascular disease

Pressure ulcer

neous abscesses have been implicated as sources of bacteremia in children with acute osteomyelitis.[12] Another risk factor for bacteremia is the long-term use of indwelling vascular access catheters for hyperalimentation or for the administration of chemotherapeutic agents.

In older adults, gram-negative organisms and *S. epidermidis* may cause osteomyelitis of the vertebral bodies. This infection may arise from primary sites in the gastrointestinal or urinary tract. A strong association has been documented between urinary tract infections and osteomyelitis of the vertebral bodies.[13] Intravenous drug use is another predisposing

factor because microorganisms can be injected into the bloodstream and cause various bacterial infections (i.e., endocarditis and osteomyelitis). Common infecting organisms include *P. aeruginosa*, *Serratia marcescens*, and *S. aureus*.[14]

Neonatal osteomyelitis also has associated risk factors. Placement of umbilical catheters following a complicated delivery or the use of frequent heel sticks to obtain blood samples for laboratory tests has preceded the development of osteomyelitis in this age group.

Osteomyelitis may also evolve from either direct bacterial inoculation (e.g., traumatic injury) or contiguous spread from an adjacent infectious focus. Direct inoculation can occur from a variety of sources, such as penetrating trauma from open injuries to bone, reduction of fractures, orthopedic and diagnostic procedures, gunshot wounds, and animal bites.[15] In many cases, the sterile bone is directly penetrated and inoculated. The pathogens may originate from the penetrating object or from the patient's skin. Osteomyelitis from a contiguous soft tissue infection is the most important type of pathogenesis in adults. The primary foci for these infections include soft tissue infections close to the bone, as in the case of osteomyelitis of the mastoid bone, which can originate from malignant otitis media or a paranasal sinus infection. Another example of contiguous osteomyelitis is mandibular osteomyelitis observed in patients with poor oral hygiene or chronic infections of the teeth. Postoperative wound infections following orthopedic correction of the skeleton, neurosurgery, median sternotomy, and oral surgery are also major sources of contiguous osteomyelitis.

Concurrent underlying diseases or conditions are recognized as predisposing risk factors to the development of osteomyelitis. Sickle cell anemia and related hemoglobinopathies are reported to predispose patients to the development of osteomyelitis due to *Salmonella* species.[16] Diabetes mellitus with vascular insufficiency often predisposes patients to chronic draining ulcers and cellulitis of feet and toes, which promotes the development of contiguous osteomyelitis.[17] Decubitus ulcers, or pressure sores, in chronically debilitated bedridden patients also are a major risk factor. Chronic osteomyelitis may develop due to inadequate or delayed management of acute osteomyelitis, unrecognized bone infection, inappropriate antibiotic pharmacology (choice, dose, duration), or inadequate surgical drainage.

PATHOPHYSIOLOGY

Animal models have long been used to explore the pathogenesis of osteomyelitis. In these studies, normal bone has been shown to be highly resistant to infection. The presence of a foreign body (e.g., a prosthetic device), trauma, or a large inoculum of microorganisms lays the groundwork for the development of osteomyelitis.[18,19]

Acute hematogenous osteomyelitis in children usually occupies the metaphysis of a long bone such as the femur. The pathogenesis is thought to involve the capillary ends of the

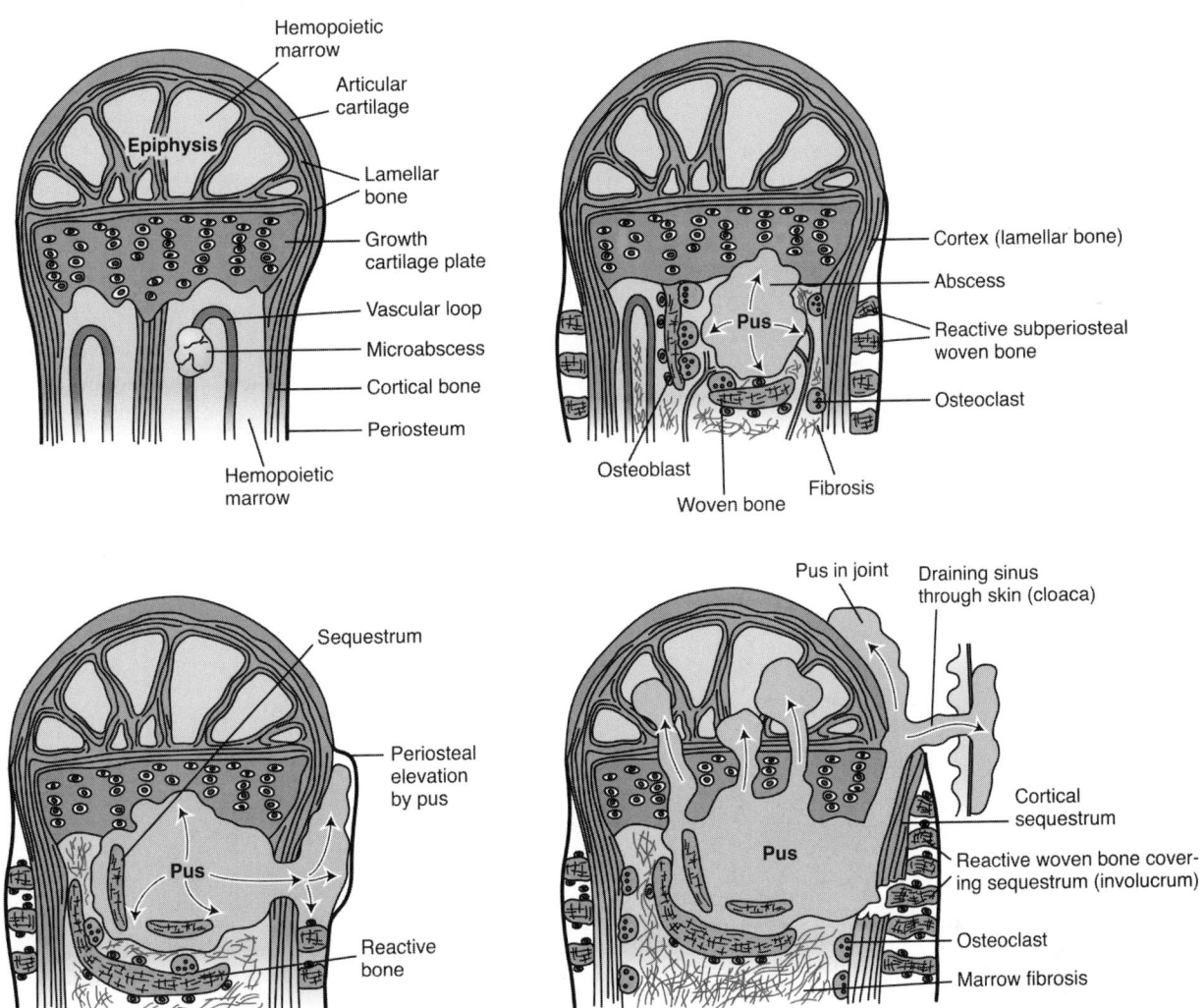

FIGURE 82.1 Pathogenesis of hematogenous osteomyelitis (*see color insert*). **A.** The epiphysis, metaphysis, and growth plate are normal. A small, septic microabscess is forming at the capillary loop. **B.** The expansion of the septic focus stimulates resorption of adjacent bony trabeculae. Woven bone begins to surround this focus. The abscess expands into the cartilage and stimulates reactive bone formation by the periosteum. **C.** The abscess, which continues to expand through the cortex into the subperiosteal tissue, shears off the perforating arteries that supply the cortex with blood, leading to necrosis of the cortex. **D.** The extension of this process into the joint space, the epiphysis, and the skin produces a draining sinus. The necrotic bone is called a sequestrum. The viable bone surrounding a sequestrum is termed the involucrum. (Image from Rubin E, Farber JL. Pathology, 3rd ed. Philadelphia: Lippincott Williams & Wilkins, 1999.)

nutrient artery, which make sharp turns under the epiphyseal growth plate and enter large venous sinusoids, where blood flow slows considerably (Fig. 82.1; *see color insert*). Also, the capillary lining lacks phagocytic cells. These anatomic and physiologic features favor the growth of microorganisms. Following hematogenous seeding of the bone, the host's inflammatory response ensues. Vascular permeability is increased, resulting in edema and an influx of polymorphonuclear leukocytes. Cytokines, toxic oxygen radicals, and proteolytic enzymes generated by the inflammatory response destroy surrounding tissue, including bone. Prostaglandins, generated in response to bone disruption, decrease the threshold for bacterial infection of the bone.[20] Intraosseous pressure

increases as pus collects and is confined within the rigid bone. In children, the cortical section of the bone and the metaphyses are much thinner than in adults. There is also less adherence of the periosteum to the underlying cortex. The culmination of these factors is extension of the suppurative process from the metaphysis through the cortex and into the subperiosteal space. The blood supply to the outer cortical bone may be further diminished due to the pressure, leading to the development of dead bone or sequestra. In adults, the infectious process usually remains intramedullary due to the thicker cortex and tightly bound periosteum.

Infecting microorganisms have attributes that aid in the development of osteomyelitis. *S. aureus*, the common etiologic agent, adheres to bone, cartilage, and prostheses via adhesions that are specific for bone components (e.g., collagen, laminin, fibronectin).[21] The ability of *S. aureus* to survive within leukocytes after phagocytosis may explain some chronic bone infections.[22]

CLINICAL PRESENTATION AND DIAGNOSIS

SIGNS AND SYMPTOMS

The diagnosis of osteomyelitis is primarily made through clinical assessment. Acute hematogenous osteomyelitis is often associated with both local and systemic symptoms. Local symptoms include pain, swelling, tenderness, decreased range of motion in an adjacent joint, and suppuration at the involved site. Systemic symptoms include fever, malaise, chills, headache, nausea, vomiting, and myalgias.

In adults, osteomyelitis secondary to hematogenous spread usually affects the vertebrae. If diagnosis is delayed, the disease may progress to vertebral destruction and paralysis.[23]

Osteomyelitis secondary to a contiguous focus usually affects the bones that are more prone to fracture or open reduction surgical procedures (e.g., femur, tibia). Fever may be present during the initial episode, but major symptoms are generally confined to the infected area and consist of pain, tenderness, swelling, and redness.

In patients with diabetes or vascular insufficiency, osteomyelitis occurs almost exclusively in the feet.[24] This population may have claudication or extremity neuropathy, which blunts both perception of local injury and the inflammatory response. Local skin infection can progress insidiously to the bone. The clinical presentation of these patients is often dichotomous. If advanced neuropathy exists, the infection is often painless. However, if acute bony destruction occurs, excruciating pain may be elicited on physical examination.[25] Other symptoms include swelling, erythema, exudative drainage, and ulceration.

Acute osteomyelitis due to hematogenous spread or a contiguous focus can progress to a chronic infection. This recalcitrant disease is characterized by repeated therapeutic failures. This type of osteomyelitis cannot be cured until the nidus of infection has been removed. The common characteristic of all types of chronic osteomyelitis is the presence of vascular thrombosis or sequestra. Sequestra provide a bacterial milieu for persistence of the infection and perpetuation of the inflammatory progress. This results in eventual vascular thrombosis and further development of necrotic bone.[26] In addition, glycocalyx formation acts as a barrier to hormonal and cellular host defenses while enhancing the attachment of microorganisms to the bone or foreign bodies.[27]

DIAGNOSIS

No single laboratory test is specific for the diagnosis of osteomyelitis, but some tests are indicative of osteomyelitis.

A definitive diagnosis can be made only with microbiologic identification of the pathogen or pathogens from a bone specimen. In acute hematogenous osteomyelitis, the diagnosis rests with isolation of the pathogen from the bone lesion or blood culture. Bone biopsies or aspirates are superior to blood cultures in yielding organisms.[28] When vertebral osteomyelitis is suspected, blood cultures and computed tomographic (CT)-guided needle biopsy have been successful in making a definitive diagnosis.[29]

Other tests that are of importance include a white blood cell count (WBC) and an erythrocyte sedimentation rate (ESR). A leukocytosis, with a left shift, may be consistent with an infectious process such as osteomyelitis. However, it has been reported that a normal WBC occurs in 40% to 75% of patients with acute osteomyelitis.[30]

Although nonspecific, ESRs are frequently elevated in excess of 20 mm per hour in acute untreated osteomyelitis. An ESR that returns to normal during therapy may be a favorable prognostic sign. The ESR is not a reliable laboratory test in patients who have inflammatory diseases, collagen vascular disease, or sickle cell disease or those receiving corticosteroids.[31]

C-reactive protein (CRP) is another nonspecific indicator of inflammation used primarily in neonates and children. The CRP level usually begins to decline within 6 hours of initiation of appropriate therapy.[32]

A culture diagnosis of contiguous osteomyelitis may be more complex. Because the infection arises from a contiguous abscess, cellulitis, or penetration of the overlying skin, culture specimens obtained from subcutaneous or other surrounding tissues may also need evaluation. The cultures may be obtained either by direct needle biopsy or at the time of surgical débridement. Caution should be used when evaluating culture specimens from draining sinus tracts because these areas may be heavily colonized. The results in this case may be misleading and not indicative of the actual pathogen at the site of infection.

In chronic osteomyelitis, blood cultures and drainage from the sinus tract are often not reliable. Needle aspiration of the subperiosteal or metaphyseal space is required if blood and tissue cultures are negative. Bone biopsy specimens should be carefully cultured and stained for aerobes, anaerobes, mycobacteria, and fungi.

A variety of imaging methods can be used in the diagnosis of osteomyelitis, but no imaging test can confirm the presence or absence of infection. Radiography is the initial imaging study of choice. Radiographic changes in the bone may lag 2 weeks behind the development of infection. With appropriate antimicrobial therapy, radiologic improvements may also lag behind clinical symptom improvement. Other imaging techniques, such as CT, magnetic resonance imaging (MRI), nuclear imaging studies (e.g., technetium or gallium), and positron emission tomography (PET), have improved disease detection and can reveal bony abnormalities even when plain radiographs are normal. These are more expensive techniques and are usually reserved for cases in which the diagnosis is equivocal.

MRI and CT have excellent resolution and can detect edema, destruction of the medulla, cortical destruction, periosteal reaction, articular damage, and soft tissue involvement even when plain radiographs are normal.[33] MRI has emerged as the preferred imaging technique for the diagnosis of osteomyelitis and soft tissue infections and is superior to CT in establishing the level of involvement of the infection. CT is preferred for establishing cortical bone destruction or sequestra as a guide for drainage or biopsy.[34] PET is another noninvasive method that assesses perfusion and metabolic states of tissue. PET enables detection and demonstration of the extent of chronic osteomyelitis with a high degree of accuracy.[35]

Technetium-99m methylene diphosphonate is the current radiopharmaceutical of choice for nuclear imaging.[36] After intravenous administration of the radionuclide, the skeletal system is imaged or scanned. Abnormal findings consistent with osteomyelitis are related to the technetium-99m uptake ability of the inflamed tissues due to increased bone activity and blood flow. This isotope is highly sensitive but not specific, so scanning studies may also be positive in the presence of other inflammatory processes such as trauma, tumor, or arthritis.[31] Gallium-67 citrate is a more selective radionuclide that is taken up by polymorphonuclear leukocytes that have mobilized to the site of bacterial infection.

TREATMENT

PHARMACOTHERAPY

Because the treatment of osteomyelitis involves a protracted commitment to antibiotic therapy, careful evaluation and diagnosis are paramount. The keys to effective treatment are initiating appropriate empiric antimicrobial therapy before the culture and sensitivity results are known, identifying the pathogens and their antibiotic sensitivities, and delivering adequate quantities of the antibiotic to the site of infection. Both parenteral and oral antibiotics are effective for the treatment of osteomyelitis, as long as serum and bone concentrations are adequate for eradication of the infecting organisms.

Parenteral Antibiotic Therapy. In uncomplicated cases of osteomyelitis, empiric antimicrobial regimens should provide adequate antistaphylococcal coverage. Additional empiric antibiotics can be initiated based on the presence of probable organisms, specific risk factors, and patient history. Initial therapy can be guided by the Gram stain results, as shown in Table 82.5. If Gram stain results are negative, broad-spectrum antibiotics should be initiated. After culture and sensitivity results are known, the therapy can be tailored to reflect the infecting organisms and their respective sensitivity profile.

Initial empiric therapy usually consists of high-dose parenteral antibiotics because these regimens achieve high

TABLE 82.5	Probable Organisms Associated With Gram Stain Results in Osteomyelitis and Infectious Arthritis
Gram Stain	**Probable Organisms**
Gram-positive cocci in clusters	S. aureus (methicillin-sensitive)
	Methicillin-resistant S. aureus (MRSA)
	Coagulase-negative staphylococci (typically methicillin-resistant, MRSE)
Gram-positive cocci in pairs/chains	S. pneumoniae
	Group A streptococci
	Group B streptococci
	Enterococci (group D streptococci)
Gram-negative bacilli	Enterobacteriaceae
	E. coli
	Enterobacter species
	Serratia species
	Salmonella species
Gram-negative diplococci	*Pseudomonas aeruginosa*
	Neisseria gonorrhoeae

steady-state bone and serum concentrations more quickly than orally administered drugs. The most commonly used empiric antimicrobial regimens based on patient age are summarized in Table 82.6.

Intravenous penicillinase-resistant penicillins (e.g., nafcillin, oxacillin) have the advantages of antistaphylococcal coverage, good bone penetration, bactericidal activity, and low cost. One disadvantage is the short half-life of these drugs, which results in a more frequent dose administration schedule. Also, the potential for penicillin-induced hypersensitivity or anaphylactic reactions exists. An alternative antibiotic is an intravenous first-generation cephalosporin such as cefazolin. Cefazolin can be used in some penicillin-allergic patients (e.g., in patients who have an inconsequential rash from penicillin) and has the advantage of good activity against *S. aureus* and some gram-negative organisms, such as *E. coli*. If a patient has had a serious allergic reaction to β-lactam antibiotics, clindamycin or vancomycin can be used in the treatment of staphylococcal osteomyelitis.

Appropriate antimicrobial therapy for polymicrobial contiguous osteomyelitis, with or without vascular insufficiency, may include an aminoglycoside (e.g., gentamicin, tobramycin) added to the antistaphylococcal regimens described earlier. Patients receiving aminoglycosides must be carefully monitored because of the potential for ototoxicity and nephrotoxicity, especially in children, older adults, and those with renal dysfunction. Alternatives include monotherapy with a broad-spectrum β-lactam antibiotic such as cefotaxime or ceftriaxone. These third-generation cephalospo-

TABLE 82.6	Empiric Antibiotic Treatment of Osteomyelitis and Infectious Arthritis Based on Patient Age	
Probable Organisms	**Antibiotic Regimen of Choice**[a]	**Alternative Antibiotics**
Neonates (<1 month)[b]		
S. aureus	Nafcillin/oxacillin 200 mg/kg/day AND	Cefazolin 100 mg/kg/day AND
Group B streptococci E. coli	Cefotaxime 100–150 mg/kg/day OR Nafcillin/oxacillin 200 mg/kg/day AND Gentamicin[c] 5–7.5 mg/kg/day	Gentamicin[c] 5–7.5 mg/kg/day Vancomycin 20–45 mg/kg/day (if methicillin-resistant S. aureus)
Infants, children, and adolescents (1 month–16 years)		
S. aureus	Nafcillin/oxacillin 50 mg/kg/dose IV q6h	Cefazolin 25 mg/kg/dose IV q6–8h
Methicillin-resistant S. aureus (MRSA)	Vancomycin[c] 10–15 mg/kg/dose IV q6h	Clindamycin 10 mg/kg/dose IV q6–8h
Group A streptococci	Penicillin G 100,000 units/kg/dose IV q6h	Clindamycin[d] 10 mg/kg/dose IV q6–8h
S. pneumoniae		
Penicillin-sensitive	Penicillin G 100,000 units/kg/dose IV q6h	Clindamycin 10 mg/kg/dose IV q6–8h
Penicillin-intermediate	Cefotaxime 50 mg/kg/dose IV q8h Ceftriaxone 50 mg/kg/dose IV q24h	Clindamycin 10 mg/kg/dose IV q6–8h
Penicillin-resistant	Vancomycin[c] 10–15 mg/kg/dose IV q6h	Clindamycin 10 mg/kg/dose IV q6–8h
Adults (>16 years)		
S. aureus	Nafcillin/oxacillin 2 g IV q6h	Cefazolin 2 g IV q8h Clindamycin 900 mg IV q8h
Methicillin-resistant S. aureus (MRSA)	Vancomycin[c] 1 g IV q12h	Clindamycin[d] 900 mg IV q8h Linezolid 600 mg IV/PO q12h
S. epidermidis (MRSE)	Vancomycin[c] 1 g IV q12h	
Group A streptococci	Penicillin G 4 million units IV q6h	Clindamycin 900 mg IV q8h
S. pneumoniae		
Penicillin-sensitive	Penicillin G 4 million units IV q6h	Clindamycin 900 mg IV q8h Ceftriaxone 1 g IV Q24h
Penicillin-intermediate	Cefotaxime 1 g IV q8h Ceftriaxone 1 g IV Q24h	Clindamycin 900 mg IV q8h
Penicillin-resistant	Vancomycin[c] 1 gram IV q12h	Levofloxacin 500 mg IV/PO daily

(continued)

TABLE 82.6	continued	
Probable Organisms	**Antibiotic Regimen of Choice**[a]	**Alternative Antibiotics**
P aeruginosa	Ceftazidime 2 g IV q8h OR Cefepime 2 g IV q12h AND Aminoglycoside[c] (gentamicin or tobramycin) 2.5 mg/kg/dose IV q8h or 4–7 mg/kg/dose IV q24h	Imipenem 500 mg IV q6h OR Piperacillin/tazobactam 3.375 g IV q6h AND Aminoglycoside
Salmonella	Ciprofloxacin 400 mg IV q12h	Third-generation cephalosporin (ceftriaxone)
E. coli	Ampicillin 1–2 g IV q6h	Cefazolin 2 g IV q8h
N. gonorrhoeae (infectious arthritis)	Ceftriaxone 1–2 g IV Q24h	Cefotaxime 1 g IV q8h
Mixed infections (aerobic and anaerobic)	Amoxicillin/clavulanate 875 mg PO q12hr (outpatient) OR Piperacillin/tazobactam 3.375 g IV q6h (hospitalized)	Imipenem 500 mg IV q6h Ampicillin/sulbactam 3 g IV q6h Ticarcillin/clavulanate 3.1 g IV q6h

[a] Based on normal renal function.

[b] Frequency determined by postnatal age and weight.

[c] Requires pharmacokinetic monitoring.

[d] Useful in community-acquired MRSA without erythromycin-inducible resistance (negative D test).

rins are highly active against *S. aureus* and common Enterobacteriaceae species. Ceftazidime, a third-generation cephalosporin, is less active against *S. aureus*, but it is the most active against *P. aeruginosa*.[37,38] Cefepime, a fourth-generation cephalosporin, has adequate *S. aureus* coverage and is active against *P. aeruginosa*. The current standard of care for the treatment of contiguous osteomyelitis, following surgical débridement, is a 4- to 6-week course of antibiotic therapy directed at organisms isolated from the culture.[39]

Anaerobic bacteria have been isolated in both acute hematogenous and contiguous osteomyelitis. Intraabdominal infections are often a source of anaerobic bacteremia. Anaerobic osteomyelitis of the mandible or the cranial and facial bones may result from the relatively high number of anaerobes present in the normal flora of the oral cavity. The most common form of osteomyelitis due to anaerobes, however, is that related to underlying peripheral vascular disease. This syndrome is almost always associated with long-standing diabetes mellitus or severe peripheral vascular disease. Patients at high risk of an anaerobic infection should be started on a broad-spectrum empiric antibiotic regimen to provide both aerobic and anaerobic coverage. Broad-spectrum agents include imipenem/cilastatin, piperacillin/tazobactam, ampicillin/sulbactam, and ticarcillin/clavulanate.

Chronic osteomyelitis is characterized by infected necrotic bone and repeated therapeutic failures. Any osteomyelitis may progress to a chronic infection. Both aggressive surgical débridement and long-term antibiotic therapy are required for the treatment of chronic osteomyelitis. Appropriate antimicrobial therapy includes a 4- to 6-week course of high-dose parenteral antibiotics specific for the microorganisms isolated from the infected bone. Oral therapy can be continued for a subsequent 2 to 4 weeks.[40] Despite adequate treatment, recurrence occurs in approximately 20% to 30% of patients.[41] When the infection relapses, prolonged oral antibiotic therapy is often used for suppression of infection rather than cure.

Special populations may require alternative therapy, such as those with nosocomial or prosthetic joint infections, intravenous drug users, or those with sickle cell disease. An empiric regimen for a patient with hemoglobinopathy would be a penicillinase-resistant penicillin plus a third-generation cephalosporin or a fluoroquinolone. Intravenous drug users should begin therapy that is active against *P. aeruginosa*, such as ciprofloxacin or levofloxacin, or the combination of an aminoglycoside plus ceftazidime, cefepime, or an extended-spectrum penicillin (e.g., piperacillin, ticarcillin). Patients with prosthetic joint devices may develop infections with organisms such as *S. epidermidis* or Propionibacterium species and may require vancomycin.

The duration of antibiotic therapy for the treatment of osteomyelitis has not been fully elucidated. The best cure rates are usually obtained when parenteral therapy is administered for a minimum of 4 to 6 weeks. However, the duration of therapy can vary depending on the etiology of the infection and host risk factors. For example, acute hematogenous osteomyelitis caused by *H. influenzae*, *Neisseria meningitidis*, and *S. pneumoniae* may be treated with shorter courses in a minimum of 14 days, whereas *S. aureus* and enteric gram-negative organisms usually require a minimum of 4 weeks.[38] Most clinicians prefer to use the amelioration of clinical signs, normalization of laboratory parameters (e.g., WBC and ESR), and improvement in radiographic findings in determining the patient-specific length of therapy for osteomyelitis from contiguous foci or chronic osteomyelitis.

The management of osteomyelitis in children and adults often includes surgery and immobilization in addition to antibiotic therapy. In neonates, surgical intervention by débridement of necrotic tissue is controversial and less frequently desired.[7]

The emergence of antibiotic resistance, especially associated with gram-positive organisms, is a growing concern in the treatment of osteomyelitis.[42] Methicillin-resistant *S. aureus* (MRSA), a common nosocomial pathogen, has become an increasing cause of community-acquired infections, especially in children. Community-acquired MRSA can develop in patients with no predisposing risk factors or history of hospitalization. Clindamycin, sulfamethoxazole-trimethoprim (with or without rifampin), and vancomycin have been used in the treatment of community-acquired MRSA osteomyelitis.[43,44] Antibiotic sensitivity testing is crucial for community-acquired MRSA infections due to the risk of inducible resistance to clindamycin in erythromycin-resistant strains. If an isolate is resistant to erythromycin but sensitive to clindamycin, further testing must be performed to determine if inducible resistance is present. Detection of inducible clindamycin resistance cannot be accomplished with routine antibiotic sensitivity panels; a disk diffusion method (D test) must be performed by the laboratory to determine its presence. The D test involves placing an erythromycin disk and a clindamycin disk close together on an agar plate and determining the shape of the clindamycin zone of inhibition.[45] If erythromycin-inducible resistance is present, the zone will appear flattened and resemble a D. If the D test is negative, clindamycin is an appropriate treatment option for community-acquired MRSA infections.

Several new antibiotics have been approved in recent years for the treatment of MRSA and vancomycin-resistant enterococci. While these newer agents have not been approved for the treatment of osteomyelitis, they have been used successfully in the treatment of osteomyelitis due to resistant gram-positive infections. Linezolid, an oxazolidinone antibiotic, can achieve therapeutic bone concentrations and it has high oral bioavailability; it is given using a twice-daily regimen.[46] Linezolid is available in equipotent intravenous and oral formulations, which aids in both inpatient and outpatient therapy. It has been used to treat prosthetic hip infections and osteomyelitis associated with diabetic foot infections caused by vancomycin-resistant *Enterococcus faecium* and MRSA.[47–49] Thrombocytopenia, anemia, and leukopenia have been associated with the use of linezolid. The development of these adverse effects is associated with prolonged therapy (more than 2 weeks). Quinupristin-

dalfopristin, a streptogramin antibiotic, is a combination of two antibiotics in a 30:70 ratio to provide synergistic activity against gram-positive bacteria. It has been used successfully to treat patients with osteomyelitis due to vancomycin-resistant *E. faecium* and MRSA.[50,51] Although it is available only as an intravenous formulation, it can be successfully administered in an outpatient setting.[51] Myalgias and arthralgias are the most frequently reported adverse effects with the use of quinupristin-dalfopristin. Daptomycin, a cyclic lipopeptide, has been used in an experimental animal model for the treatment of MRSA osteomyelitis.[52]

Oral Antibiotic Therapy. Oral antibiotics are advantageous for the long-term treatment of osteomyelitis because prolonged intravenous antibiotic therapy can be associated with iatrogenic complications (e.g., phlebitis, local and vascular infections, excess fluid administration, patient discomfort) and higher patient cost. Most clinicians recommend at least 2 weeks of parenteral therapy followed by oral therapy for the remainder of treatment.[53,54] A variety of oral agents have been used, including penicillins, cephalosporins, clindamycin, and fluoroquinolones.[55,56]

In children with hematogenous osteomyelitis, a brief course of intravenous antibiotics (typically 3 to 10 days) may be followed by oral therapy for several additional weeks.[57] The serum bactericidal titer (SBT) is reported to be a useful indicator of the adequacy of oral therapy in children with infections due to *S. aureus*.[58] The SBT assesses the ability of serial dilutions of the patient's serum to kill the infecting organism. When these tests are used, a peak serum sample is drawn and a target SBT of 1:8 or greater and a trough titer of 1:2 or greater are recommended.[58,59]

In adults, the fluoroquinolones are promising agents for the treatment of gram-negative osteomyelitis, including that due to *P. aeruginosa*. Long-term suppressive therapy with this class of drugs can attenuate the signs and symptoms of chronic refractory osteomyelitis.[60] The fluoroquinolones have shown excellent efficacy against Enterobacteriaceae. Further studies comparing the fluoroquinolones to traditional intravenous antibiotic regimens are needed before the fluoroquinolones supplant these agents in the treatment of osteomyelitis due to other organisms such as *P. aeruginosa* and *S. aureus*. The indiscriminate use of quinolones is especially worrisome, given the ability of *S. aureus* to develop resistance during treatment. However, the fluoroquinolones may be used in combination with rifampin to help minimize resistance and improve outcomes, even in patients with prostheses.[40] In children, clinicians must weigh the risks against the benefits of treating osteomyelitis with a fluoroquinolone because of the potential for arthropathy or chondrodysplasia.[61] While this adverse effect has never been reported in children, it was evident in early animal studies involving the fluoroquinolones.

Antibiotic Bone Concentrations. Debate continues over the relevance of antibiotic concentrations in infected bone. Clinical studies have failed to show that antibiotic bone concentrations considerably above the minimum inhibitory concentration (MIC) of the infecting organism are required for effective treatment of osteomyelitis.[62,63] There are several reasons for this controversy. A variety of sampling techniques and assay methods were used in these studies when bone samples were obtained from patients without bone infections who were undergoing orthopedic procedures. The vascular supply to infected bone may significantly affect the antibiotic bone concentration. Infected tissue that is highly vascularized will achieve higher antibiotic bone concentrations than an area with compromised blood flow. Animal models of bone infection are being used to clarify the relationship between antibiotic bone concentrations and the treatment of osteomyelitis.

Home Antibiotic Therapy. Administering parenteral antibiotics on an outpatient basis is an obvious alternative to hospitalization in patients who need long-term treatment of selected infectious diseases such as osteomyelitis and endocarditis. This method of treatment is a safe, efficacious, and cost-effective alternative to prolonged hospitalization.[64] A candidate for outpatient parenteral antibiotic therapy must meet three criteria: (a) the infection must require treatment beyond the expected duration of hospitalization, (b) the patient must be otherwise medically stable, and (c) there must be no equally effective and safe oral antibiotic regimen.[65] Therapy should be initiated in the hospital, where observation for untoward effects and the overall tolerability of the regimen can be assessed. Once the patient is sent home, drugs are administered through a peripheral venous access site (e.g., intermittent needle therapy), a central catheter (e.g., peripheral intravenous central catheter), or directly through a Hickman-Broviac catheter. Intermittent needle therapy has a disadvantage in that the needle must be replaced every 3 days. Also, patients often report local pain and inflammation. Central catheters generally remain in place for the duration of therapy. Hickman-Broviac catheters have the disadvantage of requiring minor surgery for placement.

To ensure the safety and efficacy of outpatient parenteral antibiotic therapy, the expertise of the physician and the pharmacist must be combined. Pharmacologic considerations include safety, efficacy, stability, and storage conditions. Patient factors include manual dexterity, the ability of a friend or family member to assist, expense, proximity to a medical center for drug supplies and follow-up, and minimal interference with activities of daily living.[66] Despite these considerations, outpatient parenteral therapy can be a cost-saving tool when compared with the expense of prolonged hospitalization.

Local Antibiotic Therapy
Antibiotic-Impregnated Beads. Antibiotic-impregnated beads may be used as an alternative treatment or in conjunction with systemic antibiotic therapy for the treatment of osteomyelitis. This form of local antibiotic therapy originated with the use of antibiotic-impregnated bone cement for the treatment of infected arthroplasties. From this concept

evolved the use of antibiotic-impregnated cement beads, which are strung on surgical wire, for the treatment of local bone and soft tissue infections. Several antibiotics, including aminoglycosides, vancomycin, penicillins, cephalosporins, clindamycin, and erythromycin, have been incorporated into cement beads. In this system, polymethyl methacrylate (PMMA) acts as a carrier for the antibiotic. The release of antibiotic from the bead follows a bimodal pattern: approximately 5% of the antibiotic is released within the first 24 hours, and the remainder is released over several weeks to months.[67]

Impregnated PMMA beads have a number of advantages over systemic antibiotic therapy. Parenteral antibiotic therapy and its associated high serum concentrations may lead to nephrotoxic, ototoxic, or allergic events. Also, due to the poor vascularization in the area of infected bone, high doses of parenteral antibiotics are often required for adequate penetration into necrotic areas. Use of impregnated beads results in local antibiotic concentrations that are 5 to 10 times higher than concentrations achieved via systemic administration.[67] The PMMA used as a carrier for the antibiotic has not been shown to significantly alter the host's normal immune response, but this remains a concern.

A number of disadvantages also exist. Not all antibiotics are suitable candidates for incorporation into cement beads. Drug characteristics that must be taken into consideration include the following: (a) the drug must be heat stable up to 100°C due to the exothermic reaction generated when mixing the bone cement, (b) the antibiotic must be water-soluble so that it can easily diffuse through the cement, (c) the antibiotic should have a low incidence of hypersensitivity reactions, and (d) the antibiotic should be bactericidal at low concentrations. An additional surgical procedure is required to remove the beads.

NONPHARMACOLOGIC THERAPY

Surgery. Infections in the bone have long been a formidable foe of orthopedic surgeons. Antimicrobials often control the disease, but surgical débridement is usually necessary to eradicate the infection. Surgical intervention should be undertaken if pus is found on bone biopsy or aspiration or if a metaphyseal cavity is seen on the initial radiograph. The surgical approach consists of draining and irrigating the abscess and sinus tracts. The procedure is supplemented by preoperative and postoperative antibiotics given systemically or locally as antibiotic-impregnated beads. If no abscess is found, antibiotic therapy alone should be effective. If a patient does not show symptomatic improvement after 36 to 48 hours of empiric antibiotic therapy, the bone may need to be reaspirated and débrided. In adult osteomyelitis, any contiguous infectious process should be evaluated for surgical drainage. Surgical débridement is required to excise avascular tissue and necrotic bone in patients with chronic infection.

Hyperbaric Oxygen. Hyperbaric oxygen (HBO) therapy has been used in the treatment of osteomyelitis.[68] HBO is administered by placing the patient in an enclosed chamber where oxygen pressure greater than sea level, usually 2 atmospheres, can be effected. Hypoxia at the site of infection results in poor wound healing. By attenuating the hypoxic environment in the infected tissues, HBO promotes the formation of a collagen matrix and subsequent angiogenesis. Increasing the oxygen tension also revives and amplifies neutrophil-mediated killing of bacteria.

Several studies have shown beneficial effects of HBO when it is used in the treatment of chronic refractory osteomyelitis.[68] However, the scarcity of well-controlled prospective studies make it difficult to support the routine use of HBO therapy. The cost-effective use of HBO as a standard regimen in the treatment of osteomyelitis is controversial. An average treatment regimen for osteomyelitis consists of 20 to 30 sessions lasting 90 minutes each, with the cost for one session between $300 and $400.[68] Adverse effects of HBO include reversible myopia, mild to moderate pain secondary to barotrauma (rupture of the middle ear, cranial sinuses, teeth, or lungs), and, rarely, self-limiting seizures.

HBO is adjunctive therapy and should always be used in conjunction with surgery and antibiotics. It should be reserved for cases of chronic refractory osteomyelitis that have not responded to standard surgical and antibiotic therapy.

IMPROVING OUTCOMES

The treatment of osteomyelitis involves prompt initiation of broad-spectrum antibiotics active against staphylococci, streptococci, and common enteric gram-negative rods as soon as possible after the onset of symptoms. This may minimize the number of patients who require extensive surgical débridement or those who develop chronic osteomyelitis. Patients with acute osteomyelitis have the best prognosis, having an approximately 80% cure rate when parenteral antibiotics are maintained for more than 4 weeks and appropriate surgical intervention is employed.[58] Children with acute osteomyelitis can expect similar results if, after initial parenteral antibiotics, oral therapy compliance can be ensured. Peak SBT values of 1:8 or greater are monitored to optimize therapy.

In chronic osteomyelitis, the prognosis is substantially less favorable. Unsuccessful results have been attributed to several factors: short-term antibiotic treatment, poor bone penetration by antibiotics, existence of bone abscess and sequestra, presence of foreign bodies, and the frequent nosocomial origin of pathogens that are often resistant to several antibiotics.[69] The combination of proper surgical débridement of dead bone and sequestra along with appropriate antibiotic treatment is critical and may increase follow-up success rates to 50%.[53] Patients for whom surgical débridement was unsuccessful or contraindicated may require long-term suppressive treatment with antibiotics to control their infections.

Outpatient intravenous antibiotic therapy represents a safe and cost-effective method for treating conditions such

TABLE 82.7	Patient Instructions for Administering Intravenous Antibiotics

1. Remove antibiotic from refrigerator and thaw (if applicable).
2. Draw heparin solution into syringe and replace needle.
3. Hang intravenous bag above arm.
4. Establish fluid level in chamber and purge air.
5. Cleanse intravenous catheter stopper with alcohol.
6. Connect intravenous tubing to catheter.
7. Establish appropriate flow rate.
8. Complete infusion and use heparin flush.
9. Carefully dispose of used materials to prevent needlestick.

as osteomyelitis and infectious arthritis.[66] Outpatient intravenous antibiotic therapy requires selection of patients who are both medically and psychologically stable. Education of patients regarding compliance with antibiotic regimen is extremely helpful in ensuring successful therapy. Patients must learn to properly manage drugs and equipment, care for their intravenous access site, administer the medications, and recognize complications. Patients are trained by a pharmacist or nurse employed by the hospital or home care pharmacy.

Administration of intravenous antibiotics in the home represents only one of several methods of administration outside of the hospital. For patients who are not candidates for home intravenous therapy, medications may be administered in a physician's office, outpatient clinic, day-stay clinic, or emergency department. Patient instructions for administration of intravenous antibiotics are listed in Table 82.7.

PHARMACOECONOMICS

The treatment of osteomyelitis often involves a protracted commitment to long-term parenteral antibiotics and surgical débridement, which can entail a major financial burden. In the era of prospective reimbursement of providers, it is not prudent to prolong hospitalization of an afebrile, stable patient for the sole purpose of administering 4 to 6 weeks of intravenous antibiotics. Outpatient parenteral antibiotic therapy, via clinic visits, home health agencies, or self-administration, can substantially reduce hospital costs. Patient education, compliance, and follow-up visits are essential for eradication of the infection.

SUMMARY

Infection of bone remains difficult to treat, despite recent advances in antimicrobial therapy, diagnostic procedures and tests, and refinements in surgical techniques. When left untreated, osteomyelitis can result in significant systemic disease and bone deformity. The medical management involves accurate classification of the disease, identification of the offending pathogen via culture, surgical débridement, radiologic procedures, laboratory studies, and prompt initiation of high-dose parenteral antibiotic therapy. Most β-lactam and aminoglycoside antibiotics penetrate normal and infected bone adequately but do not penetrate necrotic bone. Chronic osteomyelitis may require several months of treatment with intravenous and oral antibiotics and is associated with a less favorable prognosis. The majority of cases of acute osteomyelitis can be treated with monotherapy for a

minimum of 4 weeks and are associated with a favorable prognosis. The oral fluoroquinolones are probably the most promising agents for the treatment of osteomyelitis caused by gram-negative bacilli. HBO may be useful as adjunctive therapy for chronic, refractory patients. Administering antibiotics at home has been shown to be a safe and cost-effective alternative in specific patients who would otherwise need prolonged hospitalization. Oral antibiotic therapy offers advantages in terms of convenience and comfort for the patient and avoids iatrogenic disease and nosocomial superinfections, but it requires good patient compliance, careful follow-up, and laboratory monitoring.

INFECTIOUS ARTHRITIS

TREATMENT GOALS: INFECTIOUS ARTHRITIS

The treatment goals for infectious arthritis are essentially identical to those described in the osteomyelitis section.

DEFINITION

Infectious arthritis, also known as septic arthritis or pyogenic arthritis, is a serious infection of the joints affecting individuals of all ages. The infection begins acutely in a monoarticular joint and is characterized by an inflammatory reaction of the joint space, synovium, synovial fluid, and articular cartilage. Chronic monoarticular and polyarticular joint involvement is also common, depending on the causative agent. The disease is characterized as a closed-space infection with swelling, tenderness, and accumulation of pus within the joint.

When infectious arthritis is suspected in any patient, it should be considered a medical emergency because the disease may be fatal. Prompt diagnosis and treatment are also important to minimize damage to the joint or prevent spread of infection to contiguous bone and soft tissue.

Bacteria are the most common cause of joint infections, but fungi, viruses, and chlamydia have also been isolated. Viral infectious arthritis is associated with multiple joints and frequently involves inflammation without presentation of pus. Mycobacteria or fungi present as chronic granulomatous monoarticular arthritis. The distribution of these sites and organisms are shown in Table 82.8. The discussion in this chapter deals exclusively with bacterial arthritis.

EPIDEMIOLOGY

The yearly incidence of infectious arthritis is 2 to 10 per 100,000 in the general, healthy population and increases dra-

matically to 30 to 70 per 10,000 in high-risk patients, such as those with rheumatoid arthritis or joint prostheses.[70] The pathogens that cause infectious arthritis vary considerably with the age of the patient. A few bacterial species cause the majority of cases, although given the right conditions any microorganism may infect a joint.

ETIOLOGY

Infectious arthritis can be classified into nongonococcal and gonococcal etiologies. The most common bacterial causes of infectious arthritis among different age groups are listed in Table 82.9. Gram-positive organisms are the most common pathogens isolated in nongonococcal arthritis. Staphylococci, particularly *S. aureus*, are the most common etiologic organisms in people of all ages. Streptococcal species (e.g., group A, group B, and *S. pneumoniae*) are also common causes. Gram-negative enteric bacilli (e.g., *E. coli*, *Proteus* species, *Salmonella* species, and occasionally *Pseudomonas* species) cause 20% of cases of infectious arthritis in infants, children, and adults.[71] Neonates, patients greater than 60 years of age, and intravenous drug users are particularly at risk for infections due to gram-negative organisms. *S. epidermidis* is the leading cause in patients with prosthetic joints. Although rare, anaerobic infections have been isolated in patients with traumatic injuries, prosthetic joints, and diabetes. *Neisseria gonorrhoeae* remains the most common cause of infectious arthritis in young, otherwise healthy, sexually active adults. Up to 20% of clinically diagnosed cases of infectious arthritis are never confirmed with a positive synovial fluid aspirate or blood culture.[71]

TABLE 82.8	Differential Diagnosis of Arthritis Syndromes	
Acute Monoarticular Arthritis	**Chronic Monoarticular Arthritis**	**Polyarticular Arthritis**
Staphylococcus aureus	*Mycobacterium tuberculosis*	*Neisseria meningitides*
Streptococcus pneumoniae	Nontuberculous mycobacteria	*N. gonorrhoeae*
β-Hemolytic streptococci	*Borrelia burgdorferi*	Nongonococcal bacterial arthritis
Gram-negative bacilli	*Treponema pallidum*	Bacterial endocarditis
Neisseria gonorrhoeae	*Candida* species	*Candida* species
Candida species	*Sporothrix schenckii*	Poncet's disease (tuberculous rheumatism)
Crystal-induced arthritis	*Coccidioides immitis*	Hepatitis B virus
Fracture	*Blastomyces dermatitidis*	Parvovirus B19
Hemarthrosis	*Aspergillus* species	HIV
Foreign body	*Cryptococcus neoformans*	Human T lymphotropic virus type I
Osteoarthritis	*Nocardia* species	Rubella virus
Ischemic necrosis	*Brucella* species	Arthropod-borne viruses
Monoarticular rheumatoid arthritis	Legg-Calve-Perthes disease	Sickle cell disease flare
	Osteoarthritis	Reactive arthritis
		Serum sickness
		Acute rheumatic fever
		Inflammatory bowel disease
		Systemic lupus erythematosus
		Rheumatoid arthritis/Still's disease
		Other vasculitides
		Sarcoidosis

From Thaler SJ, Maguire JH. Infectious arthritis, 15th ed. New York: McGraw-Hill, 2001:1945, with permission.

RISK FACTORS

Risk factors for the development of infectious arthritis can be categorized into systemic (host) factors and local factors. Host factors, such as age, preexisting joint disease, and immunosuppression, predispose patients to develop infectious arthritis. Disorders that increase the risk of infectious arthri-tis include diabetes mellitus, preexisting rheumatoid arthri-tis, organ transplantation, liver disease, malignancy, chronic renal failure, acquired immunodeficiency syndrome, or in-travenous drug abuse.[72–74]

Local risk factors include direct joint trauma, prosthetic joints, recent joint surgery, puncture wounds (e.g., animal or human bites, stepping on a nail), intraarticular corticosteroid

TABLE 82.9	Commonly Isolated Organisms in Infectious Arthritis Based on Patient Age			
Neonates (<1 month)	**Infants and Children (1 month–5 years)**	**Children and Adolescents (5–16 years)**	**Adults (>16 years)**
S. aureus	*S. aureus*	*S. aureus*	*N. gonorrhoeae*
Group B streptococci	Group A, B streptococci	Group A streptococci	*S. aureus*
Enterobacteriaceae (particularly *E. coli*)	*S. pneumoniae*	Gram-negative bacilli	*S. epidermidis*
	Gram-negative bacilli		Enterobacteriaceae
			P. aeruginosa
			Group A, B streptococci
			S. pneumoniae

administration, rheumatoid arthritis, and osteoarthritis arising from a single joint. Approximately 2% of prosthetic joints develop an infection. One in 17,000 to 50,000 administrations of intraarticular corticosteroids leads to infectious arthritis.[75]

PATHOPHYSIOLOGY

The development of infectious arthritis is usually secondary to hematogenous spread of infection to a joint from a distant focus, or it may represent extension from infected bone. The latter is especially true in children younger than 1 year of age when the epiphyseal growth plate contains infection.

Once the organism invades the joint space, the infection usually develops in the microvasculature of the synovial membrane (Fig. 82.2; *see color insert*). At this site, the bacteria proliferate rapidly and trigger an acute inflammatory synovitis. This response is activated by bacteria engulfed by macrophages, synoviocytes, and migrating polymorphonuclear cells and is associated with the release of proteolytic enzymes, which can destroy intraarticular cartilage in as little as 3 days.[76] The infectious process induces a joint effusion, which increases intraarticular pressure, mechanically impeding blood and nutrient supply to the joint.[77] The con-

tinued inflammatory process may lead to destruction of the cartilage and invasion of the adjacent bone, causing osteomyelitis.[78]

CLINICAL PRESENTATION AND DIAGNOSIS

SIGNS AND SYMPTOMS

Nongonococcal infectious arthritis usually presents with an acute onset of a painful, swollen, and erythematous monoarticular joint. Fever in the range of 38.3 to 38.9°C, sometimes higher, and malaise usually accompany the initial onset of localized symptoms. However, patients with rheumatoid arthritis or renal or hepatic insufficiency or patients on chronic immunosuppressive therapy may not present with fever. Joint range of motion is substantially limited as a result of the swelling and tenderness. The knee is involved in most cases (40% to 50%), followed by the hip (20% to 25%), ankle, elbow, shoulder, and joints of the hand, although hip infections are more common in young children.[79,80]

A thorough inspection of all joints for erythema, swelling (90% of cases), warmth, and tenderness is essential for diagnosing infection. A hip or shoulder effusion is often difficult to detect on physical examination, so the use of imaging studies is important in establishing the diagnosis of infectious arthritis. Polyarticular arthritis is most likely to occur in patients with rheumatoid arthritis or other collagen vascular diseases, in intravenous drug users, or in patients with overwhelming sepsis.[81]

N. gonorrhoeae is the most common cause of infectious arthritis in young, otherwise healthy, sexually active adults and is a potentially serious complication of a urogenital infection. Unlike nongonococcal arthritis, gonococcal arthritis is usually polyarticular.[82] Typical symptoms of gonococcal arthritis include inflammation, swelling, warmth, redness of the overlying skin, rash, pain, and restriction of motion in the affected joints. A small number of papules that progress to hemorrhagic pustules may develop on the trunk and the distal extremities. If left untreated, 1% to 3% of infections have been reported to disseminate to the synovial fluid and cause arthritis, which can cause various degrees of joint tissue damage.[76] Women are three times more likely than men to present with disseminated gonococcal infection because their initial infection is asymptomatic and may go untreated for a longer time.

DIAGNOSIS

The definitive diagnosis of infectious arthritis requires isolation and identification of bacteria from the peripheral blood or synovial fluid by Gram stain or culture. The synovial fluid culture is positive in 90% of nongonococcal cases.[83] In gonococcal infectious arthritis, *N. gonorrhoeae* is often not recovered from the synovial fluid, and blood cultures are positive in only approximately 20% of cases. In most cases of gonococcal arthritis, the presumptive diagnosis is

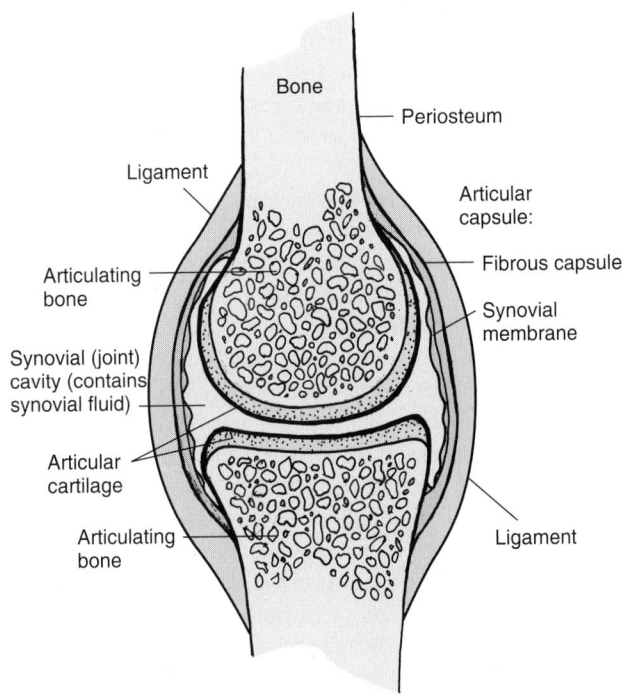

FIGURE 82.2 A typical synovial joint (*see color insert*). (From Oatis CA. Kinesiology. The Mechanics and Pathomechanics of Human Movement. Baltimore: Lippincott Williams & Wilkins, 2003.)

based on signs and symptoms and the presence of gonococci on a culture from the urogenital tract, rectum, or throat.[84] The presumptive diagnosis of infectious arthritis can be supported by the following laboratory data: (a) Gram stain of the joint fluid; (b) synovial fluid leukocytosis greater than 50,000 per mm^3 with neutrophils greater than 75%; (c) decreased synovial fluid glucose relative to the patient's serum glucose; and (d) increased synovial fluid levels of lactate dehydrogenase, protein, and lactic acid. Increases in synovial fluid lactate dehydrogenase, protein, and lactic acid are nonspecific and may be seen in inflammatory joint diseases.[76] The absence of uric acid or calcium pyrophosphate dehydrate crystals in the synovial fluid rules out gout and pseudogout, respectively. ESR and CRP are elevated in most patients and can be used to monitor therapy.

Amplification of bacterial DNA by polymerase chain reaction (PCR) is a promising technique that may be more widely used in the future to allow a more rapid and accurate diagnosis of most bacterial infections. PCR has been shown to be 96% specific and 76% sensitive in detecting *N. gonorrhoeae* DNA in the synovial fluid.[83]

Early radiologic evaluation of the joint is generally nonspecific, showing only joint effusion or soft tissue swelling with displacement of tissue. Radionuclide imaging, CT, and MRI are far more sensitive than plain films in early septic arthritis.[77]

TREATMENT

PHARMACOTHERAPY

The treatment of infectious arthritis involves microbiologic assessment, immediate antibiotic therapy, and joint aspiration. The empiric antibiotic regimen should be based on the Gram stain of aspirated fluid, as well as the patient's age and concomitant risk factors. Even if the Gram stain of aspirated fluid is negative, an empiric antibiotic regimen that covers *S. aureus* and streptococci should be initiated.[84] In these cases, infection is likely, and prompt initiation of empiric antibiotics will decrease the potential for long-term sequelae. Tables 82.7 and 82.8 outline empiric antibiotic regimens for the most common causative organisms. Modifications of the empiric antibiotic regimens can be made once definitive culture and sensitivity results are known.

Parenteral antibiotic therapy is usually administered for 2 to 4 weeks, although the optimal duration of therapy has not been extensively studied. Shorter courses of parenteral treatment with an early switch to oral antibiotics are often efficacious in adults with gonococcal arthritis or in children.[84]

Successful treatment of infectious arthritis is contingent on the antibiotic's ability to penetrate the joint space and achieve sufficient synovial concentrations. Most antibiotics (e.g., penicillin, cephalosporins, aminoglycosides, and fluoroquinolones) achieve a maximal concentration in synovial fluid several times higher than the MIC for the most common infecting organisms. Intraarticular administration of antibi-

otics is usually unnecessary and not recommended because it may cause a secondary chemical synovitis.[77] Although aminoglycosides are reported to achieve adequate concentrations in the joint fluid, their activity is diminished in acidic environments. Drainage of the infected joint is paramount when using this class of drugs.[85]

NONPHARMACOLOGIC THERAPY

As with osteomyelitis, patients with suppurative arthritis are best managed with a combination of antibiotic therapy and débridement procedures. Débridement for arthritis is done routinely with needle aspiration but may include arthroscopy and open surgical drainage with drainage tube placement. Needle aspiration is used mostly on peripheral joints such as the elbow, wrist, knee, and ankle. Axial joints such as the shoulder, sternoclavicular joint, and hip undergo open drainage.[76] Intermittent or even daily needle aspiration may be needed during the first weeks of therapy, with laboratory results of the repeated aspiration serving as a clinical indicator. Parameters to be monitored are the volume of synovial fluid, total cell count, and percentage of polymorphonuclear leukocytes, which should decrease with each aspiration.

IMPROVING OUTCOMES

The overall prognosis for infectious arthritis is generally favorable and has not changed much over the past few decades, despite more effective antibiotics and improved methods of joint drainage. Prompt use of therapeutic dosages of antibiotics administered within the first week of the infection can produce complete symptomatic recovery with little if any residual limitation of joint motion. Permanent joint damage develops in 50% of cases.[71] Nongonococcal infectious arthritis has been associated with a mortality rate of 10%.[71] The majority of deaths occur in patients with underlying risk factors such as sepsis, rheumatoid arthritis, and malignancy.

A favorable prognosis is usually contingent on several host factors. In children, the prognosis is correlated with parameters such as the particular joint involved, type of organism, adequate drainage, appropriate antibiotic coverage, and time of initiation of treatment relative to the onset of symptoms. Infections of the hip are associated with the highest rate of sequelae, and the morbidity in these cases may not be evident until months or years later. In adults, the outcome of treatment is considerably worse if the offending organism is not eradicated from the synovial fluid within 6 days of initiating therapy or if the patient is over 60 years old.[78] *S. aureus* has the greatest propensity for causing chronic problems.[86]

SUMMARY

Infectious arthritis arises from hematogenous spread of organisms through the synovial membrane or from direct extension from a contiguous infection. The most common causative organism is *S. aureus*, although other pathogens such as streptococci, Enterobacteriaceae, *P. aeruginosa*, and *N. gonorrhoeae* have also been isolated. The initial presentation is a painful, erythematous, and swollen joint. The diagnosis rests on isolation of the pathogen from joint fluid obtained during needle aspiration or débridement. Optimal treatment includes the prompt and judicious use of β-lactam antimicrobial agents coupled with drainage of the affected joint. The duration of therapy can range from 2 to 4 weeks, depending on the offending pathogen. Infectious arthritis is associated with low mortality rates and few residual symptoms if recognized and treated properly and with alacrity.

KEY POINTS

- It is important to make the diagnosis of osteomyelitis or infectious arthritis early in the course of the disease because the prognosis depends on the rapidity and adequacy of treatment
- Typical physical findings in a patient with acute hematogenous osteomyelitis include tenderness over the involved bone and decreased range of motion in adjacent joints
- Except for culture results, no single laboratory test is diagnostic of osteomyelitis or infectious arthritis. Therefore, careful monitoring of the trends of the WBC with differential, ESR, and perhaps CRP is required
- The diagnosis of infectious arthritis rests on the isolation of the pathogens from joint fluid obtained by aspiration or débridement
- Children with acute bone pain and tenderness and signs of systemic sepsis should be considered to have osteomyelitis until proven otherwise
- *S. aureus* is the most common pathogen causing both osteomyelitis and infectious arthritis, although other microbes are often found, depending on the age of the patient, concomitant disease states, and risk factors
- Young, otherwise healthy, sexually active adults who have joint pain and stiffness should be evaluated and cultured for gonococcal infection
- The basic principles for the treatment of osteomyelitis and infectious arthritis include adequate débridement followed by identification of the organism, selection of the correct antibiotic, and delivery of adequate quantities of the antibiotic to the site of infection for an extended period
- There is little difference in effectiveness between oral and intravenous antibiotics as long as they achieve serum concentrations sufficient to eradicate the pathogens
- In the treatment of osteomyelitis, oral agents may be efficacious if used in the appropriate patient population and if compliance can be ensured

- Outpatient parenteral antibiotic therapy for osteomyelitis may, in specific patients, be a cost-saving tool when compared with the expense of prolonged hospitalization for the sole purpose of administering intravenous antibiotics
- The duration of antibiotic therapy for treatment of acute osteomyelitis has not been fully elucidated; however, the best cure rates are obtained when parenteral therapy is administered for a minimum of 4 to 5 weeks. More prolonged therapy (i.e., months) may be necessary for chronic osteomyelitis

REFERENCES

1. Waldvogel FA, Medoff G, Swartz MN. Osteomyelitis: a review of clinical features, therapeutic considerations and unusual aspects (first of three parts). N Engl J Med 282:198–206, 1970.
2. Waldvogel FA, Medoff G, Swartz MN. Osteomyelitis: a review of clinical features, therapeutic considerations and unusual aspects (second of three parts). N Engl J Med 282:198–206, 1970.
3. Waldvogel FA, Medoff G, Swartz MN. Osteomyelitis: a review of clinical features, therapeutic considerations and unusual aspects (third of three parts). N Engl J Med 282:198–206, 1970.
4. Cierny G, Mader JT, Pennick JJ. A clinical staging system for adult osteomyelitis. Contemp Orthop 10:17–37, 1985.
5. David R, Barron BJ, Madewell JE. Osteomyelitis, acute and chronic. Radiol Clin North Am 25:1171–1201, 1987.
6. Mader JT, Shirtliff M, Calhoun JH. Staging and staging application in osteomyelitis. Clin Infect Dis 25:1303–1309, 1997.
7. Gentry LO. Antibiotic therapy for osteomyelitis. Infect Dis Clin North Am 3:485–499, 1990.
8. Nelson JD. Acute osteomyelitis in children. Infect Dis Clin North Am 4:513–522, 1990.
9. Gentry LO. Approach to the patient with osteomyelitis. In: Kelley WN, ed. Textbook of internal medicine, 3rd ed. Philadelphia: Lippincott-Raven, 1997:1560–1565.
10. Karwowska A, Davies HD, Jadavji T. Epidemiology and outcome of osteomyelitis in the era of sequential intravenous-oral therapy. Pediatr Infect Dis J 17:1021–1026, 1998.
11. Dirschl DR, Almekinders LC. Osteomyelitis: common causes and treatment recommendations. Drugs 45:29–43, 1993.
12. Anderson JR, Scobie WG, Watt B. The treatment of acute osteomyelitis in children: 10-year experience. J Antimicrob Chemother 7 (Suppl A):43–50, 1981.
13. Wald ER. Risk factors for osteomyelitis. Am J Med 78 (Suppl 6B):206–212, 1985.
14. Vibhagool A, Calhoun J, Mader JP, et al. Therapy of bone and joint infections. Hosp Formul 28:63–85, 1993.
15. Hass DW, McAndrew MP. Bacterial osteomyelitis in adults: evolving considerations in diagnosis and treatment. Am J Med 101:550–561, 1996.
16. Burnett MW, Bass JW, Cook BA. Etiology of osteomyelitis complicating sickle cell disease. Pediatrics 101:296–297, 1998.
17. Lipsky BA. Osteomyelitis of the foot in diabetic patients. Clin Infect Dis 25:1318–1326, 1997.
18. Norden CW. Lessons learned from animal models of osteomyelitis. Rev Infect Dis 10:103–110, 1988.
19. Belmatoug N, Cremieux AC, Bleton R, et al. A new model of experimental prosthetic joint infection due to MRSA: a microbiologic, histopathologic, and MRI characterization. J Infect Dis 174:414–417, 1996.
20. Nair SP, Meghji S, Wilson M, et al. Bacterially induced bone destruction: mechanism and misconceptions. Infect Immun 64:2371–2380, 1996.
21. Hermann M, Vandaux PE, Pittet D, et al. Fibronectin, fibrinogen and laminin act as mediators of adherence of clinical staphylococcal isolates to foreign material. J Infect Dis 158:693–701, 1988.

22. Hudson MC, Ramp WK, Nicholson NC, et al. Internalization of *S aureus* by cultured osteoblasts. Microbial Pathogenesis 19:409–419, 1995.
23. Bamberger DM. Osteomyelitis: a commonsense approach to antibiotic and surgical treatment. Postgrad Med 95:177–184, 1993.
24. Caputo GM, Cavanagh PR, Ulbrecht JS, et al. Assessment and management of foot disease in patients with diabetes. N Engl J Med 331:854–860, 1994.
25. Lew DP, Waldvogel FA. Osteomyelitis. N Engl J Med 336:999–1007, 1997.
26. Gutman L. Acute, subacute, and chronic osteomyelitis and pyogenic arthritis in children. Curr Probl Pediatrr 15:1–72, 1985.
27. Marrie TJ, Costerton JW. Mode of growth of bacterial pathogens in chronic polymicrobial human osteomyelitis. J Clin Microbiol 22:924–933, 1985.
28. Sonnen GM, Henry NK. Pediatric bone and joint infections. Diagnosis and antimicrobial management. Pediatr Clin North Am 43:933–947, 1996.
29. Howard CB, Einhorn M, Dagan R, et al. Fine-needle bone biopsy to diagnose osteomyelitis. J Bone Joint Surg [Br] 76:311–314, 1994.
30. Waldvogel FA, Papageorgiou PS. Osteomyelitis: the past decade. N Engl J Med 303:360–370, 1980.
31. Stuart J, Whicker JT. Tests for detecting and monitoring the acute phase response. Arch Dis Child 63:115–117, 1988.
32. Unkila-Kallio L, Kallio MJT, Peltola H. The usefulness of C-reactive protein levels in the identification of concurrent septic arthritis in children who have acute hematogenous osteomyelitis. A comparison with the usefulness of the erythrocyte sedimentation rate and the white blood-cell count. J Bone Joint Surg [Am] 76:848–853, 1994.
33. Schauwecker DS. The scintigraphic diagnosis of osteomyelitis. Am J Rheum 158:9–18, 1992.
34. Magid D. Computed tomographic imaging of the musculoskeletal system. Radiol Clin North Am 32:255–273, 1994.
35. Guhlmann A, Brecht-Krauss D, Suger G, et al. Chronic osteomyelitis: detection with FDG PET and correlation with histopathologic findings. Radiology 206:749–754, 1998.
36. Tumeh SS, Tohmeh AG. Nuclear medicine techniques in septic arthritis and osteomyelitis. Rheum Dis Clin North Am 17:559–583, 1991.
37. Gentry LD. Role for newer beta-lactam antibiotics in the treatment of osteomyelitis. Am J Med 78 (Suppl 6A):134–139, 1985.
38. Tice AD. Osteomyelitis. Hosp Pract 28 (Suppl 2):36–39, 1993.
39. Nelson JD, Norden C, Mader JT, et al. Evaluation of new anti-infective drugs for the treatment of acute hematogenous osteomyelitis in children. Clin Infect Dis 15 (Suppl 1):S162–S166, 1992.
40. Rissing JP. Antimicrobial therapy for chronic osteomyelitis in adults: role of the quinolones. Clin Infect Dis 25:1327–1333, 1997.
41. Ramos OM. Chronic osteomyelitis in children. Pediatr Infect Dis J 21:431–432, 2002.
42. Dagan R. Management of acute hematogenous osteomyelitis and septic arthritis in the pediatric patient. Pediatr Infect Dis J 12:88–93, 1993.
43. Martinez-Aguilar G, Hammerman WA, Mason EO, et al. Clindamycin treatment of invasive infections caused by community-acquired, methicillin-resistant and methicillin-susceptible *Staphylococcus aureus* in children. Pediatr Infect Dis J 22:593–598, 2003.
44. Adra M, Lawrence KR. Trimethoprim/sulfamethoxazole for treatment of severe *Staphylococcus aureus* infections. Ann Pharmacother 38:338–341, 2004.
45. Fiebelkorn KR, Crawford SA, McElmeel ML, et al. Practical disk diffusion method for detection of inducible clindamycin resistance in *Staphylococcus aureus* and coagulase-negative staphylococci. J Clin Microbiol 41:4740–4744, 2003.
46. Rana B, Butcher I, Grigoris P, et al. Linezolid penetration into osteo-articular tissues. J Antimicrob Chemother 50:747–750, 2002.
47. Lipsky BA, Itant K, Norden C, et al. Treating foot infections in diabetic patients: a randomized, multicenter, open-label trial of linezolid versus ampicillin-sulbactam/amoxicillin-clavulanate. Clin Infect Dis 38:17–24, 2004.
48. Bassetti M, Biagio AD, Cenderello G, et al. Linezolid treatment of prosthetic hip infections due to methicillin-resistant *Staphylococcus aureus* (MRSA). J Infection 43:143–157, 2001.
49. Till M, Wixson, RL, Pertel PE. Linezolid treatment for osteomyelitis due to vancomycin-resistant *Enterococcus faecium*. Clin Infect Dis 34:1412–1414, 2002.
50. Summers M, Misenhimer GR, Anthony SJ. Vancomycin-resistant *Enterococcus faecium* osteomyelitis: successful treatment with quinupristin-dalfopristin. South Med J 94:353–355, 2001.
51. Rehm SJ, Graham DR, Srinath L, et al. Successful administration of quinupristin/dalfopristin in the outpatient setting. J Antimicrob Chemother 47:639–645, 2001.
52. Mader JT, Adams K. Comparative evaluation of daptomycin (LY146032) and vancomycin in the treatment of experimental methicillin-resistant *Staphylococcus aureus* osteomyelitis in rabbits. Antimicrob Agents Chemother 33:689–692, 1989.
53. Mader JT, Calhoun JH. Osteomyelitis. In: Mandell GL, Douglas RG, Bennett JE Jr., eds. Principles and practice of infectious diseases. New York: Churchill Livingstone, 1995:1039–1051.
54. Cierny G, Mader JT. Adult chronic osteomyelitis. Orthopedics 7:1557–1564, 1984.
55. MacGregor RR, Graziani AL. Oral administration of antibiotics: a rational alternative to the parenteral route. Clin Infect Dis 24:457–467, 1997.
56. Black J, Hunt TL, Godley PJ, et al. Oral antimicrobial therapy for adults with osteomyelitis or septic arthritis. J Infect Dis 155:967–972, 1987.
57. Syrogiannopoulos GA, Nelson JD. Duration of antimicrobial therapy for acute suppurative osteoarticular infections. Lancet 1:37–40, 1988.
58. Marshall GS, Mudido P, Rabalais GP, et al. Organism isolation and serum bactericidal titers in oral antibiotic therapy for pediatric osteomyelitis. South Med J 89:67–70, 1996.
59. Vosti K. Serum bactericidal test: past, present, and future use in the management of patients with infections. Curr Clin Top Infect Dis 10:43–55, 1989.
60. Waldvogel FA. Use of quinolones for the treatment of osteomyelitis and septic arthritis. Rev Infect Dis 11 (Suppl 5):S1259–S1263, 1989.
61. Zabraniecki L, Negrier I, Vergne P, et al. Fluoroquinolone-induced tendinopathy: report of six cases. J Rheum 23:516–520, 1996.
62. Fitzgerald RH. Antibiotic distribution in normal and osteomyelitic bone. Orthop Clin North Am 15:537–545, 1984.
63. LeFrock J, Smith BR. The penicillins and bone penetration of antibiotics. J Foot Surg 26 (Suppl 1):S34–S41, 1987.
64. Rich D. Physicians, pharmacists, and home infusion antibiotic therapy. Am J Med 97:3–8, 1994.
65. Gilbert DN, Dworkin RJ, Raber SR, et al. Outpatient parenteral antimicrobial drug therapy. N Engl J Med 337:829–838, 1997.
66. Brown RB. Selection and training of patients for outpatient intravenous antibiotic therapy. Rev Infect Dis 13 (Suppl 2):S147–S151, 1991.
67. Henry SL, Galloway KP. Local antibacterial therapy for the management of orthopaedic infections. Clin Pharmacokinet 29:36–45, 1995.
68. Tibbles PM, Edelsberg JS. Medical progress: hyperbaric-oxygen therapy. N Engl J Med 334:1642–1648, 1996.
69. Galankis N. Giamarellou H, Moussat T, et al. Chronic osteomyelitis caused by multi-resistant gram-negative bacteria; evolution of treatment with newer quinolones after prolonged follow-up. J Antimicrob Chemother 39:241–246, 1997.
70. Garcia-De La Torre I. Advances in the management of septic arthritis. Rheum Dis Clin North Am 29:61–75, 2003.
71. Ryan MJ, Kavanaugh R, Wall PG, et al. Bacterial joint infections in England and Wales: analysis of bacterial isolates over a four year period. Br J Rheumatol 36:370–373, 1997.
72. Perez LC. Septic arthritis. Baillieres Clin Rheumatol 13:37–58, 1999.
73. Jones A, Weston V. Septic arthritis. CPD Rheumatol 1:54–8, 1999.
74. Gupta MN, Sturrock RD, Field M. Prospective comparative study of patients with culture proven and high suspicion of adult-onset septic arthritis. Ann Rheum Dis 62:327–331, 2003.
75. Duggan JM, Georgiadis GM, Kleshinski JF. Management of prosthetic joint infections. Infect Med 18:534–541, 2001.
76. Cimmino MA. Recognition and management of bacterial arthritis. Drugs 54:50–60, 1997.
77. Goldenberg DL. Septic arthritis. Lancet 351:197–202, 1998.
78. Smith JW. Infectious arthritis. Infect Dis Clin North Am 4:523–538, 1990.

79. Brooks GF, Pons VG. Septic arthritis. In: Hoeprich PD, Jordan MC, Ronald AR, eds. Infectious diseases, 5th ed. Philadelphia: Lippincott, 1994:1382–1389.

80. Morgan DS, Fisher D, Merianos A, et al. An 18-year clinical review of septic arthritis from tropical Australia. Epidemiol Infect 117: 423–428, 1996.

81. Zimmerman B 3rd, Mikolich DJ, Lally EV. Septic sacroiliitis. Semin Arthritis Rheum 26:592–604, 1996.

82. Dubost JJ, Fis I, Denis P, et al. Polyarticular septic arthritis. Medicine 72:296–310, 1993.

83. Goldenberg DL, Reed JI. Bacterial arthritis. N Engl J Med 312: 764–771, 1985.

84. Smith JM, Piercy EA. Infectious arthritis. Clin Infect Dis 20: 225–231, 1995.

85. Hamed KA, Tam JY, Prober CG. Pharmacokinetic optimisation of the treatment of septic arthritis. Clin Pharmacokinet 21:156–163, 1996.

86. Kaandorp CJE, van Schaardenburg D, Krijnen P, et al. Risk factors for septic arthritis in patients with joint disease: a prospective study. Arthritis Rheum 38:1819–1825, 1995.

Sexually Transmitted Diseases

83

Vicky Dudas

Sexually transmitted diseases (STDs), which are occasionally referred to as venereal diseases, are infections that are caused by a variety of pathogenic microorganisms, as summarized in Table 83.1. It is generally accepted that patients with one STD are at greater risk for the development of other STDs, concurrently or at some later point in time. In addition, sexual partners of patients with diagnosed STDs are at high risk for the development of STDs. Age is an important risk factor given that the incidence of STDs is much higher in persons in their teens and twenties. Although rates of STDs are higher in men than in women, it is important to remember that the usual clinical manifestations are more obvious in men, leading to a larger percentage of men seeking treatment. Over the past decade, primarily because of concern about transmission of the human immunodeficiency virus (HIV), much effort has

been directed toward changes in sexual practices to reduce the potential for transmission of disease by sexual contact.[1] In addition, because many STDs are asymptomatic, STD screening programs are a critical component in treatment and prevention of transmission.[2] Nevertheless, STDs continue to be an important public health concern, with annual costs for treatment of nonacquired immunodeficiency syndrome (AIDS) STDs in the United States of over 5 billion dollars.[3]

This chapter is organized into three general sections: (a) a review of common urethritis syndromes, (b) discussion of infections associated with genital ulceration, and (c) limited comments on less common STDs. Several diseases that are transmitted by sexual contact, such as hepatitis, HIV infection, AIDS, and parasitic infections, are discussed in other chapters of this text.

TABLE 83.1	Sexually Transmitted Pathogens and Associated Disease
Pathogens	**Corresponding Clinical Syndrome/Disease**
Bacteria	
Neisseria gonorrhoeae	Gonorrhea
Treponema pallidum	Syphilis
Haemophilus ducreyi	Chancroid
Calymmatobacterium granulomatis	Granuloma inguinale
Gardnerella vaginalis	Nonspecific vaginitis
Mycoplasma	
Ureaplasma urealyticum	Nongonococcal urethritis
Chlamydia	
Chlamydia trachomatis	Nongonococcal urethritis or lymphogranuloma venereum
Viruses	
Herpes simplex type II (or I)	Herpes genitalis
Human immunodeficiency virus	Acquired immunodeficiency syndrome (AIDS)
Hepatitis A, B, and C	Hepatitis
Human papillomavirus (HPV)	Condylomata acuminata
Poxvirus	Molluscum contagiosum
Parasites	
Trichomonas vaginalis	Trichomoniasis or nonspecific vaginitis
Giardia lamblia	Giardiasis
Entamoeba histolytica	Amebiasis
Phthirus pubis	Pediculosis
Sarcoptes scabiei	Scabies

TREATMENT GOALS: SEXUALLY TRANSMITTED DISEASES

- Prevent disease transmission.
- Completely eradicate the infectious pathogen.
- Eliminate or alleviate clinical symptoms.
- Prevent associated long-term sequelae.

PREVENTION GUIDELINES

It is the responsibility of health care professionals to educate persons at risk for acquiring an STD. It is important to detect disease in asymptomatic patients and in those who are unlikely to seek treatment to reduce transmission rates. In addition, it is important to remember that for every patient with an STD requiring therapy, there are one or more infected sexual partners who should be identified and treated regardless of the appearance of symptoms.

The most effective method of preventing the transmission of STDs (including HIV) is the use of a latex condom used consistently and correctly, with or without spermicide, with each act of sexual intercourse. Currently there is a female condom (Reality) available that is a lubricated polyurethane sheath with a diaphragmlike ring at each end. Female condoms provide an alternative for women and should reduce the risk of STDs; however, to date they have been shown to prevent the transmission of only trichomoniasis. Vaginal spermicides can reduce the risk of cervical chlamydia and gonorrhea, but their effect on preventing transmission has not been evaluated.[4] Case-control studies have shown that the use of a diaphragm protects against cervical gonorrhea, chlamydia, and trichomoniasis.[4]

The STD that is most commonly seen is urethritis, or inflammation of the urethra, which usually presents clinically as a urethral discharge that may be accompanied by dysuria (painful or difficult urination). Clinically, urethritis is usually divided into gonococcal or nongonococcal syndromes on the basis of the infecting pathogen. Nationwide, chlamydia (nongonococcal urethritis) is much more common than gonococcal urethritis (gonorrhea).[5] Although the usual clinical features of gonococcal and nongonococcal urethritis differ to some degree, there is sufficient overlap in presentation to make distinguishing between the two syndromes difficult.[6]

GONORRHEA

EPIDEMIOLOGY

Although the actual incidence of gonorrhea is unclear because of the large number of asymptomatic carriers and unreported cases, an estimated 700,000 to 800,000 new infections occur each year in the United States. It is caused by *Neisseria gonorrhoeae,* a Gram-negative aerobic coccus that usually grows in pairs (diplococci). Individuals between ages 15 and 24 years have the highest reported incidence of gonorrhea. The incidence of gonorrhea is reported to be 10 times greater in nonwhites than in whites. Other risk factors for gonorrhea include low socioeconomic status, urban residence, single marital status, and a previous history of gonococcal infections.[7,8]

PATHOPHYSIOLOGY

Gonorrhea primarily affects the epithelium and mucous membranes of the lower genital tract; however, it may also involve the eyes, oropharynx, and anus. Humans appear to be the only natural host for this intracellular pathogen. Transmission of gonorrhea is almost always by sexual intercourse, although perinatal transmission of the disease may occur. Once the gonococci are attached to the cell membranes by pili, one of the primary virulence factors, they are pinocytosed. Subsequently, polymorphonuclear leukocytes invade the tissue, leading to secretion of purulent exudates. The rate of male to female transmission of gonorrhea during sexual intercourse is reported to be higher than female to male transmission, probably because the cervix is a more accessible target. The risk of transmission from an infected female to her male partner ranges from 20% to 40% per episode of unprotected vaginal intercourse; transmission risk from an infected male to his female partner has been reported to be closer to 50% and up to 90% per episode.[7,9]

CLINICAL PRESENTATION AND DIAGNOSIS

SIGNS AND SYMPTOMS

The clinical presentation of gonorrhea varies greatly in individuals from complicated to uncomplicated and symptomatic to asymptomatic. In men, the incubation period for gonococcal urethritis is usually 2 to 7 days; the majority of patients develop symptoms within a week of the initial infection. The clinical presentation of gonorrhea is usually characterized by profuse, purulent urethral discharge that is associated with dysuria. Many cases of gonorrhea in men are asymptomatic and resolve spontaneously over the course of several weeks without specific treatment. However, up to 10% of untreated cases may be further complicated by the development of acute epididymitis, periurethral abscess, acute prostatitis, seminal vesiculitis, or urethral strictures.

In women, gonorrhea primarily involves the endocervix and the urethra. Most women develop acute symptoms within 10 days of infection, consisting of increased vaginal discharge and dysuria that are often overlooked because they tend to be nonspecific. Progression to salpingitis may occur in up to 15% of untreated women and usually is characterized by the development of acute abdominal or pelvic pain. In addition, 25% to 65% of women with gonorrhea are also coinfected with *Chlamydia trachomatis* or *Trichomonas vaginalis.*[4] Approximately 15% of women with untreated gonorrhea develop pelvic inflammatory disease, which may be associated with infertility and ectopic pregnancies if inadequately managed.

Infectious involvement of other body sites by *N. gonorrhoeae* can also be seen. Pharyngeal gonococcal infection, developed after orogenital sexual activity with an infected partner, is more common in women and homosexual men. The presentation is often asymptomatic, but symptoms resembling acute streptococcal pharyngitis may occur. Anal transmission of *N. gonorrhoeae* in women is generally by perianal contamination with vaginal discharge; in men it is usually via receptive anal intercourse with an infected partner. Most cases of anorectal gonorrhea are asymptomatic, but anal pruritus, constipation, tenesmus, and rectal bleeding have been observed in association with this condition.[7] Ocular gonococcal infection most commonly involves the conjunctiva and is often considered secondary to autoinoculation from fingers contaminated by sexual contact with an individual with urogenital gonorrhea. Gonococcal conjunctivitis may be serious and requires timely initiation of aggressive antibiotic therapy to prevent corneal ulceration. Disseminated gonococcal infection secondary to hematogenous spread is uncommon but is often considered the cause of septic arthritis in otherwise healthy young adults. Most patients with disseminated gonococcal infection do not have significant fevers or elevated white blood cell counts but commonly have monoarticular arthritic complaints in the wrist, knee, or ankle (any joint can be involved). In addition, a striking pustular, erythematous rash, located primarily on the extremities, is also common in patients with bacteremia secondary to *N. gonorrhoeae*.[4,7]

Newborns exposed to gonococci in utero or during delivery are at risk for the development of gonococcal ophthalmia neonatorum, a sight-threatening infection of the conjunctiva. Fortunately, this condition is rare today in the United States because of the use of aggressive ophthalmic prophylaxis after delivery.

DIAGNOSIS

The diagnosis of gonorrhea is best made by identification of *N. gonorrhoeae* from a specimen taken from an involved site. In women, cultures taken from the cervix produce the highest yield, but urethral cultures are also acceptable. Men should have urethral and anal cultures performed. Cultures can become positive within 24 to 48 hours. Culturing and susceptibility testing of the organism is important for diagnosis in areas where drug-resistant *N. gonorrhoeae* is a concern in determining therapeutic options.[4,10] An alternative diagnostic technique that is commonly used in clinics to evaluate the collected specimen is Gram staining. If intracellular Gram-negative diplococci are observed, a presumptive diagnosis of gonorrhea is made, pending confirmation by subsequent culture. In men, Gram-stain evaluation of the urethral discharge is highly sensitive and highly specific; therefore, culture confirmation is not considered necessary. However, the Gram stain is not considered acceptable as the sole method to diagnose gonococcal infection of the pharynx or rectum or in women with endocervical infection.[7] Rapid diagnostic tests based on detection of gonococcal antigens or cellular components do not have better sensitivity or specificity than Gram stain and culture and are, therefore, infrequently used, but they may have a role in asymptomatic individuals.

THERAPEUTIC PLAN

A number of treatment options for the management of gonococcal disease are available to the practicing clinician. Most cephalosporins and fluoroquinolones have potent in vitro and in vivo activity against *N. gonorrhoeae*. Historically, penicillins, tetracyclines, and sulfonamides were used widely as therapy for gonococcal infections, but widespread resistance now prevents their clinical use. Discovered in the 1970s, penicillinase-producing strains of *N. gonorrhoeae* make up a significant number of strains throughout the world. Table 83.2 summarizes the current Centers for Disease Control and Prevention (CDC) treatment recommendations for gonococcal infections.[10] Selection of a specific therapeutic regimen must be based on careful consideration of efficacy and safety, allergy history, age, pregnancy, patient preference, and costs.

TREATMENT

Many clinicians consider IM ceftriaxone to be the treatment of choice for noncomplicated gonorrhea; this choice is based on extensive clinical evaluations demonstrating effective clearing of gonococcal infections from all sites.[4,10] Resistance to ceftriaxone has not been reported to date, so concern about potential treatment failure is reduced. Previous CDC treatment guidelines recommended an IM ceftriaxone dose of 250 mg, but single doses as low as 62.5 mg have been reported to produce 100% cure rates in noncomplicated gonorrhea.[10] The currently recommended ceftriaxone regimen of 125 mg allows for a smaller volume for IM injection and a lower drug cost. The serum levels of ceftriaxone are well above the minimum inhibitory concentration (MIC_{90}) of the organism, as shown in Table 83.3. There are limited data suggesting that IM ceftriaxone provides adequate coverage for incubating syphilis as well, a therapeutic benefit that other treatment options do not have.[11] The most common adverse effects associated with IM ceftriaxone are pain at the injection site and gastrointestinal side effects such as nausea and diarrhea.

Cefixime is the only oral cephalosporin that is recommended by the CDC for the treatment of gonococcal infections. A cefixime dose of 400 mg is effective for urethral disease, but it has not been well studied for pharyngeal infection and does not provide activity against incubating syphilis.[12] The oral dose has been demonstrated to have cure rates of approximately 97%; however, it does not provide serum levels as high as those produced by ceftriaxone, as shown in Table 83.3. The main side effect associated with cefixime is gastrointestinal complaints such as nausea and diarrhea. Availability of cefixime has been limited because the manufacturer discontinued it in 2002; however Lupin, Ltd has received Food and Drug Administration (FDA) approval to manufacture cefixime. At the time of this publication the 400 mg tablets are not yet available; the suspension (100 mg/5 ml) is available.[8] Other oral agents approved by the FDA for gonorrhea (e.g., cefpodoxime) are less well studied.

The preferred fluoroquinolones, ciprofloxacin, levofloxacin, and ofloxacin, are also highly safe and effective single-dose oral alternatives for the treatment of uncomplicated gonorrhea, but they are contraindicated for use during preg-

TABLE 83.2	CDC Recommendations for Treatment of Gonococcal Infections		
Presentation	**Drug Regimen**	**Cost**[a]	**Alternative Regimens/Comments**
Uncomplicated gonorrhea of the cervix, urethra, rectum, and pharynx (see comments)[b]	Cefixime[c] 400 mg PO in single dose or	$ variable	Ceftizoxime 500 mg IM, cefotaxime 500 mg IM, cefotetan 1 g IM, cefoxitin 2 g IM with probenecid 1 g orally. Limited clinical experience.
	Ceftriaxone 125 mg IM in single dose or	$15.82	
	Ciprofloxacin 500 mg PO in single dose or	$5.55	Quinolones should not be used for infections acquired in HI, CA, MA, and Pacific Islands
	Ofloxacin 400 mg PO in single dose or	$6.00	
	Levofloxacin 250 mg PO in a single dose	$9.35	Quinolones and tetracyclines are contraindicated in pregnancy and children.
	PLUS (cotreatment of *Chlamydia*)		
	Doxycycline 100 mg PO bid for 7 days Or	$1.20	If first-line therapy is contraindicated, spectinomycin 2 g IM in a single dose can be used.
	Azithromycin 1 g PO in single dose	$25.58	
Disseminated gonococcal infection[d,e]	Ceftriaxone 1g IV or IM q24h or	$49.00	Cefotaxime 1 g IV q8hr. Ceftizoxime 1 g IV q8h.
	if β-lactam allergy:		
	Ciprofloxacin 400 mg IV q12h or	$30.00	
	Spectinomycin 2 g IM q12h	$34.00	
	Continue for 24–48 hr after improvement, then continue oral therapy for a total of 7 days:		
	Cefixime 400 mg PO bid or	Variable	
	Ciprofloxacin 500 mg PO bid or		
	Ofloxacin 400 mg bid		
Gonococcal conjunctivitis (adult)	Ceftriaxone 1 g IM as single dose	$49.00	Infected eye should be lavaged with saline solution one time.
Gonococcal ophthalmia neonatorum	Ceftriaxone 25–50 mg/kg IV or IM in a single dose, not to exceed 125 mg	Variable	Topical antibiotic therapy alone is inadequate and is unnecessary with systematic therapy.
Disseminated gonococcal infections in infants	Ceftriaxone 25–50 mg/kg IM or IV qd for 7 days or 10–14 days for documented meningitis	Variable	If meningitis is present, treat for 10–14 days.

[a] Based on 2004 Red Book AWP for daily drug costs or total drug costs for single-dose regimens.

[b] Patients should refer sex partners for evaluation and treatment. Patients should avoid sexual intercourse until therapy is completed and they are symptom free.

[c] Note: Pharyngeal infections are more difficult to treat. Cefixime should not be used.

[d] Gonococcal meningitis: ceftriaxone 2 g IV q12h 2 weeks.

[e] Gonococcal endocarditis: ceftriaxone 2 g IV q12–24h 4 weeks.

PO, by mouth; IM, intramuscularly; HI, Hawaii; CA, California; MA, Massachusetts; bid, twice daily; IV, intravenously; q, every; qd, every day.

TABLE 83.3	Selected Pharmacokinetics of Antibiotics Active Against *Neisseria gonorrhoeae*			
Antimicrobial Agent	**Dose/Route**	**Peak Serum Concentration (mg/L)**	**$t_{1/2}$ (hr)**	**MIC_{90} (μ g/mL)**
Cefixime	400 mg PO	3.7	3–4	< 0.03
Ceftriaxone	125 mg IM	12–15	7–8	< 0.06
Ciprofloxacin	500 mg PO	2.4	4	< 0.25
Ofloxacin	400 mg PO	2.9	4–5	< 0.625

PO, my mouth; IM, intramuscularly.
(From Judson F. Gonorrhea. Med Clin North Am 74:1353–1366, 1990, with permission.)

nancy and for children under age 18, according to the package labeling.[10] However, quinolone experience has accumulated in the adolescent population indicating that the benefit outweighs the risk.[13] Ofloxacin is more active than ciprofloxacin against *C. trachomatis* but requires prolonged dosing (7–10 days) for successful treatment of chlamydial infections (Table 83.4). Unfortunately, fluoroquinolone-resistant *N. gonorrhoeae* has become problematic in Asia, Pacific Islands (including Hawaii), California, and Massachusetts such that quinolones are no longer recommended by the CDC to treat gonococcal infections that are acquired in these locations. Resistance to the fluoroquinolones is expected to continue to spread in several other regions of the United States and around the world.[8,10] The overall prevalence of gonorrhea with decreased susceptibility to fluoro-

quinolones, except in California and Hawaii, was preliminarily reported to be 0.9% in 2003. Fluoroquinolone-resistant gonorrhea demonstrates an MIC of 1.0 μg per milliliter or greater to ciprofloxacin and 2 μg per milliliter or greater to ofloxacin.[10] The fluoroquinolones provide no activity against *Treponema pallidum*.[8,10] Considering the geographic variability in resistance, it is imperative that clinicians obtain a travel history and monitor quinolone susceptibility data. Other single-dose fluoroquinolones have been used, such as lomefloxacin 400 mg by mouth (PO), and norfloxacin 800 mg PO ; however these regimens do not offer any advantages over the other quinolones.

A single 2,000 mg oral dose of azithromycin provides a 95% cure rate for uncomplicated gonorrhea.[14] Unfortunately, at this dose azithromycin is expensive and causes

TABLE 83.4	CDC Recommendations for Treatment of Chlamydial Infections	
Presentation	**Initial Drug Regimen**	**Alternatives/Comments**
Uncomplicated urethritis, endocervical or rectal infection	Azithromycin 1 g PO as a single dose *or* Doxycycline 100 mg PO bid for 7 days	Erythromycin base 500 mg qid *or* Erythromycin ethylsuccinate 800 mg PO qid for 7 days *or* Ofloxacin 300 mg PO bid for 7 days *or* Levofloxacin 500 mg PO qd for 7 days
Urethritis during pregnancy	Erythromycin base 500 mg PO qid for 7 days *or* Amoxicillin 500 mg PO tid for 7 days	Erythromycin base 250 mg qid for 14 days Erythromycin ethylsuccinate 800 mg PO qid for 7 days Erythromycin ethylsuccinate 400 mg PO qid for 14 days *or* Azithromycin 1 g orally as single dose
Ophthalmia neonatorum	Erythromycin 50 mg/kg/day PO qid for 14 days	
Lymphogranuloma venereum	Doxycycline 100 mg PO bid for 21 days	Erythromycin base 500 mg PO qid for 21 days

Patients should refer sex partners for evaluation and treatment. Patients should avoid sexual intercourse until therapy is completed and they are symptom free.
CDC, Centers for Disease Control and Prevention; PO, by mouth; qid, four times daily; bid, twice a day.

considerable gastrointestinal intolerance such that it is not considered an option for routine treatment of gonorrhea.

Spectinomycin was once a commonly used alternative to β-lactam treatment of gonorrhea. Today it is useful only for patients with urogenital or anal infections who are unable to tolerate therapy with a cephalosporin or fluoroquinolone.[4,10]

Of importance, a regimen that is active against *C. trachomatis* should be administered following the initial treatment of gonorrhea (Table 83.2).

Disseminated gonococcal infections are best treated with a prolonged course of intravenous (IV) ceftriaxone, cefotaxime, or ceftizoxime. Therapy should be continued for 24 to 48 hours after significant clinical improvement (e.g., decrease in fever and white blood cell count), then followed with a suitable oral agent for another 7 days. Gonococcal endocarditis and meningitis require several weeks of IV antibiotic therapy.[7]

Topical therapy with 1% silver nitrate, 1% tetracycline, or 0.5% erythromycin is recommended by the American Academy of Pediatrics for immediate postpartum administration to all newborns, but it is insufficient to treat gonococcal ophthalmia neonatorum in a baby born to a mother with active gonorrhea. A single IM or IV dose of ceftriaxone (25–50 mg/kg, not to exceed 125 mg total) is thought to be adequate treatment for gonococcal ophthalmia neonatorum and gonococcal conjunctivitis in adults.[4]

IMPROVING OUTCOMES

Routine follow-up is not necessary for patients who are treated with a regimen recommended in the CDC guidelines because of the very low treatment failure rates that have been reported. Patients who are treated with alternative regimens should be evaluated within 3 to 7 days to ensure resolution of symptoms. In most cases, persistence of clinical signs and symptoms indicates reinfection rather than treatment failure or may indicate coinfection with another infectious pathogen, such as *C. trachomatis*. Any gonococci isolated after initial treatment course should be tested for antimicrobial susceptibility. In either case the patient needs another diagnostic workup along with aggressive identification and treatment of all recent sexual partners.[10]

NONGONOCOCCAL URETHRITIS

EPIDEMIOLOGY

Nongonococcal urethritis is more common than gonorrhea in the United States. The most common cause of nongonococcal urethritis, *C. trachomatis,* accounts for up to 55% of cases. An estimated 4 million Americans contract chlamydia each year. It is an obligate intracellular organism that has features of bacteria and viruses.[15,16] *Chlamydia* species, like viruses, require host cellular material for replication, yet like bacteria maintain their cellular identity. There are 15 known serovars of *C. trachomatis*. The lymphogranuloma venerum strains produce invasive infections; the remaining strains produce superficial infections of epithelial cells. It is estimated that almost 50% of individuals with gonorrhea are coinfected with *C. trachomatis*.[17] Other pathogens that can produce a urethritis syndrome include the bacterium *Ureaplasma urealyticum,* identified in approximately 20% to 40% of cases, and the parasite *T. vaginalis,* seen in fewer than 10% of patients.[15,16] However, approximately 20% to 30% of men with urethritis fail to demonstrate gonococcal or common nongonococcal pathogens on evaluation. These cases of urethritis may be due to yeasts, viruses, and other bacteria that are difficult to culture or identify.[15] Risk factors associated with chlamydial infection include change in partner, sexually active adolescents, lower socioeconomic status, and African-American race.[17]

CLINICAL PRESENTATION AND DIAGNOSIS

SIGNS AND SYMPTOMS

The clinical presentation of nongonococcal urethritis cannot be distinguished easily from the clinical features of gonococcal urethritis. Common symptoms of nongonococcal urethritis in men include dysuria, polyuria, and the presence of a mucoid urethral discharge within several weeks of exposure; however, approximately 25% of men are asymptomatic.[15] Unlike gonorrhea, the discharge seen in nongonococcal urethritis is typically mucoid or mucopurulent, and dysuria is present in fewer than 50% of cases. In addition, *C. trachomatis* is responsible for the majority of cases of acute epididymitis in men.

The majority of women with chlamydial urethral infections are clinically asymptomatic, making the identification of these individuals almost impossible.[17] Dysuria and urinary frequency are uncommon with urethral infections, but when symptoms occur, a mucopurulent discharge from the endocervicitis is most commonly seen. Symptoms associated with chlamydial infection are usually much less severe than those associated with gonorrhea. In one study, 70% of the chlamydial infections were detected during screening, at which time the women were asymptomatic.[18] Chlamydia is a major cause of pelvic inflammatory disease, which may subsequently lead to tubal infertility or ectopic pregnancy. In a manner similar to gonorrhea, chlamydia may be transmitted to an infant during vaginal delivery through an infected birth canal. The most common presentations in the neonate are conjunctivitis and nasopharyngeal infection.

DIAGNOSIS

Identification of the infecting organism for most cases of nongonococcal urethritis is hampered because the two most common pathogens, *C. trachomatis* and *U. urealyticum,* cannot be cultured by routine laboratory procedures. Therefore, the diagnosis of nongonococcal urethritis usually depends on the presence of a characteristic urethral discharge (microscopically greater than four polymorphonuclear leukocytes per oil immersion field on a smear of an intraurethral swab specimen), the exclusion of gonorrhea, and a clinical response to therapy. Serologic tests that are specific for chlamydia and tissue-culturing techniques are thought to be unnecessary for the management of STDs in general clinical practice.[15] Rapid office tests using an enzyme immunoassay for the diagnosis of chlamydia infections are now available and are reported to offer excellent sensitivity and specificity.[19] Additional tests that allow rapid identification of chlamydial antigens in genital secretions are the enzyme-linked immunoabsorbent assay (ELISA) and the direct fluorescent antibody (DFA) test. Both tests are highly sensitive and specific.[20]

THERAPEUTIC PLAN

A number of antibiotic regimens have been evaluated for the clinical management of nongonococcal urethritis. The recent CDC treatment guidelines shown in Table 83.4 recommend a regimen of doxycycline 100 mg orally twice a day for 7 days.[10] Azithromycin orally as a single 1,000 mg dose is equivalent to doxycycline in the treatment of nongonococcal urethritis.[21,22] Doxycycline and azithromycin have cure rates greater than 95% in cases of nongonococcal urethritis.[23] Doxycycline is an inexpensive 7-day regimen that requires patient compliance because of multiple daily dosing. The toxicities of doxycycline include nausea and vomiting and the potential for phototoxicity. The bioavailability of doxycycline is reduced if taken concomitantly with multivalent ions such as iron; however, it can be administered without regard to meals or dairy products. Although azithromycin is an expensive alternative, it may be useful in patients with poor compliance with treatment or minimal follow-up. A single 1,000-mg oral dose can be administered under direct patient observation to ensure compliance. Diarrhea, nausea, dizziness, and headache have been reported in fewer than 3% of treated patients. Alternative regimens that have been indicated by the CDC include erythromycin base 500 mg and erythromycin ethylsuccinate 800 mg orally four times a day for 7 days. These regimens are considered to be less efficacious than doxycycline or azithromycin.[10] Many patients cannot tolerate such high doses of erythromycin because of gastrointestinal side effects. If necessary, lower dosages of 250 mg for the base or 400 mg for the ethylsuccinate salt can be used, but the duration of treatment should be extended to 14 days.[15]

Ofloxacin has been evaluated for the treatment of nongonococcal urethritis. On the basis of the limited data available, ofloxacin appears to be similar to doxycycline in efficacy, with treatment success rates approaching 100%.[23,24] The dose of ofloxacin that has been used most often is 300 mg orally twice daily for 7 days. Larger doses (up to 400 mg twice daily) administered for shorter periods of time (5 days) have also been studied in a limited number of patients. Ofloxacin is more expensive than doxycycline, and, unlike azithromycin, it does not afford the opportunity for improved patient compliance. Ciprofloxacin has limited activity against *C. trachomatis* and should not be considered a therapeutic option for the treatment of nongonococcal urethritis.[25] Although levofloxacin has not been evaluated in clinical trials, levofloxacin 500 mg daily for 7 days may be substituted for ofloxacin, because it is the l-isomer of ofloxacin and has similar microbiologic activity.[10]

When considering therapy for pregnant women, erythromycin base should be used because doxycycline and ofloxacin are contraindicated. Doxycycline can cause permanent discoloration of the teeth during tooth development, and the quinolones have been shown to cause cartilage damage in juvenile animal species. Due to increased clinical experience, azithromycin is recommended as an alternative agent for use during pregnancy (pregnancy category B) (see Table 83.4 for treatment of pediatric infections).

IMPROVING OUTCOMES

As with the treatment of gonorrhea, no specific patient follow-up is required unless symptoms persist after completion of therapy or recur shortly thereafter. However, pregnant women should receive a follow-up test of cure 3 weeks after completion of therapy because compliance with erythromycin may be less than optimal and these regimens may not be highly efficacious.[23] Patients should be strongly encouraged to refer recent sexual partners for evaluation and treatment, regardless of the presence of clinical signs and symptoms of infection. In addition, patients should be instructed to abstain from sexual intercourse until treatment has been completed and there is evidence that the infection has been cured. An alternative to abstinence would be careful use of a condom and contraceptive foam.

PHARMACOECONOMICS

Several pharmacoeconomic studies have been done evaluating the costs of azithromycin versus doxycycline. Although the acquisition cost of azithromycin therapy is considerably higher than that of doxycycline, it offers the advantage of single-dose treatment, thereby increasing compliance. Several studies have reported that when patient compliance is considered, azithromycin may be more cost-effective than doxycycline.[26,27]

The development of genital ulcerations is associated with several STDs, particularly syphilis, genital herpes simplex infections, and chancroid. Each of these diseases is discussed separately.

SYPHILIS

EPIDEMIOLOGY

Syphilis is an important contagious disease that can have many different manifestations.[28,29] The incidence of syphilis in the United States reached a peak during World War II and then declined after the introduction of penicillin in the late 1940s. In the 1960s, the number of reported cases of syphilis rose slightly and then plateaued until the mid-1980s, when the incidence again began to rise. During 1990 to 2000, the rates of primary and secondary syphilis declined; however rates have increased again in 2001 to 2002.[30] Although syphilis continues to be more prevalent in non-Hispanic blacks, and infections are more concentrated in the southern region of the United States, during the last 12 years, the number of primary and secondary cases declined among women and non-Hispanic blacks.[30] The majority of new cases occur among individuals who are 15 to 30 years old and among men who have sex with men. Various studies have shown the prevalence of syphilis in patients with HIV infection to be as high as 36%.[31] Although syphilis is most commonly transmitted via sexual intercourse, the organism can also be transmitted through placental transfer (congenital syphilis), by the administration of fresh human blood, by kissing or touching active lesions, or by accidental inoculation.[32]

The spirochete *T. pallidum* is the causal agent of syphilis. This unicellular organism is elongated and tightly coiled and divides approximately every 30 hours. The human is the only natural host. Unfortunately, the organism cannot be grown in vitro. The disease is usually transmitted by direct contact with an active infectious lesion, which teems with approximately 10^7 organisms per gram of tissue.[29] *T. pallidum* penetrates intact skin or mucous membranes and, within hours, invades regional lymphatics and blood vessels. Dissemination throughout the body is rapid. Any organ system can be infected, including the central nervous system (CNS).

CLINICAL PRESENTATION AND DIAGNOSIS

SIGNS AND SYMPTOMS

Syphilis can be divided clinically into five stages: incubating, primary, secondary, latent, and tertiary (late) syphi-

lis.[29,30,31,33] The incubation period usually lasts about 3 weeks, appears to be directly related to the size of the inoculum, and may range from 3 days to 3 months. During this period the individual is asymptomatic and noninfectious, and serologic tests are usually negative. The hallmark of primary syphilis is the development of a painless chancre in as many as 60% of patients at the site of initial inoculation. The lesion consists of spirochetes, histiocytes, and plasma cells. Multiple chancres may occur; this feature is usually observed in HIV-infected individuals. Not all patients develop a chancre, and some chancres are atypical in appearance or so small and inconspicuous that they are undetected. Painless regional lymphadenopathy (bubo) can be present. Chancres quickly erode and ulcerate, developing a smooth base with raised borders that usually heals spontaneously within several weeks, accompanied by resolution of lymphadenopathy.

Secondary syphilis, or disseminated syphilis, is a generalized illness that develops approximately 2 to 8 weeks after contact and may begin before complete resolution of the chancre. Essentially all untreated patients progress to secondary syphilis. The presentation is most often characterized by classic lesions of the skin and mucous membranes.[31] The rash most often starts as reddish or copper-colored macular lesions appearing on the truncal extremities but may also appear maculopapular, papular, or pustular. The soles of the feet and palms of the hands are commonly involved. It is not uncommon to also detect similar nonpainful lesions on mucous membranes. These lesions usually persist for up to a week. Generalized lymphadenopathy is also often present. Constitutional symptoms are common and include headache, fever, sore throat, malaise, myalgias, arthralgias, anorexia, and weight loss. Condylomata lata are flat, hypertrophic lesions resembling warts that develop in moist areas and contain spirochetes. Involvement of other organ systems is possible and may include the development of immune-complex glomerulonephritis, syphilitic hepatitis, and synovitis. The CNS is asymptomatically involved in nearly 30% of cases of secondary syphilis. Unless there is clinical evidence of CNS infection, evaluation of the cerebrospinal fluid (CSF) is not indicated. Serologic tests are positive in 65% to 85% of cases of secondary syphilis.[31]

Latent syphilis refers to a period of time during which there are no clinical manifestations of disease but the serologic tests for syphilis are positive. Early latent syphilis, generally considered to be the first 4 years, is the time when relapses of secondary syphilis may occur, and the patient is considered to be infectious. More than 90% of relapses, most often mucocutaneous in nature, occur in the first year, and it is widely believed that each relapse is clinically less florid than the previous episode. Late latent syphilis may continue for the balance of the patient's life or may progress to tertiary syphilis.[31] During late latent syphilis, relapses are rare, and the patient is not considered to be infectious. Nevertheless, in utero transmission of disease is possible during latent syphilis.

Approximately 30% of untreated patients progress to late (tertiary) syphilis, a slowly progressive disease that can affect any system in the body years after initial infection. Clinically, late syphilis is often classified as neurosyphilis, cardiovascular syphilis, or gummatous syphilis (late benign syphilis), a condition that is characterized by the development of hyperimmune granulomas, known as gummas, which often involve the skin and the bones.

Approximately 10% of untreated patients progress to the development of neurosyphilis. As mentioned, CNS involvement is initially asymptomatic and can be detected only by evaluation of the CSF. Under ideal situations, all patients should have evaluation of the CSF at 1 year after diagnosis and treatment of syphilis to detect evidence of residual CNS disease, such as pleocytosis, increased protein, decreased glucose, or positive nontreponemal antigen test. Examination of the CSF is also indicated for all HIV-positive patients with syphilis. The clinical manifestations of symptomatic neurosyphilis may include focal or generalized seizures, visual disturbances, paresthesias, altered reflexes, speech disturbances, pupillary abnormalities, dementia, and stroke. Tabes dorsalis is a manifestation resulting from degeneration of the dorsal columns of the spinal cord; it is characterized by ataxia with a wide-based gait, impotence, urinary incontinence or retention, paroxysms of intense shooting pain (usually in the legs), and loss of reflexes.[31,32]

Congenital syphilis results from transplacental transmission of spirochetes to the fetus in utero. Babies who are born to mothers who acquire syphilis during pregnancy are at a higher risk of developing congenital syphilis than are those whose mothers acquired syphilis before pregnancy. Although nearly 75% of cases of congenital syphilis are diagnosed after age 10 years, some cases manifest very early after birth. Early cases often cause rhinitis and a diffuse maculopapular rash that may result in significant epithelial sloughing. In addition, there may be generalized osteochondritis and perichondritis, eventually leading to bone destruction. Neonatal death from congenital syphilis is usually due to pneumonia, pulmonary hemorrhage, or hepatic failure. Patients with late congenital syphilis may have Hutchinson triad, which includes Hutchinson teeth (short, narrow, barrel-shaped incisors with a central notch), interstitial keratitis (photophobia, eye pain, tearing), and nerve deafness.

DIAGNOSIS

Using dark-field microscopy, silver staining, or specific immunofluorescence or immunoperoxidase, stains of transudate or tissue from the lesion can easily identify *T. pallidum* spirochetes.

The most direct method for establishing the diagnosis of syphilis is demonstration of *T. pallidum* on dark-field microscopic examination of fluid or tissue taken from a suspicious cutaneous lesion or lymph node.[28,29,34] Because *T.*

pallidum is susceptible to environmental changes, it is recommended that any clinical specimen taken from a patient with suspected syphilis be examined immediately. Because of their highly characteristic spiral shape and motility, viable treponemes are easy to distinguish under microscopic examination. Dark-field microscopic examination of material from the oral cavity may not be useful in diagnosing syphilis because nonpathogenic spirochetes can be members of the normal oral flora. An alternative to dark-field microscopy that has been implemented in many clinical laboratories is the use of a DFA test, which has greater specificity for *T. pallidum* (DFA-TP) and does not require immediate examination.[35]

In the absence of suitable pathologic specimens to examine, the diagnosis of syphilis can be based on serologic testing.[29,36] The serologic tests that are used in the diagnosis of syphilis are classified as nontreponemal or treponemal. Two commonly used nontreponemal antibody tests, Venereal Disease Research Laboratories (VDRL) and rapid plasma reagin (RPR), are quantitative measurements of antibodies against cardiolipin. These tests report serum titers that correlate with disease activity, with higher titers consistent with more active disease. These tests are inexpensive and easy to perform and are, therefore, often used for routine screening of patients. However, the test may remain reactive at low titers after treatment (serofast state) or become negative after 5 to 10 years, even without treatment (serorevert).[36] In some patients with secondary syphilis a prozone phenomenon may occur leading to a false-negative VDRL test. This is due to an excess of antibody relative to antigen and may be corrected by dilution of the patient's serum before testing.[35] These tests can be used for patient monitoring and evaluation of therapy. Titers should fall and become nonreactive within 1 year after successful treatment of primary syphilis and within 2 years after effective treatment of secondary syphilis. Patients who are treated for late syphilis usually become nonreactive after a period of up to 5 years.[37] Other nontreponemal tests that have been used include the reagin screen test, the automated reagin test, and the unheated serum reagin test.[34]

Specific treponemal antibody tests, such as the fluorescent treponemal antibody-absorbed test (FTA-abs), are highly sensitive and specific. The positive predictive value of the FTA-abs test is 100% for the initial or any subsequent symptomatic case of syphilis. Unfortunately, because this specific treponemal test usually remains positive for life, despite treatment, it is much less reliable in the evaluation of asymptomatic patients with a previous history of treated syphilis.[30] Two additional treponemal antibody tests that are useful in the diagnosis of syphilis are the microhemagglutination assay for antibodies to *T. pallidum* (MHATP) and the hemagglutination treponemal test for syphilis (HATTS). These tests are less expensive and easier to perform than the FTA-abs test but are also somewhat less sensitive in diagnosing early syphilis.[38]

THERAPEUTIC PLAN

Four basic principles guide the current treatment strategy for syphilis: (a) the requirement of a minimum treponemicidal antibiotic concentration; (b) maintenance of continuous antibiotic concentration above this minimum inhibitory concentration; (c) adequate duration of therapy; and (d) the fact that the response to treatment is inversely related to the duration of the infection.[39] The specific CDC recommendations for the preparation, dosage, and duration of therapy are based on the stage and clinical manifestations of the disease at the time of treatment and are summarized in Table 83.5.[40]

TREATMENT

On the basis of more than 50 years of experience, the drug of choice for the treatment of all stages of syphilis is parenteral penicillin G.[40,41] *T. pallidum* is highly sensitive to the effects of penicillin. Unfortunately, there have been no adequately controlled clinical trials to clearly define the optimal penicillin regimen for the treatment of various stages of syphilis. In addition, the data addressing nonpenicillin therapy are extremely limited. The current treatment guidelines for syphilis use benzathine penicillin G as first-line therapy for primary, secondary, and latent syphilis. Alternative therapeutic options for patients with significant penicillin allergy are limited. The use of doxycycline (100 mg orally every 12 hours) or tetracycline (500 mg orally every 6 hours) is considered an acceptable alternative treatment. There is less clinical experience with doxycycline, but compliance should be better. Erythromycin (500 mg orally every 6 hours) has undergone limited evaluation but may be associated with high treatment failure rates, particularly in pregnancy.[28,40–42] The use of first-generation cephalosporins has shown limited efficacy and unacceptably high treatment failure rates. Limited clinical studies suggest that ceftriaxone may be a viable alternative. Although the optimal dose and duration of ceftriaxone have not been defined, experts recommend 1 g daily IV or IM for 8 to 10 days.[11,43] In addition, azithromycin has demonstrated promising results as a 2-g single-dose; however, reports of azithromycin treatment failures in syphilis infections are starting to arise.[44,45] Close follow-up of patients receiving ceftriaxone or azithromycin is imperative because the efficacy of these therapies has not been adequately documented.

Parenteral penicillin G is the therapy of choice because it has been demonstrated to be effective in the management of syphilis during pregnancy and for neurosyphilis; therefore, patients who are allergic to penicillin should be treated with penicillin following desensitization.[42] Patients who have positive skin tests to the major or minor determinants of penicillin allergy can usually be safely desensitized over a 4- to 6-hour period using oral penicillin V suspension as outlined in Table 83.6.[41] After they have been desensitized, patients should be maintained on penicillin continuously until completion of the treatment course. The CDC recommends ceftriaxone 2 g daily given IM or IV for 10 to 14 days as an alternative to penicillin in patients who are penicillin allergic.[40] However, the possibility of cross-reactivity between ceftriaxone and penicillin is approximately 3% to 7% in documented immunoglobulin E (IgE) mediated reactions.[46]

Many clinicians treat primary and secondary syphilis in HIV-infected patients more aggressively than in non–HIV-infected patients, using three IM doses of benzathine penicillin G administered at weekly intervals (Table 83.7).

Occasionally, within the first 24 hours of treatment for early syphilis, the patient will experience a Jarisch-Herxheimer reaction, an acute, benign, febrile episode that is commonly accompanied by myalgias, transient adenopathy, and headache lasting for several hours. This reaction is thought to be caused by release of treponemal antigens due to rapid lysis of the organism by antibiotics. It is important that the clinician recognize this reaction as being independent of the drug regimen and not consider it to be an allergic reaction to the therapeutic agent used. If necessary for patient comfort, acetaminophen or aspirin can be used for symptomatic relief.

IMPROVING OUTCOMES

The CDC recommends serologic follow-up of patients who are treated for syphilis to evaluate the therapeutic outcome. Quantitative nontreponemal tests should be performed at 6, 12, and 24 months after completion of therapy for primary, secondary, and latent syphilis.[10] For patients with neurosyphilis, the CSF should be examined every 6 months until the cell count is normal. If the cell count remains abnormal at 24 months, retreatment is suggested. A quantitative nontreponemal test every 2 to 3 months until it is nonreactive is recommended as a follow-up for congenital syphilis. The adequacy of treatment for syphilis during pregnancy should be evaluated with nontreponemal serologic testing on a monthly basis. HIV-infected patients should be evaluated clinically and serologically more frequently for treatment failure at 3, 6, 9, 12, and 24 months after therapy. Patients who fail to demonstrate a fourfold reduction in titer over a 3-month period or who show a fourfold increase in titer between tests should be retreated.

HERPES GENITALIS

Genital herpes, or herpes genitalis, is an acute inflammatory infection caused by the double-stranded DNA herpes simplex virus (HSV).[10]

EPIDEMIOLOGY

Genital herpes is the most commonly encountered cause of genital ulceration in the United States and can involve the

TABLE 83.5	Recommended Treatment Regimens for All Stages of Syphilis in Patients Not Infected with Human Immunodeficiency Virus		
Disease Stage	**Adult Regimen**	**Child Regimen**	**Adult Penicillin Allergy**
Sexual contact to infectious case of syphilis	Benzathine penicillin G, 2.4 million units IM as single-dose therapy		Doxycycline 100 mg PO bid for 14 days *or* Tetracycline, 500 mg PO qid for 14 days
Primary or secondary syphilis	Benzathine penicillin G, 2.4 million units IM as single-dose therapy	Benzathine penicillin G, 50,000 U/kg IM as single-dose therapy (max. 2.4 million units)	Doxycycline, 100 mg PO bid for 14 days *or* Tetracycline, 500 mg PO qid for 14 days
Early, latent syphilis (<1-yr duration)	Treat as primary or secondary syphilis		
Late, latent syphilis (>1-yr duration)	Benzathine penicillin G, 2.4 million units IM weekly for 3 doses	Benzathine penicillin G, 50,000 U/kg IM weekly for 3 doses (max. 2.4 million units/dose)	Doxycycline, 100 mg PO bid for 28 days *or* Tetracycline, 500 mg PO qid for 28 days
Late syphilis (not neurosyphilis)	Treat as late, latent syphilis		
Neurosyphilis	Aqueous penicillin G, 12–24 million units/day IV (administered as 2–4 million units q4hr) for 10 to 14 days *or* Procaine penicillin G, 2.4 million units IM once daily PLUS probenecid 500 mg PO qid, both for 10–14 days (acceptable regimen only if compliance can be ensured)		Desensitize; then give IV aqueous penicillin G
Syphilis in pregnancy	Treat as appropriate with parenteral penicillin		Desensitize; then give parenteral penicillin
Congenital syphilis	N/A	Aqueous penicillin G, 100,000–150,000 U/kg/day (administered as 50,000 U/kg IV q12h during the first 7 days of life, and q8h thereafter, for 10–14 days) *or* Procaine penicillin G, 50,000 U/kg IM once daily as a single dose for 10–14 days	

IM, intramuscularly; PO, by mouth; bid, twice a day; qid, four times daily; IV, intravenously; q, every hour.
(From Hook EW, Marra CM. Acquired syphilis in adults. N Engl J Med 326:1060–1069, 1992, with permission.)

TABLE 83.6	Oral Penicillin Desensitization Protocol[a]			
Dose Number for Penicillin V Suspension[b]	Suspension Concentration (U/mL)	Dose (mL)	Dose (U)	Cumulative Dose (U)
1	1,000	0.1	100	100
2	1,000	0.2	200	300
3	1,000	0.4	400	700
4	1,000	0.8	800	1,500
5	1,000	1.6	1,600	3,100
6	1,000	3.2	3,200	6,300
7	1,000	6.4	6,400	12,700
8	10,000	1.2	12,000	24,700
9	10,000	2.4	24,000	48,700
10	10,000	4.8	48,000	96,700
11	80,000	1.0	80,000	176,700
12	80,000	2.0	160,000	336,700
13	80,000	4.0	320,000	656,700
14	80,000	8.0	640,000	1,296,700

[a] The penicillin dose should be diluted in 30–45 mL of water and administered orally.
[b] The interval between individual doses is 15 minutes; therefore elapsed time for desensitization is 3 hours 45 minutes.
(From Hook EW, Marra CM. Acquired syphilis in adults. N Engl J Med 326:1060–1069, 1992, with permission.)

male and female genital tracts with equal prevalence. Studies have shown that people with multiple sexual partners have an increased chance of acquiring herpes infection. Based on serologic data, it is reported that more than 40 million Americans are currently infected with genital herpes.[10] HSV type 2 (HSV-2) is the predominant viral type associated with herpes genitalis, and HSV type 1 (HSV-1) is most closely associated with oropharyngeal disease; however, each virus can cause infections in both anatomic areas. Humans are the only reservoir for transmission to other humans. Primary

TABLE 83.7	Recommended Treatment Regimens for Syphilis in Patients Infected with Human Immunodeficiency Virus	
Disease Stage	Adult Regimen	Alternative Regimen
Primary and Secondary	Benzathine penicillin G, 2.4 million units IM as single-dose therapy (some experts suggest multiple doses)	None; must desensitize and treat with penicillin
Latent	Benzathine penicillin G, 2.4 million units IM weekly for 3 doses	None; must desensitize and treat with penicillin

IM, intramuscularly.

genital herpes develops after transmission of the virus by direct contact of the recipient's mucous membranes or skin with infected secretions or mucocutaneous surface of an infected sexual partner.[47] After inoculation there is an incubation period ranging from 2 to 20 days when the HSV replicates locally in epithelial cells, eventually causing a localized inflammatory response and ulceration. The virus also migrates via peripheral neurons to the sacral ganglia, where latency is established. After latency, a stimulus (physiologic, immunologic, or emotional factors) can produce periodic viral reactivation of symptomatic disease or asymptomatic viral shedding. The factors that contribute to this reactivation are poorly understood at present.[48] Transmission of HSV-2 often occurs in individuals who are unaware that they have the infection or are asymptomatic when transmission occurs.

CLINICAL PRESENTATION AND DIAGNOSIS

SIGNS AND SYMPTOMS

The clinical manifestations and recurrence rates of genital herpes are influenced by the viral type and numerous host-related factors, such as sex, immunocompetence, site of infection, and previous infection with HSV.[4] A significant number of HSV-2 infections are asymptomatic. First-episode infection (primary infection) occurs in individuals with HSV-1 or HSV-2 infections, in the absence of serum antibody to either type of HSV, and causes severe manifestations. Nonprimary first-episode infections tend to cause less severe manifestations because individuals already have serum antibodies to either of the herpes types; patients with serum antibodies to HSV-2 seldom develop genital HSV-1 infection.[48]

A significant percentage of patients with primary HSV infection experience a prodromal flulike syndrome with fever, headache, malaise, and diffuse myalgias. After a brief incubation period of 2 to 20 days (average 4–7 days), local symptoms develop, consisting of genital itching, tenderness, and dysuria. Typically, the lesions start as painful papules or vesicles that spread rapidly over the genital region, often clustering together to form large areas of shallow ulceration. The pain and irritation gradually increase over the first week, reaching maximum intensity between days 7 and 11 of infection, then slowly recede over the next week. Over the course of several weeks, the cutaneous ulcers crust over and eventually reepithelialize. Crusting does not occur with lesions on mucous membranes.[4,48] Viral shedding occurs during the period from development of the initial lesion until approximately the 11th or 12th day of illness. First-episode nonprimary genital herpes infections tend to be milder than primary infections. Patients experience lower incidence and shorter duration of prodromal flulike symptoms.

The symptoms of recurrent HSV infection are similar to those seen with primary episodes, without the systemic manifestations. The symptoms often appear to be more severe in women than men, possibly because of the extent of involved mucosal surface. In general, recurrent symptoms are milder than those seen with primary infection, are localized to the genital area, and usually last from 5 to 7 days.

Complications of genital herpes infection occur most commonly after primary episodes and usually result from the spread of genital disease or by autoinoculation of the virus. HSV infection of the rectum, pharynx, and eye are not unusual. CNS involvement can include aseptic meningitis, transverse myelitis, or sacral radiculopathy. Blood-borne dissemination of HSV infection may accompany primary mucocutaneous infection in immunocompromised patients or during pregnancy. HSV infection of neonates who were exposed during pregnancy or delivery is associated with extremely high morbidity and mortality, with a case-fatality rate approaching 50%.[49] Herpes infections tend to be more prolonged and severe in immunocompromised patients (e.g., HIV, solid organ transplant).

DIAGNOSIS

Because a number of other diseases are associated with genital ulceration, the diagnosis of herpes genitalis often requires laboratory testing. The easiest, but least sensitive and specific, technique is examination of cells scraped from the base of a typical lesion or ulcer (Tzanck smear) and stained by Giemsa or Papanicolaou stain.[4] Evidence of multinucleated giant cells with intranuclear inclusions is characteristic of HSV infection. Identification of HSV in tissue culture pro-

cessed from a specimen taken from a symptomatic patient is the most sensitive and specific method for confirmation of primary HSV infection but is expensive and time-consuming to perform. Serologic demonstration of HSV infection is useful for confirming the diagnosis of primary HSV infection, for determining the HSV serotype (if a serotype-specific assay is used), and for distinguishing between primary and reactivated infections, because recurrent genital herpes rarely induces a significant increase in anti-HSV antibodies.[48,49] However, therapeutic decisions should not be postponed until the results are obtained.

THERAPEUTIC PLAN

The goals in treating herpes genitalis are to decrease the duration and severity of active infection, prevent associated complications, decrease the frequency of recurrence, and reduce the period of viral shedding and infectivity.[4] It is important to remember that these drugs do not eradicate latent virus or affect the risk or severity of recurrences after the drug is discontinued. To date, acyclovir, famciclovir, and valacyclovir have been shown to be effective in the clinical management of genital herpes. These antivirals are associated with reductions in viral shedding, decreases in the severity and duration of symptoms, and accelerated lesion healing of first-episode HSV genital infections. The use of 5% acyclovir topical ointment in cases of genital herpes should be discouraged because of lack of demonstrated efficacy.[49] The recommended regimens for management of primary herpes genitalis are summarized in Table 83.8. In first-episode cases, prompt initiation of antiviral therapy is associated with reduction in symptoms within 48 hours.[4,48] Acyclovir dosages should be reduced for patients with significant renal dysfunction. There is no advantage to using parenteral acyclovir instead of oral acyclovir except for patients with severe disease or complications who require hospitalization and cannot take acyclovir orally. To decrease the frequency of recurrent genital herpes, many patients with recurrent infection may benefit from chronic administration of antiviral therapy; therefore, treatment options (episodic treatment or daily suppressive therapy) should be discussed with patients as shown in Table 83.9.

To derive benefit, episodic antiviral therapy has to be started at the beginning of the prodrome or when lesions are first noted, because recurrent episodes of genital herpes in immunocompetent patients are self-limited.[4] In patients with more than six episodes per year, daily dosing of acyclovir for chronic suppressive therapy to prevent recurrences has been reported to reduce the frequency of recurrences by nearly 75%. If suppressive therapy is started, the current recommendation is to discontinue therapy after 12 months of continuous treatment to reassess the patient's rate of recurrence.[10] Although the potential for adverse effects from

TABLE 83.8	Recommended Regimens for Treatment of Herpes Genitalis			
Type of Infection	**Recommended Regimen**	**Cost**[a]	**Alternative Regimen**	
First episode of genital herpes[b]	Acyclovir 400 mg PO tid for 7–10 days	6.50	Acyclovir 5–10 mg/kg IV q8h for 5–7 days or until clinical resolution (only for patients who require hospitalization)	
	or			
	Acyclovir 200 mg PO 5 times daily for 7–10 days	5.00		
	or			
	Famciclovir 250 mg PO tid for 7–10 days	13.00		
	or			
	Valacyclovir 1 g PO bid for 7–10 days	17.50		
First episode of herpes proctitis	Acyclovir 400 mg PO 5 times daily for 10 days[c]	10.80	As above	

[a] Based on 2004 Red Book AWP for daily drug costs.
[b] Treatment may be continued for 10 days until clinical resolution occurs.
[c] Clinical experience is lacking with famciclovir and valacyclovir, but they should be effective.
PO, by mouth; tid, three times daily; IV intravenously; q, every; bid, twice a day.

long-term acyclovir administration and the possibility of developing acyclovir-resistant strains of HSV are concerns, clinical data suggest few cumulative acyclovir toxicities and no significant changes in HSV susceptibility to acyclovir after prolonged acyclovir use for up to 6 years.[4,50] Safety and efficacy have been demonstrated among patients receiving daily therapy with valacyclovir and famciclovir for 1 year.[51,52] There have been limited reports of apparent acyclovir-resistant strains of HSV in patients with genital herpes. Foscarnet (40 mg/kg IV every 8 hours or 60 mg/kg every 12 hours) until clinical resolution, is the recommended treatment alternative in such cases.[10] Based on clinical experience, immunocompromised patients should receive higher doses of antivirals (acyclovir 400 mg three times daily, famciclovir 500 mg twice a day, valacyclovir 500 mg twice a day) for daily suppressive therapy because these patients may have more severe cases.

The safety of systemic acyclovir therapy during pregnancy has not been clearly established, although there is currently no evidence to suggest that acyclovir is teratogenic in humans.[10,49,53] Current recommendations state that oral acyclovir may be administered during pregnancy for first episode genital herpes or severe recurrent herpes and should be administered IV during pregnancy with severe HSV infection.[10,46]

TREATMENT

Acyclovir, a guanosine analog, is selectively taken up by HSV-infected cells and undergoes serial phosphorylation to the active form, acyclovir triphosphate. This triphosphorylated moiety acts to inhibit HSV DNA polymerase and viral replication. HSV-1 and HSV-2 are inhibited by concentra-

TABLE 83.9	Recommended Regimens for Recurrent Episodes of Herpes Genitalis		
Type of Infection	**Recommended Regimen**	**Type of Infection**	**Recommended Regimen**
Recurrent infection	Acyclovir 400 mg PO tid for 5 days	Daily suppressive therapy	Acyclovir 400 mg PO bid
	or		*or*
	Acyclovir 200 mg PO five times daily for 5 days		Famciclovir 250 mg PO bid
	or		*or*
	Acyclovir 800 mg PO bid for 5 days		Valacyclovir 500 mg PO qd[a]
	or		*or*
	Famciclovir 125 mg PO bid for 5 days		Valacyclovir 1,000 mg PO qd
	or		
	Valacyclovir 500 mg PO bid for 5 days		

[a] this regimen may be less effective in patients with ≥10 episodes/year.
PO, by mouth; tid, three times daily; bid, twice a day; qd, every day.

tions of acyclovir that are achieved in serum and body tissues at the currently recommended dosages.[49] Unlike acyclovir, famciclovir and valacyclovir are prodrugs. After oral administration, valacyclovir, the L-valyl ester (prodrug) of acyclovir, is hydrolyzed to acyclovir, and famciclovir is converted to its active form, penciclovir.[53,54] To exert an antiviral effect, all of these agents must become activated within the cell to a monophosphate form by thymidine kinase, an enzyme found predominantly in virally infected cells. The end result is inhibition of viral DNA synthesis. Of note, acyclovir-resistant strains of HSV and varicella-zoster virus are usually cross-resistant to penciclovir because the most common mechanism of resistance is a deficiency of thymidine kinase.

When compared with acyclovir, the pharmacokinetic profiles of the new analogs offer improved features. The oral bioavailability of acyclovir is poor, limited to only 15% to 30%; however, the bioavailability of acyclovir after valacyclovir administration is substantially increased to 54%.[53] Serum concentrations derived from 1 to 2 g of valacyclovir given orally four times daily are comparable to those achieved with administration of 5 to 10 mg per kilogram of IV acyclovir every 8 hours. Famciclovir, a prodrug, is converted to penciclovir, which has excellent oral bioavailability (77%).[54] Acyclovir and penciclovir are predominantly cleared by the kidneys. In patients with renal insufficiency, accumulation can result; therefore, reduced doses are necessary. The antivirals are well tolerated in immunocompetent patients. When compared with placebo, adverse events were similar in patients taking either agent. No differences in incidence of adverse effects between famciclovir or valacyclovir compared with acyclovir were noted in comparative genital herpes trials. The most common adverse effects in clinical trials include gastrointestinal upset, diarrhea, headache, insomnia, dizziness, and fatigue. To date, there are essentially no clinically significant drug interactions with these drugs.[53,54]

Of concern, in comparative clinical trials involving immunocompromised patients given higher doses of valacyclovir (>3 g/day), more cases of thrombotic thrombocytopenic purpura/hemolytic uremic syndrome (TTP/HUS) have been observed in patients receiving valacyclovir versus acyclovir.[55] The overall incidence of TTP/HUS in valacyclovir-treated patients is less than 3%, and the median time to occurrence of this complication is 53 days (range 8–100 days). To date, TTP/HUS has not been observed in immunocompetent patients or in immunocompromised patients given valacyclovir in doses of 3 g per day or less.[55]

Patients with genital herpes should be advised to refrain from sexual activity while genital lesions are present. In addition, sexual partners of infected individuals should be evaluated and counseled about the lifelong nature of the disease. Successful management of genital HSV infection involves educating the patient about the natural history of the infection (i.e., the potential for recurrent episodes, asymp-

tomatic viral shedding, and sexual transmission, especially because this often occurs during asymptomatic periods).

CHANCROID

EPIDEMIOLOGY

Chancroid is a STD disease caused by *Haemophilus ducreyi*, a small, Gram-negative, facultative anaerobic bacillus that is particularly hard to grow in culture. Most experts agree that genital herpes and primary syphilis are responsible for the majority of ulcerative genital lesions in developed countries, and chancroid accounts for most of the genital ulcers in developing societies.[56,57] Nevertheless, since the early 1980s, there have been several significant outbreaks of chancroid in the United States and Canada. Men, especially uncircumcised men, have a higher incidence of infection than women.[56]

For several years, the epidemiologic relationship between the presence of genital ulcers, such as chancroid, and heterosexual transmission of the HIV has been recognized, particularly in Africa. It is believed that contact between the infectious ulcer of one sexual partner and mucous membranes of the other partner leads to this viral transmission. Therefore, identification and treatment of patients with chancroid, and other infections such as genital herpes that lead to the formation of genital ulcers, are important in limiting the spread of HIV. In the United States, it has been estimated that 10% of persons with chancroid are coinfected with *T. pallidum* or HSV.[57]

CLINICAL PRESENTATION AND DIAGNOSIS

SIGNS AND SYMPTOMS

The incubation period for chancroid ranges from 3 to 10 days. The chancre starts as a tender, papule-like lesion with surrounding erythema and progresses over several days to an eroded, pustular ulcer that can be quite painful, particularly in men.[56] Many women with chancroid are asymptomatic. Over time, several of these small lesions can coalesce to form giant ulcers. The presence of painful inguinal lymphadenitis is seen concurrently in approximately 50% of cases and is often unilateral. Inflamed lymph nodes can progress to the development of formed buboes, which may rupture spontaneously in severe cases. Superinfection of the ulcerative lesions by enteric aerobic and anaerobic pathogens may further complicate the condition.[56]

DIAGNOSIS

The definitive diagnosis of chancroid is dependent on the identification of *H. ducreyi* from culture on special media from samples collected from the ulcer or bubo. Because the proper media for culture is not widely available, the diagnosis is generally made by the exclusion of other diseases that produce inguinal ulceration, such as herpes genitalis, lymphogranuloma venereum, and syphilis.[56,57]

THERAPEUTIC PLAN

The CDC recommends systemic antibiotic therapy with any one of the following regimens: azithromycin (1,000 mg orally) as a single dose, ceftriaxone (250 mg IM) as a single dose, ciprofloxacin (500 mg twice a day) for 3 days, or erythromycin base (500 mg orally) every 6 hours for 7 days.[57] Each of these regimens has proven to be highly effective in non–HIV-infected patients with chancroid. Most clinicians should not routinely recommend single-dose therapy for HIV-infected patients because of reported higher treatment failure rates.[58]

Trimethoprim plus sulfamethoxazole (cotrimoxazole) is no longer a recommended treatment option for chancroid because of reports of *H. ducreyi* developing increased resistance to this combination.[58]

Patients should be reexamined several days after starting therapy to ensure that symptomatic improvement is observed. The time for complete healing may be several weeks, and significant scarring of tissues is common. Relapse after apparent healing has been reported in up to 5% of cases.[58] All known recent sexual contacts of the patient with chancroid should be evaluated and treated if possible.

SELECTED OTHER SEXUALLY TRANSMITTED DISEASES

TRICHOMONIASIS

EPIDEMIOLOGY

Trichomoniasis is a common condition caused by the flagellated, motile protozoan *Trichomonas vaginalis*.[59] In the United States, approximately 3 million females are treated for trichomoniasis annually; the incidence among males is unknown.[60] Individuals who have multiple sexual partners or are concurrently infected with another STD appear to be at increased risk for trichomoniasis. This supports the contention that trichomoniasis is an STD. Transmission between sexual partners is further confirmed by reports of recovery of *T. vaginalis* from 66% to 100% of female sexual partners of infected men and 30% to 40% of male partners of infected women.[61] For unclear reasons, trichomoniasis appears to be less common in women who use barrier contraception or oral contraceptives. Nonvenereal transmission can also occur from contact with colonized materials, such as towels and clothing. Neonates can acquire the organism during normal vaginal delivery.[62]

CLINICAL PRESENTATION AND DIAGNOSIS

SIGNS AND SYMPTOMS
Trichomoniasis is thought to be an asymptomatic and self-limited disease in most men and neonates, often requiring no specific therapy.[63,64] Up to 50% of women with vaginal trichomoniasis are asymptomatic. However, symptoms may develop after an incubation period ranging from 1 to 4 weeks. Common complaints include malodorous grayish or yellow-green vaginal discharge, dysuria, pruritus in the genital area, and vulvovaginal tenderness. Signs and symptoms may be exacerbated during menstruation, possibly because of increased vaginal pH facilitating an increase in organism growth.[64]

DIAGNOSIS
Laboratory findings include an elevated vaginal pH (>4.5) and large numbers of neutrophils seen on microscopic evaluation on the wet mount prep of the discharge. Evaluation of a wet mount prep from a vaginal swab remains the easiest, cheapest, and most widely used diagnostic technique used.[59] Traditional stains, such as the Gram, Giemsa, and acridine orange stains, are not helpful in the diagnosis of trichomoniasis but should be done on all samples because of the high likelihood of concurrent disease in infected patients.[59] Culture of *T. vaginalis* from collected specimens is the most sensitive diagnostic technique available but requires up to 48 hours for necessary growth, reducing the clinical usefulness of culture for clinical diagnosis.[64]

THERAPEUTIC PLAN

The treatment of choice for trichomoniasis in men and women is oral metronidazole.[59,65] Although topical metronidazole gel is available and approved as a treatment for bacterial vaginosis, systemic therapy is far superior. A single 2-g oral dose of metronidazole or 500 mg orally twice daily for 7 days for women has resulted in cure rates of 90% to 95%.[59,64,65] This probably holds true for men as well, although data are lacking to confirm this belief. As with any STD, it is important to treat all sexual partners as well to prevent reinfection. When sexual partners are treated simultaneously with metronidazole, the cure rate increases to greater than 95%.[65] Infants with symptomatic trichomoniasis or with prolonged (>4 weeks) colonization after birth can be treated with parenteral metronidazole (10–30 mg/kg/day for 7 days).[64] No specific follow-up is required unless signs and symptoms of infection continue.

TREATMENT

Metronidazole therapy is associated with some well-recognized side effects, particularly mild nausea, which are more common with large single doses. Peripheral neuropathy, manifesting as numbness and paresthesias, is also associated with metronidazole therapy, especially in patients who take large doses for prolonged periods of time. Metronidazole can interfere with alcohol metabolism by blocking alcohol dehydrogenase, producing an "antabuse- like" or "disulfiram-like" reaction consisting of severe nausea, vomiting, and flushing when the two are taken concomitantly. The use of metronidazole during pregnancy is contraindicated, most importantly during the first trimester. Data suggest that metronidazole use during the second and third trimesters of pregnancy is safe; however, most clinicians do not consider specific therapy for trichomoniasis to be necessary during pregnancy unless the symptoms are severe.[64]

When the clinician is faced with an apparent failure of metronidazole, consideration must be given to the possibility of failure due to poor compliance, reinfection of the patient by an infected sexual partner, or the potential of infection by metronidazole-resistant organisms. Although *T. vaginalis* resistance to metronidazole appears to be increasing, alternative therapies are limited.[62] Current therapeutic options for infections caused by suspected or known metronidazole-resistant organisms include treatment for 7 to 10 days with daily oral doses of 2 g of metronidazole, with or without concurrent use of metronidazole 0.5% gel intravaginally.[64]

LYMPHOGRANULOMA VENEREUM

EPIDEMIOLOGY

Lymphogranuloma venereum (LGV) is caused by the invasive serotypes of *C. trachomatis,* the same pathogen that is associated with the development of nongonococcal urethritis in many patients.[66] LGV is a rare disease in the United States and must be differentiated clinically from such other conditions as lymphoma, syphilis, chancroid, plague, tularemia, and genital herpes. Like other STDs, LGV is more common among individuals with multiple sexual contacts, in urban rather than rural areas, and in lower socioeconomic populations.[67]

CLINICAL PRESENTATION AND DIAGNOSIS

SIGNS AND SYMPTOMS

The most common clinical manifestation of LGV is tender inguinal lymphadenopathy, which is most commonly unilateral. This inguinal adenopathy appears 2 to 6 weeks after the development of an unremarkable herpetiform vesicle at the site of inoculation. The initial vesicle often goes unnoticed, particularly in women. Within 2 weeks, the inflamed inguinal node (bubo) may progress to fluctuance and rupture through the skin, forming sinus tracts that are slow to heal. This occurs in fewer than 30% of cases.[67] The remaining cases slowly form firm inguinal masses without suppuration. In females and homosexual males, LGV can cause perianal or perirectal inflammation that can progress to the formation of colonic fistulas or strictures. These patients may have rectal bleeding or rectal discharge of pus. In severe cases, patients may appear systemically ill. Laboratory findings are usually nonspecific and may consist of slightly elevated white blood cell counts, elevated erythrocyte sedimentation rate, and mild increases in hepatic transaminases.

DIAGNOSIS

The diagnosis of LGV is based largely on the clinical presentation of significant inguinal adenopathy in the absence of another etiology. Isolation of *C. trachomatis* from an aspirated swollen bubo is possible in up to one third of cases but requires special culture techniques that are not available in most laboratories. Serologic documentation of antichlamydial antibodies by microimmunofluorescence or ELISA is thought to be sensitive and more specific than complement fixation but can lead to false-positive results because of the widespread prevalence of other chlamydial infections in the at-risk population.

THERAPEUTIC PLAN

The recommended treatment of choice for LGV is doxycycline, 100 mg orally twice daily for 21 days, as shown in Table 83.4.[67,68] Alternative antibiotic regimens include erythromycin, 500 mg orally four times daily for 21 days. Erythromycin is the treatment of choice for pregnant females. Although it is expected that azithromycin 1 g once weekly for 3 weeks should offer similar efficacy to that of erythromycin as alternative therapy to doxycycline, insufficient clinical data are available to support its widespread use at this time. Swollen, inflamed lymph nodes may require surgical aspiration or incision and drainage for optimal care.

In general, appropriate antibiotic therapy and surgical intervention, if necessary, cure LGV and prevent further tissue damage and scarring. However, patients should be followed clinically until resolution of signs and symptoms of the disease. Sexual partners should be evaluated and treated appropriately if urethral or cervical chlamydial infection is detected.

HUMAN PAPILLOMAVIRUS INFECTION—CONDYLOMATA ACUMINATA

EPIDEMIOLOGY

Condylomata acuminata, or genital warts, are venereal infections caused by human papillomavirus (HPV).[69] Genital HPV infection is the second most common venereal disease seen in STD clinics in the United States; it is responsible for more than 1 million office visits annually. Papillomaviruses are double-stranded DNA viruses that often produce squamous epithelial tumors. The virus has been shown to penetrate and infect the basal cell layer, the only site of actively dividing cells in the epithelium. More than 70 types of HPV have been identified; they contribute to a wide range of lesions, including plantar warts, laryngeal carcinoma, and cervical dysplasia. The HPV types that are considered to be primarily responsible for genital warts are HPV-6 and HPV-11.[69] These HPV types are easily transmitted during sexual intercourse. Genital warts are almost always the result of anal intercourse, particularly in homosexual men.

The natural history of untreated genital warts is variable. Some may grow larger, some regress, and many stay the same over time. Several years ago, it was commonly believed that, if left untreated, large genital warts would progress to malignancy. As techniques to identify particular types of HPV have become available, it has become clear that the risk of genital warts progressing to cancerous lesions is very small.[70] The HPV types that are most strongly associated with the development of cervical cancer are not the same types that are associated with genital warts. In addition, the rates of noncervical genital cancers are extremely low in the United States, whereas the prevalence of genital HPV infections is very high.

CLINICAL PRESENTATION AND DIAGNOSIS

SIGNS AND SYMPTOMS

Condylomata acuminata may be asymptomatic, with only occasional anogenital pruritus and burning.[69] These lesions are usually known as flat condylomas and are identified as shiny white plaques after the application of dilute (3%–5%) acetic acid solution to the site. The common locations for these flat warts are the penis, anus, vagina, vulva, and cervix. Large, hyperplastic, exophytic warts with raised, pinkish-colored papules are the classic condylomata acuminata.[71] These larger lesions may be associated with increased pain, bleeding, burning, and soiling of undergarments.

DIAGNOSIS

Condylomata acuminata should be differentiated from other anogenital growths, such as molluscum contagiosum, moles, and skin tags. HPV cannot be grown in tissue culture; therefore, diagnosis is based on gross clinical appearance and confirmed by biopsy.[71] Histologic evidence of koilocytosis, the characteristic finding of HPV infection, can be observed with appropriate staining techniques, such as the Papanicolaou smear. Recently, newer techniques, such as DNA hybridization and polymerase chain reaction, have expanded the ability to identify specific HPV types, but these procedures are not currently useful for clinical screening.[70]

THERAPEUTIC PLAN

Although eradication of genital HPV infection is not accomplished by any therapeutic option, the goal is to remove visible warts with the intent of inducing a wart-free period. Although aggressive techniques for removal of the warts do produce cosmetic benefits, the surrounding tissues usually remain subclinically infected with HPV. Many experts believe that recurrences of genital warts are much more commonly due to reactivation of subclinical infection than to reinfection by a sexual partner.[72] There are no definitive data to suggest that any of the available treatments are superior, therefore drug therapy should be guided by patient preference and clinician experience. The recommended regimens for external genital warts include both patient-applied and provider-administered therapy.[71]

The plant resin podophyllin, applied as a 10% to 25% solution in compound tincture of benzoin by the provider, has traditionally been the most common initial treatment. Podophyllin has been shown to inhibit mitosis, leading to cell death. Topical applications of limited amounts (<0.5 mL per application) are made to the lesions and followed by thorough washing in 1 to 4 hours.[72] Applications can be repeated weekly as needed by health care providers to avoid the possibility of complications. In several clinical trials, podophyllin treatment was associated with initial clearance of warts in 32% to 79% of patients, with recurrence within 9 months seen in 27% to 65% of patients.[70] Systemic absorption of topically applied podophyllin can occur. The use of podophyllin is contraindicated during pregnancy.

Another treatment option that is administered by the provider is trichloroacetic acid (80%–90%) applied to the genital warts followed by powdering of the area with talc or baking soda to remove excess unreacted acid. Application can be made at weekly intervals as required.[69] Cryotherapy, performed by a health care provider using liquid nitrogen or a cryoprobe, produces results similar to those reported with podofilox and podophyllin.[70] An alternative regimen is intralesional injection of interferon-a 2b for external genital warts or laser surgery. When intralesional interferon injection was combined with topical podophyllin, the response observed was superior to that seen with podophyllin alone, particularly in non–HIV-infected patients who had warts for less than 1 year. Systemic interferon administration in combination with other treatment options has not been associated with any improvement in response rates.

The preferred patient-applied preparation is podofilox (podophyllotoxin), the most biologically active component of podophyllin as a 0.5% solution or gel.[73] Limited topical application of podofilox (<0.25 mL per application) is made to warts twice daily for 3 days, followed by a 4-day period of no treatment. Treatment cycles can be repeated as needed for up to four cycles. Complete clearance of warts has been described in 45% to 88% of patients, with recurrence within 3 months observed in 33% to 60% of these patients.[70] Local irritation and mild/moderate pain are associated with the use of podofilox which appear to be more frequent than that reported with podophyllin use. Podofilox has not been approved for the treatment of perianal, rectal, vaginal, or urethral warts.

Another patient-applied treatment option is imiquimod 5% cream applied once daily at bedtime, three times a week for as long as 16 weeks. Six to 10 hours after application the treatment area should be washed with mild soap. Like podophyllin and podofilox, imiquimod is contraindicated during pregnancy. Mild to moderate local inflammatory reactions are common.

KEY POINTS

- Health care professionals have a responsibility to contribute to the efforts to reduce the ever-expanding prevalence of sexually transmitted diseases
- Infected patients and their sexual partners must be identified and treated appropriately, consistent with recently published CDC guidelines
- Infected patients and their sexual partners must be counseled about the nature of their disease and methods that can be used to reduce the transmission of all STDs
- Advances in drug therapy have led to safe and effective treatment regimens for most STDs that are also relatively inexpensive and easy to follow
- Compliance has been enhanced for several diseases through the development of regimens requiring only a single dose of medication

REFERENCES

1. Piot P, Islam MQ. Sexually transmitted diseases in the 1990s: global epidemiology and challenges for control. Sex Transm Dis 21 (Suppl 2):S7–S13, 1994.
2. Gerbase A, Rowley J, Mertens T. Global epidemiology of sexually transmitted diseases. Lancet 351:2–4, 1998.
3. Centers for Disease Control and Prevention. Addressing emerging infectious disease threats: a prevention strategy for the United States. Atlanta, GA: US Department of Health and Human Services, Public Health Service, 1994.
4. King E, Sparling FP, Holmes KK, et al. Sexually transmitted diseases. 3rd ed. New York: McGraw-Hill, 1999:433–449.
5. Centers for Disease Control and Prevention. Summary of notifiable diseases, United States, 2002. MMWR Morb Mortal Wkly Rep 51:1–84, 2004.
6. Rothenberg R, Judson FN. The clinical diagnosis of urethral discharge. Sex Transm Dis 10:24–28, 1983.
7. Handsfield HH, Sparling PF. Neisseria gonorrhoeae. In: Mandell GL, Bennet JE, Dolin R, eds. Principles and practice of infectious diseases. 5th ed. New York: Churchill Livingstone, 2000: 2242–2258.
8. Centers for Disease Control and Prevention. Increases in fluoroquinolone-resistant Neisseria gonorrhoeae among men who have sex with men—United States, 2003, and revised recommendations for gonorrhea treatment, 2004. MMWR Morb Mortal Wkly Rep. 53:335–338, 2004.
9. Judson F. Gonorrhea. Med Clin North Am 74:1353–1366, 1990.
10. Centers for Disease Control and Prevention. 2002 Guidelines for treatment of sexually transmitted diseases. MMWR Morb Mortal Wkly Rep 51:1–77, 2002.
11. Hook EW, Roddy RE, Handsfield HH. Ceftriaxone therapy for incubating and early syphilis. J Infect Dis 158:881–884, 1988.
12. Handsfield HH, McCormack WM, Hook EW, et al. A comparison of single dose cefixime with ceftriaxone as treatment for uncomplicated gonorrhea. N Engl J Med 325:1337–1341, 1991.
13. Burstein GR, Berman SM, Blumer JL, et al. Ciprofloxacin for the treatment of uncomplicated gonorrhea infection in adolescents: does the benefit outweigh the risk? Clin Infect Dis 35 (Suppl 2):S191–S199, 2004.
14. Handsfield HH, Dalu ZA, Martin DH, et al. Multicenter trial of single-dose azithromycin vs. ceftriaxone in the treatment of uncomplicated gonorrhea. Sex Transm Dis 21:107–111, 1994.
15. King E, Sparling FP, Holmes KK, et al. Sexually transmitted diseases. 3rd ed. New York: McGraw-Hill, 1999:433–449.
16. Bowie WR, Wang SP, Alexander ER, et al. Etiology of nongonococcal urethritis: evidence for Chlamydia trachomatis and Ureaplasma urealyticum. J Clin Invest 59:735–742, 1977.
17. Martin DT. Chlamydial infections. Med Clin North Am 74:1367–1388, 1990.
18. Schacter J, Stoner E, Moncada JL, et al. Screening for chlamydial infection in women attending family planning clinics: evaluation of presumptive indicators for therapy. West J Med 138:375, 1983.
19. Coleman P, Varitek V, Muchahwar IK, et al. Testpack chlamydia: a new rapid assay for the detection of Chlamydia trachomatis. J Clin Microbiol 27:2811–2814, 1989.
20. Black CM. Current methods of laboratory diagnosis of Chlamydia trachomatis infections. Clin Microbiol Rev 10:160–184, 1997.
21. Martin DH, Mroczkowski TF, Dalu ZA, et al. A controlled trial of a single dose of azithromycin for the treatment of chlamydial urethritis and cervicitis. N Engl J Med 327:921–925, 1992.
22. Whatley JD, Thin RN, Mumtaz G, et al. Azithromycin vs doxycycline in the treatment of non-gonococcal urethritis. Int J STD AIDS 2:248–251, 1991.
23. Adimora AA. Treatment of uncomplicated genital Chlamydia trachomatis infections in adults. Clin Infect Dis 35 (Supp2):S187–S190, 2002.
24. Augenbraun MH, Cummings M, McCormack WM. Management of chronic urethral symptoms in men. Clin Infect Dis 15:714–715, 1992.
25. Hooton TM, Rogers MR, Medina TG, et al. Ciprofloxacin compared with doxycycline for nongonococcal urethritis: ineffectiveness against Chlamydia trachomatis due to relapsing infection. JAMA 264:1418–1421, 1990.
26. Magid D, Douglas J, Schwartz S. Doxycycline compared with azithromycin for treating women with genital Chlamydia trachomatis infections: An incremental cost-effectiveness analysis. Ann Intern Med 124:389–399, 1996.

27. Lea A, Lamb HM. Azithromycin. A pharmacoeconomic review of its use as a single-dose regimen in the treatment of uncomplicated urogenital Chlamydia trachomatis infections in women. Pharmacoeconomics 12:596–611, 1997.
28. King E, Sparling FP, Holmes KK, et al. Sexually transmitted diseases. 3rd ed. New York: McGraw-Hill, 1999:467–509.
29. Tramont EC. Treponema pallidum (syphilis). In: Mandell GL, Bennet JE, Dolin R, eds. Principles and practice of infectious diseases. 5th ed. New York: Churchill Livingstone, 2000:2474–2490.
30. Centers for Disease Control. Primary and secondary syphilis: United States, 2002 MMWR Morb Mortal Wkly Rep 52:1117–1120, 2003.
31. Flores J. Syphilis—a tale of twisted treponemes. West J Med 163:552–559, 1995.
32. Hook EW, Marra CM. Acquired syphilis in adults. N Engl J Med 326:1060–1069, 1992.
33. Chapel TA. The signs and symptoms of secondary syphilis. Sex Transm Dis 7:161–165, 1980.
34. Fitzgerald TJ. Treponema. In: Balow A, Hausler WJ, Herrmann KL, et al., eds. Manual of clinical microbiology. 5th ed. Washington, DC: American Society for Microbiology, 1991:567–571.
35. Larsen SA. Syphilis. Clin Lab Med 9:545–557, 1989.
36. Quinn TC, Zenilman J, Rompalo A. Sexually transmitted diseases: advances in diagnosis and treatment. Adv Intern Med 39:149–196, 1994.
37. Romanowski B, Sutherland R, Fick GH, et al. Serologic response to treatment of infectious syphilis. Ann Intern Med 114:1005–1009, 1991.
38. Zenker PN, Rolfs RT. Treatment of syphilis, 1989. Rev Infect Dis 12 (Suppl 6):S590–S609, 1990.
39. Wolters EC. Treatment of neurosyphilis. Clin Neuropharmacol 10:143–154, 1987.
40. Centers for Disease Control and Prevention. 2002 Guidelines for treatment of sexually transmitted diseases. MMWR Morb Mortal Wkly Rep 51:1–77, 2002.
41. Rolfs RT. Treatment of syphilis, 1993. Clin Infect Dis 20 (Suppl 1):S23–S38, 1995.
42. Wendel GD, Stark BJ, Jamison RB, et al. Penicillin allergy and desensitization in serious infections during pregnancy. N Engl J Med 312:1229–1232, 1985.
43. Marra CM, Boutin P, McArthur JC, et al. A pilot study evaluating ceftriaxone and penicillin G as treatment agents for neurosyphilis in HIV-infected patients. Clin Infect Dis 30:540–544, 2000.
44. Augenbraun MH. Treatment of syphilis 2001:nonpregnant adults. Clin Infect Dis 35 (Suppl 2):S187–S190, 2002.
45. Centers for Disease Control and Prevention. Azithromycin treatment failures in syphilis infections–San Francisco, CA, 2002–2003. MMWR Morb Mortal Wkly Rep 53:197–198, 2004.
46. Salkind AR, Cuddy PG, Foxworth JW. Is this patient allergic to penicillin? An evidence-based analysis of the likelihood of penicillin allergy? JAMA 285:2498–2505, 2001.
47. Guinan ME, Wolinsky SN, Reichman RC. Epidemiology of genital herpes simplex virus infection. Epidemiol Rev 7:127–132, 1985.
48. Whitley R, Kimberlin D, Roizman B. Herpes simplex viruses. Clin Infect Dis 26:541–555, 1998.
49. de Ruiter A, Thin RN. Genital herpes: a guide to pharmacologic therapy. Drugs 47:297–304, 1994.
50. Fife KH, Crumpacker CS, Mertz GJ, et al. Recurrence and resistance patterns of herpes simplex virus following cessation of 6 years of chronic suppression with acyclovir. J Infect Dis 169:1338–1341, 1994.
51. Reitano M, Tyring S, Lang W, et al. Valaciclovir for the suppression of recurrent genital herpes simplex virus infection: a large scale dose range-finding study. J Infect Dis 178:603–610, 1998.
52. Diaz-Mitoma F, Sibbald G, Shafron S, et al. Oral famciclovir for the suppression of recurrent genital herpes. JAMA 280:887–892, 1998.
53. Blanchier H, Huraux JM, Hurauz-Rendu C, et al. Genital herpes and pregnancy: preventive measures. Eur J Obstet Gynecol Reprod Biol 53:33–38, 1994.
54. Perry CM, Faulds D. Valaciclovir. A review of its antiviral activity, pharmacokinetic properties and therapeutic efficacy in herpesvirus infections. Drugs 52:754–772, 1996.
55. Perry CM, Wagstaff AJ. Famciclovir: a review of its pharmacological properties and therapeutic efficacy in herpesvirus infections. Drugs 50:396–415, 1995.
56. Acyclovir product information (package insert). Data on file. Glaxo Wellcome Inc. 2003.
57. Centers for Disease Control and Prevention. 2002 Guidelines for treatment of sexually transmitted diseases. MMWR Morb Mortal Wkly Rep 51:1–77, 2002.
58. Schulte JM, Schmid GP. Recommendations for treatment of chancroid, 1993. Clin Infect Dis 20 (Suppl 1):S39–S46, 1995.
59. King E, Sparling FP, Holmes KK, et al. Sexually transmitted diseases. 3rd ed. New York: McGraw-Hill, 1999:515–523.
60. Kent HL. Epidemiology of vaginitis. Am J Obstet Gynecol 165:1168–1176, 1991.
61. Muller M, Rein ME. Trichomonas vaginalis. In: Holmes KK, Mardh PA, Sparking PF, et al., eds. Sexually transmitted diseases. 2nd ed. New York: McGraw-Hill, 1990:481–492.
62. Grossman JH, Galash RP. Persistent vaginitis caused by metronidazole-resistant trichomoniasis. Obstet Gynecol 76:521–522, 1990.
63. Kriega JN, Jenny C, Verdon M, et al. Clinical manifestations of trichomoniasis in men. Ann Intern Med 118:844–949, 1993.
64. Rein MF. Trichomoniasis vaginalis. In: Mandell GL, Bennet JE, Dolin R, eds. Principles and practice of infectious diseases. 4th ed. New York: Churchill Livingstone, 1995:2493–2497.
65. Centers for Disease Control and Prevention. 2002 Guidelines for treatment of sexually transmitted diseases. MMWR Morb Mortal Wkly Rep 51:1–77, 2002.
66. Perine PL, Osoba AO. Lymphogranuloma venereum. In: Holmes KK, Mardh PA, Sparling PF, et al., eds. Sexually transmitted diseases. 2nd ed. New York: McGraw-Hill, 1990:195–204.
67. King E, Sparling FP, Holmes KK, et al. Sexually transmitted diseases 3rd ed. New York: McGraw-Hill, 1999:423–432.
68. Centers for Disease Control and Prevention. 2002 Guidelines for treatment of sexually transmitted diseases. MMWR Morb Mortal Wkly Rep 51:1–77, 2002.
69. King E, Sparling FP, Holmes KK, et al. Sexually transmitted diseases 3rd ed. New York: McGraw-Hill, 1999:347–359.
70. Whiley DJ, Douglas J, Beutner K, et al. External genital warts: diagnosis, treatment, and prevention. Clin Infect Dis 35 (Suppl 2):S210–S224, 2002.
71. Howley PM, Schlegel R. The human papillomaviruses: an overview. Am J Med 85:155–172, 1988.
72. Centers for Disease Control and Prevention. 2002 Guidelines for treatment of sexually transmitted diseases. MMWR Morb Mortal Wkly Rep 51:1–77, 2002.
73. Podofilox for genital warts. Med Lett Drugs Ther 33:117–118, 1991.

Human Immunodeficiency Virus Infection—Antiretroviral Therapy

84

Betty J. Dong and Jennifer Cocohoba

TREATMENT GOALS

During the last decade promising evidence of immune system reconstitution and dramatic reductions in opportunistic infections, disease progression to acquired immune deficiency syndrome (AIDS), and death from the use of potent combinations of antiretroviral (ARV) agents have led to widespread enthusiasm that human immunodeficiency virus (HIV) might be eradicated.[1,2] However, the discoveries of latent, resting reservoirs of HIV that are inaccessible to current ARV agents have dampened optimism for a "cure."[3–5] Eradication of HIV is highly unlikely and chronic ARV therapy will likely be required to maintain viral suppression and reduce disease progression. During the next decade, innovative therapies aimed at blocking HIV cell entry, continued suppression of HIV replication, and ARVs targeting resting HIV reservoirs will be critical to prolong survival and renew hopes for a cure. The complete lack of efficacy of the first two phase III AIDS vaccine trials (e.g., AIDSVAX) clearly show that development of an effective AIDS vaccine is not forthcoming in the near future.[6]

- Reduce symptoms and delay disease progression to AIDS.
- Minimize AIDS-related opportunistic infections and malignancies.
- Improve quality of life and prolong survival.
- Reduce viral load to undetectable levels or lowest levels possible for as long as possible.
- Eliminate resting reservoirs of HIV.
- Increase CD4 lymphocyte count.
- Reduce viral resistance and drug failure.
- Reconstitute the immune system.
- Prevent perinatal transmission from mother to fetus.
- Prevent HIV infection from high-risk occupational or nonoccupational exposures.
- Design effective therapeutic regimens that minimize drug adherence problems.
- Reduce total pill burden and minimize interference with quality of life.

DEFINITION

A person infected with HIV is defined by the Centers for Disease Control and Prevention (CDC) as having positive antibodies against HIV (positive HIV test), with 200 or more helper T-lymphocytes (CD4 cell/mm^3), and the absence of an AIDS-defining illness.[7] By definition, an HIV-infected person with AIDS has fewer than 200 cells/mm^3 CD4 cells or the presence of an AIDS-defining illness (Table 84.1).

ETIOLOGY

HIV is a single-stranded RNA retrovirus that can be divided into types HIV-1 and HIV-2. HIV-1 is the predominant infection found in the United States and is the type addressed

TABLE 84.1	1993 AIDS-Defining Illnesses from Centers for Disease Control and Prevention

Candidiasis of esophagus, bronchi, trachea, or lungs

Cervical cancer, invasive

Coccidioidomycosis, disseminated or extrapulmonary

Cryptococcoses, extrapulmonary

Cryptosporidiosis, chronic intestinal (>1 month duration)

Cytomegalovirus disease other than liver, spleen, or nodes

Cytomegalovirus retinitis with vision loss

Encephalopathy, HIV-related

Herpes simplex: chronic ulcers (>1 month), bronchitis, pneumonitis, or esophagitis

Histoplasmosis, disseminated or extrapulmonary

Isosporiasis, chronic intestinal (>1 month)

Kaposi's sarcoma

Lymphoma Burkitt's (or equivalent term)

Lymphoma immunoblastic (or equivalent term)

Lymphoma, primary, of brain

Mycobacterium avium complex or *Mycobacterium kansasii*, disseminated or extrapulmonary

Pneumocystis jirovecii (formerly *Pneumocystis carinii*) pneumonia (PCP)

Pneumonia, recurrent

Progressive multifocal leukoencephalopathy (PML)

Salmonella septicemia, recurrent

Toxoplasmosis of the brain

Tuberculosis

Wasting syndrome, HIV-related

HIV, human immunodeficiency virus. (From Palella FJ, Delaney KM, Moorman AC, et al. Declining morbidity and mortality among patients with advanced human immunodeficiency virus infection. N Engl J Med 338:853–860, 1998,[1] with permission).

in this chapter. HIV-2 is found primarily in Africa. Both types of HIV infection deplete the helper T-lymphocytes (CD4 cell/mm^3) and other cells of the immune system, including monocytes and macrophages, resulting in continued destruction of the immune system, and leading to the occurrence of opportunistic infections and malignancies.

EPIDEMIOLOGY

Individuals who lack a coreceptor required for HIV cell entry do not acquire HIV infection despite repeated high-risk exposures.[8] HIV infection is acquired by contact with infected blood or hazardous body fluids by unprotected sexual intercourse, contact with contaminated drug paraphernalia, transfusion of infected blood products, and vertical transmission from mother to infant. Although urine, tears, and saliva can contain HIV, transmission from these nonbloody fluids is rare. Proteaselike inhibitor substances found in saliva can inhibit the ability of HIV to enter the white blood cells.[9] One case of HIV infection, reported after deep kissing, is presumed related to contact with infected blood from poor dentition and gingivitis. Experts estimate infection risks from a single unprotected sexual exposure with an infected sexual partner at 1/1,000 to 1/10,000 depending on the type of the exposure.[10] The highest probability of HIV transmission (0.8%–3.2%) is associated with unprotected receptive anal intercourse with a partner infected with HIV; lower risks are estimated with receptive vaginal intercourse (0.1%–0.2%). Rarely, HIV infection has been reported after oral sex.[11] The risk of HIV infection after a percutaneous occupational exposure to a contaminated needle is estimated to be 0.3% (1/300). The likelihood of infection is increased by a deep puncture, a device used in an artery or vein, a visibly bloody device, or exposure to a source patient who died of AIDS within 2 months. The estimated risk from bloody mucocutaneous exposures (e.g., eye or mouth splashes) is much lower at 1/1,000. The estimated HIV probability after the use of contaminated injection drug paraphernalia (0.67%) is slightly higher than that associated with a puncture in an occupational setting, which may reflect the greater volume of blood transferred when sharing. In two large trials, the risks of perinatal HIV transmission to the infant was reported to be 19% and 23%.[12,13] The greatest risk for perinatal transmission likely occurs near or during delivery. HIV can also be transmitted via breast milk (20% risk); and breastfeeding should be avoided in mothers infected with HIV. Since 1985, surveillance of U.S. blood products have significantly reduced the chance of contaminated transfusions; the risk is estimated to be 1/450,000 to 1/660,000 transfusions or two cases per million.

Worldwide in 2004, an estimated 39.4 million adults and children are living with HIV/AIDS, of whom 17.6 million are women and 2.2 million are children less than 15 years of age. The majority of infected persons reside in developing countries, including Sub-Saharan Africa, Asia, and the Pacific. In 2004 alone, a staggering 4.9 million persons (e.g., 4.3 million adults and 640,000 children) became newly infected with HIV (approximately 14,000 infections daily) while 3.1 million deaths occurred. To date, more than 20 million persons have died since the epidemic began in the 1980s.

In the United States estimates indicate that about 900,000 Americans are living with HIV infection, 25% of whom are unaware of their infection.[14] New infections continue at a rate of 40,000 infections annually in the United States, affecting men (70%) more than women (30%). Younger persons less than 25 years of age and ethnic minorities (i.e., >50% African-Americans, 18%–20% Hispanics) are disproportionately affected. African-American women account for 64% of new HIV cases. People aged 65 years or older represented approximately 2% of HIV/AIDS cases diagnosed in 2002. Although the epidemic has disproportionately affected certain ethnic minorities, ethnicity is not considered a risk factor for HIV but a marker for other factors that might be predictive of increased risk for HIV infection (e.g., low income, history of injection drug use, high-risk sex, lack of education).

In men, the primary routes of HIV transmissions are men who have sex with men (MSM 60%), intravenous drug use (25%), and heterosexual contact (15%). In women, hetero-sexual contact (75%) and intravenous drug use (IDU) (25%) represent the major routes of infection while most children are infected perinatally. AIDS constitutes the fifth leading cause of death among Americans aged 25 to 44 years, the seventh leading cause of death among those aged 15 to 24 years, and the ninth cause of death in those aged 45 to 64 years of age. It is the primary cause of death among African-American women aged 25 to 34 years of age. Since the introduction of highly active antiretroviral therapy (HAART) and prophylaxis against opportunistic infections, dramatic declines in mortality rates have been observed from 1995 to 1998 (e.g., 21.0%–47.7%); less impressive reductions were reported during 1999 to 2001 (1.9%–3.8%).

PATHOPHYSIOLOGY

The single-stranded RNA-containing HIV virus requires the creation of proviral DNA within the host to complete its life cycle and infect other cells (Fig. 84.1). The surface envelope of HIV contains a structure known as glycoprotein (gp 120 and gp 41) that binds to the CD4 receptor of the host cell. Cell entry also requires concomitant binding with chemokine coreceptors, CCR5 or CXCR4 to gp 41 to allow cell fusion and entry of viral genetic material.[8] Viral RNA is uncoated

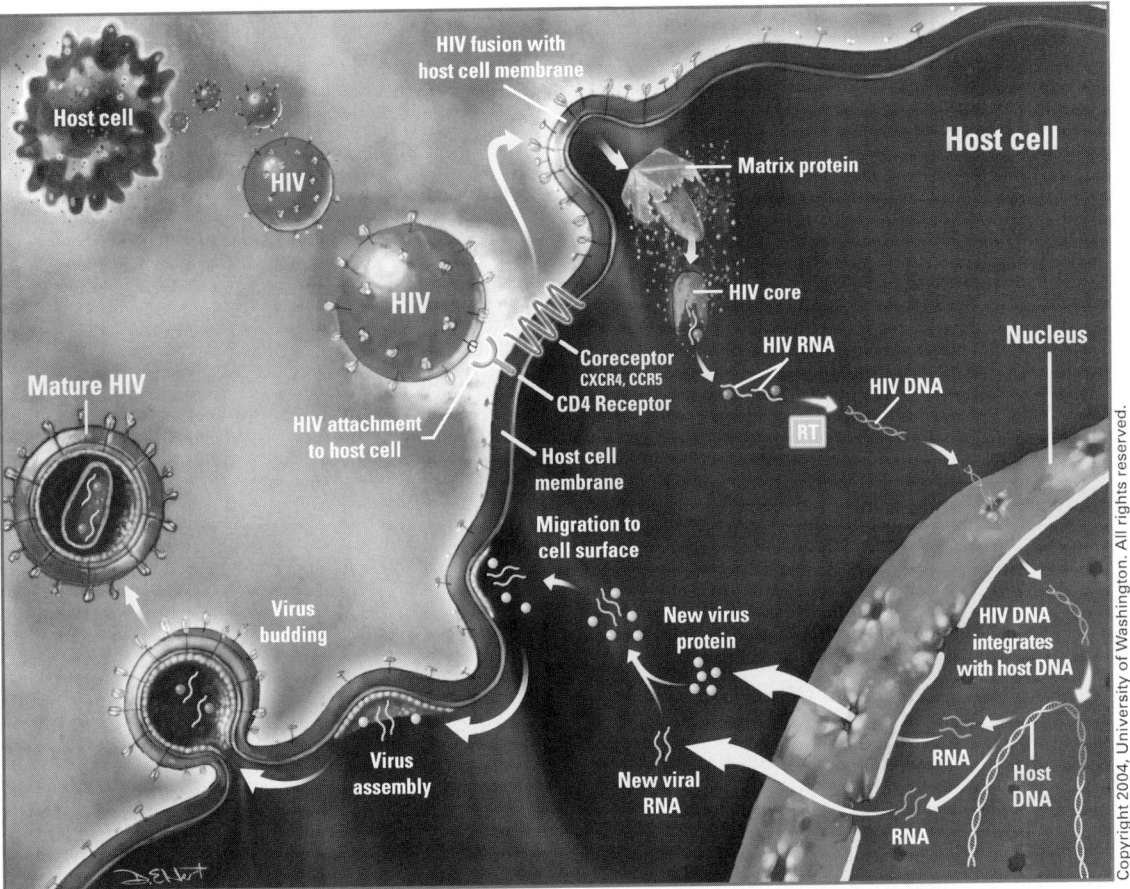

FIGURE 84.1 Life Cycle of HIV-1. (Modified from the New Mexico AIDS InfoNet.)

before being transcribed by the reverse transcriptase (RT) enzyme into proviral DNA. The proviral DNA is integrated into the host nucleus by the integrase enzyme. The integrated viral genes may remain inactive or be transcribed (tat protein) back into genomic RNA and messenger RNA, which are then translated into viral proteins. Finally, the viral proteins are cleaved by the protease enzyme into new HIV particles, assembled, and new infectious virions are released to infect other cells.

Viral kinetics, replication, and clearance have been clarified. Viral replication is an ongoing and dynamic process that results in the progressive destruction of CD4 lymphocytes and continued immune depletion. Approximately 1 to 10 billion virions are produced daily to maintain a steady-state of viral replication, even during a period of clinical latency.[15] Using mathematical modeling, the half-life of free virus is estimated to be 6 hours. Infected memory CD4 lymphocytes serve as latent reservoirs of HIV infection, making eradication difficult.[4–6] It has been estimated that effective ARV therapy would have to be maintained for a minimum of 70 years to eliminate these latent reservoirs.[16] Therefore, a cure during one's lifetime is highly unlikely.

After initial HIV infection, there is immediate widespread dissemination of the virus to other lymphatic systems and organs (e.g., brain). The majority of persons during primary infection exhibit some nonspecific symptoms of an acute viral infection. High plasma viremia (HIV RNA viral load or burden $>10^7$ copies/mL) is detected in blood and present in sexual organs and secretions. Dramatic declines in CD4 cell counts (e.g., <200 cells) can occur transiently. Infectivity is high during acute primary infection. During acute infection, the appearance of potent, cytotoxic CD8 T-lymphocytes from a highly activated immune system limits viral replication and reduces symptoms as plasma viremia declines.[17,18] In adults, a new steady-state plasma HIV RNA "viral setpoint" is established 6 months or longer after the initial infection that can remain stable for months or years before progression to AIDS. Because infected individuals have different steady-state levels of viral replication, it is important to identify their plasma HIV RNA level before starting therapy. In infants infected with HIV, the new viral setpoint is often not reached until more than a year after infection.

The time course of progression to AIDS can be quite variable in adults; however, average durations of 10 to 11 years are reported in the absence of ARV therapy. A landmark study showed that steady-state plasma HIV RNA levels are highly predictive of disease progression and can be elevated in persons with normal or low CD4 cell counts. Persons with the highest viral loads depleted CD4 cell counts quicker, had more rapid disease progression to AIDS, and died earlier than those with the lowest viral loads.[19] Approximately 5% to 10% of persons infected with HIV do not progress to AIDS and are identified as long-term nonprogressors (LTNPs). These HIV-infected LTNPs remain asymptomatic with stable CD4 counts and low plasma vire-

mia more than 15 years after their infection. It is believed that a strong cellular immune response from strong cytotoxic T-lymphocyte responses (e.g., CD8 cells) limits cell death (apoptosis) and disease progression.[20] Currently, there is no accurate commercial method to identify these LTNPs. Humoral immunity (i.e., antibodies) appears less effective in controlling viremia.

CLINICAL PRESENTATION AND DIAGNOSIS

SIGNS AND SYMPTOMS

The clinical presentation of an acute primary HIV infection can be confused with a typical viral illness; however, it should be suspected in persons with a history of high-risk behaviors or presence of sexually transmitted disease. Common signs and symptoms are nonspecific, generally occur within days to weeks after the initial exposure, and include fever, fatigue, myalgias, arthralgias, headache, lymphadenopathy, pharyngitis, and oral lesions.[21] A maculopapular rash is present in 40% to 80% of persons during the acute illness. Symptoms last approximately 10 to 14 days but may continue for several weeks; prolonged symptoms are indicative of a poorer prognosis and more rapid disease progression.

Patients with established HIV infection can remain clinically asymptomatic for many years, or develop symptomatic disease (e.g., unexplained low-grade fevers, thrush, or symptoms of AIDS) (Table 84.1).

DIAGNOSIS

Established HIV infection is diagnosed by finding antibodies to HIV in the plasma using various serological testing methods. The initial screening test for detection of anti-HIV antibodies is the enzyme-linked immunosorbent assay (ELISA). However, because a false-positive ELISA can occur in those with collagen vascular diseases, chronic hepatitis, pregnancy, and other conditions, all positive ELISA results must be confirmed by a Western blot (WB) before a diagnosis of HIV infection can be made. The accuracy of the WB is excellent, the specificity (likelihood that a person without infection will have a negative test) and sensitivity (likelihood that a person with infection will have a positive test) is greater than 99.9%. In neonates, the diagnosis of HIV infection is difficult because of the presence of passive maternal HIV antibodies, which can persist for many months. Most importantly, a false-negative test can occur in an HIV-infected person if the ELISA and WB are obtained during the "window period" or before antibody production has occurred after primary HIV infection. These routine diagnostic HIV tests may not be positive until 22 to 27 days after the acute infection.[21] In a high-risk patient with a negative WB test, elevated plasma viral RNA levels (VL) greater than 50,000 copies per milliliter or the detection of the p24 antigen can establish the diagnosis of an acute HIV infection.

Because a false-positive VL results can occur, the diagnosis of HIV infection should not be made on the basis of low viral titers (<5,000 RNA copies/mL). A positive WB is essential to confirm the existence of HIV infection. A major disadvantage of serial HIV testing by ELISA and the WB is that the 1-week to 2-week delay or more for test results has resulted in loss of infected persons for follow-up and treatment. In 2000, 31% of persons testing HIV positive and 33% of persons testing negative did not return for their results.[22]

A rapid HIV assay licensed by the Food and Drug Administration (FDA) for use with blood or oral fluids, the Ora-Quick Advance Rapid HIV1/2 Antibody test, can detect antibodies to HIV-1 and HIV-2 within 20 minutes of testing. These immediate results can improve HIV detection, particularly in persons who would have been lost to follow-up. Validation of these results in HIV-infected persons has demonstrated comparable sensitivity (99.6% for blood and 99.3% for oral fluids) and specificity (100% for blood and 99.8% for oral fluids). Therefore, no further confirmatory testing is needed if the OraQuick test is negative unless the testing is done soon after a risky exposure. However, to eliminate the possibility of a false-positive test, a positive OraQuick test should be considered inconclusive until the results are confirmed by the WB. To perform the test with oral fluids, the person uses a device to gently swab completely around the outer gums, both upper and lower, one time around before inserting the device into a vial containing a developer solution. The appearance of two reddish-purple lines in a small window in the device indicates a preliminary positive test that requires confirmation by a WB.

Urine tests for HIV infection may also be useful when collection of blood is not possible The Sentinel HIV-1 Urine EIA is a urine HIV-1 test approved by the FDA in August 1996 that is only available to health care professionals. The sensitivity and specificity of this test to detect HIV antibodies in urine (99.3%) are less than HIV tests for blood and oral specimens. A repeatedly positive urine EIA should be confirmed by a serum WB.

One home HIV-1 testing kit, Home Access HIV-1 Test System, is available in pharmacies and by mail. The advantages of home testing are confidentiality and convenience if the $40 to $50 cost is not prohibitive. Concerns about adequate pretest and posttest counseling and support for patients with positive results have not been documented. The user pricks a fingertip with the supplied lancet to collect the blood specimen, which is then sent to a central testing laboratory. The reported sensitivity and specificity is 100% provided that the specimens are collected properly. Once the specimens are received, EIA results are available by telephone within 3 to 7 days. All persons with positive or indeterminate results are referred immediately to a counselor. New home HIV tests that could provide results in less than 10 minutes are currently awaiting FDA approval and are expected on the market in the near future.

MONITORING VIRAL ASSAYS

Viral Load Assays. The ability to measure the viral load (VL) or burden (amount of virus in the blood) has revolutionized HIV care. Plasma HIV RNA assays can assess the risk of disease progression and evaluate the efficacy of ARV therapy.[19] The three RNA assays include the RT polymerase chain reaction (RT-PCR), in vitro signal amplification nucleic acid probe assay or branched DNA (bDNA), and the nucleic acid sequence-based amplification (NASBA). The NASBA and RT-PCR both amplify the viral RNA to detectable levels, whereas the bDNA technique amplifies the detection signal from the viral RNA. Plasma HIV RNA levels obtained by the RT-PCR correlate well with levels obtained by the bDNA assay and can detect levels of HIV RNA as low as 20 to 50 copies per milliliter. Results of VL testing expressed in copies per milliliter are often converted to log units to reduce variability. Therefore, one log is equivalent to a factor of 10 and a VL of 100,000 copies per milliliter would be 5 logs.

CD4 Cell Count. The CD4 cell count is the best indicator of the extent of immune damage and risk of opportunistic infections. Therefore, it is often used to determine if HAART should be started. Since CD4 cell counts are quite variable and sensitive to circadian rhythms, the CD4 percentage can fluctuate less and be more accurate but is still not the best predictor of OI (opportunistic infection) risk. Persons with CD4 counts lower than 200 cells/mm³ or less than 14% of all lymphocytes are predisposed to a variety of opportunistic infections, including *Pneumocystis jirovecii* (previously known as *carinii*) pneumonia (Table 84.1). As the CD4 counts drop below 50 cells/mm³, the prevalence of other infections, including *Mycobacterium avium-intracellulare* and *Cytomegalovirus* disease, increases.

THERAPEUTIC PLAN

National HIV disease guidelines on the use of ARV agents in adults have been published by the Department of Health and Human Services (DHHS) and the Henry J. Kaiser Family Foundation.[23] Similar recommendations for ARV therapy in adults have also been developed by the International AIDS Society, USA panel.[24] Additional guidelines for using ARV agents in pediatrics, pregnancy, and for prophylaxis after occupational and nonoccupational exposures have been developed by the CDC. Updates in these national guidelines can be obtained at the following websites: http://AIDSinfo.nih.gov, http://ucsf.edu/hivcntr, and http://hivinsite.ucsf.edu. The British HIV Association Guidelines recommend a similar approach to care of the adult infected with HIV.[25] Physicians with greater experience in the care of persons infected with HIV may be more knowledgeable about current treatment guidelines that may impact on the quality of care given.[26]

The major classes of ARV agents include the nucleoside and nucleotide RT inhibitors (NRTIs) (Table 84.2), the pro-

(text continues on page 2097)

TABLE 84.2 **NucleoSIDE and NucleoTIDE Reverse Transcriptase Inhibitors (NRTIs)**

Drug	Dosage Forms	Usual Doses	Special Administration Instructions	Selected Adverse Effects	Potential for Drug Interactions (Table 85.9)
Zidovudine (ZDV, AZT, Retrovir)	CAPS 100 mg; TABS 300 mg; Syrup 10 mg/mL IV solution: 10 mg/mL	300 mg bid or 200 mg tid (500–600 mg/day); 100 mg tid if needed to ↓ anemia; Renal dysfunction: CrCl <25 mL/min or HD 100 mg tid	Take with meals to reduce nausea	Headaches, fatigue, nausea, insomnia; bone marrow suppression: anemia, neutropenia, thrombocytopenia, hepatitis, ↑ LFT, myopathy with >6 months use, lactic acidosis with hepatic steatosis (rare)	Avoid concurrent bone marrow suppressive agents (e.g., ganciclovir induction, trimethoprim-sulfamethoxazole treatment) P-450 drug interactions unlikely.
In combination with 3TC	Combivir (3TC 150 mg + ZDV 300 mg)	Combivir: 1 tablet bid			
In combination with 3TC and ABC	Trizivir (3TC 150 mg + ABC 300 mg + ZDV 300 mg)	Trizivir: 1 tablet bid			
Didanosine (ddI, Videx EC, Videx)	Enteric coated (EC) capsules 125, 200, 250, or 400 mg; Chewable buffered TABS 25,50,100, 150, 200 mg; POWDER for oral solution 100, 167, 250 mg packets; Pediatric solution: dilute powder with antacid 10 mg/ml	(>60 kg) 400 mg daily or 200 mg bid (buffered Tablet only) (<60 kg) 250 mg daily or 125 mg bid (buffered Tablet only) (>60 kg) PWD 250 mg bid (<60 kg) 167 mg bid Renal dysfunction: CrCL (≥60 kg) (<60 kg) 30–59 200 mg qd 125 mg qd 10–29 125 mg qd 100 mg qd <10 or HD 125 mg qd 75 mg qd	Administer on an empty stomach (1 hour before or 2 hours after a meal). Can give with food if given concomitantly with tenofovir (Viread) Buffered tablets: Administer at least > 2 hours from agents whose absorption is impaired by buffer. Must chew or crush two buffered tablets/dose for adequate buffer.	Nausea, vomiting, diarrhea, painful peripheral neuropathy, pancreatitis, hyperglycemia, hyperuricemia, hypertriglyceridemia, hyperamylasemia, ↑ LFT, lactic acidosis with hepatic steatosis (rare)	Avoid or limit alcohol or other pancreatic toxins (e.g., IV pentamidine). Avoid concurrent neurotoxic agents (e.g., d4T). Dosage adjustment required if given with tenofovir

Drug	Formulations	Dosing		Adverse Effects	Drug Interactions
Stavudine (d4T, Zerit)	CAPS 15, 20, 30, 40 mg; EXTENDED Release CAPS XR 75, 100 mg (not yet marketed but FDA approved); Oral Solution: 1 mg/mL	(>60 kg) 40 mg bid or 100 mg XR daily; (<60 kg) 30 mg bid or 75 mg XR daily; Renal dysfunction CrCl 26–50 mL/min 10–25 mL/min; ≥60 kg 20 mg q12hr 20 mg daily; ≤60 kg 15 mg q12hr 15 mg daily	Take with or without meals	Painful peripheral neuropathy, insomnia, pancreatitis, ↑ LFT, lipoatrophy, lactic acidemia, lactic acidosis with hepatic steatosis (rare)	Avoid concurrent neurotoxic agents (e.g., ddI). Avoid antagonistic combination of ZDV and d4T
Lamivudine (3TC, Epivir)	TABS 150, 300 mg; 100 mg tabs (for HBV therapy, may be inadequate for HIV treatment); Oral solution 10 mg/mL syrup	300 mg daily or 150 mg bid; Renal dysfunction CrCl 30–49 mL/min 150 mg qd; 15–29 150 mg LD+ 100 mg qd; 5–14 150 mg LD+ 50 mg qd; <5 or HD 50 mg LD, then 25 mg qd	Take with or without meals	Well tolerated, headache, nausea, rash, lactic acidosis with hepatic steatosis (rare); pancreatitis in children	No significant DI. Also see interactions for individual agents
In combination with ZDV	Combivir (3TC 150 mg + ZDV 300 mg)	Combivir: 1 tablet bid			
In combination with ZDV and ABC	Trizivir (3TC 150 mg + ABC 300 mg + ZDV 300 mg)	Trizivir: 1 tablet bid			
In combination with ABC	Epzicom 3TC 300 mg + ABC 600 mg	Epzicom one tablet daily			
Emtricitabine (FTC, Emtriva)	CAPS 200 mg	200 mg daily; Renal dysfunction CrCl 30–49 mL/min 200 mg q48hr; 15–29 200 mg q72hr	Take with or without meals	Well tolerated, nausea, headache, hyperpigmentation of hands and soles (rare), lactic acidosis with hepatic steatosis (rare)	No significant DI. Also see tenofovir

(continued)

TABLE 84.2	continued			
Drug	**Dosage Forms**	**Usual Doses**	**Special Administration Instructions**	**Selected Adverse Effects**	**Potential for Drug Interactions (Table 85.9)**
In combination with tenofovir (TDF)	Truvada TDF 300 mg + FTC 200 mg	<15 or HD 200 mg q96hr Give after HD Truvada 1 tablet daily			
Abacavir (ABC, Ziagen)	TABS 300 mg; Oral solution 20 mg/mL	600 mg qd or 300 mg bid No dosage adjustment for renal dysfunction. Reduce dose to 200 mg bid in mild liver disease. Not recommended for those with moderate to severe hepatic impairment	Take with or without meals	Nausea, headache, malaise, diarrhea, abdominal pain, lactic acidosis with hepatic steatosis (rare). 3%–8% hypersensitivity reaction (rash, fever, malaise, nausea, vomiting, sore throat, cough, SOB, hepatitis, pancreatitis, weakness) which can be life threatening: Do NOT rechallenge	Alcohol can increase ABC levels by 41%, unknown clinical significance. Also see individual agents
In combination with ZDV and 3TC	Trizivir (3TC 150 mg + ABC 300 mg + ZDV 300 mg	Trizivir: 1 tablet bid			
In combination with 3TC	Epzicom 3TC 300 mg + ABC 600 mg	Epzicom: 1 tablet daily			
NucleoTIDE Reverse Transcriptase Inhibitor					
Tenofovir disoproxil fumarate (TDF, Viread)	TABS 300 mg	300 mg daily Renal dysfunction: CrCl 30–49 300 mg q48hr 10–29 300 mg twice weekly HD 300 mg once weekly	Take with or without meals	Fatigue, headache, diarrhea, nausea, vomiting, bloating, lactic acidosis with hepatic steatosis (rare), renal failure and Fanconi's syndrome (rare)	Can ↑ ddI levels and toxicity: reduce ddI dosage to 250 mg daily for ≥60 kg.
In combination with emtricitabine (FTC)	Truvada TDF 300 mg + FTC 200 mg	Truvada 1 tablet daily			Can ↓ ATZ levels, boost ATZ 300 mg with ritonavir 100 mg daily

ATZ, atazanavir; CAPS, capsules; TABS, Tablets; IV, intravenous; bid, twice a day; tid, three times daily; CrCl, creatinine clearance; HD, hemodialysis; LFT, liver function test; qd, every day; d4T, stavudine; PWD, powder; FDA, Food and Drug Administration; HBV, hepatitis B virus; LD, loading dose; DI, drug interactions; SOB, shortness of breath.

tease inhibitors (PIs) (Tables 84.3 and 84.4), the nonnucleoside RT inhibitors (NNRTIs), and the fusion inhibitors (Table 84.5).

TREATMENT

INITIATING HIGHLY ACTIVE ANTIRETROVIRAL THERAPY AND MONITORING

Before starting ARV therapy, it is essential that clinicians educate patients about the need for strict adherence to these complex regimens to minimize the potential for drug failure and drug resistance. Psychosocial barriers (e.g., housing issues, substance abuse, psychiatric issues) should be improved or removed if possible to facilitate adherence. Willingness of the patient to be responsible for therapy, and the prognosis for AIDS-free survival, should be established before starting therapy. There is general consensus that all persons with AIDS or symptomatic HIV disease should promptly receive HAART. In asymptomatic HIV-infected persons with CD4 cell counts between 200 and 350 cells/mm³ the optimal time to start ARV therapy is controversial since the benefits of early intervention are less clear, can limit future treatment options, and pose significant drug toxicity, while the risk of disease progression is low. However, it is generally accepted that treatment should be offered before immunologic and clinical deterioration occurs (i.e., CD4 <200 cells/mm³).[23,24] For asymptomatic persons with CD4 cell counts higher than 350 cells/mm³ and low viral RNA levels (i.e., <100,000 copies/mL), some but not all experts advocate delaying therapy, given that the benefits of early treatment in this cohort are unknown and the 3-year risk of developing AIDS or death is about 3.4%. Observation may be appropriate, given the complexities and toxicities of treatment and the possibility that such persons might be LTNPs. Others argue that with the availability of simplified and potentially less toxic therapy, earlier treatment is justified at these higher CD4 cell counts due to a lower risk of death or progression to AIDS and prevention of HIV transmission by reducing HIV shedding.[27] If the viral load is higher (i.e., >100,000) some experts might consider starting therapy to prevent the 30% risk of developing AIDS in 3 years although the long-term outcome is unknown. Recommendations for starting HAART by the International AIDS Society and the British HIVAIDS Association are in agreement with the DHHS guidelines.[24,25] Recommendations for starting HAART in HIV-infected women are similar to men although conflicting results exist. Some advocate that therapy should be started in women infected with HIV earlier (e.g., at lower viral loads) since they may have a 60% higher risk of progressing to AIDS than men with the same viral load. A viral load of 5,000 copies per milliliter in women was considered equivalent to 10,000 copies in men.[28] Guidelines for starting ARV therapy are summarized in Table 84.6.

Before starting ARV therapy, establishment of two baseline CD4 cell count and VL determinations are recommended to monitor the effectiveness of the ARV regimen. The baseline VL is determined by averaging at least two viral loads taken a few weeks apart that do not differ by more than 0.5 log¹⁰. Within 2 to 8 weeks after starting an ARV regimen that the virus is sensitive to, a 0.5 to 1 log (tenfold) reduction in plasma HIV RNA from baseline should be observed. A more durable ARV response is associated with a more rapid decline in VL during the first 1 to 4 weeks after starting therapy.[29,30] Although the goal of therapy is complete viral suppression or an undetectable VL (e.g., below the current assay's limits of detection), it is important to note that the maximal reduction in VL may not occur until 4 to 6 months after starting therapy. Therefore, changes in therapy before this time are not recommended if there is a consistent downward trend in VL reduction, indicating a therapeutic response. Highly experienced patients with evidence of drug resistance may never attain complete viral suppression. Complete virologic suppression is important since viral replication in the presence of ARV drugs can lead to viral resistance, and subsequently, virologic failure. Routine monitoring of VL is recommended every 3 to 6 months after starting therapy or after a change in the ARV regimen. Virologic failure in naïve persons is suggested by incomplete viral suppression (VL >400 copies/mL after 6 months or >50 copies/mL at 1 year) or more than a 0.5 log¹⁰ increase in viral load when compared with the patient's most recent VL. Therefore, before establishing treatment failure, it is imperative to eliminate any factors that might elevate plasma HIV RNA levels transiently and alter interpretation of viral loads. For example, VL should not be determined within 1 month following immunizations or treatment of concurrent infections (e.g., herpes, tuberculosis, etc.).

The CD4 cell count should be checked every 3 to 4 months. CD4 cell counts are expected to increase approximately 100 to 150 cells/mm³ in the first 3 months. Immunologic failure is defined as failure to increase the CD4 cell count 25 to 50 cells/mm³ above baseline within the first year of therapy or a reversal of CD4 cell gain above baseline. Although an inverse relationship is usually seen between viral load and CD4 cell counts, a small percentage of persons may exhibit discordance between CD4 cell counts and viral load. The significance of this discordance is unknown. Certain ARVs [e.g., didanosine ddI)] may be cytotoxic to CD4 cell increase and an ARV change may be warranted.

SELECTING ANTIRETROVIRAL THERAPY REGIMENS

The basic principles for successful ARV therapy are summarized in Table 84.7. Because the first therapeutic regimen selected in an ARV-naive person is often the most successful in achieving maximal durable viral suppression and immunologic recovery, it is a very important therapeutic decision that should be thoroughly planned. Preparing and educating the patient about the complexities of the therapeutic regimen

(*text continues on page 2101*)

TABLE 84.3	Protease Inhibitors (PIs)				
Drug	**Dosage Forms**	**Usual Doses[a] (Table 85.4 for "boosted" PI dosages)**	**Special Administration Instructions**	**Common Adverse Effects**	**Potential for Drug Interactions (Table 85.9)**
Saquinavir (HG-SAQ, Invirase)	TABS 500 mg; Hard-gel CAPS 200 mg (Likely to be discontinued)	Use only in "boosted" combination with ritonavir (RTV). Not recommended as sole PI	Take with food. Grapefruit juice ↑ SAQ absorption (variable)	Generally well tolerated. GI (diarrhea, nausea, abdominal pain), headache, elevated LFTs, hyperlipidemia, hyperglycemia, lipodystrophy	Least potent CYP3A4 enzyme inhibitor
Ritonavir (RTV) (Norvir)	CAPS 100 mg; Oral Solution 80 mg/mL (43% EtOH)	Rarely used as sole PI. Titration schedule (as sole PI) to limit GI intolerance: 300 mg bid (days 1–2) 400 mg bid (days 3–5) 500 mg bid (days 6–13) to full therapeutic dose of 600 mg bid on day 14. No titration needed if RTV used for "boosting" Use with caution in hepatic impairment	Take 6 capsules/dose or 7.5 mL bid with meals to minimize GI symptoms; can mix oral solution with Advera, chocolate milk, or Ensure. Separate administration of RTV from antacids/ddI by more than 2 hours	GI (nausea, diarrhea, vomiting, anorexia, abdominal pain), fatigue, weakness, numbness, circumoral paresthesia (tingling around the lips), change in taste, dizziness, headache, ↑ LFTs, antabuse reaction, hyperlipidemia, hyperglycemia, lipodystrophy	Potent CYP3A4, CYP2D, and other isoenzyme inhibitor; induction of glucuronosyl transferases
Indinavir (IDV, Crixivan)	CAPS 200, 333, 400 mg	800 mg q8hr ATC Dosage adjustment in liver disease/cirrhosis 600 mg q8hr. Avoid in renal failure	Take 2 X 400 mg capsules/dose q8hr on empty stomach (1 hr before or 2 hours after a meal) or with light meal (skim milk, juice, coffee, tea, dry toast, corn flakes). Avoid high fat, high caloric meal, and grapefruit juice that ↓ absorption. Hydration (minimum of 6 glasses H₂0/day) to prevent kidney stones.	Kidney stones GI (nausea, diarrhea, vomiting, abdominal pain); neurologic: headaches, insomnia, change in taste. Hyperlipidemia, hyperglycemia, ↑ LFTs, lipodystrophy. Indirect hyperbilirubinemia, hepatitis	Moderate CYP3A4 enzyme inhibitor

Drug	Formulations	Dosage	Administration	Toxicities	Metabolism/Interactions
Nelfinavir (NFV, Viracept)	TABS 625, 250 mg; Oral powder 50 mg/g	1250 mg bid or 750 mg tid. Use with caution in hepatic impairment	Separate administration of IDV from antacids/ddI by more than 2 hours. Take 2 × 625 mg tablets/dose bid with high fat meal (20% fat) or 3 × 250 mg tablets/dose tid with high fat meals (20% fat)	Diarrhea, nausea, hyperlipidemia, ↑LFTs, hyperglycemia, lipodystrophy	Moderate CYP3A4 enzyme inhibitor; induction of glucuronosyl transferases
Lopinavir/ritonavir (LPV/r, Kaletra)	TABS 200 mg LPV plus 50 mg RTV; CAPS 133.3 mg LPV plus 33.3 mg RTV; Oral solution 80 mg LPV plus 20 mg RTV per mL (contains 42% alcohol)	400/100 mg bid. Once daily 800/100 mg FDA approved for naïve persons. Use with caution in hepatic impairment. Dosage increase to 4 capsules bid if given with NVP, EFV, or in pregnancy	Take 3 capsules or 1 teaspoon oral solution bid with food. Can also be given as 6 capsules or 2 teaspoons solution ONCE daily in naïve persons	GI: nausea, vomiting, diarrhea, fatigue, ↑LFTs, hyperglycemia, hyperlipidemia, hypertriglyceridemia, lipodystrophy	Potent CYP3A4, CYP2D, and other isoenzyme inhibitor; induction of glucuronosyl transferases
Atazanavir (ATZ, Reyataz)	CAPS 100, 150, 200 mg	400 mg daily. See boosted PI dosages if given with tenofovir (Viread) or efavirenz (Sustiva). Reduce to 300 mg daily with hepatic impairment, avoid in severe hepatic disease	Take 2 capsules once daily with food	GI: nausea, vomiting, diarrhea, headache. Indirect hyperbilirubinemia, prolongation of PR interval; ↑LFTs, hyperglycemia, lipodystrophy	Moderate CYP3A4 enzyme inhibitor. Avoid concomitant use with indinavir. Cautious use with diltiazem (↓diltiazem dose by 50%), and other calcium channel blockers that can prolong PR interval
FosAmprenavir (fos-APV, Lexiva)	TABS 700 mg	1400 mg bid for ARV naïve persons. Table 85.4 for "boosted" dosages in ARV-experienced persons, and use with efavirenz (Sustiva). Reduce to 700 mg bid with hepatic impairment, avoid in severe hepatic disease	Take 2 tablets bid with or without food	GI: nausea, vomiting, diarrhea; rash, headache, oral paresthesias, ↑LFTs, hyperglycemia, hyperlipidemia, lipodystrophy	Moderate CYP3A4 enzyme inhibitor. Induction of glucuronosyl transferases

(continued)

TABLE 84.3	continued				
Drug	**Dosage Forms**	**Usual Doses**	**Special Administration Instructions**	**Selected Adverse Effects**	**Potential for Drug Interactions (Table 85.9)**
Amprenavir (APV, Agenerase)	CAPS 50 mg; Oral Solution (SOLN) 15 mg/mL. Solution and capsules not interchangeable. Avoid solution (propylene glycol) in patients with hepatic and renal failure, on disulfiram or metronidazole, in pregnancy, and in children <4 years old	(> 50 kg): CAPS 1,200 mg bid; or SOLN 1,400 mg bid (< 50 kg): CAPS 20 mg/kg bid to maximum of 2,400 mg daily; or SOLN 1.5 mL/kg bid to maximum of 2,800 mg daily. Reduce to 300–450 mg bid in hepatic impairment	(>50 kg) Take 8 tablets/dose or 6 1/4 tablespoons bid with or without meals. Avoid high fat meals	GI: nausea, vomiting, diarrhea; rash, headache, oral paresthesias, ↑ LFTs, hyperglycemia, hyperlipidemia, lipodystrophy	Moderate CYP3A4 enzyme inhibitor; induction of glucuronosyl transferases

[a] No dosage adjustment needed in renal dysfunction.

TABS, Tablets; CAPS, capsules; GI, gastrointestinal; LFT, liver function test; CYP, cytochrome; EtOH, ethyl alcohol; ATC, around the clock; bid, twice a day; tid, three times daily; FDA, Food and Drug Administration; NVP, nevirapine; EFV, efavirenz; ARV, antiretroviral.

TABLE 84.4	Common "Boosted" PI Dosing Regimens	
PI Drug Levels Enhanced	**"Boosted" Protease Regimens**	**Comment**
Atazanavir (ATZ, Reyataz)	RTV 100 mg daily + ATZ 300 mg daily	Boosted ATZ recommended for all ARV-experienced persons, and those taking concomitant efavirenz (Sustiva) or tenofovir (Viread) containing regimens. Some recommend "boosted" ATZ for HIV-infected naïve persons
Fosamprenavir (fos-APV, Lexiva)	RTV 100 mg bid + fosAPV 700 mg bid RTV 200 mg daily + fos-APV 1,400 mg daily. RTV 300 mg daily + fos-APV 1,400 mg daily (if efavirenz coadministered)	bid "boosted" fosAPV regimen recommended for ARV-experienced persons. Avoid coadministration with Kaletra until detrimental drug interactions are clarified; however, dosing of 4 Kaletra bid plus Fos-APV 1,400 mg bid has been suggested
Indinavir (IDV, Crixivan)	RTV 400 mg bid + IDV 400 mg bid RTV 200 mg bid + IDV 800 mg bid	"Boosted" IDV can be given with meals
Saquinavir (HG-SAQ Invirase)	RTV 100 mg bid + Invirase 1,000 mg bid RTV 100 mg qd + Invirase 1,600 mg qd RTV 400 mg bid + Invirase 400 mg bid	Hard-gel formulation (Invirase 500 mg tablet) preferable due to fewer GI side effects and lower pill burden

^a Take all within 2 hours of a meal to limit GI side effects.

PI, protease inhibitors; RTV, ritonavir; ARV, antiretroviral; HIV, human immunodeficiency virus; bid, twice a day; qd, every day; GI, gastrointestinal.

before initiating therapy are essential. Similarly, the ability of a regimen to achieve these goals declines as the number of failed regimens increases or as the HIV progresses. An undetectable viral load is associated with a lower risk of de novo mutations developing during selective pressure of therapy. Because the virus is error prone during viral replication, the likelihood of drug resistance is minimized if viral replication is low or undetectable. HIV must develop several mutations to become resistant to combination therapy, and mutations can only arise as a consequence of de novo mutations in the presence of ARV agents. Development of resistance can limit future treatment options, because resistance developing within a class of agents usually confers resistance to other agents within the same class (e.g., NNRTI).

The goal of treatment should be to achieve maximal and durable viral suppression (i.e., undetectable viral load for as long as possible), restore and preserve immunologic function (i.e., increase the CD4 cell count), and improve quality of life. Therefore, a potent and tolerable regimen tailored to

the patient's lifestyle should be used initially, if possible, in ARV-naive persons. The availability of once daily regimens and fixed dosage combinations that reduce pill burden and frequency of administration allow regimen simplification that may increase adherence. Consideration should also be given to how the given regimen will impact on concomitant disease states, drug interactions, and future treatment options (e.g., failure of one NNRTI confers resistance to other NNRTIs). Monotherapy or dual therapy regimens are no longer recommended, because incomplete viral suppression can encourage development of resistance. Similarly, the magnitude and durability of viral suppression is lower with dual ARV combinations than with combinations containing three or more agents.

Approximately 60% to 90% of HIV-naïve persons receiving initial HAART regimens are able to achieve and maintain complete viral suppression for more than 1 year.[31–33] In clinical trials virologic suppression has been reported for up to 6 years.[34,35] The optimal combinations of ARV agents are unknown; however, most guidelines recommend starting

TABLE 84.5	Nonnucleoside Reverse Transcriptase Inhibitors (NNRTIs) and Fusion Inhibitors				
Drug	Dosage Forms	Usual Doses	Special Administration Instructions	Common Adverse Effects	Potential for Drug Interactions (Table 9)
Nevirapine (NVP, Viramune)	TABS 200 mg; Oral suspension 10 mg/mL	200 mg daily for the first 14 days, then if no rash ↑ 200 mg bid or 400 mg daily	Take with or without meals	Skin rash (30%–50%) can be severe, headache, diarrhea, nausea; ↑ LFT, hepatitis and liver failure. Dose escalation can reduce the incidence of rash. Cross-reactivity of rash with other NNRTI	CYP3A4 enzyme inducer, including its own metabolism
Delavirdine (DLV, Rescriptor)	TABS 100, 200 mg	600 mg bid or 400 mg tid (4X 100 mg tabs in >3 oz of water to produce slurry) or 2X 200 mg intact tabs tid	Can be given with meals; separate administration by >1 hr from ddl/antacids	Rash, headaches, ↑ LFT, hepatitis. Cross-reactivity of rash with other NNRTI	CYP3A4 enzyme inhibitor
Efavirenz (EFV, Sustiva)	TABS 600 mg CAPS 50, 100, 200 mg	600 mg once daily bedtime or 200 mg tid	Can be administered at bedtime with low-fat meal	Headaches, dizziness, "disconnected" lightheadness, nightmares, rash. Avoid in pregnancy due to possible teratogenicity	CYP3A4 mixed inhibitor and inducer. Induction >inhibition
Fusion Inhibitor: Enfuviritide (T-20, Fuzeon)	Lyophilized powder 90 mg/mL (reconstitute with 1.1 mL of sterile water)	90 mg subcutaneously bid	Inject one ml under the skin twice a day. Massage site with vibrator may reduce nodule and cyst formation	Local injection site reactions: pain, redness, nodules and cysts, hypersensitivity reactions: rash, fever, nausea, vomiting, chills, hypotension, increased risk of bacterial pneumonias	No CYP3A interactions identified.

TABS, tablets; bid, twice a day; LFT, liver function test; CYP, cytochrome; ddl, didanosine.

TABLE 84.6 | **Prescribing Guidelines for Antiretroviral Agents: Initiation of Therapy**

Clinical Category	CD4 T Cell Count	HIV Viral Load	Treatment Recommendations	Treatment Regimens (Table 85.8)
Symptomatic (AIDS, thrush, unexplained fever)	Any value	Any value	Treat	2 NRTIs plus 1 PI 2 NRTIs plus 2 PIs 2 NRTIs plus 1 NNRTI 3 NRTIs (only when a PI or NNRTI-based regimen can not be used)
Asymptomatic, AIDS	CD4 count <200/mm³	Any value	Treat	Same as above
Asymptomatic	CD4 count >200/mm³ but ≤350/mm³	Any value	Offer therapy; willingness of patient to accept therapy is critical following discussion of pros and cons of therapy	Same as above
Asymptomatic	CD4 count ≥350/mm³	HIV RNA >100,000 (by RT-PCR and DNA)	Offer therapy; willingness of patient to accept therapy is critical. Benefits of therapy are unclear. Some experts recommend starting therapy because the 3-year risk of AIDS is >30% but in the absence of an elevated HIV RNA, some defer therapy since clinical outcome data is lacking	Same as above
Asymptomatic	CD4 count ≥350/mm³	HIV RNA <100,000 (by RT-PCR and DNA)	Most experts would defer therapy and observe since the risk of progression to AIDS is <15% in 3 years	
Pregnancy	Any value	Any value	Treat mother and passively treat fetus	Same as above, but ZDV should be administered during delivery if not included in the maternal ARV regimen. Addition of NVP 200 mg PO X 1 at the onset of delivery may be considered
Newborn	Not applicable	Any value	Treat all neonates if born to high risk or HIV+ mother. All infants born to HIV-infected mothers will be HIV+ due to transfer of maternal IgG antibodies through 18 months of age	For the neonate, 6 weeks of ZDV 2 mg/kg q6hr beginning within 1–8 hours of birth or +/− NVP 2 mg/kg PO X 1 within 48 hours of birth
Primary HIV infection	Any value	Any value	Offer therapy; controversial whether benefits outweigh risks of therapy	Same as above
Postexposure prophylaxis following occupational and nonoccupational risky exposures	Not applicable	Not applicable	Treat within ASAP or within 48 to 72 hours of risky exposure; benefits of treatment >72 hours not known. Consider risks vs. benefits for nonoccupational and sexual exposures from an unknown source patient	2 NRTIs (+/−) 1–2 PIs. Add PI for higher risk exposures. Avoid NNRTI Regimens should be tailored to minimize resistance and improve tolerability

HIV, human immunodeficiency virus; AIDS, acquired immune deficiency syndrome; NRTI, nucleotide reverse transcriptase inhibitors; PI, protease inhibitor; NNRTI, nonnucleoside reverse transcriptase inhibitors; RT-PCR, reverse transcriptase polymerase chain reaction; ZDV, zidovudine; ARV, antiretroviral; NVP, nevirapine; PO, by mouth; IgG, immunoglobulin G.

TABLE 84.7	Principles of Antiretroviral Therapy

- Tailoring antiretroviral therapy to the patient's lifestyle can increase therapy success.
- Adherence is critical to maintain viral suppression and minimize the emergence of viral resistance.
- Avoid monotherapy to prevent the emergence of resistance and drug failure.
- Three or more antiretroviral agents are more effective than two agents.
- The first regimen provides the best chance for complete viral suppression and immunologic recovery.
- Treatment is most effective in antiretroviral-naive compared to experienced persons.
- Never add a single agent to a failing regimen.
- Resistance to one drug is likely to confer resistance to another drug in the same class.
- Resistance testing may assist in identifying antiretrovirals that the virus will be resistant to.

with a minimum of two NRTIs plus a ''boosted'' PI or an NNRTI (Tables 84.6 and 84.8).[23,24] A durable and potent nucleoside combination that is often used initially is zidovudine (ZDV) plus lamivudine (3TC).[32–34] Better tolerated NRTI combinations include tenofovir (TDF) plus 3TC or emtricitabine (FTC). Boosted protease-containing regimens [e.g., lopinavir (LPV)/ritonavir (RTV)] appear to be more potent than single PI or NNRTI-containing combinations; therefore, they may be more appropriate for persons with symptomatic HIV disease or AIDS.[31,32] Only an efavirenz (EFV)-containing regimen has been demonstrated to be comparable to a PI-containing regimen.[32,33]EFV-containing regimens are attractive initial regimens because they can be given once daily, have a low pill burden, and can spare the PI for future use and avoid bothersome PI toxicities. Alternatively, if a PI or NNRTI-based regimen cannot be used because of toxicity, drug interactions, or intolerance, a triple NRTI-containing regimen can be considered [e.g., ZDV plus 3TC plus abacavir (ABC)] but virologic failures are more common. An AIDS Clinical Trials Group (ACTG) study A5095 that compared ZDV/3TC/ABC to EFV in ARV-naive subjects was stopped early since virologic failures occurred sooner and more often in the triple NRTI arm (21%) compared to the EFV arm (10%).[36] Higher virologic failures have also been reported with other triple NRTI-containing regimens (e.g., TDF/ABC/3TC, TDF/ddI/3TC) and these combinations should be avoided (Table 84.8).[37,38]

Clinical issues, including drug toxicity, laboratory abnormalities, medication adherence, drug to drug interactions, and impact on future treatment options should be considered before selecting any ARV regimen. These considerations are more complex when treating persons with more advanced illness on multiple drug therapies, or when there are concomitant issues such as dementia, substance abuse, psychiatric disorders, or homelessness.[39,40] Salvage regimens (e.g., for

persons failing multiple regimens) can contain more than four ARV agents, have a higher pill burden, and can include investigational agents available by expanded access from pharmaceutical companies.

Certain combinations of ARV agents should be avoided because of potential antiviral antagonism, lack of proven efficacy, or overlapping toxicity profiles (Table 84.8). Likewise, certain combinations of agents, such as boosted PI therapy, can increase effective PI levels and promote adherence by reducing the frequency and the daily number of tablets taken. In an effort to take advantage of a particular PI drug to drug interaction, a standard combination is to use a potent PI inhibitor of the cytochrome (CYP) P-450 system (e.g., RTV) to reduce the metabolism of the coadministered PI, thereby permitting lower doses of each PI to be given. A typical example is the combination of RTV increasing the drug concentrations and therefore, the activity of concomitant saquinavir (SAQ). Other examples of dual PI combination therapy are shown in Table 84.4.

Once maximal viral suppression has been achieved using an aggressive induction regimen, investigators have evaluated the feasibility of giving a less intensive ARV regimen for maintaining viral suppression. After achieving viral suppression, three studies agree that less intensive maintenance regimens are not as successful in suppressing the virus as continuation of the induction regimen.[41–43] Therefore, once maximal viral suppression occurs, the initial ARV regimen should be maintained to continue maximal viral suppression.

CHANGING ANTIRETROVIRAL THERAPY AND ANTIRETROVIRAL RESISTANCE TESTING

Changes in ARV regimens should be considered for documented treatment failures (e.g., virologic or immunlogic failures, disease progression), unmanageable drug toxicity, or patient intolerance. Treatment failures can be caused by multiple factors, including incomplete adherence, suboptimal ARV regimens, medication intolerance and toxicity, drug to drug interactions, suboptimal pharmacokinetics, use of a subpotent regimen, or other unknown reasons. Drug intolerance and poor adherence may be responsible for 28% to 40% of treatment failure and discontinuation.[44,45]

The optimal time to change therapy for virologic and immunologic failure is unclear and should be individualized depending on the likelihood for complete viral suppression and immunologic recovery. For patients with limited ARV experience and treatment options, an earlier change is reasonable to reduce the potential for further drug resistance. However, for highly experienced patients with few ARV options, maintenance of low level viremia (e.g., VL 1,000–5,000 copies/mL) may be acceptable if there is no disease progression and the patient is asymptomatic. In discordant situations where there is limited CD4 cell count re-

TABLE 84.8 | HAART Treatment Options and Regimens to Avoid

Regimens	Potential ARV Combinations (usual dosages unless specified)	Regimens/Combinations to Avoid	Comments
Preferred NNRTI regimen	(ZDV or TDF) plus (3TC or FTC) plus EFV	FTC + 3TC: no potential benefits	EFV-containing regimen compared favorably to a PI containing regimen.[127]
Preferred PI-based regimen	ZDV plus (3TC or FTC) plus LPV/r		Optimal use of 3TC or FTC is in a 3-drug suppressive regimen to avoid the emergence of 3TC/FTC resistance
Alternative NRTI Options	(FTC or 3TC) plus (ZDV or d4T or ddI or ABC or TDF)	d4T + ZDV (antagonistic) ddI +ddC (overlapping toxicity) ddI + TDF (increased ddI toxicity) Monotherapy or dual NRTI regimens	
Alternative PI Options	Table 85.4 lists boosted PIs ATZ or ATZ/RTZ with TDF Fos-APV or Fos-APV/RTV IDV/RTV SAQ/RTV NFV	IDV + ATZ (overlapping toxicity). Avoid HG-SAQ as sole PI due to poor bioavailability. IDV + SAQ (antagonistic in vitro) APV + fos-APV (duplicative therapy, no combined benefit) Kaletra + fos-APV: unclear dosing	Select PI-based on patient's ability to adhere with special administration requirements, drug-drug interactions, and toxicity profile
Alternative NNRTI Options	Nevirapine	Dual NNRTI regimens	DLV might also be effective but data limited. No head-to-head comparisons among NNRTI.
3 NRTIs	ZDV + 3TC + ABC	TDF + ABC + 3TC TDF + ddI + 3TC (high rate of virologic failure)	Data limited. Consider triple NRTI only when a NNRTI or PI-based regimen cannot be used.

HAART, highly active antiretroviral therapy; ARV, antiretroviral; NNRTI, nonnucleoside reverse transcriptase inhibitor; PI, protease inhibitor; ZDV, zidovudine; TDF, tenofovir; 3TC, lamivudine; FTC, emtricitabine; EFV, efavirenz; NRTI, nucleotide reverse transcriptase inhibitors; d4T, stavudine; ddI, didanosine; ABC, abacavir; ddC, 2'3'-dideoxycytidine; IDV, indinavir; ATZ, atazanavir; HG-SAQ, hard-gel saquinavir; RTV, ritonavir; Fos-APV, fosamprenavir; NFV, nelfinavir; DLV, delavirdine.

covery but complete viral suppression, current ARV therapy may be continued or ARVs changed if drug toxicity is of concern (e.g., ddI cytotoxicity). Changes in ARV therapy may also be considered if there is development of new opportunistic infections or evidence of disease progression. Disease progression should be distinguished from the possibility of an immune reconstitution syndrome (e.g., inflammatory reaction) that can occur within the first 3 months after starting HAART.[46]

If therapy has to be discontinued, generally all agents except for EFV and nevirapine (NVP) should be stopped simultaneously to minimize the emergence of drug resistance.[47] It has been suggested that EFV and NVP should be stopped first in a regimen while continuing the rest of the ARVs for a few more days, possibly 5 to 7 days, to reduce the risk of selection of NNRTI-resistant mutations. Preliminary pharmacokinetic data show the prolonged half-life of these NNRTIs, especially in African-Americans and Hispanic patients, and that stopping all agents simultaneously might lead to theoretical monotherapy with the NNRTI.[48,49] When selecting a new regimen for drug toxicity or intolerance, it is appropriate to substitute another agent from the same drug class responsible for causing the drug toxicity. However, if a regimen must be changed owing to treatment failure or administration of a suboptimal regimen, it is preferable that the patient receive at least three or more potent agents to minimize the development of resistance. Highly experienced patients may benefit from an optimized ARV regimen (e.g., agents selected by resistance testing) and the addition of enfuvirtide, an HIV entry inhibitor.

ARV drug resistance (Table 84.9) can be detected in vitro using commercially available phenotypic and preferred genotypic assays that may help guide ARV decisions. Genotypic assays identify specific nucleic acid changes (http://www.iasusa.org/resistance) known to cause mutations associated with resistance and cross-resistance to other ARVs; however, their results should be interpreted carefully. Phenotypic assays provide information about viral replication in the presence of the drug (e.g., median concentrations of the drug required to inhibit 50% [IC_{50}] or 90% [IC_{90}] of viral replication). Interpretation of phenotypic results are more difficult than genotypic results due to the lack of data regarding the specific inhibitory concentrations associated with drug failure. In addition, genotypic assays are less expensive to perform and results are usually available in 1 to 2 weeks while phenotypic assays are more costly and results are often not back before 3 weeks. Interpretation of either drug resistance results is most accurate when the test is performed when the VL is greater than 1,000 copies per milliliter while taking the failing ARV regimen or within 4 weeks of stopping the ARV regimen. Although genotypic assays may help identify ARV agents to avoid, they do not absolutely identify which agents may be clinically effective. Long-term studies using resistance testing are currently lacking. These assays are most beneficial in guiding ARV decisions for virologic failures in newly infected persons and during pregnancy.[50,51]

TABLE 84.9	**Primary Mutations Associated with Antiretroviral Resistance**[47]
NucleoSide and Nucleotide Reverse Transcriptase Inhibitors (NRTI)[a]	Codon Mutations
Zidovudine (ZDV) Stauvudine (d4T)	T215Y/F, M41L, D67N, K70R, L210W, K219Q (Thymidine Analog Mutations or TAMs)
Didanosine (ddI)	L74V
Tenofovir (TDF)	K65R (Presence of M41L and L210W confer cross-resistance to tenofovir)
Lamivudine (3TC) Emtricitabine (FTC)	M184V, E44D
Abacavir (ABC)	M184V, K65R, L74V, Y115F
Nonnucleoside Reverse Transcriptase Inhibitors (NNRTI)[b]	K103N, Y181CI, G190A
Nevirapine (NVP) Delavirdine (DLV) Efavirenz (EFV)	
Protease Inhibitors (PIs)[c]	
Saquinavir (SAQ)	G48V, L90M
Lopinavir/ritonavir (LPV/r)	None identified. Resistance correlates with number of mutations
Indinavir (IDV) Ritonavir (RTV)	V82I/A/T/F/S, M46I/L, I84V, L90M
Nelfinavir (NFV)	D30N, L90M
Atazanavir (ATZ)	I50L, I84V
Amprenavir (APV) Fos-Amprenavir (Fos-APV)	I50V, I84V
Tipranavir (TPV)	L33I/F/L/T, V82A/F/L/T, I84V, L90M

[a] Q151 M and T69S insertion mutation associated with NRTI class resistance.
[b] K103N, Y181C/I, Y188L, G190A, 230L confers cross-resistance to NNRTI class.
[c] V82A/F, I84V, and L90M confers cross resistance to PI class.
(From Deeks S. Treatment of antiretroviral-drug-resistant HIV-1 infection. Lancet 362:2002–2011, 2003, with permission.)

Using resistance assays in patients with chronic HIV infection appears less helpful.

PHARMACOTHERAPY IN PREGNANCY

HIV infection in pregnant women should be managed similarly to HIV infection in nonpregnant women (Table 84.6). Combination ARV therapy, similar to those for HIV-infected adults, to maximally suppress viral replication to undetectable levels are currently recommended (Table 84.8). Although pregnancy may affect the choice and timing of ARV therapy, the use of optimal suppressive regimens should not be deferred because of theoretical teratogenicity concerns. Two major therapeutic issues need to be considered when using ARV agents in pregnancy: (a) providing effective maternal ARV therapy, including dosage alterations for pregnancy-related physiologic changes; and (b) providing effective ARV chemoprophylaxis to reduce the risk of vertical transmission and minimize toxicity to the fetus and the newborn. Because the long-term impact of ARV therapy on the fetus is unknown, the decision to institute ARV therapy during pregnancy requires a discussion with the mother of the risks and benefits to her, the fetus, and her newborn. Women infected with HIV should also be counseled not to breastfeed the newborn to avoid the 20% risk of HIV transmission through breast milk.

The optimal time to start ARV prophylaxis and choice of prophylaxis are unknown although the risk of HIV transmission appears highest near the time of or during delivery. Several clinical U.S. and international trials strongly support the inclusion of ZDV as part of any maternal ARV regimen to prevent perinatal HIV transmission, even if the mother is severely immunosuppressed or harbors resistance to ZDV.[12,13] The mechanism of ZDV protection is unknown but presumed to be related to postexposure prophylaxis. Its mechanism is not entirely related to viral suppression since effective HIV prophylaxis of the newborn occurred despite detectable maternal viral loads. In 1994, a landmark trial (PACTG 076) found that ZDV alone, started orally at 14 to 34 weeks' gestation, followed by intravenous ZDV during labor, and then given orally to the newborn for the first 6 weeks of life, reduced the risk of mother-to-child HIV transmission by 66%.[12,13] The principal toxicity in the newborn was anemia that was reversible after drug discontinuation. Subsequent follow-up (mean 4.2 years) in children who received ZDV in utero and during the first 6 weeks of life revealed similar rates of congenital abnormalities and no significant adverse effects on growth, neurodevelopment, immunologic status or malignancies (i.e., up to 6 years) compared to those receiving placebo.[52] Although U.S., African, and European cohorts noted no long-term infant adverse effects, French studies report neurologic and lactic acid abnormalities in infants at 18 months after exposure in utero.[13,53]

Several international clinical trials using various treatment strategies involving a short-course antenatal ZDV (e.g., 28–36 weeks' gestation) with or without the addition of 3TC, combined with intrapartum prophylactic ZDV, and a shortened (e.g., 3–7 days) or no infant component reported a 37% to 63% risk of vertical transmission. Because the efficacy of these short-term ZDV studies in reducing vertical transmission is less than that achieved by the three-part ZDV regimen, it suggests that a longer maternal treatment period is essential to reduce the risk of vertical transmission. The addition of a single dose of NVP 200 mg to the mother at the onset of delivery plus a single 2 mg per kilogram dose

to the infant within 48 hours of delivery has been shown to provide additional efficacy in reducing perinatal transmission, but this was significant only in those mothers receiving an abbreviated ZDV regimen. However, in mothers receiving the standard three-part ZDV regimen and achieving optimal viral suppression, the addition of single-dose NVP to the mother and infant did not significantly alter the risk of HIV transmission (e.g., 1.6% in placebo vs. 1.4% in the NVP group). Therefore, the addition of NVP to a ZDV-based antenatal/intrapartum/infant prophylaxis regimen does not offer significant benefits but increases the risks of toxicity (e.g., rash, hepatitis) and NNRTI mutations that might limit future treatment options.

ZDV monotherapy is not recommended because incomplete viral suppression can lead to resistance and reduce the efficacy of future ARV agents in the mother. If ZDV is not part of the initial regimen, addition or substitution of ZDV for other NRTIs is highly recommended. EFV should be avoided in pregnancy, especially the first trimester, because it is teratogenic. Similarly, the combination of stavudine (d4T) and ddI should not be used unless the benefits outweigh the risks of fatal lactic acidosis.[13,23] "Unboosted" indinavir (IDV), SAQ, and three times daily nelfinavir (NFV) are also not recommended due to subtherapeutic levels in pregnant women compared to nonpregnant women.[13] In addition, all women should receive HIV counseling and treatment.

The CDC guidelines give several possible treatment strategies for various clinical scenarios to reduce the risk of perinatal transmission.[13] For pregnant women infected with HIV without any prior ARV therapy during the first trimester of pregnancy, decisions to delay therapy until at least after 10 to 12 weeks gestation should be entertained to reduce the risk of teratogenicity. For women infected with HIV already receiving ARV therapy during the first trimester of pregnancy, women should be counseled about the risks and benefits to themselves and their babies. Stopping therapy could lead to rebound in viral load in the mother, which could have adverse effects on the mother and the fetus. If the decision is to stop therapy during the first trimester, all ARV agents should be stopped and reintroduced simultaneously after the first trimester to avoid inducing resistance. For women in labor or for infants in whom no prior maternal ARV therapy has been administered, administration of intrapartum intravenous ZDV and the 6-week oral ZDV to the newborn is highly recommended. Scheduling an elective Cesarean section is encouraged if the maternal viral load is greater than 1,000 copies per milliliter at 38 weeks of gestation.

POSTEXPOSURE PROPHYLAXIS FOR OCCUPATIONAL AND NONOCCUPATIONAL EXPOSURES

The benefits of postexposure prophylaxis (PEP) after an occupational percutaneous exposure have been suggested. A retrospective case-control study of health care workers found that the use of ZDV alone within 2 to 4 hours of the exposure reduced the risk of HIV transmission by 80%.[54] The risk of HIV transmission is estimated to be 0.3% (1/300) from a needlestick. The highest transmission risk of HIV to the exposed person is from anal sex or sharing of intravenous drug use paraphernalia. The CDC recommends immediate initiation of two or three potent ARVs after a high-risk occupational exposure for 28 days.[54] The typical combinations are similar to those used in persons infected with HIV (Tables 84.6 and 84.8). A more complicated PEP regimen may be warranted if there is concern for transmission of a resistant virus, especially if the source is HIV positive and on an ARV regimen. The risks and benefits of PEP should be clearly explained before therapy is started. Side effects or concerns about potential side effects can limit initiation and completion of therapy. The CDC found that approximately one third of health care workers who started PEP did not complete their therapy.

CDC guidelines have also been provided for nonoccupational exposures after a risky sexual exposure or injection drug use.[55] PEP for the aforementioned exposures is recommended if the source is known to be HIV positive and care is obtained before 72 hours of the exposure. Repeated PEP is not recommended. If the HIV status of the source is unknown, PEP may be considered if the benefits of PEP outweigh the risks of drug toxicity. Two or three ARVs similar to those given for occupational exposures and HIV-infected persons are administered for 28 days.

THERAPY FOR ACUTE PRIMARY HUMAN IMMUNODEFICIENCY VIRUS INFECTION

Currently, there are no outcome data to support the use of ARV agents in the treatment of acute HIV infection; data in support of early therapy are limited.[21,23,56] Nevertheless, most experts agree that early intervention with aggressive ARV therapy appears valid. A discussion of the risks and benefits of ARV therapy is appropriate before therapy is instituted. The theoretical benefits of early ARV therapy include limiting systemic viral dissemination by suppressing the initial burst of viremia, decreasing the severity of the acute illness, changing the viral setpoint that may affect the rate of disease progression, decreasing the emergence of resistant strains by suppressing viral replication, preserving immunologic function, and reducing HIV transmission. Risks of treatment include drug toxicity, decreased quality of life, and drug resistance that may affect potency of future indicated therapies. Acute ARV therapy is warranted only after a discussion of the risks and benefits of early intervention. The therapeutic regimens are similar to those used for the treatment of HIV infection (e.g., two NRTIs and a PI). Although the duration of therapy is unknown, it is likely that chronic treatment will be required, because viral rebound has occurred after stopping treatment.

ANTIRETROVIRAL AGENTS

Current ARV agents inhibit virus replication at various points in the viral life cycle (Fig. 84.1): initial cell entry

(fusion inhibitors); viral transcription by RT enzyme (nucleoside, nucleotide, and nonnucleoside RT inhibitors); and protein cleavage by protease enzyme (PIs).

Nucleoside Reverse Transcriptase Inhibitors. The nucleoside RT inhibitors (NRTIs) are the first class of ARV agents approved for the treatment of HIV infection. There are currently seven NRTI agents available (Table 84.2), including TDF, a NRTI. Zalcitabine (ddC or Hivid) was discontinued in 2006 due to lack of use. In addition, there are four fixed dosage combination products available that can ease the pill burden and frequency of administration. NRTIs continue to be essential agents in the treatment of HIV infection, forming the ''backbone'' of HAART regimens. Generally when starting HAART, two NRTIs are used in combination with ARV agents from different classes, such as a NNRTI or a PI. All the NRTI are prodrugs that must be converted intracellularly to their active form for antiviral activity. Because the NRTI are not inducers or inhibitors of the CYP P-450 system, drug interactions are not as problematic as with the PI or NNRTI. However, non-P-450 drug interactions have been reported with ddI and TDF use (Table 85.10).[57–59] In addition, pharmacodynamic interactions should be monitored. Resistance and cross-resistance has been described for all the NRTI (Table 84.9) and develops more rapidly in patients with advanced disease and high levels of viral replication.[47] The dosage of the NRTI and their modifications in patients with renal dysfunction are shown in Table 84.2.

Although there are side effects specific to each NRTI, a class effect of the NRTI is mitochrondrial toxicity due to inhibition of the enzyme (DNA polymerase-γ) required for mitochrondrial DNA synthesis. Toxicities attributed to mitochondrial damage include lactic acidosis, hepatic steatosis, peripheral neuropathy, myopathy, pancreatitis, and likely, lipoatrophy. Studies suggest that the risk of NRTI-induced mitochondrial toxicities is greater with zalcitabine, ddI, d4T, and ZDV than with 3TC, FTC, ABC, and TDF.[58,60,61]

Zidovudine. ZDV (Retrovir) was the first FDA-approved (1987) ARV agent that was modestly effective in delaying disease progression to AIDS in those with asymptomatic HIV disease and CD4 counts less than 500 cells/mm^3 (ACTG 019). The time-limited and suboptimal benefits of ZDV monotherapy were first evident during The European Concorde Trial.[62] No difference in clinical end points were observed at the 3-year follow-up in 1,749 asymptomatic persons infected with HIV randomized to immediate or delayed ZDV therapy (begun after the development of AIDS-related symptoms). Several important trials, including the ACTG 175, Delta, and the Community Providers for Clinical Research in AIDS (CPCRA) have demonstrated the superiority of dual nucleoside analog therapy over ZDV monotherapy in delaying disease progression to AIDS or death, particularly in ARV-naive patients.[63–65] A ZDV and 3TC backbone has demonstrated durable virologic potency in combination

(*text continues on page 2112*)

TABLE 84.10 Selected Pharmacodynamic and Pharmacokinetic Drug Interactions with Selected Antiretroviral Agents

Antiretroviral Agents	Interacting Drugs	Consequence of Interaction	Recommendations
Zidovudine (ZDV)	Ganciclovir	Concomitant bone marrow suppression	Stop ZDV during ganciclovir induction therapy
	Ribavirin	May cause virologic failure by inhibiting phosphorylation of ZDV	Avoid if possible
Didanosine (ddl), stavudine (d4T)	Isoniazide, ddl, d4T, vincristine, ribavirin (↑ ddl levels)	↑ risk of peripheral neuropathy	Use cautiously and if possible, avoid coadministration
	Alcohol, systemic pentamidine, ddl, d4T, ribavirin (↑ ddl levels)	↑ risk of pancreatitis	
	ddl, d4T, ribavirin (↑ ddl levels)	↑ risk of lactic acidosis, especially in pregnancy	
Buffered ddl formulation (Videx)	Quinolones, tetracyclines, ketoconazole, itraconazole, ritonavir (RTV), indinavir (IDV), delavirdine (DLV), atazanavir (ATZ)	Impaired absorption by buffered ddl	Separate coadministration by at least 2 hours or change to enteric coated ddl (Videx EC)
		See ATZ	
Tenofovir (TDF)	ddl	↑ ddl concentrations 44%–60%; ↑ risk of ddl toxicity	↓ ddl to 250 mg qd in patients >60 kg; ↓ ddl 200 mg in patients < 60 kg
	ATZ	↓ ATZ levels 25% and loss of efficacy	Use "boosted" 300 mg ATZ plus RTV 100 mg daily
Protease Inhibitors (PIs)[a] Delavirdine (DLV)	Amiodarone, bepridil, encainide, flecainide, propafenone, quinidine	Potential for life-threatening arrhythmias and increased toxicity of drugs due to cytochrome (CYP)3A4 inhibition by PI [especially with lopinavir (LPV)/r and RTV]	Avoid coadministration.
	Triazolam, midazolam, pimozide, terfenadine, cisapride, astemizole, ergot alkaloids	Potential for increased toxicity of drugs due to CYP3A4 inhibition by PI	Avoid coadministration. Use nonsedating antihistamines (e.g., loratadine) or other sedative hypnotics (e.g., lorazepam, temazepam)
	Simvastatin, lovastatin, rosuvastatin	Risk of myositis and rhabdomyolysis	Avoid coadministration. Use pravastatin, fluvastatin, or low-dose atorvastatin
	Sidenafil, vardenafil, tadalafil	↑ serum concentrations and toxicity of erectile dysfunction agents	Use cautiously and monitor for toxicity. Start with 25 mg of sidenafil q 48 hr; vardenafil 2.5 mg q 24 hrs to a maximum of q72 hr with "boosted PI"; tadalafil 5 mg q 24hr to a max of 10 mg in 72 hr.

(continued)

TABLE 84.10 continued

Antiretroviral Agents	Interacting Drugs	Consequence of Interaction	Recommendations
PIs,[a] Nonnucleoside reverse transcriptase inhibitor (NNRTI)[b]	Rifabutin	↓ PI/NNRTI efficacy due to enzyme induction by rifabutin; ↑ rifabutin toxicity due to ↑ rifabutin level with PI and delavirdine (DLV)	When combined with LPV/r, ATZ, or "boosted PI" ↓ rifabutin to 150 mg qd or 3X/week. When combined with boosted SAQ or "unboosted" IDV, RTV, NFV, APV or fos-APV: ↓ rifabutin to 150 mg qd or 300 mg 3x/week; ↑ "unboosted" IDV to 1,000 mg q8hr or use IDV 800 mg/RTV 200 mg bid; use only NFV 1,250 mg bid. Avoid coadministration with DLV or "unboosted" saquinavir (SAQ). ↑ rifabutin dose to 450–600 mg qd or 600 mg 3x/week with standard doses of efavirenz (EFV).
PIs, NNRTI[c]	Rifampin, St. John's wort	↓ PI/NNRTI efficacy due to enzyme induction	Avoid coadministration if possible. Consider changing rifampin to rifabutin. Avoid boosted SAQ and rifampin due to ↑ risk of hepatotoxicity. With rifampin consider :↑ EFV to 600–800 mg qd
Ritonavir (RTV), nelfinavir (NFV), amprenavir (APV), fos-amprenavir (fos-APV), lopinavir (LPV)/r, nevirapine (NVP)	Oral contraceptives	↓ efficacy of oral contraceptives; ↓ APV fos-APV levels; ↑ EE levels with IDV, APV, fos-APV, ATZ, EFV, DLV	Use additional or alternative forms of contraception or change to another PI.
PIs, NNRTI	Phenytoin, phenobarbital, carbamazepine	Unknown interaction. Possible enzyme induction and potential reduction of effective PI, NNRTI, and anticonvulsant levels. Bidirectional interaction with ↓ in both LPV/r and phenytoin levels.	Use cautiously or avoid coadministration. Monitor anticonvulsant levels or change if possible to gabapentin or valproic acid.
PIs, NNRTI	Voriconazole	Potential for bidirectional interaction between voriconazole and PI/NNRTI	Monitor for toxicity. Avoid coadministration if possible.
PIs, NNRTI	Methadone	NVP and EFV cause significant ↓ methadone levels and potential narcotic withdrawal; PI can ↓ levels but narcotic withdrawal uncommon except with LPV/r.	With NVP, EFV, and LPV/r, ↑ methadone dosage to prevent narcotic withdrawal. With other PI, monitor and adjust if needed.

Drug	Interacting drug	Effect	Recommendation
Atazanavir (ATZ)	Diltiazem	Significant ↑ diltiazem levels and potential for atrioventricular block, bradycardia, and hypotension	Monitor ECG, Use cautiously, ↓ diltiazem dosage by 50%
	Clarithromycin	Significant ↑ clarithromycin levels and risk of QTc prolongation	Reduce clarithromycin dosage 50%; consider azithromycin
	H₂-receptor antagonists	↓ ATZ levels	Separate coadministration by 12 hours
	Antacids, buffered ddl	↓ ATZ levels	Give ATZ 2 hours before or one hour after; change to Videx EC
	Proton pump inhibitors	↓ ATV levels	Avoid coadministration; change to H₂ receptor antagonist.
	IDV	Additive hyperbilirubinemia	Lansoprazole may be considered.
	Irinotecan	↑ irinotecan levels	Avoid coadministration
Lopinavir (LPV)/r	EFV, NVP	Significant ↓ LPV/r levels	↑ LPV/r to 4 capsules bid
	APV, fos-APV	Bidirectional interaction with ↓ in both amprenavir/fos-APV and LPV/r levels. Preliminary data indicates Fos-APV 1,400 mg bid and Kaletra 4 capsules bid	Avoid coadministration of LPV/r and fos-APV until further data available. Optimal dosing of APV and LPV/r unclear; consider APV 600–750 mg bid and LPV/r 3–4 caps bid. Consider monitoring PI levels.
Saquinavir (SAQ), IDV, APV, fos-APV, ATZ	Efavirenz, possibly NVP	Significant ↓ PI levels if sole PI	Avoid coadministration if sole PI. Consider "boosted PI" therapy
EFV	↓ simvastatin levels 58% ↓ atorvastatin levels 43%	Insufficient lipid lowering effects	Adjust statin dosage to obtain desired lipid response

ª PI = SAQ, RTV, IDV, NFV, APV, fos-APV, ATZ, LPV/r
ᵇ NNRTI = EFV, NVP, DLV
qd, every day; qod, every other day; EKG, electrocardiograph; QTc, corrected QT.

with a PI or NNRTI in naïve persons in several clinical trials.[32–34] The combination of ZDV plus d4T should be avoided because antagonism has been demonstrated.[66] ACTG 290 found that ZDV-experienced persons who received the combination of ZDV plus d4T had an unexpected rapid decline in their CD4 cells.[67]

ZDV is a thymidine analog that requires intracellular phosphorylation to its active moiety, zidovudine triphosphate (ZDV-TP) which has a half-life of 7 hours.[68] Because of its structural similarity to thymidine triphosphate, the RT incorporates the ZDV-TP into the viral DNA copy, resulting in proviral DNA chain termination or competitive RT antagonism to block further viral replication (Fig. 84.1). ZDV is well absorbed with a bioavailability of approximately 60%. Plasma ZDV-TP concentrations are highly variable; efficacy and toxicity plasma concentrations have not been established. Higher ZDV-TP concentrations found in women and those with low CD4 counts may be responsible for greater ZDV toxicity.[68,69] Its penetration into the cerebrospinal fluid (CSF) is advantageous in the treatment of HIV-related dementia. Dosage adjustment is required in severe renal insufficiency (Table 84.2).

The toxicities of ZDV are well known (Table 84.2). During the first 6 weeks of therapy, complaints of nausea, vomiting, anorexia, bloating, headache, malaise, insomnia, confusion, or flulike symptoms should be expected. However, these bothersome and usually transient symptoms can be minimized by taking ZDV with food, analgesics (e.g., acetaminophen), and antinausea agents until their resolution in a few weeks. Hematological toxicities, including neutropenia and anemia, are less severe with the lower dosages currently used (e.g., 600 mg/day), but tend to predominate in those with advanced HIV infection or in those patients receiving concomitant marrow suppressive agents [e.g., induction doses of ganciclovir, TMP/SMX doses for treatment of *Pneumocystis carinii* pneumonia (PCP)]. Therefore, ZDV should be discontinued during induction doses of ganciclovir (Table 84.10). Anemia, which can be severe (e.g., hemoglobin 9 g/dL), can occur after 6 to 8 weeks of therapy, and responds to blood transfusions, erythropoietin, dosage reduction, or alternatively, changing to a less bone marrow suppressive ARV agent. Asymptomatic macrocytosis develops in most patients after several weeks of ZDV and is a good marker of adherence. Giving granulocyte colony-stimulating factor (G-CSF) for ZDV-induced neutropenia (e.g., 500 cells/mm³) may allow continued ZDV therapy; however, changing to an alternative ARV agent when debilitating neutropenia occurs is easier and more cost effective. Myopathy, reported in 6% to 18% of patients, occurs after prolonged therapy (e.g., 6 months) and is reversible after stopping the drug.[70] An elevated creatinine kinase (CK) level can confirm this idiosyncratic reaction in patients with symptoms of muscle pain and weakness. Hepatitis and hyperpigmentation of the nails and skin are infrequent. Although one case of cardiomyopathy and two retinal abnormalities were reported in children who received ZDV in utero, growth and develop-

ment were considered to be normal.[52] Complete blood count (CBC), platelets, and liver function tests should be monitored at baseline, then every 2 to 4 weeks for 3 months, and then every 3 months or as necessary based on symptoms.

Didanosine (Videx EC, Videx). DdI was the second NRTI approved (1991) in the United States for treatment of HIV infection in adults or children. It is typically not used as initial therapy because it is less potent and substantially more toxic than most nucleosides. Although ddI is less potent than ZDV in terms of its HIV inhibitory concentrations, ddI has improved activity within monocytes and macrophages, known reservoirs for HIV infection. Synergy of ddI with other NRTI, NNRTI, and hydroxyurea has been demonstrated. Two clinical trials of ddI versus ZDV monotherapy demonstrated the efficacy of ddI in ZDV-experienced persons. Subjects receiving ddI had a lower incidence of new AIDS-defining events or disease progression compared with those receiving ZDV, but there was no survival advantage.[71,72] A ddI plus d4T/EFV combination regimen was less effective and more toxic than a ZDV and 3TC/EFV-based regimen in a randomized double-blind trial of naïve patients.[32]

The active form of ddI, a purine nucleoside analog RT inhibitor, is dideoxyadenosine triphosphate (ddATP) whose long intracellular half-life of greater than 12 hours permits once or twice daily dosing. DdI differs considerably from ZDV in its pharmacokinetic, pharmacodynamic, and tolerability profile. Penetration of ddI into the CSF is lower than ZDV, which might limit its usefulness in HIV dementia. The CSF to plasma concentration ratio for ddI is low, 0.2 compared with 0.6 for ZDV. Various formulations of ddI are available (Table 84.2). The enteric-coated preparation, allowing once daily administration, is preferable to the less tolerable, twice daily buffered formulations. Because food can limit ddI absorption by 50%, instructions to administer all formulations on an empty stomach (1 hour before or 2 hours after meals) are critical for proper absorption. One exception is when ddI is combined with TDF, ddI can be administered with food without impairing its absorption.[57-] Approximately 50% of ddI is renally excreted and dosage reductions are warranted in those with significant renal impairment (Table 84.2).

Gastrointestinal side effects, including nausea and diarrhea, are more prominent with the buffered ddI (30%) than with the enteric coated (<10%) preparation.[73] Painful peripheral neuropathy is the most serious toxicity of ddI, affecting approximately 13% to 34% of those on therapy. Symptoms of tingling, burning, pain, numbness in distal extremities, and sensations of ''walking on golf balls'' are intermittent initially, but worsen with continued administration. Symptoms can be disabling but often resolve slowly (e.g., several weeks) after drug discontinuation. Prompt recognition of peripheral neuropathy is required to prevent irreversible neurologic damage. Neuropathy is more frequent in those with a history of neuropathy or concurrent use of neurotoxins (e.g., isoniazid). Pancreatitis has been reported in 7% of persons receiving prolonged ddI therapy. This risk increases to 27% in those with a prior history of pancreatitis. Fatalities have occurred from ddI-associated pancreatitis. Patients should be educated about the signs and symptoms of pancreatitis (e.g., anorexia, nausea, vomiting, abdominal pain), informed about the dangers of concurrent alcohol intake, and instructed to contact their pharmacist or primary physician immediately if the preceding symptoms occur. An elevated amylase level can confirm the diagnosis of pancreatitis in persons presenting with the preceding complaints. Persons with a history of pancreatitis, renal impairment, and active alcohol intake are at increased risk for pancreatitis and should be considered poor candidates for ddI therapy. Pancreatitis and peripheral neuropathy need to be distinguished from an HIV-related etiology. Rarely, elevated hepatic transaminases, rash, and hyperuricemia occur. Hematological toxicities to ddI are uncommon.

Several potential drug to drug interactions with ddI should be recognized (Table 84.10). TDF can increase the AUC (area under the curve) of ddI by 44% to 60%, necessitating a dosage reduction of ddI to 250 mg daily in persons weighing more than 60 kg to minimize ddI-induced toxicities.[57] In those weighing less than 60 kg, a dosage reduction to 200 mg daily has been suggested but requires further investigation. Despite ddI dosage adjustments, an increased risk of pancreatitis (13.3%) has been reported with the concomitant use of TDF, especially in women weighing 60 kg or less.[74] This combination may also be cytotoxic to CD4 cells, resulting in a less robust CD4 cell increase despite virologic suppression.[75] Similarly, patients receiving ddI and ribavirin therapy should be closely monitored for an increased risk of ddI toxicity; ddI dosage adjustments are unavailable.[58] Because medications that require an acidic environment for absorption can be impaired by the buffered ddI, this drug to drug interaction may be avoided by changing to the enteric coated formulation or by administering the buffered ddI at least 2 hours apart from delavirdine (DLV), RTV, IDV, quinolones, tetracyclines, ketoconazole, and itraconazole. Agents with overlapping toxicity that can increase the risk of peripheral neuropathy (e.g., isoniazid, vincristine, d4T) or pancreatitis (e.g., d4T, intravenous pentamidine) should be avoided if possible or used cautiously with ddI if the benefits outweigh the toxicity. A CBC, amylase, hepatic transaminases, and uric acid should be monitored at baseline and every 4 weeks initially during the first 3 months of therapy, and then as warranted based on symptoms.

Stavudine (Zerit). D4T is a thymidine-based nucleoside analog that received fast-track approval by the FDA in 1994 based on positive survival data from two randomized, double-blind clinical trials conducted in ZDV and ddI-experienced persons. In one trial, survival between the d4T 20-mg two times a day and 40-mg two times a day dosage regimens were comparable. With the addition of a PI or NNRTI, d4T is a potent component of a nucleoside backbone combination

that has included nucleosides such as ddI and 3TC. A 48-week trial found that a d4T/ddI or a d4T/3TC-based protease regimen was comparable or superior to a ZDV/3TC-containing protease regimen in achieving sustained virologic suppression and immunological benefits.[76,77] However, d4T is generally not recommended as initial therapy because of its significantly greater mitochondrial toxicity (e.g., lactic acidosis, lipoatrophy).[32,37,60,61] In ZDV-heavily experienced subjects, changing to an d4T backbone-based regimen did not provide additional antiviral benefits due to cross-resistance between these nucleosides.[78]

The combination of d4T and ZDV has shown antagonism in vitro and should be avoided.[66] Clinically, a decline in CD4 counts was observed in patients receiving this combination.[67] These negative effects have been attributed to competition for the same activating enzyme because d4T and ZDV share thymidine kinase for phosphorylation to the active TP moiety. In vitro data found that d4T-TP levels were reduced by more than 95% with ZDV, whereas d4T had no effect on the phosphorylation of ZDV owing to the higher affinity of ZDV than d4T for the enzyme. Preliminary data suggest that previous use of ZDV might also impair the future ARV activity of d4T. In a small group of six persons infected with HIV, the intracellular phosphorylation of d4T to the active triphosphate was impaired for several weeks following ZDV use.[66] The effects of current d4T use affecting future use of ZDV are unknown.

D4T is rapidly absorbed with a bioavailability of approximately 78% to 86%. The intracellular half-life is about 4 hours. Significant levels of d4T were attained in CSF that exceeded the in vitro IC_{50} concentrations for most wild-type HIV-1 strains, causing reduction of CSF HIV RNA concentrations.[79] Semen concentrations also approximate plasma concentrations. The FDA-approved dosage is 40 mg two times a day regardless of food for patients weighing more than 60 kg and 30 mg two times a day for those weighing less than 60 kg. Lower dosages of 20 mg two times a day for those more than 60 kg and 15 mg two times a day for those less than 60 kg are appropriate for those at an increased risk of neuropathy. An extended release once daily formulation has been FDA approved but not yet marketed (Table 84.2). Dosage reduction is required in renal insufficiency because approximately 50% of d4T is excreted unchanged in the urine (Table 84.2).

D4T is moderately well tolerated with 33% of patients discontinuing therapy due to side effects.[80] Long-term (>6 months) administration of d4T-containing regimen are more often associated with a greater risk of lipoatrophy (e.g., loss of subcutaneous fat from face, limb, and buttocks) and lactic acidosis, particularly in combination with ddI, than other NRTI.[80–82] Lipoatrophy was significantly higher (48% vs. 22%, respectively) in a d4T versus a ZDV-containing study arm and similarly, in a d4T (19%) versus a TDF (3%) arm. D4T-associated lipoatrophy is attributed to mitochrondrial toxicity and/or adipocyte apoptosis. Additional risk factors for lipoatrophy include severity of the HIV disease, increasing age, elevation of lactic acid levels, and concurrent administration of PIs. Improvement of the lipoatrophy, albeit modest, after changing d4T to other nucleosides (e.g., ABC or TDF greater than ZDV) provides further evidence implicating d4T in the pathogenesis of lipoatrophy. Reversal is often slow, taking more than 48 weeks, if at all, to see increases in subcutaneous fat.[83–87]

The incidence of peripheral neuropathy (10%–20%) is also increased with the use of d4T, particularly if it is used with ddI in those with lower CD4 cell counts.[32,61] Symptoms might resolve after drug discontinuation. In a parallel track trial, efficacy was comparable but the occurrence of neuropathy was less in those receiving d4T 20 mg two times a day (15%) compared with those receiving d4T 40 mg two times a day (21%). If neuropathy develops on traditional dosages of d4T (e.g., 40 mg twice a day), a dosage reduction to 20 mg two times a day may be warranted before stopping therapy. Other reported toxicities include gastrointestinal disturbances (e.g., nausea, vomiting), headache, insomnia, pancreatitis, transaminase elevations, and rash. Hematological toxicity is infrequent.

Lamivudine (Epivir). 3TC, a cytosine triphosphate analog, was approved in 1995 as the fourth NRTI for HIV infection. 3TC is also approved by the FDA for the treatment of hepatitis B infection in a lower dosage of 100 mg daily. Because of its favorable tolerability and potency, 3TC is often used for initial therapy and is also effective in preventing mother to child transmission.[13,23,24] The Canada, Australia, Europe, and South Africa (CAESAR) Trial was the first trial to demonstrate a survival benefit for a 3TC-containing regimen.[88] This trial randomized the addition of placebo, 3TC, or 3TC plus loviride to the underlying ARV regimen of 1,840 ARV-experienced persons with median CD4 cell counts of 126 cells/mm^3. A significant 54% reduction in the risk of disease progression occurred in those receiving 3TC. Several ARV combinations containing a 3TC and nucleoside backbone (e.g., ddI, d4T, ABC, ZDV) have been found to possess durable antiviral activity.[24,32,89] The synergistic combination of 3TC and ZDV delayed the emergence of resistance to ZDV and improved virologic and immunologic measures in four double-blind trials.[90–93] In the NUCA and the NUCB trials, the combination of ZDV plus 3TC, compared with ZDV or 3TC alone, sustained a 1-log decline in viral load and an increase of 60 to 80 CD4 cells from baseline that persisted through week 52 in ARV-naive persons. In ARV-experienced persons, the combination of ZDV plus 3TC was superior to ZDV alone, however, the effects on CD4 cell counts and viral load were less impressive. Comparable virologic and immunologic efficacy has been demonstrated in ARV-naïve persons who received a once daily compared to a twice daily 3TC-based combination regimen for 48 weeks.[94]

3TC should be used only in a fully suppressive viral regimen (e.g., combination with two or more ARV) to prevent the emergence of resistance and the loss of antiviral activity. Resistance to 3TC is associated with the M184V mutation,[47]

a mutation that results in a less fit virus and while improving antiviral drug activity, may prevent rapid viral replication (Table 84.8).

The mean oral bioavailability of 3TC is 82% and is not affected by meals. It is phosphorylated intracellularly to 3TC-TP, which has a long intracellular half-life of 10 to 15 hours. Significant concentrations of 3TC are attained in the CSF that exceeded the in vitro IC$_{50}$ concentrations for most wild-type HIV-1 strains, causing suppression of CSF HIV RNA concentrations.[79] Once daily administration of 300 mg leads to similar pharmacokinetic values as 150 mg twice daily and increases ease of use.[95] Dosage reduction is required in renal impairment because 79% of 3TC is eliminated unchanged in the urine (Table 84.2).

Several studies have demonstrated the efficacy and tolerability of 3TC as a component of a HAART.[32–34] In clinical trials, the addition of 3TC to ZDV did not increase adverse effects or laboratory abnormalities. Headache, diarrhea, and occasionally, neutropenia have been reported. No clinically significant drug to drug interactions have been reported. However, 3TC should not be used in combination with FTC because of possible antagonism. In patients with concomitant hepatitis B and HIV infection, discontinuation of the 3TC can cause a ''flare'' of the hepatitis B infection.

Emtricitabine (Emtriva). FTC was approved by the FDA in July 2003. 3TC and FTC are structurally identical except for the replacement of fluorine for the hydroxy group on the position 5 of the cytosine ring. The creation of the active form of FTC requires intracellular phosphorylation to the triphosphate moiety. Like 3TC, FTC has activity against hepatitis B DNA polymerase, though it does not currently have an FDA-approved indication for hepatitis B treatment. Because of a similar resistance pattern, patients with HIV resistant to 3TC would be resistant to FTC.[47]

Three clinical trials in the treatment of naïve HIV-infected adults have evaluated the safety and efficacy of FTC-based regimens for up to 3 years.[96–99] Patients taking FTC achieved a 1.7-log reduction in HIV-1 viral load compared to a 1.5-log reduction with 3TC during a 10-day comparative monotherapy study conducted in 81 HIV-infected patients.[96] A once daily ARV regimen of FTC, ddI, and EFV produced a 3.5-log decrease in HIV-1 viral load and an average 159 cell/μL CD4 cell increase after 24 weeks of therapy in 40 treatment-naive HIV-infected patients.[97] A randomized, double-blind, placebo-control trial (FTC-301) compared FTC with d4T against the same background of ddI plus EFV.[98] Probability of virologic failure as measured by Kaplan-Meier analysis was statistically higher in the d4T group (15.3%) compared to the FTC group (7.3%). CD4 cell count increase from baseline was statistically higher in the FTC group by intent to treat analysis. Trials in pediatric and ARV-experienced patients are under investigation.[99]

FTC is well absorbed with a bioavailability of 93% regardless of meals.[99] Its long plasma half-life (8–10 hours) allows for once daily administration. One pharmacokinetic study suggested that a 6-mg per kilogram dose would produce a similar area under the curve in children as a 200-mg dose in adults, though further studies are required to evaluate this dosing strategy.[100] The CNS penetration of FTC is unknown. Since FTC is eliminated primarily unchanged, dosing should be adjusted for patients with renal impairment (e.g., CrCl <50 mL/min).

FTC is well tolerated. Discontinuation of FTC occurred in 7.4% of patients compared to 16.6% of those receiving a d4T-based regimen.[98] Common side effects include headache, nausea, diarrhea, and rash. Hyperlactatemia, creatine kinase, and triglyceride elevations have also been reported.[99] An unusual and uncommon side effect in 3% of patients is hyperpigmentation of the skin, primarily in the palms and soles of the feet that occurs after 3 months of therapy and may resolve with continued therapy. Hyperpigmentation may be more prevalent in African-Americans. The clinical significance of this side effect is unknown.

Abacavir (Ziagen). ABC is the sixth NRTI approved in December 1998 by the FDA for use in infected adults and children. FDA approval was based on virologic and immunologic outcomes rather than survival. ABC is intracellularly phosphorylated to its monophosphate form before subsequent conversion to the active carbovir triphosphate moiety. In vitro, ABC displays synergy when combined with all other ARV classes. ABC is not recommended for initial ARV therapy but may be considered as a nucleoside component of alternative regimens.[22,23] Several triple nucleoside-only regimens containing ABC have shown virologic failures and should be avoided.[23,36–38]

The potency of ABC-containing combinations on viral suppression has been demonstrated in several clinical trials involving ARV-naive and ARV-experienced persons, including children. FDA approval was based on data showing no significant differences in viral load suppression and CD4 cell count improvements in 173 ARV-naïve, HIV-infected subjects receiving the triple NRTI combination of ABC/ZDV/3TC versus the PI-containing regimen of IDV/ZDV/3TC.[101] Another trial showed that more HIV-infected ARV-naive subjects developed virologic failure and resistant mutations on the dual 3TC/ZDV/placebo regimen compared to the triple combination of ABC/3TC/ZDV irrespective of baseline viral load.[102] In a multicenter, double-blind trial of 649 naïve HIV-infected persons, the efficacy of ABC was compared to ZDV against the same background of 3TC and EFV.[103] At 48 weeks, 70% of the ABC group compared with 69% of the ZDV group achieved viral suppression. Comparable CD4 cell counts were found. FDA approval for once daily ABC was based on a double-blind trial in 770 treatment-naïve adults that found comparable virologic suppression and CD4 increments in those receiving either once or twice daily ABC against a background of EFV and 3TC.[104]

The bioavailability of ABC is excellent (>75%) and its central nervous system (CNS) penetration is similar to ZDV.

HIV RNA levels in the CSF have declined with an ABC-containing regimen. The half-life of the ABC carbovir triphosphate is approximately 20.6 hours, permitting once daily dosing. ABC is conveniently dosed 600 mg once or 300 mg twice daily irrespective of meals. ABC is also available in several fixed combination dosage forms (Table 84.2). The majority of ABC is metabolized; only 11% to 13% of the drug is excreted unchanged. Therefore, dosing adjustments are not required in renal dysfunction but ABC should be reduced to 200 mg twice daily in mild liver impairment. Similar to other NRTI, no clinically significant drug to drug interactions have been identified. Resistance to multiple NRTI reduces the effectiveness of ABC. Patients who have had extensive exposure to ZDV, 3TC, and other NRTIs may have a minimal response to regimens containing ABC.[47]

ABC is generally well tolerated. Adverse effects include nausea, vomiting, malaise/fatigue, headache, muscle pain, abdominal pain, diarrhea, rash, and sleep disorders. Clinicians need to be aware of, and patients need to be alerted about, a potentially fatal hypersensitivity reaction that has been reported in about 2% to 11% of study subjects.[101–104] This reaction may be higher with the once daily than the twice a day dosing regimen and in those with HLA-B*5701 haplotypes.[105] Symptoms usually occur within the first 6 weeks of therapy and are heralded by the onset of fever; concomitant symptoms in about half of the subjects might include rash, nausea, oral lesions, conjunctivitis, and respiratory symptoms. Once stopped, the reaction subsides within a few days. Resuming ABC is absolutely contraindicated because fatalities have been reported on rechallenge. Patients should be instructed to contact their pharmacist or doctor if these symptoms occur. A "Medication Guide" is issued to each patient by Glaxo Smith Kline to alert patients about this potentially fatal reaction.

Tenofovir (Viread, PMPA). TDF is the first nucleotide analogue approved by the FDA in October 2001. A fixed dosage combination tablet with FTC was approved in August 2004. The disoproxil fumarate form is an esterified prodrug that enhances TDF oral bioavailability. Its long plasma (i.e., 17 hours) and intracellular half-life (i.e., >60 hours) allows for once daily dosing.[106] TDF has activity against hepatitis B virus as well as HIV, though it does not have FDA approval for treatment of hepatitis B. It can be taken without regards to meals.

TDF is a potent nucleotide analogue that reduced HIV-1 viral load 0.97 to 1.57 log copies per milliliter in eight naïve patients during a phase I/II dose ranging monotherapy study.[107] TDF (with 3TC and EFV) was found to be equivalent to d4T in a study of 602 treatment-naïve patients.[80] At 144 weeks, 73% in the TDF group versus 69% in the d4T group achieved HIV-1 RNA less than 50 copies per milliliter. Treatment-experienced patients with detectable virus achieved an additional 0.61 to 0.62-log drop in HIV-1 viral load after addition of TDF.[108,109] For reasons that are unclear, combinations of ddI/TDF and an NNRTI have shown higher rates of virologic failure and should be avoided.

Potency of TDF is decreased by accumulation of nucleoside analogue mutations, particularly M41L, L210W, and K65R.[47] K65R is of special concern because it reduces susceptibility across all nucleoside analogues. It is believed that selection of the K65R mutant by TDF is largely responsible for the virologic failures of studied once daily triple nucleoside regimens such as ABC/3TC/TDF.[110]

TDF is generally well tolerated. The most common side effects include nausea, vomiting, diarrhea, and flatulence. Renal tubular dysfunction, proteinuria, and Fanconi's syndrome associated with TDF have been reported in the literature.[111–113] A urinalysis for protein should be obtained and a creatinine clearance should be calculated prior to starting TDF; renal dosage adjustments should be made if indicated. Studies suggest that TDF has little effect on serum lipids, compared to d4T.[80]

Unlike many of the other nucleoside/tide analogues, TDF displays significant interactions with other ARVs. TDF lowers the plasma levels of the PI atazanavir (ATZ), therefore, it is recommended to use the boosted dosing of ATZ with RTV to overcome this interaction.[59] TDF significantly increases plasma concentrations of ddI.[57] Pancreatitis, lactic acidosis, and less robust CD4 responses have been reported in patients receiving this combination.[74,111] In patients weighing 60 kg or more it is recommended to lower the ddI dose to 250 mg (enteric coated) once daily when administering with TDF. In patients weighing less than 60 kg, a 200-mg ddI dosage reduction may be appropriate but further investigation is required.

PROTEASE INHIBITORS

There are eight available FDA approved PIs that differ in their pharmacokinetics, tolerability, resistance pattern, and drug interaction profile (Tables 84.3, 84.9, and 84.10). The PIs are thought to act primarily at the end of the HIV life cycle where the HIV polypeptide chains await action by the protease enzyme (Fig. 84.1). Cleavage of these polyproteins is required for the formation of infectious virions; therefore, noninfectious mature virions are produced when PIs are used.

The introduction of the PI in late 1995 revolutionized the care of persons infected with HIV and renewed hope for those affected by the HIV epidemic. These agents represent a major advance in the management of HIV disease and have dramatically altered disease progression to AIDS, reduced HIV-related hospitalizations owing to opportunistic infections, and prolonged survival.[2,3] Patients gained weight, felt stronger, and rejoined the work force. Significant improvements in CD4 cell counts and profound suppression of viral replication were observed, even in advanced HIV disease. Combining PIs (e.g., avoid monotherapy) with other ARVs is necessary to prevent the emergence of resistance and subsequent drug failure.

The combination of a boosted PI and a dual NRTI regimen is typically recommended as initial therapy.[23,24] Boosted PI therapy is a key development that improves PI bioavailability and achieves higher PI concentrations, thereby overcoming resistance or drug interactions that reduce PI levels.[114] Low-dose RTV (e.g., 100–200 mg/day), the most potent P-450 enzyme inhibitor, is typically used to boost levels of the concomitant PI, thereby allowing a smaller pill burden, less frequent dosing, and less food restrictions that may improve adherence. RTV boosted PI combinations can be dosed once or twice daily (Table 84.4).

A review of PI-containing trials, including boosted PI regimens, have been summarized.[23,24,32,114,115] These studies show single PI regimens to be comparable or inferior to NNRTI-based regimens and significantly better than NRTI-only regimens in achieving virologic suppression and immunologic benefits. The Atlantic Study, a randomized, open label trial that compared a PI-based (IDV), NNRTI-based (NVP), or triple NRTI regimen (d4T, ddI, 3TC) in treatment-naïve patients, found comparable viral suppression at 48 weeks in the IDV and NVP-containing arms (80%) compared to the NRTI arm (59%).[116] Single PI regimens are inferior to EFV or boosted PI-containing regimens.[31–33] Boosted PI regimens have been effective in achieving virologic suppression even in those failing a single PI-containing regimen.[117,118]

Despite their undisputed effectiveness, several complex clinical issues are associated with the use of these agents. Adherence is critical, as loss of antiviral efficacy has been correlated with poor pill taking and loss of viral suppression.[119] The high pill burden and coordination with meals make these agents laborious to take; proper instructions are key to improve adherence.[120] The potential for life-threatening drug to drug interactions are significant because the PI are substrates of, and are metabolized by, the CYP P-450 system (Table 84.10).[121–123] The most potent P-450 enzyme inhibitor is RTV. Moderate inhibitors include ATZ, LPV, IDV, NFV, fosamprenavir (fos-APV), and amprenavir (APV) while SAQ is considered the least potent inhibitor. Some PI (e.g., RTV, LPV, NFV, APV, fos-APV) also demonstrate enzyme-inducing characteristics, making identification of the outcome of drug interactions challenging.[124] In addition, PI drug interactions can also involve alterations in p-glycoprotein and multidrug resistance-associated proteins (MRP1 and MRP2) which are involved in the active transport of PI out of cells (e.g., CNS, gut). Drug resistance is shared among the class of PI; therefore, development of resistance to one PI can confer resistance to another (Table 84.9). Lastly, many adverse effects have been only recently identified (Table 84.11), a consequence of their rapid approval and limited knowledge about their long-term toxicity.

Since the introduction of the PI, a number of metabolic complications, including insulin resistance, diabetes, hyperlipidemia, abnormalities in fat redistribution (lipodystrophy), have emerged, increasing the risk for cardiovascular complications.[23,125–130] Additional reports of liver and bone

TABLE 84.11	Complications Associated with HAART		
Adverse Effect	**Potential Mechanism**	**Counseling**	**Treatment Recommendations**
Hyperglycemia/diabetes,	Related to insulin resistance from PI	Signs and symptoms of diabetes, Lifestyle changes: ↓ weight (wt) if obese, ↓ carbohydrate intake, ↑ exercise	Diet, weight loss, oral hypoglycemics, insulin.
Hyperlipidemia Hypercholesterolemia Hypertriglyceridemia	Unknown mechanism of action; due to PI	↓ cardiac risk factors: Lifestyle changes: ↓ wt if obese, ↑ exercise, stop smoking, good BP control	Diet, niacin, fibric acid derivatives, omega-3 fatty acids, HGMCo reductase inhibitors. Avoid simvastatin and lovastatin due to risk of rhabdomyolysis and renal failure. Consider ATZ or NNRTI if appropriate.
Abnormal fat accumulation: ↑ abdominal girth, ↑ breast size, "buffalo hump"	Unclear mechanism Abdominal fat accumulation related to PI.	Cosmetic; may reverse if change PI or NRTI. Slow resolution of lipoatrophy	Stop PI if bothersome. Growth hormone effective for fat accumulation.
Lipoatrophy and peripheral wasting	Lipoatrophy and wasting due to NRTI, especially d4T.		If appropriate, change NRTI. Consider change to ABC, ZDV, or TDF. Consider poly-L lactic injections for facial lipoatrophy
Osteoporosis	Unclear mechanism; associated with HIV infection	Lifestyle changes to increase bone density	Calcium supplementation, consider biphosphonates, calcitonin, raloxifene if fractures

HAART, highly active antiretroviral therapy; PI, protease inhibitors; BP, blood pressure; NNRTI, nonnucleoside reverse transcriptase inhibitor; NRTI, nucleotide reverse transcriptase inhibitors; d4T, stavudine; ABC, abacavir; ZDV, zidovudine; TDF, tenofovir; HIV, human immunodeficiency virus.

toxicity raise concerns about the long-term safety of PI-containing regimens.[131–135]

Lipodystrophy is characterized by an abnormal fat accumulation syndrome, including a "buffalo hump," augmented breast size, and increased abdominal girth (i.e., visceral fat) that is associated with peripheral wasting of the buttocks, face, and extremities (lipoatrophy). The prevalence is unknown due to varied criteria for the diagnosis of lipodystrophy. However, incidences of 10% to 84% have been reported.[125] These body changes are delayed, occurring after 1 to 2 years of ARV therapy, and usually associated with beneficial therapeutic effects (e.g., improved well-being, higher CD4 counts, suppressed viral load). The etiology of this syndrome is unknown. Most experts believe that the abnormal fat accumulation is related to the use of PIs, while the lipoatrophy is associated with the NRTI, particularly d4T. Additional risk factors for lipoatrophy include older age, lower body weight, an AIDS diagnosis, and lower CD4 cell count. Currently, there are no recommendations to stop PI therapy unless the lipodystrophy is of significant cosmetic concern to the patient, or if control of metabolic abnormalities is inadequate. Treatment of the abnormal fat accumulation with growth hormone (GH) 4 mg daily is effective, however, improvement is transient if the GH is stopped. Disadvantages of GH include expense, arthralgias, joint

swelling, glucose intolerance, and loss of subcutaneous fat.[125,136] Growth hormone releasing hormone (GHRH) has also been effective in reducing abdominal fat accumulation by normalization of endogenous GH levels and is better-tolerated.[137] Facial lipoatrophy can be improved by the injection of polylactic acid. Surgery can temporarily remove abnormal fat accumulations (e.g., buffalo hump). Changing the offending NRTI (e.g., d4T, ddI) to improve lipoatrophy can be considered if virologic control is not lost; however, changes in PI therapy do not improve the abnormal fat accumulation. Insulin-sensitizing agents (e.g., rosiglitazone, metformin) have not been beneficial for PI-induced lipodystrophy.

Insulin resistance is more common than diabetes.[125,128–130] The incidence of diabetes ranges from 3% to 7% and is most common in those with risk factors for diabetes (e.g., obesity, family history of diabetes, older age). The use of PI therapy was associated with a threefold increase (2.8%) in the development of diabetes in nonpregnant HIV-infected women compared to HIV-infected women on only NRTI or no ARV. PIs, particularly IDV, APV, NFV, LPV/ritonavir (LPV/r), and RTV, are believed to contribute to insulin resistance by inhibiting cellular glucose uptake mediated by GLUT-4. ATZ and SAQ might have less negative effects on insulin sensitivity.[125,130] Treatment of hyperglycemia with diet, oral hypoglycemic agents (e.g., sulfonylureas, metformin, thiazolidinediones), or insulin is effective, permitting continued use of the PI.

Hyperlipidemia is very common, occurring in 40% to 70% of patients receiving PIs. Hypertriglyceridemia can be more severe than hypercholesterolemia, particularly with LPV and RTV, and difficult to manage. Lifestyle modifications should be implemented if appropriate. HGM-CoA reductase inhibitors, niacin, cholesterol binders, ezetimibe, or fibric acid derivatives can be used. Coadministration of simvastatin or lovastatin or possibly rosuvastatin, with PI, whose metabolism is impaired by the PI, should be avoided because of the potential for rhabdomyolysis and acute renal failure. Pravastatin, atorvastatin, and fluvastatin are less likely to cause this toxic reaction and are recommended. For isolated hypertriglyceridemia, the fibric acid derivatives (e.g., gemfibrozil, fenofibrate) are indicated, but response may be poor.[138] Creatinine phosphokinase (CPK) levels should be routinely monitored, if warranted, for complaints of muscle weakness, muscle pain, or new renal dysfunction. Changing to a PI (e.g., ATZ) with a more favorable lipid profile should be considered if virologic control can be maintained.

Lipodystrophy, hypercholesterolemia, hypertriglyceridemia, and insulin resistance often occur concomitantly, raising concerns about the possibility of cardiovascular and cerebrovascular complications.[125–127] A large prospective study found that the relative risk (RR 1.26) of myocardial infarction increased with the duration of ARV therapy.[126] Data from a large retrospective VA study, however, did not find an association but the findings may have been limited by the short duration of ARV use.[127] Evaluation for concomitant cardiac risk factors (e.g., smoking, sedentary life style, obesity) should be undertaken and corrected if feasible. Changing ARVs to reduce the metabolic abnormalities may be considered as discussed previously.

Bone abnormalities, including osteoporosis, osteopenia, osteonecrosis, and compression fracture of the lumbar spine, have been reported in HIV-infected persons receiving HAART.[125,131,132] However, these bone abnormalities have been found in ARV-naïve persons, suggesting that HIV infection itself might be contributory.[139] Osteonecrosis (e.g., avascular necrosis or ischemia of the bone) often presents with hip pain but can involve other joints. In addition to HAART, risk factors associated with osteonecrosis include prolonged steroid use, chronic alcoholism, injection drug use, testosterone use, and advanced AIDS. Surgical correction of the osteonecrosis is often needed. Lifestyle modifications (e.g., exercise, cessation of smoking, restriction of alcohol), calcium supplements, and antiresorptive therapies (e.g., bisphonates, raloxifene) to prevent and treat osteopenia/osteoporosis should be implemented, if appropriate. Whether changing ARVs is beneficial is unclear as a clear association of bone abnormalities with HAART has not been proven.

Hepatotoxicity has been associated with the long-term use of PI-containing regimens. Risk factors include coexist-

ing hepatitis B or C infection, alcoholism, elevated baseline liver enzymes, and use of concomitant hepatotoxins such as the NRTI and NNRTI.[133–135] The presentation is variable; ranging from asymptomatic elevated transaminases (most commonly) to clinical jaundice. The greatest risk of hepatotoxicity is associated with full doses of RTV. The HAART regimen should be discontinued and a new regimen started after liver enzymes have normalized.[135]

Hard-Gel Saquinavir (Invirase).

The hard-gel SAQ (HG-SAQ) formulation was approved by the FDA in December 1995 as the first member of this new ARV class. It is considered the least potent of the currently approved PI and is to be used only in a boosted regimen with RTV. In 2004, a 500-mg HG-SAQ formulation was primarily approved for use in combination with RTV. RTV boosting of SAQ provide potent regimens associated with significant rises in CD4 cell counts and viral suppression.[140,141] Plasma levels of SAQ boosted by RTV are 60-fold higher than when SAQ is given alone.

FDA approval was based on favorable surrogate marker changes in three double-blind studies involving persons infected with HIV at different stages of their disease.[115] Modest increases in CD4 counts of 40 to 50 cells/mm^3 and declines in viral load of 0.5 log^{10} were found in ZDV-experienced patients who received the triple combination of HG-SAQ/ZDC/ddC compared with those receiving the dual combinations of ZDV/ddC and ZDV/HG-SAQ.[142] In ZDV-experienced patients infected with HIV, a 66% reduction in deaths and a 50% decrease in the risk of disease progression to the first AIDS-defining event occurred in those receiving HG-SAQ/ddC compared with those on ddC SAQ monotherapy. Resistance to SAQ is associated with G48V and L90M mutations (Table 84.9).

The mean absolute bioavailability of HG-SAQ is poor because of its large first-pass effect, about 4% when taken with a high-fat meal. A soft-gel SAQ formulation (Fortovase), FDA-approved in 1997, overcame the poor bioavailability of the HG-SAQ by dissolving SAQ in Capmul MCM90 to provide levels eightfold to tenfold higher than the HG-SAQ formulation.[143] Although clinical studies showed that the unboosted soft-gel SAQ-based regimen was more effective than the unboosted hard-gel regimen in achieving an undetectable viral load, tolerability of the soft-gel was poor due to gastrointestinal intolerance from the Capmul component and the large pill burden of 18 pills daily.[143,144] Because of patient intolerance, low usage of soft-gel SAQ, and preferential use of boosted SAQ, manufacture of the soft-gel formulation was discontinued in 2006.

The terminal elimination half-life of SAQ is approximately 13 hours and the drug is rapidly metabolized to inactive metabolites by the CYP P-4503A4 isoenzyme.

Medications or foods (e.g., ketoconazole, grapefruit juice, RTV) that inhibit the P-4503A4 enzyme system can significantly increase plasma concentrations of SAQ (Table 84.10). Similarly, enzyme inducers (e.g., rifampin, rifabutin, NVP,

EFV, anticonvulsants) can significantly reduce SAQ levels and should be avoided if possible. Transaminase elevations are also more frequent if SAQ is given with rifampin. RTV boosting may overcome some of the aforementioned interactions. Unboosted SAQ is reduced 60% by EFV and should be avoided. Likewise, rifabutin should only be administered with boosted SAQ to avoid reducing the steady-state AUC of SAQ by 40%. However, the combination of rifampin and boosted SAQ should be avoided due to an increased risk of hepatotoxicity. Although SAQ is not a strong enzyme inhibitor, coadministration of SAQ with cisapride, ergot alkaloids, triazolam, and midazolam should be avoided because of the increased risk of cardiac arrhythmia and excessive sedation. Garlic reduced unboosted SAQ levels by more than 50% in healthy volunteers.[145]

SAQ is generally well tolerated. Gastrointestinal effects include nausea, vomiting, diarrhea, and abdominal pain. In combination with RTV, diarrhea, cough, rash, and elevated transaminases are more frequent. Laboratory abnormalities include hyperglycemia, hypercholesterolemia, hypertriglyceridemia, and elevated transaminases and CPK levels. Complications of HAART also occur (Table 84.11).

Ritonavir (Norvir). RTV was approved by the FDA in March 1996 as the second licensed PI for use alone or in combination for treatment of HIV-infected adults. In March 1997, RTV was approved for treatment of HIV-infected children. Approval was based on the striking clinical benefits of RTV, including beneficial immunologic and virologic outcomes, improved quality of life, and reductions in disease progression and mortality. Two phase I/II trials of RTV monotherapy (1,000–1,200 mg/day) demonstrated a potent reduction in VL of 1 to 2 $\log^{10}$ and significant CD4 cell count increases of 230 cells/mm^3.[146,147] The addition of full doses of RTV 600 mg twice daily to at least two other ARVs in 1,090 persons with AIDS found approximately a 50% reduction in disease progression or death compared to placebo after 6 months.[148] Although RTV is an extremely potent PI, its poor tolerability and its extensive drug interaction profile are of concern. Therefore, RTV is rarely used in single PI-containing regimens but is typically used as a booster in low doses of 100 to 400 mg daily (Table 84.4). RTV-enhanced regimens have shown durable virologic potency and immunologic benefits.[31,35,114,117,118]

RTV is available as capsules, which require refrigeration, and as a liquid, which is stable at room temperature for 30 days. RTV is well absorbed and should be administered with food to minimize the gastrointestinal intolerance. Decreased absorption occurs when RTV is administered with antacids; therefore, patients should be instructed to separate RTV and antacids, including buffered ddI, by at least 2 hours. Of the PIs, RTV is the most potent inhibitor of the CYP 450 isoenzymes and the efflux pump P-glycoprotein.[121–123,149] Therefore, the potential for fatal drug to drug interactions is significant but are minimized when boosting dosages are used (Table 84.10). Coadministration of RTV with astemizole,

cisapride, various antiarrhythmics, simvastatin, lovastatin, several sedative-hypnotics (e.g., triazolam, midazolam), and recreational drugs is contraindicated because of the potential for cardiac arrhythmias and oversedation. Caution is also required when RTV is coadministered with a wide variety of agents, including agents for erectile dysfunction, narcotics, psychotropics, and immunosuppressants whose metabolism is inhibited by RTV. RTV can also induce glucuronosyl transferases, decreasing efficacy of oral contraceptives, thyroxine, and theophylline.[150] Alternate forms of contraception are recommended. An increase in dosage on patients receiving thyroxine and theophylline might be necessary to maintain efficacy. Enzyme inducers, including rifampin, rifabutin, and anticonvulsants, should be avoided to maintain effective RTV levels. The significant alcohol content of RTV liquid and capsules can produce a disulfiram reaction in those receiving disulfiram or metronidazole. Because of the potential for significant drug to drug interactions with RTV, pharmacists should review the patient's medication profile before starting therapy. However, this potent enzyme inhibition has been advantageous for boosted PI therapy.

RTV is the most problematic PI to administer because of its poor tolerability profile, leading to a high rate of drug discontinuation. Tolerability and drug toxicity are improved when lower boosting dosages are used. Patients should be instructed that RTV can cause frequent gastrointestinal side effects, including nausea, vomiting, anorexia, abdominal pain, diarrhea, and taste disturbances, especially during the first 2 to 4 weeks of therapy. These symptoms are correlated with high plasma concentrations of RTV, especially if full doses are used, and can be minimized by slowly escalating the dose of RTV. No dosage titration is recommended for lower boosted RTV doses. RTV induces its own metabolism, causing high, initial plasma levels to fall with continued dosing. If used as a single PI, it is recommended that RTV be started at 300 mg two times a day and increased over 1 to 2 weeks, in 100-mg increments as tolerated, to 600 mg two times a day (Table 84.3). Proper instructions to administer RTV liquid are essential to increase palatability and improve adherence. Several suggestions, including coating the tongue with peanut butter and disguising the medication with ice cream, jelly, or chocolate syrup have been recommended to improve the palatability of the liquid. Circumoral paresthesia (25%), peripheral paresthesia (5%–6%) asthenia, fatigue, and headaches are self-limiting and do not necessitate stopping the drug. Hematological toxicity is infrequent. Laboratory abnormalities include hypertriglyceridemia, hyperglycemia, hypercholesterolemia, and elevations in transaminases and CK. Triglyceride levels can exceed 1,000 mg per deciliter (11 mmol/L); however, pancreatitis is uncommon. The adverse effects of RTV on the lipid profile have raised concerns about potential long-term complications from atherosclerotic disease.[125–127] CPK should be routinely monitored for complaints of muscle weakness, muscle pain, or new renal dysfunction. Abnormal fat accumulations (e.g., lipodystrophy) and hepatitis occurs.

Indinavir (Crixivan). IDV received accelerated FDA approval in March 1996 as the third available PI. Accelerated approval was based on several studies that found impressive increases in CD4 cell counts and significant reductions in viral load in naïve persons receiving the triple combination of IDV/ZDV/3TC compared to IDV alone or a dual NRTI combination.[115,151,152] Merck 035, a double-blind trial, found that 90% of those on the triple combination achieved an undetectable viral load at 48 weeks that was sustained up to 3 years, compared with 43% for IDV alone, and 0% for the dual NRTI arm. Mean CD4 cell count increases were 100.6, 86, and 46.3 cells/mm^3 for the three respective groups. In a double-blind trial of patients with advanced HIV disease (i.e., mean CD4 cell count of 15 cells/mm^3), 65% of those on the triple combination of ZDV/3TC/IDV achieved complete viral suppression compared to 4% on IDV alone and 0% in the dual NRTI arm. Findings of a significant reduction in mortality and a 50% reduction in disease progression to AIDS led to early termination of a landmark trial that compared the triple combination of ZDV/3TC/IDV to ZDV/3TC.[153] Eight subjects in the triple combination arm died compared with 18 receiving the dual combination (*p* <0.042). RTV-boosted IDV regimens have shown comparable and superior virological and immunologic outcomes compared to a single IDV-containing regimen.[154] Enhanced IDV-containing regimens, rather than unboosted IDV regimens, may be considered as alternative regimens for initial ARV therapy.

IDV is optimally administered twice daily in combination with RTV irregardless of meals (Table 84.4). The dosage of unboosted IDV is 800 mg every 8 hours around the clock to maintain effective plasma levels. A study evaluating an unboosted IDV dosing interval of every 12 hours achieved suboptimal trough concentrations and has been abandoned. IDV is rapidly absorbed, but its bioavailability is reduced with meals. Patients should be reminded to administer unboosted IDV on an empty stomach (1 hour before meals or 2 hours after) for maximal benefit. If gastrointestinal symptoms are intolerable, unboosted IDV can also be ingested with a light, low-fat, low-protein meal. IDV has been detected in CSF, most likely related to its lower protein binding (60%) to α-₁acid glycoprotein compared with other PIs.[155] In cirrhosis, the dosage of unboosted IDV should be reduced to 600 mg every 8 hours. In patients on hemodialysis, no dosage modification is necessary if liver function is normal. Dosage adjustments are not required in renal dysfunction since only about 20% of IDV is eliminated unchanged in the urine.

Similar to RTV, drug interactions are of concern because IDV is also metabolized by the CYP3A4 isoenzyme. Coadministration of IDV with agents whose metabolism will be inhibited, including cisapride, astemizole, triazolam, midazolam, ergots, simvastatin, and lovastatin should be avoided to prevent potentially fatal complications (Table 84.10). Coadministration with rifampin, St. John's wort, anticonvulsants, garlic, and vitamin C can compromise the efficacy of IDV and should be avoided. Dosage adjustments of rifabutin, azoles, agents for erectile dysfunction, and calcium channel blockers may be needed to prevent toxicity. Decreased absorption occurs when IDV is administered with antacids; therefore, patients should be instructed to separate IDV and antacids, including ddI, by at least 2 hours.

IDV is better tolerated than RTV.[152] IDV can cause mild gastrointestinal complaints of nausea (12%–32%), vomiting (5%–12%), abdominal pain (8%–9%), diarrhea (4.5%), and symptoms of gastroesophageal reflux (2%). Headache, fatigue, and weight gain can also occur. The principal complication of IDV is nephrolithiasis, caused by crystallization of the drug in the kidney. Kidney stones have been reported in 4% to 8% of patients.[156,157] Symptoms include nausea, flank pain (with or without hematuria), dysuria, urgency, renal colic, and renal obstruction leading to renal dysfunction. Oral hydration with 1.5 to 2 L of noncaffeinated beverages daily is recommended to prevent stone formation; higher fluid intakes may be necessary in warmer climates. Patients unable (e.g., uncontrolled heart failure) or unwilling to comply with hydration should be considered poor candidates for IDV therapy. Stopping IDV therapy is not always necessary to reverse urologic symptoms or resolution of the stone. If aggressive hydration does not relieve symptoms, and renal obstruction persists, then discontinuing therapy is warranted. Asymptomatic IDV crystalluria, reported in 20% of patients receiving IDV, did not predict development of renal stones, and is not an indication for stopping therapy. Lipodystrophy, hepatitis, diabetes, dry skin, and alopecia have also been reported. Laboratory abnormalities include hyperglycemia, hyperlipidemia, and mild to moderate asymptomatic rises in the indirect bilirubin (usually >2.5 mg/dL), which usually do not require drug discontinuation. The combination of ATZ and IDV should be avoided because of additive adverse effects on hyperbilirubinemia.

Nelfinavir (Viracept). NFV was the fourth PI approved by the FDA in March 1997 for adults and children infected with HIV. Approval was based on improvement in immunologic and virologic markers but data showing a delay in disease progression or a survival advantage is lacking.[115,158] Several clinical trials show that NFV plus two NRTIs as initial therapy is superior to dual nucleosides but not to boosted PI regimens or EFV in improving CD4 cell counts and reducing viral load. A double-blind trial of 297 ARV-naive patients, randomized to ZDV/3TC plus NFV (500 or 750 mg three times daily) or the combination of ZDV/3TC and placebo, found that 75% of those receiving the higher NFV dosing regimen had undetectable viral loads compared with 60% of those on the lower dose NFV regimen. Studies also confirm that the current more convenient dosing of NFV 1,250 mg twice a day is comparable to NFV 750 mg three times daily. In a double-blind, placebo-control trial of 653-naïve subjects, 63% of subjects achieved viral suppression on a NFV-containing regimen compared to 75% of those receiving a RTV boosted PI regimen.[31] As initial therapy, an NFV-containing regimen was inferior to an EFV-based regimen in predicting successful responses to subsequent regimens.[32] Based on these studies, an NFV plus dual nucleoside regimen can be considered an alternative regimen for initial therapy.[23] Resistance occurs through the L90M or a D30N mutation that is unique to NFV (Table 84.9).

NFV is well absorbed, and plasma levels are increased two to three times when NFV is administered with a high fat meal (500 kcal). The half-life is approximately 3.5 hours and NFV undergoes metabolism by hepatic CYP3A4 and CYP2C9 isoenzymes. However, RTV boosting appears less beneficial for increasing NFV levels than other PI. Data is limited regarding the optimal dosing and efficacy of NFV boosted regimens. NFV is most similar to IDV in its drug interaction profile (Table 84.10). Like other PIs, cisapride, ergots, simvastatin, and lovastatin is contraindicated with the concomitant use of NFV. Anticonvulsants, rifampin, rifapentin, and St John's wort can significantly reduce NFV levels and coadministration is not recommended. Because NFV can reduce the efficacy of combination oral contraceptives by enzyme induction, an alternative or additional form of contraception (e.g., barrier contraceptives) is recommended. The dosages of agents for erectile dysfunction will also require a dosage reduction to prevent toxicity.

NFV is generally well tolerated. The most bothersome complaint is moderate to severe diarrhea that occurs in 15% to 32% of those receiving NFV.[158,159] The diarrhea is responsive to over-the-counter and prescription antidiarrheal agents, calcium carbonate 500 mg twice a day, and possibly L-glutamine 30 gm per day.[160] Diarrhea led to study discontinuation in less than 2% of subjects. Similar to other PI, NFV is associated with lipodystrophy, lipid abnormalities, hyperglycemia, insulin resistance, and hepatitis. Less common side effects include rash, headache, nausea, and flatulence. Laboratory abnormalities are similar to those seen with other PIs.

Amprenavir (Agenerase). APV is a "fast-track" PI that received FDA approval in April 1999 for HIV-infected adults and children.[161] Significant virologic and immunologic activity was found with the combination of APV/3TC/ZDV versus ZDV/3TC in 232 HIV-infected subjects with less than or equal to 4 weeks of prior nucleoside therapy. Using an intent-to-treat analysis, 41% of patients on the triple combination versus 3% on the dual combination achieved a undetectable viral load at 48 weeks of therapy.[162] Clinical studies indicate that antiviral activity of APV is comparable to other PIs, producing a median VL reduction of 2.65 log[10] from baseline when used in combination with other ARV agents in naïve persons. However, its high pill burden of 16 pills per day (approved dosage 1,200 mg twice a day) and poor tolerability limits its usefulness as an ARV agent. Boosting with RTV can minimize its pill burden and provide once daily administration (Table 84.4). Since the approval of its prodrug, fos-APV, APV is no longer recommended as an alternative regimen for initial therapy. Manu-

facture of the capsules stopped in December 2004 although the liquid is still available. In vitro, the principal mutation producing a twofold reduction in susceptibility to APV occurs at codon I50V, a mutation not found with other PI, making cross-resistance to other PI less likely (Table 84.9). Isolates resistant to APV showed limited cross-resistance to other PI. Additional mutations at codons M46I and I47V produced a 3-fold to 14-fold reduction in its susceptibility.

The bioavailability of APV capsules ranges from 35% to 90%. However, the bioavailability of the oral solution is 86% relative to the capsules, making doses of the two formulations not interchangeable.[161] APV is 90% protein bound to α1-acid glycoprotein and CNS penetration is limited. The half-life of APV is approximately 9 hours, permitting twice a day dosing. APV undergoes biliary excretion and its metabolites are excreted in the urine. Dosage adjustment is not required in renal dysfunction.

APV is an inhibitor of the hepatic P-450 CYP3A4 and CYP2C19 isoenzyme system. Its P-450 inhibitory potency is less than RTV, greater than those of SAQ, and similar to NFV, IDV, and ATZ. Its drug interaction profile is likely to be similar to other PI (Table 84.10). The administration of cisapride, ergots, simvastatin, lovastatin, and certain benzodiazepines is contraindicated with the concomitant use of APV. Anticonvulsants, rifampin, rifapentin, oral contraceptives and St John's wort can significantly reduce APV levels and coadministration is not recommended. The dosages of antifungal azoles and agents for erectile dysfunction will also require a dose reduction to prevent toxicity. If APV is coadministered with EFV, only the boosted APV regimens should be used to prevent virologic failure; EFV can significantly reduce unboosted APV levels.

The high pill burden of APV limits its tolerability. Adverse effects reported in more than 10% of patients receiving APV include nausea, vomiting, diarrhea, headache, fatigue, rash, and oral/perioral paresthesia.[161,162] Rarely, Stevens-Johnson syndrome has been reported. Because APV contains a sulfonamide moiety, it should be used cautiously in those with a serious sulfa allergy. Similar to other PIs, APV is associated with lipodystrophy, lipid abnormalities, hyperglycemia, insulin resistance, and hepatitis. Other reported laboratory findings include hyperbilirubinemia and elevated transaminases.

Lopinavir/Ritonavir (Kaletra). LPV was approved by the FDA in September 2000 as the sixth PI.[163] It is also the first PI coformulated with low-dose RTV to boost its own plasma concentrations. FDA approval was based on favorable results of viral suppression from a double-blind, 48-week trial of 653 ARV-naïve patients randomized to an LPV/r or an NFV-containing regimen.[31] Sixty-seven percent of those in the LPV/r group achieved complete viral suppression (e.g., VL <50 copies/mL) compared with 52% in the NFV group. In follow-up studies, virologic response to LPV/r was sustainable out to 4 years and the LPV/r group demonstrated a lower risk of virologic failure after 96 weeks, when compared to the NFV group.[35,164] Genotypic and phenotypic analyses from those that did have virologic breakthrough showed no resistance in the LPV/r group (0%, n = 51) and significant resistance (45%, n = 96) in the NFV group.[165]

An LPV/r regimen in PI-experienced patients may still be effective although the viral load and CD4 cell count response may be much less compared to naïve persons.[163,166,167] In an uncontrolled trial, 58 ARV-experienced patients with an average of four baseline protease mutations still achieved an average 1.9-log drop in their HIV-1 viral load over 48 weeks when started on an LPV/r-containing regimen.[166] Seventy NNRTI-naïve patients failing a PI-containing regimen were randomized in a double-blind trial to a regimen containing two doses of LPV, NVP, and one new nucleoside analog. Using an intent-to-treat analysis, 60% achieved complete viral suppression and there was a significant CD4 count increase of 125 cells from baseline.[167] There are no specific single-point mutations that confer resistance to LPV/r, but there is cross-resistance with other PI. A slightly higher genetic barrier to resistance may be its advantage in salvage therapy: it requires accumulation of approximately 5 to 6 protease mutations for potency to be greatly reduced.[168] The efficacy of an LPV/r regimen in deep salvage therapy is unknown.

The U.S. DHHS guidelines currently list LPV/r as the preferred PI for initiation of ARV therapy in naïve patients.[23] Kaletra is available in gel capsules containing 133.3 mg LPV with 33.3 mg RTV, tablets containing 200 mg LPV with 50 mg RTV, and in a liquid formulation (Table 84.3). The capsules and liquid expire on the manufacturer's expiration date if stored in the refrigerator. If kept out of the refrigerator, the contents should be used within 2 months.

LPV/r is usually dosed twice daily. However, in April 2005, a once daily regimen of 800/200 mg LPV/r (six capsules) received FDA approval only for HIV-naïve persons based on favorable 48-week data. In study 418, a randomized, open label, multicenter trial in 190 naïve persons, 71% of persons receiving once daily 800/200 mg LPV/r plus FTC 200 mg and TDF 300 mg achieved viral suppression compared to 65% of those receiving twice daily LPV/r plus the same NRTI. In another 48-week trial using an intent-to-treat analysis, 74% in the once daily group and 70% in the twice daily group achieved complete viral load suppression (p = 0.7); adherence was not different between the groups.[169] Once daily LPV is not indicated in treatment-experienced patients or in those receiving concomitant EFV, NVP, APV, or NFV.

LPV/r should be taken with food to increase its bioavailability.[163] Fasting reduced the AUC of the liquid and the capsule by 44% and 36%, respectively, when compared with food. Taken with a meal, the liquid and capsules are bioequivalent. LPV/r is highly protein-bound (98%–99%) and penetrates poorly into the CNS and genital tract. The half-life is approximately 4 to 6 hours. Less than 3% is excreted renally. No dosage adjustments are required in renal dysfunction.

LPV/r is an inhibitor of the CYP3A4 isozyme. Enzyme induction also occurs. Coadministration of LPV/r is contraindicated with several antiarrhythmics, cisapride, pimozide, various benzodiazepines, rifampin, ergot derivates, St. John's wort, simvastatin, and lovastatin (Table 84.10). Phenytoin and LPV/r have a bidirectional interaction, resulting in significant reductions of both drug levels.[124] The efficacy of estrogen birth control pills can be compromised, requiring alternative forms of contraception. Doses of other PIs, such as APV or SAQ, require adjustment when combined with LPV/r. EFV and NVP significantly reduce plasma levels of LPV and require a dosage increase to four capsules of LPV/r twice daily. Dosages of azoles used for fungal infections and agents for erectile dysfunction will also require adjustments (Table 84.10).

The most common side effects of LPV/r are gastrointestinal upset, nausea, vomiting, and diarrhea. Antidiarrheal agents are usually not necessary because the diarrhea is less frequent and severe compared to NFV.[159] However, diarrhea is greater with once a day dosing compared to twice a day dosing (57% vs. 35%). As with other PIs, LPV/r may also impair glucose tolerance, cause body habitus changes, and hepatitis. LPV/r can have a marked effect on serum transaminases, cholesterol, and triglycerides. Elevations in triglyceride levels can be impressive and occur within the first month of therapy. Baseline and follow-up cholesterol and fasting triglyceride screenings are recommended. Lifestyle modifications and antilipidemic medications should be instituted as appropriate to normalize lipid levels.

Fosamprenavir (Lexiva). Fos-APV was approved by the FDA in October 2003 as the seventh PI in its class. Fos-APV is a prodrug that is rapidly hydrolyzed by cellular phosphatases in the gut to its active form, APV.[170] The absolute bioavailability of APV from the oral administration of fos-APV is unknown. Cmax was 30% lower but steady-state AUCs were equivalent for fos-APV compared to APV in two pharmacokinetic studies.[171,172] As with other PIs, coadministration with low doses of RTV decreases variability in plasma APV concentrations. The pill burden associated with the prodrug fos-APV (four pills daily) is significantly improved over that of its predecessor, APV. The three FDA-approved dosing strategies for fos-APV in ARV-naïve patients are 1,400 mg twice daily, 1,400 mg once daily boosted with 200 mg of RTV, or 700 mg plus 100 mg RTV twice daily in ARV-experienced patients. It can be taken without regard to food.[172] Dosing adjustments in renal dysfunction are not required.

FDA approval was based on studies in naïve patients and in patients with previous PI exposure. In 78 PI-naïve patients with less than 4 weeks of NNRTI or NRTI therapy, fos-APV yielded an average 100 cell/mm³ increase in CD4 cell count and an approximate 2-log drop in HIV-1 RNA when given in combination with ABC and 3TC for 28 days.[171] Fos-APV (1,400 mg twice daily) compared favorably to NFV twice daily in combination with ABC and 3TC in 249 ARV-naïve patients with advanced HIV disease in the open label NEAT (APV30001) study. More patients achieved VL less than 400 copies per milliliter in the fos-APV (66%) versus the NFV (51%) groups by an intention-to-treat analysis.[173] SOLO (APV 30002) randomized 649 ARV-naïve patients to open label fos-APV 1,400 mg boosted with RTV 200 mg once daily versus NFV 1,250 mg twice daily, each in combination with ABC and 3TC twice daily. Comparable achievement of VL less than 50 copies per milliliter were observed in both groups (58% vs. 55%) at 48 weeks of therapy.[174] However, more patients receiving NFV (17%) than fos-APV (7%) experienced virologic failure. The emergence of resistance to the fos-APV and NRTI arm was significantly less than in the NFV arm (0% vs. 50%).[175] CONTEXT (APV30003) attempted to demonstrate equivalency between two boosted regimens of fos-APV versus standard dose LPV/r in 315 ARV-experienced patients. Mean CD4 cell count increases and percentage of patients achieving undetectable viral loads were higher in the LPV/r than in the fos-APV groups. Only 37% of patients in the fos-APV once daily group achieved viral loads less than 50 copies per milliliter compared to 46% and 50% in the fos-APV twice daily and LPV/r groups, respectively.[176]

Fos-APV is metabolized primarily by the liver CYP P-450 3A4. Drugs that interact with APV can also be expected to interact with fos-APV (Table 84.10). Avoid coadministration of H-2 blockers that can significantly impair APV levels.[177] If administered with EFV, the RTV boosted twice daily regimen should be used. If once daily dosing is preferable, an additional 100 mg of RTV (300 mg total per day) should be added to overcome this interaction.[178] Until further studies are completed, fos-APV should not be combined with LPV/r due to a bidirectional interaction that reduces the levels of both agents (Table 84.4).

Tolerability is significantly improved with fos-APV. Common adverse effects associated with fos-APV are gastrointestinal (diarrhea, nausea, vomiting), abdominal pain, headache, skin rash, and hypersensitivity reactions. The incidence of diarrhea was significantly lower with fos-APV compared to NFV.[173,174] Stevens-Johnson type rash was reported in less than 1% of patients.

Atazanavir (Reyataz). ATZ was approved by the FDA in June 2003 as the sixth available PI. It was the first PI to be approved by the FDA for once daily dosing. FDA approval was based on favorable results on CD4 count and viral load in ARV-naïve persons; effects on survival are unknown.[179–184] Current DHHS guidelines recommend ATZ 400 mg (2 capsules) daily as an alternative regimen for initial therapy.[23] RTV (100 mg) boosted ATZ 300 mg (2 capsules), given once daily, should be used in HIV-experienced patients and in those receiving concomitant EFV, NVP, or TDF.

Approval was based on two 48-week phase II clinical trials in ARV-naïve persons that found that 400 or 600 mg daily doses of ATV achieved a 2.31-log to 2.58-log reduction in viral load and a 208 to 243 cell/mm³ increase in CD4 cell counts that was comparable to NFV, each given in combina-

tion with d4T and ddI.[179–181] In the continuation rollover/switch study AI424–044, 83% to 87% of patients continued on ATZ or switched from NFV to ATZ (400 mg daily), maintained viral loads less than 400 copies per milliliter after 72 weeks of therapy.[180,181] A double-blind trial in ARV-naïve persons found that ATZ (400 mg once daily) and EFV (600 mg once daily), each in combination with ZDV plus 3TC, produced complete viral suppression (VL <50 copies/mL) in a comparable percentage of subjects (32% and 37%, respectively).[182] A once daily combination of 400 or 600 mg ATZ plus 1,200 mg SAQ versus RTV 400 mg/SAQ 400 mg twice daily, both with a nucleoside backbone, were compared in 82 ARV-experienced patients.[183] Patients in the ATZ/SAQ arm achieved viral load reductions of 1.19 to 1.44 logs and mean increases in CD4 cell counts of 55 to 109 cells/mm³ that were not significantly different from the RTV/SAQ comparator arm.

The signature mutation conferring resistance to ATZ is the I50L substitution.[185] The I50L is a unique mutation that causes decreased susceptibility to ATZ but increased susceptibility to other PIs. Other genotypic mutations associated with ATZ resistance include M46I, A71V, I84V, and N88S. Viral isolates resistant to one or two PIs generally remain sensitive to ATZ, however, susceptibility decreases as multiple protease resistance mutations are acquired. In an ongoing phase III open trial, boosted ATZ was virologically comparable to LPV/r; each in combination with TDF and one other NRTI, in 358 patients requiring salvage therapy.[184]

ATZ requires an acidic environment for adequate absorption. Its bioavailablility and pharmacokinetic variability are significantly improved if administered with food. The bioavailability of ATZ can increase as much as 70% if given with a light meal, or drops to 35% with a high fat meal.[184] It is highly protein bound (86%) and penetrates well into the CSF and genital tract. ATZ undergoes hepatic metabolism by CYP 3A4 and also inhibits CYP3A4 and uridine diphosphate glucuronosyl transferase 1A1 (UGT1A1) enzymes. Approximately 7% of unchanged ATV is excreted renally. Therefore, dosage adjustments in renal dysfunction are not necessary.

Common side effects of ATZ include headache, nausea, vomiting, diarrhea, abdominal pain, and rash. Clinical trials show that diarrhea is more common with NFV (50%) than ATV (20%). Unlike other PIs, elevations in low-density lipoprotein (LDL) cholesterol and triglycerides are negligible.[179–184] Significant improvements in lipid abnormalities were observed in patients changing from NFV to ATZ.[180,181] This may make it a favorable choice for patients at risk for cardiovascular disease. Similar to IDV, ATZ is associated with dose-dependant asymptomatic rises in indirect bilirubin above 2.6 times the upper limits of normal (22%–49% in clinical trials) which may result in jaundice (7%) or scleral icterus. This reaction is believed to be mediated by UGT1A1 inhibition. The hyperbilirubinemia can improve with continued drug administration, is usually not associated with elevations in transaminases, and is reversible upon discontinuation. In clinical trials, jaundice was not a major reason for drug discontinuation. Hepatitis and abnormal fat accumulations have been reported. Because of its minimal impact on lipids, the risk of cardiovascular disease is expected to be low but long-term data is lacking. Hyperglycemia might be less due to negligible effect of ATZ on insulin sensisitivity.[130] Because ATZ has the potential to prolong the PR interval, ATZ should be used with caution in those with conduction abnormalities [e.g., first-degree atrioventricular (AV) block].

Drug interactions with ATZ can be anticipated to occur through CYP3A inhibition and changes in gastric acidity (Table 84.10). Absolute contraindications are similar to those with other PI. If ATZ is to be administered with TDF, EFV, or NVP, ATZ should be boosted with RTV to maintain effective levels. DdI buffered formulations and other antacids should be separated 1 hour before or 2 hours after ATZ. Proton pump inhibitors are not recommended for coadministration due to significant decreases in ATZ levels. H-2 blockers should be administered 12 hours apart from ATZ so as not to interfere with its absorption. Calcium channel blockers (e.g., diltiazem, verapamil) that have the potential to increase PR interval, should be used with caution. If a patient is taking the aforementioned CCB a 50% dose reduction is recommended to avoid CCB-induced bradycardia and heart block. Likewise, clarithromycin dosage may need reduction by 50% to prevent excessive clarithromycin levels. ATZ increases the plasma concentrations of SAQ, though an optimal dosing strategy has not been determined. The dosages of agents for erectile dysfunction, azoles, and anticonvulsants may need to be adjusted.

Tipranavir (Aptivus). Tipranavir (TPV) is an ARV agent that is likely to be approved by the FDA in mid-2005, but it is under phase III investigation at the writing of this chapter. TPV is a novel nonpeptidic PI that was created using structure-based design.[186] It has good oral bioavailability and is pharmacokinetically enhanced by RTV. Boosting with RTV increased TPV exposure up to 70-fold.[187] The marketed preparation will likely be a twice daily preparation of 500 mg of TPV coformulated with 200 mg of RTV to reduce pill burden.

FDA approval will likely be based on the results of the RESIST-1 (620 patients enrolled from the US, Canada, and Australia) and RESIST-2 (863 patients from Europe and Latin America) open label phase 3 trials designed to compare the safety and efficacy of boosted TPV with comparator boosted PI (e.g., LPV, SAQ, APV, or IDV) in patients with documented resistance. Preliminary results indicate that approximately 41% of those receiving TPV/r compared to 15% to 22% of those receiving the comparator boosted PI achieved a 1 log or greater decrease in viral load from baseline ($p <0.0001$).

A randomized, open label, parallel design study in 31 treatment-naïve patients evaluated potential dosing strategies for TPV.[187] Groups were randomized to receive TPV (1,200 mg twice daily), TPV plus RTV (300 and 200 mg twice daily, respectively), or TPV plus RTV (1,200 and 200 mg twice daily, respectively) for 14 days. Plasma HIV-1 viral load reductions in the different treatment arms were 0.77, 1.43, and 1.64 logs, respectively.

The flexibility of the nonpeptidic chain may make TPV valuable in cases of HIV PI resistance. One published study assessed the in vitro activity of TPV against PI resistant clinical isolates.[188] Study samples had an average of 6.1 PI mutations and a minimum tenfold increase in IC50 to three out of four of the following PIs: IDV, RTV, NFV, and SAQ. Of these resistant clinical isolates, 90% (95/105) displayed phenotypic susceptibility to TPV.

Adverse events (>1%) include diarrhea, nausea, vomiting, fatigue, and headache. Mild rash occurred more often in women than men. Elevations in liver function tests, cholesterol, and triglycerides were also found.

Similar to other PI, drug interactions with TPV will also be problematic. TPV is a potent inducer of the CYP3A4 enzyme.[186] Substantial decreases in the levels of the concomitant PI, including LPV/r, SAQ, fos-APV, and APV have been observed. Antacids may reduce TPV levels by 23% while clarithromycin and fluconazole can raise TPV levels. Further studies regarding TPV drug interactions are warranted.

NONNUCLEOSIDE REVERSE TRANSCRIPTASE INHIBITORS (NNRTI)

The NNRTIs include NVP, DLV, and EFV (Table 84.5). Unlike the NRTIs, the NNRTIs do not require activation by cellular phosphorylation for its ARV activity. These agents do not have any activity against HIV-2. The NNRTIs inactivate the HIV-1 RT by noncompetitively binding directly to the HIV-RT structure, likely at amino acid positions 100 and 103 (Fig. 84.1). Substitutions of the RT amino acids residues at these positions confer resistance to their antiviral activity. All the NNRTIs bind to the same RT enzyme pocket so that cross-resistance among the NNRTIs is likely despite their structural dissimilarities (Table 84.9). K103N was the predominant viral mutant, followed by Y188L or V108I mutations, that were observed among HIV persons experiencing viral rebound on EFV monotherapy. The NNRTIs should not be used as monotherapy but should be used only in combination with other ARV agents to prevent the rapid emergence of resistance. Similar to the PI, drug interactions are of concern, since the NNRTIs are metabolized by the hepatic CYP3A4 isoenzymes and can be enzyme inducers or inhibitors (Table 84.10). Unlike most of the PIs, these agents are also attractive because they penetrate the blood to brain barrier. These agents are often used as effective protease-sparing regimens as concerns about drug resistance and new adverse effects of the PI (e.g., lipodystrophy, hyperlipidemia) emerge. Current DHHS guidelines recommend the use of EFV as a component of an initial ARV regimen.[23] Although clinical trials show NVP to be an effective ARV agent, its toxicity profile and its drug interaction profile limits its use. Data for the clinical use of delavidine are limited and is rarely used.

Nevirapine (Viramune). NVP was the first NNRTI approved by the FDA in June 1996 for treatment of HIV-infected adults. In December 1998, an FDA indication for the treatment of HIV-infected children was approved. FDA approval was based on immunologic and virologic improvements found in a controlled trial (ACTG 241) of 398 ZDV-experienced patients with mean CD4 cell counts of 140 cells/mm[3] receiving an NVP-containing regimen. After 48 weeks, a sustained 0.5-log VL reduction and improved CD4 cell count gain of 34 cells/mm[3] from baseline was noted in the group randomized to NVP/ZDV/ddI versus ZDV/ddI/placebo. However, no difference in clinical progression to AIDS or death was observed.[189] Subsequent clinical trials have shown similar beneficial responses in approximately 50% of treatment-naïve persons. In Italy, the Netherlands, Canada, Australia (INCAS trial), a double-blind study of 151 treatment-naive patients with mean CD4 cell counts of 376 cells/mm[3] found that a significant proportion of subjects achieved viral suppression ($p <0.001$), a more durable reduction in VL, and a greater increase in CD4 cell count on an NVP-containing triple regimen compared to two dual NRTIs regimens.[190] Although disease progression or death were lower for those receiving the triple combination regimen (12%), it was not significantly different from both of the dual regimens (23%, 25%, $p = 0.08$). Two trials comparing an NVP-containing regimen to two PI-based regimens (i.e., an IDV-containing regimen in ATLANTIC and to an NFV-containing regimen in COMBINE) suggest that NVP could be an effective protease-sparing regimen. The NVP-based regimens resulted in a greater proportion of subjects achieving viral load suppression (e.g., 55%, 75% of subjects, respectively) than either of the PI-containing regimens (44%, 60% of subjects, respectively).[116,191] The 2NN study, a randomized trial of 1216 HIV-infected ARV-naïve subjects, showed that the proportion of subjects achieving viral suppression (70%) was similar between those receiving an NVP-based regimen or an EFV-based regimen when each was combined with d4T and 3TC. In addition, combining the two NNRTIs did not provide additional benefits but resulted in more adverse effects.[192]

NVP is well absorbed (bioavailability of 93%) and is not affected by food or antacids.[193] Approximately 60% of NVP is protein bound, permitting NVP to penetrate the CSF, attaining levels about 50% of those achieved in the plasma. The half-life ranges from 22 to 84 hours (mean 40 hours), allowing a convenient once daily dosing regimen. Similar to the PI, NVP is metabolized by the hepatic CYP3A4 isoenzymes. NVP is an enzyme inducer and has the potential to reduce blood levels of various medications and PI (Table 84.10), including inducing its own metabolism. Metabolic autoinduction of NVP results in as much as a twofold increase in NVP systemic clearance after chronic administration of 200 to 400 mg daily for 1 to 2 weeks. With chronic

NVP administration, its half-life is shortened from 45 hours to 25 to 30 hours.[193] Therefore, an initial dose-escalation of NVP is recommended to minimize high drug concentrations and possibly, reduce adverse effects of rash and hepatitis. The dosage of NVP is 200 mg every day for the first 2 weeks to reduce the incidence of rash, and then, if no rash, the dose should be increased to 200 mg two times a day. After the initial titration period, the 2NN study demonstrated that 400 mg once daily is comparable to twice daily dosing but is associated with a higher incidence of side effects.[192]

The safety and pharmacokinetics of NVP has also been evaluated in seven HIV-1 infected pregnant women who received a single 200-mg oral dose at the onset of labor.[13] Their infants also received a single oral 2-mg per kilogram dose at 2 to 3 days of age. Although NVP elimination was impaired, the half-life of NVP was prolonged to 66 hours in the mother (compared with 45 hours in the nonpregnant female) and to 36.8 hours in the neonate (compared with 24.8 hours in children). No adverse effects were noted.

Adverse effects to NVP can be significant, causing drug discontinuation in 21.2% of patients in one study.[193] The dose-limiting side effect of NVP is a diffuse, erythematous, maculopapular rash that can occur in 30% to 50% of subjects. Rash may be seven times more frequent and more severe in women than in men.[194] The rash typically occurs within the first few weeks of administration (mean onset 11 days) and is minimized by dose escalation. If the rash does not disappear or worsens with continued NVP administration, it is prudent not to escalate the dose to twice daily administration until the rash subsides. Antihistamines or corticosteroids have been used to alleviate symptoms but worsening of symptoms can occur so that NVP should be stopped if the rash is severe or if systemic symptoms (e.g., fever, blisters, hematologic abnormalities, eosinophilia, multiple organ involvement) are present. Drug discontinuation is required in 6% of cases. Patients should be instructed about the characteristics of the rash and to contact their pharmacist or physician if the rash persists. Rarely (0.5%), life-threatening Stevens-Johnson syndrome has been reported. Prophylactic use of antihistamines or corticosteroids is not recommended since a higher occurrence of rash has been reported among those receiving prophylactic agents at the initiation of NVP therapy.

Hepatitis is a life-threatening adverse effect of NVP that has been reported in 2.5% to 11% of clinical trials. It is most common during the first 6 weeks of therapy; but can be delayed until 4 or more months after starting therapy.[195] Patients at highest risk include women, those with CD4 cell counts greater than 250 cells/mm[3], and those coinfected with hepatitis B or C. In most cases, hepatitis is reversible after stopping NVP, but fatalities have been reported, even in healthy health care workers who received NVP for postexposure prophylaxis.[23] NVP-induced hepatitis might also occur in association with rash, fever, and eosinophilia. The etiology is unknown but higher NVP serum levels might be responsible, emphasizing the need for a dosage titration period.

Asymptomatic rises in transaminases greater than five times normal have also been reported. Patients should be instructed about the signs and symptoms of hepatitis and to contact their pharmacist or physician if worrisome symptoms of fever, rash, abdominal pain, and gastrointestinal distress occur. It is prudent to stop NVP if ALT is greater than five to ten times normal, especially if in conjunction with other systemic symptoms. Hepatic transaminases should be monitored at baseline, 2 and 4 weeks, then monthly for the next 3 months, and thereafter every 3 months.[23]

Other adverse reactions reported include headache, dizziness, fever, fatigue, nausea, ulcerative stomatitis, abdominal pain, and diarrhea.

Because NVP is an enzyme inducer, drug interactions should be anticipated. NVP can reduce effective drug concentrations of several medications (e.g., voriconazole, rifampin, ethinyl estradiol, statins) leading to drug failure (Table 84.10). An increase in methadone dosage is often required to prevent narcotic withdrawal. A higher dosage of the PI (e.g., LPV/r) or RTV boosting of several PI (e.g., SAQ, IDV, APV, ATV) may be required when given in conjunction with NVP. Administration of the following agents (e.g., anticonvulsants, St. John's wort, rifampin) is not recommended to prevent reduction of effective NVP levels.

Delavirdine (Rescriptor). DLV is the second NNRTI approved in 1997 for treatment of HIV-1 infection in adults. It is a bis(heteroaryl) piperazine and is chemically distinct from NVP. Although the approval package was sent to the FDA in November of 1996, the approval of DLV by the FDA was delayed until April 1997 because of the weakness of the data presented. Protocol 017 randomized treatment-experienced patients with mean CD4 cell counts of 135 cell/mm^3 to DLV 400 mg three times a day plus ddI or ddI monotherapy. The trial was stopped at 6 months because there was no statistical difference in mortality or disease progression between the two groups. Protocol 021 randomized less experienced patients with a mean CD4 cell counts of 325 cells/mm^3 to ZDV plus DLV at doses of 200, 300, or 400 mg three times a day. Clinical data on DLV are very limited and there are no data confirming a survival advantage or delay in disease progression.[196] A phase II trial comparing a triple combination of DLV/ZDV/ddI to two drug combinations of these drugs found modest, but not always significant virologic and immunologic benefits with the triple combination.[197] DLV is not recommended for use as an initial ARV regimen. Studies are evaluating its use as an 3A4 inhibitor similar to RTV for use in boosted PI regimens.[198]

The bioavailability of DLV is 85% and can be administered without regard to meals.[193] The preferred method is to administer DLV as (600 mg; three 200-mg tablets) intact tablets twice daily. Alternatively, a slurry of four (100 mg) tablets, dissolved in 3 to 4 oz of water to improve its bioavailability by 20%, can be administered three times daily. Absorption of DLV is decreased if administered with buffered products; therefore, patients should be instructed to separate DLV and antacids, including ddI by at least 2 hours (Table

84.5). The penetration of DLV into the CNS is more limited than NVP because of DLV's higher protein binding (98%).

DLV is also metabolized by the CYP P-4503A4 system; however, unlike NVP, DLV is an enzyme inhibitor, and may inhibit its own metabolism.[196] Coadministration of DLV with cisapride, alprazolam, midazolam, triazolam, ergots, simvastatin, lovastatin, and amphetamines should be avoided because toxicity can occur from excessive blood levels of these drugs (Table 84.10). Enzyme inducers, including rifampin, St. John's wort, and the anticonvulsants (e.g., phenytoin, carbamazepine, and phenobarbital) can reduce efficacy of DLV and coadministration is not recommended. Dosages of agents used for erectile dysfunction and PI should be adjusted.

DLV's tolerability profile is very similar to NVP. A diffuse, erythematous, maculopapular, pruritic skin rash is the most frequent complaint, occurring in 20% to 40% of the study subjects.[196] The rash usually occurs during the first few weeks of DLV dosing, and it is self-limiting in 85% of patients despite drug continuation. Antihistamines can alleviate the pruritus and rash. In severe cases, the drug should be stopped to avoid progression to systemic symptoms of fever, facial swelling, mucosal involvement, or desquamation. Dose escalation of DLV is not helpful to reduce the occurrence of the rash. The cross-reactivity of rash from DLV or NVP is unknown but might be low based on its different chemical structures. Gastrointestinal side effects (nausea, diarrhea, abdominal pain) were experienced by 33% of patients in one study.[197] Other adverse effects include headaches and fatigue. Laboratory abnormalities include increased transaminases, and rarely, anemia and neutropenia.

Efavirenz (Sustiva). EFV is the third NNRTI approved by the FDA in late September 1998 for the treatment of HIV-1 infection in adults and children. Like other ARV agents, viral suppression is more pronounced in ARV-naive than in experienced patients. EFV is unique among the NNRTIs because it is the first NNRTI recommended by the DHHS guidelines as an effective "protease-sparing" agent for initial therapy.[23,24] FDA approval was based on the superiority of EFV versus IDV, each plus ZDV/3TC, in achieving virologic suppression in a large, multicenter, open label, randomized, head-to-head trial (Dupont 006) of 450 ARV-naive or minimally pretreated patients.[33] At 48 weeks, using an "intent-to-treat" analysis, 64% of those receiving the EFV triple combination achieved an undetectable viral load (<50 copies/mL) compared with 43% on the IDV regimen. (p <0.001) A higher rate of adverse effects leading to drug discontinuation occurred in the IDV (43%) arm versus the EFV (27%) arm that may have biased the results favorably toward EFV. Nevertheless, convincing data from several clinical trials show that EFV is comparable or superior to a single PI-based regimen and superior to a triple nucleoside regimen in achieving durable viral suppression and immunologic benefits when used as initial therapy.[32,33,36,80,98,103,182,192,199] A multicenter, double-blind trial in naïve persons found that EFV plus ZDV/3TC rather than d4T/ddI was superior to two NFV-based regimens containing the aforementioned NRTI.[32,199] Likewise, more complex four-drug NFV-containing or EFV-containing (QUAD) regimens did not offer additional benefits over this triple EFV (ZDV/3TC) combination in naïve persons.[32,199,200] Comparable efficacy has also been demonstrated when EFV has been combined with d4T/3TC, ABC/3TC, ddI/FTC, or TDF/3TC.[80,98,103] However, higher virologic failures have been reported with the combination of TDF/ddI/EFV and this regimen should be avoided pending further investigation.[201] The 2NN trial also demonstrated the efficacy and safety of an EFV-containing rather than an NVP-based regimen as first-line therapy.[192] An EFV-based regimen may also delay the time to virologic failure of subsequent treatment regimens.[199,202,203] Two switch studies show that substitution of EFV for a PI in patients virologically suppressed on a PI-containing regimen produced more durable viral load suppression compared to those maintained on the PI regimen. An ongoing study, comparing the addition of EFV, NFV, or EFV/NFV to new NRTIs in ARV-experienced persons, showed that the VL was undetectable in 64% on NFV, 69% on EFV, and 81% on the combination of EFV plus NFV at 16 weeks. A double-blind, multicenter study randomized 327 experienced patients on two NRTIs to IDV/placebo or to EFV plus IDV (1 g q8hr). At 24 weeks, 68.2% of those on EFV combination compared with 52.4% on the IDV combination achieved a plasma VL less than 400 copies per milliliter.[201] However, data showing a survival advantage is not yet available.

EFV can be taken with or without food; however, a high-fat meal should be avoided to limit increased absorption. Its long half-life of more than 40 hours permits once daily dosing. Therapeutic CSF concentrations of EFV have been reported, similar to other NNRTIs.

EFV is metabolized by the hepatic CYP3A4, and is an inhibitor and inducer of the P-450 system, although induction properties appear to dominate (Table 84.10). The administration of EFV with cisapride and rifampin is contraindicated. Combining EFV with a single PI regimen can produce clinically significant declines in PI concentrations, limiting use of this combination (Table 84.10). However, RTV boosting appears to overcome this interaction. For example, it is not necessary to increase the dosage of SAQ when EFV is added in persons receiving a boosted combination of SAQ (400 mg) plus RTV (400 mg) two times a day. However, some clinicians have empirically increased the dosage of SAQ to 800 mg twice a day. Data from the manufacturer of RTV reported no increase in adverse effects in HIV-negative volunteers who took RTV 400 mg two times a day and SAQ 800 mg two times a day. The metabolism of IDV as a single PI is increased about 35% by EFV, necessitating an unboosted IDV dosage increase to 1 g every 8 hours.[204] No dosage adjustment of NFV or RTV is required with EFV. It can be given at bedtime or divided into three daily doses if necessary to minimize the CNS adverse effects. Narcotic withdrawal due to lower levels should be anticipated when EFV is used with methadone.

CNS side effects from EFV can be disabling in up to 50% of patients. Typical symptoms include fatigue, dizziness, headache, insomnia, "feelings of disconnection," and impaired concentration; however, confusion, stupor, agitation, hallucinations, abnormal dreaming, euphoria, paresthesias, nervousness, and somnolence are also reported. Patients should be educated that these CNS side effects are transient and in most, resolve within 1 month with drug continuation. Instructions to take the EFV at bedtime can alleviate some of these CNS symptoms. Patients with a history of baseline altered mental status, psychiatric disturbances, or confusion may not be appropriate candidates for EFV therapy. Other side effects include nausea, headache, and a rash that usually do not require drug discontinuation; serious rash is less common than other marketed NNRTIs. In a phase II trial, adverse effects were reported in 58% (n = 54) of patients and included grade II rash (10.7%), diarrhea (6%), abdominal pain (9%), nausea (6%), headache (5%), hematuria (8%), and elevations in transaminases (5%). EFV should be avoided in pregnant women because congenital malformations (e.g. meningeomyocele) have been reported.[13] Barrier contraceptives are recommended during EFV use in women of childbearing age.

FUSION INHIBITORS

Enfuvirtide (pentafuside, T-20, Fuzeon). Enfuvirtide is the first fusion inhibitor to be approved by the FDA in March 2003. Fusion inhibitors have a unique mechanism of action, blocking glycoprotein–41-mediated binding of HIV to the host cell and preventing HIV cell entry. It also must be administered by subcutaneous injection. FDA approval was based on two studies [T-20 versus Optimized Regimen Only (TORO)] showing virologic efficacy in patients requiring salvage therapy.

TORO-1 and TORO-2 were randomized, multicenter, open label, phase III clinical trials evaluating the efficacy of T-20 against HIV-1.[205,206] To qualify, participants had a history of prior treatment with three available classes of ARVs for at least 6 months, documented ARV resistance, and an HIV-1 viral load greater than 5,000 copies per milliliter. The average baseline viral load was greater than 100,000 copies per milliliter prior to initiation of the study. The optimized regimen was selected by genotype, phenotype, or both, and consisted of three to five ARV agents. Patients in the T-20 arms of the TORO studies achieved a 1.42 to 1.69 log^{10} decrease in viral load compared to a 0.64 to 0.74 log^{10} decrease for patients on optimized regimen alone. CD4 cell count increased by 76 versus 32 cells/mm^3 in TORO-1 and 65.5 versus 38 cells/mm^3 in the TORO-2 arm for enfuvirtide and optimized regimens, respectively. Although this medication has been studied primarily in the salvage setting, some clinicians suggest it may work better when initiated at higher CD4 T-cell counts.

Subcutaneous enfuvirtide is well absorbed with an approximate bioavailability of 84.3%.[207] It is highly protein bound (92%) and has an elimination half-life of 3.8 hours, supporting twice daily dosing. Dosing adjustment is not required in renal dysfunction.[207,208] Enfuvirtide does not appear to have any significant drug interactions. It has little to no effect on drugs metabolized by the CYP P-450 3A4, 2D6, 1A2, 2E1, or 2C19 pathways.[207,209] HIV-1 strains with resistance to enfuvirtide have been selected both in vivo and in vitro. Mutations between the 36 and 45 amino acid positions in the HIV envelope glycoprotein 41 have been shown to mediate phenotypic resistance.

The most common side effect of enfuvirtide is injection site reactions. Injection-related pain, discomfort, and tenderness can be treated symptomatically with over-the-counter pain relievers. Repeated subcutaneous injections may cause formation of hard, granulated lumps of tissue around the injection sites. Massaging the injection area may decrease the formation of these lumps. Nausea, diarrhea, anorexia, fever, swelling, malaise, and flulike syndromes are other common side effects. A significant higher frequency (8X) of bacterial pneumonia has been observed. Eosinophilia without symptoms of a hypersensitivity reaction was a consistent finding in 11.2% of TORO patients. Rarely, delayed hypersensitivity reactions (e.g., rash, nausea, vomiting, fever) can occur. Desensitization may be successful for hypersensitivity reactions in those requiring enfuvirtide therapy.[210]

Enfuvirtide is dosed 90 mg subcutaneously twice daily. It is stable for 12 hours after reconstitution with sterile water for injection. Patients may mix two single-dose vials at a time and store the second one in the refrigerator for use 12 hours later. After reconstitution, patients should be instructed to inspect the vials carefully to ensure the solution is clear and particulate-free before injecting. It may take up to 45 minutes for the powder to dissolve entirely. Injection sites should be rotated but avoid the area near the umbilicus. Absorption does not differ between the injection sites of the thigh, arm, or abdomen.[207] Enfuvirtide, as Fuzeon, comes with a patient education pack that includes an instructional video on injection technique, practice injection pad, sharps container, and carrying case.

FUTURE THERAPIES

Several new agents within the existing ARV classes are under investigation (Table 84.12). Most of the investigational NRTIs, NNRTIs, and PIs under investigation have potent antiviral activity that target mutations that confer drug resistance to currently available agents. In addition, under development are improved fixed dosage combinations that

TABLE 84.12	Human Immunodeficiency Virus Antiretroviral Agents Currently in Development		
Class/Mechanism	**Name**	**Characteristics**	**Developing Company**
Nucleoside Reverse Transcriptase Inhibitors	d-d4FC (reverset)	Cytidine analogue active against viral isolates with lamivudine resistance. Possible once daily dosing.	Pharmasset/Dupont Pharmaceuticals
	SPD-754	Retains activity against some NRTI-resistant viruses. Possible once daily dosing.	Shire Pharmaceuticals
Non-Nucleoside Reverse Transcriptase Inhibitors	TMC-125 (etravirine)	Second-generation NNRTI active against resistant virus.	Tibotec/Virco
Protease Inhibitors	Tipranavir	Novel nonpeptidic protease inhibitor active against multi PI-resistant viruses. P-450 enzyme inducer	Boehringer Ingelheim
	TMC-114	Binds tightly to protease target site. Active against multi-PI resistant viruses.	Tibotec/Virco
CCR5 inhibitors	GW873140	Orally bioavailable with a unique CCR5 binding site.	GlaxoSmithKline
	SCH-D	Orally bioavailable CCR5 inhibitor well-tolerated in phase I clinical trials.	Schering-Plough
	UK 427,857	Orally bioavailable CCR5 inhibitor with a long CCR5 90% saturation time.	Pfizer Pharmaceuticals
GP 120 envelope attachment inhibitor	BMS-488043	Potent, orally bioavailable attachment inhibitor which reduced HIV1-RNA 1–2 logs during phase II monotherapy studies.	Bristol Myers Squibb
Viral maturation inhibitor	PA-457	Blocks maturation of the viral capsid precursor, resulting in noninfectious particles.	Panacos Pharmaceuticals
Anti-CD4 monoclonal antibody	TNX-355	Reduced plasma HIV1-RNA 0.56–1.1 logs when given as monotherapy; safe and well tolerated in a phase Ib clinical trial.	Tanox Pharmaceuticals

NRTI, nucleotide reverse transcriptase inhibitors; NNRTI, nonnucleoside reverse transcriptase inhibitor.

will assist in easing the pill burden (e.g., TDF/FTC/EFV, d4T/3TC/NVP).

Phase III data on clinical outcomes from interleukin-2 (IL-2) are pending. IL-2 is reported to increase the CD4 cell count when used with HAART for chronic HIV infection. However, the durability of IL-2's effect on CD4 count and its immunologic benefits have been questioned. The use of IL-2 is also limited by its adverse effects of flulike symptoms, including myalgias, fever, malaise, and fatigue. Elevations in viral load occur after IL-2 therapy so that adequate ARV therapy must occur before receiving IL-2 therapy.

Novel strategies focus on an essential step in the life cycle of HIV, that is, preventing HIV entry and infection of CD4 lymphocytes and other target cells. Oral CCR5 inhibitors (e.g., UK 427,857, SCH-D, GW873140) that inhibit cell entry by blocking interaction of the gp 120 with the CCR5 coreceptor appear promising. A gp 120 envelope attachment inhibitor, a viral maturation inhibitor, and anti-CD4 monoclonal antibody are early in the development phase. Preliminary results from French investigators report on the efficacy of a therapeutic vaccine against AIDS. In a small group of HIV-infected persons not on HAART, the vaccine suppressed 90% of the viral load at the end of one year. However, the vaccine, containing dendritic cells from the HIV-infected person, is difficult to produce and costly.[211]

Development of an effective AIDS vaccine has been disappointing. The ability of the virus to rapidly mutate and evolve is a major obstacle and challenge to the development of a vaccine. Two large phase III trials in the United States and Thailand evaluating a gp 120-envelope HIV vaccine have been halted due to dismal results.

However, several new prevention strategies in high-risk HIV-negative persons seem promising. Studies are underway to test the efficacy of once daily TDF as a prevention strategy (Project T). Several sites in the United States, South America, Caribbean, and Australia will begin recruitment for a Merck vaccine that is expected to stimulate the production of HIV killing T-cells. Results will not be available until 2010.

IMPROVING OUTCOMES

PATIENT EDUCATION

ARV agents are extremely complex regimens that need to be properly administered and taken by the patient to maximize therapeutic efficacy. Therefore, patient education and an assessment of the patient's ability to comply with therapy are essential before therapy is started. Key points for discussion include goals of ARV therapy, including the patient's objective for taking ARV; proper administration of the regimen, including the brand and generic names of the drugs, the number of pills taken per dose, the frequency of doses, total number of pills taken daily, coordination with meals; storage conditions, drug interactions, including herbal and recreational drugs; anticipated side effects and recommendations

for management; and availability of the pharmacist for consultation. The relationship between adherence, viral load response, viral resistance, drug failure, and impact on future regimens need to be emphasized. The pharmacist should ensure that the patient has a clear understanding of the information discussed. Counseling by pharmacists to increase medication adherence and knowledge about HIV disease has been effective in reducing viral load. However, detection of nonadherence is difficult. One study found that clinicians overestimated adherence on average by 9%.[212]

METHODS TO IMPROVE PATIENT ADHERENCE TO DRUG THERAPY

Reported rates of adherence to HIV therapy, defined as missed doses, incorrect dosages, or incorrect time of administration, range from 46% to 88%.[213] Using a Medication Event Monitoring System (MEMS), an ACTG study indicated that 82% of doses were taken but only 55% to 76% were taken at the right time, and 27% took the right dosage.[119] In ten ACTG clinics reporting nonadherence rates of 11% to 36%, the most common explanations given for missed dosages were forgetfulness and disruption of daily routine (e.g., being away from home, long clinic visits, and number of blood tests). Only 10% missed doses because of adverse events. Additional barriers to compliance include the patient's actual or perceived state of health (e.g., threat posed by the disease, perceived self-benefit), the complexity of the therapeutic regimen, the patient-provider relationship (e.g., mutual respect), and psychological barriers (e.g., mental disturbance; substance abuse, including alcohol; unstable living situations; lack of support system).[39,40,119,120]

Several strategies and devices can enhance medication adherence.[23,120] Because forgetfulness is common, written instructions, individualized medication organizers, and reminder devices (e.g., programmable watch, beepers, electronic pillboxes) should supplement verbal medication instructions. Pharmacists have achieved undetectable viral load by educating patients about HIV disease, simplifying the medication regimen, and using medication reminders. Once daily regimens, if appropriate, should be considered for ease of administration. Simple instruction sheets identifying the time of pill administration can be helpful. Directly observed therapy has been recommended to improve medication adherence in persons infected with HIV.

PHARMACOECONOMICS

The direct cost of care in the United States of HIV-infected patients declined from about $1,800 to less than $1,400 per patient per month (PMPM) during the first 3 years of HAART.[214] Despite the introduction of the costly ARV agents, HAART actually lowered the total cost of care by reducing hospitalization costs related to HIV and its complications. An observational cohort study conducted in HIV-positive patients in Maryland showed significantly reduced Medicaid payments for those on PI-containing regimens.[215] In 1997 mean monthly inpatient Medicaid costs for patients with CD4 counts less than 50 cells/mm^3 were $1,531 for those not receiving PIs versus $390 for those on PIs. A study conducted at the Dallas Veteran's Affairs Medical Center from January 1995 to June 1998 also found cost savings in inpatient HIV care, a reduction from $1,257.51 PMPM during the first study quarter to $1,194.44 PMPM during the second quarter.[216]

Consistent with the trend toward managing HIV as a chronic disease, outpatient visits and ARV costs have increased. In the Maryland cohort the mean monthly ARV expenditures increased across all CD4 strata, ranging from $158 in 1995 to $361 in 1997.[215] In the Dallas VA cohort, outpatient costs decreased from $1,905 to $1,090, then rose

up to $1,349 over the years 1995 to 1998. This included an increase in ARV costs from $79 to $518 PMPM.[216] A multicenter study conducted in nine HIV specialty clinics in 1999 found an association between HAART, lower inpatient costs, and higher outpatient costs ($389 and $181, respectively).[217] A random sample conducted between January 1996 and July 1998 of HIV-infected patients also found that ARV expenditures increased by 33% over the 18-month study period despite significantly decreased overall cost of HIV-related care[214] A study conducted in privately insured individuals in the year 2000 found that average drug costs ranged from $3,476 to $9,702 per year.[218]

In the United States, the major payers of ARV therapy are government funded Medicaid programs and state run AIDS Drug Assistance Programs (ADAPs). The rising cost of therapy in combination with increasing numbers of pa-

TABLE 84.13	HIV/AIDS Information Websites	
Name/Organization	URL	Description
AIDSInfo National Institutes of Health	http://www.aidsinfo.nih.gov	Houses U.S. Public Health Service HIV treatment guidelines and opportunistic infection prophylaxis guidelines. Has an antiretroviral drug database with monographs
National Clinicians' Consultation Center *University of California, San Francisco*	http://www.ucsf.edu/hivcntr	Another source for U.S. Public Health Service HIV or OI prophylaxis guidelines. "Pharmacist central" section has a downloadable antiretroviral drug chart and a chart of web references for looking up antiretroviral drug interactions
HIV Insite University of California, San Francisco	http://www.hivinsite.com	General HIV information website. Has articles on ARV therapy and an ARV drug interaction database. Also has several useful antiretroviral-related charts including renal dosing guidelines, ARV adverse effects, and OI prophylaxis and treatment adverse effects
HIV Guide Johns Hopkins University	http://www.hopkins-hivguide.org/	General HIV information website. Has antiretroviral drug monographs with an interaction tool. Also has bulleted articles on medication-related topics such as adherence, initial regimen selection
HIV Pharmacology Virology Education	http://www.hivpharmacology.com	Has antiretroviral pharmacokinetics profiles, an antiretroviral drug interaction database, and therapeutic drug monitoring guidelines
HIV Drug Interactions University of Liverpool	http://www.hiv-druginteractions.org	Has color-coded drug interaction charts
Drug Resistance Mutations International AIDS Society	http://www.iasusa.org/	Publishes a figure which delineates resistance mutations for each antiretroviral drug. Updated when new ARV agents are approved
HIV Drug Resistance Database Stanford University	http://hivdb.stanford.edu/	Website with an interactive ARV drug resistance mutation tool. Also has color coded tables (by ARV class) that show susceptibility by single mutation
HIV Tools *Pacific AIDS Education & Training Centers*	http://www.hivtools.com	Has a drug interaction tool and a therapeutic drug monitoring tool which predicts therapeutic concentrations based on an IC50

HIV, human immunodeficiency virus; AIDS, acquired immune deficiency syndrome; OI, opportunistic infections; ARV, antiretroviral.

tients and only modest corresponding increases in state budgets has placed a strain on many of these programs. Individuals who are uninsured or who do not have adequate insurance are in danger of not being able to access life-saving therapies. As of December 2004, 58 U.S. states and territories with ADAPs had 813 patients on waiting lists, despite meeting eligibility criteria.[219] In the era of ARV therapy one of the biggest global challenges will be to devise solutions that ensure all HIV-infected patients have access to these life-saving, but costly therapies.

KEY POINTS

- Management of HIV infection with HAART have dramatically reduced the progression of HIV to AIDS, reduced hospitalizations for opportunistic infections, improved overall health and well being, and prolonged survival
- Effective therapy with HAART allows discontinuation of antibiotics for primary and secondary prophylaxis of opportunistic infections
- Therapy with two nucleoside analogs and two PIs or an NNRTI is considered the standard of care for initial ARV therapy
- Once daily therapy and use of more tolerable regimens can improve HAART adherence
- Therapy is most effective in ARV-naive patients compared with experienced persons
- The goals of therapy are to improve survival by reducing the viral load to undetectable levels for as long as possible to maintain durable viral suppression, prevent the emergence of resistance, and prevent drug failure
- Patient adherence to HAART is essential to avoid the emergence of drug resistance and drug failure
- Eradication of HIV is not likely due to the presence of latent reservoirs that are inaccessible to current ARV therapy
- ARV therapy is protective against mother-to-child HIV transmission, against occupational exposures in health care workers, and against nonoccupational exposures
- Lipodystrophy, diabetes, hyperlipidemia, lactic acidosis are some disturbing side effects of HAART
- Significant drug to drug interactions with PIs and NNRTIs could be fatal and should be anticipated
- Pharmacists can take an active role in the care of HIV-infected persons through patient education, improving adherence, anticipating side effects and providing management recommendations, avoiding drug-drug interactions, and preventing ARV errors
- Because HIV is a rapidly changing area, pharmacists need to be able to access current information (Table 84.13)

SUGGESTED READINGS

Centers for Disease Control and Prevention. Public Health Service Task Force recommendations for the use of ARV drugs in pregnant women infected with HIV-1 for maternal health and for reducing perinatal HIV-1 transmission in the United States. Available at: http://aidsinfo.nih.gov. Accessed December 17, 2004.

Department of Health and Human Services and Henry J. Kaiser Family Foundation. Guidelines for the use of ARV agents in HIV-infected adults and adolescents. Available at: http://AIDSinfo.nih.gov. Accessed October 29, 2004.

Yeni PG, Hammer SM, Hirsch MS, et al. Treatment for adult HIV infection. 2004. Recommendations of the International AIDS Society-USA Panel. JAMA 292:251–265, 2004.

REFERENCES

1. Palella FJ, Delaney KM, Moorman AC, et al. Declining morbidity and mortality among patients with advanced human immunodeficiency virus infection. N Engl J Med 338:853–860, 1998.
2. Hogg RS, Heath KV, Yip B, et al. Improved survival among HIV-infected individuals following initiation of antiretroviral therapy. JAMA 279:450–454, 1998.
3. Finzi D, Hermankova M, Pierson T, et al. Identification of a reservoir for HIV-1 in patients on highly active antiretroviral therapy. Science 278:1295–1300, 1997.
4. Chun TW, Stuyver L, Mizell SB, et al. Presence of an inducible HIV-1 latent reservoir during highly active antiretroviral therapy. Proc Natl Acad Sci USA 94:13193–13197, 1997.
5. Chun TW, Engel D, Berrey MM, et al. Early establishment of a pool of latently infected, resting CD4 (%) T cells during primary HIV-1 infection. Proc Natl Acad Sci USA 95:8869–8873, 1998.
6. Garber DA, Silvestri G, Feinberg MB. Prospects for an AIDS vaccine: three big questions, no easy answers. Lancet Infect Dis 4: 397–413, 2004.
7. Centers for Disease Control and Prevention. 1993 revised classification system for HIV infection and expanded surveillance case definition for AIDS among adolescents and adults. MMWR 41(RR-17):1–19, 1992.
8. Moore JP. Co-receptors: implications for HIV pathogenesis and therapy. Science 276:51–52, 1997.
9. Rothenberg RB, Scarlett M, delRio C, et al. Oral transmission of HIV. AIDS 12:2095–2105, 1998.
10. Katz M, Gerberding JL. The care of persons with recent sexual exposure to HIV. Ann Intern Med 128:306–312, 1998.
11. Richters J, Grulich A, Ellard J, et al. HIV transmission among gay men through oral sex and other uncommon routes: case series of HIV seroconverters, Sydney. AIDS. 17:2269–71, 2003.
12. Connor EM, Sperling RS, Gelber R, et al. Reduction of maternal-infant transmission of human immunodeficiency virus type 1 with zidovudine treatment. N Engl J Med 331:1173–1180, 1994.
13. Centers for Disease Control and Prevention. Public Health Service Task Force recommendations for the use of antiretroviral drugs in pregnant women infected with HIV-1 for maternal health and for reducing perinatal HIV-1 transmission in the United States. February 24, 2005 Available at: http://aidsinfo.nih.gov. Accessed November 7, 2005.
14. CDC National Viral Statistics Reports. 11 February 52:1–48, 2004.
15. Ho DD, Neumann AU, Perelson AS, et al. Rapid turnover of plasma virions and CD4 lymphocytes in HIV-1 infection. Nature 373:123–126, 1995.
16. Ho DD. Toward HIV eradication or remission: the tasks ahead. Science 280:1866–1867, 1998.
17. Robbins PA, Roderiquez GL, Peden KW, et al. Human immunodeficiency virus type 1 infection of antigen-specific CD4 cytotoxic T lymphocytes. AIDS Res Hum Retroviruses 14:1397–1406, 1998.
18. Greenough TC, Brettler DB, Somasundaran M, et al. Human immunodeficiency virus type 1-specific cytotoxic T lymphocytes (CTL), virus load, and CD4 T cell loss: evidence supporting a protective role for CTL in vivo. J Infect Dis 176:118–125, 1997.
19. Mellors JW, Munoz AM, Giorgi VJ, et al. Plasma viral load and CD4% lymphocytes as prognostic markers of HIV-1 infection. Ann Intern Med 126:946–954, 1997.

20. Liegler TJ, Yonemoto W, Elbeik T, et al. Diminished spontaneous apoptosis in lymphocytes from human immunodeficiency virus-infected long-term nonprogressors. J Infect Dis 178:669–679, 1998.

21. Kahn JO, Walker BD. Acute human immunodeficiency virus type 1 infection. N Engl J Med 339:33–39, 1998.

22. National Center for HIV, STD, and TB Prevention. Rapid HIV testing. Available at: http://www.cdc.gov/hiv/rapid_testing. Accessed November 7, 2005.

23. Department of Health and Human Services and Henry J. Kaiser Family Foundation. Guidelines for the use of antiretroviral agents in HIV-infected adults and adolescents. October 29, 2004. Available at: http://AIDSinfo.nih.gov. Accessed November 7, 2005.

24. Yeni PG, Hammer SM, Hirsch MS, et al. Treatment for adult HIV infection. 2004. recommendations of the International AIDS Society-USA Panel. JAMA 292:251–265, 2004.

25. British HIV Association (BHIVA) BHIVA guidelines for the treatment of HIV infected adults with antiretroviral therapy. HIV Med 4 (Suppl 1):1–41, 2003. Available at: http://www.bhiva.org/guidelines/2003/hiv. Accessed November 7, 2005.

26. Kitahata MM, VanRompaey SE, Shields AW. Physician experience in the care of HIV-infected persons is associated with earlier adoption of new antiretroviral therapy. J Acquis Immune Defic Syndr 24:106–114, 2000.

27. Holmberg SD, Palella FJ, Lichtenstein KA, et al. The case for earlier treatment of HIV infection. Clin Infect Dis 39:1699–1704, 2004.

28. Farzadegan H, Hoover DR, Astemborski J, et al. Sex differences in HIV-1 viral load and progression to AIDS. Lancet 352:1510–1514, 1998.

29. Maggiolo F, Migliorino M, Pirali A, et al. Duration of viral suppression in patients on stable therapy for HIV-1 infection is predicted by plasma HIV level after 1 month of treatment. J Acquir Immune Defic Syndr 25:36–43, 2000.

30. Polis MA, Sidorov IA, Yoder C, et al. Correlation between reduction in plasma HIV-1 RNA concentration 1 week after start of antiretroviral treatment and longer-term efficacy. Lancet 358:1760–1765, 2001.

31. Walmsley S, Bernstein B, King M, et al. Lopinavir-ritonavir versus nelfinavir for the initial treatment of HIV infection. N Engl J Med 346:2039–2046, 2002.

32. Robbins GK, DeGruttola V, Shafer RW, et al. Comparison of sequential three-drug regimens as initial therapy for HIV-1 infection. N Engl J Med 349:2293–2303, 2003.

33. Staszewski S, Morales-Ramirez J, Tashima KT, et al. Efavirenz plus zidovudine and 3TC, efavirenz plus indinavir and indinavir plus zidovudine and 3TC in the treatment of HIV-1 infection in adults. Study 006 team. N Engl J Med 341:1863–1873, 1999.

34. Gulick RM, Meibohm A, Havlir D, et al. Six year follow-up of HIV-infected adults in a clinical trial of antiretroviral therapy with indinavir, zidovudine, and lamivudine. AIDS 17:2345–2349, 2003.

35. Hicks C, King MS, Gulick RM, et al. Long term safety and durable antiretroviral activity of lopinavir/ritonavir in treatment naïve patients: 4 year follow-up study. AIDS 18:775–779, 2004.

36. Gulick RM, Ribaudo HJ, Shikuma CM, et al. Triple-nucleoside regimens versus efavirenz-containing regimens for the initial treatment of HIV-1 infection. N Engl J Med 350:1850–1861, 2004.

37. Gerstoft J, Kirk O, Obel N, et al. Low efficacy and high frequency of adverse events in a randomized trial of the triple nucleoside regimen abacavir, stavudine and didanosine. AIDS 17:2045–2052, 2003.

38. Gallant JE, Rodriguez A, Weinberg W, et al. Early non-response to tenofovir DF (TDF) + abacavir (ABC) and lamivudine (3TC) in a randomized trial compared to efavirenz (EFV) + ABC and 3TC: ESS30009 unplanned interim analysis (oral presentation # H-1722a). Presented at: The 43rd Interscience Conference on Antimicrobial Agents and Chemotherapy; September 14–17, 2003; Chicago, IL.

39. Bangsberg D, Tulsky JP, Hecht RM, et al. Protease inhibitors in the homeless. JAMA 278:63–65, 1997.

40. Strathdee SA, Palepu A, Cornelisse PG, et al. Barriers to use of free antiretroviral therapy in injection drug users. JAMA 280:547–549, 1998.

41. Havlir DV, Marschner IC, Hirsch MS, et al. Maintenance antiretroviral therapies in HIV infected subjects with undetectable plasma HIV RNA after triple drug therapy. N Engl J Med 339:1261–1268, 1998.

42. Pialoux G, Raffi F, Brun-Vezinet B, et al. A randomized trial of three maintenance regimens given after three months of induction therapy with zidovudine, lamivudine, and indinavir in previously untreated HIV-1 infected patients. N Engl J Med 339:1269–1276, 1998.

43. Reijers MH, Weverling GJ, Jurriaans S, et al. Maintenance therapy after quadruple induction therapy in HIV-1 infected individuals: Amsterdam Duration of Antiretroviral Medication (ADAM) study. Lancet 352:185–190, 1998.

44. d'Arminio Monforte A, Lepri AC, Rezza G, et al. Insights into the reasons for discontinuation of the first highly active antiretroviral therapy (HAART) regimen in a cohort of antiretroviral naïve patients. I.C.O.N.A. Study Group, Italian Cohort of Antiretrovrial Naïve Patients. AIDS 14:499–507, 2000.

45. Mocroft A, Youle M, Moore A, et al. Reasons for modification and discontinuation of antiretrovirals: results from a single treatment center. AIDS 15:185–194, 2001.

46. Hirsch HH, Kaufmann G, Sendi P, et al. Immune reconstitution in HIV-infected patients. Clin Infect Dis 38:1159–1166, 2004.

47. Deeks S. Treatment of antiretroviral-drug-resistant HIV-1 infection. Lancet 362:2002–2011, 2003.

48. Muro E, Droste J, Hofstede H, et al. Nevirapine plasma concentrations are still detectable after more than 2 weeks in the majority of women receiving single-dose nevirapine: implications for intervention studies. Presented at: The 11th Conference on Retroviruses and Opportunistic Infections; February 8–11, 2004; San Francisco, CA. Abstract 891.

49. Taylor S, Allen S, Fidler S, et al. Stop study: after discontinuation of efavirenz, plasma concentrations may persist for 2 weeks or longer. Presented at: The 11th Conference on Retroviruses and Opportunistic Infections; February 8–11, 2004; San Francisco, CA. Abstract 131.

50. Cingolani A, Antinori A, Rizzo MG, et al. Usefulness of monitoring HIV drug resistance and adherence in individuals failing highly active antiretroviral therapy: a randomized study (ARGENTA). AIDS 16:369–379, 2002.

51. Tural C, Ruiz L, Holtzer C, et al. Clinical utility of HIV-1 genotyping and expert advice: the Havana trial. AIDS 16:209–218, 2002.

52. Culnane M, Fowler M, Lee SS, et al. Lack of long-term effects of in utero exposure to zidovudine among uninfected children born to HIV-infected women. JAMA 281:151–157, 1999.

53. Barret B, Tardieu M, Rustin P, et al. Persistent mitochrondrial dysfunction in HIV-1 exposed but uninfected infants: clinical screening in a large prospective cohort. AIDS 17:1769–1785, 2003.

54. Centers for Disease Control and Prevention. Updated US Public Health Service guidelines for the management of occupational exposures to HBV, HCV, and HIV and recommendations for postexposure prophylaxis. MMWR 50:1–43, 2001.

55. Recommendations from the US Department of Health and Human Services. Antiretroviral postexposure prophylaxis after sexual, injection drug-use, or other nonoccupational exposure to HIV in the United States, Centers for Disease Control and Prevention. MMWR 54:1–20, 2005.

56. Smith DE, Walker BD, Cooper DA, et al. Is antiretroviral treatment of primary HIV infection clinically justified on the basis of current evidence? AIDS 18:709–718, 2004.

57. Kearney BP, Isaacson E, Sayre J, et al. Didanosine and tenofovir DF drug-drug interaction: assessment of didanosine dose reduction. Program and abstracts of the 10th Conference on Retroviruses and Opportunistic Infections; February 10–14, 2003; Boston, MA. Abstract 533.

58. Fleischer R, Boxwell D, Sherman KE. Nucleoside analogues and mitochrondrial toxicity. Clin Infect Dis 38:e79–e80, 2004.

59. Taburet AM, Piketty C, Chazallon C, et al. Interactions between atazanavir-ritonavir and tenofovir in heavily pretreated human immunodeficiency virus-infected patients. Antimicrob Agents Chemother 48: 2091–2096, 2004.

60. Birkus G, Hitchcock MJ, Cihlar T. Assessment of mitochondrial toxicity in human cells treated with tenofovir: comparison with other nucleosides reverse transcriptase inhibitors. Antimicrob Agents Chemother 46:716–723, 2002.

61. Anderson PL, Kakuda TN, Lichtenstein KA. The cellular pharmacology of nucleoside-and nucleotide-analogue reverse-transcriptase inhibitors and its relationship to clinical toxicities. Clin Infect Dis 38:743–753, 2004.

62. Concorde Coordinating Committee. Concorde: MRC/ANRS randomized double-blind controlled trial of immediate vs. deferred zidovudine in symptom-free HIV infection. Lancet 343:871–888, 1994.

63. Hammer SM, Katzenstein DA, Hughes MD, et al. A trial comparing nucleoside monotherapy with combination therapy in HIV-infected adults with CD4 cell counts from 200 to 500 per cubic millimeter. N Engl J Med 335:1081–1090, 1996.

64. Delta Coordinating Committee. Delta: a randomized double-blind controlled trial comparing combinations of zidovudine plus didanosine or zalcitabine with zidovudine alone in HIV-infected individuals. Lancet 348:283–291, 1996.

65. Saravolatz LD, Winslow DL, Collins G, et al. Zidovudine alone or in combination with didanosine or zalcitabine in HIV-infected patients with the acquired immunodeficiency syndrome or fewer than 200 CD4 cells per cubic millimeter. Investigators for the Terry Beirn Community Program for Clinical Research on AIDS. N Engl J Med 335:1099–1106, 1996.

66. Hoggard PG, Kewn S, Barry MG, et al. Effects of drugs on 2′3′dideoxy-2′-didehydrothymidine phosphorylation in vitro. Antimicrob Agents Chemother 41:1231–1236, 1997.

67. Havlir DV, Tierney C, Friedland GH, et al. In vivo antagonism with zidovudine plus stavudine combination therapy. J Infect Dis 182:321–325, 2000.

68. Anderson PL, Kakuda TN, Kawle S, et al. Antiviral dynamics and sex differences of zidovudine and lamivudine triphosphate concentrations in HIV-infected individuals. AIDS 17:2159–2168, 2003.

69. Stretcher BN, Pesce AJ, Frame PT, et al. Correlates of zidovudine phosphorylation with markers of HIV disease progression and drug toxicity. AIDS 8:763–769, 1994.

70. Dalakas MC, Illa I, Pezeshkpour GH, et al. Mitochondrial myopathy caused by long term zidovudine therapy. N Engl J Med 322:1098–1105, 1990.

71. Kahn JO, Laggakos SW, Richman DD, et al. A controlled trial comparing continued zidovudine with didanosine in human immunodeficiency virus infection. The NIAID AIDS Clinical Trials Group. N Engl J Med 327:581–587, 1992.

72. Abrahms DI, Goldman AI, Launer C, et al. A comparative trial of didanosine or zalcitabine after treatment with zidovudine in patients with the human immunodeficiency virus infection. N Engl J Med 330:657–662, 1994.

73. Chuck SK, Areff D. Improved tolerability and adherence with enteric coated didanosine capsules (Videx-EC) versus buffered tablets (Videx). Program and abstracts of the XIV International AIDS Conference; July 7–12, 2002; Barcelona Spain. Abstract WePeB5855.

74. Martinez EM, de Lazzari E, Ravasi JL, et al. Pancreatic toxic effects associated with co-administration of didanosine and tenofovir in HIV-infected adults. Lancet 364:65–67, 2004.

75. Barrios A, Rendon A, Negredo E, et al. Paradoxical CD4 + T-cell decline in HIV-infected patients with complete virus suppression taking tenofovir and didanosine. AIDS 19:569–575, 2005.

76. Eron JJ, Murphy RL, Peterson D, et al. A comparison of stavudine, didanosine and indinavir with zidovudine, lamivudine and indinavir for the initial treatment of HIV-infected individuals: Selection of thymidine analog regimen therapy (START II). AIDS 14:1601–1610, 2000.

77. Squires KE, Gulick R, Tobas P, et al. A comparison of stavudine plus lamivudine versus zidovudine plus lamivudine in combination with indinavir in antiretroviral naïve individuals with HIV infection: selection of thymidine analog regimen therapy (START I). AIDS 14:1591–1600, 2000.

78. Joly V, Flandre P, Meiffredy V, et al. Efficacy of zidovudine compared to stavudine, both in combination with lamivudine and indinaivr, in human immunodeficiency virus-infected nucleoside-experienced patients with no prior exposure to lamivudine, stavudine, or protease inhibitors (Novavir Trial). Antimicrob Agents Chemother 46:1906–1913, 2002.

79. Foudraine NA, Hoeteimans RM, Lange JM, et al. Cerebrospinal-fluid HIV-1 RNA and drug concentrations after treatment with lamivudine plus zidovudine or stavudine. Lancet 351:1547–1551, 1998.

80. Gallant JE, Staszewski S, Pozniak A, et al. Efficacy and safety of tenofovir DF versus stavudine in combination therapy in antiretroviral-naive patients: a 3 year randomized trial. JAMA 292:191–201, 2004.

81. Bernasconi E, Boubaker K, Junghans C, et al. Abnormalities of body fat distribution in HIV-infected persons treated with antiretroviral drugs. J Acquir Immune Defic Syndr 31:50–55, 2002.

82. Joly V, Flandre P, Meiffredy V, et al. Increased risk of lipoatrophy under stavudine in HIV-1-infected patients: results of a substudy from a comparative trial. AIDS 16:2447–2454, 2002.

83. John M, McKinnon EJ, James IR, et al. Randomized controlled, 48-week study of switching stavudine and/or protease inhibitors to Combivir/abacavir to prevent or reverse lipoatrophy in HIV-infected patients. J Acquir Immune Defic Syndr 33:29–33, 2003.

84. McComsey GA, Ward DJ, Hessenthaler SM, et al. Improvement in lipoatrophy associated with highly active antiretroviral therapy in human immunodeficiency virus-infected patients switched from stavudine to abacavir or zidovudine: The results of the TARHEEL study. Clin Infect Dis 38:263–270, 2004.

85. Martin A, Smith DE, Carr A, et al. Reversibility of lipoatrophy in HIV-infected patients 2 years after switching from a thymidine analogue to abacavir: the MITOX Extension Study. AIDS 18:1029–1036, 2004.

86. Moyle GJ, Baldwin C, Langroudi B, et al. A 48-week, randomized, open label comparison of three abacavir-based substitution approaches in the management of dyslipidemia and peripheral lipoatrophy. J AIDS 33:22–28, 2003.

87. Carr A, Workman C, Smith DE, et al. Abacavir substitution for nucleoside analogs in patients with HIV lipatrophy. JAMA 288:207–215, 2002.

88. CAESAR Coordinating Committee. Randomized trial of addition of lamivudine or lamivudine plus loviride to zidovudine-containing regimens for patients with HIV-1 infection: the CAESAR trial. Lancet 349:1413–1421, 1997.

89. Dando TM, Scott LJ. Abacavir plus lamivudine: a review of their combined use in the management of HIV infection. Drugs 65:285–302, 2005.

90. Eron JJ, Benoit SL, Jemsek J, et al. Treatment with lamivudine, zidovudine, or both in HIV-positive patients with 200 to 500 CD4% cells per cubic millimeter. North American HIV Working Party. N Engl J Med 333:1662–1669, 1995.

91. Katlama C, Ingrand D, Loveday C, et al. Safety and efficacy of lamivudine-zidovudine combination therapy in antiretroviral-naive patients. A randomized controlled comparison with zidovudine. JAMA 276:118–125, 1996.

92. Staszewski S, Loveday C, Picazo JJ, et al. Safety and efficacy of lamivudine-zidovudine combination therapy in zidovudine-experienced patients: a randomized controlled comparison with zidovudine monotherapy. Lamivudine European HIV Working Group. JAMA 276:111–117, 1996.

93. Bartlett JA, Benoit SL, Johnson VA, et al. Lamivudine plus zidovudine compared with zalcitabine plus zidovudine in patients with HIV infection: a randomized, double-blind, placebo-controlled trial. North American HIV Working Party. Ann Intern Med 125:161–172, 1996.

94. DeJesus E, McCarty D, Farthing CF, et al. Once-daily versus twice-daily lamivudine, in combination with zidovudine and efavirenz, for the treatment of antiretroviral naïve adults with HIV infection: a randomized equivalence trial. Clin Infect Dis 39:411–418, 2004.

95. Bruno R, Regazzi MB, Ciappina V, et al. Comparison of the plasma pharmacokinetics of lamivudine during twice and once daily administration in patients with HIV. Clin Pharmacokinet 40:695–700, 2001.

96. Rousseau FS, Wakeford C, Mommeja-Marin H, et al. Prospective randomized trial of emtricitabine versus lamivudine short-term monotherapy in human immunodeficiency virus-infected patients. J Infect Dis 188:1652–1658, 2003.

97. Molina JM, Ferchal F, Randinan C, et al. Once-daily combination therapy with emtricitabine, didanosine, and efavirenz in human immunodeficiency virus-infected patients. J Infec Dis 182:599–602, 2000.

98. Saag MS, Cahn P, Raffi P, et al. Efficacy and Safety of emtricitabine vs stavudine in combination therapy in antiretroviral-naïve paitents. JAMA 292:180–190, 2004.

99. Modrzejewski KA, Herman RA. Emtricitabine: a once daily nucleoside reverse transcriptase inhibitor. Ann Pharmacother 38: 1006–1014, 2004.

100. Wang LH, Wizinia AA, Rathore MH, et al. Pharmacokinetics and safety of single oral doses of emtricitabine in human immunodeficiency virus-infected children. Antimicrob Agents Chemother 48: 183–191, 2004.

101. Staszewski S, Keiser P, Montaner J, et al. for the CNAAB3005 International Study Team. Abacavir-lamivudine-zidovudine vs indinavir-lamivudine-zidovudine in antiretroviral-naïve HIV-infected adults: A randomized equivalence trial. JAMA 285: 1155–1163, 2001.

102. Ait-Khaled M, Rakik A, Griffin P, et al. Mutations in HIV-1 reverse transcriptase during therapy with abacavir, lamivudine, and zidovudine in HIV-1 infected adults with no prior antiretroviral therapy. Antivir Ther 7:43–51, 2000.

103. DeJesus E, Herrera G, Teofilo E, et al. Abacavir versus zidovudine combined with lamivudine and efavirenz, for the treatment of antiretroviral-naïve HIV-infected adults. Clin Infect Dis 39:1038–1046, 2004.

104. Gazzard BG, DeJesus E, Cahn P, et al. Abacavir (ABC) once daily (OAD) plus lamivudine (3TC) OAD in combination with efavirenz (EFV) OAD is well tolerated and effective in the treatment of antiretroviral therapy (ART) naïve adults with HIV infection (ZODIAC study: CNA30021). Presented at: The 43rd Annual International Conference on Antimicrobial Agents and Chemotherapy; September 14–17, 2003; Chicago, IL. Abstract H-1722b.

105. Martin AM, Nolan D, Gaudieri S, et al. Predisposition to abacavir hypersensitivity conferred by HLA-B*5701 and a haplotypic Hsp70-Hom variant. Proc Natl Acad Sci U S A 101:4180–4185, 2004.

106. Kearney BP, Flaherty JF, Shah J. Tenofovir disoproxil fumarate: clinical pharmacology and pharmacokinetics. Clin Pharmacokinet 43:595–612, 2004.

107. Barditch-Crovo P, Deeks SG, Collier A, et al. Phase I/II trial of the pharmacokinetics, safety, and antiretroviral activity of tenofovir disoproxil fumarate in human immunodeficiency virus-infected adults. Antimicrob Agents Chemother 45:2733–2739, 2001.

108. Squires K, Pozniak AL, Pierone G Jr, et al. Tenofovir disoproxil fumarate in nucleoside-resistant HIV-1 infection: a randomized trial. Ann Intern Med 139:313–320, 2003.

109. Margot NA, Isaacson E, McGowan I, et al. Extended treatment with tenofovir disoproxil fumarate in treatment-experienced HIV-1 infected patients: genotypic, phenotypic, and rebound analyses. J Acquir Immune Defic Syndr 33:15–21, 2003.

110. Hoogewerf M, Regez RM, Schouten WE, et al. Change to abacavir-lamivudine-tenofovir combination treatment in patients with HIV-1 who had complete virological suppression. Lancet 362: 1979–1980, 2003.

111. Murphy M, Ohearn M, Chou S. Fatal lactic acidosis and acute renal failure after addition of tenofovir to an antiretroviral regimen containing didanosine. Clin Infect Dis 36:1082–1085, 2003.

112. Verhelst D, Monge M, Meynard JL, et al. Fanconi syndrome and renal failure induced by tenofovir: a first case report. Am J Kidney Dis 40:1331–1333, 2002.

113. Karras A, Lafaurie M, Furco A, et al. Tenofovir-related nephrotoxicity in human immunodeficiency virus-infected patients: three cases of renal failure, Fanconi syndrome, and nephrogenic diabetes insipidus. Clin Infect Dis 36:1070–1073, 2003.

114. King JR, Wynn H, Brundage R, et al. Pharmacokinetic enhancement of protease inhibitor therapy. Clin Pharmacokinet 43: 291–310, 2004.

115. Rana KZ, Dudley MN. Human immunodeficiency virus protease inhibitors. Pharmacotherapy 19:35–39, 1999.

116. VanLeeuwen R, Katlama C, Murphy RI, et al. A randomized trial to study first line combination therapy with or without a protease inhibitor in HIV-1 infected patients. AIDS 17:987–999, 2003.

117. Losina E, Islam R, Pollock AC, et al. Effectiveness of antiretroviral therapy after protease inhibitor failure: an analytic overview. Clin Infect Dis 38:1613–1622, 2004.

118. Hammer SM, Vaida F, Bennett KK, et al. Dual vs. single protease inhibitor therapy following antiretroviral treatment failure. A randomized trial. JAMA 288:169–180, 2002.

119. Paterson DL, Swindells S, Mohr J, et al. Adherence to protease inhibitor therapy and outcomes in patients with HIV infection. Ann Intern Med 133:21–30, 2000.

120. Chesney MA. Factors affecting adherence to antiretroviral therapy. Clin Infect Dis 30 (Suppl 2):S171–176, 2000.

121. Piscitelli SC, Gallicano KD. Interactions among drugs for HIV and opportunistic infections. N Engl J Med 344:984–996, 2001.

122. deMaat MM, Ekhart GC, Huitema AD, et al. Drug interactions between antiretroviral drugs and comedicated agents. Clin Pharmacokinet 42:223–282, 2003.

123. Izzedine H, Launay-vacher V, Baumelou A, et al. Antiretroviral and immunosuppressive drug-drug interactions: an update. Kidney Int 66:532–541, 2004.

124. Lim ML, Min SS, Eron JJ, et al. Coadministration of lopinavir/ritonavir and phenytoin results in a two-way drug interaction through cytochrome P-450 induction. J Acqui Immune Defic Syndr 36: 1034–1040, 2004.

125. Grinspoon S, Carr A. Cardiovascular risk and body-fat abnormalities in HIV-infected adults. N Engl J Med 352:48–62, 2005.

126. The Data Collection on Adverse Events of Anti-HIV Drugs (DAD) Study Group. Combination antiretroviral therapy and the risk of myocardial infarction. N Engl J Med 349:1993–2003, 2003. {Erratum N Engl J Med 350:955, 2004.}

127. Bozzette SA, Ake CF, Tam HK, et al. Cardiovascular and cerebrovascular events in patients treated for human immunodeficiency virus infection. N Engl J Med 348:702–710, 2003.

128. Yoon C, Gulick RM, Hoover DR., et al. Case-control study of diabetes mellitus in HIV-infected patients. J Acquir Immune Defic Syndr 37:1464–1469, 2004.

129. Justman JE, Benning L, Danoff A, et al. Protease inhibitor use and the incidence of diabetes mellitus in a large cohort of HIV-infected women. J Acquir Immune Defic Syndr 32:298–302, 2003.

130. Noor MA, Parker RA, O'Mara E, et al. The effects of HIV protease inhibitors atazanavir and lopinavir/ritonavir on insulin sensitivity in HIV-seronegative healthy adults. AIDS 18:2137–2144, 2004.

131. Mondy K, Tebas P. Emerging bone problems in patients infected with human immunodeficiency virus. Clin Infect Dis 36 (Suppl 2): S101–S105, 2003.

132. Miller KD, Masur H, Jones EC, et al. High prevalence of osteonecrosis of the femoral head in HIV-infected adults. Ann Intern Med 137:17–25, 2002.

133. Sulkowski MS. Drug-induced liver injury associated with antiretroviral therapy that includes HIV-1 protease inhibitors. Clin Infect Dis 38 (Suppl 2):S90–97, 2004.

134. Dore G. Antiretroviral therapy-related hepatotoxicity: predictors and clinical management. J HIV Ther 8:96–100, 2003.

135. Dieterich D. Managing antiretroviral-associated liver disease. J Acquir Immune Defic Syndr 34 (Suppl 1):S34–39, 2003.

136. Kotler DP, Muurahainen N, Grunfeld C, et al. Effects of growth hormone on abnormal visceral adipose tissue accumulation and dyslipidemia in HIV-infected patients. J Acquir Immune Defic Syndr 35:239–252, 2004.

137. Koutkia P, Canavan B, Breu J, et al. Growth hormone-releasing hormone in HIV-infected men with lipodystrophy. A randomized controlled trial. JAMA 292:210–218, 2004.

138. Miller J, Brown D, Amin J, et al. A randomized, double-blind study of gemfibrozil for the treatment of protease inhibitor-associated hypertriglyceridaemia. AIDS 16:2195–2200, 2002.

139. Lawal A, Engelson E, Wang J, et al. Equivalent osteopenia in HIV-infected individuals studied before and during the era of highly active antiretroviral therapy. AIDS 15:278–280, 2001.

140. Plosker GL, Scott LJ. Saquinavir: a review of its use in boosted regimens for treating HIV infection. Drugs 63:1299–1324, 2003.

141. Dragsted UB, Gerstoft J, Pedersen C, et al. Randomized trial to evaluate indinavir/ritonavir versus saquinavir/ritonavir in human immunodeficiency virus type 1-infected patients: theMaxCmin1 Trial. J Infect Dis 188:635–642, 2004.

142. Collier AC, Coombs R, Schoenfeld DA, et al. Treatment of human immunodeficiency virus infection with saquinavir, zidovudine, and zalcitabine. N Engl J Med 334:1011–1017, 1996.

143. Mitsuyasu RT, Skolnik PR, Cohen SR, et al. Activity of the soft gelatin formulation of saquinavir in combination therapy in antiretroviral-naïve patients. NV153355 Study Team. AIDS 12: F103–F109, 1998.

144. Figgitt DP, Plosker GL. Saquinavir soft-gel capsule: an updated review of its use in the management of HIV infection. Drugs 60: 481–516, 2000.

145. Piscitelli SC, Burstein AH, Welden N, et al. The effect of garlic supplements on the pharmacokinetics of saquinavir. Clin Infect Dis 34:234–238, 2002.

146. Markowitz M, Saag M, Powderly WG, et al. A preliminary study of ritonavir, an inhibitor of HIV-1 protease, to treat HIV-1 infection. N Engl J Med 333:1534–1539, 1995.

147. Danner SA, Carr A, Leonard JM, et al. A short-term study of the safety, pharmacokinetics, and efficacy of ritonavir, an inhibitor of HIV-1 protease. N Engl J Med 333:1528–1533, 1995.

148. Cameron W, Health-Chiozzi M, Danner S, et al. Randomised placebo-controlled trial of ritonavir in advanced HIV-1 disease. The advanced HIV disease ritonavir study group. Lancet 351:543–554, 1998.

149. Hsu A, Granneman GR, Bertz RJ. Ritonavir. Clinical pharmacokinetics and interactions with other anti-HIV agents. Clin Pharmacokinet 35:275–291, 1998.

150. Tseng A, Fletcher D. Interaction between ritonavir and levothyroxine. AIDS 12:2235–2236, 1998.

151. Gulick RM, Mellors JW, Havlir D, et al. Treatment with indinavir, zidovudine and lamivudine in adults with human immunodeficiency virus infection and prior antiretroviral therapy. N Engl J Med 337:734–739, 1997.

152. Plosker GL, Noble S. Indinavir: a review of its use in the management of HIV infection. Drugs 58:1165–1203, 1999.

153. Hammer SM, Squires KE, Hughes MD, et al. A controlled trial of two nucleoside analogues plus indinavir in persons with human immunodeficiency virus infection and CD4 cell counts of 200 per cubic millimeter or less. N Engl J Med 337:725–733, 1997.

154. Cooper CL, vanHeeswijk RPG, Gallicano K, et al. A review of low-dose ritonavir in protease inhibitor combination therapy. Clin Infect Dis 36:1585–1592, 2003.

155. Solas C, Lafeuillade A, Halfon P, et al. Discrepancies between protease inhibitor concentrations and viral load in reservoirs and sanctuary sites in human immunodeficiency virus-infected patients. Antimicrob Agents Chemother 47:238–243, 2003.

156. Daudon M, Estepa L, Viard JP, et al. Urinary stones in HIV-1 positive patients treated with indinavir. Lancet 349:1294–1295, 1997.

157. Kopp JB, Miller KD, Mican JM, et al. Crystalluria and urinary tract abnormalities associated with indinavir. Ann Intern Med 127: 119–125, 1997.

158. Bardsley-Elliot A, Plosker GL. Nelfinavir: an update on its use in HIV infection. Drugs 59:581–620, 2000.

159. Guest JL, Ruffin C, Tschampa JM, et al. Difference in rates of diarrhea in patients with human immunodeficiency virus receiving lopinavir-ritonavir or nelfinavir. Pharmacotherapy 24:727–735, 2004.

160. Turner MJ, Angel JB, Woodend K. The efficacy of calcium carbonate in the treatment of protease inhibitor-induced persistent diarrhea in HIV-infected patients. HIV Clin Trials 5:19–24, 2004.

161. Fung HB, Kirschenbaum HL, Hameed R. Amprenavir: A new human immunodeficiency virus type 1 protease inhibitor. Clin Ther 22:549–572, 2000.

162. Goodgame JC, Pottage JC Jr, Jablonowski H, et al. Amprenavir in combination with lamivudine and zidovudine versus lamivudine and zidovudine alone in HIV-1 infected antiretroviral-naïve adults. Amprenavir PROAB3001 International Study Team. Antivir Ther 5:215–225, 2000.

163. Cyetkovic RS, Goa KL. Lopinavir/ritonavir: a review of its use in the management of HIV infection. Drugs 63:769–802, 2003.

164. King MS, Bernstein BM, Walmsley SL, et al. Baseline HIV-1 RNA level and CD4 count predict time to loss of virologic response to nelfinavir but not lopinavir/ritonavir, in antiretroviral therapy-naïve patients. J Infec Dis 190:280–284, 2004.

165. Kempf DJ, King MS, Bernstein B, et al. Incidence of resistance in a double-blind study comparing lopinavir/ritonavir plus stavudine and lamivudine to nelfinavir plus stavudine and lamivudine. J Infec Dis 189:51–60, 2004.

166. Voigt E, Wasmuth JC, Vogel M, et al. Safety, efficacy and development of resistance under the new protease inhibitor lopinavir/ritonavir: 48 week results. Infection 32:82–88, 2004.

167. Benson CA, Deeks SG, Brun SC, et al. Safety and antiviral activity at 48 weeks of lopinavir/ritonavir plus nevirapine and 2 nucleoside reverse-transcriptase inhibitors in human immunodeficiency virus type 1-infected protease inhibitor-experienced patients. J Infect Dis 185:599–607, 2002.

168. Bongiovanni M, Bini T, Adorni F, et al. Virological success of lopinavir/ritonavir salvage regimen is affected by an increasing number of lopinavir/ritonavir related mutations. Antivir Ther 8: 209–214, 2004.

169. Eron JJ, Feinberg J, Kessler HA, et al. Once-daily versus twice-daily lopinavir/ritonavir in antiretroviral-naive HIV-positive patients: a 48-week randomized clinical trial. J Infect Dis 189: 265–272, 2004.

170. Chapman TM, Plosker GL, Perry CM. Fosamprenavir: a review of its use in the management of antiretroviral therapy-naive patients with HIV infection. Drugs 64:2101–2124, 2004.

171. Wood R, Arasteh K, Stellbrink HJ, et al. Six-week randomized controlled trial to compare the tolerabilities, pharmacokinetics, and antiviral activities of GW433908 and amprenavir in human immunodeficiency virus type 1-infected patients. Antimicrob Agents Chemother 48:116–123, 2004.

172. Falcoz C, Jenkins JM, Bye C, et al. Pharmacokinetics of GW433908, a prodrug of amprenavir, in healthy male volunteers. J Clin Pharmacol 42:887–898, 2002.

173. Rodriguez-French A, Boghossian J, Gray GE, et al. The NEAT study: a 48-week open-label study to compare the antiviral efficacy and safety of GW433908 versus nelfinavir in antiretroviral therapy-naïve HIV-1 infected patients. J Acquir Immune Defic Syndr 35: 22–32, 2004.

174. Gathe JC Jr, Ive P, Wood R, et al. SOLO: 48-week efficacy and safety comparison of once-daily fosamprenavir /ritonavir versus twice-daily nelfinavir in naive HIV-1-infected patients. AIDS 18: 1529–1537, 2004.

175. MacManus S, Yates PJ, Elston RC, et al. GW433908/ritonavir once daily in antiretroviral therapy-naive HIV-infected patients: absence of protease resistance at 48 weeks. AIDS 18:651–655, 2004.

176. DeJesus E, LaMarca A, Sension M, et al. The Context Study: Efficacy and safety of GW433908/RTV in PI-experienced subjects with virologic failure (24 week results). Presented at: The 10th Conference on Retroviruses and Opportunistic Infections; February 10–14, 2003; Boston, MA. Abstract 178.

177. Ford SL, Wire MB, Lou Y, et al. Effect of antacids and ranitidine on the single dose pharmacokinetics of fosamprenavir. Antimicrob Agents Chemother 49:467–469, 2005.

178. Wire MB, Ballow C, Preeston SL, et al. Pharmacokinetics and safety of GW433908 and ritonavir, with and without efavirenz, in health volunteers. AIDS 18:897–907, 2004.

179. Sanne I, Piliero P, Squires K, et al. Results of a phase 2 clinical trial at 48 weeks (AI424-007): a dose-ranging, safety, and efficacy comparative trial of atazanavir at three doses in combination with didanosine and stavudine in antiretroviral-naive subjects. J Acquir Immune Defic Syndr 32:18–29, 2003.

180. Murphy RL, Sanne I, Cahn P, et al. Dose-ranging, randomized, clinical trial of atazanavir with lamivudine and stavudine in antiretroviral-naïve subjects: 48-week results. AIDS 17:2603–2614, 2003.

181. Wood R, Phanuphak P, Cahn P, et al. Long-term efficacy and safety of atazanavir with stavudine and lamivudine in patients previously treated with nelfinavir or atazanavir. J Acquir Immune Defic Syndr 36:684–692, 2004.

182. Squires K, Lazzarin A, Gatell JM, et al. Comparison of once-daily atazanavir with efavirenz, each in combination with fixed-dose zidovudine and lamivudine, as initial therapy for patients infected with HIV. J Acquir Immune Defic Syndr 36:1011–1019, 2004.

183. Haas DW, Zala C, Schrader S, et al. Therapy with atazanavir plus saquinavir in patients failing highly active antiretroviral therapy: a randomized comparative pilot trial. AIDS 17:1339–1349, 2003.

184. Orrick JJ, Steinhart CR. Atazanavir. Ann Pharmacother 38: 1664–1674, 2004.

185. Colonno R, Rose R, McLaren C, et al. Identification of I50L as the signature atazanavir (ATV)-resistance mutation in treatment-naïve

HIV-1 infected patients receiving ATV-containing regimens. J Infect Dis 189:1802–1810, 2004.

186. Yeni P. Tipranavir: a protease inhibitor from a new class with distinct antiviral activity. J Acquir Immune Defic Syndr 34 (Suppl 1): S91–S94, 2003.

187. McCallister S, Valdez H, Curry K, et al. A 14-day dose response study of the efficacy, safety, and pharmacokinetics of the nonpeptidic protease inhibitor tipranavir in treatment-naïve HIV-1 infected patients. J Acquir Immune Defic Syndr 35:376–382, 2004.

188. Larder BA, Herlogs K, Bloor S, et al. Tipranavir inhibits broadly protease inhibitor-resistant HIV-1 clinical samples. AIDS 14: 1943–1948, 2000.

189. D'Aquila RT, Hughes MD, Johnson VA, et al. Nevirapine, zidovudine, and didanosine compared with zidovudine and didanosine in patients with HIV-1 infection. A randomized, double-blind, placebo-controlled trial. National Institute of Allergy and Infectious Disease AIDS Clinical Trials Group Protocol 241 Investigators. Ann Intern Med 124:1019–1030, 1996.

190. Montaner JSG, Reiss P, Cooper D, et al. A randomized, double-blind trial comparing combinations of nevirapine, didanosine, and zidovudine for HIV-infected patients. The INCAS Trial. JAMA 279:930–937, 1998.

191. Podzamczer D, Ferrer E, Consiglio E, et al. A randomized clinical trial comparing nelfinavir or nevirapine associated to zidovudine/lamivudine in HIV-infected naïve patients (the COMBINE study). Antivir Ther 7:81–90, 2002.

192. Van Leth F, Phanuphak P, Ruxrungtham K, et al. Comparison of first-line antiretroviral therapy with regimens including nevirapine, efavirenz or both drugs, plus stavudine and lamivudine: a randomized open label trial, the 2 NN study. Lancet 363:1253–1263, 2004.

193. Smith PF, DiCenzo R, Morse GD. Clinical pharmacokinetics of non-nucleoside reverse transcriptase inhibitors. Clin Pharmacokinet 40:893–905, 2001.

194. Bersoff-Matcha SJ, Miller WC, Aberg JA, et al. Sex differences in nevirapine rash. Clin Infect Dis 32:124–129, 2001.

195. Martinez E, Blanco JL, Arnaiz JA, et al. Hepatotoxicity in HIV-1 infected patients receiving nevirapine-containing antiretroviral therapy. AIDS 15:1261–1268, 2001.

196. Scott LJ, Perry CM. Delavirdine: a review of its use in HIV infection. Drugs 60:1411–1444, 2000.

197. Friedland GH, Pollard R, Griffith B, et al. Efficacy and safety of delavirdine mesylate with zidovudine and didanosine compared with two-drug combinations of these agents in persons with HIV disease with CD4 counts of 100 to 500 cells/mm3 (ACTG 261). ACTG 261 Team. Acquir Immune Defic Syndr 21:281–292, 1999.

198. Harris M, Alexander C, O-Shaughnessy M, et al. Delavirdine increases drug exposure of ritonavir-boosted protease inhibitors. AIDS 16:798–799, 2002.

199. Shafer RW, Smeaton LM, Robbins GK, et al. Comparison of four-drug regimens and pairs of sequential three-drug regimens as initial therapy for HIV-1 infection. N Engl J Med 349:2304–2315, 2003.

200. Orkin C, Stebbing J, Nelson M, et al. A randomized study comparing a three- and four-drug HAART regimen in first-line therapy (QUAD study). J Antimicrob Chemother 55:246–251, 2002.

201. Podzamczer D, Ferrer E, Gatell JM, et al. Early virological failure with a combination of tenofovir, didanosine and efavirenz. Antivir Ther 10:171–177, 2005.

202. Hirschel B, Flepp M, Bucher HC, et al. Switching from protease inhibitors to efavirenz: difference in efficacy and tolerance among risk groups: a case-control study from the Swiss HIV Cohort. AIDS 16:381–385, 2002.

203. Martinez E, Arnaiz JA, Podzamczer D, et al. Substitution of nevirapine, efavirenz, or abacavir for protease inhibitors in patients with human immunodeficiency virus infection. N Engl J Med 349: 1036–1046, 2003.

204. Haas DW, Fessel WJ, Delapenha RA, et al. Therapy with efavirenz plus indinavir in patients with extensive prior nucleoside reverse-transcriptase inhibitor experience: a randomized, double-blind, placebo-controlled trial. J Infect Dis 183:392–400, 2001.

205. Lalezari J, Henry K, O'Hearn M, et al. Enfuvirtide, an HIV-1 fusion inhibitor, for drug-resistant HIV-infection in North and South America. N Engl J Med 348:2175–2185, 2003.

206. Lazzarin A, Clotet B, Cooper D, et al. Efficacy of enfuvirtide in patients infected with drug-resistant HIV-1 in Europe and Australia. N Engl J Med 348:2186–2195, 2003.

207. Patel IH, Zhang X, Nieforth K, et al. Pharmacokintics, pharmacodynamics and drug interaction potential of enfuvirtide. Clin Pharmacokinet 44:175–186, 2005.

208. Leen C, Wat C, Nieforth K. Pharmacokinetics of enfuvirtide in a patient with impaired renal function. Clin Infect Dis 39:e119–e121, 2004.

209. Zhang Z, Lalezari JP, Badley AD, et al. Assessment of the drug-drug interaction potential of enfuvirtide in human immunodeficiency virus type 1-infected patients. Clin Pharmacol Ther 75: 558–568, 2004.

210. DeSimone JA, Ojha A, Pathak R, et al. Successful desensitization to enfuvirtide after a hypersensitivity reaction in an HIV-1-infected man. Clin Infect Dis 39:e110–e112, 2004.

211. Lu W, Arraes LC, Ferreira WT, et al. Therapeutic dendritic-cell vaccine for chronic HIV-1 infection. Nat Med 10:1359–1365, 2004.

212. Miller LG, Liu H, Hays RD, et al. How well do clinicians estimate patients' adherence to combination antiretroviral therapy. J Gen Intern Med 17:1–11, 2002.

213. Tseng AL. Compliance issues in the treatment of HIV infection. Am J Health Syst Pharmacists 55:1817–1824, 1998.

214. Bozzette SA, Joyce G, McCaffrey DF, et al. Expenditures for the care of HIV-infected patients in the era of highly active antiretroviral therapy. N Engl J Med 344:817–823, 2001.

215. Gebo KA, Chaisson RE, Folkemer JG, et al. Costs of HIV medical care in the era of highly active antiretroviral therapy. AIDS 13: 963–969, 1999.

216. Keiser P, Nassar N, Kvanli MB, et al. Long-term impact of highly active antiretroviral therapy on HIV-related health care costs. J Acquir Immune Defic Syndr 27:14–19, 2001.

217. HIV Research Network. Hospital and outpatient health services utilization among HIV-infected patients in care in 1999. J Acquir Immune Defic Syndr 30:21–26, 2002.

218. Hellinger FJ, Encinosa WE. Antiretroviral therapy and health care utilization: a study of privately insured men and women with HIV disease. Health Serv Res 39:949–967, 2004.

219. Henry J. Kaiser Family Foundation. Waiting for AIDS Medications in the United States: An Analysis of ADAP Waiting Lists. 2004 December. Available at: http://www.kff.org. Accessed November 7, 2005.

Human Immunodeficiency Virus Infection—Opportunistic Infections

85

Robert C. Stevens

Opportunistic infections have a profound effect on the morbidity and mortality of individuals coinfected with the human immunodeficiency virus (HIV). By definition, when a person infected with HIV develops certain opportunistic infections, that individual is diagnosed with the acquired immunodeficiency syndrome (AIDS). The quality of life of patients with AIDS can be markedly affected after developing an opportunistic infection if prolonged therapies are indicated to prevent relapse of the infection. This chapter discusses the pathophysiology, clinical presentation, and treatment of selected opportunistic infections in patients with AIDS, including *Pneumocystis jirovecii* pneumonia (PCP), toxoplasmosis encephalitis, disseminated *Mycobacterium avium* complex (MAC) infection, and cytomegalovirus (CMV) retinitis. Important opportunistic fungal infections for AIDS patients are discussed in the chapter on mycotic infections.

PNEUMOCYSTIS JIROVECII PNEUMONIA

PCP is caused by *P. jirovecii*; this organism is of low virulence in healthy persons but causes pneumonia in immunocompromised subjects. The taxonomy of the organism has changed since the previous edition of this chapter: *Pneumocystis carinii* now refers only to the species that infects rodents and *P jirovecii* refers to the distinct species that infects humans, but the abbreviation ''PCP'' remains as the acronym for *Pneumo-cystis* pneumonia. Most people in the United States are infected with *P. jirovecii* by the age of 4 years but do not develop pneumonia because of an intact host defense system.[1] Significant knowledge about this pathogen has been acquired over the past 25 years since the AIDS epidemic was first uncovered. Most notable are improved measures for prevention and alternatives for treatment of acute PCP infection.

EPIDEMIOLOGY

Early in the AIDS epidemic, PCP was the indicator disease in more than 60% of newly diagnosed AIDS cases.[1] The widespread implementation of effective preventive measures (i.e., primary drug prophylaxis) has significantly decreased the incidence of this infection. Adherence to drug treatment for PCP prophylaxis and potent antiretroviral regimens, coupled with a decrease in the number of individuals with advanced HIV infection, have had pronounced effects on reducing the overall incidence of PCP. The number of hospitalizations and in-hospital mortality for PCP in HIV-infected patients has decreased significantly over the past decade following the introduction of highly active antiretroviral therapy (HAART) in the mid-1990s. However, recent geographic (southern United States) and demographic (females, African-Americans) trends in hospitalization suggest that PCP is becoming more frequent in minority groups with less access to health care.[2]

PATHOPHYSIOLOGY

P. jirovecii is a slow-growing, unicellular eukaryote whose genetic sequence is linked to the fungal kingdom but that shares biologic characteristics with protozoa.[1] Its inability to grow on fungal media and its susceptibility to antiprotozoal agents, however, incline clinicians to view *P. jirovecii* as a parasite, despite the molecular evidence that it is a fungus. Transmittal of the organism is likely to require inhalation of an infectious inoculum. Once inhaled, the organism resides in the alveoli, generating large numbers of organisms in the setting of T-lymphocyte depletion caused by HIV. Significant production of *P. jirovecii* alters the alveolar capillary permeability, resulting in impairment of gas exchange. Poor distribution of inspired air into alveoli that are obstructed with the organism, fluid, and inflammatory mediators leads to ventilation–perfusion mismatch. This clinical description is similar to the pathogenesis of the adult respiratory distress syndrome discussed in Chapter 86.

CLINICAL PRESENTATION AND DIAGNOSIS

SIGNS AND SYMPTOMS

The primary target of infection is the lungs, with pneumonia accounting for more than 95% of *P. jirovecii* infections. More than 90% of patients have pulmonary complaints, primarily cough, shortness of breath, and tachypnea. Nonspecific constitutional symptoms such as fever, night sweats, fatigue, or weight loss also are observed. Since *P. jirovecii* is a much slower-growing organism than pyogenic bacteria, there is an indolent onset of pulmonary symptoms in persons infected with HIV. These patients may have fever and complain of lethargy and progressive onset of dyspnea on exertion over 2 to 4 weeks before seeking medical attention. The chest radiograph reveals the characteristic bilateral patchy infiltrates. Radiologic appearance lags behind clinical deterioration or improvement. Occasionally, fine basilar rales are encountered on auscultation, but otherwise physical examination of the pulmonary system is often normal.

Patients with AIDS who develop PCP often have an elevation of serum lactate dehydrogenase (LDH). The sensitivity of an elevated LDH for PCP in this population is between 83% and 100%, with greater sensitivity in critically ill patients than ambulatory patients.[1] Although serum LDH is nonspecific for PCP, it is elevated less frequently with other types of pneumonia. The value of LDH is in evaluating prognosis and response to treatment. A strong correlation exists between the degree of LDH elevation and survival. A high or rising LDH while on antipneumocystis therapy correlates with a worse prognosis, a failure of therapy, and increased mortality, whereas a low or a declining serum LDH suggests the opposite trend.

DIAGNOSIS

Individuals infected with HIV who present with pulmonary and nonspecific constitutional symptoms consistent with PCP, and with a chest radiograph revealing bilateral infiltrates, should have samples collected either by induced sputum or fiberoptic bronchoscopy with bronchoalveolar lavage to isolate the *P. jirovecii* cysts. Recovery of cysts from sputum or lungs is the definitive diagnosis.

PSYCHOSOCIAL ASPECTS

There are still occasions when the diagnosis of PCP or another opportunistic infection represents the defining moment when a patient first learns of his or her possible or probable infection with HIV. Despite widespread educational efforts promoting HIV awareness, there are still individuals who participate in high-risk behaviors relative to acquiring HIV (i.e., intravenous drug use) but do not know of their HIV status until they seek medical care for their ailing health caused by an opportunistic infection. The implications can be devastating, especially if the individual is seriously ill from the opportunistic infection. These patients require counseling about their newly diagnosed HIV status, as well as how to resolve the acute episode of PCP.

It is imperative to provide the patient with support and candid information about AIDS so that he or she will not dwell in a state of denial and thus increase the likelihood of nonadherence to therapy. The more knowledge the person has about AIDS, the more likely he or she will cope well with this infection. Pertinent advice includes information on transmission of the virus, how to discuss his or her HIV status with family and loved ones, arrangement for follow-up care in HIV clinics, and financial resources to support medical and social care.

TREATMENT

PHARMACOTHERAPY FOR ACUTE *P JIROVECII* PNEUMONIA

The selection of appropriate antipneumocystis agents for patient-specific conditions requires an understanding of the subtleties in drug selection and monitoring. The first process in drug selection involves categorizing the pneumonia into mild to moderate PCP versus severe PCP. Mild to moderate PCP is defined by a patient's Pao_2 on room air greater than or equal to 70 mm Hg or an alveolar–arterial oxygen difference [(A-a) DO_2] less than 35 mm Hg. Severe PCP is defined as a Pao_2 on room air of less than 70 mm Hg or an A-a gradient greater than or equal to 35 mm Hg. [The A-a gradient is the difference between the ideal alveolar partial pressure of oxygen (ideal Pao_2) less the measured arterial partial pressure of oxygen (measured PaO_2).] Table 85.1 lists the first-line and alternative treatment methods for PCP.

Mild to Moderate PCP. The schema for therapy of mild to moderate PCP is depicted on the left side of the algorithm in Figure 85.1. Trimethoprim-sulfamethoxazole (TMP-SMX) is widely considered the drug of choice.[3–5] No other drug or drug combination has been demonstrated to be superior to TMP-SMX in efficacy. However, TMP-SMX-in-

duced adverse events are common; therefore, TMP-SMX dosage regimen modifications or drug therapy switches are often indicated.[6]

Mutations in *P. jirovecii* associated with resistance to sulfa drugs have been documented, but their effect on therapeutic response and clinical outcome is uncertain.[7] Patients who have PCP despite TMP-SMX prophylaxis as discussed below are usually effectively treated with the standard dose of TMP-SMX listed in Table 85.1.

Commonly observed toxicities associated with TMP-SMX in persons infected with HIV include rash, gastrointestinal distress, neutropenia, thrombocytopenia, elevated liver transaminases, hyperkalemia (TMP acts akin to a potassium-sparing diuretic), hyponatremia, and renal dysfunction. Typically, these toxicities manifest within the first 1 to 2 weeks of therapy.

Morbilliform rash, the most frequent adverse event with TMP-SMX, is commonly self-limiting; rarely have patients infected with HIV developed severe skin reactions. If a patient with HIV has had a prior nondesquamating dermatologic reaction to TMP-SMX that has not involved the mucous membranes, there is no absolute contraindication to him or her receiving the drug in the future, should he or she present with acute PCP or need prophylactic treatment. In patients with AIDS who develop a rash while on TMP-SMX, it is acceptable to continue treatment provided no mucous membranes are involved and no skin has vesiculated. The mild rash or pruritus can be alleviated with antihistamines if needed.

Neutropenia is a concentration-dependent toxicity of TMP-SMX and can be minimized with appropriate dose modification. Dosing TMP-SMX at 15 mg/kg/day instead of 20 mg/kg/day, or adjusting the dose to obtain TMP concentrations of 5 to 8 µg/mL 1.5 hours after intravenous (IV) infusion or oral ingestion, has been shown to lower the incidence of neutropenia.[8] Attempts to ameliorate the bone marrow suppression with folinic acid (analogous to the ''leucovorin rescue'' practiced with methotrexate in treatment of leukemia) was associated with higher rates of therapeutic failure and death compared with placebo in AIDS patients with PCP treated with TMP-SMX.[9]

Clinicians should also be aware of the nonspecific central nervous system (CNS) adverse effects associated with TMP-SMX, including fine tremors, headache, nervousness, lightheadedness, insomnia, drowsiness, and acute psychosis. These toxicities can be concentration-dependent and appear to be more intense at daily doses of 20 mg per kg TMP.[10] Dosage reduction (12 to 15 mg/kg/day) is appropriate empirically and if CNS toxicity occurs. Clinicians may also reduce the risk of the potentiating CNS side effects by careful review and monitoring of concurrent medication use to avoid other drugs that may have a similar CNS toxicity profile.

Clearly, the toxicities associated with TMP-SMX require alternative therapies. The AIDS Clinical Trials Group (ACTG) 108 study compared oral TMP-SMX with oral TMP-dapsone and clindamycin-primaquine in 181 patients

TABLE 85.1	Treatment of *Pneumocystis jirovecii* Pneumonia in Patients With HIV		
Therapy Type	**First-Line Therapy**	**Alternative Therapy**	**Comment**
Acute infection	TMP (15 mg/kg/day) + SMX (75 mg/kg/day) divided in 3 or 4 daily doses PO/IV for 21 days	Pentamidine (4 mg/kg/day IV or IM) for 21 days	TMP-SMX is the preferred regimen.
	TMP (15 mg/kg/day PO or IV) + dapsone (100 mg/day PO) for 21 days	Atovaquone suspension (750 mg PO BID with food) for 21 days	See text and Figure 85.1 for appropriate selection of other regimens.
	Clindamycin (600 mg every 6–8 hr PO or IV) + primaquine (30 mg base PO/day) for 21 days	Alternative considerations for refractory infections or side effects with standard agents: trimetrexate (45 mg/m^2/day IV) for 21 days + leucovorin (20 mg/m^2 IV or PO q6h) for 24 days	Adverse events to sulfonamides (rash, fever, leukopenia, hepatitis, etc.) most common at 1–2 wk
			Pts w/ severe pneumonia (PaO$_2$ <70 mm Hg) should receive corticosteroids (prednisone, 40 mg PO BID for 5 days, then 40 mg/day for 5 days, then 20 mg/day until completion of treatment).
Prophylaxis	TMP-SMX (1 SS/day, 1 DS/day, or 1 DS 3 times/week)	Dapsone (50 mg BID or 100 mg/day)	Prophylaxis is indicated for any HIV-infected patient with a history of PCP, CD4+ count <200/mm^3, unexplained fever (>100°F) for >2 weeks, or a history of oropharyngeal candidiasis.
		Dapsone (50 mg/day) + pyrimethamine (50 mg/wk) + leucovorin (25 mg/wk)	
		Dapsone (200 mg/week) + pyrimethamine (75 mg/wk) + leucovorin (25 mg/wk)	Efficacy shown in controlled studies only for TMP-SMX, dapsone (± pyrimethamine), and aerosolized pentamidine
		Aerosolized pentamidine (300 mg) every month via Respirgard II nebulizer—pretreatment with β$_2$ agonist (albuterol, 2 puffs)	Aerosolized pentamidine should not be used in pts w/ CD4+ counts <100/mm^3 because of diminished efficacy.
		Pentamidine (4 mg/kg) IM or IV q2wk	

TMP, trimethoprim; SMX, sulfamethoxazole; SS, single-strength TMP-SMX tablet; DS, double-strength TMP-SMX tablet.
(Adapted from Centers for Disease Control and Prevention. Treating opportunistic infections among HIV-infected adults and adolescents: recommendations from CDC, the National Institutes of Health, and the HIV Medicine Association/Infectious Diseases Society of America. Clin Infect Dis 40 (Suppl 3):S131–S235, 2005; and from Stevens RC. Opportunistic infections in AIDS due to protozoal and *Mycobacterium avium* complex. In: Carter BL, Lake KD, Raebel MA, et al, eds. Pharmacotherapy self-assessment program, 3rd ed. Kansas City, MO: American College of Clinical Pharmacy 1998:129–130, 2000.)

infected with HIV with PCP.[11] Survival and dose-limiting toxicity (36%, 24%, and 33% for each drug combination, respectively) did not differ among the three treatment arms. Elevation of serum aminotransferase levels to more than five times the baseline value was more common in the TMP-SMX group ($p = 0.003$), and one or more serious hematologic toxicities (neutropenia, anemia, thrombocytopenia, or methemoglobinemia) occurred more frequently in the clindamycin-primaquine group ($p = 0.01$). These findings provide clinicians with a better perspective on appropriate drug selection for individual patients (Fig. 85.1).

TMP-dapsone can be used as an alternative in subjects infected with HIV who are intolerant to TMP-SMX. This regimen may have similar efficacy and perhaps fewer side

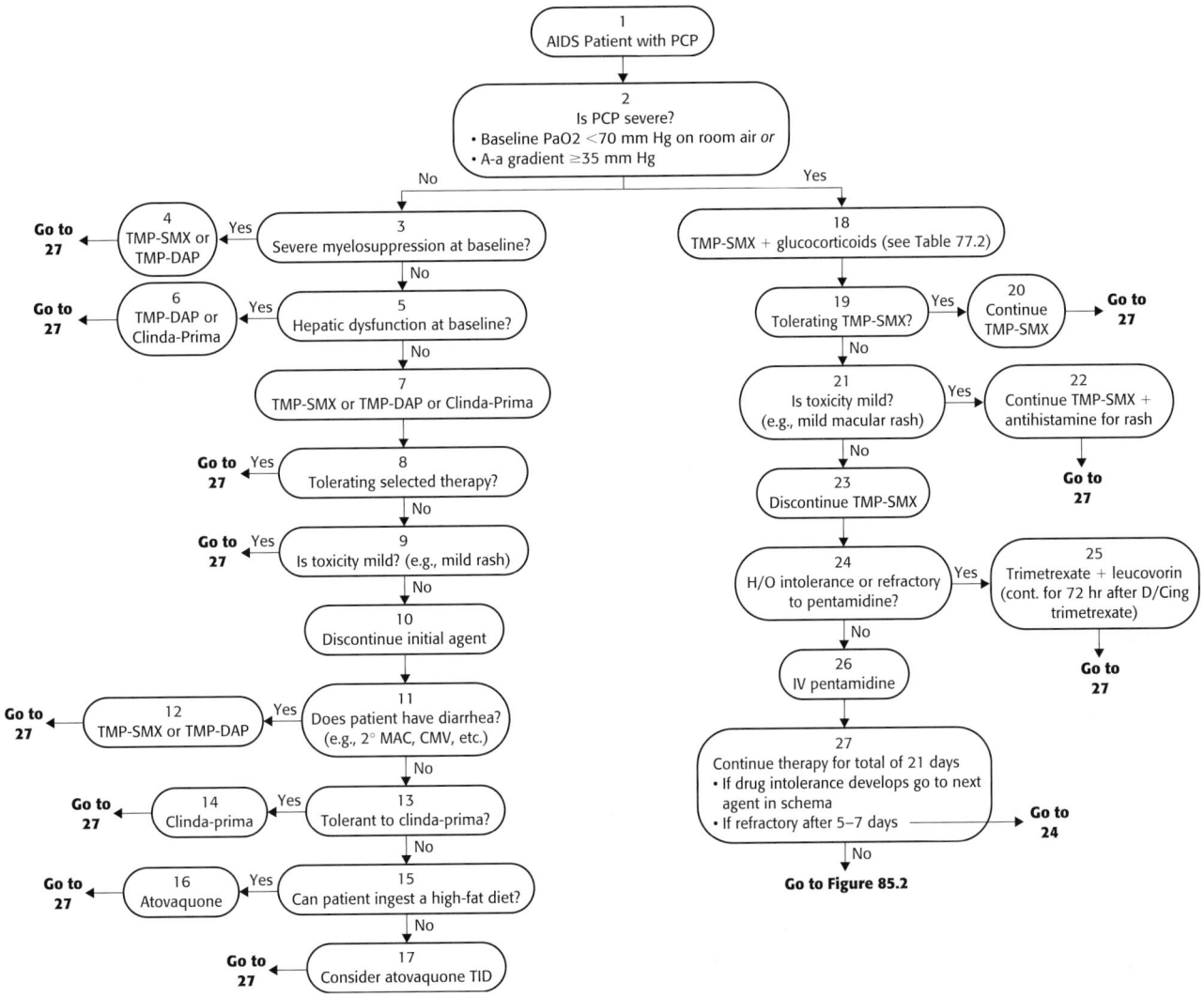

FIGURE 85.1 Algorithm for acute therapy of *Pneumocystis jirovecii* pneumonia (PCP). The schema is divided into therapies for mild to moderate pneumonia and severe pneumonia. Duration of therapy is 21 days, followed by secondary prophylaxis (Fig. 85.2). Doses are provided in Table 85.1. Atovaquone is the suspension formulation. *A-a gradient,* alveolar-arterial oxygen difference; *Clinda-Prima,* clindamycin-primaquine; *CMV,* cytomegalovirus; *MAC, Mycobacterium avium* complex; *PaO2,* arterial partial pressure of oxygen; *TMP-DAP,* trimethoprim-dapsone; *TMP-SMX,* trimethoprim-sulfamethoxazole. (Reproduced with permission from Stevens RC. Opportunistic infections in AIDS due to protozoal and *Mycobacterium avium* complex. In: Carter BL, Lake KD, Raebel MA, et al., eds. Pharmacotherapy self-assessment program, 3rd ed. Kansas City, MO: American College of Clinical Pharmacy, 1998:131.)

effects than TMP-SMX but is less convenient because of the number of pills required. Patients who develop a mild rash from TMP-SMX and are subsequently changed to TMP-dapsone also develop a rash from dapsone in up to 22% of cases.[12] Dapsone is a sulfonamide moiety and cross-sensitivity is observed. A TMP-SMX rash, presumably owing to the sulfa entity, however, does not preclude the use of dapsone.

Dapsone-induced methemoglobinemia occurs in up to two thirds of persons infected with HIV, but most individuals who are not deficient in the enzyme NADH-methemoglobin-reductase are asymptomatic. The manifestations of methemoglobinemia include cyanosis, headache, dizziness, drowsiness, stupor, fatigue, ataxia, dyspnea, tachycardia, nausea,

and vomiting. Severe methemoglobinemia can lead to hemolysis owing to a change in iron oxidation state with impairment of oxygen transport. Dapsone and other potential hemolyzing agents should be discontinued, and methylene blue (1 to 2 mg/kg in a 1% saline solution given once IV over 10 to 15 minutes) should be administered as an antidote if methemoglobin concentrations exceed 20%, or at lower concentrations of methemoglobin if patients are severely symptomatic. Dapsone can also cause hemolysis, especially in patients who are deficient in the enzyme glucose-6-phosphate dehydrogenase (G6PD).

Rash, diarrhea, bone marrow suppression, hemolysis, and methemoglobinemia have been reported with the clindamycin-primaquine combination.[11] This combination should be avoided if possible in patients with underlying diarrhea due to HIV gastroenteropathy or invasion of the gastrointestinal tract by some other diarrhea-causing opportunistic pathogen (e.g., CMV, *Cryptosporidium*, MAC).

Atovaquone, an oral agent, has been shown to be better tolerated than TMP-SMX and pentamidine in patients with mild to moderate PCP; however, it is associated with a higher rate of therapeutic failure.[13,14] In some patients, this may be explained in part by the reduced bioavailability of the drug when it is not administered with a high-fat meal. Atovaquone absorption is enhanced with fatty foods. Persons infected with HIV should be instructed to take atovaquone with fatty foods because poor absorption is considered to be the most likely explanation for its inferior therapeutic response compared with TMP-SMX. Consumption of a high-fat diet can be problematic in this patient population because they can develop diarrhea secondary to the fatty foods, and diarrhea is linked to therapeutic failure and higher mortality in atovaquone-treated patients.[12,13] Macular rash is the most common adverse effect. Hematologic toxicity from atovaquone is rare. Atovaquone is perhaps the best tolerated antipneumocystis agent, but the lower therapeutic response necessitates restricting this agent to patients with mild to moderate PCP. Atovaquone is not indicated for initial treatment of severe PCP.

Severe PCP. Severe PCP requires parenteral antipneumocystis therapy, adjunctive glucocorticoids, and aggressive supportive care (e.g., supplemental oxygen, nutritional support—low albumin is a risk factor for a poor prognosis). A patient can be switched to oral therapy once he or she is clinically stable. TMP-SMX is the first-line parenteral therapy, followed by IV pentamidine as an alternate, for treatment of severe PCP.

IV pentamidine is the most frequently prescribed alternative for TMP-SMX in patients with severe PCP who have significant intolerance to TMP-SMX, or who have not quickly responded to therapy (Fig. 85.1). In general, patients should not be labeled as TMP-SMX therapeutic failures until at least 4 to 8 days of anti-PCP treatment.[3] Patients with severe infection often deteriorate during the first few days of therapy because of worsening oxygen desaturation. This is most likely because of release of cytokines from alveolar macrophages during the acute inflammatory process and lysis of *P. jirovecii* cysts after exposure to appropriate therapy. Thus, switching to alternative therapy would be premature during this transient decompensation period.

Commonly, parenteral pentamidine causes serious side effects including nephrotoxicity, hypotension, and hypoglycemia. Other serious complications include elevations in liver transaminases, hyperkalemia, hyperglycemia, leukopenia, thrombocytopenia, acute pancreatitis, and ventricular arrhythmias. A 5-year retrospective review of the incidence of parenteral pentamidine-associated adverse effects at San Francisco General Hospital in patients infected with HIV

who received at least 5 days of pentamidine therapy found that 72% of the patients experienced an adverse effect.[15] Nephrotoxicity occurred in 45%, hypoglycemia in 24%, and pancreatitis in 9% of patients receiving pentamidine.

Nephrotoxicity caused by pentamidine is related to cumulative exposure, making renal damage unlikely in the first 5 to 7 days of therapy. Empiric dosage reduction (3 mg/kg/day) has been used in mild to moderate PCP, and especially after azotemia has developed, but the efficacy of this dosage has not been well established in severe PCP.[16] The concurrent use of other nephrotoxic drugs may increase the risk of renal injury.

Hypoglycemia caused by pentamidine, which occurs in 10% to 50% of patients with AIDS, is potentially the most dangerous toxicity because of its insidious onset. This side effect has been associated with use of higher doses, prolonged therapy, and repeated courses of IV pentamidine. A statistically significant relationship has been observed between hypoglycemia and nephrotoxicity.[15] Pentamidine exerts a lytic effect on pancreatic B cells, causing a sudden influx of insulin into the systemic circulation. No guidelines have been established for monitoring blood glucose, but daily assessment seems advisable. The optimal time for sample collection is unknown. It can be theorized that blood glucose should be ascertained within 4 hours after pentamidine infusion based on the assumption that a temporal relationship exists between lysis of the B cells and the maximum tissue drug concentration. However, fatal hypoglycemia has occurred 2 weeks after the drug was stopped, presumably owing to pentamidine's high tissue affinity and subsequent drug accumulation. In hypoglycemic patients, it would be prudent to determine blood glucose levels every 4 to 6 hours for the first 24 to 48 hours, two or three times daily for the following 10 to 14 days, then daily for the remainder of therapy. Patient-specific monitoring programs would need to be structured dependent on the patient's baseline glucose control.

The role of adjunctive corticosteroids in patients with AIDS who have severe PCP is indisputable. Several well-controlled studies indicate that pulmonary failure (PaO_2 <75 mm Hg), the need for mechanical ventilation, and mortality rates were all significantly reduced in AIDS patients with PCP randomized to receive corticosteroids.[17,18] Negative outcomes from these studies found that mild, localized, mucocutaneous, herpetic lesions were the most significant complication in the steroid-treated patients. Subsequent investigations have shown that short-course steroid use has not enhanced the risk of developing active tuberculosis or relapses of other AIDS-related infections.

These trials collectively led to a consensus statement that recommended adjunctive corticosteroids be prescribed within 72 hours of initiating antipneumocystis therapy in AIDS patients with severe PCP.[19] Dosage guidelines for prednisone, including a tapering schedule, are listed in Table 85.1. Methylprednisolone, with appropriate dosage adjustment for potency differences (i.e., 75% of the respective prednisone dose), can be used when patients cannot ingest oral prednisone.

PROPHYLAXIS PHARMACOTHERAPY

Chemoprophylaxis is either primary (directed against preventing the initial episode of clinical PCP) or secondary (directed against relapses or recurrences following treatment of an acute infection). The Department of Health and Human Services (DHHS) recommends that adults and adolescents with HIV infection should receive prophylaxis against PCP if they have a CD4 lymphocyte count of less than 200 per mm^3, unexplained fever (>100°F or >38°C) for more than 2 weeks, or a history of oropharyngeal candidiasis (Fig. 85.2). Some clinicians use a slightly higher CD4 lymphocyte count of 225 to 250 cells per mm^3 if the patient has had a downward trend pattern of the CD4 cell count over the preceding months. Any patient who has recovered from an episode of acute PCP should receive secondary prophylaxis therapy (chronic maintenance therapy).

The effect of HAART that uses triple-drug combinations on suppressing the HIV RNA viral load with immune reconstitution has been impressive. Often the HIV RNA viral load drops below the limits of assay detection (<50 copies/mL), and with it the subsequent restoration of CD4 cell counts above 200 per mm^3. As a result, PCP prophylaxis (primary or secondary) should be discontinued for patients whose CD4+ T-lymphocyte cell count has increased from below 200 cells per mm^3 to above 200 cells per mm^3 for at least 3 months as a result of HAART.[3,20] Prophylaxis should be reintroduced if the CD4 cell count decreases to below 200

cells per mm^3 or, in the setting of secondary prophylaxis, if PCP recurs at a CD4 count of above 200 cells per mm^3.[3]

TMP-SMX, dapsone monotherapy, dapsone plus pyrimethamine, and aerosolized pentamidine are the more common agents used to prevent PCP (Fig. 85.2). No single agent or combination has been shown to be superior to TMP-SMX.[21,22]

ACTG 081 was a randomized trial to evaluate three regimens for primary PCP prophylaxis: TMP-SMX, one double-strength tablet containing TMP 160 mg, and SMX 800 mg given twice daily (a high dose relative to current recommendations); dapsone 50 mg twice daily; and aerosolized pentamidine 300 mg once monthly.[21] Overall, the estimated 36-month risk of PCP was 18%, 17%, and 21%, respectively, for TMP-SMX, dapsone, and aerosolized pentamidine. These differences were not significant. However, for patients with a baseline CD4+ count less than 100 per mm^3, the risk was 33% for aerosolized pentamidine compared to 19% for TMP-SMX and 22% for dapsone ($p = 0.04$). Although aerosolized pentamidine was better tolerated compared to the systemic agents, the inhaled product had two significant limitations: (a) the aerosolized pentamidine group had increased mortality among patients who entered the study with a CD4+ count of below 100 per mm^3 and (b) the group had greater numbers of patients with toxoplasmosis. Thus, this study demonstrates the advantage of systemic chemoprophylaxis, particularly TMP-SMX, over inhalation therapy in preventing PCP.

The use of aerosolized pentamidine for prophylaxis has some limitations, including the following: (a) less efficacy

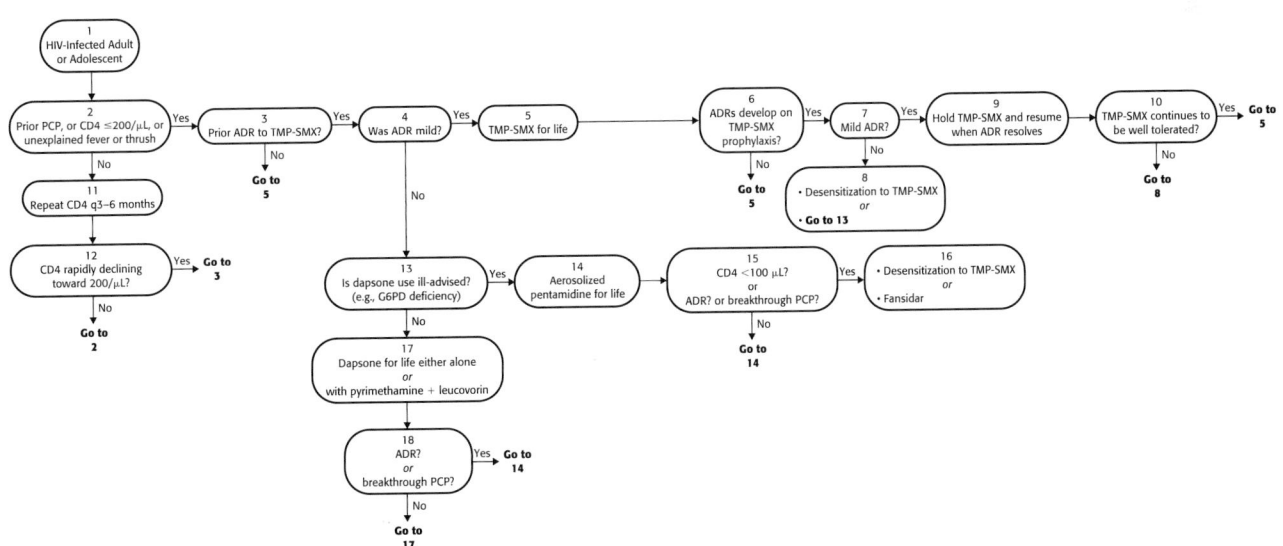

FIGURE 85.2 Algorithm for primary and secondary prophylaxis of *Pneumocystis jirovecii* pneumonia (PCP). Prophylaxis therapy should continue until immune recovery (CD4 count >200 cells/mm^3 for at least 3 months). Refer to Table 85.1 for recommended doses. *ADR*, adverse drug reaction; *CD4*, T-lymphocyte helper cells; *G6PD*, glucose-6-phosphate dehydrogenase; *TMP-SMX*, trimethoprim-sulfamethoxazole. (Reproduced with permission from Stevens RC. Opportunistic infections in AIDS due to protozoal and *Mycobacterium avium* complex. In: Carter BL, Lake KD, Raebel MA, et al., eds. Pharmacotherapy self-assessment program, 3rd ed. Kansas City, MO: American College of Clinical Pharmacy 1998:136.)

compared with TMP-SMX in controlled trials, especially in persons infected with HIV who have advanced immunodeficiency (CD4 count <100 cells/mm^3); (b) increased rates of extrapulmonary foci of *P. jirovecii* infection and pneumothorax; (c) increased risk of PCP manifesting as an upper lobe disease owing to poor distribution of the aerosolized drug to this region; (d) lack of prophylaxis against toxoplasmosis and bacterial infections; and (e) high cost.

Aerosolized pentamidine's clear advantage, however, is its minor toxicity. Side effects (primarily cough, wheezing, and dyspnea during inhalation administration) are mild and infrequent causes of drug discontinuation. These bronchoconstrictive reactions can be diminished or prevented by administration of an inhaled β_2-agonist (e.g., albuterol, two 100-μg puffs) before aerosolized pentamidine. Also, an inhaled β_2-agonist can be used as needed for bronchoconstriction during or after aerosolized pentamidine.

IMPROVING OUTCOMES

The most efficient, cost-effective method to organize treatment of PCP is not well defined, as evidenced by the geographic variation in the management and outcome of the disease. Geographic variations in mortality were accounted for by differences in the severity of illness at admission, insurance status (private versus public versus no insurance), and in-hospital patient management. The latter may be prolonged because of inefficiencies in arranging home care coordination or outpatient follow-up. Independent of the severity of illness, strategies to promote timely diagnostic testing and access to appropriate pharmaceuticals, including outpa-

tient management if the subject is clinically stable, may reduce the variability observed in outcomes.

When the desired outcomes for either acute PCP therapy or PCP prophylaxis are not achieved, then a detailed review of the patient's entire medication regimen is needed. The clinician must reassess whether the patient received optimal treatment, as well as what the new treatment options are. Specific questions that should be asked are presented algorithmically in Figure 85.1: Is the patient receiving his or her medication according to schedule? Have the dosages been adjusted for the patient's weight and renal function? (Refer to Table 85.1 for appropriate dosing regimens.) Is the patient receiving adjunctive corticosteroids if indicated for severe PCP? Does the patient have significant nausea and vomiting or diarrhea? (If so, avoid clindamycin-primaquine and atovaquone, or consider IV therapy.) Has adequate time elapsed (at least 4 to 8 days) to enable an adequate assessment of the efficacy of the regimen in question?

Without question, widespread PCP prophylaxis has had a profound effect. The most obvious effect is that the percentage of new PCP cases categorized as the initial AIDS-defining illness has decreased substantially. As health systems continue to be taxed and further strain valuable resources, it is conceivable that patients may inadvertently lose access to care or pharmaceuticals. Pharmacists are in a unique position to ensure that persons infected with HIV receive optimal prophylaxis for PCP. This is achieved through close monitoring of the patient's CD4 + lymphocyte count, selection of chemoprophylaxis based on the individual's medication history, and, perhaps most important, constant support and motivation to enhance adherence. These activities probably do more to extend the quality of life than any other intervention short of behavioral modifications and strict adherence to antiretroviral therapy.

TOXOPLASMOSIS ENCEPHALITIS

Toxoplasma gondii is a protozoal pathogen that is among the most prevalent causes of CNS infections in individuals infected with HIV. The primary disease associated with *T.*

gondii infection is toxoplasmosis encephalitis, but other sites may be affected, including the eye (retinochoroiditis), lung (pneumonitis), heart, skin, liver, or gut.[23]

TREATMENT GOALS: TOXOPLASMOSIS ENCEPHALITIS

- Design a drug treatment plan for acute opportunistic infection and prophylaxis of toxoplasmosis encephalitis (primary and secondary), as with PCP.
- Design a treatment scheme that includes appropriate monitoring parameters to assess efficacy and tolerance in a person infected with HIV and toxoplasmosis encephalitis.
- Develop an alternative treatment regimen in a patient with a history of intolerance to sulfonamides.
- Select the appropriate drug for secondary prophylaxis of *T. gondii* infection, and counsel patients on how to minimize their risk to toxoplasmosis.
- Identify subjects infected with HIV who may benefit from primary prophylaxis of toxoplasmosis.

EPIDEMIOLOGY

The prevalence of *T. gondii* antibodies among adults infected with HIV is 8% to 16% in major urban areas of the United States.[24] The prevalence is higher (≥25%) in certain ethnic groups, especially Hispanics and Haitians. Even in the HAART era, the overall prevalence of toxoplasmosis encephalitis was 26% in a European registry neuro-AIDS database; it was the most frequent neurologic disorder in the cohort.[25]

Toxoplasmosis most often occurs in persons infected with HIV when the CD4 + count is less than 100 cells per mm³. Ingestion of undercooked or raw meat containing tissue cysts and vegetables or other food products contaminated with oocysts and direct contact with cat feces are major modes of transmission of the parasite.

PATHOPHYSIOLOGY

Once *T. gondii* is ingested and reaches the systemic circulation, it has a high predilection for the CNS.[23] The response of the brain to *T. gondii* infection can vary from a granulomatous reaction to a severe focal or generalized necrotizing encephalitis.[24] Perivascular inflammatory cell infiltrates can lead to fibrosis or necrosis, which can result in hemorrhage or thrombosis, accounting for neurologic signs and symptoms. Necrotizing lesions are not dependent on the host's inflammatory response because severe necrotizing processes may occur with minimal or no inflammation, suggesting that the parasite causes lysis of infected cells.[23,24]

CLINICAL PRESENTATION AND DIAGNOSIS

SIGNS AND SYMPTOMS

The clinical presentation of toxoplasmosis encephalitis is typically a mixture of focal and generalized neurologic deficits. The presentation varies from a subacute course worsening over several weeks to a more acute fulminant process. The most frequent manifestations (usually in more than half of patients in published series) are fever, headache, disorientation, lethargy, and hemiparesis.[24] One third of patients with AIDS who have toxoplasmosis encephalitis seek medical attention because of seizures. Headache can be focal or generalized and can be relentless in intensity, with marginal relief produced by nonsteroidal anti-inflammatory agents or acetaminophen.

DIAGNOSIS

Brain imaging studies [computed tomography (CT) or magnetic resonance imaging (MRI) scans] typically reveal multiple, bilateral, hypodense, enhancing mass lesions. So classic are these findings that the presence of multiple ring-enhancing lesions on CT or MRI scans in a patient with AIDS is assumed to be indicative of clinical toxoplasmosis encephalitis until proven otherwise. A single lesion is uncharacteristic of toxoplasmosis encephalitis and more often is associated with CNS lymphoma. The presumptive diagnosis of toxoplasmosis encephalitis is thus made in persons infected with HIV with positive serology for *T. gondii* antibodies and who have CNS changes and imaging studies consistent with toxoplasmosis encephalitis as described. A brain biopsy to confirm this diagnosis is *not* typically completed unless the patient fails to improve clinically after receiving 10 to 14 days of empiric toxoplasmosis encephalitis therapy or actually clinically deteriorates over at least 3 days of therapy.[24]

TREATMENT

Pharmacologic intervention in the management of toxoplasmosis in individuals infected with HIV is divided into acute therapy, maintenance therapy (i.e., secondary prophylaxis), and primary prophylaxis (Table 85.2).

ACUTE THERAPY

Empiric, first-line therapy involves a combination of pyrimethamine and sulfadiazine plus "leucovorin rescue" for the pyrimethamine-associated toxicities (Fig. 85.3).[3] Toxoplasmosis encephalitis dosage regimens are listed in Table 85.2. The preferred alternative regimen for patients who cannot tolerate or who fail to respond to first-line therapy is pyrimethamine plus clindamycin plus leucovorin. The expert recommendation is to use pyrimethamine-sulfadiazine because of its more established use and better outcome for secondary prophylaxis or maintenance therapy.[26,27] This regimen should be continued for at least 3 weeks, and 6 weeks or more in severe episodes or in patients responding slowly (i.e., lack of or incomplete clinical or radiologic improvement). Monotherapy, which may show initial benefits, is associated with high rates of relapse, even while the drug is continued. For this reason, it is recommended that all therapeutic regimens include two drugs for the entire duration of therapy. Similar treatment scenarios should also be applied to the management of extraneuronal toxoplasmosis.

Pyrimethamine is the cornerstone for current treatment of AIDS-related CNS toxoplasmosis. It is greater than 10 times more potent than TMP in interfering with dihydrofolate synthetase. TMP-SMX was reported in a small (77 patients) randomized trial to be effective and better tolerated than pyrimethamine-sulfadiazine.[28] On the basis of less in vitro activity and fewer comparative clinical trial data, pyrimethamine plus sulfadiazine with leucovorin is the preferred therapy.[3] In the rare event of a patient having concurrent PCP and toxoplasmosis encephalitis, the combination of pyrimethamine-sulfadiazine should be prescribed. No addi-

TABLE 85.2	Treatment of *Toxoplasma gondii* Encephalitis in Patients with AIDS		
Therapy Type	**First-Line Therapy**	**Alternative Therapy**	**Comment**
Acute infection	Pyrimethamine (200 mg loading dose) then pyrimethamine (50–75 mg/day) PO for 3–6 wk + leucovorin (10–25 mg/day) PO + sulfadiazine (1 g q6h) for 3–6 wk	Pyrimethamine (200 mg loading dose) then pyrimethamine (50–75 mg/day) PO for 3–6 wk + one of the following: clindamycin (600 mg PO or IV q6h), clarithromycin (1 g PO q12h), or atovaquone suspension (750 mg PO q8h) or azithromycin (1,200–1,500 mg/day PO) or dapsone (100 mg/day PO)	All HIV-infected persons who respond to acute therapy must receive subsequent maintenance therapy
		TMP (20 mg/kg/day) + SMX (100 mg/kg/day) divided in 3 or 4 doses	TMP-SMX is inferior against *T gondii* compared to first-line therapies. Leucovorin (10–25 mg/day) should be given along with and continued for 72 h after stopping pyrimethamine. Corticosteroids are indicated only for life-threatening cerebral edema/brain mass.
Maintenance therapy	Pyrimethamine (25–75 mg/day) + leucovorin (10–25 mg/day) + sulfadiazine (500–1,000 mg PO q6h)	Pyrimethamine (50–100 mg/day) + leucovorin	Maintenance therapy with pyrimethamine-clindamycin does not provide effective prophylaxis against PCP and alternatives are needed (e.g., TMP-SMX).
	Pyrimethamine (25–75 mg/day) + leucovorin (10–25 mg/day) + clindamycin (300–450 mg PO q6-8h)	Pyrimethamine (50 mg/day) + leucovorin + one of the following: atovaquone suspension (750 mg q8h) or clarithromycin (1,000 mg q12h), or azithromycin (1,200–1,500 mg/day)	
		Pyrimethamine (25 mg) + sulfadoxine (500 mg) PO 2 times/week (equal to Fansidar 1 tablet twice weekly) + leucovorin (10–25 mg/Fansidar dose)	
Primary prophylaxis	TMP-SMX (1 DS tablet/day)	TMP-SMX (1 SS tablet/day)	Strong support for primary prophylaxis in HIV-infected pts with positive *T gondii* serology plus CD4+ count <200/mm³
		Pyrimethamine (50 mg/wk) + leucovorin (25 mg/wk) + dapsone (50 mg/day)	
		Pyrimethamine (25–75 mg/wk) + leucovorin (25 mg/wk) + dapsone (100–200 mg/wk)	

TMP, trimethoprim; SMX, sulfamethoxazole; SS, single-strength; TMP-SMX tablet; DS, double-strength TMP-SMX tablet.
(Adapted from Centers for Disease Control and Prevention. Treating opportunistic infections among HIV-infected adults and adolescents; recommendations from CDC, the National Institutes of Health, and the HIV Medicine Association/Infectious Diseases Society of America. Clin Infect Dis 40 (Suppl 3):S131–S235, 2005; and from Stevens RC. Opportunistic infections in AIDS due to protozoal and *Mycobacterium avium* complex. In: Carter BL, Lake KD, Raebel MA, et al, eds. Pharmacotherapy self-assessment program, 3rd ed. Kansas City, MO: American College of Clinical Pharmacy 1998:129–130, 2000.)

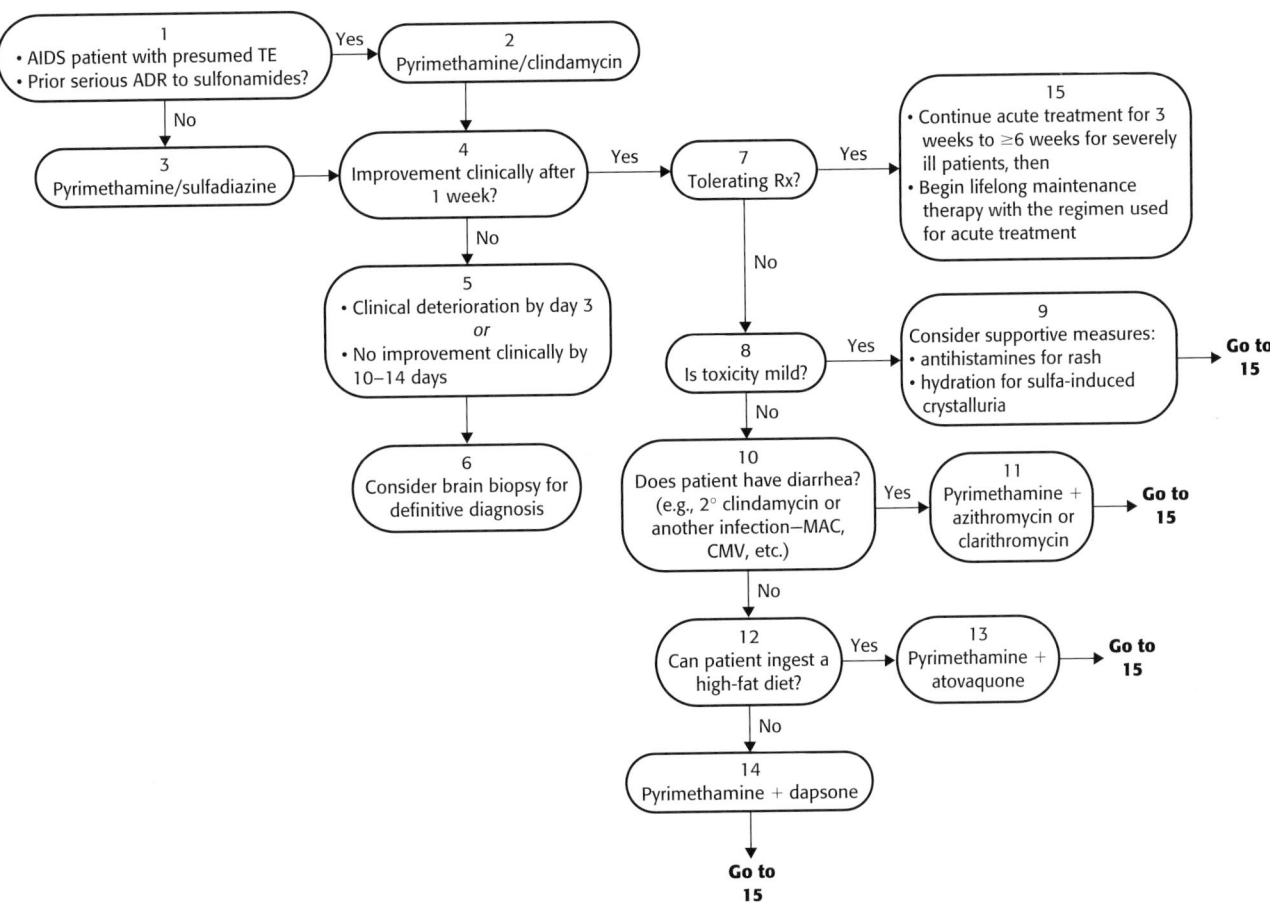

FIGURE 85.3 Algorithm for empiric treatment of toxoplasmosis encephalitis. Following acute therapy, maintenance therapy is required to prevent relapse until immune restoration has occurred. Leucovorin (folinic acid) should be administered with pyrimethamine. Atovaquone is the suspension formulation. ADR, adverse drug reaction; CMV, cytomegalovirus; MAC, *Mycobacterium avium* complex. (Reproduced with permission from Stevens RC. Opportunistic infections in AIDS due to protozoal and *Mycobacterium avium* complex. In: Carter BL, Lake KD, Raebel MA, et al., eds. Pharmacotherapy self-assessment program, 3rd ed. Kansas City, MO: American College of Clinical Pharmacy 1998:139.)

tional drugs are needed for therapy of concurrent infections from these two protozoal pathogens.

Treatment-terminating adverse reactions are experienced by up to 40% of patients.[24] The most notable toxicities of pyrimethamine are rash and dose-related bone marrow suppression that results in neutropenia, thrombocytopenia, and megaloblastic anemia. Hematologic suppression can be expected at pyrimethamine doses of 75 to 100 mg per day.

Leucovorin (folinic acid) is recommended to prevent pyrimethamine-induced ''cytopenias.'' As noted in the PCP section, concurrent use of leucovorin with TMP-SMX for acute PCP is contraindicated; however, this is not true with pyrimethamine, where ''leucovorin rescue'' is recommended. Folic acid must not be substituted for leucovorin because it is reported that folic acid will inhibit the activity of pyrimethamine against *T. gondii*.[24]

Adverse effects from sulfadiazine commonly include rash, nephrotoxicity with crystalluria, blood dyscrasias, and CNS effects. There have been few reports of life-threatening sulfadiazine-associated rashes, which should not preclude the use of sulfadiazine for patients who experience a macular rash. Crystalluria is reversed with hydration, alkalinization of the urine, and dose reduction.[29] Sulfadiazine can cause an encephalitis-like syndrome that can be clinically indistinguishable from worsening toxoplasmosis encephalitis to the clinician who is not suspicious of such toxicity.

Alternative therapies investigated in nonrandomized, uncontrolled trials include (a) atovaquone (with meals) plus pyrimethamine plus leucovorin;[30] (b) atovaquone with sulfadiazine or, for patients intolerant of both pyrimethamine and sulfadiazine, as a single agent;[30] and (c) azithromycin plus pyrimethamine plus leucovorin daily.[31,32] Relapse occurred in approximately 50% of patients in whom atovaquone was used alone for acute and subsequent maintenance therapy.[33] If atovaquone is used alone, measuring plasma levels might be useful given the high variability of drug absorption; plasma levels of at least 18.5 g per mL are associated with an improved response rate. Appropriately conducted clinical trials are needed to assess the role of these alternative combinations in treating AIDS-related toxoplasmosis encephalitis.

Adjunctive corticosteroid therapy with dexamethasone to relieve inflammation and cerebral edema frequently is required for management of patients with intracranial hypertension caused by the mass effect of *T. gondii* abscesses. The response rate, time to response, and mortality in patients who received corticosteroids was no different compared with those who did not receive steroids.[34] At present, the DHHS treatment guidelines recommend that adjunctive corticosteroids (e.g., dexamethasone) be administered when clinically indicated only for treatment of a mass effect associated with focal lesions or associated edema.[3] The dosage depends on the clinical severity, and duration should be for no more than 2 weeks if possible.[24]

MAINTENANCE THERAPY (SECONDARY PROPHYLAXIS)

The relapse rate after 12 months of toxoplasmosis encephalitis in patients with AIDS who do not receive maintenance therapy is 50% to 80%.[24] Thus, patients with AIDS who successfully complete acute toxoplasmosis encephalitis therapy must be maintained on lifelong antitoxoplasma agents. Some patients even relapse while on maintenance therapy, and undoubtedly poor adherence or drug intolerance contributes to this relapse rate. Maintenance doses are usually lower (as low as 25 mg/day) compared with those used for acute therapy (Table 85.2).

The regimen of pyrimethamine-sulfadiazine with leucovorin appears to have a lower relapse rate than other drug regimens and thus is recommended most often for maintenance therapy.[24] Unlike the efficacy of TMP-SMX given three times weekly for secondary PCP prophylaxis, pyrimethamine-sulfadiazine administered twice weekly had a high relapse rate of 30% by 12 months. The relapse rate for daily administration of pyrimethamine-sulfadiazine was only 6% by 12 months.[35] Thus, the latter regimen should be taken daily for secondary prophylaxis (maintenance therapy) of toxoplasmosis encephalitis. However, administration twice weekly may be an option in patients who cannot continue daily use because of significant drug intolerance. Importantly, patients receiving pyrimethamine-sulfadiazine for toxoplasmosis encephalitis maintenance therapy do not need further PCP prophylaxis because of activity against both pathogens with this regimen.[36]

Pyrimethamine-clindamycin is an alternative for maintenance therapy in patients with intolerance to sulfonamides because of a higher rate of relapse. Furthermore, this combination is less desirable because it does not prevent PCP. Pyrimethamine-sulfadoxine (Fansidar) is another alternative that offers the advantage of being dosed as one tablet orally twice weekly. Leucovorin (10 to 25 mg orally) should be added on the days of the week that the patient takes pyrimethamine-sulfadoxine. Side effects were relatively common (40%), with 7% of patients discontinuing therapy because of toxicity.[37] Pyrimethamine used alone at daily doses of 50 and 100 mg had relapse rates of 10% to 28% and 5%, respectively, suggesting that the higher dose may offer good protection in patients with AIDS who cannot tolerate sulfonamides, clindamycin, or any of the other less-studied agents.

PRIMARY PROPHYLAXIS

Despite the availability of effective regimens, toxoplasmosis in patients with AIDS is associated with a mortality rate of 70% by 12 months after diagnosis.[24] This statistic alone strongly supports the use of primary prophylaxis in persons infected with HIV who are at the greatest risk of toxoplasmosis encephalitis when their CD4 cell count is less than 200 per mm^3 (as is the situation in 90% of toxoplasmosis encephalitis cases). In addition, persons infected with HIV who are seronegative for *T. gondii* antibodies should receive instructions on how to protect themselves from initial inoculation or newly acquired infection. Such measures include: (a) eating meat that is well cooked (not pink or bloody); (b) avoiding touching the mouth and eyes (i.e., mucous membranes) while handling raw meat; (c) washing hands thoroughly after handling raw meat; (d) washing all kitchen utensils, cutting boards, and surfaces that come in contact with raw meat with hot soapy water; (e) washing fresh fruit and vegetables before consumption; and (f) avoiding contact, if possible, with cat feces or cat litter boxes, or wearing gloves when disposing of cat litter.

In various reports, TMP-SMX, pyrimethamine-dapsone, and pyrimethamine-sulfadoxine were effective in preventing toxoplasmosis encephalitis (Table 85.2). A randomized trial that compared TMP-SMX with pyrimethamine-dapsone indicated that both regimens were effective against toxoplasmosis.[38] However, the TMP-SMX regimen appeared to be more protective against PCP.[38,39] Between these two regimens, up to 40% to 60% of patients will experience side effects and 2% to 12% will require discontinuation of therapy. Pyrimethamine alone is not considered a first-line agent for primary prophylaxis because of its less protective effect compared with TMP-SMX.[40,41]

TMP-SMX in low doses used intermittently for PCP prophylaxis prevents toxoplasmosis in patients with AIDS with positive *Toxoplasma* antibodies.[38,39] Thus, measures to enhance TMP-SMX adherence and minimize intolerance are critical. Until other preventive agents are identified, every effort (intermittent dose schedules, desensitization protocols, use of antihistamines) should be made to maintain patients with AIDS whose CD4+ counts are less than 100 per mm^3 on TMP-SMX for prophylaxis against *P. jirovecii* and *T. gondii*.

MYCOBACTERIUM AVIUM COMPLEX

Disseminated MAC is an opportunistic infection observed in persons infected with HIV who have a more advanced stage of AIDS compared with PCP or toxoplasmosis encephalitis, as represented by a lower CD4 count. Although MAC is not yet curable in the HIV-infected host, advances in chemoprophylaxis have resulted in fewer symptoms and prolonged survival. Implementation of HAART regimens has significantly decreased the occurrence of MAC infection and underscores the importance of restoring the immune system in persons with AIDS.[42]

TREATMENT GOALS: *MYCOBACTERIUM AVIUM* COMPLEX

- Construct a treatment regimen that provides the most efficacious outcome while minimizing drug intolerance and the potential for the significant drug interactions that are associated with anti-MAC therapy.
- Identify subjects infected with HIV who may benefit from primary prophylaxis of MAC infections.
- Implement HAART regimens along with appropriate regimens against MAC as the most effective strategy for treating disseminated MAC infections.[43]
- Make certain that all anti-MAC regimens contain an extended-spectrum macrolide antibiotic (preferably clarithromycin).
- The goals for treatment of MAC are well defined: Reduce or eradicate the number of organisms, ameliorate the symptoms of infection, and enhance the quality and duration of life.

EPIDEMIOLOGY

The state of immunodeficiency in persons infected with HIV is the single most important factor that predicts the risk of MAC infection. Disseminated MAC has occurred almost exclusively in individuals with advanced HIV infection, especially in patients with CD4 + cell counts less than 50 per mm^3.[44] There is an inverse relationship between the risk of acquiring MAC and the CD4 + count: the risk is extremely high (approaches 80% by 12 months) when the CD4 + count is less than 10 per mm^3. It is hoped that this will change as more patients are exposed to the potency of HAART regimens and MAC prophylaxis. In the absence of these chemotherapeutic interventions, the yearly rate of development of MAC is 20% to 25% following an initial AIDS-defining illness and a CD4 + count less than 100 per mm^3.

PATHOPHYSIOLOGY

MAC organisms are ubiquitous environmental saprophytes found in soil, water, animals, birds, food, and tobacco. The portal of entry for MAC into the body is presumed to be the gastrointestinal tract or the lungs. Macrophages in the small bowel can be found to be teeming with mycobacterial invasion, and respiratory isolation of MAC frequently precedes disseminated disease. It is unknown whether MAC infection results primarily from acquisition of the organism from environmental exposure or reactivation of latent endogenous infection. Person-to-person transmission is unlikely, as suggested by the absence of an increased risk of developing the disease among individuals infected with HIV who are housemates or close contacts of those with MAC disease.

It is not always a given that HIV-infected patients with MAC have positive mycobacterial blood cultures.[45] MAC has also been isolated from liver, spleen, lymph nodes, lung, adrenals, colon, kidney, and bone marrow. The organism can colonize the stool, urine, or respiratory secretions, which may or may not be associated with localized symptoms.

CLINICAL PRESENTATION AND DIAGNOSIS

SIGNS AND SYMPTOMS

The disabling complications associated with MAC include fever, malaise, night sweats, severe weight loss, anemia, neutropenia, diarrhea, abdominal pain, and malabsorption. These manifestations can result in profound fatigue, weakness, and emaciation that ultimately marginalize the quality of life for these patients.

DIAGNOSIS

Special blood culture techniques for isolating mycobacteria with nearly 100% sensitivity are available. Time to culture positivity ranges from 5 to 51 days. It is uncommon for blood cultures to be negative when there is a positive histologic diagnosis from lymph node, liver, or bone marrow biopsies.

In a prospective natural history study at San Francisco General Hospital among persons infected with HIV, the following were sensitive predictors of MAC bacteremia: (a) CD4 + cell count less than 50 per mm^3; (b) history of fever for more than 30 days; (c) hematocrit less than 30%; or (d) a serum albumin level less than 3.0 g per dL.[46]

TREATMENT

PHARMACOTHERAPY

Monotherapy of MAC in patients with AIDS is not effective and should not be used.[3] Although patients may show initial improvement, symptoms subsequently recur and the organisms proliferate. This suggests that monotherapy provides only a transient benefit, organisms can re-emerge, and resistance can develop. With 1 billion-plus MAC organisms burdening the immunodeficient host, a relatively large number of resistant organisms will exist as wild-type strains. Under the selective pressure of single-drug therapy, resistant organisms will continue to proliferate in the infected tissue. Thus, the most appropriate therapy of MAC in persons infected with HIV is polypharmacy, which parallels the management of HIV and tuberculosis (Table 85.3).

Initial treatment of MAC disease should consist of two antimycobacterial drugs to prevent or delay the emergence of resistance. Clarithromycin is the preferred first agent: it has been studied more extensively than azithromycin and appears to be associated with more rapid clearance of MAC from the blood.[3,47,48] However, azithromycin can be substituted for clarithromycin when drug interactions or clarithromycin intolerance occurs. Ethambutol is the recommended second drug: it has good in vitro activity, was superior to clofazimine when each was combined with a macrolide, is generally well tolerated in the doses used clinically, and does not have the potential drug interactions associated with rifabutin.[48–50]

The addition of rifabutin should be considered in persons with advanced immunosuppression (CD4 cell count <50/mm^3), high mycobacterial loads (>2 log$_{10}$ colony-forming units/mL of blood), in the absence of effective HAART, or in settings in which mortality is increased and emergence of drug resistance is most likely.[3] If rifabutin cannot be used because of drug interactions or intolerance, a third or fourth drug may be selected from among either the quinolones (ciprofloxacin or levofloxacin) or parenteral amikacin, although data supporting a survival or microbiologic benefit when these agents are added have not been compelling.[51,52]

TABLE 85.3	Treatment of *Mycobacterium avium* Complex in Patients With AIDS		
Therapy Type	**First-Line Therapy**	**Alternative Therapy**	**Comment**
Acute infection	Multidrug regimen of at least 2 drugs: clarithromycin (500 mg PO BID) + ethambutol (15 mg/kg/day PO)	Alternative to clarithromycin Azithromycin 500–600 mg QD Alternative third or fourth drug for severe disease: Ciprofloxacin (500–750 mg PO BID), or Levofloxacin (500 mg PO QD), or Amikacin (10–15 mg/kg IV QD)	Resistance develops with monotherapy. Maintenance therapy can be discontinued in pts who complete at least 12 months of therapy, remain asymptomatic, and have a sustained (at least 6 months) CD4 count >100 cells/mm^3.
	Consider adding rifabutin 300 mg PO QD to the above regimens in pts with CD4 <50 cells/mm^3, high mycobacterial loads, or ineffective HAART options.		Mortality is higher when clarithromycin dose exceeds 1,000 mg/day.
			Mortality was increased when clofazimine was added to clarithromycin + ethambutol. Its use must be carefully weighed.
Prophylaxis	Clarithromycin (500 mg PO BID) Azithromycin (1,200 mg/wk PO)	Rifabutin (300 mg/day PO)	Prophylaxis is recommended for CD4+ counts <50/mm^3

(Adapted from Centers of Disease Control and Prevention. Treating opportunistic infections among HIV-infected adults and adolescents: recommendatoins from CDC, the National Institutes of Health, and the HIV Medicine Association/Infectious Diseases Society of America. Clin Infect Dis 40 (Suppl 3):S131–S235, 2005; and Stevens RC. Opportunistic infections in AIDS due to protozoal and *Mycobacterium avium* complex. In Carter BL, Lake KD, Raebel MA, et al, eds. Pharmacotherapy self-assessment program, 3rd ed. Kansas City, MO: American College of Clinical Pharmacy 1998:129–130.)

Approximately two thirds of patients receiving the macrolide-ethambutol regimen can be anticipated to become culture negative.[49,50] Overall, MAC colony-forming units can be expected to decrease by about 1 to 2 logs from baseline with appropriate therapy. The time course for clinical response to MAC therapy is variable, but most patients who defervesce and improve symptomatically do so after 2 weeks. The symptoms at 4 weeks should not continue at the same intensity as baseline if the patient is experiencing a beneficial response.

Alternative drugs (rifabutin, clofazimine, ciprofloxacin, and, in some situations, amikacin) for management of MAC are less than ideal, mainly due to lack of beneficial microbiologic or clinical response, drug interactions, and intolerance. With the administration of protease inhibitors and the potential for drug interactions with rifabutin, use of this antimycobacterial has become more complicated, as described in the drug interaction section below. Clofazimine has a slow onset of action and has the undesirable side effect of skin hyperpigmentation, but it is rarely the cause of severe toxicity. However, clofazimine added to a regimen of clarithromycin and ethambutol for MAC bacteremia in patients with AIDS was shown not to contribute to clinical response and was associated with higher mortality.[50] This finding provides compelling evidence to question the continued use of clofazimine in the therapy of MAC infection. High doses of ciprofloxacin (750 mg one or two times per day) may cause intolerable gastrointestinal distress. IV ciprofloxacin and IV or intramuscular amikacin should be considered in patients with severe symptomatic disease in whom gastrointestinal absorption of the oral medications may be marginal.

Adverse Effects of Anti-MAC Agents. Adverse effects associated with anti-MAC drugs are not as notorious for treatment-terminating events as are the drugs used for PCP or toxoplasmosis. The macrolides are generally well tolerated, with gastrointestinal disturbances (e.g., anorexia, diarrhea, abdominal pain) being the most common adverse effects; these can be alleviated by dividing the dose and administering it more frequently throughout the day. Taste perversion has been associated with clarithromycin.

Ethambutol can cause hyperuricemia or acute gout, but this is an infrequent observation in the HIV-infected population. Retrobulbar neuritis is rarely seen with ethambutol at the dosage recommended for MAC (15 mg/kg/day), but it is possible when dosages are not adjusted in patients with renal impairment. A pink to brownish-black discoloration of the skin is a common adverse effect of clofazimine. Other sites affected by these color changes are conjunctiva, tears, sweat, urine, feces, and nasal secretions. The discolorations are not a source of any symptoms but can be a troubling cosmetic problem. Peripheral neuropathies associated with clofazimine warrant further precaution in patients receiving antiretroviral therapy with didanosine or stavudine because these antiretrovirals can also cause peripheral neuropathy.

The high dose of ciprofloxacin recommended for MAC can result in headaches and restlessness.

Rifabutin, like rifampin, causes orange discoloration of bodily secretions, transaminase elevations, myalgias and arthralgias, rash, and hematologic toxicities. Uveitis is associated with rifabutin and appears to be a concentration-dependent toxicity.[53] Symptoms include acute onset of ocular pain, blurry vision, photophobia, and diminished visual acuity. Rifabutin should be discontinued when these symptoms occur. Ophthalmic corticosteroids or atropine drops cause rapid improvement in symptoms and clinical findings. In mild cases, rifabutin can be restarted with close monitoring for symptoms and careful review of the patient's medication profile to avoid drugs that may increase the rifabutin concentrations.

Drug Interactions Associated with Anti-MAC Agents. Drug interactions with agents used in MAC regimens are extensive, and many are clinically significant. This is a primary area in which pharmacists can provide significant input into drug selection to avoid drug interactions that may reduce efficacy or accentuate toxicity. Careful review of the patient's concurrent medications is essential to avoid drug interactions during therapy or prophylaxis of MAC.

Clarithromycin, an inhibitor of the cytochrome P450 metabolic pathway, can increase the serum concentrations of theophylline, carbamazepine, digoxin, and warfarin. Alternatively, protease inhibitors, which are potent inhibitors of the P450 3A metabolic pathway, can increase clarithromycin concentrations by over 50% in some cases. The provider needs to refer to the product label for appropriate dose reduction of clarithromycin when used with HAART regimens containing protease inhibitors.

A bidirectional drug interaction is observed between clarithromycin and rifabutin. Clarithromycin can inhibit the metabolism of rifabutin and its active metabolite. The area under the concentration–time curve (AUC) for rifabutin increased approximately twofold when co-administered with clarithromycin. The higher rifabutin concentrations may be associated with greater toxicity (e.g., uveitis). Conversely, rifabutin, an inducer of the cytochrome P450 pathway, can decrease the mean plasma concentration of clarithromycin by up to 30%. The impact of this bidirectional interaction on clinical efficacy is not known. No guidelines for dosage modifications exist, so close patient monitoring for therapeutic response and toxicity is imperative. Azithromycin may be a more suitable macrolide when combined with rifabutin because the former is not typically associated with drug interactions via P450 inhibition (e.g., unlike clarithromycin, azithromycin does not cause a clinically significant interaction with theophylline).

Rifabutin, like rifampin but to a lesser extent, is an enzyme inducer and as such can increase the hepatic metabolism of certain drugs (e.g., protease inhibitors, ketoconazole, and dapsone) used in the management of persons infected with HIV. It would seem prudent to avoid dapsone for PCP prophylaxis in patients requiring rifabutin for MAC therapy. Zidovudine's AUC can be decreased by 30% when administered with rifabutin, but the clinical significance of this potential interaction is not known. Fluconazole can increase concentrations of rifabutin and its active metabolite by at least 80%.[54] Rifabutin, unlike rifampin, does not alter fluconazole metabolism.

If coadministration of rifabutin and a protease inhibitor, especially those with pharmacokinetic enhancement with ritonavir (i.e., "boosting"), is necessary, the healthcare provider needs to consult the product label of the protease inhibitor for appropriate dose reduction of rifabutin. Ritonavir markedly inhibits the metabolism of rifabutin via the cytochrome P450 3A pathway. For example, when co-administered with lopinavir-ritonavir, dosage reduction of rifabutin by at least 75% of the usual dose of 300 mg per day is recommended (i.e., a maximum dose of 150 mg every other day or three times per week). Failure to reduce the rifabutin dose with protease inhibitors will most likely result in rifabutin toxicity.

Ciprofloxacin can increase serum concentrations of theophylline, caffeine, warfarin, and cyclosporine. Concurrent administration of cation-containing antacids will decrease ciprofloxacin absorption significantly. This can be avoided by giving the quinolone 2 hours before the antacid. Didanosine can also reduce the bioavailability of ciprofloxacin, and doses should be spaced 2 hours apart.

PROPHYLAXIS PHARMACOTHERAPY

Individuals with HIV infection should receive chemoprophylaxis against disseminated MAC disease if they have a CD4 count below 50 cells per mm[3].[44] Clarithromycin or azithromycin is the preferred prophylactic agent. The combination of clarithromycin and rifabutin is no more effective than clarithromycin alone for chemoprophylaxis and is associated with a higher rate of adverse effects than either drug alone; thus, this combination should not be used.[44,55,56]

Azithromycin may be preferred because it is often easier for patients to take medication once weekly than twice daily as with clarithromycin, drug interactions are less problematic, and it may be less costly. Patients unable to tolerate the two 600-mg tablets of azithromycin may split the regimen and take one tablet in the morning and one tablet in the evening until gastrointestinal tolerance develops. The two 600-mg tablets can be taken with or without food, unlike the capsules, which should be taken on an empty stomach. The tablets can simplify medication administration for patients receiving protease inhibitors because the latter drugs also require close attention to timing of meals.

Combined results from two randomized, placebo-controlled trials of rifabutin prophylaxis in more than 1,100 patients infected with HIV with median CD4 counts in the mid-50s showed that rifabutin 300 mg per day reduced the incidence of MAC bacteremia by one half.[57] This result was almost exclusively observed in patients with CD4 counts of 75 per mm[3] or less at study entry, and there was no benefit in patients with CD4 counts above 100 per mm[3]. Overall survival did not differ between the two groups, but the trial was not designed to show such differences.

Rifabutin is an alternative prophylactic agent in patients intolerant to macrolides (Table 85.3). Lifelong rifabutin prophylaxis may not be feasible in selected patients. Adverse effects that may limit the use of rifabutin are neutropenia, thrombocytopenia, rash, nausea, flatulence, hepatitis, and arthralgias. A red-orange discoloration of urine, tears, sweat, or other body fluids can occur; soft contact lenses may be permanently stained. Patients receiving antiretroviral therapy with protease inhibitors generally, as a precaution, should not be administered rifabutin prophylaxis. As noted previously, if coadministration is necessary, the dose of rifabutin should be reduced by 50% when given with indinavir or nelfinavir, which are the preferred protease inhibitors in this setting because ritonavir is contraindicated with rifabutin.

Primary MAC prophylaxis should be discontinued among patients who have responded to HAART with an increase in the CD4 count to above 100 cells per mm[3] for at least 3 months.[44,58] Secondary prophylaxis (chronic maintenance therapy) can be discontinued when patients have completed a course of at least 12 months of treatment for MAC, remain asymptomatic with respect to MAC disease, and have a sustained increase (e.g., at least 6 months) in their CD4 cell counts to above 100 per mm[3] after HAART.[44]

IMPROVING OUTCOMES

PATIENT EDUCATION

The effectiveness of MAC therapy or prevention involves an understanding by the person infected with HIV about the opportunistic infection and the complexity of the medications used in its management. Other therapies (e.g., antiretrovirals, PCP prophylaxis) may confuse the patient and lead to poor adherence to the prescribed medications. Another caveat is that it may be necessary to coach the patient through the first 2 to 4 weeks to adhere to the MAC regimen, because a response usually is not immediate. Mycobacteria grow slowly, symptoms are insidious, and response to treatment is slow. Therefore, patients may need to be encouraged to adhere to treatment in the first few weeks, especially if they state that the drugs are not helping them to feel better.

METHODS TO IMPROVE PATIENT ADHERENCE TO DRUG THERAPY

Without question, patient outcomes can be improved if the healthcare provider can simplify the anti-MAC drug regimen, whether it be for treatment of MAC or its prevention. Effective disease management can be promoted by simplifying anti-MAC drug regimens so that dosing schemes are convenient (once-daily dosing of azithromycin and ethambutol), drug interactions are minimized (avoid rifabutin if possible), and drugs whose bioavailability are affected by food are avoided (azithromycin capsules). Incorporating these strategies in patient care will ultimately enhance adherence and improve outcomes in persons infected with HIV with MAC infection.

CYTOMEGALOVIRUS

CMV infection is an opportunistic infection in persons with AIDS that can result in significant morbidity and diminished quality of life if not treated properly. End-organ diseases produced by CMV are retinitis, colitis, and encephalitis. This section will be limited to a discussion of CMV retinitis because this accounts for 75% to 85% of CMV disease in patients with AIDS.

TREATMENT GOALS: CYTOMEGALOVIRUS

- Use CMV treatment modalities, which have enhanced the options for therapy and prevention of this opportunistic viral infection.
- Reverse or attenuate the retinitis, which ultimately can lead to blindness. Use ganciclovir or foscarnet as first-line therapy, depending on the underlying clinical conditions in patients, while reserving the use of cidofovir to subjects with refractory CMV disease.
- Discuss with the patient the role and potential complications associated with ganciclovir intraocular implants, if clinically indicated.
- Consider ganciclovir for prevention of CMV disease in persons with advanced AIDS who are seropositive for CMV and willing to commit to prevention until restoration of immune function is achieved with HAART.

EPIDEMIOLOGY

Retinitis is the most common manifestation of CMV infection in persons with AIDS. The majority of infections result from the reactivation of latent infection. Prior to the widespread use of HAART, clinical evidence of CMV retinitis occurred in as many as 40% of subjects infected with HIV, and autopsy series have revealed that CMV retinitis was present in up to 30% of patients.[59] Persons infected with HIV who are CMV seropositive with a CD4+ cell count of less than 50 per mm^3 are at greatest risk of CMV retinitis. The profound effect of HAART therapy has reduced the occurrence of CMV disease in patients with AIDS from its peak during the mid-1990s. In one large urban HIV center, the incidence of CMV disease was reduced by 80% because of combination antiretroviral therapy.[60]

PATHOPHYSIOLOGY

Ophthalmologic examination shows large creamy to yellowish-white granular areas of retinal necrosis and edema that follow a vascular distribution and can be hemorrhagic. This observation has been dubbed a "cottage cheese and ketchup" appearance. These pathophysiologic changes may be isolated early on at the periphery of the fundus, but if left untreated the lesions progress within 2 to 3 weeks.[59] Ultimately, irreversible damage to the retina occurs, leading to diminished visual acuity and eventually blindness. Retinitis usually begins unilaterally but can progress to contralateral involvement in patients with systemic CMV viremia.

CLINICAL PRESENTATION AND DIAGNOSIS

SIGNS AND SYMPTOMS

Decreased visual acuity, the presence of floaters (spots in front of the eyes that "float" across the visual field) or light flashes, or unilateral loss of the central or peripheral visual field is the usual presenting complaint of patients with AIDS with CMV retinitis. Patients may be asymptomatic initially or may have poorly defined complaints about their vision. Photophobia or ocular pain is not associated with CMV retinitis.

Most patients with CMV retinitis have good vision at presentation, with 70% to 80% having a visual acuity of 20/40 or better.[61,62] Despite systemic therapy with ganciclovir or foscarnet, progressive visual loss occurs over time. In 287 patients with CMV retinitis, the median time to vision of 20/200 or worse in an eye with retinitis was 13.4 months;

time to bilateral vision of 20/200 or worse was 21.1 months.[61]

DIAGNOSIS

The diagnosis of CMV retinitis is clinical. Virtually all patients infected with HIV with CMV retinitis have CD4+ cell counts less than 50 per mm[3] and are seropositive for CMV. An ophthalmologist can establish the diagnosis on examination of both fundi by indirect ophthalmoscopy after pupillary dilation and finding the "cottage cheese and ketchup" appearance.

PSYCHOSOCIAL ASPECTS

Irreversible vision loss as a result of retinitis can be devastating because it affects all aspects of one's daily activities. Suddenly, what once was routine becomes dependent on others—patients may be unable to drive or complete simple errands. Reading books or watching television may no longer be possible. Obviously, it may be overwhelming to cope with the implications of such drastic alterations in lifestyle. Professional counseling can be offered, but perhaps more important is the provision of necessary support services to compensate for any lifestyle changes.

TREATMENT

The management of CMV retinitis involves two phases: (a) induction therapy for acute infection and (b) maintenance therapy (i.e., secondary prophylaxis) following completion of the induction phase pending immune recovery. More than one treatment regimen could be appropriate in most settings.

PHARMACOTHERAPY

Induction and Maintenance Therapy. The choice of initial therapy for CMV retinitis should be individualized based on the location and severity of the lesion(s), immune function, other factors such as concomitant medications that could augment drug toxicity, acceptance of parenterally administered antiviral drugs and willingness to comply, and quality of life. Oral valganciclovir, IV ganciclovir, IV ganciclovir followed by oral valganciclovir, IV foscarnet, IV cidofovir, and the ganciclovir intraocular implant coupled with valganciclovir are all effective treatments for CMV retinitis.[62–66]

The ganciclovir intraocular implant is a novel approach to drug delivery for CMV retinitis and is recommended for immediate sight-threatening lesions.[3] The implant requires intraocular surgery and is subject to surgical complications. Many patients have immediate transient blurred vision with their current glasses that resolves within a few weeks. Approximately 10% of patients who received implants complain of a vision-compromising event. The benefit of this drug delivery device is that the median time to progression

of disease (216 to 226 days) is significantly prolonged compared with the IV therapies.[63] The implant is depleted of ganciclovir after 5 to 8 months and must be replaced, which exposes the patient to subsequent risks (e.g., surgical complication, retinal detachment). The outcome of undergoing several reimplantation procedures is not known.[63] The major adverse event is retinal detachment, which can be a cause of substantial visual impairment. In addition, the local effect of the implant does not protect against disease that may develop in the contralateral eye.

Daily IV infusions of ganciclovir or foscarnet, or weekly then biweekly IV infusions of cidofovir are each appropriate initial choices for induction and maintenance therapy for CMV retinitis.[3] Induction therapy is for 14 to 21 days followed by lifelong maintenance therapy (Table 85.4). Ganciclovir and foscarnet require lifelong daily IV infusions. The cost and inconvenience of these infusions and the risk of serious infections associated with central venous catheters are problematic.[67] The prolonged dosing interval for IV cidofovir may offset the need for a central line catheter and offer the patient greater flexibility in lifestyle; however, problems with nephrotoxicity may diminish the advantage of weekly dosing. Oral valganciclovir can be used as monotherapy for induction therapy for peripheral lesions of CMV retinitis.

Numerous case series have reported that maintenance therapy can be discontinued safely among HIV-infected patients with CMV retinitis whose CD4 counts have achieved a sustained (at least 6 months) increase to above 100 to 150 cells per mm[3] in response to HAART.[44] The decision to discontinue maintenance therapy needs to be made in concert with an ophthalmologist, and it needs to be underscored that the immune recovery must be sustained and robust. Reinstitution of secondary prophylaxis should be implemented if the CD4 cell count falls below the threshold noted above.

Bone marrow suppression (neutropenia, thrombocytopenia) is the most significant adverse effect with systemic ganciclovir. Concentration-dependent neutropenia can be reversed with the use of granulocyte colony-stimulating factor, starting at a dose of 300 μg three times per week and then titrating the dose over time.[67] It is imperative to assess kidney function (estimate creatinine clearance) and adjust the dose accordingly, because ganciclovir is primarily renally eliminated as unchanged drug. The complete blood count (including white blood cells with differential) should be monitored at least weekly during induction therapy and weekly during the maintenance phase. Patients should be switched to foscarnet if neutropenia is severe (<500 to 1000 cells/mm[3]).

Dose-limiting toxicities occur in approximately 30% of patients who receive IV foscarnet and include nephrotoxicity, electrolyte imbalances, nausea, malaise, genital ulcers, and neurologic symptoms. Patients should be hydrated before and during the infusion to reduce the risk of nephrotoxicity, which can be augmented with concurrent administration of other nephrotoxic agents (e.g., amphotericin B, IV pent-

TABLE 85.4	Treatment of Cytomegalovirus Retinitis in Patients With AIDS		
Therapy Type	**First-Line Therapy**	**Alternative Therapy**	**Comment**
Induction and maintenance therapy	For immediate sight-threatening lesions: Ganciclovir intraocular implant and valganciclovir (900 mg PO QD) For peripheral lesions: Valganciclovir (900 mg PO BID for 14–21 days, then 900 mg PO QD)	Ganciclovir (5 mg/kg IV q12h) for 14–21 days, then 5 mg/kg IV QD, or Ganciclovir (5 mg/kg IV q12h) for 14–21 days, then valganciclovir 900 mg PO QD, or Foscarnet 60 mg/kg IV q8h or 90 mg/kg IV q12h for 14–21 days, then 90–120 mg/kg IV q24h, or Cidofovir (5 mg/kg IV once a week) for 2 weeks, then 5 mg/kg every other week + probenecid pretreatment (2 g given 3 h prior to infusion and 1 g at 2 h and 8 h after infusion), with hydration before each dose	Monitor white blood cell count with differential for ganciclovir-induced neutropenia. Foscarnet IV infusion is over 2h and requires 500–1,000 mL of 0.9% saline solution with each dose to minimize nephrotoxicity. Cidofovir requires premedication with probenecid to minimize nephrotoxicity. Maintenance therapy for CMV retinitis can be discontinued in pts with inactive disease and robust and sustained CD4 counts of >100–150 cells/mm^3 for at least 6 months.
Primary prophylaxis	Valganciclovir (900 mg PO QD)		Prophylaxis may be considered for HIV-infected persons who are CMV seropositive and who have CD4+ cell counts <50/mm^3.

(Adapted from Centers of Disease Control and Prevention. Treating opportunistic infections among HIV-infected adults and adolescents: recommendatoins from CDC, the National Institutes of Health, and the HIV Medicine Association/Infectious Diseases Society of America. Clin Infect Dis 40 (Suppl 3):S131–S235, 2005.)

amidine, aminoglycosides). Supplemental potassium, magnesium, and calcium are often required during foscarnet therapy. An infusion pump should be used to control the rate of infusion (2 hours). The controlled infusion rate may ameliorate renal toxicity and the infusion-related malaise and neurotoxic effects. The serum creatinine and electrolytes should be monitored at least twice weekly during induction and weekly during maintenance therapy.

Nephrotoxicity is the most serious adverse effect of cidofovir therapy and can be prolonged and irreversible.[68–70] Concurrent probenecid and hydration with normal saline is required before each dose of cidofovir to minimize renal toxicity. Other nephrotoxic drugs, including nonsteroidal anti-inflammatory drugs, should be discontinued 1 week before initiating cidofovir therapy. The dose should be modified as listed in the product labeling for changes in renal function. Other adverse effects include neutropenia, metabolic acidosis, uveitis, and ocular hypotony. The serum creatinine, urinalysis (proteinuria), and white blood cell count (with differential) should be checked within 48 hours of each dose of cidofovir. Ocular examination should be performed monthly.

IMPROVING OUTCOMES

PATIENT EDUCATION

Early recognition of CMV retinitis is most likely to occur when the patient has received information about the topic, so this is an important intervention for preventing severe CMV disease. Patients should be made aware of the significance of increased floaters in the eye and should be advised to assess their visual acuity regularly by simple techniques such as reading newsprint. Patients should be instructed to seek medical attention should any visual changes occur.

METHODS TO IMPROVE PATIENT ADHERENCE TO DRUG THERAPY

Daily IV infusions of ganciclovir or foscarnet require major adjustments in the lifestyle of patients to accommodate drug administration. This can disrupt routine activities such as work or other obligations. Alternative maintenance therapies such as oral valganciclovir or IV cidofovir should be considered with the patient.

KEY POINTS

P. JIROVECII PNEUMONIA

- TMP-SMX is the drug regimen of choice for acute therapy and prophylaxis of PCP
- Macular rash is a common adverse effect of sulfonamides in patients with AIDS but should not necessarily preclude future use of these drugs
- Adjunctive corticosteroids should be administered within 72 hours of starting antipneumocystis therapy for severe PCP, defined as a Pao_2 less than 70 mm Hg or an A-a gradient greater than 35 mm Hg
- Atovaquone is an alternative for treatment of mild to moderate PCP in patients who have no diarrhea and can ingest the oral suspension with fatty foods
- Prophylaxis with systemic agents (TMP-SMX or dapsone) is recommended in persons infected with HIV with a CD4+ count of less than 200 cells per mm^3. Aerosolized pentamidine is an alternate in patients with CD4+ counts between 100 and 200 cells per mm^3
- Patients receiving pyrimethamine-sulfadiazine for toxoplasmosis encephalitis maintenance therapy do not need further PCP prophylaxis because of activity against both pathogens with this regimen

TOXOPLASMOSIS ENCEPHALITIS

- Pyrimethamine-sulfadiazine is the preferred regimen for treating acute toxoplasmosis encephalitis and subsequent maintenance therapy (i.e., secondary prophylaxis). Patients should be well hydrated to reduce the chances of sulfadiazine-induced crystalluria
- Leucovorin (folinic acid) is recommended to prevent bone marrow suppression caused by pyrimethamine
- Patients should receive instructions on how to protect themselves from infection of newly acquired *T gondii* (e.g., eat only well-done meat, thoroughly wash fresh fruits and vegetables, wear latex gloves when handling cat litter boxes)

MYCOBACTERIUM AVIUM COMPLEX

- Treatment regimens should contain a macrolide [azithromycin or clarithromycin (preferred)] and ethambutol

- Drug interactions with anti-MAC agents are significant and require careful review of the medication profile to avoid complications, especially with clarithromycin (cytochrome P450 inhibitor) and rifabutin (cytochrome P450 inducer)
- A macrolide (azithromycin or clarithromycin) is the first-line agent for prophylaxis of MAC infection in persons infected with HIV with CD4+ cell counts less than 50 per mm^3

CYTOMEGALOVIRUS RETINITIS

- The selection of initial therapy for CMV retinitis must be individualized and can be oral valganciclovir (for peripheral lesions) or IV ganciclovir, foscarnet, or cidofovir. Neutropenia and nephrotoxicity are frequent and serious adverse effects encountered with these drugs, respectively
- The ganciclovir intraocular implant is a novel drug delivery system recommended for patients with immediate sight-threatening lesions. The implant must be replaced when the drug supply is exhausted (about 5 to 8 months), and the long-term outcome of multiple reimplantation procedures is not known
- Concurrent use of probenecid and hydration with normal saline is required before each dose of IV cidofovir to minimize renal toxicity

SUGGESTED READINGS

Centers for Disease Control and Prevention. Treating opportunistic infections among HIV-infected adults and adolescents: recommendations from CDC, the National Institutes of Health, and the HIV Medicine Association/Infectious Diseases Society of America. Clin Infect Dis 40 (Suppl 3):S131–S235, 2005.

REFERENCES

1. Stansell JD, Huang L. *Pneumocystis carinii* pneumonia. In: Sande MA, Volberding PA, eds. The medical management of AIDS, 5th ed. Philadelphia: Saunders, 1997:275–300.
2. Kelly C, Checkly W, Mannino D, et al. Hospitalizations for AIDS-related *Pneumocystis jirovecii* pneumonia in the United States from the pre-prophylaxis era through the introduction of HAART: 1986:2002. In: Program and abstracts of the 12th Conference on Retroviruses and Opportunistic Infections (Boston, MA). Alexandria, VA: Foundation for Retrovirology and Human Health, 2005:881.
3. Centers for Disease Control and Prevention. Treating opportunistic infections among HIV-infected adults and adolescents: recommendations from CDC, the National Institutes of Health, and the HIV Medicine Association/Infectious Diseases Society of America. Clin Infect Dis 40 (Suppl 3):S131–S235, 2005.
4. Klein NC, Duncanson FP, Lenox TH, et al. Trimethoprim-sulfamethoxazole versus pentamidine for *Pneumocystis carinii* pneumonia in AIDS patients: results of a large prospective randomized treatment trial. AIDS 6:301–305, 1992.
5. Fishman JA. Treatment of infection due to *Pneumocystis carinii*. Antimicrob Agents Chemother 42:1309–1314, 1998.
6. Stein DS, Stevens RC. Treatment-associated toxicities: incidence and mechanisms. In: Sattler FR, Walzer PD, eds. *Pneumocystis carinii*. London: Bailliere Tindall, 1995:505–530.
7. Navin TR, Beard CB, Huang L, et al. Effect of mutations in *Pneumocystis carinii* dihydropteroate synthase gene on outcome of P cari-

nii pneumonia in patients with HIV-1: a prospective study. Lancet 358:545–549, 2001.

8. Sattler FR, Cowan R, Nielsen DM, et al. Trimethoprim-sulfamethoxazole compared with pentamidine for treatment of *Pneumocystis carinii* pneumonia in the acquired immunodeficiency syndrome. A prospective, noncrossover study. Ann Intern Med 109:280–287, 1988.

9. Safrin S, Lee BL, Sande MA. Adjunctive folinic acid with trimethoprim-sulfamethoxazole for *Pneumocystis carinii* pneumonia in AIDS patients is associated with an increased risk of therapeutic failure and death. J Infect Dis 170:912–917, 1994.

10. Stevens RC, Laizure SC, Williams CL, et al. Pharmacokinetics and adverse effects of 20-mg/kg/day trimethoprim and 100-mg/kg/day sulfamethoxazole in healthy adult subjects. Antimicrob Agents Chemother 35:1884–1890, 1991.

11. Safrin S, Finkelstein DM, Feinberg J, et al. Comparison of three regimens for treatment of mild to moderate *Pneumocystic carinii* pneumonia in patients with AIDS. A double-blind, randomized trial of oral trimethoprim-sulfamethoxazole, dapsone-trimethoprim, and clindamycin-primaquine. ACTG 108 Study Group. Ann Intern Med 124:792–802, 1996.

12. Holtzer CD, Flaherty JF, Coleman RL. Cross-reactivity in HIV-infected patients switched from trimethoprim-sulfamethoxazole to dapsone. Pharmacotherapy 18:831–835, 1998.

13. Hughes W, Leoung G, Kramer F, et al. Comparison of atovaquone with trimethoprim-sulfamethoxazole for the treatment of *Pneumocystis carinii* pneumonia in patients with the acquired immunodeficiency syndrome (AIDS). N Engl J Med 328:1521–1527, 1993.

14. Dohn MN, Weinberg WG, Torres RA, et al. Oral atovaquone compared with IV pentamidine for *Pneumocystis carinii* pneumonia in patients with AIDS. Ann Intern Med 121:174–180, 1994.

15. O'Brien JG, Dong BJ, Coleman RL, et al. A 5-year retrospective review of adverse drug reactions and their risk factors in human immunodeficiency virus-infected patients who were receiving IV pentamidine therapy for *Pneumocystis carinii* pneumonia. Clin Infect Dis 24:854–859, 1997.

16. Conte J Jr, Chernoff D, Feigal D Jr, et al. IV or inhaled pentamidine for treating *Pneumocystis carinii* pneumonia in AIDS. A randomized trial. Ann Intern Med 113:203–209, 1990.

17. Bozzette SA, Sattler FR, Chiu J, et al. A controlled trial of early adjunctive treatment with corticosteroids for *Pneumocystis carinii* pneumonia in the acquired immunodeficiency syndrome. California Collaborative Treatment Group. N Engl J Med 323:1451–1457, 1990.

18. Gagnon S, Boota AM, Fischl MA, et al. Corticosteroids as adjunctive therapy for severe *Pneumocystis carinii* pneumonia in the acquired immunodeficiency syndrome. A double-blind, placebo-controlled trial. N Engl J Med 323:1444–1450, 1990.

19. National Institutes of Health-University of California Expert Panel for Corticosteroids as Adjunctive Therapy for *Pneumocystis* Pneumonia. Consensus statement on the use of corticosteroids as adjunctive therapy for *Pneumocystis* pneumonia in the acquired immunodeficiency syndrome. N Engl J Med 323:1500–1504, 1990.

20. Mussini C, Pezzotti P, Antinori A, et al. Discontinuation of secondary prophylaxis for *Pneumocystis carinii* pneumonia in human immunodeficiency virus-infected patients. Clin Infect Dis 36:645–651, 2003.

21. Bozzette SA, Finkelstein DM, Spector SA, et al. A randomized trial of three antipneumocystis agents in patients with advanced human immunodeficiency virus infection. N Engl J Med 332:693–699, 1995.

22. Hardy WD, Feinberg J, Finkelstein DM, et al. A controlled trial of trimethoprim-sulfamethoxazole or aerosolized pentamidine for secondary prophylaxis of *Pneumocystis carinii* pneumonia in patients with the acquired immunodeficiency syndrome. ACTG Protocol 021. N Engl J Med 327:1842–1848, 1992.

23. Montoya JG, Liesenfeld O. Toxoplasmosis. Lancet 363:1965–1976, 2004.

24. Subauste CS, Wong SY, Remington JS. AIDS-associated toxoplasmosis. In: Sande MA, Volberding PA, eds. The medical management of AIDS, 5th ed. Philadelphia: Saunders 1997:343–362.

25. Antinori A, Larussa D, Cingolani A, et al. Prevalence, associated factors, and prognostic determinants of AIDS-related toxoplasmic encephalitis in the era of advanced highly active antiretroviral therapy. Clin Infec Dis 39:1681–1691, 2004.

26. Katlama C, De Wit S, O'Doherty E, et al. Pyrimethamine-clindamycin vs. pyrimethamine-sulfadiazine as acute and long-term therapy for toxoplasmic encephalitis in patients with AIDS. Clin Infect Dis 22:268–275, 1996.

27. Dannemann BR, McCutchan JA, Israelski DM, et al. Treatment of toxoplasmic encephalitis in patients with AIDS: a randomized trial comparing pyrimethamine plus clindamycin to pyrimethamine plus sulfonamides. Ann Intern Med 116:33–43, 1992.

28. Torre D, Casari S, Speranza F, et al. Randomized trial of trimethoprim-sulfamethoxazole versus pyrimethamine-sulfadiazine for therapy of toxoplasmic encephalitis in patients with AIDS. Antimicrob Agents Chemother 42:1346–1349, 1998.

29. Becker K, Jablonowski H, Haussinger D. Sulfadiazine-associated nephrotoxicity in patients with the acquired immunodeficiency syndrome. Medicine 75:185–194, 1996.

30. Chirgwin K, Hafner R, Leport C, et al. Randomized phase II trial of atovaquone with pyrimethamine or sulfadiazine for treatment of toxoplasmic encephalitis in patients with acquired immunodeficiency syndrome. Clin Infect Dis 34:1243–1250, 2002.

31. Saba J, Morlat P, Raffi F, et al. Pyrimethamine plus azithromycin for treatment of acute toxoplasmic encephalitis in patients with AIDS. Eur J Clin Microbiol Infect Dis 12:853–856, 1993.

32. Jacobson JM, Hafner R, Remington J, et al. Dose-escalation, phase I/II study of azithromycin and pyrimethamine for the treatment of toxoplasmic encephalitis in AIDS. AIDS 15:583–589, 2001.

33. Kovacs JA. Efficacy of atovaquone in treatment of toxoplasmosis in patients with AIDS. Lancet 340:637–638, 1992.

34. Luft BJ, Hafner R, Korzun AH, et al. Toxoplasmic encephalitis in patients with the acquired immunodeficiency syndrome. N Engl J Med 329:995–1000, 1993.

35. Podzamczer D, Miro JM, Bolao F, et al. Twice-weekly maintenance therapy with sulfadiazine-pyrimethamine to prevent recurrent toxoplasmic encephalitis in patients with AIDS. Ann Intern Med 123:175–180, 1995.

36. Heald A, Flepp M, Chave JP, et al. Treatment of cerebral toxoplasmosis protects against *Pneumocystis carinii* pneumonia in patients with AIDS. Ann Intern Med 115:760–763, 1991.

37. Ruf B, Schurmann D, Bergmann F, et al. Efficacy of pyrimethamine/ sulfadoxine in the prevention of toxoplasmic encephalitis relapses and *Pneumocystis carinii* pneumonia in HIV-infected patients. Eur J Clin Microbiol Infect Dis 12:325–329, 1993.

38. Podzamczer D, Salazar A, Jimenez J, et al. Intermittent trimethoprim-sulfamethoxazole compared with dapsone-pyrimethamine for simultaneous primary prophylaxis of Pneumocystis pneumonia and toxoplasmosis in patients infected with HIV. Ann Intern Med 122:755–761, 1995.

39. Podzamczer D, Santin M, Jimenez J, et al. Thrice weekly cotrimoxazole is better than weekly dapsone-pyrimethamine for the primary prevention of *Pneumocystis carinii* pneumonia in HIV-infected patients. AIDS 7:501–506, 1993.

40. Leport C, Chene G, Morlat P, et al. Pyrimethamine for primary prophylaxis of toxoplasmic encephalitis in patients with human immunodeficiency virus infection: a double-blind, randomized trial. J Infect Dis 173:91–97, 1996.

41. Jacobson MA, Besch CL, Child C, et al. Primary prophylaxis with pyrimethamine for toxoplasmic encephalitis in patients with advanced human immunodeficiency virus disease: results of a randomized trial. J Infect Dis 169:384–394, 1994.

42. Lange CG, Woolley IJ, Brodt RH. Disseminated *Mycobacterium avium-intracellulare* complex (MAC) infection in the era of effective antiretroviral therapy: is prophylaxis still indicated? Drugs 7:679–692, 2004.

43. Wright J. Current strategies for the prevention and treatment of disseminated *Mycobacterium avium* complex infection in patients with AIDS. Pharmacotherapy 18:738–747, 1998.

44. Centers for Disease Control and Prevention. Guidelines for preventing opportunistic infections among HIV-infected persons: 2002 Recommendations of the U.S. Public Health Service and the Infectious Diseases Society of America. MMWR 51:1–60, 2002.

45. MacGregor RR, Hafner R, Wu JW, et al. Clinical, microbiological, and immunological characteristics in HIV-infected subjects at risk of disseminated *Mycobacterium avium* complex disease: an AACTG study. AIDS Res and Human Retroviruses 21:689–695, 2005.

46. Chin DP, Reingold AL, Horsburgh CR Jr, et al. Predicting *Mycobacterium avium* complex bacteremia in patients with the human immunodeficiency virus: a prospectively validated model. Clin Infect Dis 19:668–674, 1994.

47. Chaisson RE, Benson CA, Dube MP, et al. Clarithromycin therapy for bacteremic *Mycobacterium avium* complex disease. A randomized, double-blind, dose-ranging study in patients with AIDS. Ann Intern Med 121:905–911, 1994.

48. Shafran SD, Singer J, Zarowny DP, et al. A comparison of two regimens for the treatment of *Mycobacterium avium* complex bacteremia in AIDS: rifabutin, ethambutol, and clarithromycin versus rifampin, ethambutol, clofazimine, and ciprofloxacin. N Engl J Med 335:377–383, 1996.

49. Dube MP, Sattler FR, Torriani FJ, et al. A randomized evaluation of ethambutol for prevention of relapse and drug resistance during treatment of *Mycobacterium avium* complex bacteremia with clarithromycin-based combination therapy. J Infect Dis 176:1225–1232, 1997.

50. Chaisson RE, Keiser P, Pierce M, et al. Clarithromycin and ethambutol with or without clofazimine for the treatment of bacteremic *Mycobacterium avium* complex disease in patients with HIV infection. AIDS 11:311–317, 1997.

51. Cohn DL, Fisher EJ, Peng GT, et al. A prospective randomized trial of four three-drug regimens in the treatment of disseminated *Mycobacterium avium* complex disease in AIDS patients: excess mortality associated with high-dose clarithromycin. Clin Infect Dis 29:125–133, 1999.

52. Chiu J, Nussbaum J, Bozzette S, et al. Treatment of disseminated *Mycobacterium avium* complex infection in AIDS with amikacin, ethambutol, rifampin, and ciprofloxacin. Ann Intern Med 113:358–361, 1990.

53. Havlir D, Torriani F, Dube M. Uveitis associated with rifabutin prophylaxis. Ann Intern Med 121:510–512, 1994.

54. Narang PK, Trapnell CB, Schoenfelder JR, et al. Fluconazole and enhanced effect of rifabutin prophylaxis. N Engl J Med 330:1316–1317, 1994.

55. Pierce M, Crampton S, Henry D, et al. A randomized trial of clarithromycin as prophylaxis against disseminated *Mycobacterium avium* complex infection in patients with advanced acquired immunodeficiency syndrome. N Engl J Med 335:384–391, 1996.

56. Havlir DV, Dube MP, Sattler FR, et al. Prophylaxis against disseminated *Mycobacterium avium* complex with weekly azithromycin, daily rifabutin, or both. N Engl J Med 335:392–398, 1996.

57. Nightingale SD, Cameron W, Gordin FM, et al. Two controlled trials of rifabutin prophylaxis against *Mycobacterium avium* complex infection in AIDS. N Engl J Med 329:828–833, 1993.

58. Brooks JT, Song R, Hanson DL, et al. Discontinuation of primary prophylaxis against *Mycobacterium avium* complex infection in HIV-infected persons receiving antiretroviral therapy: observations from a large national cohort in the United States 1992–2002. Clin Infect Dis 41:549–553, 2005.

59. Drew WL, Stempien MJ, Erlich KS. Management of herpesvirus infections (CMV, HSV, VZV). In: Sande MA, Volberding PA, eds. The medical management of AIDS, 5th ed. Philadelphia: Saunders, 1997:381–388.

60. Moore R, Keruly JC, Gallant J, et al. Decline in mortality rates and opportunistic disease with combination antiretroviral therapy. Abstract 22374. 12th World AIDS Conference. Geneva, Switzerland, June 28–July 3, 1998.

61. Jabs DA. Ocular manifestations of HIV infection. Trans Am Ophthalmol Soc 93:623–683, 1995.

62. Studies of Ocular Complications of AIDS Research Group and the AIDS Clinical Trials Group. Foscarnet-ganciclovir cytomegalovirus retinitis trial 4: visual outcomes. Ophthalmology 101:1250–1261, 1994.

63. Musch DC, Martin DF, Gordon JF, et al. Treatment of cytomegalovirus retinitis with a sustained-release ganciclovir implant. N Engl J Med 337:83–90, 1997.

64. Martin DF, Kuppermann DB, Wolitz RA, et al. Oral ganciclovir for patients with cytomegalovirus retinitis treated with a ganciclovir implant. N Engl J Med 340:1063–1070, 1999.

65. Studies of Ocular Complications of AIDS Research Group. The AIDS Clinical Trials Group. The ganciclovir implant plus oral ganciclovir versus parenteral cidofovir for the treatment of cytomegalovirus retinitis in patients with acquired immunodeficiency syndrome. Am J Ophthalmol 131:457–467, 2001.

66. Martin DF, Sierra-Madero J, Walmsley S, et al. A controlled trial of valganciclovir as induction therapy for cytomegalovirus retinitis. N Engl J Med 346:1119–1126, 2002.

67. Whitley RJ, Jacobson MA, Friedberg DN, et al. Guidelines for the treatment of cytomegalovirus diseases in patients with AIDS in the era of potent antiretroviral therapy. Arch Intern Med 158:957–969, 1998.

68. Studies of Ocular Complications of AIDS Research Group and the AIDS Clinical Trials Group. Mortality in patients with the acquired immunodeficiency syndrome treated with either foscarnet or ganciclovir for cytomegalovirus retinitis. N Engl J Med 326:213–220, 1992.

69. Lalezari JP, Stagg RJ, Kuppermann BD, et al. IV cidofovir for peripheral cytomegalovirus retinitis in patients with AIDS. A randomized, controlled trial. Ann Intern Med 126:257–263, 1997.

70. Studies of Ocular Complications of AIDS Research Group in Collaboration with the AIDS Clinical Trials Group. Parenteral cidofovir for cytomegalovirus retinitis in patients with AIDS: the HPMPC peripheral cytomegalovirus retinitis trial. A randomized, controlled trial. Ann Intern Med 126:264–274, 1997.

Sepsis

86

Brien L. Neudeck and P. David Rogers

TREATMENT GOALS

- Immediately correct hypotension and hypoperfusion abnormalities using early goal-directed therapy and other supportive measures.
- Obtain appropriate cultures from multiple sites for identification of causative organisms and guidance of empiric therapy.
- Eradicate infectious loci using intravenous antibiotics, source control, and all other available measures.
- Attenuate the systemic inflammatory response with immunomodulatory therapies in selected patients who meet criteria.
- Achieve clinical improvement and prevent morbidity and mortality.

DEFINITION

The term *sepsis* has been historically applied to a broad array of similar but overlapping clinical syndromes. This imprecise definition not only led to confusion among practitioners but also hampered the construction of well-designed clinical trials evaluating new therapies. Thus, a consensus conference of the American College of Chest Physicians and Society of Critical Care Medicine attempted to more accurately define the term *sepsis* and related syndromes to standardize terminology, eliminate confusion among clinicians and researchers, and allow for expedited treatment based on earlier recognition of the clinical syndrome (Table 86.1).[1] Furthermore, due to the recognition that noninfectious events can trigger a similar clinical and physiologic response, the term ''systemic inflammatory response syndrome'' (SIRS) was adopted as a general description for an inflammatory process, independent of its cause.

Using these new definitions, sepsis is the systemic inflammatory response to infection and consequently a subset of SIRS (Fig. 86.1). Severe sepsis is defined as sepsis associated with organ dysfunction or hypoperfusion abnormalities. Septic shock is the most serious complication of sepsis, and these patients have the highest mortality from sepsis.

ETIOLOGY

Causative microorganisms in sepsis vary and will depend on the site of infection. The most common site of infection in patients with severe sepsis and septic shock is the lung.[2] Other sites of infection, in order of frequency, are the bloodstream, the abdomen, urinary tract, and skin and soft tissues. It is conceivable that any microorganism can cause sepsis or septic shock, including bacteria, viruses, protozoa, fungi, spirochetes, and rickettsiae. However, bacteria are the most common causes of sepsis in the United States and Europe and are responsible for greater than 90% of all cases.[3,4] In past decades, gram-negative organisms such as *Escherichia coli*, *Klebsiella pneumoniae*, and *Pseudomonas aeruginosa* were predominant among causes of sepsis (Table 86.2).[5] However, recent epidemiologic data indicate that gram-positive bacteria such as *Staphylococcus aureus*, coagulase-negative staphylococci, enterococci, and streptococci are now responsible for at least half of the infectious causes of sepsis.[4,6–8] More alarming is the fact that methicillin-resistant *S aureus* (MRSA) and methicillin-resistant *Staphylococcus epidermidis* (MRSE) infections are increasing.[9,10] Although fungal etiologies represent only 5% of all cases, the inci-

TABLE 86.1	Definitions of Sepsis and Related Disorders
Disorder	**Definition**
Systemic inflammatory response syndrome (SIRS)	The response to a variety of severe clinical insults manifested by 2 or more of the following conditions: • Temperature ≥38°C (100.4°F) or ≤36°C (96.8°F) • Heart rate ≥90 beats per minute • Respiratory rate ≥20 breaths per minute or $PaCO_2$ <32 mm Hg • White blood cell count ≥12,000/mm³ or ≤4,000/mm³, or >10% bands
Sepsis	SIRS + suspected/documented infection
Severe sepsis	Sepsis + sepsis-induced organ dysfunction
Septic shock	Sepsis-induced hypotension despite adequate fluid resuscitation, and perfusion abnormalities such as lactic acidosis, oliguria, altered mental status
Sepsis-induced hypotension	A systolic blood pressure ≤90 mm Hg or a reduction of ≥40 mm Hg from baseline in the absence of other causes of hypotension

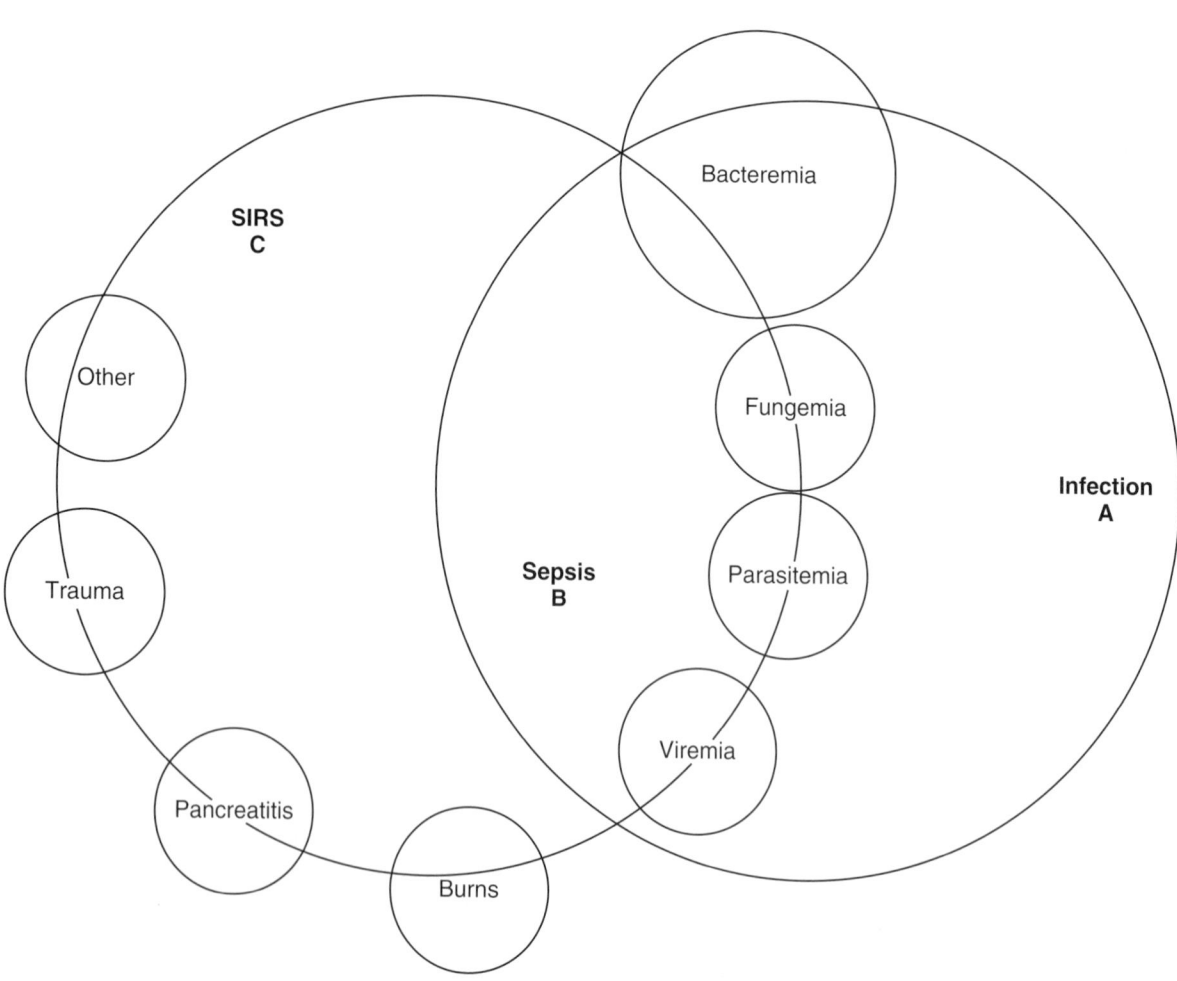

FIGURE 86.1 The relationship between systemic inflammatory response syndrome (SIRS), sepsis, infection, and bacteremia. (Adapted with permission from Bone RC, Balk RA, Cerra FB, et al. The ACCP/SCCM Consensus Conference Committee: definitions for sepsis and organ failure and guidelines for the use of innovative therapies in sepsis. Chest 101:1644–1655, 1992.)

TABLE 86.2	Frequency of Gram-Negative Isolates from 1,754 Patients with Sepsis Syndrome in 80 U.S. Hospitals

Organism	No. of Isolates (%) (N = 389)
Escherichia coli	155 (39.85)
Klebsiella spp	49 (12.6)
Enterobacter spp	29 (7.46)
Pseudomonas spp	46 (11.83)
Bacteroides spp	11 (2.83)
Proteus spp	15 (3.86)
Mixed	30 (7.71)
Miscellaneous	54 (13.88)

(From Conboy K, Welage LS, Walawander CA, et al. Sepsis syndrome and associated sequelae in patients with high risk for gram-negative sepsis. Pharmacotherapy 15:66–77, 1995.)

dence of fungal sepsis has increased threefold between 1979 and 2000.[4] Most are due to *Candida* spp, which are the fourth most common bloodstream pathogens identified in nosocomial infections.[11]

EPIDEMIOLOGY

Sepsis is an important healthcare problem and is the leading cause of death in intensive care units (ICUs).[12] Over the past two decades, the incidence of sepsis in the United States has increased consistently, with approximately 750,000 new cases of sepsis every year.[4,13] It has been estimated that 25% of ICU patients develop sepsis, whereas the incidence in non-ICU patients is 10-fold lower. Treating patients with sepsis has proved to be a difficult challenge, given the heter-

ogeneity of the patients it afflicts and the complexity of the host response. Despite supportive therapy and treatment with broad-spectrum antimicrobials, the 28-day mortality rate approaches 30%. Comparing mortality rates to other diseases, the number of deaths due to sepsis is similar to myocardial infarction and is greater than most common cancers.[14] Both the attributable mortality and existence as a modifiable disease process are unknown because sepsis is often a complication of other disease states or their treatment.

PATHOPHYSIOLOGY

INFLAMMATORY/ANTI-INFLAMMATORY CASCADE

Pathogenic microorganisms possess specific toxins and exogenous molecules that are the ultimate cause of sepsis and the sepsis syndrome. These include pathogen-associated molecular patterns (PAMPs) such as lipopolysaccharide (LPS), lipoproteins, outer membrane proteins, flagellin, fimbriae, peptidoglycan, lipoteichoic acid, and mannan, as well as internal motifs released during lysis of the pathogen, such as heat shock proteins and bacterial DNA.[15] PAMPs interface with pattern recognition receptors such as Toll-like receptors (TLRs) (for example, CD14 and TLR4 with LPS), which stimulate monocytes and macrophages to produce proinflammatory cytokines including tumor necrosis factor (TNF)-α, interleukin (IL)-1β, IL-6, and IL-8.[16–20] These cytokines produce secondary events, including upregulation of E-selectin and P-selectin on endothelial cells, anchoring and chemotaxis of neutrophils, and subsequent release of proteases and other proinflammatory products by neutrophils, all of which are part of the normal host innate immune response (Fig. 86.2; *see color insert*).[17] However, in the case of sepsis and sepsis syndrome, a pronounced proinflammatory

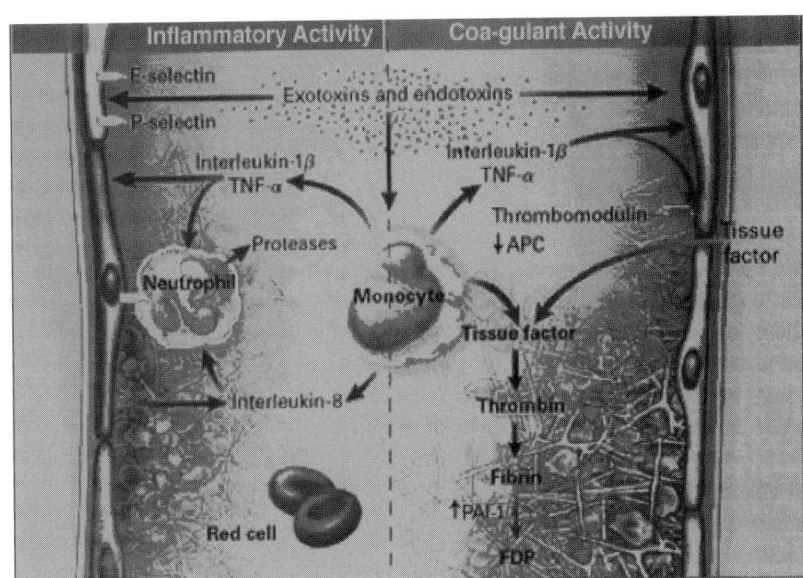

FIGURE 86.2 Mechanisms of injury to the microcirculation in severe sepsis (*see color insert*). (Adapted with permission from Matthay MA. Severe sepsis—a new treatment with both anticoagulant and anti-inflammatory properties. N Engl J Med 344:759–762, 2001.)

response contributes greatly to the deleterious clinical consequences of this disease state.

In an effort to counter the proinflammatory responses to infecting pathogens, leukocytes produce anti-inflammatory cytokines upon stimulation by TNF-α and IL-1β, which drive a counter-anti-inflammatory response. These include transforming growth factor (TGF)-β, IL-10, and IL-13, which produce anti-inflammatory effects on monocytes, macrophages, and endothelial cells.[18] Such effects include suppressed T- and B-lymphocyte function, inhibition of antigen-presenting cells, suppressed proinflammatory gene expression, and release of soluble cytokine receptors and receptor antagonists.[18,21,22] The resulting immune dysregulation impairs the ability of the host to adequately combat infection.

COAGULATION/ANTICOAGULATION CASCADE

Closely linked to the inflammatory cascade in the pathophysiology of sepsis is the coagulation cascade. Dysregulation of this cascade results in the coagulopathy associated with sepsis and the sepsis syndrome from thrombocytopenia to disseminated vascular coagulation (DIC), ultimately culminating in microvascular thrombosis with subsequent local tissue hypoxia and organ dysfunction.[23–25] TNF-α, IL-1β, and certain toxins activate the coagulation cascade through the release of tissue factor (TF) from various sources (Fig. 86.2).[17] TNF-α also reduces the expression of thrombomodulin by endothelial cells.

Thrombomodulin, along with thrombin, is critical for the activation of the circulating proenzyme protein C. Activated protein C (APC) cleaves and inhibits cofactors VIIIa and Va, thus downregulating the activity of the coagulation system.[15] In addition to its anticoagulant activity, APC also has anti-inflammatory and antiapoptotic activity.[26–28] Reduced thrombomodulin expression during sepsis results in reduced levels of APC. This, combined with reduced circulating levels of antithrombin III, results in excess thrombin being produced from TF, and ultimately the formation of fibrin clots in the microcirculation.[29] The cumulative effect of these events is tissue ischemia and organ disfunction.

Upon the formation of fibrin clots, endothelial cells produce tissue factor pathway inhibitor (TFPI), which inhibits factor VIIa complexed with TF and decreases the formation of thrombin and fibrin clots.[30] Unfortunately, full-length TFPI is limited in limited in pre-DIC conditions such as sepsis.[31] TNF-α and IL-1β also stimulate the production of excessive amounts of plasminogen-activator inhibitor type 1 (PAI-1).[32] This inhibits the normal mechanisms in place for the degradation of fibrin. Indeed, elevated PAI-1 levels are correlated with more severe organ failure and death in septic patients.[33]

CLINICAL PRESENTATION AND DIAGNOSIS

SIGNS AND SYMPTOMS

The clinical presentation of sepsis is not easily defined because of the numerous biologic mediators that are released as innate host defense mechanisms are activated as a response to inflammation. Additionally, the site of infection, duration of illness, genetic factors, degree of mediator release, and underlying comorbidities may influence the clinical presentation.[34] Symptoms may evolve rapidly from one to another, rendering the ability to make the diagnosis of sepsis on symptoms alone difficult at best. Depending on the degree of insult, patients can present with sepsis, severe sepsis, or septic shock. Fever is frequently associated with infection and is the most common indication of sepsis.[35] Other signs and symptoms suggestive of early sepsis include chills, leukocytosis, increase in immature neutrophils, hypoxia, tachycardia, hyperventilation, skin lesions, and/or changes in mental status. Immunosuppressed or elderly patients may have a blunted response, and traditional blood chemistry markers may not be elevated. Hypothermia, rather than hyperthermia, can manifest as a symptom of systemic infection and is associated with a poor prognosis.[36] Hyperventilation precedes the onset of fever and chills in many patients. As patients progress to severe sepsis and septic shock, oliguria, anuria, acidosis, elevated liver enzymes, leukopenia, DIC, adult respiratory distress syndrome, hypotension, and shock may be present.

DIAGNOSIS AND CLINICAL FINDINGS

Identification of the infectious etiology is essential for ensuring that effective and tailored antimicrobial therapy can be initiated. Early clinical suspicion should be quickly confirmed by obtaining appropriate cultures so that rapid identification and antimicrobial susceptibility of pathogens can be determined. Confirmation of the diagnosis of sepsis cannot be accomplished by relying on one diagnostic test alone. Rather, the incorporation of results from multiple diagnostic modalities as well as patient history is required and increases the likelihood of a correct diagnosis. A detailed clinical examination incorporating predisposing factors such as surgery, organ transplantation, chemotherapy, other immunocompromise, or recent trauma should be performed. These should be undertaken to provide clues to potential sources of sepsis and assist with future diagnostic strategies.

Attempts to discriminate between gram-positive and gram-negative sepsis on clinical presentation alone have not yielded consistent findings. However, incorporating the most likely site of infection allows for the refinement of potential causative organisms based on the pathogens associated with infections in those sites. Surgical sites or locations of previous traumatic injury should be examined for signs of infection. A sudden change in respiratory status should prompt the clinician to obtain cultures. In addition, vascular access sites should be evaluated for evidence of infection or colonization. Data on previous and/or current antimicrobial therapy as well as previous culture results are also useful and should be integrated into the decision-making process.

Approximately 30% to 50% of patients with severe sepsis or septic shock present with positive blood cultures.[34] Therefore, early blood cultures should be obtained in all patients with suspected sepsis, regardless of the suspected source of infection.[4,13] Several parameters have been independently correlated with the presence of bacteria in the blood, including fever, chills, leukocytosis, hypoalbuminemia, and renal failure. Two sets of blood specimens for culture should be drawn from different peripheral sites at the time of first clinical suspicion of bacteremia or sepsis.[34,37] Preferably, these should be obtained by new venipuncture, because the risk of contamination is higher if drawn through a catheter.[38–41] However, if a catheter-related infection is suspected, two sets of blood cultures should be obtained, one set from the catheter and another from a peripheral site.

Because many patients have negative blood cultures, these findings should not lessen the importance of proper clinical diagnosis and initiation of appropriate supportive therapies. Identification of other infectious loci should be vigorously attempted.

In addition to blood cultures, specimens from urine, sputum or endotracheal aspirates, and other potential sites of infection should be collected and sent expeditiously to the microbiology laboratory for culture and sensitivity determination.[34] The presence of a radiographic infiltrate and one clinical finding such as fever, leukocytosis, or purulent tracheal secretions has a high sensitivity for diagnosis of pneumonia, but the specificity is low.[42] In mechanically ventilated patients, fiberoptic bronchoscopy with protected specimen brush or bronchoalveolar lavage is useful and increases the sensitivity of the findings.[43–45] Because culture results may not be available for 24 hours, Gram stains of collected samples aid in the selection of the initial antimicrobial therapy, because they are often available within hours of collection.

Imaging studies are a valuable addition to culture collection as they can greatly assist in identifying the locus of infection. Simple chest radiographs should be performed to identify the presence of pulmonary infiltrates. Computed tomography and magnetic resonance imaging provide more detailed study of the anatomy and should be performed when greater sensitivity is required.

THERAPEUTIC PLAN

The transition from SIRS to severe sepsis and septic shock is a complex and often rapid process. Therefore, the therapeutic plan for treatment of severe sepsis must be initiated quickly if the factors leading to illness are to be corrected. Measures that should be incorporated include early and rigorous diagnostic measures, aggressive resuscitation, stabilization of respiratory function, and correction of underlying infectious processes. Stabilization of respiratory function is achieved with supplemental oxygen, close monitoring of arterial blood gases, and often mechanical ventilation.[46] Hemodynamic parameters are usually monitored by invasive means in the critically ill septic patient. This may involve the placement of an arterial line to provide continuous blood pressure monitoring and/or placement of a pulmonary artery (PA) catheter to monitor fluid status and cardiac output. Although PA catheters are useful when titrating resuscitation, their safety has been called into question and therefore their need must be carefully evaluated. Lastly, antibiotic therapy and/or immunotherapy should be initiated as soon as possible.

TREATMENT

NONPHARMACOLOGIC THERAPY

Source Control. Patients presenting with signs and symptoms of sepsis should be immediately evaluated for a source of infection.[47] If a focal source is identified, every effort should be made to remove it using drainage, débridement of necrotic tissue, or other interventional measures, keeping in mind the risk/benefit of the intervention itself. Failure to do so prolongs the pathophysiologic consequences of sepsis and ultimately leads to poor outcomes, because antibiotic therapy alone is often insufficient.

Removal of devices colonized with bacteria is another important step to ensure the efficacy of empiric antibiotics. In patients with suspected catheter-related infections, the catheter should be removed immediately and sent for culture once other intravascular access has been obtained. Culture results should be compared to those obtained from the blood to confirm the diagnosis of a catheter-related infection. If other sites of infection carry greater suspicion, it may be reasonable to leave selected intravascular catheters in place, although this is subject to debate. The removal of urinary catheters, which may predispose patients to persistent infection, may also be required and should be evaluated. Finally, radiographic studies are indispensable for determining sources of infection not identifiable on physical examination.

Renal Replacement Therapy. The incidence of acute renal dysfunction in patients with severe sepsis can be up to 70%, and some patients require temporary hemodialysis.[48–50] Because of the hemodynamic instability often present in these patients, hemofiltration techniques such as continuous venovenous hemofiltration are preferred to intermittent hemodialysis. If patients can tolerate it from a hemodynamic standpoint, intermittent dialysis may be used. Both appear to be effective, but continuous hemofiltration allows for a more careful management of fluid balance issues, which are common in critically ill patients. Although renal dosing of antibiotics may be required, clinicians should be wary of reducing doses to amounts that may not be sufficient to maintain bactericidal concentrations in target tissues.

PHARMACOTHERAPY

Initial Fluid Resuscitation and Restoration of Hemodynamic Stability. Obtaining vascular access and initiating aggressive fluid resuscitation are paramount to improving the survival of patients with severe sepsis and septic shock. Delayed resuscitation can result in sudden cardiovascular collapse, refractory tissue hypoxia, and organ dysfunction. Despite aggressive resuscitation attempts, therapy is often inadequate because the progression to severe disease is well on its way. Thus, early, goal-directed resuscitation is required immediately when severe sepsis or sepsis-induced hypotension is recognized and must not be deferred until the patient is admitted to the ICU. During the first 6 hours of resuscitation, fluids should be administered to achieve a central venous pressure of 8 to 12 mm Hg, mean arterial pressure of at least 65 mm Hg, and urine output of at least 0.5 mL/kg/hr. If the central venous oxygen saturation is 70% or less and the hematocrit is low, red cells should be transfused to achieve a hematocrit of at least 30%. In mechanically ventilated patients, a higher central venous pressure of 12 to 15 mm Hg may be required to account for increased intrathoracic pressure. In a randomized controlled trial evaluating goal-directed therapy initiated in the emergency department, patients fared better when clinicians used this approach.[51] Patients receiving early, goal-directed therapy had a lower 28-day mortality rate, a decreased incidence of multiple-organ dysfunction, and decreased use of hospital resources compared to patients receiving standard therapy.

There is controversy regarding whether crystalloids or colloids are the optimal modality for resuscitation. Both can be used to attain central venous pressure goals in critically ill septic patients. To correct hypovolemia, crystalloids can be administered at a rate of 500 to 1,000 mL every 30 minutes until goals are obtained, with the awareness that patients require monitoring to avoid complications such as fluid overload. Crystalloids, which require smaller volumes to attain hemodynamic goals, can be administered at a rate of 300 to 500 mL every 30 minutes.[52] If low cardiac output persists despite adequate fluid resuscitation, vasopressors should be initiated. Norepinephrine and dopamine are examples of agents typically administered as first-line agents. Although no high-quality, definitive studies have been completed, human and animal studies suggests that these catecholamines are better than epinephrine or phenylephrine.[53,54] Epinephrine has been associated with tachycardia and may have deleterious effects on splanchnic perfusion.[55,56] Phenylephrine, although associated with a low incidence of tachycardia, may lead to decreases in stroke volume.[56] Despite wide acceptance for decades, low-dose dopamine for renal protection should be avoided. Both individual trials and a well-designed meta-analysis conducted in critically ill patients found no evidence to support this practice.[57,58]

Transfusion of red cells is recommended if the central venous oxygen saturation is 70% or less to achieve a hematocrit of 30% or greater. If central venous pressure, mean arterial pressure, and hematocrit have been optimized and the central venous oxygen saturation still remains below 70%, an inotropic agent such as dobutamine should be started.[52,56]

Antibiotic Therapy. Unfortunately, the causative organism in sepsis is rarely known at the time when the decision to

treat presumed sepsis is made. The initial choice of antibiotic therapy in a patient with presumed sepsis is empiric in most instances and depends on several factors: (a) activity against the presumed causative pathogens; (b) the patient's history, including underlying diseases and comorbidities; (c) penetration into suspected sites of infection; (d) patient drug allergies; (e) local susceptibility patterns in the hospital or unit; and (f) formulary availability.

Several retrospective studies have shown that early, aggressive administration of antibiotics that have activity against most likely pathogens reduces mortality in severe infections.[59–61] Additional studies have shown that patients receiving at least one antibiotic having documented in vitro activity against causative bacteria have significantly reduced mortality.[62–64] In a study of over 2,000 patients with gram-negative bacteremia, patients receiving appropriate antibiotic therapy had a mortality of 18%, whereas patients receiving inappropriate therapy had a significantly higher mortality of 34%.[63] Although fewer studies have been published with sepsis specifically, it is likely that similar findings would occur. Therefore, once cultures have been obtained, intravenous (IV) broad-spectrum antibiotics directed against the most likely pathogens should be immediately initiated, preferably within 1 hour of recognizing the clinical syndrome of sepsis. Given the small margin of error in this subset of critically ill patients, oral antibiotic therapy is contraindicated at this time.

Addition of Antimicrobials With Gram-Positive Activity. Randomized controlled trials comparing empiric treatment regimens including or excluding gram-positive–active agents have not been performed in adult sepsis patients. However, given that gram-positive organisms account for approximately half of all infections in patients with sepsis, empiric treatment with antibiotics with gram-positive activity is justified until the infectious etiology can be confirmed.[8] Thus, empiric therapy should consist of antibiotics with both gram-negative and gram-positive coverage. Many of the antibiotics routinely given for empiric therapy of sepsis have a broad spectrum of activity, have gram-positive activity, and can be used to accomplish this goal.

Depending on the presumed source of infection, the local epidemiology of pathogens associated with sepsis in the hospital, and susceptibility patterns, the addition of vancomycin may be warranted. To prevent inappropriate use of vancomycin in patients with severe sepsis, its use should be limited to those with a documented hypersensitivity to β-lactams or to patients at hospitals with endemic rates of MRSA or MRSE. Nosocomial infections due to vancomycin-resistant enterococci (VRE) have increased dramatically, and the use of linezolid and quinupristin/dalfopristin may be required in some patients with severe sepsis. Empiric use of these agents should be avoided unless an infection with VRE is suspected. Linezolid has activity against both E faecium and E faecalis, whereas quinupristin/dalfopristin has activity only against E *faecium.* Both have activity against MRSA and can be used in patients with documented vancomycin hypersensitivity.

Monotherapy Versus Combination Therapy. The decision to use monotherapy or combination antibiotic therapy for severe sepsis has not been adequately addressed using clinical trials in this population. Most studies addressing this issue have been conducted in other patient populations, and therefore extrapolation of results is required. Moreover, studies comparing monotherapy to combination therapy involved relatively small sample sizes, limiting the statistical power. In the selection of broad-spectrum empiric therapy for sepsis, the debate continues regarding combination antibiotic therapy versus monotherapy. Because of the life-threatening nature of sepsis, many advocate the use of combination therapy based on multiple arguments: (a) use of combination therapy allows for the coverage of a wide range of organisms, including both gram-negative and gram-positive organisms; (b) therapy with two different antibiotics with different mechanisms of action may yield additive or synergistic effects against the pathogen; and (c) combination therapy may delay or prevent the emergence of resistance. Indeed, positive associations between the use of combination antibiotic therapy that produces synergistic effects in vitro and improved clinical results have been documented in human studies.[65,66] However, evaluation of the literature regarding antibiotic treatments for sepsis reveals little difference between monotherapy and combination therapy once a causative pathogen has been identified. One reason for these findings may be the fact that antibiotics used alone tend to be highly bactericidal, including extended-spectrum penicillins, third- or fourth-generation cephalosporins, or carbapenems. Thus, these agents alone have broad antibacterial activity and may therefore yield comparable results to combination therapy.

Another consideration relates to the choice of agent to be included in the combination therapy regimen. Aminoglycosides are frequently used in combination with β-lactam antibiotics and have been associated with higher incidences of nephrotoxicity and ototoxicity, especially when administered without appropriate serum concentration monitoring.[67,68] Careful therapeutic drug monitoring can decrease the incidence of toxicity and therefore should be used.[69,70] The added nephrotoxicity profile must be weighed against the potential for added antibacterial spectrum or decreased emergence of resistant bacteria. Fluoroquinolones may be useful if dual therapy is required but the clinician is unwilling to use an aminoglycoside. Given the diverse administration schedules of available antibiotics, it may be difficult to maintain the synergistic concentrations in the patient that were described with in vitro studies. Therefore, although it may be desirable to do so, extrapolating in vitro synergy data to the individual patient is difficult.

Specific Therapy. Depending on the infectious source (e.g., abdominal, pulmonary, urinary), empiric antibiotic treatment will vary. For specific therapies for these infections, the reader is referred to respective chapters in this textbook. Examples of initial empiric antibiotic therapy may include:

1. Extended-spectrum penicillins with antipseudomonal activity ± an aminoglycoside or antipseudomonal fluoroquinolone ± vancomycin
2. Carbapenem ± an aminoglycoside or antipseudomonal fluoroquinolone ± vancomycin
3. Third- or fourth-generation cephalosporin ± an aminoglycoside or antipseudomonal fluoroquinolone ± vancomycin
4. β-lactam/β-lactamase inhibitor combination ± an aminoglycoside or antipseudomonal fluoroquinolone

Tailoring Empiric Antibiotic Therapy and Monitoring. Once the causative pathogen has been identified, broad-spectrum therapy should be tailored toward the specific pathogen. This not only results in more specific therapy, but may also reduce the likelihood of superinfection, emergence of resistant pathogens, and cost of care. If cultures are negative and the causative agent cannot be determined, the decision to alter empiric antimicrobial therapy will default to clinician judgment and findings from ongoing diagnostics.

The recommended duration of therapy is 7 to 10 days, but this is only a guide and should be dictated by patient response. Many patients have complicated courses and require a longer duration of therapy. If patients fail to respond to empiric antimicrobial therapy within 24 to 48 hours, cultures should be repeated to confirm poor source control and antibiotic therapy should be expanded to cover additional pathogens.

Sepsis is a dynamic process, and the patient's status may change from hour to hour or day to day. Attaining therapeutic antibiotic concentrations, minimizing toxicity, and careful monitoring of drug therapy are integral for the success of the prescribed course. Hepatic and renal dysfunction is common in patients with severe sepsis.[71,72] In addition, given the large volumes of crystalloids and colloids used during resuscitation, combined with altered vascular permeability, patients typically exhibit large volumes of distributions. Therefore, adjustments to therapy may be required on an ongoing basis to maximize efficacy while limiting or preventing toxicity.

Immunotherapy of Sepsis. Advances in the understanding of the host inflammatory response to sepsis have led to considerable interest in modulating the expression and end-organ actions of systemic inflammatory mediators. Many attempts have been made to synthesize novel therapeutic entities targeted toward specific mediators important for the pathophysiology of sepsis. There have been over 70 randomized clinical trials involving immunomodulatory drugs with the hopes of decreasing mortality from sepsis. Although several animal studies have yielded impressive results, the efficacy of these agents in humans has been largely disappointing. In fact, with some immunomodulatory trials, treatment with the investigational agent resulted in increased rather than decreased morbidity and mortality.[73,74]

In all the years of sepsis research, only one novel sepsis drug has been approved by the U.S. Food and Drug Administration (FDA), while another previously approved drug has shown benefit.[75,76] This clearly illustrates the complexity of the challenge in treating patients with severe sepsis.

One of the first targets for immunotherapies was endotoxin. One early study used a polyclonal antiserum (J5 antiserum) raised by immunizing healthy human volunteers with a mutant form of endotoxin (*E coli* J5).[77] When administered to patients with gram-negative bacteremia, the mortality rate was reduced to 22% compared to 39% in the control group. Mortality was also significantly reduced in patients with severe shock compared to control patients. In a subsequent study, prophylactic administration of J5 antiserum in high-risk surgical patients also improved outcomes.[78] These were the first studies to provide clinical evidence that reduction of endotoxin in septic patients may lead to improved patient outcomes.

Although these results were favorable, the use of antiendotoxin antiserum has not been embraced because of the impracticality of obtaining sufficient numbers of volunteers to generate the antiserum and the potential for disease transmission. However, these studies generated considerable interest in mitigating the effects of endotoxin, and thus for several years multiple attempts using different strategies were tested in patients with severe sepsis. Unfortunately, none of the agents significantly reduced overall mortality.

Reasons for Failure of Immunotherapies for Sepsis. Multiple reasons have been proposed for why immunotherapies for sepsis have not met expectations in clinical trials:

- Animal models are poor predictors of human results: Many of the agents tested showed promising results in animal models and were therefore further developed for human use. Given the genetic homogeneity and lack of comorbid conditions (diabetes, cancer, heart disease, and others) of animals, the complexity of sepsis in humans is difficult to recreate.
- Complexity of host response: The innate host response to inflammatory stimuli is both extremely intricate and redundant, and therefore therapies directed against individual mediators may fall short of expectations.
- Ensuring biologic activity: Construction of recombinant proteins for sepsis trials is difficult, and ensuring biologic activity in vivo is problematic. For example, the monoclonal antibody HA-1A to endotoxin did not yield favorable results in human trials.[79] Subsequent investigation of HA-1A showed that although the antibody bound endotoxin, it did not prevent its ability to induce a cellular response.[80]
- Timing and administration: When designing clinical trials, one challenge is a lack of understanding regarding the optimal timing of therapies and the correct dose and duration of treatment. The goal is to initiate therapy early enough in the disease course when targeted mediators are present and can be effectively modulated. Administering therapy too early or late may result in the target not being present and therefore not amenable to modulation. Whereas titration of therapies such as insulin or vasopressors is common in the ICU, titration of therapy for investigational agents in sepsis has not typically been conducted. Most trials are designed so that the agent is given at a fixed dose for an arbitrary duration of time. Thus, it is likely that the therapeutic window for previous agents was often missed.
- Trial design: Mortality at 28 days is the major clinical endpoint in most sepsis trials. A frequently held belief is that reversal of pathophysiologic changes will be sustained, even though the agents are routinely administered over a very brief period. However, because approximately 40% of septic patients who are still alive remain in the ICU at day 28, many are at increased risk for recurrent disease, complications, and death. Therefore, the period over which success is evaluated may be inappropriate. Another major problem related to trial design has been the heterogeneity of the populations studied. Criteria for SIRS or sepsis syndrome, although improved from previous definitions, are still arbitrary and relatively nonspecific. Despite considerable effort, it is almost impossible to stratify extremely heterogeneous populations based on their varied clinical settings and levels of circulating proinflammatory mediators. Given the growing awareness of the importance of genetic polymorphisms in innate immunity, past trials were undoubtedly lacking in this regard.[81,82]

Recombinant Human Activated Protein C. The many beneficial effects of APC on both inflammatory and coagulation pathways led investigators to evaluate the utility of this protein as a therapeutic agent for treatment of severe sepsis. Numerous trials have documented that decreased protein C synthesis in septic patients leads to a prothrombotic state.[33,83–86] Based on its physiology, it was presumed that APC could blunt the activation of the coagulation cascade, improve fibrinolysis, and ultimately diminish the deleterious effects on organ function that result from inflammation in sepsis.[85,87,88] The PROWESS trial evaluated drotrecogin alfa, a recombinant form of human APC (rhAPC) in patients with severe sepsis.[75] Patients receiving 24 μg/kg/hr for 96 hours had significant reductions in the 28-day all-cause mortality compared to patients receiving placebo.

Based on this trial, rhAPC is now recommended for patients with severe sepsis who meet certain criteria. Specifically, those with an APACHE II score of at least 25, sepsis-induced multiple-organ failure, septic shock, or sepsis-induced acute respiratory distress syndrome should receive rhAPC, providing they do not have conditions that would result in the risks not outweighing the benefits of this therapy. Contraindications to rhAPC therapy include active internal bleeding, hemorrhagic stroke within 3 months, severe head trauma, intracranial or intraspinal surgery within 2 months, need for an epidural catheter, or other factors that would increase the likelihood of life-threatening bleeding.

Corticosteroids. During inflammation, proinflammatory mediators initially act on the hypothalamic-pituitary-adrenal axis to increase production of the stress hormone cortisol.[89] This in turn affects the inflammatory process through the secretion of cytokines, modulation of circulating immune cells, and nitric oxide production. However, in septic shock, inflammatory cytokines may actually suppress the cortisol response to adrenocorticotropin hormone, resulting in a relative adrenal insufficiency and peripheral glucocorticoid resistance.[90,91] This ultimately leads to a deregulation of the inflammatory process and negative effects on vascular tone. Several studies have shown that functional adrenal insufficiency and inability to augment adrenal cortisol release in response to ACTH stimulation are common in sepsis.[76,92] More importantly, this decreased response has been associated with poor outcomes.[93]

Early studies used high doses of corticosteroids over short periods but were not conclusive.[94] Evaluating trials of IV corticosteroids conducted after 1992, when the definitions for sepsis and septic shock were revised, however, reveals that low-dose steroids may have a role in the treatment of certain subsets of patients with sepsis. Patients with septic shock requiring vasopressors to maintain blood pressure and organ perfusion despite adequate fluid resuscitation who received low doses of corticosteroids (200 to 300 mg of hydrocortisone or equivalent in three or four divided doses) for 7 days had significant reductions in 28-day all-cause mortality and hospital mortality, in addition to significantly reversing shock.[95] Furthermore, administration of low-dose corticosteroids may reduce circulating levels of IL-6 and IL-8, as well as nitric oxide formation.

It remains unclear whether the administration of corticosteroids should be based on the results of an ACTH stimulation test to identify nonresponders. Some studies have used this test to stratify patients, but recommendations for relative adrenal sufficiency vary. Standardization of peak cortisol levels after stimulation, threshold levels of random cortisol, and combinations of these criteria is difficult. If an ACTH stimulation test cannot be obtained immediately, clinicians can still begin low-dose corticosteroids until a test can be performed. In these cases, dexamethasone rather than hydrocortisone should be administered because dexamethasone does not interfere with the cortisol assay.[52]

SUPPORTIVE PHARMACOTHERAPY

Glucose Control. Hyperglycemia associated with insulin resistance is common in critical illness in both diabetic and nondiabetic patients. Prolonged episodes of hyperglycemia are believed to place patients at risk for infectious complications, critical-illness polyneuropathy, and multiple-organ failure.[96,97] Although sliding-scale insulin therapy is the standard of care in many ICUs, recent evidence indicates that stringent glycemic control with intensive insulin therapy improves outcomes. One large trial in postoperative surgical patients found that maintaining glucose concentrations between 80 and 110 mg per dL using a continuous infusion of insulin led to significant reductions in ICU mortality compared to patients receiving standard therapy.[98] The greatest reduction in mortality was seen with deaths due to multiple-organ failure associated with sepsis. Intensive insulin therapy also led to reductions in overall hospital mortality, bloodstream infections, acute renal failure, and critical-illness polyneuropathy.

This and other studies have led to dramatic changes in how glucose control is managed in the ICU. The use of intensive insulin therapy increases the risk of hypoglycemia, so frequent glucose monitoring should accompany therapy.

Stress Ulcer Prophylaxis. Two independent risk factors for clinically significant bleeding due to stress ulcers are mechanical ventilation and coagulopathy, factors often present in sepsis patients.[99] Other factors placing patients at risk are acute renal failure, acute hepatic failure, major surgery, severe head trauma, and major burns (greater than 30% total body surface area).[99,100] Thus, all patients with severe sepsis should receive stress ulcer prophylaxis. Use of gastroprotective agents such as sucralfate and antacids has declined over the past decade due to administration issues and lack of superiority compared to antisecretory agents.[101,102] Most trials evaluating stress ulcer prophylaxis regimens have used H2-receptor antagonists, and their use has been associated with significant reductions in clinically significant bleeding versus placebo.[103]

The role of proton pump inhibitors for stress ulcer prophylaxis continues to be defined. Unfortunately, no well-designed, randomized, controlled trials comparing proton pump inhibitors to H2-receptor antagonists for stress ulcer prophylaxis have been completed. Most are small, often open-label studies, and therefore interpretation is required. However, due to their increased potency compared to H2-receptor antagonists and superiority in other acid-related disease states, it is likely that their role will continue to evolve.

As the patient's clinical condition improves, the presence of risk factors for clinically significant bleeding due to stress ulceration should be reassessed. Once patients no longer have risk factors, stress ulcer prophylaxis should be discontinued.

Deep Vein Thrombosis Prophylaxis. The incidence of deep vein thrombosis (DVT) ranges from 10% to 80% in ICU patients, and therefore patients with severe sepsis should receive DVT prophylaxis.[104] Although trials have not been specifically conducted in septic patients, several large trials evaluating DVT prophylaxis involving ICU patients included patients with sepsis, and therefore it is widely believed that the results can be extrapolated.[105–107] The most common pharmacologic prophylaxis modalities are low-dose unfractionated heparin (UFH) or low-molecular-weight heparin (LMWH). It appears that certain populations, such as those with trauma or spinal cord injury, benefit more from LMWH than UFH, and therefore careful evaluation of the patient for risk factors is warranted. Patients at a higher risk for thrombosis should receive LMWH.[104] For patients who are at high risk of bleeding, mechanical methods of prophylaxis such as intermittent compression devices can be used and are effective. Ongoing studies are evaluating the utility of combined pharmacologic and mechanical means of DVT prophylaxis.

Other Supportive Pharmacotherapy Measures. In addition to the well-characterized hemodynamic and immune consequences of SIRS, a hypermetabolic state may result, leading to a malnourished state. Nutritional support is a key component of care for patients with severe sepsis and may even modulate the immune response.[108] Enteral feeding is preferred over parenteral nutrition in light of findings that the former may better preserve gut integrity and gut-associated lymphoid tissue.[109–111]

Regardless of the route of administration, nutritional support should be initiated as soon as possible. In patients requiring parenteral nutrition, the ability to change to enteral feeding should be assessed on a daily basis.

Mechanically ventilated patients should receive sedation and analgesia. The choice between bolus sedation and continuous infusions of sedatives is the prerogative of the healthcare team; both are effective. Importantly, sedation goals using standardized sedation scales should be set for each patient. Patients receiving continuous sedation should be awakened daily or at least have sedation lightened to assist with assessment of sedation levels and the need for titration. Mechanically ventilated patients subject to sedation protocols have been shown to have significantly reduced number of days of mechanical ventilation, tracheostomy rates, and length of stay.[112] If neuromuscular blockers are required to maintain ventilatory parameters, they should be used sparingly, with strict assessment using train-of-four monitoring so that the degree of neuromuscular blockade can be assessed.

FUTURE THERAPIES

Despite therapeutic advances such as APC, the overall survival rate from severe sepsis is still poor. Additional research is required to identify therapies that will improve mortality from this disease. One area that may be exploited in the future relies on information gained from genetic association studies. It is becoming increasing clear that an individual's susceptibility to infection and his or her innate immune response to pathogens can be partially explained by genetic background. Genes encoding proteins important for inflam-

mation, coagulation, and fibrinolysis may exhibit polymorphisms, and therefore response to inflammatory stimuli may be different from patient to patient.[113,114] For example, polymorphisms in genes linked to the coagulation pathway have been described and may influence the outcome from sepsis.[115–117]

PHARMACOECONOMICS

The economic impact of sepsis is profound, with annual healthcare expenditures totaling over $16 billion in the United States.[14] Compared to patients without sepsis, direct costs are estimated to be six times higher for patients with sepsis.[118] True pharmacoeconomic evaluations of severe sepsis have been hampered by a lack of proven, life-saving therapies until recently (rhAPC, low-dose steroids). Moreover, of the studies that have been conducted, most have been performed in Europe, where practice patterns are very different, so conclusions reached in those studies may not reflect what occurs in U.S. hospitals. Another consideration when evaluating pharmacoeconomic data is that most studies are conducted in academic institutions, where hospital costs typically are significantly higher compared to nonteaching hospitals.[14]

Resource use tends to increase as patients progress from sepsis to severe sepsis to septic shock. Of the resources consumed, length of stay appears to be one of the most important factors determining the magnitude of cost of care.[119] Patient location prior to the diagnosis of sepsis is another important influence on cost. If sepsis develops prior to admission to the ICU, costs have been reported to be two to three times lower than if severe sepsis develops while the patient is in the ICU. Surgical patients, patients in the ICU, and those with organ dysfunction have higher resource use.[14]

With the high cost of newer sepsis therapies, identifying subsets of patients who will benefit is important from both economic and patient care perspectives. For example, analysis of the PROWESS trial showed that patients with an APACHE II score of at least 25 benefited from rhAPC, whereas patients with lower APACHE scores did not.

One area that will undoubtedly influence whether new therapies are cost-effective is the cost of ongoing care of patients who survive sepsis. Most clinical trials evaluating treatments for severe sepsis use the traditional 28-day mortality as a primary outcome measure, and any pharmacoeconomic analyses tend to encompass this time period. Utilization of resources after the 28-day period has not been extensively studied. If patients survive, it is likely that significant resources will be consumed, especially if the therapeutic intervention does not affect long-term survival. Limited data indicate that the cost of care for survivors of sepsis is highest in the first year after hospital discharge, with many patients requiring readmission. Patient comorbidity and the severity of illness while in the hospital appear to be two factors that heavily influence cost.[120]

KEY POINTS

■ The successful management of sepsis, with its attendant high mortality, relies on early clinical suspicion, rapid diagnosis, and appropriate choice of antimicrobial agents based on clinical presentation, the suspected source of infection, and a variety of underlying patient-specific factors

■ The use of traditional treatment modalities such as prompt fluid resuscitation and ventilatory and blood pressure support is fundamental to the clinical management of this syndrome

■ Rapid changes in the patient's condition require prompt modification of drug dosing, use of therapeutic drug monitoring, and close monitoring of the patient's hemodynamic status to adjust primary therapy as well as supportive therapy

■ Only through continued research and the proper application of the results to the management of sepsis patients can the overall outcome of this syndrome be improved

SUGGESTED READINGS

Bernard GR, Vincent JL, Laterre PF, et al. Efficacy and safety of recombinant human activated protein C for severe sepsis. N Engl J Med 344:699–709, 2001.

Dellinger RP, Carlet JM, Masur H, et al. Surviving Sepsis Campaign guidelines for management of severe sepsis and septic shock. Crit Care Med 32:858–873, 2004.

Hollenberg SM, Ahrens TS, Annane D, et al. Practice parameters for hemodynamic support of sepsis in adult patients: 2004 update. Crit Care Med 32:1928–1948, 2004.

Marshall JC. Such stuff as dreams are made on: mediator-directed therapy in sepsis. Nature Reviews Drug Discovery 2:391–405, 2003.

REFERENCES

1. Bone RC, Balk RA, Cerra FB, et al. Definitions for sepsis and organ failure and guidelines for the use of innovative therapies in sepsis. The ACCP/SCCM Consensus Conference Committee. American College of Chest Physicians/Society of Critical Care Medicine. Chest 101:1644–1655, 1992.

2. Bochud PY, Bonten M, Marchetti O, et al. Antimicrobial therapy for patients with severe sepsis and septic shock: an evidence-based review. Crit Care Med 32 (11 Suppl):S495–512, 2004.

3. Alberti C, Brun-Buisson C, Burchardi H, et al. Epidemiology of sepsis and infection in ICU patients from an international multicentre cohort study.[erratum appears in Intensive Care Med 28: 525–526, 2002]. Intensive Care Med 28:108–121, 2002.

4. Martin GS, Mannino DM, Eaton S, et al. The epidemiology of sepsis in the United States from 1979 through 2000. N Engl J Med 348:1546–1554, 2003.

5. Conboy K, Welage LS, Walawander CA, et al. Sepsis syndrome and associated sequelae in patients at high risk for gram-negative sepsis. Pharmacotherapy 15:66–77, 1995.

6. Marchetti O, Calandra T. Infections in neutropenic cancer patients. Lancet 359:723–725, 2002.

7. Vincent JL, Bihari DJ, Suter PM, et al. The prevalence of nosocomial infection in intensive care units in Europe. Results of the European Prevalence of Infection in Intensive Care (EPIC) Study. EPIC International Advisory Committee. JAMA 274:639–644, 1995.

8. Richards MJ, Edwards JR, Culver DH, et al. Nosocomial infections in medical intensive care units in the United States. National Noso-

comial Infections Surveillance System. Crit Care Med 27:887–892, 1999.

9. National Nosocomial Infections Surveillance System. National Nosocomial Infections Surveillance (NNIS) System Report, data summary from January 1992 through June 2004, issued October 2004. Am J Infection Control 32:470–485, 2004.

10. Wisplinghoff H, Seifert H, Coimbra M, et al. Systemic inflammatory response syndrome in adult patients with nosocomial bloodstream infection due to Staphylococcus aureus. Clin Infect Dis 33: 733–736, 2001.

11. Edmond MB, Wallace SE, McClish DK, et al. Nosocomial bloodstream infections in United States hospitals: a three-year analysis. Clin Infect Dis 29:239–244, 1999.

12. Riedemann NC, Guo RF, Ward PA. The enigma of sepsis. J Clin Invest 112:460–467, 2003.

13. Crowe M, Ispahani P, Humphreys H, et al. Bacteraemia in the adult intensive care unit of a teaching hospital in Nottingham, UK, 1985–1996. Eur J Clin Microbiol Infect Dis 17:377–384, 1998.

14. Angus DC, Linde-Zwirble WT, Lidicker J, et al. Epidemiology of severe sepsis in the United States: analysis of incidence, outcome, and associated costs of care. Crit Care Med 29:1303–1310, 2001.

15. Annane D, Bellissant E, Cavaillon JM. Septic shock. Lancet 365: 63–78, 2005.

16. Poltorak A, He X, Smirnova I, et al. Defective LPS signaling in C3H/HeJ and C57BL/10ScCr mice: mutations in Tlr4 gene. Science 282:2085–2088, 1998.

17. van der Poll T, van Deventer SJ. Cytokines and anticytokines in the pathogenesis of sepsis. Infect Dis Clin North Am 13:413–426, 1999.

18. van der Poll T. Immunotherapy of sepsis. Lancet Infect Dis 1: 165–174, 2001.

19. Thijs LG, Hack CE. Time course of cytokine levels in sepsis. Intensive Care Med 21 (Suppl 2):S258–263, 1995.

20. van Deventer SJ, Buller HR, ten Cate JW, et al. Experimental endotoxemia in humans: analysis of cytokine release and coagulation, fibrinolytic, and complement pathways. Blood 76:2520–2526, 1990.

21. Curfs JH, Meis JF, Hoogkamp-Korstanje JA. A primer on cytokines: sources, receptors, effects, and inducers. Clin Microbiol Rev 10:742–780, 1997.

22. Bone RC. Sir Isaac Newton, sepsis, SIRS, and CARS. Crit Care Med 24:1125–1128, 1996.

23. Rice TW, Bernard GR. Therapeutic intervention and targets for sepsis. Ann Rev Med 56:225–248, 2005.

24. Thijs LG, de Boer JP, de Groot MC, et al. Coagulation disorders in septic shock. Intensive Care Med 19:S8–15, 1993.

25. Levi M, ten CH, van der Poll T, et al. Pathogenesis of disseminated intravascular coagulation in sepsis. JAMA 270:975–979, 1993.

26. Girardin SE, Philpott DJ. Mini-review: the role of peptidoglycan recognition in innate immunity. Eur J Immunol 34:1777–1782, 2004.

27. Weijer S, Lauw FN, Branger J, et al. Diminished interferon-gamma production and responsiveness after endotoxin administration to healthy humans. J Infect Dis 186:1748–1753, 2002.

28. Fumeaux T, Pugin J. Role of interleukin-10 in the intracellular sequestration of human leukocyte antigen-DR in monocytes during septic shock. Am J Resp Crit Care Med 166:1475–1482, 2002.

29. Aird WC. Vascular bed-specific hemostasis: role of endothelium in sepsis pathogenesis. Crit Care Med 29 (7 Suppl):S28–35, 2001.

30. Broze GJ, Jr. Tissue factor pathway inhibitor and the current concept of blood coagulation. Blood Coag Fibrinolysis 6 (Suppl 1): S7–13, 1995.

31. Wesselschmidt R, Likert K, Huang Z, et al. Structural requirements for tissue factor pathway inhibitor interactions with factor Xa and heparin. Blood Coag Fibrinolysis 4:661–669, 1993.

32. van Hinsbergh VW, Kooistra T, van den Berg EA, et al. Tumor necrosis factor increases the production of plasminogen activator inhibitor in human endothelial cells in vitro and in rats in vivo. Blood 72:1467–1473, 1988.

33. Lorente JA, Garcia-Frade LJ, Landin L, et al. Time course of hemostatic abnormalities in sepsis and its relation to outcome. Chest 103:1536–1542, 1993.

34. Cohen J, Brun-Buisson C, Torres A, et al. Diagnosis of infection in sepsis: an evidence-based review. Crit Care Med 32 (11 Suppl): S466–494, 2004.

35. O'Grady NP, Barie PS, Bartlett JG, et al. Practice guidelines for evaluating new fever in critically ill adult patients. Task Force of the Society of Critical Care Medicine and the Infectious Diseases Society of America. Clin Infectious Dis 26:1042–1059, 1998.

36. Young LS. Sepsis syndrome. In: Mandell GL, Bennett JE, Dolin R, eds. Principles and practice of infectious diseases. New York: Churchill Livingstone, 2000:806–819.

37. Chandrasekar PH, Brown WJ. Clinical issues of blood cultures. Arch Intern Med 154:841–849, 1994.

38. Bates DW, Goldman L, Lee TH. Contaminant blood cultures and resource utilization. The true consequences of false-positive results. JAMA 265:365–369, 1991.

39. Bryant JK, Strand CL. Reliability of blood cultures collected from intravascular catheter versus venipuncture. Am J Clin Pathol 88: 113–116, 1987.

40. DesJardin JA, Falagas ME, Ruthazer R, et al. Clinical utility of blood cultures drawn from indwelling central venous catheters in hospitalized patients with cancer. Ann Intern Med 131:641–647, 1999.

41. Martinez JA, DesJardin JA, Aronoff M, et al. Clinical utility of blood cultures drawn from central venous or arterial catheters in critically ill surgical patients. Crit Care Med 30:7–13, 2002.

42. Wunderink RG. Clinical criteria in the diagnosis of ventilator-associated pneumonia. Chest 117 (4 Suppl 2):191S–194S, 2000.

43. Marquette CH, Herengt F, Mathieu D, et al. Diagnosis of pneumonia in mechanically ventilated patients. Repeatability of the protected specimen brush. Am Rev Resp Dis 147:211–214, 1993.

44. Timsit JF, Misset B, Francoual S, et al. Is protected specimen brush a reproducible method to diagnose ICU-acquired pneumonia? Chest 104:104–108, 1993.

45. Baughman RP. Protected-specimen brush technique in the diagnosis of ventilator-associated pneumonia. Chest 117 (4 Suppl 2): 203S–206S, 2000.

46. Light RB. Septic shock. In: Hall JB, Schmidt GA, Wood LDH, ed. Principles of critical care. New York: McGraw-Hill, 1992: 1172–1185.

47. Jimenez MF, Marshall JC, International Sepsis Forum. Source control in the management of sepsis. Intensive Care Med 27 (Suppl 1): S49–62, 2001.

48. Hoste EA, Lameire NH, Vanholder RC, et al. Acute renal failure in patients with sepsis in a surgical ICU: predictive factors, incidence, comorbidity, and outcome. J Am Soc Nephrol 14: 1022–1030, 2003.

49. Groeneveld AB, Tran DD, van der Meulen J, et al. Acute renal failure in the medical intensive care unit: predisposing, complicating factors and outcome. Nephron 59:602–610, 1991.

50. Brivet FG, Kleinknecht DJ, Loirat P, et al. Acute renal failure in intensive care units: causes, outcome, and prognostic factors of hospital mortality; a prospective, multicenter study. French Study Group on Acute Renal Failure. Crit Care Med 24:192–198, 1996.

51. Rivers E, Nguyen B, Havstad S, et al. Early goal-directed therapy in the treatment of severe sepsis and septic shock. N Engl J Med 345:1368–1377, 2001.

52. Dellinger RP, Carlet JM, Masur H, et al. Surviving Sepsis Campaign guidelines for management of severe sepsis and septic shock. Crit Care Med 32:858–873, 2004.

53. Hollenberg SM, Ahrens TS, Annane D, et al. Practice parameters for hemodynamic support of sepsis in adult patients: 2004 update. Crit Care Med 32:1928–1948, 2004.

54. LeDoux D, Astiz ME, Carpati CM, et al. Effects of perfusion pressure on tissue perfusion in septic shock. Crit Care Med 28: 2729–2732, 2000.

55. De Backer D, Creteur J, Silva E, et al. Effects of dopamine, norepinephrine, and epinephrine on the splanchnic circulation in septic shock: which is best? Crit Care Med 31:1659–1667, 2003.

56. Beale RJ, Hollenberg SM, Vincent JL, et al. Vasopressor and inotropic support in septic shock: an evidence-based review. Crit Care Med 32 (11 Suppl):S455–465, 2004.

57. Bellomo R, Chapman M, Finfer S, et al. Low-dose dopamine in patients with early renal dysfunction: a placebo-controlled randomised trial. Australian and New Zealand Intensive Care Society (ANZICS) Clinical Trials Group. Lancet 356:2139–2143, 2000.

58. Kellum JA, Decker M. Use of dopamine in acute renal failure: a meta-analysis. Crit Care Med 29:1526–1531, 2001.

59. McCabe WR, Jackson GG. Gram-negative bacteremia. Arch Intern Med 110:92–100, 1962.

60. Young LS, Martin WJ, Meyer RD, et al. Gram-negative rod bacteremia: microbiologic, immunologic, and therapeutic considerations. Ann Intern Med 86:456–471, 1977.

61. Bryant RE, Hood AF, Hood CE, et al. Factors affecting mortality of gram-negative rod bacteremia. Arch Intern Med 127:120–128, 1971.

62. Kreger BE, Craven DE, McCabe WR. Gram-negative bacteremia. IV. Re-evaluation of clinical features and treatment in 612 patients. Am J Med 68:344–355, 1980.

63. Leibovici L, Shraga I, Drucker M, et al. The benefit of appropriate empirical antibiotic treatment in patients with bloodstream infection. J Intern Med 244:379–386, 1998.

64. Ibrahim EH, Sherman G, Ward S, et al. The influence of inadequate antimicrobial treatment of bloodstream infections on patient outcomes in the ICU setting. Chest 118:146–155, 2000.

65. Anderson ET, Young LS, Hewitt WL. Antimicrobial synergism in the therapy of gram-negative rod bacteremia. Chemotherapy 24: 45–54, 1978.

66. Klastersky J, Meunier-Carpentier F, Prevost JM. Significance of antimicrobial synergism for the outcome of gram-negative sepsis. Am J Med Sci 273:157–167, 1977.

67. Swan SK. Aminoglycoside nephrotoxicity. Semin Nephrol 17: 27–33, 1997.

68. Lerner SA, Matz GJ. Aminoglycoside ototoxicity. Am J Otolaryngol 1:169–179, 1980.

69. Dahlgren JG, Anderson ET, Hewitt WL. Gentamicin blood levels: a guide to nephrotoxicity. Antimicrobial Agents Chemotherapy 8: 58–62, 1975.

70. Goodman EL, Van GJ, Holmes R, et al. Prospective comparative study of variable dosage and variable frequency regimens for administration of gentamicin. Antimicrobial Agents Chemotherapy 8: 434–438, 1975.

71. Strassburg CP. Gastrointestinal disorders of the critically ill. Shock liver. Best Practice Res Clin Gastroenterol 17:369–381, 2003.

72. Klenzak J, Himmelfarb J. Sepsis and the kidney. Crit Care Clin 21: 211–222, 2005.

73. Fisher CJ, Jr., Agosti JM, Opal SM, et al. Treatment of septic shock with the tumor necrosis factor receptor:Fc fusion protein. The Soluble TNF Receptor Sepsis Study Group. N Engl J Med 334:1697–1702, 1996.

74. Grover R, Lopez A, Lorente J, et al. Multi-center, randomized, placebo-controlled, double blind study of the nitric oxide synthase inhibitor 546C88: effect on survival in patients with septic shock. Crit Care Med 27:A33, 1999.

75. Bernard GR, Vincent JL, Laterre PF, et al. Efficacy and safety of recombinant human activated protein C for severe sepsis. N Engl J Med 344:699–709, 2001.

76. Annane D, Sebille V, Charpentier C, et al. Effect of treatment with low doses of hydrocortisone and fludrocortisone on mortality in patients with septic shock. JAMA 288:862–871, 2002.

77. Ziegler EJ, McCutchan JA, Fierer J, et al. Treatment of gram-negative bacteremia and shock with human antiserum to a mutant Escherichia coli. N Engl J Med 307:1225–1230, 1982.

78. Baumgartner JD, Glauser MP, McCutchan JA, et al. Prevention of gram-negative shock and death in surgical patients by antibody to endotoxin core glycolipid. Lancet 2:59–63, 1985.

79. McCloskey RV, Straube RC, Sanders C, et al. Treatment of septic shock with human monoclonal antibody HA-1A. A randomized, double-blind, placebo-controlled trial. CHESS Trial Study Group. Ann Intern Med 121:1–5, 1994.

80. Warren HS, Amato SF, Fitting C, et al. Assessment of ability of murine and human anti-lipid A monoclonal antibodies to bind and neutralize lipopolysaccharide. J Exp Med 177:89–97, 1993.

81. Sorensen TI, Nielsen GG, Andersen PK, et al. Genetic and environmental influences on premature death in adult adoptees. N Engl J Med 318:727–732, 1988.

82. Cooke GS, Hill AV. Genetics of susceptibility to human infectious disease. Nature Reviews Genetics 2:967–77, 2001.

83. Powars D, Larsen R, Johnson J, et al. Epidemic meningococcemia and purpura fulminans with induced protein C deficiency. Clin Infect Dis 17:254–261, 1993.

84. Boldt J, Papsdorf M, Rothe A, et al. Changes of the hemostatic network in critically ill patients: is there a difference between sepsis, trauma, and neurosurgery patients? Crit Care Med 28:445–450, 2000.

85. Fourrier F, Chopin C, Goudemand J, et al. Septic shock, multiple organ failure, and disseminated intravascular coagulation. Compared patterns of antithrombin III, protein C, and protein S deficiencies. Chest 101:816–823, 1992.

86. Boehme MW, Deng Y, Raeth U, et al. Release of thrombomodulin from endothelial cells by concerted action of TNF-alpha and neutrophils: in vivo and in vitro studies. Immunology 87:134–140, 1996.

87. Esmon CT, Taylor FB, Jr., Snow TR. Inflammation and coagulation: linked processes potentially regulated through a common pathway mediated by protein C. Thrombosis Haemostasis 66:160–165, 1991.

88. Esmon CT. The protein C anticoagulant pathway. Arteriosclerosis Thrombosis 12:135–145, 1992.

89. Chrousos GP. The hypothalamic-pituitary-adrenal axis and immune-mediated inflammation. N Engl J Med 332:1351–1362, 1995.

90. Hotta M, Baird A. Differential effects of transforming growth factor type beta on the growth and function of adrenocortical cells in vitro. Proc Natl Acad Sci USA 83:7795–7799, 1986.

91. Jaattela M, Ilvesmaki V, Voutilainen R, et al. Tumor necrosis factor as a potent inhibitor of adrenocorticotropin-induced cortisol production and steroidogenic P450 enzyme gene expression in cultured human fetal adrenal cells. Endocrinology 128:623–629, 1991.

92. Rothwell PM, Udwadia ZF, Lawler PG. Cortisol response to corticotropin and survival in septic shock. Lancet 337:582–583, 1991.

93. Keh D, Sprung CL. Use of corticosteroid therapy in patients with sepsis and septic shock: an evidence-based review. Crit Care Med 32 (11 Suppl):S527–533, 2004.

94. Lefering R, Neugebauer EA. Steroid controversy in sepsis and septic shock: a meta-analysis. Crit Care Med 23:1294–1303, 1995.

95. Annane D, Bellissant E, Bollaert PE, et al. Corticosteroids for treating severe sepsis and septic shock. Cochrane Database of Systematic Reviews (1):CD002243, 2004.

96. McCowen KC, Malhotra A, Bistrian BR. Stress-induced hyperglycemia. Crit Care Clin 17:107–124, 2001.

97. Bochicchio GV, Sung J, Joshi M, et al. Persistent hyperglycemia is predictive of outcome in critically ill trauma patients. J Trauma Injury Infection Crit Care 58:921–924, 2005.

98. van den Berghe G, Wouters P, Weekers F, et al. Intensive insulin therapy in the critically ill patient. N Engl J Med 345:1359–1367, 2001.

99. Cook DJ, Fuller HD, Guyatt GH, et al. Risk factors for gastrointestinal bleeding in critically ill patients. Canadian Critical Care Trials Group. N Engl J Med 330:377–381, 1994

100. ASHP Therapeutic Guidelines on Stress Ulcer Prophylaxis. ASHP Commission on Therapeutics and approved by the ASHP Board of Directors on Nov. 14, 1998. Am J Health-System Pharm 56: 347–379, 1999.

101. Tryba M, Cook D. Current guidelines on stress ulcer prophylaxis. Drugs 54:581–596, 1997.

102. Cook D, Guyatt G, Marshall J, et al. A comparison of sucralfate and ranitidine for the prevention of upper gastrointestinal bleeding in patients requiring mechanical ventilation. Canadian Critical Care Trials Group. N Engl J Med 338:791–797, 1998.

103. Cook DJ, Reeve BK, Guyatt GH, et al. Stress ulcer prophylaxis in critically ill patients. Resolving discordant meta-analyses. JAMA 275:308–314, 1996.

104. Geerts WH, Pineo GF, Heit JA, et al. Prevention of venous thromboembolism: the Seventh ACCP Conference on Antithrombotic and Thrombolytic Therapy. Chest 126 (3 Suppl):338S–400S, 2004.

105. Cade JF. High risk of the critically ill for venous thromboembolism. Crit Care Med 10:448–450, 1982.

106. Belch JJ, Lowe GD, Ward AG, et al. Prevention of deep vein thrombosis in medical patients by low-dose heparin. Scot Med J 26:115–117, 1981.

107. Samama MM, Cohen AT, Darmon JY, et al. A comparison of enoxaparin with placebo for the prevention of venous thromboembolism in acutely ill medical patients. Prophylaxis in Medical Patients with Enoxaparin Study Group. N Engl J Med 341:793–800, 1999.

108. Sigalet DL, Mackenzie SL, Hameed SM. Enteral nutrition and mucosal immunity: implications for feeding strategies in surgery and trauma. Can J Surg 47:109–116, 2004.

109. Wu Y, Kudsk KA, DeWitt RC, et al. Route and type of nutrition influence IgA-mediating intestinal cytokines. Ann Surg 229: 662–668, 1999.

110. King BK, Li J, Kudsk KA. A temporal study of TPN-induced changes in gut-associated lymphoid tissue and mucosal immunity. Arch Surg 132:1303–1309, 1997.

111. Wheeler AP, Bernard GR. Treating patients with severe sepsis. N Engl J Med 340:207–214, 1999.

112. Brook AD, Ahrens TS, Schaiff R, et al. Effect of a nursing-implemented sedation protocol on the duration of mechanical ventilation. Crit Care Med 27:2609–2615, 1999.

113. Lin MT, Albertson TE. Genomic polymorphisms in sepsis. Crit Care Med 32:569–579, 2004.

114. Texereau J, Pene F, Chiche JD, et al. Importance of hemostatic gene polymorphisms for susceptibility to and outcome of severe sepsis. Crit Care Med 32 (5 Suppl):S313–319, 2004.

115. Kerlin BA, Yan SB, Isermann BH, et al. Survival advantage associated with heterozygous factor V Leiden mutation in patients with severe sepsis and in mouse endotoxemia. Blood 102:3085–3092, 2003.

116. Eriksson P, Kallin B, van't Hooft FM, et al. Allele-specific increase in basal transcription of the plasminogen-activator inhibitor 1 gene is associated with myocardial infarction. Proc Natl Acad Sci USA 92:1851–1855, 1995.

117. Nicolaes GA, Dahlback B. Activated protein C resistance (FV(Leiden)) and thrombosis: factor V mutations causing hypercoagulable states. Hematol Oncol Clin North Am 17:37–61, 2003.

118. Manns BJ, Lee H, Doig CJ, et al. An economic evaluation of activated protein C treatment for severe sepsis. N Engl J Med 347: 993–1000, 2002.

119. Brun-Buisson C, Roudot-Thoraval F, Girou E, et al. The costs of septic syndromes in the intensive care unit and influence of hospital-acquired sepsis. Intensive Care Med 29:1464–1471, 2003.

120. Lee H, Doig CJ, Ghali WA, et al. Detailed cost analysis of care for survivors of severe sepsis. Crit Care Med 32:981–985, 2004.

Mycotic Infections

87

Annie Wong-Beringer

The incidence and spectrum of invasive fungal infections have increased dramatically over the past two decades.[1,2] Advances in medical technology and therapies such as bone marrow or solid-organ transplantation, use of invasive monitoring devices, mechanical ventilation, parenteral nutrition, broad-spectrum antimicrobial agents, intensive cancer chemotherapies, corticosteroids, and other immunosuppressives predispose patients to invasive fungal infections. Adding to this growing population of susceptible hosts are individuals infected with human immunodeficiency virus (HIV).[1-4]

Medically important fungi causing systemic fungal infections can be classified as endemic versus opportunistic. Endemic pathogens are those capable of causing disease in otherwise healthy individuals and in immunocompromised hosts who reside in a specific geographic location; infections tend to be more disseminated and rapidly progressive in the latter population.[5] The three major pathogens that cause endemic mycoses in North America are (a) *Coccidioides immitis*, (b) *Histoplasma capsulatum*, and (c) *Blastomyces dermatitidis*. In contrast, opportunistic pathogens such as *Candida* sp, *Aspergillus* sp, and *Cryptococcus neoformans* generally cause invasive disease in patients with overt immunosuppression.

The diagnosis of invasive fungal diseases is based on a combination of two or more of the following: careful evaluation of the clinical presentation of signs and symptoms, blood cultures, results of serologic testing, diagnostic imaging, and tissue biopsies for histopathology and cultures. Although associated mortality with invasive candidiasis and aspergillosis are extremely high in immunocompromised hosts, early diagnosis generally is difficult to establish with existing tests or studies.[6,7] Current research focuses on the development of newer methods using DNA and RNA gene probes, polymerase chain reactions (PCRs), and detection of fungal antigen and fungal metabolites in the early diagnosis and monitoring of therapeutic response of invasive fungal diseases.[7]

TREATMENT GOALS

- Determine the spectrum and severity of mycotic infections, which vary depending on the immune status of the host and pathogen.
- Understand the patient's risk factors for and etiology of immunosuppression, because the treatment goals may differ dramatically according to patient immune status and pathogen.
- Understand that immunocompetent patients usually do not require specific antifungal therapy for endemic mycoses.
- Use prolonged or lifelong secondary prophylaxis following acute initial treatment of primary fungal infections for some individuals (e.g., patients who are HIV-positive).
- Initiate antifungal therapy aggressively and promptly in patients who experience prolonged and profound neutropenia secondary to cytotoxic chemotherapy, because they are at high risk for acute life-threatening systemic opportunistic mycoses such as disseminated candidiasis and invasive aspergillosis.
- Understand that primary antifungal prophylaxis administered during the period of prolonged and profound neutropenia may improve infectious morbidity and mortality in susceptible hosts.

EPIDEMIOLOGY AND CLINICAL PRESENTATION OF ENDEMIC MYCOSES

HISTOPLASMOSIS

Histoplasmosis is an endemic mycosis caused by the pathogenic fungus, *H. capsulatum*. The organism was first described by Samuel Darling at the turn of the 20th century. Histoplasmosis occurs throughout the world; however, the geographic distribution of this fungus in the United States prevails primarily along the Mississippi and Ohio river valleys and in other central, southeastern, and mid-Atlantic states. *H. capsulatum* is a dimorphic fungus that exists as a mold in soil or culture media at temperatures of less than 37°C (98.6°F) and as budding yeasts at 37°C or higher.[8] Infection is initiated following inhalation and distribution of the spores to the lungs. The spores convert promptly to the tissue-invasive yeast form on entering the mammalian hosts.[8]

T-cell immunity appears to be most critical in determining the outcome of infection. Individuals with impaired T-cell immunity, such as those with HIV infection, succumb to the severe and disseminated form of the disease. In fact, histoplasmosis has been recognized as an AIDS-defining illness since 1987; it is the most commonly diagnosed endemic mycosis in patients with HIV.[5]

Epidemiology. Factors accounting for the specific geographic distribution of *H. capsulatum* in the United States are not fully understood. However, humid environments along fertile river valleys appear to be favorable for growth of the organism. In addition, bird or bat droppings enhance the rate of sporulation, thereby increasing the number of infectious particles. Old buildings or urban parks inhabited by birds or bats, farms, bird roosts, and caves are sources of exposure to *H. capsulatum*. Exposure to spores may result from activities such as demolishing or remodeling old structures, clearing brush from urban parks, cleaning chicken coops, and repairing damaged chimneys. Spores can be spread by wind over large areas, and can be found even 10 years after birds have abandoned their roosts.[8]

Clinical Presentation and Diagnosis. Host factors such as underlying immunosuppression and enhanced immunity from prior infection are important determinants of the outcome of infection. Environmental factors also play an important role in the severity of illness and attack rates. Exposure in enclosed areas rather than in the outdoors, for longer duration, or to high inoculum of spores usually results in more severe clinical disease.[8,9]

Signs and Symptoms

Pulmonary. The majority of symptomatic patients (80%) experience self-limiting acute disease that resembles an influenzalike illness.[7] Improvement of symptoms usually occurs within a few weeks. Inflammatory complications such as arthritis, severe arthralgia accompanied by erythema nodosum, and pericarditis may occur in up to 10% of patients. Management with anti-inflammatory agents is adequate without the need for antifungal therapy. In about 10% of symptomatic patients, histoplasmosis may present as cavitary disease resembling tuberculosis.[9] Chronic pulmonary symptoms (less severe than tuberculosis) and apical lung lesions that progress with inflammation, cavitation, and fibrosis are characteristic of this form of illness. Many such patients have underlying chronic obstructive pulmonary disease.

Disseminated. Disseminated histoplasmosis occurs rarely in patients without overt immunosuppression, at a rate of 1 in 2,000 to 5,000.[8,9] In contrast, disseminated disease occurs in 95% of cases in patients with acquired immunodeficiency syndrome (AIDS).[9] The incidence of histoplasmosis in patients with HIV residing in endemic areas is 2% to 5% versus less than 1% in nonendemic areas. Most adults present with subacute illness characterized by low-grade fever, weight loss, and fatigue.[9] Untreated illness may last up to 20 years with asymptomatic periods interrupted by clinical illness. Central nervous system (CNS) involvement in the form of lymphocytic meningitis or cerebritis may complicate 10% to 20% of those with severe underlying immunosuppression. Focal organ involvement is uncommon. In patients with AIDS, 90% of disseminated disease occurs in those with CD4 counts below 200 per microliter.[9] The majority of patients present with low-grade fever, fatigue, weight loss of 1 to 3 months' duration, and respiratory symptoms such as cough and dyspnea. Approximately 10% to 20% of patients develop a syndrome resembling septicemia with shock, respiratory insufficiency, hepatic and renal failure, and intravascular coagulation with coagulopathy.

Diagnosis. A number of tests currently are available for the diagnosis of histoplasmosis, which include serologic tests for antibodies, antigen detection, fungal cultures, and fungal stains.[5,9] In general, serologic tests for antibodies are positive in 90% of otherwise healthy patients with active symptomatic disease.[5] As for patients with AIDS who have disseminated disease, antigen detection from urine and serum is the most sensitive method for diagnosis. Cultures of bone marrow, blood, urine, and sputum are recommended for all patients suspected to have disseminated histoplasmosis; bone marrow cultures provide the highest yield with positive results in more than 75% of cases.[5,9]

BLASTOMYCOSIS

Blastomycosis is an endemic fungal infection caused by *B. dermatitidis*. Like *H. capsulatum*, this organism is a thermal dimorphic fungus that lives in the soil.[5] The geographic distribution of this organism overlaps that of *H. capsulatum* in much of the central and southeastern United States, and extends farther to the north and west, including Northern Wisconsin, northern Minnesota, and the adjacent areas of south-central Canada.[10] The United States appears to be the most heavily endemic area for *B. dermatitidis* in the world.

Blastomycosis is an uncommon disease even among residents in endemic areas and is the least common opportunistic endemic mycosis in patients with AIDS.[5] The immunologic defense to *B. dermatitidis* in normal hosts is not fully understood. It is thought that cellular and humoral immunity are important in controlling infection.[10] The disease is acquired by inhalation of conidia, with the lungs being the primary site of infection. Secondary spread to extrapulmonary sites may occur concurrent with the respiratory illness or after the respiratory illness has resolved.[10]

Epidemiology.

The precise epidemiology of blastomycosis is less well understood than other endemic mycoses such as histoplasmosis and coccidioidomycosis.[10] The lack of a reliable skin test for large-scale surveys and the difficulty in isolating *B. dermatitidis* from soil do not allow for a precise determination of the endemic area and the ecologic niche of the fungus. Current evidence suggests that nitrogen-rich soil along rivers, streams, and lakes enhances growth of the fungus. Incidentally, many sporadic cases or outbreak cases occurred in close proximity to recreational water. Sporadic cases most commonly occur in men between 25 and 50 years of age who have heavy vocational or recreational exposure to woods and streams. Unlike histoplasmosis, where virtually every resident in endemic areas has acquired primary infection (as indicated by a positive skin test), exposure and infection with blastomycosis is less universal. Late reactivation of a primary infection may occur as long as 40 years after initial exposure.[10]

Clinical Presentation and Diagnosis

Signs and Symptoms. Pulmonary blastomycosis occurs in up to 80% of all patients with a highly variable clinical presentation.[10] Five distinct symptomatology may be seen:

1. Asymptomatic illness detectable only as part of an outbreak;
2. Brief flulike illness, usually with rapid resolution;
3. Acute illness resembling bacterial pneumonia;
4. Subacute or chronic illness with a symptomatic complex resembling tuberculosis or lung cancer;
5. Fulminant infection with acute respiratory distress syndrome (ARDS).

The latter presentation, in which severe gas exchange abnormality and diffuse infiltrates are present, is associated with a mortality of more than 50%.[8] Most sporadic cases present with subacute or chronic pulmonary symptoms resembling tuberculosis or lung cancer. Approximately 25% of those patients have concurrent skin or bone involvement. Conversely, symptomatic cases that occur during point-source outbreaks tend to present with flulike illness or acute illness that resembles bacterial pneumonia.

Extrapulmonary manifestations most commonly involve the skin in the form of verrucous or ulcerative lesions, followed by bone (osteomyelitis), prostate (prostatitis), and CNS (cranial abscesses or meningitis) involvement. The CNS may be involved in 5% to 10% of disseminated cases.[10]

In general, multiple visceral organ involvement and CNS disease are common among immunocompromised patients.[5,11]

Unlike other endemic mycoses, blastomycosis occurs rarely in patients with AIDS, and 90% of those affected have advanced disease with a CD4 count of less than 200 μL.[5] Fulminant respiratory failure and ARDS occur in 20% to 30% of patients, whereas disseminated cutaneous lesions may be present in one third of patients. CNS involvement has been reported in up to 40% of patients with AIDS. Death owing to overwhelming pulmonary disease, with or without extrapulmonary manifestations, has been reported in up to 40% of patients with AIDS in contrast to a mortality rate of 2% to 3% in otherwise normal hosts. Most deaths occur within 4 weeks of diagnosis.

Diagnosis. Definitive diagnosis of blastomycosis is based on demonstration of the organism by culture or stain of body fluids or tissue specimen.[5,10–12] The easiest and most rapid method is by direct visualization of the organism in expectorated sputum or aspirated pus after 10% potassium hydroxide digestion. Cultures are positive in 90% of cases, but it may take several weeks to obtain the results. Serologic tests for antibodies are negative in most cases and a negative result does not exclude diagnosis. Reliable tests for antigen are not yet available for diagnostic purposes.

COCCIDIOIDOMYCOSIS

Coccidioidomycosis is caused by *C. immitis*, a thermal dimorphic fungus like *H. capsulatum* and *B. dermatitidis*. In soil, it grows as a mold with Arthroconidia but converts to a spherule containing 200 to 400 endospores each in host tissues. The number of multiplying coccidioidal organisms is significantly higher than *H. capsulatum* or *B. dermatitidis*, which may explain the higher incidence of clinical infection following exposure to *C. immitis*.[13] Primary pulmonary infection occurs in the susceptible host when airborne Arthroconidia generated by dust storms or strong winds are inhaled.[14] T-cell immunity is critical for control of infection. Host immune response results in the production of immunoglobulin M (IgM) and immunoglobulin G (IgG) antibodies; although they do not confer specific protection to disease development, serologic tests measuring antibody levels have diagnostic and prognostic value.[12]

Epidemiology. The geographic distribution of *C. immitis* is along the warm and dry southwestern region of the United States; the southern San Joaquin Valley of California and southern Arizona are the most heavily endemic areas.[12] Hence, the popular terms ''valley fever'' and ''desert rheumatism'' are used to describe the common manifestations of coccidioidomycosis. Dusty conditions during late summer and fall, especially following rainy winters, predispose residents or travelers in endemic areas to the acquisition of airborne Arthroconidia. Epidemiologic investigation of a recent large outbreak of coccidioidomycosis that occurred after the January 1994 Northridge earthquake in California confirms that dust cloud-generating events are significant risks for acquisition of infection.[14] Because T-cell immunity is a key defense to coccidioidal infection, patients with the following conditions are at risk for developing severe pulmonary and disseminated disease: HIV positive, AIDS, hematologic malignancies, organ transplantation, third-trimester pregnancy, and recent postpartum. In the nonimmunocompromised population, disseminated disease is more likely to occur in the very old and very young. Interestingly, for unknown reason, patients belonging to certain ethnic groups (in order of descending risk) are predisposed to the development of disseminated disease: Filipino, African-American, Native American, Hispanic, and Asian.[13]

Clinical Presentation and Diagnosis

Signs and Symptoms. The majority (60%) of patients infected with coccidioidomycosis are asymptomatic. Approximately 40% develop symptoms with a spectrum of manifestations ranging from mild to moderate influenzalike illness, pneumonia, and disseminated disease.[13,15] The incubation period for the onset of symptoms following exposure is usually 1 to 4 weeks.

Acute respiratory illness often is misdiagnosed as viral bronchitis; respiratory symptoms usually last several days and are often accompanied by myalgia, malaise, and fatigue that may persist for several weeks.[13,15] In 15% to 20% of patients, a distinctive rash develops during the acute illness, as erythema nodosum with raised painful nodules over the tibial or ankle areas or as a more diffuse erythema multiforme.[13] Arthritis of the ankle or other joints may be involved symmetrically. This is often called "desert rheumatism" and represents a self-limited immune complex reaction. A minority (5%) of acute coccidioidomycosis cases progress to complicated pulmonary disease with persistence of a pulmonary nodule or cavity.[13,15] Patients with diabetes mellitus are more likely to be affected. One third of the cavities may close spontaneously within 2 years of its discovery, whereas the remainder may be complicated by secondary bacterial infections or persistent hemoptysis that require excision.[11] Diffuse pulmonary infiltrates accompanied by respiratory failure is noted more frequently in patients with AIDS compared with individuals without AIDS, and has an associated mortality of 70%.[5]

Disseminated disease develops in approximately 1% of symptomatic patients. In contrast to the general population, about 15% of patients with AIDS develop extrapulmonary manifestations.[5] Secondary spread to virtually all organs except the gastrointestinal tract has occurred.[13,15] The most frequent extrapulmonary manifestations is the development of granulomas or abscess on the skin, followed by synovitis and osteomyelitis. Meningitis is the most severe form of dissemination and is responsible for the majority of deaths owing to coccidioidomycosis, which may occur within 2 to 3 weeks of the onset of pulmonary symptoms or may follow an asymptomatic primary infection. The course of meningitis ranges from indolent to rapidly fatal within a few days.[13,15]

Clinical presentation may be nonspecific and subtle with headache, weakness, mental status changes, weight loss, and occasional hydrocephalus. Cerebrospinal fluid (CSF) findings are marked by lymphocytic pleocytosis, elevated protein, and decreased glucose, with cultures often negative for the organism.

Diagnosis. Definitive diagnosis is made with fungal culture and stains of blood, tissue, and fluids.[7,13,15] However, blood cultures are frequently negative. Growth of the organism on appropriate media typically is apparent in 3 to 5 days. Histopathologic evidence of spherules with characteristic endosporulation also may confirm diagnosis. More than 50% of adult patients living in endemic areas have a positive reaction to the skin test, whereas a negative skin test does not rule out coccidioidomycosis.[7,13] A negative reaction in those with severe infection is a poor prognostic sign and may reflect an inability of the host to mount an adequate cell-mediated immunity.[13,15] Serologic tests measuring IgM and IgG antibodies to *C. immitis* are available commercially and are sensitive and specific.[7,13] The diagnosis of coccidioidomycosis can be confirmed by positive serologic test results in the presence of acute illness. IgM is measured by an immunodiffusion method and is reported qualitatively as positive or negative. A positive result indicates acute disease activity, either initially or during a later exacerbation. However, complement-fixing (CF) IgG antibody in serum and CSF is measured quantitatively.[11] The quantity of antibody titers parallels the antigen (fungal) load to which the antibodies are developing. High-serum IgG titers (>1:64) predict the likelihood for dissemination of infection especially with the reversal of a previously positive skin test.[13,15] In addition, serial measurement of CF IgG titers at 3- to 4-week intervals during the period of illness is useful for monitoring disease progression. A positive CF IgG test of the CSF is the most useful test for confirming the diagnosis of coccidioidal meningitis.[13,15]

EPIDEMIOLOGY AND CLINICAL PRESENTATION OF OPPORTUNISTIC MYCOSES

CRYPTOCOCCOSIS

Cryptococcus neoformans is an opportunistic fungal pathogen that causes invasive diseases primarily in patients with underlying immunodeficiency and rarely in hosts with normal defenses. It exists as an encapsulated yeast surrounded by a polysaccharide capsule and has a worldwide distribution.[16] Infection is acquired via inhalation of the spores of *C. neoformans* into the lungs. In patients with intact T-cell immunity, primary infection usually is contained within the lungs, whereas rapid dissemination to other sites, most notably the CNS, occurs in immunocompromised hosts.

Epidemiology. More than 20 species of *Cryptococcus* are known; however, *C. neoformans* is essentially the only human pathogen. The organism grows most abundantly in avian excreta, particularly pigeon droppings.[16] *C. neoformans* also has been isolated from nonavian sources such as fruits, vegetables, and dairy products. Four serotypes (A, B, C, and D) of *C. neoformans* are based on the antigenic determinants of the polysaccharide capsule.[16] The varieties of *C. neoformans* serotypes are *neoformans* and *gattii*. Epidemiologic evidence suggests differences in geographic distribution, host preference related to immune status, clinical course, and response to therapy between the two varieties.[17] Var. *neoformans* is ubiquitous, whereas var. *gattii* has geographic limitation to tropical and subtropical areas (e.g., southern California, Australia, Southeast Asia, Brazil, and Central America), particularly in the soil under eucalyptus trees. The majority (90%) of infections with *C. neoformans* var. *neoformans* occur in immunocompromised hosts, whereas var. *gattii* affects primarily immunocompetent hosts with a predilection for invasion of the CNS. Patients infected with the latter variety have more neurologic complications, such as altered mental status, papilledema, focal deficits, ataxia, and seizures. In addition, infections owing to var. *gattii* tend to have a protracted course and are less responsive to therapy.

In the pre-AIDS era, lymphoreticular malignancies, organ transplantation, diabetes, cirrhosis, malnutrition, and corticosteroid therapy were risk factors predisposed to cryptococcosis.[16] Since the beginning of the AIDS epidemic, cryptococcosis occurs primarily in patients with advanced HIV disease (CD4 count <100 cells/μL) and has become the fourth leading opportunistic infection in this population.[18,19] It is estimated that up to 10% of patients with AIDS in western countries will develop cryptococcal meningitis, whereas up to 30% of patients in sub-Saharan Africa are affected.[18,19] In a minority of patients (20%–30%) infected with *C. neoformans*, no predisposing risk factors or underlying condition are apparent.[16]

Clinical Presentation and Diagnosis
Signs and Symptoms

Pulmonary. Cryptococcal infection most often affects the lungs and CNS. Even though the lung is the portal of entry, pulmonary cryptococcosis is relatively uncommon.[16] In immunocompetent hosts, the infection is usually mild and localized with spontaneous resolution.[16,20] In contrast, the mortality rate associated with cryptococcal pneumonia in patients with AIDS exceeds 40%.[18,19] Most patients with AIDS and pulmonary cryptococcosis have disseminated disease; about 60% to 70% have concurrent meningeal involvement.[18–20] In normal hosts, concurrent CNS involvement with pulmonary disease is more likely associated with infection owing to *C. neoformans* var. *gattii*.[17] Some have suggested that all patients with pneumonia or colonization be evaluated with a lumbar puncture to rule out CNS involvement despite the absence of obvious neurologic signs or symptoms.[16]

Central Nervous System. Cryptococcal meningitis is the most common manifestation of disseminated disease. Acute presentation with neurologic sequelae is much more common in immunocompetent hosts.[16] Conversely, 75% to 90% of patients with AIDS present with subacute meningitis or meningoencephalitis characterized by fever, malaise, and headache.[18–20] Approximately 30% may present with altered mental status, confusion, lethargy, personality change, and memory loss. Overt signs of meningismus such as neck stiffness and photophobia are uncommon among patients with AIDS. Also, response to infection in CSF is usually blunted with normal protein and sugar accompanied by a mild pleocytosis. CNS complications include hydrocephalus, visual or hearing loss, cranial nerve palsies, ataxia, seizures, and dementia. Mortality rate of up to 25% has been reported with most deaths occurring within the first few weeks of illness; a recent large comparative study reported overall mortality rate as low as 6% with early appropriate treatment.[20] Various prognostic signs have been associated with poor outcomes of CNS disease in patients with AIDS (Table 87.1). Relapse rate in patients with AIDS-associated cryptococcal meningitis is as high as 37% in the absence of maintenance therapy.[20]

Other Sites. Cryptococcosis may involve other sites such as the skin, skeletal system, and prostate gland in decreased frequency.[16] Cutaneous disease may be present in 10% of the disseminated cases, appearing as papules, tumors, vesicles, abscesses, cellulitis, and lesions resembling molluscum contagiosum in patients with AIDS. More important, persistent but usually asymptomatic infection of the prostate gland may occur in as many as 29% of patients with AIDS, and serves as a source for subsequent relapse after completion of primary therapy.[16,18,19]

Diagnosis. Diagnosis of cryptococcosis is made by isolating the organism from a sterile body site, by histopathology, or by cryptococcal capsular antigen testing. Blood cultures are positive in 70% of patients with AIDS who are infected with *C. neoformans*.[18,19] India ink stain outlines the polysaccharide capsule of the yeast. Results from direct examination

TABLE 87.1	Prognostic Signs Associated With Poor Treatment Outcomes of Cryptococcal Meningitis in AIDS

Prognostic Signs

Altered mental status at presentation

Elevated opening cerebrospinal pressure

Low CSF leukocyte count (<20 cell/μL)

High CSF cryptococcal antigen titers (> 1:8)

High serum cryptococcal antigen titers (> 1:32)

AIDS, acquired immunodeficiency syndrome; CSF, cerebrospinal fluid.

of the CSF are positive for India ink stain in more than 80% of patients with AIDS and approximately 50% of the time in normal hosts with meningeal involvement.[18,19] The latex agglutination test for cryptococcal polysaccharide antigen has a sensitivity and specificity exceeding 95%.[16] Testing for antigen in serum is a useful initial screening test in patients with AIDS who present with fever and headaches. A positive serum antigen test indicates the need for lumbar puncture; about 99% of patients with cryptococcal meningitis have positive serum antigen test.[16] Secondary infection with *Trichosporon beigelii* can cause false-positive results owing to cross-reactivity with the antigen. Serial measurement of antigen titers during therapy does not appear to be helpful in monitoring disease response or predicting relapse.[16]

ASPERGILLOSIS

Aspergillosis, the most common invasive mold infection worldwide, is caused by the ubiquitous fungus *Aspergillus* spp. Approximately 150 species have been identified thus far. Pathogenic species that commonly cause invasive diseases include *A. fumigatus, A. flavus, A. niger, A. terreus,* and *A. nidulans.*[21] *A. fumigatus* is the predominant species causing invasive aspergillosis; it accounts for approximately 90% of all cases. *A. fumigatus* is the most rapidly growing species and has very small spore size, allowing deep penetration into the lungs; both characteristics are likely to contribute to its pathogenicity. The growth rate of *A. fumigatus* and *A. flavus* may be accelerated by 30% to 40% in the presence of physiologic and pharmacologic concentrations of hydrocortisone.[21] The rate of progression of invasive diseases may be closely related to the growth rate of the organisms. Macrophage ingestion and killing of the spores and extracellular killing of hyphae by neutrophils are the primary host defenses against *Aspergillus* in the lungs.[21] Corticosteroids can substantially impair the functions of macrophages and neutrophils. T-cell function is thought to be important in the more chronic forms of invasive aspergillosis.

Epidemiology. *Aspergillus* spp. are ubiquitous in the air and environment. They can be found in decomposing vegetable material, cellars, potted plants, pepper and spices, unfiltered marijuana smoke, shower heads, and hot water faucets. In addition, the release of large quantities of spores into the air is associated with local construction work, which represents a major risk factor for immunocompromised patients susceptible to the development of invasive aspergillosis.[22] Thus, the primary means of reducing the risk of acquiring the organisms for at-risk patients is the use of high-efficiency particulate air (HEPA) filtration or laminar airflow to remove *Aspergillus* spores from the air. In addition, pharmaceutical agents are used to remove *Aspergillus* from surface areas.[21-23]

Although aspergillosis has been documented in immunocompetent patients, the occurrence is unusual. Those at highest risk for acquiring invasive diseases are patients in the following categories: bone marrow and solid organ transplant recipients, people with profound neutropenia, and those with severe burns. Other at-risk groups include individuals with underlying diseases such as late-stage AIDS, chronic granulomatous disease, and diabetes mellitus.[21-23]

Clinical Presentation and Diagnosis

Signs and Symptoms. Clinical manifestations and the rate of disease progression vary among different patient groups.[21,23] Typically, individuals who are the least immunocompromised have prominent signs and symptoms with an indolent progression of disease over a 2- to 3-month period (from onset to diagnosis). In contrast, patients who are the most immunocompromised are least likely to have symptoms and may progress within 7 to 10 days from onset of disease to death. The respiratory tract is the primary portal of entry, accounting for 80% to 90% of invasive aspergillosis. Other possible sites of entry include damaged skin or operative wounds, the cornea, and the ear, which have resulted in burn-associated cutaneous aspergillosis, prosthetic valve endocarditis, keratitis, and catheter-site infection.

Aspergillosis can present as acute and chronic invasive pulmonary disease, tracheobronchitis, acute and chronic sinusitis, and disseminated disease in the form of cutaneous or cerebral infection.

Pulmonary. Acute invasive pulmonary aspergillosis occurs primarily in immunocompromised hosts. Prolonged neutropenia is a major risk factor for developing disease; as many as 70% of patients may be affected if the duration of neutropenia extends to or beyond 34 days.[22] Up to one third of patients with acute invasive pulmonary disease are asymptomatic initially.[22] As the disease progresses, early symptoms may consist of dry cough with fever and nonspecific chest pain. Dyspnea and hypoxemia with a normal white blood cell (WBC) count are characteristic of diffuse bilateral disease. Those with focal disease tend to progress slower and have a more favorable prognosis because surgical resection is a therapeutic option. Hemoptysis can occur with focal disease without warning and can be life threatening.[21] Plain chest radiographs are extremely heterogeneous but cavitated lesions or nodular shadows with and without cavitation are highly suspicious. As many as 30% of neutropenic bone marrow transplant patients with invasive aspergillosis have normal chest radiographs in the week preceding death.[21,22] More commonly, the clinical presentation of acute pulmonary aspergillosis in immunocompromised hosts is one of unremitting fever and the development of lung infiltrates despite broad-spectrum antibacterial therapy.

Chronic invasive aspergillosis occurs less frequently than acute aspergillosis.[21] Affected patients commonly have underlying conditions such as AIDS, chronic granulomatous disease, diabetes mellitus, alcoholism, and corticosteroid use. Presenting signs and symptoms are more prominent and tend to extend over weeks or months; they include chronic productive cough, mild to moderate hemoptysis, low-grade fever, malaise, and weight loss. Patients with chronic disease are usually strongly positive for antibodies to *Aspergillus*; this finding can be used to infer the diagnosis when bronchial biopsies are contraindicated or negative for *Aspergillus* hyphae.

Tracheobronchitis. Among immunocompromised patients, aspergillus tracheobronchitis occurs more commonly in patients with AIDS and lung transplant recipients.[21,23,24] Approximately 25% of the patients with tracheobronchitis have no apparent immunocompromise. Notably, in lung transplant recipients, it is difficult to differentiate *Aspergillus* colonization of the airways from infection. The majority of patients (80%) are symptomatic with cough, fever, dyspnea, chest pain, and hemoptysis. Airway disease ranges from excess mucous production and inflammation to ulceration and extensive pseudomembranous tracheobronchitis. Death usually results from respiratory insufficiency secondary to occlusion of airways or disseminated aspergillosis.

Sinusitis. Invasive aspergillus sinusitis can occur as acute rhinosinusitis or chronic invasive sinusitis.[21] *A. flavus* is more commonly a cause of sinusitis. Acute rhinosinusitis is relatively common in neutropenic patients and bone marrow transplant recipients and rare in solid organ transplant recipients. Common signs and symptoms include fever, cough, epistaxis, and headache. Sinus pain, nasal discharge, and sore throat may occur. Local extension to palate, orbit, or brain is common and may occur relatively rapidly.[21,22] Relapse of disease during episodes of neutropenia and relapses of leukemia can be expected after initial response to treatment.[21,22]

Chronic invasive sinusitis occurs in healthy or somewhat immunocompromised patients; the latter typically are those with diabetes and alcoholism.[21] The disease usually progresses over months. Signs and symptoms are typical of chronic sinusitis, such as visual (e.g., diplopia, pain in the eye) and olfactory disturbances, and headaches with absence of fever. Complications such as bony destruction and osteomyelitis of the base of the skull may occur. Management requires surgical debridement with prolonged antifungal therapy.

Disseminated. In most patients who die of invasive aspergillosis, disseminated disease is often a postmortem diagnosis, unless cutaneous or cerebral aspergillosis is suspected and diagnosed before death. Cutaneous aspergillosis most commonly is associated with the intravenous (IV)–catheter site in neutropenic patients.[21] Premature neonates and children with AIDS also may develop invasive fungal dermatitis. Surgical wounds infected with *Aspergillus* may occur preoperatively or postoperatively; occurrence in liver transplant recipients are relatively common. Cutaneous disease in burn patients tends to occur over a rapidly progressive course, typically refractory to treatment.[21] The clinical appearance of cutaneous lesions is characterized by raised erythema that rapidly increase in size with the center of the lesion changing from red to purple and finally to black with possible ulcera-

tion. The rate of progression is most rapid in those who are neutropenic. The lesions usually progress over several days in those with circulating neutrophils and are associated with pain and discomfort. In general, cutaneous aspergillosis is most responsive to antifungal therapy with the exception of burn-associated aspergillosis.[21]

Cerebral aspergillosis accounts for 10% to 20% of the cases of invasive aspergillosis.[21,22] In patients who are profoundly neutropenic, altered mental status and seizures may be the presenting signs shortly before death. Individuals who are relatively less immunocompromised may have more focal features such as headaches and occasional fever. Radiologic evidence by computed tomography (CT) scans reveals multiple hypodense lesions or ring-enhancing lesions with surrounding edema. CSF findings are abnormal but nonspecific. Definitive diagnosis is based on biopsy or aspiration of the lesion but is rarely performed because of the clinical status of the patient or coagulation problems.

Diagnosis. When aspergillosis is suspected based on clinical grounds, radiologic evaluation should be performed immediately using CT or magnetic resonance imaging (MRI).[21] Plain radiographs of chest or sinuses early in the course of disease may be falsely negative or insensitive. Surgical resection or tissue biopsy should be performed on identification of a lesion. In those who are not surgical candidates or in whom surgical resection is not possible owing to diffuse pulmonary disease, bronchoscopy and bronchoalveolar lavage are recommended.

Laboratory diagnosis of invasive aspergillosis is based on a combination of approaches including detection of organism in tissue by direct microscopic examination, isolation, and identification of pathogen in culture, and detection of an immunologic response to the pathogen or some other marker of its presence, such as metabolic product.[21,24–26] Microscopy and culture should be performed on fluids obtained from bronchoalveolar lavage or on pus obtained from aspirated pulmonary lesions, infected sinuses, or abscesses. Typically, microscopy allows direct identification of *Aspergillus* from the preceding specimens based on the presence of hyphae; however, several other fungi may have similar microscopic and histologic appearances. Hence, further confirmation of the diagnosis should be made by culture of the preceding specimens.

Detection of galactomannan, a component of the fungal cell wall and an exoantigen of *Aspergillus* by enzyme-linked immunosorbent assay has been shown to be a useful screening test for invasive aspergillosis in hematology patients and in solid organ transplant recipients.[24–26] A commercially available kit known as Platelia *Aspergillus* EIA was approved in May 2003 by the Food and Drug Administration (FDA). The assay detects galactomannan antigen in serum and body fluids with a sensitivity and specificity of 80.7% and 89.2% from serum samples. Test positivity may precede by 5 to 8 days prior to the development of clinical signs, visible radiographic findings, and positive culture. Of note, specificity of the assay is much lower in children. A negative test result does not rule out disease. False-positive reactions have been reported in 1% to 18% of the tested samples possibly related to antigenic cross reactivity with other fungi, translocation of galactomannan antigen found in food sources most notable in children, and concurrent therapy with piperacillin-tazobactam. The assay may be helpful in assessing clinical response as the titer tends to decline in case of favorable clinical response and rise in treatment failure. However, due to technical difficulties in performing the assay and interpreting results, the assay is not yet routinely performed in clinical laboratories.

Given the rapid rate of progression of invasive aspergillosis from onset to death in those profoundly immunocompromised, delayed diagnosis and treatment is usually fatal. Frequently in clinical practice, aggressive empirical therapy for acute invasive aspergillosis is initiated based on a combination of clinical, radiologic, or microbiologic features before definitive proof of a diagnosis, which is based ideally on the histologic documentation of tissue invasion by hyphae and a positive culture of *Aspergillus*.[27–30]

CANDIDIASIS

Candida sp are opportunistic pathogens that are a part of the normal human commensals. *Candida* as a cause of oral lesions was first identified in the 1840s. The appearance of all forms of *Candida* infections has arisen only following the introduction of antibiotics into clinical use in the 1940s.[1–3] Over the past decade, the incidence of infections owing to *Candida* sp has increased dramatically. Data reported to the National Nosocomial Infections Surveillance (NNIS) system from participating hospitals in the United States between 1980 and 1989, reveal an increase in the rate of nosocomial candidemia by 500% in large teaching hospitals and by 219% and 370% in small teaching hospitals and large nonteaching hospitals, respectively.[1,2] Most recent data from the NNIS system (1990–1999) indicate that *Candida* sp are now the fourth leading cause of nosocomial bloodstream infection in U.S. hospitals.[1–3] Invasive candidiasis is associated with considerable morbidity and mortality. Based on a case-control study well matched for age, sex, service, underlying diagnosis, and duration of hospital stay, nosocomial candidemia was found to result in a crude mortality of 61% compared with 12% among cases and controls respectively, with an excess mortality of 49%. Those who survived spent an extra 11 days in the hospital.[31]

Candida organisms are yeasts that exist microscopically as small (4–6 μm), thin-walled, ovoid cells that reproduce by budding. Other morphologic forms, such as pseudohyphae and hyphae, also can be seen in clinical specimens for most *Candida* sp except *C. glabrata*.[2] More than 150 *Candida* sp have been identified previously; however, approximately 10 are considered important human pathogens. The pathogenic species include *C. albicans, C. tropicalis, C. parapsilosis, C. glabrata* (formerly classified as *Torulopsis glabrata*), *C. krusei, C. guilliermondii, C. lusitaniae, C. kefyr* (*C. pseudotropicalis*), *C. rugosa, C. dubliniensis,* and *C. stellatoidea* (now considered *C. albicans*).[2] Speciation of the pathogens is important owing to the varied pathogenic potential and susceptibility to antifungal agents.[32] A rapid presumptive identification of *Candida albicans* usually can be made by performing the specific germ tube test.[2] Hyphal outgrowths from the yeast cells occur only for *C. albicans* following incubation at 37°C (98.6°F) in horse serum for 2 to 3 hours, which allows it to be differentiated from other species. Identification of a germ tube-negative *Candida* sp (presumably non-*albicans*) relies on a combination of morphologic and biochemical testing. All pathogenic species are capable of causing similar spectrums of disease ranging from mucocutaneous to disseminated disease.[2,33] Breakdown of the normal host defense mechanisms is necessary for *Candida* organisms to become pathogens. An intact integument is required for protection against cutaneous invasion. When invasion occurs, functioning neutrophils, macrophages, and lymphocytes are important host defenses against the development of systemic disease.[2,33]

Epidemiology. *Candida* sp can be found in soil, inanimate objects, hospital environments, and food.[2] More important, the organisms are normal commensals of humans and are commonly found on diseased skin, along the entire gastrointestinal (GI) tract, in expectorated sputum, along the female genital tract, and in urine in patients with indwelling Foley catheters.[2,33] A majority of the infections arise from an endogenous source, with the GI tract or skin being the most likely portals of entry. However, exogenous acquisition of the organism is possible. For example, oral thrush in a newborn can result from the acquisition of *Candida* from the vagina of the mother during birth. In addition, *Candida* balanitis can be acquired by sexual contact with a partner who has *Candida* vaginitis.

Patients at risk for the development of invasive candidiasis include cancer patients, premature neonates, heroin addicts, burn patients, patients undergoing abdominal surgery, and organ transplantation recipients.[2,33] Specifically, risk factors predisposed to the development of candidemia are prior treatment with multiple antibiotics, prolonged hospital stay, prior central venous catheterization, parenteral hyperalimentation, corticosteroid use, prior hemodialysis, and prior colonization at sites other than blood.[2,33] Antibiotics allow the proliferation of *Candida* sp in the GI tract by suppressing normal bacterial flora, whereas instrumentation with catheters or other invasive monitoring devices provide a conduit for entry of *Candida* sp into the bloodstream.

C. albicans is the predominant cause of focal and invasive infections. *C. albicans* has been reported to account for 50% to 70% or more of cases of invasive candidiasis, followed by *C. tropicalis, C. glabrata,* and *C. parapsilosis*.[2,33] Notably, recent data indicate an apparent shift to an increasing proportion of invasive infections caused by non-*albicans* species presumably related to the widespread use of antifungal agents such as fluconazole.[2,33,34] In general, non-*albicans*

TABLE 87.2	Susceptibility of Bloodstream Isolates of Non-*albicans Candida* spp. to Fluconazole
Candida spp. Isolated	**MIC$_{50}$ (μg/mL)**
C. albicans	0.25
C. tropicalis	1.0
C. parapsilosis	1.0
C. glabrata	16
C. krusei	32

(From Pfaller MA. Nosocomial candidiasis: emerging species, reservoirs, and modes of transmission. Clin Infect Dis 22 (Suppl 2):S89– S94, 1996, with permission.)

Candida sp as a group are considered less susceptible than *C. albicans* to the azoles (Table 87.2).[33]

Clinical Presentation and Diagnosis

Signs and Symptoms. Candidiasis can be broadly categorized as mucocutaneous or deep invasive infections.[2,33] The two categories of infection tend to have a distinct set of predisposing factors and diagnostic and treatment approaches. The more common forms of mucocutaneous candidiasis among susceptible patients are oropharyngeal (thrush), esophageal, and vulvovaginal candidiasis. Invasive syndromes are often hematogenous in origin ranging from catheter-related transient candidemia to acute disseminated candidiasis characterized by candidemia accompanied by simultaneous spread of the infection to one or more noncontiguous organs, and chronic disseminated candidiasis (previously known as hepatosplenic candidiasis). Focal organ involvement such as candidiasis involving the brain, heart, bone, and joint can occur and is presumably owing to hematogenous spread of the infection. Peritonitis may result from local processes and spread secondary to bowel injury.

Mucocutaneous Candidiasis
Thrush and Esophagitis
Oropharyngeal candidiasis (thrush) occurs generally among patients with disruption of local defenses or damage to the mucosal membranes resulting from radiation or cytotoxic chemotherapy and those receiving local or systemic antibiotics or corticosteroids.[2,33] In addition, the incidence of thrush is high among patients with malignancies or defects in cell-mediated immunity such as AIDS. Every year more than 60% of patients with HIV who have CD4 counts lower than 100 μL will develop disease complicated by frequent recurrences.[35] Oral thrush is characterized by creamy white, curd-like patches on the tongue and other mucosal surfaces that are removable by scraping.[2,33,35]

Esophageal involvement usually occurs by direct spread of oral disease, although a number of patients with *Candida* esophagitis have no associated oral disease.[2] Esophagitis most commonly occurs in patients receiving cytotoxic chemotherapy. In addition, approximately 10% to 20% of patients with AIDS have *Candida* esophagitis.[2,33,35] In esophagitis, white patches resembling thrush can be seen endoscopically along the esophagus. Symptoms consist of pain and difficulty swallowing, a feeling of obstruction on swallowing, and substernal chest pain. In extensive disease, bleeding and perforation may occur.[2,33,35]

Vulvovaginitis
Vulvovaginal candidiasis is estimated to occur at least once during reproductive years in 75% of women with no recognizable predisposing factors.[2,33,36] However, identifiable risk factors include broad-spectrum antibiotics, high estrogen-containing oral contraceptives, poorly controlled diabetes, and pregnancy. Among patients infected with HIV, one large cross-sectional study found similar incidence (9%) of vaginal candidiasis compared with patients who do not have HIV.[35] Clinical signs and symptoms include whitish cheesy discharge, vulvovaginal pruritus, irritation, soreness, dyspareunia, and burning on micturition.[2,33]

Deep Organ Involvement
Candidemia and Acute Disseminated Candidiasis
Candidemia is defined as the isolation of *Candida* sp from at least one blood culture. The syndromes of candidemia can be subdivided into catheter-related candidemia limited to the bloodstream and acute disseminated candidiasis with hematogenous spread of the infection to one or more noncontiguous organs.[31] Catheter-related candidemia typically occurs in medical or surgical patients with an indwelling central venous catheter. Presenting signs often include an abrupt onset of fever and local signs of inflammation at the site of the catheter. Prognosis is usually good. Prompt response can be expected with antifungal therapy and early removal of the infected catheter within 72 hours.[33,37]

Acute disseminated candidiasis is a fulminant infection most often seen in neutropenic patients, burn patients, and postoperative patients.[2,33] In the latter group, those who have had organ transplantation, heart surgery, or GI tract surgery are at greatest risk.[2] Disseminated candidiasis typically presents as overwhelming sepsis with no distinct clinical features. Multiple organs usually are involved, with formation of microabscesses, most commonly in the kidney, brain, myocardium, and eye. Endophthalmitis and macular or erythematous cutaneous lesions are suggestive signs of disseminated disease but often are absent.[33] In the neutropenic patient, the most common manifestation is persistent fever despite broad-spectrum antibiotic therapy. Prognosis of disseminated candidiasis is heavily dependent on underlying disease, physiologic status of the patient [i.e., Acute Physiologic and Chronic Health Evaluation (APACHE) II score], degree of immunosuppression, and the extent of disease when antifungal therapy is instituted.[33]

Chronic Disseminated Candidiasis
Chronic disseminated candidiasis (also known previously as hepatosplenic candidiasis) is a distinct form of hematogenous candidiasis seen almost exclusively in patients with

leukemia or bone marrow transplantation.[2,33] Infection of the liver or spleen presumably occurs during the period preceding chemotherapy-induced neutropenia. Candidemia may be detected occasionally during this period; however, the disease does not manifest itself until after neutrophil recovery. The typical patient will have persistent fever after neutrophil recovery and complain of abdominal pain. Multiple lesions are revealed on CT scans of the liver or spleen. Elevation of alkaline phosphatase and other liver function tests are usually present.[33]

Candiduria

Lower urinary tract infection is thought to occur via ascending route from the bladder. However, pyelonephritis can occur as a result of ascending or hematogenous spread.[2,33] Distinguishing infection versus colonization by the presence of *Candida* sp in the urine is difficult.[38] Unlike bacterial urinary tract infection, in candiduria the quantity of organisms and the presence of pyuria do not significantly correlate with the presence of infection.[38] In patients with an indwelling Foley catheter, colonization of the urine with *Candida* sp is common. In addition, candiduria may simply indicate the filtering of the organism during an episode of hematogenous spread in the critically ill patient and may be the only positive culture indicating disseminated disease.[2,33,39] In light of the relatively low sensitivity of blood cultures in diagnosing patients with disseminated candidiasis, a positive urine culture often poses a diagnostic and therapeutic dilemma for the clinician.

Diagnosis

Mucocutaneous Candidiasis. The diagnosis of oropharyngeal and esophageal candidiasis is based on the clinical appearance and the demonstration of hyphae, pseudohyphae, or yeast forms obtained from scraping the lesions using a 10% potassium hydroxide smear. Similarly, vulvovaginal candidiasis can be diagnosed by clinical presentation, direct microscopy using a saline solution or a 10% potassium hydroxide smear in addition to the presence of normal vaginal pH.

Deep Organ Involvement. Hematogenous spread is essential in disseminated candidiasis. Hence, prompt and accurate detection of *Candida* sp in the bloodstream is tantamount to the diagnosis of disseminated disease. However, the diagnosis of hematogenous candidiasis remains elusive because of the low sensitivity of blood cultures. Several series have reported positive blood cultures in less than 50% of patients with autopsy-proven invasive candidiasis.[2,33,39] In addition, routine blood cultures may take several days to become positive. Serologic tests based on the detection of antibodies, antigen, or metabolites of the *Candida* sp are not routinely recommended and few are commercially available.[2,33,39]

Owing to the lack of distinct clinical presentation and reliable diagnostic methods for disseminated candidiasis, some have suggested a clinical approach to aid clinicians in making the diagnosis.[39] Multiple risk factors have been shown to predict the likelihood of disseminated candidiasis

in a given patient. Based on these risk factors, disseminated candidiasis should be considered for patients who have persistent, unexplained fever in conjunction with some combination of the following: neutropenia, prolonged duration of intensive care stay (>7 days), prolonged use of multiple antibacterial agents, prolonged use of intravascular catheters, and colonization with *Candida* at one or more body sites.

TREATMENT AND OUTCOMES OF ENDEMIC MYCOSES AND OPPORTUNISTIC MYCOSES

Antifungal pharmacotherapy for systemic infections is limited to a few pharmacologic classes compared with antibacterial agents. An overview of the pharmacology of systemically available antifungal agents is provided in the following sections, which include amphotericin B, ketoconazole, itraconazole, fluconazole, 5-flucytosine, terbinafine, and two recently approved agents, caspofungin and voriconazole. The current status and utility of antifungal susceptibility testing to guide therapy are also discussed. In addition, the role in therapy for each agent is detailed with respect to endemic and opportunistic mycoses.

GENERAL TREATMENT GUIDELINES

Pharmacotherapy. The major classes of systemic antifungal agents in clinical use consist of the polyenes (amphotericin and nystatin), the azole derivatives, the allylamines-thiocarbamates (terbinafine), and the echinocandins (caspofungin). The first three antifungal classes target fungal cell membranes by interacting with or inhibiting ergosterol. The echinocandins uniquely target fungal cell wall. Table 87.3 provides a comparative table on the pharmacologic characteristics, dosage administration, and costs of the above agents.

Amphotericin B. Amphotericin B has been available for more than 40 years and served as the gold standard for the treatment of systemic fungal infections. However, its use is associated with significant toxicities. To circumvent these toxicities, three lipid-formulated products have been developed and approved for use recently based on their improved safety profile.[40,41] The optimal dosage and duration of amphotericin B deoxycholate are largely empiric; total dosage generally has been determined by patient response and tolerance. Daily dosage varies from 0.5 to 1.5 mg per kilogram depending on the host's immune status, site, severity, and type of infection.[42] An initial 1-mg test dose of amphotericin is recommended traditionally to observe for anaphylactic reaction, which occurs on rare occasions; however, recent clinical experience suggests that this practice may not be necessary and may significantly delay therapy in those who are acutely ill.[42] In fact, for life-threatening infections, many clinicians advocate that the maximum or target daily dose

TABLE 87.3	Comparative Pharmacologic Characteristics and Costs of Systemic Antifungal Agents						
	AMBd	**ABLC**	**L-AMB**	**FCZ**	**ICZ**	**VCZ**	**CAS**
Spectrum							
Aspergillus	Cidal	Cidal	Cidal	No activity	Cidal	Cidal	Static
C. albicans	Cidal	Cidal	Cidal	Static	Static	Static	Cidal
Non-*albicans* sp	Cidal	Cidal	Cidal	Limited activity	Limited activity	Static	Cidal
Proven Efficacy	IA, IC, FN	IA, IC	IA, IC, FN	IC	IC, IA, FN	IA	IA, IC
Safety							
Nephrotoxicity	23%–53%	11%–42%	0%–21%	1%–2%	5%	7%	1%–7%
IRAE	30%–87%	30%–80%	5%–30%	1%	10%	3%–13%	1%–5%
Increased LFTs	1%–16%	4%–27%	5%–26%	1%–14%	1%–7%	7%–18%	2%–8%
Visual	4%	–	–	8%	–	20%–45%	–
Rash	1%–3%	4%	2%	4%–5%	9%	6%–8%	1%–7%
DDI	Minimal	Minimal	Minimal	Low-moderate	Moderate	High	Low
Pharmacokinetics							
Oral Bioavailability	Minimal	Minimal	Minimal	>80%	20%–60%	96%	Minimal
CSF penetration	Minimal	Minimal	Minimal	>70%	Minimal	20%–50%	Unknown
Primary route of elimination	Unknown	Unknown	Unknown	Renal	Hepatic CYP450	Hepatic CYP450	Hydrolysis, N-acetylation
Dosage	0.5–1.5 mg/kg	5 mg/kg	3–6 mg/kg	400 mg QD	200 mg BID	LD: 6 mg/kg BID; MD 3–4 mg/kg BID	LD 70 mg, MD 50 mg QD
Regimen	QD	QD	QD				
AWP Cost/day[c]	$14–40	$805	$790–1,580	IV $148 PO $28	IV $310 Solution $34	IV LD $447, MD $223–298 PO $63	LD $474, MD $368

[a] Incidence varies depending on definition, daily and cumulative dosages used in the study, [b]Hepatitis (rare), [c]Cost/day based on dose/day of a 70-kg patient with normal renal and hepatic function, AWP March 2003.

AmBd, amphotericin B deoxycholate; ABLC, amphotericin B lipid complex; L-AMB, liposomal amphotericin B; FCZ, fluconazole; ICZ, itraconazole; VCZ, voriconazole; CAS, caspofungin; "cidal," fungicidal; "static," fungistatic; IA, invasive aspergillosis; IC, invasive candidiasis; FN, febrile neutropenia; IRAE, infusion related adverse effects; LFTs, liver function tests; DDI, drug-drug interactions; CSF, cerebrospinal fluid; CYP 450, cytochrome P450 enzymes; IV, intravenous; LD, loading dose; MD, maintenance dose.

(From Wong-Beringer A, Kriengkauykiat J. Systemic Antifungal Therapy: new options, new challenges. Pharmacotherapy 23:1441–1462, 2003.)

be given at initial infusion 1.0–1.5 mg per kilogram for conventional formulation and 3.0–5.0 mg per kilogram for the lipid formulations.[40] Adverse effects associated with systemic administration of amphotericin B are primarily acute infusion-related (e.g., fever, chills, rigors) and dose-limiting nephrotoxicity. Premedications with acetaminophen (10 mg/kg), diphenhydramine (50 mg), meperidine (25–60 mg) administered one half hour before amphotericin B infusions have been shown to reduce the incidence of fever and chills.[42] Hydrocortisone (25 mg) added to the infusion also has reduced febrile reactions. Thrombophlebitis can also occur and can be minimized with the use of central venous line for administration, dilute solutions (<0.1 mg/mL), or the addition of heparin 500 to 1,000 U per liter of solution. The most significant adverse effect is nephrotoxicity. Reversible nephrotoxicity develops in approximately 80% of patients with receipt of at least 500 mg total dose of amphotericin B.[42] Irreversible renal damage occurs rarely and usually does not occur unless the total dose exceeds 4 to 5 g.[42] Efforts to minimize or reverse nephrotoxicity include the

use of sodium loading, mannitol administration, and alternate-day administration. Infusion of 0.5 L of sodium chloride 0.9% over 30 minutes before and after completion of the amphotericin B infusion is advocated by some for patients at the first sign of rising serum creatinine (Scr) and blood urea nitrogen (BUN) concentrations.[42] However, caution must be exercised when liberalizing salt intake in patients with congestive heart failure (CHF), renal failure, or cirrhosis with ascites. The lipid-formulated amphotericin B products (e.g., Abelcet, Amphotec, AmBisome) have all shown a lower incidence of nephrotoxicity when compared to the conventional formulation.[41] Of note, direct comparison between Abelcet and AmBisome on safety has been evaluated in patients with febrile neutropenia. AmBisome was associated with significantly lower nephrotoxicity compared to Abelcet at 5mg/kg/day (15% vs. 42%, $p < 0.001$).[43] Clinical experience with the use of the lipid products has been primarily limited to patients who are intolerant of or refractory to amphotericin B deoxycholate. Renal tolerance is usually defined as Scr greater than or equal to 2.5 mg per deciliter or doubling of baseline Scr in compassionate use studies and clinical trials. Efficacy data from animal models of fungal infections suggest differential activity for the three commercially available lipid formulations. In addition, none of the lipid-based products demonstrates superior efficacy when prospectively compared with amphotericin B deoxycholate against invasive candidiasis and cryptococcal meningitis.[41,44] The acquisition costs of all three lipid products vary, but all are substantially higher than deoxycholate formulation. In general, use of these expensive agents should be considered for salvage therapy particularly in patients who are not expected to receive prolonged therapy or have preexisting renal dysfunction. Some experts advocate the use of lipid formulation as initial therapy based on emerging data demonstrating adverse outcomes, higher mortality, longer hospital stay, and higher cost of care associated with amphotericin B-induced nephrotoxicity.[45] Nonetheless, the recent addition of two new agents may supplant the use of amphotericin B deoxycholate and lipid formulations as new data accumulates.

Azoles. Ketoconazole, which was introduced in the 1980s, was the first systemically useful treatment alternative to amphotericin B for invasive mycoses. However, the high doses required (>800 mg/day) for treatment are associated with frequent toxicities.[40,44] Since the introduction of fluconazole and itraconazole in the 1990s, the use of ketoconazole has been replaced largely by the newer agents owing to their greater efficacy and tolerability. Fluconazole and itraconazole are available in oral and parenteral formulations. Both drugs are highly active against endemic mycoses; itraconazole is more effective than fluconazole against histoplasmosis and blastomycosis. In addition, they have variable activity against the yeasts and molds that cause invasive diseases. Non–*albicans Candida* species as a group are less susceptible to fluconazole and itraconazole, whereas *Aspergillus* spp. are susceptible only to itraconazole.[40,44] Despite the favorable adverse effect profile, itraconazole and fluconazole each has its unique limitations.[40,44] Oral absorption of itraconazole is poor and variable. The capsule formulation requires an acidic medium for drug dissolution; thus, drug absorption is problematic in patients with HIV who have achlorhydria, or in those receiving concurrent antacids or H$_2$-antagonists. A new oral solution has improved bioavailability over the capsule form. Serum levels should be measured to ensure adequate absorption. In contrast, fluconazole has excellent bioavailability and its absorption is not pH-dependent. All three azoles inhibit mammalian cytochrome P-450 enzyme families; ketoconazole is the most potent and fluconazole the least potent inhibitor.[40,44] In general, the magnitude of interaction increases when higher doses of azoles are employed. Clinically significant drug interactions have been documented when azoles are coadministered with cyclosporine, phenytoin, rifampin, terfenadine, astemizole, and cisapride; the latter three agents have been withdrawn from the market due to the occurrence of life-threatening arrhythmias. Azole-induced inhibition of cyclosporine metabolism results in an increase in cyclosporine trough concentration and area

under the curve; thus, close monitoring of cyclosporine serum concentrations and renal function is important in patients receiving both agents. In addition, rifampin and phenytoin may induce the metabolic clearance of ketoconazole and itraconazole (and, to a lesser extent, fluconazole), resulting in treatment failure of fungal infections. Phenytoin metabolism also can be inhibited by fluconazole; nystagmus and ataxia as a result of excessive phenytoin concentrations have been reported in a few patients in whom phenytoin and fluconazole were concomitantly administered.

Voriconazole is the latest addition to the azole class.[44,46] It is a congener of fluconazole available as an oral and parenteral agent. In vitro activity includes all *Candida* species (including *C. krusei* and fluconazole-resistant *C. glabrata*), *Aspergillus* spp, and other molds such as *Fusarium* sp and *Scedosporium apiospermum*.[44,46] It is available for parenteral and oral administration with a bioavailability of 96%. Like itraconazole, it is extensively metabolized hepatically with <1% excreted unchanged in the urine. Drug interaction potential is high due to its inhibitory effect on cytochrome P450 (CYP450) isoenzymes 3A4, 2C9, and 2C19.[44,47] Significant alterations in serum level of drugs undergoing CYP450 metabolism such as cyclosporine, tacrolimus, phenytoin, and warfarin are expected with concomitant administration of voriconazole. Other interactions relate to its potential to prolong the QT interval. Adverse effects most commonly relate to the GI tract (nausea, vomiting). Rash, photosensitivity, and hepatitis have been reported. In addition, voriconazole causes unique transient nonsight-threatening visual disturbances (i.e., blurred vision, color vision change) at an incidence of 20% to 45%.[44,46]

Owing to their relatively favorable safety profile compared with amphotericin B, the fluconazole and itraconazole have assumed widespread use in the treatment of candidiasis, cryptococcosis, and endemic mycosis and for primary and secondary prophylaxis. It is notable that the emergence of azole-resistant oropharyngeal isolates of *C. albicans* from patients infected with HIV is being increasingly reported, which may limit clinical utility of these drugs in the near future.[47,48] Immune reconstitution from use of highly active antiretroviral therapy (HAART) has mitigated the development of *Candida* resistance to the azoles in the HIV population as a result of better control of mucosal disease. At the same time, the superior efficacy of voriconazole in the treatment of invasive aspergillosis may supplant amphotericin B as first-line treatment.

Echinocandin. Caspofungin is the first approved drug in this new class of antifungal agents.[44,49] It acts uniquely by inhibiting the synthesis of β-(1,3)-D-glucan, a vital component of fungal cell wall. The echinocandins demonstrate fungicidal activity against all *Candida* species except for *C. parapsilosis* and *C. guillermondii* which require higher drug concentrations for inhibition. Caspofungin is fungistatic against *Aspergillus* sp and is not active against *Cryptococcus* sp. It is available only for parenteral administration. Unlike the azoles, caspofungin is metabolized via hydrolysis and N-acetylation and does not inhibit or induce CYP enzymes.

Thus, relatively few drug-drug interactions have been reported, namely cyclosporine, rifampin, efavirenz, phenytoin, dexamethasone, and carbamazepine. Due to its unique cellular target, mechanism-based toxicities are minimal. Headache, nausea, vomiting, flushing, and infusion-related adverse effects are most commonly reported at a frequency of approximately 3% in clinical trials.

Other Agents. 5-Flucytosine is a nucleoside analog with limited utility owing to its narrow spectrum of activity, its toxicities, and the rapid emergence of resistance when used alone.[50] Its role in therapy is primarily for use in combination with amphotericin B for treating cryptococcal meningitis. Maintaining a serum level of 5-flucytosine below 100 mg per milliliter is recommended to avoid dose-related bone marrow toxicities.[50] Dosage reduction is required in renal dysfunction.[50] Terbinafine is an allylamine primarily used for the treatment of dermatophytic infections of the skin and nail. It has activity against non-*fumigatus Aspergillus* sp and synergistic potential with the azoles against azole-resistant *Candida* sp.[29,30] However, its therapeutic role for invasive mycoses is uncertain in light of available new agents.

Agents under investigation in clinical trials include additional azoles (posaconazole and ravuconazole) and echinocandins (micafungin and anidulafungin). The new azoles are expected to expand treatment options against difficult to treat mold infections. In addition, new antifungal drug targets are currently under investigation.[51,52] Agents that inhibit the biosynthesis of fungal cell wall components (chitin) and fungal protein synthesis have shown broad in vitro activity against pathogenic fungi; few have shown promise in animal models of invasive mycoses and are being evaluated in early clinical trials.[51,52]

ANTIFUNGAL SUSCEPTIBILITY TESTING

The use of antifungal susceptibility testing to guide therapy may become the standard of care in the near future as the number and spectrum of fungal infections increases, reports of antifungal resistance continues, and new antifungal agents are developed. Studies correlating antifungal susceptibility testing results with in vivo outcome of fungal infections are ongoing. A reference method for in vitro susceptibility testing of yeasts has been standardized whereas in vitro testing of molds is still being developed.[32,33,53,54] Clinical correlation between in vitro results and in vivo outcome has been established for the use of azoles in the treatment of oropharyngeal candidiasis in patients infected with HIV (for itraconazole and fluconazole) and nonneutropenic patients with candidemia (for fluconazole only). Thus, interpretive breakpoints for susceptibility may not necessarily apply to the treatment of invasive candidiasis in patients with neutropenia or those infected with non-*C. albicans* species. At present, antifungal susceptibility testing is not recommended for routine use but is most useful for evaluation of cases that lack clinical response to azole therapy and to support a change from parenteral therapy to step-down oral therapy with an azole.

TREATMENT OF ENDEMIC MYCOSES

The majority of patients infected with endemic fungal pathogens (*H. capsulatum, B. dermatitidis,* and *C. immitis*) are asymptomatic or have self-limited acute pulmonary disease that does not require treatment with antifungal agents.[9,12,15] A minority of patients with the following clinical presentations may develop fulminant or chronic progressive disease requiring specific therapy: acute pulmonary disease accompanied by severe respiratory distress; chronic pulmonary cavitary disease; extrapulmonary dissemination involving skin, bone, CNS, and others.[9,12,15] Those who have underlying immunodeficiency also are candidates for antifungal therapy. Among the major endemic mycoses, coccidioidomycosis is most refractory to treatment, particularly the meningeal form of disease.[15] Lifelong maintenance therapy following acute treatment to prevent relapse is indicated in patients infected with HIV who have endemic mycoses and may be required in all patients with coccidioidal meningitis.[15,55] According to the 2002 U.S. Public Health Service Guidelines, primary prevention for histoplasmosis has been shown to reduce the frequency of disease without survival benefit; thus, primary prevention with itraconazole can be considered in residents living in endemic areas who have advanced HIV infection (CD4 count <100/μL) particularly those who are at high risk because of occupational exposure.[55] Routine prevention against primary infection with blastomycosis and coccidioidomycosis is not recommended currently for patients who are HIV-positive.[55]

Amphotericin B has been the mainstay of treatment of endemic mycoses. However, therapy often is complicated by acute infusion-related adverse effects and dose-limited nephrotoxicity. Recent introduction of the azoles provides less toxic treatment alternatives. Of note, patients who are immunocompromised or who have life-threatening or meningeal disease have been excluded from studies using the azoles. In addition, direct comparison between amphotericin B and the azole drugs has not been performed in controlled trials for endemic mycoses.[56] Nonetheless, response to treatment appears slower with the azoles by comparison with historical controls.[56] Hence, use of amphotericin B is currently indicated for treating patients with ARDS, sepsis syndrome, or other evidence of overwhelming infection with the endemic mycoses (including those with meningeal involvement, with the exception of coccidioidal meningitis).[5,9,12,15] A total dosage of 1.0 to 2.5 g of amphotericin B generally is recommended.[42] Daily dosage ranges from 0.7 to 1.5 mg per kilogram with administration of the drug until the disease is inactive or for a total of 2 to 3 months, depending on the host's response.[9,12,15,42] Therapy usually can be switched to itraconazole in patients who are clinically stable; thus, the total dosage or duration of amphotericin B may be shorter than that stated in the preceding.

Local administration via intraarticular injections of amphotericin B may be useful as a primary therapy or as an adjunct to systemic therapy or surgery in coccidioidal synovitis or osteomyelitis.[15,42] Direct lumbar or cisternal injections or intraventricular administration via an Ommaya reservoir have been used to administer the drug along with parenteral administration for the treatment of coccidioidal meninigitis.[42] Because of the serious neurologic sequelae associated with this mode of drug administration, high-dose therapy with oral fluconazole starting at 400 to 1,000 mg per day is currently preferred.[15] Some clinicians prefer to initiate oral fluconazole therapy with intrathecal administration of amphotericin B daily to weekly to achieve a faster response. The intrathecal dose of amphotericin B begins at 0.01 with gradual increase up to 1.5 mg depending on patient tolerance.[15,42]

Itraconazole is considered the drug of choice for histoplasmosis and blastomycosis in nonimmunocompromised patients who do not have life-threatening or meningeal disease.[9,12] Itraconazole administered at dosages of 200 to 400 mg daily for a duration of 6 to 24 months has been associated with a response rate of 86% and 95% for histoplasmosis and blastomycosis, respectively.[57] Treatment is recommended for 6 months, or 3 months after all lesions have resolved. Patients with chronic cavitary pulmonary histoplasmosis are less responsive to itraconazole and may require therapy for at least 1 year or longer.[9]

Acute treatment with amphotericin B followed by lifelong maintenance therapy with itraconazole 200 mg twice daily is recommended to prevent relapse in HIV-infected patients with histoplasmosis.[5,9,55] Itraconazole has been shown to be effective for induction therapy in patients who have HIV with mild to moderate disease, and as lifelong maintenance therapy. In an open-label, nonrandomized prospective trial, itraconazole therapy at 300 mg twice a day for 3 days followed by 200 mg twice a day for 12 weeks resulted in an 85% response (50/59) in patients with AIDS and disseminated histoplasmosis.[56] Patients with CNS involvement or severe clinical manifestations were excluded from the study. In a separate study involving a similar group of patients, fluconazole induction therapy at 800 mg per day for 12 weeks followed by maintenance therapy at 400 mg per day resulted in a 74% response.[58] However, the 1-year relapse rate with high-dose fluconazole therapy (800 mg/day) was substantially higher when compared with patients receiving itraconazole at 200 mg per day as maintenance therapy (47% vs. 5%).[56,58] Ketoconazole is not an acceptable treatment option in patients with AIDS owing to the low response rate of less than 20%.[9]

Fluconazole is less active than itraconazole against blastomycosis and histoplasmosis, and is considered second-line therapy.[9,12] It is indicated for patients who cannot tolerate or adequately absorb itraconazole. A minimum dosage of 400 to 800 mg per day is required for treatment over a duration of at least 6 months.[58] However, for nonmeningeal coccidioidomycosis, response rates appear similar with fluconazole and itraconazole treatment at 400 mg per day.[15] Efficacy results from a comparative trial on the treatment of progressive nonmeningeal coccidioidomycosis indicate that fluconazole 400 mg per day and itraconazole 200 mg twice daily are not statistically different, although a trend towards

slightly greater efficacy with itraconazole was observed.[59] Fluconazole is considered the drug of choice for most patients with coccidioidal meningitis, which obviates the need for intrathecal administration of amphotericin B. Fluconazole administered at 400 mg per day orally for up to 4 years resulted in a 79% (37/47) response rate.[60] Most improvement occurred within 4 to 8 months after starting therapy. Only two patients developed confusion during treatment, whereas alopecia was noted in three patients. Similarly, itraconazole treatment at 300 to 400 mg per day for a median of 10 months in eight evaluable patients with meningitis was associated with a favorable response.[61]

Despite these encouraging results with azole therapy for coccidioidal meningitis, a follow-up study on 18 patients in whom azole therapy had been discontinued because of a presumption of cure indicates that the relapse rate is unacceptably high.[62] Those patients were treated for a median duration of 37 months; 14 of 18 patients relapsed with disseminated disease, resulting in three deaths. Relapses occurred at 2 weeks to 30 months after treatment discontinued. Although the azoles appear to be safer alternatives to intrathecal administration of amphotericin, lifelong suppressive therapy is likely required for meningitis.

Specifically, for histoplasmosis, measurement of antigen levels in blood and urine samples is useful for setting treatment endpoint and detection of early relapse.[9] Treatment should continue until antigen concentrations revert to negative or at least four or less units. When measured at 3- to 4-month intervals, a relative increase in antigen levels of more than 2 U compared with previously measured levels suggests recurrence of disease. Reinduction therapy may be instituted to control this recurrence. As for coccidioidomycosis, baseline evaluation of the skin test reactivity and CF antibody titers are recommended for all patients receiving therapy to help determine the duration and the response to treatment.[13,15] Persistently negative skin test reactivity in a patient with disseminated disease is associated with high likelihood of relapse when treatment is discontinued. A decreasing CF antibody titer during the treatment course is predictive of a positive response.

TREATMENT OF OPPORTUNISTIC MYCOSES

Cryptococcosis. The choice of agent(s) for treatment of cryptococcosis depends on the anatomic sites of involvement and underlying immune status of the host. Pulmonary disease in normal hosts resolves spontaneously and can be observed without antifungal therapy along with careful follow-up. However, patients with progressive pulmonary disease, those with accompanying extrapulmonary involvement, and all immunocompromised patients should receive antifungal therapy. Amphotericin B total dosage of 1.0 to 1.5 g with or without flucytosine is recommended. The optimal total dosage and duration is unknown; however, therapy should continue until there is clinical and radiographic resolution of disease with eradication of the organisms from sputum cultures or bronchoalveolar lavage. Fluconazole therapy at 200 to 400 mg per day for a duration of 3 to 6 months

TABLE 87.4	Antifungal Therapy for Cryptococcal Meningitis
Patient Subgroups	**Antifungal Regimen**
Non-AIDS	Amphotericin B 0.3 mg/kg/day (5-flucytosine 150 mg/kg/day in four divided doses × 6 weeks
AIDS Induction	Amphotericin B 0.7 mg/kg/day ± 5-flucytosine 100 mg/kg/day in two to three divided doses × 2 weeks, then fluconazole or itraconazole 400 mg/day × 8 weeks[a]
Maintenance (lifelong)	Fluconazole 200 mg every day
Prophylaxis	*Not* recommended routinely

[a] A switch to oral azole therapy after 2 weeks is appropriate only for patients who are clinically stable or who have improved.
AIDS, acquired immunodeficiency syndrome.

may be considered for those with mild to moderately severe pulmonary disease.[20,63]

All patients with cryptococcal meningitis require treatment (Table 87.4). In patients not infected with HIV, combination therapy of amphotericin B with flucytosine for 6 weeks has been established as the regimen of choice based on two early prospective randomized comparative trials.[64,65] It is notable that the incidence of adverse effects (e.g., bone marrow suppression and liver enzyme abnormalities) owing to flucytosine 150 mg per kilogram per day was high; 30 of 194 patients developed leukopenia, 22 of 194 developed thrombocytopenia, and 13 of 194 developed hepatitis.[65] The development of toxic effects was significantly correlated with the presence of flucytosine serum concentrations of greater than or equal to 100 μg per milliliter for 2 weeks or more. Approximately 50% of the toxic reactions occurred within the first 2 weeks and more than 90% within the first 4 weeks of therapy.

Antifungal therapy in patients with AIDS has been carefully evaluated in several large comparative trials over the past 10 years. Early studies have established the superior efficacy of amphotericin B with or without flucytosine over fluconazole for the acute treatment of cryptococcal meningitis in AIDS.[66,67] Fluconazole alone compared with the combined regimen was associated with higher mortality rates during the first 2 weeks of therapy (15% vs. 8%, respectively) and a longer period to CSF sterilization (64 vs. 42 days, respectively).[67] Similarly, more failures and relapses were observed for patients receiving itraconazole compared with combination therapy of amphotericin and flucytosine in another prospective randomized comparative trial.[68] The most recent trial evaluated a two-step treatment strategy consisting of amphotericin at higher dosages (0.7 mg/kg/day) for 2 weeks (step 1) followed by 8 weeks of either itraconazole or fluconazole 400 mg per day (step 2).[69] A total of 381 patients were randomized to receive amphotericin alone

or in combination with flucytosine 100 mg/kg/day in step 1. The addition of flucytosine did not significantly improve survival at 2 weeks or shorten the time to negative CSF cultures. For the group receiving amphotericin B alone, mortality at 2 weeks was 6% with negative CSF cultures in 51% of the patients. When compared with regimens used in previous studies, the short-term use of high dosage amphotericin with or without flucytosine during initial therapy was associated with lower mortality (6% vs 14%–18%, respectively) and higher rates of CSF sterilization (50% vs. 20%, respectively) at 2 weeks. The overall efficacy (complete resolution of symptoms) for this two-step regimen was 70% at 10 weeks. Of note, the strategy of changing therapy to an azole at 2 weeks cannot be recommended for patients who did not improve or who had clinical deterioration after 2 weeks of high-dose amphotericin therapy because those patients were excluded from enrollment onto step 2 of the study.

Alternative treatment strategies also have been evaluated in a limited number of patients. The combination of fluconazole 400 mg per day with flucytosine 150 mg/kg/day for 10 weeks resulted in negative CSF cultures after a median time of 23 days in 75% of study patients.[70] Based on the shorter time to CSF sterilization, flucytosine appears to enhance the efficacy of fluconazole; however, 30% of patients had dose-limiting adverse reactions to flucytosine requiring discontinuation of the drug. In addition, the safety and efficacy of a lipid formulation of amphotericin B (i.e., Abelcet) also has been compared prospectively with conventional formulation for the treatment of cryptococcal meningitis in patients with AIDS.[71] Comparable treatment success was observed for both formulations despite the use of lipid-formulated amphotericin B at five times the treatment dosage of conventional formulation (42% vs. 50%, respectively). However, a higher number of recipients of the lipid formulation had persistent positive CSF cultures at the end of treatment despite symptom resolution. A disproportionate share of negative prognostic factors was present in the Abelcet group, suggesting that perhaps amphotericin B lipid complex may be less effective in that subgroup. In addition, the cost effectiveness of using the lipid formulations of amphotericin for this indication will need to be addressed considering the low rates of nephrotoxicity (4%) when amphotericin was given at high dosage for 2 weeks in the aforementioned trial.[69]

Similar to endemic mycoses, cryptococcosis in HIV-infected patients is associated with a high relapse rate after completion of primary therapy.[72] Patients receiving fluconazole maintenance therapy have a relapse rate of 3% versus 37% placebo from any site.[72] Hence, lifelong maintenance therapy is recommended unless immune reconstitution occurs as a result of highly active antiretroviral therapy (i.e., sustained increase of at least 6 months in their CD4 T lymphocyte counts to >100–200 cells/μL).[55] Fluconazole has been established as the maintenance treatment of choice by two controlled trials.[72,73] At daily dosages of 200 mg per day, fluconazole therapy resulted in no relapse compared with 15% in placebo patients.[74] When compared to amphotericin B (1 mg/kg per week), recipients of fluconazole 200 mg per day had fewer relapses (2% vs. 18%).[73] In addition, when administered at the same 200 mg daily dose, itraconazole was less effective than fluconazole as maintenance therapy in preventing relapses.[74]

Routine administration of fluconazole for primary prophylaxis is currently not recommended by the United States Public Health Service/Infectious Disease Society of America owing to the low incidence of disease, lack of survival benefit, concerns for development of *Candida* and *Cryptococcus* resistance, and cost.[55] Prophylaxis may be administered selectively to those who have CD4 less than 50 cells per microliter with fluconazole (100–200 mg daily) and may have a need for prophylaxis against other fungal infections.[55]

Aspergillosis. Antifungal therapy for invasive aspergillosis has been limited primarily to two agents with intrinsic activity against the organism, amphotericin B and itraconazole until recently. Therapy with either agent is associated with dismal outcomes, significant drug toxicities, and potential drug-drug interactions.

In general, treatment response for invasive aspergillosis has been disappointing with an overall response rate of 34% for amphotericin B.[75,76] Results from noncomparative open-label trials with itraconazole suggest similar response rates in immunocompromised patients.[77,78] A subset of patients who failed to respond to initial treatment with amphotericin B have responded to subsequent treatment with itraconazole or lipid-formulated amphotericin B products (e.g., Abelcet, Amphotec, AmBisome).[44,77,78] Based on available animal and uncontrolled clinical data, at least five times the daily dosages of conventional amphotericin B formulation should be used when a lipid-formulated product is used for the treatment of aspergillosis. No prospective comparative studies have been performed to address the relative efficacy among different formulations of amphotericin B thus far. It is clear that the lipid formulations of amphotericin B afford less nephrotoxicity than conventional forms, but at a much higher drug-acquisition cost. The response rate and overall mortality vary substantially among different host groups in relation to underlying disease status, site of disease, and disease management. In one review on the therapeutic outcomes of more than 1,200 cases of invasive aspergillosis involving the lungs, sinus, and brain in immunocompromised patients, the crude mortality rates (regardless of if treatment was or was not given) were 86%, 66%, and 99%, respectively.[75] Among patients who lived long enough to receive at least 14 days of therapy for pulmonary aspergillosis, bone marrow transplant and liver transplant recipients had poorer responses compared with renal and heart transplant recipients (20%–33% vs. 83%, respectively). Virtually no patients with cerebral aspergillosis survived despite treatment; however, diagnosis was first made at autopsy for the majority of the patients.[27,75] Various factors other than the host group and site of infection have been suggested to predict poor response to treatment

TABLE 87.5	Factors Predictive of Poor Response to Antifungal Therapy of Invasive Aspergillosis

Factors

Leukemic relapse

Persistent neutropenia

No reduction in immunosuppression

Diffuse pulmonary disease

Major hemoptysis

Delayed therapy

Low dosages of amphotericin B, especially during neutropenia

Undetectable or low serum itraconazole concentrations

Lack of secondary prophylaxis during another episode of neutropenia

Angioinvasion (histologically evident)

(From Denning DW. Therapeutic outcome in invasive aspergillosis. Clin Infect Dis 23:608–615, 1996, with permission.)

(Table 87.5).[75] Early diagnosis and prompt initiation of aggressive antifungal therapy are extremely important.

Until recently, amphotericin B (deoxycholate or lipid-associated formulation) was considered first-line therapy for invasive aspergillosis in immunocompromised hosts whereas itraconazole was reserved as a treatment alternative for sequential step-down therapy or those intolerant of amphotericin B toxicities.[28,44,77–80] Voriconazole, the newest approved azole agent, is the first agent to have demonstrated superior efficacy to amphotericin B as primary treatment for invasive aspergillosis. In a pivotal trial that led to drug approval, voriconazole was compared to amphotericin B in a randomized unblinded fashion in 392 patients at 92 centers in 19 countries.[81] Patients received either voriconazole (6 mg/kg IV twice daily on day 1, then 4 mg/kg IV twice daily for at least 7 days followed by oral voriconaozle 200 mg twice daily) or amphotericin B deoxycholate (1–1.5 mg/kg/day). Most patients (>80%) had hematologic underlying diseases; about 25% had allogeneic bone marrow transplantation and 40% to 45% acute leukemia. The lungs were the most common site of involvement. Patients who received voriconazole had higher overall treatment response (53% vs. 32%, respectively) and survival rates (71% vs. 58%, respectively) at week 12 compared to those receiving amphotericin B deoxycholate initially. The improvements in outcome was statistically significant. Voriconazole has also proven value as salvage therapy in patients who were intolerant of or refractory to previous therapy with amphotericin B (deoxycholate or lipid formulation) or itraconazole. A response rate of 38% to 44% was reported in those patients from two noncomparative open label studies.[82,83] Voriconazole was associated with fewer adverse events compared to amphotericin B. However, transient visual disturbances was reported in 30% to 45% of patients receiving voriconazole which were reversible on drug discontinuation with no reported long term sequelae thus far.[81–83]

Another new treatment option for invasive aspergillosis is the first marketed agent from the echinocandin class. Caspofungin received FDA approval based on favorable results on 56 patients enrolled in a compassionate use trial in which the drug was prescribed as salvage therapy for those who were intolerant of or refractory to previous therapy with amphotericin B (deoxycholate or lipid formulation) or itraconazole.[84] More than a third (39%) of the patients who were refractory to previous therapy responded favorably to caspofungin treatment. The dosage regimen administered was 70 mg IV daily on day 1, then 50 mg IV daily. The mean treatment duration was 35 days and was generally well tolerated.

In the patient who achieved initial response to therapy, secondary prophylaxis may be important to administer to prevent relapse during further episodes of immunosuppression from cancer chemotherapy or bone marrow transplantation, or during treatment of acute allograft rejection.[27] Prophylactic administration of antifungal therapy with activity against *Aspergillus* should commence immediately before or at the same time as cytotoxic chemotherapy begins, and should continue until neutrophil recovery in those with prior documentation of invasive aspergillosis is achieved.

It appears that voriconazole may supplant the role of amphotericin B as first-line therapy for the treatment of invasive aspergillosis based on the available data. Combination therapy with any two of the following agents, caspofungin, amphotericin B, and voriconazole has been described for a limited number of patients with refractory disease.[85,86] Combination therapy using agents targeting different components of the fungal cell is now possible and is supported by evidence of synergy from in vitro studies and animal models of infection.[85,86]

Candidiasis

Mucocutaneous Candidiasis. Oral thrush may be treated effectively with topical antifungal therapy; systemic therapy may be used in more extensive cases. In esophagitis, systemic therapy usually is required because of the need for longer contact time. Among the azoles, fluconazole is proven superior to ketoconazole in patients with AIDS, which is likely owing to the presence of achlorhydria and the fact that absorption of fluconazole is not dependent on an acidic pH medium. In a randomized, double-blind comparative trial, itraconazole oral solution achieved similar clinical response rates as fluconazole (94% vs. 91%, respectively).[87] Both were given at 100 to 200 mg per day for 3 to 8 weeks to patients infected with HIV. Recently, mucosal candidiasis refractory to fluconazole is an evolving problem in patients with advanced HIV disease.[35] Progressive immunosuppression and frequent exposure to antifungal agents are associated with the development of refractory disease. Some experts define fluconazole treatment failure as persistent or progressive disease after a 2-week course of fluconazole

(200 mg daily). Response rates of 64% to 80% to itraconazole solution have been reported in fluconazole-refractory patients.[33] IV therapy with amphotericin B (0.3–0.7 mg/kg/day) or caspofungin (50 mg/day) are reasonable alternatives for patients who do not respond to the above oral therapies or who have severe disease or esophageal involvement.[33] Treatment duration is based on response, but is typically 7 to 10 days for oropharyngeal and at least 21 days for esophageal disease.

A number of topical over-the-counter and systemic antifungal agents are available for treating vulvovaginal candidiasis.[33] The different formulations of topical agents that are available include creams, vaginal tablets, and suppositories; the choice of treatment is a matter of patient preference rather than a difference in efficacy. All of the azole topical agents are highly effective, resulting in cure rates exceeding 80% with no clear difference in clinical efficacy for individual agents.[33,36] Single-dose oral fluconazole or itraconazole has shown comparable efficacy with multidose conventional topical azole therapy for uncomplicated vulvovaginal candidiasis. However, patients with severe disease respond better to 7-day topical azole therapy than single-dose fluconazole. Similarly, those with a history of recurrent infection (i.e., four or more episodes of proven infection during a 12-month period) are recommended to receive a longer course of therapy (10–14 vs. 5–7 days). More than one dose of fluconazole 150 mg (given 72 hours apart) may be needed to achieve clinical and mycologic remission in this subgroup. Boric acid administered intravaginally as 600-mg gelatin capsule once daily for 14 days is also effective.[33] Topical azole therapy is associated with low incidence of local side effects and may be used in the first trimester of pregnancy.[36] Systemic azole therapy is not currently recommended for use during pregnancy. Single-dose fluconazole is infrequently associated with GI intolerance, headache, and rash.

Candiduria. Removal of an indwelling urinary catheter alone may eradicate candiduria in up to 40% of patients.[33,88] Treatment in nonneutropenic asymptomatic catheterized patients has not been proven of value.[33] However, the presence of *Candida* in the urine may be the only indication of disseminated candidiasis in neutropenic patients, critically ill patients in the intensive care units (ICUs), infants with low-birth weights, and transplant recipients.[33] Treatment is recommended for patients with the following: urinary symptoms, neutropenia, low-birth weight infants, renal allografts, and undergoing urologic manipulations.[33] Local therapy with amphotericin B, 50 mg in 1 L of sterile water as a continuous or intermittent irrigation of the bladder, has been successful in greater than 90% of the cases.[38] Fluconazole (50–200 mg/day) offers the convenience of oral administration for ambulatory patients.[33,89] Response rates are comparable to amphotericin B bladder irrigation. However, infections owing to non-*albicans Candida* have reportedly persisted or failed fluconazole therapy. Treatment of upper tract infection requires the use of systemic therapy. Surgical intervention to correct the underlying obstructive abnormalities may be necessary to eliminate recurrent *Candida* colonization and subsequent infections of the urinary tract.[33]

Candidemia And Disseminated Candidiasis. Treatment options for invasive candidiasis consist of amphotericin B (deoxycholate or lipid formulations), fluconazole, voriconazole, and caspofungin. The choice of agent depends on the clinical status of the patient (neutropenic vs. nonneutropenic), the infecting *Candida* species (*albicans* vs. non-*albicans*), the presence of organ dysfunction relative to drug toxicity, and the patient's prior exposure to antifungal agents.

Amphotericin B deoxycholate and caspofungin are both fungicidal agents against *Candida* species. The former is associated with significant nephrotoxicity, whereas the latter is a more costly alternative.[44] Amphotericin B lipid complex (ABLC) at five times the daily dose of amphotericin B deoxycholate (0.6–1.0 mg/kg/day) did not demonstrate superior efficacy (65% ABLC vs. 61% amphotericin B) when compared in a prospective, randomized trial for the treatment of invasive candidiasis.[42,90] However, caspofungin is an excellent nonnephrotoxic alternative to amphotericin B based on results from a pivotal trial leading to its approved indication for the treatment of candidemia and Candida infections (intraabdominal abscesses, peritonitis, and pleural space infections).[44,91] Study patients were randomized to receive caspofungin (70 mg once, then 50 mg daily) or amphotericin B (0.6–1.0 mg/kg/day). A majority of the patients (>80%) had candidemia, of which non-*C. albicans* species account for 50% to 60% of the cases. Other patient characteristics were similar, with 11% of patients having neutropenia. Favorable responses were observed in 73% and 62% of caspofungin versus amphotericin B-treated patients, respectively. The difference in efficacy rates was attributed to treatment failure due to toxicities requiring drug discontinuation (3% caspofungin vs. 16% amphotericin B) and not necessarily superior efficacy of caspofungin. It is notable that *C. parapsilosis* accounts for only 19% of candidemia in the caspofungin-treated group cases but was associated with 42% cases of treatment failure due to persistent fungemia. This result suggests that this species may respond less readily to the echinocandins.

Alternatively, fluconazole has been demonstrated to have comparable efficacy to amphotericin B in a large, randomized, controlled trial involving nonneutropenic, noncritically ill patients with candidemia.[92] Patients were administered either amphotericin B (0.5–0.6 mg/kg/day) or fluconazole (400 mg/day) IV then by mouth for 17 and 18 days, respectively. Treatment success was similar in both groups (79% amphotericin vs. 70% fluconazole). Catheter-related candidemia was present in 72% of the patients with *C. albicans* as the predominant pathogen. Recently, combination therapy with high-dose fluconazole (800 mg/day) plus amphotericin B (0.7 mg/kg/day for the first 5 to 6 days) did not demonstrate significant benefit compared to fluconazole alone (80

mg/day) for the treatment of invasive candidiasis in the nonneutropenic population. However, a trend towards more effective bloodstream clearance was noted.[93]

In another prospective comparative trial that included neutropenic patients, fluconazole 400 mg per day was compared with amphotericin B (25–50 mg/day up to 0.67 mg/kg/day) in the treatment of documented or presumed invasive candidiasis.[94] A total of 142 patients were evaluable; at least half in each group were neutropenic patients (<1,000 cells/μL). Approximately 40% of the patients were treated for presumed invasive candidiasis; a presumed diagnosis was made only for neutropenic and postoperative patients. Overall response rates were not different between fluconazole-treated and amphotericin-treated patients (66% vs. 64%). As in the previous study, fewer side effects were noted among fluconazole recipients compared with amphotericin B.

Voriconazole is the newest addition to the azole class of agents. It has a broad spectrum of activity to include all *Candida* species (including fluconazole-resistant *C. glabrata* and *C. krusei*).[44] Preliminary data on the use of voriconazole for refractory candidiasis appears promising.[44] Considering the increasing prevalence of non-*C. albicans* species causing candidemia and the oral availability of voriconazole, this agent may serve as an attractive treatment option for step-down therapy.

The fungicidal activity of amphotericin B deoxycholate against commonly involved Candida species and its low drug acquisition cost make it a cost-effective treatment option for invasive candidiasis in patients who do not have significant risk for nephrotoxicity. In the otherwise critically ill patients who are infected with non-*C. albicans* or those who have preexisting renal dysfunction, caspofungin is an attractive option. Fluconazole is a safe and effective alternative for infections caused by *C. albicans* in the stable and nonneutropenic population. Oral fluconazole or voriconazole may be used as step-down therapy in patients who had responded favorably to initial IV therapy; voriconazole may be considered for infections caused by *C. glabrata* or *C. krusei*.

IMPROVING OUTCOMES

Prolonged neutropenia is a significant risk factor for the development of invasive fungal infections, notably aspergillosis and candidiasis.[22] Associated mortality is high, whereas the diagnosis of invasive disease remains elusive. Thus, management strategies have included the use of antifungal prophylaxis and empiric therapy in those at high risk for developing invasive disease.[95,96]

Prophylaxis with high-dose fluconazole (400 mg/day) during prolonged neutropenia following bone marrow transplantation has been shown to decrease the incidence of invasive candidiasis and mortality in a placebo-control trial. However, routine fluconazole prophylaxis has resulted in the selection of fluconazole-resistant *Candida* spp. (i.e., *C. krusei* and *C. glabrata*) in some centers and also *Aspergillus* as the cause of superinfections.[97,98] Thus, some advocate the use of fluconazole as prophylaxis only in those patients who are likely to have profound (<100 cells/mm^3) and protracted neutropenia (>10 days), and particularly those colonized with *Candida* or *Aspergillus*.[33]

Antifungal therapy targeting candidiasis and aspergillosis should begin in patients who failed to respond to 4 to 7 days of broad-spectrum antibacterial therapy during neutropenia and continued until resolution of neutropenia. Several large, prospective, randomized trials have been conducted comparing amphotericin B deoxycholate with liposomal amphotericin and itraconazole, liposomal amphotericin B with voriconazole and caspofungin for this indication. Composite end points (e.g., defervescence, no breakthrough fungal infections, no discontinuation of drug therapy due to toxicities) were used to evaluate success in the trials. When compared to amphotericin B deoxycholate (0.5–0.7 mg/kg/day) as the reference standard, liposomal amphotericin B (3 mg/kg/day) demonstrated similar overall success, but superior safety and efficacy in preventing breakthrough infections in high-risk bone marrow transplant recipients in a large, prospective randomized trial.[99] Itraconazole administered at 200 mg IV every 12 hours initially, then switched to 400 mg daily solution achieved similar efficacy as amphotericin B deoxycholate with significantly less toxicity.[100] However, although voriconazole (6 mg/kg/day every 12 hours × 1 day, followed by 3 mg/kg every 12 hours) did not achieve noninferiority comparison to liposomal amphotericin B in an open-label randomized trial, significantly less breakthrough infections occurred in the subset of high-risk patients (allogeneic bone marrow transplant recipients and those with relapsed leukemia) receiving voriconazole.[101] It is notable that itraconazole oral absorption is less reliable compared to voriconazole. Thus, oral voriconazole may be an attractive option in patients who could tolerate oral therapy and have reversible renal dysfunction. However, in those who have a high potential for complex drug-drug interactions and/or experienced adverse events with voriconazole, caspofungin may be a reasonable alternative as demonstrated by the similar efficacy and improved safety when compared to liposomal amphotericin B in a recently completed trial.[102] Overall, amphotericin B deoxycholate appears to serve as a reference standard as empirical treatment in febrile neutropenia; treatment alternatives appear to demonstrate similar efficacy with improvements in preventing breakthrough infections in the high-risk subset of patients and less potential for adverse events at much higher costs.

KEY POINTS

- Advances in medical technology and therapies have contributed to a dramatic increase in the incidence and spectrum of invasive fungal infections over the past two decades
- Medically important fungi causing systemic fungal infections can be classified as endemic versus opportunistic, with *C. immitis*, *H. capsulatum*, and *B. dermatitidis* being the major endemic pathogens, whereas *Candida* sp, *Aspergillus* sp, and *Cryptococcus* sp are opportunistic pathogens causing invasive disease in patients with overt immunosuppression
- The majority of patients infected with endemic fungal pathogens are asymptomatic or have self-limited acute pulmonary disease that does not require treatment with antifungal agents
- Itraconazole is considered the drug of choice for histoplasmosis and blastomycosis in nonimmunocompromised patients who do not have life-threatening or meningeal disease, whereas amphotericin is the mainstay of treatment for critically ill patients with overwhelming infection
- The risk for developing invasive candidiasis and aspergillosis is directly related to the duration and degree of neutropenia
- Individuals who are the most immunocompromised are the least likely to have symptoms and have a rapidly fatal course with invasive aspergillosis
- In clinical practice, aggressive therapy for acute invasive aspergillosis is initiated based on a combination of clinical, radiologic, or microbiologic features before a diagnosis is proven definitively. Voriconazole will likely replace amphotericin B as first-line treatment based on improved efficacy and survival. Caspofungin is the first agent of a new class of compounds, the echinocandin, with proven value as salvage therapy for invasive aspergillosis
- *Candida* sp is now the fourth leading pathogen causing nosocomial bloodstream infections, with an apparent shift to an increasing proportion of infections caused by non-*albicans Candida* sp
- Speciation of *Candida* is important because of the varied pathogenic potential and susceptibility to antifungal agents; non-*albicans Candida* sp as a group are considered less susceptible than *C. albicans* to fluconazole and itraconazole
- Distinguishing infection versus colonization by the presence of *Candida* sp in the urine is difficult, particularly in patients with indwelling urinary catheters
- Disseminated candidiasis should be considered for patients who have persistent, unexplained fever in conjunction with some combination of the following: neutropenia, prolonged duration of intensive care stay (>7 days), prolonged use of multiple antibacterial agents, prolonged use of intravascular catheters, and colonization with *Candida* at one or more body sites
- Lipid-formulated amphotericin B products have not been shown superior efficacy but clearly are associated with lower incidence of nephrotoxicity in comparison to conventional deoxycholate formulation. New non-nephrotoxic treatment options for invasive aspergillosis and candidiasis include caspofungin and voriconazole

■ Fluconazole and caspofungin appear to be as efficacious as amphotericin B in the treatment of invasive candidiasis; fluconazole is an attractive treatment option for the nonneutropenic patients with catheter-related candidemia owing to *C. albicans* in stable condition, and caspofungin may be used in critically ill patients with invasive candidiasis (including those caused by non-*C. albicans* species and at high risk for developing nephrotoxicity). Fluconazole prophylaxis in neutropenic hosts may result in the selection of fluconazole-resistant *Candida* sp and also *Aspergillus* as the cause of superinfections

■ The emergence of azole-resistant *Candida* sp is being reported increasingly, particularly among oropharyngeal isolates of *C. albicans* from patients with advanced HIV disease who have received repeated courses of azole treatment for oropharyngeal candidiasis

REFERENCES

1. National Nosocomial Infections Surveillance (NNIS) System report, data summary from January 1990–May 1999, 27:520–532.
2. Fridkin SK, Jarvis WR. Epidemiology of nosocomial fungal infections Clin Microbiol Rev 9:499–511, 1996.
3. Edmond MB, Wallace SE, McCLish DK, et al. Nosocomial bloodstream infections in United States hospitals: a three-year analysis. Clin Infect Dis 29:239–244, 1999.
4. Pfaller MA, Wenzel R. The impact of changing epidemiology of fungal infections in the 1990s. Eur J Clin Microbiol Infect Dis 11:287–291, 1992.
5. Wheat J. Endemic mycoses in AIDS: a clinical review. Clin Microbiol Rev 8:146–159, 1995.
6. Rinaldi MG. Problems in the diagnosis of invasive fungal disease. Rev Infect Dis 13:493–495, 1991.
7. Yeo SF, Wong B. Current status of nonculture methods for diagnosis of invasive fungal infections. Clin Microbiol Rev 15:465–484, 2002.
8. Deepe GS Jr. Histoplasma capsulatum: darling of the river valleys. ASM News 63:599–604, 1997.
9. Wheat J, Sarosi, McKinsey D, et al. Practice guidelines for the management of patients with histoplasmosis. Clin Infect Dis 30:688–695, 2000.
10. Davies SF, Sarosi GA. Epidemiological and clinical features of pulmonary blastomycosis. Sem Respir Infect 12:206–218, 1997.
11. Pappas PG. Blastomycosis in the immunocompromised patients. Sem Respir Infect 12:243–251, 1997.
12. Chapman SW, Bradsher RW, Campbell GD, et al. Practice guidelines for the management of patients with blastomycosis. Clin Infect Dis 30:679–683, 2000.
13. Chiller TM, Galgiani JN, Stevens DA. Coccidioidomycosis. Infect Dis Clin North Am 17:41–57, 2003.
14. Schneider E, Hajjeh RA, Spiegel RA, et al. A coccidioidomycosis outbreak following the Northridge, Calif, earthquake. JAMA 277:904–908, 1997.
15. Galgiani JN, Ampel NM, Catanzaro A, et al. Practice guidelines for the treatment of coccidioidomycosis. Clin Infect Dis 30:658–661, 2000.
16. Aberg JA, Powderly WG. Cryptococcosis. Adv Pharmacol 37:215–251, 1997.
17. Peachey PR, Gubbins PO, Martin RE. The association between cryptococcal variety and immunocompetent and immunocompromised hosts. Pharmacotherapy 18:255–264, 1998.
18. Zeind CS, Cleveland KO, Menon M, et al. Cryptococcal meningitis in patients with acquired immunodeficiency syndrome. Pharmacotherapy 16: 547–561, 1996.
19. Powderly WG. Cryptococcal meningitis and AIDS. Clin Infect Dis 17:837–842, 1993.
20. Saag MS, Graybill RJ, Larsen RA, et al. Practice guidelines for the management of cryptococcal disease. Clin Infect Dis 30:710–718, 2000.
21. Denning DW. Invasive aspergillosis. Clin Infect Dis 26:781–805, 1998.
22. Gerson SL, Talbot GH, Hurwitz S, et al. Prolonged granulocytopenia: the major risk factor for invasive pulmonary aspergillosis in patients with acute leukemia. Ann Intern Med 100:345–351, 1984.
23. Warnock DW. Fungal complications of transplantation: diagnosis, treatment and prevention. J Antimicrob Chemother 36 (Suppl B): 73–90, 1995.
24. Wheat LJ. Rapid diagnosis of invasive aspergillosis by antigen detection. Transplant Infect Dis 5:158–166, 2003.
25. Herbrecht R, Letscher-Bru V, Oprea C, et al. Aspergillus galactomannan detection in the diagnosis of invasive aspergillosis in cancer patients. J Clin Oncol 21:1898–1906, 2002.
26. Hamaki T, Kami M, Kanda Y, et al. False-positive results of Aspergillus enzyme-linked immunosorbent assay in a patient with chronic graft-versus-host disease after allogeneic bone marrow transplantation. Bone Marrow Transplant 28:633–634, 2001.
27. Denning DW, Stevens DA. Antifungal and surgical treatment of invasive aspergillosis: review of 2,121 published cases. Rev Infect Dis 12:1147–1201, 1990.
28. Stevens DA, Kan VL, Judson MA, et al. Practice guidelines for diseases caused by Aspergillus. Clin Infect Dis 30:696–709, 2000.
29. Steinbach WJ, Stevens DA. Review of newer antifungal and immunomodulatory strategies for invasive aspergillosis. Clin Infect Dis 37 (Suppl 3):S157–S187, 2003.
30. Steinbach WJ, Stevens DA. Combination and sequential antifungal therapy for invasive aspergillosis: review of published in vitro and in vivo interactions and 6281 clinical cases from 1966 to 2001. Clin Infect Dis 37 (Suppl 3):S188–224, 2003.
31. Gudlaugsson O, Gillespie S, Lee K, et al. Attributable mortality of nosocomial candidemia, revisited. Clin Infect Dis 37:1172–1177, 2003.
32. Rex JH, Pfaller MA, Barry AL, et al. Antifungal susceptibility testing of isolates from a random multicenter trial of fluconazole versus amphotericin B as treatment of nonneutropenic patients with candidemia. Antimicrob Agents Chemother 39:40–44, 1995.
33. Pappas PG, Rex JH, Sobel JD, et al. Guidelines for treatment of candidiasis. Clin Infect Dis 38:161–189, 2004.
34. Pappas PG, Rex JH, Lee J, et al. A prospective observational study of candidemia: epidemiology, therapy, and influences on mortality in hospitalized adult and pediatric patients. Clin Infect Dis 37: 634–643, 2003.
35. Fichtenbaum CJ, Powderly WG. Refractory mucosal candidiasis in patients with human immunodeficiency virus infection. Clin Infect Dis 26:556–565, 1998.
36. Sobel JD, Faro S, Force RW, et al. Vulvovaginal candidiasis: epidemiologic, diagnostic, and therapeutic considerations. Am J Obstet Gynecol 178:203–211, 1998.
37. Nucci M, Anaissie E. Should vascular catheters be removed from all patients with candidemia: evidence-based review. Clin Infect Dis 34:591–599, 2002.
38. Wong-Beringer A. Treatment of funguria. JAMA 267:2780–2785, 1992.
39. Rodriguez LJ, Rex JH, Anaissie EJ. Update on invasive candidiasis. Adv Pharmacol 37:349–400, 1997.
40. Dismukes WE. Introduction to antifungal drugs. Clin Infect Dis 30:653–657, 2000.
41. Wong-Beringer A, Jacobs RA, Guglielmo BJ. Lipid formulations of amphotericin B: clinical efficacy and toxicities. Clin Infect Dis 27:608–618, 1998.
42. Gallis HA, Drew RH, Pickard WW. Amphotericin B: 30 years of clinical experience. Rev Infect Dis 12:308–329, 1990.
43. Wingard JR, White MH, Anaissie E, et al. A randomized double-blind comparative trial evaluating the safety of liposomal amphotericin B versus amphotericin B lipid complex in empiricial treatment of febrile neutropenia. Clin Infect Dis 31:1155–1163, 2000.

44. Wong-Beringer A, Kriengkauykiat J. Systemic antifungal therapy: new options, new challenges. Pharmacother 23:1441–1462, 2003.

45. Ostrosky-Zeichner L, Marr KA, Rex JH, et al. Amphotericin B: time for a new "gold standard." Clin Infect Dis 37:415–425, 2003.

46. Johnson LB, Kauffman CA. Voriconazole: a new triazole antifungal agent. Clin Infect Dis 36:630–637, 2003.

47. White TC, Marr KA, Bowden RA. Clinical, cellular, and molecular factors that contribute to antifungal drug resistance. Clin Microbiol Rev 11:382–402, 1998.

48. Kontoyiannis DP, Lewis RE. Antifungal drug resistance of pathogenic fungi. Lancet 359:1135–1144, 2002.

49. Deresinski SC, Stevens DA. Caspofungin. Clin Infect Dis 36: 1445–1457, 2003.

50. Vermes A, Guchelaar HJ, Dankert J. Flucytosine: a review of its pharmacology, clinical indications, pharmacokinetics, toxicity and drug interactions. J Antimicrob Chemother 46:171–179, 2000.

51. Kurtz MB. New antifungal drug targets: a vision for the future. ASM News 64:31–39, 1998.

52. Ernst EJ. Investigational antifungal agents. Pharmacother 21: 165S–75S, 2001.

53. Pfaller MA, Rex JH, Rinaldi MG. Antifungal susceptibility testing: technical advances and potential clinical applications. Clin Infect Dis 24:776–784, 1997.

54. Rex JH, Pfaller MA, Galgiani JN, et al. Development of interpretive breakpoints for antifungal susceptibility testing: conceptual framework and analysis of in vitro-in vivo correlation data for fluconazole, itraconazole, and candida infections. Clin Infect Dis 24: 235–247, 1997.

55. CDC. USPHS/IDSA guidelines for preventing opportunistic infections among HIV-infected persons - 2002. MMWR Morb Mortal Wkly Rep 51:1–23, 2002.

56. Wheat J, Hafner R, Korzun AH, et al. Itraconazole treatment of disseminated histoplasmosis in patients with the acquired immunodeficiency syndrome. Am J Med 98:336–342, 1995.

57. Dismukes WE, Bradsher RW Jr, Cloud GC, et al. Itraconazole therapy for blastomycosis and histoplasmosis. Am J Med 93:489–497, 1992.

58. Wheat J, MaWhinney S, Hafner R, et al. Treatment of histoplasmosis with fluconazole in patients with acquired immunodeficiency syndrome. Am J Med 103:223–232, 1997.

59. Galgiani JN, Catanzaro A, Cloud GA, et al. Comparison of oral fluconazole and itraconazole for progressive, nonmeningeal coccidioidomycosis: a randomized, double-blind trial. Ann Intern Med 133: 676–686, 2000.

60. Galgiani JN, Catanzaro A, Cloud GA, et al. Fluconazole therapy for coccidioidal meningitis. Ann Intern Med 119:28–35, 1993.

61. Tucker RM, Denning DW, Dupont B, et al. Itraconazole therapy for chronic coccidioidal meningitis. Ann Intern Med 112:108–112, 1990.

62. Dewsnup DH, Galgiani JN, Graybill JR, et al. Is it ever safe to stop azole therapy for *Coccidioides immitis* meningitis? Ann Intern Med 124:305–310, 1996.

63. Yamaguchi H, Ikemoto H, Watanabe K, et al. Fluconazole monotherapy for cryptococcosis in non-AIDS patients. Eur J Clin Microbiol Infect Dis 15:787–792, 1996.

64. Bennett JE, Dismukes WE, Duma RJ, et al. A comparison of amphotericin B alone and combined with flucytosine in the treatment of cryptococcal meningitis. N Engl J Med 301:126–131, 1979.

65. Dismukes WE, Cloud G, Gallis HA, et al. Treatment of cryptococcal meningitis with combination amphotericin B and flucytosine for four as compared with six weeks. N Engl J Med 317:334–341, 1987.

66. Larsen RA, Leal MAE, Chan LS. Fluconazole compared to amphotericin B plus flucytosine for cryptococcal meningitis in AIDS. Ann Intern Med 113:183–187, 1990.

67. Saag MS, Powderly WG, Cloud GA, et al. Comparison of amphotericin B and fluconazole in the treatment of acute AIDS-associated cryptococcal meningitis. N Engl J Med 326:83–89, 1992.

68. DeGans J, Portegeis P, Tiessens G, et al. Itraconazole compared with amphotericin B plus flucytosine in AIDS patients with cryptococcal meningitis. AIDS 6:185–190, 1992.

69. Van der Horst CM, Saag MS, Cloud GA, et al. Treatment of cryptococcal meningitis associated with the acquired immunodeficiency syndrome. N Engl J Med 337:15–21, 1997.

70. Larsen RA, Bozzette SA, Jones BE, et al. Fluconazole combined with flucytosine for treatment of cryptococcal meningitis in patients with AIDS. Clin Infect Dis 19:741–745, 1994.

71. Sharkey PK, Graybill JR, Johnson ES, et al. Amphotericin B lipid complex compared with amphotericin B in the treatment of cryptococcal meningitis in patients with AIDS. Clin Infect Dis 22: 315–321, 1996.

72. Bozzette SA, Larsen RA, Chiu J, et al. A placebo-controlled trial of maintenance therapy with fluconazole after treatment of cryptococcal meningitis in the acquired immunodeficiency syndrome. N Engl J Med 324:580–584, 1991.

73. Powderly WG, Saag MS, Cloud GA, et al. A controlled trial of fluconazole or amphotericin B to prevent relapse of cryptococcal meningitis in patients with the acquired immunodeficiency syndrome. N Engl J Med 326:793–798, 1992.

74. Saag MS, Cloud GC, Graybill JR, et al. A comparison of itraconazole versus fluconazole as maintenance therapy of AIDS-associated cryptococcal meningitis. Clin Infect Dis 1999;28:291–296.

75. Denning DW. Therapeutic outcome in invasive aspergillosis. Clin Infect Dis 23:608–615, 1996.

76. Patterson TF, Kirkpatrick WR, White M, et al. Invasive aspergillosis: disease spectrum, treatment practices, and outcomes. Medicine 79:250–260, 2000.

77. Denning DW, Lee JY, Hostetler JS, et al. NIAID Mycoses Study Group multicenter trial of oral itraconazole therapy for invasive aspergillosis. Am J Med 97:135–144, 1994.

78. Stevens DA, Lee JY. Analysis of compassionate use itraconazole therapy for invasive aspergillosis by the NIAID Mycoses Study Group Criteria. Arch Intern Med 157:1857–1862, 1997.

79. Sanchez C, Mauri E, Dalmau D, et al. Treatment of cerebral aspergillosis with itraconazole: do high doses improve the prognosis? Clin Infect Dis 21:1485–1487, 1995.

80. Schwartz S, Milatovic D, Thiel E. Successful treatment of cerebral aspergillosis with a novel Triazole (voriconazole) in a patient with acute leukemia. Br J Haematol 97:663–665, 1997.

81. Herbrecht R, Denning DW, Patterson TF, et al. Voriconazole versus amphotericin B for primary therapy of invasive aspergillosis. N Engl J Med 347:408–415, 2002.

82. Perfect JR, Marr KA, Walsh TJ, et al. Voriconazole treatment for less-common, emerging, or refractory fungal infections. Clin Infect Dis 36:1122–1131, 2003.

83. Denning DW, Ribaud P, Milpied N, et al. Efficacy and safety of voriconazole in the treatment of acute invasive aspergillosis. Clin Infect Dis 34:563–571, 2002.

84. Maertens J, Raad I, Petrikkos G, et al. Update of multicenter noncomparative study of caspofungin (CAS) in adults with invasive aspergillosis (IA) refractory (R) or intolerant (I) to other antifungal agents: analysis of 90 patients [abstract]. In: Program and abstracts of the 42nd interscience conference on antimicrobial agents and chemotherapy, San Diego, CA, September 27–30, 2002. Washington, DC: American Society of Microbiology, 2002:M-856.

85. Johnson MD, MacDougall C, Ostrosky-Zeichner L, et al. Combination antifungal therapy. Antimicrob Agents Chemother 48: 693–715, 2004.

86. Steinbach WJ, Stevens DA, Denning DW. Combination and sequential antifungal therapy for invasive aspergillosis: review of published in vitro and in vivo interactions and 6281 clinical cases from 1966 to 2001. Clin Infect Dis 37 (Suppl 3):S188–224, 2003.

87. Wilcox CM, Darouiche RO, Laine L, et al. A randomized, double-blind comparison of itraconazole oral solution and fluconazole tablets in the treatment of esophageal candidiasis. J Infect Dis 176: 227–232, 1997.

88. Fisher JF, Newman CL, Sobel JD. Yeast in the urine: solutions for a budding problem. Clin Infect Dis 20:183–189, 1995.

89. Sobel JD, Kauffman CA, McKinsey D, et al. Candiduria: a randomized, double-blind study of treatment with fluconazole and placebo. Clin Infect Dis 30:19–24, 2000.

90. Anaissie EJ, Darouiche RO, Abi-Said D, et al. Management of invasive candidal infections: results of a prospective, randomized, multicenter study of fluconazole versus amphotericin B and review of the literature. Clin Infect Dis 23:964–972, 1996.

91. Mora-Duarte J, Betts R, Rotstein C, et al. Comparison of caspofungin and amphotericin B for invasive candidiasis. N Engl J Med 347:2020–2029, 2002.

92. Rex JH, Bennett JE, Sugar AM, et al. A randomized trial comparing fluconazole with amphotericin B for the treatment of candidemia in patients without neutropenia. N Engl J Med 331: 1325–1330, 1994.

93. Rex JH, Pappas PG, Karchmer AW, et al. A randomized and blinded multicenter trial of high-dose fluconazole plus placebo versus fluconazole plus amphotericin B as therapy for candidemia and its consequences in nonneutropenic subjects. Clin Infect Dis 36: 1221–1228, 2003.

94. Anaissie EJ, Darouiche RO, Abi-Said D, et al. Management of invasive candidal infections: results of a prospective, randomized, multicenter study of fluconazole versus amphotericin B and review of the literature. Clin Infect Dis 23:964–972, 1996.

95. Lortholary O, Dupont B. Antifungal prophylaxis during neutropenia and immunodeficiency. Clin Microbiol Rev 10:477–504, 1997.

96. Gubbins PO, Bowman JL, Penzak SR. Antifungal prophylaxis to prevent invasive mycoses among bone marrow transplantation recipients. Pharmacotherapy 18:549–564, 1998.

97. Wingard JR, Merz WG, Rinaldi MG, et al. Increase in Candida krusei infection among patients with bone marrow transplantation and neutropenia treated prophylactically with fluconazole. N Engl J Med 325:1274–1277, 1991.

98. Wingard JR, Merz WG, Rinaldi MG, et al. Association of Torulopsis glabrata infections with fluconazole prophylaxis in neutropenic bone marrow transplant patients. Antimicrob Agents Chemother 37:1847–1849, 1993.

99. Walsh TJ, Finberg RW, Arndt C, et al. Liposomal amphotericin B for empirical therapy in patients with persistent fever and neutropenia. National Institute of Allergy and Infectious Diseases Mycoses Study Group. N Eng J Med 340:764–771, 1999.

100. Boogaerts M, Winston DJ, Bow EJ, et al. Intravenous and oral itraconazole versus intravenous amphotericin B deoxycholate as empirical antifungal therapy for persistent fever in neutropenic patients with cancer who are receiving broad-spectrum antibacterial therapy: a randomized control trial. Ann Intern Med 135:412–422, 2001.

101. Walsh TJ, Pappas P, Winston DJ, et al. Voriconazole compared with liposomal amphotericin B for empiric antifungal therapy in patients with neutropenia and persistent fever. N Engl J Med 346: 225–234, 2002.

102. Walsh TJ, Sable C, DePauw B, et al. A randomized, double-blind, multicenter trial of caspofungin (CAS) v liposomal Amphotericin B (LAMB) for empirical antifungal therapy of persistently febrile neutropenic patients. [abstract] In: Program and abstracts of the 43nd interscience conference on antimicrobial agents and chemotherapy, San Diego, CA, September, 2003. Washington, DC: American Society of Microbiology, 2003.

Parasitic Infections

R. Chris Rathbun

DEFINITION

Parasitic diseases are a major cause of morbidity and mortality worldwide. Parasitism involves a relationship where an animal host is injured as a result of close and prolonged contact by an infecting organism.[1] Knowledge of the parasite life cycle is critical to understanding the pathogenesis, treatment, and prevention of infection. The incidence of parasitic infections overall is increasing in the United States secondary to recent immigration trends, increased foreign travel to endemic areas, and immunosuppression secondary to human immunodeficiency virus (HIV) infection and transplantation.

This chapter covers the major parasitic infections such as protozoal infections (malaria, cryptosporidiosis, giardiasis), helminthic infections (ascariasis, enterobiasis), and ectoparasites (lice, scabies). Special emphasis is placed on diseases that occur in the United States or represent a significant threat to international travelers. Parasitic infections such as American trympanosomiasis (Chagas disease) caused by *Trympanosoma cruzi*, leishmaniasis, and amebiasis (*Entamoeba histolytica*) are not included. The reader is referred to recent reviews on these topics.[2–4]

TREATMENT GOALS

The goal of antiparasitic therapy is to eliminate disease manifestations and to prevent complications. Treatment is also used to prevent the acquisition and spread of infection to other individuals. Specific treatment goals for individual infections are as follows:

- The goal of malaria chemoprophylaxis is to prevent clinical manifestations of disease.
- Treatment of malaria is used to eliminate parasitemia and hepatic reservoirs and prevent vascular complications secondary to *Plasmodium falciparum* infection.

- Treatment of intestinal protozoa (e.g., cryptosporidia, giardia) is used to alleviate diarrheal symptoms and reduce stool passage of infective spores.
- Treatment of helminthic infections is used to decrease or eliminate worm infestation and reduce passage of infective forms (eggs, larvae, cercariae) into the environment.
- Treatment of lice and scabies is used to eliminate infestation and prevent spread to other individuals.

PROTOZOAN DISEASES

MALARIA

EPIDEMIOLOGY

Plasmodium species responsible for human malaria include *P. falciparum*, *P. vivax*, *P. malariae*, and *P. ovale*. Malaria afflicts approximately 500 million people in the world annually and causes up to 2.7 million deaths each year.[5] Plasmodium species are spread by *Anopheles* mosquitoes, which are endemic in tropical areas such as sub-Saharan Africa, Asia, Central America, South America, and portions of Turkey, Greece, and the Middle East. Other mechanisms of transmission include blood transfusions, needle sharing, and parturition. At the start of the twentieth century, more than 500,000 cases of malaria occurred annually in the United States; approximately 1,300 cases are now reported each year.[6–8]

PATHOPHYSIOLOGY

Infection is acquired from the female *Anopheles* mosquito when saliva containing sporozoites is injected during a blood meal. Sporozoites spread hematogenously to the liver, resulting in development of exoerythrocytic forms (tissue schizonts, hypnozoites) within hepatocytes. Merozoites are released from tissue schizonts into the circulation approximately 1 to 2 weeks later, leading to invasion of erythrocytes. *P. falciparum* merozoites proliferate within erythrocytes of all ages, whereas other malarial species are restricted to certain subpopulations. Within erythrocytes, merozoites consume hemoglobin and mature to ring, trophozoite, and schizont stage parasites by asexual replication or to sexual male and female gametocyte forms. Rupture of schizont-infected red cells occurs after 48 hours (72 hours with *P. malariae*), releasing merozoites that perpetuate erythrocytic invasion. Ingestion of gametocyte-infected red blood cells by *Anopheles* mosquitoes leads to fertilization of male and female forms within the mosquito gut and development of sporozoites that migrate to the mosquito's salivary glands, completing the infectious cycle. Relapse of disease does not occur with *P. falciparum* or *P. malariae* infection; however, *P. ovale* and *P. vivax* hypnozoites can become activated weeks to months following resolution of initial infection.[7,9]

CLINICAL PRESENTATION AND DIAGNOSIS

SIGNS AND SYMPTOMS

The presentation of malaria is typically nonspecific and includes fever, malaise, headache, rigors, and diaphoresis in over 80% of patients. Symptom onset commonly occurs approximately 2 weeks after exposure. Anorexia, nausea, and vomiting occur in approximately 33% of patients and diarrhea, cough, and abdominal pain in approximately 16%. Tachypnea, tachycardia, hypotension, and altered consciousness may also occur. Splenomegaly (~25%) and hepatomegaly (~20%) can develop as the disease progresses. Classic cycling of fever every 48 to 72 hours (tertian or quartan pattern) due to synchronized schizont rupture is rarely observed but may be seen with prolonged, untreated illness.[6,7,10]

Falciparum malaria can rapidly become life-threatening due to adherence of parasitized cells to vascular endothelium, producing microvascular disease secondary to flow obstruction. Acute renal failure, symmetrical encephalopathy (cerebral malaria) manifesting as seizures and coma, and pulmonary edema may occur. Severe anemia secondary to hemolysis and decreased hematopoiesis along with thrombocytopenia and hypoglycemia are common. Hyperbilirubinemia due to hemolysis may also be prominent.[11] Acidosis is a major determinant of mortality and is commonly manifested as respiratory distress.[12] Reduced deformability in nonparasitized red blood cells and parasitemia (>5%) with concomitant end-organ disease or shock are associated with a poorer prognosis.[12,13] Nonimmune individuals, pregnant women, and children living in endemic regions are at greater risk for complications.[10]

DIAGNOSIS

Microscopic evaluation of Giemsa-stained blood smears, ideally obtained at 12- to 24-hour intervals over 36 to 72 hours, is used most frequently for diagnosis.[7] Thick smears are used to optimize parasite detection. Thin smears viewed under oil immersion magnification are used to examine characteristic species morphology. A malaria diagnosis cannot be excluded unless a minimum of three negative smears are obtained within 48 hours.[10] Alternatively, rapid diagnosis (10 minutes) in the field can be made by using a finger prick test strip containing monoclonal antibody to *Plasmodium* histidine-rich protein 2 or parasite lactate dehydrogenase isoenzymes.[14] Buffy coat examination with acridine dye staining, DNA hybridization, or DNA or mRNA amplification by polymerase chain reaction can also be used.[6,15] Antibody testing for most species is also available from the Centers for Disease Control and Prevention.[15]

TREATMENT

PHARMACOTHERAPY

Uncomplicated *P. vivax*, *P. malariae*, *P. ovale*, and chloroquine-sensitive *P. falciparum* infections should be treated with oral chloroquine. Chloroquine dosage is routinely expressed as the amount of chloroquine phosphate or chloroquine base and should be carefully noted because dosages can vary significantly. A loading dose of chloroquine base 600 mg (10 mg base/kg for children) followed by 300 mg (5 mg base/kg for children) at 6, 24, and 48 hours should be used.[13,15] Pruritus is common in dark-skinned individuals.

Hydroxychloroquine sulfate may be substituted for chloroquine base (200 mg hydroxychloroquine salt = 155 mg chloroquine base) if chloroquine phosphate (250 mg salt = 156 mg base) is not available. Defervescence and resolution of symptoms and parasitemia should occur within 72 hours of treatment initiation. To prevent relapse, patients with *P. vivax* and *P. ovale* infection living in nonendemic areas should also receive a 2-week "terminal prophylaxis" course of primaquine 30 mg daily (0.6 mg base/kg for children) to eradicate hepatic hypnozoites.[13,15]

Patients with mild glucose-6-phosphate dehydrogenase (G6PD) deficiency, defined as 10% to 60% residual enzyme activity, should alternatively receive primaquine 45 mg once weekly (0.8 mg base/kg for children) for 8 weeks to minimize development of hemolytic anemia. Primaquine should not be used in patients with severe G6PD deficiency (<10% residual enzyme activity) or during pregnancy.[15,16]

Patients with suspected chloroquine-resistant falciparum malaria should receive oral quinine in combination with a second agent. For infections acquired in Africa or South America, quinine sulfate 650 mg every 8 hours (25–30 mg/kg/day in three divided doses for children) for 3 days in conjunction with doxycycline 100 mg twice daily (2–4 mg/kg/day divided twice daily for children) for 7 days is recommended. Quinine treatment should be extended to 7 days for infections acquired in Southeast Asia. Doxycycline should begin 2 to 3 days after quinine to allow discrimination between quinine and doxycycline-related side effects.[15,17] Cinchonism (tinnitus, nausea, headache, blurred vision) and cor-

rected QT (QTc) interval prolongation can occur with quinine. For pregnant women or children less than 8 years old, quinine should be used in combination with clindamycin 900 mg three times daily (20 to 40 mg/kg/day in three divided doses) for 5 to 7 days.[15,17] Single-dose sulfadoxine/pyrimethamine (3 tablets in adults; see weight-based dosing for children in Table 88.1) can be used if clindamycin is not tolerated and should be administered on the last day of quinine. Atovaquone/proguanil for three consecutive days (four 250 mg/100 mg tablets daily in adults) is an alternative to quinine-based therapies provided it was not used for chemoprophylaxis and can also be used for presumptive self-treatment during travel.[15,16] If severe nausea ensues, the daily dose can be divided in half and taken twice daily.[15] Single-dose mefloquine 750 mg (15 mg base/kg in children) followed by a second dose of 500 mg (10 mg base/kg in children) 6 to 8 hours later in nonimmune patients is also effective for drug-resistant falciparum malaria; however, neurologic toxicities make it less desirable as a first-line or second-line therapy.[13,15,18]

Patients with severe malaria should be treated with intravenous quinidine gluconate. A loading dose of 10 mg salt per kilogram (maximum 600 mg, 6.25 mg base/kg) in 250 mL of normal saline infused over 1 to 2 hours should be given followed by a continuous infusion at 0.02 mg salt/kg/min (0.0125 mg base/kg per minute) for a minimum of 24 hours. If mefloquine or quinine was recently used, consideration should be given to omitting the loading dose because of additive cardiac conduction effects.[15] Quinidine serum concentrations should be maintained between 3 to 8 mg per liter and the dose decreased or interrupted if: (a) the QRS interval increases by 50% or greater, (b) the QT interval exceeds 0.6 seconds, (c) the QTc interval becomes prolonged by more than 25% from its baseline value, or (d) severe hypotension develops.[13,15] When parasite density falls below 1%, therapy can be continued with quinine sulfate to complete a 3-day course for chloroquine-resistant falciparum malaria and a 7-day course for multidrug-resistant falciparum malaria in combination with 7 days of doxycycline (as noted above).[15,18]

Artemisinin and its derivatives (e.g., artesunate, artemether) are widely used as alternatives to quinine for drug-resistant falciparum malaria in Asia and Africa. Advantages of these agents are their rapid parasite clearance, low cost, and apparent lack of resistance to date by *P. falciparum*.[19–21] Combination therapy with a second agent (e.g., mefloquine) for 3 to 5 days is typically necessary in multidrug-resistant areas to prevent relapse because of the short half-life of artemisinin compounds.[20,21] Oral, suppository, and injectable formulations have been developed but are not currently approved in the United States.[20] Neurotoxicity has been observed in animal models but not in humans when artemisinin drugs are used as monotherapy.[19,20]

Chemoprophylaxis is indicated in all nonimmune individuals traveling to malarious areas where mosquito exposure is likely. A summary of dosing guidelines and side

TABLE 88.1	Adult and Pediatric Dosing for Atovaquone/Proguanil and Sulfadoxine/Pyrimethamine for Treatment of Malaria	
Drug	**Adult Dose**	**Pediatric Dose**
Atovaquone/Proguanil[a,b] (250 mg/100 mg adult tablet, 62.5 mg/25 mg pediatric tablet)	4 adult tablets (1,000 mg/400 mg) daily for 3 days	5–8 kg: 2 pediatric tablets (125 mg/50 mg) daily for 3 days 9–10 kg: 3 pediatric tablets (187.5 mg/75 mg daily) for 3 days 11–20 kg: 1 adult tablet (250 mg/100 mg) daily for 3 days 21–30 kg: 2 adult tablets (500 mg/200 mg) daily for 3 days 31–40 kg: 3 adult tablets (750 mg/300 mg) daily for 3 days >40 kg: adult dose
Sulfadoxine/Pyrimethamine[a,c] (500 mg/25 mg tablet)	3 tablets (1,500 mg/75 mg) ×1	5–10 kg: ½ tablet (250 mg/12.5 mg) ×1 11–14 kg: ¾ tablet (375 mg/19 mg) ×1 15–20 kg: 1 tablet (500 mg/25 mg) ×1 21–30 kg: 1½ tablets (750 mg/37.5 mg) ×1 31–40 kg: 2 tablets (1,000 mg/50 mg) ×1 41–50 kg: 2½ tablets (1,250 mg/62.5 mg) ×1 >50 kg: 3 tablets ×1 (adult dose)

[a] Take with food. [b] Daily dose can be divided in half and taken twice daily to decrease nausea. [c] Taken on the last day of quinine treatment. (From Centers for Disease Control and Prevention. Treatment of malaria (guidelines for clinicians). http://www.cdc.gov/malaria/pdf/highres-treatmenttable.pdf. Accessed Apr. 27, 2004, with permission.)

effects for individual agents is listed in Table 88.2. Chloroquine is the drug of choice in geographic areas with low resistance.[17,22] Side effects with chloroquine are common and can be minimized by splitting the weekly dose in half and taking twice a week.[11] In areas where chloroquine-resistant *P. falciparum* exists, mefloquine, doxycycline, or atovaquone/proguanil can be used.[22] Neuropsychiatric effects are the primary reason for discontinuation of mefloquine therapy and are more common in women.[23] A loading dose comprised of 250 mg once daily for 3 days followed by weekly dosing can be used by travelers to rapidly obtain therapeutic concentrations and allow assessment of side effects prior to departure.[24] In areas where mefloquine resistance is high or therapy is contraindicated, doxycycline should be used.[25,26] Atovaquone/proguanil is an effective alternative to doxycycline for falciparum malaria and appears to be effective for vivax malaria.[22,27] Azithromycin can be used in place of doxycycline in children older than 8 years of age and in pregnant women, but it is less effective.[28] Terminal prophylaxis with primaquine for 14 days on departure from a malarious region endemic for *P. ovale* or *P. vivax* should be considered for individuals with extended stays (e.g., missionaries, peace corp volunteers).[22] Primary prophylaxis with primaquine should be reserved for individuals who cannot take other agents and taken only under the advice of a malaria expert.[22]

NONPHARMACOLOGIC THERAPY

Exchange transfusions are controversial because of insufficient evidence to support an impact on mortality but are generally recommended for nonimmune patients with severe falciparum malaria where parasitemia exceeds 15% and should be considered in patients with 5% to 10% parasitemia or with altered mental status, renal, or pulmonary complications.[13,29,30] Volume expansion with 0.9% sodium chloride or 4.5% albumin improves organ dysfunction and acidosis.[12] Hemodialysis or peritoneal dialysis may be necessary in patients who develop renal failure.

FUTURE THERAPIES

Tafenoquine is a primaquine analogue with an extended plasma half-life (2–3 weeks) that has the potential to improve adherence because of the ability to administer it on an extended dosing schedule. A single loading dose over 3 days may also be sufficient to provide protection for short-term travel (<1 month) in malarious areas.[31] Malarial proteases are central to invasion of erythrocytes and subsequent release of merozoites. Synthetic peptide inhibitors of plasmodial cysteine and aspartic proteases are in early stages of development.[32] Inhibitors of plasmodial farnesyl transferase, cyclin-dependent kinases, and choline transporters are also being examined.[33] Efficacy studies of a recombinant circumsporozoite protein vaccine are currently ongoing.[12]

TABLE 88.2	Malaria Chemoprophylaxis			
Drug	**Adult Dose**	**Pediatric Dose**	**Adverse Effects**	**Comments**
Atovaquone/Proguanil (250 mg/100 mg tablet, 62.5 mg/25 mg pediatric tablet)	250 mg/100 mg PO beginning 1–2 days before departure and continuing for 1 week after leaving malarious area	11–20 kg: 62.5 mg/25 mg 21–30 kg: 125 mg/50 mg 31–40 kg: 187.5 mg/75 mg >40 kg: adult dose	Common: diarrhea, abdominal pain, headache, dizziness Less common: rash, photophobia, urticaria, alopecia, mouth ulcers Rare: erythema multiforme, Stevens-Johnson syndrome, hematuria	• Alternative to doxycycline • Take with food or milk • Pregnancy Category C • Side effects are typically mild • Contraindications: renal impairment (CrCl <30 mL/min) • Children: tablets can be pulverized and placed in gelatin capsules
Chloroquine phosphate (250 mg, 500 mg)	300 mg base (500 mg salt) PO once/week beginning 1–2 weeks before departure and continuing for 4 weeks after leaving malarious area	5 mg/kg base (8.3 mg/kg salt) (maximum: 300 mg base)	Common: pruritus, nausea, headache Less common: photophobia, reversible corneal opacities, partial alopecia Rare: nerve deafness, blood dyscrasia, nail/mucous membrane discoloration, retinopathy, myopathy, psychosis	• Take with food • Safe for use in pregnancy • May exacerbate psoriasis
Doxycycline (100 mg tablet, capsule)	100 mg PO once daily beginning 1–2 days before departure and continuing for 4 weeks after leaving malarious area	≥8 yr: 2 mg/kg/day (maximum: 100 mg)	Common: GI upset, photophobia, vaginal candidiasis Less Common: azotemia in renal disease Rare: allergic reactions, blood dyscrasias	• Not for use in pregnancy or children <8 yr
Hydroxychloroquine sulfate (200 mg tablet)	310 mg base (400 mg salt) PO once/week beginning 1–2 weeks before departure and continuing for 4 weeks after leaving malarious area	5 mg/kg base (6.5 mg/kg salt) (maximum: 310 mg base)	(Same as chloroquine)	• Alternative to chloroquine • Take with food • Safe for use in pregnancy • May exacerbate psoriasis
Mefloquine (250 mg tablet)	228 mg base (250 mg salt) PO once/week beginning at least 2 weeks before departure and continuing for 4 weeks after leaving malarious area	15–19 kg: ¼ tablet/wk 20–30 kg: ½ tablet/wk 31–45 kg: ¾ tablet/wk >45 kg: adult dose	Common: nausea, diarrhea, headache, dizziness, strange dreams, insomnia Rare: seizures, psychosis	• Pregnancy Category C • Contraindications: history of psychosis, epilepsy, cardiac conduction abnormalities
Primaquine phosphate (15 mg base tablet)	*Terminal prophylaxis:* 30 mg base PO once daily for 14 days after departure from malarious area *Primary prophylaxis:* 30 mg base (52.6 mg salt) PO once daily beginning 1 day before departure and continuing for 1 week after leaving malarious area	0.6 mg/kg base (1.0 mg/kg salt) (maximum: 30 mg) 0.6 mg/kg base (1.0 mg/kg salt) (maximum: 30 mg)	Common: abdominal pain, nausea, vomiting, methemoglobinemia Less Common: hemolytic anemia (G6PD deficiency) Rare: leukopenia	• Terminal prophylaxis indicated for individuals with prolonged exposure in areas endemic for *P. vivax* or *P. ovale*; primary prophylaxis reserved for instances when other drugs cannot be taken • Not for use in pregnancy • Rule out G6PD deficiency

PO, by mouth; CrCl, creatinine clearance; GI, gastrointestinal; G6PD, glucose-6-phosphate dehydrogenase.
(From Kain KC, Keystone JS. Malaria in travelers: epidemiology, disease, and prevention. Infect Dis Clin North Am 12:267–284, 1998; Wyler DJ. Malaria: overview and update. Clin Infect Dis 16:449–458, 1993; National Center for Infectious Diseases, Centers for Disease Control and Prevention. Travelers' health, malaria. Available at: http://www.cdc.gov/travel/diseases/malaria/index.htm. Accessed Apr. 27, 2004, with permission.)

CRYPTOSPORIDIOSIS, ISOSPORIASIS, MICROSPORIDIOSIS, CYCLOSPORIASIS

EPIDEMIOLOGY

The intestinal spore-forming protozoa include cryptosporidia, isospora, microsporidia, and cyclospora. Principal species infecting humans include *Cryptosporidium parvum* (genotypes 1 and 2), *Isospora belli*, *Cyclospora cayatanensis*, and the microsporidia species *Enterocytozoon bieneusi* and *Encephalitozoon intestinalis* (formerly *Septata intestinalis*).[34–36] Fecal-oral spread is the predominant route of transmission; however, ingestion of fecally-contaminated water or food has also led to widespread community outbreaks.[34,35,37] In Milwaukee, an estimated 403,000 people developed symptomatic cryptosporidia infection secondary to contamination of the municipal water supply.[38] Infection is more common in developing countries where sanitation is poor; however, seroprevalence rates of approximately 30% have been reported in adults and children in the United States.[36] Predilection for symptomatic infection in immunocompromised patients [acquired immune deficiency syndrome (AIDS), organ transplant] is apparent.[34,36,37,39]

PATHOPHYSIOLOGY

The life cycles of cryptosporidia, isospora, microsporidia, and cyclospora are similar in that infection occurs by ingestion of spores. Sporozoites are released from ingested spores by contact with bile salts and pancreatic enzymes. Invasion of intestinal epithelium in the small bowel follows, resulting in marked distortion of the villus architecture in some patients. Malabsorption of vitamin B_{12}, D-xylose, and fat may occur with more severe infection. Asexual reproduction (schizogony) leads to the formation of merozoites which reinfect the host's intestinal lining and perpetuate infection. Other merozoites develop into sexual forms, resulting in formation of oocysts (or spores). Oocysts are excreted in the stool or may sporulate and release their sporozoites within the host, causing autoinfection.[34] *Encephalitozoon* spp. also infect macrophages, leading to secondary infections in the kidney, liver, brain, and sinuses.[39] Infection with *I. belli*, *C. cayatanensis*, and microsporidia species is limited to humans; however, *C. parvum* causes disease in humans and animals.[34,36]

CLINICAL PRESENTATION AND DIAGNOSIS

SIGNS AND SYMPTOMS

Diarrhea with or without abdominal cramping is the primary clinical manifestation and may occasionally be accompanied by nausea, vomiting, and fever. Symptoms typically occur 7 to 10 days following ingestion of oocysts. Disease severity varies considerably among patients such that stool frequency may be intermittent versus continuous, watery, and high volume (12–17 L/day). Immunocompetent patients typically have acute, self-limiting disease lasting 3 to 25 days; although disease can last for months to years in some patients. Immunocompromised patients [e.g., AIDS, cancer, immunoglobulin A (IgA) deficiency] are more prone to chronic, life-threatening diarrhea, malabsorption, and dehydration. Biliary tract invasion has been described with cryptosporidia, microsporidia, and isospora in patients with AIDS. Hepatitis, nephritis, peritonitis, pneumonia, keratoconjunctivitis, and encephalitis with seizures may develop with disseminated *Encephalitozoon intestinalis* infection.[34,39]

DIAGNOSIS

Diagnosis is routinely established on the basis of stool smears for cysts. Oocyst size and shape are used to differentiate among organisms. Modified, acid-fast stains are effective for detecting cryptosporidia, isospora, and cyclospora. Sensitivity can be improved by stool concentrating techniques or using a cryptosporidial immunofluorescent stain.[34] Enzyme immunoassays are now available commercially for detection of *C. parvum*.[40] Microsporidia are best visualized in body fluids using a modified trichrome or fluorochrome stain; however, small bowel biopsy tends to be more sensitive for intestinal disease. Absence of fecal leukocytes and erythrocytes differentiates infection with other intestinal pathogens. Centrifugation enhances detection of microsporidia in respiratory secretions and urine.[34]

TREATMENT

PHARMACOTHERAPY

Palliative therapy with antidiarrheal agents (bismuth subsalicylate, loperamide, kaolin and pectin, diphenoxylate) can be used to provide temporary relief of symptoms. In general, no antiparasitic therapy is indicated for asymptomatic or immunocompetent patients with cryptosporidiosis due to the self-limiting nature of the infection in these individuals.[37] If antiparasitic treatment is initiated, a 3-day course of nitazoxanide (500 mg tablets twice daily for adults, 200 mg twice daily for children 4–11 years old, and 100 mg twice daily for children 1–3 years old using the 100 mg/5 mL oral suspension) should be used.[17] Common side effects include abdominal pain, diarrhea, vomiting, and headache and are generally mild. Reversible scleral icterus has been observed in rare instances.[41] Infection with cyclospora in immunocompetent patients should be treated with trimethoprim/sulfamethoxazole (TMP/SMX) 160 mg/800 mg (1 double-strength [DS] tablet) twice daily for 7 to 10 days.[17] For patients with isospora, 1 DS tablet twice daily for 10 days should be used.[17] Patients with HIV infection should receive 1 DS tablet four times daily for 10 days for cyclospora and isospora; chronic suppressive therapy with 1 DS tablet three times weekly is routinely necessary because relapses are common.[42,43] Pyrimethamine 50 to 75 mg with folinic acid 10 mg daily can be used to treat isospora in HIV-infected patients with sulfonamide allergy, followed by pyrimethamine 25 mg and folinic acid 5 mg daily indefinitely until sufficient immune reconstitution occurs.[44] Ciprofloxacin 500 mg twice daily for 7 days followed by 500 mg three times weekly as suppressive therapy is another alternative to TMP-SMX for sulfonamide allergic HIV-infected patients but is less effective than TMP-SMX.[45]

For patients with chronic cryptosporidial infection who are immunocompromised, no uniformly effective therapy has been identified.[36,37] In HIV-infected patients, initiation of highly active antiretroviral therapy is most consistently associated with resolution of symptoms secondary to improved immune function.[37] In the absence of antiretroviral therapy, nitazoxanide 500 to 1,000 mg twice daily for 14 days may improve or eliminate diarrhea and oocyst excretion, particularly in patients with CD4 counts above 50 cells per microliter; however, longer treatment courses may be necessary to achieve resolution in some patients.[46] Paromomycin 500 mg three to four times daily for 2 to 4 weeks is effective in decreasing stool frequency in approximately 66% of patients and may reduce or eliminate oocyst shedding but does not prevent biliary tract invasion in HIV-infected patients.[47] Relapse is common following discontinuation of therapy, necessitating suppressive therapy with 500 mg twice daily. Azithromycin 900 mg daily demonstrated improvement in oocyst shedding and clinical endpoints (decreased stool frequency and weight loss) in a double-blind, placebo-control trial.[48] Azithromycin serum concentrations correlated with treatment response, suggesting that doses greater than 900 mg per day may be necessary. Combination therapy with paromomycin (1 g twice daily) and azithromycin (600 mg daily) for 4 weeks followed by paromomycin alone for 8 weeks was more effective than either drug alone in a small, open-label trial but was not a placebo-control trial.[49] Biological immunomodifiers (e.g., hyperimmune bovine colostrum, oral bovine transfer factor) that contain antibodies to cryptosporidia are variably effective in eradicating oocyst shedding and have limited availabilty.[48,50]

Albendazole displays in vivo activity against microsporidia species, with the exception of *Enterocytozoon bieneusi*. For *Encephalitozoon intestinalis*, albendazole 400 mg orally twice daily for 2 to 4 weeks produces clinical improvement and eradicates intestinal spore shedding.[17,51] Chronic suppressive therapy with 400 mg twice daily may be necessary to prevent relapse in HIV-infected patients. Fumagillin, an antibiotic produced by *Aspergillus fumigatis*, has been used topically for keratoconjunctivitis secondary to *Encephalitozoon* species.[52] For ocular infections, a combination of oral albendazole (400 mg twice daily) and fumagillin eyedrops is currently recommended.[17] Fumagillin 20 mg three times daily by mouth for 2 to 3 weeks is effective for treatment

of *Enterocytozoon bieneusi*-induced diarrhea in patients with AIDS, but is associated with thrombocytopenia.[37,53]

Primary prophylaxis to prevent symptomatic infection with spore-forming protozoa is not currently recommended in HIV-infected patients; however, prophylaxis for *Mycobacterium avium* complex with clarithromycin 500 mg twice daily or rifabutin 300 mg daily is associated with a lower incidence of symptomatic cryptosporidiosis.[54] Initiation of highly active antiretroviral therapy for HIV infection has significantly diminished the overall frequency of symptomatic protozoal infections in this population.[39,55,56]

NONPHARMACOLOGIC THERAPY

Fluid and electrolyte replacement is the mainstay of therapy in patients with severe dehydration.[37] Diets consisting of medium-chain triglycerides may help decrease the severity of diarrhea.[57] Parenteral nutrition may be necessary in patients with prolonged malabsorption. Cholecystectomy or sphinterotomy and stent placement may be necessary in patients with biliary tract disease.[47]

FUTURE THERAPIES

β-Cyclodextrin is an excipient for other drugs that has been observed to have activity against cryptosporidia in animal models and warrants further investigation.[58] TNP-470 (AGM-1470) is an investigational semisynthetic fumagillin analogue that appears to be less toxic than fumagillin and may prove to be useful for treatment of microsporidia.[59]

GIARDIASIS

EPIDEMIOLOGY

Giardia lamblia (also known as *G. duodenalis* or *intestinalis*) is a flagellated, intestinal protozoan that is a common cause of diarrheal illness worldwide. Numerous waterborne outbreaks have been documented in mountainous regions throughout the United States. Infection occurs through ingestion of fecally contaminated food or water or by fecal-oral contact. Infection rates are high in day care settings and among homosexual males.[60,61]

PATHOPHYSIOLOGY

Exposure of ingested cysts to gastric acid and pancreatic enzymes releases pear-shaped trophozoites that colonize and replicate in the small bowel. Trophozoites attach to the intestine by means of an adhesive disk. Encystation by trophozoites follows within the ileum.[62] Disruption of the brush border membrane may occur; however, mucosal invasion is rare. Small bowel biopsy may appear normal or reveal sprue-like lesions.[61]

CLINICAL PRESENTATION AND DIAGNOSIS

SIGNS AND SYMPTOMS

Acute, self-limiting diarrhea lasting 1 to 3 weeks occurs in 25% to 50% of infected patients. Symptoms begin 1 to 2 weeks following ingestion of cysts. Stools are typically greasy and foul smelling but may be watery and profuse at symptom onset. Significant weight loss ($\geq$10 lb) occurs in over half of patients. Malaise, nausea, abdominal cramping, bloating, and flatulence are also common. Gastric infection may develop in patients with achlorhydria. A subset of patients develop chronic diarrhea associated with protein, D-xylose, and vitamins A and B_{12} malabsorption. Steatorrhea may also be observed. Lactose intolerance lasting several weeks is commonly observed following resolution of infection. Children are frequently more symptomatic than adults.[60–62]

DIAGNOSIS

Examination of fresh, iodine-stained stool or preserved (10% buffered formalin), trichrome or iron hematoxylin-stained stool for cysts is routinely used. Sensitivity approaches 90% with three stool samples. Occasionally, motile trophozoites can be visualized in feces by saline wet mount. Fecal leukocytes are typically absent. In difficult cases, proximal jejunal biopsy by endoscopy may be necessary. Alternatively, the Enterotest (Hedeco, Mountain View, CA) can be used where a gelatin capsule containing a nylon string is anchored in the mouth, ingested, and allowed to pass into the jejunum. After 4 to 6 hours, the string is removed and examined for presence of trophozoites within the adsorbed mucous.[61] Commercial enzyme immunoassays are now available with 100% sensitivity and 98% to 100% specificity.[40]

TREATMENT

PHARMACOTHERAPY

Oral metronidazole 250 mg three times daily for 5 to 7 days in adults or 5 mg per kilogram three times daily for 7 days in children is the treatment of choice for *Giardia* and is 80% to 95% effective.[17,61] Side effects include metallic taste, nausea, dizziness, headache, and a disulfuram reaction when taken with alcohol. Reversible neutropenia may occur rarely. Alternatively, nitazoxanide oral suspension (100 mg/5 mL) can be used in children at a dose of 100 mg every 12 hours (ages 1–3 years) or 200 mg every 12 hours (ages 4–11 years) for 3 days and is comparable to metronidazole.[17,63] Furazolidone 100 mg four times daily for 7 to 10 days in adults and 2 mg per kilogram four times a day for 10 days in children (>1 month) is less effective but available in an oral suspension (50 mg/15 mL). Side effects include nausea, vomiting, brown discoloration of the urine, and mild hemolysis in G6PD-deficient patients.[61] Albendazole 400 mg daily for 5 days or bacitracin 120,000 U [United States Pharmacopeia (USP)] for 10 days is also reportedly effective.[17] Treatment is typically deferred during pregnancy; however, if disease severity warrants, paromomycin 25 to 30 mg/kg/day in three divided doses for 5 to 10 days during the first trimester or metronidazole during the second or third trimester carries a low teratogenic risk.[17,61]

HELMINTHIC DISEASES

EPIDEMIOLOGY

Helminthic parasites consist of the nematodes (roundworms; e.g., *Ascaris*, *Enterobius*, *Trichuris*), trematodes (flukeworms; e.g., *Schistosoma*), and cestodes (tapeworms; e.g., *Taenia*). Over 25% of the world's population is infected with helminthic parasites. In the United States, *Enterobius* affects approximately 50 million people, *Ascaris* 4 million people, and *Trichuris* 2.2 million people. Approximately 400,000 immigrants from endemic areas are infected with *Schistosoma* in the United States. Fecal-oral spread is the predominant means of transmission for intestinal nematodes and cestode larvae. Infection with adult cestodes (e.g., *Taenia*) and tissue nematodes (e.g., *Trichinella*) is acquired by eating raw or undercooked meat.[64] Trematode infection (e.g., *Schistosoma*) occurs by contact with fresh water inhabited by larval forms.

PATHOPHYSIOLOGY

Given the complex life cycle of helminths, most adult worms do not multiply within humans. Therefore, infestation with multiple worms is the result of separate infection events. Exceptions to this are seen when the organism life cycle is completed within the human host (e.g., *Strongyloides*) or when infection occurs during the organism's larval stage (e.g., larva migrans, cysticercosis, hydatidosis).[65]

Roundworm infection occurs through ingestion of parasite eggs (*Enterobius*, *Trichuris*, *Ascaris*) or from external skin penetration by larvae (hookworm, *Strongyloides*). Adult worms of *Trichuris* and *Enterobius* mature in the large intestine and cecum, respectively, from larvae released from ingested eggs. *Ascaris* larvae burrow through the small intestine and spread hematogenously to the lungs, where they penetrate the alveolar space, migrate up the trachea, are swallowed, and mature to adult worms within the small intestine. After skin penetration, hookworm and *Strongyloides* larvae reach the small intestine in a similar manner.[66]

Beef, pork, or fish tapeworm (*Taenia saginata, Taenia solium, Diphyllobothrium latum*) infection occurs from ingestion of cyst-infected tissue where excystation in the gut leads to development of a mature tapeworm in the intestine. Gravid proglottids are released into the intestinal lumen, depositing numerous eggs in the feces. Incidental ingestion of eggs by animal hosts or humans leads to larval tissue invasion and cyst formation [e.g., cysticerus (*T. solium*), hydatid cyst (*Echinococcus*)].[67]

Schistosoma infection occurs from fresh water exposure when cercariae penetrate the skin and migrate to the lungs and liver where they mature to adult worms. Adult worms ultimately descend to the urinary bladder or portal venous system and release eggs into the urine or feces. Miracidia hatch from eggs in fresh water and infect the species-specific snail host, leading to cercariae formation.[68]

CLINICAL PRESENTATION AND DIAGNOSIS

SIGNS AND SYMPTOMS

Disease severity is related to the intensity of infection within the affected tissue. Asymptomatic infection is common with low organism burdens. In patients who are symptomatic, nocturnal anal pruritus is characteristic of enterobiasis. Diarrhea, weight loss, protein and iron malabsorption occur with hookworm. Heavy infection with *Trichuris* can result in bloody diarrhea, mild anemia, growth retardation, or rectal prolapse.[66] Abdominal cramping, vomiting, and diarrhea caused by intestinal or biliary obstruction can occur with heavy *Ascaris* or *T. saginata* infections.[66,67] Migration of hookworm, *Ascaris*, and *Strongyloides* larvae can cause pulmonary infiltration and eosinophilia (''Löffler-like'' syndrome), and localized skin erythema, rash, and pruritus at the site of larval skin entry. Strongyloidiasis in immunocompromised individuals can be life-threatening due to larval dissemination throughout the body (''hyperinfection syndrome''), resulting in secondary Gram-negative sepsis.[66] Acute *Schistosoma* infection can cause a serum sickness-like illness (Katayama fever) due to intravascular egg deposition. Long-term infection can result in species-specific, chronic granuloma formation in venules of the portal, genitourinary, and pulmonary systems, leading to obstructive manifestations such as portal hypertension.[68] Seizures, hydrocephalus, coma, and death can result from cysticerci in the brain (neurocysticercosis).[68,69]

DIAGNOSIS

Definitive diagnosis is commonly made by microscopic examination of fecal specimens collected over several days for eggs or intact proglottids. Stool concentration techniques can increase the sensitivity of *Schistosoma* egg and *Strongyloides* larvae detection. Transparent adhesive tape applied to the perianal region in the morning is useful for detecting adult female pinworms (*Enterobius*). The Enterotest can be used to detect *Strongyloides* larvae in duodenal fluid. Computed tomography and magnetic resonance imaging are used to detect neurocysticerci and hydatid cysts. Eosinophilia is more commonly observed with ascariasis, hookworm, strongyloidiasis, and occasionally taeniasis. Serologic tests are of limited use due to lack of standardization.[66–69]

TREATMENT

PHARMACOTHERAPY

Treatment of helminthic infection is indicated in all patients, regardless of the degree of symptoms. Mebendazole 100 mg twice daily for 3 days or a single 500 mg dose (for mass treatment programs) is used for trichuriasis, ascariasis, and hookworm. Expulsion of worms through the nose and mouth can occur with heavy *Ascaris* infections. Patients should be advised to drink fruit juices to minimize worm adherence to mucous membranes. A single dose of mebendazole (100 mg), albendazole (400 mg), or pyrantel pamoate [11 mg/kg base (maximum 1 g)] repeated several times at 1 to 2 week intervals is typically necessary to cure *Enterobius*.[17,70] Close family members should be treated concurrently to minimize reinfection. Albendazole (400 mg daily for 3 days) is 80% curative for trichuriasis.[70] A single 400 mg dose is as effective as mebendazole for ascariasis, more effective against hookworm, and better tolerated.[71] Alternatively, pyrantel pamoate 11 mg per kilogram (base) as a single daily dose (maximum 1 g) for 1 and 3 days can be used to treat *Ascaris* and hookworm, respectively.[17]

Single-dose ivermectin (200 μg/kg for 1–2 days) is the treatment of choice for uncomplicated strongyloidiasis (cure rate 83%–100%).[17,72] Thiabendazole (25 mg/kg twice daily, maximum 3 g/day for 2 days) can also be used; however, gastrointestinal and central nervous system side effects are common.[17,70] Albendazole in doses ranging from 400 to 800 mg per day for 3 days is less effective (cure rate 38%–95%) but better tolerated than thiabendazole, making it an attractive alternative.[70] Thiabendazole remains the preferred agent for disseminated strongyloidiasis; experience with ivermectin is currently limited.[65]

Praziquantel is highly effective for most tapeworm and flukeworm infections and is the drug of choice for schistosomiasis.[70] Single-dose therapy (5–10 mg/kg) is effective for *T. saginata, T. solium,* and *D. latum.* Flukeworm infections are treated with 25 mg per kilogram three times daily for 1 to 2 days. For schistosomiasis, 20 mg per kilogram two to three times daily for 1 day is used.[65] For treatment of cysticercosis, 50 to 100 mg/kg/day in three divided doses for 30 days or albendazole 400 mg (7.5 mg/kg) twice daily for 8 to 30 days is recommended.[17] Corticosteroid and antiepileptic administration to reduce adverse reactions from cyst rupture can decrease praziquantel serum concentrations, and may necessitate higher doses.[69] Albendazole is considered preferable for neurocysticercosis; however, the role of antiparasitic therapy remains controversial due to uncertain clinical benefit and concern for neurologic sequelae.[17,69,70]

Side effects are uncommon with mebendazole and albendazole due to poor bioavailability (<10%) and include abdominal pain, nausea, vomiting, headache, dizziness, and rare allergic reactions. Liver function abnormalities, alopecia, and leukopenia can occur with prolonged therapy at high doses. Both agents should be avoided during the first trimester of pregnancy and can be dosed the same in adults and children when treating intestinal nematodes. Albendazole serum concentrations can be increased fivefold when taken with a fatty meal. Mebendazole and albendazole come in 100 mg and 200 mg chewable tablets, respectively. Tablets may be chewed, crushed and mixed with food, or swallowed whole.[70] Pyrantel pamoate is available over the counter in 180 mg capsules, 50 and 144 mg per milliliter oral solutions, and a 50 mg per milliliter oral suspension. Side effects are mild due to poor absorption and include nausea, vomiting, anorexia, and diarrhea. Praziquantel comes in 600 mg tri-scored tablets. Adverse effects are mild and include headache, dizziness, malaise, nausea, vomiting, and abdominal pain.[70] Ivermectin comes in 6 mg tablets and is associated with pruritus, dizziness, fever, edema, and postural hypotension.[70] Coadministration of cimetidine with mebendazole, albendazole, or praziquantel leads to higher serum concentrations and greater efficacy for extraintestinal helminth infections.[70]

ECTOPARASITES

EPIDEMIOLOGY

Lice infestation (pediculosis) is caused by *Pediculus humanus* var. *corporis* (human louse), var. *capitis* (head louse), and *Phthirus pubis* (pubic or crab louse). Head lice outbreaks are common among school-age children. Human scabies is highly infectious and is caused by the itch mite, *Sarcoptes scabiei* var. *hominis*. Institutional outbreaks can occur in hospitals and nursing homes. Norwegian (crusted) scabies is a severe variant of scabies that typically occurs in immunocompromised or institutionalized individuals. Lice and scabies mites are distributed worldwide.[73,74]

PATHOPHYSIOLOGY

Adult female lice lay fertilized eggs (nits) on hair shafts or clothing fibers. Nymphs emerge 7 to 10 days later and obtain a blood meal. Saliva injected during the meal causes a localized hypersensitivity reaction within the skin. Adult female scabies mites lay two to three eggs daily for 4 to 6 weeks within narrow burrows in the stratum corneum layer of the epithelium. Larvae emerge in approximately 3 days. Localized hypersensitivity develops to dead mites, eggs, larvae, and their excrement. Infestation is generally limited to 5 to 10 mites in immunocompetent hosts versus greater than 10,000 in individuals with Norwegian scabies.[73,75]

CLINICAL PRESENTATION AND DIAGNOSIS

Pruritic, erythematous lesions are characteristic of lice infestation. Head lice are typically localized within the temporal and occipital areas but can involve the entire scalp. Body lice reside predominantly in the seams of clothing and produce small macules and papules on the trunk. Crab lice are found on pubic, axillary, or truncal hair, or eyelashes, and cause pruritus of affected areas and distinctive small bluish lesions (maculae ceruleae). Adult lice are difficult to see; however, nits are readily visible on hair shafts.[73] Scabies is characterized by intensely pruritic, erythematous papules. Classic linear burrows may be observed within interdigital web spaces or on wrists and ankles. Norwegian scabies produces generalized, crusted nodules and plaques, frequently involving the nails. Wet mount evaluation of skin scrapings can reveal presence of organisms, eggs, or fecal pellets.[74] Secondary bacterial infections may develop with pediculosis or scabies.

TREATMENT

PHARMACOTHERAPY

Topical permethrin (1%) is the treatment of choice for head and crab lice.[17] After shampooing and towel drying, the hair and scalp are saturated with permethrin 1%, wrapped in a towel for 10 minutes, and then rinsed thoroughly. Nits can be removed by applying an equal parts vinegar-water solution to the hair and using a fine-toothed comb dipped in vinegar. One application is 97% to 99% effective but should be repeated after 1 week if lice and nits remain. For crab lice, permethrin 1% should be applied to affected areas in a similar fashion, except the eyelids where a thin layer of petrolatum should be placed. Sexual contacts should be treated concurrently. Pubic lice should be treated with permethrin 5% or a single oral dose of ivermectin 200 μg per kilogram.[17] Body lice can be eliminated by laundering clothing in hot water and ironing seams.[73] When resistance to permethrin or other pediculicides is strongly suspected, malathion 0.5% should be used.[76] Disadvantages of malathion are its longer application period (8–12 hours), flammable nature, and severe respiratory depressant effect if inadvertently ingested.[77] Reapplication after 7 to 10 days may be necessary to treat newly hatched nymphs.[77]

Permethrin 5% cream is the preferred treatment for scabies. One application is massaged into the entire skin surface except the face and washed off after 8 to 14 hours. Household and sexual contacts should be treated at the same time. For Norwegian scabies, permethrin should be applied following a 10-minute lukewarm bath, applied again in 12 hours, and rinsed off after 12 more hours. This should be repeated in 1 week. Clothing and bed linen should be cleaned in hot, soapy water and dried in the dryer's hot cycle.[74] Lindane 1% is also effective against lice and scabies but is associated with severe side effects (aplastic anemia, seizures) due to systemic absorption and is less effective than permethrin. In addition, lindane-resistant lice and scabies have been reported.[78] Side effects associated with permethrin include pruritus, mild burning or stinging, tingling, numbness, and rash. Permethrin is contraindicated in patients with known hypersensitivity to chrysanthemums, pyethrins, or pyethrinoids. Other alternatives to permethrin include topical pyethrins and piperonyl butoxide or single-dose oral ivermectin (200 μg/kg). Systemic antihistamines and antibiotics are used to relieve pruritus and treat secondary bacterial infections.[17,79]

PSYCHOSOCIAL ASPECTS

Cultural beliefs regarding acquisition of parasitic infections influence the utility of preventive strategies and use of appropriate therapy in developing countries. Herbal remedies and spiritualists are commonly used in endemic malarial areas.[80] Travelers' misconceptions about disease risk and severity can produce complacency about using chemoprophylaxis and seeking medical attention.[81] The common misconception that head lice infestation is related to poor personal hygiene can lead to poor self-image in affected children. Institutionalized individuals may refuse presumptive therapy during scabies outbreaks because of denial.

IMPROVING OUTCOMES

PATIENT EDUCATION

The most effective means of managing parasitic infections is disease prevention. Travelers in developing countries or wilderness areas can avoid infection by treating water with iodine, boiling for 1 minute, or drinking canned or bottled beverages. Chloride water treatment alone is ineffective against *G. lamblia* and *C. parvum*.[82] Microfilters with pore sizes less than 1 μm can also be used to filter water for small

volume use.[36] When traveling in endemic malarial areas, preventive measures such as wearing long-sleeved shirts and pants, applying insect repellent containing DEET (diethylmetatoluamide), spraying aerosolized pyrethrins in living and sleeping areas, and sleeping in properly screened or enclosed areas should be utilized to minimize mosquito exposure. Travelers can obtain updated information from the Centers for Disease Control and Prevention (CDC) web site (http://www.cdc.gov), CDC's annual pamphlet entitled "Health Information for International Travel," or from their local health department.[82]

DISEASE MANAGEMENT STRATEGIES TO IMPROVE PATIENT OUTCOMES

Patient adherence is critical to maintaining the activity of antimalarial therapies and in preventing disease onset. It is estimated that 1% to 7% of individuals will discontinue chemoprophylaxis prematurely, in part due to side effects.[24] Chemoprophylaxis regimens should be begun prior to departure to endemic malarial areas so that side effects can be managed effectively and therapeutic drug concentrations are achieved within the individual. Travelers should be informed of the importance of adhering to chemoprophylaxis regimens throughout their stay and on their return and to take precautionary measures to avoid mosquito exposure. Given the magnitude of helminthic infection worldwide, the World Health Organization has recommended that community-wide treatment be performed in endemic areas to prevent ongoing dissemination of infection. Improvement in growth and academic performance has been observed in treated children.[70] Simultaneous administration of anthelmintics has also been advocated to treat coinfection with multiple organisms.[70]

PHARMACOECONOMICS

Chemoprophylaxis is a cost-effective approach to decreasing the morbidity and mortality associated with malaria; however, in areas where attack rates are low, presumptive therapy may be preferred when the incidence of adverse effects with chemoprophylaxis exceeds the incidence of disease.[81] When chemoprophylaxis is indicated, once-weekly agents (mefloquine, chloroquine) are preferable to those administered daily (doxycycline, atovaquone/proguanil). Annual mass treatment programs for geohelminths and schistosomiasis have been demonstrated to be cost-effective in developing countries by decreasing disease manifestations and transmission. Despite its lower effectiveness for strongyloidiasis, albendazole is more cost-effective than thiabendazole for mass treatment programs due to better tolerance and improved patient adherence.[70] Similarly, mebendazole is less effective than albendazole for hookworm; however, generic mebendazole is significantly lower in cost, making it attractive for mass treatment programs targeting mixed helminthic infections.[71]

KEY POINTS

- The goals of antiparasitic therapy are to treat disease symptoms, minimize complications, and reduce disease transmission.

- Malaria is caused by *Plasmodium* spp. transmitted by *Anopheles* mosquito vectors.

- Selection of appropriate chemoprophylaxis, minimizing mosquito exposure, and patient adherence are critical to malaria prevention.

- Falciparum malaria can become rapidly life-threatening; therefore, prompt institution of appropriate antiprotozoal therapy and supportive treatment is necessary.

- Poor sanitation and fecal-oral spread can lead to infection with intestinal protozoans (cryptosporidia, microsporidia, isospora, cyclospora, giardia) and intestinal helminths.

- Asymptomatic infection or mild symptoms are common with intestinal protozoans and low density helminthic infection.

- Individuals with HIV infection are more prone to developing chronic diarrhea and extraintestinal infection with intestinal protozoans.

- Intestinal infection with *G. lamblia* ranges from asymptomatic cyst passage to acute, self-limited diarrhea to chronic, severe diarrhea associated with significant weight loss, malabsorption, and lactose intolerance.

- Effective treatments for cyclospora, isospora, and microsporidia are available; however, only recovery from immunosuppression is reliable in relieving symptoms from chronic cryptosporidia infection.

- Treatment strategies for helminthic infections are directed at decreasing symptomatology, reducing worm burdens, and preventing spread of infection.

- Benzimidazoles and pyrantel pamoate are preferred agents for intestinal roundworms whereas praziquantel is used for tapeworms, flukeworms, and schistosomes.

- Metronidazole is the drug of choice for Giardia; however, furazolidone is frequently used in children due to ease of administration and mild side effects.

- Lice and scabies infestation are characterized by development of pruritic, erythematous skin lesions secondary to localized skin hypersensitivity.

- Topical permethrin (1% and 5%, respectively) is the treatment of choice for lice and scabies.

SUGGESTED READINGS

Chen X, Keithly J, Paya C, et al. Cryptosporidiosis. N Engl J Med 346: 1723–1731, 2002.

de Silva N, Guyatt H, Bundy D. Anthelmintics: a comparative review of their clinical pharmacology. Drugs 53:769–788, 1997.

Ortega YR, Adam RD. Giardia: overview and update. Clin Infect Dis 25:545–549, 1997.

Suh KN, Kain KC, Keystone JS. Malaria. CMAJ 170:1693–1702, 2004.

White NJ. Antimalarial drug resistance. J Clin Invest 113:1084–1092, 2004.

REFERENCES

1. Markell EK, Voge M, John DT. Medical parasitology. 8th ed. Philadelphia: W.B. Saunders Company, 1999:7.
2. Barrett MP, Burchmore RJ, Stich A, et al. The trypanosomiases. Lancet 362:1469–1480, 2003.
3. Berman J. Current treatment approaches to leishmaniasis. Curr Opin Infect Dis 16:397–401, 2003.
4. Stanley SL Jr. Amoebiasis. Lancet 361:1025–1034, 2003.
5. World Health Organization. World malaria situation in 1994. Wkly Epidemiol Rec 72:269–276, 1997.
6. Kain KC, Keystone JS. Malaria in travelers: epidemiology, disease, and prevention. Infect Dis Clin North Am 12:267–284, 1998.
7. Wyler DJ. Malaria: overview and update. Clin Infect Dis 16: 449–458, 1993.
8. Shah B, Filler S, Causer LM, et al. Malaria Surveillance—United States 2002. In: CDC Surveillance Summaries (April 30, 2004). MMWR Morb Mortal Wkly Rep 53:21–34, 2004.
9. Schwartz E, Parise M, Kozarsky P, et al. Delayed onset of malaria—implications for chemoprophylaxis in travelers. N Engl J Med 349:1510–1516, 2003.
10. Suh KN, Kain KC, Keystone JS. Malaria. CMAJ 170:1693–1702, 2004.
11. Krogstad DJ, Plasmodium species (malaria). In: Mandell GL, Bennett JE, Dolin R. Principles and practice of infectious diseases. 5th ed. New York: Churchill Livingstone, 2000:2824, 2827.
12. Maitland K, Phillip B, Newton CRJC. Malaria. Curr Opin Infect Dis 16:389–935, 2003.
13. White NJ. The treatment of malaria. N Engl J Med 335:800–806, 1996.
14. Palmer CJ, Lindo JF, Klaskala WI, et al. Evaluation of the OptiMAL test for rapid diagnosis of *Plasmodium vivax* and *Plasmodium falciparum* malaria. J Clin Micro 1998;36:203–206, 1998.
15. Centers for Disease Control and Prevention. Treatment of malaria. Available at: http://www.cdc.gov/malaria/diagnosis_treatment/tx_clinicians.htm. Accessed 5/25/2004.
16. Lee LH, Caserta MT: Malaria: update on treatment. Ped Infect Dis J 17:342–343, 1998.
17. Anonymous. Drugs for parasitic infections. Med Letter 1127:1–12, 2002. Available at: http://www.medletter.com/freedocs/parasitic.pdf. Accessed 4/27/2004.
18. Barat LM, Bloland PB. Drug resistance among malaria and other parasites. Infect Dis Clin North Am 11:969–987, 1997.
19. Haynes RK. Artemisinin and derivatives: the future for malaria treatment? Curr Opin Infect Dis 14:719–726, 2001.
20. McIntosh HM, Olliaro P. Artemisinin derivatives for treating uncomplicated malaria [review]. Cochrane Database Syst Rev CD000256, 2000.
21. White NJ. Antimalarial drug resistance. J Clin Invest 113: 1084–1092, 2004.
22. National Center for Infectious Diseases, Centers for Disease Control and Prevention. Travelers' health, malaria. Available at: http://www.cdc.gov/travel/diseases/malaria/index.htm. Accessed 4/27/2004.
23. Schlagenhauf P, Tschopp A, Johnson R, et al. Tolerability of malaria chemoprophylaxis in non-immune travellers to sub-Saharan Africa: multicentre, randomised, double blind, four arm study. BMJ 327:1078, 2003.
24. Kain KC, Shanks GD, Keystone JS. Malaria chemoprophylaxis in the age of drug resistance. I. Currently recommended drug regimens. Clin Infect Dis 33:226–234, 2001.
25. Ohrt C, Richie TL, Widjaja H, et al. Mefloquine compared with doxycycline for the prophylaxis of malaria in Indonesian soldiers. A randomized, double-blind, placebo-controlled trial. Ann Intern Med 126:963–972, 1997.
26. Wolfe MS. Protection of travelers. Clin Infect Dis 25:177–184, 1997.
27. Ling J, Baird KJ, Fryauff DJ, et al. Randomized, placebo-controlled trial of atovaquone/proguanil for the prevention of *Plasmodium falciparum* or *Plasmodium vivax* malaria among migrants to Papua, Indonesia. Clin Infect Dis 35:825–833, 2002.
28. Andersen SL, Oloo AJ, Gordon DM, et al. Successful double-blinded, randomized, placebo-controlled field trial of azithromycin and doxycycline as prophylaxis for malaria in western Kenya. Clin Infect Dis 26:146–150, 1998.

29. Panosian CB. Editorial Response: exchange blood transfusion in severe falciparum malaria—the debate goes on. Clin Infect Dis 26:853–854, 1998.
30. Riddle MS, Jackson JL, Sanders JW, et al. Exchange transfusions as an adjunct therapy in severe *Plasmodium falciparum* malaria: a meta analysis. Clin Infect Dis 34:1192–1198, 2002.
31. Shanks GD, Kain KC, Keystone JS. Malaria chemoprophylaxis in the age of drug resistance. II. Drugs that may be available in the future. Clin Infect Dis 33:381–385, 2001.
32. Rosenthal PJ. Proteases of malaria parasites: new targets for chemotherapy. Emerg Infect Dis 4:49–57, 1998.
33. Go ML. Novel antiplasmodial agents. Med Res Rev 23:456–487, 2003.
34. Goodgame RW. Understanding intestinal spore-forming protozoa: cryptosporidia, microsporidia, isospora, cyclospora. Ann Intern Med 124:429–441, 1996.
35. Guerrant RL. Cryptosporidiosis: an emerging, highly infectious threat. Emerg Infect Dis 3:51–57, 1997.
36. Leav BA, Mackay M, Ward HD. Cryptosporidium species: new insights and old challenges. Clin Infect Dis 36:903–908, 2003.
37. Chen X, Keithly J, Paya C, et al. Cryptosporidiosis. N Engl J Med 346:1723–1731, 2002.
38. MacKenzie WR, Hoxie NJ, Proctor ME, et al. A massive outbreak in Milwaukee of cryptosporidium infection transmitted through the public water supply. N Engl J Med 331:161–167, 1994.
39. Didier ES: Microsporidiosis. Clin Infect Dis 27:1–8, 1998.
40. Katanick MT, Schneider SK, Rosenblatt JE, et al. Evaluation of ColorPAC *giardia/cryptosporidium* rapid assay and ProSpec T *giardia/cryptosporidium* microplate assay for detection of *giardia* and *cryptosporidium* in fecal specimens. J Clin Micro 39:4523–4525, 2001.
41. Anonymous. Nitazoxanide (Alinia)—a new anti-protozoal agent. Med Letter 45:29–31, 2003.
42. Pape JW, Verdier RI, Boney M, et al. Cyclospora infection in adults infected with HIV: clinical manifestations, treatment, and prophylaxis. Ann Intern Med 121:654–657, 1994.
43. Pape JW, Verdier RI, Johnson WD. Treatment and prophylaxis of *Isospora belli* infection in patients with the acquired immunodeficiency syndrome. N Engl J Med 320:1044–1047, 1989.
44. Ackers JP. Gut coccidia—isospora, cryptosporidium, cyclospora, and sarcocystis. Semin Gastrointest Dis 8:33–44, 1997.
45. Verdier RI, Fitzgerald DW, Johnson WD, et al. Trimethoprim-sulfamethoxazole compared with ciprofloxacin for treatment and prophylaxis of *Isospora belli* and *Cyclospora cayetanensis* infection in HIV-infected patients: a randomized, controlled trial. Ann Intern Med 132:885–888, 2000.
46. Rossignol JF, Hidalgo H, Feregrino M, et al. A double-blind placebo-controlled study of nitazoxanide in the treatment of cryptosporidial diarrhea in AIDS patients in Mexico. Tran R Soc Trop Med Hyg 92:663–666, 1998.
47. Hashmey R, Smith NH, Cron S, et al. Cryptosporidiosis in Houston, Texas. A report of 95 cases. Med 76:118–139, 1997.
48. Ritchie DJ, Becker ES. Update on the management of intestinal cryptosporidiosis in AIDS. Ann Pharmacother 28:767–778, 1994.
49. Smith NH, Cron S, Valdez LM, et al. Combination therapy for cryptosporidiosis in AIDS. J Infect Dis 178:900–903, 1998.
50. Gomez M, Pozio E. Humoral and cellular immunity against cryptosporidium infection. Curr Drug Targets Immune Endocr Metabol Disord 2:291–301, 2002.
51. Molina JM, Chastang C, Goguel J, et al. Albendazole for treatment and prophylaxis of microsporidiosis due to *Encephalitozoon intestinalis* in patients with AIDS: a randomized double-blind controlled trial. J Infect Dis 177:1373–1377, 1998.
52. Diesenhouse MC, Wilson LA, Corrent GF, et al. Treatment of microsporidial keratoconjunctivitis with topical fumagillin. Am J Ophthalmol 115:293–298, 1993.
53. Molina JM, Goguel J, Sarfati C, et al. Potential efficacy of fumagillin in intestinal microsporidiosis due to *Enterocytozoon bineusi* in patients with HIV infection: results of a drug screening study. AIDS 11:1603–1610, 1997.
54. Holmberg SD, Moorman AC, Von Bargen JC, et al. Possible effectiveness of clarithromycin and rifabutin for cryptosporidiosis chemoprophylaxis in HIV disease. JAMA 279:384–386, 1998.
55. Carr A, Marriott D, Field A, et al. Treatment of HIV-1-associated microsporidiosis and cryptosporidiosis with combination antiretroviral therapy. Lancet 351:256–261, 1998.
56. Miao YM, Awad-El-Kariem FM, Franzen C, et al. Eradication of cryptosporidia and microsporidia following successful antiretroviral therapy. J Acquir Immun Defic Syndr 25:124–129, 2000.
57. Wanke CA, Plesko D, DeGirolami PC, et al. A medium chain triglyceride-based diet in patients with HIV and chronic diarrhea reduces diarrhea and malabsorption: a prospective, controlled trial. Nutrition 12:766–771, 1996.
58. Chappell CL, Okhuysen PC. Cryptosporidiosis. Curr Opin Infect Dis 15:523–527, 2002.
59. Coyle C, Kent M, Tanowitz HB, et al. TNP-470 is an effective antimicrosporidial agent. J Infect Dis 177:515–518, 1998.
60. Thielman NM, Guerrant RL. Persistent diarrhea in the returned traveler. Infect Dis Clin North Am 12:489–501, 1998.
61. Hill DR, *Giardia lamblia*. In: Mandell GL, Bennett JE, Dolin R, eds. Principles and practice of infectious diseases. 5th ed. New York: Churchill Livingstone, 2000:2888–2892.
62. Ortega YR, Adam RD. Giardia: overview and update. Clin Infect Dis 25:545–549, 1997.
63. Ortiz JJ, Ayoub A, Gargala G, et al. Randomized clinical study of nitazoxanide compared to metronidazole in the treatment of symptomatic giardiasis in children from Northern Peru. Aliment Pharmacol Ther 15:1409–1415, 2001.
64. VandeWaa EA, Henderson JD, White GL Jr, et al. Common helminth infections: battling wormlike parasites in primary care. Clin Rev 8:75–92, 1998.
65. Liu LX, Weller PF. Antiparasitic drugs. N Engl J Med 334:1178–1184, 1996.
66. Mahmoud AAF, Intestinal nematodes (roundworms): In: Mandell GL, Bennett JE, Dolin R, eds. Principles and practice of infectious diseases. 5th ed. New York: Churchill Livingstone, 2000:2939–2943.
67. King CH, Cestodes (tapeworms). In: Mandell GL, Bennett JE, Dolin R, eds. Principles and practice of infectious diseases, 5th ed. New York: Churchill Livingstone, 2000:2950–2955.
68. Mahmoud AAF, Trematodes (schistosomiasis) and other flukes. In: Mandell GL, Bennett JE, Dolin R, eds. Principles and practice of infectious diseases. 5th ed. New York: Churchill Livingstone, 2000:2956–2964.
69. White AC. Neurocysticercosis: a major cause of neurological disease worldwide. Clin Infect Dis 24:101–113, 1997.
70. de Silva N, Guyatt H, Bundy D. Anthelmintics: a comparative review of their clinical pharmacology. Drugs 53:769–788, 1997.
71. Albonico M, Smith PG, Hall A, et al. A randomized controlled trial comparing mebendazole and albendazole against Ascaris, Trichuris, and hookworm infections. Trans R Soc Trop Med Hyg 88:585–589, 1994.
72. Gann PH, Neva FA, Gam AA. A randomized trial of single- and two-dose ivermectin versus thiabendazole for treatment of strongyloidiasis. J Infect Dis 169:1076–1079, 1994.
73. Mathieu ME, Wilson BB. Lice (pediculosis): In: Mandell GL, Bennett JE, Dolin R, eds. Principles and practice of infectious diseases. 5th ed. New York: Churchill Livingstone, 2000:2972–2974.
74. Mathieu ME, Wilson BB. Scabies. In: Mandell GL, Bennett JE, Dolin R, eds. Principles and practice of infectious diseases. 5th ed. New York: Churchill Livingstone, 2000:2974–2976.
75. Mackey SL, Wagner KF. Dermatologic manifestations of parasitic diseases. Infect Dis Clin North Am 8:713–743, 1994.
76. Hansen RC, and Working Group on the Treatment of Resistant Pediculosis. Guidelines for the treatment of resistant pediculosis. Contemp Pediatr 17 (Suppl):1–10, 2000.
77. Frankowski BL, Weiner LB. Committee on School Health and the Committee on Infectious Diseases, American Academy of Pediatrics. Head Lice. Pediatrics 110:638–643, 2002.
78. Brown S, Becher J, Brady W. Treatment of ectoparasitic infections: review of the English–language literature, 1982–1992. Clin Infect Dis 20 (Suppl 1):S104–109, 1995.
79. Meinking TL, Taplin D, Hermida JL, et al. Treatment of scabies with ivermectin. N Engl J Med 333:26–30, 1995.
80. Ahorlu CK, Dunyo SK, Afari EA, et al. Malaria-related beliefs and behavior in southern Ghana: implications for treatment, prevention and control. Trop Med Int Health 2:488–499, 1997.
81. Schlagenhauf P, Steffen R, Tschopp A, et al. Behavioral aspects of travelers in their use of malaria presumptive therapy. Bull WHO 73:215–221, 1995.
82. Centers for Disease Control and Prevention, Health information for international travel 2003–2004, DHHS, Atlanta, GA. 2003.

Surgical Infections and Antibiotic Prophylaxis

89

Ronald L. Braden

DEFINITION

Surgical antibiotic prophylaxis is the appropriate use of pre-operative and postoperative antibiotics to decrease the incidence of postoperative wound infections.

TREATMENT GOALS: SURGICAL ANTIBIOTIC PROPHYLAXIS

- Decrease the incidence of postoperative wound infections.
- Decrease the incidence of adverse drug effects in surgical patients.
- Decrease the cost of care for surgical patients.
- Minimize the adverse effects of prophylactic antibiotics on the microflora of the patient and the overall bacterial resistance patterns in a particular institution.

SURGICAL INFECTIONS

EPIDEMIOLOGY

Twenty-five percent of all nosocomial infections are post-operative wound infections.[1] Haley et al[2] demonstrated that surgical wound infections can be responsible for an additional week of hospitalization and an increase by approximately 20% in the overall cost of care. This cost is estimated to exceed $1.5 billion per year in the United States. Administration of prophylactic antibiotics in certain surgical procedures can decrease postoperative infections, decrease length of hospital stay, and reduce the overall cost of care.

Inappropriate or indiscriminate use of prophylactic antibiotics can increase cost of care by increasing drug cost, increasing drug toxicity, increasing bacterial resistance, and increasing laboratory costs. Prophylactic antibiotics can account for 30% to 40% of total antibiotic usage in some hospitals and inappropriate usage remains a significant problem. Pharmacy practitioners must become more astute in the development and implementation of cost-control measures in prevention of postoperative wound infections.[3]

PATHOPHYSIOLOGY

Surgical wound infection does not necessarily follow bacterial contamination. The predominant organisms involved are the endogenous microflora at the surgical site. The development of a surgical wound infection is dependent on a complex interaction between the patient's host-defense response, intrinsic bacterial factors, and local tissue factors.[4,5] Factors which increase the risk of surgical wound infection are as follows:

1. Host-Defense Response Factors: Patients with an underlying host-defense deficit are at increased risk of surgical wound infection (extremes of age, malnutrition, diabetes, corticosteroid therapy, other immunologic deficiency)
2. Bacterial Factors
   a. Degree of wound contamination
   b. Bacterial virulence
   c. Microbial resistance to prophylactic antibiotics
3. Local Tissue Factors
   a. Blood supply and tissue hypoxia
   b. Presence of necrotic material
   c. Presence of hematoma
   d. Presence of a foreign body

CLASSIFICATION OF SURGICAL WOUNDS

The Ad Hoc Committee of the Committee on Trauma of the National Research Council developed a standard classification of surgical wounds in 1964.[6] This classification identified four basic categories of wound contamination and the resultant postoperative infection rate expected within each category (Table 89.1).

RISK FACTORS

The risk of postoperative infection is dependent on patient factors, intraoperative factors, and perioperative management. Factors that have been identified as increasing the risk of postoperative infection are listed in Table 89.2. Regardless of the wound classification, emergency surgical procedures have a higher postoperative infection rate than the same elective operative procedure. Institutions in which a high volume of an operative procedure is performed have a lower postoperative infection rate than those institutions where the operative procedure is performed less frequently.[7] Operative procedures that last longer have a higher postoperative infection rate regardless of their wound classification.

SURGICAL ANTIBIOTIC PROPHYLAXIS

PRINCIPLES

Prophylactic antibiotics are indicated when the risk of postoperative infection is high or when the consequence of infection is excessive morbidity or mortality.[8] Antibiotic selection should be based on spectrum of antimicrobial activity, pharmacokinetic profile, drug toxicity, and positive results from well-controlled clinical trials. The benefit of the prophylactic antibiotic must always clearly outweigh its risks.

ANTIMICROBIAL SPECTRUM

The antimicrobial agent chosen for an individual patient should have activity against the most common pathogens which cause surgical wound infections (Table 89.3).

TABLE 89.1	National Research Council Wound Classification Criteria
Classification	**Criteria**
Clean (<2%)[a]	Elective (not urgent or emergency), primarily closed; no acute inflammation or transection of gastrointestinal, oropharyngeal, genitourinary, biliary, or tracheobronchial tracts; no surgical technique break (e.g., elective inguinal herniorrhaphy)
Clean-contaminated (<10%)[a]	Urgent or emergency procedure that is otherwise clean; elective gastrointestinal, oropharyngeal, biliary, or tracheobronchial tracts; minimal spillage and/or minor technique break; reoperation via clean incision within 7 days; blunt trauma, intact skin, negative exploration (e.g., vagotomy and pyloroplasty)
Contaminated (20%)[a]	Acute, nonpurulent inflammation; major break in surgical technique or major spill from hollow organ; penetrating trauma <4 hr old; chronic open wounds to be grafted or covered (e.g., acute, nonperforated, nongangrenous appendicitis)
Dirty (40%)[a]	Purulence or abscess; preoperative perforation of gastrointestinal, oropharyngeal, biliary, or tracheobronchial tracts; penetrating trauma >4 hr old (e.g., perforated appendicitis with abscess)

[a] Wound infection rates appear in parentheses
(From Page CP, Bohnen JM, Fletcher JR, et al. Antimicrobial prophylaxis for surgical wounds. Guidelines for clinical care. Arch Surg 128:79–88, 1993, with permission.)

TABLE 89.2	Factors Associated with Increased Risk of Postoperative Infection	
Patient Factors	**Perioperative Factors**	**Intraoperative Factors**
Extremes of age	>48 hr preoperative hospitalization	Intraoperative contamination
Malnutrition	No preoperative shower	Lengthy operation
Obesity	Early shaving of site (>4 hr)	Excessive electrocautery
Associated problems	Hair removal	Prosthetic material
Diabetes	Prior antibiotic therapy	Wound drainage
Hypoxemia		Bloody wound fluid drainage
Previous infection		Epinephrine wound injection
Corticosteroid therapy		Intraoperative hypotension
Recent operation		Massive transfusion
Chronic inflammation		Skin preparation with alcohol/hexachlorophene
Prior site irradiation		

(From Page CP, Bohnen JM, Fletcher JR, et al. Antimicrobial prophylaxis for surgical wounds. Guidelines for clinical care. Arch Surg 128:79–88, 1993, with permission.)

The agent does not need to possess antibacterial activity against all of the endogenous microbial flora at the surgical site; the use of agents with an excessively broad spectrum of activity increases the risk of microbial resistance and superinfection without an improvement in effectiveness. Third-generation cephalosporins exemplify this point. Despite their increased antimicrobial activity, these agents have not proven superior to first-generation cephalosporins in any operative procedure.[9]

PHARMACOKINETICS

The pharmacokinetic profile of the prophylactic agent is also an extremely important factor. Burke[10] demonstrated the importance of adequate serum concentrations of the prophylactic antibiotic at the time of surgical incision in an experimental animal model. Most antibiotics used in surgical prophylaxis distribute rapidly into tissue compartments after intravenous administration, therefore, total body clearance and volume of distribution become the most important pharmacokinetic variables. Intraoperative factors such as blood loss, fluid replacement, and alteration of blood flow to the liver and kidneys may cause significant alterations in the clearance and volume of distribution of prophylactic antibiotics.[11] Guglielmo et al[12] demonstrated a significant increase in volume of distribution and elimination half-life of cefamandole in patients undergoing elective vascular surgery. The increased volume of distribution resulted in low serum concentrations of the antibiotic at the time of prosthetic graft placement, which would theoretically place the patient at increased risk of postoperative infection.

TIMING OF ANTIBIOTIC ADMINISTRATION

The most common error encountered in surgical prophylaxis is in the timing of antibiotic administration. As previously stated, Burke[11] demonstrated the importance of adequate serum concentrations of the prophylactic antibiotic at the time of incision in experimental animals. Polk and Lopez-Mayor[11]

confirmed this finding in a prospective clinical trial where inappropriate time of drug administration was an independent risk factor for postoperative infection. Classen et al[13] prospectively monitored the timing of antibiotic prophylaxis and studied the occurrence of surgical wound infections in patients undergoing elective clean or clean-contaminated surgical procedures. Patients receiving prophylactic antibiotics during the 2 hours prior to the initial surgical incision had the lowest overall surgical wound infection rate. "On call" dosing of prophylactic antibiotics may result in early drug administration due to an unforeseen delay in the beginning of the operative procedure and may result in inadequate tissue concentrations of the drug at the time of the initial surgical incision. Therefore, this practice should be strongly discouraged.

DURATION OF PROPHYLAXIS

Antibiotic administration should be continued for the shortest duration established to decrease the risk of postoperative infections. Antibiotic administration continued beyond 24 hours has not been shown to be superior to shorter duration antibiotic prophylaxis in most surgical procedures. Antibiotic prophylaxis continued beyond 24 hours increases cost, alters the patient's microflora, and adversely affects the bacterial resistance patterns of the institution.[14] Single-dose antibiotic prophylaxis provides the optimal balance of reducing wound infections in most operative procedures while decreasing adverse drug effects.[15]

SUGGESTED ANTIBIOTIC REGIMENS FOR SELECTED SURGICAL PROCEDURES

CARDIAC OPERATIONS

Cardiac operations are classified as clean surgical procedures and pose a low risk of surgical wound infection. Car-

TABLE 89.3	Recommendations for Prophylactic Antibiotic Agents for Adults		
Procedure	**Bacteria**	**Antibiotic Agent**	**Dose**
Cardiac: all procedures with cardiopulmonary bypass	S. aureus, S. epidermidis, diphtheroids, Gram-negative enterics	Cefazolin[a] or cefuroxime	1–2 g preinduction, 1 g every 8 hr for 48 hr
Gastroduodenal: Esophageal, gastroduodenal procedures in patients treated with H_2 blockers, bleeding duodenal ulcer, gastric cancer	Oropharyngeal flora and Gram-negative enterics, S. aureus	Cefazolin[a]	1–2 g preinduction
Biliary: all open and laparoscopic procedures	Gram-negative enterics, S. aureus, Enterococcus faecalis, clostridia	Cefazolin[a]	1–2 g preinduction
Colorectal: operations that involve the colon and/or rectum	Enteric aerobes and anaerobes	Oral neomycin/ erythromycin	See below[b]
Appendectomy: simple appendicitis	Enteric aerobes and anaerobes	Cefoxitin[c]	1 g preinduction
	Enteric Gram-negative aerobes, enterococci		
Genitourinary: High-risk only	Enteric aerobes and anaerobes, E. faecalis, group B streptococci	Ciprofloxacin	500 mg PO or 400 mg IV
Gynecologic and Obstetric: Cesarean section	Enteric aerobes and anaerobes, E. faecalis, group B streptococci	Cefazolin[a]	1 g after umbilical cord is clamped
Hysterectomy		Cefazolin[a]	1 g preinduction
Head and neck: procedures involving transection of the oropharyngeal mucosa (see text)	Oral aerobes and anaerobes, Enteric Gram-negative bacilli, S. aureus	Cefazolin[a] + clindamycin	1–2 g preinduction + 600 mg preinduction for up to 24 hr
Neurosurgery	S. aureus, S. epidermidis	Cefazolin[a]	1–2 g preinduction
Orthopaedic: insertion of prosthetic joints, open operations	S. aureus, S. epidermidis	Cefazolin[a]	1 g preinduction
Vascular: aortic resection or prosthetic bypass	S. aureus, S. epidermidis, diphtheroids, Gram-negative enterics	Cefazolin[a]	1–2 g preinduction, 1 g every 8 hr for 24 hr

[a] Vancomycin 1 g IV can be substituted for patients with life-threatening type 1 β-lactam allergies.
[b] Oral neomycin 1 g and erythromycin base 1 g PO given the day before surgery at 1, 2, and 11 PM, + cefoxitin[c] 1 g IV preinduction.
[c] Cefoxitin, cefotetan, or cefmetazole.
IV, intravenous; PO, by mouth.

diac operative procedures such as pacemaker or defibrillator placement pose a low postoperative infection risk and require single-dose antibiotic prophylaxis only. However, in cardiac operations that involve placement of prosthetic material, such as prosthetic valve replacement, the excessive morbidity and mortality of endocarditis and mediastinitis mandate the use of prophylactic antibiotics. The pathogens most commonly responsible for postoperative infection include *Staphylococcus aureus*, *Staphylococcus epidermidis*, and diphtheroid species. In most institutions, first-generation cephalosporins possess good activity against these pathogens and have remained the standard against which other antibiotics are compared. Cefazolin, a first-generation cephalosporin with a relatively long elimination half-life, has

remained the most commonly prescribed prophylactic agent. Several investigations have compared newer cephalosporins with varying results. Slama et al[16] compared cefamandole, cefazolin, and cefuroxime. Their results indicate cefamandole and cefuroxime are both superior to cefazolin in overall wound infection rates; however, other investigators have been unable to reproduce these results and the choice of agent remains an area of controversy.[17,18] The choice of agent in this setting should be based on the individual institution's sensitivities, however, the literature supports cefazolin as the prophylactic agent of choice in most cardiothoracic operations. Some practitioners recommend prolonged postoperative prophylactic antibiotics if the patient has been in the hospital awaiting surgery for greater than 48 hours. This practice has not been shown to be more effective in reducing postoperative infection rates and increases the risk of colonization of the patient with multidrug resistant microorganisms.[19] This practice should be strongly discouraged.

GASTRODUODENAL PROCEDURES

Surgical wound infection rates of the upper gastroduodenal tract (esophageal and gastroduodenal procedures) have been documented to be a function of gastric pH. Disease states or drugs that increase pH are well known to increase the incidence of postoperative infection.[20] The predominate pathogens in gastroduodenal procedures are normal mouth flora, skin flora, and to a lesser extent, bowel flora. Several cephalosporins have been proven effective in reducing postoperative infection rates, and cefazolin has been studied in a single-dose regimen and appears to have equal efficacy to that of multidose regimens. The preferred regimen is cefazolin 1 or 2 g as a single dose at the induction of anesthesia.[21,22]

BILIARY TRACT OPERATIONS

The postoperative infection rate of biliary tract procedures is directly related to the presence or absence of microorganisms in the bile. The infection rate of patients with positive bile cultures is reported to be approximately 36% whereas the infection rate of patients with sterile bile is less than 5%.[23,24] Risk factors for positive bile cultures include acute cholecystitis, biliary tract obstruction, and age greater than 70 years.[25] The most common organisms found in biliary tract surgery are *Escherichia coli*, *Klebsiella* species, *Enterococci*, *Streptococci*, and *Staphylococci*. Cephalosporins have shown good activity in biliary tract surgery and a meta analysis by Meijer et al[26] concluded that perioperative antibiotics should be used in all patients undergoing biliary tract surgery. Although patients with sterile biliary tracts appear to gain little or no benefit, preoperative identification of these patients is not possible. Cefazolin is the preferred agent and should be given as a single preinduction dose.

APPENDECTOMY

The incidence of surgical wound infections following appendectomy is highly variable and is dependent on the status of the appendix at the time of surgery. In uncomplicated appendicitis the infection rate is reported to be 4% to 9% without perioperative antibiotics and 1% to 5% with antibiotics.[27] The most common pathogens isolated after appendectomy are anaerobic organisms such as *Bacteroides fragilis*, and aerobic Gram-negative organisms such as *E. coli*. *Streptococci*, *Staphylococci*, and *Enterococci* are identified less frequently but may be associated with antibiotic treatment failure. Antibiotic regimens found to be effective in significantly reducing postoperative complications have included cefoxitin, cefotaxime, mezlocillin, piperacillin, and clindamycin.[28-30] The first-generation cephalosporins, cefazolin and cephalothin, have not been proven effective in reducing postoperative infections and do not appear to be appropriate

prophylactic agents.[29,31] Cefoxitin, cefotetan, or cefmetazole given as a single-dose preinduction regimen appear to be the preferred regimen in uncomplicated appendicitis.[28] Antibiotic use in complicated appendicitis is classified as treatment, not prophylaxis, and is therefore not included in the discussion.

COLORECTAL PROCEDURES

Surgical wound infections are responsible for excessive morbidity and mortality following elective colorectal surgery, which mandates the use of effective prophylactic antibiotics. Risk factors for postoperative infections include impaired host defenses, age greater than 60 years, hypoalbuminemia, inadequate bowel preparation, and spillage of colonic contents with bacterial contamination of the surgical wound.[32] The goal of surgical prophylaxis in colorectal surgery is to reduce the risk of wound contamination by bacteria spilled from the colon and rectum during the surgical procedure. This is accomplished most effectively by use of mechanical bowel preparation, preoperative oral antibiotics, and parenteral perioperative antibiotics.[33] Mechanical bowel preparation reduces fecal bulk but does not significantly alter the concentration of microorganisms in the stool and does not decrease surgical wound infection rates.[33] The addition of oral antibiotics (e.g., erythromycin and neomycin) to mechanical bowel preparation decreases postoperative infections and the addition of a perioperative parenteral cephalosporin, (e.g., cefoxitin, cefotetan, or cefmetazole) can further decrease postoperative infection rate to less than 10% for elective colorectal procedures.[34] The preferred prophylactic regimen would include the following: (a) 4 L of a polyethylene glycol-electrolyte lavage solution given the day prior to surgery, plus, (b) oral neomycin sulfate 1 g and erythromycin base 1 g given after the bowel preparation is completed at 1, 2, and 11 PM the day prior to surgery, plus, (c) cefoxitin, or similar agent, at induction of anesthesia.

GENITOURINARY PROCEDURES

Genitourinary procedures can be divided into two major classifications; transurethral procedures, and procedures performed through the abdomen or perineum. Transurethral procedures include: transurethral resection of the prostate (TURP), urethral dilatation, and renal calculi removal. Prostatectomy performed through the abdomen and perineum involve organisms similar to those encountered in colorectal procedures (refer to the Colorectal Procedures section for appropriate recommendations). The most common organisms encountered in transurethral procedures include enteric Gram-negative aerobes and enterococci. The most common postoperative infections in these procedures involve bacteriuria, and rarely bacteremia.[35] Numerous prophylactic antibiotics directed at enteric Gram-negative aerobes and enterococci have demonstrated efficacy in decreasing postoperative bacteriuria, including trimethoprim-sulfamethoxazole, fluorquinolones, cephalosporins, and aminoglycosides.[36] The current literature supports use of prophylactic antibiotics in high-risk patients with positive urine cultures or preoperative urinary catheters only.[37] Trimethoprim-sulfamethoxazole and the fluroquinolones appear to be equal to more broad-spectrum agents and should be used as first-line prophylactic agents. Duration of prophylaxis should be limited to one dose given orally 2 hours before the procedure.[38,39]

GYNECOLOGIC AND OBSTETRIC PROCEDURES

Cesarean Section. The risk of postoperative infection in cesarean section appears to be related to host factors and can be divided into high risk and low risk populations. High-risk patients are women who have not received prenatal care, are undernourished, undergo multiple vaginal examinations, have prolonged labor, and have undergone frequent invasive monitoring. The risk of postpartum endometritis is reported as high as 85% in the high-risk patient as opposed to 5% to 10% for the low-risk patient.[40] Appropriate prophylactic antibiotics can reduce the incidence of postoperative infection by 50% to 70% as documented by controlled clinical trials.[41] The preferred prophylactic regimen is cefazolin 1 g given after umbilical cord clamping. Administration of the drug after cord clamping is intended to minimize toxicity to the infant.

Hysterectomy. The incidence of postoperative infection following vaginal hysterectomy without prophylactic antibiotics is reported to be as high as 40%, whereas appropriate prophylactic antibiotics can reduce this incidence to less than 10%.[42] Risk factors for postoperative infection include: low socioeconomic status, extremes of age, obesity, diabetes, and prior instrumentation of the genitourinary tract. Postoperative infections are caused by a variety of aerobic and anaerobic organisms, with *Bacteroides* species being the predominant anaerobe. However, single-dose cefazolin has proven as effective as extended spectrum cephalosporins and is the preferred prophylactic agent.[42]

HEAD AND NECK PROCEDURES

Head and neck procedures should be divided into two categories: clean procedures where no transection of the oropharyngeal mucosa occurs, and clean-contaminated procedures where transection of the oropharyngeal tract does occur. Clean procedures include parotidectomy, thyroidectomy, and submandibular-gland excision. The infection rate for these procedures is low and routine prophylactic antibiotics are not recommended.[43] Clean-contaminated procedures performed without prophylactic antibiotics have produced surgical wound infection rates of 24% to 87% and appropriate perioperative antibiotics have been shown to reduce the postoperative infection rate by approximately 50%.[44] The predominate pathogens in clean-contaminated head and neck procedures are the normal flora of the mouth and oropharynx. Multiple prophylactic antibiotic regimens have been proven effective in reducing surgical wound infection rates; however, the preferred regimens are cefazolin 1 or 2 g plus clindamycin or clindamycin plus gentamicin. Metronidazole appears to be as effective against anaerobic bacteria as clindamycin and may be substituted. Ampicillin/sulbactam has been shown to be equal to standard regimens, although further study is required to identify the most optimal antibiotic prophylaxis in these operative procedures.[45] Duration of prophylactic antibiotics should not exceed 24 hours in these clean-contaminated cases.[46]

NEUROSURGICAL PROCEDURES

The benefit of prophylactic antibiotics has not been well documented in clean neurosurgical operations without shunt placement, but the practice is common. *S. aureus* and *S. epidermidis* are the predominant pathogens, with Gram-negative aerobes being somewhat more common in cerebrospinal fluid (CSF) shunt infections. A review of the literature published by Haines[47] supports the use of prophylactic antibiotics including cefazolin, cloxacillin, and vancomycin as monotherapy, and cefazolin plus gentamicin, and gentamicin plus vancomycin as combination therapy. These agents have been shown to reduce postoperative infection rates, but the choice of the most effective prophylactic agent remains difficult and should be based on the individual institution's antimicrobial sensitivities.[47–50] Limited data are available regarding CSF shunt procedures, but applying knowledge from other procedures involving prosthetic material would mandate the use of prophylactic antibiotics due to the extreme morbidity and mortality of postoperative infections associated with these procedures. From the available literature, cefazolin monotherapy appears effective in reducing the surgical wound infection rate in neurosurgical operations and should be considered the preferred prophylactic agent.

ORTHOPAEDIC PROCEDURES

As with the previously described operative procedures, orthopaedic procedures are clean and pose a low risk of infection; therefore no antibiotic prophylaxis is necessary in most operative procedures. However, the morbidity and mortality associated with prosthetic joint infections is extremely high and warrants the use of prophylactic antibiotics whenever prosthetic joints are placed. The most common pathogens are *S. aureus* and *S. epidermidis*. Cefazolin is the prophylactic agent of choice. It has significantly reduced postoperative infections, demonstrated adequate tissue and bone concentration, and posses a low risk of toxicity.[51] Duration of antibiotic prophylaxis is somewhat controversial, but prophylaxis greater than 48 hours after prosthetic device implantation offers no added benefit, therefore single-dose or short-term antibiotic prophylaxis is indicated.[51,52]

VASCULAR PROCEDURES

Like cardiac operations, noncardiac vascular procedures are classified as clean. The most common pathogens are *S. aureus* and *S. epidermidis*. The incidence of postoperative infection is increased with insertion of vascular prosthesis or in procedures involving the groin.[53–55] Several authors have demonstrated the efficacy of three-dose cefazolin prophylaxis and cefazolin remains the prophylactic agent of choice in these procedures.[54,55] Prophylactic antibiotics have not been shown to improve outcomes for carotid endarterectomy or brachial artery repair when prosthetic material is not inserted. Therefore, prophylactic antibiotics are not indicated for these operative procedures.[56,57] In institutions with a significant incidence of methicillin-resistant *S. aureus*, vancomycin is an acceptable alternative agent but Centers for Disease Control and Prevention (CDC) criteria should be followed.[58]

FUTURE THERAPIES

Our understanding of the issues of surgical antibiotic prophylaxis has increased significantly over the past 30 years. Issues remaining to be resolved include development of a better risk stratification system to identify those patients at highest risk of postoperative infections and improved therapeutic plans for those patients.[59] Further research is required to adequately assess the impact of surgical prophylaxis on the development of bacterial resistance.

IMPROVING OUTCOMES

Prophylactic antibiotics play a significant role in the perioperative management of surgical patients. The resultant decrease in postoperative infections serves to decrease morbidity and mortality, which in turn can limit the length of the hospital stay and decrease health care delivery costs in general. In utilizing antibiotic prophylaxis, however, several criteria should be emphasized to extend its safety and efficacy. First, pharmacists should actively involve themselves in the process to ensure the antibiotic's benefit outweigh the risk of treatment. Second, the pharmacist must be aware of the individual institution's bacterial resistance patterns to base antibiotic selection on appropriate spectrum of antimicrobial activity. Third, antibiotic administration should be scheduled so adequate tissue concentrations are achieved during the critical period, and postoperative duration of prophylaxis is limited to the shortest effective duration. By being aware of the above considerations and being actively involved in the medication use process, the pharmacist is well positioned to improve surgical antibiotic prophylaxis and help to ensure that a successful surgical result is realized.

KEY POINTS

- Identification of patients at risk for postoperative infection should be based on the surgical wound classification and the patient's specific risk factors for infection
- Antibiotics should be chosen that possess an antimicrobial spectrum of activity which adequately covers the microflora for each operative procedure

- Antimicrobial agents should be chosen which achieve adequate tissue concentrations at the surgical site and are effective against the most common pathogens
- The antimicrobial agent should be administered to maintain therapeutic tissue concentrations for the duration of the surgical procedure
- The timing of antimicrobial prophylaxis administration is critical. Antimicrobial agents should not be given as "on call" doses, but administered at the induction of anesthesia to provide effective concentrations during the procedure
- Antimicrobial agents should be administered for the shortest period of time proven effective in decreasing the rate of postoperative infections

REFERENCES

1. McGowan JE Jr. Cost and benefit of perioperative antimicrobial prophylaxis: methods for economic analysis. Rev Infect Dis 13 (Suppl 10): S879–S889, 1991.
2. Haley RW, Schaberg DR, Crossley KB, et al. Extra charges and prolongation of stay attributable to nosocomial infections: a prospective interhospital comparison. Am J Med 70:51–58, 1981.
3. Haley RW. Measuring the costs of nosocomial infections: methods for estimating economic burden on the hospital. Am J Med 91: 32S–38S, 1991.
4. Kernodle DS, Kaiser AB. Postoperative infections and antimicrobial prophylaxis. In: Mandell GL, Bennett JE, Dolin R. Principles and practice of infectious disease. 4th ed. New York: Churchill Livingstone, 1995:2742–2756.
5. Nichols RL. Surgical infections and choice of antibiotics. In: Sabiston DC. Sabiston's essentials of surgery. 1st ed. Philadelphia: W.B. Saunders Company, 1997:141–168.
6. Ad Hoc Committee of the Committee on Trauma, Division of Medical Sciences, National Academy of Sciences, National Research Council: Postoperative wound infections: the influence of ultraviolet irradiation of the operating room and various other factors. Ann Surg 160 (Suppl 2):23, 1964.
7. Farber BF, Kaiser DL, Wenzel RP. Relation between surgical volume and incidence of postoperative wound infection. N Engl J Med 305:200–204, 1981.
8. Page CP, Bohnen JM, Fletcher JR, et al. Antimicrobial prophylaxis for surgical wounds. Guidelines for clinical care. Arch Surg 128: 79–88, 1993.
9. DiPiro JT, Bowden TA Jr., Hooks VH III. Prophylactic parenteral cephalosporins in surgery. Are the newer agents better? JAMA 252: 3277–3279, 1984.
10. Burke JF. Effective period of preventive antibiotic action in experimental incisions and dermal lesions. Surgery 50:161, 1961.
11. Polk HC, Lopez-Mayor JF. Postoperative wound infection: a prospective study of determinant factors and prevention. Surgery 66: 97–103, 1969.
12. Guglielmo BJ, Salazar TA, Rodondi LC, et al. Altered pharmacokinetics of antibiotics during vascular surgery. Am J Surg 157: 410–412, 1989.
13. Classen DC, Evans RS, Pestotnik SL, et al. The timing of prophylactic administration of antibiotics and the risk of surgical-wound infection. N Engl J Med 326:281–286, 1992.
14. Guglielmo BJ, Hohn DC, Koo PJ, et al. Antibiotic prophylaxis in surgical procedures. A critical analysis of the literature. Arch Surg 118:943–955, 1983.
15. DiPiro JT, Cheung RP, Bowden TA Jr, et al. Single dose systemic antibiotic prophylaxis of surgical wound infections. Am J Surg 152: 552–559, 1986.
16. Slama TG, Sklar SJ, Misinki J, et al. Randomized comparison of cefamandole, cefazolin, and cefuroxime prophylaxis in open-heart surgery. Antimicrob Agents Chemother 29:744–747, 1986.

17. Conklin CM, Gray RJ, Neilson D, et al. Determinants of wound infection incidence after isolated coronary artery bypass surgery in patients randomized to receive prophylactic cefuroxime or cefazolin. Ann Thorac Surg 46:172–177, 1988.
18. Gentry LO, Zeluff BJ, Cooley DA. Antibiotic prophylaxis in openheart surgery: a comparison of cefamandole, cefuroxime, and cefazolin. Ann Thorac Surg 46:167–171, 1988.
19. Niederhauser U, Vogt M, Vogt P, et al. Cardiac surgery in a highrisk group of patients: is prolonged postoperative antibiotic prophylaxis effective? J Thorac Cardiovasc Surg 114:162–168, 1997.
20. Gatehouse D, Dimock F, Burdon DW, et al. Prediction of wound sepsis following gastric operations. Br J Surg 65:551–554, 1978.
21. Pories WJ, Van RA, Burlingham BT, et al. Prophylactic cefazolin in gastric bypass surgery. Surgery 90:426–432, 1981.
22. Lewis RT, Goodall RG, Marien B, et al. Efficacy and distribution of single dose preoperative antibiotic prophylaxis in high-risk gastroduodenal surgery. Can J Surg 34:117–122, 1991.
23. Cainzos M, Potel J, Puente JL. Prospective randomized controlled study of prophylaxis with cefamandole in high risk patients undergoing operations upon the biliary tract. Surg Gynecol Obstet 160:27–32, 1985.
24. Stone HH, Hooper CA, Kolb LD, et al. Antibiotic prophylaxis in gastric, biliary and colonic surgery. Ann Surg 184:443–452, 1976.
25. Chetlin SH, Elliot DW. Preoperative antibiotics in biliary surgery. Arch Surg 107:319–323, 1973.
26. Meijer WS, Schmitz PI, Jeekel J. Meta-analysis of randomized, controlled clinical trials of antibiotic prophylaxis in biliary tract surgery. Br J Surg 77:283–290, 1990.
27. Bauer T, Vennits B, Holm B, et al. Antibiotic prophylaxis in acute nonperforated appendicitis. The Danish Multi-center Study Group III. Ann Surg 209:307–311, 1989.
28. Winslow RE, Dean RE, Harley JW. Acute nonperforating appendicitis. Efficacy of brief antibiotic prophylaxis. Arch Surg 118:651–655, 1983.
29. Donovan IA, Ellis D, Gatehouse D, et al. One-dose antibiotic prophylaxis against wound infection after appendicectomy: a randomized trial of clindamycin, cefazolin sodium and a placebo. Br J Surg 66:193–196, 1979.
30. Salam IM, Abu Galala KH, el Ashaal YI, et al. A randomized prospective study of cefoxitin versus piperacillin in appendectomy. J Hosp Infect 26:133–136, 1994.
31. Panichi G, Pantosti AL, Marsiglio F, et al. Cephalothin or cefoxitin in appendectomy? J Antimicrob Chemother 6:801–804, 1980.
32. Nichols RL. Prophylaxis for elective bowel surgery. In: Wilson SE, Williams RA, Finegold S. Intra-abdominal infections. New York: McGraw Hill, 1982:267–285.
33. Bartlett JG, Condon RE, Gorbach SL, et al. Veterans Administration Cooperative Study on bowel preparation for elective colorectal operations: impact of oral antibiotic regimen on colonic flora, wound irrigation cultures and bacteriology of septic complications. Ann Surg 188:249–254, 1978.
34. Stellato TA, Danziger LH, Gordon N, et al. Antibiotics in elective colon surgery: a randomized trial of oral, systemic, and oral/systemic antibiotics for prophylaxis. Am Surg 56:251–254, 1990.
35. Taha SA, Sayed AAK, Grant C, et al. Risk factors in wound infection following urologic operations: a prospective study. Int Surg 77:128–130, 1992.
36. Hall JC, Christiansen KJ, England P, et al. Antibiotic prophylaxis for patients undergoing transurethral resection of the prostate. Urology 47:852–856, 1996.
37. Berry A, Barratt A. Prophylactic antibiotic use in transurethral prostatic resection: a meta-analysis. J Urol 167:571–577, 2002.
38. Antimicrobial prophylaxis in surgery. Treatment Guidelines from The Medical Letter 2:27–32, 2004.
39. ASHP therapeutic guidelines on antimicrobial prophylaxis in surgery. American Society of Health-System Pharmacists Best Practices for Health-System Pharmacy, 2003–2004 ed. Bethesda, MD, 2004:405–452.
40. Anstey JT, Sheldon GW, Blyth JG. Infectious morbidity after primary cesarean section in a private institution. Am J Obstet Gynecol 136:205–210, 1980.
41. Mugford M, Kingston J, Chalmers I. Reducing the incidence of infection after caesarean section: implications of prophylaxis with antibiotics for hospital resources. BMJ 299:1003–1006, 1989.
42. Soper DE, Yarwood RL. Single-dose antibiotic prophylaxis in women undergoing vaginal hysterectomy. Obstet Gynecol 69:879–882, 1987.
43. Johnson JT, Wagner RL. Infection following uncontaminated head and neck surgery. Arch Otolaryngol Head Neck Surg 113:368–369, 1987.
43. Friberg D, Lundberg C. Antibiotic prophylaxis in major head and neck surgery when clean-contaminated wounds are established. Scand J Infect Dis (Suppl 70):87–90, 1990.
45. Weber RS. Wound infection in head and neck surgery: implications for perioperative antibiotic treatment. Ear Nose Throat J 76:795–798, 1997.
46. Righi M. Short-term versus long-term antimicrobial prophylaxis in oncologic head and neck surgery. Head Neck 18:399–404, 1996.
47. Haines SJ. Efficacy of antibiotic prophylaxis in clean neurosurgical operations. Neurosurgery 24:401–405, 1989.
48. Geraghty J, Feely M. Antibiotic prophylaxis in neurosurgery. A randomized control trial. J Neurosurg 60:724–726, 1984.
49. Bullock R, van Dellen JR, Ketelbey W, et al. A double-blind placebo-controlled trial of perioperative prophylactic antibiotics for elective neurosurgery. J Neurosurg 69:687–691, 1988.
50. van Ek B, Dijkmans BA, van Dulken H, et al. Effect of cloxacillin prophylaxis on the bacterial flora of craniotomy wounds. Scand J Infect Dis 22:345–352, 1990.
51. Van Meirhaeghe J, Verdonk R, Verschraegen G, et al. Flucloxacillin compared with cefazolin in short-term prophylaxis for clean orthopaedic surgery. Arch Orthop Trauma Surg 108:308–313, 1989.
52. Nelson CL. Prevention of sepsis. Clin Orthop 222:66–72, 1987.
53. Szilagyi DE, Smith RF, Elliott JP, et al. Infection in arterial reconstruction with synthetic grafts. Ann Surg 186:321–333, 1972.
54. Goldstone J, Moore WS. Infection in vascular prostheses: clinical manifestations and surgical management. Am J Surg 128:225–233, 1974.
55. Landreneau MD, Raju S. Infections after elective bypass surgery for lower limb ischemia: the influence of preoperative transcutaneous arteriography. Surgery 90:956–961, 1981.
56. Kaiser AB, Clayson KR, Mulherin JL Jr, et al. Antibiotic prophylaxis in vascular surgery. Ann Surg 188:283–289, 1978.
57. Pitt HA, Postier RG, MacGowan AW, et al. Prophylactic antibiotics in vascular surgery: topical, systemic, or both? Ann Surg 192:356–364, 1980.
58. Mangram AJ, Horan TC, Pearson ML, et al. Guidelines for the prevention of surgical site infection, 1999. Infect Control Hosp Epidemiol 20:247–278, 1999.
59. Nichols RL. Surgical infections: prevention and treatment 1965 to 1995. Am J Surg 172:68–74, 1996.

Infections in the Immunocompromised Patient

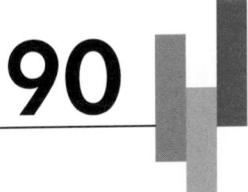

90

Russell E. Lewis

Infectious complications remain a significant cause of morbidity and death in the immunocompromised population. The risk of infection in the immunocompromised patient is largely determined by (a) the net state of immunosuppression, (b) epidemiologic exposures encountered by the patient, and (c) consequences of procedures and drug therapies to which the patient is subjected. This chapter will highlight the general concepts and the approaches toward the management of infection in the immunocompromised host. Special focus will be directed at pathogens that arise with various types of immune suppression as well as empiric strategies for managing these infections.

TREATMENT GOALS

- Identify inherited and acquired risk factors for infection in the immunosuppressed patient.
- Identify the most common bacterial, viral, and fungal pathogens in immunocompromised patients.
- Describe the temporal pattern of opportunistic infections in febrile neutropenia and after solid organ or hematopoietic stem cell transplantation.
- Understand general principles of antiinfective therapy in the immunocompromised patient.
- Provide specific indications requiring modification of empiric antibacterial, antifungal, or antiviral therapy.
- Describe indications for prophylactic or preemptive versus empiric therapy in immunocompromised hosts.

Advances in the fields of oncology, transplantation, and critical care have made possible the support of critically ill and severely immunosuppressed patients for progressively longer periods of time. With this improved prognosis, however, comes an increased opportunity for patients to acquire life-threatening infections from a widening spectrum of bacterial, viral, and fungal pathogens. Consequently, infection remains the most formidable complication encountered in immunocompromised patients. Experience gained over the past half-century in the diagnosis, prevention, and treatment of infections in patients with inherited or acquired immunodeficiency has clarified the relationship between the type and degree of immunosuppression and the most likely pathogens. Indeed, the tempo, timing, and susceptibility of immunocompromised patients to infection can often be anticipated and treated empirically to reduce the patient's risk of dying from an undiagnosed infection. This chapter will highlight the general concepts and treatment approach toward empiric therapy of infection in the immunocompromised host. Special emphasis will be placed on pathogens associated with specific types of immune deficits in patients.

DEFINING IMMUNOSUPPRESSION

Infection is the result of a negative balance between the capacity of host immune defenses and the virulence of invading microorganisms.[1] An intact immune system provides protection against most microbial invaders through a coordinated and highly interrelated system of mucocutaneous barriers, specialized immune cells, and soluble factors that compose the innate and adaptive arms of the host immune response. An immunocompromised state arises when these protective barriers are breached and/or essential immune cells are absent or functionally impaired. The most common factors leading to defective immune cell responses include inherited or acquired diseases of the immune system, cancer and its treatment, infection, poor nutritional status or metabolic disturbances, and immunosuppressive drug therapy (Fig. 90.1).

Theoretically, impairment of a specific component of the immune system should predispose a patient to the very pathogens that are eradicated by that particular host defense mechanism.[1] However, isolated defects in the immune system are the exception rather than the rule. Therefore, the first step in evaluating the risk of an immunocompromised host for infection is to define the "net immunosuppressive state" of the patient.[2] For most patients, the net immunosuppressive state is a function of (a) the dose, duration, and sequence of immunosuppressive drug therapy, (b) the presence or absence of leukopenia, (c) breaches to the integrity of the mucocutaneous barriers to infection, (d) the presence of devitalized tissue or undrained fluid collections, (e) the presence or absence of protein-calorie malnutrition, uremia, hyperglycemia, or acidosis, and (f) the presence or absence of infection with at least of the known immunomodulating viruses (cytomegalovirus, herpesvirus, Epstein-Barr virus, hepatitis B or C, and HIV).[2] Defining the net immunosuppressive state of the patient allows a clinician to devise an appropriate differential diagnosis of potential pathogens, which can be reconciled with the patient's signs and symptoms (if present) and possible epidemiologic exposures to provide appropriate antimicrobial therapy.

As the net state of immunosuppression increases, the spectrum of potential pathogens widens, as does the difficulty in establishing an early and accurate diagnosis of infection. Severely immunocompromised patients often present with multiple infections during a single clinical episode that may not be initially detectable by laboratory and radiographic studies. Broad empiric therapy, accomplished with

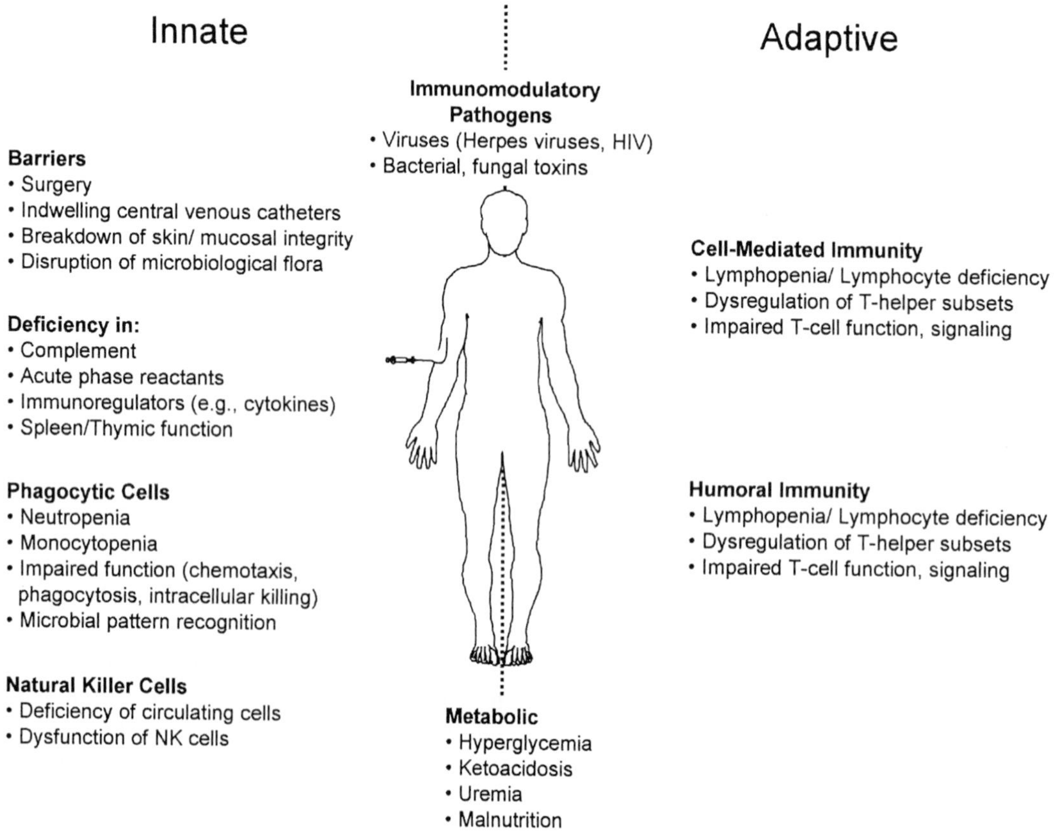

Innate

Adaptive

Immunomodulatory Pathogens
- Viruses (Herpes viruses, HIV)
- Bacterial, fungal toxins

Barriers
- Surgery
- Indwelling central venous catheters
- Breakdown of skin/ mucosal integrity
- Disruption of microbiological flora

Deficiency in:
- Complement
- Acute phase reactants
- Immunoregulators (e.g., cytokines)
- Spleen/Thymic function

Phagocytic Cells
- Neutropenia
- Monocytopenia
- Impaired function (chemotaxis, phagocytosis, intracellular killing)
- Microbial pattern recognition

Natural Killer Cells
- Deficiency of circulating cells
- Dysfunction of NK cells

Cell-Mediated Immunity
- Lymphopenia/ Lymphocyte deficiency
- Dysregulation of T-helper subsets
- Impaired T-cell function, signaling

Humoral Immunity
- Lymphopenia/ Lymphocyte deficiency
- Dysregulation of T-helper subsets
- Impaired T-cell function, signaling

Metabolic
- Hyperglycemia
- Ketoacidosis
- Uremia
- Malnutrition

FIGURE 90.1 Types of host immunosuppression.

combinations of antibacterial, antifungal, and antiviral agents, may be necessary in patients with the most severe and complex immune deficits.

OVERVIEW OF COMPONENTS OF IMMUNE DYSFUNCTION AND INFECTION

THE INTEGUMENT AND MUCOCUTANEOUS BARRIERS TO INFECTION

The skin, respiratory tract, ears, conjunctiva, and alimentary and genitourinary tracts are in constant contact with the environment and serve as the first line of defense against microbial invasion. This defense is accomplished through several mechanisms, including colonization with commensal bacteria and fungi that compete for nutrients and space with more virulent organisms (colonization resistance); maintenance of an acidic environment in the stomach, vagina, and outer skin layers; production of saliva, mucus, digestive enzymes, bile salts, and secreted immunoglobulins (IgA) that enhance the trapping, killing, and removal of organisms from mucocutaneous barriers; and the continuous mechanical measures (mucociliary clearance, sneezing, coughing, peristalsis, micturition) that aid in elimination of unattached microorganisms. Breaches of the mucocutaneous barriers are often iatrogenic due to medical devices (central venous catheters, Foley catheters, and endotracheal tubes), procedures (surgery), and therapies (chemotherapy and radiation) that damage mucosal barriers.

The use of indwelling central venous catheters has increased considerably over the past two decades, and they are considered an essential component in the care of patients undergoing intensive medical or surgical procedures.[3] The benefits and convenience of prolonged indwelling central venous access, however, are offset by an increased risk of bloodstream infection with skin flora, especially *Staphylococcus* spp, that readily colonize the catheter hub and lumen.[3] Catheter-related bloodstream infections (CRBSI) affect 4% to 8% of all patients with indwelling central venous catheters; this is one of the most common sites of infection in immunocompromised patients.[3]

Once established, CRBSI are difficult to treat without removal of the catheter, especially if the catheter is colonized with *Staphylococcus aureus*, *Candida* spp, or *Pseudomonas aeruginosa*.[4] Colonization of catheters and/or infection with lower-virulence organisms such as coagulase-negative staphylococcus or *Corynebacterium* may be amenable to antibiotic therapy alone without catheter removal.[4] However, relapse is seen in up to 20% of patients with CRBSI caused by less virulent organisms, thus underscoring the need to restore normal protective barriers to prevent recurrent infection.[5]

Chemotherapy and radiation therapy are especially damaging to host integument and mucosal barriers.[6] This damage may range from superficial hair loss, skin dryness, and de-

creased sweat production to direct and extensive injury of the mucocutaneous barrier in the oral cavity and gastrointestinal (GI) and respiratory tract. Mucositis is a clinical manifestation of chemotherapy or radiation-induced mucosal barrier injury in the oral cavity and GI tract. Damage to the mucosal barrier in these areas allows the direct invasion of endogenous microflora of the upper GI tract, including *Viridans* streptococci and Enterobacteriaceae as well as lower GI organisms such as anaerobes (*Clostridium* spp, *Bacteroides* spp), *Enterococcus* spp, *Stomatococcus mucilaginosa*, and *Capnocytophaga gingivalis* into the bloodstream and internal organs.[1,6] Chemotherapy- and radiation-induced damage to mucosal barriers can also induce reactivation of latent herpesvirus infection and ulceration, which serves as an additional portal of invasion for the endogenous flora (Table 90.1).

NEUTROPENIA

Neutrophils form the major type of leukocytes in peripheral blood, with counts ranging between 40% to 70% of leukocytes under normal conditions.[7] Neutrophils are also called polymorphonuclear (PMN) leukocytes or granulocytes, but the latter designation also includes neutrophilic granulocytes (neutrophils), eosinophilic granulocytes (eosinophils), and basophilic granulocytes (basophils). Neutrophils protect the human body from bacterial and fungal infections.[7] For neutrophils to be effective, they must be generated and released from the bone marrow in adequate numbers, migrate to the site of infection, and efficiently phagocytose and kill invading organisms.

Neutropenia ($<$1,000 cells/mm^3) due to underlying disease or the myelotoxic effects of chemotherapy is one of the most common forms of immunosuppression that predisposes patients to infection. The potential for infection is proportional to the rate and degree of decline of the absolute neutrophil count (ANC), which is obtained by multiplying the number of leukocytes by the percentage of circulating neutrophils. As the total neutrophil count falls below 500 cells per mm^3, the risk of infection increases (Fig. 90.2, Table 90.2).[8] A rapid drop in neutrophil counts is frequently associated with life-threatening bacterial or fungal infection.[8,9] As the duration of neutropenia increases (i.e., ANC $<$100 cells/mm^3 for $>$10 days), the spectrum and severity of infections also increase. Prolonged episodes of drug-induced myelosuppression (neutropenia lasting $>$27 days) are most commonly seen in patients receiving accelerated, salvage chemotherapy for either relapsed or refractory cancer.[10] These patients are at a high risk for death due to bacterial or fungal infection.

Functional defects in neutrophil migration, phagocytosis, and killing can also be inherited (i.e., chronic granulomatous disease) or arise secondary to drug and/or radiation therapy. Despite increasing peripheral neutrophil counts, adrenal corticosteroids are known to impair many aspects of neutrophil function, including migration, phagolysosome fusion, and intracellular killing.[7,11] Other factors such as prolonged hy-

TABLE 90.1	Defects in Host Immunity and Their Common Associated Infections	
Component	**Common Defects or Conditions**	**Increased Susceptibility to Infections Caused by:**
Anatomic barriers		
Skin	*Primary defects*: tumors, skin diseases	*Staphylococcus* spp. *Streptococcus* spp. *Corynebacterium*
	Secondary defects: skin puncture, surgery, vascular catheters, wound dressing, radiation therapy, trauma (hematoma), burns	*Pseudomonas aeruginosa* *Candida* spp
Mucous membranes	*Primary defects:* tumors, ulceration (aphthae, mucositis, herpes virus infection, adenovirus) *Secondary defects:* chemotherapy, radiation therapy, bleeding, surgery, urinary tract catheters, esophageal stents, loss of gag reflex	*Viridans* streptococci Coagulase-negative staphylococci *Enterococcus* spp Anaerobes, including *Clostridium difficile* Enterobacteriaceae *Pseudomonas* spp Herpes simplex virus *Candida* spp
Innate Immunity Complement	Primary complement deficiencies or plasma/membrane protein regulating complement activation	*Streptococcus pneumoniae* *Haemophilus influenzae* *Neisseria meningitidis* *Staphylococcus aureus* *Pseudomonas aeruginosa*
Cells Leukocytes	*Quantitative defects* (granulocytopenia <1,000/mL): cyclic neutropenia, aplastic anemia, myelodysplastic syndromes, hypersplenism *Iatrogenic quantitative defects*: chemotherapy, radiation therapy, immune-mediated (drugs, leukemia, lymphoma)	*Viridans* streptococci *Staphylococcus aureus* Coagulase-negative staphylococci Gram-negative bacilli (Enterobacteriaceae, *Pseudomonas* spp) *Candida* spp *Aspergillus* spp and other molds
	Primary qualitative defects: diabetes mellitus, leukocyte adhesion deficiency, chronic granulomatous disease, Chediak-Higashi syndrome, Job syndrome, various deficiencies of oxidative and nonoxidative killing mechanisms	Similar to quantitative defects
	Secondary qualitative defects: High-dose corticosteroid therapy, chemotherapy, radiation therapy	Similar to quantitative defects
Adaptive immunity Cellular immunity	*Primary defects:* Severe combined immunodeficiency (SCID), bare lymphocyte syndrome, CD3$^+$, CD4$^+$, and CD8$^+$ deficiency, natural killer cell deficiency, T-cell signaling deficiency, Wiskott-Aldrich syndrome, malignancies	Bacteria: *Mycobacterium tuberculosis* Atypical mycobacteria *Legionella* spp *Listeria monocytogenes* *Salmonella typhi* Viruses: Herpes simplex virus Varicella virus Cytomegalovirus Epstein-Barr virus Adenovirus Fungi: *Candida* spp Endemic fungi (*Histoplasma capsulatum,* *Blastomycosis dermatitidis,* *Coccidioidomycosis immitis*), *Cryptococcus neoformans* *Pneumocystis jirovecii* (*carinii*) Parasites: *Toxoplasma gondii* *Cryptosporidium* spp *Leishmania*
	Secondary defects: Immunosuppressive therapy (corticosteroids, cyclosporine, tacrolimus, methotrexate, antithymocyte globulin, anti-T-cell monoclonal antibodies, tumor necrosis factor blockers), viral infections (HIV, CMV, EBV, HHV-6, influenza, RSV, measles), parasite infections (leishmaniasis, leprosy, malaria), chemotherapy, bone marrow transplantation, therapy, malnutrition	

(continues)

TABLE 90.1	continued	
Component	Common Defects or Conditions	Increased Susceptibility to Infections Caused by:

Humoral immunity	*Primary defects*
	X-linked agammaglobulinemia
	Hypogammaglobinemia
	Severe combined immunodeficiency
	Wiskott-Aldridge syndrome
	Selective IgA and IgG deficiency
	Secondary defects
	Malignancies (multiple myeloma, Waldenström
	  disease, chronic lymphocytic leukemia, lymphoma,
	  nephritic syndromes, severe burns, splenectomy,
	  hematopoietic cell transplantation
		Streptococcus pneumoniae
		Other streptococci
		Haemophilus influenzae
		Neisseria meningitidis

poxia, acidosis, hypovolemic states, and hyperglycemia can result in dysfunctional neutrophils and increase the risk of infection.[12,13] Recovery of neutrophil counts and function is essential for full recovery from infection in neutropenic hosts.[8,9]

The most prevalent causes of infection in neutropenic patients vary with the duration of neutropenia (Table 90.1). In early phase of neutropenia (<10 days), bacteremia arising from endogenous colonized sources, including the central venous catheter and/or damaged GI mucosa, is the most likely source of infection. Historically, gram-negative bacteria represented over 70% of infections associated with neutropenic fever.[9,14,15] The widespread use of antibacterial prophylactic regimens with activity against gram-negative bacteria, particularly fluoroquinolones or trimethoprim-sulfamethoxazole (TMP-SMX), however, shifted the spectrum of bloodstream pathogens towards gram-positives as the most common bloodstream pathogens.[14,16] *S. aureus*, coagulase-negative staphylococcus, and α-hemolytic streptococci are now the predominant bacteria isolated from the bloodstream in neutropenic patients.[17,18] Occasionally, resistant gram-positive (i.e., vancomycin-resistant enterococci) or gram-negative organisms (*Stenotrophomonas maltophilia*) may arise following prophylactic use of broad-spectrum antimicrobials.[16] Therefore, prior antibiotic therapy must always be considered with the possible etiologies

of infection in a neutropenic patient on broad-spectrum prophylaxis.

During the second and third weeks of neutropenia (phase II), yeasts emerge as a prominent cause of infection in patients who are not receiving fluconazole prophylaxis.[16,18] Even in patients who do receive prophylaxis, breakthrough infections with non-*albicans* species that are less susceptible (*C. glabrata*) or inherently resistant to fluconazole (*C. krusei*) are possible. Less commonly, amphotericin B-resistant yeasts such as *Trichosporon beigelii*, *Rhodotorula* spp, and *Clavispora* are seen. *Candida* is the fourth most common bloodstream pathogen in U.S. hospitals and is associated with higher rates of crude mortality than common bacterial species, including *P. aeruginosa*.[19] Although *Candida* are not particularly fastidious organisms, the sensitivity of blood cultures is relatively poor (<60%) and a negative culture does not rule out infection. Therefore, empiric antifungal therapy is generally recommended in neutropenic patients with persistent fever and neutropenia lasting more than 10 days.[16]

As neutropenia extends beyond the third week (phase III), opportunistic mold infections such as invasive aspergillosis, invasive fusariosis, or zygomycosis become more prominent.[16,20] Patients with prolonged neutropenia and long-term exposure to high dosages of adrenal corticosteroids are at the highest risk for developing infections with invasive molds due to deficient or poorly functioning lines of cellular defense in the lung.[21,22] Specifically, pulmonary alveolar macrophages are needed to clear fungal conidia that are ubiquitous in the environment and continuously inhaled by patients.[21,22] Conidia that are not cleared by macrophages can germinate into hyphal forms that invade blood vessels or contiguous tissues or bone (if in the sinuses), resulting in hemorrhage and/or infarction, and coagulative necrosis. Neutrophils are essential for killing and controlling the hyphal form of invasive molds in tissue. Without neutrophils, hyphae can spread in the bloodstream to distal organs including the skin, brain, liver, kidney, and heart.[23] Mortality rates of invasive mold infections approach 100% in patients who do not recover from neutropenia during active infection.[24,25] Management of invasive mold infections is complicated by

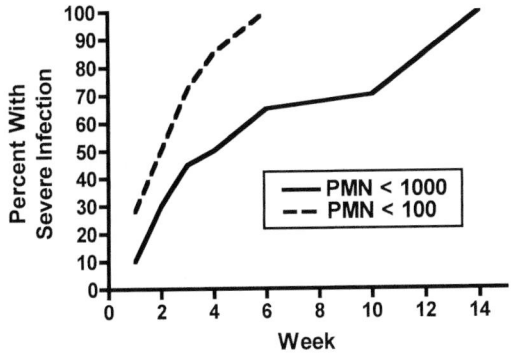

FIGURE 90.2 Relationship of neutrophil count and infection.

TABLE 90.2	Frequency of Clinical Manifestation of Infection Related to Absolute Neutrophil Count (ANC)		
Signs and Symptoms	ANC <100/mm³	ANC 101–1,000/mm³	ANC >1,000/mm³
Fever	98	90	76
Fluctuance	6	36	52
Fissure/Ulceration	21	42	54
Exudate	11	64	91
Purulent sputum	8	67	84
Pyuria	11	63	97

(Adapted from Burroughs L, Storb R. Low-intensity allogeneic hematopoietic stem cell transplantation for myeloid malignancies: separating graft-versus-leukemia effects from graft-versus-host disease. Curr Opin Hematol 12:45–54, 2005.)

the difficulty in establishing a definitive diagnosis, which requires a tissue biopsy of the lung, that is not medically feasible in many neutropenic patients with thrombocytopenia. Respiratory cultures and high-resolution computed tomographic (CT) scanning (to look for early evidence of hemorrhagic necrosis) are used to detect early forms of fungal pneumonia. In some centers, non-culture-based diagnostic strategies such as detection of *Aspergillus* cell wall antigens (i.e., galactomannan, β1,3 glucan) or fungal nucleic acid detection by polymerase chain reaction (PCR) are used as an aid to early diagnosis.[26] However, culturing is still required to confirm the mold species. Some *Aspergillus* spp, *Fusarium* spp, and Zygomycetes exhibit resistance to commonly used antifungals such as amphotericin B, caspofungin, itraconazole, and voriconazole.[26] Because of the high mortality associated with these infections, immunocompromised patients on fluconazole with sinus or pulmonary disease consistent with hemorrhage and necrosis are often considered to have invasive mold infections until proven otherwise.

DEFECTS IN CELL-MEDIATED IMMUNITY

Defects in the interaction of thymus-derived lymphocytes (T lymphocytes) and cells of the mononuclear phagocytic system (monocytes, macrophages, and dendritic cells) can predispose patients to severe and recurrent infections with viruses, facultative intracellular bacteria, fungi, and certain parasites (Table 90.1).[1,20] As with neutrophils, impairments in cell-mediated immune function can be quantitative (i.e., absolute lymphopenia secondary to chemotherapy or AIDS) or qualitative (defective cytokine production, antigen presentation). Inherited defects in cell-mediated immunity, such as severe combined immunodeficiency syndrome (SCID), often present shortly after birth with recurrent infections, failure to thrive, and unexpected infections after vaccination of the infant with attenuated live-virus vaccines. Certain cancers such as lymphocytic leukemia, Hodgkin's disease, hairy cell leukemia, lymphoma, and adult T-cell leukemia predispose patients to cellular immune dysfunction. Antineoplastic chemotherapy, particularly with the lymphoablative agents fludarabine, cladribine, and anti-T-cell antibodies (e.g.,

antithymocyte globulin, alemtuzumab), profoundly and persistently suppress T-cell function.[6] Adrenal corticosteroids and drugs used to prevent rejection of transplanted organs (cyclosporine, tacrolimus, mycophenolate) or graft-versus-host disease (GvHD) following allogeneic hematopoietic stem cell transplantation (Allo-HSCT) act primarily by suppressing the T-cell signaling necessary for antigen-specific cell-mediated immune response. In general, the patient's risk of developing opportunistic infections can largely be predicted by the dose, duration, and sequence of drug therapies required after transplantation to manage organ rejection or GvHD.

Because of the critical role of CD4+/CD8+ T-helper lymphocytes in the control of viral infection, patients with cell-mediated immune dysfunction are at high risk for reactivation of viral hepatitis and herpesvirus.[20] Patients with hematologic malignancies or with high-grade relapsed lymphoma frequently experience reactivation of herpes simplex type 1 or 2 virus (HSV), which can lead to severe buccal or perianal mucocutaneous ulcers that serve as a portal of entry for GI flora colonizing the mucosal surfaces.[27–29] The use of prophylactic acyclovir (or other similar antivirals) during periods of anticipated lymphopenia has been shown to reduce morbidity associated with HSV reactivation.[30] Reactivation of varicella-zoster virus (VZV; herpesvirus 3) may occur in patients with Hodgkin's disease receiving chemotherapy and radiation therapy and is associated with a meningoencephalitis-type presentation.[31,32] Reactivation of Epstein-Barr virus (EBV; herpesvirus 4) is less common, although viral shedding can be detected after HSCT transplantation.[33] On the other hand, cytomegalovirus (CMV; herpesvirus 5) infections are common and typically present as an interstitial pneumonia or enterocolitis.[27,34] In patients with AIDS, the most common form of CMV disease is retinitis. Although several antivirals with good activity against CMV are available (i.e., ganciclovir, foscarnet, cidofovir), treatment outcomes of CMV are generally poor once infection is established in the lungs. Therefore, management of CMV infection emphasizes a prophylactic or preemptive treatment approach based on the detection of viral antigen (pp65) of CMV or nucleic acid by PCR assay in the bloodstream of patients with suppressed cellular immunity during a period of viral shedding or replication before the infection reaches the target organ.[34] Antiviral therapy is generally initiated at the first sign of antigen or PCR positivity to suppress viral replication before development of a severe infection. This preemptive therapeutic approach also minimizes patient exposure to antivirals that are toxic to the bone marrow (ganciclovir) or kidneys (foscarnet, cidofovir).

Other herpesviruses are occasionally encountered after transplantation. Reactivation of human herpesvirus 6 (HHV 6; cause of exanthem subitum or sixth disease in children) is associated with encephalitis and possibly pneumonitis in transplant recipients.[20,27] Reactivation of herpesvirus 8 in patients with AIDS is associated with the development of Kaposi's sarcoma.[20,27]

Depending on the time of year and exposures, patients with impaired cellular immunity can develop severe pneumonia caused by community respiratory viruses including influenza, parainfluenza, and respiratory syncytial virus (RSV).[35] Typically, patients with upper respiratory symptoms are screened by nasal aspirate or wash and examination for viral respiratory antigens. If viral antigens are detected, antiviral therapy for influenza A and B (e.g., oseltamivir + rimantadine) or RSV (ribavirin ± palivizumab) is initiated to reduce the risk of severe lower respiratory tract infection. In the case of an influenza or RSV epidemic, antiviral therapy prophylaxis may be administered to select high-risk patients.[35]

Primary infection or reactivation of adenovirus as well as JC and BK polyomaviruses has been reported more frequently in oncology transplantation centers with the increasing use of lymphoablative chemotherapy.[36,37] Adenovirus and BK virus have been associated with acute hemorrhagic cystitis following HSCT.[36] JC virus infection is associated with a demyelinating disease in the cerebral hemispheres called progressive multifocal leukoencephalopathy (PML). Unfortunately, antiviral therapy has not been shown to be particularly effective for adenovirus or polyomavirus infections, although cidofovir is often administered based on in vitro studies and clinical case reports.[38]

Mycobacterial infections are another common pathogen complication in patients with prolonged lymphopenia, and may present in a similar fashion to fungal infections. Persistent fever is often the only clinical marker of disseminated infection caused by M. tuberculosis, M. avium-intracellulare complex, M. kansasii, or M. cheloni.[39,40] The most common sites of infection include the lung, liver, spleen, and bone marrow.[39] The standard approach for screening patients for exposure to M. tuberculosis, the tuberculin skin test, is unlikely to be positive in patients with impaired cellular immunity despite active infection.

Impaired cellular immune defenses can also predispose patients to fungal infections caused by Cryptococcus neoformans and molds. Candida infections may also appear but are typically restricted to mucosal disease.[22] Mold infections generally begin with paranasal sinus infection or in the lung with peripheral, pleural-based dense alveolar infiltrates or nodules accompanied by fever. Dissemination to the skin or brain is not uncommon and is associated with high mortality.[20] As discussed previously, diagnosis of the mold to the species level is critical for the selection of appropriate antifungal therapy.[41] Profound defects in cellular immunity also predispose patients to pulmonary Pneumocystis jirovecii (formally carinii) pneumonia (PCP). Progressive dyspnea with exertion, nonproductive cough, and interstitial infiltrates are the hallmarks of PCP.[42] The diagnosis is typically established by bronchioalveolar lavage, where the cyst form of the organisms can be easily recovered. Although P. jirovecii is classified as a fungus, the treatment of choice is high-dose (15 mg/kg/day) TMP-SMX and corticosteroids in patients with severe (Pao_2 <70 mm Hg) hypoxia.[43]

Nocardia spp (N. asteroides, N. brasiliensis, N. nova, N. farcinica) are acid-fast gram-positive rods from the soil that can cause infection in patients with suppressed cellular immunity, especially following prolonged, high-dose adrenal corticosteroid therapy.[44] Nocardiosis generally presents as an ill-defined lung nodule accompanied by fever. Dissemination to the central nervous system (CNS) is not uncommon and can result in single or multiple brain abscesses.[44] Bacteremia with N. asteroides can be associated with a high mortality rate, with nearly one third of patients having concurrent gram-negative bacteremia.[45] TMP-SMX or carbapenems with or without amikacin are considered first-line treatment options for nocardiosis, although minocycline and linezolid also have activity and the latter agent is a useful alternative in patients with CNS disease who cannot tolerate sulfa drugs.[44]

Listeriosis is an infrequent but serious infection in patients with impaired cellular immunity caused by the facultative bacterium Listeria monocytogenes.[46,47] The most common presentation is bacteremia; however, meningitis and meningoencephalitis are also seen in patients with cellular defects due to cancer chemotherapy, malnutrition, or an immature immune system (i.e., neonates).[46,47] Importantly, L. monocytogenes is not covered by empiric cephalosporin or carbapenem therapy. High-dose TMP-SMX and ampicillin plus gentamicin are considered first-line therapies for listeriosis.[48]

DEFECTS IN HUMORAL IMMUNITY

Immunoglobulins play a critical role in combating infections against encapsulated bacteria such as Streptococcus pneumonia, Neisseria meningitidis, and Haemophilus influenzae by binding to organisms and rendering them susceptible to phagocytosis.[49] Immunoglobulins also induce lysis of S. aureus and Streptococcus pyogenes by interacting with complement that becomes deposited on the bacterial cell wall. Immunoglobulins can also activate lymphocytes via the FC receptor to initiate a process called antibody-dependent cellular cytotoxicity, which plays a key role in eliminating cells infected with facultative organisms or parasites.[49] Patients with primary immunoglobulin deficiencies or B-cell cancers (multiple myeloma, Waldenström's macroglobulinemia) are susceptible to fulminant infection caused by encapsulated organisms (Table 90.1).[50] Hypogammaglobinemia is also seen in patients with chronic lymphocytic leukemia or following allo-HSCT. Occasionally gram-negative organisms such as *Salmonella* spp and *Campylobacter* spp cause life-threatening sepsis in patients with hypogammaglobinemia.[20,50]

Splenectomy is often indicated in patients with traumatic injury to the spleen, immune thrombocytopenic purpura (ITP) unresponsive to medical management, or hematologic malignancies resulting in massive splenomegaly. The spectrum of infections following splenectomy is essentially identical to patients with hypogammaglobinemia (Table 90.1).[20,50]

SOLID ORGAN TRANSPLANTATION

The incidence of infection following solid organ transplantation varies widely depending on the type of organ transplanted, the technical or surgical complexity of the transplant surgery, and the need for additional antirejection therapy.[51] Another major factor in the development of infection is the possible exposure to a donor pathogen when the recipient is at risk for primary infection (e.g., develops primary CMV infection from a donor organ). The timing of infection after organ transplantation is generally determined by several factors, including surgical complications, level of immunosuppression, and environmental and epidemiologic exposures. The risk periods for infection can be classified into three phases: the first month (early postoperative period), the second to the sixth month, and the late posttransplant period.[51]

Most infections in the first month after transplantation are related to surgical complications (Fig. 90-3A). They include bacterial and *Candida* wound infections, pneumonia, urinary tract infections, intravascular catheter sepsis, infections of biliary, chest, and other drainage catheters, and *Clostridium difficile* colitis. Reactivation of HSV in individuals who are seropositive is also widespread during the first month, but the use of prophylactic acyclovir can reduce the risk of infection during this period.[52]

The period from the second to sixth month is when classic opportunistic infections begin to arise secondary to the immunosuppression used to prevent organ rejection.[51] Opportunistic pathogens and latent infections including viruses (CMV, hepatitis B and C, EBV, HHV-6, adenovirus), fungi (PCP, invasive aspergillosis, endemic mycoses), and bacterial pathogens associated with T-cell dysfunction (*Listeria, Nocardia, Mycobacteria*) begin to manifest.[51]

After 6 months, most solid organ transplant recipients do fairly well and develop infections similar to healthy patients in the community. If patients have had frequent and recurrent rejection episodes or require chronic immunosuppressive therapy to prevent chronic rejection, the risk of infections caused by pathogens in months 2 to 6 may persist for more than a year.[51]

In transplant patients undergoing retransplantation, the timetable of infections may be altered, with infections characteristic of any given time period occurring simultaneously and with increased severity.[51] Retransplantation itself significantly increases the risk of infection due to the need for more complex surgical procedures and prior immunosuppressive therapy.

HEMATOPOIETIC STEM CELL TRANSPLANTATION

HSCT has become a lifesaving treatment for lymphohematopoietic, immunologic, metabolic, and other inherited disorders.[53] The risk of infection early in the course of HSCT is largely driven by neutropenia and mucosal barrier injury caused by the conditioning chemotherapy used to ablate marrow cells in preparation for stem cell engraftment (Fig. 90-3B). Consequently, bacterial and fungal infections dominate the early transplant period, along with reactivation of latent herpesviruses.[54] For this reason, antibacterial (e.g., fluoroquinolone ± TMP-SMX) and antifungal prophylaxis (fluconazole or itraconazole) along with therapy to suppress herpesvirus replication (acyclovir or valacyclovir) is required. The neutropenia seen with conditioning chemotherapy may last 2 to 5 weeks or more, depending on the source of stem cells (bone marrow, peripheral blood, or umbilical cord) used for transplant and the degree of histocompatibility mismatch between donor and recipient.[53–55] However, advances in stem cell collection techniques and the use of recombinant myeloid growth factors (granulocyte-colony stimulating factor, G-CSF; granulocyte-macrophage colony stimulating factor, GM-CSF) have decreased the duration of neutropenia following HSCT. In older patients, nonmyeloablative conditioning chemotherapy (also known as a "mini-transplant") may be used to avoid excessive organ toxicities and delayed engraftment secondary to high-dose conditioning chemotherapy.[6]

The risk of infection after stem cell engraftment depends on the type of transplant and the corresponding risk for the development of GvHD. Because the cells used in autologous (recipient is the donor of stem cells) and syngeneic (identical twin is the source) transplantation have a perfect histocompatibility match, GvHD and the associated infections seen with its treatment do not occur. Allogeneic transplantation (donor is not the recipient), on the other hand, is hampered by the development of GvHD, which is arbitrarily categorized as acute or chronic depending on its occurrence before or after day 100, respectively, following transplantation (Fig. 90-3B). GvHD is the result of alloreactive cytotoxic T lymphocytes in the graft attacking host tissues that they recognize as foreign.[56] The severity is determined by the histocompatibility or human leukocyte antigen (HLA) match of stem cells transplanted to the host. Patients who received stem cells from matched, unrelated or non-HLA-identical siblings or umbilical cord blood are at the highest risk for developing severe acute and chronic GvHD.[56] The most

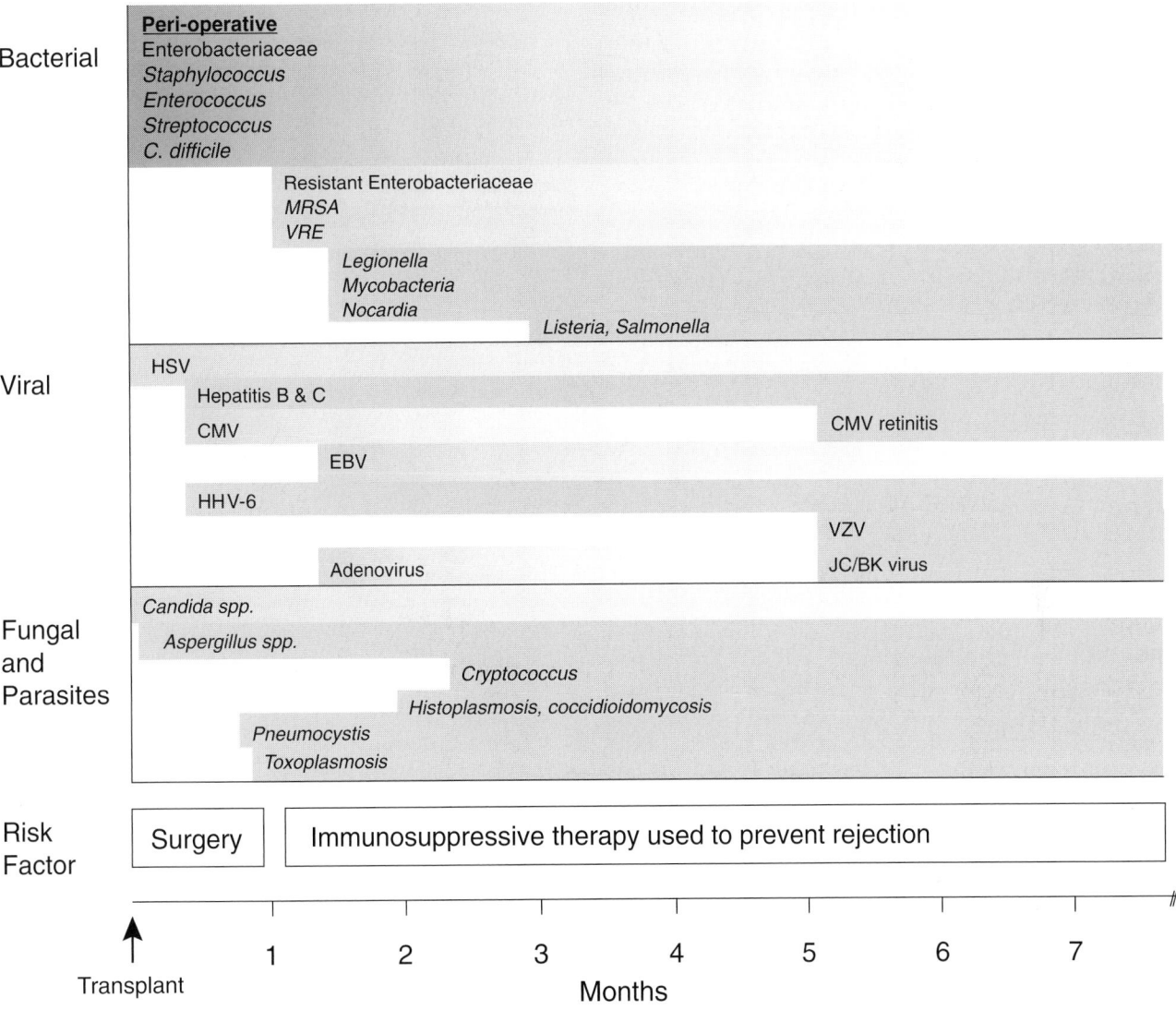

Bacterial

Peri-operative
Enterobacteriaceae
Staphylococcus
Enterococcus
Streptococcus
C. difficile

Resistant Enterobacteriaceae
MRSA
VRE

Legionella
Mycobacteria
Nocardia

Listeria, Salmonella

Viral

HSV
Hepatitis B & C
CMV
CMV retinitis
EBV
HHV-6
VZV
Adenovirus
JC/BK virus

Fungal and Parasites

Candida spp.
Aspergillus spp.
Cryptococcus
Histoplasmosis, coccidioidomycosis
Pneumocystis
Toxoplasmosis

Risk Factor

Surgery | Immunosuppressive therapy used to prevent rejection

1   2   3   4   5   6   7

Transplant   Months

FIGURE 90.3 Timing of infections following solid organ transplantation (**A**) (*continues*)

commonly affected tissues are the skin, upper and lower GI tract, the liver, and occasionally the eye and oral mucosa.[56] The severity of GvHD is generally graded on a scale of I to IV (less severe to more severe) according to the degree of skin involvement, liver, and gut (diarrhea) involvement.

Management of GvHD requires the administration of high dosages of corticosteroids (e.g., 2 mg/kg methylprednisolone) and/or in refractory cases antithymocyte globulin, pentostatin, or monoclonal antibodies directed against interleukin-2 (IL-2) or tumor necrosis factor-α (infliximab) to halt excessive organ toxicity.[56–58] These therapies profoundly and persistently suppress antigen-specific T-cell-mediated immunity and therefore predispose the patient to severe infections caused by viruses, facultative bacteria including mycobacteria, and fungi (Fig. 90-3B).[20]

Despite the immune dysregulation associated with GvHD after transplantation, patients who develop this complication often have lower relapse rates of their underlying malignancy and improved disease-free survival, provided the excessive morbidity and infectious risks can be controlled.[59] The lower relapse rate is thought to be the result of alloreactive cytotoxic T cells attacking malignant cells in the host. Optimization of this "graft-versus-malignancy" effect of transplantation has become an increasingly important component of HSCT.[59] Indeed, patients who exhibit early signs of relapse after allo-HSCT may be given infusions of donor lymphocytes in an attempt to induce a graft-versus-malignancy effect. As a result, these patients also develop severe GvHD that must be treated with immunosuppressive therapy to prevent excessive organ damage. Therefore, management of these patients becomes a delicate balance between attacking the underlying malignancy and avoiding excessive damage to the host and excessive immunosuppression and infectious morbidity.

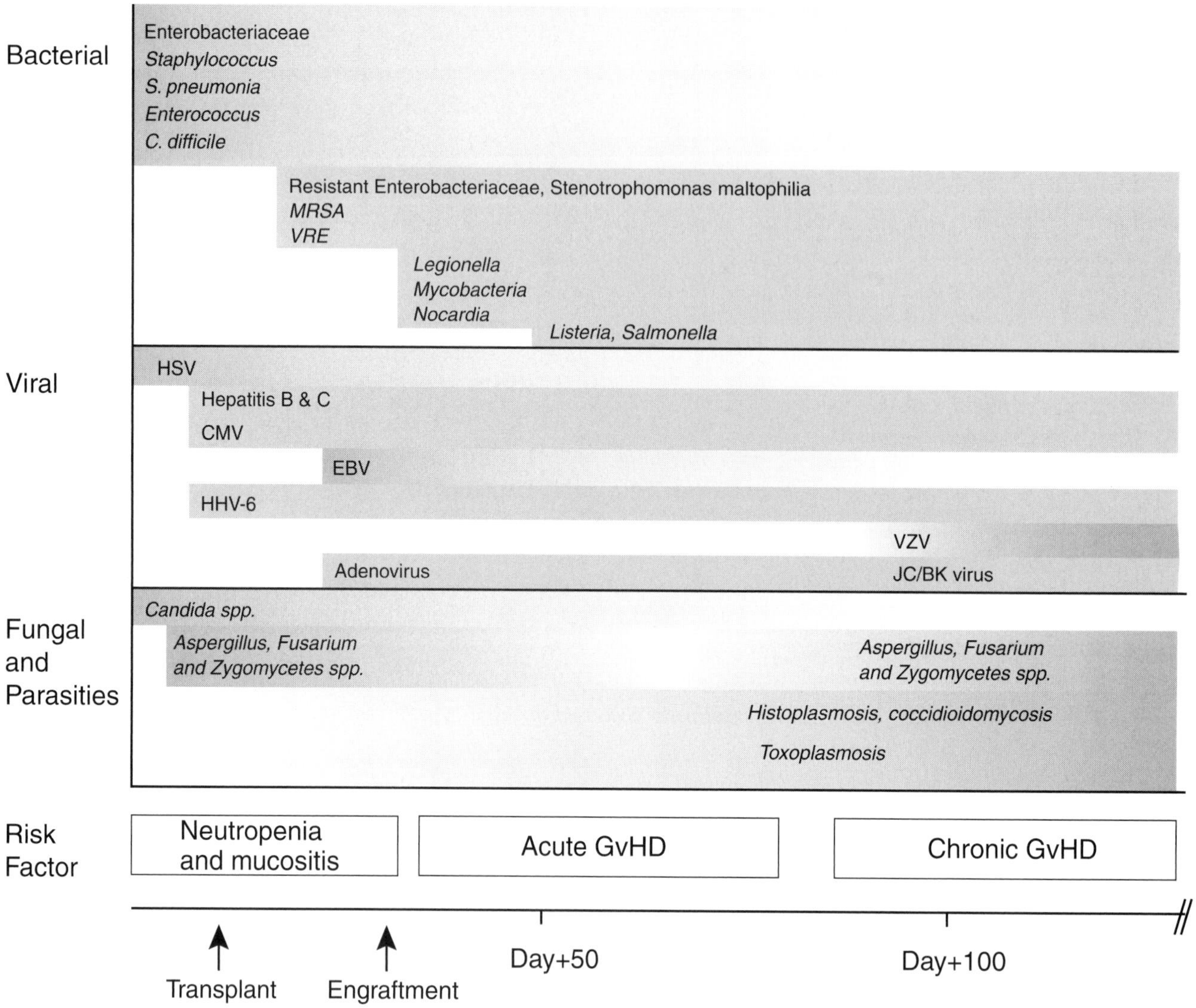

Bacterial	Enterobacteriaceae *Staphylococcus* *S. pneumonia* *Enterococcus* *C. difficile*		

Resistant Enterobacteriaceae, Stenotrophomonas maltophilia
MRSA
VRE

Legionella
Mycobacteria
Nocardia
Listeria, Salmonella

Viral — HSV
Hepatitis B & C
CMV
EBV
HHV-6
VZV
Adenovirus
JC/BK virus

Fungal and Parasities — *Candida spp.*
Aspergillus, Fusarium and Zygomycetes spp.
Aspergillus, Fusarium and Zygomycetes spp.
Histoplasmosis, coccidioidomycosis
Toxoplasmosis

Risk Factor — Neutropenia and mucositis | Acute GvHD | Chronic GvHD

Transplant   Engraftment   Day+50   Day+100

FIGURE 90.3 (*continued*) and allogeneic hematopoietic stem cell transplantation (**B**).

CLINICAL PRESENTATION AND DIAGNOSIS

The principal challenge in managing infections in the immunocompromised patient is early and accurate diagnosis of infection.[16] Depending the type and degree of immunosuppression, the spectrum of potential pathogens can be very broad and include true primary pathogens (e.g., *S. aureus, Mycobacterium tuberculosis*), opportunistic pathogens (e.g., *Aspergillus* spp and other molds), and microorganisms that occasionally act as pathogens (e.g., atypical rapidly growing *Mycobacteria*). Chronic, progressing viral infections (e.g., hepatitis C, EBV, CMV) are also seen at a higher frequency in immunocompromised hosts. Therefore, as discussed earlier, the "net immunosuppressive state" of the host needs to be considered during the clinical workup and selection of antimicrobial therapy. Localizing clinical signs and symptoms of infection that allow identification of the source of

infection (e.g., fluctuance, fissure or ulceration, exudates, pyuria) are often absent and radiographic findings are typically blunted in immunosuppressed patients.[60] This attenuation of clinical signs and symptoms of infections is most obvious in patients with neutropenia, who will often have fever as the only sign of an active infection (Table 90.2).[60] Unfortunately, fever is not a specific sign of infection, as fever may arise from the underlying malignancy, blood transfusions, biologic agents, chemotherapy, contrast dyes used in radiography, or procedures. Medications can cause, or in the case of antipyretics and corticosteroids, suppress fever in immunocompromised hosts. Antibiotics are a notorious cause of drug fever, especially in patients receiving broad-spectrum empiric coverage with multiple agents. It has been estimated that once a patient is receiving more than three antimicrobial agents simultaneously, the risk of fever due to antimicrobial therapy exceeds 30%.[61] However, antibiotic-related fever is generally a diagnosis of exclusion

TABLE 90.3	Common Antimicrobial Treatment Regimens Used for Treatment of Severe Infections in Immunocompromised Hosts
Pathogen	**Intravenous Therapies**[a]
Bacterial	
Gram-positive cocci S. aureus, S. epidermidis, S. pneumoniae, Viridans	*Empiric:* Vancomycin 0.5–1 g q6–12h; nafcillin 1–2 g q4–6h if MRSA rates are low
Streptococci E, faecalis, E. faecium	*Definitive:* According to culture and sensitivity results
Gram-negative aerobic bacilli (Enterobacteriaceae, *Pseudomonas aeruginosa, Haemophilus influenzae*)	*Empiric:* Cefepime 2 g IV q8h; piperacillin/tazobactam 3.5–4.6 g q6h, imipenem 500–1,000 mg q6h; meropenem 1 g q8h; with or without aminoglycoside;[b] ciprofloxacin 400 q8–12h or levofloxacin 750 mg q24h or aztreonam 1 g q8h with or without aminoglycoside in penicillin-allergic patients *Definitive:* According to culture and sensitivity results
Legionella spp.	Azithromycin 500 mg daily; levofloxacin 750 mg q24h; gatifloxacin 400 mg q24h; moxifloxacin 400 mg q24h
Listeria monocytogenes	Ampicillin 1–2 g q4–6h + gentamicin[b] or TMP-SMX 4 mg/kg q12h
Nocardia spp	TMP-SMX 7.5 mg/kg q12h; imipenem 500 mg q6h + amikacin 7.5 mg/kg IV q12h
Fungal	
Candida	Amphotericin B 0.7–1 mg/kg or lipid AMB formulation 3–5 mg/kg q24h Caspofungin 70 mg day #1, then 50 mg q24h Fluconazole 6–12 mg/kg q24h Voriconazole 3–6 mg/kg q12h
Cryptococcus neoformans	Meningitis: amphotericin B 1 mg/kg or liposomal amphotericin B 5 mg/kg + flucytosine orally q24h or fluconazole 400 mg q24h Pulmonary: fluconazole 400 mg q24h
Aspergillus spp.	Voriconazole 6 mg/kg q12h for 48 h, then 4 mg/kg q12h; lipid AMB formulation 5 mg/kg q24h; caspofungin 70 mg day #1, then 50 mg q24h; caspofungin + voriconazole
Fusarium spp, 2000.	Lipid AMB formulation 5–10 mg/kg q24h or voriconazole 4–6 mg/kg q12h
Zygomycetes	Lipid AMB formulation 5–10 mg/kg q24h; posaconazole[c] orally 200 mg PO four times daily
Pneumocystis jirovecii	TMP-SMX 5 mg/kg q6h; atovaquone PO 750 mg q12h; pentamidine 4 mg/kg q24 hours; dapsone orally 100 mg/day + TMP 5 mg/kg q6h; clindamycin 450–600 mg q6h + primaquine 15 mg daily
Viral	
Herpes simplex virus	Acyclovir 5–10 mg/kg q8h; foscarnet 40 mg/kg q8h
Cytomegalovirus	Ganciclovir 5 mg/kg q12h; foscarnet 60 mg/kg q8h; intravenous immune globulins 100–500 mg/kg every 1–2 weeks; Cidofovir 5 mg/kg every week + probenecid
Varicella-zoster virus	Acyclovir 10 mg/kg q8h; foscarnet 40 mg/kg q8h
Epstein-Barr virus	No effective therapy
Papovaviruses (BK, JC)	No effective therapy. Anecdotal: Cidofovir 5 mg/kg every week + probenecid
Protozoal/Parasites	
Toxoplasma gondii	Oral pyrimethamine 50–100 mg daily + sulfadiazine 1 g q4–6h;[d] oral pyrimethamine 50–100 mg daily + clindamycin 400–600 mg q6h[d]
Strongloides stercoralis	Thiabendazole 25 mg/kg q12h (max 3 g/day)

[a] General dosing recommendations in patients with typical body habitus and kidney function. Dosages may require adjustment in individualized patients. All doses are intravenous unless otherwise indicated.

[b] Gentamicin or tobramycin 2 mg/kg loading dose followed by maintenance dose determined by serum drug level monitoring. Alternatively, 5–7 mg/kg once-daily dose followed by maintenance dose determined by serum drug level monitoring.

[c] Investigational; only triazole with activity against Zygomycetes.

[d] Folinic acid (5–10 mg/day) recommended with pyrimethamine-containing regimens to reduce bone marrow toxicity.

and is considered only after a thorough patient workup is done and diagnostic procedures repeatedly yield no source of infection.

Although some clinicians believe that infections can be categorized based on fever patterns, prospective studies have not been able to demonstrate a consistent pattern that differentiates infection etiology.[62] Nevertheless, sustained fever may be more common in patients with gram-negative pneumonia or CNS infections.[62] High fevers (>40.5°C) are also frequently seen with *Clostridium difficile* colitis.[63]

Immunocompromised patients with suspected infection require a careful clinical examination and history. Patients are generally stratified according the risk of infection based on the net immunosuppressive state. Following transplantation, infections often follow a consistent timetable (Fig. 90.3). However, exceptions to the timetable are common and serve as an important clue for excessive epidemiologic exposure. Therefore, a careful patient history is critical in all patients with suspected infection. In general, this history should include (a) recent illnesses or past history of infection, (b) travel history and region or locality of residence, (c) exposure to pets or other animals, (d) gardening or other environmental exposures, (e) dietary exposures, including drinking and bathing water, (f) possible community or hospital exposures to sick individuals, (g) recent antimicrobial therapy, and (h) the tempo (onset of symptoms) of the current illness.[2,16]

Physical and laboratory assessment of immunocompromised patients is essential at first suspicion and throughout the treatment of infection. Patients should be carefully examined for focal signs and symptoms of infection that can narrow the initially large list of pathogens and possible sites of infection. Suspected bloodstream infections should be evaluated by blood culture. At least two specimens are sent for culture and examination, and culture is repeated every 2 to 3 days if the patient is febrile. Patients with indwelling central venous catheters should have blood samples taken through each lumen as well as from a peripheral vein to rule out the possibility of CRBSI. CRBSI is strongly suggested if the culture density from the catheter lumen is two to five times higher than simultaneous peripheral vein cultures.[4] If bacteremia persists longer than 24 to 48 hours after the institution of antimicrobial therapy, consideration must be given to an infected thrombus or endocarditis. Doppler ultrasonography or transthoracic/transesophageal echocardiography, respectively, can help identify the presence of an infected thrombus or vegetation on a heart valve. Large vegetations on the heart valve may be uncommon, however, in patients who are profoundly thrombocytopenic.

The upper and lower respiratory tract is the most common site of infection in immunocompromised patients, and careful physical and radiographic examination is required. The sinuses should be examined radiographically, and where indicated, brushings or endoscopically aspirated secretions should be obtained and examined by culture. Careful lung examinations are essential, including auscultation of the chest for the presence of rales, rhonchi, and wheezes, adventitious sounds, or a pleural friction rub. However, these signs may be absent in the immunocompromised host. Radiographic studies of the lungs are typically required to look for focal or diffuse parenchymal changes. In the neutropenic patient, these changes may not be evident on plain radiographs of the lung and high-resolution CT or magnetic resonance imaging (MRI) of the thorax may be necessary to detect small focal areas of infection.[16] Diffuse pneumonitis or diffuse patchy infiltrates may be more suggestive of acute viral pneumonia such as CMV or possibly PCP.[20] Therefore, the sputum should be examined microscopically and by culture, but specimens of pulmonary secretions are best obtained by bronchoalveolar lavage. In some situations, transbronchial or transthoracic needle biopsy or open lung biopsy may be required for definitive diagnosis if the patient's condition permits. Because prior antimicrobial therapy decreases the yield of organisms from clinical specimens, serologic studies or PCR detection of bacterial, viral, or fungal nucleic acid may be clinically indicated to aid diagnosis.[16]

The mouth and oropharynx should be examined for vesicles or ulcers and gingivitis. If present, lesions are swabbed or biopsied for direct staining or culture of bacteria, viruses, or fungi. Plaques in the oropharynx are often indicative of herpesvirus infection and should prompt serologic studies of viral antigens. Mucocutaneous candidiasis is also common and may cause retrosternal discomfort, pain, or dysphagia that should be evaluated by endoscopy.

Careful examination of the skin and nail beds, including palpation, can provide important clues to infection caused by bacterial, viral, and fungal pathogens, as the appearance of cutaneous lesions is highly suggestive of certain pathogens. For example, necrotic lesions with a center sunken eschar (ecthyma gangrenosum) are highly suggestive of disseminated *Pseudomonas* or mold infection.[64,65] Therefore, all suspicious lesions or rashes should be biopsied and cultured.

Diarrhea is common in hospitalized patients, particularly patients receiving chemotherapy or broad-spectrum antibiotics, and is not necessarily indicative of infection. However, special attention must be paid to the possibility of *C. difficile* colitis, which may or may not be accompanied by fever. All immunocompromised patients with diarrhea should have their stools tested for *C. difficile* toxin, and empiric treatment with metronidazole with or without vancomycin may be considered if diarrhea continues. Perianal lesions may also develop with pain, induration, discharge, and bleeding. Smears and culture of discharge are used to identify possible causes.

Typhlitis is a necrotizing inflammation of the cecum, appendix, and/or ileum that is seen most commonly in patients with leukemia during neutropenia. The inflammation is likely caused by infection due to CMV and bacterial invasion, which can evolve into perforation of the colon and sepsis. The mortality rate averages 40% to 50%, and death is usually caused by cecal perforation, bowel necrosis, and sepsis.[66,67] The infection typically presents with right lower quadrant pain and fever. Typhlitis is diagnosed by ultrasound and MRI of the abdomen to detect decreased peristalsis and hypervascularity of the bowel wall and mucosa. Most patients can be treated conservatively with intravenous fluids and antibiotics, although surgery may be necessary if complications arise.[66,67]

Although colonization of the urine by Enterobacteriaceae and *Candida* is likely in immunocompromised patients who are catheterized, midstream specimens of urine and catheter drainage should still be collected and cultured in a patient with suspected infection. Radiographic scans of the kidneys may also show evidence of obstructing lesions or focal renal enlargement. Infections involving the liver are often suspected on the basis of elevated serum chemistry levels (serum transaminases, bilirubin) and ultrasonographic examination and/or radiographic scans that demonstrate hepatic enlargement with or without focal lesions. Pronounced increases in serum alkaline phosphatase accompanied by diffuse abdominal symptoms in patients recovering from neutropenia are suspicious for hepatosplenic candidiasis. Generally, abdominal CT scans will reveal multiple well-defined lucencies in the liver, spleen, and occasionally the kidneys that are highly suggestive of infection in a patient with a compatible clinical history.[68] Prolonged treatment courses with antifungal therapy are needed to treat hepatosplenic candidiasis, and resolution of fever may require several weeks despite adequate antifungal therapy.[68]

Infections of the skeletal system, particularly osteomyelitis, are often detected by plain radiography, CT or MRI scans. Further information can be derived from technetium (^{99m}Tc) bone scans or radiolabeled white blood cell scans. Septic arthritis of the joints can develop following bacteremia and is diagnosed by aspiration of the joint fluid, culture, and Gram staining.

Meningitis and encephalitis can present as focal or diffuse CNS infections and generally require CT and/or MRI scans of the brain for diagnosis. If intracranial pressure permits, cerebrospinal fluid should be collected for Gram staining, chemistries, microscopy, serologic examination, and PCR testing of potential viral pathogens. If present, focal lesions in the brain may require stereotactic biopsy for definitive diagnosis.

TREATMENT

GENERAL PRINCIPLES

Because of the difficulties associated with the diagnosis of infection in immunocompromised patients, empiric antimicrobial therapy is indicated to prevent death from infection.[16,69] Ideally, antimicrobial therapy is selected on the basis of the most likely pathogens and local antimicrobial susceptibility patterns and individualized to the patient's underlying immunosuppression, clinical history and presentation, past antibiotic exposure, and current organ function.[16]

Antimicrobials used to treat infections in immunocompromised patients should be broad-spectrum, should have rapidly lethal mechanisms of action, should be safe for prolonged administration, and should be well tolerated. Antimicrobials that are convenient to administer (i.e., once or twice daily), available as intravenous or oral formulations, and inexpensive are also desirable, especially for treatment of the lower-risk patient outside the hospital.

EMPIRICAL THERAPY IN NEUTROPENIC PATIENTS

An example of an initial empirical therapy approach for a patient with fever and neutropenia (ANC $<500/\text{mm}^3$) as recommended by the Infectious Diseases Society of America is presented in Figure 90.4.[16] Patients are initially assessed on the basis of the severity of immunosuppression and the expected duration of neutropenia. Higher-risk patients, or those with evidence of severe infection, significant mucosal barrier injury, and/or comorbidities including cardiovascular instability, changing mental status, hemorrhage, or liver/renal dysfunction, should be treated in the hospital or possibly the intensive care unit with high-dose, intravenous antimicrobial therapy tailored to the patient's microflora and local susceptibility patterns.

Typically, therapy is directed at the most likely pathogens in the initial phases of neutropenia: Enterobacteriaceae and *P. aeruginosa*, *Streptococcus*, and *Staphylococcus* spp. Core antibiotics used to cover these pathogens include antipseudomonal β-lactam antibiotics, third- or fourth-generation antipseudomonal cephalosporins, and carbapenems (excluding ertapenem, which lacks anti-*Pseudomonas* activity), possibly in combination with vancomycin with or without an aminoglycoside. First-line use of vancomycin in febrile neutropenic patients is controversial, as no survival benefit was demonstrated in prospective randomized trials that included vancomycin as part of an initial empiric regimen during the first 72 hours of therapy.[70] Moreover, routine widespread use of vancomycin has been associated with an increased risk of acquiring vancomycin-resistant *Enterococcus*.[71,72] Nevertheless, many experts feel that including vancomycin in an empiric regimen is justified in patients with suspected catheter infection, mucositis, cellulitis, or known colonization with methicillin-resistant *S. aureus* or penicillin-resistant *S. pneumonia*, or in any patient who appears to be clinically unstable (e.g., hypotensive).[16] Patients with necrotizing or marginal gingivitis should also receive antimicrobials with anti-anaerobic activity (e.g., metronidazole, clindamycin, or carbapenems), as these infections are seen in patients with bad dentition.

The necessity of double coverage for gram-negative bacteremia, particularly *P. aeruginosa*, continues to be debated, even though success rates for antipseudomonal β-lactams, cephalosporins, as well as antipseudomonal carbapenem monotherapy appear to be similar to combinations of these agents with aminoglycosides.[73] In general, the most important factors governing the effectiveness of antibacterial regimens for gram-negative bacteremia are the timing of therapy

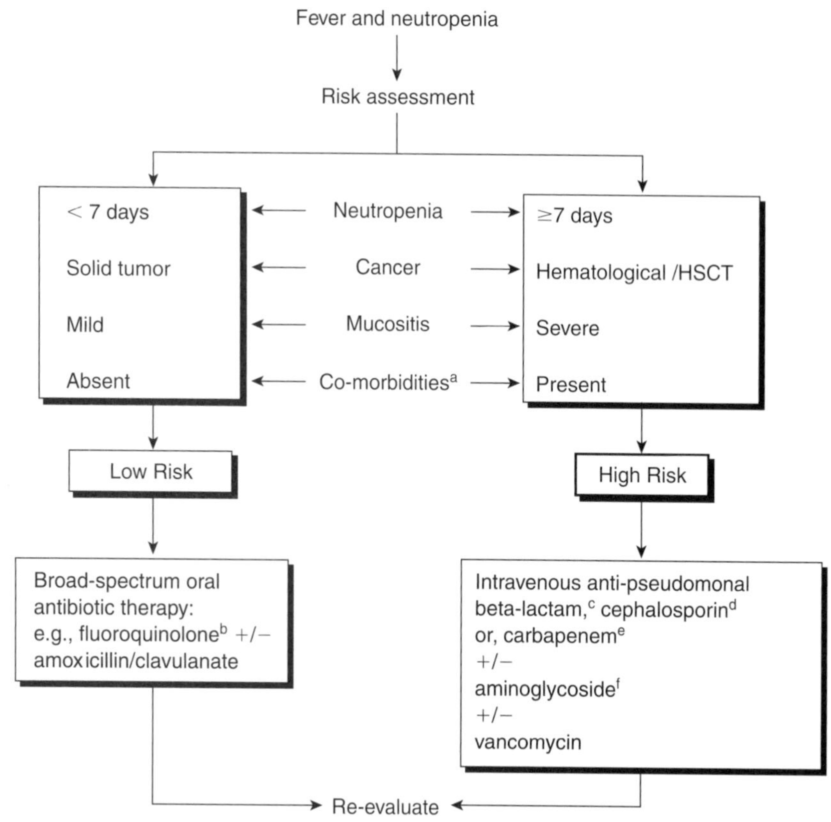

Fever and neutropenia

↓

Risk assessment

< 7 days	←	Neutropenia	→	≥7 days
Solid tumor	←	Cancer	→	Hematological /HSCT
Mild	←	Mucositis	→	Severe
Absent	←	Co-morbidities[a]	→	Present

Low Risk

High Risk

Broad-spectrum oral antibiotic therapy: e.g., fluoroquinolone[b] +/− amoxicillin/clavulanate

Intravenous anti-pseudomonal beta-lactam,[c] cephalosporin[d] or, carbapenem[e] +/− aminoglycoside[f] +/− vancomycin

→ Re-evaluate ←

[a] hypotension, altered mental status, new neurologic changes, respiratory failure, abdominal pain, hemorrhage, cardiac compromise or new arrhythmia, catheter tunnel infection, extensive cellulits, acute renal or liver failure
[b] ciprofloxacin, levofloxacin, gatifloxacin or, moxifloxacin
[c] piperacillin/tazobactam, ticarcillin/clavulanate
[d] ceftazidime, cefepime₌ imipenem/cilastatin, meropenem
[f] gentamicin, tobramycin, amikacin

FIGURE 90.4 Management of febrile episodes in neutropenic cancer patients.

(i.e., any delay adversely affects outcome) and the susceptibility of the organisms to the non-aminoglycoside component of the therapeutic regimen.[74] Adding an aminoglycoside is often prudent, however, in patients with gram-negative bacteremia until sterilization of the blood and documentation of susceptibility to the non-aminoglycoside component of the regimen can be confirmed.

Therapeutic modifications to empiric antimicrobial regimens are often made upon receiving culture results. However, it is not uncommon for culture studies to come back negative. If the patient defervesces rapidly after initiating antibiotics, therapy does not need to be continued for more than 7 days.[16] Persistent fever after 72 hours of empirical antimicrobial therapy, however, may indicate a persistent untreated infection or a pathogen that is resistant to the empiric antimicrobial regimen. If patients are clinically stable and underlying risk factors for infection such as neutropenia are resolved, it is appropriate to continue the initial antimicrobial regimen, as more than 50% of patients require more than 72 hours to defervesce on appropriate antimicrobial therapy.[16] If vancomycin has not been added, it should be empirically started in patients with 72 hours of persistent

fever. If the patient is persistently neutropenic, the possibility of an occult fungal infection due to *Candida* species or *Aspergillus* becomes more likely. Approximately 10% to 40% of patients who die with neutropenic fever have evidence of an invasive fungal infection at autopsy.[75] Therefore, initiation of empiric antifungal therapy directed at yeast (*Candida* spp) or both yeast and molds (*Candida* and *Aspergillus* principally, depending on the patient risk factors and epidemiology) is recommended.[16]

PERSISTENT INFECTION IN THE IMMUNOCOMPROMISED HOST

Persistent fever is the most common sign of an inadequately treated occult infection in the immunocompromised host. Typically persistent fever requires a broadening of empiric antimicrobial coverage, especially in critically ill patients. Addition of TMP-SMX and fluoroquinolones to empiric antibacterial coverage may be considered initially to pick up coverage of organisms such as *Mycoplasma, Legionella* spp, *Listeria monocytogenes, Nocardia* spp, and the carbapenem-resistant gram-negative *Stenotrophomonas maltophilia*, all of which are not sufficiently covered by standard antipseudomonal β-lactams, cephalosporins, and aminoglycoside regimens (Table 90.3). However, empiric expansion of antibacterial, antiviral, and antifungal coverage should occur only after further workup of the persistent fever.

The general approach toward working up persistent fever can be summarized by the acronym "FAIL." The "F" stands for false diagnosis. Chronic viral syndromes are common causes of persistent fever in patients with suppressed cell-mediated immunity. Alternatively, fever due to underlying disease (e.g., tumor fever) or tissue damage (e.g., atelectasis in the lung) is also a common component of false diagnosis. Unfortunately, a diagnosis of noninfectious causes of fever can be made only after an extensive workup and exclusion of infectious causes. In the case of tumor fever, a short trial of naproxen may attenuate the fever and is strongly suggested as a noninfectious cause for persistent fever.[76–78] The second principle in the workup of persistent fever is "A," or allergic causes of fever. As mentioned earlier, medications, particularly antibiotics, but also other drug therapies, are common causes of persistent fever in immunocompromised patients. If fever is due to antimicrobial therapy, it will generally resolve within 72 hours after discontinuation of the offending agent, provided the patient does not have concurrent rash or other allergic manifestations.[79] The third consideration is "I," or the presence of intercurrent infections. These are typically caused by less virulent but more antimicrobial-resistant pathogens that start as superinfections but then invade internal organs and the bloodstream. Multi-drug-resistant Enterobacteriaceae, *S. maltophilia*, vancomycin-resistant *Enterococcus*, rapidly growing *Mycobacteria*, and some fungi are pathogens that frequently start as superinfections before causing intercurrent illness (often simultaneously with a separate infection). Therefore, in the setting of persistent fever, these organisms need to be considered and where possible empirically covered until a more definitive diagnosis is possible.

The last component that should be considered in persistent fever is "L," or localized problems that are slow in responding to therapy. Undrained fluid collections including abscesses, infected prosthetic materials, endovascular infections, and septic thrombi are all examples of localized problems that can contribute to prolonged fevers in immunocompromised hosts.[2] Correction of these factors often leads to a prompt response to medical therapy.

ADJUNCTIVE THERAPIES

Because host immunodeficiency is the critical risk factor for the development of infection as well as the most important variable in treatment outcome, strategies that focus on boosting immune deficiencies would appear to be critical for reducing infection morbidity and mortality. Protective environmental isolation in laminar airflow rooms with high-efficiency particular air filters (e.g., HEPA filters) can help reduce bacterial and fungal exposure to the host. However, it is not an effective long-term solution for patients with persistent immunosuppression. Proper nutrition is also essential to improve the likelihood of immune system reconstitution and to enhance the patient's response to stress and infection.

Stimulation of the immune system with recombinant hematopoietic cell growth factors or cytokines such as G-CSF and GM-CSF has become standard therapy in neutropenic patients and patients undergoing allo-HSCT, although their routine use has not demonstrated convincing reductions in infectious mortality.[80] Intriguing preclinical data suggest that quantitative and qualitative deficiencies in host cellular immune responses can be blunted or reversed with adjunctive cytokine therapy such as γ-interferon or a combination of various cytokines plus infusions of host effector cells (e.g., γ-interferon plus granulocyte transfusions).[81,82] In patients with neutrophil defects such as chronic granulomatous disease, administration of γ-interferon reduces the frequency of recurrent bacterial infections and hospitalization needed to manage infectious complications.[83–85] However, the effectiveness of γ-interferon for improving cell-mediated immunodeficiency in other disease states is less well studied.

Direct infusions of granulocytes are sometimes considered in patients with severe infection who are 1 to 2 weeks from neutrophil recovery. This strategy has been reported to have efficacy rates between 30% and 85% in patients with persistent bacteremia of fungal infections.[86,87] Although granulocyte transfusion therapy has become more feasible since the introduction of G-CSF/corticosteroid mobilization into the donor leukocyte collection process, patients may require a minimum of 1×10^{10} neutrophils per day or every other day to see substantial benefits in the treatment of infection. Therefore, granulocyte transfusions are often not logistically possible for more than two weeks. Adverse effects include acute toxicities such as fever, chills, and urticaria, which can be minimized by premedication with antipyretics, antihistamines, and slowing of the infusion.[86,87] In rare cases, patients develop severe reactions associated with antileukocytic antibody reactions. Respiratory distress and the appearance of pulmonary infiltrates were described in the early 1980s for granulocyte transfusions administered during amphotericin B therapy.[86] However, later reports have failed to confirm the interaction between granulocyte transfusions and amphotericin B in causing lung injury. Granulocyte transfusions have also been reported to delay bone marrow engraftment and host–donor chimerism after HSCT.[88] Humoral defenses can be supplemented by administration of pooled immune globulin or hyperimmune globulin in the case of active herpesvirus infections.

Although many immunocompromised patients are still candidates for vaccination, the effectiveness of vaccines is often diminished, and live-virus vaccines should be avoided in these populations.[54]

PROPHYLAXIS

Prevention of infection in immunocompromised patients is always better than treatment of an active infection. Prophylaxis can be distinguished from empiric therapy in that antimicrobial agents are administered prior to the appearance of any sign or symptom of active infection. A similar but different strategy for initiating therapy before documented infection is the use of *preemptive* therapy. Preemptive therapy is the administration of an antimicrobial at the first detection of some marker of impending infection, but before signs and symptoms of infection develop.[89] For example, antiviral therapy for CMV infection is often initiated at the first sign of viral shedding (as determined by detection of the pp65 viral antigen coat in leukocytes) but before the development of active pneumonia or colitis in immunocompromised patients.[34] Sensitive and selective diagnostic tests are required to use antimicrobial therapy in a preemptive fashion, and because such tests are not widely available for all of the common infections in immunocompromised patients, antimicrobial prophylaxis based on the most likely pathogens and underlying immunosuppression is still required to reduce infectious morbidity and mortality.

Effective prophylactic strategies in immunocompromised patients often share several features. First, there must be a high background incidence of infection caused by the particular pathogen or group of pathogens to justify the need for prophylaxis. Second, an effective therapy must be available for treatment of the specific pathogens. Third, the therapy must be well tolerated with minimal to no toxicity. Fourth, the therapy should be convenient and available as an oral therapy so prolonged administration is feasible. Several therapies meet this requirement for protecting severely immunocompromised patients against bacterial, viral, and fungal pathogens.

In terms of bacterial infections, prophylaxis aimed at gram-negative organisms is common in patients with neutropenia. Fluoroquinolones are typically the preferred agents and have been shown in prospective clinical trials to reduce the frequency of serious gram-negative infections.[16,54] Although newer fluoroquinolones (gatifloxacin, moxifloxacin, gemifloxacin) also have enhanced coverage against many gram-positive pathogens and anaerobes, they may not have sufficient coverage against *Viridans* streptococci. Therefore, vancomycin or occasionally penicillin is added in patients who are expected to develop severe mucositis. Routine vancomycin prophylaxis is not recommended, however, to prevent bloodstream infections caused by *Staphylococcus* and *Enterococcus*, as this practice was not shown to result in consistent mortality benefits and may increase the risk of severe infections caused by vancomycin-resistant enterococci.[16]

Persistent neutropenia is associated with a significant risk of invasive fungal infections caused by *Candida*, and if neutropenia persists beyond 2 to 3 weeks, *Aspergillus* spp and

other molds. Fluconazole 200 to 400 mg per day has been shown in two prospective randomized studies to reduce the incidence of both superficial and invasive candidiasis among patients undergoing HSCT.[90–92] Similar prophylaxis studies in high-risk leukemia patients showed that the regimen caused some reduction in infections but did not improve overall mortality.[93,94] The variable activity of fluconazole against more resistant non-*albicans* species, particularly *C. glabrata* and *C. krusei*, however, has led some centers to use intermittent low-dose amphotericin B deoxycholate or liposomal amphotericin B. Several studies have shown that itraconazole solution 200 mg taken two or three times daily is an alternative to fluconazole and also an effective strategy for reducing the frequency of infections due to *Aspergillus*. However, 20% to 30% of patients taking itraconazole prophylaxis discontinue therapy due to GI side effects.[95–98] Studies are underway to assess the efficacy of oral voriconazole, posaronazole, and inhaled lipid amphotericin B formulations (lung transplantation) in the prevention of *Aspergillus* infections among high-risk populations.

Pulmonary infections with *P. jirovecii* are relatively uncommon but may occur in patients with persistent lymphopenia or profound cell-mediated immunodeficiency. Prophylactic use of TMP-SMX (one double-strength table three times weekly or one single-strength tablet daily) is recommended as prophylaxis for most transplant recipients.[6,54]

Recurrent viral infections are problematic in patients with suppressed cellular immunity. Prophylaxis with acyclovir (250 mg/m^2 or 200 to 400 mg orally two to four times a day) has been proven to be an effective strategy for preventing viral shedding and clinical symptoms of HSV reactivation in seropositive patients undergoing HSCT.[6,54] Although acyclovir is generally less expensive, the acyclovir prodrug valacyclovir (500 mg daily) can also be used and is more convenient. Acyclovir prophylaxis may also have an added benefit of reducing CMV replication, although these agents are not effective treatments for active CMV disease.[34] Patients who develop breakthrough infections on acyclovir can still be treated with acyclovir, but at much higher dosages (e.g., 10 mg/kg intravenously every 8 hours). Foscarnet is the drug of choice for HSV that does not respond to acyclovir. However, foscarnet has a much higher potential for nephrotoxicity and is typically reserved for patients with acyclovir-refractory dT infection.[54]

CMV prophylaxis strategies have been studied extensively in HSCT recipients due to the high morbidity and mortality associated with CMV pneumonitis. If possible, CMV patients should receive stem cells and supportive blood products from CMV-negative seropositive donors only.[54] However, CMV-seropositive patients are not at higher risk for CMV reactivation if they receive products from CMV-seropositive donors. Ganciclovir was shown to be an effective agent to reduce CMV replication in patients, but it failed to show a survival benefit as a prophylaxis strategy in patients undergoing HSCT.[34] This failure was attributed in part to the myelosuppressive effects of ganciclovir therapy, which prolonged engraftment and increased the risk of infection due to other pathogens. As a result, ganciclovir prophylaxis is often reserved for patients at extremely high risk for primary CMV infection (i.e., mismatched allo-HSCT from a CMV-positive donor to a CMV-negative recipient) after engraftment of the donor cells. Preemptive administration of ganciclovir or foscarnet, with the onset of viral shedding as detected by the pp65 CMV antigen in peripheral leukocytes, has become the predominant strategy for treating and preventing pneumonitis in high-risk populations.[34]

KEY POINTS

- Infections remain the most important cause of excessive morbidity and mortality in immunocompromised patients. The most likely causes of infection can be anticipated based on the patient's net immunosuppressive state, past epidemiologic exposures, and prior exposure to medical procedures and/or antimicrobial therapy
- Disruption of mucocutaneous barriers predisposes patients to infection caused by bacterial microflora in the gut and reactivation of herpesviruses. This microflora includes gram-negative Enterobacteriaceae, *Pseudomonas aeruginosa,* as well as gram-positive organisms including *Staphylococcus epidermidis, Staphylococcus aureus, Viridans* streptococci, and *Enterococcus* spp
- Central venous catheters are one of the most common portals and/or reservoirs for infection into the bloodstream for gram-positive organisms as well as *Candida* species
- Neutropenia predisposes patients to potentially life-threatening infections with bacteria and fungi depending on the rate and extent of neutrophil decline and time to neutrophil recovery
- Cell-mediated immunodeficiency predisposes patients to reactivation of viral infections, severe infections caused by *Mycobacteria* and other facultative organisms, as well as endemic and opportunistic fungal pathogens
- Defects in humoral immunity are predominately associated with recurrent infections caused by encapsulated bacteria
- Most infections in immunocompromised patients require empiric therapy due to the difficulties associated with diagnosis of infection in the immunocompromised host. Fever is often the only consistent sign of infection
- In immunocompromised patients with persistent fever, the ''FAIL'' principle can be applied for further workup of infection
- Antimicrobial prophylaxis is an essential strategy for the reduction of infectious morbidity and mortality in select groups of immunocompromised patients. To be effective, a nontoxic therapy must be available and a high background incidence of infection must be present to justify routine prophylaxis

ACKNOWLEDGMENT

The author acknowledges Dr. Dimitrios P. Kontoyiannis, MD, ScD, FACP, FIDSA, for his advice and excellent suggestions for organizing this chapter.

REFERENCES

1. Donnelly JP, De Pauw BE. Infections in the immunocompromised host. In: Mandell GL, Bennet JE, Dolin R, eds. Principles and practice of infectious diseases, vol. 2, 6th ed. Philadelphia: Elsevier; 2005.
2. Rubin RH, Schaffner A, Speich R. Introduction to the Immunocompromised Host Society consensus conference on epidemiology, prevention, diagnosis, and management of infections in solid-organ transplant patients. Clin Infect Dis 33 (Suppl 1):S1–4, 2001.
3. Mermel L. Infections related to central venous catheters in US intensive-care units. Lancet 361:1562, 2003.
4. Mermel LA, Farr BM, Sherertz RJ, et al. Guidelines for the management of intravascular catheter-related infections. Clin Infect Dis 32: 1249–1272, 2001.
5. Raad I, Davis S, Khan A, et al. Impact of central venous catheter removal on the recurrence of catheter-related coagulase-negative staphylococcal bacteremia. Infect Control Hosp Epidemiol 13:215–221, 1992.
6. O'Brien SN, Blijlevens NM, Mahfouz TH, et al. Infections in patients with hematological cancer: recent developments. Hematology (Am Soc Hematol Educ Program) 438–472, 2003.
7. Kuijpers TW, Roos D. Neutrophils: the power within. In: Kaufmann SHE, Medzhitov R, Gordon S, eds. The innate immune response to infection. Washington DC: American Society for Microbiology Press, 2004.
8. Bodey GP, Buckley M, Sathe YS, et al. Quantitative relationships between circulating leukocytes and infection in patients with acute leukemia. Ann Intern Med 64:328–340, 1966.
9. Bodey GP. The treatment of febrile neutropenia: from the Dark Ages to the present. Support Care Cancer 5:351–357, 1997.
10. Kim SK, Demetri GD. Chemotherapy and neutropenia. Hematol Oncol Clin North Am 10:377–395, 1996.
11. Baltch AL, Hammer MC, Smith RP, et al. Comparison of the effect of three adrenal corticosteroids on human granulocyte function against *Pseudomonas aeruginosa.* J Trauma 26:525–533, 1986.
12. Delamaire M, Maugendre D, Moreno M, et al. Impaired leucocyte functions in diabetic patients. Diabet Med 14:29–34, 1997.
13. Gallacher SJ, Thomson G, Fraser WD, et al. Neutrophil bactericidal function in diabetes mellitus: evidence for association with blood glucose control. Diabet Med 12:916–920, 1995.
14. Pizzo PA. Fever in immunocompromised patients. N Engl J Med 341:893–900, 1999.
15. Todeschini G, Franchini M, Tecchio C, et al. Improved prognosis of *Pseudomonas aeruginosa* bacteremia in 127 consecutive neutropenic patients with hematologic malignancies. Int J Infect Dis 3:99–104, 1998.
16. Hughes WT, Armstrong D, Bodey GP, et al. 2002 guidelines for the use of antimicrobial agents in neutropenic patients with cancer. Clin Infect Dis 34:730–751, 2002.
17. Jones RN. Contemporary antimicrobial susceptibility patterns of bacterial pathogens commonly associated with febrile patients with neutropenia. Clin Infect Dis 29:495–502, 1999.
18. Wisplinghoff H, Seifert H, Wenzel RP, et al. Current trends in the epidemiology of nosocomial bloodstream infections in patients with hematological malignancies and solid neoplasms in hospitals in the United States. Clin Infect Dis 36:1103–1110, 2003.
19. Wisplinghoff H, Bischoff T, Tallent SM, et al. Nosocomial bloodstream infections in US hospitals: analysis of 24,179 cases from a prospective nationwide surveillance study. Clin Infect Dis 39: 309–317, 2004.

20. Safdar A, Armstrong D. Infectious morbidity in critically ill patients with cancer. Crit Care Clin 17:531–570, vii–viii, 2001.
21. Latge JP, Calderone R. Host-microbe interactions: fungi invasive human fungal opportunistic infections. Curr Opin Microbiol 5:355–358, 2002.
22. Romani L. Immunity to fungal infections. Nat Rev Immunol 4:1–23, 2004.
23. Latge JP. *Aspergillus fumigatus* and aspergillosis. Clin Microbiol Rev 12:310–350, 1999.
24. Denning DW. Therapeutic outcome in invasive aspergillosis. Clin Infect Dis 23:608–615, 1996.
25. Lin SJ, Schranz J, Teutsch SM. Aspergillosis case-fatality rate: systematic review of the literature. Clin Infect Dis 32:358–366, 2001.
26. Marr KA, Patterson T, Denning D. Aspergillosis. Pathogenesis, clinical manifestations, and therapy. Infect Dis Clin North Am 16:875–894, vi, 2002.
27. Wingard JR. Viral infections in leukemia and bone marrow transplant patients. Leuk Lymphoma 11 (Suppl 2):115–125, 1993.
28. Machado CM, Vilas Boas LS, Dulley FL, et al. Herpes simplex virus shedding in bone marrow transplant recipients during low-dose oral acyclovir prophylaxis. Braz J Infect Dis 1:27–30, 1997.
29. Morfin F, Bilger K, Boucher A, et al. HSV excretion after bone marrow transplantation: a 4-year survey. J Clin Virol 30:341–345, 2004.
30. Gluckman E, Lotsberg J, Devergie A, et al. Prophylaxis of herpes infections after bone-marrow transplantation by oral acyclovir. Lancet 2:706–708, 1983.
31. Koc Y, Miller KB, Schenkein DP, et al. Varicella zoster virus infections following allogeneic bone marrow transplantation: frequency, risk factors, and clinical outcome. Biol Blood Marrow Transplant 6:44–49, 2000.
32. Steer CB, Szer J, Sasadeusz J, et al. Varicella-zoster infection after allogeneic bone marrow transplantation: incidence, risk factors and prevention with low-dose acyclovir and ganciclovir. Bone Marrow Transplant 25:657–664, 2000.
33. Skinhoj P. Herpesvirus infections in the immunocompromised patient. Scand J Infect Dis Suppl 47:121–127, 1985.
34. Boeckh M, Nichols WG, Papanicolaou G, et al. Cytomegalovirus in hematopoietic stem cell transplant recipients: current status, known challenges, and future strategies. Biol Blood Marrow Transplant 9:543–558, 2003.
35. Hicks KL, Chemaly RF, Kontoyiannis DP. Common community respiratory viruses in patients with cancer: more than just "common colds." Cancer 97:2576–2587, 2003.
36. Mylonakis E, Goes N, Rubin RH, et al. BK virus in solid organ transplant recipients: an emerging syndrome. Transplantation 72:1587–1592, 2001.
37. Priftakis P, Bogdanovic G, Kokhaei P, et al. BK virus (BKV) quantification in urine samples of bone marrow transplanted patients is helpful for diagnosis of hemorrhagic cystitis, although wide individual variations exist. J Clin Virol 26:71–77, 2003.
38. Gonzalez-Fraile MI, Canizo C, Caballero D, et al. Cidofovir treatment of human polyomavirus-associated acute haemorrhagic cystitis. Transplant Infect Dis 3:44–46, 2001.
39. Phillips MS, von Reyn CF. Nosocomial infections due to nontuberculous mycobacteria. Clin Infect Dis 33:1363–1374, 2001.
40. Sepkowitz KA. Opportunistic infections in patients with and patients without acquired immunodeficiency syndrome. Clin Infect Dis 34:1098–1107, 2002.
41. Wiederhold NP, Lewis RE, Kontoyiannis DP. Invasive aspergillosis in patients with hematologic malignancies. Pharmacotherapy 23:1592–1610, 2003.
42. Roblot F, Le Moal G, Godet C, et al. *Pneumocystis carinii* pneumonia in patients with hematologic malignancies: a descriptive study. J Infect 47:19–27, 2003.
43. Dykewicz CA. Hospital infection control in hematopoietic stem cell transplant recipients. Emerg Infect Dis 7:263–267, 2001.
44. Torres HA, Reddy BT, Raad II, et al. Nocardiosis in cancer patients. Medicine (Baltimore) 81:388–397, 2002.
45. Kontoyiannis DP, Ruoff K, Hooper DC. *Nocardia* bacteremia. Report of 4 cases and review of the literature. Medicine (Baltimore) 77:255–267, 1998.
46. Safdar A, Armstrong D. Listeriosis in patients at a comprehensive cancer center, 1955–1997. Clin Infect Dis 37:359–364, 2003.
47. Safdar A, Papadopoulous EB, Armstrong D. Listeriosis in recipients of allogeneic blood and marrow transplantation: thirteen-year review of disease characteristics, treatment outcomes and a new association with human cytomegalovirus infection. Bone Marrow Transplant 29:913–916, 2002.
48. Safdar A, Armstrong D. Antimicrobial activities against 84 *Listeria monocytogenes* isolates from patients with systemic listeriosis at a comprehensive cancer center (1955–1997). J Clin Microbiol 41:483–485, 2003.
49. Frank MM, Joiner K, Hammer C. The function of antibody and complement in the lysis of bacteria. Rev Infect Dis 9 (Suppl 5):S537–545, 1987.
50. Calandra T. Practical guide to host defense mechanisms and predominant infections encountered in immunocompromised hosts. In: Glauser MP, Pizzo PA, eds. Management of infections in the immunocompromised host. London: Harcourt, 2000.
51. Snydman DR. Epidemiology of infections after solid-organ transplantation. Clin Infect Dis 33 (Suppl 1):S5–8, 2001.
52. Balfour HH J., Chace BA, Stapleton JT, et al. A randomized, placebo-controlled trial of oral acyclovir for the prevention of cytomegalovirus disease in recipients of renal allografts. N Engl J Med 320:1381–1387, 1989.
53. Wingard JR, Vogelsang GB, Deeg HJ. Stem cell transplantation: supportive care and long-term complications. Hematology (Am Soc Hematol Educ Program) 422–444, 2002.
54. Dykewicz CA. Preventing opportunistic infections in bone marrow transplant recipients. Transplant Infect Dis 1:40–49, 1999.
55. Chanock SJ, Pizzo PA. Infectious complications of patients undergoing therapy for acute leukemia: current status and future prospects. Semin Oncol 24:132–140, 1997.
56. Couriel D, Caldera H, Champlin R, et al. Acute graft-versus-host disease: pathophysiology, clinical manifestations, and management. Cancer 101:1936–1946, 2004.
57. Antin JH, Chen AR, Couriel DR, et al. Novel approaches to the therapy of steroid-resistant acute graft-versus-host disease. Biol Blood Marrow Transplant 10:655–668, 2004.
58. Couriel D, Saliba R, Hicks K, et al. Tumor necrosis factor-alpha blockade for the treatment of acute GVHD. Blood 104:649–654, 2004.
59. Burroughs L, Storb R. Low-intensity allogeneic hematopoietic stem cell transplantation for myeloid malignancies: separating graft-versus-leukemia effects from graft-versus-host disease. Curr Opin Hematol 12:45–54, 2005.
60. Sickles EA, Greene WH, Wiernik PH. Clinical presentation of infection in granulocytopenic patients. Arch Intern Med 135:715–719, 1975.
61. O'Hanley P, Easaw J, Rugo H, et al. Infectious disease management of adult leukemic patients undergoing chemotherapy: 1982 to 1986 experience at Stanford University Hospital. Am J Med 87:605–613, 1989.
62. Musher DM, Fainstein V, Young EJ, et al. Fever patterns. Their lack of clinical significance. Arch Intern Med 139:1225–1228, 1979.
63. Mylonakis E, Ryan ET, Calderwood SB. *Clostridium difficile*-associated diarrhea: a review. Arch Intern Med 161:525–533, 2001.
64. D'Antonio D, Pagano L, Girmenia C, et al. Cutaneous aspergillosis in patients with haematological malignancies. Eur J Clin Microbiol Infect Dis 19:362–365, 2000.
65. van Burik JA, Colven R, Spach DH. Cutaneous aspergillosis. J Clin Microbiol 36:3115–3121, 1998.
66. Lea JW Jr, Masys DR, Shackford SR. Typhlitis: a treatable complication of acute leukemia therapy. Cancer Clin Trials 3:355–362, 1980.
67. Varki AP, Armitage JO, Feagler JR. Typhlitis in acute leukemia: successful treatment by early surgical intervention. Cancer 43:695–697, 1979.
68. Kontoyiannis DP, Luna MA, Samuels BI, et al. Hepatosplenic candidiasis. A manifestation of chronic disseminated candidiasis. Infect Dis Clin North Am 14:721–739, 2000.
69. Schimpff SC. Empiric antibiotic therapy for granulocytopenic cancer patients. Am J Med 80:13–20, 1986.
70. Vancomycin added to empirical combination antibiotic therapy for fever in granulocytopenic cancer patients. European Organization for Research and Treatment of Cancer (EORTC) International Antimicrobial Therapy Cooperative Group and the National Cancer Insti-

tute of Canada-Clinical Trials Group. J Infect Dis 163:951–958, 1991.

71. Polk R. Vancomycin prescribing in the era of vancomycin-resistant enterococci. Pharmacotherapy 15:682–683, 1995.

72. Shay DK, Goldmann DA, Jarvis WR. Reducing the spread of antimicrobial-resistant microorganisms. Control of vancomycin-resistant enterococci. Pediatr Clin North Am 42:703–716, 1995.

73. Klastersky J. Science and pragmatism in the treatment and prevention of neutropenic infection. J Antimicrob Chemother 41 (Suppl D): 13–24, 1998.

74. Rolston KVI. Infections in patients with solid tumors. In: Glauser MP, Pizzo PA, eds. Management of infections in the immunocompromised host. London: WB Saunders, 2000.

75. Glauser MP, Calandra T. Infections in patients with hematological malignancies. In: Glauser MP, Pizzo PA, eds. Management of infections in the immunocompromised host. London: WB Saunders, 2000.

76. Chang JC, Hawley HB. Neutropenic fever of undetermined origin (N-FUO): why not use the naproxen test? Cancer Invest 13: 448–450, 1995.

77. Tsavaris N, Zinelis A, Karabelis A, et al. A randomized trial of the effect of three non-steroid anti-inflammatory agents in ameliorating cancer-induced fever. J Intern Med 228:451–455, 1990.

78. Chang JC. NSAID test to distinguish between infectious and neoplastic fever in cancer patients. Postgrad Med 84:71–72, 1988.

79. Foster FP, Beard RW. Fever from antibiotics: some lessons drawn from 25 cases. Med Clin North Am 47:532–539, 1963.

80. Ozer H, Armitage JO, Bennett CL, et al. 2000 update of recommendations for the use of hematopoietic colony-stimulating factors: evidence-based, clinical practice guidelines. American Society of Clinical Oncology Growth Factors Expert Panel. J Clin Oncol 18: 3558–3585, 2000.

81. Roilides E, Lamaignere CG, Farmaki E. Cytokines in immunodeficient patients with invasive fungal infections: an emerging therapy. Int J Infect Dis 6:154–163, 2002.

82. Rosenzweig SD, Holland SM. Phagocyte immunodeficiencies and their infections. J Allergy Clin Immunol 113:620–626, 2004.

83. Ohga S, Okamura J, Nakayama H, et al. Interferon-gamma therapy for infection control in chronic granulomatous disease. Acta Paediatr Jpn 37:315–320, 1995.

84. Bemiller LS, Roberts DH, Starko KM, et al. Safety and effectiveness of long-term interferon gamma therapy in patients with chronic granulomatous disease. Blood Cells Mol Dis 21:239–247, 1995.

85. Curnutte JT. Conventional versus interferon-gamma therapy in chronic granulomatous disease. J Infect Dis 167 (Suppl 1):S8–12, 1993.

86. Hubel K, Dale DC, Engert A, et al. Current status of granulocyte (neutrophil) transfusion therapy for infectious diseases. J Infect Dis 183:321–328, 2001.

87. Hubel K, Dale DC, Liles WC. Granulocyte transfusion therapy: update on potential clinical applications. Curr Opin Hematol 8: 161–164, 2001.

88. Adkins D, Spitzer G, Johnston M, et al. Transfusions of granulocyte-colony-stimulating factor-mobilized granulocyte components to allogeneic transplant recipients: analysis of kinetics and factors determining posttransfusion neutrophil and platelet counts. Transfusion 37:737–748, 1997.

89. Rex JH, Sobel JD. Prophylactic antifungal therapy in the intensive care unit. Clin Infect Dis 32:1191–1200, 2001.

90. Ellis ME, Clink H, Ernst P, et al. Controlled study of fluconazole in the prevention of fungal infections in neutropenic patients with haematological malignancies and bone marrow transplant recipients. Eur J Clin Microbiol Infect Dis 13:3–11, 1994.

91. Goodman JL, Winston DJ, Greenfield RA, et al. A controlled trial of fluconazole to prevent fungal infections in patients undergoing bone marrow transplantation. N Engl J Med 326:845–851, 1992.

92. Marr KA, Seidel K, Slavin MA, et al. Prolonged fluconazole prophylaxis is associated with persistent protection against candidiasis-related death in allogeneic marrow transplant recipients: long-term follow-up of a randomized, placebo-controlled trial. Blood 96: 2055–2061, 2000.

93. Bohme A, Ruhnke M, Buchheidt D, et al. Treatment of fungal infections in hematology and oncology: guidelines of the Infectious Diseases Working Party (AGIHO) of the German Society of Hematology and Oncology (DGHO). Ann Hematol 82:S133–S140, 2003.

94. Marr KA. Issues in the design of the fluconazole prophylaxis trials in patients undergoing hematopoietic stem cell transplantation. Clin Infect Dis 39 (Suppl 4):S170–175, 2004.

95. Glasmacher A, Molitor E, Hahn C, et al. Antifungal prophylaxis with itraconazole in neutropenic patients with acute leukemia. Leukemia 12:1338–1343, 1998.

96. Marr KA, Crippa F, Leisenring W, et al. Itraconazole versus fluconazole for prevention of fungal infections in patients receiving allogeneic stem cell transplants. Blood 103:1527–1533, 2004.

97. Winston DJ, Busuttil RW. Randomized controlled trial of oral itraconazole solution versus intravenous/oral fluconazole for prevention of fungal infections in liver transplant recipients. Transplantation 74: 688–695, 2002.

98. Winston DJ, Maziarz RT, Chandrasekar PH, et al. Intravenous and oral itraconazole versus intravenous and oral fluconazole for long-term antifungal prophylaxis in allogeneic hematopoietic stem-cell transplant recipients: a multicenter, randomized trial. Ann Intern Med 138:705–713, 2003.

Skin and Soft Tissue Infections

91

Jeanne Hawkins Van Tyle and Cindy C. Selzer

The skin is the largest organ system of the human body. As long as it is healthy, the skin is an effective physical barrier against invasion and infection. Bacteria normally colonize the skin without causing infection. Normal skin flora includes a variety of aerobic and anaerobic bacteria and fungi (Table 91.1). The body's best defense against bacterial infection is an intact skin barrier. A variety of bacterial infections of the skin may occur (Table 91.2). Infections may be primary or secondary. The common etiologic agents and empiric treatment options vary depending on the infection, as summarized in Table 91.2. This chapter will discuss a number of the more common skin infections, including cellulitis, impetigo, erysipelas, periorbital cellulitis, decubitus ulcers, and infected diabetic foot ulcers.

TABLE 91.1	Microorganisms Commonly Found on the Human Skin (Normal Flora)

Bacteria

    Staphylococcus epidermidis[a]

    Diphtheroids

        Corynebacterium spp[a]

        Propionibacterium acnes[a]

    Staphylococcus aureus

    Streptococcus spp

        Streptococcus pyogenes

    Peptococcus

    Mycobacterium spp

    Bacillus spp

Fungi

    Malassezia furfur[a]

    Candida spp

[a] Most common organisms.

TABLE 91.2	Common Bacterial Infections of the Skin	
Lesion	**Common Etiologic Agents**	**Treatment Options**
Primary Infections		
Cellulitis	Group A Streptococcus; Straphylococcus aureus	Penicillinase-resistant synthetic penicillin, amoxicillin/clavulanate, first-gen. cephalosporin, azithromycin, clarithromycin, ciprofloxacin, gatifloxacin, levofloxacin, moxifloxacin
	MRSA	Vancomycin, daptomycin, linezolid, dalfopristin-quinupristin, tigecycline
Impetigo	Group A Streptococcus; Straphylococcus aureus	Oral first- or second-gen. cephalosporin, amoxicillin-clavulanate, erythromycin, azithromycin, clarithromycin, mupirocin
Erysipelas	Group A Streptococcus	Penicillin G, penicillinase resistant synthetic penicillin, cefazolin, amoxicillin-clavulanate, azithromycin, cephalexin
Periorbital cellulitis	Group A Streptococcus Staphylococcus aureus	Penicillinase-resistant synthetic penicillin, ticarcillin-clavulanate, ampicillin-sulbactam, amoxicillin-clavulanate, first-, second-, or third-gen. cephalosporin
	Streptococcus pneumoniae	Ceftriaxone, vancomycin
Secondary Infections		
Chronic ulcers (decubitus)	Polymicrobic: can include coliform bacteria, Peptostreptococci, Enterococci, *Bacteroides* spp, *Proteus* spp, *Clostridium perfringens, Pseudomonas aeruginosa*	Cefoxitin + antipseudomonal aminoglycoside, imipenem-cilastatin, ticarcillin-clavulanate, piperacillin-tazobactam, ciprofloxacin, gatifloxacin, levofloxacin, or moxifloxacin + clindamycin or metronidazole
Diabetic foot ulcers	Polymicrobic: can include *Staphylococcus aureus, S. epidermidis, Bacteriodes fragilis, Clostridium perfringens, Pseudomonas aeruginosa,* Peptostreptococcus, Enterococci, *Proteus* spp, *Klebsiella* spp	Imipenem-cilastatin, meropenem, ertapenem, ticarcillin-clavulanate, piperacillin-tazobactam ciprofloxacin + clindamycin, levofloxacin + metronidazole, cefepime + metronidazole

CELLULITIS

> **TREATMENT GOALS: CELLULITIS**
>
> - Modify risk factors to prevent recurrence.
> - Provide appropriate antimicrobial therapy.
> - Prevent complications such as osteomyelitis or bacteremia.
> - Treat signs and symptoms of systemic illness.

DEFINITION

Cellulitis is defined as an acute infection of the skin with extension into the subcutaneous tissues.[1]

EPIDEMIOLOGY

Although cellulitis may affect patients of all ages, most patients have risk factors. Lymphedema, site of entry (leg ulcer, traumatic wound, fissured toe webs), venous insufficiency, leg edema, and being overweight are independent risk factors for the development of cellulitis.[2] The presence of a foreign body, such as an intravenous catheter, also increases the risk of developing cellulitis.

PATHOPHYSIOLOGY

Cellulitis may occur when the barrier is broken, as in a cut, bite, or abrasion. Other etiologies of cellulitis include infection from a contiguous site (e.g., osteomyelitis) or due to hematogenous spread.[1,3]

Commonly observed bacterial etiologies of cellulitis are group A streptococci and *Staphylococcus aureus*.[1,3] However, the most likely organism may vary depending on the age of the patient and concomitant diseases such as diabetes mellitus or human immunodeficiency virus (HIV) infection (Table 91.3).

CLINICAL PRESENTATION AND DIAGNOSIS

Cellulitis may affect any area of the body but most commonly affects the face and lower extremities.[2,4]

SIGNS AND SYMPTOMS

Patients with cellulitis may present with local and/or systemic features. The most common local signs and symptoms include pain, tenderness, erythema, swelling, and warmth at the site of infection.[1,3] Less frequently, cellulitis causes localized symptoms such as lymphangitis (streaks of erythema spreading from the area of cellulitis) and enlarged and tender lymph nodes. Some patients may experience a prodrome, which includes chills, malaise, anorexia, nausea, and vomiting. Fever and an elevated white blood cell count may occur.[1,3]

DIAGNOSIS

Cellulitis is clinically diagnosed by the combination of local and systemic features. All patients should be evaluated for risk factors. To determine a microbial etiology, blood or skin cultures are not generally useful or reliable because no pathogen is typically found. Empiric therapy should target the most likely organisms.[3] Cultures should be considered (a) if the infection is considered complex; (b) if there is an increased risk of complications, such as in very young or elderly patients, in patients with diabetes or peripheral vascular disease, or in immunosuppressed patients; and (c) for those who have failed to respond to a standard course of appropriate antibiotics.[5–7] Radiologic examination is not necessary in most patients with cellulitis but may be valuable in patients with suspected subadjacent osteomyelitis or necrotizing fasciitis.[3]

TABLE 91.3	Common Microorganisms Causing Cellulitis in Specific Populations
Normal healthy population	Group A streptococcus
	Staphylococcus aureus
Children	Group A streptococcus
	Staphylococcus spp
	Haemophilus influenzae
Diabetic patients	*Staphylococcus* spp
	Streptococcus spp
	Aerobic gram-negative organisms (*Enterobacteriaceae, P. aeruginosa, Acinetobacter*)
	Anaerobic organisms (Bacteroides, Peptococcus)
Hospitalized patients	*Staphylococcus* spp (including coagulase-negative staphylococci)
	Streptococcus spp, gram-negative organisms (*Haemophilus* spp, *Escherichia coli, Klebsiella, Pseudomonas*)

TREATMENT

PHARMACOTHERAPY

Choosing the optimal antibiotic for the treatment of cellulitis is based on a number of factors, including the most likely causative organism, penetration of the antibiotic to the site of infection, current medications, medication allergies, patient compliance, and cost.

Depending on the severity, extent, and location of the infection, the patient may be treated with oral antibiotics as an outpatient or with intravenous antibiotics as an inpatient. Empiric therapy of uncomplicated cellulitis should be effective against *Streptococcus* and *Staphylococcus* species. An antistaphylococcal penicillin, such as dicloxacillin, or a first-generation cephalosporin, such as cephalexin, is a reasonable empiric choice for oral use. Table 91.4 summarizes commonly used outpatient antibiotic regimens in the treatment of uncomplicated cellulitis.

Initial treatment with intravenous antibiotics should be given in patients with rapidly spreading lesions, a prominent systemic response (chills and fever), or clinically significant coexisting medical conditions, such as neutropenia, preexist-

ing edema, or renal insufficiency.[3] If intravenous therapy is indicated, empiric therapy with an antistaphylococcal penicillin, such as nafcillin or oxacillin, or a first-generation cephalosporin, such as cefazolin, may be used. Once the patient becomes afebrile and lesions have begun to improve (usually 3 to 5 days), patients may be switched to oral antibiotics to complete the course of treatment.

A variety of the newer antibiotics have been evaluated in the treatment of cellulitis. Oral fluoroquinolones, such as moxifloxacin,[8] gatifloxacin,[9] ciprofloxacin, and levofloxacin,[10,11] have shown efficacy in the treatment of uncomplicated skin and soft tissue infections. β-lactam antibiotics, such as ceftriaxone,[12] ampicillin–sulbactam,[13] piperacillin–tazobactam, and ticarcillin–clavulanate,[14] have also been used successfully in the treatment of cellulitis. Although many of the newer agents have shown efficacy equivalent to that of traditional therapies of cellulitis, their cost is generally higher, and this should be taken into account when selecting these newer agents. In addition, the antibiotic that is most active against the causative agent and has the narrowest spectrum should be chosen so as not to promote the development of antimicrobial resistance.

TABLE 91.4	Commonly Used Outpatient Oral Antibiotic Regimens in the Treatment of Uncomplicated Cellulitis		
Generic Name	Brand Name	Adult Dose	Pediatric Dose
Penicillin Antibiotics			
Penicillin V	Pen-Vee K, V-Cillin K, others	250–500 mg q6–8h	15–62.5 mg/kg/day divided q6–8h
Dicloxacillin	Dynapen, Pathocil, others	125–250 mg q6h	12–25 mg/kg/day divided q6h
Amoxicillin/clavulanate	Augmentin	250–500 mg (of amoxicillin) q8h 500–875 mg q12h	20–40 mg/kg/day (of amoxicillin) divided q8h
First-Generation Cephalosporin Antibiotics			
Cephalexin	Keflex, Keftabs, others	250–500 mg q6–12h	25–50 mg/kg/day divided q6–12h
Cefadroxil	Duricef, Ultracef	1 g as single dose or divided q12h	30 mg/kg/day divided q12h
Cephradine	Velosef	250–500 mg q6–12h	25–50 mg/kg/day divided q6–12h
Macrolide Antibiotics			
Erythromycin	ERYC, Ery-Tab, EES, others	250–500 mg q6–12h 333 mg q8h	30–50 mg/kg/day divided q6h
Clarithromycin	Biaxin	250 mg q12h	15 mg/kg/day divided q12h
Azithromycin	Zithromax	500 mg, then 250 mg daily on days 2 to 5	10 mg/kg on day 1; 5 mg/kg on days 2 to 5
Fluoroquinolone Antibiotics			
Ciprofloxacin	Cipro	500 mg twice daily	Not recommended
Gatifloxacin	Tequin	400 mg daily	Not recommended
Levofloxacin	Levaquin	500 mg daily	Not recommended
Moxifloxacin	Avelox	400 mg daily	Not recommended
Other Antibiotics			
Clindamycin	Cleocin, others	150–450 mg q6h	20–30 mg/kg/day divided q6h

Methicillin-resistant *S. aureus* (MRSA) is an increasing cause of community-acquired cellulitis. MRSA should be suspected in patients who were previously colonized, recently hospitalized, have a delayed response to therapy, or live in an area with a high prevalence. Most community-acquired strains of MRSA can be treated with clindamycin, trimethoprim–sulfamethoxazole, or a fluoroquinolone with enhanced gram-positive coverage (gatifloxacin, levofloxacin, or moxifloxacin). Cultures and susceptibilities, if available, should dictate the antibiotic chosen for the treatment of a community-acquired strain of MRSA. However, vancomycin is the treatment of choice for severe infections due to MRSA. Alternatives to vancomycin include daptomycin and linezolid.[3,4,15]

Patients at risk for complicated infections (diabetic patients, patients with a prolonged hospital stay, or immunocompromised patients) should be started on empiric, broad-spectrum therapy that covers the likely pathogens. Broad-spectrum coverage may be initiated with monotherapy or combination therapies. Broad-spectrum β-lactam antibiotics with anaerobic activity are reasonable choices for monotherapy in the treatment of complicated infections and include piperacillin–tazobactam, ticarcillin–clavulanate, ampicillin–sulbactam, ertapenem, imipenem–cilastatin, and meropenem. High-dose levofloxacin (750 mg/day) showed therapeutic equivalence to ticarcillin–clavulanate in the treatment of complicated skin and soft tissue infections and therefore is also a reasonable empiric choice.[16] To improve gram-negative coverage, an aminoglycoside such as gentamicin or tobramycin may be added to an antistaphylococcal penicillin or first-generation cephalosporin. If anaerobic organisms are suspected, clindamycin or metronidazole may be added to the antibiotic regimen.

The total duration of therapy for antimicrobials in the treatment of cellulitis is usually 7 to 14 days. If patients have continued signs of cellulitis at the end of treatment, antibiotics should be continued until all erythema is resolved. Daily prophylaxis with oral amoxicillin or penicillin G may be initiated in patients who have more than two episodes of cellulitis in the same area.[3]

NONPHARMACOLOGIC THERAPY

Nonpharmacologic therapy of cellulitis consists of rest and elevation of the affected area and the application of cool sterile dressings. Existing tinea pedis infections should be treated with topical antifungals. These infections may provide entry for infecting bacteria and should be treated until cleared.[3] Surgery may be necessary if an abscess is present.

IMPETIGO

TREATMENT GOALS: IMPETIGO

- Initiate appropriate antimicrobial therapy.
- Provide local wound care.
- Provide education to prevent recurrence and transmission.

DEFINITION

Impetigo is one of the most common, contagious, superficial bacterial skin infections and occurs predominantly in children.[17] Initially, impetigo presents as vesicles, which become pustules that rupture and form honey-crusted lesions. The vesicles usually occur on exposed areas of the skin such as the face and extremities after trauma.

PATHOPHYSIOLOGY

The most common causative organism is group A streptococci, although *S. aureus* may be present. It is unclear whether *S. aureus* is a primary cause or represents a secondary invader of the infected site.

CLINICAL PRESENTATION

Conditions in which there is a break in the skin such as chickenpox, abrasions, and burns are predisposing factors to the development of impetigo. The nose and the perioral region are also common sites for lesions. Diagnosis can be made by history and examination, but for definitive diagnosis a culture must be obtained from the base of a lesion that has had the crust removed.

TREATMENT

PHARMACOTHERAPY

The most effective therapy for impetigo remains controversial.[18] Although some investigators claim that systemic therapy is necessary, others argue that topical therapy is sufficient. Penicillin therapy has long been considered the drug of choice,[1] but this is being questioned.[18–20] In one study, only 53% of patients responded to oral penicillin V therapy, whereas cloxacillin therapy was effective in 100%.[20] Consequently, a 7-day course of therapy with a β-lactamase-resistant antibiotic (cloxacillin, cephalexin, cefaclor, cefadroxil, amoxicillin–clavulanic acid, erythromycin, azithromycin or clarithromycin) aimed at both group A streptococci and *S. aureus* may be preferred.[20–25] Cephalexin appears to be the drug of choice for oral treatment of children with impetigo. Erythromycin therapy should be avoided in geographic areas where there is a high rate of erythromycin-resistant *S. aureus*.

Mupirocin (Bactroban), a topical antibiotic,[26] has activity against gram-positive organisms, including group A streptococci and *S. aureus*.[27,28] In localized cases, mupirocin 2% ointment applied three times daily for 7 to 10 days is sufficient. A number of studies[21,24,25,29–31] comparing oral erythromycin to topical mupirocin have supported the efficacy of topical mupirocin. Consequently, topical mupirocin may be the treatment of choice in patients whose lesions are not widespread.[32]

Regardless of the agent used, impetigo should respond to treatment within 7 days. If no improvement is seen, antimicrobial resistance or noncompliance with the prescribed regimen should be considered.

NONPHARMACOLOGIC THERAPY

Patients should be counseled on the importance of hygiene in preventing recurrence and transmission of impetigo. Improved hygiene is a mainstay of therapy. Bed sheets and clothing should be disinfected.

ERYSIPELAS

TREATMENT GOALS: ERYSIPELAS

- Administer appropriate antimicrobial therapy.
- Prevent complications.
- Reduce recurrence.

DEFINITION

Erysipelas is a superficial skin infection that presents with the abrupt onset of a fiery red rash. Fever is usually apparent some hours before the skin signs and symptoms appear.[33]

PATHOPHYSIOLOGY

The most common etiology of erysipelas is group A streptococci, but other streptococci, *Haemophilus influenzae*, and staphylococci have been implicated. Bacteria enter through a break in the skin such as a scratch, cut, or lesion such as a chickenpox lesion.[34] Facial erysipelas may occur following a streptococcal upper respiratory tract infection.[23] Patients often develop blisters, and malaise, myalgia, chills, fever, nausea, and vomiting may be present. Diagnosis is made by examination of the rash and on clinical appearance.

CLINICAL PRESENTATION AND DIAGNOSIS

The rash typically occurs in the lower extremities but may also occur on the face, ears, or arms.[35] The leg is involved in erysipelas 90% of the time.[33] It affects people of all ages but appears to be more prevalent in neonates, infants, and the elderly. It occurs more commonly in patients with underlying diseases but can occur in previously healthy individuals.[36]

TREATMENT

PHARMACOTHERAPY

Penicillin is the drug of choice for erysipelas.[37] It may be administered orally or intravenously, depending on the severity of the infection. Other agents that may be used include ampicillin, amoxicillin, nafcillin, oxacillin, dicloxacillin, erythromycin, clindamycin, and cephalosporins such as cefazolin, cephalexin, cefadroxil, cefuroxime axetil, or cefaclor.[36,38] In nonimmunized children, empiric therapy with a second-generation cephalosporin such as cefaclor, cefuroxime axetil, or cephradine may be necessary to ensure adequate treatment for *H. influenzae* in addition to streptococci.[36] Oral antibiotics should be continued for 10 to 14 days or until the rash has resolved.[39,40]

The recurrence rate in erysipelas is relatively high. Recurrence is more common in immunocompromised patients and in patients with a history of venous insufficiency. Erysipelas does not always recur in the same site. Although it is unknown why recurrence occurs, there may be an association with pharyngeal carriage of group A streptococci. Prophylactic antibiotics (penicillin V orally or benzathine penicillin intramuscularly) have been used to reduce the rate of recurrence and may be considered in patients with a high rate of recurrence.[41,42]

NONPHARMACOLOGIC THERAPY

Although nonpharmacologic therapy (bedrest, elevation of the affected area, and cool, moist dressings) is helpful, antibiotic therapy is the mainstay of therapy. Without antibiotics, the mortality rate may be as high as 80% in neonates.[35]

PERIORBITAL CELLULITIS

TREATMENT GOALS: PERIORBITAL CELLULITIS

- ■ Initiate appropriate antimicrobial therapy.
- ■ Minimize complications such as meningitis.
- ■ Manage systemic signs and symptoms.

DEFINITION

Periorbital (preseptal) cellulitis involves the superficial area around the eye and may be a medical emergency. The eyelid is edematous, erythematous, warm, and tender. Systemic signs of illness, such as fever and leukocytosis, are more commonly observed in patients with periorbital cellulitis resulting from pneumococcal bacteremia.[43–45]

CLINICAL PRESENTATION AND DIAGNOSIS

Periorbital cellulitis is an infection that most commonly affects infants and children. Periorbital cellulitis is often preceded by an upper respiratory tract infection, sinusitis, or conjunctivitis. At other times, it may be posttraumatic, following a scratch, abrasion, or insect bite. The most common causative organisms are *Staphylococcus* and *Streptococcus* species.[45] Although it was once a common causative organism, the incidence of *H. influenzae* periorbital cellulitis has dramatically declined in recent years due to the routine administration of *H. influenzae* type b vaccine.

Traditionally, the aggressive diagnostic workup required for periorbital cellulitis involved hospitalization for blood cultures, lumbar puncture, and intravenous antibiotics. This approach was advocated primarily due to the high incidence of *H. influenzae* and its invasive nature, resulting in high morbidity and mortality. Lumbar punctures and blood cultures are still routinely performed, especially in young children and nontraumatic cases, because the likelihood of meningitis increases with systemic illness and bacteremia. However, admission to the hospital and intravenous antibiotics may not be necessary in uncomplicated posttraumatic cases.[45,46]

TREATMENT

PHARMACOTHERAPY

Empiric antibiotic therapy should be effective against the most likely pathogens. Streptococcus and Staphylococcus should be covered in all infants and children. In addition, *H. influenzae* may be an important pathogen in nonimmunized infants and children. Posttraumatic periorbital cellulitis is usually caused by *S. aureus* or *Streptococcus pyogenes*. Uncomplicated posttraumatic cases can generally be treated with an oral antibiotic, such as cephalexin, dicloxacillin, or clindamycin.[45]

If intravenous antibiotics are warranted, penicillins, such as nafcillin, oxacillin, or ampicillin–sulbactam, or a first-generation cephalosporin, such as cefazolin, are effective against *Streptococcus* and most *Staphylococcus* species. Second-generation cephalosporins, such as cefuroxime, are effective against *H. influenzae* in addition to streptococci and staphylococci. In patients with signs of systemic illness and without evidence of trauma, *Streptococcus pneumoniae* is the most likely pathogen. In these patients, a lumbar puncture is recommended due to the increased risk of meningitis, and treatment with ceftriaxone and/or vancomycin should be initiated quickly.

A clinical response such as reduction in fever and resolution of symptoms typically occurs within 24 to 72 hours. Following such a response, oral antibiotic therapy with amoxicillin-clavulanic acid, trimethoprim–sulfamethoxazole, cefadroxil, or a broad-spectrum cephalosporin should be continued for a total course of 10 days.[43,45]

NONPHARMACOLOGIC THERAPY

Topical wet compresses may provide some symptomatic relief.

PRESSURE SORES (DECUBITUS ULCERS, BEDSORES)

TREATMENT GOALS: PRESSURE SORES

- Relieve pressure and pain.
- Provide adequate nutritional support.
- Remove devitalized tissues.
- Promote granulation and re-epithelization of tissue.
- Eliminate sources of moisture such as fluids from incontinence, perspiration, or wound drainage.

DEFINITION

Pressure sores[46–55] result from ischemic necrosis and ulceration of tissues overlying a bony prominence that has been subjected to prolonged pressure against an external object such as a bed, wheelchair, cast, or splint. This pressure may be sufficient to occlude small vessels and result in irreversible ischemic changes. These lesions often develop into infected ulcers.

EPIDEMIOLOGY

Pressure ulcers are a serious problem; they affect approximately 9% of all hospitalized patients and 23% of all nursing home patients, according to the Agency for Health Care Research and Quality (AHRQ, formerly AHCPR).[46]

PATHOPHYSIOLOGY

Immobility is the most important risk factor. Four factors critical to formation of pressure sores are pressure, shearing forces, friction, and moisture. Shearing forces relate to the sliding of parallel surfaces of tissue in unequal fashion, as when the head of the bed is raised and the patient slides toward the foot of the bed. Friction generated by pulling a patient across a bed sheet may result in tissue trauma and development of an ulcer. Moisture from perspiration or incontinence may lead to maceration and skin irritation, which weaken the epidermal barrier. These lesions are most often seen in patients who have diminished or absent sensation, patients with spinal cord injury[56] or degenerative neurologic disease, or those who are debilitated, demented, emaciated, or paralyzed.[57] Other risk factors for the development of pressure sores include advanced age,[58] poor nutrition, and low arteriolar pressure.

CLINICAL PRESENTATION AND DIAGNOSIS

CLINICAL FINDINGS

Pressure sores most commonly occur in tissues over the sacrum and the heels and may involve skin, muscle, and bone. More than 95% of pressure sores are located on the lower body.

CLASSIFICATION

Clinical staging[46] or grading helps to guide management (Table 91.5). Stage I lesions involve only the epidermis,

TABLE 91.5	Classification of Pressure Sores	
Stage	**Description**	**Treatment**
I	Lesion involves only the epidermis; nonblanchable erythema of the intact skin	Relief of pressure and local wound care
II	Partial-thickness loss; ulcer extends into the dermis	Relief of pressure and local wound care
III	Full-thickness loss; deep ulcer extends into the subcutaneous tissue and fascia	Relief of pressure and surgery and systemic antibiotics if needed
IV	Ulcer extends into muscle, bone, or joint	Radical surgery and systemic antibiotics to treat osteomyelitis if present

This classification for pressure ulcers has been recommended by the National Pressure Ulcer Advisory Panel.

stage II ulcers extend into the dermis, stage III ulcers are deep lesions that extend into the subcutaneous tissues, and stage IV lesions extend into muscle and bone. Deep lesions frequently require months to heal and extensive surgical treatments. Figure 91.1 illustrates the classification of lesions based on depth and tissue involvement.

DIAGNOSIS

Identification of patients who are at increased risk is essential to the prevention of pressure sores. Nursing personnel have primary responsibility for the skin care of patients.[59] Several authors have proposed risk assessment scales.[60–63] One such scale, the Braden Scale,[60–64] comprises six subscales: sensory perception, skin moisture, activity level, mobility, nutritional status, and friction and shear. A score of 16 or less out of a possible 23 points predicts development of an ulcer.

The Braden Scale has shown high reliability with different assessors, including nurses' aides, licensed practical nurses, and registered nurses. The size, number, and location of pressure ulcers need to be documented to allow evaluation of the effectiveness of treatment.

The keys to prevention are early recognition of predisposing factors and measures to prevent pressure on sensitive areas, frequent position changes, frequent visual skin inspection, and keeping the predisposed skin areas clean and dry. Durable medical goods and special supplies are useful in these patients. The use of sheepskin or ''egg-crate'' mattresses has been proposed, but objective data suggest that they do not lower pressures sufficiently to prevent pressure sores. Many institutions have nursing policies that combine air mattresses with frequent repositioning to assist in preventing pressure ulcers.

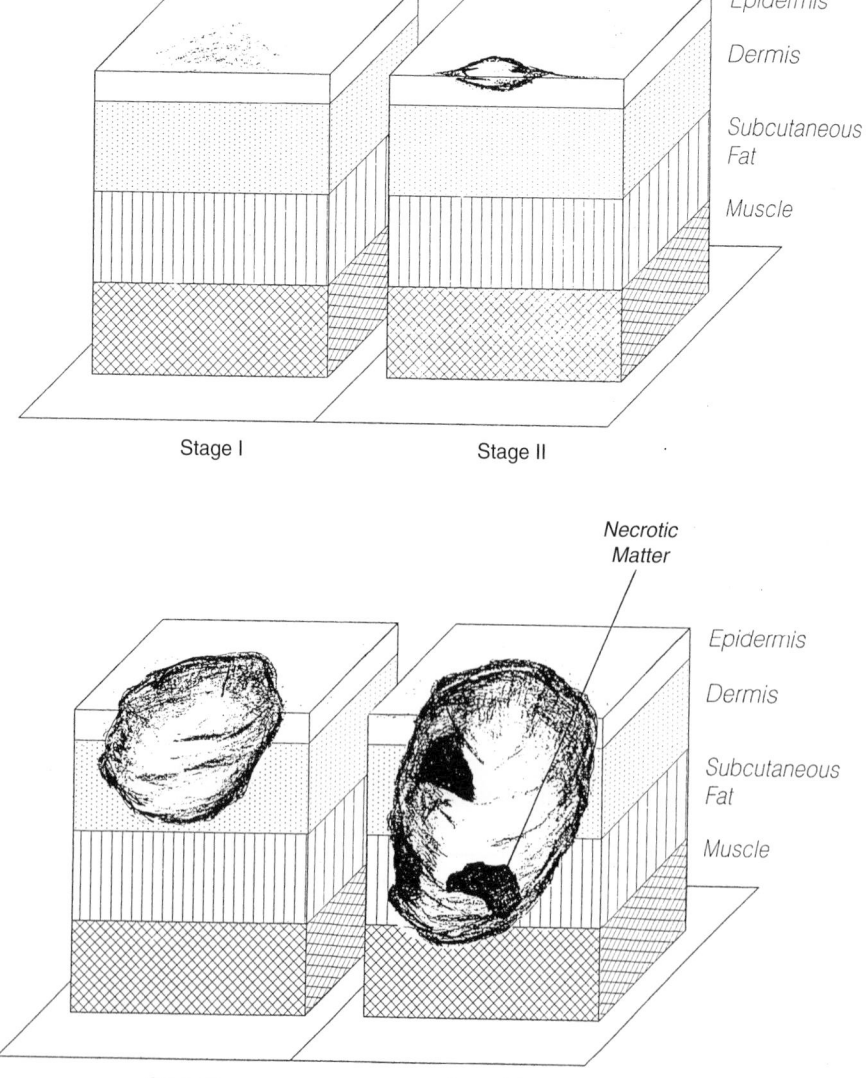

FIGURE 91.1 Classification of pressure sores.

Quigley and Curley[65] developed a pediatric scale called the Braden Q scale. The adverse effects of immobility and physiologic problems present serious issues even in young patients in the pediatric intensive care unit. The performance of the Braden Q scale in a pediatric population was similar to the Braden Scale in adult patients.

PSYCHOSOCIAL ASPECTS

All individuals being treated for pressure ulcers should undergo a psychosocial assessment to determine their ability to comprehend information and their motivation to adhere to the treatment program. The assessment should, at a mini-

mum, include mental status, learning ability, and signs of depression.

THERAPEUTIC PLAN

Ulcer treatment must be planned with the understanding that ulcers are much like an iceberg, with a small visible surface but an extensive unknown base. Many treatments for pressure ulcers have been recommended without adequate evidence to support their use. The treatment of stage I and stage II lesions is primarily local. If the patient cannot adequately oxygenate the tissue, systemic antibiotics are unlikely to have high penetration into the area. Figure 91.2 is an algo-

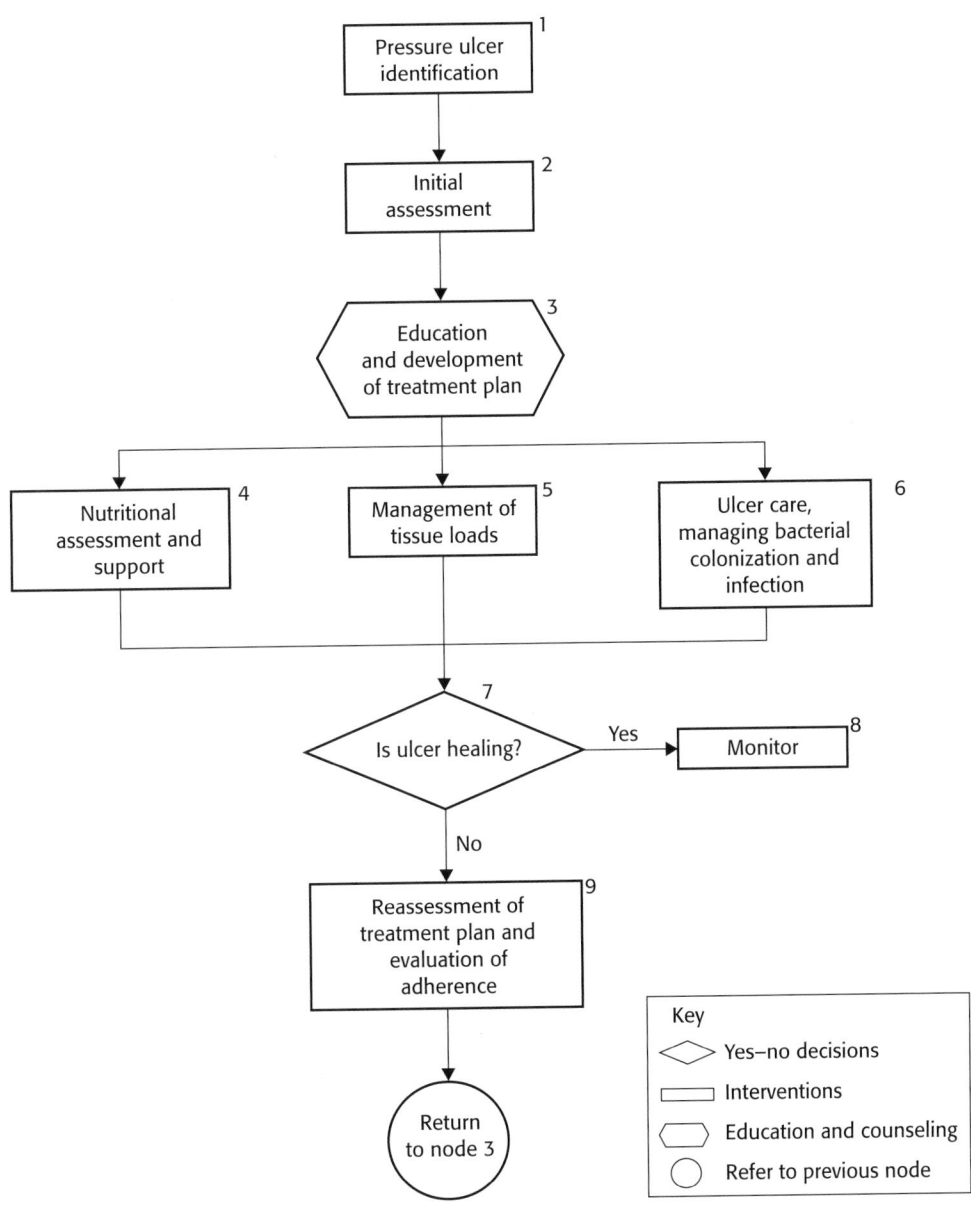

FIGURE 91.2 Algorithm for the management of pressure ulcers: overview. (Reproduced with permission of AHRQ.)

rithm that provides an overview of the activities related to pressure ulcer treatment.[46]

TREATMENT

PHARMACOTHERAPY

Local Therapy. The role of pharmaceutical débriding agents in the care of pressure ulcers is not well defined. Many products that are used as débriding agents are applied to the wound on gauze. Mechanical débridement through the use of gauze dressings may allow earlier development of granulation tissue. However, mechanical débridement with wet-to-dry dressings is painful and may also traumatize the wound.[66] Wet-to-moist or wet-to-wet débridement may accomplish the same result while causing less discomfort. Gauze interacts physically with the wound surface and can cause débridement by dry-to-dry débridement, wet-to-dry débridement, or wet-to-wet débridement. In addition, gauze may harbor bacteria.

Absorbent materials such as dextranomer (Debrisan) microbeads have been used on moist ulcers. Dextranomer is a sterile, chemically inert, hydrophilic substance that removes exudate from the wound surface via an osmotic pressure mechanism. It is available as a paste or bead preparation. When sprinkled onto open wounds, these products are thought to act through the formation of a gel that removes fluids, microbes, and debris from the wound through capillary forces.

Enzymatic débridement has been used to clean pressure sores that are covered with eschar. Eschar is the scab or slough produced by the wound. A moist environment is necessary for optimal enzymatic activity. The wound is cleaned and irrigated with normal saline. A thin layer of enzymatic ointment is applied to the site and covered with a moist dressing. The site should be cleansed and redressed three or four times a day for best results. The action of the enzyme is impaired by certain agents such as benzalkonium chloride, hexachlorophene, nitrofurazone, and thimerosal, which may be used as preservatives in other products. Antibiotics such as penicillin, neomycin, and streptomycin do not affect the enzyme activity. Collagenase–Santyl is collagenase in white petrolatum. Collagenase can dissolve undenatured collagen fibers that retard healing. Collagenase is effective within a narrow pH range of 6 to 8. Collagenase ointment is applied directly to deep wounds with a tongue depressor or onto sterile gauze. In the presence of an infection, the topical antibiotic should be applied first. It is used once daily and is compatible with neomycin–polymyxin B–bacitracin ointment.

It is doubtful whether antiseptics (Table 91.6) have any beneficial effects on open ulcers. The contact time between antiseptic and microbe is too brief for bactericidal effects, and antiseptics may inhibit wound healing locally. The topi-

TABLE 91.6 | Topical Antiseptic Agents

Generic Name	Trade Name	Comments
Chlorhexidine	Hibiclens	Associated with corneal opacification
Povidone–iodine	Betadine	Associated with hypothyroidism
Hydrogen peroxide	Various	Cytotoxic; may impair healing; no longer recommended
Acetic acid	Various	Cytotoxic; may impair healing; no longer recommended
Sodium hypochlorite	Dakin's solution	Cytotoxic; may impair healing; no longer recommended

Chemicals used as antiseptics may kill the microflora in a wound but may also damage delicate, newly forming skin. The AHRQ Clinical Practice guidelines do not recommend any topical antiseptic.

cal use of disinfecting agents may also be counterproductive. These solutions are cytotoxic to granulating tissues and impair wound healing.[67] The clinical practice guidelines published by AHRQ specifically state that antiseptics should not be used in the treatment of pressure sores. Normal saline is the recommended cleansing solution for most pressure ulcers.

The topical antibiotics (Table 91.7) do not penetrate deeper tissues. Antibiotic dressings may not enhance healing and may induce microbial resistance. Neomycin-based products may produce allergic reactions. Infected pressure sores require culture and susceptibility testing with appropriate parenteral antibiotics if bacterial infection is documented.[68] Figure 91.3 guides the clinician through a preferred pathway for managing bacterial colonization and local and systemic infection. A 2-week trial of topical antibiotics (e.g., silver sulfadiazine) for clean pressure ulcers that are not healing should be considered. Silver sulfadiazine is a broad-spectrum agent with activity against

TABLE 91.7 | Topical Antibiotic Agents

Suggested role in pressure ulcers with purulent drainage and/or foul odor:

Silver sulfadiazine

Gentamicin

Bacitracin

Mupirocin (Bactroban)

Metronidazole gel (MetroGel) (not FDA approved)

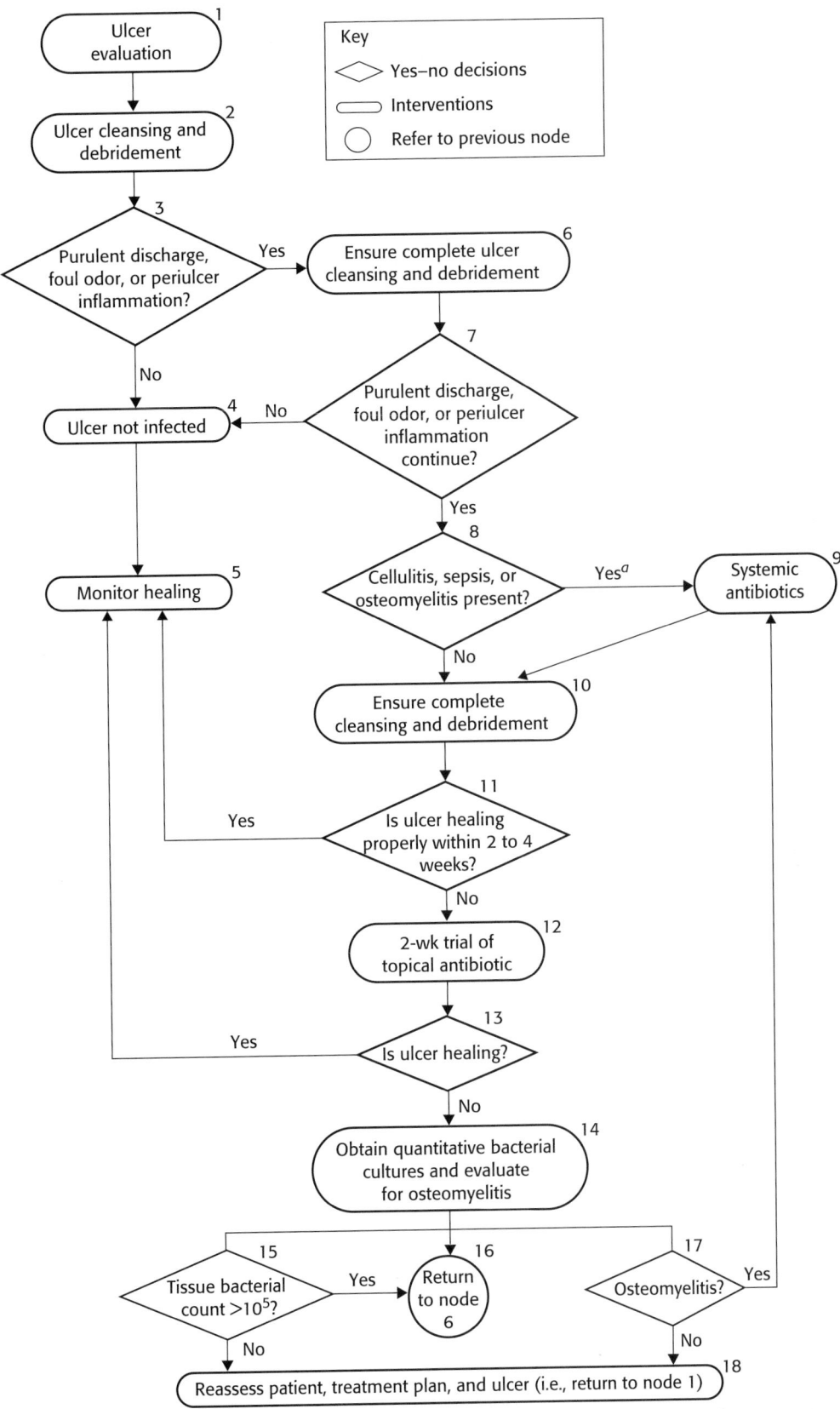

^aSuspicion of sepsis warrants urgent medical evaluation and treatment. Sepsis treatment is not discussed in this guideline.

FIGURE 91.3 Algorithm for managing bacterial colonization and infection. (Reproduced with permission of AHRG.)

gram-positive and gram-negative bacteria. It has been used in pressure ulcers and infected leg ulcers.[69] Topical metronidazole may be effective on infected ulcers that produce a characteristic foul odor. A few studies[70–72] have used once- or twice-daily application of topical metronidazole with promising results, but this is not an indication approved by the U.S. Food and Drug Administration (FDA). In a study by Pierleoni,[72] 1% topical metronidazole was applied to sterile gauze in infected decubitus ulcers every 8 hours. Microbiologic efficacy was documented. It may be combined with oral therapy in suspected or documented susceptible anaerobic infections. A commercially available gel contains metronidazole 0.75% in a water-soluble gel (MetroGel Curatek).

Systemic Therapy. Systemic antibiotics[73] are indicated only when there is evidence of advancing cellulitis, sepsis, bacteremia, or osteomyelitis. Because ulcer débridement results in transient bacteremia in about 50% of patients, prophylaxis for bacterial endocarditis seems prudent in patients with artificial heart valves.

NONPHARMACOLOGIC THERAPY

Nutrition. Attention to nutritional status is essential in the management of pressure ulcers at all stages.[74] Figure 91.4 provides an algorithm to help clinicians ensure that the diet of the patient with a pressure ulcer contains nutrients that are adequate to support healing.[46] Hypoalbuminemic patients have been shown to be at higher risk

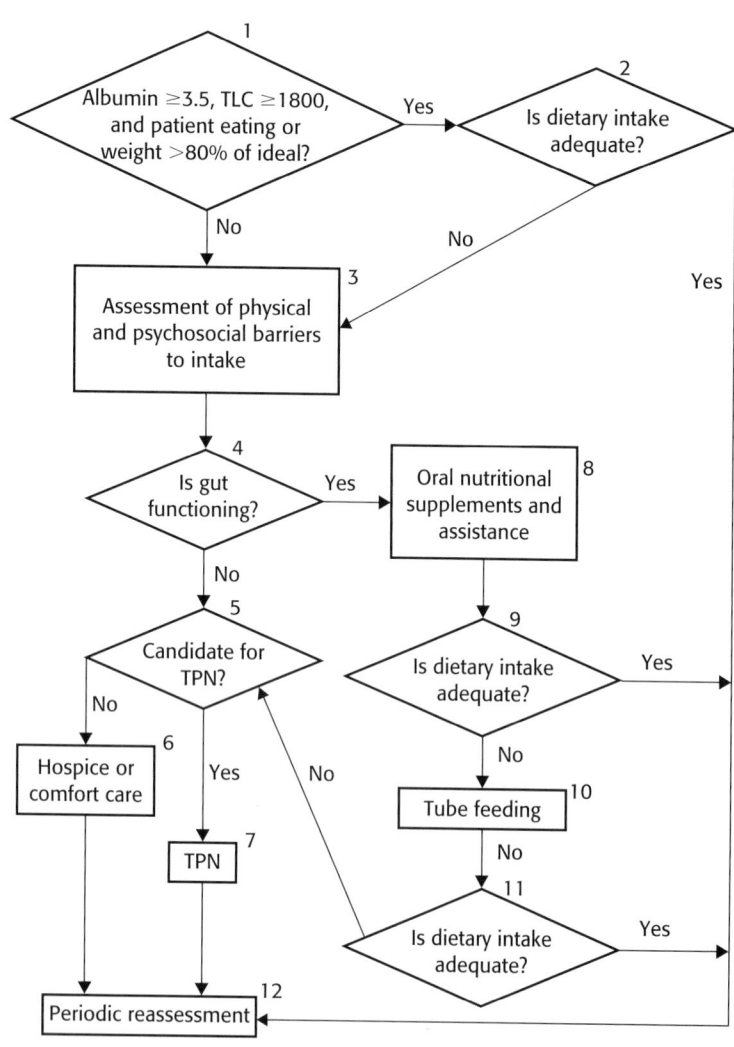

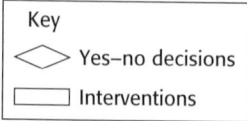

FIGURE 91.4 Algorithm for nutritional assessment and support of patients with pressure sores. (Reproduced with permission of AHRQ.)

TABLE 91.8	Local Wound Therapy for Pressure Ulcers	
Therapy	**Examples**	**Comments**
Cleanse with normal saline or lactated Ringer's		Avoid antiseptic solutions.
Moist environment dressings	AlgiSite M, Cutinova hydro	For moderately to highly exuding wounds
Enzymatic débridement	Collagenase Santyl, Gladase	May also damage healing tissue
Skin barrier products (used primarily with stage I and II ulcers)	Polyurethane: OpSite, Tegaderm, Bioclusive, Acu-Derm	Transparent dressing
	Hydrogel: Biolex, Carrasyn, Flexigel, Solosite, IntraSite, Tegagel	Dressings interact with wound exudate, producing a soft moist gel that enables removal of the dressings with little damage to the newly formed tissue. Dressings stay in place for 1 to 7 days.
	Hydrocolloid: Duoderm, Comfeel, Restore, Tegasorb, NuDerm	Opaque and impermeable to oxygen and water. For heavily draining wounds
	Hydrocellular (foam): Allevyn, Biatain	Can stay in place for up to 7 days. Capable of handling large amounts of exudate

for the development of pressure sores and exhibit slower rates of healing. Nutritional monitoring with attention to dietary protein is essential. In addition, supplementation with ascorbic acid (500 mg twice daily) and zinc sulfate has been suggested, but study flaws make interpretation of this treatment difficult.

Local Care. The mainstay of therapy is local care.[75] Managing an established ulcer involves treatment of underlying medical conditions, proper nutrition and hydration, and the use of dressings or procedures that facilitate repair of tissue. The goal of therapy is to produce a local wound environment that enhances wound healing. Table 91.8 summarizes local wound therapies for pressure ulcers. The environment to promote wound healing is one that is warm, moist, and clean and has an adequate blood supply. This promotes wound healing by permitting the formation of healthy granulation tissue. Polyurethane films such as Tegaderm or OpSite may help to reduce friction between skin and bed sheets and may prevent further skin maceration. OpSite is a semipermeable, gas-permeable, transparent, polyurethane film that permits evaporation of perspiration but is impermeable to bacterial entry. DuoDerm is an impermeable, opaque, hydrocolloid dressing that forms a gel-like wound covering on absorption of wound exudate. This is helpful to prevent and treat stage I lesions.

SURGICAL MANAGEMENT

Débridement is the process of cleaning an open wound by removing foreign material and dead tissue so that healing may occur. Removing dead tissue is necessary to prevent the dead tissue from promoting infection and to start re-epithelialization of the area. Figure 91.5 outlines initial care of the pressure ulcer, including débridement and wound care.[46] Extensive necrotic material can be removed rapidly and effectively by surgical débridement.

HUMAN SKIN EQUIVALENTS AND GROWTH FACTORS

Advances in our understanding of chronic wound biology have led to the development of new treatments. It is hypothesized that lack of cellular and molecular signals required for normal wound repair may be a contributing factor to poor wound healing. Cytokine growth factors provide many of the cellular and molecular signals necessary for normal healing that may be deficient in pressure wounds.[76–80]

IMPROVING OUTCOMES

PATIENT EDUCATION

Educational programs for the prevention of pressure ulcers should include information on risk factors, assessment of common areas, and the importance of reducing pressure, friction, and shear. Because many of the patients are elderly, it is important to carefully assess mental status and cognitive abilities. Family members or the caregiver should attend educational programs as well.

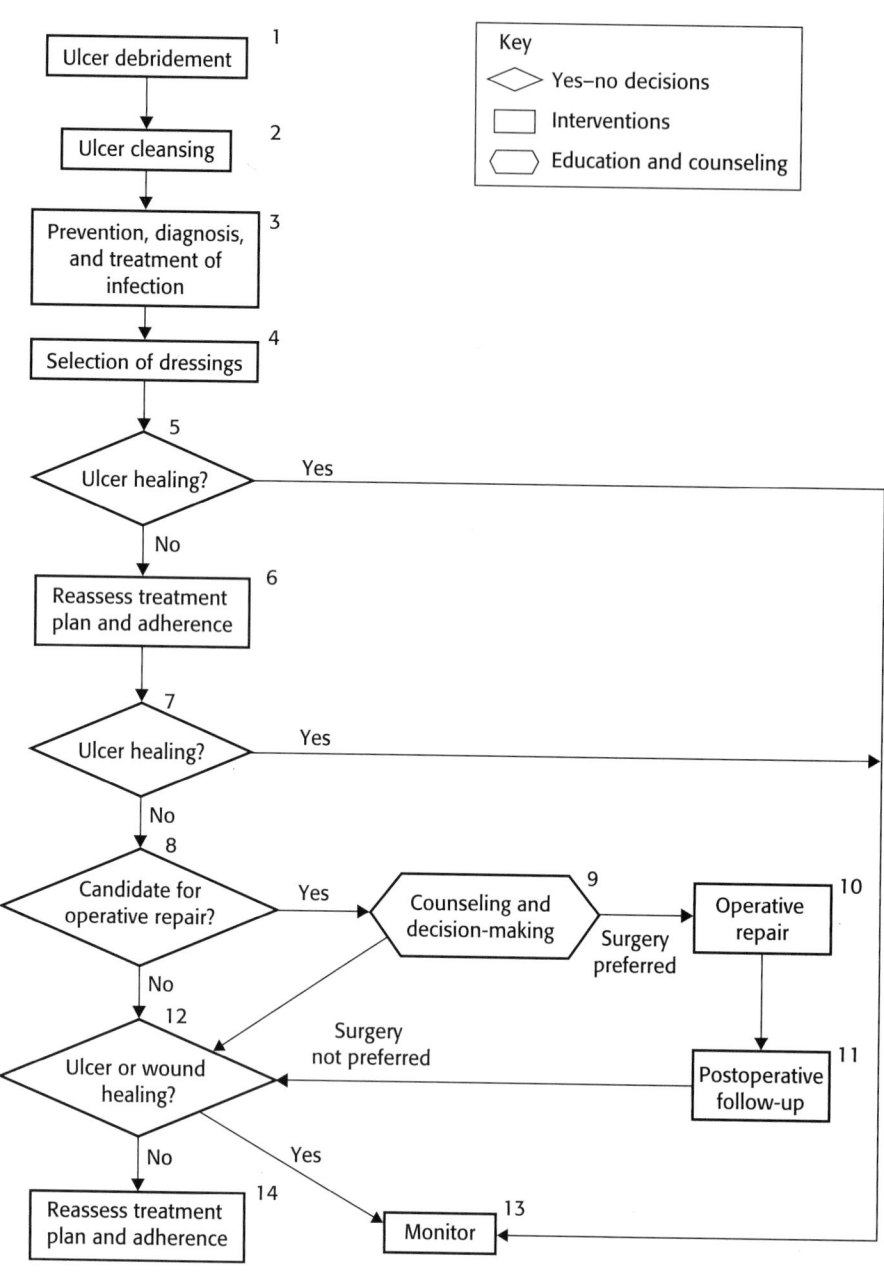

Key
◇ Yes–no decisions
▭ Interventions
⬡ Education and counseling

1. Ulcer debridement
2. Ulcer cleansing
3. Prevention, diagnosis, and treatment of infection
4. Selection of dressings
5. Ulcer healing? — Yes
   No
6. Reassess treatment plan and adherence
7. Ulcer healing? — Yes
   No
8. Candidate for operative repair? — Yes → 9. Counseling and decision-making — Surgery preferred → 10. Operative repair → 11. Postoperative follow-up
   No   Surgery not preferred
12. Ulcer or wound healing?
    No   Yes
14. Reassess treatment plan and adherence   13. Monitor

FIGURE 91.5 Algorithm for pressure ulcer care. (Reproduced with permission of AHRQ.)

BACTERIAL DIABETIC FOOT INFECTIONS

TREATMENT GOALS: BACTERIAL DIABETIC FOOT INFECTIONS

- Control hyperglycemia.
- Administer appropriate antimicrobial therapy.
- Provide local wound care.
- Avoid weight bearing and/or reduce pressure over areas of ulceration.
- Evaluate vascular supply.
- Educate the patient in prevention and follow-up care.

DEFINITION

A diabetic foot infection is defined as a polymicrobial infection of the bones and soft tissues of the lower extremities of a patient with diabetes.[81]

ETIOLOGY

Diabetic patients often have several risk factors for the development of ulcers. Peripheral neuropathy, peripheral vascular disease, edema, and deformity are important components in causing ulceration. Trauma is another contributing factor and is usually associated with inappropriate footwear. Neuropathy, deformity, and trauma are the triad observed in almost two thirds of patients with foot ulcers.[82] Prolonged and excessive pressure over bony prominences of the foot results in callus formation. The callus eventually separates from the underlying dermis and forms an ulcer. These lesions may go unnoticed in patients with peripheral neuropathies due to decreased sensation in the area. Ulceration results in the loss of the protective skin barrier, and when combined with the warm, moist environment of the shoe, infection may spread quickly.[82,83]

EPIDEMIOLOGY

Foot ulcers are a common problem encountered in the management of patients with diabetes. Foot ulcers develop in approximately 15% of diabetic patients and are the leading cause of hospitalization. The annual incidence of diabetic foot ulcers is 2% to 3%; this figure increases to 5% to 7.5% in patients with concomitant neuropathy.[82] Half of the amputations performed in the United States occur in patients with diabetes. Foot ulceration precedes 85% of the nontraumatic lower limb amputations. The first amputation required in a diabetic is a poor prognostic sign; the patient's risk for a second amputation and 5-year mortality rates range from 28% to 51% and 39% to 68%, respectively.[83]

PATHOPHYSIOLOGY

Many factors are involved in the development of diabetic foot ulcers; three major factors are neuropathy, vascular insufficiency, and immunologic defects. Neuropathy, which includes sensory disturbances and autonomic neuropathy with anhidrosis, vasodilation, edema, and erythema, causes structural and functional changes in the foot that alter weight bearing, muscle function and support, and normal pain sensations. Classic neuropathic ulcers occur most frequently on the plantar surfaces of the foot. Vascular insufficiency and angiopathy are risk factors for foot infections, and a decreased blood supply impairs healing in these infections.

Finally, diabetics are impaired hosts. Granulocytes from poorly controlled diabetics exhibit defects in phagocytosis.

These ulcers may involve only superficial tissues or may involve deeper tissues and structures.[82–85] Many classification systems have been reported in the literature to evaluate the ulceration. One of the most frequently cited is a grading system using a 6-point scale (0 to 5) proposed by Wagner; it evaluates the depth and appearance of the wound.[86] Another system, the University of Texas Wound Classification System, evaluates the size and depth of the ulcer, ischemia, and infection. This system appears to be a good outcome predictor.[87]

CLINICAL PRESENTATION AND DIAGNOSIS

SIGNS AND SYMPTOMS

Local signs and symptoms of infection include purulence, cellulitis, and lymphangitis. Systemic signs are more common with severe infection and include fever, leukocytosis, and clinical septicemia. Typical symptoms of pain may not be present because neuropathy can render infection and gangrene relatively painless in a patient with diabetes. For this reason, prophylactic foot care is essential.[82,88,89]

DIAGNOSIS

The commonly accepted definition of foot infection is the presence of systemic signs of infection (fever, leukocytosis), purulent secretions, or two or more local signs/symptoms (redness, warmth, induration, pain, or tenderness).[82,88] Infection should be classified as mild, moderate, or severe, based on the clinical presentation.[90] If infection is suspected, a deep tissue specimen for culture should be obtained aseptically. All skin wounds harbor microorganisms, so swab cultures are not useful or reliable. Urgent diagnosis and appropriate treatment are required due to the limb-threatening potential of diabetic foot infections. Patients with diabetic foot infections should also be evaluated for osteomyelitis, as up to two thirds of patients also have osteomyelitis on presentation.

Aerobic gram-positive organisms most commonly cause superficial infections. *S. aureus* is a frequently isolated microorganism in an infection in which a single pathogen is recovered. Bacteriologic investigations from deep, penetrating ulcers typically reveal polymicrobial isolates, including aerobic and anaerobic species. Commonly isolated gram-positive organisms include *S. epidermidis*, enterococci, Corynebacterium, and group B streptococci. *Pseudomonas aeruginosa*, *Proteus* species, *Klebsiella* species, *Enterobacter* species, and *Escherichia coli* are among the most frequently reported gram-negative organisms. *Bacteroides* species, *Clostridium* species, *Peptococcus*, and *Peptostreptococcus* are regularly encountered anaerobic isolates when an appropriate collection technique is used.[82,88,90–94]

PSYCHOSOCIAL ASPECTS

Management is facilitated when diabetic patients are properly educated to make decisions about their daily care. Patients should have a full psychosocial assessment to determine their ability to comprehend information. A minimum assessment of mental status, learning ability, and psychological well-being can help practitioners understand patient education needs. Diabetic patients require many medications and medical supplies. Issues such as costs and transportation can play an important role in the therapeutic outcome. Visual changes and sensory changes also have a major impact on prevention, recognition, and treatment. Patients with concomitant diabetes and neuropathy have an increased risk of depression. Patients should be routinely screened for depression, as poor foot care and an increased risk of ulcers are more common in patients who are depressed.

THERAPEUTIC PLAN

Diabetic foot infections are commonly treated with a combination of local wound care, surgery, and systemic antimicrobials. Preserving the limb and its function and preventing spread of the infection are primary goals of therapy.[88]

Local wound care consists of foot elevation, elimination of weight-bearing activities, topical antibiotics, and wound dressings. Removing pressure from the affected limb may be accomplished by a variety of methods: casts or boots, sandals, half-shoes, and felted foam dressings. Patient compliance with off-loading (prevention of repetitive trauma associated with walking) is critical in improving ulcer healing. Topical antimicrobials, such as bacitracin and silver sulfadiazine, stimulate healing by eliminating bacteria on the surface of the wound and may be used as adjunctive therapy. Treatment with topical antimicrobials should not exceed 2 weeks to reduce the risk of developing antimicrobial resistance.[95,96]

A moist environment that is free of external contamination assists in healing of the wound and may be accomplished by the use of dressings. Normal saline moist-to-dry dressings are commonly used in the United States. However, disadvantages of moist-to-dry dressings are lack of a sufficiently moist environment and the possibility of nonselective tissue destruction. Many commercially available occlusive dressings are available and include hydrocolloids, alginates, foams, and films. Each of these options has advantages and disadvantages. The appropriate dressing is determined by wound location, depth, condition of wound margins, amount of exudate, presence of infection, need for adhesiveness, and conformability of the dressing.[82,88,95,96]

Surgical measures include débridement, drainage, and if necessary amputation. Débridement is the process of removing necrotic tissue, foreign material, and/or infected tissue from the wound. To promote healing and enhance the effectiveness of other treatment measures, débridement is critical. Some of the available débridement techniques are autolytic, enzymatic, chemical, or sharp. The most thoroughly studied method is sharp débridement, which involves removal of the callus with a scalpel and forceps.[82,88,95,96]

In addition, the patient must monitor and control his or her blood glucose levels to achieve maximum therapeutic benefit, as chronic hyperglycemia impairs leukocyte function. Patients should also be counseled on the importance of smoking cessation. Smoking affects vascular factors and also increases the rates of incisional wound infections when compared to nonsmokers.[82,88]

TREATMENT

PHARMACOTHERAPY

In the treatment of infected diabetic foot ulcers, objective data from randomized trials are lacking, and strategies for appropriate antibiotic therapy are largely based on clinical experience. Determination of the optimal antibiotic is based on factors such as suspected bacterial flora, appearance of the infected site, history of the lesion, and the patient's clinical condition[88] (Table 91.9). The antibiotic that is most active against the causative agent and has the narrowest spectrum should be chosen so as not to promote the development of antimicrobial resistance.

Oral antimicrobial therapy is acceptable for the treatment of mild, superficial lesions in the early stages of infection, with minimal drainage, and in the absence of gangrene and systemic symptoms. In a prospective study of outpatient oral treatment of mild diabetic foot infections with a 2-week course of either cephalexin (500 mg four times daily) or clindamycin (300 mg four times daily), Lipsky et al[92] found that both agents were effective and produced comparable rates of cure/improvement (96% clindamycin vs. 86% cephalexin). Other commonly used oral antibiotics are ciprofloxacin, levofloxacin, and amoxicillin–clavulanate. If no improvement is observed after 48 to 72 hours, intravenous therapy should be initiated.[88] Empiric intravenous antibiotics are recommended in serious infections when there is evidence of cellulitis, septicemia, or osteomyelitis.[88,97,98]

Because diabetics are impaired hosts and have granulocyte defects, bactericidal antibiotics are preferred, and prolonged courses of treatment may be necessary. The recommended length of therapy for soft tissue infection is 1 to 2 weeks. Osteomyelitis may require more than 6 weeks of therapy. The appropriate time to switch from intravenous to oral antimicrobial therapy varies. These infections are presumed to be polymicrobic with aerobes and anaerobes. Empiric therapy should provide broad coverage until culture results are available. The higher incidence of renal insufficiency in diabetic patients requires cautious use and careful monitoring of nephrotoxic agents such as the aminoglycosides. Ampicillin–sulbactam, ticarcillin–clavulanate, piperacillin–tazobactam, meropenem, imipenem–cilastatin, and ertapenem are reasonable choices for monotherapy because

TABLE 91.9	Antibiotic Regimens for Infected Diabetic Ulcers	
Appearance	**Microbiology**	**Possible Treatment Regimen**
Limited in extent	Aerobic gram-positive cocci	Oral clindamycin
		Oral (first-gen. cephalosporin) cephalexin
		Oral amoxicillin − clavulanate
		Intravenous cefazolin
		Oral ciprofloxacin + clindamycin
		Oral trimethoprim–sulfamethoxazole
Chronic, recurrent limb-threatening	Polymicrobic (aerobes and anaerobes)	Cefoxitin
		Oral ciprofloxacin + clindamycin
	If septic	Imipenem–cilastatin
		Meropenem
		Ertapenem
		Ticarcillin–clavulanate
		Piperacillin–tazobactam
		Ampicillin–sulbactam
		Cefepime + metronidazole
		Vancomycin + metronidazole + aztreonam
		Ampicillin + antipseudomonal aminoglycoside + clindamycin
		Penicillinase-resistant synthetic penicillin + antipseudomonal aminoglycoside + clindamycin

of their broad spectrum of activity against most anticipated organisms. Table 91.9 lists agents that may be useful in the treatment of diabetic foot infections. Even with careful treatment and monitoring, however, amputation may be necessary under certain conditions.

Diabetic foot ulcers can take a long time to heal because of the underlying poor circulation and tissue oxygenation. Nutritional monitoring and support are essential. Anemia should be corrected to enhance tissue oxygenation.

ADJUNCTIVE THERAPY

Recombinant platelet-derived growth factor (becaplermin; Regranex, Ortho-McNeil) was the first growth factor approved by the FDA for the treatment of neuropathic foot ulcers in patients with diabetes. The most successful of the four placebo-controlled trials resulted in a moderate improvement in the rate of healing at 20 weeks (50% in the growth factor patients vs. 35% in the placebo patients).[82] Although other growth factors have failed to demonstrate improved healing, a recent review concluded that platelet-derived growth factor may be useful as adjunctive therapy in the treatment of chronic neuropathic ulcers that do not respond to conventional therapies.[99] Tissue engineered skin (Apligraf, Organogenesis) and dermis derived from human fibroblasts (Dermagraft, Smith and Nephew) are additional adjunctive therapies that are associated with faster healing. Patients who do not experience a reduction in ulcer size after 4 weeks of conventional therapy should be considered for adjunctive therapies. However, current adjunctive therapies are significantly limited by their substantial costs.[82] Electrical stimulation, administration of hyperbaric oxygen, and hydrotherapies are other adjuvant therapies that may be used.

IMPROVING OUTCOMES

PATIENT EDUCATION

The patient and caregivers need to learn the basics of foot care. In patients with reduced vision secondary to retinopathy, the role of the family and caregivers becomes very important. The patient should be instructed to follow a program of proper footwear, education, and regular foot care. Diabetic education programs can be an important source of information, resulting in better glycemic control and fewer lower extremity infections.

KEY POINTS

■ Skin and soft tissue infections are common. Treatment demands knowledge of the anticipated flora and the host's normal defense mechanisms. The infections result in morbidity and extended healthcare needs

- Decubitus ulcers and diabetic foot ulcers result from an interplay of the host factors and tissue invasion that result in chronic care dilemmas
- Healthcare practitioners should be knowledgeable about the therapeutic management issues of skin and soft tissue infections

SUGGESTED READINGS

Bonnetblanc JM, Bedane C. Erysipelas: recognition and management. Am J Clin Dermatol 4:157–163, 2003.

Boulton AJM, Kirsner RS, Vileikyte L. Neuropathic diabetic foot ulcers. N Engl J Med 351:48–55, 2004.

Brown J, Shriner DL, Schwartz RA, Janniger CK. Impetigo: an update (review). Int J Dermatol 42:251–255, 2003.

Givner LB. Periorbital versus orbital cellulitis. Pediatr Infect Dis J 21:1157–1158, 2002.

Lyder CH. Pressure ulcer prevention and management. JAMA 289:223–226, 2003.

Swartz MN. Cellulitis. N Engl J M ed 350:904–912, 2004.

REFERENCES

1. Swartz MN. Cellulitis and subcutaneous tissue infections. In: Mandell GL, Bennett JE, Dolin R, eds. Principles and practice of infectious diseases, 5th ed. Philadelphia: Churchill Livingstone, 2000: 1037–1057.
2. Dupuy A, Benchikhi H, Roujeau JC, et al. Risk factors for erysipelas of the leg (cellulitis): case-control study. Br Med J 318: 1591–1594, 1999.
3. Swartz MN. Cellulitis. N Engl J Med 350:904–912, 2004.
4. Vinken AG, Li JZ, Balan DA, et al. Comparison of linezolid with oxacillin or vancomycin in the empiric treatment of cellulitis in US hospitals. Am J Ther 10:264–274, 2003.
5. Sachs MK. The optimum use of needle aspiration in the bacteriologic diagnosis of cellulitis in adults. Arch Intern Med 150: 1907–1912, 1990.
6. Lindbeck G, Powers R. Cellulitis. Hosp Pract (Off Ed) 28 (suppl 2): 10–14, 1993.
7. Perl B, Gottehrer NP, Raveh D, et al. Cost effectiveness of blood cultures for adult patients with cellulitis. Clin Infect Dis 29: 1483–1488, 1999.
8. Parish LC, Routh HG, Miskin B, et al. Moxifloxacin versus cephalexin in the treatment of uncomplicated skin infections. Int J Clin Pract 54:497–503, 2000.
9. Preston SL, Drusano GL. Gatifloxacin: a new fluoroquinolone for use in community-acquired pneumonia and other infections. Formulary 34:1002–1015, 1999.
10. Nichols RL, Smith JW, Gentry LO, et al. Multicenter, randomized study comparing levofloxacin and ciprofloxacin for uncomplicated skin and skin structure infections. South Med J 90:1193–1200, 1997.
11. Nicodemo AC, Robledo JA, Jasovich A, et al. A multicentre, double-blind, randomised study comparing the efficacy and safety of oral levofloxacin versus ciprofloxacin in the treatment of uncomplicated skin and skin structure infections. IJCP 52:69–74, 1998.
12. Gainer RB. Ceftriaxone in the treatment of serious infections. Skin and soft tissue infections. Hosp Pract (Off Ed) 26 (suppl 5):24–30, 1991.
13. Campoli-Richards DM, Brogden RN. Sulbactam/ampicillin. A review of its antibacterial activity, pharmacokinetic properties, and therapeutic uses. Drugs 33:577–609, 1987.
14. Tan JS, Wishnow RM, Talan DA, et al. The piperacillin/ tazobactam skin and skin structure study group. Treatment of hospitalized patients with complicated skin and skin structure infections: double-blind, randomized, multicenter study of piperacillin-tazobactam versus ticarcillin-clavulanate. Antimicrob Agents Chemother 37: 1580–1586, 1993.
15. Choice of antibacterial drugs. Medical Letter 2:13–26, 2004.
16. Graham DR, Talan DA, Nichols RL, et al. Once-daily, high dose levofloxacin versus ticarcillin-clavulanate alone or followed by amoxicillin-clavulanate for complicated skin and skin-structure infections: a randomized, open-label trial. Clin Infect Dis 35:381–389, 2002.
17. Brown J, Shriner DL, Schwartz RA, et al. Impetigo: an update (review). Int J Dermatol 42:251–255, 2003.
18. Dagan R. Impetigo in childhood: changing epidemiology and new treatments. Pediatr Ann 22:235–40, 1993.
19. Demidovich CW, Wittler RR, Ruff ME, et al. Impetigo: current etiology and comparison of penicillin, erythromycin and cephalexin therapies. Am J Dis Child 144:1313–1315, 1990.
20. Dagan R, Bar-David Y. A double-blind study comparing erythromycin and mupirocin for treatment of impetigo in children: implication of a high prevalence of erythromycin-resistant *Staphylococcus aureus* strain. Antimicrob Agents Chemother 36:287–290, 1992.
21. Jacob RF, Brown WD, Chartrand S, et al. Evaluation of cefuroxime axetil and cefadroxil suspension for the treatment of pediatric skin infections. Antimicrob Agents Chemother 36:1614–1618, 1992.
22. Blumer JL, Lemon E, O'Horo J, et al. Changing therapy for skin and soft tissue infections in children: have we come full circle? Pediatr Infect Dis J 6:117–122, 1987.
23. Bisno AL, Stevens DL. Streptococcal infections of skin and soft tissues. N Engl J Med 334:240–245, 1996.
24. Sadick NS. Current aspects of bacterial infections of the skin. Dermatol Clin 15:341–349, 1997.
25. Goldfarb J, Crenshaw D, O'Hord J, et al. Randomized clinical trial of topical mupirocin versus oral erythromycin for impetigo. Antimicrob Agents Chemother 32:1780–1783, 1988.
26. Gisby J, Bryant J. Efficacy of a new cream formulation of mupirocin: comparison with oral and topical agents in experimental skin infections. Antimicrob Agents Chemother 44:255–260, 2000.
27. Leyden JJ. Review of mupirocin ointment in the treatment of impetigo. Clin Pediatr 31:549–553, 1992.
28. Bass JW, Chan DS, Creamer KM, et al. Comparison of oral cephalexin, topical mupirocin, and topical bacitracin for treatment of impetigo. Pediatr Infect Dis 16:708–710, 1997.
29. Britton JW, Fajardo JE, Krafte-Jacos B. Comparison of mupirocin and erythromycin in the treatment of impetigo. J Pediatr 117: 827–829, 1990.
30. McLinn S. Topical mupirocin vs systemic erythromycin treatment for pyoderma. Pediatr Infect Dis J 7:785–790, 1988.
31. McLinn S. A bacteriologically controlled, randomized study comparing the efficacy of 2% mupirocin ointment (Bactroban) with oral erythromycin in the treatment of patients with impetigo. J Am Acad Dermatol 22:883–885, 1990.
32. Barton LL, Friedman AD, Sharky AM, et al. Impetigo contagiosa, III: comparative efficacy of oral erythromycin and topical mupirocin. Pediatr Dermatol 6:134–138, 1989.
33. Bonnetblanc JM, Bedane C. Erysipelas: recognition and management. Am J Clin Dermatol 4:157–163, 2003.
34. Canoso JJ, Barza M. Soft tissue infections. Rheum Dis Clin North A 19:293–307, 1993.
35. Fekety FR Jr. Erysipelas. In: Demis DJ, ed. Clinical dermatology, volume 3, section 16. Philadelphia: JB Lippincott, 1992:1–4.
36. Ben-Amitai D, Ashkenazi S. Common bacterial skin infections in childhood. Pediatr Ann 22:225–233, 1993.
37. Gilbert DN, Moellering RC Jr, Eliopoulos GM, et al, eds. The Sanford guide to antimicrobial therapy, 34th ed. Vermont: Antimicrobial Therapy, 2004:36–37.
38. Kahn RM, Goldstein EJC. Common bacterial skin infections. Postgrad Med 93:175–182, 1993.
39. Bratton RL, Nesse RE. St. Anthony's fire: diagnosis and management of erysipelas. Am Fam Physician 51:401–404, 1995.
40. Eriksson B, Jorup-Rönström C, Karkkonen K, et al. Erysipelas: clinical and bacteriologic spectrum and serological aspects. Clin Infect Dis 23:1091–1098, 1996.
41. Sjöblom AC, Eriksson B, Jorup-Rönström C, et al. Antibiotic prophylaxis in recurrent erysipelas. Infection 21:390–393, 1993.
42. Kremer M, Zuckerman R, Avraham Z, et al. Long-term antimicrobial therapy in the prevention of recurrent soft-tissue infections. J Infect 22:37–40, 1991.

43. Malinow I, Powell KR. Periorbital cellulitis. Pediatr Ann 22: 241–246, 1993.
44. Givner LB. Pneumococcal facial cellulitis in children. Pediatrics 106:e61, 2000.
45. Givner LB. Periorbital versus orbital cellulitis. Pediatr Infect Dis J 21:1157–1158, 2002.
46. Schwartz GR, Wright SW. Changing bacteriology of periorbital cellulitis. Ann Emerg Med 28:617–620, 1996.
46. Panel for the Prediction and Prevention of Pressure Ulcers in Adults. Pressure ulcers in adults: prediction and prevention. Clinical Practice Guideline, Number 3. AHCPR Publication No. 92–0047. Rockville, MD: Agency for Health Care Policy and Research, Public Health Service, U.S. Department of Health and Human Services. May 1992 (reviewed 2002).
47. Bergstrom N, Bennett MA, Carlson CE, et al. Treatment of pressure ulcers. Clinical Practice Guideline, No. 15. Rockville, MD: U.S. Department of Health and Human Services, Public Health Service, Agency for Health Care Policy and Research. AHCPR Publication. No. 95–0652, December 1994 (reviewed 2000).
48. National Pressure Ulcer Advisory Panel. Pressure ulcer prevalence, cost and risk assessment. Consensus development conference statement. Decubitus 2:24–28, 1989.
49. Brandeis GH, Morris JN, Nash DJ, et al. The epidemiology and natural history of pressure ulcers in elderly nursing home residents. JAMA 264:2905–2909, 1990.
50. Young JB, Dobrzanski S. Pressure sores: epidemiology and current management concepts. Drugs Aging 2:42–57, 1992.
51. Lyder CH. Pressure ulcer prevention and management. JAMA 289: 223–226, 2003.
52. Lyder CH, Preston J, Grady JN, et al. Quality of care for hospitalized Medicare patients at risk for pressure ulcers. Arch Intern Med 161:1549–1554, 2001.
53. Leigh IH, Bennett G. Pressure ulcers: prevalence, etiology, and treatment modalities. Am J Surg 167 (1A Suppl):25S–30S, 1994.
54. Longe RL. Current concepts in clinical therapeutics: pressure sores. Clin Pharm 5:669–681, 1986.
55. Spoelhof GD, Ide K. Pressure ulcers in nursing home patients. Am Fam Physician 47:1207–1215, 1993.
56. Ditunno JF Jr, Formal CS. Chronic spinal cord injury. N Engl J Med 330:550–556, 1994.
57. Hunter SM, Cathcart-Silberberg T, Langemo DK, et al. Pressure ulcer prevalence and incidence in a rehabilitation hospital. Rehab Nurs 17:239–242, 1992.
58. Allman RM. Pressure ulcers among the elderly. N Engl J Med 320: 850–853, 1989.
59. Young ZF, Evans A, Davis J. Nosocomial pressure ulcer prevention: a successful project. JONA 33:380–383, 2003.
60. Gosnell DJ. Assessment and evaluation of pressure sores. Nurs Clin North Am 22:339–415, 1987.
61. Bergstrom N, Braden BJ, Laguzza A, et al. The Braden scale for predicting pressure sore risk. Nurs Res 36:205–210, 1987.
62. Bergstrom N, Demuth PJ, Braden BJ. A clinical trial of the Braden scale for predicting pressure sore risk. Nurs Clin North Am 22: 417–428, 1987.
63. Bergstrom N, Braden B. A prospective study of pressure sore risk among institutionalized elderly. J Am Geriatr Soc 40:747–758, 1992.
64. Bergstrom N, Braden BJ. Predictive validity of the Braden Scale among black and white subjects. Nurs Res 51:398–403, 2002.
65. Curley MAQ, Razmus IS, Roberts KE, et al. Predicting pressure ulcer risk in pediatric patients. The Braden Q Scale. Nurs Res 52: 22–33, 2003.
66. Stuzin J, Engrav L, Buehler P. Care of open wounds. Compr Ther 8:32–34, 1982.
67. Takahashi PY, Kiemele LJ, Jones JP. Wound care of elderly patient: advances and clinical applications for practicing physicians. Mayo Clin Proc 79:260–267, 2004.
68. Rogers KG. The rational use of antimicrobial agents in simple wounds. Emerg Med Clin North Am 10:753–766, 1992.
69. Payne CM, Bladin C, Colchester AC, et al. Argyria from excessive use of topical silver sulphadiazine [letter]. Lancet 340:126, 1992.
70. Jones PH, Willis AT, Ferguson IR. Treatment of anaerobically infected pressure sores with topical metronidazole. Lancet 8057: 213–214, 1978.
71. Young JB, Dobrzanski S. Pressure sores. Epidemiology and current management concepts. Drugs Aging 2:42–57, 1997.
72. Pierleoni EE. Topical metronidazole therapy for infected decubitus ulcers. J Am Geriatr Soc 32:775–781, 1984.
73. Leaper DJ. Prophylactic and therapeutic role of antibiotics in wound care. Am J Surg 167 (1A Suppl):15S–19S, 1994.
74. Telfer NR, Moy RL. Drug and nutrient aspects of wound healing. Dermatol Clin 11:729–737, 1993.
75. Howell JM. Current and future trends in wound healing. Emerg Med Clin North Am 10:655–663, 1992.
76. Payne WG, Ochs DE, Meltzer DD, et al. Long-term outcome of growth factor-treated pressure ulcers. Am J Surg 181:81–86, 2001.
77. Robson MC, Hill DP, Smith PD, et al. Sequential cytokine therapy for pressure ulcers: clinical and mechanistic response. Ann Surg 231:600–611, 2000.
78. Bello YM, Phillips TJ. Recent advances in wound healing. JAMA 283:716–718, 2000.
79. Brem H, Balledux J, Bloom T, et al. Healing of diabetic foot ulcers and pressure ulcers with human skin equivalent: a new paradigm in wound healing. Arch Surg 135:627–634, 2000.
80. Kallianinem LK, Hirshberg J, Marchant B, et al. Role of platelet-derived growth factor as an adjunct to surgery in the management of pressure ulcers. Plast Reconstr Surg 106:1243–1248, 2000.
81. Taber's electronic dictionary. FA Davis, 2001.
82. Boulton AJM, Kirsner RS, Vileikyte L. Neuropathic diabetic foot ulcers. N Engl J Med 351:48–55, 2004.
83. Culleton JL. Preventing diabetic foot complications. Postgrad Med 106:74–83, 1999.
84. Caputo GM, Cavanagh PR, Ulbrecht, et al. Assessment and management of foot disease in patients with diabetes. N Engl J Med 331: 854–860, 1994.
85. Caputo GM, Joshi N, Weitekamp MR. Foot infections in patients with diabetes. Am Fam Physician 56:195–202, 1997.
86. Wagner FW. The dysvascular foot: a system for diagnosis and treatment. Foot Ankle 2:64–122, 1981.
87. Armstrong DG, Lavery LA, Harkless LB. Validation of a diabetic wound classification system: the contribution of depth, infection and ischemia to risk of amputation. Diabetes Care 21:855–859, 1998.
88. West NJ. Systemic antimicrobial treatment of foot infections in diabetic patients. Am J Health Syst Pharm 52:1198–1207, 1995.
89. Watkins PJ. The diabetic foot. Br Med J 326:977–979, 2003.
90. Shea KW. Antimicrobial therapy for diabetic foot infections. Postgrad Med 106:85–94, 1999.
91. Peterson LR, Lissack LM, Canter K, et al. Therapy of lower extremity infections with ciprofloxacin in patients with diabetes mellitus, peripheral vascular disease, or both. Am J Surg 86:801–808, 1989.
92. Lipsky BA, Pecoraro RE, Larson SA, et al. Outpatient management of uncomplicated lower-extremity infections in diabetic patients. Arch Intern Med 150:790–797, 1990.
93. Wheat LJ, Allen SD, Henry M, et al. Diabetic foot infections. Arch Intern Med 146:1935–1940, 1986.
94. Mertz PM, Ovington LG. Wound healing microbiology. Dermatol Clin 11:739–747, 1993.
95. Millington JT, Norris TW. Effective treatment strategies for diabetic foot wounds. J Family Practice 49:S40–S48, 2000.
96. Muha J. Local wound care in diabetic foot complications. Postgrad Med 106:97–102, 1999.
97. Gentry LO. Therapy with newer oral beta-lactam and quinolone agents for infections of the skin and skin structures: a review. Clin Infect Dis 14:285–297, 1992.
98. Leichter SB, Schaefer JC, O'Brian JT. New concepts in managing diabetic foot infections. Geriatrics 46:24–30, 1991.
99. Bennett SP, Griffiths GD, Schor AM, et al. Growth factors in the treatment of diabetic foot ulcers. Br J Surg 90:133–146, 2003.

CASE STUDIES

CASE 30

TOPIC: Ventilator-Associated Pneumonia (VAP)

THERAPEUTIC DIFFICULTY: Level 3
Brian M. Hodges and Douglas Slain

Chapter 75: Pneumonia

■ Scenario

Patient and Setting: GL, a 57-year-old female; surgical intensive care unit (SICU)

Chief Complaint: Fever, increasing ventilatory support needs, and production of purulent sputum

■ History of Present Illness

GL has developed a fever and a new infiltrate is noted in the right middle and lower lobes on a portable chest radiograph; has required suctioning every hour due to copious production of green sputum; minute ventilation has increased substantially, requiring more ventilatory support to maintain adequate gas exchange

Past Medical History: Admitted to the SICU 6 days ago following a subarachnoid hemorrhage due to a ruptured intracranial aneurysm; underwent aneurysm coiling 16 hours after admission; has remained mechanically ventilated in the SICU since the operation, having only exhibited a partial neurologic recovery; does not follow commands; has become agitated on several occasions; urine analysis on ICU day 3 revealed the presence of bacteria, and the patient was prescribed ciprofloxacin, despite a lack of definitive culture data, fever, or leukocytosis confirming the presence of a urinary tract infection; treated for hypercholesterolemia as an outpatient

Past Surgical History: Tonsillectomy at age 8 and laparoscopic cholecystecomy at age 49

Family/Social History: Family History: No relatives known with ruptured aneurysms
Social History: Smoked 1 pack cigarettes/day for the last 40 years, two alcoholic beverages/week (per family report)

Medications:
Ciprofloxacin, 400 mg IV q12h
Fentanyl infusion, 30 μg/hour
Propofol infusion, 25 μg/kg/min
Phenytoin, 100 mg IV q8h
Famotidine, 20 mg IV q12h
Nimodipine, 60 mg OG q4h
Senna liquid, 5 mL OG BID
Docusate liquid, 100 mg OG BID
Albuterol/ipratropium MDI, 5 puffs q4h and PRN

Allergies: Sulfonamides (rash)

■ Physical Examination

GEN: Well-developed, well-nourished white female appears in moderate distress due to respiratory difficulty
VS: BP 110/65, RR 24, HR 120, T 39.3°C, Wt 65 kg, Ht 165 cm
HEENT: Airway suctioning reveals purulent green sputum, orogastric tube present
COR: Normal S_1 and S_2, no murmurs, rubs, or gallops
CHEST: Bilateral rales and rhonchi, greater on the right
ABD: WNL
GU: Foley catheter in place, urine clear yellow
RECT: WNL
EXT: Clean, dry and intact; sequential compression devices on bilateral lower extremities, right subclavian triple-lumen catheter noted (placed 3 days ago), site nonerythematous
NEURO: Glasgow Coma Scale (with propofol/fentanyl held) E3 V1(intubated) M4

■ Results of pertinent Laboratory Tests, Serum Drug Concentrations, and Diagnostic Tests

Na 137 (137)	Hct 0.33 (33)	AST 0.5 (30)
K 3.9 (3.9)	Hgb 110 (11.0)	ALT 0.67 (40)
Cl 100 (100)	Lkcs 19.1 × 10⁹ (19.1 × 10³)	Glu 6.1 (110)
HCO₃ 23 (23)	Plts 240 × 10⁹ (240 × 10³)	TG 1.36 (120)
BUN 5.7 (16)		
CR 80 (0.9)		

Lkc differential: PMN 0.85 (85%), bands 0.09 (9%), lymphs 0.06 (6%)
ABG $F_iO_2 = 0.5$ (50%): PO_2 90, PCO_2 47, pH 7.36
Urine culture: 1,000–10,000 mixed gram-positive cocci
Chest x-ray: new infiltrates noted in RLL, RML consistent with pneumonia

■ Problem List

Identify principal problems from the scenario in priority order (see Answers in back of book for correct list of problems).

■ SOAP Note

To be completed by the student (see Answers in back of book for correct SOAP Note).

■ QUESTIONS

(See Answers in back of book for correct responses.)

1. Which of the following pathogens is the most likely cause of GL's pneumonia? (EO-1, 3)
   a. *Moraxella catharralis*
   b. *Pseudomonas aeruginosa*
   c. *Haemophilus influenzae*
   d. *Staphylococcus epidermidis*

2. List three common methods for lower respiratory tract specimen collection that should be considered when attempting to identify a pathogen in GL. (EO-5)

3. Which of the following classes of antibiotics should be avoided in designing an empiric regimen to treat GL's pneumonia? (EO-1, 4, 8)
   a. Carbapenems
   b. Aminoglycosides
   c. Beta-lactam/beta-lactamase inhibitors
   d. Fluoroquinolones

4. List the antibiotics (drug, route, and dosing interval) you would recommend empirically for GL. (EO-4, 6, 8, 11)

5. Explain how optimizing GL's analgesic and sedative therapy can affect the development of ventilator-associated pneumonia (VAP). (EO-9, 10, 12)

6. Explain how maintaining euglycemia from admission to the ICU benefits patients like GL. (EO-9, 10, 12)

7. What laboratory tests and physical signs and symptoms indicate that GL has VAP? (EO-2, 5)

8. If vancomycin is indicated to treat GL's VAP, what is the goal trough concentration ? (EO-4, 6, 12)
   a. 0–5 μg/mL
   b. 5–10 μg/mL
   c. 10–15 μg/mL
   d. 15–20 μg/mL

9. If, on day 4 of therapy, GL's infiltrates are no longer present on x-ray, she is no longer febrile, and a noninfectious cause of her symptoms is identified, what is the most appropriate course of action? (EO-2, 5, 9, 10, 11)
   a. Switch to cefazolin monotherapy
   b. Complete her current course of therapy
   c. Resume her ciprofloxacin therapy
   d. Discontinue all antibiotics

10. If GL is found to have *K. pneumoniae* VAP susceptible to an agent in your empiric regimen and has symptom resolution by day 4 of therapy, what total duration of antibiotic treatment is recommended? (EO-5, 8, 11)
    a. 4 days
    b. 8 days
    c. 14 days
    d. 21 days

11. If GL is found to be infected with an ESBL producing strain of *K. pneumoniae*, which of the following antimicrobials is the most appropriate choice of therapy? (EO-5, 8, 11)
    a. Cefuroxime
    b. Ceftazidime
    c. Meropenem
    d. Levofloxacin

12. Explain how knowing local susceptibility patterns would affect the choice of empiric antibiotics for GL. (EO-8, 11)

13. Evaluate the pharmacoeconomic considerations relative to GL's plan of care. (EO-17)

14. Synthesize etiology, pathophysiology, epidemiology, therapeutic, and disease management concepts for VAP using a key points format. (EO-18)

CASE 31

TOPIC: Tuberculosis

THERAPEUTIC DIFFICULTY: Level 3
Helene Hardy and Caroline S. Zeind

Chapter 76: Tuberculosis
Chapter 84: HIV Infection-Antiretroviral Therapy

■ Scenario

Patient and Setting: SV, 65-year-old Haitian female; infectious diseases clinic

Chief Complaint: Reports that she has experienced two near syncopal episodes in the last several weeks; each time she reports a dizzy sensation prior to her symptoms; denies any chest pain (CP), palpitations, shortness of breath (SOB), tremors, tongue biting, or loss of bowel or bladder continence; complains of ongoing lethargy, poor appetite (25-lb weight loss in the past 3 months), nausea, intermittent headaches, and joint pain

■ History of Present Illness

Poor historian; speaks mainly French Creole; most of her current symptoms predate both diagnosis and treatment of tuberculosis (TB); she was taken off antiretroviral therapy (ARVT) 1 month ago in order to initiate antituberculosis treatment. Today she has a 1-month clinic follow-up appointment postinitiation of treatment for TB, and her doctor would like to evaluate when she can restart ARVT. She missed her appointment 2 weeks after initiation of treatment for TB.

Medical History: Diagnosed with HIV/AIDS in 1995 (risk factor: heterosexual contact); *Pneumocystis carinii* pneumonia (PCP) prophylaxis since 1995; history of herpes simplex virus (HSV) type 2 (diagnosed in 1999, last recurrence in 2004); herpes zoster diagnosed in 2000; hypertension (HTN) diagnosed in 1995; partial seizure disorder diagnosed in 2003; active TB was diagnosed 1 month ago; depression diagnosed in 1999

Surgical History: None

Family/Social History: Family History: noncontributory
Social History: lives alone in the Boston area; has three sons that are involved in her medical care; does not smoke or drink; does not use recreational drugs

Medication History:
Current antiretroviral therapy (ARVT): none
Past ARVT:
  1996 zidovudine (stopped due to anemia)
  1996–1998 stavudine, lamivudine, indinavir
  1998–2000 didanosine, stavudine, saquinavir (unable to tolerate due to GI effects)
  8/31/00 abacavir, lamivudine, efavirenz (discontinued due to dizziness after 2 doses)
  9/00–9/01 nevirapine, didanosine, zidovudine (therapy failure, poor medication adherence, lactic acidosis)
  9/01–11/02 zidovudine/lamivudine, lopinavir/ritonavir (unable to tolerate lopinavir/ritonavir due to GI adverse effects); changed to tenofovir and zidovudine/lamivudine (intermediate adherence to therapy, discontinued in 2005—treatment failure)
Antituberculosis therapy:
Started 4-drug regimen 1 month ago:
  Rifampin, 600 mg PO QD
  Isoniazid, 300 mg PO QD, along with supplementation with pyridoxine (vitamin B6) 25 mg PO QD
  Pyrazinamide, 1,500 mg PO QD
  Ethambutol, 1,200 mg PO QD

Additional medications:
  Atenolol, 25 mg PO QD
  Dapsone, 100 mg PO QD
  Ensure liquid supplement; 1 can PO TID
  Mirtazapine, 30 mg; 1 PO QD at 9 PM
  Diphenhydramine, 25 mg 50 mg PO BID
  Hydrocortisone cream 0.5%, apply to face BID
  Phenytoin, 150 mg PO TID

Allergies: Abacavir (pruritis)

■ Physical Examination

GEN: Ill-appearing female but well hydrated and in no acute distress
VS: BP 125/76, Pulse rate 67, RR 22, T 37.5°C, Wt 134 lbs, Ht 163 cm, O$_2$ sat 99
HEENT: Bilateral horizontal nystagmus
COR: RRR
CHEST: No rales, rhonchi, or wheezes but chest x-ray taken 1.5 months ago was suggestive of a hilar lesion, which was followed up with a CT thorax, demonstrating a pulmonary mass with associated adenopathy
ABD: Soft, nontender, no masses, bowel sounds normal
LYMPHATIC: No cervical, axillary, inguinal adenopathy, mild swelling of lymph nodes
SKIN: No rashes, lesions, or ulcerations, no subcutaneous nodules or induration, no jaundice
NEURO: Alert but confused on today's date and unable to recall clearly what she did this week

■ Results of Pertinent Laboratory Tests, Serum Drug Concentrations, and Diagnostic Tests

Na 137 (137)	Hgb 100.8 (10.8)	LDH 3.65 (219)
K 3.7 (3.7)	Lkc 3.4 × 10⁹	Alk Phos 3.05 (183)
Cl 104 (104)	(3.4 × 10³)	Alb 25 (2.5)
HCO₃ 24 (24)	Plts 267 × 10⁹	T Bili 18 (1.0)
BUN 8.21 (23)	(267 × 10³)	Glu 6.1 (110)
CR 79.6 (0.9)	ALT 1.75 (105)	AST 1.46 (88)
Hct 0.29 (29)		

CD4: 88 cells/mm³
CD4 %: 6
HIV viral load: 224,136 copies/mL (b-DNA)
PPD tuberculin skin test: positive (1.5 months ago), negative in 2000 when she immigrated to the United States
AFB smear (1.5 months ago): positive for mycobacteria
Sputum (× 3) and bronchoalveolar lavages (1 month ago) grew *Mycobacterium tuberculosis* (culture positive); sensitive to first-line antituberculosis agents
Phenytoin serum concentration: 59.4 μmol/L (15 μg/mL)

■ Problem List

Identify principal problems from the scenario in priority order (see Answers in back of book for correct list of problems).

■ SOAP Note

To be completed by the student (see Answers in back for book for correct SOAP Note).

■ QUESTIONS

(See Answers in back of book for correct responses.)

1. SV acquired tuberculosis: (EO-1)
   a. Via heterosexual transmission
   b. By inhalation of airborne particles of *Mycobacterium tuberculosis* from an individual with active tuberculosis
   c. By touching an animal with active tuberculosis
   d. By touching the skin of an individual with active tuberculosis

2. Discuss the epidemiology of latent TB infection versus active TB disease in HIV-infected persons. (EO-3)

3. Analyze factors that should be considered when choosing an antiretroviral regimen for SV. (EO-8)

4. Which of the following statements is true regarding potential drug-drug interactions? (EO-9)
   a. Isoniazid is metabolized via cytochrome P-450 and inhibits metabolism of phenytoin and may increase serum phenytoin levels.
   b. Rifampin is metabolized via cytochrome P-450 and inhibits metabolism of phenytoin and may increase serum phenytoin levels.
   c. Isoniazid is not metabolized via cytochrome P-450 and does not interact with phenytoin.
   d. Rifampin is not metabolized via cytochrome P-450 and does not interact with phenytoin.

5. SV presents with hepatitis. Describe potential causes of drug-induced hepatitis and appropriate monitoring of this adverse effect. (EO-5, 10)

6. SV's serum albumin concentration is low. How will this affect the phenytoin serum concentration? Calculate the adjusted phenytoin serum concentration. (EO-4, 5, 6)

7. Which of the following statements regarding ethambutol is true? (EO-4, 6, 9)
   a. Ethambutol is an inhibitor of cytochrome P-450.
   b. The most toxic effect of this agent is optic neuritis, and SV should be questioned monthly regarding possible visual disturbances.
   c. Ethambutol is an inducer of cytochrome P-450.
   d. Ethambutol may cause an orange/brown discoloration of bodily fluids (urine, sweat, and tears).

8. SV is receiving supplementation with pyridoxine while taking isoniazid. Explain the rationale. (EO-9, 10)

9. Which statement is correct regarding agents within the rifamycin class?
   a. Rifampin has the longest half-life.
   b. Rifabutin is the most potent inducer of cytochrome P-450.
   c. All agents in this class can cause orange discoloration of bodily fluids.
   d. The most toxic effect of rifampin is cardiomyopathy.

10. Develop a detailed education plan for SV addressing goals of antituberculosis therapy and adherence strategies and describe the role of the pharmacist. (EO-14, 16)

11. Describe the pharmacist's role relative to the proposed psychosocial factors identified. (EO-16)

12. Evaluate the pharmacoeconomic considerations relative to SV's plan of care. (EO-17)

13. Summarize therapeutic, pathophysiologic, and disease management concepts for tuberculosis utilizing a key points format. (EO-18)

CASE 32

TOPIC: **Urinary Tract Infections**

THERAPEUTIC DIFFICULTY: Level 1
Snehal H. Bhatt

Chapter 77: Urinary Tract Infections

■ Scenario

Patient and Setting: KD, a 55-year-old female; primary care physician's office

Chief Complaint: Increased urinary urgency, frequency, fever, and lower back pain

■ History of Present Illness

Presents to her primary care physician's office with increased urine frequency, urgency, and lower back pain; claims that she was in her usual state of health until about 2 days ago, when she first noticed an increased frequency and urgency to use the bathroom. She attributed her symptoms to trying a different brand of coffee. She became more concerned when she began experiencing a slight fever and lower back pain (5/10) yesterday evening; now presents to her primary care physician's office for further evaluation.

Medical History: Hypertension (HTN) for 10 years; type 2 diabetes mellitus for 8 years; history of nephrolithiasis

Family/Social History: Family History: Father died of myocardial infarction (MI) age 70
Social History: Occasional alcohol use on weekends, no history of smoking

Medication History:
Atenolol, 25 mg PO QD
Metformin, 500 mg PO BID
Enteric-coated aspirin, 325 mg PO QD
Multivitamin, 1 tablet PO QD
Calcium carbonate + Vitamin D, 500 mg PO BID

Allergies: No known drug allergies

■ Physical Examination

GEN: Pleasant woman in mild discomfort
VS: T 37.5°C, BP 146/90, HR 70, RR 20, O$_2$ Sat 98% RA, Wt 58 kg, Ht 158 cm
HEENT: PERRLA, EOMI
COR: RRR, normal S1, S2, no M/R/G
CHEST: Lungs CTA Bilaterally
ABD: Soft NTND, (+) BS
EXT: Warm, no C/C/E
NEURO: A and O × 3

■ Results of Pertinent Laboratory Tests, Serum Drug Concentrations, and Diagnostic Tests

Na: 140 (140) Hct: 0.35 (35) HBA1c 0.078 (7.8%)
K: 4.1 (4.1) Hgb: 135 (13.5)
Cl: 100 (100) Lkcs: 14.1 × 10^9 (14.1 × 10^3)
HCO$_3$: 24 (24) Plts: 330 × 10^9 (330 × 10^3)
BUN: 4.99 (14)
SCr: 88.4 (1.0)
Glucose: 13.3 (240)

Urinalysis
WBC 3 +
Gram (−) rods >10^5 CFU/mL
(+) Hematuria
(+) Nitrite
Blood Cultures: Pending

■ Problem List

Identify principal problems from the scenario in priority order (see Answers in back of book for correct list of problems).

■ SOAP Note

To be completed by the student (see Answers in back of book for correct SOAP Note).

■ QUESTIONS

(*See Answers in back of book for correct responses.*)

1. Which organism is the most prevalent in urinary tract infections (UTIs)? (EO-1, 3)
   a. *Klebsiella spp*
   b. *Proteus mirabilis*
   c. *Escherichia coli*
   d. *Staphylococcus saprophyticus*

2. What is the most common route of organism entry into the urinary tract?
   a. Via contaminated food
   b. Via an ascending route from the urethra into the bladder
   c. Via a descending route from the kidney into the bladder
   d. Clearance of a systemic infection into the bladder

3. KD most likely has what type of UTI? EO-6)
   a. Acute uncomplicated cystitis
   b. Acute uncomplicated pyelonephritits
   c. Acute complicated pyelonephritis
   d. Nosocomial UTI

4. Why did the medical team obtain blood cultures? (EO-3, 5)

5. According to the IDSA Guidelines, empiric treatment with TMP/SMX is not recommended in areas in which *E. coli* resistance is greater than: (EO-3, 5)
   a. 0%
   b. 20%
   c. 30%
   d. 50%

6. If KD's medical team wanted to initiate treatment with Gentamicin, which of the following dosing regimens represents the **best option** for KD? (EO-6)
   a. Gentamicin 100 mg IV q12h × 10 days
   b. Gentamicin 50 mg IV q12h × 10 days
   c. Gentamicin 50 mg IV q8h × 5 days
   d. Gentamicin 100 mg IV q12h × 3 days

7. KD is discharged from the hospital and given a prescription for Levofloxacin 500 mg PO QD × 10 days. As the pharmacist dispensing this prescription to KD, what are some important patient counseling points that you should mention to KD? (EO-9, 10, 12)

8. If the medical team diagnosed KD with a noso-comial UTI, which organism would be the most concerning? (EO-1, 3)
   a. *E. coli*
   b. *S. saprophyticus*
   c. *Pseudomonas aeruginosa*
   d. *Klebsiella*

9. Which of the following represents the **best choice** for the initial management of a nosoco-mial UTI?
   a. Gentamicin IV + piperacillin/tazobactam IV
   b. Imipenem IV
   c. Oxacillin IV
   d. Ceftazidime IV + ticarcillin/clavulanate IV

10. What is the **most appropriate** target gentamicin peak and trough concentration in the initial management of nosocomial UTIs?
   a. Peak: 4–5 μg/mL and trough: 1–2 μg/mL
   b. Peak: 6–8 μg/mL and trough: 2–4 μg/mL
   c. Peak: 8–10 μg/mL and trough: 2–4 μg/mL
   d. Peak: 8–10 μg/mL and trough: 1–2 μg/mL

11. If KD develops frequent UTIs, what alternative therapies exist to decrease the frequency of UTI recurrence? (EO-11, 12)

12. Summarize therapeutic, pathophysiologic, and disease management concepts for the treatment of UTI using the key points format. (EO-18)

CASE 33

TOPIC: Infective Endocarditis

THERAPEUTIC DIFFICULTY: Level 2
Dorothea Rudorf

Chapter 80: Infective Endocarditis

■ Scenario

Patient and Setting: AM, a 56-year-old male; walk-in clinic of local hospital

Chief Complaint: Fatigue, fever, night sweats, weakness, dyspnea, anorexia, 6 kg weight loss

■ History of Present Illness

Complains of persistent low-grade fever (ranging from 37.9°C to 38.8°C), fatigue, and increasing overall weakness, making it difficult for him to work for several weeks; took ibuprofen but the drug did not seem to alleviate his symptoms. Lately has experienced night sweats and short-ness of breath. He also noticed a decreased appe-tite and a 6 kg weight loss over the last month; he believes onset of most of his problems started shortly after the extraction of 2 wisdom teeth 1 1/2 months ago.

Medical History: Rheumatic fever at age 8; mitral valve prolapse, diagnosed 2 years ago. Other: hy-pertension × 10 years; prostatic hypertrophy with occasional urinary tract infections (UTIs) (last one 9 months ago); hearing deficit in left ear.

Surgical History: Extraction of two wisdom teeth 1 1/2 months ago; appendectomy 5 years ago

Family/Social History: Family History: Father died of myocardial infarction (MI); mother alive with cardiac disease
Social History: Married × 30 years with two grown children; works as construction manager; alcohol use only at social occasions; no tobacco or illicit drug use

Medications:
Metoprolol, 50 mg PO BID
Hydrochlorothiazide, 25 mg PO QD
Aspirin, 81 mg PO QD
Ibuprofen, 200–400mg PO q4–6h PRN
Vitamin C, 1,000 mg QD

Allergies: Penicillin (rash "many years ago")

■ Physical Examination

GEN: Pleasant, cachectic, ill-appearing man in no acute stress
VS: T 38.7°C, BP 150/89, HR 80, RR 21, O$_2$ sat 98% RA, Wt 67 kg, Ht 172.5 cm
HEENT: PERRLA, EOMI, conjunctival petechiae, hearing deficit in left ear
COR: Diastolic murmur with mitral regurgitation, normal S1 and S2
CHEST: Clear to auscultation and percussion
ABD: Soft, NT/ND, normal BS, no HSM
GU: Prostatic hypertrophy, otherwise normal
RECTAL: WNL
EXT: No C/C/E, splinter hemorrhages in fingertips, petechiae noted on lower legs
NEURO: A and O × 3, CN II-XII intact, normal re-flexes

■ Results of Pertinent Laboratory Tests, Serum Drug Concentrations, and Diagnostic Tests

Lkcs 15.5 × 10⁹
(15.0 × 10³)
Diff: 76% N,
  4% bands, 14 %
  L, 4% M, 2% E

Na 137 (137)
K 3.5 (3.5)

Ca 2.20 (8.9)
Glucose 7.49 (135)
PO₄ 1.10 (3.4)

Mg 1.05 (2.1)
Hct 0.33 (33)
Hgb 114 (11.4)
Plts 145 × 10⁹
(145 × 10³)

Cl 105 (105)
HCO₃ 23 (23)
BUN 10.8 (30)
Cr 159 (1.8)

ESR 66
Rheumatoid factor: positive

Urinanalysis: pH 7.4, clear, 1+ protein, 5 RBCs/HPF, 5 WBC/HPF, nitrite neg, few gram-negative organisms

Chest x-ray: normal

Transesophageal echocardiogram: moderate mitral regurgitation/flail mitral leaflet; vegetation 1 × 1.5 cm located on mitral valve

Blood culture and sensitivity tests: pending

■ Problem List

Identify principal problems from the scenario in priority order (see Answers in back of book for correct list of problems).

■ SOAP Note

To be completed by the student (see Answers in back of book for correct SOAP Note).

■ QUESTIONS

(See Answers in back of book for correct responses.)

1. Which of the following is *not* a risk factor for infective endocarditis in AM? (EO-1, 3)
   a. Previous dental procedure
   b. Hypertension
   c. Mitral valve regurgitation
   d. Rheumatic fever

2. Which pathogen is most likely the cause for AM's infective endocarditis? (EO- 1, 3, 5)
   a. Enterococci
   b. *Staphylococcus aureus*
   c. *Streptococcus viridans*
   d. Gram-negative bacilli

3. Various pathophysiologic factors are necessary for infective endocarditis to develop. Identify the *correct* sequence of events that lead to endocarditis and the formation of vegetations and refer to patient AM. (EO-1)

4. Discuss general pharmacologic principles and goals for the optimal treatment of a patient with infective endocarditis. (EO-8, 11, 12)

5. Which of the following statements is *not correct* regarding infective endocarditis in IVDAs? (EO-1, 3, 5, 8, 12)
   a. Primarily caused by staphylococci
   b. Usually causes right-sided (tricuspid valve) endocarditis
   c. Should be treated with 2-week course of nafcillin and gentamicin
   d. Should be treated with 2-week course of cefazolin or vancomycin

6. Which of the following options would you consider as the *most appropriate* empiric treatment for AM? (EO-4, 8, 12)
   a. An optimal therapy would consist of 2 weeks of IV gentamicin plus 2 weeks of IV penicillin.
   b. The patient should receive IV ceftriaxone for 4 weeks.
   c. The patient should receive IV vancomycin for 2 weeks.
   d. AM should receive IV cefazolin plus IV gentamicin for 2 weeks.

7. Explain the rationale for combination therapy with an aminoglycoside, especially during the initial treatment of infective endocarditis? (EO-7, 8, 11, 12)

8. Two days after starting empiric therapy, AM's blood culture report indicates *S. viridans* with relative resistance to penicillin (MIC 0.3μg/mL). Which of the following regimens would be appropriate for AM at this time? (EO-8, 11, 12)
   a. Vancomycin IV for 4 weeks
   b. Ampicillin IV plus gentamicin IV for 4–6 weeks
   c. Penicillin IV for 4 weeks with gentamicin for the first 3–5 days
   d. Vancomycin plus gentamicin for 4–6 weeks

9. Independent of which regimen is chosen, what specific problems should AM be monitored for? (EO-2, 10)
   a. Hepatotoxicity and nephrotoxicity
   b. CNS reactions, hypersensitivity, and hepatotoxicity
   c. Hepatotoxicity and hypersensitivity reactions
   d. Nephrotoxicity, ototoxicity, and hypersensitivity reactions

10. If AM were to receive gentamicin or vancomycin, what would be the appropriate doses and how should they be determined? (EO-6, 8, 10, 12)

11. Two days after initiating appropriate therapy for *S. viridans* endocarditis, AM feels much better, but his blood culture is still positive. What

should his further management be? (EO-8, 11, 12)

a. The regimen chosen is not effective and should be changed.

b. It is not unusual a patient to remain bacteremic for 5–7 days after initiation of therapy, and another blood culture should be taken in 1–2 days.

c. The patient most likely has a superimposed infection and should be reevaluated.

d. The patient most likely has developed resistance to the current regimen, and therefore it should be changed.

12. AM is planning to soon undergo a prostatectomy to relieve the symptoms associated with his prostatic hypertrophy. Which of the following is *not correct* regarding prevention of infective endocarditis associated with this procedure? (EO-8, 10, 12)

a. There are no good clinical studies in humans regarding prophylaxis and most data is based on animal studies.

b. Prophylaxis for AM should consist of amoxicillin (2 g PO given 1 hour before the procedure), as he is a high-risk patient.

c. AM's prophylaxis may consist of IV gentamicin plus ampicillin (given 30 min prior to the procedure), followed by either PO amoxicillin or IV ampicillin (6 hours later).

d. AM could receive IV vancomycin plus gentamicin (infusions to be completed 30 minutes prior to the procedure).

13. Identify psychosocial issues that may affect AM's adherence to therapy and describe the pharmacist's role relative to those. (EO-15, 16)

14. Summarize therapeutic, pathophysiologic, and disease management concepts for the treatment of infective endocarditis utilizing the key points format. (EO-18)

CASE 34

TOPIC: Bacterial Meningitis

THERAPEUTIC DIFFICULTY: Level 3
Susan Crecco

Chapter 81: Central Nervous System Infections

■ Scenario

Patient and Setting: SB, a 10-year-old female; emergency department (ED)

Chief Complaint: Fever, headache, neck pain, vomiting

■ History of Present Illness

SB has a 2-day history of fever, headache, neck stiffness, vomiting, and a rash on her legs. All of these symptoms developed after she finished her 5-day course of azithromycin that was prescribed to treat an ear infection about 7 days ago. Her mom states she went to wake her up this morning and she was very difficult to arouse.

Medical History: Asthma diagnosed at age 5, sickle cell anemia, history of recurrent otitis media

Surgical History: S/p splenectomy 4 years ago

Family/Social History: Lives at home with her parents and 4-year-old brother, is in the fourth grade

Medications:
Advair 100/50, 1 inhalation PO twice a day
Singulair, 5 mg PO once a day
Folic acid, 1 mg PO once a day
Albuterol inhaler, 1 to 2 puffs q6h PRN wheezing
Multivitamin, 1 tablet PO once a day
Penicillin VK, 250 mg PO twice a day

Immunizations: *Haemophilus influenzae* B, Influenzae

Allergies: No known drug allergies

■ Physical Examination

GEN: WDWN female who is in respiratory distress and nonresponsive
VS: BP 80/40, HR 115, RR 31, T 38.9°C, Wt 35 kg, Ht 137 cm
HEENT: Poorly reactive pupils, no papilledema, + Kernig's sign, decreased neck movement
COR: RRR, no m/r/g
CHEST: CTA
ABD: Soft NTND
NEURO: A and O × 1, reflexes symmetrical
EXT: Purpuric rash on lower extremities

■ Results of Pertinent Laboratory Tests, Serum Drug Concentrations, and Diagnostic Tests

Na 130 (130)	CR 133 (1.5)	Lkcs 19 × 10⁹ (19 × 10³)
K 4.8 (4.8)	Glu 4.4 (80)	Mg 0.9 (1.8)
Cl 101 (101)	Hgb 100 (10)	Alb 3.5 (3.5)
HCO₃ 26 (26)	Hct 0.30 (30)	
BUN 12.5 (35)	Plt 270 × 10⁹ (270 × 10³)	

LP: cloudy fluid with a glucose of 20 mg/dL, protein of 150 mg/dL, WBC 18.5 × 10³, 93% PMN
CSF: Gram stain: gram-positive cocci in pairs and chains
Blood and CSF cultures pending

■ Problem List

Identify principal problems from the scenario in priority order (see Answers in back of book for correct list of problems).

■ SOAP Note

To be completed by the student (see Answers in back of book for correct SOAP Note).

■ QUESTIONS

(See Answers in back of book for correct responses.)

1. List the predisposing factors for SB's bacterial meningitis. (EO-3)

2. List SB's signs and symptoms of meningitis. (EO-2)

3. Which of the following organisms is most likely to be the cause of meningitis in SB? (EO-1, 3, 4, 5)
   a. *Neisseria meningitides*
   b. *Staphylococcus epidermidis*
   c. *Streptococcus pneumoniae*
   d. *Haemophilus influenzae*

4. Explain what a positive Kernig's sign is and how to interpret it. (EO-1, 2)

5. Identify the factors that influence the ability of an antimicrobial to cross the blood brain barrier (BBB). (EO-6)

6. Which of the following is considered first-line empiric treatment for SB's meningitis? (EO-8, 12)
   a. Vancomycin
   b. Vancomycin + ceftriaxone or cefotaxime
   c. Ceftriaxone
   d. Ampicillin

7. What would be the duration of SB's antimicrobial therapy if there were no complications? (EO-12)
   a. 10 to 14 days
   b. 7 to 10 days
   c. More than 14 days
   d. 21 days

8. What is the *major* consideration when recommending SB's antimicrobial regimen? (EO-8)
   a. Liver function
   b. Drug allergies
   c. Renal function
   d. Drug interactions

9. Explain if SB would be a good candidate to receive adjuvant dexamethasone. (EO-8)

10. Which of the following is the most appropriate preventative measure that should be given to SB? (EO-14)
    a. Her prophylactic dose of PCN VK should be increased to 500 mg PO BID.
    b. Her prophylactic dose of PCN VK should be discontinued to decrease the risk of her developing resistant organisms.
    c. She should be given the meningococcal vaccine only.
    d. She should be given the 23-valent pneumococcal polysaccharide, meningococcal, and 7-valent conjugate pneumococcal vaccines.

11. Describe why penicillin is no longer used as first-line empiric therapy for meningitis. (EO-11, 12)

12. If SB was prescribed adjuvant dexamethasone, it should be administered: (EO-7, 11)
    a. Prior to her first dose of antibiotics
    b. After her first dose of antibiotics because it may decrease the permeability of the BBB
    c. It doesn't matter as long as she gets it
    d. It should be started only when the cultures come back and if they show *H. influenzae*

13. What would be the appropriate monitoring parameters if vancomycin was initiated in SB? (EO-10)
    a. Peak (goal 35–40 µg/mL), trough (goal 10–20 µg/mL), BUN, SCr, urine output
    b. Peak (goal 20–30µg/mL), trough (goal 5– µg/mL), LFTs, BUN, SCr
    c. Peak (goal 6–12 µg/mL), trough (goal <2 µg//mL), lactate, BUN, SCr
    d. Peak (goal 25–35 µg/mL), trough (goal 10–15 µg/mL), BUN, T. Bili, stool output

14. Which one of the following is *not* a risk factor for developing penicillin resistance: (EO-11)
    a. Age <5 years old
    b. Frequent antibiotic use
    c. Use of appropriate vaccinations
    d. Use of prophylactic antibiotics to prevent chronic infections

15. Summarize pathophysiologic, therapeutic, and disease management concepts for central nervous system (CNS) infections utilizing a key points format. (EO-18)

CASE 35

TOPIC: Bone and Joint Infections

THERAPEUTIC DIFFICULTY: Level 2
Kalen B. Porter

Chapter 82: Bone and Joint Infections

■ Scenario

Patient and Setting: EP, a 48-year-old male, emergency department

Chief Complaint: Pus coming from "wound on foot," redness and swelling around wound, increased pain upon walking

■ History of Present Illness

Foot ulcer appeared 1 month ago secondary to stepping on a rock while walking barefoot in his backyard; seen in diabetes clinic following trauma; treated with amoxicillin/clavulanate 875 mg PO BID for 2 weeks; did not return for follow-up clinic appointment 2 weeks ago; symptoms started 5 days ago

Medical History: Type 2 diabetes × 12 years, mild renal insufficiency (SCr 1 month ago = 1.5 mg/dL), obesity, hypertension

Surgical History: Tonsillectomy at age 15

Family/Social History: Family History: Father died 40 years ago in an automobile accident; mother alive S/P 3 previous transient ischemic attacks (TIAs)
Social History: Married × 20 years, 2 children, smoked 1 pack/day of cigarettes until 12 years ago, drinks 3–4 glasses of wine or beer per week, denies illicit drug use

Medications:
Metformin, 850 mg PO BID
Glimepiride, 1 mg PO BID
Hydrochlorothiazide (HCTZ), 12.5 mg PO QD

Allergies: Bactrim (rash)

■ Physical Examination

GEN: Obese male in no apparent distress
VS: BP 138/82, HR 80, RR 19, T 37.6°C, Wt 110 kg, Ht 175 cm
HEENT: PERRLA, EOMI, no hemorrhages or exudates on fundoscopic exam
COR: RRR, normal S_1 and S_2
CHEST: CTA, no congestion, no wheezing
ABD: Nondistended, +BS, no guarding or tenderness
GU: Deferred
EXT: 3 cm wide × 3 cm deep ulcer on inferior surface of right foot with yellowish-green drainage and a foul smell, no edema, decreased sensation to light touch (both feet), normal range of motion, minor pain upon palpation of area surrounding ulcer
NEURO: A and O × 3

■ Results of Pertinent Laboratory Tests, Serum Drug Concentrations, and Diagnostic Tests

Na 138 (138)	Lkcs 17 × 10⁹ (17 × 10³)
K 4 (4)	Hgb 130 (13)
Cl 100 (100)	Hct 0.38 (38)
HCO₃ 20 (20)	Plts 350 × 10⁹ (350 × 10³)
BUN 7.5 (21)	ESR 72 (72)
SCr 150 (1.7)	CRP 12.6
Glu 10.3 (185)	HbA₁c 0.103 (10.3%)

Lkc differential: PMN 0.70 (70%), bands 0.08 (8%), lymphs 0.06 (6%)
Gram stain (wound culture): Aerobic gram-positive cocci in pairs, anaerobic gram-positive cocci, gram-negative rods; cultures pending
Blood culture pending
X-ray of foot indicates soft tissue swelling and periosteal swelling consistent with osteomyelitis

■ Problem List

Identify principal problems from the scenario in priority order (see Answers in back of book for correct list of problems).

■ SOAP Note

To be completed by the student (see Answers in back of book for correct SOAP Note).

■ QUESTIONS

(See Answers in back of book for correct responses.)

1. EP's clinical presentation is consistent with which category of osteomyelitis? (EO-1)

a. Acute hematogenous osteomyelitis
b. Contiguous osteomyelitis without vascular insufficiency
c. Contiguous osteomyelitis with vascular insufficiency
d. Chronic osteomyelitis

2. Which of the following is FALSE regarding the epidemiology of acute hematogenous osteomyelitis? (EO-3)
   a. Neonates are at highest risk for the development of osteomyelitis due to *Pseudomonas aeruginosa*.
   b. The most common organism seen in sickle cell patients with hematogenous osteomyelitis is *Salmonella*.
   c. Elderly patients are at high risk for the development of vertebral osteomyelitis.
   d. The most common organism isolated from adults with hematogenous osteomyelitis is *Staphylococcus aureus*.

3. The majority of cases of infectious arthritis in adults are caused by which of the following organisms?
   a. *Pseudomonas aeruginosa*
   b. *Haemophilus influenzae*
   c. *Neisseria gonorrhoeae*
   d. *Staphylococcus epidermidis*

4. Which of the following is the appropriate antibiotic selection for a patient with contiguous osteomyelitis due to methicillin-resistant *Staphylococcus aureus*? (EO-12)
   a. Nafcillin 2 g IV q6h
   b. Vancomycin 1 g IV q12h
   c. Ceftriaxone 1 g IV q24h
   d. Penicillin G 4 million U IV q6h

5. The most common organism associated with osteomyelitis in patients with prosthetic joints is:
   a. *Staphylococcus aureus*
   b. *Staphylococcus epidermidis*
   c. *Pseudomonas aeruginosa*
   d. *Haemophilus influenzae*

6. Which of the following empiric antibiotic regimens is appropriate for polymicrobial osteomyelitis involving both aerobic and anaerobic bacteria? (EO-8, 12)
   a. Levofloxacin
   b. Vancomycin + clindamycin
   c. Imipenem
   d. Nafcillin + gentamicin

7. Which of EP's signs and symptoms are consistent with a diagnosis of osteomyelitis? (EO-2)

8. Describe the important differences between ESR and CRP and why each is monitored during an infection due to osteomyelitis. (EO-5)

9. Discuss the factors that should be considered in choosing appropriate pharmacologic and nonpharmacologic treatment for EP. (EO-8)

10. Discuss the appropriate use of oral antibiotic therapy in the treatment of osteomyelitis. (EO-8)

11. List appropriate antibiotic agents that can be used in the treatment of community-acquired-methicillin-resistant *Staphylococcus aureus*. Include advantages and disadvantages of using each agent. (EO-12)

12. Summarize therapeutic, pathophysiologic, and disease management concepts for osteomyelitis utilizing a key points format. (EO-18)

CASE 36

TOPIC: Cellulitis

THERAPEUTIC DIFFICULTY: Level 1
Cindy C. Selzer and Jeanne H. Van Tyle

Chapter 91: Skin and Soft Tissue Infections

■ Scenario

Patient and Setting: AC, a 45-year-old male; emergency department

Chief Complaint: Increasing redness, swelling, warmth, and tenderness in his right arm; fevers and chills

■ History of Present Illness

AC was helping to build his new home and noticed a splinter in his right arm approximately 7 days ago. He removed the splinter completely but was seen by his primary physician in an outpatient clinic 2 days ago for redness and warmth surrounding the splinter site. Cellulitis was diagnosed and he was started on cephalexin 500 mg PO every 6 hours. The cellulitis has continued to worsen despite patient compliance with antibiotic therapy. In addition, AC has developed a red, itchy rash over his chest and neck and has been febrile with chills over the past day.

Medical History: Type 2 diabetes for 1 year; seasonal allergies

Surgical History: Noncontributory

Family/Social History: Family History: Mother, HTN; father, died at age 71 due to coronary artery disease (CAD)
Social History: Occasional ethanol intake (1 drink/month); no history of smoking

Medications:
Metformin, 1 g PO BID for 8 months
Glipizide XL, 5 mg PO daily for 6 months
Aspirin enteric-coated, 81 mg PO daily for 8 months

Allergies: Penicillin (rash)

■ Physical Examination

GEN: Well-developed, well-nourished man
VS: BP 128/78, HR 73, RR 18, T 39.1°C, Wt 95 kg, Ht 182.88 cm
HEENT: WNL
COR: RRR
CHEST: Maculopapular rash that extends from the neck to the chest
ABD: WNL
GU: Deferred
RECT: Deferred
EXT: Warmth, redness, swelling, and tenderness in right lower arm extending to upper arm
NEURO: A and 0 × 4

■ Results of Pertinent Laboratory Tests, Serum Drug Concentrations, and Diagnostic Tests

(Fasting)	HCO_3 26 (26)	Hct 0.48 (48)	Plts 231 × 10⁹ (231 × 10³)
Na 137 (137)	BUN 6.4 (18)	Hgb 150 (15)	
K 4.3 (4.3)	Cr 133 (1.5)	Lkcs 18.5 × 10⁹ (18.5 × 10³)	A1C 6.8%
Cl 100 (100)	Glu 8.05 (145)		

■ Problem List

Identify principal problems from the scenario in priority order (see Answers in back of book for correct list of problems).

■ SOAP Note

To be completed by the student (see Answers in back of book for correct SOAP Note).

■ QUESTIONS

(See Answers in back of book for correct responses.)

1. What is the most probable cause for AC's cellulitis? (EO-1)

2. List signs and symptoms of cellulitis. (EO-2)

3. List the physical assessment and laboratory findings in AC consistent with cellulitis. (EO-5)

4. Describe the natural progression of cellulitis if untreated. (EO-1)

5. List the most common etiologies of cellulitis in AC. (EO-1)

6. Discuss appropriate treatment options for AC's cellulitis and include rationale for medications that should be avoided in this patient. (EO-8, EO-11)

7. List your treatment option for cellulitis including dose, route, dosing interval, and duration of therapy. Justify your choice. (EO-11)

8. The patient is started on vancomycin 1,250 mg every 12 hours (0900 and 2100) as an IV infusion over 1 hour. When levels are determined with the third dose, the following are returned: peak 37 μg/mL 1 hour after a 1-hour infusion (1100) and a trough of 20.1 μg/mL 30 minutes prior to the next dose (2050). Evaluate this regimen and adjust the dose appropriately if needed. The physician has asked you, the pharmacist, for the appropriate vancomycin dose for this patient and his disease state. (EO-6)

9. List your goals of therapy with vancomycin, including physical, laboratory, and pharmacokinetic parameters. (EO-12)

10. List the monitoring parameters for cellulitis in AC. (EO-5)

11. What is the most probable cause of AC's rash? (EO-1)

12. List pharmacologic and nonpharmacologic treatment options for AC's rash. (EO-11)

13. Develop a detailed patient education plan for AC's rash and infection. (EO-14)

14. What is the most probable cause of AC's hyperglycemia? (EO-1)

15. Discuss treatment options for the management of AC's hyperglycemia and include rationale for medications that should be avoided in this patient. (EO-11)

16. Summarize therapeutic, pathophysiologic, and disease management concepts for cellulitis utilizing a key points format. (EO-18)

Supportive Care Therapies for Patients with Cancer

92

Kimberly Bardel Whitlock

OVERVIEW

Supportive care therapies are critical to the physical and emotional well-being of the patient with cancer who is undergoing treatment. Supportive care agents increase the chance that chemotherapy and radiation can be administered on schedule at the optimal dose. These therapies are also crucial in minimizing the severity of side effects that may diminish the patient's quality of life and compliance with future cancer treatment. The use of supportive care therapy has become even more important with recent advances in the management of cancer. These therapies have allowed increases in the dose intensity of cancer therapies (e.g., high-dose chemotherapy for bone marrow transplantation), new chemotherapy combinations that previously were associated with intolerable side effects, or high-dose radiation. Increased dose intensity is associated with an improved survival rate for patients with certain cancers, and for some tumor types, it can improve the chance for a cure.

Supportive care agents are used to prevent and manage chemotherapy and radiation-related toxicities in treatment phases that range from initial diagnosis to management of recurrent disease or palliative treatment. This chapter discusses the agents used to prevent gastrointestinal complications such as mucositis, xerostomia, constipation, diarrhea, and nausea and vomiting. It also discusses the hematologic complications such as anemia, neutropenia, and thrombocytopenia. Cytoprotective agents to prevent specific chemotherapy-induced toxicities are also covered.

Additional therapeutic modalities discussed in other chapters that are important to consider in the overall management of a patient with cancer include nutritional support, management of fever and infection in immunocompromised patients, behavioral health (e.g., anxiety and depression), pain management, and cancer treatment-induced bone loss.

ORAL COMPLICATIONS

MUCOSITIS

Each year there are approximately 400,000 cases of treatment-induced damage to the oral cavity.[1] Oral complications that arise as a result of cancer therapy, particularly chemotherapy and localized radiation therapy, include mucositis; xerostomia (dry mouth); bacterial, fungal, or viral infection; dental caries; loss of taste; trismus (spasm of the mastication muscles); and osteoradionecrosis (necrosis

of the bone secondary to radiation).[2] Because severe oral injury occasionally results in life-threatening complications, effective supportive therapies to prevent and treat mucosal damage are vital to the positive clinical outcome of cancer patients.

Mucositis is generalized inflammation of the oral mucosal membranes and typically manifests as erythema or ulcerations. This is an important complication to address, as it can be a dose-limiting toxicity for both chemotherapy and radiotherapy.

TREATMENT GOALS: MUCOSITIS

- Avoid the complications associated with mucositis, including local and systemic infections.
- Provide pain relief.
- Promote healing.[3]
- Help patients to complete their scheduled cancer therapy on time, improve their therapeutic outcomes, and maintain a good quality of life during treatment.

EPIDEMIOLOGY

The likelihood of developing mucositis depends on treatment- and patient-related factors. Approximately 40% of patients treated with standard chemotherapy develop mucositis, compared with 76% of patients who receive high-dose chemotherapy and undergo bone marrow transplantation. Between 30% and 60% of patients receiving radiation therapy for cancer of the head and neck develop mucositis, and greater than 90% of patients receiving concomitant chemotherapy and localized radiation therapy will be affected.[1,4] There are patient-related and treatment-related risk factors that may predict which patients are more likely to develop mucositis (Table 92.1).[4] Patients with risk factors should be followed closely and preventive measures should be used to diminish the incidence and severity of mucositis.

PATHOPHYSIOLOGY

The development of mucositis occurs through two mechanisms. The first mechanism is through the direct effect of the

chemotherapy or radiation therapy on the oral mucosa (direct stomatotoxicity). The second mechanism is through the indirect result of myelosuppression (indirect stomatotoxicity).

DIRECT STOMATOTOXICITY

The oral mucosal epithelial cells undergo rapid turnover, usually every 7 to 14 days, which makes these cells particularly susceptible to the effects of cytotoxic therapy.[4] Both chemotherapy and localized radiation therapy can cause direct stomatotoxicity by interfering with cellular growth and maturation, such that the ability of the oral mucosa to regenerate is compromised.[4] The incidence and severity of chemotherapy-induced mucositis depend on the specific agent, the dose, and the method and rate of drug administration (i.e., intravenous bolus versus intravenous infusion). The severity of radiation-induced mucositis depends on the type of radiation, the volume of irradiated tissue, the daily fraction, and the cumulative dose.[4]

The onset of mucositis can also vary. Patients who receive some types of standard-dose chemotherapy develop mucositis within 5 to 7 days after the administration of chemother-

TABLE 92.1	Risk Factors for the Development of Mucositis

Factor	Comments
Hematologic malignancy	Oral complications may be associated with the underlying hematologic malignancy, particularly if the patient has severe neutropenia.*
Younger age	There is a higher incidence of hematologic malignancy in younger patients. Additionally, younger patients have a higher mucosal turnover rate than do elderly patients.
Poor oral hygiene (dental caries, gingival disease, chronic oral infection)	If these patients receive aggressive mouth care, they can diminish their chances of oral complications.
Poor nutritional status	Malnutrition interferes with tissue repair and thus impairs mucosal healing.
Seropositive for herpes simplex virus or history of flare	Prophylactic acyclovir or valacyclovir should be considered for patients at high risk for reactivation.
Stomatotoxic chemotherapy (alkylating agents, antimetabolites, hydroxyurea, procarbazine)	Drugs differ in their ability to cause mucositis; furthermore, stomatotoxicity can be dose-related. Methotrexate and 5-fluorouracil are among the most stomatotoxic agents.
Radiation therapy	Radiation therapy to the head and neck region (4,000 to 5,000 cGy) and total body irradiation increase the risk for developing mucositis.
Concomitant chemotherapy and radiotherapy	Combined modality therapy may accelerate the onset and increase the incidence and severity of oral complications.
Tobacco smoking	

* National Institutes of Health. Oral complications of cancer therapies: diagnosis, prevention, and treatment. NIH Consensus Statement 7:1–11, 1989.

apy.[5] Patients undergoing bone marrow transplantation often exhibit oral complications approximately 10 days after the treatment regimen has started,[6] whereas radiation-induced mucositis usually appears during the third to the fifth week of radiation therapy.[5] Mucositis is generally self-limiting, and in nonmyelosuppressed patients whose oral lesions are not complicated by fungal, bacterial, or viral infection, healing occurs within 2 to 3 weeks.[4,7] The sites most often affected include the lips, cheeks, soft palate, floor of the mouth, and the ventral surface of the tongue.[1,4]

INDIRECT STOMATOTOXICITY

Gram-negative bacteria such as *Pseudomonas aeruginosa* and fungi such as *Candida albicans* in the oral cavity may directly invade the oral mucosa and indirectly cause mucositis.[8] Patients are at increased risk for oral infections when they are neutropenic (<500 neutrophils/μL), and this is also when indirect stomatotoxicity usually appears. The onset of mucositis secondary to myelosuppression varies depending on the timing of the neutrophil nadir associated with the chemotherapy agent administered, but it typically develops 10 to 21 days after chemotherapy administration.[5]

CLINICAL PRESENTATION AND DIAGNOSIS

Before cancer therapy is initiated, patients should be screened to identify risk factors for developing mucositis

and should have a comprehensive dental evaluation. Risk factors for developing mucositis include a seropositive status for herpes simplex virus, poor nutritional status, use of smoked tobacco, and a history of poor oral hygiene or preexisting periodontal disease. Use of certain chemotherapy agents and radiation regimens may also put a patient at higher risk for developing mucositis (Table 92.2). A comprehensive dental evaluation is useful in documenting baseline parameters, identifying related risk factors for the development of mucositis, and developing strategies to diminish oral complications during and after therapy.

Patients with mucositis can have many symptoms. Mucositis usually begins with swelling, redness, and erythema of the mucosal membranes followed by the development of white elevated desquamative areas that progress to painful pseudomembranous lesions.[4] Once the mucosal surface is damaged, patients are more susceptible to both local secondary infection and systemic infection; therefore, the oral lesions of patients with febrile neutropenia should be cultured to rule out bacterial, fungal, or viral infection.

Patients may complain of pain, dry mouth, and burning and/or tingling of the lips.[9] The pain associated with mucositis is often intense and can be exacerbated by attempts to eat, drink, swallow, or speak. The pain may be so severe that it limits adequate nutritional and liquid intake, thus putting patients at increased risk for dehydration and malnutrition.

In assessing mucositis, a complete history of the patient's complaints and risk factors should be obtained, with particu-

TABLE 92.2	Chemotherapy Agents and Radiation Therapy Associated With the Development of Mucositis

Chemotherapy Agents:

Bleomycin	Docetaxel	Methotrexate
Busulfan	Doxorubicin	Mitomycin
Capecitabine	Etoposide (doses >10 mg/kg)	Thiotepa
Cyclophosphamide	5-Fluorouracil	Trimetrexate
Dactinomycin	High-dose cytarabine	Vinorelbine
Daunorubicin	Hydroxyurea	

Radiation Therapy[a]:

Concurrent or sequential chemotherapy/radiation

Radiation therapy to head and neck region above 40 to 50 Gy (including hyperfractionation)

Total body irradiation

Radiation to major salivary glands

[a] The severity of mucositis caused by radiation depends on the total dosage and length of treatment.

(Source: National Oncology Alliance Treatment Guideline for Mucositis, updated 2005.)

lar attention paid to the onset and duration of the lesions, the presence and severity of pain or fever, aggravating or relieving factors, and the patient's ability to eat, drink, and talk. A thorough oral examination to evaluate the appearance of the mucositis (lesion numbers, size, and locations) is also important. The National Cancer Institute has established a grading system for documenting mucositis severity (grades 1 to 4) as part of the Common Terminology Criteria Report for Adverse Events (CTCAE); Table 92.3 lists the grading criteria. A number of laboratory parameters should be ob-

tained to rule out infection or dehydration (i.e., complete blood count, platelet count, electrolyte panel, blood urea nitrogen, and serum creatinine).

PSYCHOSOCIAL ASPECTS

Mucositis adversely affects the patient's quality of life. Patients may be frustrated or embarrassed by the difficulty associated with performing the most basic functions, such as speaking, eating, and controlling saliva. In some cases, the symptoms may be so unbearable that patients may not continue with the remainder of their cancer therapy.

PREVENTION

One of the most important measures taken to prevent mucositis is strict adherence to a meticulous oral care regimen. Patients and their family members should be thoroughly counseled on the importance of maintaining good oral hygiene (Table 92.4).

The prophylactic therapies most commonly used include rinses to remove debris and soothe tissues, chlorhexidine gluconate oral rinse to diminish plaque accumulation, and oral cryotherapy before 5-fluorouracil (5-FU) administration (Table 92.5). Cryotherapy (ice chips) temporarily vasoconstricts the mucosal vasculature, thus decreasing the direct toxic effects of 5-FU. Patients should avoid commercial rinses containing alcohol or phenol because they can be drying to the mucosal tissue and result in further irritation. There are numerous other prophylactic approaches including sucralfate suspension, allopurinol mouthwash to lessen the severity of 5-FU–induced mucositis, chamomile mouthwash, and antimicrobial agents (i.e., PTA lozenges consisting of polymyxin B, tobramycin, and amphotericin B) to

TABLE 92.3	National Cancer Institute CTCAE Grading System for Mucositis			
	Grade 1	Grade 2	Grade 3	Grade 4
Functional/symptomatic evaluation for upper aerodigestive tract sites	Minimal symptoms, normal diet; minimal respiratory symptoms but not interfering with function	Symptomatic but can eat and swallow modified diet; respiratory symptoms interfering with function but not interfering with ADL	Symptomatic and unable to adequately aliment or hydrate orally; respiratory symptoms interfering with ADL	Symptoms associated with life-threatening consequences
Clinical examination	Erythema of the mucosa	Patchy ulcerations or pseudomembranes	Confluent ulcerations or pseudomembranes; bleeding with minor trauma	Tissue necrosis; significant spontaneous bleeding; life-threatening consequences

ADL, activities of daily living.

(Source: National Cancer Institute CTCAE v 3.0, Dec. 12, 2003.)

TABLE 92.4	Oral Maintenance to Prevent Mucositis

Refer patient to a dentist for a comprehensive examination to identify and correct any potential complications *before* cancer therapy is initiated. The identification of infection requires prompt therapy with the appropriate antimicrobial agent to prevent systemic infection.

Encourage patients to seek professional dental care throughout cancer therapy as necessary.

Instruct patients to brush teeth with a soft-bristle toothbrush and fluoridated toothpaste after every meal and before bedtime (patients may use a sponge dipped in chlorhexidine gluconate 0.12% oral rinse if unable to brush); the toothbrush should be changed monthly.

Recommend that patients floss teeth daily (avoid in the presence of severe pain).

Encourage good nutrition with adequate protein and fluid intake (2 L of fluid daily) and recommend avoidance of spicy, acidic, hot, or irritating foods.

prevent infection. The data, however, supporting the use of these agents are either inconclusive or lacking, and thus they cannot be recommended as a standard of care. To lessen the impact of radiation therapy, patients should have radiation stents placed in the mouth to protect normal dentition or appropriate radiation shields to protect dental implants. Furthermore, patients should be discouraged from wearing dentures once radiation therapy begins, especially at night.

Patients should be instructed to use a soft-bristle toothbrush three or four times daily to cleanse the mouth of debris, and to floss with unwaxed dental floss (if tolerated). The toothbrush should be changed monthly.

Patients who are at high risk for developing mucositis and have a herpes simplex virus seropositive status should receive daily prophylaxis with an oral antiviral agent, such as acyclovir or valacyclovir.

In patients receiving chemotherapy regimens associated with prolonged neutropenia and a high risk of mucositis, systemic antifungal prophylaxis may be considered with an oral agent such as fluconazole.

Palifermin (Kepivance), a recombinant keratinocyte growth factor, is the first agent approved by the U.S. Food and Drug Administration (FDA) for the prevention of mucositis. It has an indication that applies to a small subset of patients with cancer receiving treatment. Palifermin is approved for use to decrease the incidence and duration of severe mucositis in patients with hematologic malignancies receiving high-dose chemotherapy prior to stem cell transplant. Its role in the treatment of patients with nonhematologic malignancies has not yet been established. In a clinical trial, palifermin was shown to reduce the incidence of grade 3 or 4 mucositis from 98% when no treatment with palifermin was administered to 63% when palifermin was administered. Palifermin was also shown to reduce the duration of grade 3 or 4 mucositis from an average of 9 days in untreated patients to an average of 6 days

TABLE 92.5	Prevention of Mucositis

Measure	Administration
Saline rinse	At least four times daily, dissolve 1/2 tsp sodium chloride in 8 oz of water; swish in oral cavity for at least 2 to 3 minutes and expectorate.
Sodium bicarbonate rinse	At least four times daily, dissolve 1 tsp sodium bicarbonate (baking soda) in 8 oz of warm water; swish in oral cavity for at least 2 to 3 min and expectorate.
Sodium chloride and sodium bicarbonate combination rinse	At least four times daily, dissolve 1 tsp baking soda in 8 oz sterile saline; swish in oral cavity for at least 2 to 3 min and expectorate.
Cold water rinse	Swish in oral cavity for at least 2 to 3 minutes at least four times daily.
Chlorhexidine gluconate 0.12% oral rinse	Swish in oral cavity for 30 sec and expectorate 2 to 4 times daily (for patients undergoing treatment for leukemia or bone marrow transplantation).
Cryotherapy	Beginning 5 minutes before 5-fluorouracil administration, continuously swish ice chips in the mouth for 30 minutes.[*,†]

* Mahood DJ, Dose AM, Loprinzi CL, et al. Inhibition of fluorouracil-induced stomatitis by oral cryotherapy. J Clin Oncol 9:449–452, 1991.

† Rocke LK, Loprinzi CL, Lee JK, et al. A randomized clinical trial of two different durations of oral cryotherapy for the prevention of 5-fluorouracil–related stomatitis. Cancer 72:2234–2238, 1993.

[a] A trial comparing the efficacy of 30 versus 60 minutes of cryotherapy showed no significant difference in outcome.

in patients receiving palifermin therapy.[10] Unlike many of the topical or oral agents used for the prevention of mucositis, palifermin is administered intravenously for 6 consecutive days.

TREATMENT

With the exception of the recently approved palifermin, there are a lack of effective therapeutic strategies to reduce the severity or duration of mucositis once it develops. Difficulties associated with evaluating published studies include large variability in the patient populations studied, numerous types of cancer treatment, and lack of a universally accepted grading system to document the severity of mucositis. Much of the available treatment information is anecdotal, and the efficacy and safety of the majority of mucositis therapy regimens have not yet been established.

The treatment of mucositis is primarily palliative and focused on symptom management. For mild to moderate mucositis, ice chips or Popsicles may provide adequate pain relief for some patients.[3] The mainstays of therapy for mucositis are oral rinses or mouthwashes that cleanse the mucosa and provide pain relief. Rinses can be those used for prophylaxis of mucositis or those containing a coating agent or local anesthetic (Tables 92.5 and 92.6). Sucralfate has been evaluated with mixed results. Sucralfate forms an ionic bond with tissue proteins, creating a protective barrier, and may also stimulate the production of prostaglandin E_2, which increases blood flow to the oral mucosa.[4] Oral rinses can be made from a single agent or a combination of several agents from different therapeutic categories, and may include an antifungal or corticosteroid; however, there are no controlled trials documenting the efficacy of combination rinses (the topical antifungal agents used in combination rinses are not potent enough to treat an active fungal infection; in these cases, systemic therapy is warranted). Patients should be instructed to use rinses as needed for pain and before eating to diminish the pain associated with swallowing.

Oral rinses used to treat mucositis are generally not associated with significant side effects; however, there are several important points of caution. Viscous lidocaine 2% and dyclonine hydrochloride 0.5% to 1% may cause numbing of the oral cavity, which can make swallowing difficult and put some patients at risk for aspiration.[11] Although diphenhydramine does not cause numbing of the oral cavity, it can cause sedation and unwanted anticholinergic effects such as dry mouth if it is ingested.[3] For pain associated with severe mucositis, oral or parenteral narcotics may be required (refer to Chapter 64 for pain management strategies).[12]

If mucositis interferes with nutritional intake or reduces the patient's quality of life, the dose of chemotherapy may need to be decreased in future cycles or the schedule of radiotherapy may need to be delayed until adequate healing has occurred. This is undesirable, as decreasing the intensity of cancer therapy may have a negative impact on the patient's ultimate outcome, namely response and survival. Furthermore, if patients experience severe fluid or weight loss, oral supplementation or intravenous hydration may be necessary.

Patients receiving therapy for mucositis should be regularly assessed for their ability to eat, drink, and talk; any changes in body weight or temperature; and the degree of pain in the oral mucosa. They should also be monitored for viral, bacterial, or fungal infections as clinically indicated. Use of anticholinergic agents (e.g., tricyclic antidepressants and some types of antipsychotics and antihistamines) should

TABLE 92.6	Pharmacologic Management of Mucositis
Agent	**Dosing Recommendation**
Coating agents:	
Magnesium and aluminum-based antacids (e.g., Maalox, Mylanta), Kaopectate	Used in various amounts in combination mouthwashes to provide a soothing effect
Sucralfate slurry	1 g swished for 2 minutes four to six times daily
Local anesthetics:	
Lidocaine viscous 2%	5–15 mL swished and expectorated q2–3h PRN
Dyclonine HCl 0.5 or 1% solution	5–15 mL swished and expectorated q2–3h PRN
Diphenhydramine	12.5 mg swished and expectorated QID (dissolve 25 mg in approximately 45 mL warm water)[3]
Benzocaine 20% spray	One or two sprays PRN
Benzocaine in Orabase gel	Apply to affected (localized) lesions q2–3h PRN
Cetacaine (benzocaine, butyl aminobenzoate tetracaine, & benzalkonium Cl) spray	One spray PRN

PRN, as needed; QID, four times a day.

be avoided in patients with mucositis, if possible, due to their drying effects on the mucosa.

FUTURE THERAPIES

Clinicians are beginning to understand more about mucositis on a molecular level, and new approaches to the prevention and treatment of mucositis are being explored. The following agents are in various stages of development or are in clinical trials.

AES-14 is a topical agent designed to deliver L-glutamine to the oral mucosa. The delivery system of AES-14 circumvents the problems inherent with glutamine, namely poor solubility and limited uptake by endothelial cells. L-glutamine is thought to reduce mucosal damage by acting as a nutrient for mucosal epithelial cells and lymphocytes, and it acts to transfer nitrogen between tissues. A recent phase III trial of AES-14 included over 2,000 women with breast cancer receiving anthracycline and cyclophosphamide-based therapy. Patients who developed mucositis as a result of therapy were then randomized to receive AES-14 or placebo. In the group treated with AES-14, the duration of oral mucositis was reduced by 29%. In addition, the progression to severe mucositis was reduced by 80% compared with the arm receiving no therapy.[13] This agent is now being studied for the management of mucositis in other tumor types.

Amifostine is an agent being studied in trials for prevention of mucositis in patients with head and neck cancers receiving chemotherapy and radiotherapy. Early studies suggest that this agent may decrease the severity and duration of mucositis when administered before radiotherapy compared with patients receiving no cytoprotection.[14,15] Amifostine can also be used to reduce the incidence of mucositis in patients receiving radiation therapy or radiation combined with chemotherapy. It is also being studied for the prevention of mucositis in patients receiving high-dose chemotherapy for hematologic tumors. For example, in a recent retrospective study, patients with multiple myeloma treated with vincristine, doxorubicin, and dexamethasone (VAD), high-dose melphalan, and an autologous stem cell transplant received amifostine or no amifostine prior to transplant. The occurrence of grade 3 or 4 mucositis was significantly decreased in the group receiving amifostine compared to the control group. Supportive care requirements were different between the two groups; opioid pain relief was required in 20% of patients who received amifostine compared with 69% of patients who received no amifostine. Importantly, disease response to antineoplastic therapy did not differ between groups, suggesting that amifostine does not interfere with the desired effects of chemotherapy.[16]

Other new approaches to the management of mucositis include biologically active factors that inhibit cellular regeneration, such as tumor growth factor-β and epidermal growth factor. The rationale is that mucositis appears to be related to the rate of epithelial proliferation, and these growth factors are shown to be negative regulators of epithelial cell proliferation. Other treatment modalities that may show promise in the management of mucositis include capsaicin and laser therapy. Some other agents have been studied for the management of mucositis; however, owing to a lack of convincing data, they are not currently considered the standard of care and in some cases are experimental. Examples include hematologic and keratinocyte growth factors, allopurinol mouthwash, leucovorin, uridine, propantheline, vitamin E, vitamin C and glutathione, azelastine hydrochloride, β-carotene, Kamillosan liquid (chamomile; not available in the United States), aspirin, silver nitrate, prostaglandins, indomethacin, benzydamine (not available in the United States), corticosteroids, Oratect gel, and sodium alginate.

IMPROVING OUTCOMES

Patient understanding and compliance with proper mouth care regimens are critical to minimizing the morbidity associated with mucositis (Table 92.7). Effectively managing the adverse effects of cancer therapy decreases the costs associated with caring for the patient and can substantially improve the patient's quality of life. Furthermore, if mucositis can ultimately be prevented, clinicians may be able to increase the dose intensity of chemotherapy and radiotherapy regimens to improve patient outcome.

XEROSTOMIA

Xerostomia, or dryness of the mouth, is commonly associated with radiation therapy for head and neck cancer. Because xerostomia can be uncomfortable as well as increase the risk for additional oral complications, it is important that it be diagnosed and appropriately managed.

TABLE 92.7	**Mucositis Patient Education**

Rinse with a mild, nonirritating solution five or six times daily (especially after meals) to decrease food particles remaining in the mouth and to help prevent infection.

Cleansing rinses should be swished in the mouth for 2 to 3 minutes (or as long as tolerated), then expectorated.

Strict compliance with oral care is essential.

Keep oral tissues, including lips, moist.

Maintain a bland diet and avoid spicy or acidic foods.

Avoid or diminish alcohol consumption and smoking.

Use ice chips or popsicles to relieve pain and discomfort.

Notify healthcare provider for fever or an inability to take food or medications by mouth.

TREATMENT GOALS: XEROSTOMIA

- Stimulate salivary flow.
- Replace lost secretions.
- Protect the dentition.
- Prevent complications associated with xerostomia, such as mucositis.[4]

PATHOPHYSIOLOGY

Healthy adults secrete up to 1.5 L of saliva daily.[6] Saliva is important in maintaining mucosal health: it moistens the oral cavity and clears it of debris and oral flora, is an integral component of digestion, and is important for normal speaking and swallowing.[4,6] Radiation therapy administered for head and neck cancers damages the salivary glands, thus decreasing saliva production. One study found that the average salivary flow rate decreased 57% after 1 week of radiation, 67% after 6 weeks of radiation therapy, and 95% 3 years after treatment was completed.[1] There is a relationship between the dose and location of radiation, the volume of irradiated tissue, and the extent of damage to the salivary glands. Generally, damage is reversible in patients who receive radiation doses less than 6,000 cGy, whereas changes may be permanent in patients who receive greater than 6,000 cGy.[4] There may be additional causes that exacerbate the radiation-induced xerostomia, such as concomitant medications that have anticholinergic or diuretic properties (tricyclic antidepressants, antipsychotics, antihistamines, antihypertensives), concurrent illnesses (diabetes mellitus and interstitial nephritis), and vitamin A and nicotinic acid deficiencies.[4] It is important to thoroughly investigate and eliminate, if possible, all potential causes of xerostomia, as they predispose the patient with cancer to more serious oral complications such as mucositis, oral infection, dental caries and decalcification, periodontitis, gingival erosion, and abscesses.[4]

CLINICAL PRESENTATION AND DIAGNOSIS

The National Cancer Institute has published a grading scale (grades 1 to 3) for documenting the severity of xerostomia (Table 92.8). It is important to document all patient-reported signs and symptoms, including their severity and duration. Patients primarily complain of dryness in the mouth. As eating and swallowing become more difficult, patients may experience loss of appetite and weight loss.

TREATMENT

Keeping the mouth moist is the most important aspect of managing xerostomia. This can be achieved using pharmacologic and nonpharmacologic interventions (Table 92.9). Oral pilocarpine (Salagen) 5 mg, given three times a day, has been shown to stimulate salivary secretion and relieve symptoms in patients who have residual salivary function after radiation therapy.[17–19] The major side effect associated with pilocarpine is sweating. There are also several saliva substitutes that are commercially available; however, most patients find that these substitutes do not work well and can be costly.[6] Water rinses may be more acceptable to patients and should be used before and during meals and additionally as needed. Other measures that patients may try include sugarless gum and hard candy, sucking on ice chips, or use of a humidifier in their living spaces.[1] Use of anticholinergic

---

TABLE 92.8	**National Cancer Institute CTCAE Grading System for Xerostomia**		
	Grade 1	**Grade 2**	**Grade 3**
Subjective & objective parameters	Symptomatic (dry or thick saliva) without significant dietary alteration; unstimulated saliva flow >0.2 mL/min	Symptomatic and significant oral intake alteration (e.g., copious water, other lubricants, diet limited to purees and/or soft, moist foods); unstimulated saliva 0.1 to 0.2 mL/min	Symptoms leading to inability to adequately aliment orally; IV fluids, tube feedings, or total parenteral nutrition indicated; unstimulated saliva < 0.1 mL/min

(*Source*: National Cancer Institute CTCAE v 3.0, Dec. 12, 2003.)

TABLE 92.9	Management of Xerostomia

Maintain good oral hygiene.

Débride the tongue using a soft toothbrush.

Use saliva substitutes or water rinses four to six times daily to keep the mouth moist and aid in swallowing.

Drink liquids frequently (avoid caffeinated beverages).

Eat moistened or pureed foods.

Use sugar-free candy (i.e., lemon candy) or gum PRN.

Apply lubrication to the lips (e.g., Blistex or Aquaphor).

Discontinue or decrease alcohol consumption and smoking.

agents (e.g., tricyclic antidepressants, some types of antipsychotics and antihistamines) should be avoided in patients with xerostomia, due to their drying effects on the mucosa.

Intravenous amifostine is FDA approved to reduce the incidence of moderate to severe xerostomia in patients undergoing postoperative radiation treatment for head and neck cancer, where the radiation port includes a substantial portion of the parotid glands. A study of standard fraction-ated radiation with or without amifostine administration prior to each fraction showed that the incidence of grade 2 or higher acute (90 days or less from the start of radiation) xerostomia was significantly reduced in patients receiving amifostine (51% with amifostine versus 78% in the control group). The rate of late xerostomia (9 to 12 months following radiation) was also significantly reduced in the arm receiving amifostine versus the control group (35% versus 57%, respectively). Furthermore, at 1 year following radiation, the median saliva production was higher in the patients who received amifostine (0.26 g versus 0.1 g).[20]

CONSTIPATION AND DIARRHEA

Lower gastrointestinal toxicity, including constipation and diarrhea, is common in patients with cancer undergoing treatment. Approximately 4% to 10% of patients with cancer who are undergoing treatment develop diarrhea (this increases to 43% after bone marrow transplantation), and greater than 50% of patients referred to a palliative care setting, or hospice, suffer from constipation.[21,22]

TREATMENT GOALS: CONSTIPATION AND DIARRHEA

- Prevent the development of constipation and diarrhea.
- If constipation or diarrhea develops, treat promptly to prevent associated complications.

PATHOPHYSIOLOGY

Although numerous etiologies may contribute to the development of diarrhea and constipation in patients with cancer, there are several causes that are specific to this population (Tables 92.10 and 92.11). For example, the cells of the gastrointestinal tract (as with the oral mucosa) proliferate rapidly and thus are at increased risk of damage from chemotherapy or radiation therapy.

Irinotecan (CPT-11), a chemotherapy agent used to treat colon and rectal cancers, is commonly associated with severe diarrhea. There are two types of diarrhea associated with irinotecan: early onset (within 24 hours of administration) and late onset (>24 hours after administration). Early diarrhea is due to cholinergic causes and is generally self-limiting. The mechanism of late diarrhea is not well understood but appears to be related to a secretory process, activated by the cytotoxic effect of irinotecan on the mucosal layer of the gastrointestinal tract. Late diarrhea can be prolonged and may be associated with significant morbidity due to dehydration and electrolyte abnormalities.

Vincristine, a chemotherapy agent used in the treatment of several tumors, including lymphomas, is associated with constipation due to neurotoxic side effects of the vinca alkaloid drug class. Patients are usually begun on a bowel regimen for the prevention of constipation when vincristine therapy is initiated.

CLINICAL PRESENTATION AND DIAGNOSIS

In general, the approach to the management of diarrhea and constipation is no different from that of patients without cancer. The patient evaluation for diarrhea should include an evaluation of medications and radiation therapies, a history of bowel habits, and a physical examination to assess vital signs and hydration status. The workup may include stool cultures, if appropriate, to rule out an infectious etiology. Abdominal, rectal, and stool examinations may be performed.

The evaluation for constipation should include a history of any changes in bowel habits, any personal changes (emo-

TABLE 92.10	Possible Causes of Diarrhea in the Patient With Cancer

Antacids containing magnesium

Antibiotic use

Bile salts

Caffeine

Cancer-related:
  Carcinoid syndrome
  Colon cancer (partial bowel obstruction by tumor)
  Endocrine tumors
  VIPoma
  Malignant carcinoid tumor
  Gastrinoma
  Medullary carcinoma of the thyroid
  Lymphoma
  Pancreatic cancer (islet cell tumors)
  Pheochromocytoma

Cancer therapy-related: Chemotherapy
  Capecitabine
  Cisplatin
  Cytosine arabinoside
  Cyclophosphamide
  Daunorubicin
  Docetaxel
  Doxorubicin
  5-Fluorouracil
  Gefitinib (doses ≥500 mg)
  Imatinib
  Interferon
  Irinotecan
  Leucovorin
  Methotrexate
  Oxaliplatin
  Paclitaxel
  Topotecan

Colchicine

Enteral nutrition

Graft-versus-host disease

Infection

Nonsteroidal anti-inflammatory drugs (NSAIDs)

Potassium chloride

Prokinetic agents (e.g., metoclopramide)

Radiation therapy to abdomen, lumbar, para-aortics, pelvis

Supportive therapy agents

Surgical-related:
  Celiac plexus block
  Cholecystectomy
  Esophagogastrectomy
  Gastrectomy
  Whipple procedure
  Intestinal resection
  Vagotomy

Thyroid hormone

(*Sources:* Cox GJ, Matsui SM, Lo RS, et al. Etiology and outcome of diarrhea after bone marrow transplantation: a prospective study. Gastroenterology 107:1398–1407, 1994; Mercadante S. Diarrhea, malabsorption, and constipation. In: Berger A, Portenoy RK, Weissman DE, eds. Principles and practice of supportive oncology. Philadelphia: Lippincott-Raven, 1998:191.)

tional state, activity level, dietary intake), and a thorough review of medications. An abdominal examination can help to establish the presence of bowel sounds, and a rectal examination will assess for external hemorrhoids, scars, fistulas, or fissures.

The National Cancer Institute has published a grading scale (grades 1 to 4) for documenting the severity of both constipation and diarrhea (Table 92.12). The Rome II Criteria are also used to assess for constipation in adults (Table 92.13).

TREATMENT

For a detailed treatment plan for the assessment and management of patients with diarrhea or constipation, refer to Chapter 48.

DIARRHEA

Irinotecan-induced diarrhea is so prevalent that drugs to treat and prevent it have been standardized and should be administered to all patients. Because the early-onset diarrhea is cholinergic in nature, intravenous atropine 0.25 to 1 mg should be administered (after ruling out a history of cardiac disease) prior to irinotecan therapy. At the first sign of late-onset diarrhea, patients should be given oral loperamide 4 mg, followed by 2 mg every 2 hours (not to exceed 16 mg/24 hours) until the patient does not experience diarrhea for at least 12 hours.[23] Patients may take 4 mg every 4 hours during the night. If grade 2, 3, or 4 late-onset diarrhea occurs, subsequent doses of irinotecan within the cycle should be decreased.

For persistent chemotherapy- or radiation-induced diarrhea that has failed to respond to first-line options, intravenous fluid/electrolyte replacement and octreotide therapy may be started. The actions of octreotide mimic those of the natural hormone somatostatin. Octreotide is FDA approved for the symptomatic management of patients with carcinoid tumors and vasoactive intestinal peptide tumors, where it suppresses or inhibits the severe diarrhea associated with the disease. It has been studied in patients refractory to loperamide who were receiving chemotherapy regimens consisting of fluorouracil, leucovorin, irinotecan, cyclophosphamide, methotrexate, and cisplatin.[24] When administered at a dose of 100 μg subcutaneously three times daily for 3 days, it was shown to be both effective primary treatment and second-line therapy (after loperamide failure). If there is no improvement in the diarrhea after 24 hours, the dosage may be increased to 300 to 500 μg subcutaneously three times daily. Octreotide may be discontinued 24 hours after the end of diarrhea and upon reestablishment of a normal diet.

Diarrhea secondary to graft-versus-host disease, occasionally seen in patients undergoing allogeneic stem cell

TABLE 92.11 | Possible Causes of Constipation in the Patient With Cancer

Bowel obstruction by tumor

Cancer therapy (vinca alkaloids, thalidomide)

Opioid therapy

Nonsteroidal anti-inflammatory drugs

5HT-3 receptor antagonists (ondansetron, granisetron, palonosetron)

Hypercalcemia

Other patient-related risk factors (e.g., elderly, diabetes mellitus, hypothyroidism, uremia)

Antimuscarinic agents (anticholinergics, antihistamines, tricyclic, antidepressants, antipsychotics)

Calcium channel blockers (verapamil)

Cationic agents (aluminum, calcium, iron)

Central alpha-adrenergic agents (clonidine)

Decreased mobility

Malnutrition/dehydration

(*Sources:* Mercadante S. Diarrhea, malabsorption, and constipation. In: Berger A, Portenoy RK, Weissman DE, eds. Principles and practice of supportive oncology. Philadelphia: Lippincott-Raven, 1998:191; Bruera E, Suarez-Almazor M, Velasco A, et al. The assessment of constipation in terminal cancer patients admitted to a palliative care unit: a retrospective review. J Pain Symptom Manage 9:515–519, 1994.)

TABLE 92.12 | CTCAE Grading Criteria for Constipation

Grade 1	Grade 2	Grade 3	Grade 4
Occasional or intermittent symptoms; occasional use of stool softeners, laxatives, dietary modifications, or enema	Persistent symptoms with regular use of laxatives or enemas indicated	Symptoms interfering with activities of daily living; obstipation with manual evacuation indicated	Life-threatening consequences (e.g., obstruction, toxic megacolon)

TABLE 92.13 | Rome II Criteria for Constipation in Adults

Two or more of the following for at least 12 weeks (not necessarily consecutive) in the preceding 12 months:

Straining during >25% of bowel movements

Lumpy or hard stools for >25% of bowel movements

Sensation of incomplete evacuation for >25% of bowel movements

Sensation of anorectal blockage for >25% of bowel movements

Manual maneuvers to facilitate >25% of bowel movements (e.g., digital evacuation or support of pelvic floor)

<3 bowel movements weekly

Loose stools not present, and insufficient criteria for irritable bowel syndrome met

(*Source:* Lembo A, Camilleri M. Chronic constipation. N Engl J Med 349:1360, 2003.)

transplantation, can also be treated with subcutaneous or intravenous octreotide.

CONSTIPATION

For patients scheduled to receive opioid or vinca alkaloid therapy, a stool softener (docusate sodium) and laxative (e.g., magnesium hydroxide, lactulose, senna, bisacodyl) should be started at the onset of therapy. Use of a stool softener alone in this setting is usually not sufficient due to decreased bowel motility with the use of opioid or vinca alkaloid agents.

Treatment for acute or chronic constipation may involve the use of agents such as magnesium hydroxide, lactulose, senna, bisacodyl, or magnesium citrate. Suppositories and enemas should be avoided in patients who are neutropenic or thrombocytopenic due to the risk of tearing the gastrointestinal mucosa, thereby introducing an infection or causing rectal bleeding. Magnesium and phosphate salts should be avoided in patients with renal insufficiency to prevent electrolyte disturbances.

TREATMENT-INDUCED NAUSEA AND VOMITING

According to data collected in 1983,[25] patients with cancer expressed that their two most significant concerns regarding the adverse side effects of chemotherapy were nausea and vomiting. Vomiting was the number-one concern of patients, and nausea was second. In 1999,[26] several years after the development of newer antiemetic therapies, vomiting disappeared from the top-five list of patient concerns, yet nausea continued to be the number-one fear.[27]

It is extremely distressing and debilitating for patients with cancer to experience severe nausea and vomiting secondary to chemotherapy, especially with the current use of combination chemotherapy and dose-intensified regimens. Known complications of protracted emesis include dehydration, electrolyte and acid–base imbalances, esophageal tearing or rib fracture, aspiration pneumonitis, impaired nutritional state, and the potential inability to continue chemotherapy.[28] It is therefore essential that effective antiemetic therapy be used to provide positive outcomes for patients.

TREATMENT GOALS: TREATMENT-INDUCED NAUSEA AND VOMITING

- Use antiemetic agents with proven effectiveness, at the correct dose, given in appropriate combinations, and properly timed, to eliminate nausea and/or vomiting and allow continuation of chemotherapy as planned.
- Use aggressive antiemetic therapy to eliminate the cost of treating any complication secondary to protracted nausea or vomiting.
- Provide total symptom management to ensure comfort and quality of life for the patient.

EPIDEMIOLOGY

The incidence and severity of nausea and/or vomiting depend on both drug- and patient-related factors. Hesketh et al[29] have tabulated the emetogenic potential of antineoplastic agents alone and ranked them into levels of emetogenicity (Table 92.14). In the Hesketh classification, antineoplastic agents are categorized into five levels:

Level 1: Agents in this class are not really considered emetogenic. There is a less than 10% risk of acute (≤ 24 hours after chemotherapy) emesis without antiemetic prophylaxis.

Level 2: Agents in this class cause acute emesis in 10% to 30% of patients.

Level 3: Agents in this class cause acute emesis in 30% to 60% of patients.

Level 4: Agents in this class cause acute emesis in 60% to 90% of patients.

Level 5: Nearly all patients (>90%) will experience an emetic episode if routine antiemetic therapy is not provided.

Although this classification provides an estimate of the emetogenicity of any particular agent, in many cases, antineoplastics are administered in combination. Thus, the Hesketh classification also includes a set of rules to assist in classifying the emetogenicity of combination chemotherapy. The steps involved in determining a regimen's emetogenic potential can be described as follows:

1. Identify the most emetogenic agent in the combination.
2. Assess the relative contribution of the other agents to the overall emetogenicity of the combination. When considering other agents, the following "rules" apply:

- Level 1 agents do not contribute to the emetogenicity of a given regimen.
- Adding one or more level 2 agents increases the emetogenicity of the combination by one level greater than the most emetogenic agent in the combination.
- Adding level 3 or 4 agents increases the emetogenicity of the combination by one level per agent.

It is also important to recognize the patient-related risk factors for postchemotherapy nausea and vomiting (Table 92.15). In providing optimal care for patients with cancer, risk factors must be carefully reviewed and evaluated before any treatment is begun. This provides a means to deliver effective symptom management while maintaining the highest quality of life possible.[30]

PATHOPHYSIOLOGY

Previously, the path for drug-induced emesis was believed to be a simple one, in which bloodborne agents act directly on the chemoreceptor trigger zone (CTZ) located in the area postrema of the fourth ventricle of the brain.[31] The CTZ then stimulates the vomiting center (VC) found on the dorsal lateral reticular formation of the medulla. Once triggered, the

TABLE 92.14	Hesketh Level, by Chemotherapy Agent

Emetogenic Level	Agent	
5	Carmustine >250 mg/m^2	Lomustine >60 mg/m^2
	Cisplatin ≥50 mg/m^{2a}	Mechlorethamine
	Cyclophosphamide >1,500 mg/m^{2a}	Pentostatin (doses of 10 mg/m^2)
	Dacarbazine ≥1,000 mg/m^2/dose	Streptozocin
	Etoposide 60 mg/kg (high dose for BMT)	
4	Amifostine >500 mg/m^2	Daunorubicin >50 mg/m^2
	Carboplatin ≥300 mg/m^2 or AUC ≥3	Doxorubicin >60 mg/m^{2a}
	Carmustine ≤250 mg/m^2	Epirubicin >90 mg/m^2
	Cisplatin <50 mg/m^2	Melphalan (IV) ≥50 mg/m^{2a}
	Cyclophosphamide >750 to ≤1,500 mg/m^{2a}	Methotrexate >1,000 mg/m^2
	Cytarabine >1,000 mg/m^2	Mitoxantrone ≥15 mg/m^2
	Dactinomycin	Procarbazine (oral)
3	Aldesleukin	Epirubicin ≤90 mg/m^2
	Amifostine >300 to ≤500 mg/m^2	Gemtuzumab ozogamicin
	Arsenic trioxide	Hexamethylmelamine (oral)
	Carboplatin <300 mg/m^2 or AUC ≤2	Idarubicin
	Cyclophosphamide ≤750 mg/m^{2a}	Ifosfamide
	Cyclophosphamide (oral)	Irinotecan
	Cytarabine ≤1,000 mg/m^2	Lomustine ≤60 mg/m^2
	Dacarbazine 150–200 mg/m^2	Methotrexate 250–1,000 mg/m^2
	Daunorubicin ≤50 mg/m^2	Mitoxantrone <15 mg/m^2
	Doxorubicin 20–60 mg/m^{2a}	Oxaliplatin
2	Amifostine ≤300 mg/m^2	Liposomal daunorubicin
	Capecitabine	Methotrexate >50 to <250 mg/m^2
	Cytarabine 100–200 mg/m^2	Mitomycin
	Docetaxel	Paclitaxel
	Doxorubicin <20 mg/m^2 or CIVI	Pemetrexed
	Etoposide	Temozolomide
	5-Fluorouracil <1,000 mg/m^2	Teniposide
	Gemcitabine	Thiotepa
	Liposomal doxorubicin	Topotecan
1	Alemtuzumab	Imatinib
	Androgens	Interferon-α-2a
	Asparaginase	Letrozole
	Bevacizumab	Melphalan (oral)
	Bexarotene (oral)	Mercaptopurine
	Bleomycin	Methotrexate ≤50 mg/m^2
	Bortezomib	Pegaspargase
	Busulfan (oral, 4 mg/kg/day)	Pentostatin 4–5 mg/m^2
	Cetuximab	Rituximab
	Chlorambucil	Tamoxifen
	Cladribine	Thalidomide
	Cytarabine 100 mg/m^2 CIVI	Thioguanine (oral)
	Denileukin diftitox	Tositumomab
	Estramustine	Trastuzumab
	Fludarabine	Tretinoin
	Gefitinib	Vinblastine
	Hydroxyurea	Vincristine
	Ibritumomab tiuxetan	Vinorelbine

CIVI, continuous intravenous infusion; AUC, area under the time–concentration curve.

^{a} Agents known to cause delayed nausea and vomiting.

To identify regimen Hesketh level: 1. Take the most highly emetogenic agent in the regimen as your starting point. 2. Make no adjustments for level 1 agents. 3. Increase Hesketh level by one level if one or more level 2 agents are included. 4. Increase by one level for *each* level 3 or 4 agent included.

(*Source:* National Oncology Alliance Treatment Guideline for Antiemetic Therapy, updated 2005.)

TABLE 92.15	Risk Factors for Postchemotherapy Nausea and Vomiting

Highly emetogenic, high-dose, or combination chemotherapy

Multiple cycles of chemotherapy

Longer infusion time for chemotherapy

Concurrent radiation therapy

Prechemotherapy nausea or vomiting

History of nausea and/or vomiting with chemotherapy

Increased level of apprehension and/or anxiety

Sensitivity to motion sickness or history of pregnancy-related morning sickness

Younger age (<50 years)

Female sex

Note: In general, men, patients older than 50 years, and those with a history of heavy alcohol use (>100 g/day for several years) have a decreased risk of postchemotherapy nausea and vomiting.

VC then initiates the body's act of emesis by integrating the actions of several organs and systems (Fig. 92.1). Because dopamine is a major neurotransmitter between the CTZ and the VC, most antiemetic agents used had traditionally been antagonists of the dopamine type 2 receptor (D_2), such as the phenothiazines (prochlorperazine) or the butyr-phenones (haloperidol or droperidol). Prochlorperazine is still considered by many to be an effective general antiemetic agent.

From work in animals, it is known that stimulation of the VC is a very complex process that derives inputs from several areas: the CTZ, vestibular apparatus, periphery, and higher cortical centers.[32] Although it can aggravate nausea and vomiting secondary to chemotherapy when the patient is driving home after treatment, input from the vestibular apparatus is not believed to play a primary role in chemotherapy-induced emesis.

The introduction of the antineoplastic cisplatin allowed the discovery of new stimulatory pathways to the VC, as it induced a different type of severe emesis. Acute cisplatin-induced emesis was refractory to even the most aggressive use of standard dopamine antagonists; thus, it currently serves as a standard to test the efficacy of new antiemetic agents and treatment strategies.[33] Metoclopramide, when administered intravenously every 2 hours in very high doses (1 to 3 mg/kg), is effective against cisplatin-induced emesis.

Studies in animals indicated that complete surgical ablation of the CTZ failed to block emesis due to cisplatin. This understanding initiated the search for other inputs (ones from the periphery) that feed into the VC and could stimulate emesis after antineoplastic therapy. This led to an understanding of the role that serotonin plays in emesis and how metoclopramide in high doses acts as a weak serotonin antagonist.[33,34]

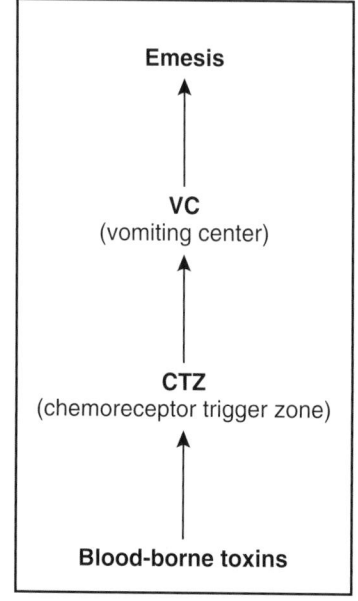

Historical single pathway for the stimulation of emesis.

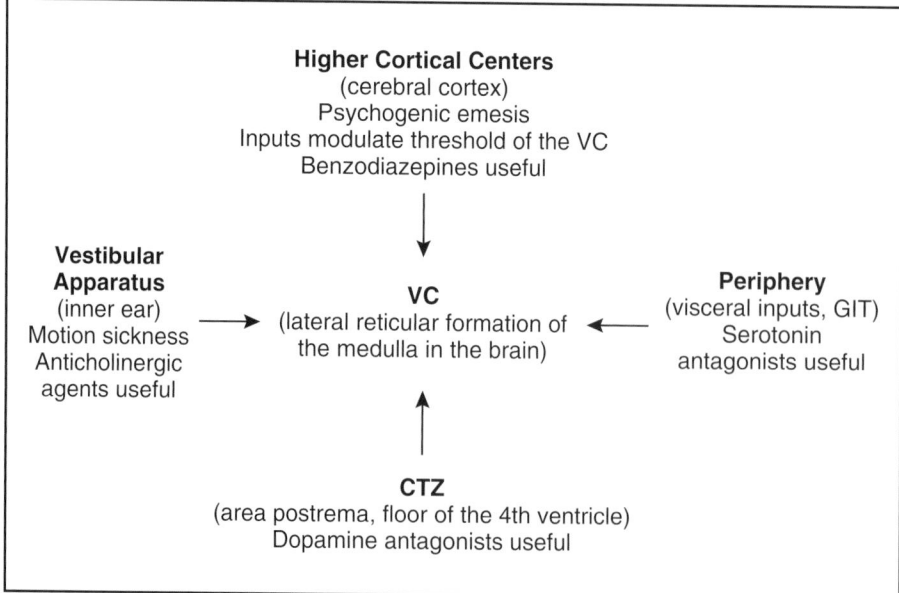

Current known pathways for emesis. A variety of neurotransmitters are involved.

FIGURE 92.1 Emetogenic pathways. CTZ, chemoreceptor trigger zone; GIT, gastrointestinal tract; VC, vomiting center.

The role of serotonin is not fully understood, but it is believed that chemotherapeutic agents such as cisplatin cause enterochromaffin cells within the gastrointestinal tract to secrete serotonin. This neurotransmitter then stimulates emesis via multiple pathways both peripherally and centrally (either via vagal afferents or via direct action on the CTZ and VC). The serotonin type 3 receptor blocking agents (5-HT-3 antagonists) are the most effective class of pharmacologic agents against chemotherapy-induced emesis to date, as they not only block the action of serotonin but also inhibit further release of serotonin from the enterochromaffin cells.

These blocking agents do not have a linear response curve but actually exhibit a saturation or plateau phenomena.[35] Thus, higher doses of 5-HT-3 antagonists do not necessarily provide an enhanced antiemetic response. Recent studies have shown that significantly decreased doses of these agents can be used without affecting desired patient outcomes and overall antiemetic response. The synergistic effect demonstrated by combining 5-HT-3 antagonists and dexamethasone and the use of higher dexamethasone doses allows an even further reduction of the 5-HT-3 antagonist dose and the overall cost of treatment.[36]

Additional reductions in treatment cost can also be realized with the combined use of oral 5-HT-3 receptor antagonists and dexamethasone, all of which possess good oral bioavailability and efficacy. With enterochromaffin cells located within the gastrointestinal tract, oral 5-HT-3 agents offer the additional effect of blocking local serotonin receptors and thus reducing serotonin secretion.[37]

CLINICAL PRESENTATION AND DIAGNOSIS

It is extremely important to determine the exact etiology of nausea and vomiting in a patient with cancer before using an antiemetic agent for symptom management (Table 92.16). For example, obstruction of the gastrointestinal tract secondary to tumor invasion or heavy use of opiates or increased intracranial pressure from metastatic processes to the brain may be the true cause of nausea and protracted vomiting.[38] In these cases, the use of an antiemetic agent is of limited benefit compared to correction of the primary problem.

Chemotherapy-related nausea and vomiting can present in three different ways: acute, delayed, and anticipatory. Nausea and vomiting are normally classified as acute and take place within the first 24 hours after the administration of antineoplastic agents, peaking between 2 and 6 hours and then diminishing thereafter.[39] Some agents can also produce a phenomenon of delayed nausea, classically observed with cisplatin or high-dose cyclophosphamide chemotherapy, which begins after the first 24 hours and can last for several days.[33] Anticipatory nausea and vomiting is a conditioned or learned response that usually follows one or more courses of emetogenic chemotherapy where there was poor control fcof acute or delayed emesis.[32] Anticipatory nausea

| TABLE 92.16 | Initial Workup and Diagnosis |

Risk factors for postchemotherapy nausea and vomiting

Other nonchemotherapy etiologies (e.g., acute abdominal emergencies, central nervous system disorders, acute systemic infections, fluid/electrolyte imbalances)

Fluid status (check hydration: skin turgor, weight, creatinine, blood urea nitrogen)

Comprehensive metabolic panel

Hepatic function panel (rule out electrolyte imbalance, electrolyte depletion, and renal/hepatic dysfunction)

Vital signs (rule out fever, dehydration)

Orientation/mentation (rule out central nervous system disorder)

Evaluation of medications (e.g., opioids, digoxin, theophylline, oral antibiotics)

(*Source:* National Oncology Alliance Treatment Guideline for Antiemetic Therapy, updated 2005.)

vomiting have no relation to chemotherapy administration and can be triggered by a variety of associated sights or smells.[38]

The National Cancer Institute has published a grading scale (grades 1 to 4) for documenting the severity of nausea and vomiting (Table 92.17).

ACUTE NAUSEA AND VOMITING

Defined as emesis within the first 24 hours after chemotherapy, acute emesis is best controlled with prophylactic combinations of oral and intravenous antiemetics. Usually a 5-HT-3 receptor antagonist combined with a steroid such as dexamethasone works well to prevent acute emesis when given 30 minutes prior to chemotherapy administration. The use of oral or intravenous dexamethasone has been shown to greatly enhance the efficacy of any antiemetic agent.[33] Because of its relatively low cost (compared to the 5-HT-3 antagonists) and low potential for side effects, the current recommendation is to give a 20-mg oral or intravenous dose of dexamethasone for maximum protection with highly emetogenic chemotherapy. The dose of 5-HT-3 agent administered should be stratified according to the particular chemotherapeutic agent and dose used. The majority of the 5-HT-3 agents have half-lives of less than 10 hours, thus requiring repeated dosing, but the newest agent, palonosetron, has a half life of about 40 hours, necessitating only a single dose. Careful examination of antiemetic dose requirements will minimize treatment cost while providing optimal patient coverage. Table 92.18 lists commonly used agents and dos-ing regimens for the prevention of acute nausea and vomiting.

In patients receiving highly emetogenic chemotherapy, where both acute nausea and delayed nausea are of particular concern, aprepitant may be considered as preventive therapy

TABLE 92.17	National Cancer Institute CTCAE Grading Systems for Nausea and Vomiting			
	Grade 1	Grade 2	Grade 3	Grade 4
Nausea	Loss of appetite without alteration in eating habits	Oral intake decreased without significant weight loss, dehydration, or malnutrition; IV fluids indicated <24 hours	Inadequate oral caloric or fluid intake; IV fluids, tube feedings, or total parenteral nutrition indicated ≥24 hours	Life-threatening consequences
Vomiting	1 episode in 24 hours	Two to five episodes in 24 hours; IV fluids indicated <24 hours	Six or more episodes in 24 hours; IV fluids, or total parenteral nutrition indicated ≥24 hours	Life-threatening consequences

(*Source*: National Cancer Institute CTCAE v 3.0, Dec. 12, 2003.)

in combination with a 5-HT-3 antagonist and dexamethasone. The mechanism and use of aprepitant are discussed later in the section on ''Delayed Nausea and Vomiting.''

If breakthrough nausea or emesis occurs within the first 24 hours of chemotherapy administration despite preventive antiemetic therapy for acute emesis, treatment options include agents such as metoclopramide, phenothiazines, or lorazepam. Table 92.19 details recommendations for management in patients who experience nausea and vomiting despite preventative pharmacologic therapy for acute emesis.

DELAYED NAUSEA AND VOMITING

Studies have shown that delayed nausea and vomiting is frequently seen after the intravenous administration of high doses of cisplatin and cyclophosphamide.[34,38–41] Other agents associated with delayed nausea and vomiting include carboplatin, doxorubicin, ifosfamide, dacarbazine, and high-dose melphalan. The nausea and vomiting begin 1 or 2 days after treatment and can last several days. The exact cause for delayed nausea and vomiting is poorly understood, but it appears to be mediated in part by the neurokinin neuropeptide substance P, and this syndrome is rather difficult to treat.[42]

There are currently two agents that are FDA approved for the prevention of delayed nausea and vomiting associated with the administration of chemotherapy. Aprepitant, an oral neurokinin-1 (NK-1) receptor antagonist, was approved for the prevention of delayed nausea and vomiting associated with highly emetogenic chemotherapy when used in combination with a steroid and 5-HT-3 receptor antagonist. Aprepitant is thought to block the normal activity of endogenous substance P at the NK-1 receptor, thus preventing emesis. Aprepitant is a moderate inhibitor of cytochrome P450 3A4, so dose adjustments of a patient's concomitant medications may be needed. Aprepitant, for example, inhibits the metabo-lism of warfarin and can result in a patient's prothrombin time/International Normalized Ratio rising to supratherapeutic levels if the dose of warfarin is not reduced.

Palonosetron, a 5-HT-3 receptor antagonist, is FDA approved for the prevention of delayed nausea and vomiting associated with moderately emetogenic chemotherapy. The additional benefit gained from adding a corticosteroid to palonosetron for the prevention of delayed nausea and vomiting has not yet been clearly established.

Other agents have been used in the setting of delayed nausea and vomiting, but they have limited effectiveness. They include metoclopramide, lorazepam, haloperidol, and a short-acting 5-HT-3 receptor antagonist in combination with a steroid.[33,43–47] Table 92.19 describes the common dosing regimens of agents used to prevent delayed nausea and vomiting.

Despite the use of agents to prevent delayed nausea and vomiting, breakthrough episodes may occur. Several of the agents used to manage breakthrough emesis with acute emesis are also used in treatment for delayed nausea and vomiting. Agents include metoclopramide, phenothiazines, lorazepam, dronabinol, and scopolamine patches (Table 92.19).

ANTICIPATORY NAUSEA AND VOMITING

Anticipatory nausea and vomiting is a conditioned response that is learned after one or more courses of emetogenic chemotherapy during which the patient has experienced nausea or vomiting.[35] The stimulus in this case comes from the higher or cortical centers of the brain transmitting impulses directly into the vomiting center, thereby greatly lowering the normal threshold for emesis. Triggers for this can be numerous, from the mere smell of isopropyl alcohol, to the reddish color of doxorubicin, to the sight of a chemotherapy nurse in public. All can elicit profound nausea and possibly immediate emesis.[39]

Anticipatory nausea and vomiting can be approached in two ways. The first is to aggressively treat the patient with adequate antiemetics to prevent a distressing experience from ever happening. The second is to use agents such as benzodiazepines to calm the patient and induce antegrade amnesia. Benzodiazepines act not only to calm and relax the patient, but also to elevate the emesis threshold back to normal. With the antegrade amnesia induced by the benzodiazepines, the patient may not remember enough to form a conditioned response.[48] Lorazepam is commonly adminis-

| TABLE 92.18 | Prevention of Acute and Delayed Nausea and Vomiting |

Highly Emetogenic Chemotherapy (Hesketh Level 5): Regimens Containing Cisplatin Doses ≥50 mg/m²

Acute	Delayed		
Day 1	Day 2	Day 3	Day 4
• Aprepitant 125 mg PO Plus	Aprepitant 80 mg PO	Aprepitant 80 mg PO	
• 5-HT₃ IV (each day of highly emetogenic chemo <u>except</u> palonosetronª (see below for doses) Plus	Plus	Plus	
• Dexamethasone 12 mg IV	Dexamethasone 8 mg PO	Dexamethasone 8 mg PO	Dexamethasone 8 mg PO

Subscript note: 5-HT$_3$; doses given as cisplatin ≥50 mg/m^2.

Highly Emetogenic Chemotherapy (Hesketh Level 5): Non–Cisplatin-Containing Regimens or Combination Regimens Including Cisplatin Doses <50 mg/m²

Day 1	Day 2–4
• 5-HT₃ IV (each day of highly emetogenic chemotherapy <u>except</u> palonosetronª (see below for doses) *plus*	<u>Option 1:</u> • Dexamethasone 8 mg PO/IV BID ± Metoclopramide 20–40 mg PO/IV q6h
• Dexamethasone 20 mg IV	*or*
	<u>Option 2:</u> • Dexamethasone 8 mg PO/IV BID ± 5-HT₃-RA (daily)ª
	With or without:
With or without:	• Aprepitant[b] 80mg PO Days 2, 3
• Aprepitant[b] 125 mg PO Day 1	

Moderately Emetogenic Chemotherapy (Hesketh Level 3 and 4)

Acute (0–24 hours after chemotherapy)

• 5-HT₃-RA IV Day 1 (see below for doses). If the regimen causes acute and delayed nausea and vomiting, should give palonosetron in the acute setting

plus

• Dexamethasone 8 mg IV Day 1

Delayed (24–120 hours after chemotherapy)

• Palonosetron 0.25 mg IV Day 1 (Palonosetron is the only 5-HT₃-RA that is FDA approved for the prevention of delayed nausea and vomiting associated with moderately emetogenic chemotherapy).ª

+/–

Dexamethasone 8 mg PO QD Day 2–4

Alternatives include the following, which should be initiated 24 hours after the last dose of chemotherapy (agents are listed in order of preference):

• Metoclopramide 30–40 mg PO QID, with diphenhydramine 25–50 mg IV/PO q4–6h and dexamethasone 8 mg PO BID for 2–4 days. Avoid metoclopramide in patients experiencing diarrhea.

• Lorazepam 0.5–2 mg PO/SL q6h (as an adjunctive agent)

• Haloperidol 0.5–1 mg PO q6h

• Other 5-HT₃ on Days 2–4 in combination with dexamethasone

Low Emetic Risk Chemotherapy (Hesketh Level 2)

Each Day of Chemotherapy

• Dexamethasone 4–8 mg PO/IV *AND/OR*

• Promethazine 12.5–50 mg PO q6h PRN

• Prochlorperazine 10 mg PO q6h or 15 mg Spansule PO q12h *OR*

• Metoclopramide 20–40 mg PO q6h PRN ± Diphenhydramine 25–50 mg PO q6h PRN

• Lorazepam 0.5–2 mg PO/SL q4–6h PRN (as an adjunctive agent)

(continues)

TABLE 92.18	continued	
Drug	**Dose**	**Route**
5-HT₃ Choices:		
Dolasetron	100 mg or 1.8 mg/kg	IV
	100 mg	PO
Granisetron	1 mg (or 10 μg/kg)	IV
	1 mg BID	PO
Ondansetron	8 mg or 0.15 mg/kg	IV
	16 mg	PO
Palonosetron[a]	0.25 mg	IV

[a] If palonosetron was prescribed as part of the prophylaxis against acute nausea and vomiting, a 5-HT₃ should not be readministered for delayed prophylaxis due to the long half-life of palonosetron.
[b] Consider adding aprepitant, particularly if the patient has a history of carboplatin, ifosfamide, and so forth. When aprepitant is used, the dose of dexamethasone administered should be halved.
BID, twice a day; IV, intravenous; PO, orally; QD, daily; QID, four times a day; SL, sublingual carboplatin.
(*Source:* National Oncology Alliance Treatment Guideline for Antiemetic Therapy, updated 2005.)

TABLE 92.19	**Treatment of Breakthrough Nausea and Vomiting**

Options include the following (choose agents that were not used in the prophylaxis strategy):

Metoclopramide[a] 0.5–1 mg/kg PO/IV q4–6h for 24–48 hours ±

Diphenhydramine 25–50 mg PO/ IV q4–6h for 24–48 hours (for dystonia or akathisia)

For <u>delayed breakthrough nausea and vomiting,</u> use the following:

Dexamethasone 8 mg PO/IV BID for 2–4 days

Metoclopramide[a] 0.5 mg/kg PO/IV QID for 48–96 hours ±

Diphenhydramine 25–50 mg PO/IV QID for 48–96 hours

Other Alternatives Include:

Phenothiazines:

Prochlorperazine 10–20 mg PO/IV q4–6h or 25 mg PR[b] q12h for 24–48 hours

Promethazine 12.5–25 mg PO/IV or 25 mg PR[b] q4–6h for 24–48 hours

Lorazepam 0.5–2 mg PO/SL/IV q4–6h PRN. (Use as adjunctive agent.)

Haloperidol 0.5–1 mg PO/IV q6h for 24–48 hours

[a] Avoid if patient is experiencing diarrhea.
[b] Avoid PR route of administration in neutropenic patients.
Source: National Oncology Alliance Treatment Guideline for Antiemetic Therapy, updated 2005.

tered sublingually at a dose of 1 or 2 mg to prevent anticipatory nausea and vomiting.

Benzodiazepines are also useful in reducing the level of fear and anticipation when the patient receives treatment. Fear can also cause significant stress for the patient and decrease the threshold for nausea and vomiting. Use of benzodiazepines the night before to induce sleep not only serves to provide a good night's rest but also calms the patient before treatment. Table 92.20 summarizes some of the commonly used pharmacologic approaches to the prevention of anticipatory nausea and vomiting.

Patients with a history of anticipatory nausea and vomiting may also benefit from behavioral interventions such as relaxation techniques, guided imagery, distraction (music, books-on-tape, video games), or massage therapy.

PSYCHOSOCIAL ASPECTS

It is extremely difficult for patients to deal with both a diagnosis of cancer and its many treatments. Surgery, radiation

TABLE 92.20	**Prevention of Anticipatory Nausea and Vomiting**

• Prevention/treatment of acute nausea and vomiting is imperative in the prevention of anticipatory nausea and vomiting.

• Provide extensive education before chemo administration to alleviate patient fears.

• Lorazepam (Ativan) 1–2 mg PO at bedtime, then 1–2 mg PO/SL/IV on arrival to office

• Alprazolam (Xanax) 0.5–2 mg PO at bedtime and again upon arrival to office

(*Source:* National Oncology Alliance Treatment Guideline for Antiemetic Therapy, updated 2005.)

therapy, and chemotherapy are all associated with a wide variety of feared complications and side effects. The situation can be made more distressing if the patient also suffers from severe nausea and vomiting secondary to chemotherapy.

Both nausea and vomiting have a direct impact on patients and their sense of well-being and control. They also have a detrimental impact and toll on family, friends, and coworkers. Severe nausea and vomiting may prevent the patient from participating in family activities and continuing to play a vital role in the workplace or community. There is also a significant impact on the physical, psychological, social, and spiritual dimensions of the patient's quality of life.[49]

Dietary or behavioral interventions can assist with minimizing nausea or vomiting. Avoiding spicy, greasy, or strong smelling foods and eating smaller, more frequent meals can help. The timing of chemotherapy may also be important; some patients favor treatment on an empty stomach first thing in the morning after a good night's sleep. Acupressure (sea sickness bands), herbal remedies (oral ginger supplements/teas, use of lavender-scented oils), distraction (watching videos, playing video games, or using imagery), or self-hypnosis can also assist in minimizing nausea and vomiting in some patients without the need for prescription medications.[50,51]

TREATMENT

Tables 92.18 to 92.20 give evidence-based recommendations used in the prevention and treatment of acute, anticipatory, and delayed nausea and vomiting.

Many dosing recommendations for the 5-HT-3 receptor antagonists are reported as a range in milligrams. Studies such as those by Seynaeve et al[52] showed how both the dose and cost of 5-HT-3 antagonists could be reduced significantly without compromising overall patient outcome. A total of 535 chemotherapy-naive patients who received cisplatin (50 to 120 mg/m^2)-containing regimens participated in a randomized, double-blind, parallel study and were given single doses of ondansetron 8 or 32 mg intravenously or a bolus dose of 8 mg followed by continuous infusion of 1 mg per hour for 24 hours (total 32 mg). Complete and major control (less than two episodes) of acute emesis was achieved by 78% of patients in the 32-mg group, 74% of patients in the 8-mg group, and 74% of patients in the bolus plus infusion group. The investigators thus concluded that a single intravenous dose of ondansetron 8 mg given before chemotherapy was as effective as a 32-mg daily dose in the prophylaxis of acute cisplatin-induced emesis.

To track the outcome of antiemetic therapy, it is important to use standardized measurement tools such as the National Cancer Institute CTCAE scale (Table 92.17). These measurements should be taken from patient interviews and documented after each cycle of treatment to determine whether antiemetic therapy was successful or whether a change in

| TABLE 92.21 | Other Causes of Persistent Nausea and Vomiting |

Acute abdominal emergencies (acute appendicitis, acute cholecystitis, intestinal obstruction, pancreatitis, or acute peritonitis)

Infections (bacterial, fungal, or viral) (acute systemic infections; infections of the gastrointestinal tract, possibly parasitic; or inner ear infections)

Central nervous system disorders (e.g., increased intracranial pressure due to neoplasms, meningitis, bleeding)

Medication-related (opioid side effects, oral antibiotic side effects, digoxin toxicity, theophylline toxicity)

drug selection or dose is required. Patient-reported symptoms should also include an assessment of potential antiemetic-related toxicity, the most common being dystonic reactions secondary to agents such as phenothiazines. Appropriate medications can be prescribed if these side effects occur.

If symptoms of nausea and vomiting persist despite the use of proper antiemetics, it may be warranted to reevaluate the patient for an alternative etiology for continued nausea and vomiting. These include acute abdominal emergencies, various infections, disorders of the central nervous system, and possibly toxicity due to other medications being taken (Table 92.21). Patients with persistent nausea and vomiting should be monitored for fluid status, changes in heart rate and blood pressure, mental status changes, and electrolyte disturbances.

IMPROVING OUTCOMES

The aggressive use of potent and effective antiemetics improves overall outcome for the patient by allowing treatment to proceed as planned with the doses of antineoplastic agents necessary to achieve a desired response.[53] Patients can quickly return to normal family, work, and community activities and avoid the need for additional interventions because of the complications of nausea and vomiting.

With the advent of 5-HT-3 receptor antagonists and their enhanced efficacy combined with dexamethasone, chemotherapy-induced nausea and vomiting can easily be prevented or greatly minimized. Today, there is a better understanding of emetic pathways and a wide selection of antiemetic agents to choose from. Optimal use of these agents has made the treatment of cancer tolerable and the completion of therapy more likely. With the newly found use of NK-1 receptor antagonists such as aprepitant, both acute and delayed emesis can now be readily managed.

TREATMENT-INDUCED MYELOSUPPRESSION

To assist patients in recovering from some of the hematologic toxicities of cancer chemotherapy, several proteins have been developed that stimulate various steps of hematopoiesis; they are designated as growth factors or stimulatory cytokines. These proteins are produced in vivo and bind to specific cell receptors to stimulate stem cell proliferation and differentiation. Hematopoiesis proceeds from a pluripotent stem cell (one that can differentiate into any of the hematopoietic cell-lines) in an orderly, timed fashion to mature cells (Fig. 92.2).

TREATMENT-INDUCED NEUTROPENIA

Many chemotherapy agents can have toxic effects on the bone marrow. An infection resulting from chemotherapy-induced neutropenia (CIN) is the primary life-threatening event of any chemotherapy course. Patients experience severe CIN when the absolute neutrophil count (ANC) falls below 500 per μL. At this time, patients are most vulnerable to bacterial, fungal, and viral infections.

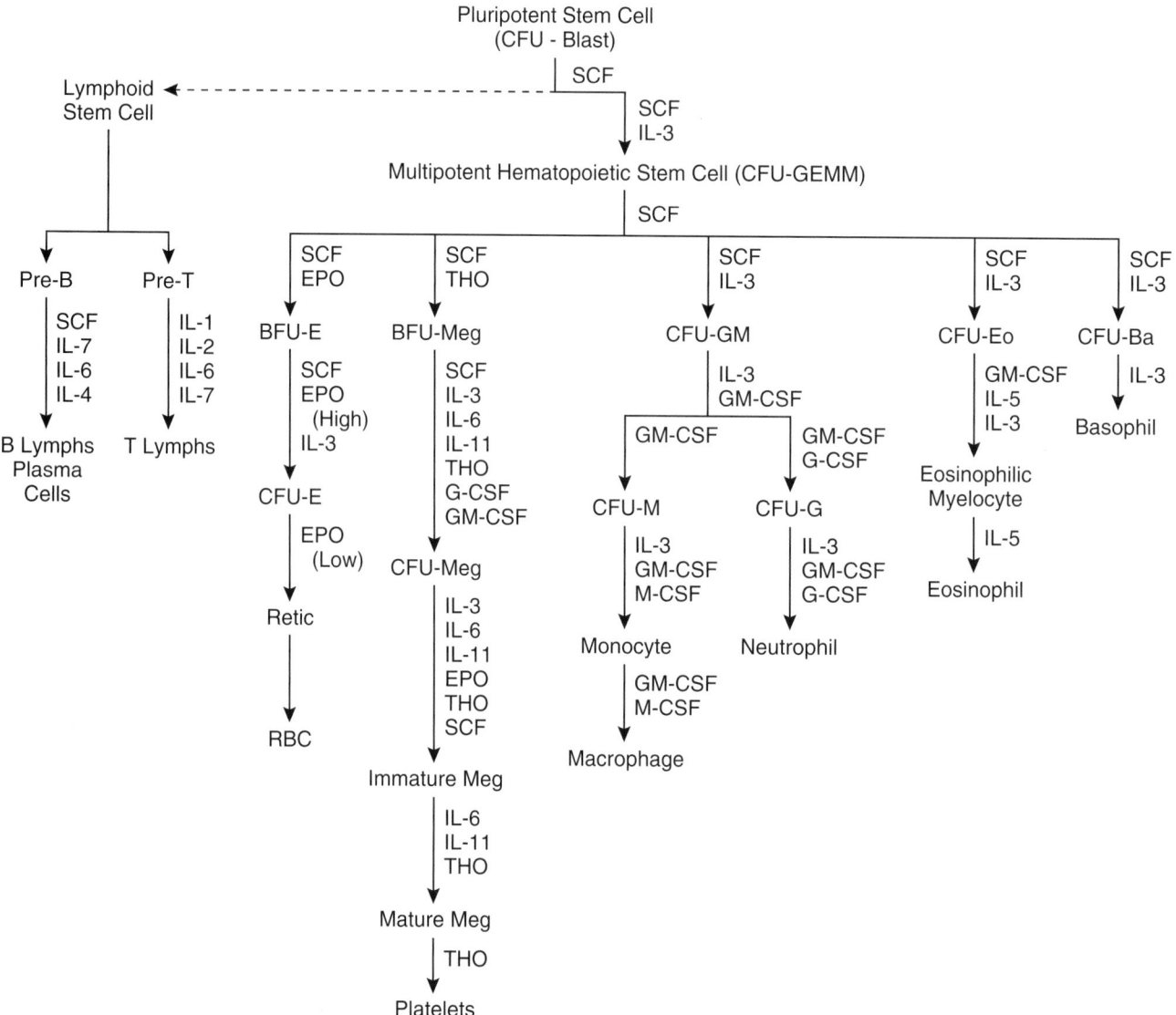

FIGURE 92.2 Hematopoiesis. Ba, basophil; BFU, blast-forming unit; CFU, colony-forming unit; CSF, colony-stimulating factor; E, erythroid; Eo, eosinophil; EPO, erythropoietin; G, granulocyte; GEMM, granulocyte, erythroid, macrophage, megakaryocyte; GM, granulocyte-macrophage; IL, interleukin; Lymphs, lymphocytes; M, macrophage; Meg, megakaryocyte; Retic, reticulocyte; SCF, stem cell factor/steel factor; THO, thrombopoietin.

TREATMENT GOALS: TREATMENT-INDUCED NEUTROPENIA

Prevent prolonged duration of CIN and its associated infection risk by administering primary and secondary prophylactic myelopoietic cytokines with standard-dose chemotherapy and high-dose cytotoxic therapy associated with bone marrow transplantation (BMT).

PATHOPHYSIOLOGY

Chemotherapy-induced neutropenic infections are the primary life-threatening event of any chemotherapy course. The duration and severity of CIN are the most important predictors of infection risk. Myelopoietic growth factors decrease the time that granulocyte counts remain below 500 per μL, decrease the incidence of febrile neutropenia, and decrease the number of infectious complications in patients receiving high-dose autologous BMT or allogeneic BMT. Growth factors are also effective for mobilizing progenitor cells into the peripheral blood so that they can be harvested for autologous or allogeneic transplantation.

TREATMENT

WHITE BLOOD CELL GROWTH FACTORS

There are three exogenous growth factor agents commonly used for the management of chemotherapy-induced neutropenia: recombinant human granulocyte–macrophage colony stimulating factor (GM-CSF or sargramostim), recombinant human granulocyte colony-stimulating factor (G-CSF or filgrastim), and a covalent conjugate of rhu-G-CSF and monomethoxypolyethylene glycol, commonly referred to as pegylated G-CSF or pegfilgrastim. Although these agents do not uniformly prevent neutropenia after the administration of myelosuppressive therapy, they have been found to shorten the duration of neutropenia. They are also effective in accelerating neutrophil recovery after BMT and can increase the yield of peripheral blood stem cells collected by leukophoresis for use in peripheral blood stem cell transplantation.

GM-CSF is a 127-amino acid glycosylated protein derived from yeast cultures. GM-CSF has multilineage effects on granulopoiesis, stimulating both primitive and terminal differentiation of neutrophils, macrophages, and eosinophils (Fig. 92.2).

G-CSF is a 175-amino acid nonglycosylated protein derived from *Escherichia coli* cultures. Unlike GM-CSF, the actions of G-CSF are limited to the terminal differentiation of neutrophils. There are no comparative trials evaluating the efficacy of G-CSF versus GM-CSF in CIN.

Pegylated G-CSF is produced by covalently binding a 20-KD monomethoxypolyethylene glycol molecule to the N-terminal methionyl residue of filgrastim. Its action as a colony-stimulating factor is like that of G-CSF, but pegylation results in reduced renal clearance and a prolonged persistence in vivo compared with G-CSF.

American Society of Clinical Oncology (ASCO) guidelines for the use of hematopoietic growth factors (HGFs) or colony-stimulating factors (CSFs), as they are also called, recommend primary prophylactic (with the first course of chemotherapy) use of CSFs if the expected incidence of febrile neutropenia with a chemotherapy regimen is 40% or greater. Special circumstances that support CSF use in primary prophylaxis with chemotherapy regimens for which the incidence of febrile CIN is less than 40% are patients receiving dose-intensive chemotherapy, poor performance status (Eastern Cooperative Oncology Group score $\geq$2), age more than 65 years, advanced cancer (metastatic disease, having received multiple chemotherapy regimens), preexisting neutropenia secondary to disease, extensive prior chemotherapy, previous radiation to the pelvis (as this area contains a large amount of bone marrow), open wounds and active tissue infections, decreased immune function (human immunodeficiency virus infection, acquired immunodeficiency syndrome, cytopenias, diabetes mellitus), history of recurrent febrile neutropenia with previous chemotherapy of similar or lesser myelosuppressive potential, or serum albumin level of 3.5 g per dL or less in patients with non-Hodgkin's lymphoma or multiple myeloma.[54,55]

Secondary prophylaxis with CSF is defined as use after a previous febrile CIN episode or previous CIN when dose reduction or delay is not appropriate [e.g., in curable tumors such as germ cell (testicular) cancers, intermediate/high-grade non-Hodgkin's lymphoma, and Hodgkin's lymphoma] and for patients being treated in the adjuvant or neoadjuvant setting. Silber et al[56] correlated first-cycle ANC nadirs with a predicted need for CSF in subsequent chemotherapy courses. Their mathematical model is complex, but soon guidelines using first-cycle nadir counts can be used to select patients who should receive CSF with subsequent cycles for chemotherapy dose maintenance.

The use of CSFs for the treatment of febrile neutropenia is recommended only if serious prognostic comorbidities are present. Studies have not yet supported a decrease in the number of neutropenic days or duration of hospitalization beyond antibiotics and/or antifungal therapy alone. Serious concomitant illnesses include pneumonia, hypotension, and multiorgan dysfunction.

Pharmacokinetics. G-CSF absorption and distribution follow first-order pharmacokinetics. The volume of distribution is 150 mL/kg and the serum half-life is approximately

3.5 hours after either subcutaneous or intravenous administration. GM-CSF absorption and distribution also follow first-order pharmacokinetics. The half-life after intravenous administration is 60 minutes; that after subcutaneous administration is 162 minutes. Thus, daily administration is recommended for filgrastim and sargramostim. Pegfilgrastim, in contrast, has a half-life that ranges from 15 to 80 hours after subcutaneous injection, thus requiring less frequent dosing compared with filgrastim and sargramostim. Pegfilgrastim is administered once per chemotherapy treatment cycle.

Dosing. The ANC after G-CSF use is discontinued falls rapidly for 1 to 3 days before a new, lower baseline level is maintained. The time to reach a desired ANC with GM-CSF may be 1 day longer, but the ANC levels are more sustained, with little or no decrease after discontinuation. Filgrastim and sargramostim dosing (Table 92.22) should begin 24 to 72 hours after chemotherapy and continue daily past the ANC nadir. Pegfilgrastim, in contrast, is administered once per cycle (24 hours after chemotherapy is given in the cycle) and should not be administered in the period between 14 days before and 24 hours after cytotoxic chemotherapy is administered. Administration within this time period may have the undesired effect of increasing the sensitivity of rapidly dividing myeloid cells to chemotherapy.

The original recommendations for filgrastim and sargramostim use were to treat until an ANC of 10,000 per μL was reached, but most clinicians now treat until the ANC is greater than 1,500 to 2,500 per μL for 2 consecutive days or for a maximum of 14 days. Filgrastim and sargramostim should be discontinued at least 24 hours before the next chemotherapy course. Discontinuation of the agents 48 hours before the next cycle of chemotherapy has also been shown to decrease the chance of worsening CIN with subsequent cycles.[57]

Side Effects. Particular side effects of the CSFs that should be managed appropriately include temperature elevation, local injection site reactions, and bone pain or arthralgias. Body temperature elevation can occur 30 minutes to 4 hours after injection and usually peaks at 38°C or less. Patients can be given acetaminophen or ibuprofen before injection to prevent this reaction. If temperature rises above 38.2°C or does not respond to antipyretics, an underlying infection must be considered. Site reactions are typically localized and caused by the injection technique.

The injection sites should be rotated, and the CSF should be injected at room temperature. It is often helpful to cool the skin with ice for a few minutes before injection. Medullary bone pain and arthralgias are common reactions and can be treated with analgesics. The pain can be severe but usually resolves 1 to 3 days after CSF use is discontinued. Capillary leak syndrome previously reported with molgramostim (not available in the United States) is rarely associated with the yeast-derived GM-CSF (sargramostim) product that is currently available.[58,59]

There are several precautions with CSF use. Administration with combined chemotherapy and radiotherapy has not been studied, and the use of CSF with daily radiation therapy may worsen neutropenia or damage the bone marrow. Lithium results in rapid release of neutrophils as they develop; thus, close monitoring is warranted in patients receiving concomitant lithium and CSF therapy. Lower CSF doses and/or a shorter duration of therapy may be required when concomitant lithium therapy is being administered. Sargramostim is contraindicated in patients sensitive to yeast-derived products, whereas filgrastim is contraindicated in patients sensitive to *E. coli*-derived products.

TREATMENT-INDUCED ANEMIA

Anemia in patients with cancer may have several potential causes.[60] The causes must be differentiated to make sure that all treatable causes are identified. Cancer may cause anemia directly by acute or chronic blood loss, intratumor bleeding, erythrophagocytosis, splenomegaly, and bone marrow replacement. Anemia also results from inhibitory cytokines produced by the cancer or physiologic effects of the cancer. This anemia may, in part, be similar to the anemia of chronic disease. Mechanisms involve abnormalities of iron usage and/or blunted erythropoietic bone marrow response by inhibitory cytokines. A few such cytokines are tumor necrosis factor-α, interleukin-6, interleukin-1, and interferon-γ. Immune hemolytic anemias, microangiopathic hemolysis, primary bone marrow failure, and nutritional deficiencies also must be considered before labeling anemia in a patient with cancer as a cancer- or chemotherapy-induced anemia.

TABLE 92.22	**Myelopoietic Cytokines**		
	GM-CSF (sargramostim)	**G-CSF (filgrastim)**	**Pegylated G-CSF (pegfilgrastim)**
Dose	250 μg/m²/day (rounded to the nearest 50 μg)	5 μg/kg/day [rounded to the nearest vial size (300 or 480 μg)] ≤70 kg = 300-μg vial	6 mg fixed dose
Route & frequency	Subcutaneous or IV daily	Subcutaneous or IV daily	Subcutaneous once per chemotherapy cycle

TREATMENT GOALS: TREATMENT-INDUCED ANEMIA

- Maintain hemoglobin (Hgb) at a target range of 11 to 13 g per dL during chemotherapy and/or radiation therapy.
- Decrease the sequelae of anemia such as fatigue, shortness of breath, and requirements for blood transfusions.
- Improve the patient's quality of life.

PATHOPHYSIOLOGY

The most common cause of anemia in a patient with cancer is chemotherapy or radiotherapy. Therapy-induced anemia is caused by stem cell death, committed progenitor cell death, blockage or delay in hematopoiesis cell cycling, or damage to mature red blood cells. Patients at highest risk for therapy-induced anemia are those who were anemic before therapy or who undergo combined modality (chemotherapy plus radiotherapy) treatment.

CLINICAL PRESENTATION AND DIAGNOSIS

Patients with chemotherapy-induced anemia may differ in clinical presentation. Patients with mild anemia [National Cancer Institute (NCI) definition Hgb >10 g/dL] may have fatigue or may be asymptomatic. Patients with moderate to severe anemia (NCI definition Hgb 8 to 10 g/dL and <8 g/dL, respectively) can have weakness, vertigo, concentration impairment, dyspnea, headaches, or irritability. [61]

Treatment Guidelines from the National Comprehensive Cancer Centers (NCCN) and the National Oncology Alliance (NOA) recommends therapeutic intervention for patients with Hgb <11 g/dL and for patients who have Hgb between 11-13 g/dL and are either symptomatic or have risk factors for developing symptomatic anemia.[61,62] Symptoms related to mild and moderate anemia for which erythropoietic therapy is warranted include dyspnea on exertion, chest pain, peripheral edema, sustained tachycardia, severe fatigue, and dizziness.

Risk factors and comorbidities that warrant consideration for therapy include blood product transfusions in the past 6 months, a history of radiation therapy to greater than 20% of the skeleton, advanced age, a cardiac history, chronic pulmonary distress, cerebrovascular disease, and use of highly myelosuppressive chemotherapy.

TREATMENT

RED BLOOD CELL TRANSFUSION

Patients who require immediate correction of their Hgb (e.g., an elderly patient with severe symptoms) may receive a blood product transfusion in addition to management with pharmacologic therapy. Patients who are mildly symptomatic may be started on drug therapy alone, consisting of recombinant human erythropoietin (rhuEPO).

RED BLOOD CELL GROWTH FACTORS

rhuEPO mimics the actions of endogenous erythropoietin and is the primary drug treatment for patients with chemotherapy-induced anemia. The endogenous hormone erythropoietin is a glycoprotein produced and secreted by the kidney in response to low oxygen tension. On release into the bloodstream, erythropoietin migrates to its site of action within the bone marrow, where it is responsible for the amplification and terminal differentiation of erythroid progenitors and precursors for the formation of new red blood cells (Fig. 92.2). rhuEPO administration in patients undergoing cancer chemotherapy and radiotherapy results in a 40% to 70% response rate, as measured by a minimum Hgb increase of 2 g per dL.[63] Likewise, it has also been shown to decrease the need for red blood cell transfusions by 30% to 80%.[64] An increased Hgb has been associated with improved quality of life.[65,66]

Currently two forms of rhuEPO are available for use in the U.S. market, epoetin alfa and darbepoetin alfa. The two agents differ primarily in their half-life, so the drugs are administered on different dosing schedules.

Epoetin alfa, the first agent marketed, is a 165-amino acid glycoprotein derived from mammalian cells. It is identical to isolated natural erythropoietin. It demonstrates first-order pharmacokinetics after intravenous administration. Epoetin alfa is most often administered subcutaneously; subcutaneous administration results in peak serum concentrations in 12 to 24 hours that decline slowly thereafter, with a half-life of 7 to 18 hours.[66] Following intravenous administration, patients with normal renal function exhibit an epoetin alfa half-life that is 20% shorter compared with subcutaneous administration of the drug. The half-life in patients with chronic renal failure is 4 to 13 hours and is not affected by dialysis. For patients with chemotherapy-induced anemia, epoetin alfa may be administered subcutaneously on a schedule of 40,000 units weekly or 150 units per kilogram three times weekly.

Darbepoetin alfa is very similar in structure to epoetin alfa, but it contains five N-linked oligosaccharide chains, compared to the three in the epoetin structure. The addition of these carbohydrate chains results in a longer half-life compared with epoetin alfa. For example, when administered intravenously, the terminal half-life of darbepoetin alfa is three times that of epoetin alfa.

The FDA-approved dosing for darbepoetin alfa is 2.25 μg per kg subcutaneously once a week. Several studies have also shown efficacy in the treatment of chemotherapy-induced anemia when the agent is administered at a fixed dose of 200 μg subcutaneously every 2 weeks, and efficacy is similar to that of epoetin alfa.[67–69]

Before rhuEPO therapy is started in any of these scenarios, adequate levels of vitamin B_{12}, folate, and iron should be confirmed by laboratory tests, and any deficiencies should be addressed.

Once patients are begun on rhuEPO therapy, Hgb, reticulocyte counts, iron, transferrin, and ferritin are monitored at 4-week intervals. Dosage decreases of rhuEPO are warranted if Hgb rises too quickly (e.g., if transfusion-independent Hgb rises more than 1 g/dL in any 2-week period or exceeds 13 g/dL). In clinical studies, increases in Hgb greater than approximately 1 g per dL during any 2-week period with use of rhuEPO were associated with an increased incidence of cardiac arrest, neurologic events (including seizures and stroke), congestive heart failure, exacerbations of hypertension, vascular thrombosis/ischemia/infarction, acute myocardial infarction, and fluid overload/edema.[70] Conversely, if patients fail to show an Hgb increase of at least 1 g per dL after 4 to 6 weeks of rhuEPO therapy, a dose increase is warranted. Once the target Hgb range of 11 to 13 g per dL is obtained, a maintenance dose is used to keep the patient within the desired range. Table 92.23 lists initial doses and dose adjustments for rhuEPO agents.

Several investigators have tried to determine predictive factors for chemotherapy-induced anemia responsive to rhuEPO. There are no reliable predictive factors; even pre-erythropoietin levels of several hundred units/L (normal 10 to 20 units/L) do not predict unresponsiveness. Some investigators do not use rhuEPO if endogenous erythropoietin levels are 1,000 units per L or greater, whereas other investigators use cutoff levels of 500 units per L or greater. More information is needed in this area. At present, a therapeutic trial is the only way to determine responsiveness.

The etiology of failures, if all other causes of anemia are eliminated, is generally unknown. A small group of failures, though, may be related to functional iron deficiency.[71] This is caused by impaired bone marrow utilization of iron stores. Early evidence shows that administration of intravenous iron, when transferrin saturation is 15% or less or ferritin is

TABLE 92.23 | Erythropoietic Growth Factor Dosing

Agent	Initial Dose & Schedule	Dose Adjustments
Darbepoetin alfa	2.25 μg/kg subcutaneously weekly or 200 μg subcutaneously every other week	**Upward Dose Titration** After 6 weeks, if <1 g/dL increase in Hgb, increase dose as follows: – If previous dose was 2.25 μg/kg, increase to 4.5 μg/kg weekly. – If previous dose was 200 μg every other week, increase to 300 μg every other week. If after an additional 4–6 weeks of therapy, the patient fails to respond, discontinue therapy unless there is clear evidence that the patient is benefiting from therapy.
Epoetin alfa	150 units/kg subcutaneously three times a week or 40,000 units subcutaneously weekly	**Upward Dose Titration** After 4 weeks, if <1 g/dL increase in Hgb, increase dose as follows: – If previous dose was 40,000 units weekly, increase to 60,000 units weekly. – If previous dose was 150 units/kg three times a week, increase to 300 units/kg three times a week. If after an additional 4–6 weeks of therapy, the patient fails to respond, discontinue therapy unless there is clear evidence that the patient is benefiting from therapy. **Downward Dose Titration, either agent** – If transfusion-independent Hgb increases by >1 g/dL in any 2-week period, or if Hgb is >12 g/dL, decrease erythropoietic dose by 25%. – If Hgb is >13 g/dL, hold dose until Hgb falls below 12 g/dL. Then reinitiate with a 25% dose reduction.

Source: National Oncology Alliance Treatment Guidelines for Anemia, Updated 2005.

100 ng per mL or less, improves the response to rhuEPO response and allows decreased doses of rhuEPO to be administered in patients with renal failure.[72–74]

The side effects of rhuEPO are minimal. Medullary bone pain is reported most commonly. The hypertension from increased red blood cell mass seen in patients with renal failure is rare in patients with cancer.

TREATMENT-INDUCED THROMBOCYTOPENIA

Chemotherapy-induced thrombocytopenia is a significant and increasing problem in patients with cancer. Of patients with solid tumors who are undergoing chemotherapy, 25% develop thrombocytopenia with platelet counts less than 50×10^9 per liter, whereas 10% to 15% have platelet counts less than 20×10^9 per liter.[75–79] Both the severity and duration of thrombocytopenia are correlated with serious bleeding. Patients with a platelet count less than 20×10^9 per liter for 7 days have a 10% risk of bleeding, whereas patients with similar low counts for 14 days have a 60% risk.[80] With the availability of G-CSF and GM-CSF to prevent neutropenia, thrombocytopenia is now often the dose-limiting toxicity related to chemotherapy administration with agents such as gemcitabine, carboplatin, 5-FU, mitomycin-C, and thiotepa. A delayed onset of thrombocytopenia, due to cumulative toxicity, can also be seen with agents such as carmustine, fludarabine, and lomustine.

TREATMENT GOALS: TREATMENT-INDUCED THROMBOCYTOPENIA

- Prevent chemotherapy-induced thrombocytopenia through use of thrombopoietic cytokines.
- Decrease the risk of serious bleeding complications, decrease the need for platelet transfusions, and allow chemotherapy administration to proceed on schedule.

PATHOPHYSIOLOGY

Platelets, like the other components of the blood, develop from hematopoietic stem cells through a series of cell divisions. Several growth factors/cytokines are required to support thrombopoiesis (Fig. 92.2). Interleukin-3, G-CSF, GM-CSF, and stem cell factor (SCF) function at the progenitor cell stage, and interleukin-6 has a role late in maturation. Thrombopoietin (TPO) and interleukin-11 stimulate all stages of megakaryocytopoiesis, including proliferation of progenitors, and the development and maturation of megakaryocytes. In addition, TPO acts with erythropoietin to stimulate the growth of erythroid progenitor cells and, with interleukin-3 or SCF, stimulates the replication and prolongs the survival of hematopoietic stem cells and all types of blood cell progenitors. TPO also has some role in regulating neutrophil activation. It can sensitize platelets to various agonists and may predispose them to thrombosis when given therapeutically.

TREATMENT

Currently, platelet transfusions are the primary treatment for the management of severe thrombocytopenia. However, platelet transfusions come with the increased risk of infections and alloimmunization, as well as increased healthcare costs.

The only product that is currently FDA approved for the treatment of thrombocytopenia is oprelvekin (interleukin-

11). Interleukin-11 primarily has maturational effects on megakaryocytes, but with interleukin-3 and SCF it enhances the proliferation of early progenitors as well (Fig. 92.2).[78] Oprelvekin is a nonglycosylated, 177-amino acid protein, produced in *E. coli*. The terminal half-life is approximately 7 hours. There is no accumulation with daily administration at either the 25- or 50-μg/kg doses.

Oprelvekin has been shown to increase platelet counts at the chemotherapy nadir and decrease the need for platelet transfusions when used in patients with severe thrombocytopenia from a previous chemotherapy course.[79] It has also been shown (compared with placebo) to decrease platelet transfusions and speed platelet recovery with initial dose-intense chemotherapy.[80] In clinical studies, administration of oprelvekin resulted in significant clinical benefit; however, 30% of patients still required at least one platelet transfusion.

Oprelvekin is given at a daily dose of 50 μg per kilogram subcutaneously starting the day after chemotherapy and continued for 10 to 21 days. Platelet counts increase within 5 to 9 days and can continue to increase for up to 7 days after injections are discontinued. Treatment with oprelvekin should be discontinued at least 2 days before the next chemotherapy administration.

Side effects of oprelvekin are minimal. Plasma volume expansion can occur and cause dyspnea, peripheral edema, and transient atrial arrhythmias. These side effects are usually self-limiting and are reversible after discontinuation. Transient atrial arrhythmias have occurred at the 50 μg/kg/day dose and greater and have been characterized as brief and without sequelae. Oprelvekin is not directly arrhythmogenic, and atrial arrhythmias are likely to be associated with increased plasma volume. Thiazide diuretics can be used to decrease plasma volume expansion. Minor arthralgias, skin rash, conjunctival redness, and fatigue can also occur. Oprelvekin has been used with G-CSF and GM-CSF without any evidence of adverse reactions, pharmacokinetic profile change, or altered therapeutic benefit.

Cytokine support of thrombopoiesis is evolving. Much effort has been directed at the use of recombinant TPO for the management of thrombocytopenia after myelosuppressive chemotherapy. TPO is the major regulator of megakaryocyte development and subsequent platelet production. Although early studies of the full-length molecule showed enhanced platelet recovery and reduced thrombocytopenia with moderately myelosuppressive chemotherapy, the results were not duplicated in patients receiving intensive chemotherapy regimens, despite multiple postchemotherapy doses. In addition, the risk of development of neutralizing antibodies was of concern. A recent study suggests that the administration of TPO before *and* after chemotherapy may be associated with improved platelet nadirs and recovery after intensive chemotherapy.[81] Randomized trials are ongoing to determine the importance of the TPO schedule around multiple chemotherapy regimens.

TREATMENT-INDUCED ORGAN TOXICITY

There are now three established drugs used in conjunction with chemotherapy to reduce the severity of or prevent specific organ toxicity. Two of these agents allow for the use of dose-intense chemotherapy while protecting an organ from the toxic effects of therapy. Mesna and dexrazoxane protect against specific side effects (ifosfamide-induced hemorrhagic cystitis and doxorubicin-induced cardiotoxicity, respectively). The third agent, amifostine, is a general cytoprotectant. It is approved for cisplatin-induced renal toxicity, mucositis, or xerostomia related to treatment of head and neck cancer, and prevention of bone marrow toxicity.

TREATMENT GOALS: TREATMENT-INDUCED ORGAN TOXICITY

- Administer cytoprotective agents with chemotherapy to reduce or prevent specific chemotherapy-induced organ toxicities.
- Enable continuation of scheduled chemotherapy.

TREATMENT

MESNA

Cyclophosphamide and ifosfamide can cause hemorrhagic cystitis and fibrosis due to the metabolite acrolein. Mesna (sodium-2-mercaptoethane sulfonate) protects the uroepithelium by binding acrolein to its free sulfhydryl groups, thus forming a nontoxic, stable compound. Mesna can also bind other metabolites of ifosfamide such as 4-hydroxy-ifosfamide and chloracetaldehyde. It has been shown to be superior to hydration and urinary alkalinization in preventing hemorrhagic cystitis.[82,83]

Mesna is oxidized to dimesna in the circulation. Approximately 50% is glomerularly filtered and converted back to mesna by renal tubular glutathione reductase and is available in urine as intact mesna with free sulfhydryl groups. Mesna has a short plasma half-life compared to ifosfamide and is water-soluble, with little tissue penetration. The efficacy of ifosfamide is not altered by mesna.

Mesna is available in an intravenous as well as an oral formulation. Intravenous dosing results in urinary concentrations twice those of oral administration. Urinary excretion of an intravenous dose is complete in 4 hours, but orally administered doses result in urinary levels that last for at least 8 hours. Intravenous mesna must be given frequently (every 4 hours) to protect the uroepithelium after ifosfamide dosing. Mesna is given at 60% of the ifosfamide dose in three equal doses: just before chemotherapy and then 4 hours and 8 hours after chemotherapy. An alternative method of administration uses a 200-mg loading dose of mesna followed by a constant infusion of mesna with ifosfamide over 24 hours. With the constant infusion, the mesna dose is equivalent to the ifosfamide dose.

Adverse reactions to mesna are minor and include nausea, diarrhea, headache, and fatigue.

DEXRAZOXANE

Dexrazoxane (Zinecard) is a dioxopiperazine analogue of EDTA that is hydrolyzed intracellularly to its active form. It then binds iron and prevents iron-mediated free radical formation responsible for doxorubicin-induced cardiotoxicity.[84]

Doxorubicin is a highly active chemotherapy agent used to treat many malignancies; it is included in first-line regimens for breast cancer, many lymphomas, sarcomas, and small cell lung cancer. Doxorubicin use is limited by cardiotoxicity in patients who have received a cumulative dose of 300 mg per m^2. Use of dexrazoxane has been shown to allow higher cumulative doses of doxorubicin to be given. In clinical trials, 90% less cardiotoxicity was observed with cumulative doxorubicin doses up to 750 mg per m^2.[85]

Dexrazoxane administration must be completed 30 minutes before doxorubicin administration at a dose ratio of 10:1. Slow intravenous push or rapid infusion is recommended. Adverse reactions include enhanced myelosuppression and pain at the injection site. Several other side effects reported in studies are most likely caused by doxorubicin: alopecia, nausea, vomiting, fatigue, and anorexia. The myelosuppression appears to be dose-related and is more common at doses of 600 mg per m^2 and higher. Studies have shown that the pharmacokinetic profile of doxorubicin is not altered by the concurrent administration of dexrazoxane. Dexrazoxane itself can be myelosuppressive. There are no reported cumulative toxicities with dexrazoxane.[86]

Doxorubicin is an important chemotherapy agent, and amelioration of its dose-limiting toxicity is an important advance. It is unknown how useful dexrazoxane is with other anthracyclines such as epirubicin, idarubicin, and daunorubicin or the anthracenedione, mitoxantrone.

AMIFOSTINE

Amifostine was initially developed by Walter Reed Medical Center as a cell protector from radiation associated with nuclear war. It has been investigated more recently as a cytoprotector from the effects of certain chemotherapy agents and radiotherapy.

Amifostine is a phosphorylated aminothiol drug metabolized to free thiol by alkaline phosphatase enzyme in the cell membrane of normal tissue. This allows selective action on normal tissue versus malignant tissue, which has lower activity of this cell membrane-associated enzyme. The increased free thiol concentration intracellularly binds free radicals generated by certain chemotherapy agents or radiation therapy and protects the normal cell tissue.

Amifostine is a broad-range cytoprotectant. Clinical studies in ovarian cancer and non-small cell lung cancer have consistently shown decreases in mucositis, renal toxicity, bone marrow suppression, and neurologic toxicity with platinum-based chemotherapy regimens.[87] Amifostine is FDA approved for use in the reduction of cumulative renal toxicity associated with repeated administration of cisplatin in patients with advanced ovarian or non-small cell lung cancer. Decreased effectiveness against tumors has not been seen in those cancer types. In head and neck cancer, a decreased incidence of mucositis and xerostomia due to radiation therapy has also been documented.[88] Amifostine is also FDA approved to reduce the incidence of moderate to severe xerostomia in patients undergoing postoperative radiation treatment for head and neck cancer where the radiation port includes a substantial portion of the parotid glands. Amifostine has also been shown to protect the bone marrow better than G-CSF after carboplatin therapy.[89] In early studies, amifostine has shown beneficial effects in myelodysplastic syndromes.[90] Three- and 5-day regimens at 200 mg per m^2 have improved platelet counts, ANCs, and Hgb. This effect could be important in a disease with few therapeutic options.

Amifostine has a short half-life (α half-life <1 minute and β half-life of 8 minutes) and is 90% cleared from the plasma in 6 minutes. It is given intravenously over less than 10 minutes, 30 minutes before chemotherapy. It is not effective if given after chemotherapy. The dose originally studied and approved for use was 910 mg per m^2, but current recommendations are to give only 740 mg per m^2 before cisplatin or carboplatin. In patients undergoing radiation therapy, 200 mg/m^2/day given over 3 minutes has been shown to protect against xerostomia and mucositis.

Amifostine has several side effects that may limit its use. During intravenous administration, hypotension can be significant (a 20-mm drop in systolic blood pressure is average). This effect can be reduced by prehydrating the patient and by limiting the infusion time to 10 minutes or less. Intake of any antihypertensive medication should be delayed until 24 hours after amifostine is administered. Prehydrating the patient with 1 L of intravenous fluids 2 hours before amifostine and having the patient remain supine for 30 minutes after the infusion has decreased the incidence of this side effect. Blood pressure should be monitored every 5 minutes during amifostine infusion, at the completion of infusion, and as clinically indicated thereafter. If hypotension occurs, the amifostine infusion should be discontinued. The baseline blood pressure usually returns to normal in 5 minutes, and then amifostine administration can be resumed. The guidelines for quantitative blood pressure changes and altered infusion rates are detailed in the prescribing information.

Nausea with or without vomiting, another common side effect, can be prevented with premedications: dexamethasone and a 5-HT-3 receptor antagonist. These antiemetics should be administered at least 1 hour before amifostine. Adequate hydration prior to amifostine administration and the brief supine positioning of the patient during the infusion can also reduce the incidence of nausea and vomiting. Other adverse reactions reported include allergic reactions and decreased calcium levels.

Amifostine is an effective cytoprotectant and can be used in many chemotherapy and radiotherapy protocols. The side effects of hypotension and nausea/vomiting limited its initial use. The new lower dosing recommendations, combined with hydration, antiemetics, and limited infusion time, have controlled these side effects. Amifostine is an effective protectant of hematopoiesis, peripheral nerves, oral/esophageal mucosa, and nephrotoxicity.

KEY POINTS

■ When used appropriately, supportive care for the patient with cancer diminishes some of the complications associated with chemotherapy and radiation. It increases the chances that cancer therapy will be delivered at the optimal dosage intensity and on schedule; it improves quality of life, both physically and emotionally; and in some cases it allows for increased chemotherapy dose intensity, which may improve survival for patients with some cancers

■ Recently, great strides have been made in the development of supportive care strategies in terms of identifying, preventing, and treating the complications associated with the delivery of chemotherapy and radiation. While the search continues for effective therapies for some of the complications of chemotherapy, pharmacologic therapies have vastly improved for the treatment of others. The discovery of the 5-HT-3 antagonists has dramatically decreased the incidence and severity of nausea and vomiting. Furthermore, the hematologic support agents have improved the outcomes in patients receiving cancer therapy that may cause neutropenia (CSFs), anemia (rhuEPO), and thrombocytopenia (oprelvekin). There are also a number of cytoprotective agents that can be used to diminish the incidence of particular side effects: mesna for ifosfamide-induced hemorrhagic cystitis, dexrazoxane for doxorubicin-induced cardiotoxicity, and amifostine for a broad range of toxicities

■ There is intensive ongoing research devoted to the identification of supportive care therapies that will improve outcomes in terms of quality of life and survival rates for cancer patients

SUGGESTED READINGS

Devita VT, Hellman S, Rosenberg SA. Cancer: principles and practice of oncology, 7th ed. Philadelphia: Lippincott Williams & Wilkins, 2004.

Otto SE, ed. Oncology nursing clinical reference, 4th ed. St. Louis: CV Mosby, 2003.

REFERENCES

1. Dose AM. The symptom experience of mucositis, stomatitis, and xerostomia. Semin Oncol Nurs 11:248–255, 1995.
2. Zlotolow IM. General considerations in prevention and treatment of oral manifestations of cancer therapies. In: Berger A, Portenoy RK, Weissman DE, eds. Principles and practice of supportive oncology. Philadelphia: Lippincott-Raven, 1998:237.
3. Kinzie BJ. Treatment of stomatitis associated with antineoplastic-drug therapy. Clin Pharm 7:14–17, 1988.
4. Berger AM, Kilroy TJ. Oral complications. In: DeVita VT Jr, Hellman S, Rosenberg SA, eds. Principles and practice of oncology, 5th ed. Philadelphia: Lippincott-Raven, 1997:2714.
5. Verdi CJ. Cancer therapy and oral mucositis. Drug Saf 9:185–195, 1993.
6. Carl W. Oral complications of local and systemic cancer treatment. Curr Opin Oncol 7:320–324, 1995.
7. Haskell CM. Principles of cancer chemotherapy. In: Haskell CM, ed. Cancer treatment, 4th ed. Philadelphia: WB Saunders, 1995:42.
8. Loprinzi CL, Foote RL, Michalak J. Alleviation of cytotoxic therapy-induced normal tissue damage. Semin Oncol 22 (2, Suppl 3): 95–97, 1995.
9. Solomon MA. Oral sucralfate suspension for mucositis. N Engl J Med 315:459–460, 1986.
10. Palifermin prescribing information. Available at http://www.kepivance.com/pi.jsp. Accessed May 8, 2005.
11. Epstein JB. The painful mouth. Infect Dis Clin North Am 2: 103–202, 1988.
12. Berger AM, Kilroy TJ. Oral complications of cancer therapy. In: Berger A, Portenoy RK, Weissman DE, eds. Principles and practice of supportive oncology. Philadelphia: Lippincott-Raven, 1998:223.
13. Peterson DE, Petit RG. Phase III study: AES-14 in patients at risk for mucositis secondary to anthracycline-based chemotherapy [abstract 8008]. Proc Am Soc Clin Oncol 22:14S, 2004.
14. Patni N, Patni S, Bapna A, et al. The role of amifostine in prophylaxis of radiotherapy induced mucositis and xerostomia in head and neck cancer [abstract 5568]. Proc Am Soc Clin Oncol 22:14S, 2004.
15. Martin LM, Moran A, Damour MD, et al. Amifostine (A) reduces acute mucosal toxicity of accelerated radiotherapy (ART) and carboplatin (CBP) in locally advanced head and neck cancer (HNSC) [abstract 5566]. Proc Am Soc Clin Oncol 22:14S, 2004.
16. Ferrero JM, Weber B, Lepille D, et al. Carboplatin (PA) and pegylated liposomal doxorubicin (CA; PACA regimen) in patients with advanced ovarian cancer in late (>6 months) relapse (AOCLR): survival results of a GINECO phase II trial [abstract 5022]. Proc Am Soc Clin Oncol 22:14S, 2004.
17. Fox PC, Atkinson JC, Macynski AA, et al. Pilocarpine treatment of salivary gland hypofunction and dry mouth (xerostomia). Arch Intern Med 151:1149–1152, 1991.
18. Greenspan D, Daniels TE. Effectiveness of pilocarpine in postradiation xerostoma. Cancer 59:1123–1125, 1987.
19. Johnson JT, Ferretti FA, Nethery J, et al. Oral pilocarpine for postirradiation xerostomia in patients with head and neck cancer. N Engl J Med 329:390–395, 1993.
20. Amifostine prescribing information. Available at http://www.ethyol.com/products/ethyol/index.asp. Accessed May 8, 2005.
21. Cox GJ, Matsui SM, Lo RS, et al. Etiology and outcome of diarrhea after bone marrow transplantation: a prospective study. Gastroenterology 107:1398–1407, 1994.
22. Mercadante S. Diarrhea, malabsorption, and constipation. In: Berger A, Portenoy RK, Weissman DE, eds. Principles and practice of supportive oncology. Philadelphia: Lippincott-Raven, 1998:191.
23. Rothenberg ML, Eckardt JR, Kuhn JG, et al. Phase II trial of irinotecan in patients with progressive or rapidly recurrent colorectal cancer. J Clin Oncol 14:1128–1135, 1996.
24. Zidan J, Haim N, Beny A, et al. Octreotide in the treatment of severe chemotherapy-induced diarrhea. Ann Oncol 12:227–229, 2001.
25. Coates A, Abraham S, Kaye SB, et al. On the receiving end: patient perception of the side effects of cancer chemotherapy. Eur J Cancer 19:203–208, 1983.
26. Griffin AM, Butow PN, Coates AS, et al. On the receiving end. V: patient perceptions on the side effects of cancer chemotherapy in 1993. Ann Oncol 7:189–195, 1996.
27. Lindley C, McCune JS, Thomason TE, et al. Perception of chemotherapy side effects cancer versus noncancer patients. Cancer Pract 7:59–65, 1999.
28. Graves T. Emesis as a complication of cancer chemotherapy: pathophysiology, importance, and treatment. Pharmacotherapy 12: 337–345, 1992.
29. Hesketh PH, Kris MG, Grunberg SM, et al. Proposal for classifying the acute emetogenicity of cancer chemotherapy. J Clin Oncol 15: 103–109, 1997.
30. Osaba D, Zee B, Pater J, et al. Determinants of postchemotherapy nausea and vomiting in patients with cancer. J Clin Oncol 15: 116–123, 1997.
31. Borrison HL, Wang SC. Physiology and pharmacology of vomiting. Pharmacol Rev 5:193–230, 1953.
32. Grunberg SM, Hesketh PJ. Control of chemotherapy-induced emesis. N Engl J Med 329:1790–1796, 1993.
33. Gralla RJ, Rittenberg C, Peralta M, et al. Cisplatin and emesis: aspects of treatment and a new trial for delayed emesis using oral dexamethasone plus ondansetron beginning at 16 hours after cisplatin. Oncology 53:86–91, 1996.

34. Del Favero A, Roila F, Tonato M. Reducing chemotherapy-induced nausea and vomiting: current perspectives and future possibilities. Drug Saf 9:410–428, 1993.

35. Grunberg SM. Antiemetic drugs: essential pharmacology. In: Tonato M, ed. Antiemetics in the supportive care of cancer patients. Berlin: Springer Verlag, 1996:25–33.

36. Pectasides D, Mylonakis A, Varthalitis J, et al. Comparison of two different doses of ondansetron plus dexamethasone in the prophylaxis of cisplatin-induced emesis. Oncology 54:1–6, 1997.

37. Blaver P. A pharmacological profile of oral granisetron (Kytril tablets). Semin Oncol 22 (Suppl 10):3–5, 1995.

38. Lichter I. Nausea and vomiting in patients with cancer. Hematol Oncol Clin North Am 10:207–220, 1966.

39. ASHP therapeutic guidelines on the pharmacologic management of nausea and vomiting in adult and pediatric patients receiving chemotherapy or radiation therapy or undergoing surgery. Am J Health Syst Pharm 56:729–764, 1999.

40. Stewart A. Optimal control of cyclophosphamide-induced emesis. Oncology 53 (Suppl 1):32–38, 1996.

41. Martin M. The severity and pattern of emesis following different cytotoxic agents. Oncology 53 (Suppl 1):26–31, 1996.

42. Hesketh PJ, Van Belle S, Aapro M, et al. Differential involvement of neurotransmitters through the time course of cisplatin-induced emesis as revealed by therapy with specific receptor antagonists. Eur J Cancer 39:1074–1080, 2003.

43. Bountra C, Gale JD, Gardner CJ, et al. Towards understanding the etiology and pathophysiology of the emetic reflex: novel approaches to antiemetic drugs. Oncology 53 (Suppl 1):102–109, 1996.

44. Lakhbir S, Field MJ, Hughes J, et al. The tachykinin NK1 receptor antagonists PD 154075 blocks cisplatin-induced delayed emesis in the ferret. Eur J Pharmacol 321:209–216, 1997.

45. Hesketh P. Management of cisplatin-induced delayed emesis. Oncology 53 (Suppl 1):73–77, 1996.

46. Tavorath R, Hesketh PJ. Drug treatment of chemotherapy-induced delayed emesis. Drugs 52:639–648, 1996.

47. Kris MG, Roila F, De Mulder PHM, et al. Delayed emesis following anticancer chemotherapy. Support Care Cancer 6:228–232, 1998.

48. Laszlo J, Clark RA, Hanson DC, et al. Lorazepam in cancer patients treated with cisplatin: a drug having antiemetic, amnesic and anxiolytic effects. J Clin Oncol 3:864–869, 1985.

49. Grant M. Introduction: nausea and vomiting, quality of life, and the oncology nurse. Oncol Nurs Forum 24:5–7, 1997.

50. King CR. Nonpharmacologic management of chemotherapy-induced nausea and vomiting. Oncol Nurs Forum 24:41–47, 1997.

51. Suekawa M, Ishige A, Yuasa K, et al. Pharmacological studies on ginger. I. Pharmacological actions of pungent constituents, (6)-gingerol and (6)-shogaol. J Pharmacobiodyn 7:836–848, 1984.

52. Seynaeve C, Schuller J, Buser K, et al. Comparison of the antiemetic efficacy of different doses of ondansetron, given as either a continuous infusion or a single intravenous dose, in acute cisplatin-induced emesis. A multicentre, double-blind, randomised, parallel group study. Br J Cancer 66:192–197, 1992.

53. Marty M. Future trends in cancer treatment and emesis control. Oncology 50:159–162, 1993.

54. Rowe JM, Anderson JW, Mazza JJ, et al. A randomized placebo-controlled phase III study of granulocyte-macrophage colony-stimulating factor in adult patients: a study of the Eastern Cooperative Oncology Group (E1490). Blood 86:457–462, 1995.

55. Ozer H, Armitage JO, Bennett CL, et al. 2000 update of recommendations for the use of hematopoietic colony-stimulating factors: evidence-based, clinical practice guidelines. American Society of Clinical Oncology Growth Factors Expert Panel. J Clin Oncol 18: 3558–85, 2000.

56. Silber JH, Fridman M, DiPaola RS, et al. First-cycle blood counts and subsequent neutropenia, dose reduction, or delay in early stage breast cancer therapy. J Clin Oncol 16:2392–2400, 1998.

57. Vivianne CG, Tijan-Heijnen, Biesma B, et al. Enhanced myelotoxicity due to granulocyte colony stimulating factor administration until 48 hours before the next chemotherapy course in patients with small cell lung carcinoma. J Clin Oncol 16:2708–2714, 1998.

58. Groppman JL, Itri LM. Chemotherapy-induced anemia in adults: incidence and treatment. JNCI 91:1616–1634, 1999.

59. Bunn PA, Crowley J, Kelly K, et al. Chemoradiotherapy with or without granulocyte-macrophage colony-stimulating factor in the treatment of limited-stage small-cell lung cancer: a prospective phase III randomized study of the Southwest Oncology Group. J Clin Oncol 13:1632–1641, 1995.

60. Ludwig H, Fritz E. Anemia in cancer patients. Semin Oncol 25 (Suppl):2–6, 1998.

61. National Comprehensive Cancer Center Practice Guidelines in Oncology. Cancer- and treatment-related anemia, v2.2005. Available at: www.nccn.org. Accessed Dec. 21, 2005.

62. National Oncology Alliance Treatment Guidelines: Anemia v1.2004. Available at: www.noainc.com. Accessed Dec. 21, 2005.

63. Glaspy J, Bukowski R, Steinberg D, et al. Impact of therapy with epoetin alpha or clinical outcomes in patients with nonmyeloid malignancies during cancer chemotherapy in community oncology practice. J Clin Oncol 15:1218–1234, 1997.

64. Cascinu S, Fedeli A, Del Ferro E, et al. Recombinant human erythropoietin treatment in cisplatin-associated anemia: a randomized, double-blind trial with placebo. J Clin Oncol 12:1058–1062, 1997.

65. Cella D. Factors influencing quality of life in cancer patients: anemia and fatigue. Semin Oncol 25 (Suppl 7):43–46, 1998.

66. Leitgeb C, Pecherstorfer M, Fritz E, et al. Quality of life in chronic anemia of cancer during treatment with recombinant human erythropoietin. Cancer 73:2535–2542, 1994.

67. Kaufman JS, Reda DJ, Fye CL, et al. Subcutaneous compared with intravenous epoetin in patients receiving hemodialysis. N Engl J Med 339:578–583, 1998.

68. Glaspy JA, Tchekmedyian NS. Darbepoetin alfa administered every 2 weeks alleviates anemia in cancer patients receiving chemotherapy. Oncology (Huntingt) 16 (10 Suppl 11):23–29, 2002.

69. Schwartzberg L, Yee L, Senecal F, et al. Darbepoetin alfa (DA) 200 mcg every 2 weeks (Q2W) vs epoetin alfa (Epo) 40,000 U weekly (QW) in anemic patients (pts) receiving chemotherapy (ctx) [abstract 8063]. Proc Am Soc Clin Oncol 22:14S, 2004.

70. Aranesp Prescribing Information. Available at: http://www.aranesp.com/pdf/aranesp PI.pdf. Accessed Nov. 1, 2004.

71. Weinberh ED. The role of iron in cancer. Eur J Cancer Prev 5: 19–36, 1996.

72. Henry D, Mason B, Staddon A, et al. Efficacy of Infed plus recombinant human erythropoietin (rhuEPO) in treating anemia in cancer patients with suboptimal response to rhuEPO: a pilot study [abstract 230]. Proc Am Soc Clin Oncol 17:59a, 1998.

73. Adamson JW. The relationship of erythropoietin and iron metabolism to red blood cell production in humans. Semin Oncol 21 (Suppl 13):9–15, 1994.

74. Fishbane S, Frei GL, Maesaka J. Reduction in recombinant human erythropoietin doses by the use of chronic intravenous iron supplementation. Am J Kidney Dis 26:41–46, 1995.

75. Dutcher J, Schiffer C, Aisner J, et al. Incidence of thrombocytopenia and serious hemorrhage among patients with solid tumors. Cancer 53:557–562, 1984.

76. Rebulla P, Finazzi G, Marangoni F, et al. The threshold for prophylactic platelet transfusions in adults with acute myeloid leukemia. N Engl J Med 337:1870–1875, 1997.

77. Kaushansky K. Thrombopoietin. N Engl J Med 339:746–754, 1998.

78. Du X, Williams DA. Interleukin II: review of molecular, cell biology and clinical use. Blood 89:3897–3908, 1997.

79. Tepler I, Elias L, Smith JW, et al. A randomized placebo-controlled, trial of recombinant human interleukin-11 in cancer patients with severe thrombocytopenia due to chemotherapy. Blood 87:3607–3614, 1996.

80. Issacs C, Robert NJ, Bailey A, et al. Randomized placebo-controlled study of recombinant human interleukin-II to prevent chemotherapy induced thrombocytopenia in patients with breast cancer receiving dose-intensive cyclophosphamide and doxorubicin. J Clin Oncol 15: 3368–3377, 1997.

81. Vadhan-Raj S, Patel S, Bueso-Ramos C, et al. Importance of predosing of recombinant human thrombopoietin to reduce chemotherapy-induced early thrombocytopenia. J Clin Oncol 21:3158–3167, 2003.

82. Schoenike SE, Dana WJ. Ifosfamide and mesna. Clin Pharm 9: 179–191, 1990.

83. Goren MP. Oral administration of mesna with ifosfamide. Semin Oncol 23 (Suppl 16):91–96, 1996.

84. Seifert CF, Nesser ME, Thompson DF. Dexrazoxane in the preven-

tion of doxorubicin-induced cardiotoxicity. Ann Pharmacother 28: 1063–1072, 1994.

85. Speyer JL, Green, MD, Felerluch-Jacquotte A, et al. ICRF-187 permits longer treatment with doxorubicin in women with breast cancer. J Clin Oncol 10:117–127, 1992.

86. Hellman K. Cardioprotection by dexrazoxane (Cardioxane; ICRF-187): progress in supportive care. Support Care Cancer 4:305–307, 1996.

87. Capizzi RL. Amifostine: the preclinical basis for broad-spectrum selective cytoprotection of normal tissues from cytotoxic therapies. Semin Oncol 23:2, 1996.

88. Buntzel J, Schuth J, Kuttner K, et al. Radiochemotherapy with amifostine cytoprotection for head and neck cancer. Support Care Cancer 6:155–160, 1998.

89. Anderson H, Mercer V, Thatcher N. A phase III randomized trial of carboplatin and amifostine versus carboplatin and G-CSF in patients with inoperable non-small cell lung cancer (NSCLC) [abstract 1787]. Proc Am Soc Clin Oncol 17:465a, 1998.

90. List AF, Farah B, Heaton R, et al. Stimulation of hematopoiesis by amifostine in patients with myelodysplastic syndrome. Blood 90: 3364–3369, 1997.

Chronic Leukemias

93

Courtney W. Yuen

Chronic myelogenous leukemia (CML) and chronic lymphocytic leukemia (CLL) are hematologic malignancies that occur primarily in older adults. Patients usually survive several years beyond the diagnosis of leukemia, even in the absence of treatment. Over time, the chronic leukemias become more aggressive and less responsive to treatment. CML is curable only with an allogeneic hematopoietic cell transplant (AHCT), which is available to about 20% to 30% of patients. CLL is incurable at this time.

New therapies are emerging that contribute to prolonged survival and may possibly lead to a cure for patients with chronic leukemia. Patients with chronic leukemia are benefiting from the knowledge and application of new therapeutic approaches, including the use of biologic agents, advances in hematopoietic cell transplants (HCTs), new effective chemotherapy, and improved supportive care. As these advances in treatment are made available for patients, care must be taken to safeguard patient quality of life. The new approaches under development will warrant evaluations of cost to benefit ratios.

CHRONIC MYELOGENOUS LEUKEMIA

CML is a hematologic malignancy originating from a leukemic transformation in a clonal pluripotent stem cell. Ninety-five percent of patients display a characteristic t(9; 22) chromosome translocation, the Philadelphia chromosome. The disease progresses through three distinct phases.[1] The first stage, lasting from 3 to 5 years, is an early chronic phase in which the patient is minimally symptomatic. At this point, there is usually less than 5% immature or blast cells present in the bone marrow. In this early phase of the disease, the leukemic cells retain the ability to differentiate and mature into granulocytes. The leukemia may then go through a transition phase or accelerated phase (5%–30% blast cells) of several months' duration, in which the symptoms are more pronounced and more refractory to medication. Finally, CML invariably progresses to a blast phase (>30% blast cells), which causes a fatal leukemic blast crisis, unless the leukemic clone has been eradicated and normal hematopoiesis is restored. Blast crisis is characterized by fevers and bleeding complications, similar to the presentation of acute leukemia, and unless the patient receives treatment, the risk of mortality is extremely high. At this time, the only potential cure for CML is an AHCT.

TREATMENT GOALS: CHRONIC MYELOGENOUS LEUKEMIA

- Provide curative therapy by eradicating the leukemic cells and restoring normal hematopoiesis. A cure for CML is currently available only by allogeneic bone marrow (or hematopoietic stem cell) grafts, which are available for about 20% to 30% of patients with CML.
- For patients who are not candidates for allogeneic stem cell grafting, prolong the chronic phase of the disease as long as possible to prolong survival with minimal symptoms.

EPIDEMIOLOGY

CML accounts for approximately 20% of all cases of leukemia with an incidence of 1 to 1.5 cases per 100,000 population. The median age at diagnosis is 67 years, although patients may be diagnosed at any age.[2] There is a slight male to female predominance in a ratio of about 1.5:1.[3]

The etiology of the leukemogenic transformation is unclear. There appears to be no hereditary component. Chemical leukemogens have not been distinctly identified, but may include benzene and chemotherapy. No role for viral involvement has been observed. Exposure to ionizing radiation appears to have an etiologic role in some cases. Survivors of atomic bomb explosions, radiologists, and patients exposed to large amounts of radiation have an increased incidence of CML.[4]

PATHOPHYSIOLOGY

The key event in the evolution of CML appears to be the translocation of the proto-oncogene c-ABL located on the long arm of chromosome 9 to the BCR gene on the long arm of chromosome 22. A reciprocal translocation occurs, and the BCR gene on chromosome 22 is translocated to chromosome 9. A BCR-ABL gene is formed on chromosome 22, and an ABL-BCR gene is formed on chromosome 9. The BCR-ABL gene is transcribed into an 8.5-kb mRNA, which is translated into a 210-kD protein. The expression of the BCR-ABL gene to the p210BCR/ABL tyrosine kinase protein is linked to the oncogenic transformation to CML. The BCR-ABL fusion produces an abundance of tyrosine kinase that results in the deregulation of cellular proliferation and reduction in apoptosis to mutagenic stimuli.[5] The resultant t(9; 22) chromosomal translocation is named the "Philadelphia (Ph)" chromosome (Fig. 93.1).

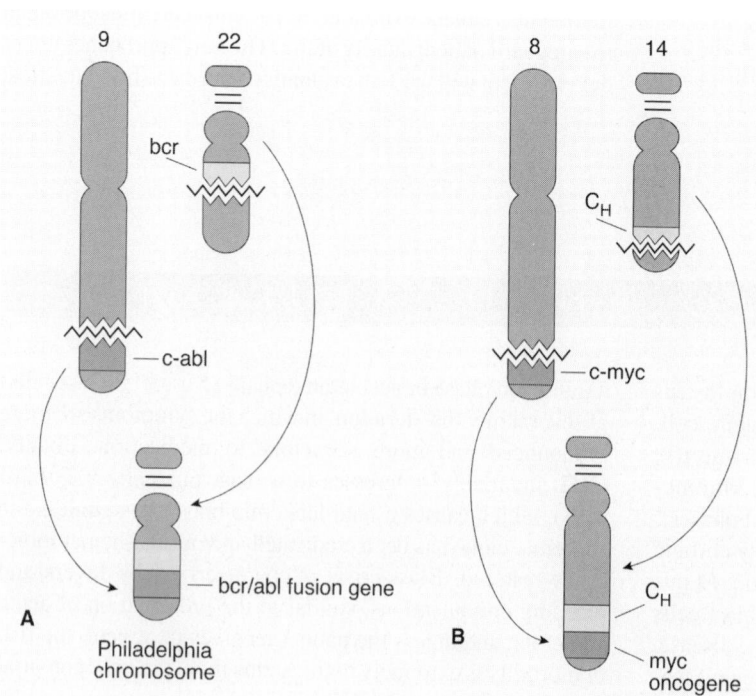

FIGURE 93.1 Oncogene activation by chromosomal relocation. **A.** Chronic myelogenous leukemia. Breaks at the ends of the long arms of chromosomes 9 and 22 allow reciprocal translocations to occur. The c-abl proto-oncogene on chromosome 9 is translocated to the breakpoint region (bcr) of chromosome 22. The result is the Philadelphia chromosome, which contains a new fusion gene coding for a hybrid oncogenic protein (BCR-ABL), presumably involved in the pathogenesis of chronic myelogenous leukemia. **B.** Burkitt lymphoma. In this disorder, chromosomal breaks involve the long arms of chromosomes 8 and 14. The c-myc gene on chromosome 8 is translocated to a region on chromosome 14 adjacent to the gene coding for the constant region of an immunoglobulin heavy chain (CH). The expression of c-myc is enhanced by its association with the promoter/enhancer regions of the actively transcribed immunoglobulin genes. (From Rubin E, Farber JL. Pathology, 3rd ed. Philadelphia: Lippincott Williams & Wilkins, 1999, with permission.)

Further chromosomal abnormalities occur as the disease progresses to the accelerated and blast phase. Examples of these acquired abnormalities include trisomy 8, an additional Ph chromosome, and isochromosome 17q.[6]

CLINICAL PRESENTATION AND DIAGNOSIS

SIGNS AND SYMPTOMS

Chronic Phase. The onset of symptoms is usually gradual. Common presenting symptoms are fatigue, weight loss, anorexia, abdominal fullness, early satiety, and sweating. Physical findings commonly include splenomegaly, hepatomegaly, sternal tenderness, pallor, and palpable lymph nodes. Laboratory findings include an elevated white blood cell (WBC) count, often greater than 100×10^9 per liter. Basophilia, eosinophilia, and monocytosis are typical. Most patients have normochromic, normocytic anemia. Many patients have thrombocytosis. The lactic acid dehydrogenase (LDH), uric acid, and serum vitamin B_{12} levels are usually above normal. The leukocyte alkaline phosphatase level is almost always low. The bone marrow is hypercellular.[3,4,6]

Progression to Accelerated and Blast Phases. The disease may progress from the chronic phase to the accelerated phase and then to blast crisis or may move directly from the chronic phase to the blast phase. The transition may occur at any time in the course of the disease. Although the chronic phase usually lasts several years, there is no guarantee that the CML will not rapidly advance to blast crisis. As the disease moves into the accelerated phase, medication is no longer as effective as in the chronic stage and laboratory test results and clinical findings will worsen. New cytogenetic abnormalities will appear. Patients entering the accelerated phase may report fever, night sweats, weight loss, myalgias, and arthralgias.

Patients in the blast phase of CML have signs and symptoms of acute leukemia. Many patients will present with fever (with or without infection), bone pain and enlarged spleen. Often infection and bleeding occur due to bone marrow failure. CML will evolve to acute myeloid leukemia (AML) in about two thirds of patients and to acute lymphocytic leukemia (ALL) in about one third. The acute leukemic phase of CML is more refractory to therapy than is de novo acute leukemia. CML that transforms into ALL is more responsive to therapy than CML that transforms into AML.[3,4,6]

DIAGNOSIS

CML is commonly diagnosed incidentally after the detection of a high WBC count on routine screening. The patient with symptoms most frequently reports asthenia, abdominal discomfort, weight loss, and fever. On physical examination, the majority of patients have splenomegaly. Hepatomegaly is also common. The WBC count is elevated in more than 90% of patients, with many having a WBC count greater

than 100×10^9 per liter. Anemia and thrombocytosis are usually present. The bone marrow shows hyperplasia of myeloid cells. Analysis generally shows less than 5% blasts. Cytogenetic analysis, an examination of the chromosomes in metaphase in the leukemic cells, is necessary to confirm the presence of the Ph chromosome.[3,4,6]

PSYCHOSOCIAL ASPECTS

CML is usually diagnosed when patients have few symptoms. They will be told that they have leukemia that is incurable without an AHCT and that the chance of a successful HCT is greatest if it is performed during the chronic phase and within the first year of diagnosis. Therefore, at a time in their disease when they are feeling well, patients have to choose between the possibility of their CML remaining in the chronic phase for 3 to 5 years with a decreased chance of cure or undergoing an early HCT with its attendant risk of early death but with the chance of cure. If the patient chooses to wait for disease progression before undergoing HCT, the likelihood of cure with HCT is reduced. Family members may feel guilty if they are not eligible as bone marrow donors. If the patient undergoes a HCT and dies from transplant-related complications, the related donor may feel that he or she contributed to patient harm. Patients who are too old for transplant or without suitable donors will be faced with the knowledge that the leukemia is incurable.

THERAPEUTIC PLAN

The only curative therapy available for a patient with CML is allogeneic bone marrow or stem cell transplant. This approach is available only to patients who have a suitable donor and who are young enough to tolerate the procedure and the subsequent toxic effects of allogeneic transplant. All patients with chronic-phase CML who are younger than 50 years of age with a matched sibling donor should undergo HCT. Although the upper age limit at which a HCT is too dangerous is controversial, it has been advancing over the years because supportive care has led to improved survival even in older patients. The decision to perform a HCT in patients older than 50 years of age may be based on the patient's functional status and overall health and not on age alone. Treatment decisions are complicated more due to ever increasing treatment options such as nonmyeloablative preparative regimens and imatinib (see below). The timing of the transplant is also controversial. Survival is markedly improved if the transplant is performed during the chronic phase of CML and in the first year from diagnosis. However, the patient is often asymptomatic or minimally symptomatic during this time, and it may be difficult for the patient to decide to undergo a life-threatening procedure when he or she feels well.[3–6]

The patient variables considered in treatment decisions include patient age, patient functional status, phase of disease (chronic versus blast crisis), and donor availability. Treatment options include chemotherapy and/or interferon (INF-α), imatinib, AHCT with a matched sibling donor, AHCT with an unrelated donor, nonmyeloablative AHCT, or experimental autologous HCT.

TREATMENT

CHRONIC PHASE

If CML is in the chronic phase and an AHCT is unavailable or inappropriate because of the patient's age or performance status, the standard treatment options are busulfan, hydroxyurea, IFN-α, or imatinib alone or in combination with other chemotherapy regimens. The goal of therapy for CML in the chronic phase is to prolong survival and minimize symptoms by achieving a complete hematologic response and a complete cytogenetic response. Complete hematologic response is generally defined as the return to normal hematologic laboratory values and the absence of any signs or symptoms of CML. A complete cytogenetic response is the disappearance of the Ph chromosome, also described as the absence of all Ph-positive metaphases. A partial cytogenetic response has been variously defined. A useful definition is the presence of the Ph chromosome in less than 35% of the metaphases.[4] Busulfan, hydroxyurea, INF-α, and imatinib usually provide a complete hematologic response. A cytogenetic response is rarely, if ever, achieved with busulfan or hydroxyurea. Interferon can provide a complete cytogenetic response in 9% to 26% of patients and a partial cytogenetic response in about the same percentage. Imatinib may also produce a complete cytogenetic response, but the impact on overall survival is still debatable due to the development of resistance and its potential for making future stem cell transplant less effective.

Busulfan. Busulfan was at one time the most effective agent available for the chronic phase of CML, but its use has been supplanted by agents with less toxicity and more efficacy. Busulfan is an alkylsulfonate alkylating agent, which is not cell cycle specific. It is well absorbed orally. The half-life in adults is 2.1 to 2.6 hours. Busulfan is metabolized in the liver, and the metabolites are renally cleared. The primary effect at low doses is to suppress granulocytopoiesis. Busulfan use may lead to a delayed, prolonged, and profound myelosuppression. This effect requires that patients receiving busulfan be carefully monitored so that the dose can be decreased or the drug stopped before the target WBC count is reached. Because blood counts continue to drop after busulfan is discontinued, the drug must be stopped at about double the desired WBC count to prevent dangerously low WBC counts. Pancytopenia from busulfan is frequently fatal. Skin hyperpigmentation is common. An infrequent but serious complication of chronic busulfan therapy

is pulmonary fibrosis. The initial symptoms include fever, dry cough, and dyspnea. Busulfan should be discontinued while other possible causes of pulmonary symptoms, such as infection, are ruled out. If the patient is thought to have busulfan-induced pulmonary dysplasia, further therapy with busulfan is absolutely contraindicated. No effective treatment for the pulmonary complications of busulfan is known. The patient may develop pulmonary failure, which usually results in death within 6 months of the onset of pulmonary symptoms. An Addison-like syndrome can rarely develop with chronic busulfan therapy with symptoms of anorexia, weakness, hypotension, and fatigue.[7–10]

Busulfan is commercially available as 2-mg tablets (Table 93.1). It may be given daily or intermittently. On the intermittent schedule, the usual dose is 0.1 mg/kg/day orally (PO).[4] Once the WBC count decreases by half, the dose should be reduced by half. When the WBC count falls below 20×10^9 per liter, busulfan should be stopped and restarted when the WBC rises to 50×10^9 per liter. Alternatively, busulfan can be given as a 4-mg per day dose, holding the dose when the WBC falls below 10×10^9 per liter.[3] Advantages to the use of busulfan in chronic-phase CML are that it is effective in most patients in achieving a hematologic remission, it is given orally, it is inexpensive, and it is generally well tolerated. Busulfan's role in the treatment of chronic-phase CML has been largely replaced by hydroxyurea, which has fewer side effects, has a dose that is easier to titrate, and may result in improved survival.

Hydroxyurea. Hydroxyurea is a ribonucleotide diphosphate reductase inhibitor. Ribonucleotide reductases catalyze the conversion of ribonucleotides to deoxyribonucleotides. Hydroxyurea may have other mechanisms of action as well. Hydroxyurea is cell cycle specific for the S phase, causing cell arrest at G_1 to S.[7–11] Its oral bioavailability is 73% to 127%.[12,13] The half-life is about 3.5 to 4.5 hours. Hydroxyurea is hepatically metabolized and renally excreted. The usual dose is 20 to 30 mg/kg/day or 1.5 to 2 g per day (Table 93.1). The drug is commercially available in 500-mg capsules and 1,000-mg tablets. The dose should be adjusted downward for patients with leukopenia or thrombocytopenia. The primary adverse effect is bone marrow

TABLE 93.1	Agents Used in Chronic Myelogenous Leukemia

Summary of Suggested Dosing for Agents Used in CML

Busulfan[3,4]	4 mg/day PO
Hydroxyurea[7–11]	20–30 mg/kg/day PO in divided dose (500 mg tid, 1,000 mg bid)
Alpha Interferon[17,18]	5 million units/m²/day Sq daily
Imatinib[43,44]	400–800 mg/day PO

CML, chronic myelogenous leukemia; PO, by mouth; tid, three times daily; bid, twice a day; Sq, subcutaneous.

suppression. Gastrointestinal effects are uncommon at usual doses.[7–11]

An unusual and infrequent complication of chronic hydroxyurea use is the development of cutaneous leg ulcers. The ulcers are usually painful and may be numerous. The ulcers heal or markedly improve after hydroxyurea is discontinued.[14]

Hydroxyurea is used in chronic-phase CML to control blood counts. It does not delay or prevent the transition to blast crisis. It has few side effects, and the dose is easily titrated. It is preferred over busulfan because of its greater tolerability, no severe adverse effects, ease of dose adjustment, and it appears to provide a survival advantage compared to busulfan.[15] It may be used as a single agent or combined with INF-α or other agents.

Interferon-α. INF-α has been found to be useful in patients with CML for inducing a complete hematologic remission and a major or complete cytogenetic response.[16,17] Because INF-α does not benefit all patients, is expensive, and has side effects that may make it difficult for patients to continue therapy, careful attention to patient selection and monitoring is important to achieve the best response with the least toxicity.

The side effects of INF-α may decrease the patient's sense of well-being. These side effects include flu-like symptoms of malaise, fever, chills, and aching. The symptoms are sometimes relieved by acetaminophen. Tachyphylaxis to these side effects usually develops within weeks. Anorexia, nausea, and diarrhea are common. Fatigue and depression may be significant. INF-α should be avoided in patients with clinical depression.[17,18]

In general, the recommended dose of INF-α is 5 million units/m^2/day, adjusted to the patient's tolerance of side effects (Table 93.1). In at least one study, a dose lower than 5 million units/m^2/day subcutaneously was used and equal efficacy was reported[19]; however, other studies have observed a dose-response effect, suggesting a better response with the standard dose (Table 93.2 lists interferon administration recommendations).[17,18]

The best time to begin therapy for optimal response is in the early chronic phase when the patient has more Ph-negative polyclonal hematopoiesis. Most patients achieving a hematologic response will do so within the first 3 months of therapy. Most patients who achieve a cytogenetic response will do so within the first 12 months of treatment, but it may take as long as 18 months.[20]

For patients with chronic-phase CML, there is an improved 5-year survival rate when INF-α is used, compared to chemotherapy.[20] A comparison of INF-α to busulfan in the early chronic phase found a 54% predicted survival rate at 5 years for patients receiving INF-α and a 32% predicted 5-year survival rate for those receiving busulfan.[21]

In a meta-analysis of seven randomized trials, the 5-year survival rate with INF-α was 57% compared to 42% with chemotherapy.[20] However, in some studies, no survival ad-

TABLE 93.2	Recommendations for Interferon Administration

In general, the recommended dose of INF-α is 5 million units/m^2/day, adjusted to the patient's tolerance of side effects.

Try to give the full dose of INF-α if possible, adjusting to patient tolerance, to side effects, and effect on quality of life.

Begin the INF-α at a low dose for several days to allow the patient time to adjust to the side effects. A reasonable beginning dose is 3 million units subcutaneously daily, then increase toward the intended dose.

Add hydroxyurea 0.5–2 g orally daily to decrease the WBC count to 10–20 × 10^9 per liter. It is reasonable to continue both agents. If one drug needs to be stopped because of a low WBC count, discontinue the hydroxyurea before altering the INF-α.

Give INF-α at bedtime.

Instruct the patient to take acetaminophen with each dose to decrease fever and myalgias.

INF-α, interferon alpha; WBC, white blood cell.

vantage of INF-α over hydroxyurea was seen. One study found no advantage in survival for the combination of INF-α and hydroxyurea compared to hydroxyurea alone.[22] Low-dose INF-α (3 million units subcutaneously 5 days/week) was used. The survival of the INF-α group was similar to that seen in other studies. The hydroxyurea group showed better survival than that seen in other studies. The German CML Study Group also found no difference in survival between hydroxyurea and INF-α groups,[23] while the Italian Cooperative Study Group found a significant survival advantage with the use of INF-α.[24] A comparison of the German and Italian studies suggested that the different findings are based on differences of study design and that the combination of INF-α and hydroxyurea is more effective than either agent used alone.[25] The potential benefits of the combination of INF-α and hydroxyurea include possible additive effects that may provide a survival advantage and earlier hematologic remission, and therefore, earlier relief of disease symptoms for the patient. A long-term follow-up of the Italian Cooperative Study Group reported that the significant improvement in survival seen in the INF-α study arm compared to the chemotherapy arm was maintained over time. Of 218 patients, 26% achieved a complete or major cytogenetic response. In nine (4%) patients, the complete cytogenetic response has continued for more than 8 years.[26] The German CML Study Group found that INF-α 5 million units/m^2/day plus hydroxyurea 40 mg/kg/day was associated with a long-term survival advantage over hydroxyurea monotherapy in patients with chronic phase CML.[27]

In one study, the combination of low-dose cytarabine and INF-α appeared to increase survival in patients with chronic-phase CML compared to treatment with INF-α alone.[28] The dose of INF-α used was 5 million units/m²/day, and the dose of cytarabine was 20 mg/m²/day for 10 days out of every month. Patients also were given hydroxyurea 50 mg/kg/day until complete hematologic remission was obtained. There was an increase in hematologic and cytogenetic remissions. However, there were more side effects in the combination treatment group. Cytarabine contributed thrombocytopenia, nausea, vomiting, diarrhea, mucositis, weight loss, asthenia, and skin rashes to the usual side effects of INF-α therapy. About one half of the patients in the study receiving the combination therapy discontinued treatment because of side effects compared to one third of patients treated with INF-α alone. Patient quality of life or functional status between combination therapy and INF-α alone was not compared. Because of the observed increase in cytogenetic response and improved survival, it is reasonable to provide combination therapy with low-dose cytarabine and INF-α, despite the increase in side effects.

It appears that INF-α probably prolongs the survival of patients who achieve a major cytogenetic response. However, it may take more than 12 months for the cytogenetic response to occur, and it would be useful to be able to make an early prediction about which patients are likely to eventually respond to continued INF-α therapy. Some investigators have attempted this. Preliminary guidelines based on a large, single-institution study have been developed (Table 93.3).[29] The authors recommend that INF-α therapy should be continued in patients who have more than a 10% chance of achieving a major cytogenetic response if an allogeneic transplant is not available to them. They found that pretreatment risk factors for a low chance of response are a spleen size more than 5 cm below the costal margin and platelet count greater than 700×10^9 per liter. The decision algorithm appears to be fairly complex. At 3 months, interferon should be discontinued in patients who achieve no better than a partial hematologic response and have pretreatment

TABLE 93.3	Treatment Continuation/Discontinuation Algorithm for Interferon-α in Patients with Chronic Myelogenous Leukemia	
Evaluation Time from Start of IFN-α	**Patient Characteristics**	**IFN Therapy Decision**
3 mo	Less than or equal to a partial hematologic response and poor pretreatment risk factors (splenomegaly ≥5 cm below the costal margin or pretreatment platelet count ≥700 × 10⁹/L)	Discontinue IFN-α
6 mo	Less than or equal to a partial hematologic response and poor pretreatment risk factors	Discontinue IFN-α
	Complete hematologic response, no cytogenetic response, and no pretreatment risk factors	
	or	
	Complete hematologic response, no cytogenetic response, and poor pretreatment risk factors (splenomegaly ≥ 5 cm below the costal margin or pretreatment platelet count ≥ 700 × 10⁹/L)	Continue IFN-α
12 mo	Less than or equal to a partial hematologic response	
	or	
	Complete hematologic response, no cytogenetic response, and poor pretreatment risk factors (splenomegaly ≥ 5 cm below the costal margin or pretreatment platelet count ≥ 700 × 10⁹/L)	Discontinue IFN-α
	Complete hematologic response, no cytogenetic response, and no poor pretreatment risk factors	May offer to continue IFN-α for 6 mo

risk factors (splenomegaly or thrombocytosis). At 6 months, patients with a complete hematologic response and a minor cytogenetic response have a 60% chance of achieving a major cytogenetic response. Patients with a complete hematologic response and no cytogenetic response and no pretreatment risk factors have a 38% to 45% chance of achieving a major cytogenetic response. Both of these groups should continue INF-α therapy. Patients with no cytogenetic response at 6 months and pretreatment risk factors of thrombocytosis or splenomegaly have a less than 10% chance of achieving a major cytogenetic response. INF-α should be stopped and other treatment options offered. At 12 months, if patients with pretreatment risk factors have no cytogenetic response, INF-α therapy should be stopped. However, patients with no cytogenetic response at 12 months, but with a complete hematologic response and no pretreatment risk factors, have a 16% to 26% chance of achieving a major cytogenetic response and can be offered INF-α therapy for another 6 months. It is believed that achieving a major cytogenetic response confers a survival advantage.[17]

These findings have been supported by a single institution trial reporting that failure to have a hematologic response at 3 months predicted a low probability of a cytogenetic response to INF-α and that a major or complete cytogenetic response to INF-α is associated with prolonged survival.[30]

It is not known if patients with a long-term complete cytogenetic response from INF-α can be considered cured. Patients may have no detectable Ph chromosome, yet still have residual *BCR-ABL* transcript. The absence of the *BCR-ABL* transcript is a molecular complete remission, which may be associated with a decreased relapse rate.[31] Molecular complete remissions have been observed in recipients of HCTs. There are some patients with a long-term complete cytogenetic response from INF-α who also have been observed to have nondetectable *BCR-ABL*.[27,32] It is possible that these patients have been cured of CML without a HCT, but further follow-up is required.

The cost-effectiveness of INF-α has been determined by two investigators.[32,33] For a therapy to be considered worthwhile, the marginal cost-effectiveness should be less than $50,000 per quality-adjusted life year (QALY). One trial found the marginal cost-effectiveness to be $34,800 per QALY saved.[33] The model used $1,500 as the estimated drug cost for INF-α for 1 month at a dose of 5 million units/m²/day. A second trial estimated the marginal cost-effectiveness to be $89,500 or $63,000 per QALY saved, depending on the scenario.[34] The authors estimated the monthly cost of INF-α to be $2,750 for a mean dose of 8 million units/m²/day. In the second analysis, therefore, INF-α was not found to be a cost-effective therapy. Both groups of authors reported that the models are most sensitive to manipulation of drug cost.

Imatinib. Imatinib is a tyrosine kinase inhibitor that shows promise in CML. The *BCR-ABL* transcript of CML has tyrosine kinase activity, which is necessary for its ability to cause leukemic transformation. Imatinib is an *ABL* protein tyrosine kinase inhibitor. Imatinib is available as 100-mg PO capsules or 400-mg PO tablets. The parent compound has a half-life of 18 hours, while its active N-demethyl metabolite has a half-life of 40 hours. It is primarily metabolized by CYP 3A4 enzymes. Imatinib is also a potent CYP3A4 inhibitor, and interactions with other drugs must be considered. Significant side effects include neutropenia, fatigue, fluid retention, dermatologic reactions, nausea, vomiting, and muscle cramps.[35] A phase I study showed that patients with chronic phase CML, who had failed treatment with interferon, demonstrated a 98% (53/54) hematologic response rate for 4 weeks.[36] In a phase II trial, 532 patients who had failed interferon were placed on imatinib 400 mg PO once daily. Complete hematologic response was found in 95% of patients and 60% had a major cytogenetic response.[37]

The International Randomized study of Interferon and Imatinib compared imatinib 400 mg PO daily versus interferon 5 million units/m²/day + cytarabine 20 mg/m²/day × 10 days every month in 1,106 newly diagnosed patients. The imatinib arm showed significance in all end points including complete hematologic response (97% vs. 69%), major cytogenetic response (87% vs. 35%), and complete cytogenetic response (76% vs. 14%).[38] Long-term survival benefits have recently been shown in follow-up studies. In newly diagnosed patients, survival was estimated at 15.3 years in patients who were treated with imatinib versus 9.07 years in those who received interferon and cytarabine.[39] One study looked at 261 patients who had failed interferon therapy and were subsequently treated with imatinib. After a median follow-up of 45 months, 73% had a major cytogenetic response and 63% had a complete cytogenetic response, and an estimated 4-year survival of 86%.[40]

Although the current recommended dose of imatinib for chronic phase CML is 400 mg per day (Table 93.1) and 600 mg per day for CML in transformation, some studies suggest that a higher starting dose of imatinib 400 mg twice a day may offer better disease control and a reduction in the emergence of imatinib-resistant CML clones.[41] Higher doses lead to earlier and more profound reduction in the *BCR-ABL* transcript levels, which was associated with a higher probability of progression free survival.[42] Newer studies will better determine the role of a higher dose imatinib. In addition, there are new tyrosine kinase inhibitors in phase II and early phase III trials. These ''super imatinibs'' are approximately 100 times more potent than imatinib.

ACCELERATED PHASE

Patients with CML in the accelerated phase have a 6- to 18-month average survival. There is no standard therapy for accelerated-phase CML. The treatment goal is to provide symptom palliation and a return to chronic-phase CML. Generally, each patient must be assessed and treated with an individualized treatment plan that is modified for disease response and patient tolerance. A patient with accelerated-phase CML has circulating blasts, and these blasts can be immunophenotyped to determine if the CML is transforming into a myeloid or lymphoid blast crisis phase with associated development of AML or ALL. The patient may then receive treatment appropriate for the associated acute leukemia. Imatinib has been used in patients with accelerated phase CML with modest results. One study evaluating 200 patients showed a clinical response of 90% and a complete cytogenetic response in 24%.[43] Patients receiving a HCT during the accelerated phase have a much lower survival rate than during the chronic phase.

BLAST PHASE

Patients with blast-phase CML have an expected average survival of 2 to 3 months. The goal of treatment is to provide symptom palliation and a return to chronic-phase CML. Patients should be managed with therapy for acute leukemia. Many patients have disease that is resistant to this therapy. Patients with a lymphoid blast crisis are more likely to respond than patients with a myeloid blast crisis. HCT during a blast crisis provides a 0% to 20% chance for long-term survival. For some patients with blast-phase CML, a second chronic phase may be achieved, in which case a HCT should be performed if there is an available donor. Patients in blast crisis may benefit from imatinib. One study looking at 260 patients with CML in blast crisis, demonstrated a 52% hematologic response while on 400 to 600 mg of imatinib. In addition, 31% of patients had a sustained response for at least 4 weeks and 8% had a complete hematologic response.[44]

BONE MARROW TRANSPLANT

Allogeneic Hematopoietic Cell Transplant. AHCT has the potential to cure CML and is the treatment of choice for young patients with chronic-phase CML. A human leukocyte antigen (HLA)-matched sibling donor is available for only 20% to 25% of patients with CML. HLA matching helps determine the chance of acceptance of the donor cells by the recipient. A matched HLA sibling donor has the highest chance of success, however, if a HLA-matched sibling is not available, a matched unrelated donor may be used, but with a higher risk of rejection. The probability of long-term survival for patients receiving a HCT in the chronic phase is 60% to 80%, but it is less than 20% for patients in blast crisis. Survival outcomes appear to be more favorable if the patient receives a HCT within 1 year of diagnosis. Younger patients have better outcomes, but the upper age limit is controversial and is advancing as supportive care improves.[2]

A retrospective study compared survival after HLA-identical AHCT versus treatment with INF-α or hydroxyurea. The group included patients from 15 to 55 years of age. The study described better survival with INF-α or hydroxyurea in the first 18 months from diagnosis. Survival figures for the HCT group did not surpass those of the hydroxyurea/INF-α group until 5.5 years from the initial diagnosis. If HCT was delayed for more than 1 year after diagnosis, the survival advantage from HCT decreased. At

7 years, the survival probability in the transplant group was 58% and in the hydroxyurea/INF-α group the survival probability was 32%.[45] Table 93.4 shows the recommendations for stem cell transplantation by age. The usual preparative regimens (treatment that the patient receives prior to transplant) for HCT in patients with CML are cyclophosphamide and total body irradiation or cyclophosphamide and busulfan. Modified preparative regimens with less toxic effects and equal efficacy continue to show promise in reducing the mortality from HCT, making it available to an older age group.[46]

Unrelated Donor Hematopoietic Cell Transplant. The use of unrelated bone marrow donors for HCT carries increased risk for the patient. More failure to engraft the new marrow is seen, and graft-versus-host disease (GVHD) occurs more frequently and is more severe. Because of the increased risk with unrelated donor HCTs, the decision to perform this type of transplant in a patient with CML who is feeling well can be difficult.[47,48]

Most recommendations for unrelated donor transplants for CML have included an upper age limit for patients of 35 to 45 years. It is possible that this age limit may be raised. A review of unrelated donor transplants for CML showed a 74% 5-year survival rate for patients younger than 50 years who received matched unrelated donor transplants within the first year of diagnosis.[48] This high survival rate may reflect improved supportive care, including antiviral and antifungal prophylaxis.

A decision analysis for unrelated donor HCT compared transplant within the first year from diagnosis (early transplant), delayed transplant, and no transplant.[47] The study concluded that unrelated donor transplant performed within the first year was superior in quality-adjusted expected survival to no transplant, but that it takes 4 years before survival for patients receiving an early transplant is improved over that for patients with no transplant. Delayed transplant (i.e., transplant later than 1 year from diagnosis) also showed increased quality-adjusted expected survival compared to no transplant, although it took 6 years to realize this difference.

A model of the cost-effectiveness of unrelated donor HCT compared to therapy with INF-α or hydroxyurea has been developed.[49] Compared to INF-α therapy, the cost-effectiveness ratio for an unrelated donor HCT is $51,800 for each QALY gained and compared to hydroxyurea it is $55,000. When the model parameter estimates were manipulated to simulate changes in clinical scenarios, the cost-effectiveness ratio ranged from $32,600 to $126,800 QALY. The authors concluded that while unrelated donor HCT is very expensive, it is cost-effective for a carefully selected patient population in whom it can significantly prolong life.

A patient with chronic-phase CML who is younger than 50 years old and who lacks a matched sibling donor should be offered a matched, unrelated donor transplant, if a donor is available, and the institution is experienced in performing unrelated donor marrow transplants. Older patients in the same situation should be given a trial of imatinib. Alterna-

TABLE 93.4	Summary of Treatment Options: Chronic Myelogenous Leukemia

Treatment Options for CML Chronic Phase

Young (<50)

Option 1	Option 2
HLA-matched sibling HSCT (Patients may be started on imatinib while searching for donor)	Imatinib[a]
If no HLA-matched sibling donor, a MUD should be considered	If no response to imatinib, consider HLA-matched sibling donor
If no response to transplant, consider experimental agents.	If no HLA-matched sibling donor, a MUD should be considered
	If no response to transplant, consider experimental agents.

Age 50–60

Option 1	Option 2
HLA-matched sibling HSCT (Patients may be started on imatinib while searching for donor)	Imatinib[a]
If no response to HLA-matched transplant, consider experimental agents	If no response to imatinib, consider HLA-matched sibling donor
	If no response to HLA-matched transplant, consider experimental agents

MUDs are usually not recommended for patients over the age of 50, however, a nonmyeloablative transplant may be indicated.

Older (>60)

Option 1	Option 2
Nonmyeloablative transplant	Imatinib
If no response to transplant, consider experimental agents	If poor response, consider nonmyeloablative transplant or experimental agents

[a] First-line treatment will depend on age of patient, staging of disease (chronic, acute, blast), and availability of HLA-matched donor. First-line therapy is still controversial. Recent data suggest that imatinib should be first-line therapy, however there is still no long-term survival data, curative ability is still unknown and there is a concern regarding resistance.

CML, chronic myelogenous leukemia; HLA, human leukocyte antigen; HSCT, hematopoietic stem cell transplant; MUD, matched unrelated donor.

tively, nonmyeloablative HCT regimens may be considered (see below).

Nonmyeloablative Hematopoietic Cell Transplant. An important change in the philosophy of preparative regimens for allogeneic transplant is the realization that ablative regimens may not be absolutely necessary. Engraftment can be accomplished by using less intensive and toxic regimens. This translates into a decrease in treatment related mortality, which has been the major concern for patients older than 50 years of age.[50] Nonmyeloablative regimens rely more on the graft versus leukemic effect than the cytotoxic effects of the traditional preparative regimens. Experience is limited, and more trials are warranted.

Relapse After Hematopoietic Stem Cell Transplant. Relapse after HCT may be hematologic or cytogenetic. It is common for the Ph chromosome to be detectable for several months after the transplant. This does not necessarily herald relapse. The persistence of the Ph chromosome for more than 6 months after transplant, the reappearance of the Ph chromosome after it has disappeared, or a rising proportion of Ph-positive metaphases are triggers to begin therapy for relapse. Several approaches that have been successful for treating CML relapse after HCT are donor lymphocyte infusion (DLI), and the use of INF-α or imatinib. DLI appears to be more effective in eradicating the Ph chromosome compared to INF-α; however, there is significant toxicity in the form of loss of engraftment or severe GVHD, with as much as a 20% mortality rate. INF-α appears to provide cytogenetic remission in a significant number of patients with cytogenetic relapse, without causing life-threatening toxic effects.[51,52] A reasonable strategy may be to offer INF-α therapy to patients with cytogenetic relapse, and if they do not have remission within 1 year, to offer DLI. Patients with hematologic relapse may receive either INF-α or DLI. There may be a role for combination therapy using a modified dose of DLI and INF-α.[52] There are also reports of patients who have failed INF-α and DLI who have responded to imatinib. Twenty-eight patients with CML, who relapsed after an allogeneic stem cell transplant, were placed on 400 to 1,000 mg imatinib daily. The overall response rate was 79% with a 35% complete cytogenetic response rate. The 1-year survival rate was 74%.[53]

Autologous Hematopoietic Stem Cell Transplant. It may be possible to obtain long-term survival in patients by using an infusion of Ph chromosome-negative autologous peripheral blood progenitor cells.[54] Some investigators have reported that treatment in the early chronic phase, before initiation of INF-α therapy, may allow for collection of more Ph-negative stem cells. In one study, patients received a course of intensive conventional chemotherapy, followed by granulocyte colony-stimulating factor. Peripheral blood progenitor cells were pheresed (removed) when blood count results were beginning to improve. These patients then received preparative regimens of high-dose chemotherapy with or without total body irradiation, followed by infusion of the previously mobilized stem cells. Half of the patients achieved Ph-negative marrow, but follow-up has been short.[55] With AHCT, the duration of remission seems to depend on the graft-versus-leukemia (GVL) effect. With the GVL effect, the donor hematopoietic cells recognize persistent leukemia cells as foreign and act to eradicate them. This effect is absent in autograft recipients. It may be necessary to provide posttransplant maintenance therapy such as INF-α to patients receiving autografts. Autografting may prove useful for patients without matched donors or who are outside the age limit to tolerate allogeneic grafting. This procedure is investigational and should be performed in the context of a clinical trial.

Hematopoietic Stem Cell Versus Imatinib. To date, only an allogeneic hematopoietic stem cell offers cure to a patient with CML, however data from imatinib is revolutionizing treatment. Data suggests quick and reliable decreases in surrogate markers traditionally associated with outcomes in patients treated with interferon, but not yet proven with imatinib.[56] Long-term outcomes are unknown in patients treated with imatinib alone. Currently, there are two approaches to the management of a newly diagnosed CML patient: (a) to offer a trial of imatinib and offer a hematopoietic stem cell transplant to those who fail imatinib treatment, or (b) to continue to discuss transplant up front to those for whom a more aggressive therapy is thought to be appropriate.[57]

CHRONIC LYMPHOCYTIC LEUKEMIA

CLL is a slowly progressing leukemia that may be quiescent for years and occurs primarily in older adults. It is not curable, but in many patients does not decrease survival compared to the normal population. Therefore, CLL is usually not treated unless the patient is symptomatic or the rate of disease progression increases.

CLL is a malignancy of monoclonal small mature lymphocytes that have prolonged survival and which proliferate and accumulate in the blood, bone marrow, lymph nodes, spleen, and liver. Ninety-five percent of patients have B-cell CLL and 5% have T-cell CLL.

TREATMENT GOALS: CHRONIC LYMPHOCYTIC LEUKEMIA

The treatment goal is to prolong survival and palliate disease symptoms, while maintaining good quality of life.[58] There is no known curative therapy for CLL. Aggressive therapy with HCT may be an appropriate consideration in younger patients with risk factors for poor survival, but this approach is investigational.

EPIDEMIOLOGY

The cause of CLL is unknown. Radiation and drug exposure do not seem to be risk factors. There may be an increased risk with industrial exposure for agricultural and asbestos workers.[59] CLL is primarily a disease of older adults, and its incidence increases with age. The median age at diagnosis is 65 years.[58] More men than women are affected by a ratio of about 2:1. CLL is the most commonly occurring leukemia in Western Europe and North America, but it is uncommon in Japan and China. Immigrants from Japan to the West do not acquire an increased risk for the disease.[59]

PATHOPHYSIOLOGY

CLL may result from a mutational change that prevents normal programmed cell death (apoptosis), rather than from increased cell proliferation.[60] It is speculated that a normal

CD5-positive lymphocyte is transformed via multiple mutational steps into a monoclonal leukemic cell line that lacks normal apoptotic mechanisms, which then accumulates.[58] Most CLL cells (about 95%) are in the quiescent G_0 stage of the cell cycle. Symptoms of CLL arise from accumulation of leukemic lymphocytes in organs and tissues and from immune dysfunction.

CLINICAL PRESENTATION AND DIAGNOSIS

SIGNS AND SYMPTOMS

Patients are often asymptomatic at diagnosis, with the diagnosis being made when a routine complete blood count is done. Patients with symptoms may report typical ''B'' symptoms of weight loss, fever, fatigue, and night sweats. They may experience early satiety or a feeling of abdominal fullness from splenomegaly or hepatomegaly. They may notice enlarged lymph nodes and may report frequent infections.

DIAGNOSIS

The diagnosis of CLL is based on an absolute lymphocyte count in the blood of 5×10^9 per liter. The leukemic cells are normal-appearing small mature lymphocytes. They have monoclonal expression of either κ or λ light chains. There is a smaller than normal amount of surface immunoglobulin.[61] B lymphocytes in CLL express surface antigens CD5, CD19, CD20, and CD23. If a bone marrow aspirate and biopsy are performed, more than 30% of nucleated cells must be lymphoid for a diagnosis of CLL.

There are two staging systems for CLL: (a) the Rai system[62] and (b) the Binet system.[63] The Rai system is used primarily in the United States and the Binet system is used mostly in Europe. Both systems are useful and either can be applied. The two systems stage CLL based on evidence of lymphocyte infiltration into tissue and organs and on evidence of impaired bone marrow function, as seen by anemia or thrombocytopenia. Patients with low-risk disease exhibit lymphocytosis only and have a median survival of longer than 10 years. Patients with high-risk disease have lymphocytosis with anemia or thrombocytopenia and have a median

TABLE 93.5	Staging Systems Used for Chronic Lymphocytic Leukemia				
System and Risk	**Stage**	**Definition**	**Percentage of Patients With CLL in Stage**	**Survival**	
				Median (yr)	**10-Year (%)**
Rai staging system					
Low	0	Lymphocytosis only	31	>10	59
Intermediate	I	Lymphocytosis and lymphadenopathy	35	9	
	II	Lymphocytosis and splenomegaly with or without lymphadenopathy or hepatomegaly	26	5	10
High	III	Lymphocytosis and anemia, with or without organomegaly	6	2	10
	IV	Lymphocytosis, anemia, and thrombocytopenia, with or without organomegaly	2	2	10
Binet staging system					
Low	A	Lymphocytosis, with enlargement of < lymphoid areas[a]	63	>10	51
	A'	Stage A with lymphocyte count of ≤ 30,000/mm³ and hemoglobin concentration of ≥120 g/L	49	>10	56
	A''	Stage A with lymphocyte count of >30,000/mm³, hemoglobin concentration of <20 g/L, or both	14	7	38
Intermediate	B	Lymphocytosis, with enlargement of ≥ lymphoid areas	30	5	
High	C	Lymphocytosis and anemia, or thrombocytopenia, or both	7	2	

[a] The following lymphoid areas are included: cervical, axillary, and inguinal (unilateral or bilateral), spleen, and liver.

survival of 2 years (Table 93.5).[64] One useful prognostic indicator is lymphocyte doubling time. A lymphocyte doubling time of less than 1 year is associated with a much worse prognosis. The typical patient with CLL usually develops a higher stage of disease slowly over several years. The patient then requires more treatment, and the treatment gradually needs to be more aggressive to control symptoms, bringing with it more side effects of therapy.

In a small percentage of patients CLL may transform abruptly into a large-cell non-Hodgkin lymphoma that is resistant to treatment. This is called Richter transformation or Richter syndrome. The patient will have fever, increased lymphadenopathy, a rising LDH level, and widespread tissue infiltration of lymphoma cells. It occurs in 3% to 15% of patients with CLL. Few patients with Richter transformation survive longer than 6 to 8 months. There is controversy over whether the lymphoma arises from the original malignant clone or is from a separate, distinct clone. It appears that the lymphoma arises from the original clone in at least two thirds of patients.[59,65]

Patients with CLL may develop autoimmune reactions against hematopoietic cells. Autoimmune hemolytic anemia is estimated to occur in 5% to 37% of patients with CLL.[66] Pure red cell aplasia may be present in 6% of patients. Idiopathic thrombocytopenia occurs in 2% to 3% of patients. The cause of the autoimmune dysfunction is not well understood.

The immune dysfunction seen in patients with CLL contributes significantly to the morbidity of the disease. The mechanism for the immune dysfunction is multifaceted and includes impairment in humoral and cell-mediated immune function.[67] The malignant CLL B-cell functions poorly as an antigen-presenting cell. The B-cell to T-cell interaction is weakened. There are a decreased number of normal B-cells, and their immune function may be down regulated by cytokine production from the malignant B-cell clone. This may contribute to the low levels of immunoglobulin usually seen in patients with CLL. T cells in patients with CLL may be anergic. Natural killer (NK) cells have a decreased ability to become activated and to lyse target cells. NK cell mediation of antibody-dependent cell-mediated cytotoxicity is decreased. There is a proposed mechanism in which the dysfunction of the NK cells and T cells in patients with CLL may lengthen the survival of the malignant B-cell clone and so contribute to the progression of the disease.

Infectious complications are a major manifestation of the immune dysfunction seen in CLL. The majority of deaths in patients with CLL are actually due to bacterial infections. The usual infecting organisms are *Staphylococcus aureus, Streptococcus pneumoniae, Haemophilus influenzae, Escherichia coli, Klebsiella pneumoniae,* and *Pseudomonas aeruginosa.* With the recent increased use of purine analogs such as fludarabine, cladribine, and pentostatin, new pathogens have been observed.[68] These include *Listeria* sp, *Pneumocystis carinii, Mycobacterium tuberculosis, Nocardia* sp, *Candida* sp, *Aspergillus* sp, and herpes viruses. The risk for these infections increases if the patient receives corticosteroids concurrently or before purine analog therapy.[69]

PSYCHOSOCIAL ASPECTS

Patients may be told that they have incurable leukemia and that they do not need treatment. This confuses most patients. Patients with low-stage disease may have no symptoms or have symptoms that are controlled with an oral medication taken once or twice a month. The change to a more aggressive disease will develop gradually, usually over several years. The patient is usually elderly and may have other medical problems, some of which may be more life threatening or may affect the person's quality of life more distinctly than does CLL. If the patient is young with high-risk disease, he or she may be faced with a choice between a HCT with its multiple risks, which has not yet been shown to improve survival, but may ultimately control the leukemia, or standard therapy, which is usually well tolerated, but does not prolong survival.

TREATMENT

Patients with CLL are usually only treated if they develop uncomfortable symptoms, such as increasing adenopathy, or constitutional symptoms, such as fatigue and weight loss, develop significant anemia or thrombocytopenia, or show evidence of more rapid disease progression, such as a lymphocyte doubling time of less than 1 year.

PHARMACOTHERAPY

Alkylating Agents. When the decision is made to treat a patient with CLL, the initial therapy is usually chlorambucil, an oral alkylating agent. It may be given at 0.1 mg per kilogram daily, or at 4 mg per kilogram every 2 to 4 weeks, or as a 0.7 mg per kilogram total dose over 4 days every month (Table 93.6). It is available as a 2-mg tablet and is well absorbed orally. Chlorambucil is hepatically metabolized with hepatic and renal clearance of the metabolites. The half-

TABLE 93.6	Agents used in Chronic Lymphocytic Leukemia
Summary of Suggested Dosing for Agents Used in CLL	
Chlorambucil[59]	0.1 mg/kg/day PO
Cyclophosphamide[73]	1–2 mg/kg/day PO
Fludarabine[74]	25 mg/m² /day IV over 30 minutes × 5 days every 4 weeks
Cladribine[83]	0.1 mg/kg/day continuous IV infusion over 24 hours,
Rituximab[92]	375 mg/m² /day IV once every 4 weeks
Alemtuzumab[95]	Dose escalation to 30 mg IV three times weekly for 16 weeks

CLL, chronic lymphocytic leukemia; PO, by mouth, IV, intravenously.

life is 2 to 8 hours. The dose is adjusted for disease response and myelosuppression. Chlorambucil is well tolerated and has mild side effects other than myelosuppression. The use of chlorambucil in patients with CLL does not prolong survival, but does control disease symptoms. It has been shown to be as effective as more aggressive and more toxic combinations of chemotherapy such as cyclophosphamide, vincristine, and prednisone (CVP) or cyclophosphamide, melphalan, and prednisone.[70–72] No advantage has been found for starting chlorambucil therapy in patients in the early stage of disease.[64] Prednisone may be added to chlorambucil at a dose of 40 mg/m^2/day PO for 5 days every month. Other schedules have also been used. The addition of prednisone to chlorambucil does not prolong survival, but may increase symptom improvement in lymphadenopathy and splenomegaly. It appears to have particular value in patients who have immune-mediated anemia or thrombocytopenia. Because of emerging evidence suggesting that prior steroid therapy may contribute to the risk of opportunistic infection in patients who eventually receive one of the purine analogs, such as fludarabine, an attempt should be made to limit the use of prednisone to those patients who show response of CLL-related anemia or thrombocytopenia to steroid therapy. Cyclophosphamide, another alkylating agent, appears to have efficacy similar to that of chlorambucil. The usual dose is 1 to 2 mg/kg/day. There is no clear advantage when cyclophosphamide is given in combination with other chemotherapy agents compared to chlorambucil alone.

The alkylating agent (chlorambucil or cyclophosphamide) is usually continued until the patient's symptoms have responded and no additional improvement is seen or until the patient experiences myelotoxicity.[73] The drug can then be stopped. If the patient's disease symptoms recur or worsen after therapy is discontinued, it is reasonable to renew treatment with the same agent. If the disease progresses while the patient is receiving therapy, the alkylating agent should be discontinued, and another agent, such as a purine analog, should be started.

Purine Analogs. Three purine analogs that have shown efficacy in CLL include (a) fludarabine, (b) cladribine, and (c) pentostatin. The most experience is with fludarabine. It has been approved for use in the treatment of CLL refractory to alkylating agents. Cladribine has also been shown to be effective for this indication. Pentostatin has not been used as extensively, and may be less effective than fludarabine or cladribine in the treatment of CLL. There appears to be cross-resistance between fludarabine and cladribine. A patient whose disease is refractory to one of these agents is unlikely to respond to the other.

Fludarabine phosphate is a water soluble analog of adenosine and a fluorinated analog of the antiviral drug, vidarabine. It is resistant to adenosine deaminase. Fludarabine is first dephosphorylated to 2-fluoro-ara-adenine, and is then converted intracellularly to 2-fluoro-ara-adenosine triphosphate (ATP), which is the active form. It inhibits DNA polymerase, and ribonucleotide reductase. Fludarabine is also effective against the nonproliferating cells of CLL, possibly

by inducing apoptosis. The half-life of 2-fluoro-ara-adenine is about 10 hours, with a clearance of 8.9 L/hr/m^2 and a volume of distribution of 98 L/m^2.[74] Fludarabine is primarily cleared renally, and the dose should be adjusted for renal impairment, although exact guidelines are not available. The usual dose for the treatment of B-cell CLL is 25 mg/m^2/day intravenously (IV) over 30 minutes daily for 5 days every 4 weeks (Table 93.6). The drug should be continued for three cycles after the maximal response has been achieved.[8,9,75] It should be discontinued for disease progression or for the development of hemolytic anemia. The usual and expected side effect is myelosuppression, which may be cumulative. Following fludarabine, colony-stimulating factors may be useful in reducing the myelosuppression, allowing for the administration of fludarabine therapy to continue as planned. The use of colony-stimulating factors may also decrease infections.[76] At high doses of fludarabine, severe irreversible neurotoxicity has been observed, but these doses are no longer used.[77] Rarely, patients may develop interstitial pneumonitis. Opportunistic infections are common, especially in patients who have had extensive prior therapy or have received steroids. Patients may even develop infections after the first dose of fludarabine without a history of corticosteroid use.[78] Patients should be carefully monitored for infection, and care must be taken not to miss infections such as *P. carinii* pneumonia (PCP), listeriosis, tuberculosis, herpes infections, and *Candida* or *Aspergillus* infections.[79,80] Consideration should be given for the use of PCP prophylaxis in all patients receiving fludarabine. It should be required in patients with CLL who have a current or previous history of corticosteroid use. The role for prophylaxis against herpes and fungal infections has not been determined.

There may be an increased risk of hematologic immune manifestations such as hemolytic anemia in fludarabine-treated patients. Although hemolytic anemia is common in patients with CLL, the purine analogs appear to further promote its occurrence. A causal relationship has not been firmly established. Most patients with fludarabine-associated hemolytic anemia have a recurrence if the drug is given again, which carries a high risk of mortality. Patients who develop hemolytic anemia with any of the purine analogs should not receive further therapy with any drug in this class.[80,81]

In previously treated patients with high Rai-stage disease, the response rate to fludarabine is 31% to 36%.[82] The response rate is improved in patients who receive fludarabine as first-line therapy and has been reported to be as high as 78% in one series.[83] Although fludarabine is effective in achieving a response, there is no evidence that its use as first-line therapy instead of chlorambucil improves overall survival. It is also unknown if there are quality of life differences between treatment with chlorambucil and fludarabine regimens.

Cladribine is a chlorinated analog of adenosine. It is resistant to adenosine deaminase. Deoxycytidine kinase phosphorylates cladribine intracellularly to 2-Cd-adenosine monophosphate (2-Cd-AMP), which is then converted to 2-Cd-

ATP. 2-Cd-AMP is incorporated into DNA. 2-Cd-ATP inhibits ribonucleotide reductase. Cladribine also shows activity in resting cells by depleting nicotinamide adenine dinucleotide levels. Ultimately, the activity of cladribine results in apoptosis, even in quiescent lymphocytes.[8,9] The half-life is 5 to 6 hours; plasma clearance is about 980 mL/hr/kg, with a large amount of variability. The volume of distribution is about 9 L per kilogram. It is not known how cladribine is cleared from the body, but there is some renal clearance. Although approved for use in hairy cell leukemia where it is the drug of choice, it has also shown substantial activity in CLL.[84,85] The usual dose is 0.1 mg/kg/day as a continuous IV infusion daily for 7 days every 4 weeks (Table 93.6). Other similar schedules have been used in clinical studies with a usual maximum dose of 0.7 mg per kiolgram per cycle (e.g., 0.12 mg/kg/day IV over 2 hours daily for 5 days).[86] Bone marrow suppression is the usual and expected side effect. As with fludarabine, infections are a common occurrence, and patients should be monitored closely. Fever, even without infection, is common. Nausea may occur, but it is usually mild. High doses of cladribine, which are not in clinical use, have produced neurotoxicity. Immune hematologic effects have occurred with the use of cladribine in patients with CLL. Cladribine has been associated with an increased risk of hemolytic anemia, which may be fatal.[87] If hemolytic anemia develops while the patient is receiving therapy, the drug should be discontinued, and the patient should not be given additional therapy with cladribine or another purine analog. If the patient has a history of disease (CLL)-related autoimmune hemolytic anemia, it is appropriate to attempt therapy with a purine analog, as some patients have shown resolution of disease-related autoimmune hemolytic anemia when treated with fludarabine or cladribine. At this time, pentostatin for CLL should be reserved for use in the context of a clinical trial.

Therapy for patients with CLL for whom treatment is indicated should begin with chlorambucil. If the patient has a good performance status and is young, the use of fludarabine as first-line therapy may be considered because it may provide a higher response rate and a longer remission. However, it has more severe and dangerous side effects, requires IV administration, and is expensive compared to chlorambucil. It is not known if fludarabine improves survival compared to chlorambucil. If a patient receiving chlorambucil fails to respond or has disease progression, the patient should be treated with fludarabine or cladribine, because these agents are less toxic than combination therapy such as cyclophosphamide, doxorubicin (Adria), and prednisone (CAP) or cyclophosphamide, hydroxydaunorubicin, vincristine (Oncovin), and prednisone (CHOP) and may be more effective.[88] At this time, fludarabine should probably be chosen over cladribine for CLL, as their efficacy and safety profile are similar, but fludarabine is approved for the indication, is easier to administer, and is less expensive. If a patient fails to respond to a purine analog or shows disease progression while receiving therapy, combination therapy such as

CHOP may be considered. Careful consideration must be given to the patient's quality of life and performance status before initiating therapy that will not prolong survival and that has significant toxic effects in elderly, heavily pretreated patients.

Intravenous Immunoglobulin. Hypogammaglobulinemia is a frequent finding in patients with CLL and may contribute to the incidence of bacterial infections. The administration of IV immunoglobulin was found to reduce the incidence of bacterial infections but not to prolong survival. The study used immunoglobulin 400 mg per kilogram IV every 3 weeks. A lower dose may also provide a similar benefit. In general, IV immunoglobulin is not recommended as standard therapy for patients with CLL. It may be appropriate in a patient with advanced disease and low immunoglobulin levels who has frequent bacterial infections requiring hospitalization.[89] IV immunoglobulin may be useful in the management of autoimmune hemolytic anemia. One recommended dosing schedule is 400 mg/kg/day IV for 5 days, repeated as needed.[90]

Monoclonal Antibodies

Rituximab. Monoclonal antibodies have been used for the treatment of CLL. Rituximab is a monoclonal antibody against cell surface antigen CD20. It is currently approved for the treatment of B-cell non-Hodgkin lymphoma, but has also been used for a variety of CD20-positive B-cell lineage tumors. Studies have looked at rituximab in previously untreated CLL[91] and relapsed or refractory disease.[91] Although there are no randomized comparative trials, initial reports indicated a reasonable response rate with rituximab (51%)[90] compared to treatments with fludarabine(63%),[86] and with less toxicities. More recently, the combination of fludarabine with rituximab given concurrently or sequentially was found to prolong progression free and overall survival in previously untreated CLL.[91] Generally, rituximab is well tolerated, however, there have been reports of deaths, hypotension, and tumor lysis syndrome with the use of this agent.[92,93] This happens more often with the initial dose of rituximab. It is recommended that patients be premedicated with acetaminophen and diphenhydramine prior to each infusion to minimize risk. For rituximab dosing refer to Table 93.6. Overall, rituximab may have a role in the treatment of CLL patients who cannot tolerate traditional chemotherapy.

Alemtuzumab. Alemtuzumab is a human anti-CD52 monoclonal antibody. CD52 antigen is expressed on the surface of more than 95% of human B and T lymphocytes. There appears to be some activity of alemtuzumab even in heavily pretreated patients with CLL, including patients who have received purine analogs.[94–96] Some patients have achieved a complete response to this agent. Alemtuzumab has been used in combination with fludarabine with some success.[97] In patients with bulky lymphadenopathy, alemtuzumab was not as effective, suggesting a potential role in postremission therapy,[98] but to date, there are no set guidelines. The primary toxic effect is immune suppression and a high frequency of infections is seen with this agent. The use of fluconazole, acyclovir, and trimethoprim/sulfamethoxazole for prophylaxis has minimized infectious complications. For alemtuzumab dosing refer to Table 93.6. Hypersensitivity is also a risk and premedication with acetaminophen and diphenhydramine is recommended.

BONE MARROW TRANSPLANT

The role of HCT in the management of CLL is controversial. The age of most patients with CLL is above the limit for AHCT. The value of autologous HCT in a disease in which the bone marrow is heavily infiltrated with disease may be limited. Patients with low-stage disease often have the same life expectancy as age-matched control subjects. No survival advantage has yet been demonstrated using HCT in patients with CLL. Nevertheless, in patients younger than 55 years of age with good performance status and Rai stage III or IV disease, AHCT may be considered.[99,100] In patients between 55 and 65 years of age with good performance status and high Rai stage disease, an autologous HCT may be appropriate. Several investigators have reported the feasibility of transplant under these conditions, reporting a high percentage of patients achieving a complete response, and in some studies, low transplant-related mortality.[101-103] One study reported that prior treatment with fludarabine might reduce the incidence of GVHD, owing to its immunosuppressive effects.[104] Patients undergoing autologous or AHCT for CLL should be treated within the framework of a clinical study.

An exciting new development is the use of nonablative and less toxic preparative regimens for AHCT. This approach harnesses the GVL effect to provide the antileukemic response, instead of relying on the intensity of the chemotherapy and radiation therapy to eradicate the leukemic cells. This milder preparative regimen decreases the toxic risks of transplantation, making it more tolerable for older patients.[105]

NONPHARMACOLOGIC THERAPY

Patients may sometimes benefit from the removal of their spleen. In particular, patients with refractory anemia or thrombocytopenia often show improvement after splenectomy.[106] Splenic radiation has also been of value for patients with symptomatic splenomegaly that does not respond to drug therapy.

IMPROVING OUTCOMES

Infection is the leading cause of death in patients with CLL. Many of the infections are common bacterial infections that can be treated with standard antibiotics. Patients need to be educated about the signs and symptoms of infections and instructed to seek medical evaluation when these signs and symptoms occur.

KEY POINTS

CHRONIC MYELOGENOUS LEUKEMIA

- The earlier an allogeneic transplant is performed in the course of CML, the better the chance for long-term disease-free survival
- Patients with chronic-phase CML who are younger than age 50 years with a matched sibling donor should undergo an AHCT within the first year following diagnosis
- Patients without a donor for a HCT and patients who are older and in poor health are not candidates for HCT
- There are many patients with CML who do not fit into the above categories. Making decisions about treatment of these patients is difficult and should be done on a case-by-case basis
- Imatinib may be used as initial treatment in some patients, however, its exact place in overall management is still under investigation
- Patients without a matched sibling donor or patients who are older than age 50 years should be given a trial of imatinib. In the absence of a complete cytogenetic response, AHCT should be offered if age and functional status allow and a donor is available

CHRONIC LYMPHOCYTIC LEUKEMIA

- CLL is incurable at this time
- Many patients with CLL do not require treatment. Patients with low-stage disease do not benefit from the addition of drug therapy
- Patients are at high risk for infection from the disease and from drug therapy and, therefore, require careful monitoring
- Autoimmune hematologic disease is common
- Aggressive therapy, such as HCT, should be reserved for patients with good performance status and progressive disease

ACKNOWLEDGMENT

The author acknowledges the contribution of Betsy Aulthaus, Pharm. D., who authored the corresponding chapter in the Seventh Edition. Portions of that chapter have been used in this edition.

SELECTED READINGS

Athens J. Chronic myelogenous leukemia. In: Lee GR, Bithell TC, Foerster JW, et al. Wintrobe's clinical hematology. 9th ed. Philadelphia: Lea and Febiger, 1993:1969–1998.

Byrd JC, Stilgenbauer S, Flinn IW. Chronic lymphocytic leukemia. Educational program. Am Soc Hematol 1:163–183, 2004.

Deisseroth AB, Kantarjian H, Andreeff M, et al. Chronic leukemias. In: Devita VT, Hellman S, Rosenberg RA. Cancer principles and practice of oncology. 5th ed. Philadephia: Lippincott-Raven 1997: 2321–2338.

Foester J. Chronic lymphocytic leukemia. In: Lee GR, Bithell TC, Foerster JW, Luekn JN. Wintrobe's clinical hematology, 9th ed. Philadelphia: Lea and Febiger, 1993:2034–2053.

Melo JV, Hughes TP, Apperley JF. Chronic myeloid leukemia. Educational program. Am Soc Hematol 1:132–152, 2003.

REFERENCES

1. Sokal JE, Baccarani M, Russo D, et al. Staging and prognosis in chronic myelogenous leukemia. Semin Hematol 25:49–61, 1988.
2. Lee SJ, Anasetti C, Horowitz MM, et al. Initial therapy for chronic myelogenous leukemia: playing the odds [editorial]. J Clin Oncol 16:2897–2903, 1988.
3. Athens JW. Chronic myeloid leukemia. In: Lee GR, Bithell TG, Foerster J, et al. Wintrobe's clinical hematology. 9th ed. Philadelphia: Lea & Febiger, 1993:1969–1998.
4. Cortes JE, Talpaz M, Kantarjian H. Chronic myelogenous leukemia: a review. Am J Med 100:555–570, 1996.
5. DeiningerWM, Goldman JM, Melo JV. The molecular biology of chronic myeloid leukemia. Blood 96:3343–3356, 2000.
6. Ferrajoli A, Fizzotti M, Liberati AM, et al. Chronic myelogenous leukemia: an update on the biological findings and therapeutic approaches. Crit Rev Oncol Hematol 22:151–174, 1996.
7. Hardman JG, Limbird LE, Molinoff PB, et al. Goodman & Gilman's the pharmacological basis of therapeutics. 9th ed. New York: McGraw-Hill, 1996.
8. Dorr RT, Von Hoff DD. Cancer chemotherapy handbook. 2nd ed. Norwalk, CT: Appleton & Lange, 1994.
9. Chabner BA, Longo DL. Cancer chemotherapy and biotherapy. 2nd ed. Philadelphia: Lippincott-Raven, 1996.
10. Package labeling. Busulfan. Research Triangle Park, NC: Glaxo-Wellcome, 1996.
11. Package labeling. Hydroxyurea. New Jersey: Bristol Laboratories, 1996.
12. Gwilt PR, Tracewell WG. Pharmacokinetics and pharmacodynamics of hydroxyurea. Clin Pharmacokinet 34:347–358, 1998.
13. Rodriguez GI, Kuhn JG, Weiss GR, et al. A bioavailability and pharmacokinetic study of oral and intravenous hydroxyurea. Blood 91:1533–1541, 1998.
14. Best PJ, Daoud MS, Pittelkow MR, et al. Hydroxyurea-induced leg ulceration in 14 patients. Ann Intern Med 128:29–32, 1998.
15. Hehlmann R, Heimpel H, Hasford J, et al. Randomized comparison of busulfan and hydroxyurea in chronic myelogenous leukemia: prolongation of survival by hydroxyurea. Blood 82:398–407, 1993.
16. Wetzler M, Kantarjian H, Kurzrock R, et al. Interferon-α therapy for chronic myelogenous leukemia. Am J Med 99:402–410, 1995.
17. Kantarjian HM, Smith TL, O'Brien S, et al. Prolonged survival in chronic myelogenous leukemia after cytogenetic response to interferon-α therapy. Ann Intern Med 122:254–261, 1995.
18. Deisseroth AB, Kantarjian H, Andreef M, et al. Chronic leukemias. In: DeVita VT, Hellman S, Rosenberg SA, eds. Cancer: principles and practice of oncology. 5th ed. Philadelphia: Lippincott-Raven, 1997.
19. Schofield JR, Robinson WA, Murphy JR, et al. Low doses of interferon-α are as effective as higher doses in inducing remissions and prolonging survival in chronic myeloid leukemia. Ann Intern Med 121:736–744, 1994.
20. Chronic Myeloid Leukemia Trialists' Collaborative Group. Interferon alfa versus chemotherapy for chronic myeloid leukemia: a meta-analysis of seven randomized trials. J Natl Cancer Inst 89: 1616–1620, 1997.
21. Ohnishi K, Ohno R, Tomonaga M, et al. A randomized trial comparing interferon-α with busulfan for newly diagnosed chronic myelogenous leukemia in chronic phase. Blood 86:906–916, 1995.
22. The Benelux CML Study Group. Randomized study on hydroxyurea alone versus hydroxyurea combined with low-dose interferon-α 2b for chronic myeloid leukemia. Blood 91:2713–2721, 1998.
23. Hehlmann R, Heimpel H, Hossfield DK, et al. Randomized study of the combination of hydroxyurea and interferon alpha versus hydroxyurea monotherapy during the chronic phase of chronic myelogenous leukemia (CML Study II). Bone Marrow Transplant 17(Suppl 3):S21–S24, 1997.
24. The Italian Cooperative Study Group on Chronic Myeloid Leukemia. Interferon alfa-2a as compared with conventional chemotherapy for the treatment of chronic myeloid leukemia. N Engl J Med 330:820–825, 1994.
25. Hasford J, Baccarani M, Hehlmann R, et al. Interferon-α and hydroxyurea in early chronic myeloid leukemia: a comparative analysis of the Italian and German chronic myeloid leukemia trials with interferon-α. Blood 87:5384–5391, 1996.
26. The Italian Cooperative Study Group on Chronic Myeloid Leukemia. Long-term follow-up of the Italian trial of interferon-α versus conventional chemotherapy in chronic myeloid leukemia. Blood 92:1541–1548, 1998.
27. Hehlmann R, Berger U, Pfirrmann M, et al. Randomized comparison of interferon alfa and hydroxyurea with hydroxyurea monotherapy in chronic myeloid leukemia (CML-study II): prolongation of survival by the combination of interferon alfa and hydroxyurea. Leukemia 17:1529–1537, 2003.
28. Guilhot F, Chastang C, Michallet M, et al. Interferon alfa-2b combined with cytarabine versus interferon alone in chronic myelogenous leukemia. N Engl J Med 337:223–229, 1997.
29. Sacchi S, Kantarjian HM, Smith TI, et al. Early treatment decisions with interferon-alfa therapy in early chronic-phase chronic myelogenous leukemia. J Clin Oncol 16:882–889, 1998.
30. Mahob FX, Fabres C, Pueyo S, et al. Response at three months is a good predictive factor for newly diagnosed chronic myeloid leukemia patients treated by recombinant interferon-α. Blood 92: 4059–4065, 1998.
31. Hochhaus A, Reiter A, Saussele S, et al. Molecular heterogeneity in complete cytogenetic responders after interferon-alpha therapy for chronic myelogenous leukemia: low levels of minimal residual disease are associated with continuing remission. Blood 95:62–66, 2000.
32. Kurzrock R, Estrov Z, Kantarjian H, et al. Conversion of interferon-induced, long-term cytogenetic remissions in chronic myelogenous leukemia to polymerase chain reaction negativity. J Clin Oncol 16:1526–1531, 1998.
33. Kattan MW, Inoue Y, Giles FJ, et al. Cost-effectiveness of interferon-α and conventional chemotherapy in chronic myelogenous leukemia. Ann Intern Med 125:541–548, 1996.
34. Liberato NL, Quaglini S, Barosi G. Cost-effectiveness of interferon alfa in chronic myelogenous leukemia. J Clin Oncol 15: 2673–2682, 1997.
35. Package Labeling. Gleevec, New Jersey: Novartis Pharmaceutical Corp. 2004
36. Drucker BJ, Talpaz M, Resta DJ et al. Efficacy and safety of a specific inhibitor of BCR-ABL tyrosine kinase in chronic myelogenous leukemia. N Engl J Med 344:1031–1037, 2001.
37. Kantarjian H, Sawyers C, Hochhaus A, et al. Hematologic and cytogenetic responses to imatinib mesylate in chronic myelogenous leukemia. N Engl J Med 346:645–652, 2002.
38. Kantarjian HM, Cortes JE, O'Brien S, et al. Imatinib mesylate therapy in newly diagnosed patients with Philadelphia chromosome positive chronic myelogenous leukemia: high incidence of early complete and major cytogenetic responses. Blood 101:97–100, 2003.
39. Anstrom KJ, Reed SD, Glendenning GA, et al. Long term survival estimates for imatinib versus interferon alpha plus low dose cytarabine for patients with newly diagnosed chronic-phase chronic myeloid leukemia. Cancer 101:2584–2592, 2003.
40. Kantarjian HM, Cortes JE, O'Brien S, et al. Long-term survival benefit and improved complete cytogenetic and molecular response rates with imatinib mesylate in Philadelphia chromosome-positive chronic phase chronic myeloid leukemia after failure with interferon-alpha. Blood 104:1979–1988, 2004.
41. Kantarjian H, Talpaz M, O'Brien S, et al. High dose imatinib mesylate therapy in newly diagnosed Philadelphia chromosome positive chronic phase chronic myeloid leukemia. Blood 103:8, 2004.
42. Merk K, Muller MC, Kreil S, et al. Early reduction of BCR-ABL transcript levels predicts cytogenetic response in chronic phase CML patients treated with imatinib after failure of interferon alpha. Leukemia 16:1579–1583, 2002.
43. Kantarjian HM, O'Brien S, Cortes JE, et al. Treatment of Philadelphia chromosome positive, accelerated phase chronic myeloid leukemia with imatinib mesylate. Clin Cancer Res 8:2167–2176, 2003.

44. Drucker BJ, Sawyer CL, Kantarjian H, et al. Activity of specific inhibitor of BCR-ABL tyrosine kinase in the blast crisis of chronic myeloid leukemia and acute lymphoblastic leukemia with Philadelphia chromosome. N Engl J Med 344;1038–1042, 2001.

45. Gale RP, Hehlmann R, Zhang M, et al. Survival with bone marrow transplantation versus hydroxyurea or interferon for chronic myelogenous leukemia. Blood 91:1810–1819, 1998.

46. Keleman E, Masszi, Renenyi P, et al. Reduction in the frequency of transplant-related complications in patients with chronic myeloid leukemia undergoing HCT preconditioned with a new, nonmyeloablative drug combination. Bone Marrow Transplant 21: 747–749, 1998.

47. Lee SJ, Kuntz KM, Horowitz MM, et al. Unrelated donor bone marrow transplantation for chronic myelogenous leukemia: a decision analysis. Ann Intern Med 127:1080–1088, 1997.

48. Hansen JA, Gooley TA, Martin PJ, et al. Bone marrow transplants from unrelated donors for patients with chronic myeloid leukemia. N Engl J Med 338:962–968, 1998.

49. Lee SJ, Anasetti C, Kuntz KM, et al. The costs and cost-effectiveness of unrelated donor bone marrow transplantation for chronic phase chronic myelogenous leukemia. Blood 92:4047–4052, 1998.

50. Uzunel M, Mattsson J, Brune M, et al. Kinetics of minimal residual disease and chimerism in patients with chronic myeloid leukemia after nonmyeloablative conditioning and allogeniec stem cell transplantation. Blood 101:469–472, 2003.

51. Higano CS, Chielens D, Raskind W, et al. Use of α-2a-interferon to treat cytogenetic relapse of chronic myeloid leukemia after bone marrow transplantation. Blood 90:2549–2554, 1997.

52. Steegman JL, Casado F, Granados E, et al. Treatment of chronic myeloid leukemia relapsing after allogeneic bone marrow transplantation: the case for giving interferon [correspondence]. Blood 91: 2617–2618, 1998.

53. Kantarjian HM, O'Brien S, Cortes JE, et al. Imatinib mesylate therapy for relapse after allogeneic stem cell transplantation for chronic myelogenous leukemia. Blood 100:1590–1595, 2002.

54. McGlave PH, De Fabritiis P, Deisseroth A, et al. Autologous transplants for chronic myelogenous leukemia: results from eight transplant groups. Lancet 343:1486–1491, 1994.

55. Carella AM, Cunningham I, Lerma E, et al. Mobilization and transplantation of Philadelphia-negative peripheral-blood progenitor cells early in chronic myelogenous leukemia. J Clin Oncol 15: 1575–1582, 1997.

56. Bonifazi F, de Vivo A, Rosti G, et al. Chronic myeloid leukemia and interferon-alpha: a study of complete cytogenetic responders. Blood 98:3074–3081, 2001.

57. Melo JV, Hughes TP, Apperley JF. Chronic myeloid leukemia. Educational program. Am Soc Hematol 1:132–152, 2003.

58. Rozman C, Montserrat E. Chronic lymphocytic leukemia. N Engl J Med 333:1052–1057, 1995.

59. Flinn IW, Grever M. Chronic lymphocytic leukemia. Cancer Treat Rev 22:1–13, 1996.

60. Reed JC. Molecular biology of chronic lymphocytic leukemia. Semin Oncol 25:11–18, 1998.

61. Cheson BD, Bennett JM, Grever M, et al. National Cancer Institute-sponsored working group guidelines for chronic lymphocytic leukemia: revised guidelines for diagnosis and treatment. Blood 87: 4990–4997, 1996.

62. Rai KR, Sawitsky A, Cronkite EP, et al. Clinical staging of chronic lymphocytic leukemia. Blood 46:219–234, 1975.

63. Binet JL, Auquier A, Dighiero G, et al. A new prognostic classification of chronic lymphocytic leukemia derived from a multivariate survival analysis. Cancer 48:198–206, 1981.

64. Dighiero G, Maloum K, Desablens B, et al. Chlorambucil in indolent chronic lymphocytic leukemia. N Engl J Med 338:1506–1514, 1998.

65. Giles FJ, O'Brien SM, Keating MJ. Chronic lymphocytic leukemia in (Richter's) transformation. Semin Oncol 25:117–125, 1998.

66. Diehl LF, Ketchum LH. Autoimmune disease and chronic lymphocytic leukemia: autoimmune hemolytic anemia, pure red cell aplasia, and autoimmune thrombocytopenia. Semin Oncol 25: 80–97, 1998.

67. Bartik MM, Welker D, Kay NE. Impairments in immune cell function in B cell chronic lymphocytic leukemia. Semin Oncol 25: 27–33, 1998.

68. Morrison VA. The infectious complications of chronic lymphocytic leukemia. Semin Oncol 25:98–106, 1998.

69. Anaissie EJ, Kontoyiannis DP, O'Brien S, et al. Infections in patients with chronic lymphocytic leukemia treated with fludarabine. Ann Intern Med 129:559–566, 1998.

70. Raphael B, Anderson JW, Silber R, et al. Comparison of chlorambucil and prednisone versus cyclophosphamide, vincristine, and prednisone as initial treatment of chronic lymphocytic leukemia: long-term follow-up of an Eastern Cooperative Oncology Group randomized clinical trial. J Clin Oncol 9:770–776, 1991.

71. French Cooperative Group on chronic lymphocytic leukemia: a randomized clinical trial of chlorambucil vs COP in stage B chronic lymphocytic leukemia. Blood 75:1422–1425, 1990.

72. Montserrat E, Alcala A, Alonso C, et al. A randomized trial comparing chlorambucil plus prednisone versus cyclophosphamide, melphalan, and prednisone in the treatment of chronic lymphocytic leukemia stages B and C. Nouv Rev Fr Hematol 30:429–432, 1998.

73. Faguet GB. Chronic lymphocytic leukemia: an updated review. J Clin Oncol 12:1974–1990, 1994.

74. Package labeling. Fludarabine. Richmond, CA: Berlex Laboratories, 1996.

75. O'Brien S, Kantarjian H, Beran M, et al. Fludarabine and granulocyte colony-stimulating factor (G-CSF) in patients with chronic lymphocytic leukemia. Leukemia 11:1631–1635, 1997.

76. Cheson BD, Vena DA, Foss FM, et al. Neurotoxicity of purine analogs: a review. J Clin Oncol 12:2216–2228, 1994.

77. Hequet O, de Jaureguiberry JP, Jaubert D, et al. Listeriosis after fludarabine treatment of chronic lymphocytic leukemia. Hematol Cell Ther 39:89–91, 1997.

78. Byrd JC, Hargis JB, Kester KE, et al. Opportunistic pulmonary infections with fludarabine in previously treated patients with low-grade lymphoid malignancies: a role of *Pneumocystis carinii* pneumonia prophylaxis. Am J Hematol 49:135–142, 1995.

79. Cheson BD. Infectious and immunospuppressive complications of purine analog therapy. J Clin Oncol 13:2431–2448, 1995.

80. Weiss R, Freiman J, Kweder SL, et al. Hemolytic anemia after fludarabine therapy for chronic lymphocytic leukemia. J Clin Oncol 16:1885–1889, 1998.

81. Sorenson MJ, Vena DA, Fallavollita A, et al. Treatment of refractory chronic lymphocytic leukemia with fludarabine phosphate via the group C protocol mechanism of the National Cancer Institute: five-year follow-up report. J Clin Oncol 15:458–465, 1997.

82. Keating MJ, O'Brien S, Lerner S, et al. Long-term follow-up of patients with chronic lymphocytic leukemia (CLL) receiving fludarabine regimens as initial therapy. Blood 92:1165–1171, 1998.

83. Tallman MS, Hakiman D, Zanzig C, et al. Cladribine in the treatment of relapsed or refractory chronic lymphocytic leukemia. J Clin Oncol 13:983–998, 1995.

84. Juliusson G, Liliemark J. Long-term survival following cladribine (2-chlorodeoxyadenosine) therapy in previously treated patients with chronic lymphocytic leukemia. Ann Oncol 7:373–379, 1996.

85. Robak T, Blasinska-Morawiec M, Krykowski E, et al. Intermittent 2-hour intravenous infusions of 2-chlorodeoxyadenosine in the treatment of 110 patients with refractory or previously untreated B-cell chronic lymphocytic leukemia. Leuk Lymphoma 22:509–514, 1996.

86. Robak T, Blasinska-Morawiec M, Krykowski E, et al. Autoimmune haemolytic anaemia in patients with chronic lymphocytic leukaemia treated with 2-chlorodeoxyadenosine (cladribine). Eur J Haematol 58:109–113, 1997.

87. Johnson S, Smith AG, Loffler H, et al. Multicentre prospective randomised trial of fludarabine versus cyclophosphamide, doxorubicin, and prednisone (CAP) for treatment of advanced-stage chronic lymphocytic leukaemia. Lancet 347:1432–1438, 1996.

88. Cooperative group for the study of immunoglobulin in chronic lymphocytic leukemia. N Engl J Med 319:902–907, 1988.

89. Flores G, Cunningham-Rundles C, Newland AC, et al. Efficacy of intravenous immunoglobulin in the treatment of autoimmune hemolytic anemia: results in 73 patients. Am J Hematol 44:237–242, 1993.

90. Hainsworth JD, Litchy S, Barton JH, et al. Single agent rituximab as first line and maintenance treatment for patients with chronic lymphocytic leukemia or small lymphocytic lymphoma: A phase II

trial of the Minnie Pearl Cancer Research Network. J Clin Oncol 21:1746–1757, 2003.

91. Byrd JC, Rai K, Bercedis L, et al. Addition of rituximab to fludarabine may prolong progression-free survival and overall survival in patients with previously untreated chronic lymphocytic leukemia: an updated retrospective comparative analysis of CALGB9712 and CALGB 9011. Blood 105;49–53, 2005.

92. Huhn D, von Schilling C, Wilhelm M, et al. Rituximab therapy of patient with B-cell chronic lymphocytic leukemia. Blood 98: 1326–1331, 2001.

93. Yang H, Rosove MH, Figlin RA, Tumor lysis syndrome occurring after the administration of rituximab in lymphoproliferative disorders: high grade non-hodgkin's lymphoma and chronic lymphocytic leukemia. Am J Hematol 62;247–250, 1999.

94. Osterberg A, Dyer MJS, Bunjes D, et al. Phase II multicenter study of human CD52 antibody in previously treated chronic lymphocytic leukemia. J Clin Oncol 54:1567–1574, 1997.

95. Rai KR, Freter CE, Mercier RJ, et al. Alemtuzumab in previously treated chronic lymphocytiuc leukemia patinets who also had received fludarabine. J Clin Oncol 20:3891–3897, 2002.

96. Dyer MJ, Kelsey SM, Mackay HJ, et al. In vivo 'purging' of residual disease in CLL with Campath-1H. Br J Haematol 97:669–672, 1997.

97. Kennedy B, Rawstron A, Carter C, et al. Campath-1H and fludarabine in combination are highly active in refractory chronic lymphocytic leukemia Blood 99:2245–2247, 2002.

98. O'Brien SM, Kantarjian HM, Thomas DAQ, et al. Alemtuzumab as treatment for residual disease after chemotherapy in patients with chronic lymphocytic leukemia Cancer 98;2657–2663, 2003.

99. Flinn IW, Vogelsang G. Bone marrow transplant for chronic lymphocytic leukemia. Semin Oncol 25:60–64, 1998.

100. Michallet M, Archimbaud E, Bandini G, et al. HLA-identical sibling bone marrow transplantation in younger patients with chronic lymphocytic leukemia. Ann Intern Med 124:311–315, 1996.

101. Rabinowe SN, Soiffer RJ, Gribben JG, et al. Autologous and allogeneic bone marrow transplantation for poor prognosis patients with B-cell chronic lymphocytic leukemia. Blood 82:1366–1376, 1993.

102. Khouri IF, Keating MJ, Vriesendorp HM, et al. Autologous and allogeneic bone marrow transplantation for chronic lymphocytic leukemia: preliminary results. J Clin Oncol 12:748–758, 1994.

103. Dreger P, von Neuhoff N, Kuse R, et al. Early stem cell transplantation of chronic lymphocytic leukaemia: a chance for cure? Br J Cancer 77:2291–2297, 1998.

104. Khouri IF, van Besien, et al. Allogeneic blood or marrow transplantation for chronic lymphocytic leukaemia: timing of transplantation and potential effect of fludarabine on acute graft-versus-host disease. Br J Hematol 97:466–473, 1997.

105. Khouri IF, Keating M, Korbling M, et al. Transplant-lite: induction of graft-versus-malignancy using fludarabine-based nonablative chemotherapy and allogeneic blood progenitor-cell transplantation as treatment for lymphoid malignancies. J Clin Oncol 16: 2817–2824, 1998.

106. Cusack JC Jr, Seymour JF, Lerner S, et al. Role of splenectomy in chronic lymphocytic leukemia. J Am Coll Surg 185:237–243, 1997.

Acute Leukemia

94

John N. McCormick, Tammi T. Miyahara, and Jennifer L. Pauley

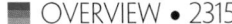
OVERVIEW

The leukemias are a group of neoplastic diseases of the blood-forming cells of the bone marrow that result in the proliferation and accumulation of immature and generally defective blood cells in both the bloodstream and the bone marrow.[1] This may result in anemia, thrombocytopenia, and granulocytopenia. There may also be infiltration of other sites such as lymph nodes, kidney, spleen, testes, and the central nervous system (CNS). The cells involved are usually leukocytes, but several different forms of the disease may be manifested according to which leukocyte cell line is involved. The leukemias are universally fatal if untreated, generally due to complications resulting from leukemic infiltration of the bone marrow and replacement of normal hematopoietic precursor cells. These fatal complications are usually hemorrhage and infection.[1] The natural history of untreated leukemia has led to the classifications of "acute" and "chronic" leukemia, referring to the rapidity of death, with average survival for untreated acute leukemia of about 3 months. Patients with chronic leukemia generally have more differentiated types of malignant cells and survive longer without treatment.

TREATMENT GOALS

Therapy depends on a number of factors, including morphology, biologic markers, immunology, genetic alterations, and other known risk factors of the leukemia.

- Rapidly achieve a complete clinical and hematologic remission with the use of multidrug combination chemotherapy. Remission is generally defined as a normocellular bone marrow with less than 5% blasts, normal hematopoiesis (absolute granulocyte count $>0.5 \times 10^9$/L and platelet count $>100 \times 10^9$/L), and a normal performance status.

- Maintain complete remission by eradicating any residual, undetectable disease with the use of radiation, CNS therapy, and adjuvant multidrug chemotherapy, considering maximum effect and reduction of late toxic effects.
- Provide supportive care to manage the toxic effects of therapy, and provide a good quality of life during and after leukemia therapy.

DEFINITION

The acute leukemias are cancers of the blood-forming cells that are rapidly progressive and uniformly fatal if not treated quickly. Acute leukemias are classified according to the predominant cell type involved and are divided into two predominant types: acute lymphoblastic leukemia (ALL) and acute myelogenous leukemia (AML). There are significant differences in age distribution, response to treatment, and prognosis associated with the different types of leukemia. In this chapter, ALL and AML will be discussed separately with regard to pathophysiology, treatment, and prognosis. Acute promyelocytic leukemia (APL) is a unique form of AML and will also be discussed separately.

EPIDEMIOLOGY

Approximately 16,000 new cases of acute leukemia are identified each year in the United States, according to the National Cancer Institute's Surveillance, Epidemiology and End Results (SEER) program.[2] Of those, approximately 4,000 are ALL and 12,000 are AML. Of the 1,368,030 Americans diagnosed with cancer in 2004, the acute leukemias accounted for only 1% of the total but 2% of the total cancer-related deaths. Despite the overall low incidence rate in children younger than 15 years of age, the acute leukemias are the most common malignancy and rank second only to accidents in mortality for this age group.[3]

ETIOLOGY

The causes of acute leukemias are generally not known. Viruses have been shown to produce some types of leukemia in animals (e.g., feline leukemia), and the Epstein–Barr virus has been implicated as the causative agent of Burkitt's lymphoma in Africans and of some types of nasopharyngeal carcinoma.[4] Persons who have previously been exposed to radiation, with or without antineoplastic drugs, are also at greater risk of developing leukemia. In addition, numerous genetic derangements (particularly Down syndrome), exposure to benzene, pesticides, and smoking have been associated with a higher incidence of acute leukemia.[5] In most children and adults, the cause of leukemia cannot be identified. There are probably numerous factors that interact to result in the malignant condition.

PATHOPHYSIOLOGY

Despite differences in appearance and clinical behavior, all hematologic neoplasms have in common the fact that they are clonal; that is, all cells composing the malignant population in a given patient are derived from a single mutant precursor cell.[6] The neoplastic clones have two important features compared to normal cells. First, they appear to possess an advantage over normal hematopoietic clones that results in growth of the malignant population at the expense of normal cells. Second, there is an imbalance between proliferation and differentiation. Most malignant populations are made up of poorly differentiated cell types that ordinarily would not proliferate or be found in the bloodstream in large numbers. However, the malignant transformation of these cells results in immature cell types that proliferate but do not further differentiate into mature cell lines.

It is useful to review the process of normal production of cellular blood elements. Pluripotent stem cells originating from the bone marrow differentiate (change), mature (grow), and proliferate (divide) to form mature cells that exist in the peripheral circulation. These stem cells have virtually unlimited potential for self-renewal. They are capable of responding to physiologic needs by inducing production of progenitor cells or precursor cells committed to mature separately into lymphoid cells or myeloid cells. The myeloid cells differentiate to form erythrocytes (red blood cells), megakaryocytes (precursors of platelets), granulocytes, and monocytes (white blood cells that help fight infection), whereas the lymphoid cells form circulating B and T lymphocytes. As maturation proceeds in the various cellular lineages, the proliferative capacity becomes progressively restricted until eventually it is lost completely. Therefore, mature cells must be continually replaced as they complete their life cycle. Various stimulatory factors, such as erythropoietin, thrombopoietin, and colony-stimulating factors, regulate the proliferation and differentiation of committed precursor cells, derived from the pluripotent stem cells. Leukemia cells do not undergo terminal differentiation and thus do not lose their proliferative potential. The leukemic cell population continues to expand and normal bone marrow elements may be "crowded out," resulting in the characteristic signs of bone marrow failure, which generally bring patients to medical attention.

CLASSIFICATIONS OF ACUTE LEUKEMIAS

Acute leukemias are classified depending on the cell type of origin. However, additional classifications of leukemia have been developed to further identify differences in the clinical course, response to treatment, and prognosis of various types of acute leukemia. An important development introduced in the 1970s is the French-American-British (FAB) system of nomenclature that was widely used for nearly three decades to classify the morphologic subgroups of acute leukemias.[7] Although the FAB classification recognizes the morphologic heterogeneity of AML, it does not adequately reflect the genetic or clinical diversity of the disease. Therefore, the World Health Organization (WHO) recently published a newer classification for myeloid malignancies incorporating not only the morphologic heterogeneity of AML but also the importance of genetic features, prior therapies that may contribute to the development of AML, and any prior history of myelodysplasia. These factors have shown to have a significant impact on the clinical behavior of AML but do not always nicely correlate with the FAB classification. The WHO classification divides AML into four groups: (a) AML with recurrent cytogenetic translocations; (b) AML with myelodysplasia-related features; (c) therapy-related AML and myelodysplastic syndrome (MDS); and (d) AML not otherwise specified[8] (Table 94.1).

In addition to classification schemas, immunologic and biochemical markers and specific genetic abnormalities are used to classify and identify subtypes of leukemia cells. Moreover, these genetic abnormalities are important in determining the prognosis of the various types of acute leukemias. Immunologic "markers" refer to the surface immunoglobulin found on the cell membrane of malignant leukocytes or to their cytoplasmic immunoglobulins. As normal cells undergo differentiation, these markers change and may be used to determine the degree of differentiation achieved by the malignant cell line. This permits identification of the type of cell involved and leads to further classification. Genetic alterations (e.g., chromosomal translocations, deletions or inactivation of tumor-suppressor genes, and chromosomal gains or losses, resulting in hyperdiploidy or hypodiploidy, respectively) are found in most patients with lymphoid leukemia.[9]

The development of hybridoma techniques (which is a hybrid cell that results from the fusion of a lymphocyte and a tumor cell used to culture a specific monoclonal antibody and produce unlimited quantities of specific monoclonal antibodies against malignant cell markers) has led to more precise identification of specific immunologic markers in the classification of ALL and to a revised immunologic classification system (Table 94.2). Because leukemic lymphoblasts lack specific morphologic or cytochemical features, immunophenotyping or immunologic testing is necessary for diagnosis. Although monoclonal antibodies against 166 different clusters of differentiation (CD) molecules on human leukocytes exist, only a few are truly lineage-specific.[10] T-lineage ALL is documented based on a positive reaction with the highly sensitive monoclonal antibody CD7 plus the highly specific monoclonal antibody CD3. B-lineage ALL can be confirmed based on positive reactions with antibodies CD19 and CD79a.[11] The B-lineage classification includes three major subtypes: B-cell (expression of surface immunoglobulin heavy chains and either κ or λ light chains), pre-B (presence of cytoplasmic immunoglobulin), and early pre-B (no surface and cytoplasmic immunoglobulins). Transitional B cells, which express cytoplasmic and surface immunoglobulin chains and surrogate light-chain proteins, appear to define a clinically distinct form of ALL. T cells may also be classified according to the degree of differentiation (early, intermediate, or late), but this classification of T-cell ALL has limited clinical significance.[12] The prognosis associated with these various subgroups of ALL will be discussed later.

Biochemical markers refer to the altered concentrations of intracellular enzymes found in various forms of leukemia. Terminal deoxynucleotidyl transferase is an intracellular enzyme that is generally not detected in mature lymphocytes but is found in most patients with ALL, excluding those with the B-cell subtype. It may also be found in up to 5% of patients with AML. Reactions with myeloperoxidase and Sudan black stain, on the other hand, are positive predominantly in AML. The periodic acid-Schiff reaction is positive in ALL and is useful in differentiating it from AML.[13]

In actual practice, the classification of acute leukemia in a particular patient is based on the combination of morphology and immunologic and biochemical studies. These studies generally correlate with one another and are used to confirm the suspected classification in a patient.

Genetic abnormalities in patients with acute leukemia have contributed greatly to the understanding of the pathogenesis of the disease. Alterations in the *p53* suppressor gene are found in acute leukemia. Normal *p53* allows cells to stop in the G_1 phase of the cell cycle. Inactivation of *p53* allows cells to proliferate unregulated, which occurs in acute leukemia.[14] Mutations of the *ras* gene may lead to unregulated proliferation and differentiation, a characteristic of acute leukemia.[15] Several chromosomal translocations are well documented in acute leukemia and provide information on risk and prognosis of disease. Mixed lineage leukemia (MLL) gene rearrangements located on chromosome 11q23, positive Philadelphia chromosome translocation on chromosome 9;22, and alterations in chromosome 4;11 confer a poor prognosis. However, an excellent outcome is expected in patients who have the *TEL-AML1* fusion on chromosome 12;21.[16]

CLINICAL PRESENTATION AND DIAGNOSIS

SIGNS AND SYMPTOMS

The initial presenting symptoms of acute leukemia differ very little for ALL and AML. The complaints that most often

TABLE 94.1	The French-American-British (FAB) Cooperative Group Classification of Acute Leukemias and World Health Organization (WHO) Classification of Acute Myeloid Leukemia

FAB Designation	Common Terms (Abbreviations) for Leukemic Subgroups	Predominant Cell Type	Unique Clinical or Laboratory Features
L1	Acute lymphoblastic leukemia, childhood (ALL)	Microlymphoblasts	
L2	ALL, adult	Mixed lymphoblasts, prolymphoblasts	
L3	Burkitt's-type leukemia	Lymphocytes	
M0	Minimal myeloid differentiation	Undifferentiated	Blasts often express CD34 and terminal deoxynucleotidyl transferase.
M1	Acute myelocytic leukemia (AML), undifferentiated; acute myelogenous, acute granulocytic	Myeloblasts	
M2	AML, differentiated	Mixed myeloblasts, promyelocytes	Myeloblastomas (especially orbital)
M3	Acute progranulocytic leukemia	Hypergranular promyelocytes	Disseminated intravascular coagulation
M4	Acute myelomonocytic leukemia (AMML)	Mixed myelocytes, monocytes	Infants, extramedullary leukemia
M5	Acute monocytic leukemia (AMOL)	Monocytes	Infants, extramedullary leukemia, second leukemia after epipodophyllotoxins
M6	Erythroleukemia	Mixed erythroblasts, erythrocytes, myelocytes	
M7	Megakaryoblastic leukemia	Megakaryoblasts	Down syndrome

WHO Classification	Description
AML with recurrent cytogenetic translocations	
AML with multilineage dysplasia	With prior myelodysplastic syndrome
	Without prior myelodysplastic syndrome
AML, therapy-related	Alkylating agent-related
	Epipodophyllotoxin-related
	Other
AML, not otherwise specified	AML, minimally differentiated
	AML without maturation
	AML with maturation
	Acute myelomonocytic leukemia
	Acute monocytic leukemia
	Acute erythroid leukemia
	Acute megakaryocytic leukemia
	Acute basophilic leukemia
	Acute panmyelosis with myelofibrosis

bring patients to medical attention are fatigue, weight loss, fever, pallor, purpura, and pain.[17] These symptoms result from bone marrow failure. Anemia occurs because of inadequate erythrocyte production, infections are caused by inadequate neutrophil production, and bleeding is the result of inadequate platelet production. In addition, infiltration of leukemia cells into the liver, spleen, or lymph nodes may result in hepatosplenomegaly, lymphadenopathy, and bone and joint pain. Table 94.3 lists the frequency of presenting complaints among patients with ALL. These complaints may be present for a few days or even a few weeks; rarely, there may be a history of these symptoms for several months before diagnosis. The most common symptom at diagnosis is the presence of fever, occurring in about 60% of patients.

TABLE 94.2	Classification of Acute Lymphoblastic Leukemia by Morphologic Characteristics, Immunophenotype, and Chromosome Number[a]

Category	Frequency (%)
FAB morphologic classification system	
L1	80
L2	17
L3	3
Immunophenotype	
Early pre-B	57
Pre-B	25
Transitional pre-B	1
B-cell	2
T-cell	15
Ploidy	
Hypodiploid (<45 chromosomes)	7
Diploid (normal 46 chromosomes)	8
Pseudodiploid (46 chromosomes, with abnormalities)	42
Hyperdiploid (47–50 chromosomes)	15
Hyperdiploid (>50 chromosomes)	27
Triploid/tetraploid	1

FAB, French-American-British.

[a] On the basis of 500 consecutive patients with newly diagnosed disease (age <18 years) treated at St. Jude Children's Research Hospital (From Altman AJ, Schwartz AD. Malignant diseases of infancy, childhood and adolescence. Philadelphia: WB Saunders, 1983:187–238[6]; Bennett JM, Catovsky D, Daniel M-T, et al. Proposals for the classifications of the acute leukemias; French-American-British (FAB) co-operative group. Br J Haematol 33:451–458, 1976.[7]).

TABLE 94.3	Frequency of Common Presenting Complaints Among Children With Acute Lymphoblastic Leukemia

Finding	Percentage
Fever	61
Pallor	55
Hemorrhage	52
Anorexia	33
Fatigue	30
Bone pain	23
Abdominal pain	19
Joint pain	15
Lymphadenopathy	15
Weight loss	13

Although patients may be neutropenic at diagnosis, fever appears to be due to the leukemia itself, as 70% of these patients become afebrile within 72 hours of beginning initial chemotherapy without antibiotics.[18] Nevertheless, empiric antibiotic therapy is usually begun in febrile, neutropenic patients at the diagnosis of leukemia because the risk of serious systemic infections in such patients cannot be ignored.

Patients with newly diagnosed leukemia may have a total white blood cell (WBC) count that is markedly elevated, normal, or markedly depressed. A very high circulating WBC count (hyperleukocytosis) is associated with a poorer prognosis. This condition can also be life-threatening because blasts (immature WBCs) can occlude small vessels in vital organs. Additionally, most of the white cells in the circulation are immature blast forms; therefore, they cannot mount a response to bacterial infections. Thus, most patients with leukemia have an increased risk of opportunistic infections at diagnosis.

DIAGNOSIS/CLINICAL FINDINGS

The diagnosis of acute leukemia is not usually difficult to establish. A bone marrow aspirate and biopsy with cytogenetic evaluation is performed to allow examination of the cellular elements of the bone marrow. It is often hypercellular, with 60% to 100% blast cells. A minimum of 20% blast cells is considered adequate to establish the diagnosis of acute leukemia, but most commonly this is an all-or-none diagnosis and the pattern is obvious. Abnormal cells found in the peripheral blood may be suggestive of acute leukemia but usually are not considered diagnostic because bizarre mononuclear cells may be seen in the blood of patients with viral illnesses. If blasts or other unidentified cells are seen in the peripheral blood, the diagnosis must be confirmed by a bone marrow examination.

THERAPEUTIC PLAN

The modern cure-oriented approach to the treatment of any malignant condition usually involves some combination of surgery, radiation, and chemotherapy. Although surgery is important in the treatment of solid tumors, it is impossible to surgically remove tumor tissue in leukemia, and therefore surgery has a minor supportive role.

Radiation therapy has a larger role in leukemia, but it is not used alone as a curative modality. It is important in the treatment of either occult or overt leukemia in the CNS. High-dose radiotherapy is also used to obliterate functional bone marrow as part of the preparation for bone marrow transplantation. It may also be used in individual patients to reduce the size of an infiltrative leukemic mass, particularly when functional impairment of an organ or joint is involved.

TREATMENT

Drug therapy remains the primary modality for the treatment of acute leukemias, with the goal of treatment for both AML and ALL being the complete eradication of any detectable disease. Beginning with the use of aminopterin in childhood ALL in 1948,[19] additional effective agents have been identified and introduced into routine clinical use. The clinical indications and common toxic effects of the drugs routinely used to treat acute leukemia today are summarized in Table 94.4.

For all phases of acute leukemia, it has been clearly shown that drugs used in combination are superior to monotherapy. The rationale for combination therapy is that several effective agents with different mechanisms of action are more likely to destroy different subpopulations of leukemia cells and reduce the potential for development of drug resistance. The practical problem in the design of clinical treatment programs is determining the optimal number of agents in the most effective doses and sequence. Several principles guide the use of combination chemotherapy for malignant diseases: (a) each of the drugs used should have demonstrated single-agent activity against the tumor; (b) the drugs should have different mechanisms of action; (c) the drugs used should have minimally overlapping toxicities; and (d) the maximal optimal doses should be used, with administration scheduled with respect to specific tumor cell kinetics.

The optimal use of anticancer drugs is limited by our incomplete understanding of their mechanisms of action and mechanisms of resistance to them and their interactions. In addition, our understanding of the biology of tumors and the factors that control their growth is incomplete. Current research directed at elucidating the cellular mechanisms that govern both the reproduction of malignant cells and their response to anticancer drugs is expected to improve our use of the drugs currently available as well as to lead to the development of new agents.

ACUTE LYMPHOBLASTIC LEUKEMIA

Childhood ALL represents one of the cancer treatment success stories of recent years. Long-term event-free survival rates in children receiving modern therapy are now approximately 80%.[20] In adults, however, survival rates are only 30% to 40%.[21] Several distinct phases of therapy, each with a specific rationale, have been developed, and current efforts to improve the cure rate of ALL have focused on refining and optimizing therapy for each of these phases. The first phase of treatment, which is intended to produce a complete remission (CR) of the leukemia, is called induction therapy. Induction therapy is followed by consolidation therapy. Consolidation therapy is then followed by maintenance therapy to ensure that the leukemia does not return.

The objectives of initial remission induction are to (a) eradicate as many leukemia cells as possible, within the limits of biologic tolerance, and (b) reestablish normal hematopoiesis and general good health. "Standard" remission induction therapy generally consists of two or more drugs. Prednisone and vincristine are almost always used, and this combination produces a CR in more than 90% of patients. However, the intensity of the initial treatment influences the duration of remission, and addition of a third agent, either asparaginase or an anthracycline (daunorubicin or doxorubicin), appears to increase the fraction of patients who remain in continuous complete remission (CCR) and are eventually cured.[22–24] Therefore, induction regimens for both children and adults generally include at least three drugs: prednisone, vincristine, and either asparaginase or an anthracycline.

TREATMENT

INDUCTION THERAPY

CR, defined as the complete eradication of all detectable disease, may be obtained in at least 95% of children[20] and 80% to 85% of adults[21] with ALL following induction therapy. Patients in CR have no evidence of leukemia and may lead relatively normal lives while in remission. However, patients in remission may have as many as 10^8 leukemia cells in their bodies, even though this mass of cells remains clinically undetectable. Remission induction therapy is capable of eradicating up to 99.9% of the total body burden of malignant cells, but because patients may have 10^{10} to 10^{12} leukemia cells at diagnosis, a substantial number of cells remain to be eliminated after patients achieve a clinical CR.

CONSOLIDATION THERAPY

Consolidation therapy refers to a period of intensive therapy administered after CR is achieved. The purpose of consolidation therapy is to secure the CR by eradicating as many of the remaining leukemic cells as possible, within the limits of biologic tolerance. Consolidation therapy may consist of different combinations of agents or repeated courses of the regimen used to achieve the initial clinical remission.

CENTRAL NERVOUS SYSTEM THERAPY

An important site of initial relapse in patients who achieve a CR is the CNS. After conventional induction therapy alone, up to 60% of patients may have their initial reappearance

TABLE 94.4	Principal Toxic Effects and Clinical Indications for Drugs Used to Treat Leukemia		
Drug	**Acute**	**Delayed**	**Indications**
Plant alkaloids			
Etoposide	Nausea and vomiting; hypotension with rapid administration; hypersensitivity reactions (2%–20%); vesicant with extravasation	Bone marrow depression; alopecia, oral ulceration	AML (induction 200 mg/m^2 CI for 3 days) ALL (150–300 mg/m^2 weekly pairs)
Vincristine	Vesicant reaction with extravasation; mild emetogenicity	Neurotoxicity; peripheral neuropathy, jaw pain, paralytic ileus, foot drop, decreased reflexes, constipation; alopecia; bone marrow depression	ALL (remission induction and continuation: 1–1.5 mg/m^2 weekly pairs)
Topotecan	Nausea, vomiting, diarrhea, rash	Myelosuppression	AML (salvage therapy) 1.25 mg/m^2 CIV Days 1–5
Antimetabolites			
Cladribine (2-CDA)	Mild nausea and vomiting; rash	Bone marrow depression; immunosuppression	AML 8.9 mg/m^2/day for 5 days CI
Cytarabine	Nausea, vomiting, diarrhea, rash	Bone marrow depression; CNS toxicity; interstitial pneumonitis; pulmonary capillary leak (high dose)	ALL (200–300 mg/m^2 weekly or alternating pairs); if intrathecally: 28–36 mg AML (100 mg/m^2 CI Days 1–7 or 250 mg/m^2 CIV Days 1–5) AML high dose: 2–3 g/m^2 IV q12h Days 1, 3, and 5 or Days 1–3 AML intermediate dose: 1–1.5 g/m^2/day for 4–6 doses
Fludarabine	Nausea and vomiting	Bone marrow depression; megaloblastosis; oral ulceration; fever and arthralgias; diarrhea; alopecia; rash on soles and palms	AML 50–150 mg/m^2/day for 5 days over 30 minutes IV
Mercaptopurine	Occasional nausea and vomiting	Bone marrow depression; liver damage	ALL (continuation therapy: 75–100 mg/m^2/day)
Methotrexate	Dose-related nausea and vomiting; diarrhea (usually mild); rash	Bone marrow depression; oral and gastrointestinal ulceration; nephrotoxicity (high doses); hepatic cirrhosis (low dose) and elevated liver transaminases; pulmonary infiltration (fibrosis/pneumonitis); CNS toxicity (high-dose and intrathecal therapy)	ALL (intrathecal 6–12 mg, low doses orally or IV 40 mg/m^2 dose, high doses IV 1,500–5,000 mg/m^2 over 2–24 hours)
Thioguanine	Occasional nausea and vomiting 1 or 2 days after administration	Bone marrow depression	AML (100 mg/m^2 daily to twice daily Days 1–7)
Antibiotics			
Daunorubicin	Nausea and vomiting; diarrhea; vesicant local reactions at infiltration site; red urine, 1 or 2 days after administration	Bone marrow depression; cardiotoxicity; stomatitis; alopecia; potentiation of radiation	AML (45–60 mg/m^2 CI over 3 days) Doses may be decreased to 30 mg/m^2 in older adults. ALL (25 mg/m^2 IV once a week for 2–3 weeks)

(continues)

TABLE 94.4	continued		

Drug	Acute	Delayed	Indications
Doxorubicin	Nausea and vomiting; diarrhea; local reactions at infiltration site; red urine, 1 or 2 days after administration	Bone marrow depression; cardiotoxicity; stomatitis; alopecia; potentiation of radiation	
Idarubicin	Nausea and vomiting; diarrhea; local reactions at infiltration site; red urine, 1 or 2 days after administration	Bone marrow depression; cardiotoxicity; stomatitis; alopecia; potentiation of radiation	AML 12 mg/m^2 for 2 or 3 days
Mitoxantrone	Nausea and vomiting; diarrhea; local reactions at infiltration site; bluish-green urine, 1 or 2 days after administration	Bone marrow depression; cardiotoxicity; stomatitis; alopecia; potentiation of radiation	AML 12 mg/m^2 for 2 or 3 days
Alkylating agents			
Cyclophosphamide	Nausea and vomiting (sometimes delayed)	Bone marrow depression; immunosuppression; alopecia; hemorrhagic cystitis; sterility; secondary malignancies; SIADH	ALL (150–300 mg/m^2 IV alternating weekly pairs)
Miscellaneous			
Asparaginase	Nausea and vomiting; fever; anaphylaxis; local reaction	Hepatotoxicity; hyperglycemia; pancreatitis; abdominal pain; coagulation defects; CNS depression	ALL induction (10,000 U/m^2/day IM QOD to weekly for 6–9 doses)
All-*trans* retinoic acid	Fever; progressive increase in WBC without symptoms ATRA syndrome: increased WBC count with symptoms of fever, respiratory distress, weight gain, lower extremity edema, pleural effusions, hypotension, and sometimes renal failure	Increase in transaminases; increase in triglycerides; bone pain; headaches; increased calcium; dry lips and mucosa; pseudotumor cerebri	AML (M3)-APL (45 mg/m^2/day) To reduce side effects, doses of 25 mg/m^2/day have been effective.
Gemtuzumab	Fever, chills, nausea, vomiting, thrombocytopenia, neutropenia, asthenia, diarrhea, abdominal pain, headache, epistaxis, stomatitis, dyspnea, hypokalemia	Liver function abnormalities, specifically veno-occlusive disease	AML: 9 mg/m^2 IV over 2 hours for 2 doses on Day 1 and Day 8 or 14
Arsenic trioxide	Hyperleukocytosis, fever, rigors, chest pain, nausea, vomiting, diarrhea, constipation, abdominal pain, fatigue, edema, cough, rash, headaches, dizziness, hyperglycemia	Cardiac problems have been reported; therefore, monitor patients carefully, checking for hypokalemia and hypomagnesemia. Avoid agents that prolong the QT interval.	APL remission induction: 0.15 mg/kg daily until remission (total induction dose should not exceed 60 doses) APL consolidation: 0.15 mg/kg daily for 5 days each week (Monday through Friday) for 5 weeks for a total of 25 doses

ATRA, all-*trans* retinoic acid; AML, acute myelogenic leukemia; ALL, acute lymphoblastic leukemia; APL, acute promyelocytic leukemia; CI, continuous infusion; CIV, continuous intravenous infusion; CNS, central nervous system; IV, intravenous; QOD, every other day; SIADH, syndrome of inappropriate secretion of diuretic hormone; WBC, white blood cell.

of malignant blast cells in the CNS,[25] probably because of poor penetration across the blood–brain barrier by the drugs used to induce remission. The precise definition of CNS disease has been controversial. The two most commonly accepted definitions of CNS disease are (a) a total cerebrospinal fluid (CSF) WBC count greater than 5 cells per mm^3 and the presence of blast cells in the CSF or with cranial nerve palsy and (b) the presence of any number of blasts regardless of cell counts in the CSF.

The CNS, which is considered a ''pharmacologic sanctuary'' for patients with ALL, has led to the recognition that specific CNS therapy is an essential component of treatment for this disease. Proposed by George and Pinkel in the 1960s,[26] CNS therapy has reduced the CNS relapse rate to less than 10%.[27] The mainstay of CNS therapy has been either spinal irradiation or intrathecal administration of methotrexate. The dose of radiation originally used was 2,400 cGy delivered over 2 to 3 weeks, but more recently it has been shown that 1,800 cGy provides adequate treatment, with less toxicity and morbidity.[28] Intrathecal methotrexate has been used with success in place of spinal irradiation, resulting in less myelosuppression and growth abnormalities.[29] The usual dose for patients older than 3 years of age is 12 mg.[30] Cytarabine or hydrocortisone, or both, may be added to methotrexate to further improve the effectiveness of CNS therapy. Recent data have suggested that the treatment for CNS disease should be intensified based on prognostic factors as well as on the CNS disease at diagnosis, reserving cranial irradiation and multiple intrathecal doses for those at greater risk for relapse. Therefore, patients with non–T-cell, non–B-cell ALL who have less than 5 cells per mm^3 in the CSF, regardless of blasts, would receive less CNS prophylaxis and no irradiation in the context of highly effective chemotherapy.[25,31]

Another approach to CNS treatment is the use of high-dose methotrexate intravenously, without irradiation.[32] This therapy consists of methotrexate in doses of 500 mg per m^2 or more, infused over 24 hours. The long infusion time is intended to improve the penetration of methotrexate across the blood–brain barrier. Although CSF methotrexate concentrations are typically only 1% or less of the concurrent plasma concentrations,[33] use of high-dose methotrexate allows prolonged high plasma concentrations to achieve cytocidal methotrexate concentrations in the CSF. Leucovorin ''rescue'' is then administered to prevent excessive and intolerable toxicity to normal tissues. High-dose intravenous methotrexate may be combined with intrathecal methotrexate to further boost CSF concentrations. Doses as high as 33.6 g per m^2 have been used[34] to achieve CSF concentrations of 10 μM from intravenous methotrexate alone. However, no improvement in overall survival has been shown as a result of using this approach. In general, high-dose methotrexate may result in a slightly higher CNS relapse rate than cranial irradiation with intrathecal methotrexate,[32] but overall disease-free survival does not appear to be different. This

suggests that high-dose methotrexate may improve control of disease in the bone marrow as well. In addition, cranial irradiation may result in more significant long-term sequelae associated with therapy than does methotrexate. This may include leukoencephalopathy, deficits in intellectual function, memory loss, secondary cancers, endocrinopathy, and craniofacial deformities.[21]

The optimal dose of high-dose methotrexate in the treatment of ALL has not been defined. One study[33] identified a relationship between the plasma methotrexate concentration and the probability of relapse. Patients received 15 courses of methotrexate 1,000 mg per m^2, given as a loading dose of 200 mg per m^2, followed by 800 mg per m^2 over 24 hours. This therapy was delivered as CNS therapy during the first 75 weeks of continuation therapy. Patients who achieved steady-state plasma concentrations greater than 16 μM for at least half their courses were more likely to remain in CCR than patients whose plasma concentrations were lower. The variability in plasma concentrations was due solely to interpatient differences in drug elimination, because all patients were treated with identical methotrexate doses. This study provides insight into how best to use methotrexate for ALL and offers guidance in selecting a dose of methotrexate that will yield optimal cytotoxic exposure and the best results. The study also cites the potential role of prospective pharmacokinetic monitoring of high-dose methotrexate to improve its therapeutic benefit in ALL patients.

Monitoring methotrexate serum concentrations is warranted in all patients receiving high doses. The leucovorin rescue dose should be adjusted based on the patient's clearance of the methotrexate and the measured serum levels. Aggressive hydration with alkalinization improves clearance of methotrexate, while leucovorin should prevent many of the unwanted side effects of methotrexate. The amounts of fluid, alkalinization, and leucovorin are increased with delayed clearance as defined by the elevated methotrexate level.

The preceding data for the use of CNS prophylaxis and high-dose methotrexate for control or prevention of CNS disease and/or relapse is in the context of intense systemic therapy. Data suggest that the addition of epipodophyllotoxins to the systemic therapy may result in better CNS cytotoxicity because of documented CNS penetration.[35] However, these agents have also been associated with the development of secondary leukemia, primarily AML. Another approach to improving control of CNS disease is the use of dexamethasone instead of prednisone during maintenance therapy.[36]

MAINTENANCE THERAPY

Of patients who have achieved a CR, only a few (perhaps 15%) will be long-term survivors if no additional therapy is administered.[37] Continuation, or maintenance, therapy appears to be necessary to eradicate the remaining leukemia cells that are undetectable during remission. The growth fraction of leukemia cells is relatively small, and the cell cycle time is fairly long. Therefore, only a small fraction of the total number of leukemia cells is susceptible at any given time to the effects of most anticancer drugs that are cell cycle phase-specific agents. Hence, a prolonged period of exposure to anticancer drugs is necessary to further reduce the malignant population. The most common maintenance therapy has consisted of a two-drug combination of mercaptopurine and methotrexate.[37] Mercaptopurine is given orally in doses of 50 to 90 mg/m^2/day, and methotrexate can be given orally, intravenously, or intramuscularly at doses of 15 to 30 mg/m^2/week.

The optimal duration of maintenance therapy is not known, and current guidelines are based on empiric trial-and-error approaches. Most treatment programs use 2 to 6 years of maintenance therapy. In determining the length of maintenance therapy, the risk of off-therapy relapses must be considered in comparison to the risks of undesirable toxic effects of the therapy. Therapy may be stopped after 30 months of CCR or at least 12 months of continuous remission after an isolated nonmedullary relapse (CNS or testes). Results of several large long-term studies indicate that 70% of patients who elect to have therapy stopped in this fashion will remain disease-free and be long-term survivors.[37]

Although maintenance therapy is well tolerated, there are risks associated with continual therapy. Development of resistance to standard agents or poor compliance with therapy may result in relapse. In addition, maintenance therapy is immunosuppressive and associated with the risk of opportunistic infections. Other complications such as avascular necrosis of bone, osteoporosis, and cardiomyopathy may occur during maintenance therapy. Therefore, alternative strategies have been used to overcome the development of resistance and to reduce the risk of infections and other complications.

Approaches to prevent bone marrow relapse during remission have included increasing the number of drugs administered during remission, periodic repetition of the agents used to induce the initial remission (referred to as "reinforcement" pulses), and intermittent rather than continuous chemotherapy. Use of more than two agents simultaneously does not appear to improve the rate of disease-free survival, but it does increase the toxicity of the therapy.[38] A recent approach to improving event-free survival includes a delayed reintensification phase, or reinduction.[25]

One approach to the maintenance therapy of ALL is rotational use of non–cross-resistant anticancer drugs early in therapy. This concept is based on the somatic mutation theory of Luria and Delbrück[39] and its further development by Goldie and Coldman.[40,41] This hypothesis states that intense early therapy and sequential or rotational use of multiple non–cross-resistant agents during maintenance therapy will reduce the likelihood of the emergence of a drug-resistant subpopulation of leukemia cells. Patients who have bone marrow relapses during this phase of therapy account for the largest fraction of patients who die of ALL, undoubtedly because of development of resistance, either by mutation or by selection, to the methotrexate–mercaptopurine combination usually administered during this phase of therapy. The rationale for administering additional non–cross-resistant agents during maintenance therapy is to reduce the opportunity for resistance to be manifested to the primary drug combination. Therefore, other effective agents such as etoposide, cyclophosphamide, cytarabine, teniposide, asparaginase, or additional anthracyclines may be administered during the maintenance phase of therapy in addition to the more customary methotrexate and mercaptopurine. However, the negative aspect is the increase in toxicity that may be encountered with some of these other agents. Because up to 50% of patients may be cured with the relatively well-tolerated methotrexate–mercaptopurine combination, the addition of more toxic drugs during continuation therapy may result only in more morbidity for patients who may be cured with less aggressive therapy. This dilemma points out the need to develop a better understanding of the various subtypes of ALL and significant prognostic factors to more readily identify those patients who would be expected to do well with less intense therapy.

Pharmacogenetics also plays an important role in the efficacy and toxicity of chemotherapy. One example is the polymorphisms in the gene for thiopurine methyltransferase, which render the protein susceptible to degradation. This enzyme catalyzes S-methylation (inactivation) of mercaptopurine. Approximately 10% of patients carry at least one such variant allele for this gene, which leads to accumulation of high levels of active metabolites of mercaptopurine (thioguanine nucleotides). When these patients are treated with the standard dose of mercaptopurine, they have an increased risk of acute hematologic toxic effects.[20]

Cytochrome P-450 enzymes are also involved in the activation of many anticancer drugs (e.g., epipodophyllotoxins and cyclophosphamide) or their inactivation (e.g., vincristine and glucocorticoids). Levels of cytochrome P-450 enzymes are directly affected by drugs used in the supportive care of patients with leukemia. Specifically, phenytoin and phenobarbital, both used for the long-term treatment of seizures, increase the levels of these enzymes and may adversely affect the outcome of therapy for ALL, whereas azole antifungal agents (e.g., fluconazole, itraconazole, voriconazole, and ketoconazole) inhibit these enzymes, increasing the toxicity of the anticancer agent.[20]

HEMATOPOIETIC STEM CELL TRANSPLANTATION

Hematopoietic stem cell transplantation (HSCT) is a treatment modality that has an important role in the treatment of ALL. Recent studies indicate that certain ALL patients may benefit from HSCT and exhibit improved survival. Induction failures, infants, Ph+ ALL, and adults in second remission are groups in whom increased survival rates after HCST have been reported.[42–44] This procedure typically includes total body irradiation, with or without high-dose chemotherapy (cyclophosphamide, cytarabine, busulfan, and etoposide have all been used), to kill residual leukemia cells and produce irreversible bone marrow suppression. Bone marrow stem cells are obtained from either the bone marrow or peripheral blood from a human leukocyte antigen (HLA)-matched donor (allogeneic), an identical twin (syngeneic), or a patient in remission (autologous). Bone marrow is harvested from the iliac crest of the donor or obtained from peripheral blood and then intravenously infused into the patient. Engraftment, or the ability of the bone marrow to produce cells, usually occurs in about 2 to 3 weeks following infusion of the stem cells. HSCT may also be associated with a number of risks. Graft-versus-host disease (GVHD), which results from the T lymphocytes in the donor marrow reacting against host tissue, may occur after allogeneic transplantation. Patients are at increased risk of infection as a result of profound immunosuppression due to the preparative regimen. Viral and fungal infections are especially common and difficult to treat. Veno-occlusive disease (VOD) of the liver, a fibrous obliteration (either partial or complete) of small hepatic venules, may develop and lead to thrombosis, endophlebitis, fibrosis, and portal hypertension with ascites. Unfortunately, the risk of relapse of leukemia, despite the intensive therapy, remains a possibility.

PROGNOSIS

Numerous variables are associated with the prognosis of patients with ALL (Table 94.5). Age at diagnosis is important: children younger than 2 years and those older than 10 years have a higher mortality rate with current standard therapy. Several studies have shown that males have a slightly greater risk of relapse than females, even after accounting for nonmedullary relapses in the testes, which apparently act as a pharmacologic sanctuary from systemic anticancer drugs. WBC count at diagnosis is universally recognized as an important prognostic factor, because higher WBC counts represent a greater tumor burden and are associated with a poorer outcome. T-cell and mature B-cell leukemias are associated with a poorer prognosis than leukemia expressing other surface immunoglobulins. Many studies have shown that nonwhite patients may have a poorer prognosis, although there has been speculation that this may be due, at least in part, to socioeconomic factors that cause delays in diagnosis and treatment. A thymic or mediastinal mass on chest roentgenograms is a feature of high-risk disease, although this is often associ-

TABLE 94.5	Adverse Prognostic Factors at Diagnosis of Acute Lymphoblastic Leukemia	
Age	Hematologic findings
<2 years	Elevated WBC count
>10 years	Elevated hemoglobin
Sex	Decreased platelet count
Male	FAB morphology
Race	L2, L3
Nonwhite	Immunologic markers
Physical findings	T-cell or B-cell leukemia
Hepatosplenomegaly	Cytogenetics
Lymphadenopathy	DNA index <1.16
Mediastinal mass (on chest x-ray)	Translocations
	Philadelphia chromosome
Lymphoblasts in CNS	

CNS, central nervous system; WBC, white blood cell; FAB, French-American-British.

ated with T-cell disease. Patients with lymphoblasts detectable in the CSF at diagnosis have a poorer prognosis.

Genetic characteristics, in addition to clinical factors, also have prognostic significance. Ploidy, defined as the number of chromosomes present in leukemic clones, is an established prognostic factor. The types and frequency of various ploidies are summarized in Table 94.2. Leukemic cell clones with more than 53 chromosomes or a ratio of DNA content greater than 1.15 times normal (sometimes referred to as the DNA index) are more responsive to treatment, and this type of disease has a better prognosis.[45] Cytogenetic studies have shown that leukemic clones that exhibit various types of translocations are associated with a poorer prognosis. For example, in children younger than 1 year of age, 70% to 80% have rearrangement of the *MLL* gene, indicative of a poor prognosis.[46] In adolescent and adult patients, poor prognostic factors include the frequency of *MLL* rearrangements and the presence of the Philadelphia chromosome.[11]

These risk factors are not necessarily independent; patients with T-cell leukemia often have a high WBC count, for example. Therefore, none of these factors should be regarded as having completely independent prognostic value, and any treatment plan that uses these factors to individualize therapy should consider how these factors interact and correlate with one another. It appears likely that as our understanding of the molecular biology of leukemia improves, the genetically oriented prognostic factors will gradually replace the more traditional clinical factors in assigning risk categories and designing treatment regimens. On the other hand, any prognostic factor is important relative only to the treatment currently used. If a major new treatment advance is found, all currently used prognostic factors could lose their predictive value.

AML differs in many respects from ALL, particularly with regard to its age distribution and prognosis. Whereas ALL is primarily a childhood disease, AML is primarily a disease of adults. In addition, it has proved much more resistant to treatment: to achieve a cure, most patients require much more intense, toxic, and myelosuppressive therapy than that required for ALL. The most successful treatment programs available today result in cure rates of no more than about 40% of all patients with AML. Moreover, approximately 80% of relapses occur within the first year after treatment. Furthermore, the more intense therapy results in greater morbidity and mortality, particularly in older patients, and may limit the amount of effective therapy that can be administered. HSCT has a well-established role in the treatment of AML for patients who have an acceptably matched donor.

TREATMENT

REMISSION INDUCTION THERAPY

Although early attempts to treat AML used the same drugs that had been found to be successful in ALL, the two diseases are quite different in their biologic characteristics and their responses to therapy. The goal of therapy in the management of AML is to achieve a complete response, defined as less than 5% blast cells in the marrow, a neutrophil count greater than 1 to 1.5×10^9 per liter, and a platelet count greater than 100×10^9 per liter.

Therapy for AML is divided into two phases: remission induction and postremission therapy. Remission induction is generally initiated prior to knowledge of any cytogenetic abnormalities; therefore, treatment is based primarily on age, performance status, and history of any other hematologic disease. Almost all current treatment protocols administer 7 to 10 days of cytarabine by continuous infusion, in conjunction with an anthracycline (e.g., daunorubicin or idarubicin), or mitoxantrone, which is administered daily for 2 or 3 days. This standard induction combination, known as 7 + 3, results in CR in 64% to 75% of patients.[47–50] Recent research replacing daunorubicin with idarubicin has resulted in not only a higher CR rate but also longer remission and survival.[51–53] Suppression of the WBCs and platelets appears to be greater with the idarubicin and cytarabine combination.[51] The Children's Cancer Group and the Australian Leukemia Study Group recently reported that intensification of induction chemotherapy prolongs remissions in both children and adults with AML. These data are consistent with the concept that early leukemia cell kill prevents the emergence of drug-resistant leukemia clones.[54]

Recent data also suggest that high-dose cytarabine (HiDAC) at 3 g per m^2 administered on alternate days for eight doses compared with conventional doses of cytarabine will significantly prolong remission and disease-free survival; however, this generally results in prolonged myelosuppression.[55] Therefore, growth factor support with granulocyte colony-stimulating factor (G-CSF) is commonly given if counts remain low 14 to 21 days following therapy and/or if the patient is febrile.

The challenge in the treatment of AML is to maintain remission. Relapses are usually due to resistant disease in the bone marrow; isolated extramedullary relapses are uncommon. In addition, relapses occur earlier than with ALL, generally during the first year after diagnosis. Therefore, most current treatment regimens have emphasized early intense therapy but use a shorter duration of therapy relative to that for ALL.

CENTRAL NERVOUS SYSTEM THERAPY

Treatment of the CNS is of lesser importance in AML because the primary reason for treatment failure is bone marrow relapse. Although lymphoblasts are found in the CSF more frequently in AML than in ALL, treatment of the CNS is often limited to intrathecal drugs, with radiation administered at the end of therapy to patients with CNS disease at diagnosis. Intrathecal therapy usually consists of methotrexate, cytarabine, and hydrocortisone.

POSTREMISSION THERAPY

Once a CR is obtained, further intensive therapy is required to prevent relapse. Thus, postremission consolidation with either HSCT or chemotherapy is an integral component of the management of patients with AML. Without continued therapy, survival rates are less than 30% at 5 years. The decision as to the appropriate postremission therapy is typically determined by the patient's risk of relapse and age-specific factors. Whether autologous HSCT or HiDAC-based chemotherapy is better has been a controversial issue for a number of years, with no clinical trials showing a significant overall survival advantage for either. Another avenue of consideration is allogeneic HSCT; however, the transplant-related morbidity and mortality associated with this option tend to offset its benefits. In general, patients with good-risk AML in first CR should proceed to HiDAC-based therapy, as these patients have a greater chance of rescue with an allogeneic HSCT should they subsequently relapse. In patients with standard/intermediate-risk or poor-risk disease who are younger than 60 years of age, the use of allogeneic HSCT with a matched sibling donor is the preferred consolidation treatment, as its benefits may outweigh the potential risks of toxicity and mortality.

Allogeneic HSCT from an HLA-matched family donor was evaluated in young adults with AML in first remission as an alternative to continued chemotherapy.[56–58] The early results were quite favorable compared with chemotherapy, with leukemia-free survival rates of 50% to 65% at 5 years.

However, in subsets of older patients and those with unfavorable cytogenetic abnormalities, these rates decreased.[59] Cassileth et al[60] reviewed patients between 16 and 55 years of age and compared HiDAC, allogeneic HSCT, and autologous HSCT as postremission therapy. Each group received one course of postremission chemotherapy consisting of idarubicin and cytarabine and then was given one of the previous three treatment modalities. The results revealed superior survival for patients receiving chemotherapy over those receiving autologous HSCT. A marginal advantage was observed in those receiving chemotherapy compared with those receiving allogeneic HSCT. The use of matched, unrelated, or mismatched family donors should be reserved for the patient in a second or subsequent remission. HSCT is complicated by the occurrence of both acute and chronic GVHD, which results from the T lymphocytes in the donor marrow reacting against host tissue, and only a few patients with AML (25% to 40%) have compatible donors. Therefore, HSCT does not offer a universal cure for this disease.

SALVAGE THERAPY

Despite the intense upfront therapies that AML patients receive, disease recurrence is common, and overcoming treatment failure is crucial in improving the outcome associated with this disease. When treatment fails, further therapeutic options are typically determined by the patient's age and the duration of the first remission. Patients who are refractory to initial therapies, those who never achieve a CR, or those whose CR lasts less than 1 year carry the worst prognosis and should be offered new therapeutic options through clinical trials. Reinduction with HiDAC-based therapy may offer significant response rates for patients under the age of 60 whose CR is greater than 1 year; however, a large majority of AML patients are older than 60 years of age, which presents clinicians with a treatment dilemma. Because older patients cannot typically tolerate intensive therapies, less intensive but effective options are needed. Recently, the U.S. Food and Drug Administration (FDA) approved gemtuzumab ozogamicin (Mylotarg), an antibody-targeted agent consisting of a humanized anti-CD33 monoclonal antibody linked to calicheamicin, for the treatment of older patients with AML in first relapse. This accelerated approval was based on a clinical trial in 142 patients with relapsed AML, 30% of whom obtained a CR.[61] Better descriptions of the molecular abnormalities associated with AML have led to the identification of new classes of agents with potential activity. Investigations are underway evaluating agents that reverse multidrug resistance, agents that modulate cell signaling pathways such as farnesyl transferase inhibitors, and antiangiogenic agents including bevacizumab, a vascular endothelial growth factor (VEGF) inhibitor, to name a few.

ACUTE PROMYELOCYTIC LEUKEMIA

TREATMENT

REMISSION INDUCTION THERAPY

APL is a type of AML characterized by the t(15;17) genotype or the promyelocytic leukemia/retinoic acid receptor alfa positive (PML-RAR alfa+) genetic rearrangement; it was previously referred to as AML-M3 in the FAB classification. Remission induction strategies for patients with APL are quite different and use all-*trans* retinoic acid (ATRA), generally in combination with an anthracycline, although the anthracycline of choice has not been clearly defined. Prior to the introduction of ATRA, traditional cytarabine-based chemotherapy regimens similar to those used for AML were used. However, evidence suggests that APL is particularly sensitive to anthracycline therapy and that the role of cytarabine is limited. Although cytarabine-based combinations generated CR rates in the range of 65% to 80% of newly diagnosed cases, the remaining patients died early, primarily as a result of bleeding due to the coagulopathy commonly associated with APL. The introduction of ATRA into the treatment of these patients increased the CR rates to 80% to 90%, however, patients who obtained a CR and were maintained on either ATRA alone or low-dose chemotherapy typically relapsed quickly. The European APL group conducted a prospective phase III clinical trial comparing ATRA plus concurrent chemotherapy with a sequential approach of ATRA followed by chemotherapy. The event-free survival (EFS) times at 2 years were 84% and 77% respectively, which was attributed to a significantly decreased risk of relapse in the concurrent group (6% versus 16%, $P = 0.04$). Furthermore, disease-free survival rates as high as 75% to 81%, with CR rates of 90%, have been achieved with ATRA combined with chemotherapy.[62–67] Thus, the approach of concurrent ATRA plus chemotherapy has become the standard by which the majority of APL patients are treated.[68] This approach offers the added benefit of reducing the incidence of the retinoic acid syndrome (RAS) associated with ATRA therapy from approximately 25% to 10%. The use of ATRA alone frequently results in RAS, which is characterized by low-grade fever, aches, respiratory distress, weight gain, lower extremity edema, pleural or pericardial effusions, and episodic hypotension. For APL patients unable to tolerate an anthracycline, clinical trials are combining ATRA with gemtuzumab or arsenic trioxide. The results of these clinical trials are forthcoming and may eventually offer added treatment options in the APL armamentarium.

POSTREMISSION THERAPY

The primary goal of postremission therapy in APL is eradication of the leukemic clones [e.g., t(15,17) and PML-RAR]. Therefore, patients should be routinely monitored during therapy for these abnormalities. A positive PML-RAR test is predictive of a subsequent hematologic relapse and requires early salvage chemotherapy prior to the emergence of overt disease. Most studies have used anthracycline-based therapy, generally in combination with cytarabine. However, just as the role of cytarabine in induction therapy appears limited, emerging data suggest that there is little role for cytarabine in postremission therapy. A study by the Spanish Cooperative Group PETHEMA (Programa de Estudio y Tratamiento de las Hemopatias Malignas) suggests that patients receiving cytarabine do as well as those not receiving cytarabine as part of APL postremission therapy.[69] Although the ideal number of cycles of postremission therapy is not known, it has become customary to administer at least two cycles after remission induction with ATRA plus an anthracycline.

The value of maintenance therapy in patients with APL is controversial. Preliminary results of two randomized trials suggested that 2 years of maintenance therapy with intermittent ATRA and low-dose chemotherapy may be of benefit in patients with APL.[68,69] However, long-term follow-up of these trials yielded conflicting results, primarily in those who were PML-RAR negative after consolidation therapy.[70,71] Thus, at present it appears that patients receiving more intensive consolidation therapy and who are PML-RAR negative after consolidation may not require maintenance therapy, whereas patients receiving less intensive consolidation therapy may benefit from 2 years of ATRA and low-dose chemotherapy.

SALVAGE THERAPY

If relapse occurs in patients with APL, therapeutic options are typically based on the timing of the recurrence. In general, if the relapse occurs more than 1 year after ATRA plus anthracycline, a second CR can be achieved in 85% to 90% of patients with ATRA as reinduction therapy. However, patients who relapse within 1 year of ATRA may be resistant to its use as reinduction because of potential mutations in the RAR moiety of PML-RAR. It is in these patients that the use of arsenic trioxide has shown benefit. A recent multicenter trial evaluated the use of single-agent arsenic trioxide in 40 relapsed APL patients (21 in first CR, 19 in second CR or more). Arsenic trioxide 0.15 mg/kg/day was administered until there were no detectable leukemic cells in the bone marrow. Patients who achieved a CR were given one cycle of consolidation with arsenic trioxide at the same dose for as long as 25 days and could receive up to four more doses repeated every 25 days as maintenance therapy. Arsenic trioxide therapy resulted in a CR rate of 85%, with a median time to bone marrow remission of 35 days and overall survival of 66%.

Moreover, all patients who achieved a clinical CR also showed evidence of the elimination of the t(15;17) chromosomal abnormality, the hallmark cytogenetic abnormality associated with APL. Thus, therapy with arsenic trioxide is now considered a highly effective therapy for relapsed APL.[72]

PROGNOSIS

Prognostic factors for AML are less well defined than for ALL, primarily because the overall survival is much poorer. Nevertheless, a number of variables have been identified that are associated either with a poor likelihood of achieving a CR or with a short remission (Table 94.6). Patients may be classified as having a favorable prognosis, standard prognosis, or poor prognosis, primarily defined by the cytogenetic abnormalities present at diagnosis as well as other variables including age, performance status, WBC count at diagnosis, the presence or absence of an antecedent hematologic disorder, and the presence of the multidrug resistant (MDR) protein. Variables associated with a poor prognosis in AML are advancing age, a high WBC count at diagnosis, and a high degree of bone marrow involvement. In general, the risk of recurrence for APL is categorized based on the presenting WBC and platelet counts:

TABLE 94.6	Prognostic Factors at Diagnosis of Acute Myelocytic Leukemia (AML)
Favorable Prognosis	Cytogenetics: t(8;21), inv 16, or t(16;16) FAB morphology
Standard Prognosis	Cytogenetics: normal, t(9;11), +8
	Age <65 years
	Good performance status
	No history of antecedent hematologic disorder
	No prior chemotherapy or radiation therapy
	WBC count $<20 \times 10^9$/L
Poor Prognosis	Cytogenetics: monosomies of 5 or 7; 7q-, 5q-, complex karyotypes (≥3 abnormalities), t(6;9), 11q23, 20q-, Ph(+) [e.g., t(9;22)]
	Age >65
	Poor performance status
	Presence of MDR1 protein
	Any abnormal blood counts more than 6 months prior to AML diagnosis; history of myelodysplastic syndrome or any antecedent hematologic disorder
	WBC count $>100 \times 10^9$/L
	HIV positive

- Low risk: WBC count less than 10×10^9 per L, platelet count 40×10^9 per L or more
- Intermediate risk: WBC count less than 10×10^9 per L, platelet count less than $40 \times 10^9/$ per L
- High risk: WBC count above 10×10^9 per L

Cytogenetic studies are becoming increasingly important for prognosis as well as treatment selection.[73,74]

KEY POINTS

- Tremendous advances have been made in the treatment of the acute leukemias over the past 10 years, and the successes that have been achieved in the treatment of childhood ALL serve as a model for treatment of other malignancies
- Today, acute leukemias are potentially curable diseases in many patients, and considerable prolongation of a useful and productive life can be achieved in many others
- Current research efforts in immunology and molecular biology are likely to lead to powerful new treatments
- AML is typically a disease of adults, whereas ALL is a disease of children
- AML is generally more resistant to treatment than ALL
- Initial presenting symptoms result from bone marrow failure and include fatigue, weight loss, fever, pallor, purpura, and pain
- A diagnosis of acute leukemia is made by performing a bone marrow biopsy, which contains a minimum of 20% blast cells
- The primary treatment modality is chemotherapy for both AML and ALL
- Transplantation plays an important role in the treatment of AML
- The treatment phases involved in ALL therapy are induction, consolidation, CNS therapy, and maintenance treatment
- The treatment phases for AML are remission induction and postremission therapy with either chemotherapy or transplantation
- ALL induction therapy involves the use of prednisone, vincristine, and either asparaginase or an anthracycline
- The 7 + 3 regimen (cytarabine plus daunorubicin) is the standard of care in AML for remission induction

SUGGESTED READINGS

DeVita V, ed. Cancer: principles and practice of oncology, 7th ed. Philadelphia: Lippincott Wilkins & Wilkins, 2005.
DiPiro J, ed. Pharmacotherapy: a pathophysiologic approach, 6th ed. New York: McGraw-Hill, 2005.

REFERENCES

1. Clarkson B. The acute leukemias. In: Thorn GW, Adams RD, Braunwald E, et al, eds. Harrison's principles of internal medicine, 8th ed. New York: McGraw-Hill, 1977:1767–1777.
2. Ries LAG, Eisner MP, Kosary CL, et al, eds. SEER Cancer Statistics Review, 1975–2000. National Cancer Institute, Bethesda, MD. Available at: http://seer.cancer.gov/csr/1975_2000, 2003.
3. Wingo PA, Tong T, Bolden S. Cancer statistics. CA Cancer J Clin 45:8–30, 1995.
4. Gallo RD, Wong-Staal F. Retroviruses as etiologic agents of some animal and human leukemias and lymphomas and as tools for elucidating the molecular mechanism of leukemogenesis. Blood 60:545–556, 1982.
5. Sandler DP, Ross JA. Epidemiology of acute leukemia in children and adults. Semin Oncol 24:3–16, 1997.
6. Altman AJ, Schwartz AD. Malignant diseases of infancy, childhood and adolescence. Philadelphia: WB Saunders, 1983:187–238.
7. Bennett JM, Catovsky D, Daniel M-T, et al. Proposals for the classifications of the acute leukemias; French-American-British (FAB) cooperative group. Br J Haematol 33:451–458, 1976.
8. Harris NL, Jaffe ES, Diebold J, et al. World Health Organization of neoplastic diseases of the hematopoietic and lymphoid tissues; report of the clinical advisory committee meeting, Airlie House, VA, November 1997. J Clin Oncol 17:3835–3849, 1999.
9. Pui C-H. Acute lymphoblastic leukemia. Pediatr Clin North Am 44:831–846, 1997.
10. Kishimoto T, Goyert S, Kikutani H, et al. CD antigens 1996. Blood 89:3502, 1997.
11. Pui C-H, Evans W. Acute lymphoblastic leukemia. N Engl J Med 339:605–615, 1998.
12. Pui C-H. Childhood leukemias (Medical Progress). N Engl J Med 332:1618–1630, 1995.
13. Pui C-H, Behm FG, Crist WM. Clinical and biologic relevance of immunologic marker studies in childhood acute lymphoblastic leukemia. Blood 82:343–362, 1993.
14. Marks DI, Kurz BW, Link MP, et al. High incidence of potential p53 inactivation in poor outcome childhood acute lymphoblastic leukemia at diagnosis. Blood 87:1155–1161, 1996.
15. Cline MJ. The molecular basis of leukemia. N Engl J Med 330:328–336, 1994.
16. Rubnitz JE, Downing JR, Pui C-H, et al. TEL gene rearrangement in acute lymphoblastic leukemia: a new genetic marker with prognostic significance. J Clin Oncol 15:1150–1157, 1997.
17. Fernbach DJ. Natural history of acute leukemia. In: Sutow WW, Fernbach DJ, Vietti TJ. Clinical pediatric oncology, 3rd ed. St. Louis: CV Mosby, 1984:332–377.
18. Freeman AI, Pantazopoulos N, DeCastro L, et al. Infections in children with acute leukemia. Med Pediatr Oncol 1:67–73, 1975.
19. Farber S, Diamond LK, Mercer RD, et al. Temporary remissions in acute leukemia in children produced by folic antagonist 4–amethopteroylglutamic acid (aminopterin). N Engl J Med 238:787–793, 1948.
20. Pui CH, Relling MV, Downing JR. Acute lymphoblastic leukemia. N Engl J Med 350:1535–1548, 2004.
21. Hoelzer D, Gokbuget N, Ottmann O, et al. Acute lymphoblastic leukemia. Hematology (Am Soc Hematol Educ Program) 162–192, 2002.
22. Jacquillat C, Weil M, Gemon MF, et al. Combination therapy in 130 patients with acute lymphoblastic leukemia (protocol 06 LA 66–Paris). Cancer Res 33:3278–3284, 1973.
23. Ortega JA, Nesbit ME Jr, Donaldson MH, et al. L-Asparaginase, vincristine and prednisone for induction of first remission in acute lymphocytic leukemia. Cancer Res 37:535–540, 1977.
24. Sackman JF, Pavlovsky S, Penalver JA, et al. Evaluation of induction of remission, intensification and central nervous system prophylactic treatment in acute lymphoblastic leukemia. Cancer 34:418, 1974.
25. Tubergen DG, Gilchrist GS, O'Brien RT, et al. Improved outcome with delayed intensification for children with acute lymphoblastic leukemia and intermediate presenting features: a Children's Cancer Group phase III trial. J Clin Oncol 11:527–537, 1993.

26. George P, Pinkel D. CNS radiation in children with acute lympho-cytic leukemia in remission [abstract]. Proc Am Assoc Cancer Res 6:22, 1965.

27. Aur RJA, Simone JV, Hustu HO, et al. A comparative study of cen-tral nervous system irradiation and intensive chemotherapy early in remission of childhood acute lymphocytic leukemia. Cancer 29:381, 1972.

28. Nesbit ME, Robison LL, Littman PS, et al. Presymptomatic central nervous system therapy in previously untreated childhood acute lymphoblastic leukaemia: comparison of 1800 rad and 2400 rad. A report for Children's Cancer Study Group. Lancet 1:461, 1981.

29. Aur RJA, Hustu HO, Verzosa MS, et al. Comparison of two meth-ods of preventing central nervous system leukemia. Blood 42: 349–357, 1973.

30. Bleyer WA. Clinical pharmacology of intrathecal methotrexate. II. An improved dosage regimen derived from age-related pharmacoki-netics. Cancer Treat Rep 61:1419–1425, 1977.

31. Gilchrist GS, Tubergen DG, Sather HN, et al. Low numbers of CSF blasts at diagnosis do not predict for the development of CNS leuke-mia in children with intermediate-risk acute lymphoblastic leukemia: a Children's Cancer Group report. J Clin Oncol 12:2594–2600, 1994.

32. Freeman AI, Weinberg V, Brecher ML, et al. Comparison of inter-mediate-dose methotrexate with cranial irradiation for the post-induc-tion treatment of acute lymphocytic leukemia in children. N Engl J Med 308:477–484, 1983.

33. Evans WE, Crom WR, Yalowich JC. Methotrexate. In: Evans WE, Schentag JJ, Jusko WJ, eds. Applied pharmacokinetics; principles of therapeutic drug monitoring, 2nd ed. Spokane: Applied Therapeutics 1986:1009–1056.

34. Balis FM, Savitch JL, Bleyer WA, et al. Remission induction of me-ningeal leukemia with high-dose intravenous methotrexate. J Clin Oncol 3:485–489, 1985.

35. Relling MV, Mahmoud H, Pui C-H, et al. Intravenous etoposide ther-apy achieves potentially cytotoxic concentrations in cerebrospinal fluid of children with acute lymphoblastic leukemia [abstract]. Proc Annu Meet Am Assoc Cancer Res 35:A1438, 1994.

36. Jones B, Freeman AI, Shuster JJ, et al. Lower incidence of menin-geal leukemia when prednisone is replaced by dexamethasone in the treatment of acute lymphocytic leukemia. Med Pediatr Oncol 19: 269–275, 1991.

37. Simone JV, Rivera G. Management of acute leukemia. In: Sutow WW, Fernbach DJ, Vietti TJ, eds. Clinical pediatric oncology, 3rd ed. St. Louis: CV Mosby, 1984:378–402.

38. Aur RJA, Simone JV, Verzosa JS, et al. Childhood acute lympho-cytic leukemia: study VIII. Cancer 42:2123–2134, 1978.

39. Luria SE, Delbrück M. Mutations of bacteria from virus sensitivity to virus resistance. Genetics 28:491–511, 1943.

40. Goldie JH, Coldman AJ. A mathematical model for relating the drug sensitivity of tumors to their spontaneous mutation rate. Cancer Treat Rep 63:1727–1733, 1979.

41. Goldie JH, Coldman AJ, Gudauskas GA. Rationale for the use of al-ternating non-cross-resistant chemotherapy. Cancer Treat Rep 66: 439–449, 1982.

42. Biggs JC, Horowitz MM, Gale RP, et al. Bone marrow transplants may cure patients with acute leukemia never achieving remission with chemotherapy. Blood 80:1090–1093, 1992.

43. Forman SJ, Schmidt GM, Nademanee AP, et al. Allogeneic bone marrow transplantation as therapy for primary induction failure for patients with acute leukemia. J Clin Oncol 9:1570–1574, 1991.

44. Arico M, Valsecchi MG, Camitta B, et al. Outcome of treatment in children with Philadelphia chromosome-positive acute lymphoblastic leukemia. N Engl J Med 342:998–1006, 2000.

45. Williams DL, Tsiatis A, Brodeur GM, et al. Prognostic importance of chromosome number in 136 untreated children with acute lymph-oblastic leukemia. Blood 60:864–871, 1982.

46. Pui C-H, Kane JR, Crist WM. Biology and treatment of infant leuke-mia. Leukemia 9:762–769, 1995.

47. Lister TA, Rohatiner AZS. The treatment of acute myelogenous leu-kemia in adults. Semin Hematol 19:172–192, 1982.

48. Gale RP. Advances in the treatment of acute myelogenous leukemia. N Engl J Med 300:1189–1199, 1979.

49. Gale RP, Foon KA, Cline M, et al. Intensive chemotherapy for acute myelogenous leukemia. Ann Intern Med 94:753–757, 1981.

50. Mayer RJ, Davis RB, Schiffer CA, et al. Intensive post-remission chemotherapy in adults with acute myeloid leukemia. N Engl J Med 3331:896–903, 1994.

51. Wiernik PH, Banks PC, Case DC, et al. Cytarabine plus idarubicin or daunorubicin as induction and consolidation therapy for previ-ously untreated adults with acute myeloid leukemia. Blood 79: 313–319, 1992.

52. Berman E, Heller G, Santorsa J, et al. Results of a randomized trial comparing idarubicin and cytosine arabinoside with daunorubicin and cytosine arabinoside in adult patients with newly diagnosed acute myelogenous leukemia. Blood 77:1666–1674, 1991.

53. Vogler WR, Velez-Garcia E, Omura G, et al. A phase 3 trial com-paring daunorubicin or idarubicin combined with cytosine arabino-side in acute myelogenous leukemia. J Clin Oncol 10:1103–1111, 1992.

54. Woods W, Kobrinsky N, Buckley J, et al. Timed-sequential induc-tion therapy improves post-remission outcome in acute myeloid leu-kemia: a report from the Children's Cancer Group. Blood 87: 4979–4989, 1996.

55. Bishop JF, Matthews JP, Youg GA, et al. A randomized study of high-dose cytarabine in induction in acute myeloid leukemia. Blood 87:1710–1717, 1996.

56. Sanders JE, Thomas ED, Buckner CE, et al. Marrow transplantation of children in first remission of acute nonlymphoblastic leukemia: an update. Blood 66:460–462, 1985.

57. Woods W, Kobrinsky N, Neudorf S, et al. Intensively timed induc-tion therapy followed by autologous or allogeneic bone marrow transplantation for children with acute myeloid leukemia or myelo-dysplastic syndrome: a Children's Cancer Group pilot study. J Clin Oncol 11:1448–1457, 1993.

58. McGlave PB, Haake RJ, Bostrom BC, et al. Allogeneic bone mar-row transplantation for acute nonlymphocytic leukemia in first remis-sion. Blood 72:1512–1517, 1988.

59. Leith CP, Kopecky KJ, Godwin J, et al. Acute myeloid leukemia in the elderly: assessment of multidrug resistance (MDR1) and cytoge-netics distinguishes biologic subgroups with remarkably distinct re-sponses for standard chemotherapy: a Southwest Oncology Group study. Blood 89:3323–3329, 1997.

60. Cassileth PA, Harrington DP, Appelbaum FR, et al. Chemotherapy compared with autologous or allogeneic bone marrow transplanta-tion in the management of acute myeloid leukemia in first remis-sion. N Engl J Med 339:1649–1656, 1998.

61. Sievers EL, Larson RA, Stadtmauer EA, et al. Efficacy and safety of gemtuzumab ozogamicin in patients with CD33-positive acute myeloid leukemia in first relapse. J Clin Oncol 19:3244–3254, 2001.

62. Chessells JM, O'Callaghan U, Hardisty RM. Acute myeloid leuke-mia in childhood: clinical features and prognosis. Br J Haematol 6: 555–564, 1986.

63. Creutzig U, Ritter J, Schellong G. Identification of two risk groups in childhood acute myelogenous leukemia after therapy intensifica-tion in study AML-BFM-83 as compared with study AML-BFM-78. Blood 75:1932–1940, 1990.

64. Ravindranath Y, Steuber CP, Krischer H, et al. High-dose cytarabine for intensification of early therapy of childhood acute myeloid leuke-mia: a Pediatric Oncology Group study. J Clin Oncol 9:572–580, 1991.

65. Tallman M, Anderson J, Schiffer C, et al. Phase III randomized study of all-trans-retinoic acid (ATRA) vs. daunorubicin and cyto-sine arabinoside as induction therapy and ATRA vs. observation as maintenance therapy for patients with previously untreated acute pro-myelocytic leukemia [abstract]. Blood 86:125, 1995.

66. Wells R, Woods W, Lamphin B, et al. Impact of high-dose cytara-bine and asparaginase intensification on childhood acute myeloid leu-kemia: a report from the Children's Cancer Group. J Clin Oncol 11: 538–545, 1993.

67. Kanamaru A, Takemoto Y, Tanimoto M, et al. All-trans retinoic acid for the treatment of newly diagnosed acute promyelocytic leuke-mia. Blood 85:1202–1206, 1995.

68. Fenaux P, Chastang C, Chevret S, et al. A randomized comparison of all transretinoic acid (ATRA) followed by chemotherapy and ATRA plus chemotherapy and the role of maintenance therapy in newly diagnosed acute promyelocytic leukemia. Blood 94: 1192–1200, 1999.

69. Sanz MA, Martin G, Rayon C, et al. A modified AIDA protocol with anthracycline-based consolidation results in high antileukemic efficacy and reduced toxicity in newly diagnosed PML/RARα positive acute promyelocytic leukemia. Blood 94:3015–3021, 1999.

70. Giuseppe A, Petti M, Lo Coco F, et al. AIDA: the Italian way of treating acute promyelocytic leukemia (APL), final act. Blood 102: abstract 487, 2003.

71. Bourgeois E, Chevret S, Sanz M, et al. Long-term follow-up of APL treated with ATRA and chemotherapy (CT) including incidence of late relapses and overall toxicity. Blood 102:abstract 483, 2003.

72. Soignet S, Frankel S, Douer D, et al. United States multicenter study of arsenic trioxide in relapsed acute promyelocytic leukemia. J Clin Oncol 19:3852–3860, 2001.

73. Arthur DC, Berger R, Golomb HM, et al. The clinical significance of karyotype in acute myelogenous leukemia. Cancer Genet Cytogenet 40:203–216, 1989.

74. Fourth International Workshop on Chromosomes in Leukemia 1982. Clinical significance of chromosomal abnormalities in acute non-lymphoblastic leukemia. Cancer Genet Cytogenet 11:332–350, 1984.

Lymphomas

95

Rebecca S. Finley

TREATMENT GOALS

- The goal of treatment for Hodgkin's disease is to cure with minimal long-term sequelae.
- Cure is possible for patients with early stage indolent non-Hodgkin's lymphomas (NHL) with radiation therapy (RT). Cure is less frequently achieved in more advanced indolent NHL, and the goal of therapy is generally to prolong survival and minimize toxicities and maintain quality of life.
- Cure is the goal for many aggressive and highly aggressive NHLs.
- For patients with treatment-refractory lymphomas, the goals of additional therapy are to minimize symptoms of disease, maintain quality-of-life, and prolong survival.

DEFINITION

Lymphoid malignancies may manifest in the bone marrow and peripheral blood or in other tissue where lymphocytes may aggregate. When they present as extramedullary tumors arising primarily in the lymph nodes or other sites, these tumors are called lymphomas; when the bone marrow is the predominant site of the disease, they are classified as leukemias. Lymphomas are generally separated into Hodgkin's disease (HD) and non-Hodgkin's lymphomas (NHLs). The term "non-Hodgkin's lymphomas" represents multiple diseases with diverse morphologic, immunophenotypic, cytogenetic, and clinical features.

PATHOPHYSIOLOGY

ANATOMY AND PHYSIOLOGY OF THE LYMPHORETICULAR SYSTEM

The lymphoreticular system constitutes the anatomic basis of cellular and humoral immunity. Lymphocytes are the principal cellular component of the lymphoreticular system and are widely distributed in the body individually and in aggregated centers (most commonly the lymph nodes). Reticulum cells and cells of the monocyte-macrophage series are also included in this system. Lymphoid cells originate in the bone marrow, undergo differentiation, and migrate, by way of the blood and lymphatic vessels to populate the

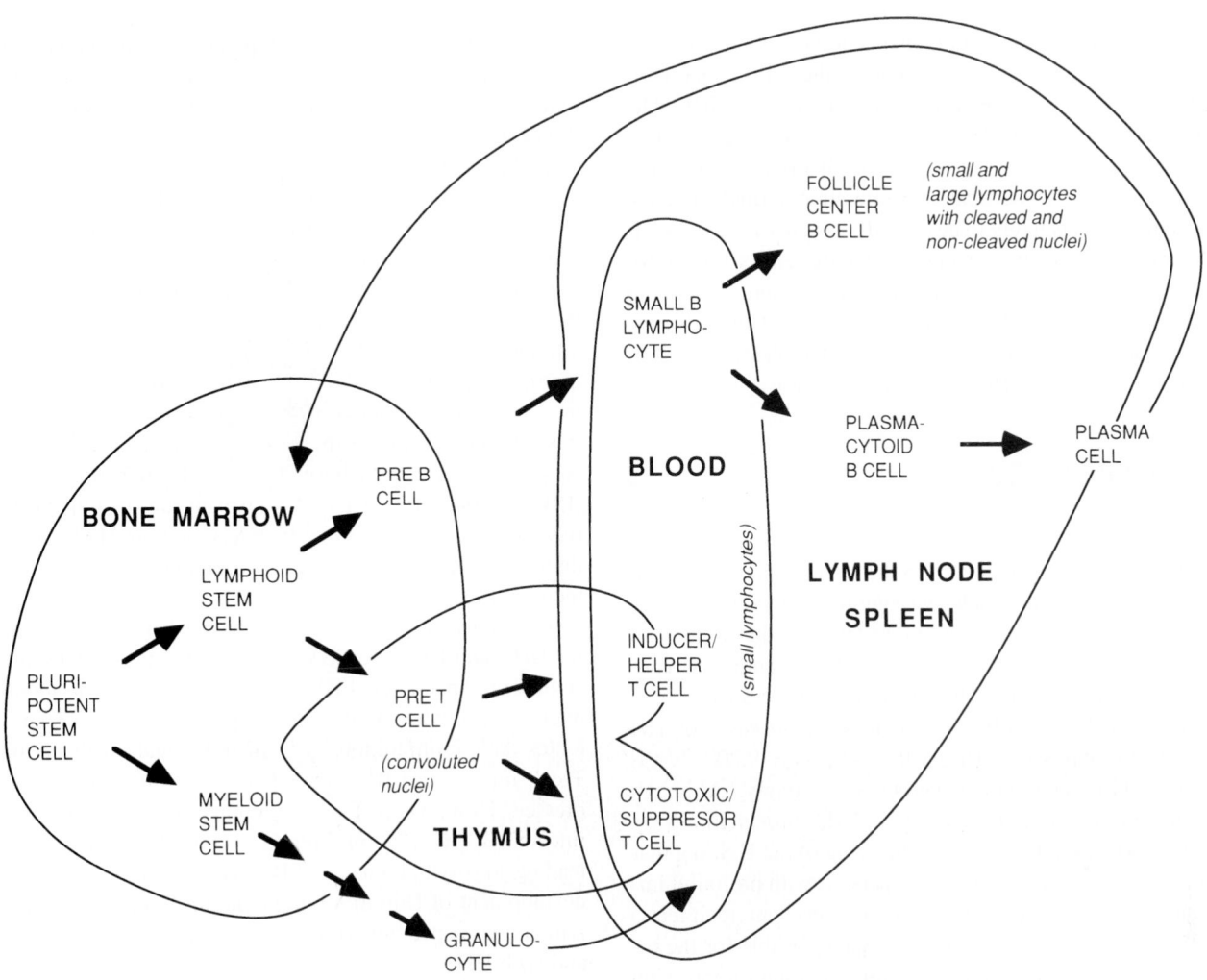

FIGURE 95.1 Tissue distribution of lymphocytes. (From Aisenber AC. Cell lineage in lympho-proliferative disease. Am J Med 74:680, 1983, with permission.)

other lymphoreticular tissues (Fig. 95.1). As lymphocytes differentiate, their morphologic appearance changes, and they sequentially express different antigens on the cell surface. T lymphocytes are processed by the thymus gland and are responsible for cell-mediated immunity. T lymphocytes are the predominant lymphocytes in peripheral blood and occupy the deep cortex of the lymph nodes. B lymphocytes are derived from the bone marrow and confer humoral immunity. B lymphocytes constitute only 10% to 15% of circulating lymphocytes and predominate in the follicles of the lymph nodes.

MALIGNANT TRANSFORMATION

Most lymphomas can be classified by the cell of origin, however, the precise cellular origin of HD is often difficult to establish. Two types of cells are characteristic of HD. These are mononuclear Hodgkin's cells (HC) and poly-nucleated Reed-Sternberg (R-S) cells. In recent years, newly identified immunophenotype characteristics have confirmed that in the vast majority of patients with HD, the characteris-

tic cells, the R-S cells, are clonal lymphoma cells derived from B cells. They have somatic mutations that prevent immunoglobulin expression that B cells normally demonstrate. Other typical B-cell markers are also absent on the R-S cells. In rare cases, HD appears to be derived from T cells.[1] Although genetic alterations are common in HC and R-S cells, no specific chromosomal aberration has been defined.[2]

NHLs result from the malignant transformation of normal lymphoid cells at specific stages of differentiation. Like other malignancies, cytogenetic abnormalities have been identified that are associated with specific types of NHLs. In contrast to many other types of malignancies, however, most NHLs have only one or a very few cytogenetic changes. The most common type of changes is oncogenes activated by chromosomal translocations or tumor suppressor genes inactivated by chromosomal deletions or mutations.[3] After the malignant transformation, there is a clonal expansion of the malignant cells. Although some NHL cells may morphologically resemble the normal lymphocyte or lymphocyte precursor at the stage when the transformation occurred, others may appear quite different. However, lymphoma cells tend to retain the same immunophenotype as their normal counterparts, and thus, assessment of the cell surface antigens may be used to determine the exact type of NHL. The clinical course of the NHL is influenced by the stage at which the malignant transformation occurs. If the transformation occurs in a stage where rapid proliferation normally occurs, the lymphoma is likely to be a rapidly progressive disease. If the transformation occurs in more mature cells or progenitor resting stages, the lymphoma is likely to progress more slowly. In developed countries, such as the United States, most adult NHLs are derived from B lymphocytes (85%), whereas only about 15% are of T-cell origin.

EPIDEMIOLOGY

INCIDENCE

The incidence of lymphomas in the United States increased steadily for several decades through the late 1980s or early 1990s, however, it has appeared to level off during the late 1990s.[4] Through the 1980s, the most substantial increase were in cases of NHL. The American Cancer Society estimated that during 2005 there will be 7,350 cases of HD and 56,390 cases of NHL, with 1,410 and 19,200 deaths attributed to each lymphoma group, respectively.[5] Although the precise reason for the increase in NHL through the 1980s and 1990s was unknown, both the aging of the U.S. population and the increased number of persons with profound immunosuppression (e.g., HIV, organ transplant recipients) were believed to be at least partially responsible for the increase. Support for this relationship to immunosuppression was demonstrated by the disproportionate occurrence of acquired immunodeficiency syndrome (AIDS)-related NHL among young to middle-aged persons during the 1980s which has now decreased sharply due to the availability of effective human immunodeficiency virus (HIV) therapies.[4,6] Most epidemiologic studies report that the incidence of NHL increases steadily from childhood to age 80, is higher in males than females, and higher in whites than African-Americans, and recent data suggest an increasing rate of NHL among African-Americans of several age groups.[4] Throughout the 1970s and 1980s, the incidence of NHL increased dramatically in older Americans. This rate of increase appears to have slowed significantly, however, the explanation for this change is not readily apparent.[4] Further analyses of these changes in the demographics of NHL will hopefully further elucidate the risk factors and etiology of this group of diseases.

HD exhibits a bimodal incidence curve, with the first peak occurring in the late 20s, after which there is a decline in the incidence until about age 50. After age 45 to 50, there is another smaller peak.[1] HD is also more common in males than females[7] and more common in whites than African-Americans.

ETIOLOGY

Although the etiology of most lymphomas is unknown, several factors have been associated with an increased risk. Patients with immunodeficiency disorders, acquired (e.g., AIDS or caused by immunosuppressive therapies) or congenital (e.g., Wiskott-Aldrich syndrome, ataxia-telangiectasia), appear to have an increased risk of NHL.[3,8–10] Patients receiving chronic immunosuppressive therapy after organ transplantation to prevent graft rejection have a substantial risk. It has been estimated that 2% of patients with renal transplants and 5% of patients with heart transplants will ultimately develop NHL.[11] Patients who undergo allogeneic marrow or peripheral blood stem cell transplants are also at increased risk.[11] In each of these cases, it appears that the risk correlates with the severity of posttransplant immunosuppression. Individuals who were Epstein-Barr Virus (EBV) seronegative prior to transplant are also at greater risk.[3] Chronic autoimmune disorders such as Hashimoto's thyroiditis, Sjögren's syndrome, or rheumatoid arthritis also increase the risk of NHL.[9,10,12,13]

Infectious etiologies have been suggested for many years for NHL and HD. The EBV has been the most extensively studied viral pathogen. EBV is the cause of infectious mononucleosis and when it infects B lymphocytes in vitro, it stimulates their proliferation.[3,11,14] In individuals with normal T-cell immunity, EBV-induced B-cell proliferation is suppressed. However, if T-cell immunity is depressed, EBV-infected B cells may proliferate uncontrollably, ultimately leading to a lymphoma.[3,14] EBV has been linked with the development of Burkitt's lymphoma in African children,[15] lymphomas in patients with underlying immunodeficiencies, and with HD.

There has been a small (threefold), but consistent, increased risk of HD among persons who have had infectious mononucleosis.[1] Also, in some series, the proportion of patients with HD who have elevated titers of antibody against EBV is larger than expected and enhanced activation of EBV may precede the development of HD.[16] An important finding is that DNAs of EBV and EBV-encoded genes[17,18] have been detected in R-S cells[19]; however, at least 50% of patients with HD in the United States and other developed countries show no evidence of EBV. Interestingly, more than 90% of HD patients in developing countries have been reported to carry the virus.[1] Evidence suggests that infection of the B lymphocyte with EBV may "hide" it from immune surveillance, creating an antiapoptotic scenario and promoting proliferation that may lead to the lymphoma.[1] It is not clear whether EBV has a direct role in the development of HD or if EBV infection is a result of decreased underlying immune competency that is linked to the pathogenesis of HD. Also, because of the high prevalence of EBV in the general population, coincidence cannot be entirely ruled out. Some epidemiologic studies of HD have reported a correlation of HD in younger patients with a higher level of maternal education, fewer siblings and playmates, early birth order, and residence in a single family dwelling during early childhood.[1] These links have led some investigators to postulate that HD may occur as a host response to an infection because individuals, who as children, were less likely to be exposed to infectious pathogens seem to have an increased risk of HD. Overall, however, there is no evidence to support the hypothesis that HD is transmitted by person-to-person contact.

A number of studies have suggested familial links or genetic predisposition to HD. There does appear to be an increased risk in first-degree relatives, while siblings have a twofold to fivefold risk.[1,20] There is also an association of HD with certain leukocyte antigens.[21]

Besides EBV, other viruses have also been associated with several types of NHL. Human T-cell lymphotropic virus type 1 (HTLV-1) is transmitted by sexual contact, infected blood products, breast feeding, and has been isolated from adult T-cell lymphoma/leukemias.[22] A herpes virus, HHV-8, that was initially isolated from Kaposi's sarcoma lesions has also been found in some patients with AIDS-related lymphomas, many of whom also have EBV.[23] It has been suggested that HHV-8 may be required for the EBV-initiated malignant transformation in some lymphomas.[3,24] Chronic hepatitis C virus infection has also been linked to B-cell NHL in some studies. It is believed that the chronic viral infection may cause chronic antigen stimulation of B cells leading to malignant transformation.[3]

Gastric infection with *Helicobacter pylori* has been implicated in the pathogenesis of primary gastric lymphomas. The chronic gastritis that results from the infection leads to antigen stimulation and the eventual development of malignant B cells in the form of gastric mucosa-associated lymphoid tissue (MALT) lymphoma.[25]

Other environmental, occupational, and therapeutic exposures associated with an increased risk of NHL include herbicides, pesticides, solvents, woodworking, and some cancer chemotherapeutic drugs.[3,26] Ionizing radiation may also induce lymphoma, as evidenced by the increased incidence in survivors of Hiroshima and patients irradiated for ankylosing spondylitis.[27] Patients who have previously been treated for HD also have a significantly increased risk of developing NHL.[28] Chronic phenytoin use may lead to a condition known as ''lymphoid hyperplasia'' or ''pseudolymphoma.'' In most cases, this condition regresses when the phenytoin is discontinued.[29]

PATHOLOGY

Although the diagnosis and classification of many lymphomas can be made by biopsy and histopathologic examination under a light microscope, the application of immunophenotypic and cytogenetic assessments have become increasingly important in differentiating the various subtypes of lymphomas and determining the most appropriate therapies.

A biopsy specimen of HD reveals a heterogenous cellular population of normal-appearing lymphocytes (predominantly helper T cells), eosinophils, plasma cells, and a relatively few number of the malignant R-S cells. These R-S cells, the characteristic malignant cells of HD, are multinucleated giant cells that are usually required to make a pathologic diagnosis. The normal appearing host inflammatory cells that surround the R-S cells are the body's response to the tumor. Although 35% to 40% of patients with HD have cytogenetic abnormalities, no specific chromosomal marker has been identified. Several classifications have been used to categorize HD into various subtypes. The Rye classification (based on morphology) was widely used in the past, but the availability of more immunologic and molecular information has resulted in a newer classification by the International Lymphoma Study Group. This system makes an important distinction between nodular lymphocyte-predominant HD (NLPHD) and the other subtypes, which are often called classic HD. More recently the World Health Organization (WHO) has also offered a classification that takes into account the immunologic and molecular characteristics (Table 95.1).[30–32]

NLPHD represents about 5% of all HD cases. It differs morphologically and immunologically from classic HD in that the R-S cells have vesicular, polylobulated nuclei resembling popcorn. As the name implies, a nodular pattern is almost always present and the background (infiltrate surrounding the R-S cells) is predominantly lymphocytes. The immunophenotype of NLPHD lacks the HD-associated antigens, CD15 and CD30, but expresses CD 45, B-cell associated antigens (CD19, CD20, CD22, and CD79a), and CD57 positive T cells are often present.[1] NLPHD is often diagnosed while in the early stages (I or II) of disease. Most patients have a complete response (CR) to therapy with 90% of patients surviving more than 10 years.[1] However, patients with NLPHD have a higher risk of developing NHL than those with other subtypes of HD and, in fact, NHL is often the eventual cause of death for these patients.[1,33]

Classic HD is defined by the presence of R-S cells with a nodular sclerosis, mixed cellularity, lymphocyte depletion, or lymphocyte-rich background. Immunologically, cells are CD15-positive and CD30-positive, and commonly lack T-cell and B-cell antigens. Although most patients have cytogenetic abnormalities, no specific abnormality is characteristic for the disease.

The mixed-cellularity subtype contains an infiltrate of lymphocytes, epithelioid histiocytes, eosinophils, neutrophils, and plasma cells. It represents 15% to 30% of all cases and may be seen at any age. Patients may be diagnosed at any clinical stage, with abdominal lymph node and splenic involvement being relatively common.

Lymphocyte-depleted HD is characterized by a predominance of variant R-S cells with a hypocellular background. This subtype is the least common, accounting for less than

TABLE 95.1	Classification of Hodgkin's Lymphomas	
Rye Classification	**REAL Classification**	**WHO Classification**
Lymphocyte predominant	Nodular lymphocyte predominant	Lymphocyte predominant, nodular
	Classic HL	Classic HL
	Lymphocyte-rich classic HL	Lymphocyte-rich classic HL
Nodular sclerosis	Nodular sclerosis	Nodular Sclerosis
Mixed cellularity	Mixed cellularity	Mixed cellularity
Lymphocyte depleted	Lymphocyte depleted	Lymphocyte depleted
		Unclassifiable HL

REAL, Revised European-American Lymphoma; WHO, World Health Organization; HL, Hodgkin's lymphoma.

1% of cases and is most commonly seen in older patients and HIV-positive patients. Patients with the lymphocyte-depleted subtype often have symptomatic and disseminated disease.

Nodular-sclerosing HD is characterized by a nodular pattern with fibrous bands separating the nodules. The background contains lymphocytes, histiocytes, plasma cells, neutrophils, and eosinophils. Necrosis is frequently seen. This is the most common type of HD, accounting for 60% to 80% of all cases. It most frequently occurs in adolescents and young adults, but it can occur at any age. It is associated with a good prognosis, especially if the disease is localized.

Lymphocyte-rich HD is a recently described subtype of HD that is characterized by a background of lymphocytes with very few eosinophils. About 5% of classic HDs are classified as lymphocyte-rich. Patients are frequently diagnosed with the disease in its early stages and symptoms are rare. The age at diagnosis is typically older than seen with nodular sclerosing and the prognosis is quite good.

Occasionally, patients will present with mixed HD and NHL. In these cases, the NHL is usually of B-cell derivation. As mentioned earlier, patients who have been successfully treated for HD are at a higher risk of developing NHL later.[33]

The classification of NHLs are based on their cellular origin (and at what point during lymphocyte differentiation the malignant transformation occurred), and the morphologic, cytogenetic, and immunologic characteristics of the malignant cells. Many different histologic classification systems have been used over the years. In the past, the Rappaport system, first described in 1966, based solely on morphology, was the most commonly used. With the availability of more sophisticated immunophenotypic and cytogenetic techniques, several revised classification systems have developed that incorporate the morphology, immunophenotype, cytogenetics, and clinical features. In 1999, the European and American Hematologic Societies published the WHO classification of hematologic malignancies that is widely used today[32,34,35] (Table 95.2). This system recognizes three major groups of lymphomas: B-cell, T-cell, or

NK cell, and HD. Within these three groups, there are more than 30 individual disease entities. Over the years it has become increasingly apparent that the NHLs represent a very diverse group of diseases with a wide range of cellular characteristics and clinical features. In the past, the NHLs were grouped according to their aggressiveness or propensity to proliferate (i.e., indolent or low grade, intermediate grade or aggressive, and high grade or highly aggressive). However, it is now realized that this grouping did represent an accurate prediction of each individual disease entity. An international study[36] confirmed that the clinical characteristics and prognoses of many NHLs could not be accurately predicted based on these older disease groupings and other factors are important in predicting a patient's clinical course.[1] To date, most clinical trials have used inclusion criteria based on the histology and the corresponding propensity of aggressiveness typically associated with it, according to the older classification system, and are, therefore, referred to as such in the following sections.

Many of the more indolent lymphomas have a follicular or nodular histologic pattern, where bands of connective tissue create a nodular pattern throughout the involved lymph nodes. Commonly, indolent lymphomas are not diagnosed until they are stage III or IV because patients may be relatively asymptomatic until that time. They are characterized by a slow clinical progression with only moderate sensitivity to conventional cytotoxic drugs. Patients are rarely cured, although some survive for many years with active disease. Many of the aggressive and highly aggressive lymphomas have a diffuse pattern on pathology, where the disease completely replaces the normal architecture of the lymph node. The aggressive lymphomas have a more rapid clinical course and if untreated, patients usually die within 3 to 6 months. These lymphomas are much more sensitive to conventional cytotoxic drugs; many patients experience prolonged disease-free intervals and approximately 35% to 40% are cured. Patients with highly aggressive lymphomas will die within several weeks if effective treatment is not initiated. The mor-

TABLE 95.2	Comparison of Classification Systems for NHL

Rappaport	Working Formulation	Revised European-American Lymphoma (REAL)/World Health Organization
Lymphocytic, well-differentiated	**Low Grade**	**B-Cell Neoplasms**
Nodular (follicular) lymphocytic, poorly differentiated	A. Small lymphocytic consistent with chronic leukemia; plasmacytoid	*Precursor B-cell neoplasm*
Nodular (follicular) histiocytic	B. Follicular, predominantly small cleaved by diffuse areas; sclerosis	Precursor B-lymphoblastic leukemia/lymphoma
Diffuse lymphocytic, poorly differentiated	C. Follicular mixed, small cleaved and large cell sclerosis	*Mature (peripheral) B-cell neoplasms*
Diffuse mixed, lymphocytic and histiocytic	**Intermediate Grade**	Chronic lymphocytic leukemia/B-cell small lymphocytic lymphoma
Diffuse histiocytic (with or without sclerosis)	D. Follicular, predominantly large-cell diffuse areas sclerosis	B-cell prolymphocytic lymphoma
Lymphoblastic (with or without convoluted cells)	E. Diffuse small cleaved cell sclerosis	Splenic marginal zone B-cell lymphoma
Diffuse, undifferentiated (Burkitt's and non-Burkitt's type)	F. Diffused mixed, small and large cell sclerosis, epithelioid cell component	Hairy cell leukemia
	G. Diffuse large cell cleaved cell, noncleaved cell sclerosis	Plasma cell myeloma
	High Grade	Extranodal marginal zone B-cell lymphoma
	H. Large cell, immunoblastic plasmacytoid clear cell polymorphous epithelioid cell component	Nodal marginal zone B-cell lymphoma
	I. Lymphoblastic convoluted cell, nonconvoluted cell	Follicular lymphoma
	J. Small cleaved, Burkitt's tumor; follicular areas	Mantle cell lymphoma
		Diffuse large B-cell lymphoma
		Burkitt's lymphoma/leukemia
		T and NK-cell Neoplasms
		Precursor T-cell neoplasm
		Precursor T-lymphoblastic leukemia/lymphoma
		Blastoid NK cell lymphoma
		Mature (peripheral) T-cell neoplasms
		T-cell prolymphocytic leukemia
		T-cell large granular lymphocytic leukemia
		Aggressive NK cell leukemia
		Adult T-cell lymphoma/leukemia (HTLV 1+)
		Extranodal NK/T-cell lymphoma, nasal type
		Enteropathy-type T-cell lymphoma
		Hepatosplenic T-cell lymphoma
		Subcutaneous panniculitis-like T-cell lymphoma
		Mycosis fungoides/Sezary syndromes
		Primary cutaneous anaplastic large cell lymphoma
		Peripheral T-cell, not otherwise specified.
		Angioimmunoblastic T-cell, lymphoma
		Primary systemic anaplastic large cell lymphoma.

HTLV, human T-cell lymphotropic virus type 1. (From references 32, 34, and 35.)

TABLE 95.3	Morphologic and Clinical Characteristics of Selected Non-Hodgkin's Lymphomas	
REAL Classification	**Morphology**	**Clinical Characteristics**
Indolent		
Follicle center lymphoma, follicular	Cleaved and large noncleaved follicle center cells; pattern of growth is at least partially follicular and diffuse areas may be present; 40%–60% progress to diffuse large B-cell lymphoma	Most common adult lymphoma in US, comprising 35%–40% of all NHL and 75%–80% of indolent B-cell lymphomas; affects mostly older adults; spleen and bone marrow frequently involved along with many lymph nodes
Mantle cell lymphoma	Small to medium sized lymphoid cells with slightly irregular or "deaved" nuclei	About 5% of adult NHL in US: affects mostly older adults; patients usually have widespread disease
Aggressive		
Diffuse large B-cell lymphoma	Large cells that resemble centroblasts or immunoblasts; some may be rich in small T lymphocytes or histiocytes	Accounts for 30%–40% of adult NHL; may be seen in any age group, but primarily adults; often presents with single or multiple rapidly enlarging masses; up to 40% occur extranodally (e.g., stomach, CNS, bone, kidney)
Peripheral T-cell lymphomas, unspecified	Mixture of small and large atypical cells; diffuse or occasionally interfollicular proliferation that ranges from atypical small cells to medium size or large cells	Less than 15% of lymphomas in US; most frequently affects adults; may be accompanied by eosinophilia, pruritus, or hemophagocytic syndromes; may involved lymph nodes, skin, liver, spleen, and other viscera
Highly aggressive/acute lymphomas/leukemias		
Precursor T-lymphoblastic lymphoma, leukemia	Lymphoblasts slightly larger than small lymphocytes but smaller than cells or large B-cell lymphoma	40% of childhood lymphomas and 15% of acute lymphoblastic leukemia; patients predominantly adolescent and young adult males; mediastinal masses and peripheral lymphadenopathy common, CNS involvement also common
Burkitt's lymphoma	Medium-sized cells with round nuclei, multiple nucleoli, and basophilic cytoplasm; extremely high rate of cell proliferation	Most common in children; rare in adults and often associated with AIDS; most present in abdomen, ovaries, or kidneys, rarely seen as acute leukemia with circulating turnor cells

NHL, non-Hodgkin's lymphoma; CNS, central nervous system; AIDS, acquired immunodeficiency syndrome.

phologic, histologic, and clinical features of some of the NHLs are described in Table 95.3.

CLINICAL PRESENTATION AND DIAGNOSIS

SIGNS AND SYMPTOMS

General. Most patients with lymphomas have superficial lymphadenopathy. Although superficial lymphadenopathy in adults is most frequently related to an acute infectious process, a biopsy should be performed on discrete hard lymph nodes, particularly if they are fixed or matted. The cervical nodes are the most common site of presentation in HD (65%–80%), but this presentation is less common in NHL (30%–40%). HD is believed to be unifocal in origin, probably beginning with a single lymph node. Spread occurs to adjacent nodes via lymph node channels, by direct extension into adjacent organs, or by blood vessel invasion with dissemination to the spleen, bone marrow, liver, bone, and other organs.[1] Supraclavicular and mediastinal lymphadenopathy are also common in HD.

In NHL, with disease initially limited to the lymph nodes, the disease tends to spread to contiguous lymphatic sites or occasionally to adjacent extranodal sites. In contrast to HD, many types of NHL spread more rapidly to distant nodal and extranodal sites via the bloodstream, similar to the metastatic dissemination of many other solid tumors. The presentation of NHL depends on the specific type of NHL. Some typically are more indolent, presenting with slowly progressive, non-tender peripheral lymphadenopathy that may wax and wane spontaneously, whereas other types of NHL have a much more aggressive course. The natural history of some more indolent lymphomas is progression to a more aggressive pattern with actual changes in the histologic appearance from small, relatively slowly proliferating cells to large, more rapidly dividing cells.

Disease occurring only outside the lymph nodes appears in 20% to 35% of patients with NHL. The majority of the extranodal lymphomas exhibit a diffuse histology pattern. The most commonly involved extranodal site is the head and neck area, followed by the gastrointestinal tract. Other primary extranodal sites include the skin, central nervous system (CNS), liver, lungs, testes, and bone marrow. When bone marrow involvement occurs, half of the patients show some evidence of disease dissemination in the blood.[37]

In rare situations, HD may present with massive mediastinal adenopathy, causing superior vena cava obstruction accompanied by headache; congestion of the face; subcutaneous edema involving the face, neck, and thorax; and cough and dyspnea (see ''Complications'' below). Lymphoblastic lymphoma may also present with mediastinal adenopathy, which may also produce vena cava obstruction. NHL, and less commonly HD, may present with massive retroperitoneal adenopathy that may obstruct the ureters or the inferior vena cava, giving rise to ascites and edema in the lower extremities.

At initial presentation, 20% of patients with NHL and 30% to 40% of patients with HD experience systemic or constitutional symptoms (fever, night sweats, weight loss, and pruritus).[1,3] These symptoms may develop about the same time as the lymph node enlargement or may occasionally precede the detection of lymphadenopathy. They generally subside rapidly with treatment, and their reappearance at any time in the course of the disease represents an unfavorable prognostic sign. In patients with HD, the frequency of systemic symptoms increases with the stage of the disease, age of the patient, and unfavorable histologic subtype.

Lymphomas Associated with Human Immunodeficiency Virus Infection. After the AIDS epidemic began in 1981, the number of reports of lymphomas in patients with AIDS and HIV infection increased steadily. The Centers for Disease Control and Prevention (CDC) includes large cell lymphomas, small noncleaved cell NHL, and primary CNS lymphomas as AIDS-defining conditions. The majority of AIDS-related NHLs are also EBV-related, and it is believed that the effect of EBV on infected lymphocytes is involved with the malignant transformation.[38]

The incidence of lymphoma associated with HIV infection is not unexpected because various other immunodeficiency disorders are also associated with an increased incidence of lymphomas.[1,8–13] The risk of lymphoma in this population correlates with the degree of immunosuppression (i.e., CD4 count).[38] Several types of NHL and HD have been reported in patients with AIDS. Although HD is not considered an AIDS-defining illness, its prevalence is increased up to tenfold among HIV-positive patients.[39] Most

lymphomas in this population present at advanced stages with unusual clinical features including prodromal manifestations, a high frequency of extranodal and CNS involvement, and usually a poorer prognosis as compared to immunocompetent patients with the same type of lymphoma. However, the inclusion of antiretroviral therapy and prophylactic antibiotics have improved outcomes.[3] Although the disease may appear at any site, gastrointestinal, bone marrow, central nervous system, and hepatic involvement are far more common than in non–HIV-infected patients with NHL and HD.[1,38,40] It is estimated that about 15% of HIV-associated NHLs are primary lymphomas of the CNS.[1]

DIAGNOSIS AND STAGING

Decisions regarding appropriate therapy for a patient with a lymphoma depend on the correct diagnosis and accurate assessment of the extent of disease. Diagnosis of lymphoma requires histopathologic confirmation of lymph node biopsy. When lymphadenopathy is present, one or more complete lymph nodes must be excised. Needle biopsies are generally not adequate. When primary extranodal lymphoma presents with regional or distant adenopathy, both sites should be examined histologically to ensure a correct diagnosis. Extranodal disease is sometimes mistaken for solid tumors in certain sites (e.g., stomach, breast, or testicle), and it is not until surgical removal and pathologic examination that the tumor is discovered to be a lymphoma.

Hodgkin's Disease. Staging systems have been developed to facilitate therapeutic planning and communication of data concerning the natural history of the disease and treatment outcomes. The Ann Arbor staging system was developed in 1971 for use in HD and was revised in 1989. The current staging system is called the Ann Arbor or Cotswold Staging Classification for Hodgkin's Lymphoma (Table 95.4).[41] This staging system has been reproducible and predictive of response to therapy. The Cotswold Staging Classification is divided into four stages, and each stage is further subdivided into A (asymptomatic) and B (symptomatic) groups. As the disease progresses from stage I to stage IV, the prognosis becomes worse. The presence of symptoms (designated B) also confers a worse prognosis. The clinical symptoms associated with HD are general, rather than specific and include unexplained weight loss, fever with temperature above 38°C (100.4°F), and night sweats. A patient may experience additional symptoms such as pruritus or alcohol-induced pain, but they generally do not correlate with the severity of disease and are not considered in the staging evaluation.

When localized extranodal disease is contiguous to involved lymph nodes (often in the lungs or vertebrae adjacent to involved lymph nodes), staging is based on the appropriate lymph node involvement followed by the subscript ''E,'' which denotes direct extension. This type of disease confers a more favorable prognosis than clearly disseminated (stage IV) disease. In general, the ''E'' designation is used in pa-

TABLE 95.4	Ann Arbor (Cotswold) Classification for the Staging of Hodgkin's Disease
Stage I	Disease involvement of a single lymph node region (I) or lymphoid structure (e.g., spleen, thymus) or a single localized extrnodal organ or site (I_E)
Stage II	Disease involvement of two or more lymph node regions on the same side of the diaphragm (II); localized contiguous involvement of one extranodal organ or site and lymph node region on the same side of the diaphragm (II_E); the number of anatomic sites is indicated by a subscript (e.g., II_3)
Stage III	Disease involvement of lymph node regions on both sides of the diaphragm (III); may also be accompanied by localized involvement of an extralymphatic organ or site (III_E) or by involvement of the spleen (III_S), or both (III_{SE})
	III_1 indicates with or without involvement of splenic, hilar, celiac, or portal nodes
	III_2 indicates involvement of para-aortic, iliac, or mesenteric nodes
Stage IV	Diffuse or disseminated disease involvement of one or more extranodal organs or tissues, with or without associated lymph node enlargement
Designations applicable to any stage of disease	
A	Asymptomatic
B	Symptomatic: weight loss 10% of body weight, unexplained fever with temperature above 38°C (100.4°F), and night sweats
X	Designates bulky disease as >1/3 widening of the mediastinum or >10 cm maximum dimension of nodal mass
E	Involvement of a single extranodal site that is contiguous or proximal to the known nodal site
Staging should be identified as clinical stage (CS) or pathologic stage (PS)	

tients with extranodal disease that is so limited in extent and location that it can be easily irradiated.

The diaphragm has key significance in the staging of HD. It is the reference point from which the extent (or stage) of HD is measured. If the disease is confined to lymph nodes on only one side (above or below) of the diaphragm, the disease is considered to be localized, and the prognosis is generally better than if the disease were disseminated and present on both sides of the diaphragm.

Procedures necessary for the accurate clinical staging of HD are listed in Table 95.5. A detailed patient history is obtained, making note of the presence or absence of symptoms, and a thorough physical examination must be performed, giving particular attention to areas of bone tenderness and the size of the liver and spleen. Laboratory tests and procedures are used to detect clinical abnormalities that may implicate a specific organ or organ system to where the HD has spread. Further pathologic staging is then necessary to definitively diagnose HD in tissues that have been implicated by the clinical staging procedures. Pathologic staging involves biopsy and microscopic examination of the suspect tissue. More aggressive staging techniques have included laparotomy and splenectomy. In the past, these procedures made significant contributions in staging accuracy and knowledge of the natural history of HD. Improved radiologic and radioisotopic technologies provide vastly improved diagnostic information over what was previously available. Current recommendations specify that laparotomy should be performed only if treatment decisions depend on the identification of abdominal disease, and in some of these situations,

laparoscopy combined with needle biopsies of bone marrow may substitute for this procedure. Laparotomy is of most value in identifying those patients who appear to have stage I or II disease by other diagnostic criteria and who might, therefore, be eligible for treatment with RT alone (i.e., pa-

TABLE 95.5	Procedures Commonly Recommended for the Staging of Hodgkin's Disease and Non-Hodgkin's Lymphoma

Required procedures:

1. Detailed history with special attention to the presence (and duration) or absence of systemic symptoms (i.e., fever, unexplained sweating, unexplained weight loss)
2. Careful physical examination with special attention to all lymph node areas; size of liver and spleen
3. Adequate surgical biopsy reviewed by an experienced hemopathologist with immunophenotyping
4. Routine laboratory testing including complete blood count, erythrocyte sedimentation rate, liver and renal function tests, serum uric acid
5. Radiologic examination of the chest; Computed tomography (CT) of the chest, abdomen, and pelvis

Procedures necessary under certain circumstances:

1. Bilateral bone marrow biopsy
2. Positron emission tomography
3. Lumbar puncture
4. Brain magnetic resonance image (MRI) or head CT

tients with negative laparotomy results verifying pathologic stage I or II disease).[42] If systemic chemotherapy is already considered essential to the patient's management, based on noninvasive studies such as computed tomography (CT) or magnetic resonance imaging (MRI), then staging laparotomy becomes inconsequential. Although the overall morbidity is low, laparotomy plus splenectomy increases the risk of sepsis from encapsulated organisms (i.e., *Streptococcus pneumoniae, Haemophilus influenzae*), varicella zoster reactivation, and bowel obstruction resulting from adhesions among the intestinal loops. Therefore, the decision to perform such a staging procedure must be carefully weighed, especially because a CT or MRI scan is easy to administer and is noninvasive.[43] Gallium scanning or positron emission tomography (PET) may also be used in combination with CT scans for initial evaluation of disease below the diaphragm. More data is necessary to determine their value in disease above the diaphragm.[1]

Non-Hodgkin's Lymphoma. NHLs are not as predictable in their patterns of involvement, nor do they reflect discrete changes in their prognosis with changes in stages, as seen with HD. In spite of these limitations, the Cotswold staging system has been widely used for defining patient groups in clinical trials. Much effort has been spent on identifying other factors that have prognostic significance for patients with NHL. Such factors relate to the extent of the lymphoma (lactate dehydrogenase, β_2-microglobulin, stage, number of disease sites, extent of extranodal disease, and bone marrow involvement), the patient's response to the disease (performance status and B symptoms), and the patient's ability to tolerate therapy (age, performance status, and bone marrow involvement).[3,44] Other disease-related variables, such as the rate of proliferation of tumor cells, the immunophenotype, and cytogenetic abnormalities, also have been reported to correlate with survival, and it is likely that they will soon be widely used to establish prognosis.

In contrast to those with HD, patients with NHL are more likely to have disseminated disease, so local therapeutic options such as surgery and RT are less commonly used. Therapeutic options in NHL are also more likely to be limited because of the advanced age or comorbid conditions of the patient. Because of the diverse clinical features of patients with NHL, no rigid or routine staging plan is appropriate for all patients. Many of the staging procedures used in HD (Table 95.5) are used for the NHLs, although they are less applicable because of the high prevalence of extranodal disease. These staging procedures should be carefully considered with regard to the histologic subtype, the individual patient, and the anticipated and available therapeutic options. Extensive staging procedures should be reserved for clinical trials or for patients in whom a specific therapeutic alternative, such as RT, is available.

As in HD, a thorough physical examination and routine laboratory tests are aimed at the detection of potential sites of involvement, the rate of lymph node enlargement, and the presence of B symptoms. Renal and hepatic function should also be evaluated to assess for signs of organ involvement and to ascertain the patient's ability to tolerate aggressive therapy. Although the bone marrow is frequently involved in NHL, peripheral blood abnormalities are uncommon. Bilateral bone marrow aspirations and biopsies are generally indicated for patients with indolent follicular lymphomas or clinically advanced aggressive subtypes. The frequency of bone marrow involvement ranges from 5% to 15% in patients with diffuse B-cell lymphoma to 55% to 85% of patients with follicular lymphomas. Although relatively uncommon in diffuse large B-cell lymphoma, bone marrow involvement may predict CNS involvement, and patients with this finding should receive a lumbar puncture with examination of the cerebrospinal fluid.

Gastrointestinal studies are indicated in patients with abdominal symptoms or masses and in patients with nasopharyngeal lymphomas to obtain prognostic information, to plan therapy, and to establish involvement or impending obstruction of the gastrointestinal or genitourinary tract. A chest x-ray or chest CT scan is usually done to identify hilar and mediastinal lymphadenopathy and effusions. Abdominal CT scans are used for assessment of retroperitoneal and intraabdominal disease. In the past, [67]Gallium scans were also done to identify sites of disease, however, PET scans have been found to be more sensitive and reliable in the initial staging and subsequent assessments for relapse or disease progression.[45–48] As in HD, there is no justification for routine staging laparotomy, and this procedure should be used only when it will influence management decisions.

TREATMENT

TREATMENT PRINCIPLES

The treatment of lymphomas primarily includes RT and chemotherapy. Surgery, although useful in the management of many other malignancies, does not play a major role. The only roles for surgery in lymphomas are (a) initial staging and diagnostic procedures; (b) relief of obstruction related to a localized lymph node enlargement not responding to therapy; (c) management of a gastrointestinal lymphoma, to reduce the rate of perforation or hemorrhage; and (d) management of complications of lymphomas such as hypersplenism.

Radiation Therapy. Lymphomas were recognized early on as being very responsive to RT. Over the past few decades, improvements have been made in defining appropriate fields or ports for radiation, optimal doses, and delivery techniques that minimize risk to surrounding normal tissues. RT essentially has the same effect on cellular biochemistry as the alkylating cytotoxic chemotherapy agents. DNA replication is prevented by interference with the cross-links necessary to maintain the double-helix DNA molecule. Proliferating tissue, characteristic of malignancies, is especially radiosensitive because of its constant DNA production necessary for cell division. The epithelial lining of the gastrointestinal tract is also rapidly dividing tissue. Frequently encountered side effects with RT include radiation-induced pharyngitis, esophagitis, and gastroenteritis. The rapid production of cells in the bone marrow makes this site very susceptible to radiation-induced bone marrow suppression. It is important that vital, uninvolved organs and viscera be shielded during RT to minimize radiation-induced toxicities. Possible radiation fields for the treatment of lymphomas are described in Table 95.6.

Chemotherapy. The use of drugs in the management of neoplastic diseases was developed after the end of World War II, and lymphomas and leukemias were among the first tumors to respond to such chemotherapy. In general, single-drug therapy with conventional cytotoxic drugs, produces CR rates rarely exceeding 20% to 30%, so the treatment of lymphomas requires the use of drug combinations. Combination chemotherapy uses drugs with different mechanisms of action that attack proliferating cells at different stages of cell replication.

Although most cytotoxic drugs can produce responses in lymphomas, it was in 1970 with the four-drug regimen known as MOPP (mechlorethamine or Mustargen, vincristine or Oncovin, prednisone, and procarbazine) that DeVita et al[49] showed that chemotherapy could induce a high rate of complete remission in patients with advanced HD. Later, the ability of chemotherapy to produce long-term remissions (i.e., cure) in patients with HD and certain NHL histologic subtypes was confirmed. Today, more than 30 years later, many of the patients treated on the initial MOPP clinical trial are alive and free of HD. Over the past decade, the use of monoclonal antibodies targeted to specific cell surface antigens and radioisotopes attached to monoclonal antibodies also have played a major role in the treatment of lymphomas. All of these therapies are discussed in more detail in the following sections.

After RT or chemotherapy has been administered to a patient with lymphoma, the patient's response to treatment must be assessed. Standard criteria are generally used for the objective evaluation of treatment response (Table 95.7) so that various therapies may be compared in a consistent manner. Objective reduction of disease manifestations usually begins within the first month after the start of treatment. However, this depends on the type of lymphoma, and is usually more rapid in HD than in NHL.

Selection of the most appropriate type of therapy depends on confirmation of the histologic subtype and the extent of the disease, and any patient-specific factors (e.g., age or concomitant illness) that may influence the patient's ability to withstand treatment. With few exceptions, the initial approach to managing malignant lymphomas is to cure the patient, regardless of the disease stage and histologic type.

HODGKIN'S DISEASE

Since the 1970s, it has been recognized that HD is very sensitive to the lethal effects of chemotherapy and radiation. Chemotherapy regimens discussed in the following sections with or without RT have demonstrated impressive rates of complete responses with more than 50% of patients in most studies ultimately achieving long-term disease-free survival or cure. However, there has always existed a subset of patients who do not respond to therapy or relapse following disease remission. In addition, the early generation of chemotherapy regimens has been linked to several serious

---

TABLE 95.6	Radiation Therapy Fields Used in the Management of Lymphomas

Mantle: Encompasses mediastinal, hilar, and bilateral supraclavicular, infraclavicular, cervical, and axillary node chains, with lead shields shaped to lungs, heart, and spinal cord.

Inverted-Y: Encompasses splenic or splenic pedicle, para-aortic, iliac, inguinal, and femoral node chains, with lead shields for rectum and bladder, iliac and upper femoral bone marrow, and "gap" at junction with mantle fields.

Para-aortic/hepatic: Encompasses splenic hilar and para-aortic node chains and entire right lobe of liver, usually joined across another "gap" by a separate pelvic field.

Waldeyer: Encompasses preauricular nodes and lymphatic tissues of Waldeyer's ring when clinically involved or when adenopathy is present in high cervical nodes.

Total nodal: Encompasses all lymph node regions above the diaphragm (cervical, supra- and infraclavicular, axillary, mediastinal) and all lymph node regions below the diaphragm (periaortic, retroperitoneal, inguinal, and splenic regions).

Subtotal nodal: Encompasses the mantle plus para-aortic, spleen and pedicle fields.

Involved field: Encompasses only the known involved sites.

Extended field: Encompasses known involved sites plus contiguous uninvolved regions.

TABLE 95.7	Criteria for Treatment Response

Complete response (CR): Disappearance of all signs and symptoms of the disease; this includes the return to normal of all previously abnormal parameters and a negative second biopsy of known involved extranodal sites.

Partial response (PR): A reduction of 50% in the product of the longest perpendicular diameters of all measurable lesions.

Minimal response (MR) or no change: A reduction of <50% in the product of the longest perpendicular diameters of all measurable lesions.

Treatment failure (TF): Increase in size of any lesion and/or appearance of new lesion(s).

late complications, such as sterility and acute leukemia, and very significant acute toxicities in the days and weeks following each treatment. Therefore, research over the past 30 years has focused on improving the initial success by increasing the proportion of patients who are cured and identifying regimens with improved long-term safety.

Early Stage (I and II) Hodgkin's Disease. Decades of experience has demonstrated that stages I and II HD are very amenable to radical external beam RT (i.e., high doses of radiation with curative intent), because in these stages, the disease is present in a few well-defined, focal areas.[50] Radiation treatment may be limited to the known involved sites [i.e., involved field (IF)], given to only the known involved sites plus contiguous uninvolved regions [i.e., extended field (EF)], or delivered to all major lymphoid regions [i.e., total nodal irradiation (TNI)]. However, as more patients have become long-term survivors of HD, more late complications of the treatment have become apparent. This is true for radiation and chemotherapy. For this reason, investigators in recent years have focused on the development of equally effective therapeutic strategies that carry less long-term risks and the evaluation of prognostic factors that will help to identify patients at greatest risk of treatment failure who may warrant more aggressive and toxic therapies. Prognostic factors for stages I and II HD that have been associated with worse outcome include advanced age, male sex, mixed cellularity subtype, B symptoms, large mediastinal mass, greater number of involved lymph node regions, elevated erythrocyte sedimentation rate, anemia, and low serum albumin.[1] Strategies that have been evaluated to lessen the long-term treatment risks while maintaining the exceptional long-term disease-free survival rates have included reduced dose or field size of radiation, shorter and less toxic chemotherapy regimens, and chemotherapy alone for stage I or II disease.

With either TNI or subtotal nodal irradiation (sTNI), the 10-year relapse-free survival rate (which is often equated to cure) in patients with pathologic (confirmed by laparotomy) stages I and II HD is 75% to 80%.[51–53] However, as discussed previously, most patients do not undergo staging laparotomy and the concern is that occult intraabdominal disease may not be adequately treated with this approach. Thus, unless a staging laparotomy is performed, combined modality therapy with radiation and chemotherapy appears to provide the greatest benefit. Therefore, most research in recent years has focused on developing effective combined modality regimens that have minimal long-term risks.

For patients with stage I or II HD without adverse prognostic factors, the National Comprehensive Cancer Network (NCCN) Practice Guidelines[54] recommend combined modality therapy with chemotherapy and involved field radiation for most patients. This approach provides irradiation to the obvious site of the disease and systemic chemotherapy to manage occult disease and the identifiable site of disease. Most agree that four cycles of the ABVD chemotherapy regimen that combines doxorubicin (Adriamycin), *b*leomycin, *v*inblastine, and *d*acarbazine is the treatment of choice for initial systemic treatment of favorable prognosis, stage

I or II disease (Table 95.8). If combined with radiation (20–30 Gy), four cycles of chemotherapy appear to be sufficient for patients with favorable prognostic factors. Recently, several clinical trials have evaluated an even lower number of chemotherapy cycles in this patient group. These trials compared standard combined modality therapy to less intense or shorter regimens such as two courses of ABVD plus sTNI, three cycles of doxorubicin and vinblastine plus sTNI and splenic irradiation, or a relatively short course (8 weeks total) of an intensive regimen that includes mechlorethamine, doxorubicin, vinblastine, prednisone, vincristine, bleomycin, and etoposide. This latter regimen is often referred to as the Stanford V regimen and is considered an acceptable alternative to ABVD by the NCCN.

For patients who are unable to tolerate chemotherapy, subtotal nodal irradiation may be given alone and if radiation is contraindicated, chemotherapy may be given alone, however, six cycles of ABVD are generally recommended.

For patients with unfavorable prognostic signs, the NCCN recommends initiating chemotherapy followed by involved field radiation plus inclusion of tissues surrounding bulky disease sites (large tumor masses) and bilateral supraclavicular areas. In this situation, the recommended radiation dose (30–36 Gy) is higher than in patients with favorable prognostic indicators and up to six courses of ABVD or 12 weeks of the Stanford V chemotherapy regimen are given.[54] In patients with large (greater than one third of the largest transverse chest diameter) mediastinal masses or other bulky disease, the relapse rate is significant (approximately 50%) if patients are treated only with radiation.

Advanced Stage (III and IV) Hodgkin's Disease. Chemotherapy with or without RT is the treatment of choice for patients with stage III or IV HD. Stage IV HD is not well suited for RT because many different sites throughout the body may be involved and localized radiation to each site cannot be effectively administered. Parenchymal organs cannot tolerate curative doses of radiation, and the presence of HD in these organs precludes the use of radical radiation. Stage IV disease is, therefore, treated primarily with systemic chemotherapy, which reaches all sites of disease. "Spot" radiation is recommended for bulky sites of disease and for palliative treatment to anatomical areas of disease that are not responding to chemotherapy or that are causing pain, tenderness, or obstruction.

The drug combination that was first successful in producing long-term remissions in HD is MOPP. Pioneered by DeVita et al,[49] the MOPP regimen produced complete remissions (CR) in 159 (80%) of the 198 patients initially treated, with 54% of these patients still disease free 20 years after completion of therapy. Subsequent trials using this combination and similar regimens reported long-term disease-free survival in at least 50% of patients.[1] In an effort to improve the long-term disease-free survival rate and reduce the risk of serious long-term complications, Bonadonna et al[55] first described the use of the ABVD regimen in patients who had relapsed after receiving MOPP therapy and subsequently compared MOPP plus extended field radiation to ABVD

TABLE 95.8	Combination Chemotherapy Regimens Used in Hodgkin's Disease			
Acronymcles	Drugs	Dose and Route	Treatment Days	Frequency of Cy-
MOPP	Mechlorethamine	6 mg/m² IV	1, 8	Every 28 day
	Vincristine (Oncovin)	1.4 mg/m² IV (max: ² mg)	1, 8	
	Procarbazine	100 mg/m² PO	1–14	
	Prednisone	40 mg/m² PO	1–14, cycles 2 and 4	
ABVD	Doxorubicin	25 mg/m² IV	1, 15	Every 28 days
	Bleomycin	10 mg/m² IV	1, 15	
	Vinblastine	6 mg/m² IV	1, 15	
	Dacarbazine	375 mg/m² IV	1, 15	
MOPP/ABV	Mechlorethamine	6 mg/m² IV	1	Every 28 days
	Vincristine	1.4 mg/m² IV (max: 2 mg)	1	
	Prednisone	40 mg/m² PO	1–14	
	Procarbazine	100 mg/m² PO	1–7	
	Doxorubicin	35 mg/m² IV	8	
	Bleomycin	10 mg/m² IV	8	
	Vinblastine	6 mg/m² IV	8	
Stanford V (12 week schedule)	Vinblastine	6 mg/m² IV	1, 15, 29, 43, 57, 71	One 12 week cycle
	Doxorubicin	25 mg/m² IV	1, 15, 29, 43, 57, 71	
	Vincristine	1.4 mg/m² IV	8, 22, 36, 50, 64, 78	
	Bleomycin	5 mg/m² IV	8, 22, 36, 50, 64, 78	
	Mechlorethamine	6 mg/m² IV	8, 29, 57	
	Etoposide	60 mg/m² IV	15, 43, 71	
	Prednisone	40 mg/m² PO	Every other day until, 71, then taper	

IV, intravenously; PO, by mouth.

plus extended field radiation.[1] They reported a significantly superior freedom from disease progression rate in patients receiving ABVD. After their very positive results, they undertook a prospective study to compare MOPP versus MOPP alternating with ABVD.

Goldie and Coldman[56] proposed that during treatment malignant cells may mutate and become resistant to therapy. The use of alternating, noncross-resistant chemotherapy regimens has been suggested as a possible means of improving the CR rate and lengthening the median duration of disease-free survival by exposing tumor cells to an increased number of cytotoxic drugs. This strategy offers the possibility of reducing treatment failures caused by the overgrowth of singly, doubly, or even multiresistant phenotypes. The ABVD regimen consists of drugs that are individually noncross-resistant with the agents in the MOPP regimen. In the trial comparing MOPP alone to cycles of MOPP alternating with ABVD (MOPP/ABVD), the rates of both CR (89% vs. 74%) and 8-year relapse-free survival for patients achieving a CR (73% vs. 45%) were significantly better for the MOPP/

ABVD regimen, with a similar incidence of serious toxic reactions.[57,58]

Over the years, several groups have evaluated various hybrid regimens that include many of the drugs in the MOPP and ABVD regimens (MOPP/ABV). Similar CR and survival rates to ABVD alone have been reported with these hybrids, however, the MOPP/ABV and similar regimens have often times been associated with significantly more serious hematologic and nonhematologic toxicities including treatment-related deaths and secondary malignancies.[1,59] Following this series of trials, ABVD became the clear-cut standard for initial treatment of HD against which new regimens should be compared. Based on impressive efficacy and less apparent risk of infertility, secondary malignancies, and cumulative dose-related cardiac (doxorubicin) and pulmonary (bleomycin) toxicities, the NCCN also supports the use of 12 weeks of the Stanford V regimen.[54] BEACOPP [bleomycin, etoposide, doxorubicin (Adriamycin), cyclophosphamide, vincristine (Oncovin), procarbazine, and prednisone] is also recommended for selected patients with poor prognostic indicators.[48] Whereas ABVD is often given alone to patients who do not have bulky tumor masses, RT is recommended for similar patients receiving Stanford V. RT to involved sites is generally recommended in combination with chemotherapy for all patients with bulky disease.[48] After the initial four cycles of ABVD or BEACOPP, each patient should undergo a restaging evaluation to assess the impact of treatment. If the patient has achieved a CR, two more cycles of ABVD or four more cycles of BEACOPP should be administered. Occasionally, one or two additional cycles of ABVD (maximum of eight total cycles) may be given, if the CR was achieved late. When Stanford V is used, restaging is done following the 12-week course of therapy. Following completion of any of these regimens, there is no advantage in prolonging therapy or administering any type of maintenance therapy.

As described above, it has become apparent that several factors negatively influence the overall prognosis and likelihood of treatment success for HD. After treatment is initiated, the rate of tumor regression and the dose intensity (i.e., amount of drug administered per unit of time) also appear to influence the duration of response and survival.[60,61] Because the most common dose-limiting toxicity of many of the HD regimens has been myelotoxicity, the use of erythropoietin and myeloid colony stimulating factors may allow for a higher dose intensity (i.e., administration of all planned doses on time).

Following completion of treatment, patients who achieve a CR should undergo repeat CT scans, chest x-ray, complete blood counts, serum chemistries, and physical examination every 3 to 6 months for the first 2 to 5 years, then annually thereafter.

Relapsed or Refractory Hodgkin's Disease. Despite the success of first-line therapies for HD, 10% to 50% of patients (depending on prognostic factors), will have disease that is initially refractory to primary treatment or will have a relapse after primary treatment. For patients with early stage disease who might have received RT alone as initial treatment, the success rate with subsequent chemotherapy is very good.

The optimal management for patients who have a relapse after an initial chemotherapy-induced CR or for those in whom initial chemotherapy failed to produce a CR, the optimal treatment is less well defined. Evidence does suggest that a significant number of these patients may still achieve a long-term benefit from subsequent therapies. In general, the longer the duration of the first CR, the greater the likelihood of a favorable response to further treatment. If patients do not respond to initial chemotherapy or if they relapse after a brief remission ($\leq$1 year), high-dose chemotherapy (HDCT) followed by autologous stem cell transplantation appears to be superior to additional conventional dose chemotherapy.[62–64] Several randomized trials have demonstrated superior relapse-free survival following HDCT versus conventional dose chemotherapy with similar drugs[62,63] and other nonrandomized studies have reported similar outcomes. Disease-free or event-free survival 3 or 4 years following HDCT has been reported to be approximately 30% to 53% in most studies.[1] The use of HDCT with stem cell transplantation for patients who have had a longer remission following initial treatment is more controversial. Several decades of experience with these patient groups has demonstrated that as many as 40% to 55% of patients who relapse more than a year after initial CR may achieve a second CR and long-term survival following additional conventional dose chemotherapy. However, at least one randomized trial has demonstrated superior long-term outcomes with HDCT.[63] Allogeneic stem cell transplant is not usually recommended for patients with HD because of the high risk of serious graft versus host toxicity and associated mortality rates of up to 75%.

If patients refuse HDCT or are not considered candidates for this aggressive approach, conventional dose chemotherapy may be beneficial. If the remission was longer than 1 year in duration, patients may be treated with the same chemotherapy or with a noncross-resistant regimen. If patients received ABVD as initial therapy, care should be taken to ensure that maximum recommended cumulative doses of doxorubicin and bleomycin are not exceeded, due to the risks of cardiac and pulmonary toxicity, respectively. Other salvage chemotherapy regimens may include drugs such as etoposide, ifosfamide, cisplatin, cytarabine, carmustine, melphalan, gemcitabine, vinorelbine, and idarubicin.

NON-HODGKIN'S LYMPHOMA
The management of NHL depends on many factors, including the age of the patient, presence of concomitant disease, and the stage and histologic subgroup of the primary disease.

Indolent Non-Hodgkin's Lymphoma.
Stage I and Stage II Indolent Non-Hodgkin's Lymphoma. Only about 20% of patients with the indolent subtypes of NHL (Table 95.2) have localized disease (i.e., stage I or II) at the time of diagnosis.[65] Local and regional RT is generally very effective in achieving disease control in the irradiated areas and as many as 50% of patients will have long-term disease free survival.[65,66] Unfortunately, approximately 50% of these patients will have a recurrence of the disease within 10 years, and in most cases the disease will have disseminated to multiple sites at the time of relapse.[65,67] Although early clinical trials evaluating the effectiveness of nonanthracycline-based chemotherapy in combination with RT failed to show any advantage over radiation alone, Seymour et al[43] reported an impressive 76% disease-free survival with a median follow-up of 10 years. This was not a randomized trial, however the 10-year disease-free survival rate appears to be superior when compared to historical controls. In this trial, patients with stage I or II low-grade lymphomas received cyclophosphamide, vincristine, prednisone, and bleomycin or the same regimen with added doxorubicin plus 30 to 40 Gy of IF RT. Additional clinical trials will be helpful in defining the optimal role of chemotherapy in early stage indolent lymphomas. Currently, the NCCN Clinical Practice Guidelines for NHL recommend

either RT to the involved areas or chemotherapy followed by RT in this situation.[68]

Stage III and Stage IV Indolent Non-Hodgkin's Lymphomas. More than 50% to 75% of patients with low-grade lymphomas have stage III or IV disease at the time of initial diagnosis. Only a small proportion of these patients can be cured, and therefore, treatment selection is somewhat controversial. In this situation, treatment options may include RT to the involved areas (IF) or all lymph node regions in the body (TNI), single-agent or combination chemotherapy, targeted therapy with a monoclonal antibody or a radioimmunoconjugate, or combined modality therapy with two or more of these approaches. Because of the indolent nature of this disease, some patients may not require immediate therapy at the time of initial diagnosis. Clinicians who have advocated the no immediate treatment strategy emphasize that close monitoring is always necessary and that therapy can be delayed until the disease progresses and the patient becomes symptomatic. This observational approach is appealing, especially in older patients who are less likely to tolerate the side effects of chemotherapy or radiation. Several randomized trials have evaluated if initiating therapy immediately after diagnosis is superior to this "watch and wait approach," and the results have not established a clearcut superiority in terms of overall survival for either approach. French investigators, the National Cancer Institute (NCI), and researchers at Stanford University reported comparable survival rates following the observational approach or immediate intervention.[69–71] Currently, the NCCN Guidelines recommend that observation only is appropriate for patients who do not have any of the following disease-related clinical findings: symptoms, threatened function of a major organ, cytopenia, bulky disease, or evidence of steady disease progression.[68] These guidelines also indicate that if a patient prefers to receive immediate therapy, that treatment would be acceptable. If patients have any of the above disease-related findings, initiation of therapy with single or combination drug therapy or RT (for palliation of local symptoms) is recommended.[68] Because advanced stage indolent NHL are not considered curable and the overall long-term survival rates have not significantly improved over the past 30 years, enrollment of patients with advanced disease on clinical trials is also highly recommended.

Over the past 30 years, many conventional cytotoxic drugs and several biological agents have been shown to have significant activity against the indolent lymphomas. Although CR rates as high as 65% have been reported with some single agents and the duration of relapse-free survival may be up to several years, this type of therapy is not considered to be curative. With the use of molecular biology diagnostic techniques, it appears that many patients with follicular NHL who appear to be in CR still have cells containing cytogenetic evidence of the disease.[72] In an attempt to improve results observed with single-agent therapy, many combination chemotherapy regimens have been evaluated. Initially, one of the most widely studied and used regimens was the cyclophosphamide, vincristine, prednisone (CVP)

combination. Although studies with this regimen suggested higher CR rates than those observed with single-agent therapy, the overall disease-free survival and survival rates were not significantly improved. More aggressive chemotherapy regimens that included doxorubicin, bleomycin, methotrexate, fludarabine, mitoxantrone, and other active agents have also failed to improve overall survival.

The CD20 antigen is expressed on the surface of more than 90% of the B-cell lymphomas. Because the antigen does not shed, modulate, or internalize, it is an ideal target for antibody therapy. If the antigen were shed from the surface, the monoclonal antibody would bind to it in the serum and never reach the tumor cell. Likewise, if the antigen was altered or internalized within the cell, the antibody would not recognize or could not reach its target. Initial trials with the chimeric human-mouse anti-CD20 monoclonal antibody, rituximab (Rituxan) demonstrated biological efficacy in producing transient depletion of B-cells and a good safety profile.[73] After binding to the CD20 antigen, rituximab induces lysis of the cell. A multicenter, single-agent trial reported a 48% response rate in 166 patients with low-grade or follicular lymphomas who had progressive disease that had relapsed or failed to respond to previous conventional chemotherapy. Although most of the responses were partial, the median duration of response was projected to be 10 to 12 months.[74] Other trials have evaluated rituximab as first-line therapy and reported 1-year progression-free survival rates of 69% and 77%, suggesting that initial rituximab is comparable to other single agents or combinations as initial therapy.[75,76] After the marketing of the product in 1998, the manufacturer did report that several deaths had been reported in patients with bulky disease that were presumably related to a massive cell lysis and metabolic complications within several hours after the initial dose. Therefore, it is recommended that patients with high tumor burdens be closely monitored during and after therapy until the risk of such a reaction has passed.

The highest response rates to initial therapy for advanced indolent lymphomas appear to be achieved with the use of rituximab plus combination chemotherapy. Czuczman et al[77] reported an overall response rate of 95% (55% CR) in 40 patients who received six infusions of rituximab (375 mg/m^2) in combination with *c*yclophosphamide, *h*ydroxydaunorubicin, vincristine (*O*ncovin), and *p*rednisone (CHOP) chemotherapy (cyclophosphamide, doxorubicin, vincristine, and prednisone). Thirty-one of these patients had not received any prior therapy. The combination of CHOP plus rituximab (CHOP-R) did not appear to cause any additional toxicity over what would be anticipated with the individual regimens.

In an effort to improve disease-free and overall survival, maintenance therapy with rituximab following chemotherapy or induction therapy with rituximab has been evaluated.[76,78] Hainsworth et al[78] randomized 90 patients who had responded to rituximab therapy to receive rituximab maintenance with standard 4-week courses given every 6 months or no further rituximab until the time of disease progression.

They reported that patients who received the rituximab maintenance had a significantly longer progression-free survival (31.4 vs. 7.4 months; $p = 0.007$), however, patients who received rituximab only at disease progression had a similar duration of benefit (interval until they failed rituximab therapy) as the group who received maintenance therapy. There was no significant difference in 3-year overall survival. Further trials will therefore be necessary to determine the value of maintenance rituximab.

Radioimmunotherapy is a relatively new strategy which uses monoclonal antibodies to carry lethal radioisotopes directly to the tumor cells. The emission of the radiation is also able to damage nearby cells that may not express the target antigen (innocent bystander effect). Two radioimmunoconjugates, iodine-131 tositumomab (Bexxar) and ytriumm-90 ibritumomab (Zevlin) are available for the treatment of refractory low-grade NHL. In patients who were refractory to rituximab, Witzig et al[79] reported a 74% response rate (15% CR, 59% PR). Similarly impressive overall response rates ranging from 47% to 68% with CR rates ranging from 20% to 38% have been reported in patients who were refractory to either chemotherapy, rituximab or both with the use of tositumomab.[80–83] Approximately 30% of these patients appear to have a durable remission lasting from 1 to 10 years (median 60 months).[84] These results led investigators to study iodine-131 tositumomab as first-line therapy for low grade or follicular lymphomas. Kaminski et al[85] reported that 95% of the 76 patients initially treated with iodine-131 tositumomab responded with 75% achieving a complete response. After a median follow-up of 5.1 years, the actuarial 5-year progression-free survival for all patients was 59% and the median progression-free survival for the responding patients was 6.1 years. Of the 57 patients who achieved a CR, 40 remained in CR for 4.3 to 7.7 years.

Preparation and administration of each of these radioimmunoconjugates requires specialized expertise and facilities. Ibritumomab tiuxetan therapy is preceded by infusions of rituximab 1 week and immediately prior to the ibritumomab tiuxetan to eliminate CD20 positive cells from the circulating blood and therefore reduce the risk of radiation delivery to unintended sites due to the radioimmunoconjugate binding to circulating blood cells. In the case of tositumomab, a dose of the monoclonal antibody without the radioisotope is administered prior to the actual therapeutic dose. Both of these agents have been associated with serious infusion reactions and severe and prolonged myelosuppression, in some cases. Patients who receive these therapies may also not be able to tolerate subsequent myelotoxic therapies as well as patients who had received prior cytotoxic therapy. Occasional cases of acute leukemia or myelodysplastic syndrome have also been reported. Therefore, despite the impressive response rates, the decision to use radioimmunotherapy must be carefully balanced with the potential risks.

HDCT with autologous stem cell transplantation with or without RT has also been used for patients who fail to achieve a CR or relapse. To date, only one randomized trial has been reported, however, these investigators described a

TABLE 95.9	National Comprehensive Cancer Network Suggested Regimens for Advanced Indolent Lymphomas

First-Line Therapy

Rituximab

Chlorambucil

Cyclophosphamide

Cyclophosphamide, vincristine, and prednisone (CVP) ± rituximab

Fludarabine ± rituximab

Fludarabine, mitoxantrone, dexamethasone ± rituximab

Cyclophosphamide, doxorubicin, vincristine, and prednisone (CHOP) ± rituximab

Second-Line Therapy

Radioimmunotherapy

High-dose chemotherapy with autologous stem cell transplant

Chemo-immunotherapy

significantly longer progression-free and overall survival for patients who received HDCT versus chemotherapy alone.[86] Several other groups have also reported relapse-free survival of longer than 3 to 4 years and a retrospective analysis done by the International Bone Marrow Transplant Registry reported a 5-year probability of survival of 62% and 55% in patients receiving HDCT with or without purging of the stem cells infusate to remove residual tumor cells, respectively.[87] Allogeneic transplants are usually not recommended because of the reported high rate of transplant-related mortality.[3]

Currently, the NCCN supports the use of single-agent chemotherapy or rituximab or several combination regimens in the first-line treatment of advanced indolent NHL (Table 95.9). Patients who do not achieve a CR after initial therapy or eventually relapse, often receive various palliative therapies for many years. For patients who have relapsed following chemotherapy or rituximab, radioimmunotherapy, HDCT with stem cell transplantation or combinations of chemotherapy with immunotherapy may be used.[68] The optimal therapy for a patient should take into consideration their age, comorbidities, and performance status that may impact their ability to tolerate aggressive regimens. Unfortunately, many patients with indolent lymphomas cannot be cured and typically receive multiple different treatment regimens throughout the duration of their disease. These patients eventually die of unrelated causes, toxicity due to the therapy, progressive disease, or transition to a more aggressive type of lymphoma.

Aggressive Non-Hodgkin's Lymphoma.
Localized (Stages I and II) Aggressive Non-Hodgkin's Lymphoma. Although in the past, patients with stage I and stage II aggressive histologic subtypes were often managed with RT, randomized studies have confirmed that combina-

tion chemotherapy produces superior 5-year disease-free survival rates versus radiation alone.[88,89] Several studies have also shown that patients with bulky and nonbulky disease benefit from IF RT in combination with chemotherapy.[90,91] The NCCN guidelines recommend six to eight cycles of CHOP-R followed by IF RT for patients with bulky disease or other adverse prognostic factors such as age older than 60 years, stage II disease, poor performance status, or elevated lactate dehydrogenase (LDH).[68]

Advanced Stage III and Stage IV Aggressive Non-Hodgkin's Lymphoma. Combination chemotherapy is also indicated for all patients with stage III or IV aggressive NHL. Unlike the indolent nature of many of the follicular histologic subtypes, patients with the more aggressive histologic subtypes may succumb to their disease rapidly, unless they receive and respond to appropriate therapy. For more than 25 years, it has been recognized that many patients with aggressive lymphomas can be cured with chemotherapy, and more recently it has become more widely accepted that the addition of rituximab may further increase the cure rate.

CHOP is a first-generation regimen that has been widely used and accepted as the standard for aggressive lymphomas for the past 2 decades. Numerous clinical trials have confirmed that approximately 40% of patients with advanced aggressive lymphomas are cured following six to eight courses of CHOP therapy. With the goal of increasing the percentage of long-term, disease-free survivors, researchers have evaluated several different strategies including: (a) increasing the intensity of CHOP or similar regimens by dose escalation or administering cycles more frequently (i.e., every 2 weeks vs. every 4 weeks); (b) adding other active chemotherapy agents such as cytarabine, bleomycin, etoposide, or methotrexate; (c) administering HDCT followed by autologous stem cell transplant; or (d) adding rituximab to CHOP or other conventional chemotherapy regimens. While some trials have reported improvements in subgroups of patients receiving intensified chemotherapy regimens or with the addition of other active agents, overall, the benefits have been inconsistent and no strategy has universally emerged as preferred over standard CHOP. Over time, the importance of maintaining the planned dose intensity of the selected chemotherapy regimen has been emphasized. Although regimens like CHOP are effective, they also produce serious side effects. In patients experiencing toxic reactions, it is often tempting to allow more recovery time (i.e., delay the next scheduled dose). However, the specified schedule must be adhered to, whenever possible, to produce the best results. The use of myeloid colony-stimulating factors has reduced the incidence of serious neutropenia associated with many of these regimens and enabled planned dose intensity to be safely delivered.

The addition of rituximab to standard CHOP therapy has appeared to have the most significant impact of all the strategies evaluated to improve long-term outcomes achieved with the CHOP regimen. Coiffier et al[92–94] have reported the results of a large phase III study that compared CHOP to CHOP-R in 399 patients aged 60 to 80 years. In this elderly,

high-risk patient group, the addition of rituximab to CHOP improved the 3-year event-free (53% vs. 35%; $p = 0.00008$) and overall survival (62% vs. 51%; $p = 0.008$), and reduced the risk of treatment failure or death without clinically significant increases in serious adverse effects. The NCCN guidelines now recommend six to eight cycles of CHOP-R for all patients with stage III or IV aggressive NHL who are over age 60 and state that rituximab may be considered for patients under age 60.

For patients with aggressive NHL, only those patients who achieve a CR will have a long, disease-free survival. The International Non-Hodgkin's Lymphoma Prognostic Factors Project report that risk correlates with the number of adverse prognostic signs which include age over 60 years, serum LDH level greater than 1 times normal, poor performance status, stage III or IV disease, or more than one extranodal site of disease. Because major prognostic factors have been identified, it has been suggested that patients with more favorable prognostic factors may be safely treated with less aggressive treatment. This strategy is commonly referred to as "risk-related therapy." Although it is recommended that all patients without high-risk adverse prognostic factors receive a minimum of six to eight courses of CHOP (or similar chemotherapy) with rituximab, more aggressive therapies have been evaluated for patients with high-risk disease.

If the disease responds favorably to a conventional regimen (e.g., CHOP), it is deemed to be chemotherapy-sensitive. Because there is a close dose-response relationship for the sensitive aggressive lymphomas, the use of HDCT with autologous stem cell support has been postulated to offer a greater chance of cure for high-risk patients. A potential advantage of this approach is that tumor cells are not exposed to repeated chemotherapy and, therefore, have little chance to develop acquired resistance. HDCT followed by autologous stem cell transplantation is standard therapy for many younger patients with aggressive NHL who relapse or are refractory to CHOP.[95] The use of this aggressive strategy as part of the initial treatment for aggressive NHL has also been studied but is considered controversial.[95,96] Most of the trials that have evaluated early HDCT with autologous stem cell transplant have included younger patients with adverse prognostic factors such as multiple extranodal sites or evidence of heavy disease burden (i.e., elevated LDH), however several trials have also included lower risk patients. Although the methodology has differed among the randomized trials, most have compared conventional chemotherapy with conventional dose regimens followed by the HDCT if the patient's disease appeared to be chemosensitive (i.e., they had at least a minor response to the conventional dose regimen). The consensus of trial results is that, overall, there does not seem to be any benefit to add HDCT with autologous stem cell support to conventional combination regimens.[97–100] Some trials did report that HDCT might provide benefit for carefully selected subsets of patients, and therefore, research continues in this area. Trials are underway, specifically, to identify if early transplant provides better long-term outcomes than initial treatment with conventional therapy and salvage HDCT with transplant at the time of first relapse.

Salvage Therapy for Relapsed or Refractory Aggressive Non-Hodgkin's Lymphomas. As mentioned above, HDCT followed by autologous stem cell transplantation is standard therapy for many younger patients with aggressive NHL who relapse or are refractory to CHOP chemotherapy.[68,95] The patients who are mostly likely to benefit are those with chemotherapy-sensitive relapsed disease or those who achieved at least a partial response to initial therapy. A prospective randomized trial of 215 patients with relapsed NHL initiated therapy with two cycles of cisplatin, dexamethasone, and cytarabine. Patients who responded to this initial salvage therapy were then randomized to continue this same regimen or receive HDCT with autologous stem cell support. Both 5-year and 8-year posttreatment evaluations have shown a significant benefit for the use of HDCT.[101,102] At 5-years follow-up, the event-free survival was 46% for those who received HDCT versus 12% for those who received conventional therapy ($p = 0.001$) and at 8-years the event-free survival was 36% for the HDCT group and 11% for the conventional therapy group ($p <0.002$). Although the long-term survival rate for patients who achieve a complete response with HDCT after relapse is approximately 50%, it is also important to remember that only a relatively small portion of patients are eligible for this aggressive treatment approach. Therefore, the identification of more effective conventional chemotherapy and biologic therapies is also very important.

Salvage conventional chemotherapy regimens that have been most successful include dexamethasone, cisplatin, and cytarabine (DHAP); etoposide, methylprednisolone, cytarabine, and cisplatin (ESHAP); and ifosfamide, carboplatin, and etoposide (ICE) (Table 95.10). Although the overall response rate with these regimens is generally quite high (approximately 65%–75%), only 20% to 40% of patients typically will achieve a CR. A small subset (5%–10%) of the patients who achieve a CR remain disease-free at 5 years and may be considered cured.[103] More recently, the addition of rituximab to salvage regimens has been investigated. Initial trials which added rituximab to salvage regimens have reported an apparent increase in the percentage of patients who achieved a complete response, however, large randomized trials evaluating second-line treatment with rituximab in patients who received rituximab as part of their initial therapy (current standard) have not been reported.

Highly Aggressive Non-Hodgkin's Lymphoma. Precursor lymphoblastic lymphoma/leukemia (T-cell type) generally occurs in adolescents and young adults. These patients are more likely to have bone marrow, mediastinal, and CNS involvement than those with other lymphomas. Encouraging results have been reported with regimens similar to those used to treat acute lymphoblastic leukemia with CNS prophylaxis and maintenance chemotherapy.

TABLE 95.10	Combination Chemotherapy Regimens for the Treatment of Aggressive Non-Hodgkin's Lymphomas			
Acronym	**Drugs**	**Dose (mg or gm/m²) Route (unless otherwise specified)**	**Treatment Days**	**Frequency of Cycle**
CHOP-R	Cyclophosphamide	750 mg/m² IV	1	Every 21 days
	Doxorubicin	50 mg/m² IV	1	
	Vincristine	1.4 mg/m² IV (max: 2mg)	1	
	Prednisone	100 mg/m² PO	1–5	
	Rituximab	375 mg/m² IV	1	
ICE	Ifosfamide	5 gm/m² IV	24-hour continuous infusion on day 2	Every 21 days
	Carboplatin	AUC of 5	2	
	Etoposide	100 mg/m² IV	1–3	
DHAP	Dexamethasone	40 mg PO or IV	1–4	Every 21–28 days
	Cytarabine	2 gm/m² IV Q12	2	
	Cisplatin	100 mg/m² IV	24-hour continuous infusion on day 1	
ESHAP	Etoposide	40 mg IV	1–4	Every 21–28 days
	Methylprednisolone	250–500 mg total	1–5	
	Cytarabine	2 gm/m² IV	5	
	Cisplatin	25 mg/m² IV	1–4	

IV, intravenously; PO, by mouth; AUC, area under the curve.

Burkitt's lymphoma is a highly aggressive B-cell lymphoma that accounts for about 40% of all childhood NHL worldwide. An endemic form is relatively common in African children, and is almost always associated with EBV infection. Sporadic cases are also seen in adults, however, most do not seem to be associated with EBV infection. Burkitt's lymphoma often presents with extranodal disease involvement, including the CNS. Systemic chemotherapy is the treatment of choice for Burkitt's lymphoma. Although chemotherapy regimens have achieved durable systemic remissions, many patients have relapses in the CNS. Therefore, such regimens should be augmented with intermittent intrathecal methotrexate or cytarabine prophylaxis. Initial selection of chemotherapy is based on risk factors such as serum LDH level and the presence of intraabdominal masses. In patients with an elevated serum LDH level or an intraabdominal mass, additional agents such as rituximab, ifosfamide, and high-dose cytarabine may be added to the standard Burkitt's regimens of an anthracycline, high-dose methotrexate, cyclophosphamide, and vincristine.[68] With these regimens, approximately 90% of patients with localized disease and 50% of patients with extensive disease are cured.[3] Notably, standard regimens used for the aggressive lymphomas (e.g., CHOP) do not adequately control this disease.

OTHER LYMPHOMAS

Cutaneous T-cell lymphoma (CTCL) is a malignancy of T lymphocytes that presents predominantly in the skin. It may have very diverse presentation and thus for many decades a number of distinct entities were described (e.g., Mycoses fungoides, Sézary syndrome, reticulum cell sarcoma of the skin) which are now all considered to be included within CTCL. While this disease primarily involves cutaneous lymphocytes, these cells may travel via the blood to involve other sites in the body.[104]

Early stage disease that is confined to the skin is treated with local approaches and the cure rate is high, however, if the disease has advanced to involve other organs, it is rarely cured and treatment mostly provides palliative benefit.

Therapies used for localized skin involvement only of CTCL include external beam radiation, topical bexarotene gel, carmustine in an ointment-based preparation, topical mechlorethamine, and phototherapy with psoralen and ultraviolet light. These therapies destroy cutaneous T-cells and many of them interfere with the local production of cytokines that are required for T-cell proliferation and survival.[104]

Extracorporeal photochemotherapy (ECP), oral bexarotene, denileukin diftitox (Ontak), interferon, and systemic chemotherapy all are used in the management of advanced or systemic CTCL. ECP involves removing white blood cells from the patient's blood and exposing them to radiation in the presence of psoralen. When the cells are reinfused back into the patient, they appear to stimulate the immune system to recognize and destroy the malignant cells. Evidence suggests that ECP prolongs the median survival of patients with advanced CTCL from approximately 30 to 60 months.[105,106]

Bexarotene (Targretin) is an oral retinoid that selectively binds to and activates the retinoid X receptor. Response rates to bexarotene range from 40% to 60%, depending on the stage of the disease at diagnosis and responses appear to be durable over several years.[107] Hypertriglyceridemia is the most common adverse effect and most patients require concomitant therapy with a lipid-lowering agent.

Denileukin diftitox is approved for the treatment of persistent or recurrent CTCL when malignant cells express the CD25 subunit of the interleukin-2 (IL-2) receptor. Denileukin diftitox is a fusion protein containing part of the diphtheria toxin and IL-2. It is designed to direct the cytocidal action of diphtheria toxin to cells that express the IL-2 receptor. After binding with the receptor on the cell surface, cellular protein synthesis is inhibited, resulting in cell death within hours. Subunits of the IL-2 receptor are found on many CTCL cells; however, before denileukin diftitox therapy, malignant cells must be tested for CD25 expression. The recommended treatment regimen is 9 or 18 μg/kg/day via intravenous infusion over at least 15 minutes for 5 consecutive days every 21 days. Overall response rates of approximately 30% have been reported.[108]

Interferon alfa has also been reported to produce responses in many patients with advanced CTCL. The rate and extent of response and the duration of response appear to correlate with the extent of disease and prior therapies, with heavily treated patients who experience more advanced disease having worse outcomes. In such patients the expected CR rate is less than 30% with a median duration of approximately 6 months.[104] The toxicities associated with interferon alfa must be carefully considered with respect to the anticipated benefits. Systemic chemotherapy also produces CRs in approximately 30% to 50% of patients, however, the duration of response is generally short.[104]

Human Immunodeficiency Virus-Associated Lymphomas. For patients with AIDS-related lymphomas, the presentation is often more widespread and the course of the disease is often more aggressive than patients with similar histologic subtypes who are not infected with HIV. The availability of effective antiretroviral therapies has dramatically improved the patients' ability to tolerate systemic lymphoma therapies and the outcomes of therapy. Currently, chemotherapy regimens for AIDS-related lymphomas are similar to those used in non-HIV positive patients (e.g., CHOP), however, antiretrovirals, myeloid colony stimulating factors, and intrathecal therapy are usually recommended, as well.[68] Although outcomes for HIV-positive patients are inferior, some do appear to have long-term benefits.[109] Some also recommend the use of prophylactic chemotherapy and rituximab, however, at least one randomized trial has reported an increased incidence of infection in patients receiving rituximab.[110] For patients with relapsed or refractory disease, the use of HDCT with autologous stem cell support is also being studied.

TREATMENT COMPLICATIONS

Patients with malignant lymphomas may experience a wide variety of complications, which may be secondary to the disease or the therapy (Table 95.11). Although many of the disease-related complications have been reduced or eliminated with the use of more effective therapies, the use of more aggressive treatment regimens has resulted in more treatment-related complications. In addition, the increased cure rate for HD and many of the NHLs has stimulated concern of late and long-term treatment associated complications.

Many disease-related complications result from infiltration or obstruction of organs, tissues, or blood vessels by the lymphoma. Rapidly growing lymphomas (e.g., nodular sclerosing HD and lymphoblastic lymphoma) may produce obstruction of the superior vena cava. Patients with this complication frequently exhibit shortness of breath; swelling of the face, neck, and upper extremities; headache; and sensations of choking. The occurrence of superior vena cava syndrome should be considered an oncologic emergency. Therapy must often be initiated before a tissue diagnosis is made (if this is the initial presentation of the lymphoma) and includes immediate RT to the mass, diuretics, and combination chemotherapy.

TABLE 95.11	Serious Complications Associated with Lymphomas (and the Treatment of Lymphomas)

Disease-related

Superior vena cava obstruction

Spinal cord compression

Central nervous system infiltration

Renal failure

Immunologic abnormalities

Pleural effusion

Hemolytic anemia

Treatment-related

Chemotherapy-related

  Granulocytopenia and infection

  Tumor lysis syndrome

  Gonadal injury/sterility

  Secondary leukemia

  Organ damage (e.g., renal, hepatic, cardiac) secondary to specific agents

Radiation therapy-related

Tumor lysis syndrome

Pneumonitis

Pericarditis

Hypothyroidism

Lymphoma masses may occasionally cause compression of the spinal cord. At initial diagnosis, this is generally more common with HD than NHL; however, it is more common overall in patients with relapsed or refractory NHL and HIV-associated lymphomas. The most common presenting symptom is central back pain. As the degree of compression progresses, other neurologic symptoms develop (e.g., motor dysfunction, paresthesias, and incontinence) and paraplegia may result if no treatment is given. Appropriate therapy depends on the extent of compression. If detected early enough, chemotherapy and/or RT may elicit a rapid improvement. In some, patients with more advanced spinal cord compressions, emergency surgery (laminectomy) followed by RT may be required. Corticosteroids are also used to prevent edema or promote its resolution. These agents may also have a direct cytotoxic effect as well.

Some lymphomas may infiltrate the CNS and develop meningeal seeding (leptomeningeal involvement). Signs of this complication include headache, nausea and vomiting, and lethargy. Confirmation of meningeal involvement is made by examination of the cerebrospinal fluid, and treatment includes corticosteroids and intrathecal chemotherapy agents (e.g., methotrexate and cytarabine) and RT. Intracerebral lymphomas may also occur, but these are generally primary tumors (now most commonly seen in patients with HIV) and not complications of other systemic disease.

Renal failure may be caused by infiltration of the kidneys or obstruction of the ureters by the lymphoma. Infiltration of the kidneys is usually treated with systemic therapy (although low-dose, local RT may occasionally be used), and urethral obstruction may be treated with local RT combined with systemic chemotherapy.

Tumor lysis syndrome (TLS) is characterized by hyperkalemia, hyperphosphatemia, secondary hypocalcemia, and hyperuricemia. Some patients may also develop acute renal failure due to intravascular volume depletion and precipitation of uric acid and calcium phosphate in the renal tubules. Patients with bulky, highly proliferating (aggressive or highly aggressive) lymphomas, including HD are most at risk for this complication which results from the rapid release of intracellular contents following cytotoxic therapy. It most commonly occurs following the first dose of therapy when the tumor burden is greatest. For patients at risk of TLS, it is recommended that aggressive hydration, allopurinol, and oral phosphate binders be started prior to therapy. If TLS occurs, aggressive measures, including hemodialysis, if necessary, should be taken to avoid life-threatening or permanent complications due to electrolyte disturbances or renal failure.

As would be anticipated from the nature of the disease, immunologic abnormalities commonly occur in patients with malignant lymphomas. Abnormalities in delayed hypersensitivity, particularly cutaneous anergy, develop with extensive involvement of lymphatic tissues or severe lymphocytopenia. Depressed cell-mediated immunity (T lymphocyte) is associated with a high risk of opportunistic infections, including tuberculosis, salmonellosis, toxoplasmosis, and herpes zoster. This is particularly true in patients with HD. In some cases, infection may precede the diagnosis of the disease.[111] Furthermore, patients may continue to have an underlying T-cell function deficit that persists after their disease is in remission.[112] Radiation and chemotherapy also contribute to decreased immunologic function and subsequent infectious complications.

Granulocytopenia secondary to myelosuppressive chemotherapy also predisposes patients to serious infections with both Gram-positive and Gram-negative pathogens. As chemotherapy regimens became more aggressive (especially those used in NHL) the degree and duration of granulocytopenia has increased, placing more patients at risk for infectious complications. The availability of the myeloid colony stimulating factors ameliorated the risk substantially and the use of these agents is now widely accepted. Acute and chronic adverse effects associated with combination chemotherapy are determined by the individual drugs used in the treatment regimen. In addition to myelosuppression, these may include nausea and vomiting, mucositis, neurotoxicity, cardiotoxicity, skin changes, and pulmonary toxicity. Many of these toxic reactions are avoidable or reversible if the clinicians managing the patient are familiar with the agents being used and their associated risks. The major long-term complications of chemotherapy are sterility and risk of secondary malignancies.

Testicular function in adult men is particularly susceptible to injury by many chemotherapeutic agents. As discussed earlier, permanent sterility associated with the MOPP regimen for HD was one of the factors that stimulated the development of new regimens. A comparison of the MOPP and ABVD regimens revealed that azoospermia occurred in 100% of MOPP-treated men but in only 15% to 35% of those receiving ABVD therapy. In addition, spermatogenesis almost always recovers in the ABVD-treated men.[113] This information may be very important in planning treatment for men with HD who are concerned about preservation of fertility after treatment. Gonadal injury also occurs in women after combination chemotherapy. Ovarian failure is associated with arrest of follicular maturation or frank destruction of ova and follicles. Persistent amenorrhea also appears to be less common after ABVD than after MOPP therapy.[113]

The potential of myelodysplastic syndrome and second malignancies, particularly acute nonlymphocytic leukemia, are well-documented complications associated with HD and/or its therapies. Several studies have provided convincing evidence that the risk of leukemia varies markedly with the form of therapy for HD. The well-substantiated risk of secondary leukemia in patients receiving MOPP therapy with or without RT also stimulated the development of alternative, safer therapies. The risk of acute leukemia after ABVD is negligible. Patients with HD are also at increased risk of developing NHL.[114] NHLs apparently occur more frequently after combined modality therapy with RT and chemotherapy

and are frequently similar to NHL seen in immunosuppressed patients. Patients with HD may also have a slightly increased risk of developing solid tumors. In particular, an increased risk of lung cancer has been noted in HD patients who smoke and an increased risk of breast cancer has been reported in women who received radiation at a young age.[115,116]

Complications after RT are largely related to the field that has been irradiated, although fatigue generally occurs in most patients. Nausea, vomiting, mucositis/esophagitis, diarrhea, and anorexia commonly occur after abdominal radiation, while dryness of the mouth and throat, dysphagia, alteration in taste, and increased dental caries may occur after irradiation of the head and neck regions. Bone marrow suppression may occur during abdominal-pelvic irradiation and may require interruption of treatment. In addition to these acute side effects, long-term complications may pose more serious problems. Long-term effects are usually related to the volume of normal tissue that has been irradiated, the total dose given, and the size of the daily dose administered. They include radiation pneumonitis, pericarditis, nephritis, hepatitis, growth retardation (in children), and hypothyroidism.

PATIENT EDUCATION

The aggressive therapies used to treat many of the lymphomas may be associated with complications that may be acutely life-threatening, cause chronic health problems, and negatively impact quality of life. Like many other malignancies, however, advances in the prevention and treatment of these complications have dramatically reduced the negative impact that they have on patients. It is important that patients and their caregivers be familiar with the risks associated with therapies and clearly understand when medical intervention is necessary such as fever during episodes of neutropenia or bleeding. As noted previously, several of the drugs used in the management of lymphomas may be associated with late toxicities such as secondary malignancies. The risk of such late complications should be carefully explained to patients and like all toxicities, in the context of potential risk versus benefit. Patients should also be educated regarding disease-related complications that may require immediate intervention such as severe headaches, difficulty walking, new onset of severe back pain, and swelling of the face and neck. Most importantly, patients must understand the planned treatment course and be instructed regarding the correlation of adhering to the treatment plan and positive outcomes. Lymphomas are very dose-responsive malignancies and, as described throughout this chapter, cure and meaningful prolongation of survival are realistic goals in most cases. Adherence to planned treatment regimens has been associated with higher cure rates in several of subtypes of lymphomas, and therefore, patients must understand the planned treatment schedule and the importance of following it.

IMPROVING OUTCOMES

Advanced diagnostic techniques such as the use of PET scans have facilitated more accurate and less invasive staging procedures. In addition, routine immunophenotyping or identification of molecular markers on the surface of lymphoma cells has resulted in the effective application of targeted therapies. Such molecular markers also are providing improved prognostic information about lymphomas and guiding treatment decisions, including when very aggressive interventions such as stem cell transplants are worthwhile. Evidence-based clinical practice guidelines such as those published by the NCCN are also tools that assist clinicians and patients in understanding the most appropriate therapeutic interventions for specific types of lymphomas.

The use of colony stimulating factors, erythropoietin, and combination antiemetics have reduced the toxic sequelae associated with chemotherapy and radiation and facilitated the administration of full-dose chemotherapy on the recommended schedules. Supportive interventions such as these have also significantly improved quality of life, reduced symptoms associated with therapy, and the need for hospitalization.

EMERGING THERAPIES

Immunostimulatory DNA sequences (ISS) are short sequences of DNA that have been shown to have effects on the immune system including B-cell proliferation and production of immunoglobulins, secretion of various cytokines, expression of costimulatory molecules, and antigen-presenting cell activity of lymphoma cells. It is believed that by increasing the antigen expression, the lymphoma cells may have increased sensitivity to monoclonal antibody therapies such as rituximab. In addition to rituximab, other monoclonal antibodies are also being developed to treat lymphomas.

CONCLUSION

Most lymphomas are sensitive to RT and many chemotherapy agents. Combination chemotherapy regimens are curative in many patients with HD and chemotherapy in combination with rituximab has significantly increased the proportion of patients with many types of NHL who are cured. In addition, many other patients experience a significant prolongation of disease-free survival after treatment. HDCT with stem cell support and the monoclonal antibody, rituximab have assumed more prominent roles in the management of lymphomas in recent years. Well-accepted prognostic factors, disease cytogenetics, and immunophenotype now play a more important role in the selection of therapies. Comprehensive, evidence-based guidelines are available from the NCCN to guide therapeutic decisions for HD and NHL.

Management of patients with lymphomas requires not only an understanding of the disease process and its appropriate therapy but also an understanding of the complications that may arise secondary to the disease or its therapy. These complications include opportunistic infections, obstruction by the tumor, tumor lysis syndrome, second malignancies, and chemotherapy-, biologic-, or radiation-associated toxicities. Anticipation and appropriate management of these complications can greatly reduce the overall morbidity experienced by the patient.

KEY POINTS

■ Lymphoid malignancies that present as extramedullary tumors arising primarily in the lymph nodes are called lymphomas, whereas lymphoid malignancies occurring predominantly in the bone marrow are leukemias

■ Lymphomas are divided into HD and NHLs. Each of these groups includes various subtypes distinguished by morphologic, immunophenotypic, cytogenetic, and clinical features

■ Treatment is determined by the classification and stage of the lymphoma at diagnosis and patient-specific factors that influence a patient's ability to tolerate therapy. Evidence-based clinical practice guidelines published by the NCCN are available to guide treatment decisions

■ Although some patients with early stage HD can be successfully treated with RT, chemotherapy with or without RT is now recommended for most patients. The ABVD and Stanford V regimens are the most widely used regimens for management of HD. Additional cycles of chemotherapy are recommended for patients with more extensive disease

■ RT to the involved areas or chemotherapy followed by RT is recommended for potentially curable localized indolent NHL. Because advanced stage indolent NHLs are not considered curable, observation until symptoms or disease complications are apparent is appropriate for many patients. Single-agent chemotherapy with a cytotoxic drug or rituximab or combination chemotherapy are recommended for patients with symptomatic disease

■ CHOP plus rituximab is generally the treatment of choice for aggressive NHL

■ HDCT with stem cell support is a widely used strategy to treat patients with relapsed or refractory HD or NHL

SUGGESTED READINGS

Diehl V, Harris NL, Mauch PM. Hodgkin's lymphoma. In: Devita VT, Hellman S, Rosenberg SA, eds. Cancer. Principles and practice of oncology. 7th ed. Philadelphia: Lippincott, Williams & Wilkins, 2005:2020–2075.

Fisher RI, Mauch PM, Harris NL, et al. Non-Hodgkin's Lymphomas. In: Devita VT, Hellman S, Rosenberg SA, eds. Cancer. Principles and practice of oncology. 7th ed. Philadelphia: Lippincott, Williams & Wilkins, 2005:1957–1997.

Mauch PM, Armitage JO, Harris NL, Dalla-Favera R, Coiffier B, eds. Non-Hodgkin's lymphomas. Philadelphia: Lippincott, Williams & Wilkins, 2003.

REFERENCES

1. Diehl V, Harris NL, Mauch PM. Hodgkin's lymphoma. In: Devita VT, Hellman S, Rosenberg SA, eds. Cancer. Principles and practice of oncology. 7th ed. Philadelphia: Lippincott, Williams & Wilkins, 2005:2020–2075.
2. Thangavelu M, Le BM. Chromosomal abnormalities in Hodgkin's disease. Hematol Oncol Clin North Am 3:221–236, 1989.
3. Fisher RI, Mauch PM, Harris NL, et al. Non-Hodgkin's lymphomas. In: Devita VT, Hellman S, Rosenberg SA, eds. Cancer. Principles and practice of oncology. 7th ed. Philadelphia: Lippincott, Williams & Wilkins, 2005:1957–1997.
4. Clarke CA, Glaser SL. Changing incidence of non-Hodgkin's lymphoma in the United States. Cancer 94:2015–2023, 2002.
5. American Cancer Society. Cancer Statistics 2005. New York: American Cancer Society, 2005. Available at: http://www.cancer.org/docroot/STT/stt 0.asp. Accessed November 9, 2005.
6. Clarke CA. Changing incidence of Kaposi's sarcoma and non-Hodgkin's lymphoma among young men in San Francisco. AIDS 15:1913–1915, 2001.
7. MacMahon B. Epidemiological evidence of the nature of Hodgkin's disease. Cancer 10:1045–1054, 1957.
8. Filipovich AH, Mathur A, Kamat D, et al. Primary immunodeficiencies: genetic risk factors for lymphoma. Cancer Res 52: 5465s–5467s, 1992.
9. Wolfe F, Fries JF. Rate of death due to leukemia/lymphoma in patients with rheumatoid arthritis. Arthritis Rheum 48:2694–2695, 2003.
10. Gelfand JM, Berlin J, Van Voorhees A, et al. Lymphoma rates are low but increased in patients with psoriasis: results from a population-based cohort study in the United Kingdom. Arch Dermatol 139:1425–1429, 2003.
11. Levine AM. Lymphoma complicating immunodeficiency disorders. Ann Oncol 5:29–35, 1994.
12. Voulgarelis M, Moutsopoulos HM. Malignant lymphoma in primary Sjögren's syndrome. Isr Med Assoc J 3:761–766, 2001.
13. Royer B, Cazals-Hatem D, Sibilia J, et al. Lymphomas in patients with Sjögren's syndrome are marginal zone B-cell neoplasms, arise in diverse extranodal and nodal sites, and are not associated with viruses. Blood 90:766–775, 1997.
14. Cohen JI. Benign and malignant Epstein-Barr virus-associated B-cell lymphoproliferative diseases. Semin Hematol 40:116–123, 2003.
15. Reedman BM, Klein G. Cellular localization of an Epstein-Barr virus (EBV)-associated complement fixing antigen in producer and nonproducer lymphoid cell lines. Int J Cancer 11:499–520, 1973.
16. Mueller N, Evans A, Harris NL, et al. Hodgkin's disease and Epstein-Barr virus. Altered antibody pattern before diagnosis. N Engl J Med 320:689–695, 1989.
17. Pallesen G, Hamilton-Dutoit SJ, Rowe M, et al. Expression of Epstein-Barr virus latent gene products in tumour cells of Hodgkin's disease. Lancet 337:320–322, 1991.
18. Herbst H, Raff T, Stein H. Phenotypic modulation of Hodgkin's and Reed-Sternberg cells by Epstein-Barr virus. J Pathol 179: 54–59, 1996.
19. Weiss LM, Movahed LA, Warnke RA, et al. Detection of Epstein-Barr viral genomes in Reed-Sternberg cells of Hodgkin's Disease. N Engl J Med 320:502–506, 1989.
20. Grufferman S, Cole P, Smith PG et al. Hodgkin's disease in siblings. N Engl J Med 296;248–250, 1977.
21. Prazak J, Hermanska Z. Study of HLA antigens in patients with Hodgkin's disease. Eur J Haematol 43:50–53, 1989.
22. Reitz M. Human T-cell leukemia virus, type 1, and human leukemia and lymphoma. In: Cossman J, ed. Molecular genetics in cancer diagnosis. New York: Elsevier, 1990:163–172.
23. Antman K, Chang Y. Kaposi's sarcoma. N Engl J Med 342: 1027–1038, 2000.
24. Sun Q, Matta H, Chaudhary PM. The human herpes virus 8–encoded viral FLICE inhibitory protein protects against growth factor withdrawal–induced apoptosis via NF-kappa B activation. Blood 101:1956–1961, 2003.
25. Zucca E, Bertoni F, Roggero E, et al. Molecular analysis of the progression from Helicobacter pylori–associated chronic gastritis to mucosa-associated lymphoid-tissue lymphoma of the stomach. N Engl J Med 338:804–810, 1998.
26. Rabkin CS, Devesa SS, Zahm SH, et al. Increasing incidence of non-Hodgkin's lymphoma. Semin Hematol 30:286–296, 1993.
27. Anderson RD, Nishiyama H, Yohei I, et al. Pathogenesis of radiation related leukemia and lymphoma. Speculations based primarily on experience of Hiroshima and Nagasaki. Lancet 1:1060–1062, 1972.
28. Ng AK, Bernardo MP, Weller E, et al. Long-term survival and competing causes of death in patients with early-stage Hodgkin's disease treated at age 50 or younger. J Clin Oncol 20:2101–2108, 2002.
29. Olsen JH, Boice JD, Jensen JP, et al. Cancer among epileptic patients exposed to anticonvulsant drugs. J Natl Cancer Instit 81: 803–808, 1989.
30. Lukes RJ, Craver LF, Hall TC, et al. Report of the nomenclature committee. Cancer Res 26:1311, 1966.
31. Harris NL, Jaffe ES, Stein H, et al. A revised European-American classification of lymphoid neoplasms: a proposal from the International Lymphoma Study Group. Blood 84:1361–1392, 1994.
32. Harris NL, Jaffe ES, Diebold J, et al. World Health Organization classification of neoplastic diseases of the hematopoietic and lymphoid tissues: Report of the Clinical Advisory Committee Meeting—Arlie House, Virginia, November, 1997. J Clin Oncol 17:3835–3849, 1999.
33. Bennett M, MacLennan K, Vaughn Hudson G, et al. Non-Hodgkin's lymphoma arising in patients treated for Hodgkin's disease in the BNLI: a 20-year experience. British National Lymphoma Investigation. Ann Oncol 2:83–92, 1991.
34. Rappaport H. Tumors of the hematopoietic system. In: Atlas of Tumor Pathology. Section III, Fascicle 8. Washington DC: Armed Forces Institute of Pathology, 1966.
35. National Cancer Institute sponsored study of classification of non-Hodgkin's lymphomas. Summary and description of a working formulation for clinical usage. Cancer 49:2112–2135, 1982.
36. Armitage JO, Weisenburger DD. New approach to classifying non-Hodgkin's lymphomas: clinical features of the major histologic subtypes. Non-Hodgkin's Lymphoma Classification Project. J Clin Oncol 16:2780–2795, 1998.
37. Foucar K. Incidence and patterns of bone marrow and blood involvement by lymphoma in relationship to the Lukes-Collins classification. Blood 54:1417–1422, 1979.
38. DeMario MD, Liebowitz DN. Lymphoma in the immunocompromised patient. Semin Oncol 25:492–502, 1998.
39. Frisch M, Biggar RJ, Engels EA, et al. Association of cancer with AIDS-related immunosuppression in adults. JAMA 285: 1736–1745, 2001.
40. Glaser S, Clarke CA, Gulley ML, et al. Population-based patterns of human immunodeficiency virus-related Hodgkin's lymphoma in the greater San Francisco bay area, 1988–1998. Cancer 98: 300–309, 2003.
41. Lister T, Crowther D, Sutcliffe SB, et al. Report of a committee convened to discuss the evaluation and staging of patients with Hodgkin's disease: Cotswolds meeting. J Clin Oncol 7:1630–1636, 1989.
42. Ng AK, Weeks JC, Mauch PM, et al. Laparotomy versus no laparotomy in the management of early-stage, favorable-prognosis Hodgkin's disease: a decision analysis. J Clin Oncol 17:241–252, 1999.
43. Seymour JF, Pro B, Fuller LM, et al. Long-term follow-up of a prospective study of combined modality therapy for stage I-II indolent non-Hodgkin's lymphoma. J Clin Oncol 21:2115–2122, 2003.

44. Ship MA. Prognostic factors in aggressive non-Hodgkin's lymphoma: who has "high-risk" disease? Blood 83:1165–1173, 1994.

45. Friedberg JW, Chengazi V. PET scans in the staging of lymphoma: current status. Oncologist 8:438–447, 2003.

46. Kostakoglu L, Leonard JP, Kuji I, et al. Comparison of fluorine-18 fluorodeoxyglucose positron emission tomography and Ga-67 scintigraphy in evaluation of lymphoma. Cancer 94:879–888, 2002.

47. Van Den Bossche B, Lambert B, DeWinter F, et al. [18]FDG PET versus high-dose ^{67}Ga scintigraphy for restaging and treatment follow-up of lymphoma patients. Nuclear Med Comm 23:1079–1083, 2002.

48. Kostakoglu L, Leonard JP, Coleman M, et al. The role of FDG-PET imaging in the management of lymphoma. Clin Adv Hematol Oncol 2:115–121, 2004.

49. DeVita VT, Serpick A, Carbone P. Combination chemotherapy in the treatment advanced Hodgkin's disease. Ann Intern Med 73:881–895, 1970.

50. Hoppe RT. Radiation therapy in the management of Hodgkin's disease. Semin Oncol 17:704–715, 1990.

51. Leslie NT, Mauch PM, Hellman S. Stage IA to IIB supradiaphragmatic Hodgkin's disease: long-term survival and relapse frequency. Cancer 55:704–715, 1985.

52. Lee CK, Aeppli DM, Bloomfield CD, et al. Curative radiotherapy for laparotomy-staged IA, IIA, IIIA Hodgkin's disease: an evaluation of the gains achieved with radical radiotherapy. Int J Radiat Oncol Biol Phys 19:547–549, 1990.

53. Farah R, Ultmann J, Griem M, et al. Extended mantle radiation therapy for pathologic stage I and II Hodgkin's disease. J Clin Oncol 6:1047–1058, 1998.

54. National Comprehensive Cancer Network. Clinical practice guidelines in oncology. Hodgkin's Disease, version 2.2005. Available at: http://www.nccn.org/professionals/physician gls/PDF/Hodgkin'ss.pdf. Accessed November 9, 2005.

55. Bonadonna G, Zucali R, Monfardini S, et al. Combination chemotherapy of Hodgkin's disease with Adriamycin, bleomycin, vinblastine, and imidazole carboxamide versus MOPP. Cancer 36:252–259, 1957.

56. Goldie JH, Coldman AJ. A mathematic model for relating the drug sensitivity of tumors to their spontaneous mutation rate. Cancer Treat Rep 63:1727–1733, 1979.

57. Santoro A, Bonadonna G, Bonfante V, et al. Alternating drug combinations in the treatment of advanced Hodgkin's disease. N Engl J Med 306:770–775, 1982.

58. Bonadonna G, Valgussa P, Santoro A. Alternating non-cross-resistant combination chemotherapy or MOPP in stage IV Hodgkin's disease. Ann Intern Med 104:739–746, 1986.

59. Jones S, Haut A, Weick JK, et al. Comparison of Adriamycin-containing chemotherapy (MOP-BAP) with MOPP-bleomycin in the management of advanced Hodgkin's disease. A Southwest Oncology Group Study. Cancer 51:1339–1347, 1983.

60. Longo DL, Young RC, Wesley M, et al. Twenty years of MOPP therapy for Hodgkin's disease. J Clin Oncol 4:1295–1306, 1986.

61. Carde P, MacKikntosh FR, Rosenberg SA. A dose and time response analysis of the treatment of Hodgkin's disease with MOPP chemotherapy. J Clin Oncol 1:146–153, 1983.

62. Linch D, Winfield D, Goldstone AH, et al. Dose intensification with autologous bone-marrow transplantation in relapsed and resistant Hodgkin's disease: results of a NLI randomised trial. Lancet 341:1051–1054, 1993.

63. Schmitz N, Sextro M, Pfistner B. HDR-1: high-dose therapy (HDT) followed by hematopoietic stem cell transplantation (HSCT) for relapsed chemosensitive Hodgkin's disease (HD): final results of a randomized GHSG and EBMT trial (HD-R1) [abstract]. Proc Am Soc Clin Oncol (Suppl 5):18, 1999.

64. Josting A, Reiser M, Rueffer U, et al. Treatment of primary progressive Hodgkin's and aggressive non-Hodgkin's lymphoma: is there a chance for cure? J Clin Oncol 18:332–339, 2000.

65. Archuleta TD, Armitage JO. Advances in follicular lymphoma. Semin Oncol 31:66–71, 2004.

66. Wilder RB, Jones D, Tucker SL, et al. Long term results with radiotherapy for stage I-II follicular lymphoma. Int J Radiat Oncol Biol Phys 51:1219–1227, 2001.

67. MacManus MP, Hoppe R. Is radiotherapy curative for stage I and II low-grade follicular lymphomas? Results of a long-term follow-up study of patients treated at Stanford University. J Clin Oncol 14:1282–1298, 1996.

68. National Comprehensive Cancer Network. Clinical practice guidelines in oncology. Non-Hodgkin's Lymphoma. Version 1.2005. Available at: http://www.nccn.org/professionals/physician_gls/PDF/nhl.pdf. Accessed November 9, 2005.

69. Brice P, Bastion Y, Lepage E, et al. Comparison of low-tumor burden follicular lymphomas between an initial no-treatment policy, prednimustine, or interferon alfa: a randomized study from the Groupe d'Etude des Lymphomes Folliculaires. Groupe d'Etude des Lymphomes de l'Adulte. J Clin Oncol 15:1110–1117, 1997.

70. Young RC, Longo DL, Glatstein E, et al. Watchful-waiting VS aggressive combined modality therapy in the treatment of stage III–IV indolent non-Hodgkin's lymphoma [abstract]. Proc Am Soc Clin Oncol 1987;6:200.

71. Horning S, Rosenberg S. The natural history of initially untreated low-grade non-Hodgkin's lymphomas. N Engl J Med 311:1471–1475, 1984.

72. Gribben JG, Freeman AS, Woo SD, et al. All advanced stage non-Hodgkin's lymphomas with polymerase chain reaction amplifiable breakpoint of bcl-2 have residual cells containing the bcl-2 rearrangement at evaluation and after treatment. Blood 78:3275–3280, 1991.

73. Maloney DG, Liles TM, Czerwinski DK, et al. Phase I clinical trial using escalating single-dose infusion of chimeric anti-CD20 monoclonal antibody (IDEC-C2B8) in patients with recurrent B-cell lymphoma. Blood 84:2457–2466, 1994.

74. McLaughlin P, Grillo-Lopez AJ, Link BK, et al. Rituximab chimeric anti-CD20 monoclonal antibody therapy for relapsed indolent lymphoma: half of patients respond to a four-dose treatment program. J Clin Oncol 16:2825–2833, 1998.

75. Hainsworth JD, Burris HA, Morrissey LH, et al. Rituximab monoclonal antibody therapy as initial systemic therapy for patients with low-grade non-Hodgkin's lymphoma. Blood 95:3052–3056, 2000.

76. Hainsworth JD, Litchy J, Burris HA, et al. Rituximab as first-line and maintenance therapy for patients with indolent non-Hodgkin's lymphoma. J Clin Oncol 20:4261–4267, 2002.

77. Czucaman MS, Grillo-Lopez AJ, White CA, et al. Treatment of patients with low-grade B-cell lymphoma with the combination of chimeric anti-CD20 monoclonal antibody and CHOP chemotherapy. J Clin Oncol 17:268–276, 1999.

78. Hainsworth JD, Litchy S, Shaffer DW, et al. Maximizing therapeutic benefit of rituximab: maintenance therapy versus re-treatment at progression in patients with indolent non-Hodgkin's lymphoma-a randomized phase II trial of the Minnie Pearl Cancer Research Network. J Clin Oncol 23:1088–1095, 2005.

79. Witzig TE, Flinn IW, Gordon LI, et al. Treatment with ibritumomab tiuxetan radioimmunotherapy in patients with rituximab-refractory follicular non-Hodgkin's lymphoma. J Clin Oncol 20:3262–3269, 2002.

80. Kaminski MS, Estes J, Zasadny KR, et al. Radioimmunotherapy with iodine (131)I tositumomab for relapsed or refractory B-cell non-Hodgkin's lymphoma: updated results and long-term follow-up or the University of Michigan experience. Blood 96:1259–1266, 2000.

81. Vose JM, Wahl RI, Saleh M, et al. Multicenter phase II study of iodine-131 tositumomab for chemotherapy-relapsed/refractory low-grade and transformed low-grade B-cell non-Hodgkin's lymphomas. J Clin Oncol 18:1316–1323, 2000.

82. Kaminski MS, Zelentz AD, Press OW, et al. Pivotal study of iodine I 131 tositumomab for chemotherapy-refractory low-grade or transformed low-grade B-cell non-Hodgkin's lymphomas. J Clin Oncol 19:3918–3928, 2001.

83. Horning SJ, Younes A, Lucas J, et al. Rituximab treatment failures: tositumomab and iodine I 131 tositumomab (Bexxar) can produce meaningful durable responses [abstract]. Blood 100 (Suppl):357a, 2002.

84. Coleman M, Kaminski MS, Knox SJ, et al. The BEXXAR therapeutic regimen (tositumomab and iodine I 131 tositumomab) produced durable complete remissions in heavily pretreated patients with non-Hodgkin's lymphoma (NHL), rituximab-relapsed refractory disease, and rituximab-naïve disease [abstract]. Blood 102 (Suppl):29a, 2003.

85. Kaminski MS, Tuck M, Estes J, et al. ^{131}I-tositumomab therapy as initial treatment for follicular lymphoma. N Engl J Med 352:441–449, 2005.

86. Schouten HC, Qian W, Kvaloy S, et al. High-dose therapy improves progression-free survival and survival in relapsed follicular non-Hodgkin's lymphoma: results from the randomized European CUP trial. J Clin Oncol 21:3918–3927, 2003.

87. van Besien K, Loberiza FR Jr, Bajorunaite R, et al. Comparison of autologous and allogeneic hematopoietic stem cell transplantation for follicular lymphoma. Blood 102:3521–3529, 2003.

88. Monfardini S, Banfi A, Bonadonna G, et al. Improved five year survival after combined radiotherapy-chemotherapy for stage I-II non-Hodgkin's lymphoma. Int J Radiat Oncol Biol Phys 6:125–134, 1980.

89. Nissen NI, Ersboll J, Hansen HS, et al. A randomized study of radiotherapy versus radiotherapy plus chemotherapy in stage I-II non-Hodgkin's lymphoma. Cancer 52:1–7, 1983.

90. Horning S, Glick J. Final report of E1484: CHOP v CHOP + radiotherapy for limited stage diffuse aggressive lymphoma [abstract]. Blood 98:724a, 2001.

91. Miller TP, Dahlberg S, Cassady JR, et al. Chemotherapy alone compared with chemotherapy plus radiotherapy for localized intermediate- and high-grade non-Hodgkin's lymphoma. N Engl J Med 339:21–26, 1998.

92. Coiffier B, Lepage E, Herbrecht R, et al. MabThera (rituximab) plus CHOP is superior to CHOP alone in elderly patients with diffuse large B-cell lymphoma (DLCL): interim results of a randomized GELA trial [abstract]. Blood 96:223a, 2000.

93. Coiffier B, Lepage E, Briere J, et al. CHOP chemotherapy plus rituximab compared with CHOP alone in elderly patients with diffuse large-B-cell lymphoma. N Engl J Med 346:235–242, 2002.

94. Coiffier B, Herbrecht R, Morel P, et al. GELA study comparing CHOP and R-CHOP in elderly patients with DLCL: 3-year median follow-up with an analysis according to co-morbidity factors [abstract]. Hematol J 4:111, 2003.

95. Coiffier B. Effective immunochemotherapy for aggressive non-Hodgkin's lymphoma. Semin Oncol 31 (Suppl 2):7–11, 2004.

96. Fisher RI. Autologous stem-cell transplantation as a component of initial treatment for poor-risk patients with aggressive non-Hodgkin's lymphoma: resolved issues versus remaining opportunity. J Clin Oncol 20:4411–4412, 2002.

97. Haioun C, Lepage E, Gisselbrecht C, et al. Comparison of autologous bone marrow transplantation with sequential chemotherapy for intermediate and high-grade non-Hodgkin's lymphoma in first complete remission: a study of 465 patients. J Clin Oncol 12:2543–2551, 1994.

98. Martelli M, Gherlinzoni F, DeRenzo A, et al. Early autologous stem-cell transplantation versus conventional chemotherapy as front-line therapy in high-risk, aggressive non-Hodgkin's lymphoma: an Italian multicenter randomized trial. J Clin Oncol 21:1255–1262, 2003.

99. Kaiser U, Uebelacker I, Abel U, et al. Randomized study to evaluate the use of high-dose therapy as part of primary treatment for "aggressive" lymphoma. J Clin Oncol 20:4413–4419, 2002.

100. Kluin-Nelemans HC, Zagonel V, Anastasopoulou A, et al. Standard chemotherapy with or without high-dose chemotherapy for aggressive non-Hodgkin's lymphoma: randomized phase III EORTC study. J Natl Cancer Inst 93:22–30, 2000.

101. Philip T, Guglielmi C, Hagenbeek A, et al. Autologous bone marrow transplantation as compared with salvage chemotherapy in relapses of chemotherapy-sensitive non-Hodgkin's lymphoma. N Engl J Med 333:1540–1545, 1995.

102. Philip T, Gomez F, Gugliemi C, et al. Long-term outcome of relapsed non-Hodgkin's lymphoma (NHL) patients included in the Parma trial: incidence of late relapses, long-term toxicity and impact of the International Prognostic Index (IPI) at relapse [abstract]. Proc Am Soc Clin Oncol 17;16a, 1998.

103. Gisselbrecht C, Mounier N. Improving second-line therapy in aggressive non-Hodgkin's lymphoma. Semin Oncol 31 (Suppl 2):12–16, 2004.

104. Wilson L, Jones GW, Girardi M, et al. Cutaneous T-cell lymphomas. In: Devita VT, Hellman S, Rosenberg SA, eds. Cancer. Principles and practice of oncology. 7th ed. Philadelphia: Lippincott, Williams & Wilkins, 2005:1998–2011.

105. Heald PW, Rook A, Perez M, et al. Treatment of erythrodermic cutaneous T-cell lymphoma patients with photopheresis. J Am Acad Dermatol 27:427, 1992.

106. Heald P, Laroche L, Knobler R. Photoinactivated lymphocyte therapy of cutaneous T-cell lymphoma. Dermatol Clin 12:443, 1994.

107. Duvic M, Hymes K, Heald P, et al. Worldwide Study Group. Bexarotene is effective and safe for treatment of refractory advanced-stage cutaneous T-cell lymphoma: multinational phase II–III trial results. J Clin Oncol 19:2456–2471, 2001.

108. Olsen E, Duvic M, Frankel A, et al. Pivotal phase III trial of two dose levels of denileukin diftitox for the treatment of cutaneous T-cell lymphoma. J Clin Oncol 9:376–388, 2001.

109. Spina M, Carbone A, Vaccher E, et al. Outcome in patients with non-Hodgkin's lymphoma with or without human immunodeficiency virus infection. Clin Infect Dis 38:142–144, 2004.

110. Kaplan LD, Lee J, Scadden DT. No benefit from rituximab in a randomized phase III trial of CHOP with or without rituximab for patients with HIV-associated non-Hodgkin's lymphoma: updated data from AIDS Malignancies Consortium study 010 [abstract]. Blood 102:409a, 2003.

111. Hohl RJ, Shilsky RL. Nonmalignant complications of therapy for Hodgkin's disease. Hematol Oncol Clin North Am 3:331–343, 1989.

112. Vanhaelan CPJ, Fisher RI. Increased sensitivity of T cells to regulation by normal suppressor cells persists in long-term survivors with Hodgkin's disease. Am J Med 72:385–390, 1982.

113. Santoro A, Viviani S, Zucali R, et al. Comparative results and toxicity of MOPP vs ABVD combined with radiotherapy in PS IIB, III Hodgkin's disease [abstract]. Proc Am Soc Clin Oncol 2:223, 1983.

114. Krikorian JG, Burke JS, Rosenberg SA, et al. Occurrence of non-Hodgkin's lymphoma after therapy for Hodgkin's disease. N Engl J Med 300:452–458, 1979.

115. van Leeuwen FE, Klokman WJ, Stovall M, et al. Roles of radiation dose, chemotherapy, and hormonal factors in breast cancer following Hodgkin's disease. J Natl Cancer Inst 95:971–980, 2003.

116. Behringer K, Josting A, Schiller P, et al. Solid tumors in patients treated for Hodgkin's disease: a report from the German Hodgkin's Lymphoma Study Group. Ann Oncol 15:1079–1085, 2004.

Breast Cancer

96

Suzanne Fields Jones and Howard A. Burris III

TREATMENT GOALS

- The treatment of breast cancer varies by disease stage at diagnosis and patient-specific prognostic factors.
- The goal of treatment for early-stage disease is cure, achieved with a combination of surgery, radiation, hormonal therapy, or chemotherapy.
- The combination of surgery, radiation, chemotherapy, and hormonal therapy is also used for locally advanced disease and may result in disease cure or palliation.
- The goals of treatment of metastatic disease are symptom palliation and prolonged survival. Chemotherapy, hormonal therapy, and/or radiation therapy are used in this setting.

EPIDEMIOLOGY

INCIDENCE AND MORTALITY

Breast cancer is the most common malignancy diagnosed in women in the United States and is the second most common cause of cancer death in women, surpassed only by lung cancer. Approximately 217,440 new cases of breast cancer were diagnosed in the United States during 2004, and an estimated 40,580 people died due to breast cancer in 2004.[1] The incidence of breast cancer continues to increase annually, but at a slower rate than in previous years. The mortality rate from breast cancer appears to be declining, which may be due to detection of disease at an earlier stage and improvements in adjuvant treatment.

ETIOLOGY

The etiology of breast cancer is unknown, but several predisposing risk factors for the disease have been determined. These factors can be divided into three major categories: genetic or familial, endocrine, and environmental (Table 96.1).

Women who have a first-degree relative (mother or sister) with breast cancer have a twofold to threefold increased risk of developing breast cancer.[2,3] This risk may be increased further if more than one first-degree relative is diagnosed with the disease, the relative is of a young age at the time of diagnosis, or the relative has bilateral breast cancer.[4] Women who have a personal history of breast cancer have a higher probability than the average woman of developing primary breast cancer in the contralateral breast.[3]

A small percentage of breast cancers can be classified as hereditary cancers. The majority of these hereditary cancers are caused by mutations in the BRCA1 and BRCA2 genes, and a small percentage are associated with other rare cancer syndromes such as Li-Fraumeni syndrome or Cowden disease.[5] It is estimated that the risk of developing breast cancer in women who carry BRCA1 mutations is 73% and the risk of developing a second primary breast cancer (contralateral) is 41% by age 70.[6] As a result, many women may want to undergo genetic testing for breast cancer. However, the interpretation of the genetic test results and the management of patients with positive results are controversial. Although women who test positive for BRCA1 and BRCA2 are at increased risk for the development of breast cancer, the appropriate management of these patients remains a challenge for physicians. Women who test positive for BRCA1 and

TABLE 96.1	Risk Factors for Breast Cancer Development

Personal history of breast cancer

Family history of breast cancer in first-degree relative BRCA1/BRCA2 mutation

Proliferative benign breast disease

Early menarche, late menopause

Nulliparity

First pregnancy after age 35

Exogenous hormones (postmenopausal hormone replacement therapy, oral contraceptives)

Obesity

Sedentary lifestyle

Dietary factors: alcohol, high-fat diet

Radiation

Smoking

BRCA2 should be encouraged to practice intensified early-detection methods for breast cancer such as monthly breast self-examinations, clinician breast examination every 6 to 12 months, and annual mammography beginning between ages 25 and 35 years.[5] Prophylactic mastectomy and chemoprevention with tamoxifen remain controversial in this patient population. A case-control study estimates that bilateral prophylactic mastectomy reduces the risk of breast cancer in women with BRCA1 and BRCA2 mutations by approximately 90%.[7] In a large prospective study in women diagnosed with breast cancer with BRCA1 or BRCA2 mutation (n = 491), the 10-year actuarial risk of contralateral breast cancer was 30% and was reduced in women who underwent contralateral mastectomy or oophorectomy (bilateral removal of the ovaries) or who received tamoxifen.[8]

Patients with benign breast disease have an increased risk of developing breast cancer if they have proliferative lesions with atypical hyperplasia.[2,3] Their risk is increased further if there is also a positive family history for breast cancer. Patients in these higher-risk groups may warrant close monitoring for breast cancer development, but other patients with benign breast disease (e.g., fibrocystic or ''lumpy'' breasts) should be treated similar to the general population.

Both endogenous and exogenous hormones have also been associated with an increased risk for breast cancer. The incidence of breast cancer is thought to correlate with prolonged high levels of estrogen in the bloodstream, such as in women with long menstrual histories. As a result, women with early menarche (age less than 12) or late menopause (age greater than 55) are at higher risk for the development of breast cancer.[9,10] Women who have never been pregnant are also at a greater risk for breast cancer than women who have given birth. However, the age at which a woman experiences her first full-term pregnancy also influences her risk of developing breast cancer. A first full-term pregnancy after age 35 increases the risk for breast cancer because of hormonal changes and latent breast tissue differentiation that occurs during pregnancy, particularly during the first pregnancy.[3,9] Theoretically, increasing the number of menstrual cycles with oral contraceptive use could be associated with an increased risk of breast cancer. However, the studies that have been published in this area show conflicting results. Most studies have been conducted retrospectively with numerous hormone preparations and have shown no relation between oral contraceptives and breast cancer. A meta-analysis of 54 studies (>150,000 women) showed a slightly increased risk of having breast cancer diagnosed in women currently using combined oral contraceptives or women who have used them in the past 10 years.[11] There was no increased risk of having breast cancer diagnosed after 10 or more years after cessation of use. However, the studies in the meta-analysis were conducted prior to 1996 and used older contraceptive preparations (higher estrogen content). In a more recent population-based, case-control study among women 35 to 64 years of age, current or former oral contraceptive use was not associated with a significantly increased risk of breast cancer.[12]

The knowledge base regarding the risk of breast cancer in women receiving hormone replacement therapy (HRT) has grown tremendously over the last decade. In 1997, the Collaborative Group on Hormonal Factors in Breast Cancer published a reanalysis of 51 epidemiologic studies that found that the risk of having breast cancer diagnosed was increased in women using HRT, and this risk increased with increasing duration of use of HRT.[13] Subsequent cohort studies conducted in the United States and Europe confirmed the increased risk of breast cancer with HRT and also determined that the risk was greater for estrogen–progestin combinations than other types of HRT.[14,15] The increased risk of breast cancer in postmenopausal women receiving estrogen–progestin HRT has also been confirmed in a placebo-controlled randomized clinical trial conducted by the Women's Health Initiative.[16] The trial was stopped prematurely after a mean follow-up of 5 years because the test statistic for invasive breast cancer exceeded the stopping boundary and the global index statistic indicated that the risks of treatment exceeded the benefits. As a result, HRT should be discouraged and alternative therapeutic options (i.e., clonidine, antidepressants, vaginal estrogen preparations, bisphosphonates, selective estrogen-receptor modulators, and HMG CoA reductase inhibitors) should be used for women presenting with new postmenopausal-related symptoms or health problems.

Based on the variable incidence rates of breast cancer in various countries, it is thought that environmental factors contribute to the development of breast cancer in women. Western countries such as the United States have high breast cancer rates, whereas Eastern countries such as Japan have a low incidence of the disease. The difference in breast cancer rates is thought to be partially due to dietary differences between the two populations, specifically the amount of fat consumed in the diet. A recent prospective analysis in pre-menopausal women enrolled in the Nurse's Health Study II showed that increased fat intake was associated with an increased risk of breast cancer.[17] Obesity has also been associated with an increased risk of breast cancer in postmenopausal women, possibly due to the concomitant alterations in ovarian hormones, glucose metabolism, and breast cancer growth factors.[2,18,19] Women who are physically active have a decreased risk of developing breast cancer, possibly due to anovulatory menstrual cycles and maintaining a lean body weight.[19] Alcohol consumption has been associated with an increased risk of developing breast cancer. In a large reanalysis of data from 53 epidemiologic studies correlating alcohol, tobacco, and breast cancer, the relative risk of breast cancer increased by 7.1% for each additional 10 g per day intake of alcohol.[20] Clinical trials have shown increased concentrations of circulating hormones in both pre- and postmenopausal women who consumed alcohol, suggesting that higher concentrations of circulating estrogens could contribute to the increased risk of breast cancer.[21,22] Although the large data reanalysis did not find an increased risk of breast cancer associated with smoking, data from the California Teachers Study would suggest differently. In this large prospective analysis of 116,544 teachers, an increased risk of breast cancer that increased with smoking intensity and duration was observed in active smokers.[23] As diet, exercise, alcohol consumption, and smoking are all lifestyle choices that have been associated with breast cancer risk, behavioral modifications aimed at altering these detrimental lifestyles could lead to a decreased incidence of breast cancer.

Survivors of the atomic bomb blasts during World War II have experienced an increased incidence of breast cancer due to radiation exposure.[24] Similar breast cancer incidence rates have also been reported in women treated with radiation for mastitis, women receiving multiple fluoroscopies for the treatment of tuberculosis, and women receiving mantle radiation for the treatment of Hodgkin's disease. Some physicians have expressed concern about the use of repeated screening mammographies in women due to the link between radiation exposure and breast cancer. However, the amount of radiation a woman is exposed to during a mammogram is extremely low, and there have been no reports to date of breast cancer development secondary to mammography screening.

PATHOPHYSIOLOGY

BREAST ANATOMY AND TUMOR DEVELOPMENT
Human breast tissue is composed primarily of connective tissue and fat. There is also an elaborate duct system within the breasts that is used during lactation. Breast tissue has an abundant blood supply and an extensive lymphatic network. Lymphatic drainage of the mammary tissues flows into the axillary, interpectoral, and internal mammary lymph nodes. This is important because breast cancer commonly spreads via the lymphatic system, and metastatic disease is often discovered in the regional lymph nodes at the time of diagnosis (Fig. 96.1; *see color insert*).

A woman's breast tissue and glands begin to develop around the time of puberty due to the influence and interaction of sex hormones. However, the amount of breast development occurring at puberty is limited and the majority occurs during the first pregnancy. The large amounts of estrogen and progesterone produced by the ovaries during pregnancy stimulate rapid growth and terminal differentiation of immature breast tissue. A delay in the terminal differentiation of breast tissue until a later age may help explain why women who become pregnant for the first time after age 35 have an increased risk for breast cancer development, because immature cells are more susceptible to cycling estrogen effects and estrogens are known to initiate tumor growth.[25]

PATHOGENESIS OF BREAST CANCER
The development of breast cancer occurs when breast cells lose their normal differentiation and proliferation controls. Various hormones, oncogenes, and growth factors influence the proliferation of these abnormal or tumor cells. There is strong evidence to suggest that estrogen directly and indirectly stimulates the growth of tumor cells.[26] Furthermore, numerous growth factors that also play a role in tumor development are secreted by the breast cancer cells themselves. These factors can be classified as either autocrine (if they stimulate their own growth) or paracrine (if they have an effect on other cells). Examples of the autocrine growth factors include transforming growth factor alpha (TGF-α) and insulin-like growth factors I and II (IGF-I and IGF-II). Transforming growth factor beta (TGF-β), platelet-derived growth factor (PDGF), and procathepsin D (52K protein) are all paracrine growth factors. The exact mechanism of tumor development is not completely understood, but tremendous progress has been made in this area with the discovery of the autocrine and paracrine growth factors. The mechanism of action of several of the hormonal agents used for the treatment of breast cancer involves the alteration of the growth factors involved in tumor development. Trastuzumab, a monoclonal antibody that binds specifically to growth factor receptors on the malignant cell surface, has been approved by the U.S. Food and Drug Administration (FDA) for use in metastatic disease.

CLINICAL PRESENTATION AND DIAGNOSIS

SIGNS AND SYMPTOMS
Breast cancer masses tend to be painless, solitary, unilateral, hard, irregular, and nonmobile. Patients may also have skin changes, nipple discharge, or axillary lymphadenopathy. On presentation, any woman with suspected benign or malignant breast disease should have a mammogram.

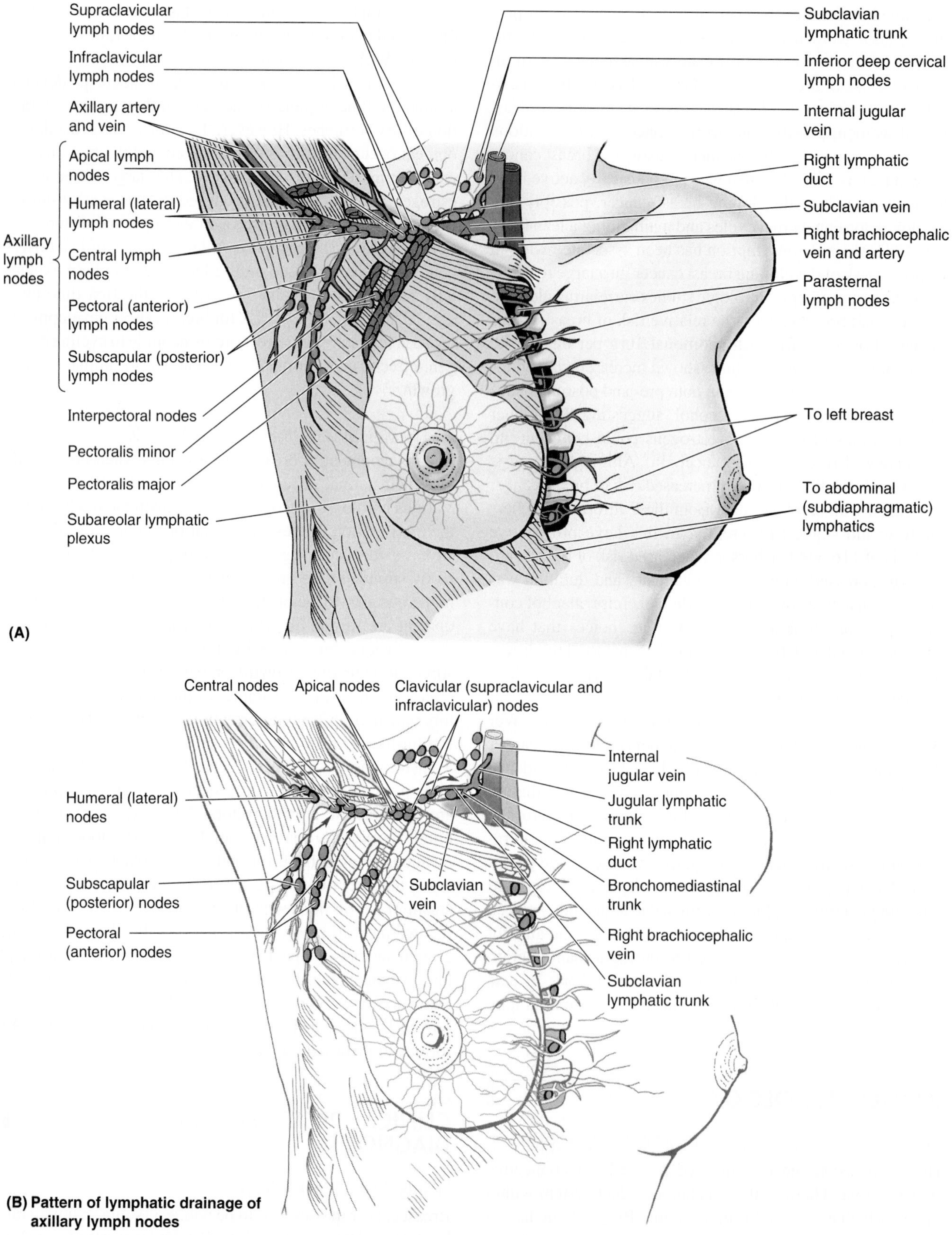

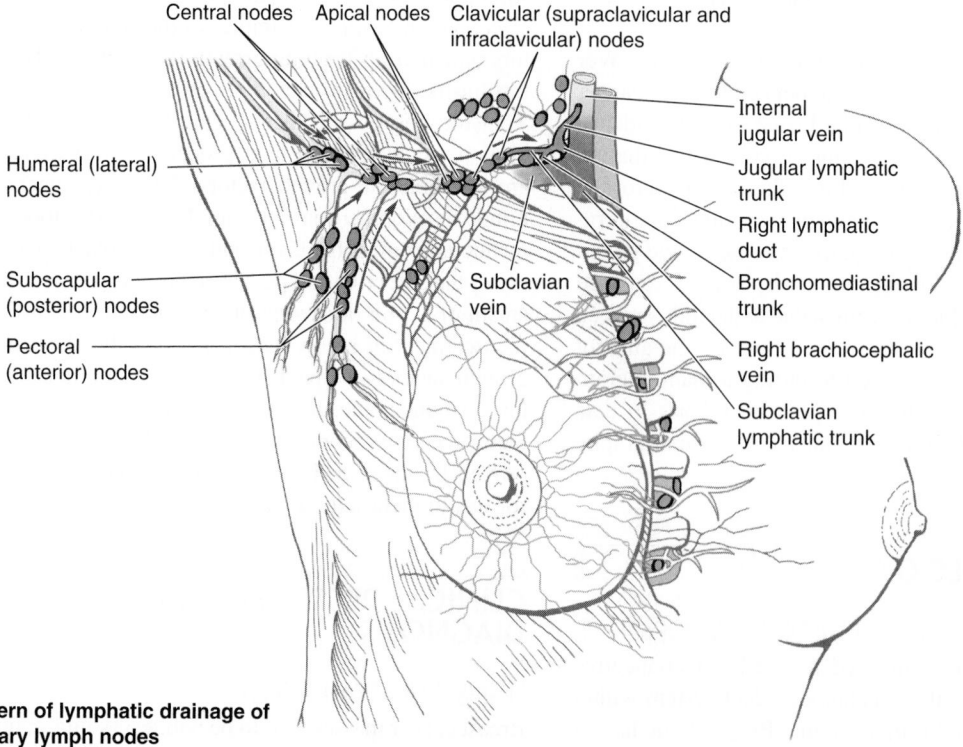

(A)

(B) Pattern of lymphatic drainage of axillary lymph nodes

FIGURE 96.1 Breast tissue drainage and its relationship to tumor metastases (*see color insert*). (From Moore KL, Dalley AF. Clinical oriented anatomy, 4th ed. Baltimore: Lippincott Williams & Wilkins, 1999.)

SCREENING AND DIAGNOSIS

Early detection of breast cancer is critical because patients with limited-stage disease have a better prognosis. Table 96.2 lists the American Cancer Society (ACS) Guidelines for Breast Cancer Screening. The term ''screening'' refers to the testing of asymptomatic individuals for the detection of occult disease. It is recommended that patients periodically undergo physical examinations by a trained physician as well as regular mammograms for early detection and diagnosis of nonpalpable and palpable breast cancers. However, screening will not benefit all patients who are diagnosed with breast cancer and may even be harmful in some women who undergo biopsies for breast abnormalities detected at screening that are not breast cancer. Any breast mass that is suggestive of malignancy by mammography or physical examination should be biopsied by fine-needle aspiration, core-needle biopsy, incisional biopsy, or excisional biopsy. Although needle aspirations and core biopsies provide enough evidence for a histologic diagnosis of breast cancer, they do not delineate the size of the tumor or allow determination of the tumor's estrogen receptor (ER) status.

Many breast tumors are discovered incidentally by the patient. In the past, it was recommended that women perform monthly breast self-examinations (BSE) to detect palpable tumors earlier. However, the studies on the effectiveness of BSE for early detection of tumors have found no direct benefit and a high rate of benign biopsies.[27] As a result, patients are now encouraged to perform BSE to develop an awareness of their normal breast composition so that they may have a heightened awareness of any changes that may be detected.

The ACS recommends that women have a clinical breast examination (CBE) conducted by a trained physician as part of their periodic health examination for breast cancer screening. Although mammography is more sensitive for detecting small breast tumors than physical examination, a small percentage of palpable masses are missed by mammography. Clinical trials have shown the value of CBE in combination with mammography, but these studies were conducted before the development of the high-quality mammography equipment used today for breast imaging.[27] As a result, the contribution of CBE to early breast cancer detection deserves reevaluation in the era of modern technology.

The ACS guidelines regarding mammography screening have also been revised. It is now recommended that women at average risk begin screening at age 40 with repeat examinations annually. This recommendation is based on a meta-analysis of eight randomized controlled trials evaluating screening mammography versus routine care in combination with data evaluating the impact of community screening programs. The meta-analysis showed a 16% decrease in breast cancer mortality among women 40 to 74 years of age who underwent screening mammography.[28] The decrease in mortality was even greater in the subset of patients older than 50 (22% decrease). Data from breast cancer screening programs corroborate the mortality reduction observed in randomized controlled trials.[27]

The benefits of early detection by mammography have begun to be realized, as shown by the increased incidence of breast cancer detection and the declining breast cancer mortality rate. The elderly population (older than 65) in the United States is growing exponentially, and the incidence and mortality of breast cancer increase with increasing age. As a result, clinicians and patients will be faced with decisions regarding the efficacy of screening mammography in this population. The majority of randomized clinical trials evaluating screening mammography did not include patients older than 65 years of age, but the risk of breast cancer mortality was reduced by 22% to 32% in two trials that included patients 65 to 74 years of age.[28] Based on these data, no upper age limit should be placed on screening mammography. Instead, the decision to continue mammography screening should be based on the risks and benefits of the procedure in the individual patient.

TABLE 96.2	American Cancer Society Guidelines for Early Breast Cancer Detection, 2003

Begin mammography at age 40.

For women in their 20s and 30s, clinical breast examination should be part of a periodic health examination, preferably at least every 3 years. Asymptomatic women aged 40 and over should continue to receive a clinical breast examination as part of a periodic health examination, preferably annually.

Beginning in their 20s, women should be told about the benefits and limitations of breast self-examination (BSE). The importance of prompt reporting of any new breast symptoms to a health professional should be emphasized. Women who choose to do BSE should receive instruction and have their technique reviewed on the occasion of a periodic health examination. It is acceptable for women to choose not to do BSE or to do BSE irregularly.

Women should have an opportunity to become informed about the benefits, limitations, and potential harms associated with regular screening.

BREAST CANCER STAGING

The TNM classification system is the most commonly accepted staging system for breast cancer. Tumor size (T) is described on a scale of 0 to 4 based on characteristics of the primary tumor. Extent of lymph node involvement (N), based on location and palpability, and the presence or absence of distant metastases (M), are also included in the system. In January 2003, a revised TNM staging system for breast cancer was adopted for use in tumor registries.[29] One change in the revised staging system is the definition of the lower size limit of micrometastases due to the availability of immunohistochemical (IHC) technology and molecular biologic techniques. The revised staging system is also different regarding nodal involvement. Because prognosis and treatment correlate with extent of disease, the new system differentiates patients according to the number of positive lymph nodes. The use of an identifier to designate sentinel lymph node detection has also been added. Because of the poorer prognosis in patients with infraclavicular, supraclavicular, or internal mammary lymph node involvement, metastasis to any of these nodal areas has been reclassified in the revised system. The changes in the new staging system will have an impact on the stage-specific survival of breast cancer patients.[30] As a result, clinicians must use caution when comparing survival from studies using the new staging system with historical data. Table 96.3 gives the revised American Joint Committee on Cancer TNM staging system for breast cancer.

PSYCHOSOCIAL ASPECTS

In addition to the physical changes that occur in a woman's life as a result of breast cancer treatment, she must also cope with many psychosocial issues. The changes in appearance that occur due to surgery (breast removal) or chemotherapy (alopecia) may create problems with self-image or perceived acceptance by family and friends. It may also be difficult for healthy women diagnosed with breast cancer to make the transition from the role of caregiver in the family to the role of "care receiver." The possible inability to continue working plus the costs of treatment may place additional financial burdens on families during this time. Many women may find it difficult to deal with the numerous added stresses associated with a cancer diagnosis and should be encouraged to participate in support groups to address these and many other issues.

THERAPEUTIC PLAN

The goal of treatment in breast cancer varies by the stage of disease at diagnosis and patient-specific prognostic factors. Most breast cancer disease (excluding metastatic disease) is treated with the intent to cure the patient. Some patients with isolated metastases that can be resected may also be treated for cure. Most often, if the disease recurs it is nonresectable, making the goal of cure nearly impossible. When cure is not possible, the goals of treatment are to prolong survival and palliate symptoms.

NONINVASIVE BREAST CANCER

The increased use of mammography, with the subsequent increase in suspicious breast masses, has led to more frequent diagnosis of lobular carcinoma in situ (LCIS). LCIS is confined to the lobules and terminal ducts, is nonpalpable, and is not detected by mammography.[3] It is most often diagnosed incidentally in premenopausal women and is not considered a malignancy in and of itself, but its presence may predispose women to the development of breast cancer in

the future. Standard treatment for LCIS consists of close observation of the patient after the excisional biopsy with regular physical examinations and mammograms.

The increased use of mammography has also led to an increase in the diagnosis of ductal carcinoma in situ (DCIS).[31] Patients with DCIS are managed with mastectomy or breast-conservation treatment (partial mastectomy or lumpectomy with radiation therapy). No studies directly comparing the two procedures have been conducted. However, the National Surgical Adjuvant Breast and Bowel Project (NSABP) has conducted a trial comparing lumpectomy and lumpectomy plus radiation in patients with DCIS.[32] At 8-year follow-up, patients who received lumpectomy plus radiation had a decreased incidence of both invasive and noninvasive ipsilateral (same-side) breast cancers compared with patients who received lumpectomy alone, suggesting that lumpectomy plus radiation is sufficient treatment for most patients with DCIS. The addition of tamoxifen to the combination of lumpectomy and radiation therapy in patients with DCIS provided a reduction in the risk of developing both ipsilateral and contralateral breast cancer events, so the risks and benefits of tamoxifen therapy should be thoroughly evaluated in patients with DCIS.[33]

EARLY-STAGE BREAST CANCER

Approximately 75% to 80% of women diagnosed with breast cancer have stage I or II disease at diagnosis. In the early days of breast cancer management, the primary mode of treatment was a radical mastectomy. The goal of this treatment was to remove the breast, underlying tissues, and regional lymph nodes. However, as surgical skills and patient management improved, the modified radical mastectomy, which spares the pectoralis muscles and some high axillary lymph nodes, became acceptable for the treatment of primary disease, and patients were spared the sequelae associated with a radical mastectomy. *Breast-conservation treatment* is defined as lumpectomy or partial mastectomy accompanied by node dissection and followed by radiation therapy. Six randomized trials have found no difference in overall survival and disease-free survival between patients who underwent total mastectomy or breast-conservation treatment.[34] Although the addition of radiation to surgery does not improve survival compared to surgery alone, the rate of local recurrence is reduced threefold in patients who receive combination surgery and radiation.[35] These findings suggest that the combination of lumpectomy and radiation is appropriate therapy for patients with early-stage breast cancer.

The need for axillary node dissection in patients with early-stage breast cancer is a controversial issue. With the increased use of mammography, the number of primary breast tumors smaller than 1 cm in diameter that have not spread to the lymph nodes (node negative) at diagnosis has increased dramatically. Furthermore, the use of adjuvant systemic therapy in node-negative patients, as well as node-positive patients, shifts the purpose of axillary node dissec-

TABLE 96.3	**TNM Staging System for Breast Cancer**

Primary Tumor (T)

Tx	Primary tumor cannot be assessed
T0	No evidence of primary tumor
Tis	Carcinoma in situ
Tis (DCIS)	Ductal carcinoma in situ
Tis (LCIS)	Lobular carcinoma in situ
Tis (Paget)	Paget's disease of the nipple with no tumor
T1	Tumor ≤2 cm in greatest dimension
T1mic	Microinvasion ≤0.1 cm in greatest dimension
T1a	Tumor >0.1 cm but not >0.5 cm in greatest dimension
T1b	Tumor >0.5 cm but not >1 cm in greatest dimension
T1c	Tumor >1 cm but not >2 cm in greatest dimension
T2	Tumor >2 cm but not >5 cm in greatest dimension
T3	Tumor >5 cm in greatest dimension
T4	Tumor of any size with direct extension to (a) chest wall or (b) skin, only as described below:
T4a	Extension to chest wall, not including pectoralis muscle
T4b	Edema (including peau d'orange) or ulceration of the skin of the breast or satellite skin nodules confined to the same breast
T4c	Both T4a and T4b
T4d	Inflammatory carcinoma

Note: Paget's disease associated with a tumor is classified according to the size of the tumor.

Regional Lymph Nodes (N)

Nx	Regional lymph nodes cannot be assessed (e.g., previously removed)
N0	No regional lymph node metastasis
N1	Metastasis in movable ipsilateral axillary lymph node(s)
N2	Metastasis in ipsilateral axillary lymph nodes fixed or matted, or in clinically apparent* ipsilateral internal mammary nodes in the absence of clinically evident axillary lymph node metastasis
N2a	Metastasis in ipsilateral axillary lymph nodes fixed to one another (matted) or to other structures
N2b	Metastasis only in clinically apparent* ipsilateral internal mammary nodes and in the absence of clinically evident axillary lymph node metastasis
N3	Metastasis in ipsilateral infraclavicular lymph node(s), or in clinically apparent* ipsilateral internal mammary lymph node(s) and in the presence of clinically evident axillary lymph node metastasis; or metastasis in ipsilateral supraclavicular lymph node(s) with or without axillary or internal mammary lymph node involvement
N3a	Metastasis in ipsilateral infraclavicular lymph node(s) and axillary lymph node(s)
N3b	Metastasis in ipsilateral internal mammary lymph node(s) and axillary lymph node(s)
N3c	Metastasis in ipsilateral supraclavicular lymph node(s)

Regional Lymph Nodes (pN)±

pNx	Regional lymph nodes cannot be assessed (e.g., previously removed, or not removed for pathologic study)
pN0	No regional lymph node metastasis histologically, no additional examination for isolated tumor cells^φ
pN0(i−)	No regional lymph node metastasis histologically, negative IHC
pN0(i+)	No regional lymph node metastasis histologically, positive IHC, no IHC cluster >0.2 mm
pN0(mol−)	No regional lymph node metastasis histologically, negative molecular findings (RT-PCR)
pN0(mol+)	No regional lymph node metastasis histologically, positive molecular findings (RT-PCR)
pN1mi	Micrometastasis (>0.2 mm, none >2 mm)

(continues)

TABLE 96.3	continued

pN1	Metastasis in one to three axillary lymph nodes and/or in internal mammary nodes with microscopic disease detected by sentinel lymph node dissection but not clinically apparent[§]
pN1a	Metastasis in one to three axillary lymph nodes
pN1b	Metastasis in internal mammary nodes with microscopic disease detected by sentinel lymph node dissection but not clinically apparent[§]
pN1c	Metastasis in one to three axillary lymph nodes and in internal mammary lymph nodes with microscopic disease detected by sentinel lymph node dissection but not clinically apparent[§, ‖]
pN2	Metastasis in four to nine axillary lymph nodes or in clinically apparent* internal mammary lymph nodes in the absence of axillary lymph node metastasis
pN2a	Metastasis in four to nine axillary lymph nodes (at least one tumor deposit >2 mm)
pN2b	Metastasis in clinically apparent* internal mammary lymph nodes in the absence of axillary lymph node metastasis
pN3	Metastasis in 10 or more axillary lymph nodes, or in infraclavicular lymph nodes, or in clinically apparent* ipsilateral internal mammary lymph nodes in the presence of one or more positive axillary lymph nodes; or in more than three axillary lymph nodes with clinically negative microscopic metastasis in internal mammary lymph nodes; or in ipsilateral supraclavicular lymph nodes
pN3a	Metastasis in 10 or more axillary lymph nodes (at least one tumor deposit >2 mm), or metastasis to the infraclavicular lymph nodes
pN3b	Metastasis in clinically apparent* ipsilateral internal mammary lymph nodes in the presence of one or more positive axillary lymph nodes; or in more than three axillary lymph nodes and in internal mammary lymph nodes with microscopic disease detected by sentinel lymph node dissection but not clinically apparent[§]
pN3c	Metastasis in ipsilateral supraclavicular lymph nodes

Distant Metastasis (M)

MX	Distant metastasis cannot be assessed.
M0	No distant metastasis
M1	Distant metastasis

Stage Grouping

Stage 0	Tis	N0	M0	Stage IIIA	T0	N2	M0
Stage I	T1[a]	N0	M0		T1[a]	N2	M0
Stage IIA	T0	N1	M0		T2	N2	M0
	T1[a]	N1	M0		T3	N1	M0
	T2	N0	M0		T3	N2	M0
Stage IIB	T2	N1	M0	Stage IIIB	T4	N0	M0
	T3	N0	M0		T4	N1	M0
					T4	N2	M0
				Stage IIIC	Any T	N3	M0
				Stage IV	Any T	Any N	M1

IHC, immunohistochemistry; RT-PCR, reverse transcriptase polymerase chain reaction.

[a] T1 includes T1mic.

* "Clinically apparent" is defined as detected by imaging studies (excluding lymphoscintigraphy) or by clinical examination.

± Classification is based on axillary lymph node dissection with or without sentinel lymph node dissection. Classification based solely on sentinel lymph node dissection without subsequent axillary lymph node dissection is designated (sn) for "sentinel node" (e.g., pN0(I+0(sn)).

ɸ Isolated tumor cells are defined as single tumor cells or small cell clusters not greater than 0.2 mm, usually detected only by immunohistochemical or molecular methods but which may be verified on hematoxylin and eosin stains. Isolated tumor cells do not usually show evidence of metastatic activity (e.g., proliferation or stromal reaction).

§ "Not clinically apparent" is defined as not detected by imaging studies (excluding lymphoscintigraphy) or by clinical examination.

‖ If associated with more than three positive axillary lymph nodes, the internal mammary nodes are classified as pN3b to reflect increased tumor burden.

(From the American Joint Committee on Cancer (AJCC), Chicago, Illinois with permission. The original source for this material is the AJCC Cancer Staging Manual, 6th ed. New York: Springer-Verlag, 2002.)

tion at diagnosis to a prognostic indicator only. Finally, the elimination of the lymph node dissection from breast-conservation treatment would significantly decrease the morbidity of the surgical procedure (specifically the lymphedema and limitation of arm motion and strength). In light of these facts, researchers recently presented preliminary results from the International Breast Cancer Study Group Trial evaluating the feasibility of omitting axillary lymph node dissection in older patients (60 years and up) with breast cancer.[36] There was no difference in disease-free or overall survival between the two groups, but quality of life was improved in patients who did not have axillary dissection.

Researchers are investigating the use of sentinel lymph node detection as a possible alternative to lymph node dissection for detecting lymph node metastases. The sentinel lymph node is the first node that receives lymphatic drainage from a tumor. It can be detected by injecting a blue dye or radioactive colloid around the primary tumor and following the drainage pathway of the dye or colloid. The sentinel node can then be biopsied to determine the presence or absence of lymphatic metastases. Randomized clinical trials comparing sentinel node biopsy/dissection and axillary lymph node dissection are ongoing. In the only small randomized trial published to date (n = 516), the number of positive sentinel nodes found was the same in the two groups.[37] Patients who underwent sentinel node biopsy experienced fewer postoperative side effects and slightly better disease-free survival. Preliminary results from the Axillary Lymphatic Mapping Against Nodal Axillary Clearance (ALMANAC) Trial were recently reported.[38] Axillary metastases were detected in 22% of patients undergoing sentinel node biopsy and 20% undergoing standard axillary treatment. Sentinel node biopsy was also associated with less arm morbidity and better quality of life and was more cost-effective. Randomized clinical trial data showing comparable long-term survival rates with sentinel lymph node dissection are warranted before axillary dissection is abandoned, but the widespread acceptance of sentinel lymph node dissection as standard of care will make these trials difficult if not impossible to perform.

In the setting of breast cancer, adjuvant therapy is chemotherapy or hormonal therapy that is administered in an attempt to eliminate the residual micrometastatic disease that remains after surgery.

The Early Breast Cancer Trialists' Collaborative Group (EBCTCG) published a meta-analysis summarizing the results of all randomized adjuvant chemotherapy trials that began before 1990.[39] The results of this large meta-analysis have helped define the use of adjuvant chemotherapy in women with stage I or II disease. It has also helped identify deficiencies in the currently available data that should be addressed in subsequent randomized trials.

Because the 5-year and 10-year disease-free survival rate in node-negative patients receiving no adjuvant therapy ranges from 70% to 90%, many physicians question whether patients with node-negative disease with tumors less than 1 cm in diameter should receive adjuvant therapy. Further-

more, the acute and delayed toxicities, as well as the direct cost and cost-effectiveness of the therapy, must be considered. Indirect costs in the form of drug toxicities and decreased quality of life during therapy are difficult to quantitate but should be included when weighing the risks and benefits of adjuvant therapy. In some clinical trials, acute toxicities, such as nausea, vomiting, mucositis, and myelosuppression, resulted in death in a small percentage of patients. Long-term toxicities in the form of secondary malignancies (leukemia following alkylating agents and endometrial cancers following tamoxifen therapy), venous and arterial thrombosis, and congestive heart failure secondary to anthracycline administration were not observed due to the relatively short follow-up period. These delayed toxicities, however, are increasingly important when the survival benefits associated with adjuvant therapy are minimal or nonexistent, as in patients with node-negative tumors smaller than 1 cm. Due to the limited number of patients older than 70 with early-stage breast cancer who have participated in clinical trials, there are insufficient data to make recommendations for adjuvant chemotherapy for this patient subset. The decision to administer adjuvant chemotherapy to these women must be made on an individual basis, with comorbid medical conditions being taken into consideration.

A recent study evaluated quality of life in women with early-stage breast cancer who received adjuvant treatment 2 to 5 years previously.[40] The self-rated quality of life was generally favorable, with less than one third of patients reporting moderate to severe symptoms. Sexual function did appear to be compromised following adjuvant therapy. Another interesting finding from the study was that 65% of patients stated that they were willing to undergo 6 months of chemotherapy for a 5% increase in likelihood of cancer cure. Another survey of breast cancer survivors found a similar willingness to receive chemotherapy for a low degree of benefit.[41] The women surveyed would have undergone chemotherapy for a median life expectancy improvement of 3 to 6 months or an improvement of less than 1% in the risk of recurrence. However, this survey also revealed that many women are incompletely informed about their prognosis and the impact of adjuvant therapy. Women appear to overestimate the risk of early relapse and the effectiveness of adjuvant therapy.

In the EBCTCG, combination chemotherapy improved long-term relapse-free and overall survival rates in women up to 70 years of age irrespective of nodal status or ER status. Based on this analysis and the National Institutes of Health Consensus Statement, several generalizations regarding adjuvant chemotherapy can be made.[39,42] The use of polychemotherapy (two or more drugs) appears superior to single agents, and four to six cycles of treatment (3 to 6 months) appears to be optimal. A randomized trial conducted by the Cancer and Leukemia Group B (CALGB 8541) determined that dose and dose intensity are important for disease-free and overall survival.[43] As a result, clinicians should try to avoid chemotherapy dose reductions in the adjuvant setting so that the maximal benefit of therapy may be achieved. The availability of hematopoietic growth factors makes this more feasible.

Although combination chemotherapy regimens have proven to be more effective than single-agent therapy, the optimal combination chemotherapy regimen has not been determined. Table 96.4 describes some of the combination regimens used in the treatment of breast cancer. The combination of cyclophosphamide, methotrexate, and fluorouracil (CMF) was historically used extensively as adjuvant chemotherapy. However, in the EBCTCG meta-analysis, anthracycline-containing regimens (either doxorubicin or epirubicin) improved survival compared to non-anthracycline regi-

mens.[39] Two randomized studies, NSABP-15 and NSABP-23, found that four cycles of doxorubicin/cyclophosphamide (AC) were equivalent to six cycles of conventional CMF, so AC was readily adopted as a standard adjuvant regimen in the United States.[44,45] Another cooperative group trial, CALGB 9344, found that increasing the dose of doxorubicin in the AC regimen did not improve disease-free or overall survival when compared to the standard dose of 60 mg per m^2.[46] In Europe and Canada, epirubicin-containing regimens are used more commonly as adjuvant therapy.

The taxanes (docetaxel, paclitaxel) were not available at the time of the EBCTCG meta-analysis. These drugs have shown the most activity as single agents or in combination

TABLE 96.4	Combination Chemotherapy Regimens Used in the Treatment of Breast Cancer
Regimen	**Drug**	**Dose**
CMF (oral cyclophosphamide)	Cyclophosphamide	100 mg/m^2/day PO Days 1–14
Repeat every 28 days.	Methotrexate	40 mg/m^2 IV Days 1 and 8
	Fluorouracil	600 mg/m^2 IV Days 1 and 8
CMF (IV cyclophosphamide)	Cyclophosphamide	600 mg/m^2 IV Day 1
Repeat every 21 days.	Methotrexate	40 mg/m^2 IV Day 1
	Fluorouracil	600 mg/m^2 IV Day 1
AC	Doxorubicin	60 mg/m^2 IV Day 1
Repeat every 21 days.	Cyclophosphamide	600 mg/m^2 IV Day 1
FAC or CAF	Fluorouracil	500 mg/m^2 IV Day 1
Repeat every 21 days.	Doxorubicin	50 mg/m^2 IV Day 1
	Cyclophosphamide	500 mg/m^2 IV Day 1
TAC	Docetaxel	75 mg/m^2 IV Day 1
Repeat every 21 days.	Doxorubicin	50 mg/m^2 IV Day 1
	Cyclophosphamide	500 mg/m^2 IV Day 1
AC → T	Doxorubicin	60 mg/m^2 IV Day 1
Repeat AC every 21 days ×4 then	Cyclophosphamide	600 mg/m^2 IV Day 1
repeat T every 21 days ×4.	followed by	followed by
	Paclitaxel	175 mg/m^2 IV Day 1
CEF	Fluorouracil	500 mg/m^2 IV Days 1 & 8
Repeat every 28 days.	Epirubicin	60 mg/m^2 IV Days 1 & 8
	Cyclophosphamide	75 mg/m^2 PO Days 1–14
TCH	Paclitaxel	200 mg/m^2 IV Day 1
Repeat every 21 days.	Carboplatin	AUC 6 IV Day 1
	Trastuzumab	8 mg/kg then 6 mg/kg
TCH	Paclitaxel	80 mg/m^2 IV
Repeat weekly for 3 out of every 4 weeks.	Carboplatin	AUC 2
	Trastuzumab	4 mg/kg then 2 mg/kg weekly continuously
Gemcitabine/Paclitaxel	Gemcitabine	1,250 mg/m^2 IV Days 1 & 8
Repeat every 21 days.	Paclitaxel	175 mg/m^2 IV Day 1
Docetaxel/Capecitabine	Docetaxel	75 mg/m^2 IV Day 1
Repeat every 21 days.	Capecitabine	1,250 mg/m^2 PO BID Days 1–14

regimens in patients with metastatic breast cancer.[47] As a result of this activity, numerous trials using these agents in the adjuvant setting have been completed or are ongoing. Two large cooperative group trials, CALGB 9344 and NSABP B-28, found that four cycles of AC followed by four cycles of every-3-week paclitaxel resulted in improved disease-free survival and equivalent (NSABP B-28) or improved (CALGB 9344) overall survival compared to AC alone.[46,48] These trials, however, have been criticized for the longer duration of treatment in the AC-plus-paclitaxel arms compared to the AC arm. Concurrent anthracycline/taxane administration was also explored in a randomized trial conducted by the Breast Cancer International Research Group (BCIRG 001 trial). In this study, node-positive patients were randomized to receive six cycles of standard fluorouracil, doxorubicin, and cyclophosphamide (FAC) or six cycles of docetaxel, doxorubicin, and cyclophosphamide (TAC).[49] Patients who received TAC had an improved disease-free and overall survival compared to patients who received FAC.

For many antineoplastic agents there is a linear relationship between dose and tumor response, but the toxic effects of the drug on the bone marrow limit the dose that can be administered. High-dose chemotherapy intensification with or without autologous bone marrow or peripheral blood stem cell support has been extensively investigated as adjuvant therapy for patients with high-risk breast cancer (more than four positive lymph nodes). The results from 10 randomized trials indicate that high-dose chemotherapy does not significantly prolong disease-free or overall survival compared to standard therapy, so this adjuvant treatment modality is no longer being pursued.[50]

Although increasing dose intensity by increasing the doses of chemotherapy has not been successful at improving survival, preliminary data exploring dose density (i.e., decreasing the time interval between treatment cycles) appears to improve treatment outcomes. A randomized trial (CALGB 9741) was conducted to compare sequential and concurrent administration of doxorubicin, paclitaxel, and cyclophosphamide and to determine whether dose density of the regimens (every-2-week versus every-3-week treatment cycles) improves survival.[51] Patients receiving dose-dense therapy also received filgrastim to enable 2-week treatment cycling. There was no difference in efficacy between sequential and concurrent chemotherapy dosing. However, the dose-dense regimens (every-2-week dosing) showed a significant improvement in both disease-free and overall survival compared to the standard regimens (every-3-week dosing).

Patients who have hormone-responsive disease and poor prognostic factors may benefit from the addition of hormonal therapy to adjuvant systemic chemotherapy. Many clinical trials empirically incorporated tamoxifen either concurrently or sequentially with chemotherapy in patients whose tumors were ER positive. To determine the proper timing for chemotherapy and tamoxifen administration, researchers randomized postmenopausal, node-positive, hormone-receptor-positive patients to receive cyclophosphamide, doxorubicin,

and fluorouracil (CAF) plus either concurrent or sequential tamoxifen or single-agent tamoxifen.[52] Both CAF regimens were superior to tamoxifen alone in terms of disease-free survival. The sequential administration of tamoxifen after CAF completion was also superior to concurrent CAF and tamoxifen, with an estimated disease-free survival advantage of 18%. Currently available data would support delaying the start of hormonal therapy until the adjuvant chemotherapy treatment is completed.

Adjuvant hormonal therapy should be offered to any patient whose tumor overexpresses hormone receptors [either ER or progesterone (PgR)], regardless of patient age, nodal status, or menopausal status. Tamoxifen, a selective estrogen-receptor modulator (SERM), has been the adjuvant hormonal therapy most commonly used. In the meta-analysis performed by the EBCTCG of all randomized trials started before 1990, tamoxifen therapy showed a significant reduction in the annual odds of breast cancer recurrence and mortality.[53] Data from the meta-analysis showed that 5 years of tamoxifen was superior to 1 to 2 years of tamoxifen. A subsequent study (NSABP B-14) showed that 10 years of tamoxifen was inferior to 5 years, so it is recommended that tamoxifen be discontinued after 5 years.[54] However, the benefits of tamoxifen must be weighed against the side effects of treatment, particularly when the drug is being used in the adjuvant setting. The most common side effects of tamoxifen include hot flashes and vaginal discharge, but an increased risk of thromboembolic events and endometrial cancer can also occur.

The aromatase inhibitors (letrozole, anastrazole, and exemestane), which interfere with the final step of estrogen biosynthesis, are another class of compounds used as hormonal therapy in patients with metastatic breast cancer. Recent data suggest that these agents are also effective in the adjuvant setting. The ATAC (Arimidex, Tamoxifen Alone or in Combination) Trialists' Group found superior disease-free survival for anastrozole as adjuvant therapy in postmenopausal women with hormone-sensitive disease when compared to tamoxifen or the combination of tamoxifen and anastrozole.[53] As a result, anastrozole was granted accelerated approval as adjuvant therapy for breast cancer.

Researchers are also investigating the sequential use of tamoxifen and aromatase inhibitors in the adjuvant setting. In the Intergroup Exemestane Study, patients who were switched to exemestane therapy after 2 to 3 years of tamoxifen had significantly improved disease-free survival compared with the standard 5 years of tamoxifen.[55,56] In another double-blind trial, postmenopausal women who had completed 5 years of adjuvant tamoxifen were randomized to receive 5 years of letrozole or placebo (National Cancer Institute of Canada MA17 Trial).[57] Patients who received 5 additional years of letrozole experienced a 40% decrease in the risk of distant breast cancer recurrence and a 39% reduction in mortality.[58] The emerging data for the use of aromatase inhibitors in the adjuvant setting are encouraging, but continued follow-up of these trials is critical to establish the long-term safety of these drugs, particularly with regard to bone and lipid metabolism.

In the past, ovarian ablation via surgery or radiation has been used as adjuvant therapy and first-line therapy of metastatic disease in premenopausal women with breast cancer. However, the development of pharmacologic agents that block estrogen binding or produce medical castration allows drug therapy to be used in this setting and avoids the morbidity and mortality associated with surgery or radiation. Large randomized trials have shown that treatment with a luteinizing hormone-releasing hormone (LHRH) agonist (i.e., goserelin) with or without antiestrogen therapy (i.e., tamoxifen) is equivalent to cytotoxic chemotherapy (i.e., CMF) in premenopausal women with hormone-sensitive disease.[59-62] The sequential administration of goserelin with or without tamoxifen after completion of cytotoxic chemotherapy produces a modest benefit in disease-free and overall survival compared to chemotherapy alone in premenopausal women with hormone-sensitive disease. Estrogen suppression is a critical component of adjuvant therapy in premenopausal and perimenopausal women, so the use of LHRH agonists alone or in combination should be considered in this population.

The presence or absence of prognostic and predictive factors and the patient's desire to receive treatment should influence the physician's final judgment concerning adjuvant therapy. It is also imperative that physicians try to improve the education of patients regarding the risk of disease relapse, as well as the potential benefits of adjuvant therapy. To determine optimal adjuvant therapy regimens and treatment durations, all physicians should encourage patients receiving adjuvant therapy to participate in clinical trials when they are available. Adjuvant therapy should be tailored to the individual characteristics of the patient, and the benefits must be weighed against the risks of treatment, recognizing that the threshold for derived benefit of therapy varies between individual patients. The American Society of Clinical Oncology (ASCO) has issued recommended breast cancer surveillance guidelines.[63] Generally, women with a history of breast cancer should perform monthly BSE and undergo annual mammography of both the preserved and contralateral breast. The patient should also have a complete history and physical examination every 3 to 6 months for the first 3 years after diagnosis, then every 6 to 12 months for 2 years, and then annually. ASCO does not recommend bone scans, chest radiographs, blood counts, tumor markers, liver ultrasonograms, or computed tomography scans as part of routine follow-up.

LOCALLY ADVANCED BREAST CANCER

Patients diagnosed with locally advanced breast cancer [stage III disease or inflammatory breast cancer (IBC)] have tumors larger than 5 cm or direct tumor involvement of the skin or underlying chest wall. These patients also have extensive lymph node involvement. Because of the bulk of disease at the time of diagnosis, surgical management is generally not feasible. Furthermore, standard treatment modalities are minimally effective, resulting in poor survival rates. In an attempt to improve the overall survival rates in women with locally advanced disease, researchers began to use combined modality therapy consisting of radiation therapy, systemic chemotherapy, and surgery. Preoperative (primary or neoadjuvant) systemic therapy involves the use of chemotherapy before surgery to decrease the size of the tumor and improve resectability. Other advantages of preoperative chemotherapy include earlier treatment of micrometastatic disease, intact tumor vasculature resulting in improved drug delivery, the ability to determine the tumor's responsiveness to chemotherapy in vivo, and the ability to customize postsurgical systemic therapy based on this response. After preoperative chemotherapy, patients may receive radiation therapy, surgery alone, or a combination of the two modalities.

Nine-year follow-up data from the NSABP B-18 trial showed a significant correlation between primary tumor response and long-term outcome.[64] Patients who have a pathologic complete response (pCR) to preoperative chemotherapy have significantly improved disease-free and overall survival rates; thus, this level of response is now frequently used as a surrogate marker for prognosis when evaluating new agents or regimens in this treatment setting.

Both anthracycline- and taxane-based regimens have been used as preoperative chemotherapy.[65,66] Recent trials have also shown that sequential docetaxel following anthracycline-based therapy results in increased pathologic response rates and 5-year survival.[67,68] Trials exploring the optimal dose and scheduling of preoperative chemotherapy (including dose-dense regimens) and the value of postoperative adjuvant therapy are ongoing. The availability of pre- and post-treatment tumor biopsy samples and the surrogate marker for prognosis (pCR) make the preoperative treatment setting attractive for evaluating the activity of novel chemotherapy drugs and molecularly targeted therapies.

METASTATIC BREAST CANCER

Radiation therapy, hormonal therapy, and chemotherapy have all been used in the treatment of metastatic breast cancer to palliate the patient and possibly prolong survival. Because palliation is the primary goal of therapy at this point, the easiest, least toxic treatment that can provide the best possible response is generally preferred. Breast cancer can metastasize to virtually any site, but the most common sites include bone, lung, pleura, liver, soft tissue, and the central nervous system. The choice of therapy for metastatic disease is based on the site of disease involvement and the presence or absence of certain patient characteristics. For example, patients who experience a longer disease-free survival (2 years or longer), have disease that is primarily located in bone or soft tissue, have responded to primary endocrine therapy, and are late premenopausal or postmenopausal will most likely respond to endocrine therapy. The most important factor predicting response to hormonal therapy, however, is the presence of ER and PgR on tumor tissues. From

50% to 60% of ER-positive patients and 75% to 85% of ER- and PgR-positive patients have a chance of responding to hormonal therapy, whereas those with no hormone receptors have a 90% chance of failure with hormone therapy.[2] Chemotherapeutic drugs are most commonly used as palliative therapy in patients who would not be expected to respond to hormonal therapy (i.e., patients with rapidly progressive lung, liver, or bone marrow disease, patients with ER/PgR-negative disease) or patients who have failed to respond to initial treatment with endocrine therapy.

Radiation therapy is primarily used to control symptomatic disease such as bone metastases, metastatic brain lesions, and spinal cord compressions. Both brain and spinal cord metastases seldom respond to chemotherapy and hormonal manipulations, but they do respond somewhat to irradiation.

The goal of hormonal therapy is to reduce the stimulation of the tumor cells by estrogen. Historically, the antiestrogen tamoxifen was the backbone of hormonal therapy. However, the partial agonist activity of tamoxifen, resulting in an increased incidence of thromboembolic disease and endometrial cancer, as well as the development of drug resistance has prompted the development of alternative agents. The third-generation aromatase inhibitors have been extensively studied as first- and second-line therapy for metastatic breast cancer.[69] Fulvestrant, an injectable pure estrogen antagonist, has also shown activity in patients with hormone-receptor-positive disease progressing on hormonal therapy. The choice of hormonal therapy is patient-specific and may be influenced by prior therapy in the adjuvant setting, toxicity profiles, cost, and ease of administration. The recommended doses, routes of administration, and side effects reported with the hormonal therapies used for breast cancer are listed in Table 96.5.

If a patient fails to respond to initial hormonal therapy or progresses during therapy after an initial response, an alternative hormonal manipulation should be attempted because multiple responses may occur. The median duration of response to the first attempt at hormonal manipulation is usually in the range of 9 to 12 months, and the duration of any subsequent responses is generally shorter. First-line hormonal therapy should be administered for at least 6 to 8 weeks before disease response is assessed. After initiation of therapy, some patients may experience a flare (or worsening) of their disease that may or may not be accompanied by hypercalcemia. Therapy may need to be withheld or decreased during this initial period, but treatment can usually continue. Furthermore, 5% to 10% of patients may actually experience regression of their tumor when therapy is withdrawn.[70,71] If a patient becomes refractory to hormonal therapy at any time, chemotherapy should be given.

Patients with rapidly progressive disease, those who do not fulfill the criteria for treatment with hormonal therapy, or those who fail to respond to hormonal therapy should receive chemotherapy. The agents that have demonstrated activity in the treatment of breast cancer are described in Table 96.6. Historically, the combination regimens listed in Table 96.4, as well as numerous ad hoc combination regimens, have been used in the metastatic disease setting because of the presumed increase in activity with combination therapy. However, some clinicians prefer to use sequential single-agent therapy rather than combination regimens.[6]

The taxanes, both paclitaxel and docetaxel, have been extensively studied as single agents and in combination regimens for the treatment of breast cancer.[47] In a randomized trial comparing docetaxel and paclitaxel in patients with anthracycline-resistant metastatic breast cancer, docetaxel produced a higher overall response rate and superior disease-free and overall survival. However, grade 3 to 4 treatment-related toxicities were also increased with docetaxel compared to paclitaxel.[72] Alternative taxane dosing schedules including weekly drug administration, sequential dosing,

TABLE 96.5	Hormonal Therapies Used for Breast Cancer		
Class	Drug	Dose	Side Effects
Antiestrogen	Tamoxifen	20 mg PO qd	Disease flare, hot flashes, nausea, vomiting, edema, vaginal discharge; rare: thrombophlebitis, ocular abnormalities, endometrial cancer
	Toremifene	60 mg PO qd	
LHRH Agonists	Leuprolide	7.5 mg SQ q28 days	Amenorrhea, hot flashes, occasional nausea
	Goserelin	3.6 mg SQ q28 days	
Aromatase Inhibitors First Generation	Aminoglutethimide (must also give hydrocortisone 40 mg/d)	250 mg PO BID ×2 wks then QID	Lethargy, skin rash, ataxia, nystagmus, postural dizziness, diarrhea, asthenia, nausea, headache, hot flashes
Third Generation	Anastrozole	1 mg PO qd	Hot flashes, nausea, vomiting, headache, fatigue; rare: fractures, musculoskeletal disorders
	Letrozole	2.5 mg PO qd	
	Exemestane	25 mg PO qd	
Pure Estrogen Antagonist	Fulvestrant	250 mg IM q month	Hot flashes, headache, nausea, vomiting, injection site reactions

TABLE 96.6	Toxicities of Commonly Used Breast Cancer Agents
Drug	**Toxicity**
Cyclophosphamide	Myelosuppression, nausea/vomiting, alopecia, hemorrhagic cystitis, stomatitis
Methotrexate	Myelosuppression, mucositis, diarrhea, nausea/vomiting, hepatic dysfunction, nephrotoxicity
Fluorouracil (5FU)/ capecitabine	Myelosuppression, mucositis, alopecia, nausea/vomiting, diarrhea, skin hyperpigmentation/photosensitivity, cerebellar ataxia (5FU only), hand–foot syndrome
Vinblastine/vinorelbine	Neurotoxicity, constipation, alopecia, myelosuppression, injection site reactions, skin necrosis after extravasation, peripheral neuropathy
Doxorubicin/Epirubicin	Myelosuppression, nausea/vomiting, alopecia, stomatitis, radiation recall, skin necrosis after extravasation, cardiotoxicity (occurs more frequently with cumulative doses)
Paclitaxel/Docetaxel	Myelosuppression, hypersensitivity reactions (require premedications), paresthesia/neuropathy, myalgias and arthralgias (greater with paclitaxel), nausea, vomiting, diarrhea, alopecia, fluid retention (docetaxel), cutaneous reactions (docetaxel)
Trastuzumab	Fever, chills, diarrhea, cardiac dysfunction

and dose-dense regimens are being explored in the adjuvant, preoperative, and metastatic disease settings. Recent data indicate that increased dose intensity (paclitaxel 210 or 250 mg/m^2) does not improve response rate or survival in women with metastatic breast cancer compared to standard dosing (paclitaxel 175 mg/m^2).[73] However, weekly lower-dose taxane administration significantly improves treatment-related toxicities while maintaining or increasing antitumor activity, making this mode of administration particularly attractive for palliative treatment in the metastatic setting or for frail or elderly patients.[74] Because of significant antitumor activity, the anthracycline/taxane combination regimen is frequently used in the adjuvant setting. As a result, alternative, non–cross-resistant treatment regimens are necessary for women who develop disease recurrence after receiving anthracycline/taxane adjuvant therapy.

Capecitabine is a prodrug that is converted to fluorouracil after oral administration. The convenience of oral administration makes capecitabine an attractive agent in the metastatic disease setting because the primary goal of treatment is palliation. The drug is approved by the FDA as a single agent for the treatment of patients with anthracycline/taxane-resistant metastatic breast cancer at a dose of 2,500 mg/m^2/day administered orally twice daily with food for 2 consecutive weeks followed by 1 week of rest (21-day cycles). However, in clinical practice many physicians choose to initiate treatment with reduced doses (approximately a 20% decrease) from the FDA-approved dose to improve treatment tolerability. The most common toxicities associated with therapy include diarrhea, nausea, vomiting, stomatitis, and hand–foot syndrome. The combination of capecitabine and docetaxel is also approved for patients with metastatic breast cancer who have failed to respond to prior anthracycline-based therapy. In a large randomized trial, the combination of capecitabine and docetaxel resulted in a significantly superior response rate, time to disease progression, and overall survival compared with single-agent docetaxel.[75]

Gemcitabine, a nucleoside analogue with a unique mechanism of action, was also recently approved by the FDA in combination with paclitaxel as first-line therapy for patients with metastatic breast cancer who failed to respond to adjuvant anthracycline therapy. In a large randomized phase III trial, the combination of gemcitabine and paclitaxel resulted in a statistically significant improvement in response rate and time to disease progression compared to single-agent paclitaxel.[76] At interim analysis, the combination also showed a strong trend toward improved survival compared to paclitaxel alone.

HER2 overexpression has been correlated with decreased disease-free and overall survival in breast cancer patients, and approximately 20% to 25% of breast tumors overexpress HER2.[77] Trastuzumab, a humanized monoclonal antibody that binds to the HER2 receptor, was the first targeted therapy approved by the FDA. The drug is approved as a single agent or in combination with paclitaxel for the treatment of patients with metastatic breast cancer whose tumors overexpress the HER2 protein. Further data analysis indicates that patients who show 3+ overexpression of HER2 by IHC or HER2 gene amplification by fluorescent in situ hybridization (FISH) testing are more likely to respond to trastuzumab.[77] Trastuzumab appears to be well tolerated overall, with infusion-related fever and chills being the most commonly reported side effects. Cardiac dysfunction, manifested as a decrease in left ventricular ejection fraction that may or may not be associated with symptoms of heart failure, has also been reported with trastuzumab treatment.[78] Retrospective review indicates that patient age, prior anthracycline exposure, and the presence of cardiac risk factors are predisposing factors for trastuzumab-associated cardiac dysfunction. The majority of patients who develop symptomatic cardiac dysfunction respond to standard measures used in the management of congestive heart failure (i.e., diuretics, angiotensin-converting enzyme inhibitors, and cardiac glycosides) and may not worsen with continued trastuzumab therapy. The

FDA-approved dose of trastuzumab is a loading dose of 4 mg per kg followed by weekly dosing at 2 mg per kg. Subsequent trials have shown that trastuzumab has a terminal half-life of more than 18 days, so many clinicians are using every-3-week dosing (6 mg/kg) for improved patient convenience.[79] Additional data also show that the combination of docetaxel and trastuzumab significantly improves response rate, time to disease progression, and estimated median survival compared to docetaxel alone in patients with HER2-overexpressing metastatic breast cancer.[80] The addition of a platinum compound to the taxane and trastuzumab combination has also been evaluated. In a randomized phase III trial, the triple combination of trastuzumab, paclitaxel, and carboplatin significantly improved response rate and time to progression, with a trend toward improved overall survival, compared to the trastuzumab and paclitaxel combination in women with previously untreated metastatic breast cancer.[81] A second trial conducted by the NCCTG (protocol 98-32-52) compared weekly and every-3-week paclitaxel, carboplatin, and trastuzumab.[82] The response rates and time to progression data echoed the data for the triplet combination reported by Robert et al, but the weekly schedule was superior to the every-3-week schedule for response rate, time to progression, and survival. These data, however, must be interpreted with caution, as this was a relatively small trial with too few patients to be powered for statistical superiority.

The anthracyclines have shown significant activity in the adjuvant treatment of breast cancer and in the treatment of metastatic disease. Unfortunately, however, anthracycline dosing is limited by the development of cardiomyopathy, which occurs with cumulative lifetime doses of greater than 400 mg per m^2 for doxorubicin and 900 mg per m^2 for epirubicin. As a result, patients commonly cannot be retreated with anthracyclines when they develop metastatic disease because of the doses they received in the adjuvant setting. Dexrazoxane is an intracellular chelating agent that interferes with the generation of iron-mediated free radicals, which are thought to be responsible for anthracycline-induced cardiotoxicity. The drug is approved for the reduction of the incidence and severity of cardiomyopathy associated with doxorubicin administration in women with metastatic breast cancer who have received a cumulative doxorubicin dose of 300 mg per m^2. Although the use of dexrazoxane would allow patients to receive higher cumulative lifetime doses of doxorubicin, many clinicians choose to use alternative agents in the setting of metastatic disease.

The use of pamidronate and zoledronic acid, bone resorption inhibitors or bisphosphonates, for the treatment of osteolytic bone metastases is another advance in the management of patients with metastatic breast cancer. The administration of 90 mg of pamidronate intravenously over 2 hours or zoledronic acid 4 mg over 15 minutes every 3 to 4 weeks in conjunction with standard chemotherapy or hormonal therapy decreases the number of skeletal complications in women with metastatic disease.[83] The role of bisphosphonates in the adjuvant setting is also being explored. Premeno-pausal women receiving adjuvant chemotherapy frequently develop ovarian failure or premature menopause, which leads to accelerated bone loss and osteoporosis. The use of aromatase inhibitors in the adjuvant and metastatic disease setting is also associated with bone loss and increased fracture risk. As a result, women with a history of breast cancer should regularly undergo bone mineral density screening for osteoporosis and adopt a lifestyle for maintaining bone health (i.e., adequate calcium and vitamin D intake, exercising regularly, and avoiding smoking). The use of intravenous or oral bisphosphonates as preventive therapy is also being explored in this setting.

In summary, the goal of treatment of metastatic disease is palliation. As a result, patient quality of life should play a role in treatment decisions. The newer agents approved for metastatic breast cancer, such as gemcitabine, trastuzumab, and capecitabine, offer alternatives for patients with anthracycline- or taxane-resistant disease. However, the data on the use of these drugs as single agents or in combination regimens are limited, so additional clinical trials are warranted. The optimal duration of treatment in women with metastatic disease also remains to be determined.

PROGNOSIS

The natural history of breast cancer varies greatly among patients. Some patients have extremely aggressive disease that progresses rapidly; in others the disease follows a more indolent course. Because of these variations, the ability to predict which patients will experience a better prognosis is extremely important. Table 96.7 lists some of the prognostic factors determined in breast cancer patients to date. The most commonly assessed prognostic factors include nodal status, tumor size, hormone receptor status, histologic grade, and cell proliferation indices. The remaining prognostic factors are still considered investigational until there are sufficient data to support their clinical utility.

The single most important prognostic factor at the time of diagnosis is the extent of axillary lymph node involvement. Numerous studies have confirmed the significance of nodal involvement for predicting disease recurrence and survival. The number of affected nodes is directly related to disease recurrence and indirectly related to survival. In patients with no nodal involvement at diagnosis, the 10-year survival rate is approximately 75%. As nodal involvement increases to one to three nodes and four to nine nodes, the 10-year survival rate decreases to 62% and 42%, respectively.[84] When 10 or more nodes are involved, the 10-year survival rate decreases dramatically to only 20%. The increased acceptance of sentinel node mapping with omission of axillary node dissection may diminish the importance of nodal status as a prognostic factor for the use of adjuvant therapy.

Tumor size at the time of diagnosis is also an important prognostic factor for breast cancer.[85] Although large tumors have a greater tendency to metastasize to axillary lymph

TABLE 96.7	Prognostic Factors in Breast Cancer	
Prognostic Factor	**Favorable**	**Unfavorable**
Nodal involvement	Absent	Present
Tumor size	Small	Large
Histologic grade	Well differentiated	Poorly differentiated
Estrogen receptor	Positive	Negative
Progesterone receptor	Positive	Negative
S-phase fraction	Low	High
Mitotic index	Low	High
Ploidy	Diploid	Aneuploid
Thymidine labeling index	Low	High
HER2/neu (c-erbB-2)	Absent	Present
p53	Absent	Present
Cyclin E	Low	High
UPA/PAI-1	Low	High
Stat 5	Activated	Inactive
Isolated bone marrow disease	Absent	Present

nodes, tumor size is also an independent predictor for breast cancer recurrence. Patients with well-differentiated tumors also have a better prognosis than patients with poorly differentiated tumors, making histologic grade an important prognostic factor as well.

Another important prognostic factor is ER and PgR status. Women with ER/PgR-positive tumors have a better prognosis than women with ER/PgR-negative or ER-positive/PgR-negative tumors.[86] Furthermore, PgR status significantly improves the accuracy of predicting responsiveness to hormonal therapy, with patients with ER/PgR-positive tumors experiencing the greatest benefit and patients with ER-positive/PgR-negative tumors experiencing less benefit from adjuvant hormonal therapy. As a result, patients with ER-positive/PgR-negative tumors should probably receive adjuvant chemotherapy followed by hormonal therapy. Preliminary data also suggest that HER2 and AIB1 (an estrogen receptor coactivator) overexpression may also predict responsiveness to hormonal therapy.[77,87]

The rate of tumor cell proliferation has also shown prognostic significance in breast cancer recurrence. The rate of cell proliferation can be determined using either the tritiated thymidine labeling index or DNA flow cytometry, which determines the percentage of tumor cells actively dividing in the S phase of the cell cycle. Both techniques indicate that patients with rapidly proliferating tumors (high S-phase fraction, high mitotic index) have a decreased disease-free survival compared with patients with slowly proliferating tumors.[88,89] In addition, flow cytometry can detect the presence of abnormal DNA content, or aneuploidy, in breast

cancer cells. Patients with aneuploid tumors also appear to have a decreased disease-free survival.[89]

Tumor concentrations of breast cancer growth factors and their receptors have also been measured to determine prognostic significance. Increased levels of the HER2/neu (c-erbB-2) oncogene, a protein that promotes tumor cell development, have been correlated with decreased disease-free and overall survival in patients with node-positive disease.[77] Expression of the tumor suppressor gene p53 may also predict prognosis. Patients with node-negative breast cancer who express p53 appear to have a decreased disease-free and overall survival rate compared with patients who do not express the p53 gene.[84] High levels of cyclin E, a regulator of the cell cycle, has been correlated with decreased survival in patients with breast cancer.[90] High levels of urokinase-type plasminogen activator (uPA) and its inhibitor (PAI-1), two critical components of tumor invasion and metastasis, have also been correlated with decreased relapse-free and overall survival.[91] More recently, activation of Stat5 (signal transducer and activator of transcription-5), a breast epithelial differentiation factor, predicted a favorable prognosis in patients with node-negative breast cancer.[92]

Detection of isolated tumor cells in the bone marrow at the time of diagnosis has been shown to be a predictor for future systemic relapse and death from breast cancer.[93] Many researchers are also investigating the predictive value of gene expression profiling for prognosis and survival.[94,95] As a result, a test that measures genes from standard pathology blocks and estimates the risk of relapse for node-negative patients receiving tamoxifen is now commercially available. Preliminary data also suggest that gene expression profiling may be used clinically to predict response to specific chemotherapy regimens.[96]

Predicting disease recurrence in patients with breast cancer is a difficult task, especially in patients with negative nodes at diagnosis. The ability to determine prognostic factors for disease recurrence would be extremely useful clinically, because patients with a poor prognosis could be treated more aggressively initially in an attempt to prolong survival, and patients with a very low risk of recurrence could avoid unnecessary adjuvant systemic therapy. The ability to predict response to treatment would also be extremely useful clinically. The presence of hormone receptors on tumor cells predicts which patients are more likely to respond to hormonal therapy. The discovery of predictive factors for response to other treatment modalities would allow clinicians to tailor treatment regimens for individual patients based on predicted efficacy. Genomic profiling may be the tool that will lead to new clinically useful predictive and prognostic factors for patients diagnosed with breast cancer.

FUTURE THERAPIES

Although progress has been made in the treatment of breast cancer, further improvements in therapy are necessary. Current avenues of research include new methods of administration for commercially available drugs, the development of new drugs, and the search for synergistic drug combination using conventional and new therapeutic agents. It is hoped that new combination regimens will increase response rates and overall survival. The use of the newer therapies such as the aromatase inhibitors and trastuzumab in the adjuvant setting are being explored.

Multiple targeted therapies, or therapies directed against a critical molecular mechanism, are currently in development for the treatment of breast cancer.[97,98] It is hoped that these therapies can eventually be designed to be specific for tumor cell targets, rather than targets that are found on both tumor and normal cells, so that treatment-related toxicities can be minimized. The epidermal growth factor receptor has an established role as an oncogene in the development and progression of breast cancer. The development of monoclonal antibodies and small-molecule tyrosine kinase inhibitors that target the epidermal growth factor are being investigated as therapy for breast cancer. Several novel agents targeting the vascular endothelial growth factor (VEGF) and natural angiogenesis inhibitors are also in clinical development, because angiogenesis is known to play such an important role in tumor progression.

PREVENTION

Tamoxifen has been shown to decrease the risk of developing a second primary carcinoma in the contralateral breast in women diagnosed with breast cancer.[53] Data from the Breast Cancer Prevention Trial conducted by NSABP and the National Cancer Institute also supported this finding, which resulted in the FDA approval of tamoxifen for reducing the incidence of breast cancer in women at high risk for developing the disease.[99] Currently, four randomized chemoprevention trials with tamoxifen have been conducted and produce a pooled estimate of a 38% reduction in breast cancer incidence (specifically, ER-positive tumors).[100] Although the benefit of tamoxifen administration outweighs the risk of treatment in women at high risk for breast cancer, the increased risk of thromboembolic events and endometrial cancer associated with tamoxifen hinder its use in a broader patient population. Raloxifene is a SERM approved for the treatment of osteoporosis that has estrogenic effects on bone and lipids and antiestrogenic effects on the endometrium (in contrast to tamoxifen). A lower incidence of breast cancer was reported in postmenopausal women receiving raloxifene for prevention and treatment of osteoporosis [MORE trial (Multiple Outcomes of Raloxifene Evaluation)].[101] These data were recently updated and included data from the follow-up protocol for the MORE trial [CORE (Continuing Outcomes Relevant to Evista)], which allowed patients to continue raloxifene or placebo for a total of 8 years.[102] Compared to placebo, a 59% reduction in breast cancer incidence was reported for patients receiving raloxifene. Two addi-

tional trials, RUTH (Raloxifene Use for the Heart) and STAR (Study of Tamoxifen and Raloxifene), will also evaluate the breast cancer-preventive effects of raloxifene in over 29,000 additional postmenopausal women. The STAR trial will enroll 19,000 postmenopausal women at increased risk for breast cancer and will directly compare tamoxifen and raloxifene in this setting. Trials are also ongoing comparing anastrozole, a third-generation aromatase inhibitor, with tamoxifen or placebo as chemoprevention in postmenopausal women at high risk for breast cancer development. The long-term effects of anastrozole on bone health will be particularly important to evaluate because the trial is being conducted in the chemoprevention setting. Longer follow-up of the current studies and data obtained from additional studies may support chemoprevention in the general patient population in the future.

CONCLUSION

Advances in the areas of early detection, genetic testing, primary surgical treatment, radiation therapy, and chemotherapy or hormonal therapy for adjuvant and metastatic disease have occurred due to the willingness of both physicians and patients to participate in randomized, controlled clinical trials and the long-term analysis of these trial results. However, many unanswered questions remain regarding the etiology, detection, treatment, and prevention of breast cancer, so continued intensive research is warranted.

KEY POINTS

■ Noninvasive breast cancer (LCIS and DCIS) is generally easily controlled with surgery alone or surgery plus radiation

■ Early-stage breast cancer (stages I and II) is most often managed with breast-conserving surgery and radiation. Adjuvant hormonal therapy or chemotherapy is indicated and the treatment approach depends on nodal and ER status

■ Locally advanced breast cancer (stage III) is most effectively managed with combined-modality therapy. Pathologic complete response to preoperative chemotherapy correlates with disease-free and overall survival and may be used as a surrogate marker for prognosis when evaluating treatment regimens in this setting

■ The goals of treatment for metastatic breast cancer are to prolong survival and palliate symptoms. The choice of therapy depends on the site of disease involvement and patient characteristics. Although patients with metastatic breast cancer will most likely die of their disease, many patients can achieve durable responses to treatment that allow them to lead prolonged lives with good quality

■ Many new therapies, including targeted monoclonal antibodies and the taxanes, have helped prolong survival in patients with metastatic disease and may also be beneficial in the treatment of earlier-stage disease

SUGGESTED READINGS

Wood WC, Muss HB, Solin LJ, et al. Malignant tumors of the breast. In: DeVita VT, Hellman S, Rosenberg SA, ed. Cancer principles & practice of oncology, 7th ed. Philadelphia: Lippincott Williams & Wilkins, 2005:1415–1477.

www.nci.nih.gov/cancertopics/pdq/treatment/breast/healthprofessional

REFERENCES

1. Jemal A, Tiwari RC, Murray T, et al. Cancer statistics, 2004. CA Cancer J Clin 54:8–29, 2004.
2. Hutchins L, Broadwater R Jr, Lang NP, et al. Breast cancer. Dis Mon 36:63–125, 1990.
3. Abeloff MD, Lichter AS, Niederhuber JE, et al. Breast. In: Abeloff MD, Armitage JO, Lichter AS, et al., eds. Clinical oncology. New York: Churchill Livingstone, 1995:1617–1714.
4. Anderson DE. A genetic study of human breast cancer. J Natl Cancer Inst 48:1029–1034, 1972.
5. Mincey BA. Genetics and the management of women at high risk for breast cancer. The Oncologist 8:466–473, 2003.
6. Brose MS, Rebbeck TR, Calzone KA, et al. Cancer risk estimates for BRCA1 mutation carriers identified in a risk evaluation program. J Natl Cancer Inst 94:1365–1372, 2002.
7. Rebbeck TR, Friebel T, Lynch HT, et al. Bilateral prophylactic mastectomy reduces breast cancer risk in BRCA1 and BRCA2 mutation carriers: the PROSE study group. J Clin Oncol 22:1055–1062, 2004.
8. Metcalfe K, Lynch HT, Ghadirian P, et al. Contralateral breast cancer in BRCA1 and BRCA2 mutation carriers. J Clin Oncol 22:2328–2335, 2004.
9. Henderson DE. Endogenous and exogenous endocrine factors. Hematol Oncol Clin North Am 3:577–598, 1989.
10. Jawed Iqbal M, Taylor W. Hormonal and reproductive factors: new evidence. In: Stoll BA, ed. Women at high risk to breast cancer. Dordrecht: Kluwer Academic, 1989:41–46.
11. Collaborative Group on Hormonal Factors in Breast Cancer. Breast cancer and hormonal contraceptives: collaborative reanalysis of individual data on 53,297 women with breast cancer and 100,239 women without breast cancer from 54 epidemiological studies. Lancet 347:1713–1727, 1996.
12. Marchbanks PA, McDonald JA, Wilson HG, et al. Oral contraceptives and the risk of breast cancer. N Engl J Med 346:2025–2032, 2002.
13. Collaborative Group on Hormonal Factors in Breast Cancer. Breast cancer and hormone replacement therapy: collaborative reanalysis of data from 51 epidemiological studies of 52,705 women with breast cancer and 108,411 women without breast cancer. Lancet 350:1047–1059, 1997.
14. Schairer C, Lubin J, Troisi R, et al. Menopausal estrogen and estrogen–progestin replacement therapy and breast cancer risk. JAMA 283:485–491, 2000.
15. Million Women Study Collaborators. Breast cancer and hormone-replacement therapy in the Million Women Study. Lancet 362:419–427, 2003.
16. Writing Group for the Women's Health Initiative investigators. Risks and benefits of estrogen plus progestin in healthy postmenopausal women. Principal results from the Women's Health Initiative randomized controlled trial. JAMA 288:321–333, 2002.
17. Cho E, Spiegelman D, Hunter DJ, et al. Premenopausal fat intake and risk of breast cancer. J Natl Cancer Inst 95:1079–1085, 2003.
18. Endogenous Hormones Breast Cancer Collaborative Group. Body mass index, serum sex hormones, and breast cancer risk in postmenopausal women. J Natl Cancer Inst 95:1218–1226, 2003.
19. McTiernan A. Behavioral risk factors in breast cancer: can risk be modified. The Oncologist 8:326–334, 2003.
20. Collaborative Group on Hormonal Factors in Breast Cancer. Alcohol, tobacco, and breast cancer: collaborative reanalysis of individual data from 53 epidemiological studies including 58,515 women with breast cancer and 95,067 women without the disease. Br J Cancer 87:1234–1245, 2002.
21. Reichman ME, Judd JT, Longcope C, et al. Effects of alcohol consumption on plasma and urinary hormone concentrations in premenopausal women. J Natl Cancer Inst 85:722–727, 1993.
22. Dorgan JF, Baer DJ, Albert PS, et al. Serum hormones and the alcohol–breast cancer association in postmenopausal women. J Natl Cancer Inst 93:710–715, 2001.
23. Reynolds P, Hurley S, Goldberg DE, et al. Active smoking, household passive smoking, and breast cancer: evidence from the California Teachers Study. J Natl Cancer Inst 96:29–37, 2004.
24. Goss PE, Sierra S. Current perspectives on radiation-induced breast cancer. J Clin Oncol 16:338–347, 1998.
25. Pike MC, Krailo MD, Henderson DE, et al. Hormonal risk factors, breast tissue age and age-incidence of breast cancer. Nature 303:676–770, 1983.
26. Osborne CK, Arteaga CL. Autocrine and paracrine growth regulation of breast cancer: clinical implications. Breast Cancer Res Treat 15:3–11, 1990.
27. Smith RA, Saslow D, Sawyer KA, et al. American Cancer Society guidelines for breast cancer screening: update 2003. CA Cancer J Clin 54:141–169, 2003.
28. Humphrey LL, Helfand M, Chan BKS, et al. Breast cancer screening: a summary of the evidence for the U.S. Preventive Services Task Force. Ann Intern Med 137:347–360, 2002.
29. Singletary SE, Allred C, Ashley P, et al. Revision of the American Joint Committee on Cancer staging system for breast cancer. J Clin Oncol 20:3628–3636, 2002.
30. Woodward WA, Strom EA, Tucker SL, et al. Changes in the 2003 American Joint Committee Cancer staging for breast cancer dramatically affect stage-specific survival. J Clin Oncol 21:3244–3248, 2003.
31. Morrow M, Strom EA, Bassett LW, et al. Standard for the management of ductal carcinoma in situ of the breast (DCIS). CA Cancer J Clin 52:256–276, 2002.
32. Fisher B, Dignam J, Wolmark N, et al. Lumpectomy and radiation therapy for the treatment of intraductal breast cancer: findings from National Surgical Adjuvant Breast and Bowel Project B-17. J Clin Oncol 16:441–452, 1998.
33. Fisher B, Dignam J, Wolmark N, et al. Tamoxifen in the treatment of intraductal breast cancer: National Surgical Adjuvant Breast and Bowel Project B-24 randomized controlled trial. Lancet 353:1993–2000, 1999.
34. Morrow M, Strom EA, Bassett LW, et al. Standard for breast conservation therapy in the management of invasive breast carcinoma. CA Cancer J Clin 52:277–300, 2002.
35. Early Breast Cancer Trialists' Collaborative Group. Effects of radiotherapy and surgery in early breast cancer. An overview of the randomized trials. N Engl J Med 333:1444–1455, 1995.
36. Holmberg SB, Crivellari D, Zahrieh D, et al. A randomized trial comparing axillary clearance versus no axillary clearance in older patients (≥60 years) with breast cancer: first results of International Breast Cancer Study Group Trial 10-93. Proc Am Soc Clin Oncol 22:4 (Suppl;abstr 505), 2004.
37. Veronesi U, Paganelli G, Viale G, et al. A randomized comparison of sentinel-node biopsy with routine axillary dissection in breast cancer. N Engl J Med 349:546–553, 2003.
38. Mansel RE, Goyal A, Fallowfield L, et al. Sentinel node biopsy in breast cancer: the first results of the randomized multicenter ALMANAC trial. Proc Am Soc Clin Oncol 22:4 (Suppl;abstr 506), 2004.
39. Early Breast Cancer Trialists' Collaborative Group. Polychemotherapy for early breast cancer: an overview of the randomised trials. Lancet 352:930–942, 1998.
40. Lindley C, Vasa S, Sawyer WT, et al. Quality of life and preferences for treatment following adjuvant therapy for early-stage breast cancer. J Clin Oncol 16:1380–1387, 1998.
41. Ravdin PM, Siminoff LA, Harvey JA. Survey of breast cancer patients concerning their knowledge and expectations of adjuvant therapy. J Clin Oncol 16:515–521, 1998.

42. Adjuvant therapy for breast cancer. NIH Consensus Statement 2000, Nov. 1–3; 17:1–35.

43. Wood WC, Budman DR, Korzun AH, et al. Dose and dose intensity of adjuvant chemotherapy for stage II, node-positive breast carcinoma. N Engl J Med 330:1253–1259, 1994.

44. Fisher B, Brown AM, Dimitrov NV, et al. Two months of doxorubicin–cyclophosphamide with and without interval reduction therapy compared with 6 months of cyclophosphamide, methotrexate, and fluorouracil in positive-node breast cancer patients with tamoxifen-nonresponsive tumors: results from National Surgical Adjuvant Breast and Bowel Project B-15. J Clin Oncol 8:1483–1496, 1990.

45. Fisher B, Anderson S, Tan-Chiu, et al. Tamoxifen and chemotherapy for axillary node-negative, estrogen receptor-negative breast cancer: findings from National Surgical Adjuvant Breast and Bowel Project B-23. J Clin Oncol 19:931–942, 2001.

46. Henderson IC, Berry DA, Demetri GD, et al. Improved outcomes from adding sequential paclitaxel but not from escalating doxorubicin dose in an adjuvant chemotherapy regimen for patients with node-positive primary breast cancer. J Clin Oncol 21:976–983, 2003.

47. Crown J, O'Leary M, Ooi WS. Docetaxel and paclitaxel in the treatment of breast cancer: a review of clinical experience. The Oncologist 9 (Suppl 2):24–32, 2004.

48. Mamounas EP, Bryant J, Lembersky BC, et al. Paclitaxel (T) following doxorubicin/cyclophosphamide (AC) as adjuvant chemotherapy for node-positive breast cancer: results from NSABP B-28. Proc Am Soc Clin Oncol 22:4 (abstr 12), 2003.

49. Martin M, Dienkowski T, Mackey T, et al. TAC improves disease free survival and overall survival over FAC in node positive early breast cancer patients BCIRG001: 55 months follow-up. 26th Annual Meeting of the San Antonio Breast Cancer Symposium; Dec. 5, 2003, San Antonio, TX (abstr 43).

50. Hortobagyi GN. What is the role of high-dose chemotherapy in the era of targeted therapies? J Clin Oncol 22:2263–2266, 2004.

51. Citron ML, Berry DA, Cirrincione C, et al. Randomized trial of dose-dense versus conventionally scheduled and sequential versus concurrent combination chemotherapy as postoperative adjuvant treatment of node-positive primary breast cancer: first report of Intergroup Trial C9741/Cancer and Leukemia Group B Trial 9741. J Clin Oncol 21:1431–1439, 2003.

52. Albain KS, Green SJ, Ravdin PM, et al. Adjuvant chemohormonal therapy for primary breast cancer should be sequential instead of concurrent: initial results from Intergroup Trial 0100 (SWOG-8814). Proc Am Soc Clin Oncol 21:37a (abstr 143), 2002.

53. Early Breast Cancer Trialists' Collaborative Group. Tamoxifen for early breast cancer: an overview of the randomized trials. Lancet 351:1451–1467, 1998.

54. Fisher B, Dignam J, Bryant J, et al. Five versus more than five years of tamoxifen for lymph node negative breast cancer: updated findings from the National Surgical Adjuvant Breast and Bowel Project B-14 randomized trial. J Natl Cancer Inst 93:684–690, 2001.

55. The ATAC (Arimidex, Tamoxifen Alone or in Combination) Trialists' Group. Anastrozole alone or in combination with tamoxifen versus tamoxifen alone for adjuvant treatment of postmenopausal women with early breast cancer: first results of the ATAC randomised trial. Lancet 359:2131–2139, 2002.

56. Coombes RC, Hall E, Gibson LJ, et al. A randomized trial of exemestane after two to three years of tamoxifen therapy in postmenopausal women with primary breast cancer. N Engl J Med 350:1081–1092, 2004.

57. Goss PE, Ingle JN, Martino S, et al. A randomized trial of letrozole in postmenopausal women after five years of tamoxifen therapy for early-stage breast cancer. N Engl J Med 349:1793–1802, 2003.

58. Goss PE, Ingle JN, Martino S, et al. Updated analysis of the NCIC CTG MA.17 randomized placebo (P) controlled trial of letrozole (L) after five years of tamoxifen in postmenopausal women with early stage breast cancer. Proc Am Soc Clin Oncol 22:88 (Suppl; abstr 847), 2004.

59. Jakesz R, Hausmaninger H, Kubista E, et al. Randomized adjuvant trial of tamoxifen and goserelin versus cyclophosphamide, methotrexate, and fluorouracil: evidence for the superiority of treatment with endocrine blockade in premenopausal patients with hormone-responsive breast cancer-Austrian Breast and Colorectal Cancer Study Group Trial 5. J Clin Oncol 20:4621–4627, 2002.

60. Kaufmann M, Jonat W, Blamey R, et al. Survival analysis from the ZEBRA study. Goserelin (Zoladex) versus CMF in premenopausal women with node-positive breast cancer. Eur J Cancer 39:1711–1717, 2003.

61. Davidson NE, O'Neill A, Yukov A, et al. Chemohormonal therapy in premenopausal node-positive. receptor-positive breast cancer: an Eastern Cooperative Oncology Group phase III intergroup trial (E5188, INT-0101). Proc Am Soc Clin Oncol 22:5 (abstr 15), 2003.

62. International Breast Cancer Study Group. Adjuvant chemotherapy followed by goserelin versus either modality alone for premenopausal lymph node-negative breast cancer: a randomized trial. J Natl Cancer Inst 95:1833–1846, 2003.

63. Smith TJ, Davidson NE, Schapira DV, et al. American Society of Clinical Oncology 1998 Update of Recommended Breast Cancer Surveillance Guidelines. J Clin Oncol 17:1080–1082, 1999.

64. Wolmark N, Wang J, Mamounas E, et al. Preoperative chemotherapy in patients with operable breast cancer: nine-year results from National Surgical Adjuvant Breast and Bowel Project B-18. J Natl Cancer Inst Monogr 30:96–102, 2001.

65. Kaufmann M, von Minckwitz G, Smith R, et al. International expert panel on the use of primary (preoperative) systemic treatment of operable breast cancer: review and recommendations. J Clin Oncol 21:2600–2608, 2003.

66. Cristofanilli M, Buzdar AU, Hortobagyi GN. Update on the management of inflammatory breast cancer. The Oncologist 8:141–148, 2003.

67. Bear HD, Anderson S, Brown A, et al. The effect on tumor response of adding sequential preoperative docetaxel to preoperative doxorubicin and cyclophosphamide: preliminary results from National Surgical Adjuvant Breast and Bowel Project Protocol B-27. J Clin Oncol 21:4165–4174, 2003.

68. Hutcheon AW, Heys SD, Sarkar TK, et al. Docetaxel primary chemotherapy in breast cancer: a five-year update of the Aberdeen trial. Breast Cancer Res Treat 82 (Suppl 1):S9 (abstr 11), 2003.

69. Campos SM. Aromatase inhibitors for breast cancer in postmenopausal women. The Oncologist 9:126–136, 2004.

70. Buzdar AU. Advances in endocrine treatments for postmenopausal women with metastatic and early breast cancer. The Oncologist 8:335–341, 2003.

71. Buzdar AU. Current status of endocrine treatment of carcinoma of the breast. Semin Surg Oncol 6:77–82, 1990.

72. Jones S, Erban J, Overmoyer B, et al. Randomized trial comparing docetaxel and paclitaxel in patients with metastatic breast cancer. Breast Cancer Res Treat 82 (Suppl 1):S9 (abstr 10), 2003.

73. Winer EP, Berry DA, Woolf S, et al. Failure of higher-dose paclitaxel to improve outcome in patients with metastatic breast cancer: Cancer and Leukemia Group B trial 9342. J Clin Oncol 22:2061–2068, 2004.

74. Seidman AD, Berry D, Cirrincione C, et al. CALGB 9840: phase III study of weekly paclitaxel via 1-hour infusion versus standard 3-hour infusion every third week in the treatment of metastatic breast cancer (MBC), with trastuzumab (T) for HER2 positive MBC and randomized for T in HER2 normal MBC. Proc Am Soc Clin Oncol 22:6 (Suppl;abstr 512), 2004.

75. O'Shaughnessy J, Miles D, Vukelja S, et al. Superior survival with capecitabine plus docetaxel combination therapy in anthracycline-pretreated patients with advanced breast cancer: phase III trial results. J Clin Oncol 20:2812–2823, 2002.

76. Albain KS, Nag S, Calderillo-Ruiz G, et al. Global phase III study of gemcitabine plus paclitaxel vs. paclitaxel as frontline therapy for metastatic breast cancer: first report of overall survival. Proc Am Soc Clin Oncol 22:5 (Suppl;abstr 510), 2004.

77. Ross JS, Fletcher JA, Linette GP, et al. The HER-2/neu gene and protein in breast cancer 2003: biomarker and target of therapy. The Oncologist 8:307–325, 2003.

78. Seidman A, Hudis C, Pierri MK, et al. Cardiac dysfunction in the trastuzumab clinical trials experience. J Clin Oncol 20:1215–1221, 2002.

79. Leyland-Jones B, Gelman K, Ayoub JP, et al. Pharmacokinetics, safety, and efficacy of trastuzumab administered every three weeks in combination with paclitaxel. J Clin Oncol 21:3965–3971, 2003.

80. Extra JM, Cognetti F, Chan S, et al. First-line trastuzumab (Herceptin) plus docetaxel versus docetaxel alone in women with HER-2 positive metastatic breast cancer (MBC): results from a randomized phase II trial (M77011). Breast Cancer Res Treat 82 (Suppl 1):S47 (abstr 217), 2003.

81. Robert NJ, Leyland-Jones B, Asmar LJ, et al. Randomized phase III study of trastuzumab, paclitaxel, and carboplatin versus trastuzumab and paclitaxel in women with HER-2 overexpressing metastatic breast cancer: an update including survival. Proc Am Soc Clin Oncol 22:20 (Suppl;abstr 573), 2004.

82. Perez EA, Rowland KM, Suman VJ, et al. N98-32-52: efficacy and tolerability of two schedules of paclitaxel, carboplatin, and trastuzumab in women with HER2 positive metastatic breast cancer: a North Central Cancer Treatment Group randomized phase II trial. Breast Cancer Res Treat 82 (Suppl 1):S47 (abstr 216), 2003.

83. Hillner BE, Ingle JN, Chlebowski RT, et al. American Society of Clinical Oncology 2003 update of the role of bisphosphonates and bone health issues in women with breast cancer. J Clin Oncol 21: 4042–4057, 2003.

84. Fisher BR, Anderson S, Redmond C, et al. Pathologic findings from the National Surgical Adjuvant Breast Project Protocol B-06: 10-year pathologic and clinical prognostic discriminants. Cancer 71:2507–2514, 1993.

85. Carter Cl, Allen C, Henson DE. Relation of tumor size, lymph node status, and survival in 24,740 breast cancer cases. Cancer 63: 181–187, 1989.

86. Bardou VJ, Arpino G, Elledge R, et al. Progesterone receptor status significantly improves outcome prediction over estrogen receptor status alone for adjuvant endocrine therapy in two large breast cancer databases. J Clin Oncol 21:1973–1979, 2003.

87. Osborne CK, Bardou V, Hopp TA, et al. Role of the estrogen receptor coactivator AIB1 (SRC-3) and HER-2/neu in tamoxifen resistance in breast cancer. J Natl Cancer Inst 95:353–361, 2003.

88. Silvestrini R, Daidone MG, Valagussa P, et al. 3H-thymidine labeling index as a prognostic indicator in node-positive breast cancer. J Clin Oncol 8:1321–1326, 1990.

89. Clark GM, Dressler LG, Owens MA. Prediction of relapse or survival in patients with node-negative breast cancer by DNA flow cytometry. N Engl J Med 320:627–633, 1989.

90. Keyomarsi K, Tucker SL, Buchholz TA, et al. Cyclin E and survival in patients with breast cancer. N Engl J Med 347:1566–1575, 2002.

91. Look MP, van Putten WLJ, Duffy MJ, et al. Pooled analysis of prognostic impact of urokinase-type plasminogen activator and its inhibitor PAI-1 in 8377 breast cancer patients. J Natl Cancer Inst 94:116–128, 2002.

92. Nevalainen MT, Xie J, Torhorst J, et al. Signal transducer and activator of transcription-5 activation and breast cancer prognosis. J Clin Oncol 22:2053–2060, 2004.

93. Wiedswang G, Borgen E, Karesen R, et al. Detection of isolated tumor cells in bone marrow is an independent prognostic factor in breast cancer. J Clin Oncol 21:3469–3478, 2003.

94. Van de Vijver MJ, He YD, van't Veer LJ, et al. A gene expression signature as a predictor of survival in breast cancer. N Engl J Med 347:1999–2009, 2002.

95. Paik S, Shak S, Tang G, et al. Multi-gene RT-PCR assay for predicting recurrence in node negative breast cancer patients: NSABP studies B-20 and B-14. Breast Cancer Res Treat 82 (Suppl 1):S10 (abstr 16), 2003.

96. Ayers M, Symmans WF, Stec J, et al. Gene expression profiles predict complete pathologic response to neoadjuvant paclitaxel and fluorouracil, doxorubicin, and cyclophosphamide chemotherapy in breast cancer. J Clin Oncol 22:2284–2293, 2004.

97. Schneider BP, Houck WA, Sledge G. Targeted therapy in breast cancer. Disease of the Breast Updates 6:1–16, 2003.

98. Nahta R, Hortobagyi GN, Esteva FJ. Growth factor receptors in breast cancer: potential for therapeutic intervention. The Oncologist 8:5–17, 2003.

99. Fisher B, Costantino JP, Wickerham DL, et al. Tamoxifen for prevention of breast cancer: report of the National Surgical Adjuvant Breast and Bowel Project P-1 Study. J Natl Cancer Inst 90: 1371–1388, 1998.

100. Martino S, Costantino J, McNabb M, et al. The role of selective estrogen receptor modulators in the prevention of breast cancer: comparison of the clinical trials. The Oncologist 9:116–125, 2004.

101. Cauley JA, Norton L, Lippman ME, et al. Continued breast cancer risk reduction in postmenopausal women treated with raloxifene: 4-year results from the MORE trial. Multiple Outcomes of Raloxifene Evaluation. Breast Cancer Res Treat 65:125–134, 2001.

102. Martino S, Cauley JA, Barrett-Connor E, et al. Incidence of invasive breast cancer following 8 years of raloxifene therapy in postmenopausal women with osteoporosis: results from the Continuing Outcomes Relevant to Evista (CORE) trial. Proc Am Soc Clin Oncol 22:97 (Suppl;abstr 1000), 2004.

Liver Tumors

97

Robert J. Stagg

OVERVIEW

Liver tumors are classified as being either primary tumors, those arising from the hepatobiliary system, or secondary tumors, those metastasizing to the liver from a primary tumor of extrahepatic origin, and as being either benign or malignant. Liver tumors, as a group, are one of the most common malignancies in the world. In Europe and North America, metastatic adenocarcinomas are the most common liver tu-mors; in Southeast Asia and Africa, primary hepatocellular carcinoma (HCC) is the most prevalent hepatic malignancy. Primary and metastatic liver tumors account for approxi-mately 20% of cancer-related deaths in the United States. Because of the liver's vital physiologic role, hepatic tumors often govern patient survival, even in the presence of extra-hepatic tumor. Primary and metastatic liver tumors will be discussed separately because of their distinct biologic and clinical features.

ANATOMY AND PHYSIOLOGY OF THE LIVER

The liver is a wedge-shaped organ that is suspended from the diaphragm and lies in the right upper quadrant of the abdomen (Fig. 97.1). The liver consists of three lobes: the right lobe, which is the largest; the left lobe; and the caudate lobe, which is the smallest lobe and is located on the dorsal aspect of the liver. The right lobe is subdivided into the anterior and posterior segments, and the left lobe is subdivided into the medial and lateral segments.

The liver has a dual blood supply, coming from both the portal vein and the hepatic artery. Normal hepatic parenchyma receives the majority of its blood supply from the portal vein, whereas hepatic tumors receive the majority of their blood supply from the hepatic artery.[1] Several of the modalities used to treat hepatic tumors exploit this unique finding. The blood from both the portal vein and the hepatic artery is drained from the liver by the hepatic vein, which returns it to the inferior vena cava, immediately below the right atrium. The vena cava lies in a groove on the dorsal aspect of the liver. Each segment of the liver has its own biliary system; these systems join intrahepatically to form the right and left hepatic ducts and then unite as they exit the liver to form the common bile duct. The hepatic artery and portal vein enter and the bile duct exits the liver at the hilum in a region known as the porta hepatis.

The liver performs a number of critical physiologic functions, including producing and excreting bile (including bilirubin), synthesizing proteins (including albumin, gamma globulins, and several clotting factors), and metabolizing food, drugs, and toxins. Hepatic tumors may interfere with these physiologic functions. When a healthy liver is damaged by surgical resection, disease, or a toxic insult, it is capable of regenerating to its original size. However, an impaired liver, such as a cirrhotic liver, may not be able to regenerate after such an insult. Liver regeneration occurs through hypertrophy of the remaining liver parenchyma and appears to be regulated by a variety of growth factors, including epidermal growth factor (EGF), hepatocyte growth factor (HGF), transforming growth factor α and β (TGF-α and TGF-β), fibroblast growth factor (FGF), interleukin 1-α (IL-1), interleukin-6 (IL-6), cardiotrophin-1, hepatic stimulation factor, and hepatopoietin-B. The precise interactive role of each of these growth factors in initiating and subsequently terminating liver regeneration has not been fully elucidated. The liver's ability to regenerate enables it to tolerate several of the treatment modalities that are commonly used to treat liver tumors, such as surgical resection, radiofrequency ablation, and chemoembolization. Patients with cirrhosis of the liver may not tolerate these therapies as well.

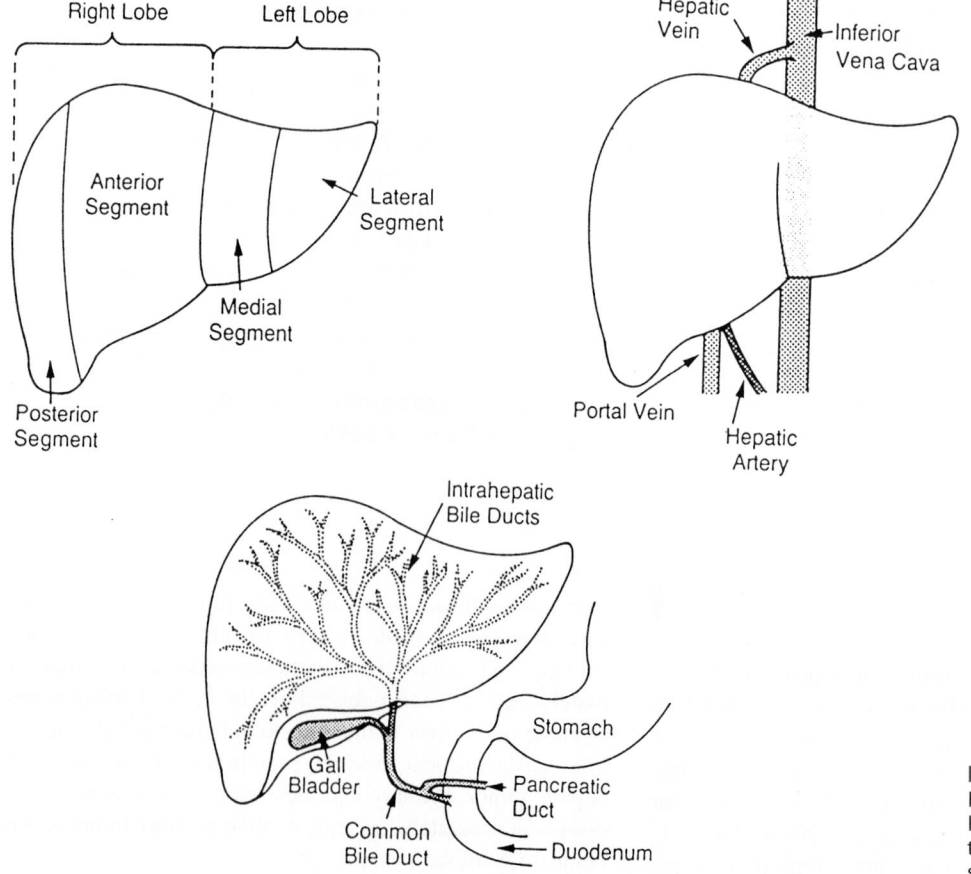

FIGURE 97.1 Schematic of the liver. *Left:* right and left hepatic lobes. *Center:* hepatobiliary system. *Right:* hepatic blood supply.

Table 97.1 lists the various types of benign and malignant primary liver tumors.

BENIGN PRIMARY LIVER TUMORS

Benign tumors of the liver include cavernous hemangioma, infantile hemangioendothelioma, hepatic cell adenoma, and focal nodular hyperplasia. Of these, cavernous hemangioma is the most prevalent, occurring in up to 7% of the population.

CAVERNOUS HEMANGIOMA

Cavernous hemangioma is a hypervascular tumor that most commonly occurs in women in the fourth, fifth, or sixth decade of life. It increases in size during pregnancy or estrogen administration. Hemangiomas are usually asymptomatic and are most often discovered incidentally at autopsy. Occasionally, patients develop symptoms, including right upper quadrant pain, fever, early satiety, or vomiting. While the exact indication for treatment remains unclear, typically only severely symptomatic patients and those with large lesions who are at risk for intraperitoneal hemorrhage should be treated. For such patients, surgical resection is the treatment of choice.[2] Additional therapeutic modalities that have been used include steroids, radiation, hepatic arterial ligation, embolization, and radiofrequency ablation.[3]

INFANTILE HEMANGIOENDOTHELIOMA

Infantile hemangioendothelioma is a benign tumor of vasculoendothelial origin that occurs in the first 6 months of life.

TABLE 97.1	Primary Liver Tumors	
Benign	**Malignant**
Infantile hemangioendothelioma	Hepatocellular carcinoma
Cavernous hemangioma	Hepatoblastoma
Hepatic cell adenoma	Intrahepatic cholangiocarcinoma
Focal nodular hyperplasia	Angiosarcoma
	Epithelioid hemangioendothelioma
	Undifferentiated sarcoma

Because of the vascular nature of this tumor, a bruit can sometimes be heard over the liver. Approximately half of the patients also present with a 2- to 15-mm, red to blue black papular hemangioma involving the skin. In addition, patients may have hepatomegaly, congestive heart failure secondary to arteriovenous shunting, thrombocytopenia, or microangiopathic hemolytic anemia, and up to one third of patients have hemolytic jaundice.[4] Asymptomatic patients can be followed without treatment because spontaneous regression of the tumor may occur within 1 year. However, patients with symptomatic congestive heart failure should be managed medically with diuretics and inotropic agents. If medical management is unsuccessful, symptoms may be controlled with steroids, vincristine, radiotherapy, hepatic arterial ligation, or embolization.[5] Surgical resection or more rarely liver transplantation may also be used in patients with intractable cardiac failure or refractory consumptive coagulopathy.[6]

HEPATIC CELL ADENOMA

Hepatic cell adenoma occurs primarily in young women of childbearing age and usually manifests as a large solitary mass in the liver. Oral contraceptives, anabolic steroids, and type 1 glycogen storage disease have been implicated in the etiology of hepatic adenoma.[7] It is not known whether the development of hepatic cell adenoma in women taking oral contraceptives is due to the estrogen or progesterone component and whether the reduction in the estrogen content of many oral contraceptives will decrease the incidence of this tumor. Complete spontaneous regression, as well as progression, has been noted in women after discontinuation of oral contraceptive use. Rare cases of malignant transformation of hepatic cell adenoma to HCC have been reported.[8] Surgical resection of a persistent hepatic cell adenoma is the standard treatment because of its propensity to rupture and the possibility of malignant transformation. Radiation and chemotherapy do not play a role in the management of this disease. Oral contraceptives and anabolic steroids should be strictly avoided in all patients with a history of hepatic cell adenoma.

FOCAL NODULAR HYPERPLASIA

Focal nodular hyperplasia is a hypervascular tumor that occurs most often in females and presents as an asymptomatic hepatic mass. It can occur at any age, including childhood. The etiology is largely unknown, but oral contraceptives have been reported to be a possible cause.[9] Patients often have coexisting congenital heart disease or other tumors, including cavernous hemangiomas, glioblastomas, astrocytomas, pheochromocytomas, and multiple endocrine neoplasias.[9] Treatment is generally not indicated because this tumor is rarely symptomatic and is not premalignant, but surgical resection has been successful in symptomatic patients.[10] The long-term prognosis of this tumor is excellent.

MALIGNANT PRIMARY LIVER TUMORS

HCC is the most prevalent malignant tumor of the liver and will be the major focus of this section. Other primary malignant tumors are rare but warrant mention.

HEPATOBLASTOMA

Hepatoblastoma is the most common primary malignant liver tumor in young children, affecting approximately 1 child per 100,000. It is typically diagnosed before age 5 but has also rarely been diagnosed in adults. It may be familial and occurs twice as frequently in males than in females. The exact etiology is unknown, but recent data suggest that genetic alterations, including the hypermethylation of the p16 gene resulting in the lack of p16 expression, might play an important role in the tumorigenesis of hepatoblastoma.[11] It may occur in conjunction with congenital anomalies such as tetralogy of Fallot, persistent ductus arteriosus, or extrahepatic biliary atresia. Hepatoblastoma usually presents as a solitary mass that may be encapsulated. The most common presenting symptom is abdominal swelling. Serum α-fetoprotein (AFP) levels are elevated in most cases.

If untreated, hepatoblastoma is uniformly fatal. Approximately 30% to 50% of patients with hepatoblastoma are cured by surgical resection, which is the treatment of choice whenever feasible. Preoperative chemotherapy, chemoembolization, or radiation may reduce tumor bulk, allowing removal of an originally unresectable tumor.[12] Postoperative adjuvant chemotherapy has also been administered to patients with hepatoblastoma, but its utility remains unclear.[13] Encouraging results have also been obtained with neoadjuvant chemotherapy followed by liver transplantation, although further study is needed to determine its role.[14] Chemoembolization has also produced promising results in small numbers of patients.[15] Systemic chemotherapy, typically with a cisplatin-, carboplatin-, or doxorubicin-based regimen, can be used in patients with an unresectable hepatic tumor or extrahepatic disease, but it is generally not curative. Irinotecan may also be useful in the treatment of patients who have hepatoblastoma that has relapsed multiple times.[16]

INTRAHEPATIC CHOLANGIOCARCINOMA

Intrahepatic cholangiocarcinoma, a tumor arising from the intrahepatic bile ducts, is the second most common malignant primary tumor of the liver. Occasionally, tumors contain a mixture of cholangiocarcinoma and HCC. Intrahepatic cholangiocarcinoma may arise from a peripheral bile duct or a major intrahepatic duct and has a low tendency to metastasize. Cholangiocarcinomas arising from the intrahepatic bile ducts in the hilum of the liver are known as Klatskin tumors. Patients with Crohn's disease, sclerosing cholangitis, biliary atresia, ulcerative colitis, and hepatolithiasis are at increased risk for developing cholangiocarcinoma.

The median survival of untreated patients is approximately 6.5 months, although patients who have small peripheral tumors may survive much longer. Surgical resection is occasionally curative and should be performed whenever possible.[17] Liver transplant has also been used to treat perihilar cholangiocarcinoma. Heimbach et al reported on 28 patients who underwent neoadjuvant chemoradiotherapy followed by liver transplantation.[18] Patient survival was 82% at 5 years. Patients with intrahepatic cholangiocarcinoma have a poor outcome following liver transplant, and it should be considered a contraindication for this procedure. Systemic chemotherapy is given to patients with unresectable or metastatic disease. A partial response rate of 31% was reported with intravenous 5-fluorouracil (5-FU), mitomycin, and doxorubicin in combination.[19] Responses have also been observed with intraarterial chemotherapy.[20]

ANGIOSARCOMA

Angiosarcoma, though uncommon, is the most frequently occurring sarcoma of the liver. It grows rapidly and is often accompanied by thrombocytopenia. Approximately 40% of cases are associated with exposure to a carcinogen, specifically thorium oxide (Thorotrast), vinyl chloride, arsenic, or radium.[21] There can be a latency period of up to 40 years from the carcinogen exposure to the development of the angiosarcoma.[22] It is a rapidly progressive tumor that often metastasizes to the lungs, porta hepatis, lymph nodes, or spleen. Angiosarcomas occasionally rupture, leading to intraabdominal bleeding. Resection offers the only potential for cure and is the treatment of choice whenever feasible. Radiation or chemotherapy, frequently consisting of doxorubicin and ifosfamide, may produce partial responses in unresectable lesions, although experience with these modalities is limited. Patients with unresectable angiosarcoma usually survive less than 1 year.

EPITHELIOID HEMANGIOENDOTHELIOMA

Epithelioid hemangioendothelioma is a rare vascular tumor of the liver.[23] It occurs primarily in middle age and more frequently in women than in men. In some patients, the development of epithelioid hemangioendothelioma appears to be causally related to the use of oral contraceptives. Epithelioid hemangioendothelioma causes hepatic fibrosis and frequently infiltrates the hepatic and portal veins. Patients typically present with an enlarged painful liver, high blood pressure, impaired liver function, ascites, and jaundice. The prognosis and clinical course of this malignancy are highly variable. Various treatments have been used, including liver transplantation, partial hepatectomy, chemotherapy, and radiation. It can be very slow-growing, with 25% of patients with an unresectable tumor surviving longer than 5 years from diagnosis.

HEPATOCELLULAR CARCINOMA

TREATMENT GOALS: HEPATOCELLULAR CARCINOMA

- Patients with HCC confined to the liver who are deemed to be candidates for surgical removal of their tumor should have their HCC removed by surgical resection or, in certain cases, liver transplantation, as these are potentially curative modalities.
- If surgical removal is not feasible but the disease is predominately confined to the liver, a local ablative treatment such as radiofrequency ablation or locally administered chemotherapy such as chemoembolization should be administered, as these approaches locally treat the tumor and thus are typically associated with better efficacy and fewer toxicities than systemic treatment.
- Patients with significant extrahepatic disease should be treated with systemic chemotherapy, as this is the only approach that will treat all sites of disease.

DEFINITION

HCC, also known as hepatoma, accounts for 40% of childhood and 90% of adult malignant primary tumors of the liver. It is more common in males than in females. HCC rarely occurs in adults before age 40 and increases in frequency thereafter, with the peak incidence occurring in the sixth decade of life.

ETIOLOGY

HCC is typically caused by preexisting liver disease. In the United States, approximately 45% of patients with HCC have underlying hepatitis C, approximately 15% to 20% of patients have underlying hepatitis B, 5% of patients have underlying hepatitis B and C, and the majority of the remaining patients have underlying cirrhosis secondary to alcohol abuse, postnecrotic cirrhosis, or hemochromatosis.[26] Primary biliary cirrhosis and the cirrhosis associated with Wilson's disease do not appear to significantly predispose patients to developing HCC. It is estimated that approximately 5% of all patients with cirrhosis will eventually develop HCC.

UNDIFFERENTIATED SARCOMA

Undifferentiated (embryonal) sarcoma of the liver is a term used to describe a group of very rare pediatric sarcomas of the liver that defy categorization since they lack cellular differentiation.[24] The tumor rarely metastasizes but spreads by direct invasion into adjacent organs. If untreated it is usually rapidly fatal. Surgical resection with or without prior neoadjuvant chemotherapy is potentially curable for patients with locally confined disease.[25] Radiation and chemotherapy have been used in the treatment of unresectable lesions and metastatic disease, but their utility is unclear.

Chronic active hepatitis B infection is the most important predisposing factor worldwide.[27,28] Epidemiologic studies reveal a high incidence of HCC in patients living in areas where hepatitis B is endemic. Patients chronically infected with hepatitis B have a 10- to 390-fold increased risk of developing HCC. The method by which chronic hepatitis B infection causes hepatic oncogenesis is not completely understood, but three possible mechanisms have been proposed. The first postulates that viral infection results in chronic inflammation and hepatocyte regeneration, leading to random mutations in the host genome and malignant transformation. The second theory postulates that there is targeted integration of hepatitis B regulatory genes adjacent to specific sites in the host genome, resulting in activation of host proto-oncogenes or inactivation of tumor suppressor genes and subsequent malignant transformation. The final theory postulates that random integration of the hepatitis B genome into the host genome occurs and that malignant transformation is a direct result of the oncogenic action of the integrated viral genes or viral gene products. Whatever the mechanism, approximately 80% of HCC cases worldwide are thought to be the result of prior hepatitis B infection. Thus, the hepatitis B virus appears to rank in importance with tobacco as a human carcinogen.

Hepatitis C infection also predisposes patients to developing HCC.[29] Hepatitis C infection is present in about 35% to 40% of HCC patients in the United States and 76% of patients in Japan.[30,31] Little is known about the exact mechanism by which hepatitis C produces hepatic oncogenesis.

Aflatoxin B1, a toxin produced by *Aspergillus flavus,* has also been implicated as a possible cause of HCC.[32] It appears to cause HCC by producing distinct point mutations in the p53 tumor suppressor gene. Aflatoxins are present on several foods consumed in large quantities in parts of the world that have a high incidence of HCC. These include rice, peanuts, soybeans, corn, wheat, bread, milk, and cheese, especially when they are stored in unrefrigerated conditions.

Case reports in the literature suggest an association between hormone exposure and the development of HCC. Women and men have developed HCC after exposure to oral contraceptives and androgens, respectively.[33,34] However, it remains to be determined whether the ingestion of hormones is causally related to the development of HCC.

Finally, certain inherited metabolic disorders, including hemochromatosis, glycogen storage disease, α_1-antitrypsin deficiency, and tyrosinemia, predispose patients to develop HCC.

EPIDEMIOLOGY

HCC is relatively uncommon in the United States, although the incidence is increasing in the United States due to the increasing incidence of hepatitis C over the past decade, with approximately 8,000 to 10,000 cases of HCC diagnosed annually.[26] However, it is one of the most prevalent cancers in the world due to its high prevalence in Asia, sub-Saharan Africa, and the South Pacific islands. HCC is estimated to cause approximately 1.25 million deaths worldwide each year.

PATHOPHYSIOLOGY

HCC is a grayish-white to bright yellow tumor that is usually not encapsulated. Occasionally, however, encapsulated HCC is found in older patients; it is a slower-growing and less invasive tumor than typical HCC.[35] Three major categories of HCC have been described based on macroscopic appearance. The most common type is the nodular form, in which the liver is studded with tumor. The second is the massive type, which manifests as a large mass and is sometimes associated with small satellite lesions. The last type is the diffuse form, which is the rarest and manifests as scattered tumor throughout the liver. The diffuse form always occurs in association with cirrhosis.

Eight different histologic subtypes of HCC have been identified based on the microscopic appearance of the tumor (Table 97.2). The hepatic variant, also known as the trabecu-

TABLE 97.2	Histologic Variants of Hepatocellular Carcinoma
Hepatic or trabecular	Giant cell
Pleomorphic	Clear cell
Adenoid or acinar	Fibrolamellar
Sclerosing	Mixed

lar variant, is the most common. The fibrolamellar variant is noteworthy because it is usually solitary and has a better prognosis than the other types.[36] It occurs primarily in women between ages 15 and 30 and is not associated with cirrhosis. The clear cell variant may also be associated with a better prognosis.

HCC often infiltrates the diaphragm and invades the intrahepatic portal veins. Less often the tumor invades the hepatic vein or bile duct. Frequently, regional lymph nodes are involved with tumor, but unless this occurs in the porta hepatis, such involvement usually does not alter the clinical course. At autopsy, 40% to 50% of patients with HCC are found to have distant metastases. The lung is the most common site of metastases, although almost any organ can be involved. The presence of metastatic disease rarely alters the patient's outcome because the tumor burden in the liver usually determines the duration of survival.

CLINICAL PRESENTATION AND DIAGNOSIS

SIGNS AND SYMPTOMS

Unfortunately, HCC is not typically symptomatic until there is advanced disease. The most common symptoms are abdominal pain, abdominal distention, fatigue, anorexia, weight loss, and fevers. On examination, most patients have hepatomegaly. Less often, patients have ascites, edema, or jaundice. Rarely, patients have hemorrhage secondary to esophageal varices. Although uncommon in North American patients, patients in Asia and Africa sometimes (10% to 20%) have spontaneous rupture of their HCC with intraperitoneal hemorrhage.

Many laboratory abnormalities may be present in a patient with HCC. Levels of the hepatic transaminases and alkaline phosphatase are usually elevated, and the bilirubin level is elevated in up to 50% of patients. Because of the decreased synthetic ability of the liver and the cachectic state of patients, the albumin level is often decreased, and the prothrombin time (PT) and partial thromboplastin time (PTT) may be elevated. A mild anemia and a reactive leukocytosis frequently occur. Rarely, erythrocytosis is present in patients having HCC with underlying cirrhosis. Hypoglycemia occurs in two distinct subpopulations of patients with HCC. The first group consists of patients with good performance status who have an acquired form of glycogen storage disease, secondary to their tumor, with reduced hepatocellular levels of glucose 6-phosphatase and a phosphorylase required for the breakdown of glycogen. The second group consists of terminal patients in whom hepatic gluconeogenesis is impaired. Approximately one third of patients have high serum cholesterol levels. Finally, some patients have hypercalcemia due to either bone metastases or a parathormone-like substance produced by the tumor.

DIAGNOSIS AND CLINICAL FINDINGS

The diagnostic workup of a patient suspected of having HCC generally proceeds from the physician's clinical suspicion based on the presenting signs and symptoms, to laboratory tests, to noninvasive radiologic studies, and then to tissue biopsy. The clinician usually first suspects a hepatic malignancy when the patient reports right upper quadrant pain or an enlarged liver is detected on physical examination. When these signs and symptoms occur in a patient with a history of hepatitis B or cirrhosis, a diagnosis of HCC must be considered.

Laboratory tests may be helpful in the diagnosis, but most are nonspecific. Liver function tests are typically elevated, although their utility is limited, as elevation occurs in many other diseases as well. The most useful laboratory test in the diagnosis of HCC is the AFP level.[37] AFP is a glycoprotein synthesized by fetal liver, fetal intestine, and yolk sac cells. Levels are very high before birth and fall to normal adult levels of less than 10 ng per mL after delivery. AFP levels can also be elevated in patients with underlying hepatitis B or C with or without HCC being present. Thus, a patient with hepatoma and underlying viral hepatitis who has a slightly elevated AFP level may or may not have an AFP-producing hepatoma. Recently, it has been determined that there are three different glycoforms of AFP: AFP-L1, AFP-L2, and AFP-L3. AFP-L1 is the major glycoform found in the serum of patients with hepatitis, while AFP-L3 appears to be a specific marker for HCC. Thus, when necessary, testing for the specific glycotype of AFP can assist with the determination of whether a patient has an AFP-producing HCC. AFP levels are elevated due to the tumor (greater than 100 ng/mL) in about 75% to 90% of patients who have HCC.[31] Although levels are elevated in a few other malignant conditions, the frequency of elevated levels in patients with HCC makes this a useful initial test. When elevated, the AFP level can also be used to follow a patient's clinical course because it usually falls with response to therapy and rises with progressive disease. Ferritin levels are also elevated in patients with HCC; however, ferritin levels are elevated in most patients with uncomplicated cirrhosis, so it lacks specificity.[38] In addition, ferritin levels do not correlate with therapeutic response, as does AFP.

Several radiologic tests may be used to confirm the presence of a hepatic mass and to follow the course of the disease. Arteriography may be used to assist in the diagnosis of HCC when other radiographic techniques fail. On arteriographic examination, HCC typically has a dilated feeding artery with a hypervascular tumor bed. Radionuclide liver–spleen scanning with technetium sulfur colloid is simple to perform, inexpensive, and not associated with morbidity, but it is rarely used because it cannot image the rest of the abdomen. Ultrasound is similarly inexpensive and is not associated with morbidity, but it cannot detect hepatic lesions smaller than 1 cm and has limited utility in determining the presence of extrahepatic tumor. Although they are more expensive, computed tomography (CT) and magnetic resonance imaging (MRI) are the most frequently used methods for imaging a hepatic malignancy. These techniques are more sensitive than ultrasound and allow visualization of the entire abdomen. However, the most sensitive radiographic technique for detecting a hepatic lesion is intraoperative ultrasound. This procedure should be performed whenever hepatic resection is contemplated because it is even more sensitive for detecting lesions than the surgeon's visual and tactile inspection of the liver.[39]

These radiographic techniques are useful for documenting the presence of a hepatic mass and following the course of disease once the diagnosis has been confirmed and therapy has been instituted, but by themselves they do not provide a definitive diagnosis of HCC. This requires pathologic examination of a tissue specimen. Tissue specimens may be obtained by percutaneous biopsy, peritoneoscopy with directed needle biopsy, or open biopsy at laparotomy.

PREVENTION

Because very few patients with HCC are cured, prevention of HCC is the most appealing approach to decreasing the incidence of HCC.[40] As previously discussed, hepatitis B appears to be a major etiologic cause of HCC. Vertical transmission from mother to infant is the most common method of hepatitis B transmission in endemic areas. Therefore, vaccination of newborns should prevent vertical transmission and thus eliminate the predisposition for subsequently developing HCC.[41] Pilot data from Shanghai and Gambia have shown that such a strategy is effective in preventing transmission of hepatitis B in endemic areas.[42,43] In addition, a universal hepatitis B vaccination program in Taiwan found a significant decline in the incidence of HCC.[44] A cost/benefit analysis of newborn vaccination has shown that it is justifiable even in areas with intermediate to high endemicity.[45] It is estimated that worldwide vaccination against hepatitis B could reduce the incidence of HCC by up to 60%.[40] In addition, the risk of patients with chronic active hepatitis B developing HCC may be reduced by the administration of α-interferon.[46] Other factors that may reduce the incidence of HCC include reducing alcohol intake, reducing exposure to aflatoxin B1, and decreasing the incidence of hepatitis C infection.[47]

SCREENING

Theoretically, screening patients who are at high risk for developing HCC (i.e., patients with chronic viral hepatitis or cirrhosis from any cause) should result in the detection of the malignancy earlier, thus allowing potentially curative surgical resection or liver transplantation to be performed in more patients. While screening patients with AFP or ultrasound is capable of detecting some early HCCs, no definitive outcome advantage has been observed.[48–51]

PSYCHOSOCIAL ASPECTS

The diagnosis of HCC has a major impact on patients and their family members. Patients have to cope with the diagnosis of a potentially rapidly fatal illness, as well as the anxiety of contemplating the aggressive surgical and medical treatments used in this disease. Thus, patients and their family members must be educated about HCC and its treatment options, as well as assisted with the emotional impact of the diagnosis itself.

Since HCC often occurs in immigrants from areas such as Asia, patients and their family members may not always speak fluent English. In such cases, it is essential that translators assist with the education of the patient and family members. In addition, cultural differences should be taken into consideration when caring for these patients. For instance, in some Asian countries, patients are often not informed that they have terminal cancer. As a result, it is not uncommon to have family members request that the patient not be fully informed regarding the diagnosis and prognosis. This situation requires discussion with the family so that an approach can be agreed on that allows the patient to be appropriately informed of treatment options.

PROGNOSIS

HCC is an aggressive malignancy that carries a grave prognosis unless the tumor can be cured by surgical resection, liver transplantation, or a local ablative therapy. The reported median survival in untreated patients from the time of diagnosis varies from 1 to 6 months. Several factors are of prognostic importance (Table 97.3).[52] The most important of these is the resectability of the tumor. Surgical removal offers the only potential cure for HCC.

A patient's performance status is of prognostic significance, with ambulatory patients surviving longer than those who are bedridden. The percentage of liver involved with tumor at the time of presentation is inversely related to the duration of survival. Also, the location of tumors within the liver can alter outcome. Patients with tumor near the porta hepatis may deteriorate rapidly because a small increase in tumor volume may cause compression of the inferior vena cava, portal vein, hepatic artery, and bile duct, leading to ascites, edema, and jaundice.

The patient's baseline liver function is also important: patients with normal liver function tests, bilirubin, albumin, and PT and PTT have the best prognosis. Patients presenting with ascites, edema, or esophageal varices have a poorer

TABLE 97.3	Prognostic Variables in Patients With Hepatocellular Carcinoma	
Factor	**Favorable**	**Unfavorable**
Resectability	Yes	No
Liver function	Normal LFTs	Abnormal LFTs
	Bilirubin ≤36 μmol/L	Bilirubin >36 μmol/L
	Normal albumin	Hypoalbuminemia
	Normal PT, PTT	Abnormal PT, PTT
	No ascites	Ascites
	No portal hypertension	Portal hypertension
Metastases	No	Yes
Performance status	Ambulatory	Bedridden
Age	≤45 years	>45 years
Sex	Female	Male
Country	North American	African, Asian
Histology	Fibrolamellar variant	Remaining histologies
	Clear cell variant	
Tumor encapsulation	Encapsulated tumor	Nonencapsulated tumor
Cirrhosis	No	Yes

LFTs, liver function tests; PT, prothrombin time; PTT, partial thromboplastin time

prognosis. Patients having the fibrolamellar or clear cell variants of HCC and those with encapsulated tumors generally survive longer. Although metastatic disease itself rarely determines outcome, its presence suggests a more aggressive tumor and is associated with a shorter survival.

Other important prognostic factors include the patient's age, sex, country of origin, and the presence or absence of cirrhosis. Patients 45 years of age or younger have a better prognosis than those over 45, and female patients survive longer than their male counterparts. Patients with otherwise normal livers survive longer and respond better to chemotherapy than those with cirrhosis.

Several staging systems have been used to categorize patients according to their prognosis, including the Okuda staging system and the Cancer of Liver Italian Program (CLIP) prognostic score.[53] Most recently, the Chinese University prognostic index (CUPI) has been proposed as the most accurate method for determining the prognosis of a HCC patient.[54] This staging system assigns a prognostic score based on the patient's TNM staging, total bilirubin value, presence or absence of ascites, alkaline phosphatase value, AFP value, and the presence or absence of symptomatic disease upon presentation. However, the CUPI needs to be validated using additional cohorts of patients before it can be recommended for general use.

THERAPEUTIC PLAN

Surgical resection and orthotopic liver transplantation are potentially curative modalities for locally confined disease and thus should be used whenever feasible. For patients with severe underlying cirrhosis, liver transplantation may be the preferred modality, as it has the potential to treat the underlying liver disease as well as cure the HCC. Local ablative therapies (to be described later), such as radiofrequency ablation, microwave coagulation therapy, laser-induced interstitial thermotherapy, cryosurgery, percutaneous ethanol injection, and percutaneous acetic acid injection, can also provide good local control for patients with potentially resectable HCCs who are not candidates for surgical resection because of underlying liver disease, comorbid illnesses, or minimal extrahepatic disease. Patients with unresectable but liver-predominant disease are frequently treated with intraarterial chemotherapy with or without Lipiodol, or chemoembolization. Other alternatives for these patients include hepatic artery ligation, embolization, and radiation (external beam radiation or radioimmunotherapy). Systemic chemotherapy is the only alternative for patients who have significant extrahepatic tumor.

TREATMENT

NONPHARMACOLOGIC TREATMENT

Surgical Treatment. Surgical resection and liver transplantation are potentially curative modalities but are typically used only in the few patients who have three or fewer lesions and whose disease is confined to the liver. Liver transplantation is also reserved for patients with relatively small-volume disease confined to the liver, although it can be undertaken in patients with more significant underlying liver disease, such as cirrhotic patients. However, the shortage of available liver donors limits the use of this modality, and tumor progression while the patient is awaiting a donor can lead to ineligibility for transplantation.

Surgical Resection. Surgical resection of HCC is the most widely used modality that offers a potential for cure. Partial hepatectomy is a relatively safe procedure with a low mortality rate when performed by an experienced hepatic surgeon and limited to patients with small-volume disease with relatively normal underlying hepatic parenchyma. However, it is associated with more significant morbidity and mortality (up to 15%) when performed in patients with significant underlying liver disease.[55-76] Unfortunately, the majority of patients are not candidates for surgical resection because their intrahepatic tumor is too extensive, their underlying liver disease limits their ability to withstand the surgical

procedure, or they have extrahepatic disease. Approximately one third of patients are considered candidates for resection after preoperative staging of their tumor; of those, approximately two thirds are found to be unresectable at surgery because of the presence of extrahepatic tumor or previously undiagnosed additional intrahepatic tumor. Thus, only about 10% to 15% of patients with HCC have resectable disease. Occasionally, unresectable HCC may be rendered resectable with a prior treatment modality, such as chemoembolization.[77]

Table 97.4 summarizes the results of surgical resection for HCC. The 5-year survival rates for patients undergoing a potentially curative resection ranged from 15% to 65%, with recent series reporting 5-year survival rates between 37% and 65% in patients with small-volume HCC. Approximately 20% of the 5-year survivors ultimately die of recurrent disease; thus, approximately 30% to 50% of the resected patients are cured of HCC. Factors associated with an increased likelihood of cure include having adequate hepatic function to withstand the surgery, having relatively normal underlying hepatic parenchyma, tumor size 5 cm or smaller, negative resection margins, a well-differentiated tumor, an encapsulated tumor, lack of vascular invasion, or having the

TABLE 97.4	Results of Surgical Resection for Hepatocellular Carcinoma			
Author/Year	Number of Patients	Perioperative Mortality (%)	5-Year Survival (%)	Reference
Toshihara/1990	119	15	33	55
Choi/1990	174	13	15	56
Yamanaka/1990	128	6	54	57
Kobayashi/1990	180	3	49	58
Tsuzuki/1990	119	15	39	59
Iwatsuki/1991	76	6	33	60
Gozzetti/1993	168	8	36	61
Kawarada/1994	149	4	39	62
Tani/1997	90	4	38	63
Yamasaki/1991	427	3	41	64
Nagashima/1996	50	12	53	65
Takenaka/1996	280	2	50	66
Chen/1997	382	4	46	67
Makuuchi/1998	352	1	47	68
Takayama/1998	163	1	51	69
Lise/1998	100	11	38	70
Philosophe/1998	67	4	38	71
Grazi/2001	264	5	41	72
Kanematsu/2002	303	2	51	73
Belghiti/2002	328	6	37	74
Mo/2003	121	0	65	75
Shimozawa/2004	135	2	55	76

fibrolamellar variant of HCC.[38,72] In addition, patients without viral hepatitis are at a decreased risk for recurrence of HCC.

The role of adjuvant chemotherapy after resection has not been fully elucidated. Data from a small study in Asia suggest that adjuvant intraarterial chemotherapy may improve disease-free and overall survival of patients with HCC.[78] However, a recent randomized study comparing surgical resection with or without adjuvant chemotherapy reported a higher incidence of overall recurrence and extrahepatic recurrence and a shorter disease-free survival for the group that received adjuvant intraarterial chemotherapy.[79]

Liver Transplantation. Orthotopic liver transplantation (OLT) is performed in selected cirrhotic patients who have HCC confined to the liver and a limited volume of disease.[80–82] While surgical resection continues to be the mainstay of surgical intervention for HCC patients, the potential advantages of OLT in patients with significant underlying liver disease include complete resection of all hepatic tumor and elimination of the underlying liver disease. OLT is typically limited to cirrhotic patients with HCC confined to the liver; a single tumor no larger than 5 cm or up to three tumors, none larger than 3 cm; no macroscopic vascular invasion or thrombosis; and a well-differentiated histology. Using these patient selection criteria, known as the Milan criteria, 5-year survival rates of about 60% have been reported after OLT. Factors that limit the utility of OLT include a shortage of donor livers and long waiting periods, which allow time for progression of the HCC and the underlying liver disease. Because of these issues, an increasing number of HCC patients who are eligible for transplantation are transplanted with the right or left hepatic lobe from a living donor.

Hepatic Artery Ligation. Surgical ligation of the hepatic artery has been performed in patients who have HCC without significant extrahepatic involvement in an attempt to produce tumor necrosis secondary to ischemia. This approach has been used as a single modality and in combination with chemotherapy.[83,84] Responses with hepatic arterial ligation are often transient because extrahepatic collateral arteries develop rapidly, reperfusing the tumor.[85] This procedure is generally well tolerated, with hepatic pain, fever, and elevated hepatic enzymes being the most prevalent adverse events. Rarely, hepatic artery ligation causes hepatic necrosis, resulting in death. Patients with severely compromised hepatic function or portal vein thrombosis should not undergo this procedure. Although frequently used in the past, hepatic artery ligation is rarely used today because occlusion of the hepatic artery can be accomplished radiologically (i.e., embolization), and permanent loss of the hepatic artery precludes its use for other liver-directed treatments, such as intraarterial chemotherapy or chemoembolization. Ligation of the hepatic artery has also been used to stop intraabdominal bleeding from a ruptured HCC,[86] but this can also be

accomplished angiographically with coiling or embolization;[87] thus, it is rarely used for this purpose.

Local Ablative Therapies. Local ablative therapies may be used to treat small HCCs (generally 5 cm or smaller) in patients who are not candidates for surgical removal of their tumor due to underlying cirrhosis from hepatitis B, hepatitis C, or alcohol abuse. Local ablative therapies include radiofrequency ablation, microwave coagulation therapy, laser-induced interstitial thermotherapy, cryosurgery, percutaneous ethanol injection, and percutaneous acetic acid injection. Of these modalities, radiofrequency ablation is the preferred approach due to its large ablation volume, few treatment sessions, and predictable ablation size.

Radiofrequency Ablation. Radiofrequency ablation, which uses radiofrequency energy to heat the tumor above 60°C, resulting in coagulation and necrosis of the tumor, is currently the most widely used local ablative treatment for HCC.[88] It is accomplished by percutaneously inserting a needle into the hepatic tumor under ultrasound or magnetic resonance guidance and then passing radiofrequency energy through the needle. Tumor size and the degree of underlying cirrhosis appear to be the major determinants of outcome, with the best results achieved in patients with Child-Pugh class A cirrhosis and tumors 3 cm or smaller. In a study by Tarantino et al, 84 patients with HCC and underlying cirrhosis were treated with radiofrequency ablation. Complete necrosis of the tumor was observed in 95% of the tumors smaller than 3 cm, 71% of those 3.1 to 5 cm, and 12% of those larger than 5 cm.[89] In another study, 65 HCC patients were treated with radiofrequency ablation and complete necrosis was observed in 91%, 74%, and 36% of tumors that were smaller than 3 cm, 3 to 5 cm, and larger than 5 cm, respectively, after the first treatment.[90] The complete necrosis rates increased to 100%, 93%, and 64% after multiple treatments. No local recurrences were noted in patients with HCCs smaller than 4 cm. After 3 years, the survival rates were 83% in Child-Pugh class A cirrhotic patients and 31% in Child-Pugh class B patients. Surgical resection was found to be superior to radiofrequency ablation in a recent trial that retrospectively compared the outcome of 79 patients treated with radiofrequency ablation to 79 patients treated with surgical resection.[91] The 1- and 3-year survival rates were 83% and 65% for the patients undergoing surgical resection compared to 78% and 33% for the patients treated with radiofrequency ablation.

Cryosurgery. Cryosurgery uses a probe circulating liquid nitrogen through its tip, which is inserted into a tumor under intraoperative ultrasound guidance to induce freezing temperatures within a tumor, resulting in necrosis. The use of multiple freeze–thaw cycles increases the percentage of tumor cells killed.[92] Cryosurgery is relatively well tolerated. However, in the largest published experience to date, only 12 of 60 (20%) patients were alive 3 years after cryosurgery.[93] It may be most useful in patients with resectable disease who are not candidates for partial hepatectomy due to underlying liver disease, such as cirrhosis.

Microwave Coagulation Therapy and Laser-Induced Interstitial Thermotherapy. Microwave coagulation therapy and laser-induced interstitial thermotherapy are relatively new thermal ablative techniques for treating HCC. Dong et al treated 234 patients with microwave coagulation therapy, and complete necrosis was observed in 89% of the treated lesions; the 5-year survival rate was 57%.[94] Similar results have also been reported in smaller numbers of HCC patients treated with laser-induced interstitial thermotherapy.[95] Currently, the utility of these techniques is limited due to the relatively small area of thermal necrosis around the interstitial probes, but design modifications and new equipment may ultimately lead to an expanded role for these two modalities in the future.

Percutaneous Alcohol Injection. Percutaneous injection of absolute ethyl alcohol directly into a tumor under ultrasound guidance is capable of producing histologically confirmed complete responses in small HCCs by inducing dehydration and intracellular coagulation, leading to necrosis, vascular occlusion, and fibrosis. The volume of ethyl alcohol injected depends on the size of the tumor and its vascularity, but it is generally 2 to 8 mL. The distribution of alcohol within the tumor during the injection is evaluated by ultrasound. In various studies, percutaneous alcohol injection for small, typically solitary, HCCs resulted in a 3-year survival of 55% to 70%.[96–98] Castells et al[96] compared the outcome of 30 patients treated with percutaneous alcohol injection with 33 patients treated with surgical resection. Two years after the procedure, 66% of the group treated with percutaneous alcohol, compared with 45% of the surgical resection group, had recurrence of their tumor, although the survival rates were similar for the two groups. As with cryosurgery and radiofrequency ablation, percutaneous alcohol injection appears to be most useful in the patient who has potentially resectable HCC but is not a good candidate for surgical resection because of underlying liver disease.

Percutaneous Acetic Acid Injection. Recently, percutaneous injection of acetic acid directly into HCCs has also been performed, and the results appear to be comparable to percutaneous alcohol injection.[99]

Radiotherapy
External Beam Radiotherapy. Standard external radiation is of limited benefit in the management of HCC because of the inherent intolerance of normal liver parenchyma to radiation. Specifically, doses in excess of 3,000 rads produce radiation hepatitis in a significant number of patients.[100] Patients with underlying liver disease develop radiation hepatitis at even lower doses. Some partial responses to external beam radiation at doses of 2,000 to 3,000 rads fractionated over 7 days have been reported, although survival does not appear to be extended.[101] Three-dimensional radiation treatment can minimize the radiation dose to the

liver and allow a higher dose of radiation to be delivered to the HCC than conventional external beam radiation.[102,103] Whether this approach will improve on the results obtained with standard external beam radiation remains to be determined.

Regionally Administered Radiotherapy. Because the normal liver parenchyma has a limited ability to tolerate radiation, approaches that deliver radiotherapy directly to the tumor while minimizing exposure to the normal liver tissue have been explored. One such approach is the administration of radioimmunoglobulin targeted to a tumor antigen. Initial studies of iodine-131 polyclonal antiferritin antibody plus chemotherapy and external beam radiation produced encouraging results, but a subsequent randomized trial comparing this approach to chemotherapy alone failed to show a survival advantage.[104] In addition, significant myelosuppression was observed.

Two additional methods of delivering regional radiotherapy are the administration of intraarterial iodine-131–labeled Lipiodol and the delivery of neutron-activated yttrium-90 containing glass microspheres.[105–107] In one study, 48% of patients treated with intraarterial iodine-131–labeled Lipiodol had a response to treatment and 60% were alive at 3 years.[106]

Intraarterial yttrium-90 glass microspheres is the only treatment of HCC approved by the U.S. Food and Drug Administration. In a recent study, 18 of 65 patients treated with this modality had a partial response.[107] The principal toxicities include nausea, abdominal pain, fatigue, lymphopenia, and transient hyperbilirubinemia.

PHARMACOTHERAPY
Systemic Chemotherapy. Intravenous chemotherapy is of limited benefit in altering the natural history of HCC. However, it is the only therapeutic option for patients with widely metastatic disease. The experience with single-agent chemotherapy is summarized in Table 97.5. Doxorubicin is the agent with the most reproducible activity, producing responses in approximately 10% to 20% of patients. It is usually administered intravenously in doses of 50 to 75 mg per m^2 every 21 days.[108–116] Because doxorubicin is cleared by the hepatobiliary system, the dose of doxorubicin must be reduced in HCC patients with hyperbilirubinemia. Epirubicin and mitoxantrone also appear to have activity against HCC.[117–121] 5-FU has been administered both orally[110,122,123] and intravenously[123–126] to patients with HCC. By both routes, the response rates have been low. Amsacrine, etoposide, cisplatin, oxaliplatin, and α-interferon have all produced occasional responses, but the overall response rates with these agents have been low.[112,127–139]

Historically, combination chemotherapy has not improved the results obtained with single-agent therapy. However, recently, the combination of cisplatin, doxorubicin, 5-FU, and α-IFN (PIAF) produced higher response rates than single-agent chemotherapy in small phase 2 studies.[140]

TABLE 97.5	Results of Single-Agent Intravenous Chemotherapy for Hepatocellular Carcinoma

Drug	Number of Patients	Responses	Response Rate (%)	Reference
Doxorubicin	41	6/41	15	108
	44	14/44	32	109
	57	9/57	16	110
	74	22/74	30	111
	28	8/28	29	112
	35	3/35	9	113
	52	6/52	11	114
	45	11/45	24	115
	109	11/109	10	116
	485	**91/485**	**19**	
Mitoxantrone	22	6/22	27	117
	20	0/20	0	118
	42	**6/42**	**14**	
4′-Epidoxorubicin	18	3/18	17	119
	13	3/13	23	120
	33	3/33	9	121
	64	**9/64**	**14**	
5-Fluorouracil	12	6/12	50	122
	48	0/48	0	110
	21	0/21	0	123
	10	1/10	10	124
	8	0/8	0	125
	15	1/15	7	126
	114	**8/114**	**7**	
Amsacrine	23	3/23	13	127
	16	0/16	0	128
	20	1/20	5	129
	35	1/35	3	130
	94	**5/95**	**5**	
Dichloro-methotrexate	14	0/14	0	131
	7	3/7	43	132
	21	**3/21**	**14**	
Etoposide	24	3/24	13	133
	38	7/38	18	112
	62	**10/62**	**16**	
Cisplatin	13	1/13	8	134
	26	4/26	15	135
	39	**5/39**	**13**	
Interferon	28	2/28	7	136
	25	2/25	8	137
	53	**4/53**	**8**	
Oxaliplatin	14	1/14	7	138
Gemcitabine	48	1/48	2	139

As a result of these encouraging data, a phase 3 randomized study is currently assessing the relative efficacy of single-agent doxorubicin versus PIAF in previously untreated hepatoma patients. Unfortunately, early results from this study suggest that while the response rate was higher (20% versus 11%) with PIAF therapy, survival was not significantly different (8.4 versus 7.1 months) between the two arms, and the toxicity was substantially higher in the PIAF arm. Thus, single-agent doxorubicin appears to still represent the gold standard for systemic treatment of HCC.

Intraarterial Chemotherapy. Because of the discouraging results obtained with intravenous chemotherapy, administration of chemotherapy directly into the hepatic artery has been used to increase the drug exposure (concentration versus time) to the tumor and thus enhance efficacy.[141,142] The drug exposure is most dramatically increased when the agent being administered has a rapid total body clearance, because intraarterial infusion enables the drug to be delivered in a high concentration to the tumor before it is eliminated from the body. An additional benefit is derived from intraarterial administration when the agent has a high first-pass hepatic extraction. The high first-pass hepatic extraction of the drug leads to a lower systemic drug exposure than with intravenous administration and thus fewer adverse effects.

Table 97.6 lists the total body clearance rates and hepatic extraction ratios of chemotherapeutic agents commonly used to treat hepatic malignancies.[143–149] Floxuridine, 5-FU, and doxorubicin have rapid total body clearance and high hepatic extraction ratios. Therefore, the intraarterial administration of these agents results in a substantial increase in drug exposure at the tumor site and a decrease in systemic exposure. In contrast, cisplatin, oxaliplatin, and mitomycin C have relatively slow total body clearance and low hepatic extraction ratios. Thus, intraarterial administration of these agents produces less exposure time at the tumor site and more systemic drug exposure.

In the past, hepatic intraarterial chemotherapy was most commonly administered via a radiographically placed transcutaneous catheter inserted into the hepatic artery via the

TABLE 97.6	Total Body Clearances and Hepatic Extractions of Drugs Administered by Hepatic Intraarterial Infusion

Drug	Total Body Clearance (mL/min)	Hepatic Extraction Ratio (%)	Reference
Floxuridine	4800	95	143
Doxorubicin	2000	50	144
5-Fluorouracil	1000	80	145, 146
Cisplatin	600	24	147
Mitomycin C	575	10	148
Oxaliplatin	250	47	149

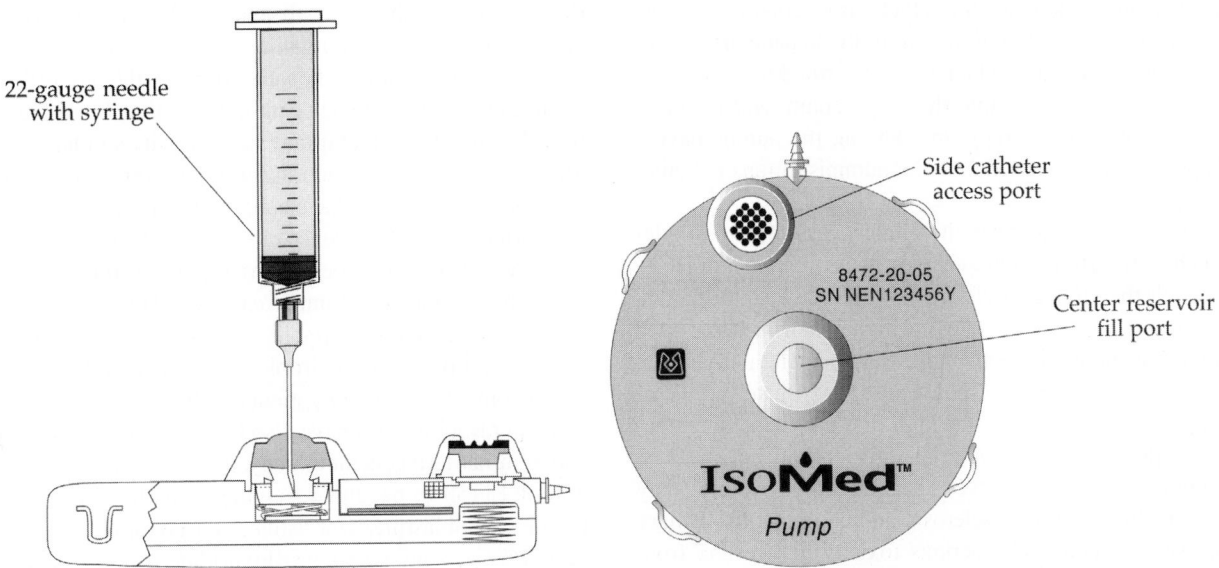

FIGURE 97.2 Medtronics (Minneapolis, MN) IsoMed implantable pump (*left*) and cross section of implantable pump (*right*). (Reprinted with permission from Medtronic, Inc., 2006.)

femoral or brachial artery. This can be successfully accomplished in approximately 80% of patients but is associated with several complications, including catheter migration, drug misperfusion, infection, catheter thrombosis, hepatic arterial thrombosis, and arterial emboli. To avoid catheter migration, transcutaneous catheters may be surgically placed and secured in the hepatic artery. Although this approach prevents catheter migration, the other difficulties of a transcutaneous catheter remain.

The advent of totally implantable ports and pumps in the early 1980s made the administration of long-term hepatic intraarterial chemotherapy feasible. Implanted ports are sur-

gically placed into a subcutaneous pocket, and the catheter is inserted in a ligated gastroduodenal artery, with the tip at the hepatic artery. Implanted ports are most useful for the administration of bolus chemotherapy. Continuous-infusion chemotherapy via implanted ports requires the use of an external infusion device and is therefore technically cumbersome.

Totally implantable pumps have made it feasible to administer infusional hepatic intraarterial chemotherapy in the outpatient setting (Fig. 97.2). Table 97.7 lists the characteristics of the various constant-flow and programmable implantable pumps. The pumps, like the ports, are placed into a

TABLE 97.7	Implantable Pumps						
Device	**Diameter**	**Weight**	**Volume**	**Flow Rate**	**Side Port**	**Battery**	**Alarms**
Constant Flow							
Codman (Model 3000-16)	61 mm	98 g	16 mL	1.0 mL/d	No[a]	No	No
Codman (Model 3000-30)	78 mm	137 g	30 mL	1.2 mL/d	No[a]	No	No
Codman (Model 3000-50)	86 mm	173 g	50 mL	2.5 mL/d	No[a]	No	No
Medtronic (IsoMed)	77 mm	113–120 g	20, 35, 60 mL	0.3–4 mL/day	Yes	No	No
Programmable							
Medtronic (SynchroMed)	87.5 mm	165–185 g	20, 40 mL	0.048–24 mL/day	Yes	Yes	Low volume, end of service, pump stall, memory error

[a]Acess into pump and hepatic intraarterial catheter achieved via the same central port using different needles.

subcutaneous pocket, and the catheter is inserted in a ligated gastroduodenal artery with the tip in the hepatic artery. All the devices have a drug chamber that is filled by percutaneously passing a needle into the inlet septum and injecting the next course of therapy. In addition, the pumps have a side port that may be used for bolus administration of chemotherapy.

Table 97.8 summarizes the clinical results with single-agent hepatic arterial chemotherapy in the treatment of HCC. Although the clinical trials are few and have small patient populations, the response rates are higher than those reported with intravenous chemotherapy. Single-agent intraarterial floxuridine produces a response in approximately 55% of patients.[125,150] Because of the high first-pass hepatic extraction of floxuridine, intraarterial infusions do not produce systemic toxicity. However, hepatobiliary toxicity may occur, including biliary sclerosis and cholecystitis. Biliary sclerosis is a potentially serious toxicity that results from floxuridine-induced inflammation and subsequent thrombosis of the peribiliary vascular plexus, which causes ischemic damage to the bile duct.[151] Serious biliary toxicity can usually be prevented with careful monitoring and appropriate dosage adjustments. Prophylactic cholecystectomy is recommended if repeated courses of hepatic intraarterial floxuridine are to be administered. Also, gastritis and gastroduodenal ulceration have occurred as a result of misperfusion of

floxuridine into the stomach and duodenum. This can be prevented by surgically ligating the arterial feeders to the stomach arising from the hepatic artery. Although 5-FU has not been tested as a single agent in the United States, results from Japan indicate that it may have activity similar to floxuridine when administered intra-arterially for HCC.[152] Doxorubicin also appears to have enhanced activity when infused intra-arterially, with response rates of 40% to 50%.[111,153–156] Mitomycin C has also been reported to have significant efficacy when administered intraarterially.[32] However, detailed response data are not available. Finally, hepatic intraarterial cisplatin, mitoxantrone, epirubicin, and ifosfamide have produced some responses in patients with HCC.[157–163]

High response rates have also been reported with combination intraarterial chemotherapy. Responses were observed in 8 of 15 (53%) patients receiving intraarterial mitomycin C, 5-FU, vinblastine, vincristine, and doxorubicin;[164] 8 of 12 (67%) patients receiving floxuridine, doxorubicin, and mitomycin C;[165] and 8 of 13 (61%) patients receiving floxuridine, leucovorin, doxorubicin, and cisplatin.[154] It remains unclear whether combination intraarterial chemotherapy is superior to single-agent intraarterial chemotherapy.

Intraarterial Lipiodol Chemotherapy. Lipiodol is an ethyl ester of the fatty acid of poppyseed oil, containing 38% iodine by weight; it is used as lymphangiogram dye. After intraarterial injection, Lipiodol concentrates in HCC. As a result of this finding, lipophilic chemotherapeutic agents have been administered intra-arterially in conjunction with Lipiodol in an attempt to facilitate the delivery of the chemotherapeutic agent into the tumor cell. The drugs most commonly combined with Lipiodol are doxorubicin and styrene-maleic acid-neocarzinostatin (SMANCS). SMANCS is a conjugation of neocarzinostatin, a proteinaceous antitumor antibiotic, and copolystyrene-maleic acid, a drug used to treat hepatic malignancies in Asia. Studies with intraarterial Lipiodol and doxorubicin, cisplatin, FUDR, and/or SMANCS have reported responses in 30% to 40% of patients.[164–169] In one study, intraarterial Lipiodol and SMANCS produced an overall response rate of 40% (27% complete response rate) in 30 HCC patients.[165] A randomized study comparing hepatic intraarterial cisplatin and doxorubicin to hepatic intraarterial cisplatin, doxorubicin, and Lipiodol failed to show an advantage for the Lipiodol-containing regimen.[166] Thus, further comparative studies are needed to ascertain whether Lipiodol has a role in the management of HCC.

Antiangiogenic Therapy. Because HCC is a hypervascular tumor, antiangiogenic agents might be expected to have some degree of therapeutic activity against this malignancy. Seventeen of 112 (15%) HCC patients who were treated with the antiangiogenic agent thalidomide responded to treatment.[170] In addition, one response has been reported in five evaluable HCC patients treated with bevacizumab.[171] While these early data are encouraging, additional studies with anti-

TABLE 97.8	Results of Single-Agent Intraarterial Chemotherapy for Hepatocellular Carcinoma			
Drug	Number of Patients	Responses	Response Rate (%)	Reference
Floxuridine	16	9	56	125
	28	15	54	150
	44	**24**	**55**	
Fluorouracil	9	2	22	152
Doxorubicin	10	4	40	121
	13	6	46	153
	2	1	50	154
	6	3	50	155
	19	8	42	156
	19	8	42	152
	69	**30**	**44**	
Cisplatin	16	3	19	157
	33	18	55	158
	10	4	40	159
	59	**25**	**42**	
Mitoxantrone	22	6	27	160
	23	6	26	161
	45	**12**	**27**	
Epirubicin	53	8	15	162
Ifosfamide	16	6	38	163

angiogenic agents need to be performed to determine their ultimate role in the therapeutic armamentarium for HCC.

Hormonal Therapy. Hormonal agents such as tamoxifen citrate and megestrol acetate (Megace) have been investigated for the treatment of HCC because some HCCs are estrogen-receptor positive, as are some breast cancers.[172] Based on this finding, patients with HCC have been treated with Megestrol or tamoxifen citrate. Although occasional responses have been reported with tamoxifen citrate, four well-designed, multicenter studies have found that it is comparable to placebo for the treatment of HCC.[173–176] Megestrol has also been reported to produce some benefit in HCC patients, although this has not been confirmed in large randomized studies.[177–179]

Embolization and Chemoembolization. Embolization and chemoembolization are frequently used to treat unresectable but liver-predominant HCC. Embolization of HCC involves radiographic placement of a percutaneous catheter into the hepatic artery and injection of an embolizing substance that occludes the arterial blood flow at the tumor capillary level, thus producing tumor ischemia. Embolizing substances that have been administered include Ethibloc (Ethicon, Hamburg, Germany), Gelfoam powder (50 to 300 microns; Pfizer), Gelfoam cubes (1 to 3 mm; Pfizer), Ivalon particles (150 to 500 microns) (Unipoint Lab, High Point, NC), and autologous blood clot. The various embolizing substances achieve different levels and durations of arterial blockade; the optimal embolizing substance has yet to be determined. Embolization is preferred over hepatic artery ligation because it is nonsurgical and is associated with fewer collateral arteries. In one study of HCC patients who had failed to respond to hepatic arterial chemotherapy, six of nine patients responded to embolization.[180] In Japan, 120 patients with HCC were treated with Gelfoam embolization, and 90% responded, with 1-, 2-, and 3-year survival rates of 44%, 29%, and 15%, respectively.[181]

Chemoembolization combines the tumor ischemia produced by embolization with prolonged high intratumoral concentrations of chemotherapy. This is accomplished by infusing embolizing microspheres that contain chemotherapeutic agents or a mixture of concentrated chemotherapy with an embolizing substance into the hepatic artery. In two studies, biodegradable albumin microspheres containing mitomycin C were used to embolize patients with HCC, and responses were observed in 7 of 7 (100%) patients and 15 of 20 (75%) patients.[182,183] In another study, chemoembolization with Gelfoam and doxorubicin, mitomycin C, and cisplatin produced responses in 12 of 50 (24%) patients and liquefaction necrosis in 70% of patients.[184] Additional studies using mitoxantrone, epirubicin, doxorubicin, and Lipiodol chemoembolization obtained similar response rates.[185,186] In a study comparing cisplatin chemoembolization to supportive care, chemoembolization reduced tumor size and AFP levels but did not affect overall survival.[187] However, in two recent studies comparing chemoemboliza-

tion to supportive care, chemoembolization resulted in a statistically significant prolongation of survival.[188,189] In addition, another recent trial showed that chemoembolization was superior to intraarterial chemotherapy plus Lipiodol: the comparative response rates were 73% and 51% and the comparative median survival times were 3.1 years and 2.5 years, respectively.[190]

Both embolization and chemoembolization are generally well tolerated, with liver pain, fever, and elevated liver function enzymes being the most prevalent adverse events. Recently, the coadministration of lidocaine has been reported to minimize the pain associated with chemoembolization.[191] Rare cases of acute renal failure, necrosis of the bile ducts or gallbladder, and hemoperitoneum have been reported. Also, if the embolizing substance is inadvertently injected into an area other than the tumor capillary bed, necrosis of that region may result.

ALTERNATIVE THERAPIES

Complementary and alternative therapies that may be pursued by HCC patients include herbal therapy, nutritional/special diet therapy, manipulation, massage, mind–body approaches, energy therapy, and biologic/organic therapy. Herbal medicine is the most common form of alternative therapy that is pursued by these patients. Some herbal medicines have been shown to contain substances that are cytotoxic to hepatoma cells in vitro.[192,193] While there are limited clinical trial data regarding the use of herbal medicine for the treatment of HCC, one randomized study comparing chemoembolization versus chemoembolization plus the herbal medicine gan'ai number I and number II reported that the combination was superior to chemoembolization alone.[194]

Another viable alternative for some patients who present with or develop metastatic disease is no therapy. This decision may be arrived at by the patient due to the limited utility of current therapies for metastatic disease, the toxicities of these treatments, and the desire to focus on quality of life. In such cases, this decision should be honored as long as the patient arrived at this decision after being fully informed of all potential treatment options.

FUTURE THERAPIES

Future therapies for HCC may include the development of novel methods of regionally treating the tumor with newer ablative techniques or chemotherapeutic agents. In addition, gene therapy may ultimately play a role in the treatment of HCC.[195] Finally, new chemotherapeutic or biologic agents with activity against HCC may emerge. Five investigational agents are being studied in the treatment of HCC. MTC-Dox consists of iron particles adsorbed to doxorubicin. MTC-Dox is administered intra-arterially under fluoroscopic guidance. The drug is then targeted to the tumor by an externally positioned magnet. In a phase 1/2 study, eight HCC patients were treated with escalating doses of intraarterial MTC-Dox.[196] The drug was successfully targeted to the tumor in all patients, with two of the patients having a partial response. Currently, a phase 2/3 trial of MTC-Dox versus doxorubicin in HCC patients is being conducted.

In a phase 2 study, intravenous T67, an irreversible antitubulin agent, produced a response rate of 6% in previously untreated HCC patients.[197] A randomized phase 2/3 trial of T67 versus intravenous doxorubicin is ongoing. Similar activity has been observed with intravenous Thymitaq, and a phase 3 randomized trial comparing its activity to intravenous doxorubicin is also ongoing.[198] Bay 49-4006, a ras-kinase inhibitor and vascular endothelial growth factor receptor inhibitor, has demonstrated activity against a variety of tumor types in early clinical trials and is being tested in a phase 2 study for its activity against HCC.[199] Finally, polyethylene glycol arginine has been reported to have activity against HCC in early clinical trials. Arginine is a nonessential amino acid for normal human cells. However, it has been determined in in vitro studies that HCC cells rely on arginine for growth because of loss of expression of arginosuccinate synthetase, the rate-limiting enzyme in the conversion of citrulline to arginine. Thus, the arginine-degrading enzyme polyethylene glycol arginine deiminase is potentially capable of causing cell death in HCC cells without significantly affecting normal cells. In a phase 2 study, polyethylene glycol deiminase produced responses in previously untreated patients with very little toxicity.[200] Two phase 3 trials of polyethylene glycol deiminase in HCC patients are ongoing.

IMPROVING OUTCOMES

PATIENT EDUCATION

Educating patients in high-risk areas about the methods of hepatitis B and C transmission and the benefits of hepatitis B vaccination should ultimately lead to a decrease in the incidence of HCC, although this decrease will take decades to become evident. In addition, educating high-risk patients (e.g., those with chronic viral hepatitis) about the importance of screening for HCC to detect the disease at an early stage may improve outcomes.

METHODS TO IMPROVE ADHERENCE TO DRUG THERAPIES

Most HCC patients who desire treatment are highly motivated to comply with their therapy, given that this is a life-threatening illness. In addition, these treatments are typically administered by healthcare professionals rather than the patient, so adherence is rarely a problem. Every attempt should be made to minimize treatment side effects through the use of appropriate premedication and so forth, as this will help maintain the patient's desire to continue treatment over time.

DISEASE MANAGEMENT STRATEGIES TO IMPROVE PATIENT OUTCOMES

Until pharmacologic agents are identified that can cure patients with HCC, the key to improving outcomes will remain the prevention of the disease through vaccination programs in regions having a high incidence of hepatitis B and diagnosing the disease early so that surgical removal can be performed. In addition, the continued refinement of local ablative techniques may improve patient outcomes, as will the development of more active chemotherapeutic or biologic agents for the treatment of patients with metastatic disease.

PHARMACOECONOMICS

The chemotherapeutic agents, such as doxorubicin, that are currently used in the treatment of HCC are generic and are thus moderately priced. Newer agents, such as polyethylene glycol arginine deiminase, will likely be priced at a premium compared to these agents. These agents will have to be substantially more efficacious or less toxic to justify such an increase in price.

SECONDARY MALIGNANT LIVER TUMORS

Liver metastases may occur from virtually any malignancy. Of all organs in the body, the liver is the most common site of bloodborne metastases. In an autopsy series of 9,497 cancer patients, 8,055 (84.8%) had metastatic disease, and 4,444 (46.8%) had liver metastases.[180] Liver metastases may manifest as the only site of metastatic disease or may be part of a more widely metastatic process. Hepatic metastases occur most frequently in patients with primary tumors originating in organs drained by the portal vein, including tumors of the stomach, small intestine, colon, pancreas, gallbladder, and extrahepatic biliary tract. However, some malignancies, such as breast cancer, lymphomas, testicular cancer, and ocular melanoma, which arise in organs having nonportal sources of venous drainage, are also associated with a high incidence of liver metastases.

The factors contributing to the high incidence of liver metastases in cancer patients are complex and not fully understood. On an ultrastructural level, the sinusoidal fenestrations of the liver may be more permeable to metastatic cells than the capillary endothelium of other organs. Further, the liver has relatively little connective tissue, which in other organs may act as a physical barrier to metastatic cells. From a physiologic standpoint, the liver, as the organ that filters the blood, may inherently be more efficient than other organs at removing metastatic cells from the blood. Last, in patients with tumors originating in organs drained by the portal circulation, the liver is the first organ encountered by the meta-

static cells after their release into the bloodstream and thus is the organ presented with the highest burden of metastatic cells. The remainder of the discussion on liver metastases will focus on colorectal cancer because it is the most common tumor that metastasizes to the liver.

COLORECTAL CANCER METASTATIC TO THE LIVER

TREATMENT GOALS: COLORECTAL CANCER METASTATIC TO THE LIVER

- For patients with resectable disease confined to the liver, undertake surgical removal in an attempt to cure the patient.
- Treat patients with unresectable liver-predominant disease with locally ablative therapy, hepatic intraarterial chemotherapy, or systemic chemotherapy.
- For patients with significant extrahepatic involvement, treat with systemic chemotherapy in an attempt to improve survival without significantly impairing the patient's quality of life.

DEFINITION

Colorectal cancer affects about 1 person out of every 20 in the United States and most Westernized countries. At the time of diagnosis, approximately 15% to 25% of these patients have metastatic disease in the liver, and another 25% of patients develop metastasis later during the course of disease. The liver is the most common site of metastatic involvement, followed by the lung.

ETIOLOGY

For a full discussion of the etiology of colorectal cancer, the reader is referred to Chapter 98. Liver metastases are believed to be the most common site of metastatic disease because the blood that is drained from the colon and rectum enters the portal vein and is filtered by the liver on its way back to the heart. Thus, the liver is the first organ that is exposed to bloodborne tumor cells from colorectal cancer.

EPIDEMIOLOGY

For a discussion of the epidemiology of colorectal cancer, the reader is referred to Chapter 98.

PATHOPHYSIOLOGY

For a discussion of the pathophysiology of colorectal cancer, the reader is referred to Chapter 98.

CLINICAL PRESENTATION AND DIAGNOSIS

SIGNS AND SYMPTOMS
Often liver metastases are diagnosed incidentally during surgery in patients without signs or symptoms suggestive of hepatic involvement or during routine follow-up. The most common complaints in patients with symptomatic liver metastases include abdominal pain, abdominal distention, anorexia, weight loss, fatigue, jaundice, and unexplained fever.

DIAGNOSIS AND CLINICAL FINDINGS
The diagnosis of a patient suspected of having liver metastases generally proceeds from the physical examination, to laboratory tests, to radiographic imaging, and then to tissue biopsy. The most common finding on physical examination is hepatomegaly. In patients with advanced hepatic metastases, the tumor may occlude the bile duct, portal vein, or inferior vena cava, resulting in jaundice, portal hypertension (ascites, esophageal varices), or lower extremity edema, respectively. Some patients with primary colorectal cancer have synchronous liver metastases; in other cases, the liver metastases may appear months to years after the initial diagnosis of the primary tumor.

Approximately 60% of patients with hepatic metastases have elevated levels of alanine aminotransferase (ALT), aspartate aminotransferase (AST), lactic dehydrogenase (LDH), or alkaline phosphatase (AP).[201] In addition, serum bilirubin levels are often elevated in patients with advanced hepatic metastases. The greater the extent of liver involvement, the more likely these levels will be elevated. No single liver enzyme test is superior to the others for detecting liver metastases. Although hepatic enzyme elevations can be useful in identifying patients with liver metastases, elevations can occur in patients without liver metastases, and thus these tests lack specificity.

Another laboratory test that is helpful in diagnosing colorectal cancer is the carcinoembryonic antigen (CEA) level. CEA is a glycoprotein that is produced in small amounts by normal columnar epithelial cells (normal value is less than 4 ng/mL). CEA levels are elevated in 60% to 80% of patients with colorectal cancer. The CEA level tends to fall with tumor regression and to rise with disease progression. Although colorectal cancer at any site may produce CEA, levels greater than 20 ng per mL are most frequently associated with liver metastases.[202,203] Approximately 70% of patients with colorectal cancer metastatic to the liver have elevated CEA levels. However, because CEA is elevated in a variety of other malignant and nonmalignant conditions, it lacks diagnostic specificity. Thus, its major role lies in screening patients for recurrent disease and monitoring patients known to have metastases who are receiving treatment.

Several radiographic techniques are helpful in diagnosing liver metastases.[204,205] CT and MRI are the two preferred radiographic techniques for detecting liver metastases. These methods are more expensive than others, but they can accurately detect small lesions, are more reproducible, and allow for simultaneous imaging of the remainder of the abdomen. Ultrasound is inexpensive and does not expose patients to radiation, but intestinal gas, excessive fat, and overlying ribs can interfere with imaging; thus, small lesions may go undetected. Radionuclide liver–spleen scanning using technetium sulfur colloid is simple to perform but is associated with high false-positive and false-negative results, cannot image extrahepatic tumor, and often does not detect lesions smaller than 2 cm. Gamma camera imaging after the administration of indium-111 satumomab pendetide can be used in addition to other radiographic techniques to detect colorectal cancer metastatic to the liver.[206]

When liver-associated laboratory tests and radiographic techniques are used together, the combined sensitivity in diagnosing liver metastases increases to 90%, whereas alone the sensitivities are 60% and 80%, respectively.[207]

Taking a tissue biopsy to confirm liver metastases is usually unnecessary in colorectal cancer patients because data from the patient's history, physical examination, laboratory tests, and radiographic studies are usually sufficient to make the diagnosis. If a tissue specimen is required to confirm the diagnosis, it may be obtained by percutaneous biopsy, peritoneoscopy with needle-directed biopsy, or open biopsy at laparotomy.

PSYCHOSOCIAL ASPECTS

Patients with synchronous liver metastases must cope with the diagnosis and treatment of their primary colorectal cancer as well as their liver metastases. Typically, treatment of the primary tumor involves surgical resection of the tumor in the colon or rectum. If a colostomy is performed, this represents an additional psychological issue for the patient. The liver metastases may be treated with surgery, local ablative therapy, or regional or systemic chemotherapy. After surgery, patients must cope with their prognosis, which can range from a high likelihood of cure to a projected survival of only a few months.

Patients who develop metachronous liver metastases must cope with the recurrence of their disease. In addition, as with patients who have synchronous metastases, they must cope with the surgical or medical treatment being undertaken, as well as their prognosis.

PROGNOSIS

In general, colorectal cancer metastatic to the liver has a poor prognosis. Because of this, studies have been performed to identify prognostic factors that may further define indications for resection. Although data remain inconclusive, regional lymph node involvement, CEA level, tumor size and location, and positive liver resection margins are consistent with poor outcome.[208–211] The most important prognostic factor by far is the resectability of the hepatic metastases. Surgical resection is the only potentially curative modality for liver metastases and should be performed whenever possible. The most important prognostic factor in patients with unresectable tumor is the extent of hepatic involvement.[212] The survival in untreated patients ranges from 2 to 22 months (median of 8 to 10 months); patients who have the smallest amount of tumor survive the longest. Another important factor is the degree of histologic differentiation. Patients with well-differentiated tumors survive longer than those with poorly differentiated tumors.[213] In addition, patients with a poor performance status, significant weight loss, low albumin level, ascites, elevated hepatic enzymes, or elevated bilirubin levels have a shorter survival.

THERAPEUTIC PLAN

TREATMENT

Several modalities have been used, either alone or in combination, for the treatment of colorectal cancer metastatic to the liver, including surgical resection, radiotherapy, local ablative therapies, hepatic arterial ligation, intravenous chemotherapy, hepatic intraarterial chemotherapy, cryotherapy, and gene therapy. The following is a discussion of the results obtained with each of these modalities.

NONPHARMACOLOGIC THERAPY

Surgical Resection. Surgical resection offers a potential cure for patients with colorectal cancer metastatic to the liver and thus should be performed whenever removal of all the apparent metastatic disease can be safely accomplished. Surgical resection is typically undertaken in patients having disease confined to the liver and three or fewer nodules in the liver; thus, resection has historically been feasible in only approximately 15% of patients.

However, the use of preoperative neoadjuvant chemotherapy in appropriately selected patients may render some previously unresectable tumors resectable and thus increase the total percentage of patients with liver metastases that can be treated by surgical resection.[214,215] The results of surgical resection are summarized in Table 97.9.[216–243] The operative mortality rate in these studies ranged from 0% to 8%, with rates of 1% to 4% in most recent studies. The operative mortality rate is highest in patients who undergo extensive resections and those with a significant comorbid illness. The 5-year survival rate ranged between 18% and 51%. Patients with solitary metastases, those without extrahepatic disease, those who are female, those with synchronous metastases (compared with those who develop metachronous metastases), those with clear margins of resection, and those whose primary originated in the colon (compared with the rectum) survive longer after resection.

Intraoperative ultrasound with palpation is commonly used in an attempt to identify and resect any disease that was not apparent on preoperative radiographic imaging. In one study, detection of hepatic lesions by intraoperative ultrasound had a 97% accuracy rate compared with a 78% accuracy rate when preoperative radiographic imaging, surgical inspection, and palpation were used.[207] Also, radioimmunoguided surgery has been used in an attempt to identify and resect inapparent hepatic tumor. The impact of intraoperative ultrasound and radioimmunoguided surgery on survival after resection is yet to be determined. Adjuvant chemotherapy is not routinely used after the surgical removal of hepatic metastases from colorectal cancer, but results from pilot studies suggest that it may be beneficial.[244,245]

Hepatic Arterial Ligation. As with HCC, ligation of the hepatic artery has been performed in patients with liver metastases from colorectal cancer in an attempt to produce tumor necrosis secondary to ischemia.[246] Symptomatic improvement is observed in some patients after hepatic arterial ligation, but it is usually transient. In addition, ligation of the hepatic artery prevents its future use for other liver-directed therapies, such as intraarterial chemotherapy.

Local Ablative Therapies. Several local ablative therapies, including radiofrequency ablation, cryotherapy, laser thermotherapy, and microwave coagulation, have been used in the treatment of unresectable but locally confined liver metastases from colorectal cancer.

Radiofrequency Ablation. Radiofrequency ablation is currently the most widely used local ablative technique used to treat liver metastases from colorectal cancer. In one study, 88 patients with a total of 134 liver metastases were treated with radiofrequency ablation.[247] Complete necrosis of all lesions was obtained in 53 of the 88 (60%) patients, and 30% of the 53 patients had remained disease-free at the time of publication. In addition, encouraging results have recently been reported with radiofrequency ablation plus surgical resection in patients with otherwise unresectable disease.[248]

Cryotherapy. Cryotherapy is another therapeutic alternative for patients with colorectal cancer metastatic to the liver. In various studies, 20% to 51% of patients were alive without evidence of disease at median follow-ups of 14 to 36 months after cryotherapy.[243,244,250] In one study, 136 patients with unresectable disease who underwent cryosurgery had a median survival of 30 months.[251] In a trial in which cryotherapy plus postoperative regional chemotherapy was used to treat residual disease after resection in 20 patients, the median survival was 32 months.[252]

Laser Thermotherapy. Laser-induced interstitial thermotherapy is another local ablative therapy that has recently been used in the treatment of metastatic colorectal cancer confined to the liver. In one study, 603 patients were treated with laser thermotherapy, and the recurrence rate ranged from 1.9% for patients with small tumors (smaller than 2 cm) to 4.4% for patients with the largest lesions (larger than 4 cm).[253] The median survival from the date of treatment was 2.9 years.

TABLE 97.9	Results of Surgical Resection for Colorectal Cancer Metastatic to the Liver				
Author/Year	Number of Patients	Operative Mortality (%)	3 year	5 year	Reference
Choti/2002	133	—	—	58%	237
Yokoi/2002	116	2	—	51%	238
Belli/2002	181	—	—	40%	239
Minagawa/2003	304	—	51%	36%	240
Bramhall/2003	212	3	54%	28%	241
Cavallari/2003	246	—	75%	47%	242
Shimada/2004	161	—	—	47%	243

Microwave Coagulation. Microwave coagulation therapy is yet another local ablative modality that has been used in the treatment of metastatic colorectal cancer to the liver. One study compared the outcome of patients treated with microwave coagulation alone, microwave coagulation plus surgical resection, or surgical resection alone.[254] The 5-year survival rates for these three modalities were 20%, 24%, and 24%, respectively.

Radiation Therapy. External beam radiation currently plays a very limited role in the management of liver metastases from colorectal cancer because of the liver's inherent radiosensitivity. As mentioned earlier, lifetime doses of greater than 3,000 rads are associated with a high incidence of radiation hepatitis.[100] Fractionated doses of 1,800 to 2,400 rads can provide pain relief for patients with symptomatic metastases. However, external beam radiotherapy does not prolong survival.[255] Radiotherapy has been used in combination with chemotherapy, although it is unclear whether the outcome is superior to that obtained with chemotherapy alone.[256] Recent advances in tumor imaging, external beam radiotherapy techniques that allow for high-precision treatment, and the development of novel radiation sensitizers may improve the outcome of patients treated with external beam radiation in the future.[257] In addition, radioimmunotherapy may ultimately play a role in the treatment of metastatic colorectal cancer to the liver, as some activity has recently been reported with the use of this modality in patients with small-volume disease.[258]

PHARMACOTHERAPY

Systemic Chemotherapy and Biologic Therapy. There have been several recent advances in the systemic treatment of metastatic colorectal cancer. These include the recent approvals of oxaliplatin, the anti-vascular endothelial growth factor monoclonal antibody bevacizumab, and cetuximab, an anti-epidermal growth factor monoclonal antibody. These agents are being used in combination with 5-FU plus leucovorin, capecitabine, irinotecan, mitomycin C, and/or lomustine (CCNU) and are producing response rates of about 40%. Chapter 98 gives a full description of the systemic treatment of metastatic colorectal cancer.

Hepatic Intraarterial Chemotherapy. Hepatic intraarterial chemotherapy has been widely used in the treatment of colorectal cancer metastatic to the liver. (A complete discussion of the rationale for intraarterial chemotherapy is given in the ''Intraarterial Chemotherapy'' section earlier in this chapter.) Table 97.10 summarizes the phase 2 results with single-agent hepatic intraarterial chemotherapy. The most commonly administered agent is floxuridine, in part because it is available in a convenient formulation for use in an implantable pump. It has produced partial responses ranging from 29% to 88% and median survivals ranging from 13 to 26 months.[259–266] In an attempt to augment the activity of intraarterial floxuridine, the addition of intraarterial leucovorin was studied, but the regimen resulted in pro-

hibitive hepatobiliary toxicity.[267] A phase 2 study of intraarterial floxuridine, leucovorin, and dexamethasone showed that the addition of dexamethasone helped to reduce the biliary sclerosis.[268] 5-FU has also been administered by hepatic intraarterial infusion, with response rates ranging from 34% to 67% and a median survival of 9 to 14.3 months.[269–274] The lower solubility of 5-FU (relative to floxuridine) prevents its use in the implantable pump; thus, an external pump and a radiographically placed percutaneous catheter are required to administer the drug by continuous infusion. Recently, small trials have also been conducted with hepatic intraarterial oxaliplatin or irinotecan, resulting in response rates of 46% and 14% to 33%, respectively.[275–278]

To improve on the results obtained with single-agent intraarterial chemotherapy, various combination regimens have been investigated (Table 97.11).[279–293] Unfortunately, the results have been similar to those obtained with single-agent intraarterial therapy, with response rates ranging from 20% to 83% and median survival times ranging from 8 to 22 months.

Seven randomized trials have been conducted comparing hepatic intraarterial floxuridine with systemic chemotherapy or no treatment (Table 97.12).[294–300] All studies showed a

TABLE 97.10	Results of Single-Agent Intraarterial Chemotherapy for Colorectal Cancer Metastatic to the Liver

Drug	Number of Patients	Response Rate (%)	Median Survival (months)	Reference
5-Fluorouracil	145	34	14.3	274
Oxaliplatin	17	46	19	275
Irinotecan	12	33	—	276
	22	14	—	277
	12	42	—	278

TABLE 97.11	Results of Combination Intraarterial Chemotherapy for Colorectal Cancer Metastatic to the Liver

Drug	Number of Patients	Response Rate (%)	Median Survival (months)	Reference
Oxaliplatin+ 5-fluorouracil+ leucovorin	18	59	—	291
Irinotecan+ 5-fluorouracil+ leucovorin	15	38	—	292
5-fluorouracil+ mitomycin C	56	46	—	293

TABLE 97.12	Results of Randomized Trials Comparing Intravenous to Hepatic Intraarterial (IA) Chemotherapy for Colorectal Cancer Metastatic to the Liver			
Author/Year	Number of Patients	Response Rate[a]	Survival (months)[a]	Reference
Lorenz/2000	168	45%/43%/20%	18.7/12.7/17.6	300

[a]Data presented for the IA 5-FU/leucovorin, IA FUDR, and IV 5-FU leucovorin arms of the study, respectively.

significantly higher response rate in the patients treated with intraarterial therapy, and two of the studies reported a survival benefit with intraarterial chemotherapy.[298,299] The two largest studies,[294,295] neither of which found a survival advantage for intraarterial therapy, allowed patients on the intravenous arm to receive intraarterial therapy at the time of hepatic tumor progression, thus confounding the survival analyses. A meta-analysis of the data from six of these seven trials revealed that hepatic intraarterial chemotherapy produced a modest survival advantage compared with intravenous chemotherapy.[301]

Gene Therapy. Recently gene therapy, including mutant gene correction, prodrug activation, immune stimulation, and genetically modified oncolytic viruses, has been explored in the treatment of colorectal cancer. Hepatic intraarterial p53 gene therapy has been investigated for the treatment of colorectal cancer metastatic to the liver. Venook et al[302] administered a single dose of recombinant adenovirus encoding the human wild-type p53 gene by hepatic intraarterial infusion to 16 patients with colorectal cancer metastatic to the liver whose tumor had a mutant p53 gene. Although the single-dose treatment was well tolerated, with fevers being the principal toxicity, no responses were observed. The failure of this and other gene therapies to produce a therapeutic effect in patients with liver metastases from colorectal cancer may be due to poor targeting selectivity of the vectors and inefficient gene transfer.[303] It remains to be seen whether gene therapy will ultimately play a role in the treatment of this disease once improved techniques to enhance the targeting and delivery of gene therapy are available.

ALTERNATIVE THERAPIES

Some patients will take alternative therapies either alone or in combination with standard treatment for liver metastases from colorectal cancer. Several alternative therapies may be pursued, including herbal therapy, nutritional/special diet therapy, manipulation and/or body-base massage, mind–body approaches, energy therapy, and biologic/organic therapy. However, limited clinical trial data exist on the potential benefits and risks of these modalities.

Finally, at some point in the course of disease, a patient with unresectable liver metastases from colorectal cancer may opt not to undergo any further treatment. If the patient has arrived at this decision after being well informed about the various treatment options, this request should be honored. Such patients should be offered supportive care and ultimately directed to a hospice organization at the appropriate time to ensure that they remain as comfortable as possible throughout the remainder of their life.

FUTURE THERAPIES

For a discussion of potential future systemic therapies for colorectal cancer, including liver metastases from colorectal cancer, the reader is referred to Chapter 98. Other potential therapies for colorectal cancer metastatic to the liver may include the development of novel ablative techniques or new approaches to regionally administering existing chemotherapeutic agents. In addition, novel chemotherapeutic agents with demonstrated activity against colorectal cancer may be given regionally to patients with liver metastases. Finally, gene therapy may ultimately play a role in the treatment of colorectal cancer metastatic to the liver.

IMPROVING OUTCOMES

PATIENT EDUCATION

Educating patients about the etiology of colorectal cancer should lead to a decrease in its incidence, although this will take decades to become evident. In addition, education of high-risk patients (e.g., those with ulcerative colitis or familial polyposis) about the importance of screening colonoscopies should result in a decreased incidence of the disease.

Patients with incurable liver metastases should be educated about all the therapeutic alternatives and should be made aware of all the possible adverse effects of treatment; this will help the patient to choose the optimal treatment and will improve patient compliance.

METHODS TO IMPROVE ADHERENCE TO DRUG THERAPIES

Most patients with colorectal cancer metastatic to the liver who desire treatment are highly motivated to comply with their therapy, given that this is a life-threatening illness. In addition, these treatments are typically administered by healthcare professionals rather than the patient, so adherence to the treatment is typically not a problem. Every attempt should be made to minimize the side effects of treatment through the use of appropriate premedications and so forth, as this will improve the acceptability of the treatment to the patient and ensure that the optimal dose intensity can be administered.

DISEASE MANAGEMENT STRATEGIES TO IMPROVE PATIENT OUTCOMES

Until pharmacologic agents are identified that can cure patients with unresectable liver metastases, the key to significantly improving the outcome will remain prevention of the disease and early diagnosis so that surgical removal or ablation can be performed. Finally, for patients with incurable liver metastases, patient outcome should be optimized by educating the patient about all aspects of treatment and ensuring that any adverse events are ameliorated by the use of prophylactic or therapeutic supportive care.

PHARMACOECONOMICS

Agents such as 5-FU (typically administered with leucovorin), floxuridine, and mitomycin C that have activity against liver metastases for colorectal cancer have been commercially available for several years and are relatively inexpensive; however, these agents are also relatively ineffective when administered systemically as single agents. The newer agents, such as irinotecan, oxaliplatin, bevacizumab, and cetuximab, are substantially more expensive. The current pharmacologic treatment of unresectable colorectal cancer metastatic to the liver involves either administering a combination of these drugs or regionally administering these chemotherapeutic agents. Both of these approaches are costly, but these expenses are warranted given the fact that these therapies prolong survival or, in the case of regionally administered chemotherapy, minimize systemic toxicity.

KEY POINTS

- Liver tumors are a diverse group of benign and malignant tumors comprising primary tumors, which arise from the hepatobiliary system, and secondary tumors, which metastasize to the liver from neoplasms elsewhere in the body
- The most prevalent primary malignancy of the liver is HCC, also referred to as hepatoma, and the most common source of hepatic metastases is colorectal cancer
- Complete surgical removal by resection or, for primary malignant tumors, liver transplantation offers a potential for cure of malignant liver tumors and should be performed whenever feasible
- Unfortunately, surgical removal is feasible in only approximately 10% to 15% of patients; of those patients, only approximately 30% are cured

- Cryosurgery, radiofrequency ablation, and percutaneous alcohol injection are three modalities that are useful in patients with potentially resectable disease who are not candidates for surgical removal because of underlying liver disease, such as cirrhosis
- Several therapies have been used to treat patients with unresectable malignant liver tumors. Radiotherapy has been used, but it is of limited benefit because of the inherent intolerance of the normal hepatic parenchyma to radiation. Systemic chemotherapy has been used, but it produces responses in only 15% to 35% of patients
- In patients who have liver-predominant disease, more encouraging results have been obtained with liver-directed therapies such as hepatic intraarterial chemotherapy with or without Lipiodol and chemoembolization
- Further research is required to develop more efficacious therapies for liver tumors
- HCC is the most common primary malignant tumor of the liver in adults. It is relatively uncommon in the United States but is very prevalent in Asia, sub-Saharan Africa, and the South Pacific islands
- HCC is frequently associated with preexisting liver disease. Chronic active hepatitis B infection is the most important predisposing factor worldwide. In addition, hepatitis C infection, exposure to aflatoxin B1 or sex hormones, and certain inherited metabolic disorders predispose patients to developing HCC
- Whenever feasible, the goal of HCC therapy should be to cure the patient by surgical removal via either resection or transplantation or locally ablating the tumor via an approach, such as radiofrequency ablation
- When cure of HCC is not feasible, either because of extensive hepatic involvement or the presence of extrahepatic metastases, the goal of treatment should be to treat patients desiring therapy with a modality that has a reasonable chance of producing a response while maintaining the patient's quality of life. Patients with disease predominately confined to the liver may be treated with either liver-directed therapies, such as chemoembolization or hepatic intraarterial chemotherapy, or systemic chemotherapy. Patients with significant extrahepatic disease may be treated with systemic chemotherapy
- Colorectal cancer is the most common metastatic tumor to the liver
- Whenever feasible, the goal of therapy for patients with colon cancer metastatic to the liver should be to cure the patient by surgical removal with or without adjuvant chemotherapy or a treatment modality that causes local tumor necrosis, such as radiofrequency ablation
- When cure is not feasible for patients with colorectal cancer metastatic to the liver, either because of extensive hepatic involvement or the presence of extrahepatic metastases, the goal of treatment should be to treat patients desiring therapy with a modality that has

a reasonable chance of producing a response while maintaining the patient's quality of life. Patients with metastatic disease confined to the liver may be treated with hepatic intraarterial chemotherapy or systemic chemotherapy. Patients with significant extrahepatic disease may be treated with systemic chemotherapy

SUGGESTED READINGS

Allegra CJ, Lawrence TS. Metastatic cancer to the liver. In: DeVita VT, Hellman S, Rosenberg SA, eds. Cancer: principles and practice of oncology, 6th ed. Philadelphia: Lippincott Williams & Wilkins, 2001: 2690–2713.

Fong Y, Kemeny N, Lawrence TS. Cancer of the liver and biliary tree. In: DeVita VT, Hellman S, Rosenberg SA, eds. Cancer: principles and practice of oncology, 6th ed. Philadelphia: Lippincott Williams & Wilkins, 2001:1162–1203.

REFERENCES

1. Bierman HR, Byron RL Jr, Kelly LH, et al. Studies on the blood supply of tumors in man: III. Vascular patterns of the liver by hepatic arteriography in vivo. JNCI 12:107–227, 1951.
2. Tsai HP, Jeng LB, Lee WC, et al. Clinical experience of hepatic hemangioma undergoing hepatic resection. Dig Dis Sci 48: 916–920, 2003.
3. Zagoria RJ, Roth TJ, Levine EA, et al. Radiofrequency ablation of a symptomatic hepatic cavernous hemangioma. AJR Am J Roentgenol 182:210–212, 2004.
4. Yohannan MD, Abdulla AM, Patel PJ. Neonatal hepatic hemangioendothelioma: presentation with jaundice and microangiopathic hemolytic anemia. Eur J Pediatr 149:804–805, 1990.
5. Warmann S, Bertram H, Kardorff R, et al. Interventional treatment of infantile hepatic hemangioendothelioma. J Pediatr Surg 38: 1177–1181, 2003.
6. Samuel M, Spitz L. Infantile hepatic hemangioendothelioma: the role of surgery. J Pediatr Surg 30:1425–1429, 1995.
7. Nichols FC, van Heerden JA, Weiland LH. Benign liver tumors. Surg Clin North Am 69:297–314, 1989.
8. Gordon SC, Reddy KR, Livingstone AS, et al. Resolution of a contraceptive steroid-induced hepatic adenoma with subsequent evolution into hepatocellular carcinoma. Ann Intern Med 105:547–549, 1986.
9. Wanless JR, Mawdsley C, Adams R. On the pathogenesis of focal nodular hyperplasia of the liver. Hepatology 5:1194–1200, 1985.
10. Landen S, Siriser F, Bardoxoglou E, et al. Focal nodular hyperplasia of the liver. A retrospective review of 20 patients managed surgically. Acta Chir Belg 93:94–97, 1993.
11. Shim TH, Park HJ, Choi MS, et al. Hypermethylation of the p16 gene and lack of p16 expression in hepatoblastoma. Mod Pathol 16:430–436, 2003.
12. Seo T, Ando H, Watonabe Y, et al. Treatment of hepatoblastoma: less extensive hepatic resection after effective preoperative chemotherapy with cisplatin and Adriamycin. Surgery 123:407–414, 1998.
13. Evans AE, Land VJ, Newton WA, et al. Combination chemotherapy (vincristine, Adriamycin, cyclophosphamide, 5-fluorouracil) in the treatment of children with hepatoblastoma. Cancer 50:821–826, 1982.
14. Cillo U, Ciarleglio FA, Bassanello M, et al. Liver transplantation for the management of hepatoblastoma. Transplant Proc 35: 2983–2985, 2003.
15. Xianliang H, Jianhong L, Xuewu J, et al. Cure of hepatoblastoma with transcatheter arterial chemoembolization. J Pediatr Hematol Oncol 26:60–63, 2004.
16. Palmer RD, Williams DM. Dramatic response of multiply relapsed hepatoblastoma to irinotecan (CPT-11). Med Pediatr Oncol 41: 78–80, 2003.
17. Kondo S, Hirano S, Ambo Y, et al. Forty consecutive resections of hilar cholangiocarcinoma with no postoperative mortality and no positive ductal margins: results of a prospective study. Ann Surg 240:95–101, 2004.
18. Heimbach JK, Gores GJ, Haddock MG, et al. Liver transplantation for unresectable perihilar cholangiocarcinoma. Semin Liver Dis 24: 201–207, 2004.
19. Harvey JH, Smith FP, Schein PS. 5-Fluorouracil, mitomycin, and doxorubicin (FAM) in carcinoma of the biliary tract. J Clin Oncol 2:1245–1248, 1984.
20. Smith GW, Bukowski RM, Hewlett JS, et al. Hepatic artery infusion of 5-fluorouracil and mitomycin C in cholangiocarcinoma and gallbladder carcinoma. Cancer 54:1513–1516, 1984.
21. Locker GY, Doroshow JG, Zwelling LA, et al. The clinical features of hepatic angiosarcoma: a report of four cases and a review of the English literature. Medicine (Balt) 58:48–64, 1979.
22. Azodo MV, Gutierrez OH, Greer T. Thorotrast-induced ruptured hepatic angiosarcoma. Abdom Imaging 18:78–81, 1993.
23. Dean PJ, Haggett RC, O'Hara CJ. Malignant epithelioid hemangioendothelioma of the liver in young women. Relationship to oral contraceptive use. Am J Surg Pathol 9:695–704, 1985.
24. Walker NI, Horn MJ, Strong RW, et al. Undifferentiated (embryonal) sarcoma of the liver. Pathologic findings and long-term survival after complete surgical resection. Cancer 69:52–59, 1992.
25. Kim DY, Kim KH, Jung SE, et al. Undifferentiated (embryonal) sarcoma of the liver: combination treatment by surgery and chemotherapy. J Pediatr Surg 37:1419–1423, 2002.
26. Jemal A, Tiwari RC, Murray T. Cancer statistics, 2004. CA Cancer J Clin 54:8–29, 2004.
27. Moertel CG. The liver. In: Holland JF, Frei E III, eds. Cancer medicine. Philadelphia: Lea & Febiger, 1973:1541–1547.
28. Popper G, Gerber MA, Thung SN. The relation of hepatocellular carcinoma to infection with hepatitis B and related viruses in man and animals. Hepatology 2:1S–9S, 1982.
29. Zala G, Havelka J, Altorfer J, et al. Hepatitis C and hepatoma. Schweiz Med Wochenschr 122:194–197, 1992.
30. Hassan F, Jeffers LJ, De Medina M, et al. Hepatitis C-associated hepatocellular carcinoma. Hepatology 12:589–591, 1990.
31. Kiyosawa K, Sodeyama T, Tanaka E, et al. Interrelationship of blood transfusion, non-A non-B hepatitis and hepatocellular carcinoma: analysis by detection of antibody to hepatitis C virus. Hepatology 12:671–675, 1990.
32. Gerbes AL, Caselmann WH. Point mutations of the p53 gene, human hepatocellular carcinoma and aflatoxins. J Hepatol 19: 312–315, 1993.
33. Palmer JR, Rosenberg L, Kaufmann DW, et al. Oral contraceptive use and liver cancer. Am J Epidemiol 130:878–882, 1989.
34. Farrell GC, Uren RF, Perkins RW, et al. Androgen induced hepatoma. Lancet 1:430–431, 1975.
35. Okuda K, Musha H, Nakajima Y, et al. Clinicopathologic features of encapsulated hepatocellular carcinoma: a study of 26 cases. Cancer 40:1240–1245, 1977.
36. Ruffin MT. Fibrolamellar hepatoma. Am J Gastroenterol 85: 577–581, 1990.
37. Li D, Mallory T, Satomura S. AFP-L3: a new generation of tumor marker for hepatocellular carcinoma. Clin Chim Acta 313; 215–219, 2001.
38. Okuda K, Ohtsuki T, Obata H. Natural history of hepatocellular carcinoma and prognosis in relation to treatment. Study of 850 patients. Cancer 56:918–928, 1985.
39. Salminen PM, Hockerstedt K, Edgren J, et al. Intraoperative ultrasound as an aid to surgical strategy in liver tumors. Acta Chir Scand 156:329–332, 1990.
40. Stuver SO. Toward global control of liver cancer? Semin Cancer Biol 8:299–306, 1998.
41. Xu ZY, Liu CB, Francis DP, et al. Prevention of perinatal acquisition of hepatitis B virus carriage using vaccine: preliminary report of a randomized, double-blind placebo-controlled and comparative trial. Pediatrics 76:713–718, 1985.
42. Sun ZT, Zhu Y, Stjernsward, et al. Design and compliance of HBV vaccination trial on newborns to prevent hepatocellular carcinoma and 5-year results of its pilot study. Cancer Detect Prev 15: 313–318, 1991.

43. Fortuin M, Chotard J, Jack AD, et al. Efficacy of hepatitis B vaccine in the Gambian expanded programme on immunization. Lancet 341:1129–1131, 1993.
44. Chang MH, Chen CK, Lai MS, et al. Universal hepatitis B vaccination in Taiwan and the incidence of hepatocellular carcinoma in children. Taiwan Childhood Hepatoma Study Group. N Engl J Med 336:1855–1859, 1997.
45. Ginsburg GM, Shouval D. Cost benefit analysis of a nationwide neonatal inoculation programme against hepatitis B in an area of intermediate endemicity. J Epidemiol Commun Health 46:587–594, 1992.
46. Ikeda K, Saitoh S, Suzuki Y, et al. Interferon decreases hepatocellular carcinogenesis in patients with cirrhosis caused by the hepatitis B virus: a pilot study. Cancer 82:827–835, 1998.
47. Recommendations for prevention and control of hepatitis C virus (HCV) infection and HCV-related chronic disease. Centers for Disease Control and Prevention. MMWR Morb Mortal Wkly Rep 47:1–39, 1998.
48. McMahon BJ, London T. Workshop on screening for hepatocellular carcinoma. J Natl Cancer Inst 83:916–919, 1991.
49. Dodd GD, Miller WJ, Baron RL, et al. Detection of malignant tumors in end-stage cirrhotic livers: efficacy of sonography as a screening technique. AJR Am J Roentgenol 159:727–733, 1992.
50. Nguyen MH, Keeffe EB. Screening for hepatocellular carcinoma. J Clin Gastroenterol 35 (5 Suppl 2):S86–91, 2002.
51. Arguedas MR. Screening for hepatocellular carcinoma: why, when, how? Curr Gastroenterol Rep 5:57–62, 2003.
52. Okuda K and the Liver Tumor Study Group of Japan. Primary liver cancers in Japan. Cancer 45:2663–2669, 1980.
53. Prospective validation of the CLIP score: a new prognostic system for patients with cirrhosis and hepatocellular carcinoma. The Cancer of the Liver Italian Program (CLIP) Investigators. Hepatology 31:840–845, 2000.
54. Leung TW, Tang AM, Zee B, et al. Construction of the Chinese University Prognostic Index for hepatocellular carcinoma and comparison with the TNM staging system, the Okuda staging system, and the Cancer of the Liver Italian Program staging system: a study based on 926 patients. Cancer 94:1760–1769, 2002.
55. Toshihara T, Sugioka A, Veda M, et al. Hepatic resection for hepatocellular carcinoma. Surgery 107:551–560, 1990.
56. Choi TK, Edward CS, Fan ST, et al. Results of surgical resection for hepatocellular carcinoma. Hepatogastroenterology 37:172–175, 1990.
57. Yamanaka N, Okamoto, E, Toyosaka A, et al. Prognostic factors after hepatectomy for hepatocellular carcinomas. A univariate and multivariate analysis. Cancer 65:1104–1110, 1990.
58. Kobayashi N, Kumada K, Yamaoka Y, et al. The outcomes of the operated hepatocellular carcinoma patients. Nippon Geka Hokan 59:369–376, 1990.
59. Tsuzuki T, Sugioka A, Ueda M, et al. Hepatic resection for hepatocellular carcinoma. Surgery 107:511–520, 1990.
60. Iwatsuki S, Starzl TW, Sheahan DG, et al. Hepatic resection versus transplantation for hepatocellular carcinoma. Ann Surg 214:221–229, 1991.
61. Gozzetti G, Mazziotti A, Grazi GL, et al. Surgical experience with 168 primary liver cell carcinomas treated with hepatic resection. J Surg Oncol 3 (Suppl):59–61, 1993.
62. Kawarada Y, Ito F, Sakurai H, et al. Surgical treatment of hepatocellular carcinoma. Cancer Chemother Pharmacol 33:S7–S12, 1994.
63. Tani M, Edamoto Y, Kawai S, et al. Results of 90 consecutive hepatectomies for hepatocellular carcinoma: a multivariate analysis of survival. Semin Oncol 24:S6–S16, 1997.
64. Yamasaki S, Makuuchi M, Hasegawa H. Results of hepatectomy for hepatocellular carcinoma at the National Cancer Center Hospital. HPB Surg 3:235–249, 1991.
65. Nagashima I, Hamada C, Naruse K, et al. Surgical resection for small hepatocellular carcinoma. Surgery 119:40–45, 1996.
66. Takenaka K, Kawahara N, Yamamoto K, et al. Results of 280 liver resections for hepatocellular carcinoma. Arch Surg 131:71–76, 1996.
67. Chen MF, Jeng LB. Partial hepatic resection for hepatocellular carcinoma. J Gastroenterol Hepatol 12:S329–S334, 1997.
68. Makuuchi M, Takayama T, Kubota K, et al. Hepatic resection for hepatocellular carcinoma: Japanese experience. Hepatogastroenterology 45:1267–1274, 1998.
69. Takayama T, Makuuchi M, Yamasaki S, et al. Systemic resection for hepatocellular carcinoma. Nippon Geka Gakkai Zasshi 99:241–244, 1998.
70. Lise M, Bacchetti S, Da Pian PD, et al. Prognostic factors affecting long-term outcome after liver resection for hepatocellular carcinoma. Cancer 82:1028–1036, 1998.
71. Philosophe B, Greig PD, Hemming AW, et al. Surgical management of hepatocellular carcinoma: resection or transplantation? J Gastrointest Surg 2:21–27, 1998.
72. Grazi GL, Ercolani G, Pierangeli F, et al. Improved results of liver resection for hepatocellular carcinoma on cirrhosis give the procedure added value. Ann Surg 234:71–78, 2001.
73. Kanematsu T, Furui J, Yanaga K, et al. A 16-year experience in performing hepatic resection in 303 patients with hepatocellular carcinoma: 1985–2000. Surgery 131 (1 Suppl):S153–158, 2002.
74. Belghiti J, Regimbeau JM, Kianmanesh AR, et al. Resection of hepatocellular carcinoma: a European experience of 328 cases. Hepatogastroenterology 49:41–46, 2002.
75. Mo QG, Liang AM, Yang NW, et al. Surgery-predominant comprehensive therapy for 134 patients with small hepatocellular carcinoma. Ai Zheng 22:189–191, 2003.
76. Shimozawa N, Hanakaki K. Long-term prognosis after hepatic resection for small hepatocellular carcinoma. J Am Coll Surg 198:356–365, 2004.
77. Ramsey DE, Kernagis LY, Soulen MC, et al. Chemoembolization of hepatocellular carcinoma. J Vasc Interv Radiol 13:S211–221, 2002.
78. Nakashima K, Kim Y, Okada K, et al. Prophylactic chemotherapy by regional arterial infusion in resected hepatoma patients. Gan To Kagaku Ryoho 19 (Suppl):1489–1492, 1992.
79. Lai EC, Lo CM, Fan ST, et al. Postoperative adjuvant chemotherapy after curative resection of hepatocellular carcinoma: a randomized controlled trial. Arch Surg 133:183–188, 1998.
80. Mazzaferro V, Regalia E, Doci R, et al. Liver transplantation for the treatment of small hepatocellular carcinomas in patients with cirrhosis. N Engl J Med 334:693–699, 1996.
81. Vauthey JN, Ajani JA. Liver transplantation and hepatocellular carcinoma biology: beginning of the end of the era of educated guesses. J Clin Oncol 21:4265–4266, 2003.
82. Yoo HY, Patt CH, Geschwind JF, et al. The outcome of liver transplantation in patients with hepatocellular carcinoma in the United States between 1987 and 2001: 5-year survival has improved significantly with time. J Clin Oncol 21:4329–4335, 2003.
83. Lee YT, Irwin L. Hepatic artery ligation and Adriamycin infusion chemotherapy for hepatoma. Cancer 41:12459–12555, 1978.
84. Nagasue N, Inokuchi K, Kobayashi M, et al. Serum alpha-fetoprotein levels after hepatic artery ligation and postoperative chemotherapy: correlation with clinical status in patients with hepatocellular carcinoma. Cancer 40:615–618, 1997.
85. Charnsangavej C, Chuang VP, Wallace S, et al. Angiographic classification of hepatic arterial collaterals. Radiology 144:485–494, 1982.
86. Chearanai O, Plengvanit U, Asavanich C, et al. Spontaneous rupture of primary hepatoma: report of 63 cases with particular reference to the pathogenesis and rationale treatment by hepatic artery ligation. Cancer 51:1532–1536, 1983.
87. Soyer P, Levesque M, Zeittoun G, et al. Hemoperitoneum caused spontaneous rupture of hepatocellular carcinoma. Role of hepatic artery embolization in the therapeutic procedure. J Radiol 72:287–290, 1991.
88. Lewin JS, Connell CF, Duerk JL, et al. Interactive MRI-guided radiofrequency interstitial thermal ablation of abdominal tumors: clinical trial for evaluation of safety and feasibility. J Magn Reson Imaging 8:40–47, 1998.
89. Tarantino GA, de Stefano G, Scala V, et al. Percutaneous sonographically guided saline-enhanced radiofrequency ablation of hepatocellular carcinoma. AJR Am J Roentgenol 181:479–484, 2003.
90. Ruzzenente GA, Battocchia A, Tonon A, et al. Radiofrequency ablation of hepatocellular carcinoma in cirrhotic patients. Hepatogastroenterology 50:480–484, 2003.

91. Vivarelli M, Guglielmi A, Ruzzenente, et al. Surgical resection versus percutaneous radiofrequency ablation in the treatment of hepatocellular carcinoma on cirrhotic liver. Ann Surg 240:102–107, 2004.

92. Ravikumar TS, Steele GS. Hepatic cryosurgery. Surg Clin North Am 69:433–440, 1989.

93. Zhou XD, Tang ZY, Yu YQ, et al. Clinical evaluation of cryosurgery in the treatment of primary liver cancer. Cancer 61:1889–1892, 1988.

94. Dong B, Liang P, Yu X, et al. Percutaneous sonographically guided microwave coagulation therapy for hepatocellular carcinoma: results in 234 patients. AJR Am J Roentgenol 180:1547–1555, 2003.

95. Chistophi C, Muralidharan V. Treatment of hepatocellular carcinoma by percutaneous laser hyperthermia. J Gastroenterol Hepatol 16:548–552, 2001.

96. Castells A, Bruix J, Bru C, et al. Treatment of small hepatocellular carcinoma in cirrhotic patients: a cohort study comparing surgical resection and percutaneous ethanol injection. Hepatology 18:1121–1126, 1993.

97. Ebara M, Kita K, Nagato Y, et al. Percutaneous ethanol injection for small hepatocellular carcinoma. Gan To Kagaku Ryoho 20:884–888, 1993.

98. Isobe H, Sakai H, Imari Y, et al. Intratumor ethanol injection therapy for solitary minute hepatocellular carcinoma. A study of 37 patients. J Clin Gastroenterol 18:122–126, 1994.

99. Huo TI, Huang YH, Wu JC, et al. Comparison of percutaneous acetic acid injection and percutaneous ethanol injection for hepatocellular carcinoma in cirrhotic patients: a prospective study. Scand J Gastroenterol 38:770–778, 2003.

100. Ingold JA, Reed GB, Kaplan HS, et al. Radiation hepatitis. AJR Am J Roentgenol 93:200–208, 1965.

101. Phillips R, Murikama K. Primary neoplasms of the liver. Results of radiation therapy. Cancer 4:714–720, 1960.

102. Lawrence TS, Tesser RJ, Ten Haken RK. An application of dose volume histograms to the treatment of intrahepatic malignancies with radiation therapy. Int J Radiat Oncol Biol Phys 20:555–561, 1991.

103. Robertson JM, Lawrence TS, Dworzanin LM, et al. Treatment of primary hepatobiliary cancers with conformal radiation therapy and regional chemotherapy. J Clin Oncol 11:1286–1293, 1993.

104. Order S, Pajak T, Leibel S, et al. A randomized prospective trial comparing full dose chemotherapy to 131 I antiferritin: an RTOG study. Int J Radiat Oncol Biol Phys 20:953–963, 1991.

105. Leung WT, Lau WY, HO S, et al. Selective internal radiation therapy with intraarterial 131-iodine-Lipiodol in inoperable hepatocellular carcinoma. Proc Am Soc Clin Oncol 13:202, 1994.

106. Boucher EJ, Marchetti C, Roland R, et al. Curative intraarterial 131-iodine-labeled lipiodol: an alternative for patients with hepatocellular carcinoma. Proc Am Soc Clin Oncol 20:665, 2001.

107. Carr BI. Advanced, unresectable hepatocellular carcinoma (HCC): responses and long-term survival after 90-Yttrium microspheres (Theraspheres) treatment in 80 patients. Proc Am Soc Clin Oncol 23:4085, 2004.

108. Vogel CL, Bayley AC, Brockes RJ. A phase II study of Adriamycin in patients with hepatocellular carcinoma from Zambia and the United States. Cancer 39:1923–1929, 1977.

109. Johnson PJ, Williams R, Thomas H, et al. Induction of remission in hepatocellular carcinoma with doxorubicin. Lancet 1:1006–1009, 1978.

110. Falkson G, Lavin P, Moertel CG, et al. Chemotherapy studies in primary liver cancer: a prospective randomized clinical trial. Cancer 42:2149–2156, 1978.

111. Olweny CLM, Katongole-Mbidde E, Bahendeka S, et al. Further experience in treating patients with hepatocellular carcinoma in Uganda. Cancer 46:2717–2722, 1980.

112. Melia WM, Johnson PJ, Williams R. Induction remission in hepatocellular carcinoma: a comparison of VP-16 with Adriamycin. Cancer 51:206–210, 1983.

113. Yang P, Sheu J, Chen D, et al. Systemic chemotherapy of hepatocellular carcinoma with Adriamycin alone and FAM regimen. In: Chemotherapy of hepatic tumors. Tokyo: Excerpta Medica, 1984:41–47.

114. Chlebowski RT, Brezechwa-Asjukiewicz A, Cowdon A, et al. Doxorubicin for hepatocellular carcinoma: clinical and pharmacokinetic results. Cancer Treat Rep 68:487–491, 1984.

115. Choi TK, Lee NW, Wong J, et al. Chemotherapy for advanced hepatocellular carcinoma: clinical and pharmacokinetic results. Cancer Treat Rep 68:487– 491, 1984.

116. Sciarrino E, Simonetti RG, Moli SL, et al. Adriamycin treatment for hepatocellular carcinoma: experience with 109 patients. Cancer 56:2751–2755, 1985.

117. Dunk AA, Scott SC, Johnson PJ, et al. Mitoxantrone as single agent therapy in hepatocellular carcinoma: a phase II study. J Hepatol 1:395–404, 1985.

118. Lai KH, Tsai YT, Lee SD, et al. Phase II study of mitoxantrone in unresectable primary hepatocellular carcinoma following hepatitis B infection. Cancer Chemother Pharmacol 23:54–56, 1989.

119. Hochester HS, Green MD, Speyer J, et al. 4'-Epidoxorubicin (epirubicin) activity in hepatocellular carcinoma. J Clin Oncol 3:1525–1540, 1985.

120. Tan YO, Lim F. 4'-Epidoxorubicin as a single agent in advanced primary hepatocellular carcinoma: a preliminary experience. Ann Acad Med Singapore 15:169–171, 1986.

121. Shiu W, Leung N, Li M, et al. The efficacy of high dose 4'-epidoxorubicin in hepatocellular carcinoma. Jpn J Clin Oncol 18:235–237, 1988.

122. Kennedy PS, Lehane DE, Smith FE, et al. Oral fluorouracil therapy of hepatoma. Cancer 39:1930–1935, 1977.

123. Link JS, Bateman JR, Paroly WS, et al. 5-Fluorouracil in hepatocellular carcinoma: report of 21 cases. Cancer 39:1936–1939, 1977.

124. Davis HL, Ramirez H, Ansfield FJ. Adenocarcinomas of the stomach, pancreas, liver, and biliary tracts: survival of 328 patients treated with fluoropyrimidine therapy. Cancer 33:193–197, 1974.

125. Al-Sarraf M, Go TS, Kithier K, et al. Primary liver cancer: a review of the clinical features, blood groups, serum enzymes, therapy and survival of 65 cases. Cancer 33:574–582, 1974.

126. Tetef M, Doroshow J, Akman S, et al. 5-Fluorouracil and high-dose calcium leucovorin for hepatocellular carcinoma: a phase II trial. Cancer Invest 13:460–463, 1995.

127. Bukowski RM, Legna S, Saidi J, et al. Phase II trial of m-AMSA in hepatocellular carcinoma: a Southwest Oncology Group Study. Cancer Treat Rep 66:1651–1652, 1982.

128. Cheng E, Lightdale C, Young C, et al. Phase II trial of (m-AMSA) 4'-9 (acridinylamino)-methane-sulfon-m-aniside in primary liver cancer. Am Clin Oncol 6:211–213, 1983.

129. Amrein PC, Richards F, Coleman M, et al. Phase II trial of Amsacrine in patients with hepatoma: a Cancer and Leukemia Group B study. Cancer Treat Rep 68:923–924, 1984.

130. Falkson G, Coetzer B, Klaasen DJ. A phase II study of m-AMSA in patients with primary liver cancer. Cancer Chemother Pharmacol 8:305–310, 1982.

131. Vogel CL, Adamson RH, DeVita VT, et al. Preliminary clinical trials of dichloromethotrexate (NSC-29630) in hepatocellular carcinoma. Cancer Chemother Rep 56:249–258, 1972.

132. Tester WJ, Donehower RS, Eddy JL, et al. Evaluation of weekly escalating doses of dichloromethotrexate in patients with hepatocellular carcinoma and other solid tumors. Cancer Chemother Pharmacol 8:305–310, 1982.

133. Cavalli F, Rosenzweig M, Renard J, et al. A phase II study of oral VP-16-213 in patients with hepatocellular carcinoma. Proc Am Soc Clin Oncol 22:457, 1981.

134. Melia WM, Westaby D, Williams R. Diaminodichloride platinum (cisplatinum) in treatment of hepatocellular carcinoma. Clin Oncol 7:275–280, 1981.

135. Okada S, Okazaki N, Nose H, et al. A phase 2 study of cisplatin in patients with hepatocellular carcinoma. Oncology 50:22–26, 1993.

136. Gastrointestinal Tumor Study Group. A prospective trial of recombinant human interferon 2B in previously untreated patients with hepatocellular carcinoma. Cancer 66:135–139, 1990.

137. Lai LL, Wu PL, Lok AS, et al. Recombinant alpha-2-interferon is superior to doxorubicin for inoperable hepatocellular carcinoma: a prospective randomized trial. J Pharmacokinet Biopharm 2:257–285, 1974.

138. Yen T, Doroshow J, Leong L, et al. Phase II study of oxaliplatin in patients with unresectable, metastatic or recurrent hepatocellular carcinoma. Proc Am Soc Clin Oncol 23:4169, 2004.

139. Guan Z, Wang Y, Maoleekoonpairoj S, et al. Prospective randomized phase II study of gemcitabine at standard or fixed dose rate

schedule in unresectable hepatocellular carcinoma. Br J Cancer 89: 1865–1869, 2003.

140. Yeo W, Zee B, Leung WT, et al. A phase III study of doxorubicin (A) versus cisplatin (P), interferonα-2b (I), doxorubicin (A), fluorourial (F) combination chemotherapy for inoperable hepatocellular carcinoma (HCC). Proc Am Soc Clin Oncol 23:4026, 2004.

141. Eckman WW, Patlak CS, Fenstermacher JD. A critical evaluation of the principles governing the advantages of intraarterial infusions. J Pharmacokinet Biopharm 2:257–285, 1974.

142. Chen HG, Gross JF. Intraarterial infusion of anticancer drugs: theoretical aspects of drug delivery and review of responses. Cancer Treat Rep 64:31–40, 1980.

143. Ensminger WS, Rosowsky A, Raso V, et al. A clinical pharmacologic evaluation of hepatic arterial infusions of 5-fluoro-2′-deoxyuridine and 5-fluorouracil. Cancer Res 38:3784–3792, 1978.

144. Garnick MB, Ensminger WD, Israel M. A clinical pharmacologic evaluation of hepatic arterial infusion of Adriamycin. Cancer Res 39:4105–4110, 1979.

145. Fraile RJ, Baker LH, Buroker TR, et al. Pharmacokinetics of 5-fluorouracil administered orally, by rapid intravenous and by slow infusion. Cancer Res 40:2223–2228, 1980.

146. Ensminger W, Stetson P, Gyves J, et al. Dependence of hepatic arterial fluorouracil pharmacokinetics on dose, route and duration of infusion. Proc Am Soc Clin Oncol 2:25, 1983.

147. Campbell TN, Howell SB, Pfeifle CE, et al. Clinical pharmacokinetics of intraarterial cisplatin in humans. J Clin Oncol 12: 755–762, 1983.

148. Gyves JL, Ensminger W, Stetson P, et al. Clinical pharmacology of mitomycin C by hepatic arterial infusion. Proc Am Soc Clin Oncol 2:25, 1983.

149. Guthoff I, Lotspeich E, Fester C, et al. Hepatic artery infusion using oxaliplatin in combination with 5-fluorouracil, folinic acid and mitomycin C: oxaliplatin pharmacokinetics and feasibility. Anticancer Res 23:5203–5208, 2003.

150. Wellwood JM, Cady B, Oberfield RA. Treatment of primary liver cancer: response on regional chemotherapy. Clin Oncol 5:25–31, 1979.

151. Ludwig J, Kim CH, Wiesner RH, et al. Floxuridine-induced sclerosing cholangitis: an ischemic cholangiopathy. Hepatology 9: 215–219, 1989.

152. Doci R, Bignami P, Bozzetti F, et al. Intrahepatic chemotherapy for unresectable hepatocellular carcinoma. Cancer 61:1983–1987, 1988.

153. Bern MM, McDermott W, Cady B. Intraarterial hepatic infusion and intravenous Adriamycin for treatment of hepatocellular carcinoma: a clinical and pharmacology report. Cancer 42:399–406, 1978.

154. Urist MM, Balch CM. Intraarterial chemotherapy for hepatoma using Adriamycin administered via an implantable infusion pump. Proc Am Soc Clin Oncol 3:146, 1983.

155. Shepherd FA, Evans WK, Fine S, et al. Hepatic arterial infusion of mitoxantrone and Adriamycin in the treatment of primary hepatocellular carcinoma. Proc Am Soc Clin Oncol 4:95, 1985.

156. Ukeda H, Kuroda S, Ohnoshi T, et al. Intraarterial Adriamycin for patients with hepatocellular carcinoma and metastatic carcinoma. Gan To Kagaka Ryoho 11:2579–2584, 1984.

157. Cheng E, Watson RC, Fortner J, et al. Regional intraarterial infusion of cisplatin in primary liver cancer. Proc Am Soc Clin Oncol 1:179, 1982.

158. Onohara S, Kobayashi H, Itoh Y, et al. Intraarterial cisplatinum infusion with sodium thiosulfate protection and angiotensin II-induced hypertension for treatment of hepatocellular carcinoma. Acta Radiol 29:197–202, 1988.

159. Kajanti M, Riassanen P, Kirkkunen P, et al. Regional intraarterial infusion of cisplatin in primary hepatocellular carcinoma. A phase II study. Cancer 58:2386–2388, 1986.

160. Shepherd FA, Evan WK, Blackstein ME, et al. Hepatic artery infusion of mitoxantrone in the treatment of primary hepatocellular carcinoma. J Clin Oncol 5:635–640, 1987.

161. Shepherd FA, Evans WK, Blackstein ME, et al. Hepatic arterial infusion of mitoxantrone in the treatment of primary hepatocellular carcinoma. J Clin Oncol 5:635–640, 1987.

162. Ando K, Kirai K, Kubo Y, et al. Intraarterial administration of epirubicin in the treatment of nonresectable hepatocellular carcinoma.

Epirubicin Study Group for Hepatocellular Carcinoma. Cancer Chemother Pharmacol 19:183–189, 1987.

163. Malik IA, Khan WA, Haq S, et al. A prospective phase II trial to evaluate the efficacy and toxicity of hepatic arterial infusion of ifosfamide in patients with inoperable localized hepatocellular carcinoma. Am J Clin Oncol 20:289–292, 1997.

164. Douglas CC. Prolongation of survival with periodic percutaneous multidrug arterial infusions in patients with primary and metastatic gastrointestinal carcinoma to the liver. Proc Am Soc Clin Oncol 21:416, 1980.

165. Patt YZ, Chuang VP, Wallace S, et al. Hepatic artery chemotherapy and occlusion for palliation of primary hepatocellular and unknown primary neoplasms in the liver. Cancer 51:1359–1363, 1983.

166. Patt YZ, Charnsangavej C, Lawrence D, et al. Hepatic arterial infusion for FUDR, leucovorin, Adriamycin, and Platinol: effective palliation for nonresectable hepatocellular carcinoma. Proc Am Soc Clin Oncol 11:165, 1992.

167. Kanematsu T, Matsumata T, Furuta T, et al. Lipiodol drug targeting in the treatment of primary hepatocellular carcinoma. Hepatogastroenterology 37:442–444, 1990.

168. Okusaka T, Okada S, Ishii H, et al. Transarterial chemotherapy with zinostatin stimalamer for hepatocellular carcinoma. Oncology 55:276–283, 1998.

169. Carr B, Iwatsuki S, Baron R. Intrahepatic arterial cisplatinum and doxorubicin with or without Lipiodol for advanced hepatocellular carcinoma: a prospective randomized study. Proc Am Soc Clin Oncol 12:219, 1993.

170. Hsu C, Chen LT, Lai MY, et al. Comparison of the antitumor activity of thalidomide between hepatitic B and hepatitis C-related hepatocellular carcinoma. Proc Am Soc Clin Oncol 23:4198, 2004.

171. Schwart JD, Schwartz M, Goldman J, et al. Bevacizumab in hepatocellular carcinoma in patients without metastases and without invasion of the portal vein. Proc Am Soc Clin Oncol 23:4088, 2004.

172. Friedman MA, Demanes DJ, Hoffman PG. Hepatomas: hormone receptors and therapy. Am J Med 73:362–366, 1982.

173. Paliard P, Clement G, Saez S, et al. Treatment of hepatocellular carcinoma with tamoxifen [letter]. Gastroenterol Clin Biol 8: 680–681, 1984.

174. Riestra S, Rodriquez M, Delgado M, et al. Tamoxifen does not improve survival of patients with advanced hepatocellular carcinoma. J Clin Gastroenterol 26:200–203, 1998.

175. Chow PK, Tai BC, Tan CK, et al. High-dose tamoxifen in the treatment of inoperable hepatocellular carcinoma: a multicenter randomized controlled trial. Hepatology 36:1221–1226, 2002.

176. Barbare JC, Milan C, Bouche O, et al. Treatment of advanced hepatocellular carcinoma with tamoxifen: a phase III trial in 420 patients. Proc Am Soc Clin Oncol 21:551, 2002.

177. Villa E, Ferretti I, Grottola A, et al. Hormonal therapy with megestrol in inoperable hepatocellular carcinoma characterized by variant oestrogen receptors. Br J Cancer 84:881–885, 2001.

178. Chao Y, Chan WK, Wang SS, et al. Phase II study of megestrol acetate in the treatment of hepatocellular carcinoma. J Gastroenterol Hepatol 12:277–281, 1997.

179. Chao Y, Chan WK, Wang SS, et al. Phase II study of megestrol acetate in the treatment of hepatocellular carcinoma. J Gastroenterol Hepatol 12:277–281, 1997.

180. Wallace S, Charnsangavej C, Carrasco H, et al. Infusion-embolization. Cancer 54:2751–2765, 1984.

181. Yamada R, Sato M, Kawabata M, et al. Hepatic artery embolization in 120 patients with unresectable hepatoma. Radiology 148: 397–401, 1983.

182. Fujimoto S, Miyazaki M, Endoh F, et al. Biodegradable mitomycin C microspheres given intraarterially for operable hepatic cancer. Cancer 56:2404–2410, 1985.

183. Ohnishi K, Tsuchiya S, Nakayama T, et al. Arterial chemoembolization of hepatocellular carcinoma with mitomycin C microcapsules. Radiology 152:51–55, 1984.

184. Venook A, Stagg R, Lewis B, et al. Chemoembolization for hepatocellular carcinoma. J Clin Oncol 8:1108–1114, 1990.

185. Civalleri D, Pellicci R, Decaro G, et al. Palliative chemoembolization of hepatocellular carcinoma with mitoxantrone, Lipiodol, and Gelfoam. A phase II study. Anticancer Res 16:937–941, 1996.

186. Kawai S, Tani M, Okamura J, et al. Prospective and randomized trial of Lipiodol–transcatheter arterial chemoembolization for treatment of hepatocellular carcinoma: a comparison of epirubicin and doxorubicin (second cooperative study). The Cooperative Study Group for Liver Cancer Treatment of Japan. Semin Oncol 24:S6-38–S6-45, 1997.

187. Groupe d'Etude et de Traitement du Carcinome Hepatocellulaire. A comparison of Lipiodol chemoembolization and conservative treatment for unresectable hepatocellular carcinoma. N Engl J Med 332:1256–1261, 1995.

188. Llovet JM, Real MI, Montana X, et al. Arterial embolisation or chemoembolisation versus symptomatic treatment in patients with unresectable hepatocellular carcinoma: a randomised controlled trial. Lancet 59:1734–1739, 2002.

189. Lo CM, Ngan H, Tso WK, et al. Randomized controlled trial of transarterial lipiodol chemoembolization for unresectable hepatocellular carcinoma. Hepatology 35:1164–1171, 2002.

190. Ikeda M, Maeda S, Shibata J, et al. Transcatheter arterial chemotherapy with and without embolization in patients with hepatocellular carcinoma. Oncology 66:24–31, 2004.

191. Romano M, Giojelli A, Tamburrini O, et al. Chemoembolization for hepatocellular carcinoma: effect of intraarterial lidocaine in peri- and postprocedural pain and hospitalization. Radiol Med (Torino) 105:350–355, 2003.

192. Chou CC, Pan SL, Teng CM, et al. Pharmacological evaluation of several major ingredients of Chinese herbal medicines in human hepatoma Hep3B cells. Eur J Pharm Sci 19:403–412, 2003.

193. Li XR, Zhang D, Qi YF. Experimental study on xiaoliu pingyi mixture with medicated serum in inducing apoptosis of human hepatocellular carcinoma cell line H-7402 Zhongguo Zhong Xi Yi Jie He Za Zhi 21:684–687, 2001.

194. Shao ZX, Cheng ZG, Yin X. Clinical study on treatment of middle–advanced stage liver cancer by combined treatment of hepatic artery chemoembolization with gan'ai no. I and no. II Zhongguo Zhong Xi Yi Jie He Za Zhi 21:168–170, 2001.

195. Iimuro Y, Fujimoto J. Strategy of gene therapy for liver cirrhosis and hepatocellular carcinoma. J Hepatobiliary Pancreat Surg 10: 45–47, 2003.

196. Li H, Qin S, Ye SL, et al. A phase 1/2 study of hepatic delivery of doxorubicin adsorbed to magnetic targeted carriers (MTC–dox) in patients with unresectable HCC. Proc Am Soc Clin Oncol 22:1422, 2003.

197. Leung TW, Feun L, Posey J, et al. A phase II study of T138067–sodium in patients with unresectable hepatocellular carcinoma. Proc Am Soc Clin Oncol 21:572, 2002.

198. Gall J. Nolatrexed dichloride vs. doxorubicin, a clinical update of a multicenter randomized phase II study (014) in ethnic Chinese subjects with unresectable or metastatic HCC. Proc Am Soc Clin Oncol 23:4262, 2004.

199. Lee JT, McCubrey JA. BAY-43-9006 Bayer/Onyx. Curr Opin Investig Drugs 4:757–763, 2003.

200. Curley SA, Bomalaski JS, Ensor CM, et al. Regression of hepatocellular cancer in a patient treated with arginine deiminase. Hepatogastroenterology. 50:1214–1216, 2003.

201. Beck PR, Belfield A, Spooner RJ, et al. Serum enzyme elevations in colorectal cancer. Cancer 43:1772–1776, 1979.

202. Kemeny MM, Sugarbaker PH, Smith TJ, et al. A prospective analysis of laboratory tests and imaging studies to detect hepatic lesions. Ann Surg 195:163–167, 1982.

203. Szymendera JJ, Nowacki MP, Szawlowski AW, et al. Predictive value of plasma CEA levels: preoperative and postoperative monitoring of patients with colorectal carcinoma. Dis Colon Rectum 25: 46–52, 1982.

204. Gunven P, Makuuchi M, Takayasu K, et al. Preoperative imaging of liver metastases. Comparison of angiography, CT scan, and ultrasound. Ann Surg 202:573–579, 1985.

205. Schreve RH, Terpstra OT, Ausema L, et al. Detection liver metastases. A prospective study comparing liver enzymes, scintigraphy, ultrasonography, and computed tomography. Br J Surg 71:947–949, 1984.

206. Domingues JM, Wolff BG, Nelson H, et al. 111In-CYT-103 scanning in recurrent colorectal cancer: does it affect standard management? Dis Colon Rectum 39:514–519, 1996.

207. Knol JA, Marn CS, Francis IR, et al. Comparisons of dynamic infusion and delayed computed tomography, intraoperative ultrasound, and palpation in the diagnosis of liver metastases. Am J Surg 165: 81–87, 1993.

208. Rosen CB, Nagomey DM, Taswell HF, et al. Perioperative blood transfusions and determinants of survival after liver resection for metastatic colorectal carcinoma. Ann Surg 216:493–505, 1992.

209. Cady B, Stone MD, McDermott WV, et al. Technical and biological factors in disease-free survival after hepatic resection for colorectal cancer metastases. Arch Surg 127:561–569, 1992.

210. Hughes KS. Resection of the liver for colorectal carcinoma metastases: a multi-institutional study of indications for resection. Surgery 103:278–288, 1988.

211. Scheele J, Stangl R, Altendorf-Hormann A, et al. Indicators of prognosis after hepatic resection for colorectal secondaries. Surgery 110:13–29, 1991.

212. Pettavel J, Morgenthaler F. Protracted arterial chemotherapy of the liver tumors: an experience of 107 cases over a 12-year period. Prog Clin Cancer 7:217–233, 1978.

213. Goslin R, Steele G, Zamcheck N, et al. Factors influencing survival in patients with hepatic metastases from adenocarcinoma of the colon or rectum. Dis Colon Rectum 25:749–754, 1982.

214. Bismuth H, Adam R, Levi F, et al. Resection of nonresectable liver metastases from colorectal cancer after neoadjuvant chemotherapy. Ann Surg 224:509–522, 1996.

215. Pozzo C, Basso M, Cassano A, et al. Neoadjuvant treatment of unresectable liver disease with irinotecan and 5-fluorouracil plus folinic acid in colorectal cancer patients. Ann Oncol 15:933–939, 2004.

216. Hughes K, Schilel J, Sugerbaker P, et al. Surgery for colorectal cancer metastatic to the liver. Surg Clin North Am 69:339–359, 1989.

217. Adloff M, Arnaud JP, Thebault Y, et al. Hepatic metastases of colorectal cancer. Should it be treated surgically? Report of 55 cases. Chirurgie 116:144–149, 1990.

218. Doci R, Genarri L, Bignami P, et al. One hundred patients with hepatic metastases from colorectal cancer treated by resection: analysis of prognostic determinants. Br J Surg 78:797–801, 1991.

219. Pettrelli N, Gupta B, Piedmonte M, et al. Morbidity and survival of liver resection for colorectal adenocarcinoma. Dis Colon Rectum 34:899–904, 1992.

220. Nakamura S, Yokoi Y, Suzuki S, et al. Results of extensive surgery for liver metastases in colorectal carcinoma. Br J Surg 79: 35–38, 1992.

221. Rosen CB, Nagorney DM, Taswell HF, et al. Perioperative blood transfusions and determinants of survival after liver resection for metastatic colorectal carcinoma. Ann Surg 216:493–505, 1992.

222. van Ooijen B, Wiggers T, Meijer S, et al. Hepatic resections for colorectal metastases in The Netherlands. A multiinstitutional 10–year study. Cancer 70:28–34, 1992.

223. Gayowski TJ, Iwatsuki S, Madariaga JR, et al. Experience in hepatic resection for metastatic colorectal cancer: analysis of clinical and pathologic risk factors. Surgery 116:703–710, 1994.

224. Fuhrman GM, Curley SA, Hohn DC, et al. Improved survival after resection of colorectal liver metastases. Am Surg Oncol 2: 537–541, 1995.

225. Jatzko GR, Lisborg, PH, Stettner HM, et al. Hepatic resection for metastases from colorectal carcinoma: a survival analysis. Eur J Cancer 31A:41–46, 1995.

226. Scheele J, Stang R, Altendorf-Hofmann A, et al. Resection of colorectal liver metastases. World J Surg 19:59–71, 1995.

227. Scott S, Carty N, Anderson L, et al. Liver resection for colorectal liver metastases. Eur J Surg Oncol 21:33–35, 1995.

228. Nordlinger B, Guiguet M, Vaillant JC, et al. Surgical resection of colorectal carcinoma metastasized to the liver. A prognostic scoring system to improve case selection, based on 1568 patients. Cancer 77:1254–1262, 1996.

229. Fong Y, Cohen AM, Fortner JG, et al. Liver resection for colorectal metastases. J Clin Oncol 15:938–946, 1997.

230. Marmorale C, Miconi G, De Luca S, et al. Surgical treatment of hepatic metastatic colorectal cancer. Ann Ital Chir 67:245–249, 1996.

231. Jenkins LT, Millikan KW, Bines SD, et al. Hepatic resection for metastatic colorectal cancer. Am Surg 63:605–610, 1997.

232. Rees M, Plant G, Bygrave S. Late results justify resection for multiple hepatic metastases from colorectal cancer. Br J Surg 84: 1136–1140, 1997.

233. Shirabe K, Takenaka K, Gion T, et al. Analysis of prognostic risk factors in hepatic resection for metastatic colorectal carcinoma with special reference to the surgical margin. Br J Surg 84:1077–1080, 1997.

234. Taylor M, Forster J, Langer B, et al. A study of prognostic factors for hepatic resection for colorectal metastases. Am J Surg 173:467–471, 1997.

235. Elias D, Cavalcanti A, Sabourin JC, et al. Results of 136 curative hepatectomies with a safety margin of less than 10 mm for colorectal metastases. J Surg Oncol 69:88–93, 1998.

236. Ohlsson B, Stenram U, Tranberg KG. Resection of colorectal liver metastases: 25-year experience. World J Surg 22:268–277, 1998.

237. Choti MA, Sitzmann JV, Tiburi MF, et al. Trends in long–term survival following liver resection for hepatic colorectal metastases. Ann Surg 235:759–66, 2002.

238. Yokoi Y, Suzuki S, Nakamura S. The impact of hepatic resection on metastatic colorectal cancer. Gan To Kagaku Ryoho 29:848–855, 2002.

239. Belli G, Agostino A, Ciciliano F, et al. Liver resection for hepatic metastases: 15 years of experience. J Hepatobiliary Pancreat Surg 9:607–661, 2002.

240. Minagawa M, Makuuchi M. Surgical treatment of colorectal liver metastases. Nippon Geka Gakkai Zasshi 104:721–729, 2003.

241. Bramhall SR, Gur U, Coldham C, et al. Liver resection for colorectal metastases. Ann R Coll Surg Engl 85: 334–339, 2003.

242. Cavallari A, Vivarelli M, Bellusci R, et al. Liver metastases from colorectal cancer: present surgical approach. Hepatogastroenterology 50:2067–2071, 2003.

243. Shimada H, Tanaka K, Masui H, et al. Results of surgical treatment for multiple (≥5 nodules) bilobar hepatic metastases from colorectal cancer. Langenbecks Arch Surg 389:114–121, 2004.

244. Curley SA, Roh MS, Chase JL, et al. Adjuvant hepatic arterial infusion chemotherapy after curative resection of colorectal liver metastases. Am J Surg 166:743–746, 1993.

245. Bolton JS, O'Connell MJ, Mahoney MR, et al. Final results of hepatic intraarterial infusion plus systemic chemotherapy after multiple metastasectomy in patients with colorectal carcinoma metastatic to the liver. A North Central Cancer Treatment Group phase II study. Proc Am Clin Oncol 3527, 2004.

246. Evans JT. Hepatic artery ligation in hepatic metastases from colon and rectal malignancies. Dis Colon Rectum 22:370, 1979.

247. Livraghi T, Solbiati L, Meloni F, et al. Percutaneous radiofrequency ablation of liver metastases in potential candidates for resection: the ''test of time approach.'' Cancer 97:3027–3035, 2003.

248. Pawlik TM, Izzo F, Cohen DS, et al. Combined resection and radiofrequency ablation for advanced hepatic malignancies: results in 172 patients. Ann Surg Oncol 10:1002–1004, 2003.

249. Seifert JK, Junginger T, Morris DL. A collective review of the world literature on hepatic cryotherapy. J R Coll Surg Edinb 43:141–154, 1998.

250. Seifert JK, Junginger T. Cryotherapy for liver tumors: current status, perspectives, clinical results, and review of literature. Technol Cancer Res Treat 3:151–163, 2004.

251. Weaver ML, Ashton JG, Zemel R. Treatment of colorectal liver metastases by cryotherapy. Semin Surg Oncol 14:163–170, 1998.

252. Hewitt PM, Dwerryhouse SJ, Zhao J, et al. Multiple bilobar liver metastases: cryotherapy for residual lesions after liver resection. J Surg Oncol 67:112–116, 1998.

253. Vogel TJ, Straub R, Eichler K, et al. Colorectal carcinoma metastases in the liver: laser-induced interstitial thermotherapy—local tumor control rate and survival data. Radiology 230:450–458, 2004.

254. Morita T, Shibata T, Okuyama M, et al. Microwave coagulation therapy for liver metastases from colorectal cancer. Gan To Kagaku Ryoho 31:695–699, 1998.

255. Borgelt BB, Gelber R, Brady LW, et al. The palliation of hepatic metastases: results of Radiation Therapy Oncology Group pilot study. Int J Radiat Oncol Biol Phys 7:587–591, 1981.

256. Barone RM, Byfield JE, Goldfarb PB, et al. Intraarterial chemotherapy using an implantable infusion pump and liver irradiation for the treatment of hepatic metastases. Cancer 50:850–862, 1982.

257. Dawson LA, Lawrence TS. The role of radiotherapy in the treatment of liver metastases. Cancer J 10:139–144, 2004.

258. Behr TM, Liersch T, Greiner-Bechert L, et al. Radioimmunotherapy of small–volume disease of metastatic colorectal cancer. Cancer 94 (4 Suppl):1373–1381, 2002.

259. Balch CM, Urist MM, Soong SJ, et al. A prospective phase II clinical trial of continuous FUDR regional chemotherapy for colorectal metastases to the liver using a totally implantable pump. Ann Surg 198:567–573, 1983.

260. Niederhuber JE, Ensminger W, Gyves J, et al. Regional chemotherapy of colorectal cancer metastatic to the liver. Cancer 53:1336–1343, 1984.

261. Reed ML, Vaitkevicius VK, Al-Sarraf M, et al. The practicality of chronic hepatic artery infusion therapy of primary and metastatic hepatic malignancies: ten-year results in 124 patients in a prospective protocol. Cancer 47:402–409, 1981.

262. Weiss GR, Garnick MB, Osteen RT, et al. Long-term hepatic arterial infusion of 5-fluorodeoxyuridine for liver metastases using an implanted infusion pump. J Clin Oncol 1:337–344, 1983.

263. Kemeny MM, Goldberg DA, Browning S, et al. Experience with continuous regional chemotherapy and hepatic resection as treatment of hepatic metastases from colorectal primaries. A prospective randomized study. Cancer 55:1265–1270, 1985.

264. Kemeny N, Daly J, Oderman P, et al. Hepatic artery pump infusion: toxicity and results in patients with metastatic colorectal carcinoma. J Clin Oncol 2:595–600, 1984.

265. Riether RD, Khubchandani IT, Sheets JA, et al. A prospective study of continuous hepatic perfusion with implantable pump. Dis Colon Rectum 28:24–26, 1985.

266. Kemeny N, Seiter K, Niedzwiecki D, et al. A randomized trial of intrahepatic infusion of fluorodeoxyuridine with dexamethasone versus fluorodeoxyuridine alone in the treatment of metastatic colorectal cancer. Cancer 69:327–333, 1991.

267. Hohn DC, Roh M, Chase J, et al. Prohibitive toxicity with hepatic arterial infusion of low-dose floxuridine and folinic acid for colorectal liver metastases. Proc Am Soc Clin Oncol 10:459, 1991.

268. Kemeny N, Conti JA, Cohen A, et al. Phase II study of hepatic arterial floxuridine, leucovorin, and dexamethasone for unresectable liver metastases from colorectal carcinoma. J Clin Oncol 12:2288–2295, 1994.

269. Tandon RN, Bunnell IL, Cooper RG. The treatment of metastatic carcinoma of the liver by the percutaneous selective hepatic artery infusion of 5-fluorouracil. Surgery 73:118–121, 1973.

270. Ansfield FJ, Ramirez G. The clinical results of 5-fluorouracil intrahepatic arterial infusion in 528 patients with metastatic cancer to the liver. Prog Clin Cancer 7:201–206, 1978.

271. Petrek JA, Minton JP. Treatment of hepatic metastases by percutaneous hepatic arterial infusion. Cancer 43:2182–2188, 1979.

272. Grage TB, Vassilopoulos PP, Shingleton WW, et al. Results of a prospective randomized study of hepatic arterial infusion with 5-fluorouracil versus intravenous 5-fluorouracil in patients with hepatic metastases from colorectal origin. Surgery 86:550–555, 1979.

273. Berger M. Hepatic infusion for metastatic colorectal cancer in a community hospital setting [abstract]. Proc Am Soc Clin Oncol 22:456, 1981.

274. Van Riel JM, van Groeningen CJ, Albers SH, et al. Hepatic arterial 5-fluorouracil in patients with liver metastases from colorectal cancer: single-centre experience in 145 patients. Ann Oncol 11:1563–1570, 2000.

275. Mancuso A, Giuliani R, Accettura C, et al. Hepatic arterial infusion (HACI) of oxaliplatin in patients with unresectable liver metastases from colorectal cancer. Anticancer Res 23:1917–1922, 2003.

276. Fiorentini G, Rossi S, Dentico P, et al. Irinotecan hepatic arterial infusion chemotherapy for hepatic metastases from colorectal cancer: a phase II clinical trial. Tumori 89:382–384, 2003.

277. Van Riel JM, van Groeningen CJ, di Greve J, et al. Continuous infusion of hepatic arterial irinotecan in pretreated patients with colorectal cancer metastatic to the liver. Ann Oncol 15:59–63, 2004.

278. Hu G, Estrov Z, Barber D, Mavligit GM. 40% response rate after hepatic arterial infusion of CPT-11 in patients with colorectal cancer metastatic to the liver. Proc Am Soc Clin Oncol 20:2174, 2001.

279. Adson MA, van Heerden JA, Adson MH, et al. Resection of hepatic metastases from colorectal cancer. Arch Surg 119:647–651, 1984.

280. Oberfield RA, McCafferreu JA, Polio J, et al. Prolonged and continuous percutaneous intraarterial hepatic infusion chemotherapy in ad-

vanced metastatic liver adenocarcinoma from colorectal primary. Cancer 44:414–423, 1979.

281. Stagg RJ, Venook AP, Chase JL, et al. Alternating hepatic intra–arterial floxuridine and fluorouracil: a less toxic regimen for treatment of liver metastases from colorectal cancer. J Natl Cancer Inst 83:423–428, 1991.

282. Patt Y, Mavligit GM, Chuang VP, et al. Percutaneous hepatic arterial infusion of mitomycin C and floxuridine: an effective treatment for metastatic colorectal cancer to the liver. Cancer 46:261–265, 1980.

283. Shepard KV, Levin B, Karl RC, et al. Therapy for metastatic colorectal cancer with hepatic artery infusion chemotherapy using a subcutaneous implanted pump. J Clin Oncol 3:161–169, 1985.

284. Hatfield AK, Krammer BA, Danley RA, et al. Intermittent hepatic artery perfusions for symptomatic metastatic colon carcinoma [abstract]. Proc AM Soc Clin Oncol 1:102, 1981.

285. Theodors A, Bukowski RM, Lavery I, et al. Hepatic artery infusion with 5-fluorouracil and mitomycin-C in metastatic colorectal carcinoma phase II study. Med Pediatr Oncol 10:463–470, 1982.

286. Isenberg J, Fischback R, Kruger I, et al. Treatment of liver metastases from colorectal cancer. Anticancer Res 16: 1291–1295, 1996.

287. Patt YZ, Boddie AW, Jr, Charnsangavej C, et al. Hepatic arterial infusion with floxuridine and cisplatin: overriding importance of antitumor effect versus degree of tumor burden as determinants of survival among patients with colorectal cancer. J Clin Oncol 4: 1356–1364, 1986.

288. Cohen AM, Schaeffer N, Higgins J. Treatment of metastatic colorectal cancer with hepatic arterial combination chemotherapy. Cancer 57:1115–1117, 1986.

289. Wils J, Schlangen J, Naus A. Phase II study of hepatic artery infusion with 5-fluorouracil, Adriamycin, and mitomycin C in liver metastases from colorectal carcinoma. Cancer Chemother Pharmacol 12:215–217, 1984.

290. Kemeny N, Cohen A, Seiter K, et al. Randomized trial of hepatic arterial floxuridine, mitomycin, and carmustine versus floxuridine alone in previously treated patients with liver metastases from colorectal cancer. J Clin Oncol 11:330–335, 1993.

291. Kern W, Beckert B, Lang N, et al. Phase 1 and pharmacokinetic study of hepatic arterial infusion with oxaliplatin in combination with folinic acid and 5-fluorouracil in patients with hepatic metastases from colorectal cancer. Ann Oncol 12:599–603, 2001.

292. Melichar B, Dvorak J, Jandik P, et al. Regional administration of irinotecan in combination with 5-fluorouracil and leucovorin in patients with colorectal cancer liver metastases: a pilot experience. Hepatogastroenterology 48:1721–1726, 2001.

293. Liu LX, Zhang WH, Jiang HC, et al. Arterial chemotherapy of 5-fluorouracil and mitomycin C in the treatment of liver metastases of colorectal cancer. World J Gastroenterol 8:663–667, 2002.

294. Kemeny N, Reichman B, Oberfield P, et al. Update of randomized study of intrahepatic vs. systemic fluorodeoxyuridine in patients with liver metastases from colorectal cancer. Proc Am Soc Clin Oncol 5:89, 1986.

295. Hohn DC, Stagg RJ, Friedman MA, et al. A randomized trial of continuous intravenous verus hepatic intraarterial floxuridine in patients with liver colorectal cancer metastatic to the liver: the Northern California Oncology Group Trial. J Clin Oncol 7:1646–1654, 1989.

296. Chang AE, Schneider PD, Sugarbaker PH, et al. A prospective randomized trial of regional versus systemic continuous infusion 5-fluorodeoxyuridine chemotherapy in the treatment of colorectal liver metastases. Ann Surg 206:685–693, 1987.

297. Martin JK, O'Connell MJ, Wieand HS, et al. Intraarterial floxuridine vs. systemic fluorouracil for hepatic metastases from colorectal cancer. Arch Surg 125:1022–1027, 1990.

298. Rougier P, LaPlanche A, Huguier M, et al. Hepatic arterial infusion of floxuridine in patients with liver metastases from colorectal carcinoma: long-term results of a prospective randomized trial. J Clin Oncol 10:1112–1118, 1992.

299. Allen-Mersh TG, Earlam S, Fordy C, et al. Continuous hepatic artery floxuridine infusion prolongs overall and normal-quality survival in colorectal liver metastases patients. Proc Am Soc Clin Oncol 1:202, 1994.

300. Lorenz M, Muller HH. Randomized, multicenter trial of fluorouracil plus leucovorin administered either via hepatic arterial or intravenous infusion versus fluorodeoxyuridine administered via hepatic arterial infusion in patients with nonresectable liver metastases from colorectal cancer. J Clin Oncol 18:243–254, 2000.

301. Harmantas A, Rotstein LE, Langer B. Regional versus systemic chemotherapy in the treatment of colorectal carcinoma metastatic to the liver. Is there a survival difference? Meta-analysis of the published literature. Cancer 78:1639–1645, 1969.

302. Venook AP, Begsland EK, Ring E, et al. Gene therapy of colorectal liver metastases using a recombinant adenovirus encoding WT P53 (SCH 58500) via hepatic artery infusion: a phase I study [abstract]. Proc Am Soc Clin Oncol 17:1661, 1998.

303. Kerr D, Seymour L, Maruta F. Gene therapy for colorectal cancer. Expert Opin Biol Ther 3:779–788, 2003.

Gastrointestinal Cancers

98

Judy L. Chase, Kristin L. Hennenfent,

Richard D. Lozano, and Dina K. Patel

The gastrointestinal (GI) system is one of the most common sites of cancer in humans. This chapter will focus on colorectal, pancreatic, and gastric cancer. Hepatocellular (primary liver cancer) is discussed in detail in Chapter 97. Other GI cancers that occur less frequently and that are not covered in this chapter include esophageal, biliary, small intestine, gall bladder, and appendiceal neoplasms.

TREATMENT GOALS: GASTROINTESTINAL CANCERS

- In general, surgery is the primary treatment and usually the only curative modality currently available.
- Early-stage disease can be treated with curative intent.
- Advanced, surgically unresectable disease is treated with palliative chemotherapy, radiation, or both.
- Response rates and survival of patients with advanced disease have improved, but remain relatively poor.

COLORECTAL CANCER

EPIDEMIOLOGY

ETIOLOGY

A specific cause of colorectal cancer has not been identified. Clinical risk factors include dietary practices, genetic factors, familial syndromes, other preexisting diseases, and advancing age (Table 98.1). Epidemiology and animal studies have determined that diets rich in animal fats and poor in fiber are associated with an increase in the risk of the disease.[1] Dietary fat may enhance colorectal carcinogenesis by a number of mechanisms. Dietary fat increases the production of secondary bile acids that promote tumorigenesis and increase the proliferative activity of intestinal crypt cells.[2] Dietary fat may also enhance the damaging activity of intraluminal free fatty acids to the intestinal epithelium.[3]

Another correlate of dietary fat intake and the risk of colorectal cancer is meat consumption. In industrialized countries, including the United States, meat is the major source of dietary fat, and high-fat diets tend to be high in meat intake. It is still unclear whether the association of meat with colorectal cancer reflects the effect of fat, meat in general, or certain types of meat.

A number of animal, human case-control, and epidemiologic studies have assessed the influence of dietary fiber on the risk of developing colorectal cancer. The majority of studies have found dietary fiber to be protective. The most widely accepted mechanism reflects the stool-bulking characteristics of dietary fiber. By increasing stool bulk, the concentration of potentially carcinogenic or epithelium-damaging agents are diluted out in the bowel lumen.[4] A second explanation involves dietary fiber enhancing fermentation by gut bacteria. This fermentation produces short-chain fatty acids that decrease the intraluminal pH, which may decrease the solubility and ionization of free bile acids and free fatty acids, thus reducing the risk of colorectal cancer.[5] Third, some dietary fiber metabolites, such as butyrate, may have antineoplastic properties of their own.[6] However, a recent prospective study of 88,757 women by Fuchs et al[7] concluded that their data did not support the existence of an important protective effect of dietary fiber against colorectal cancer. Other dietary factors, such as alcohol intake, have been studied and have produced conflicting data. Several epidemiologic studies have reported a direct association between alcohol ingestion and colorectal cancer, whereas other studies have found minimal or no association. A meta-analysis concluded that alcohol consumption and the increased risk of colorectal cancer was at best small, and no clear causative role could be established.[8]

Multiple genetic factors have been implicated in the development of colorectal cancer. First-degree relatives of persons with colorectal cancer have a threefold increased risk of developing the disease, thereby conferring a genetic etiology. Familial adenomatous polyposis is a rare inherited condition characterized by hundreds of large intestinal polyps. The majority of patients with this disease develop colorectal cancer by age 30. The extent to which other genetic factors, in isolation or combined with environmental factors, contribute to the development of colorectal cancer requires continued research.

INCIDENCE

In the United States, more than 145,000 new cases of colorectal cancer occurred in 2004, representing approximately 11% of all cancer diagnoses. Incidence rates for colorectal cancer have continued to decline from a high of 53 per 100,000 in 1985 to 34 per 100,000 in 2004.[9] Cancers of the colon and rectum are the third most commonly diagnosed cancers among men and women, and are the third most common cause of cancer death in both sexes. Overall, in the United States, it is estimated that approximately 1 in 17 people will develop colorectal cancer in their lifetime. North America, Australia, New Zealand, and portions of Europe have the highest incidence of the disease. Africa and other underdeveloped countries tend to have a low incidence of colorectal cancer. In the United States, the median age at diagnosis is 70 for men and 73 for women with the age-specific incidence rising steeply from the fourth to the eighth decades of life. Approximately 50,000 deaths per year are attributed to colorectal cancer in the United States, accounting for about 10% of cancer deaths.[9] The incidence appears to be relatively equally distributed between the sexes, with a slight male predominance. Colorectal cancer rates, unlike those for cancers of the lung, cervix, and prostate, show little

TABLE 98.1	Risk Factors for Colorectal Cancer
Dietary	High animal fats and meat
	Low fiber
Genetic	Familial adenomatous polyposis syndrome
	Gardner, Oldfield, or Turcot syndrome
Familial	Familial colorectal cancer syndrome
	Hereditary adenocarcinomatosis syndrome
	Family history of colorectal cancer
Preexisting Disease	Inflammatory bowel disease
	Colorectal cancer
	Pelvic irradiation for cancer
	Neoplastic colorectal polyps
General	All men and women over age 40
	Previous cholecystectomy
	Previous ureterosigmoidostomy

socioeconomic correlation in the United States and other developed countries.

In the United States, the Seventh Day Adventists and Mormon religious groups have a diminished risk for colorectal cancer. The 20% to 50% reduction in risk is probably attributed to religious practices prohibiting alcohol and tobacco use and promoting some form of dietary moderation.[10,11]

PATHOPHYSIOLOGY

Approximately 70% of all colorectal cancers occur in the sigmoid colon and rectum. The remainder occur in decreasing frequency in the ascending colon (16%), the transverse colon and splenic flexure (8%), and the descending colon (6%). Histologically, adenocarcinoma accounts for 90% to 95% of colorectal tumors. The remaining 5% to 10% of large bowel tumors are squamous cell carcinomas, undifferentiated carcinomas, rectal carcinoid, or, very rarely, sarcomas. The adenocarcinomas are further classified by grade. The grade is based on the degree of tumor differentiation, reflected by structural and cytologic features of the tumor specimen. Grade 1 is the most differentiated, with well-formed tubules and the least nuclear polymorphism and mitoses. Grade 3 is the least differentiated, with only occasional glandular structures, and grade 2 is intermediate between grades 1 and 3. Poorly differentiated tumors are associated with a poor prognosis. Two histologic subtypes of colorectal adenocarcinoma, colloid, or mucinous, adenocarcinoma and signet ring cell carcinoma are associated with a more aggressive clinical course. They tend to occur more frequently in individuals less than 40 years of age. They also tend to be poorly differentiated and associated with a poor prognosis.

Colorectal adenocarcinomas tend to remain superficial for a long time, growing first into the lumen of the bowel and then slowly invading the deeper layers of the intestinal wall. The extent of tumor invasion into the bowel wall correlates with the presence of lymph node metastases and, ultimately, patient survival. Colorectal cancer may spread by direct invasion of adjacent tissues and metastasize via lymphatic and hematogenous routes. The liver is the most common site of hematogenous metastases, followed by the lung. Involvement of other sites in the absence of liver or lung metastases is rare.

CLINICAL PRESENTATION AND DIAGNOSIS

SIGNS AND SYMPTOMS
The signs and symptoms of colorectal cancer are often subtle and nonspecific. Many patients may be completely asymptomatic and have colorectal cancer detected via routine screening procedures. The symptoms that are most commonly associated with colorectal cancer are the passage of

blood around the stool or on toilet paper; abdominal pain, which is frequently crampy and intermittent; and a change in bowel habits. The passage of bright red blood is most often seen with cancers of the rectum or sigmoid colon. Melena may result from right-sided colon tumors or obstructing tumors that retard the passage of fecal contents. Unexplained iron deficiency anemia may be the first sign in otherwise asymptomatic patients, especially in tumors located in the proximal colon. Any persistent change in bowel habits should be considered suspicious and deserves further evaluation. Such a change may be newly developed diarrhea, constipation, rectal pressure, or a change in stool caliber. These symptoms may mimic those of other bowel disorders such as diverticular disease, irritable bowel disease, or inflammatory bowel disease. More advanced colorectal cancer may produce unexplained weight loss. When compared with proximal colon cancers, left-sided tumors typically cause obstructive symptoms earlier in the disease course because stool in the distal colon is more solid and, therefore, less likely to pass easily through a narrowed lumen. Conversely, right-sided tumors can grow larger and into advanced disease and remain virtually asymptomatic.

Physical examination is usually unrevealing in early colorectal cancer. In advanced disease, a palpable abdominal mass, signs of bowel obstruction or perforation, hepatomegaly, or ascites may be present.

SCREENING
The natural history of colorectal cancer often involves a prolonged period of growth whereby many patients remain asymptomatic until advanced disease is present. Colorectal cancer presents a major health risk to the population, and routine screening of asymptomatic patients with the hope of early detection is recommended. The primary care physician should develop a colorectal screening strategy for adult patients as part of an annual physical examination. The screening program should include stool guaiac testing, digital rectal examination, and a flexible sigmoidoscopy. The routine screening procedures are listed in Table 98.2. Stool guaiac

TABLE 98.2	Screening Recommendations for Colorectal Cancer for General Population Starting at Age 50
Procedure	**Frequency**
Fecal Occult Blood Test	Annually
Sigmoidoscopy	Every 5 years
OR colonoscopy	Every 5–10 years
OR double contrast barium enema	Every 5–10 years
Digital rectal examination	Every 5–10 years at time of each screening sigmoidoscopy, colonoscopy, or double contrast barium enema

for occult blood may be useful as a means of early detection. Stool guaiac testing is not without problems. A negative test does not assure the absence of large bowel cancer and, therefore, should not be relied on as the sole screening test. Colonoscopy should be used for screening purposes in high-risk patients. Routine screening of individuals at average risk should begin at age 50. The American Cancer Society guidelines recommends that, at age 50, men and women have a fecal occult blood test yearly; have a sigmoidoscopy every 5 years, or a colonoscopy or double contrast barium enema every 5 to 10 years; and have a digital rectal exam every 5 to 10 years at the time of each screening sigmoidoscopy, colonoscopy, or barium enema. Although these are the published screening guidelines, colonoscopies are usually performed in clinical practice in place of sigmoidoscopy because sigmoidoscopy may miss up to 50% of potential lesions. If not performed initially, any positive result should be followed by a colonoscopy.[12] The frequency of screening may be determined based on the results of the baseline screening exam and physician recommendations. Individuals with high-risk factors (personal past history of colorectal cancer or adenomas, a family history of colorectal cancer or adenomas, or inflammatory bowel disease) should begin screening at an earlier age. Children of a parent with a history of colorectal cancer should begin screening at an age equal to 10 years prior to the age of the parent at diagnosis. Colonoscopy or barium enema may be justified at age 40 or less in first-degree relatives. Patients with signs or symptoms of colorectal cancer should be referred for a definitive examination and evaluation of their entire large bowel.

DIAGNOSIS

Patients with any symptoms suggestive of colorectal cancer or a history of polyps should proceed with specific studies to establish a definitive diagnosis. The most widely used diagnostic tests are double-contrast barium enema and colonoscopy.[13] Colonoscopy is somewhat more sensitive than the barium enema and offers the advantages of direct visualization of the tumor and the ability to biopsy lesions for immediate tissue diagnosis. However, colonoscopy tends to be more expensive than a barium enema. The double-contrast barium enema involves the rectal administration of barium combined with distension of the bowel lumen with air. The barium outlines the colonic wall and may reveal lesions as small as 1 to 2 cm. However, a barium enema often cannot differentiate an early colon cancer from a benign polyp. The barium enema may be helpful in assessing the remainder of the bowel in patients in whom the colonoscope cannot be passed beyond the tumor because of a narrowed bowel lumen. Therefore, a barium enema and colonoscopy are often used together.

No blood tests are effective in identifying colorectal cancer. Carcinoembryonic antigen (CEA) is a tumor marker that can be measured in the blood and may be elevated in colorectal cancer. It is not specific to colorectal cancer because it may be elevated in other GI and non-GI malignancies and is not quantitative. However, a marked elevation in CEA may indicate metastatic disease, especially to the liver, and may warrant further workup.[14] A normal or low preoperative level does not guarantee a small or localized primary lesion. CEA may be useful in screening after curative resection and in monitoring response to treatment; however, it should not be used as the sole screening or monitoring method. Other laboratory tests that should be included in the workup are not specific to colorectal cancer and include the usual preoperative evaluations such as complete blood count, differential, platelets, serum chemistry, liver panel, electrolytes, and coagulation profile. Chest x-ray is often requested as a part of the standard preoperative workup but is not required for diagnosis. It may be used to rule out metastatic disease to the lung in patients with an already confirmed diagnosis of colorectal cancer. Patients with a recently diagnosed colorectal cancer may also undergo computed tomography (CT) or ultrasound of the abdomen to assess the presence or absence of liver metastases. However, this is not required as part of the standard diagnostic workup, but is used in selected patients with symptoms or laboratory test suggestive of liver metastases. A CT scan of the pelvis is recommended for large, palpable abdominal masses or rectal tumors that may be associated with genitourinary involvement. Endorectal ultrasound is a relatively new procedure that may provide more accurate assessment of the depth of invasion into the bowel wall and the nodal status of patients with rectal tumors. Thus endorectal ultrasound may be able to determine the stage of rectal tumors before surgery.

STAGING AND PROGNOSIS

The staging of colorectal cancer has been complicated by the development of multiple staging systems, many of which use the same descriptors to represent different stages. The Dukes staging system was used in the past, however, the tumor-node-metastasis (TNM) system is the most common staging system currently used (Table 98.3). Recently, a new TNM strategy to further classify patients with node-positive (stage III) rectal cancer was implemented.[15] Greene et al[16] conducted a retrospective analysis that demonstrated a significant difference in overall survival between the three subsets of stage III disease. Subclassifying traditional stage III patients with rectal cancer is clearly of prognostic value. Most investigators agree that the single most important prognostic factor for survival or recurrence after curative surgical resection is stage of the cancer. The 5-year survival rate for stage I disease is 85% to 95%, stage II disease 60% to 80%, stage III disease 30% to 60%, and stage IV disease less than 5%.[17] Stage is determined by the depth of tumor penetration through the bowel wall, the presence and number of positive lymph nodes (lymph nodes with tumor involvement), and the presence of distant metastatic disease (colon cancer that has spread to other sites such as the liver and lungs). Other factors that have a negative influence on prognosis include lymphatic vessel invasion, blood vessel invasion, mucinous or signet cell tumor type, colonic obstruction or perforation,

TABLE 98.3	TNM Staging Classification for Colorectal Cancer

Primary Tumor (T)

TX	Primary tumor cannot be assessed.
T0	No evidence of primary tumor.
Tis	Carcinoma in situ.
T1	Tumor invades submucosa.
T2	Tumor invades muscularis propria.
T3	Tumor invades through the muscularis propria into the subserosa, or into nonperitonealized pericolic or perirectal tissues.
T4	Tumor directly invades other organs or structures and/or perforates visceral peritoneum.

Regional Lymph Nodes (N)

NX	Regional nodes cannot be assessed.
N0	No regional lymph node metastasis.
N1	Metastasis in one to three regional lymph nodes.
N2	Metastasis in four or more regional lymph nodes.

Distant Metastasis (M)

MX	Distant metastasis cannot be assessed.
M0	No distant metastasis.
M1	Distant metastasis.

Stage Grouping

0	Tis	N0	M0
I	T1	N0	M0
	T2	N0	M0
IIA	T3	N0	M0
IIB	T4	N0	M0
IIIA	T1 or T2	N1	M0
IIIB	T3 or T4	N1	M0
IIIC	Any T	N2	M0
IV	Any T	Any N	M1

lack of rectal bleeding, age under 40, male sex, symptomatic at diagnosis, high-grade tumors, tumors located in the rectosigmoid area, and elevated preoperative CEA levels.[18]

TREATMENT

STAGES I, II, AND III COLORECTAL CANCER

Surgery. Surgery with curative intent is the primary treatment modality for stages I, II, and III colorectal cancers. Cancers of the colon are removed by a wide resection of the primary lesion together with all surrounding tissue that contains lymph nodes to which the tumor is likely to spread.[19] The specific surgical procedure used depends on the location of the primary tumor and its corresponding lym-

phatic drainage. A standard procedure for tumors of the right colon (i.e., cecum and ascending colon) is a right hemicolectomy, for left-sided tumors (i.e., transverse and descending colon), a left hemicolectomy, and for sigmoid tumors, a sigmoid colectomy. Tumors in the upper portion of the rectum are usually treated with a low anterior resection with reanastomosis. Low rectal tumors often require an abdominoperineal resection and colostomy. Based on historical concerns of early local recurrence and inadequacy of tumor clearance, an open resection surgical technique is most often preferred over laparoscopic resection. However, surgeons have continued to evaluate the laparoscopic technique based on the benefits of better postoperative recovery and reduced surgical complications. Leung et al[20] recently evaluated laparoscopic resection of rectosigmoid carcinoma compared to open resection in a prospective randomized trial. The results of this study indicate that the laparoscopic technique did not adversely impact disease control or overall survival, and it may decrease postoperative complications. Which technique is used will continue to be based on surgeon preference and on the perceived value of improving postoperative complications. If the tumor involves adjacent organs such as the small bowel, bladder, uterus, or ovaries, an en bloc resection of the entire area is indicated.

Resection of the primary tumor is often warranted in patients with incurable metastatic disease found operatively or postoperatively. Resection of the primary tumor is intended to avoid local complications of cancer growth such as bleeding or hemorrhage, obstruction or perforation, and pain. Resection of the primary tumor in this setting has no impact on survival but may be associated with an improved quality of life. Patients with rectal cancer and distant metastatic disease at the time of diagnosis may receive palliative radiotherapy to the primary lesion instead of surgical resection.

Adjuvant Therapy

Rationale. The administration of treatments aimed at occult microscopic disease that may remain after complete surgical resection of all gross disease is termed adjuvant therapy. The goal of treatment when no disease is visually present is to decrease the risk of recurrence and ultimately prolong survival. Adjuvant therapy may involve systemic therapy with chemotherapy, local-regional therapy with radiation, or both, depending on the natural history and location of the primary neoplastic disease being treated. It is indicated when there is a high likelihood of recurrence and the potential benefit outweighs the risk of morbidity and cost. To obtain maximal benefit, the adjuvant therapy should be administered when the potential tumor burden is minimal (i.e., as soon as feasible after the primary surgical treatment), and it must be administered in maximally tolerated doses.[21] For adjuvant chemotherapy, only agents with proven efficacy against measurable disease should be used because there is no way to evaluate efficacy in the adjuvant setting when no measurable disease exists.

As discussed, surgical excision is the primary treatment of colorectal cancer, with approximately 80% of patients diagnosed at a stage when all gross tumor can be surgically removed. However, nearly 50% of patients develop recurrent disease and ultimately succumb to metastatic disease. In such patients, cure with surgery alone is unlikely due to residual microscopic disease. Therefore, treatment directed at occult disease after complete surgical resection of the primary disease is warranted. The risk of recurrence and subsequent death is highly dependent on stage. Without adjuvant therapy, the range of recurrence rates for a stage I lesion is 0% to 13%; 11% to 61% for stage II lesions; and 32% to 88% for stage III lesions.[22] Approximately 60% to 84% of recurrences become apparent within 2 years, and treatment depends on location, size, patient performance status, and prior therapy. Because the risk of recurrence after resection of a stage I colorectal tumor is low, the cost-benefit ratio does not warrant adjuvant therapy for these patients. Adjuvant therapy for stage II and stage III lesions is discussed in the following section. Because there are anatomic, natural history, and therapeutic differences between colon and rectal tumors, adjuvant therapy for each is addressed separately.

Adjuvant Therapy for Colon Cancer. Initially, adjuvant therapy after potentially curative surgical resection for large bowel cancer was attempted using alkylating agents, nitrogen mustard, and thiotepa. These drugs have not been shown to have activity in advanced colorectal cancer, and it is, therefore, not surprising that they were ineffective in the adjuvant treatment of colorectal cancer. Subsequent trials focused on the use of 5-fluorouracil (5-FU) and fluorodeoxyuridine because these drugs had produced some responses in patients with metastatic disease. These drugs were first used alone and then in combination with other agents, including semustine, vincristine, and the Bacillus of Calmette and Guerin (BCG) vaccine. None of the single-agent or combination trials resulted in decreased recurrence rates or improved survival compared with untreated controls.[23]

Levamisole, an anthelmintic agent, attracted interest for cancer therapy because of its presumed immunomodulatory activity. In the early 1980s, a small nonrandomized trial reported levamisole to have activity in the adjuvant setting for colon cancer.[24] Subsequent trials investigated levamisole alone and in combination with 5-FU in the hope of achieving additive activity. In the IMPACT trial, levamisole combined with 5-FU was found to significantly reduce the recurrence rate by 40% and death rate by 33% compared with no adjuvant therapy in patients with stage III disease.[25] On the basis of these results, a Consensus Panel convened by the National Institutes of Health in 1990 recommended levamisole plus 5-FU as standard adjuvant treatment for patients with stage III colon cancer.[26]

More recently, 5-FU and leucovorin (LV) have been extensively studied in the treatment of metastatic colorectal cancer. The addition of LV to 5-FU increased the response rates compared with 5-FU alone in the metastatic setting.

This prompted an extensive investigation into the role of LV plus 5-FU and the combination of LV plus levamisole plus 5-FU in colon cancer adjuvant trials. Multiple studies have since compared 5-FU plus levamisole and 5-FU plus levamisole and LV in the adjuvant setting. Overall, LV-containing regimens produced an improvement in overall survival compared to 5-FU and levamisole alone. These studies also demonstrated that 12 months of treatment did not provide any additional benefit over a 6-month period of therapy.[27] Later, data emerged suggesting that the addition of levamisole to 5-FU and LV did not produce improvements in survival compared to 5-FU and LV alone.[28,29] Thus, combination therapy with 5-FU and LV emerged as the standard treatment after surgical resection of the primary tumor in patients with stage III disease and remains the standard for these patients currently. As will be discussed in more detail later in the chapter, Capecitabine (Xeloda) is an orally administered prodrug of 5-FU and may be used in the adjuvant setting in place of 5-FU/LV. Studies are underway to confirm its efficacy in this role.

With stage II disease, the benefit of adjuvant therapy remains controversial. A meta analysis of data from approximately 1,000 stage II patients showed improvement in event-free 5-year survival and overall survival, however, the results did not reach statistical significance.[30] Thus, it has not been recommended to administer adjuvant chemotherapy to all patients with stage II disease, but rather only to those patients with stage II disease at high risk for recurrence (e.g., tumor perforation, adherence to or invasion of adjacent organs, involved resection margins, or unfavorable cellular kinetic pattern).[31]

Recently, combination regimens using irinotecan or oxaliplatin combined with 5-FU and LV have been investigated in the adjuvant setting. As will be discussed later, these regimens have been shown to be highly active in the metastatic setting and improve response rate, time to progression, and overall survival when compared to 5-FU and LV alone. A recent European study documented improvement in 3-year disease-free survival when oxaliplatin was added to infusional 5-FU and LV.[32] Oxaliplatin plus infusional 5-FU and LV (FOLFOX) regimens are now considered the standard for adjuvant therapy of stage III colorectal cancer. Adjuvant therapy of stage II colorectal cancer is not as clear as for stage III disease. Most clinicians recommend adjuvant chemotherapy for stage II patients at high risk of recurrence, but there is not a clear standard of care and the choice of regimen is at the discretion of the treating physician. Research continues to evaluate the different regimens and duration of adjuvant treatments. Common chemotherapy regimens used in the adjuvant setting are detailed in Table 98.4.

Adjuvant Therapy for Rectal Cancer. Rectal cancer, which should be distinguished from colon cancer, is characterized by an increased risk of local recurrence and a comparable risk for distant metastases compared with colon cancer. The risk of local recurrence after surgical resection of a rectal

TABLE 98.4	Adjuvant Therapy for Stage III Colon Cancer
Regimen	**Dosage**
Fluorouracil + Leucovorin (Mayo Clinic Regimen)	Fluorouracil 425 mg/m² IV, days 1–5
	Leucovorin 20 mg/m² IV, days 1–5
	Repeat every 28 days x 6 cycles
Fluorouracil + Leucovorin (Roswell Park Cancer Institute Regimen)	Fluorouracil 500 mg/m² IV weekly x 6 weeks
	Leucovorin 500 mg/m² IV weekly x 6 weeks
	Repeat every 8 weeks x 4 cycles
FOLFOX4	Oxaliplatin 85 mg/m² IV, day 1
	Leucovorin 200 mg/m² IV, days 1 and 2
	Fluorouracil 400 mg/m² IV, days 1 and 2
	Fluorouracil 600 mg/m² Continuous IV infusion over 22 hours, days 1 and 2
	Repeat every 14 days x 12 cycles
Capecitabine (Xeloda)	Capecitabine 1,000–1,250 mg/M² PO bid (total dose = 2,000–2,500 mg/M²/day) days 1–14
	Repeat every 21 days x 8 cycles

IV, intravenously; PO, by mouth; bid, twice a day.

tumor depends on disease extension beyond the rectal wall and the presence of lymph node involvement. Patients with tumor confined to the rectal wall and nodal involvement have a local recurrence rate of 20% to 40%. In patients with tumor extending beyond the rectal wall and negative lymph nodes, the recurrence rate is approximately the same (20%–30%). In contrast, patients with the tumor extending beyond the rectal wall and positive lymph nodes have a recurrence rate that is almost double (40%–70%).[33] Because of an increased risk of local recurrence with rectal cancer compared to colon cancer, clinicians have placed an increased emphasis on local-regional treatment with radiation therapy in the adjuvant setting. The addition of chemotherapy during radiation therapy (i.e., chemoradiation) appears to improve local response rates and, therefore, is increasing in practice.

There is some controversy regarding the sequencing of surgery, radiation therapy, and chemotherapy. Preoperative treatment appears to be equally beneficial and perhaps less toxic.[34] Preoperative radiation has been shown to improve resectability rates of patients with inoperable rectal cancer and to improve overall survival compared to surgery alone.[35] Postoperative radiation without chemotherapy has been shown to improve local control, but 15% to 20% of patients

still experience local recurrence.[36–38] Multiple trials have suggested that using a combined modality approach of postoperative irradiation and a 5-FU–based chemotherapy regimen has been shown to improve local control and survival of resected high-risk rectal cancer patients.[38–40] Based on these results, it is currently suggested that any patient with rectal cancer in which the tumor penetrates through the bowel wall or has positive lymph nodes should receive adjuvant chemotherapy and radiation. Systemic adjuvant chemotherapy with 5-FU/LV or 5-FU/LV and oxaliplatin may be recommended by some clinicians depending on pathologic findings at the time of surgery.[41] Whether radiation therapy is best administered preoperatively or postoperatively requires continued evaluation in clinical trials.

METASTATIC COLORECTAL CANCER (STAGE IV)

In contrast to the different treatment approaches used in the adjuvant setting, stage IV colon and rectal cancers are treated in the same manner.

Single-Agent Chemotherapy. Chemotherapy is usually the only feasible approach to controlling advanced (stage IV) colorectal cancer. Ten to 15% of patients present with metastatic disease, while as many as two thirds of all patients may develop disease at metastatic sites.[42] The liver and lungs are the most common sites of disease spread, while metastases to the brain or bone is less common. Historically, median survival of patients with advanced disease has ranged from 6 to 10 months. For the most part, the treatment of advanced colorectal cancer is considered palliative. A few patients with small isolated liver metastases may undergo surgical resection or radiofrequency ablation, but this results in cure or long-term disease-free survival in only a small percentage of patients. The majority of patients with metastatic colorectal cancer receive systemic chemotherapy that has no curative potential in an attempt to decrease symptoms and ultimately prolong survival. For most of the past 40 years, 5-FU has remained the mainstay of therapy for advanced colorectal cancer, initially alone and later in combination with LV. Most recently, 5-FU is used in combination with oxaliplatin, irinotecan, or bevacizumab.

5-FU is an antimetabolite that inhibits the formation of the DNA-specific nucleoside base thymidine. The main mechanism of action is believed to be inhibition of thymidylate synthase by 5-fluoro-2′-deoxyuridine 5′-phosphate (FdUMP), the active metabolite of 5-FU. 5-FU exerts its major cytotoxicity during the S phase of the cell cycle. The plasma half-life of 5-FU is only 10 to 20 minutes, and the inhibition of thymidylate synthase after a bolus dose is also short.[43,44] Thus, only a small fraction of cancer cells are susceptible to the toxic effects of 5-FU after bolus administration. This may theoretically limit the efficacy of 5-FU when administered by intravenous bolus. Infusional schedules have been investigated as a means to overcome this limitation. 5-FU infusion durations ranging from 24 hours to greater than 10 weeks have been explored in clinical trials.

Infusional 5-FU/LV is superior to bolus 5-FU/LV for improved efficacy and reduced toxicities.[45–48] The dose-limiting toxicity of infusional 5-FU is usually mucositis, but may also include diarrhea or dermatitis; the dose-limiting toxicity of bolus 5-FU is usually myelosuppression, but may include mucositis and diarrhea. A distinct type of dermal toxicity, termed "palmar-plantar erythrodysesthesia," or hand-foot syndrome, may be seen in up to 30% of patients treated with prolonged infusions of 5-FU. This syndrome causes painful swelling and erythema of the hands and feet and may progress to painful desquamation. It is managed by prompt discontinuation of the 5-FU infusion at the onset of symptoms and reinstitution of treatment at reduced dosage after complete recovery from toxicity.

Biochemical Modulation of 5-FU. Aside from fluorouracil, the lack of available agents with activity against colorectal cancer has stimulated the search for methods to improve response rates with 5-FU. One method of overcoming the schedule dependence of 5-FU is to prolong the inhibition of thymidylate synthase by the coadministration of a reduced folate. LV has been successfully used for this purpose. LV stabilizes the covalent bond between thymidylate synthase and FdUMP and thus increases the cytotoxicity of 5-FU.[49] A meta analysis demonstrated the superiority of 5-FU/LV over bolus 5-FU alone in terms of response rate (23% vs. 11%, respectively), but there was no difference in median survival. There did appear to be a trend towards improved survival, however. Despite the lack of a clear-cut survival advantage, 5-FU plus LV has been considered standard therapy for advanced colorectal cancer by most oncologists for much of the last decade.

Doses for LV have ranged from 15 to 500 mg/m^2/day, but data demonstrate that a LV dose of 20 mg/m^2/day effectively enhances 5-FU efficacy and is associated with less toxicity compared with high-dose LV regimens.[50] The most commonly accepted dosing schedule of 5-FU/LV incorporates the lower doses of LV. It should be noted that, because of its mechanism of modulation, LV should always be administered before or concomitantly with the 5-FU. The toxicity of the 5-FU and LV combinations is qualitatively different from the bolus or infusional 5-FU alone. In general, myelosuppression is not increased over what would be expected with 5-FU alone. However, lower doses of 5-FU are usually used when combined with LV. GI toxicity in the form of diarrhea and mucositis is significantly increased with the addition of LV and can produce life-threatening dehydration if not treated promptly. Hand-foot syndrome, which is rarely seen with bolus 5-FU, has been reported to occur frequently with the LV plus 5-FU combination, even with bolus dosing.[49] A variety of other agents have been used to modulate the activity of 5-FU, including, but not limited to, methotrexate, interferon-α, dipyridamole, N-phosphonoacetyl-l-aspartate (PALA), and uridine.[51–54] All of these modulators have shown poorer response rates and increased toxicity compared to LV as a modulating agent and, therefore, are not used in clinical practice.

Combination Chemotherapy. Numerous combinations of chemotherapeutic agents have been explored in colorectal cancer. Most of these have combined one or more agents with 5-FU in an attempt to improve response rates. Drugs used in combination regimens in the past have included 5-FU, cisplatin, semustine, mitomycin C, cyclophosphamide, dimethyltriazenyl imidazole carboxamide (DTIC), hydroxyurea, methotrexate, vincristine, and doxorubicin.[55] None of these combination chemotherapy regimens have been shown to be superior to 5-FU alone. In recent years, irinotecan and oxaliplatin have demonstrated activity in colorectal cancer and have shown increased response rates when administered in combination with 5–FU-based chemotherapy regimens for metastatic disease.

Irinotecan (CPT-11,Camptosar), a semisynthetic derivative of camptothecin, is a potent inhibitor of topoisomerase I. Irinotecan blocks DNA replication and causes DNA strand breaks and cell death. Phase II trials with irinotecan as first-line therapy for colorectal cancer revealed response rates of 19% to 32% and response rates of 13% to 25% as second-line treatment of 5-FU–resistant colorectal carcinoma.[56] Multiple phase III trials in patients that had previously failed 5-FU therapy have demonstrated significant improvement in overall survival compared to supportive care or infusional 5-FU/LV alone.[57,58] Recently, the FOLFIRI regimen consisting of biweekly irinotecan in combination with bolus and infusional 5-FU/LV, improved response rates after fluorouracil or 5-FU/oxaliplatin failure.[59] Irinotecan was approved by the Food and Drug Administration (FDA) as the standard second-line treatment for patients with advanced colorectal carcinoma. The approved dose is 125 mg/m^2 intravenously (IV) weekly for 4 weeks, followed by a 2-week rest period.[60] An alternative dosing schedule of 350 mg/m^2 IV every 3 weeks was also approved for use in the United States. Efficacy with this regimen is similar to the weekly schedule. The main toxicities associated with irinotecan are diarrhea (acute and delayed), myelosuppression, and nausea. Diarrhea generally occurs within the first two cycles of treatment, often requiring treatment with atropine and/or loperamide, and in severe cases may require dose or schedule modification of irinotecan.[61,62] Weekly administration tends to result in an increased rate of diarrhea.[63]

Irinotecan has also been studied in the first-line treatment of metastatic colorectal cancer. A variety of combination regimens containing irinotecan and 5-FU have been evaluated.[64] Irinotecan in combination with either infusional (e.g., FOLFIRI) or bolus 5-FU (e.g., IFL) resulted in statistically significant improvements in response rate and overall survival compared to 5-FU/LV alone.[65,66] Common chemotherapy regimens containing irinotecan for metastatic disease are presented in Table 98.5, associated toxicities are presented in Table 98.6.

TABLE 98.5	Therapy for Metastatic (Stage IV) Colon Cancer
Regimen	**Drug Doses and Schedules**
IFL	Irinotecan 100–125 mg/m² IV over 90 minutes weeks 1, 2, 3, and 4
	Leucovorin 20 mg/m² IV weeks 1, 2, 3, and 4
	Fluorouracil 425–500 mg/m² IV weeks 1, 2, 3, and 4
	Repeat every 6 weeks.
FOLFIRI	Irinotecan 180 mg/m² IV over 90 minutes day 1
	Leucovorin 400 mg/m² IV over 2 hours day 1
	Fluorouracil 400 mg/m² IV bolus day 1
	Fluorouracil 2,400 mg/m² CI over 46 hours
	Repeat every 14 days.
FOLFIRI *(Douillard)*	Irinotecan 180 mg/m² IV over 90 minutes day 1
	Leucovorin 200 mg/m² IV over 2 hours days 1 and 2
	Fluorouracil 400 mg/m² IV bolus days 1 and 2
	Fluorouracil 600 mg/m² CI over 22 hours days 1 and 2
	Repeat every 14 days.
FOLFOX4	Oxaliplatin 85 mg/m² IV over 2 hours day 1
	Leucovorin 200 mg/m² over 2 hours days 1 and 2
	Fluorouracil 400 mg/m² IV bolus days 1 and 2
	Fluorouracil 600 mg/m² CI over 22 hours days 1 and 2
	Repeat every 14 days.
FOLFOX6	Oxaliplatin 100 mg/m² IV day 1
	Leucovorin 400 mg/m² over 2 hours day 1
	Fluorouracil 400 mg/m² IV bolus day 1
	Fluorouracil 2,400–3,000 mg/m² CI over 46 hours
	Repeat every 14 days.
IROX	Irinotecan 200 mg/m² IV day 1
	Oxaliplatin 85 mg/m² IV day 1
	Repeat every 21 days.
Bevacizumab + 5-FU/LCV	Bevacizumab 5 mg/kg IV every 2 weeks
	Fluorouracil 500 mg/m² IV on weeks 1, 2, 3, 4, 5, and 6
	Leucovorin 500 mg/m² IV over 2 hours weeks 1, 2, 3, 4, 5, and 6
	Repeat every 8 weeks.
Bevacizumab + IFL	Bevacizumab 5 mg/kg IV every 2 weeks
	IFL (as regimen previously described in chart)
	Repeat every 6 weeks.
Capecitabine	Capecitabine 1,000–1,250 mg/m² PO bid (total dose = 2,000–2,500 mg/m²/day) days 1–14
	Repeat every 21 days.
XELOX *(CAPOX)*	Oxaliplatin 130 mg/m² IV day 1
	Capecitabine 1,000 mg/m² PO bid (total dose = 2,000 mg/m²/day) days 1–14
	Repeat every 21 days.
XELIRI *(CAPIRI)*	Capecitabine 1,000 mg/m² PO bid (total dose = 2,000 mg/m²/day) days 1–14
	Irinotecan 200–250 mg/m² IV day 1 *OR* 80 mg/m² IV days 1 and 8
	Repeat every 21 days.
Cetuximab	Cetuximab 400 mg/m² IV loading dose, then 250 mg/m² IV weekly
Irinotecan + Cetuximab	Irinotecan 100–125 mg/m² IV weeks 1, 2, 3, and 4
	or
	Irinotecan 200–250 mg/m² IV every 3 weeks
	Cetuximab 400 mg/m² IV loading dose then 250 mg/m² IV weekly

IV, intravenously; PO, by mouth; bid, twice a day; IFL, Irinotecan, Flurouracil, and Leucovorin; CI, continuous infusion.

TABLE 98.6	Toxicities of Therapeutic Agents Used in Colorectal Cancer
Agent	**Toxicities**
5-fluorouracil (5-FU)	Nausea, vomiting, diarrhea, stomatitis, dermatitis, myelosuppression, palmar-plantar erythrodysesthesia
Leucovorin (Folinic acid)	Increased diarrhea and mucositis when administered with 5-FU
Irinotecan (CPT-11; Camptosar)	Diarrhea (acute and delayed), myelosuppression, nausea
Oxaliplatin (Eloxatin)	Peripheral neuropathy, mild myelosuppression, nausea, vomiting
Capecitabine (Xeloda)	Similar to those seen with 5-FU
Bevacizumab (Avastin)	Hypertension, minor bleeding, poor wound healing
Cetuximab (Erbitux)	Acneform rash, asthenia, fatigue, and diarrhea

Oxaliplatin (Eloxatin) is a third-generation platinum complex that cross-links DNA and induces cell death. Compared to cisplatin, this agent exhibits increased therapeutic activity with reduced toxicity. Oxaliplatin and 5-FU work synergistically. Early studies evaluating oxaliplatin as a single agent produced a response rate of 10% in patients with tumors resistant to fluorouracil.[67] As second-line therapy, different schedules of oxaliplatin plus 5-FU and LV have generated response rates ranging from 18% to 46%.[68,69] The FDA approved oxaliplatin in combination with infusional 5-FU and LV for treatment of patients whose disease has recurred or progressed during or within 6 months of completing first-line therapy with bolus 5-FU/LV and irinotecan.[70] Since its FDA approval, oxaliplatin has demonstrated improvements in response rates and overall survival as frontline treatment of metastatic disease. The most common side effects include a reversible, acute peripheral neuropathy that is enhanced by exposure to cold and a dose-limiting cumulative peripheral sensory neuropathy that usually improves after treatment discontinuation.[69] Oxaliplatin lacks nephrotoxicity, which is commonly associated with cisplatin and carboplatin, and it has limited hematologic toxicity.[69]

Since its FDA approval, oxaliplatin has been investigated in a number of clinical trials for its activity in the frontline treatment of metastatic colorectal cancer. Recent data demonstrated the superiority of oxaliplatin in combination with 5-FU/LV in terms of progression-free survival and response rate compared to 5-FU and LV alone. However, it did not show a significant improvement in overall survival.[71] Multiple randomized trials evaluating oxaliplatin with different schedules of 5-FU/LV had similar findings.[72,73] Recently, however, oxaliplatin in combination with infusional

5-FU has been shown to significantly improve overall survival compared to irinotecan and bolus 5-FU.[74] Whether the difference is related to the method of 5-FU administration or the addition of oxaliplatin requires continued evaluation in clinical trials. Tournigard et al[59] attempted to answer this question in a recent study comparing oxaliplatin to irinotecan, in which both agents were given in combination with infusional 5-FU. Overall survival, response rates, or progression-free survival did not differ significantly in either group.

Combination therapy with irinotecan, oxaliplatin, 5-FU, and LV has also been evaluated and preliminary results suggest that combination therapy resulted in similar efficacy and safety when compared to irinotecan plus 5-FU/LV.[72] Thus, multiple trials suggest that irinotecan or oxaliplatin in combination with infusional 5-FU are efficacious in the first-line setting. Common chemotherapy regimens containing oxaliplatin for metastatic disease are presented in Table 98.5, associated toxicities are presented in Table 98.6.

Capecitabine (Xeloda) is an orally administered prodrug of 5-FU. Capecitabine passes through the intestinal mucosa as an intact molecule and is then activated by a cascade of three enzymes that results in the intracellular release of 5-FU. This tumor-specific activation allows for higher concentrations of 5-FU to be achieved in the tumor cells compared to normal tissue, thereby reducing systemic toxicities. Results from multiple clinical trials indicate that capecitabine significantly improves response rates and results in equivalent time to progression and overall survival compared to 5-FU. In addition, capecitabine was better tolerated and more convenient for patients compared to intravenous therapy. Currently, investigators are conducting phase II trials evaluating capecitabine in combination with oxaliplatin or irinotecan.[75–77] Side effects and toxicities of capecitabine are similar to those seen with infusional 5-FU (hand-foot syndrome, diarrhea, nausea and vomiting, mucositis, and neutropenia). Common chemotherapy regimens containing capecitabine for metastatic disease are presented in Table 98.5, associated toxicities are presented in Table 98.6.

Biologic Agents. Therapies targeting specific activities of tumor cells are now being used to improve response rates to systemic chemotherapy even further and ultimately extend overall survival. Investigators hope that targeted therapy may improve the efficacy of standard treatment without adversely affecting the safety profiles. Theoretically, normal tissues will not be affected by these agents.

One innovative approach to the treatment of metastatic colorectal cancer involves therapeutic agents that inhibit angiogenesis, or the formation of new blood vessels from the existing vasculature. Angiogenesis ensures continued delivery of nutrients and is seen in tumor growth, wound healing, and ovulation. It is not necessary for most normal tissues. There is strong evidence to link angiogenesis with tumor growth and metastases, therefore antiangiogenic therapy has gained considerable interest. One of the angiogenic factors, vascular endothelial growth factor (VEGF), has recently been recognized as an important regulator of this process. Bevacizumab (Avastin), a recombinant monoclonal antibody that inhibits VEGF, has been evaluated in several phase II and phase III clinical trials. In phase II studies, bevacizumab has been used in combination with 5-FU/LV at various doses and in combination with irinotecan, 5-FU, and LV with response rates ranging from 24% to 40% for first-line treatment of patients with metastatic disease.[78,79] Based on these promising results, bevacizumab has been further evaluated in combination with IFL in a large phase III trial (n = 925) in the first-line metastatic setting. The authors reported an improvement in median overall survival, overall response rate, and progression-free survival compared to IFL alone that reached statistical significance.[80] Other clinical trials are investigating this agent in the second-line setting as well. The FDA recently approved bevacizumab for the management of previously untreated metastatic colorectal cancer in combination with any intravenous 5-FU–containing chemotherapy regimen. The recommended dose is 5 mg per kilogram IV every 2 weeks. The most common side effects seen with this agent have been hypertension, minor bleeding, and poor wound healing. There was an increased incidence of thromboembolic events and GI perforations in bevacizumab clinical trials, although neither reached statistical significance.[81] Common chemotherapeutic regimens using bevacizumab are presented in Table 98.5.

Epidermal growth factors have also been implicated in the development of malignancy. The epidermal growth factor receptor (EGFr) is commonly expressed on tumor cell surfaces and appears to be related to cell growth, differentiation, and proliferation. Cetuximab (Erbitux) is a monoclonal antibody directed against the binding site of EGFr. Clinical studies have been performed to investigate its role as a single agent or in combination with irinotecan for patients with irinotecan-refractory or oxaliplatin-refractory colorectal cancer that express EGFr. Combination therapy with cetuximab and irinotecan demonstrated a significant improvement in overall response rate and time to progression.[82] The FDA recently approved this agent as a single agent or in combination with irinotecan for the treatment of EGFr-expressing, metastatic colorectal cancer in patients who are refractory to irinotecan-based chemotherapy. The recommended dose, as monotherapy or in combination, is 400 mg/m^2 IV as an initial loading dose followed with 250 mg/m^2 IV every week. Due to its black box warning for infusion-related reactions, premedication with an H$_1$-antagonist is recommended. Common side effects include an acneform rash, asthenia, fatigue, and diarrhea.[83] Common chemotherapeutic regimens utilizing cetuximab are presented in Table 98.5.

Regional Chemotherapy. Regional chemotherapy for the treatment of colorectal cancer usually refers to hepatic arterial infusion of chemotherapy for the treatment of liver metastases. This approach offers the advantage of substantially increasing the intensity of drug delivery to the liver while minimizing the systemic side effects. It is indicated in pa-

tients who have liver-only metastases and a good performance status. Hepatic arterial infusion for colorectal liver metastases is discussed in more detail in Chapter 97.

FUTURE THERAPIES

The introduction of irinotecan and oxaliplatin significantly improved the treatment of advanced colorectal cancer. Targeted therapy with bevacizumab and cetuximab appears to be a major breakthrough as well. Determining the most efficacious sequence of therapeutic agents requires further investigation. In addition, continued research involving new targeted therapies may expand treatment options further.

CONCLUSION

Colorectal cancer is one of the most common malignancies and is a major health problem in the United States. Prevention and early detection programs have received attention in recent years as the incidence continues to rise, with a large proportion of patients diagnosed with already advanced disease. Prognosis has been directly associated with the depth of tumor invasion into or through the bowel wall, the presence of lymph node involvement, and presence of distant metastatic disease. The initial treatment for colorectal cancer is surgery to remove the primary lesion and surrounding tissue. Adjuvant therapy for patients with localized disease has been shown to decrease recurrence rates and prolong survival. Adjuvant therapy is currently recommended for patients with stage III colon cancer and standard treatment is considered by most to be the FOLFOX regimen for all patients that can tolerate it. Alternatively, in patients unable to tolerate FOLFOX, a 5-FU plus LV regimen or capecitabine is acceptable. Stage II patients at high risk of recurrence may also receive adjuvant chemotherapy at the discretion of the treating physician. Many other agents and combinations continue to be investigated for their role in the adjuvant treatment of colon cancer. Adjuvant treatment for locally advanced (stage III) rectal cancer includes concomitant 5-FU and LV (or capecitabine) with radiation therapy. Depending on pathologic findings at the time of surgery, systemic chemotherapy with 5-FU/LV with or without oxaliplatin may be recommended. Treatment of advanced disease (stage IV) with chemotherapy remains palliative, but the introduction of new therapeutic agents have expanded treatment options and improved survival. The fluoropyrimidines continue to be the mainstay in the treatment of colorectal cancer. Biochemical modulation of 5-FU with LV and identification of new agents such as irinotecan, oxaliplatin, bevacizumab, and cetuximab have increased response rates and improved survival. First-line treatment of metastatic disease currently includes 5-FU, LV, and oxaliplatin or irinotecan. Many clinicians would recommend adding bevacizumab to this frontline chemotherapy regimen. Second-line chemotherapy regimens would incorporate these same agents, substituting irinotecan for oxaliplatin or vice versa depending on the initial treatment choice. Third-line regimens may include cetuximab monotherapy or irinotecan and cetuximab combination therapy. Despite substantial progress in treatment options, future research will focus on how best to sequence these agents and on potential sites for additional targeted therapies.

PANCREATIC CANCER

EPIDEMIOLOGY

INCIDENCE

Pancreatic cancer is a relatively rare malignancy, with an estimated 31,860 new cases in the United States in 2004.[9] The incidence has decreased slightly over the last two decades, primarily due to a steady decline in the rate for white men.[9,84,85] Carcinoma of the pancreas is mainly a disease of the elderly. More than 80% of cases occur between the ages of 60 and 80, and cases below age 40 are very rare.[9,85] There had been a slight male preponderance in the incidence, with the male to female ratio being 1.7:1.0 in older epidemiologic studies.[84] This ratio has gradually equalized because the incidence rate has declined significantly in men since 1974.[9] Racial differences in incidence and mortality rates from pancreatic cancer have also been observed. Incidence and mortality rates in African-Americans of both sexes are higher than in whites and other ethnic groups.[9] The incidence is higher in urban than in rural areas and higher in industrialized nations implying that environmental factors may play a role in the etiology.[86] Countries with a high incidence include Denmark, Sweden, Finland, Ireland, Austria, Czechoslovakia, Hungary, and certain areas of Canada.[86–88]

In the United States, approximately 31,270 deaths in 2004 were attributed to pancreatic cancer, making it the fourth most common cause of cancer death.[9] Prognosis is dismal for patients diagnosed with pancreatic cancer, with median survival from the time of diagnosis being only 6 months.[84] Less than 5% of patients survive 5 years.[9] Carcinoma of the pancreas is one of the most aggressive solid tumors, representing a major public health problem and a significant clinical challenge.

ETIOLOGY

Many dietary and environmental factors have been implicated as possible etiologic factors in the development of pancreatic cancer, but definite causal relationships have not been established in the majority of cases. The strongest evidence points to cigarette smoking as a risk factor associated with pancreatic cancer. Results from animal studies suggest that nitrosamines in tobacco smoke are carcinogenic to the pancreas. Several case-control studies found a twofold to threefold increase in risk in smokers compared with nonsmokers.[89–93] Occupational exposure to certain chemicals has also been linked to an excess of pancreatic carcinoma.

Employees of petroleum and chemical industries appear to be at especially high risk. Workers exposed to industrial solvents or petroleum products for more than 10 years have up to a fivefold increase in the incidence of pancreatic cancer.[94] Stone miners, cement workers, gardeners, textile workers, and leather tanners are also among the high-risk group of patients.[85,95] Numerous studies have examined the causative role of nutrition in the development of pancreatic cancer with inconsistent results. Some found a positive correlation with total energy intake, carbohydrate ingestion, or meat consumption.[85,90,92] Others suggested a protective effect of diets high in fiber, fruits, and vegetables.[85] An increased risk for pancreatic cancer has also been attributed to alcohol or coffee consumption; however, evidence is weak and inconsistent.[88,89]

A connection between pancreatic malignancy and a number of medical conditions, such as diabetes mellitus and chronic pancreatitis, has long been suspected. Approximately 15% of patients diagnosed with pancreatic cancer have a history of diabetes mellitus, implying a causal relationship between diabetes mellitus and the development of pancreatic cancer.[96] However, in more than half of these patients, the onset of clinical diabetes preceded the diagnosis of pancreatic cancer by only a few months. This suggests that the cancer may cause insulin insufficiency, and diabetes manifesting many years before the diagnosis of pancreatic cancer would be better evidence for an etiologic correlation.[97] However, this line of reasoning has been counterbalanced by the argument that although the clinical diagnosis of diabetes was made very recent to the diagnosis of pancreatic cancer, undiagnosed diabetes may well have preceded the cancer by many years.[98] With regard to chronic inflammation of the pancreas, the issue remains controversial as well. Some studies have proposed a causal relationship between chronic pancreatitis and the development of pancreatic cancer.[99,100] However, others suggest that the long-term risk of pancreatic cancer in patients with chronic pancreatitis may actually be related to alcohol consumption, smoking, and selection bias.[101]

Recent advances in the understanding of human genetics have brought about an increasing appreciation for the hereditary influence on the etiology of pancreatic cancer. Abnormal changes in K-*ras,* an oncogene, or p53, p16, DPC4, and BRCA2, the tumor suppressor genes, have been linked with carcinoma of the pancreas.[102,103] Several genetic syndromes associated with pancreatic cancer, including hereditary pancreatitis, ataxia-telangiectasia, hereditary nonpolyposis colorectal cancer, familial atypical multiple mole-melanoma, Peutz-Jeghers, and familial breast cancer, have been described.[102,104,105] Identification of familial clusters of pancreatic cancer also facilitates genetic study of the disease. Although the overall percentage of pancreatic carcinoma that shows familial clustering remains uncertain, a crude estimate suggests that as many as 3% to 5% of all pancreatic cancers have a hereditary origin.[106]

PATHOPHYSIOLOGY

The pancreas lies transversely in the posterior part of the upper abdomen (Fig. 98.1; *see color insert*). The head of the pancreas is on the right side of the abdomen and rests against the curve of the duodenum. The body of the pancreas lies beneath the stomach, and the tail of the pancreas extends across the abdomen to the left side. The pancreas is virtually surrounded by other organs in the upper abdomen. However, unlike other organs, it cannot be palpated because of its posterior location. Because of its position and large functional reserve, symptoms of pancreatic disease, including cancer, often do not appear until the disorder is far advanced.

The pancreas is an endocrine and an exocrine organ. Most tumors (95%) occur in the exocrine portion. Tumors of the endocrine portion are usually benign, whereas only 2% of tumors arising in the exocrine portion of the pancreas are benign. Malignant tumors may arise from pancreatic ductal epithelial cells, acinar cells, connective tissue, or lymphatic tissue. Histologically, ductal adenocarcinoma accounts for

more than 80% of all pancreatic malignancies. The head of the pancreas is the site for approximately 60% of all pancreatic tumors, with 15% occurring in the body and tail, and 20% diffusely involving the gland.[107]

On gross examination, tumors of the pancreas usually appear hard, gritty, and whitish. The surrounding tissue often displays evidence of chronic pancreatitis. Tumors in the head of the pancreas are usually less than 5 cm in diameter at diagnosis and are often associated with pancreatic and common bile duct obstruction, adjacent duodenum invasion, and portal vein or superior mesentery artery occlusion. Tumors occurring in the tail of the pancreas are usually larger (5–10 cm) at the time of diagnosis and associated with splenic vein obstruction (Fig. 98.2; *see color insert*). Early subclinical metastases are characteristic of pancreatic cancer. Less than 20% of patients have disease confined to the pancreas at the time of diagnosis. Forty percent of patients have locally advanced (regional lymph nodes, adjacent organs) disease, whereas more than 40% have distant metastases at diagnosis.[9] The most commonly involved distant organ is the liver, followed by lung, bone, and brain.

CLINICAL PRESENTATION AND DIAGNOSIS

SIGNS AND SYMPTOMS

The early symptoms of pancreatic cancer tend to be very nonspecific and insidious in nature, thus delaying diagnosis in 80% to 90% of patients. Pain is the single most common presenting symptom, which is usually the reason why patients seek medical attention. Pain, described as dull, constant, and radiating to the middle and upper back, is attrib-

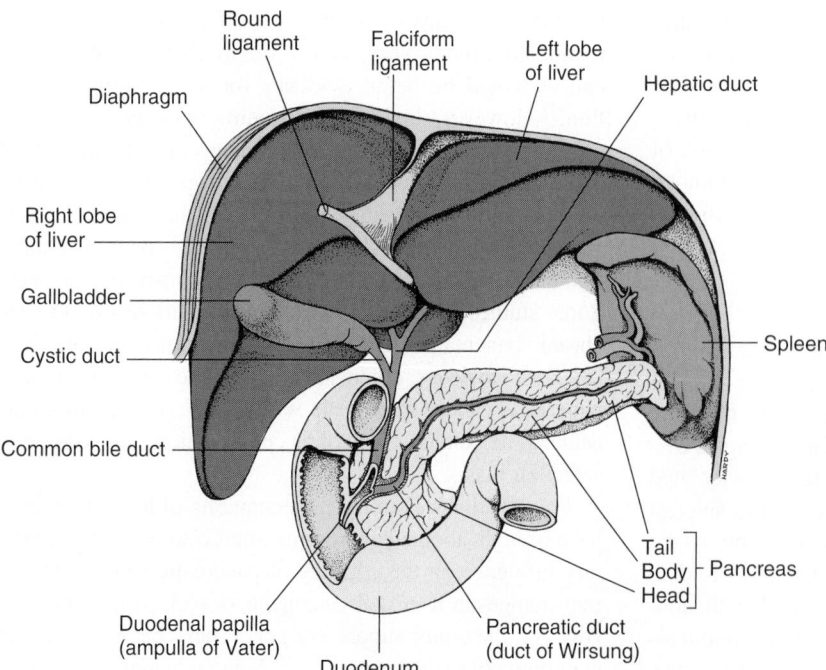

FIGURE 98.1 Pancreatic anatomy (*see color insert*). (From Stedman's Medical Dictionary, 27th ed. Baltimore: Lippincott Williams & Wilkins, 2000, with permission.)

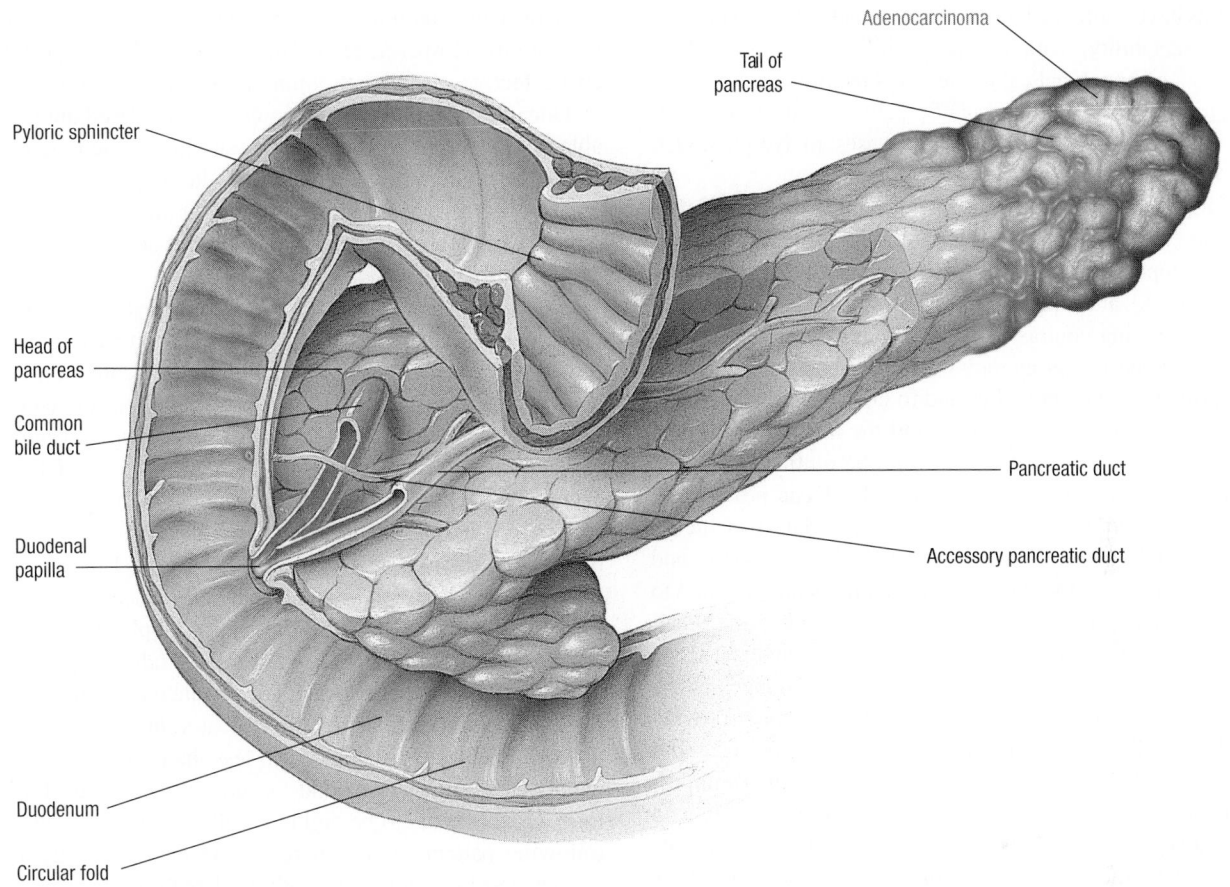

FIGURE 98.2 Pancreatic tail lesion (*see color insert*). (Asset provided by the Anatomical Chart Co., with permission.)

uted to tumor invasion of the celiac and mesenteric plexus.[108–110] Because most tumors arise in the ductal system, biliary obstruction is common. Obstructive jaundice occurs in approximately 50% of all patients with pancreatic cancer, and in up to 90% of patients with tumors in the head of the pancreas.[111] Obstructive jaundice is generally associated with less advanced disease because it forces patients to seek medical attention when the tumor is still localized and potentially resectable. Nausea, anorexia, weight loss, and fatigue are among the common complaints at presentation and can be attributed to biliary obstruction and GI obstruction.[108,111] Pancreatic endocrine and exocrine insufficiency have also been reported, causing glucose intolerance, malabsorption, and steatorrhea.

Pancreatic cancer may spread by invading surrounding tissues or by metastasizing to distant sites. Direct invasion into the abdominal lymph nodes, liver, and gastroduodenum is often present at diagnosis. The natural history of pancreatic cancer is highlighted by the early development of widespread metastatic disease, and death is often secondary to liver failure and malnutrition.[84]

DIAGNOSIS

Because the symptoms of pancreatic cancer tend to be nonspecific and are often attributed to other medical conditions,

a high index of suspicion is necessary to make an accurate and timely diagnosis. Pancreatic cancer should be included in the differential diagnosis of any patient with unexplained jaundice, pancreatitis, weight loss, and nonspecific upper abdominal or back pain. The goal of medical evaluation in a patient with suspected pancreatic cancer is to establish the presence or absence of a primary tumor, and if one is present to determine the extent of local and metastatic disease. The diagnostic evaluation usually begins with a physical examination to establish clinical correlation such as jaundice, weight loss, palpable mass, ascites, or metastatic disease. Blood tests are obtained to help evaluate jaundice, liver function, and pancreatic function. Serum amylase, lipase, alkaline phosphatase, and leucine aminopeptidase levels may be increased in patients with pancreatic cancer. If the tumor involves the liver, levels of lactic dehydrogenase and the transaminases may also be elevated.

The diagnostic workup continues with noninvasive radiologic studies and then, if necessary, proceeds to more invasive radiologic and endoscopic procedures, and eventually to tissue biopsy. Currently, contrast-enhancing helical CT is considered the mainstay imaging modality for diagnostic and staging workup of pancreatic cancer.[112] The primary goals of a CT scan are to detect the suspected pancreatic mass and to determine the resectability of the identified tumor. Many studies have confirmed the accuracy of helical CT in predicting resectability, with the resectability rate approaching 80%.[113] Although helical CT remains the preferred imaging test for diagnosis and staging of pancreatic cancer, it has its limitation in detecting small metastases to lymph nodes, liver, and peritoneum.[114]

More invasive procedures to aid in the diagnosis of pancreatic cancer include angiography, endoscopic retrograde cholangiopancreatography (ERCP), endoscopic ultrasonography (EUS), and laparoscopy. Angiography is an x-ray procedure utilizing contrast material for examining blood vessels. In the past, angiography was performed preoperatively to define vascular anomalies and to determine the anatomic relationship between the tumor and the major surrounding vessels. Currently, it has no place in the routine workup of pancreatic malignancy because helical CT can provide the same information.[114] An ERCP is a procedure in which a long flexible scope is passed through the esophagus and stomach and into the duodenum. This procedure is used to visualize the common bile duct is connected to the small intestine. Contrast material can be injected through the scope into the common bile duct to visualize x-ray images of the common bile and pancreatic ducts. ERCP does not provide additional diagnostic information if a pancreatic mass has been identified on CT. However, it still maintains an important role in the differential diagnosis of those patients who have a typical history of pancreatic cancer but do not have a pancreatic mass on CT.[84,114] In the absence of gall stones or a history of pancreatitis, obstructive lesions of the intrapancreatic portion of the common bile duct are almost always secondary to malignancy. Another role of ERCP is to place a stent to relieve obstructive jaundice in symptomatic patients who are not to be bypassed or resected shortly. A metal or plastic stent can be placed in the common bile duct during an ERCP. The procedure is fairly simple and can be performed under conscious sedation. EUS is a relatively new diagnostic tool developed for a staging workup of pancreatic cancer. Using the wall of the stomach and duodenum as an acoustic window, EUS produces detailed images of the pancreas and can be helpful in detecting small intrapancreatic masses missed by CT. Its role in assessing vascular involvement is still controversial. EUS may also be used as a means of obtaining tissue biopsy and instituting celiac plexus neurolysis, commonly known as a nerve block for pain management.[115] The role of EUS in the management of patients with pancreatic cancer has not yet been established. Some authors have advocated laparoscopy with peritoneal washing for cytology to further increase the resectability rate predicted by helical CT.[114,116] During a laparoscopic procedure, the surgeon typically makes a small incision to insert a scope to visualize the area in question and also the surrounding tissue and organs. The peritoneum is the second most common site for pancreatic metastases; however, peritoneal seeding, typically a few millimeters in diameter, most likely fails to be detected by CT. Direct laparoscopic visualization of the peritoneum, omentum, and liver surface for tumor implants can potentially spare patients from an unnecessary laparotomy. However, more data are required to support the cost-effectiveness of the routine use of this procedure.

Once a suspected pancreatic mass is considered unresectable or if metastatic disease is present, histologic diagnosis should be obtained by direct fine-needle biopsy of the pancreas or percutaneous biopsy of a liver metastasis. If the tumor is considered resectable, the patient should be evaluated for surgery.

A variety of biologic substances identified in the serum of patients with pancreatic cancer may be considered tumor markers. At the current time, a number of potential markers have been identified, including CEA, tumor-associated carbohydrate antigen (CA 19-9), CA 125 antigen, and monoclonal antibody products (DUPAN-2, SPAN-1).[117] CEA is elevated in approximately 50% of patients with pancreatic cancer, but it is also increased in many other benign and malignant GI diseases.[117] CA 19-9 is elevated in approximately 80% of patients with pancreatic cancer. Although there are some limitations to the clinical application of CA 19-9, reasonable data from worldwide studies support its promising role in the management of pancreatic cancer as a diagnostic adjunct, a prognostic indicator, and a monitoring tool.[118,119] CA 125 is elevated in less than 50% of patients with pancreatic cancer and is not clinically useful.[117] DUPAN-2 appears to be highly specific for identifying and following patients with pancreatic cancer, but it may also be elevated in patients with other GI malignancies or diseases.[120] Further investigation into the development of more specific and sensitive tumor markers in pancreatic cancer is required before they will be considered to be consistently clinically useful.

STAGING AND PROGNOSIS

The American Joint Committee on Cancer (AJCC) has developed staging criteria for adenocarcinoma of the pancreas.[121] This system, also known as the TNM staging system, is based on the extent of the primary tumor, regional lymph nodes, and metastatic disease.[120] The TNM staging system is presented in Table 98.7. Unfortunately, this staging system is not clinically useful. It is difficult to apply because the lymph node status is difficult to assess without surgery. Moreover, the TNM stage does not correlate well with treatment or prognosis. Instead, for prognosis prediction and therapy decision, most centers rely on the clinical or radiographic staging system[84] (Table 98.8). It classifies pancreatic cancer into three groups: stage I disease is localized to the pancreas and is surgically resectable; stage II disease is locally advanced and not surgically resectable; stage III disease has metastatic spread. Obviously, patients with stage I disease have the best prognosis and are the only patients in whom the disease is curable. Unfortunately, less than 15 % of patients are in stage I at the time of presentation. Most patients present with advanced disease stage II or III, and are considered unresectable and incurable. These patients

TABLE 98.7 | TNM Staging System for Pancreatic Cancer

Primary tumor (T)

TX:	Primary tumor cannot be assessed
T0:	No evidence of primary tumor
Tis:	Carcinoma in situ
T1:	Tumor limited to the pancreas, ≤2 cm in greatest dimension
T2:	Tumor limited to the pancreas, >2 cm in greatest dimension
T3:	Tumor extends beyond the pancreas but without involvement of the celiac axis or the superior mesenteric artery
T4:	Tumor involves the celiac axis or the superior mesenteric artery (unresectable primary tumor)

Regional lymph nodes (N)

NX:	Regional lymph nodes cannot be assessed
N0:	No regional lymph node metastasis
N1:	Regional lymph node metastasis

Distant metastasis (M)

MX:	Distant metastasis cannot be assessed
M0:	No distant metastasis
M1:	Distant metastasis

AJCC stage groupings

Stage 0	Tis, N0, M0
Stage IA	T1, N0, M0
Stage IB	T2, N0, M0
Stage IIA	T3, N0, M0
Stage IIB	T1, N1, M0
	T2, N1, M0
	T3, N1, M0
Stage III	T4, any N, M0
Stage IV	Any T, any N, M1

AJCC, American Joint Committee on Cancer.

TABLE 98.8 | Clinical/Radiographic Staging of Pancreatic Cancer

Potentially resectable

Defined (roughly) as pancreatic cancer including no evidence of extrapancreatic involvement of the tumor, demonstration of fully patent superior mesenteric/portal veins, and showing no evidence of encroachment ("encasement") by the tumor on the arterial celiac axis or the superior mesenteric artery.

Locally advanced

Tumor includes evidence of arterial encroachment (celiac axis or superior mesenteric artery) or venous occlusion (superior mesenteric/portal veins).

Metastatic

This stage includes evidence of metastatic spread (typically to the liver, peritoneum, or lung).

LOCALIZED, RESECTABLE PANCREATIC CANCER (STAGE I)

Cancer of the pancreas usually manifests in advanced stages with local invasion into vital structures, making curative surgery an option for only a small number of patients. Before modern imaging technologies became available, laparotomy often revealed that the pancreatic malignancy was actually more advanced than what had been apparent on preoperative studies. Therefore, many patients ended up with incomplete tumor removal or palliative surgery. Unfortunately, data have shown that positive-margin resection does not provide additional survival benefit beyond what can be achieved with palliative chemoradiation alone.[122,123] Moreover, laparotomy carries with it a significant morbidity rate of 20% to 30% and a mean hospital stay of 3 to 4 weeks.[84]

Recently, high-quality helical CT has significantly increased the resectability rate, presuming strict observation of resectability criteria. For a resectable mass located in the head of the pancreas, a pancreaticoduodenectomy (Whipple procedure) is considered standard care.[124] This operation involves the en bloc removal of the distal stomach and duodenum, the first portion of the jejunum, and the head and part of the body of the pancreas (Fig. 98.3; *see color insert*). Despite successful surgery with curative intent, the prognosis remains unfavorable even in this selected group of patients with only 10% to 30% 5-year survival rates.[122] Long-term postoperative morbidity further reduces quality of life, with hemorrhage, infection, pancreatic fistula, and nutritional problems being the commonly encountered complications. Therefore, surgical procedures continue to be modified with an effort to improve the cure rate and reduce morbidity. Currently, about one third of all pancreatic surgeons in the United States advocate the pylorus-preserving Whipple procedure, in which the stomach and the pylorus are retained.[125] The potential advantage of this modification is that the nutritional sequelae of the standard pancreaticoduodenectomy, such as food dumping syndrome and diarrhea,

have a very poor prognosis with less than 10% of them surviving 1 year after diagnosis.

TREATMENT

Surgery, radiation therapy, and chemotherapy are treatment options for patients with pancreatic cancer. Primary treatment goals vary with stage. For those patients with stage I disease, therapy is aimed toward a cure. With more advanced disease, the objectives of medical management are to prolong survival, palliate symptoms, and improve quality of life. Unfortunately, the available treatment options for this patient population have not significantly altered the natural history of the disease.

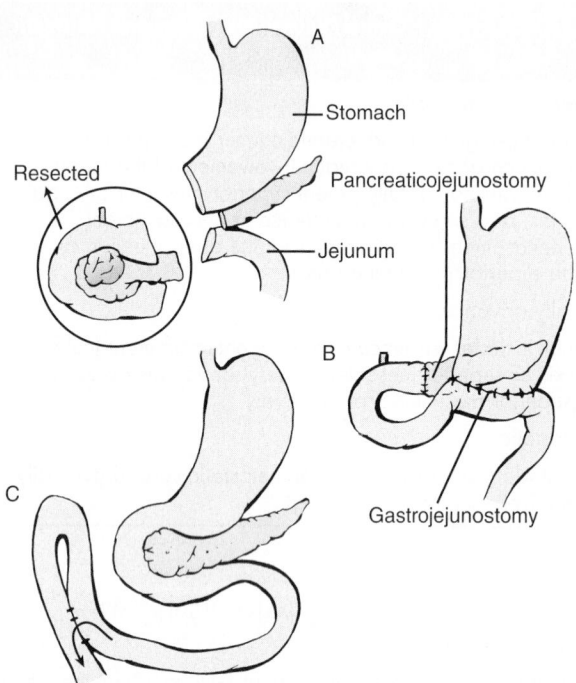

FIGURE 98.3 Whipple procedure (*see color insert*). (From Nettina SM. The Lippincott Manual of Nursing Practice. 7th ed. Baltimore: Lippincott Williams & Wilkins, 2001, with permission.)

can be avoided. So far, there is no evidence suggesting a survival disadvantage associated with this new surgical technique. Another surgical alternative is a total pancreatectomy,[126,127] which may have the advantage of preventing local recurrence. However, long-term survival rate after total pancreatectomy was not different from the Whipple procedure. Moreover, there are disadvantages associated with complete removal of the pancreas, such as pancreatic exocrine insufficiency and permanent diabetes mellitus requiring lifelong insulin replacement therapy.

The incidence of local tumor recurrence after curative resection is 50% to 80%. Patients who undergo pancreaticoduodenectomy alone have a median survival of 12 months. It is currently recommended that patients receive adjuvant treatment with chemoradiation to improve local-regional control. External-beam radiation therapy (EBRT) and concomitant 5-FU have been demonstrated to improve survival after curative resection by the Gastrointestinal Tumor Study Group (GITSG). The standard care at the present is the delivery of 40 Gy in a split-course fashion plus 5-FU at 500 mg/m^2/day IV bolus for 3 days concurrently with each 20-Gy segment of radiation therapy. Split-course radiation signifies administering 2 weeks of radiation followed by 2 weeks of rest followed by another 2 weeks of radiation. The 5-FU regimen is then continued weekly, beginning 1 month after completion of radiation, for a full 2 years. Median survival was 20 months with the multimodality approach compared with 11 to 12 months with surgery alone.[128,129]

Despite the clinical benefit of adjuvant chemoradiation, the delivery of multimodality therapy is delayed or omitted in 25% of patients due to prolonged recovery after pancreaticoduodenectomy.[130] This stems the interest in neoadjuvant chemoradiation. Preoperative chemoradiation offers several potential advantages. First, radiation appears to be more effective on well-oxygenated cells that have not been devascularized by surgery. Second, peritoneal tumor cell implantation due to surgical manipulation may be prevented by preoperative chemoradiation. Third, patients with disseminated disease evident on restaging after chemoradiation will not be subjected to laparotomy. Fourth, because chemoradiation is given first, delayed postoperative recovery will have no effect on the delivery of multimodality therapy.[84,131] Spitz et al[130] have compared the neoadjuvant approach to the standard adjuvant chemoradiation. Preoperative radiotherapy was delivered at 50.4 Gy in standard split course over 5.5 weeks or 30 Gy as rapid fractionation over 2 weeks. Rapid fraction radiation involves administering a smaller amount of radiation over a shorter course of time in hopes of minimizing toxicity while still achieving the same efficacy. Postoperative irradiation was given to a total dose of 50.4 Gy in standard fractionation. Preoperative and postoperative radiotherapy were carried out concomitantly with continuous-infusion 5-FU at 300 mg/m^2/day for 5 days weekly. At a median follow-up of 19 months, it was found that the delivery of preoperative and postoperative chemoradiation in patients who underwent potentially curative surgery for pancreatic adenocarcinoma led to similar treatment toxicity, patterns of tumor recurrence, and survival. This represents an approach to maximize the proportion of patients who receive all components of multimodality therapy and avoids the toxicity of pancreaticoduodenectomy in patients found to have metastatic disease at the time of restaging. Formal evaluation of neoadjuvant chemoradiation for locally advanced pancreatic cancer in the clinical trials setting is warranted.

A novel approach of delivering chemoradiation involves the use of gemcitabine, a pyrimidine antimetabolite, as a radiosensitizer. Evidence supporting gemcitabine's efficacy in the treatment of advanced pancreatic cancer, and its activity as a radiosensitizing agent, provides the rationale for the ongoing multiinstitutional phase II study of preoperative EBRT and concomitant gemcitabine for patients with resectable adenocarcinoma of the pancreas.[131–134] Wolff et al[135] at The University of Texas M.D. Anderson Cancer Center have presented preliminary results from their trial of preoperative gemcitabine-based chemoradiation for resectable pancreatic cancer. Eighty-six patients with potentially resectable adenocarcinoma of the pancreatic head or uncinate process received 7 weekly infusions of gemcitabine (400 mg/m^2) and 30 Gy of EBRT delivered as 3 Gy per fraction every Monday to Friday over 2 weeks beginning 3 days after the first dose of gemcitabine. Eighty-three patients underwent restaging evaluation 4 to 6 weeks after the last dose of gemcitabine (3 patients were still awaiting restaging).

Twelve (14%) patients did not undergo surgery, 7 of these 12 patients had disease progression at time of restaging. Seventy-one (86%) patients underwent laparotomy, 10 (12%) of which had metastatic disease while 61 (73%) underwent a successful pancreaticoduodenectomy (Whipple procedure).

Another alternative to postoperative adjuvant chemoradiation is the use of electron-beam intraoperative radiation therapy (EB-IORT). EB-IORT is delivered after resection of the specimen but before initiating GI reconstruction. Of note, EB-IORT prolongs the surgical procedure by only an additional 30 to 40 minutes. The dose of EB-IORT ranges from 10 to 15 Gy. Initial results support the safety of adjuvant EB-IORT and suggest improved rates of local-regional control.[136,137] EB-IORT has also been added to preoperative chemoradiation and pancreaticoduodenectomy with good result. Pisters et al[138] reported a median survival of 25 months at a median 37-month follow-up in the group of patients treated with preoperative chemoradiation, pancreaticoduodenectomy, and EB-IORT.

With better local-regional control using neoadjuvant or adjuvant chemoradiation, disease recurrence usually manifests as distant metastases. Prognosis remains dismal. The major barrier to progress in the treatment of pancreatic cancer lies in the absence of effective systemic therapies. Innovative therapeutic approaches continue to be developed and investigated in clinical trials, which will hopefully result in newer and more efficacious strategies to alter the natural history of the disease.

LOCALIZED, UNRESECTABLE PANCREATIC CANCER (STAGE II)

Patients who are found to have locally advanced unresectable disease at the time of operation can undergo palliative surgical bypass to correct impending biliary or GI obstruction. These operations do not prolong survival, but they usually improve the quality of life for these patients. For treatment, patients with stage II disease can receive 5–FU-based chemoradiation or gemcitabine.

Based on the results of a GITSG trial completed in 1981, patients with locally advanced pancreatic cancer who receive 5–FU-based chemoradiation have a median survival of about 10 months compared with 6 months in those who receive radiation alone.[139] Of note, the clinical benefit of chemoradiation is primarily limited to patients with good performance status. The optimal chemoradiation regimen is yet to be determined. In the GITSG trial, a split-course radiotherapy was delivered to a total dose of 40 to 60 Gy in combination with 5-FU at 500 mg/m^2/day IV bolus for the first 3 days of each 20 Gy course. Weekly maintenance was 5-FU then followed at 500 mg/m^2 IV bolus for 2 years or until tumor progression. Several other combinations have also been used. With concurrent radiation, combination chemotherapy has not been proven to be superior to 5-FU alone[140,141]; therefore, it cannot be recommended. Many investigational radiotherapy techniques are currently being tested, including EB-IORT, high-energy particle-beam irra-

diation, and interstitial implantation of iodine-125.[136,137,142] Radiosensitizers other than 5-FU, such as bromodeoxyuridine, paclitaxel, cisplatin, gemcitabine, and even a monoclonal antibody against VEGF, such as bevacizumab, have also been investigated.[132–134,143–145] However, no randomized trials have been conducted to confirm the superiority of any of these modifications over the original regimen reported by the GITSG.

Gemcitabine, a pyrimidine antimetabolite, has been approved by the FDA as first-line therapy for locally advanced and metastatic adenocarcinoma of the pancreas.[146–149] Gemcitabine is dosed at 1,000 mg/m^2/week for 7 weeks followed by 1-week rest; each subsequent cycle is dosed at 1,000 mg/m^2/week for 3 weeks followed by 1-week rest.[146] The advantage of gemcitabine in treating advanced pancreatic cancer lies in the clinical benefits it offers to patients with significant symptomatology. A randomized single-blinded phase III trial was conducted to compare the clinical benefit of 5-FU and gemcitabine in treating patients with advanced disease. The primary end point in this trial was the clinical benefit response measured by pain control, functional improvement, and weight gain.[150–152] Other secondary end points included time to tumor progression, median survival, and 1-year survival rate. At the conclusion of the trial, a significantly higher percentage of patients receiving gemcitabine experienced clinical benefit compared with those treated with 5-FU. Patients in the gemcitabine arm also had longer median survival and higher probability to survive 1 year than patients in the 5-FU arm. Toxicity was generally tolerable in both arms, with myelosuppression being the dose-limiting side effect for gemcitabine.[152] Because the major advantage of gemcitabine is symptomatic relief, it is reasonable to use gemcitabine in patients with poor performance status or with significant pain as an alternative to chemoradiation.

METASTATIC PANCREATIC CANCER (STAGE III)

For patients with metastatic pancreatic cancer, systemic chemotherapy is the only treatment option. Until recently, the mainstay of therapy has been 5-FU, with a modest response rate and little clinical benefit.[153] Several 5-FU doses and schedules have been used to treat metastatic carcinoma of the pancreas. To date, there is no consensus regarding the optimal dosing regimen for 5-FU in this clinical setting. Refer to Table 98.9 for commonly used dosing schedules, side effects, and monitoring parameters of 5-FU.

Attempts to modulate single-agent 5-FU activity with LV, methotrexate, and interferon alpha have failed to demonstrate additional therapeutic advantage.[154] To improve on the disappointing results obtained with single-agent 5-FU, combination chemotherapy has also been tried. Response rates with these combination regimens have ranged from 2% to 40% (median 20%).[155] Some of the combinations included 5-FU plus doxorubicin and mitomycin c, and cyclophosphamide plus methotrexate, vincristine, and mitomycin c. This is not substantially different from the results seen with single-agent 5-FU.

TABLE 98.9	Commonly Used Chemotherapeutic Agents in Pancreatic Cancer		
Agent and Commonly Used Schedules	**Side Effects**	**Monitoring Parameters**	**Comments**
5-FU (bolus) 400–500 mg/m^2/day × 5 days, repeated monthly	Nausea/vomiting	Control of nausea/vomiting	Hesketh level II emetogen. Premedicate with phenothiazine antiemetic; have antiemetic available as needed
	Myelosuppression (primarily neutropenia)	CBC with differential and platelet	
		Signs and symptoms (S/S) of infection or bleeding	
	Mucositis	S/S of mucositis	Ensure good mouth care
		Pain level	
		Nutrition	
	Diarrhea	Fluid and electrolytes	Instruct patients to report if three or more loose stools per day
		Bowel habit	
		S/S of dehydration	
	Photosensitivity		Instruct patients about photosensitivity
	Hair loss, nailbed changes		Usually partial hair loss
	Inflammation of tear ducts and lacrimal glands (dacryocystitis)		Instruct patients to report if eye problems occur
			Topical steroid may be useful for dacryocystitis
	Neurotoxicity	S/S such as headache, ataxia, confusion, nystagmus	Rare
			Discontinue 5-FU
Gemcitabine 1,000 mg/m^2 weekly for 7 weeks followed by 1 week rest, then 1,000 mg/m^2 weekly for 3 weeks, repeated monthly	Nausea/vomiting	Control of nausea/vomiting	Hesketh Level II emetogen
			Premedicate with phenothiazine antiemetic; have 5HT$_3$-RA antiemetic available as needed
	Acute infusion-related reactions (flushing, dyspnea, facial swelling, hypotension)		Slowing of infusion rate may be helpful
	Rash		Systemic steroid may be helpful
	Hair loss		Usually partial hair loss
	Myelosuppression (primarily neutropenia)	CBC with differential and platelet	Dosing adjustment based on severity of neutropenia is required
		S/S of infection or bleeding	
	Proteinuria and hematuria	Urinalysis	Instruct patients to report change in color of urine or difficulty passing urine
		S/S of hematuria	

FU, fluorouracil; CBC, complete blood count.

Gemcitabine has provided some hope for patients with metastatic pancreatic cancer (Table 98.9). Despite its modest impact on survival, gemcitabine has been shown to significantly palliate pain and improve performance status. Due to its clinical benefit on symptomatology, gemcitabine has evolved to become the standard of care for patients with metastatic pancreatic cancer.[152]

Pharmacokinetic data from gemcitabine has incited an interest in the concept of a fixed-dose rate (FDR) infusion which supports the idea that the active metabolite, gemcitabine triphosphate, could be accumulated more effectively by a longer infusion allowing for greater inhibition of DNA synthesis and subsequent cell death.[156] A phase II trial in which 92 patients with locally advanced or metastatic pancreatic cancer were randomized to receive either 2,200 mg/m^2 of gemcitabine administered as a standard 30-minute infusion, or 1,500 mg/m^2 given at a FDR of 10 mg/m^2/min.[157] The median survival for all patients was 5 months in the standard infusion arm and 8 months in the FDR arm (P = 0.13). For patients with metastatic disease, the median survival was 4.9 months in the standard infusion arm and 7.3 months in the FDR arm (P = 0.094).[157]

Other strategies to improve the activity of gemcitabine have involved the use of gemcitabine-based combination regimens. Gemcitabine plus 5-FU was studied in a series of phase II and phase III trials but the results were not very encouraging. The interest in 5–FU-based combination regimens has generally decreased based on potentially more promising data with other agents.

Gemcitabine in conjunction with cisplatin has shown activity in many other tumors thereby spurring interest for this combination in pancreatic cancer. Results from two phase II trials indicate that gemcitabine plus cisplatin is more effective at producing tumor responses when compared to single-agent gemcitabine without significantly compromising tolerability.[158,159]

Irinotecan, a topoisomerase I inhibitor, has also been evaluated in combination with gemcitabine for the treatment of unresectable or advanced pancreatic cancer. One phase II single-arm trial treated 45 patients with gemcitabine 1,000 mg/m^2 over 30 minutes followed by irinotecan 100 mg/m^2 over 90 minutes given IV on days 1 and 8 every 21 days.[160] The results indicated a 20% response rate with a median survival of 6 months and a median time to tumor progression of 2.9 months. The regimen was well tolerated with minimal grade 3 and 4 toxicities.

Oxaliplatin has clinical activity in a number of GI tumors, especially colorectal cancer. A number of combination regimens with gemcitabine and oxaliplatin are being studied. A phase II multicenter trial of previously untreated patients with unresectable or metastatic pancreatic cancer enrolled patients to receive gemcitabine 1,000 mg/m^2 as a 10-mg/m^2/min infusion on day 1 and oxaliplatin 100 mg/m^2 as a 2-hour infusion on day 2 repeated every 2 weeks. The response rate was 30.6% (95% confidence interval 19.7%–42.3%). Forty percent of the patients had clinical benefit demonstrated by improved pain and/or performance status for at least 4 consecutive weeks. The median progression-free survival and median overall survival was 5.3 and 9.2 months, respectively.[161]

A number of other agents have also been studied in combination with gemcitabine including docetaxel and pemetrexed. In phase II trials to date, the response rate for gemcitabine-based combinations have generally been higher than with single-agent gemcitabine, however, no randomized phase III trial has yet established a survival benefit for combination therapy compared to gemcitabine alone.

FUTURE DIRECTIONS

With better local-regional control with chemoradiation, treatment failure and disease recurrence in patients with stage I or stage II disease are mostly secondary to distant metastases. Unfortunately, the available systemic chemotherapy has not significantly modified the natural history of the disease, necessitating the development of newer and more efficacious agents.

Dolastatin 10 is a potent antimitotic that binds to tubulin and inhibits the polymerization of purified tubulin, thus disrupting microtubule assembly. The exact binding site of the drug on tubulin has not been identified, but it is probably located near the vinca alkaloid binding sites. In vitro studies have demonstrated potent antiproliferative activity in a number of leukemias, lymphomas, and solid tumor cell lines. Phase I trials to define the maximal tolerated dose have been completed, with myelosuppression found to be the dose-limiting toxicity. Phase II studies with dolastatin are currently being conducted in patients with metastatic pancreatic cancer.[162–165]

Novel treatment strategies that use gene transfer technology open up a new frontier in cancer therapy. A number of genetic abnormalities have been detected in pancreatic tumor cells, and gene therapy may be a promising alternative to conventional approaches in treating pancreatic cancer. Approximately 60% of pancreatic cancer specimens have abnormalities in the p53 tumor suppressor gene,[102,166,167] and gene therapy targeting this genetic lesion is currently being investigated. Intratumoral injection with adenovirus ONYX-015, alone and in combination with gemcitabine, is under phase I study in patients with unresectable pancreatic tumors. ONYX-015 is an attenuated adenovirus that efficiently replicates in and lyses tumor cells deficient in the p53 gene.[163,168,169]

Another area that has generated tremendous interest is biological targeted therapy. The concept of combining cytotoxic therapy with agents that aim at molecular tumor targets is being explored with immense optimism. Trials with several biological agents have been conducted in pancreatic cancer. Examples of some areas of interest include inhibition of members of the ErbB family of receptors, ErbB-1 (epidermal growth factor receptor) and ErbB-2 (HER2), with monoclonal antibodies. Gemcitabine has been combined with trastuzumab, which is a monoclonal antibody to HER2 and also with cetuximab, a humanized monoclonal antibody to an EGFr. Preliminary results from these trials are very promising.[170] Bevacizumab is a recombinant humanized monoclonal antibody to VEGF. Bevacizumab is also being studied in combination with gemcitabine for advanced pancreatic cancer and again, preliminary results are very encouraging.[171]

IMPROVING OUTCOMES

The clinical course of pancreatic cancer is characterized by significant symptomatology with survival usually measured in weeks to months. To date, the available treatment options have not significantly improved survival. Given this scenario, supportive care of the patient with pancreatic cancer often becomes more important than treatment of the primary disease. Supportive care for this patient population includes, but is not limited to, pain control, amelioration of psychosocial issues, nutritional support, relief of obstructive jaundice, and control of GI symptoms (nausea, vomiting, constipation, GI obstruction, etc.).[111,172,173]

Obstructive jaundice and GI obstruction can be managed by invasive measures. Biliary decompression can be achieved with nonoperative percutaneous or endoscopic stenting with low complication rates. However, in the long run, recurrent jaundice due to stent collapse can be a problem.[172] Development of self-expanding metallic stents may prolong the duration of stent patency.[174] Because of the higher complication rate, surgical biliary bypass is usually reserved for patients who also require bypass surgery to palliate impending GI obstruction.[172] To manage GI obstruction, a palliative gastrojejunostomy can be done.[172] Postoperative use of an H_2-antagonist is required to reduce the risk of stomal ulceration. Again, due to higher mortality and morbidity of major surgery in this patient population, nonoperative duodenal stenting is currently under investigation.

Pain is another supportive care issue that demands appropriate attention and management.[108,109] Effective pain control measures should be comprehensive, including a pharmacologic approach, invasive techniques, and a strong support group. For pharmacologic management of pain, the World Health Organization three-step analgesic ladder and the guidelines from the Agency for Health Care Policy and Research represent good community practice standards.[172,173,175–178]

Invasive measures, such as chemical or surgical splanchnicectomy, which is the removal or resection of the splanchnic nerves or percutaneous celiac plexus block better known as a nerve block procedure, can be performed to complement opioid-based treatment.[179,180]

Psychosocial issues, typically described as depression, anxiety, and a feeling of doom, are commonly observed in patients with pancreatic cancer.[173] Psychological and behavioral studies suggest higher rates of depression in this patient population than in those with other neoplasms.[181,182] Etiology of such depressive and anxiety symptoms is comprehensive, including the chemical imbalance secondary to the disease itself and the contribution of pain, terminal illness, and other life stressors. If such psychosocial issues are present, they must be taken seriously and treatment should be considered. The use of psychotherapy, cognitive-behavioral techniques, and psychotropic medications concomitant with proper management of other symptomatology can significantly abate depression and anxiety to enhance quality of life.[173]

CONCLUSION

Pancreatic cancer is a relatively rare but highly lethal disease resulting in the death of more than 95% of patients within 5 years of diagnosis. The symptoms of this disease are vague and often attributed to more benign conditions, allowing the disease to progress to advanced stages before diagnosis. Only patients with very early disease are potentially curable, and the treatment of choice is surgical resection plus neoadjuvant or adjuvant radiation and chemotherapy. Effective treatments for advanced disease are still being sought. Because there is no consistently effective treatment for advanced disease, these patients should be entered into clinical trials whenever possible. Most patients experience progressive deterioration, and supportive care often becomes the mainstay of therapy. Patients often require supportive care that includes control of GI symptoms (nausea, vomiting, diarrhea, constipation, and obstruction), pain control, and nutritional support.

GASTRIC CANCER

EPIDEMIOLOGY

INCIDENCE

Gastric cancer was the leading cause of cancer deaths worldwide until the late 1980s.[183] In the United States, the estimated total number of new gastric cancer cases in 2004 was approximately 22,710 (13,640 men and 9,070 women, and approximately 11,780 will die from this disease).[184] Over the last 60 years the incidence of gastric cancer in the United States has been declining. Worldwide, the most prevalent areas for gastric cancer are Japan, South America (particularly Chile and Costa Rica), and Eastern Europe. Japan has the highest incidence by far, and it is the number one cause of death in that country.[183] The male to female ratio for gastric cancer in the United States is 2–3:1, and the median age at diagnosis is 70 years for men and 74 years for women. African-Americans,

Hispanic Americans, and Native Americans are 1.5 to 2.5 times more likely to develop gastric cancer than are whites.[185]

ETIOLOGY

The risk factors for the development of gastric cancer are believed to be associated with the environment. Diet is probably the most commonly postulated environmental factor studied in relation to gastric cancer. Diets including high concentrations of nitrates/nitrites, high salt intake, inappropriate food storage, food spoilage/fermentation, and other factors fostering nitrosamine formation have been related to increasing the risk of developing gastric cancer.[186] Diets that are rich in vitamin A and vitamin C lower the risk of gastric cancer.[187] Therefore, one proposed chemopreventive agent is ascorbic acid (vitamin C). The mechanism of action of ascorbic acid is thought to be by this vitamin's ability to prevent the reduction of nitrous acid to N-nitroso compounds. These N-nitroso compounds are carcinogenic in the stomach.[188,189]

Another factor that may increase the risk of gastric cancer is chronic infection with *Helicobacter pylori*. *H. pylori* is commonly present in patients with severe gastritis and chronic atrophic gastritis. It is a common infection, with approximately 50% of adults over age 50 in North America and virtually 100% of adults in some developing or newly industrialized countries infected.[186] It is estimated that the incidence of gastric cancer is six times higher in a 100%-infected population when compared with a noninfected population.[190] Still, only a small percentage of the total number of patients infected with *H. pylori* develop gastric cancer.[191] Infection with *H. pylori* indirectly causes gastric cancer. The chronic gastritis secondary to *H. pylori* leads to an increase in cell turnover and intestinal metaplasia development.[192] Other risk factors increasing the occurrence of gastric cancer include family history, individuals from blood group A, and individuals with pernicious anemia, atrophic gastritis, prior gastric surgery, gastric polyps, or achlorhydria.[193] Individuals from lower socioeconomic classes tend to be at increased risk for the development of gastric cancer. This increased risk is thought to be secondary to dietary and environmental factors common in this population.

Obesity is also being linked to increased gastric cancer incidence.[194] Smoking has also been associated with increased risk of gastric cancer. However, alcohol consumption has not been shown to increase the risk of gastric cancer.

PATHOPHYSIOLOGY

The majority of malignant gastric cancers are adenocarcinomas, accounting for approximately 84% of all gastric neoplasms. The incidence of other less common histologic classifications include signet ring cell tumors (8%), mucinous adenocarcinomas (3%), and diffuse type adenocarcinoma, intestinal type adenocarcinoma, papillary adenocarcinoma, undifferentiated carcinoma, adenosquamous carcinoma, and tubular adenocarcinoma, each identified in less than 2% of patients.[195]

Approximately 30% of primary gastric cancers occur in the upper third of the stomach, 14% in the middle third, and 26% in the lower third. The incidence in the gastric cardia (upper third) and involving the gastroesophageal junction has been increasing over the last 15 years.[196] The entire stomach may be involved in up to 10% of patients.[195] Gastric cancer has four major patterns of spread: (a) direct extension into the surrounding tissues and organs such as the liver, diaphragm, pancreas, spleen, biliary tract, and transverse colon; (b) nodal metastases, both local (perigastric, celiac axis, porta hepatis, retroperitoneal) and distant (Virchow node, left axillary nodes); (c) hematogenous spread to liver, lung, bone, and brain; and (d) intraperitoneal dissemination in the pelvis.[193] Intraperitoneal spread may be evidenced by the presence of peritoneal implants or ascites.

CLINICAL PRESENTATION AND DIAGNOSIS

SIGNS AND SYMPTOMS

Patients with early gastric cancer are typically men who are 44 to 70 years of age, 80% of which are asymptomatic. By the time gastric cancer is diagnosed in the United States, it is usually advanced. This is primarily because the signs and symptoms of early gastric cancer are vague and nonspecific and similar to those of peptic ulcer disease. The first signs and symptoms that patients may have are mild epigastric pain and dyspepsia. Approximately 40% of patients experience nausea and vomiting. Persistent vomiting may be associated with a distal cancer obstructing the pylorus. Patients with proximal lesions or lesions involving the gastroesophageal junction may have dysphagia as their primary symptom. When gastric cancer is still in the early stages, weight loss is minimal, in spite of anorexia. Only one fourth of patients with early gastric cancer demonstrate signs and symptoms of upper GI bleeding with associated anemia. Once the disease has advanced, patients complain of significant weight loss (more than 10 pounds), abdominal pain, anorexia, hematemesis, guaiac-positive stools, and anemia. Other physical changes that might suggest advanced gastric cancer when observed in conjunction with the previous signs include palpable lymph nodes, palpable ovarian mass (Krukenberg tumor), hepatomegaly, palpable abdominal mass, ascites, jaundice, and cachexia.[197]

Many patients report experiencing the symptoms of mild epigastric pain for 21 to 36 months. Patients with advanced gastric cancer often relate having experienced symptoms for at least the previous 6 to 8 months. In general, the abdominal pain and discomfort experienced with early or advanced gastric cancer is not relieved by food or antacids.[197]

A study to better understand gastric cancer was undertaken in the late 1980s by the American College of Surgeons.[195] The study included 18,365 patients. Men outnum-

TABLE 98.10	Common Presenting Signs/Symptoms of Gastric Cancer
Weight loss	Dysphagia
Abdominal pain	Melena
Nausea	Early satiety
Anorexia	Ulcer-type pain

bered women in this study (63% and 37%, respectively). The median age of men was 68.4 years, and the median age of women was 71.9 years. The presenting features of these patients were evaluated and are listed in Table 98.10. The most common symptoms observed in more than 50% of the patients were weight loss and abdominal pain. Other frequently encountered symptoms included nausea, anorexia, dysphagia, and melena.

DIAGNOSIS

The differential diagnosis between peptic ulcer disease and gastric cancer must be made in these patients because the presenting signs and symptoms are so similar. Currently, no blood test is available for the definitive diagnosis of gastric cancer. Blood tests that may be useful in determining the extent of disease include complete blood count, liver function tests (bilirubin, alkaline phosphatase, lactate dehydrogenase [LDH], alanine aminotransferase [ALT], aspartate aminotransferase [AST]), and CEA. CEA is not used as a diagnostic tool because it is elevated in only 15% to 30% of patients with advanced disease.[198] CEA may be useful in assessment of response to treatment or evaluating recurrence after potentially curative surgical resection.

Historically, the diagnostic procedure performed on patients with upper GI complaints has been the upper GI series/ barium swallow. However, upper GI endoscopy [esophagogastroduodenoscopy (EGD)] is the diagnostic procedure of choice in the diagnosis of gastric symptomatology. The increase in the use of endoscopy demonstrates the usefulness of direct visualization of the stomach with an additional advantage of obtaining biopsy specimens. Thus, EGD has become the diagnostic procedure of choice.[195] CT scan has become an integral part of the staging of gastric cancer, primarily if advanced disease is suspected.[193]

EUS can also be performed to diagnose gastric cancer and the extent of disease. The main use of EUS is in preoperative staging by enabling evaluation of the depth of cancer invasion into the gastric wall. EUS has a 91% accuracy rate in evaluating depth of invasion and may also be useful in diagnosing perigastric metastatic lymph nodes.[199] Proper staging is the cornerstone to determining the proper treatment. Positron emission tomography (PET) and PET CT are still under investigation and may be beneficial to determine the response to chemotherapy or extent of distant metastasis.[200] Laparoscopy, even though it is more invasive than CT or EUS, has an advantage of directly visualizing local lymph nodes, the peritoneum, and the liver for determining the extent of disease and the possibility of resection. Laparoscopy is usually done when all other studies indicate localized disease.[201]

Screening for early gastric cancer is currently being conducted in areas associated with a high risk of gastric cancer, primarily Japan, South America, and Eastern Europe. Again, EGD is the diagnostic procedure used in these areas.[197] Screening programs in Japan have increased the number of patients diagnosed with an early-stage gastric cancer by up to 40%.[202]

STAGING AND PROGNOSIS

The staging of gastric cancer depends on the extent of the disease. This information is obtained during the diagnostic period for the patient (endoscopic procedures, radiology examinations). The TNM classification is used to describe the stage of gastric cancer as recommended by the AJCC (Table 98.11).[193] The percentage of patients diagnosed at various stages are stage I (<5%), stage II (10%–15%), stage III (17%–20%), and stage IV (72%).[202]

The prognostic factors found to be most significant in predicting poor prognosis are depth of invasion and presence of lymph node metastasis.[203,204] The 5-year survival of patients with tumors invading only the mucosa is 91%; in comparison, the 5-year survival of patients with tumors invading adjacent organs is 6.6%. In patients with more than three positive lymph nodes, the 5-year survival is approximately 20%. Other factors that may have some role in predicting outcome include favorable histology (mucinous adenocarcinoma 5-year survival 38.6%) and location of the tumor (whole stomach 5-year survival 20%, upper third of stomach 5-year survival 29.1%). Overall, the prognosis for patients diagnosed with gastric cancer is poor, mainly because only a few patients are diagnosed with early-stage disease. The overall survival is strongly correlated with stage at diagnosis. The 5-year survival rate for stage I gastric cancer is 90%; stage II, 70%; stage III, 45%; and stage IV, less than 10%.[203]

TREATMENT

SURGERY

Surgery is the only therapeutic option that offers a potential cure for gastric cancer patients, especially in combination with adjuvant chemotherapy.[205] The amount of stomach removed should be enough to allow ample tumor-free margins with the regional lymph nodes also being removed. Extension of the surgical margins into the adjacent organs should be done only if necessary, and a controversy surrounds the prophylactic removal of other lymph nodes (i.e., those not directly involved regionally).[206–211] To ensure tumor-free margins, a subtotal or total gastrectomy will be performed based on the location of the tumor in the stomach and on the pattern of spread of the tumor within the stomach. In general, tumors in the distal portion of the stomach can be

TABLE 98.11	American Joint Committee on Cancer (AJCC) TNM Staging Classification for Carcinoma of the Stomach

Primary Tumor (T)

TX	Primary tumor cannot be assessed
T0	No evidence of primary tumor
Tis	Carcinoma in situ: intraepithelial tumor without invasion of the lamina propria
T1	Tumor invades lamina propria or submucosa
T2	Tumor invades muscularis propria or subserosa[a]
T2a	Tumor invades muscularis propria
T2b	Tumor invades subserosa
T3	Tumor penetrates serosa (visceral peritoneum) without invasion of adjacent structures[b]
T4	Tumor invades adjacent structures[b]

Regional Lymph Nodes (N)

NX	Regional lymph node(s) cannot be assessed
N0	No regional lymph node metastasis[c]
N1	Metastasis in 1–6 regional lymph nodes
N2	Metastasis in 7–15 regional lymph nodes
N3	Metastasis in >15 regional lymph nodes

Distant Metastasis (M)

MX	Distant metastasis cannot be assessed
M0	No distant metastasis
M1	Distant metastasis

Histologic Grade (G)

GX	Grade cannot be assessed
G1	Well differentiated
G2	Moderately differentiated
G3	Poorly differentiated
G4	Undifferentiated

Stage Grouping

Stage 0	Tis	N0	M0
Stage IA	T1	N0	M0
Stage IB	T1	N1	M0
	T2a/b	N0	M0
Stage II	T1	N2	M0
	T2a/b	N1	M0
	T3	N0	M0
Stage IIIA	T2a/b	N2	M0
	T3	N1	M0
	T4	N0	M0
Stage IIIB	T3	N2	M0
Stage IV	T4	N1–3	M0
	T1–3	N3	M0
	Any T	Any N	M1

[a] A tumor may penetrate the muscularis propria with extension into the gastrocolic or gastrohepatic ligaments, or into the greater or lesser omentum, without perforation of the visceral peritoneum covering these structures. In this case, the tumor is classified as T2. If there is perforation of the visceral peritoneum covering the gastric ligaments or the omentum, the tumor should be classified as T3. [b]The adjacent structures of the stomach include the spleen, transverse colon, liver, diaphragm, pancreas, abdominal wall, adrenal gland, kidney, small intestine, and retroperitoneum. Intramural extension to the duodenum or esophagus is classified by the depth of the greatest invasion in any of these sites, including the stomach. [c]A designation of pN0 should be used if all examined lymph nodes are negative, regardless of the total number removed and examined. (From AJCC Cancer Staging Manual. 6th ed. New York: Springer-Verlag, 2002.)

best treated with a radical subtotal gastrectomy. Tumors in the middle third of the stomach, or linitis plastica, often require a total gastrectomy. Tumors located in the proximal portion of the stomach and the cardia require a total gastrectomy, with the margins often extending into the distal esophagus.[212,213] However, complete resection of all gross disease with negative margins is still associated with a high rate of recurrent disease.

If a patient has locally advanced (invading other organs) or metastatic gastric cancer, surgery would only be considered with a palliative intent. The symptoms most commonly palliated include pain, hemorrhage, dysphasia, nausea, vomiting, and weight loss. Again, this could be a subtotal or total gastrectomy depending on the location of the obstruction. Currently, palliation from symptom-producing gastric obstruction may also be achieved with endoscopic laser surgery. This often provides recanalization with minimal morbidity and mortality.[213]

RADIATION

Radiation therapy alone has a limited role in the treatment of advanced gastric cancer. However, when combined with chemotherapy, in the treatment of locally advanced gastric cancer and in the adjuvant setting, it has demonstrated improvement in survival. In the palliative setting, radiotherapy my provide relief from bleeding, obstruction, and pain in patients with advanced disease.[214–216]

CHEMOTHERAPY

Neoadjuvant Chemotherapy. The goal of neoadjuvant chemotherapy is to improve resectability of tumors in patients with locally advanced disease by decreasing the tumor burden and, therefore, increasing the survival time. Gastric cancer patients who are candidates for neoadjuvant chemotherapy are those patients who have locoregional extension of disease (stage II and stage III) and are considered unresectable at diagnosis or those patients who are potentially resectable, but have bulky disease or other poor prognostic factors (cardial location or enlarged lymph nodes). The advantages of giving chemotherapy to these groups of patients before surgery are to (a) promote tumor regression; (b) increase local control rate; (c) allow for more conservative surgical procedures; and (d) define postoperative chemotherapy regimens for patients who have responded to chemotherapy preoperatively. Problems with neoadjuvant chemotherapy include (a) development of resistant clones to chemotherapy; (b) delay of local control measures (i.e., surgery); and (c) increased risk of metastatic spread.[217]

Many of the combinations of drugs used in the treatment of advanced disease have been used in the neoadjuvant setting. Currently, two randomized trials have compared neoadjuvant chemotherapy versus surgery alone. In the first trial, from Korea, patients with locally advanced gastric cancer were randomized to preoperative chemotherapy with cisplatin, etoposide, and 5-FU (PEF) followed by surgery versus surgery alone. The curative resection rate was 79% for

treated patients versus 61% for the surgery alone patients.[218] In a trial from Japan, patients with advanced gastric cancer (stage IV) were randomized to preoperative chemotherapy with cisplatin, etoposide, mitomycin C, and tegafur plus uracil (UFT) (1:4 molar ratio, not available in the United States) followed by surgery versus surgery alone. The curative resection rate was 38% for treated patients and 15% for the surgery alone patients. The median survival was 17 months and 8 months, respectively.[219] Randomized trials are now being conducted to clearly confirm the benefit of preoperative therapy.[217,220–222]

Adjuvant Chemotherapy. Many trials with adjuvant chemotherapy regimens have been investigated in an effort to improve survival rates in resected gastric cancer patients. These adjuvant regimens have been compared with surgery alone. Single agents that have been used as adjuvant chemotherapy in separate trials include thiotepa, floxuridine, and high-dose mitomycin C.[223] Only mitomycin C demonstrated an increase in survival when compared with surgery alone.[224]

With the advent of combination chemotherapy regimens for the treatment of unresectable gastric cancer, combination regimens in the adjuvant chemotherapy setting have increased in use. GITSG reported a survival benefit in the group of patients receiving adjuvant chemotherapy with 5-FU and methyl-CCNU.[225] These results, however, were not able to be duplicated in two separate confirmatory trials.[226,227] 5-FU, doxorubicin, and mitomycin C (also known as the ''FAM regimen'') is a regimen that has been tested extensively for the treatment of advanced disease. Two separate trials have evaluated FAM in the adjuvant setting compared with surgery alone. Neither study demonstrated a survival advantage for adjuvant therapy over surgery alone. Other variations of the FAM regimen, and other combination chemotherapy regimens, have been studied in the adjuvant setting, again without affecting survival.[228]

The Intergroup INT-0116 trial randomized 603 patients following curative resection to surgery alone versus surgery plus adjuvant therapy. The treatment group received bolus 5-FU/LV × 1 cycle, then chemoradiotherapy with 5-FU/LV and 45 Gy in 25 fractions followed by one more cycle of 5-FU/LV. The median relapse free survival was 19 months for the surgery alone group and 30 months for the chemoradiotherapy group ($P < 0.001$). The median survival was 27 months for the surgery alone and 36 months for the chemoradiotherapy group ($P = 0.005$). As a result of this trial this treatment has been adopted in the adjuvant setting in the United States.[215]

Chemotherapy of Advanced Disease. Numerous single agents have been tested for the treatment of advanced gastric cancer.[229] Of these agents tested, 5-FU, doxorubicin, mitomycin C, cisplatin, and more recently paclitaxel and docetaxel, have demonstrated activity as single agents. Because of this single-agent activity, investigators have combined these agents in a number of varying regimens.[230–232]

One of the first combinations used in advanced gastric cancer was the FAM regimen. In the initial study of the FAM regimen, a 42% partial response (PR) rate was reported with no complete responses (CRs) observed. The median survival of responding patients was 12.5 months, compared with 5.5 months for all patients.[233] Experience with the combination has since increased, and approximately 650 patients in various studies have received treatment with a FAM regimen. The overall response rate in these studies is approximately 30% (2% CR) (median survival time 6.9 months).[229]

Numerous other combination regimens have been compared with FAM. All regimens produced a response rate that was comparable to FAM with no difference in survival. The North Central Cancer Treatment Group (NCCTG), a clinical trials organization including several teaching institutions, concluded after studying FAM versus single-agent 5-FU that 5-FU should be considered the standard treatment for advanced gastric cancer, because less expense and toxicities were observed with comparable response rates.[234] Other studies have not been able to document a statistically significant survival advantage of one treatment over another.[235,236]

In the late 1980s many attempts were made to improve on the efficacy of combination chemotherapy for advanced gastric cancer. The combination of high-dose methotrexate, 5-FU, and doxorubicin (FAMTX), produced a promising initial response rate of 63%. A direct comparison was done in a multicenter randomized trial of FAMTX versus FAM. The response rate for FAMTX in this trial was 41% versus 9% for FAM, and the overall median survival for FAMTX was 10.5 months versus 7 months for FAM. Moreover, the toxicities of the two arms were comparable. Mucositis was more often observed in the FAMTX arm; thrombocytopenia was a cumulative toxicity of FAM. FAMTX became the treatment of choice for metastatic gastric cancer.[237] Multiple modifications of the FAMTX regimen have been reported; some of these modifications have included altering drug doses, substituting drugs, or adjusting the dosing schedule. None of these modifications has provided survival or response advantages over other combination chemotherapy regimens.[238–240]

Numerous other combinations have been developed using various known active drugs in gastric cancer. Table 98.12 shows many of these trials and indicates response rates and survival information. ELF chemotherapy is a combination of LV, 5-FU, and etoposide. The original ELF regimen produced a 48% overall response rate (12% CR).[241] Modifications (l-leucovorin for d,l-leucovorin; oral etoposide for intravenous etoposide) of the ELF regimen have not affected the overall response rate.[242–243] PELF chemotherapy (cisplatin, epirubicin, LV, 5-FU) has been compared to an FAM regimen. Patients receiving PELF demonstrated a higher overall response rate (43%) than the patients in the FAM arm. However, more grade 3 and 4 toxicities were reported in the PELF arm, and there was no survival advantage with PELF.[244]

Another combination chemotherapy regimen studied extensively in advanced gastric cancer has been etoposide, doxorubicin, and cisplatin (EAP) (Table 98.12). Response rates

TABLE 98.12	Clinical Trials in Metastatic Gastric Cancer	
Regimen	Response Rate (%)	Overall Median Survival (months)
ELF[249]	48	11
PELF[244]	43	8.1
EAP[245]	53	6
ECF[250]	45	8.9
DCF[251]	44.1	10.2
Irinotecan/Cisplatin[252]	58	5
FOLFOX 6[254]	44	8.6

ELF, leucovorin (LV), 5-fluorouracil (5-FU), etoposide; PELF, cisplatin, epirubicin, LV, 5-FU; EAP, etoposide, doxorubicin, cisplatin; ECF, epirubicin, cisplatin, continuous infusion 5-FU; DCF, docetaxel, cisplatin, 5-FU; FOLFOX, Oxaliplatin plus infusional 5-FU, leucovorin.

using this combination of agents have ranged from 20% to 72%.[245–248] Toxicities observed with EAP chemotherapy were leukopenia, thrombocytopenia, and mucositis.[246] In a comparison trial of EAP versus FAMTX, both regimens produced similar response rates and toxicities; however, the toxicities associated with EAP therapy were more severe and required longer hospitalizations.[247]

In the 1990s a combination of epirubicin, cisplatin, and continuous infusion 5-FU (ECF) had impressive response rates as high as 71%.[249] When compared to FAMTX in a randomized trial, a higher response rate (45% vs. 21%) and improved overall survival (8.9 vs. 5.7 months) was observed.[250] Currently this is the treatment of choice in Europe.

More recently, several different drugs have demonstrated activity in gastric cancer including the taxanes (paclitaxel and docetaxel), irinotecan, and oxaliplatin. A phase III trial comparing docetaxel, cisplatin, 5-FU (DCF) versus 5-FU, cisplatin demonstrated a significant increased response rate (39% vs. 23%) and overall survival (10.2 vs. 8.5 months).[251] Irinotecan as a single agent has demonstrated a response rate of 20% in gastric cancer. When combined with cisplatin, response rates improved to 51%.[252] Even in second-line therapy, the combination of irinotecan and cisplatin produced a response rate of 31% and overall survival of 5 months.[253] A phase II trial of FOLFOX 6 (oxaliplatin, 5-FU, LV) demonstrated a response rate of 44% and overall survival of 8.6 months.[254]

Overall, the use of combination chemotherapy has improved the response rate in advanced gastric cancer patients; however, patient survival has demonstrated little improvement. New agents are continuously being screened for the treatment of advanced gastric cancer. Outside of a clinical trial, the least toxic chemotherapy regimens should be used in the treatment of advanced gastric cancer. A summary of chemotherapy agents and toxicities currently used in the treatment of gastric cancer appears in Table 98.13.

TABLE 98.13	Toxicities of Chemotherapeutic Agents Used in Gastric Cancer
Agent Toxicities	
Cisplatin	Nausea, vomiting, diarrhea, nephrotoxicity, myelosuppression, peripheral neuropathy, ototoxicity
5-Fluorouracil	Nausea, vomiting, stomatitis, diarrhea, dermatitis, myelosuppression, palmar-plantar erythrodysesthesia, photosensitivity
Leucovorin	Increased diarrhea and stomatitis when used with 5-fluorouracil
Etoposide	Myelosuppression, nausea, vomiting, alopecia, hypotension
Doxorubicin	Myelosuppression, nausea, vomiting, alopecia, cardiotoxicity, mucositis
Mitomycin C	Myelosuppression (delayed), nausea, vomiting, pulmonary toxicity, hemolytic uremic syndrome
Methotrexate	Myelosuppression, nausea, vomiting, diarrhea, stomatitis, malaise, fatigue, alopecia
Paclitaxel	Myelosuppression, peripheral neuropathy, nausea, vomiting, alopecia, hypersensitivity reaction
Docetaxel	Myelosuppression, paresthesia, nausea, vomiting, hypersensitivity reaction, alopecia, fluid retention, rash, stomatitis, diarrhea
Irinotecan	Diarrhea, myelosuppression, nausea, vomiting
Oxaliplatin	Allergic/infusion related reactions, neuropathy, cold hypersensitivity, nausea, vomiting, anorexia, myelosuppression,
Epirubicin	Discolored urine (red, orange, pink), myelosuppression, diarrhea, mucositis, alopecia

CONCLUSION

Because the signs and symptoms of early gastric cancer are so similar to those of peptic ulcer disease, gastric cancer is usually diagnosed in advanced stages. The treatment of gastric cancer depends on the stage of disease. As with other cancers of the GI tract, surgery is the only means to achieve a cure. Patients who are able to undergo surgery for curative purposes are those with early-stage disease (stages I and II). In patients with locally advanced or metastatic disease, surgery is performed only as a palliative therapy. The role of neoadjuvant chemotherapy with or without radiation therapy must be explored further. The use of adjuvant chemotherapy is currently the standard in the United States. Multiple combination chemotherapy regimens have been used in the treatment of unresectable gastric cancer, each providing the patient with varying response rates and toxicities. Unfortunately, overall survival continues to be poor. Because of this, new agents and combinations continue to be studied in the treatment of gastric cancer.

KEY POINTS

- Of the GI tumors, those arising from the colon and rectum are most common
- The prognosis for colorectal cancer is completely dependent on the depth of tumor invasion into or through the bowel wall
- Early-stage GI tumors can be cured with surgical resection, but advanced disease treatment remains palliative
- Pancreatic cancer, although relatively rare in the United States, is one of the most lethal malignancies, resulting in death of more than 95% of patients within 5 years of diagnosis
- Most patients with pancreatic disease have advanced disease at diagnosis, leading to poor outcomes
- Because there is no truly effective treatment for advanced pancreatic cancer, patients should be encouraged to participate in clinical trials
- Gastric cancer, like pancreatic cancer, is often diagnosed late in the course of the disease
- With all of the GI tumors, surgery is the only modality that is currently curative
- New agents and combinations are needed before significant progress can be made in curing advanced GI tumors

SUGGESTED READINGS

Libutti SK, Saltz LB, Tepper JE. Cancers of the gastrointestinal tract: cancer of the colon. In: DeVita VT, Hellman S, Rosenberg SA, eds. Cancer principles and practice of oncology. 7th ed. Philadelphia: Lippincott Williams & Wilkins, 2005:1061–1109.

Pisters PWT, Kelsen DP, Powell SM, et al. Cancers of the gastrointestinal tract: cancer of the stomach. In: DeVita VT, Hellman S, Rosenberg SA, eds. Cancer Principles and Practice of Oncology, 7th ed. Philadelphia: Lippincott Williams & Wilkins 2005:909–944.

Yeo CJ, Yeo TP, Hruban RH, et al. Cancers of the gastrointestinal tract: cancer of the pancreas. In: DeVita VT, Hellman S, Rosenberg SA, eds. Cancer principles and practice of oncology. 7th ed. Philadelphia: Lippincott Williams & Wilkins, 2005:945–985.

REFERENCES

1. Ziegler RG, Devesa SS, Fraumeni JF, et al. Epidemiology pattern of colorectal cancer. In: DeVita VT, Hellman S, Rosenberg SA, eds. Important advances in oncology. Philadelphia: JB Lippincott, 1986:209–232.

2. Deschner EE, Cohen BI, Raicht RF. Acute and chronic effect of dietary cholic acid on colonic epithelial cell proliferation. Digestion 21:290–296, 1981.
3. Newmark HL, Wargovich MJ, Bruce WR. Colon cancer and dietary fat, phosphate, and calcium: a hypothesis. J Natl Cancer Inst 72:1323–1325, 1984.
4. Kritchevsky D. Dietary fiber and cancer. Nutr Cancer 6:213–219, 1985.
5. Yang CS, Newmark HL. The role of micronutrient deficiency in carcinogenesis. CRC Crit Rev Oncol Hematol 7:267–287, 1987.
6. Eastwood M. Dietary fiber and risk of cancer. Nutr Rev 45:193–198, 1977.
7. Fuchs CS, Giovannucci EL, Colditz GA, et al. Dietary fiber and the risk of colorectal cancer and adenoma in women. N Engl J Med 340:169–171, 1999.
8. Longnecker MP, Orza MJ, Adams ME, et al. A metaanalysis of alcoholic beverage consumption in relation to risk of colorectal cancer. Cancer Causes Control 1:59–68, 1990.
9. Jemal A, Tiwari RC, Murray T, et al. Cancer statistics, 2004. CA Cancer J Clin 54:8–29, 2004.
10. Phillips RL, Kuzma JW, Lotz TM. Cancer mortality among comparable members versus non-members of the Seventh Day Adventist Church. In: Cairns J, Lyon JL, Skolnick M, eds. Cancer incidence in defined populations. Cold Spring Harbor, NY: Cold Spring Laboratory, 1980:83–102.
11. Enstrom JE. Health and dietary practices and cancer mortality among California Mormons. In: Cairns J, Lyon JL, Skolnick M, eds. Cancer incidence in defined populations. Cold Spring Harbor, NY: Cold Spring Laboratory, 1980:69–90.
12. American Cancer Society. ACS cancer detection guidelines. Available at: http://www.ACS.com. Accessed 2004 May.
13. Margulis AR, Thoeni RF. The present status of the radiologic examination of the colon. Radiology 167:1–5, 1988.
14. O'Dwyer PT, Mojzcsk C, McCabe DP. Reoperation directed by carcinoembryonic antigen level: the importance of a thorough preoperative evaluation. Am J Surg 155:227–231, 1988.
15. Fleming ID, Cooper JS, Henson DE, et al. AJCC Cancer Staging Manual. 5th ed. Philadelphia, PA: Lippincott-Raven Publishers, 1997.
16. Greene FL, Stewart AK, Norton HJ. New tumor-node-metastasis staging strategy for node-positive (stage III) rectal cancer: an analysis. J Clin Oncol 22:1778–1784, 2004.
17. MacDonald JS. Adjuvant therapy of colon cancer. CA Cancer J Clin 49:202–219, 1999.
18. Bond JH. Screening and early detection. In: Wanebo JH, ed. Colorectal cancer. St. Louis: Mosby, 1993:149–157.
19. Enker WE, Loffer UT, Block GE. Enhanced survival of patients with colon and rectal cancer is based upon wide anatomic resection. Ann Surg 190:350–360, 1979.
20. Leung KL, Kwok SPY, Lam SCW, et al. Laparoscopic resection of rectosigmoid carcinoma: prospective randomized trial. Lancet 363:1187–1192, 2004.
21. Steele G, Posner MR. Adjuvant treatment of colorectal adenocarcinoma. Curr Probl Cancer 17:223–229, 1993.
22. Devasa JM, Morales V, Enriques JM. Colorectal cancer: the basis for a comprehensive follow-up. Dis Colon Rectum 31:636–652, 1988.
23. Moertel CG. Accomplishment in surgical adjuvant therapy for large bowel cancer. Cancer 70:1364–1371, 1992.
24. Verhaegen H, DeCree J, DeCock W, et al. Levamisole therapy in patients with colorectal cancer. In: Terry WD, Rosenberg SA, eds. Immunotherapy of human cancer. New York: Excerpta Medica, 1982:222–229.
25. Moertel CG, Fleming TR, MacDonald JS, et al. Fluorouracil plus levamisole as effective adjuvant therapy after resection of stage III colon carcinoma: a final report. Ann Intern Med 122:321–326, 1995.
26. NIH Consensus Conference. Adjuvant therapy for patients with colon and rectal cancer. JAMA 264:1444–1450, 1990.
27. O'Connell MJ, Mailliard JA, Kahn MJ, et al. Controlled trial of fluorouracil and low-dose leucovorin given for 6 months as postoperative adjuvant therapy for colon cancer. J Clin Oncol 15:246–250, 1997.
28. Haller DG, Catalano PJ, Macdonald JS, et al. Fluorouracil, leucovorin and levamisole adjuvant therapy for colon cancer: five year final report of INT-0089 [abstract 982]. Proc Am Soc Clin Oncol 17:256a, 1998.
29. Wolmark N, Rockette H, Mamounas E, et al. Clinical trial to assess the relative efficacy of fluorouracil and leucovorin, fluorouracil and levamisole, and fluorouracil, leucovorin, and levamisole in patients with Dukes' B and C carcinoma of the colon: results from National Surgical Adjuvant Breast and Bowel Project C-04. J Clin Oncol 17:3553–3559, 1999.
30. Efficacy of adjuvant fluorouracil and folinic acid in B2 colon cancer. International Multicentre Pooled Analysis of B2 Colon Cancer Trials (IMPACT B2) investigators. J Clin Oncol 17:1356–1363, 1999.
31. Cascinu S, Georgoulias V, Kerr D, et al. Colorectal cancer in the adjuvant setting: perspectives on treatment and the role of prognostic factors. Ann Oncol 14 (Suppl 2):ii25–ii29, 2003.
32. Andre T, Boni C, Mounedji-Boudiaf L, et al. Oxaliplatin, fluorouracil, and leucovorin as adjuvant treatment for colon cancer. N Engl J Med 350:2343–2351, 2004.
33. Gunderson LL, Martenson JA. Colrectal cancer: radiotherapy. In: Brain MC, Carbone PC, eds. Current therapy in hematology-oncology. 5th ed. St. Louis: Mosby, 1995:371–384.
34. Rougier P, Nordinger B. Larger scale trial for adjuvant treatment in high risk resected colorectal cancers. Rationale to test the combination of loco-regional and systemic chemotherapy and to compare l-leucovorin + 5-FU to levamisole + 5-FU. Ann Oncol 2:21–28, 1993.
35. Midgley R, Kerr D. Colorectal cancer. Lancet 353:391–399, 1999.
36. Gastrointestinal Study Group. Prolongation of the disease-free interval in surgically treated rectal cancer. N Engl J Med 312:1465–1472, 1985.
37. Douglass HO, Mayer RJ, Thomas PRM, et al. Survival after postoperative combination treatment of rectal cancer [letter]. N Engl J Med 315:1294, 1986.
38. Krook J Moertel C, Gunderson LL, et al. Effective surgical adjuvant therapy for high-risk rectal carcinoma. N Engl J Med 324:709–714, 1991.
39. Weaver D, Lindblad AS. Gastrointestinal Tumor Study Group: radiation therapy and 5-fluorouracil (5-FU) with or without MeCCNU for the treatment of patients with surgically adjuvant adenocarcinoma of the rectum [abstract 106]. Proc Am Soc Clin Oncol 9:106, 1990.
40. O'Connell M, Wieand HS, Krook J, et al. Lack of value for methyl-CCNU as a component of effective rectal cancer surgical adjuvant therapy: interim analysis of intergroup protocol 86-47-51 [abstract 134]. Proc Am Soc Clin Oncol 10:134, 1991.
41. National Comprehensive Cancer Network Clinical Practice Guidelines in Oncology, Rectal Cancer. Version 4.2004. *National Comprehensive Cancer Network.* http://www.nccn.org/physician_gls/f_guidelines.html
42. Skibber JM, Minsky BD, Hoff PM. Cancer of the Colon. In: DaVita VT, Hellman S, Rosenberg SA, et al., eds. Cancer principles & practice of oncology. 6th ed. Philadelphia: Lippincott Williams & Wilkins; 2001:1216–1262.
43. Macmillan WE, Wolberg WH, Welling PG. Pharmacokinetics of fluorouracil in humans. Cancer Res 38:3479–3482, 1978.
44. Washtien WL, Santi DV. Intracellular free and macromolecular-bound metabolites of 5-fluorodeoxyuridine and 5-fluorouracil. Cancer Res 39:3397–3404, 1979.
45. Rougier P, Mitry E. Epidemiology, treatment and chemoprevention in colorectal cancer. Ann Oncol 14 (Suppl 2):ii3–ii5, 2003.
46. Braun AH, Achterrath W, Wilke H, et al. New systemic frontline treatment for metastatic colorectal carcinoma. Cancer 100:1558–1577, 2004.
47. Seifert P, Baker LH, Reed MD, et al. Comparison of continuously infused 5-fluorouracil with bolus injection in patients with colorectal adenocarcinoma. Cancer 36:123–128, 1975.
48. Ardalan B, Singh G, Silberman H. A randomized phase I and II study of short-term infusion of high-dose fluorouracil with and without N-(phosphonacetyl)-L-aspartic acid in patients with advanced pancreatic and colorectal cancers. J Clin Oncol 6:1053–1058, 1988.

49. Evans RM, Laskin JD, Hakala MT. Effect of excess folates and deoxyinosine on the activity and site of action of 5-fluorouracil. Cancer Res 41:3283–3295, 1981.

50. Poon MA, O'Connell MJ, Moertel CG, et al. Biochemical modulation of fluorouracil: evidence of significant improvement of survival and quality of life in patients with advanced colorectal carcinoma. J Clin Oncol 7:1407–1408, 1989.

51. Wadler SW, Schwartz EL, Goldman M, et al. Fluorouracil and recombinant alfa-2a-interferon: an active regimen against advanced colorectal carcinoma. J Clin Oncol 7:1769–1775, 1998.

52. Ardalan B, Singh G, Silberman H. A randomized phase I and II study of short-term infusion of high-dose fluorouracil with or without N-(phosphonacetyl)-L-aspartic acid in patients with advanced pancreatic and colorectal cancer. J Clin Oncol 7:1053–1058, 1988.

53. Grem JL, Fischer PH. Enhancement of the antitumor activity of 5-fluorouracil's anticancer activity by dipyridamole. Pharmacol Ther 40:349–371, 1989.

54. Klubes P, Leyland-Jones B. Enhancement of the antitumor activity of 5-fluorouracil by uridine rescue. Pharmacol Ther 41:289–302, 1989.

55. Ahlgren JD. Colorectal cancer: chemotherapy. In: Ahlgren JD, Macdonald JS, eds. Gastrointestinal oncology. Philadelphia: JB Lippincott, 1992:339–357.

56. Punt CJA. New drugs in the treatment of colorectal carcinoma. Cancer 83:679–689, 1998.

57. Rougier P, Van Cutsem E, Bajetta E, et al. Randomised trial of irinotecan versus fluorouracil by continuous infusion after fluorouracil failure in patients with metastatic colorectal cancer. Lancet 355: 1407–1412, 1998.

58. Cunningham D, Pyrhonen S, James RD, et al. Randomised trial of irinotecan plus supportive care versus supportive care alone after fluorouracil failure for patients with metastatic colorectal cancer. Lancet 352:1413–1418, 1998.

59. Tournigand C, Andre T, Achille E, et al. FOLFIRI followed by FOLFOX6 or the reverse sequence in advanced colorectal cancer: a randomized GERCOR study. J Clin Oncol 22:229–237, 2004.

60. Camptosar package insert. Kalamazoo, MI: Pharmacia & Upjohn Co., 2002 May.

61. Bugat R, Rougier P, Douillard JY, et al. Efficacy of irinotecan HCl (CPT11) in patients with metastatic colorectal cancer after progression while receiving a 5-FU based chemotherapy. Proc Am Soc Clin Oncol 14:A567, 1995.

62. Abigerges D, Chabot GG, Armand JP, et al. Phase I and pharmacologic studies of the camptothecin analog irinotecan administered every 3 weeks in cancer patients. J Clin Oncol 13:210–221, 1995.

63. Folprecht G, Kohne CH. The role of new agents in the treatment of colorectal cancer. Oncology 66:1–17, 2004.

64. Missel JL. Oxaliplatin in practice. Br J Cancer 77 (Suppl 4):4–7, 1998.

65. Doulliard JY, Cunningham D, Roth AD, et al. Irinotecan combined with fluorouracil compared with fluorouracil alone as first-line treatment for metastatic colorectal cancer: a multicentre randomized trial. Lancet 355:1041–1047, 2000.

66. Saltz LB, Cox JV, Blanke C, et al. Irinotecan plus fluorouracil and leucovorin for metastatic colorectal cancer. N Engl J Med 343: 905–914, 2000.

67. Machover D, Diaz-Rubio E, de Gramont A, et al. Two consecutive phase II studies of oxaliplatin for treatment of patients with advanced colorectal carcinoma who were resistant to previous treatment of fluoropyrimidines. Ann Oncol 7:95–98, 1996.

68. Maindrault-Goebel F, Louver C, Andre T, et al. Oxaliplatin added to the simplified bimonthly leucovorin and 5-fluorouracil regimen as second-line therapy for metastatic colorectal cancer (FOLFOX6). Eur J Cancer 35:1338–1342, 1999.

69. Rothenberg ML, Oza AM, Bigelow RH, et al. Superiority of oxaliplatin and fluorouracil-leucovorin compared with either therapy in patients with progressive colorectal cancer after irinotecan and fluorouracil-leucovorin: interim results of a phase II trial. J Clin Oncol 21:2059–2069, 2003.

70. Eloxatin package insert. New York, NY: Sanofi-Synthelabo, Inc., 2004 Jan.

71. de Gramont A, Figer A, Seymour M, et al. Leucovorin and fluorouracil with or without oxaliplatin as first-line treatment in advanced colorectal cancer. J Clin Oncol 18:2938–2947, 2000.

72. Giacchetti S, Perpoint B, Zidani R, et al. Phase III multicenter randomized trial of oxaliplatin added to chronomodulated fluorouracil-leucovorin as first-line treatment of metastatic colorectal cancer. J Clin Oncol 18:136–147, 2000.

73. Grothey A, Deschler B, Kroening H, et al. Phase III study of bolus 5-fluorouracil(5-FU)/folinic acid (FA) (Mayo) versus weekly high-dose 24 h 5-FU infusion/FA + oxaliplatin (FUFOX) in advanced colorectal cancer. Proc Am Soc Clin Oncol 21:129a, 2002.

74. Goldberg RM, Sargent DJ, Morton RF, et al. A randomized controlled trial of fluorouracil plus leucovorin, irinotecan, and oxaliplatin combinations in patients with previously untreated metastatic colorectal cancer. J Clin Oncol 22:23–30, 2004.

75. Van Cutsem E, Hoff PM, Harper P, et al. Oral capecitabine versus intravenous 5-fluorouracil and leucovorin: integrated efficacy data and novel analyses from two large, randomized, phase III trials. Br J Cancer 90:1190–1197, 2004.

76. Van Cutsem E, Twelves C, Tabernero J, et al. XELOX: mature results of a multinational, phase II trial of capecitabine plus oxaliplatin, an effective first line option for patients with metastatic colorectal cancer [abstract 1023]. Proc Am Soc Clin Oncol 22:255, 2003.

77. Patt YZ, Lin E, Liebman J, et al. Capecitabine plus irinotecan: a highly active first-line treatment for metastatic colorectal cancer [abstract 228]. Paper presented at: 2004 Gastrointestinal Cancers Symposium: Current Status and Future Directions for Prevention and Management; January 22–24, 2004; San Francisco, CA.

78. Kabbinavar F, Hurwitz HI, Fehrenbacher L, et al. Phase II, randomized trial comparing bevacizumab plus fluorouracil (FU)/leucovorin (LV) with FU/LV alone in patients with metastatic colorectal cancer. J Clin Oncol 21:60–65, 2003.

79. Giantonio BJ, Levy D, O'Dwyer PJ, et al. Bevacizumab plus IFL as front-line therapy for advanced colorectal cancer: results from the Eastern Cooperative Oncology Group study E2200 [abstract 1024]. Proc Am Soc Clin Oncol 22:255, 2003.

80. Hurwitz H, Fehrenbacher L, Novotny W, et al. Bevacizumab plus irinotecan, fluorouracil, and leucovorin for metastatic colorectal cancer. N Engl J Med 350:2335–2342, 2004.

81. Avastin package insert. South San Francisco, CA: Genentech, 2004 Feb.

82. Cunningham D, Humblet Y, Siena S, et al. Cetuximab monotherapy and cetuximab plus irinotecan in irinotecan-refractory metastatic colorectal cancer. N Engl J Med 351:337–345, 2004.

83. Erbitux package insert. Princeton, NJ: Bristol-Myers Squibb, 2004 Jun.

84. Evans DB, Abbruzzese JL, Rich TA. Cancer of the pancreas. In: DeVita VT Jr, Hellman S, Rosenberg SA, eds. Cancer: principles and practices of oncology. 5th ed. Philadelphia: Lippincott-Raven, 1997.

85. Gold EB, Goldin SB. Epidemiology of and risk factors for pancreatic cancer. Surg Oncol Clin North Am 7:67–88, 1998.

86. Parkin DM, Pisani P, Ferlay J. Global cancer statistics. CA Cancer J Clin 49:33–64, 1999.

87. Tominaga S, Kuroishi T. Epidemiology of pancreatic cancer. Semin Surg Oncol 15:3–7, 1998.

88. Ahlgren JD. Epidemiology of and risk factors in pancreatic cancer. Semin Oncol 23:241–250, 1996.

89. Silverman DT, Dunn JA, Hoover RN, et al. Cigarette smoking and pancreas cancer: a case-control study based on direct interviews. J Natl Cancer Inst 86:1510–1516, 1994.

90. La Vecchia C, Boyle P, Franceschi S, et al. Smoking and cancer with emphasis on Europe. Eur J Cancer 27:94–104, 1991.

91. Mack TM, Yu MC, Hanisch R, et al. Pancreas cancer and smoking, beverage consumption, and past medical history. J Natl Cancer Inst 76:49–60, 1986.

92. Zheng W, McLaughlin JK, Gridley G, et al. A cohort of smoking, alcohol consumption, and dietary factors for pancreatic cancer (United States). Cancer Causes Control 4:477–482, 1993.

93. Olsen GW, Mandel JS, Gibson RW, et al. A case-control study of pancreatic cancer and cigarettes, alcohol, coffee and diet. Am J Public Health 79:1016–1019, 1989.

94. Mancuso TF, El-Attar AA. Cohort study of workers exposed to betanaphthylamine and benzidine. J Occup Med 9:277–285, 1967.

95. Pietri F, Clavel F. Occupational exposure and cancer of the pancreas: a review. Br J Ind Med 48:583–587, 1991.

96. Karmody A, Kyle J. The association between carcinoma of the pancreas and diabetes mellitus. Br J Surg 56:362–364, 1969.

97. Gullo L, Pezzilli R, Morselli-Labate AM. Diabetes and the risk of pancreatic cancer. N Engl J Med 331:81–84, 1994.

98. Jones SC. Pancreatic cancer and diabetes [letter]. N Engl J Med 331:1526–1528, 1994.

99. Lowenfels AB, Maisonneuve P, Cavallini G, et al. Pancreatitis and the risk of pancreatic cancer. N Engl J Med 328:1433–1437, 1993.

100. Ekbom A, McLaughlin JK, Karlsson BM, et al. Pancreatitis and pancreatic cancer: a population-based study. J Natl Cancer Inst 86: 625–627, 1994.

101. Karlson BM, Ekbom A, Josefsson S, et al. The risk of pancreatic cancer following pancreatitis: an association due to confounding? Gastroenterology 113:587–592, 1997.

102. Hruban RH, Petersen GM, Ha PK, et al. Genetics of pancreatic cancer: from genes to families. Surg Oncol Clin North Am 7:1–23, 1998.

103. Nomoto S, Nakao A, Ando N, et al. Clinical application of K-ras oncogene mutations in pancreatic carcinoma: detection of micrometastases. Semin Surg Oncol 15:40–46, 1998.

104. Goldstein AM, Fraser M, Struewing JP, et al. Increased risk of pancreatic cancer in melanoma-prone kindreds with p16^{INK4} mutations. N Engl J Med 333:970–974, 1995.

105. Whelan AJ, Bartsch D, Goodfellow PJ. Brief report: a familial syndrome of pancreatic cancer and melanoma with a mutation in the CDKN2 tumor-suppressor gene. N Engl J Med 333:975–977, 1995.

106. Lynch HT, Smyrk T, Kern SE, et al. Familial pancreatic cancer: a review. Semin Oncol 23:251–275, 1996.

107. Wilentz RE, Hruban RH. Pathology of cancer of the pancreas. Surg Oncol Clin North Am 7:43–63, 1998.

108. Krech RL, Walsh D. Symptoms of pancreatic cancer. J Pain Symptom Manage 6:360–367, 1991.

109. Kelsen DP, Portenoy RK, Thaler HT, et al. Pain and depression in patients with newly diagnosed pancreas cancer. J Clin Oncol 13: 748–755, 1995.

110. Passik SD, Breitbart WS. Depression in patients with pancreatic carcinoma: diagnostic and treatment issues. Cancer 78:625–626, 1996.

111. Lillemoe KD, Pitt HA. Palliation. Cancer 78:605–614, 1996.

112. Bluemke DA, Fishman EK. CT and MR evaluation of pancreatic cancer. Surg Oncol Clin North Am 7:103–124, 1998.

113. Furhman GM, Charnsangavej C, Abbruzzese JL, et al. Thin-section contrast enhanced computed tomography accurately predicts resectability of malignant pancreatic neoplasms. Am J Surg 167: 104–113, 1994.

114. Steinberg WM, Barkin J, Bradley EL III, et al. Controversies in clinical pancreatology. Pancreas 17:24–30, 1998.

115. Stevens PD, Lightdale CJ. The role of endosonography in the diagnosis and management of pancreatic cancer. Surg Clin North Am 7:125–133, 1998.

116. Fernandez-del Castillo, Warshaw AL. Laparoscopic staging and peritoneal cytology. Surg Oncol Clin North Am 7:135–142, 1998.

117. Posner MR, Mayer RJ. The use of serologic tumor markers in gastrointestinal malignancies. Hematol Oncol Clin North Am 8: 533–552, 1994.

118. Ritts RE, Pitt HA. CA 19-9 in pancreatic cancer. Surg Oncol Clin North Am 7:93–101, 1998.

119. Nakao A, Oshima K, Nomoto S, et al. Clinical usefulness of CA 19-9 in pancreatic carcinoma. Semin Surg Oncol 15:15–22, 1998.

120. Kiriyama E, Hayakawa T, Kondo T, et al. Usefulness of a new tumor marker, span-1, for the diagnosis of pancreatic cancer. Cancer 65:1557–1561, 1990.

121. American Joint Committee on Cancer. Exocrine pancreas. In: Fleming ID, Cooper JS, Henson DE, et al., eds. AJCC cancer staging manual. 5th ed. Philadelphia: Lippincott-Raven, 1997.

122. Nitecki SS, Sarr MG, Colby TV, et al. Long-term survival after resection for ductal adenocarcinoma of the pancreas. Is it really improving? Ann Surg 221:59–66, 1995.

123. Whittington R, Bryer MP, Haller DG, et al. Adjuvant therapy of resected adenocarcinoma of the pancreas. Int J Radiat Oncol Biol Phys 21:1137–1143, 1991.

124. Reber HA. Pancreas. In: Schwartz SI, Shires GT, Spencer FC, et al., eds. Principles of surgery. 7th ed. New York: McGraw-Hill, 1999.

125. Yeo CJ. Pylorus-preserving pancreaticoduodenectomy. Surg Oncol Clin North Am 7:143–156, 1998.

126. Brooks JR, Brooks DC, Levine JD. Total pancreatectomy for ductal cell carcinoma of the pancreas. Ann Surg 209:405–410, 1989.

127. Van Heerden JA, McIlrath DC, Ilstrup DM, et al. Total pancreatectomy for ductal cell carcinoma of the pancreas: an update. World J Surg 12:658–662, 1988.

128. Gastrointestinal Tumor Study Group. Further evidence of effective adjuvant combined radiation and chemotherapy following curative resection of pancreatic cancer. Cancer 59:2006–2010, 1987.

129. Kalser MH, Ellenberg SS. Pancreatic cancer: adjuvant combined radiation and chemotherapy following curative resection. Arch Surg 120:899–903, 1985.

130. Spitz FR, Abbruzzese JL, Lee JE, et al. Preoperative and postoperative chemoradiation strategies in patients treated with pancreaticoduodenectomy for adenocarcinoma of the pancreas. J Clin Oncol 15:928–937, 1997.

131. Miller AR, Robinson EK, Lee JE, et al. Neoadjuvant chemoradiation for adenocarcinoma of the pancreas. Surg Oncol Clin North Am 7:183–197, 1998.

132. Lawrence T, Chang E, Hahn T, et al. Radiosensitization of pancreatic cancer cells by 2′,2′-difluoro-2′-deoxycytidine. Int J Radiol Oncol Biol Phys 34:867–872, 1996.

133. Robertson JM, Shewach DS, Lawrence TS. Preclinical studies of chemotherapy and radiation therapy for pancreatic carcinoma. Cancer 78:674–679, 1996.

134. Hidalgo M, Castellano D, Paz-Ares L, et al. Phase I-II study of gemcitabine and fluorouracil as a continuous infusion in patients with pancreatic cancer. J Clin Oncol 17:585–592, 1999.

135. Wolff RA, Evans DB, Crane CH, et al. Initial results of preoperative gemcitabine (GEM)-based chemoradiation for resectable pancreatic adenocarcinoma [abstract]. Proc Am Soc Clin Oncol 21: 130a, 2002.

136. Roldan GE, Gunderson LL, Nagorney DM, et al. External beam versus intraoperative and external beam irradiation for locally advanced pancreatic cancer. Cancer 61:1110–1116, 1988.

137. Shibamoto Y, Manabe T, Baba N, et al. High dose, external beam and intraoperative radiotherapy in the treatment of resectable and unresectable pancreatic cancer. Int J Radiol Oncol Biol Phys 19: 605–611, 1990.

138. Pisters PWT, Abbruzzese JL, Janjan NA, et al. Rapid-fractionation preoperative chemoradiation, pancreaticoduodenectomy, and intraoperative radiation therapy for resectable pancreatic adenocarcinoma. J Clin Oncol 16: 3843–3850, 1998.

139. Moertel CG, Frytak S, Hahn RG, et al. Therapy of locally unresectable pancreatic carcinoma: a randomized comparison of high dose (6000 rads) radiation alone, moderate dose radiation (4000 rads) plus 5-FU, and high dose radiation plus 5-FU: the gastrointestinal tumor study group. Cancer 48:1705–1710, 1981.

140. Gastrointestinal Tumor Study Group. Treatment of locally unresectable carcinoma of the pancreas: comparison of combined-modality therapy (chemotherapy plus radiotherapy) to chemotherapy alone. J Natl Cancer Inst 80:751–755, 1988.

141. Boz G, De Paoli A, Roncandin M, et al. Radiation therapy combined with chemotherapy for inoperable pancreatic carcinoma. Tumori 77:61–64, 1991.

142. Dobelbower RR Jr, Merrick H, Ahuja R, et al. I-125 interstitial implant, precision high-dose external beam therapy, and 5-FU for unresectable adenocarcinoma of pancreas and extrahepatic biliary tree. Cancer 58:2185–2195, 1986.

143. Safran H, King TP, Choy H, et al. Paclitaxel and concurrent radiation for locally advanced pancreatic and gastric cancer: a phase I study. J Clin Oncol 15:901–907, 1997.

144. Robertson JM, Ensminger WD, Walker S, et al. A phase I trial of intravenous bromodeoxyuridine and radiation therapy for pancreatic cancer. Int J Radiol Oncol Biol Phys 37:331–335, 1997.

145. Crane CH, Ellis LM, Xiong H, et al. Preliminary results of a phase I study of rhuMab VEGF (bevacizumab) with concurrent radiotherapy (XRT) and capecitabine (CAP). Proc Am Soc Clin Oncol Gastrointestinal Cancers Symposium 2004 (abstr 85).

146. Gemzar (Gemcitabine HCl) injection, package insert. Indianapolis, IN: Eli Lilly and Co., 1996.

147. Noble S, Goa KL. Gemcitabine: a review of its pharmacology and clinical potential in non-small cell lung cancer and pancreatic cancer. Drugs 54:447–472, 1997.

148. Moore M. Activity of gemcitabine in patients with advanced pancreatic carcinoma. Cancer 78: 633–638, 1996.

149. Casper ES, Green MR, Kelsen DP, et al. Phase II trial of gemcitabine (2,2′-difluorodeoxycytidine) in patients with adenocarcinoma of the pancreas. Invest New Drug 12:29–34, 1994.

150. Burris III HA. Objective outcome measure of quality of life. Oncology 11:131–135, 1996.

151. Rothenberg ML, Abbruzzese JL, Moore M, et al. A rationale for expanding the endpoints for clinical trials in advanced pancreatic carcinoma. Cancer 78: 627–632, 1996.

152. Burris III HA. Improvements in survival and clinical benefit with gemcitabine as first-line therapy for patients with advanced pancreas cancer: a randomized trial. J Clin Oncol 15:2403–2413, 1997.

153. Schnall SF, McDonald JS. Chemotherapy of adenocarcinoma of the pancreas. Semin Oncol 23:220–228, 1996.

154. DeCaprio, JA, Mayer RJ, Gonin R, et al. Fluorouracil and high dose leucovorin in previously untreated patients with advanced adenocarcinoma of the pancreas: results of a phase II trial. J Clin Oncol 9:2128–2133, 1991.

155. The Gastrointestinal Tumor Study Group. Phase II studies of drug combinations in advanced pancreatic carcinoma: fluorouracil plus doxorubicin plus mitomycin C and two regimens of streptozocin plus mitomycin C plus fluorouracil. J Clin Oncol 4:1794–1798, 1986.

156. Grunewald R, Abbruzzese JL, Tarassoff P, et al. Saturation of 2′2′-difluorodeoxycytidine 5′-triphosphate accumulation by mononuclear cells during a phase I trial of gemcitabine. Cancer Chemother Pharmacol 27:258–262,1991.

157. Tempero M, Plunkett W, Ruiz van Haperen V, et al. Randomized phase II comparison of dose-intense gemcitabine: thirty-minute infusion and fixed dose rate infusion in patients with pancreatic adenocarcinoma. J Clin Oncol 21:3402–3408, 2003.

158. Heinemann V, Wilke H, Mergenthaler HG, et al. Gemcitabine and cisplatin in the treatment of advanced or metastatic pancreatic cancer. Ann Oncol 11:1399–1403, 2000.

159. Philip PA, Zalupski MM, Vaitkevicius VK, et al. Phase II study of gemcitabine and cisplatin in the treatment of patients with advanced pancreatic carcinoma. Cancer 92:569–577, 2001.

160. Rocha Lima CM, Savarese D, Bruckner H, et al. Irinotecan plus gemcitabine induces both radiographic and CA19-9 tumor marker responses in patients with previously untreated advanced pancreatic cancer. J Clin Oncol 20:1182–1191, 2002.

161. Louvet C, André T, Lledo G, et al. Gemcitabine combined with oxaliplatin in advanced pancreatic adenocarcinoma: final results of a GERCOR multicenter phase II study. J Clin Oncol 20:1512–1518, 2002.

162. Bai R, Pettit GR, Hamel E, et al. Binding of dolastatin 10 to tubulin at a distinct site for peptide antimitotic agents near the exchangeable nucleotide and vinca alkaloid sites. Biochem Pharmacol 39:1941–1949, 1990.

163. Von Hoff DD, Goodwin AL, Garcia L, et al. Advances in the treatment of patients with pancreatic cancer: improvement in symptoms and survival time. Br J Cancer 78:9–13, 1998.

164. Bagniewski PG, Pitot HC. Pharmacokinetics of dolastatin 10 in adult patients with solid tumors [abstract]. Proc Ann Am Assoc Cancer Res 38:A1492, 1997.

165. Cascinu S, Silva RR, Barni S, et al. Gemcitabine and 5-FU in advanced pancreatic cancer: a GISCAD phase II study [abstract]. Proc Am Soc Clin Oncol 17:264a, 1998.

166. Clary BM, Lyerly HK. Gene therapy and pancreatic cancer. Surg Oncol Clin North Am 7:217–237, 1998.

167. Takeda S, Nakao A, Miyoshi K, et al. Gene therapy for pancreatic cancer. Semin Surg Oncol 15:57–61, 1998.

168. Ganly I, Kirn D, Rodriguez GI, et al. Phase I trial of intratumoral injection with an E1B-attenuated adenovirus, ONYX-015, in patients with recurrent p53(!) head and neck cancer [abstract]. Proc Am Soc Clin Oncol 16:382, 1997.

169. Heise C, Sampson-Johannes A, Williams A, et al. ONYX-015, an E1B-attenuated adenovirus, causes tumor-specific cytolysis and antitumoral efficacy that can be augmented by standard chemotherapeutic agents. Nat Med 3:639–645, 1997.

170. Abbruzzese JL, Rosenberg A, Xiong Q, et al. Phase II study of anti-epidermal growth factor receptor (EGFR) antibody Cetuximab (IMC-C225) in combination with gemcitabine in patients with advanced pancreatic cancer [abstract]. Proc Am Soc Clin Oncol 20130a, 2001.

171. Kindler HL, Friberg G, Stadler WM, et al. Bevacizumab plus gemcitabine is an active combination in patients with advanced pancreatic cancer: interim results of ongoing phase II trial from the University of Chicago Phase II Consortium [abstract 86]. Proc Am Soc Clin Oncol Gastrointestinal Cancers Symposium 2004.

172. Lillemoe KD. Palliative therapy for pancreatic cancer. Surg Oncol Clin North Am 7:199–217, 1998.

173. Alter CL. Palliative and supportive care of patients with pancreatic cancer. Semin Oncol 23:229–240, 1996.

174. Davids PH, Groen AK, Rauws EA, et al. Randomized trial of self-expanding metal stents versus polyethylene stents for distal malignant biliary obstruction. Lancet 340:1488–1492, 1992.

175. Caraceni A, Portenoy RK. Pain management in patients with pancreatic carcinoma. Cancer 78:639–653, 1996.

176. Lebovitz AH, Lefkowitz M. Pain management of pancreatic carcinoma: a review. Pain 36:1–11, 1989.

177. World Health Organization. Cancer pain relief and palliative care. Geneva: World Health Organization, 1990.

178. Agency for Health Care Policy and Research. Management of cancer pain: clinical practice guideline, number 9. Washington, DC: US Department of Health and Human Services, Agency for Health Care Policy and Research, 1994.

179. Lillemoe KD, Cameron JL, Kaufman HS, et al. Chemical splanchnicectomy in patients with unresectable pancreatic cancer: a prospective randomized trial. Ann Surg 217:447–457, 1993.

180. Kawamata M, Ishitani K, Ishikawa K, et al. Comparison between celiac plexus block and morphine treatment on quality of life in patients with pancreatic cancer pain. Pain 64:597–602, 1996.

181. Holland JC, Korzun AH, Tross S, et al. Comparative psychological disturbance in patients with pancreatic and gastric cancer. Am J Psychiatry 143:982–986, 1996.

182. Fras I, Litin EM, Pearson JS. Comparison of psychiatric symptoms in carcinoma of the pancreas with those in some other intra-abdominal neoplasm. Am J Psychiatry 123:1553–1562, 1967.

183. Boring C, Squires T, Tong J. Cancer statistics 1991. CA Cancer J Clin 41:19–36. Erratum in: CA Cancer J Clin 1991 Mar–Apr; 41(2):111.

184. Jemal A, Tiwari RC, Murray T, et al. Cancer statistics, 2004. CA Cancer J Clin 54:8–29, 2004.

185. Wiggins CL, Becker TM, Key CR, et al. Stomach cancer among New Mexico's American Indians, Hispanic Whites, and non-Hispanic whites. Cancer Res 49:1595–1599, 1989.

186. Hwang H, Swyer J, Russell RM. Diet, *Helicobacter pylori* infection, food preservation and gastric cancer risk: are these new roles for preventive factors. Nutr Rev 52:75–83, 1994.

187. Hotz J, Goebell H. Epidemiology and pathogenesis of gastric carcinoma. In: Meyer HJ, Schnoll HF, Hotz J, eds. Gastric carcinoma. New York: Springer-Verlag, 1989:3.

188. Tannenbaum SR, Wishnok JS, Leaf CD. Inhibition of nitrosamine formation by ascorbic acid. Am J Clin Nutr 53 (Suppl): 247S–250S, 1991.

189. Schorah CJ, Sobala GM, Sanderson M, et al. Gastric juice ascorbic acid: effects of disease and implications for gastric carcinogenesis. Am J Clin Nutr 53:287S–293S, 1991.

190. Eurogast. An international association between *Helicobacter pylori* infection and gastric cancer. Lancet 341:1359–1362, 1993.

191. Parsonnett J, Friedman GD, Vandersteen DP, et al. *Helicobacter pylori* infection and the risk of gastric carcinoma. N Engl J Med 325: 1127–1131, 1991.

192. Graham DY. Benefits from elimination of *Helicobacter pylori* infection include major reduction in the incidence of peptic ulcer disease, gastric cancer, and primary gastric lymphoma. Prev Med 32: 712–716, 1994.

193. Macdonald JS, Hill MC, Roberts IM. Gastric cancer: epidemiology, pathology, detection, and staging. In: Ahlgren J, Macdonald J, eds. Gastrointestinal oncology. Philadelphia: JB Lippincott, 1992: 151–158.

194. Lagcragren J, Bergstrom R, Nyren O. Association between body mass and adenocarcinoma of the esophagus and gastric cardia. Ann Intern Med 130:883–890, 1999.

195. Wanebo HJ, Kennedy BJ, Chmiel J, et al. Cancer of the stomach: a patient care study by the American College of Surgeons. Ann Surg 218:583–592, 1993.

196. Salvon-Harman JC, Nikulasson S, Stone MD, et al. Shifting proportions of gastric adenocarcinomas. Arch Surg 129:381–388, 1994.

197. Farley DR, Donohue JH. Early gastric cancer. Surg Clin North Am 72:401–421, 1992.

198. Ellis DJ, Spevis C, Kingston RD, et al. Carcinoembryonic antigen levels in advanced gastric carcinoma. Cancer 42:623–625, 1978.

199. Caletti G, Ferrari A, Brocchi E, et al. Accuracy of endoscopic ultrasonography in the diagnosis and staging of gastric cancer and lymphoma. Surgery 113:14–27, 1993.

200. Ott K, Sendler A, Becker K, et al. Neoadjuvant chemotherapy with cisplatin, 5-FU, and leucovorin (PLF) in locally advanced gastric cancer: a prospective phase II study. Gastric Cancer 6:159–163, 2003.

201. Pollack BJ, Chak A, Sivak MV Jr: Endoscopic Ultrasonography. Semin Oncol 23:336–346, 1996.

202. Kaneko E, Nakamura T, Umeda N, et al. Outcome of gastric carcinoma detected by gastric mass survey in Japan. Gut 18:626–630, 1977.

203. Kim JP, Kim YW, Yang HK, et al. Significant prognostic factors by multivariate analysis of 3926 gastric cancer patients. World J Surg 18:872–878, 1994.

204. Lee WJ, Lee Ph, Yue SC, et al. Lymph node metastases in gastric cancer: significance of positive number. Oncology 52:45–50, 1995.

205. Macdonald JS, Smalley SR, Beneditti J, et al. Chemoradiotherapy after surgery compared with surgery alone for adenocarcinoma of the stomach or gastroesophageal junction. N Engl J Med 345:725–730, 2001.

206. Boddie AW Jr. The role of lymphadenectomy in cancer, with particular reference to gastric cancer. Int Surg 79:6–10, 1994.

207. Behrns KE, Dalton RR, van Heerden JA, et al. Extended lymph node dissection for gastric cancer: is it of value? Surg Clin North Am 72:433–443, 1992.

208. Bonenkamp JJ, Van de Velde CJH, Sasako M, et al. R2 compared with R1 resection for gastric cancer: morbidity and mortality in a prospective, randomized trial. Eur J Surg 158:413–418, 1992.

209. Robertson CS, Chung SCS, Woods SDS, et al. A prospective randomized trial comparing R1 subtotal gastrectomy with R3 total gastrectomy for antral cancer. Ann Surg 220:176–182, 1994.

210. Bunt AMG, Hermans J, Boon MC, et al. Evaluation of the extent of lymphadenectomy in a randomized trial of Western-versus Japanese-type surgery in gastric cancer. J Clin Oncol 12:417–422, 1994.

211. Pacelli F, Doglietto GB, Ballantone R, et al. Extensive versus limited lymph node dissection for gastric cancer: a comparative study of 320 patients. Br J Surg 80:1153–1156, 1993.

212. Smith JW, Brennan MF. Surgical treatment of gastric cancer: proximal, mid and distal stomach. Surg Clin North Am 72:381–399, 1992.

213. Vezeridis MP. Wanebo HJ. Gastric cancer: surgical approach. In: Ahlgren J, Macdonald J, eds. Gastrointestinal oncology. Philadelphia: JB Lippincott, 1992:159–170.

214. Moertel CG, Childs DS Jr, Reitemeier RJ et al. Combined 5-fluorouracil and supervoltage radiation therapy for locally unresectable gastrointestinal cancer. Lancet 2 (7276): 865–867.

215. Macdonald JS, Smalley SR, Beneditti J, et al. Chemoradiotherapy after surgery compared with surgery alone for adenocarcinoma of the stomach or gastroesophageal junction. N Engl J Med 345:725–730, 2001.

216. Myint AS. The role of radiotherapy in the palliative treatment of gastrointestinal cancer. Eur J Gastroenterol Hepatol 12:381–390, 2000.

217. Rougier P. Lasser P, Ducreux M, et al. Preoperative chemotherapy of locally advanced gastric cancer. Ann Oncol 5 (Suppl 3): S59–S68, 1994.

218. Kang YK, Choi DW, Im YH, et al. A phase III randomized comparison of neoadjuvant chemotherapy followed by surgery for locally advanced stomach cancer [abstract]. Proc Am Soc Clin Oncol 15:215, 1996.

219. Yonemura Y, Sawa T, Kinoshita K, et al. Neoadjuvant chemotherapy for high-grade advanced gastric cancer. World J Surg 17:256–262, 1993.

220. Alexander HR, Grem JL, Pass HI, et al. Neoadjuvant chemotherapy of locally advanced gastric cancer. Oncology 7:37–41, 1993.

221. Kelsen D. Neoadjuvant therapy for gastrointestinal cancers. Oncology 7:25–31, 1993.

222. Leichman L, Silberman H, Leichman CG, et al. Preoperative systemic chemotherapy followed by adjuvant postoperative intraperitoneal therapy for gastric cancer: a University of Southern California pilot program. J Clin Oncol 10:1933–1942, 1992.

223. Agboola O. Adjuvant treatment in gastric cancer. Cancer Treat Rev 20:217–240, 1994.

224. Grau JJ, Estape J, Alcobendas F, et al. Positive results of adjuvant mitomycin C in resected gastric cancer: a randomized trial on 134 patients. Eur J Cancer 29A:340–342, 1993.

225. Gastrointestinal Tumor Study Group. Controlled trial of adjuvant chemotherapy following curative resection for gastric cancer. Cancer 49:1116–1122, 1982.

226. Engstrom PF, Lavin PT, Douglass HO Jr, et al. Postoperative adjuvant 5-fluorouracil plus methyl-CCNU for gastric cancer patients: Eastern Cooperative Oncology Group Study (EST 3275). Cancer 55:1868–1873, 1985.

227. Higgins GA, Amadeo JH, Smith DE, et al. Efficacy of prolonged intermittent therapy with combined 5-FU and methyl-CCNU following resection for gastric carcinoma. A Veterans Administration Surgical Oncology Group report. Cancer 52:1105–112, 1983.

228. Douglass HO Jr. Gastric cancer: current status of adjuvant therapy. Oncology 3:61–66, 1989.

229. Kelsen D. The use of chemotherapy in the treatment of advanced gastric and pancreas cancer. Semin Oncol 21 (Suppl 7):58–66, 1994.

230. Macdonald JS, Gastric cancer: chemotherapy of advanced disease. Hematol Oncol 10:37–42, 1992.

231. Ajani JA, Fairweather J, Dumas P, et al. A phase II study of Taxol in patients with advanced untreated gastric carcinoma [abstract]. Proc Ann Soc Clin Oncol 16:A933, 1997.

232. Taguchi T. A late phase II study of docetaxel in patients with gastric cancer [abstract]. Proc Ann Soc Clin Oncol 16:A934, 1997.

233. Macdonald JS, Schein PS, Woolley PV, et al. 5-fluorouracil, doxorubicin, and mitomycin (FAM) combination chemotherapy for advanced gastric cancer. Ann Intern Med 93:533–536, 1980.

234. Cullinan SA, Moertel CG, Fleming TR, et al. A comparison of three chemotherapeutic regimens in the treatment of advanced pancreatic and gastric carcinoma. Fluorouracil vs. fluorouracil and doxorubicin vs. fluorouracil, doxorubicin and mitomycin. JAMA 253: 2061–2067, 1985.

235. Figoli F. Galligioni E, Crivellari D, et al. Evaluation of two consecutive regimens in advanced gastric cancer. Cancer Invest 93: 257–262, 1991.

236. Kim NY, Park YS, Heo DS, et al. A phase III randomized study of 5-fluorouracil, doxorubicin, and mitomycin C versus 5-fluorouracil alone in the treatment of advanced gastric cancer. Cancer 71: 3813–3818, 1993.

237. Wils JA, Klein HO, Wagener DJT, et al. Sequential high-dose methotrexate and fluorouracil combined with doxorubicin a step ahead in the treatment of advanced gastric cancer: a trial of the European Organization for Research and Treatment of Cancer Gastrointestinal Tract Cooperative Group. J Clin Oncol 9:827–831, 1991.

238. Murad AM, Santiago FF, Petroianu A, et al. Modified therapy with 5-fluorouracil, doxorubicin, and methotrexate in advanced gastric cancer. Cancer 72:37–41, 1993.

239. Pyrhonen S, Kuitunen T, Nyandoto P, et al. Randomized comparison of fluorouracil, epidoxorubicin and methotrexate plus supportive care with supportive care alone in patients with non-resectable gastric cancer. Br J Cancer 71:587–591, 1995.

240. Roelofs EMJ, Wagener DJY, Conroy T, et al. Phase II study of sequential high-dose methotrexate and 5-fluorouracil alternated with epirubicin and cisplatin in advanced gastric cancer. Ann Oncol 4: 426–428, 1993.

241. Wilke H, Preusser P, Fink U, et al. High dose folinic acid, etoposide and 5-fluorouracil in advanced gastric cancer. A phase II study in elderly patients or patients with cardiac risk. Invest New Drugs 8:65–70, 1990.

242. DiBartolomeo M, Bajetta E, deBraud F, et al. Phase II study of the etoposide, leucovorin and fluorouracil combination for patients

with advanced gastric cancer unsuitable for aggressive chemotherapy. Oncology 52:41–44, 1995.

243. Taal BG, Teller FGM, ten Bokkel Huinink WW, et al. Etoposide, leucovorin, 5-fluorouracil combination chemotherapy for advanced gastric cancer: experience with two treatment schedules incorporating intravenous or oral etoposide. Ann Oncol 5:90–92, 1994.

244. Cocconi G, Bella M, Zironi S, et al. Fluorouracil, doxorubicin, and mitomycin combination versus PELF chemotherapy in advanced gastric cancer: a prospective randomized trial of the Italian Oncology Group for Clinical Research. J Clin Oncol 12:2687–2693, 1994.

245. Preusser P, Wilke H, Achterrath W, et al. Phase II study with the combination of etoposide, doxorubicin, and cisplatin in advanced measurable gastric cancer. J Clin Oncol 7:1310–1317, 1989.

246. Bajetta E, diBartolomeo M, deBraud F, et al. Etoposide, doxorubicin, and cisplatin treatment in advanced gastric cancer: a multicentre study of the Italian Trials in Medical Oncology (ITMO) Group. Eur J Cancer 30A:596–600, 1994.

247. Kelsen D, Atiq OT, Saltz L, et al. FAMTX versus etoposide, doxorubicin and cisplatin: a random assignment trial in gastric cancer. J Clin Oncol 10:541–548, 1992.

248. Haim M, Tsalik M, Robinson E. Treatment of gastric adenocarcinoma with the combination of etoposide, Adriamycin and cisplatin: comparison between two schedules. Oncology 51:102–107, 1994.

249. Findlay M, Cunningham D, Norman A, et al. A phase II study in advanced gastro–esophageal cancer using epirubicin and cisplatin in combination with continuous infusion 5-fluorouracil (ECF). Ann Oncol 5:609–616, 1994.

250. Webb A, Cunningham D, Scarffe JH, et al. Randomized trial comparing epirubicin, cisplatin, and 5-fluorouracil, vs. fluorouracil, doxorubicin and methotrexate in advanced esophagogastric cancer. J Clin Oncol 15:261–267, 1997.

251. Ajani JA, VanCutgem E, Moiseyenko V, et al. Docetaxel, cisplatin, 5-fluorouracil compare to cisplatin and 5-fluorouracil for chemotherapy naïve patients with metastatic or locally advanced or locally recurrent unresectable gastric carcinoma (MGC): Interim results of a randomized phase III trial (V325) [abstract]. Proc Am Soc Clin Oncol 22:2–9, 2003.

252. Shirao K, Shimada Y, Kondo H, et al. Phase I-II study of irinotecan hydrochloride combined with cisplatin in patients with advanced gastric cancer. J Clin Oncol 15:921–927, 1997.

253. Ajani JA, Baker J, Pisters PW, et al. Irinotecan plus cisplatin in advanced gastric or gastroesophageal junction carcinoma. Oncology (Huntington) 16 (35 Supple 5):52–54, 2002.

254. Louvet C, Andre T, Tiguad JM, et al. Phase II Study of oxaliplatin, fluorouracil and folinic acid in locally advanced or metastatic Gastric Cancer Patients. J Clin Oncol 20:4543–4548, 2002.

255. Fujimoto S, Takahashi M, Kobayashi K, et al. Relation between clinical and histologic outcome of intraperitoneal hyperthermic perfusion for patients with gastric cancer and peritoneal metastasis. Oncology 50:338–343, 1993.

256. Tsujitani D, Okuyama T, Watanabe A, et al. Intraperitoneal cisplatin during surgery for gastric cancer and peritoneal seeding. Anticancer Res 13:1831–1834, 1993.

257. Jones AI, Trott P, Cunningham D, et al. A pilot study of intraperitoneal cisplatin in the management of gastric cancer. Ann Oncol 5:123–125, 1994.

Lung Cancer

99

Kristan M. Augustin, Jody Sheehan Garey,

and Timothy J. Heuring

TREATMENT GOALS

- For patients with early-stage lung cancer, when treatment is curative in nature, the goal is to eradicate disease, minimize toxicity from treatment, and prevent disease recurrence both locally and at distant sites.
- For patients with advanced or metastatic lung cancer, the goal is to prolong survival, minimize toxicity from treatment, and control symptoms such as shortness of breath, pain, and cough in order to improve quality of life.

Lung cancer is the leading cause of cancer death in both men and women in the United States. It is estimated that in 2004, 173,770 new cases of lung cancer were diagnosed and approximately 160,440 deaths will be related to this disease.[1] Lung cancer is divided into two distinct classes that have important prognostic and therapeutic implications. Approximately 80% of new cases diagnosed will be of non-small cell lung cancer (NSCLC) histology, whereas only a minority of cases will be of small cell lung cancer (SCLC) histology. Although vast improvements in diagnosis, treatment, and prevention of lung cancer have been made over the past few years, prognosis is poor, with survival of less than 20% 5 years after diagnosis. In addition to the poor outcome of these patients, this disease is costly, with an estimated $5 billion dollars spent annually, representing about 9% of all cancer costs in the United States.[2,3]

EPIDEMIOLOGY AND ETIOLOGY

In 2004, approximately 173,700 persons were diagnosed with lung cancer in the United States. The incidence of new cases of lung cancer ranges between 50 and 90 persons annually per 100,000 population. The incidence rates of lung cancer trended upward through the early 1990s but have declined or leveled off since this time.[1] Historically, lung cancer was a disease that primarily affected men. Unfortunately, the annual incidence of women diagnosed with lung cancer has increased substantially since the 1930s due to increased smoking rates in women. In addition, the declining smoking rates observed in the 1990s have not been as pronounced among women.[4] Blacks have the highest rates of lung cancer compared to other races. In 2001, black men had the highest incidence of lung cancer (>100 cases per 100,000 population) followed by white men (80 cases per 100,000 population). In 2001, women had lower incidence rates of lung cancer regardless of race (50 cases per 100,000 population).[1] Currently, lung cancer is the leading cause of cancer death for men and women regardless of race or gender in the United States.[5] More than 160,000 persons died of progressive lung cancer in 2004.

Lung cancer is largely a preventable disease. Cigarette smoking remains the most important risk factor associated with lung cancer. More than 80% of patients with lung cancer have a history of smoking cigarettes. Smoking prevalence in the United States has decreased by almost 50% in men since the 1960s but by only 25% in women.[6] These trends likely are due to advertisements targeted at young women, peer pressure, and a belief that smoking helps control weight gain.[1] Despite stabilization in female smoking rates in the United States, aggressive promotional techniques in Africa and Asia have caused a 100% increase in smoking rates among young women in those areas. The effect that these increased smoking rates may have on the incidence of lung cancer in these developing areas is not yet known.

Women may be more susceptible to the harmful effects of smoking, although this hypothesis is controversial.[7-9] It is well established that women are more likely to be diagnosed with adenocarcinoma, whereas men are more likely to develop squamous cell carcinoma. Adenocarcinoma is the most common form of lung cancer in nonsmokers, women regardless of smoking status, and young persons.[10] This suggests that the pathophysiology of lung cancer may differ based on sex, likely due to genetic susceptibility and changes due to cigarette smoke.[5]

Regardless of gender, years of cigarette smoking is far more important than the number of cigarettes smoked per day in predicting a person's risk for lung cancer.[11] The first study to report this finding was the British Physician Male Cohort Study, a large study of over 30,000 male British physicians followed for 20 years and published in the late 1970s.[12] The findings from this study established that smoking duration was a much more important risk factor than smoking intensity. Recently, these results were supported by another large cohort study sponsored by the American Cancer Society starting in 1982.[11] This study also suggested that smoking may influence cancer pathogenesis at multiple pathways due to different risks within different age groups. In both studies, intensity of smoking was identified as a risk factor, although a lesser risk factor than smoking duration. Thus, pack-year history, which includes both smoking duration and intensity, is an important tool to monitor the patient's risk of lung cancer.[13]

In 2004, the British Male Physician Cohort Study published its 50-year findings.[14] The purpose of this study was to assess the overall mortality of men born in different periods by smoking habit. Men born in 1900 to 1930, who smoked only cigarettes and continued smoking, died on average about 10 years younger than lifelong nonsmokers. An increased life expectancy was observed regardless of the age when a person quit smoking. Smoking cessation at age 60, 50, 40, or 30 years gained about 3, 6, 9, or 10 years of life expectancy, respectively. The cigarette smoker versus nonsmoker probabilities of dying between the ages of 35 and 69 years were 42% versus 24% for those born in 1900 to 1909 and 43% versus 15% for those born in the 1920s. These results highlight and confirm the risks of smoking as well as showing the benefits from smoking cessation, especially early smoking cessation.

Environmental tobacco smoke, also known as second-hand smoke, has also been identified as a risk factor for lung cancer.[15] It is defined as exposure by persons who live with a smoker or are exposed to at least 20 cigarettes a day. Over 50 studies involving more than 7,300 lung cancer cases in nonsmokers have shown approximately a 25% increase in lung cancer in persons exposed to second-hand tobacco smoke. Recently, a pooled analysis of 1,263 lung cancer patients who never smoked compared to 2,740 controls who never smoked investigated the risk of lung cancer following exposure to second-hand smoke while adjusting for potential confounders.[15] Increased risk of lung cancer ranged from 13% to 23% and did not significantly vary depending on site of exposure (spouse, workplace, or social sources), occupation, or nutritional assessment. Odds ratios also increased significantly with increased years of exposure to second-hand smoke.

Asbestos and radon are two occupational risk factors correlated with lung cancer. Lung cancer was first noted in mine, mill, insulation, textile, and shipyard workers exposed to asbestos. Those exposed had a relative risk eight times that of nonexposed workers. In workers exposed to both asbestos and cigarette smoke, the risk increases to 45 times that of a nonexposed worker.[16]

Radon has been known to cause respiratory problems and death in silver miners since the 16th century. It may leak indoors through the soil, basements, and crawl spaces. This inert gas decomposes and emits alpha particles, which damage cells in the lung. Uranium miners exposed to the gas and particles are believed to be at increased risk, but the cases are complicated by exposure to other substances, including arsenic, silica, and tobacco. In combination with tobacco smoke, radon poses an even greater risk of lung cancer.

Other substances postulated to increase the risk of lung cancer include arsenic, formaldehyde, ether, chromium, polycyclic aromatic hydrocarbons, nickel, and silica. Case reports also suggest that lung cancer may develop secondary to interstitial fibrosis caused by tuberculosis, chronic fibrosis, and chronic obstructive pulmonary disease.

HISTOPATHOLOGY

Lung malignancies are categorized as either NSCLC or SCLC (Fig. 99.1). By classifying the type of lung cancer, clinicians can better determine treatment strategies and prognosis. NSCLC accounts for more than 80% of cases diagnosed each year. NSCLC does not proliferate as rapidly as SCLC and can be characterized as one or more histologic types, including adenocarcinoma, squamous cell, and large cell carcinoma. Adenocarcinoma is the most common histologic type of NSCLC and typically presents as a small peripheral coin-like lesion (<4 cm), with metastases occurring early, often before diagnosis. This type of NSCLC is more likely to occur in nonsmokers and women than the other types of lung cancer. Squamous cell carcinoma, most often observed in men and smokers, is a rapidly growing tumor that presents in the central or hilar regions of the lung. It may remain localized and cavitate, or it may spread to regional lymph nodes. Large cell carcinoma is an anaplastic tumor that generally presents as a large and bulky peripheral lesion. It is known to rapidly proliferate and metastasize to both local and distant sites.

SCLC is a rapidly growing and aggressive tumor. It typically arises from the central region of the lung but occasionally appears in the periphery. Early metastases are common, with a majority occurring outside the hemithorax.

Adenocarcinoma

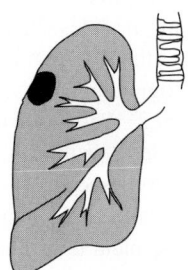

Peripheral Coinlike
Lesion

Large Cell Carcinoma

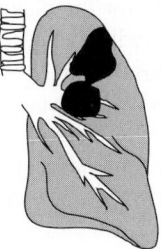

Variable (peripheral
or central)

Squamous Cell

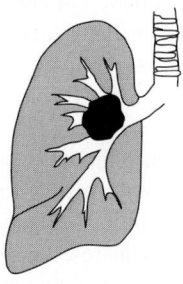

Hilar Region

Small Cell

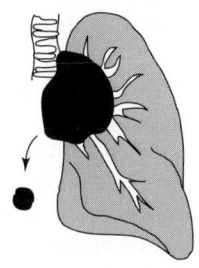

Central Region, Nodal
Metastasis

FIGURE 99.1 Size and location of each cellular type of lung cancer. (Adapted from Harvey JC, Beattie EJ. Lung cancer. Clin Symp 45:2–34, 1993.)

TABLE 99.1	Clinical Signs and Symptoms Associated With Anatomic Site of Involvement	
Primary Tumor	**Intrathoracic Spread**	**Systemic Metastases**
Cough	Hoarseness	Bone pain
Dyspnea	Shortness of breath	Weakness
Hemoptysis	Shoulder and arm pain	Weight loss
Chest discomfort	Ptosis	Headache
	Myosis	Nausea/vomiting
	Ipsilateral anhidrosis	Seizures
	Nonspecific chest wall pain	Confusion
	Pleuritic chest pain	Personality changes
	Facial swelling	Lymphadenopathy
	Tamponade	
	Difficulty swallowing	

CLINICAL PRESENTATION

The anatomic location of the lesion and the extent of disease usually determine how this carcinoma will present (Table 99.1). Tumors in the periphery of the lung are typically asymptomatic and discovered secondary to a chest radiograph obtained for some other medical condition. Centrally located tumors usually present earlier, with nonspecific symptoms that often are mistaken for other respiratory disorders, including pneumonia. Cough is the most common symptom in patients with lung cancer. However, this symptom may be present for years before diagnosis, as many of these patients have a history of smoking. The patient needs to be questioned about a change in frequency, productivity, and severity of coughing because it usually worsens as the tumor progresses. Dyspnea is also a nonspecific symptom that may worsen with obstruction. Hemoptysis may present as one of the first new symptoms, but it is also nonspecific and often confused with other respiratory conditions, including tuberculosis, bronchitis, and aspergillosis. Invasion of the left recurrent laryngeal nerve may cause compression and vocal cord paralysis, resulting in hoarseness. Postobstructive pneumonia, fatigue, and anorexia with weight loss may also be present.

Pancoast's, Horner's, and superior vena cava syndromes sometimes are present at diagnosis. Compression of the brachial plexus causing shoulder and arm pain is referred to as Pancoast's syndrome. Facial swelling often is a sign that the tumor is compressing or invading the superior vena cava and is characterized as superior vena cava syndrome. Horner's syndrome may be present secondary to the invasion of the sympathetic ganglia, resulting in ptosis (inability to lift the eyelid and uncover the eye completely), myosis (constriction of the pupil), and ipsilateral anhidrosis (lack of perspiration).

Paraneoplastic syndromes often present in patients with NSCLC and SCLC. These syndromes can produce signs and symptoms at a site distant from the primary lesion and metastases. Paraneoplastic syndromes associated with NSCLC include hypercalcemia, digital clubbing, and hypertrophic osteoarthropathy. Hypercalcemia, present in up to 15% of patients with NSCLC, is frequently associated with bony metastases or the production of ectopic parathyroid hormone-related peptide. Digital clubbing and hypertrophic osteoarthropathy may develop due to a possible neurogenic, hormonal, or vascular mechanism associated with NSCLC. Digital clubbing is a condition associated with abnormal proliferation of connective tissue in the fingers and toes, resulting in thickening of the extremities of those digits. A less common sequela, hypertrophic osteoarthropathy, occurs in less than 5% of patients with NSCLC as a painful symmetrical arthropathy in bone and joints, clubbing, and elevation in alkaline phosphatase levels; it may resolve after surgical resection of the primary tumor.

Syndrome of inappropriate antidiuretic hormone (SIADH), Cushing syndrome, Lambert–Eaton myasthenic syndrome, cerebellar degeneration, and encephalomyelitis are paraneoplastic syndromes associated with SCLC. SIADH may be seen in up to 50% of the patients with SCLC. Severe dilutional hyponatremia may cause confusion, seizures, and coma in patients if not promptly treated. Cushing syndrome is the result of ectopic adrenocorticotropic hormone secretion. Lambert–Eaton myasthenic syndrome is a rare but damaging neurologic paraneoplastic syndrome. It results from impaired acetylcholine release at the neuromuscular junction and may produce profound muscular weakness. Paraneoplastic cerebellar degeneration and paraneoplastic encephalomyelitis may also occur, resulting in various neuromuscular and neurologic sequelae.

Approximately one third of patients present with symptoms of extrathoracic disease. A complete evaluation to determine the exact stage of disease and appropriate treatment is necessary. Common sites of distant metastases include the bone, liver, adrenal glands, brain, bone marrow, contralateral lung, and lymph nodes. Twenty-five percent of patients will present with bone metastases, most commonly involving the axial skeleton and proximal long bones, resulting in bone pain, with a possible pleuritic component if there is rib involvement. Weakness and weight loss are the most common presenting symptoms associated with hepatic metastasis. The results of liver function tests are generally elevated only in the setting of numerous or large metastases. Signs and symptoms of adrenal insufficiency and para-aortic lymph node involvement are rarely seen at initial presentation; if present, they are usually discovered during staging. Ten percent of patients with lung cancer present with headache, nausea, vomiting, focal neurologic signs or symptoms, seizures, confusion, and personality changes consistent with brain or spinal cord metastases. Palpable lymphadenopathy of the supraclavicular fossa is involved in 15% to 20% of lung cancer cases during the course of the disease.

DIAGNOSIS

Careful evaluation of the clinical signs and symptoms is important. A complete physical examination and medical history provide valuable information for assessing the patient, as well as determining the best treatment approach for each individual patient. Blood chemistries and a complete blood count should be obtained to evaluate for abnormalities. Symptomatic patients at risk for lung cancer should get a chest radiograph to look for pulmonary nodules, mediastinal widening, pleural effusions, and potential osseous metastases. A spiral computed tomographic (CT) scan with intravenous contrast dye extending to include the liver and adrenal glands is recommended for staging purposes. If the CT scan is negative for metastatic disease in NSCLC patients, positron emission tomography (PET) with 18-fluorodeoxyglucose (FDG) is recommended to evaluate for the presence of extrathoracic disease.

In patients suspected of having lung cancer based on clinical and radiographic findings, histologic or cytologic diagnosis should be performed using at least one of six methods, depending on the size and anatomic location of the tumor.[17] Sputum collection for cytology may be performed, but sensitivity is low and generally multiple sputum collections are

needed. Therefore, a bronchoscopy is performed in patients with central lesions. Transthoracic needle aspiration is preferred for the diagnosis of peripheral lung nodules. In patients with mediastinal lymph nodes larger than 1 cm, mediastinoscopy may be performed for histologic diagnosis and for additional staging information (Fig. 99.2). Patients with pleural effusions should undergo thoracentesis or thoracoscopy (an endoscopic procedure in which a thoracoscope is inserted into the chest wall) to better visualize and obtain biopsy samples from the pleural nodules, pleural surface, and ipsilateral lymph nodes. Thoracotomy (an invasive procedure in which a large incision is made into the chest wall to gain direct access to the lung) may be used as an alternative diagnostic tool if less invasive methods for diagnosis are negative for disease. In patients with a solitary extrathoracic site of disease, a fine-needle aspiration or biopsy of that site may be suitable for diagnosis. Evaluation of distant metastases usually is performed only in symptomatic patients or those with advanced disease. In patients with locally advanced disease, when the treatment goal is curative, magnetic resonance imaging (MRI) of the brain should be obtained to rule out central nervous system metastases.

If surgical resection is a treatment option, a thorough preoperative physiologic evaluation must be performed to prevent perioperative and long-term complications. Reduction of functioning lung tissue following surgical resection of the whole or part of the lung may be complicated by acute hypercapnia, mechanical ventilation lasting greater than 48 hours, arrhythmias, pneumonia, pulmonary emboli, and myocardial infarction. A perioperative assessment considers the risk of comorbid cardiopulmonary status and long-term pulmonary disability after resection. Pulmonary function tests are obtained to identify those at risk for perioperative and postoperative complications. The most common procedure is the forced expiratory volume in 1 second (FEV_1) technique. Patients with an FEV_1 greater than 1.5 liters or a predicted FEV_1 greater than 80% are at low risk for developing postoperative complications.[18] With the high probability of interstitial lung disease in these patients due to their smoking history, other pulmonary function tests may need to be performed to determine a patient's perioperative risk. Diffusing capacity of the lung for carbon monoxide (DLCO) greater than 80% predicted and oxygen saturation/oxygen desaturation greater than 4% from resting values are markers for increased perioperative morbidity and mortality.[19,20] Pulmonary function tests used to predict postoperative lung function include percentage predicted postoperative FEV_1, maximal oxygen consumption, and stair climbing/walking tests. Perioperative and postoperative risks may be minimized in patients with poor lung function if lung volume reduction surgery along with lung cancer resection and smoking cessation is considered before surgery.[21,22]

STAGING

Lung cancer may be staged both clinically and pathologically. Clinical staging takes into account the results of noninvasive tools (i.e., physical examination, past medical history,

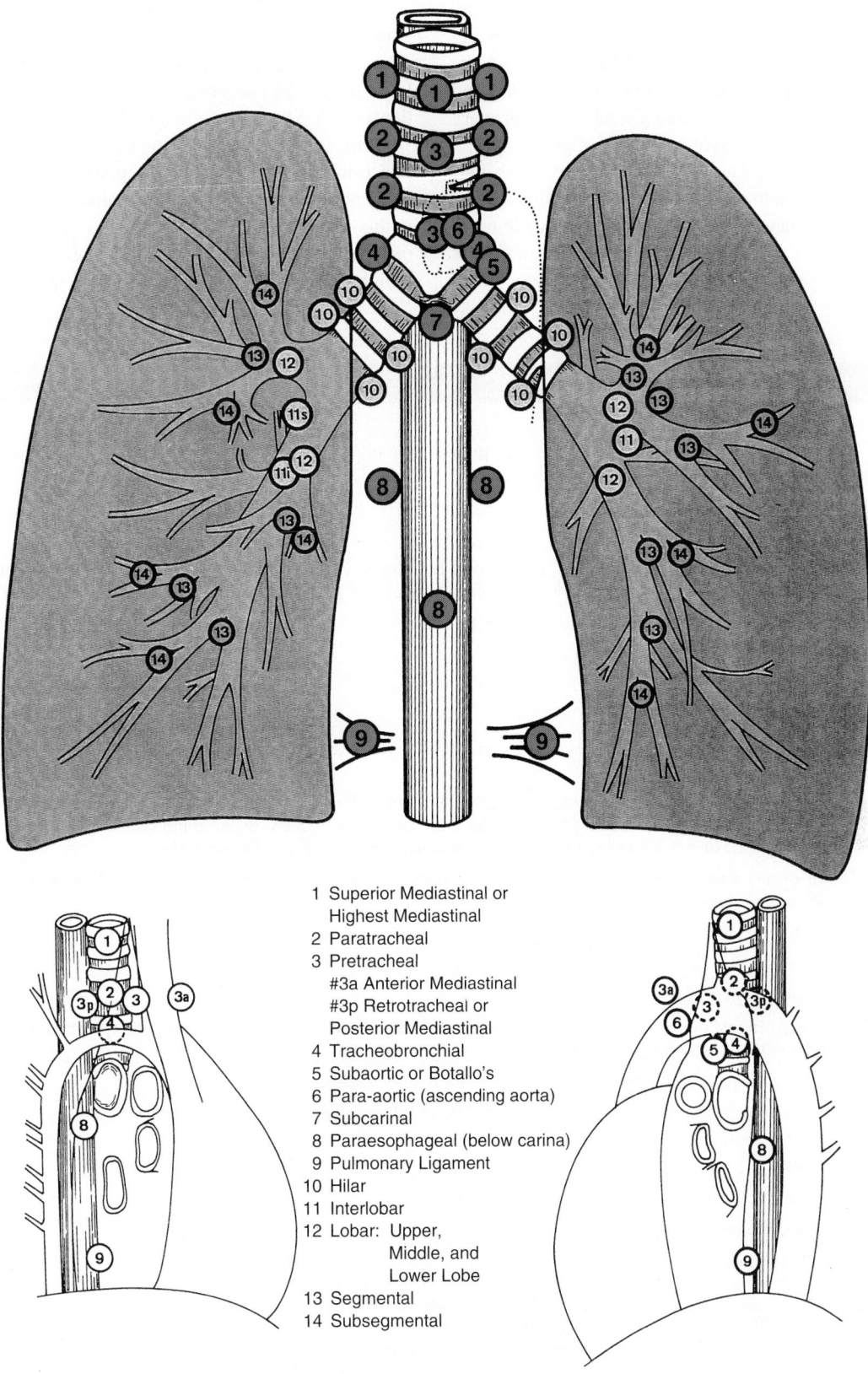

1 Superior Mediastinal or
   Highest Mediastinal
2 Paratracheal
3 Pretracheal
   #3a Anterior Mediastinal
   #3p Retrotracheal or
   Posterior Mediastinal
4 Tracheobronchial
5 Subaortic or Botallo's
6 Para-aortic (ascending aorta)
7 Subcarinal
8 Paraesophageal (below carina)
9 Pulmonary Ligament
10 Hilar
11 Interlobar
12 Lobar: Upper,
         Middle, and
         Lower Lobe
13 Segmental
14 Subsegmental

FIGURE 99.2 Thoracic lymph node map. (From Naruke T, Suemasu K, Ishikawa S. Surgical treatment for lung cancer with metastasis to mediastinal lymph nodes. J Thorac Cardiovasc Surg 71:279–285, 1976.)

laboratory studies, and imaging studies) and invasive procedures.[23] Pathologic staging occurs after the surgically resected specimen is evaluated. The TNM classification is used for the staging of lung cancer (Tables 99.2 and 99.3).[24,25] *T* refers to the size and extent of the primary tumor, *N* represents the involvement of regional lymph nodes, and *M* denotes distant metastatic disease. It is a universally accepted system that groups patients with a similar extent of disease to determine prognosis and facilitate treatment decisions. It is also used to group patients with similar characteristics together for analysis in clinical trials.

Although the TNM system is used for all histologies, it is more applicable to NSCLC. SCLC can be staged according to this system, but few patients are candidates for pathologic staging by surgery at the time of diagnosis. Thus, patients with SCLC are classified as having ''limited'' or ''extensive'' disease according to the Veterans Administration Lung Cancer Therapy Group system.[26,27]

Limited SCLC is defined as a tumor that may be treated within a single, tolerable radiotherapy port. This definition includes tumors restricted to one hemithorax with regional lymph node metastases, including hilar, ipsilateral, and con-

TABLE 99.2	TNM Classification of Lung Cancer
Primary tumor (T)	
TX	Primary tumor cannot be assessed or tumor proven by malignant cells present in sputum or bronchial washings but not visualized by imaging or bronchoscopy
T0	No evidence of primary tumor
T_{is}	Carcinoma in situ
T1	Tumor ≤3 cm in greatest dimension, surrounded by lung or visceral pleura, without bronchoscopic evidence of invasion more proximal than the lobar bronchus[a] (i.e., not the main bronchus)
T2	Tumor with any of the following features of size or extent: >3 cm in greatest dimension Involves the main bronchus, ≥2 cm distal to the carina Invades the visceral pleura Associated with atelectasis or obstructive pneumonitis that extends to the hilar region but does not involve the entire lung
T3	Tumor of any size that directly invades the chest wall (including superior sulcus tumors), diaphragm, mediastinal pleura, or parietal pericardium; tumor in the main bronchus <2 cm distal to the carina but without involvement of the carina; or associated atelectasis or obstructive pneumonitis of the entire lung
T4	Tumor of any size that invades the mediastinum, heart, great vessels, esophagus, vertebral body, carina, or tumor with a malignant pleural effusion[b]
Regional lymph nodes (N)	
NX	Regional lymph nodes cannot be assessed.
N0	No regional lymph node metastasis
N1	Metastasis to ipsilateral peribronchial or ipsilateral hilar lymph nodes and intrapulmonary nodes involved by direct extension of the primary tumor
N2	Metastasis to ipsilateral mediastinal or subcarinal lymph node(s)
N3	Metastasis to contralateral mediastinal, contralateral hilar, ipsilateral or contralateral scalene, or supraclavicular lymph node(s)
Distant metastasis (M)	
MX	Presence of distant metastasis cannot be assessed.
M0	No distant metastasis
M1	Distant metastasis present[c]

(From the American Joint Committee on Cancer (AJCC), Chicago, IL, with permission. The original source for this material is the *AJCC Cancer Staging Manual*, 6th ed. (2002) published by Springer-Verlag New York, www.springer-ny.com.)

[a] The uncommon superficial tumor of any size with its invasive component limited to the bronchial wall, which may extend proximal to the main bronchus, is also classified T1.

[b] Most pleural effusions associated with lung cancer are caused by tumor. However, in a few patients, multiple cytopathologic examinations of pleural fluid show no tumor. In these cases, the fluid is nonbloody and is not an exudate. When these elements and the clinical judgment dictate that the effusion is not related to the tumor, the effusion should be excluded as a staging element and the patient's disease should be staged T1, T2, or T3. Pericardial effusion is classified according to the same rules.

[c] Separate metastatic tumor nodule(s) in the ipsilateral nonprimary lobe(s) of the lung are classified as M1.

				5-Year Survival Rate After Treatment (%)			
				NSCLC			SCLC
Stage	T	N	M	Squamous Cell	Adenocarcinoma	Large Cell	
0	T_{is}	N0	M0	NR	NR	NR	NR
I				38	53	36	15
IA	T1	N0	M0				
IB	T2	N0	M0				
II				25	25	23	12
IIA	T1	N1	M0				
IIB	T2	N1	M0				
	T3	N0	M0				
III							
IIIA	T3	N1	M0	10	13	11	8
	T1	N2	M0				
	T2	N2	M0				
	T3	N2	M0				
IIIB	T4	N0	M0	5	4	5	6
	T4	N1	M0				
	T4	N2	M0				
	T1	N3	M0				
	T2	N3	M0				
	T3	N3	M0				
	T4	N3	M0				
IV	Any T	Any N	M1	2	1	1	1

TABLE 99.3 | Stage Grouping (TNM) and 5-Year Survival Rates of Lung Cancer

T, primary tumor; N, regional lymph nodes; M, distant metastasis; NR, not reported.
(From Mountain CF. Staging classification of lung cancer. A critical evaluation. Clin Chest Med 23:103–121, 2002; and Lung. In: AJCC cancer staging manual, 6th ed. New York: Springer-Verlag, 2002:167–177.)

tralateral mediastinal nodes; ipsilateral and contralateral supraclavicular nodes; and with ipsilateral pleural effusion, independent of whether the cytology findings are positive or negative, in order to correspond to the TNM classification stages I through III.[28]

Approximately two thirds of patients at diagnosis have a tumor burden exceeding that of limited disease and are classified as having extensive disease. Patients with extensive disease, or a pleural effusion, are treated as having stage IV disease according to the TNM classification schema.

TREATMENT

NON-SMALL CELL LUNG CANCER

NSCLC represents more than 80% of the lung cancer cases diagnosed. Despite aggressive treatment, overall survival at 5 years remains just 14%.[29] Tumor stage, poor performance status, and weight loss of more than 5% have a negative impact on survival.[30] Early-stage patients have the greatest chance for long-term survival with surgical intervention. Advances in the treatment of locally advanced NSCLC now allow for definitive-intent treatment strategies with multimodal therapy. Once metastatic disease is radiographically evident, however, treatment goals become palliative, focusing on improving symptoms and quality of life and prolonging survival.

Stages I and II. Less than 20% of all lung cancer patients present with stage I or II disease. Surgical resection is the standard of care for treating these patients. The preferred surgical procedure for patients in good physical condition is a lobectomy with hilar and mediastinal lymph node dissection. Limited resection for patients with T1-2 tumors, such as a segmentectomy or a wedge resection, compromises the prognosis of these patients.[31,32] A randomized trial of patients with T1 tumors compared lobectomy to limited resection and found no difference in perioperative morbidity or mortality; however, there was an increase in the local recurrence rate and decreased survival after limited resection.[33]

Although surgery is performed with the intent to eradicate disease, patients often relapse both locally and at distant sites and subsequently die of their cancer. Adjuvant therapy refers to the use of either radiation or chemotherapy administered after surgery to eradicate residual micrometastatic disease or prevent recurrence.

Adjuvant radiation currently has no role in the treatment of stage I NSCLC outside the context of a clinical trial. In some instances postoperative radiotherapy has been shown to reduce the incidence of local recurrence, but has no impact on overall survival.[34] A large meta-analysis evaluating more than 2,000 patients with stage I to III disease from nine randomized trials showed a decrease in survival, particularly for patients with stage I disease, who received radiation after surgical resection.[35] The data evaluating adjuvant radiation therapy for stage II patients are similar. Multiple studies suggest that patients receiving postoperative radiotherapy have a decrease in local recurrence rate but no improvement in overall survival.[36,37] With the currently available data, patients with stage I and II NSCLC should not receive adjuvant radiation except in the context of a clinical trial or where surgical margins are positive for residual disease.

Thus far, trials evaluating adjuvant radiation therapy have failed to show any improvement in overall survival. A potential reason for this is that disease is controlled locally but recurs at distant sites. One thought is that by giving adjuvant systemic chemotherapy treatment, we may be able to eliminate micrometastatic disease and prolong survival. Many studies have evaluated this theory, but the results have been conflicting.[38–43] Older trials used chemotherapeutic regimens based on alkylating agents. Some trials used three-drug combinations that added to the toxicity of the regimens. Many of the studies have contained sample sizes too small to detect a benefit of adding adjuvant chemotherapy. Due to inadequate sample size, a large meta-analysis was reported in 1995 based on previously conducted randomized clinical trials.[33] The results noted an absolute benefit in overall survival of 5% at 5 years for those who received adjuvant cisplatin-based chemotherapy. Based on the results of this meta-analysis, several prospective randomized trials were initiated. One study compared three or four cycles of adjuvant cisplatin-based chemotherapy to observation alone after complete surgical resection.[44] The study included 1,867 stage I to III patients and, similar to the meta-analysis, showed a 4.1% improvement in overall survival at 5 years independent of the stage of disease. Several additional trials confirmed these results.[45,46] Winton et al treated stage IB patients with carboplatin-based chemotherapy and found an improvement in overall survival of 12% at 4 years.[46] Based on these results, adjuvant chemotherapy after complete surgical resection has become standard of care for early-stage patients and should be recommended to patients who can tolerate the treatment.

Complete resection is contraindicated in patients with compromised pulmonary function, those older than 70 years, those with a medical condition that prohibits surgery, and those who refuse surgery. In these patients, a segmentectomy or wedge resection may be performed in an attempt to prolong survival. Radiation therapy is an alternative modality used in an attempt to improve local control of the tumor and possibly prolong survival in patients with medically inoperable stage I/II lung cancer. Radiation doses of at least 60 Gy are administered with minimal complications and result in a 13% to 17% overall survival rate. Patients who are younger, have tumors less than 4 cm, have tumors with squamous cell histology, and are asymptomatic at diagnosis have a better prognosis after radiotherapy than other patients with unresectable NSCLC.

Stage III. Stage III, or locally advanced, NSCLC incorporates several different scenarios based on the staging characteristics. Staging divides patients into stage IIIA and IIIB. Stage IIIB NSCLC is generally considered inoperable, although exceptions do exist. Furthermore, patients with malignant pleural effusion, despite being included in stage IIIB, are treated like stage IV NSCLC patients. Stage IIIA patients must be divided into potential surgical candidates versus nonsurgical candidates based on T and N status.

Surgery is the treatment of choice for patients with T3N1 disease. Postoperative radiation therapy is often used in patients with positive margins, but no compelling evidence supports its use. Studies have shown, as with early disease, that adjuvant radiation therapy decreases the local recurrence rate but has no impact on overall survival.[35] Adjuvant chemotherapy, similar to that used for stage I/II disease, should be offered to patients based on improvement in overall survival at 5 years (Table 99.4).[44]

Treatment of N2 disease is very controversial. When surgery is possible, complete surgical resection provides good local control. However, most patients recur with systemic metastases, and 5-year survival is less than 20%. Patients who have multiple N2 lymph nodes or bulky N2 lymphadenopathy are usually not surgical candidates. If complete resection is not feasible, then surgery as a treatment modality should be abandoned and nonsurgical approaches pursued. Because the 5-year survival with surgery alone is disappointing, it seems logical that postoperative radiation and/or chemotherapy would prevent disseminated recurrences and prolong survival. Adjuvant radiotherapy or adjuvant chemotherapy as a single modality added to primary surgical resection has been previously discussed, and the utility of these modalities does not change in N2 disease. However, several clinical trials comparing adjuvant radiation alone to adjuvant chemoradiotherapy in patients with N2 disease have failed to show a prolonged survival or time to recurrence.[47–49]

Neoadjuvant, or induction, chemotherapy is an option under investigation for use in improving overall survival after surgical resection. The goal of preoperative therapy is to reduce the size of the tumor, improve the chance for a

TABLE 99.4 Selected Chemotherapy Regimens for the Primary Treatment of NSCLC

Regimen	Dose	Schedule	Recurrence Rate (%)	Median Progression-Free Survival (mo)	Median Survival (mo) Overall	Reference(s)
Paclitaxel + carboplatin	Paclitaxel 175–225 mg/m^2 IV over 3 hours followed by carboplatin AUC 6 IV over 30–60 minutes	Repeat cycle every 21 days (total six cycles).	25–32	4–6.5	8.6–11.4	J Clin Oncol 19:3210–3218, 2001 Ann Oncol 11:799–805, 2000
Docetaxel + carboplatin	Docetaxel 75 mg/m^2 IV over 1 hour followed by carboplatin AUC 6 IV over 30–60 minutes	Repeat cycle every 21 days (total six cycles).	24	5	9.4	J Clin Oncol 21:3016–3024, 2003
Docetaxel + cisplatin	Docetaxel 75 mg/m^2 IV over 1 hour followed by cisplatin 75 mg/m^2 IV over 2 hours	Repeat cycle every 21 days (total six cycles).	17–31	3.7–5.5	7.4–11.3	J Clin Oncol 21:3016–3024, 2003 N Engl J Med 346:92–98, 2002
Cisplatin + gemcitabine	Cisplatin 60–100 mg/m^2 IV over 2 hours on Day 1 and gemcitabine 1,000 mg/m^2 IV over 30 minutes on Days 1 and 8	Repeat cycle every 21 days (total six cycles).	22–30	4.2–5.7	8–9.5	N Engl J Med 346:92–98, 2002 J Clin Oncol 18:122–130, 2000 J Clin Oncol 21:3025–3034, 2003
Carboplatin + gemcitabine	Carboplatin AUC 5 IV over 30–60 minutes on Day 1 and gemcitabine 1,000–1,200 mg/m^2 IV over 30 minutes on Days 1 and 8	Repeat cycle every 21 days (total six cycles).	29.2	4.75	8	Lung Cancer 41:321–331, 2003
Gemcitabine + vinorelbine	Gemcitabine 800–1,200 mg/m^2 IV over 30 minutes and vinorelbine 25–30 mg/m^2 IV over 10 minutes on Days 1 and 8	Repeat cycle every 21 days.	21–25	4.25–4.75	7.5–8	J Clin Oncol 16:3025–3034, 2003 J Natl Cancer Inst 95:362–372, 2003

AUC, area under the curve; GFR, glomerular filtration rate. Dose calculated using the Calvert equation [AUC (GFR + 25)].

complete resection, downstage the tumor, decrease the chance of local relapse, and treat any micrometastatic disease that may be present in locally advanced but potentially resectable disease. Studies indicate that induction chemotherapy is feasible, toxicity is acceptable, and response rates range from 50% to 80%.[50] In a nonrandomized trial, Martini et al evaluated mitomycin C, vindesine or vinblastine, and high-dose cisplatin administration before surgery.[51] Overall survival at 5 years was 17%, with a median survival of 19 months. Survival was improved in patients who had complete resection, with a 5-year survival rate of 26%. Kirn et al[52] found similar results from a nonrandomized trial evaluating platinum-based regimens followed by surgical resection. Patients with complete resections appeared to benefit from neoadjuvant chemotherapy, with a 2-year survival rate of 67%.

More recent trials have used the same approach with newer chemotherapy combinations. Van Zandwijk et al[53] treated 47 patients with N2 disease with induction cisplatin and gemcitabine prior to surgery. The overall response rate after three cycles was 70%, with 71% of patients able to undergo complete resection. In two small randomized trials, chemotherapy administered before surgical resection was compared with surgery alone. Roth et al[54] randomized 60 patients to receive either three courses of preoperative cyclophosphamide, etoposide, and cisplatin or resection alone. Patients who responded to neoadjuvant chemotherapy and had a complete resection were given three additional courses of chemotherapy. A survival advantage for patients receiving preoperative chemotherapy was observed, with 3- and 5-year survival rates of 43% and 36%, respectively. Rosell et al[55] compared the combination of mitomycin, ifosfamide, and cisplatin as neoadjuvant therapy to surgery alone in 60 patients. Median survival time and 3- and 5-year survival rates were significantly higher in the chemotherapy group than in those treated with surgery alone. In contrast to these results, a large phase III trial was conducted by Depierre et al[56] evaluating preoperative chemotherapy with mitomycin, ifosfamide, and cisplatin compared to surgery alone in stage I to IIIa patients. There was a statistically significant improvement in overall survival for patients with stage I and II disease who received neoadjuvant chemotherapy. However, although there was a trend toward prolonged survival for stage IIIa patients, it was not a statistically significant difference. Two reasons may account for this fact: small numbers of patients with stage IIIa disease and lower doses of chemotherapy that may have been ineffective. Despite the seeming controversy, the data in support of neoadjuvant chemotherapy are significant, and results of future trials are needed to confirm the survival advantage of induction chemotherapy.

Not all patients who present with N2 disease can undergo surgery. In fact, most patients are deemed inoperable because the likelihood of complete surgical resection is poor. Patients with inoperable stage IIIA and stage IIIB disease (without malignant effusion) are treated with a combination of chemotherapy and radiation. Historically, patients were treated with radiation alone; however, local recurrences occurred and few patients achieved long-term survival.[57,58] A landmark trial by Dillman et al[59] randomized patients with stage III disease to receive either three cycles of cisplatin and vinblastine followed by radiation, or radiation therapy alone. Response rates were higher in the group who received combined treatment (56% versus 43%, respectively; $p = 0.092$). After a 7-year follow-up, median survival was longer for patients receiving chemotherapy and radiation (13.7 months versus 9.6 months, respectively; $p = 0.012$). These results were confirmed in a phase III intergroup trial in which both median survival and 5-year survival were improved using a combined approach versus single-modality radiation therapy (13.2 months versus 11.4 months and 8% versus 5%, respectively).[60] Although not all studies have shown an advantage to chemotherapy plus radiation,[61] several trials evaluating chemotherapy with radiation have been positive in favor of a combined modality approach.[62–65]

Chemotherapy and radiation may be given sequentially (chemotherapy followed by radiation) or concurrently (both treatment modalities given at the same time). The optimal sequence of combination treatment has yet to be determined. A few large trials have directly compared sequential to concurrent treatment. Furuse et al evaluated 320 patients randomized to receive cisplatin (80 mg/m^2 on days 1 and 29), vindesine (3 mg/m^2 on days 1, 8, 29, and 36), and mitomycin (8 mg/m^2 on days 1 and 29) concurrently with radiation therapy or the same chemotherapy followed by radiation.[66] Response rate, median survival time, and 3- and 5-year overall survival were superior in the concurrent arm (84% versus 66%, 16.5 months versus 13.3 months, 22.3% versus 14.7%, and 15.8% versus 8.9%, respectively). The Radiation Therapy Oncology Group (RTOG) also conducted a phase III study investigating concurrent chemoradiotherapy with cisplatin and vinblastine compared to sequentially administered chemotherapy followed by radiation. Median survival time and the 4-year survival rate were improved with the combined approach (17 months versus 14.6 months, 21% versus 12%, respectively; $p = 0.046$).[67]

Other areas of debate include whether to add induction chemotherapy before concomitant treatment or to add consolidation chemotherapy after definitive treatment. The Southwest Oncology Group (SWOG) conducted a phase II study to evaluate concurrent chemoradiation followed by three cycles of consolidation docetaxel (75 mg/m^2 every 3 weeks) in patients with stage IIIB NSCLC.[68] Median progression-free survival was 16 months, median overall survival was 26 months, and 1-, 2-, and 3-year survival rates were 76%, 54%, and 37%, respectively. The Locally Advanced Multimodality Protocol randomized 276 patients to receive arm 1, sequential chemotherapy (two cycles of carboplatin AUC 6 and paclitaxel 200 mg/m^2) followed by radiation; arm 2, the same chemotherapy followed by concurrent weekly chemotherapy (paclitaxel 45 mg/m^2 and carboplatin AUC 2) and radiation; or arm 3, concurrent weekly chemoradiotherapy followed by consolidation chemotherapy (two cycles of carboplatin AUC 6 and paclitaxel 200 mg/m^2).[69] At a median follow-up of 26 months, the median survival time was prolonged in arm 3 versus arm 1 or 2 (16.1 months versus 12.5 months or 11 months, respectively).

Induction chemotherapy was again evaluated in a phase III trial by Vokes et al.[70] The study involved 366 patients with stage III NSCLC who were randomly assigned to receive weekly chemotherapy and concomitant radiation (Con) or induction chemotherapy followed by the same concurrent treatment (Ind/Con). Median survival in the Con arm versus the Ind/Con arm was 11.4 months versus 14 months ($p = 0.154$). One-year survival estimates were 48% and 54%, respectively. This study failed to support the use of induction chemotherapy followed by concurrent chemoradiation for treatment of stage III patients. Future studies will continue to investigate the addition of induction or consolidation chemotherapy to the current standard of concurrent chemotherapy and radiation.

Stage IV. Stage IV NSCLC is defined as any disease that has escaped regional involvement. It may include a metastatic lesion in the ipsilateral or contralateral lung, as well as distant organ involvement. Once stage IV disease is diagnosed, treatment goals change: treatment in this setting is palliative. The focus becomes prolonging survival and, importantly, maximizing quality of life. Approximately 50% of patients diagnosed with NSCLC present with stage IV disease.[71] Untreated, median survival is approximately 4 to 6 months; 1-year survival is 10%.

Chemotherapy is the standard treatment for stage IV NSCLC. Palliative radiation is incorporated for symptomatic treatment of brain or bone metastasis. The use of chemotherapy has been controversial because the toxicity associated with chemotherapy was thought to outweigh the minimal benefits it produced. However, trials have shown that chemotherapy can offer improvement in not only survival but also quality of life.[33,72–74] Unfortunately, the survival benefit is modest, with chemotherapy improving median survival time by 2 to 4 months and 1-year survival by 10% to 20%. In addition, chemotherapy has been shown to be a cost-effective way of treating advanced NSCLC because it reduces symptoms, number and duration of hospitalizations, and number of palliative radiation treatments administered.[75,76]

There are many agents with activity against NSCLC. Active single agents have response rates greater than 15%. Up until the 1990s, cisplatin remained the preferred agent by which to compare other single agents and combination regimens because it was thought to be the most active. Typical combination regimens added etoposide, vindesine, vinblastine, and mitomycin-C to cisplatin. These combinations were not proven superior to single-agent cisplatin, and toxicity was far greater with combination therapy.[77–79] Cisplatin/etoposide showed a 1-year survival rate of 25% and for a

time became a widely used regimen.[80] After the development of several new agents such as gemcitabine, paclitaxel, docetaxel, irinotecan, and vinorelbine, combination chemotherapy was investigated again. Studies suggested that newer combination chemotherapy could be delivered with minimal additive toxicity while improving response rates and median survival versus cisplatin alone.[81–83]

Carboplatin is more easily tolerated than cisplatin due to a decreased incidence of adverse effects such as nephrotoxicity, neurotoxicity, ototoxicity, nausea, and vomiting. Thus, it has been substituted into combination chemotherapy regimens with the hope that patients will better tolerate treatment while maintaining the activity of cisplatin-based chemotherapy. Early comparisons of cisplatin versus carboplatin showed little if any difference in response rates or median survival.[84–86] Therefore, carboplatin has largely replaced cisplatin in treatment of stage IV disease. However, recent trials investigating modern agents with cisplatin versus carboplatin raise the question of cisplatin superiority over carboplatin.[87,88] Rosell et al compared the combinations of paclitaxel/cisplatin versus paclitaxel/carboplatin.[88] Although the response rate was similar between the two regimens (28% versus 25%, respectively; $p = 0.45$), patients on the cisplatin arm had a longer median overall survival and an improvement in 2-year survival (9.8 months versus 8.2 months, $p = 0.019$, and 15% versus 9%, respectively). Because the margin of benefit with cisplatin appears small and has not been consistently reported, the choice of platinum compounds remains controversial and treatment decisions need to be based on individual patient characteristics, including performance status.

There have been thousands of trials investigating chemotherapy response rates against advanced NSCLC. In 2000 one of these trials compared a modern regimen against the former commonly used regimen cisplatin/etoposide.[89] Cisplatin/paclitaxel showed an improvement in median survival time as well as 1-year survival rate (9.9 months versus 7.6 months and 38.9% versus 31.8%, $p = 0.048$, respectively) versus cisplatin/etoposide. Other investigators have found similar outcomes with varying modern regimens, but few studies have compared modern regimens to each other.[87,90–92] Schiller et al compared four modern chemotherapy combinations (paclitaxel/cisplatin, docetaxel/cisplatin, paclitaxel/carboplatin, gemcitabine/cisplatin) in the treatment of advanced NSCLC.[93] Response rates (19%), median survival (7.9 months), and 1-year survival (33%) did not significantly differ between the regimens. The authors concluded that none of the regimens differed significantly from each other. Because of these conclusions, the decision of which chemotherapy regimen to use is based on individual patient characteristics and the predicted toxicity profile associated with the regimen. The only standard of care is that patients should receive a platinum-based doublet therapy, an opinion backed by the American Society of Clinical Oncology (ASCO).[94]

Duration of chemotherapy has been an area of controversy as well. Trials have shown that prolonged chemotherapy does not improve responses or prevent progression.[95,96] ASCO recommends four cycles of chemotherapy in patients with stable disease and a maximum of six cycles for responding patients.[94]

RECURRENT OR REFRACTORY DISEASE

Second-line therapy for patients who fail to respond to initial platinum-based therapy is used frequently, as virtually every patient with advanced NSCLC will recur or progress at some point (Table 99.5). Doublet therapy has not been proven in this setting; therefore, single-agent chemotherapy is the standard of care. Many agents, such as gemcitabine, vinorelbine, and irinotecan, have been studied in this setting with limited success. Gemcitabine has been associated with response rates varying from 6% to 20%, but its effect on survival has not been evaluated.[97,98] Similarly, vinorelbine has reported response rates of 0% to 20% when evaluated in the second-line setting, but there are no data evaluating survival.[99] Several randomized studies have shown that docetaxel has utility in the second-line setting. Shepherd et al evaluated single-agent docetaxel (75 mg/m^2) compared to best supportive care in previously treated patients.[100] Docetaxel had a response rate of 7.1% and improved both median survival and 1-year survival versus best supportive care (7 months versus 4.6 months, $p = 0.047$, and 37% versus 11%, $p = 0.03$, respectively). Fossella et al compared two different doses of docetaxel (100 mg/m^2 and 75 mg/m^2) to vinorelbine or ifosfamide in a phase III randomized trial.[101] Patients receiving docetaxel at either dose had a significantly higher response rate than patients who received vinorelbine or ifosfamide. Overall survival was similar between the arms, but 1-year survival was improved in the docetaxel arms (32% versus 19% for docetaxel 100 mg/m^2 and 75 mg/ m^2, respectively, $p = 0.025$). Due to unacceptable rates of fever, neutropenic fever, and toxicity-related treatment discontinuation for patients receiving docetaxel 100 mg/m^2, the recommended dose of docetaxel is 75 mg/m^2. These two trials provided the evidence needed to support docetaxel as the first U.S. Food and Drug Administration (FDA)-approved second-line therapy for NSCLC.

In 2004, pemetrexed, a multitargeted antifolate compound, was approved for second-line treatment of NSCLC. A phase III trial compared pemetrexed to docetaxel in patients who failed to respond to platinum-based therapy.[102] Although response rates, median survival, and 1-year survival were similar between the two arms, pemetrexed was better tolerated.

Durability with second-line chemotherapy responses is generally short-lived. Once a patient progresses on second-line therapy, there are few data to support continued chemotherapy. Until recently, there have been limited options for patients with adequate performance status whose disease continues to progress on chemotherapy. Targeted therapy has been an active area of research in many tumor types,

including lung cancer. The concept is to develop a compound that may target molecular abnormalities involved in the pathogenesis of the disease.[103-105] The epithelial growth factor receptor (EGFR) is the best-studied target in lung cancer. The first compound in this class of agents, gefitinib, was approved by the FDA for treatment of NSCLC after failure of both platinum-based and docetaxel chemotherapy. This is an orally available compound given on a daily basis; it produces response rates of 12% to 19%.[106,107] Results of a recent trial comparing gefitinib to best supportive care for refractory NSCLC failed to show a survival advantage for gefitinib. Given the results of this phase III trial, the role of gefitinib in NSCLC is left in question. A derivative of gefitinib, erlotinib, has shown a survival benefit over best supportive care.[108] The advantage of this class of compounds is the toxicity profile, which has few to none of the adverse effects of traditional cytotoxic therapy. The class effects include a rash resembling acne, and diarrhea.[106-108]

Despite these advances, survival for patients with NSCLC remains grim. Therapeutic advances have been made in locally advanced NSCLC, but researchers continue to look for ways to improve disease-free survival. In addition, treatment for stage IV lung cancer remains disappointing. Interested patients are encouraged to participate in clinical trials. Future directions include molecularly targeted approaches, including protein kinase C, cyclooxygenase pathways, antiangiogenesis pathways, and farnesyl transferase.

SMALL CELL LUNG CANCER

SCLC differs from NSCLC in its histology, propensity for early widespread metastatic dissemination, and sensitivity to chemotherapeutic agents. It accounts for 15% to 25% of all lung cancers and can be attributed to cigarette smoking in most patients. SCLC is an aggressive tumor: most patients present with locally bulky disease, mediastinal lymph nodes, and either subclinical or detectable metastases at diagnosis. This malignancy often occurs later in life, making aggressive therapy difficult to tolerate. Patients presenting with extensive disease, a weight loss of greater than 5%, male gender, and elevated LDH levels often have a poorer prognosis, once again limiting the usefulness of aggressive regimens in patients with comorbidities.

The treatment goals for patients with SCLC are to cure the few patients who present with limited-stage disease through a combination of surgery, radiation, and chemotherapy. In patients with extensive disease, platinum-based chemotherapy should be offered in an attempt to prolong life and palliate symptoms. Untreated, the median survival time of patients with SCLC is between 2 and 4 months.

Limited Disease. SCLC is sensitive to chemotherapy and radiotherapy, but as monotherapy each cures only a small number of patients with limited disease. Two meta-analyses evaluating the addition of thoracic irradiation to chemotherapy found that the two modalities in combination produced initial response rates of 80% to 100%, improved local con-

| TABLE 99.5 | Selected Chemotherapy Regimens for the Salvage Treatment of NSCLC |

Regimen	Dose	Schedule	Recurrence Rate (%)	Median Time to Progression (mo)	Median Overall Survival (mo)	Reference(s)
Docetaxel	Docetaxel 75 mg/m^2 IV over 1 hour	Repeat cycle every 21 days.	6.7–7.1	2.6–2.1	5.7–7	J Clin Oncol 18:2095–2103, 2000 J Clin Oncol 18:2354–2362, 2000
Gemcitabine	Gemcitabine 1,000 mg/m^2 IV over 30 minutes Days 1, 8, and 15	Repeat cycle every 21–28 days.	6–19	NA	4	Lung Cancer 29:67–73, 2000 J Clin Oncol 17:2081–2085, 1999
Gefitinib	Gefitinib 250 mg PO daily	Continuous administration	12–18.4	2.7–7	7–7.6	J Clin Oncol 21:136–144, 2003 JAMA 290:2149–2158, 2003
Vinorelbine	Vinorelbine 25–30 mg/m^2 IV over 10 minutes Days 1, 8, and 15	Repeat cycle every 21–28 days.	0–20	NA	3.2	Lung Cancer 29:91–104, 2000
Irinotecan	Irinotecan 80–100 mg/m^2 IV over 90 minutes Days 1, 8, and 15	Repeat cycle every 21–28 days.	31	3.75	10.5	J Clin Oncol 10:16–20, 1992

trol, and increased the 2- and 3-year survival rate by 5%.[109,110] However, using chemoradiation limits the chemotherapy regimens that can be administered. Doxorubicin is a radiosensitizer and anthracycline-based regimens produce significant toxicity. The administration of this agent results in drug interruptions or dose reductions, thus preventing the completion of the planned therapy. In addition, regimens containing an anthracycline had no impact on survival compared to modern platinum-based chemotherapy regimens in combination with irradiation.[111–115] Platinum-based regimens are better tolerated when given in combination with radiotherapy, making them the preferred regimens.[116–118] Common regimens used include cisplatin plus etoposide, and carboplatin plus etoposide (Table 99.6). In chemotherapy-naïve patients, the combination of carboplatin and etoposide appears to minimize toxicity without diminishing efficacy.[119–121] Thus, this regimen may be a suitable alternative to cisplatin plus etoposide in older adults or medically compromised patients.

The manner in which radiotherapy is administered with chemotherapy has been studied, but trial design, chemotherapy regimens, and the dose and fractionation of radiation therapy differed. Despite these limitations, concurrent radiotherapy appears to be superior to sequential therapy and is the preferred way to administer radiotherapy in combination with chemotherapy.[122] Although the combination of cisplatin plus etoposide and concurrent thoracic irradiation is the cornerstone of treatment in limited-disease SCLC, it confers significant toxicity, including weight loss, esophagitis, and pulmonary dysfunction compared with either modality alone. The median duration of response with combined modality therapy ranges from 6 to 8 months, and it produces median survival rates of 14 to 20 months.[122]

Several years ago surgery was considered the treatment of choice for SCLC, but a study conducted by the British Medical Research Council concluded that surgery was inferior to radiotherapy in promoting long-term survival.[123] This resulted in the abandonment of surgery as the primary treatment modality in SCLC. However, a few years later, in a retrospective trial conducted by the Veterans Administration Surgical Oncology Group, patients with very limited disease (T1N0M0 and possibly T1N1M0 or T2N0M0) benefited from potentially curative resection, with a reduction in local recurrences observed.[124] Thus, in patients with clinical stage T1-2N0 tumors who are good surgical candidates, a mediastinoscopy should be performed to rule out lymph node involvement, followed by surgical resection and chemotherapy.[122]

Extensive Disease. Most patients with SCLC will present with extensive disease. Platinum-based chemotherapy is the treatment of choice, and regimens similar to those administered in limited disease are used.[121,125–127] Initially, four cycles of chemotherapy should be administered, with an additional two cycles given to patients responding to therapy.

Although chemotherapy will produce initial responses in most patients, the duration of progression-free survival is approximately 4 months. Future clinical trials evaluating the combination of existing chemotherapeutic agents, along with the development of new treatment modalities, may result in new regimens that have a positive impact on the outcome of patients with extensive disease.

Prophylactic Cranial Irradiation. The incidence of brain metastases in patients with SCLC is higher than that with other histologic types. The probability of developing brain metastases increases as survival is prolonged with multimodality treatment. Central nervous system (CNS) metastases are present in greater than 50% of patients surviving more than 2 years or at autopsy despite treatment.[128–131] Once brain metastases occur, the symptoms can be devastating and often result in death. Treatment with cranial irradiation and corticosteroids, surgical resection of a solitary lesion, or stereotactic radiosurgery often improves neurologic symptoms and may result in a partial or complete response, but long-term survival is rare.[132,133]

Prevention of CNS metastases is the goal, but it is difficult to achieve. Prophylactic cranial irradiation (PCI) has been widely studied in both retrospective reviews and prospective clinical trials. These studies concluded that the development of brain metastases was significantly reduced in patients receiving PCI, but only a modest survival advantage was observed. Furthermore, some patients develop brain metastases despite PCI. Although data for improvement in overall survival are modest, the incidence of CNS metastases is reduced, and PCI is recommended for patients with limited disease who achieve a complete response after initial therapy.[122,134] For patients with extensive disease who achieve a complete response, PCI should be considered. In this circumstance, the optimal timing of PCI administration and the dose of radiation have yet to be established.

PCI is not without complications. Acute toxicities are often mild and include alopecia, headaches, fatigue, skin erythema, as well as disturbances in taste, appetite, and hearing. In long-term survivors, delayed complications are the most devastating and are a reason for controversy. Several clinical trials report conflicting results of the neuropsychological effects of PCI compared to no PCI.[135–140] Gradual intellect decline, short-term memory loss, optic atrophy, fine motor skills impairment, gait difficulty, and speech impairment are frequently reported. Diffuse cerebral atrophy, white matter abnormalities, and ventricular enlargement are often noted on CT and MRI scans. Overall, several studies concluded that the neurotoxicity associated with PCI produces minimal impairment and should not prohibit the administration of PCI in patients who completely respond to therapy.

There are a few alternatives to PCI. For patients who fail to achieve a complete remission with initial therapy, have baseline mental deficits, or have a poor performance status, a watch-and-wait policy may be recommended. Combination chemotherapy regimens including agents that penetrate the

TABLE 99.6 Selected Chemotherapy Regimens for the Primary Treatment of SCLC

Regimen	Dose	Schedule	Recurrence Rate (%)	Median Time to Progression (mo)	Median Overall Survival (mo)	Reference(s)
Carboplatin/etoposide	Carboplatin AUC 5–6 IV over 30–60 minutes on day 1 and etoposide 100 mg/m^2 IV over 4 hours on days 1–3	Repeat cycle every 21 days.	75–93	6.4–10.5	10.8–17.5	Ann Oncol 12:1231–1238, 2001 J Clin Oncol 17:3540–3545, 1999
Cisplatin/etoposide	Cisplatin 60–100 mg/m^2 IV over 2 hours on day 1 and etoposide 80–120 mg/m^2 IV over 4 hours on days 1–3	Repeat cycle every 21 days.	78–87	6.4	9.9–23	N Engl J Med 340:265–271, 1999 J Natl Cancer Inst 83:855–861, 1991
Cisplatin/irinotecan	Cisplatin 60 mg/m^2 IV over 2 hours on day 1 and irinotecan 60 mg/m^2 IV over 90 minutes on days 1, 8, and 15	Repeat cycle every 21 days.	84.4	6.9	12.8	N Engl J Med 346:85–91, 2002

TABLE 99.7	Selected Chemotherapy Regimens for the Salvage Treatment of SCLC					
Regimen	Dose	Schedule	Recurrence Rate (%)	Median Time to Progression (mo)	Median Overall Survival (mo)	Reference(s)
Topotecan	Topotecan 1.5 mg/m² IV over 30 minutes daily for 5 days	Repeat cycle every 21 days.	6.4–37.8	3.3–7.6	4.6–6.9	J Clin Oncol 17:658–667, 1999 J Clin Oncol 15:2090–2096, 1997
Cyclophosphamide/ doxorubicin (Adriamycin)/ vincristine	Cyclophosphamide 1,000 mg/m² IV over 2 hours, doxorubicin 45 mg/m² IV, and vincristine 2 mg IV	Repeat cycle every 21 days.	18.3	3.1	6.2	J Clin Oncol 17:658–667, 1999
Docetaxel	Docetaxel 75 mg/m² IV over 90 minutes	Repeat cycle every 21 days.	23	3	9	Cancer J Sci Am 5:237–241, 1999
Paclitaxel	Paclitaxel 175 mg/m² IV over 3 hours	Repeat cycle every 21 days.	29	2.1	3.3	Br J Cancer 77:347–351, 1998

blood–brain barrier, resection of an isolated lesion, and whole brain or stereotactic radiation are therapies that may be implemented when brain metastases occur in an attempt to provide symptomatic relief and prolong survival.

Refractory or Recurrent Disease. Although many patients with SCLC respond initially to therapy, progression-free survival is often brief. Patients relapsing greater than 3 months after therapy may be retreated with their initial induction regimen. Patients whose response lasts less than 3 months are considered refractory, and alternative therapy should be offered. Regimens containing topotecan, irinotecan, docetaxel, and paclitaxel produce responses in some patients but have little impact on lengthening survival (Table 99.7).

Elderly. Nearly one quarter of all patients diagnosed with SCLC are older than 70 years of age. In the past it was thought that these patients could not tolerate aggressive treatment regimens due to poor performance status and/or concomitant illnesses. However, this aging population has the same prognosis as younger patients, and failure to treat with combination chemotherapy and possibly radiotherapy diminishes the chance for long-term survival.[141–144] Thus, physiologic age, comorbid conditions, and functional status must be taken into account when outlining the treatment course of elderly patients with SCLC.

In healthy older patients with a good performance status, a platinum-based regimen should be administered. The myelosuppression and organ toxicity encountered may be increased, resulting in the need for greater supportive care, dose reductions, and treatment delays. Chemotherapeutic agent selection is key. Carboplatin offers several advantages in the elderly population compared to cisplatin, including ease of administration and reduced nonhematologic toxicities. Furthermore, the dose is calculated based on the area under the curve and thus is individualized by taking into account the declining renal function of aging patients. Finally, in healthy older SCLC patients, combined modality therapy (chemotherapy and radiotherapy) may be considered. In elderly patients with a poor performance status or in poor health, chemotherapy is still a consideration. Abbreviated chemotherapy regimens, enrollment onto a clinical trial, and newer combination regimens are acceptable options.[145–148] In all elderly patients achieving a complete response, PCI should be offered.[122]

TREATMENT COMPLICATIONS

Many complications may occur during the administration of chemotherapy (Table 99.8). Frequently, the regimen-related toxicities are tolerable and self-limiting, but occasionally long-term effects occur that may compromise the patient's health and quality of life. Often the gastrointestinal tract is affected by the drugs administered. Nausea and vomiting commonly occurs; it varies in intensity and may require antiemetics. The emesis may occur acutely or it may be delayed, as is frequently observed with agents such as cisplatin and cyclophosphamide. Diarrhea, stomatitis, and anorexia may complicate the patient's health. Supplemental nutrition, antidiarrheals, hydration, and pain control may be necessary, as well as implementing good oral hygiene to avoid infections. Myelosuppression, including neutropenia and thrombocytopenia, may result, but usually does not require administration of a colony-stimulating growth factor. Anemia may occur with certain chemotherapy regimens, and the administration of an erythropoietic colony-stimulating factor may be appropriate. Cardiotoxicity often appears as congestive heart failure or as a cardiomyopathy requiring symptomatic treatment. Patients who develop a fever during therapy will require broad-spectrum antibiotics regardless of the results of microbiology cultures. Laboratory abnormalities may occur, including electrolyte disturbances requiring supplementation. Laboratory results may also indicate hepatic dysfunction or renal failure. Cisplatin frequently causes hypomagnesemia and other electrolyte alterations. Renal tubular damage, peripheral neuropathy, and ototoxicity are other potential side effects of cisplatin and may not be reversible. Although carboplatin may cause these toxicities to a lesser extent, it has a profound effect on reducing the platelet count. Other treatment-related toxicities include pulmonary toxicity, hemorrhagic cystitis, rash, and neurotoxicity.

Radiation therapy produces several acute and delayed side effects (Table 99.9).[149,150] Side effects that occur within 90 days of completing radiotherapy are labeled acute and reflect local damage to tissue. Fatigue and myelosuppression are common after completion of treatment, and rarely adult respiratory distress syndrome may occur. Erythema and tissue desquamation may present acutely, whereas fibrosis and telangiectasia occur months and even years after radiotherapy. Mucositis and esophagitis are common during and after radiotherapy. This is generally self-limited and may be treated with analgesics and by maintaining good oral hygiene. Late esophageal strictures may require repeated endoscopic dilatation; rarely, fistulas and perforation occur. Pericarditis may occur within the first 90 days after treatment. It is generally self-limited and can be treated with analgesics, antipyretics, and occasionally antiarrhythmic agents. Heart failure and coronary stenosis may occur months after treatment. Radiation pneumonitis occurs in 5% to 15% of patients within 1 to 4 months after therapy. It typically presents with dyspnea, cough, low-grade fever, and pleuritic chest pain. Steroid administration and supportive care should be offered to patients in an attempt to prevent progression to fibrosis. Pulmonary fibrosis generally presents 3 to 18 months after completion of radiotherapy. Patients may be asymptomatic, and treatment is supportive care only.

As previously discussed, chemotherapy and radiotherapy are often combined in multimodality regimens. These combinations may potentiate the toxicities observed with either chemotherapy or radiation alone, increasing the morbidity associated with each individual treatment plan. Care should be taken to minimize these effects in patients receiving aggressive therapy.

TABLE 99.8	Chemotherapeutic Agents and Selected Toxicities for Treating NSCLC and SCLC	
Chemotherapy Agent	**Common Adverse Drug Events**	**Monitoring Parameters**[a]
Carboplatin	Myelosuppression, nausea and vomiting, mucositis, stomatitis, alopecia, peripheral neuropathy, hypomagnesemia, hyponatremia, hypokalemia, hypocalcemia, liver function test elevations, hemorrhagic complications, asthenia, and pain at injection site	CBC w/ differential, magnesium, sodium, potassium, calcium, total bilirubin, alkaline phosphatase, SGPT, LDH, pain, urine output, and weight
Cisplatin	Nephrotoxicity, acute and delayed nausea and vomiting, high-frequency hearing loss, hyperuricemia, myelosuppression, peripheral neuropathy, hypomagnesemia, hypokalemia, hyponatremia, hypocalcemia, hypophosphatemia, and mild alopecia	BUN, creatinine, CBC w/ differential, magnesium, potassium, sodium, calcium, inorganic phosphorus, uric acid, urine output, and weight
Cyclophosphamide	Myelosuppression, cardiotoxicity, alopecia, mucositis, nausea and vomiting, anorexia, diarrhea, stomatitis, hemorrhagic cystitis, jaundice, amenorrhea, and renal tubular necrosis	CBC w/ differential, creatinine, urine output, weight, pain, and urinalysis as indicated
Docetaxel	Myelosuppression, nausea and vomiting, mucositis, diarrhea, fluid retention, rash, alopecia, hypotension, increased liver function tests, flushing, peripheral neuropathies, angioedema, pleural effusions, and fever	CBC w/ differential, total bilirubin, LDH, alkaline phosphatase, SGPT, pain, blood pressure, temperature, urine output, and weight
Doxorubicin	Cardiotoxicity, nausea and vomiting, myelosuppression, anorexia, mucositis, stomatitis, esophagitis, diarrhea, alopecia, necrosis of colon, and discoloration of urine	CBC w/ differential, pain, urine output, weight, and baseline electrocardiogram and echocardiogram
Erlotinib	Diarrhea, rash, acne, dry skin, fatigue, anorexia, and nausea and vomiting	Weight
Etoposide	Myelosuppression, nausea and vomiting, infusion-related hypotension, mucositis, stomatitis, alopecia, diarrhea, anorexia, metallic taste, and fatigue	CBC w/ differential, weight, pain, and blood pressure
Gefitinib	Diarrhea, rash, acne, dry skin, fatigue, anorexia, and nausea and vomiting	Weight
Gemcitabine	Myelosuppression, nausea and vomiting, diarrhea, constipation, stomatitis, pain, alopecia, elevated liver function tests, fever, rash, peripheral edema, proteinuria, hematuria, dyspnea, and elevated BUN	CBC w/ differential, BUN, total bilirubin, LDH, SGPT, alkaline phosphatase, pain, and temperature
Ifosfamide	Myelosuppression, nausea and vomiting, hemorrhagic cystitis, nephrotoxicity, neurotoxicity (including lethargy, ataxia, mental status changes, disorientation, seizures, hallucinations), alopecia, stomatitis, anorexia, diarrhea, constipation, metabolic acidosis, and transient elevations in liver function tests	CBC w/ differential, serum electrolytes, urinalysis as indicated, BUN, creatinine, total bilirubin, LDH, SGPT, alkaline phosphatase, weight, and pain
Irinotecan	Myelosuppression, diarrhea, abdominal pain, nausea and vomiting, vasodilation, dizziness, rhinitis, dyspnea, cough, insomnia, fever, alopecia, and weakness	CBC w/ differential, and pain
Mitomycin C	Myelosuppression, nausea and vomiting, stomatitis, diarrhea, hemolytic-uremic syndrome, creatinine elevation, alopecia, pulmonary toxicity, hepatotoxicity, anorexia, and extremity paresthesia	CBC w/ differential, total bilirubin, alkaline phosphatase, LDH, SGPT, chest radiograph as indicated, BUN, creatinine, pain, and weight

(continues)

TABLE 99.8	continued	
Chemotherapy Agent	**Common Adverse Drug Events**	**Monitoring Parameters**[a]
Paclitaxel	Hypersensitivity reactions, hypotension, myelosuppression, mucositis, nausea and vomiting, diarrhea, peripheral neuropathy, alopecia, myalgia, abnormal liver function tests, and abnormal electrocardiogram	CBC w/ differential, pain, total bilirubin, alkaline phosphatase, LDH, and SGPT
Pemetrexed	Myelosuppression, nausea and vomiting, fatigue, elevated creatinine, fever, infection, stomatitis, and rash	CBC w/ differential, creatinine, temperature, microbiology cultures, pain, and weight
Topotecan	Myelosuppression, diarrhea, nausea and vomiting, dyspnea, asthenia, paraesthesias, headache, and alopecia	CBC w/ differential
Vinblastine	Myelosuppression, alopecia, nausea and vomiting, anorexia, stomatitis, metallic taste, and abdominal cramps	CBC w/ differential, pain, and weight
Vincristine	Myelosuppression, constipation, peripheral neuropathy, paralytic ileus, neuromuscular difficulties, mental status changes, alopecia, orthostatic hypotension, hypertension, seizures, headache, fever, rash, and hyperuricemia	CBC w/ differential, uric acid, temperature, and blood pressure
Vinorelbine	Myelosuppression, nausea and vomiting, constipation, diarrhea, stomatitis, abdominal cramps, anorexia, peripheral neuropathy, myalgia, arthralgia, alopecia, metallic taste, and fatigue	CBC w/ with differential, pain, and weight

[a] Patients should be monitored clinically for symptomatic toxicities.
CBC, complete blood count; SGPT, serum glutamic-pyruvic transaminase; LDH, lactate dehydrogenase; BUN, blood urea nitrogen.

PATIENT EDUCATION

Upon diagnosis, patients should be counseled on the means of treating their disease, relieving the symptoms, and preventing recurrence. Reviewing treatment options and the toxicities of each therapy will assist the patient in better understanding the expectations associated with each modal-

TABLE 99.9	Complications Associated With Radiotherapy

Fatigue

Myelosuppression

Adult respiratory distress syndrome

Mucositis

Esophageal strictures, fistulas, and perforation

Skin erythema and desquamation

Skin fibrosis and telangiectasia

Pericarditis

Heart failure and coronary stenosis

Pneumonitis

Pulmonary fibrosis

ity chosen. Smoking cessation should be strongly encouraged in patients who currently smoke.[151,152] Not only will it assist in relieving symptoms, but it may also prevent additional primary tumors from occurring. Nicotine and bupropion are often used to assist in breaking this habit. Nicotine is available in a wide variety of formulations, including gum, patch, inhaler, and nasal spray. Enrollment in programs that offer counseling, behavioral modification therapies, and support, in addition to medication, may further benefit a patient's effort to stop smoking. Refer to Chapter 60 for further discussion.

CHEMOPREVENTION

Interventions aimed at reducing the incidence of lung cancer include tobacco cessation and abstinence, early detection, and chemoprevention. Chemoprevention is the administration of specific natural or synthetic compounds to reverse or stop the progression of premalignant cells or inhibit the development of cancer by blocking DNA damage.[152] Primary chemoprevention trials in patients with known risk factors produced surprising results. Two large randomized clinical trials, the ATBC and CARET, evaluating the effects of alpha-tocopherol, beta-carotene, and vitamin A on the incidence of lung cancer, showed that these supplements have no benefit and may actually increase the risk of lung cancer in smokers.[153,154] In patients with known lung cancer precursors, no large randomized clinical trials evaluating secondary chemoprevention defined lung cancer incidence as an endpoint. Tertiary chemoprevention trials evaluating isotretinoin, retinyl palmitate, or retinyl palmitate plus n-acetylcysteine in patients with a prior cancer diagnosis treated with a curative intent failed to show an effect on the development of secondary cancers.[155,156]

Potential new agents and approaches include other retinoids, selenium, vitamin E in combination with 13-cis-retinoic acid, cyclooxygenase-2 inhibitors, and inhaled retinoids. Administration of antibodies or small molecules that inhibit HER2 or EGFR, which are significantly expressed in patients with bronchial preneoplasia, may be of benefit. Finally, the evaluation of sputum cytology in high-risk individuals may identify patients at risk earlier, allowing further clinical trials involving chemoprevention.[157] Outside the context of a clinical trial, however, chemoprevention should not be recommended.

PSYCHOSOCIAL ASPECTS OF DISEASE

Upon learning of the diagnosis of lung cancer, patients exhibit a wide variety of emotions and behaviors. Anger, shock, fear, and sadness are common terms that describe their feelings at diagnosis. Guilt is often present, as many patients feel that their lung cancer was caused by their lifestyle. Once patients begin to deal with their diagnosis and potential approaching death, some may become depressed, whereas others will exhibit signs of denial. Furthermore, the quality of life these patients possess is greatly affected by their illness and may further contribute to their physical and psychological well-being. Symptoms may affect their ability to complete daily activities by interfering with physical and psychological functions, as well as their social, sexual, occupational, and spiritual interactions. In addition to the physical ailments associated with lung cancer, the psychological, emotional, and social concerns of these patients and their families need to be addressed and treated accordingly. Support groups, counseling, medications, and religion often provide comfort to patients and their families, as well as improving the patient's quality of life.

CONCLUSION

Lung cancer continues to be the leading cause of cancer death among men and women worldwide. This disease primarily affects patients with a history of cigarette smoking and therefore may be highly preventable. Accurate histologic confirmation and staging is important in determining both prognosis and treatment options. NSCLC is not as aggressive

as SCLC and is classified into adenocarcinoma, squamous cell, and large cell carcinoma. SCLC is an aggressive and rapidly proliferating tumor with metastases often detectable at diagnosis. Despite the many diagnostic and therapeutic improvements over the past few years, the prognosis for patients with lung cancer is still poor. New agents, combination regimens, targeted therapies, and newer selective approaches need further investigation in an attempt to improve response rates and prolong survival. Until further therapeutic breakthroughs occur, though, prevention is the only means of controlling this disease.

KEY POINTS

- Complete surgical resection with adjuvant chemotherapy should be offered to patients with stage I and II NSCLC who can tolerate treatment
- Patients with stage IIIA NSCLC should be treated with surgery and chemotherapy if feasible, or with combined chemotherapy and radiation
- Treatment of stage IIIB NSCLC consists of multimodality therapy with chemoradiotherapy
- Stage IV NSCLC is considered unresectable; chemotherapy and/or radiotherapy in a clinical setting is generally offered as palliative therapy
- Chemoradiation with a platinum-based regimen is the standard of care for patients with limited SCLC
- Surgery may be indicated in a subgroup of patients with very limited SCLC (no lymph node involvement) who are in good health
- Patients who present with extensive SCLC should be offered platinum-based chemotherapy
- Prophylactic cranial irradiation is indicated in patients with SCLC who achieve a complete remission after primary therapy

SUGGESTED READINGS

Cersosimo RJ. Lung cancer: a review. Am J Health Syst Pharm 59:611–642, 2002.
Pfister DG, Johnson DH, Azzoli CG, et al. American Society of Clinical Oncology treatment of unresectable non-small-cell lung cancer guideline: update 2003. J Clin Oncol 22:330–353, 2004.
Simon GR, Wagner H. Small cell lung cancer. Chest 123:259S–271S, 2003.
Spira A, Ettinger DS. Multidisciplinary management of lung cancer. N Engl J Med 350:379–392, 2004.

REFERENCES

1. Jemal A, Tiwari RC, Murray T, et al. Cancer statistics, 2004. CA Cancer J Clin 54:8–29, 2004.
2. Brown ML, Lipscomb J, Snyder C. The burden of illness of cancer: economic cost and quality of life. Annu Rev Public Health 22:91–113, 2001.
3. Brown ML, Riley GF, Schussler N, et al. Estimating health care costs related to cancer treatment from SEER-Medicare data. Med Care 40:IV-104–117, 2002.

4. US Department of Health, Education, and Welfare. Smoking and Health Report of the Advisory Committee to the Surgeon General of the Public Health Service. Rockville, MD: US Department of Health, Education, and Welfare, Public Health Service, PHS pub no. 1103, 1964.

5. Patel JD, Bach PB, Kris MG. Lung cancer in US women: a contemporary epidemic. JAMA 291:1763–1768, 2004.

6. Giovino GA. Epidemiology of tobacco use in the United States. Oncogene 21:7326–7340, 2002.

7. Bain C, Feskanich D, Speizer FE, et al. Lung cancer rates in men and women with comparable histories of smoking. J Natl Cancer Inst 96:826–834, 2004.

8. Tanoue LT. Cigarette smoking and women's respiratory health. Clin Chest Med 21:47–65, viii, 2000.

9. Halpern MT, Gillespie BW, Warner KE. Patterns of absolute risk of lung cancer mortality in former smokers. J Natl Cancer Inst 85:457–464, 1993.

10. Muscat JE, Wynder EL. Lung cancer pathology in smokers, ex-smokers and never smokers. Cancer Lett 88:1–5, 1995.

11. Flanders WD, Lally CA, Zhu BP, et al. Lung cancer mortality in relation to age, duration of smoking, and daily cigarette consumption: results from Cancer Prevention Study II. Cancer Res 63:6556–6562, 2003.

12. Doll R, Peto R. Cigarette smoking and bronchial carcinoma: dose and time relationships among regular smokers and lifelong nonsmokers. J Epidemiol Community Health 32:303–313, 1978.

13. Bach PB, Kattan MW, Thornquist MD, et al. Variations in lung cancer risk among smokers. J Natl Cancer Inst 95:470–478, 2003.

14. Doll R, Peto R, Boreham J, et al. Mortality in relation to smoking: 50 years' observations on male British doctors. Br Med J 2004; 328:1519, 2004.

15. Brennan P, Buffler PA, Reynolds P, et al. Secondhand smoke exposure in adulthood and risk of lung cancer among never smokers: a pooled analysis of two large studies. Int J Cancer 109:125–131, 2004.

16. Selikoff IJ, Hammond EC, Churg J. Asbestos exposure, smoking, and neoplasia. JAMA 204:106–112, 1968.

17. Rivera MP, Detterbeck F, Mehta AC. Diagnosis of lung cancer: the guidelines. Chest 123:129S–136S, 2003.

18. Beckles MA, Spiro SG, Colice GL, et al. The physiologic evaluation of patients with lung cancer being considered for resectional surgery. Chest 123:105S–114S, 2003.

19. Ferguson MK, Little L, Rizzo L, et al. Diffusing capacity predicts morbidity and mortality after pulmonary resection. J Thorac Cardiovasc Surg 96:894–900, 1988.

20. Ninan M, Sommers KE, Landreneau RJ, et al. Standardized exercise oximetry predicts postpneumonectomy outcome. Ann Thorac Surg 64:328–332, 1997.

21. DeMeester SR, Patterson GA, Sundaresan RS, et al. Lobectomy combined with volume reduction for patients with lung cancer and advanced emphysema. J Thorac Cardiovasc Surg 115:681–688, 1998.

22. DeRose JJ, Jr., Argenziano M, El-Amir N, et al. Lung reduction operation and resection of pulmonary nodules in patients with severe emphysema. Ann Thorac Surg 65:314–318, 1998.

23. Mountain CF. Staging classification of lung cancer. A critical evaluation. Clin Chest Med 23:103–121, 2002.

24. Lung. In: AJCC cancer staging manual, 6th ed. New York: Springer-Verlag, 2002:167–177.

25. Fry WA, Phillips JL, Menck HR. Ten-year survey of lung cancer treatment and survival in hospitals in the United States: a national cancer data base report. Cancer 86:1867–1876, 1999.

26. Hyde L, Yee J, Wilson R, et al. Cell type and the natural history of lung cancer. JAMA 193:52–54, 1965.

27. Stitik FP. The new staging of lung cancer. Radiol Clin North Am 32:635–647, 1994.

28. Stahel RA, Ginsberg RJ. Staging and prognostic factors in small cell lung cancer: a consensus report. Lung Cancer 5:119–126, 1989.

29. Spira A, Ettinger DS. Multidisciplinary management of lung cancer. N Engl J Med 350:379–392, 2004.

30. Lau CL, D'Amico TA, Harpole DH Jr. Clinical and molecular prognostic factors and models for non-small cell lung cancer. In: Pass HI, Mitchell JB, Johnson DH, et al., eds. Lung Cancer, Principles and Practice, 2nd ed. Philadelphia: Lippincott Williams & Wilkins, 2000:602–611.

31. Smythe WR. Treatment of stage I and II non-small-cell lung cancer. Cancer Control 8:318–325, 2001.

32. Korst RJ, Ginsberg RJ. Appropriate surgical treatment of resectable non-small-cell lung cancer. World J Surg 25:184–188, 2001.

33. Chemotherapy in non-small cell lung cancer: a meta-analysis using updated data on individual patients from 52 randomised clinical trials. Non-small Cell Lung Cancer Collaborative Group. Br Med J 311:899–909, 1995.

34. Granone P, Trodella L, Margaritora S, et al. Radiotherapy versus follow-up in the treatment of pathological stage Ia and Ib non-small cell lung cancer. Early stopped analysis of a randomized controlled study. Eur J Cardiothorac Surg 18:418–424, 2000.

35. Postoperative radiotherapy in non-small-cell lung cancer: systematic review and meta-analysis of individual patient data from nine randomised controlled trials. PORT Meta-analysis Trialists Group. Lancet 352:257–263, 1998.

36. Stephens RJ, Girling DJ, Bleehen NM, et al. The role of postoperative radiotherapy in non-small-cell lung cancer: a multicentre randomised trial in patients with pathologically staged T1-2, N1-2, M0 disease. Medical Research Council Lung Cancer Working Party. Br J Cancer 74:632–639, 1996.

37. Weisenburger TH. Effects of postoperative mediastinal radiation on completely resected stage II and stage III epidermoid cancer of the lung. LCSG 773. Chest 106:297S–301S, 1994.

38. Wada H, Hitomi S, Teramatsu T. Adjuvant chemotherapy after complete resection in non-small-cell lung cancer. West Japan Study Group for Lung Cancer Surgery. J Clin Oncol 14:1048–1054, 1996.

39. Scagliotti GV, Fossati R, Torri V, et al. Randomized study of adjuvant chemotherapy for completely resected stage I, II, or IIIA non-small-cell Lung cancer. J Natl Cancer Inst 95:1453–1461, 2003.

40. Shields TW, Higgins GA, Jr., Humphrey EW, et al. Prolonged intermittent adjuvant chemotherapy with CCNU and hydroxyurea after resection of carcinoma of the lung. Cancer 50:1713–1721, 1982.

41. Holmes EC. Surgical adjuvant therapy for stage II and stage III adenocarcinoma and large cell undifferentiated carcinoma. Chest 106:293S–296S, 1994.

42. Figlin RA, Piantadosi S. A phase 3 randomized trial of immediate combination chemotherapy vs. delayed combination chemotherapy in patients with completely resected stage II and III non-small cell carcinoma of the lung. Chest 106:310S–312S, 1994.

43. Feld R, Rubinstein L, Thomas PA. Adjuvant chemotherapy with cyclophosphamide, doxorubicin, and cisplatin in patients with completely resected stage I non-small-cell lung cancer. The Lung Cancer Study Group. J Natl Cancer Inst 85:299–306, 1993.

44. Arriagada R, Bergman B, Dunant A, et al. Cisplatin-based adjuvant chemotherapy in patients with completely resected non-small-cell lung cancer. N Engl J Med 350:351–360, 2004.

45. Winton TL, Livingston D, Johnson J. A prospective randomized trial of adjuvant vinorelbine (VIN) and cisplatin (CIS) in completely resected stage 1B and II non small cell lung cancer (NSCLC) Intergroup JBR.10. Proc Am Soc Clin Oncol Abstract 7018, ASCO 2004.

46. Strauss GM, Herndon J, Maddaus MA. Randomized clinical trial of adjuvant chemotherapy with paclitaxel and carboplatin following resection in Stage IB non-small cell lung cancer (NSCLC): Report of Cancer and Leukemia Group B (CALGB) Protocol 9633. Proc Am Soc Clin Oncol Abstract 7019, ASCO 2004.

47. Lad T. The comparison of CAP chemotherapy and radiotherapy to radiotherapy alone for resected lung cancer with positive margin or involved highest sampled paratracheal node (stage IIIA). LCSG 791. Chest 106:302S–306S, 1994.

48. Keller SM, Adak S, Wagner H, et al. A randomized trial of postoperative adjuvant therapy in patients with completely resected stage II or IIIA non-small-cell lung cancer. Eastern Cooperative Oncology Group. N Engl J Med 343:1217–1222, 2000.

49. Pisters KM, Kris MG, Gralla RJ, et al. Randomized trial comparing postoperative chemotherapy with vindesine and cisplatin plus thoracic irradiation with irradiation alone in stage III (N2) non-small cell lung cancer. J Surg Oncol 56:236–241, 1994.

50. Rosell R, Lopez-Cabrerizo MP, Astudillo J. Preoperative chemotherapy for stage IIIA non-small cell lung cancer. Curr Opin Oncol 9:149–155, 1997.
51. Martini N, Kris MG, Flehinger BJ, et al. Preoperative chemotherapy for stage IIIa (N2) lung cancer: the Sloan-Kettering experience with 136 patients. Ann Thorac Surg 55:1365–1374, 1993.
52. Kirn DH, Lynch TJ, Mentzer SJ, et al. Multimodality therapy of patients with stage IIIA, N2 non-small-cell lung cancer. Impact of preoperative chemotherapy on resectability and downstaging. J Thorac Cardiovasc Surg 106:696–702, 1993.
53. Van Zandwijk N, Smit EF, Kramer GW, et al. Gemcitabine and cisplatin as induction regimen for patients with biopsy-proven stage IIIA N2 non-small-cell lung cancer: a phase II study of the European Organization for Research and Treatment of Cancer Lung Cancer Cooperative Group (EORTC 08955). J Clin Oncol 18: 2658–2664, 2000.
54. Roth JA, Atkinson EN, Fossella F, et al. Long-term follow-up of patients enrolled in a randomized trial comparing perioperative chemotherapy and surgery with surgery alone in resectable stage IIIA non-small-cell lung cancer. Lung Cancer 21:1–6, 1998.
55. Rosell R, Gomez-Codina J, Camps C, et al. Preresectional chemotherapy in stage IIIA non-small-cell lung cancer: a 7-year assessment of a randomized controlled trial. Lung Cancer 26:7–14, 1999.
56. Depierre A, Milleron B, Moro-Sibilot D, et al. Preoperative chemotherapy followed by surgery compared with primary surgery in resectable stage I (except T1N0), II, and IIIa non-small-cell lung cancer. J Clin Oncol 20:247–253, 2002.
57. Damstrup L, Poulsen HS. Review of the curative role of radiotherapy in the treatment of non-small cell lung cancer. Lung Cancer 11:153–178, 1994.
58. Perez CA, Pajak TF, Rubin P, et al. Long-term observations of the patterns of failure in patients with unresectable non-oat cell carcinoma of the lung treated with definitive radiotherapy. Report by the Radiation Therapy Oncology Group. Cancer 59:1874–1881, 1987.
59. Dillman RO, Herndon J, Seagren SL, et al. Improved survival in stage III non-small-cell lung cancer: seven-year follow-up of cancer and leukemia group B (CALGB) 8433 trial. J Natl Cancer Inst 88:1210–1215, 1996.
60. Sause W, Kolesar P, Taylor SI, et al. Final results of phase III trial in regionally advanced unresectable non-small cell lung cancer: Radiation Therapy Oncology Group, Eastern Cooperative Oncology Group, and Southwest Oncology Group. Chest 117:358–364, 2000.
61. Blanke C, Ansari R, Mantravadi R, et al. Phase III trial of thoracic irradiation with or without cisplatin for locally advanced unresectable non-small-cell lung cancer: a Hoosier Oncology Group protocol. J Clin Oncol 13:1425–1429, 1995.
62. Albain KS, Crowley JJ, Turrisi AT, 3rd, et al. Concurrent cisplatin, etoposide, and chest radiotherapy in pathologic stage IIIB non-small-cell lung cancer: a Southwest Oncology Group phase II study, SWOG 9019. J Clin Oncol 20:3454–3460, 2002.
63. Byhardt RW, Scott C, Sause WT, et al. Response, toxicity, failure patterns, and survival in five Radiation Therapy Oncology Group (RTOG) trials of sequential and/or concurrent chemotherapy and radiotherapy for locally advanced non-small-cell carcinoma of the lung. Int J Radiat Oncol Biol Phys 42:469–478, 1998.
64. Kim TY, Yang SH, Lee SH, et al. A phase III randomized trial of combined chemoradiotherapy versus radiotherapy alone in locally advanced non-small-cell lung cancer. Am J Clin Oncol 25: 238–243, 2002.
65. Le Chevalier T, Arriagada R, Quoix E, et al. Radiotherapy alone versus combined chemotherapy and radiotherapy in nonresectable non-small-cell lung cancer: first analysis of a randomized trial in 353 patients. J Natl Cancer Inst 83:417–423, 1991.
66. Furuse K, Fukuoka M, Kawahara M, et al. Phase III study of concurrent versus sequential thoracic radiotherapy in combination with mitomycin, vindesine, and cisplatin in unresectable stage III non-small-cell lung cancer. J Clin Oncol 17:2692–2699, 1999.
67. Curran WJ, Scott CB, Langer CJ. Long-term benefit is observed in a phase III comparison of sequential vs. concurrent chemoradiation for patients with unresected stage III NSCLC: RTOG 9410. Proc Am Soc Clin Oncol Abstract 2499, ASCO 2003.
68. Gandara DR, Chansky K, Albain KS, et al. Consolidation docetaxel after concurrent chemoradiotherapy in stage IIIB non-small-cell lung cancer: phase II Southwest Oncology Group Study S9504. J Clin Oncol 21:2004–2010, 2003.
69. Choy H, Curran WJ, Scott CB. Preliminary report of locally advanced multimodality protocol (LAMP): ACR 427: a randomized phase II study of three chemo-radiation regimens with paclitaxel, carboplatin, and thoracic radiation (TRT) for patients with locally advanced non small cell lung cancer (LA-NSCLC). Proc Am Soc Clin Oncol Abstract 1160, ASCO 2002.
70. Vokes EE, Herndon JE, Kelley MJ. Induction chemotherapy followed by concomitant chemoradiotherapy (CT/XRT) versus CT/XRT alone for regionally advanced unresectable non-small cell lung cancer (NSCLC): initial analysis of a randomized phase III trial. Proc Am Soc Clin Oncol Abstract 7005, ASCO 2004.
71. Cersosimo RJ. Lung cancer: a review. Am J Health Syst Pharm 59:611–642, 2002.
72. Gridelli C. The ELVIS trial: a phase III study of single-agent vinorelbine as first-line treatment in elderly patients with advanced non-small cell lung cancer. Elderly Lung Cancer Vinorelbine Italian Study. Oncologist 6 (Suppl 1):4–7, 2001.
73. Souquet PJ, Chauvin F, Boissel JP, et al. Meta-analysis of randomised trials of systemic chemotherapy versus supportive treatment in non-resectable non-small cell lung cancer. Lung Cancer 12 (Suppl 1):S147–154, 1995.
74. Thongprasert S, Sanguanmitra P, Juthapan W, et al. Relationship between quality of life and clinical outcomes in advanced non-small cell lung cancer: best supportive care (BSC) versus BSC plus chemotherapy. Lung Cancer 24:17–24, 1999.
75. Dranitsaris G, Cottrell W, Evans WK. Cost-effectiveness of chemotherapy for non-small-cell lung cancer. Curr Opin Oncol 14: 375–383, 2002.
76. Evans WK. Cost-effectiveness of gemcitabine in stage IV non-small cell lung cancer: an estimate using the Population Health Model lung cancer module. Semin Oncol 24:S7-56–S7-63, 1997.
77. Lilenbaum RC, Langenberg P, Dickersin K. Single agent versus combination chemotherapy in patients with advanced non-small cell lung carcinoma: a meta-analysis of response, toxicity, and survival. Cancer 82:116–126, 1998.
78. Ruckdeschel JC, Finkelstein DM, Mason BA, et al. Chemotherapy for metastatic non-small-cell bronchogenic carcinoma: EST 2575, generation V: a randomized comparison of four cisplatin-containing regimens. J Clin Oncol 3:72–79, 1985.
79. Ruckdeschel JC, Finkelstein DM, Ettinger DS, et al. A randomized trial of the four most active regimens for metastatic non-small-cell lung cancer. J Clin Oncol 4:14–22, 1986.
80. Bonomi P. Platinum/etoposide therapy in non-small cell lung cancer. Oncology 49 (Suppl 1):43–50, 1992.
81. Wozniak AJ, Crowley JJ, Balcerzak SP, et al. Randomized trial comparing cisplatin with cisplatin plus vinorelbine in the treatment of advanced non-small-cell lung cancer: a Southwest Oncology Group study. J Clin Oncol 16:2459–2465, 1998.
82. Sandler AB, Nemunaitis J, Denham C, et al. Phase III trial of gemcitabine plus cisplatin versus cisplatin alone in patients with locally advanced or metastatic non-small-cell lung cancer. J Clin Oncol 18:122–130, 2000.
83. Gatzemeier U, von Pawel J, Gottfried M, et al. Phase III comparative study of high-dose cisplatin versus a combination of paclitaxel and cisplatin in patients with advanced non-small-cell lung cancer. J Clin Oncol 18:3390–3399, 2000.
84. Paccagnella A, Favaretto A, Oniga F, et al. Cisplatin versus carboplatin in combination with mitomycin and vinblastine in advanced non-small cell lung cancer. A multicenter, randomized phase III trial. Lung Cancer 43:83–91, 2004.
85. Klastersky J, Sculier JP, Lacroix H, et al. A randomized study comparing cisplatin or carboplatin with etoposide in patients with advanced non-small-cell lung cancer: European Organization for Research and Treatment of Cancer Protocol 07861. J Clin Oncol 8:1556–1562, 1990.
86. Mazzanti P, Massacesi C, Rocchi MB, et al. Randomized, multicenter, phase II study of gemcitabine plus cisplatin versus gemcitabine plus carboplatin in patients with advanced non-small cell lung cancer. Lung Cancer 41:81–89, 2003.
87. Fossella F, Pereira JR, von Pawel J, et al. Randomized, multinational, phase III study of docetaxel plus platinum combinations ver-

sus vinorelbine plus cisplatin for advanced non-small-cell lung cancer: the TAX 326 study group. J Clin Oncol 21:3016–3024, 2003.

88. Rosell R, Gatzemeier U, Betticher DC, et al. Phase III randomised trial comparing paclitaxel/carboplatin with paclitaxel/cisplatin in patients with advanced non-small-cell lung cancer: a cooperative multinational trial. Ann Oncol 13:1539–1549, 2002.

89. Bonomi P, Kim K, Fairclough D, et al. Comparison of survival and quality of life in advanced non-small-cell lung cancer patients treated with two dose levels of paclitaxel combined with cisplatin versus etoposide with cisplatin: results of an Eastern Cooperative Oncology Group trial. J Clin Oncol 18:623–631, 2000.

90. Cardenal F, Lopez-Cabrerizo MP, Anton A, et al. Randomized phase III study of gemcitabine-cisplatin versus etoposide-cisplatin in the treatment of locally advanced or metastatic non-small-cell lung cancer. J Clin Oncol 17:12–18, 1999.

91. Bonomi P, Kim K, Kusler J, et al. Cisplatin/etoposide vs paclitaxel/cisplatin/G-CSF vs. paclitaxel/cisplatin in non-small-cell lung cancer. Oncology 11:9–10, 1997.

92. Grigorescu AC, Draghici IN, Nitipir C, et al. Gemcitabine (GEM) and carboplatin (CBDCA) versus cisplatin (CDDP) and vinblastine (VLB) in advanced non-small-cell lung cancer (NSCLC) stages III and IV: a phase III randomised trial. Lung Cancer 37:9–14, 2002.

93. Schiller JH, Harrington D, Belani CP, et al. Comparison of four chemotherapy regimens for advanced non-small-cell lung cancer. N Engl J Med 346:92–98, 2002.

94. Pfister DG, Johnson DH, Azzoli CG, et al. American Society of Clinical Oncology treatment of unresectable non-small-cell lung cancer guideline: update 2003. J Clin Oncol 22:330–353, 2004.

95. Smith IE, O'Brien ME, Talbot DC, et al. Duration of chemotherapy in advanced non-small-cell lung cancer: a randomized trial of three versus six courses of mitomycin, vinblastine, and cisplatin. J Clin Oncol 19:1336–1343, 2001.

96. Socinski MA, Schell MJ, Peterman A, et al. Phase III trial comparing a defined duration of therapy versus continuous therapy followed by second-line therapy in advanced-stage IIIB/IV non-small-cell lung cancer. J Clin Oncol 20:1335–1343, 2002.

97. Sculier JP, Lafitte JJ, Berghmans T, et al. A phase II trial testing gemcitabine as second-line chemotherapy for non-small cell lung cancer. The European Lung Cancer Working Party. Lung Cancer 29:67–73, 2000.

98. Crino L, Mosconi AM, Scagliotti G, et al. Gemcitabine as second-line treatment for advanced non-small-cell lung cancer: a phase II trial. J Clin Oncol 17:2081–2085, 1999.

99. Barr F, Clinthorne HMD, Burris H. A phase II study of gemcitabine and vinorelbine salvage chemotherapy for taxane-resistant non-small cell lung cancer (NSCLC). Proc Am Soc Clin Oncol Abstract 496, ASCO 1999.

100. Shepherd FA, Dancey J, Ramlau R, et al. Prospective randomized trial of docetaxel versus best supportive care in patients with non-small-cell lung cancer previously treated with platinum-based chemotherapy. J Clin Oncol 18:2095–2103, 2000.

101. Fossella FV, DeVore R, Kerr RN, et al. Randomized phase III trial of docetaxel versus vinorelbine or ifosfamide in patients with advanced non-small-cell lung cancer previously treated with platinum-containing chemotherapy regimens. The TAX 320 Non-Small Cell Lung Cancer Study Group. J Clin Oncol 18:2354–2362, 2000.

102. Fossella FV. Pemetrexed for treatment of advanced non-small cell lung cancer. Semin Oncol 31:100–105, 2004.

103. Salgia R, Skarin AT. Molecular abnormalities in lung cancer. J Clin Oncol 16:1207–1217, 1998.

104. Dy GK, Adjei AA. Novel targets for lung cancer therapy: part II. J Clin Oncol 20:3016–3028, 2002.

105. Dy GK, Adjei AA. Novel targets for lung cancer therapy: part I. J Clin Oncol 20:2881–2894, 2002.

106. Kris MG, Natale RB, Herbst RS, et al. Efficacy of gefitinib, an inhibitor of the epidermal growth factor receptor tyrosine kinase, in symptomatic patients with non-small cell lung cancer: a randomized trial. JAMA 290:2149–2158, 2003.

107. Fukuoka M, Yano S, Giaccone G, et al. Multi-institutional randomized phase II trial of gefitinib for previously treated patients with advanced non-small-cell lung cancer. J Clin Oncol 21:2237–2246, 2003.

108. Shepherd FA, Pereira J, Ciuleanu TE. A randomized placebo-controlled trial of erlotinib in patients with advanced non-small cell

lung cancer (NSCLC) following failure of 1st-line or 2nd-line chemotherapy. A National Cancer Institute of Canada Clinical Trials Group (NCIC CTG) trial. Proc Am Soc Clin Oncol Abstract 7022, ASCO 2004.

109. Warde P, Payne D. Does thoracic irradiation improve survival and local control in limited-stage small-cell carcinoma of the lung? A meta-analysis. J Clin Oncol 10:890–895, 1992.

110. Pignon JP, Arriagada R, Ihde DC, et al. A meta-analysis of thoracic radiotherapy for small-cell lung cancer. N Engl J Med 327:1618–1624, 1992.

111. Perry MC, Herndon JE, 3rd, Eaton WL, et al. Thoracic radiation therapy added to chemotherapy for small-cell lung cancer: an update of Cancer and Leukemia Group B Study 8083. J Clin Oncol 16:2466–2467, 1998.

112. Murray N, Coy P, Pater JL, et al. Importance of timing for thoracic irradiation in the combined modality treatment of limited-stage small-cell lung cancer. The National Cancer Institute of Canada Clinical Trials Group. J Clin Oncol 11:336–344, 1993.

113. Gregor A, Drings P, Burghouts J, et al. Randomized trial of alternating versus sequential radiotherapy/chemotherapy in limited-disease patients with small-cell lung cancer: a European Organization for Research and Treatment of Cancer Lung Cancer Cooperative Group Study. J Clin Oncol 15:2840–2849, 1997.

114. Lebeau B, Urban T, Brechot JM, et al. A randomized clinical trial comparing concurrent and alternating thoracic irradiation for patients with limited small cell lung carcinoma. "Petites Cellules" Group. Cancer 86:1480–1487, 1999.

115. Work E, Nielsen OS, Bentzen SM, et al. Randomized study of initial versus late chest irradiation combined with chemotherapy in limited-stage small-cell lung cancer. Aarhus Lung Cancer Group. J Clin Oncol 15:3030–3037, 1997.

116. Tsukada H, Yokoyama A, Goto K, et al. Concurrent versus sequential radiotherapy for small cell lung cancer. Semin Oncol 28:23–26, 2001.

117. Skarlos DV, Samantas E, Briassoulis E, et al. Randomized comparison of early versus late hyperfractionated thoracic irradiation concurrently with chemotherapy in limited disease small-cell lung cancer: a randomized phase II study of the Hellenic Cooperative Oncology Group (HeCOG). Ann Oncol 12:1231–1238, 2001.

118. Jeremic B, Shibamoto Y, Acimovic L, et al. Initial versus delayed accelerated hyperfractionated radiation therapy and concurrent chemotherapy in limited small-cell lung cancer: a randomized study. J Clin Oncol 15:893–900, 1997.

119. Ellis PA, Talbot DC, Priest K, et al. Dose intensification of carboplatin and etoposide as first-line combination chemotherapy in small cell lung cancer. Eur J Cancer 31A:1888–1889, 1995.

120. Bishop JF, Raghavan D, Stuart-Harris R, et al. Carboplatin (CBDCA, JM-8) and VP-16–213 in previously untreated patients with small-cell lung cancer. J Clin Oncol 5:1574–1578, 1987.

121. Kosmidis PA, Samantas E, Fountzilas G, et al. Cisplatin/etoposide versus carboplatin/etoposide chemotherapy and irradiation in small cell lung cancer: a randomized phase III study. Hellenic Cooperative Oncology Group for Lung Cancer Trials. Semin Oncol 21:23–30, 1994.

122. Simon GR, Wagner H. Small cell lung cancer. Chest 123:259S–271S, 2003.

123. Fox W, Scadding JG. Medical Research Council comparative trial of surgery and radiotherapy for primary treatment of small-celled or oat-celled carcinoma of bronchus. Ten-year follow-up. Lancet 2:63–65, 1973.

124. Shields TW, Higgins GA Jr, Matthews MJ, et al. Surgical resection in the management of small cell carcinoma of the lung. J Thorac Cardiovasc Surg 84:481–488, 1982.

125. Chute JP, Chen T, Feigal E, et al. Twenty years of phase III trials for patients with extensive-stage small-cell lung cancer: perceptible progress. J Clin Oncol 17:1794–1801, 1999.

126. Pujol JL, Carestia L, Daures JP. Is there a case for cisplatin in the treatment of small-cell lung cancer? A meta-analysis of randomized trials of a cisplatin-containing regimen versus a regimen without this alkylating agent. Br J Cancer 83:8–15, 2000.

127. Noda K, Nishiwaki Y, Kawahara M, et al. Irinotecan plus cisplatin compared with etoposide plus cisplatin for extensive small-cell lung cancer. N Engl J Med 346:85–91, 2002.

128. Komaki R, Cox JD, Whitson W. Risk of brain metastasis from small cell carcinoma of the lung related to length of survival and prophylactic irradiation. Cancer Treat Rep 65:811–814, 1981.

129. Nugent JL, Bunn PA Jr, Matthews MJ, et al. CNS metastases in small cell bronchogenic carcinoma: increasing frequency and changing pattern with lengthening survival. Cancer 44:1885–1893, 1979.

130. Hirsch FR, Paulson OB, Hansen HH, et al. Intracranial metastases in small cell carcinoma of the lung: correlation of clinical and autopsy findings. Cancer 50:2433–2437, 1982.

131. Cox JD, Yesner RA. Adenocarcinoma of the lung: recent results from the Veterans Administration Lung Group. Am Rev Respir Dis 120:1025–1029, 1979.

132. Kurtz JM, Gelber R, Brady LW, et al. The palliation of brain metastases in a favorable patient population: a randomized clinical trial by the Radiation Therapy Oncology Group. Int J Radiat Oncol Biol Phys 7:891–895, 1981.

133. Sause WT, Crowley JJ, Morantz R, et al. Solitary brain metastasis: results of an RTOG/SWOG protocol evaluation surgery + RT versus RT alone. Am J Clin Oncol 13:427–432, 1990.

134. Auperin A, Arriagada R, Pignon JP, et al. Prophylactic cranial irradiation for patients with small-cell lung cancer in complete remission. Prophylactic Cranial Irradiation Overview Collaborative Group. N Engl J Med 341:476–484, 1999.

135. Arriagada R, Le Chevalier T, Borie F, et al. Prophylactic cranial irradiation for patients with small-cell lung cancer in complete remission. J Natl Cancer Inst 87:183–190, 1995.

136. Catane R, Schwade JG, Yarr I, et al. Follow-up neurological evaluation in patients with small cell lung carcinoma treated with prophylactic cranial irradiation and chemotherapy. Int J Radiat Oncol Biol Phys 7:105–109, 1981.

137. Frytak S, Shaw JN, O'Neill BP, et al. Leukoencephalopathy in small cell lung cancer patients receiving prophylactic cranial irradiation. Am J Clin Oncol 12:27–33, 1989.

138. Lee JS, Umsawasdi T, Lee YY, et al. Neurotoxicity in long-term survivors of small cell lung cancer. Int J Radiat Oncol Biol Phys 12:313–321, 1986.

139. Lishner M, Feld R, Payne DG, et al. Late neurological complications after prophylactic cranial irradiation in patients with small-cell lung cancer: the Toronto experience. J Clin Oncol 8:215–221, 1990.

140. Gregor A, Cull A, Stephens RJ, et al. Prophylactic cranial irradiation is indicated following complete response to induction therapy in small cell lung cancer: results of a multicentre randomised trial. United Kingdom Coordinating Committee for Cancer Research (UKCCCR) and the European Organization for Research and Treatment of Cancer (EORTC). Eur J Cancer 33:1752–1758, 1997.

141. Girling DJ. Comparison of oral etoposide and standard intravenous multidrug chemotherapy for small-cell lung cancer: a stopped multicentre randomised trial. Medical Research Council Lung Cancer Working Party. Lancet 348:563–566, 1996.

142. Shepherd FA, Amdemichael E, Evans WK, et al. Treatment of small cell lung cancer in the elderly. J Am Geriatr Soc 42:64–70, 1994.

143. Siu LL, Shepherd FA, Murray N, et al. Influence of age on the treatment of limited-stage small-cell lung cancer. J Clin Oncol 14:821–828, 1996.

144. Souhami RL, Spiro SG, Rudd RM, et al. Five-day oral etoposide treatment for advanced small-cell lung cancer: randomized comparison with intravenous chemotherapy. J Natl Cancer Inst 89: 577–580, 1997.

145. Westeel V, Murray N, Gelmon K, et al. New combination of the old drugs for elderly patients with small-cell lung cancer: a phase II study of the PAVE regimen. J Clin Oncol 16:1940–1947, 1998.

146. Steele JP. Gemcitabine/carboplatin versus cisplatin/etoposide for patients with poor-prognosis small cell lung cancer: a phase III randomized trial with quality-of-life evaluation. Semin Oncol 28: 15–18, 2001.

147. Murray N, Grafton C, Shah A, et al. Abbreviated treatment for elderly, infirm, or noncompliant patients with limited-stage small-cell lung cancer. J Clin Oncol 16:3323–3328, 1998.

148. Matsui K, Masuda N, Fukuoka M, et al. Phase II trial of carboplatin plus oral etoposide for elderly patients with small-cell lung cancer. Br J Cancer 77:1961–1965, 1998.

149. Van Houtte P, Danhier S, Mornex F. Toxicity of combined radiation and chemotherapy in non-small cell lung cancer. Lung Cancer 10 (Suppl 1):S271–280, 1994.

150. Machtay M, Friedberg JS. The role of radiation therapy in the management of non-small cell lung cancer. Semin Thorac Cardiovasc Surg 9:80–89, 1997.

151. Dragnev KH, Stover D, Dmitrovsky E. Lung cancer prevention: the guidelines. Chest 123:60S–71S, 2003.

152. Kelley MJ, McCrory DC. Prevention of lung cancer: summary of published evidence. Chest 123:50S–59S, 2003.

153. The effect of vitamin E and beta carotene on the incidence of lung cancer and other cancers in male smokers. The Alpha-Tocopherol, Beta Carotene Cancer Prevention Study Group. N Engl J Med 330:1029–1035, 1994.

154. Omenn GS, Goodman GE, Thornquist MD, et al. Effects of a combination of beta carotene and vitamin A on lung cancer and cardiovascular disease. N Engl J Med 334:1150–1155, 1996.

155. Lippman SM, Lee JJ, Karp DD, et al. Randomized phase III intergroup trial of isotretinoin to prevent second primary tumors in stage I non-small-cell lung cancer. J Natl Cancer Inst 93:605–618, 2001.

156. van Zandwijk N, Dalesio O, Pastorino U, et al. EUROSCAN, a randomized trial of vitamin A and N-acetylcysteine in patients with head and neck cancer or lung cancer. For the European Organization for Research and Treatment of Cancer Head and Neck and Lung Cancer Cooperative Groups. J Natl Cancer Inst 92:977–986, 2000.

157. Kennedy TC, Proudfoot SP, Franklin WA, et al. Cytopathological analysis of sputum in patients with airflow obstruction and significant smoking histories. Cancer Res 56:4673–4678, 1996.

Prostate Cancer

Carol Balmer

DEFINITION

Carcinoma of the prostate gland is a malignancy of the male genitourinary tract and the most common cancer in men in the United States.

TREATMENT CONSIDERATIONS

Prostate cancer is a disorder of older men. It usually is a slowly growing cancer, and in many men it never becomes clinically evident. Because of the age of patients at diagnosis and the characteristic slow growth of prostate cancer, it is much more common to die of other causes, with a diagnosis of prostate cancer, than to die directly from prostate cancer. This has led to much controversy about whether prostate cancer should be treated at all in patients with short life expectancy. Treatment decisions in prostate cancer, more than any other cancer, depend on the patient's age and medical condition. These factors combine to determine the treatment goals for patients with prostate cancer.

TREATMENT GOALS: PROSTATE CANCER

- Attempt curative interventions for patients with localized disease who have symptoms of prostate cancer or who are likely to live for more than 10 years after diagnosis.
- Avoid treatment interventions that increase morbidity without a corresponding increase in length or quality of life.
- Preserve sexual, bladder, and bowel function and quality of life.
- Relieve symptoms of localized and metastatic disease.
- Minimize the side effects of treatment.

EPIDEMIOLOGY

INCIDENCE

The estimated incidence of prostate cancer in 2005 is approximately 232,000 men in the United States. This figure represents 33% of new cancers in men. Prostate cancer is the most common cancer in men excluding nonmelanoma skin cancers, and it is also the most common cancer overall in the United States. About 30,350 deaths from prostate cancer occur each year, accounting for 10% of cancer deaths in men.[1] Only lung cancer is responsible for more cancer deaths.[1] The disparity between the number of men diagnosed with prostate cancer and the number who die from it each year, approximately a 7 to 1 ratio, supports some of the difficulties that are faced in making treatment decisions for individual patients, discussed later in this chapter.[2]

The incidence of prostate cancer has increased dramatically in the past 20 years (Table 100.1). This is likely due to a combination of factors: aging of the American population, improved screening tests that can detect prostate cancer long before it produces symptoms, and the impact of changes in dietary or other environmental factors. Current trends in incidence are expected to be sustained, because the first "baby boomers" are entering their 60s, the beginning of the age range during which prostate cancer is most typically diagnosed. However, advances in prostate cancer prevention may negate some of the projected increases.

In Table 100.1, note that the incidence of prostate cancer appeared to increase very rapidly during the late 1980s and early 1990s, more than doubling within a few years. During that time period, prostate-specific antigen (PSA) blood testing became widely used as a screening test for prostate cancer. This resulted in the diagnosis of prostate cancer in many thousands of men, most at an earlier age and earlier stage of disease than previously had been possible. It is likely that

TABLE 100.1	Incidence of Prostate Cancer and Prostate Cancer Deaths, Based on Annual Predictions	
Year	Incidence	Deaths
1984	76,000	25,000
1989	103,000	28,500
1991	122,000	32,000
1993	165,000	35,000
1995	244,000	40,400
1997	317,000	41,800
Adjustment	209,900	—
1999	179,300	37,000
2001	198,100	31,500
2003	220,900	28,900
2005	232,000	30,350

without PSA testing, most of these men would have remained undiagnosed for years or might never have been diagnosed.[1,2]

Despite the great changes in the incidence estimates for prostate cancer, the predicted number of deaths remained fairly stable for several years and now are decreasing. Decreasing death rates from prostate cancer are generally attributed to progress in treatment methods, and also to earlier detection that permits diagnosis of prostate cancer in earlier more curable stages. Before PSA testing became widespread, only about two thirds of men had clinically localized prostate cancer at diagnosis; now more than 95% of men are diagnosed before their cancer has spread. This "stage migration" has a strong impact on overall survival because the 5-year survival is now nearly 100% for men diagnosed with localized disease, and about 33% for those diagnosed with metastatic or distant disease.[1,2]

The wide discrepancy between prostate cancer incidence and mortality has raised questions about the clinical significance of early stage prostate cancer. It has fueled controversies about the need for widespread screening and the need to treat patients with early stage disease.

ETIOLOGY

Precise determination of the cause of prostate cancer in any individual is not yet possible, although research studies continue to contribute to the understanding of prostate cancer etiology. Some facts and associations are well established.

Effects of Age. Prostate cancer is a disease of older men, with the mean age at presentation about 70 years when diagnosed by the presence of symptoms. Use of PSA testing permits the diagnosis of prostate cancer several years before symptoms appear, effectively lowering the average age at diagnosis. Even with PSA testing, more than 70% of all prostate cancers are diagnosed after age 65.[1] During 1999 to 2001, the last period for which data are available, the probability of developing prostate cancer was about 1 in 10,000 for men less than 39 years of age, 1 in 39 for men aged 40 to 59, and 1 in 7 for those aged 60 to 79. The lifetime risk is estimated at 1 in every 6 men, or approximately 18%.[1]

Racial Factors. The risk of developing prostate cancer is affected by racial and environmental factors. The worldwide incidence is highest in North America and Western Europe, but low in Asia and in South America. African-American men and Jamaican men of African descent have the highest incidences of prostate cancer in the world.[1] In the United States, the incidence of prostate cancer in African-American men is about 50% higher than in white men. Prostate cancer is also diagnosed at a younger age in African-American men, and is more deadly in African-Americans than in white men. In contrast, Asian-American men develop prostate cancer at only half of the rate of whites.[1,3,4]

A variety of reasons have been proposed to account for the differences in prostate cancer incidence among African-American, white, and Asian-American men. Socioeconomic factors such as access to health care, attitudes about care, or education may play a role. Hormonal, dietary, and genetic differences are also believed to be significant. Testosterone levels, or more importantly, the levels of the enzyme 5-alpha reductase that converts testosterone to dihydrotestosterone (DHT), the active form in prostate cells, vary by ethnicity. Several genes involved in pathways that are relevant to prostate cancer biology have alleles that vary in frequency between white and African-American men.[4–6]

Family History. Family history is strongly associated with prostate cancer incidence. The magnitude of familial risk increases with the number of first-degree relatives who are affected, and also if the affected relative is diagnosed with prostate cancer at an early age. The risk of developing prostate cancer is doubled or tripled by having one first-degree relative with prostate cancer. With two or more relatives affected, the risk is increased by 5 to 11 times over men in the general population. Genetic changes may contribute to the increased risk associated with family history. True familial prostate cancer is believed to account for 5% to 10% of new cases, especially those diagnosed in men less than 50 years of age.[2,6]

The strongest risk factors for development of prostate cancer are age, ethnicity, and family history.

Dietary Factors. It is also very likely that dietary factors play an important role in prostate cancer risk. The strongest dietary association is with increased meat and animal fat intake. Prostate cancer risk has been inversely associated with several dietary components, including the essential non-metallic trace element selenium, lycopene (a component of tomato products), the antioxidant vitamin E (alpha-tocopherol), and 1,25-dihydroxyvitamin D.[6] High calcium intake has been correlated with increased prostate cancer risk in some studies, with a proposed mechanism of a calcium-mediated decrease in the formation of 1,25-dihydroxyvita-min D. However, a randomized trial of oral calcium supplementation showed no increase in the number of prostate cancer cases diagnosed during a 4-year period of supplementation, and suggested, instead, the possibility of a protective effect.[7]

Obesity. Obesity has been associated with poor outcomes in prostate cancer treatment, although the association with prostate cancer incidence is less strong. Two recent population-based case-control trials have failed to show a correlation between increasing body mass index (BMI) and prostate cancer risk. One study showed an inverse or protective relationship; that the risk of prostate cancer was less in men with higher BMIs.[8,9] Whether the impact of high fat diets and obesity are independent or interdependent in their impact on prostate cancer risk remains to be determined. It is clear that the interactions of dietary factors on prostate cancer risk are complex, but modification of diet may prove to be an effective means of reducing risk.

Gene expression. For prostate cancer to develop, a variety of genetic, hormonal, and environmental factors must alter the expression of specific genes. No single genetic change can account for cancer development, and no major susceptibility gene has yet been proven to be clinically significant for prostate cancer development. However, several chromosomal alterations are associated with an inherited predisposition to prostate cancer and/or prostate cancer development. Two prostate cancer susceptibility genes that have been identified are the *RNASEL* and *MSR1* genes, both of which are associated with response to infections. *RNASEL* encodes a ribonuclease that can induce apoptosis (programmed cell death) during viral infections of the prostate. *MSR1* is macrophage-scavenger receptor-1, and is involved with the function of macrophages found in the prostate gland during inflammation. The association with these genetic changes has fueled investigation of possible links between prostate infection or inflammation as potential triggers of carcinogenesis.

Loss of so called "caretaker genes" such as glutathione S-transferase pi-1 (*GSTP1*) may make the cell more susceptible to carcinogenic insults. *GSTP1* protects the genome against stress at sites of damage from carcinogens or from inflammation. Other genetic changes may modulate the expression or function of the androgen receptor (AR), or the progression of prostate cancer.[6] One of the best established genetic changes affecting the AR gene is the number of "CAG repeats." CAG is the trinucleotide sequence involving cytosine, adenine, and guanine. A lower number of CAG repeats is associated with increased risk of developing prostate cancer. Other chromosomal alterations may be important in prostate carcinogenesis, particularly loss or inactivation of tumor suppressor genes, such as phosphatase and tensin (PTEN) homologue deleted from chromosome 10, which normally prevent cancerous growth. Investigation of genetic determinants of prostate cancer susceptibility remains an important avenue for investigation.[10,11]

Miscellaneous Factors. Epidemiologic evidence in the past suggested a slightly higher risk for developing prostate cancer in men who had undergone vasectomy. The increase in risk has not been validated, and vasectomy is no longer considered to be a risk factor. Prostate cancer is not associated with tobacco smoking or alcohol intake. No occupational exposures have been convincingly linked with prostate cancer development, nor has presence of benign prostatic hypertrophy (BPH), the normal overgrowth of the prostate that occurs with age. Sexual activity is not associated with prostate cancer.[2,3,6]

PATHOPHYSIOLOGY

NORMAL ANATOMY

The prostate is a small, heart-shaped gland about an inch and a half in diameter. It is located at the base of the urinary bladder and completely surrounds the first inch of the ure-

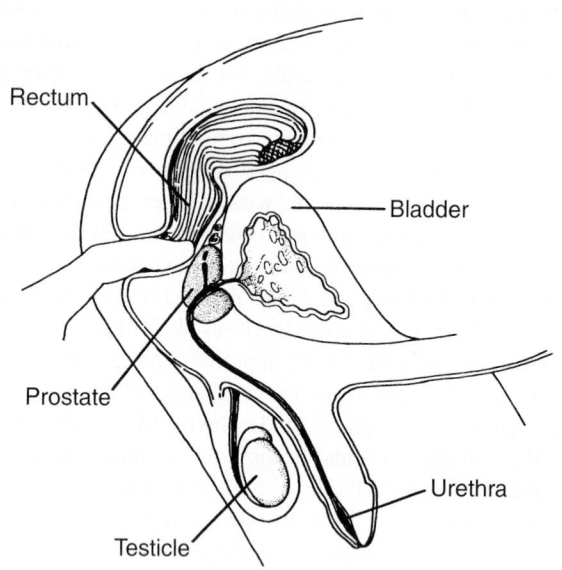

Rectum

Bladder

Prostate

Urethra

Testicle

FIGURE 100.1 Male anatomy and digital rectal exam.

TABLE 100.2	*Clinical Uses of Prostate-Specific Antigen Measurements*

Screening asymptomatic populations, in combination with digital rectal exam

Assessing clinical importance of biopsy-detected cancers

Assessing disease prognosis

Selecting appropriate candidates for expectant management

Assessing efficacy of radical prostatectomy or radiation therapy

Monitoring patients for disease recurrence after surgery or radiation

Determining timing for retreatment in intermittent ADT, or for treatment in deferred ADT

Evaluating objective response to ADT or chemotherapy

ADT, androgen deprivation therapy.

thra. It lies slightly above the rectum (Fig. 100.1). Anatomically, the prostate gland is divided into three zones: (a) transitional (surrounding the urethra), (b) central, and (c) peripheral. Most prostate cancers arise in the peripheral zone of the prostate, in the posterior lobe. The prostate gland is surrounded by a thin fibrous capsule and is composed primarily of glandular tissue. The cavernous nerves that control penile erection are contained in neurovascular bundles that lie in grooves along the surface of the prostate gland, just outside the fibrous capsule. The normal function of the prostate is the production of a milky secretion called prostatic fluid that adds to the volume of the ejaculate during sexual intercourse. Normal growth and also the growth of malignant prostate tissues are controlled by androgens. Although testosterone has some effect on prostate tissue, DHT formed from testosterone is the primary androgen that controls prostate cell growth and differentiation.[2,3,10]

PATHOLOGY

About 98% of prostate cancers arise from glandular tissues and are pathologically classified as adenocarcinomas. A precursor lesion, prostatic intraepithelial neoplasm (PIN) is typically detectable in the prostate for several years before invasive prostate cancer is detectable. Prostate cancers are graded pathologically by their degree of differentiation, that is, how much (well differentiated) or how little (poorly differentiated) they resemble normal prostate tissue. This grading has very important prognostic value because well-differentiated tumors tend to grow more slowly and behave less aggressively than poorly differentiated tumors. The most widely used pathology grading system is the Gleason grading system. In this system, cancers are assigned two scores based on the most dominant pathologic pattern, and on the next most dominant pattern. Each pattern is graded from 1 to 5. Gland sections assigned grades of 1 must have closely

packed, single, separate uniform glands; grades of 5 represent tissue with few or no visible glands, but with masses or sheets of tumor cells. The two scores are added to make a total grading score from 2 (very well differentiated) to 10, which indicates a very poorly differentiated carcinoma.[3,10] Most prostate cancers are graded as intermediate (Gleason grade 5–7), 11% are well differentiated (Gleason grade 2–4), and only 4% are poorly differentiated (Gleason grade 8–10).[12]

Normal and malignant prostate tissues produce PSA, a glycoprotein with serine protease activity. Because PSA is produced exclusively by prostatic tissue and circulates in the blood, it has become an important tumor marker for prostate tissue growth. However, PSA is produced by normal and hypertrophied prostate tissue (BPH) and malignant tissue, so it is not a specific marker for prostate cancer. PSA levels are somewhat quantitative, and very generally correlate with the volume of prostate tissue present in the body. Prostate cancer cells generally produce more PSA than do nonmalignant prostate cells. However, poorly differentiated prostate tumors may have lost the ability to produce PSA. In this case, even patients with high tumor burdens may have low PSA levels. The absolute PSA level and the rate of increase (PSA velocity), reflect the activity of the prostate tissue growth process. PSA has many roles in prostate cancer screening, diagnosis, monitoring, and management (Table 100.2). Unfortunately, the correlations of PSA with objective tumor responses are not completely consistent. Because of this, PSA can only be considered a surrogate marker of tumor response. More definitive markers such as clinical benefit, survival, and shrinkage of soft tissue masses should be used to evaluate treatment efficacy when available.[3,13]

CLINICAL PRESENTATION AND DIAGNOSIS

Prostate cancer is usually a slow-growing cancer with a long doubling time that may exceed 2 years. Although most prostate cancers grow slowly, if it does become clinically active, the cancer will progress relentlessly in the absence of treatment and eventually will threaten the patient's life.

Prostate cancer always begins in the prostate gland. It can spread locally by direct extension, penetrating the fibrous prostate capsule to invade adjacent structures such as the seminal vesicles and bladder wall. The most serious sequelae of local spread is urinary obstruction, which can result from compression of the urethra or the bladder neck.

Prostate cancer may also spread through the lymphatic system or through the blood. Blood-borne metastatic spread carries prostate cancer cells primarily to the bones, the most common site of metastases. The bones that are located near the prostate, that is, those of the lower spine, pelvis, and proximal femurs, are the most common early sites of bony spread, although prostate cancer typically affects many bones in its advanced stages. Bone metastases are typically osteoblastic (tumor that builds onto bone) or a combination of osteoblastic and osteolytic (bone dissolving) lesions. Osteoblastic tumor masses that grow on spinal bones may compress the spinal cord. Resulting spinal cord compression can produce lower extremity weakness or paralysis, or loss of bowel or bladder control. Other metastatic sites of spread are lungs, liver, and soft tissue, especially pelvic lymph nodes.[3]

SIGNS AND SYMPTOMS

The anatomy and natural history of prostate cancer account for its presenting signs and symptoms. Prostate cancer usually is asymptomatic in its early stages because tumor growth within the prostate is small at first and is usually located near the periphery of the gland. Larger tumor masses may produce urinary obstructive symptoms. Because the prostate physically surrounds the urethra, overgrowth of prostate tissue can compress the urethra and compromise urine flow. Because most prostate cancers grow in the outer areas of the prostate, urinary obstructive symptoms are much less commonly caused by prostate cancer than by noncancerous overgrowth of prostate tissue, or BPH, in which the tissue overgrowth typically is in the central area of the prostate gland. However, when obstructive symptoms result from prostate cancer, they are indistinguishable from symptoms produced by BPH. Symptoms include difficulty in initiating the urine stream, urgency, frequency, nocturia, dribbling, and incomplete bladder emptying.[2,3]

Prostate cancer may spread before it produces serious local symptoms. The presenting symptoms of metastatic diseases usually result from spread to the bones, particularly low back pain. Prostate cancer is so common that evaluating unexplained low back pain in men older than 50 years should include a PSA measurement. In patients with advanced metastatic disease, the presenting symptoms may be those of spinal cord compression. Prostate cancer in these patients must be treated as a medical emergency. Anemia, weakness, or weight loss may also be presenting signs of advanced disease. Fortunately, with improved techniques for early de-

tection of prostate cancer, currently less than 10% of men have metastatic prostate cancer at diagnosis.[1,2]

SCREENING

Cancer screening refers to testing asymptomatic people who are at risk for a specific cancer. Because prostate cancer usually is asymptomatic in its early and most curable stages, significant public health efforts have been devoted to widespread screening of populations at risk. However, despite the lifesaving potential of prostate cancer screening, whether men should be screened for prostate cancer is controversial.

Some of the controversy can be explained by the natural history of prostate cancer. One of the most unusual features of prostate cancer, and one that still is not fully understood, is that the histologic prevalence of prostate cancer is much greater than its clinical incidence. Autopsy series evaluating prostates from men who died of unrelated causes have demonstrated microscopic cancer in about 30% of men over age 50 and in 67% of men in their 80s. These figures represent more than 10 million men in the United States who have cancer foci physically present in their prostate glands. In contrast, the 232,000 new patients diagnosed in 2005 represent only about 2% of these men. Most histologically detectable cancers do not progress within the lifetime of the host and are called latent or clinically unimportant cancers. Those that threaten the life or well-being of the host are called clinically important. One of the most important challenges in effective prostate cancer control and screening is to find objective criteria to distinguish between these two forms of prostate cancer.[2,14,15]

The foundation of the controversy about widespread screening programs for asymptomatic men is that most prostate cancers that are detected by screening are likely to remain latent and will never cause clinical symptoms during that person's lifetime. Because of the advanced age of most patients with prostate cancer, even those in whom the disease becomes clinically evident are statistically more likely to die of causes other than prostate cancer. The argument continues that diagnosing a patient with prostate cancer may lead to costly treatments that may be unnecessary in that patient but produce well-defined morbidity. Opponents of screening say that this violates the medical principle to "do no harm." Supporters of screening programs argue that PSA screening programs have resulted in an increase in the proportion of men who are diagnosed with localized, curable cancers rather than late-stage metastatic disease, and have also resulted in an increase in the proportion of well-differentiated cancers that are diagnosed. There is also some evidence that the screening tests used, PSA and digital rectal exam (DRE) have limited use in detecting latent cancers. Most cancers detected by screening programs have proved to be clinically important in follow-up and probably would have progressed if left untreated. In this context, widespread screening, particularly of younger patients with a greater than 10-year life expectancy, is seen as an ethical and economical public health initiative because treating early-stage disease is less costly than treating advanced disease. To reduce prostate cancer mortality, men who are most likely to suffer with and die from prostate cancer must be diagnosed and treated.[14,15]

Until the value, or lack of value, of widespread screening for prostate cancer can be objectively determined from the outcomes of large prospective randomized trials, a conservative approach to screening is recommended by the American Cancer Society. They recommend that annual PSA testing and DRE should be offered to men, beginning at age 50, who have a life expectancy of at least 10 years. Testing should be offered beginning at age 45 for men who are at high risk for developing prostate cancer. This includes all African-American men and men with strong family histories of prostate cancer. Men should receive information about the potential benefits and limitations of early detection and treatment, so that each man can make an informed decision about whether or not to be tested.[1]

Newer refinements of PSA measurements continue to add to the specificity and clinical utility of PSA testing. Examples are PSA velocity, which indicates the rate of rise of PSA from year to year, PSA density, which compensates for the size of the prostate gland, use of age-specific values (Table 100.3), comparisons of free and total forms of PSA, and measurement of membrane-bound forms of PSA.[14,16]

DIAGNOSIS

The tests most widely used in screening, PSA and DRE, are also cornerstone tests for prostate cancer diagnosis. Although PSA testing is not specific for prostate cancer, it is the single most accurate method for prostate cancer detection. Patients with PSA levels greater than 4 ng per milliliter, or greater than age-specific values listed in Table 100.3, should be evaluated with DRE. Because most prostate cancers arise in the posterior lobe of the prostate, which can be palpated through the rectal wall (Fig. 100.1), DRE has long been a clinically useful diagnostic tool. Prostate cancers are felt as hard nodules in the otherwise rubbery glandular tissue. DRE

may also detect extension of cancerous growth into tissues adjacent to the prostate. Suspicious or equivocal results after PSA and DRE are evaluated further using transrectal ultrasound (TRUS), which can visualize prostate size, nodules, and invasion of periprostatic tissues.[3]

TRUS is also used to guide prostate biopsy, the definitive diagnostic test. Current standards of practice for prostate biopsy use high-speed, spring-loaded, gun-like biopsy devices to take needle biopsy samples of the prostate through the rectal wall. At least six needle cores of tissue, distributed throughout the gland, usually are taken. Use of high-speed biopsy devices has made this an outpatient procedure with little discomfort and very low morbidity, and has increased the reliability of tissue sampling. Repeat biopsies are recommended when initial biopsies fail to show tumor in the presence of a palpable mass.[16]

STAGING

Once prostate cancer has been detected, the Gleason grade, PSA, and clinical stage are assessed and used as indicators of prognosis. A variety of molecular and genetic indicators are under evaluation to assist with clinical decision-making. A limited metastatic workup, including bone scan, chest radiograph, and liver function tests, is also performed to assess extent and stage of disease. Pelvic imaging studies to evaluate lymph node involvement may be performed but do not reliably detect small lymph nodes.

Two staging systems for prostate cancer are in widespread use and have important prognostic significance. They are outlined in Table 100.4. The American Urologic Association Whitmore-Jewett staging system, which uses an A, B, C, D classification, is still used, but is being replaced in clinical practice with the tumor, node, and metastasis (TNM) staging system. This system stages prostate cancer based on the size of the primary tumor (T), lymph node involvement (N), and presence or absence of distant metastases (M). Patients are grouped into stages I to IV based on their TNM classifications. It is a much more precise system than the A, B, C, D classification, and it permits development of more accurate prognostic information for individual patients. The TNM system also includes classifications for cancer that is diagnosed only by PSA testing, and for PIN, a precursor to prostate cancer.[17] Survival of patients with prostate cancer is closely tied to stage of disease. Fortunately, most men are now diagnosed with localized rather than advanced disease.[2]

TABLE 100.3	Guide to Interpreting Prostate-Specific Antigen (PSA) Values
Value (ng/mL)[a]	**Interpretation**
0–4	Normal range, age nonspecific
0–2.5	Age-specific normal range, ages 40–49
0–3.5	Age-specific normal range, ages 50–59
0–4.5	Age-specific normal range, ages 60–69
0–6.5	Age-specific normal range, ages 70–79
4–10	Overlap area of BPH and prostate cancer
>10	High likelihood of prostate cancer
<0.2	Expected level after radical prostatectomy or radiation

[a] Hybritech Tandem assay.
BPH, benign prostatic hypertrophy.

PSYCHOSOCIAL ASPECTS

Psychosocial issues are important in prostate cancer screening and treatment decisions. Until the mid-1980s prostate cancer was poorly addressed in the United States. Perhaps because of the close association of prostate function and male sexual performance, many men were unwilling to discuss prostate function or to undergo the rectal examinations needed for screening. As a result of focussed public educa-

TABLE 100.4	Staging Classification Systems for Prostate Cancer			
AUA	**Description**		**TNM**	**Description**
			TX	Primary tumor cannot be assessed.
			T_0	No evidence of primary tumor.
A	No palpable tumor.		T_1	Clinically inapparent tumor, not palpable or visible by imaging.
A_1	Focal.		T_{1a}	5% or less of tissue.
A_2	Diffuse.		T_{1b}	More than 5% of tissue.
			T_{1c}	Tumor identified by needle biopsy because of elevated prostate-specific antigen.
B	Confined to prostate.		T_2	Tumor confined within the prostate but detectable clinically.
B_1	Small, discrete nodule.		T_{2a}	Tumor involves half of a lobe or less.
B_2	Large or multiple nodules.		T_{2b}	Tumor involves more than half of a lobe but not both lobes.
			T_{2c}	Tumor involves both lobes.
C	Localized to periprostatic area.		T_3	Tumor extends through capsule.
C_1	No involvement of seminal vesicles.		T_{3a}	Extracapsular extension on one side.
			T_{3b}	Extracapsular extension on both sides.
C_2	Involvement of seminal vesicles.		T_{3c}	Tumor invades seminal vesicles.
			T_4	Tumor fixed or invades adjacent structures other than those listed in T_3.
D	Metastatic disease.		N_1	Metastasis in a single lymph node, ≤ 2 cm.
D_1	Pelvic lymph node metastases.		N_2	Metastasis in single lymph node, >2 cm but <5 cm, or multiple lymph nodes none >5 cm.
			N_3	Metastasis in lymph node >5 cm.
D_2	Metastases to bone or distant lymph nodes or other organs.		M_1	Distant metastases.

AUA, American Urologic Association; TNM, tumor, node, and metastasis.
(From Anonymous. Genitourinary sites. In: Greene FL, Page DL, Fleming ID, eds. AJCC cancer staging manual. 6th ed. New York: Springer, 2002:309–316, with permission.)

tion and public awareness efforts, the willingness of men to undergo prostate cancer testing and treatment has increased. Today, most older men know their PSA value, as they may know their blood pressure or lipid levels, and talk freely about prostate cancer issues.

There are other important psychosocial considerations. Prostate cancer can significantly shorten lifespan. Although treatments for localized prostate cancer continue to improve, as recently as the 1990s, men with clinically localized prostate cancer, the most favorable form, lost an estimated 33%

of their remaining life expectancy.[18] The life expectancy of men with advanced prostate cancer is even more severely compromised. Most of this time sacrificed to prostate cancer occurs during the typical retirement years, the time during which most men plan to enjoy life. Treatments for prostate cancer commonly produce impotence, incontinence, feminization, bone density loss, and weakness, and can discourage men from selecting the most effective or potentially curative treatments. It is important that public education issues be continued, targeted at populations at highest risk for prostate cancer and those most likely to benefit from early treatment.[19]

THERAPEUTIC PLAN

Prostate cancer treatment has been outlined by health care organizations. Two algorithms are presented: (a) treating patients with clinically localized disease (Fig. 100.2) and treating patients with advanced disease (Fig. 100.3).[2,3,20]

TREATMENT

CLINICALLY LOCALIZED DISEASE

There are several primary treatment options for cancer that is clinically localized to the prostate gland (stages I and II or A and B): surgery, radiation therapy with or without androgen deprivation therapy (ADT), cryotherapy, or close observation without treatment.

Surgery. The standard of treatment is radical prostatectomy, or surgical removal of the prostate gland, plus pelvic lymph node dissection. This procedure offers the best chance to eradicate cancer that is confined to the prostate. PSA levels decline rapidly to undetectable levels (<0.2 ng/mL) after successful removal of all prostatic tissue with this surgery. PSA nadir levels are reached within 6 weeks. Survival at 15 years is approximately 90%. Radical prostatectomy has been technically improved in recent years, but it still entails significant risks of morbidity and related mortality up to 1%. The most common complications are impotence, with an incidence of 40% to 60% or greater, and some degree of urinary incontinence (2%–10%).[21,22]

Impotence was nearly universal with early radical prostatectomy techniques. The cavernous neurovascular bundles that carry the innervation for erectile control run in channels along each side of the prostate gland. Using the standard radical prostatectomy technique, the neurovascular bundles are removed with the prostate. Nerve-sparing surgical techniques can preserve one or both neurovascular bundles and are feasible when the cancer does not involve these structures. Return of erections sufficient for penetration and intercourse depends on the patient's age, extent of tumor, and their erectile capability before surgery. Best success is achieved when both neurovascular bundles are preserved in younger men with good erectile function before surgery.[21–23] Potency lost from the effects of surgery, and from other prostate cancer treatments, may be restored pharmacologically with oral phosphodiesterase-5 inhibitors such as sildenafil.[24]

Urinary incontinence is a less common but also very troublesome consequence of radical prostatectomy. The section of the urethra that passes through the prostate is removed during surgery, and the urinary sphincter muscles at the base of the bladder are damaged. Continence tends to improve gradually over time and is dependent on the surgical technique and the surgeon's experience. In large controlled series, 90% to 98% of men recover normal urinary continence or report only stress-induced spotting within 2 years after surgery. The remainder need pads to keep their outer garments dry or are totally incontinent.[2,21–23] Urinary incontinence can be treated with pelvic floor muscle exercises, anticholinergic or α-adrenergic agonists, antiincontinence clamps, injection of sphincter bulking devices, or with artificial sphincters. Other surgical complications include blood loss, urethral stricture, rectal injury, thromboembolism, and wound infection. Surgery-related death occurs in less than 1% of patients in controlled series.[21,22]

Complication rates are expected to be reduced by the increasingly widespread application of laparoscopic "key-

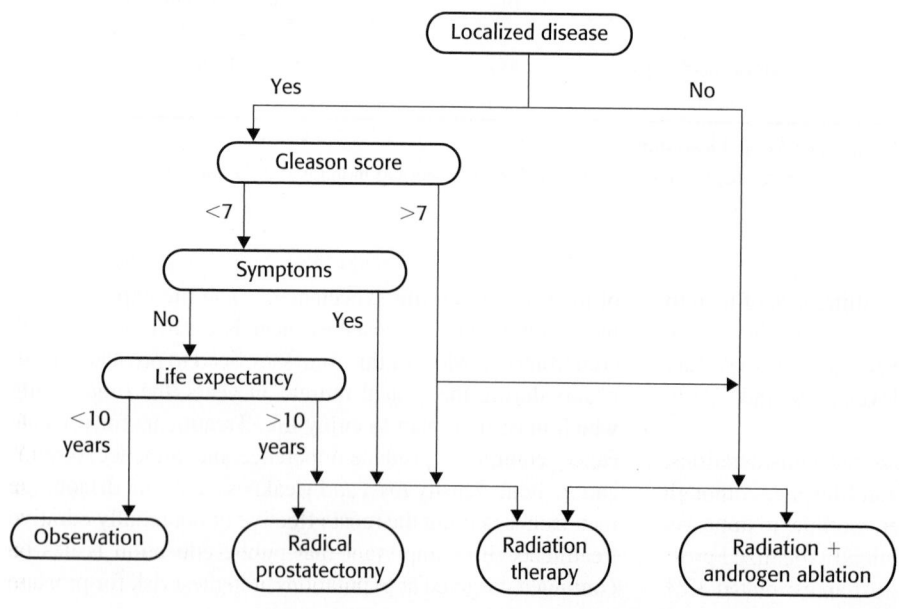

FIGURE 100.2 Treatment algorithm for patients with localized prostate cancer.

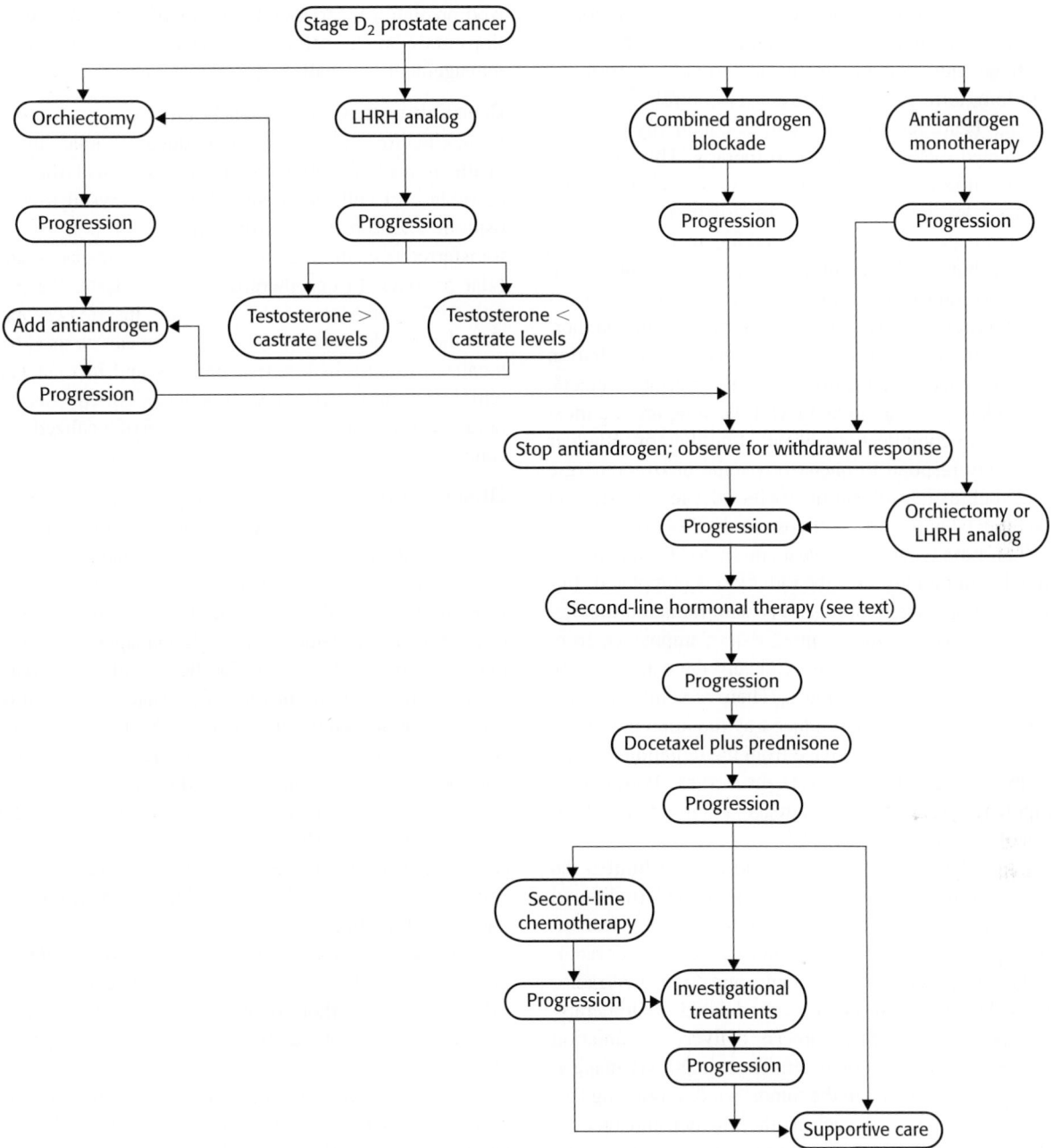

FIGURE 100.3 Treatment algorithm for patients with advanced disease.

hole'' techniques for radical prostatectomy. Surgery is performed through small incisions rather than the traditional open technique. The results of large, randomized controlled trials are needed to provide true evidence-based comparison of the effectiveness and acute and chronic complications of laparoscopic prostatectomy compared with traditional surgical approaches.[25]

Radiation. Destruction of the prostate with radiation therapy is an alternative to radical prostatectomy. Radiation may be accomplished by external beam irradiation that uses high-energy photon beams produced from linear accelerators, or by permanent implantation of seeds of radioactive sub-

stances (Iodine-125 or Palladium-103). Use of implanted sources of radiation is called interstitial radiation or brachytherapy.[3,23]

Until the last decade, radiation therapy was reserved for men with localized prostate cancer who were not good surgical candidates because of advanced age or concomitant health problems, because long-term cancer control with radiation was inferior to what could be achieved with surgery. However, improved radiation therapy techniques permitting higher radiation doses, combinations of external beam and implanted radiation techniques, and the use of hormonal therapies with radiation in selected patients has improved the effectiveness of radiation therapy. Using contemporary techniques and higher doses, radiation therapy has been proven to be equivalent in effectiveness to radical prostatectomy in long-term local prostate cancer control.[2,23]

External beam radiation is the most commonly used and best evaluated method of radiation therapy. This generally entails radiation therapy sessions 5 days a week for 7 to 8 weeks. PSA levels drop much more slowly after radiation therapy than after surgery, often taking many months to reach nadir, but usually are ultimately reduced to undetectable levels. Administering androgen deprivation therapy (discussed later) before and during external beam radiation therapy results in higher disease-free survival than radiation alone in patients with locally advanced prostate cancers. Rectal or bladder irritation and rectal bleeding are the most common acute complications of radiation therapy. Bladder irritation may respond to phenazopyridine or α-adrenergic blockers such as tamsulosin hydrochloride; rectal irritation may be relieved with rectal corticosteroids. Proctitis or cystitis persist for many months or years in 3% to 8% of patients, and may begin months after the radiation is completed. Impotence develops much more slowly with radiation therapy than with surgery, but the eventual risk of impotence from external beam radiation is approximately the same as with nerve-sparing surgical techniques. There is some evidence that the sexual dysfunction produced by radiation therapy is the result of blood vessel damage from the radiation therapy rather than damage to the cavernous nerves. Fortunately, the impotence from radiation damage usually responds to pharmacologic management.[2,23,26]

Radiation damage to the rectum and bladder limited the dose of radiation that could be administered with traditional radiation therapy techniques, and also limited the effectiveness of radiation in destroying prostate cancer. Newer radiation techniques, such as three-dimensional conformal radiotherapy (3D-CRT) and intensity-modulated radiotherapy (IMRT), permit much more precise delivery of radiation doses to the prostate tumor itself. These methods make it possible to increase doses to the tumor, while producing less damage to nearby organs such as the bladder and rectum. Use of higher radiation doses using these methods has made radiation therapy comparable in effectiveness to radical prostatectomy, in terms of cure rates.[23,26]

Brachytherapy, also called ''interstitial'' or ''implanted radiation therapy,'' delivers a high dose of radiation directly to the prostate with relative sparing of nearby normal tissue. The greatest advantage of radiation implants over external beam radiation techniques is that the radiation procedure is accomplished as a 1-day outpatient procedure rather than with weeks of daily radiation therapy visits. Improved techniques for identifying the optimal location for implantation of the radioactive seeds have improved the efficacy of brachytherapy and reduced its toxicity, by minimizing the radiation dose delivered to surrounding tissues. With current techniques, brachytherapy is considered comparable to external beam radiation for management of patients with local-

ized prostate cancer. Combinations of external beam radiation and brachytherapy are also used effectively for management of localized prostate cancer.[23,26]

Cryoablation. Cryoablation is the process of destroying tissues by freezing. Freezing produces cellular injury and death by a combination of direct mechanical shock (such as rupture of cell membranes from ice crystal formation), osmotic shock resulting from cell dehydration as water is transferred from intracellular to extracellular spaces, and cellular hypoxia. In cryotherapy of the prostate, the prostate tissue is frozen by means of perineally inserted cryoprobes. Cryotherapy destruction of the prostate can be used to treat localized tumors in low-risk patients and to treat patients with local tumor recurrence. It is not as effective as surgery or radiation therapy in long-term control of localized prostate cancer.[2]

Observation. The fourth modality for management of patients with localized prostate cancer is observation, also called ''watchful waiting,'' ''expectant management,'' and ''active surveillance.'' This has been a much-debated issue. Prostate cancer is the only curable cancer in which a lack of treatment is considered a viable management option for many patients. The rationale for the lack of active treatment is based on the natural history of prostate cancer and on the average age of patients at diagnosis. Prostate cancer usually is slow-growing and occurs late in life, so that many men diagnosed with prostate cancer die of unrelated causes, whether or not their cancer is treated. Treating localized prostate cancer is costly and can result in long-term complications such as impotence, incontinence, and rectal pain that compromise quality of life. Yet 30,000 men still die of this painful, debilitating disease each year. Clearly the difficulty lies in accurate patient selection, to be able to determine prospectively which patients with prostate cancer can be safely observed without treatment, and which patients must be treated to prevent the prostate cancer from compromising their life expectancy.[2,27-29]

Observation with careful follow-up is considered an appropriate decision choice for men who have a life-expectancy of less than 10 years and who have low-grade, localized prostate cancers. With this combination of factors, it is unlikely that the cancer will become clinically active and result in the patient's death before he dies of other causes.[2,3,28] It is not a recommended option for all men. The risk of progression to metastatic disease is significantly greater in men with localized prostate cancer who are managed with observation than in those managed with surgery.[27] Younger men with a longer projected period of risk should be offered potentially curative treatment. Men who elect to forego surgery, radiation, or cryotherapy should have active surveillance. They should be monitored closely using the PSA doubling time (PSADT), an indicator of the rate of rise of the man's PSA. If a patient's PSADT is short in comparison to his life expectancy, prostate biopsy should be performed and definitive treatment should be offered if indicated.[28] Prostate cancer progression rates do not increase after 15 years in men managed with observation.[29]

In summary, patients with localized prostate cancer have several treatment options:

- Radical prostatectomy is the most effective local therapy, but carries significant risks of impotence and incontinence.
- External beam radiation is equivalent to surgery when higher doses are used.
- Radiation produces slower PSA responses and entails 6 to 8 weeks of daily treatment.
- Interstitial radiation with implanted radioisotope seeds produces results comparable to those of external beam radiation in men with low-risk prostate cancer. The implantation is a 1-day outpatient procedure.
- Prostate cryotherapy is not as effective as surgery and radiation therapy, but appears to produce acceptable results in men with low-risk disease.
- Observation is a feasible option in men with low-grade, well-localized tumors who have a life expectancy of less than 10 years. Careful follow-up is needed.

LOCALLY ADVANCED DISEASE

It is unlikely that patients with prostate cancer that has penetrated the prostate capsule and spread locally (Stage C or III disease) will be cured by radical prostatectomy or radiation therapy. Most of these patients have clinically undetectable micrometastases at the time of diagnosis that eventually cause disease recurrence.

External beam radiation therapy is the most commonly used treatment for patients with locally advanced prostate cancer. However, as a single therapy it is limited in its ability to provide long-term control of locally extensive prostate cancer. Neoadjuvant hormonal therapy, administered before and during radiation therapy to decrease the size of the cancerous prostate, decreases the local prostate cancer recurrence rate and results in longer disease-free survival over radiation therapy alone.[30,31] Continuation of hormonal therapy after completion of radiation therapy provides additional survival benefit and has been shown to improve overall survival.[32] However, addition of hormonal therapy increases the risk of late rectal toxicity from radiation therapy.[32,33] Long-term administration after completion of radiation therapy is more accurately termed adjuvant rather than neoadjuvant therapy. The administration of cytotoxic chemotherapy in combination with radiation therapy is under investigation.[34] Hormonal therapy and cytotoxic chemotherapy are discussed more fully below.

METASTATIC DISEASE

Hormonal therapy is the cornerstone of metastatic prostate cancer treatment. Prostate tissue growth is fed by androgens, the male sex hormones. This applies to normal prostate tissue, to BPH, and to prostate cancers, although the androgen sensitivity of individual cells or cell clones within a tumor mass may vary. Prostate cancer masses are heterogeneous; that is, all of the cells are not identical. Some are hormone dependent. These cells die when androgenic hormones are withdrawn. Hormone-sensitive cells stop growing until resupplied with androgen. Some prostate cancer cells are hormonally independent and are unaffected by the presence or absence of androgen.[35,36]

The goal of all hormonal interventions for prostate cancer management is androgen deprivation, sometimes called androgen ablation. Both terms refer to eliminating the stimulatory effects of male hormones from prostate cancer cells. There are many ways to accomplish this goal (Table 100.5). To put androgen deprivation interventions in context, it is necessary to review the normal regulation of male hormone secretion.[2,35–37] These relationships are illustrated in Figure 100.4.

Testosterone is the primary androgen. About 95% of circulating androgens are produced by the testes; the balance is produced by the adrenal glands.[2] This proportion varies from patient to patient, and in some patients the adrenal gland is a very important source of androgens. Androgen production is regulated by a negative feedback system that includes the hypothalamus and the pituitary, in addition to the testes and adrenal glands.[35–37]

Secretion of testosterone by the testes is regulated in the brain. The hypothalamus acts as a sensor that registers changes in circulating levels of hormones. When it detects low levels of testosterone, the hypothalamus secretes luteinizing hormone-releasing hormone (LHRH). This is also called gonadotropin-releasing hormone (GnRH). Under the stimulation of LHRH, the pituitary gland secretes luteinizing hormone (LH), a gonadotropin. LH stimulates the Leydig cells of the testes to secrete testosterone. A similar feedback loop controls steroid hormone production in the adrenal glands. The adrenals cannot produce testosterone directly but produce androgenic precursors that can be enzymatically converted to testosterone in many peripheral tissues.[2,35,36]

Testosterone is the main circulating androgen, but within the prostate, it is transformed into DHT by 5-α reductase. Although testosterone and DHT can stimulate the same ARs in the prostate, DHT has more than twice the affinity of testosterone for these receptors. DHT's actions within prostate cells are believed to be similar to those of other steroid hormones: DHT binds to specific receptors in the cytoplasm and is transferred to the nucleus, where the hormone-induced effects on gene transcription ultimately result in the synthesis of proteins that produce the hormone's biologic effects.[35,36]

Guidelines for Hormonal Therapy. Hormonal interventions for prostate cancer control are possible at every site in the hypothalamic-pituitary-gonadal-adrenal axis, at the point of conversion of testosterone to DHT, and at the hormone receptor level. Interventions differ in their mechanisms, advantages, and disadvantages, but some general guidelines apply broadly to their application in the treatment of prostate cancer.[2,3,35–38]

TABLE 100.5	Hormonal Agents for Managing Prostate Cancer		
Classification	**Drug Name**	**Usual Dosing**	**Monitoring Parameters**
Antiandrogens	Bicalutamide	50 mg PO/day	Monitor LFTs (first 2 months of therapy); diarrhea, gynecomastia
	Flutamide	250 mg PO q8h	Same as bicalutamide
Adrenal enzyme inhibitors	Aminoglutethimide	250 mg PO 4 × daily	Rash, sedation, somnolence or lethargy, steroid replacement with dexamethasone needed, drug interactions.
	Ketoconazole	400 mg q8h	Nausea and vomiting, monitor LFTs, gynecomastia, may need corticosteroid replacement therapy, caution: drug interactions.
Corticosteroids	Prednisone	5–10 mg/day	Fluid retention, impaired glucose control, mood changes, gastrointestinal bleeding, opportunistic infections.
LHRH agonists	Goserelin	3.6 mg/28 days SC[a]	Flare reactions first 1–2 weeks, hot flashes, anemia, osteoporosis, impotence.
	Leuprolide	7.5 mg/month. SC, IM, and implanted formulations[a]	Same as goserelin.
	Triptorelin	3.75 mg/28 days IM[a]	Same as goserelin.
LHRH Antagonist	Abarelix	100 mg/28 days SC[b]	Hypersensitivity reactions, other side effects as LHRH agonists with exception of flare reactions (do not occur with abarelix).
Progestins	Megestrol	160 mg PO/day in 2–4 divided doses	Weight gain, impaired glucose control, fluid retention.

[a] Depot formulations for multiple-month (3- and/or 4-month) dosing are available. Leuprolide implanted formulation is replaced yearly.
[b] Give additional dose on day 15 of first month of treatment.
Disease response is monitored in all patients by prostate-specific antigen measurements, pain and other symptoms, bone scans, and radiographic studies of soft tissue masses if present. Impotence is common from androgen ablative therapies. Usual doses and specific monitoring parameters are noted in the table, but should not be considered a guide for dosing. Check individual product information provided by manufacturer. PO, by mouth; LFTs, liver function tests; SC, subcutaneously; IM, intramuscularly; LHRH, luteinizing hormone-releasing hormone.

■ The goal of all hormonal therapy for prostate cancer is androgen deprivation, to eliminate the growth stimulatory effects of androgens.

■ About 85% of patients with metastatic prostate cancer have an objective or subjective response (relief of symptoms) to first-line hormonal therapy.

■ With a few qualifications, all of these hormonal interventions are effective and have comparable response rates.

■ Choice of ADT depends on patient and physician preference, cost considerations, concomitant medical conditions, and rapidity of response needed.

■ ADT is palliative. It does not cure patients with prostate cancer, although disease-free survival is lengthened. ADT produces small improvements in overall survival.

■ The average duration of response to first-line ADT is 1 to 2 years if the patient already has symptoms when hormonal therapy is started. If treatment is started based on increasing PSA blood levels in the absence of symptoms, response times are longer. This probably reflects "lead time bias."

■ The likelihood of response, and the duration of response decrease with successive ADT interventions.

■ ADTs all produce symptoms of the androgen deprivation syndrome to varying degrees. Common symptoms include impotence, loss of libido, hot flashes, fatigue, anemia, loss of bone and muscle mass, and weight gain. Some produce feminizing effects such as gynecomastia and loss of male-distributed body hair.

First-line Androgen Deprivation Therapies

Orchiectomy. Huggins et al[39] were the first investigators to recognize the hormonal dependence of prostate cancer in the early 1940s and to treat it with an ADT. They noted dramatic improvement in prostate cancer patients after surgical removal of the patients' testes, or castration. More than 6 decades later, surgical removal of the testes, now called orchiectomy, remains the standard against which other hormonal therapies are evaluated. It is still a widely used first-line treatment for metastatic prostate cancer. The external location of the testes makes orchiectomy an outpatient surgical procedure with very low physical morbidity. Castration re-

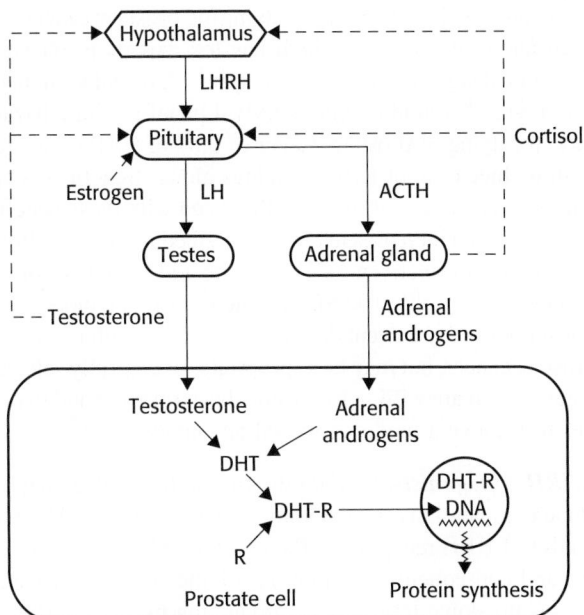

FIGURE 100.4 Influence of endocrine system on prostate cell growth. ACTH, adenocorticotropic hormone; DHT, dihydro-testosterone; LH, luteinizing hormone; LHRH, luteinizing hormone-releasing hormone; R, receptor.

lieves prostate cancer symptoms very rapidly; patients may report relief of pain from bone metastases within hours of the procedure. This makes it the hormonal intervention of choice in emergent situations such as impending paralysis from spinal cord metastases. Other advantages are its cost-effectiveness and lack of compliance issues. Subcapsular orchiectomy, in which the testes are excised but the scrotal sac remains, helps overcome the cosmetic disadvantages of this surgery, but despite this, removal of the testes remains unacceptable to many patients. Orchiectomy carries negative psychologic and gender-related associations and is not reversible. It produces impotence and loss of libido in nearly 100% of patients. Hot flashes, weight gain, and other symptoms of androgen deprivation are very common.[2,3,35,37]

Medical Interventions. There are several medical alternatives that result in the same low "castrate" levels of androgens that is achieved by orchiectomy. The reversibility of these pharmacologic methods has made prostate cancer treatment more acceptable to many patients.

Estrogens were the first form of so called "medical castration" and were widely used as androgen deprivation therapy in patients with prostate cancer in the 1960s and 1970s. Estrogens have many hormonal effects but primarily interfere with the release of LHRH from the hypothalamus. This decreases LH production, and eliminates the hormonal signal for testosterone production by the testes.[35,36]

Estrogens. Diethylstilbestrol (DES) has been the most widely used estrogen in prostate cancer therapy. Its use and dosing were studied in a series of Veterans Administration Urological Research Group (VACURG) trials.[40] The first

VACURG trial proved that 5 mg DES per day was as effective as orchiectomy in treating metastatic prostate cancer, but was also more toxic, causing an excess of cardiovascular deaths. The next VACURG trial compared several DES doses. Without strong objective data, an empiric 3-mg dose became the standard of practice. At this dose, the incidence of serious thromboembolic cardiovascular adverse effects remained very high. Estrogens as a means of first-line medical castration therapy went out of favor with the advent of the LHRH analogs. Manufacture of oral DES has been discontinued in the United States. Other estrogens probably would produce similar clinical and toxic effects but have not been widely studied in patients with prostate cancer. Currently, estrogens are not recommended as ADT.[20,35,38]

LHRH Analogs. The use of LHRH analogs or agonists (Table 100.5) to treat an androgen-dependent disorder such as prostate cancer seems counter to the logic of ADT because it is LHRH that begins the cascade of signals that results in testosterone production. An LHRH analog can theoretically increase testosterone and stimulate the growth of prostate cancer. This is exactly what happens during the first two weeks of LHRH agonist administration. Symptoms of prostate cancer such as bone pain, and urinary obstruction may increase. This is called the "flare phenomenon." However, chronic administration disrupts the normal pulsatile release of LHRH and down regulates LHRH receptors in the pituitary. This suppresses LH production and, ultimately, testosterone production. Castrate levels of testosterone are achieved within 4 weeks.[2,35,41]

LHRH analogs are as effective as orchiectomy or DES in treating metastatic prostate cancer, without the cardiovascular complications that estrogens produce. Disadvantages are high cost, lack of oral formulations, high incidence of hot flashes and other symptoms of androgen deprivation syndrome, and risk of tumor flare. Flare symptoms occur in up to 10% of patients. Although they usually manifest as a manageable increase in bone pain, flare can be very serious in patients with tumor masses near the spinal cord or obstructing urine flow. Tumor flare can be prevented by administering an antiandrogen (discussed below) with the initiation of LHRH analog therapy. The main advantage of LHRH analogs over orchiectomy is reversibility of their effects, although it may take several months for testosterone levels to return to normal if LHRH analog therapy is stopped. The LHRH agonists are the most commonly used medical interventions in the hormonal management of patients with prostate cancer.[35,36,41] Orchiectomy and LHRH analog therapy are considered standard first-line hormonal therapies (Fig. 100.3).[20,38]

Other Medical Interventions. Orchiectomy or LHRH analog therapy meets the needs of most patients with newly diagnosed metastatic hormonally responsive prostate cancer, but each method of ADT has limitations. Other medical options exist that may be appropriate for selected patients.

Antiandrogen Monotherapy. Antiandrogens are AR antagonists that competitively inhibit the uptake and binding of testosterone and DHT to nuclear receptors. This blocks the growth-stimulatory effects of androgens on prostate cancer cells. Two nonsteroidal antiandrogens are available in the United States: flutamide and bicalutamide (Table 100.5). Because testosterone production is not decreased by antiandrogens, sexual interest and physical capacity for sexual intercourse are generally preserved. Other complications of ADT therapy such as bone loss and fatigue are also avoided, although gynecomastia and breast tenderness are common, and hepatotoxicity can occur. High serum testosterone levels may override competitive androgen blockade produced by antiandrogens, and for that reason they are not currently approved as single-agent therapy. Administration of higher doses of antiandrogens, such as 150 mg of bicalutamide, may prevent the competitive override of antiandrogen effects by testosterone. Single-agent therapy using nonsteroidal antiandrogens has been compared with orchiectomy, and been shown to produce equivalent survival in one meta analysis. Additional evidence is needed before antiandrogen monotherapy can be considered first-line hormonal intervention, but it is a reasonable option in well-informed men who refuse other hormonal therapies to avoid compromising sexual functioning.[20,38,42]

Combined Androgen Blockade. Orchiectomy and LHRH analogs effectively eliminate testicular androgens. Neither intervention affects adrenal androgens, which normally account for 5% to 10% of male androgen production. Even this low level of androgens can stimulate prostate cancer growth. Combined androgen blockade (CAB), also called total or maximal androgen blockade, refers to combination therapies designed to eliminate the effects of testicular and adrenal androgens. Orchiectomy or an LHRH analog is combined with an antiandrogen to prevent any physiologic effects from adrenally produced androgens.

CAB was the most commonly used hormonal intervention for men requiring ADT during the 1990s. A landmark controlled trial (Southwest Oncology Group Intergroup Study 0036), which randomized patients to leuprolide plus flutamide or placebo, was published in 1989.[43] This study demonstrated a 7-month survival advantage for patients on the combination therapy arm. Analysis of a small subset of patients with minimal metastatic disease and good performance status showed greater benefit, with a remarkable 20-month survival advantage at 5 years. This was the first time that hormonal therapy had been proven to prolong survival in patients with metastatic prostate cancer.[43]

After that study was published, many large randomized trials were performed in attempts to reproduce its findings. No study has shown a dramatic difference in favor of CAB or testicular suppression alone, nor have they shown differential responses for patients with good performance status and minimal disease. However, it is now established that CAB produces small, statistically significant survival benefits compared with testicular suppression alone. The benefit

in absolute risk reduction for dying of prostate cancer has been about 3% overall, which has led experts to question the clinical significance of the benefit.[38] A recent systematic trial review[44] found a larger survival benefit, with a hazard ratio for dying of prostate cancer of 0.87 of CAB compared with orchiectomy or LHRH analogs alone. Benefit was apparent after 5 years of therapy. Balanced with these benefits are substantial increases in costs, described as ''extraordinarily poor cost-effectiveness''[38] and the added toxicity of the antiandrogen (Table 100.5). Complete androgen blockade is not supported by current data for all patients with metastatic prostate cancer, but may be appropriate for carefully selected patients who are willing to assume the extra costs and toxicities to achieve a modest survival advantage.[21,38,45]

LHRH Antagonists. In 2004 the first LHRH antagonist became commercially available in the United States. Abarelix binds to LHRH receptors in the pituitary, blocking the binding and consequently the pharmacologic actions of LHRH. This shuts down testosterone production by the testes very rapidly, without the initial increase in testosterone secretion that is caused by LHRH analogs. Because no flare reaction occurs, abarelix can be used without risk of temporarily stimulating prostate cancer growth. However, it causes a high (nearly 4%) risk of immediate onset hypersensitivity reactions, which have included urticaria, hypotension, or syncope. Because of this serious risk, the use of abarelix is restricted to patients with metastatic prostate cancer who refuse orchiectomy and who are not appropriate candidates for LHRH agonist therapy. Patients must sign a statement indicating their understanding of the risks and benefits of abarelix treatment before beginning treatment. It can only be prescribed by physicians enrolled with the manufacturer (Plenaxis PLUS Program).[46,47]

Scheduling Issues in First-Line Hormonal Therapy. Other important considerations in hormonal prostate cancer management are the questions of intermittent compared with continuous ADT and of immediate versus deferred treatment.

Intermittent ADT. Administering ADT intermittently, with off-therapy periods between periods of active treatment, has two goals. The first goal of intermittent ADT is to help maintain the hormonal responsiveness of prostate cancers by delaying the progression of the patient's cancer from the usual initial state of androgen dependence to androgen independence. The second goal is to reduce the symptoms of androgen deprivation syndrome to improve quality of life.[48]

In intermittent ADT, patients are treated with hormonal therapy, usually LHRH analogs or CAB, until the patient's PSA nadirs. ADT is stopped until the PSA begins to rise again, as a result of tumor regrowth. When the PSA reaches a specified level, ADT is restarted. For most, but not all patients, the tumor will respond to reinstitution of therapy and PSA will decline again. On the average, patients on intermittent ADT spend one third to one half of their time off treatment. Because testosterone levels rise when the patient is off therapy, many of the side effects of ADT, which are related to castrate levels of testosterone, are reduced or eliminated. Quality of life improves significantly and costs of treatment may be reduced. However, the objective impact of intermittent ADT on overall survival, time to progression, development of androgen resistance, and quality of life are not yet known. Two large randomized trials designed to answer these questions are underway. Until that information is available, intermittent ADT should be considered investigational.[38,48]

Immediate Versus Deferred ADT. Deferring ADT until a patient develops symptoms from metastatic prostate cancer is based on the general principle that treatment is palliative rather than curative in patients with advanced cancer. Palliation traditionally is viewed as relief of symptoms, so from this perspective it is not reasonable to treat unless the patient has symptoms that can be improved. This is the most cost-effective way to administer ADT, because some patients may never develop symptoms, or may progress slowly to development of symptoms. Deferring ADT also defers the onset of symptoms of androgen deprivation therapy, and may preserve quality of life. Opponents of deferred treatment argue that palliation must be viewed in a broader scope of lengthening symptom-free intervals to improve quality of life. Early treatment with LHRH analogs has been shown to provide a small increase in overall survival and to delay the time to progression to symptoms, which may reduce serious complications of prostate cancer. However, the studies on which this information is based were performed before PSA testing was widely used. Until better evidence is available on which to base decisions, patients should be informed of the risks and benefits of early versus deferred treatment. Antiandrogen monotherapy should not be used for deferred treatment.[38,41,49]

SECOND AND THIRD-LINE INTERVENTIONS

About 15% to 20% of patients with metastatic prostate cancer do not respond to first-line ADT and are considered androgen-resistant. All other patients who do not die of other causes will eventually become refractory to first-line ADT. Second-line hormonal interventions have lower response rates, shorter durations of effects, and in general, greater toxicity than the first-line therapies outlined earlier. Second-line and third-line therapies include first-line options that were not used initially, manipulation of antiandrogens, progestins, and adrenal enzyme inhibitors. No uniform sequence of second-line and third-line ADT can be recommended because of the variety of first-line options and individual patient characteristics. Testosterone levels should be measured in patients who have progressed on treatment with LHRH analogs. Patients who do not have castrate testosterone levels may benefit from orchiectomy; see Figure 100.3.[2,3,20,35]

Manipulation of Antiandrogens. Adding antiandrogens should be considered in patients who have not previously received them. Testicular suppression therapy should be continued. Upon further progression, the antiandrogen should be stopped to assess for a withdrawal response. About one third of patients whose prostate cancer progresses during therapy that includes an antiandrogen will benefit from stopping the antiandrogen. This is called antiandrogen withdrawal syndrome. Antiandrogens may begin to act as androgens rather than antiandrogens during prolonged therapy, because of mutational changes in ARs. Patients may also respond to a different antiandrogen after progression on one drug in that class.[20,35,50,51]

Aminoglutethimide or Ketoconazole. Adrenal androgen production can be suppressed with the aromatase inhibitor aminoglutethimide or with ketoconazole, an antifungal agent (Table 100.5). Both agents are adrenal enzyme inhibitors that block adrenal steroid production by blocking cytochrome P-450; ketoconazole also interferes with testicular steroid production. Glucocorticoid replacement is necessary with aminoglutethimide treatment and sometimes with ketoconazole. Aminoglutethimide is used as second-line or third-line treatment in patients who have progressed after other agents.[52] Ketoconazole lowers serum testosterone levels very rapidly and is a short-term alternative in patients with impending spinal cord compression. High doses are needed and may produce severe hepatitis.[35]

Corticosteroids. Corticosteroids decrease PSA by more than 50% in about one third of patients with hormone-refractory progressive prostate cancer. They may act in part by suppressing adrenal androgen production through feedback effects on adrenocorticotropic hormone (ACTH) production, although other mechanisms appear to be involved as well. Only low doses (5 to 20 mg prednisone daily) are needed.[2,35]

Progestins. Megestrol acetate is a progestin that inhibits pituitary LH secretion and is also weakly antiandrogenic. Side effects associated with its use include fluid retention, impaired glucose control, and weight gain.[35]

Cytotoxic Chemotherapy. Traditionally, cytotoxic chemotherapy has been viewed as having little value for treatment of prostate cancer. Prostate cancer cells are resistant to most conventional cytotoxic agents. The long doubling time of prostate cancer cells may partially account for this low level of efficacy, because conventional cytotoxic chemotherapy agents have their greatest effects against rapidly dividing cells.[53] However, there have been several important developments in the treatment of metastatic prostate cancer with cytotoxic chemotherapy within the past few years. Chemotherapy is now recommended treatment for patients whose prostate cancer is no longer responsive to hormonal interventions, and has been proven to increase survival, which is the most stringent measure of efficacy in oncology.

Some of this change can be attributed to changes in how drug efficacy is measured. Most patients with androgen independent prostate cancer (AIPC), also called hormone refractory prostate cancer (HRPC) have bone metastases as their major or only metastatic site, but no current assessment methods satisfactorily measure changes in prostate cancer bone metastases. Only 10% of patients with HRPC have measurable soft tissue disease, and objective response rates in these patient subsets cannot be directly extrapolated to patients with bone metastases. A decrease in PSA levels is often used as a surrogate indicator of response but does not uniformly correlate with tumor response. For these reasons, clinical benefit response, which is defined by changes in quality of life indicators of response such as pain relief, decreased use of analgesics, and improvements in performance status, is accepted by the U.S. Food and Drug Administration (FDA) as evidence of efficacy in patients with advanced prostate cancer.[2,3]

Based on clinical benefit response, the cytotoxic chemotherapy regimen of mitoxantrone plus prednisone was demonstrated to be more effective than prednisone alone in palliating symptoms of AIPC, and was approved by the FDA in the mid-1990s for this indication. In a carefully controlled trial, 29% of patients on mitoxantrone plus prednisone experienced significant pain relief, compared with 12% of patients on prednisone alone ($P = 0.01$). Duration of palliative response was also significantly longer, 43 weeks versus 18 weeks ($P < 0.0001$), although there was no difference in overall survival.[54]

Over the past several decades, chemotherapy for patients with AIPC has focused primarily on combinations of antimicrotubule agents: the taxanes, vincas, and estramustine. Estramustine is an unusual oral agent that combines an alkylating agent with an estrogen. It was designed as a means of targeting the alkylator to hormone-sensitive cells. However, estramustine works neither as an alkylator nor as an estrogen. It is now recognized to work as an antimitotic agent with antimicrotubule effects. Although the estrogenic component does not appear to contribute to estramustine's efficacy, it contributes to toxicity. Estramustine shares the thromboembolic and cardiovascular side effects of estrogens.[55]

In 2004, with the publication of two large randomized controlled trials, chemotherapy was proven for the first time to extend survival in men with AIPC.[56,57] In both studies, docetaxel-based regimens were compared against the combination regimen of mitoxantrone plus prednisone approved by the FDA. The randomization and eligibility criteria were very similar between the two studies.

The first study (TAX 327), compared two administration schedules of docetaxel plus prednisone: (a) weekly or every 3 weeks docetaxel plus prednisone or (b) mitoxantrone plus prednisone administered every three weeks. The every 3-week docetaxel regimen decreased the risk of death by 24% (hazard ratio 0.76) and increased survival by 2.4 months compared with the mitoxantrone regimen. Differences were statistically significant. Declines in serum PSA levels, reduction of pain, and improvements in quality of life were also significant compared with the mitoxantrone control arm. The weekly docetaxel regimen produced intermediate changes

in these parameters; changes in survival were not statistically significant with the weekly regimen. Toxicity was greater in both docetaxel arms than with mitoxantrone, with the exception of cardiac events. Toxicity was not reduced by weekly docetaxel administration.[56]

In the second study, Southwest Oncology Group (SWOG) 99-16, every 3-week docetaxel plus estramustine was compared with mitoxantrone plus prednisone on the standard every 3-week schedule. Survival was increased by about 2 months, and the risk of death was decreased by 20% (hazard ratio for death of 0.80) with docetaxel, compared with mitoxantrone. The median time to disease progression was nearly doubled (6.3 vs. 3.2 months). Toxicity was also greater in the docetaxel plus estramustine arm: neutropenic fevers, cardiovascular events, nausea and vomiting, metabolic disturbances, and neurologic events were significantly increased.[57]

Although both studies demonstrated improved survival in comparison with the previous standard of mitoxantrone plus prednisone, the improvement produced by docetaxel plus prednisone was greater than the improvement produced by docetaxel plus estramustine. Serious toxicities, especially cardiovascular events, were also less. On that basis, in 2004, docetaxel was approved by the FDA in combination with prednisone for the management of patients with AIPC. This regimen has rapidly become the standard of care for patients with metastatic prostate cancer who no longer respond to hormonal therapies.[56,57]

NONPHARMACOLOGIC THERAPY FOR ADVANCED PROSTATE CANCER

The major form of nonpharmacologic therapy for patients with advanced prostate cancer is orchiectomy, discussed earlier as a first-line androgen ablative therapy. Radiation therapy plays an important role in managing pain secondary to bone metastases. It is administered by external beam techniques to palliate isolated painful bony sites. Patients who have too many painful bony sites to make external beam radiation therapy feasible may be radiated systemically using parenterally administered bone-targeting radioisotopes. Two products are currently available: strontium-89 and samarium-153. These agents accumulate in bone at sites of increased turnover, such as metastatic tumor sites, and release low levels of radiation to nearby tissues. Onset of pain relief is gradual, with improvements occurring over several weeks, but persists for several months. The main toxicity is bone marrow suppression from incidental radiation damage to the bone marrow.[58]

COMPLEMENTARY AND ALTERNATIVE THERAPIES

Although treatment options continue to improve for men with AIPC, advanced prostate cancer remains an incurable disease. Several complementary and alternative medical

(CAM) therapies have been widely used by men with AIPC to help provide additional options. Others are used by men at risk of prostate cancer, as preventative therapy.

The most widely publicized CAM therapy for prostate cancer was the proprietary combination of eight Chinese herbal agents known as PC-SPES (Table 100.6). ''PC'' is an abbreviation for prostate cancer; ''SPES'' is Latin for hope. This product was available through Internet sales from BotanicLab in California from the mid-1990s through 2002.[59] Use of PC-SPES became very popular after a small clinical trial, published as the lead article in the *New England Journal of Medicine* in 1998, demonstrated effectiveness comparable to the best treatments for metastatic prostate cancer available at that time. In that report, six of eight men with advanced prostate cancer responded to PC-SPES treatment, achieving castrate testosterone levels. PSA decreased in all eight patients.[60] Subsequent larger studies demonstrated PSA declines of more than 50% in approximately half of the patients treated, some of whom had received many previous treatments. Although PC-SPES was promoted as a nonestrogenic treatment, it was proven to have estrogenic properties, and produced common estrogenic side effects: gynecomastia, breast tenderness, leg cramps, and thromboembolic effects.[59,60] However, the individual herbal components of PC-SPES also had nonestrogenic pharmacologic activities that potentially contributed to its anticancer effects.

Because of the documented efficacy in small trials, a prospective, multicenter, randomized phase II trial was initiated that compared PC-SPES with DES in men with AIPC.[61] Patients in both arms also received 2 mg of warfarin daily to decrease thromboembolic risks. Preliminary responses verified improved efficacy of PC-SPES compared with DES, but the study was closed prematurely when analysis of study supplies of PC-SPES showed contamination of PC-SPES study supplies with the estrogens DES and ethinyl estradiol.

At about the same time, there were case reports of bleeding in patients receiving PC-SPES. Warfarin contamination was detected in some lots. Other lots were contaminated with indomethacin. A public health advisory was issued early in 2002, advising patients to discontinue use of PC-SPES. BotanicLab issued a product recall and moved production to China; however, the quality was unsatisfactory, and BotanicLab closed later that year.[59–62]

Although PC-SPES is no longer available, several similar products (PC Hope, PC Care, and others) continue to be marketed. Research continues into the components of PC-SPES, to determine the basis of the product's therapeutic activity. Other CAM products relatively specific to prostate cancer patients include selenium, vitamin E, and lycopene, discussed below.

FUTURE THERAPIES

Despite the availability of many palliative treatments for prostate cancer, more than 30,000 men die of prostate cancer each year, enduring disease courses that are often relentless, painful, and debilitating. Although substantial progress has been made in hormonal and chemotherapy treatments, more effective and less toxic treatments are needed. The remarkable successes of the last decade have generated a great deal of interest and have resulted in increased funding for prostate cancer research. Many avenues of research are being investigated. Some of these are summarized in Table 100.7.[63–66]

IMPROVING OUTCOMES

Outcome evaluation in prostate cancer is complicated by the advanced age of most patients and the slow growth of the disease. It is one of the few cancers in which treatment may not be necessary for all patients. In some cases, the best outcomes are achieved with no treatment.

PATIENT EDUCATION

It is only since the early 1990s that prostate cancer has been openly discussed in the lay press. Significant changes in public awareness have taken place in a short time, but much education is still needed. It is still common for the lay public to be confused about precisely what the prostate is, where it is located, differences between prostatectomy and orchiectomy, and the management of side effects associated with prostate cancer therapies. Decision-making about the best choice of local treatment and hormonal interventions requires detailed patient information about the risks and benefits of the available options. Excellent patient education materials are available through the American Cancer Society and the National Cancer Institute.

METHODS TO IMPROVE ADHERENCE TO DRUG THERAPY

One method to improve adherence to drug therapy is to simplify dosage regimens. Use of the once daily antiandrogen

TABLE 100.6	Components of PC-SPES
Scientific Name	**Common Name**
Dendranthema morifolium	Chrysanthemum
Isatis indigotica	Dyer's Woad
Glycyrrhiza glabra	Licorice
Ganoderma lucidum	Reishi
Panax pseudo ginseng	Ginseng
Rabdosia rubescens	Rabdosia
Serenoa repens	Saw Palmetto
Scutellaria baicalensis	Baikal Skullcap

PC-SPES, eight Chinese herbal agents known as PC-SPES. "PC" is an abbreviation for prostate cancer; "SPES" is Latin for hope.
(From Kosty MP. PC-SPES: hope or hype (editorial)? J Clin Oncol 22:3657–3659, 2004; Wilkinson S, Chodak GW. Critical review of complementary therapies for prostate cancer. J Clin Oncol 21:2199–2210, 2003, with permission.)

TABLE 100.7	Investigational Therapies for Androgen-Independent Prostate Cancer	
Category	**Agents**	**Rationale**
Docetaxel plus other agents	Vinorelbine Diethylstilbestrol Bortezomib Capecitabine	Building on known efficacy of docetaxel with other agents with single agent efficacy
Epothilones	Ixabepilone (BMS-247550) EPO906	New class of antimicrotubule agents, with mechanism of action similar to taxanes
New platinum agents	Satraplatin	Oral platinum agent that has shown efficacy in prostate cancer patients in a randomized trial
Vitamin D	Calcitriol	May induce cell cycle arrest and apoptosis
Angiogenesis inhibitors	Thalidomide	Interferes with tumor necrosis factor (TNF) alpha, which promotes growth of new blood vessels needed for tumor growth
	Bevacizumab	Targets VEGF (vascular endothelial growth factor) needed for new blood vessel growth
	Atrasenten	Antagonizes endothelin receptor involved in new blood vessel growth
Vaccines	APC8015	Patient's antigen-presenting cells are "taught" to attack cells that express prostatic acid phosphatase.
	GVAX	Tumor cells that are modified to secrete GM-CSF, which has several antitumor effects
	PSA-based vaccines	Designed to target PSA-producing cells
Monoclonal antibodies	J591 (MLN591)	Targets prostate-specific membrane antigen (PSMA). Can be used to carry radioisotopes to prostate cancer cells.
Apoptosis inhibitors	Cis-retinoic acid Interferon Bcl–2 Antisense Oligonucleosides	These agents target Bcl-2 expression in different ways. Bcl–2 is overexpressed in AIPC and causes resistance to apoptosis.
Growth factor receptor signaling inhibitors	Gefitinib Imatinib	Interfere with growth factors such as epidermal growth factor (EGF) that stimulate prostate cancer growth.
Gene therapy	Various	Many approaches such as introducing tumor suppressor genes, controlling cancer cell growth, stimulating the immune system to destroy the tumor, or interfering with new blood vessel growth

GM-CSF, granulocyte-macrophage colony-stimulating factor; PSA, prostate-specific antigen; AIPC, androgen independent prostate cancer.

bicalutamide may improve adherence, compared with the every 8-hour dosing regimen dictated by the short half-life of flutamide. LHRH analogs are the most commonly used drugs for prostate cancer treatment, but must be administered parenterally. Extended-depot formulations that release drug over 3-month or 4-month periods have been available since the late 1990s. Once yearly formulations are now available. Patient reminders to schedule clinic visits for repeat injections may help improve adherence.

Treatment adherence can also be improved by preventing or managing undesirable side effects of treatment. Quality of life issues are extremely important because prostate cancer treatment often continues for many years. Most surgical, radiation, and hormonal interventions for prostate cancer produce impotence. Loss of sexual functioning can have a serious negative impact on quality of life and treatment satisfaction and can adversely affect patient willingness to initiate or continue therapy. Availability of oral phosphodiesterase-5 inhibitors has made prostate cancer therapy more acceptable to many patients.[24]

Vasoactive flushes, or hot flashes, are a common and troublesome side effect of surgical castration and LHRH analogs. Vasoactive flushes are centrally mediated and produce sensations of heat and sweating that persist for several minutes. They can be controlled in about 75% of patients with low doses of progestin, megestrol acetate, or with antidepressant agents such as venlafaxine hydrochloride.[67]

Gynecomastia is a very common side effect of antiandrogens. The feminizing effect of breast enlargement can be very disturbing to men, whose masculinity is compromised by prostate cancer treatments. The antiestrogen tamoxifen, with or without breast irradiation, has been proven to prevent breast enlargement and breast pain caused by antiandrogens.[68]

Osteoporosis is an important adverse outcome of chronic ADT, because maintenance of bone density depends on androgens. Screening men at risk and instituting prophylactic measures such as calcium and vitamin D supplementation, or bisphosphonates, can reduce the morbidity of bone density loss.[69]

DISEASE MANAGEMENT STRATEGIES TO IMPROVE PATIENT OUTCOMES

Several disease management interventions for prostate cancer in the last few years have improved outcomes for patients with localized disease and with advanced prostate cancer. The management of localized disease has been improved by more specific dosing techniques that permit use of higher more effective radiation doses and combinations of ADT with radiation. Both interventions have improved local control rates. Less invasive surgical techniques, such as laparoscopic prostatectomy, are expected to reduce morbidity of surgical treatments. Increasing use of monotherapies rather than combination regimens for androgen-dependent disease decreases toxicity of hormonal therapies. Use of docetaxel-based chemotherapy regimens marks the first time that chemotherapy has been proven to prolong survival for patients with AIPC.

PREVENTION

Improved understanding of factors that affect prostate cancer growth has important implications for prostate cancer prevention. The Prostate Cancer Prevention Trial (PCPT), evaluated long-term treatment with the 5-α reductase inhibitor, finasteride compared with placebo in 18,000 men at high risk of developing prostate cancer. Finasteride prevents the conversion of testosterone to DHT, the androgen with the greatest effect on prostate cells. Finasteride administration decreased the incidence of prostate cancer by 24.8% compared with placebo ($P < 0.001$). One very concerning finding was that cancers that did occur were more likely to be a higher Gleason grade, indicating more aggressive cancers than in the placebo group. Impaired sexual function was more common in the finasteride group, but urinary symptoms were more common in the placebo group, because finasteride is effective in treating symptoms of BPH.[70]

Another very large prostate cancer prevention trial is underway. The Selenium and Vitamin E Chemoprevention Trial (SELECT) has randomized more than 30,000 men to selenium, vitamin E, both, or neither, in a blinded format. Results are expected in 2013.[71] The most promising dietary intervention to decrease the risk of prostate cancer is ingestion of diets high in lycopene that is present in tomato products. Other potential chemopreventive agents include: soy

isoflavones, nonsteroidal anti-inflammatory drugs, antiandrogens, antiestrogens, vitamin D, and difluoromethylornithine (DFMO).[72]

PHARMACOECONOMICS

Prostate cancer carries a significant economic burden to individuals and society. The course of disease often spans 10 years or more with the greatest expenses incurred in the first year after diagnosis and after development of metastatic disease.

During the first year, costs for management of localized disease are incurred. Observation is the most economical management approach for localized disease, although active surveillance includes the costs of close patient follow-up. Of definitive interventions, newer advances in therapy generally increase the cost of the intervention, but decrease costs of complications from the intervention.[73] This is true for laparoscopic surgical techniques compared with traditional open incision surgical procedures and of three-dimensional conformal radiation therapy compared with standard external beam techniques. The cost of delivering three-dimensional conformal radiation therapy at typical doses is approximately 2.5 times the cost of conventional external beam radiotherapy for early stage prostate cancer.[74] Despite this, three-dimensional conformal techniques are favored over conventional techniques in cost-effectiveness analyses, which take overall costs rather than just procedural costs into consideration.[75]

Drug therapy is an important cost factor in prostate cancer management. The cost of LHRH analog therapy for ADT is several thousand dollars per year, and the therapy is usually administered for several years. The surgical alternative of orchiectomy is much less expensive (less than one fifth of the cost of 30 months of LHRH analog treatment in one study),[73] however, patient acceptance of medical management is greater.[76]

The new standard of docetaxel-based chemotherapy treatment for patients with AIPC will add substantial additional cost to management of prostate cancer, but also increases survival. The cost-effectiveness of docetaxel-based regimens is being determined. The previous chemotherapy standard, mitoxantrone and prednisone, improved quality of life but did not extend survival. Despite this, the total cost of care was decreased slightly compared with prednisone alone, establishing that treatments that reduce symptoms and improve quality of life can reduce overall costs of care, even in the absence of objective survival benefits.[77]

KEY POINTS

■ Prostate cancer is a disease of older men and is the most common cancer in men

- The apparent incidence of prostate cancer has increased because of the availability of PSA testing; most cancers are diagnosed when the cancer is still localized
- The cause of prostate cancer is unknown, although race, family history, and genetic changes are known to increase risk
- Early diagnosis offers the best opportunity for cure, but the value of screening programs remains controversial because many prostate cancers are biologically latent and would not produce symptoms within the lifetime of the patient
- Prognosis is determined by Gleason pathologic grade and stage of disease
- Treatment options for patients with localized prostate cancer include radical prostatectomy, three-dimensional conformal radiation therapy, or brachytherapy. Observation is a management option in patients with low-grade tumors and a life expectancy of less than 10 years
- Combinations of ADTs with radiation therapy increase duration of response and progression-free survival
- Androgen deprivation therapy is the cornerstone of treatment for metastatic prostate cancer. It is palliative rather than curative
- First-line hormonal treatments for metastatic prostate cancer include orchiectomy or an LHRH analog. Combined androgen blockade, monotherapy with antiandrogens, or LHRH antagonists are acceptable alternatives in selected patients. The choice of hormonal therapy depends on patient preference, costs, and other medical conditions
- Options for second-line hormonal therapy include antiandrogen addition or withdrawal, progestins, corticosteroids, aminoglutethimide, ketoconazole, or estrogens
- Chemotherapy with docetaxel plus prednisone has been proven to increase survival and progression-free survival and to improve symptoms in men with AIPC, and is now considered standard therapy for men with AIPC
- The Chinese herbal product, PC-SPES, was proven to be effective in men with androgen dependent or independent prostate cancer, but was removed from the market because of product contamination. Similar products remain available
- Economic evaluations have demonstrated the value of widespread screening, new technologies for management of localized disease, and drug therapies
- Future directions include combinations of antimicrotubule agents, and the development of targeted agents, prostate cancer vaccines, apoptosis-inducing agents, and gene therapy

SUGGESTED READINGS

Bostwick DG, Burke HB, Djakiew D, et al. Human prostate cancer risk factors. Cancer 92:2371–2490, 2004.

Nelson WG, DeMarzo AM, Isaacs WB. Prostate cancer. N Engl J Med 349:366–381, 2003.

Peschel RE, Colbert JW. Surgery, brachytherapy, and external-beam radiotherapy for early prostate cancer. Lancet Oncology 4:233–241, 2003.

Scher HI, Leibel SA, Fuks Z, et al. Cancer of the prostate. In: DeVita VT, Hellman S, Rosenberg S, eds. Cancer: principles and practice of oncology. 7th ed. Philadelphia: Lippincott, Williams & Wilkins, 2005:1192–1267.

REFERENCES

1. American Cancer Society. Cancer facts and figures 2005. Atlanta: American Cancer Society, 2005.
2. Scher HI, Leibel SA, Fuks Z, et al. Cancer of the prostate. In: DeVita VT, Hellman S, Rosenberg S, eds. Cancer: principles and practice of oncology. 7th ed. Philadelphia: Lippincott, Williams & Wilkins, 2005:1192–1267.
3. Oh WK, Hurwitz M, D'Amico AV, et al. Neoplasms of the prostate. In: Kufe DW, Pollock RE, Weichselbaum RR, et al., eds. Cancer medicine. 6th ed. Hamilton, ON: BC Decker, 2003:1707–1740.
4. Freedland SJ, Isaacs WB. Explaining racial differences in prostate cancer in the United States: sociology or biology? Prostate 62:243–252, 2005.
5. Hsieh k, Albertsen PC. Populations at high risk for prostate cancer. Urol Clin North Am 30:669–676, 2003.
6. Bostwick DG, Burke HB, Djakiew D, et al. Human prostate cancer risk factors. Cancer 92:2371–2490, 2004.
7. Baron JA, Beach M, Wallace K, et al. Risk of prostate cancer in a randomized controlled trial of calcium supplementation. Cancer Epidemiol Biomarkers Prev 14:586–589, 2005.
8. Porter MP, Stanford JL. Obesity and the risk of prostate cancer. Prostate 62:316–321, 2005.
9. Kane CJ, Bassett WW, Sadetsky N, et al. Obesity and prostate cancer clinical risk factors at presentation: data from CaPSURE. J Urol 173:732–736, 2005.
10. Nelson WG, DeMarzo AM, Isaacs WB. Prostate cancer. N Engl J Med 349:366–381, 2003.
11. Visakorpi T. The molecular genetics of prostate cancer. Urology 62:3–10, 2003.
12. Ohori M, Scardino PT. Localized prostate cancer. Curr Probl Surg 39:833–957, 2002.
13. Balk SP, Ko Y-J, Bubley GJ. Biology of prostate-specific antigen. J Clin Oncol 21:383–391, 2003.
14. Wilson SS, Crawford ED. Screening for prostate cancer. Urol Clin North Am 31:219–226, 2004.
15. Postma R, Schroder FH. Screening for prostate cancer. Eur J Cancer 41:825–833, 2005.
16. Djavan B, Milani S, Remzi M. Prostate biopsy: who, how, and when. An update. Can J Urol 12 (Suppl 1):44–48, 2005.
17. Anonymous. Genitourinary sites. In: Greene FL, Page DL, Fleming ID, et al., eds. AJCC cancer staging manual. 6th ed. New York: Springer, 2002:309–316.
18. Abbas F, Scardino PT. The natural history of clinical prostate cancer (editorial). Cancer 80:827–833, 1997.
19. Talcott Ja, Clark JA. Quality of life in prostate cancer. Eur J Cancer 41:922–931, 2005.
20. NCCN Guidelines: Prostate Cancer, v2.2005. National Comprehensive Cancer Network. Available at: http://www.nccn.org/professional/physicians_gls/PDF/prostate.pdf. Accessed August 13, 2005.
21. Maroni PD, Crawford ED. Surgical management of prostate cancer: optimizing patient selections and clinical outcome. Surg Oncol Clinics North Am 14:301–319, 2005.
22. Saranchuk JW, Kattan MW, Elkin E, et al. Achieving optimal outcomes after radical prostatectomy. J Clin Oncol 23:4146–4151, 2005.
23. Peschel RE, Colbert JW. Surgery, brachytherapy, and external-beam radiotherapy for early prostate cancer. Lancet Oncology 4:233–241, 2003.

24. Kendirci M, Hellstrom WJ. Current concepts in the management of erectile dysfunction in men with prostate cancer. Clin Prostate Cancer 3:87–92, 2004.
25. Trabulsi EJ, Guillonneau B. Laparoscopic radical prostatectomy. J Urol 173:1072–1079.28, 2005.
26. Miller DC, Sanda MG, Dunn RL, et al. Long-term outcomes among localized prostate cancer survivors: health-related quality-of-life changes alter radical prostatectomy, external radiation, and brachytherapy. J Clin Oncol 23:2772–2780, 2005.
27. Holmberg L, Bill-Axelson A, Helgesen F, et al. A randomized trial comparing radical prostatectomy with watchful waiting in early prostate cancer. N Engl J Med 347:781–789, 2002.
28. Parker C. Active surveillance: towards a new paradigm in the management of early prostate cancer. Lancet Oncol 5:101–106, 2004.
29. Albertsen PC, Hanley JA, Fine J. 20-year outcomes following conservative management of clinically localized prostate cancer. JAMA 293:2095–2101, 2005.
30. Bolla M, Gonzalez D, Warde P, et al. Improved survival in patients with locally advanced prostate cancer treated with radiotherapy and goserelin. N Engl J Med 337:295–300, 1997.
31. Jani AB, Kao J, Hellman S. Hormone therapy adjuvant to external beam radiotherapy for locally advanced prostate carcinoma. Cancer 98:2351–2361, 2003.
32. Hanks GE, Pajak TF, Porter A, et al. Phase III trial of long-term adjuvant androgen deprivation after neoadjuvant hormonal cytoreduction and radiotherapy in locally advanced carcinoma of the prostate: the radiation therapy oncology group protocol 92-02. J Clin Oncol 21:3972–3978, 2003.
33. Liu M, Pickles T, Agranovich A, et al. Impact of neoadjuvant androgen ablation and other factors on late toxicity of external beam radiotherapy. Int J Radiat Oncol Biol Phys 58:59–67, 2004.
34. Kumar P, Perrotti M, Weiss R, et al. Phase I trial of weekly docetaxel with concurrent three-dimensional conformal radiation therapy in the treatment of unfavorable localized adenocarcinoma of the prostate. J Clin Oncol 22:1909–1915, 2004.
35. Denmeade SR, Isaacs JT. Androgen deprivation therapies in the treatment of advanced prostate cancer. In: Kuffe DW, Pollock RE, Weichselbaum RR, et al, eds. Cancer Medicine 6. Hamilton, ON: BC Decker Inc, 2003:967–979.
36. Ellis MJ, Swain SM. Steroid hormone therapies for cancer. In: Chabner BA, Longo DL, eds. Cancer chemotherapy and biotherapy: principles and practice. 3rd ed. Philadelphia: Lippincott Williams & Wilkins, 2001:85–138.
37. Downing AJ, Tannock IF. Systemic treatment for prostate cancer. Cancer Treat Rev 24:283–301, 1998.
38. Loblaw DA, Mendelson DS, Talcott JA, et al. American Society of Clinical Oncology recommendations for the initial hormonal management of androgen-sensitive metastatic, recurrent, or progressive prostate cancer. J Clin Oncol 22:2927–2941, 2004.
39. Huggins C, Stevens R, Hodges C. The effect of castration on advanced carcinoma of the prostate gland. Arch Surg 43:209–223, 1941.
40. Blackard CE. The Veterans' Administration cooperative urological research group studies of carcinoma of the prostate: a review. Cancer Chemother Rep 59:225–227, 1975.
41. Marks LS. Luteinizing hormone-releasing hormone agonists in the treatment of men with prostate cancer: timing, alternatives, and the 1-year implant. Urology 62 (Suppl 1):36–42, 2003.
42. Baltogiannis D, Giannacopoulos X, Charalabopoulos K, et al. Monotherapy in advanced prostate cancer: an overview. Experimental Oncol 26:185–191, 2004.
43. Crawford ED, Eisenberger MA, McLeod DG, et al. A controlled trial of leuprolide with and without flutamide in prostatic carcinoma. N Engl J Med 321:419–424, 1989.
44. Samson DJ, Seidenfeld J, Schmitt B, et al. Systematic review and meta-analysis of monotherapy compared with combined androgen blockade for patients with advanced prostate carcinoma. Cancer 95:361–376, 2002.
45. Prostate Cancer Trialists' Collaborative Group. Maximum androgen blockade in advanced prostate cancer: an overview of the randomized trials. Lancet 355:1491–1498, 2000.
46. Anonymous. Abarelix (Plenaxis) for advanced prostate cancer. Med Lett Drugs Ther 46:22–23, 2004.
47. Mongeat-Artus P, Teillac P. Abarelix: the first gonadotropin-releasing hormone antagonist for the treatment of prostate cancer. Expert Opin Pharmacother 5:2171–2179, 2004.
48. Bouchot O, Lenomand L, Karam G, et at. Intermittent androgen suppression in the treatment of metastatic prostate cancer. Eur Urol 38:543–549, 2000.
49. Wilt T, Nair B, MacDonald R, et al. Early versus deferred androgen suppression in the treatment of advanced prostate cancer. The Cochrane Library (1 ed Issue 4). Oxford, Update Software, 2003.
50. Scher HI, Kelly WK. Flutamide withdrawal syndrome: its impact on clinical trials in hormone-refractory prostate cancer. J Clin Oncol 11:1566–1572, 1993.
51. Culig Z, Bartsch G, Hobisch A. Antiandrogens in prostate cancer endocrine therapy. Curr Cancer Drug Targets 4:455–461, 2004.
52. Kruit WH, Stoter G, Klijn JG. Effect of combination therapy with aminoglutethimide and hydrocortisone on prostate-specific antigen response in metastatic prostate cancer refractory to standard endocrine therapy. Anticancer Drugs 15:843–847, 2004.
53. Tannock IF. Is there evidence that chemotherapy is of benefit to patients with carcinoma of the prostate? J Clin Oncol 3:1013–1021, 1985.
54. Tannock IF, Osaba D, Stockler MR, et al. Chemotherapy with mitoxantrone plus prednisone or prednisone alone for symptomatic hormone-resistant prostate cancer: a Canadian randomized trial with palliative end points. J Clin Oncol 14:1756–1764, 1996.
55. Bergenheim AT, Henriksson R. Pharmacokinetics and pharmacodynamics of estramustine phosphate. Clin Pharmacokinet 34:163–172, 1998.
56. Tannock IF, deWit R, Berry WR, et al. Docetaxel plus prednisone or mitoxantrone plus prednisone for advanced prostate cancer. N Engl J Med 351:1502–1512, 2004.
57. Petrylak DP, Tangen CM, Hussain MHA, et al. Docetaxel and estramustine compared with mitoxantrone and prednisone for advanced refractory prostate cancer. N Engl J Med 351:1513–1520, 2004.
58. Mertens WC, Filipczak LA, Ben-Josef E, et al. Systemic bone-seeking radionuclides for palliation of painful osseous metastases: current concepts. CA Cancer J Clin 48:361–374, 1998.
59. Kosty MP. PC-SPES: hope or hype (editorial)? J Clin Oncol 22:3657–3659, 2004.
60. DiPaola RS, Zhang H, Lambert GH, et al. Clinical and biologic activity of an estrogenic herbal combination (PC-SPES) in prostate cancer. N Engl J Med 339:785–791, 1998.
61. Oh WK, Kantoff PW, Weinberg V, et al. Prospective, multicenter, randomized phase II trial of the herbal supplement, PC-SPES, and diethylstilbestrol in patients with androgen-independent prostate cancer. J Clin Oncol 22:3705–3712, 2004.
62. Wilkinson S, Chodak GW. Critical review of complementary therapies for prostate cancer. J Clin Oncol 21:2199–2210, 2003.
63. Ryan CW, Vogelzang NJ. Management of hormone refractory prostate cancer. In: Crawford ED, ed. Prostate cancer annual update 2005. Clinical Care Options 2005:71–96.
64. Petrylak DP. Future directions in the treatment of androgen-independent prostate cancer. Urology 65 (Suppl 6):8–12, 2005.
65. Foley R, Lawler M, Hollywood D. Gene-based therapy in prostate cancer. Lancet Oncol 5:469–479, 2004.
66. Papatsoris AG, Karamouzis MV, Papavassiliou AG. Novel biological agents for the treatment of hormone-refractory prostate cancer. Curr Med Chem 12:277–296, 2005.
67. Spetz AC, Zetterlund EL, Varenhorst E, et al. Incidence and management of hot flashes in prostate cancer. J Supportive Oncol 1:263–266, 269–270, 2003.
68. Perdona S, Autorino R, DePlacido S, et al. Efficacy of tamoxifen and radiotherapy for prevention and treatment of gynaecomastia and breast pain caused by bicalutamide in prostate cancer: a randomized controlled trial. Lancet Oncol 6:295–300, 2005.
69. Diamond TH, Higano CS, Smith MR, et al. Osteoporosis in men with prostate carcinoma receiving androgen-deprivation therapy: recommendations for diagnosis and therapies. Cancer 100:892–899, 2004.
70. Thompson IM, Goodman PJ, Tangen CM, et al. The influence of finasteride on the development of prostate cancer. N Engl J Med 349;215–224, 2003.
71. Parnes HL, Thomson IM, Ford LG. Prevention of hormone-related cancers: prostate cancer. J Clin Oncol 23:368–377, 2005.

72. Parnes HL, House MG, Kagan J, et al. Prostate cancer chemoprevention agent development: the National Cancer Institute, Division of Cancer Prevention portfolio. J Urol 171:S68–75, 2004.

73. Hummel S, Paisley S, Morgan A, et al. Clinical and cost-effectiveness of new and emerging technologies for early localized prostate cancer. Health Technol Assess 7:1–157, 2003.

74. Poon I, Pintilie M, Potvin M, et al. The changing costs of radiation treatment for early prostate cancer in Ontario: a comparison between conventional and conformal external beam radiotherapy. Canadian J Urol 11:2125–2132, 2004.

75. Ruchlin HS, Pellissier JM. An economic overview of prostate cancer. Cancer 92:2796–2810, 2001.

76. Chon JK, Jacobs SC, Naslund MJ. The cost value of medical versus surgical hormonal therapy for metastatic prostate cancer. J Urol 164: 735–737, 2000.

77. Bloomfield DJ, Krahn MD, Neogi T, et al. Economic evaluation of chemotherapy with mitoxantrone plus prednisone for symptomatic hormone-resistant prostate cancer: based on a Canadian randomized trial with palliative end points. J Clin Oncol 16: 2272–2279, 1998.

Pediatric Solid Tumors

101

Susannah E. Motl and Deborah A. Ward

In 2005, approximately 9,510 children in the United States under the age of 15 will be diagnosed with cancer and about 1,585 will die from the disease.[1] Despite this low incidence, cancer is the second leading cause of death after accidents in children ages 1 to 14 years, making it the leading cause of death attributed to disease in this population.[2] The incidence of all cancers in this age group is slightly greater in males than females (1.13:1).[3–5] The causes of childhood cancers remain largely unknown, although specific chromosomal abnormalities and ionizing radiation exposure may explain a small percent. Over the past 20 years, while there has been an increase in the incidence (11.5–14.6 cases/100,000 children in 1975–2002, respectively) death rates declined dramatically, and 5-year survival rates increased for most childhood cancers (combined rates increased from 55.9% in 1974–1976 to 78.6% in 1995–2001[6] (Tables 101.1 and 101.2). For childhood brain tumors, the overall incidence rose from 2.3 to 3.5 per 100,000 from 1975 to 2002, with the greatest increase occurring from 1983 to 1986. However, these data may reflect more advanced imaging capabilities made possible by the use of magnetic resonance imaging (MRI), which may not have been previously detected with older equipment.[1]

Increases in survival rates are attributed to the use of a more effective combination chemotherapy regimens given as adjuvant therapy; dose-intensified chemotherapy regimens with improvements in supportive care; and refined diagnostic, surgical, and radiotherapy techniques to treat tumors. Long-term survivors of childhood cancer may experience treatment-related side effects several months or years after they have been cured of their disease, which includes organ malfunction and increased risk of secondary cancers. Solid tumors account for more than 40% of all pediatric malignancies[3] and peak incidence varies with tumor type. For example, neuroblastoma (NB), retinoblastoma (RB), rhabdomyosarcoma (RMS), and Wilms' tumor (WT) are more common in infants and toddlers, whereas osteosarcoma (OS) and Ewing's sarcoma (ES) have their peak incidence during adolescence.[3] Treatment of solid tumors, unlike hematologic malignancies, requires one or more of the following: surgery, radiation, multiagent chemotherapy, and immunotherapy. Thus the organization of efforts from the pediatric oncologist, radiation oncologist, pathologist, radiologist, surgeon, and other health care professionals, such as nurses, pharmacists, dietitians, psychologists, and social workers, is vital to achieving the stated treatment goals.

TABLE 101.1	Current Incidence of Solid Tumors in the United States[a]	
Type	1975–1981 Rate[b]	1996–2002 Rate[b]
Neuroblastoma	7.7	8.6
CNS tumor	23.6	28.7
Retinoblastoma	2.7	3.1
Soft-tissue sarcoma	9.9	2.6
Renal	6.3	7.1
Malignant bone tumors	8	8.6
Osteosarcoma	4	4.9
Ewing's sarcoma	3	2.9

[a] Includes all races, males and females, ages 0–19 compared with 1975–1981.
[b] Per one million U.S. children.
CNS, central nervous system.
(From Ries LAG, Eisner MP, Kosary CL, et al. SEER Cancer Statistics Review, 1975–2002. National Cancer Institute, Bethesda, MD, 2005, with permission.)

TABLE 101.2	5-Year Relative Survival Rates for Children Ages 0–19
Site	5-Year Relative Survival Rates 1985–2001
CNS	69.1
Retinoblastoma	95.5
Neuroblastoma	66.3
Soft tissue sarcoma	71.2
Renal tumors	89.9
Malignant Bone tumor	65.4
Osteosarcoma	64.3
Ewing's Sarcoma	61.5

CNS, central nervous system.
(From Ries LAG, Eisner MP, Kosary CL, et al. SEER Cancer Statistics Review, 1975–2002. National Cancer Institute, Bethesda, MD, 2005.)

This chapter introduces the reader to the more common pediatric solid tumors. An overview of epidemiology, clinical presentation, diagnosis, and prognosis is given for each tumor type. Treatment modalities and supportive care issues relating to pharmaceutical care encountered in clinical practice are emphasized. Where appropriate, the reader is referred to primary literature for more detailed information.

TREATMENT GOALS: PEDIATRIC TUMORS

- Eradicate the primary tumor and systemic disease.
- Minimize and treat toxicities relating to therapy.
- Identify and manage long-term sequelae of therapy.
- Use a multidisciplinary approach incorporating multimodal therapy to achieve treatment goals.

OVERVIEW

TREATMENT MODALITIES

The four major modalities used in patients with solid tumors are (a) surgery, (b) radiation therapy, (c) chemotherapy, and (d) immunotherapy. Surgery remains the primary treatment for most solid tumors and serves three functions:

1. Diagnosis and staging
2. Treatment
3. Prevention

Visual inspection and tissue sampling for pathologic evaluation can provide the basis for staging, which in turn can facilitate the determination of subsequent therapy. Total resection, debulking, metastatic resection, palliation, and reconstruction procedures are examples of the role of surgery in treatment. The goal of surgery is maximal tumor resection while minimizing the chance of deformities and harm to normal surrounding tissues, vessels, and organ systems.

Maximizing the local control of a tumor is the goal of radiation therapy. Radiotherapy is usually administered as a series of small exposures (fractions) delivered over a few minutes. Typically, radiotherapy is scheduled to last 1 to 7 weeks with administration occurring once or twice a day for 5 days per week. Radiation works by damaging cellular DNA (by causing ionization of atoms and the formation of free radicals), and cell death occurs when irradiated cells attempt to replicate. The effects of radiation therapy are most pronounced on rapidly dividing cells, making malignancies an excellent target for this treatment modality. However, rapidly dividing healthy cells (namely bone marrow stem cells and gastrointestinal cells) are often damaged by radiation therapy, and significant toxicities (neutropenia, thrombocytopenia, nausea, vomiting, diarrhea, mucositis, etc.) are the result. Fractionated radiation and dose reductions used in combination with chemotherapy have decreased radiation-related toxicities.[7] Long-term toxicities from radiation therapy include cardiac toxicity; learning disabilities; and impaired development of soft tissues, teeth, and visual structures resulting in decreased muscle mass and cosmetic deformities.[8]

The majority of pediatric malignancies are chemosensitive. Chemotherapy can be administered before surgery or radiation (neoadjuvant therapy), concurrently with radiotherapy, or as adjuvant therapy following other treatment modalities. It is also used as the primary modality to treat unresectable metastatic disease. Chemotherapy regimens used in pediatric solid tumors consist of multiple agents. The rationale of combination chemotherapy, with different adverse effect profiles, is that using numerous agents with different mechanisms of action allows for synergistic or additive effects, while minimizing the likelihood of drug resistance and toxicities.[9] In addition, studies using dose-intensive therapies, regimens in which agents are given at higher doses over shorter intervals, have demonstrated promising results.[10] Multidrug resistance (MDR) is beginning to be identified in pediatric patients with solid malignancies. The identification of p-glycoprotein-mediated MDR is currently a controversial issue, with conflicting reports validating the need for additional research.[11] Agents most commonly used in solid tumors are summarized in Table 101.3 and are discussed in more detail throughout the chapter.

Autologous hematopoietic stem cell rescue following myeloablative chemotherapy (with or without radiotherapy) continues to be a subject of investigation. This process involves the collection of hematopoietic stem cells from a patient before the administration of lethal doses of chemotherapy or radiation, which produces profound myelosuppression. After the administration of the chemotherapy regimen that is intended to ablate residual tumor, the collected stem cells are reinfused to restore the patient's bone marrow. This technique has been studied in patients in whom

TABLE 101.3 | Commonly Used Chemotherapeutic Agents in Pediatric Solid Malignancies

Drug	Class	Spectrum of Use	Route	Common Toxicities	Key Monitoring Parameters
Methotrexate (MTX)	Antimetabolite	Osteosarcoma Medulloblastoma	IV, PO, IT	Myelosuppression, mucositis, nausea, vomiting, diarrhea, rash, alopecia, hepatotoxicity, renal (high doses)	CBC, lytes, liver enzymes, SCr, BUN, UOP
Cyclophosphamide (Cytoxan) (CTX)	Alkylator	Rhabdomyosarcoma Ewing's sarcoma Neuroblastoma Wilms' tumor	IV, PO	Myelosuppression, nausea, vomiting, diarrhea, hemorrhagic cystitis, alopecia, SIADH, cardiac toxicity (high doses)	CBC, lytes, Scr, BUN, UOP, UA, I/O
Ifosfamide (Ifex) (IFOS)	Alkylator	Rhabdomyosarcoma Osteosarcoma Ewing's sarcoma Neuroblastoma	IV	Myelosuppression, nausea, vomiting, diarrhea, hemorrhagic cystitis, neurotoxicity, alopecia, renal tubular acidosis, electrolyte disturbances	CBC, lytes, SCr, BUN, UOP, UA, I/O
Cisplatin (Platinol) (CDDP)	Alkylator	Brain tumors Osteosarcoma Neuroblastoma Germ cell tumors	IV	Myelosuppression, nausea, vomiting, renal toxicity, electrolyte disturbances, ototoxicity, anaphylaxis, neurotoxicity	CBC, lytes, SCr, BUN, UOP, I/O
Carboplatin (Paraplatin) (CBDCA)	Alkylator	Brain tumors Osteosarcoma Neuroblastoma	IV	Myelosuppression, nausea, vomiting, hepatotoxicity, electrolyte abnormalities	CBC, liver enzymes, lytes, renal function
Doxorubicin (Adriamycin) (DOX, ADR)	Antitumor antibiotic	Most solid tumors	IV	Myelosuppression, nausea, vomiting, diarrhea, alopecia, radiation recall reaction, cardiotoxicity	CBC, lytes, bilirubin (for dose adjustments), injection site (vesicant)
Dactinomycin (Cosmegen)	Antitumor antibiotic	Wilms' tumor Ewing's sarcoma Rhabdomyosarcoma	IV	Myelosuppression, nausea, vomiting, diarrhea, alopecia, radiation recall reaction, photosensitizer, hepatotoxicity	CBC, lytes, liver panel, skin (previously irradiated areas) Ascites, bilirubin
Mechlorethamine (Mustargen)	Alkylator	Brain tumors	IV	Myelosuppression, nausea, vomiting, hyperuricemia, anaphylaxis	CBC, lytes, uric acid
Lomustine (CeeNU) (CCNU)	Alkylator	Brain tumors	PO	Myelosuppression, nausea, vomiting, hepatotoxicity, neurotoxicity, alopecia	CBC, lytes, liver panel
Procarbazine (Matulane)	Alkylator	Brain tumors	PO	Myelosuppression, nausea, vomiting, diarrhea, alopecia, neurotoxicity	CBC, lytes
Dacarbazine (DTIC-Dome) (DIC)	Alkylator	Brain tumors	IV	Myelosuppression, nausea, vomiting, flu-like symptoms, photosensitizer	CBC, lytes
Vincristine (Oncovin) (VCR)	Vinca alkaloid	Most solid tumors	IV (NEVER IT)	Neurotoxicity, peripheral neuropathy, constipation, alopecia, SIADH, hypotension	Lytes, blood pressure, bowel movements, extremities (tingling, foot drop)
Etoposide (VePesid) (VP-16)	Topoisomerase inhibitor	Brain tumors Neuroblastoma Ewing's sarcoma Rhabdomyosarcoma	IV, PO	Myelosuppression, nausea, vomiting, mucositis, alopecia, hypotension (IV formulation), anaphylaxis	CBC, lytes, blood pressure

IV, intravenously; PO, by mouth; CBC, complete blood cell count with differential; lytes, electrolyte panel; SCr, serum creatinine; BUN, blood urea nitrogen; UOP, urine output; SIADH, syndrome of inappropriate antidiuretic hormone; UA, urinalysis; I/O, ins/outs.
(From Pizzo PA, Poplack DG, eds. The principles and practice of pediatric oncology. 4th ed. Philadelphia, Lippincott, Williams and Wilkins, 2001, with permission).

survival is estimated to be less than 30%, and, although mixed results have been reported, some patients have shown significant benefit.[12–14] This therapy may gain a more defined role in the future after additional studies are performed.

Immunotherapy is another treatment modality in pediatric solid malignancies. Immunotherapy, which includes growth-differentiating agents, gene therapy, and biologic therapy, is used to augment the patient's own immune system or can be used to directly transfer immunity by the incorporation of physiologic proteins in the defense of cancer. Interferons, interleukins, monoclonal antibodies, and retinoids are examples of such agents. This area of therapy continues to be one of great interest, and the exact role of these agents in solid tumors has yet to be clearly defined.

SUPPORTIVE CARE

With the introduction of dose-intensive chemotherapy regimens, the frequency and severity of side effects have increased. Some of the most common adverse reactions encountered include severe myelosuppression, mucositis, nausea, and vomiting. Delays in subsequent cycles of chemotherapy can result due to hospitalization for management of febrile neutropenia and dehydration. Resultant delays in subsequent chemotherapy (inability to maintain dose density), and chemotherapy dose reductions (failure to maintain dose intensity) can adversely affect overall tumor response and survival.

Recent advances in supportive care therapies have allowed more patients to remain on schedule with fewer side effects. Granulocyte colony-stimulating factor (G-CSF, filgrastim, pegfilgrastim) and granulocyte-macrophage colony-stimulating factor (GM-CSF, sargramostim) are growth factors that stimulate the production of white blood cells. These agents have demonstrated benefit in cancer management by shortening the period and degree of neutropenia in some patients. Improvements in nausea control have been made possible with the use of the nonsedating serotonin (5-HT$_3$) receptor antagonists (ondansetron, granisetron, dolasetron, palonosetron). When compared to the phenothiazines (prochlorperazine and chlorpromazine) and the dopamine receptor antagonist metoclopramide, administered in high doses, they provide effective control of nausea and vomiting with fewer side effects, particularly the extrapyramidal side effects seen more frequently in children.[15] Other supportive measures in the pediatric population include blood products (red blood cells and platelets), hyperalimentation, broad-spectrum antibiotics, pain management, and fluid and electrolyte replacement.

CLINICAL TRIALS AND RESEARCH

The National Cancer Institute (NCI) has supported national and international collaborations devoted to studying cancer etiologies in children. By monitoring U.S. and international trends in incidence and mortality, patterns may emerge providing information on the causes and control of cancer. By studying the biology of childhood cancer, such as cellular processes, signal transduction, cell cycle control, and tumor suppressor gene inactivation, new targeted treatment strategies may be developed. Each year about 4,000 children enter into ongoing clinical trials sponsored by the NCI and conducted by several cooperative groups. The Children's Oncology Group (COG) is composed of more than 200 institutions throughout the United States, Canada, Europe, and Australia. COG was formed in 2000 by the merger of four pediatric cancer cooperative groups to accelerate curative research and to provide equal access to therapy and medical expertise in pediatric oncology. Another group working together is the Pediatric Brain Tumor Consortium (PBTC).The goal of the PBTC is to conduct phase I and phase II clinical trials in new drug development, drug delivery systems (i.e., intrathecal administration), biologic therapies, and radiation treatments in children with primary central nervous system (CNS) malignancies.

Members of these organizations meet periodically within their groups to review current data, revise treatment standards based on their data, and discuss future therapeutic plans. Conducting studies at several institutions allows for greater patient accrual, and they can expedite the research process and validate results that can be put into clinical practice more quickly. In addition, these patients are more likely to receive follow-up care that is meticulously documented, allowing for the observation of delayed effects following treatments and determination of appropriate interventions and treatments for these long-term sequelae. Therefore, enrollment of children in clinical studies should be strongly encouraged.

LONG-TERM SEQUELAE AND SECONDARY MALIGNANCIES

There are an estimated 270,000 childhood cancer survivors in the U.S. population or 1 in 640 people aged 18 to 45. Because the majority of children treated for a childhood malignancy become long-term survivors, late effects and secondary malignancies are a concern for the clinician.[16–18] Secondary malignancies are estimated to occur in 3% to 12% of patients within 20 years of diagnosis and are most frequently associated with alkylating agents, nitrosoureas, and epipodophyllotoxins.[19–21] The actual manifestations of delayed toxicities following chemotherapy or radiotherapy and their appropriate management should remain an integral part of the therapeutic plan for each patient. Common complications following treatment are summarized in Table 101.4.[17,20,21]

The Childhood Cancer Survivor Study, an NCI-funded retrospective cohort study initiated in 1993 and completed in 2004, collected outcome information from 14,000 childhood

TABLE 101.4	Long-Term Effects After Treatment for Childhood Malignancies		
Organ System	**Offending Agent(s)**	**Manifestations**	**Monitoring Parameters**
Endocrine	Radiation therapy to the head, neck, or central nervous system or chemotherapy to the central nervous system	Impaired growth Abnormal pubertal progression Hypothyroidism	Height, weight, growth velocity, scoliosis examination Growth velocity and development Thyroid-stimulating hormone and T4 measurements, size of thyroid
Reproductive	Males: radiation to the testes or central nervous system, nitrosoureas, alkylators, procarbazine	Azoospermia, oligospermia, decreased testicular size	Testosterone, follicle-stimulating hormone, luteinizing hormone, testicular volume, semen analysis
	Females: radiation to the pelvis, nitrosoureas, alkylators, procarbazine	Amenorrhea, oligomenorrhea, precocious puberty, ovarian dysfunction	Estrogen, follicle-stimulating hormone, luteinizing hormone, menstrual history
Renal	Nephrectomy (Wilms' tumor), cisplatin, cyclophosphamide, ifosfamide	Decreased glomerular filtration rate, chronic cystitis, tubular necrosis, Fanconi's syndrome, vesicoureteral reflux	Serum creatinine, blood urea nitrogen, electrolytes, urinalysis, blood pressure, possible renal ultrasound
Cardiac	Radiation to the thorax, anthracyclines, high-dose cyclophosphamide	Left ventricular dysfunction, coronary artery disease, congestive heart failure, arrhythmias	Chest x-ray, electrocardiogram, echocardiogram, lipid profile, consider exercise testing or radionuclide angiocardiogram (baseline and serial measurements for life)
Pulmonary	Whole-lung irradiation, bleomycin, nitrosoureas, busulfan, methotrexate, cyclophosphamide	Decreased lung volume, restrictive airway disease, decreased cardiac output diffusion, decreased exercise tolerance	Chest x-ray, pulmonary function tests
Liver	Radiation to the abdomen, methotrexate, 6-mercaptopurine	Elevation of bilirubin and liver enzymes, liver fibrosis, hepatitis, cirrhosis	Liver enzyme panel, serologies for hepatitis, imaging studies
Central nervous system	Cranial irradiation and central nervous system chemotherapy	Decreased attention span, memory loss, leukoencephalopathy, brain necrosis, seizures, cerebrovascular accident	Cognitive learning tests, computed tomography, MRI, EEG

MRI, magnetic resonance imaging; EEG, electroencephalography.

cancer survivors diagnosed before the age of 20 between 1970 and 1986. A total of 3,500 siblings of the survivors served as the controls. Data were collected from 26 participating institutions within the United States and one in Canada. The most frequently occurring tumor types were studied: leukemia, lymphoma, brain tumors, osteosarcoma, WT, NB, and soft-tissue sarcomas.

The aim of the study was to learn about the long-term effects of cancer and its therapy to design future treatment protocols tested by clinical trials and identify interventional strategies that increase survival and minimize harmful ef-

fects. High-risk groups and several key findings have been identified. Mortality due to recurrent disease occurs within 10–15 years of diagnosis, whereas late mortality (approximately 30 years from diagnosis) is due to cardiac/pulmonary events and the development of a second malignancy (SMN). Childhood cancer survivors have a sixfold increased risk of developing a new cancer, with a higher risk in females versus males, and in those patients who had received prior radiation therapy. The most common SMNs include bone, breast, thyroid, and CNS tumors. Multiple publications based on this study are now available.[22]

BRAIN TUMORS

Primary neoplasms of the brain are second only to leukemia in their frequency during childhood, and are the most common solid tumors in children under 15 years of age. A multidisciplinary approach is required to meet the challenges encountered when taking care of the pediatric brain tumor patient secondary to acute and long-term disease and treatment-related morbidity. Members of the team should include psychologists; physical, occupational, and speech therapists; clinical nutritionists; medical oncologists, neuro-surgeons, radiation oncologists, and radiologists. Improvements in diagnostic, surgical, and radiation techniques, chemotherapeutic regimens, and drug delivery methods have allowed for an improvement in the overall 5-year survival rates from 35% in the early 1960s to better than 60% in the early 1990s.[2] Brain tumors are a heterogeneous group of neoplasms, with tissue type and site of tumor incidences varying with the patient's age.

TREATMENT GOALS: PEDIATRIC BRAIN TUMORS

The initial management of the child with a brain tumor is surgery is to establish a diagnosis, reduce tumor burden, and potentially cure the patient. Gross total resection (GTR) is the treatment of choice for *accessible* tumors, those that can be removed without causing severe neurological damage. Tumor location, morphologic features, growth potential, extent of invasion, and tendency for progression and recurrence will determine the therapeutic treatment plan.[23]

■ Improve cure rates while minimizing the acute toxicity of therapy and significant late treatment effects.

EPIDEMIOLOGY

All CNS tumors account for approximately 20% of cancers in children under the age of 15 years. The incidence of brain tumors in males is slightly greater than in females (1.13:1), and whites have a higher incidence than African-Americans (1.25:1).[3] Incidence peaks in the first decade of life, and then decreases until a second peak occurs in older adulthood. In the early 1990s, the incidence appeared to be increasing, however, increased use of MRI at the time allowed for better evaluation and confirmation of CNS lesions. Also, the World Health Organization (WHO) changed the classification of some tumors from benign to malignant.[24] Cerebral lesions are most common in the first 2 years of life, while cerebellar lesions are more common up to age 10. Most frequently encountered tumor types are medulloblastomas, supratentorial primitive neuroectodermal tumors (sPNETs), and pineoblastomas. Unlike adults, high-grade gliomas are much less common in children. The only two factors consistently shown to place a child at increased risk of developing a brain tumor are various genetic disorders and exposure to ionizing radiation.[25,26]

CLINICAL PRESENTATION AND DIAGNOSIS

SIGNS AND SYMPTOMS

Initially, clinical manifestations of brain tumors are nonspecific. Generalized symptoms, such as nausea, vomiting, and headaches, are commonly mistaken for evidence of an infectious etiology, migraine, or tension headache. Clinical presentation depends on tumor location, age, and developmental level. Increases in intracranial pressure (ICP), as a result of compression of structures or obstruction of cerebral spinal fluid flow, initially present as declining academic performance, fatigue, personality changes, and headaches, which worsen in the morning and are accompanied by emesis in school-aged children. Infants and young children present with irritability, anorexia, failure to thrive, and possible loss of developmental milestones. Localizing symptoms may include gait disturbances and ataxia, seizures, visual field defects, neuroendocrine abnormalities, facial and extraocular muscle palsies, and hemiparesis. Unlike adults, a seizure seldom indicates the presence of a mass in children. However, all seizure activity in a child mandates imaging of the brain with computed tomography (CT) or MRI. Nonlocalizing signs and symptoms include changes in affect, energy level, motivation, or behavior.[23]

DIAGNOSIS

Preoperative assessment of tumor type and extent by imaging with MRI or CT is used to diagnose the presence of a CNS lesion based on location, tissue characterization, and enhancement pattern, along with a clinical history. MRI and CT are also performed postoperatively to assess for the presence of residual tumor. For tumors with a high propensity for metastasis into the cerebrospinal fluid (CSF), such as medulloblastoma, posterior-fossa ependymoma, and germ-cell tumors, spinal MRI and a cytologic examination of CSF are performed for staging purposes. To achieve sharp images, movement during MRI and CT must be kept to a minimum; thus children are often immobilized and sedated before the examination.

Tumors are commonly classified by their location and are broadly divided into two categories: (a) supratentorial neoplasms, including cerebral hemispheric and midline tumors; and (b) infratentorial neoplasms, including brain stem and cerebellar tumors (Table 101.5).[27] Unlike adults, in whom most brain tumors are located supratentorially near the cerebral hemispheres, 45% to 60% of CNS tumors in children older than 1 year arise infratentorially in the posterior fossa. The most prevalent histology is glial in origin and includes a broad variety of tumor types, most commonly low-grade astrocytoma. The medulloblastoma, of primitive neuroectodermal origin, is a malignant cerebellar tumor that has a marked propensity to invade the meninges and parenchymal tissue and is the most common tumor type of childhood brain neoplasms. Midline tumors, such as craniopharyngiomas and pineal tumors, occur near the optic chiasm and often cause visual field defects, hydrocephalus, and extraocular muscle palsies.[23]

TREATMENT

SURGERY

The specific management of brain malignancies depends on tumor type and location. To make a histologic diagnosis and reduce tumor burden, surgery is often the first treatment modality of a series of interventions. The goal is to remove as much tumor as is safely possible. However, surgical cure is often not an obtainable goal because of the anatomic location of many tumors, which may not allow for total resection. A limitation to complete resection is the infiltration of the neoplasm into normal surrounding tissue. Unlike other solid, non-CNS tumors, a resection with clean margins is rarely feasible due to the unacceptable risk of producing irreversible neurologic deficits. Short-term external ventricular drains or long-term internal ventriculoperitoneal shunts are often placed to drain CSF in patients with obstructive hydro-

TABLE 101.5	Distribution of Common Brain Tumors in Children According to Location and Histologic Appearance
Location and Type of Tumor	**Percentage of All Brain Tumors**
Infratentorial	
Primitive neuroectodermal tumor (medulloblastoma)	20–25
Low-grade astrocytoma, cerebellar	12–18
Ependymoma	4–8
Malignant glioma, brainstem	3–9
Low-grade astrocytoma, brainstem	3–6
Other	2–5
Total	**45–60**
Supratentorial hemispheric	
Low-grade astrocytoma	8–20
Malignant glioma	6–12
Ependymoma	2–5
Mixed glioma	1–5
Ganglioglioma	1–5
Oligodendroglioma	1–2
Choroid-plexus tumor	1–2
Primitive neuroectodermal tumor	1–2
Meningioma	0.5–2
Other	1–3
Total	**25–40**
Supratentorial midline	
Suprasellar	
Craniopharyngioma	6–9
Low-grade glioma, chiasmatic-hypothalamic	4–8
Germ-cell tumor	1–2
Pituitary adenoma	0.05–2.5
Pineal region	
Low-grade glioma	1–2
Germ-cell tumor	0.05–2
Pineal parenchymal tumor	0.05–2
Total	**15–20**

(From Pollack IF. Brain tumors in children. N Engl J Med 331:1500–1510, 1994, with permission.)

cephalus. Table 101.6 summarizes the perioperative supportive care issues often seen in clinical practice when treating patients with brain tumors.[27]

RADIOTHERAPY

Brain tumors have customarily been treated with maximum tolerated doses of 5,000 to 6,000 cGy administered in once

| TABLE 101.6 | Common Perioperative Problems of Childhood Brain Tumors with Pharmacologic or Surgical Solutions |

Perioperative Problem	Type of Tumors Involved	Preoperative and Intraoperative Management	Postoperative Management
Peritumoral edema	Large tumors; smaller tumors in critical areas such as the brainstem	Corticosteroids (e.g., dexamethasone [Decadron] at a dose of 0.05–0.1 mg/kg or body weight 4 times daily) are administered.	Corticosteroids are tapered within several days of surgery, particularly if tumor resection is extensive.
Obstructive hydrocephalus	Intraventricular or periventricular tumors	An external ventricular drain is placed before tumor resection is begun.	If the tumor resection opens the cerebrospinal fluid pathways, drainage established by ventriculostomy can often be discontinued within several days of surgery. Patients in whom progressive ventriculomegaly develops or who have an enlarging pseudomeningocele require definitive diversion of cerebrospinal fluid. Although a shunt poses a theoretical risk of peritoneal seeding of the tumor, this has not been confirmed in studies.
Seizures	Tumors of the cerebral hemispheres; tumors that will require cerebral retraction during their removal	An anticonvulsant agent, such as phenytoin (Dilantin), is started preoperatively and continued during surgery.	In children without prior seizures, anticonvulsant drugs can generally be stopped within several months of surgery. In patients with a history of preoperative seizures who undergo complete tumor removal and are rendered seizure free, anticonvulsant agents can often be discontinued within several months of surgery.
Hypothalamic-pituitary hormonal insufficiency	Tumors arising in and around the hypothalamus	An evaluation of endocrine function is useful if the child is clinically stable. "Stress" doses (doses several times the normal maintenance dose) of a corticosteroid, such as hydrocortisone, are administered before and during surgery. Because diabetes insipidus may develop during surgery, fluid balance must be monitored closely.	Doses of corticosteroids can be decreased to maintenance levels during the first postoperative week. Fluid balance and electrolyte levels are monitored closely and controlled by administration of appropriate fluids and, if indicated, vasopressin. Detailed postoperative and, follow-up endocrine testing is required to determine long-term needs for hormonal replacement.

(From Pollack IF. Brain tumors in children. N Engl J Med 331:1500–1510, 1994, with permission.)

daily fractions of 180 to 200 cGy over 5 to 6 weeks. Radiation hyper-fractionation, the administration of larger numbers (twice daily doses) of smaller fractions of radiotherapy over an equivalent period, may allow for higher total doses with less morbidity and intensified tumor kill.[29] Results of studies in brain stem gliomas have been mixed.[30] By combining the advances in imaging with technology, conformal radiation therapy targets the radiation dose to the tumor while minimizing exposure to normal brain structures.[31,32] Brain stem tumors are often surgically inaccessible; therefore, primary treatment is radiotherapy with or without combination chemotherapy.[27] For neoplasms that have a propensity to metastasize throughout the neuraxis, craniospinal irradiation may be indicated.[28]

The responses of brain tissues to radiation are classified into three groups: (a) acute (occurring during treatment), (b) early delayed/subacute (occurring a few weeks up to 3 months after treatment), and (c) late delayed reactions. Acute adverse effects of brain irradiation include transient exacerbation of local neurologic signs; radiation sickness with symptoms of nausea, vomiting, loss of appetite, drowsiness, and irritability; xerostomia and sialadenitis (inflammation of the salivary glands); hair loss; bone marrow suppression in those receiving craniospinal irradiation; skin erythema, breakdown, and hyperpigmentation; and the somnolence syndrome, a period of extreme drowsiness that may occur 4 to 8 weeks after the completion of a course of treatment with recovery in 1 to 2 weeks thereafter. Late side effects include focal radiation necrosis, postirradiation diffuse white-matter injury, leukoencephalopathy, secondary tumors, and late neurological effects, which includes intellectual impairment, memory deficits, and inability to acquire new knowledge.[24]

Radiation-induced brain injury is regarded as one of the most serious complications of radiation therapy, limiting the dose of irradiation administered. Brain development is most rapid in the first 3 years of life, slows after age 6, and reaches maturation in puberty. Therefore, impairment in cognition is worse in children irradiated younger than age 4 to 7 and for those patients who receive whole-brain or supratentorial irradiation.[24]

CHEMOTHERAPY

The presence of the blood–brain barrier (BBB) prevents the ability to achieve therapeutic antineoplastic drug concentrations in the brain. Determinants of BBB penetration embody physiochemical and pharmacokinetic drug properties and pathophysiology of the tumor itself. Chemotherapeutic agents of low molecular weight, of high lipid solubility, and that unionize at physiologic pH have the highest chance of crossing the BBB. Pharmacokinetic properties such as low serum protein binding and a long elimination half-life may also improve drug entrance into the brain. The pathophysiology of large CNS masses creates a paradoxical situation in which permeability of the BBB is enhanced at the necrotic center, but reduced around the viable periphery of the tumor where antineoplastic effects are desired. However, clinical trials have demonstrated that some water-soluble agents (platinum analogs and classical alkylators) have significant activity in certain brain tumors that may be a result of increased BBB permeability induced by the malignancy. The efficacy of chemotherapy agents also depends on tumor growth kinetics.

The use of high-dose chemotherapy followed by autologous bone marrow or peripheral blood stem cell rescue is

aimed at overcoming these limitations. The nitrosoureas were the first class of agents studied because of their lipid solubility. However, dose escalation was not possible secondary to excessive neurotoxicity. More recent trials have used combinations of cyclophosphamide, melphalan, and thiotepa, with or without etoposide. However, no specific regimen can be considered standard for any tumor types. Therefore, the NCI established the PBTC from within nine institutions that collectively diagnose and treat primary brain tumors in children. Their objectives are to rapidly develop pilot data about new therapeutic agents, neuroimaging techniques, and perform biologic studies of brain tumor specimens. Results will then be made available to the COG and other international cooperative groups for testing in larger phase II and phase III studies.

Primary chemotherapy is indicated in children less than 3 years of age due to their increased risk of developing severe long-term neurological deficits from irradiation. Published results of infant brain tumor trials have demonstrated that the use of up-front chemotherapy, with delayed or lower-dose radiation, show similar survival rates to those seen in older children.

Drug delivery directly into the intrathecal space, through a lumbar puncture or a ventricular reservoir, is currently under investigation. As the volume of the CSF is small, this allows for higher concentrations of drug with lower doses. Agents investigated include mafosfamide and topotecan.[33] Mafosfamide, is the preactivated derivative of the prodrug cyclophosphamide. Topotecan is a water soluble analog of camptothecin and is an inhibitor of topoisomerase I. Temozolomide, an orally administered alkylating agent with the same active metabolite as dacarbazine, is approved by the Food and Drug Administration (FDA) for the treatment of adult brain tumors, and is currently under clinical investigation in children.[34] Table 101.7 summarizes some common chemotherapy combinations (and their acronyms) that have been used in brain tumors.[35]

FUTURE THERAPIES

On-going clinical trials are evaluating drug therapies aimed at specific molecular targets involved in promoting apoptosis (programmed cell death) or inhibiting cellular proliferation. For example, understanding cell signaling pathways via the epidermal growth factor receptor (EGFR), its expression patterns, and correlation with clinical outcomes has led to several studies investigating the role of the tyrosine kinase inhibitors, gefitinib, lapatinib, and erlotinib.

Several studies are underway to determine whether or not chemotherapy, given concurrently or following radiation therapy, will make the tumor more responsive (i.e., more radiosensitive) to the effects of radiation, resulting in greater tumor cell kill.

TABLE 101.7	Chemotherapy Combinations for Pediatric Brain Tumors	
Regimen	**Dosage/Route**	**Comments**
"PCV"		
CCNU	100 mg/m² PO, day 1 or day 2	Every 6 weeks × 8 cycles (1 year)
Vincristine[a]	1.5 mg/m² IV (max 2 mg), days 1, 8, 15	
Prednisone	40 mg/m² PO, days 1–14	
OR		
Procarbazine	100 mg/m² PO days 1–14	
"MOPP"		
Nitrogen Mustard	6 mg/m² IV, days 1, 8	Every 4 weeks × 12 cycles (1 year)
Vincristine[a]	1.4–1.5 mg/m² IV (max 2 mg), days 1, 8	
Procarbazine	100 mg/m² PO, days 1–14	
Prednisone	40 mg/m² PO, days 1–14	
"8-in-1"		
Vincristine[a]	1.5 mg/m² IV, hour 0	Every 4–6 weeks × 10–24 cycles
CCNU	100 mg/m² PO, hour 0	
Procarbazine	75 mg/m² PO, hour 1	
Hydroxyurea	1500–3000 mg/m² PO, hour 2	
Cisplatin	60–90 mg/m² IV, hours 3–9	
Ara-C	300 mg/m² IV, hour 9	
Cyclophosphamide	300 mg/m² IV, hour 12	
OR		
Dacarbazine	150 mg/m² IV, hour 12	
Methylprednisolone	300 mg/m² IV, hours 0, 6, 12	
Cisplatin Combinations		
Cisplatin with Vincristine[a]	90–100 mg/m² IV, day 1 1.5 mg/m² IV, day 1	Every 3–4 weeks Various combinations with cisplatin, which is a very active agent in medulloblastoma and ependymoma
OR		
Etoposide	150 mg/m² IV, day 3 and 4	
OR		
Cyclophosphamide	1000 mg/m² IV, day 1	

[a] Maximum dose 2 mg.
PO, orally; IV, intravenously; CCNU, lomustine; MOPP, *mechlorethamine or Mustargen, vincristine or Oncovin, prednisone, and procarbazine.*

Continued data collection, and further evaluation of the data collected as part of the Childhood Cancer Survivor Study, will help identify the patients at greatest risk of developing acute and long-term treatment-related complications. Maximizing drug and radiation delivery techniques, coupled with surgical advances, may help to minimize or alleviate the physical, medical, cognitive, and psychosocial adverse outcomes commonly associated with CNS neoplasms.

PROGNOSIS

The 5-year survival rate is best in children with cerebellar astrocytomas and worse for those with brain stem gliomas. Less than one third of patients in poor risk categories (high-grade astrocytomas, including glioblastoma multiforme, unresectable medulloblastomas, anaplastic ependymomas, unresectable brain stem tumors, and in children

<4 years of age) become long-term survivors. Even when therapy is successful, brain tumor survivors suffer physical, cognitive, neurologic, endocrinologic, and other deficits as a result of their disease and its treatment.[36]

Social, physical, and intellectual function is lower than their peers, resulting in a poorer quality of life. Patients must also be followed closely for possible disease relapse.

NEUROBLASTOMA

NB is the most common extracranial solid tumor in children, accounting for 8% to 10% of all childhood cancers. It is the most common cancer diagnosed during infancy with a median age at diagnosis of 17.3 months. The neuroblastic tumors (including NB, ganglioneuroblastoma, and ganglioneuroma) are derived from primordial neural crest cells that ultimately give rise to the sympathetic ganglia, adrenal medulla, and other sites.[37] Spontaneous regression of NB is occasionally observed in young infants; it is extremely rare in older children. Furthermore, the tumor may undergo differentiation to a more mature and benign tumor type classified as a ganglioneuroma. Tumors with mixed pathologic characteristics (benign and malignant cells) are termed "ganglioneuroblastoma."[38] A small, round, blue-cell tumor, NB consists of uniformly sized cells with dense, hyperchromatic nuclei and scant cytoplasm. It is important for the pathologist to differentiate between NB and other small, round-cell tumors such as ES, lymphoma, RMS, and Askin's tumor.

EPIDEMIOLOGY

There are approximately 600 new cases of NB per year in the United States, occurring in 1 of every 7,000 live births. NB rarely occurs after 10 years of age. There is little difference in the incidence between males and females. Whites are more likely to develop NB than African-Americans (1.31:1). Genetic abnormalities associated with NB include deletions on the short arm of chromosome 1 and N-*myc* oncogene (also known as *MYCN*) amplification (found in 5%–10% of low stage disease vs. 30%–40% of advanced disease).[37] Amplification of N-*myc* is associated with advanced stages of disease, rapid tumor progression, and a poor prognosis. Etiology is unknown in most cases. No prenatal or postnatal exposure to drugs, chemicals, viruses, environmental factors, or radiation has been associated strongly, consistently, or unequivocally with an increased incidence of NB.

CLINICAL PRESENTATION AND DIAGNOSIS

SIGNS AND SYMPTOMS

Since NB can arise from any site along the sympathetic nervous system chain, locations of primary tumors vary and

change with age. The most common site of the primary tumor is in the abdomen [adrenal gland (40%) or a retroperitoneal paraspinal ganglion (25%)], thoracic cavity (15%), or pelvis (5%). Infants have more thoracic and cervical primaries than children. Metastatic disease, via lymphatic and hematogenous spread, is identified in 41% of infants and 80% in older children at diagnosis. The most common sites of metastases are lymph nodes, bone marrow, bone, liver, and subcutaneous tissue.

Signs and symptoms at presentation depend on the location of the primary tumor and metastatic sites. Patients with abdominal disease will have complaints of fullness, discomfort, and rarely, obstruction. A fixed, hard abdominal mass is palpated on physical exam. Compression of venous and lymphatic drainage from the lower extremities due to large primary or metastatic abdominal masses may lead to painful scrotal and lower extremity edema. Sudden increases in abdominal girth may be a result of spontaneous hemorrhage into the tumor. Thoracic NB presents as a posterior mediastinal mass and may be found coincidentally on a chest x-ray obtained during an evaluation for trauma or infection. Mechanical obstruction from large thoracic tumors may result in superior vena cava syndrome. High thoracic and cervical masses can be associated with Horner's syndrome, which consists of unilateral ptosis, myosis, and anhydrosis. Paraspinal tumors may extend into neuronal foramina of the vertebral bodies and result in symptoms related to compression of nerve roots and the spinal cord. The range of symptoms includes radicular pain, subacute paraplegia, and bowel and bladder dysfunction. Constitutional symptoms include weight loss, anorexia, intermittent fever, hypertension (due to compression of the renal vasculature), secretory diarrhea (due to tumor secretion of vasoactive intestinal peptide), and irritability.[37]

Ferritin levels may be increased in actively growing tumors and have been associated with worse prognosis. Increased lactase dehydrogenase (LDH) levels indicate rapid cellular turnover or a large tumor burden. Signs and symptoms associated with metastatic disease include: proptosis (protruding eyes) and periorbital ecchymoses (tumor infiltrating periorbital bones); limping and irritability from bone pain; anemia, bleeding and increased risk of infection due to bone marrow replacement with malignant cells; and skin involvement (blue subcutaneous nodules).

TABLE 101.8	International Neuroblastoma Staging System and Treatment Summary			
Stage	**Staging Criteria**	**Incidence**	**Treatment**	**Survival at 5 Years**
I	Localized tumor confined to the area of origin, complete gross excision with or without microscopic residual disease; identifiable ipsilateral and contralateral lymph nodes negative microscopically,	5%	Surgery alone, chemotherapy with recurrence	90% or greater
IIa	Localized tumor with incomplete gross excision; representative ipsilateral nonadherent lymph nodes negative for tumor microscopically	10%	Surgery plus postoperative chemotherapy with 5 courses of cyclophosphamide plus doxorubicin	70%–80%
IIb	Unilateral tumor with complete or incomplete gross excision; with positive ipsilateral regional lymph nodes: identifiable contralateral lymph nodes negative microscopically	10%	Surgery plus postoperative chemotherapy with 5 courses of cyclophosphamide plus doxorubicin	70%–80%
III	Tumor infiltrating across the midline with or without regional lymph node involvement; or, midline tumor with bilateral regional lymph node involvement	25%	Surgery plus postoperative chemotherapy with 5 courses of cyclophosphamide plus doxorubicin	40%–70% (depending on completeness of surgical resection)
IV	Dissemination of the tumor to distant lymph nodes, bone, bone marrow, liver, or other organs (except as defined in stage IVs)	60%	Aggressive chemotherapy with cyclophosphamide plus doxorubicin then cisplatin plus teniposide plus radiotherapy; consider dose intensification with ABMT for older children	More than 60% if age at diagnosis is younger than 1 year; 20% if age at diagnosis is older than 1 year and under 2 years; 10% if age at diagnosis is over 2 years
IVs	Localized primary tumor as defined for stage 1 or 2 with dissemination limited to liver, skin, or bone marrow.	5%	Individualized therapy, not standardized	More than 80%

ABMT, allogenic bone marrow transplantation.

DIAGNOSIS

A definitive diagnosis is made under one of the following circumstances: (a) an unequivocal pathologic diagnosis made from tumor tissue by light microscopy with or without immunohistology, electron microscopy, or increased serum or urine catecholamines or metabolites; or (b) bone marrow aspirate or trephine biopsy containing tumor cells and increased serum or urine catecholamines or metabolites.[37]

Metastatic workup should include plain radiographs to detect a calcified abdominal or mediastinal mass; bone scintigraphy and skeletal survey to detect bone metastases; abdominal ultrasound and CT to rule out lymph node and liver involvement; head CT or MRI to detect skull, orbital, mandible, or brain metastasis; bone marrow aspirates and biopsies (one of each on either side of the iliac crest).

In 1987, the International Neuroblastoma Staging System (INSS) was proposed that would lead to uniformity in staging patients with NB for clinical trials and biologic studies worldwide. The INSS combines features from two other widely used staging systems used by the former Children's Cancer Study Group (CCG) (Evans' staging system) and the Pediatric Oncology Group (POG), which are detailed elsewhere.[39] Table 101.8 summarizes the INSS along with treatment and prognosis for each stage of disease.[40] Clinical, radiographic, and surgical evaluation of the child with NB forms the foundation for the INSS.

TREATMENT

The treatment of NB is a combination of surgery, radiotherapy, and chemotherapy. The stage of the tumor, age of the patient, and biologic features of the tumor determine the role of each treatment modality. Infants less than 1 year of age commonly have a small primary tumor and metastases to the skin, liver, or bone marrow (stage IVs). Their disease often regresses spontaneously, and only supportive care may be necessary.[38] Chemotherapy remains the backbone of the multimodality treatment plan. The same tests used to determine extent of disease at diagnosis and should be used to assess response to treatment. Evaluations are usually done at the end of induction therapy (after 3–4 months), at the end of treatment, before and after surgical procedures, and as clinically indicated.

SURGERY

Surgery is an important treatment modality in NB for diagnosis and treatment. The goals of surgery are to establish the diagnosis, provide tissue samples for pathologic and biologic evaluation, stage the patient, and completely resect the tumor without injury to vital structures. Those patients with localized disease (stages I and II) require no additional treatment after surgery. In patients with large abdominal primary tumors, surgery is often delayed until after several cycles of chemotherapy have been administered (neoadjuvant chemotherapy). As these tumors may encircle the celiac axis and the superior mesenteric vessels, chemotherapy may decrease the vascularity and friability of the tumor. Complications from surgical procedures are relatively uncommon (5%–25%) and occur most frequently with abdominal tumors and in infants. Complications include nephrectomy, hemorrhage, adhesions, renal failure, and neurologic deficits.

RADIOTHERAPY

NB is considered a radiosensitive tumor. Tumoricidal doses of 15 to 30 cGy (dose dependent on age, tumor volume, and location) are generally used to treat residual tumor after surgery or chemotherapy. Radiotherapy is also used in palliation of symptoms for end-stage disease. Radioactive-labeled meta-iodobenzylguanidine (MIBG) has been studied in Europe and the United States for diagnostic and therapeutic purposes. MIBG is taken up by catecholamine-secreting tumors, such as pheochromocytomas and immature NB cells. Using this specificity, MIBG radiolabeled with ^{125}I and ^{131}I has been used for detection of NB and evaluated for antitumor activity in small phase I and phase II studies. MIBG may be ultimately useful for the treatment of advanced stage or residual tumor following surgery in stage III patients or palliation of bone pain. Use of this therapy may advantageously decrease the patient's overall exposure to radiation while increasing the total dose of radiation delivered to the tumor. The myelosuppressive effects of MIBG on tumor-infiltrated bone marrow have been problematic. Future studies will better define its role in the diagnosis and therapy of NB.[41,42]

CHEMOTHERAPY

The primary treatment modality for intermediate or high-risk NB is chemotherapy. A number of agents have demonstrated activity in NB in several single-agent phase II trials. Examples of these agents, which have yielded response rates of 34% to 45%, include cyclophosphamide, cisplatin, doxorubicin, vincristine, etoposide, and teniposide.[39] Combination chemotherapy has been shown to be more effective than single-agent therapy. Dose-intensified regimens have produced excellent local responses, but the duration of response has been limiting. High-dose chemotherapy followed by purged autologous stem cell rescue, after initial induction chemotherapy, has produced promising results in patients with advanced disease.[43,44]

Topotecan, a topoisomerase I inhibitor, has shown activity in disseminated, recurrent, and refractory NB.[45,46] Clinical trials are underway evaluating its role in combination therapy with agents such as cyclophosphamide.

BIOLOGIC THERAPY

Because NB cells are known at times to undergo spontaneous regression or maturation to benign tumors, indicating that these cells may be regulated by natural defense mechanisms, newer research strategies are focusing on biologic manipulation of minimal residual disease. These strategies include exploitation of the body's own defense system with interleukin–2-stimulated natural killer cells and attempts to achieve tumor maturation with the use of vitamin B_{12} and retinoic acid.[40,47] In several randomized trials, isotretinoin (13-*cis*-retinoic acid) was found to significantly improve event-free survival in high-risk NB patients when administered after intensive chemotherapy alone or after intensive chemoradiotherapy supported by purged autologous bone marrow transplantation. Based on these results, it is recommended that isotretinoin is used as part of the standard therapy for minimal residual disease after consolidation therapy is complete. The dose is 160 mg/m²/day administered orally twice daily for 14 consecutive days in a 28-day cycle repeated for six cycles.[44,48] Another area of exploration is eradication of disease via monoclonal antibodies against the cell surface diganglioside antigen, G_{D2}, specifically located on NB cells. Radioactive ^{131}I-coupled G_{D2} antibodies have been administered as therapy for NB. Responses have been seen in patients with disseminated disease, but those with large tumor masses were resistant to this therapy. Monoclonal antibodies may also be useful in purging tumor cells from bone marrow ex vivo before reinfusion of autologous marrow after dose-intensive therapy.[37]

IMPROVING OUTCOMES

The New Approaches to Neuroblastoma Therapy Consortium (NANT) is a collaborative effort of clinical investigators and laboratory programs from university and children's hospitals, funded by the NCI, which tests promising new therapies and combinations of existing therapies for the treatment of NB on a national level via clinical trials.

Some new therapeutic strategies currently under investigation include the role of tyrosine kinase inhibitors, as NBs have been shown to express the Trk family tyrosine kinase receptors, which regulate growth, differentiation, and cell death. Newer retinoids are also being developed for use in NB, and targeted delivery of radiation to NB cells using radionuclides attached to MIBG.

With a greater understanding of the genetic and biologic features of NB, coupled with risk stratification according to prognostic indicators (such as N-*myc* amplification), clinicians will be able to determine the most appropriate type and intensity of treatment to optimize cure while minimizing side effects.

PROGNOSIS

The most important prognostic factors for NB are age of the patient at the time of diagnosis, stage at diagnosis, and the site of the primary tumor. Patients with primary tumors of the adrenal gland appear to have a poorer prognosis than patients with tumors originating at other sites, particularly the thorax. The survival of patients with a localized, surgically resected tumor without distant metastasis is 75% to 90%; however, patients greater than age 1 year with distant metastasis at presentation have only a 10% to 30% 2-year

TABLE 101.9	**Factors Associated with a Poor Prognosis in Neuroblastoma**

Age > 1 year

Advanced disease (stage 3 or 4)

Urinary catecholamine ratio of VMA/HVA ≤1

Serum ferritin >143 ng/mL (321 pmol/L)

Lactate dehydrogenase >1500 U/L

Neuron-specific enolase >100 ng/mL

N-*myc* oncogene amplification

Diploid karyotype (DNA index = 1)

Allelic loss or deletion associated with chromosome 1

disease-free survival rate.[38,49] Infants tend to have a better prognosis than do older children. The presence of the N-*myc* oncogene is found predominantly in patients with advanced disease and is associated with a rapid tumor progression and a poor prognosis.[50] Indicators associated with a poor prognosis in NB are listed in Table 101.9.[39,49,50]

WILMS' TUMOR

WT, also known as "nephroblastoma" or "renal embryoma," is the most common renal neoplasm in children. This tumor, which was first extensively described by Max Wilms more than 100 years ago, has a peak incidence during the second and third year of life and rarely occurs after age 6. Several genetic anomalies have been identified in patients with WT, including germline mutations within the WT1 gene. However, the precise etiology of WT remains unclear.

TREATMENT GOALS: WILMS' TUMOR

- The treatment of WT relies on the coordination of multidisciplinary efforts from the surgeon, radiation oncologist, and medical oncologist.
- A complete surgical excision of the tumor to cure the patient is the primary goal of treatment.
- Adjuvant radiation and chemotherapy are added to some treatment courses in patients in whom benefit has been previously demonstrated; thus the therapeutic approach to the child with WT depends on several factors.

EPIDEMIOLOGY

WT accounts for approximately 6.1% of all childhood cancers in the United States or 500 to 600 cases per year.[51] Males, females, African-Americans, and whites have a similar incidence, although previous evidence suggested that girls and African-American children were more likely to develop WT compared to boys and white children respectively.[3,51] Boys are more likely than girls to develop WT at a younger age; and bilateral disease, which accounts for approximately 4% to 8% of cases, more frequently occurs in the younger child. Several carcinogens during the prenatal period have been implicated in the development of WT, although definitive correlation is lacking. Examples of these exposures include cigarette smoking, alcohol, coffee, pesticides, oral contraceptive use, hair dyes, ionizing radiation, and industrial hydrocarbons.[52]

When WT occurs in the child with no genetic predisposition or family history, it is termed "sporadic." "Familial" WT is reserved for those patients with a genetic predisposition to the development of WT or when WT occurs as a feature of a specific genetic disorder. Several syndromes and related genes are associated with the development of WT. These include the WAGR syndrome (WT, aniridia, genitourinary anomalies, and mental retardation) and the WT1 gene on chromosome 11, the Denys-Drash syndrome and the WTI gene on chromosome 11, and the Beckwith–Weidemann syndrome and IGF2, H19, p57 genes on chromosome 11.[53,54] Other associated genes include the WT2, FWT1, and FWT2 genes.

CLINICAL PRESENTATION AND DIAGNOSIS

SIGNS AND SYMPTOMS

Most children are found to have nontumor-specific abdominal swelling or an asymptomatic palpable mass upon examination. Other symptoms, which occur in 20% to 30% of patients, are fever, malaise, abdominal pain, nausea, vomiting, and gross or microscopic hematuria. Approximately 25% of patients have hypertension as a result of increased renin activity and 10% have coagulopathy. Metastatic disease at the time of presentation is rare (15% of patients) and usually occurs in the lung (85%), the liver (7%), or both sites (8%).[53,55]

DIAGNOSIS

Diagnostic techniques are directed toward the primary goal of verifying the presence of WT and differentiating it from NB that can also present as a palpable abdominal mass. WT arises intrarenally and distorts the calyceal region of the kidney. NB occurs extrarenally and displaces rather than distorts cells in the kidney. In general, an abdominal ultrasound is sufficient for providing proper evaluation of the kidney in determining whether the mass is cystic or solid. Extrarenal involvement of other abdominal organs can be verified by CT; however, the benefit of this diagnostic technique in the child with WT is lacking because the decision to perform a laparotomy is usually supported by results from the ultrasound.[56] A chest x-ray can verify the presence of metastasis.

The physical examination should include a careful exploration to locate and size the tumor. Any movement during respiration should be carefully noted. These findings assist the physician in distinguishing WT from NB or splenomegaly. Laboratory evaluation should include a complete blood cell count with differential, liver function tests, serum calcium, blood, urea, nitrogen (BUN), serum creatinine, and urinalysis. When the diagnosis of WT is confirmed, the child

TABLE 101.10 | **Staging of Wilms' Tumor (NWTS-4)**

I. Tumor limited to the kidney and completely excised. The surface of the renal capsule is intact. The tumor was not ruptured before or during removal. There is no residual tumor apparent beyond the margins of excision.

II. Tumor extends beyond the kidney, but is completely excised. There is regional extension of the tumor (i.e., penetration through the outer surface of the renal capsule into the perirenal soft tissues). Vessels outside the kidney substance are infiltrated or contain tumor thrombus. The tumor may have been biopsied or there has been local spillage of tumor confined to the flank. There is no residual tumor apparent at or beyond the margins of excision.

III. Residual nonhematogenous tumor confined to the abdomen. Any of the following may occur:

a. Lymph nodes on biopsy are found to be involved in the hilus, the periaortic chains, or beyond.

b. There has been diffuse peritoneal contamination by the tumor such as by spillage of tumor beyond the flank before or during surgery, or by tumor growth that has penetrated through the peritoneal surface.

c. Implants are found on the peritoneal surface.

d. The tumor is not completely resectable because of local infiltration into vital structures.

IV. Hematogenous metastases. Deposits beyond stage III (e.g., lung, liver, bone, and brain).

V. Bilateral renal involvement at diagnosis. An attempt should be made to stage each side according to the above criteria on the basis of extent of disease before therapy.

NWTS, National Wilms' Tumor Study.
(From Kalapurakal JA, Dome JS, Perlman EJ, et al. Management of Wilms' tumour: current perspective and future goals. Lancet Oncol 5:37–46, 2004, with permission.)

is staged accordingly (Table 101.10).[4] The therapeutic plan is based on the stage of disease and by the histology of the tumor (patients are classified as favorable or anaplastic).[54] Approximately 10% of patients have anaplastic disease (characterized by enlarged polyploid nuclei), which is associated with chemotherapy resistance and historically has poorer outcomes compared to favorable histologies.

TREATMENT

Research in the area of WT has been facilitated via the formation of the National Wilms' Tumor Study Group (NWTSG). Increased survival rates have been achieved primarily by the multidisciplinary efforts of several institutions in four separate collaborations from 1969 (NWTS-1) to 1994 (NWTS-4). Each study yielded important findings that have molded current therapeutic practices to provide the most effective and economical treatment to the WT patient while reducing treatment-related morbidity and mortality. A summary of significant findings from each collaboration appears in Table 101.11.[55,57–61] The NWTS-5 study recently closed and results are currently being analyzed.

SURGERY

Surgery is an essential component of treatment in WT with the primary goal of complete excision of the tumor. Surgery facilitates proper staging and provides an opportunity to assess tumor location and spread. Inspection of the contralateral kidney for WT, which may have been missed on diagnostic evaluation, is imperative during surgery. The surgeon also looks for invasion or thrombosis of the renal artery and vein. After the tumor is excised, the surgeon inspects the liver to determine if there is any tumor involvement. Finally, lymph node sampling is performed to determine the possibility of hematogenous seeding.[55] Partial nephrectomies, as opposed to complete resection, remain controversial in small tumors and are not recommended at this time.

RADIOTHERAPY

WT is a radiosensitive tumor; however, not every patient will benefit from radiotherapy, as demonstrated by the NWTS-1, NWTS-2, and NWTS-3 trials.[56–59] For patients who are diagnosed with stage I or II WT with favorable histology, radiation therapy is not indicated if vincristine and dactinomycin are administered. For those patients with stage III WT with favorable histology, a dose of 1,000 cGy is effective if given in combination with vincristine, dactinomycin, and doxorubicin. If tumor spillage occurs during surgery and is confined to the flank, radiation is not advocated. However, if spillage occurs throughout the abdomen, radiation therapy is given. For patients with pulmonary metastases visible on plain chest radiographs, whole-lung irradiation (dose of 1,200 cGy) is recommended.[55] The advent of three-dimensional technologies will likely impact the delivery of radiation.

CHEMOTHERAPY

The first pediatric solid tumor found to be responsive to chemotherapy (dactinomycin) was WT. In general, chemotherapy is initiated soon after surgery. Preoperative chemotherapy is reserved for those patients with very large tumors requiring debulking before surgery. The NWTS-1, NWTS-2, and NWTS-3 demonstrated that combination chemotherapy was superior to single-agent therapy. First-line therapy of WT generally includes a combination of dactinomycin and vincristine, with or without doxorubicin. Other chemotherapeutic agents that are used in relapsed or nonresponders include combinations of cyclophosphamide, ifosfamide, carboplatin, and etoposide.[54]

The NWTS-4 determined that ''pulse-intensive'' therapy was as effective as standard chemotherapy regimens and patients with stage II, III, or IV WT with favorable histology do not achieve a greater benefit with 15 months of therapy than with 6 months of therapy. Pulse-intensive therapy regimens allow for dactinomycin and doxorubicin to be given as a single dose rather than smaller, divided doses. This

TABLE 101.11	Summary of Significant Findings in the NWTS Collaborations
Study (Registration Dates)	**Significant Conclusions**
NWTS-1 (1969–1973)	1. In children less than 2 years old with stage I favorable histology, postoperative radiation had no benefit.
	2. The combination of vincristine and dactinomycin was more effective than either drug alone in stage II or III disease.
NWTS-2 (1974–1978)	1. For children with stage I favorable histology, 15 months of vincristine and dactinomycin was no more effective than 6 months of therapy.
	2. The addition of doxorubicin to vincristine and dactinomycin improve relapse-free survival rates in stage II–IV disease.
NWTS-3 (1979–1986)	1. For stage I disease, 11 weeks of vincristine and dactinomycin without radiation is effective therapy.
	2. For stage II favorable histology disease, vincristine and dactinomycin without radiation for 15 months was equivalent to vincristine and dactinomycin with radiation or with doxorubicin.
	3. For patients with stage II favorable histology, the addition of abdominal radiation did not improve survival.
	4. 1,000 cGy abdominal radiation was equivalent to 2,000 cGy in stage III favorable histology.
	5. For stage III favorable histology, the addition of doxorubicin to vincristine and dactinomycin was more beneficial than vincristine and dactinomycin together.
	6. The addition of cyclophosphamide to vincristine, dactinomycin, and doxorubicin did not improve survival in stage IV favorable histology, but the addition of cyclophosphamide to the three-drug regimen may benefit those patients with stage II–IV anaplastic histology.
NWTS-4 (1986–1994)	1. Pulse-intensive chemotherapy regimens are as effective as standard regimens.
	2. For stage II–IV favorable histology, 6 months of chemotherapy is as effective as 15 months.

NWTS, National Wilms' Tumor Study.

form of chemotherapy also has proven to be of economical benefit. The regimens studied in the NWTS are detailed elsewhere.[55,62,63]

FUTURE THERAPIES

The NWTS-5 opened in 1995 as a single-arm trial to examine biologic features of WT in an effort to predict outcome. Specifically, investigators will evaluate the prognostic value of DNA ploidy and the loss of heterozygosity of chromosomes 1p and 16q. The planned treatment regimen did not change from previous recommendations (i.e., 18-week regimen of pulse-intensive dactinomycin and vincristine) for older patients, large tumors, stage I anaplastic disease, and stage II favorable histology. Patients with stage III or IV WT with favorable histology and focal anaplasia stage II, III, or IV patients will receive radiation therapy in addition to 24 weeks of pulse-intensive dactinomycin, vincristine, and doxorubicin. New chemotherapy regimens involving etoposide and carboplatin in addition to radiation will be analyzed for those patients designated as high risk.[61]

Several questions have already been answered, including the efficacy of managing patients under the age of 2 with a stage I WT with a favorable histology and tumors weighing less than 550 g with surgery alone. Green et al[64] showed that these patients had a 13.2% risk of relapse 2 years after surgery, which exceeded the study stopping rule. Therefore, surgery alone in these patients is not recommended.

IMPROVING OUTCOMES

For patients who receive radiation therapy during their treatment, dose reductions of chemotherapeutic agents are often necessary. Dactinomycin and doxorubicin are known to have two types of interactions with radiotherapy, enhancement of radiation effects and a "radiation recall" reaction.[65–67] Radiation recall, or reactivation, is a recurrence of the effects of radiation, especially in mucous membranes and the skin, for up to several weeks after radiation following the administration of chemotherapy. To decrease the likelihood of occurrence in patients requiring radiation, doses of dactinomycin and doxorubicin should be decreased by 50% during and for up to 6 weeks after radiotherapy.

Pulse-intensive therapy has shown great benefit in patients with WT. The NWTS-4 provided evidence that patients experienced less hematologic toxicity than previously reported despite the administration of myelosuppressive chemotherapy in higher doses.[63] However, the regimens studied in the NWTS-4 were not free of side effects. Dactinomycin is associated with hepatotoxicity causing transient elevations in liver function tests. The NWTS-4 demonstrated an increase in the incidence of hepatotoxicity (and the observation of acute veno-occlusive disease) when compared with the NWTS-3. The initial dactinomycin pulse-intensive dose of 60 mg per kilogram was thought to be excessive and was reduced to the 45 mg per kilogram dose. However, follow-up analysis has found the current pulse-intensive regimen (i.e., 45 mg/kg) and the standard dose of 15 mg/kg/day for 5 days to have more hepatotoxicity than that reported in the NWTS-3. The pathogenesis of these observations remains unknown.[68,69] It is important for health care professionals to recognize this condition, which usually occurs within the first 3 months after diagnosis and not confuse it with other causes for liver dysfunction. Liver enzymes usually return to baseline values within 2 weeks of discontinuing therapy. A reduction in dactinomycin dose should be made if a patient's liver function tests are elevated. If laboratory values are greater or continue to rise, dactinomycin should be held until values return to a range that is more appropriate for its use.

The dose of dactinomycin used in patients with WT illustrates an important concept in pediatric oncology. The dose of this chemotherapeutic agent is expressed as an amount (milligram) per amount of body weight (kilogram) rather than amount per body surface area (square meters) that is usually seen with other protocols. After analysis of data from NWTS-2, it was noted that an unusually large number of infants died from regimen-related toxicities.[70] Doses in the NWTS-4 for this same age group were reduced by 50%. Results were more favorable with fewer toxicities without compromise in therapeutic efficacy.[71] These findings illustrate the need for alternative dosing methods in infants, which is most likely due to the fact that infants, when compared with children and adults, have a larger body surface area to weight ratio. An approximate conversion of a dose per square meter to a dose per kilogram can be made by dividing the dose per square meter by 30, which is based on the assumption that the average 30-kg child has a body surface area of 1 m^2.

The current literature suggests that successfully treated WT children can also have a number of adverse treatment-related sequelae.[54] The type and severity depend on the kind of chemotherapy, extent of surgery and radiation, and age and sex of the child. Organ systems to be monitored for several years after therapy include the kidneys, heart, lungs, and gonads. Common causes of renal failure include bilateral nephrectomy and radiation complications. Cumulative doses of doxorubicin are known to cause congestive heart failure, and effects may be delayed by as much as 20 years. Radiation to the lungs can affect pulmonary function and decrease vital capacity up to 70% after bilateral therapy. Patients are also at risk of developing secondary malignancies. A higher risk is seen in patients that receive large radiation doses, are exposed to broad areas or breast and thyroid tissue, and those that receive alkylating agents.

PROGNOSIS

Children diagnosed with WT have an excellent overall survival rate, and more than 90% of these patients achieve a cure. Through the collaborative research efforts of several institutions in the NWTS, tumor histology has emerged as the most important prognostic indicator. Based on the appearance of the tumor tissue, patients are broadly classified as favorable histology or anaplastic histology. Approximately 85% of patients with WT are classified as favorable

histology, and 4-year overall survival rates for these patients, as demonstrated in the NWTS-5, are significant: stage I (98%), stage II (96%), stage III (95%), and stage IV (90%).[72] Additional factors linked to prognosis are lymph node involvement and distant metastasis.

SARCOMAS

A sarcoma is a malignant neoplasm formed by proliferation of embryonic mesenchymal cells, which normally give rise to connective tissue, including blood, bone, cartilage, and muscle tissue. Sarcomas in children can be divided into two principal categories, bone sarcomas and soft tissue sarcomas, which are further subdivided into various tumor types. Bone sarcomas occur with a peak incidence in adolescents and most commonly include osteosarcoma and ES. Soft tissue sarcomas are made up of a multitude of histologic types, of which the subtype RMS makes up at least one half of all cases. A more detailed pathologic description of pediatric soft tissue tumors is described elsewhere.[73]

RHABDOMYOSARCOMA

RMS, a very aggressive tumor first described by Weber in 1854,[74] is thought to arise from primitive mesenchymal tissue that mimics immature striated muscle. The two major histologic subtypes of RMS are embryonal (70%) and alveolar (20%). Embryonal cells, which resemble striated muscle, are more commonly found in younger children with involvement in the head and neck or genitourinary tract. Alveolar cells, which resemble lung parenchymal cells, occur more frequently in adolescents, usually involve the trunk or extremities, and are more likely to have metastasized on diagnosis.[75] An alveolar histology is a negative prognostic factor.

TREATMENT GOALS: RMS

■ The two main treatment goals for RMS are to cure the cancer and to retain as much function of the affected area(s) as possible. Therefore, treatment strategies for RMS encompass several therapeutic modalities.
■ Surgery, if feasible without causing disfigurement or disability, is directed at removing as much tumor as possible. Even if the entire tumor is removed, chemotherapy is still required. Chemotherapy and radiation may be given before or after surgery.

EPIDEMIOLOGY

RMSs accounts for approximately 7.4% of all childhood cancers in the United States or 300 cases per year.[76] Boys have a slightly higher incidence than girls and African-Americans are more likely to develop RMS than whites.[76] The majority of RMSs are seen in children under age 6; however, a second peak in incidence occurs in late adolescence (15–19 years). RMS has been associated with an increased incidence of maternal breast cancer and an increased number of cancers in siblings.[77] This familial manifestation is referred to as the "Li- Fraumeni cancer family syndrome" and may be associated with alterations in the p53 tumor suppressor gene.[78] In addition, a strong correlation exists between alveolar RMS and translocations on chromosomes 2 and 13.[79]

CLINICAL PRESENTATION AND DIAGNOSIS

SIGNS AND SYMPTOMS
Presenting symptoms of RMS are widely variable because this tumor can arise anywhere in the body. The most common sites for occurrence depend on the tumor histology.[76] The four most common sites of embryonal disease are (a) head and neck (excluding the orbit) accounting for 29% of all cases, (b) genital (18%), (c) pelvic soft tissue (11%), or (d) orbital (11%). Alveolar RMS is most likely to present in extremities (39%), head and neck (excluding the orbit) (22%), and pelvic soft tissues (11%). Table 101.12 lists some common signs and symptoms for selected locations of RMS.[75]

The natural progression of RMS involves local invasion of adjacent organs or structures, and distant metastases by

TABLE 101.12	Signs and Symptoms of Rhabdomyosarcoma Based on Tumor Location
Tumor Location	**Signs and Symptoms**
Head and neck region	Nausea, vomiting, headache, cranial nerve palsies, hypertension, proptosis, ophthalmoplegia, epistaxis, sinus obstruction with or without nasal discharge
Genitourinary tract	Hematuria, urinary obstruction, constipation, vaginal discharge, painless scrotal or inguinal enlargement
Extremities	Swelling of the affected site, possibly accompanied by pain, tenderness, and redness

(From Wexler LH, Helman LJ. Rhabdomyosarcoma and the undifferentiated sarcomas. In: Pizzo PA, Poplack DG, eds. Principles and practice of pediatric oncology. 2nd ed. Philadelphia: Lippincott-Raven, 1997:799–829, with permission.)

lymphatic and hematogenous spread. The most common sites of metastases include the lungs, liver, bone and bone marrow, and CNS.

DIAGNOSIS

Techniques commonly used in the diagnosis of RMS include biopsies, radiographic studies, CT, and MRI. Biopsies are essential for histologic diagnosis, and radiographic evaluation assist in determining the location of lesions and the extent of metastasis, if applicable. Preoperative CT with or without contrast, which historically has been considered the imaging modality of choice, enables the radiation therapist to ascertain the extent of tumor involvement and plan treatment fields accordingly. More recently, MRI has become popular because of the ability to provide superior soft tissue contrast when compared with CT imagery. Bone marrow involvement can be confirmed with bone marrow aspirates and biopsies. Lumbar puncture is necessary for all cases of parameningeal involvement and in some primary tumors involving sites in the head and neck.[75]

Precise determination of the location and amount of disease is critical in treating a patient with RMS as staging directs therapy and predicts prognosis. Today, the Soft Tissue Sarcoma Children's Oncology Group (STS COG), a pediatric cancer cooperative subgroup of the COG, assigns patients to treatment using a risk classification scheme that combines two different staging systems. Patients are treated as low risk, intermediate, or high risk based on the amount of disease present after surgery (the Intergroup RMS's surgicopathological staging system) and their pretreatment status [the site-based tumor-node-metastasis (TNM) staging system]. The former system categorizes patients as group I, II, III, or IV based on the amount of tumor following surgery and the degree of tumor dissemination. Because surgery

techniques vary among surgeons, this system is often criticized for its lack of consistency. In addition, important prognostic factors, such as tumor size and location, are not incorporated in the CG system. The latter staging system is used in adult patients with RMS. Here, patients are classified as stages I, II, III, or IV, based on pretreatment status of disease.

TREATMENT

SURGERY

Patients with completely resected tumors have the best prognosis. However, most patients with RMS do not have tumors that are completely resectable because of their location (e.g., cosmetic disfigurement) or due to extensive invasion into surrounding tissues, blood vessels, or nerves. Thus, primary excisions are rare. In most cases, incisional biopsies are conducted first, followed by other treatment modalities. Secondary excision may be feasible after tumor debulking with chemotherapy with or without radiotherapy. Occasionally, second-look procedures after chemotherapy alone may spare a patient from radiation treatments if no residual tumor is present. This hypothesis is currently being studied in the IRS-V study to see how second-look surgeries impact local control in intermediate-risk patients.

RADIOTHERAPY

Although radiation therapy is an important treatment modality in the childhood treatment of RMS, many late adverse effects are associated with radiation. The place of radiotherapy in RMS treatment regimens is heavily debated for this reason. Studies have shown that patients with completely resected tumors (group I) with an embryonal histology do not need radiation after chemotherapy.[80] In contrast, several studies have shown that group I patients with an alveolar histology have a high rate of local relapse, necessitating the need for radiation.[81] Another area of debate on the use of radiation includes patients that have residual disease after surgery and at the start of chemotherapy, but obtain an apparent complete response after chemotherapy.

In general, the radiation dose depends on the amount of residual tumor following surgery and/or chemotherapy. Average doses are between 4,000 and 5,000 cGy, as unacceptable long-term side effects have been seen with total doses greater than 6,000 cGy.[82] Therapy is usually administered every weekday for 5 to 6 weeks after or during chemotherapy. Hyperfractionated (>1 dose/day) radiation initially was hypothesized to decrease toxicity, especially bone growth retardation. However, studies have shown that twice daily radiation is difficult to administer to pediatric patients and does not improve local control.[83] For this reason, conventional radiation should be considered as the standard of care. Brachytherapy, the delivery of radiation to a carefully restricted volume via an implanted radioactive device, may be indicated for critically located, incompletely resected tumors. This internal radiation strategy may lower the radiation fibrosis in adjacent normal structures associated with external radiotherapy that inherently allows more radiation scatter.[75]

CHEMOTHERAPY

Due to the high risk of disseminated disease and the high degree of chemosensitivity, all RMS patients will receive chemotherapy, regardless of stage. Chemotherapy also plays an integral role in local control and may reduce the need for radiation in some patients. Treatment length varies with stage; patients with stage I disease usually require 1 year of therapy, whereas patients with stage II, III, or IV disease require at least 2 years of therapy because the majority of relapses occur within 2 years of starting therapy. The prototypic chemotherapy regimen used in RMS is vincristine, dactinomycin, and cyclophosphamide (VAC). Doxorubicin was used in early trials (RMS-I and RMS-II) in combination with VAC; however, its use has declined because its addition to VAC did not improve overall survival and it was found to be associated with serious delayed cardiotoxicity in approximately 2% of patients.[84,85] An ongoing trial sponsored by the European Pediatric Soft-tissue Sarcoma Study Group seeks to gain more evidence on the anthracycline controversy by treating high-risk RMS patients with doxorubicin, ifosfamide, vincristine, and dactinomycin.[80]

Another area of debate has been the choice of alkylating agent; cyclophosphamide versus ifosfamide. To address this question, the IRS-IV study randomized 883 untreated RMS patients to one of three arms: (a) VAC, (b) vincristine, etoposide, ifosfamide, or (c) vincristine, dactinomycin, ifosfamide.[86] No statistically significant difference was seen in 3-year failure-free survival rates between any of the arms and VAC remains the standard of care for most groups of patients.

Newer combinations of agents, including etoposide, ifosfamide, cisplatin, and melphalan, have been compared with VAC therapy in more recent studies (IRS-III and IRS-IV).[87,88] These studies also explored giving dose-intensive chemotherapy (involving dose escalations of cyclophosphamide and ifosfamide) early in therapy to improve outcome while sparing patients surgical procedures and excessive radiation treatments. Melphalan was found to be an active agent in previously untreated patients but was highly myelosuppressive. Ifosfamide and etoposide have demonstrated favorable activity in pilot studies. Therapy complications following chemotherapy have included hemorrhagic cystitis, Fanconi's syndrome, and secondary neoplasms.

FUTURE THERAPIES

Currently, the IRS-V, a study that is assigning patients to one of four histologic subgroups and is exploring risk-directed therapy, is using G-CSF with combination chemotherapy to reduce the duration of neutropenia after highly myelosuppressive regimens. Other agents, topotecan and irinotecan, are being evaluated for utility in RMS. In addition, the European Pediatric Soft-Tissue Sarcoma group is exploring the value of maintenance chemotherapy for high-risk patients that have achieved a complete response by the use of oral cyclophosphamide and vinorelbine.[89]

IMPROVING OUTCOMES

PATIENT MONITORING

As mentioned previously, ifosfamide is commonly used in the treatment of RMS. This is an alkylating agent with significant renal and neurologic toxicities. After the administration of ifosfamide, myelosuppression ensues and granulocytes reach their nadir in 10 to 14 days with recovery occurring in 3 weeks. Thrombocytopenia is more commonly associated with higher doses. Hemorrhagic cystitis is common and requires judicious hydration of the patient before and for up to 72 hours after ifosfamide infusions. Administration of mesna serves as an uroprotectant and should accompany the infusion of ifosfamide and continue for 24 hours after its completion. The total dose of mesna is generally 60% to 120% of the ifosfamide dose on a weight-per-weight basis.

Fanconi's syndrome, or proximal renal tubular acidosis, which is characterized by tubular wasting of glucose, protein, sodium, potassium, calcium, phosphate, and bicarbonate, is a significant dose-dependent nephrotoxicity after the administration of ifosfamide. An increase in serum creatinine is also characteristic of renal damage from ifosfamide. Other predisposing factors for developing Fanconi's syndrome are young age, unilateral nephrectomy, cumulative dose of ifosfamide, and concomitant administration of platinum chemotherapy.[90,91] The total dose of ifosfamide is also a risk factor in the development of Fanconi's syndrome. Once a cumulative dose of 60 g/m^2 is achieved, a change in therapy (to cyclophosphamide) should be considered to decrease the likelihood of adverse reactions.

Neurologic toxicities are common with higher doses of ifosfamide and generally manifest as somnolence, confusion, and disorientation. Nausea and vomiting can be a significant problem after the administration of ifosfamide, but generally is well controlled with the use of antiemetics. Because ifosfamide undergoes hepatic activation, mild, transient increases in liver enzymes have been reported. Monitoring parameters in patients receiving ifosfamide include serum creatinine, BUN, complete blood cell count with differential, electrolytes, calcium, phosphorus, liver enzymes, urinalysis, and urine output.

PATIENT EDUCATION

The importance of hydration and adequate urine output should be emphasized. Oral hydration to ensure continued diuresis at home should be encouraged. The patient should be made aware of manifestations of hemorrhagic cystitis, and any blood or clots in the urine should be reported immediately. Drugs that are inducers of P-450 enzymes have the potential to interact with ifosfamide, and their use should be carefully monitored.

Trimethoprim/sulfamethoxazole (TMP/SMX, Bactrim, Septra) administration is strongly suggested to prevent *Pneumocystis carinii* infections. Regimens reviewed in the IRS studies can be profoundly myelosuppressive and warrant prophylactic antibiotic administration. Several dosing regimens for TMP/SMX are used in clinical practice; a widely accepted regimen is 5 mg/kg/day (based on the trimethoprim component) divided two times per day given on Monday, Wednesday, and Friday. Patients and their caregivers should be counseled to maintain adequate fluid intake and avoid prolonged sun exposure while on therapy. A rash that develops during therapy should be reported to a health care professional immediately.

PROGNOSIS

Several prognostic indicators have been elucidated in RMS.[75,92] The extent of tumor at the time of diagnosis appears to be the most important and the strongest predictor of outcome. Patients with metastasis have a poorer prognosis than patients with localized disease. Total surgical resection of tumor confers a better prognosis than residual disease. The tumor's histopathologic subtype is a useful prognostic indicator (embryonal has a better prognosis than alveolar); however, research suggests that tumor location is the more important tumor characteristic in predicting outcome. The tumor's primary site is important because it affects the length of time before a diagnosis is made, the feasibility of surgical resection, and the likelihood of metastasis. Sites with a favorable prognosis are orbit, paratesticular, gastrointestinal, prostate, and genitourinary tract; sites with an unfavorable prognosis are the extremities, retroperitoneum, intrathoracic, head and neck, trunk, perineal, ear, and sinuses.[93] Younger age and early response to chemotherapy are additional favorable prognostic indicators. Finally, initial treatment can affect the outcome of RMS patients. A comparison of 5-year survival data from two large scale pediatric cooperative clinical trials (i.e., MMT-89 and IRS-IV) has shown a significant event-free survival (EFS) and overall survival advantage for patients that receive upfront local therapy via radiation as studied in the IRS-IV trial rather than postponing local therapy as studied in the MMT-89 study.[94,95] Specifically, the IRS-IV trial demonstrated a 5-year EFS rate of 78% and a 5-year overall survival rate of 84% versus the MMT-89 trial with an EFS rate of 57% and an overall survival rate of 71%.

OSTEOSARCOMA

Osteosarcoma (OS), the most common bone neoplasm occurring in children, accounts for 5% of all childhood tumors with approximately 400 cases per year in the United States.[96] It is a primary malignant tumor of mesenchymal origin characterized by the production of osteoid tissue (immature bone) by the malignant proliferating spindle cell stroma.[97] The past three decades have produced more favorable treatment outcomes; however, up to one half of all patients diagnosed with OS do not realize a cure. Despite a more detailed understanding of the pathophysiology of OS, questions revolving around therapy remain, and, as research continues, determination of these answers is anticipated in the near future.[97,98]

TREATMENT GOALS: OSTEOSARCOMA

- The goals of therapy for OS are local control of the primary tumor and eradication of distant microscopic disease, which is always assumed to be present at diagnosis.
- Because radiation is ineffective, surgery and chemotherapy are the two treatment modalities used to manage patients.

EPIDEMIOLOGY

Osteosarcoma is primarily a cancer of adolescence, and peak incidence occurs during the second decade of life (age 14 years for males and age 13 years for females) and then again in adults older than 65 years of age.[99] The current overall incidence of OS in children fewer than 15 years old is slightly greater in females than in males (1:0.97); however, historically, more males develop OS than females. Racial differences in OS are not varied, with the rate of OS in African-American children slightly exceeding the rate in white children (1:0.87).[3] The exact incidence and sex and racial differences of OS are debated because SEER data are restricted to persons less than 15 years old.[100]

The growth spurt seen during puberty is probably the basis for peak incidence during adolescence, suggesting a relation of the development of malignancy to rapid bone proliferation. In fact, the most likely sites of tumor are the distal femur, proximal tibia, and proximal humerus, all of which are the metaphyseal portions of bones, which undergo the most rapid growth during adolescence. Predisposing factors to OS have not been identified in children, although previous ionizing radiation and Paget's disease have been implicated in older patients. Children with hereditary RB have a significantly greater chance of later developing OS, suggesting a genetic predisposition in some patients. Deregulation of the p53 tumor suppressor gene also appears to be important in the development of OS.[97,98]

CLINICAL PRESENTATION AND DIAGNOSIS

SIGNS AND SYMPTOMS

OS can occur in any bone, but approximately one half of tumors arise in the femur.[100] Eighty percent of these cases arise adjacent to the knee joint. Other major sites include the humerus, tibia, fibula, jaw, and ribs. The majority of patients have a chief complaint of pain over the site of disease. A soft tissue mass is not present in all cases. Symptoms usually occur a few weeks to several months before medical evaluation is conducted. If symptomatology is thought to be secondary to injury, evaluation can be furthered delayed. Fever, weight loss, and adenopathy, all of which are more suggestive of advanced disease, may also be present. At the time of diagnosis, most patients have micrometastatic disease and up to 20% of patients have visible signs of distant metastasis, usually appearing as tumors in the lung. The second most common place for metastatic spread is to another bone. Lymph node spread in OS is rare because bones lack a lymphatic system.[97,100]

DIAGNOSIS

Radiographic evaluation plays a pivotal role in OS. It not only determines the presence of disease, but it can be helpful, although not definitive, in assisting the clinician in assessing tumor response to chemotherapy. Plain film radiographs are part of the initial series of studies ordered and allow the clinician to determine the extent of bone involvement and the presence of any pathologic fractures. The exact location of tumor is best made with the aid of MRI and CT. CT can also detect pulmonary metastasis. Radionuclide bone scans are used to identify the extent of the primary tumor and are instrumental in determining the presence of metastatic disease.

Laboratory evaluation in the patient with OS is limited. Serum alkaline phosphatase can be elevated in up to 40% of patients. Although it is a poor indicator of the extent of tumor, it can be used as a prognostic indicator. Serum LDH is another laboratory marker that can be elevated in patients.

A universal staging system is not used in the diagnosis of OS because most tumors are considered high grade. The only delineation made in patients with OS is local disease versus metastatic disease.[85]

TREATMENT

SURGERY

Because radiation therapy is not active in OS, surgery is the only means of local control of tumor. For the best chance at proper resection, it is essential that the initial evaluation be completed by an orthopedic oncologist. Past surgical techniques were limited to limb amputation, and outcomes were poor despite these radical procedures. Fewer than 25% of patients lived several years beyond surgery. Today surgical techniques have been refined to include limb-sparing techniques. These procedures are made possible with the use of neoadjuvant chemotherapy and incorporate CT and MRI diagnostic procedures early in the treatment process. Clinical trials have shown no difference in overall survival between limb-sparing procedures and amputations in patients with OS of the limb that have received neoadjuvant chemotherapy.[101] However, wide surgical margins must be achieved to gain long-term survival. Other surgical procedures include resection of pulmonary nodules in patients with limited lung disease, which may provide long-term survival results in some patients.[97,100]

CHEMOTHERAPY

The importance of chemotherapy in OS is evident, as less than 20% of patients survive with surgery alone. Administration of chemotherapy can occur before or after surgery. Adjuvant chemotherapy is generally administered for 6 to 9 months after surgery and has increased disease-free survival rates and overall survival rates significantly to more than 65% and approximately 50%, respectively, in patients with nonmetastatic disease.[102–104] Neoadjuvant chemotherapy has gained popularity in the past decade and offers several advantages. It allows the surgeon more time to develop a plan and to construct prosthetic devices for the patient, facilitating limb-salvage techniques. Metastatic disease is treated earlier in the disease course, and, by administering chemotherapy as first-line therapy, tumor response can be assessed, which can then be correlated with outcome. When neoadjuvant chemotherapy is administered, the amount of tumor necrosis observed postoperatively can serve as a predictive factor of local recurrence, overall survival, and disease-free survival.

Because OS is a relatively drug-resistant tumor, patients require intensive doses of active agents given over a specified time (dose-intensive chemotherapy). Agents with demonstrated activity in OS include cisplatin,[102–104] doxorubicin,[10,102–104] ifosfamide,[105] methotrexate with leucovorin rescue,[106] cyclophosphamide,[107] carboplatin,[108] and etoposide.[107] Ifosfamide has demonstrated the most beneficial effects in patients with very large tumor burdens.[109] High-dose methotrexate (HDMTX) regimens involve the administration of methotrexate in doses of up to 12 g/m^2 over 4 to 6 hours followed by the administration of leucovorin 24 hours after methotrexate until a desired concentration of methotrexate is achieved (<0.1 μmol/L). Because methotrexate is renally eliminated, measures are used by the clinician to enhance its excretion and decrease the likelihood of toxicities. These methods include adequate hydration (2–3.5 L/m^2/day) to ensure diuresis and administering sodium bicarbonate [orally (PO) or intravenously (IV)] or acetate (IV) to alkalinize the urine, which promotes excretion of methotrexate metabolites. When these prophylactic measures are instituted, side effects from methotrexate, which include nausea, vomiting, mucositis, stomatitis, rash, and myelosuppression, are minimized. Certain drugs are avoided during methotrexate therapy to minimize methotrexate accumulation and direct insult to the kidney. Examples of other nephrotoxic drugs include cisplatin, amphotericin B, aminoglycosides, and cyclosporine. Nonsteroidal anti-inflammatory drugs and TMP/SMX administration should be avoided because these agents compete with methotrexate for renal tubular excretion and can lead to prolonged elevations in methotrexate serum concentrations.[110]

FUTURE THERAPIES

Muramyl-tripeptide conjugated with phosphatidyl ethanolamine (MTP-PE) may have a role in the future treatment of OS. A derivative of bCG vaccine, MTP-PE is encapsulated into liposomes that facilitates its delivery and promotes the in vitro activation of monocytes. These activated monocytes have a tumoricidal effect against OS. Preliminary data show that it is safe for administration to humans.[97] Results from a phase III trial sponsored by the COG and the POG suggested the MTP-PE might enhance EFS, however, an interaction with ifosfamide make results difficult to interpret.[111] The investigators concluded that MTP-PE requires additional laboratory and clinical investigation.

IMPROVING OUTCOMES

PATIENT MONITORING

With respect to HDMTX therapy, monitoring serum methotrexate levels is the pharmacist's primary concern. Serial methotrexate levels should be obtained at designated times after the infusion of the dose. Based on the concentration at a designated period, leucovorin dosing may need modification to reach the desired end point. Recommendations for leucovorin adjustments are described in more detail elsewhere.[110,112] Renal function should be monitored as well. Serum creatinine and BUN should be followed to assess renal function. Urine output should be noted as well to determine if diuresis is adequate (usually a goal of 2–3 mL/kg/hour). Monitoring urine pH (to maintain above 6.5–7) is also advisable to ensure alkalinization of the urine. Although mild myelosuppression is common, it can be monitored by serial complete blood cell counts with differentials. Significant but reversible elevations in liver transaminases and increases in bilirubin and prothrombin time are not uncommon, and the monitoring of liver chemistries is warranted. Nausea, vomiting, mucositis,

and stomatitis should be noted for two reasons. First, electrolyte disturbances can occur with vomiting, and replacement therapy via adequate hydration is common. Second, if oral intake is limited or impaired, oral medications may need to be switched to the intravenous route to prevent a compromise in patient care.

PATIENT EDUCATION

It is important to educate patients and their families with regard to adequate hydration while on an HDMTX protocol. Vigorous intravenous hydration is given before and in the hours after the methotrexate infusion. Patients should be encouraged to drink plenty of fluids to ensure adequate hydration and diuresis. Patients should report nausea and vomiting that interferes with their ability to take oral medications, particularly if they are receiving leucovorin as tablets. Because methotrexate can cause a rash, patients should be advised to remain out of the sun for prolonged periods of time, and they should be educated on protective methods to avoid sunburn. Key drug to drug interactions should be explained to patients and their temporary avoidance should be stressed.

PROGNOSIS

Prognostic indicators in OS have been reported in the literature with varied implications and interpretations. Some indicators that confer a poorer prognosis are male sex, large tumor burden, a shorter time interval from disease to treatment, elevated alkaline phosphatase and LDH, and tumors located at the proximal femur, humerus, and axial skeleton.[113,114] Age was once considered a prognostic indicator (with young age having a poorer outcome) but must be further evaluated because many trials exclude older children and young adults.[98] Tumor necrosis of greater than 90% to 95% after neoadjuvant chemotherapy appears to be the most important characteristic in children with favorable clinical outcomes.[100] Despite the identification of these prognostic factors, patients should not be stratified to receive a particular treatment regimen based on the presence or absence of these factors.[100]

EWING'S SARCOMA

First described in 1921 by James Ewing, ES is the second most common primary bone cancer diagnosed in children. In the United States, there are approximately 200 new cases per year.[96] ES is a small round-cell neoplasm belonging to a family of tumors of neural histogenesis. Although it usually arises in the bone, up to 40% of ES may originate in soft tissue. Treatment of ES more closely parallels RMS than that of OS. Also included in this family, but excluded from this discussion, is peripheral primitive neuroectodermal tumor.

TREATMENT GOALS: EWING'S SARCOMA

- The treatment goals of ES are similar to those of OS, and include local control of tumor and management of micrometastatic disease
- Surgery and chemotherapy are used to achieve these goals. Radiation therapy is an effective tool for the treatment of ES.

EPIDEMIOLOGY

The peak incidence of ES occurs in the second decade of life and rarely occurs before age 5 or after age 30.[3,115] In children less than age 15 years, the incidence in males is similar to that in females (1.08:1) and both sexes have a peak incidence at age 13 years. However, there are striking differences in the high incidence in white children when compared with African-American children of the same age (11:1). In fact, ES is the childhood malignancy with the most remarkable difference in racial incidence.[3]

The exact cause of ES has yet to be determined. ES is not associated with familial cancer syndromes and does not appear to be inherited or associated with other congenital diseases of childhood. Radiation exposure does not appear to contribute to the development of ES. Cytogenetic studies in children with ES have produced valid associations with certain genetic rearrangements. The most common genetic anomalies in ES include the t(11;22) translocation and the t(21;22) translocation. As a result, molecular assays are being used to aid the clinician in diagnosing ES.[116]

CLINICAL PRESENTATION AND DIAGNOSIS

SIGNS AND SYMPTOMS

Approximately 60% of ES arises in the bones; with most cases arising in the distal skeleton followed by the proximal, pelvis, chest, spine, and skull. More than 90% of children have pain and swelling at the site of tumor. The pain may be intermittent at first, which may delay medical evaluation, but usually progresses to being persistent and severe. A palpable mass is not always present at diagnosis, and patients rarely have paraplegia. Fever is present in approximately 20% of patients. When fever is accompanied by leukocytosis, an infectious etiology is usually suspected, and an incorrect diagnosis, such as osteomyelitis, may be made. Other presenting findings that have been reported are weight loss and an increase in erythrocyte sedimentation rate.[115–117]

DIAGNOSIS

A variety of diagnostic tests are performed on the patient with suspected ES to define the exact location of the tumor, estimate the size of the tumor, and determine the presence of metastasis. ES primarily affects long tubular bones of the lower extremities, especially the femur. The most common axial site of involvement is the pelvis. Unlike OS, which primarily damages the ends of bones, ES causes damage to bones in more central locations between the diaphysis and metaphysis. Plain radiographs can easily demonstrate the damage caused by ES, which is referred to as "onion skinning." CT and MRI are used to complement one other. MRI is more sensitive than CT for detecting abnormalities, but can overestimate tumor involvement, which necessitates confirmatory studies by CT.[115–117]

Clinically detectable metastatic disease is present in approximately 20% of patients at the time of diagnosis. The most common site of metastasis is the lung (50% of patients). Other locations for metastatic ES are bone (25% of patients), bone marrow (10%–20% of patients), and rarely the liver and lymph nodes. Because there is a high rate of metastatic disease at the time of presentation, diagnostic procedures including CT of the chest, bone scan, and bone marrow aspirate and biopsy should be performed. There is no definitive tumor marker in ES; however, one half of all patients with ES have an elevated erythrocyte sedimentation rate. An elevated LDH is a common finding as well. There is no universal staging schema for ES; the only delineation made at the time of diagnosis is local disease versus metastatic disease for bone disease.[115–117] Soft-tissue disease is categorized using the RMS staging system where tumors are classified as group I, II, or III based on tumor excision status.[118]

TREATMENT

ES is a radiosensitive tumor. Local control is achieved via surgery or radiation, and chemotherapy is always given adjuvantly to treat microscopic metastatic disease either before or after local control measures.

LOCAL CONTROL

Radiation therapy is reserved for those patients with small tumors. Doses of radiation used to control ES are fairly high (5,500–6,000 cGy), and, until recently, radiation was given over the entire affected bone. However, improved techniques are being used to deliver radiation over more refined fields, which can decrease the toxicity of this therapy. Radiation is advantageous in ES because it can significantly decrease the soft tissue component before chemotherapy or surgery. However, doses greater than 6,000 cGy have been associated with up to a 20% risk of developing secondary malignancies, compared to a 5% incidence for exposure of 4,800 to 6,000 cGy, and no incidence with less than 4,800 cGy.[119]

Surgery is reserved for larger tumors because it has been demonstrated that applying radiation to these tumors is associated with higher local failure rates. Surgery may be a better option for local control in cases where radiation would cause significant morbidity. Such cases include the presence of small rib lesions; cases in which the primary tumor occurs in expendable bones, such as the clavicle, body of the scapula, and proximal tibia, and in small well-confined lesions of the ileum; and cases in which the tumor involves weight-bearing bones or major growth sites.[115]

CHEMOTHERAPY

Vincristine, dactinomycin, and cyclophosphamide have been recognized as single agents with activity in ES since the early 1960s. As a result, their use in combination (VAC) was one of the first therapeutic regimens used in patients with ES. Doxorubicin was found to have activity in ES in the 1970s, and several institutions added it to the VAC regimen (VACAdr).[117] The benefit of the addition of doxorubicin was investigated by a collaborative study, the Intergroup ES Study I (IESS-I), in the United States. This study compared the VAC regimen with the VACAdr regimen and found the latter regimen to be superior. The study also demonstrated the importance of dose-intensive chemotherapy in ES, in that the administration of VACAdr at 3-week intervals versus 6-week intervals was associated with less incidence of relapse.[120] A recent study examining these regimens in extraosseous ES showed no difference in response rates between these regimens; however, these results must be interpreted with caution because identification of patients with extraosseous ES has become more precise.[116,121] A second study (IESS-II) using the VACAdr regimen confirmed the importance of dose intensity by demonstrating the superiority of high-dose intermittent cyclophosphamide over moderate-dose continuous cyclophosphamide.[122]

More recently, the roles of ifosfamide and etoposide in the treatment of ES have been investigated. Ifosfamide has been substituted for cyclophosphamide in the VACAdr regimen with mixed results.[123,124] The addition of ifosfamide and etoposide alternating with the VACAdr regimen has been shown to produce higher response rates when compared with VACAdr alone, particularly for those patients with localized tumors and good prognostic indicators at the time of diagnosis.[125-128] The 5-year event-free survival rate for patients with nonmetastatic disease at diagnosis treated on the standard VACAdr regimen was 54% compared with 69% for patients who received the addition of ifosfamide and etoposide to their chemotherapy. Overall survival was also significantly better in the ifosfamide, etoposide arm (72% vs. 61%, $p = 0.01$). However, the addition of ifosfamide or etoposide is associated with more adverse effects and significantly more morbidity than the VACAdr regimen. In addition, patients who presented with metastatic disease had no disease-free or survival improvements with the ifosfamide, etoposide arm.[128,129]

FUTURE THERAPIES

Collaborative research continues in determining the most appropriate chemotherapy regimen for ES. The current COG protocol is randomizing nonmetastatic ES patients to receive alternating treatment of the VACAdr regimen with ifosfamide, etoposide, and filgrastim to a 14-day or 21-day schedule to investigate the benefit of increasing the dose intensity and reducing the interval between cycles.[130] Another promising treatment modality in ES is the use of autologous stem cell transplantation. This process allows the administration of large doses of chemotherapy to patients followed by the reinfusion of previously collected stem cells as "rescue" therapy. Patients with high-risk ES have been successfully treated with stem cell transplantation after the failure of conventional therapy.[12,131] Additional studies involving larger patient cohorts are necessary before the exact role of stem cell transplantation can be determined.

IMPROVING OUTCOMES

PATIENT MONITORING

Doxorubicin is known to cause congestive heart failure, however, cardiac effects may be delayed by as much as 20 years. Recognized risk factors for the development of anthracycline-induced cardiac toxicity are mediastinal radiation and cumulative doxorubicin dose. Patients should be monitored accordingly for several years after therapy.[132-136] In addition, many ES treatment modalities are associated with an increased risk of developing secondary malignancies, specifically large doses of radiation and dose-intensive chemotherapy regimens. Patients need to be closely monitored for secondary malignancies for the rest of their lives.

PROGNOSIS

Several prognostic indicators have been identified for patients with ES. The following are suggestive of a poor prognosis at the time of diagnosis: increased LDH levels, large tumor size (>8 cm), the presence of constitutional symptoms, metastatic disease, older age, and a primary tumor site that is axial (pelvic).[116,117] Other poor prognostic indicators that have been recently identified and warrant additional investigation for their confirmation are an increased serum albumin and the presence of tumor cells in the bone marrow but not in the blood.[137,138] Almost 70% of patients who present with local disease will achieve a cure. In contrast, of the approximately 20% of patients who are diagnosed with metastatic disease, only a third will achieve a cure.[139]

RETINOBLASTOMA

RB, the most common intraocular tumor in children, is a malignant tumor of the embryonic neural retina. The majority of RB appears sporadically, however, there is also an inherited form of the disease. Therefore, RB serves as the prototype and model for understanding the heredity and genetics of childhood cancer. RB is usually white-gray with a chalky appearance, a soft friable consistency, and made of packed, round, undifferentiated small cells with darkly stained nuclei and scant cytoplasm.[140] Tumors can originate from single or multiple foci in one or both eyes. When detected and treated early, overall survival is excellent. However, treatment of patients with advanced disease still remains a challenge. In addition, 25% to 40% of patients who survive bilateral RB will develop a second cancer in the future.

TREATMENT GOALS: RETINOBLASTOMA

- As RB affects primarily younger children, primary treatment goals include cure and vision preservation.
- Although a radiosensitive tumor, delaying or preventing radiation exposure will help to minimize the risk of long-term morbidities and mortality, such as facial deformities and the development of a secondary malignancy.
- The use of chemotherapy as initial management of RB, combined with local therapies, may help prevent or delay the onset of metastatic disease.

EPIDEMIOLOGY

In the United States, an estimated 200 children per year develop RB, or 1 in 14,000 to 18,000 live births, of which 20% to 30% are bilateral. Eighty percent of cases are diagnosed before the age of 4 (median 2 years) and rarely after 6 years of age.[141] Bilateral disease, which is usually multifocal involving numerous tumors in both eyes, is often diagnosed earlier. There are no racial or sex predilections. Sixty percent of cases are nonhereditary and unilateral (affecting one eye), 15% are hereditary and unilateral, and 25% are hereditary and bilateral.

Forty percent of children are born with a germ-line mutation of the RB1 gene and develop multiple, bilateral RBs at an earlier age. The presence of deletions on chromosome 13 involving the two RB alleles localized to the 13q14 region was the first evidence supporting an inherited mechanism of tumor development. Thus bilateral disease is always inherited.[140]

This deletion places the patient at increased risk of developing second primary tumors, particularly osteogenic sarcoma. Siblings of a child with bilateral disease have a 45% chance of developing RB when there is a positive family history. Therefore, any child born to a survivor of RB or who has a sibling who has the disease, should have eye examinations beginning at birth and every 4 to 6 weeks until the age of 3 years.

CLINICAL PRESENTATION AND DIAGNOSIS

Most commonly, a parent or relative of an affected child notices an abnormality of the eye, prompting physician evaluation. Most cases of RB in the United States are diagnosed while the tumor is confined to the intraocular space without local invasion or distant metastases. The most common route of spread is by invasion through the optic nerve, which can then infiltrate the subarachnoid space and subsequently the CSF, brain, and spine. Primary RBs of the pineal and parasellar sites have been called "trilateral retinoblastomas," a highly fatal disease associated with a family history of RB and appearing several years after successful treatment of intraocular RB. This differs from metastatic RB, which usually presents as multiple, undifferentiated tumors within the first 2 years of initial treatment. Other sites of metastatic disease include bone and bone marrow via hematogenous seeding. Lymphatic extension is less common because the eye does not have significant lymphatic drainage and tumors must first spread into the conjunctiva, eyelids, or extraocular tissues in order to disseminate.[140]

SIGNS AND SYMPTOMS

Signs and symptoms are dependent on tumor size and position. The most common presenting symptom is leukocoria (also called cat's eye reflex or white eye), which develops as a result of retinal detachment, making the mass visible through the pupil. Strabismus occurs secondary to pressure from the tumor. Less common signs and symptoms include heterochromia (different color for each iris), rubeosis iridis (neovascularization of the surface of the iris), hyphema (blood in the anterior chamber of the eye), and glaucoma. Intraocular tumors are not associated with eye pain unless secondary glaucoma or inflammation is present. Metastatic disease may be associated with anorexia, nausea, vomiting, weight loss, and headache.[140]

DIAGNOSIS

Ophthalmoscopic examination looking for leukocoria can suffice to make the clinical diagnosis of RB. However, retinal detachment and vitreous hemorrhage can make examination difficult; thus dilation and examination under anesthesia is necessary to fully evaluate the patient's retina. Unlike most malignancies, tissue biopsy confirmation is unnecessary. Ultrasound and CT of the orbit are used to confirm the diagnosis, while ruling out any pineal or other CNS involvement. Metastatic workup also includes MRI, lumbar puncture for CSF evaluation, and bone marrow aspirate and biopsy to confirm the presence of bone marrow involvement.[142] Following diagnosis, the patient is staged accordingly. The Reese-Ellsworth staging system, introduced in 1963, is the widely accepted classification schema used in clinical practice today (Table 101.13).[143] This classification system, which groups eyes according to tumor size, number, location, and associated features, is used to predict chances of salvaging the affected eye and not systemic prognosis. Each eye is independently staged.

TABLE 101.13	Reese–Ellsworth Staging Classification of Retinoblastoma

Group 1 (very favorable)

Solitary tumor, smaller than 4 disk diameters[a] at or behind the equator. Multiple tumors, none larger than 4 disk diameters, all at or behind the equator.

Group 2 (favorable)

Solitary tumor, 4–10 disk diameters in size, at or behind the equator. Multiple tumors, 4–10 disk diameters in size, behind the equator.

Group 3 (doubtful)

Any lesion anterior to the equator. Solitary tumors larger than 10 disk diameters behind the equator.

Group 4 (unfavorable)

Multiple tumors, some larger than 10 disk diameters. Any lesion extending anteriorly to the ora serrata.

Group 5 (very unfavorable)

Tumors involving more than half the retina. Vitreous seeding.

[a] 1 disk diameter = 1.5 mm.
(From Arrigg PG, Hedges TR III, Char DH. Computed tomography in the diagnosis of retinoblastoma. Br J Ophthalmol 67:588–591, 1983, with permission.)

TREATMENT

The management of RB is dependent on many factors: size and location of the tumor, associated features such as vitreous or subretinal seeds, retinal detachment, neovascular glaucoma, patient age, tumor laterality, and anticipation of new tumors based on the family history. Historically, enucleation (removal of the intact eye without seeding the malignancy into the orbit) and various forms of radiotherapy have been the mainstay of treatment for advanced RB, with an overall survival rate of 90% to 95%. However, success rates are tempered by long-term morbidity, especially related to external beam radiation (EBR), such as radiation-induced chronic dry eye, retinopathy, optic neuropathy, cataracts, midfacial deformities, and an increased risk of developing a second malignancy. EBR has been shown to significantly increase the risk of secondary malignancies in patients who carry the RB1 germline mutation. Preservation of the globe or vision is a priority in patients with a good long-term prognosis and has led to a more conservative approach to treatment.

SURGERY

Surgical techniques have extended beyond enucleation to include cryotherapy and photocoagulation. Enucleation remains the best therapeutic option for advanced RB when there is concern for tumor invasion and little hope for salvage of useful vision in the affected eye. In the 1970s, 96% of eyes with unilateral RB were enucleated, compared to 75% in the 1980s. This trend stabilized in the 1990s secondary to earlier diagnosis and improved conservative (nonenucleation) treatment methods, such as chemoreduction and radiotherapy. Removal of the globe should be accompanied by resection of an adequate length of the optic nerve to ensure a free margin. Children can be fitted with an artificial eye as early as 6 weeks after this generally painless procedure. CT and MRI allow for detection of tumor recurrence despite the presence of an implant.

Cryotherapy and photocoagulation are techniques used to manage small tumors (usually less than 4 disc diameters) or tumors that appear after radiotherapy. Cryotherapy is most useful in managing equatorial and peripheral RB. This technique uses a small probe placed directly on the conjunctiva or sclera that ultimately interrupts the microvascularization of the tumor when intracellular ice crystals are produced. One or two sessions at 1-month intervals are required for tumor destruction. Photocoagulation, used in managing small tumors located in the posterior retina, involves an argon laser that encircles the tumor, coagulates all blood supply to the tumor, resulting in its ischemic necrosis. A 70% tumor control rate can be achieved.

RADIOTHERAPY

RB is a radiosensitive tumor. EBR delivers whole-eye irradiation to treat advanced RB, particularly when there is diffuse vitreous seeding. Delivery of 4,500 to 5,400 cGy over

4.5 to 6 weeks, given as 180 to 200 cGy daily 5 days per week, is the dose widely used in practice, although the optimum fractionation and total dose warrants further investigation. The experiences from St. Jude Children's Research Hospital suggest that a total dose of 4,000 cGy may provide the maximal benefit because doses beyond this do not confer greater benefit and are associated with an increase in morbidity.[144] Patients with brain metastases receive full cranial or craniospinal radiation as well. Complications of therapy are atrophy of the orbital bone, vitreous hemorrhage, optic neuropathy, retinopathy, glaucoma, and cataracts.[145] EBR may induce a second cancer in the radiation field, with a 35% 30-year cumulative incidence versus 6% for those who did not receive radiation. EBR use has declined recently secondary to these long-term complications and the improvement and success of newer methods.[146] Methods to decrease complications from radiation therapy are delivery of localized therapy, using smaller fractions of radiation per dose, and using radioactive plaques. Radioactive plaques deliver radioactive isotopes (e.g., cobalt 60) directly to small tumors located in the posterior retina.[147]

CHEMOTHERAPY

Until recently, chemotherapy for the treatment of RB had primarily been used when the disease had spread into the choroids, optic nerve or orbit, and distant extraocular sites. However, within the last decade, it has become important in the initial management of RB, and is now the leading conservative method of treatment. The goals of chemoreduction are to avoid enucleation and the need for EBR by combining chemotherapy with focal treatments to induce complete remission. Chemoreduction may also prevent or delay the onset of pinealoblastoma and other CNS malignancies. Multiple clinical trials have evaluated the role of combination chemotherapy with agents, such as vincristine and carboplatin, with or without etoposide as these agents have demonstrated activity in other neuroectodermal tumors.[146,148–150] Chemoreduction successfully preserves 50% of affected eyes, with greater results in less advanced disease (RE groups I–IV). Recurrence, a main concern, usually occurs within vitreous or subretinal implants, areas of difficult access for antineoplastic drugs.

Although RB is a fast-growing tumor, which, logically, would make it an excellent target for chemotherapy, this tumor type commonly expresses the multidrug-resistant P-glycoprotein efflux pump, a factor that seems to correlate with treatment failures. Cyclosporine, when given in combination with chemotherapy, could potentially abrogate the efflux of drugs from the cancer cells to reverse the effects of the MDR gene. However, this theory has not been proven in clinical trials.[150]

Several agents have been found to be effective in treating patients with metastatic RB. They include cyclophosphamide, doxorubicin, vincristine, epipodophyllotoxins, and platinum-based compounds. Combination chemotherapy has produced mixed results, and duration of response has ranged from 1 to 5 months.

Because RB presents primarily in younger children, close monitoring is required during administration of cytotoxic chemotherapy secondary to immature hepatic and renal function, primary routes of drug activation and elimination, respectively.

FUTURE THERAPIES

Recently developed laboratory models for RB will help scientists understand the basic biology of tumor cells and help to create therapy targeted to specific pathways and proteins. Studies such as those mentioned previously will be continued in the future to determine the precise role of chemoreduction in the management of patients with RB. Subconjunctival administration of carboplatin, which is enhanced by the disruption of the blood-vitreous barrier and after cryotherapy, has shown encouraging preclinical results but additional studies are required to determine its safety and efficacy.[151] Topotecan, a topoisomerase I inhibitor, has demonstrated efficacy in RB and current clinical trials are underway evaluating its use.[152] Refined radiation techniques and the use of heavy-particle radiation are also newer treatment modalities. High-dose chemotherapy followed by autologous stem cell rescue remains an experimental therapeutic approach in patients with advanced disease and has shown promise in patients with bone or bone marrow involvement.[153] Gene therapy directed at the RB1 gene is a distant but probable treatment modality.

IMPROVING OUTCOMES

The formation of the Retinoblastoma Study Group, a joint effort of the American College of Surgeons Oncology Group and the COG, will aid in performing clinical trials addressing diagnostic and therapeutic questions in this very rare disease.

Genetic testing and subsequent counseling should be performed to determine whether or not the germ-line mutation is present. Continued monitoring and long-term follow-up are crucial in the patient with RB, particularly those patients with the hereditary form of the disease. Frequent eye examinations under anesthesia should be performed until age 5. Additional eye examinations and physicals should continue indefinitely at the discretion of the physician.

PROGNOSIS

When RB is detected early, the prognosis for complete recovery is excellent, with survival exceeding 90% in those patients with limited disease confined to the globe. Extension beyond the orbit or metastases to the brain or bone marrow confers a poor prognosis. The survival rate in these patients is reported to range from 35% to 80%.[118]

KEY POINTS

■ Although childhood cancer is rare, mortality from this disease is second only to accidents as a cause of death in children under age 15 years

■ Survival outcomes for children with solid tumors have been greatly improved over the last three decades by a multimodal approach and intensive combination chemotherapy, and for many patients there is now hope for long-term survival. More than 60% of children diagnosed with cancer achieve a cure

■ Intense treatment regimens to invoke cure, however, are more toxic than past therapies, and management of patients requires extensive supportive care by a team of dedicated health care professionals. With children often surviving into adulthood, long-term follow-up of these patients is crucial to assess and ultimately prevent chronic toxicities of therapy

■ Solid tumors account for approximately 40% of pediatric malignancies

■ Enrollment of children in clinical trials is strongly encouraged to allow for greater patient accrual, more rapid reporting of research results, and an increased likelihood of long-term monitoring of patients

■ Secondary malignancies and late side effects following chemotherapy are a concern in pediatric patients, and appropriate monitoring should be part of routine physicals

■ Pediatric brain tumors are a heterogeneous group of neoplasms, and treatment is highly individualized based on patient age and tumor type and location

■ The management of NB, the most common extracranial solid tumor in children, involves a combination of surgery, radiotherapy, chemotherapy, and immunotherapy

■ Several recent advances have been made in the treatment of WT, the most common renal neoplasm occurring in children, conferring an overall survival rate of more than 90%

■ In children, sarcomas, which are characterized by proliferation of embryonic mesenchymal cells, can be divided into two broad categories (bone and soft tissue), although treatment of each type is highly specific

■ RB serves as the prototype and model for understanding genetics in childhood cancer, because many patients survive the initial diagnosis of RB but are at an increased risk of developing a second neoplasm, most notably OS

SUGGESTED READINGS

Devita VT, Hellman S, Rosenberg SA, eds. Cancer: Principles and Practice of Oncology, 7th ed. Philadelphia: Lippincott Williams & Wilkins, 2004.

Perry MC, ed. Chemotherapy Source Book, 3rd ed. Philadelphia: Lippincott Williams & Wilkins, 2001.

REFERENCES

1. National Cancer Institute Research on Childhood Cancers, Cancer Facts 6.4. Available at: http://www.cancer.gov/cancertopics/factsheet/Sites-Types/childhood. Accessed November 10, 2005.
2. Landis SH, Murray T, Bolden S, et al. Cancer statistics, 1998. CA Cancer J Clin 48:6–29, 1998.
3. Gurney JG, Severson RK, Davis S, et al. Incidence of cancer in children in the United States: sex-, race-, and 1-year age-specific rates by histology type. Cancer 75:2168–2195, 1995.
4. Kenney LB, Miller BA, Gloeckler Reis LA, et al. Increased incidence of cancer in infants in the US: 1980-1990. Cancer 82:1396–1400, 1998.
5. Gurney JG, Davis S, Severson RK, et al. Trends in cancer incidence among children in the US. Cancer 78:532–541, 1996.
6. Ries LAG, Eisner MP, Kosary CL, et al. SEER Cancer Statistics Review, 1975-2002. National Cancer Institute, Bethesda, MD, 2005
7. Trott KR. Chronic damage after radiation therapy: challenge to radiation biology. Int J Radiat Oncol Biol Phys 10:907–913, 1984.
8. Kun LE. General principles of radiation therapy. In: Pizzo PA, Poplack DG, eds. Principles and practices of pediatric oncology. 3rd ed. Philadelphia: Lippincott-Raven, 1997:289–321.
9. Goldie JH, Coldman AJ. The genetic origin of drug resistance in neoplasms: implications for systemic therapy. Cancer Res 44:3643–3653, 1984.
10. Kawai A, Sugihara S, Kunisada T, et al. The importance of doxorubicin and methotrexate dose intensity in the chemotherapy of osteosarcoma. Arch Orthop Trauma Surg 115:68–70, 1996.
11. Kuttesch JF Jr. Multidrug resistance in pediatric oncology. Invest New Drugs 14:55–67, 1996.
12. Burdach S, Jurgens H, Peters C, et al. Myeloablative radiochemotherapy and hematopoietic stem-cell rescue in poor-prognosis Ewing's sarcoma. J Clin Oncol 11:1482–1488, 1993.
13. Atra A, Pinkerton R. Autologous stem cell transplantation in solid tumors of childhood. Ann Med 28:159–164, 1996.
14. Graham-Pole J, Gee A, Emerson S, et al. Myeloablative chemoradiotherapy and autologous bone marrow infusions for treatment of neuroblastoma: factors influencing engraftment. Blood 78:1607–1614, 1991.
15. Jacobson SJ, Shore RW, Greenberg M, et al. The efficacy and safety of granisetron in pediatric cancer patients who had failed standard antiemetic therapy during anticancer chemotherapy. Am J Pediatr Hematol Oncol 16:231–235, 1994.
16. Mike V, Meadows AT, Zimmerman LE. Incidence of second malignant neoplasms in children: results of an international study. Lancet 2:1326–1331, 1982.
17. Marina N. Long-term survivors of childhood cancer: the medical consequences of cure. Pediatr Clin North Am 44:1021–1042, 1997.
18. Smith MB, Xue H, Strong L, et al. Forty-year experience with second malignancies after treatment of childhood cancer: analysis of outcome following the development of the second malignancy. J Pediatr Surg 28:1342–1349, 1993.
19. DeLaat CA, Lampkin BC. Long-term survivors of childhood cancer: evaluation and identification of sequelae of treatment. CA Cancer J Clin 42:263–282, 1992.
20. Dennis M, Hetherington CR, Spiegler BJ. Memory and attention after childhood brain tumors. Med Pediatr Oncol 26 (Suppl 1):25–33, 1998.
21. Hopewell JW. Radiation injury to the central nervous system. Med Pediatr Oncol 26 (Suppl 1):1–9, 1998.
22. The Childhood Cancer Survivor Study. Available at http://www.cancer.umn.edu/ltfu#CCSS. Accessed November 10, 2005.
23. Pollack IF. Brain tumors in children. N Engl J Med 331:1500–1507, 1994.
24. Pizzo PA, Poplack DG. Principles and practice of pediatric oncology. Tumors of the central nervous system, 4th ed. Philadelphia: Lippincott Williams & Wilkins, 2001:751–808.
25. Bunin G. What causes childhood brain tumors? Limited knowledge, many clues. Pediatr Neurosurg 32:321–326, 2000.
26. Preston-Martin S. Epidemiology of primary CNS neoplasms. Neurol Clin 14:273–290, 1996.
27. Pollack IF. Brain tumors in children. N Engl J Med 331:1500–1510, 1994.

28. Albright AL. Pediatric brain tumors. CA Cancer J Clin 43: 272–288, 1993.
29. Lassoff SJ, Allen J, Epstein F, et al. Advances in surgery: brain stem and spinal cord tumors in children. In: Bleyer A, Packer R, eds. Pediatric neuro-oncology: new trends in clinical research. New York: Hardwood Academic, 1992:278–297.
30. Packer RJ, Boyett JM, Zimmerman RA, et al. Hyperfractionated radiation therapy (72 Gy) for children with brain stem gliomas. a Childrens Cancer Group phase I/II trial. Cancer 72:1414–1421, 1993.
31. Kirsch DG, Tarbell NJ. Conformal radiation therapy for childhood CNS tumors. The Oncologist 9:442–450, 2004.
32. Habrand JL, Abdulkarim B, Roberti H. Critical review. radiotherapeutic innovations in pediatric solid tumors. Pediatr Blood Cancer 43:622–628, 2004.
33. Blaney SM, Boyett J, Friedman H, et al. Phase I Clinical Trial of mafosfamide in infants and children Aged 3 years or younger with newly diagnosed embryonal tumors: a pediatric brain tumor consortium study (PBTC-001) J Clin Oncol 23: 525–531, 2005.
34. Broniscer A, Iacona L, Chintagumpala M, et al. Role of temozolomide after radiotherapy for newly diagnosed diffuse brainstem glioma in children. Results of a multi-institutional study. (SJHG-98). Cancer 103:133–139, 2005.
35. Lanzkowsky P. Central nervous system malignancies. In: Lanzkowsky P, ed. Manual of pediatric hematology and oncology. 2nd ed. New York: Churchill Livingstone, 1995:397–417.
36. Gurney JG, Kaden-Lottick NS, Packer RJ, et al. Endocrine and cardiovascular late effects among adult survivors of childhood brain tumors. Childhood Cancer Survivor Study. Cancer 97:663–673, 2003.
37. Brodeur GM, Maris JM. Neuroblastoma. In: Pizzo PA, Poplack DG, eds. Principles and practice of pediatric oncology. 4th ed. Philadelphia: Lippincott-Raven, 2001.
38. Carlsen NLT. Neuroblastoma: epidemiology and pattern of regression. Am J Pediatr Hematol Oncol 14:103–110, 1992.
39. Brodeur GM, Castleberry RP. Neuroblastoma. In: Pizzo PA, Poplack DG, eds. Principles and practice of pediatric oncology. 3rd ed. Philadelphia: Lippincott-Raven, 1997:761–797.
40. Philip T. Overview of current treatment of neuroblastoma. Am J Pediatr Hematol Oncol 14:97–102, 1992.
41. Niethammer D, Handgretinger R. Clinical strategies for the treatment of neuroblastoma. Eur J Cancer 31A:568–571, 1995.
42. DuBois SG, Messina J, Maris JM, et al. Hematologic Toxicity of high-dose Iodine-131-Metaiodobenzylguanine therapy for advanced neuroblastoma. J Clin Oncol 22:2452–2460, 2004
43. Matthay KK, Harris R, Reynolds CP, et al. Improved event-free survival (EFS) for autologous bone marrow transplantation (ABMT) vs. chemotherapy in neuroblastoma: a phase III randomized Childrens Cancer Group (CCG) study [abstract]. Proc Am Soc Clin Oncol 17:525a, 1998.
44. Matthay KK, Villablanca JG, Seeger RC, et al. Treatment of high-risk neuroblastoma with intensive chemotherapy, radiotherapy, autologous bone marrow transplantation, and 13-cis-retinoic acid. N Engl J Med 341:1165–1173, 1999.
45. Kretschmar CS, Kletzel M, Murry K, et al. Response to paclitaxel, topotecan, and topotecan/cylcophosphamide in children with untreated disseminated neuroblastoma treated in an upfront phase II investigational window: a pediatric oncology group study. J Clin Oncol 22:4119–4126, 2004.
46. Garaventa A, Luksch R, Biasotti S, et al. A phase II study of topotecan with Vincristine and doxorubicin in children with recurrent/refractory neuroblastoma. Cancer 98:2488–2494, 2003.
47. Israel MA. Disordered differentiation as a target for novel approaches to the treatment of neuroblastoma. Cancer 71:3310–3313, 1993.
48. Reynolds CP, Villablanca JG, Stram DO, et al. 13-cis-retinoic acid after intensive consolidation therapy for neuroblastoma improves event-free survival: a randomized Childrens Cancer Group (CCG) study [plenary session 5]. Proc Am Soc Clin Oncol 17:2a, 1998.
49. Evans AE, D'Angio GJ, Propert K, et al. Prognostic factors in neuroblastoma. Cancer 59:1853–1859, 1987.
50. Look AT, Hayes FA, Shuster JJ, et al. Clinical relevance of tumor cell ploidy and N-myc amplification in childhood neuroblastoma. A Pediatric Oncology Group study. J Clin Oncol 9:581–591, 1991.
51. Bernstein L, Linet M, Smith MA, et al. Renal Tumors. In: Ries LAG, Smith MA, Gurney JG, et al. Cancer incidence and survival among children and adolescents: United States SEER program 1975–1995, National Cancer Institute, SEER Program. NIH Pub. No. 99-4649. Bethesda, MD, 1999.
52. Olshan AF, Breslow NE, Falletta JM, et al. Risk factors for Wilms' tumor. Report from the National Wilms' Tumor Study. Cancer 72:938–944, 1993.
53. Petruzzi MJ, Green DM. Wilms' tumor. Pediatr Clin North Am 44: 939–952, 1997.
54. Kalapurakal JA, Dome JS, Perlman EJ, et al. Management of Wilms' tumour: current perspective and future goals. Lancet Oncol 5: 37–46, 2004.
55. Green DM, Coppes MJ, Breslow NE, et al. Wilms' tumor. In: Pizzo PA, Poplack DG, eds. Principles and practice of pediatric oncology. 3rd ed. Philadelphia: Lippincott-Raven, 1997:733–759.
56. Green DM, D'Angio GJ, Beckwith JB, et al. Wilms' tumor. CA Cancer J Clin 46:46–63, 1996.
57. D'Angio GJ, Evans AE, Breslow N, et al. The treatment of Wilms' tumor. Results of the National Wilms' Tumor Study. Cancer 38: 633–646, 1976.
58. D'Angio GJ, Evans A, Breslow N, et al. The treatment of Wilms' tumor. Results of the Second National Wilms' Tumor Study. Cancer 47:2302–2311, 1981.
59. D'Angio GJ, Breslow N, Beckwith JB, et al. Treatment of Wilms' tumor. Results of the Third National Wilms' Tumor Study. Cancer 64:349–360, 1989.
60. Green D, Breslow N, Beckwith J, et al. A comparison between single dose and divided dose administration of dactinomycin and doxorubicin. A report from the National Wilms' Tumor Study Group [abstract]. Proc ASCO 15:460, 1996.
61. Wiener JS, Coppes MJ, Ritchey ML. Current concepts in the biology and management of Wilms' tumor. J Urol 159:1316–1325, 1998.
62. Mehta MP, Bastin KT, Wiersma SR. Treatment of Wilms' tumor. Current recommendations. Drugs 42:766–780, 1991.
63. Green DM, Breslow NE, Evans I, et al. The effect of chemotherapy dose intensity on the hematologic toxicity of the treatment of Wilms' tumor. A report from the National Wilms' Tumor Study. Am J Pediatr Hematol Oncol 16:207–212, 1994.
64. Green DM, Breslow NE, Beckwith JB, et al. Treatment with nephrectomy only for small, stage I/favorable histology Wilms' tumor: a report from the National Wilms' Tumor Study Group. J Clin Oncol 19:3719–3724, 2001.
65. D'Angio GJ, Farber S, Maddock CL. Potentiation of x-ray effects by actinomycin D. Radiology 73:175–177, 1959.
66. Donaldson SS, Glick GM, Wilbur JR. Adriamycin activating a recall phenomenon after radiation therapy. Ann Intern Med 81: 407–408, 1974.
67. Greco FA, Bereton HD, Kent H, et al. Adriamycin and enhanced radiation reaction in normal esophagus and skin. Ann Intern Med 85:294–298, 1976.
68. Green DM, Finklestein J, Norkool P, et al. Severe hepatic toxicity after treatment with single-dose dactinomycin and vincristine. A report of the National Wilms' Tumor Study. Cancer 62:270–273, 1988.
69. Green DM, Norkool P, Breslow NE, et al. Severe hepatic toxicity after treatment with vincristine and dactinomycin using single-dose or divided dose schedules. A report from the National Wilms' Tumor Study. J Clin Oncol 8:1525–1530, 1990.
70. Jones B, Breslow N, Takashima J, et al. Toxic deaths in the Second National Wilms' Tumor Study. J Clin Oncol 2:1028–1033, 1984.
71. Morgan E, Baum E, Breslow N, et al. Chemotherapy-related toxicity in infants treated according to the Second National Wilms' Tumor Study. J Clin Oncol 6:51–55, 1988.
72. Green DM, Breslow NE, Beckwith JB, et al. Comparison between single-dose and divided-dose administration of dactinomycin and doxorubicin for patients with Wilms' tumor: a report from the National Wilms' Tumor Study Group. J Clin Oncol 16:237–245, 1998.
73. Coffin CM, Dehner LP. Pathologic evaluation of pediatric soft tissue tumors. Am J Clin Pathol 109 (Suppl 1):S38–S52, 1998.

74. Pappo AS, Shapiro DN, Crist WM. Rhabdomyosarcoma. Biology and treatment. Pediatr Clin North Am 44:953–972, 1997.

75. Wexler LH, Helman LJ. Rhabdomyosarcoma and the undifferentiated sarcomas. In: Pizzo PA, Poplack DG, eds. Principles and practice of pediatric oncology. 2nd ed. Philadelphia: Lippincott-Raven, 1997:799–829.

76. Gurney JG, Young JL, Roffers SD, et al. Soft tissue sarcomas. In: Ries LAG, Smith MA, Gurney JG, et al. Cancer incidence and survival among children and adolescents: United States SEER program 1975–1995, National Cancer Institute, SEER Program. NIH Pub. No. 99-4649. Bethesda, MD, 1999.

77. Hartley AL, Birch JM, Blair V, et al. Patterns of cancer in the families of children with soft tissue sarcoma. Cancer 72:923–930, 1993.

78. Malkin D, Li FP, Strong LC, et al. Germ line p53 mutations in a familial syndrome of breast cancer, sarcomas, and other neoplasms. Science 250:1233–1238, 1990.

79. Pappo AS, Shapiro DN, Crist WM, et al. Biology and therapy of pediatric rhabdomyosarcoma. J Clin Oncol 13:2123–2139, 1995>.

80. Stevens MG. Treatment of childhood rhabdomyosarcoma: the cost. Lancet Oncol 6:77–84, 2005.

81. Wolden SL, Anderson RJ, Crist WM, et al. Indications for radiotherapy and chemotherapy after complete resection in rhabdomyosarcoma: a report from the Intergroup Rhabdomyosarcoma Studies I to III. J Clin Oncol 17:3468–3475, 1999.

82. Tefft M, Lattin PB, Jereb B, et al. Acute and late effects on normal tissues following combined chemo- and radiotherapy for childhood rhabdomyosarcoma and Ewing's sarcoma. Cancer 37 (Suppl 2): 1201–1217, 1976.

83. Donaldson SS, Meza J, Anderson JR, et al. Results from the IRS-IV randomized trial of hyperfractionated radiotherapy in children with rhabdomyosarcoma- a report from the IRSG. Int J Radiat Oncol Biol Phys 51:718–728, 2001.

84. Maurer HM, Beltangady M, Gehan EA, et al. The Intergroup Rhabdomyosarcoma Study–I. A final report. Cancer 61:209–220, 1988.

85. Maurer HM, Gehan EA, Beltangady M, et al. The Intergroup Rhabdomyosarcoma Study–II. Cancer 71:1904–1922, 1993.

86. Christ WM, Anderson JR, Meza JL, et al. The Intergroup Rhabdomyosarcoma Study-IV: results for patients with nonmetastatic disease. J Clin Oncol 19:3091–3102, 2001.

87. Crist W, Gehan EA, Ragab AH, et al. The Third Intergroup Rhabdomyosarcoma Study. J Clin Oncol 13:610–630, 1995.

88. Ruymann F, Crist W, Wiener E, et al. Comparison of two doublet chemotherapy regimens and conventional radiotherapy in metastatic rhabdomyosarcoma: improved overall survival using ifosfamide/etoposide compared to vincristine/melphalan in IRSG-IV [abstract]. Proc Am Soc Clin Oncol 16:521a, 1997.

89. Casanova M, Ferrari A, Bisogno G, et al. Vinorelbine and low-dose cyclophosphamide in the treatment of pediatric sarcomas: pilot study for the upcoming European Rhabdomyosarcoma Protocol. Cancer 101:1664–1671, 2004.

90. Skinner R, Sharkey IM, Pearson ADJ, et al. Ifosfamide, mesna, and nephrotoxicity in children. J Clin Oncol 11:173–190, 1993.

91. Loebstein R, Koren G. Ifosfamide-induced nephrotoxicity in children: critical review of pediatric risk factors. Pediatrics 101:E8, 1998.

92. Rodary C, Gehan EA, Flamant F, et al. Prognostic factors in 951 nonmetastatic rhabdomyosarcoma in children: a report from the International Rhabdomyosarcoma Workshop. Med Pediatr Oncol 19: 89–95, 1991.

93. Tsokos M, Webber B, Parham DM, et al. Rhabdomyosarcoma. A new classification scheme related to prognosis. Arch Pathol Lab Med 116:847–855, 1992.

94. Donaldson SS, Anderson JR. Rhabdomyosarcoma: many similarities, a few philosophical differences. J Clin Oncol 23:2586–2587, 2005.

95. Raney BR, Anderson JR, Barr FG, et al. Rhabdomyosarcoma and undifferentiated sarcoma in the first two decades of life: a selective review of intergroup rhabdomyosarcoma study group experience and rationale for intergroup rhabdomyosarcoma study V. J Ped Hematol Oncol 23:215–220, 2001.

96. Gurney JG, Swensen AR, Bulterys M. Malignant bone tumors. In: Ries LAG, Smith MA, Gurney JG, et al. Cancer incidence and survival among children and adolescents: United States SEER program 1975–1995, National Cancer Institute, SEER Program. NIH Pub. No. 99-4649. Bethesda, MD, 1999.

97. Link MP, Eilber F. Osteosarcoma. In: Pizzo PA, Poplack DG, eds. Principles and practice of pediatric oncology. 3rd ed. Philadelphia: Lippincott-Raven, 1997:889–920.

98. Whelan JS. Osteosarcoma. Eur J Cancer 33:1611–1619, 1997.

99. Miller RW, Boise JD, Curtis FE. Bone cancer. In: Schottenfeld D, Fraumeni JF, eds. Cancer epidemiology and prevention. 2nd ed. New York: Oxford University Press, 1996:971–983.

100. Meyers PA, Gorlick R. Osteosarcoma. Pediatr Clin North Am 44: 973–989, 1997.

101. Bacci G, Ferrari S, Lari S, et al. Osteosarcoma of the limb. Amputation or limb salvage in patients treated by neoadjuvant chemotherapy. J Bone Joint Surg Br 84:88–92, 2002.

102. Eilber F, Giuliano A, Eckardt J, et al. Adjuvant chemotherapy for osteosarcoma: a randomized prospective trial. J Clin Oncol 5: 21–26, 1987.

103. Winkler K, Beron G, Delling G, et al. Neoadjuvant chemotherapy of osteosarcoma: results of a randomized cooperative trial (COSS-82) with salvage chemotherapy based on histological tumor response. J Clin Oncol 6:329–337, 1988.

104. Link MP, Goorin AM, Miser AW, et al. The effect of adjuvant chemotherapy on relapse-free survival in patients with osteosarcoma of the extremity. N Engl J Med 314:1600–1606, 1986.

105. Harris MB, Cantor AB, Goorin AM, et al. Treatment of osteosarcoma with ifosfamide: comparison of response in pediatric patients with recurrent disease versus patients previously untreated: a pediatric oncology group study. Med Pediatr Oncol 24:87–92, 1995.

106. Goorin A, Strother D, Poplack D, et al. Safety and efficacy of l-leucovorin rescue following high-dose methotrexate for osteosarcoma. Med Pediatr Oncol 24:362–367, 1995.

107. Cassano WF, Graham-Pole J, Dickson J. Etoposide, cyclophosphamide, cisplatin, and doxorubicin as neoadjuvant chemotherapy for osteosarcoma. Cancer 68:1899–1902, 1991.

108. Meyer WH, Pratt CB, Poquette CA, et al. Carboplatin / ifosfamide window therapy for osteosarcoma: results of the St. Jude Children's Research Hospital OS-91 trial. J Clin Oncol 19:171–182, 2001.

109. Voute PA, van den Berg H, Behrendt H. Ifosfamide in the treatment of pediatric malignancies. Semin Oncol 23 (Suppl 7):8–11, 1996.

110. Chu E, Allegra C. Antifolates. In: Chabner BA, Longo DL, eds. Cancer chemotherapy and biotherapy. 2nd ed. Philadelphia: Lippincott-Raven, 1996:109–148.

111. Meyers PA, Schwartz CL, Krailo M, et al. Osteosarcoma: a randomized, prospective trial of the addition of ifosfamide and/or muramyl tripeptide to cisplatin, doxorubicin, and high-dose methotrexate. J Clin Oncol 23:2004–2011, 2005.

112. Ackland SP, Schilsky RL. High-dose methotrexate: a critical reappraisal. J Clin Oncol 5:2017–2031, 1987.

113. Hudson M, Jaffe MR, Jaffe N, et al. Pediatric osteosarcoma: therapeutic strategies, results, and prognostic factors derived from a 10-year experience. J Clin Oncol 8:1988–1997, 1990.

114. Davis AM, Bell RS, Goodwin PJ. Prognostic factors in osteosarcoma: a critical review. J Clin Oncol 12:423–431, 1994.

115. Horowitz ME, Tsokos MG, DeLaney TF. Ewing's sarcoma. CA Cancer J Clin 42:300–332, 1992.

116. Grier HE. The Ewing family of tumors. Ewing's sarcoma and primitive neuroectodermal tumors. Pediatr Clin North Am 44: 991–1004, 1997.

117. Horowitz ME, Malawer MM, Woo SY, et al. Ewing's sarcoma family of tumors: Ewing's sarcoma of the bone and soft tissue and the peripheral primitive neuroectodermal tumors. In: Pizzo PA, Poplack DG, eds. Principles and practice of pediatric oncology. 3rd ed. Philadelphia: Lippincott-Raven, 1997:831–863.

118. Raney RB, Asmar L, Newton WA, et al. Ewing's sarcoma of soft tissues in childhood: a report from the Intergroup Rhabdomyosarcoma Study, 1972 to 1991. J Clin Oncol 1997; 15: 574–582.

119. Kuttesch JF, Wexler LK, Marcus RB, et al. Second malignancies after Ewing's sarcoma: radiation dose-dependency of secondary sarcomas. J Clin Oncol 14:2818–2825, 1996.

120. Nesbit ME, Gehan EA, Burgert EO Jr, et al. Multimodal therapy for the management of primary, nonmetastatic Ewing's sarcoma of

bone: a long-term follow-up of the first intergroup study. J Clin Oncol 8:1664–1674, 1990.

121. Raney RB, Asmar L, Newton WA Jr, et al. Ewing's sarcoma of soft tissues in childhood: a report from the Intergroup Rhabdomyosarcoma Study, 1972 to 1991. J Clin Oncol 15:574–582, 1997.

122. Burgert EO Jr, Nesbit ME, Garnsey LA, et al. Multimodal therapy for the management of nonpelvic, localized Ewing's sarcoma of bone: Intergroup Study IESS-II. J Clin Oncol 8:1514–1524, 1990.

123. Jurgens H, Exner U, Kuhl J, et al. High-dose ifosfamide with mesna uroprotection in Ewing's sarcoma. Cancer Chemother Pharmacol 24 (Suppl 1):S40–S44, 1989.

124. Oberlin O, Habrand JL, Zucker JM, et al. No benefit of ifosfamide in Ewing's sarcoma: a nonrandomized study of the French Society of Pediatric Oncology. J Clin Oncol 10:1407–1412, 1992.

125. Grier H, Krailo M, Link M, et al. Improved outcome in non-metastatic Ewing's sarcoma and PNET of bone with the addition of ifosfamide and etoposide to vincristine, cyclophosphamide, adriamycin, and actinomycin: a Childrens Cancer Group and Pediatric Oncology Group report [abstract]. Proc Am Soc Clin Oncol 13: 421, 1994.

126. Grier H, Krailo M, Tarbell N, et al. Adding ifosfamide and etoposide to vincristine, cyclophosphamide, adriamycin, and actinomycin improves outcome in non-metastatic Ewing's and PNET: update of CCG/POG study. Med Pediatr Oncol 27:259–265, 1996.

127. Wexler LH, DeLaney TF, Tsokos M, et al. Ifosfamide and etoposide plus vincristine, doxorubicin, and cyclophosphamide for newly diagnosed Ewing's sarcoma family of tumors. Cancer 78:901–911, 1996.

128. Grier HE, Krailo MD, Tarbell NJ, et al. Addition of ifosfamide and etoposide to standard chemotherapy for Ewing's sarcoma and primitive neuroectodermal tumor of the bone. N Engl J Med 348: 694–701, 2003.

129. Miser JS, Krailo, MD, Tarbell NJ, et al. Treatment of metastatic ewing's sarcoma or primitive neuroectodermal tumor of the bone: evaluation of ifosfamide and etoposide-a children's cancer group and pediatric oncology group study. J Clin Oncol 22:2873–2876, 2004.

130. Womer RB, Daller RT, Fenton JG, et al. Granulocyte colony stimulating factor permits dose intensification by interval compression in the treatment of Ewing's sarcomas and soft tissue sarcomas in children. Eur J Cancer 36:87–94, 2000.

131. Atra A, Whelan JS, Calvagna V, et al. High-dose busulphan/melphalan with autologous stem cell rescue in Ewing's sarcoma. Bone Marrow Transplant 20:843–846, 1997.

132. Von Hoff DD, Layard MW, Basa P, et al. Risk factors for doxorubicin-induced congestive heart failure. Ann Intern Med 91: 710–717, 1979.

133. Goorin AM, Borrow RW, Goldman A, et al. Congestive heart failure due to adriamycin cardiotoxicity: its natural history in children. Cancer 47:2810–2816, 1981.

134. Steinherz LJ, Steinherz PJ, Tan CTC, et al. Cardiac toxicity 4 to 20 years after completing anthracycline therapy. JAMA 266: 1672–1677, 1991.

135. Hausdorf G, Morf G, Beron G, et al. Long term doxorubicin cardiotoxicity in childhood: non-invasive evaluation of the contractile state and diastolic filling. Br Heart J 60:309–315, 1988.

136. Steinherz LJ, Graham T, Hurwitz R, et al. Guidelines for cardiac monitoring of children during and after anthracycline therapy: report of the cardiology committee of the Childrens Cancer Study Group. Pediatrics 89:942–949, 1992.

137. Aparicio J, Munarriz B, Pastor M, et al. Long-term follow-up and prognostic factors in Ewing's sarcoma. A multivariate analysis of 116 patients from a single institution. Oncology 55:20–26, 1998.

138. Fagnou C, Michan J, Peter M, et al. Presence of tumor cells in bone marrow but not blood is associated with adverse prognosis in patients with Ewing's tumor. J Clin Oncol 16:1707–1711, 1998.

139. Sandoval C, Meyer WH, Parham DM, et al. Outcome in 43 children presenting with metastatic Ewing sarcoma: the St. Jude Children's Research Hospital experience, 1962 to 1992. Med Pediatr Oncol 26:180–185, 1996.

140. Hurwitz RL, Shields CL, Shields JA, et al. Retinoblastoma. In: Pizzo PA, Poplack DG, eds. Principles and practice of pediatric oncology. 4th ed. Philadelphia: Lippincott Williams & Wilkins, 2002: 825–841.

141. Ries LAG, Eisner MP, Kosary CL, et al. SEER Cancer Statistics review, 1975–2002. National Cancer Institute, Bethesda, MD, 2005.

142. Arrigg PG, Hedges TR III, Char DH. Computed tomography in the diagnosis of retinoblastoma. Br J Ophthalmol 67:588–591, 1983.

143. Reese AB, Ellsworth RM. The evaluation and current concept of retinoblastoma treatment. Trans Am Acad Ophthalmol Otolaryngol 65:169–172, 1963.

144. Fontanesi J, Pratt CB, Hustu HO, et al. Use of irradiation for therapy of retinoblastoma in children more than 1 year old: the St. Jude Children's Research Hospital experience and review of literature. Med Pediatr Oncol 24:321–326, 1995.

145. Pradhan DG, Sandridge AL, Mullaney P, et al. Radiation therapy for retinoblastoma: a retrospective review of 120 patients. Int J Radiat Oncol Biol Phys 39:3–13, 1997.

146. Beck MN, Balmer A, Dessing C, et al. First line chemotherapy with local treatment can prevent external-beam irradiation and enucleation in low stage intraocular retinoblastoma. J Clin Oncol 18: 2881–2887, 2000.

147. Donaldson SS, Egbert PR, Newsham I, et al. Retinoblastoma. In: Pizzo PA, Poplack DG, eds. Principles and practice of pediatric oncology. 3rd ed. Philadelphia: Lippincott-Raven, 1997:699–715.

148. Shields CL, et al. Chemoreduction for unilateral retinoblastoma. Arch Ophthal 120:1653–1658, 2002.

149. Shields CL, Mashayekhi A, Demirici H, et al. Practical approach to management of retinoblastoma. Arch Ophthal 122: 729–735, 2004.

150. Rodriguez-Galindo C, Wilson MW, Haik BG, et al. Treatment of intraocular retinoblastoma with Vincristine and Carboplatin. J Clin Oncol 21:2019–2025, 2003.

151. Abramson DH, Frank CM, Dunkell IJ, et al. A phase I/II study of subconjunctival Carboplatin for intraocular retinoblastoma. Ophthalmology 106:1947–1950, 1999.

152. Chantada GL, Fandion AC, Casak SJ, et al. Activity of topotecan in retinoblastoma. Ophthalmic Genet 25:37–43, 2004.

153. Namouni F, Doz F, Tanguy ML, et al. High-dose chemotherapy with carboplatin, etoposide and cyclophosphamide followed by a haematopoietic stem cell rescue in patients with high-risk retinoblastoma: a SFOP and SFGM study. Eur J Cancer 33:2368–2375, 1997.

Gynecologic Cancers

102

Dayna L. McCauley

TREATMENT GOALS

- Prevent gynecologic cancers by recognizing and avoiding identified risk factors.
- Detect gynecologic cancer early; cervical cancer in particular has an effective screening tool and early detection improves survival.
- Cure the patient. Most gynecologic cancers are curable in early stages. Cure is still a goal for patients with advanced disease, but is less likely.
- Prolong survival.
- Improve, maintain, or prevent deterioration of the patient's functional status and quality of life.
- Relieve disease-related symptoms.

GYNECOLOGICAL CANCERS

DEFINITION

The gynecologic cancers are cancers of the female reproductive tract and include ovarian, endometrial, cervical, vaginal, vulvar cancers, and gestational trophoblastic disease. The most common of these include ovarian cancer, cervical cancer, and endometrial cancer, and will be the topics of this chapter. To find information regarding other gynecologic cancers not covered here, please refer to selected readings at the end of this chapter.

OVARIAN CANCER

DEFINITION

Epithelial ovarian cancer is a cancer that results from malignant transformation of the epithelial ovarian surface cells. Other ovarian tumor types include tumors of uncertain malignant potential (low-malignant potential or borderline malignancies) and ovarian germ cell tumors. This section will focus on the diagnosis, staging, and management of epithelial ovarian cancer. Importantly, although fallopian tube cancer and primary peritoneal cancer are separate and distinct pathologic entities, their clinical management is identical to epithelial ovarian cancer. Thus, the treatments discussed in this chapter for ovarian cancer can also be applied to the management of fallopian tube and primary peritoneal cancers.

ETIOLOGY

The exact cause of sporadic ovarian cancer is unknown, but is likely a combination of endocrine and environmental factors acting on a genetically susceptible host.[1] Sporadic, or nonhereditary ovarian cancer is the most common type, accounting for 85% to 90% of all epithelial ovarian cancers in the United States. Familial and hereditary syndromes are less common, and account for 10% to 15% of all ovarian cancers. The "incessant ovulation" theory states that a woman's risk of developing ovarian cancer is related to her number of ovulatory cycles. Ovulation results in disruption and repair of the epithelial lining of the ovary. An aberrant repair process is proposed to be one origin of sporadic ovarian cancer. Tumor suppressor genes, such as BRCA-1, BRCA-2, and p53, are thought to play a role in approximately 5% to 10% of ovarian cancer cases. Mutations of these genes results in unregulated production of mutant proteins and progression toward malignancy. Ovarian cancer also occurs in 5% to 10% of patients known to have rare hereditary cancer syndromes such as hereditary nonpolyposis colorectal cancer (HNPCC), Lynch II, and other rare syndromes.

EPIDEMIOLOGY OF OVARIAN CANCER

Epithelial ovarian cancer is the leading cause of death from gynecologic cancer in the United States. It is the fourth most frequent cause of cancer death in women. The lifetime risk of developing ovarian cancer is about 1.6%. The estimated number of new ovarian cancer cases in 2005 is approximately 22,211 while the estimated number of deaths from ovarian cancer is 16,210. Ovarian cancer is primarily a postmenopausal disease. The peak incidence for epithelial ovarian cancer is 65 to 69 years of age, but can occur in women as young as 18 to 20 years of age. Ovarian cancer is more common in whites than African-American women. Except for Japan, where the incidence is low, ovarian cancer is more common in developed countries.[1-3]

RISK FACTORS

Factors known to increase the frequency or duration of ovulation are associated with an increased risk of ovarian cancer: early menarche, late menopause, and nulliparity (due to increased number and/or duration of ovulatory cycles).[1,4] Other risk factors include increased age, white race, and residence in North America or Northern Europe. The role of ovulatory-stimulating drugs, environmental and dietary factors, and hormone replacement therapy remain highly controversial.[5,6]

By far the greatest risk factor for the development of ovarian cancer in any woman is a personal family history of ovarian cancer. The lifetime risk of a woman developing ovarian cancer increases to 4% to 5% if she has one first-degree relative with ovarian cancer, and 7% if she has two affected first-degree relatives. Genetically susceptible, or hereditary ovarian cancer syndromes accounts for less than 10% of all ovarian cancers. Two tumor suppressor genes have been identified that increase a woman's risk of breast and/or ovarian cancer. These genes are referred to as the breast cancer 1 and 2 genes (BRCA-1 and BRCA-2 genes, respectively). Under normal conditions, BRCA-1 and BRCA-2 suppress tumor growth. Normally, these genes produce proteins that control cell division. When a mutation occurs in a tumor suppressor gene, control of cell division is lost and a tumor can form. BRCA-1 mutations are associated with a 25% to 45% increased risk of developing ovarian cancer. BRCA-2 mutations are associated with a 27% increased risk. However, survival appears to be better in ovarian cancer patients with BRCA-1 or BRCA-2 mutations compared to those with sporadic ovarian cancer.

Factors that reduce the number of ovulatory cycles are associated with a reduced risk for developing ovarian cancer. These include multiple pregnancies and breast-feeding (although these are not fully protective), tubal ligation, prophylactic oophorectomy, and prolonged use of oral contraceptives. Oral contraceptive pill (OCP) use decreases a woman's risk of developing ovarian cancer by more than 50% after 5 years of use.

SCREENING AND PREVENTION

SCREENING

There is no effective screening test for ovarian cancer at this time, although large scale screening studies are underway in Europe and the United States.[1,7–9] Previously, pilot studies looking at transvaginal ultrasound, pelvic examination and/or CA-125 have not been sensitive or specific enough to warrant large scale screening programs. Current recommendations for screening women at low or standard risk (not familial or hereditary) include an annual physical and pelvic examination.[1,7] Recommendations for screening women at high risk (hereditary ovarian cancer, patients who are BRCA-1 or BRCA-2 positive) include pelvic examination, transvaginal ultrasound, and CA-125 every 6 to 12 months starting at age 25 to age 35 years. These patients should also undergo coun-

seling regarding the use of birth control pills and/or prophylactic bilateral oophorectomy on a case-by-case basis.[7]

Analysis of serum protein patterns (a technique known as proteomics) is promising as a screening tool for the early detection of ovarian cancer.[10] In the first proteomics studies in ovarian cancer, Petricoin, et al[10] used mass spectroscopy to identify unique protein patterns in the serum of 50 women with known ovarian cancer. These protein patterns were compared to 50 women without ovarian cancer. They found that the assay exhibited a sensitivity of 100%, a specificity of 95%, and a positive predictive value of 94%. Large scale validation studies are currently in progress. When this test is approved by the Food and Drug Administration (FDA) it will be marketed under the trade name OvaCheck.

PREVENTION

Oral contraceptives have been used to prevent the development of ovarian cancer in high risk patients.[11,12] Oral contraceptive use for 5 or more years decreases the risk of ovarian cancer by 50% or more. Prophylactic oophorectomy also decreases the risk of ovarian cancer in high-risk patients (BRCA mutations) and is used as a prevention strategy in these women. Prophylactic oophorectomy is not recommended for patients in low-risk categories. Importantly, prophylactic oophorectomy does not protect against the risk of developing primary peritoneal carcinoma in patients with BRCA-1 or BRCA-2 mutations.

PATHOPHYSIOLOGY

Ovarian cancer originates from a malignant transformation of the ovarian surface epithelium (Fig. 102.1). What causes this malignant transformation is unknown, but it likely in-

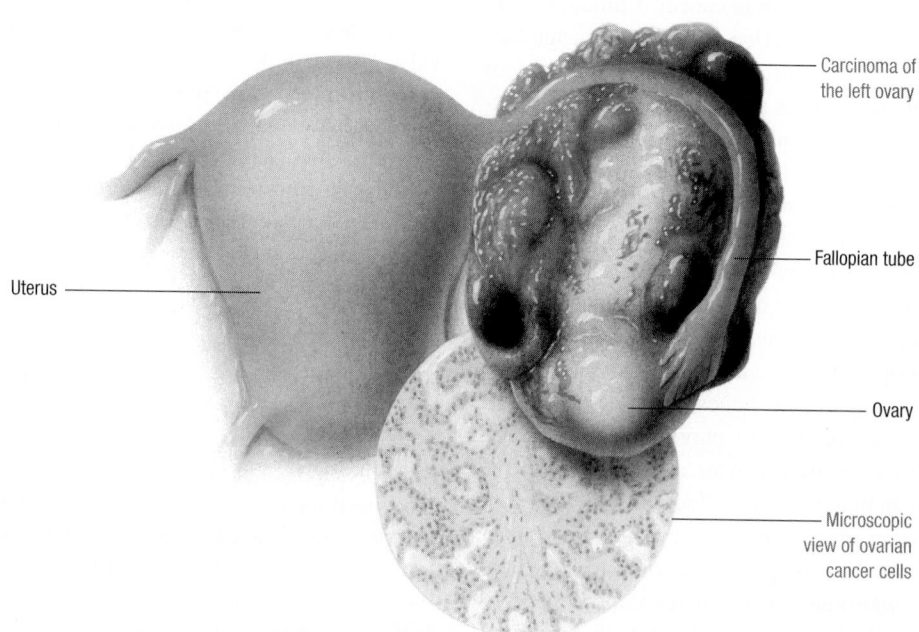

Uterus —

Carcinoma of the left ovary —

Fallopian tube —

Ovary —

Microscopic view of ovarian cancer cells —

FIGURE 102.1 Ovarian cancer. (From Anatomical Chart Co.)

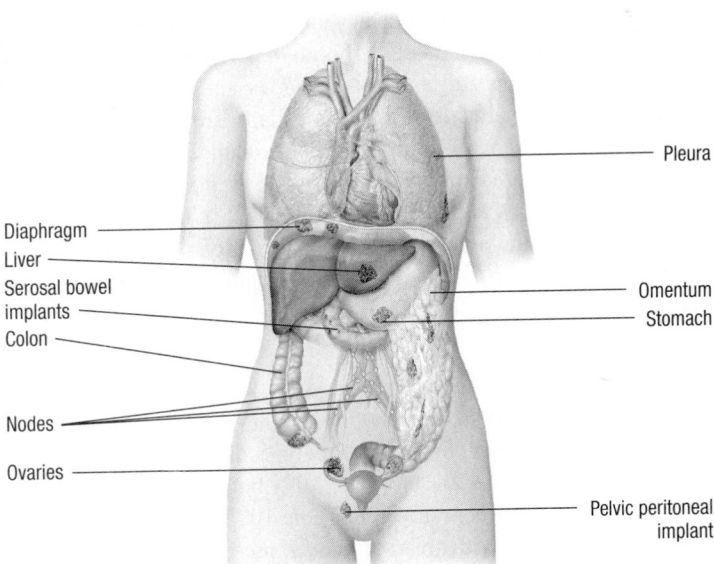

FIGURE 102.2 Likely metastatic sites for ovarian cancer. (From Anatomical Chart Co.)

volves alterations in cellular oncogene activity and/or growth factor signals. As the tumors grow, they penetrate the ovarian capsule. The most common mechanisms of spread are direct extension and peritoneal seeding of tumor cells (Fig. 102.2). Direct extension occurs when tumor cells invade adjacent tissues and organs, including the fallopian tubes, uterus, cervix, bladder, and rectosigmoid and pelvic peritoneum. Hematogenous spread of ovarian cancer is rare. These cells are carried by the peritoneal fluid to sites on the peritoneal surfaces where they form micrometastases. Free-floating tumor cells are removed from the peritoneal cavity by lymphatic channels in the diaphragm. Tumor spread also occurs via the lymphatics from the ovary. Therefore, common sites of tumor spread include the peritoneum, diaphragm, omentum, bowel surfaces, and retroperitoneal lymph nodes. Distant organs at risk include the liver, lungs, pleura, kidneys, bone, adrenal glands, bladder, and spleen in decreasing order of frequency. Impaired pleural lymphatic drainage may result in malignant pleural effusions, which can be the first extraperitoneal sign of ovarian cancer.

HISTOLOGY

Ovarian cancer is comprised of several diverse pathologic entities. Epithelial adenocarcinoma makes up more than 90% of all cases of ovarian cancer and is the subject of this chapter. The most common histopathologic subtype of epithelial ovarian cancer is a serous subtype. Others include mucinous, endometrioid, clear-cell (most virulent), and Brenner histologies (very rare). Low malignant potential or borderline malignancies are associated with a good prognosis and can often be cured with surgery alone. Ovarian germ cell tumors are rare and often highly aggressive. Germ cell tumors include dysgerminoma, endodermal sinus tumor, malignant teratoma, embryonal carcinoma, and primary choriocarci-

noma of the ovary. The treatment of these tumors is beyond the scope of this chapter. Ovarian sex-cord stromal tumors are often hormone producing and include granulosa cell tumors, Sertoli-Leydig tumors, and others. Lastly, ovarian malignancies can also manifest as metastases from other primary sites (most commonly breast and colon cancer).

Epithelial ovarian cancers are assigned a histologic grade based on the characterization of the cell architecture. Grade 1 tumors are well differentiated; grade 2 tumors are moderately differentiated, and grade 3 tumors are poorly differentiated. Histologic grading is especially important in the management of early stage (stages I and II) ovarian cancers.

CLINICAL PRESENTATION AND DIAGNOSIS

SIGNS AND SYMPTOMS

Ovarian cancer is often asymptomatic in early stages, however, only 15% to 20% of patients present with early stage disease. Because the ovaries are in a spacious pelvic cavity, the tumor can grow considerably before producing symptoms. When symptoms do develop, they are usually a sign of advanced stage disease and may include nausea, dyspepsia, vaginal bleeding, abdominal distention, or nonspecific intermittent lower abdominal discomfort. Unilateral or bilateral, solid, cystic and/or complex pelvic or adnexal masses are usually present on radiologic examination. The CA-125 is frequently highly elevated (normal CA-125 = 0–35 units/mL).

DIAGNOSIS AND STAGING

DIAGNOSIS

The findings of an adnexal mass concurrent with an elevated CA-125 in a postmenopausal woman should be considered suspicious for an ovarian malignancy until proven otherwise. The diagnostic workup includes a thorough pelvic examination, an imaging study to assess the ovaries and abdomen [an abdominal or pelvic ultrasound is usually sufficient; a computed tomography (CT) or magnetic resonance imaging (MRI) are considered optional], a CA-125 if not already drawn, a chest x-ray, complete blood cell count (CBC) with platelets, differential and chemistries, and finally, a barium enema or colonoscopy if the differential diagnosis includes colon cancer.

STAGING

Cancer of the ovary is staged according to the recommendations of the International Federation of Gynecology and Obstetrics (FIGO) (Table 102.1).[1,7] The distribution by stage at the time of diagnosis is shown in Table 102.2. As can be seen, most patients with ovarian cancer present with advanced stage (III or IV) disease. Lack of a sensitive and specific early tumor marker precludes diagnosis in early stages at this time.

TREATMENT OF OVARIAN CANCER

SURGERY

Ovarian cancer treatment requires a combination of surgery and chemotherapy to affect the best patient outcomes. Complete surgical staging (determining the breadth and severity of the tumor), preferably by a specially trained gynecologic oncologist, forms the foundation for the treatment plan. Further decisions regarding the use and/or duration of chemotherapy and the patient's ultimate prognosis are dictated by the findings at the time of initial surgery. All patients with a suspected ovarian malignancy should undergo comprehensive surgical staging that includes a total abdominal hysterectomy and bilateral salpingo-oophorectomy, omentectomy, pelvic and paraaortic lymph node sampling, appendectomy, peritoneal biopsies, cytologic washings, complete abdominal exploration, and intact tumor removal if possible. Patients found to have stage IA disease (Table 102.1) that desire future fertility may opt to undergo a unilateral salpingo-oophorectomy and full staging procedure, although this recommendation remains controversial. For patients with advanced disease at presentation, the surgical goal is to remove as much gross disease as possible, preferably to microscopic disease. Approximately 20% to 25% of patients with ovarian cancer require bowel resections resulting in the need for a temporary or permanent colostomy. Surgical removal of gross disease is referred to as "debulking" surgery. Patients who have more than 2 cm of residual tumor remaining at the conclusion of surgery are termed "suboptimally" debulked while patients with less than 2 cm of residual disease remaining are termed "optimally" debulked. The presence of bulky residual disease at the end of surgery is a poor prognostic sign.[13,14] Patients undergoing optimal

TABLE 102.1	International Federation of Gynecology and Obstetrics Staging for Carcinoma of the Ovary
Stage I	Tumor limited to the ovaries.
Stage IA	Tumor limited to one ovary; capsule intact, no tumor on ovarian surface. No malignant cells in ascites or peritoneal washings.
Stage IB	Tumor limited to both ovaries; capsules intact, no tumor on ovarian surface. No malignant cells in ascites or peritoneal washings.
Stage IC	Tumor limited to one or both ovaries with ruptured capsule, tumor on ovarian surface, or malignant cells in ascites or peritoneal washings.
Stage II	Tumor involving one or both ovaries with pelvic extension.
Stage IIA	Extension or metastases on the uterus or tubes. No malignant cells in ascites or peritoneal washings.
Stage IIB	Extension to other pelvic tissues. No malignant cells in ascites or peritoneal washings.
Stage IIC	Tumor is stage IIA or IIB with malignant cells in ascites or peritoneal washings.
Stage III	Tumor involving one or both ovaries with microscopically confirmed peritoneal metastasis outside the pelvis or regional lymph node metastasis. Any liver capsule metastasis.
Stage IIIA	Microscopic peritoneal metastasis beyond the pelvis.
Stage IIIB	Macroscopic peritoneal metastasis beyond the pelvis 2 cm or less in the greatest dimension.
Stage IIIC	Peritoneal metastasis beyond the pelvis more than 2 cm in the greatest dimension or regional lymph node metastasis.
Stage IV	Distant metastasis (excludes peritoneal metastasis). Any liver parenchymal metastasis. If pleural effusion is present, it must have positive cytology.

surgical debulking to less than 2 cm of residual disease have a mean survival advantage of 22 months compared to patients with gross residual disease (>2 cm).[1,13,14]

Following surgery, the current practice is to initiate early oral feeding with or without oral pain medications.[15,16] Using these practices, the length of stay in the hospital for a patient following surgery for ovarian cancer is approximately 3 to 4 days.

TABLE 102.2	Distribution of Cases by Stage at Time of Diagnosis for Ovarian Cancer

Stage	Frequency
I	20%–25%
II	10%–15%
III	45%
IV	15%

CHEMOTHERAPY FOR EARLY STAGE DISEASE (STAGES I AND II)

Patients with surgical stage I or stage II disease are those whose cancer is limited to one or both ovaries and has not undergone extension to other pelvic structures (Table 102.1) The cancer is then further defined by its pathologically favorable and/or unfavorable features (Table 102.3). The recommendations for treatment with chemotherapy for early stage disease are based on these features.

Favorable Features of Early Stage Disease. In the United States, the National Comprehensive Cancer Center Network (NCCN) and Society of Gynecologic Oncologists (SGO) consensus guidelines for patients with stage IA or IB grade 1 cancer recommend comprehensive surgical debulking and staging followed by no further therapy.[7] These patients have an excellent prognosis and an estimated 5-year survival of 90% to 95%.

Unfavorable Features of Early Stage Disease. All patients with early stage disease and unfavorable features should undergo comprehensive surgical debulking and staging followed by combination chemotherapy with paclitaxel 175 mg/m² over 3 hours plus carboplatin (AUC = 6) every 3 weeks for six cycles.[7] Historically, studies have shown that adjuvant therapy with melphalan or cisplatin improved survival compared to no further treatment in early stage ovarian cancer patients with unfavorable features (high risk of recurrence).[17,18] The current recommendation for the use of paclitaxel plus carboplatin is extrapolated from the current standard of care for treatment of advanced stage ovarian cancer.

The question of if fewer cycles of chemotherapy is adequate treatment for early stage disease has been studied in

TABLE 102.3	Pathologic Classification for Early Stage Ovarian Cancer

Favorable Features	Unfavorable Features
Stage IA or IB grade 1	Stage IA or IB grade 2 or grade 3
	Stage IC
	Stage II with ascites, ruptured capsule, clear cell histology

the United States by the Gynecologic Oncology Group (GOG-157), a national clinical trials organization devoted exclusively to gynecologic cancer studies.[19] In this trial, 457 women with early stage ovarian cancer and unfavorable features were randomized to receive paclitaxel 175 mg/m² over 3 hours and carboplatin (AUC = 7.5) every 3 weeks for three or six cycles. After adjusting for stage and grade, the recurrence rate was found to be 33% lower in patients treated with six cycles. Because this difference did not reach statistical significance, six cycles of combination chemotherapy with paclitaxel plus carboplatin remains the standard of care in this patient population in this country.

Results of two recent large, randomized, multicenter European trials in early stage ovarian cancer have complicated interpretation of current treatment recommendations. In one trial, 477 patients were randomized following surgery to receive six cycles of platinum-based chemotherapy [single-agent carboplatin, cyclophosphamide, doxorubicin (Adria), and prednisone (CAP), or other combinations] or observation.[20] This trial, known as the International Collaborative Ovarian Neoplasm Trial I (ICON-1 trial), included patients with grade 1 tumors, which are not currently treated with chemotherapy in the United States. Results demonstrated a significant improvement in both the progression-free survival (73% vs. 62%) and the overall 5-year survival (79% vs. 70%) for patients treated with chemotherapy compared to observation alone, respectively. This trial supports the role of adjuvant treatment for all patients with early stage ovarian cancer.

The second trial, known as the Adjuvant Chemotherapy in Ovarian Neoplasm (ACTION) trial,[21] excluded patients with favorable features (stage IA or IB well-differentiated tumors). Following surgery, 448 patients with early stage high-grade tumors were randomized to receive four cycles of platinum-based chemotherapy (single-agent carboplatin or cisplatin and cyclophosphamide) or no further therapy. At a median follow-up of 5.5 years, no statistically significant difference in overall survival or progression-free survival was noted between the two arms. A statistically significant survival benefit has only been demonstrated in a subgroup analysis of patients who did not undergo optimal surgical staging. Thus, in contrast to current recommendations, results of this trial imply that adjuvant therapy for high-risk early stage cancer patients may not be of benefit unless the patients have not been adequately staged surgically. In addition, this trial also suggests that if patients do undergo therapy that four cycles of single-agent carboplatin may be sufficient therapy. Indeed, this regimen is widely used throughout Europe.

CHEMOTHERAPY FOR ADVANCED STAGE DISEASE (STAGES III AND IV)

While the initial goal remains curing the patient, the probability of cure decreases in patients with stage IV or surgically unresectable disease. Following complete surgical staging, the current recommendation for first-line treatment of advanced ovarian cancer is six cycles of adjuvant chemotherapy with paclitaxel 175 mg/m^2 intravenously (IV) over 3 hours plus carboplatin (AUC = 5–7.5) every 3 weeks for six cycles (see addendum at the end of the chapter for updated recommendations for the treatment of first-line advanced stage disease).[1,7,22] This recommendation is based on an evolution of clinical trials. First, platinum-based regimens have been shown to be superior to nonplatinum regimens in the treatment of ovarian cancer.[23,24] Second, treatment beyond six cycles of chemotherapy appears to offer no additional benefit in the adjuvant setting.[25,26] Third, carboplatin has been proven to be equal in efficacy to cisplatin with a more favorable toxicity profile.[27–29] As these trials evolved, cyclophosphamide plus carboplatin, administered on an outpatient basis was the standard until the early 1990s when paclitaxel became available for use. Due to its exceptional activity in the treatment of multiply relapsed and platinum refractory ovarian cancer, clinical trials were initiated looking at paclitaxel-containing regimens as first-line therapy. The seminal trial establishing its role in first-line treatment of ovarian cancer was the GOG 111 trial.[30] This trial compared cyclophosphamide 750 mg/m^2 plus cisplatin 75 mg/m^2 to paclitaxel 135 mg/m^2 IV over 24 hours plus cisplatin 75 mg/m^2 in 410 patients with stage III and stage IV ovarian cancer. All patients had "suboptimal" disease and a greater than 2-cm residual disease following surgery. The complete response rates, progression-free survival, and overall survival were all significantly improved in patients treated with paclitaxel plus cisplatin compared to patients treated with cyclophosphamide plus cisplatin (51% vs. 31%, 18 vs. 13 months, and 38 vs. 24 months, respectively). A similar trial that was completed in Europe (OV-10 trial)[31] substantiated the survival benefit of paclitaxel plus cisplatin compared to the old standard using cyclophosphamide. An important difference is noted in the toxicity profiles of these trials, however. The OV-10 trial combined paclitaxel 175 mg/m^2 IV over 3 hours with cisplatin 75 mg/m^2. This administration regimen resulted in substantially greater peripheral neurotoxicity (18%) than the comparable regimen with paclitaxel administered over 24 hours. Thus, doses of paclitaxel of 175 mg/m^2 or greater are not recommended for administration over 3 hours if combined with cisplatin.

After publication of the GOG-111 and OV-10 trials, paclitaxel plus cisplatin became the new standard for first-line treatment of ovarian cancer following surgery. A series of studies in the United States and Europe then substantiated that carboplatin could be substituted for cisplatin to improve toxicity without compromising efficacy.[22,23] In the pivotal U.S. trial (GOG-158), 802 patients with stage III and stage IV ovarian cancer were randomized following surgery to receive cisplatin 75 mg/m^2 plus paclitaxel 135 mg/m^2 over 24 hours or carboplatin (AUC = 7.5) plus paclitaxel 175 mg/m^2 over 3 hours for six cycles each.[22] There was no difference between the two arms in terms of complete response or overall survival. Hematologic toxicity was manageable, and the nonhematologic toxicity was significantly reduced in the carboplatin-containing arm. A second large

trial in Europe confirmed these findings.[32] With publication of these two trials, paclitaxel 175 mg/m^2 plus carboplatin (AUC = 5–7.5) every 3 weeks for six cycles became the new and current standard of care for first-line treatment of advanced stage ovarian cancer. Although the original trials were conducted using an AUC = 7.5, subsequent trials use lower AUC dosing (5–6). Most clinicians have moved to dosing carboplatin with an AUC = 5–6. This reduces platelet and neutrophil toxicity and chemotherapy dose delays.

Although the current recommendation is for six cycles of therapy, some patients experience a slow decline in the tumor marker for ovarian cancer, known as CA-125. Ideally, the CA-125 is normal (<35 U/mL) at the end of six cycles of combination chemotherapy. However, if the CA-125 is declining, but has not normalized, and the patient is not experiencing significant toxicity most clinicians continue administering first-line therapy and treat for one or two cycles past a normal CA-125. This may require several additional cycles of treatment, and the exact number can be tailored to the patient.

The most troublesome and potentially long-term complication associated with paclitaxel administered over 3 hours is peripheral nerve damage. This is usually manifest as bilateral numbness or tingling in the hands and feet that can progress to permanent sensory loss and impaired motor function. Newer agents are being investigated to attempt to reduce this complication. Recent data suggests that if docetaxel is substituted for paclitaxel in combination with carboplatin, response rates and survival remains equivalent but neurotoxicity is significantly reduced.[33] The trial investigating this theory is a European trial known as the SCOTROC trial. In this trial 1,077 patients with previously untreated, stage IC-IV ovarian or primary peritoneal cancers were randomized following surgery to receive docetaxel 75 mg/m^2 plus carboplatin (AUC = 5) or paclitaxel 175 mg/m^2 over 3 hours plus carboplatin (AUC = 5) for six cycles. There was no significant difference in progression-free or overall survival between the two groups. The regimens have offsetting significant toxicities, resulting in no difference in the global quality of life scores between the two regimens. Docetaxel plus carboplatin is associated with significantly more grade 3 to 4 neutropenia and fever, although this is transient. Paclitaxel plus carboplatin causes significantly more neurotoxicity. Based on the results of this study, docetaxel plus carboplatin can be considered a reasonable alternative first-line therapy for the treatment of ovarian cancer.

Alternative regimens that can be used as first-line therapy and that further reduce toxicity are outlined in Table 102.4. Use of lower dose, weekly therapy reduces hematologic and neurotoxicity. Alopecia may be reduced or avoided with the use of lower doses of paclitaxel. In addition, the fluid retention syndromes associated with higher doses of docetaxel are not seen when it is administered in lower weekly doses. Weekly regimens may be especially attractive for older patients who are less able to tolerate toxicity in standard regimens.

| TABLE 102.4 | Regimens for First-line Treatment of Ovarian Cancer |

Regimen	Comments
Paclitaxel 175 mg/m^2 IV over 3 hours plus Carboplatin (AUC = 5–7.5) IV every 21 days for six cycles	Current standard in the United States. Most centers use an AUC of 5–6 now. Outpatient regimen, very well tolerated
Paclitaxel 135 mg/m^2 IV over 24 hours plus Cisplatin 75 mg/m^2 IV every 21 days for six cycles	Equally efficacious to paclitaxel plus carboplatin. Administration schedule mandates 2-day admission to hospital, which is not feasible under most insurance plans
Docetaxel 75 mg/m^2 IV over 1 hour plus Carboplatin (AUC = 5) IV every 21 days for six cycles	The SCOTROC regimen. Associated with significant hematologic toxicity but reduced neurotoxicity
Paclitaxel 60–80 mg/m^2 IV over 1 hr plus Carboplatin (AUC = 2) IV weekly days 1,8,15. Repeat every 28 days for six cycles	Weekly dosing reduces neurologic and hematologic toxicity
Docetaxel 25–30 mg/m^2 IV over 1 hr plus Carboplatin (AUC = 2) IV weekly days 1,8,15. Repeat every 28 days for six cycles	Weekly dosing reduces hematologic toxicity and fluid retention

Large multicenter randomized trials are ongoing in the United States (GOG-182) and Europe (ICON-5) to ascertain if the addition of newer agents (e.g., liposomal doxorubicin or gemcitabine) or sequential doublets and triplets improves response rates when compared to paclitaxel plus carboplatin.

DOSE INTENSITY

Although this is still controversial, ovarian cancer is generally not considered to be a dose-responsive malignancy. Randomized trials comparing combination chemotherapy with cisplatin 50 to 100 mg/m^2 have failed to show an improvement in survival for patients treated with higher doses. Higher doses, do however, cause more toxicity.[34–36] In addition, randomized trials comparing combination chemotherapy with carboplatin (AUC = 4–12) failed to show an improvement in survival, while again, higher doses resulted in greater toxicity.[37,38] However, there is a modest dose response with paclitaxel. Evidence from one trial indicated that paclitaxel 175 mg/m^2 was associated with significantly longer progression-free survival when compared to doses of 135 mg/m^2 in patients with recurrent disease (19 vs. 14 weeks, respectively).[39] However, the clinical significance of this remains unknown and unproven in large randomized trials in the adjuvant setting.

There is limited data to support the role of hematopoietic stem cell transplantation in the treatment of ovarian cancer. The series of trials published to date are phase II trials with small numbers of patients with chemotherapy sensitive disease.[34,40,41] Response rates are high (60%–80%), but the duration of response is limited. A phase III trial was initiated by the GOG to address the role of stem cell transplantation compared to standard dose therapy. This study was closed for failure to recruit sufficient numbers of patients. At this time, there is no data to support the role of stem cell transplantation outside of a clinical trial.

NEOADJUVANT CHEMOTHERAPY

Neoadjuvant chemotherapy is the use of chemotherapy prior to surgery to reduce or eliminate sites of tumor before the surgeon removes the remaining tumor. Typically, paclitaxel plus carboplatin will be administered every 3 weeks for three to six cycles, followed by cytoreductive or interval surgery. Additional cycles of chemotherapy may be administered postoperatively. This strategy is especially useful in patients who are initially considered to be medically inoperable. Chemotherapy reduces tumor volume and allows successful interval surgery without compromising overall survival.[1,42]

SECOND-LOOK SURGERY

A second-look surgery (referred to as second-look laparotomy, or SLL) is sometimes completed at the end of six cycles of first-line therapy in patients who have achieved a clinical complete remission (normal CA-125 and physical examination). The purpose of the surgery is to visually explore the abdominal cavity for residual disease and perform multiple peritoneal and abdominal biopsies. If the biopsies are negative, the patient is considered to be in a pathologic complete response. These patients are then identified as being especially responsive to chemotherapy and may be considered for further therapy (referred to as consolidation therapy) while in complete remission. Intraperitoneal (IP) chemotherapy, if used, is usually reserved for this select subset of patients. Conversely, if visually gross residual disease is found at the time of second surgery, some consider it useful to perform a secondary cytoreductive procedure. In theory, this would allow removal of residual disease and improve response rates to salvage chemotherapy. The benefit of SLL remains widely controversial. To date, there have been no randomized trials that have proven a survival benefit in patients undergoing second-look surgeries. Furthermore, 80% to 85% of patients with advanced stage ovarian cancer ultimately relapse from their disease and require additional therapy irrespective of whether they achieve an initial complete clinical or pathologic response to front-line therapy. Thus, at this time, there are little data to support the routine use of second-look surgeries outside the setting of a clinical trial.

CONSOLIDATION THERAPY

Consolidation chemotherapy refers to the administration of additional chemotherapy after a complete clinical remission is obtained. The drugs may be the same as those administered during first-line therapy or may be noncross resistant. The purpose of continuation, or consolidation therapy, is to help maintain the complete clinical remission. The role of consolidation therapy for epithelial ovarian cancer is controversial due to its lack of evidence for improving patient care outcomes.[7] The need for additional therapy is rarely in dispute; as mentioned previously, eventually 70% to 80% of patients will recur with ovarian cancer and require additional therapy. The question surrounds the timing for initiation of additional chemotherapy (i.e., at the time of first clinical complete remission, or at first relapse).

A large study was undertaken specifically to address the question of whether consolidation therapy improves survival for patients in complete remission following six cycles of standard therapy (GOG-178/SWOG-9701).[43] Patients with advanced ovarian, fallopian tube, or primary peritoneal carcinoma achieving a clinical complete remission following platinum/paclitaxel-based therapy were randomized to paclitaxel 175 mg/m^2 over 3 hours for 3 or 12 additional months. The study was closed early when an interim analysis discovered a statistically significant improvement in progression-free survival in patients randomized to 12 months of therapy (28 vs. 21 months). There was no difference in overall survival at the time of the analysis, and likely never will be, as patients randomized to 3 months of therapy were subsequently allowed to crossover to the 12-month arm. Quality of life was not measured in this study. However, the dose of paclitaxel was reduced to 135 mg/m^2 midway in the study when a large number of patients randomized to 12 months of therapy developed grades 3 and 4 peripheral neuropathy.

INTRAPERITONEAL CHEMOTHERAPY

IP chemotherapy has been used as treatment for ovarian cancer because the disease spreads primarily within the peritoneal cavity. Chemotherapy is instilled directly into the peritoneal cavity through a special catheter. The chemotherapy is diluted in a large volume of fluid (1–3 L) and allowed to "dwell" in the peritoneal cavity for several hours. The patient may need to be rotated from side to side during administration to ensure adequate distribution of drug throughout the peritoneal cavity. In theory, IP chemotherapy should provide very high concentrations of drug locally at the site of disease, while sparing the patient systemic side effects. Optimal agents for IP therapy have a high molecular weight, low lipid solubility, are cleared slowly from the peritoneal cavity and are minimally toxic to the peritoneum. Cisplatin is the drug of choice for this use, as it meets these criteria and has excellent activity in ovarian cancer.

A study comparing IP and intravenous cisplatin, both in combination with intravenous cyclophosphamide, in optimally debulked stage III ovarian cancer patients showed a higher response rate in the IP arm (47% vs. 36%) and an 8-month survival advantage.[44] In addition, there were significantly fewer toxic effects in patients receiving IP therapy. At the time of publication in 1996 the results of this trial were largely discounted by the medical community, as paclitaxel had replaced cyclophosphamide in the treatment of ovarian cancer. Recently, a trial evaluating IP therapy in combination with paclitaxel for the treatment of first-line advanced stage, optimally surgically treated patients has been published and demonstrates a significant survival advantage in favor of the IP arm. This trial, and the results of others including those cited in reference 44, form the basis for an NCI clinical announcement recommending IP therapy as first-line treatment for select patients with ovarian cancer. At this time, IP therapy has a major role in the first-line treatment of advanced stage disease. Outside of a clinical trial, there is no role for the use of IP therapy in the treatment of recurrent disease. The reader is referred to the addendum published at the end of this chapter for a full discussion of this topic.

MONITORING PLAN

Patients receiving first-line therapy for ovarian cancer should undergo the following monitoring plan: a pelvic examination should be completed at least every two cycles of chemotherapy. A CA-125 should be drawn prior to each cycle (if used as a marker) to assess response to chemotherapy. Ideally, the CA-125 should return to normal (0–35 units/mL) following the third cycle of chemotherapy.[45] A slow response or failure to normalize the CA-125 level after six cycles of chemotherapy is associated with a worse prognosis. A rising CA-125 in the middle of primary therapy indicates that the patient is a primary nonresponder and mandates a change in therapy (see Refractory and Relapsed Disease). There is lab to lab variation in CA-125 assays. Thus, to accurately interpret the results of a CA-125 value, the patient should obtain this test at the same laboratory every month.

Other laboratory studies that should be obtained prior to each cycle of treatment include a CBC with differential, platelets, and chemistries. Imaging studies should only be performed in patients with disease that cannot be measured by physical examination (e.g., paraaortic lymph nodes or hepatic metastases) and where CA-125 is not an adequate marker.

At the completion of primary therapy, patients should begin surveillance examinations including a complete physical and pelvic examination and CA-125 level every 3 to 4 months for 2 years. After 2 years, the frequency can be reduced to every 6 months for 3 more years. At the end of 5 years, if the patient remains in remission, then surveillance examinations can be completed annually. A rising CA-125 level at any time during surveillance examinations is the most sensitive indicator that the patient has recurrent disease.

TREATMENT OF RECURRENT DISEASE

GENERAL PRINCIPLES

Ultimately, 70% to 80% of all patients with ovarian cancer relapse from their disease and require salvage chemotherapy. At this point, the goal of treatment is no longer curative. Instead, the goals shift to improving or eliminating symptoms, achieving an objective response, improving quality of life, delaying time to symptomatic disease, and prolonging survival if possible.

As a general rule, once a patient has relapsed, the length of subsequent remissions is shorter than the initial remission (e.g., length of first remission > length of second remission > length of third remission, etc.). Decisions regarding choice of therapy should include factors such as length of initial remission, patient or family member convenience, prior patient toxicity, insurance coverage, and overall quality of life.

There is no ''standard therapy'' for recurrent ovarian cancer. Once therapy has been initiated, it is usually continued for as long as the patient is responding and has not developed unacceptable toxicity. Stable disease is a reasonable end point and a reason to continue therapy. If a second complete remission is achieved, the decision to continue or stop therapy is individualized. Patients with recurrent ovarian cancer often remain on chemotherapy for the rest of their lives.

A patient's prognosis and treatment decisions are defined by response to initial chemotherapy.[1] Platinum-sensitive disease refers to patients whose initial response to platinum (and paclitaxel) was greater than 6 months. The longer the initial remission, the greater the likelihood of responding to second-line and third-line therapies. The probability of response to salvage chemotherapy in a patient with platinum-sensitive disease is 30% or more. Platinum-resistant disease refers to patients whose initial response to platinum (and paclitaxel) is less than 6 months. Platinum-resistant disease carries a poor prognosis with the likelihood of response to salvage chemotherapy in this patient population being 10% to 15%. Median survival is approximately 9 months. Platinum/paclitaxel-refractory disease (also referred to as primary progressive disease) refers to patients who fail to respond or experience progression of disease during primary therapy with platinum/paclitaxel, respectively. This characteristic is associated with the worst prognosis. The probability of responding to salvage chemotherapy is less than 10% in these patients and median survival is less than 6 months.

RECURRENT DISEASE

Table 102.5 outlines treatment options for patients with recurrent ovarian cancer. The timing of the use of these agents varies. For example, the most likely choices for the treatment of platinum-sensitive ovarian cancer in first relapse are retreatment with paclitaxel and/or carboplatin, alone or in combination. These two agents are the two most active agents in ovarian cancer and both are well tolerated as single agents. A recently completed large European randomized trial demonstrated that retreatment with combination therapy containing paclitaxel and carboplatin significantly improves progression-free and overall survival in a select subset of patients with chemotherapy-sensitive disease and a long initial remission (>12 months).[48] Unless patient specific factors preclude combination therapy, retreatment with paclitaxel plus carboplatin should be offered to all women with platinum-sensitive ovarian cancer in first relapse. On second and subsequent relapse, any of the other agents listed in Table 102.5 can be used.

There is no preferred agent for the treatment of platinum-resistant ovarian cancer. Carboplatin and paclitaxel would not be reinitiated in this patient population at time of first recurrence. A randomized trial comparing topotecan to liposomal doxorubicin showed a nonsignificant survival advantage for patients treated with topotecan.[52] Topotecan and liposomal doxorubicin are the two agents most widely used in the management of patients with platinum-resistant or refractory ovarian cancer in first recurrence. Liposomal doxorubicin is better tolerated, although weekly dosing of topotecan improves patient tolerability.

Patients with primary progressive disease should strongly be urged to enroll in an ongoing clinical trial. If the patient declines, then treatment with topotecan or liposomal doxorubicin is warranted. Patients who progress on two consecutive single-agent regimens are unlikely to respond to further therapy. Hospice and/or a clinical trial should be considered.

RADIATION THERAPY

Radiation may be used as primary adjuvant therapy (additional therapy administered after the primary tumor mass has been eliminated by the initial treatment modality) after surgery in patients with stage I or early stage II ovarian cancer, or in a study setting after a negative second-look surgery in advanced disease. Radiation must be directed to the pelvis and the upper abdomen to prevent relapses throughout the peritoneal cavity. Many normal tissues such as the kidney and liver are also radiosensitive, a situation that limits the dose of radiation that can be administered safely. The dose of radiation depends on the size of the tumor and is fractionated into multiple doses delivered over several weeks. The overall toxicity and complexity of whole-abdomen radiation and the effectiveness of chemotherapy have limited its usefulness for early stage ovarian cancer, and its role has declined in the United States in recent years. In advanced disease, radiation is usually reserved for inoperable tumors that are unresponsive to chemotherapy or as salvage therapy for persistent or symptomatic disease. It is also being explored in combination with chemotherapy in advanced and optimally debulked disease.[1,66]

TABLE 102.5	Salvage Single-agents and Doublet Regimens for Recurrent Ovarian Cancer	
Agent	**Dose/Schedule**	**Comments**
Carboplatin[46]	AUC = 5–7.5 IV every 28 days	Used alone or in combination with paclitaxel for treatment of platinum-sensitive recurrence. No alopecia. Minimal nausea or vomiting; very well tolerated
Paclitaxel[47]	135–175 mg/m² IV over 3 hours; repeat every 21–28 days	Used alone or in combination with carboplatin for treatment of platinum-sensitive recurrence
Paclitaxel + Carboplatin[48–51]	Same as above; repeated every 21 days	Combination therapy improves survival compared to single-agent platinum in patients with a long (duration of first remission >12 months. Not recommended for patients with second or subsequent relapse.
Liposomal doxorubicin (Doxil)[52,53]	40 mg/m² IV every 28 days	Well tolerated. Dose limited by stomatitis and hand-foot syndrome. Randomized trial versus topotecan shows improved survival for Doxil in platinum-sensitive patients only.[47]
Topotecan[52,54,55]	1.25 mg/m²/day IV × 5 days; repeat every 21–28 days or 3–4 mg/m² IV Day 1,8,15 repeat every 28 days	Hematologic toxicity dose limiting. Reduce dose for decreased renal function. Weekly regimen has less hematologic toxicity. Better tolerated if patient is not heavily pretreated
Docetaxel[56]	75–100 mg/m² IV day 1, repeat every 21 days or 30 mg/m² IV days 1,8,15 repeat every 28 days	Significantly less neutropenia, alopecia, or fluid retention with weekly dosing; useful in patients who have progressed on paclitaxel (noncross resistant)
Gemcitabine[57,58]	600–1,000 mg/m² IV Day 1,8,15 repeat every 28 days	Clinically necessary to reduce dose significantly in heavily pretreated patients.
Gemcitabine + cisplatin[59,60]	Gemcitabine 600–750 mg/m² IV + Cisplatin 30 mg/m² IV days 1 and 8, repeat every 21 days	Gemcitabine shown to overcome cisplatin resistance intracellularly. Combination therapy more toxic than single agent
Etoposide (oral)[61]	50 mg/m²/day orally, days 1–21; repeat every 28 days	Expensive
Altretamine (Hexalen)[62]	260 mg/m²/day, orally, divided tid days 1–14; repeat every 28 days	Side effects include nausea/vomiting, myelosuppression, and neurotoxicity.
Vinorelbine[63,64]	30 mg/m² IV Days 1, 8 repeat every 21 days	Hematologic toxicity is dose-limiting. Reduce day 8 dose for granulocyte and platelet toxicity. Reduce dose for elevated bilirubin.
Tamoxifen[65]	20 mg bid orally daily	Oral therapy. Minimal side effects; excellent QOL. Consider for patients with chemical recurrence only with no gross evidence of disease or for consolidation therapy.

IV, intravenously; bid, twice a day; tid, three times daily; QOL, quality of life.

The most common side effect of radiation therapy for ovarian cancer is radiation enteritis. This syndrome is dose-related and may include diarrhea, nausea, vomiting, and weight loss. These gastrointestinal symptoms usually subside a few weeks after therapy is completed. Radiation-induced hepatitis and nephritis can occur with doses greater than 3,500 cGy, especially if precautions have not been taken to minimize organ exposure during treatment. The most serious complication is small bowel obstruction, which usually warrants surgical correction. Radiation may also cause bone marrow suppression with a subsequent reduction in peripheral blood counts, which usually return to normal after therapy cessation. Irradiated bone marrow can remain impaired for extended periods of time, which should be a consideration for patients who may later receive myelosuppressive chemotherapy.

Radioactive phosphorus (^{32}P) or chromic phosphate is a radioisotope that emits beta particles with a tissue penetration range of 1 to 2 mm and has a half-life of 14.3 days. IP ^{32}P instillation can sterilize microscopic peritoneal tumor but cannot effectively treat larger tumors.[1] Unfortunately, distribution may be quite variable within the peritoneal cavity because of adhesions or loculations that are secondary to surgery. Side effects include abdominal pain (15%–20%), peritonitis (2%–3%), and small bowel obstruction (5%–10%). Because of its low toxicity, it can be useful as adjuvant therapy in patients with negative second-look surgeries. Difficulty of administration, uneven distribution of radioisotopes, and the incidence of late bowel complications have reduced the enthusiasm for the use of ^{32}P in early stage ovarian cancer. In addition, ^{32}P therapy does not have a survival advantage over cisplatin-based chemotherapy.[66]

PROGNOSIS

The stage of disease at diagnosis is the single most important prognostic factor for ovarian cancer survival.[1] The 5-year survival declines substantially from 90% for patients with stage I disease to less than 5% for patients with suboptimal (gross residual disease >2 cm following surgery) stage IV disease. As discussed previously, other important factors include the amount of residual disease after initial surgical resection and histologic subtype. Patients with suboptimal surgical cytoreduction and/or serous and other high-grade histologies have the worst prognosis. The role of histologic grading is especially important in assessing prognosis for patients with early stage disease.

CERVICAL CANCER

DEFINITION

Cervical cancer is a cancer arising from a premalignant lesion in the cervix. This section outlines the diagnosis, staging, and management of invasive cervical cancer. Surgery and radiation comprise the most commonly used treatments. While these are discussed briefly, a more thorough discussion of these topics can be found elsewhere.[67] This section does not cover the diagnosis or treatment of cervical sarcomas or other unusual histologic subtypes.

ETIOLOGY

Invasive cervical cancer is, theoretically, a preventable disease. Cervical dysplasia (hyperplastic, abnormal cells) is a precursor of cervical cancer. The risk of progression to invasive cervical cancer increases with the grade of dysplasia (Table 102.6).[68] Early detection and appropriate treatment of cervical dysplasia can stop progression to cervical cancer.

EPIDEMIOLOGY

Globally, cervical cancer is the third most common malignancy in women and the second most frequent cause of cancer-related death. It is estimated that 371,000 cases and 190,000 deaths occur annually, overwhelmingly in developing countries. It is estimated that 12,200 new cases of cervical cancer and 4,100 deaths will occur in the United States in 2004.[2,69] A substantial decline in mortality has occurred in developed countries due to effective screening programs. Cervical cancer is more common in Latin America, and is less frequent among Jewish and European women.

RISK FACTORS

The most important risk factor for the development of cervical cancer is infection with the human papilloma virus (HPV). HPV has been identified in more than 90% of invasive cervical cancers. Of the more than 20 different HPV types identified in the human genital tract, types 16 and 18

TABLE 102.6	Likelihood of Progression of Lesions to Cervical Cancer		
Pap Results	Regress to Normal (%)	Progress or Persist as HSIL in 24 Months (%)	Progress to Invasive Cancer in 24 Months (%)
ASCUS	68.19	7.13	0.25
LGSIL	47.39	20.81	0.15
HGSIL	35.03	23.37	1.44

ASCUS, abnormal squamous cells of undetermined significance; LSIL, low-grade squamous intraepithelial lesion; HGSIL, high-grade intraepithelial lesion.

are the most common.[70] Other risk factors include early onset of intercourse (coitarche), multiple sexual partners, multiparity, a history of sexually transmitted diseases, smoking, immunocompromised state (e.g., human immunodeficiency virus, transplant recipient), lower socioeconomic status, poor diet, (e.g., vitamin deficiency), and alcoholism. Factors associated with a decreased risk of cervical cancer include nulliparity and sexual inactivity.

PATHOPHYSIOLOGY

As mentioned above, cervical cancer is causally related to infection with HPV. The HPV infects the epithelium of the lower anogenital tract, including the cervical squamocolumnar junction. This is a site of continuous metaplastic change. The precursor lesion is called dysplasia or cervical intraepithelial neoplasia (CIN), which precedes the development of invasive cervical cancer. CIN is characterized by cellular immaturity and disorganization and increased mitotic change. Progression from CIN to invasive disease can be quite long with 66% of all patients developing invasive carcinoma within 10 years. The tumor becomes invasive when it breaks through the basement membrane into the underlying tissue. Cervical cancer usually progresses in a predictable manner, and tumor dissemination generally is a function of the extent of local tumor invasion. The disease can spread by direct extension into the vagina or endometrium, then to the walls of the pelvis, the bladder, and the rectum. In addition to local invasion, tumor spread can occur through the rich lymphatic network of the cervix, which anastomoses with those of the lower uterus. It spreads initially to lymph nodes in the pelvis, then to the paraaortic lymph nodes, and distant sites. The most common sites of distant spread are the lung, extrapelvic nodes, liver, and bone.[67]

HISTOLOGY

Squamous cell carcinoma makes up 80% to 90% of all cervical cancers. These are further differentiated into large cell keratinizing, large cell nonkeratinizing, and small cell nonkeratinizing cell types. Adenocarcinomas make up approximately 10% of cases, with most subtypes containing glandular features. Adenosquamous cell and small cell carcinomas are rare.[71] Invasive tumors usually are defined as exophytic or endophytic (endocervical) lesions. Exophytic lesions protrude from the cervix into the vagina, are friable, and bleed easily. They may be less extensive than they appear on first examination. Endophytic lesions are located in the endocervical canal of a normal-appearing cervix and can be more extensive than they appear. These lesions may become large enough to distend the cervix and create barrel-shaped lesions.[67]

TABLE 102.7	American Cancer Society Guidelines for Cervical Cancer Screening

3 years after first intercourse, but no later than age 21 in all women

Annually with a regular PAP or every other year with a liquid-based PAP test (e.g., Thin-Prep)

Starting at age 30, if a woman has no risk factors and three normal PAP tests in a row, then screening can:

  Decrease to every 2–3 years with a regular PAP or liquid-based prep or

  Decrease to once every 3 years and include a regular or liquid-based PAP plus HPV–DNA test

Annually for life in any woman with risk factors

Annually for life in any woman with a personal history of cervical cancer and/or HIV disease

Screening may be stopped if a woman has had a TAH/BSO including removal of the cervix. (EXCEPTION: women undergoing a TAH/BSO for the treatment of cervical cancer

HPV, human papilloma virus; HIV, human immunodeficiency virus; TAH/BSO, total abdominal hysterectomy plus bilateral salpingo-oophorectomy.

SCREENING AND PREVENTION

Prevention is aimed at avoiding risk factors (e.g., delay onset of coitarche, minimizing number of sexual partners, avoid smoking, etc.). Mass population screening with pap smears is effective at reducing the mortality from cervical cancer worldwide. The American Cancer Society Guidelines for cervical cancer screening and frequency of Papanicolaou (PAP) tests is listed in Table 102.7.

CLINICAL PRESENTATION AND DIAGNOSIS

SIGNS AND SYMPTOMS

Patients with preinvasive disease are often completely asymptomatic and the disease is only detected with routine screening by a PAP test. Frequently, the first manifestation of early invasive disease is abnormal vaginal bleeding (e.g., postcoital bleeding, intermenstrual bleeding). As the lesion progresses, the vaginal discharge becomes more pronounced and can be a serosanguinous or yellowish vaginal discharge that is frequently foul-smelling. Other symptoms of advanced disease may include anemia, weight loss, fatigue, lumbosacral or gluteal pain, and lower extremity swelling. Advanced stage cervical cancer may present with urinary or rectal symptoms, including uremia progressing to coma. These symptoms are caused by tumor that extends into the vagina, paracervical tissues, bladder, rectum, or lymph nodes.

DIAGNOSIS AND STAGING

If abnormal findings are discovered on the PAP smear, a procedure known as colposcopy should be performed to identify abnormal areas that warrant biopsy and to determine the extent of the lesion. The colposcope is a low-power magnification device that allows visualization of mucosal abnormalities. All visible or suspicious lesions should be biopsied deeply enough to assess for invasion.

Patients with a biopsy positive for invasive cervical cancer should undergo one or more of the following tests to complete a clinical staging workup: a careful physical examination, including bimanual and rectovaginal examinations (may require examination under anesthesia), CBC, SMA-12, chest x-ray, and an intravenous pyelogram.[72] A CT or MRI may be used but only if the presence or absence of hydronephrosis or hydroureter affects stage. A cystosigmoidoscopy or proctoscopy to look for disease extension into the rectum or the bladder may be required for locally advanced disease. An exam under anesthesia (EUA), positron emission tomography (PET) scan, or lymphangiogram are considered optional. All these tests are completed to determine the extent of disease. Decisions regarding further therapy are based on the clinical stage. Cervical cancer is staged clinically according to the criteria outlined by FIGO (Table 102.8).

TREATMENT

GENERAL PRINCIPLES

The goal of primary treatment is to cure the patient. This is an achievable goal for early stage disease. It is also possible to cure patients that present with advanced stage disease, although it is less likely. Treatment is based on the clinical stage and individual patient characteristics. Primary therapeutic modalities include surgery and radiation. The type of surgery and radiation used varies between institutions, as may the sequencing of these therapies.

In general, the treatment of early stage disease (stage I and stage IIA) focuses on surgery or radiation. In terms of survival, surgery is equivalent to radiation, but surgery is favored because it has fewer side effects. Reproductive function can be preserved and vaginal atrophy and stenosis can be avoided with a surgical approach. Primary treatment may include surgery and radiation if the surgical findings leave the patient at high risk of developing recurrent disease (e.g., positive surgical margins or positive lymph nodes).

For patients with advanced stage disease (bulky stages IIB, III, and IVA), surgery no longer plays a primary role in the primary treatment. Instead, primary treatment is focused on radiation. Types of radiation include whole pelvic radiotherapy (WPRT), intracavitary radiotherapy (ICRT) and high-dose rate radiotherapy (HDRT). Intracavitary radiation involves the placement of radiation seeds directly into the cervix (see below). Table 102.9 outlines the primary treatment for cervical cancer by stage.

TABLE 102.8	International Federation of Gynecology and Obstetrics Staging for Carcinoma of the Cervix
Stage I	Tumor confined to the uterus (extension to corpus should be disregarded)
Stage IA	Invasive carcinoma diagnosed only by microscopy
Stage IA$_1$	Tumors with stromal invasion 3 mm or less in depth taken from the base of the epithelium and 7 mm or less in horizontal spread
Stage IA$_2$	Tumors with stromal invasion more than 3 mm and not more than 5 mm with a horizontal spread 7 mm or less
Stage IB	Clinically visible lesion confined to the cervix or microscopic lesion greater than a stage IA2
Stage IB$_1$	Clinically visible lesion 4 cm or less in greatest dimension
Stage IB$_2$	Clinically visible lesion more than 4 cm in greatest dimension
Stage II	Tumor invades beyond the uterus but not to the pelvic wall or to the lower third of the vagina
Stage IIA	Tumor without parametrial invasion
Stage IIB	Tumor with parametrial invasion
Stage III	Tumor extends to the pelvic wall, involves the lower third of the vagina, or causes hydronephrosis or a nonfunctioning kidney
Stage IIIA	Tumor involves the lower third of the vagina, no extension to the pelvic wall.
Stage IIIB	Tumor extends to the pelvic wall or causes hydronephrosis or a nonfunctioning kidney
Stage IV	Tumor extension beyond the true pelvis
Stage IVA	Tumor invades the mucosa of the bladder or rectum
Stage IVB	Distant metastasis

CHEMOTHERAPY

Chemosensitization. Chemosensitization refers to the use of chemotherapy just prior to radiation to sensitize the patient to the effects of radiation. In the treatment of cervical cancer, the use of cisplatin-containing chemotherapy concurrent with radiation improves response rates and survival. Proposed mechanisms whereby cisplatin increases the effectiveness of radiation include a complementary action by working on different phases of the cell cycle, direct cell cytotoxicity, tumor cell synchronization and/or, inhibition of sublethal radiation repair.

Five large randomized trials comparing radiation to radiation plus concurrent chemotherapy demonstrate that the risk

TABLE 102.9	Summary of Primary Treatment for Cervical Cancer by Stage[67,72]	
Stage	**Surgery**	**Radiation**
IA$_1$	Cone biopsy (to preserve fertility) or extrafascial hysterectomy	ICRT
IA$_2$, IB$_1$, IIA	RAH/BSO/BLPLND	WPRT/ICRT with chemosensitization
IB$_2$	RAH/BSO/BLPLND or extrafascial hysterectomy following RT	WPRT/ICRT with chemosensitization
IIB, IIIA, IIIB		WPRT/ICRT with chemosensitization
IVA	Pelvic exenteration (if vesico- or rectovaginal fistula present)	WPRT/ICRT with chemosensitization
IVB		Radiation therapy with chemosensitization (palliative)

ICRT, cervical brachytherapy; WPRT, whole pelvic radiation therapy; RAH/BSO/BLPLND, radical abdominal hysterectomy, bilateral salpingo–oophorectomy, bilateral pelvic lymph node dissection.

of death from cervical cancer is decreased by 30% to 50% with concurrent chemoradiation (Table 102.10).[73] Based on these results, radiation therapy plus concurrent cisplatin-based chemotherapy is considered the standard of care for advanced stage cervical cancer. Adjuvant chemoradiation using a cisplatin-containing regimen is also recommended for patients with early stage disease treated with a radical hysterectomy who have surgical findings that place them at high risk of recurrence (i.e., positive lymph nodes or positive surgical margins).

The combination of chemotherapy plus radiation is more toxic than either therapy given alone. Patients being treated with chemosensitization should undergo a weekly CBC, differential, platelets and blood urea nitrogen/creatine ratio

(BUN/CR). Both radiation and cisplatin should be held for an ANC less than 1,500/mm^3, and platelets less than 100,000/mm^3. Cisplatin should be held for a serum creatinine greater than 1.5 mg per deciliter ($>$132.6 μmol/L). A dose reduction by 50% should be considered for a rapid change in serum creatinine, even if it is still reported as ''within normal limits'' [e.g., increased from 0.6 (53 μmol/L) to 1.2 mg/dL (106 μmol/L) in 1 week]. Patients that are most at risk for cisplatin-toxicity are patients that present with bulky stage IIIB disease where enlarged lymph nodes may compress the ureters and impair kidney function.

A pain assessment should also be completed intermittently after radiation begins for any patient that presents with pain. Frequently, pain intensifies when radiation is initiated

TABLE 102.10		Summary of Trials Referenced in the National Institutes of Health Consensus Statement		
Ref	**N**	**Stage**	**Control arm**	**Experimental Arm**
74	369	Bulky 1B ($>$4cm)	XRT	XRT + cisplatin 40 mg/m^2 IV once weekly for 6 weeks
75	368	IIB, III, IVA	XRT + hydroxyurea 80 mg/kg PO 2x/wk	XRT + cisplatin 50 mg/m^2 IV Days 1, 29 + 5-FU 1 g/m^2/day IV via continuous infusion Days 2–5 and 30–33.
76	526	IIB, III, IVA and IIA with poor pathologic prognostic findings	XRT + hydroxyurea 3 g/m^2 PO twice weekly	XRT + cisplatin 40 mg/m^2 IV weekly x 6; or XRT + cisplatin 50 mg/m^2 IV Days 1, 29 + 5-FU 1 g/m^2/d IV via continuous infusion days 1–4, 29–33 + hydroxyurea 2 g/m^2 PO twice weekly for 6 weeks
77	386	IIB, III, IVA, IB and IIA with poor pathologic prognostic findings	XRT (pelvic + paraaortic)	XRT + cisplatin 75 mg/m^2 IV Day 1 + 5-FU 1g/m^2/day Days 1–5 repeat every 3 weeks × 3
78	243	IA$_2$, IB, IIA, all with poor pathologic prognostic findings	XRT	XRT + cisplatin 70 mg/m^2 IV + 5-FU + g/m^2/d IV via continuous infusion days 1–4; repeat every 3 weeks × 4

XRT, pelvic radiation; IV, intravenous; PO, by mouth; 5-FU, fluorouracil.

(due to tumor swelling), then markedly decreases once the radiation becomes effective. Patients can successfully be weaned off narcotics in this setting.

Chemotherapy for Recurrent Disease. Recurrent disease is defined as reappearance of tumor more than 6 months after treatment.[67] At this point, curative therapy is unlikely. Treatment should be focused on palliation of symptoms and pain management. If feasible, treatment with radiation therapy and concurrent cisplatin-based chemotherapy is preferred. A procedure known as a pelvic exenteration, whereby a complete surgical removal of all pelvic organs (uterus, fallopian tubes, ovaries, cervix, vagina, bladder, and rectum) is followed by reconstruction, is a possibility in highly selected patients with central recurrences following radiation therapy. This offers the potential for long-term cure, although few patients qualify based on the pattern of recurrence.

Palliative chemotherapy should be considered for patients who are not candidates for radiation or surgery. Because the number of chemotherapy options is limited, patients should be encouraged to consider enrollment in clinical trials.

Table 102.11 describes single-agent chemotherapy options for recurrent cervical cancer. Response rates ranging from 10% to 20% are typically reported for single-agent chemotherapy. Median survival following recurrence is approximately 12 months. Patients whose disease recurs within a radiation field respond poorly to chemotherapy. Conversely, patients who recur outside the radiated field are more likely to respond. Treatment with any agent is continued indefinitely for as long as the patient responds and does not develop therapy-limiting toxicity.

Combination chemotherapy incorporates the most active agent (cisplatin) with newer agents to enhance response rates. Compared to single-agent therapy, combination chemotherapy improves response rates, but also increases toxicity. Only one trial has demonstrated a survival benefit for combination therapy compared to single-agent therapy in recurrent disease.[87] In the GOG-179 trial, 364 patients with primary stage IVB or recurrent or persistent cervical cancer were randomized to one of three chemotherapy regimens: (a) single-agent cisplatin 50 mg/m^2, versus (b) cisplatin 50 mg/m^2 plus topotecan 0.75 mg/m^2 IV (Day 1–3) or (3) methotrexate, vinblastine, doxorubicin, and cisplatin (MVAC). All cycles were repeated every 21 days for six cycles. The MVAC arm was closed early due to excessive toxicity at an interim analysis. The progression-free survival and overall survival were significantly improved in the patients treated with cisplatin plus topotecan compared to cisplatin alone (19% vs. 14% and 19% vs. 11%, respectively). The regimen was well tolerated. Therefore, cisplatin plus topotecan should be considered as the most active regimen for the treatment of primary advanced or recurrent cervical cancer. Table 102.12 details combination chemotherapy used in the treatment of recurrent cervical cancer.

SURGERY

Surgery is the therapy of choice in early invasive cervical cancer. Patients with stage 1A$_1$ tumors have a low risk of

TABLE 102.11	Single-agent Chemotherapy for Recurrent Cervical Cancer			
Agent	**Dose**	**Response**	**Comments**	
Paclitaxel[79]	135 mg/m^2 IV over 3 or 24 hr	17%	Minimal bone marrow toxicity with 3-hr treatment; tolerated well by patients pretreated with pelvic XRT	
Cisplatin[80]	50–100 mg/m^2 IV every 21 days	20%–30%	Most active single agent. No advantage for higher doses, just more toxicity. N/V decreased with slower infusion rates	
Carboplatin[81]	400 mg/m^2 (or AUC = 5–7.5) IV every 28 days	15%	Not as active as cisplatin	
Vinorelbine[82,83]	30 mg/m^2 IV weekly	12%–18%	Patients with prior radiation require dose reduction. 40%–60% of patients require dose reduction without a break; suggest 30 mg/m^2 Days 1, 8 repeat every 21 days. More active in squamous cell cancers; activity limited in nonsquamous histologies.	
Topotecan[84,85]	1.5 mg/m^2/day x 5 days; repeat every 21–28 days	18%	68% of patients experience grade 4 neutropenia at these doses. Patients with prior pelvic XRT require empiric dose reduction; patients with impaired renal function require dose reduction	
Docetaxel[86]	100 mg/m^2 IV every 21 days	30%	Dose response not proven. Doses of 75 mg/m^2 cause less hematologic toxicity	

TABLE 102.12	Combination Chemotherapy for Recurrent Cervical Cancer	
Agents	**Doses**	**Response**
Cisplatin plus Topotecan[87,88]	Cisplatin 50 mg/m^2 IV day 1; Topotecan 0.75 mg/m^2 IV days 1–3; repeat every 21 days	31%
Cisplatin plus Paclitaxel[89]	Paclitaxel 135 mg/m^2 IV over 24 hr day 1; cisplatin 50 mg/m^2 IV day 2; repeat every 21 days	46%
Cisplatin plus Vinorelbine[90]	Cisplatin 50 mg/m^2 IV day 1; Vinorelbine 30 mg/m^2 IV days 1, 8; repeat every 21 days	64%
Cisplatin plus Gemcitabine[91]	Cisplatin 50 mg/mg^2 IV day 1; Gemcitabine 1250 mg/m^2 IV days 1, 8; repeat every 21 days	41%

IV, intravenously.

lymph node metastases and a recurrence rate of only 4.2%. A total abdominal hysterectomy without lymph node resection is recommended for these patients with what is now called microinvasive carcinoma of the cervix. Patients with stage IA$_2$, IB$_1$, or IIA disease have a higher incidence of lymph node metastases, and a radical hysterectomy with pelvic lymph node dissection is recommended.[92] A 5-year survival rate of more than 90% in stage IA disease and 80% to 90% in stage IB or IIA disease can be achieved after surgery or radiation alone. Survival drops to approximately 45% for patients with stage IB or IIA disease who have pelvic lymph node involvement. The reader is referred elsewhere for a detailed discussion regarding surgical or radiotherapy options.[67,72]

RADIATION

Radiation therapy is appropriate in the management of all stages of cervical cancer. External beam radiation therapy can be administered in combination with cisplatin as primary therapy for advanced stage disease or patients with early stage disease who are medically inoperable. Radiation plus cisplatin may also be administered following surgery in patients with lymphovascular space invasion or positive lymph nodes.

Intracavity radiation, or brachytherapy, can be used to treat stage IA disease, or in combination with external beam radiation. Brachytherapy involves the administration of radiation directly into the cervix and paracervical tissues. Applicators are placed surgically into the vagina and then loaded with radioactive cesium or iridium. These applications may be repeated more than once. The use of brachytherapy and the doses of radiation used vary widely between institutions.

MONITORING AND FOLLOW-UP

Following primary therapy, a patient should undergo a history, physical, and PAP test every 3 months for 1 year, then every 6 months for 3 years, then annually thereafter.[72] A chest x-ray should be obtained annually to screen for recurrent pulmonary disease. Other optional monitoring tests include a CBC, BUN/Cr every 6 months and a CT or other imaging study for patients with advanced disease.

PROGNOSIS WITH TREATMENT

The prognosis and 5-year survival for cervical cancer decrease with increased stage. For example, in patients who undergo treatment, the 5-year survival for stage I disease is approximately 85%. Conversely, the 5-year survival for patients undergoing treatment of stage IV disease is 11%. Other prognostic factors include tumor size, depth of invasion, vascular space invasion, and lymph node involvement.[93]

ENDOMETRIAL CANCER

DEFINITION

Endometrial carcinoma, also known as uterine cancer, refers to cancer that arises from the endometrium. Although there are several histologic subtypes, this section will only cover the diagnosis and management of adenocarcinomas, the most common histologic type of endometrial cancer. The diagnosis and management of uterine sarcomas will not be addressed.

EPIDEMIOLOGY

Endometrial cancer is the most common gynecologic cancer and the fourth most common cancer occurring in women in the United States. It is estimated that approximately 40,100 new cases and 8,100 deaths occurred in 2004.[2] Seventy-five percent of women with uterine cancer are postmenopausal and the median age of diagnosis is 63 years. The incidence is age-dependent (e.g., 12 cases per 100,000 women at 40 years of age and 84 cases per 100,000 women at 60 years of age). Endometrial cancer is more common in North America. Whites are almost twice as likely to develop uterine cancer as blacks, however, the mortality rate for blacks is higher than whites.[2,94,95]

ETIOLOGY

The endometrium is a complex tissue that is responsive to endogenous and exogenous hormone fluctuations. Estrogen is a growth-stimulating hormone to the endometrium. Estrogen can cause proliferation of endometrial tissue (hyperplasia). Conversely, progesterone blocks estrogen-mediated growth and may cause a hyperplastic endometrium to revert to a secretory endometrium. The "Classic Pathway" proposes that endometrial cancer arises from a precursor lesion (atypical endometrial hyperplasia) in an estrogen-rich environment. This is thought to be the most common pathway for carcinogenesis. Body weight and high-estrogen risk factors contribute to this pathogenesis. Estrogen-dependant malignancies are often well differentiated and associated with a low nuclear grade.

The "Alternative Pathway" is proposed to be the etiology for the development of serous tumors of the endometrium. This pathway is less common, not dependent on estrogen, and is not linked to body weight or fat intake. Malignancies that are not related to estrogen overstimulation are usually poorly differentiated and associated with a high nuclear grade.[94,96]

RISK FACTORS

Factors associated with an increased risk of endometrial cancer are related to excessive or unopposed estrogenic stimulation of the endometrium and include: nulliparity, early menarche, late menopause, and anovulatory or oligoovulatory syndromes (polycystic ovary disease, estrogen-secreting granulosa cell tumors).[94,96] Obesity predisposes a woman to endometrial cancer by increasing the production of estrogen from peripheral adipose tissue. Compared to women with normal body weight, women 9 to 22 kg above ideal body weight are three times as likely to develop uterine cancer. Women greater than 22 kg above ideal body weight have a ninefold greater risk for developing uterine cancer. Other risk factors include use of unopposed estrogen and tamoxifen. In two large trials comparing tamoxifen to placebo in women with breast cancer, the use of tamoxifen was associated with a three-fold to four-fold increase in the incidence of uterine cancer compared to placebo.[97,98]

Prolonged use of oral contraceptives decreases the risk of endometrial cancer. Use of the OCP for at least 12 months reduces the risk of uterine cancer by 40%. This protection persists for several years after use.[99]

PATHOPHYSIOLOGY

Endometrial cancer arises in the glandular component of the uterine lining. It progresses from an abnormal proliferation of endometrial cells known as endometrial hyperplasia. Endometrial hyperplasia is classified as simple, complex, and/or atypical. Complex atypical hyperplasia (CAH) is most likely a precursor lesion for endometrial cancer. The risk of hyperplasia progressing to cancer increases from 1% for simple hyperplasia without atypia to 29% for CAH.[96]

Endometrial carcinomas are usually friable with focal areas of ulceration or hemorrhage. Local extension accounts for disease in the ovary, vagina, or cervix. Invasion into the myometrium can also occur, resulting in spread to adjacent tissues such as the bladder or fallopian tubes. Because of the rich lymphatic network of the uterus, nodal metastases can occur in the pelvic, paraaortic, and superficial inguinal nodes. Hematogenous spread is uncommon, and sites of distant metastasis can include lung, liver, bone, and the brain.[96]

HISTOLOGY

The most common endometrial cancer cell type is adenocarcinoma, which accounts for approximately 75% to 80% of all cases. Major subtypes include papillary, secretory, ciliated, and adenocarcinoma with squamous differentiation. Less common and more aggressive cell types include papillary serous, mucinous, clear cell, squamous cell, mixed, and undifferentiated.

Tumors are graded based on their degree of nuclear differentiation. Grade 1 lesions are well differentiated and associated with a better prognosis. Grade 3 lesions are poorly differentiated and associated with a poorer prognosis.

SCREENING AND PREVENTION

There is no effective noninvasive screening test to identify precursor lesions. There are no specific tumor markers and PAP smears are not reliable as a screening tool for endometrial cancer. Thus, recommendations for screening in healthy women include an annual pelvic examination only. The use of transvaginal ultrasound or endometrial sampling is only recommended in women that experience abnormal bleeding. Routine screening with endometrial biopsies are not recommended for women on tamoxifen, either. In a retrospective review of tamoxifen users and nonusers who underwent screening endometrial sampling, only women with simultaneous vaginal bleeding developed uterine cancer.[100] Therefore, the American College of Obstetricians and Gynecologists recommends that women on tamoxifen should undergo endometrial sampling only if they become symptomatic (i.e., develop abnormal bleeding).[101]

Performing a hysterectomy in women with CAH will effectively prevent the development of endometrial cancer.

Alternatively, women with CAH may undergo a progesterone challenge. The use of progesterone may counteract the hyperplasia caused by estrogenic overstimulation and effectively prevent the progression to endometrial carcinoma.

CLINICAL PRESENTATION AND DIAGNOSIS

SIGNS AND SYMPTOMS

Postmenopausal bleeding is the most common clinical feature. Abnormal vaginal bleeding is the initial symptom in 90% of patients. Because it is a disease of postmenopausal women, this is usually recognizable, but the diagnosis should be considered in premenopausal women with heavy or prolonged bleeding. Less than 2% of uterine cancers are diagnosed incidental to other procedures or findings (e.g., PAP smear showing abnormal endometrial cells). Pain can also be reported, but this usually signifies advanced disease. Occasionally, asymptomatic women with endometrial cancer have abnormalities detected by cervical cytology, but less than 50% of women have an abnormal PAP smear.[94,96]

DIAGNOSIS

Diagnosis of endometrial cancer requires pathologic analysis of an endometrial tissue sample.[102] A high suspicion for uterine cancer may occur as a result of a transvaginal ultrasound that indicates a thickened endometrium. However, this test alone is not sufficient for a diagnosis of endometrial cancer. A biopsy of the endometrium must be obtained in the office by endocervical curettage or in the operating room through formal dilatation and curettage (D & C). A complete history and physical exam with careful examination of lymph nodes, a CBC, chemistries, chest x-ray, and current PAP test should be obtained to complete the staging workup.[96,102] A CA-125 is usually only ordered preoperatively if extrauterine, clear cell, or papillary serous tumors are suspected (more likely to be elevated in stage III or IV disease, or high grade tumors).

STAGING

The staging for endometrial cancer is based on FIGO and is depicted in Table 102.13.[96,102] This staging system is defined by surgical and pathologic evaluation of removed tissue.

TREATMENT

GENERAL PRINCIPLES

The goal of initial therapy is to cure the patient. The primary treatment(s) for early stage endometrial cancer is surgery, radiation, or a combination of both. There are many variations on type and extent of radiation depending on the stage of disease (e.g., whole abdomen, pelvic, intracavitary, vagi-

TABLE 102.13	International Federation of Gynecology and Obstetrics Staging for Endometrial Carcinoma
Stage I	Tumor confined to the corpus uteri
Stage IA	Tumor limited to the endometrium
Stage IB	Tumor invades one half of the myometrium or less
Stage IC	Tumor invades more than one half of the myometrium
Stage II	Tumor invades the cervix but does not extend beyond the uterus
Stage IIA	Endocervical glandular involvement only
Stage IIB	Cervical stromal invasion
Stage III	Local or regional spread
Stage IIIA	Tumor involves the serosa or adnexa (direct extension or metastasis) or cancer cells in ascites or peritoneal washings
Stage IIIB	Vaginal involvement (direct extension or metastasis)
Stage IIIC	Metastasis to the pelvic area or paraaortic lymph nodes
Stage IV	Extension beyond the true pelvis
Stage IVA	Tumor invades the bladder or bowel mucosa
Stage IVB	Distant metastasis, including metastasis to intraabdominal lymph nodes other than paraaortic or inguinal lymph nodes

nal cuff). For a full listing and discussion of options, the reader is referred elsewhere.[96,102]

In general, chemotherapy plays a limited role in the treatment of endometrial cancer. Its use is confined to first-line treatment of advanced (stage III or IV) disease in patients whose potential for cure by radiation or surgery alone or in combination is poor, or in the setting of recurrent cancer, any stage, that has failed surgery or radiation. The number of chemotherapeutic drugs active in the treatment of endometrial cancer is limited. Hormonal therapy plays an important role in the treatment of well or moderately differentiated tumors. Hormonal therapy is used less commonly in the management of poorly differentiated cancers, or those with serous, or clear cell histologies.

EARLY STAGE DISEASE (STAGES I AND II)

The primary therapy for the treatment of early stage endometrial cancer is surgery or radiation. Surgery can include a total abdominal hysterectomy (complete removal of the uterus) plus bilateral salpingo-oophorectomy (TAH/BSO) (removal of both ovaries) or a radical abdominal hysterectomy (stage II disease). Lymph node sampling or dissection or omentectomy should be performed on patients with grade

2 to 3 lesions. Laparoscopy-assisted vaginal hysterectomy and BSO and node dissection should be performed in the context of a clinical trial. Extended surgical staging, including multiple peritoneal biopsies and omentectomy, may be beneficial for patients with high-grade lesions such as papillary serous or clear cell cancers.

Whether to initiate estrogen replacement therapy (ERT) postoperatively in women with endometrial cancer is controversial. Because these cancers are often estrogen or progesterone-receptor positive, there is significant concern if use of ERT will increase the risk of recurrent disease. A randomized phase III trial evaluating the role of estrogen-replacement therapy versus placebo in patients with stage I or stage II endometrial cancer following surgery, has recently been completed. Until results are published, therapy should be individualized and undertaken only after counseling regarding the potential risks and benefits of ERT.

Primary radiation is an option for patients who are not surgical candidates because of severe medical problems or who refuse surgery. Adjuvant radiation therapy may be used following surgery in order to reduce the risk of recurrence. The use of adjuvant therapy varies widely between institutions and by stage and grade and surgical prognostic factors. In general, patients with stage I well differentiated tumors do not require postoperative or adjuvant therapy. Patients with stage I or II disease and high-grade tumors and/or adverse risk factors require some form of postoperative radiation (type varies).

Chemotherapy is of no benefit in the adjuvant setting for patients with stage I or II disease.[103] In a randomized trial, 181 women with high-risk stage I or II endometrial cancer were treated with surgery (TAH/BSO) and postoperative radiation. Patients were then randomized to adjuvant chemotherapy with doxorubicin or no further therapy. At 5 years, there was no difference in survival between the groups.

ADVANCED STAGE DISEASE (STAGES III AND IV)

In the majority of patients with advanced stage disease, surgery is still a component of their primary therapy. Surgery still includes a TAH/BSO, but should also include an omentectomy and lymph node dissection to complete the surgical staging. The role of tumor debulking (removing all visibly accessible tumor) in the management of endometrial cancer is controversial. Almost all patients require postoperative adjuvant therapy of some type (possible exception, stage IIIA, grade 1–2 lesions). However, there is significant disagreement among experts regarding optimal postoperative adjuvant therapy. Radiation is the mainstay, but the type of radiation (external beam, vaginal cuff, whole abdomen, or brachytherapy) varies. The role of chemotherapy in the adjuvant management of endometrial cancer, with or without radiation, is also considered controversial.[102] Ongoing clinical trials are evaluating the role of chemotherapy in the adjuvant setting for patients at high risk of recurrence.

PRIMARY ADVANCED OR RECURRENT DISEASE

The following discussion pertains to patients with primary advanced disease (stage III or IV) that are considered unlikely to be cured by surgery, radiation, or both, and for all patients whose cancer recurs.

Treatment options for patients with primary advanced or recurrent endometrial cancer are limited. Therefore, all patients should be considered for enrollment in clinical trials. Radiation is useful only in patients with an isolated recurrence that has not received prior radiation. Surgery has a very limited role in the management of recurrent disease. Its use is primarily restricted to highly select patients with an isolated metastasis.

The use of endocrine therapy (progestins and tamoxifen) is the mainstay in the management of recurrent endometrial cancer. Progestins (e.g., megestrol and medroxyprogesterone acetate) and tamoxifen act as antiestrogens. Due to their tolerable side effect profile, they are the agents of choice in patients with long disease-free intervals, well differentiated, and estrogen and/or progesterone-receptor positive tumors. There is no dose response for these agents (Table 102.14). The overall response rates are approximately 25%. The median duration of remission is approximately 4 months and overall survival is 12 months.

Cisplatin, carboplatin, doxorubicin, and paclitaxel are the most active single agents in the treatment of recurrent endometrial cancer (Table 102.15). Overall response rates for all agents are approximately 25%. Therapy is initiated and then continued indefinitely until clinical complete remission

TABLE 102.14	Endocrine Therapy for Recurrent Endometrial Cancer	
Agent	**Dose**	**Comments**
Medroxyprogesterone acetate (Provera)[104–106]	Dose range = 200–1,000 mg PO every day or every week;	Most common dose is Depo–Provera 150 mg IM monthly or Provera 200 mg PO daily for 14 days; repeat monthly; may alternate with tamoxifen
Megestrol acetate (Megace)[96]	160–320 mg PO daily	Give in divided doses. Most common oral progesterone used clinically
Tamoxifen[106–108]	20–40 mg PO daily	May alternate with Provera

PO, by mouth; IM, intramuscularly.

TABLE 102.15	Single-agent Therapy for Recurrent Endometrial Cancer		
Agent	**Dose**	**Overall Response**	**Comments**
Cisplatin[109–110]	50–60 mg/m^2 IV every 21 days	25%–40%	
Carboplatin[111–112]	AUC=5; repeat every 21–28 days	25%–30%	
Doxorubicin[113]	45–60 mg/m^2 IV; repeat every 21 days	25%–35%	Initial dose should be lowered in patients who have received whole abdominal radiation
Paclitaxel[114]	135–250 mg/m^2 IV over 3 hours; repeat every 21 days	25%–35%	Higher doses cause more neurotoxicity. No evidence that higher doses improve survival. A dose of 135–175 mg/m^2 is recommended
Liposomal doxorubicin (Doxil)[115]	40–50 mg/m^2 IV every 28 days	10%	Dose reduction to 40 mg/m^2 recommended to reduce toxicity. Not active in patients treated with prior anthracyclines. Activity modestly better for first line treatment of recurrent disease

(rare), development of intolerable side effects, or disease progression. In the absence of significant side effects, therapy is continued indefinitely in responding patients (partial response or stable disease).

Combination chemotherapy has been evaluated in an attempt to improve response rates by combining two or more active agents with nonoverlapping toxicity profiles. Doxorubicin plus cisplatin (AP) has been proven to be more effective (in terms of higher response rates) than either agent alone.[116,117] Compared to single-agent therapy, AP results in higher overall response rates (45%–50%), more toxicity, and a slight survival advantage (clinical significance unknown). No advantage has been shown to adding cyclophosphamide to doxorubicin plus cisplatin (CAP).

Recently, due to its significant single-agent activity in the management of endometrial cancer, paclitaxel has been added to AP to assess additional response. In a trial known as GOG-177, 273 patients with primary stage III or IV or recurrent endometrial carcinoma were randomized to treatment with doxorubicin 60 mg/m^2 on day 1 plus cisplatin 50 mg/m^2 on day 1 versus doxorubicin 45 mg/m^2 on day 1 plus cisplatin 50 mg/m^2 on day 1 plus paclitaxel 160 mg/m^2 over 3 hours on day 2.[118] Both regimens were repeated every 21 days for 7 cycles and growth factor support with filgrastim or peg-filgrastim were used to prevent febrile neutropenia.

The results of this study demonstrated an improved response rate, improved progression-free survival, and slight improvement in overall survival favoring the AP-T arm. However, more toxicity (especially neurotoxicity) was found

with the AP-T arm. Based on this study, the GOG now considers AP-T to be the standard first-line combination chemotherapy regimen for advanced stage or recurrent endometrial cancer. A study comparing AP-T to paclitaxel plus carboplatin is currently in progress.

In summary, recurrent or advanced endometrial cancer is considered incurable. Thus, enrollment on a clinical trial should be considered for all patients with recurrent endometrial cancer. For patients who decline and are appropriate candidates, first-line treatment with progestins provides the best quality of life. Combination chemotherapy provides higher response rates and more toxicity than single-agent chemotherapy. The current recommendation for combination chemotherapy (AP-T) requires growth factor support and is toxic and more expensive. Irrespective of the regimen chosen, responses are short, and median survival is less than 2 years.

MONITORING PLAN

Patients being treated for early stage endometrial cancer should have a history and physical exam every 3 to 5 months for 2 years, then 6 to 12 months thereafter at the conclusion of their primary therapy. A CA-125 should be obtained at each visit only if it was initially elevated. A PAP smear should be obtained every 6 months for 2 years, then annually thereafter.[102]

Patients being treated for recurrent disease should be evaluated at least every two cycles of chemotherapy with a complete physical examination. Imaging studies should only be obtained if there is no disease on physical examination. The choice of agent dictates what other laboratory studies or chemistries are indicated.

PROGNOSIS

Overall, endometrial carcinoma is the most curable gynecologic cancer. However, this is due to a preponderance of stage I cancers being detected by early symptoms of vaginal bleeding. Stage-for-stage, the 5-year survival rates for uterine cancer are comparable to other gynecologic cancers. For example, the 5-year survival rates for stage I, stage II, stage III, and stage IV endometrial cancer are approximately, 85% to 95%, 75%, 50%, and 25%, respectively.[96]

There are several disease-related prognostic factors associated with a poor prognosis.[94,96] Serous and clear cell histologies are the most likely to metastasize. Five-year survival for stage I and stage II papillary serous carcinoma is 36% to 40%, respectively, and <5% for advanced stage disease. The histologic grade (or degree of differentiation) also affects prognosis. High grade or poorly differentiated tumors carry a worse prognosis than low-grade, well-differentiated tumors.

Other poor prognostic signs include myometrial invasion (>50% of myometrial invasion is associated with a high rate of spread to extrauterine tissue [metastases]), extension of disease to the cervix, vascular space invasion, positive peritoneal cytology, and pelvic and/or paraaortic lymph node involvement.

KEY POINTS

- There is no effective screening tool to date for ovarian cancer
- The most identifiable risk factors for ovarian cancer are a family history, nulliparity or low parity, and unsuppressed ovulation
- Chemotherapy is the most common form of therapy for patients with ovarian cancer, and the first-line regimen consists of a platinum-based compound and paclitaxel
- Cervical cancer can be curable if detected early by a PAP smear performed during routine pelvic examinations
- The biggest risk factor for cervical cancer is HPV, and the disease occurs most often in women who experience sexual intercourse at a younger age, have multiple sexual partners, have multiple pregnancies, or become pregnant at a younger age
- Most patients with cervical cancer are treated with surgery or radiation therapy, although, recent studies have demonstrated significant improvement in overall survival with combination chemotherapy and radiation therapy for patients with locally advanced disease
- Endometrial cancer usually is curable because of early detection due to unusual vaginal bleeding in postmenopausal women
- Major risk factors for endometrial cancer included unopposed estrogen exposure, nulliparity or low parity, early menarche, and late menopause
- Surgery is the treatment of choice for patients with endometrial cancer; chemotherapy is reserved for women with advanced disease, and responses are usually partial and short in duration
- New chemotherapeutic agents and multimodality therapy are improving the outcome for patients with advanced gynecologic cancer

ADDENDUM

Recommendations for first-line treatment of women with ovarian cancer were modified in January 2006 based on a seminal article evaluating the role of intraperitoneal cisplatin and paclitaxel in the treatment of ovarian cancer.[1] In this trial, 415 women with stage III ovarian or primary peritoneal carcinoma who underwent optimal surgical cytoreduction (residual tumor mass less than 1 cm) were randomly assigned to receive paclitaxel 135 mg/m^2 intravenously over 24 hours (day 1) followed by either cisplatin 75 mg/m^2 intravenously (day 2) or cisplatin 100 mg/m^2 IP (day 2) and paclitaxel 60 mg/m^2 IP Day 8 (IP therapy treatment group). Results of this trial demonstrate a statistically significant difference in median overall survival in the IP treatment arm (49.7 months vs. 65.6 months; $p = 0.03$). These impressive survival statistics were demonstrated despite the fact that only 42% of the 205 patients randomized to the IP arm were able to complete all six cycles of therapy. The IP arm was associated with significantly more grade 3 and grade 4 toxicities of all organ systems and patients who were unable to tolerate IP therapy were allowed to cross over to the IV treatment arm to complete therapy.

Concurrent with publication of the above trial, the NCI issued a clinical announcement on the treatment of ovarian cancer. The announcement, available on the NCI website (www.cancer.gov), summarizes the randomized trials on IP therapy for ovarian cancer and updates recommendations to offer IP therapy as first-line therapy to select women with ovarian cancer. Patients suitable for consideration of IP therapy include patients with ovarian, primary peritoneal and fallopian tube carcinomas with stage III, optimally reduced (residual disease at surgery <1.0 cm) who have not had bowel resection surgery. Patients with advanced stage IV, or suboptimal surgical resection, are not considered candidates. Other patients who may not be eligible is any woman who has a high likelihood of having intra-abdominal scarring or adhesions for other surgeries of disease processes. Collectively, these characteristics can result in inadequate drug distribution in the peritoneal cavity and greater toxicity. Patients who are not considered candidates for IP therapy should continue to be treated with six cycles of a taxane/platinum therapy. For more details on the administration, toxicity and unanswered questions about IP therapy for ovarian cancer, the reader is referred to the NCI clinical announcement.

REFERENCES FOR ADDENDUM

1. Armstrong DK, Bundy B, Wenzel L, et al. Intraperitoneal cisplatin and paclitaxel in ovarian cancer. N Engl J Med 354:34–43, 2006.

SUGGESTED READINGS

Berek JS. Epithelial ovarian cancer. In: Berek JS, Hacker NF, eds. Practical gynecologic oncology. 4th ed. Phildelphia, PA: Phildelphia, PA: Lippincott Williams & Wilkins, 2005:443–509.

Hacker NF. Cervical cancer. In: Berek JS, Hacker NF, eds. Practical gynecologic oncology. 4th ed. Phildelphia, PA: Lippincott Williams & Wilkins, 2005:337–395.

Hacker NF. Uterine cancer. In: Berek JS, Hacker NF, eds. Practical gynecologic oncology. 4th ed. Phildelphia, PA: Lippincott Williams & Wilkins. 2005:397–442.

REFERENCES

1. Ozols RF, Rubin SC, Thomas GM, et.al. Epithelial ovarian cancer. In: Hoskins WJ, Perez CA, Young RC, eds. Principles and practice of gynecologic oncology. 3rd ed. Phildelphia, PA: Lippincott Williams & Wilkins, 2000:981–1053.

2. Brinton LA, Hoover RN. Epidemiology of gynecologic cancers. In: Hoskins WJ, Perez CA, Young RC, eds. Principles and practice of gynecologic oncology. 3rd ed. Phildelphia, PA: Lippincott Williams & Wilkins, 2000:3–27. Available at: www.cancer.org. Accessed October 3, 2004.

4. Daly M, Obrams GI. Epidemiology and risk assessment for ovarian cancer. Semin Oncol 25:255–264, 1998.

5. Lucey JV, Mink PJ, Lubin JH, et al. Menopausal hormone replacement therapy and risk of ovarian cancer. JAMA 288:334–41, 2002.

6. Anderson GL, Judd HL, Kaunitz AM, et al. Effects of estrogen plus progestin on gynecologic cancers and associated diagnostic procedures. JAMA 290;1739–1748, 2003.

7. National Comprehensive Cancer Network (NCCN) Guidelines. Practice Guidelines. Ovarian Cancer.v.1.2003. Available at: www.nccn.org. Accessed November 8, 2005.

8. UK Collaborative Trial of Ovarian Cancer Screening (protocol). Gynaecology Cancer Research Unit, St Bartholomew's and the London School of Medicine and Dentistry, London, United Kingdom, 2000.

9. Gohagan JK, Prorok PC, Hayes RB, et.al. The prostate, lung, colorectal and ovarian (PLCO) cancer screening trial of the National Cancer Institute: history, organization, and status. Control Clin Trials 21 (Suppl.):251S–272S, 2000.

10. Petricoin EF, Ardekani AM, Hitt BA, et al. Use of proteomic patterns in serum to identify ovarian caner. Lancet 359:572–577, 2002.

11. Gross TP, Schlesselman JJ. The estimated effect of oral contraceptive use on the cumulative risk of epithelial ovarian cancer. Obstet Gynecol 83:419–424, 1994.

12. Franceschi S, Parazzini F, Negri E, et al. Pooled analysis of three European case–control studies of epithelial ovarian cancer III. Oral contraceptive use. Int J Cancer 49:61–65, 1991.

13. Curtin JP, Malik R, Venkatraman ES, et al. Stage IV ovarian cancer: impact of surgical debulking. Gynecol Oncol 64:9–12, 1997.

14. Bristow RE, Montz FJ, Lagasse LD, et al. Survival impact of surgical cytoreduction in stage IV epithelial ovarian cancer. Gynecol Oncol 72:278–287, 1999.

15. Pearl ML, Frandina M, Mahler L, et al. A randomized controlled trial of a regular diet as the first meal in gynecologic oncology patients undergoing intra–abdominal surgery. Obstet Gynecol 196:765–780, 2002.

16. Pearl ML, McCauley DL, Thompson J, et al. A randomized controlled trial of early oral analgesia in gynecologic oncology patients undergoing intra–abdominal surgery. Obstet Gynecol 99:704–708, 2002.

17. Young RC, Walton LA, Ellenberg SS, et al. Adjuvant therapy in stage I & stage II epithelial ovarian cancer: results of two prospective randomized trials. N Engl J Med 322:1021–1027, 1990.

18. Bolis G, Colombo N, Pecorelli S, et al. Adjuvant treatment for early epithelial ovarian cancer: results of two randomized clinical trials comparing cisplatin to no further treatment or chromic phosphate (^{32}P). Ann Oncol 6:887–893, 1995.

19. Young RC, Bell JG, Lage J, et al. A randomized phase III trial of carboplatin (AUC 7.5) and paclitaxel 175 mg/m2 Q 21 days x 3 courses versus the same regimen x 6 courses, in patients with selected stage IC and II (A,B,C) and selected IA and IB ovarian cancer [abstract]. Gynecol Oncol 88:156, 2003.

20. International Collaborative Ovarian Neoplasm Trial I: A randomized trial of adjuvant chemotherapy in women with early–stage ovarian cancer. J Natl Cancer Inst 95:125–132, 2003.

21. Trimbos JB, Vergote I, Bolis G, et al. Impact of adjuvant chemotherapy and surgical staging in early–stage ovarian carcinoma: European Organisation for Research and Treatment of Cancer–Adjuvant Chemotherapy in Ovarian Neoplasm Trial. J Natl Cancer Inst 95:113–125, 2003.

22. Ozols RF, Bundy BN, Fowler J, et al. Randomized phase III study of cisplatin/paclitaxel versus carboplatin/paclitaxel in optimal stage III epithelial ovarian cancer: A Gynecologic Oncology Group trial (GOG–158). J Clin Oncol 21:3194–3200, 2003.

23. Decker DG, Fleming TR, Malkasian GD, et al. Cyclophosphamide plus cisplatinum in combination: treatment program for stage III or IV ovarian carcinoma. Obstet Gynecol 60:481–487, 1982.

24. Omura G, Blessing JA, Ehrlich CE, et al. A randomized trial of cyclophosphamide and doxorubicin with or without cisplatin in advanced ovarian carcinoma. Cancer 57:1725–1730, 1987.

25. Bertelsen K, Jakobsen A, Stroyer I, et al. A prospective randomized comparison of 6 and 12 cycles of cyclophosphamide, Adriamycin, and cisplatin in advanced epithelial ovarian cancer: a Danish Ovarian Study Group Trial (DACOVA).Gynecol Oncol 49:30–36, 1993.

26. Howell SB, Zimm S, Markman M, et al. Long–term survival of advanced ovarian refractory ovarian carcinoma patients with small-volume disease treated with intraperitoneal chemotherapy. J Clin Oncol 5:1607–1612, 1987.

27. Meerpohl HG, Sauerbrei W, Kuhnle H, et al. Randomized study comparing carboplatin/cyclophosphamide and cisplatin/cyclophosphamide as first-line treatment in patients with stage III/IV epithelial ovarian cancer and small volume disease. Gyn Oncol 66:75–84, 1997.

28. Swenerton K, Jeffrey J, Stuart G, et al. Cisplatin-cyclophosphamide versus carboplatin-cyclophosphamide in advanced ovarian cancer: a randomized phase III study of the National Cancer Institute of Canada clinical trials group. J Clin Oncol 10:718–726, 1992.

29. Alberts DS, Green S, Hannigan EV, et al. Improved therapeutic index of carboplatin plus cyclophosphamide versus cisplatin plus cyclophosphamide: a final report by the Southwest Oncology Group of a phase III randomized trial in Stages III and IV ovarian cancer. J Clin Oncol 10:706–717, 1992.

30. McGuire WP, Hoskins WJ, Brady MF, et al. Cyclophosphamide and cisplatin compared with paclitaxel and cisplatin in patients with stage III and stage IV ovarian cancer. N Engl J Med 334:1–6, 1996.

31. Piccart MJ, Bertelsen K, James K, et al. Randomized intergroup trial of cisplatin-paclitaxel versus cisplatin-cyclophosphamide in women with advanced epithelial ovarian cancer. J Natl Cancer Inst 92:699–708, 2000.

32. DuBois A, Leuck HJ, Meier W, et al. Arbeitsgemein–chaft gynaekologische onkologie Ovarian Cancer Study Group. A randomized clinical trial of cisplatin/paclitaxel versus carboplatin/paclitaxel as first–line treatment of ovarian cancer. J Natl Cancer Inst 95:1320–1329, 2003.

33. Vasey PA, Jayson GC, Gordon A, et al. Phase III randomized trial of docetaxel–carboplatin versus paclitaxel-carboplatin as first-line chemotherapy for ovarian cancer. J Natl Cancer Inst 96:1682–1691, 2004.

34. Thigpen T. Dose-intensity in ovarian carcinoma: hold, enough? J Clin Oncol 15:1291–1292, 1997.

35. McGuire WP, Hoskins W, Brady M, et al. Assessment of dose-intensive therapy in suboptimally debulked ovarian cancer: a Gynecologic Oncology Group study. J Clin Oncol 13:1589–1599, 1995.

36. Conte P, Bruzzone M, Carnino F, et al. High-dose versus low-dose cisplatin in combination with cyclophosphamide and epidoxorubicin in suboptimal ovarian cancer: a randomized study of the Gruppo Oncologico Nord-Ovest. J Clin Oncol 13:351–356, 1996.

37. Jakobsen A, Bertelsen K, Andersen JE, et al. Dose-effect study of carboplatin in ovarian cancer: a Danish Ovarian Cancer Group Study. J Clin Oncol 15:193–198, 1997.

38. Gore M, Mainwaring P, A'Hern R, et al. Randomized trial of dose-intensity with single-agent carboplatin in patients with epithelial ovarian cancer. London Gynaecological Oncology Group. J Clin Oncol 16:2426–2434, 1998.

39. Eisenhauer EA, ten Bokkel Huinink WW, Swenerton KD, et al. European–Canadian randomized trial of paclitaxel in relapsed ovar-

ian cancer: high-dose versus low-dose and long versus short infusion. J Clin Oncol 12:2654–2666, 1994.

40. Stiff PJ, Bayer R, Kerger C, et al. High-dose chemotherapy with autologous transplantation for persistent/relapsed ovarian cancer: a multivariate analysis of survival for 100 consecutively treated patients. J Clin Oncol 15:1309–1317, 1997.

41. Legros M, Dauplat J, Fleury J. High–dose chemotherapy with hematopoietic rescue in patients with stage III to IV ovarian cancer: long-term results. J Clin Oncol 15:1302–1308, 1997.

42. Schwartz PE, Rutherford TJ, Chambers JT, et al. Neoadjuvant chemotherapy for advanced ovarian cancer: long–term survival. Gynecol Oncol 72:93–99, 1999.

43. Markman M. Phase III randomized trial of 12 months vs. 3 months of paclitaxel in patients with advanced ovarian, fallopian tube or primary peritoneal cancer who attain a clinically defined complete response (CR) following platinum/paclitaxel–based chemotherapy. Annual Meeting [abstract]. Soc Gynecol Oncol 3:479, 2002.

44. Alberts DS, Liu PY, Hannigan EV, et al. Intraperitoneal cisplatin plus intravenous cyclophosphamide versus intravenous cisplatin plus intravenous cyclophosphamide for stage III ovarian cancer. N Engl J Med 335:1950–1955, 1996.

45. Fayers PM, Rustin G, Wood R, et al. The prognostic value of serum CA 125 in patients with advanced ovarian carcinoma: an analysis of 573 patients by the Medical Research Council Working Party of Gynaecological Cancer. Int J Gynecol Cancer 3:285–292, 1993.

46. Bolis G, Scarfone G, Villa A, et al. Carboplatin alone vs carboplatin plus epidoxorubicin as second-line therapy for cisplatin or carboplatin-sensitive ovarian cancer. Gynecol Oncol 91:3–9, 2001.

47. Cantu MG, Buda A, Parma G, et al. Randomized controlled trial of single–agent paclitaxel versus cyclophosphamide, doxorubicin and cisplatin in patients with recurrent ovarian cancer who responded to first–line platinum–based regimens. J Clin Oncol 20: 1232–1237, 2002.

48. Parmar MK, Ledermann JA, Colombo N, et al. Paclitaxel plus platinum-based chemotherapy versus conventional platinum-based chemotherapy in women with relapsed ovarian cancer: the ICON4/ AGO–OVAR–2.2 trial. Lancet 361:2099–2106, 2003.

49. Havrilesky LJ, Alvarez AA, Sayer RA, et al. Weekly low-dose carboplatin and paclitaxel in the treatment of recurrent ovarian and peritoneal cancer. Gynecol Oncol 88:51–57, 2003.

50. Rose P, Fusco N, Fluellen L, et al. Second–line therapy with paclitaxel and carboplatin for recurrent disease following first–line therapy with paclitaxel and platinum in ovarian or peritoneal carcinoma. J Clin Oncol 16:1494–1497, 1998.

51. Gronlund B, Hogdall C, Hansen HH, et al. Results of reinduction therapy with paclitaxel and carboplatin in recurrent epithelial ovarian cancer. Gynecol Oncol 83:128–134, 2001.

52. Gordon AN, Fleagle JT, Guthrie D, et al. Recurrent epithelial ovarian carcinoma: a randomised phase III study of pegylated liposomal doxorubicin versus topotecan. J Clin Oncol 19:3312–3322, 2001.

53. Muggia FM, Hainsworth JD, Jeffers S, et al. Phase II study of liposomal doxorubicin in refractory ovarian cancer: antitumor activity and toxicity modification by liposomal encapsulation. J Clin Oncol 15:987–993, 1997.

54. Ten Bokkel Huinink W, Gore M, Carmichael J, et al. Topotecan versus paclitaxel for the treatment of recurrent epithelial ovarian cancer. J Clin Oncol 15:2183–2193, 1997.

55. McGuire WP, Blessing JA, Bookman MA, et al. Topotecan has substantial antitumor activity as first line salvage therapy in platinum–sensitive epithelial ovarian carcinoma: a Gynecologic Oncology Group Study. J Clin Oncol 18:1062–1067, 2000.

56. Kaye SB, Piccart M, Aapro M, et al. Phase II trials of docetaxel in advanced ovarian cancer—an updated overview. Eur J Cancer 33: 2167–2170, 1997.

57. Markman M, Webster K, Zanotti K, et al. Phase 2 trial of single-agent gemcitabine platinum-paclitaxel refractory ovarian cancer. Gynecol Oncol 90:593–596, 2003.

58. D'Agostino G, Amant F, Berteloot P, et al. Phase II study of gemcitabine in recurrent platinum- and paclitaxel-resistant ovarian cancer. Gynecol Oncol 88:266–269, 2003.

59. Nagourney RA, Brewer CA, Radecki S, et al. Phase II trial of gemcitabine plus cisplatin repeating doublet therapy in previously treated, relapsed ovarian cancer patients. Gynecol Oncol 88:35–39, 2003.

60. Rose PG, Mossbruger K, Fusco N, et al. Gemcitabine reverses cisplatin resistance: demonstration of activity in platinum and multidrug-resistant ovarian and peritoneal carcinoma. Gynecol Oncol 88: 17–21, 2003.

61. Rose PG, Blessing JA, Mayer AR, et al. Prolonged oral etoposide as second line therapy for platinum-resistant and platinum-sensitive ovarian carcinoma: A Gynecologic Oncology Group Study. J Clin Oncol 16:405–410, 1998.

62. Vergote I, Himmelmann A, Frankendal B, et al. Hexamethylmelamine as second-line therapy in platinum-resistant ovarian cancer. Gynecol Oncol 47:282–286, 1992.

63. Gershenson DM, Burke TW, Morris M, et al. A phase I study of a daily x 3 schedule of intravenous vinorelbine for refractory epithelial ovarian cancer. Gynecol Oncol 70:404–409, 1998.

64. Burger RA, DiSaia PJ, Roberts JA, et al. Phase II trial of vinorelbine in recurrent and progressive epithelial ovarian cancer. Gynecol Oncol 72:148–153, 1999.

65. Markman M, Iseminger KA, Hatch KD, et al. Tamoxifen in platinum–refractory ovarian cancer: a Gynecologic Oncology Group ancillary report. Gynecol Oncol 62:4–6, 1996.

66. Lanciano R, Reddy S. Update on the role of radiotherapy in ovarian cancer. Semin Oncol 25:361–371, 1998.

67. Stehman FB, Perez CA, Kurman RJ, et al. Uterine cervix. In: Hoskins WJ, Perez CA, Young RC, eds. Principles and practice of gynecologic oncology. 3rd ed. Phildelphia, PA: Lippincott Williams & Wilkins, 2000:841–918.

68. Melinkow J, Nouvo J, Willan AR, et al. Natural history of cervical squamous intraepithelial lesions: a meta–analysis. Obstet Gynecol 92:727–735, 1998.

69. Jemal A, Murray T, Samuels A, et al. Cancer statistics. 2003. CA Cancer J Clin 53:5–26, 2003.

70. Lombard I, Vincent–Salomon A, Validire P, et al. Human papillomavirus genotype as a major determinant of the course of cervical cancer. J Clin Oncol 16:2613–2619, 1998.

71. Benda JA. Pathology of cervical carcinoma and its prognostic implications. Semin Oncol 21:3–11, 1994.

72. NCCN Clinical Practice Guidelines in Oncology. Cervical Cancer. V.1.2003. Available at: www.nccn.org. Accessed November 8, 2005.

73. Concurrent chemoradiation for cervical cancer. Clinical Announcement. National Cancer Institute. February 1999.

74. Keys HM, Bundy BN, Stehman FB, et al. Cisplatin, radiation, and adjuvant hysterectomy compared with radiation and adjuvant hysterectomy for bulky stage IB cervical carcinoma. N Engl J Med 340: 1154–1161, 1999.

75. Whitney CW, Sause W, Bundy BN, et al. Randomized comparison of fluorouracil plus cisplatin vs. hydroxyurea as an adjunct to radiation therapy in stage IIB–IIIA carcinoma of the cervix with negative para–aortic lymph nodes: a Gynecologic Oncology Group and Southwest Oncology Group Study. J Clin Oncol 17:1339–1348, 1999.

76. Rose PG, Bundy BN, Watkins EB, et al. Concurrent cisplatin-based radiotherapy and chemotherapy for locally advanced cervical cancer. N Engl J Med 340:1144–1153, 1999.

77. Morris M, Eifel PJ, Lu J, et al. Pelvic radiation with concurrent chemotherapy compared with pelvic and para-aortic radiation for high-risk cervical cancer. N Engl J Med 340:1137–1143, 1999.

78. Peters WA, Liu PY, Barrett RJ, et al. Concurrent chemotherapy and pelvic radiation therapy compared with pelvic radiation therapy alone as adjuvant therapy after radical surgery in high-risk early-stage cancer of the cervix. J Clin Oncol 18:1606–1613, 2000.

79. McGuire WP, Blessing JA, Moore D, et al. Paclitaxel has moderate activity in squamous cervix cancer: a Gynecologic Oncology Group study. J Clin Oncol 14:792–795, 1996.

80. Bonomi P, Blessing JA, Stehman FB, et al. Randomized trial of three cisplatin dose schedules in squamous cell carcinoma of the cervix: a Gynecologic Oncology Group study. J Clin Oncol 3: 1079–1985, 1985.

81. McGuire WP, Arseneau J, Blessing JA, et al. A randomized comparative trial of carboplatin and iproplatin in advanced squamous carcinoma of the uterine cervix: a Gynecologic Oncology Group study. J Clin Oncol 7:1462–1468, 1989.

82. Morris M, Brader KR, Levenback C, et al. Phase II study of vinorelbine in advanced and recurrent squamous cell carcinoma of the cervix. J Clin Oncol 16:1094–1098, 1998.

83. Lhomme C, Vermorken JB, Mickiewicz E, et al. Phase II trial of vinorelbine in patients with advanced and/or recurrent cervical carcinoma: an EORTC Gynaecological Cancer Cooperative Group Study. Eur J Cancer 36:194–199, 2000.

84. Muderspach LI, Blessing JA, Levenback C, et al. A phase II study of topotecan in patients with squamous cell carcinoma of the cervix. Gynecol Oncol 81:213–215, 2001.

85. Bookman MA, Blessing JA, Hanjani P, et al. Topotecan in squamous cell carcinoma of the cervix: a phase II study of the Gynecologic Oncology Group. Gynecol Oncol 77:446–449, 2000.

86. Vallejo CT, Machiavelli MR, Perex JE, et al. Docetaxel as neoadjuvant chemotherapy in patients with advanced cervical carcinoma. Am J Clin Oncol 26:477–482, 2003.

87. Long HJ, Grendys EC, Benda J, et al. A randomized phase III study of cisplatin versus cisplatin plus topotecan versus MVAC in stage IVB, recurrent or persistent squamous cell carcinoma of the cervix. Presented at: Annual Meeting for the Society of Gynecologic Oncologists; March 2004; San Diego, CA.

88. Fiorica J, Grendys E, Holloway R, et al. Phase II trial of topotecan combined with cisplatin in squamous and non-squamous cervical cancer: Preliminary results (letter). Proc Am Soc Clin Oncol 18: 373a, 1999.

89. Rose PG, Blessing JA, Gershenson DM, et al. Paclitaxel and cisplatin as first–line therapy in recurrent or advanced squamous cell carcinoma of the cervix: a Gynecologic Oncology Group study. J Clin Oncol 17:2676–2680, 1999.

90. Pignata S, Silvestro G, Ferrari E, et al. Phase II study of cisplatin and vinorelbine as first-line chemotherapy in patients with carcinoma of the uterine cervix. J Clin Oncol 17:756–760, 1999.

91. Burnett AF, Roman LD, Garcia AA, et al. A phase II study of gemcitabine and cisplatin in patients with advanced, persistent, or recurrent squamous cell carcinoma of the cervix. Gynecol Oncol 76: 63–66, 2000.

92. Sevin BU, Nadji M, Averette HE, et al. Microinvasive carcinoma of the cervix. Cancer 70:2121–2128, 1992.

93. Benedet JL, Odicino F, Maisonneuve P, et al. Carcinoma of the *cervix uteri*. J Epidemiol Biostat 6:5–44, 2001.

94. Irvin WP, Rice LW, Berkowitz RS. Advances in the management of endometrial adenocarcinoma. J Reprod Med 47:173–190, 2002.

95. Brinton LA, Hoover RN. Epidemiology of gynecologic cancers. In: Hoskins WJ, Perea CA, Young RC, eds. Principles and practice of gynecologic oncology. 3rd ed. Phildelphia, PA: Lippincott Williams & Wilkins, 2000:3–27.

96. Barakat RR, Grigsby PW, Sabbatini P, et al. Corpus: epithelial tumors. In: Hoskins, WJ, Perez CA, Young RC, eds. Principles and practice of gynecologic oncology. 3rd ed. Phildelphia: Lippincott Williams & Wilkins, 2000:919–959.

97. Fisher B, Constantino JP, Redmond CH, et al. Endometrial cancer in tamoxifen-treated breast cancer patients: Findings from the National Surgical Adjuvant Breast and Bowel Project B-14. J Natl Cancer Inst 86:527–537, 1994.

98. Rutqvist LE, Johansson H, Signomklao T, et al. Adjuvant tamoxifen therapy for early stage breast cancer and second primary malignancies. J Natl Cancer Inst 87:645–651, 1995.

99. Cancer and Steroid Hormone Study of the Centers for Disease Control and Human Development: Combination oral contraceptive use and the risk of endometrial cancer. JAMA 257:796–800, 1987.

100. Gibson LE, Barakat RR, Venkatraman ES, et al. Endometrial pathology at dilatation and curettage in breast cancer patients: A comparison of tamoxifen users and nonusers. Cancer J Sci Am 2: 35–38, 1996.

101. American College of Obstetricians and Gynecologists Committee on Gynecologic Practice: Tamoxifen and endometrial cancer. Washington, DC. ACOG 169, 1996.

102. Uterine Cancers. National Comprehensive Cancer Center Network Practice Guidelines. V.1.2003. Available at: www.nccn.org. Accessed November 8, 2005.

103. Morrow C, Bundy B, Homesley H, et al. Doxorubicin as an adjuvant following surgery and radiation therapy in patients with high–risk endometrial carcinoma, stage I and occult stage II: a Gynecologic Oncology Group study. Gynecol Oncol 36:166–171, 1990.

104. Podratz KC, O'Brien PC, Malkasian GD Jr, et al. Effects of progestational agents in the treatment of endometrial carcinoma. Obstet Gynecol 66:106–110, 1985.

105. Thigpen JT, Blessing J, DiSaia P. Oral medroxyprogesterone acetate in advanced or recurrent endometrial carcinoma: results of therapy and correlation with estrogen and progesterone levels. The gynecologic oncology experience. In: Baulieu EE, Slocabelli S, McGuire WL, eds. Endocrinology of malignancy. Park Ridge, NJ: Parthenon, 1986:446.

106. Whitney CW, Brunetto VL, Zaino RJ, et al. Phase II study of medroxyprogesterone acetate plus tamoxifen in advanced endometrial carcinoma: a Gynecologic Oncology Group study. Gynecol Oncol 92:4–9, 2004.

107. Bonte J, Ide P, Billiet G, et al. Tamoxifen as a possible chemotherapeutic agent in endometrial adenocarcinoma. Gynecol Oncol 11: 140–161, 1981.

108. Slavik M, Petty WM, Blessing JA, et al. Phase II clinical study of tamoxifen in advanced endometrial adenocarcinoma: a Gynecologic Oncology Group study. Cancer Treat Rep 68:809–811, 1984.

109. Deppe G, Cohen CJ, Bruckner HW. Treatment of advanced endometrial adenocarcinoma with cisplatin after intensive prior therapy. Gynecol Oncol 10:51–54, 1980.

110. Seski JC, Edwards CL, Herson J, et al. Cisplatin chemotherapy for disseminated endometrial cancer. Obstetric Gynecol 59:225–228, 1982.

111. Burke TW, Munkarah A, Kavanagh JJ, et al. Treatment of advanced or recurrent endometrial carcinoma with single-agent carboplatin. Gynecol Oncol 51:397–400, 1993.

112. Green JB III, Green S, Alberts DS, et al. Carboplatin therapy in advanced endometrial cancer. Obstet Gynecol 75:696–700, 1990.

113. Thigpen JT, Buchsbaum HJ, Mangan C, et al. Phase II trial of Adriamycin in the treatment of recurrent endometrial carcinoma: A Gynecologic Oncology Group study. Cancer 63:21–27, 1979.

114. Ball HG, Blessing JA, Lentz SS, et al. A phase II trial of Taxol in advanced and recurrent adenocarcinoma of the endometrium: A Gynecologic Oncology Group study. Gynecol Oncol 62:278–281, 1996.

115. Muggia FM, Blessing JA, Jorosky J, et al. Phase II trial of the pegylated liposomal doxorubicin in previously treated metastatic endometrial cancer: a Gynecologic Oncology Group Study. J Clin Oncol 20:2360–2364, 2002.

116. Thigpen T, Blessing J, Homesley H, et al. Phase III trial of doxorubicin +/–cisplatin in advanced or recurrent endometrial carcinoma: A Gynecologic Oncology Group study [abstract]. Proc Am Soc Clin Oncol 12:261, 1993.

117. Burke TW, Stringer CA, Morris M, et al. Prospective treatment of advanced or recurrent endometrial carcinoma with cisplatin, doxorubicin and cyclophosphamide. Gynecol Oncol 40:264–267, 1991.

118. Fleming GF, Brunetto VL, Cella D, et al. Phase III trial of doxorubicin plus cisplatin with or without Paclitaxel plus filgrastim in advanced Endometrial carcinoma: A Gynecologic Oncology Group Study. J Clin Oncol 22:2159–2166, 2004.

Skin Cancers and Melanomas

VanAnh Trinh

The skin is the largest organ in the human body. It comprises the epidermis, dermis, and subcutaneous tissues. Skin performs many functions, including protection from the environment, synthesis of vitamin D, thermoregulation, and sensations of touch and temperature. Several different cell and tissue types make up the skin and its appendages (hair follicles and apocrine, eccrine, and sebaceous glands). These components can transform to produce many different benign and malignant tumors.[1] This chapter focuses on the most common skin neoplasms (basal cell and squamous cell carcinoma) and the most life-threatening skin cancer (cutaneous melanoma). Tumor registries divide skin cancers into two broad categories: nonmelanoma skin cancer (NMSC) and melanoma.

TREATMENT GOALS

- For the vast majority of patients with nonmelanoma skin cancer, the treatment goal is to cure the patient.
- The treatment goal for melanoma in its early stages (stages I and II) is to cure the patient.
- In stage III melanoma, the goal is to prolong survival and prevent metastasis.
- In patients with metastatic melanoma, the focus is on palliating symptoms, improving quality of life, and prolonging life.

EPIDEMIOLOGY

INCIDENCE

NMSC is the most common cancer in the United States and many other countries (e.g., Australia, New Zealand, United Kingdom). In the United States, basal cell carcinoma (BCC) and squamous cell carcinoma (SCC) are estimated to account for more than 1.3 million new cases and 2,200 deaths annually.[2] These numbers are believed to be grossly underestimated due to the fact that most cases of skin cancer are managed in a private clinic setting and are subsequently not recorded with tumor registries. Studies designed to investigate underreporting have been performed in Australia and the United Kingdom and indicate that the incidence of NMSC is significantly underestimated in these countries.[3–5]

ETIOLOGY

Ultraviolet Radiation and Skin Type. Several factors have been determined to influence the incidence of skin cancer (Table 103.1). Two major factors are ultraviolet (UV) radiation exposure and skin type. UV light is subdivided by wavelength into UV-A, UV-B, and UV-C (Fig. 103.1). This figure also depicts the depth of penetration by each type of UV light and the protective role of the ozone layer. UV-A and UV-B are considered harmful to humans, but their effects on biologic systems are still being characterized. UV-B radiation consists of short wavelengths, absorbed by the skin and responsible for sun-induced erythema, photoaging, and photocarcinogenesis. UV-A light is not absorbed by the ozone layer, and it penetrates deep into the dermal layer of the skin, producing erythema, immediate pigment darkening, delayed melanogenesis, and elastosis and other dermal connective tissue damage.

UV-B energy can be absorbed by many cellular components, including DNA, lipids, and proteins.[6] DNA absorbs strongly in the UV-B spectrum, partially governing the nature of damage produced by sunlight. UV-A radiation exerts its genotoxic effects indirectly, possibly through production of reactive oxygen species.[6] Effects of UV radiation on other cellular components, including the immune system and DNA-repair mechanisms, may also play a major role in skin

TABLE 103.1	**Risk Factors Associated with Nonmelanoma Skin Cancer**
Ultraviolet radiation	Immunosuppression
Chemicals[a]	Viruses[a]
Chronic inflammation	Genetic factors

[a] Questionable etiologic relationship with nonmelanoma skin cancer (see text).

carcinogenesis.[7] Tumor cell initiation, represented by DNA damage, may be induced by UV radiation, as well as other compounds and exposures.[1] Effects on surrounding normal cells allow for clonal expansion of the initiated cells, a process termed *tumor cell promotion*. Both initiation and promotion are required for carcinogenesis to occur. UV radiation may also act as a promoter in skin, inducing apoptosis in surrounding normal cells and allowing space for expansion of tumor cells.[1]

The amount of UV light reaching the earth's surface at any given place depends on several factors (Table 103.2). The ozone layer determines the amount of UV-B light that penetrates the atmosphere. Many theories attribute the rise in skin cancer incidence over the past two decades to the depletion of the ozone layer and the change in lifestyle seen in modern society (i.e., increased recreational sun exposure and decreased clothing requirements).[3] Geographic location, age at time of exposure, and the amount and type of UV exposure appear to play an important role in the epidemiology of skin cancer. There are numerous studies in the literature investigating this topic, most of which are retrospective reviews. Although there is consensus that UV exposure is an important factor in determining risk, there is little consensus regarding age at time of exposure and amount and type of exposure in relation to predisposition.[8,9]

Skin type influences the effects of UV radiation in humans. Skin types are divided into six types based on sunburning and suntanning history (Table 103.3).[1] Types I and II are at highest risk for skin cancers. Skin cancers are rare in African Americans, with SCCs being more prevalent than BCCs in this population.[10] There is evidence to support an increased risk of both BCC and SCC in people of older age, with freckling skin, and with blue eyes.[3] SCC and BCC are most common on sun-exposed areas of the body (e.g., head, neck, and dorsum of the hands).[1] Although older age is associated with an increased risk of NMSC, as chronic sun exposure has shifted from occupational to recreational, the incidence of skin cancer in younger patients is increasing. Increases in recreational UV radiation exposure are believed to contribute to the rising incidence of skin cancer in the United States, but decreased clothing requirements and a societal focus on tanning have also influenced the incidence of skin cancer in most countries.

Chemical Carcinogenesis. Carcinogenesis is a process generally occurring over a span of 10 to 50 years and progressing from initiation through promotion and ultimately to carcinogenesis. Basic changes in DNA configuration take place in cells during initiation (i.e., purine and pyrimidine substitutions, dimers, deletions). At this point, cells may progress to malignancy (if promoted effectively) or remain unchanged for life. Cells must be completely initiated for promotion to occur. Promoters cause reversible inflamma-

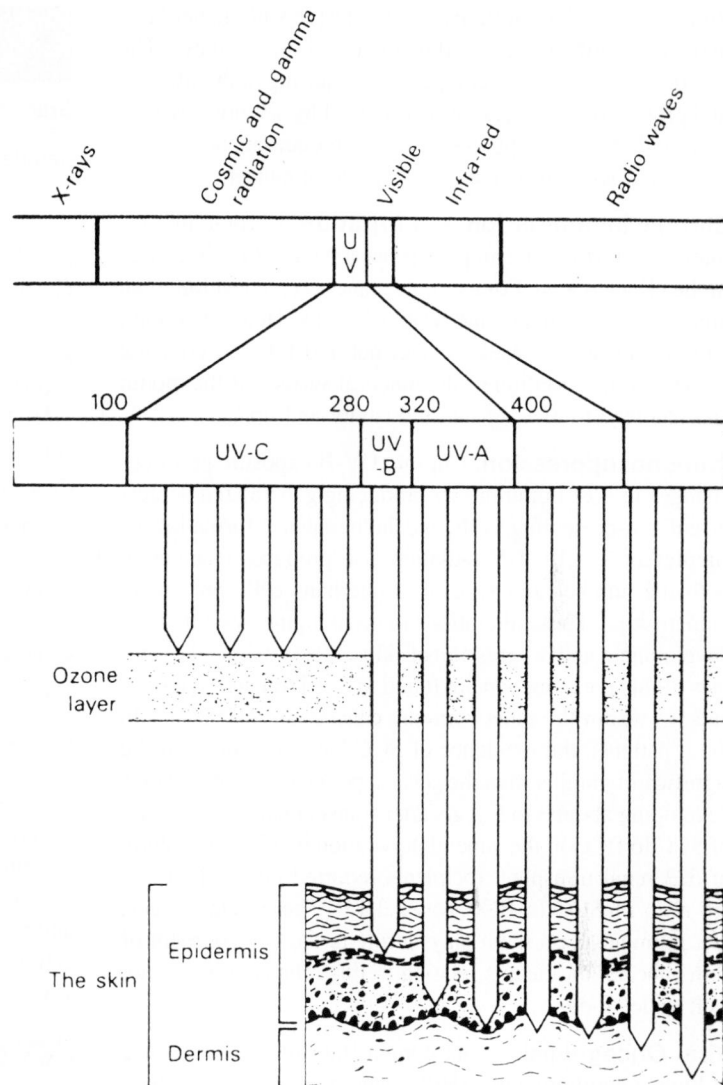

FIGURE 103.1 Solar electromagnetic spectrum showing depth of penetration of radiation into the skin. (Reprinted with permission from Emmett AJJ, O'Rourke MGE, eds. Malignant skin tumours. New York: Churchill Livingstone, 1991:24.)

tion and hyperplasia, allowing for clonal expansion of initiated cells, which leads to carcinogenesis in cells that have been completely initiated.[1] Chemical carcinogenesis was first reported in chimney sweeps of the 1700s who acquired scrotal SCC secondary to the arsenic present in the soot of chimneys.[11] Most chemical carcinogenesis data since this time have been established in laboratory animals and cannot be directly applied to humans. Several chemicals act as initi-

ators and promoters that may influence the risk of cancer. Tar, a compound containing polycyclic aromatic hydrocarbons used to treat psoriasis, acts as an initiator. Benzoyl peroxide, used to treat acne, is a known promoter. Many other agents used to treat skin disorders are initiators and

TABLE 103.2	Factors Influencing Ultraviolet Radiation Exposure
Amount of ozone	Season of the year
Latitude	Occupation
Altitude	Recreational activities
Reflective surfaces	Clothing requirements (styles)
Time of day	

TABLE 103.3	Skin Types	
Skin Type	Suntanning and Sunburning History	Skin Color
I	Always burns, never tans	White
II	Always burns, minimal tan	White
III	Burns often, tans gradually	Light brown
IV	Burns minimally, tans well	Moderate brown
V	Burns rarely, tans profusely	Dark brown
VI	Never burns, deeply pigmented	Black

promoters, but long-term use of these agents has never been associated with an increased incidence of malignancy.[1] The "two-hit" theory of carcinogenesis, requiring both initiation and promotion, is a hypothesis accepted by scientists worldwide and seems to explain why these products are not always associated with an increased incidence of cancer.

Chronic Inflammation and Irritation. Chronic inflammation and irritation can predispose a patient to skin cancer in the affected area. For example, cancers can develop in an area of chronic ulcers and scars of burns. Heavy smoking and alcohol use as well as betel nut and tobacco chewing cause chronic irritation of the mucosal surface of the mouth and can lead to SCC of the oral cavity and lip.[1]

Immunosuppression. Chronic UV-B exposure produces changes in host immunity by producing generalized defects in antigen-presenting cells and inducing the formation of suppressor T cells. UV radiation also produces changes in both the number and type of Langerhans cells present in human skin.[1] These alterations in the immune system allow development and progression of skin cancers. Clinical examples of this phenomenon are found in renal transplant recipients, in whom the most common cancers are NMSCs.[12] In these patients, the incidence of SCC has been shown to be significantly higher than the general population, with lesions developing about 3 to 5 years after transplantation. The ratio of SCC to BCC in the general population is 0.2:1. In a study of 523 renal transplant recipients reported out of Toronto, the ratio of SCC to BCC was 2.3:1.[13] These data suggest that immunosuppression plays a role in the development of skin cancers, but details relating to this relationship are not well understood.

Viral Oncogenesis. Data demonstrate that the presence of human papillomavirus (HPV) may be associated with an increased risk of cutaneous malignancies. HPV types 5, 8, 14, 16, 17, and 33 have been associated with various epidermal carcinomas and carcinoma of the cervix.[1] These viruses appear to be oncogenic, but conclusive evidence of causation is not available.

Genetic Factors. Many genetic syndromes are associated with an increased incidence of skin neoplasms. These genodermatoses are listed in Table 103.4. Patients with xeroderma pigmentosum are known to be extremely susceptible to UV radiation-induced cancers secondary to a defect in the DNA-excision repair mechanism. This supports the theory that photodamage to DNA plays a major role in UV radiation-induced carcinogenesis.[1]

The tumor suppressor gene, p53, has been shown to be mutated in 90% of SCCs of the skin and 50% of BCCs.[7] Mutations in p53 are uniformly secondary to UV radiation exposure and can lead to the development of skin cancers.[8] Recently, loss of heterozygosity at chromosome 9q22 has been identified in patients with basal cell nevus syndrome and in 30% of cases of sporadic BCCs.[8] Region 9q22 is the location of the PTCH (patched tumor suppressor gene) tumor

TABLE 103.4	Genodermatoses Associated with Cancers of the Skin
Genodermatoses	**Associated Skin Cancers**
Xeroderma pigmentosum	Basal cell and squamous cell carcinomas
	Malignant melanoma
Basal cell nevus syndrome	Basal cell carcinomas
Familial atypical mole and melanoma syndrome	Malignant melanoma
Multiple self-hearing epithelioma of Ferguson-Smith	Squamous cell carcinoma
Torre's syndrome	Sebaceous adenomas
Cowden's syndrome	Hair follicle tumors
Gardner's syndrome	Cutaneous cysts (may progress to carcinoma)
Carney's syndrome	Myxomas (benign connective tissue tumor)
Oculocutaneous albinism	Basal cell and squamous cell carcinoma
	Malignant melanoma

suppressor gene, which plays a role in regulating cell proliferation and differentiation.[8] Recently it has been found that the ras oncogene is mutated in 10% to 40% of NMSCs,[14] and many other chromosomal regions are lost in SCCs and actinic keratoses (AKs), including, but not limited to, 9q, 13q, 17p, 17q, and 3p.[7]

BASAL CELL CARCINOMA

BCC represents approximately 80% of all reported cases of NMSC in the United States.[1] BCC is generally less invasive than SCC and rarely metastasizes, with a mortality rate of 0.05%.[15] However, the morbidity from BCC may profoundly affect the lives of patients, with disfiguring lesions and scars from treatment. BCC is rare before age 20, and occurs more frequently in men than in women.[8]

CLINICAL PRESENTATION AND DIAGNOSIS

SIGNS AND SYMPTOMS
BCC arises from the basal layer of cells in the epidermis and its appendages. Malignant basal cells cannot mature into keratinocytes and retain their ability to divide beyond the basal layer, becoming a bulky neoplasm. BCC generally begins as a slow-growing, shiny, skin-colored to pink, firm, well-circumscribed, raised, dome-shaped papule. As the nodule increases in size, its center may become ulcerated,

surrounded by a pearly, rolled border. Telangiectasias are often seen on the surface of the lesion. Classification of these lesions is a complex process that lacks uniformity and clear definition. The World Health Organization (WHO) classification contains 10 variations and is based on histopathologic features. A simplified schema has been suggested by a number of authors, basing the classification of lesions on generally recognized forms of growth pattern: (a) nodular, including micronodular; (b) infiltrative, including morphea; (c) superficial, apparently multicentric; and (d) mixed, including a combination of any two or all of these types.[16] Use of this classification system allows for appropriate decisions to be made regarding prognosis and treatment. Also, it is reproducible and fairly easy to use. However, because of the lack of uniformity across studies and reports, discrepancies still exist.

Nodular BCC represents approximately 50% of all BCCs.[16] Peripheral palisading of nuclei (the arrangement of peripheral cell nuclei side by side in rows, like pickets in a fence), a phenomenon characteristic of BCC, is prominent in the nodular type and produces an effect on the surrounding stroma that is required to allow for expansion of malignant cells.[1,16] These lesions have a nodular clinical appearance and may have central necrosis with cyst or microcyst formation. The size of the nodules in the dermis may determine prognosis. Micronodular BCC (15%), consisting of small nodules less than 0.15 mm in diameter, is a subgroup that is more likely to recur.[17] The most common site of nodular BCC is the head and neck area.[1] Multiple lesions may appear simultaneously on any part of the body.[1,10] Figure 103.2 shows this type of BCC.

Infiltrative BCC represents approximately 10% to 20% of all BCCs. The important feature in its presentation appears to be the shape of the cells in the dermis. Groups of cells vary in size and have irregular spiky projections, and palisading is poorly developed or absent. Larger groups are located centrally and superficially, with smaller groups in the periphery of the dermis, where they infiltrate between collagen. In a subvariant termed *morphea* type (5%), all cell groups are small, the stroma is densely sclerotic and fibrous, and irregular islands and cords of cells infiltrate the stroma in a configuration that appears parallel to the skin surface.[15] In other classification schemes, this is often referred to as the sclerosing or morphea-type lesion.[1] They usually manifest as a yellow, sclerotic, scar-like patch with indistinct margins. These typically appear on the face and neck areas and may go undetected for a long time.[1] Morphea-type BCCs tend to be more aggressive.[8]

Superficial, apparently multifocal lesions represent approximately 15% of all BCCs.[15] They are termed this because of the small buds of cells that grow down from the dermis into the superficial dermis while remaining attached to the base of the epidermis. This often occurs over a wide area of skin and is intermittently separated by normal epidermis. Although the downgrowths appear to be separated by normal epidermis, this is in fact one lesion, with the groups of cells being interconnected at the epidermal basal layer.[16] This type of growth is often referred to as multifocal and may be more deeply invasive. Clinically, these appear as a flat, erythematous, scaly patch surrounded by a fine, thread-like pearly border.[1] These lesions most commonly occur on the trunk and, to a lesser degree, on the extremities.[16]

Mixed histology represents approximately 10% to 15% of all BCCs. Superficial and infiltrative patterns of growth often occur in combination and are seen at either the lateral or deep margins of the lesion and may increase the risk of incomplete removal.

Pigment may be present in any of these lesions and may facilitate removal of the lesion, secondary to the obvious appearance of the resected specimen margins.[18] This occurs most commonly in nodular or superficial types of lesions. Only 2% of all lesions are pigmented in the white population, but this incidence is much higher in black[19] and Japanese[20] populations.

Basosquamous cell carcinomas appear to have biologic behavior and pathologic features that represent both BCC and SCC.[1,16] Consensus is lacking regarding what constitutes this definition. If a lesion within this category exhibits a prominent squamous component, it may be more likely to recur and metastasize.

STAGING

Staging for NMSCs is based on the tumor-node-metastasis (TNM) staging system adopted by the American Joint Committee on Cancer (AJCC). Because BCC so rarely metastasizes even to local lymph nodes, size has been the most important factor for prognosis and treatment planning (Table 103.5).[21] Most BCCs manifest as T1 lesions (2 cm or less). Secondary to neglect, some lesions grow to be very large (T3, greater than 5 cm) and may invade underlying structures (T4). On entering the bone or blood circulation, BCCs metastasize. There have been approximately 300 reported cases of metastatic BCC in the world literature to date.[1]

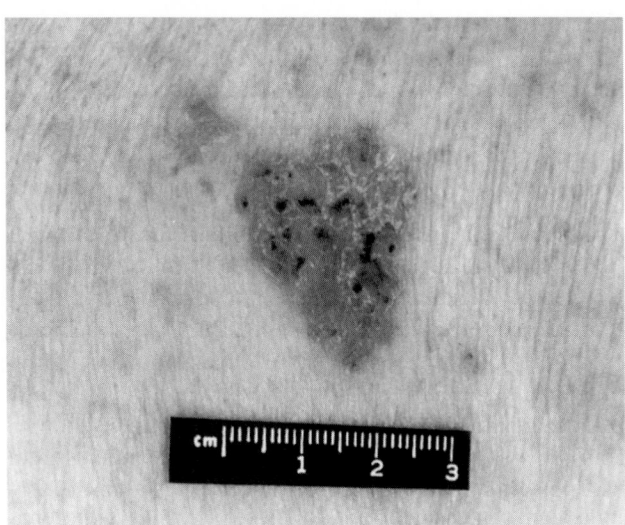

FIGURE 103.2 Nodular basal cell carcinoma.

TABLE 103.5	American Joint Committee on Cancer Staging for Basal Cell Carcinoma and Squamous Cell Carcinoma

Stage	Tumor (T)[a]	Nodes (N)[b]	Metastases (M)[c]
0	T_{is}	N0	M0
I	T1	N0	M0
II	T2	N0	M0
	T3	N0	M0
III	T4	N0	M0
	Any T	N1	M0
IV	Any T	Any N	M1

Note: If multiple simultaneous tumors are identified, the tumor with the highest T category is classified and the number of separate tumors are indicated in parentheses–for example, T2(5).
[a] T_{is} = carcinoma in situ; T1 = ≤2 cm; T2 = >2 cm and ≤5 cm; T3 = >5 cm; T4 = invades deep extradermal structures (cartilage, skeletal muscle, or bone).
[b] N0 = no regional lymph node metastases; N1 = regional lymph node metastases.
[c] M0 = no distant metastases; M1 = distant metastases.

PROGNOSIS

The incidence of recurrent lesions depends on the size and number of lesions and the length of follow-up. Large BCCs (greater than 2 cm) have a higher recurrence rate than smaller tumors. One study reported that 33% of BCC recurrences occurred within 1 year after treatment, 66% within 3 years, and 82% within 5 years.[22] Of these recurrences, 18% did not become apparent until 5 to 10 years later, emphasizing the need for long-term follow-up. Up to 70% of metastases occur in regional lymph nodes that can be surgically removed; however, distant metastases may occur in lungs, bones, liver, and other viscera.[1] The median survival of patients with distant metastases is approximately 10 to 14 months.[1] Primary tumor size and resistance of the primary tumor to surgery and radiation increase the propensity for metastasis.

The histologic type of lesion and the ability to completely resect the lesion are thought to be important factors in determining prognosis. Infiltrative and micronodular tumors are more likely to be incompletely excised.[16] Superficial, apparently multifocal tumors may be incompletely excised without demonstrating tumor cells at the surgical margins. Complete resection is key in determining the likelihood of recurrence. Incompletely excised tumors have a recurrence rate of 33% to 39%, compared with a recurrence rate of 1% for tumors that are thought to be completely excised.[23,24]

SQUAMOUS CELL CARCINOMA

SCC is the second most common skin cancer and represents approximately 20% of all reported cases.[1] SCC is more inva-

sive and has a greater propensity to metastasize than BCC. One literature review noted a weighted average metastatic rate of 2.3% or 5.2%, depending on follow-up of less than or greater than 5 years, respectively.[25] SCCs are most common in whites, with the incidence being higher in males than females.[9]

The presence of AKs is a risk factor for SCC. AKs are the most common premalignant skin lesions and have histologic similarities to SCC in situ (see the section on Pathophysiology). Untreated AKs can spontaneously remit, remain stable, or progress to SCC. Studies have estimated that up to 20% of AK lesions eventually develop into SCC.[9] There is a great deal of controversy regarding the rate of malignant transformation, and as many as 25% of lesions may spontaneously remit. However, 60% of newly diagnosed SCCs occur at the site of a previous AK.[26–28] These studies controlled for as many risk factors as possible, but the number of known risk factors makes trial design complex and difficult to analyze.

PATHOPHYSIOLOGY

SCC is a tumor of keratinizing cells, arising from stratified squamous epithelium and growing to invade the dermis. Confined to the epidermal layer, these tumors are defined as SCC in situ, referred to as Bowen's disease. Once they have invaded the dermis, they can track along tissue planes, perichondrium, or periosteum. SCC grows more rapidly than BCC but has similar invasive characteristics, causing tissue destruction. In contrast to BCC, SCC has a much greater potential for regional and distant metastasis.[1]

CLINICAL PRESENTATION AND DIAGNOSIS

SIGNS AND SYMPTOMS

SCC appears as a flesh-colored or erythematous raised, firm papule.[9] It may be crusted with keratin products and may ulcerate and bleed in later stages. SCCs in the area of an AK have somewhat different characteristics from those that appear on normal skin (de novo SCC). With an SCC that arises from an AK, the lesion appears as a plaque or a nodule with a warty scale covering. These lesions bleed easily with minor trauma and may have telangiectasias on their surface.[1] De novo SCC may have a slightly raised, indurated border (Fig. 103.3). Invasion can occur and manifests as a firm, erythematous nodule with a center core that may be ulcerated. The surface may be smooth or warty and papillomatous and may contain telangiectasias.[1] Infiltrative lesions are often attached to underlying tissues and cartilage; this is a sign of aggressive tumor growth. SCC occurs most commonly on the head and neck, followed by the upper extremities and trunk.[9] SCC may also occur on mucous membranes.

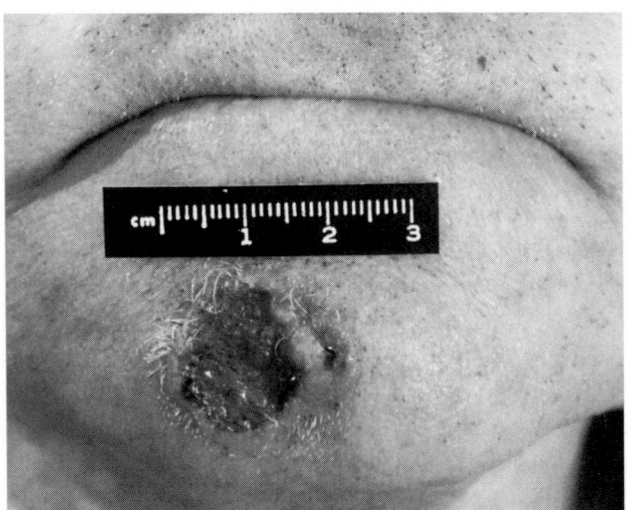

FIGURE 103.3 De novo squamous cell carcinoma (arising from normal tissue).

These lesions may appear in the oral cavity and lip, can invade other structures of the face, and are more likely to metastasize.

STAGING

The AJCC has identified the TNM staging system as the system to be used for all skin cancers (Table 103.5).[21] For SCC this is inadequate because of the lack of inclusion of key prognostic variables. The TNM system takes into account the diameter and depth of invasion, as well as the involvement of cartilage, muscle, or bone, but fails to consider anatomic site, etiology, and host immunosuppression, among other prognostic factors.

PROGNOSIS

The frequency of metastasis depends on anatomic site, histologic features, etiology, host immunosuppression, diameter, depth of invasion, neurotropism (the quality of having a special affinity for nervous tissue), and prior treatment. Some factors have more prognostic significance than others. Mucosal SCC is more aggressive than cutaneous SCC and metastasizes more frequently.[29] SCC of the lip has a worse prognosis than cutaneous SCC but a better prognosis than SCC of the penis, scrotum, or anus.[29] Histologic features that determine levels of differentiation have been shown to be of prognostic significance. Tumors with a greater percentage of well-differentiated cells have a better prognosis than those with a greater percentage of poorly differentiated cells.[9,29]

The etiology of SCC also determines prognosis. Lesions that occur secondary to immunosuppressive disorders are more likely to metastasize than lesions appearing secondary to UV light exposure.[9] SCCs that arise from chronic lesions, such as scars or ulcers, are associated with higher rates of metastasis than lesions found on normal skin.[9]

Generally, larger and deeper primary lesions are more likely to metastasize. According to some reports, lesions greater than 2 cm in diameter make up the majority of metastatic cases, and lesions larger than 1 cm in diameter make up the majority of recurring SCCs.[29] A report based on the size and depth of invasion found a risk of metastasis of 1.4% with T1 lesions, 9.2% with T2 lesions, and greater than 13% with T3 or T4 lesions.[30] In this study, SCCs with a depth of less than 2 mm never metastasized. Those with a depth between 2 and 6 mm had a metastatic rate of 4.5%, and those with a depth greater than 6 mm had a 15% metastatic rate.[30]

Depth of skin cancers can also be classified by level of anatomic invasion. Clark's levels (I through V), which were initially developed for cutaneous melanomas, have been used to study SCC (see discussion of Clark's levels in melanoma section).[29] Penetration to Clark's level IV (the reticular dermis) has been associated with a greater potential for metastasis.

Perichondrial, periosteal, and perineural invasion correlates with poor prognoses.[29] Lesions exhibiting perineural invasion typically have higher recurrence rates. However, with the acceptance of Mohs' surgery (see discussion of Mohs' surgery later in this chapter), this rate has decreased significantly but is still higher than lesions lacking this characteristic.[31] Recurrent lesions are historically more difficult to treat than primary lesions, showing the importance of aggressive first-line treatment when the opportunity for cure is optimal. Metastases most commonly occur to the parotid lymph nodes from primary lesions on the temple or ear.[31] If treated aggressively and early, multimodality therapy including surgery, chemotherapy, or radiation therapy can produce cure rates of more than 50%.[31] If the nodal metastases measure less than 3 cm or are confined to the superficial parotid nodes, cure rates can reach 85% to 95%.[31] The 5-year disease-free survival (DFS) figures for SCC are listed in Table 103.6.

TREATMENT OF NONMELANOMA SKIN CANCERS

Once the diagnosis of NMSC is confirmed with a biopsy, the treatment planning begins. Planning requires consideration of the type of skin cancer; anatomic location; size; general health and age of the patient; and whether the lesion is primary, recurrent, or metastatic. SCCs require that a wide margin be removed or treated because of their aggressive nature.[1,31] Smaller BCC lesions can be treated with curettage and electrodesiccation (defined below).[1] The anatomic location of the lesion also influences the rate of recurrence. Lesions located along the embryonal fusion planes (the midface under the eyes; periauricular and postauricular areas; the paranasal, nasolabial, and inner canthal areas) have the potential for deep invasion and higher recurrence rates.[1] Cos-

TABLE 103.6	Management of Nonmelanoma Skin Cancer

Method	Indications	5-Year Disease-Free Survival	Comments
Curettage and electrodesiccation	Nodular BCC Anatomic areas with low recurrence rates	77%–97% (BCC)	Skilled, experienced practitioners' cure rates are 95%–97%
Cryotherapy	Best for nodular and recurrent BCC Best anatomic locations are eyelid, nose, ear, chest, back, or tip of the nose	95%–99% (BCC) 90% (AK)	Lack specimen for pathologic review to check margins. Best results with very small tumors (<0.5 cm).
Surgical excision	Best for aggressive or large lesions Wider margins required for SCC, morphea-type, and recurrent BCC	96% (all nonmelanoma skin cancers)	Skin grafts may be required for wound closure.
Mohs' micrographic surgery	Lesions that do not have well-defined border Recurrent or morphea-type tumors Large tumors (>2 cm) Incompletely excised tumors Tumors within radiation dermatitis Anatomic areas with high recurrence rates	98% (BCC) 96.5% (recurrent BCC) 93% (SCC)	Very complex, time-consuming procedure. Only done at a few institutions. Highest disease-free survival.
Radiation	Reserved for treatment of lesions not amenable to other treatment modalities Lesions along the embryonal fusion plane Good for lesions on eyelids, periorbital region, medial triangle of cheek, earlobe, and nose	96.4% (BCC) 91.9% (SCC)	Areas of radiation are at higher risk of developing other cutaneous malignancies.
Photodynamic therapy	Not a treatment of choice yet Investigational treatment	CR 88%–100% (Photophrin)	Persistent photosensitivity for 8–10 weeks.
Topical imiquimod	Superficial BCC	Await data from long-term follow-up	2-year clearance rate: 70%–80% Used when surgery is medically less appropriate
Chemotherapy Topical	5-FU only approved agent Treatment of choice for multiple AK Very small superficial BCC (not amenable to other treatment modalities) Older adult patients not eligible for other treatments	79% (superficial BCC)	If used after curettage, recurrence rate is decreased. Not generally used as single-modality therapy.
Systemic	Neoadjuvant combination chemotherapy has been investigated	CR 26% PR 54% (SCC skin or lip)	Not commonly used for nonmelanoma skin cancer; less effective. Used in conjunction with other treatments (e.g., radiation therapy).

AK, actinic keratosis; BCC, basal cell carcinoma; CR, complete response; PR, partial response; SCC, squamous cell carcinoma.

metic results of treatment are also considered during planning. A lesion located on the eyelids or the tip of the nose requires a tissue-sparing approach (i.e., radiation therapy or Mohs' micrographic surgery).[1] Cryotherapy (freezing of the lesion) and topical fluorouracil treatments are also effective for BCC but generally are associated with lower cure rates.[1] Mohs' micrographic surgery is generally used for BCC le-

sions that have poorly defined margins or for recurrent lesions.

The general health of the patient is key in treatment planning. Unless the disorder can be corrected before surgery, patients with coagulopathies require a less invasive procedure to decrease the risk of bleeding. If travel is a problem (e.g., older adults, debilitated patients, or those without transportation), procedures requiring one or two office visits are better than those requiring 10 to 15 office visits. The chance of infection is higher in immunosuppressed patients and should be considered if compliance and cleanliness are of concern.[1]

Treatment choices include curettage with electrodesiccation, cryotherapy, surgical excision (including Mohs' micrographic surgery), radiation therapy, topical imiquimod, and chemotherapy (topical and systemic). These options are listed in Table 103.6.

CURETTAGE AND ELECTRODESICCATION

Curettage is performed with a curet, a pencil-like instrument with a round or oval tip, sharpened on one side. The tumor is debulked down to the normal tissue, using differences in texture and sound reflection to distinguish between normal tissue and tumor. The tumor is removed with a 2- to 3-mm margin of normal tissue. Electrodesiccation may follow curettage, destroying any tumor cells remaining at the base and periphery of the excision site and producing hemostasis. This procedure uses an electrical current to produce sufficient heat, causing tissue damage at the point of contact. Increasing the amperage (current) causes more heat, deeper penetration, and more tissue damage and scarring.[1]

The overall DFS rate with this procedure is 77% to 97%.[1] The rate of recurrence depends on patient selection and the practitioner's skill in performing the procedure. Skilled, experienced practitioners produce DFS rates as high as 95% to 97%; less experienced dermatology residents have higher recurrence rates.[1] Lesions with more aggressive histology, larger size, longer history, or locations in high-risk anatomic areas are not candidates for this procedure as primary treatment. Use of this procedure is reserved for minimally invasive BCCs and SCC in situ lesions. The disadvantage to this procedure is the lack of margin control. Many clinicians believe that the cure rates published in the literature (as high as 99%) are actually much lower, due to careful patient selection and a high degree of skilled practitioners used in the published studies.[31]

CRYOTHERAPY

Cryotherapy uses liquid nitrogen ($-195.5°C$) to freeze viable tissue. Freezing causes the formation of extracellular and intracellular ice, abnormal concentration and crystallization of electrolytes, and denaturation of lipoprotein complexes that are lethal to the cells.[1] A 3- to 5-mm margin is required to maximize cure rates.[1] The temperature of the tissue is measured with a thermocoupler inserted underneath the tumor. A temperature sufficient for cell death is at least $-50°C$.[1] The tissue is allowed to thaw, and then the procedure is repeated for best results.[1]

This technique is best suited for patients who have pacemakers or are poor surgical candidates. Cryotherapy is most effective for lesions that are less than 2 cm and are located on the eyelid, nose, ear, chest, back, or tip of the nose.[1] This is the recommended procedure for recurrent BCCs and tumors with well-defined margins.[1,31] Studies with cryotherapy of SCC are limited, and cryotherapy is not routinely used for invasive lesions of this type.[31] Cryotherapy is contraindicated in morphea-type BCCs, patients with cold intolerance (e.g., cryoglobulinemia, Raynaud's disease), lesions in certain anatomic locations (free margin of eyelid, vermilion border of the lip, ala nasi, anterior and posterior ear, or scalp), or tumors larger than 3 cm.[1] The adverse reactions related to cryotherapy include edema, oozing, erosions, hemorrhaging, and secondary infections. Re-epithelialization may take as long as 10 weeks.[32] The cosmetic results obtained with cryotherapy are very good, with the exception of hypopigmentation and hyperpigmentation. Hyperpigmentation usually fades within a few months after the procedure.[1]

The DFS rates achieved with cryotherapy are very high. One study reported a 99% 5-year DFS rate using cryotherapy in extremely small BCCs (most tumors were 0.5 cm or smaller).[33] Most studies report a recurrence rate of less than 5% when skilled, experienced practitioners perform the procedure.[31] One disadvantage is the lack of pathologic evidence of tumor-free margins. The margins are determined by sight only. Tumor cells could be left behind, predisposing the patient to recurrence; therefore, only very superficial lesions should be treated with this technique.[1,10,29] The use of cryotherapy for AKs is effective in patients with few individual lesions and has a very low recurrence rate (10%), but it is not recommended for those with multiple AKs.[34]

SURGERY

Surgical excisions use a scalpel to make an elliptical incision, removing the entire tumor with a 3- to 5-mm margin for BCC and a margin of 4 to 6 mm for SCC.[1,31] The optimal tumor-free margin required for SCC has not been determined, but it is well accepted that wider margins than for BCCs are needed. For recurrent or morphea-type BCC, a wide margin is required (e.g., 1 cm).[1] Large tumors with deep invasion also require wider surgical margins. Regional lymph node dissection is required only when lymph nodes are clinically palpable. Skin grafts are occasionally required for wound closure. These grafts take 5 to 7 days to be accepted and 2 to 3 months to become mature and cosmetically acceptable.[1] A skin flap is a piece of tissue that is attached on one side to the donor area and carries its own blood supply, and is an option for wound closure.[1] The decision to perform a surgical excision is made after evaluating all other treatment options. DFS rates with surgery alone for NMSC have been reported to be 96%.[10,29] Surgical excisions are contraindicated in patients with coagulation disorders, unless they can be corrected before surgery.

MOHS' MICROGRAPHIC SURGERY

Frederick Mohs first described this technique for tumor removal in 1930.[1,32] The procedure is depicted in Figure 103.4. A scalpel is used to make a saucer-shaped excision with a 45-degree angle to provide a specimen with a beveled edge. A map is drawn to correspond to the specimen removed. The specimen is then divided, numbered, and color-coded on the edges. Corresponding numbers and color codes are marked on the map. Serial frozen sections are performed. The saucer shape and the angled edge allow for viewing of all surfaces. Any remaining tumor is marked on the map, and excision is repeated until the tumor is completely excised. With this procedure, minimal normal skin is sacrificed and cosmetic results are usually very good, depending on the size of the area excised and the anatomic location of the tumor. Occasionally skin grafts or flaps are required for coverage of very large lesions, but these are not needed as often as with surgical excisions.[1,31]

Mohs' micrographic surgery is indicated if the tumor recurrence rate is high (embryonal fusion planes of the midface, nasal area, or periauricular areas), if the tumor borders are not well defined, if the tumors are recurrent, in morphea-type BCC, for incompletely excised or large tumors (larger than 2 cm), and for tumors within radiation dermatitis. Infiltrative, micronodular, and multifocal BCCs are most appropriately managed with Mohs' micrographic surgery if possible.[16] Five-year DFS rates with Mohs' micrographic surgery are higher than with any other treatment modality (98% for primary BCC, 96.5% for recurrent BCC, and 93% for SCC).[35,36] This treatment approach is now recognized as the standard method of excision for primary and recurrent NMSCs.

RADIATION

BCCs and SCCs are radiosensitive tumors. Because of the lack of pathologic confirmation of clear margins and radiation-related morbidity, this method is reserved for lesions that are not amenable to other treatment modalities. Patients with tumors located on the eyelids; periorbital region; and medial triangle of the cheek, earlobe, and nose are good candidates for radiotherapy. Skin cancers along the embryonal fusion plane can be successfully treated with radiation. This method of treatment is not recommended for use in tumors located on the trunk, extremities, dorsum of the hands, or scalp or those arising in sweat and sebaceous glands. It is also not recommended for tumors greater than 8 cm in diameter, morphea-type BCC, intraoral lesions, or tumors that occur on the upper lip growing into a nostril. Radiation is a good choice for patients who are poor surgical candidates and for palliation of very large tumors in older adults.[36] DFS rates with this treatment modality are 96.4%

for BCC and 91.9% for SCC.[1] Immediate sequelae are erythema, loss of eyelashes when treating the eyelids, and mucositis when treating the nose. Long-term sequelae include radiation dermatitis, which may manifest as atrophy, telangiectasias, hyperpigmentation or hypopigmentation, and precancerous lesions.[1] Radiated areas have a higher risk for the development of other skin neoplasms.[1,32] These reasons contribute to the decision to reserve radiation for lesions not amenable to other treatment modalities.

PHOTODYNAMIC THERAPY

Photodynamic therapy (PDT) is a new technique for the treatment of superficial BCCs. This technique uses tumor-sensitizing drugs to selectively target tumor cells in the skin. A light is required to activate the drugs to produce free radical formation and tissue damage. Many agents are under investigation, including porphyrin-, chlorine-, and phthalocyanine-containing substances that produce free radicals when subjected to certain wavelengths of light. The first compound approved by the U.S. Food and Drug Administration (FDA) is a hematoporphyrin derivative (HPD, Photophrin). It is given intravenously and is preferentially taken up by tumor cells. When exposed to laser light, the drug is activated and the tumor is killed. Photophrin is approved for the treatment of esophageal cancer only. One study reported a complete response rate of 88% to 100% when treating primary and recurrent BCCs, depending on the dose received by the tumor bed and the nature of the lesion.[37] Retreatment of recurrences resulted in a 100% complete response rate. SCC lesions appear to respond to PDT, but at a lower rate than BCC, requiring higher doses to achieve acceptable results.[38] Complete response rates with skin metastases have been reported to be 74% with lesions from a variety of primary sites.[39] Patients with multiple lesions or large areas that are affected are particularly suited for PDT.[38] Generalized photosensitivity for 8 to 10 weeks after administration of this agent is a major concern.[37] Newer agents have been developed to circumvent these problems. One agent, 5-aminolevulinic acid (ALA), can be applied topically to skin cancer lesions and illuminated with different types of light sources.[38,40]

PDT is not yet the treatment of choice for any cancer, with higher recurrence rates making it inferior to other proven modalities of treatment. However, future investigations may target difficult-to-treat or recurrent lesions, as well as patients with multiple or large affected areas. Further clinical studies must be done to identify the role of photodynamic therapy in the treatment of primary and secondary skin cancers.

TOPICAL IMIQUIMOD

Imiquimod is an immune response modifier that stimulates monocytes, macrophages, and dendritic cells to produce cy-

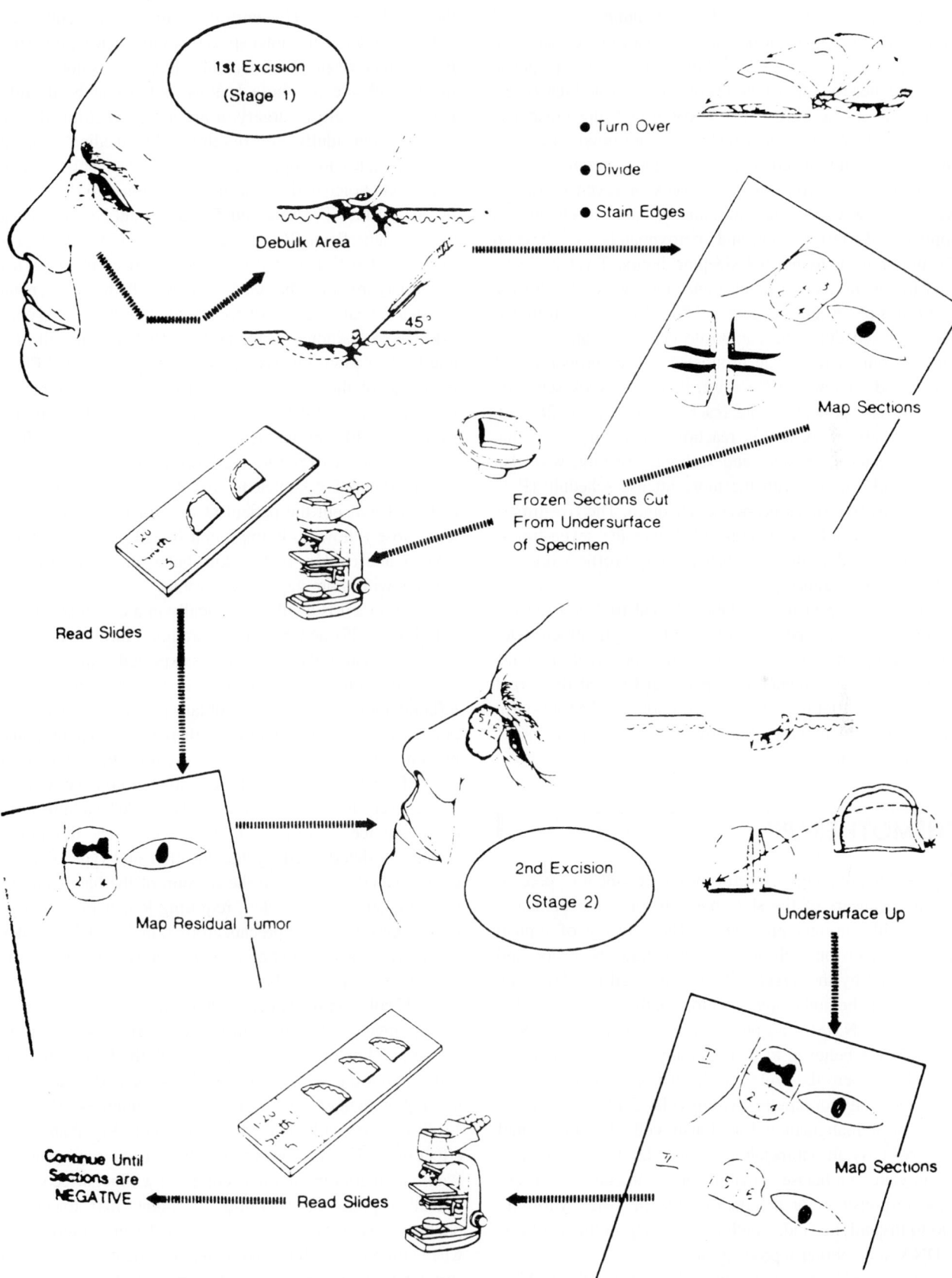

FIGURE 103.4 Techniques of Mohs' micrographic surgery. (Reprinted with permission from Safai B. Cancers of the skin. In: DeVita VT, Hellman S, Rosenberg SA, eds. Cancer: principles and practice of oncology, 4th ed. Philadelphia: Lippincott, 1993:1602.)

tokines necessary for cell-mediated immunity.[41] A topical preparation of this agent has been shown to be effective in clearing AKs and BCCs.[41,42] Among BCCs, the response rate is higher for superficial lesions than for nodular types.

In two double-blind, vehicle-controlled, dose-response clinical trials, 724 patients with biopsy-confirmed superficial BCC were randomized to receive topical imiquimod 5% cream or vehicle five times per week or seven times per week for 6 weeks.[41] The imiquimod cream or vehicle was applied to the target tumor and approximately 1 cm beyond the tumor prior to normal sleeping hours. Twelve weeks after treatment, composite clearance rates were 75% for the five-times-per-week schedule and 73% for the seven-times-per-week schedule; the composite clearance rate was 2% for the combined vehicle groups. A higher proportion of imiquimod patients on the seven-times-per-week schedule experienced application site reactions (44.1% vs. 28.1%). The intensity of local skin reactions, including erythema, edema, vesicles, erosion, and scabbing/crusting, was also significantly higher with the more intense schedule (P < 0.05 versus five-times-per-week schedule). The five-times-per-week schedule is recommended over the seven-times-per-week schedule due to a better safety profile without a reduction in clearance rates.

An ongoing 5-year open-label clinical trial is assessing the recurrence of superficial BCC following treatment with topical imiquimod 5% cream, five times per week. Patients with no clinical evidence of superficial BCC at the target site 12 weeks after treatment were eligible for the long-term study. After 24 months of follow-up, 79% of patients remained clinically clear.[43]

CHEMOTHERAPY

Topical chemotherapy is useful for the treatment of precancers and cancers of the skin, but cure rates are generally higher with surgical procedures. The efficacy of topical agents depends on their ability to penetrate the lesion and be absorbed by the target cells. Fluorouracil (5-FU) is the only topical chemotherapy agent to date that has shown efficacy against NMSC and precancerous lesions (e.g., AKs). This agent is believed to preferentially penetrate sun-damaged skin, where the protective layer is deficient. Because of its selectivity for rapidly dividing cells, 5-FU has a greater effect on premalignant and malignant cells than on normal cells. 5-FU is an antimetabolite that inhibits the action of thymidylate synthetase. Thymidylate synthetase is the enzyme responsible for the methylation of 2-deoxyuridylic acid to thymidylic acid, which is a key step in the synthesis of DNA and cellular reproduction.

Topical 5-FU is the treatment of choice for multiple AKs. It must be applied to the entire area of skin and should not be used to "spot treat" small areas of AKs.[44] A patient with AKs on the face must have the entire face treated, not just

the visible lesions. This ensures treatment of occult lesions in the affected area. Under special circumstances, superficial BCC can be treated with topical 5-FU. This is not the treatment of choice for these lesions, but it can be useful in patients who refuse surgery or are not good surgical candidates.[1] Older adults with multiple other medical problems are candidates for topical 5-FU. One disadvantage of this treatment choice is the lack of penetration into deep tissues of the dermis. The reported 5-year cumulative recurrence rate for superficial BCC treated with 5-FU topical therapy alone is 21%.[45] This can be improved if curettage is used as primary treatment before 5-FU to debulk the tumor, resulting in a 5-year cumulative recurrence rate of 6%.[45] Topical 5-FU is contraindicated for nodular BCC and for all SCCs due to their more invasive characteristics. Use of 5-FU for treatment of these lesions should be reserved for patients who are not candidates for other therapies. Optimal areas for use of 5-FU are the facial areas, the dorsum of the hand, and the lower extremities. A biopsy should be performed after treatment is complete to ensure that there are no hidden cells that will put the patient at risk for recurrence. Long-term close follow-up is important for all patients with precancers and cancers of the skin, but is most important for patients with more aggressive lesions.

Fluorouracil is available topically in a cream or solution (Efudex) in 2% and 5% concentrations. Inflammation is a clinical indicator of efficacy and is expected in the cancerous or precancerous area (not in normal skin). Mild to moderate inflammation is sufficient to obtain results. An increase in potency of the agent is required if there is insufficient inflammation at the treatment site. There are no clinical data showing a difference between these available concentrations if adequate erythema is achieved. 5-FU should be administered once or twice a day for 2 to 10 weeks.[44] The duration of therapy is determined by the location and type of lesion being treated. Lesions on the dorsum of the hands and the forearms tend to be thicker, requiring longer treatment periods. Certain types of precancerous skin disorders are more aggressive, have a higher rate of recurrence, and require longer treatment periods.

5-FU solution is applied with a soft brush and the cream with a fingertip. Using a plastic occlusive dressing can increase the time of contact of 5-FU with the lesion, theoretically increasing the response.[44] This method is useful in treating more aggressive lesions. Concomitant use of topical 13-all-*trans*-retinoic acid (tretinoin, Retin-A) enhances the effect of 5-FU.[44] Steroid cream can be used to alleviate inflammation after treatment is complete without affecting the overall response of the tumor.[44] Patients may experience photosensitivity when using 5-FU, which can be more severe when combined with tretinoin cream. Patients should be instructed to use a sunscreen and to cover with clothing when exposed to the sun to prevent severe sunburns. Contact hypersensitivity to the vehicle and the 5-FU has been reported.[44] This reaction differs from the expected erythema in that vesicles are seen in the area of contact and itching is reported. The usual manifestations associated with the expected erythema produced by 5-FU are described as burning or stinging, *not* itching.[44] Extemporaneous compounding of 5-FU with a different vehicle may prevent recurrence of this problem. 5-FU can cause severe irritation of the conjunctiva or nares if allowed to enter the eyes or nose.[46] Therefore, contact with these areas should be avoided. Patients should wash their hands carefully after applying 5-FU, with instructions not to touch the eyes or nasal membranes while the fingers are still contaminated with 5-FU.

Systemic administration of 5-FU alone or with cisplatin has not been effective in the treatment of BCC. *Neoadjuvant therapy* is defined as any treatment used before definitive local therapy in hopes of (a) determining sensitivity of the lesion to chemotherapy and (b) decreasing the size of the lesion, allowing for tissue-sparing procedures. Large SCCs (greater than 5 cm) have been treated with neoadjuvant combination chemotherapy. A study using CFB [cisplatin 100 mg/m^2 on day 1, 5-FU 650 mg/m^2/day continuous infusion for 5 days, and bleomycin 15 mg IV bolus on day 1 followed by continuous-infusion bleomycin (16 mg/m^2/day) for 5 days] showed complete response rates of 26% and partial response rates of 54% in patients with SCC of the skin or lip greater than 5 cm in diameter.[47] This strategy, when combined with surgical excision, may be useful in downstaging lesions, improving cosmetic results, and limiting the need for reconstruction.

CUTANEOUS MELANOMA

EPIDEMIOLOGY AND RISK FACTORS

INCIDENCE

Melanoma is now the fifth most common malignancy in men and the sixth most common in women, with approximately 59,580 new cases (4% of all cancers in the United States) and 7,770 deaths in 2005 (1.4% of all cancer deaths in the United States).[48] Melanoma has increased at a rate faster than that of any other cancer over the past 30 years. In 1935, the estimated lifetime risk of developing melanoma was 1 in 1,500. In 2004, this lifetime risk is projected to be 1 in 65 (Fig. 103.5).[49,50] This increase in incidence is exponential, whereas the increase in mortality has been linear.[51]

Whether this melanoma epidemic is "real" has been a heated debate.[52] Some have argued that the rise in incidence rate is simply due to early detection secondary to screening programs, which have led to an increase in the diagnosis of earlier-stage lesions and clinically insignificant tumors.[53] These patients are highly curable, which positively influences overall survival. In contrast, others have pointed out that the incidence of localized, regional, and metastatic melanomas has gone up altogether. Additionally, there is a comparable increase across all Breslow tumor thickness levels among localized lesions.[54–56] These data strongly refute the belief that the rise in incidence is just an artifact of heightened surveillance and early detection. In fact, it suggests

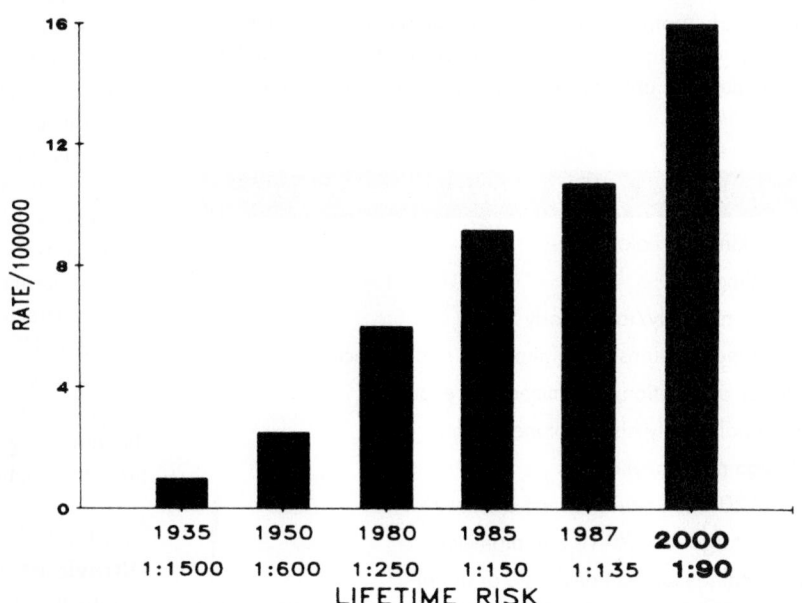

FIGURE 103.5 Past, current, and projected lifetime risk of a person in the United States developing malignant melanoma. (Adapted from Rigel DS, Kopf AW, Friedman RJ. The rate of malignant melanoma in the US: are we making an impact? J Am Acad Dermatol 17:1050, 1987.)

that the melanoma epidemic may actually represent a true increase in the number of invasive melanomas, reflecting increased exposure to the damaging effects of UV radiation.

Invasive melanoma affects all age groups, even though it is rare in childhood (less than 15 years old). The risk of developing the disease escalates with age, with the median age at diagnosis ranging between 40 and 50 years, much younger than most other cancers.[57] In fact, melanoma is the most common cancer in young adults between 20 and 30 years of age.[58] Overall, melanoma incidence is slightly higher in men than in women, with a male to female ratio of about 1.2:1.[48] Males have a greater incidence of melanoma on the trunk or the head and neck and females on the lower extremities.[54] Melanoma is mostly a disease of whites, with rates being 10 times higher in whites than in African Americans.[2] Table 103.7 lists the risk factors associated with cutaneous malignant melanoma.

RISK FACTORS

The risk for developing melanoma is determined by a number of host and environmental factors. Certain nevi phenotypes are major host-related risk factors. Lentigines (freckles) are considered clones of mutated melanocytes and their presence is associated with a higher risk of developing invasive melanoma.[57,59] Benign melanocytic nevi (moles) are no longer believed to be premalignant lesions. However, the number, size, and type of nevi play an important role in risk assessment.[59] The data equating a relationship between the number of benign melanocytic nevi and an associated increased incidence of melanoma are controversial. Different measures and combinations of number and size of lesions have been applied, and no consensus has been developed to assist in analyzing risk. One study showed a significantly increased risk of nonfamilial melanoma developing in persons with more than 120 small (less than 5 mm in diameter) nevi, more than five large (5 to 10 mm in diameter) nevi, and at least one atypical-appearing nevus.[60] All nevi should be closely monitored for changes that may indicate increased growth or malignant potential. Atypical (dysplastic) melanocytic nevi are characteristically different from benign mela-

TABLE 103.7	Risk Factors for Melanoma

Fair skin/hair coloring

Freckling

Sunburns easily/tans poorly

Blistering sunburns in childhood or adolescence

Indoor occupation/intermittent sun exposure

Personal/family history of melanoma

Benign melanocytic nevi

   >120 small nevi (<5 mm diameter)

   >5 large nevi (5–10 mm diameter)

Atypical (dysplastic) nevi (one or more)

nocytic nevi and are thought to be associated with a much higher incidence of melanoma (see etiology section).[59,61]

Skin, hair, and eye color have been recognized as historically classic risk determinants for melanoma. In a review of the literature, Armstrong and English found a relative risk of developing melanoma ranging from one to three for persons with "light" skin color.[62] In this same review, they found that red hair, compared with dark brown to black hair, confers a twofold to fourfold increase in risk and fair hair confers less than a twofold increase in risk.[62] The skin's reaction to sunlight is also important in determining risk. People who burn easily rather than tan after relatively short exposures to UV light are at increased risk (types I and II; Table 103.3). With the exception of lentigo maligna melanoma, people with outdoor occupations do not appear to have an increased risk of melanoma. The only form of melanoma associated with cumulative (chronic) sun exposure has been lentigo maligna melanoma.[63] All other forms of melanoma have been associated with intermittent sun exposure, especially during childhood. A history of blistering sunburns during childhood or adolescence has been associated with an increased risk of developing melanoma.[63,64]

People who have had a previous melanoma are at increased risk of developing a second primary melanoma.[57,63] Patients with familial melanoma are at greater risk of developing multiple primary melanomas. However, only 4% to 10% of melanoma patients describe a history of melanoma in a first-degree relative, showing that familial melanoma is uncommon.[63,65] Atypical mole syndrome (AMS) is now used to describe dysplastic nevus syndrome. The classic AMS describes patients who have at least 100 nevi, 1 or more of which are 8 mm or larger in diameter and displays clinically atypical features.[61] AMS can be either sporadic or familial. Because most families with AMS also have members with melanoma, the syndrome is now referred to as familial atypical mole and melanoma syndrome (FAMMS).[66] FAMMS occurs when two or more family members have melanoma within a family of individuals with AMS.[67] FAMMS kindreds with dysplastic nevi have a lifetime risk of developing melanoma approaching 100%.[68] An unconfirmed linkage analysis appears to correlate FAMMS to the short-arm region of chromosome 1 (locus 1p36).[68,69] Many other studies show linkage to the 9p21 locus on chromosome 9.[68,69] The inheritance patterns for FAMMS are being actively investigated.

Xeroderma pigmentosum, a rare autosomal recessive disorder characterized by deficient repair of DNA damage caused by UV-B light, is associated with more than a 1,000-fold increase in the incidence of skin cancer, including melanoma.[62,68] It is believed that a relationship exists between the immune system and genetics, which determines the reactions to melanoma antigens (see etiology section).

ETIOLOGY

Ultraviolet Radiation. The precise cause of melanoma is unknown, but host factors and environmental exposures have been most extensively studied. UV radiation is suggested to be the most important etiologic agent responsible for the development of cutaneous melanoma. Epidemiologic studies show a strong association between melanoma development and intermittent sun exposure, especially in early childhood.[70,71] Additionally, melanoma tends to occur more frequently in sun-protected skin areas with intermittent exposure, such as the trunk in men and lower extremities in women.[72] People with light coloring (skin, hair, eyes) are at increased risk of developing melanoma, indicating that pigmentation plays a role in protecting the skin from the effects of UV radiation.

Experiments using animal models to establish a direct causal effect of UV-B in melanoma formation have not always been successful. In fact, many studies attempting to induce melanoma in animals with UV radiation have failed, except for one conducted in opossums and another in fish.[63,72–74] However, due to structural differences between animal and human skin, it is difficult to extrapolate the findings from animal models to humans. In 1998, Atillasoy et al used an experimental system of immunodeficient mice bearing newborn human skin grafts to investigate the role of UV-B in the development of melanoma.[75] Atypical hyperplasia was found in 73% of all UV-B-exposed xenografts. One graft exposed to both UV-B and 7,12-dimethyl(a)benzanthracene (a carcinogen) developed nodular melanoma. This study was the first to prove that exposure to UV-B, with or without a carcinogen, can induce atypical melanocytic lesions and malignant melanoma in human skin.

Although most clinicians accept the role of sun exposure in the etiology of melanoma, the exact mechanism by which UV radiation induces melanoma is still being investigated. As mentioned in the NMSC section, UV-B radiation has been most commonly linked to skin cancers and is responsible for the erythematous reaction of the skin after excessive sun exposure. UV-B irradiation can induce DNA adducts such as cyclobutane-pyrimidine dimers and pyrimidine-pyrimidone photoproducts.[72,76] Incorrect repair of these lesions leads to DNA mutations. The extent of involvement of UV-A radiation in the development of melanomas has not been fully elucidated. UV-A irradiation can cause oxidative DNA damage and induce immunosuppression, which may fail to reject early clones of skin cancers.[72,76,77]

Melanocytes are pigmented cells that produce melanin, which provides photoprotection to the skin. With intense intermittent sun exposure, melanocytes cannot instantly synthesize adequate amount of melanin to protect the skin from UV light, allowing DNA adducts to occur. Typically, if DNA lesions are not properly repaired, cells harboring mutated DNA will likely undergo apoptosis (programmed cell death). Interestingly, melanocytes, which contain high levels of anti-apoptotic proteins such as bcl-2, tend to resist apoptosis and survive to mutate and proliferate.[72,76] In fact, freckles are considered clones of mutated melanocytes, and their presence is associated with a higher risk of developing invasive melanoma.[57,59]

Recently, mutations of the B-raf protooncogene have been identified as a common event in melanocytic nevi and primary melanomas.[72,78,79] Pollock et al reported that B-raf mutations were present in 82% of melanocytic nevi, 80% of primary melanomas, and 68% of melanoma metastases. Normal B-raf gene encodes a protein kinase that plays an important role in regulating melanocyte proliferation and survival.[78] Mutations in B-raf lead to the production of an aberrant protein product with much higher kinase activity, thus signaling uncontrolled cell growth.[78] The exact impact of B-raf mutation in the process of melanoma tumorigenesis is being actively investigated.

Genetics. Genetics plays a major role in certain types of melanoma, especially the familial form mentioned earlier. Also, individuals with a personal history of melanoma are at increased risk of developing a second lesion. This indicates the presence of a genetic predisposition. At least three genes, 1p36, 9p21, and 12q14, have been linked to familial melanoma.[68,69] The gene p16^{INK4a}, also known as CDKN2A, CDKN2, and INK4A, has been mapped to the locus 9p21. P16^{INK4a} encodes for two proteins, p16 and p19, both involved in cell cycle regulation.[68] Germline p16 mutations were identified in 37% of 150 familial melanoma families.[68,80] Ongoing studies are evaluating the relationship between genetic predispositions and the incidence of melanoma. More than likely, multiple genetic lesions, in conjunction with other host and environmental factors, are responsible for the biologic progression of a normal melanocyte to a malignant melanoma.

Other Etiologic Factors. The effects of hormonal manipulations on the incidence of melanoma have been studied. These studies stem from the observation that nevi often undergo changes in appearance during pregnancy and puberty. This observation was attributed to changes in hormone levels in the body, especially increases in circulating estrogen. Oral contraceptives have been associated with an increased incidence of melanoma in only a few studies, and in all of these, the increase could be attributed to chance due to the small number of cases and the lack of control for other well-documented risk factors (e.g., sun exposure).[81,82] The same situation exists for exogenous estrogen replacement therapy.[83–85]

Other factors have been studied, including the effects of alcohol, tobacco, coffee, tea, dietary fat, parity, age at first pregnancy, hair dyes, surgery, prior skin problems, and viruses. None of these factors has been proven to have a consistent relationship with the risk of developing melanoma.[62]

PATHOPHYSIOLOGY

Melanomas arise from melanocytes that are located in the epidermal–dermal junction of the skin and the choroid of the eye. Melanocytes can also be found in the meninges (of the brain and spinal cord), mucosa of the alimentary and

TABLE 103.8	Differential Diagnosis of Pigmented Cutaneous Lesions
Common Lesions	**Uncommon Lesions**
Seborrheic keratosis	Hemangioma
Subungual hematoma	Pigmented basal cell carcinoma
Compound nevus	Blue nevus
Junctional nevus	Pigmented dermatofibroma
Lentigo	Kaposi's sarcoma
	Cutaneous T-cell lymphoma
	Tattoo

respiratory tracts, and lymph node capsules. Melanocytes are dendritic pigmented cells that produce melanin. These cells arise from the neural crest early in fetal development. It usually takes 4 to 6 weeks for the melanocytes to migrate to their final destinations.

Melanin is produced in melanosomes (organelles located in the cytoplasm of melanocytes) and is derived from tyrosine. There are several types of melanin, ranging from black (eumelanin) to red-yellow (pheomelanin). Skin color is dependent on the type of melanin and melanosomes produced and their interactions with neighboring keratinocytes, not the density of melanocytes in the skin.[86] The differences in genetics that determine skin color, and therefore the type of melanosomes and melanin produced, are not yet entirely identified. However, it is generally accepted that many different genes collaborate to determine skin color, texture, and anomalies.

The most important proteins used to identify melanomas are S-100, HMB-45, and MART-1.[87] S-100 is expressed by nearly all melanomas, but it is also expressed by sarcomas, nerve sheath tumors, and a subset of carcinomas; therefore, it displays excellent sensitivity but lacks specificity.[87] HMB-45 is more specific for melanoma cells but is not always present in metastatic melanomas, thus restricting its clinical utility.[59] MART-1 has been shown to be more sensitive and specific than HMB-45 for the diagnosis of both primary and metastatic melanoma, with higher diagnostic accuracy than either S-100 or HMB-45.[88,89] These proteins are used most effectively when applied together with a panel of markers specialized to identify and differentiate melanomas.

Several types of pigmented lesions must be differentiated from melanoma lesions (Table 103.8). Normal epidermal melanocytes accumulate to develop into common acquired nevi. This occurrence is thought be related to sun exposure. Common acquired nevi are benign and in small numbers do not impose an increased risk of melanoma. These lesions mature through characteristic phases of growth and development, beginning as flat, focal proliferations of melanocytes within the epidermis, and occasionally progress to include the dermis.[86] Atypical (dysplastic) nevi do not go through these predictable developmental stages. They manifest as asymmetric, irregularly shaped, hazy-bordered, irregularly pigmented lesions and may range in diameter from 2 mm to greater than 6 mm.[61,90] It has been reported that most primary cutaneous melanomas arise from an atypical nevus. However, the vast majority of atypical nevi do not progress to melanoma.[91] Histopathologic confirmation must be obtained for any lesion with the aforementioned characteristics.

Melanoma cells differ from normal epidermal melanocytes in their ability to grow independent of exogenous growth factors, invade into tissues, and metastasize.[85] Melanoma cells usually have marked chromosomal anomalies, with two general phases of growth. The radial growth phase is the early phase of horizontal growth, with little invasion into surrounding tissue. This phase of growth is characteristically slow, but it is most noticeable by the examiner's eye. In contrast, the vertical growth phase is not recognized by examination, due to changes taking place beneath the epidermal layer of skin. Vertical growth is expressed in later phases of melanoma progression and is required for extension into the dermal or subcutaneous layers of the skin or metastases to other organs.

Clark et al[92] proposed a model for tumor progression from normal melanocyte to melanoma (Fig. 103.6). This theory begins with a benign nevus undergoing atypical changes (distortion of the cell architecture). Most of these atypical lesions spontaneously regress over time, as is typical for most precancerous lesions, but they occasionally undergo transformation into an upregulated proliferation of melanocytes confined solely to the epidermal layer of the skin (melanoma in situ). During the radial growth phase, primary melanomas may develop the characteristics to invade the basement membrane of the epidermis, but they usually do not have the capacity to survive in the new dermal environment. These thin lesions, when removed surgically, have a very high cure rate. If left intact, these lesions may develop the capacity to survive in the dermal layer and potentially metastasize and survive in other tissues. Nodular melanomas

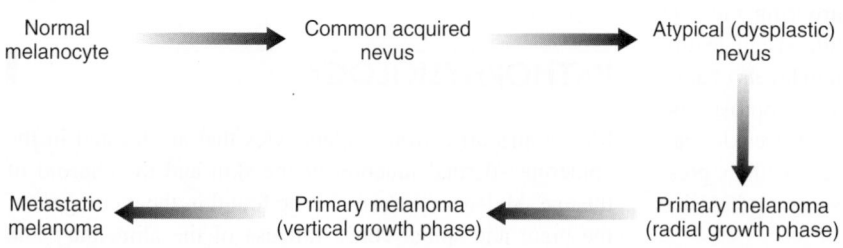

FIGURE 103.6 Clark's model of tumor progression from normal melanocyte to melanoma. (Adapted from Balch CM, Houghton AN, Peters LJ. Cutaneous melanoma. In: DeVita VT, Hellman S, Rosenberg SA, eds. Cancer: principles and practice of oncology, 4th ed. Philadelphia: Lippincott, 1993:1615.)

do not exhibit a radial growth phase and have a greater potential for metastasis from their onset. These lesions are the only exceptions to the progression theory.[93]

Normal melanocytes require growth factors from other cells (paracrine growth factors) for proliferation. Some of these substances have been identified and include basic fibroblast growth factor (bFGF), insulin, insulin-like growth factor (IGF-1), hepatocyte growth factor (HGF), and c-kit ligand.[93,94] Melanoma cells can proliferate without the need for exogenous growth factors. This led to the discovery that melanomas can produce autocrine growth factors that would otherwise be supplied by the cellular environment. Several autocrine growth factors have been identified in cell culture systems of melanoma cells. The production of bFGF by melanoma cell lines in vitro has been well characterized and seems to be an early event in the progression of melanoma cells.[86] Melanocyte growth-stimulating activity (MGSA), platelet-derived growth factor (PDGF), transforming growth factor alpha (TGF-α), interleukin-6 (IL-6), and interleukin-8 (IL-8) are also thought to be autocrine growth factors produced by melanoma cells but are less well characterized.[86,93] Expression of only one of these factors is not sufficient to cause malignant transformation to melanoma. Transforming growth factor beta (TGF-β) and possibly interleukin-1 (IL-1) are believed to prevent the growth of melanoma cell lines in vitro.[86,93] The relatively quiescent nature of normal melanocytes leads to the assumption that numerous negative control mechanisms are working in concert to control growth. These mechanisms would need to be turned off for transformation into a highly invasive melanoma.[93] Paracrine factors seem to play a role in melanoma growth and differentiation, including insulin-like growth factor and epidermal growth factor, which have been shown to stimulate growth of melanoma cells.[86,93] Inhibitory factors (TGF-β, IL-6) may play a role in confining early melanomas to the epidermal layer.[91] Resistance to these factors emphasizes an important aspect of melanoma progression in that later stages of the disease are biologically and genetically different from earlier-stage lesions.[91]

Adhesion molecules and angiogenesis factors are being investigated to define their role in the evolution of melanoma cells, enabling them to exist in foreign environments (e.g., other tissue sites) and metastasize.[93] Cadherins are cell-surface glycoproteins that control cell–cell adhesion. In normal skin tissue, E-cadherin, which is normally expressed by melanocytes and keratinocytes, promotes cellular communication, prevents melanocytes from uncontrolled division, and maintains homeostasis in the skin. However, E-cadherin expression is turned off during malignant transformation.[72,95] On melanoma cells, E-cadherin is replaced by N-cadherin, which allows the malignant cells to adhere to fibroblasts and vascular endothelial cells. This is thought to facilitate the migration of melanoma cells through the dermis and into the circulation. Besides the E-cadherin to N-cadherin switch, changes in other cell adhesion receptors, such as the integrins, have been linked to melanoma progression.

For example, upregulation of the integrin $\alpha_v\beta_3$ has been shown to increase melanoma's invasive ability, mediating the transition of primary melanoma from the radial growth phase to the vertical growth phase.[72,96]

It is rapidly becoming evident that there are complex cellular systems involved in the growth and progression of melanoma. These interactions are being investigated for the development of prognostic indicators, therapeutic interventions, and predictors of response.

Many suppressor genes and oncogenes have been investigated in relation to growth stimulation and inhibition. Chromosomes 1, 6, and 9 are most often found to contain abnormalities in melanomas.[68,69,93] Melanoma cells have been found to abnormally express common tumor suppressor genes identified for other cancers, including p53, NF1 (neurofibromatosis-1 tumor suppressor gene), nm 23 (metastasis suppresser gene), and c-kit (oncogene expression is diminished in melanomas). Familial melanoma has been studied extensively to reveal the genetic link that increases these patients' susceptibility to melanoma, implicating both chromosome 1 and 9 as possible loci for genes involved in susceptibility to familial melanoma.[68,69]

CLINICAL PRESENTATION AND DIAGNOSIS

SIGNS AND SYMPTOMS

Melanomas can occur anywhere on the body but are most commonly found on the lower extremities in women and the trunk in men. Typical features of cutaneous melanoma are variegation, irregular raised surface, irregular border with indentations, and ulceration of the surface. The American Cancer Society has developed the ABCD rules for identification of suspected lesions.[97] These rules incorporate the aforementioned features into an easily remembered acronym:

Asymmetry
Border irregularity
Color variegations
Diameter greater than 6 mm (the size of a pencil-tip eraser)

The key in diagnosing melanoma is recognizing that *any change* in a pigmented lesion is significant. Any pigmented lesion that undergoes a change in size, shape, color, texture, or sensation should be biopsied to rule out melanoma. This includes lesions that lose color and become amelanotic. Itching, burning, or pain in a pigmented lesion should always arouse suspicion of melanoma. However, most patients have none of these symptoms.[59,98]

Four major histologic classifications exist for melanomas: superficial spreading, nodular, lentigo maligna, and acral lentiginous (Fig. 103.7 and Table 103.9). Superficial spreading melanomas are the most common variety, making up 70% of all melanomas.[59] These lesions usually arise from a preexisting nevus and evolve slowly over 1 to 5 years, but

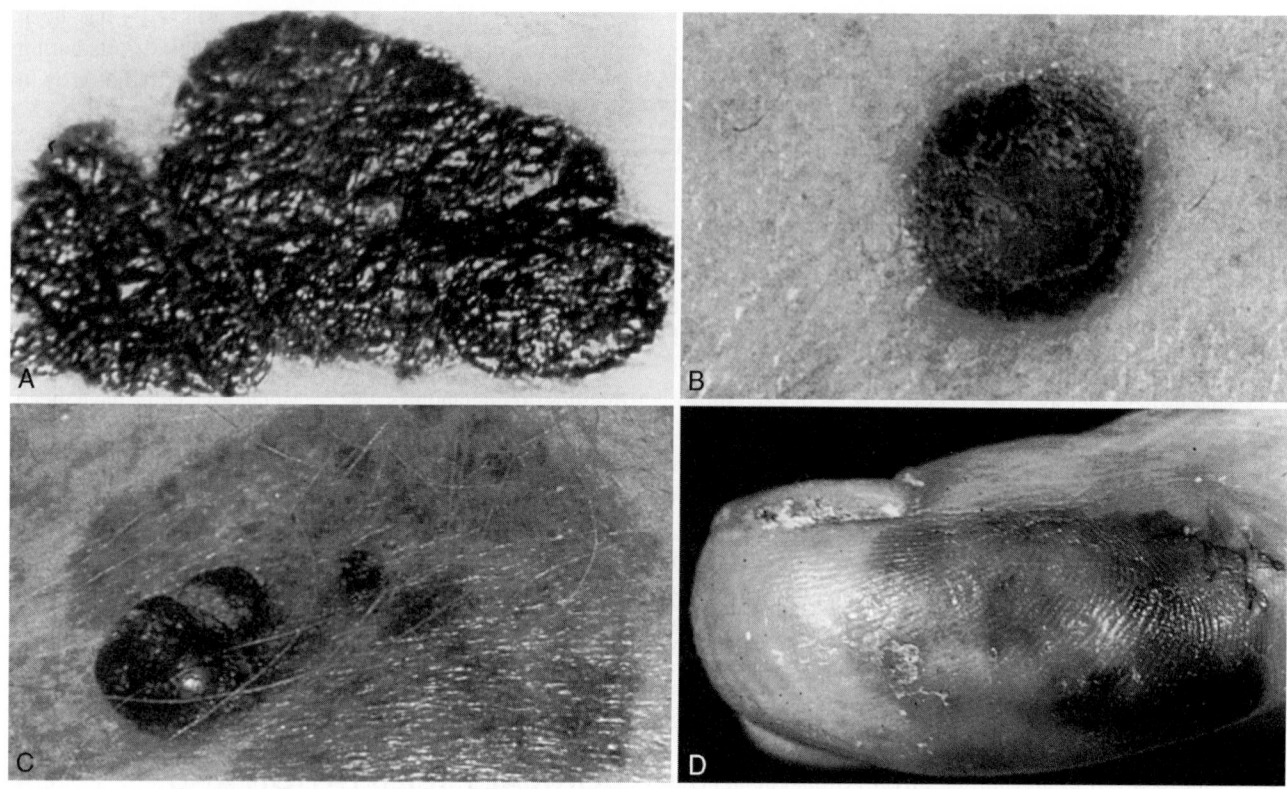

FIGURE 103.7 Four major histologic classifications of melanomas. **A.** Superficial spreading melanoma. **B.** Nodular melanoma. **C.** Lentigo maligna melanoma. **D.** Acral lentiginous melanoma. (Reprinted with permission from Balch CM, Houghton AN, Peters LJ. Cutaneous melanoma. In: DeVita VT, Hellman S, Rosenberg SA, eds. Cancer: principles and practice of oncology, 4th ed. Philadelphia: Lippincott, 1993:1615.)

they also can manifest after only a few months. These lesions spend the majority of their existence in the radial growth phase, eventually progressing to the vertical phase of growth, invading the dermis and other underlying tissues and acquiring the capacity to metastasize.[59] Some lesions never progress to the vertical growth phase, but determining which lesions will progress is not currently possible. These lesions occur at any age after puberty and are more common in women than men.[59] The ABCD rules apply most appropriately to superficial spreading melanomas.[97]

Nodular melanoma is the second most common subset of melanomas, accounting for 15% to 30% of all melanomas.[59] These lesions are more aggressive, lacking a radial growth phase and growing undetected vertically into the underlying structures. The undetected growth of these lesions predisposes them to late diagnosis, with regional spread more likely evident at presentation.[59] These lesions tend to arise from normal skin rather than preexisting nevi and can occur anywhere on the body. The most common areas are the trunk, head, and neck, and they are true to their name, having a dome shape with sharply demarcated borders.[59] Nodular melanomas are typically diagnosed between 40 and 50 years of age, but they can occur at any age and are more common in men than women.[59] Nodular melanomas are usually 1 to 2 cm in diameter but can be much larger. They are characteristically dark brown to black and can have shades of blue

color but are amelanotic (lacking pigment) in approximately 5% of cases.[59] The ABCD rules do not apply to these characteristic lesions.[97]

Lentigo maligna melanoma arises from the precursor or in situ lesion (lentigo maligna), which is light brown and flat with markedly irregular borders, usually appearing on sun-exposed areas of skin in older adults.[59] If invasion is documented within a lentigo maligna, the lesion is considered to be lentigo maligna melanoma.[59] These lesions are closely related to cumulative lifetime UV radiation exposure. The radial growth phase can last for 5 to 15 years or more before converting to the vertical growth phase, which manifests as a nodule or papule within the lentigo maligna lesion. This form of melanoma is less common than superficial spreading melanoma or nodular melanoma and has less of a propensity to metastasize. Lentigo maligna melanoma represents only 4% to 10% of all cutaneous melanomas.[59] These lesions are usually located on the face, with the nose and cheeks most commonly affected. The average age at diagnosis is 70 years; it is very uncommon in those younger than 50.[59] Lentigo malignas tend to be large (greater than 3 cm), and changes within the lesion are often overlooked because of their slow-growing nature. If neglected, they have the potential to spread and become aggressive. The diagnosis requires that sun-related changes be evident in the dermis and epidermis.[59]

TABLE 103.9	Classification of Cutaneous Malignant Melanoma	

Subtype	Percent of All Melanomas	Characteristics
Superficial spreading	70	1. Initial phase of radial growth 2. Progresses to predominantly vertical growth
Nodular	15–30	1. Rapid growth (over weeks to months) 2. Uniformly blue-black, dome-shaped nodule (amelanotic variants exist) 3. No discernible phase of radial growth
Lentigo maligna	4–10	1. Primarily on sun-exposed skin of older adults, most often on face 2. Closely linked to cumulative sun exposure 3. Arise from lentigo ("age spots") 4. After decades of radial growth develop nodular areas
Acral-lentiginous	2–8 (in whites)	1. Most often found on palms, soles, nail beds, and mucous membranes 2. Sunlight not a factor 3. More common in African Americans, Asians, and Hispanics

Acral lentiginous melanomas are the most common melanomas in dark-skinned people such as African Americans, Asians, and Hispanics, representing 35% to 60% of melanomas diagnosed, but they make up only 2% to 8% of melanomas in whites.[59] These lesions arise on the palms and soles, beneath the nail plate, or in the mucous membranes, and they are large, with the average diameter at diagnosis being 3 cm.[59] These lesions appear to have little correlation with exposure to UV radiation. They occur most commonly in older people (average age in the 60s).[59] Acral lentiginous melanoma is present an average of 2.5 months before diagnosis, showing its more aggressive nature. These lesions often are confused with lentigo maligna melanoma because of their light-brown, flat appearance. The growth can be deceptive, growing undetected vertically with little evidence of change from the surface. These lesions are more aggressive than superficial spreading melanoma or lentigo maligna melanoma and therefore have a poorer prognosis.[59] Subungual melanoma is one particular type of acral lentiginous melanoma. The median age at diagnosis is 55 to 65 years, and it is equally common in males and females.[59]

Melanoma can metastasize anywhere in the body, with the most common sites of metastases at first relapse being the skin, subcutaneous tissue, and distant lymph nodes.[59] Lung, liver, brain, and the gastrointestinal tract are the next

most common sites. In-transit metastases are defined as lesions located between the primary site of the lesion and the first major regional lymph node basin.[59] These lesions are thought to originate from cells trapped in the lymphatics. They are usually observed in the subcutaneous or intracutaneous layer of the skin (i.e., satellitosis). Local recurrences are defined as any tumor that occurs within 5 cm of the scar of a previously excised melanoma.[99]

Patients with stage I, II, or III melanoma rarely have changes in radiographic evaluation if micrometastases are present, but instead have symptoms.[98] Particular attention should be paid to signs or symptoms of central nervous system involvement. Also, blood in the stool and gastrointestinal symptoms can be possible indicators of metastatic disease. Although some patients remain stable for months, others have rapid progression of disease, with clinical deterioration within weeks. The clinical course of any individual patient is difficult to predict and should be followed carefully by close monitoring of symptoms and signs relevant to the most common sites of metastases, as well as any other change in symptoms.

STAGING AND PROGNOSIS

If melanoma is suspected, biopsy is required for diagnosis. Several characteristics must be considered when determining biopsy technique. Microstaging, to determine the full thickness of the lesion, is essential and must be performed with the initial biopsy. Therefore, excisional biopsy (removing the entire lesion) is the optimal biopsy procedure for lesions suspected of being melanoma.[63] Other characteristics that must be considered are the location of the lesion (amount of tissue coverage) and the size of the lesion. It is difficult to completely excise a large lesion on the face with acceptable cosmetic results. In these cases, a punch biopsy can be done in the most raised, deeply pigmented portion of the lesion, reaching its full depth. Another alternative is an incisional biopsy. Shave, needle, curettage, and saucerization biopsies are contraindicated for any primary pigmented lesion suspected of being melanoma because these procedures may compromise the integrity of the histologic confirmation. The needle biopsy technique may be useful to document nodal metastases of melanoma.[63]

Microstaging, an integral part of staging and management of melanoma (Fig. 103.8), is traditionally accomplished using two methods: Breslow's tumor thickness measurement and Clark's level of invasion. Breslow's method uses an ocular micrometer to measure the total height (not just depth) of the lesion from the granular layer to the area of deepest penetration.[100] If the lesion is ulcerated, measurements are made from the base of the ulcer to the deepest portion of the lesion; if it is raised above the normal surface of the skin, the measurements are taken from the highest point to the deepest point of the lesion. The original Breslow's classification is listed in Table 103.10. Clark et al[101] developed microstaging levels based on the depth of invasion into the skin rather than the thickness of the lesion (Table 103.10).

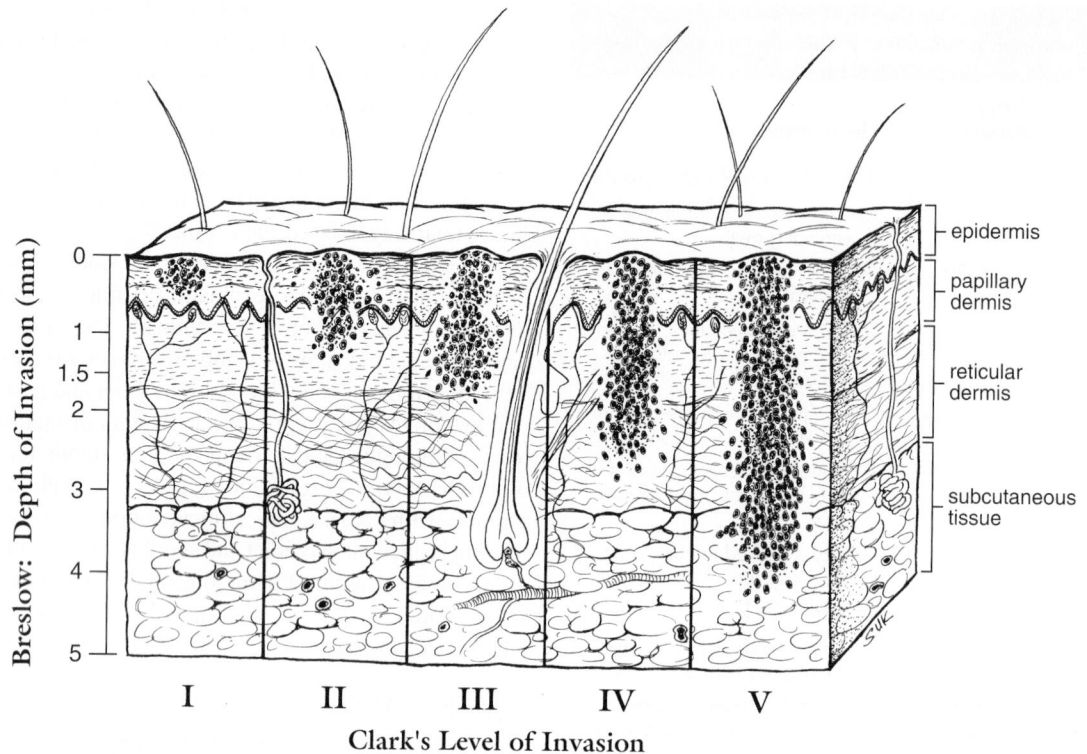

FIGURE 103.8 Pathologic microstaging of melanoma. Breslow's levels measure tumor thickness in millimeters and are shown on the left side of the figure. Clark's levels measure the depth of invasion by tissue level of deepest penetration and are depicted across the bottom of the figure.

However, several studies evaluating the prognostic significance of these two methods have established that Breslow's measures of tumor thickness are more accurate and reproducible in predicting the risk for metastasis.[102–104] Also, it is recognized that the relationship between tumor thickness and melanoma mortality is a continuum, with no specific biologic breakpoints.[104,105] Therefore, the thickness thresholds have been redefined using the simplest best fit statistical model (Table 103.11) and incorporated into the new TNM staging system as the primary criterion to stage primary mel-

anoma lesions (Tables 103.12 and 103.13).[104–107] On the other hand, Clark's levels of invasion provide additional prognostic information only for patients with thin melanoma (1 mm or less) and are merely used to subcategorize T1 lesions in the current staging system (Tables 103.12 and 103.13).[104–107]

The revised TNM staging system for melanoma published in 2002 also integrates other prognostic factors to assist clinicians in determining survival outcome and planning treatment (Tables 103.12 and 103.13; Fig. 103.9).[107] Tumor thickness (measured in millimeters) is the single most important prognostic factor for patients with stage I and II

TABLE 103.10	Pathologic Microstaging for Cutaneous Malignant Melanoma

Breslow's Levels[a]	Clark's Levels	
≤ 0.75 mm	I	Confined to the epidermis
0.76–1.49 mm	II	Extends into the papillary dermis
1.50–2.49 mm	III	Up to but not extending into the reticular dermis
2.50–3.99 mm	IV	Extending into the reticular dermis
≥4 mm	V	Extending into the subcutaneous tissue

[a]Uses an ocular micrometer to measure the total height of the lesion from the granular layer to the area of deepest penetration

TABLE 103.11	New Cut-Off Points of Microstaging for Cutaneous Melanoma

Breslow's Thickness	Clark's Levels	
≤ 1mm	I	Confined to the dermis
1.01–2 mm	II	Extends into the papillary dermis
2.01–4 mm	III	Up to but not extending into the reticular dermis
>4 mm	IV	Extending into the reticular dermis
	V	Extending into the subcutaneous tissue

TABLE 103.12	Melanoma TNM Classification	
T		
	Thickness	**Ulceration**
T1	≤1 mm	a: No ulceration
		b: Ulceration or Clark's level IV/V
T2	1.01–2 mm	a: No ulceration
		b: Ulceration
T3	2.01–4 mm	a: No ulceration
		b: Ulceration
T4	>4 mm	a: No ulceration
		b: Ulceration
N		
	Number of Positive Nodes	**Extent of Nodal Involvement**
N1	1	a: Micrometastasis
		b: Macrometastasis
N2	2 or 3	a: Micrometastasis
		b: Macrometastasis
		c: In-transit metastasis/satellite without positive nodes
N3	≥4, or matted nodes, or in-transit metastasis/satellite with positive nodes	
M		
	Site	**Serum LDH**
M1a	Distant skin, subcutaneous tissue, or nodal metastases	Normal
	Lung metastases	Normal
M1b	Other visceral metastases	Normal
M1c	Any distant metastases	Elevated

LDH, lactate dehydrogenase.

TABLE 103.13	Pathologic Stage Grouping for Cutaneous Melanoma		
0	Tis (in situ)	N0	M0
IA	T1a	N0	M0
IB	T1b	N0	M0
IIA	T2a	N0	M0
IIB	T2b	N0	M0
IIC	T3a	N0	M0
IIIA	T3b	N0	M0
IIIB	T4a	N0	M0
IIIC	T4b	N0	M0
IV	T1–4a	N1a	M0
	T1–4a	N2a	M0
	T1–4b	N1a	M0
	T1–4b	N2a	M0
	T1–4a	N1b	M0
	T1–4a	N2b	M0
	Any T	N2c	M0
	T1–4b	N1b	M0
	T1–4b	N2b	M0
	Any T	N3	M0
	Any T	Any N	M1

melanomas. Clark's levels of invasion are of prognostic significance only to patients with thin melanoma (T1 lesions). Besides tumor thickness, ulceration of the primary lesion (defined as the absence of an intact epidermis overlying a major portion of the primary melanoma) is the second most powerful predictor of survival for patients with stage I and II melanomas.[104–107] Additionally, ulceration is the only primary lesion characteristic that can adversely influence the prognosis of stage III disease.[104–107] For stage I and II lesions, patients with lesions on the extremities have a better survival rate than those with lesions on the trunk or head and neck.[104] Gender is also an independent prognostic factor for early-stage disease, with women having a better survival rate than men.[104] Increasing age unfavorably affects survival outcome, with older patients having a worse prognosis than younger patients.[104] There is also evidence to suggest that certain growth patterns of the primary tumor may influence prognosis, with lentigo maligna melanoma associated with a better outcome and acral lentiginous melanoma with a poorer prognosis compared to superficial spreading and nodular melanoma (Fig. 103-9).[106]

For patients with stage III disease, three factors that most significantly affect survival are the number of metastatic lymph nodes, the extent of nodal tumor involvement (microscopic versus macroscopic), and the ulceration status of the primary lesion.[104–107] A method of lymphatic mapping and sentinel node biopsy has recently been developed as a relatively noninvasive means of staging the nodal basin. Coupling this technique with serial sectioning, advances in immunohistochemistry, and new molecular markers (e.g., polymerase chain reaction for tyrosinase) improves the ability to stage nodal status and identify patients who can benefit from complete lymphadenectomy and possibly adjuvant therapy.[108] Less important prognostic variables for stage III melanomas are the location of the primary lesion and the patient's age.[104]

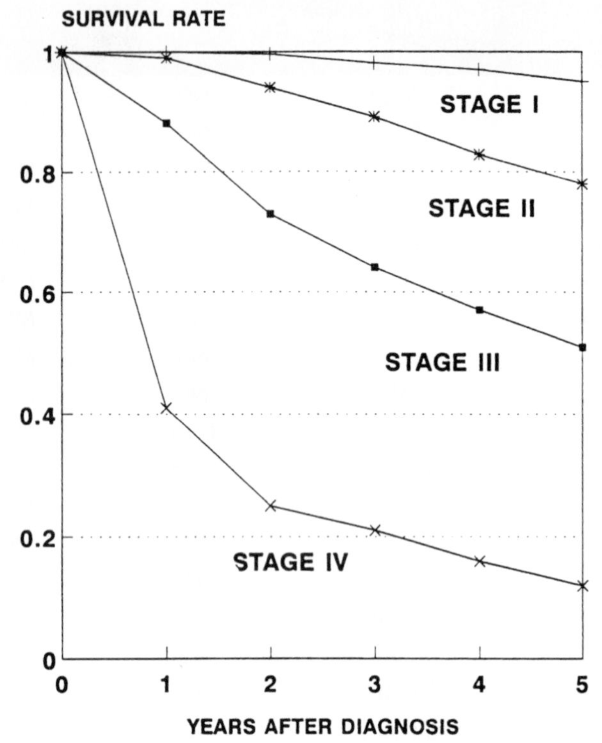

FIGURE 103.9 Relative survival rates according to the stage of disease. Data taken from 8,479 patients who were diagnosed between 1977 and 1982. Patients are listed in the Surveillance, Epidemiology, and End Results (SEER) program of the National Cancer Institute. Stage I comprises 4,286 patients, stage II 3,328, stage III 648, and stage IV 216. (Reprinted with permission from American Joint Committee on Cancer. Manual for staging of cancer, 4th ed. Philadelphia: Lippincott, 1995:144.)

The single most important prognostic variable for patients with stage IV (distant metastases) disease is the anatomic sites of metastases. Patients with nonvisceral involvement (skin, subcutaneous, and distant lymph nodes) tend to fare better than those with visceral disease. Among patients with visceral metastases, individuals with lung involvement have a better prognosis than those with metastases to any other visceral sites.[104–107] Elevated serum lactate dehydrogenase (LDH) levels above the upper limits of normal, based on two or more laboratory samples obtained at least 24 hours apart to avoid the chance of false positivity, also indicate an unfavorable survival outcome.[104–107]

TREATMENT

For melanoma, surgical excision is generally the most effective treatment modality. Even in selected cases of metastatic disease, the optimal palliative treatment includes surgical resection of the lesions. Metastatic lesions are generally not responsive to other treatment modalities and should be considered relatively resistant to radiotherapy and chemotherapy. Much of the research with melanoma lies in the arena of systemic therapy for metastatic melanoma and adjuvant treatment of patients after removal of involved lymph nodes by several different modalities. Patients with advanced disease have a poor prognosis; therefore, any treatment modality recommendation must emphasize the importance of an acceptable quality of life.

SURGERY

Excision of Primary Melanoma. For stage I and II melanomas, the treatment of choice is surgical excision of the primary lesion, down into the subcutaneous tissue, plus a radius of normal-appearing skin.[109] Due to the theoretical concern of residual microscopic disease in the vicinity of the primary tumor, a 4- to 5-cm margin was historically advocated for all melanoma lesions to prevent local recurrences. Local relapse in melanoma is generally considered a bad prognostic sign because it is associated with both an increased risk of regional and systemic metastases as well as a higher rate of mortality.[110,111] However, such radical excisions necessitate the use of split-thickness skin grafting to close the surgical defect and can cause unacceptable cosmetic disfigurement, significant morbidity, and prolonged hospitalization.[112] Better understanding of the influence of tumor thickness on the likelihood of local recurrence has prompted many investigators to prove that narrower margins are appropriate for thinner lesions without compromising overall survival, rate of metastasis, or incidence of local relapse. Data from five prospective randomized trials (Table 103.14)[111,113–116] helped establish a rational evidence-based guideline regarding the surgical excision margin for primary melanomas up to 4 mm in thickness. Excisional requirements for thicker lesions (larger than 4 mm) have not been studied in a randomized, controlled manner, but the current recommendations are to excise these lesions with at least a 2-cm margin.[109,117]

Regardless of these guidelines, it is crucial to procure a histologically negative margin. For example, if there are melanoma cells at the excision border after a 2-cm margin is obtained, further excision must be done to achieve a negative margin. The anatomic location of the primary lesion should also be taken into consideration when determining the extent of surgery. If a 2-cm margin can potentially cause significant cosmetic disfigurement or functional impairment, a 1-cm margin is acceptable as long as it is histologically negative. Table 103.15 outlines margin treatment recommendations for melanoma.

For primary cutaneous melanomas on the fingers or toes, digital amputation is required. It is important to preserve enough of the digit to ensure adequate functioning, but without compromising sufficient margin.[109] The ear can usually be partially amputated or wedge resected, reserving complete amputation for recurrent lesions or widespread disease. Ear prostheses are available for patients requiring this type of surgery.[109]

Elective Lymph Node Dissection. Removal of normal-appearing regional lymph nodes in hopes of decreasing the

| TABLE 103.14 | Surgical Trials Evaluating Excision Margin |

Trial	Tumor Thickness	No. Pts.	Margins (cm)	Median Follow-Up	Results/Conclusion
French Cooperative Study	≤2 mm	326	2 vs. 5	16 yr	DFS: ND; OS: ND Margin >2 cm not necessary for lesions ≤2 mm
WHO Melanoma Program	<2 mm	612	1 vs. 3	7.5 yr	LR: ND; OS: ND Total LR for lesions 1–2 mm higher with 1-cm margin vs. 3-cm margin (5 vs.1) but not statistically significant 1-cm margin safe for lesions <2 mm *Others are concerned about the trend toward increased LR with 1-cm margin for lesions 1–2 mm*
Intergroup Melanoma Trial	1–4 mm	486	2 vs. 4	10 yr	LR: ND; OS: ND; skin graft: higher with 4-cm margin; hospital stay: longer with 4-cm margin LR associated with high mortality rate LR increased with increased tumor thickness and presence of ulceration 2-cm margin safe for lesions <4 mm *In the subgroup of 1- to 2-mm lesions, LR rate 0.6 mm with 2-cm margin vs. 4.5% for lesions of same thickness receiving 1-cm margin in the WHO trial*
Swedish Melanoma Study Group	0.8–2 mm	989	2 vs. 5	11 yr	LR: ND; OS: ND 2-cm margin safe for lesions 0.8–2 mm
UK Melanoma Study Group	≥2 mm	900	1 vs. 3	5 yr	OS: ND Regional recurrence significantly higher with 1-cm margin Surgical complications significantly higher with 3-cm margin 1-cm margin should be avoided for lesions ≥2 mm

DFS, disease-free survival; OS, overall survival; ND, no statistically significant difference; LR, local recurrence.

incidence of distant failure is termed *elective lymph node dissection* (ELND). In the past, ELND was advocated for both staging and therapeutic purposes in patients with clinically negative lymph nodes but at a high risk of regional metastasis. However, ELND is a controversial procedure and

| TABLE 103.15 | Recommended Excision Margins for Primary Cutaneous Melanoma |

Tumor Thickness	Recommended Margins
In situ	0.5 cm
≤1 mm	1 cm
1.01–2 mm	1–2 cm
2.01–4 mm	2 cm
>4 mm	2 cm

It is crucial to procure a histologically negative margin. Margins may be modified for anatomic or cosmetic reasons.

may or may not be associated with improved survival. This procedure is based on the belief that melanoma metastasizes sequentially, first spreading to the regional lymph nodes and then to distant sites. Thus, ELND supporters hypothesize that early removal of clinically negative lymph nodes harboring microscopic disease can ultimately halt the systemic dissemination of tumor cells and potentially prolong survival.[118] Opponents of the procedure note the successes with surgical excision of the primary alone for stage I and II patients as reasons not to inflict this type of morbidity on patients who may not have microscopic disease in the lymph nodes.[119]

To date, four randomized prospective trials[120–123] evaluating ELND versus wide local excision of the primary alone have been completed. None of these studies showed that routine ELND altered overall survival for patients with clinically negative lymph nodes. However, the Intergroup Melanoma Surgical trial revealed that ELND did benefit the subgroup of patients 60 years of age or younger with tumor thickness of 1 to 2 mm and without ulceration. The 5-year survival rate for this group was reported to be 97% with ELND compared to 87% for those patients with similar characteristics receiving wide local excision alone.[123] Subgroup analysis of the WHO Melanoma Group trial 14 pointed out that the survival rate for patients with microscopic nodal involvement undergoing ELND was superior to that of patients treated with delayed lymphadenectomy for clinically positive nodal recurrence (48% versus 26.6% at 5 years, respectively).[121] This result did reiterate the need for an adequate staging workup to identify patients with occult nodal involvement early in the course of the disease.

One resolution for this controversy is a new procedure that can accurately stage the suspected lymph node basin without requiring full dissection. This technique is termed *intraoperative lymphatic mapping and sentinel lymph node biopsy* (IOLM/SLNB).[124] IOLM/SLNB is based on the observation that the lymphatic channels from a specific region of the skin are highly predictable and ultimately converge in a specific lymph node (the sentinel lymph node) within the regional nodal basin.[124] Therefore, the sentinel lymph node is most likely to harbor tumor cells in the event of lymphatic metastasis, and its pathologic examination can determine the histologic status of the entire nodal basin. In IOLM/SLNB, a vital blue dye (isosulfan blue) and a technetium sulfur colloid are injected into the dermis at the site of the primary melanoma lesion. A hand-held gamma probe is then used to track the lymphatic drainage and to identify the location of the sentinel lymph node. Subsequently, a small incision is made at the site of the radioactivity to harvest the node for serial sectioning and histopathologic analysis.[125] If this node is positive for microscopic disease, a complete lymphadenectomy will follow. However, if the node is negative, the procedure can be halted and the patient is spared an unnecessary surgery. The identification rate with this procedure is reported to be 90% or higher, with low false-negative rate.[125,126]

With recent recognition of the prognostic significance of the sentinel lymph node status, IOLM/SLNB has been widely accepted as a standard staging method to select the group of patients with nodal involvement who will most likely benefit from therapeutic lymphadenectomy and adjuvant therapy. However, the true impact of this procedure on overall survival remains unknown. The Multicenter Selective Lymphadenectomy Trial is ongoing to compare the difference in long-term outcome of wide local excision alone versus wide local excision plus IOLM/SLNB, followed by complete nodal dissection only in patients with occult metastasis.[127]

Therapeutic Lymph Node Dissection. Lymphadenectomy performed when clinically apparent nodes are found is termed *therapeutic dissection.* Clinically evident regional lymph node involvement (stage III) is managed primarily with surgical resection. Long-term disease-free survival after lymphadenectomy is predicted to be 20% to 40% for stage III melanoma patients. The adverse effects of lymphadenec-

tomy depend on the site of resection. The ilioinguinal lymph node basins drain the lower extremities. After resection of these basins, there is noticeable edema in approximately 26% of patients at long-term follow-up, but only 5% and 3% of patients, respectively, report pain and functional deficit.[59] Leg exercises, elastic stockings, diuretics, and perioperative antibiotics have been shown to prevent edema in these patients. Complications with axillary node dissection are infections (7%), seroma (27%), hemorrhage (1%), and arm edema (1%).[59] Cervical and parotid lymph nodes can also be removed with similar complications. Nerve damage occurring in the location of these lymph nodes (close proximity to the cranial nerves) is rarely seen but is always a possibility.[59]

Surgical Management of Metastases. Patients with distant metastases have a poor prognosis, with a median survival of 5 to 8 months and a 5-year survival rate of less than 5%. Resection of metastatic lesions can offer palliation of symptoms but rarely affects survival rates. Resection of isolated pulmonary or subcutaneous metastases is associated with prolonged survival in 15% to 30% of patients.[128,129] At this point in the disease process, emphasis is placed on quality of life rather than longevity.

RADIATION

Radiotherapy for Primary Melanomas. The use of radiation for the treatment of melanoma is controversial. Initial reports of complete radioresistance in all melanomas have been challenged. With early stages of melanoma, surgery alone is the standard of care, with very high cure rates (greater than 95%). Treatment of primary melanomas with conventional radiation is limited to large facial lentigo maligna lesions, which may require extensive reconstruction if surgery is performed. Radiotherapy can be useful for these patients with little morbidity and very good clinical and cosmetic results. In one series, using fractionated doses of radiation to treat 28 patients with lentigo maligna, only 2 patients experienced recurrence, but some lesions took as long as 24 months to fully regress after radiation.[130] The long-term adverse effects with radiation are skin pallor, telangiectasias, and atrophy in the area of treatment (approximately 10%).[130] Adjuvant irradiation of the primary site after wide local excision has not been adequately studied; therefore, its use cannot be routinely recommended at this time.[131] However, adjuvant radiotherapy may be justified if concern for local recurrence is high, such as in the cases of thick primary lesions (more than 4 mm) with ulceration or satellitosis (the presence of satellite metastases within 2 cm of the primary melanoma), close or positive margins when further resection is not practical, or locally recurrent disease.[131]

Adjuvant Radiotherapy for Regional Lymph Nodes. For patients with stage III melanoma, the overall risk of regional recurrence after a therapeutic lymphadenectomy is about 15%.[131,132] However, this number dramatically increases to 30% to 50% when the lymphatic metastases show high-risk features such as positive nodes in the cervical nodal basin, extracapsular extension, four or more positive lymph nodes, an involved lymph node 3 cm in size or larger, and recurrent nodal disease. Data from prospective series and retrospective analyses suggest that adjuvant irradiation to the regional nodal basin could improve regional control when the risk for local relapse is high.[133–135] Survival was at least equal to that seen with conventional approaches. Postoperative nodal radiation is generally well tolerated and does not significantly worsen the overall morbidity, with mild to moderate lymphedema or loss of subcutaneous fat occurring in a minority of patients.[131] Randomized, controlled studies must be done to better identify the role for adjuvant radiotherapy, either to the primary sites or to the nodal basins.

Radiotherapy for Distant Metastases. Distant sites of metastases may be treated with radiation. The most common indications for radiotherapy are treatment of subcutaneous, dermal, lymph node, brain, or bone metastases. Palliation of symptoms can often be accomplished with radiotherapy directed toward the specific site of involvement. Spinal cord compression or symptomatic visceral involvement not amenable to surgery can also be radiated for palliation.[132]

ISOLATED LIMB PERFUSION

Isolated limb perfusion (ILP) with and without hyperthermia has been studied, particularly in patients with multiple le-

sions on an isolated extremity (Fig. 103.10). The goal of limb perfusion is to maximize the concentration of drug in the affected limb while minimizing the systemic side effects of chemotherapy. The rationale behind the addition of hyperthermia to this procedure is that hyperthermia in the range of 40° to 45°C is cytotoxic to melanoma cells.[136] Moreover, drug uptake by tumor tissues has been shown to be greater at temperatures higher than 37°C.[137] Many agents have been used either alone or in combination, such as melphalan, actinomycin-D, mechlorethamine, dacarbazine, cisplatin, carboplatin, tumor necrosis factor (TNF), interferon (IFN)-β, and IFN-γ. The drug most studied and most effective is melphalan, which has complete response rates of about 54% (range 26% to 81%).[138]

ILP was used in the past to prevent or to treat in-transit metastases (lesions more than 2 cm from the primary tumor) in the limbs. However, the intergroup trial randomizing 832 patients with high-risk primary limb melanoma (1.5 mm or larger) to wide local excision with or without prophylactic ILP failed to show a survival benefit from the combined approach.[139] Also, ILP is a costly procedure with significant morbidity; therefore, it is no longer recommended in the adjuvant setting. For management of bulky or extensive in-transit metastases confined to a limb, this treatment modality is very encouraging and should be considered the standard of care, especially as an alternative to amputation. Even though ILP can achieve high rates of complete remission

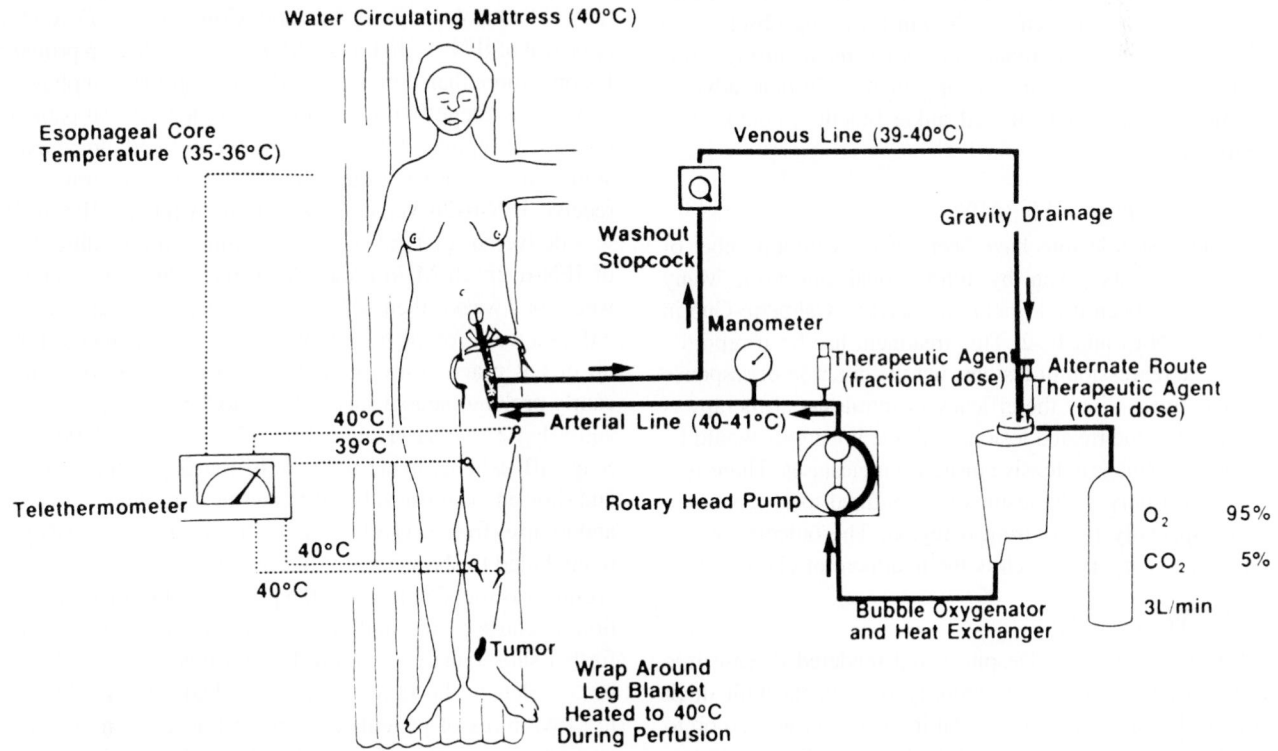

FIGURE 103.10 Isolated limb perfusion with hyperthermia for lower limb melanoma. (Reprinted with permission from Krementz ET, Ryan RF, Muchmore JH, et al. Hyperthermic regional perfusion for melanoma of the limbs. In: Balch MC, Houghton AN, Milton GW, et al, eds. Cutaneous melanoma, 2nd ed. Philadelphia: Lippincott, 1992:405.)

with current techniques and cytotoxic agents, local relapse is inevitable.[140] Thus, improving the rate and duration of tumor response to ILP with melphalan has been the objective of current research activities. The addition of hyperthermia was shown to induce higher complete response rates (up to 80%) at the expense of increased regional toxicity.[141,142]

Cytokines such as TNF-α or IFN-γ have also been used in adjunctive therapy with melphalan. An early trial evaluating the combination of all three agents reported a complete response rate of 90%, with acceptable regional and systemic toxicity.[143] However, subsequent data failed to substantiate that initial impressive result. The American College of Surgeons Oncology Group (ACOSOG) is currently conducting a study randomizing patients with extensive in-transits to receive either ILP with hyperthermia and melphalan, or ILP with hyperthermia, melphalan, and TNF-α to validate the response rates previously described and to determine their durability. The result of this trial is eagerly awaited.[127]

ILP is a complicated and costly procedure that requires an experienced team of experts to maximize benefits and minimize the toxicity associated with the procedure. ILP with melphalan can cause considerable side effects both systemically and regionally. Systemic toxicity is generally mild, but it can become severe if there is substantial leakage of perfusate into the systemic circulation, especially when TNF-α is combined with melphalan. Regional adverse effects are more worrisome and can limit the use of this procedure. Acute regional toxicities include pain, edema, and erythema, which usually resolve within 2 to 3 weeks. More serious events can occur, with skin blistering observed in 15% of patients and compartment syndrome requiring fasciotomy or amputation in 5% of patients. Chronic adverse reactions consist of restricted ankle function, edema, and neuropathy.[144,145]

INTRALESIONAL THERAPY

Metastatic skin lesions have been treated with a number of different agents given by intralesional injection. Many agents have been used, including bacillus Calmette-Guérin (bCG), IFN-α, and IL-2. This treatment has been reported to induce regression of lesions, but the duration of response is short-lived. Since the efficacy of intralesional therapy is restricted to the treated lesion, multiple injections would be needed to manage extensive in-transit metastases. Therefore, it is useful only if the lesions are confined to a very small area, especially in the truncal region. The outcome is not superior to surgery, which is the treatment of choice.[146]

SYSTEMIC THERAPY

Adjuvant Therapy. Despite being rendered disease-free with definitive surgery, a majority of patients with thick primary lesions or positive nodal involvement will go on to develop distant metastases and die from the disease. Therefore, the search for effective adjuvant therapy to minimize the risk of recurrence has been ongoing over the past two decades. Unfortunately, postoperative treatment with non-

specific immunostimulants such as bCG, *Corynebacterium parvum,* and levamisole showed no survival advantage over surgery alone for stage I, II, and III melanoma.[147] Results with chemotherapy, including high-dose chemotherapy with autologous bone marrow transplantation, were also disappointing.[147,148] To date, adjuvant high-dose IFN-α remains the only agent with significant effect on the survival of melanoma patients. Trials with other cytokines and vaccines in the adjuvant setting are underway.

Interferon-α. Numerous adjuvant trials using IFN-α have been carried out. All of the trials used different dosing schedules, route of administration, duration of therapy, and type of IFN. The risk groups enrolled in the trials were slightly different, and this may have affected the overall results (Table 103.16).

The North Central Cancer Treatment Group (NCCTG) conducted the first randomized adjuvant trial using high-dose IFN. In this study, IFN-α-2a (Roferon-A), given at 20 MU/m^2/day intramuscularly three times a week for 12 weeks, was compared to observation.[149] Patients with resected stage IIA/B melanoma of depth greater than 1.69 mm or stage III disease were studied. No significant impact on overall survival or relapse-free interval was noted when the entire study population was analyzed, but a trend toward benefit was noted among patients with stage III disease.

The ECOG 1684 trial (E1684) is the only trial to date to show an overall survival benefit when used in the adjuvant setting for melanoma and was the primary study used by the FDA Oncologic Drug Advisory Committee (ODAC) for approval of IFN-α-2b (Intron-A). Patients with deep primary lesions (more than 4 mm, stage IIB) or regional lymph node metastases (stage III) were enrolled in the trial. All patients underwent regional lymphadenectomy and wide local excision. After curative surgery, patients were randomized to receive IFN-α-2b versus observation. Adjuvant IFN-α-2b was delivered for 1 full year and comprised a loading dose of IFN-α-2b 20 MU/m^2/day given intravenously 5 days a week for 4 weeks, then 10 MU/m^2/day given subcutaneously 3 days a week for the next 48 weeks.[150] At a median follow-up of 6.9 years, adjuvant IFN-α-2b was shown to significantly prolong median survival (2.8 to 3.8 years, $p = 0.02$) and relapse-free survival (1.0 to 1.7 years, $p = 0.002$).[150] Stage III patients made up 89% of the population studied and showed the greatest benefit in terms of prolonged overall and relapse-free survival.[151] A small subset of stage IIB patients failed to show benefit, but imbalance in the treatment groups was found in terms of the presence of primary ulceration. Because of the small numbers of patients in this group, further subset analysis, controlling for ulceration, could not be completed. This treatment regimen had substantial toxicity: two thirds of patients experienced at least one grade 3 or 4 adverse event, and more than 50% of patients required dosage adjustment or discontinuation of therapy.

Concerns regarding quality of life and cost have been addressed in two subsequent analyses of these data for qual-

TABLE 103.16	Adjuvant Interferon-α Trials

Study	IFN Type	Dose and Schedule	Impact on DFS and OS	Pt. Population
High-Dose IFN				
NCCTG	IFN-α–2a	Arm 1: 20 MU/m²/day IM TIW for 12 wk Arm 2: Observation	DFS and OS: NS	T >1.69 mm or positive regional nodes (n = 262)
ECOG 1684	IFN-α-2b	Arm 1: 20 MU/m²/day IV, 5 days/wk for 4 wk, then 10 MU/m²/day SC TIW for 48 wk Arm 2: Observation	DFS: 1.7 yr vs. 1 yr (p = 0.002) OS: 3.8 yr vs. 2.8 yr (p= 0.02)	T >4 mm or positive regional nodes (n = 287)
ECOG 1690	IFN-α-2b	Arm 1: 20 MU/m²/day IV, 5 days/wk for 4 wks, then 10 MU/m²/day SC TIW for 48 wk Arm 2: 3 MU SC TIW for 2 yr Arm 3: Observation	Arm 1 vs. arm 3: DFS: Increased (p = 0.03) OS: NS	T >4 mm or positive regional nodes (n = 642)
Low-Dose Interferon				
WHO #16	IFN-α-2a	Arm 1: 3 MU SC TIW for 3 yr Arm 2: Observation	DFS and OS: NS	Positive regional nodes (n = 444)
ECOG 1690	IFN-α-2b	As above	Arm 2 vs. arm 3: DFS and OS: NS	T >4 mm or positive regional nodes (n = 642)
Scottish Melanoma	IFN-α-2b	Arm 1: 3 MU SC TIW for 6 mo Arm 2: Observation	DFS and OS: NS	T >3 mm or positive regional node (n = 95)
UKCCCR	IFN-α-2a	Arm 1: 3 MU SC daily for 2 yr Arm 2: Observation	DFS and OS: NS	T ≥4 mm or positive regional nodes (n = 674)
EORTC 18871	IFN-α-2b	Arm 1: 1 MU SC QOD for 1 yr Arm 2: IFN-γ Arm 3: Iscador M (mistletoe extract) Arm 4: Observation	Arm 1 vs. arm 4: DFS and OS: NS	T >3 mm or positive regional nodes (n = 830)
Austrian Intergroup	IFN-α-2a	Arm 1: 3 MU SC daily for 3 wk, then 3 MU SC TIW for 1 yr Arm 2: Observation	DFS: Increased (p = 0.02) OS: NS	T ≥1.5 mm and clinically negative nodes (n = 311)
French Cooperative	IFN-α-2a	Arm 1: 3 MU SC TIW for 18 mo Arm 2: Observation	DFS: Increased (p = 0.035) OS: NS	T >1.5 mm and clinically negative nodes (n = 489)
Intermediate-Dose Interferon				
EORTC 18952	IFN-α-2b	Arm 1: 10 MU SC, 5 days/wk for 4 wk, then 10 MU SC TIW for 12 mo Arm 2: 10 MU SC, 5 days/wk for 4 wk, then 5 MU SC TIW for 24 mo Arm 3: Observation	Data not yet available	T >4 mm or positive regional nodes (n = 1,418)
Scandinavian Cooperative	IFN-α-2b	Arm 1: 10 MU SC, 5 days/wk for 4 wk, then 10 MU SC TIW for 12 mo Arm 2: 10 MU SC, 5 days/wk for 4 wk, then 10 MU SC TIW for 24 mo Arm 3: Observation	Data not yet available	T >4 mm or positive regional nodes (n = 575)

IM, intramuscularly; TIW, three times/wk; DFS, disease-free survival; OS, overall survival; NS, no statistically significant difference; T, thickness; IV, intravenously; SC, subcutaneously; QOD, every other day.

ity-of-life-adjusted survival time and cost of quality-adjusted life-year gained. In the Q-TWIST study, investigators compared the time patients gained without relapse and overall survival between the treatment and observation groups.[152] The IFN group gained a median of 8.9 months without relapse and 7 months of overall survival time. The treated group experienced severe treatment-related side effects for an average of 5.8 months. The net result was that patients in the IFN-treated group had more quality-adjusted survival time than the observation group. This analysis was retrospective and relied on the clinicians' reporting of side effects experienced when determining time with symptoms.

Cost analysis of the data also determined that benefits of IFN over a lifetime yielded incremental cost per life-year or quality-adjusted life-year of less than $16,000 for both.[153] This compares favorably with the Canadian benchmark of $20,000 per quality of life-year gained, identifying a meaningful intervention.

To confirm the positive result of ECOG 1684 as well as to explore the benefit of low-dose IFN-α-2b, a prospective, randomized, three-arm, multi-institutional trial (ECOG 1690) was carried out.[154] After surgical resection, 642 patients with stage IIB or III melanoma were randomly assigned to receive high-dose IFN-α-2b for 1 year (same regimen as in ECOG 1684), low-dose IFN-α-2b at 3 MU given subcutaneously three times a week for 2 years, or observation. Unlike ECOG 1684, patients with T4 lesions (more than 4 mm thick) and clinically negative nodal disease were not required to undergo lymphadenectomy. At a median follow-up of 4 years, adjuvant high-dose IFN-α-2b continued to show a relapse-free survival benefit compared to observation, but the positive impact on overall survival previously observed in ECOG 1684 was lost. The improvement in relapse-free survival was seen regardless of nodal status. In contrast to high-dose IFN-α-2b, the low-dose regimen did not influence relapse-free or overall survival compared to observation. Of note, patients in the observation arm in ECOG 1690 lived significantly longer than those in ECOG 1684, with median overall survival of 6 years versus 2.8 years, respectively. The reasons for this striking difference could be more accurate staging methods, improved surgical management initially or at relapse, and better post-relapse systemic therapies.[154] These variations could explain the loss of survival advantage of high-dose IFN-α-2b in ECOG 1690.

A pooled analysis of these two ECOG trials was performed using data updated to April 2001.[155] This evaluation confirmed the relapse-free survival benefit associated with high-dose IFN-α-2b for high-risk patients with melanoma. Again, the overall survival outcome was not improved compared to observation. Of interest, statistical evaluation of these two studies also suggested that most clinical benefit of high-dose IFN-α might be obtained from the intravenous induction phase. Therefore, trials have been initiated to test this theory, comparing 1 month of intravenous IFN-α-2b to either observation or 1-year of high-dose interferon (ECOG regimen) in similar patient populations.

High-dose IFN-α is a toxic treatment regimen. Toxicities occurring in more than 20% of patients receiving high-dose IFN in the ECOG regimen consisted of fatigue (96%), neutropenia (92%), fever (81%), myalgia (75%), anorexia (69%), vomiting/nausea (66%), increased serum glutamic-oxaloacetic transaminase (SGOT) levels (63%), headache (62%), chills (54%), depression (40%), diarrhea (35%), alopecia (29%), altered taste sensation (24%), dizziness/vertigo (23%), and anemia (22%).[150] Severe, life-threatening toxicities (ECOG grade 3 or 4) occurring in greater than 10% of patients included neutropenia/leukopenia (26%), fatigue (23%), fever (18%), myalgia (17%), headache (17%), chills (16%), and increased SGOT (14%).[150] Management of these side effects is crucial in maintaining quality of life for the patient and requires an intimate knowledge of the characteristics and treatment of events that can positively affect quality of life.

In summary, it is clear that adjuvant high-dose IFN-α-2b (ECOG regimen) has a positive impact on relapse-free survival in high-risk patients, but it is difficult to determine whether it improves the overall survival outcome of these patients. Considering the serious toxicities associated with high-dose IFN-α-2b, oncologists are still debating whether adjuvant IFN-α-2b should be part of the standard of care for patients with thick primary melanomas (more than 4 mm) or positive nodal involvement. However, since the FDA has not withdrawn the indication for postoperative IFN-α-2b in high-risk patients with melanoma, it is prudent for the clinicians to discuss this option with patients when developing a treatment plan.

To avoid the serious toxicities of high-dose IFN-α, many investigators have examined the role of a low-dose regimen (1 to 3 MU given subcutaneously three times a week) in the adjuvant setting. Low-dose IFN has fewer adverse events and is tolerated by most patients. Adverse events occurring most frequently with low-dose IFN are mild to moderate in severity and include flu-like symptoms (fever, headache, chills, myalgia) and fatigue.

The WHO Melanoma Programme Trial 16 randomized 426 patients with resected nodal disease to receive IFN-α-2a 3 MU subcutaneously three times a week for 3 years or observation.[156] Initial results indicated a relapse-free survival benefit, but on further follow-up, relapse-free and overall survival rates were no different between the treatment and observation arms. As expected, low-dose IFN was well tolerated, with no grade 3 or 4 toxicity. Similar findings were reported by three other European studies evaluating postoperative low-dose IFN in a high-risk population.[157–159] As mentioned before, the low-dose regimen influenced neither relapse-free nor overall survival compared to observation in the ECOG 1690 trial.[153]

Two European trials examined the role of adjuvant low-dose IFN-α in patients with intermediate-risk melanoma.[160,161] Both of these studies showed a beneficial effect of low-dose IFN therapy on relapse-free survival but not on overall survival. These results have led to the approval of low-dose IFN for intermediate-risk patients with melanoma in Europe. However, the FDA did not approve this regimen for the same indication based on the lack of overall survival benefit.[162]

In general, it is agreed that adjuvant low-dose IFN is not superior to observation alone in patients with high-risk melanoma. However, it may serve to delay disease recurrence in intermediate-risk patients, even though this relapse-free survival benefit does not translate into an overall survival advantage.

Because high-dose IFN has significant toxicities and low-dose IFN regimens lack clinical benefit, investigators are now examining the intermediate dose range of IFN in the adjuvant treatment of melanoma patients. Two phase III trials are being conducted by the European Organization for the Research and Treatment of Cancer (EORTC) and the Scandinavian Melanoma Cooperative Group.[162,163] Patients in these trials are randomized to observation or IFN at 10 MU given subcutaneously five times a week for 1 month followed by 5 to 10 MU given subcutaneously three times a week for 12 to 24 months. Results from these trials are forthcoming.

Pegylated IFN-α is a covalent conjugate of straight-chain polyethylene glycol and recombinant IFN-α. Linkage with polyethylene glycol reduces the clearance of IFN-α and may enhance its efficacy due to more prolonged exposure. The EORTC is conducting a randomized controlled trial to examine the efficacy of 5-years of pegylated IFN-α-2b versus observation in node-positive patients.

Adjuvant Biochemotherapy. Biochemotherapy is a combination of chemotherapy with the biologicals IL-2 and IFN-α. It will be discussed in detail under the management of metastatic melanoma. Recently, a phase III trial comparing adjuvant biochemotherapy to high-dose IFN-α in high-risk patients with melanoma (stage IIIB-C) has completed recruitment. Until there are conclusive data to establish the benefit of adjuvant biochemotherapy, this treatment regimen is considered investigational and should not be offered to patients outside a clinical trial setting.

Granulocyte/Macrophage Colony-Stimulating Factor. Granulocyte/macrophage colony-stimulating factor (GM-CSF, Sargramostim) is a hematopoietic growth factor that preferentially stimulates the granulocyte/macrophage progenitor cells. Recombinant GM-CSF is currently used clinically to shorten the time to neutrophil recovery and reduce the incidence of severe and life-threatening infections following myelosuppressive chemotherapy. Also, there is evidence that GM-CSF can potentiate the cytotoxicity of monocytes and macrophages as well as enhance antigen presentation by dendritic cells.

An open-label, multicenter, phase II trial was carried out to examine the role of this cytokine as adjuvant therapy to prolong survival in patients with stage III or IV malignant melanoma.[164] Forty-eight patients who were clinically disease-free as a result of surgical resection of nodal or meta-

static disease received GM-CSF at 125 μg per m² given subcutaneously daily for 14 days followed by 14 days of rest for a total of 1 year or until disease recurrence. Treatment result was compared to matched historical controls. The median survival was significantly longer in patients who received GM-CSF compared to the control group (37.5 months and 12.2 months; $p < 0.001$) with 1-year survival rates of 89% versus 45% ($p < 0.001$) and 2-year survival rates of 64% versus 15% ($p < 0.001$), respectively. These rates remained significant when patients were stratified according to disease stage. GM-CSF was well tolerated, with adverse events including transient myalgias, weakness, mild fatigue, rash, and mild erythema at the injection site.

Because of the potential bias associated with the use of historical controls in that study, a phase III randomized controlled trial has been initiated to evaluate the benefit of GM-CSF at a similar dosing schedule in patients with resected stage III or IV disease.

Melanoma Vaccines. Melanoma is the tumor type most likely to undergo spontaneous regression (up to 3% to 4% of lesions), leading to the belief that the body has an antitumor defense mechanism that is functional against some melanomas. This has led researchers to investigate the immune system as a potential target for therapy and modulation of the natural history of this disease. Development of melanoma vaccines represents one approach in this vast area of research.

The goal of a vaccine is to stimulate the host's immune system to reject the targeted diseased cell, in this case melanoma cells (specific immunotherapy). Nonspecific immunotherapy uses agents such as intact microorganisms, haptens, or protein products to stimulate the immune system without targeting specific tumor antigens (termed an *adjuvant*). Specific and nonspecific immunotherapeutics are often given together to maximize immune response.[145] The number and type of potential antigen targets present on the melanoma cell surface varies between patients and between cells within the same tumor nodule.[145] This fact makes the development of a specific vaccine that would be generally applicable a very difficult task. The identification of several cell-surface melanoma antigens has allowed for expansion of this technology.

Various forms of vaccines are under investigation, ranging from complex mixtures of antigens, such as whole-cell vaccines, to purified single antigens. Whole-cell vaccines may be derived from autologous or allogeneic (pooled) tumor cells and can be intact or lysed. Newer vaccine approaches include DNA vaccines and dendritic cell vaccines. DNA vaccines are nucleic acid sequences encoding for tumor antigen proteins that can be administered alone as naked DNA or incorporated into viral vectors. Dendritic cells are powerful antigen-presenting cells that can effectively activate T lymphocytes. Dendritic cell vaccines are made by in vitro loading of the dendritic cells with tumor antigens.[165]

CancerVax is a whole-cell vaccine that is made of three irradiated allogeneic melanoma cell lines. Positive results from early phase II studies have prompted two ongoing phase III trials, one for patients with resected stage III disease and the other for those with resected stage IV disease. In both studies, patients are randomized to receive either CancerVax with BCG or BCG alone.[165]

Melacine is a lysate vaccine consisting of two allogeneic melanoma cell lines. The result of a large phase III trial (n = 689) using this immunotherapeutic agent was recently reported by the Southwest Oncology Group (SWOG).[166] Patients with clinically or pathologically node-negative melanoma with tumor thickness 1.5 to 4 mm were randomized to either observation or Melacine with DETOX. DETOX, used as an immunologic adjuvant, is a mixture of monophosphoryl lipid A and mycobacterial cell wall skeleton in an oil-in-water emulsion. After a median follow-up of 5.6 years, no difference in disease-free survival was found between the two treatment arms. Overall survival data were not mature enough to be evaluated at the time of publication. Of interest, the SWOG investigators also carried out a separate prospectively planned analysis to examine the association between patients' HLA phenotypes and clinical responses to Melacine.[167] Compared with the observation group, a significant improvement in relapse-free survival was noted in vaccine-treated patients who expressed at least two of the following HLA class I antigens: HLA-A2, HLA-A28, HLA-B44, HLA-B45, and HLA-C3 (5-year disease-free survival 83% versus 59%, $p = 0.0002$). This result has driven the SWOG to plan another phase III trial to re-examine the benefit of Melacine in this specific patient subgroup.

Melacine was also compared to combination chemotherapy (cisplatin, dacarbazine, carmustine, and tamoxifen, also known as the Dartmouth regimen) in patients with metastatic disease.[168] Melacine (plus DETOX) was administered as a two-shot vaccination given intramuscularly once a week for 5 weeks, with a 2-week break, and then a repeat of the weekly vaccinations for 5 weeks. Responders could receive maintenance therapy of one vaccination per month. Cyclophosphamide at 300 mg per m² given intravenously was given 3 days before immunization on weeks 1 and 8. No difference in survival outcome was observed between the two groups. However, quality-of-life measures were significantly better in the vaccine-treated group because Melacine induced much less toxicity than chemotherapy. This led to the approval of Melacine for the treatment of metastatic melanoma in Canada.

Autologous vaccine is composed of irradiated tumor cells harvested from the patient's own tumor. This approach has the advantage of eliciting an immune response against unique melanoma antigens caused by mutations specific to the patient's tumor. However, this vaccine type is not very immunogenic because autologous tumor antigens may have already escaped the surveillance of the patient's own immune system. Another limitation is that the tumor must be surgically accessible to harvest, and large enough for suffi-cient vaccine production. Furthermore, the preparation process is logistically and technically complex, making large-scale clinical testing difficult. To date, results from small phase II trials are mixed regarding to the impact of autologous vaccines on survival outcome.[165]

Gangliosides are glycosphingolipids present in the plasma membrane. Purified GM2, the most immunogenic ganglioside commonly expressed on melanoma cells, can be used as a melanoma vaccine. Early studies showed that GM2 vaccine given in conjunction with BCG could induce antibody responses in most patients. More importantly, seropositivity was associated with improved disease-free and relapse-free survival rates.[169] To enhance the vaccine's immunogenicity, GM2 was attached to a carrier protein called keyhole limpet hemocyanin (KLH) and combined with the adjuvant QS-21. This new formulation was referred to as the GMK vaccine. In 1996, a large randomized trial was launched to compare the efficacy of GMK vaccine to high-dose IFN-α-2b (ECOG regimen) in approximately 800 patients with thick primary lesions (more than 4 mm) or nodal disease.[170] The trial was closed early when the interim analysis indicated that both disease-free and overall survival rates were inferior in the vaccine-treated group.

Metastatic Melanoma

Chemotherapy. Currently, the only role for systemic chemotherapy in melanoma is for treatment of metastatic disease. Conventional chemotherapy has little activity against melanoma. Many agents have minimal activity, with response rates of 10% to 20%. Dacarbazine (DTIC) is the most active single-agent chemotherapy for melanoma, with responses seen in 20% of patients.[147] Median duration of response is approximately 4 to 6 months. Although prolongation of survival is questionable with chemotherapy, palliation of symptoms can be accomplished in some patients, improving their quality of life if the chemotherapy is tolerable.

DTIC is a severe emetogenic agent, with up to 90% of patients vomiting in the absence of premedication with strong antiemetics before treatment. Serotonin antagonists have improved this toxicity, and the addition of dexamethasone to the antiemetic regimen decreases nausea and emesis further. A flu-like syndrome can occur with large single doses of dacarbazine, manifesting as fever, myalgia, and malaise. The onset is within 7 days, and it can last up to 3 weeks.[171] Myelosuppression is mild to moderate and dose-related and predominantly affects the granulocytes and platelets. Alopecia, facial flushing, facial paresthesias, and hepatic toxicity are rarely reported.[164]

DTIC may be given in a number of different schedules and dosages. The most common regimens are (a) 800 to 1,000 mg per m² as a bolus injection given once and (b) 250 mg/m²/day for 5 days as daily bolus injections. These treatment regimens are repeated every 3 to 4 weeks. There is no difference in response rates with these schedules, but there is less nausea and vomiting with lower, daily doses.

Temozolomide, an oral derivative of dacarbazine, has recently been approved for the treatment of refractory anaplastic astrocytoma. Compared to dacarbazine, temozolomide has excellent oral bioavailability and improved penetration of the central nervous system, with equal efficacy and activity. The clinical activity of temozolomide against melanoma was confirmed in a large randomized study, when patients were treated with a 5-day schedule of either dacarbazine or temozolomide.[172] Also, phase I/II studies with temozolomide have shown that significantly higher doses of temozolomide could be administered using the protracted dose schedules, such as daily doses for 21 days every 4 weeks or for 6 weeks repeated every 8 weeks.[173] Temozolomide is also being actively studied for the prevention and treatment of central nervous system involvement from malignant melanoma. In the above-mentioned randomized phase III trial comparing temozolomide and dacarbazine in patients with advanced metastatic melanoma, patients who responded to temozolomide had a four times lower incidence of melanoma relapse in the brain than did patients who responded to dacarbazine.[174] In two additional studies, the ability of temozolomide to prevent relapse in the central nervous system was again shown in patients with advanced melanoma receiving treatment regimens incorporating temozolomide.[175,176] More importantly, the clinical utility of temozolomide against intracranial melanoma extends beyond prevention of relapse in the central nervous system: remarkable responses in the brain and meninges have been observed in a number of patients with metastatic melanoma.[177-180]

Nitrosoureas are less active than DTIC but are widely used in combination regimens. Carmustine (BCNU), lomustine (CCNU), and semustine (methyl-CCNU) are most extensively studied in melanoma. These agents are lipid-soluble and cross the blood–brain barrier, but they usually lack significant activity against melanoma brain metastases.[147] In contrast, fotemustine, a new nitrosourea, has induced some measurable responses in melanoma brain lesions. In two phase II trials, 184 patients were treated with fotemustine; 40 (22%) responses were noted, including 4 complete responses, and 11 of the responses were in brain metastases.[181,182]

Vinca alkaloids have been shown to have some activity against melanoma and are often used in combination regimens. Vindesine is used largely in Europe, where it is commercially available, and vinblastine is more commonly used in the United States.[147]

Among the platinum-based agents, cisplatin is a common component of various combination chemotherapy regimens for metastatic melanoma. Cisplatin, in standard doses (50 to 100 mg/m^2), has shown only minimal responses, but in higher doses (60 to 150 mg/m^2) with amifostine (WR2721, Ethyol), response rates of 53% were seen.[183] However, the median duration of response was 4 months, and no complete responses were shown. Carboplatin, a derivative of cisplatin, has shown minimal activity (11% response rate) against melanoma as a single agent.[184]

Paclitaxel appears to have fairly promising activity against melanoma. In a review of clinical phase II studies of paclitaxel in metastatic melanoma, 73 patients were evaluable, with overall response rates of 16% and stable disease in an additional 14% of patients.[185] The median duration of response was approximately 5 months (range 1 to 17 months), no different from historical controls. Docetaxel, a derivative of paclitaxel, has been evaluated in a phase II trial and showed a 17% response rate (5 partial responses out of 30 patients).[186]

Combination Chemotherapy. Various combination chemotherapy regimens have been explored in the treatment of metastatic melanoma during the past 25 years. Some common regimens that show activity are listed in Table 103.17. Despite their improved response rates of 30% to 40%,[147] none of these regimens are superior to dacarbazine alone in improving overall survival. Moreover, the utility of these regimens is often limited by the short duration of responses, low complete-response rates, and significant toxicity.

High doses of chemotherapy with autologous bone marrow support have been investigated for metastatic melanoma. Overall responses have ranged from 40% to 65%, with complete response rates around 10%.[147] Unfortunately, this approach has shown no survival advantage. The toxicity of these regimens makes the risk-to-benefit ratio unacceptable at this time, preventing the endorsement of such treatment outside the context of a clinical trial.

Immunotherapy. Melanoma is the tumor type most likely to undergo spontaneous regression (up to 3% to 4% of lesions), leading to the belief that the body has an antitumor defense mechanism that is functional against some melanomas. This has directed researchers to investigate the immune system as a potential target for therapy and modulation of the natural history of this disease.

IFN-α was one of the first immunotherapies developed to augment the body's immune system. The mechanism of its antitumor activity is complex, including a direct cytostatic property, an antiangiogenic effect, and immunostimulatory activity.[187] Initial results with natural purified IFN-α showed infrequent responses, but responses with recombinant human IFN-α have been much better (average 20%).[147] The best results are seen with doses in the range of 10 to 12 MU/m^2/day, given intravenously, intramuscularly, or subcutaneously.[147]

The most common adverse effects associated with IFN-α are a flu-like syndrome consisting of myalgias, fever, headache, chills, and anorexia. With continued treatment, patients generally experience a decrease in these symptoms. Premedication with acetaminophen has proven to be helpful in tolerating standard doses (3 to 6 MU/m^2). With high doses (greater than 6 MU/m^2), these effects are intensified and prolonged, leading to less symptom relief with acetaminophen premedication. Neutropenia and increases in serum transaminases occur infrequently but may require discontinuation of therapy. In contrast to the adjuvant data discussed

TABLE 103.17	Commonly Used Chemotherapy for Metastatic Melanoma	
Regimen	**Agents**	**Dose and Schedule**
Dacarbazine	Dacarbazine	850–1,000 mg/m^2 IV on day 1, every 3 wk
Temozolomide	Temozolomide	200 mg/m^2/day for 5 days, every 4 wk
CVD	Cisplatin	20 mg/m^2/day IV for 4 days, days 2–5
	Vinblastine	1.6 mg/m^2/day IV for 5 days, days 1–5
	Dacarbazine	800 mg/m^2/day for 1 day, day 1
		Repeat every 3–4 wk.
CBDT (Dartmouth)	Cisplatin	25 mg/m^2/day IV for 3 days, days 1–3
	BCNU	150 mg/m^2/day IV for 1 day, day 1, given every other cycle
	DTIC	220 mg/m^2/day IV for 3 days, days 1–3
	Tamoxifen	20 mg PO daily continuously
		Repeat every 3 weeks (except BCNU, give every other cycle).
Temozolomide/ Thalidomide	Temozolomide Thalidomide	75 mg/m^2/day PO daily for 6 wk, followed by 2-wk rest 100 mg PO daily escalated to 200 mg PO daily continuously (patients 70 yr of age) or 200 mg PO daily escalated to 400 mg PO daily continuously (patients <70 yr)
Biochemotherapy	Cisplatin	20 mg/m^2/day IV for 4 days, days 1–4
	Vinblastine	1.5 mg/m^2/day IV for 4 days, days 1–4
	Dacarbazine	800 mg/m^2/day for 1 day, day 1
	Interleukin-2	9 MU/m^2/day IVCI for 4 days, days 1–4
	Interferon-α-2b	5 MU/m^2/day SC for 5 days, days 1–5
High-dose IL-2	IL-2	600,000–720,000 units/kg IV bolus q8h for max 14 doses per cycle

IV, intravenous; PO, oral; IVCI, intravenous continuous infusion; SC, subcutaneous.

earlier, the different types of IFN-α (2a, 2b) seem to have similar activity against metastatic melanoma.

IL-2, initially referred to as T-cell growth factor, is produced by lymphocytes and is responsible for many immunoregulatory functions. IL-2 can amplify immune responses by promoting growth of activated T-cells and natural killer (NK) cells, resulting in enhancement of both specific and nonspecific antitumor cytotoxicity. Specific antitumor cytotoxicity is T-cell-mediated, whereas nonspecific antitumor cytotoxicity is mediated by NK cells. Also related to the amplification of the immune response is the induction of other cytokines, including TNF-α and IFN-γ. IL-2 does not have any direct antitumor activity, but rather acts through immunologic modulation to kill cancer cells. This was the first agent to show that an immunologic intervention can induce significant anticancer effects.

High-dose bolus IL-2 is the only biologic agent approved by the FDA for the treatment of metastatic melanoma, based on the result of a single-arm study conducted by Rosenberg et al.[188,189] In this trial, patients with stage IV disease received IL-2 at 720,000 IU per kg intravenously every 8 hours for a maximum of 14 doses per cycle. Overall and complete response rates were 17% and 7%, respectively. More re-

markable was the fact that most of these complete responses were durable.[188,189] Responses to IL-2 may be delayed, with initial increases in tumor volume secondary to inflammation. Of these responses, a greater proportion (usually one third) are complete compared with conventional chemotherapy.

Although no direct comparisons have been performed, in general the response rates, quality, and duration of responses are superior with high-dose IL-2 compared with lower-dose regimens. In a report of the experience of the NCI Surgery Branch with the use of high-dose IL-2, tumor response appeared to correlate with the amount of IL-2 delivered.[190] Different doses, schedules, and routes of IL-2 have been investigated to try to maximize the antitumor response while minimizing toxicity. Low-dose bolus injections, continuous infusion, or subcutaneous administration have all been attempted, but the response duration appears to be shorter, with fewer complete responses.[191]

High-dose IL-2 is a highly toxic regimen, with a mortality rate of up to 4% when it was introduced into clinical practice.[192] Life-threatening multiple-organ system toxicity is commonly associated with high-dose IL-2, requiring specialized units capable of providing intensive care and management of these toxicities. Table 103.18 is a partial list of the

TABLE 103.18	Adverse Events Associated with High-Dose Interleukin-2	
Adverse Event	**Associated Symptoms**	**Management**
Capillary leak syndrome	Fluid retention, weight gain, pulmonary edema, hypotension	Administer vasopressors (pure α-sympathomimetic agent) and fluid support for hypotension
Cardiac	Arrhythmias, decreased myocardial contractility, angina, myocardial infarction	Manage capillary leak and treat any arrhythmias appropriately
Neurologic	Paresthesias, constipation, confusion, agitation, hallucinations, lethargy, somnolence, seizures, coma	May have to discontinue therapy; may take a few days to reverse after discontinuation, but are fully reversible
Renal dysfunction	Oliguria, azotemia	Renal-dose dopamine to enhance renal blood flow
Gastrointestinal	Nausea, vomiting, diarrhea, stomatitis	Prophylactic antiemetics (nausea/vomiting), diphenoxylate+atropine (diarrhea), and histamine-2 blockers (gastrointestinal ulceration/ bleeding
Elevations in liver function tests	Transient increases in aminotransferases, alkaline phosphatases, and total bilirubin	May require discontinuation of therapy; usually return to normal a few days after discontinuation
Hematologic	Anemia, thrombocytopenia, leukopenia in first few days (secondary to demargination); then rebound leukocytosis	Monitor for signs/symptoms of infections, especially related to central venous access devices; erythropoietin may be beneficial for anemia.
Constitutional symptoms	Fever, chills, myalgias, arthralgias, fatigue	Premedicate with acetaminophen or indomethacin[a]
Other	Hypothyroidism, rash	May require discontinuation of therapy; rash seen with subcutaneous administration at injection site

[a] Indomethacin may exacerbate the renal dysfunction associated wtih interleukin-2 and may be detrimental to the patient.

most common toxicities associated with high-dose IL-2 and their management. The toxicity profile of this agent is believed to be mediated by lymphoid infiltration, capillary leak syndrome, and the local effects of secondary cytokines.[192] Although corticosteroids can ameliorate IL-2 toxicity, they may also diminish its antitumor effects and thus are contraindicated in patients receiving IL-2.[191] Low-dose dopamine has been used to prevent IL-2-induced renal insufficiency, but its actual benefit remains an area of debate.[191,192] Careful patient selection and a knowledge of the details of administration and toxicity management are required to improve the therapeutic index of this regimen.[192] Nevertheless, many patients cannot tolerate the toxicity and prefer to discontinue therapy, while some patients develop severe, life-threatening toxicity that mandates discontinuation. With a better understanding of the incidence and management of IL-2-associated adverse events, these regimens can now be safely administered by experienced clinicians.[193]

Combination Immunotherapy. Combining IL-2 and IFN has been largely unsuccessful, resulting in short responses in 8% to 15% of patients. An exception to this has been the regimen developed by Keilholz et al,[194] consisting of "decrescendo" IL-2 and IFN. In the decrescendo schedule, IL-2 was delivered at 18 MU per m^2 over 6 hours, followed by 18 MU per m^2 over 12 hours, then 18 MU per m^2 over 24 hours, and thereafter 4.5 MU/m^2/day for 3 consecutive days. This regimen used a fixed dose of IFN-α (10 MU/m^2/ day given subcutaneously for 5 days). A 41% response rate

was found with the "decrescendo" schedule compared with a fixed dose of IL-2 at 18 MU/m^2/day for 5 days of 18%. Although this was not a randomized comparison, these results are intriguing. In a prospective randomized trial comparing IL-2 alone versus IL-2 plus IFN-α-2a, no significant improvement in response was found with the addition of IFN.[195]

Combination Biochemotherapy. Single-agent chemotherapy is minimally effective against metastatic melanoma, and combination chemotherapy regimens have not proven better than single-agent dacarbazine. The potential advantage in combining chemotherapy with immunotherapy lies in the hope that different mechanisms of action will enhance the rate and duration of responses. Many different combinations of chemo- and immunotherapy have been investigated around the world. In early phase II studies, biochemotherapy resulted in response rates in the range of 50% to 60%, with about 7% to 15% complete responses; this was much higher than chemotherapy or biotherapy alone (historical controls).[196,197] However, the impact of biochemotherapy on survival remains controversial.

Eton et al conducted a prospective randomized trial comparing chemotherapy with sequential biochemotherapy (Table 103.19) in patients with metastatic melanoma.[198] The response rate in the biochemotherapy-treated group was superior (48% versus 25%, $p = 0.001$), but this higher response rate did not translate into an overall survival advantage. Median survival was 11.9 months with biochemo-

TABLE 103.19	Legha Biochemotherapy Sequential Regimen							
	CVD				**Biotherapy**			
Cisplatin	20 mg/m²/day IV × 4 days			IFN-α	5 MU/m² SC × 5 days			
Vinblastine	1.6 mg/m²/day IV × 5 days			IL-2	3 MU/m² IV CI over 24 hr × 4 days			
Dacarbazine	800 mg/m²/ IV × 1 day							
DAY:	**1–5**	**6–11**	**12–16**	**17–22**	**23–26**	**27–32**	**33–42**	**43–48**
	CVD Course 1	BIO	Break	BIO	CVD	BIO	Break	CVD Course 2

Only sequential therapy (CVD followed by BIO), shown here, has been superior to CVD alone.
BIO, biotherapy; CI, continuous infusion; IFN-α, interferon-α; IL-2, interleukin-2; IV, intravenous; MU, million units; SC, subcutaneous.

therapy versus 9.2 months with chemotherapy alone ($p = 0.06$). Biochemotherapy marginally improved time to disease progression (4.9 months versus 2.4 months, $p = 0.008$).

A large phase III trial was carried out by the U.S. Intergroup to examine the role of biochemotherapy in the management of stage IV melanoma.[199] Patients were randomly assigned to receive chemotherapy (CVD) alone or concurrent with IL-2 and IFN-α. No statistically significant differences in response rate, progression-free survival, and overall survival were noted between the two arms.

It is important to mention that biochemotherapy is a toxic regimen, requiring hospital admission for treatment delivery. Severe, life-threatening side effects (ECOG grade 3 or 4) include hypotension (39%), fluid retention (11%), nausea (25%), fever above 40°C (24%), neutropenia (100%), anemia (68%), and thrombocytopenia (89%).[198] Considering the cost and the toxicity of this regimen in the absence of convincing benefit on survival outcome, most oncologists remain reluctant to accept biochemotherapy as the standard of care for stage IV melanoma.

Other Agents. Thalidomide is a compound with many potential mechanisms of action. It was first used as a sedative in the 1950s but was withdrawn in 1961 because of teratogenic effects. Recently, thalidomide has been shown to interfere with the expression or release of several angiogenic factors, including TNF-α and IL-6, from renal cells and may interfere indirectly with vascular endothelial growth factor (VEGF) and bFGF in the rabbit corneal micropocket assay.[200,201] Besides its antiangiogenic activity, thalidomide exerts several immunomodulatory effects. These include alteration of adhesion molecule expression, increased production of IL-10, and enhancement of cell-mediated immunity via direct co-stimulation of T-cells, resulting in increased IFN-γ and IL-12 production.[202,203]

With antiangiogenic and immunomodulatory activities, thalidomide may theoretically have a role in the management of melanoma. In fact, thalidomide was reported to induce a complete response in a 63-year-old patient with in-transit metastases localized to the scalp.[204] Unfortunately, the clinical activity of single-agent thalidomide in melanoma was shown to be marginal at best.[205]

Despite its modest activity against melanoma, because of its antiangiogenic and immunomodulatory properties, thalidomide has the potential to enhance the therapeutic efficacy of other agents. For example, thalidomide has been combined with temozolomide in a phase II trial involving 38 chemotherapy-naïve patients with unresectable stage III or IV melanoma without brain metastases.[206] Temozolomide was given at 75 mg/m²/day for 6 weeks every 8 weeks. Thalidomide was initiated at 100 mg per day and increased to a maximum daily dose of 250 mg in patients 70 years of age and up. Younger patients were started at 200 mg of thalidomide daily with dose escalation up to 400 mg per day. Twelve objective tumor responses (1 complete, 11 partial) were observed. Five of the 11 partial responses were later converted to complete responses surgically. Median duration of response was 5 months (range 2 to 25 + months). Overall median survival was 9.5 months (range 3 to 21.7 months). Of note, in this trial, brain metastases developed in 24% of the patients, a rate that compared quite favorably to the historical incidence of brain involvement of about 50%.[207] More remarkable, this combination has been shown to induce central nervous system responses in patients with metastatic melanoma.[208,209]

Thalidomide, up to 400 mg daily, is generally well tolerated, with common side effects including somnolence, dizziness, headache, and constipation. These side effects can be minimized by slow escalation of the dose, bedtime administration, and use of stool softeners and/or a mild laxative. Dryness of the mouth, skin rash, weight gain, personality changes, and thromboembolic events have also been observed.[210] Peripheral neuropathy may occur, with symptoms of paresthesias of the hands and feet, pallor and coldness of fingers and toes, and extremity cramps. Resolution of side effects usually occurs when therapy is discontinued, but symptoms have persisted in a few cases.[210]

The bcl-2 gene product is a 239 amino acid integral-membrane mitochondrial protein that inhibits apoptosis.[211,212] It has been shown to mediate the growth and development of a number of solid tumors as well as to confer chemoresistance to cancer cells.[213,214] In melanoma, overexpression of Bcl-2 has been shown in primary and metastatic lesions.[215] This phenotype has also been linked to tumor progression.[215]

Antisense oligonucleotides are synthetic oligonucleotides that are complementary to specific mRNA transcripts. Antisense oligonucleotides form high-affinity covalent bonds with mRNA, inhibiting RNA splicing, impeding translation, and rendering the complex susceptible to degradation by RNAse-H.[216] G3139 (Oblimersen, Genasense) is an 18-mer phosphorothioate oligonucleotide that targets the first six codons of the bcl-2 mRNA open reading frame to form a DNA/RNA duplex.[217] RNAse-H recognizes the duplex, cleaves the bcl-2 mRNA strand, and renders the message nontranslatable. bcl-2 mRNA fragments are subsequently destroyed by ribonucleases.

Preclinical studies both in vitro and in vivo have shown that bcl-2 mRNA and protein are specifically downregulated by G3139, an effect not observed with reverse control or two-base-mismatch control oligonucleotides.[218,219] More importantly, biologic and antitumor activity of G3139 has been observed at submicromolar concentrations (e.g., 170 nanomolar), which are easily achieved in the plasma of patients treated systemically.[220]

Antitumor activity of G3139 in combination with standard-dose dacarbazine (DTIC) has been shown in 24 patients with advanced metastatic melanoma.[217] Daily intravenous infusion of G3139 at doses ranging from 1.7 to 7 mg/kg/day led to a decreased bcl-2 protein level (median reduction of 40%) by day 5 of treatment based on Western blots of serially biopsied malignant lesions. In the first 14 patients evaluable for response, the clinical response rate was 43%, with one complete response and two partial responses. Of note, most patients entered the study with progressive disease after receiving first-line systemic DTIC or other therapy. The median survival has not been reached at the time of publication, but it is estimated to exceed 12 months, which compares favorably to the 4-month median survival reported in a recent multicenter trial for patients who failed to respond to first-line chemotherapy.

An open-label, multicenter phase III trial was conducted to confirm the clinical usefulness of G3139 in the management of unresectable stage III or stage IV melanoma.[221] Almost 800 patients were randomized to receive dacarbazine 1,000 mg/m² every 3 weeks alone or combined with G3139. In this trial, G3139 was administered at 7 mg/kg/day as a continuous infusion over a period of 5 days before DTIC. After a median follow-up of 7 months, pretreatment with bcl-2 antisense significantly improved the response rate (11.7% versus 6.8%, $p = 0.019$) and prolonged progression-free survival (74 days versus 49 days, $p = 0.0003$) compared to DTIC alone. Overall survival was not different between the two groups. For patients followed more than 18 months, median survival was significantly longer for patients in the combination arm (302 days versus 238 days, $p = 0.04$).[222]

Treatment with G3139 was well tolerated. Common side effects included transient fever, flushing sensation, rash, and fatigue. The fever and flushing resolved with oral acetaminophen despite continuation of G3139. Rash typically responded to antihistamines and recovered completely after temporary discontinuation of G3139. Liver function abnormalities, nonfasting hyperglycemia, and prolonged partial thromboplastin times occurred infrequently, were not clinically significant, and resolved within 1 week after the end of therapy. Hematologic toxicities, typically mild to moderate, were more likely secondary to concurrent cytotoxic agents.[217,221]

Recently, reactive oxygen species generated by monocytes and macrophages have been shown to inhibit IL-2-induced activation and proliferation of NK cells and T lymphocytes.[223] Histamine, acting via H-2 receptors on monocytes and macrophages, can prevent the production and release of oxygen free radicals.[224] Therefore, it can block or reverse the state of immunosuppression induced by oxidative stress.

Results of phase II studies suggested that histamine, when combined with IL-2 and/or IFN-α, could improve overall survival of patients with metastatic melanoma.[225,226] A phase III multicenter trial was initiated to compare the clinical benefit of histamine plus IL-2 versus IL-2 alone in the management of advanced melanoma.[227] About 300 patients were randomly assigned to IL-2 with or without histamine. In this trial, IL-2 was administered at 9 MU per m² given subcutaneously twice a day on days 1 and 2 of weeks 1 and 3 plus 2 MU per m² given subcutaneously twice a day on days 1 to 5 of weeks 2 and 4. Patients in the combination arm also received histamine at 1 mg given subcutaneously twice a day on days 1 to 5 of weeks 1 to 4. There was no difference in overall survival between the two treatment groups. However, subgroup analysis suggested a survival improvement in patients with liver metastases receiving the IL-2 and histamine combination. Adverse reactions specific to histamine were mild to moderate, consisting of flushing, palpitations, headache, injection site reactions, mild hypotension, and dyspepsia. Studies to further examine the role of histamine with IL-2 in patients with stage IV melanoma involving the liver are ongoing.

NO TREATMENT

Dismal responses to conventional treatment regimens and short survival spans bring to light the question of risks versus benefits. The treatment regimens being investigated carry considerable toxicity, especially regimens including high-dose IL-2. If the benefits of these regimens do not include increased overall survival with a good quality of life, the benefits may not be worth the risks. In fact, many clinicians would consider no treatment a reasonable option for patients with metastatic melanoma. Treatment with an investigational regimen in a controlled clinical trial is the only way to ensure that the options these patients have continue to expand.

SCREENING AND PREVENTION

A key factor in increasing overall survival with all types of skin cancer is early diagnosis, improving the odds of the patient evading subclinical metastases at the time of diagnosis. This is particularly true for melanoma, which, if detected early in its radial phase, is curable, but in its later stages is deadly. Key issues that make screening for a disease successful are (a) a sensitive and specific screening tool; (b) disease prevalence that is high enough to warrant screening; (c) potential outcomes that are serious enough to warrant the expense and effort of screening; (d) a disease that is relatively slow-growing and not immediately life-threatening; (e) a screening tool that is simple, inexpensive, and acceptable to the population being screened; (f) early diagnoses that result in better overall survival rates and improved prognoses; and (g) the screening should lead to more effective treatment at an earlier stage.[228] Skin cancer is one disease that meets all these criteria.

Screening for skin cancer consists of visual inspection of the skin and subsequent referral for biopsy and histologic evaluation of any suspicious lesion. For average-risk patients, the use of monthly self-examinations is adequate with self-referral to a physician if any suspicious lesion is found. For high-risk patients, a professional examination with mole mapping, documentation, and following of all skin lesions is key for early detection and a positive impact on mortality. The prevalence of skin cancer is obviously high enough to warrant mass screening. Free mass screening has been endorsed by the American Academy of Dermatology and the American Cancer Society. For example, in 2002, over 1 million individuals were screened, leading to the identification of 160,000 suspicious lesions, among which 15,550 were suggestive of melanomas. However, the efficacy of screening or early detection programs has not been tested in randomized trials.[229]

In conjunction with disease screening, public education efforts should bring together more effective prevention programs. Preventive medicine is based on the premise that the natural history of disease can be interrupted at three major points, preventing progression to the more severe stages of disease.[230] Primary prevention focuses on improving overall health and risk reduction. Secondary prevention in relation to cancer includes tools for screening and early diagnosis to detect early, more curable stages of cancer. Tertiary prevention refers to treatment of cancer patients to avoid complications and recurrences.

Since UV radiation exposure has been associated with skin cancer of all kinds, limiting exposure to UV radiation constitutes the first-line of defense. Ways to protect the skin from the damaging effects of solar UV radiation include wearing protective clothing and hats that cover the head, trunk, arms, and legs; seeking shade whenever possible; avoiding being outdoors during periods of peak sunlight (10 AM to 4 PM); and using a sunscreen with a sun protection factor (SPF) of 15 or higher.[231] However, photoprotection programs have not been proven unequivocally to decrease the incidence of skin cancer in humans. In Australia, the "Slip, Slop, Slap" campaign and SunSmart program have been linked to a reduction in BCC incidence in people less than 50 years of age.[232]

Chemoprevention is defined as the use of chemicals to interrupt the carcinogenic process. To date, the bulk of skin cancer chemoprevention data have been generated from trials using systemic and topical retinoids to target individuals at risk for developing NMSC. Prevention of new skin cancer lesions has been reported with oral isotretinoin, oral etretinate, and topical tretinoin in people with genetic dermatoses such as xeroderma pigmentosum and nevoid BCC syndrome.[233] The doses required to maintain prevention are high, and withdrawal of therapy leads to regression and loss of preventive activity.[233] Results from several phase III studies using lower-dose retinoids in lower-risk people have been inconsistent.

The Skin Cancer Prevention—Actinic Keratoses (SKICAP-AK) trial is a large, randomized, placebo-controlled study of chemoprevention with retinol in a moderate-risk population of 2,297 participants.[234] Oral retinol was given for 3 to 5 years at a dose of 20,000 IU daily. Patients enrolled had at least 10 AKs within the past year or no more than two prior SCCs or BCCs, resided in Arizona for at least 5 years, had a daily dietary intake of vitamin A of 10,000 IU or less, and did not have a diagnosis of xeroderma pigmentosum or basal cell nevus syndrome. A significant reduction in SCC but not BCC was noted in the retinol-treated group. The total number of new diagnoses of SCC was 113 in the retinol group and 136 in the placebo group [hazard ratio (HR) >0.74; 95% confidence intervals (CI) >0.56 to 0.99; $p > 0.04$]. Differences in the number of new diagnoses of BCC did not reach statistical significance between the retinol and placebo arms (HR >1.06; 95% CI >0.86 to 1.32; $p > 0.36$). The incidence of adverse events was not clearly outlined in this trial. The authors stated that the drug was well tolerated.

The Skin Cancer Prevention—Squamous Cell Skin Cancer and Basal Cell Skin Cancer (SKICAP-S/B) trial was a randomized, double-blind, controlled study assessing the effect of retinol and isotretinoin on the incidence of NMSC in 525 high-risk individuals.[235] Patients were randomly assigned to retinol (25,000 units daily), isotretinoin (5 or 10 mg daily based on weight), or placebo. Participants had at least four or more cutaneous BCCs or SCCs, with the most recent lesion diagnosed in the past year. Also, they could not have a diagnosis of xeroderma pigmentosum or basal cell nevus syndrome and must have planned to live in Arizona for the succeeding 3 years. There were no differences between the three arms with regard to time to the first new occurrence or to the total number of NMSC lesions.

Promising agents that have been tested in clinical trials for NMSC chemoprevention include difluoromethylornithine (DFMO),[236] Dimericine (T4 endonuclease V liposome lotion),[237] and topical diclofenac.[238] Studies with vitamin E, β-carotene, and selenium did not demonstrate significant protective effect in humans.[239,240] Numerous chemicals, such as polyphenolic antioxidants (major constituents of green tea or grape seed extracts), isoflavones (found in soybeans), and curcumin (ingredient of curry powder) are undergoing preclinical testing.[241]

CONCLUSION

In summary, the first-line defense against skin cancer development is avoidance of unprotected sun exposure. Regular screening to identify early lesions is also recommended. To date, the bulk of skin cancer chemoprevention data have been generated from trials focusing on NMSC. For NMSC, the role of chemoprevention remains unclear. Studies with positive results primarily target premalignant lesions (e.g., actinic keratoses), suggesting that chemoprevention may be more effective when initiated at the precancerous stage. Chemoprevention of melanoma continues to be an unexplored area.[242]

KEY POINTS

- Skin cancer is often a "forgotten cancer" because of its generally benign nature. However, the incidence and importance of this set of diseases is profound
- NMSC is not extremely threatening in terms of mortality, but it is highly detrimental in terms of morbidity and number of patients affected
- Melanoma is extremely life-threatening, especially in its later stages, and poses a great threat to the general population secondary to its rapidly increasing incidence

MANAGEMENT OF NMSC
- Treatment planning should take into account the type of skin cancer; anatomic location; size; general health and age of the patient; and whether the lesion is primary, recurrent, or metastatic
- SCCs generally require that a wider margin of normal tissue be removed to ensure optimal treatment
- Smaller BCC lesions may be removed with curettage followed by electrodesiccation
- Other treatment modalities are also used in some circumstances, including cryotherapy, Mohs' micrographic surgery, radiation, topical imiquimod, and chemotherapy (topical or systemic)
- Therapy for melanoma is more controversial, aggressive, and multidisciplinary

MANAGEMENT OF MELANOMA
- Surgical excision is the mainstay of therapy for all stages of melanoma

- Wide surgical margins are required for most lesions, with 1- to 2-cm margins being adequate for most primary lesions
- Elective lymphadenectomy is a controversial procedure and may not be associated with improved survival. Lymphatic mapping with sentinel lymph node biopsy and selective lymphadenectomy is often used to determine the nodal status of the area surrounding the tumor bed
- In addition to appropriate systemic therapy, surgical resection of involved lymph nodes and solitary visceral metastases is indicated in most cases
- Adjuvant therapy with IFN-α is FDA-approved for patients with thick primary lesions (more than 4 mm) or clinically positive lymph nodes after complete surgical resection of the primary lesion and any involved lymph nodes. However, its impact on survival remains debatable. The approved dose of IFN-α for adjuvant therapy of melanoma consists of a prolonged regimen with high doses that are associated with significant toxicity
- The most active single chemotherapy agent for the treatment of melanoma is dacarbazine. Temozolomide, an oral derivative of dacarbazine, has excellent oral bioavailability and improved penetration into the central nervous system, with equal efficacy and activity. A striking response in the central nervous system with a combination of temozolomide and thalidomide has been observed
- Combination chemotherapy has not shown superior efficacy compared with single-agent chemotherapy
- High-dose IL-2 is approved by the FDA for the treatment of metastatic melanoma. Durable responses are seen in a small number of patients. This regimen is highly toxic, requiring careful patient selection and vigilant monitoring
- Combination biochemotherapy has shown significantly greater activity compared with historical data for other types of treatment regimens. However, in phase III trials, its clinical benefit in terms of survival is marginal at best. Biochemotherapy is extremely toxic and often requires hospitalization for administration
- The detrimental outcome seen with lesions not amenable to surgery provides the impetus for the development of many new treatment modalities. These include new immunotherapies, chemotherapies, bcl2-antisense, and vaccines
- In conjunction with the search for novel therapies, the emphasis on prevention and screening is imperative

SUGGESTED READINGS

Balch CM, Reintgen DS, Kirkwood JM, et al. Cutaneous melanoma. In: DeVita VT, Hellman S, Rosenberg SA, eds. Cancer: principles and practice of oncology, 5th ed. Philadelphia: Lippincott-Raven, 1997: 1947–1994.

Brown CK, Kirkwood JM. Medical management of melanoma. Surg
Clin North Am 83:283–322, 2003.
Safai B. Management of skin cancer. In: DeVita VT, Hellman S, Rosen-
berg SA, eds. Cancer: principles and practice of oncology, 5th ed.
Philadelphia: Lippincott-Raven, 1997:1883–1933.

REFERENCES

1. Safai B. Management of skin cancer. In: DeVita VT, Hellman S,
Rosenberg SA, eds. Cancer: principles and practice of oncology,
5th ed. Philadelphia: Lippincott-Raven, 1997:1883–1933.
2. American Cancer Society. Cancer facts and figures 2004. Available
at http://www.cancer.org/docroot/STT/stt_0.asp.
3. Osterlind A. Etiology and epidemiology of melanoma and skin neoplasms. Curr Opin Oncol 3:355–359, 1991.
4. Roberts DL. Incidence of nonmelanoma skin cancer in West Gla-
morgan, South Wales. Br J Dermatol 122:399–404, 1990.
5. Emmett AJJ, O'Rourke MGE, eds. Malignant skin tumours. New
York: Churchill Livingstone, 1991:24.
6. Griffiths HR, Mistry P, Herbert KE, et al. Molecular and cellular
effects of ultraviolet light-induced genotoxicity. Crit Rev Clin Lab
Sci 35:189–237, 1998.
7. Brash DE. Molecular biology of skin cancer. In: DeVita VT, Hellman S, Rosenberg SA, eds. Cancer: principles and practice of oncology, 5th ed. Philadelphia: Lippincott-Raven, 1997:1879–1883.
8. Wong CSM, Strange RC, Lear JT. Basal cell carcinoma. Br Med J
327:794–798, 2003.
9. Alam M, Ratner D. Cutaneous squamous-cell carcinoma. N Engl J
Med 344:975–983, 2001.
10. Hacker SM, Browder JF, Ramos-Caro FA. Basal cell carcinoma:
choosing the best method of treatment for a particular lesion. Postgrad Med 93:101–111, 1993.
11. Potter M. Percival Pott's contribution to cancer research. Natl Cancer Inst Monogr 10:1, 1963.
12. Dreno B, Mansat E, Legoux B, Litoux P. Skin cancers in transplant patients. Nephrol Dial Transplant 13:1374–1379, 1998.
13. Gupta AK, Cardella CJ, Haberman HF. Cutaneous malignant neoplasms in patients with renal transplants. Arch Dermatol 122:
1288–1293, 1986.
14. Ananthaswamy HN, Pierceall WE. Molecular mechanisms of ultraviolet radiation carcinogenesis. Photochem Photobiol 52:1119,
1990.
15. Weinstock MA, Bogaars HA, Ashley M, et al. Nonmelanoma skin
cancer mortality: a population-based study. Arch Dermatol 127:
1194–1197, 1991.
16. Rippey JJ. Why classify basal cell carcinoma? Histopathology 32:
393–398, 1998.
17. Hendrix JD Jr, Parlette HL. Micronodular basal cell carcinoma.
Arch Dermatol 132:295–298, 1996.
18. Maloney ME, Jones DB, Sexton FM. Pigmented basal cell carcinoma: investigation of 70 cases. J Am Acad Dermatol 27:74–78,
1992.
19. Abreo F, Sanusi ID. Basal cell carcinoma in North American
blacks: clinical and histopathologic study of 26 patients. J Am
Acad Dermatol 25:1005–1011, 1991.
20. Kikuchi A, Shimizu H, Nishikawa R. Clinical and histopathological characteristics of basal cell carcinoma in Japanese patients.
Arch Dermatol 132:320–324, 1996.
21. American Joint Committee on Cancer. AJCC cancer staging manual, 6th ed. New York: Springer-Verlag, 2002:231–235.
22. Rowe DE, Carroll RJ, Day CL. Long-term recurrence rates in previously untreated (primary) basal cell carcinoma: implications for patient follow-up. J Dermatol Surg Oncol 15:315–328, 1989.
23. Pascal RR, Hobby LW, Lattes R, et al. Prognosis of "incompletely
excised" versus "completely excised" basal cell carcinoma. Plast
Reconstr Surg 41:328–332, 1968.
24. Gooding CA, White G, Yatsuhashi M. Significance of marginal extension in excised basal cell carcinoma. N Engl J Med 273:
923–924, 1965.
25. Rowe DE, Carroll RJ, Day CL. Prognostic factors for local recurrence, metastasis, and survival rates in squamous cell carcinoma of
the skin, ear, and lip: implications for treatment modality selection.
J Am Acad Dermatol 26:976–990, 1992.
26. Stern RS, Laird N. The carcinogenic risk of treatments for severe
psoriasis. Photochemotherapy Follow-up Study. Cancer 73:
2759–2764, 1994.
27. Marks R, Foley P, Goodman G, et al. Spontaneous remission of
solar keratoses: the case for conservative management. Br J Dermatol 115:649–655, 1986.
28. Marks R, Rennie G, Selwood T. Malignant transformation of solar
keratoses to squamous cell carcinoma. Lancet 1:795–797, 1988.
29. Kwa RE, Campana K, Moy RL. Biology of cutaneous squamous
cell carcinoma. J Am Acad Dermatol 26:1–26, 1992.
30. Breuninger H, Black B, Rassner G. Microstaging of squamous cell
carcinomas. Am J Clin Pathol 94:624–627, 1990.
31. Goldman GD. Squamous cell cancer: a practical approach. Semin
Cutaneous Med Surg 17:80–95, 1998.
32. Vargo NL. Basal and squamous cell carcinomas: an overview.
Semin Oncol Nurs 7:13–25, 1991.
33. Kuflik EG, Gage AA. The five-year cure rate achieved by cryosurgery for skin cancer. J Am Acad Dermatol 24:1002–1004, 1991.
34. Hacker SM, Flowers FP. Squamous cell carcinoma of the skin: will
heightened awareness of risk factors slow its increase? Postgrad
Med 93:115–126, 1993.
35. Lawrence CM. Mohs surgery of basal cell carcinoma: a critical review. Br J Plast Surg 46:599–606, 1993.
36. Albright SD. Treatment of skin cancer using multiple modalities. J
Am Acad Dermatol 7:143–171, 1982.
37. Wilson BD, Mang TS, Stoll H, et al. Photodynamic therapy for the
treatment of basal cell carcinoma. Arch Dermatol 128:1597–1601,
1992.
38. Allison RR, Mang TS, Wilson BD. Photodynamic therapy for the
treatment of nonmelanomatous cutaneous malignancies. Semin Cutaneous Med Surg 17:153–163, 1998.
39. Cairnduff F, Stringer MR, Hudson EJ, et al. Superficial photodynamic therapy with topical 5-aminolevulinic acid for superficial primary and secondary skin cancer. Br J Cancer 69:605–608, 1994.
40. Svanberg K, Andersson T, Killander D, et al. Photodynamic therapy of nonmelanoma malignant tumours of the skin using topical
amino levulinic acid sensitization and laser irradiation. Br J Dermatol 130:743–751, 1994.
41. Geisse J, Caro I, Lindholm J, et al. Imiquimod 5% cream for the
treatment of superficial basal cell carcinoma: results from two
phase III, randomized, vehicle-controlled studies. J Am Acad Dermatol 50:722–733, 2004.
42. Lebwohl M, Dinehart S, Whiting D, et al. Imiquimod 5% cream
for the treatment of actinic keratosis: results from two phase III,
randomized, double-blind, parallel group, vehicle-controlled trials.
J Am Acad Dermatol 50:714–721, 2004.
43. Aldara product information, 2004.
44. Cullen SI. Topical fluorouracil therapy for precancers and cancers
of the skin. J Am Geriatr Soc 12:529–535, 1979.
45. Epstein E. Fluorouracil paste treatment of thin basal cell carcinomas. Arch Dermatol 121:207–213, 1985.
46. Dillaha CJ, Jansen GT, Honeycutt WM, et al. Selective cytotoxic
effect of topical 5-fluorouracil. Arch Dermatol 88:247–256, 1963.
47. Sadek H, Azli N, Wendling JL, et al. Treatment of advanced squamous cell carcinoma of the skin with cisplatin, 5-fluorouracil, and
bleomycin. Cancer 66:1692–1696, 1990.
48. Jemal A, Tiwari RC, Murray T, et al. Cancer statistics, 2004. CA
Cancer J Clin 54:8–29, 2004.
49. American Academy of Dermatology. 2004 melanoma fact sheet.
Available at: http://www.aad.org/magmel.html
50. Lens MB, Dawes M. Global perspectives of contemporary epidemiological trends of cutaneous malignant melanoma. Br J Dermatol
150:179–185, 2004.
51. Incidence of and mortality from melanoma of the skin, 1975–2000.
J Natl Cancer Inst 95:933, 2003.
52. Beddingfield III, FC. The melanoma epidemic: res ipsa loquitur.
Oncologist 8:459–465, 2003.
53. Swerlick R, Chen S. The melanoma epidemic: more apparent than
real? Mayo Clin Proc 72:559–564, 1997.
54. Hall HI, Miller DR, Rogers JD, et al. Update on the incidence and
mortality from melanoma in the United States. J Am Acad Dermatol 40:35–42, 1999.
55. Jemal A, Devesa SS, Hartge P, et al. Recent trends in cutaneous
melanoma incidence among whites in the United States. J Natl Cancer Inst 93:678–683, 2001.

56. Dennis LK. Analysis of the melanoma epidemic, both apparent and real. Arch Dermatol 135:275–280, 1999.

57. Desmond RA, Soong S. Epidemiology of malignant melanoma. Surg Clin North Am 83:1–29, 2003.

58. Melanoma Research Foundation. Melanoma fact sheet. Available at: http://www.melanoma.org/mrf_facts.pdf

59. Lotze MT, Dallal RM, Kirkwood JM, et al. Cutaneous melanoma. In: DeVita VT, Hellman S, Rosenberg SA, eds. Cancer: principles and practice of oncology, 6th ed. Philadelphia: Lippincott-Raven, 2001:2012–2069.

60. Grob JJ, Gouvernet J, Aymar D, et al. Count of benign melanocytic nevi as a major indicator of risk for non-familial nodular and superficial spreading melanoma. Cancer 66:387–395, 1990.

61. Naeyaert JM, Brochez L. Dysplastic nevi. N Engl J Med 349: 2233–2240, 2003.

62. Armstrong BK, English DR. Epidemiologic studies. In Balch CM, Houghton AN, Milton GW, et al, eds. Cutaneous melanoma, 2nd ed. Philadelphia: Lippincott, 1992:12–26.

63. Koh HK. Cutaneous melanoma. N Engl J Med 325:171–182, 1991.

64. MacKie RM. Incidence, risk factors and prevention of melanoma. Eur J Cancer 34 (Suppl 3):S3–S6, 1998.

65. Kopf AW, Hellman LJ, Rogers GS, et al. Familial malignant melanoma. JAMA 256:1915–1919, 1986.

66. Margolin KA, Sondak VK. Melanoma and other skin cancer. In Pazdur R, Hoskins WJ, Coia LR, et al, eds. Cancer management handbook: a multidisciplinary approach, 7th ed. New York: Oncology Group, 2003:507–536.

67. Lee JE. Factors associated with melanoma incidence and prognosis. Semin Surg Oncol 12:379–385, 1996.

68. Halpern AC, Altman JF. Genetic predisposition to skin cancer. Curr Opin Oncol 11:132–138, 1999.

69. Greene MH. Genetics of cutaneous melanoma and nevi. Mayo Clin Proc 72:467–474, 1997.

70. Nelemans PJ, Groenendal H, Kiemeney LA, et al. Effect of intermittent exposure to sunlight on melanoma risk among indoor workers and sun-sensitive individuals. Environ Health Perspect 101: 252–255, 1993.

71. Whiteman DC, Whiteman CA, Green AC. Childhood sun exposure as a risk factor for melanoma: a systematic review of epidemiologic studies. Cancer Causes Control 12:69–82, 2001.

72. Perlis C, Herlyn M. Recent advances in melanoma biology. Oncologist 9:182–187, 2004.

73. Ley RD, Applegate LA, Padilla RS, et al. Ultraviolet radiation-induced malignant melanoma in *Monodelphis domestica*. Photochem Photobiol 50:1–5, 1989.

74. Setlow RB, Grist E, Thompson K, et al. Wavelengths effective in induction of malignant melanoma. Proc Natl Acad Sci USA 90: 6666–6670, 1993.

75. Atillasoy ES, Seykora JT, Soballe PW, et al. UVB induces atypical melanocytic lesions and melanoma in human skin. Am J Pathol 152:1179–1186, 1998.

76. Gilchrest BA, Eller MS, Geller AC, et al. The pathogenesis of melanoma induced by ultraviolet radiation. N Engl J Med 340: 1341–1348, 1999.

77. Drolet BA, Connor MJ. Sunscreens and the prevention of ultraviolet radiation-induced skin cancer. J Dermatol Surg Oncol 18: 571–576, 1992.

78. Pollock PM, Harper UL, Hansen KS, et al. High frequency of BRAF mutations in nevi. Nat Genet 33:19–20, 2003.

79. Uribe P, Wistuba II, Gonzalez S. BRAF mutation: a frequent event in benign, atypical, and malignant melanocytic lesions of the skin. Am J Dermatopathol 25:365–370, 2003.

80. Haluska FG, Hodi FS. Molecular genetics of familial cutaneous melanoma. J Clin Oncol 16:670–682, 1998.

81. Ramcharan S, Pellegrin FA, Ray R, et al. The Walnut Creek Contraceptive Drug Study. Vol III. An interim report. NIH pub no 81-564. Washington, DC: US Government Printing Office, 1981.

82. Holly EA, Weiss NS, Liff JM. Cutaneous melanoma in relation to exogenous hormones and reproductive factors. J Natl Cancer Inst 70:827–831, 1983.

83. Holman CDJ, Armstrong BK, Heenan PJ. Cutaneous malignant melanoma in women: exogenous sex hormones and reproductive factors. Br J Cancer 50:673–680, 1984.

84. Beral V, Evans S, Shaw H. Oral contraceptive use and malignant melanoma in Australia. Br J Cancer 50:681–685, 1984.

85. Beral V, Ramcharan S, Faris R. Malignant melanoma and oral contraceptive use among women in California. Br J Cancer 36: 804–809, 1977.

86. Herlyn M, Houghton AN. Biology of melanocytes and melanoma. In: Balch CM, Houghton AN, Milton GW, et al, eds. Cutaneous melanoma, 2nd ed. Philadelphia: Lippincott, 1992:82–92.

87. Zubovits J, Buzney E, Yu L, et al. HMB-45, S-100, NK1/C3, and MART-1 in metastatic melanoma. Hum Pathol 35:217–223, 2004.

88. Fetsch PA, Marincola FM, Filie A, et al. Melanoma-associated antigen recognized by T cells (MART-1): the advent of a preferred immunocytochemocal antibody for the diagnosis of metastatic malignant melanoma with fine-needle aspiration. Cancer 87:37–42, 1999.

89. Shidham VB, Qi DY, Acker S, et al. Evaluation of micrometastases in sentinel lymph nodes of cutaneous melanoma. Am J Surg Pathol 25:1039–1046, 2001.

90. Crutcher WA, Cohen PJ. Dysplastic nevi and malignant melanoma. Am Fam Physician 42:372–385, 1990.

91. Albino AP, Reed JA, McNutt NS. Molecular biology of cutaneous malignant melanoma. In: DeVita VT, Hellman S, Rosenberg SA, eds. Cancer: principles and practice of oncology, 5th ed. Philadelphia: Lippincott-Raven, 1997:1935–1946.

92. Clark WH Jr, Elder ED, Guerry D IV, et al. The precursor lesions of superficial spreading and nodular melanoma. Hum Pathol 15: 1147–1165, 1984.

93. Lu C, Kerbel RS. Cytokines, growth factors and the loss of negative growth controls in the progression of human cutaneous malignant melanoma. Curr Opin Oncol 6:212–220, 1994.

94. Slominski A, Wortsman J, Carlson AJ, et al. Malignant melanoma: an update. Arch Pathol Lab Med 125:1295–1306, 2001.

95. Satyamoorthy K, Herlyn M. Cellular and molecular biology of human melanoma. Cancer Biol Therapy 1:14–17, 2002.

96. Hsu MY, Shih DT, Meier FE, et al. Adenoviral gene transfer of β_3 integrin subunit induces conversion from radial to vertical growth phase in primary human melanoma. Am J Pathol 153:1435–1442, 1998.

97. Friedman RJ, Rigel DS, Kopf AW. Early detection of malignant melanoma: the role of physician examination and self-examination of the skin. CA Cancer J Clin 35:130–151, 1985.

98. Fitzpatrick TB, Milton GW, Balch CM, et al. Clinical characteristics. In: Balch CM, Houghton AN, Milton GW, et al, eds. Cutaneous melanoma, 2nd ed. Philadelphia: Lippincott, 1992:223–233.

99. Balch CM, Reintgen DS, Kirkwood JM, et al. Cutaneous melanoma. In: DeVita VT, Hellman S, Rosenberg SA, eds. Cancer: principles and practice of oncology, 5th ed. Philadelphia: Lippincott-Raven, 1997:1947–1994.

100. Breslow A. Thickness, cross-sectional areas and depth of invasion in the prognosis of cutaneous melanoma. Ann Surg 172:902–908, 1970.

101. Clark WH Jr, Ainsworth AM, Bernardino EA, et al. The developmental biology of primary human malignant melanomas. Semin Oncol 2:83–103, 1975.

102. Balch CM, Murad TM, Soong SJ, et al. A multifactorial analysis of melanoma: prognostic histopathological features comparing Clark's and Breslow's staging methods. Ann Surg 188:732–742, 1978.

103. Breslow A, Cascinelli N, Van der Esch E, et al. Stage I melanoma of the limbs: assessment of prognosis by levels of invasion and maximum thickness. Tumori 64:273–284, 1978.

104. Balch CM, Soong SJ, Gershenwald JE, et al. Prognostic factors analysis of 17,600 melanoma patients: validation of the American Joint Committee on Cancer melanoma staging system. J Clin Oncol 19:3622–3634, 2001.

105. Balch CM, Buzaid AC, Atkins MB, et al. A new American Joint Committee on Cancer staging system for cutaneous melanoma. Cancer 88:1484–1491, 2000.

106. Balch CM, Buzaid AC, Soong SJ, et al. Final version of the American Joint Committee on Cancer staging system for cutaneous melanoma. J Clin Oncol 19:3635–3648, 2001.

107. Balch CM. Cutaneous melanoma. In: Greene FL, Page DL, Fleming ID, et al, eds. AJCC cancer staging manual, 6th ed. New York: Springer-Verlag, 2002:209–217.

108. Shen J, Wallace AM, Bouvert M. The role of sentinel lymph node biopsy for melanoma. Semin Oncol 29:341–352, 2002.
109. Ross MI, Balch CM. Surgical treatment of primary melanoma. In: Balch CM, Houghton AN, Sober AJ, et al, eds. Cutaneous melanoma, 3rd ed. St. Louis: Quality Medical Pub, 1998:141–153.
110. Urist MM, Balch CM, Soong S, et al. The influence of surgical margins and prognostic factors predicting the risk of local recurrence in 3445 patients with primary cutaneous melanoma. Cancer 55:1398–1402, 1985.
111. Balch CM, Soong S, Smith T, et al. Long-term results of a prospective surgical trial comparing 2 cm vs. 4 cm excision margins for 740 patients with 1- to 4-mm melanomas. Ann Surg Oncol 8:101–108, 2001.
112. Balch CM, Urist MM, Karakousis CP, et al. Efficacy of 2-cm surgical margins for intermediate-thickness melanomas (1 to 4 mm): results of a multi-institutional randomized surgical trial. Ann Surg 218:262–269, 1993.
113. Khayat D, Rixe O, Martin G, et al. Surgical margins in cutaneous melanoma (2 cm versus 5 cm for lesions measuring less than 2.1 mm thick). Cancer 97:1941–1946, 2003.
114. Veronesi U, Cascinelli N. Narrow excision (1 cm): a safe procedure for thin cutaneous melanoma. Arch Surg 126:438–441, 1991.
115. Cohn–Cedermark G, Rutqvist LE, Anderson R, et al. Long-term results of a randomized study by the Swedish Melanoma Study Group on 2-cm versus 5-cm resection margins for patients with cutaneous melanoma with a tumor thickness of 0.8–2.0 mm. Cancer 89:1495–1501, 2000.
116. Thomas JM, Newton-Bishop J, A'Hern R, et al. Excision margins in high-risk malignant melanoma. N Engl J Med 350:757–766, 2004.
117. National Comprehensive Cancer Network. Clinical practice guidelines in oncology: melanoma, version 1.2004. Available at: http://www.nccn.com/professionals/physician_gls/f_guidelines.asp#site
118. Gumport SL, Harris MN. Results of regional lymph node dissection for melanoma. Ann Surg 179:105–108, 1974.
119. Crowley NJ. The case against elective lymphadenectomy. Surg Oncol Clin North Am 1:223–243, 1992.
120. Veronessi U, Adamus J, Bandiera DC, et al. Inefficacy of immediate node dissection in stage I melanoma of the limbs. N Engl J Med 297:627–630, 1977.
121. Cascinelli N, Morabito A, Santinami M, et al. Immediate or delayed dissection of regional nodes in patients with melanoma of the trunk: a randomized trial. Lancet 351:793–796, 1998.
122. Sim FH, Taylor WF, Pritchard DJ, et al. Lymphadenectomy in the management of stage I malignant melanoma: a prospective randomized study. Mayo Clin Proc 61:697–705, 1986.
123. Balch CM, Soong S, Ross MI, et al. Long-term results of a multi-institutional randomized trial comparing prognostic factors and surgical results for intermediate thickness melanomas (1.0 to 4.0 mm). Ann Surg Oncol 7:87–97, 2000.
124. Morton DL, Wen DR, Wong JM. Technical details of intraoperative lymphatic mapping for early stage melanoma. Arch Surg 127:392–399, 1992.
125. Leong SPL. Selective sentinel lymphadenectomy for malignant melanoma. Surg Clin North Am 83:157–185, 2003.
126. Morton DL, Thompson JF, Essner R, et al. Validation of the accuracy of intraoperative lymphatic mapping and sentinel lymphadenectomy for early-stage melanoma: a multicenter trial. Multicenter Selective Lymphadenectomy Trial Group. Ann Surg 230:453–463, 1999.
127. Bedrosian I, Gershenwald JE. Surgical clinical trials in melanoma. Surg Clin North Am 83:385–403, 2003.
128. Ollila DW, Hsueh EC, Stern SL, et al. Metastasectomy for recurrent stage IV melanoma. J Surg Oncol 71:209–213, 1999.
129. Karakousis CP, Velez A, Driscoll DL, et al. Metastasectomy in malignant melanoma. Surgery 115:295–302, 1994.
130. Harwood AR. Conventional fractionated radiotherapy for 51 patients with lentigo maligna and lentigo maligna melanoma. Int J Radiat Oncol Biol Phys 9:1019–1021, 1983.
131. Ballo MT, Ang KK. Radiotherapy for cutaneous malignant melanoma: a rationale and indications. Oncology 18:99–114, 2004.
132. Ballo MT, Ang KK. Radiation therapy for malignant melanoma. Surg Clin North Am 83:323–342, 2003.
133. Ang KK, Peters LJ, Weber RS, et al. Postoperative radiotherapy for cutaneous melanoma of the head and neck region. Int J Radiat Oncol Biol Phys 30:795–798, 1994.
134. O'Brien CJ, Petersen-Schaefer K, Stevens GN, et al. Adjuvant radiotherapy following neck dissection and parotidectomy for metastatic malignant melanoma. Head Neck 19:589–594, 1997.
135. Ballo MT, Strom EA, Zagars GK, et al. Adjuvant irradiation for axillary metastases from malignant melanoma. Int J Radiat Oncol Biol Phys 52:964–972, 2002.
136. Schmidt-Ullrich RK, Johnson CR. Role of radiotherapy and hyperthermia in the management of malignant melanoma. Semin Surg Oncol 12:407–415, 1996.
137. Omlor G, Gross G, Ecker KW, et al. Optimization of isolated hyperthermic limb perfusion. World J Surg 16:1117–1119, 1993.
138. Hohenberger P, Kettelhack C. Clinical management and current research in isolated limb perfusion for sarcoma and melanoma. Oncology 55:89–102, 1998.
139. Koops HS, Vaglini M, Suciu S, et al. Prophylactic isolated limb perfusion for localized, high-risk limb melanoma: results of a multicenter randomized phase III trial. European Organization for Research and Treatment of Cancer Malignant Melanoma Cooperative Group Protocol 18832, the World Health Organization Melanoma Program Trial 15, and the North American Perfusion Groups Southwest Oncology Group 8593. J Clin Oncol 16:2906–2912, 1998.
140. Thompson JF, Hunt JA, Shannon KF, et al. Frequency and duration of remission after isolated limb perfusion for melanoma. Arch Surg 132:903–908, 1997.
141. Storm FK, Morton DL. Value of therapeutic hyperthermic limb perfusion in advanced recurrent melanoma of the lower extremity. Am J Surg 150:32–35, 1985.
142. Kroon BBR, Klaase JM, Van Geel AN, et al. Application of hyperthermia in regional isolated perfusion for melanoma of the limbs. Reg Cancer Treat 4:223–226, 1992.
143. Lienard D, Lejeune FJ, Ewalenko P. In transit metastases of malignant melanoma treated by high-dose rTNF alpha in combination with interferon-gamma and melphalan in isolation perfusion. World J Surg 16:234–240, 1992.
144. Lens MB, Dawes M. Isolated limb perfusion with melphalan in the treatment of malignant melanoma of the extremities: a systematic review of randomized controlled trials. Lancet 4:359–364, 2003.
145. Noorda EM, Takkenberg B, Vrouenraets BC, et al. Isolated limb perfusion prolongs the limb recurrence-free interval after several episodes of excisional surgery for locoregional recurrent melanoma. Ann Surg Oncol 11:491–499, 2004.
146. Eggermont AMM, van Geel AN, de Wilt JHW, et al. The role of isolated limb perfusion for melanoma confined to the extremities. Surg Clin North Am 83:371–384, 2003.
147. Brown CK, Kirkwood JM. Medical management of melanoma. Surg Clin North Am 83:283–322, 2003.
148. Agarwala SS, Kirkwood JM. Adjuvant therapy with melanoma. Semin Surg Oncol 14:302–310, 1998.
149. Creagan ET, Dalton RJ, Ahmann DL, et al. Randomized, surgical adjuvant clinical trial of recombinant interferon alfa-2a in selected patients with malignant melanoma. J Clin Oncol 13:2776–2783, 1995.
150. Kirkwood JM, Strawderman MH, Ernstoff MS, et al. Interferon alfa-2b adjuvant therapy of high-risk resected cutaneous melanoma: the Eastern Cooperative Oncology Group trial EST 1684. J Clin Oncol 14:7–17, 1996.
151. Kirkwood JM, Strawderman MH, Ernstoff MS, et al. Adjuvant therapy of high-risk melanoma: the role of high-dose interferon alfa-2b. In: Salmon S, ed. Adjuvant therapies of cancer, VIII. Philadelphia: Lippincott-Raven, 1997:251–257.
152. Cole BF, Gelbert RD, Kirkwood JM, et al. A quality-of-life–adjusted survival analysis of interferon alfa-2b adjuvant treatment for high-risk resected cutaneous melanoma: an Eastern Cooperative Oncology Group study (E1684). J Clin Oncol 14:2666–2673, 1996.
153. Hillner BE, Kirkwood JM, Atkins MB, et al. Economic analysis of adjuvant interferon alfa-2b in high-risk melanoma based on projections from Eastern Cooperative Oncology Group 1684. J Clin Oncol 15:2351–2358, 1997.
154. Kirkwood JM, Ibrahim JG, Sondak VK, et al. High- and low-dose interferon alfa-2b in high-risk melanoma: first analysis of Inter-

group trial E1690/S9111/C9190. J Clin Oncol 18:2444–2458, 2000.

155. Kirkwood JM, Manola J, Ibrahim J, et al. A pooled analysis of Eastern Cooperative Oncology Group and Intergroup trials of adjuvant high-dose interferon for melanoma. Clin Cancer Res 10: 1670–1677, 2004.

156. Cascinelli N, Belli F, Mackie RM, et al. Effect of long-term adjuvant therapy with interferon alpha-2a in patients with regional node metastases from cutaneous melanoma: a randomized trial. Lancet 358:866–869, 2001.

157. Cameron DA, Cornbleet MC, Mackie RM, et al. Adjuvant interferon alpha 2b in high risk melanoma: the Scottish study. Br J Cancer 84:1146–1149, 2001.

158. Kleeberg UR, Suciu S, Brocker EB, et al. Final results of the EORTC 18871/DKG 80-1 randomised phase III trial: rIFN-α2b versus rIFN-γ versus ISCADOR M® versus observation after surgery in melanoma patients with either high-risk primary (thickness > 3mm) or regional lymph node metastasis. Eur J Cancer 40: 390–402, 2004.

159. Hancock BW, Wheatley K, Harris S, et al. Adjuvant interferon in high-risk melanoma: the AIM HIGH study–United Kingdom Coordinating Committee on Cancer Research randomized study of adjuvant low-dose extended-duration interferon alfa-2a in high-risk resected malignant melanoma. J Clin Oncol 22:53–61, 2004.

160. Pehamberger H, Soyer HP, Steiner A, et al. Adjuvant interferon alfa-2a treatment in resected primary stage II cutaneous melanoma. J Clin Oncol 16:1425–1429, 1998.

161. Grob JJ, Dreno B, de la Salmoniere P, et al. Randomised trial of interferon α-2a as adjuvant therapy in resected primary melanoma thicker than 1.5 mm without clinically detectable node metastasis. Lancet 351:1905–1910, 1998.

162. Eggermont AMM, Kleeberg UR, Ruiter DJ, et al. European Organization for Research and Treatment of Cancer Melanoma Group trial experience with more than 2,000 patients, evaluating adjuvant treatment with low or intermediate doses of interferon alpha-2b. In: Perry MC, ed. American Society of Clinical Oncology 2001 Educational Book. Baltimore: Lippincott Williams & Wilkins, 2001: 88–93.

163. Kirkwood, JM. Adjuvant therapy of high-risk resected melanoma: relapse-free and overall survival effects of high-dose interferon alpha-2b in randomized controlled multicenter trials E1684 and E2696 and Intergroup trials E1690 and E1696. In: Perry MC, ed. American Society of Clinical Oncology 2001 Educational Book. Baltimore: Lippincott Williams & Wilkins, 2001:94–101.

164. Spitler LE, Grossbard ML, Ernstoff MS, et al. Adjuvant therapy of stage III and IV malignant melanoma using granulocyte–macrophage colony-stimulating factor. J Clin Oncol 18:1614–1621, 2000.

165. Haigh PI, DiFronzo LA. Vaccine therapy for patients with melanoma. Oncology 13:1561–1574, 1999.

166. Sondak VK, Liu PY, Tuthill RJ, et al. Adjuvant immunotherapy of resected, intermediate-thickness, node-negative melanoma with an allogeneic tumor vaccine: overall results of a randomized trial of the Southwest Oncology Group. J Clin Oncol 20:2058–2066, 2002.

167. Sosman JA, Unger JM, Liu PY, et al. Adjuvant immunotherapy of resected, intermediate-thickness, node-negative melanoma with an allogeneic tumor vaccine: impact of HLA class I antigen expression on outcome. J Clin Oncol 20:2067–2075, 2002.

168. Mitchell MS, Von Eschen KB. Phase III trial of Melacine melanoma theraccine vs. combination chemotherapy in the treatment of stage IV melanoma. Proc Am Soc Clin Oncol 16:1778, 1997.

169. Livingston PO, Wong Gy, Adluri S, et al. Improved survival in stage III melanoma patients with GM2 antibodies: a randomized trial of adjuvant vaccination with GM2 ganglioside. J Clin Oncol 12:1036–1044, 1994.

170. Kirkwood JM, Ibrahim JG, Sosman JA, et al. High-dose interferon alfa-2b significantly prolongs relapse-free and overall survival compared with the GM2-KLH/QS-21 vaccine in patients with resected stage IIB-III melanoma: results of intergroup trial E1694/S9512/ C509801. J Clin Oncol 19:2370–2380, 2001.

171. Dorr RT, Von Hoff DD. Cancer chemotherapy handbook, 2nd ed. CT: Appleton & Lange, 1994:343–349.

172. Middleton MR, Grob JJ, Aaronson N, et al. Randomized phase III study of temozolomide versus dacarbazine in the treatment of pa-

173. Brock CS, Newlands ES, Wedge SR, et al. Phase I trial of temozolomide using an extended continuous oral schedule. Cancer Res 58: 4363–4367, 1998.

174. Summers Y, Middleton M, Calvert H, et al. Effect of temozolomide on CNS relapse in patients with advanced melanoma. Proc Am Soc Clin Oncol 18:2048, 1999.

175. Atkins MB, Gollob JA, Sosman JA, et al. A phase II pilot trial of concurrent biochemotherapy with cisplatin, vinblastine, temozolomide, interleukin 2, and interferon α2b in patients with metastatic melanoma. Clin Cancer Res 8:3075–3081, 2002.

176. Hwu WJ, Krown SE, Menell JH, et al. Phase II study of temozolomide plus thalidomide for the treatment of metastatic melanoma. J Clin Oncol 21:3351–3356, 2003.

177. Franke W, Neumann NJ, Richter-Hintz D, et al. Temozolomide: a promising agent in the therapy of brain metastases in malignant melanoma. Proc Am Soc Clin Oncol 19:2268a, 2000.

178. Hwu WJ. New approaches in the treatment of metastatic melanoma: thalidomide and temozolomide. Oncology 14 (12 Suppl 13): 25–28, 2000.

179. Hwu WJ, Raizer J, Panageas KS, et al. Treatment of metastatic melanoma in the brain with temozolomide and thalidomide. Lancet Oncol 2:634–635, 2001.

180. Bafaloukos D, Gogas H. Georgoulias V, et al. Temozolomide in combination with docetaxel in patients with advanced melanoma: a phase II study of the Hellenic Cooperative Oncology Group. J Clin Oncol 20:420–425, 2002.

181. Jacquillat C, Khayat D, Banzet P, et al. Final reports of the French multicenter phase II study of the nitrosourea fotemustine in 153 patients with disseminated malignant melanoma including patients with brain metastases. Cancer 66:1873–1878, 1990.

182. Flakson CI, Falkson G, Flakson HC. Phase II trial with fotemustine in patients with metastatic malignant melanoma. Invest New Drugs 12:251–254, 1994.

183. Glover D, Glick JH, Weiler C, et al. WR 2721 and high-dose cisplatin: an active combination in the treatment of metastatic melanoma. J Clin Oncol 5:574–578, 1987.

184. Chang A, Hunt M, Parkinson DR, et al. Phase II trial of carboplatin in patients with metastatic malignant melanoma: a report from the Eastern Cooperative Oncology Group. Am J Clin Oncol 16:152–155, 1993.

185. Weirnik PH, Enzig AI. Taxol in malignant melanoma. Monogr Natl Cancer Inst 15:185–187, 1993.

186. Aamdal S, Wolff I, Kaplan S, et al. Docetaxel (Taxotere) in advanced malignant melanoma: a phase II study of the EORTC Early Clinical Trials Group. Eur J Cancer 30A:1061–1064, 1994.

187. Jonash E, Haluska FG. Interferon in oncological practice: review of interferon biology, clinical applications, and toxicities. Oncologist 6:34–55, 2001.

188. Rosenberg SA, Yang JC, Topalian SL, et al. Treatment of 283 consecutive patients with metastatic melanoma or renal cell cancer using high-dose bolus interleukin 2. JAMA 271:907–913, 1994.

189. Atkins MB, Lotze MT, Dutcher JP, et al. High-dose recombinant interleukin 2 therapy for patients with metastatic melanoma: analysis of 270 patients treated between 1985 and 1993. J Clin Oncol 17:2105–2116, 1999.

190. Royal RE, Steinberg SM, White D, et al. Correlates of response of IL-2 therapy in patients treated for metastatic renal cell cancer and melanoma. Cancer J Sci Am 6:91–98, 1996.

191. Schwartzentruber DJ, Rosenberg SA. Interleukins. In: Balch CM, Houghton AN, Sober AJ, et al, eds. Cutaneous melanoma, 3rd ed. St. Louis: Quality Medical Publishing, Inc, 2003:623–643.

192. Schwartz RN. Managing toxicities of high-dose interleukin-2. Oncology 16 (Suppl 11):11–20, 2002.

193. Kammula US, White DE, Rosenberg SA. Trends in the safety of high-dose bolus interleukin-2 administration in patients with metastatic melanoma. Cancer 83:797–805, 1998.

194. Keilholz U, Scheibenbogen C, Brossart P, et al. Interleukin-2-based immunotherapy and chemoimmunotherapy in metastatic melanoma. Recent Results Cancer Res 139:383–390, 1995.

195. Sparano JA, Fisher RI, Sunderland M, et al. Randomized phase III trial of treatment with high-dose interleukin-2 either alone or in

combination with interferon alfa-2a in patients with advanced melanoma. J Clin Oncol 11:1969–1977, 1993.

196. Legha SS, Ring S, Bedikian A, et al. Treatment of metastatic melanoma with combined chemotherapy containing cisplatin, vinblastine and dacarbazine (CVD) and biotherapy using interleukin-2 and interferon-alpha. Ann Oncol 7:827–835, 1996.

197. Legha SS, Ring S, Eton O, et al. Development of a biochemotherapy regimen with concurrent administration of cisplatin, vinblastine, dacarbazine, interferon-alpha and interleukin-2 for patients with metastatic melanoma. J Clin Oncol 16:1752–1759, 1998.

198. Eton O, Legha SS, Bedikian AY, et al. Sequential biochemotherapy versus chemotherapy for metastatic melanoma: result from a phase III randomized trial. J Clin Oncol 20:2045–2052, 2002.

199. Atkins MB, Lee S. Flaherty LE, et al. A prospective randomized phase III trial of concurrent biochemotherapy with cisplatin, vinblastine, dacarbazine (CVD), interleukin-2 and interferon alpha-2b versus CVD alone in patients with metastatic melanoma (E3695): An ECOG-coordinated intergroup trial. Proc Am Soc Clin Oncol 22:708, 2003.

200. D'Amato RJ, Loughnan MS, Flynn E, et al. Thalidomide as an inhibitor of angiogenesis. Proc Natl Acad Sci USA 91:408–4085, 1994.

201. Kruse FE, Joussen AM, Rohrschneider K, et al. Thalidomide inhibits corneal angiogenesis induced by vascular endothelial growth factor. Graefes Arch Clin Exp Ophthalmol 236:461–466, 1998.

202. Geitz H, Handt S, Zwingenberger K. Thalidomide selectively modulates the density of cell surface molecules involved in the adhesion cascade. Immunopharmacology 31:213–221, 1996.

203. Haslett PA, Corral LG, Albert M, et al. Thalidomide co-stimulates primary human T lymphocytes, preferentially inducing proliferation, cytokine production, and cytotoxic responses in the CD8+ subset. J Exp Med 187:1885–1892, 1998.

204. Kudva GC, Collins BT, Dunphy FR. Thalidomide for malignant melanoma. N Engl J Med 16:1214–1215, 2001.

205. Eisen T, Boshoff C, Mak I, et al. Continuous low-dose thalidomide: a phase II study in advanced melanoma, renal cell, ovarian and breast cancer. Br J Cancer 82:812–817, 2000.

206. Hwu WJ, Krown SE, Menell JH, et al. Phase II study of temozolomide plus thalidomide for the treatment of metastatic melanoma. J Clin Oncol 21:3351–3356, 2003.

207. Amer MH, Al-Sarraf M, Baker LH, et al. Malignant melanoma and central nervous system metastases: incidence, diagnosis, treatment and survival. Cancer 42:660–668, 1978.

208. Hwu WJ. New approach in the treatment of metastatic melanoma: thalidomide and temozolomide. Oncology 14 (Suppl 13):25–28, 2000.

209. Hwu WJ, Raizer J, Panageas KS, et al. Treatment of metastatic melanoma in the brain with temozolomide and thalidomide. Lancet Oncol 2:634–635, 2001.

210. Celgene Corporation. Thalomid® product information, 1998.

211. Hockenbery D, Nunez G, Milliman C, et al. Bcl-2 is an inner mitochondrial membrane protein that blocks programmed cell death. Nature 348: 334–336, 1990.

212. Chen-Levy Z, Nourse J, and Cleary ML. The bcl-2 candidate proto-oncogene product is a 24-kilodalton integral membrane protein highly expressed in lymphoid cell lines and lymphomas carrying the t(14;18) translocation. Mol Cell Biol 9: 701–710, 1989.

213. Chandler D, el Naggar AK, Brisbay S, et al. Apoptosis and expression of bcl-2 proto-oncogene in the fetal and adult human kidney: evidence for the contribution of bcl-2 expression to renal carcinogenesis. Hum Pathol 25: 789–796, 1994.

214. Reed JC. Bcl-2: prevention of apoptosis as a mechanism of drug resistance. Hematol Oncol Clin North Am 9: 451–474, 1995.

215. Polsky D, Cordon-Cardo C. Oncogenes in melanoma. Oncogenes 22:3080–3091, 2003.

216. Hodges D, Crooke ST. Inhibition of splicing of wild-type and mutated luciferase-adenovirus pre-mRNAs by antisense oligonucleotides. Mol Pharmacol 48: 905–918, 1995.

217. Jansen B, Wacheck V, Heere-Ress E, et al. Chemosensitisation of malignant melanoma by bcl-2 antisense therapy. Lancet 356: 1728–1733, 2000.

218. Kitada S, Miyashita T, Tanaka S, et al. Investigations of antisense oligonucleotides targeted against bcl-2 RNAs. Antisense Res Dev 3:157–169, 1993.

219. Jansen B, Schlagbauer-Wadl H, Brown BD, et al. Bcl-2 antisense therapy chemosensitizes human melanoma in SCID mice. Nat Med 4:232–234, 1998.

220. Fingert HJ, Klem RE. Clinical pharmacokinetics and pharmacodynamics of G3139 (Genta Incorporated) antisense oligonucleotide targeting bcl-2. Clin Cancer Res 5:3847s, 1999.

221. Millward MJ, Bedikian AY, Conry RM, et al. Randomized multiinstitutional phase III trial of dacarbazine with or without bcl-2 antisense (oblimersen sodium) in patients with advanced melanoma: analysis of long-term survival. J Clin Oncol 22:7505, 2004.

222. Bedikian A. Personal communication, 2005.

223. Kono K, Salazar-Onfray F, Peterson M, et al. Hydrogen peroxide secreted by tumor-derived macrophages downmodulates signal-transducing zeta molecules and inhibits tumor-specific T cell- and natural killer cell-mediated cytotoxicity. Eur J Immunol 26: 1308–1313, 1996.

224. Hansson M, Hermodsson S, Brune M, et al. Histamine protects T cells and natural killer cells against oxidative stress. J Interferon Cytokine Res 19:1135–1144, 1999.

225. Hellstrand K, Naredi P, Lindner P, et al. Histamine in immunotherapy of advanced melanoma: a pilot study. Cancer Immunol Immunother 39:416–419, 1994.

226. Hellstrand K, Hermodsson S, Brune M, et al. Histamine in cancer immunotherapy. Scand J Clin Lab Invest 57:193–202, 1997.

227. Agarwala SS, Glaspy J, O'Day SJ, et al. Results from a randomized phase III study comparing combined treatment with histamine dihydrochloride plus interleukin-2 versus interleukin-2 alone in patients with metastatic melanoma. J Clin Oncol 20:125–133, 2001.

228. Cole P, Morrison AS. Issues in population screening for cancer. J Natl Cancer Inst 64:1263–1272, 1980.

229. Swetter SM. Dermatological perspectives of malignant melanoma. Surg Clin North Am 83:77–95, 2003.

230. Bal DG, Nixon DW, Foerster SB, et al. Cancer prevention. In: Murphy GP, Lawrence W, Lenhard SE, eds. American Cancer Society textbook of clinical oncology, 2nd ed. Atlanta: American Cancer Society, 1995:40–63.

231. American Academy of Dermatology. 2004 melanoma fact sheet. Available at: http://www.aad.org/magmel.html

232. Staples M, Marks R, Giles G. Trends in the incidence of non-melanocytic skin cancer treated in Australia 1985–1995: are primary prevention programs starting to have an effect? Int J Cancer 78: 144–148, 1998.

233. Peck GL. Topical tretinoin in actinic keratosis and basal cell carcinoma. J Am Acad Dermatol 15:829–835, 1986.

234. Moon TE, Levine N, Cartmel B, et al. Effect of Retinol in preventing squamous cell skin cancer in moderate-risk subjects: a randomized, double-blind, controlled trial. Cancer Epidemiol Biomark Prev 6:949–956, 1997.

235. Levine N, Moon TE, Cartmel B, et al. Trial of Retinol and Isotretinoin in skin cancer prevention: a randomized, double-blind, controlled trial. Cancer Epidemiol Biomark Prev 6:957–961, 1997.

236. Alberts DS, Dorr RT, Einspar LG, et al. Chemoprevention of human actinic keratoses by topical 2-(difluoromethyl)-dl-ornithine. Cancer Epidemiol Biomark Prev 9:1281–1286, 2000.

237. Yarosh D, Klein J, O'Connor A, et al. Effect of topically applied T4 endonuclease V in liposomes on skin cancer in xeroderma pigmentosum: a randomized study. Lancet 357:926–929, 2001.

238. Peterson SR, Goldberg LH. New and emerging treatments for non-melanomas and actinic keratoses. J Drugs Dermatol 2:429–432, 2002.

239. Weringhaus K, Meydani M, Bhawan J, et al. Evaluation of the photoprotective effect of oral vitamin E supplementation. Arch Dermatol 130:1257–1261, 1994.

240. Greenberg ER, Baron JA, Stukel TA, et al. A clinical trial of beta-carotene to prevent basal cell and squamous cell cancers of the skin. N Engl J Med 323:789–795, 1990.

241. Clark LC, Combs GF, Turnbull BW, et al. Effects of selenium supplementation for cancer prevention in patients with carcinoma of the skin. JAMA 276:1957–1963, 1996.

242. Demierre MF, Nathanson L. Chemoprevention of melanoma: an unexplored strategy. J Clin Oncol 21:158–165, 2003.

CASE 37

TOPIC: Acute Leukemia

THERAPEUTIC DIFFICULTY: Level 3
Maryann Cooper

Chapter 94: Acute Leukemias

■ Scenario

Patient and Setting: SS, a 52-year-old female; hospitalized

Chief Complaint: Fever, rigors, diarrhea, mouth pain

■ History of Present Illness

SS is a 52-year-old female newly diagnosed with acute myelogenous leukemia (AML). She was in her usual state of health until approximately 1 week prior to admission when she presented to her primary care physician complaining of fever, fatigue, night sweats, and easy bruising. At this time she was found to be pancytopenic. A bone marrow aspirate and biopsy revealed a hypercellular marrow with 60% blasts. She was subsequently diagnosed with AML. She is now day 14 status postinduction chemotherapy with idarubicin and ARA-C. Overnight, she spiked a fever to 39°C. She is now complaining of fever, rigors, diarrhea, and mild mouth pain. She states she is still able to swallow liquids and solids.

Medical History: Hypertension × 5 years; hypothyroidism × 20 years; status postuterine fibroids

Surgical History: Status post-total abdominal hysterectomy and bilateral salpingo-oophorectomy for uterine fibroids; status postcentral line placement

Family/Social History: No family history of cancer; SS works as a social worker; she uses alcohol rarely; denies tobacco use or illicit drug use

Medications:
Levothyroxine, 112 μg PO daily
Atenolol, 25 mg PO daily
Levofloxacin, 500 mg PO daily
Acyclovir, 400 mg PO TID
Allopurinol, 300 mg PO daily
Fluonazole, 200 mg PO daily

Allergies: Bactrim

■ Physical Examination

GEN: Thin woman in no acute distress
VS: T 39°C, BP 130/80, HR 65, RR 18, O_2 sat 99% RA, Wt 55 kg, Ht 157.5 cm
HEENT: PERRLA, EOMI, no sclera icterus, posterior oropharyngeal erythema with mild ulceration
NECK: Supple, no LAD, no thyromegaly
COR: RRR, normal S1, S2, no M/R/G
CHEST: CTA bilaterally, no rales/rhonchi
ABD: Soft, NT/ND, no HSM, hyperactive bowel sounds
EXT: Thin, no C/C/E, Central line without erythema, pain, oozing
NEURO: A and O × 3, CN II–CXII intact

■ Results of Pertinent Laboratory Tests, Serum Drug Concentrations, and Diagnostic Tests

Lkc 0.3 × 10⁹ (0.3 × 10³)
diff: N 0.53 (53); P 0.34 (34); M 0.06 (6); E 0.02 (2); B 0 (0); bands 0.05 (5)

Hct 0.30 (30)	Na 139 (139)	AST 0.32 (19)	PT 11.9
Hgb 90 (9)	K 3.8 (3.8)	ALT 0.32 (18)	PTT 23
Plts 44 × 10⁹	Cl 104 (104)	LDH 2.6 (153)	INR 0.9
(44 × 10³)	HCO₃ 29 (29)	ALP 0.98 (59)	uric acid 113 (1.9)
	BUN 6.5 (18)	T.bili 3.42 (0.2)	TSH 4 (4)
	SCr 53 (0.6)	Alb 41 (4.1)	
	Mg 1.1 (2.2)		
	PO₄ 0.9 (2.8)		

Bone marrow aspirate: hypocellular bone marrow; 5% blasts
Peripheral smear: no blasts
Cytogenetics: t(8;21)
Chest CT: clear, no change from previous
Blood culture: no growth to date
Stool culture: positive for *Clostridium difficile* toxin

■ Case Problem List

Identify principal problems from the scenario in priority order (see Answers in back of book for correct list of problems).

■ SOAP Note

To be completed by the student (see Answers in back of book for correct SOAP Note).

■ QUESTIONS

(See Answers in back of book for correct responses.)

1. What is the most likely cause of acute respiratory distress, pleural effusion, fever, weight gain, and hypotension in a patient receiving induction chemotherapy with idarubicin and ATRA for APL? (EO-2, 5, 10)
   a. Pulmonary toxicity secondary to idarubicin
   b. Retinoic acid syndrome secondary to ATRA
   c. Tumor lysis syndrome secondary to induction chemotherapy
   d. Pneumonia secondary to myelosuppression

2. Which of the following cytogenetic findings is associated with a poor prognosis in patients with ALL? (EO-1, 5)
   a. inv 16
   b. t(9:11)
   c. t(9;22)
   d. Normal cytogenetics

3. Which of the following pairs of chemotherapeutic agents is most commonly used as maintenance therapy in the treatment of ALL? (EO-12)
   a. Fludarabine, cyclophosphamide
   b. Mercaptopurine, methotrexate
   c. Vincristine, imatinib
   d. Daunorubicin, gemtuzumab ozogamicin

4. Describe how pharmacokinetic changes due to aging could potentially affect the choice of postremission therapy if SS were elderly at the time of diagnosis. (EO-4, 6, 8)

5. Which prophylactic medication must be given with HiDAC and why? (EO-11, 12)
   a. Lactulose to prevent constipation
   b. Prednisone to prevent neurotoxicity
   c. Steroid ophthalmic drops to prevent ocular toxicity
   d. Levofloxacin to prevent infection

6. What is the mechanism of action of methotrexate? (EO-7)
   a. Methotrexate prevents cellular division by cross-linking DNA strands.
   b. Methotrexate promotes the assembly of microtubules to inhibit mitosis.
   c. Methotrexate inhibits topoisomerase II to cause single- and double-stranded DNA breaks.
   d. Methotrexate inhibits dihydrofolate reductase to inhibit DNA synthesis.

7. Describe measures needed to prevent unnecessary toxicity in patients receiving high-dose methotrexate as CNS prophylaxis for the treatment of ALL. (EO-5, 6, 9, 12)

8. Which of the following complications of allogeneic hematopoietic stem cell transplantation results from the T lymphocytes of the donor reacting against the host tissue? (EO-1, 7, 10)
   a. Graft versus host disease
   b. Veno-occlusive disease
   c. Graft failure
   d. Infection

9. What are the pharmacoeconomic considerations in utilizing colony-stimulating factors in patients with AML? (EO-17)

10. Which of the following medications is given to prevent tumor lysis syndrome? (EO-8, 12)
    a. Ibuprofen
    b. Filgrastim
    c. Cyclosporine
    d. Allopurinol

11. Which of the following is an adverse prognostic factor at diagnosis of ALL? (EO-1, 3)
    a. White race
    b. Age less than 2 years
    c. Low white blood cell count
    d. Female sex

12. Describe psychosocial factors that hematopoietic stem cell transplant patients and their families may experience and describe the role of the caregiver relative to these factors. (EO-15, 16)

13. Summarize therapeutic, pathophysiologic, and disease management concepts for acute leukemia utilizing a key points format. (EO-18)

CASE 38

TOPIC: Non-Hodgkin's Lymphoma

THERAPEUTIC DIFFICULTY: Level 2
Rebecca Finley

Chapter 95: Lymphomas

■ **Scenario**

Patient and Setting: LF, a 64-year-old man; outpatient

Chief Complaint: Night sweats, occasional fevers, mild difficulty swallowing

■ History of Present Illness

LF is a 64-year-old man with newly diagnosed diffuse, large B-cell lymphoma who had been experiencing night sweats and occasional fevers for approximately 2 months. He saw his internist approximately 2 weeks ago when he began having some difficulty swallowing. The internist noted several enlarged cervical lymph nodes but no pharyngeal erythema or apparent swelling. A biopsy of one of the lymph nodes revealed diffuse, large B-cell lymphoma (CD20 +) and LF was referred to a medical oncologist for evaluation and treatment. CT and PET scans revealed widespread bulky lymphadenopathy and involvement of Waldeyer's ring. Bone marrow biopsy was also positive and LF is scheduled to begin chemotherapy tomorrow.

Medical History: Hypertension $\times$ 18 years; type 2 diabetes $\times$ 3 years; hyperlipidemia $\times$ 10 years

Family/Social History: Family History: No family history of cancer
Social History: Retired businessman; 2 or fewer beers per week; denies any tobacco or illicit drug use

Medications:

Candesarten, 16 mg PO QD
Hydrochlorothiazide, 25 mg PO QD
Metformin, 1,000 mg PO BID
Rosiglitazone, 2 mg PO BID
Atorvastatin, 20 mg PO QD

Allergies: No known drug allergies

■ Physical Examination

GEN: White male in no obvious distress
VS: T 98.6°F, BP 148/70, RR 16, HR 88, Wt 78.6 kg, Ht 177.8 cm
HEENT: PERRLA; no oropharyngeal masses; no stomatitis or erythema
NECK: Supple with 2 enlarged cervical LN
COR: RRR, no m/r/g
CHEST: Lungs CTA
ABD: Soft nontender, nondistended, no hepatomegaly; spleen palpable below costal margin, normal BS
MS/EXT: No edema, erythema, or cyanosis, normal ROM, pulses intact, strength 5/5
NEURO: A and O $\times$ 3, CN II–XII intact, DTR 2+ throughout, Babinski negative bilaterally

■ Results of Pertinent Laboratory Tests, Serum Drug Concentrations, and Diagnostic Tests

Lkcs 3.8 $\times$ 10^9 (3.8 $\times$ 10^3); diff: N 0.58 (58); bands 0.03 (3); lymph 0.28 (28); M 0.04 (4); E 0.07 (7); B 0 (0); P 0 (0)

Hct 0.36 (36)	Na 138 (138)	AST 0.46 (28)
Hgb 114 (11.4)	K 4.4 (4.4)	ALT 0.5 (30)
Plts 210 $\times$ 10^9	Cl 102 (102)	LDH 4.9 (293)
(210 $\times$ 10^3)	HCO$_3$ 26 (26)	ALP 1.2 (72)
MCV 90 (90)	BUN 6.4 (18)	T.bili 10.3 (0.6)
MCHC 317 (31.7)	SCr 108 (1.2)	Alb 46 (4.6)
EPO 45	Mg 1.0 (1.9)	Uric acid 360 (6)
PO$_4$ 1.4 (4.3)	Ca 2.2 (8.8)	

Bilateral posterior iliac bone marrow aspirate and biopsies: bilateral evidence of diffuse lymphoma
Peripheral blood smear: normochromic, normocytic; no blasts
ABD, pelvis, chest, H and N CT: widespread lymphadenopathy; 4 lymph nodes >4 cm in diameter noted in abdomen
^{18}FDG PET: multiple areas of uptake throughout abdomen, chest, and neck, including Waldeyer's ring; evidence of bone marrow involvement
MUGA: WNL

■ Problem List

Identify principal problems from the scenario in priority order (see Answers in back of book for correct list of problems).

■ SOAP Note

To be completed by the student (see Answers in back of book for correct SOAP Note).

■ QUESTIONS

(See Answers in back of book for correct responses.)

1. Approximately what percent of adult lymphomas in the United States are derived from B lymphocytes? (E0-3)
   a. 15
   b. 30
   c. 50
   d. 85

2. The risk of non-Hodgkin's lymphoma is increased in individuals who: (EO-3)
   a. Are receiving phenytoin therapy
   b. Have rheumatoid arthritis
   c. Have few or no siblings
   d. Have undergone coronary bypass surgery

3. Reed-Sternberg cells are characteristically seen in: (EO-1)
   a. Diffuse large B-cell lymphomas
   b. Mucosa-associated lymphoid tissue lymphomas
   c. Adult T-cell lymphomas
   d. Hodgkin's disease

4. Describe why the prognosis of indolent non-Hodgkin's lymphomas (NHL) is often considered to be worse than the prognosis of aggressive NHLs. (EO-1)

5. The subscript "B" following the stage designation of a NHL (e.g., IV_B) indicates that: (EO-1, 2)
   a. The patient has a mediastinal disease.
   b. The disease is relapsed following initial therapy or was refractory to initial therapy.
   c. The patient has constitutional symptoms, including fever, night sweats, weight loss, and pruritis.
   d. The disease is bulky.

6. Lymphomas that are considered AIDS-defining conditions include: (EO-1, 2)
   a. Hodgkin's disease, primary CNS lymphomas, and large cell lymphomas
   b. Primary CNS lymphomas, large cell lymphomas, and Burkitt's lymphoma
   c. Large cell lymphomas, small noncleaved cell NHL, and primary CNS lymphomas
   d. Hodgkin's disease, Burkitt's lymphoma, and primary CNS lymphomas

7. Describe why ABVD replaced MOPP as the clear-cut standard for initial treatment for HD even though many patients who received MOPP therapy are alive and well more than 20 years later. (EO-11)

8. Deaths in patients with bulky lymphomas that occurred within hours of initial doses of rituximab have been attributed to: (EO-10)
   a. Massive cell lysis and metabolic complications
   b. Cardiac arrhythmias
   c. Allergic reactions
   d. Thrombotic complications

9. Rituximab is given 1 week and immediately prior to ibritumomab tiuxetan (Zevlin) in order to: (EO-6, 7)
   a. Sensitize lymphoma cells to the radioimmunocojugate
   b. Predict the likelihood that a patient will respond
   c. Reduce treatment-related cell lysis syndrome
   d. Reduce the risk of radiation delivery to unintended sites

10. A patient with a stage IV diffuse large B-cell lymphoma has completed two cycles of chemotherapy with the CHOP regimen. Following the second course of therapy she experienced an episode of febrile neutropenia that required 3 days of hospitalization. The patient would like to delay the third cycle of chemotherapy by 2 weeks and then receive lower doses to avoid further infectious complications. Discuss whether this is a reasonable option. (EO-12)

11. Adverse prognostic signs for aggressive NHL include: (EO-3, 4)
    a. Age over 60, LDH greater than normal range, more than one extranodal site of disease
    b. Age over 60, more than one extranodal site of disease, serum creatinine greater than 1.5
    c. More than one extranodal site of disease, LDH greater than normal range, serum creatinine greater than 1.5
    d. Serum creatinine greater than 1.5, age over 50, poor performance status

12. For patients more than 60 years of age with stage III or IV diffuse large B-cell NHL, the National Comprehensive Cancer Network (NCCN) recommends: (EO-12)
    a. ABVD + rituximab
    b. CHOP
    c. CHOP + rituximab
    d. BEACOPP

13. For treatment of aggressive NHL, the greatest benefit of high-dose chemotherapy followed by autologous stem cell transplantation has been reported: (EO-6, 12)
    a. Immediately following first-line CHOP therapy in younger patients
    b. In younger patients with relapsed disease that is chemosensitive
    c. Patients who relapse within 6 months of receiving CHOP therapy
    d. Younger patients with relapsed disease that is refractory to conventional chemotherapy

14. In addition to combination chemotherapy, patients with Burkitt's lymphoma should receive: (EO-8, 12)
    a. Radiation to all disease sites
    b. Total nodal irradiation
    c. CNS prophylaxis
    d. Radioimmunoconjugate

15. Hypertriglyceridemia is the most common adverse effect associated with: (EO-10)
    a. Ibritumomab tiuxetan
    b. Denileukin difitox
    c. Rituximab
    d. Bexarotene

16. Describe why new onset of back pain is considered to be an emergency situation in a patient with a lymphoma, and why it is important to initiate treatment immediately. (EO-2, 11)

17. Summarize therapeutic, pathophysiologic, and disease management concepts for the treatment of non-Hodgkin's lymphoma using the key points format. (EO-18)

CASE 39

TOPIC: Breast Cancer

THERAPEUTIC DIFFICULTY: Level 2
Maryann Cooper

Chapter 96: Breast Cancer

■ Scenario

Patient and Setting: KF, a 62-year-old African American female; hematology/oncology clinic

Chief Complaint: Hip pain, fatigue, anorexia, constipation, confusion

■ History of Present Illness

KF presents with severe (7 out of 10) pain in her right hip. She began noticing the pain about a month ago and has been treating it herself with over-the-counter pain medications that are no longer working; also complains of a decreased appetite over the past few weeks and increasing fatigue. Her husband also states that he has noticed that KF has been more forgetful lately and is sometimes confused.

Medical History: Breast cancer: Stage IIB infiltrating ductal carcinoma of the right breast diagnosed 6 years ago. Originally, the tumor was ER+/PR+ and did not overexpress HER-2/*neu*. The tumor was staged as T2N1M0. She received a lumpectomy with axillary lymph node dissection plus breast irradiation, 6 cycles of AC, and tamoxifen for 5 years
Other: first menarche at 13 years, menopause at 55 years, type 2 diabetes mellitus × 7 years; depression

Surgical History: Lumpectomy with axillary lymph node dissection 6 years ago

Family/Social History: One child s/p childhood ALL, sister with bilateral breast cancer. Married, mother of 3 grown children, retired librarian, 20 packs per year tobacco history, quit when diagnosed with breast cancer, no alcohol use

Medications:
Metformin, 1,000 mg PO BID
Rosiglitazone, 4 mg PO daily
Lisinopril, 10 mg PO daily
Paroxetine, 20 mg PO daily
Ibuprofen, 200–400mg PO q4–6h PRN
Calcium carbonate, 1,000 mg PO TID with meals

Allergies: No known drug allergies

■ Physical Examination

GEN: Pleasant, slightly confused, overweight woman
VS: T 37°C, BP 110/70, HR 80, RR 20, O_2 sat 98% RA, Wt 72 kg, Ht 160 cm
HEENT: PERRLA, EOMI
NECK: Supple, no LAD, no thyromegaly
COR: RRR, normal S1, S2, no M/R/G
CHEST: Well-healed scar on right breast, no erythema or oozing, lungs clear with decreased BS at right base
ABD: Soft, NT/ND, no HSM, normal BS
GU: Deferred
RECTAL: Deferred
EXT: Warm, no C/C/E
NEURO: A and O × 3, CN II–XII intact

■ Results of Pertinent Laboratory Tests, Serum Drug Concentrations, and Diagnostic Tests

Lkcs 6.0 × 10⁹ (6.0 × 10³) | Na 137 (137) | Ca 3.13 (12.5) | HbA₁c 7
Hct 0.38 (38) | K 3.7 (3.7) | Mg 1.1 (2.2)
Hgb 140 (14) | Cl 107 (107)
Plts 150 × 10⁹ (150 × 10³) | HCO₃ 26 (26)
| BUN 7.5 (21)
| SCr 88.4 (1.0)
| Glucose 6.1 (110)

CT scan of chest: solitary nodule in right lung base
Lung biopsy: metastatic adenocarcinoma consistent with breast primary
Bone scan: Multiple metastases to the right pelvis
MRI: no lesions in the brain
Echocardiogram: LVEF >55%

■ Problem List

Identify principal problems from the scenario in priority order (see Answers in back of book for correct list of problems).

■ SOAP Note

To be completed by the student (see Answers in back of book for correct SOAP Note).

■ QUESTIONS

(See Answers in back of book for correct responses.)

1. Which of the following is a negative prognostic factor in this patient? (EO-1)
   a. Estrogen receptor status
   b. Progesterone receptor status
   c. HER-2/*neu* status
   d. Nodal involvement

2. KF's albumin level comes back at 30 (3.0). What is her corrected calcium level? (EO-5)
   a. 3.23 (12.9)
   b. 3.28 (13.1)
   c. 3.33 (13.3)
   d. 3.43 (13.7)

3. KF asks you if she can take black cohosh to help with her new hot flashes. What is the most appropriate response to this request? (EO-9, 10)
   a. No, you should not take black cohosh because it has not been shown to help decrease hot flashes in any setting.
   b. No, you should not take black cohosh because its estrogen-like properties can decrease the efficacy of your anastrozole.
   c. No, you should not take black cohosh because you should never take one drug to treat the side effects of another drug.
   d. No, you should not take black cohosh because it is an herbal product that is not regulated by the Food and Drug Administration (FDA).

4. Describe how drug therapy is selected in a patient with metastatic breast cancer. (EO-8)

5. Shortly after starting anastrozole therapy for metastatic breast cancer, KF's calcium level increases and her bone pain worsens. What is the most likely explanation for these findings? (EO-10)

6. KF did not demonstrate an adequate response to endocrine therapy. She is to be started on chemotherapy with doxorubicin and paclitaxel. Her pretreatment ejection fraction is 40%, she has bilateral lower leg edema, and crackles in both lungs. What is the most appropriate action to take with regard to KF's treatment plan? (EO-2, 5, 8, 11)
   a. Add dexrazoxane
   b. Discontinue doxorubicin
   c. Reduce the dose of doxorubicin
   d. Discontinue paclitaxel

7. KF presents to the clinic for her third cycle of CMF. She complains of shortness of breath and is found to have a new pleural effusion. Describe how the pharmacokinetics of her chemotherapy will change with this finding. (EO-4, 5, 6)

8. According to the American Cancer Society Guidelines, which of the following statements regarding breast cancer screening is correct? (EO-3, 5)
   a. Begin annual mammography at age 40
   b. Women aged 20–39 years should receive a clinical breast exam every 5 years.
   c. Asymptomatic women ≥40 years should receive a clinical breast exam every 3 years.
   d. Breast self-examinations are not recommended for any women.

9. Describe the pharmacoeconomic impact of the early detection of breast cancer. (EO-17)

10. What is the mechanism of action of cyclophosphamide? (EO-7)
    a. Prevents cell division by cross-linking DNA strands
    b. Promotes the assembly of microtubules
    c. Inhibits DNA synthesis by intercalation between base pairs
    d. Competitively binds to estrogen receptors

11. Which of the following is an adverse reaction of paclitaxel? (EO-10)
    a. Hypersensitivity reactions
    b. Cardiomyopathy
    c. Hemorrhagic cystitis
    d. Nephrotoxicity

12. During the administration of doxorubicin, a patient begins to complain of severe pain at the injection site and it is found that some of the chemotherapy has extravasated. What is the most appropriate action to take? (EO-8, 10)
    a. Slow the chemotherapy infusion
    b. Aspirate any drug, consult a plastic surgeon, apply a cold compress, apply 1/6 or 1/3 M sodium thiosulfate
    c. Aspirate any drug, consult a plastic surgeon, apply a cold compress, apply DSMO topical solution
    d. Aspirate any drug, consult a plastic surgeon, apply a warm compress

13. Analyze psychosocial factors that affect women with breast cancer and describe the pharmacist's role in maintaining patient compliance with treatment. (EO-15, 16)

14. Summarize therapeutic, pathophysiologic, and disease management concepts for the treatment of breast cancer utilizing the key points format. (EO-18)

CASE 40

TOPIC: Prostate Cancer

THERAPEUTIC DIFFICULTY: Level 2
Karen W. Lee and Phillip Wizwer

Chapter 100: Prostate Cancer

■ Scenario

Patient and Setting: BV, a 65-year-old African American male; urologist office visit

Chief Complaint: Increasing nocturia with weak urine stream over the past year; complains of not being able to get "a good night's rest" because he wakes up at least twice during the night with both lower back pain and the urge to go to the bathroom; also has episodes of urge incontinence during the day with possible overflow during the night.

■ History of Present Illness

Complaints of "urine pain" from a possible "urinary tract infection (UTI)"; resolved 3 months ago after therapy with 10 days of sulfamethoxazole/trimethoprim. U/A had not been performed at that time. Recently, BV's primary care physician (PCP) noted a moderately enlarged tender prostate according to a digital rectal exam (DRE) during a regular visit. BV's PCP ruled out another UTI. BV's PCP referred BV to a urologist whom BV is visiting today for further workup of his urinary complaints. Approximately 1.5 years ago, BV was initiated on terazosin HCl 1mg PO QHS with success; however, he was switched to finasteride 6 months ago due to worsening of night symptoms. BV has used Tylenol intermittently for about 25 years for his wrist joint pain. Tylenol helps relieve the recent pain in his back minimally. He wears a "heating patch" on the lower back throughout the day that does not give him good relief. Additionally, BV shares with you that he has experienced "erectile problems" during the past year, but, he has not informed his PCP of this new complaint.

Medical History: Worsening benign prostate hypertrophy (BPH) for 12 years; urinary tract infection (UTI); osteoarthritis (wrist)

Family/Social History: Family History: Mother died at age 72 due to cardiac failure, father died at age 50 with undetermined etiology, brother died at age 75 secondary to prostate cancer

Social History: single; current high-fiber diet; cigarette smoker 2 packages/day for 20 years; no alcohol intake; recent forced retirement from his full-time job as a butcher at a local meat market

Medications:
Finasteride, 5 mg PO QD (started 6 months ago)
Zolpidem, 5 mg PO QHS (started 6 months ago)
Docusate sodium, 100 mg PO BID (started 3 yrs ago)
Acetaminophen, 500 mg PO q6h PRN (started 25 years ago)
Terazosin HCl, 1 mg PO QHS (started 1.5 yrs ago; discontinued 6 months ago)
Sulfamethoxazole/trimethoprim, 800/160 mg PO BID × 10 days (started 3 months ago; discontinued after 10 days)

Allergies: NSAID—anaphylaxis

■ Physical Examination (from Urologist Consult)

GEN: Elderly, slightly overweight, African American man in considerable discomfort from urinary-related issues.
VS: T 98.6°F, BP 132/86, HR 68, RR 28, Wt 195 lb, Ht 5'10"
HEENT: PERRLA, EOMI, no hemorrhages, exudates, or A-V nickings
COR: RRR, normal S_1 and S_2, no m/r/g
CHEST: Clear to A and P bilaterally
ABD: Soft, NT/ND, (+) bowel sounds
GU: External male genitalia normal
RECT: Tender, moderately enlarged prostate
EXT: No edema
NEURO: Alert, 0 × 4, CN II–XII intact, sensory and motor normal, (−) Babinski

■ Results of Pertinent Laboratory Tests, Serum Drug Concentrations, and Diagnostic Tests (from PCP Visit)

Labs from 2 days ago (fasting):
LDL 3.3 (129)
HDL 1.08 (42)
Triglycerides 1.72 (152)
Total cholesterol (5.2) 201
Labs from 1 year ago:
BUN 6.4 (18)
CR 123.8 (1.4)
Glu (fasting) 4.8 (87)
TSH 4.0 (4.0)
All other labs WNL (1 yr ago)
Additional labs/tests: (from urologist consult)
Serum testosterone: Normal
DRE: Tender, moderately enlarged prostate
PSA: (8 µg/L) 8 ng/mL; 1 year ago: (5 µg/L) 5ng/mL
U/A: No bacteria; no WBC
TRUS /BIOPSY: Pending scheduled appointment

■ **Problem List**

Identify principal problems from the scenario in priority order (see Answers in back of book for correct list of problems).

■ **SOAP Note**

To be completed by the student (see Answers in back of book for correct SOAP Note).

■ **QUESTIONS**

(See Answers in back of book for correct responses.)

1. Which of the following are risk factors that most likely contribute to BV's suspected prostate cancer? (EO-3)
   a. High-protein diet
   b. African American
   c. Erectile dysfunction
   d. Benign prostatic hypertrophy

2. Which of the following signs and symptoms are unique to various stages of prostate cancer and not benign prostatic hypertrophy? (EO-2)
   a. Lower back pain
   b. Enlarged prostate
   c. Weak urine stream
   d. Elevated PSA levels

3. Describe the significance of the PSA level in terms of diagnosing prostate cancer. (EO-5)

4. How prevalent are UTIs in males? Why was BV prescribed sulfamethoxazole/trimethoprim for treatment of his UTI? (E0-1, 8, 11)

5. How common is prostate cancer, and what is the mortality rate once one has been diagnosed with prostate cancer? (EO-3)

6. When should men be screened for prostate cancer? (EO-5)

7. Assuming that BV has advancing prostate cancer, what would be the best treatment options? (EO-12)

8. What are some of the promising therapies on the horizon for those individuals with hormone-refractory prostate cancer? (EO-3, 8, 12)

9. Describe the role of the pharmacist in management of a patient with prostate cancer. (EO-16)

10. According to the results of the transrectal ultrasound (TRUS)-guided biopsy of prostate tissue, BV's urologist stages the cancer as: $T_2N_0M_0$; with a Total Gleason Score: 4, right lobe 2 (1 +1); left lobe 2 (1+1). Six months later, the urologist ordered a follow-up PSA that came back 9 µg/L (9 ng/mL). As a result, the urologist performed a follow-up TRUS/Biopsy that showed a Gleason Score of 6. The prostate remained tender and enlarged but there were no significant nodules on palpitation. Describe the most appropriate treatment for BV's stage of cancer that is least likely to worsen BV's erectile dysfunction. (EO-5, 12)

11. After initiating the appropriate therapy for controlling BV's prostate cancer, his PSA levels fall to 4.0 ng/mL after 8 months of aggressive treatment. However, BV complains about worsening urge incontinence that requires him to wear diapers throughout the day. This urge incontinence is affecting his quality of life. BV's urologist has determined that BV's bladder is functioning properly (i.e., complete void of urine) based on a cytoscopy. What medication would you recommend to better control BV's urge incontinence? (EO-12)

12. After several years of aggressive treatment, BV's prostate cancer has resolved. BV is interested in initiating an over-the-counter product (i.e., vitamin, mineral, herbal) in his diet in hopes of reducing his risk of prostate cancer reoccurring in the future. Which of the following over-the-counter products may reduce the risk of prostate cancer? (EO-11)
    a. Vitamin E
    b. Saw palmetto
    c. Zinc supplement
    d. L-alanine supplement

13. What are the possible nonpharmacologic and/or pharmacologic treatments that may help to minimize the risk factors of developing prostate cancer in the future? (EO-4)

14. Synthesize pathophysiology, therapeutic, and disease management concepts for prostate cancer utilizing a key points format. (EO-18)

CASE STUDY ANSWERS

CASE 1 ANSWERS

■ PROBLEM LIST

1. New-onset hypersensitivity syndrome (evidenced by diffuse skin rash with fever, mucosal lesions, arthralgias, eosinophilia, and elevated liver function tests)
2. Poorly controlled high blood pressure
3. Gout
4. Renal insufficiency

■ SOAP NOTE

S: "I have a rash all over my body that looks like measles and is very itchy. I also have a fever and my body aches like I have the flu."

O: Diffuse, symmetrical maculopapular rash; conjunctival and oral lesions; fever of 39°C; urticarial plaques; elevated liver function tests; leukocytosis with eosinophilia; low complement 4 concentration, elevated ESR; elevated BUN and SCr; no evidence of infection or autoimmune markers; has taken indomethacin periodically for the past 6 months for gouty attacks; on HCTZ for HBP and recently discontinued lisinopril on his own; one new medication: allopurinol

A: PROBLEM 1: New-onset hypersensitivity syndrome potentially related to initiation of new medication (allopurinol)

PROBLEM 2: Poorly controlled HBP potentially related to the abrupt discontinuation of lisinopril and the use of NSAID therapy

PROBLEM 3: Gout: currently controlled with no evidence of acute or chronic pain and normal uric acid concentration

PROBLEM 4: Renal insufficiency potentially related to hypersensitivity syndrome

P: PROBLEM 1: Hypersensitivity Syndrome

- Discontinue allopurinol.
- Treat pruritus with H1 blocker such as diphenhydramine 25–50 mg PO q6h.
- Interview the patient for information regarding OTC, homeopathic, and other complementary drug therapies as potential causes of the adverse event.
- Administer ocular lubricant.

- Administer hydrogen-peroxide gargle, antiseptic mouthwash (chlorhexidine), and an anesthetic (benzocaine spray) for oral lesions.
- Initiate high-dose steroids (1 mg/kg/day prednisone or equivalent) to limit progression of hypersensitivity syndrome.
- If other potential causes are ruled out, update patient's allergy history to include allopurinol-related hypersensitivity syndrome.
- Monitor rash, LFTs, and renal function for progression/resolution of the event.

PROBLEM 2: High Blood Pressure

- Discontinue lisinopril due to chronic, unrelenting cough.
- Discontinue HCTZ due to frequency of gouty attacks.
- Initiate therapy with an angiotensin receptor blocker (e.g., losartan) or a calcium channel antagonist (e.g., amlodipine).
- Counsel the patient on the need for compliance with his medications and for periodic measurements of BP.
- Advise patient on the DASH diet.
- Monitor BP daily during hospital stay.

PROBLEM 3: Gout

- Discontinue allopurinol.
- Advise the patient to resume use of a NSAID (indomethacin) upon onset of an acute gouty episode.
- Recommend a balanced, low-fat diet to reduce gout episodes.
- Educate patient to limit alcohol intake to reduce gouty attacks.
- Monitor the number and frequency of gouty attacks.

PROBLEM 4: Renal Insufficiency

- Initiate IV hydration with normal saline solution to maintain renal perfusion and urine output.
- Obtain prior renal indices (BUN and SCr) to identify whether current renal indices reflect acute or chronic renal insufficiency.
- Ensure appropriate renal dosing of drugs.
- Limit use of medications that can further decrease renal function or are dependent on renal elimination.

■ CASE QUESTIONS

1. Eosinophilia and reduced serum concentration of complement 4. Eosinophils are recruited by interleukin-5, particularly when IgE is activated by an antigen–antibody reaction. Hypocomplementemia usually indicates increased breakdown or depletion of complement due to stimulation of the immune system. The presence of skin rash may or may not be related to an immune reaction. Fever may or may not be indicative of an allergic reaction.

2. c. MM has increased concentrations of circulating inflammatory proteins.

3. b. The reaction is most likely a predictable effect of an opioid on the GI mucosa.

4. Based on a calculated creatinine clearance of 41 mL per min, the answer is B, 200 mg PO QD.

5. a. Acute cytotoxic liver injury

   The patient had elevations in the serum transaminases only, which indicates the release of intracellular enzymes from hepatocytes. Other liver tests such as alkaline phosphatase and total bilirubin, which are markers of bile duct obstruction (cholestatic injury), were within normal limits. Since the liver test elevations have occurred within the past 90 days, the adverse event is considered acute.

6. d. Indomethacin

7. d. Cetirizine

8. b. Predictable reaction

   Cough is related to the pharmacologic effects of the ACE inhibitor on the metabolism of bradykinin. Thus, the adverse effect is considered predictable.

9. The monitoring plan should include SCr, BUN, and serum potassium concentration. The patient should be counseled regarding facial edema, itchy lips, or difficulty swallowing.

10. The presence of mucosal lesions in the mouth and conjunctiva is indicative of a severe systemic hypersensitivity reaction rather than an isolated skin reaction. Mucous membrane involvement of the lips, eyes, nasal cavity, and genitalia indicate progression of the rash to a systemic condition such as Stevens-Johnson syndrome. Other markers of a systemic reaction include elevations in liver tests and elevated renal indices.

11. Thiazide diuretics have been shown to competitively inhibit the proximal tubular secretion of uric acid and increase the reabsorption of uric acid in the proximal tubule.

12. The risk of a cross-reaction to ceftriaxone is less than 5%.

13. **KEY POINTS**
    - The majority of adverse drug reactions are predictable and can be anticipated based on the drug's pharmacology and pharmacokinetic properties. Prevention of these adverse reactions can be best achieved by knowledge of the pharmacology and pharmacokinetics of the drugs that we dispense and recommend.
    - Hypersensitivity (allergic) drug reactions vary in severity from relatively mild, localized skin rashes to severe, multisystem events. Clinical markers of a severe hypersensitivity syndrome include mucous membrane lesions (of the lips, oral cavity, nasal cavity, conjunctiva, and genitalia), elevations in liver tests, and elevations in renal indices.
    - Hypersensitivity (allergic) drug reactions vary in the time of onset. Some hypersensitivity reactions may be evident within hours to several days of drug initiation, whereas others may not manifest until several months after drug initiation.
    - Regardless of the mechanism by which a drug causes an adverse reaction, all severe events (e.g., those requiring treatment, hospitalization, or extended hospital stay) should be well documented in the patient's medical record.

CASE 2 ANSWERS

■ PROBLEM LIST

1. Hypertension
2. Depression
3. Adverse effects to hepatitis C treatment
4. Chronic hepatitis C
5. Hyperlipidemia

■ SOAP NOTE

S: ''I have been doing pretty well with my new injection medicine. I have noticed that I'm very tired, irritable, and feel edgy as well as aching all over. I'm also having headaches. These have been doing better since I started using Extra-Strength Tylenol. I take two tablets about four times a day or so almost every day. I've also noticed I don't sleep too well. This is all making me feel kind of depressed.''

O: African American male in no apparent distress, complaining of numerous constitutive symptoms including HA, insomnia, and body aches; BP 156/92, HR 78, RR 18, T 37°C, Wt 95 kg, Ht 178 cm; mild AV nicking; splenomegaly; Glu 127, LDL 132, HCV RNA 2,100; all other labs WNL

A: PROBLEM 1: Hypertension uncontrolled (goal <140/90) on current therapy, possibly due to the fact that ACE inhibitors are generally less effective in African Americans as well as the fact that many individuals require combination therapy for adequate treatment of hypertension

PROBLEM 2: Depression possibly due to pegylated interferon alfa-2b therapy, as this adverse effect occurs in as many as 40% of patients on this therapy

PROBLEM 3: Adverse effects (insomnia, fatigue, body aches) due to pegylated interferon alfa-2b therapy, as these effects occur in as many as 66% of patients on this therapy; patient is at increased risk of acetaminophen toxicity due to self-administration of excessive daily dose

PROBLEM 4: Chronic hepatitis C receiving appropriate treatment but not yet at therapeutic endpoint of HCV RNA at an undetectable level

PROBLEM 5: Hyperlipidemia not yet at LDL goal value of less than 100 (10-year risk for CHD >20%) on current pharmacotherapy; simvastatin contraindicated in patient with active liver disease

P: PROBLEM 1: Hypertension

- Add hydrochlorothiazide 12.5 mg PO QD to further reduce BP as well as to mitigate the reduced response seen with ACE inhibitors in African Americans.
- Have patient monitor BP between visits (home monitor, pharmacy, or fire station) and bring log of measurements to next clinic visit.
- Stress importance of smoking cessation.
- Encourage adherence to low-fat diet for weight loss.
- Encourage exercise.

PROBLEM 2: Depression

- Add amitriptyline 25 mg PO QHS for treatment of insomnia and depression; start with lower dose, as African American patients show higher blood levels and faster therapeutic response as well as manifesting a greater degree of toxic effects.
- Monitor patient weekly by a visit or by phone for suicidal and homicidal ideations.
- If depression worsens, decrease interferon dose by 50%.

PROBLEM 3: Interferon Adverse Effects

- Continue acetaminophen therapy but counsel patient regarding maximum dosage of acetaminophen of 2 g per day.
- Amitriptyline should aid in resolution of insomnia.
- Monitor for worsening of anticholinergic symptoms such as dry mouth or urinary retention.

PROBLEM 4: Chronic Hepatitis C

- Continue current therapy with ribavirin and pegylated interferon alfa-2b for a minimum of 6 months of therapy.
- Monitor HCV RNA for response at 6 months.
- Monitor triglycerides, leukocytes, neutrophils, hemoglobin, platelets, thyroid function, bilirubin, uric acid, and liver enzymes.

PROBLEM 5: Hyperlipidemia

- Discontinue simvastatin, as it is contraindicated in patients with active liver disease.
- Add ezetimibe 10 PO QD.
- Check fasting lipid profile 6 weeks after change in therapy.

■ CASE QUESTIONS

1. d. Asians
2. c. CYP2D6
3. d. Asians
4. a. Diuretics
5. d. Asians
6. c. No differences in protein binding
7. a. Greater in women than in men
8. b. Cardiovascular and central nervous system agents
9. Some commonly prescribed medications that are metabolized via N-acetylation in-

clude isoniazid, sulfonamides, procainamide, phenelzine, clonazepam, and hydralazine.

10. Racial and ethnic groups with the lowest incidence of slow acetylators include Canadian Eskimos, Japanese, and those from mainland China (5%–15%), while an intermediate incidence is seen in Caucasians and African Americans (50%), with the highest incidence occurring in Egyptians and Moroccans (80%–90%).

11. With tricyclic antidepressant use, African Americans demonstrate higher steady-state plasma concentrations and more rapid clinical improvement compared to Caucasians. Asians also have significantly higher plasma concentrations and lower clearance rates than Caucasians, leading to the need for lower doses. Hispanics appear to experience more side effects overall associated with antidepressants.

12. Women show greater improvement in response to chlorpromazine therapy than men. Depressed women with panic attacks respond better to monoamine oxidase inhibitors, while men with the same disorder respond better to tricyclic antidepressants. Men also respond better to imipramine in general; specifically, unipolar and bipolar men respond better than depressed women. Women eliminate oxazepam and temazepam more slowly than men. However, renal clearance of alprazolam and diazepam is higher in women than in men. The renal clearance of triazolam and lorazepam is equal in women and men.

13. **KEY POINTS**
    - Therapeutic response, metabolism, and side effects may differ with various medicines because of racial, ethnic, and gender differences.
    - Genetically controlled differences in the way individuals metabolize drugs are major determinants of racial and ethnic differences in response to medicines.
    - When used as monotherapy to treat African American hypertensive patients, diuretics and calcium channel blockers tend to produce a greater reduction in blood pressure than beta-blockers and ACE inhibitors.
    - African Americans, in general, respond better than Caucasians to antidepressants, have higher plasma levels, and show a greater degree of adverse effects.

CASE 3 ANSWERS

■ PROBLEM LIST

1. Fever, rash, and malaise
2. Suspected phenytoin toxicity
3. Hypotension
4. Hypercholesterolemia

■ SOAP NOTE

S: "I get over my bladder infection and now this rash starts. I was out gardening a few days ago, got dizzy, and fell into a patch of weeds that I'm afraid was poison ivy or something like that. I've been using some lotion, but it's not helping."

O: T 38.1°C; maculopapular rash; BP 142/94, HR 62; phenytoin serum concentration 25.3 μg per mL; new medications: topical diphenhydramine and calamine; short-course SMX/TMP completed 1 day prior

A: PROBLEM 1: Erythema multiforme secondary to SMX/TMP

PROBLEM 2: Ataxia: Phenytoin toxicity secondary to interaction with SMX/TMP

PROBLEM 3: Hypertension secondary to chronic use of pseudoephedrine

PROBLEM 4: Hypercholesterolemia, control of which is lessened due to interaction with simvastatin and phenytoin

P: PROBLEM 1: Erythema Multiforme

- Continue diphenhydramine and calamine lotion applications PRN.
- Initiate prednisone 60 mg PO QD × 10 with subsequent taper.
- Begin diphenhydramine 30–60 mg PO q4–6h PRN for itching.
- Apply cold compresses PRN to rash areas.
- Counsel JA never to re-initiate SMX/TMP or other sulfonamide antibiotics.
- Counsel JA to always report a sulfonamide allergy.
- If rash continues to worsen, consider hospitalization for IV corticosteroids and further supportive care.

PROBLEM 2: Phenytoin Toxicity

- Hold phenytoin doses until serum concentration drops below 79.28 (20 μg/mL).
- No other intervention is necessary, as SMX/TMP treatment is already complete.
- Continue to monitor for seizure activity.

PROBLEM 3: Hypertension

- Discontinue cetirizine/pseudoephedrine.
- Instruct JA to take antihistamine without decongestant component, and only during periods of allergic symptoms.
- Recheck BP during corticosteroid therapy and once corticosteroid taper is complete.
- If JA remains hypertensive, increase lisinopril dose.

PROBLEM 4: Hypercholesterolemia

- Change simvastatin to non-cytochrome P450-metabolized HMG CoA reductase inhibitor (e.g., pravastatin, atorvastatin).
- Confirm patient's understanding of proper diet and exercise regimen.
- Discuss need for smoking cessation.
- Recheck cholesterol panel in 6 weeks.

■ CASE QUESTIONS

1. a. Erythema multiforme associated with sulfamethoxazole/trimethoprim.

2. d. NSAIDs

3. Erythema multiforme—lesions have iris or target appearance, erythematous plaques; sites generally are peripheral, may be associated with post-inflammatory hyperpigmentation; fade after 1 to 2 weeks.

   Stevens-Johnson syndrome—bullous or vesicular lesions, often in conjunction with mucosal or conjunctival involvement; lesions affect less than 10% of body surface area; generally heal within 6 weeks.

   Toxic epidermal necrolysis—early lesions are small, dusky, necrotic macules; early, extensive involvement of periorificial areas and mucous membranes; lesions enlarge to produce large areas of necrosis with extensive subepidermal sloughing of more than 30% of body surface area.

4. Photosensitivity, Stevens-Johnson syndrome, toxic epidermal necrolysis, drug hypersensitivity syndrome (DRESS)

5. Mucosal and conjunctival lesions, high fever, arthralgias, myalgias, vomiting, diarrhea, keratitis, conjunctival scarring and blindness, esophagitis, pneumonia

6. c. Lingering effects of drug interaction with sulfamethoxazole/trimethoprim

7. Nystagmus, dysarthria, ataxia, lethargy, serum phenytoin concentration in excess of 20 μg per mL; free phenytoin concentration in excess of 1.6 μg per mL

8. b. Simvastatin

9. d. Phenytoin induction of object drug's metabolism

10. c. Pseudoephedrine

11. d. Discontinuation of simvastatin and initiation of atorvastatin

12. a. <100 mg/dL

13. **KEY POINTS**
    - Although allergy is suspected in many cases, the specific allergen may be difficult to identify in allergic dermatologic reactions.
    - Drug-induced skin diseases tend to be acute and resolve, particularly when the offending agent is removed. However, some cutaneous reactions to drugs result in serious medical conditions that require prompt treatment.
    - Atopic dermatitis, contact dermatitis, and idiopathic urticaria tend to be more chronic, with exacerbations and remissions.
    - Topical corticosteroids, occasional short-term systemic corticosteroids in severe conditions, and antihistamines are the mainstay of drug therapy, in addition to other nonspecific topical treatments.

CASE 4 ANSWERS

■ PROBLEM LIST

1. Falls secondary to drowsiness/dizziness
2. Pain management
3. Glaucoma

■ SOAP NOTE

S: "I was making my bed this morning when I just felt dizzy and went down. . . .The doctor said I didn't break anything, but I really banged my arms and legs. I've actually done this two or three times in the last couple of weeks. . . . I've been having a real problem with staying awake after I take all my medicine. Now they are giving me more things to take!"

O: Bilateral tenderness and bruising lower and upper extremities; recent addition of tramadol prescription consistent with apparent timing of drowsiness/dizziness complaints

A: PROBLEM 1: Repeated bouts of dizziness and falls likely secondary to medications

Potential causes of ML's dizziness/drowsiness that must be ruled out include (a) cardiovascular, (b) neurologic, or (c) other unknown. According to ML, this has been a problem only for the past 2 weeks. As cardiovascular and neurologic exams currently are normal, most likely due to tramadol. Early-morning administration of timolol eyedrops must also be considered due to potential for systemic side effects.

PROBLEM 2: Pain management therapy for osteoarthritis

This is likely contributing to Problem 1; recent addition of tramadol questioned by ML. Now, ML unsure whether she is to continue taking this medication.

PROBLEM 3: Medication management for glaucoma

Current IOP measurement unknown, other than last one listed as "good" by her ophthalmologist. Must consider timolol's systemic effects contributing to Problem 1. ML is not following dosing recommendations of her physician by using this in the morning. Again, ML is unsure whether she is to continue the timolol with the addition of the new medication latanoprost.

P: PROBLEM 1: Fall Secondary to Drowsiness/ Dizziness

- Discontinue tramadol and timolol eyedrops as potential causes; replace therapy with new prescription for latanoprost and monitor as discussed below.
- Short-term pain management with ibuprofen as prescribed appropriate for swelling; monitor for potential side effects, including drowsiness.
- Monitor for improvement in dizziness or drowsiness.
- Follow-up workup by family physician in 1 week if symptoms of drowsiness or dizziness do not improve after changing therapy.

PROBLEM 2: Pain Management

- As above, discontinue tramadol; patient previously maintained with acetaminophen; ensure patient understands to discontinue tramadol.
- Topical therapy with capsaicin could be added if necessary.

- For optimal pain-relieving benefits, ensure acetaminophen dosing is maintained at 1,000 mg PO q6h versus PRN dosing.
- Monitor liver function tests quarterly for signs of acetaminophen toxicity; assess renal function every 6 months to annually.
- Documented pain scale scores by nurses at skilled care facility may be useful to follow pain relief over time.
- Suggest initiation of nonpharmacologic therapy including heat or light exercise involving low impact to maintain range of motion.

PROBLEM 3: Glaucoma

- As above, discontinue tramadol eyedrops due to potential to produce systemic adverse effects, including low BP, dizziness, or drowsiness; ensure patient understands to discontinue.
- Begin latanoprost 1 drop both eyes at bedtime; monitor for IOP measurements consistent with previous therapy with timolol. Typical goal IOP measurement in range of 10 to 15 mm Hg should be obtainable with therapy if previously maintained with timolol alone.
- Ensure proper administration technique; if ML cannot properly administer, suggest help from nursing services available at skilled care facility.

■ **CASE QUESTIONS**

1. c. Secondary to timolol or tramadol

2. d. No signs or symptoms reported

3. (a) Open-angle glaucoma typically presents "silently" until late in the course of disease. For this reason, most patients do not realize they have open-angle glaucoma until screening tests reveal increased IOP. In patients with normal-tension glaucoma, changes in the optic nerve are often first evident after serial ocular studies (ophthalmoscopy). Later in the course of disease, the following may occur: gradual loss of peripheral vision (over months to years); persistent elevation of IOP; optic nerve degeneration; retinal nerve atrophy; edema of the cornea; cataracts; trabecular meshwork degeneration.

(b) Angle-closure glaucoma presents rapidly, with the following signs and symptoms common: blurred vision; severe ocular pain and congestion; conjunctival redness; cloudy cornea; moderately dilated pupil; poor pupil response to light; IOP markedly elevated;

nausea and vomiting. Complete blindness can occur in 2 to 5 days if left untreated.

4. a. Incorrect use of timolol eyedrops

5. c. BP 130/70 (sitting), 125/65 (standing)

6. b. Decrease in IOP

7. Administration of eyedrops should include several steps: handwashing, checking the solution for any discoloration or expiration date, shaking vials if medication is in suspension, not touching the dropper tip to the skin, tilting back the head, pulling down the lower lid, and administering the correct number of drops. It is important to stress that (1) the patient should either close the eye or place an index finger over the tear duct for 3 to 5 minutes (termed "nasolacrimal occlusion") to minimize the amount of medication that reaches the systemic circulation, and (2) drops of differing types of medication should be spaced apart by at least 10 minutes. Ideally, the health care provider should also observe the patient demonstrate the procedure after instruction to verify the patient's understanding and manual dexterity.

8. b. Determine appropriateness of frequency of medication refills

9. d. Untreated angle-closure glaucoma

10. Psychosocial factors that should be discussed when a patient presents to the pharmacy with therapy for newly diagnosed open-angle glaucoma include:

    ■ Discussion that in most cases open-angle glaucoma is "silent."
    ■ Description of goals of therapy to lower IOP in effort to reduce likelihood of further damage to the optic nerve and later complications.
    ■ Determination of ability to obtain, pay for, and properly administer medical therapy for glaucoma.

11. c. Blindness due to changes of the optic nerve

12. **KEY POINTS**
    ■ Increased IOP is the most important risk factor for progression of glaucomatous damage to the optic nerve.
    ■ The patient's complete medical regimen should be evaluated to avoid medical therapy that may worsen the glaucoma.

■ A target IOP is established based on the patient's current IOP and risk factors for progression of end-organ damage, with the goal to prevent initial or worsening ocular damage.
■ Reduction of IOP should be attempted using topical medications with low systemic effects. Typically, beta-blocking agents are the agents first chosen, unless otherwise contraindicated.
■ Other medication classes, such as miotics, sympathomimetics, carbonic anhydrase inhibitors, and prostaglandin analogs, have all been useful to decrease IOP. Each medication class has unique properties and side effect profiles that should be considered prior to initiating therapy.
■ The patient should use combination therapy only after monotherapy proves unsuccessful or is not tolerated.
■ One of the most important factors in successful glaucoma therapy is compliance with medical regimens.
■ Health care providers should monitor for effectiveness and adverse events, and surgical correction should be attempted only if medical therapy is not tolerated or is unsuccessful at maintaining the target IOP.

CASE 5 ANSWERS

■ PROBLEM LIST

1. Pneumatosis
2. Central venous catheter (CVC) extravasation
3. PN-associated liver disease
4. PN dependency
5. Metabolic bone disease
6. Nystagmus

■ SOAP NOTE

S: "Patient is extremely irritable; upper right arm is swollen, warm to touch; infusion pump pressure alarms require resetting more frequently; emesis appears to be worse when feedings advanced; overall skin color appears more jaundiced than normal. Nystagmus resolving, able to fix on objects."

O: KUB film: stacked, dilated bowel loops, predominately in right upper abdomen; evidence of pneumatosis; positive evidence of intramural air; chest x-ray films show evidence of osteopenia and beading along ribs; CVC tip in brachiocephalic vein; increased abdominal girth; PN dependent, intolerant of enteral feedings; infusion pump settings on maximum setting, bilious vomiting ×5; fever; labs: fecal fat 2+, glucose 179, total bili 15, direct bili 8.1, C-reactive protein (CRP) 1.2, calcium 7.8, ALT 244, alk phos 735, albumin 2, GGT 266, hematocrit 26, hemoglobin 9, platelets 60, white blood cell count 17

A: PROBLEM 1: Pneumatosis secondary to necrotizing enterocolitis

PROBLEM 2: CVC extravasation due to malposition of catheter through which a hypertonic fluid had been infused

PROBLEM 3: PN-associated liver disease due to prolonged PN use

PROBLEM 4: PN dependency secondary to bowel rest and inability to transition to enteral feedings

PROBLEM 5: Metabolic bone disease secondary to aluminum contamination and suboptimal calcium and phosphorus composition of PN

PROBLEM 6: Nystagmus due to malabsorption of thiamine

P: PROBLEM 1: Pneumatosis

- Hold enteral feedings until pneumatosis resolves.
- Maximize PN to provide 100% total calories.
- Repeat KUB.
- Guaiac all stools.
- Monitor temperature, BP, and respiratory rate.
- Bowel decompression with NG tube
- Maximize IV fluids (in combination with PN).
- Ensure adequate IV access for both PN and IV antibiotics.
- Initiate antibiotic therapy (piperacillin/tazobactam 150 mg IV q12h).
- Consider percutaneous drainage at bedside.
- Obtain an upper GI series prior to resuming enteral feedings.
- Restart enteral feedings slowly.
- Monitor for residuals, increased abdominal girth, and bloody stools.

PROBLEM 2: CVC Extravasation

- Evaluate site for extent of tissue damage.
- Consult with Plastic Surgery if damage extensive.
- Obtain CXR to verify proper catheter tip placement.
- Rewire/replace CVC if necessary.
- Consider removing access device.

- Consider needle aspiration of fluid from tissue space to reduce tension.
- Consider hyaluronidase injections around area of infiltration (administer hyaluronidase within the first few minutes to 1 hour after the extravasation is recognized); dose 0.2 mL of 15 units per mL hyaluronidase in five separate subcutaneous or intradermal injections around site of extravasation.
- Elevate extremity.
- Apply warm compresses to affected area.
- If the IV access device is removed, consider impact on PN/fluid therapy.

PROBLEM 3: PN-Associated Liver Disease

- Monitor total/direct bilirubin and LFTs.
- Check hepatic ultrasound for evidence of sludging.
- Encourage resumption of enteral feedings as soon as safe.
- Consider alternatives to parenteral fat emulsion to minimize phytosterol exposure.
- Reduce hepatotoxic trace elements in PN.
- Cycle PN to reduce number of hours of PN therapy per day without jeopardizing calories.
- Cover PN and lipids with UV-protective/light-sensitive bag.
- Ensure that current PN is compounded with a taurine-containing amino acid solution.
- Initiate therapy with ursodeoxycholic acid 30 mg/kg/day.
- Avoid overfeeding of macronutrients in PN: dextrose less than 15 mg/kg/min, protein (amino acids) less than 3 g/kg/day, fat emulsion less than 3 g/kg/day.
- Minimize future septic events by appropriately treating pneumatosis and using aseptic technique when handling the CVC and parenteral medications/PN.

PROBLEM 4: PN Dependency

- Assess weights and vital signs daily.
- Monitor fluid balance.
- Plot length, weight, head circumference on appropriate growth curves (premature, male infant, 0–12 months)
- Check serum electrolytes daily until stable.
- Check access site for redness and leaks.
- Check PN solution for particulate matter.
- Monitor CVC function for sluggishness and resistance to flushing.
- Check visceral protein status to ensure that appropriate protein dose is being delivered.
- Monitor blood sugar and urine sugar to assess tolerance to glucose dose.

- Monitor serum triglycerides to assess tolerance to lipid emulsion.
- Monitor for signs and symptoms of essential fatty acid deficiency, including rash and elevated triene:tetraene ratio.

PROBLEM 5: Metabolic Bone Disease

- Maximize calcium and phosphorus in PN solution.
- Monitor serum aluminum for toxicity.
- Monitor ionized calcium rather than serum calcium.
- Minimize sources of aluminum (goal <5 μg/kg/day).
- Monitor serum alkaline phosphatase, vitamin D, and parathyroid hormone levels.
- Ensure adequate calcium and phosphorus when resuming enteral feedings.
- Consider DEXA scans of long bones to monitor for evidence of osteopenia.

PROBLEM 6: Nystagmus

- Review medication list for possible drug-induced causes of nystagmus.
- Obtain baseline serum thiamine, pyruvate, and lactate levels.
- Administer test dose of parenteral thiamine and perform a 24-hour urine thiamine collection to assess thiamine stores.
- Monitor erythrocyte transketolase activity before and after administration of thiamine.
- Monitor for signs and symptoms associated with thiamine deficiency, including neurologic and cardiac.

■ **CASE QUESTIONS**

1. The complications associated with PN therapy include:

   Mechanical
   Catheter-related
   - Malposition
   - Pneumothorax
   - Hemothorax
   - Blockage/thrombosis
   - Embolization

   Infusate-related
   - Superficial extravasation
   - Deep extravasation

   Infectious complications
   - Foreign body in bloodstream
   - Mucosal atrophy
   - Poor aseptic technique when caring for CVC
   - Contaminated infusate

   Metabolic complications
   - Azotemia
   - Electrolyte imbalances
   - Glucose intolerance
   - Cholestasis
   - Metabolic bone disease
   - Urolithiasis

2. PN liver disease is associated with prolonged use of parenteral nutrition (i.e., >2 weeks) in the absence of enteral feedings. Its etiology is multifactorial. In addition to the lack of enteral feedings, other risk factors include prematurity, sepsis, multiple surgical procedures, and toxicity due to the PN components. Phytosterols contained in the lipid emulsion have been implicated. Management of the patient with PN liver injury includes the use of trophic feedings, removal of the hepatic-eliminated trace elements (copper and manganese), cycling of the PN solution, and protecting the PN and lipids from ambient light. Patients with PN liver disease have an elevated serum bilirubin (>2 mg/dL) as well as an increase in CRP and hepatic enzymes. In addition to initiation of enteral feedings and cycling, other interventions that have been somewhat successful include ursodeoxycholic acid, phenobarbital, and cholecystokinin therapies, although the evidence supporting their efficacy is mixed.

3. In the pediatric patient, levels of calcium, phosphorus, and magnesium are interrelated. Inadequate intake of each may result in osteopenia of prematurity, fractures, failure of appropriate bone mineralization, and reduced linear growth. During fetal development, these minerals begin to be accrued at approximately 25 weeks' gestation, with peak accretion at 36 to 38 weeks. As a result, premature infants have considerably less mineral stores in comparison to term infants. Nearly all the body's calcium stores are located in bones. Serum levels serve as an indirect measurement of total body stores. Moreover, as almost 50% of serum calcium is protein bound, the total serum calcium level is affected by the patient's albumin status. Ionized calcium, the most biologically active form of calcium, is a more accurate measurement of calcium status.

   Relatively high amounts of calcium and phosphorus are needed in the preterm infant to match in-utero mineral accretion rates. It is a challenge to formulate a solution that can accomplish this task, given the solubility limitations of calcium and phosphorus. Solutions must be of a relatively low pH to accommodate the high neonatal requirements. Typically, neonates weighing less than 2 kg require 3 to 4.5 mEq/kg/day (50–80 mg/kg/day) of elemental calcium (as calcium gluconate) and 1.5 to 2.25 mM/kg/day of phosphorus to achieve acceptable accretion rates. Infants weighing more than 2 kg require 2 to 3 mEq/kg/day (40–60 mg/kg/day) of elemental calcium and 1 to 2 mM/kg/day of phosphorus. This is equivalent to a calcium:phosphate ratio of 1.3:1 and 1.7:1 by weight (mg:mg) or 1:1 and 1.3:1 by molar ratio. A normal calcium:phosphorus ratio promotes optimal bone mineralization due to increased retention versus urinary losses. Inverted ratios can lead to hypocalcemia and an increase in parathyroid hormone secretion that can lead to increased urinary phosphorus losses and osteopenia.

4. The ideal location for a CVC tip is at the junction of the right atrium and superior vena cava. Venous flow rate is maximal in this large-diameter vessel, an important consideration when one is infusing a hypertonic solution such as PN. The maximum osmolarity that can be infused through a non-central catheter is 900 mOsm per L. Catheter tip placement should be verified by a chest x-ray prior to being used to ensure it is indeed central.

5. The exact etiology of pneumatosis intestinalis is unknown. Ischemia, infection, and hyperosmolar enteral feedings can contribute to the development of necrotizing enterocolitis. Complications of pneumatosis include strictures, enterocyst formation, malabsorption, inflammatory polyps, and enteric fistulas.

6. JL's stool was positive for fecal fat, suggesting that he is still malabsorbing the fat contained in his enteral formula. Once his current bout of pneumatosis resolves and he resumes enteral feedings, a formula low in long-chain fats (e.g., Neocate or EleCare) should be considered. The formula selected should have a fair amount of medium-chain triglycerides (MCT), as this source of fat is well absorbed through the basolateral wall of the intestinal enterocytes and into the portal venous circulation. However, MCT oils contain no essential fatty acids, so these fats cannot be the sole source of fat. Since his

stool is negative for reducing substances, he can tolerate the carbohydrate source in the formula.

7. JL's current PN is too hypertonic to be infused through a peripheral line. It should also be noted that his most recent blood sugar was 179, suggesting he may not be tolerating the current concentration of dextrose in his PN. Now that he is NPO, the calories from his enteral nutrition, as well as the fluid volume, must be provided by his PN and intravenous fat emulsion. Previously he was receiving 150 mL/kg/day total fluids from both enteral formula (115 mL/kg/day) and PN (35 mL/kg/day).

    Since all calories and fluid will be delivered to the patient, the total fluid volume should be reduced to 120 mL/kg/day (378 mL at weight 3.15 kg).

    To provide a PN with adequate calories (goal: 110 cal/kg/day, or 350 cal/day) as well as meet JL's fluid needs and not exceed an osmolarity of 900 mOsm per L, the following PN solution could be used:
    Intralipid 20% 2 mL per hour for 24 h (provides 48 mL fluid, 96 calories fat, 3 g/kg/day fat)
    PN formulation to be delivered in 330 mL per day or 13.8 mL per hour for 24 h:

    Dextrose 33 g (112 calories)
    Amino acids 6.6 g (26.4 calories, 2 g/kg/day protein)
    Sodium 10 mEq
    Potassium 6 mEq
    Calcium 6 mEq
    Magnesium 1.6 mEq
    Phosphorus 5 mM
    Pediatric trace elements 2 mL per L
    Pediatric MVI 5 mL per day

    The overall osmolarity of this fluid is 842 mOsm per L, suitable for peripheral infusion. Unfortunately, it does not contain the same caloric density as the previous regimen (total of 234 calories from this solution), so it will be necessary to reestablish central access as soon as possible if the NPO status is prolonged. Increasing the fat calories is not an option as it increases the risk of fat overload syndrome, characterized by metabolic acidosis and respiratory distress.

8. Aluminum toxicity is associated with impaired bone mineralization. Aluminum is deposited in the bone-osteoid surface, result-

ing in decreased bone formation. Since calcium gluconate salts are a large source of aluminum contamination, neonates are at great risk for developing aluminum toxicity due to their high calcium requirements. Calcium acetate salts have been used to minimize this risk, but they are less soluble than calcium gluconate and there are few published compatibility data to support their routine use.

Signs and symptoms of aluminum-induced osteomalacia include:
- Bone pain
- Osteoporosis
- Patchy osteomalacia
- Reduced bone disposition rate

9. In addition to impaired bone mineralization, aluminum toxicity is associated with renal insufficiency and neurotoxicity. Patients with aluminum toxicity may also develop a hypochromic microcytic anemia.

10. Recent evidence demonstrates that lipids are metabolized differently depending on their route of administration. Enteral lipids are absorbed by the enterocyte in the form of a micelle and packaged into chylomicrons for ultimate disposal in the liver. Once in the bloodstream, these particles rapidly acquire apolipoproteins from circulating high-density lipoproteins and can subsequently be metabolized by the liver. The emulsified particles of commercially made and intravenously administered lipid emulsions, such as Intralipid, mimic the size and structure of chylomicrons but differ in their content. In contrast to chylomicrons, artificial lipid particles primarily contain essential fatty acids and ω-6 triglycerides and are devoid of cholesterol or protein. Recent studies suggest that these ω-6 fatty acid-containing emulsions are dependent on lipoprotein lipase, apolipoprotein E, and low-density lipoprotein receptors for clearance and are metabolized with less lipolysis and release of essential fatty acids than chylomicrons. In fact, it appears that they may be cleared as whole particles by tissues other than the liver. These factors may account for the increased incidence of steatohepatitis associated with intravenous administration of Intralipid.

11. Amino acid solutions designed for infants have markedly different amino acid compositions than those for older children and adults due to the different requirements in in-

fants. Pediatric solutions contain more cysteine, taurine, glutamic acid, and aspartic acid than those for adults, as well as lower concentrations of methionine, glycine, and phenylalanine.

12. Nutrition assessment in the PN infant must begin immediately when the decision to start PN is made. Initial nutritional assessment includes accurate determination of gestational age and degree of prematurity, as well as an accurate measurement of birth weight, length, and head circumference. A variety of intrauterine and postnatal growth curves are available. The Babson and Lubchenco growth curves, the most commonly used, are based on the gold standard that postnatal growth in the premature infant should follow the expected rate of weight gain seen in utero. The Ehrenkranz longitudinal charts are also useful for tracking day-to-day changes, taking into account physiologic weight loss, and are often used in conjunction with the aforementioned growth curves. Once an infant has reached 40 weeks postconceptional age, anthropometric data should be plotted on the National Center for Health Statistics curves using the infant's corrected age (i.e., chronologic age adjusted by the number of weeks of prematurity).

Physical assessment should include daily weight as a rough estimate of overall fat and muscle stores. Initially, when calculating fluid and nutrient requirements, most practitioners prefer to use the infant's birth weight until the infant regains birth weight. Daily weights, when available, should be used thereafter. In some instances, an infant may be too frail to be weighed daily. In such situations, a "dosing weight" that all practitioners agree upon is used for calculations.

In addition to the physical assessment, laboratory studies should be obtained at baseline. Albumin is a poor marker of malnutrition due to its long half life (>14 days) but is useful when assessing other electrolyte values, such as serum calcium and magnesium. Prealbumin, with a half-life of only 72 hours, is a more sensitive marker of acute malnutrition and subsequent response to therapy.

13. JL's serum calcium is only 7.8 (normal 8–10.5). His serum albumin is 2 g per dL. Since serum albumin status affects the interpretation of serum calcium levels, a cor-

rected calcium calculation should be performed:

Corrected total calcium = total serum calcium + (0.8 (4 - measured albumin)) = 7.8 + (0.8 (4−2)) = 9.4

As the corrected serum calcium is WNL, no additional calcium supplementation is needed. Ideally, an ionized calcium that is not affected by albumin status should be used to monitor calcium stores.

14. When compounding a solution with such high amounts of calcium and phosphorus, in addition to ensuring that the pH is low enough to optimize solubility, the additions of calcium and phosphorus salts must be done in the correct order. According to the FDA Safety Alert, calcium should always be the last additive. Phosphorus salts should be one of the first additives so that they are well diluted prior to the addition of the calcium. Furthermore, some practitioners suggest that PN solutions be formulated so that the final concentration of protein is at least 1% so that both calcium and phosphorus salts may be safely added. These recommendations do not apply to total nutrient admixtures (TNA), since calcium and phosphorus solubility is lower in these lipid-containing admixtures. Furthermore, the higher pH requirements needed to ensure stable TNA further affects the ability to provide adequate amounts of calcium and phosphorus in the pediatric patient, thus supporting the recommendations of the ASPEN safe practice guidelines that two-in-one formulations with a separate lipid infusion be used for infants.

Currently, calcium gluconate is the preferred salt for use in PN solutions since it dissociates less than chloride salts and thereby remains in solution more readily. Some practitioners use calcium acetate salts for PN compounding in the hopes of minimizing aluminum contamination. Unfortunately, there are few published stability data using this form of calcium, and its routine use cannot be advocated without further research.

The factors that must be considered to avoid calcium phosphate precipitation are:

- Addition of phosphorus before calcium
- Solubility of calcium should be calculated from the volume of the solution at the time the calcium is added, not the final volume

- Low pH amino acids
- Increased amino acid concentration
- Lower final pH
- Reduced storage temperature (4°C)
- Use of calcium gluconate or acetate salts

The administration of cysteine HCl has been used to improve calcium and phosphate solubility by decreasing the pH of the PN solution. This can increase the risk of the development of a metabolic acidosis as well as a potential leaching of calcium salts from bone.

15. Essential fatty acid deficiency (EFAD) typically occurs when less than 1% to 2% of total calories are provided as essential fatty acids in children. Due to their limited fat stores, premature infants may develop EFAD in less than 1 week when total calories are less than 4% to 5% of essential fatty acids. EFAD is also seen in patients with chronic malnutrition or malabsorption, and in patients receiving prolonged courses of PN without adequate fat calories, as in this case report.

Provided that the serum triglyceride is less than 200 mg per dL, a minimum of 2% to 4% of nonprotein calories is administered as fat (approximately 0.5 g/kg/day) to provide sufficient essential fats to prevent EFAD.

Signs and symptoms of EFAD:

- Abnormal platelet aggregation
- Decreased resistance to infection
- Diarrhea
- Growth failure
- Impaired wound healing
- Increased red blood cell fragility
- Prostaglandin abnormalities
- Thrombocytopenia
- Scaly dermatitis

16. Yes, all IV fat emulsions are isotonic and can be infused through a peripheral line, as the osmolarity is less than 900 mOsm per L.

17. Patients with short bowel syndrome who do not receive any parenteral multivitamins are at risk for malabsorption of orally administered vitamins, whether they are included in their enteral formula or provided as a supplement. Thiamine deficiency has been described in these patients despite receiving adequate intake of oral multivitamins. In some instances, patients must receive paren-

teral multivitamins to ensure that their needs are met.

Signs and symptoms of thiamine deficiency:

- Fatigue
- Irritation
- Sleep disturbances
- Precordial pain
- Anorexia
- Abdominal discomfort
- Constipation
- Peripheral neurologic changes
    - Paresthesias of the toes
    - Burning of the feet
    - Muscle cramps in the calves
- Cerebral beriberi (Wernicke-Korsakoff syndrome)
    - Mental confusion
    - Aphonia
    - Confabulation
    - Nystagmus
    - Total ophthalmoplegia
    - Coma
- Cardiovascular (wet) beriberi (Shoshin beriberi)
    - High cardiac output
    - Vasodilation
    - Warm extremities
    - Tachycardia
    - Wide pulse pressure
    - Sweating
    - Lactic acidosis
    - Heart failure
    - Orthopnea
    - Pulmonary and peripheral edema

18. **KEY POINTS**
    - In addition to meeting their basic metabolic needs, children requiring specialized nutritional support need additional calories in order to grow and develop.
    - Infants and children with short bowel syndrome and evidence of fat malabsorption are at risk for vitamin and essential fatty acid deficiency.
    - PN-associated liver disease is multifactorial in etiology. Treatment options have variable rates of success; however, patients who can be transitioned off PN and maintained exclusively on enteral feedings can recover from this complication.
    - Calcium and phosphorus requirements are higher in infants and children receiving PN, and care must be taken to provide a solution that meets their nutritional requirements and is chemically stable.

- Infants maintained on PN are at increased risk of metabolic bone disease and fractures because they often cannot receive sufficient calcium and phosphorus in their PN; calcium gluconate often contains high levels of aluminum that can also contribute to metabolic bone disease.

CASE 6 ANSWERS

■ PROBLEM LIST

1. Hypertension, possible preeclampsia
2. Nausea and vomiting
3. Smoking
4. Caffeine use
5. Hemorrhoids
6. Obesity
7. Depression

■ SOAP NOTE

S: Thirty-five-year-old smoker presenting with severe headaches and constant nausea and vomiting for 48 hours

O: BP 158/102, HR 100, 2+ edema bilateral LE, 1+ protein, headaches, N/V, obesity, Na^+ 134

A: PROBLEM 1: Preeclampsia secondary to 5-year history of HTN; BP 158/102, 2+ edema, headaches, HR 100

PROBLEM 2: N/V secondary to headaches or normal part of pregnancy

PROBLEM 3: Smoking secondary to discontinuation of antidepressant

PROBLEM 4: Caffeine secondary to discontinuation of antidepressant

PROBLEM 5: Hemorrhoids associated with normal course of pregnancy; found on rectal exam

PROBLEM 6: Obesity due to poor nutrition or secondary to smoking cessation; Wt 81 kg, Ht 163 cm

PROBLEM 7: Worsening depression status, as stated by CC; smoking and caffeine intake increase

P: PROBLEM 1: Preeclampsia (Mild)

- Goal is to decrease BP, prevent seizures, and deliver viable baby.

Treatment of BP:
    Patient put on bed rest to delay need for delivery (either induction or cesarean)
    Daily urine protein measurements
    BID BP monitoring
    Diuresis within 48 hours
    If BP increases above 160/110 or protein in urine exceeds +2, then patient must be hospitalized and IV/IM magnesium sulfate started
Prevent seizures:
    IM magnesium sulfate is drug of choice to prevent seizures
    Monitor for toxicity (serum conc. 4–7 mEq/L)
Deliver viable baby:
    Preparation for delivery must be made if severe preeclampsia develops
■ Consider adding methyldopa for better control of BP once preeclamptic crisis has subsided
■ Limit sodium intake to 2 g per day
■ Discuss the importance of smoking cessation for healthier baby and lifestyle
■ Discuss the importance of better nutrition for healthier baby and mother; recommend mother with child aerobics

PROBLEM 2: Nausea and Vomiting

■ Goal is to eliminate symptoms, improve quality of life, minimize harm to fetus, and prevent hyperemesis gravidarum
    If symptoms are related to HA associated with increased BP, then N/V should subside once BP is stable
    Check pyridoxine level for deficiency. If low, then supplement
    Nonpharmacologic therapy
        Eat small, frequent, high-carbohydrate meals
        Avoid spicy and noxious odors
        Pressure-regulated wrist bands are also safe
        If symptoms do not subside, consider giving meclizine 25 to 50 mg per day

PROBLEM 3: Smoking

■ Since CC has ceased once, then she can cease again
    Use the 5 A's: Ask, Advise, Assess, Assist, Arrange
    Recommend smoking-cessation program
    Teach cognitive and behavioral strategies
    Provide information about harm to fetus and mother

PROBLEM 4: Caffeine Use

■ Limit or discontinue intake. Positive correlation exists between heavy caffeine intake and smoking. Use the 5 A's

PROBLEM 5: Hemorrhoids

■ Goal is to reduce symptoms and development
    If constipation is underlying issue, consider adding a bulk-forming laxative
    Recommend sitz bath
    Consider external topical product such as witch hazel pads to alleviate discomfort
    Limit sitting time on toilet to reduce strain to the anal area

PROBLEM 6: Obesity

■ This part of therapy is recommended only if CC's BP is under control.
■ Goal is to develop a healthier lifestyle for both mother and baby
    Smoking cessation
    Limit caffeine intake. Recommend sports drinks and flavored water instead of cola-type products.
    Recommend low-impact water aerobics or mother with child aerobics
    CC's BMI is 30; recommended BMI is 22 to 25

PROBLEM 7: Depression

■ Refer for psychosocial exam
■ Nonpharmacologic therapy, including journal writing, group meetings, couples therapy sessions
■ Pharmacologic therapy

■ CASE QUESTIONS

1. BP 158/102, 2+ edema bilateral LE, urinalysis 2+ protein

2. Concerns to mother: risk of seizures

3. Concerns to baby: consequences of decreased blood flow via hypertension or decreased oxygen delivery during seizures

4. d. Decreased birth weight

5. Psychosocial factors
    Issues CC must address: obesity, issues surrounding depression, desire to deliver healthy newborn
    Barriers: depression itself, smoking addiction

6. c. Sertraline

7. c. Sertraline

8. Risk factors: pregnancy, obesity

9. c. Clindamycin

10. Methyldopa
    Pros: improve blood flow to fetus by reducing BP
    Cons: have not been shown to improve perinatal outcomes, potential for fetal defects

11. History of depression, marital discord, or unwanted pregnancy; need to discuss with patient

12. **KEY POINTS**
    - Treatment decisions regarding this patient's hypertension, as with all medications, need to be made with both mother and fetus in mind
    - Treatment decisions regarding this patient's depression, with the fetus/neonate in mind, may be different during and after pregnancy
    - Pregnant patients need to be educated regarding the importance of asking before taking any medications, including OTC medications
    - Lifestyle measures that can be taken to improve outcome in the fetus/neonate need to be encouraged by all health care providers

CASE 7 ANSWERS

■ PROBLEM LIST

1. CHF exacerbation
2. Drug interactions:
   Amiodarone and Coumadin
   Amiodarone and digoxin
3. Poorly controlled BP
4. Chronic renal insufficiency
5. DM type 2

■ SOAP NOTE

S: "I am having increasing difficulty breathing, swollen legs, weakness, and weight gain. This all started 2 weeks ago when my furosemide dose was decreased."

O: SOB; 3+ ankle edema; 7 kg weight gain; BP 153/91; CR 1.9; BUN 32; urinalysis: 2+ protein; chest x-ray: enlarged cardiac silhouette; left ventricular ejection fraction (LVEF) 15%, +S1, S2

A: PROBLEM 1: HF exacerbation secondary to decreased dose of furosemide

PROBLEM 2: Drug interaction with amiodarone and digoxin: dose adjustment needed for digoxin.

PROBLEM 3: Poorly controlled BP

PROBLEM 4: Chronic renal insufficiency secondary to heart failure

PROBLEM 5: Poorly controlled DM type 2

P: PROBLEM 1: CHF Exacerbation

- Increase furosemide daily dose: add PM dose; change regimen to 80 mg PO QAM and 40 mg PO QPM.
- Monitor weight q24h.
- Monitor K+ level.
- Discuss importance of daily weights (same time of day, preferably on arising, in similar clothes); maintain a diary of weights and report increases in weight.
- Analyze dietary intake of sodium and use of potassium-containing salt substitutes. Discuss importance of adhering to dietary restrictions; praise and encourage to continue sodium-restricted diet (2 g Na/day).
- Assess adherence to entire heart failure medication regimen.
- If heart failure continues to worsen, consider adding nitrates or α blocker.

PROBLEM 2: Drug Interactions: Coumadin/Amiodarone; Digoxin/Amiodarone

- Monitor interaction with amiodarone and coumadin; INR stable; no need to adjust dose
- Decrease dose of digoxin by 50%: change regimen to 0.125 mg PO Q 3 days
- Continue digoxin; monitor digoxin level (goal: 1 ng/mL). Counsel regarding need to report nausea, blurred vision
- Monitor INR (goal: 2–3)

PROBLEM 3: Poorly Controlled BP

- Goal BP for adult hypertensive diabetic patients is below 130/80
- Add ARB (ACE inhibitor induced cough). Add Cozaar CHF: initial, 12.5 mg orally PO once daily; titrate at 7-day intervals to 25 mg, then 50 mg daily (based on response)
- If BP remains elevated with increases in furosemide and addition of Cozaar, add a nitrate

PROBLEM 4: Chronic Renal Insufficiency Secondary to Congestive Heart Failure

- No interventions needed at this time
- Use caution with renally cleared medications; doses should be adjusted for decreased renal function
- Consider metolazone if renal function becomes markedly reduced

PROBLEM 5: Poorly Controlled DM Type 2

- Add glyburide 5 mg PO QD.
- Rule out use of metformin due to increased SCr level (>1.5).
- Discontinue Avandia 8 mg QD due to possible fluid retention

■ CASE QUESTIONS

1. b. Decrease in furosemide dose

2. b. Shortness of breath

3. c. Altered mental status

4. c. Hypertension

5. b. Increased age

6. b. <130/80

7. Factors to be considered when choosing current medication therapy for WJ:

   a. Diuretic = loop because CrCl is below 50 mL per min

   b. Spironolactone added because still symptomatic

   c. ARB not ACE inhibitor because of cough from ARB

   d. ASA for coronary artery disease

   e. Add sulfonylurea due to poor control of blood sugar; avoid metformin due to serum creatinine above 1.5. Consider discontinuation of Avandia due to risk of edema

8. c. Spironolactone

9. A. Avandia: member of the thiazolidinedione class of antidiabetic agents; improves glycemic control by improving insulin sensitivity. Rosiglitazone is a highly selective and potent agonist for the peroxisome proliferator-activated receptor-γ (PPARγ). In humans, PPAR receptors are found in key target tissues for insulin action such as adipose tissue, skeletal muscle, and liver. Activation of PPARγ nuclear receptors regulates the transcription of insulin-responsive genes involved in the control of glucose production, transport, and utilization. In addition, PPARγ-responsive genes also participate in the regulation of fatty acid metabolism.

   B. Spironolactone: steroid with a structure resembling that of the natural adrenocortical hormone aldosterone, acts on the distal portion of the renal tubule as a competitive antagonist of aldosterone. It acts as a potassium-sparing diuretic, increasing sodium and water excretion and reducing potassium excretion.

   C. Carvedilol: nonselective β-adrenergic blocking agent with α-1 blocking activity, moderate membrane-stabilizing activity (MSA), no intrinsic sympathomimetic activity (ISA), and high lipid solubility

   D. Coumadin: acts by inhibiting the synthesis of vitamin K-dependent clotting factors, which include factors II, VII, IX, and X, and the anticoagulant proteins C and S

   E. Amiodarone: classified as a class III antiarrhythmic agent, but it is now most appropriate to suggest that it encompasses the entire spectrum of antiarrhythmic classification. Amiodarone slows intraventricular conduction by blocking the sodium channel, slows the heart rate, and impedes AV node conduction by blocking β-adrenergic receptors and calcium channels, and it prolongs atrial and ventricular repolarization by inhibiting potassium channels.

   F. Furosemide: a short-acting sulfonamide loop diuretic. Believed to reversibly bind to the sodium, potassium, chloride cotransport mechanism on the luminal side of the ascending loop of Henle, thereby inhibiting the active reabsorption of these ions; also inhibits reabsorption of sodium and chloride in the proximal and distal tubules.

   G. Digoxin: inhibits sodium-potassium ATPase, an enzyme that regulates the quantity of sodium and potassium inside cells. Inhibition of the enzyme leads to an increase in the intracellular concentration of sodium and thus (by stimulation of sodium–calcium exchange) an increase in the intracellular concentration of calcium. The beneficial effects of digoxin result from direct actions on cardiac muscle, as well as indirect actions on the cardiovascular system mediated by effects on the autonomic nervous system. Positive inotropic and negative chronotropic effects.

10. Exacerbation of heart failure due to inappropriate therapy/dose of furosemide. Increase furosemide dose.

    a. Poorly controlled hypertension. Based on JNC-VII, the patient's goal BP is 130/80 mm Hg because she also has diabetes. Consider adding ARB agent rather than an ACE inhibitor due to ACE inhibitor-induced cough

    b. Poorly controlled type 2 DM. Consider adding a secretagogue such as glyburide or repaglinide. Avoid adding biguanide due to renal insufficiency

    c. Hepatomegaly. While the amount of ETOH currently consumed by WJ might not be cause for alarm, with hepatomegaly and the number of medications currently being used, consider a discussion about decreased ETOH consumption

11. A. Patient issues

    1. Reduced activity due to current symptoms

    2. Number and complexity of current medication therapy

    3. Dietary restrictions due to current complications may be difficult

    4. Cost of medications: assess patient's health care coverage and ability to pay for medications

    B. Potential emotional issues: Based on the number of issues and number of medications being taken, monitor:

    1. Anxiety

    2. Panic disorders

    3. Depression

    C. Other barriers

    1. Unknown family dynamics and support; needs further analysis

    2. Assess other potential stressors in WJ's life at this time

3. Ability to travel to and from pharmacy or to and from clinic for follow-up

12. **KEY POINTS**
    - The JNC-VII defines hypertension as a systolic BP greater than 140 mm Hg or a diastolic BP greater than 90 mm Hg.
    - The pathogenesis of essential hypertension remains unknown. BP is controlled through a multifaceted interplay of neuro-hormonal, renal, vascular, adrenal, and genetic manipulations.
    - Target organ disease from arterial hypertension can be cardiac, cerebrovascular, peripheral vascular, renal, and ocular.
    - The treatment of hypertension requires a multi-intervention approach that encompasses nonpharmacologic treatments such as weight reduction through appropriate physical activity and dietary habits, dietary sodium reduction, and moderate alcohol consumption as well as the appropriate individualization of pharmacotherapy.
    - Comorbid treatment options consist of:

Heart failure	ACE inhibitor, loop diuretic, β-blocker, spironolactone
Status post-MI	β-blocker
DM type 2 with microalbuminuria	ACE inhibitor, ARB
DM with microalbuminuria	ACE inhibitor
Chronic kidney disease	ACE inhibitor

CASE 8 ANSWERS

■ PROBLEM LIST

1. Coronary artery disease (ischemic heart disease)
2. Coronary artery disease (post-MI/secondary prevention)
3. Heart failure
4. Hypertension
5. Dyslipidemia
6. Renal insufficiency
7. Allergic rhinitis

■ SOAP NOTE

S: AD complaining of increased chest pain after climbing two flights of stairs or walking three blocks; also complains of leg edema, nocturia, and shortness of breath; all episodes of chest pain are relieved by sublingual nitroglycerin.

O: Wt 80 kg, Ht 158 cm, calculated BMI ~32, ECG shows occasional premature ventricular contractions. Positive S3, positive S4 with gallop, positive JVD, hepatomegaly, bilateral rales, and 1+ ankle edema, BP 145/105, AV nicking and narrowing, retinal exudates; SCr 177 mmol/L (2.0 mg/dL), BUN 8.57 mmol/L (24 mg/dL)

    Cholesterol Panel (7 months ago)
    TC: 249 mg/dL
    LDL-C: 155 mg/dL
    HDL-C: 38 mg/dL
    TG: 280 mg/dL

A: PROBLEM 1: Coronary artery disease/chronic stable angina: AD currently receiving atenolol (in addition to providing protection from sudden cardiac death post-MI), nifedipine XL chronically, and sublingual nitroglycerin acutely for anginal symptoms; complaining of increased chest pain after climbing two flights of stairs or walking several blocks; episodes of chest pain are relieved by nitroglycerin; also complaining of new-onset heart failure symptoms. Both increased chest pain and heart failure symptoms can be suggestive of worsening ischemia. Atenolol is appropriate treatment for preventing angina in patients with coronary disease but is not indicated to treat heart failure, which is now likely present in AD. Available choices are metoprolol XL, carvedilol, and bisoprolol (although bisoprolol is not approved in the United States for heart failure treatment). Goal resting heart rate is 50 to 60 bpm; current resting heart rate is 85 bpm. Nifedipine XL is reasonable choice for preventing angina (and treating hypertension) but does not reduce the risk of future events in a patient with a history of MI, nor do any data exist regarding its use in patients with heart failure. In addition, nifedipine XL is associated with a high incidence of peripheral edema If a dihydropyridine calcium channel blocker is desired, either amlodipine or felodipine would be more appropriate as both have been used safely in heart failure patients. AD appears to be taking the sublingual nitroglycerin appropriately, as it is relieving her symptoms.

PROBLEM 2: Coronary artery disease/post-MI/secondary prevention: In addition to treatment of her underlying angina secondary to her coronary artery disease, AD requires therapy to reduce the risk of a second MI or death secondary to coronary artery disease; currently receiving aspirin and atenolol for this purpose. However, other drugs are indicated for this purpose that she is not receiving, including ACE inhibitors, aldoste-

rone antagonists, and HMG CoA-reductase inhibitors (statins). Because she likely has left-ventricular systolic dysfunction, the ACE inhibitor is indicated, although the use of an aldosterone antagonist (e.g., eplerenone) is controversial and less clear. Statins are discussed below in Problem 4, dyslipidemia.

AD is receiving estrogen replacement therapy for an unknown reason, either treatment of dyslipidemia or postmenopausal symptoms. Data suggest that hormone replacement therapy is indicated only for reducing postmenopausal symptoms, not for the prevention of future coronary events or dyslipidemia. These agents should be used for the shortest possible duration due to their risk of increasing vascular events in patients with vascular disease. The issue of dyslipidemia will be addressed in Problem 4.

Finally, based on the American College of Cardiology/American Heart Association 2002 guidelines, the approach to coronary artery disease (chronic stable angina/post-MI/secondary prevention) should follow the mnemonic ABCDE: A (anti-anginals and aspirin), B (β-blockers and blood pressure), C (cholesterol and cigarettes), D (diet and diabetes treatment), and E (education and exercise). Given AD's underlying conditions (obesity as defined by BMI >30, hypertension, and dyslipidemia) and behaviors (smoking), these should be addressed; she also requires appropriate education regarding her disease and drug regimen and the importance of exercise.

PROBLEM 3: Heart failure: AD's heart failure is secondary to coronary artery disease/acute MI and longstanding hypertension; she complains of new symptoms associated with heart failure. Given previous MI history, it is presumed to be associated with systolic dysfunction. However, evaluation of systolic function (ejection fraction measurement) is essential to determine appropriate therapy. The following discussion of treatment will be based on the assumption that reduced left-ventricular systolic function has been observed.

Given the appearance of heart failure symptoms, she is currently receiving suboptimal diuretic therapy with HCTZ. Diuretic therapy likely is suboptimal for several reasons: first, estimated CrCl of ~25 mL per min, and second, thiazide diuretics usually do not provide adequate control of heart failure symptoms except in patients with mild heart failure. Given the dose of HCTZ that she is currently receiving (50 mg BID), increasing the dose is not an option. Most heart failure patients require loop diuretic therapy to reduce heart failure symptoms. Because of the presence of reduced renal function she may require higher doses of loop diuretics than would be required in patients with normal renal function.

AD is not receiving ACE inhibitor therapy, which should be initiated and titrated to the target dose immediately. The selection of one particular ACE inhibitor over another is most likely not important in terms of clinical benefits, although regimen and cost are important issues to consider. The addition of ACE inhibitor therapy will also be beneficial in treating the patient's hypertension and for reducing remodeling following an acute MI.

As described above, since heart failure symptoms are present, β-blocker therapy should be changed to either metoprolol XL or carvedilol, since all β-blockers are effective for reducing ischemia, but only carvedilol and metoprolol XL are approved for treating heart failure.

Given the discussion above regarding nifedipine XL, other dihydropyridine calcium channel blockers are more appropriate in a patient with concomitant heart failure, namely amlodipine or felodipine. The ACE inhibitor and the increase in β-blocker dose will replace the nifedipine for hypertension treatment. If AD continues to have anginal symptoms on the β-blocker therapy alone, either addition of a long-acting nitrate or appropriate calcium channel blocker (felodipine or amlodipine) will be necessary.

PROBLEM 4: Hypertension: Longstanding, uncontrolled HTN. End-organ damage is evidenced by AV nicking and narrowing, retinal exudates, and poor renal function. Given the accompanying coronary artery disease, the JNC-VII guidelines suggest a goal BP of 130/85 to 140/90 mm Hg. However, because of the accompanying reduced renal function, the JNC-VII recommendations suggest the goal BP is below 130/80 mm Hg. The current therapy is suboptimal and requires considerable attention. See above discussion about antihypertensive therapy in the heart failure section; ultimate goal in this patient is to use therapies to manage the hypertension that benefit the concomitant disorders that are present, particularly heart failure and coronary artery disease. Currently AD is receiving a β-blocker (dose to be increased), an ACE inhibitor (drug added) and furosemide (HCTZ discontinued).

PROBLEM 5: Dyslipidemia: Lipoprotein analysis was obtained in the clinic 1 month prior to AD's

MI. Based on the most recent update of the National Cholesterol Education Program guidelines and recent clinical trials, her current goal for LDL-C is at least 100 mg per dL and perhaps less than 70 mg per dL. Given her LDL-C of 155 mg per dL prior to her MI, intensive therapy is required to lower her LDL-C by 35% to 55%. Only statin therapy (either alone or in combination) can achieve those goals. Statins are also desirable as they reduce morbidity and mortality. To accurately determine the appropriate treatment strategy, a fasting lipoprotein analysis should be obtained. Baseline AST and ALT levels have been documented.

PROBLEM 6: Renal insufficiency: Estimated CrCl of ~25 mL per min secondary to poorly controlled hypertension. Renal insufficiency can affect the dosing of medication excreted unchanged by the kidneys.

PROBLEM 7: Allergic rhinitis: Well controlled.

P: PROBLEM 1: Coronary Artery Disease (Ischemic Heart Disease)

- Change atenolol 50 mg daily to metoprolol XL 50 mg daily and titrate to goal of 100 to 200 mg daily (based on heart failure symptoms) and/or heart rate of 50 to 60 bpm at rest (ischemic heart disease).
- Discontinue nifedipine XL.
- Educate AD regarding cardiovascular risk factor reduction: HTN treatment, cholesterol management, dietary modification, exercise, and smoking cessation.
- Educate about the risk factors of coronary artery disease and stress smoking cessation, weight control, and medication compliance.
- Continue sublingual nitroglycerin as needed.
- Remind AD to continue to keep track of the number of anginal attacks and the number of weekly sublingual nitroglycerin tablets used.
- If exhibiting anginal symptoms on current β-blocker therapy, consider adding a long-acting nitrate (ISDN 10 mg tid, NTG patch daily, ISMN 20 mg bid, etc.); coordinate hypertension and anginal symptom control by using agents that benefit both disease states.

PROBLEM 2: Coronary Artery Disease (Post-M Secondary Prevention)

- See plan for Problem 1 above.
- Change EC ASA from 325 mg to 81 m
- See ACE inhibitor therapy below.
- See lipid-lowering therapy below.

PROBLEM 3: Heart Failure

- Discontinue HCTZ; start furosemide 40 mg QAM.
- Discontinue Procardia XL.
- Start enalapril 2.5 mg BID (or captopril 12.5 mg TID or lisinopril 5 mg QD). Since it is likely that all ACE inhibitors are effective in this area, choice of one agent should be based on compliance (once daily versus multiple doses), cost, and other issues.
- Assess ACE inhibitor therapy in 1 week; measure BP and serum K, BUN, and Cr and adjust therapy accordingly. Goal doses: enalapril 5 mg PO BID; lisinopril 10 mg daily; captopril 25 mg TID (due to reduced renal function), and the dose should be titrated up over several weeks.
- Discontinue the potassium supplement due to ACE inhibitor therapy in a patient with renal insufficiency; consider need for chronic potassium therapy when the goal dose of ACE inhibitor is achieved.

PROBLEM 4: HTN

- Goal BP more aggressively due to presence of renal dysfunction and numerous other risk factors.
- Control HTN with heart failure and coronary artery disease medications.

PROBLEM 5: Dyslipidemia

- Discontinue hormone replacement therapy (conjugated estrogen/medroxyprogesterone acetate).
- Obtain fasting lipoprotein analysis.
- Initiate simvastatin 40 mg daily or atorvastatin 20 mg daily in the evening.
- Explain to patient that the most common adverse effects of statins are GI related, such as diarrhea, nausea, vomiting, and flatulence.
- Counsel AD to report muscle pain, tenderness, or weakness, especially if accompanied by fever malaise.
- in 4 to 6 weeks with lipoprotein analy- function testing.
- lifestyles diet and lifestyle ribed above.

of all medications as

itis
led.

■ CASE QUESTIONS

1. AV nicking and narrowing, renal insufficiency, and left-ventricular hypertrophy

2. a. Bilateral rales

3. a. Coronary artery disease

4. c. Lisinopril 20 mg daily

5. c. D/C enalapril and initiate valsartan therapy.

6. a. ECG findings of old Q waves in leads V1–V4

7. a. <70 mg per dL

8. a. Carvedilol

9. b. 0.125 mg daily

10. b. Weight gain of 2 to 3 pounds in 1 week

11. AD should be provided with the following information for using her nicotine gum correctly:
   a. The nicotine gum is used to help you stop smoking. It has a better efficacy rate if you enroll in a stop-smoking program.
   b. The gum should never be swallowed.
   c. Chew one piece of gum whenever you have the urge to smoke.
   d. Chew the gum very slowly until the taste of nicotine or a slight tingling in the mouth is perceived (about 15 chews). Then stop chewing the gum and put it to the side of your mouth.
   e. Once the tingling in the mouth is gone (usually about 1 minute), the chewing procedure should be repeated. This cycle should be repeated intermittently for about 30 minutes, and then the gum should be thrown away.
   f. To get the best results from the gum, follow the instructions carefully. Do not chew as you would regular gum.
   g. Do not use more than 30 pieces of gum per day. (Average daily use is 10 to 12 pieces.)

12. There is much information for AD to learn about the correct use of nitroglycerin (NTG). Present the information before she is to be discharged, along with a written copy of the instructions.
   a. When experiencing chest pain, AD should sit down and dissolve one NTG tablet under her tongue. The tablet should not

be swallowed, and she should not have food in her mouth at the same time.

b. Sublingual NTG rapidly relieves the chest pain, usually within 3 to 5 minutes. She should take one tablet; if the pain has not resolved in 5 minutes, she should take another tablet. If the pain has not resolved in an additional 5 minutes, AD should take a third NTG tablet and proceed to an emergency room. Educate AD and her family regarding the new American Heart Association guidelines, which recommend that patients take one NTG dose sublingually in response to chest discomfort/pain. If chest discomfort/pain is unimproved or worsening 5 minutes after one NTG dose has been taken, the patient or family member/friend should call 911 immediately to access EMS.

c. When she takes NTG, AD may get a headache, which may be relieved with acetaminophen (she should take the acetaminophen after the episode of chest pain has resolved).

d. The NTG may make AD dizzy and light-headed and increase her heart rate, so she should sit down when taking the medication.

e. The NTG may produce a burning sensation under the tongue. This is not an indication of potency.

f. AD may take the NTG prophylactically 5 to 10 minutes before activities that usually precipitate anginal attacks (e.g., climbing stairs).

g. AD should have her NTG with her at all times.

h. After each use, the cap of the bottle should immediately be closed tightly.

i. The cotton filler should be discarded after the initial opening of the bottle.

j. The NTG should be kept away from hot, humid places to prevent loss of potency.

k. The NTG should be kept in the original container, without other medications in the same bottle.

l. AD should get a new bottle of NTG 6 months after opening the bottle for the first time.

13. Summarize the risk-factor reduction therapies for this patient's ischemic heart disease:
    a. Correction and treatment of all modifiable cardiovascular risk factors is essential in an effort to reduce the risk for future vascular events.

    b. Risk-factor reduction should focus on hypertension management, smoking cessation, lipid-lowering therapy, antiplatelet therapy, cardiac rehabilitation, and exercise.

    c. Treatment of HTN reduces cardiovascular morbidity and mortality.

    d. Smoking cessation is especially important in patients with ischemic heart disease. Smoking is associated with increased morbidity and mortality, silent ischemia, arrhythmias, and coronary vasospasm in patients with coronary artery disease. Pharmacologic and nonpharmacologic approaches are available for assisting patients with smoking cessation.

    e. Lipid-lowering drug therapy in patients with angina and/or prior MI with average and elevated serum cholesterol concentrations has been shown to reduce cardiovascular morbidity and mortality.

    f. Exercise training reduces cardiovascular mortality, improves functional capacity, and attenuates myocardial ischemia and thus is an important lifestyle modification.

    g. Other cardiovascular risk factor reductions should include weight loss if overweight, alcohol use only in moderation.

14. Summarize the nonpharmacologic treatment options for this patient's heart failure.

    a. Patient/family education
       1) Discussions/pamphlets on signs and symptoms of heart failure and medications
       2) Emphasis on compliance with complete treatment agenda
       3) Instructions on when to contact health care providers

    b. Diet
       1) Daily weight chart
       2) Individualized diet according to needs/preferences/lifestyle
       3) Sodium restriction: mild (<3 g/day) or moderate (<2 g/day)
       4) Information regarding sodium and potassium content in foods
       5) Alcohol restriction
       6) Fluid restriction: ~ 2 L per day
       7) Nutritional supplements (e.g., vitamins)
       8) Emphasize importance of com

    c. Pharmacologic treatment of hy
       emia and hypertension

d. Exercise program

e. Intensive follow-up: telephone calls, home visits, outpatient clinic visits

15. **KEY POINTS**
   ■ Heart failure

   a. Heart failure is a clinical syndrome that progresses to worsening symptoms and death largely as a consequence of maladaptive effects triggered by neuro-hormones and cytokines.

   b. Heart failure can result from abnormalities in either systolic or diastolic dysfunction.

   c. Participation in cardiac rehabilitation programs can improve exercise tolerance and quality of life and may reduce mortality in heart failure patients.

   d. Patient education is extremely important, especially with respect to facilitating compliance with dietary and medication treatment plans.

   e. Based on their ability to consistently improve both the clinical status of patients and their longevity, ACE inhibitors are considered first-line therapy in the management of heart failure patients. ACE inhibitor therapy should begin with low doses that are slowly titrated to target doses.

   f. Alternative vasodilator therapy such as ARBs or the combination of nitrates plus hydralazine should be reserved for patients intolerant of ACE inhibitors.

   g. The use of β-blockers is currently advocated in the management of all stable heart failure patients based on their ability to reduce mortality and hospitalization rates. β-blocking therapy begins with low doses that are slowly and carefully increased. Since this patient has ⟨...⟩ these agents are particularly ⟨...⟩ he prevention of anginal epi-

   ⟨...⟩ he management
   ⟨...⟩ eve symptoms.

   ⟨...⟩ d safely in most pa-
   ⟨...⟩ ailure due to systolic
   ⟨...⟩ n target serum digoxin
   ⟨...⟩ between 0.7 and 1.2 ng

j. Anticoagulant therapy is indicated in heart failure patients with coexisting atrial fibrillation or other conditions that predispose them to thromboembolic conditions.

■ Status post-MI

   a. MI is one of the most common reasons for hospitalization in the Western world. The actual mortality rate is about 15%; approximately 10% of patients will die during the first year after their acute MI.

   b. Short-term and long-term survival depends on the extent and location of the coronary obstructive lesions and the prompt correction of post-MI complications.

   c. Information about the presence or absence of mechanical, electrical, ischemic, and vascular abnormalities is needed to institute approximate medical and/or surgical treatment.

   d. Correction and treatment of all modifiable cardiovascular risk factors is essential in an effort to reduce the risk for future vascular events.

   e. Risk factor reduction should focus on hypertension management, smoking cessation, lipid-lowering therapy, antiplatelet therapy, and cardiac rehabilitation and exercise.

   f. Treatment of hypertension reduces cardiovascular morbidity and mortality.

   g. Smoking cessation is especially important in patients with ischemic heart disease. Smoking is associated with increased morbidity and mortality, silent ischemia, arrhythmias, and coronary vasospasm in patients with coronary artery disease. Pharmacologic and non-pharmacologic approaches are available for assisting patients with smoking cessation.

   h. Lipid-lowering drug therapy in patients with angina and/or prior MI with average and elevated serum cholesterol concentrations has been shown to reduce cardiovascular morbidity and mortality.

   i. Exercise training reduces cardiovascular mortality, improves functional capacity, and attenuates myocardial ischemia and thus is an important lifestyle modification.

j. Other cardiovascular risk factor reductions should include weight loss if overweight, alcohol use only in moderation.

CASE 9 ANSWERS

■ PROBLEM LIST

1. Pneumonia
2. Acute renal dysfunction
3. VTE prophylaxis

■ SOAP NOTE

S: Patient has no current complaints.

O: Chest x-ray LLL infiltrate, diffuse rales bilaterally, diminished breath sounds, RR 18, Lkcs 10 × 10^9 (10 × 10^3), T 37°C, BUN 14 (38), CR 168 (1.9)

A: PROBLEM 1: Pneumonia

PROBLEM 2: Acute renal dysfunction due to dehydration from N/V

PROBLEM 3: DVT prophylaxis required secondary to hospital stay and immobility

P: PROBLEM 1: Pneumonia

- Continue IV moxifloxacin 400 mg daily for 10 to 14 days.
- Change IV moxifloxacin to PO once N/V has resolved and patient is afebrile for 24 to 48 h.
- Monitor temp q24h.
- Monitor Lkcs q24h.

PROBLEM 2: Acute Renal Dysfunction due to Dehydration From N/V

- Continue IV fluids.
- Encourage slow PO intake.
- Monitor I and O.
- Monitor BUN and Cr q24h.
- Goal is to return Cr to baseline and hydrate patient to BUN/Cr ratio less than 20:1.

PROBLEM 3: VTE Prophylaxis Required Secondary to Hospital Stay and Immobility

- Patient is at risk for VTE due to age and immobility in the hospital.
- Check baseline aPTT, PT, hemoglobin, hematocrit, and complete blood count (platelets).
- Add unfractionated heparin starting with an IV bolus 80 units per kg (5,000 units) followed by IV infusion of 1,000 units per hour to prevent VTE until patient is ambulating.
- Avoid using LMWH as patient has renal dysfunction.
- Monitor aPTT 4 to 6 hours after beginning infusion to a goal of 1.5 to 2.5 times the control.
- Continue to monitor aPTT q6h for 24 h and then q24h.
- Continue to monitor PT, hemoglobin, hematocrit, and complete blood count (platelets) q24h.
- Monitor for signs and symptoms of bleeding and VTE q24h, including calf pain/tenderness, LE swelling, venous distention and Homans sign, dyspnea, tachypnea, sinus tachycardia, and pleuritic chest pain.
- Alternative therapy VFH 5000 units SQ BID-TID until ambulating.

■ CASE QUESTIONS

1. a. Venous stasis as a result of hospitalization

2. DVT: calf pain/tenderness, LE swelling, venous distention and Homans sign; Pulmonary embolism: dyspnea, tachypnea, sinus tachycardia; pleuritic chest pain

3. Age, prolonged immobility due to hospitalization

4. DVT: Compression ultrasonography; Pulmonary embolism; no one test is preferred; test of choice is based on presence of risk factors

5. b. LMWHs do not require any laboratory monitoring.

6. c. Warfarin efficacy is monitored with an INR.

7. c. Warfarin interferes with clotting factors II, VII, IX, and X.

8. Support garments including elastic stockings or intermittent compression devices; surgery; avoid prolonged sitting, leg crossing; constrictive garments.

9. c. Thrombocytopenia

10. d. 40 mg SQ q24 hrs

11. a. Protamine sulfate

12. **KEY POINTS**
   - Hospitalized patients who are n[ot ambulat]ing are at an increased risk fo[r developing] VTE.

- There are several medication treatment options, including UFH, LMWHs, and warfarin, with different advantages and disadvantages. Use should be tailored to individual patients.
- UFH can be administered SQ or IV and has a quick onset of action. The IV infusion allows for quick titration and ability to stop drug quickly. aPTT should be monitored when using UFH.
- LMWHs can be administered BID or once daily and do not require laboratory monitoring due to a predictable dose-response. LMWHs should be used cautiously in patients with renal dysfunction.
- Warfarin is available orally. Warfarin's antithrombotic effects may take up to 4 days, so its administration should be overlapped with another agent with a quick onset of action such as UFH or LMWH. Warfarin's effects are influenced by many factors that are variable, including patient diet, liver function, and drug–drug interactions; INR should be monitored carefully.

CASE 10 ANSWERS

■ PROBLEM LIST

1. Septic shock
2. Anion gap metabolic acidosis
3. Pneumonia
4. Traumatic brain injury (TBI)
5. Risk of seizures
6. Altered metal status, sedation
7. Electrolyte abnormalities
8. Risk of deep vein thrombosis (DVT)
9. Risk of stress ulcer
10. Asthma

■ SOAP NOTE

...nt appears unarousable.

...rterial pH 7.16, HCO_3 14.2 mmol/L, ...i 150,000 CFU/mL, *S. aureus* ...nytoin level 5 mg/L, albumin ...om 11i on previous ...$^{++}$ 1.5 mg/dl, PO_4

...s evidenced by the ...py and likely related ...py. Adequate antibi- ...otrecogin alfa therapy ...ed secondary to TBI.

PROBLEM 2: Calculated anion gap of 18. Anion gap acidosis likely caused by lactic acidosis secondary to tissue hypoxia from septic shock and should respond to improved oxygen delivery.

PROBLEM 3: Untreated pneumonia as *A. baumannii* is generally resistant to piperacillin/tazobactam and tobramycin. There is also the possibility of undertreated *S. aureus* pneumonia if vancomycin levels are not optimized. Optimized antibiotic therapy is required.

PROBLEM 4: Resolving TBI as indicated by positive loss of consciousness, subdural hematoma on CT, admission GCS below 10, and improved GCS on day 9 of 11 intubated.

PROBLEM 5: Received greater than 7 days of seizure prophylaxis without witnessed seizure activity. Additionally, adjusted phenytoin level is subtherapeutic (8 mg/L). Seizure prophylaxis is no longer warranted.

PROBLEM 6: Decline in mental status is likely related to septic shock but could also be due to excessive administration of analgesics and/or anxiolytics. A less likely possibility is an abrupt worsening of his subdural hematoma. Correction of underlying etiology should improve his mental status.

PROBLEM 7: Hypokalemia, hypomagnesemia, and hypophosphatemia are related to critical illness and should respond to replacement by IV boluses of these electrolytes.

PROBLEM 8: Potential problem of DVT secondary to trauma, respiratory failure, and immobility related to cervical vertebrae fractures, moderate TBI, and ICU status. The subdural hematoma and spleen laceration are stable and would not likely contribute to future risk of bleeding.

PROBLEM 9: Potential problem of stress ulcers secondary to risk factors such as trauma, mechanical ventilation, and septic shock.

PROBLEM 10: History of mild intermittent asthma. Mechanical ventilation may act as a trigger for an asthma attack.

P: PROBLEM 1: Septic Shock

- Continue IV crystalloids (NS).
- Initiate norepinephrine at 1 μg per min and titrate to MAP above 70 or dopamine at 2 μg/kg/min and titrate to MAP above 70.
- Drotrecogin alfa is contraindicated.

- Initiate insulin continuous infusion.
- Maintain blood glucose between 80 and 100 mg per dL (4.5 to 6.1 mmol/L).
- Monitor MAP closely.
- Monitor urine output.
- Monitor respiratory status.
- Monitor mental status.
- Monitor temperature of extremities.
- Monitor WBC, SCr, and BUN.
- Monitor blood glucose hourly.
- Monitor core body temperature.

PROBLEM 2: Anion Gap Metabolic Acidosis

- Improve oxygen delivery with plan from Problem 1.

PROBLEM 3: Pneumonia

- Discontinue piperacillin/tazobactam.
- Discontinue tobramycin.
- Continue vancomycin (linezolid 600 mg IV q12h is an alternative).
- Start imipenem/cilastatin 500 mg IV q6h or 1,000 mg IV q8h.
- Start amikacin 425 mg IV q8h.
- Monitor amikacin peak and trough with third dose.
- Monitor vancomycin peak and trough.
- Monitor renal function (urine output, SCr).

PROBLEM 4: TBI

- No interventions

PROBLEM 5: Risk of Seizures

- Seizure prophylaxis is no longer warranted.
- Discontinue phenytoin.
- Continue to monitor for any seizure activity.

PROBLEM 6: Altered Mental Status, Sedation

- Hold all sedation and analgesia until SAS improves.
- Discontinue morphine.
- Use hydromorphone 0.5 mg IV q4h for analgesia.
- Monitor for improvement in mental status.

PROBLEM 7: Electrolyte Abnormalities

- Give magnesium sulfate 4 g IV over 4 hours.
- Give potassium phosphate 30 mmol IV over 4 hours.
- Give additional potassium chloride 40 mEq IV over 4 hours after potassium phosphate infusion is complete.
- Monitor renal function.
- Monitor electrolytes for response to therapy.

PROBLEM 8: Risk of DVT

- Continue enoxaparin 30 mg SQ q12h.
- Add intermittent pneumatic compression devices.
- Monitor for signs of bleeding.
- Monitor renal function.

PROBLEM 9: Risk of Stress Ulcer

- Continue ranitidine 50 mg IV q8h.
- Monitor renal function.

PROBLEM 10: Asthma

- Continue albuterol.
- Add nebulized ipratropium if JS has an acute worsening of respiratory function.
- Monitor SaO_2.
- Monitor PO_2.
- Monitor for wheezing.

■ CASE QUESTIONS

1. c. Haloperidol

2. d. 9%–30%

3. b. Imipenem/cilastatin

4. d. Norepinephrine

5. a. Hypomagnesemia

6. b. Maintain blood glucose between 80–110 mg/dL (4.5–6.1 mmol/L).

7. d. PPIs have equal or better pH control compared to H2 antagonists.

8. d. Binds and covers damaged gastric mucosa

9. c. 8 mg/L

10. Hypophosphatemia can weaken JS's ability to breathe on his own by impairing diaphragmatic contractility. It can also diminish oxygen delivery by reducing the amount of 2,3-diphosphoglycerate (2,3-DPG), which in turn increases the affinity of hemoglobin for oxygen. Increased oxygen affinity by hemoglobin prevents unloading of oxygen at the periphery.

11. Severe sepsis is defined as sepsis with accompanying acute organ dysfunction is defined as systemic inflammatory sponse to infection. JS has three S ponents, a documented infection markers of organ dysfunction. O listed below:

a. SIRS: HR ≥90 bpm (115 bpm), Temp >38°C (39°C), WBC ≥12 × 10^3/mm^3 (22 × 10^3/mm^3)

b. Infections: BAL with *A. baumannii* 150,000 CFU/mL and *Staphylococcus aureus* 100,000 CFU per mL

c. Acute organ dysfunction: PaO_2/FiO_2 <250 (229), MAP <70 (57)

The relative contraindication for JS is his subdural hematoma.

12. JS would be considered at particularly high risk for deep vein thrombosis secondary to having sustained a traumatic injury plus having multiple other risk factors such as respiratory failure, surgery, immobility secondary to spinal column fractures, head injury, and ICU status.

13. Oxygen delivery (DO_2) is the product of cardiac output (CO) and blood oxygen content (CaO_2). The determinants of CaO_2 are partial pressure of arterial oxygen (PaO_2), Hgb concentration, and the percentage of arterial Hgb saturated with oxygen (SaO_2). As the amount of oxygen dissolved in the plasma (PaO_2) is less than 2%, altering this would not significantly contribute to DO_2. It is then possible to improve DO_2 by improving each significant component. This means improving CO, Hgb, and SaO_2. Packed red blood cells (PRBCs) can be used to increase Hgb and improve oxygen carrying capacity. Improving SaO_2 can be achieved by increasing the amount of inspired oxygen (FiO_2). Finally, CO can be increased with agents that have inotropic activity (e.g., dopamine, norepinephrine, dobutamine).

14. JS has an MRSA pneumonia, which would require a higher vancomycin peak and trough secondary to poor penetration into the lung parenchyma. Based on JS's vanco-
in levels, the adjusted peak and trough
ximately 23 μg per mL and 5 μg
tively. Other pharmacokinetic
le: ke = 0.126 h^{-1}, t½ = 5.5
and Vd = 51 L (0.6
acokinetic pa-
osing of his
comycin peaks
g per mL and
mL, JS should re-
ancomycin dosing.
vancomycin 1,500
an estimated peak and

trough of 35 μg per mL and 15 μg per mL, respectively.

15. Medication recommendations:
a. Discontinue morphine, as a possibly active metabolite morphine-6-glucuronide can accumulate in renal failure.
b. Use hydromorphone or fentanyl instead of morphine.
c. Continue midazolam as JS's mental status returns toward normal.
d. Extend enoxaparin dosing interval to q24h as indicated in package insert.
e. Adjust ranitidine dosing interval to q24h or choose alternative agent that is not renally eliminated (i.e., pantoprazole 40 mg IV q12–24h).
f. Hold vancomycin and monitor level. Vancomycin will likely need to be given intermittently as indicated by levels. Linezolid 600 mg IV q12h may be an alternative.
g. Discontinue piperacillin/tazobactam, as it is likely ineffective against *A. baumannii.*
h. Begin imipenem/cilastatin 250 to 500 mg IV q12h depending on sensitivity of *A. baumannii* (package insert). Some clinicians would recommend using meropenem 500 mg IV q12h or ampicillin/sulbactam 3 g IV q12h, as these agents have a lower incidence of seizure activity related to accumulation in renal dysfunction.
i. Hold tobramycin.
j. Monitor sensitivity of *A. baumannii* to tobramycin.
k. Consider pulse-dose amikacin, as it is more likely to be effective against *A. baumannii.*
l. Discontinue phenytoin because JS has received greater than 7 days of therapy without seizure activity. JS is not likely to benefit from continuing therapy.
m. Continue albuterol therapy.
n. Consider adding ipratropium 0.02% via nebulizer q4–6h if albuterol is not sufficient.

16. **KEY POINTS**
■ Provision of adequate analgesia and sedation is essential in the supportive care of virtually all critically ill patients.
■ Mechanical ventilation is frequently required in critically ill patients and is associated with numerous complications requiring pharmacologic intervention.
■ Use of prophylactic heparin or LMWH should be considered in all critically ill pa-

tients deemed to be at risk for deep vein thrombosis.

- Stress ulcer prophylaxis should be considered in all critically ill patients deemed to be at risk for stress-related mucosal bleeding.
- Use of prophylactic phenytoin should be considered for patients with mild to moderate traumatic brain injury.

CASE 11 ANSWERS

■ PROBLEM LIST

1. Liver transplant
2. Metabolic alkalosis
3. Hypokalemia
4. Hyperglycemia
5. Postoperative pain

■ SOAP NOTE

S: Patient is awake and alert.

O: Intubated, jaundiced, mildly distended abdomen, 3+ bilateral LE edema. K 3.4, Glu 164, Ca 7.4, Alb 2.4, Tbili 8.4, AST 439, ALT 362, alk phos 50, LDH 665, tacrolimus level <3, pH 7.51, pCO_2 40, serum CO_2 35. Afebrile, BP 116/55, HR 76, RR 12 (on vent), Wt 75 kg, Ht 168 cm. Meds: tacrolimus 2 mg NG bid, methylprednisolone IV taper, valganciclovir 900 mg NG QD, sulfamethoxazole/trimethoprim 800/160 mg NG QD, nystatin 500,000 units to oral cavity QID, lansoprazole 30 mg NG QD, ursodiol 300 mg NG TID, hydromorphone IV infusion, regular insulin IV infusion

A: PROBLEM 1: Received a liver transplant for HCV cirrhosis

PROBLEM 2: Metabolic alkalosis secondary to multiple factors, including NG suction, blood transfusions during the transplant surgery (citrate used for blood product anticoagulation is converted to bicarbonate by liver), lactate produced from anaerobic metabolism during surgery (lactate is converted to bicarbonate by the liver), and/or postoperative fluid restriction and diuretics (done to prevent hepatic congestion, but may result in volume depletion and a resulting contraction alkalosis)

PROBLEM 3: Hypokalemia secondary to metabolic alkalosis

PROBLEM 4: Hyperglycemia secondary to methylprednisolone and tacrolimus administration

PROBLEM 5: Postoperative pain due to large abdominal incision

P: PROBLEM 1: Liver Transplant

- Continue tacrolimus and methylprednisolone for immunosuppression.
- Although the tacrolimus trough is below the target blood level, no dose increase is warranted. MH received his transplant yesterday and therefore received his first dose of tacrolimus last night. This level reflects only one dose, and a dose titration at this time would be premature.
- Continue valganciclovir, sulfamethoxazole/trimethoprim, and nystatin for prophylaxis of CMV, PCP, and oral thrush.
- Continue lansoprazole for prevention of gastric ulcers.
- Continue ursodiol to improve bile flow.
- Efficacy monitoring: liver function tests (should improve daily), trough tacrolimus levels (titrate dose to achieve a target of 8–10 ng/mL), signs and symptoms of infection (including fever, leukopenia, leukocytosis, oral thrush), GI upset
- Toxicity monitoring: electrolytes (watch for hyperkalemia, hypomagnesemia, and hypophosphatemia), renal function tests (watch for elevated BUN and SCr, CBC (watch for leukopenia and thrombocytopenia), finger sticks (watch for hyperglycemia), fasting lipid panel, tremor, headache, seizures, GI upset
- Counsel MH about the importance of compliance with his drug regimen. Being immunosuppressed puts MH at higher risk of infections and certain types of cancers, so he should take proper precautions. He may take tacrolimus with or without food but must be consistent to ensure consistent systemic exposure. On days of his laboratory blood draws, blood should be taken immediately before a scheduled tacrolimus dose to ensure a 12-hour trough. Advise him to alert his physician if he develops any unusual symptoms such as diarrhea, severe headaches, tremors, or sore throat. He is encouraged to monitor his own BP (and blood sugar if necessary) at home.

PROBLEM 2: Metabolic Alkalosis

- Administer 300 mL 0.1 N HCl solution over 12 hours into a central venous catheter to treat the metabolic alkalosis and facilitate prompt extubation.
  Note on calculations:
  First, calculate the HCl deficit.
  For MH: [103–99 mmol/L] × 75 kg × 0.2 = 60 mmol HCl deficit

Then, determine the amount of HCl to administer:

Give 50% of the deficit (for MH: 30 mmol) over 12–24 hours

Finally, calculate the volume of HCl solution that you will need to infuse:

Using a 0.1 N (100 mmol HCl/L) solution, you will need 300 mL.

Using a 0.2 N (200 mmol HCl/L) solution, you will need 150 mL.

- Efficacy monitoring: Check arterial blood gas and electrolytes q4h
- Toxicity monitoring: Watch infusion site for skin necrosis or phlebitis, check a CBC before and during infusion (watch for hemolysis)

PROBLEM 3: Hypokalemia

- Refrain from administering exogenous potassium in this case. Serum potassium levels should self-correct as MH's metabolic alkalosis resolves. (In metabolic alkalosis, K^+ is exchanged for H^+ in an attempt to buffer and decrease the pH.)
- Monitor serum potassium level.

PROBLEM 4: Hyperglycemia

- Continue regular insulin infusion for blood-sugar management.
- Monitor fasting blood sugar and finger sticks four to six times daily. Track daily insulin requirements.
- Over the next week (as the methylprednisolone taper ends), use QID finger sticks and insulin requirements to determine whether the patient has developed posttransplant diabetes mellitus. If so, initiate patient education on diabetes care, blood-sugar management, insulin administration, and use of a blood glucose monitor.

PROBLEM 5: Postoperative Pain

- Continue hydromorphone infusion for pain control.
- Consider docusate sodium 100 mg PO BID and senna alkaloids 1 tab PO QD for constipation.
- Efficacy monitoring: BP, HR, pain control per pain scale, medication requirements
- Toxicity monitoring: RR, assess for pruritus and regularity of bowel movements

■ CASE QUESTIONS

1. a. Dehydration, hypokalemia, metabolic acidosis.

   Sodium, potassium, bicarbonate, and water are lost in the stool. A patient with diarrhea may become dehydrated and hypokalemic. In severe cases, metabolic acidosis may develop.

2. Hypomagnesemia refers to serum concentrations below 0.8 mmol per L (1.6 mEq/L), and hypophosphatemia refers to serum concentrations below 0.8 mmol per L (2.5 mg/dL). It would be appropriate to treat when serum levels fall below these thresholds. Because this electrolyte disorder is anticipated to be a chronic problem (a side effect of a medication that will not be discontinued), oral replacement would be the best choice for long-term management. Oral replacement might include magnesium oxide 400 mg PO BID and K Phos Neutral 250 mg PO BID, but the doses must be titrated depending on the severity of the electrolyte deficiency. All oral phosphorus replacements contain potassium in varying amounts, so the medication must be carefully selected according to a patient's potassium needs.

3. a. Diarrhea

   Magnesium is a saline cathartic, and exogenous replacement may cause diarrhea.

4. d. No treatment is necessary.

   Calcium is protein bound and the serum calcium level may be artificially low in a patient with low serum albumin. MH's measured serum calcium must be corrected as follows:
   Corrected serum calcium = [4 g/dL–2.4 g/dL]0.8 + 7.4 mg/dL = 8.7.
   This corrected calcium level is within normal limits, and treatment is not required.

5. You must know the arterial pH, partial pressure of CO_2 (pCO$_2$), and plasma HCO_3 (CO$_2$).

6. d. There is no respiratory compensation because the mechanical ventilation does not allow him to hypoventilate.

   The compensatory mechanism for a metabolic alkalosis is respiratory acidosis, and this can be achieved by hypoventilating and thereby retaining CO_2. MH is currently on a mechanical ventilator that is preventing him from hypoventilating. If he were extubated at this time, he would likely go into severe respiratory depression in an attempt to minimize CO_2 loss. His normal pCO$_2$ of 40 demonstrates that does not have a respiratory compensation.

7. MH is a patient with severe hepatic insufficiency. He continues to experience third-spacing, as evident by ascites and LE edema

present on physical exam. This is most likely due to his low albumin, which is typical of patients with liver disease. As a result, the volume of the third space expands at the expense of the intravascular volume. MH, however, is not hypovolemic (BP and HR are within normal limits), and therefore he has a total body water overload.

8. c. He has a total body water overload, and 0.9% NaCl would exacerbate it.

   MH has a total body water overload (see #7). Normal saline is a poor choice for management of metabolic alkalosis in patients with a total body water overload because they cannot tolerate the sodium load and excess fluid.

9. b. Patients with symptomatic hypokalemia should receive IV rather than oral potassium replacement.

   Symptomatic hypokalemia should be managed with IV potassium. The oral liquid offers a more rapid onset of action compared to the wax matrix tablet. The maximum rate of peripheral infusion is 10 mmol per hour; higher infusion rates are associated with pain and phlebitis at the infusion site. Infusions into a central line can be administered as fast as 40 mmol per hour. Potassium must ALWAYS be diluted before administration and cannot be given via IV push.

10. c. Kayexalate can be used to increase potassium excretion.

    Kayexalate (in addition to loop diuretics and hemodialysis) corrects hyperkalemia by removing potassium from the body. IV calcium salts can be used in severe hyperkalemia: They work by stabilizing cellular membranes. The remaining treatment options include insulin (followed by glucose to prevent hypoglycemia), β-2 agonists (albuterol), and sodium bicarbonate, which work by driving potassium into the cell.

11. b. 100 mL/hr

    MH weighs 75 kg. His daily fluid maintenance needs are as follows:
    100 mL per kg for the first 10 kg = 1,000 mL
    50 mL per kg for the next 10 kg = 500 mL
    20 mL per kg for the remaining 55 kg = 1,100 mL
    TOTAL = 2,600 mL per 24 h or ~100 mL per hour

12. Crystalloids (i.e., 0.9% NaCl, 0.45% NaCl, 0.2% NaCl, Lactated Ringer's) are aqueous solutions that contain electrolytes. Colloids (i.e., plasma protein fraction, albumin, hetastarch) are solutions containing plasma proteins or other colloidal materials.

13. The cost of an ICU bed may be thousands of dollars per day. Conditions such as metabolic alkalosis can delay extubation and discharge, resulting in profound increases in cost. Interventions that facilitate extubation and lead to an earlier transfer out of the ICU can result in substantial cost savings. Costs associated with medication administration are relatively low in comparison.

14. **KEY POINTS**
    - It is imperative to correctly identify the underlying pathology to appropriately triage and manage an acid/base or electrolyte disorder.
    - In many cases, optimal treatment involves correcting the underlying cause of the disorder.
    - Careful monitoring of pertinent endpoints after a therapeutic intervention is necessary to ensure adequate treatment and prevent overcompensation.
    - Interventions must be patient-specific, taking into consideration factors such as organ function, body size, disease states, and concomitant medications.

CASE 12 ANSWERS

■ PROBLEM LIST

1. Weight loss
2. Depression
3. Fatigue

■ SOAP NOTE

S: Daughter states on visiting her father she found him "not himself." He appeared visibly depressed; states he has not really eaten well in a while and has no appetite or desire to eat. He states he is always tired and has not left his apartment in days; admits that he has stopped taking his Zoloft when it ran out about 2 months ago. She is concerned for his health and welfare and didn't want him to end up "like last time"; thus, she brought him to the ER.

O: History of depression episode with anorexia and weight loss approximately 2 years ago, sertraline 50 mg daily, acetaminophen 650 mg PO q4-6h PRN, T 37°C, BP 118/72, HR 72, RR 18, O$_2$ sat 99% RA, Wt 55 kg, Ht 175 cm, abdomen soft, NT/ND and no BS, A and O × 3, Lkcs 6.0 × 10^9 (6.0 × 10^3), Hct 0.48 (48), Hgb 160 (16), Plts 200 × 10^9 (200 × 10^3), Na 148 (148), K 3.5 (3.5), Cl 110 (110), HCO$_3$ 22 (22), Ca 2.25 (4.5), Mg 1.1 (2.2), PO$_4$ 0.65 (2.0), albumin 34 (3.4), BUN 8.5 (24), SCr 97.2 (1.1), Glucose 3.9 (70).

A: PROBLEM 1: Weight loss with electrolyte imbalances

PROBLEM 2: Depression with sertraline therapy (currently noncompliant)

PROBLEM 3: Fatigue

P: PROBLEM 1: Weight Loss With Electrolyte Imbalance

- Obtain skinfold measurements of triceps and calf areas.
- Give *Candida* and mumps skin test to assess immune status.
- Monitor vital signs and I and O daily as indicators for fluid overload and sepsis.
- Monitor weight q24h.
- Obtain baselines for sodium, potassium, magnesium, calcium, phosphorus, BUN, creatinine, and prealbumin. Monitor daily or every other day.
- Monitor BUN and creatinine for assessment of tolerance to protein load.
- Assess access site daily for signs and symptoms of infection, infiltration, or phlebitis.
- Reevaluate calorie and protein requirements periodically as JN's status indicates.

PROBLEM 2: Depression

- Resume sertraline 50 mg daily; may need to increase to 100 mg daily.
- Monitor for trends toward normalization of sleep pattern, with increases in energy and appetite.
- Increase socialization and communication with family and friends.
- Toxicity monitoring: GI complaints including nausea, diarrhea, dyspepsia, nervousness, insomnia, headache, fatigue, and sexual dysfunction
- Counsel JN that continued therapy is needed to show improvement, and he should not discontinue medication without first consulting his doctor or pharmacist.

PROBLEM 3: Fatigue

- Minimize daytime naps and staying up late at night.
- Increase nutritional calories as noted above.
- Begin multivitamin with minerals when tolerated.
- Monitoring: Ca, albumin, phosphate, K, Mg, Na, hydration status: BUN, SCr, BP, HR, I and O, appetite
- Counsel patient that fatigue is likely due to decreased appetite and depression associated with loss of job. He should minimize daytime naps and staying up late in an attempt to normalize sleeping patterns. He will receive a short course of parenteral nutrition to help provide calories and restore energy. Goal is to return to several small meals day (approximately five or six a day).

■ CASE QUESTIONS

1. a. Marasmus (normal serum protein concentrations and intact immune status)

2. b. 1,367 BEE = 66.4730 + 13.7516(55) + 5.0033 (175) − 6.7550 (49)

3. JN's starting daily water requirement during nutrition support is between 30 and 35 mL/kg/day. Using his actual body weight of 55 kg and an average 32.5 mL/kg/day, a target range of 1,787 mL or ~1,800 mL total volume is chosen. Total daily calorie requirements for JN, who presents with little physical stress, should start at 25 kcal/kg/day, or target approximately 1,375 kcal per day.

4. Parenteral nutrition can be administered via peripheral or central veins. Peripheral solutions should be no greater than 900 mOsm per L, but the risk of phlebitis increases over 600 mOsm per L. Central administration requires a minor but nonetheless invasive procedure to place a catheter in a major vein (usually the superior vena cava). Peripheral access is often used for short-term therapy, while central access is for much longer periods of time. The length of time for JN's nutritional support appears to be limited and with a functional GI tract, peripheral access with or without oral supplementation is the best access type for JN.

5. c. Prealbumin. Because of a short half-life and relatively small body pool, prealbumin is quite sensitive to nutritional fluctuations.

6. c. 350 mL. 350 mL of 70% dextrose provides 245 g. With each gram of dextrose supplying 3.4 kcal, the total energy from dextrose is approximately 833 kcal.

7. a. 366 mL. 366 mL of 15% amino acids provides 55 g. With each gram of amino acid supplying 4 kcal, the total energy from protein is approximately 220 kcal.

8. Sodium and chloride serum values are slightly elevated, while magnesium and phosphate concentrations are low. Electrolyte supplementation to provide adequate homeostasis for JN might start with the following daily amounts: Na 40 mEq, K 40 mEq, Ca 25 mEq, Mg 20 mEq, Phos 15 mM.

9. Nitrogen balance is determined by subtracting nitrogen output from nitrogen input during a 24-hour period. JN received 55 g of protein (approximately 16% nitrogen) during the past 24 hours and excreted in urine 6.5 g during the same time period. If insensible nitrogen loss is estimated at 4 g, his nitrogen balance would be (55 g/6.25) − (6.5 g + 4 g) = −1.7 g. This value suggests that nitrogen balance has been attained but is borderline. JN's nitrogen balance should be re-evaluated after an additional 1 to 2 days of continued PN therapy.

10. A multidisciplinary nutrition support team can consist of several practitioners, including a physician, pharmacist, nurse, and dietitian. The pharmacist's role will be to assist the prescribing process by providing nutrient formulation information, educate practitioners about compatibilities and drug–nutrient interactions, monitor JN's metabolic and/or mechanical complications, if any, and ensure proper PN compounding involving both sterility and stability concerns.

11. c. Prepare as a TNA (3-1 solution) and administer peripherally. The combined osmolarity for this solution is 874 mOsm per L and below the threshold limit of 900 mOsm. While it is possible to run this emulsion separately, a second access line would be needed or the PN would need to be clamped off during its infusion. Other benefits include decreased nursing time and financial savings (one pump, tubing). Filtration with a 1.2-μm filter is required.

12. **KEY POINTS**
    - In general, parenteral and/or enteral nutrition replenishes undernourished patients; maintains nutritional status during times of stress; achieves appropriate fluid, electrolyte, trace element and vitamin balance; allows for wound healing in GI surgery patients; and improves quality of life.
    - Total calories are usually dosed at 25 kcal/kg/day for adults with little stress, 30 kcal/kg/day for patients with infections, 35 kcal/kg/day for major trauma patients, and 40 kcal/kg/day for burn patients.
    - Guidelines for protein replacement range clinically from 0.6 to 2.2 g/kg/day, but rarely is more than 2 g/kg/day required. Carbohydrate replacement should not exceed 5 mg/kg/min (25 kcal/kg/day). Most clinicians use between 3 and 4 mg/kg/min (15–20 kcal/kg/day). Intralipid (fats) are usually dosed at 0.5 to 1 g/kg/day with a maximum of 2.5 g/kg/day.
    - PN can be administered via peripheral or central veins. Peripheral solutions should be no greater than 900 mOsm per L. Peripheral access is often used for short-term therapy, whereas central access is for much longer periods of time.
    - Complications of parenteral and enteral nutrition can include infection, technical or mechanical problems, metabolic imbalances, and GI and/or pulmonary complications. Daily monitoring of these patients by the pharmacist and the rest of the nutritional team will minimize the chance for complications and maximize therapy.

CASE 13 ANSWERS

■ PROBLEM LIST

1. Dehydration
2. Vitamin B_{12} deficiency
3. Involuntary weight loss
4. Bedsore
5. Constipation
6. Gout
7. Nonadherence

■ SOAP NOTE

S: Complains of pain and tingling in her lower extremities, shortness of breath, fatigue, increased anxiety, difficulty sleeping, and constipation

O: BP 126/80, HR 75, RR 14, T 37.8°C, Wt 50 kg, pale conjunctiva, pale and dry mucous membranes; bilateral wheezes; guaiac-negative stool;

slow capillary refill with slightly pale nail beds and palms of hands, dry and flaky skin, level 2 bedsore noted slightly below the lower back area Labs: Na 147 (147), Hgb 100 (10), MCV 110 (110), serum B_{12} 97.8 (133), albumin 31 (3.1), uric acid 428 (7.2), Ca 2.1 (8.4), Cr 97.2 (1.1), BUN 8.9 (25) Peripheral blood smear shows normochromic, macrocytic RBCs.

A: PROBLEM 1: Dehydration due to bedsore, failure to thrive

PROBLEM 2: Vitamin B_{12} deficiency due to a combination of medication and poor dietary intake

PROBLEM 3: Involuntary weight loss due to poor dietary intake, bedsore

PROBLEM 4: Bedsore due to immobilization and decreased blood flow to the necrotic area

PROBLEM 5: Constipation due to poor dietary intake; medications may be contributory

PROBLEM 6: Gout flare may be a result of the dehydration

PROBLEM 7: Nonadherence may be due to immobility, constipation, lack of social support (family, friends, and finances)

P: PROBLEM 1: Dehydration

- Encourage oral liquids such as water, Pedialyte, and Ensure.
- Monitor I and O daily.
- Monitor weight, physical signs, and vital signs weekly.
- Monitor electrolytes biweekly.
- Avoid alcohol use.

PROBLEM 2: Vitamin B_{12} Deficiency

- Start Vitamin B_{12} therapy (not in priority order). Option 1—Oral: Adequate absorption 1 to 10 μg daily; malabsorption 1,000 μg daily
  Option 2—Parenteral: 500 to 1,000 μg daily for 1 week, then weekly for 1 month, then monthly for life OR 1,000 μg weekly for 4 weeks, then every month for life OR 100 μg daily for 1 week, then every other day for seven doses, then every month for life
  Option 3—Intranasal: 500 μg once a week
- Use the lowest dose possible of medications that could increase risk, such as colchicine and Pepcid. Consider having the patient use Tums instead of Pepcid to control her symptoms.
- Increase the amount of vitamin B_{12}-rich foods in her diet (fresh liver, eggs, meat, kidney, milk, dairy products, fish, and shellfish).

- Monitor vitamin B_{12} and iron levels, response to therapy: signs and symptoms, complications of therapy.
- Recheck levels in 1 month.

PROBLEM 3: Involuntary Weight Loss

- Assess dentition and swallowing to ensure that this is not the cause. If so, then address the problem as needed.
- Assess current eating patterns and ways to enrich foods eaten.
- May need to connect her to a delivery meal service that will bring her meals at home, such as a Meals-on-Wheels program.
- Institute nutritional support that includes macro- and micronutrients such as Ensure, a multivitamin, and so forth. The amount of servings daily would be based on her current eating patterns. If finances are also a problem, check with community resources for seniors, which may provide vouchers.
- Consider short-term therapy with an appetite stimulant such as Remeron, Marinol, megestrol acetate, or cyproheptadine.
- Avoid alcohol.

PROBLEM 4: Bedsore

- Continue dressing changes per nursing.
- Institute nutritional support that includes macro- and micronutrients such as Ensure and multivitamins.
- Increase fluid intake.
- Ensure proper positional rotation to help prevent a lack of blood supply to the area.

PROBLEM 5: Constipation

- Assess current frequency and consistency along with her regular pattern.
- Recommend Bisacodyl for immediate relief and then Colace 100 mg BID.
- Increase fluid intake to eight 8-oz glasses of water a day.
- Increase fiber/grains, fruits, and vegetables.
- Monitor for frequency, consistency, and symptoms of constipation.

PROBLEM 6: Gout Flare

- For flare, take two tabs, then one tab every 1 to 2 hours until relief or maximum of 8 mg is taken.
- Discourage alcohol use.
- Check for adherence; if patient has not taken the medications, encourage her to do so in the future.

- Encourage adequate fluid intake (eight glasses a day).
- Monitor uric acid level, response to therapy: signs and symptoms.
- Consider risk versus benefit of drug therapy in an older patient.

PROBLEM 7: Nonadherence

- Review current medications and assess for any type of pattern regarding which medications she is more adherent with versus not (e.g., taking half the dose, skipping certain days, frequent/recent regimen changes, and so forth).
- Asses reasons for nonadherence: financial, cannot organize the medications, cannot remember to take the medications, confused as to which medications to take, needs assistance in obtaining the medications from the pharmacy.
- Assess community resources and insurance limitations and possibly locate a pharmacy that will blister pack her medications and deliver them to her. If not possible, then teach the patient to pre-fill a pill box to help her remember to take her medications for the day. If delivery is a problem and a pharmacy that delivers can't be found, check community resources for seniors, which may be able to deliver her medications to her.
- Discourage alcohol use.

■ CASE QUESTIONS

1. c. Elderly

2. d. Increased MCV level

3.
   - Inadequate dietary intake
   - Malabsorption: consider potential causes including low intrinsic factor, disorders of the terminal ileum, drugs
   - Transcobalamin II deficiency (impairs B_{12} transport)
   - Drug-induced causes

4. d. Pale nail beds

5. Fatigue, shortness of breath, tingling of extremities

6. a. Colchicine

7. c. Cobalt

8. d. Liver

9. Treatment options (not in priority order):

   a. Oral vitamin B_{12} 1,000 μg daily
   Advantages: Cost-effective, self-administered
   Disadvantages: Erratic absorption, poor adherence, due to age would want higher dosing regimen

   b. Parenteral vitamin B_{12}
   Advantages: More predictable levels, increased adherence with home visit
   Disadvantages: Varied recommended doses, decreased lean muscle mass of elderly, pain on injection, possible allergic reaction, cost of home health visit

   c. Intranasal vitamin B_{12}
   Advantages: Three times a week, self-administered, well tolerated
   Disadvantages: Costly, long-term data lacking

10. Education plan for vitamin B_{12} therapy
    a. Lifestyle changes: improving diet, eating habits
    b. Medication counseling: therapy is for life, importance of adherence
       i. Oral: Take daily
       ii. Parenteral: Pain at injection site, keep area clean
       iii. Intranasal: Lightly clean the area

11. Psychosocial factors that may affect adherence
    a. Patient-specific factors: Assess how such things as her immobility, lack of socialization, and limited finances are affecting her quality of life and might affect her adherence. Also consider how her new dietary suggestions could affect her limitations.
    b. Disease factors
       i. Depression: Assess how this could be affected by her current state (e.g., immobility, finances)
       ii. Anxiety: Assess how this could be affected by her current state (e.g., immobility, finances)
       iii. Sleep disturbances: Assess how this could be affected by her current state (e.g., immobility, finances)
    c. Others
       i. Supply EC with an advocate since she has no family in the area.
       ii. Assist EC in finding financial resources as well as resources with meals, supplements, and so forth.

12. Health care provider's role
    a. Assist in the follow-through and adjustment of her plan (both pharmacologic and nonpharmacologic aspects).
    b. Maintain close follow-up/contact with the patient; develop a good relationship.
    c. Educate the patient on her disease states.
    d. Counsel the patient on medications.
    e. Encourage the patient and provide positive reinforcement.
    f. Make referrals as needed.

13. Pharmacoeconomic considerations
    a. Cost of therapeutic options
    b. Cost of managing the disease at home versus at a hospital or skilled nursing facility
        i. Institution personnel, overhead, treatment, complications, and so forth
        ii. EC's decreased productivity and quality of life, pain and suffering

14. **KEY POINTS**
    - Anemias are often indicative of another underlying pathology, so a complete evaluation of the cause is necessary.
    - Symptoms of anemia include fatigue, shortness of breath, and neurologic symptoms.
    - Inadequate intake and decreased absorption are two potential cause of vitamin B_{12} deficiency; therefore, consider evaluating nutrition and the potential effects of other medications on absorption of vitamin B_{12}.
    - Response to therapy may occur in the first week, but correction of the anemia may take longer.
    - Assessments for potential causes of macrocytic anemia include an evaluation of lean body mass, factors that may decrease GI absorption, and economic constraints, particularly in the elderly population.
    - Adherence to pharmacologic and nonpharmacologic interventions should be encouraged and frequently evaluated.

CASE 14 ANSWERS

■ PROBLEM LIST

1. Asthma exacerbation
2. Sinus infection
3. Elevated BP intermittently controlled

4. Osteoporosis
5. Use of conjugated estrogens (Premarin) and medroxyprogesterone acetate

■ SOAP NOTE

S: "I am having trouble breathing and my albuterol inhaler is not working. I have had a sinus headache for the past week with a lot of post-nasal drip."

O: Bilateral inspiratory and expiratory wheezes, sinuses tender to palpation, BP 150/92

A: PROBLEM 1: Asthma exacerbation secondary to sinus infection

PROBLEM 2: Sinus infection probably associated with poor control of seasonal allergic rhinitis

PROBLEM 3: Elevated BP and lack of good control secondary to prednisone use and family history

PROBLEM 4: Osteoporosis secondary to prednisone use

PROBLEM 5: Increased risk of cardiovascular events secondary to use of conjugated estrogens (Premarin) and medroxyprogesterone acetate with strong family history of stroke

P: PROBLEMS 1 and 2: Asthma Exacerbation Secondary to sinus infection

- Treat sinus infection with amoxicillin/clavulanate 250 to 500 mg TID for 3 weeks.
- Increase prednisone to 40 mg PO BID for 7 days for asthma symptoms.
- Add albuterol 2.5 mg by nebulization TID or QID for 7 days for asthma symptoms.
- Return to clinic in 7 days for spirometry recheck.
- Consider adding omalizumab, weaning patient off prednisone, and decreasing Advair dose over the next 6 to 12 months.

    This patient should have a reassessment of the following factors: environmental control (allergenic and nonallergic triggers, including second-hand smoke), inhalation technique with Diskus as well as MDI, treatment regimen for allergic rhinitis (add intranasal corticosteroids), and rule out GERD.

PROBLEM 3: Elevated BP and lack of good control secondary to prednisone use

- Consider adding omalizumab with goal to decrease or discontinue treatment with prednisone over the next 6 to 12 months. Then attempt to decrease Advair dose (the fluticasone propionate component of Advair).

■ Recheck BP as patient is weaned off prednisone.

PROBLEM 4: Osteoporosis Secondary to prednisone use and high advair dose

■ Increase dose of alendronate to 5 mg QD for treatment (versus prevention) of osteoporosis.
■ Consider adding omalizumab with the goal of decreasing or discontinuing treatment with prednisone over the next 6 to 12 months.
■ If BP comes under better control, maintain thiazide therapy preferentially as it decreases urinary excretion of calcium and can provide adjunctive control of osteoporosis.
■ Recheck BMD in 1 year if omalizumab is started and prednisone dose is reduced/discontinued. Then attempt to decrease the Advair dose.
■ Reduce caffeine intake.
■ Increase weight-bearing and resistance exercises.
■ Add calcium carbonate 500 mg PO TID.

PROBLEM 5: Increased risk of cardiovascular events secondary to use of conjugated estrogens (Premarin) and medroxyprogesterone acetate with strong family history of stroke

■ Discontinue conjugated estrogens (Premarin) and medroxyprogesterone acetate.

■ CASE QUESTIONS

1.
   ■ HPA axis suppression
   ■ Linear growth velocity reduction
   ■ Bone mineral density reduction
   ■ Weight gain
   ■ Cushing syndrome
   ■ Mood swings, psychosis
   ■ Hypokalemia
   ■ Hyperglycemia
   ■ Dermal thinning and skin bruising
   ■ Glaucoma
   ■ Adrenal insufficiency and crisis
   ■ Growth suppression
   ■ Failure to attain expected adult height
   ■ Osteoporosis and fractures
   ■ Cataracts

2.
   ■ Significantly reduces coordination required
   ■ Improves pulmonary drug deposition
   ■ Reduces risk for adverse effects

3.
   ■ Prednisone: reduces inflammation in the airways
   ■ Advair: fluticasone reduces inflammation in the airways; salmeterol provides smooth muscle relaxation in the airways
   ■ Albuterol: provides smooth muscle relaxation in the airways
   ■ Amoxicillin/clavulanate: antibiotic
   ■ Alendronate: bisphosphonates bind to exposed hydroxyapatite crystals on resorption surface of bone and inhibit osteoclastic activity without an effect on osteoblastic activity
   ■ Hydrochlorothiazide: promotes diuresis
   ■ Enalapril: blocks the production of angiotensin II, a potent vasoconstrictor and stimulant of aldosterone secretion
   ■ Conjugated estrogens (Premarin): reduces bone loss following the onset of menopause
   ■ Omalizumab: a monoclonal antibody that binds to IgE molecules free (not bound to mast cells) in the serum

4.
   ■ Remove cap.
   ■ Shake canister.
   ■ Exhale (to functional residual capacity or fully if slow exhalation).
   ■ Hold MDI upright.
   ■ Place lips around mouthpiece, or
   ■ Place mouthpiece ~2 inches or 2 fingerwidths from mouth, or
   ■ Place lips around spacer mouthpiece (if using a spacer device).
   ■ Start to inhale slowly (≤30 L/min) immediately before actuation.
   ■ Actuate MDI while continuing to inhale.
   ■ Inhale completely and hold breath for 10 seconds (or at least 4 to 5 seconds).
   ■ Wait 1 minute.
   ■ Repeat above steps if more than one inhalation prescribed.
   ■ For inhaled steroids, rinse mouth with water or mouthwash and expel contents.

5.
   ■ When given orally, much smaller doses must be used compared with the inhaled route.
   ■ Inhaled route provides more rapid onset of action and fewer systemic adverse effects.

6.
   ■ Nausea
   ■ Esophageal reflux
   ■ Gastritis

7. b. Currently being managed with prednisone and/or high-dose inhaled corticosteroids

8. b. Forceful and deep inhalation

9.
   ■ Severe wheezing and shortness of breath
   ■ Unable to speak more than a few words without taking a breath
   ■ Decreased FEV_1, FVC, and peak flow

10. Patients who are younger; who have higher scores for depression on certain scales; who feel ashamed, embarrassed, or angry about their disease; and who are concerned about side effects of corticosteroids and becoming addicted to their medications have poorer adherence to therapy.

11.
   ■ Diarrhea
   ■ Hypersensitivity

12.
   a. Therapy with prednisone
      i. Low cost of drug
      ii. Serious adverse effects can occur with long-term treatment, which may increase heath care costs significantly.
         1. Osteoporosis: drug treatment, treatment for hip fractures
         2. Hypertension: long-term consequences of hypertension
         3. Diabetes: long-term consequences of diabetes
         4. Cataracts and costs of treatment
         5. Adrenal insufficiency or crisis
   b. Therapy with omalizumab
      i. Very expensive annual cost
      ii. If patient can reduce or discontinue prednisone use, then the above long-term sequelae are averted.
      iii. Could reduce the number of ED visits and hospitalizations
      iv. Is primarily for patients who have frequent hospitalizations and ED visits despite optimal management. For these patients, it is cost-effective.
   c. Discontinuation of therapy with conjugated estrogens (Premarin)
      i. Reduced risk of stroke and long-term sequelae

13. **KEY POINTS**
   ■ Asthma is a respiratory disease in which airflow obstruction is caused by airway inflammation and smooth muscle bronchoconstriction.

   ■ Treatment of airway inflammation includes use of inhaled corticosteroids, oral corticosteroids, anti-IgE therapy, or leukotriene modifiers. Long-acting β_2-agonists are used chronically in combination with an inhaled corticosteroid; they are not to be used as monotherapy or for relief of acute symptoms. Short-acting β_2-agonists are used as needed to prevent or relieve symptoms, and the frequency of use can be included in an assessment of overall asthma control.

   ■ A goal of long-term management is to reduce the dose of oral and inhaled corticosteroids to the lowest effective dose to minimize adverse effects from long-term use of corticosteroids. The addition of NSAIDs such as omalizumab or leukotriene modifiers, or of long-acting β_2-agonists may allow lower doses of corticosteroids to be used.

CASE 15 ANSWERS

■ PROBLEM LIST

1. Poorly controlled type 2 diabetes mellitus (DM)
2. Hypertension
3. Proteinuria
4. Dyslipidemia
5. Nicotine addiction
6. Diabetic peripheral neuropathy
7. Depression
8. Peripheral arterial disease
9. Coronary artery disease (history of angina prior to CABG)

■ SOAP NOTE

S: "I am having tingling sensations in both of my hands, and my feet are numb."

O: A1C 9.5%, FBG 195, BP 148/92, 1+ ankle edema, protein 1+, 118 kg BW, diminished pedal pulses (1 of 2+), nonresponse to 10-g monofilament, Cr 1.4, BUN 27, uric acid 7.6, TC 255, LDL 177, HDL 31, TG 235, ABI 0.65 (L), 0.75 (R), MI × 1, metformin for DM, propranolol and HCTZ for HTN, NTG for angina (PRN), self-treatment with niacin for dyslipidemia

A: PROBLEM 1: Poorly controlled type 2 DM due to suboptimal therapies (metformin dose too low, too much HCTZ, monotherapy approach, and advanced diabetes)

PROBLEM 2: HTN due to suboptimal therapy and the presence of type 2 DM

PROBLEM 3: Proteinuria due to type 2 DM

PROBLEM 4: Dyslipidemia due to poorly controlled type 2 DM and secondary causes

PROBLEM 5: Nicotine addiction

PROBLEM 6: Peripheral neuropathy due to poorly controlled type 2 DM

PROBLEM 7: Depression due to having chronic disease (type 2 DM) and MI

PROBLEM 8: Peripheral arterial disease due to atherosclerosis accelerated by type 2 DM and HTN

PROBLEM 9: Coronary artery disease (angina) due to atherosclerosis accelerated by type 2 DM and HTN

P: PROBLEM 1: Poorly controlled Type 2 DM

- Titrate metformin carefully to 1,000 mg BID.
- Consider initiation of a basal insulin (e.g., insulin glargine, NPH) and/or addition of a sulfonylurea.
- Consider initiation of a thiazolidinedione (third line) if insulin or a sulfonylurea is not started.
- Change HCTZ to 25 mg BID (doses >50 mg/d are associated with insulin resistance).
- Initiate low-dose ASA therapy (75–325 mg).
- Monitor serum creatinine (metformin is contraindicated with SCr 1.5 or higher in males).
- Regular self-monitoring of blood glucose.
- Repeat A1C in 3 months.
- Refer for diabetes education, preferably by a certified diabetes educator.
- Discuss importance of regular physical activity (exercise) with physician oversight.
- Refer to dietitian who specializes in diabetes.
- Monitor medication compliance.
- Ensure dilated ophthalmologic exam once yearly.

PROBLEM 2: HTN Due to suboptimal therapy and presence of Type 2 DM

- ADA-recommended BP goal is below 130/80 mm Hg.
- More stringent BP goal of 125/75 if patient has kidney disease with proteinuria (>1 g/24 h).
- Initiate ACE inhibitor (ACE inhibitor plus HCTZ for BP control; ACE inhibitor is beneficial post-MI).
- If ACE inhibitor + HCTZ do not control BP, then consider adding non-dihydropyridine calcium channel blocker (ACE inhibitors and ARBs may

not be as effective in lowering BP in African Americans, but this lack of efficacy may be negated by the addition of a diuretic).
- Monitor electrolytes (ACE inhibitor/HCTZ can alter electrolytes, in particular K^+, so be cautious about the use of potassium-containing salt substitutes).
- Monitor for ACE inhibitor–induced cough (switch to ARB if ACE inhibitor intolerable).
- Decrease HCTZ to 25 mg BID (doses >50 mg/day are associated with hyperglycemia).
- Discontinue propranolol (associated with depression, adverse lipid effects, making of hypoglycemia, and heart rate <60 bpm).
- ASA therapy as above

PROBLEM 3: Proteinuria Due to Type 2 DM

- Reassess with timed collection (e.g., 4 hour), 24-hour collection, or albumin to creatinine ratio (spot) (two of three specimens collected within a 3- to 6-month period should be abnormal before being classified as having microalbuminuria/macroalbuminuria).
- Refer patient to a physician experienced in diabetic kidney disease (e.g., nephrologist).
- Add ACE inhibitor or ARB (see Problem 2 above).
- Continued surveillance of parameters of kidney disease (microalbuminuria, serum creatinine)
- Avoid nephrotoxic medications.

PROBLEM 4: Dyslipidemia

- Screen for and modify, if possible, secondary causes of dyslipidemia [thiazide diuretics can increase LDL, β-blockers without ISA can increase triglycerides and decrease HDL, smoking decreases HDL, diabetes (uncontrolled hyperglycemia) decreases HDL and increases triglycerides, excessive alcohol intake increases triglycerides, kidney disease can increase triglycerides].
- Discontinue β-blocker therapy and add ACE inhibitor (see Problem 2 above).
- Decrease thiazide diuretic dose (see Problem 2 above).
- Tight glycemic control
- Medical nutritional therapy and physical activity
- Lifestyle modification (smoking cessation, decrease alcohol intake, weight loss)
- Discontinue OTC niacin (associated with hyperglycemia and increased uric acid levels; increases LFTs).
- Add a high-potency HMG-CoA reductase inhibitor to achieve a standard LDL cholesterol goal of below 100 mg per dL, with an optimal goal of

less than 70 mg per dL (continue to monitor LFTs closely).
- Fasting lipid profile baseline, 6 to 8 weeks after medication and/or dosage change and every 6 to 12 months when stable
- LFTs baseline, 6 to 8 weeks after medication and/or dosage change and every 6 to 12 months when stable
- Educate regarding signs and symptoms of myopathy and rhabdomyolysis.

PROBLEM 5: Nicotine addiction

- Recommend smoking cessation counseling.
- Assess level of nicotine dependence.
- Consider use of nicotine replacement therapy.
- ASA therapy as above (diabetes, smoking, HTN, and dyslipidemia places patient at increased risk for thrombosis)

PROBLEM 6: Peripheral neuropathy due to poorly controlled Type 2 DM
- Reinforce importance of glycemic control and its relationship to neuropathic symptoms.
- Consider pharmacologic management such as amitriptyline, venlafaxine, or duloxetine (may also improve depressive symptoms).
- Stress importance of foot care and self-care behaviors.

PROBLEM 7: Depression associated with having chronic disease (Type 2 DM) and MI

- Recommend pharmacotherapy and/or psychotherapy.
- Pharmacotherapy may include use of a dual norepinephrine/serotonin reuptake inhibitor such as duloxetine or venlafaxine to assist with neuropathy control.
- Monitor depression and consider referral to psychiatrist.
- Assess compliance with medications and other lifestyle practices, as depression is associated with suboptimal self-care attitudes and practices.

PROBLEM 8: Peripheral artery disease due to atherosclerosis accelerated by Type 2 DM, smoking, dyslipidemia, and HTN

- ASA therapy as above
- Reassess 3 to 6 months after lipid, BP, blood glucose, and smoking cessation approaches have been initiated.

PROBLEM 9: Coronary artery disease (Angina) Due to atherosclerosis accelerated by Type 2 DM and HTN

- Adequately controlled at present
- Refill nitroglycerin q 6 months once bottle opened or once yearly for unopened bottles.
- If symptoms return, the addition of a non-dihydropyridine calcium channel blocker can help control angina (see Problem 2 above).

■ **CASE QUESTIONS**

1. c. Poorly controlled diabetes

2. Hypoglycemia:
    - Feeling weak or dizzy
    - Nervousness
    - Tremor
    - Confusion
    - Increased sweating
    - Tachycardia/palpitations
    - Hunger
    - Irritability

    Hyperglycemia:
    - Hunger
    - Increased thirst
    - Frequent urination
    - Blurred vision
    - Fatigue
    - Weight loss
    - Poor wound healing

3. d. <0.9

4. LFTs, blood glucose levels, uric acid levels

5. Decreased gluconeogenesis/glycogenolysis in the liver and increased peripheral uptake and utilization of glucose into skeletal muscles

6. Kidney disease, development of rhabdomyolysis, ACE inhibitor therapy

7. Counseling points:
    - Can be taken without regard to meals or time of day (atorvastatin longer half-life)
    - Headache and GI upset are most common. If GI upset is an issue, take with food.
    - Educate regarding signs/symptoms of myopathy and rhabdomyolysis (e.g., bilateral muscle pain, weakness, and/or tenderness, especially if accompanied by fever or malaise).
    - If you miss a dose, take it as soon as you can. If it is almost time for your next dose, take only that dose. Do not take double or extra doses.
    - Keep out of the reach of children in a container that small children cannot open.

- Store at controlled room temperature between 20°C and 25°C (68°F to 77°F). Keep container tightly closed. Throw away any unused medicine after the expiration date.

8. a. Duloxetine

9. b. Ibuprofen

10. d. 80 mg

11. a. Pima Indians

12. a. Niacin/thiazide diuretic

13. Serum creatinine 1.5 or more in males, 1.4 or more in females; sepsis; kidney failure; cardiogenic shock; administration of IV iodinated contrast material

14. c. Nonproductive cough

15. Psychosocial factors include:
    - Depression
    - Chronic diseases
    - Lives alone/limited support system
    - Physical activity may be impaired due to smoking and alcohol consumption.

16. Health care provider's role includes:
    - Detailed treatment, monitoring, and education plan
    - Referral to appropriate specialists, which may include endocrinologist, nephrologist, ophthalmologist, psychologist/psychiatrist, and podiatrist
    - Referral to certified diabetes educator, dietitian, and smoking cessation program

17. **KEY POINTS**
    - Diabetes is for the most part an incurable disease, so the overall goals of treatment include maintaining blood-sugar levels in the normal or near-normal range and preventing the short- and long-term complications associated with this disease.
    - Type 1 diabetes is seen primarily in children and adolescents, whereas type 2 diabetes most commonly affects those over age 45. However, with the increase in adolescent obesity, type 2 diabetes is becoming more common in younger individuals.
    - Measuring glycosylated hemoglobin (A1C) is the gold standard for monitoring patients with diabetes, and all patients with diabetes should have this test performed one to four times yearly.
    - Self-monitoring of blood glucose should be performed by most patients with diabe-

tes, and the results should be reviewed regularly with a health care professional.
    - Uncontrolled diabetes results in kidney, eye, and nerve disease that greatly compromises the quality of life of patients with diabetes, so normalization or near-normalization of blood glucose is a primary treatment goal.
    - Educating the patient with diabetes is critical to the successful management of this chronic disease.
    - In addition to insulin, the therapeutic options to control diabetes include an array of agents that have various effects on the pancreas, muscle, and liver.
    - The successful treatment of diabetes requires a team approach that incorporates the expertise of physicians, nurses, pharmacists, and dietitians, among others.

CASE 16 ANSWERS

■ PROBLEM LIST

1. Hypothyroidism
2. Rule out amiodarone-induced hypothyroidism
3. Potential drug interaction: calcium carbonate (Tums) and levothyroxine
4. Hypertension

■ SOAP NOTE

S: Fatigue, weight gain, menstrual irregularities, cold intolerance

O: TSH 54 mU per L (elevated); free T_4 51 pmol per L; total T_3 1.3 nmol per L, BP 145/88

A: PROBLEM 1: Hypothyroidism

PROBLEM 2: Rule out amiodarone-induced hypothyroidism

PROBLEM 3: Potential interaction between calcium carbonate (Tums) and levothyroxine

PROBLEM 4: Hypertension

P: PROBLEM 1: Hypothyroidism

- Start thyroid replacement therapy. Per the American Thyroid Association of Clinical Endocrinologists, levothyroxine is the drug of choice. Given KZ's age, the most appropriate dose would be 50 µg; however, because she has a past medical history of ventricular tachycardia, the most appropriate initial dose would be 25 µg.

- Based on the guidelines, KZ should have her TSH rechecked in 6 weeks.

PROBLEM 2: Potential Amiodarone-induced hypothyroidism

- Confirm amiodarone-induced hypothyroidism.
- Typical thyroid function tests in euthyroid individuals receiving amiodarone include a reduction in FT_4 and a transient elevated TSH for the first 2 months of therapy. Monitor the FT_4 and TSH every 6 months.
- No intervention needed at this time.

PROBLEM 3: Potential interaction between tums and levothyroxine

- Assess the patient's use of antacids and consider a nonantacid regimen.
- Consider use of an H2 antagonist or a proton pump inhibitor.
- Counsel patient on the interaction between levothyroxine and calcium carbonate-containing products and the need to space administration times by 4 hours.

PROBLEM 4: Hypertension

- Consider increasing the lisinopril dose to 20 mg QD or adding an additional agent (e.g., hydrochlorothiazide 12.5 mg PO QD).
- Lifestyle modifications should be reinforced with the patient, and the patient's adherence with medications should be assessed.

■ CASE QUESTIONS

1. d. Graves' disease
2. b. Amiodarone use
3. a. 25 μg
4. b. 50
5. a. Separate the levothyroxine dose from Tums
6. d. 6 weeks
7. c. Decrease the dose by 25 μg
8. b. IV levothyroxine
9. Hypothyroidism is a life-threatening condition that requires pharmacologic management. Levothyroxine is the drug of choice. Young patients, such as KZ, and patients who do not have any cardiac disease should be started on 50 μg. KZ has a history of ven-

tricular tachycardia and therefore should be started on 25 μg.

10. Signs and symptoms of hypothyroidism include dry skin, cold intolerance, weight gain, constipation, weakness, changes in menstruation, lethargy, fatigue, loss of energy, depression, bradycardia, muscle cramps, and myalgia. KZ presents with fatigue, weight gain, menstrual irregularities, and cold intolerance.

11. Amiodarone's effect on thyroid function:
- Amiodarone can induce a hypothyroid state (incidence from 1%–9.8%).
- No correlation with cumulative dosage or duration of therapy.
- Usually develops within first 2 years of therapy.
- Amiodarone-induced hypothyroidism is confirmed by:
  - Elevated TSH (>10 mIU/L)
  - Reduced FT_4 levels
- Routine monitoring at initiation of amiodarone and every 6 months is recommended.

12. **KEY POINTS**
- The classic symptoms of hypothyroidism include weakness, fatigue, lethargy, cold intolerance, constipation, and weight gain.
- Marked physical findings of hypothyroidism include a puffy and masklike facies, edematous eyelids, thickened and doughy skin changes, hair loss from the lateral aspects of the eyebrows, a large tongue, cardiomegaly, and a yellowish tint of the skin.
- The American Thyroid Association of Clinical Endocrinologists has published guidelines for the treatment of hypothyroidism.
- Practitioners should be alert to drugs that cause thyroid illness, interfere with proper laboratory interpretation, or interact with effective medical management.
- TSH is the most sensitive test for monitoring thyroid function.
- L-thyroxine is the preparation of choice for managing hypothyroidism.
- The dosage of L-thyroxine can be adjusted based on symptoms or TSH and FT_4 levels after 6 to 8 weeks. Trough TSH levels should be obtained to minimize transient high peak FT_4 levels and suppressed TSH levels, for proper interpretation of laboratory results. Once the dos-

age has been established, therapy should be evaluated on an annual basis.

CASE 17 ANSWERS

■ PROBLEM LIST

1. Chronic kidney disease
2. Joint pain and renal osteodystrophy
3. Poorly controlled HTN
4. Poorly controlled diabetes and worsening diabetic nephropathy
5. Anemia

■ SOAP NOTE

S: Complains of increasing joint pain for several weeks and fatigue

O: BP 154/90, HR 85, RR 18, T 37.8°C, Wt 59 kg, Ht 162 cm
Medications: Humulin 70/30 20 units AM and 30 units PM; HCTZ 50 mg PO QD; lisinopril 20 mg PO QD; calcium carbonate 1,500 mg PO TID with meals; calcitriol 0.25 mcg PO QD; APAP 650 mg ii tabs q6h PRN for joint pain
Trace ankle edema bilaterally; good distal pulses; restricted ROM in joints; pain assessment 7/10
BUN 10 (28), Cr 167 (1.9), Hct 0.28 (28), Hgb 90 (9.0), Glu 14.4 (260), Ca 2.0 (8.0), PO_4 2.1 (6.4), Alb 37 (3.7)
Ferritin: Pending
Serum Iron: Pending
TSAT: Pending
Urinalysis: + protein, hyaline casts
Estimated GFR = 29 mL/min/1.73 m^2

A: PROBLEM 1: Chronic kidney disease

PROBLEM 2: Joint pain secondary to renal osteodystrophy

PROBLEM 3: Poorly controlled HTN

PROBLEM 4: Poorly controlled DM and progressive diabetic nephropathy

PROBLEM 5: Anemia

P: PROBLEM 1: Chronic Kidney Disease

- Estimated GFR = 29 mL/min/1.73 m^2 (steady-state SCr 1.9)
- Patient has signs and symptoms of progressive chronic kidney disease (e.g., proteinuria, edema, development of secondary complications—anemia, renal osteodystrophy)
- Discontinue thiazide diuretic (HCTZ).

- Initiate loop diuretic (furosemide) and titrate dose to effect.
- Continue ACE inhibitor (lisinopril).
- Rule out renal artery stenosis and monitor serum K.
- Avoid nephrotoxic drugs (e.g., NSAIDs, aminoglycosides).
- Adjust renally eliminated drugs according to kidney function.
- Monitor serum K and maintain at below 5 mEq per L.
- Monitor daily I and O and ankle edema.
- Monitor serum electrolytes, weight, BP, and kidney function [include assessment of spot urine albumin-SCr ratio (mg/g)].
- Assess medication adherence to antihypertensives and insulin.
- Counsel patient on the importance of strict BP and glucose control to delay progression of chronic kidney disease to end-stage kidney disease.
- Educate patient about dialysis (patients with stage 4 chronic kidney disease require early education about the future need for dialysis).
- Counsel patient on home BP and blood glucose monitoring.
- Consider risk versus benefit of protein restriction (benefit: potentially delay progression to end-stage disease; risk: malnutrition).

PROBLEM 2: Joint pain associated with renal osteodystrophy

- Monitor ROM and pain severity (scale 1–10).
- Measure iPTH to evaluate degree of secondary hyperparathyroidism (elevated iPTH is likely if patient has developed renal osteodystrophy at this stage of chronic kidney disease).
- Correct hyperphosphatemia:
  - Restrict dietary phosphorus intake to 800 to 1,000 mg per day.
  - Assess patient's adherence with phosphate binder (calcium carbonate) and vitamin D supplementation.
- Adjust phosphate binder to achieve normal calcium and phosphorus levels; consider the effect of vitamin D therapy on calcium.
- Consider measuring vitamin D levels (25-hydroxyvitamin D and 1,25-dihydroxyvitamin D) to determine if supplementation of the precursor (ergocalciferol) or active vitamin D (calcitriol) or a vitamin D analog (doxercalciferol or paricalcitol) is warranted.
- Adjust vitamin D therapy based on assessment of vitamin D status, iPTH level (goal PTH 70–110 pg/mL), calcium, and phosphorus.

- Perform routine radiographic evaluation of long and short bones.
- Counsel patient to avoid NSAIDs and use acetaminophen to control pain (do not exceed 4 g/day).
- Physical and occupational therapy as necessary
- Recommend exercise according to physical ability.

PROBLEM 3: HTN

- Assess compliance with antihypertensive medications and diet.
- Replace thiazide diuretic with loop diuretic.
- Continue ACE inhibitor and titrate dose according to BP.
- Add a β-blocker or nondihydropyridine calcium channel blocker if needed to achieve goal BP.
- JNC-VII guidelines recommend BP below 130/80 in patients with chronic kidney disease and overt proteinuria.
- Monitor BP, weight, serum K, Na, BUN, and SCr.
- Dietary consult
- Inform patient to limit daily intake of sodium to less than 2 g.
- Assess lipid panel and rule out dyslipidemia.

PROBLEM 4: Diabetic Nephropathy

- Lack of adequate blood glucose control (HgA1c 12%).
- Rule out all causes of hyperglycemia.
- Optimize BP and blood glucose control with diet and medication.
- Assess adherence to insulin and dietary compliance.
- Instruct patient to monitor fasting blood sugar and preprandial blood glucose daily and keep diary.
- Adjust insulin doses according to blood glucose level.
- Increase blood glucose monitoring to seven times daily on sick days.
- Quantitative assessment of proteinuria (monitor periodically) [include assessment of spot urine albumin-SCr ratio (mg/g)].
- Continue ACE inhibitor and adjust dose according to proteinuria and BP.

PROBLEM 5: Anemia

- Rule out folate and vitamin B_{12} deficiency.
- Assess iron body stores (serum iron, TIBC, transferrin saturation, and ferritin).
- Establish an appropriate iron supplementation or maintenance dose.

- Options: oral iron to provide 200 mg elemental iron per day (monitor for side effects and drug interaction with calcium); IV as sodium ferric gluconate, iron sucrose, or iron dextran if oral iron does not meet goal iron indices
- Consider the appropriate initial dose of a erythropoietic agent (SC route of administration preferred): epoetin alfa (80–120 units/kg per week SC or 120–180 units/kg per week IV administered in 1–3 divided doses) or darbepoetin alfa (0.45 μg/kg SC or IV administered once weekly).
- Achieve target goal of Hgb 11 to 12 g per dL (adjust dose of erythropoietic agent accordingly).
- Monitor Hgb, Hct, iron studies, BP, and weight.
- Failure to respond to erythropoietic therapy requires evaluation of factors causing resistance, such as iron deficiency (primary cause), infection, inflammation, chronic blood loss, aluminum toxicity, hemoglobinopathies, malnutrition, and hyperparathyroidism.
- Goal TSAT and ferritin for chronic kidney disease patient on erythropoietic therapy: TSAT 20% to 50%, ferritin 100 to 800 ng per mL

■ CASE QUESTIONS

1. Longstanding HTN and DM

2. c. Stage 4

3. Thiazides may be less effective in stage 4 chronic kidney disease (GFR <30 mL/min). Patients with stage 4 disease may require a loop diuretic. Assessment of urine output and BP is needed to determine response and appropriateness of therapy.

4. The decline in kidney function with chronic kidney disease decreases phosphorus excretion and leads to an increase in serum phosphorus levels and a reciprocal decrease in serum calcium concentrations. Hypocalcemia is the primary stimulus for release of PTH. Decreased conversion of vitamin D to its active form (1,25-dihydroxyvitamin D_3) in the kidney also contributes to hypocalcemia and increased production of PTH. Sustained hyperparathyroidism can lead to renal osteodystrophy if not corrected. Dietary phosphorus restriction and phosphate binding agents are needed to control serum phosphorus. Initially a calcium-containing phosphate binder (e.g., calcium carbonate, calcium acetate) may be used to help lower phosphorus and correct calcium concentrations; however, the risk of hypercalcemia must be considered

with long-term therapy. Vitamin D deficiency is treated through supplementation of the vitamin D precursor (ergocalciferol), active vitamin D (calcitriol), or a vitamin D analog (doxercalciferol or paricalcitol), depending on vitamin D levels and the stage of kidney disease. [Refer to the NKF-K/DOQI guidelines for bone metabolism and disease: *Am J Kidney Dis.* 2003;42(4 Suppl 3):1–201].

5. Sevelamer and lanthanum are alternates to calcium-containing phosphate binders in the management of hyperphosphatemia in the chronic kidney disease population. These agents do not contain calcium, aluminum, or magnesium and may be used in patients who become hypercalcemic (serum Ca >10.2 mg/dL) on conventional therapy with calcium-containing phosphate binders.

6. In the presence of kidney dysfunction, opiates may be used short term to control pain. Use the lowest effective dose of opiate according to kidney function, and do not exceed recommended doses provided by the manufacturer. Meperidine is not recommended as a first-line analgesic agent in patients with kidney disease because serum levels of its inactive metabolite, normeperidine, may accumulate and increase the risk of seizures.

7. b. iPTH 70–110 pg/mL

8. ACE inhibitors have been shown to delay the progression of kidney disease even in the absence of HTN in clinical trials. The K/DOQI Clinical Practice Guidelines for patients with stage 1 to 4 chronic kidney disease recommend ACE inhibitors to decrease proteinuria. The ADA recommends that all type I diabetics with microalbuminuria or proteinuria take an ACE inhibitor whether or not they are hypertensive. The goal of therapy is to decrease BP to less than 130/80 mm Hg, decrease proteinuria, slow the progression of kidney disease, and reduce the risk of cardiovascular disease.

9. b. 11–12 g/dL

10. Serum ferritin (assessment of storage iron), transferrin saturation (assessment of iron readily available for erythropoiesis), Hgb, Hct

11. Available agents in the United States are epoetin alfa and darbepoetin alfa. Starting doses of epoetin alfa are 80 to 120 units/kg per week SC or 120 to 180 units/kg per week IV administered in 1 to 3 divided doses. The starting dose of darbepoetin alfa is 0.45 μg per kg SC or IV administered once weekly.

12. Dose adjustments of erythropoietic agents are based on the Hgb/Hct response and should not be made more frequently than every 4 to 6 weeks based on the time required for production of mature RBCs (i.e., the pharmacodynamic response). The dose of erythropoietin or darbepoetin may be increased by 25% if there is an inadequate response (e.g., hemoglobin increase <1 g/dL in a 4-week period) or decreased by 25% if the rise in hemoglobin is excessive (e.g., hemoglobin increases by >1 g/dL in a 2-week period). The goal of therapy is to achieve the target hemoglobin of 11 to 12 g per dL. Failure to respond to erythropoietic therapy requires evaluation of factors causing resistance, such as iron deficiency (primary cause), infection, inflammation, chronic blood loss, aluminum toxicity, hemoglobinopathies, malnutrition, and hyperparathyroidism.

13. Lack of interest, lack of knowledge about progressive kidney disease, chronic pain and tiredness, failure to comply with dietary restrictions, adverse drug reactions

14.
- Educate the patient about chronic kidney disease and how strict blood glucose and BP control can delay progression to end-stage kidney disease; also educate the patient about dialysis.
- Educate the patient about secondary complications of chronic kidney disease, such as anemia and renal osteodystrophy.
- Provide prefilled syringes of insulin by the pharmacy.
- Provide pill boxes and instructions on how to administer insulin injections.
- Provide instructions on how to manage missed doses.
- Provide instructions on how to monitor blood glucose (include times) and BP.
- Provide patient with a checklist on dietary intake and medication administration, and have the patient keep a diary.
- Quiz patient on proper techniques and medication administration times.

15. **KEY POINTS**

- Chronic kidney disease is a progressive disease leading to end-stage kidney disease and the need for dialysis.
- The two leading causes of chronic kidney disease are DM and HTN.
- ACE inhibitor or ARB therapy has been shown to delay the progression of chronic kidney disease in patients with type 1 DM or type 2 DM and in patients with proteinuria.
- Renal osteodystrophy is a complication of progressive kidney disease from longstanding metabolic abnormalities (hypocalcemia, vitamin D deficiency) that lead to secondary hyperparathyroidism.
- Prevention of ROD includes controlling hyperparathyroidism and the associated metabolic abnormalities of chronic kidney disease (hyperphosphatemia, hypocalcemia, vitamin D deficiency) with phosphate binders and vitamin D supplementation.
- Sevelamer and lanthanum are non-calcium-containing phosphate binders that may be used in patients who are hypercalcemic on conventional calcium-containing phosphate-lowering treatment. These agents may be useful in limiting blood vessel calcification in patients on longstanding calcium supplements.
- Supplementation of vitamin D with a vitamin D precursor (ergocalciferol) in patients with early-stage chronic kidney disease or with active vitamin D (calcitriol) or a vitamin D analog (doxercalciferol, paricalcitol) is necessary based on the stage of kidney disease and vitamin D status.
- Anemia is another complication of CKD that occurs due to erythropoietin deficiency (hormone produced by the kidney).
- Iron deficiency is the main cause of hyporesponsiveness to erythropoietic agents such as erythropoietin alfa or darbepoetin alfa.
- Before prescribing an erythropoietic agent, iron deficiency anemia must be corrected with an oral or IV iron product.
- Target goals of Hgb (11–12 g/dL) and Hct (33%–36%) should be maintained while treating anemia with iron and erythropoietic agents in patients with chronic kidney disease.
- Patient education is important to improve adherence with medication and nonpharmacologic therapy and to increase the patient's knowledge of chronic kidney disease and the associated secondary complications (and dialysis options for patients in later stages of disease).

CASE 18 ANSWERS

■ PROBLEM LIST

1. Peritonitis
2. Hyperglycemia
3. Inadequate dialysis
4. Hyperparathyroidism and associated metabolic abnormalities
5. Hyperlipidemia

■ SOAP NOTE

S: Painful CAPD exchanges for 4 days; "hazy" dialysate fluid, abdominal tenderness, fatigued, fever for 2 days, decreased appetite, "I cannot do all my exchanges—I feel too bad," ankle edema, decreased motivation to continue peritoneal dialysis per spouse

O: T 38° C; few rales in lower third of lung fields; 1+ edema in ankles
BUN (98), Cr (6.8), Glu (190), HgA$_{1C}$ 0.062 (6.2), Ca (9.8), PO$_4$ (6.9), total cholesterol (240), LDL cholesterol (184), HDL cholesterol (28), triglycerides (140), intact PTH (450); dialysate effluent: WBC 200/mm^3, neutrophils 110/mm^3; measured Kt/V = 1.1; weekly creatinine clearance = 45 L/1.73 m^2; urine volume in 24 h = 300 mL
Dextrose content for CAPD increased 2 weeks ago

A: PROBLEM 1: Peritonitis, possibly secondary to nonadherence with aseptic technique during CAPD exchanges—one episode of peritonitis per year; current symptoms preventing patient from completing exchanges as prescribed and contributing to inadequate dialysis

PROBLEM 2: Hyperglycemia despite scheduled NPH insulin; absorption of glucose from dialysate solution and infection are contributing factors

PROBLEM 3: Inadequate dialysis therapy as assessed by weekly Kt/V <2.0, creatinine clearance <60 L per 1.73 m^2, and symptoms consistent with fluid accumulation; noncompliance with dialysis prescription a contributing factor

PROBLEM 4: Hyperparathyroidism and associated metabolic abnormalities (hyperphosphatemia, abnormal calcium) as secondary complication of end-stage kidney disease; inadequate suppression of PTH despite calcitriol therapy; inadequate control of phosphorus with phosphate binder therapy, calcium carbonate as the current phosphate binder and calcitriol therapy are both contributing to hypercalcemia (corrected calcium = 10.1 mg/dL, Ca × P = 69.7 mg^2/dL^2)

PROBLEM 5: Hyperlipidemia with total cholesterol 240 mg per dL, LDL 184 mg per dL

P: PROBLEM 1: Peritonitis

- Perform two or three rapid dialysis exchanges (20 minutes each).
- Discuss technique of peritoneal dialysis exchanges.
- Start empiric antibiotics: cefazolin 15 mg per kg (approximately 1,200 mg) in one 2-L bag of dialysate solution QD and gentamicin 0.6 mg per kg (approximately 50 mg) in one 2-L bag QD.
- Adjust antibiotics based on culture and sensitivity results.
- Monitor temperature, WBCs, color of effluent, pain during exchanges, abdominal pain.
- Consider switching to hemodialysis if peritoneal dialysis technique deemed inappropriate (i.e., nonadherence with aseptic technique) and patient remains unmotivated to do exchanges.
- Temporary switch to hemodialysis may be warranted based on culture results (e.g., Pseudomonas or fungal infections).
- If continuing CAPD, educate BC about strategies to prevent infections (aseptic technique with demonstration by patient).
- Determine prior sources of infection in BC. If multiple S aureus, consider intranasal mupirocin 2% ointment BID for 5 days every month.
- If hemodialysis initiated, educate BC and family about process.
- Goals: Treat peritonitis with appropriate antibiotics, minimize the risk of subsequent infections, provide most appropriate dialytic therapy

PROBLEM 2: Hyperglycemia

- Determine history of glucose control (home monitoring, glucose during prior visits) and dietary intake.
- Assess the continued need for increased dextrose in the dialysate solution.
- Determine if dwell times are prolonged.
- Cure infection as soon as possible.
- Add regular insulin to each 2-L dialysate bag (4 units per bag).
- Monitor glucose several times daily (q4-6h) to determine need for alteration in insulin regimen.
- Educate patient about importance of regular glucose monitoring, hyperglycemia and hypoglyce-

mia, insulin use during sick days, and appropriate adjustments in insulin doses.
- Consider adjustments in insulin requirements with changes in dialysis prescription.
- Goal: Prevent hyperglycemia and hypoglycemia

PROBLEM 3: Inadequate Dialysis

- Discuss technique of peritoneal dialysis exchanges.
- Evaluate all factors contributing to decreased Kt/V and creatinine clearance (decrease in residual kidney function, noncompliance with exchanges, change in permeability of peritoneal membrane).
- Educate patient on the consequences of nonadherence with peritoneal exchanges (inadequate dialysis, possible need to switch to hemodialysis).
- Present hemodialysis as an alternative if a viable candidate.
- Assess BP and evaluate BC for resolution of edema (fluid overload) as changes are made to his dialysis regimen (i.e., as regular CAPD exchanges are done or if hemodialysis becomes necessary based on interventions required to treat peritonitis).
- Goal: Determine the optimal modality of renal replacement therapy consistent with management of end-stage kidney disease and lifestyle

PROBLEM 4: Hyperparathyroidism and Associated Metabolic Abnormalities

- Discontinue calcium carbonate and switch to a non-calcium-containing phosphate binder (e.g., sevelamer 1,600 mg TID with meals or lanthanum carbonate 500 mg TID with meals) to lower phosphorus and minimize the risk of hypercalcemia. Sevelamer may be preferred over lanthanum as it also reduces total cholesterol and LDL.
- Assess dietary phosphorus intake and counsel BC on restricting phosphorus (consult with renal dietitian).
- Discontinue calcitriol until Ca × P at goal (<55); consider initiation of a vitamin D analog (e.g., doxercalciferol or paricalcitol, since they are available in an oral formulation) once calcium and phosphorus are better controlled in an effort to minimize the risk of hypercalcemia and hyperphosphatemia while controlling PTH.
- Start cinacalcet 30 mg PO QD to suppress PTH secretion and potentially lower calcium.
- Monitor phosphorus, calcium, PTH, alkaline phosphatase.

▪ Educate patient on importance of adherence with medications and use of phosphate binder with meals.
▪ Goals: intact PTH 150 to 300 pg per mL, phosphorus below 5.5 mg per dL, calcium 9.2 to 9.6, Ca × P below 55

PROBLEM 5: Hypercholesterolemia

▪ Educate on diet modification as appropriate in patient with end-stage kidney disease to minimize intake of saturated fats and cholesterol.
▪ LDL is above 130 mg per dL; begin drug therapy with an HMG-CoA reductase inhibitor such as simvastatin 5 to 10 mg PO QHS or lovastatin 20 mg PO QHS. Monitor hepatic function.
▪ Monitor total cholesterol and lipid profile every 3 to 6 months.
▪ Goals: Lower LDL to below 100 mg per dL with diet and drug therapy, reduce risk of cardiovascular events, minimize adverse effects of therapy (follow K/DOQI Guidelines for Management of Dyslipidemias in Chronic Kidney Disease)

▪ CASE QUESTIONS

1. a. Subjective: Painful CAPD exchanges for 4 days; "hazy" dialysate fluid, fatigued, fever for 2 days

    b. Objective: T 38°; abdominal tenderness and guarding

    Dialysate effluent: WBC 200/mm³, neutrophils 110/mm³
    Dialysate culture (if positive)

2. a. Cefazolin + gentamicin

3. c. *S epidermidis*

4. b. Is the preferred method of administration

5. c. Ceftazidime + gentamicin

6. Options for prevention of CAPD infections in BC include:

    a. Strict adherence to aseptic technique when performing CAPD exchanges
    b. Regular patient and family education regarding technique of CAPD exchanges
    c. Pharmacologic: Intranasal mupirocin 2% ointment BID for 5 days every month to reduce risk of nasal carriage of *S aureus* OR rifampin 300 mg BID for 5 days every 12 weeks based on potential causative organism

7.

▪ Measured weekly Kt/V <2.0
▪ Creatinine clearance <60 L per 1.73 m²
▪ Elevated BUN and serum creatinine
▪ Mild elevation in potassium (generally, hyperkalemia is not as common with peritoneal dialysis as it is with hemodialysis; supports inadequate dialysis in peritoneal dialysis)

8. a. <100 mg per dL

9. c. Bioavailability

10. b. AV fistula

11. BC's current regimen for management of the anemia of chronic kidney disease:
    ▪ Current dose of epoetin alfa is appropriate: Hgb/Hct in target range (Hgb 11–12 g/dL, Hct 33%–36%).
    ▪ SC administration is ideal compared to IV in peritoneal dialysis population.
    ▪ Oral administration of iron requires monitoring for potential drug interactions (i.e., oral antibiotics, phosphate binders).
    ▪ Periodic assessment of iron status is warranted.
    ▪ Darbepoetin alfa administered SC is an alternative erythropoietic agent available for treatment of anemia of chronic kidney disease that may result in decreased frequency of administration. A conversion chart is available providing dosing recommendations for conversion from epoetin alfa to darbepoetin alfa.

12. Pharmacoeconomic factors to consider include:
    ▪ Influence of CAPD schedule on work schedule
    ▪ Financial burden if unable to work
    ▪ Increased cost associated with peritonitis
    ▪ Cost effectiveness of adequate training for peritoneal dialysis exchanges to minimize risk of infection (decreased cost of hospitalization and drug therapy for treatment of peritonitis)
    ▪ Cost associated with change from CAPD to hemodialysis if peritonitis episodes prohibit continuation of CAPD as dialysis modality

13. Psychosocial factors that may influence BC's adherence with his exchanges include:
    ▪ Social activities: may find CAPD restrictive to lifestyle
    ▪ Family network: time and effort of strict adherence requires strong family support

- Education: requires an understanding of the importance of adherence with CAPD prescription and adherence to aseptic technique
- Demanding CAPD schedule
- Acceptance by others: may view CAPD dialysis as less acceptable
- Attitude: if BC is depressed he may be less likely to adhere to all aspects of CAPD

14. **KEY POINTS**
    - Peritonitis occurs at a rate of one or two episodes per patient-year and is the predominant reason patients switch from peritoneal dialysis to hemodialysis.
    - Prevention of peritonitis requires strict adherence to aseptic technique during exchanges.
    - Peritonitis is diagnosed based on the presence of two of the following: abdominal pain, more than 100 WBC per mm³ of peritoneal fluid (with >50% neutrophils), and a positive dialysate culture.
    - Common organisms associated with peritonitis include *Staphylococcus spp* (gram-positive) and *Enterobacteriaceae*, *Pseudomonas spp*, and *Acinetobacter spp* (gram-negative).
    - Treatment is initially empiric, with use of more appropriate antibiotics once the organism is identified.
    - Strategies to prevent CAPD infection are essential for successful therapy and reduction in risk of CAPD-related morbidity.

CASE 19 ANSWERS

■ PROBLEM LIST

1. Peptic ulcer secondary to *H. pylori* infection
2. Suboptimal control of allergic rhinitis
3. Exercise-induced asthma (stable)
4. Menstrual migraine (stable)

■ SOAP NOTE

S: Patient states, "I've been having some stomach pain for a few weeks now. At first I thought it was just due to stress from midterms, but antacids aren't helping like they usually do. It's definitely worse at night and between meals, and actually does seem a little better after I eat. It feels like someone's lighting a match inside my stomach, right here (points to epigastric area)." Also notes some mild abdominal cramping.

O: Epigastric tenderness; serology positive for *H. pylori*; CBC WNL; sinus tenderness, nose moderately congested, fair amount of clear discharge bilaterally, turbinates pale pink and mildly swollen; penicillin allergy; occasional alcohol use; continuous-use oral contraceptive for migraine prevention; sumatriptan for migraine treatment; ibuprofen used only occasionally for mild pain; loratadine for allergic rhinitis; albuterol for exercise-induced asthma

A: PROBLEM 1: Peptic ulcer secondary to *H. pylori* infection in penicillin-allergic patient. Rare NSAID use not likely to contribute. *H. pylori* eradication regimens with three or four drugs have better efficacy than those using only two drugs; compliance is better with two or three drugs. Will avoid amoxicillin-containing regimens due to cross-reactivity with penicillin. Side effects more likely with bismuth subsalicylate-containing regimens; will avoid as first-line therapy. Antibiotics decrease intestinal flora and therefore may decrease absorption of oral contraceptives; barrier methods for contraception should be used during any cycle in which drugs are taken that can make oral contraceptives less effective. Per manufacturer of Seasonale, barrier method should be used throughout course of antibiotics and for an additional 7 days (21 days total). Clarithromycin, metronidazole, and omeprazole are all CYP 3A4 inhibitors; metronidazole also inhibits CYP 2C9/10, and omeprazole is also a CYP 1A2 inducer, a CYP 2C8/9 inhibitor, and a substrate and inhibitor of CYP 2C18/19; therefore, medications metabolized by these enzymes should be avoided or the dose adjusted if started during *H. pylori* therapy.

PROBLEM 2: Suboptimal control of allergic rhinitis despite routine antihistamine use. Symptoms are predominately nasal/sinus. Patient notes previous use of Allegra was not any more helpful, and Zyrtec caused excessive sedation.

PROBLEM 3: Exercise-induced asthma stable with pre-exercise use of short-acting β-agonist. If exercising for longer durations, may consider use of long-acting β-agonist as alternative.

PROBLEM 4: Menstrual migraine stable with continuous-use oral contraceptive to decrease frequency and triptan for acute migraine

P: PROBLEM 1: Peptic Ulcer

- Initiate *H. pylori* eradication regimen: clarithromycin 500 mg PO BID for 14 days, metronidazole 500 mg PO BID for 14 days, and omeprazole 20 mg BID for 14 days.

- Goals of therapy: eradicate *H. pylori* infection and treat duodenal ulcer. Patient's symptoms should resolve.
- Counsel patient to take medications with food, which will decrease the GI adverse effects of clarithromycin and enhance the activity of omeprazole.
- Emphasize importance of completing regimen as prescribed (even if feeling better); noncompliance increases risk of antibiotic resistance to metronidazole, clarithromycin, or both.
- Counsel patient regarding need to avoid consuming ethanol beverages or products containing ethanol while taking metronidazole and for at least 3 days after the discontinuation of metronidazole treatment.
- Counsel patient that antibiotics can decrease the efficacy of oral contraceptives; advise patient to use barrier method of contraception during course of antibiotics and for one week after
- Counsel patient about common adverse effects of her treatment regimen: GI side effects with clarithromycin. Metronidazole and omeprazole are generally well tolerated, especially with short courses of therapy.
- Counsel patient about need to report rash, shortness of breath, and other signs of drug allergy; also advise patient to report intolerable side effects.
- Avoid (or adjust dose of) medications metabolized by CYP 1A2, 2C8/9/10, 2C18/19, and 3A4 enzyme due to potential for drug–drug interactions with omeprazole, clarithromycin, and metronidazole.
- Discuss risk of NSAID use with ulcers, although occasional low-dose use in an otherwise healthy patient is unlikely to be problematic.
- Monitor symptoms of ulcer (epigastric pain, cramping). Notify provider if symptoms persist or redevelop. Notify provider immediately if black tarry stools, coffee-ground emesis, bleeding, vomiting, or severe abdominal pain develops.
- If verification of *H. pylori* eradication is desired (not indicated for first-episode of uncomplicated peptic ulcer disease), the urea breath test is recommended; use at least 4 weeks after completion of therapy to avoid confusing bacterial suppression with eradication. Serology is not effective for follow-up because antibody titers remain elevated even after successful treatment.
- If symptoms of ulcer persist or redevelop or urea breath test is positive despite complete regimen, antibiotic resistance should be considered and cultures (via endoscopy) may be warranted to determine antibiotic sensitivity. If ulcer is re-

fractory to multiple courses of therapy, other causes of peptic ulcer disease should be considered; long-term acid suppression may be warranted in some individuals.

PROBLEM 2: Allergic Rhinitis

- Add nasal corticosteroid, such as Flonase, 50 μg per actuation, two sprays in each nostril daily.
- Discuss use of nasal saline as well.
- Counsel on appropriate technique with nasal sprays.
- Counsel on environmental management to decrease exposure to allergens.
- Patient should monitor symptoms of allergic rhinitis and follow up if no improvement.

PROBLEM 3: Exercise-Induced Asthma

- No interventions needed at this time
- Consider long-acting β-agonist (salmeterol or formoterol) if needed for extended durations of exercise.
- Consider adding an inhaled corticosteroid if asthma symptoms occur more frequently.

PROBLEM 4: Menstrual Migraine

- No interventions needed at this time

■ CASE QUESTIONS

1. c. *H. pylori*

2. Epigastric pain (burning, gnawing) worse at night and between meals, somewhat relieved with food and antacids, mild cramping sensation; epigastric tenderness on physical exam

3. a. Serology (antibody detection)

4. Pharmacologic mechanisms of action:
    - Clarithromycin: macrolide antibiotic that binds to the 50S subunit of the bacterial ribosome and inhibits bacterial protein synthesis; antibacterial activity against *H. pylori*.
    - Metronidazole: nitroimidazole antibiotic that actually has a limited spectrum of activity against most gram-negative bacteria, such as *H. pylori*; the complete mode of action of metronidazole has not been fully elucidated, particularly in aerobic bacteria; used as part of two-antibiotic regimen for treatment of *H. pylori* infection
    - Omeprazole: proton pump inhibitor that becomes active when it enters the parietal cell; irreversibly binds with H^+/K^+-ATPase

(the "proton pump"); inhibits both basal and stimulated gastric acid secretion, irrespective of the source of stimulation (acetylcholine, gastrin, or histamine). Omeprazole (monotherapy) also reduces the colonization of *H. pylori* in the gastric antrum, but once it is stopped, *H. pylori* colonization returns to pretreatment levels. Omeprazole (when administered by routes that allow direct mucosal contact, such as oral, intragastric, or intraduodenal) may also have a cytoprotective effect, although the mechanism of action for this is unknown.

5. Factors to consider when selecting the optimal treatment regimen:
   - Two or three antimicrobial agents (including bismuth compounds) are required to achieve sustained cure rates of more than 80% to 90%. Regimens containing a single antibiotic are less effective and increase the risk of antibiotic resistance.
   - Consider past antibiotic use (may be associated with antibiotic resistance).
   - Consider local bacteria resistance patterns.
   - Regimens should also include an antisecretory agent to speed relief of symptoms and ulcer healing, and also to increase the efficacy of bacterial eradication with antibiotics.
   - Efficacy rates are generally better with treatment regimens of 10 to 14 days compared to 7 days or less.
   - Assess patient's drug allergies.
   - Assess potential drug interactions.
   - Agents with significant side effects (especially bismuth compounds) or regimens with complicated dosing regimens or high cost that could decrease compliance should not be used as first-line treatment.
   - Patients should be counseled to complete the full course of therapy to maximize efficacy.

6. Potential/actual drug interactions:
   - Drug–drug interactions with substrates of CYP 1A2, 2C9/10, 2C8/9, and 3A4; inducers or inhibitors of CYP 2C18/19; oral contraceptives may have decreased efficacy with antibiotic administration
   - Drug–food interactions with ethanol; omeprazole should be taken with food to increase effectiveness
   - Drug–test interactions with omeprazole and urea breath test; need to wait at least

4 weeks after omeprazole use before administering urea breath test

7. a. Paroxetine

8. c. GI side effects

9. d. Endoscopy and bacteria culture to determine antibiotic sensitivity

10. b. When taking oral contraceptives, barrier contraceptive methods should be used during course of antibiotics and for 1 week after.

11. Psychosocial factors that may affect EC's adherence to both pharmacologic and nonpharmacologic therapy are:
    - Issues that patient must address
      - Activity/quality of life possibly affected by symptoms
      - Dietary changes: although ethanol and caffeine/cola consumption have not been proven to cause peptic ulcers, ingestion may cause increased symptoms if ulcer is present
      - Medication compliance required
    - Emotional disorders
      - Psychological stress: again, this is controversial, but increased emotional stress may have some role in causing/exacerbating peptic ulcer
    - Other barriers
      - Cost of medications may be burdensome.

12. The health care provider's role relative to the proposed psychosocial factors identified is to:
    - Emphasize limited duration of therapy to enhance compliance with pharmacologic and nonpharmacologic plan.
    - Provide patient education and positive reinforcement.
    - Investigate medical assistance if appropriate.

13. b. Travel, lost wages for frequent office visits (direct nonmedical)

14. **KEY POINTS**
    - Peptic ulcer disease is a disorder characterized by the presence of ulcers in any portion of the GI tract exposed to acid in sufficient duration and concentration.
    - *H. pylori* infection and NSAID use are the most common etiologies of peptic ulcer disease. It is suggested that *H. pylori* infection contributes to gastric mucosal injury

by direct mechanisms, alterations in the immune/inflammatory response, and hyperergastrinemia leading to increased acid secretion. The ulcerogenic effects of NSAIDs are thought to be related to direct/topical irritation of the gastric epithelium and systemic inhibition of prostaglandin synthesis, thereby weakening endogenous GI mucosal defenses.

■ The goals of treatment for peptic ulcer disease are to relieve pain, enhance ulcer healing, prevent primary complications such as GI bleeding or perforation, and prevent ulcer recurrence.

■ Antiulcer and antibiotic therapy can effectively treat and reduce the recurrence of peptic ulcer disease when *H. pylori* infections are present. NSAID-induced ulcers can be treated by discontinuing the ulcerogenic drug (if possible) and/or using agents that prevent gastric acid secretion (H2-receptor antagonists, PPIs) or protect the stomach mucosa (sucralfate, misoprostol) with NSAIDs in high-risk patients.

■ Nonpharmacologic modifications such as smoking cessation, reduction of psychological stress, and avoidance of food/beverages that exacerbate ulcer symptoms may be beneficial with active and/or chronic ulcer disease.

CASE 20 ANSWERS

■ PROBLEM LIST

1. Ulcerative colitis
2. Anemia
3. Electrolyte disturbance, nutrition
4. DVT
5. Asthma
6. Contraception

■ SOAP NOTE

S: "I have stomach pain that gets better after I have a bowel movement. I need to go to the bathroom at least six times a day now, and it has blood and mucus in it." Denies travel, hospitalizations, or recent antibiotics. Obese, tired-appearing female. Quit smoking 2 months ago.

O: BP 110/68, HR 85, RR 20, T 37.2°C, Wt 75 kg (2 months earlier 79 kg), Ht 160 cm
+BS, NTND, no masses, no hepatosplenomegaly
Na 137 (137), Hct 0.311 (31.1), AST 0.53 (32), K 3.3 (3.3), Hgb 100 (10.0), ALT 0.47 (28), Cl 97 (97), Lkcs 8.2 × 10^9 (8.2 × 10^3), Plts 455 × 10^9(455 ×

10^3), BUN 3.9 (11), MCV 78 (78), Alb 30 (3.0), Cr 97 (1.1), MCH 24 (24), PT 12.7, INR 2.7, ANA +, ESR 70
Stool: RBC, WBC, culture negative
Sigmoidoscopy: granular, edematous, and friable mucosa with continuous ulcerations extending from anus to 20 cm proximally; barium enema shows confluent disease extending from rectum to transverse colon.
Asthma Step 2: Mild Persistent by National Heart, Lung and Blood Institute; FEV1 82%, PEF 25%
GU: WNL, no lesions

A: PROBLEM 1: Newly diagnosed active ulcerative colitis, moderate disease affecting rectum to transverse colon requiring local and systemic treatment

PROBLEM 2: Microcytic, hypochromic anemia from iron deficiency likely secondary to GI blood losses

PROBLEM 3: Dehydration, electrolyte disturbance, weight loss (malnutrition) secondary to ulcerative colitis

PROBLEM 4: DVT secondary to risk factors such as past smoking and use of oral contraception and potentially ulcerative colitis; currently treated therapeutically with warfarin

PROBLEM 5: Asthma appearing controlled with current therapy.

PROBLEM 6: Contraception methods inadequate to prevent further STDs; contraindicated with history of DVT

P: PROBLEM 1: Ulcerative Colitis

■ Sulfasalazine 500 mg BID with food and water
■ Increase dose every 2 days in increments of 500 mg per day to target dose of 3 to 4 g per day. Continue for 4 weeks, re-evaluate for improvement. If improved, reduce dose to 2 g per day split TID-QID.
■ Monitor disease activity: stool frequency, pain, stool contents (blood, mucus), weight, fever.
■ Monitor side effects of medication: fever, nausea/vomiting, diarrhea, rash, headache, malaise, bruising.
■ Repeat CBC in 4 weeks and liver enzymes and serum creatinine in 6 months or sooner if side effects occur.
■ Loperamide 4 mg PO initially, followed by 2 mg after each unformed stool. Do not exceed 16 mg

per day. Discontinue in 2 days if no improvement.
■ Mesalamine enema 4 g per 60 mL qhs pr; retain for 8 hours. Continue 2 weeks, re-evaluate for improvement. Monitor for rectal or anal irritation. Empty bowel prior to use.
■ Refer for psychosocial support.
■ Supplement with folic acid 1 mg QD.

PROBLEM 2: Anemia

■ Obtain baseline serum iron and TIBC.
■ If iron deficient, ferrous sulfate 325 mg tid on empty stomach for 2 to 3 months; repeat CBC, iron indices.
■ Monitor blood in stool, dizziness, fatigue, HR.
■ Monitor side effects of medication: nausea, constipation, dark stools.
■ If nausea occurs, may take medication with light snack, but do not take with dairy, antacids, vitamins.

PROBLEM 3: Electrolyte Disturbance, Nutrition

■ Increase fluid intake.
■ Identify foods that exacerbate ulcerative colitis and eliminate from diet.
■ Monitor dizziness, muscle cramps, weight, electrolytes, albumin.

PROBLEM 4: DVT
■ Continue warfarin 5 mg QD. Recheck PT/INR in 1 week. Dose may need to be decreased. Goal INR is 2.0 to 3.0.
■ Continue warfarin for 1 more month.
■ Monitor leg swelling, pain, shortness of breath, bleeding, stool guaiac.
■ Counsel patient on vitamin K in diet.

PROBLEM 5: Asthma

■ Continue current therapy.
■ Monitor shortness of breath, need for rescue albuterol.

PROBLEM 6: Contraception

■ Counsel patient about the use of barrier methods (condoms) to prevent future STDs.
■ Discontinue current estrogen-containing oral contraceptive; consider nonestrogen methods of birth control: injectable progestin, oral progestin, IUD, or diaphragm with condoms.

■ Counsel on other STD testing (HIV).

■ CASE QUESTIONS

1. b. Age of onset
2.
 ■ Diffuse continuous involvement of the colon and rectum; absence of fistula, cobblestoning, strictures, and transmural involvement.
 ■ Presence of abdominal pain, bloody diarrhea, weight loss, and fever
 ■ Elevated ESR, ANA +
3. Cigarette smoking increases the risk of Crohn's disease. Patients who smoke cigarettes and have Crohn's disease have more severe disease, require more immunosuppressive therapy, and have a higher likelihood of disease recurrence after surgery. In contrast, smoking appears to reduce the risk of ulcerative colitis; however, former smokers are at increased risk of ulcerative colitis compared to a person who has never smoked. It appears to be the nicotine that acts as a protectant to ulcerative colitis. TA was a former smoker and quit 2 months prior to her disease outbreak. Her recent smoking cessation could have contributed to her onset of disease.
4. c. Moderate continuous disease affecting the rectum and distal colon
5. a. Toxic megacolon
6. Induce remission, maintain remission, prevent complications, maintain quality of life, prevent hospitalizations
7. d. Sulfasalazine
8. Sulfasalazine (SASP) is an azo-bond prodrug consisting of a sulfapyridine group bound to the active moiety 5-aminosalicylic acid. The majority of the orally ingested prodrug remains intact in the colon, where colonic bacteria cleave the azo-bond and release 5-ASA from the sulfapyridine group. The 5-ASA acts topically likely by interfering with arachidonic acid metabolism and acting as a free radical scavenger. The sulfapyridine group is absorbed, metabolized, and excreted in the urine.
9. b. Decreased cost of sulfasalazine
10. d. Fever
11. b. Increase; protein displacement

12.

- SASP: Dose-dependent: Nausea, vomiting, dyspepsia, diarrhea, anorexia, headache, malaise, male infertility

  Dose-independent: fever, skin rash, hemolytic anemia, agranulocytosis, hepatitis, pancreatitis, neurologic toxicity, aplastic anemia

  Monitor CBC, creatinine, liver transaminases.

- Mesalamine: fever, skin rash, nausea, diarrhea, pancreatitis, hepatitis, nephrotoxicity, headache, alopecia

  Monitor CBC, creatinine, liver transaminases.

- Balsalazide: Headache, abdominal pain, dyspepsia, nausea, diarrhea, dizziness

  Monitor CBC, creatinine, liver transaminases.

- Corticosteroids: infection, hypertension, psychosis, hypokalemia, hyperglycemia, osteoporosis, cataracts, glaucoma, Cushing's disorder, acne, hirsutism, HPA axis suppression, weight gain, easy bruising

  Monitor DEXA scan, electrolytes, glucose.

- Azathioprine/6-MP: nausea, diarrhea, fever, skin rash, infection, arthralgias, hepatitis, pancreatitis

  Monitor liver transaminases, CBC, creatinine.

- Cyclosporine: tremor, paresthesias, headache, nausea, anorexia, gingival hyperplasia, nephrotoxicity, hypertension

  Monitor CBC, creatinine, electrolytes, albumin, cholesterol, liver transaminases, cyclosporine trough concentrations.

13. b. Provide symptomatic relief in mild chronic IBD

14. Surgery can be a curative measure in ulcerative colitis but should be reserved for patients who fail to respond to drug therapy or those with actual or impending complications and to reduce the risk of colorectal cancer in patients with precancerous biopsies. This is opposed to surgical procedures in Crohn's disease. The disease often recurs after surgery, so surgery should be limited to patients with intestinal complications. Increased small bowel losses from surgical resection result in limited absorptive surfaces and often lead to malnutrition and malabsorption.

15. IBD is a chronic relapsing disease that can dramatically affect a patient's quality of life. It may impair a patient's physical, emotional, social, professional, and educational activities. Anxiety and depression often coincide, and stress is often linked to disease exacerbations. Health-related quality of life questionnaires have been developed to assess the impact of IBD on a patient's perception of psychosocial well-being. Health care practitioners should be cognizant of the impact of pharmacologic and nonpharmacologic treatment modalities. Psychosocial plans should include patient education, coping skills, stress-reduction techniques, medication adherence plans, and family/social support. Referral to self-help groups and psychological therapy should be made when appropriate.

16. Corticosteroids should be used sparingly in patients with ulcerative colitis. They should be used only in patients with moderate to severe disease to induce remission. They should not be used for maintenance therapy. In patients with severe disease in whom disease activity is refractive to steroids, other immunosuppressants can be used to control disease activity. Cyclosporine and tacrolimus can be used acutely for disease management but should not be used long term because of side effects and toxicities. Azathioprine/6-MP can be used as maintenance treatment to reduce steroid doses or in patients who are refractory to steroids. The onset of action may be delayed for several weeks.

17. **KEY POINTS**
- The goal of medical therapy in IBD is to improve quality of life. This is best accomplished by inducing and maintaining remission, controlling symptoms, and preventing or controlling complications.
- Drug selection, dose, and route of administration is determined by the location, extent, and severity of intestinal involvement.
- Psychosocial factors are an important component of treatment in IBD and should constitute a part of the daily care plan.

- Antidiarrheals should be used with caution in severe IBD because they may precipitate toxic megacolon.
- ASA/6-MP should be used to treat steroid-dependent or refractory ulcerative colitis, Crohn's disease, and fistulizing Crohn's disease.
- A colectomy is curative in ulcerative colitis and may rid the patient of systemic complications. Surgery in Crohn's disease is not curative; the decision is influenced by response to drug therapy and impending complications.
- Patient education and improvement in health-related quality-of-life parameters contribute to improvement in IBD patient outcomes.

CASE 21 ANSWERS

■ PROBLEM LIST

1. Severe depression
2. Chronic hepatitis B infection
3. Increased LFTs
4. Mild anemia

■ SOAP NOTE

S: Patient presented to doctor's office for physical exam. Patient cancelled last scheduled exam. She complains of significant fatigue and appears very depressed. She states she can find no pleasure in the activities she normally enjoys and gets easily irritated, even with her grandchildren. This frustration with her grandchildren results in feelings of guilt. She was weeping during the exam.

O: Serology indicates that chronic hepatitis B persists; 2-kg weight gain since last visit; elevated LFTs; mild anemia

A: PROBLEM 1: Severe depression. This patient's depression appears to be related to the use of interferon, as she has had no prior history of depression and her depression began about 3 weeks into the interferon course. Patient has been self-administering St. John's Wort, 300 mg three times daily, for 2 weeks. Recommend stopping interferon, as severe depression can be a very serious and dangerous adverse effect of that medication. Suicides have been reported in patients with interferon-associated depression. She is very depressed, but not currently suicidal. Recommend stopping St. John's Wort and starting the patient on Zoloft, 50 mg QD. Other SSRIs could also be

considered. Since initiation of SSRIs in depressed patients can increase the suicide risk, close monitoring of the patient is needed. Also recommend close monitoring of the patient to determine if Zoloft can be discontinued in a few months after the effects of the interferon have resolved.

PROBLEM 2: Hepatitis B infection. The patient has been on interferon α-2b, 5 million IU SQ daily. The patient has completed 8 weeks of a 16-week course. The presence of HBe and viral DNA indicates active viral replication that requires continued treatment with an antiviral agent. Recommend discontinuation of the interferon (due to the depression that appears to be related to its use) and start patient on lamivudine 100 mg orally daily for 52 weeks. Lamivudine was chosen due to its low side-effect profile compared with interferon and its lower cost compared with adefovir. One of the concerns with lamivudine is the high incidence of resistance. Although adefovir is very costly, it does have a much lower incidence of resistance.

PROBLEM 3: Elevated LFTs. The patient's rise in LFTs may be due to the interferon. Discontinuation of interferon may resolve this problem if the interferon is its underlying cause. Recommend continued monitoring of LFTs after interferon discontinuation and the initiation of lamivudine.

PROBLEM 4: Mild anemia. The patient's anemia appears to be related to the interferon, as she has had no prior history of this problem. Discontinuation of the interferon may resolve this problem. Recommend monitoring of this patient's Hgb and Hct to ensure that this problem is resolved after the discontinuation of interferon.

P: PROBLEM 1: Severe Depression

- Start patient on Zoloft 25 mg QD. This medication is recommended due to its low incidence of side effects compared to tricyclic antidepressants and its reduced cost when this dose is taken as half a 50-mg tablet daily.
- Instruct patient to discontinue use of St. John's Wort.
- Monitor liver function monthly, as Zoloft should be used with caution in patients with liver dysfunction.
- Counsel patient to avoid grapefruit juice due to the drug–food interaction between Zoloft and grapefruit juice. Counsel patient to take medication with food to reduce possibility of nausea as a side effect; advise patient that efficacy may be delayed several weeks.

- Schedule follow-up to assess depression in 1 week. Depression treatment is optimized by combining medications with therapy.

PROBLEM 2: Chronic Hepatitis B Infection

- Change interferon α-2b to lamivudine 100 mg orally daily for 52 weeks.
- Instruct patient that lamivudine should not be discontinued without doctor's advice due to the potential for severe acute exacerbations of hepatitis and emergence of resistant HBV variants.
- Advise patient to contact doctor if the following side effects occur:
  - Allergic reaction
  - Extreme weakness, tiredness, or confusion
  - Lightheadedness or fainting
  - Numbness, tingling, burning, or pain in hands or feet
  - Rapid breathing, trouble breathing, or N/V
  - Unusual bleeding, bruising, or weakness
- Schedule a follow-up appointment in 1 month to assess viral load.

PROBLEM 3: Increased LFTs

- Discontinuation of interferon may address this mild elevation in LFTs, which may be due to the interferon or the hepatitis B.
- Encourage patient to minimize use of acetaminophen. Instruct patient to take no more than 2 g per day to minimize acetaminophen's potential hepatotoxic effects.
- Evaluate liver function at follow-up visit in 1 month.
- Remind the patient of the importance of avoiding ethanol.

PROBLEM 4: Mild Anemia

- Discontinuation of interferon may resolve this problem, as the anemia appears to be temporally related to the use of interferon.
- Evaluate anemia at follow-up visit in 1 month. If Hct and Hgb are still low at this follow-up, assume anemia is related to interferon use and investigate the cause more thoroughly.

■ CASE QUESTIONS

1. d. HBc IgG
2. c. Two Extra-Strength Tylenol PO q6h PRN
3. d. Interferon alpha-2b
4. c. 100 mg first dose, then 25 mg once daily
5. c. Depression

6. d. Ribavirin
7. a. Take the interferon before bed
8. The most significant risk factor for HBV infection in this patient is the fact that she was potentially exposed via a blood transfusion. Being of Alaskan heritage is also considered a risk factor.
9. The HBV polymerase is both a reverse transcriptase and a DNA polymerase. As a reverse transcriptase, it synthesizes the negative DNA strand from the viral genomic RNA. The HIV reverse transcriptase inhibitor lamivudine appears to have activity against the HBV reverse transcriptase.
10. Epivir-HBV (lamivudine 100 mg), for hepatitis B virus infection, contains a lower dose of lamivudine than Epivir (lamivudine 150 mg), for HIV infection. If Epivir-HBV is administered to a patient with unrecognized/untreated HIV infection, rapid emergence of HIV resistance is likely because of subtherapeutic doses and inappropriate monotherapy (product information for Epivir-HBV, 2001).
11. Compensated liver disease
    - HBV replication
    - HBsAg positive (assuming this has been ongoing for at least 6 months)
    - HBeAg positive
    - Increased ALT level
    - No hepatic encephalopathy, variceal bleeding, or ascites
    - Normal bilirubin, albumin, PT, WBC, and platelets
12. Severe depression is the main factor indicating that this medication is no longer appropriate for this patient. She is also suffering from mild drug-induced anemia and a spike in LFTs that is not unusual at this point in the interferon treatment.
13. **KEY POINTS**
    - Patients must be carefully monitored to ensure that interferon α-2b is not causing severe adverse events.
    - The side effects of interferon α-2b may be dose-limiting and dictate the discontinuation of the drug.
    - Medications used to treat the side effects of interferon α-2b must be used judiciously to prevent their potential contribution to liver dysfunction.

■ Several agents are available for treating chronic HBV. Weighing the risks versus benefits for HBV treatment is an essential first step in the process of HBV treatment. Medications currently approved by the FDA for use in treating HBV include α-interferon, lamivudine, and adefovir.

CASE 22 ANSWERS

■ PROBLEM LIST

1. Bipolar I disorder, currently depressed
2. Hepatitis C
3. Degenerative joint disease
4. Hypertension
5. Benign prostatic hypertrophy
6. History of opiate dependence
7. Seasonal allergies

■ SOAP NOTE

S: "I am more tired and less motivated to do things. I do feel better than when I was off of sertraline, but not as good as when I was taking 250 mg."

O: The patient's affect is sad with decreased range. Speech is slowed.

A: PROBLEM 1: Bipolar I disorder, currently depressed. Recent restart of sertraline 200 mg has not resolved depressed mood.

PROBLEM 2: Hepatitis C. Currently does not require treatment

PROBLEM 3: Degenerative joint disease

PROBLEM 4: Hypertension

PROBLEM 5: Benign prostatic hypertrophy

PROBLEM 6: History of opiate dependence

PROBLEM 7: Seasonal allergies

P: PROBLEM 1: Bipolar I Disorder

■ Increase sertraline to 250 mg q AM.
■ Continue with risperidone 5 mg QHS and gabapentin 600 mg BID.
■ Monitor for depressive symptoms.
■ Monitor for any onset of manic symptoms.
■ Monitor for dystonia or akithisia.
■ If depressive symptoms persist 6 weeks later, consider switching sertraline to citalopram.
■ If carbamazepine replaces risperidone, then sertraline doses will have to be increased due to in-

duction of CYP450 3A4. A rare but possible side effect is hepatotoxicity, and this patient may be more at risk due to his hepatitis.
■ Lithium use in this patient will result in multiple drug changes for other disease states (see below).
■ Lamotrigine may be an option for this patient. If lamotrigine is started, the patient must be monitored closely due to the risk of rash and the potential for drug interactions. Sertraline inhibits the metabolism of lamotrigine, putting the patient at greater risk of lamotrigine adverse effects (including rash).

PROBLEM 2: Hepatitis C

■ Continue to monitor LFTs.
■ If signs and symptoms worsen, then consider instituting antiviral therapy.
■ If the patient's liver function deteriorates, then the metabolism of risperidone and sertraline may be decreased and dose reductions will be necessary.
■ If the patient is started on interferon for hepatitis C, then the patient's bipolar disorder is likely to worsen, so monitoring for such changes is necessary. Treatment for this is not well documented, but more aggressive therapy and the addition of olanzapine during interferon therapy may be necessary.
■ Valproic acid has been shown to cause hepatotoxicity and should probably not be used in this patient.
■ Olanzapine has caused hepatotoxicity in a few published case reports. It is also common to see transient increases in LFTs when starting olanzapine, but these are benign.

PROBLEM 3: Degenerative Joint Disease

■ Continue with ibuprofen 600 mg TID PRN.
■ Continue with APAP/codeine 1 tab BID PRN. Dose of opiate should be carefully followed with no early refills due to past history of opiate dependence.
■ If the patient is to start on lithium, then he will no longer be able to use ibuprofen. A relatively safe alternative is aspirin, and an even safer choice is acetaminophen; however, the patient has hepatitis C, and the risk of APAP toxicity or worsening hepatitis exists if the patient were to switch to APAP.

PROBLEM 4: Hypertension

■ Continue with HCTZ 12.5 mg q AM.
■ Continue with lisinopril 10 mg BID.

- Monitor electrolytes and kidney function.
- If the patient is to switch to lithium, then both the lisinopril and HCTZ should be changed. A safe diuretic with lithium is furosemide, but no ACE inhibitor or ARB is safe with lithium.
- Verapamil and nimodipine have been shown to help control moods in bipolar patients, although there are not very compelling data.

PROBLEM 5: Benign Prostatic Hypertrophy

- Continue with terazosin 2 mg QHS.
- Monitor for nighttime urinary frequency.

PROBLEM 6: History of Opiate Dependence

- Continue with meetings for substance abuse.
- Carefully monitor use of APAP/codeine for treatment of patient's pain. This patient needs to be monitored very closely for misuse of codeine.

PROBLEM 7: Seasonal Allergies

- No current treatment necessary as patient has no current symptoms
- Consider loratadine 10 mg QD if symptoms emerge.
- The patient should be counseled not to use vasoconstrictors for rhinitis, as these may (with frequent use) increase the risk of having a manic episode.

■ CASE QUESTIONS

1. d. Will dramatically increase risperidone serum levels

   Paroxetine is a potent inhibitor of CYP450 2D6, the metabolic pathway for risperidone. There have been numerous case reports of emerging toxicity and one fatality when paroxetine was added to risperidone.

2. d. Hepatitis C

   Valproic acid has a black box warning regarding the risk of causing hepatitis.

3. b. Lisinopril

4. a. Lithium

   Ibuprofen taken for more than 3 days can increase serum lithium levels.

5. d. Rash

6. a. Sertraline

   Sertraline is metabolized via CYP 450 3A4. Carbamazepine is a potent inducer of that particular metabolic pathway.

7. a. Some open-label studies show efficacy, but more controlled studies have shown no efficacy in bipolar I disorder.

8. a. A sustained increase in theophylline dose

   Chronic theophylline use will lead to an increase in lithium excretion, resulting in subtherapeutic levels and a risk of a manic or depressed episode.

9. c. Agranulocytosis

10. HCTZ will cause an increase in Na excretion in the distal tubule. The kidneys react to this by increasing Na resorption in the proximal tubule. This results in reabsorption of both Na and lithium, so serum lithium levels could increase.

11. A mixed episode is defined as (a) Criteria are met both for a manic episode and for a major depressive episode (except for duration) nearly every day during at least a 1-week period; (b) The mood disturbance is sufficiently severe to cause marked impairment in occupational functioning or in usual social activities or relationships with others, or to necessitate hospitalization to prevent harm to self or others, or there are psychotic features; (c) The symptoms are not due to the direct physiological effects of a substance (e.g., a drug of abuse, a medication, or other treatment) or a general medical condition (e.g., hyperthyroidism).

    Rapid cycling is four or more episodes (manic, major depressive, mixed or hypomanic) within the past 12 months.

12. Pancreatitis due to valproic acid occurs extremely rarely, but due to the risk of death there is a black box warning listed for all valproate products. Monitoring parameters for this event involve assessing for symptoms of abdominal pain, nausea, vomiting, and anorexia. If these symptoms occur, then serum levels for amylase and lipase are warranted.

13. Bipolar I disorder is diagnosed when a patient has had a manic episode or mixed episode. Bipolar II disorder is diagnosed when a patient has had a hypomanic episode and a depressed episode.

14. 1. An explanation of the lifelong, intermittent course of the disease

    2. A description of the symptoms of a manic and depressed episode so that patients can recognize when they may be cycling into an

episode and try to prevent it from becoming overwhelming

3. Recognizing side effects of medication and how to manage them

4. A list of support groups for bipolar disorder

15. **KEY POINTS**
■ Bipolar disorder is defined by mood fluctuations that are excessive compared to the norm and result in occupational, social, and academic hardships. Patients may have different subtypes of bipolar disorder, but all patients will have at least one mixed, manic, or hypomanic episode either with (bipolar I, bipolar NOS, bipolar II) or without (bipolar I, bipolar NOS) a major depressive episode.
■ Many theories exist regarding the pathophysiology of the disease, but none has yet to be fully elucidated.
■ Pharmacologic treatment involves choosing medications that are similar to ones that have already proven effective (antipsychotics, anticonvulsants, lithium).
■ The goals of therapy are to reduce the number of episodes (manic, hypomanic, mixed, and depressed) that occur per year and to reduce the intensity and duration of these episodes when they do occur. Secondary goals are to improve family/social interactions and work-related behavior and outcomes, and reduce comorbidities, particularly substance use and abuse.
■ The choice of mood stabilizer to use in a bipolar patient very much depends on tolerability of the medication, as these medications frequently have harsh side effects or unacceptable adverse effects (e.g., lithium and hypothyroidism).
■ Medication choice is also determined by the patient's concurrent medication list and medical comorbidities. These factors frequently outweigh the difference in efficacy among the mood-stabilizer options.
■ Adherence to therapy is difficult in this population due to medication side effects and reduction in hypomania. Hypomania is a desirable condition in bipolar patients and they are reluctant to give it up, particularly if the medication causes weight gain or fatigue. Substance misuse, which occurs in over 50% of this population, adds to the risk of nonadherence.

■ Although elimination of episodes is the goal of therapy, this is frequently not attained. A realistic goal is a 50% reduction in frequency and intensity of episodes, along with improved social interaction. Since this is a chronic disorder, lifelong therapy is the norm. This is frequently difficult for a 20-year-old to accept (most first episodes occur before the age of 25). Therefore, patient–clinician rapport is critical, along with good medication knowledge, to maximize the success of therapy in this population.

CASE 23 ANSWERS

■ PROBLEM LIST

1. Acute psychotic episode of schizophrenia
2. Water intoxication/psychogenic polydipsia leading to hyponatremia
3. Hepatitis C
4. HTN
5. Smoking

■ SOAP NOTE

S: Positive for auditory hallucinations and paranoid delusions, agitated and aggressive; has been drinking excessive amounts of colas and coffee over previous week or so; multiple hospitalizations over past 22 years; father diagnosed with bipolar disorder, paternal grandmother had unknown mental illness; prior history of IV heroin use but none in more than 5 years; mildly enlarged liver noted, no tenderness

O: BP 148/92; Wt 88 kg (1 month earlier 76 kg); current cigarette smoker, 2 packs a day for 20 to 25 years

Hepatitis panel (drawn upon admission): anti-HAV negative, anti-HBc negative, anti-HCV positive; hepatitis C labs (drawn 2 weeks ago): HCV RNA positive, genotype 3A; Na 132; T Bili 34.2

A: PROBLEM 1: Acute psychotic episode of schizophrenia secondary to patient's medication noncompliance with olanzapine due to weight gain

PROBLEM 2: Water intoxication/psychogenic polydipsia leading to hyponatremia

PROBLEM 3: Hepatitis C secondary to IV drug abuse

PROBLEM 4: HTN

PROBLEM 5: Smoking: 40- to 50-pack year history

P: PROBLEM 1: Acute psychotic episode of schizophrenia

- Olanzapine was discontinued and clozapine was added recently; need to titrate dose to clinical effect.
- Continue oral haloperidol while tapering clozapine upwards; reconsider need for haloperidol once clozapine has begun to take effect.
- Continue clonazepam, benztropine, and propranolol for sedation and adverse effects of the antipsychotics as needed; consider removing benztropine and propranolol if haloperidol is discontinued, as these medications may no longer be needed.
- Continue oral and IV PRN medications for agitation/psychosis; if being used regularly for symptoms, increase standing dose of medications accordingly. Once patient is stable and no longer needs them, discontinue these PRN medications as well.
- Monitor for symptom improvement (decreased hallucinations, delusions, paranoia, aggression) and increased functionality.
- Monitor for adverse effects, such as extrapyramidal symptoms (parkinsonism, dystonia, akathisia), sedation, anticholinergic adverse reactions, and other medication-specific adverse reactions.
- Monitor CBC weekly for first 6 months of clozapine therapy, then every other week for 6 months, then monthly, for signs and symptoms of agranulocytosis/neutropenia.
- Monitor patient's weight weekly for first month, then monthly; serum glucose and lipids every 3 to 6 months; and LFTs every 3 to 6 months.
- Discuss importance of compliance with medication regimen and role of medication in treating the patient's mental illness.
- If noncompliance continues, consider switching to a long-acting injectable antipsychotic, such as risperidone or haloperidol decanoate.

PROBLEM 2: Water intoxication/psychogenic polydipsia leading to hyponatremia

- Place patient on fluid restriction while on the unit.
- Increase clozapine to effective dose; published data show some efficacy for this agent in psychogenic polydipsia.
- Monitor serum sodium levels at least weekly (more often if levels drop below 130) and maintain above 135; monitor other serum electrolytes also.
- Monitor daily fluid intake and keep below 2 L per day.
- Consider temporary discontinuation of HCTZ, especially if serum sodium drops below 130.
- Consider sodium supplementation if needed to correct hyponatremia.

PROBLEM 3: Hepatitis C

- Initiate treatment with peg-interferon alfa-2b and ribavirin for 6-month course of therapy, as viral genotype is one that is susceptible to this therapy.
- Monitor LFTs and physical signs (e.g., liver tenderness, jaundice, abnormal bleeding) for signs of efficacy.
- Monitor CBC for agranulocytosis/neutropenia, particularly in light of concurrent clozapine therapy.

PROBLEM 4: HTN

- No interventions needed at this time
- Monitor fluid and electrolyte status, as fluid overload may be contributing to increased BP.
- Consider adding β-blocker (either propranolol at therapeutic dose for HTN if still being used, or metoprolol) if HTN is not under control after stabilization of fluid status.

PROBLEM 5: Smoking

- Work with patient to consider quitting; provide patient education.
- If patient is agreeable to quitting, counsel on smoking cessation products and determine appropriate method.

■ CASE QUESTIONS

1. c. Serotonin and dopamine

2. "Positive"—auditory hallucinations, paranoid delusions, disorganized bizarre behavior; "negative"—attention impairment

3. Smoking has been found to increase the metabolism of clozapine through cytochrome P450 1A2 by as much as 50% to 150%. When JD stops smoking, this effect will be lost, thereby reducing the clearance of clozapine over the next several weeks as the enzyme returns to normal levels. As this happens, the effective clozapine concentrations will increase, perhaps leading to increased adverse effects. Serum clozapine concentrations can be monitored if deemed necessary, but close monitoring of JD for signs and

symptoms of increased adverse effects is more important. A clozapine dose reduction may be needed if the clinical picture warrants it.

4. Common adverse effects of clozapine therapy include sedation, orthostasis, weight gain, dry mouth, blurred vision, constipation, urinary retention, glucose regulation impairment, and elevated triglycerides. Seizures and agranulocytosis are not common adverse effects of clozapine treatment but are serious and must be monitored for as well.

5. Counseling for JD should be done in a manner that conveys the adverse effects to him in basic terms (third-grade level), how they are being monitored for, and what he should do if he notices one of these adverse effects. Merely describing the adverse effects will only scare him and increase his risk of noncompliance, even while on the inpatient unit. Complete counseling on adverse effects must be done.

6. a. Orthostasis

7. Clozapine: Beneficial: Dopamine-2 blockade (helps positive symptoms), serotonin-2 blockade (helps negative symptoms and decreases risk of extrapyramidal symptoms); Detrimental: Anticholinergic, α-1 blockade, antihistamine (all can cause adverse effects of different types)

   Haloperidol: Beneficial: Dopamine-2 blockade (helps positive symptoms); Detrimental: Dopamine-2 blockade (causes extrapyramidal symptoms and prolactin problems)

   Clonazepam/Lorazepam: Beneficial: Benzodiazepine receptor agonism (calming/sedating effects); Detrimental: Benzodiazepine receptor agonism (possible oversedating effects)

   Benztropine: Beneficial: Anticholinergic (alleviates acute extrapyramidal symptoms); Detrimental: Anticholinergic (causes anticholinergic adverse effects)

8. b. Complete blood count (weekly), fasting serum glucose (monthly), serum lipid panel (every 3 months)

9. d. Clozapine has been shown to reduce hospitalization rates and costs, a major component of total illness costs.

10. b. Pseudoparkinsonism

11. The prevention or treatment of weight gain with the use of clozapine (as well as other antipsychotics) has been difficult. Some data, however, show that diet and exercise modification, particularly early on in treatment, has some benefit. JD should be counseled on watching what he eats and making a conscious effort not to eat more than is necessary, select foods that are more nutritionally sound (not pizza and burgers every day), and increase his physical activity. JD's weight should be monitored regularly, weekly for several months and then monthly after that, as part of the regular monitoring for his medication regimen. If any weight gain is noted, then the diet and exercise counseling should be restated.

12. b. Meeting with JD's family to discuss his illness and how it is being treated

13. He is not an appropriate candidate at this time, but only in one respect. Since he has just started clozapine treatment, he has not had a full trial with this agent. He is not yet titrated to a therapeutic dose and has not been given at least 6 weeks at this dose, perhaps even longer. However, given JD's history of noncompliance with oral medications, it may only be a matter of time before he is noncompliant with his current regimen, which would then most likely make him a candidate for a long-acting IM antipsychotic. Given JD's history of akathisia to antipsychotics, the use of haloperidol or fluphenazine decanoate might not be the best choice. We would need to review JD's past oral risperidone trial to determine what happened with that agent. If JD did not have any type of serious adverse reaction to the oral risperidone, he could be a candidate for the long-acting IM form of the drug at a starting dose of 25 mg IM every 2 weeks. If we were to use haloperidol or fluphenazine, we would need to stabilize JD on an oral form of one of these two agents and then convert him over to an equivalent dose of the decanoate injection.

14. **KEY POINTS**
   - Schizophrenia is a chronic psychiatric disorder affecting approximately 1% of the U.S. population. Patients exhibit signs and symptoms of abnormal thoughts, perceptions, and interactions.
   - Although historically this disorder was thought to be due to a dopaminergic dys-

function in the brain, the role of serotonin (and perhaps other neurotransmitters) has become better elucidated in recent years.

■ Pharmacologic management of schizophrenia is integral to the treatment of this disorder. Nonpharmacologic treatment, such as psychosocial counseling, also plays an important role in overall treatment. Compliance with treatment is of immense importance in this disorder, and numerous factors can affect compliance to varying degrees.

■ The discovery of the newer atypical class of antipsychotics has dramatically changed how schizophrenia is treated. With the improvements provided by this class of medications versus the older, conventional antipsychotics (e.g., lower rates of extrapyramidal symptoms, improvement in negative symptoms), the overall treatment of schizophrenia has been advanced.

■ While the atypical antipsychotics have become the mainstay of treatment for schizophrenia, they have also presented new problems in the management of patients, including weight gain, glucose and lipid irregularities, and other adverse effects not seen to any large degree with the older antipsychotics.

CASE 24 ANSWERS

■ PROBLEM LIST

1. ADHD
2. Comorbid depression
3. Uncontrolled epilepsy

■ SOAP NOTE

S: "He (JP) never listens or sits down and disrupts class regularly. . . What do we do to get him to behave?"

O: Nine-year-old boy presents with hyperactivity, impulsivity, inattention, and regular episodes of depression. Symptoms are present at school, home, and play, and behavioral symptoms interfere with academic performance and peer relationships. Behavioral symptoms presented before school age (4 years of age or earlier). Theophylline [300 mg at HS (12.5 mg/kg/d), plasma concentration 11 mg per L (10–20 mg/L)] is controlling JP's nocturnal asthma symptoms. Seizure fre-

quency is one seizure per month with average doses of gabapentin (38 mg/kg/d). Blood lead concentration is below 10 μg per dL.

A: PROBLEM 1: ADHD. Potential causes of JP's behavioral symptoms include (a) seizures (complex partial or absence), (b) psychological (including ADHD, depression), or (c) environmental (medication, environmental toxin exposures, social/familial environments). According to JP's parents and teachers, his behavioral symptoms have been present before age 6 years and occur in multiple settings to a degree that they affect functioning. JP's father has symptoms suggestive of childhood ADHD, and heritability for ADHD is rather high (0.75 to 0.91). Although not a proven risk factor, low birth weight and prematurity have been associated with ADHD. The onset, frequency, and duration of symptoms are too frequent to be seizures. JP's theophylline is at the lower range of the effective concentration, so symptoms are not likely due to theophylline toxicity. Likewise, JP's gabapentin was started after behavior symptoms were evident, which argues against its role as an etiologic factor. Environmental lead is also an unlikely cause. Although JP's family environment as a contributing factor cannot be ruled out, it is less likely to be the primary cause of his behavioral symptoms in that symptoms occur in multiple settings. His symptoms are consistent with DSM-IV-TR ADHD and his symptoms are significant enough to warrant medication and behavioral therapy.

PROBLEM 2: Comorbid depression. JP has symptoms of withdrawal and sadness that are significant. ADHD and anxiety and ADHD and depression coexist in children (ADHD and anxiety in 20%–25%, ADHD and depression in 15%–20%). Currently, these symptoms are not being treated, so medication and behavioral therapy/psychotherapy should be initiated.

PROBLEM 3: Uncontrolled epilepsy. Often underappreciated, epilepsy occurs in 30% to 40% of patients with the combined hyperactive/impulsive type of ADHD. Many seizure medications, including gabapentin, have been associated with behavioral symptoms, so clinicians need to be aware of this phenomenon when treating patients with epilepsy and/or ADHD. JP is not seizure-free and is without medication side effects on an average gabapentin dose, so his therapy is not optimal and should be adjusted until he is seizure-free or there are medication-associated side effects.

P: PROBLEM 1: ADHD

- Obtain baseline behavioral symptoms using appropriate rating scales (e.g., Conners Parent Rating Scale, Conners Teacher Rating Scale).
- Screen for cardiac history.
- Identify target symptoms to assess therapy.
- Start stimulant therapy; examples of appropriate therapy include:
  - Methylphenidate IR 5 mg at breakfast, 5 mg at noon; increase by 5 to 10 mg per day every 5 to 7 days until symptoms improve or side effects occur, or until maximum dose is reached (2 mg/kg/d or 90 mg/d). Switch to extended- or sustained-release dosage form when optimal dose is defined.
  - Concerta 18 mg at breakfast. Increase by 18 mg per day each week until optimal dosage defined or maximum dose of 54 mg per day is reached.
  - Dextroamphetamine 5 mg at breakfast, 5 mg at noon; increase by 5 to 10 mg per day every 5 to 7 days until symptoms improve or side effects occur, or until maximum dose is reached (40 mg/d). Switch to extended- or sustained-release dosage form when optimal dose is defined.
  - Adderall XR 5 to 10 mg at breakfast; increase by 5 to 10 mg per day each week up to a maximum of 30 mg per day.
- Counsel child, parents, and teachers on medications and need for follow-up, particularly the use of ADHD scales.
- Monitor for insomnia, height, weight loss/appetite changes, irritability, BP changes.
- Refer to psychologist or psychiatrist regarding behavioral interventions/therapy.
- Follow up in 2 weeks to assess therapy and presence of side effects.
- Suggest a support group such as CHADD (Children and Adults with Attention Deficit/Hyperactivity Disorder) and provide contact information to the family.

PROBLEM 2: Comorbid Depression

- As above, refer to psychologist or psychiatrist for appropriate counseling.
- Obtain baseline ECG.
- Consider a tricyclic antidepressant (imipramine 1 mg/kg/d at HS; increase weekly to maximum dose of 4 mg/kg/d in one or two divided doses).
- Counsel on side effects [sleepiness/dizziness, decreased urine output, dry mouth, decreased stool, possible increase in seizures, and changes in heart activity (arrhythmia)].

- Obtain follow-up ECG at maintenance dose and annually while on imipramine therapy.

PROBLEM 3: Uncontrolled Epilepsy

- Increase gabapentin by 10 mg/kg/d per week until seizures are controlled or side effects occur, up to 50 mg/kg/d.
- Consider changing anticonvulsants if the above is ineffective, avoiding medications that are overly sedating (benzodiazepines, phenobarbital, phenytoin, topiramate, zonisamide) or associated with hyperactivity (benzodiazepines, phenobarbital).
- Encourage the parents to keep a seizure diary with attention to side effects (including behavior).

■ **CASE QUESTIONS**

1. d. ADHD
2. d. Behavioral symptoms occurring in more than one setting
3. ADHD is a neurodevelopmental disorder with symptoms occurring before the age of 7 years with symptoms lasting at least 6 months with a severity that impairs functioning. Behavioral symptoms cannot be explained by another condition (mood or pervasive developmental disorder or other psychiatric condition) and must occur in more than one setting (home, school, work, play). Medication-induced causes and toxin exposures should also be excluded. Patients must exhibit six or more symptoms in hyperactivity/impulsivity domain, inattentive domain, or both and display them often. Patients may have comorbid conditions that are not considered diagnostic but influence the medication selection, need for adjunctive therapy, and monitoring.
4. c. Genetic heritability
5. a. Adderall XR
6. c. Stimulants increase dopamine, while atomoxetine increases norepinephrine.
7. Long-acting: Adderall XR, Concerta, Dexedrine Spansule,* Metadate CD,* Metadate ER, Methylin ER, Ritalin LA,* Ritalin SR (*can be opened and placed in food)
8. a. Look at improvements in JP's academic performance and teacher and parents rating scales

9. b. JP's classmates should all be informed he has ADHD so as to help him.

10.
- Discuss that ADHD is a neurodevelopmental disorder and that in some cases it persists into adulthood; for some patients this means life-long therapy.
- Discuss that it is important to obtain behavioral therapy, and this may include other family members as well.
- Provide information regarding support groups (e.g., CHADD).
- Explain the side effects that are common to stimulants (decrease in appetite, irritability, stomach upset, rarely heart problems/blood pressure changes).
- Stress that stimulants used in children with ADHD do not result in addiction, tic disorders, or short stature and do not always cause behavioral rebound.
- Educate about compliance; emphasize that medications are to be used solely by JP.
- Determine the ability of the family to obtain (pay for) and properly administer medical therapy for ADHD.

11. d. Schizophrenia

12. **KEY POINTS**
- ADHD is a neurodevelopmental disorder with significant effects on psychological, social, functional, and academic or work performance.
- ADHD is a dysfunction of dopaminergic/norepinephrine neurotransmission that produces symptoms of hyperactivity/impulsivity and/or inattention; for diagnosis, the symptoms must be present before the age of 7 years and must occur in more than setting.
- ADHD has a strong genetic component and tends to run in families. Many things may seem to induce similar symptoms and must be ruled out before a diagnosis of ADHD is made.
- Treatment should include both medication and behavioral interventions, which should be tailored to the patient's symptoms. For most patients, stimulants remain the first line of therapy, and at least two should be tried before another class of medications is considered.
- Stimulants may be associated with changes in appetite/weight loss, irritability, insomnia, and rarely cardiac problems. They do not produce addiction or short stature and only in some cases do they induce or worsen tics.

- Patients with depression may benefit from a tricyclic antidepressant or bupropion, and those with tics or conduct disorders may require clonidine.
- Follow-up should include interventions by multiple sources (parents, teachers, caregivers) and should focus on target ADHD/behavioral symptoms.

CASE 25 ANSWERS

■ PROBLEM LIST

1. Carbamazepine toxicity
2. Hyponatremia/SIADH
3. Neutropenia
4. Refractory epilepsy
5. Pneumonia
6. Hypertension
7. Congestive heart failure
8. Depression

■ SOAP NOTE

S: "I feel woozy and then I don't remember much. This happened last week four times and gets worse when I don't sleep. . . . I can't seem to get over this cold."

O: Sixty-eight-year-old man with mild to moderate confusion, Wt 105 kg, Ht 170 cm, T 40°C, BP 140/90, RR 25, O_2 at 92% on nasal cannula. Complex partial seizures with secondary generalization two or three per week every few months (seizure duration 5–7 minutes).
Labs: Na 115 (115), Cl 104 (104), K 4.0 (4.0), Glu 5.9 (107), HCO_3 28 (28), BUN 12.5 (35), SCr 106 (1.2), WBC 2.1×10^3 (2.1×10^3). Differential: Lymphs 65, PMN 15, Mono 15, Bands 5. Hct 0.40 (40), Plts 300×10^9 (300×10^3), Hgb 130 (13), serum osmolarity 248 (248), urine Na 30 (30), urine osmolality 150 (150). Carbamazepine 80.4 (19) (6-hour post-dose concentration).
EEG shows mild diffuse encephalopathy with spikes arising from the temporoparietal regions independently bilaterally. Chest x-ray shows consolidation of right superior and inferior lobes, mild cardiac enlargement. Sputum and blood cultures are pending.
For epilepsy: carbamazepine (generic) 300 mg PO QID, lamotrigine 200 mg BID, oxcarbazepine 1,200 mg PO TID. For depression: citalopram 30 mg PO HS, amitriptyline 150 mg HS. For cardiac/hypertension/heart failure: metoprolol (Toprolol XL) 300 mg PO QD, hydrochlorothiazide 50 mg HS, aspirin 325 mg PO QD. For infection: erythromycin 400 mg BID. He has a penicillin allergy (rash).

A: PROBLEM 1: Carbamazepine-induced CNS toxicity associated with supratherapeutic plasma concentration. Most likely due to carbamazepine–erythromycin drug–drug interaction.
Carbamazepine concentration (>12 mg/L) with CNS side effects

PROBLEM 2: Symptomatic hyponatremia/SIADH that is induced either by oxcarbazepine (more commonly) or carbamazepine as indicated by the low serum sodium (Na <125 mEq/L), normal urine sodium (Na >20) with undiluted urine (urine osmolarity >50 mOsm/kg). Hyponatremia associated with oxcarbazepine is more commonly found in the elderly and in those receiving thiazide diuretics and SSRI antidepressants. Other risk factors include the use of phenothiazides, NSAIDs, or other sodium-depleting medications.

PROBLEM 3: Neutropenia induced by carbamazepine and/or oxcarbazepine (WBC 2.1 × 10³; ANC 420)

PROBLEM 4: Refractory epilepsy: still experiencing seizures after exposure to three anticonvulsants with adequate doses (four anticonvulsants total in lifetime)

PROBLEM 5: Pneumonia, partially treated

PROBLEM 6: Hypertension uncontrolled with current regimen

PROBLEM 7: Congestive heart failure uncontrolled with current regimen

PROBLEM 8: Depression controlled with current regimen

P: PROBLEM 1: Carbamazepine-induced CNS toxicity

- Discontinue erythromycin.
- Begin third-generation cephalosporin and vancomycin or fluoroquinolone and vancomycin pending culture results.
- Abruptly discontinue carbamazepine because of likelihood it is contributing to Problems 1, 2, and 3.
- Reduce dose of lamotrigine by 20% empirically to prevent increases in lamotrigine concentration following removal of carbamazepine.
- Limit patient mobility and start cardiac monitoring.

PROBLEM 2: Symptomatic hyponatremia/SIADH

- Discontinue carbamazepine and reduce dose of oxcarbazepine.
- Administer 3% saline to correct sodium to 125 mEq per L.

- Restrict fluids to 800 to 1,000 mL per day and consider oral Na replacement.
- Switch hydrochlorothiazide to a loop diuretic (bumetanide 1–2 mg QD).
- Continue to monitor plasma Na.
- If Na fails to correct, consider discontinuing oxcarbazepine or amitriptyline and administering demeclocycline 1,200 mg per day.

PROBLEM 3: Neutropenia, induced by carbamazepine and/or oxcarbazepine

- Discontinue carbamazepine as above and consider discontinuing oxcarbazepine.
- Repeat CBC with differential until ANC >500 and WBC 1.2 × 10³/mm³.
- If there is no improvement in WBC, consider GCF.
- Continue antibiotic coverage.

PROBLEM 4: Refractory epilepsy

- Start therapy with levetiracetam 500 mg PO BID, with increases of 500 to 1,000 mg per day each week.
- Lorazepam 2 to 4 mg IV PRN seizure >5 minutes
- Counsel patient/daughter on medication compliance and avoidance of seizure triggers (lack of sleep). Introduce compliance aids (pill box) and consider skilled care, assisted living, or visiting nurse to encourage compliance.
- Remind of seizure precautions and need to keep a seizure diary.
- Make certain patient can afford/has access to medications.

PROBLEM 5: Pneumonia, partially treated

- Continue broad-spectrum antibiotics until cultures return and narrow if possible.
- Administer acetaminophen 500 mg PO/PR PRN fever.
- Monitor for fever curve, WBC, differential, ANC (>500), cultures, new signs/symptoms of infection.
- Avoid other sick contacts. Wash hands frequently. Wear a mask and gloves when out of the hospital room.

PROBLEM 6: Hypertension, uncontrolled with Current regimen

- Begin therapy with lisinopril 10 mg PO QD.
- Encourage smoking cessation and weight loss.
- Counsel on need to avoid getting up rapidly to avoid dizziness/imbalance.
- Continue to monitor BP.

PROBLEM 7: Congestive heart failure, uncontrolled with current regimen

■ Begin therapy with lisinopril 10 mg PO QD.
■ Encourage smoking cessation and weight loss.
■ Counsel on need to avoid getting up rapidly to avoid dizziness/imbalance and signs/symptoms of worsening heart failure (shortness of breath, peripheral edema).
■ Consider switching metoprolol to amlodipine.

PROBLEM 8: Depression, controlled with current regimen

■ Maintain current regimen; consider switch to monotherapy with citalopram or amitriptyline if possible.

■ CASE QUESTIONS

1. b. Carbamazepine-induced neutropenia with secondary pneumonia

2. b. Failure to respond to two or more anticonvulsants

3. c. Azithromycin

4. Lamotrigine is significantly affected by medications that inhibit or increase metabolism through UGT phase II metabolism. Enzyme-inducing medications such as carbamazepine, phenobarbital, and phenytoin decrease the lamotrigine concentration by increasing hepatic metabolism. In contrast, inhibitors of UGT metabolism (valproic acid) significantly decrease lamotrigine's elimination (increase lamotrigine concentrations). In contrast, there are many anticonvulsants that do not affect the UGT system significantly (gabapentin, pregabalin, levetiracetam, tiagabine, oxcarbazepine, topiramate, zonisamide) and therefore would not affect lamotrigine's metabolism. In the case described, removal of carbamazepine would result in delayed increases in lamotrigine concentrations and a reduction in lamotrigine dose should be considered. Risk factors for lamotrigine-induced rash include high dose at initiation, rapid titration, concurrent use of valproic acid, and use in pediatric patients.

5. b. Discontinue carbamazepine, start levetiracetam

6. c. Voltage-gated Na-channel inhibition

7. c. Plasma Osmolarity >280 mOsm

8. Restrict fluids, discontinue hydrochlorothiazide and carbamazepine, reduce dose of oxcarbazepine, change to loop diuretic (bumetanide 1–2 mg QD), reduce dose of oxcarbazepine. JA is symptomatic, so 3% saline along with fluid restriction to 800 to 1,000 mL per day should be used to correct sodium to 125 mEq per L. Continue to monitor plasma Na every 12 to 24 hours. If Na fails to correct, consider discontinuing oxcarbazepine or citalopram and administration of demeclocycline 1,200 mg per day.

9. JA lives alone, and it is uncertain whether he regularly takes his medication. Counseling him on the need for compliance is needed, along with ensuring that his home is arranged to minimize the risk for falls. Encouragement about good sleep hygiene is needed (going to bed at a regular time, performing relaxing things before bedtime, decreasing/eliminating caffeine intake). Review the use of a seizure diary and inquire about his ability to pay for medications. His daughter should have seizure first aid reviewed, and arrangements for other caregivers (visiting nurse or neighbor visit) or assisted living should be considered. Smoking cessation and weight loss programs should also be encouraged.

10. d. Complex partial seizure

11. a. Citalopram

12.

■ The incidence of epilepsy follows a bimodal distribution, with the frequency increased in children and the elderly. Typically, the elderly have complex partial seizures secondary to etiologies such as stroke or CNS lesion.
■ Selection of anticonvulsants in the elderly shares some of the considerations of other age groups, such as frequency of use (ideally dosing once or twice per day), pharmacokinetics and drug interaction potential (renal elimination, minimal or no hepatic metabolism), and ease of administration (availability of crushable or liquid dosage forms) for those unable to take solid tablets.
■ For patients receiving more than one anticonvulsant, medications with different side effect profiles and mechanisms of action should be used.
■ Drug–drug, drug–food, and drug–disease interactions should be reviewed regularly.

This can be compared against seizure occurrence and side effects or changes in concurrent disease states.

- The elderly are more prone to CNS side effects and may have prolonged elimination and reduced protein binding. Anticonvulsants should be started at low doses and increased slowly.
- Seizures in this population can be mistaken for confusion, medication side effects, delirium, psychiatric disorder, or dementia. The risk for injury following a seizure is also higher in this population, so the home environment and household contacts/caregivers need to be prepared.
- Costs of medication and compliance with therapy need to be assessed early in the course of therapy and continued throughout treatment. Nonseizure/nonepileptic symptoms need to be clearly distinguished from those associated with a seizure/epilepsy.
- Patients started on anticonvulsants following a stroke or trauma should have a regular reassessment of the need for continued anticonvulsant therapy, particularly if the patient is seizure-free.

13. **KEY POINTS**
- Refractory epilepsy remains a significant clinical problem in approximately 30% of patients, even with polytherapy.
- Patients with refractory seizures are at risk of many medication-associated side effects and drug–drug interactions. Selection of anticonvulsants should focus on differences in side effects, drug interaction potential, dosage form, and mechanism of action. In this case, oxcarbazepine and carbamazepine have similar mechanisms of action and toxicities.
- Carbamazepine can be associated with early, brief asymptomatic decreases in neutrophil counts in 8% to 20% of patients. In these instances, indices return to normal without clinical intervention. WBC decreases can persist, but they do not decrease to levels that warrant concern (WBC <4K/mm^3). Data regarding a dose- or concentration-effect relationship and decreases in blood cell counts are conflicting. Blood cell counts (CBC with differential) should be done at baseline and then at 1, 3, and 6 months of therapy. If WBC counts decrease to below 3.5K per mm^3 or ANC <1.2K per mm^3, then carbamaze-

pine doses should be decreased. If blood counts fail to recover or if they decrease further, then carbamazepine should be discontinued.
- In the case of most postsymptomatic epilepsies, seizures are most commonly partial-onset seizures.
- Medication compliance, maintenance of a seizure diary, and recognizing and being able to act in the case of a seizure should be emphasized to patients with epilepsy and their family members and caregivers.
- Many anticonvulsants (carbamazepine, oxcarbazepine, valproate) can cause blood dyscrasias, including neutropenia and most severely agranulocytosis. Management of mild neutropenia includes dose reduction, with more severe cases necessitating therapy discontinuation.
- Oxcarbazepine more commonly causes SIADH/hyponatremia than carbamazepine. The incidence is higher in the elderly. Concurrent use of thiazide diuretics, antipsychotics (especially phenothiazides), and antidepressants increases the risks. Management may include reducing the oxcarbazepine or carbamazepine dose, fluid restriction, and possible administration of saline. Initial management for mild symptomatic hyponatremia caused by either carbamazepine or oxcarbazepine should include a dose reduction with fluid restriction and possibly oral sodium replacement. If symptoms fail to resolve, then the offending medication should be discontinued. In patients with more severe symptoms, demeclocycline and/or intravenous Na replacement may be needed (goal Na = 125 mEq/L).

CASE 26 ANSWERS

■ PROBLEM LIST

1. Parkinson's disease with motor fluctuations ("wearing off")
2. BLE rash and ankle edema

■ SOAP NOTE

S: "I feel great. For the most part, my symptoms are controlled, but only until about 1 hour before my next dose of carbidopa/levodopa."

O: No apparent distress; mild rest tremor (R > L); rigidity with "cogwheel" or "ratchet" quality in

BUE (R > L); slow finger taps and leg mobility (R > L); no weakness; micrographia; mild difficulty standing from a seated position; slow, shuffling gait; reduced bilateral arm swing (R > L); no postural instability; reddish-purple, fishnet-patterned mottling in BLE; bilateral ankle edema

A: PROBLEM 1: Moderate PD with end-of-dose wearing-off effect of carbidopa/levodopa

PROBLEM 2: Amantadine-associated livedo reticularis

P: PROBLEM 1: Moderate PD with Carbidopa/Levodopa end-of-dose wearing-off effect

- Switch from carbidopa/levodopa 25 per 100 mg to carbidopa/levodopa/entacapone 25/100/200 mg PO TID for patient convenience and adherence. Alternatively, may add entacapone separately as 200 mg PO TID.
- Avoid carbidopa/levodopa CR due to unsatisfactory patient response in past.
- Avoid addition of selegiline because it has a mechanism of action similar to that of rasagiline.
- Due to risk of worsening LE edema, avoid dopamine agonist until edema resolves.
- If addition of entacapone is not tolerated, increase carbidopa/levodopa to QID.
- Provide patient education on Stalevo regimen.
- Counsel on potential side effects associated with addition of entacapone, including diarrhea, dizziness, dyskinesia, hallucinations, lightheadedness, nausea, and urine discoloration.
- Educate patient on other management techniques for "wearing off."
- Monitor for improvement of symptoms of PD and wearing-off fluctuations.

PROBLEM 2: Amantadine-Associated Livedo Reticularis

- Gradually taper off amantadine by reducing by 100 mg per day every 3 days until discontinued.
- Inform patient that the rash and edema will resolve upon discontinuation of amantadine.
- Monitor for worsening of symptoms of PD.

■ CASE QUESTIONS

1. c. Idiopathic

2. Rest tremor, muscle rigidity, and bradykinesia

3. d. Facial rigidity

4. b. Acts as a dopamine precursor

5. c. Deep brain stimulation

6. The key differences between immediate-release and controlled-release carbidopa/levodopa:

Feature	Immediate-Release	Controlled-Release
Bioavailability	99%	71%
Dosing with regard to food	Take on an empty stomach	Take with food
Initial duration of effect	Up to 4 hours	Up to 6 hours
May be crushed, chewed, or dissolved	Yes	No
Onset of effect	30 minutes	60 minutes

7. d. Trimethobenzamide

8. a. It is a selective MAO-B inhibitor

9. a. Quetiapine

10. d. Metoclopramide

11. The mechanism by which levodopa causes nausea:
    Dopa decarboxylase in the periphery converts levodopa to dopamine, which stimulates the chemoreceptor trigger zone, thereby resulting in nausea.

12. b. A predictable waning of levodopa benefit resulting in return of symptoms prior to the next dose

13. b. Dyskinesia

14. c. Antidyskinetic agent

15. c. Carbidopa/levodopa to reduce wearing-off symptoms

16. **KEY POINTS**
    - PD is a common movement disorder characterized by the presence of tremor, rigidity, bradykinesia, and postural instability as well as mental and autonomic changes. The resulting symptoms have profound effects on quality of life for both patients and caregivers.
    - The causes of PD remain obscure. However, environmental factors and genetic predisposition are believed to play a role in promoting oxidant stress and accumulation of intracellular toxic proteins, with subsequent neurodegeneration and depletion of nigrostriatal dopamine.
    - Initiate putative neuroprotective therapy as early as possible.
    - The initiation of symptomatic therapy should be based on the patient's level of functional impairment and quality of life. For example, hand tremor in a retiree, although a nuisance, may not interfere with

daily activities but may endanger the livelihood of a dentist.

- Anticholinergic agents should be considered for younger patients (<65 years of age) if tremor is the predominant symptom. Avoid anticholinergic agents in the elderly or patients with memory problems.
- For mild bradykinesia and rigidity, consider amantadine or selective MAO-B inhibitors. As the signs and symptoms worsen, add a dopamine receptor agonist or carbidopa/levodopa.
- Carbidopa/levodopa is the most effective oral agent for treatment of PD.
- If cognitive or memory impairment is present, give preference to carbidopa/levodopa over amantadine, anticholinergics, dopamine receptor agonists, or selective MAO-B inhibitors because these latter agents tend to exacerbate underlying memory problems more than levodopa.
- Younger patients face a greater duration of disease and are more likely to develop levodopa-related motor complications. Give preference to neuroprotective agents and use of non-levodopa products (e.g., amantadine, dopamine receptor agonists, selective MAO-B inhibitors). As the disease progresses, all patients will eventually require carbidopa/levodopa.
- Addition of a COMT inhibitor or a selective MAO-B inhibitor should be considered for managing motor fluctuations (i.e., "wearing-off" effect).
- Subcutaneous apomorphine provides consistent and rapid onset of "on time" in patients experiencing frequent "off" episodes despite optimized pharmacotherapy.
- Amantadine is useful for management of levodopa-related dyskinesias.
- Low doses of an atypical antipsychotic, such as quetiapine, are well tolerated and effective for managing hallucinations and psychosis in PD.
- Surgery should be considered for patients with idiopathic PD and disabling dyskinesias, motor fluctuations, or tremors despite optimized medical therapy.

CASE 27 ANSWERS

■ PROBLEM LIST

1. Rheumatoid arthritis, uncontrolled with progressive disease

2. Anemia of chronic disease (mild)
3. Age-associated changes in vision (mild)
4. Perennial seasonal rhinitis (inactive)
5. History of allergic reaction to "sulfa" drugs and penicillin
6. Family history of DM type 2, dyslipidemia, osteoporosis

■ SOAP NOTE

S: Chronic fatigue; joint swelling in hands, wrists, and feet; morning stiffness for months despite increasing the ibuprofen dose to 600 mg QID. Able to perform essentially all of her daily activities but is in chronic pain and discomfort.

O: 2+ swelling and tenderness of MCPs, PIPs, MTPs, and wrists; RF +, ESR 45. Hand x-rays reveal swelling and erosions. Hct 33%, MCV 88. No evidence of skin, lung, kidney, ocular, or vessel involvement.

A: PROBLEM 1: Rheumatoid arthritis: early, progressive moderately severe disease despite high-dose NSAID therapy, functional class I

PROBLEM 2: Anemia of chronic disease due to rheumatoid arthritis (mild)

PROBLEM 3: Age-associated visual changes (mild)

PROBLEM 4: Perennial seasonal rhinitis (no current symptoms)

PROBLEM 5: History of allergy to "sulfa" drugs and penicillin

PROBLEM 6: Family history of DM type 2, dyslipidemia

P: PROBLEM 1: Rheumatoid Arthritis Progression, Moderate Severity

- Continue ibuprofen 600 mg PO QID.
- Add methotrexate 7.5 mg PO once weekly and folic acid 1 mg daily.
- Add physical therapy (range-of-motion exercises), rest periods during the day if needed.
- Monitor joint swelling, joint pain, morning stiffness, fatigue, and ability to function.
- Monitor CBC, LFTs, lungs, skin and mucous membranes, and signs/symptoms of infections in 2 weeks, 4 weeks, then every 4 to 6 weeks.
- Discuss importance of no excess use of alcohol and the potential for liver toxicity from methotrexate, but can continue drinking one glass of wine daily.

PROBLEM 2: Anemia of Chronic Disease

- Treat the rheumatoid arthritis; no other therapy is needed at this time.

- Monitor Hct, Hgb, MCV, fatigue.
- Consider workup for iron-deficiency anemia if symptoms worsen or persist despite improvement in the patient's rheumatoid arthritis.

PROBLEM 3: Age-Associated Visual Changes

- No therapy recommended, except the use of reading glasses or corrective lenses

PROBLEM 4: Perennial Seasonal Rhinitis

- No therapy is needed at this time.
- Continue the use of loratadine 10 mg PO QD PRN.
- If symptoms persist, consider intranasal cromolyn.

PROBLEM 5: History of Allergy to "Sulfa" Drugs and Penicillin

- Avoid "sulfa" drugs and penicillins.

PROBLEM 6: Family History of DM Type 2, Dyslipidemia, Osteoporosis

- Maintain a healthy diet, weight control, and exercise regimen.
- Continue calcium carbonate 500 mg 2 PO QAM.

■ CASE QUESTIONS

1. Anemia of chronic disease, fatigue, and morning stiffness

    She does not have evidence of other extra-articular manifestations such as depression, anxiety, rheumatoid lung, vasculitis, rheumatoid nodules, wasting, cardiac or renal dysfunction, Felty's syndrome (leukopenia with splenomegaly), and so forth.

2. d. GI ulceration is the most likely long-term adverse effect in patients on chronic, high-dose NSAIDs.

3. c. Bony erosions seen on joint x-rays are the evidence for progressive disease listed. The other measures demonstrate acute activity.

4. a. Anemia and stomatitis are less common in patients on methotrexate who also receive folic acid.

5. The major mechanism for the development of NSAID-induced renal, platelet, and GI adverse effects is inhibition of prostaglandin synthesis. Patients with some degree of car-

diovascular compromise secrete prostaglandins to dilate renal arteries and maintain renal perfusion. Most, but not all, NSAIDs can block the synthesis of those prostaglandins and result in a decrease in renal blood flow and the glomerular filtration rate. Platelets aggregate in part to the release of thromboxane, a prostaglandin, by platelets. Many NSAIDs inhibit the production of thromboxane and therefore lead to a decrease in platelet aggregation, which may increase the risk for bleeding or hemorrhagic stroke or may decrease the risk for cardiovascular events. Prostaglandin E-1 has gastroprotective actions, but those actions are inhibited by various degrees by all NSAIDs, resulting in an increased risk for GI ulceration, bleeding, and perforation.

6. Both methotrexate and etanercept are highly effective in the treatment of rheumatoid arthritis, but etanercept may have a slight advantage. Methotrexate has a longer history of use, safety, and efficacy. The adverse effect profiles of these agents differ, except for the increase in the rate of infections seen with both. Methotrexate may be associated with more specific organ damage (liver, lungs, bone marrow), but etanercept may be associated with an increased risk of cancers and some organ toxicity (heart). Etanercept is much more expensive than methotrexate and is generally reserved for patients who have not adequately responded to methotrexate.

7. a. Cause osteoporosis and hypothalamic-pituitary-adrenal axis suppression

8. c. Celecoxib and sulfasalazine have "sulfa" moieties as part of their chemical structure. Based on this patient's history, it is unlikely that celecoxib would cause a serious allergic reaction.

9. d. Sulfasalazine

10. a. Depression

11. b. Adalimumab. However, one must look at the overall cost of the drugs (adverse effects, monitoring) and benefits (functionality).

12. In progressive disease in a patient already on a moderately to highly effective disease-modifying antirheumatic drug, combination DMARD therapy is indicated. In this case,

the most likely DMARDs to add would include etanercept, infliximab, adalimumab, and possibly sulfasalazine, cyclosporine, anakinra, and so forth. Low-dose oral corticosteroids should generally be avoided due to the risk for chronic adverse effects, but they may provide a relatively rapid response in patients who have severe, acute disease and need to be highly functional.

13. **KEY POINTS**
   - Rheumatoid arthritis is generally a progressive disorder that leads to acute inflammatory symptoms, disability, diminished quality of life, extra-articular manifestations, and shortened life span.
   - Progressive rheumatoid arthritis requires aggressive therapy with moderately to highly effective disease-modifying antirheumatic drugs. Methotrexate is generally accepted as the initial DMARD of choice due to its efficacy, safety, and cost. However, combination DMARDs and/or tumor necrosis factor inhibitors are also possible as initial therapies.
   - Nondrug therapy is important in the treatment of rheumatoid arthritis and includes exercise, physical therapy (at least range of motion), rest, diet, and education.
   - Both NSAIDs and DMARDs may cause significant short-term and long-term adverse effects. Appropriate patient education, drug selection, and drug and disease monitoring are important in managing patients with rheumatoid arthritis.

CASE 28 ANSWERS

■ PROBLEM LIST

1. Osteoarthritis, active
2. Nausea and RUQ abdominal pain
3. Osteoporosis
4. Obesity
5. Insomnia/irritability

■ SOAP NOTE

S: "I have nausea and pain in the upper right side of my abdomen. I have an aching pain in my left knee that will not go away." New onset of joint swelling in the past week; difficulty sleeping; irritable for 6 weeks; lives alone, refuses assistance, eats "fast food" four or five times a week; two glasses of sherry a night

O: Limited range of motion of L knee with mild swelling, tenderness, and warmth; elderly, obese woman (Wt 60 kg, Ht 153 cm); kyphosis in back; RUQ tenderness; mild guarding; alert, oriented ×3; laboratory tests WNLL. Chest x-ray shows increased width of intervertebral spaces; L knee x-ray shows joint space narrowing; DXA-T score −1.2

A: PROBLEM 1: Active osteoarthritis despite PRN use of acetaminophen and ibuprofen and recent use of propoxyphene napsylate/acetaminophen

PROBLEM 2: Nausea and RUQ abdominal pain due to osteoarthritis medications, osteoporosis medications, or peptic ulcer disease

PROBLEM 3: Osteoporosis: significant osteopenia shown by decreased height, DXA, and chest x-ray

PROBLEM 4: Obesity secondary to sedentary lifestyle and "fast food" diet

PROBLEM 5: Insomnia/irritability despite use of triazolam; assess use and patient adherence

P: PROBLEM 1: Osteoarthritis, Active

- Discontinue propoxyphene napsylate/acetaminophen combination tablets.
- Initiate regular use of acetaminophen 1 g QID or as extended-release product 1,300 mg TID; monitor LFTs and signs/symptoms of hepatotoxicity.
- Discontinue ibuprofen.
- Initiate capsaicin (high potency): apply to L knee QID.
- Administer triamcinolone acetonide 40 mg intra-articular injection into L knee in 1 month if problems persist.
- Discuss need for left knee replacement.
- Discuss need to lose weight (refer also to Problem 4); emphasize proper balance of rest and exercise, as well as proper nutrition.
- Discuss need for temporary family assistance.
- Educate patient and family members about osteoarthritis and refer to support groups if not done previously.

PROBLEM 2: Nausea and RUQ Abdominal Pain

- Discontinue ibuprofen and propoxyphene napsylate/acetaminophen.
- Continue to monitor LFTs and signs/symptoms of hepatotoxicity since patient will be taking acetaminophen for osteoarthritis.
- Switch alendronate to risedronate 35 mg once weekly with water first thing in the morning at least 30 minutes before food, beverage, or other

medications. Remain standing for 30 minutes after administration.
- Initiate proton pump inhibitor (e.g., rabeprazole 20 mg QAM 30 minutes before breakfast).
- Initiate lifestyle changes: use decaffeinated tea, lose weight, no alcohol, no eating at bedtime, and no reclining after eating.
- Re-evaluate in 1 to 2 months for signs and symptoms of peptic ulcer disease.

PROBLEM 3: Osteoporosis

- Continue calcium carbonate and vitamin D.
- Continue bisphosphonate (switch to risedronate).
- Initiate precautionary measures for falls to prevent fractures.
- Re-evaluate bone mineral density and/or DXA in 6 months.
- Educate about osteoporosis and proper posture.
- Evaluate nutrition.

PROBLEM 4: Obesity

- Lose weight—counseling by a nutritionist; discontinue "fast food."
- Monitor weight weekly and at each doctor visit.
- Initiate exercise regimen (aerobics, possibly in a heated pool).

PROBLEM 5: Insomnia/Irritability

- Assess adherence to triazolam; encourage use of medication at bedtime as needed and re-evaluate.
- Discontinue caffeinated tea.
- Discontinue alcohol use, especially at bedtime.
- Encourage regular sleeping pattern.
- Re-evaluate in 1 month.

■ CASE QUESTIONS

1. b. Frequent heavy, weight-bearing activities such as mowing the lawn, bowling, and vacuuming

2. b. Crepitus

3.
   - Chronic pain from osteoarthritis
   - Anxiety due to increased osteoarthritis pain
   - Anxiety and depression due to husband's death
   - Anxiety and depression due to inability to participate in activities of daily living
   - Reverse effect of alcohol each evening

- Caffeinated tea daily
- Lack of use of triazolam

4.
   - Use of alcohol and caffeinated tea
   - Increase in activity
   - Lives alone
   - Denial of pain due to desire to remain independent
   - Use of pain medicine at time of activity

5. c. Acetaminophen

6. a. Alcohol consumption

7. Nonpharmacologic:
   - Patient education regarding disease and medications
   - Support groups
   - Assistive devices: use of knee support and cane/walker
   - Exercise: mobility enhancement
   - Diet: weight loss
   - Physical and occupational therapy
   - Thermal modalities
   - Rest: appropriate length of time daily

   Pharmacologic:
   - NSAIDs: prostaglandin inhibition
   - Analgesics: central-acting pain relief
   - Benzodiazepine: adjunctive pain relief as an antianxiety agent

8. a. Use of the minimum effective dose

9. d. Acetaminophen therapy is inadequate in the treatment of osteoarthritis

10. c. Age

11. d. Triamcinolone acetonide 40 mg intra-articular injection

12. Direct costs: Medications, office visits, hospitalizations, laboratory tests, x-rays
    Indirect costs: Care if relatives not available; cost to get to activities

13.
   - For external use only
   - Will take 2 to 4 weeks for maximum effect
   - Wash hands immediately after application
   - Discontinue if severe burning or itching occurs.

14. b. Initiate concomitant therapy with rabeprazole 20 mg daily 30 minutes before breakfast

15. **KEY POINTS**
  - Osteoarthritis patients need to be treated for pain relief.
  - Nonpharmacologic therapy should be implemented for all patients with osteoarthritis.
  - Analgesics are the most effective agents for patients with osteoarthritis.
  - Acetaminophen at appropriate doses should be used to treat patients with osteoarthritis; NSAIDs may be used for patients who do not obtain adequate pain relief.
  - Hyaluronic acid, intra-articular corticosteroids, opioids, and tramadol are also used to treat patients with osteoarthritis.

CASE 29 ANSWERS

■ PROBLEM LIST

1. Confusion and lethargy
2. Polypharmacy
3. Occult blood in stool

■ SOAP NOTE

S: Noted to be lethargic and not oriented to time or place; complains of not having a good appetite; 3-lb weight loss over past 14 days

O: BP 110/70; HR 80; Wt 93.5 lb (42.5 kg); Ht 155 cm; S_3 heart sound present; thin skin, skin tear on right forearm, poor skin turgor; seborrheic lesions on scalp and face; oriented ×2; kyphosis; stool, occult blood positive. Labs: Glu (fasting) 7.8 (140), K 4.8 (4.8), CR 120 (1.4), Hct 0.36 (36), Hgb 118 (11.8), digoxin level 3 months prior 2.3 (1.8)

A: PROBLEM 1: Confusion and lethargy secondary to excess dosage and/or impaired clearance of diazepam, lorazepam, diphenhydramine, and trazodone; anticholinergic effects and sedation due to diphenhydramine and ingredients in NyQuil (acetaminophen, dextromethorphan, doxylamine, pseudoephedrine, alcohol, high-fructose corn syrup)

PROBLEM 2: Polypharmacy; multiple drug therapies for cardiovascular disease (digoxin, hydrochlorothiazide, potassium chloride, and lisinopril); multiple sedating therapies (diazepam, lorazepam, diphenhydramine, trazodone); multiple analgesic therapies (nabumetone and multiple sources of acetaminophen); no indication in medical record for use of sertraline

PROBLEM 3: Occult blood in stool possibly secondary to GI irritation due to potassium chloride, nabumetone, ferrous sulfate, and/or aspirin

P: PROBLEM 1: Confusion and Lethargy

  - Evaluate cold symptoms and discontinue NyQuil. Counsel SM on seeking advice from a pharmacist for treatment of future cold symptoms to avoid anticholinergic agents, drug duplication (acetaminophen), and alcohol.
  - Discontinue diphenhydramine for allergy symptoms. Consider nonsedating antihistamine such as loratadine 10 mg QD and/or nasal steroid such as fluticasone two sprays each nostril QD.
  - Discontinue diazepam for anxiety. Change to lorazepam 0.25 mg BID and discontinue PRN lorazepam. Evaluate need for routine use of trazodone 100 mg every night for insomnia. Educate SM on changing sleep patterns with aging and consider PRN use of trazodone at a dose of 25 to 50 mg HS.

PROBLEM 2: Polypharmacy

  - Evaluate continued need for the combination cardiovascular therapy of digoxin, hydrochlorothiazide, potassium chloride, and lisinopril. Consider discontinuing digoxin, hydrochlorothiazide, and potassium chloride and manage HTN and heart failure with lisinopril 10 mg PO QD. Monitor BP, signs and symptoms of heart failure, and electrolytes.
  - Discontinue scheduled acetaminophen for pain. Change acetaminophen to PRN and follow patient for effectiveness of nabumetone for osteoarthritis pain (see recommendation on nabumetone in Problem 3).
  - For multiple sedating medications, see plan for Problem 1.
  - Discontinue sertraline and monitor patient for signs/symptoms of depression.

PROBLEM 3: Occult Blood in Stool

  - Evaluate continued need for ferrous sulfate for treatment of anemia, as Hgb and Hct are WNL. If indication remains, decrease dose to BID or QD or change to ferrous gluconate 240 mg BID to decrease the chance of GI irritation.
  - Due to high normal K+ level, discontinue potassium chloride and monitor.
  - If potassium supplement is prescribed, change to a dosage form of potassium that is protective to the GI tract.
  - Discontinue nabumetone. Change to celecoxib 200 mg BID and monitor for pain relief.

■ CASE QUESTIONS

1. b. Living in the community

2. d. Acetaminophen

3. c. Anorexia

4. Dandruff or seborrheic dermatitis. Signs and symptoms include greasy scales in the scalp or eyebrows and around the ears and nose. FDA agents approved as safe and effective for nonprescription treatment include coal-tar preparations, pyrithione zinc, salicylic acid, selenium sulfide, and sulfur; prescription products are selenium sulfide and fluocinolone. Shampoo lather should be left on the affected areas for at least 10 minutes and rinsed thoroughly. Hair should dry naturally.

5. d. Regular exercise

6. c. Flurazepam 30 mg PO QHS

7. a. Renal function

8. c. Lethargy

9. No; an elderly patient presenting with recent-onset confusion should be worked up for a reversible cause of the confusion, such as medications, electrolyte imbalance, or another medical cause. Medication therapy should be reserved for cognitive dysfunction due to probable Alzheimer's disease.

10. Calculate SM's creatinine clearance using the Cockroft-Gault formula:

$$CrCl = 0.85 \times \frac{IBW\ in\ Kg \times (140 - age)}{CR \times 72}$$

$$CrCl = 0.85 \times \frac{(42.5) \times (54)}{(1.4) \times (72)}$$

$$CrCl = 0.85 \times \frac{2,295}{100.8}$$

$$CrCl = 19.35\ mL/min$$

11. Therapies other than NSAIDs or COX-2 inhibitors that may be useful for the symptoms associated with osteoarthritis:

   ▪ Acetaminophen in doses up to 4 g per day
   ▪ Topical therapies such as counterirritants or salicylic acid
   ▪ Physical therapy
   ▪ Exercise therapy

12. Signs and symptoms of depression in a geriatric patient:
   ▪ Continuing sadness or anxiety
   ▪ Tiredness, lack of energy
   ▪ Loss of interest or pleasure in everyday activities, including sex
   ▪ Sleep problems, including trouble getting to sleep, very early morning waking, and sleeping too much
   ▪ Eating more or less than usual
   ▪ Crying too often or too much
   ▪ Aches and pains that don't go away when treated
   ▪ Difficulty focusing, remembering, or making decisions
   ▪ Feeling guilty, helpless, worthless, or hopeless
   ▪ Irritability
   ▪ Thoughts of death or suicide; a suicide attempt

13. Psychosocial factors that may affect SM's adherence to both pharmacologic and nonpharmacologic therapy:
   a. Issues that patient must address
      1. Chronic medications require compliance.
      2. Complex medication regimen
      3. Propensity to self-medicate
      4. Dependence on daughter as caregiver
   b. Other barriers
      1. Family dynamics
      2. Limited financial resources

14. b. Increased total body fat

15. a. Reduced hepatic blood flow

16. d. Cephalosporins

17. **KEY POINTS**
   ▪ Polypharmacy, especially by older people with chronic health problems, is an important drug safety issue.
   ▪ In geriatric patients, drug therapies should address specific problems or symptoms and should be continued only as long as effective, then discontinued.
   ▪ Doses of medications should be based on individual pharmacokinetic parameters and pharmacodynamic responses in geriatric patients.
   ▪ Due to the many possibilities for age-related change and medication actions and adverse effects, the design of therapeutic regimens for geriatric patients can be complicated and unpredictable.

CASE 30 ANSWERS

■ PROBLEM LIST

1. Ventilator-associated pneumonia
2. Neurologic impairment secondary to subarachnoid hemorrhage (SAH)
3. Respiratory failure
4. Pain
5. Anxiety
6. Immobility
7. Nutritional failure
8. Bacteriuria

■ SOAP NOTE

S: Patient 6 days s/p SAH, 5 days s/p aneurysm coiling, appears to be in moderate distress due to respiratory difficulty. Green sputum visible in endotracheal tube.

O: Increasing ventilatory support, elevated minute ventilation; RR 24; T 39.3°C; hourly suctioning of purulent sputum; bilateral rales and rhonchi, R > L. Urine clear yellow, culture negative for UTI (1,000–10,000 mixed gpc). GCS 8 (intubated) with sedation and analgesia held. Lkcs 19.1 × 10^9 (19.1 × 10^3), PMN 0.85 (85%), bands 0.09 (9%). 50% F$_i$O$_2$ P$_{o2}$ 90/P$_{co2}$ 47/pH 7.36. Infiltrates in RML, RLL on CXR. Medications include ciprofloxacin for bacteria in urine, fentanyl for pain, propofol for anxiety in patient requiring frequent neurologic examinations, phenytoin for seizure prophylaxis, famotidine for stress ulcer prophylaxis, senna and docusate for stimulant and stool softening in patient receiving continuous narcotic analgesics.

A: PROBLEM 1: Ventilator-associated pneumonia, late onset. GL at risk for infection with multi-drug-resistant pathogens.

PROBLEM 2: Neurologic impairment secondary to SAH

PROBLEM 3: Respiratory failure secondary to neurologic impairment worsened by ventilator-associated pneumonia. Puts patient at risk for stress-related gastric mucosal disease.

PROBLEM 4: Pain associated with aneurysm, surgery, immobility, and invasive medical devices

PROBLEM 5: Anxiety related to impaired neurologic status, SICU environment, respiratory distress, drugs, and invasive medical devices

PROBLEM 6: Immobility due to neurologic impairment, mechanical ventilation, and sedation. Puts patient at risk for deep venous thrombus formation.

PROBLEM 7: Nutritional failure due to patient's neurologic status and mechanical ventilation. No indication of intestinal dysfunction. Patient is at risk for impaired motility secondary to the use of narcotic analgesics.

PROBLEM 8: Bacteriuria being treated on the basis of prior urinalysis. Antimicrobial therapy is not necessary to manage this problem.

P: PROBLEM 1: Ventilator-Associated Pneumonia

- Perform lower respiratory tract sputum sampling via protected brush specimen (PSB), blind or bronchoscopic bronchoalveolar lavage (BAL) specimen, or quantitative tracheal aspirate. Send specimen for quantitative culture and sensitivity analysis.
- Send blood for culture and sensitivity analysis.
- Initiate broad-spectrum antimicrobial therapy with piperacillin/tazobactam 4.5 g IV q6h, tobramycin 450 mg IV q24h for 5 days, and vancomycin 1 g IV q12h.
- If Gram stain/culture results warrant continuing vancomycin, monitor trough concentration before third dose, with a goal of 15 to 20 μg per mL.
- Continue antibiotics for 8-day course if patient achieves clinical symptom resolution, or 14 days or longer if symptoms persist or patient is infected with non-lactose-fermenting gram-negative rods.
- Monitor sputum and blood culture and sensitivity results.
- Follow temperature curve, leukocyte count, differential, sputum production, arterial blood gases, and chest x-ray as markers of clinical recovery.
- Monitor SCr, BUN, urine output, CBC as markers of potential drug toxicity.
- Streamline therapy as soon as appropriate.
- Continue preinfection preventive measures: chlorhexidine mouth care, intermittent subglottic suctioning, maintain patient at semi-recumbent 30- to 45-degree position, scheduled daily cessation of sedative drugs.

PROBLEM 2: Neurologic Impairment Secondary to SAH

- Perform frequent neurologic examinations using the GCS.
- Use the minimum effective doses of opioids and sedatives.
- Monitor closely for delayed ischemic deficit (vasospasm) and intracranial hypertension.

- Maintain patient semirecumbent at 30 to 45 degrees.
- Continue nimodipine to decrease risk of delayed ischemic deficit for a total of 21 days of therapy.
- Continue phenytoin to prevent seizure activity for 7 days.
- Monitor effects of nimodipine on systemic blood pressure; consider changing dose to 30 mg q2h if clinically significant.

PROBLEM 3: Respiratory Failure

- Continue monitoring and adjusting ventilatory support to optimize ventilation and oxygenation.
- Monitor arterial blood gases to determine acid/base and ventilatory status.
- Continue famotidine to prevent gastric stress-related mucosal disease.
- Continue albuterol/ipratropium therapy.
- Continue intensive nursing/respiratory therapy.

PROBLEM 4: Pain

- Continue minimum effective doses of fentanyl to keep patient comfortable.
- Monitor pain using a behavior-physiologic scale.
- Continue stool softener/stimulant laxative therapy with docusate and senna to minimize opioid-induced bowel dysfunction.
- Consider adding fentanyl IV bolus PRN for any painful procedures or invasive device placements.
- Reposition patient frequently, if possible, to minimize discomfort from prolonged immobility.

PROBLEM 5: Anxiety

- Decrease disorienting environmental factors (loud alarms, bells, loud talking, bright lights) to minimum necessary to maintain patient safety.
- Allow comforting environmental factors (friends, family, music), as possible without inhibiting care.
- Reorient and reassure frequently.
- Use minimum effective doses of propofol to allow frequent neurologic examinations and minimize anxiety.
- Continue to monitor triglycerides while GL is receiving propofol.
- Monitor sedation using Sedation-Agitation Scale (SAS), with a goal of 4 (calm and cooperative) as neurologic status improves.

PROBLEM 6: Immobility

- Consider physical therapy to maintain passive range of motion, if not contraindicated.
- Continue sequential compression devices to prevent DVT.
- Continue intensive nursing care to ensure good skin care.
- Reposition patient frequently, if not contraindicated.

PROBLEM 7: Nutritional Failure

- Initiate enteral nutrition via OG tube.
- Consider 24-hour urine collection to estimate patient's urinary nitrogen excretion.
- Monitor GL's nutritional status using nitrogen balance, prealbumin.
- Monitor electrolytes daily.
- Monitor serum blood glucose q6h, with a goal in the normal range (80–110).
- Monitor gastric residual concentrations q4–6h. If gastric residual is above 200 mL or patient's abdomen becomes distended or patient vomits, consider adding metoclopramide or erythromycin or placing a nasojejunal feeding tube.
- Modify nutritional plan to account for fat calories provided by lipid emulsion vehicle for propofol.

PROBLEM 8: Bacteriuria

- Discontinue ciprofloxacin.

■ CASE QUESTIONS

1. b. *Pseudomonas aeruginosa*

2. Bronchoscopic bronchoalveolar lavage, blind bronchoalveolar lavage, protected specimen brush

3. d. Fluoroquinolones

4. Piperacillin/tazobactam 4.5 g IV q6h, tobramycin 450 mg IV q24h, and vancomycin 1 g IV q12h (combination of an antipseudomonal carbapenem or β-lactam/β-lactamase inhibitor or antipseudomonal cephalosporin plus an aminoglycoside plus vancomycin or linezolid)

5. Providing the lowest effective doses and scheduling periods of sedative cessation have been shown to decrease the duration of mechanical ventilation, which decreases the likelihood of developing ventilator-associated pneumonia. Also, the use of propofol/fentanyl will allow frequent neurologic examinations.

6. Maintaining euglycemia in critically ill patients has been shown to decrease mortality, decrease prolonged exposure to antimicrobials, decrease the incidence of sepsis, pre-

vent secondary brain injury following stroke, and decrease prolonged periods of mechanical ventilation.

7. Elevated respiratory rate, fever, sputum production, bilateral rales and rhonchi, elevated Lkcs, Lkc differential, multilobar infiltrate on chest x-ray

8. d. 15–20 μg/mL

9. d. Discontinue all antibiotics

10. b. 8 days

11. c. Meropenem

12. Knowing local susceptibility patterns helps determine, along with patient-related factors, the risk of developing ventilator-associated pneumonia due to a multi-drug-resistant organism and allows the clinician to choose the most likely effective agents for the organisms occurring most often within a hospital or ICU.

13. Pharmacoeconomic considerations:
    Costs of VAP therapy
      Direct medical
        Hospital personnel and overhead
        Preventive measures preinfection
        Infection control processes
        Treatment and complications
          Method of diagnosis (e.g., bronchoscopy vs. tracheal aspiration)
          Adequate vs. inadequate initial treatment
          Susceptible vs. resistant pathogen
          Antibiotic de-escalation and discontinuation
          Length of therapy
      Direct nonmedical
        Travel, hotel, meals (family)
        Lost wages (family/patient)
      Indirect personal
        Decreased productivity
        Quality of life
      Intangible personal
        Pain/anxiety/air hunger/suffering

14. **KEY POINTS**
    - Ventilator-associated pneumonia is a disease state in which an invasive lower respiratory tract infection occurs in a patient who has required mechanical ventilation for at least 48 to 72 hours.
    - Pharmacologic and nonpharmacologic measures shown to decrease the development of ventilator-associated pneumonia

should be used. These include semirecumbent positioning, subglottic suctioning, scheduled cessation of sedative drugs, oral care with chlorhexidine, minimizing the duration of mechanical ventilation, minimizing red blood cell transfusion, maintaining euglycemia, and possible use of sucralfate to prevent stress-related mucosal disease.

- Lower respiratory tract specimens and quantitative or semiquantitative cultures are needed to identify the pathogens involved and guide appropriate antibiotic therapy.
- Appropriate empiric antibiotic therapy decreases mortality due to ventilator-associated pneumonia, so broad-spectrum antibiotic therapy should be given. This therapy should include the combination of an antipseudomonal carbapenem or a β-lactam/β-lactamase inhibitor or antipseudomonal cephalosporin plus an aminoglycoside or antipseudomonal fluoroquinolone plus vancomycin or linezolid in patients with risk factors for MRSA or in institutions with a high prevalence of MRSA.
- De-escalation of antibiotic therapy in ventilator-associated pneumonia based on cultures and susceptibility results is associated with positive clinical outcomes and pharmacoeconomic benefits and should be used whenever appropriate.
- A 7- or 8-day course of antibiotic therapy is adequate in patients who are receiving appropriate empiric coverage and who exhibit clinical improvement but who are not infected with nonfermenting gram-negative bacilli. This practice also leads to decreased development of resistance or superinfection.

CASE 31 ANSWERS

■ PROBLEM LIST

1. Phenytoin intoxication: syncope, dizziness, confusion
2. Drug-induced hepatitis
3. Active tuberculosis
4. Advanced HIV disease/AIDS
5. Partial seizure disorder
6. Polyarthralgias
7. Herpes simplex virus type 2
8. Herpes zoster

9. Hypertension
10. Depression
11. *Pneumocystis carinii* pneumonia prophylaxis

■ SOAP NOTE

S: "I am feeling weak and tired and my appetite has not improved after starting treatment for TB. I feel dizzy at times and have worsening pain in all my joints. I try to do my best taking my medicines but it makes my heartburn worse, and I have difficulty sleeping at night."

O: SV with advanced HIV disease (high viral load and low T-cell count: CD4 count is <200, AIDS diagnosis). Started antituberculosis therapy 1 month ago (positive PPD skin test, abnormal CXR, positive AFB smear and cultures); since then she has developed abnormal liver function tests, low WBC, and polyarthralgias. Phenytoin serum concentration when adjusted for a low plasma albumin level is above the therapeutic range.

A: PROBLEM 1: Confusion, syncope as a result of phenytoin intoxication

PROBLEM 2: Hepatitis; most likely drug-induced; potential additive effects of several agents that can cause hepatitis (i.e., isoniazid, rifampin, pyrazinamide, and phenytoin)

PROBLEM 3: TB diagnosed about 1.5 months ago; patient has been on therapy for about 1 month

PROBLEM 4: AIDS; diagnosed with HIV infection in 1995, now with advanced disease; has received many different antiretroviral agents in combination and has not been on antiretroviral therapy since the past month; high viral load and low CD4 cell count

PROBLEM 5: Partial seizure disorder since 2003; has been taking phenytoin; currently has phenytoin intoxication

PROBLEM 6: Polyarthralgias; likely to be drug-induced and most likely causative agent is pyrazinamide

PROBLEM 7: HSV II; currently latent; last recurrence in 2004

PROBLEM 8: Herpes zoster since 2000; currently suppressed

PROBLEM 9: Hypertension; currently on atenolol and under control

PROBLEM 10: Depression; currently on mirtazapine

PROBLEM 11: Pneumocystis carinii pneumonia prophylaxis; currently receiving dapsone prophylactic therapy

P: PROBLEM 1: Phenytoin Intoxication

- Calculate phenytoin plasma level taking into account SV's low albumin using the following formula: Adjusted phenytoin concentration = Measured total concentration ÷ [(0.2 × albumin) + 0.1]. SV's adjusted phenytoin serum concentration is approximately 25 µg per mL.
- Hold phenytoin doses and check phenytoin level at 24 hours (target serum concentration 10–20 µg per mL with adjustment for low albumin). Once within the therapeutic range, consider restarting phenytoin (extended release) at a dosage of 400 mg PO QHS or lower. This approach will simplify SV's phenytoin dosing regimen and promote adherence. Monitoring for increase in GI intolerance needs to be done with once-daily dosing of phenytoin. Repeat a phenytoin serum concentration in 5 to 7 days and then again in about 14 days (target 10–20 µg/mL once adjusted for low plasma albumin level). If free phenytoin levels are obtainable at institution, obtain free phenytoin serum concentrations (target 1–2 µg/mL) rather than total serum concentrations.
- Monitor whether nystagmus improves on a weekly basis and improvement in dizziness and syncope.
- Monitor for seizure activity.
- Monitor closely LFTs (i.e., at least every 2 weeks); her recent increase in aminotransferase levels may be a sign of hepatitis. Hepatitis can lead to slower clearance of phenytoin and therefore increased toxicity from the drug.
- Reassess adherence to medications; SV is currently confused, poor historian; difficult to know how she has been taking her medications; provide her with a pill box and ask her to come back to the clinic on a weekly basis for refill of her pill box.
- Be aware of possible drug interactions between phenytoin and the other medications SV takes that may complicate the management of her seizure disorder (i.e., isoniazid, inhibitor of phenytoin metabolism, and rifampin, inducer of phenytoin metabolism; generally, the induction effect of rifampin outweighs the inhibition effect of isoniazid).
- If managing phenytoin serum concentration is difficult because of multiple drug interactions, consider switching SV from rifampin to rifabutin after she completes her 2-month induction treat-

ment phase for TB (rifabutin is a less potent inducer of cytochrome P450 than rifampin and may be a better option in combination with ARVT).

PROBLEM 2: Hepatitis

- New onset of hepatitis. Assess the etiology of this process (drug-related hepatitis vs. constitutional).
- Review SV's medications, particularly those recently started that could cause hepatitis: isoniazid (INH), pyrazinamide (PZA), rifampin. Hepatotoxicity observed with PZA is dose-dependent and usually observed with doses above 3 g per day. Since SV takes 1.5 g a day, it is unlikely that PZA is directly responsible for the increased LFTs. Hepatotoxicity observed with INH is rare and increases with the age of the patient and when administered in combination with rifampin. SV's age (65) is a risk factor. Hepatotoxicity observed with rifampin is rare and usually occurs within the first 8 weeks of TB therapy (SV has been on therapy for about 1 month), but with the concomitant use of other medications for TB, there is an increased risk. Phenytoin may cause hepatitis (may be an additive effect with other medications, since SV has been on this medication for some time).
- INH, rifampin, and PZA are first-line agents for treatment of TB. Currently SV has asymptomatic hepatitis. SV should continue this combination for at least another 4 weeks (i.e., until she reaches the continuation phase) with careful monitoring.
- Serum aminotransaminases (ALT, AST) and bilirubin should be monitored at 4, 6, and 8 weeks of treatment (in addition to baseline and week 2) because the majority of patients have onset of symptoms of liver injury after week 4 of therapy. However, patients should be monitored throughout the entire course of treatment. Many clinicians will discontinue use of rifampin, INH, and PZA if the following findings occur in a patient: (1) aminotransferase (AST, ALT) greater than five times the upper limit of normal range in an asymptomatic person, (2) aminotransferase greater than 5 times the normal range when accompanied by symptoms of hepatitis, or (3) a serum bilirubin concentration greater than the normal range, whether or not symptoms are present. Since SV is asymptomatic (no jaundice) and aminotransferase levels are increased but remain below five times the upper limit of normal, continue to monitor LFTs, but there is no

need to discontinue rifampin, INH, or PZA therapy at this time.
- Advise SV against the concurrent use of potentially hepatotoxic drugs, including OTC drugs such as acetaminophen.
- SV should be reassessed by a health care provider at week 6 and 8 of treatment for adherence, tolerance, and adverse effects. She should also have been seen at week 2 but missed her appointment.

PROBLEM 3: Active TB

- Since susceptibility test results indicate that the organism is sensitive to all antituberculosis drugs that SV is currently on, ethambutol can be discontinued at this time.
- Pyridoxine has been added to the antituberculosis regimen (25 mg/day) to reduce the occurrence of INH-induced side effects in both the central and peripheral nervous system (e.g., peripheral neuropathy), especially in patients such as SV who are at increased risk for such side effects due to HIV/AIDS.
- SV should continue INH, rifampin, and PZA for another 4 weeks; preferable to have her continue on daily dosing of each medication because her T-cell count is below 100 cells per mm^3 and therefore she is at increased risk for development of rifamycin resistance. Directly observed therapy (DOT) should be re-emphasized.
- Monitor LFTs, CBC, and serum creatinine every 2 weeks until week 8 of therapy. A serum uric acid should also be measured since SV is on PZA (the drug inhibits renal tubular secretion of uric acid; asymptomatic hyperuricemia is frequent). Adjustment in dosages might be necessary on the basis of the lab values obtained.
- A sputum specimen for AFB smear and culture should be obtained monthly until two consecutive specimens are negative on culture. If drug resistance is not demonstrated, treatment should be continued with DOT.
- Since SV is currently completing her first month of TB treatment and the organism is pan-sensitive, may want to consider switching her to a combination preparation to help minimize development of drug resistance by decreasing pill burden and therefore enhancing adherence. Regular adherence reinforcements should be provided to SV at each clinic visit. Fixed-dose combination and DOT can be used during the continuation phase.
- Consider switching rifampin to rifabutin as a reasonable alternative if there are drug–drug inter-

action concerns with the antiretroviral treatment regimen selected.

- After the end of the 8-week induction phase, culture results and CXR will need to be reassessed to determine whether SV should continue therapy with INH and rifampin for another 4 to 7 months.

PROBLEM 4: Advanced HIV Disease: AIDS

- SV has now been off ARVT for several months and her viral load is quite elevated. ARVT should be restarted as soon as possible. However, given that SV is on an antituberculosis regimen that includes rifampin, there is a concern for interaction with protease inhibitors (PI) and non-nucleoside reverse transcriptase inhibitors (NNRTIs). Before designing an HIV regimen, assess whether SV could be switched from rifampin to rifabutin to decrease the risk for complex interactions. Rifapentine is not an option in HIV-infected patients because of its unacceptably high rate of relapse. Updated HIV guidelines no longer recommend discontinuation of all PI-containing ARVT regimens to allow for use of rifampin for TB treatment for patients with HIV-related TB. The PI that can be used in combination with rifampin is lopinavir/ritonavir, with dosage adjustment due to rifampin's induction effects. Treatment options are available that enable continued ARVT during treatment of TB. As mentioned, rifabutin exhibits fewer induction effects and is a reasonable alternative to rifampin in TB treatment regimens in patients with HIV infection.
- Several considerations should be taken into account when designing the ARVT regimen: prior exposure of SV to antiretroviral agents and tolerance/susceptibility history; interactions with TB regimens and in particular interactions between rifamycins and HIV medications and phenytoin and HIV medications; need for dose adjustment of HIV medications or rifamycins secondary to these interactions; pill burden; complexity of the regimen (dosing frequency, administration requirements); and overlapping side effects (e.g., peripheral neuropathy).
- Once initiated, close monitoring of HIV drug concentrations (PI or NNRTI) is advised. HIV-1 RNA and CD4 counts should be measured monthly for the first 3 months and every 3 months thereafter if the patient is stable.

PROBLEM 5: Partial Seizure Disorder

- Diagnosed in 2003; evaluation by a neurologist is necessary. Assess SV and monitor phenytoin

therapy (see Problem 1). Careful monitoring of phenytoin is necessary while SV is receiving rifampin and other medications metabolized via cytochrome P450 (including antiretrovirals once ARVT is restarted).

PROBLEM 6: Polyarthralgias

- Since this problem is of recent onset, it may be drug-induced. Upon reviewing SV's medication list, it appears that PZA is the drug most commonly associated with this type of side effect.
- Monitor intensity of pain using a standardized pain scale at each clinic visit.
- Initiate a trial of aspirin or other NSAID. Start with a low dose and taper up as needed.
- Should be able to discontinue PZA after 2 months of therapy if organisms remain sensitive to the TB drugs (i.e., INH and rifampin). Upon discontinuation of PZA, polyarthralgias should diminish.

PROBLEM 7: Herpes Simplex Virus Type 2

- Monitor for recurrence.

PROBLEM 8: Herpes Zoster

- If persistent postherpetic neuralgia, consider tricyclic antidepressants, gabapentin (Neurontin) 30 to 600 mg PO tid and/or OxyContin SR 10 to 20 mg PO bid with topical medications similar to those used in acute disease (i.e., corticosteroids).
- Consider counseling with a psychiatrist if recurrent excruciating pain occurs due to postherpetic neuralgia.
- Consultation with an anesthesiologist in a pain clinic may be warranted in severe cases of postherpetic neuralgia.

PROBLEM 9: HTN

- Currently receiving atenolol. Continue to monitor BP routinely.

PROBLEM 10: Depression

- Currently receiving mirtazapine for depression; with TB diagnosis, SV should be reassessed with careful monitoring for depression.

PROBLEM 11: *Pneumocystis carinii* Pneumonia Prophylaxis

- Currently receiving dapsone for prophylaxis. Monitor for adverse effects.

■ CASE QUESTIONS

1. b. By inhalation of airborne particles of *Mycobacterium tuberculosis* from an individual with active tuberculosis

2. TB disease develops rapidly after initial infection with *M. tuberculosis* in HIV-infected patients with severe immunosuppression (CD4 cell count <100); up to 50% of patients with a CD4 cell count below 100 develop TB disease within 2 years if not given preventive therapy (in contrast to 10% of individuals in the general population). An individual infected with latent TB (infected but not treated) who acquires HIV infection will develop TB at a rate of 5% to 12% per year.

3. Factors to consider before selecting antiretroviral treatment regimens:
   - Prior exposure of SV to antiretroviral agents
   - Tolerance to past antiretroviral agents
   - Review of past genotype and phenotype to assess drug susceptibility of HIV in SV
   - Drug interactions with regimen for TB and in particular interactions between rifamycins and HIV medications and phenytoin and HIV medications; need for dose adjustment of HIV medications or rifamycins secondary to these interactions
   - Pill burden, complexity of the regimen (dosing frequency, administration requirements)
   - Overlapping side effects (e.g., peripheral neuropathy caused by more than one agent)
   - SV's perceived barriers to adherence and strategies to overcome them

4. a. Isoniazid is metabolized via cytochrome P450 and inhibits the metabolism of phenytoin and may increase serum phenytoin levels.

5. Potential causes of drug-induced hepatitis: INH, PZA, rifampin, and phenytoin are potential causes of hepatitis. Hepatitis observed with PZA is dose-dependent and usually observed with doses above 3 g per day. Since SV takes 1.5 g a day, it is unlikely that this drug is solely responsible for increased LFTs; hepatitis with INH is rare and risk increases with age of patient and when administered in combination with rifampin. SV's age (65) is a risk factor; hepatitis observed with rifampin is rare and usually occurs within the first 8 weeks of TB therapy (SV has been on therapy for about 1 month), but with concomitant use of other medications for TB, there is an increased risk. Phenytoin may cause hepatitis (may be an additive effect with other medications since SV has been on this medication for some time).

Currently SV has asymptomatic hepatitis. SV should continue this combination for at least another 4 weeks (i.e., until she reaches the continuation phase) with careful monitoring. Serum aminotransaminases (ALT, AST) and bilirubin should be monitored at 4, 6, and 8 weeks of treatment (in addition to baseline and week 2) because the majority of patients have onset of symptoms of liver injury after week 4 of therapy. However, patients should be monitored throughout the entire course of treatment. Many clinicians will discontinue use of rifampin, INH, and PZA if the following findings occur in a patient: (1) aminotransferase (AST, ALT) greater than five times the upper limit of normal range in an asymptomatic person, (2) aminotransferase greater than five times the normal range when accompanied by symptoms of hepatitis, or (3) a serum bilirubin concentration greater than the normal range, whether or not symptoms are present. Since SV is asymptomatic (no jaundice) and aminotransferase levels are increased but remain below five times the upper limit of normal, continue to monitor LFTs, but there is no need to discontinue rifampin, INH, or PZA therapy at this time.

Advise SV against the concurrent use of potentially hepatotoxic drugs, including OTC drugs such as acetaminophen.

SV should be reassessed in person by a health care provider at week 6 and 8 of treatment for adherence, tolerance, and adverse effects. She should also have been seen at week 2 but missed her appointment.

6. A change in the albumin concentration alters the fraction unbound and the apparent volume of distribution of phenytoin. Calculate the phenytoin plasma level, taking into account SV's low albumin using the following formula: Adjusted phenytoin concentration = Measured total concentration ÷ [(0.2 × albumin) + 0.1]. In this patient the phenytoin adjusted level is approximately 25 µg per mL.

7. b. The most toxic effect of this agent is optic neuritis, and SV should be questioned monthly about visual disturbances.

8. Peripheral neuropathy, although uncommon at the dosages used of INH used to treat TB, it is most likely caused by INH-induced depletion of pyridoxine stores or competitive inhibition with pyridoxine in its role as a cofactor in the synthesis of synaptic neurotransmitters. Pyridoxine (25 mg/day) should be given with INH to persons who have conditions in which neuropathy is common (e.g., diabetes, uremia, alcoholism, or malnutrition). Persons with HIV infection/AIDS, such as SV, who are undergoing TB treatment with INH should also receive supplementation with pyridoxine to reduce the occurrence of INH-induced side effects in both the central and peripheral nervous systems.

9. c. All agents in this class can cause orange discoloration of bodily fluids.

10. The detailed education plan:
    ▪ Review goals of therapy using SV's information (e.g., labs, symptoms) and explain treatment strategies.
    ▪ Review impact of partial/poor adherence with SV on the overall health outcomes. Use lay terms to review these concepts and ask SV to reflect on the issues discussed. Identify SV's barriers to adherence and engage SV in identifying strategies to manage each barrier to adherence. Offer SV a number of adherence tools that might assist her in taking the medications (e.g., beeper watch, pill box, written schedule).
    ▪ Review each medication name, dose, dosing frequency, administration requirements, and storage requirements.
        ▪ Rifampin: GI reactions (nausea, vomiting, abdominal pain, anorexia), hypersensitivity reaction, influenza-like syndrome, hepatotoxicity, orange discoloration of bodily fluids, neutropenia, and so forth
        ▪ INH: hepatitis (malaise, fatigue, weakness, nausea or anorexia, jaundice), peripheral neuropathy, hallucinations, convulsions, rash, and so forth
        ▪ PZA: hepatotoxicity, polyarthralgia, hyperuricemia, and so forth
    ▪ Ethambutol: retrobulbar neuritis, GI intolerance, neuritis, hyperuricemia, hypersensitivity reaction, and so forth

The pharmacist's key medication counseling responsibilities include:

▪ Ensuring that SV can describe how she takes her medications and can identify what each medication is being used for in terms of her treatment
▪ Reviewing dosing, administration requirements (with food or no food), dosing frequency, and so forth
▪ Addressing possible side effects and discussing with SV ways to manage side effects. Inform SV's physician about your findings after discussing side effects; side effects are commonly responsible for partial adherence. The need for referrals to other providers to address the management of these side effects should also be discussed with SV.
▪ Screening for possible drug–drug or drug–food interactions

11. The pharmacist's role relative to the proposed psychosocial factors identified includes:

    ▪ Create an individualized plan for SV: both pharmacologic and nonpharmacologic.
    ▪ Provide compassionate care.
    ▪ Offer support services to the patient and be a liaison to the other caregivers to provide information on adherence to antidepressant therapy.
    ▪ Monitor for adverse effects of mirtazapine.
    ▪ Continue to monitor SV's depression carefully while she is receiving treatment (i.e., anxiety, fear, or feelings of isolation are present); refer for psychosocial support, psychiatry. Depression may have a negative impact on adherence to therapies.

12. Pharmacoeconomic considerations relative to SV's plan of AIDS and TB care may include:

    ▪ Cost of treating drug-sensitive TB versus multi-drug-resistant TB; cost of treating drug-sensitive HIV-1 virus versus HIV-1 resistant virus
        ▪ Cost of treating TB and AIDS
    ▪ Direct medical
        ▪ Hospital personnel and overhead
        ▪ Treatment, including implementation of DOT for TB and managing complications
    ▪ Direct nonmedical
        ▪ Lost wages (family/patient)
        ▪ Travel, hotels, meals
    ▪ Indirect personal

- Inability to work during infectious period (TB)
- Quality of life
- Intangible personal
  - Suffering related to the diseases, including emotional suffering

13. **KEY POINTS**
- TB is a disease that can affect the lungs as well as extrapulmonary sites. It progresses much more rapidly in immunocompromised patients.
- The epidemiology of TB is influenced by two important factors:
  - Exposure to TB in the environment. Risk factors for exposure include living in the household of a TB case, immigration from endemic area, exposure to untreated TB cases in congregate living facilities (prisons, shelters, and health care facilities), older age, residence in inner cities.
  - Susceptibility to disease after infection occurs. A number of conditions that are associated with altered host cellular immunity increase the risk of development of active TB (e.g., HIV infection, old age, end-stage renal disease, cancer, diabetes, severe malnutrition).
- Therapy for active TB must contain multiple drugs to which the organisms are susceptible to be effective; the drugs must be taken regularly and treatment must continue for a sufficient period of time (duration is defined by the rapidity with which sputum cultures become negative for AFB and the CXR improves). If the sputum culture remains positive after 4 months of therapy, the patient is defined as having failed therapy and the regimen will need to be adjusted (i.e., include at least three new TB drugs) based on the susceptibility results.
- Treatment of latent TB infection is not an infectious stage (positive PPD but normal CXR). For persons suspected of having latent TB infection, treatment should not begin until active TB disease has been excluded. Persons suspected of having TB disease should receive the recommended multidrug regimen for treatment of disease until the diagnosis is confirmed or ruled out.
- Directly observed therapy (DOT) is the standard of care for TB treatment. In DOT, a trained health care worker monitors the patient taking each dose of antituberculo-

sis medication. When TB patients receive all medications as prescribed under a program of DOT, both patients and communities benefit.

CASE 32 ANSWERS

■ PROBLEM LIST

1. Acute complicated pyelonephritis
2. Type 2 diabetes mellitus
3. Hypertension

■ SOAP NOTE

S: Increased urinary urgency, frequency, back pain (5/10)

O: Wt 58 kg, Ht 158 cm, BP 146/90, T 37.5°C. Urinalysis: WBC 3 +; Gram (-) rods >10^5 CFU/mL; (+) Hematuria; (+) Nitrite, HBA1c 0.078 (7.8%), Lkcs: 14.1×10^9 (14.1×10^3). Glucose 13.3 (240). Meds: atenolol 25 mg PO QD, metformin 500 mg PO BID, enteric-coated aspirin 325 mg PO QD, multivitamin 1 tablet PO QD, calcium carbonate + vitamin D 500 mg PO BID

A: PROBLEM 1: Acute complicated pyelonephritis with fever, lower back pain, elevated WBC requiring initial hospitalization and immediate treatment

PROBLEM 2: Type 2 diabetes mellitus: currently not at HBA1c goal and optimal drug therapy

PROBLEM 3: Hypertension stage I, currently not at target BP goal or appropriate drug therapy based on JNC-VII guidelines

P: PROBLEM 1: Acute Complicated Pyelonephritis
- Begin therapy with levofloxacin 500 mg IV q24h.
- Transition to levofloxacin 500 mg PO QD for a total of 10 to 14 days once patient is stable and can be discharged.
- Treatment can be modified once urine and blood cultures and sensitivity data are clarified.
- Efficacy monitoring: resolution of urinary urgency, frequency, lower back pain, fever; normalization of WBC count and urinalysis
- Toxicity monitoring: side effects of levofloxacin include rash, nausea, photosensitivity, headache, increasing fever, WBC, persistent lower back pain, urinary urgency and frequency
- Counsel KD about separating levofloxacin from her calcium and multivitamin. She should take levofloxacin at least 2 hours before or 2 hours

after her calcium and multivitamin. She should take levofloxacin daily, not skip doses, and complete the entire prescription, even if she feels better before completing her course. Educate her about potential side effects and how to manage them. She may experience transient diarrhea, but if it becomes severe, she should call her doctor and not take loperamide or other anti-diarrheal agents. She should wear a sunscreen to prevent sunburn, as levofloxacin can cause photosensitivity.

PROBLEM 2: Type 2 Diabetes Mellitus

- Although we are not sure whether KD's blood glucose is fasting glucose, her type 2 diabetes could be better controlled, as her HBA1c is 0.078 (7.8%). Metformin is a good choice for initial management, and treatment should be maximized before starting additional agents.
- Increase metformin to 850 mg PO BID.
- Keep enteric-coated aspirin 325 mg PO QD, as this is recommended for all patients with type 2 diabetes.
- Discontinue atenolol and start an ACE inhibitor. Lisinopril or any once-a-day ACE inhibitor should be initiated to enhance compliance. Current guidelines recommend that all patients with HTN and diabetes be treated with ACE inhibitors to prevent complications associated with both disease states. Based on recent clinical trial results, an angiotensin II receptor blocker (ARB) could also be justified and recommended for KD.
- Efficacy monitoring: KD should check her blood glucose at least three times a day, preferably four times a day. She should have her HBA1c checked again in 3 months. If she cannot check her blood sugar that many times per day, she should at least check a fasting blood glucose in the morning and an evening glucose. She should use a blood glucose meter and be taught how to use the meter appropriately.
- KD should inform other health care providers that she is on metformin. Metformin has many absolute contraindications, and health care providers need to be aware that she is taking metformin so that they can manage her appropriately.
- Toxicity monitoring: Side effects of metformin can include nausea, diarrhea, abdominal bloating, and flatulence. SCr should be monitored, as metformin is absolutely contraindicated in women with an SCr of 123 (1.4) or higher. Starting an ACE inhibitor can also cause a slight rise in SCr.

PROBLEM 3: Hypertension

- KD's blood pressure is not at goal (<130/80) for patients with HTN and type 2 diabetes.
- Discontinue atenolol and start an ACE inhibitor. Lisinopril or any once-a-day ACE inhibitor should be initiated to enhance compliance. Current guidelines recommend that all patients with HTN and diabetes be treated with ACE inhibitors to prevent complications associated with both disease states. Based on recent clinical trial results and the JNC-VII guidelines, an ARB could also be justified and recommended for KD.
- Efficacy monitoring: BP
- Toxicity monitoring: SCr, potassium, BP for signs of hypotension, chronic dry cough, and angioedema
- Counsel KD on signs and symptoms of hypotension, such as dizziness and light-headedness. Tell her that she might feel dizzy when she rises out of bed or gets up from a chair when she first starts taking lisinopril. If those symptoms persist, she should call her doctor. KD should also be aware of hyperkalemia. She should call her doctor if she experiences any unusual muscle pain, weakness, or cramping. Dry, irritating cough can occur in patients taking lisinopril and is thought to be due to bradykinin accumulation. It is often described by patients as a "tickle" in the back of the throat. The side effect is not dose-related and occurs anywhere from 1 week to 6 months after initiating ACE inhibitors. If the cough persists, she could be switched from lisinopril to another ACE inhibitor, or to an ARB. Angioedema is a rare but life-threatening anaphylactoid reaction associated with ACE inhibitors. Common signs and symptoms of angioedema include swelling of the face and lips and difficulty breathing. If these symptoms occur, she should discontinue lisinopril immediately and go to the emergency room. Cross-reactivity has been reported in some patients when switched from an ACE inhibitor to an ARB, but cases of successful switching without cross-reactivity have also been reported.

■ CASE QUESTIONS

1. c. *Escherichia coli*

2. b. Via an ascending route from the urethra into the bladder. The organisms mostly originate from the bowel. In women, these organisms colonize the vaginal vitreous and the

vagina, allowing for easy entry into the urethra and bladder.

3. c. Acute complicated pyelonephritis. KD's presentation of fever and lower back pain along with past medical history of type 2 diabetes and history of nephrolithiasis is typical of a complicated UTI.

4. In patients with complicated UTI accompanied by fever, it is important to obtain blood cultures to rule out urosepsis. Given KD's presentation and history of nephrolithiasis, she is at higher risk for developing urosepsis.

5. b. 20%

6. a. Gentamicin 100 mg IV q12h for 10 days. The recommended length of therapy for acute complicated cystitis is 7 to 14 days. In addition, giving KD a 50-mg gentamicin dose would not achieve the appropriate gentamicin peak concentrations necessary to treat acute complicated pyelonephritis.

7. Counsel KD about separating levofloxacin from her calcium and multivitamin. She should take levofloxacin at least 2 hours before or 2 hours after her calcium and multivitamin. She should take levofloxacin daily, should not skip doses, and should complete the entire prescription, even if she feels better before completing her course. Educate her about potential side effects and how to manage them. She may experience transient diarrhea, but if it becomes severe, she should call her doctor and not take loperamide or other antidiarrheal agents. She should wear a sunscreen to prevent sunburn, as levofloxacin can cause photosensitivity.

8. c. *Pseudomonas aeruginosa* is the most concerning organism for nosocomial UTI.

9. a. Gentamicin IV + piperacillin/tazobactam IV. Until cultures and sensitivities return, we must assume that the patient's infection is due to *Pseudomonas aeruginosa*. Given the serious resistance patterns of *P. aeruginosa*, appropriate empiric therapy consists of two antibiotics, each with different mechanisms of action, with hopes that *Pseudomonas* is sensitive to at least one antibiotic.

10. d. Peak: 8–10 μg/mL and trough: 1–2 μg/mL. Given that we are initially suspecting *P. aeruginosa* infection, we should target peaks of 8 to 10 μg per mL. Gentamicin trough concentrations should always be less than 2 μg per mL to minimize the risk of aminoglycoside-induced acute tubular necrosis.

11. Cranberry juice has been associated with decreased incidence of UTIs. It is believed that the high levels of proanthocyanidins in cranberry juice inhibit UPEC adherence to the urinary endothelium. Various formulations of lactobacillus have also been studied with the rationale that normalization of vaginal flora will result in less frequent UTIs. However, clinical trial results have failed to show effective results.

12. **KEY POINTS**
    - UTIs can involve the bladder, kidneys, or other urinary structures. Young to middle-aged women have the highest prevalence of UTIs.
    - Uncomplicated UTIs occur in otherwise healthy individuals, whereas complicated UTIs occur in patients with structural, functional, or immunologic abnormalities.
    - *E. coli* and other bowel organisms are the most common cause of UTIs, and the most common route of infection is ascending from the urethra into the bladder.
    - Uncomplicated cystitis can be treated effectively with a 3-day course in healthy women, uncomplicated pyelonephritis can be treated for 7 to 10 days, and complicated infections should be treated for 7 to 14 days.
    - TMP/SMX or a fluoroquinolone is a good empiric treatment option. However, TMP/SMX should not be used empirically in areas where *E. coli* resistance exceeds 20%.

CASE 33 ANSWERS

■ PROBLEM LIST

1. Infective endocarditis
2. Anemia
3. Renal insufficiency
4. Hypertension
5. Prostatic hypertrophy
6. Hearing deficit

■ SOAP NOTE

S: Fatigue, fever, night sweats, weakness, dyspnea, anorexia, 6-kg weight loss over past month

O: Cachectic, ill-appearing man; history of mitral valve prolapse and rheumatic fever; recent dental procedure. T 38.7°C, BP 150/89, HR 80, Wt 65 kg. Conjunctival petechiae and embolic lesions in extremities; hearing deficit in left ear; heart murmur and mitral regurgitation. TEE: (+) vegetation. Prostatic hypertrophy. Lkcs 15.5×10^9 with abnormal differential (76% N; 14% L); Hct 0.33 (33); Hgb 114 (11.4); BUN 10.8 (30); Cr 159 (1.8); ESR 66; (+) Rheumatoid factor; urinalysis slightly abnormal; blood cultures pending. Meds: metoprolol 50 mg BID; hydrochlorothiazide 25 mg PO QD; aspirin 81 mg PO QD; ibuprofen 200 to 400 mg PO q4–6h PRN; vitamin C 1,000 mg QD

A: PROBLEM 1: Infective endocarditis in high-risk patient after dental procedure

PROBLEM 2: Anemia secondary to endocarditis and poor nutrition

PROBLEM 3: Renal insufficiency (likely prerenal azotemia) secondary to dehydration, long-standing hypertension, or endocarditis

PROBLEM 4: Uncontrolled hypertension secondary to nonadherence to drug regimen, disease worsening, or metabolic stress in association with infection

PROBLEM 5: Prostatic hypertrophy with potential need for surgery

PROBLEM 6: Hearing deficit

P: PROBLEM 1: Infective Endocarditis

- Ask patient for more specific information about his penicillin hypersensitivity reaction in the past (severity, date).
- If mild reaction, start empiric therapy with ceftriaxone 2 g IV once daily.
- Monitor patient for potential drug hypersensitivity reaction.
- Monitor for cardiac (e.g., CHF or MI) and extracardiac (other embolic events) complications.
- Obtain LFTs.
- Check temperature (every shift).
- Daily WBC (with differential)
- Daily BUN and Cr
- Await results of blood culture and sensitivity tests and modify drug regimen accordingly.
- Monitor for clinical improvement of AM's signs and symptoms.
- Obtain daily follow-up blood cultures.
- Obtain follow-up TEE.
- Consider future mitral valve replacement (after endocarditis has subsided).

- Counsel patient regarding the need for prophylaxis with recommended drug regimens for certain dental and most surgical procedures.

PROBLEM 2: Anemia

- Ask patient about his recent diet.
- Start multivitamin 1 tablet PO QD.
- Obtain serum iron, TIBC, ferritin, and folate levels.
- Start $FeSO_4$ 325 mg PO TID.
- Counsel patient regarding adverse reactions with iron supplements.
- If low folate level, start folic acid 1 mg PO QD.
- Monitor Hct and Hgb.
- Encourage good nutrition (low in salt).

PROBLEM 3: Renal Insufficiency

- Ask patient about history of renal disease.
- Obtain renal baseline level from primary care provider (if possible).
- Start gentle IV hydration (e.g., 1 L normal saline with 20 mEq of KCl, infused at 100 cc/h).
- Monitor daily electrolytes.
- Monitor daily I and O.
- Monitor vital signs (especially BP) every shift.
- Monitor daily BUN and Cr.
- Avoid use of nephrotoxic drugs (especially prolonged use of aminoglycosides).
- Calculate CrCl and adjust doses of renally excreted drugs accordingly.

PROBLEM 4: Hypertension

- Ask patient about BP and HR baseline values and control.
- Investigate drug adherence or reasons for nonadherence.
- Re-evaluate BP after stabilization of patient and control of his infection.
- Suggest changing metoprolol 50 mg BID to 100 mg QD dosing (or to extended-release form Toprol XL) to enhance adherence.
- Monitor BP and HR every shift.
- Counsel patient regarding adverse drug reactions, adherence, and low-salt diet.

PROBLEM 5: Prostatic Hypertrophy

- Ask patient regarding efficacy of vitamin C as prophylaxis against UTIs.
- Continue vitamin C 1,000 mg QD.
- Encourage sufficient daily fluid intake and efficient voiding.
- Monitor renal function.
- Monitor urinalysis periodically for infection.
- Patient may need prostatectomy in the future.

PROBLEM 6: Hearing Deficit

- Ask patient for cause of his hearing deficit.
- Obtain baseline hearing test.
- Avoid ototoxic drugs (e.g., aminoglycosides) if possible.

■ CASE QUESTIONS

1. b. Hypertension

2. c. *Viridans streptococci*

3. Sequence of events that lead to endocarditis and the formation of vegetations:
    - Previous damage to cardiac valve (in this case, mitral valve prolapse, rheumatic fever) resulting in hemodynamic alterations and collagen exposure
    - Platelet-fibrin deposition and thrombus formation (NBTE)
    - Bacteremia from another source of infection, colonization, or dental or surgical procedures (in this case, tooth extraction)
    - Bacterial adherence; exponential growth of organisms reaching high inoculum
    - Vegetation formation and enlargement due to further platelet-fibrin deposition; sequestration of infecting organisms from leukocytes; prolonged and continuous bacteremia

4. General pharmacologic principles and treatment goals for infective endocarditis:
    - Use of bactericidal antibiotics to sterilize affected valve and surrounding tissues
    - Use of high antibiotic doses to penetrate vegetation
    - Preference for parenteral drug administration
    - Treatment for prolonged duration (4–6 weeks) to eradicate infection
    - Empiric treatment based on most likely source of bacteremia and associated micro-organisms
    - Consideration of institution's or community's resistance patterns
    - Monitoring for drug toxicity and embolic complications
    - Prevention of further disease in at-risk patients

5. d. Should be treated with a 2-week course of cefazolin or vancomycin

6. b. The patient should receive IV ceftriaxone for 4 weeks.

7. The rationale for combination therapy of penicillin, ampicillin, or vancomycin with an aminoglycoside is synergistic killing of organisms commonly associated with endocarditis. However, especially in the treatment of enterococci, gentamicin susceptibility tests should be performed to determine whether synergy with ampicillin, penicillin, or vancomycin will be achieved. In the treatment of staphylococcal endocarditis, the addition of aminoglycosides has been found beneficial for the first 3 to 5 days only to achieve a more rapid clearance of bacteremia and shorten the patient's febrile phase.

8. a. Vancomycin IV for 4 weeks

9. d. Nephrotoxicity, ototoxicity, and hypersensitivity reactions

10. Appropriate doses for gentamicin and vancomycin and monitoring:
    AM's actual body weight (ABW): 67 kg; height: 172.5 cm (5 foot 9)

    a. Calculate IBW: IBW = 50 + 2.3 × (inches >5 feet)
    For AM   IBW = 50 + 2.3 × 9 = 70.7 kg
    IBW >ABW; therefore we need to use ABW for calculating CrCl and doses

    b. Calculate CrCl (Cockroft-Gault method):
    Problem: It is unclear whether Cr (1.8) is AM's baseline or at steady state; most likely the patient is dehydrated (due to anorexia, fever) and Cr may decrease with hydration; reassess Cr after 1 to 2 days and adjust drug doses accordingly.

    CrCl: (140 - age) × IBW / Cr × 72 mL/min
    For AM: (140 = 56) × 67 / 1.8 × 72 mL/min = 43.4 mL/min

    c. Gentamicin dose: 1 mg/kg IV q8h = 67 mg, rounded to 70 mg IV q8h as initial dose; maintenance dose depends on renal function (determine percentage of loading dose based on CrCl and dosage interval ranges according to Hull and Sarrubi aminoglycoside nomogram); dose needs to be adjusted for target peak of ~3 μg per mL, trough <0.5 μg per mL.

    d. Vancomycin dose: 15 mg per kg IV q12h = 1,005 mg = 1 g IV q12h; maintenance dose depends on renal function and needs to be adjusted for target peak of ~30 to 45 μg per mL, trough ~10 to 15 μg per mL.

11. b. It is not unusual for a patient to remain bacteremic for 5 to 7 days after initiation of

therapy, and another blood culture should be taken in 1 to 2 days.

12. b. Prophylaxis for AM should consist of amoxicillin (2 g PO given 1 hour before the procedure), as he is a high-risk patient.

13. Potential psychosocial issues for the patient: Reduced quality of life due to:

Adherence to complex drug regimen
▪ Prolonged medication use
▪ Reduced activity due to parenteral drug administration
▪ Adverse drug effects
▪ Limited financial resources: unable to afford long-term antibiotic therapy and potential home health care

Emotional issues
▪ Prolonged illness and hospitalization
▪ Absence from work and potential loss of income
▪ Fear of complications and repeated disease
▪ Fear of future surgical interventions
▪ Potential limited family support

Pharmacist's role:
▪ Individualize overall treatment plan for patient (pharmacologic and nonpharmacologic).
▪ Provide patient education, counseling, and positive reinforcement.
▪ Emphasize need for prevention and prophylaxis.
▪ Facilitate home health care treatment.

14. **KEY POINTS**
▪ Infective endocarditis is a serious infectious disease with significant mortality that requires aggressive and long-term therapy for a successful outcome.
▪ Antibiotics need to be given in high doses, in parenteral form, and usually for several weeks to sufficiently penetrate into the vegetation, provide effective killing of the high inoculum of microorganisms, and reduce their low metabolic state at the site of infection.
▪ Combination therapy with aminoglycosides is often necessary to achieve synergistic killing or shorten the overall duration of therapy.
▪ Prevention of future disease is essential for patients at risk who are undergoing certain dental and surgical procedures, and guidelines regarding appropriate prophylactic regimens are published.

CASE 34 ANSWERS

▪ PROBLEM LIST

1. Bacterial meningitis
2. Acute renal insufficiency
3. Lack of appropriate vaccinations given
4. Asthma
5. Sickle cell disease
6. Recurrent otitis media

▪ SOAP NOTE

S: SB's mother states SB has had a 2-day history of fever, headache, neck stiffness, vomiting, and a rash on her legs. All of these symptoms developed after she was treated with azithromycin for acute otitis media about 7 days ago. SB was very difficult to awake this morning.

O: Respiratory distress and nonresponsive, BP 80/40, HR 115, RR 31, T 38.9°C, poorly reactive pupils, + Kernig's sign, decreased neck movement, A and O ×1, purpuric rash on lower extremities. Labs: Cr 133 (1.5), Glu 4.4 (80), Lkcs 19 × 10^9 (19 × 10^3). LP: cloudy fluid with a glucose of 20 mg per dL, protein of 150 mg per dL, WBC 18.5 × 10^3, 93% PMNs, CSF Gram stain: gram-positive cocci in pairs and chains

A: PROBLEM 1: Bacterial meningitis as evidenced by finding on LP

PROBLEM 2: Acute renal insufficiency that may be the result of SB's fever and vomiting

PROBLEM 3: Lack of appropriate immunizations for SB due to her history of a splenectomy

PROBLEM 4: Asthma (controlled)

PROBLEM 5: Sickle cell disease (stable)

PROBLEM 6: Recurrent otitis media (stable)

P: PROBLEM 1: Bacterial Meningitis

▪ Start ceftriaxone 1 g IV q12h and vancomycin 500 mg IV q6h since it is presumed SB has pneumococcal meningitis as evidenced by Gram stain and past medical history of sickle cell disease (risk of infection with encapsulated organisms) and has not received the pneumococcal vaccine
▪ Since SB is in the ED and hasn't received any antibiotics, may also start dexamethasone 5 mg IV q6h for 2 to 4 days or until cultures come back (if positive with either *Haemophilus influenzae* or *Streptococcus pneumoniae*, continue for

2–4 days; if not, discontinue), to be given either 10 to 20 minutes before or with the first dose of antibiotics
- Monitor renal function (creatinine probably increased due to dehydration), BUN, SCr, urine output.
- Monitor for red-man syndrome with infusion of vancomycin; if it occurs, either decrease the rate of the infusion or give diphenhydramine 12.5 to 25 mg PRN.
- Monitor for nephrotoxicity (BUN, SCr, urine output) and ototoxicity (vancomycin).
- Monitor vancomycin level peak 35 to 40 mg per dL (to be checked 1 hour after an hour infusion) and trough 10 to 20 mg per dL (right before the next dose is given) with the third dose unless SB's creatinine continues to rise; if so, check level before administering the next dose.
- Discuss whether a vancomycin peak is necessary.
- Discuss whether vancomycin is still considered to have a severe risk of nephrotoxicity.
- Monitor WBC, differential, CSF, and blood cultures.
- Once the organism is identified, change antibiotic therapy as necessary and determine duration of treatment (if pneumococcal, 10–14 days).

PROBLEM 2: Acute Renal Insufficiency
- Probably due to dehydration from her fever and vomiting (BUN:SCr ratio >20:1); monitor BUN, SCr, and urine output.
- Consider calculating CrCl using the Schwartz equation: k (constant based on age) × ht (in cm)/SCr = 0.55(137)/1.5 = 50 (mL/min/1.73m^2).
- Give a fluid bolus of 10 mL per kg until her BP increases, then start fluids at maintenance D5W NS to be run at 60 mL per hour.
- Monitor Na, K, Cl, CO_2, BUN, SCr, and Glu q12h.

PROBLEM 3: Lack of Appropriate Immunizations
- Counsel caregivers on the importance of SB receiving her immunizations since she has had her spleen removed.
- Give SB the 23-valent and 7-valent pneumococcal vaccines and the meningococcal vaccine when meningitis has resolved. Note: administration of the 7-valent and 23-valent pneumococcal vaccine should be separated by at least 8 weeks.

PROBLEM 4: Asthma
- No intervention needed at this time
- Make sure SB is using her inhalers appropriately and rinsing her mouth after using the steroid inhaler.

PROBLEM 5: Sickle Cell Disease
- See Problem 3.
- No further intervention needed at this time

PROBLEM 6: Recurrent Otitis Media
- Appropriate vaccinations may be helpful.
- May consider placing bilateral tympanostomy tubes

■ CASE QUESTIONS

1. History of sickle cell disease, lack of appropriate immunizations, recent otitis media infection
2. Vomiting, rash on her legs, fever, headache, neck stiffness, positive Kernig's sign, decreased neck movement
3. c. *Streptococcus pneumoniae*
4. When placing the patient in the supine position, flexing the thigh with the knee also in the flexed position, and then extending the leg; the leg resists extension because of the increased pressure due to inflammation
5. Lipophilicity, molecular weight, degree of ionization, protein binding
6. b. Vancomycin + ceftriaxone or cefotaxime
7. a. 10 to 14 days
8. c. Renal function
9. SB would be a good candidate for adjuvant dexamethasone since antibiotics have not already been started and there is a very high likelihood that her meningitis is caused by *S. pneumoniae*. Although the use of steroids is controversial in pediatrics, there is evidence in adults to support steroid use in *S. pneumoniae* meningitis, since it is proven to reduce the incidence of morbidity and mortality. In this case, the benefits would outweigh the risks.
10. d. She should be given the 23-valent pneumococcal polysaccharide, meningococcal, and 7-valent conjugate pneumococcal vaccines.
11. Because of the high rates of penicillin resistance that result from alterations in the penicillin-binding proteins of the bacterial cell wall, empiric therapy should include vancomycin + ceftriaxone or cefotaxime. SB specifically has a number of risk factors for

resistant organisms, such as frequent antibiotic use and the use of prophylactic antibiotics.

12. a. Prior to her first dose of antibiotics

13. a. Peak (goal 35–40 μg/mL), trough (goal 10–20 μg/mL), BUN, SCr, urine output

14. c. Use of appropriate vaccinations

15. **KEY POINTS**
    ■ Empiric antibiotic therapy should be directed by the Gram stain of CSF (if available) and the patient's age and underlying health status. Empiric regimens usually contain a third-generation cephalosporin (e.g., ceftriaxone) with or without additional antibiotics (ampicillin, vancomycin).
    ■ Corticosteroids should be used in childhood *H. influenzae* meningitis and should be considered in *S. pneumoniae* meningitis (pediatric or adult) to decrease the incidence of long-term neurologic deficits, specifically hearing loss.
    ■ Contacts exposed to meningitis index cases with *H. influenzae* and *Neisseria meningitidis* may require chemoprophylaxis.
    ■ Vaccines are available to decrease the incidence of disease, and therefore perhaps meningitis, due to *H. influenzae*, *N. meningitidis*, and *S. pneumoniae* in at-risk populations.

CASE 35 ANSWERS

■ PROBLEM LIST

1. Contiguous osteomyelitis with vascular insufficiency
2. Poorly controlled diabetes
3. Chronic renal insufficiency
4. Hypertension
5. Obesity

■ SOAP NOTE

S: "I have pus coming from the wound on my foot, which is also red and swollen. It hurts when I walk on my injured foot. I hurt my foot 1 month ago."

O: Three-cm wide × 3-cm deep ulcer on inferior surface of right foot with yellowish-green drainage and a foul smell; decreased sensation to light touch (both feet); normal range of motion. BP 138/82, T 37.6°C, Wt 110 kg. WBC 17 (70 PMNs, 8 bands, 16 lymphs, 6 monos), ESR 72, CRP 12.6, HbA$_{1c}$ 10.3%, Glu 183, BUN 21, SCr 1.7. Gram stain (wound culture): aerobic gram-positive cocci in pairs, anaerobic gram-positive cocci, gram-negative rods. X-ray of foot indicates soft tissue swelling and periosteal swelling consistent with osteomyelitis.

A: PROBLEM 1: Osteomyelitis secondary to acute injury 1 month ago with inappropriate follow-up; vascular insufficiency secondary to poorly controlled diabetes; Gram stain indicates polymicrobial bone infection; consider *Pseudomonas aeruginosa*, *Staphylococcus aureus*, and anaerobes

PROBLEM 2: Uncontrolled diabetes on current therapy (goal A1C <7%) and inappropriate oral therapy considering renal insufficiency

PROBLEM 3: Chronic renal insufficiency secondary to uncontrolled diabetes (SCr increased from 1.5 to 1.7 mg per dL in 1 month)

PROBLEM 4: Hypertension uncontrolled (goal <130/80) on current therapy

PROBLEM 5: Obesity with no evaluation of lipid profile

P: PROBLEM 1: Contiguous Osteomyelitis with Vascular Insufficiency

■ Admit to hospital and begin IV antibiotic therapy with imipenem 500 mg IV q8h (dose adjusted for reduced CrCl of 65 mL/min) as empiric therapy while awaiting culture results.
■ Consider adding vancomycin 1 g IV q12h if there is a concern for methicillin-resistant *S. aureus*. A trough level should be obtained prior to the third dose with a goal of 5 to 15 μg per mL.
■ Once the culture and sensitivity results are known, adjust antibiotic therapy as needed.
■ Monitor CRP for response to antibiotic therapy.
■ Monitor SCr to determine if further dosage adjustments need to be made based on renal function.

PROBLEM 2: Uncontrolled Diabetes

■ Discontinue metformin due to renal insufficiency. Metformin is contraindicated in males with an SCr of 1.5 mg per dL or higher.
■ Begin rosiglitazone 4 mg PO BID to achieve an A1c below 7%.
■ Monitor LFTs every 2 months for the first year in a patient started on thiazolidinedione therapy.
■ Change glimepiride to glipizide due to renal impairment. Glimepiride is renally eliminated and

glipizide is a better choice for a sulfonylurea in a patient with renal insufficiency. Begin Glucotrol XL 10 mg PO QD.
- Educate the patient on the importance of self-monitoring of blood glucose levels and close follow-up.
- DASH diet
- Recommend obtaining a fasting lipid profile to evaluate for hypercholesterolemia.

PROBLEM 3: Chronic Renal Insufficiency

- Continue to monitor SCr and BUN while patient is hospitalized and receiving an antibiotic that is renally eliminated.
- Recommend a urinalysis to detect the presence of proteinuria.
- Begin lisinopril 10 mg PO QD to help preserve glomerular filtration rate and decrease proteinuria.

PROBLEM 4: Hypertension

- Since BP is near goal of below 130/80 and lisinopril is to be added to the regimen as per the above recommendations, no further pharmacotherapy is recommended at this time. Consider increasing the HCTZ to 25 mg PO QD if there is no response to lisinopril in 1 month.
- Encourage adherence to the DASH diet for appropriate weight loss.
- Encourage physical activity even while the patient is hospitalized for osteomyelitis.

PROBLEM 5: Obesity

- Encourage adherence to the DASH diet for appropriate weight loss and control of blood glucose.
- Encourage physical activity even while the patient is hospitalized for osteomyelitis.
- Recommend a fasting lipid profile to evaluate for hypercholesterolemia.

■ **CASE QUESTIONS**

1. c. Contiguous osteomyelitis with vascular insufficiency

2. a. Neonates are at highest risk for the development of osteomyelitis due to *Pseudomonas aeruginosa*.

3. c. *Neisseria gonorrhoeae*

4. b. Vancomycin 1 g IV q12h

5. b. *Staphylococcus epidermidis*

6. c. Imipenem

7. Elevated ESR and CRP, high WBC count, pain upon palpation, redness and swelling around wound

8. ESR and CRP are both nonspecific markers of inflammation. Increases in both ESR and CRP can be seen with bone and joint infections. These lab tests can be useful in monitoring the response to therapy in a patient with osteomyelitis. CRP is a more specific and sensitive marker of acute inflammation. The CRP level can decrease within 6 hours of beginning appropriate therapy. It is most often used in infections in neonates and children. The ESR decreases over time and is a better marker of chronic inflammatory processes rather than acute inflammation.

9. Factors to consider when choosing pharmacologic and nonpharmacologic treatment include type of bone/joint infection, local antibiotic resistance patterns, cost of therapy, toxicity of therapy, patient risk factors, need for parenteral versus oral antibiotic therapy, need for surgical intervention, antibiotic coverage and bone penetration, duration of antibiotic therapy (including when it is appropriate to change from a parenteral to an oral agent), and preventing long-term complications.

10. Oral antibiotic therapy is advantageous in the long-term treatment of bone and joint infections to avoid the potential complications from prolonged courses of IV therapy. Most clinicians recommend at least 2 weeks of parenteral therapy before switching to an appropriate oral agent. Patients selected for oral antibiotic therapy should have had a clinical response to parenteral antibiotic therapy and should be able to be compliant with the oral therapy selected. Oral agents that have been found to be effective include dicloxacillin, cephalexin, amoxicillin-clavulanate, and fluoroquinolones.

11. Community-acquired methicillin-resistant *Staphylococcus aureus* is becoming much more prevalent. However, compared to hospital-acquired methicillin-resistant *S. aureus*, it is sensitive to several antibacterial agents, including trimethoprim/sulfamethoxazole ± rifampin, clindamycin, linezolid, vancomycin, fluoroquinolones, and tetracyclines. Advantages and disadvantages of each agent are listed below.

- Trimethoprim/sulfamethoxazole
    Advantages: Oral formulation for outpatient therapy, well tolerated, limited toxicity, low cost
    Disadvantages: Limited amount of evidence showing its efficacy in MRSA, needs to be combined with rifampin for synergistic effect, bacteriostatic
- Clindamycin
    Advantages: Coverage includes gram-positive and anaerobic organisms, equipotent IV and PO formulations for convenient inpatient to outpatient dosing, low cost
    Disadvantages: Possibility of development of pseudomembranous colitis, poor palatability of oral suspension, potential for inducible resistance
- Linezolid
    Advantages: Equipotent IV and PO formulations for convenient inpatient to outpatient dosing, twice-daily dosing schedule, expanded coverage against resistant gram-positive organisms, limited toxicity, well tolerated
    Disadvantages: Potential for thrombocytopenia, cost, bacteriostatic
- Vancomycin
    Advantages: Standard of care for MRSA infections
    Disadvantages: IV is the only available formulation, need for monitoring therapeutic drug levels, potential for toxicity
- Fluoroquinolones
    Advantages: Equipotent IV and PO formulations for convenient inpatient to outpatient dosing, well tolerated, limited toxicity, twice-daily dosing schedule
    Disadvantages: Potential for development of resistance, drug interaction profile, cost
- Tetracyclines
    Advantages: Low cost, PO formulation
    Disadvantages: Must be dosed frequently, drug interaction profile, adverse effects, bacteriostatic, potential for development of resistance

12. **KEY POINTS**
    - It is important to make the diagnosis of osteomyelitis early in the course of the disease because the prognosis depends on the rapidity and adequacy of treatment.
    - Except for culture results, no single laboratory test is diagnostic for osteomyelitis.

Therefore, careful monitoring of the trends in CBC with differential, ESR, and CRP is required.
- *S. aureus* is the most common pathogen isolated, although other organisms can be present, depending on the age and risk factors of the patient.
- Treatment of osteomyelitis includes adequate débridement, identification of the organism, selection of the correct antibiotic, and delivery of adequate quantities of antibiotic to the site of infection for an extended period of time.
- Oral agents may be efficacious if used in the appropriate patient population and if compliance can be ensured.

CASE 36 ANSWERS

■ PROBLEM LIST

1. Inpatient admission for cellulitis
2. Rash
3. Elevated fasting blood glucose

■ SOAP NOTE

S: "I am having increasing redness and tenderness in my right arm, even though I have been taking my medication. I had a fever of 100° last night and this morning with chills. I also have this red, itchy rash on my chest that is driving me crazy."

O: Warm, red, swollen, tender right lower arm with progression to the upper arm; maculopapular rash on chest and neck. T 39.1°C, WBC 18.5 × 10^3, Glu 145, A1C 6.8%. New medications: cephalexin with known penicillin allergy.

A: PROBLEM 1: Worsening cellulitis despite cephalexin therapy

PROBLEM 2: Rash appeared after initiation of cephalexin—allergic reaction; patient has known allergy to penicillin

PROBLEM 3: Glucose acutely elevated in setting of acute illness and infection

P: PROBLEM 1: Progressing Cellulitis

- Discontinue cephalexin.
- Initiate IV antibiotics due to lack of response to oral medications, patient's fever, and elevated WBC count.

- Initiate vancomycin due to possibility of community-acquired methicillin-resistant *Staphylococcus aureus* and allergy to β-lactam antibiotics. May also broaden antimicrobial spectrum to include gram-negative organisms by adding fluoroquinolone (ciprofloxacin, gatifloxacin, levofloxacin, and moxifloxacin) or aztreonam.
- Monitor for resolution of warmth, redness, swelling, and tenderness in right lower arm and upper arm.
- Monitor WBC count q24h.
- Monitor BP, heart rate, and fever q8h.
- Monitor BUN and SCr q24h.
- Obtain vancomycin serum concentrations with third dose and weekly with therapy greater than 7 days.

PROBLEM 2: Rash

- Discontinue cephalexin.
- Provide supportive care with antihistamines and topical creams.
- Educate patient on new medication allergy.
- Make sure patient understands importance of discontinuing cephalexin and need to dispose of any remaining cephalexin.

PROBLEM 3: Elevated Fasting Blood Glucose

- A1C is currently below 7, showing that glucose levels were within the desired range for the past 3 months.
- Continue metformin 1 g PO BID and glipizide XL 5 mg PO daily.
- Monitor blood glucose three or four times per day.
- If blood glucose remains elevated, consider increase of metformin 850 mg PO TID or glipizide XL to 10 mg PO daily, or provide inpatient coverage with sliding-scale insulin.
- BP is currently below goal of 130 per 80.
- Monitor BP and heart rate q8h.
- Consider evaluating for microalbuminuria to assess for diabetic nephropathy due to elevated SCr. Addition of ACE inhibitor may be warranted if micro- or macroalbuminuria is present.
- Continue ASA 81 mg EC PO daily for cardioprotective effects.

■ CASE QUESTIONS

1. Cellulitis may occur when the skin barrier is broken, as in a cut, bite, or abrasion. The patient's splinter in his right arm broke the skin barrier and resulted in cellulitis.

2. Patients with cellulitis may present with local and/or systemic features. Common local signs and symptoms include pain, tenderness, erythema, swelling, and warmth at the site of infection. Less frequently, localized symptoms such as lymphangitis and enlarged and tender lymph nodes may occur. Fever, chills, and an elevated WBC count may also occur in some patients.

3. Warmth, redness, swelling, and tenderness in the right lower arm extending to upper arm; temperature 39.1°C, Lkcs 18.5 × 10^9 (18.5 × 10^3).

4. Local symptoms of untreated cellulitis are increases in warmth, tenderness, redness, edema, lymphangitis, and possibly osteomyelitis. Systemic symptoms that may result are an elevated WBC count, fever, chills, mental status changes, hypotension, and sepsis.

5. Group A streptococci and *S. aureus*

6. Antistaphylococcal penicillins (e.g., oxacillin, nafcillin), amoxicillin/clavulanate, ampicillin/sulbactam, first-generation cephalosporins (cefazolin, cephalexin), azithromycin, clarithromycin, ciprofloxacin, gatifloxacin, levofloxacin, and moxifloxacin are antibiotics that are indicated in the treatment of skin and soft tissue infections. If methicillin-resistant *S. aureus* (MRSA) is suspected, vancomycin, daptomycin, and linezolid are treatment options. However, β-lactam antibiotics are not appropriate in AC due to his report of penicillin allergy and new-onset rash to cephalexin therapy. IV antibiotics should be initiated empirically since the patient did not respond to oral antibiotics and the cellulitis is progressing. In addition, the patient is not responding to appropriate empiric therapy with cephalexin, so resistant and/or gram-negative organisms should be suspected. Due to the increasing incidence of community-acquired MRSA and the severity of infection, vancomycin should be initiated as empiric therapy due to the severity of AC's infection. Daptomycin and linezolid are treatment options for MRSA but are more expensive and should be reserved for patients who are not candidates for vancomycin therapy. AC is at risk for a complicated infection since he has diabetes, but his A1C reflects tight glucose control. If suspected, gram-negative coverage may also be initiated with the addition of a fluoroquinolone (ciprofloxa-

cin, gatifloxacin, levofloxacin, or moxifloxacin) or aztreonam. An aminoglycoside antibiotic (tobramycin, gentamicin) is another option for gram-negative coverage. However, aminoglycoside antibiotics should be used with caution in patients with diabetes and concomitant renal impairment.

7. (Vancomycin 1,250 mg IV q12h) ± (ciprofloxacin 400 mg IV q8–12h or gatifloxacin 400 mg IV daily or levofloxacin 500–750 mg IV daily or moxifloxacin 400 mg IV daily or aztreonam 1–2 g IV q8–12h). Total duration of therapy in the treatment of cellulitis is usually 7 to 14 days. Once AC becomes afebrile and lesions have begun to improve (usually 3–5 days), he may be switched to an oral antibiotic with a similar spectrum of activity to complete his course of treatment. If patients have continued signs of cellulitis at the end of treatment, antibiotics should be continued until all erythema is resolved.

8. Patient data:

    45-year-old male
    95 kg (IBW 77.7 kg)
    Ht 6-foot-0
    SCr 1.5 mg/dL
    BSA 2.19 m^2
    Dosing weight = 84.6 kg
    Observed peak 37 μg/mL/mL
    Observed trough 20.1 μg/mL/mL
    Elapsed time = 9.5 h

$$\textit{Estimated } k_{el} = \frac{\ln(20.1/37)}{9.5 hr} = -0.064 h^{-1}$$

Estimated T1/2 = 10.79 hr

Estimated Vd = (0.7 L / kg * 84.7 Kg) = 59.2L

Goals of therapy: Target peak = 40 μg per mL and target trough = 12 μg per mL using an infusion length of 1 hour

$$\textit{Idea Tau} = \frac{\ln(12/40)}{0.064 h^{-1}} = 18.8 h$$

Now need to design a new dosing regimen:

$$\textit{New Dose} = \frac{(Vd)(\textit{des } Cp^{ss} \max - \textit{des } Cp^{ss} \min)}{(S)(F)}$$

Substituting in the patient values:

$$\textit{New Dose} = \frac{(59.2L)(40 \textit{ mcg}/mL - 12 mcg/mL)}{(1)(1)}$$
$$= \textbf{1,657.6 } \textit{mg required}$$

Suggest a dose of 1,500 mg q24h. Begin new

dosing regimen 24 h after the last dose of 1,250 mg was given.

9. Goals of vancomycin therapy: Peak of 30 to 40 μg per mL and trough of 5 to 15 μg per mL. The ideal vancomycin dosing regimen is one that results in adequate peak concentrations in the range of 30 to 40 μg per mL and trough concentrations in the range of 5 to 15 μg per mL. There is considerable controversy regarding the validity of dosing vancomycin and monitoring therapy. It is important to discuss the role of the infusion time on pharmacokinetic calculations and for the student to see the rationale for the delayed draw time relative to the distribution of the drug. In this patient, vancomycin is an appropriate therapy choice because he is showing signs of systemic infection—chills and fever with temperature >100.5°F (38.5°C) in a diabetic patient. He was empirically started as an outpatient on an oral first-generation cephalosporin. He has not responded to the therapy and has subsequently developed a rash. Since he also reports rash with penicillin, vancomycin is the choice for this potential involvement of community-acquired MRSA infection.

    Physical signs to monitor are resolution of signs and symptoms of cellulitis, including pain, redness, warmth, or edema at the site of the cellulitis. Monitor for evidence of phlebitis and a histamine reaction that may be related to the vancomycin infusion time. Follow his fever curve and monitor for defervescence within 24 to 48 hours. If physical signs of the infection are not improving, therapy should be reevaluated.

    Laboratory monitoring: Because he has an SCr of 1.5, it would be wise to follow his SCr and renal function every 24 hours initially. Monitor WBC and differential daily as a sign of improvement.

    Pharmacokinetic monitoring: Monitor vancomycin serum concentrations with the third dose after the regimen change for optimal levels and then weekly with therapy greater than 7 days.

10. Cellulitis: redness, swelling, warmth, and progression/resolution of cellulitis on right arm, fever, BP, heart rate, WBC count

11. Cross-tolerance of cephalosporin allergy in AC, who is allergic to penicillin

12. Nonpharmacologic: cold compresses to affected areas; pharmacologic: topical or systemic antihistamines to relieve itching

13. Rash due to cephalosporin and penicillin allergy: Avoid these medications completely. Inform all health care providers of this allergy, including physicians, nurses, dentists, and pharmacists. When in doubt, contact a pharmacist before taking any medication. AC must also dispose of any remaining cephalexin. Cool sterile compresses, topical creams such as diphenhydramine, and/or antihistamines such as loratadine or diphenhydramine may help with itching and rash.

Cellulitis: Cool compresses and limb elevation may provide symptomatic relief. Be sure to clean and dry all cuts, scrapes, and abrasions and watch closely for signs/symptoms of infection.

14. A1C reflects tight glucose control over the past 2 to 3 months. AC's infection and acute illness are the most likely causes of his hyperglycemia.

15. The maximum daily dose of metformin is 2,550 mg; therefore, the metformin could be increased to 850 mg PO TID. The glipizide XL could also be increased to 10 mg PO daily. Another reasonable option is to provide coverage during AC's acute illness with sliding-scale insulin in addition to his home regimen. An example of a insulin subcutaneous sliding-scale regimen is to administer 2 units of regular insulin for glucose levels of 150 to 200 mg per dL; 4 units of regular insulin for glucose levels of 201 to 250 mg per dL; 6 units of regular insulin for glucose levels of 251 to 300 mg per dL; 8 units of regular insulin for glucose levels of 301 to 350 mg per dL; call physician for glucose levels above 350 mg per dL. Most importantly, any changes in the patient's regimen should be monitored with blood glucoses three or four times daily. These changes/additions for hyperglycemia may not be needed upon discharge once the infection is resolving. Assess need for increased doses of home medications upon discharge and resolution of AC's cellulitis.

16. **KEY POINTS**
    ■ Cellulitis is an acute infection of the skin with extension into the subcutaneous tissues that may occur when the protective barrier of the skin is broken, as in a cut, bite, or abrasion.
    ■ Commonly observed bacterial etiologies of cellulitis are group A streptococci and

S. aureus. Patients with cellulitis may present with local and/or systemic features.
    ■ Cellulitis is clinically diagnosed by the combination of local and/or systemic features. Empiric therapy should target the most likely organisms because blood or skin cultures are not usually reliable. Optimal antimicrobial treatment for cellulitis is based the most likely causative organism, penetration of the antibiotic to the site of infection, current medications, medication allergies, patient compliance, and cost. The severity, extent, and location of the infection dictate whether the patient may be treated with oral antibiotics as an outpatient or as an inpatient using IV antibiotics.
    ■ Total duration of therapy for antimicrobials in the treatment of cellulitis is usually 7 to 14 days. If the patient has continued signs of cellulitis at the end of treatment, antibiotics should be continued until all erythema is resolved.
    ■ Nonpharmacologic therapy of cellulitis consists of rest and elevation of the affected area and the application of cool sterile dressings.

CASE 37 ANSWERS

■ PROBLEM LIST

1. Fever of neutropenia
2. *Clostridium difficile* infection
3. Pain/grade I mucositis
4. Acute myelogenous leukemia (AML)
5. Hypertension
6. Hypothyroidism

■ SOAP NOTE

S: Fever, rigors, diarrhea, mild mouth pain, able to swallow liquids and solids

O: Age 52, day 14 s/p induction chemotherapy with idarubicin and ARA-C, levothyroxine 112 μg PO daily, atenolol 25 mg PO daily, levofloxacin 500 mg PO daily, acyclovir 400 mg PO TID, allopurinol 300 mg PO daily, fluconazole 200 mg PO daily, Bactrim allergy. T 39°C, BP 130/80, HR 65. Posterior oropharyngeal erythema with mild ulceration, no thyromegaly, chest CTA bilaterally, no rales/rhonchi, hyperactive bowel sounds. Central line without erythema, pain, oozing. Lkc 0.3×10^9 (0.3×10^3), diff: N 0.53 (53), P 0.34 (34), M 0.06

(6), E 0.02 (2), B 0 (0), bands 0.05 (5), ANC 174, Hct 0.30 (30), Hgb 90 (9), Plts 44 × 10^9 (44 × 10^3), BUN 6.5 (18), SCr 53 (0.6), LDH 2.6 (153), uric acid 113 (1.9), TSH 4 (4). Bone marrow biopsy: hypocellular bone marrow. Peripheral smear: no blasts. Chest CT: clear, no change from previous. Blood culture: no growth to date. Stool culture: positive for Clostridium difficile toxin.

A: PROBLEM 1: Fever of neutropenia secondary to myelosuppressive chemotherapy

PROBLEM 2: Clostridium difficile infection secondary to chemotherapy and/or prophylactic antibiotics

PROBLEM 3: Pain secondary to grade I mucositis, which is secondary to chemotherapy

PROBLEM 4: AML, controlled with current regimen

PROBLEM 5: Hypertension, controlled with current regimen

PROBLEM 6: Hypothyroidism, controlled with current regimen

P: PROBLEM 1: Fever of Neutropenia

- Begin therapy with cefepime 2 g IV q8h and vancomycin 1 g IV q12h. Vancomycin is warranted because the patient received quinolone prophylaxis and has mucositis. Discontinue vancomycin if blood cultures remain negative after 3 days or if cultures grow gram-negative organisms or penicillin-sensitive gram-positives and the patient is afebrile without severe mucositis.
- Discontinue levofloxacin.
- Continue acyclovir, fluonazole.
- Ensure that SS is in an isolated hospital room.
- Consider adding a colony-stimulating factor if marrow recovery is not evident by day 21 or if infection significantly worsens.
- Efficacy monitoring: improvement in fever curve, rigors, WBC, differential, ANC, clearing of cultures
- Toxicity monitoring: worsening of fever curve, rigors, WBC, differential, ANC, cultures, new signs/symptoms of infection, signs/symptoms of anaphylaxis with first dose of cefepime, rash, pruritus, SCr, BUN, urine output, facial/upper body erythema (red-man syndrome), platelets, Hgb/Hct, vancomycin trough if long-term therapy needed, and LFTS
- Counsel SS to report any worsening or new signs/symptoms of infection. Follow a neutropenic diet (e.g., no fresh fruit/vegetables). Try to avoid getting cuts (do not shave with a razor).

Avoid invasive procedures if possible. Avoid other sick contacts. Wash hands frequently. Wear a mask and gloves when out of the hospital room. Based on time frame from chemotherapy, neutropenia should resolve in about 2 weeks.

PROBLEM 2: *Clostridium difficile* Infection

- Begin therapy with metronidazole 500 mg PO TID. Therapy may be changed to IV if the patient cannot tolerate PO medications due to worsening mucositis.
- Place patient on contact precautions.
- Continue other antibiotics, as the risk for severe systemic infection in a neutropenic patient outweighs the risk of continuing antibiotics in a patient with *C. difficile*. May consider changing antibiotics to a quinolone plus aminoglycoside if infection persists despite treatment. However, the patient spiked a fever while on quinolone prophylaxis, so changing therapy for the treatment of neutropenic fever from a quinolone to another drug class was warranted.
- Efficacy monitoring: resolution of diarrhea, improvement in fever curve, WBC, differential
- Toxicity monitoring: worsening of diarrhea, fever curve, WBC, differential, stool cultures for sensitivity, adverse reactions of metronidazole: nausea, vomiting, anorexia, metallic taste, disulfiram-like reaction, dark urine, neuropathy
- Counsel SS to report any worsening of symptoms. Avoid alcohol or medications that contain alcohol while on metronidazole. The medication may cause the urine to turn dark or reddish-brown. The medication may cause a metallic taste and can be taken with food to reduce upset stomach. Report any tingling or numbness of the extremities.

PROBLEM 3: Pain/Grade I Mucositis

- Begin therapy with oxycodone 5 to 10 mg PO q3–4h PRN pain. The opiate may be switched to a more potent drug and can be given IV as pain worsens. Do not initiate a bowel regimen, as the patient has diarrhea.
- Ensure proper mouth hygiene with soft sponge and fluoride toothpaste. Rinse mouth with normal saline or nonalcoholic mouthwash.
- Consider adding topical products (i.e., Gelclair) if ulcers worsen.
- Monitoring efficacy: decreased pain, decreased erythema/ulceration, opiate requirement
- Monitoring toxicity: increased pain, worsening erythema/ulceration, opiate requirement, decreased ability to swallow, side effects of oxyco-

done: nausea, vomiting, itching, constipation, confusion, sedation, respiratory rate
- Counsel SS that mucositis will typically resolve when the WBC recovers. Report any worsening of symptoms or difficulty swallowing. It is very important to maintain proper oral hygiene to prevent infection. Avoid eating foods that can irritate the ulcers. Other medications can be added if the oxycodone does not work. She may experience nausea, vomiting, sedation, confusion, constipation, or itching. All these adverse events, except constipation, will go away as her body gets used to the medication. Report any prolonged adverse events, severe confusion/lightheadedness, or difficulty breathing to the physician.

PROBLEM 4: AML

- SS has responded to induction chemotherapy, as evidenced by the hypocellular bone marrow and absence of blasts. Plan is to await bone marrow recovery [absolute granulocyte count $>0.5 \times 10^9$ (0.5×10^3) and platelet count $>100 \times 10^9$ (100×10^3)] and then initiate post-remission therapy. Based on SS's favorable cytogenetics, she will receive chemotherapy with high-dose cytarabine (HiDAC) 3 g per m^2 IV q12h on days 1, 3, and 5 for four cycles.
- Discontinue allopurinol as SS is no longer at risk for tumor lysis syndrome.
- Consider adding a colony-stimulating factor if marrow recovery is not evident by day 21 or if infection significantly worsens.
- Transfuse blood and platelets as needed until recovery.
- Monitoring efficacy: signs/symptoms of recovery: increased WBC, ANC, Hgb, Hct, platelets, improvement in mucositis
- Monitoring toxicity: signs/symptoms of marrow failure: WBC, ANC, Hgb, Hct, platelets, signs/symptoms of infection, fever, blast count
- Counsel SS that bone marrow recovery should occur within the next 2 weeks. Once the bone marrow recovers, she will be ready for post-remission chemotherapy with the goal of maintaining remission. For post-remission therapy she will receive four cycles of high-dose cytarabine. Some adverse events associated with this therapy include myelosuppression, nausea/vomiting, elevated LFTs, cerebellar dysfunction, conjunctivitis (prevented with steroid eye drops), mucositis, rash, and pulmonary edema. Measures will be taken to prevent these adverse events. In the meantime, report any bleeding,

bruising, fever, or symptoms of infection to the physician.

PROBLEM 5: Hypertension

- Continue atenolol 25 mg PO daily.
- Monitoring efficacy: BP, heart rate
- Monitoring toxicity: BP, heart rate, dizziness, light-headedness, fatigue, and depression
- Counsel SS to continue BP medication unless otherwise directed. Remind her of the importance of weight control/low-sodium diet in the treatment of hypertension. Remind her to maintain all follow-up appointments for hypertension. Report any dizziness or light-headedness to the physician.

PROBLEM 6: Hypothyroidism

- Continue levothyroxine 112 μg PO daily.
- Monitoring efficacy: thyroid function tests once yearly
- Monitoring toxicity: signs/symptoms of hypothyroidism (e.g., weakness, cold intolerance, constipation, weight gain, thinning hair and nails), signs/symptoms of hyperthyroidism (e.g., heat intolerance, weight loss, diarrhea, palpitations, irritability), BP, heart rate, and LFTs
- Counsel SS to continue thyroid replacement unless otherwise directed. Maintain all follow-up appointments for hypothyroidism. Report any new symptoms of hypo- or hyperthyroidism to the physician.

■ CASE QUESTIONS

1. b. Retinoic acid syndrome secondary to ATRA

2. c. t(9;22)

3. b. Mercaptopurine, methotrexate

4. Although age is not a contraindication to therapy for AML, many factors related to age must be considered before deciding on a treatment plan. Most oncologists believe in aggressive induction therapy in elderly patients, as rapid death is imminent without it. Post-remission therapy is more of a challenge, as pharmacokinetic changes due to age can increase the risk of morbidity and mortality in elderly patients. There is also a lack of clinical trial data to aid in decision making. Declining renal function can predispose the patient to cerebellar dysfunction from HiDAC. Myeloablative stem cell transplant is contraindicated in patients above 60

years as the risks of the procedure outweigh the potential benefits. The ultimate decision for post-remission therapy is based on what will be tolerated by the patient. Careful evaluation of organ function and performance status is crucial to design a plan that will benefit the patient without exposing him or her to unnecessary toxicity.

5. c. Steroid ophthalmic drops to prevent ocular toxicity

6. d. Methotrexate inhibits dihydrofolate reductase to inhibit DNA synthesis.

7. Measures include:
   ■ Check CrCl: Methotrexate is renally excreted. Decreases in renal function warrant dose reductions to prevent toxicity.
   ■ Ensure that the patient does not have any fluid accumulations (e.g., ascites, pleural effusions): Methotrexate accumulates in fluid collections. If the patient has a fluid collection, the drug will migrate to this area and slowly leak out over time, causing significant toxicity.
   ■ Alkalinize the urine with NaHCO$_3$: Methotrexate is a weak acid. Alkalinizing the urine prevents precipitation of methotrexate in the renal tubules and maximizes elimination. Adjust bicarbonate dose to achieve a urine pH above 7.0.
   ■ Avoid interacting medications: NSAIDs increase and prolong methotrexate levels, organic acids (salicylates, sulfonamides, probenecid, penicillins) compete with methotrexate for elimination, cyclosporine may compete for elimination, and acidic drugs/foods can acidify the urine and prevent excretion of methotrexate.
   ■ Administer leucovorin rescue starting 24 hours after the start of the methotrexate infusion: Leucovorin will selectively rescue normal cells over cancer cells from the toxic effects of methotrexate.
   ■ Monitor levels: Always treat the number, not the patient. Leucovorin doses should be adjusted based on the level. Leucovorin must be continued until the methotrexate level is below 0.05 uM per L.

8. a. Graft-versus-host disease

9. Myelosuppression is a universal adverse reaction to induction and intense post-remission chemotherapy for the treatment of AML. Infectious complications lead to prolonged hospitalization, increased antibiotic use, and increased morbidity and mortality. Filgrastim (G-CSF) and sargramostim (GM-CSF) have been shown in clinical trials to modestly reduce the duration of neutropenia in patients with AML (by 2–6 days). Most studies also showed a modest reduction in hospital stay and antibiotic use, but research has inconstantly shown an impact on overall survival. The benefits of these cytokines have been greatest in patients older than 55 years of age. Since the colony-stimulating factors are expensive, the benefits of using the medication must outweigh the cost of administering it. In other words, the potential decrease in hospitalization must be balanced against the cost of the medication. Careful consideration of individual patient characteristics can help make this decision. For example, patients who have received prior myelosuppressive chemotherapy or those who were infected at diagnosis may be potential candidates. The American Society of Clinical Oncology (ASCO) has developed an evidence-based guideline to aid in the appropriate use of these agents. ASCO states that these agents can be used in patients over 55 years of age after induction chemotherapy, but that the potential benefits should outweigh the costs.

10. d. Allopurinol

11. b. Age less than 2 years

12. Patients receiving a hematopoietic stem cell transplant, as well as their families, may experience many psychosocial stressors during the transplant period. The patient may experience decreased self-esteem due to hair loss, severe mucositis, and weakness from the treatment. The family members may experience significant stress if they are not an HLA match and cannot donate stem cells. Stress due to financial concerns can be a significant issue, considering the time the patient will spend away from work while he or she is in the hospital. Patients with young children may experience emotional stress because they will not be able to visit with their children at this time. Young adults may experience anxiety about fertility issues. Concerns may exist about the possibility of secondary malignancies. Both patients and family members may experience fear of what is to come, not knowing what complications may occur or whether the treatment will be a success. During this time, the health care provider must carefully explain

each step of the procedure and what is to be expected. If complications arise, explain to the patient and the family what the expected outcome and time frame for recovery is. The health care provider can also arrange for support groups for the patient and family.

13. **KEY POINTS**
   - Over the past decade, advances have been made in the treatment of acute leukemias. The successes made in the treatment of childhood ALL serve as a model for the treatment of other human malignancies.
   - Acute leukemias are potentially curable. Prolongation of a useful and productive life can be achieved for many others.
   - Immunology and molecular biology are likely to lead to new treatments.
   - AML is typically a disease of adults, while ALL is a disease of childhood.
   - AML is generally more resistant to treatment than ALL.
   - Initial presenting symptoms (fatigue, weight loss, fever, pallor, purpura, and pain) result from bone marrow failure.
   - A diagnosis of acute leukemia is made when a bone marrow biopsy contains at least 20% blast cells.
   - The primary treatment modality for acute leukemia is chemotherapy.
   - Transplantation plays an important role in the treatment of AML.
   - Childhood ALL represents one of the success stories of cancer treatment.
   - The treatment phases involved in ALL therapy include induction, consolidation, central nervous system therapy, and maintenance treatment.
   - The treatment phases for AML include remission induction and post-remission therapy with either chemotherapy or transplantation.
   - ALL induction therapy involves the use of prednisone, vincristine, and either asparaginase or an anthracycline.
   - The 7+3 regimen (cytarabine + daunorubicin) is the standard of care in AML for remission induction.

CASE 38 ANSWERS

■ PROBLEM LIST

1. Stage IV, diffuse, B-cell lymphoma (bulky disease)
2. Mild, normochromic, normocytic anemia

3. Type 2 diabetes mellitus
4. Hypertension
5. Hyperlipidemia

■ SOAP NOTE

S: Recent onset of mild difficulty swallowing and a 2+-month history of night sweats and occasional fevers

O: Sixty-four-year-old man recently referred for evaluation and treatment of diffuse large B-cell lymphoma confirmed by biopsy of cervical lymph node. Meds: candesartan 16 mg PO QD, hydrochlorothiazide 25 mg PO QD, metformin 1,000 mg PO BID, rosiglitazone 2 mg PO BID, atorvastatin 20 mg PO QD. Vital signs WNL, no obvious distress. Wt 78.6 kg, Ht 177.8 cm, BSA = 1.95 m^2. No oropharyngeal erythema or swelling, positive cervical lymphadenopathy, chest CTA, no rales/rhonchi, abdomen soft, nontender without obvious distention, spleen palpable slightly below costal margin, no other palpable abdominal masses, bowel sounds normal, extremities normal. A and O ×3, neuro intact. Hct 0.36 (36), Hgb 114 (11.4), MCV 90 (90), MCHC 317 (31.7), Lkcs 3.8 × 10^9 (3.8 × 10^3), diff: 0.58, bands 0.03 (3), lymph 0.28 (28), M 0.04 (4), E 0.07 (7), B 0 (0), P 0 (0); BUN 6.4 (18), SCr 108 (1.2), uric acid 360 (6), K 4.4 (4.4), PO$_4$ 1.4 (4.3). Cervical lymph node biopsy: diffuse large B-cell lymphoma, CD20+. Bone marrow biopsy: consistent diffuse lymphoma. Peripheral blood smear: normochromic, normocytic anemia. Abdominal, chest, neck CT and PET: widespread, bulky enlarged lymph nodes.

A: PROBLEM 1: Stage IV$_{BX}$ diffuse large B-cell lymphoma

PROBLEM 2: Normochromic, normocytic anemia secondary to lymphoma and bone marrow infiltration (asymptomatic)

PROBLEM 3: Type 2 diabetes mellitus, controlled with current regimen

PROBLEM 4: Hypertension, controlled with current regimen

PROBLEM 5: Hyperlipidemia, status unknown at present

P: PROBLEM 1: Stage IV$_{BX}$ Diffuse Large B-Cell Lymphoma

   - Begin chemotherapy with CHOP-R: cyclophosphamide 750 mg per m^2 = total 1,460 mg IV in 1 L D5W on day 1, doxorubicin 50 mg per m^2 =

97.5 mg IVP on day 1, vincristine 2 mg IVP on day 1, prednisone 100 mg per m^2 = 200 mg PO on days 1 through 5 (total 5 days), rituximab 375 mg per m^2 = 730 mg IV on day 1. Cycles to be repeated every 21 days for six to eight cycles.

- Administer prophylactic antiemetics prior to chemotherapy with aprepitant 125 mg PO on day 1, then 80 mg PO daily on days 2 and 3 plus ondansetron 24 mg PO plus dexamethasone 20 mg IV; prescriptions for ondansetron 8 mg PO daily for breakthrough emesis.
- Begin allopurinol 300 mg PO QD for 10 days for prevention of hyperuricemia due to cell lysis.
- Consider adding colony-stimulating factor if fever and neutropenia occur following first course of chemotherapy.
- Therapeutic monitoring: Repeat CT and PET 2 weeks after third cycle of chemotherapy; continue regimen for six courses if evidence of response; if no response or progressive disease, consider alternative regimen
- Toxicity monitoring: Evidence of infusion reaction during rituximab administration (hypotension, hypoxia, bronchospasm); evidence of tumor lysis syndrome, repeat in 24 to 48 hours BUN, SCr, uric acid, K, PO_4, Ca; hydration and correction of electrolyte imbalances, if needed; signs and symptoms of hyperglycemia secondary to corticosteroids, in patient with diabetes (see below); severity of nausea and vomiting episodes; if vomiting occurs, monitor for evidence of dehydration, electrolyte imbalances; CBC with differential on days 7 and 14; signs and symptoms of infection; vincristine neurotoxicity, especially after repeat courses of drug; repeat MUGA after six courses of doxorubicin
- Counsel patient regarding symptoms of rituximab infusion reaction (shortness of breath, difficulty swallowing, heart palpitations; alert nurse immediately); call clinic immediately for more than three episodes of vomiting within 24 hours.
- Educate patient regarding infectious risk and prevention and instruct to seek medical attention for fever above 100.4°F or any signs of bleeding, including nose bleed, oozing gums, blood in stool, urine, or vomitus; report any new onset of dizziness, shortness of breath, or headache.

PROBLEM 2: Normochromic, Normocytic Anemia

- Assess reticulocyte count, serum ferritin, and transferrin.

- Consider initiating epoetin alfa 40,000 U SC weekly or darbepoetin alfa 2.25 μg per kg SC weekly, because anemia is unlikely to resolve until completion of chemotherapy and may worsen.
- Therapeutic monitoring of epoetin alfa or darbepoetin alfa with supplemental iron: increased reticulocyte count by day 10, increase in Hgb and Hct by 2 to 4 weeks; if no increase, consider dose escalation; after target Hgb and Hct are reached, reduce dose to lowest effective dose
- Toxicity monitoring: BP, nausea, vomiting, and constipation secondary to iron therapy; increase of Hgb above 1.0 during any 2-week period increases the risk of thrombotic events
- Counsel patient regarding symptoms of anemia and toxicities of iron and epoetin alfa, including thrombosis.

PROBLEM 3: Type 2 Diabetes Mellitus

- Continue metformin 1,000 mg PO BID and rosiglitazone 2 mg BID; initiate insulin if glucose remains persistently highly following prednisone.
- Monitoring efficacy: serum glucose; glycosylated hemoglobin
- Monitoring toxicity: serum glucose
- Counsel patient to continue medications; however, serum glucose is likely to increase significantly while on prednisone therapy; contact clinic if glucose exceeds 350 while on prednisone or if glucose does not return to normal range within 5 days of completion of prednisone.
- Remind patient of importance of monitoring weight and diet; report significant changes in weight.

PROBLEM 4: Hypertension

- Continue hydrochlorothiazide 25 mg PO daily and candesartan 16 mg PO daily.
- Monitoring efficacy: BP, heart rate
- Monitoring toxicity: BP, heart rate, dizziness
- Counsel patient to continue BP medications unless instructed otherwise. Report headaches, dizziness, or lightheadedness to physician.

PROBLEM 5: Hyperlipidemia

- Continue atorvastatin 20 mg PO daily.
- Monitoring efficacy: serum lipid levels to assess current control
- Monitoring toxicity: headache, myalgias
- Counsel patient to continue minimizing saturated fat in diet and to report any new onset of muscle aches, soreness, or weakness.

■ CASE QUESTIONS

1. d. 85

2. b. Have rheumatoid arthritis

3. d. Hodgkin's disease

4. Indolent lymphomas are often not diagnosed until they are in advanced stages because many patients do not experience symptoms. They are only moderately sensitive to most conventional cytotoxic drugs, and even though their progression is slow, patients are rarely cured unless the disease is diagnosed in the early stages. Although the aggressive lymphomas characteristically progress rapidly (rapid cell division, high percentage of cells are actively dividing), they are very sensitive to the effects of conventional cytotoxic drugs, and many patients are cured or experience long disease-free intervals.

5. c. The patient has constitutional symptoms, including fever, night sweats, weight loss, and pruritus.

6. c. Large cell lymphomas, small noncleaved cell NHL, and primary CNS lymphomas

7. Even though the MOPP regimen produced a complete response rate of 80% in many trials and a 20-year disease-free survival rate of more than 50%, MOPP and MOBB hybrid regimens have been associated with high rates of hematologic and nonhematologic toxicities, including treatment-related deaths and second malignancies such as refractory leukemias. ABVD has produced similar efficacy rates in terms of progression-free survival and disease-free survival rates with significantly fewer acute and long-term toxicities, including leukemias.

8. a. Massive cell lysis and metabolic complications

9. d. Reduce the risk of radiation delivery to unintended sites

10. Aggressive NHLs are very sensitive to cytotoxic chemotherapy regimens, and cure is a realistic goal; however, evidence strongly supports the importance of maintaining the planned dose-intensity of the selected chemotherapy regimen. Although regimens like CHOP are effective, they also produce serious side effects. In patients experiencing toxic reactions, it is often tempting to allow more recovery time (i.e., delay the next scheduled dose). However, the specified schedule must be adhered to, whenever possible, to produce the best results. The use of myeloid colony-stimulating factors has reduced the incidence of serious neutropenia associated with many of these regimens and enabled planned dose-intensity to be safely delivered.

11. a. Age over 60, LDH greater than normal range, more than one extranodal site of disease

12. c. CHOP + rituximab

13. b. In younger patients with relapsed disease that is chemosensitive

14. c. CNS prophylaxis

15. d. Bexarotene

16. Lymphoma masses may cause compression of the spinal cord, and the most common presenting symptom is central back pain. As the degree of compression progresses, other neurologic symptoms develop (e.g., motor dysfunction, paresthesias, and incontinence), and paraplegia may result if no treatment is given. The more severe the impairment, the less likely that normal neurologic function can be restored. Appropriate therapy depends upon the extent of compression. If detected early enough, chemotherapy and/or radiation therapy may elicit a rapid improvement. In some patients with more advanced spinal cord compressions, emergency surgery (laminectomy) followed by radiation therapy may be required. Corticosteroids are also used to prevent edema or promote its resolution. These agents may also have a direct cytotoxic effect as well.

17. **KEY POINTS**
    ■ The use of advanced diagnostic techniques such as PET scans has facilitated more accurate and less invasive staging procedures, and routine immunophenotyping or identification of molecular markers on the surface of lymphoma cells has resulted in the effective application of targeted therapies. Such molecular markers also are providing improved prognostic information about lymphomas and guiding treatment decisions, including when very aggressive interventions such as stem cell transplants are worthwhile.

■ Treatment is determined by the classification and stage of the lymphoma at diagnosis as well as patient-specific factors that influence a patient's ability to tolerate therapy. Evidence-based clinical practice guidelines published by the National Comprehensive Cancer Network are available to guide treatment decisions.

■ CHOP plus rituximab is generally the treatment of choice for aggressive NHL.

■ Management of patients with lymphomas requires not only an understanding of the disease process and its appropriate therapy but also an understanding of the complications that may arise secondary to the disease or its therapy. These complications include opportunistic infections, obstruction by the tumor, tumor lysis syndrome, second malignancies, and chemotherapy-, biologic-, or radiation-associated toxicities.

■ The use of colony-stimulating factors, erythropoietin, and combination antiemetics have reduced the toxic sequelae associated with both chemotherapy and radiation and facilitated the administration of full-dose chemotherapy on the recommended schedules.

CASE 39 ANSWERS

■ PROBLEM LIST

1. Recurrent breast cancer metastatic to lung/bone
2. Bone pain
3. Hypercalcemia of malignancy
4. Type 2 diabetes mellitus
5. Depression

■ SOAP NOTE

S: Severe (7 out of 10) hip pain, decreased appetite, fatigue, more forgetful, confused

O: History of stage IIB infiltrating ductal carcinoma of the right breast, ER+/PR+, does not overexpress HER-2/neu. BP 110/70, HR 80, RR 20, O_2 sat 98% RA, Wt 72 kg, Ht 160 cm. Well-healed scar on right breast, no erythema or oozing. Decreased BS at right base. A and O ×3. BUN 7.5 (21), SCr 88.4 (1.0), calcium 3.13 (12.5), magnesium 1.1 (2.2), glucose 6.1 (110), HbA_{1C} 7. CT scan of chest: solitary nodule in right lung base. Lung biopsy: metastatic adenocarcinoma consistent with breast primary. Bone scan: multiple metastases to the right pelvis. MRI: no lesions in the brain. Echocardiogram: LVEF >55%. Meds: metformin 1,000 mg PO BID, rosiglitazone 4 mg PO QD, lisinopril 10 mg PO QD, paroxetine 20 mg PO QD, ibuprofen 200 to 400 mg PO q4–6h PRN, calcium carbonate 1,000 mg PO TID with meals.

A: PROBLEM 1: Recurrent breast cancer metastatic to lung and bone requiring palliative care

PROBLEM 2: Severe (7 out of 10) bone pain secondary to bony metastases

PROBLEM 3: Hypercalcemia of malignancy secondary to bony metastases

PROBLEM 4: Type 2 diabetes mellitus, controlled with current regimen

PROBLEM 5: Depression, controlled with current regimen

P: PROBLEM 1: Recurrent Breast Cancer Metastatic to Lung/Bone

■ Begin therapy with anastrozole 1 mg PO daily.
■ Obtain baseline LFTs.
■ Efficacy monitoring: monitor disease response in 6 to 8 weeks: decrease in pain scale, decrease in tumor size, no further spread of tumors, improvement in lung sounds
■ Toxicity monitoring: Ca level during initial disease flare, increase in pain scale, increase in tumor size, further spread of disease, worsening of lung sounds, hot flashes, nausea, vomiting, headache, fatigue, LFTs
■ Counsel KF about aromatase inhibitor adverse events, including hot flashes, nausea, vomiting, headache, and fatigue. If the medication causes nausea/vomiting, she can take it with food. Report any unresolved adverse events to her physician. KF may experience an increase in bone pain at the initiation of therapy as this class of medications can cause an initial disease flare. This should go away with time, but if it does not, the dose of the medication can be reduced or it can be stopped. If the medication needs to be stopped or she does not respond in 6 to 8 weeks, other medications can be tried. It is important to keep all follow-up appointments to have her blood tested and bones checked for fractures. It is important to take this medication every day even if she feels well.

PROBLEM 2: Bone Pain

■ Since the pain is 7 out of 10, initiate morphine sulfate immediate release 15 mg PO q3–4h.

When her opiate requirement is determined she should be switched to a sustained-release formulation with immediate release for breakthrough pain. Start senna 1 tablet PO BID and docusate sodium 100 mg PO BID. Start scheduled ibuprofen 800 mg q8h with food. Initiate pamidronate 90 mg IV over 2 hours every 4 weeks. Check SCr prior to each dose of pamidronate.

- Efficacy monitoring: decrease in pain scale, opiate requirement
- Toxicity monitoring: increase in pain, opiate requirement, nausea, vomiting, itching, BP, constipation, confusion, sedation, respiratory rate, renal function, platelets, Hct/Hgb, signs and symptoms of bleeding, calcium, magnesium, phosphate
- Counsel KF that the pain may not completely resolve but that it should substantially decrease and she should notice an improvement in mobility. She may experience nausea, vomiting, sedation, confusion, constipation, or itching. All these adverse events, except constipation, will go away as her body gets used to the medication. She should take the senna and docusate sodium every day to prevent constipation from morphine. It is important to take the pain medication around the clock to prevent the pain from recurring. Report any prolonged adverse events, severe confusion/lightheadedness, or difficulty breathing to the physician.

PROBLEM 3: Hypercalcemia of Malignancy

- Obtain albumin level, phosphate level, and EKG.
- Hold calcium carbonate supplement.
- Administer 1 to 2 L normal saline; after she is rehydrated, initiate furosemide 20 to 40 mg PO or IV q2–4h. Initiate pamidronate 90 mg IV over 2 hours.
- Maintain other electrolytes as needed.
- Monitoring: Ca level, albumin, phosphate level, calcium/phosphate product, K level, Mg level, Na level, hydration status: BUN, SCr, BP, heart rate, I and O, confusion, appetite, constipation
- Counsel patient that confusion, decreased appetite, and constipation are likely due to a high calcium level. She should stop taking her calcium supplement until cleared by her physician. She will receive some IV medications to help decrease her calcium level and correct the resultant dehydration. She may experience nausea/vomiting with the IV pamidronate. Eat small frequent meals to help with the nausea/vomiting.

PROBLEM 4: Type 2 Diabetes Mellitus

- Continue current regimen. If patient requires hospitalization for worsening dehydration or if renal function declines further, hold metformin.
- Efficacy monitoring: blood glucose, HbA1C in 3 months
- Toxicity monitoring: signs and symptoms of hypoglycemia, signs and symptoms of volume overload/CHF, LFTs, SCr, and K
- Counsel KF to continue diabetes medications and self-monitoring. Remind her of the importance of diet/exercise in the treatment of diabetes. Remind her to maintain all follow-up appointments for diabetes. Report any shortness of breath or swelling in the legs to the physician.

PROBLEM 5: Depression

- Continue current regimen.
- Monitoring parameters: signs and symptoms of depression; depression may worsen with new diagnosis and prognosis, adverse events of paroxetine: nausea, vomiting, constipation/diarrhea, sexual dysfunction
- Counsel KF to continue depression medication unless otherwise directed by her physician. She should seek a psychologist to discuss her new diagnosis. She should report any new/worsened depression symptoms to her physician.

■ CASE QUESTIONS

1. d. Nodal involvement

2. c. 3.33 (13.3)

3. b. No, you should not take black cohosh because its estrogen-like properties can decrease the efficacy of your anastrozole.

4. The goals of treatment for a patient with metastatic breast cancer are palliation and prolongation of life. Since cure is not the goal in this setting, the easiest, least toxic treatment regimen should be chosen. Agent selection is based on disease location, symptoms, hormone receptor status, and HER-2/neu status. Radiation therapy can be used to treat symptomatic disease of the bones, brain, or spinal cord. Hormone receptor-positive patients with bone, soft tissue, or asymptomatic visceral involvement may be treated with endocrine therapy alone. Hormone receptor-negative patients or patients with

symptomatic visceral disease should receive chemotherapy. Patients with tumors that overexpress HER-2/neu should receive trastuzumab in addition to chemotherapy.

5. KF is experiencing a disease flare secondary to the initiation of an aromatase inhibitor. If symptoms continue or worsen, she may require dose reduction or discontinuation of the medication. Most patients can continue therapy despite an initial disease flare.

6. b. Discontinue doxorubicin

7. Chemotherapeutic agents may migrate to and remain in fluid collections such as pleural effusions. This phenomenon is well documented with the administration of methotrexate. Slow leakage of methotrexate from third spaces prolongs the duration of action of the drug, predisposing the patient to increased toxicity. Fluid collections should be drained before the administration of methotrexate.

8. a. Begin annual mammography at age 40

9. The early detection of breast cancer will improve pharmacoeconomic outcomes by increasing the likelihood of curing the disease in early stages; decreasing the costs associated with complications of more advanced surgery; decreasing costs associated with extensive chemotherapy and its complications; and decreasing costs associated with lost productivity seen with advanced disease.

10. a. Prevents cell division by cross-linking DNA strands

11. a. Hypersensitivity reactions

12. c. Aspirate any drug, consult a plastic surgeon, apply a cold compress, apply DSMO topical solution

13. Breast cancer patients may experience many psychosocial changes and stressors associated with a cancer diagnosis that may affect compliance with therapy. Women may experience decreased self-esteem due to physical changes such as the removal of the breasts and hair loss from chemotherapy. Women also experience a transition in roles from caregiver to care-receiver. Women may not be able to continue working due to treatment and are faced with many costs associated with treatment. The pharmacist as well as other caregivers should be supportive and explain all aspects of treatment, includ-

ing the positives and negatives. Caregivers should encourage patients to join support groups to deal with the many stressors associated with this time in their life.

14. **KEY POINTS**
■ In general, noninvasive breast cancer (LCIS, DCIS) is controlled with surgery with or without radiation.
■ Early-stage disease (stage I, II) is treated with breast-conserving surgery and radiation. Patients should receive adjuvant therapy with hormonal agents and chemotherapy based on their nodal and hormone receptor status.
■ Locally advanced disease (stage III) is treated with combined modality therapy. A pathologic complete response to neoadjuvant (preoperative) chemotherapy is used as a surrogate marker for prognosis in this setting, as it correlates well with disease-free and overall survival.
■ Prolongation of life and palliation are goals of therapy in the metastatic setting. Treatment selection is based on the site of metastases and patient characteristics. Many patients with metastatic breast cancer will die from the disease. Despite this, many patients will achieve a durable response with treatment, allowing them to have a prolonged life with good quality.

CASE 40 ANSWERS

■ PROBLEM LIST

1. Benign prostatic hypertrophy (BPH)
2. Possible prostate cancer
3. Lower back pain
4. Erectile dysfunction

■ SOAP NOTE

S: "Over the past month, I have not been able to get 'a good night's rest' since I wake up frequently during the night from both lower back pain and trips to the bathroom and when I go, I usually dribble. During the day, I always feel like I have to go to the bathroom but either I can't go or I only urinate in small amounts often followed by dribbling down my legs."

O: Tender, moderately enlarged prostate on DRE; PSA 8 (5, 1 year ago); external genitalia normal.

BUN 18, CR 1.4, Glu (fasting) 87, TSH 4.0, serum testosterone Nl. BPH for 3 years; impotence over the past year; brother died secondary to prostate cancer; 2 pack/day cigarette smoker for 20 years. Recent forced retirement from full-time job. Slightly overweight (195lb).

Meds: terazosin HCl (discontinued) and finasteride for BPH. APAP used for wrist osteoarthritis as well as for complaints of back pain; it has produced minimal results, leading to the use of heating patches (not much benefit); zolpidem for sleep; docusate sodium for bowel management, sulfamethoxazole/trimethoprim for UTI

A: PROBLEM 1: BPH: poorly controlled urinary symptoms secondary to further enlargement of the prostate and worsening of BPH, supported by a recent change in therapy from terazosin to finasteride, primarily due to worsening of night symptoms

PROBLEM 2: Possible prostate cancer, supported by progressive worsening of urinary symptoms, erectile dysfunction, and recent onset of increased back pain, which may indicate metastases

PROBLEM 3: Lower back pain. Etiology is unclear; potential bone metastases from possible prostate cancer, disk-related problem, or worsening of job-related stress.

PROBLEM 4: Erectile dysfunction. Impotence secondary to possible new onset of prostate cancer.

P: PROBLEM 1: BPH

- Repeat PSA in 6 months.
- Since initial treatment with an α-blocker (terazosin) did not reduce BV's BPH-related symptoms, including improvement in his flow rate and worsening of his incontinence, BV was switched to finasteride.
- If no improvement in symptoms is noted in 6 months to 1 year and/or there is a worsening of the PSA, may consider a free PSA level with a possible TRUS/biopsy.
- If there is no change in the biopsy but the symptoms worsen, may consider a transurethral resection of the prostate (TURP).
- Efficacy monitoring: for improvement in BV's symptoms, flow rate or urge to go to the bathroom in 6 months to 1 year; monitor if there is any improvement in the AUA (American Urological Association) Symptom Index Evaluating BPH
- Toxicity monitoring: monitor for worsening of impotence, decreased libido, or ejaculation problems (finasteride)

- Patient education: Reinforce the need to adhere to a diet that is rich in unprocessed foods (e.g., fruits, whole grains, soy products) along with refraining from refined sugars, fried foods, and caffeine. Counsel BV to minimize use of OTC medications such as cough/cold or allergy medications without seeking the advice of a pharmacist (i.e., avoid medications that are strongly anticholinergic).

PROBLEM 2: Possible Prostate Cancer

- Repeat PSA in 6 months along with a DRE.
- If the PSA increases with or without worsening of symptoms, obtain a free PSA to better assess the need for a TRUS/biopsy (NCCN staging and workup may be done to assess for possible prostate cancer).
- If the NCCN workup and biopsy are positive, the type of treatment/management will vary depending on the degree of invasion, metastasis, and predicted life expectancy. Possible treatment modalities are (1) do nothing; (2) prostatectomy, either radical or TURP; (3) cryosurgery; (4) radiation therapy (external beam or brachytherapy); (5) hormone therapy; or (6) chemotherapy.
- Efficacy monitoring: reduction in prostate size, reduction in PSA, reduction in symptoms, improved biopsy
- Toxicity monitoring: depends on modality of treatment; constipation, worsening of constipation, nausea/vomiting, loss of libido, "hot flashes," hepatic dysfunction, change in mental status, gynecomastia, bone marrow suppression, hematologic complications such as cytopenia or, specifically, neutropenia
- Patient education: Explain the pros/cons of each type of intervention. Discuss the importance of maintaining a good healthy diet.

PROBLEM 3: Lower Back Pain

- Using a 10-point pain scale, assess the severity of BV's lower back pain.
- Obtain bone scan and chest radiograph if TRUS/biopsy shows possible cancer.
- Avoid NSAIDs and COX-2 inhibitors due to past allergic reaction.
- If back pain is graded 5 or less out of 10, initiate APAP 300 mg per codeine phosphate 30 mg 1 PO q4–6h PRN lower back pain.
- If back pain is graded 6 or higher out of 10, initiate oxycodone/APAP 5 mg per 325 mg 1 or 2 PO q6h. If no relief or worsening occurs over the next several weeks, consider morphine sulfate immediate release 15 mg PO q3–4h. When his opiate requirement is determined, switch BV

to the sustained-release formulation with immediate release for breakthrough pain. Discontinue docusate sodium and start combination product with senna and docusate sodium 1 tablet PO BID.

▪ Efficacy monitoring: decrease in pain scale; opiate requirement

▪ Toxicity monitoring: increase in pain, opiate requirement, nausea, vomiting, itching, BP, constipation, confusion, sedation, respiratory rate, LFTs (if initiating APAP/codeine). Monitor for anemia, weakness, and weight loss to monitor for signs of advanced prostate cancer and possible metastases.

▪ Patient education: Counsel BV on the purpose of around-the-clock pain medication versus medication for breakthrough pain. Counsel BV on possible nausea, sedation, vomiting, and constipation. Explain the purpose of the stool softener/laxative medication for bowel management. Increase the docusate to TID if stools become more difficult to pass secondary to hard dry stools. Counsel BV to report signs and symptoms of jaundice or itching if APAP/codeine is started. Counsel BV to stop the medication immediately and call his physician if he notices any signs and symptoms of an allergic reaction or any intolerable side effect.

PROBLEM 4: Erectile Dysfunction

▪ Assess BV's complaint of erectile dysfunction using the International Index of Erectile Function (IIEF), a 15-item questionnaire, or the abbreviated version called the Erectile Dysfunction Inventory for Treatment Satisfaction, a 5-item questionnaire.

▪ Inform BV that his ED could be a direct result of his past medication history of discontinued use of terazosin and current use of finasteride.

▪ Begin therapy with sildenafil 25mg PO 1 hour before sexual activity since patient is 65 years of age. Titrate upward slowly if necessary. Do not initiate androgen therapy, since testosterone levels are reported normal.

▪ Efficacy monitoring: Monitor onset of effects within 30 to 60 minutes; duration of medication effects should last 4 to 6 hours. Monitor for improved quality of life. If the number of ED episodes does not decrease, investigate alternate causes such as depression from BV's recent forced retirement.

▪ Toxicity monitoring: number of episodes of erectile dysfunction, LFTs during medication use due to hepatic metabolism of initiated drug, renal function with CrCl and SCr, reported signs

and symptoms characterizing priapism (prolonged erection for >4 hours)

▪ Patient education: Counsel BV to space sildenafil away from meals and grapefruit juice due to potential decreased absorption of sildenafil in the body. Mention possible adverse effects of sildenafil such as headache, flushing, dyspepsia, any vision changes, and priapism. Counsel BV on modifiable risk factors for erectile dysfunction such as cigarette smoking, stress from retirement, obesity, and uncontrolled prostate problems and depression (if applicable). Inform BV of drug-induced causes of ED, such as use of various OTC products such as cimetidine and various antihistamines. Counsel BV on postural hypotension if BV's physician restarts BV on an α-blocker; avoid sildenafil for 4 hours after taking the α-blocker. Counsel BV on a balanced diet and exercise to promote appropriate weight management. Recommend penile vacuum device or support sleeve if necessary.

▪ CASE QUESTIONS

1.   b. African American

2.   a. Lower back pain

3.   PSA stands for prostate-specific antigen. It is a protein manufactured in the prostate and is found in no other organ in the body. It is the best test currently available for early detection, not diagnosis, of prostate cancer, but elevated levels are not necessarily indicative of prostate cancer. Upon detection of increased levels of PSA (4.0–10 ng/mL) over a period of 6 months to a year, follow-up examinations are typically performed (e.g., DRE, biopsy), which can better depict a case of prostate cancer. The measurement of PSA levels is only a moderately sensitive test for detecting prostate cancer. This means that the positive predictive value is not very high, leading to many false-positive interpretations relative to prostate cancer. However, when PSA levels are greater than 10 ng per mL, the test is more accurate relative to prostate cancer. Refinements to PSA measurements are made possible by evaluating PSA velocity and density. Suspicious or equivocal results obtained from a PSA and DRE are confirmed with a transrectal ultrasound (TRUS). PSA exists in a bound as well as an unbound form (free PSA). During the early 1990s, it was noted that measuring the "free" PSA could help distinguish prostate

cancer from benign prostate disease. Measuring free PSA levels is very helpful in patients such as BV who have PSA levels between 4 and 10 ng per mL. It has been shown that patients with a PSA above 10 ng per mL have a greater than 50% chance of having prostate cancer when there is a negative DRE; on the other hand, patients with a free PSA level above 25% and a negative DRE have a lower probability of having prostate cancer. Patients with a 0% to 10% free PSA level have a greater than 56% probability of having prostate cancer, whereas a free PSA level of 10% to 15% corresponds to a probability of 28% for prostate cancer. In summary, as the free PSA level rises above 25%, the probability of having prostate cancer drops to below 8%. It is important to note that there are other reasons for an elevated PSA level, such as BPH. It is now suggested that a free PSA be performed in patients with negative DREs and elevated PSAs before repeat biopsies are done if they have been negative in the past. Unfortunately, there is no reliable way to determine in advance which cancers need to be treated or which ones will be harmful or advance. In assessing the PSA level, a clinician must pay attention to factors that may affect the lab value. For instance, a patient such as BV taking finasteride may experience a falsely lowered PSA level. On the contrary, recent ejaculations secondary to sexual activity during the past 48 hours may raise PSA values.

4. Women develop UTIs much more frequently than men. If a man has a UTI, it needs to be aggressively investigated. Most UTIs in men are due to anatomic abnormalities or due to a prostate infection best treated with medications that can cross the prostate membrane, such as sulfamethoxazole/trimethoprim. Often when the prostate becomes inflamed or infected, there is a rise in the PSA level.

5. There is a slightly higher risk of developing prostate cancer versus breast cancer, according to the American Cancer Society (ACS) estimated statistics for 2005 (232,000 vs. 211,000 estimated case predictions for 2005); however, the mortality rate was estimated to be higher for breast cancer than prostate cancer (40,400 vs. 30,300 individuals). This needs to be contrasted with lung cancer, in which the mortality rate was estimated to be approximately 95%, as compared to 13% for prostate cancer or 19% for breast cancer; the

colon/rectal cancer mortality rate was estimated to be 37% in 2005. The mortality rate for African American men is two to three times higher than that for Caucasian men. Prostate cancer is potentially curable if it is confined to the prostate gland and has not spread through the outer layer of the prostate to the surrounding tissues and the lymph nodes. If it metastasizes, the mortality rate becomes about 30%.

6. Screening for prostate cancer is controversial, but if a patient has a family history, as seen in BV's case, such screening should be started early (late 30s or early 40s). Generally, the PSA should be monitored yearly in all men after the age of 50. Some experts argue that screening should be initiated possibly even earlier, but many do not think that a PSA is needed unless the physician feels an abnormal prostate on DRE. On the other hand, PSA levels are useful if they are followed over a period of years. Any significant elevation from a previous PSA would warrant a further workup and biopsy. It is, however, strongly recommended that early screening be performed in African Americans or in patients with a family history of prostate cancer. There is now evidence that high normal PSA at an early age may be a predictor of prostate cancer later in life.

7. Most urologists or oncologists follow the NCCN practice guidelines, which base treatment options on the degree of advancement/progression and a patient's life expectancy. For example, if the tumor is still small and the Gleason score is below 7, radical prostatectomy may be an option. Most patients, however, are treated by a combination of androgen ablation, cryosurgery, radiotherapy, and/or chemotherapy, in addition to an initial prostatectomy. BV should not be taken off the finasteride since there is now evidence that this drug may help to reduce the mortality by helping to prevent prostate cancer. For example, administration of finasteride 5 mg QD significantly reduced the 7-year prevalence of prostate cancer from 24.9% to 18.4%. However, there is the possibility that it may affect the growth of the prostate cancer (see Unger J. Cancer, April 1, 2005).

8. In May 2003 the FDA approved the drug docetaxel injection (Taxotere) for patients who may have hormone-refractory metastatic

prostate cancer. This agent has been used successfully to treat locally advanced or metastatic breast cancer after failure of prior chemotherapy. The FDA approved in November 2003 the use of abarelix (Plenaxis) in men who refuse surgical castration and who risk neurologic compromise due to metastasis. Three promising therapies that are close to FDA approval as of June 2005 are (1) atrasentan (Xinlay), indicated for the treatment of metastatic hormone-refractory prostate cancer, is a selective endothelin-A receptor antagonist; (2) satraplatin, which is in phase III trials as of March 2005 for the second-line treatment of hormone-refractory prostate cancer; this medication will be formulated as a capsule to be given orally and will not be given IV, as most other agents are; and (3) Provenge, which has been developed for the treatment of asymptomatic metastatic hormone-refractory prostate cancer. As of April 2005 it has been in phase III trials and is also being fast-tracked by the FDA. It is designed to stimulate the immune system to attack cells that express prostatic acid phosphatase (PAP), a protein expressed in approximately 95% of prostate cancer cells.

9. The pharmacist may play a great role in encouraging men over 50, especially those with a high risk for developing prostate cancer such as African Americans and men with a family history of cancer, to get an annual check of their prostate via DRE and a PSA. Pharmacists are in an excellent position to educate men that prostate cancer is treatable and curable if caught early enough. Men need to know, however, that if they are treated with surgery or radiation, they may have a high probability of developing impotence as well as experiencing a decrease in sexual functioning. The pharmacist will need to be able to discuss treatment options to help overcome these adverse effects.

10. Gleason scores help determine how likely it is that a cancer will grow and spread based on how abnormal the cancer cells appear under a microscope compared to normal prostate cells. Based on BV's first prostate cancer grading of $T_2N_0M_0$, his cancer is confined to the prostate (i.e., T_2) and cancer cells have not spread beyond the pelvic area or to other parts of the body (i.e., M_0). BV's first total Gleason score of 4 shows that the cells are well differentiated, which carries a better prognosis due to slower-growing

tumor cells. BV's subsequent Gleason score of 6 shows moderately poorly differentiated cells consistent with cancer tissue findings. Even without any treatment, worsening prostate cancer may lead to ED due to spreading nerve damage. Any prostate cancer treatment has the potential to cause impotence or ED. Blood vessels and nerves involved in an erection may be damaged by any external radiation, internal radiation (i.e., brachytherapy), or surgery (e.g., cryosurgery, radical prostatectomy). Hormone therapy may also lead to ED. A nerve-sparing procedure, in which the surgeon identifies the cavernous nerves and avoids them, may reduce the damage to the nerves, but it may still take over a year for BV to regain an adequate erection. At this time, any of these therapies are appropriate for BV. Prolonged preservation of erectile function may be seen with watchful waiting, radiation, or nerve-sparing radical prostatectomy. However, if BV does experience worsening ED, he may be initiated on oral medicines, intraurethral suppositories, intercavernosal injections, or vacuum devices, and/or undergo a penile implant.

11. To treat urge incontinence, patients are typically prescribed medications aimed at relaxing the involuntary contraction of the bladder. Some examples include anticholinergic/antimuscarinic/antispasmodic agents (e.g., tolterodine, oxybutynin, propantheline, dicyclomine) and tricyclic antidepressants (e.g., imipramine, doxepin). When initiating these medications, it is important to counsel the patient about worsening of anticholinergic effects, such as hardening of stools leading to difficulty in passing stools, as in BV's case. When initiating this anticholinergic, it is important to closely monitor BV's complaints of problems with urination in the morning, which may indicate the need for surgery or catheterization to resolve his bladder complications. Tamsulosin would be initiated only if BV were not completely voiding during urination; this medication would work to promote complete voiding to lessen the chance of bladder infection and damage to the kidneys.

12. a. Vitamin E

13. Selenium, found in fish, grain, meat, and poultry, may help prevent prostate cancer. A very low-fat diet (dietary fat of 10% of total

calories) along with exercise and foods like broccoli or the nutrient lycopene from tomato products may help keep early-stage prostate cancer from worsening. It is also possible that high doses of extract from pomegranate juice might stop the growth of prostate cancer, as it has been noted in laboratory cultures. It has been reported that nutritional vitamin E (γ-tocopherol) may kill prostate cancer cells. At the April 2005 96th annual meeting of the American Association for Cancer Research, it was noted that the use of preparations containing polyphenols that are extracted from green tea have shown the potential to prevent progression of prostate cancer in men at high risk of prostate cancer. The use of finasteride may cut the risk of developing prostate cancer by 25%. At the May 2005 meeting of the American Society of Clinical Oncology, evidence showed that statins may reduce the incidence of prostate cancer by 54%.

14. **KEY POINTS**
    - Advanced age (>50 years old), ethnicity (African American and Jamaican), and family history (prostate cancer in younger relative) are the greatest risk factors for prostate cancer.
    - Screening for prostate cancer is controversial due to possible latency of the cancer and the reliability of detection tests such as PSA and DRE; however, African American men or men who have a family history of prostate or any other form of cancer should have PSA testing by the age of 40. The general male population should have their PSA checked by the age of 50. A free PSA test may be valuable if the PSA is under 10 and there has been a negative DRE.
    - Treatment options for patients with localized prostate cancer include radical prostatectomy, 3-D radiation therapy, or brachytherapy. Observation may be an option for patients with low-grade tumors and a life expectancy of less than 10 years.
    - The gold standard for palliative treatment for a patient with metastatic prostate cancer is androgen deprivation therapy with orchiectomy or an LHRH analog.
    - Second-line hormonal therapies include antiandrogen addition or withdrawal, progestins, corticosteroids, aminoglutethimide, ketoconazole, or estrogens.
    - When a patient is on a viable therapeutic regimen for prostate cancer management, the most common adverse effects with such therapies should be considered to maintain treatment adherence: sexual function, vasoactive flushes, gynecomastia, and osteoporosis.

Note: Page numbers in italics indicate illustrations; those followed by t indicate tables.

for diabetes, 440–441
drug selection for, 435–436, 436t, 437t
epidemiology of, 434–435
for epilepsy, 441–442
for heartburn, 442
for hemorrhoids, 442
for hypertension, 442–444
information sources for, 435, 435t
nausea and vomiting, 444
HIV and, 2106–2108
hypertension in, 475–476
hyperthyroidism in, 1002
immunizations and, 1876–1877
inflammatory bowel disease and, 8
isotretinoin therapy during, 214
lithium in, 1426
nutrition in, 724
seizure and, 1619–1620
smoking in, 445, 1555
STDs in, 2077
TB and, 1962
termination, contraception and, 430
treatment of
asthma in, 436–437
coagulation disorders during, 437–438
common cold during, 438
constipation during, 438–439
urinary tract infections in, 1969–1970, 1979
Prekallikrein (PK), 632
Premature ventricular contractions, 562–563
Premenstrual
asthma, 882
dysphoric disorder, 376, 377t, 379t
Premenstrual syndrome, 376–380, 377t, 379t
PREMIER trial, 465
Prerenal azotemia, 1108–1109, 1109t, *1110*
in renal failure, 1127
Pressure sores
clinical presentation/diagnosis of, 2241–2243, 2241t, *2242*
definition of, 2241
epidemiology of, 2241
improving outcomes for, 2247
key points on, 2251–2252
pathophysiology of, 2241
psychosocial aspects of, 2243
therapeutic plan for, *2243*, 2243–2244
treatment for, 2241
nonpharmacologic therapy, *2246*, 2246–2247, 2247t, *2248*
pharmacotherapy, 2244–2246, 2244t, *2245*
Priapism, drug-induced, 1422
Principle of superposition, 9, *9*
Prinzmetal's angina, 579
Problem-oriented method, in critical care, 656
Proctitis, 4. See also Inflammatory bowel disease
Proctosigmoiditis, 4. See also Inflammatory bowel disease

Proinflammatory antigenic triggers, in inflammatory bowel disease, 1–2
Projectile vomiting. See Vomiting
Promyelocytic leukemia/retinoic acid receptor alfa positive (PML-RAR alfa +), 2327
Prophylactic cranial irradiation, 2452
Proptosis, in Graves disease, 996
Prospective Randomized Amlodipine Survival Evaluation (PRAISE), 470
Prospective Study of Pravastatin in the Elderly at Risk (PROSPER), 1078
PROSPER. See Prospective Study of Pravastatin in the Elderly at Risk
Prostaglandins, pain and, 1675, 1675t
Prostatic intraepithelial neoplasm (PIN), 2466
Prosthetic valve endocarditis, 2016, 2021t–2022t
Prostate cancer
alternative/complementary therapies for, 2478–2479, 2479t
androgen independent, 2477–2478
clinical presentation/diagnosis of, 2466–2468, 2468t, 2469t
definition of, 2463
epidemiology of, 2464–2465, 2464t
etiology of, 2464–2465, 2464t
future therapies for, 2479, 2480t
hormone refractory, 2477–2478
improving outcomes for, 2479–2481
key points on, 2481
pathophysiology of, 2465–2466, 2466t
pharmacoeconomics of, 2481
prevention of, 2481
psychosocial aspects of, 2468–2470
therapeutic plan for, 2470, *2470, 2471*, 2474t, *2475*
treatment of, 2463, 2470–2478
goals for, 2463
Prostate Cancer Prevention Trial, 2481
Protease inhibitors (PIs), 2093–2097, 2098t–2100t, 2101t, 2116–2124, 2117t
Protein(s)
binding
clearance and, 13–14
low-extraction drugs and, *19*, 19–20, *20*
C, deficiency in, 854–855
acquired, 857–858
improving outcomes for, 857
management of, 856–857
monitoring of, 857
presentation/diagnosis of, 855
treatment of, 855–856
C-reactive, 602
glycated serum, 1053
in infant formulas, 352–354, 353t, 354t
measurement of, 102–103
metabolism, 1049
nutritional assessment and, 751–752

in nutritional support, 751–752, 754, 754t
in parenteral nutrition formulas, 755–756, 755t
recommended intakes of, 268
in burns, 268
S, deficiency in, 859–860
serum, 102–103
measurement of, 102–103
in urine, 1124–1125
Protein binding
clearance and, 13–14
low-extraction drugs and, *19*, 19–20, *20*
Protein C, deficiency in, 854–855
acquired, 857–858
improving outcomes for, 857
management of, 856–857
monitoring of, 857
presentation/diagnosis of, 855
treatment of, 855–856
Protein kinase C (PKC), 1054
Protein production, recombinant DNA technology and
host systems for, 132–133
transgenic systems for, 133
Protein S, deficiency in, 859–860
Proteinuria
in acute renal failure, 1124, 1124t
in chronic kidney disease, 1145–1146, 1158–1159, 1158t
Proteomics, biotechnology and, 153–154
Proteus mirabilis, in urinary tract infections, 1968, 1968t
Prothrombin time, 111
Proton pump inhibitors, 1227, 1243–1244, 1245t–1246t
Protozoan diseases
fecal, 2199–2200
giardiasis, 2200–2201
malaria, 2195–2197, 2197t, 2198t
PROWESS trial, 2168
PRP-OMP. See Meningococcal Protein Conjugate
PRP-T. See Tetanus Protein Conjugate
Pruritus, 184, *185*, 200t
burns and, 261
in chronic kidney disease, 1153, 1153t, 1170–1171, 1171t
in end-stage renal disease, 1201
Pseudocyst, 1373
Pseudomonas aeruginosa, 1851, 1928, 2217
in urinary tract infections, 1968–1969, 1968t
Pseudoparkinsonism, antipsychotics and, 1436, 1436t
Psoriasis, *235*, 235–248, *236, 237, 238*, 241t, 243–246
Psoriatic arthritis, 237
Psychogenic vomiting, 1298
Psychophysiologic insomnia, 1450
Psychosis, 1432. See also Schizophrenia
insomnia and, 1449
treatment of, in elderly, 1840–1841, 1841t
Psychotherapy, for depression, 1423

DRUG INDEX

Note: Page numbers in italics indicate illustrations; those followed by t indicate tables.

for infections, 1850
interaction of, 64
    with benzodiazepines, 1403
in prostate cancer, 2477
for seborrheic dermatitis, 234
sexual dysfunction and, 43
as substrate of Pgp, 54*t*
Ketoprofen
    CYP450 and, 61*t*
    for dysmenorrhea, 375*t*
    headaches and, 1594
    for pain, 1689, 1690
Ketorolac
    in critical care, 659, 661*t*
    headaches and, 1590*t*–1592*t*
    in nonsteroids, 171*t*
    ophthalmic, 285*t*
    for pain, 1689
    platelet dysfunction and, 838
Ketotifen, CYP450 and, 61*t*
KH3, for Cushing syndrome, 968

Labetalol
    in critical care, 666
    CYP450 and, 61*t*
    effects of, racial/ethnic differences in,
        120*t*, 121
    for geriatric patients, 1834*t*
    for hypertension, 16, 476, 478*t*–479*t*
    in pregnancy and lactation, 443
β-lactam
    for infective endocarditis, 947, 951
    for pneumonia, 1921*t*
    for sepsis, 2165
β-lactam antibiotic, as drug-transporter,
    52*t*–53*t*
Lactic acid
    for photoaging, 223
    for psoriasis, 239
Lactobionic acid, for photoaging, 223
Lactose, antibiotic-associated diarrhea/
    clostridium difficile and, 2010
Lactulose
    in cirrhosis, 1352*t*–1353*t*
    for constipation, 1309*t*, 1310
    constipation and, 2277
    for hepatic encephalopathy, 1358–1359
LAIV. *See* Live attenuated influenza
    vaccine
Lamivudine
    as drug-transporter, 52*t*–53*t*
    for hepatitis B, 1339
    for HIV, 2094*t*–2096*t*, 2114
    pharmacoeconomics of, 1342
Lamotrigine
    CYP450 and, 61*t*
    for depression, 1427
    headaches, 1601
    for pain, 1691
    in pregnancy and lactation, 441, 442
    for seizure disorders, 1615–1616,
        1615*t*, 1622*t*–1623*t*, 1633–1635
Lansoprazole
    CYP450 and, 57*t*–59*t*
    gastroesophageal reflux disease and,
        1245*t*–1246*t*

Lanthanum, in kidney disease, 1167,
    1168*t*, 1169
Laronidase, biotechnology and, 136*t*
Lassar's paste, for psoriasis, 239
Latanoprost, for glaucoma, 299*t*, 304, 306
Laxatives, 1307, 1308*t*–1309*t*
    antibiotic-associated diarrhea/
        clostridium difficile and, 2010
    bulk-forming, 1310
    diabetes and, 1057*t*
    emollient, 1310
    for geriatric patients, 1831*t*, 1833*t*
    hyperosmotic, 1310
    in pregnancy and lactation, 438
    saline, 1311
    stimulant, 1311
Lecithin, for Alzheimer disease, 1818
Leflunomide
    for rheumatoid arthritis, 1717, 1718,
        1721, 1729
    for transplant immunosuppression, 691
Lepirudin
    in critical care, 668
    for platelet disorders, 839
    for venous thromboembolism, 644–645
Leptin, 1498
Letrozole, in breast cancer treatment,
    2369*t*
Leucovorin
    in colorectal cancer, 2396*t*, 2411,
        2412*t*, 2414*t*–2415*t*, 2416
    diarrhea and, 2276*t*
    in gastric cancer, 2431, 2432*t*
    for hepatocellular carcinoma, 2390
    in osteosarcomas, 2507
    for rheumatoid arthritis, 1720
    for toxoplasmosis encephalitis, 2146*t*,
        2147
Leukotriene
    for asthma, 886, 898, 903–904
    ophthalmic, 286
    for premenstrual asthma, 882
    for rheumatoid arthritis, 1726
Leuprolide
    in breast cancer treatment, 2369*t*
    for endometriosis, 382*t*, 383
    osteoporosis and, 1791
    for premenstrual syndrome, 379, 379*t*
Levalbuterol
    for asthma, 896
    for chronic obstructive pulmonary
        disease, 927
Levamisole, in colorectal cancer, 2411
Levetiracetam
    headaches, 1601
    for seizure disorders, 1615*t*, 1617,
        1622*t*, 1637–1638
Levobunolol, for glaucoma, 299*t*, 300,
    300*t*
Levocabastine, 165
    for allergic conjunctivitis, 279
    in antiallergy agents, 171*t*
    ophthalmic, 285*t*
Levodopa
    CYP450 and, 60*t*
    as drug-transporter, 52*t*–53*t*
    hyperuricemia and, 1755

interactions
    with amoxapine, 1661*t*
    with chlorpromazine, 1661*t*
    with cyclopropane, 1661*t*
    with droperidol, 1661*t*
    with fluphenazine, 1661*t*
    with haloperidol, 1661*t*
    with halothane, 1661*t*
    with iron, 1661*t*
    with mesoridazine, 1661*t*
    with methyldopa, 1661*t*
    with metoclopramide, 1661*t*
    with perphenazine, 1661*t*
    with phenelzine, 1661*t*
    with pimozide, 1661*t*
    with prochlorperazine, 1661*t*
    with pyridoxine, 736
    with thioridazine, 1661*t*
    with thiothixene, 1661*t*
    with tranylcypromine, 1661*t*
    with trifluoperazine, 1661*t*
    with trifluopromazine, 1661*t*
    for Parkinsonism, 1656*t*, 1657–1661
Levofloxacin
    as antibacterial, 170*t*
    for cellulitis, 2235*t*, 2237, 2237*t*
    for diabetic foot ulcers, 2235*t*, 2250
    for gonorrhea, 2071, 2072*t*, 2073,
        2073*t*, 2075
    for intraabdominal infections, 1994
    for osteomyelitis, 2056*t*–2057*t*
    for pneumonia, 1921*t*, 1930, 1932*t*
    for pressure sores, 2235*t*
    for rhinosinusitis, 1888*t*
    for travelers diarrhea, 1320
    for urinary tract infections, 1976*t*, 1977
Levonorgestrel, as contraceptive, 420*t*,
    426–427
Levorphanol, for pain, 1685*t*, 1686
    in cancer, 1681
Levothyroxine, for geriatric patients, 1834
Lexipafant, for pancreatitis, 1376
Li gan pian, for liver disease, 1341
Licorice, for Addison disease, 973
Lidocaine
    for acute myocardial infarction, 620
    for burns, 264
    in critical care, 658
    CYP450 and, 57*t*–59*t*
    dosage adjustments for, 9
    for focal atrial tachycardias, 554
    for geriatric patients, 1834*t*
    headaches and, 1588, 1590*t*–1592*t*
    interactions of, 64
    for mucositis, 2272*t*
    for pain, 1691
        in burns, 261
    for postherpetic neuralgia, 1683
    as substrate of Pgp, 54*t*
    for sudden cardiac death, 566
    torsades de pointes, 565
    for ventricular tachyarrhythmias, 537,
        537*t*, 538, 538*t*, 539*t*
    for ventricular tachycardia, 564
Lindane
    for ectoparasites, 2204
    seizure disorders and, 1610

Nicardipine
in critical care, 666
for hypertension, 478t–479t
juices and, 66t
for post-transplant hypertension, 693
Nicotine
diabetes and, 1048t–1049t
in drug addiction, 1538t, 1539–1540
gastroesophageal reflux disease and, 1232t
gum, 1563t–1564t, 1565
inhalation system, 1563t–1564t, 1566–1567
lozenge, 1563t–1564t, 1566
nasal spray, 1563t–1564t, 1565–1566
pregnancy and, 1555
replacement therapy, 1561–1564
transdermal, 1563t–1564t, 1564
in small cell lung cancer, 2457
smoking and, 10t–11t, 1560
Nicotinic acid, hyperuricemia and, 1755
Nifedipine
for acute myocardial infarction, 617, 618
in critical care, 666
CYP450 and, 57t–59t
drug interactions of, 1954t–1955t
effects of, racial/ethnic differences in, 120t, 121–122
elimination routes for, 13
genetic polymorphisms and, 118t
for geriatric patients, 1834t
for ischemic heart disease, 587, 589t
juices and, 66t
in pregnancy and lactation, 443
as substrate of Pgp, 54t
Nilutamide, CYP450 and, 57t–59t
Nimodipine
headaches and, 1593t–1594t
juices and, 66t
Nisoldipine
CYP450 and, 57t–59t
juices and, 66t
Nitazoxanide
for cyclosporiasis, 2200
for giardiasis, 2201
for infectious diarrhea not due to *clostridium difficile*, 2008t, 2009
for parasitic infections, 2199
Nitrates
for acute myocardial infarction, 605–606
adverse effects of, 585
gastroesophageal reflux disease and, 1232t
for glaucoma, 293
for heart failure, 499t, 502, 504, 523
for ischemic heart disease, 583–585, 584t, 589–591
Nitrazepam, 127
for seizure disorders, 1615
Nitrendipine, CYP450 and, 57t–59t
L-nitroarginine methyl ester (L-NAME), gastroesophageal reflux disease and, 1232t
Nitrofurantoin
hepatotoxicity of, 1334t–1335t

nephrotoxicity and, 41t
pulmonary disease and, 42t
for urinary tract infections, 1976, 1976t, 1977, 1978t, 1979t
Nitrofurazone, for burns, 264, 265
Nitrogen mustard, in pediatric brain tumors, 2495t
Nitroglycerin
absorption of, 328
for acute myocardial infarction, 603, 604, 605–606
buccal, for ischemic heart disease, 584–585
in critical care, 665
CYP450 and, 60t
for gastrointestinal bleeding, 1357
for geriatric patients, 1834t
for hypertension, 478t–479t
for ischemic heart disease, 578, 583, 589, 591
synergistic interactions with, 63
Nitroprusside
for acute myocardial infarction, 605–606
for hypertension, 472, 478t–479t
hypothyroidism from, 1009t
in pregnancy and lactation, 443
Nitrosourea
for cutaneous melanoma, 2573
for platelet disorders, 839
pulmonary disease and, 42t
Nitrous oxide
in drug addiction, 1545t
for pain management, in burns, 261
vitamin B_{12} deficiency and, 789
Nizatidine, gastroesophageal reflux disease and, 1245t–1246t
NNRTIs. *See* Nonnucleoside reverse transcriptase inhibitors
Nonalbuterol, for asthma, 896
Nonbarbiturate nonbenzodiazepines, for insomnia, 1452
Nonnucleoside reverse transcriptase inhibitors (NNRTIs), for HIV, 2109t–2110t, 2124–2127
Nonsteriodal anti-inflammatory drugs (NSAIDs)
acute renal failure and, 1108, 1117
adverse effects of, in acute renal failure, 5t, 1111, 1112, 1113
for airway inflammation, in cystic fibrosis, 970
for Alzheimer disease, 1824
cardiovascular effects of, 42
in critical care, 661
for dysmenorrhea, 374–375, 375t
for endometriosis, 381, 382t
gastroesophageal reflux disease and, 1232t, 1236–1237, 1250–1251
genetic polymorphisms and, 118
in geriatric therapy, 1831t, 1833t, 1834t, 1841–1842
for gout, 1171, 1759–1760, 1760t
for heart failure, 498
for hemophilia, 860
inflammatory bowel disease and, 1257
kidney disease exacerbation by, 1148t

for lupus, 1777–1778
nephrotoxicity and, 41–42, 41t
for osteoarthritis, 1743t, 1744
for pain, 1689
in cancer, 1681
in pancreatitis, 1379
in sickle cell disease, 1684
for painful crises, 809
pulmonary disease and, 42t
for rheumatoid arthritis, 1716, 1722–1726, 1722t, 1724t
sexual dysfunction and, 43
Nonsteroidal anti-inflammatory drugs (NSAIDs)
for episcleritis/scleritis, 280
ophthalmic, 286
Norepinephrine
in critical care, 669
for depression, 1419
as drug-transporter, 52t–53t
for gastrointestinal bleeding, 1357
for glaucoma, 302
for hepatorenal syndrome, 1360
Norethindrone
as contraceptive, 420t, 424
CYP450 and, 57t–59t
Norfloxacin
as antibacterial, 170t
in common eye disorders, 169, 283–284, 284t
CYP450 and, 57t–59t
for peritonitis, 1992
for spontaneous bacterial peritonitis, 1355
for travelers diarrhea, 1320
for urinary tract infections, 1976t, 1977, 1978t, 1979t
Norfluoxetine, CYP450 and, 57t–59t
Norgestimate, as contraceptive, 420t
Norgestrel, as contraceptive, 424
Normeperidine
adverse effects of, in chronic kidney disease, 1172
seizure disorders and, 1610
Nortriptyline
CYP450 and, 57t–59t, 60t
for depression, 1419t, 1420
in Alzheimer disease, 1821
drug interactions of, 1954t–1955t
effects of, racial/ethnic differences in, 118t, 123, 123t
headaches and, 1593t–1594t
for insomnia, in Alzheimer disease, 1821
for pain, 1690t
in pregnancy and lactation, 440
smoking and, 1568
NSAIDs. *See* Nonsteriodal anti-inflammatory drugs
Nucleotide reverse transcriptase inhibitor, for HIV, 2094t–2096t
Nystatin
for burns, 265
for candidiasis, 387, 387t, 388t
for transplant infections, 691

Oat bran, for diarrhea, 1317t
Octreotide
in cirrhosis, 1352t–1353t